THE HEART Arteries and Veins

EIGHTH EDITION

Editors

Robert C. Schlant, M.D.

Professor of Medicine (Cardiology)
Emory University School of Medicine
and
Chief of Cardiology, Grady Memorial Hospital
Atlanta, Georgia

R. Wayne Alexander, M.D.

R. Bruce Logue Professor of Medicine
Director, Division of Cardiology
Emory University School of Medicine
and
Chief of Cardiology, Emory Hospital and Emory Clinic
Atlanta, Georgia

Associate Editors

Robert A. O'Rourke, M.D.

Charles Conrad Brown Distinguished Professor in Cardiovascular Disease
Director of Cardiology, The University of Texas Health Science Center Teaching Hospitals
San Antonio, Texas

Robert Roberts, M.D.

Professor of Medicine and Cell Biology
Chief of Cardiology, Baylor College of Medicine
Director, Center of Research in Heart Failure
Director, Bugher Foundation Center for Molecular Biology of the Cardiovascular Diseases
Houston, Texas

Edmund H. Sonnenblick, M.D.

Olson Professor of Medicine
Chief, Division of Cardiology
Albert Einstein College of Medicine
Bronx, New York

McGRAW-HILL, INC.
Health Professions Division
New York St. Louis San Francisco Auckland Bogotá
Lisbon London Madrid Mexico City Montreal New Delhi Paris
San Juan Singapore Sydney Tokyo Toronto

1 2 3 4 5 6 7 8 9 0 DOWDOW 9 8 7 6 5 4 3

ISBN 0-07-055417-X 1 VOL EDITION
ISBN 0-07-911046-0 2 VOL SET EDITION
ISBN 0-07-055418-8 VOLUME ONE
ISBN 0-07-055419-6 VOLUME TWO

This book was set in Sabon by Monotype Composition Company, Inc.
The editors were J. Dereck Jeffers and Steven Melvin;
the production supervisor was Richard Ruzycka;
the text designer was José Fonfrias; the cover designer was Michele Simari.
R.R. Donnelley & Sons Company was printer and binder.

Cover illustration reproduced with permission from S. B. King and J. S. Douglas, "Coronary Arteriography and Angioplasty," Copyright © 1985, McGraw-Hill, N.Y. Illustration by Michael Budowick, Medical Artist, Emory University School of Medicine, Office of Medical Illustration.

Library of Congress Cataloging-in-Publication Data

Hurst's the heart : arteries and veins.—8th ed./ editors, Robert C. Schlant, R. Wayne Alexander ; associate editors, Robert A. O'Rourke, Robert Roberts, Edmond H. Sonnenblick.
p. cm.
Rev. ed. of: The Heart / editor-in-chief, J. Willis Hurst. 7th ed. c1990.
Includes bibliographical references and index.
ISBN 0-07-055417-X (1 v. ed.) : — ISBN 0-07-911046-0 (2 v. set) : — ISBN 0-07-055418-8 (v. 1). — ISBN 0-07-055419-6 (v. 2)
1. Cardiovascular system—Diseases. I. Hurst, J. Willis (John Willis), date. II. Schlant, Robert C., date. . . III. Alexander, R. Wayne. IV. Title: Heart.
[DNLM: 1. Cardiovascular Diseases. WG 100 H9664 1994]
RC667.H42 1994
616.1—dc20
DNLM/DLC
for Library of Congress

93-21271
CIP

THE HEART

Arteries and Veins

NOTICE

Medicine is an ever-changing science. As new research and clinical experience broaden our knowledge, changes in treatment and drug therapy are required. The editors and the publisher of this work have checked with sources believed to be reliable in their efforts to provide information that is complete and generally in accord with the standards accepted at the time of publication. However, in view of the possibility of human error or changes in medical sciences, neither the editors nor the publisher nor any other party who has been involved in the preparation or publication of this work warrants that the information contained herein is in every respect accurate or complete, and they are not responsible for any errors or omissions or for the results obtained from use of such information. Readers are encouraged to confirm the information contained herein with other sources. For example and in particular, readers are advised to check the product information sheet included in the package of each drug they plan to administer to be certain that the information contained in this book is accurate and that changes have not been made in the recommended dose or in the contraindications for administration. This recommendation is of particular importance in connection with new or infrequently used drugs.

To

Mia, Stephanie, Christiane, and Timothy (R.C.S.)

and

Dorothy and Henry Alexander (R.W.A.)

and all of our other teachers

Contents

Contributors

George S. Abela, M.D. M.Sc. [72] Associate Professor of Medicine, Harvard Medical School; Director of Interventional Research, New England Deaconess Hospital, Boston, Massachusetts

Masood Akhtar, M.D. [46] Professor of Medicine, Associate Chief, Cardiovascular Disease Section, University of Wisconsin Medical School, Milwaukee Clinic Campus; Director for Arrhythmia Services, Sinai Samaritan Medical Center, Milwaukee, Wisconsin

E. Pendleton Alexander, M.D. [39] Assistant Professor of Surgery, George Washington University School of Medicine; Chief, Cardiothoracic Surgery, Washington D.C. Veterans Affairs Medical Center, Washington, D.C.

James K. Alexander, M.D. [104] Professor of Medicine (Cardiology), Baylor College of Medicine, Houston, Texas

R. Wayne Alexander, M.D. [2, 20, 56, 58, 60] R. Bruce Logue Professor of Medicine, Director, Division of Cardiology, Department of Medicine, Emory University School of Medicine; Chief of Cardiology, Emory Hospital and Emory Clinic, Atlanta, Georgia

Joseph S. Alpert, M.D. [49, 100] Robert S. and Irene P. Flinn Professor of Medicine and Head, Department of Medicine, University of Arizona College of Medicine, Tucson, Arizona

W. Banks Anderson, Jr., M.D. [12] Professor of Ophthalmology, Duke University School of Medicine, Durham, North Carolina

Numbers in brackets refer to chapters written or cowritten by the contributor.

Alan Appelbe, M.B.B.S. [131] Department of Cardiology, Geelong Hospital, Geelong, Victoria, Australia

Robert J. Bache, M.D. [57] Professor of Medicine, University of Minnesota School of Medicine, Minneapolis, Minnesota

Kenneth M. Baker, M.D. [6B] Associate Professor of Medicine, Thomas Jefferson University School of Medicine, Philadelphia, Pennsylvania; Staff Scientist, Weis Center for Research; Staff Cardiologist, Geisinger Clinic, Danville, Pennsylvania

Arthur C. Beall, Jr., M.D. [123] Professor of Surgery, Baylor College of Medicine, Houston, Texas

Richard C. Becker, M.D. [49] Assistant Professor of Medicine; Director, Coronary Care Unit; Director, Thrombosis Research Center, University of Massachusetts, Worcester, Massachusetts

J. Thomas Bigger, Jr., M.D. [34] Professor of Medicine and Pharmacology, Department of Medicine, Columbia University College of Physicians and Surgeons, New York, New York

Margaret E. Billingham, M.D. [32] Professor of Pathology, Director of Cardiac Pathology Laboratory, Stanford University School of Medicine, Stanford, California

Peter C. Block, M.D. [86] Associate Director, The Heart Institute, St. Vincent Hospital, Portland, Oregon

Harisios Boudoulas, M.D. [50] Professor of Medicine and Pharmacology, Division of Cardiology, Colleges of Medicine and Pharmacy, Ohio State University, Columbus, Ohio

Michael R. Bristow, M.D., Ph.D. [89] Professor of Medicine, Head, Division of Cardiology, University of Colorado School of Medicine, Denver, Colorado

Ross Brooks, M.D. [42] Instructor in Medicine, Harvard Medical School; Assistant Physician, Massachusetts General Hospital, Boston, Massachusetts

Bruce H. Brundage, M.D. [135] Professor of Medicine and Radiological Services, University of California at Los Angeles School of Medicine; Chief, Division of Cardiology, Harbor–UCLA Medical Center, Torrance, California

Peter M. Buttrick, M.D. [135] Associate Professor of Medicine (Cardiology), Albert Einstein College of Medicine; Assistant Professor of Physiology, Montefiore Medical Center, Bronx, New York

Louis R. Caplan, M.D. [122] Professor and Chairman, Department of Neurology, Tufts University School of Medicine; Neurologist-in-Chief, New England Medical Center, Boston, Massachusetts

Agustin Castellanos, M.D. [13, 36] Professor of Medicine (Cardiology), Director, Clinical Electrophysiology, University of Miami School of Medicine, Miami, Florida

Nisha Chibber Chandra, M.D. [52] Associate Professor of Medicine, Johns Hopkins University School of Medicine; Director, Coronary Care Unit, Francis Scott Key Medical Center, Baltimore, Maryland

Kanu Chatterjee, M.B. [18] Professor of Medicine, Lucie Stern Professor of Cardiology; Associate Chief, Division of Cardiology, University of California San Francisco School of Medicine; Director, Coronary Care Unit, H.C. Moffitt and J. Long Hospitals, San Francisco, California

Melvin D. Cheitlin, M.D. [107] Professor of Medicine, University of California San Francisco School of Medicine; Chief of Cardiology, San Francisco General Hospital, San Francisco, California

James T.T. Chen, M.D. [14] Professor of Radiology; Former Director, Cardiopulmonary Radiology, Duke University Medical Center, Durham, North Carolina

Leonard A. Cobb, M.D. [51] Professor of Medicine, University of Washington School of Medicine; Attending Cardiologist, Harborview Medical Center; Medical Director, Seattle Medic One, Seattle, Washington

Jay N. Cohn, M.D. [26, 30] Professor of Medicine, Head, Cardiovascular Division, University of Minnesota Medical School, Minneapolis, Minnesota

Lawrence H. Cohn, M.D. [79, 80] Professor of Surgery, Harvard Medical School; Chief, Division of Cardiac Surgery, Brigham and Women's Hospital, Boston, Massachusetts

Dèsirè Collen, M.D., Ph.D. [69] Professor of Medicine; Director, Center for Thrombosis and Vascular Research; University of Leuven, Leuven, Belgium

Mark W. Connolly, M.D. [31, 141] Assistant Professor of Surgery, Emory University School of Medicine, Atlanta, Georgia

C. Richard Conti, M.D. [72] Professor of Medicine, Palm Beach Heart Association Eminent Scholar (Cardiology), Director, Division of Cardiovascular Medicine, University of Florida College of Medicine, Gainesville, Florida

Denton A. Cooley, M.D. [111] Clinical Professor of Surgery, University of Texas Medical School; Surgeon-in-Chief, Texas Heart Institute; Chief, Cardiovascular Surgery, St. Luke's Episcopal Hospital, Houston, Texas

James L. Cox, M.D. [44] Evarts A. Graham Professor of Surgery, Chief, Division of Cardiothoracic Surgery, Washington University School of Medicine, St. Louis, Missouri

Joseph M. Craver, M.D. [31, 85] Professor of Surgery, Emory University School of Medicine, Atlanta, Georgia

Michael H. Crawford, M.D. [132] Robert S. Flinn Professor and Chief, Division of Cardiology, University of New Mexico School of Medicine, Albuquerque, New Mexico

I. Sylvia Crawley, M.D. [110] Clinical Professor of Medicine (Cardiology), Emory University School of Medicine, Atlanta, Georgia

Michael D. Dake, M.D. [126] Assistant Professor of Radiology and Medicine, Stanford University School of Medicine; Chief, Cardiovascular and Interventional Radiology, Stanford University Hospital, Stanford, California

James E. Dalen, M.D. [100] Professor, Internal Medicine; Vice Provost for Health Sciences, Dean, College of Medicine, University of Arizona College of Medicine, Tucson, Arizona

Michael J. Davies, M.D. [55] British Heart Foundation Professor of Cardiovascular Pathology, Honorary Consultant Cardiovascular Pathologist, SW Thames Regional Cardiothoracic Unit, St. Georges Hospital Medical School, London, England

John E. Deanfield, M.B., B.Ch. [98] Senior Lecturer, Institute of Child Health; Consultant Cardiologist, Hospital for Sick Children; Consultant Cardiologist, St. Bartholomew's Hospital, London, England

Michael E. DeBakey, M.D. [123] Chancellor Distinguished Service Professor, Department of Surgery, Baylor College of Medicine, Houston, Texas

Regis A. deSilva, M.D. [41] Assistant Clinical Professor of Medicine, Harvard Medical School; Section of Cardiology, New England Deaconess Hospital, Boston, Massachusetts

Thomas F. Dodson, M.D. [125] Assistant Professor of Surgery, Emory University School of Medicine, Atlanta, Georgia

John S. Douglas, Jr., M.D. [70, 71, 138] Associate Professor of Medicine (Cardiology), Assistant Professor of Radiology (Cardiac Radiology), Emory University School of Medicine, Atlanta, Georgia

David T. Durack, M.B., Ph.D. [94] Professor of Medicine and Microbiology; Chief Director of Infectious Disease and International Health, Duke University School of Medicine, Durham, North Carolina

Jesse E. Edwards, M.D. [81, 82, 97] Professor of Pathology, University of Minnesota; Senior Consultant, Registry of Cardiovascular Disease, United Hospital, St. Paul, Minnesota

Robert S. Eliot, M.D. [117] Clinical Professor of Medicine (Cardiology), Department of Medicine, University of Nebraska Medical Center, Omaha, Nebraska

Stephen M. Factor, M.D. [57] Professor of Pathology, Professor of Medicine (Cardiology), Vice Chairman for Anatomic Pathology, Albert Einstein College of Medicine; Director, Pathology Bronx Municipal Hospital Center, Bronx, New York

Frederick S. Fein, M.D. [102] Associate Professor of Medicine, Albert Einstein College of Medicine, Bronx, New York

Joel M. Felner, M.D. [15] Professor of Medicine (Cardiology), Associate Dean (Clinical Education), Emory University School of Medicine, Atlanta, Georgia

M. Irenè Ferrer, M.D. [142] Professor Emeritus of Clinical Medicine, College of Physicians and Surgeons, Columbia University, New York, New York

Charles Fisch, M.D. [37] Distinguished Professor Emeritus of Medicine, Krannert Institute of Cardiology, Indiana University School of Medicine, Indianapolis, Indiana

Alfred P. Fishman, M.D. [99] William Maul Measey Professor of Medicine, University of Pennsylvania School of Medicine; Senior Attending Physician, Hospital of the University of Pennsylvania, Philadelphia, Pennsylvania

Gerald F. Fletcher, M.D. [16] Professor and Chairman, Department of Rehabilitation Medicine; Professor of Medicine (Cardiology); Medical Director, Emory Health Enhancement Program, Emory University School of Medicine, Atlanta, Georgia

Ross D. Fletcher, M.D. [39, 48] Associate Professor of Medicine, Georgetown University School of Medicine; Chief, Cardiology Section, Veterans Affairs Medical Center, Washington, D.C.

Noble O. Fowler, M.D. [24] Emeritus Professor of Medicine and Pharmacology and Cell Biophysics, University of Cincinnati College of Medicine, Cincinnati, Ohio

Robert H. Franch, M.D. [138] Professor of Medicine (Cardiology), Emory University School of Medicine, Atlanta, Georgia

O. Howard Frazier, M.D. [111] Professor of Surgery, University of Texas at Houston Medical School; Chief of Cardiovascular Surgery, Hermann Hospital; Director of Cardiovascular and Thoracic Surgery, University Texas Medical Center; Chief, Transplant Service, St. Luke's Hospital; Surgical Director, Texas Heart Institute, Houston, Texas

Gottlieb C. Friesinger, M.D. [61] Betty and Jack Bailey Professor of Cardiology, Vanderbilt University School of Medicine, Nashville, Tennessee

William H. Frishman, M.D. [66] Professor of Medicine, Epidemiology and Social Medicine, Albert Einstein College of Medicine; Director of Medicine, Hospital of the Albert Einstein College of Medicine/ Montefiore Medical Center, Bronx, New York

Edward D. Frohlich, M.D. [75] Professor of Clinical Medicine and Adjunct Professor of Pharmacology, Tulane University School of Medicine; Professor of Medicine and Physiology, Louisiana State University School of Medicine; Alton Ochsner Distinguished Scientist and Vice President for Academic Affairs, Alton Ochsner Medical Foundation, New Orleans, Louisiana

Valentin Fuster, M.D., Ph.D. [68] Mallinckrodt Professor of Medicine, Harvard Medical School; Chief, Division of Cardiology, Massachusetts General Hospital, Boston, Massachusetts

William H. Gaasch, M.D. [80] Professor of Medicine, University of Massachusetts Medical School; Chief of Cardiology, The Medical Center of Central Massachusetts, Worcester, Massachusetts

Bernard J. Gersh, M.B., Ch.B., Ph.D. [98] W. Proctor Harvey Teaching Professor of Cardiology, Chief, Division of Cardiology, Georgetown University School of Medicine, Washington, D.C.

Ray W. Gifford, Jr., M.D. [77] Senior Physician, Department of Hypertension and Nephrology; Vice Chairman, Division of Medicine, The Cleveland Clinic Foundation, Cleveland, Ohio

Edward M. Gilbert, M.D. [89] Associate Professor of Medicine; Director, Heart Failure Treatment Program; Director, Coronary Care Unit, University of Utah Medical School, Salt Lake City, Utah

Emilio B. Gonzalez, M.D. [103] Associate Professor, Division of Rheumatology, Department of Medicine, Emory University School of Medicine; Chief, Rheumatology Service, Grady Memorial Hospital, Atlanta, Georgia

John Parker Gott, M.D. [84] Assistant Professor of Surgery, Emory University Hospital, Atlanta, Georgia

Antonio M. Gotto, Jr., M.D., D.Phil. [53] Professor and Chairman, Department of Medicine, Baylor College of Medicine; Chief, Internal Medicine, The Methodist Hospital, Houston, Texas

Kathy Griendling, Ph.D. [2] Assistant Professor of Medicine, Division of Cardiology, Emory University School of Medicine, Atlanta, Georgia

Robert F. Grover, M.D., Ph.D. [120] Professor Emeritus of Medicine, University of Colorado School of Medicine, Denver, Colorado

Scott M. Grundy, M.D., Ph.D. [65] Professor of Internal Medicine and Biochemistry, Director, Center for Human Nutrition, and Chairman, Department of Clinical Nutrition, University of Texas Southwestern Medical Center at Dallas, Dallas, Texas

Robert A. Guyton, M.D. [84, 141] Professor of Surgery, Chief, Division of Cardiothoracic Surgery, Emory University School of Medicine, Atlanta, Georgia

Robert J. Hall, M.D. [111] Clinical Professor of Medicine, Baylor College of Medicine and The University of Texas Medical School at Houston Director of Education, Cardiology, Texas Heart Institute and St. Luke's Episcopal Hospital, Houston, Texas

W. Dallas Hall, M.D. [76] Professor of Medicine, Director, Division of Hypertension, Emory University School of Medicine, Atlanta, Georgia

Peter H. Jones, M.D. [53] Assistant Professor of Medicine, Section of Atherosclerosis and Lipid Research, Department of Medicine, Baylor College of Medicine Houston, Texas

John W. Joyce, M.D. [124] Associate Professor of Medicine, Mayo Medical School, Rochester, Minnesota

William B. Kannel, M.D., M.P.H. [8] Professor of Medicine and Public Health, Section of Preventive Medicine and Epidemiology, Boston University School of Medicine, Boston, Massachusetts

Edward L. Kaplan, M.D. [78] Professor of Pediatrics, School of Medicine; Professor, School of Public Health, University of Minnesota, Minneapolis, Minnesota

Joel A. Kaplan, M.D. [140] Horace W. Goldsmith Professor and Chairman of Anesthesiology, Mt. Sinai Medical Center, New York, New York

Robert B. Karp, M.D. [82] Professor of Surgery, Chief, Cardiac Surgery, University of Chicago School of Medicine, Chicago, Illinois

Nevin M. Katz, M.D. [81] Professor of Surgery, Georgetown University School of Medicine, Washington, D.C.

Kenneth M. Kessler, M.D. [13, 36] Professor of Medicine, Associate Director, Division of Cardiology, University of Miami School of Medicine; Chief, Cardiology Section, Department of Veterans Affairs Medical Center, Miami, Florida

Deepak Kikeri, M.D. [108] Assistant Professor of Medicine, Emory University School of Medicine, Atlanta, Georgia

Spencer B. King, III, M.D. [70, 71, 138] Professor of Medicine, (Cardiology), Professor of Radiology, Emory University School of Medicine, Atlanta, Georgia

Juha P. Kokko, M.D., Ph.D. [29] Asa G. Candler Professor of Medicine; Chairman, Department of Medicine, Emory University School of Medicine, Atlanta, Georgia

Lynn M. Kutsche, M.D. [95] Associate Professor of Pediatrics, University of Florida, Gainesville, Florida

E. William Hancock, M.D. [83] Professor of Medicine (Cardiovascular), Stanford University School of Medicine, Stanford, California

Laurence A. Harker, M.D. [7] Blomeyer Professor of Medicine, Director, Division of Hematology and Oncology, Emory University School of Medicine, Atlanta, Georgia

W. Procter Harvey, M.D. [119] Professor of Medicine (Cardiology), Georgetown University School of Medicine, Washington, D.C.

Charles R. Hatcher, Jr., M.D. [74] Professor of Surgery (Cardiothoracic), Emory University School of Medicine; Vice President for Health Affairs, Director, Robert W. Woodruff Health Sciences Center, Atlanta, Georgia

Bernadine P. Healy, M.D. [103] Immediate-Past Director, National Institutes of Health; Staff, The Cleveland Clinic Foundation, Cleveland, Ohio

Eric C. Honig, M.D. [17] Associate Professor of Medicine, Assistant Professor of Anesthesiology, Emory University School of Medicine; Chief, Pulmonary Services, Grady Memorial Hospital, Atlanta, Georgia

Sharon Hunt, M.D. [32] Clinical Professor of Medicine, Division of Cardiology, Stanford University School of Medicine, Stanford, California

J. Willis Hurst, M.D. [9B, 119] Consultant to the Division of Cardiology; Former Professor and Chairman, Department of Medicine, Emory University School of Medicine, Atlanta, Georgia

Joanne S. Ingwall, Ph.D. [6A] Professor of Medicine (Physiology), Harvard Medical School; Director, Nuclear Magnetic Resonance Laboratory of Physiological Chemistry; Senior Biochemist, Brigham and Women's Hospital, Boston, Massachusetts

Lynne L. Johnson, M.D. [134] Professor of Medicine and Radiology, University of Alabama, Birmingham, Alabama

Ellis L. Jones, Jr., M.D. [74] Professor of Surgery, Emory University School of Medicine, Atlanta, Georgia

Thierry H. LeJemtel, M.D. [28] Professor of Medicine, Albert Einstein College of Medicine, Bronx, New York

E. Douglas Lewandowski, Ph.D. [6A] Assistant Professor of Radiology, Harvard Medical School; Director, Nuclear Magnetic Resonance Biochemistry Laboratory, Massachusetts General Hospital, Boston, Massachusetts

Richard P. Lewis, M.D. [50] Professor of Medicine, Ohio State University College of Medicine, Columbus, Ohio

Joseph Lindsay, Jr., M.D. [123] Professor of Medicine, The George Washington University School of Medicine; Director, Section of Cardiology, Washington Hospital Center, Washington, D.C.

Floyd D. Loop, M.D. [73] Chairman, Board of Governors and Executive Vice President, The Cleveland Clinic Foundation, Cleveland, Ohio

Bernard Lown, M.D. [41] Professor of Cardiology Emeritus, Harvard School of Public Health; Senior Physician, Brigham and Women's Hospital, Boston, Massachusetts

Jerre F. Lutz, M.D. [33] Assistant Professor of Medicine (Cardiology); Medical Director, Cardiac Transplant Program, Emory University School of Medcine, Atlanta, Georgia

Douglas D. Mair, M.D. [98] Professor of Pediatrics and Associate Professor of Internal Medicine, Mayo Medical School, Rochester, Minnesota

Frank I. Marcus, M.D. [27, 116] Distinguished Professor of Medicine, University of Arizona College of Medicine; Director, Electrophysiology, University of Arizona Health Sciences Center, Tucson, Arizona

Barry J. Maron, M.D. [90] Director, Cardiovascular Research, Minneapolis Heart Institute Foundation, Minneapolis, Minnesota

Randolph P. Martin, M.D. [131] Professor of Medicine (Cardiology), Associate Dean for Clinical Development, Emory University School of Medicine; Director of Non-invasive Cardiology, Emory University Hospital, Atlanta, Georgia

Jay W. Mason, M.D. [87] Professor of Medicine, Chief, Division of Cardiology, University of Utah Medical School, Salt Lake City, Utah

Hugh A. McAllister, Jr., M.D. [111] Clinical Professor of Pathology, Baylor College of Medicine; Adjunct Professor, Pathology and Laboratory Medicine, University of Texas Medical School, Houston, Texas; Chief, Department of Pathology, St. Luke's Episcopal Hospital and Texas Heart Institute; Consultant, Department of Pathology, Texas Children's Hospital, Houston, Texas

John H. McAnulty, M.D. [113] Professor of Medicine, Oregon Health Sciences University, Portland, Oregon

James Metcalfe, M.D. [113] Professor of Medicine, Oregon Health Sciences University; Associate Chief of Staff for Extended Care, Portland Veterans Affairs Medical Center, Portland, Oregon

Joseph I. Miller, M.D. [93] Professor of Surgery, Emory University School of Medicine, Atlanta, Georgia

William E. Mitch, M.D. [108] Garland Herndon Professor of Medicine, Director, Renal Division, Department of Medicine, Emory University School of Medicine, Atlanta, Georgia

Harry G. Mond, M.D. [40] Physician to Pacemaker Clinic, Royal Melbourne Hospital, Melbourne, Victoria, Australia

Howard E. Morgan, M.D. [6B] Senior Vice President for Research, Geisinger Clinic, Danville, Pennsylvania

Hugo M. Morales-Ballejo, M.D. [117] Associate Medical Director, Schering Plough Research Institute, Kenilworth, New Jersey

Douglas C. Morris, M.D. [9B, 60] Professor of Medicine (Cardiology), Director, Emory Heart Center, Emory University School of Medicine; Director, Carlyle Fraser Heart Center, Director of Cardiology Section, Crawford W. Long Hospital, Atlanta, Georgia

Robert J. Myerburg, M.D. [13, 36] Professor of Medicine and Physiology, Director, Division of Cardiology, University of Miami School of Medicine, Jackson Memorial Medical Center, Miami, Florida

John H. Newman, M.D. [101] Elsa S. Hanigan Chair in Pulmonary Medicine, Professor of Medicine, Vanderbilt University School of Medicine; Chief of Pulmonary Medicine, St. Thomas Hospital, Nashville, Tennessee

Steven E. Nissen, M.D. [133] Vice Chairman, Department of Cardiology, Section Head, Clinical Cardiology, Cleveland Clinic Foundation, Cleveland, Ohio

R. Joe Nobel, M.D. [45] Clinical Professor of Medicine, Indiana University School of Medicine; St. Vincent Hospital and Health Care Center, Indianapolis, Indiana

Paul E. Nolan, Pharm.D. [116] Associate Professor, College of Pharmacy; Associate Clinical Scientist, University Heart Center; Cardiovascular Clinical Pharmacist, University of Arizona Medical Center, Tucson, Arizona

Elizabeth W. Nugent, M.D. [97] Associate Professor of Pediatrics (Cardiology), Emory University School of Medicine, Atlanta, Georgia

John B. O'Connell, M.D. [88] Professor and Chairman, Department of Medicine, University of Mississippi School of Medicine, Jackson, Mississippi

Robert A. O'Rourke, M.D. [9A, 10, 19, 80] Charles Conrad Brown Distinguished Professor of Medicine, Director of Cardiology, The University of Texas Health Science Center at San Antonio; Chief of Cardiology, University of Texas Health Science Center Teaching Hospitals, San Antonio, Texas

Lionel H. Opie, M.D., Ph.D. [109] Professor of Medicine, University of Cape Town; Director, Hypertension Clinic, Groote Schuur Hospital, Cape Town, South Africa

Josef Patsch, M.D. [53] Professor, Head, Division of Clinical Atherosclerosis Research; Chairman, Department of Medicine, University of Innsbruck, Innsbruck, Austria

Alan S. Pearlman, M.D. [130] Professor of Medicine (Cardiology), University of Washington School of Medicine, Seattle, Washington

Roderic I. Pettigrew, Ph.D., M.D. [136] Associate Professor of Radiology, Emory University School of Medicine; Director, Cardiovascular Imaging Research, Emory University Hospital, Atlanta, Georgia

Claude A. Piantadosi, M.D. [120] Associate Professor of Medicine, Duke University School of Medicine; Director, F. G. Hall Hypo/Hyperbaric Center, Duke University Medical Center, Durham, North Carolina

William H. Plauth, Jr., M.D. [97] Professor of Pediatrics, Emory University School of Medicine; Cardiologist, The Children's Heart Center, Atlanta, Georgia

Gerald M. Pohost, M.D. [60] Mary Gertrude Waters Professor of Cardiovascular Medicine, University of Alabama at Birmingham School of Medicine; Director, Division of Cardiovascular Disease, University of Alabama Hospitals, Birmingham, Alabama

Craig Pratt, M.D. [60] Professor of Medicine, Baylor College of Medicine; Director, Coronary Care Unit, Methodist Hospital, Houston, Texas

Charles F. Presti, M.D. [132] Private Practice; Attending Physician, Parkview Memorial Hospital, Lutheran Hospital, St. Joseph's Medical Center, Fort Wayne, Indiana

Charles E. Rackley, M.D. [62, 79, 80, 81, 82] Professor of Medicine, Georgetown University School of Medicine; Director of Lipid Disorder Center, Georgetown University Medical Center, Washington, D.C.

B. Ashok Raj, M.D. [118] Associate Professor of Psychiatry, Chief, Division of Geriatric Psychiatry, University of South Florida College of Medicine; Director, Senior Adult Unit, University of South Florida Psychiatry Center, Tampa, Florida

Elliot Rapaport, M.D. [79] Professor of Medicine, William Watt Kerr Professor of Clinical Medicine, Associate Dean for San Francisco General Hospital, University of California, San Francisco, School of Medicine, San Francisco, California

David P. Rardon, M.D. [37] Associate Professor of Medicine, Krannert Institute of Cardiology, Indiana University School of Medicine, Indianapolis, Indiana

John T. Reeves, M.D. [120] Professor of Medicine and Pediatrics, University Colorado School of Medicine, Denver, Colorado

Timothy J. Regan, M.D. [105] Professor of Medicine, Director, Division of Cardiovascular Diseases, University of Medicine and Dentistry of New Jersey, New Jersey Medical School, Newark, New Jersey

David L. Reich, M.D. [140] Assistant Professor of Anesthesiology, Director of Cardiothoracic Anesthesia, Mt. Sinai Medical Center, New York, New York

Dale G. Renlund, M.D. [88] Associate Professor of Medicine, University of Utah School of Medicine; Medical Director, University of Utah Affiliated Hospitals Cardiac Transplant Program, Salt Lake City, Utah

Robert Roberts, M.D. [1, 21, 60, 96] Professor of Medicine and Cell Biology, Chief of Cardiology; Director, Bugher Foundation Center for Molecular Biology of the Cardiovascular Diseases; Director, Specialized Center of Research in Heart Failure, Baylor College of Medicine, Houston, Texas

William C. Roberts, M.D [90] Executive Director, Baylor Cardiovascular Institute, Baylor University Medical Center, Dallas, Texas

Thom W. Rooke, M.D. [129] Assistant Professor of Medicine, Mayo Medical School, Rochester, Minnesota

John Ross, Jr., M.D. [23] Professor of Medicine, Co-Director for Scientific Affairs, Division of Cardiology, University of California, San Diego, La Jolla, California

Joseph C. Ross, M.D. [101] Professor of Medicine, Associate Vice Chancellor for Health Affairs, Vanderbilt University Medical Center, Nashville, Tennessee

Russell Ross, Ph.D. [54] Professor and Chairman, Department of Pathology; Adjunct Professor, Department of Biochemistry; Director, Center for Vascular Biology, University of Washington School of Medicine, Seattle, Washington

Loring B. Rowell, Ph.D. [120] Professor of Physiology/Biochemistry, Professor of Medicine (Cardiology), University of Washington School of Medicine, Seattle, Washington

Marschall S. Runge, M.D., Ph.D. [7] Associate Professor of Medicine, Emory University School of Medicine, Atlanta, Georgia

Jeremy N. Ruskin, M.D. [42] Associate Professor of Medicine, Harvard Medical School; Director, Cardiac Arrhythmia Service, Massachusetts General Hospital, Boston, Massachusetts

Elliot L. Sagall, M.D. [143] Assistant Clinical Professor of Medicine, Harvard Medical School, Boston, Massachusetts

Rosemarie, Salerni, M.D. [11] Associate Professor of

Medicine, Univeristy of Pittsburgh, Pittsburgh, Pennsylvania

Herbert A. Saltzman, M.D. [120] Professor of Medicine, Duke University School of Medicine, Durham, North Carolina

Robert C. Saunders, M.D. [48] Northwest Hospital, Seattle, Washington

Stephen F. Schaal, M.D. [50] Professor of Medicine, Colleges of Medicine and Pharmacy, The Ohio State University; Director, Electrophysiology Laboratory, Ohio State University Hospitals, Columbus, Ohio

Melvin M. Scheinman, M.D. [43] Professor of Medicine, University of California, San Francisco School of Medicine; Chief, Electrocardiography and Clinical Cardiac Electrophysiology Section, H.C. Moffitt and J. Long Hospitals, San Francisco, California

Heinrich R. Schelbert, M.D. [137] Professor of Molecular and Medical Pharmacology and Professor of Radiological Sciences; Vice Chair, Department of Molecular and Medical Pharmacology; Principal Investigator, Laboratory of Structural Biology and Molecular Medicine, University of California at Los Angeles School of Medicine, Los Angeles, California

James Scheuer, M.D. [114] Professor of Medicine, Physiology and Biophysics, Baumritter Professor and Chairman of the Department of Medicine, Albert Einstein College of Medicine, Bronx, New York

Robert C. Schlant, M.D. [4, 5, 10, 16, 22, 25, 58, 103, 110, 139] Professor of Medicine (Cardiology), Emory University School of Medicine; Chief of Cardiology, Grady Memorial Hospital, Atlanta, Georgia

John S. Schroeder, M.D. [32] Professor of Medicine, Cardiovascular Medicine Division, Stanford University School of Medicine, Stanford, California

Steven P. Schulman, M.D. [115] Assistant Professor of Medicine, Johns Hopkins University School of Medicine; Director, Coronary Care Unit, Johns Hopkins Hospital, Baltimore, Maryland

Ralph Shabetai, M.D. [91, 92] Professor of Medicine, University of California San Diego School of Medicine; Chief, Cardiology Section, San Diego Veterans Affairs Medical Center, San Diego, California

James A. Shaver, M.D. [11] Professor of Medicine and Director, Division of Cardiology, University of Pittsburgh School of Medicine, Pittsburgh, Pennsylvania

David V. Sheehan, M.D. [118] Professor of Psychiatry, University of South Florida College of Medicine; Professor of Psychology, University of South Florida College of Social and Behavioral Sciences; Director, Office of Research, University of South Florida Psychiatry Center, Tampa, Florida

Benjamin Signer, M.D. [126] Fellow in Radiology, Stanford University School of Medicine, Stanford, California

Mark E. Silverman, M.D. [10] Professor of Medicine (Cardiology), Emory University School of Medicine; Chief of Cardiology, Piedmont Hospital, Atlanta, Georgia

Robert B. Smith, III, M.D. [125] Professor of Surgery and Head, General Vascular Surgery, Emory University School of Medicine, Associate Medical Director, Associate Chief of Surgery, Emory University Hospital, Atlanta, Georgia

Edmund H. Sonnenblick, M.D. [5, 22, 25, 26, 28, 66, 67, 102] Olson Professor of Medicine; Chief, Division of Cardiology; Director, Cardiovascular Center, Albert Einstein College of Medicine, Bronx, New York

Michael C. Soulen, M.D. [128] Assistant Professor of Radiology and Surgery, University of Pennsylvania School of Medicine, Philadelphia, Pennsylvania

Renate L. Soulen, M.D. [128] Professor of Radiology, Wayne State University School of Medicine; Director, Magnetic Resonance Center, Harper Hospital, Detroit, Michigan

Bernardo Stein, M.D. [21, 68] Assistant Professor of Medicine, Baylor College of Medicine; Director, Cardiac Catheterization Laboratories and Interventional Cardiology, Veterans Affairs Medical Center, Houston, Texas

Gary L. Stiles, M.D. [3] Professor of Medicine and Pharmacology, Chief, Division of Cardiology, Duke University School of Medicine, Durham, North Carolina

John H. Stone, M.D. [106] Professor of Medicine (Cardiology), Associate Dean, Emory University School of Medicine, Atlanta, Georgia

D. Eugene Strandness, Jr., M.D. [127] Professor of Surgery and Chief, Division of Vascular Surgery, University of Washington School of Medicine; Medical Director, Vascular Diagnostic Service, University of Washington Medical Center, Seattle, Washington

Panagiotis N. Symbas, M.D. [112] Professor of Surgery, Emory University School of Medicine, Atlanta, Georgia

Pierre Théroux, M.D. [59] Professor of Medicine, University of Montreal School of Medicine; Chief, Coronary Care Unit, Montreal Heart Institute; Chief, Clinical Research, Montreal Heart Institute, Montreal, Quebec, Canada

Thomas J. Thom, B.A. [8] Statistician, Division of Epidemiology and Clinical Applications, National Heart, Lung, and Blood Institute, National Institutes of Health, Bethesda, Maryland

Jeffrey A. Towbin, M.D. [96] Associate Professor of Pediatrics (Pediatric Cardiology), Institute for Molecular Genetics; Baylor College of Medicine; Director, Phoebe Willingham Muzzy Pediatric Molecular Cardiology Laboratory; Medical Director, Pediatric Cardiac Transplant Service, Texas Children's Hospital, Houston, Texas

Elbert P. Tuttle, Jr., M.D. [76] Professor of Medicine, Emeritus, Emory University School of Medicine, Atlanta, Georgia

Kent Ueland M.D. [113] Professor Emeritus, Department of Gynecology and Obstetrics, Stanford University School of Medicine, Stanford, California

Lodewyk H. S. Van Mierop, M.D. [95] Graduate Research Professor, Pediatric Cardiologist, University of Florida College of Medicine, Gainesville, Florida

Marc Verstraete, M.D., Ph.D. [69] Professor of Medicine, Director, Center for Thrombosis and Vascular Research, University of Leuven, Leuven, Belgium

Albert L. Waldo, M.D. [35] Walter H. Prichard Professor of Cardiology and Professor of Medicine; Case Western Reserve University School of Medicine; Director, Cardiac Arrhythmia Service, University Hospital of Cleveland, Cleveland, Ohio

Robert B. Wallace, M.D. [81] Chairman and Professor of Surgery, Georgetown University School of Medicine, Washington, D.C.

Bruce F. Waller, M.D. [4, 64] Clinical Professor of Pathology and Medicine, Indiana University School of Medicine; Director, Cardiovascular Pathology, St. Vincent Hospital, Indianapolis, Indiana

Paul F. Walter, M.D. [47] Professor of Medicine (Cardiology), Emory University School of Medicine, Atlanta, Georgia

David Waters, M.D. [59] Professor of Medicine (Cardiology), Director of Cardiology, University of Connecticut, School of Medicine, Hartford, Connecticut

Myron L. Weisfeldt, M.D. [52, 115] Professor and Chairman, Department of Medicine, Robert L. Levy Professor of Cardiology, College of Physicians and Surgeons, Columbia University, New York, New York

Arnold M. Weissler, M.D. [50] Professor of Medicine, Mayo Medical School; Consultant in Cardiovascular Diseases, Mayo Clinic, Rochester, Minnesota

Nanette Kass Wenger, M.D. [63, 121] Professor of Medicine (Cardiology), Emory University School of Medicine; Director, Cardiac Clinics, Grady Memorial Hospital, Atlanta, Georgia

Lewis Wexler, M.D. [126] Professor of Radiology and Medicine (Cardiology), Stanford University School of Medicine, Stanford, California

Joseph A. Wilber, M.D. [142] Clinical Associate Professor of Medicine, Emory University School of Medicine; Former Vice President of Georgia International Life Insurance Company, Atlanta, Georgia

Willis H. Williams, M.D. [97] Professor of Surgery (Cardiothoracic), Emory University School of Medicine; Chief of Cardiothoracic Surgery, Egleston Children's Hospital at Emory, Atlanta, Georgia

Marc Wish, M.D. [39] Assistant Professor of Medicine, Georgetown University School of Medicine, Washington, D.C.; Director, Pacing and Electrophysiology Laboratory, Veterans Affairs Medical Center, Washington, D.C.

Andrew L. Wit, Ph.D. [35] Professor of Pharmacology, College of Physicians and Surgeons of Columbia University, New York, New York

Gary L. Wollam, M.D. [76] Formerly Associate Professor of Medicine, Emory University School of Medicine; Medical Director, Cobb Hospital Dialysis Center, Austell, Georgia

Raymond L. Woosley, M.D., Ph.D. [38] Professor of Medicine and Pharmacology, Chairman, Department of Pharmacology, Georgetown University School of Medicine, Washington, D.C.

Douglas P. Zipes, M.D. [45] Professor of Medicine, Indiana University School of Medicine, Indianapolis, Indiana

Joel Zonszein, M.D. [102] Associate Professor of Medicine, Director, Division of Endocrinology and Metabolism, The Bronx Lebanon Hospital Center, Albert Einstein College of Medicine, New York, New York

Preface

The basic objectives of this eighth edition of *The Heart* remain the same as those of the previous seven editions: to provide a practical, authoritative, up-to-date guide to the daily practice of cardiology, closely integrated with the basic science foundations on which such practice is based. This edition is published with a strong appreciation of two major influences of cardiology. The first is an explosive growth in cardiovascular basic science, diagnostic procedures, and therapeutic alternatives. The second new major force impinging on cardiology is the increasing importance of cost-effective considerations in both the diagnosis and management of patients with cardiovascular disorders. These two forces are revolutionizing the practice of cardiology and undoubtedly will be of increasing importance in future years. The eighth edition has been extensively revised with the objective of integrating, when appropriate, clinically applicable basic science into a discussion of pathophysiology and therapeutics.

We would like to express our appreciation to J. Willis Hurst, the senor editor and editor-in-chief of the previous seven editions. His continued and enthusiastic support has been of great value in the completion of the eighth edition. We feel honored to carry on the tradition of *The Heart*.

We would like to thank our many contributors for their superb efforts. We thank our students, residents, and fellows for their continued curiosity and questioning, which provide a constant source of stimulation.

Many colleagues at Emory have helped directly and indirectly in the completion of this edition, including Dr. Daniel Arensberg, Dr. Charles B. Treasure, and Dr. Larry Klein.

Special thanks and appreciation are due to Mr. Dereck Jeffers at McGraw-Hill, Inc., who has served as sponsoring editor for five editions of *The Heart*. His great wisdom and advice have been invaluable. Mr. Steven Melvin has been a superb editing supervisor, to whom we are deeply indebted.

This edition would not have been possible without the extensive contributions and personal sacrifices of a number of individuals including Shirley Ballou, Amanda Morris, William Payne, Barbara Merchant, Larkin O'Donohue, Cynthia Painter, Linda Markwell, Jeff Clark, and Eddie Jackson. Their efforts made this edition possible.

Finally, we would like to acknowledge the inestimable personal sacrifices made by members of our families to make this volume possible. They remain our constant support and strength. They include Maria Ellingsen-Schlant, Stephanie St. Onge, and Christiane Abel, as well as Jane W. Alexander and Kate, Melissa, and David Alexander.

PART I

Basic Foundations of Cardiology

Chapter 1

Introduction to the Techniques of Molecular Biology and the Molecular Basis for Cardiac Growth

Robert Roberts, M.D.

The application of the techniques of recombinant DNA to cardiovascular disorders appears to be both essential and ideally suited to overcome several of the major obstacles to future progress.[1-3] The heart exhibits three characteristic adaptive responses to changes in its environment: The constitutive adaptive mechanism—namely, myofibril stretch that regulates cardiac output on a beat-to-beat basis (Starling's Law)[4]; modulation of excitation contraction coupling through intramyofibril calcium; and the long-term adaptation of compensatory growth (see Chap. 5). The first two adaptations have been extensively characterized in this century through the development, refinement, and application of hemodynamic techniques. To understand the long-term adaptive mechanism of cardiac growth requires an elucidation of its molecular genetic basis, particularly if one desires to intervene therapeutically and modulate growth. Similarly, elimination of restenosis after angioplasty will probably require disruption of the smooth-muscle growth response,[6-8] and to unravel the molecular basis for hereditary cardiac disorders, including the cardiomyopathies, will definitely require molecular genetics[9,10] (see Chap. 96).

Application of the techniques of molecular biology to cardiology occurred only recently; nevertheless, progress has been rapid. For example, recombinantly made tissue plasminogen activator (rt-PA) initiated in 1983[11] became part of a paradigmatic shift in the therapy of myocardial infarction, which was quickly followed by recombinantly made hirudin, superoxide dismutase, urokinase, prourokinase, and multiple mutant forms of rt-PA.[12]

Historical Perspective of Molecular Biology

In 1953, Watson and Crick[13,14] proposed the double helix model for DNA structure based on the results of X-ray diffraction by Franklin and Wilkins.[15,16] The implications of DNA being a double helix were evident; namely, that one strand could serve as a template for the synthesis of new strands, thus providing the means whereby genetic information could be perpetuated from parent to offspring. In 1957, Kornberg[17] described DNA polymerase, the enzyme necessary for the synthesis of DNA that was essential to recombinant DNA technology. Marmor and colleagues[18] showed that the double helix of DNA could be separated by high temperatures[19] into its separate strands (denatured) and that decreasing the temperature resulted in the strands reannealing, or hybridizing, thus, returning to their previous double-stranded nature. This specific hybridization, or "recombination" of complementary nucleotide strands, provides both the rationale and the practical basis for much of recombinant DNA technology. Crick had suggested correctly that the genetic code would be written in codons of three nucleotides for each amino acid.[14] The specific combination of three nucleotides that code for each amino acid was unravelled by Nirenberg, Khorana and colleagues.[20,21] Several other necessary components were discovered subsequently including the enzyme DNA ligase, which joins DNA fragments together.[22] All of this information was known in the 1960s and the complete DNA code, together with its cytoplasmic mediator RNA provided communication with the protein synthetic apparatus, had been elucidated; but recombinant technology was not yet born and, in fact, for the next few years did not appear promising.

Many important discoveries, including those from the 1950s, played a role in recombinant technology, but four that really brought it to fruition and made possible modern molecular biology occurred between the years 1970 and 1977. A major obstacle to the manipulation of DNA was its size and our inability to cut it into smaller pieces of known specific size. This obstacle was overcome by the discovery of restriction endonucleases that made it possible to cut DNA into smaller pieces in a predictable fashion.[23,24] These endonucleases, more commonly referred to as restriction enzymes, recognize specific sequences of DNA consisting of anywhere from three to eight nucleotides and specifically cut the DNA molecules at their recognition sites, making it possible to utilize and manipulate DNA fragments in a variety of procedures and reactions. In 1972, the enzyme, reverse transcriptase, was discovered by two investigators simultaneously,[25,26] making it possible to translate messenger RNA (mRNA) into its complementary DNA (cDNA). Around this time the group at Stanford[27] cloned the first molecule and the recombinant technique was born. Modern molecular biology rapidly accelerated into reality and development has continued to accelerate. In 1977, Sanger et al.[28] and Maxim and Gilbert[29] developed techniques for the rapid sequencing of DNA and RNA. In addition to these four developments, the recent development of polymerase chain reaction (PCR), a technique that can be used to amplify rapidly small amounts of DNA or RNA several millionfold, is having a revolutionary effect on the application of these techniques in medicine and other fields.

NUCLEIC ACIDS

The Essentials of Nucleic Acids

The human genome is known to contain about three billion base pairs, which contain information that would more than fill a 500,000 page textbook. It is estimated that the DNA molecules present in a single human being joined together head to tail would reach from the earth to the moon 8000 times. The immensity of the DNA molecules and their massive size was a major deterrent to the development of recombinant DNA techniques. The DNA is contained in 46 chromosomes consisting of 44 autosomal and two sex chromosomes, but each chromosome is one continuous DNA molecule. The smallest chromosome, twenty-one, has more than 50 million base pairs, while chromosome one, the largest, has over 250 million base pairs. There is enough DNA to form about 10 million genes; however, it is estimated that only about 30,000 to 50,000 genes are required to code for a human being. This would indicate that less than 1% of our DNA is used to code for protein.

DNA consists of four building blocks—the nucleotides, often referred to as merely as bases. There are two purine bases (adenine and guanine) and two pyrimidine bases (cytosine and thymine) (Fig. 1-1). A nucleotide consists of a base joined to the 5-carbon sugar, deoxyribose, together with a phosphate group attached to the 5′ carbon (Fig. 1-2). DNA is a double-stranded molecule forming a spiral right-handed helix with the two chains in opposite direction (Fig. 1-3). The backbone of the molecule, formed by the sugar and phosphate molecules, is exposed to the outside of the double helix. The center of the molecule consists of the bases which face inward and are opposite to each other. This arrangement provides for the hydrogen bonding between the bases that keeps the two strands together. The hydrogen bonds are perpendicular to the helical axis. The directionality of the strands is referred to as 5′ to 3′ or 3′ to 5′, which refers to the position of the carbons in the sugar. The sugars are joined together by bonding between the 5′ carbon via the phosphate group to the 3′ carbon of the adjacent sugar. The end of the molecule with a phosphate or hydroxyl group on the 5′ carbon, is termed the 5′ end, whereas a free terminal 3′ carbon, is referred to as the 3′ end. It is important to distinguish the two ends since DNA replication always proceeds from the 5′ to the 3′ end, and the sequences essential to gene regulation (discussed later) are located on the 5′ or 3′ ends of the

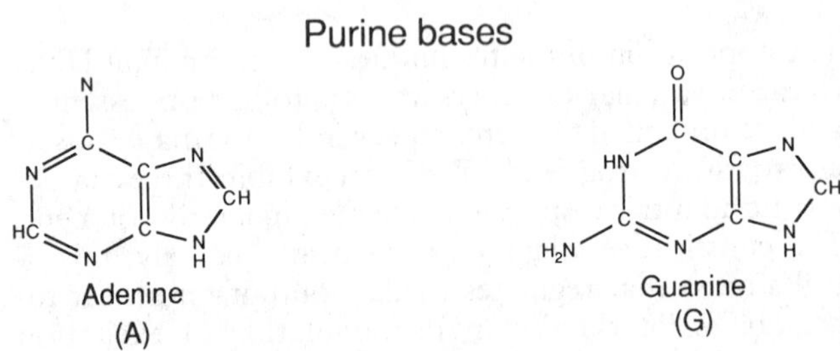

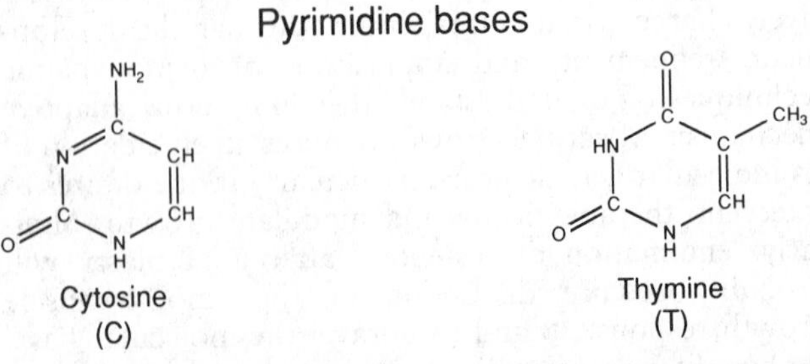

FIGURE 1-1 The common purine and pyrimidine bases found in DNA. Uracil is substituted for thymine in RNA. *(From Mares A Jr., Towbin J, Bies RG, Roberts R: Molecular biology for the cardiologist. Curr Probl Cardiol 1992; 17: 9–72. Reproduced with permission from the publisher and authors.)*

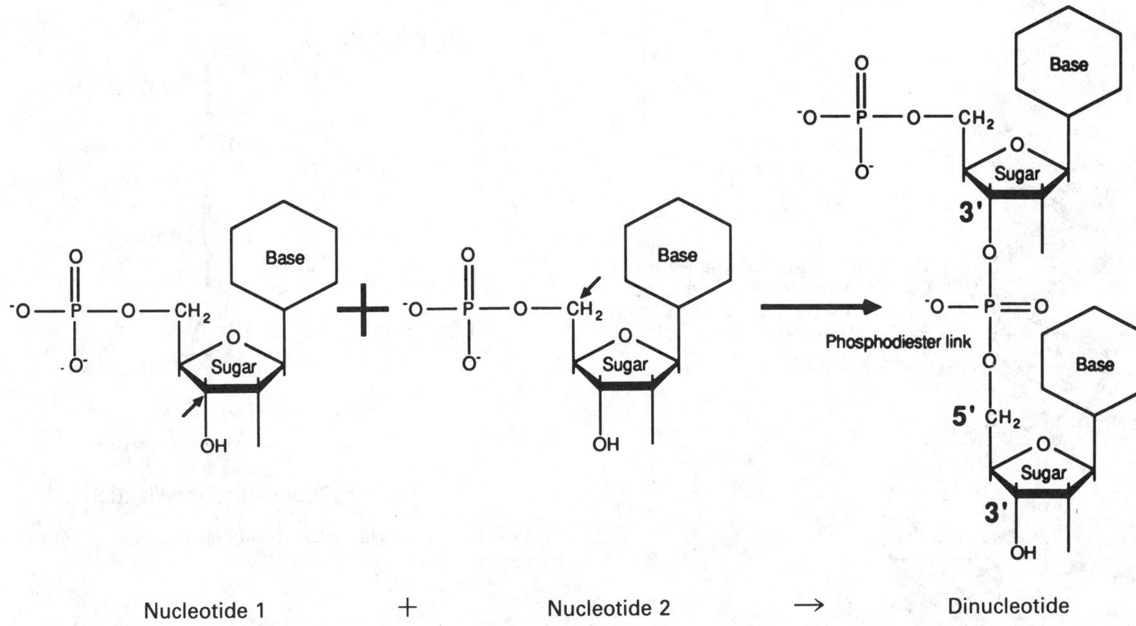

FIGURE 1-2 Formation of polynucleotides from nucleotide precursors. Nucleotides are joined together by a phosphodiester linkage to form a nucleic acid. Arrows indicate the carbon atoms of deoxyribose that are joined by phosphodiester bonds to form polynucleotides. Note that the bases are attached to 1′ carbon position of the sugar molecule and face the interior of the molecule. The backbone is formed by the sugar linked by phosphate groups binding to 5′ and 3′ carbons of the sugar. *(From Mares A Jr., Towbin J, Bies RG, Roberts R: Molecular biology for the cardiologist. Curr Probl Cardiol 1992; 17: 9–72. Reproduced with permission from the publisher and authors.)*

gene. There seem to be no constraints on which bases can be adjacent to each other; however, the hydrogen pairing between the bases of the two chains is highly specific, as adenine (A) always pairs with thymine (T), and guanine (G) always pairs with cytosine (C). The specificity of this "base pairing" is the basis of the ability of DNA to replicate itself and pass on the characteristics of genotype, as well as the basis for the specificity of essentially all of the procedures used in recombinant DNA technology. During the process of DNA replication, the strands separate and new strands form complementary to the original strands resulting in two additional identical molecules.

Transcription

The central dogma of molecular biology is that DNA produces RNA, which in turn produces proteins, the latter being the molecules that provide the cytoskeleton and perform the functions of the cell (Fig. 1-4). The genetic information inherited by each individual is encoded by the DNA (the genotype), which is translated into proteins and provides the observable characteristics of the individual (the phenotype). This overall process from DNA to protein, however, must first go through the intermediary step of RNA. The process whereby messenger RNA (mRNA) is synthesized using DNA as the template is referred to as transcription (Fig. 1-5). Transcription and the processing of mRNA occurs in the nucleus of the cell, separated by the nuclear membrane from the cytoplasm of the cell. The process of transcription is initiated by the attachment of the enzyme RNA polymerase II to specific recognition sites where the DNA is double-stranded, but, upon activation by the enzyme, the strands now selectively unwind and separate (Fig. 1-6). The binding site for RNA polymerase II is always located on the 5′ end of the gene, and the enzyme remains attached to a single strand of DNA as it travels in the 3′ direction. The DNA immediately in front of it separates into two strands with just one strand of DNA (antisense) acting as a template for the synthesis of mRNA. Thus, in contrast to DNA, mRNA is a single-stranded polynucleotide. Messenger RNA also differs from DNA in that deoxyribose, the sugar found in DNA, is replaced by ribose, and uracil (U) replaces thymine (T) which, like thymine, exclusively pairs with adenine (A). Thus, by this mechanism each adenine (A) of DNA pairs with uracil (U) of RNA; each cytosine (C) of DNA pairs with guanine (G) of RNA; each thymine (T) of DNA pairs with adenine (A) of RNA; and each guanine (G) of DNA pairs with cytosine (C) of RNA.

The mRNA, as transcribed from the DNA, is referred to as the primary transcript, or sometimes as immature mRNA, and is a complementary copy of the DNA (Fig. 1-7). Since protein synthesis occurs in the cytoplasm, the mRNA must exit the nucleus, but prior to transport, it undergoes extensive posttranscriptional processing. The three main events in mRNA processing are the addition of a cap to the 5′ end, a poly (A) tail to the 3′ end, and the specific resplicing of the exons. (1) The addition of a methylated guanosine (7-methylguanosine residue) to the 5′ end, which is referred to as a cap, is important in the initiation of translation. (2) The addition of a long tail of repeated adenine nucleotides, called the poly (A) tail, to the 3′ region of the mRNA, appears to be essential for subsequent stability of the message in the cytoplasm. In the nucleus, the poly (A) tail is approximately 250 nucleotides long but decreases with the age of the mRNA

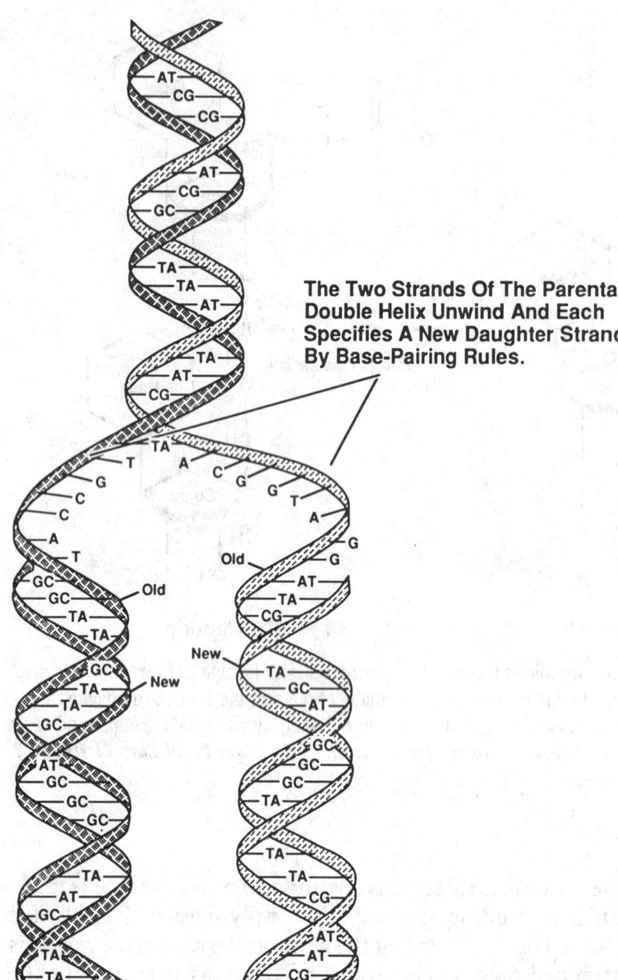

FIGURE 1-3 DNA replication conserves the nucleotide sequence. DNA is a double-stranded helical molecule bound together by the nucleotide bases contained on each individual strand. During cell division two identical copies of the original parental strand are made by unwinding the DNA, then synthesizing a complementary second strand to make two identical new daughter strands.

in the cytoplasm. (3) The primary transcript, which contains introns and exons, undergoes a specific splicing process whereby the introns are removed and the exons are properly respliced together prior to exit from the nucleus as mature mRNA. The process of splicing is, in part, performed by molecules referred to as small nuclear ribonucleoproteins (snRNPs), which consist of RNA molecules tightly associated with a group of about 10 different proteins. Exons consist of DNA coding for

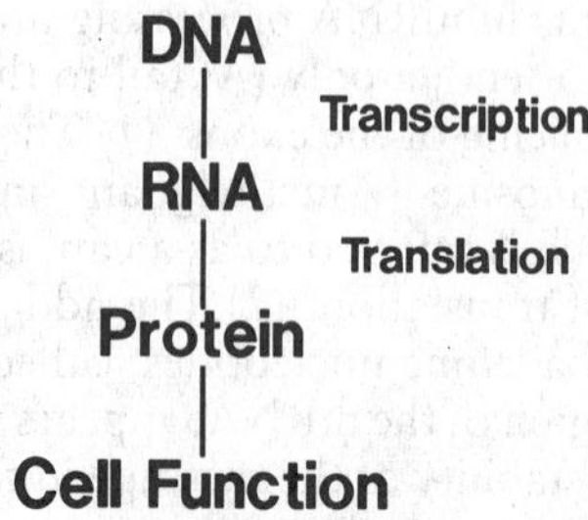

FIGURE 1-4 Central dogma of molecular biology.

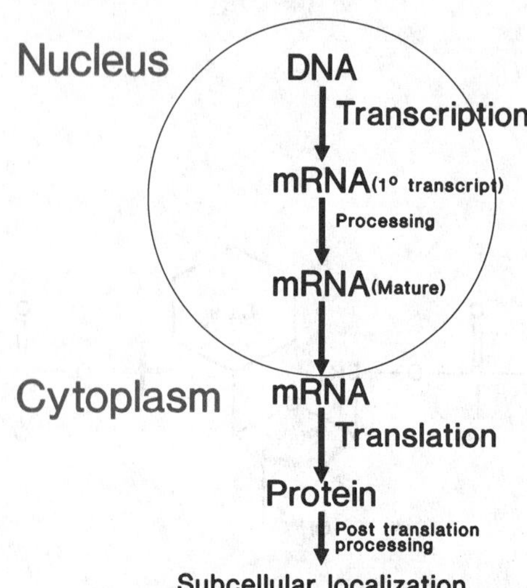

FIGURE 1-5 Schematic localization of the processes of transcription and translation.

RNA that survives the mRNA processing and exits the nucleus as part of the mature mRNA. Exons generally occupy three distinct regions of the mRNA. The first is not translated into protein but signals the beginning of mRNA transcription and contains sequences that direct the mRNA to the ribosome in the cytoplasm for protein synthesis. The exons in the second region, sometimes referred to as the coding region, contain the information that is translated into the amino acid sequence of the protein. The exons of the third region do not code for protein but code for the signals for the termination of translation and the addition of the poly (A) tail. Introns are portions of the gene that code for mRNA and are included in the primary transcript, but are spliced out so

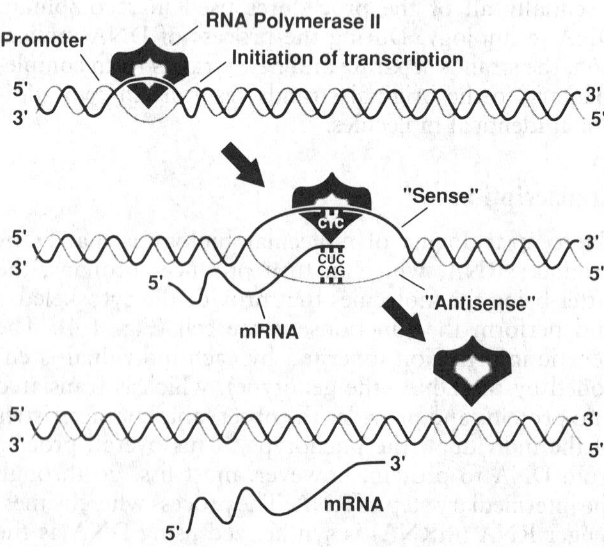

FIGURE 1-6 Illustration of how RNA polymerase II interacts with DNA and the promoter to generate a single-stranded mRNA. RNA Polymerase II attaches to the initiation site promoted by the 5′ promoter sequence. mRNA is synthesized in the 5′ to 3′ direction from just one strand, the antisense strand. The specificity of base pairing between mRNA and the antisense strand provides for a mRNA with sequences complementary to that of the antisense and identical to that of the sense strand.

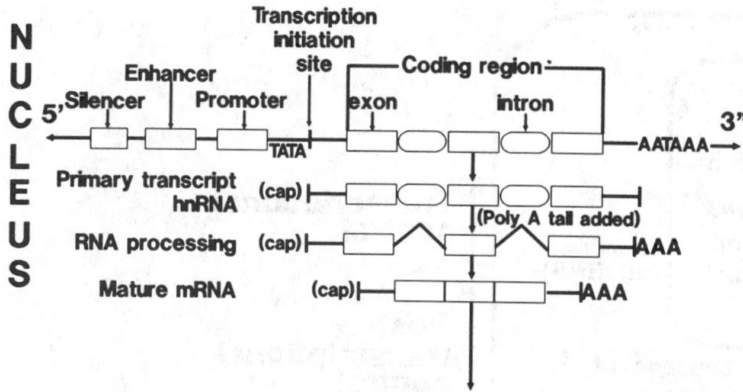

FIGURE 1-7 Transcription. Transcription occurs in the nucleus, producing mRNA, which is processed into mature mRNA and transported to the cytoplasm. In the cytoplasm, translation occurs with the mRNA coding for specific amino acids, which are linked together to form a polypeptide and, ultimately, to form a mature protein. *(From Mares A Jr., Towbin J, Bies RG, Roberts R: Molecular biology for the cardiologist. Curr Probl Cardiol 1992; 17: 9–72. Reproduced with permission from the publisher and authors.)*

they do not appear in the mature mRNA. The process of splicing out of introns and the rejoining of exons is an important means of introducing genetic diversity and will be discussed further under gene regulation. The primary transcript undergoes extensive shortening such that the mature mRNA may represent only 5% to 10% of the primary transcript. The different species of mRNA produced during the process of splicing within the nucleus are sometimes referred to as heterogeneous nuclear mRNA; hence, the term hnmRNA. Once mRNA processing is complete, the mature mRNA rapidly exits the nucleus through nuclear pores and enters the cytoplasm where it attaches to a ribosome to initiate protein synthesis.

Translation

The final process whereby the nucleic acids of the mRNA code for a specific polypeptide is referred to as translation. This process is the most complex of the various processes that occur in the flow from genomic DNA (gene) to that of the fully mature protein. The alphabet of the mRNA is, of course, the nucleotide (base), while that of the protein is the amino acid. In 1961 Crick[13] showed that the genetic code was written in triplets with each amino acid being encoded by three base pairs referred to as a *codons* and that the specificity is determined by the sequence of the base pairs in the codon. The mRNA codons dictate which amino acids are to be selected and the order of the codons dictates the sequence of the amino acids in the protein. The definition of the codons for each amino acid was completed in 1966. There are four different nucleotides to form the triplets; thus, the number of combinations (4^3) is 64, but there are only 20 amino acids. There is considerable redundancy referred to as degeneracy, which results in several of the amino acids having more than one codon. In addition to codons for each amino acid, there is also the codon AUG, which is the start codon that initiates protein synthesis, and also codes for methionine. To stop translation, there are three codons, UAA, UAG, and UGA, which signal the end of a particular polypeptide. The mRNA, after exiting the nucleus, recognizes the ribosome, which is the site of protein synthesis. The ribosome moves along a mRNA molecule translating each of its triplet code words, or codons, in a 5′ to 3′ direction to assemble the polypeptide from its amino (N-terminal) to its carboxy (C-terminal) ends (Fig. 1-8).

The mRNA does not interact directly with amino acids but rather through adaptor molecules—referred to as transfer RNA (tRNA)—to which amino acids are joined by a highly specific enzyme (aminoacyl tRNA synthetase) via an energy-rich covalent bond. There is at least one tRNA species corresponding to each of the 20 naturally occurring amino acids. The aminoacyl tRNA synthetase performs a special function of activating the amino acids and assuring that each amino acid is joined to its tRNA and to no other. The structure of tRNA is now known in great detail and its specificity is attributed to the sequence of three nucleotides complementary to the codon exposed at one end of the folded tRNA molecule, which, on the tRNA, is referred to as the *anticodon.* The amino acid receptor site is exposed at the other end. Amino acids are, thus, specified at two recognition steps: one in which a specific enzyme joins the amino acid to a specific tRNA and the other in which the tRNA serving as an adaptor molecule joins the amino acid to the ribosomal-mRNA complex through a codon-anticodon specific-base-pairing interaction between the mRNA and the tRNA. Once the amino acid has been activated and the process of protein synthesis initiated, the large structural ribosomal RNA (rRNA) moves along the mRNA joining the amino acids via peptide bonds in the sequence specified by the mRNA to form the mature polypeptide. The process of protein synthesis from this complex of mRNA and ribosomal RNA involves over 100 enzymes. The steps involved consist of initiation, elongation, and termination of the polypeptide with each process having its own enzymes.

The mature polypeptide consists of amino acids joined together by peptide bonds; however, the mature protein often consists of multiple covalently-bound polypeptides and many undergo other modifications referred to as posttranslational changes. A more detailed analysis of protein synthesis is discussed in Chap. 6B. Encoded in the polypeptide are other features that have been determined by the mRNA; namely, leader sequences that will direct the protein to either intracellular membranes, the plasma membrane, or to organelles, such as the mitochondria. There is also considerable proteolytic activity following entry of the molecule into its organelle, or membrane, as the leader sequences are removed. There are also the processes whereby disulfhydryl bonds are formed or glycosylation occurs (in the Golgi apparatus) (Fig. 1-8). The mRNAs generally are not long-lived due to their rapid degradation by RNAses and so may last from only a few minutes to many hours. A single mRNA may code for only a few copies of the polypeptide, or it may encode for several thousand, which on the average is estimated to be 1400. In contrast, rRNAs and tRNAs are much less rapidly degraded and, therefore, have acquired the name, “stable” RNAs. Their relative concentration in the cell, in large part, reflect their stability with 80 percent being rRNA, 15 percent tRNA, and less than 5 percent mRNA.

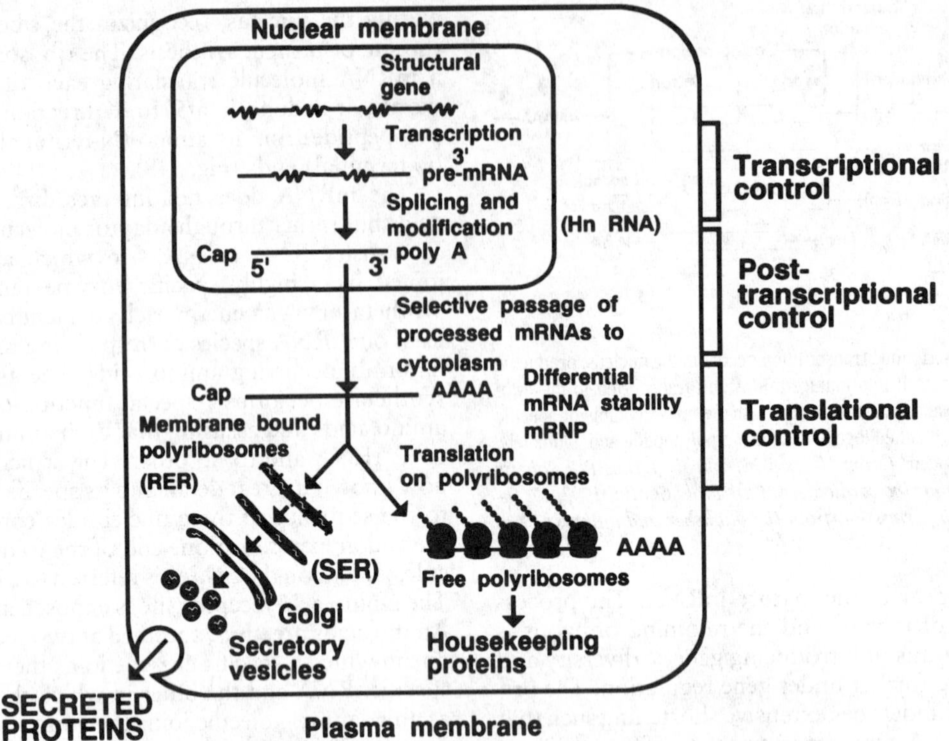

FIGURE 1-8 A summary of the multiple steps involved in gene expression from the genomic DNA to the protein. Note the protein destined for secretion follows a systematic path different from those destined to remain in the cytoplasm. *(From Nucleic acids and protein biosynthesis. PN Campbell, AD Smith (eds) Biochemistry Illustrated 2d ed. New York, Churchill Livingston, 1988:111. Reproduced with permission from the publisher.)*

Gene Structure, Expression and Its Regulation

The concept that one gene leads to one protein remains basic to the central dogma of molecular biology, but does need to be modified in view of recent observations. A gene consists of a discrete unit of DNA that encodes for either a ribonucleic acid or a protein and may give rise to more than one unique polypeptide. In the classical description, one envisions the gene encoding only for protein, but we now know certain genes encode for the ribonucleic acid of rRNA, tRNA, and snRNA, that are essential for the synthesis of proteins. They are the products of transcription rather than translation, and act directly in performing their specific function of assisting in the expression of genes that encode for proteins. The other class of genes, those that encode for proteins, do so through mRNA. It is now known that a single gene, as a result of rearrangement of the exons, may give rise to several mRNAs, which in turn translate into several unique polypeptides rather than a single polypeptide as originally envisioned. The following discussion will address the regulation of those genes that encode for proteins.

Gene expression refers to all of the processes required to go from DNA to protein, from the initial unfolding of the nuclear chromatin in preparation for transcription until the mature protein emerges following completion of posttranslational changes. Regulation of this process occurs at all levels in response to signals both from within the cell and from the environment. The latter mechanism is of particular interest as it represents one of the major areas of research in molecular biology and cardiology, and it is also an area which has great potential for therapeutic intervention. The cell maintains its integrity and responds to external stimuli through signals that activate receptors (generally in the cell membrane). These in turn use signaling proteins to transfer the message to the nucleus or cytoplasm, which in some way modifies gene expression. Delineation of the receptor, the signaling proteins, and where and how gene expression is altered is of prime importance.

The most fundamental level of gene regulation involves cell differentiation. The body contains approximately 200 different types of cells that have been programmed by their genes to perform highly specialized functions. All cells have the same DNA and the same genes, but only those genes that are expressed (produce protein) determine the cell's phenotype. Cardiac myocytes, for example, are characterized by a set of proteins that specialize in contractile activity while hepatocytes specialize in the synthesis and catabolism of proteins. Selective gene expression is the basis of cell differentiation. Cell growth and replication occur in what is termed the undifferentiated cell, but, through complex mechanisms, give rise to cells that cease to replicate and are programmed to take on specialized functions (cell differentiation). In the process of cell differentiation, genes—particularly those concerned with cell proliferation and undifferentiated functions—are down-regulated, while those genes coding for the proteins that perform the specialized functions are up-regulated. Once cells are differentiated, protein synthesis, however, remains a dynamic process to maintain cell integrity. Most of gene regulation is concerned with the maintenance of cellular integrity, and the genes responsible for this basal function are referred to as housekeeping genes. Housekeeping genes are constitutively regulated, as opposed to genes responsible for cell differentiation and growth that are developmentally regulated. It is estimated that organs utilize about 10,000 genes (constitutive) to maintain their integrity, with one exception—the brain, which is estimated to utilize around 20,000 genes. The expression of a gene may be regulated at any stage from chromatin rearrangement to the final subcellular localization of the mature protein. Regulation may be classified under the following headings: pretranscription, transcription, posttranscription, translation, and posttranslation.[30]

Pretranscriptional regulation refers to the decompaction of the DNA and exposure of the region about to undergo transcription. The total DNA of a single cell would measure about one meter in length; yet, in the nucleus it is markedly compacted and is folded around specific proteins, the dominant one being histone. The coiling of the DNA appears to be in domains that can be exposed when transcription is activated. It is also at this level that methylation plays a role, in that heavily methylated genes tend not to be transcribed, while other areas sensitive to digestion by the enzyme DNase appear to be very active in transcription. The precise mechanisms that regulate vulnerability to digestion by various DNases and the factors involved with chromatin conformational changes or exposure of the gene for transcription are, at present, relatively unknown. There is evidence, however, that methylation is involved in regulating cell differentiation.

Transcription is regulated by the enzyme RNA polymerase II, which determines genes that will be transcribed, and the rate of transcription; thus, the rate-limiting step to gene expression. Transcription is catalyzed by the enzyme RNA polymerase II, but the enzyme by itself cannot initiate transcription and acts only with the help of additional factors. These essential factors involve DNA sequences that, in conjunction with their corresponding DNA binding proteins, act as either promoters, enhancer, or silencers of transcription, and will be subsequently defined (Fig. 1-9). Each gene consists of a coding region comprised of exons and introns, and a regulatory region flanking the noncoding sequences on the 3′ and 5′ ends of the gene referred to as downstream and upstream sequences, respectively (Fig. 1-9). The 5′ upstream region, immediately adjacent to the transcription initiation site and including the area that binds RNA polymerase II, is referred to as the promoter region. The presence of a promoter is an absolute requirement for initiation of transcription. Thus, promoters may be defined as a sequence, or sequences, of DNA that must be in a relatively fixed location with respect to the starting point of transcription. In simplistic terms, the promoter acts by catalyzing the binding of the RNA polymerase to its binding site near the start codon. A promoter is only active when its sequences are bound by the appropriate protein. The protein that binds to the DNA promoter sequence is referred to as a transcription factor. The promoter sequences are often referred to as cis-acting sequences since they are on the same DNA molecule on which they act. The transcription factors (also referred to as DNA-binding proteins) are referred to as trans-

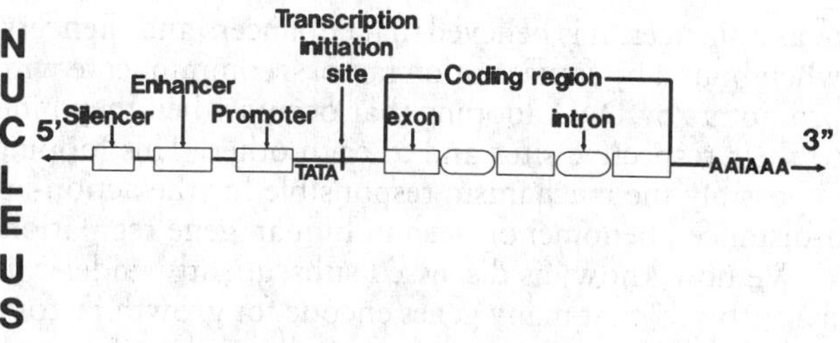

FIGURE 1-9 Structure of a gene. These small functional units within the nucleus contain the coding information for the synthesis of a polypeptide and, on its 5′ end, have regulatory sequences that include silencers, enhancers, and promoters. The coding region consisting of exons (code for protein) as well as intervening noncoding sequences (introns) is followed by a 3′ non-coding region which is translated into the mRNA. The 3′ end appears important for exit of the mRNA from the nucleus and its stability in the cytoplasm but does not code for protein. The TATA is the initiation site for polymerase and is present in most eukaryotes at about 10 to 30 bp 5′ from the start codon (TAC) of the coding region. The AATAAA will become the recognition site on the mRNA to which attaches an enzyme that cleaves the 3′ region and replaces the distal portion with a poly A tail. *(From Mares A Jr., Towbin J, Bies RG, Roberts R: Molecular biology for the cardiologist. Curr Probl Cardiol 1992; 17: 9–72. Reproduced with permission from the publisher and authors.)*

acting factors (acting at a distance) since they are encoded by DNA molecules removed from the genes they control. The average promoter consists of several hundred base pairs grouped into motifs of 6 to 10 base pairs and are active only in the 5′ to 3′ direction. They are usually within 1000 to 2000 base pairs of the beginning of the coding region.[31,32] It is hypothesized that all of the motifs have to be bound by transcription factors of the appropriate nature and in the appropriate sequence for transcription to occur.

It is generally accepted that the initiation of transcription always requires multiple factors other than RNA polymerase II. The promoters and their corresponding DNA-binding proteins may act ubiquitously or may be tissue-specific. The recently discovered myo-D protein, which induces skeletal muscle differentiation, is not expressed during cardiac muscle development. It is also believed that certain promoters and/or trans-acting factors enhance the transcription of classes of genes rather than a single gene. Certain promoter sequences are consistently present upstream of the start site of RNA polymerase II, one of which is the consensus sequence of 5′-TATA-3′ located 25 to 31 base pairs upstream from the transcription initiation site (Fig. 1-9). Another type of DNA sequence that enhances the initiation of transcription is that of an enhancer. These differ from promoter sequences in that they may be upstream or downstream from the coding region, can be separated by several thousand base pairs, and will work whether in the 5′ to 3′ or 3′ to 5′ direction. An example is the DNA sequence that enhances expression of the gene for hemoglobin that is located more than 1,000,000 base pairs from the transcription initiation site. These enhancers, like promoters, consist of several small motifs of 6 to 10 base pairs and, when bound by their corresponding DNA binding proteins (transcription factors), have a positive influence on gene transcription. Another regulatory DNA sequence that is similar to enhancers in size and location but exerts a negative influence on transcription is referred to as a silencer. It is believed that enhancers and silencers, when bound by transcription factors, communicate with promoters by DNA looping that occurs when they bind to their respective sites and to each other. This looping is possibly the mechanism responsible for the action-at-a-distance phenomenon seen in human gene regulation.

We now know, as discussed subsequently under cardiac growth, that many genes encode for growth factors, growth factor receptors, and intracellular signalling proteins that relay growth signals from the extracellular milieu to transcription factors that regulate RNA polymerase and selectively induce or down-regulate gene expression.[33] There are at least three major classes of DNA-binding proteins (transcription factors) (Fig. 1-10): the zinc fingers, leucine zippers, helix-loop-helix, and the helix-turn-helix proteins. The zinc finger type is utilized by circulating hormones, including the glucocorticoids, progesterones, androgens, mineralocorticoids, estrogen, thyroxine, vitamin D_3, and retinoic acid. These hormones are known to penetrate the cell membrane and to activate an intracellular receptor or nuclear receptor, which, in turn, activates gene expression through the zinc-finger transcription proteins. Many of the growth-related signalling proteins, such as c-*fos*, c-*myc*, and c-*jun*, products of oncogenes, dimerize through the leucine zippers prior to binding to DNA. For example, c-*fos* dimerizes with c-*jun* and subsequently binds to DNA.[34] Transcription factors such as myo-D, which is believed to be a master gene for inducing differentiation of skeletal muscle, acts through a helix-loop-helix mechanism. The helix-turn-helix proteins are trans-acting factors that bind to a binding site on the DNA referred to as a homeodomain, and are important in prokaryotes and eukaryotes.

Another level at which gene expression may be regulated is that of mRNA processing, whereby the introns are removed and the exons spliced together to provide the mature mRNA. In the majority of instances, each exon present in the gene is incorporated into a mature mRNA via ligation of consecutive pairs of exons with removal of all introns. This constitutive splicing process produces a single gene product from each transcriptional unit, even when the coding sequence is split into many separated exons. In other instances, however, nonconsecutive exons (or splice sites) are joined in the processing of some gene transcripts, and this alternative pattern of primary mRNA splicing can exclude individual exons from mature mRNA in some transcripts and include them in others. The use of such differential splicing patterns creates mRNAs that generate a variety of proteins from a single gene. Differential splicing is particularly prevalent in genes of muscles and has been shown to occur in four of the eight major sarcomeric proteins studied thus far—myosin heavy chains, alkali myosin light chains, tropomyosin, and troponin T (skeletal and cardiac) (Fig. 1-11).

The 3′ non-protein-coding region of the mature mRNA contains the poly (A) tail which is essential for message stability. It is believed that protein synthesis is, in part, regulated on the basis of alterations in message stability. The mechanism whereby a mRNA is induced to remain stable and encode for several thousand polypeptides as opposed to being extremely unstable and encoding for only a few molecules is unknown. Nevertheless, it is likely to be an important step in regulating the response to cytoplasmic signals that require rapid synthesis of a particular polypeptide. Synthesis of a poly-

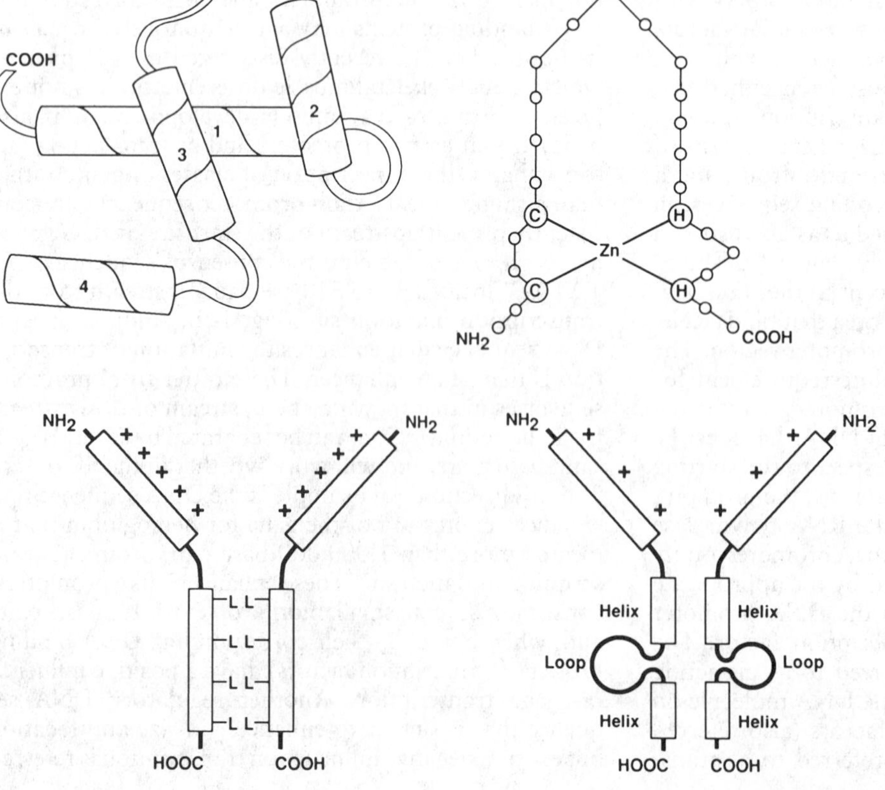

FIGURE 1-10 Type of transcription factors that affect gene activation. Schematic representation of the shape of four types of protein transcription factors that bond to DNA and influence gene activation. Helix-turn-helix is a protein with two α-helices separated by a β-turn. Leucine zippers are protein dimers with entering leucine amino acids. Zinc fingers have a peptide loop connected at the base by a zinc ion tetrahedran between cysteine and/or histidine in amino acids. The helix-loop-helix consists of α-helix but utilizes leucine zippers and has a loop between the α-helices. The darkened areas are believed to be the regions of the protein which interact with the DNA to modulate transcription.

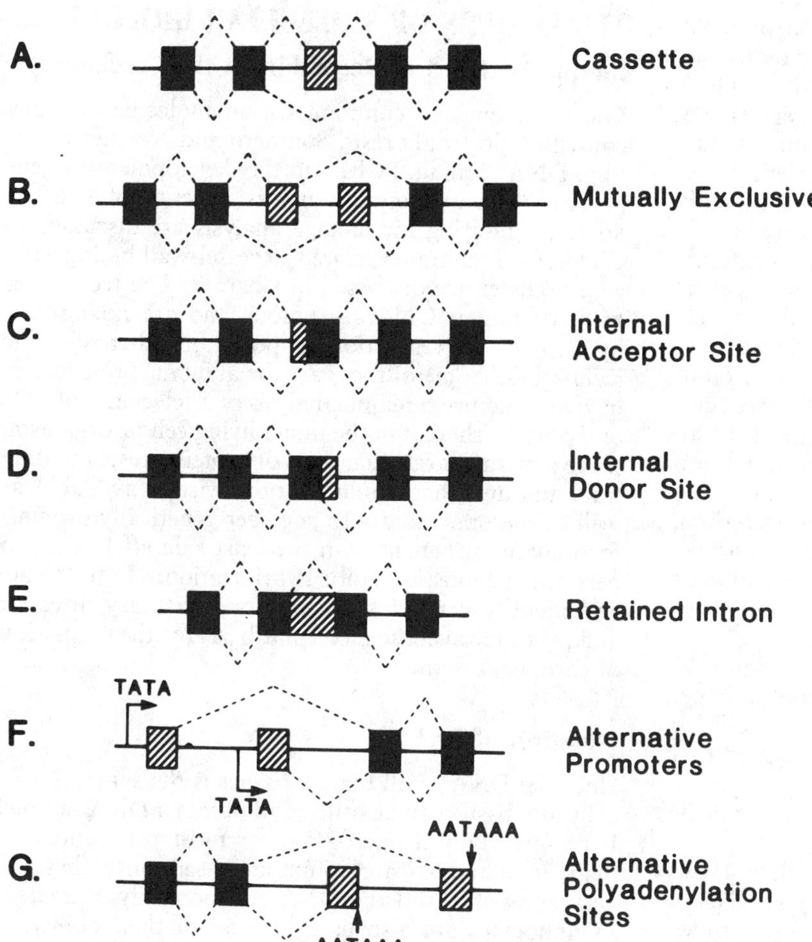

FIGURE 1-11 Patterns of alternative RNA splicing. Constitutive exons (black), alternative sequences (striped), and introns (solid lines) are spliced according to different pathways (dotted lines), as described in the text. Alternative promoters (TATA) and polyadenylation signals (*AATAAA*) are indicated. (*From Breitbant RE, Andreadis A, Nadel-Ginard B: Ann. Rev. Biochem* 1987: 56:467. *Reproduced with permission from the publisher.*)

peptide initiated via transcription is estimated to take several minutes while synthesis of a protein initiated through translation requires only seconds. Regulation of gene expression also occurs at the translational and post-translational levels. Proteins are often translated as precursors which must undergo proteolytic cleavage. Others must undergo cleavage of leader sequences attached to direct them to their particular subcellular compartment. Other posttranslational modifications include protein glycosylation, or the addition of lipids, polysaccharides, and the formation of disulfide bonds. Finally, polypeptides often require polymerization into complex tertiary structures to form the mature proteins. Regulation of gene expression at the protein synthesis level is more fully discussed in Chap. 6B.

Basis for Recombinant DNA Technology

The four major discoveries in the 1970s, as previously discussed, are regarded by many as having been pivotal in launching modern molecular biology that is based on the techniques of recombinant DNA. Since DNA consists simply of four nucleotides joined together, it is a monotonous, repetitive molecule that, at first glance, offers no landmarks to recognize that a particular segment of DNA codes for a particular mRNA. The discovery of the restriction endonucleases provided the genetic scalpel to cut DNA into smaller pieces of predictable size, which could be utilized in a variety of procedures. The unique feature of these enzymes is that each recognizes a specific sequence of DNA of three to eight base pairs and cleaves the molecule at that particular site. Thus, one knows precisely where the enzyme cuts and, using a variety of different enzymes, one can identify the site and number of recognition sites for each enzyme in a fragment of DNA of interest and develop what is referred to as a restriction map. These enzymes also made it possible to cut DNA from different sources in a predictable manner in preparation for ligating them together into a recombinant molecule. Restriction endonucleases have now been obtained from over 400 strains of bacteria that recognize more than 100 different cleavage sites. A restriction endonuclease is named after the bacterium from which it is isolated, taking the first letter of genus of the bacterium, the first two letters of the species, and the first letter of the strain. An example of this would be an enzyme from hemophilus influenza referred to as Hind-*III*. The *III* simply refers to the third restriction endonuclease enzyme isolated from that particular species of bacteria. Thus, the availability of restriction endonucleases made it possible to digest DNA into smaller molecules that could be manipulated and utilized in a variety of reactions, and to develop a restriction map as well as develop chimeric DNA molecules, the latter being the essence of recombinant DNA technology.

The discovery, in retroviruses of an enzyme reverse

transcriptase, which catalyzed the formation of DNA using mRNA as the template, revolutionized molecular biology. The resulting so-called complementary DNA (cDNA) (represented by the appropriate complementary bases for the mRNA except, of course, with thymine replacing uracil) will then bind to the nucleotide sequences from which the particular mRNA was originally derived (Fig. 1-12). Messenger RNA, as discussed previously, upon exit from the nucleus codes for a specific polypeptide and was derived from a discrete, specific unit of DNA referred to as a gene. Thus, radioactively labelling a cDNA derived from mRNA provides an extraordinarily powerful tool to develop known chromosomal landmarks and to isolate and identify particular genes. The reverse transcriptase makes it possible to clone a gene. The cDNA, which can be reinserted into the genome of a vector (virus or plasmid) and subsequently into an appropriate host, such as a bacterium, can be cloned. The labelled cDNA, referred to as a probe, is a routine, essential tool of the molecular biologist used to identify and isolate DNA or RNA fragments of interest.

Development of rapid-sequencing techniques[29,30] made it possible to sequence 100 to 200 base pairs per day, and with more automated types, it is possible to sequence up to 2000 bases per day. It is expected that for the Human Genome Project, the ability to sequence up to 10,000 or even 100,000 bases per day will be developed.

One feature of DNA recognized in the late 1950s needs to be highlighted. This is the property of DNA to denature and anneal, or hybridize. The double-stranded DNA held together by hydrogen bonding of the bases will, upon exposure to high temperatures (95°C), separate into two strands and, under appropriate conditions, the complementary strands will again anneal to their corresponding base pairs (55°C) precisely as in the original molecule and return to its normal double-stranded state. The process of separating into separate strands is referred to as denaturation and the recombining process as annealment or hybridization, with the latter term preferred if the two DNA fragments are from different sources. This property of DNA to denature and again reanneal is essential to most recombinant techniques.

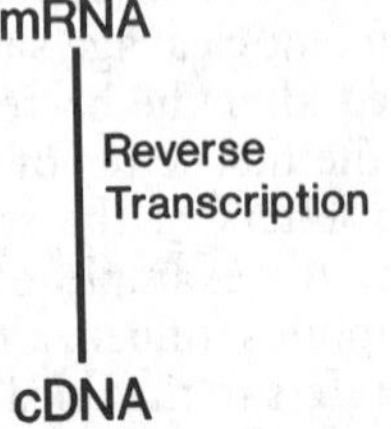

FIGURE 1-12 Generation of a complementary DNA (cDNA). Taking advantage of the enzyme, reverse transcriptase, mRNA is converted to DNA, referred to as complementary DNA or cDNA. The DNA is single-strand and complementary to the sequence of RNA, except that thymine now replaces uracil. Utilizing DNA polymerase, one can then make the single-strand DNA into double-strand cDNA. The cDNA can be used as a probe to identify specific sequences or genes of the genomic DNA, or it can be inserted into vectors to be cloned or expressed in a variety of hosts.

TECHNIQUES OF MOLECULAR BIOLOGY

Unique Features of Recombinant DNA Technology

The techniques of common use in molecular biology consist of electrophoresis, Southern and Northern blotting, DNA cloning, PCR, and the development of gene libraries. Other techniques such as detection of RFLP by Southern blotting for linkage analysis are discussed in Chap. 96. Techniques related to vessel-wall biology and gene transfer are discussed in Chap. 2. The techniques of recombinant DNA are unique and are not limited by some of the restrictions imposed on other scientific techniques.[3] Some of these are the ability (1) to perform in vivo structure function analysis of a selected molecule or a portion thereof in the intact living cell or organism; (2) to generate large quantities of protein present in only trace amounts that would not otherwise be available, as well as the opportunity to engineer genetically proteins for maximum benefit with the least side effects; (3) to perform diagnostic in situ hybridization; (4) to isolate and identify genes responsible for hereditary diseases; and (5) to unravel the molecular basis for the regulation of cardiac growth.

Isolation of DNA

Since the DNA of all human tissues is the same, practically any tissue can be utilized to obtain a DNA sample. It requires only a microgram for most procedures. In man, lymphocytes are commonly used since they are very accessible and the DNA can be easily extracted. Lymphocytes are also used because of their ability to be transfected with Epstein-Barr virus to produce an immortal cell line that can provide a continuous, renewable source of DNA. A blood sample of 10 to 15 mL of whole blood would typically yield about 50 to 100 μg of genomic DNA. If one's interest is restricted to DNA that is expressed, then one would isolate mRNA and employing the enzyme reverse transcriptase derive from the mRNA its complementary DNA (cDNA). cDNA molecules represent the expressed form of a gene and, thus, can be used as probes to select the specific genomic DNA segments from which the mRNA was transcribed. Myocardial biopsies provide adequate tissue for most DNA or RNA analysis.

Digestion and Electrophoretic Separation of DNA

One of the important physical properties of the DNA molecule is that each individual nucleotide possesses a net negative charge resulting from the phosphate group. Thus, fragments of different sizes exposed to an electric field tend to migrate toward the positive electrode at differential rates depending upon their size, with small fragments migrating faster than larger ones. This process of separation based on electric charge is called electrophoresis.[35] The DNA sample, after being digested into fragments of different size by a restriction endonuclease, is added to a support medium such as agarose or acrylamide. After electrophoresis, the pattern of the DNA can be visualized under a UV lamp after staining with a fluorescent dye such as ethidium bromide[36] (Fig. 1-13). Agarose gel electrophoresis will separate fragments from

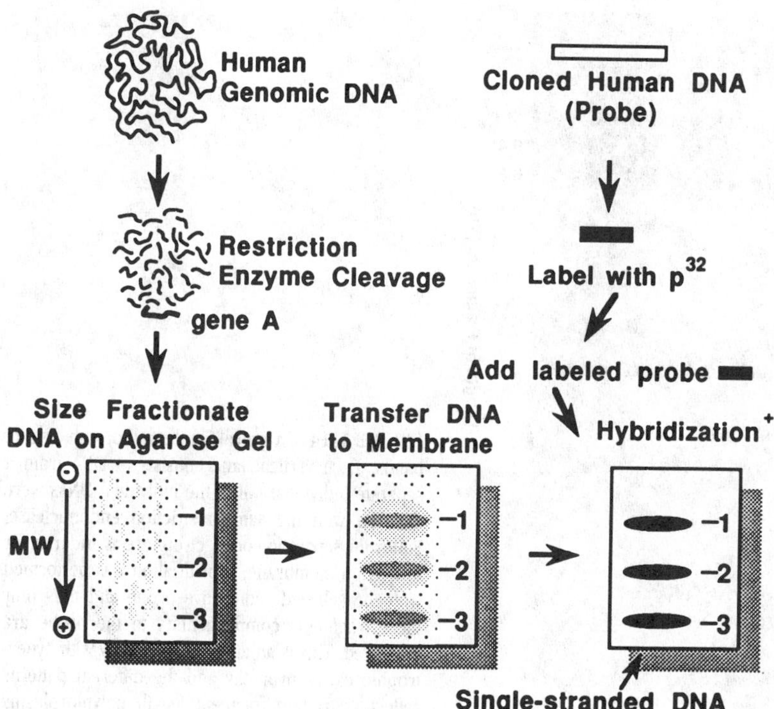

FIGURE 1-13 Southern blotting technique. The DNA is cleaved with an appropriately selected restriction endonuclease. The digested fragments are separated according to molecular weight by electrophoresis on agarose-gel, and the fragments of gene A are located at positions 1, 2, and 3, but cannot be seen against the background of many other randomly occurring DNA fragments. The DNA is denatured and transferred to a membrane in an identical pattern to what it was on the agarose gel. It is difficult to manipulate anything on a soft gel or to remove it. Once transferred to the membrane (filter), a solid support system, the DNA is much easier to handle. A DNA probe (cDNA) which has been labeled with ^{32}P is hybridized to its complementary DNA and visualized after exposure of the nylon membrane to an autoradiograph. The transfer of the DNA from the gel to the membrane developed by Southern was a major innovation. *(From Mares A Jr., Towbin J, Bies RG, Roberts R: Molecular biology for the cardiologist. Curr Probl Cardiol 1992; 17: 9–72. Reproduced with permission from the publisher and authors.)*

100 base pairs to 60,000 base pairs (60 kb) in size and polyacrylamide gels effectively separate fragments smaller than 1000 base pairs (1 kb). Until recently, resolution of large fragments was not possible, but the recent development of pulse-field-gel electrophoresis (PFGE) has made possible the separation of DNA fragments even up to 2 kb. In this technique the electric field is alternated in different directions forcing the molecules of DNA to reorient between each pulse, or surge, of electric current. Thus, this technique is particularly suitable for isolating and characterizing large segments of DNA, such as genomic fragments, to identify a known gene.

As noted previously, prior to electrophoresis, the DNA must be digested with one of the restriction endonucleases. The size of the fragments resulting from digestion will depend on the type of restriction endonuclease utilized, as to whether they recognize a 3, 4, 5, 6, or 8 base pair sequence. Enzymes recognizing a 4-base pair sequence will cut the DNA into much smaller fragments than one that recognizes an 8-base pair sequence.

Development of a DNA Probe

A nucleic acid probe is a fragment of nucleic acid to which has been attached a label such as a radioisotope, or a fluorescent compound, making it possible to easily detect and recognize the desired fragment among other complex native DNA molecules. The fragment labeled is usually cDNA or a synthetic oligonucleotide, although it could be RNA. It is now possible to synthesize DNA fragments of up to 30 to 40 base pairs referred to as an oligonucleotide that, with an attached label, can be used as probes to identify complementary DNA in the human genome or that of mRNA. This takes advantage of the fact that at high temperatures, the double-stranded oligonucleotide probe and that of the native DNA will separate into separate strands. On recombining at random, the labeled oligonucleotide will bind not only to its original complementary strand, but also equally well to that of the native DNA that is complementary to the probe, and thus provide a means of isolating a fragment of native genomic DNA. A probe is necessary in most recombinant DNA procedures to detect the molecule of interest following electrophoresis.

Southern and Northern Blotting

The procedure to separate and detect specific DNA fragments, which is now referred to as Southern blotting, is named after E. M. Southern, who developed it in 1975.[37] Genomic DNA is isolated, digested, and electrophoresis performed as described previously. Following separation, DNA fragments are denatured into single-strand fragments. Southern developed a technique whereby these separated single-strand fragments can be transferred by capillary action to a solid support medium (nylon or cellulose membrane) and permanently fixed by heating. The pattern on the membrane reflects identically the pattern induced by electrophoresis. The process used to produce a Southern blot is illustrated schematically in Fig. 1-13. The nylon membrane and its attached single-strand DNA fragments are then incubated with a radioactively labeled complementary probe. The hybridized radioactive, double-strand product, upon exposure to X-ray film (autoradiography), will exhibit the pattern of the radiolabeled DNA fragments (Fig. 1-14). In summary, the electrophoretic separation of DNA followed by its transfer to a nylon membrane for subsequent identification by radioactive hybridization is referred to as Southern blotting, and the autoradiogram as a Southern blot. The same approach to detect mRNA is referred to as Northern blotting. This procedure can also be used for detection of proteins, in which case it is referred to as Western blotting (Table 1-1). The only significant

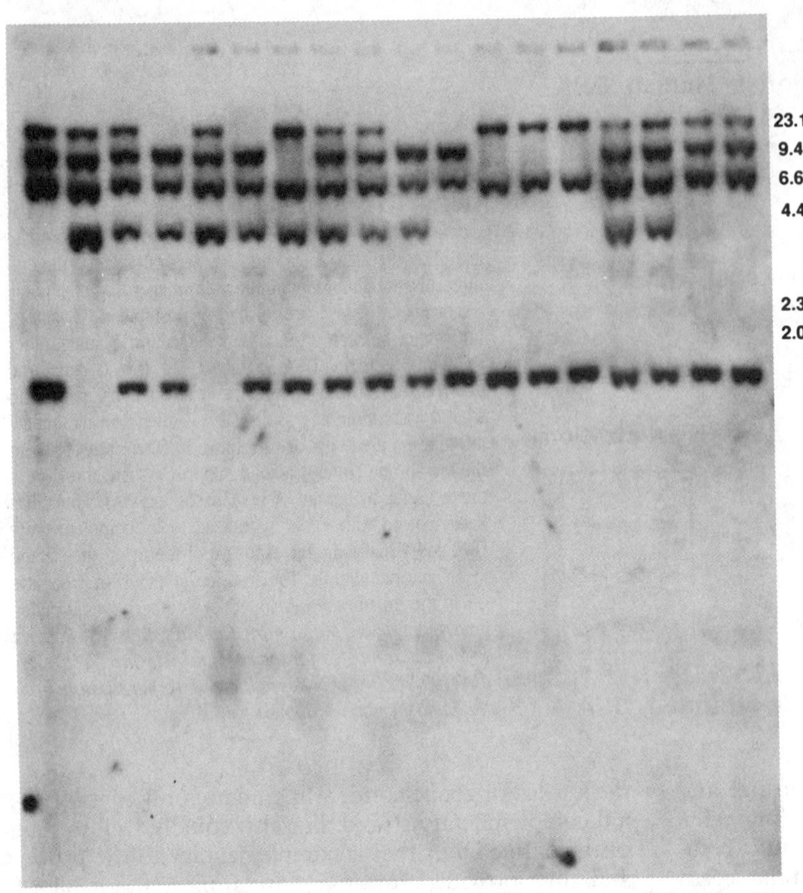

FIGURE 1-14 A typical Southern blot with distinct bands. Each vertical lane consists of DNA from a separate individual. All of the individual DNAs were digested with the same restriction endonuclease. Following separation on electrophoresis and transfer to a nylon membrane, hybridization was performed with the selected radioactive probe and thus only those fragments complementary to the probe are visualized. This is an analysis of a family with hypertrophic cardiomyopathy and the different patterns reflect restriction fragment length polymorphisms (RFLP) characteristic of the marker locus that is linked to the disease locus. *(From Mares A Jr, Towbin J, Bies, RD, Roberts R: Molecular biology for the cardiologist. Curr Probl Cardiol 1992; 17: 9–72. Reproduced with permission from the publisher and authors.)*

difference in detecting protein versus nucleic acid by this procedure is the probe, which is an antibody rather than an oligonucleotide, or cDNA. However, as in Southern and Northern blotting, the probe may be labelled with a radioactive isotope, a fluorescent tag, or some visual colorimetric substance.

DNA Cloning

DNA cloning is a technique used to produce large quantities of a specific DNA fragment of interest.[38] It is generally quite feasible to produce a million copies of a DNA fragment by routine bacterial cloning techniques. The DNA fragment of interest (insert) is inserted into DNA of a vector, and the vector amplified in an appropriate host cell. The host provides amplification of the DNA of both the vector and the foreign insert. The prerequisites for cloning are (1) isolation of the DNA fragment of interest; (2) a vector, which is often an extra chromosomal segment of DNA with the ability to propagate independently of the host DNA; (3) a restriction endonuclease to digest both the insert and the vector so the DNA ends will be compatible for ligation as illustrated in Fig. 1-15; (4) a DNA ligase to ligate the insert into the vector; (5) a means to introduce the vector into the host cell; and (6) a means to differentiate the host cells that have incorporated the vector from those that have not. Standard vectors used in cloning fall into three classes: (1) plasmids harvested from bacterial cells; a plasmid is an extra chromosomal segment of DNA present in bacteria that is self-replicating and on which are located certain genes that express resistance to ampicillin or other antibiotics; (2) bacteriophage, commonly referred to as merely a phage, which are viruses that invade and multiply in bacterial cells; (3) an artificially developed vector referred to as a cosmid. The insert and vector are enzymatically ligated together by DNA ligase, and the recombinant product (hence the name recombinant) is incorporated into a host such as a bacterium or a mammalian cell for amplification (Fig. 1-16). In order to identify whether or not the particular DNA of interest has been replicated in the host, a so-called reporter gene, such as one responsible for ampicillin resistance, is incorporated into the vector. The bacteria are grown in media containing ampicillin, so only those that have the resistance gene will survive. Since the resistance gene is attached to the DNA fragment of interest, it indicates that colonies (bacteria) or plaques (phage) that survive must contain the gene of interest. The size of the insert is a limitation in cloning. Plasmids can only accommodate inserts up to approximately 15,000 bp, phage up to 25,000 bp, and cosmids up to 45,000 bp. This limitation

TABLE 1-1
Procedure for Identification of Separate Molecules

Procedure	Target	Labeled Probe
Southern blotting	DNA	DNA or cDNA
Northern blotting	RNA	DNA or cDNA
Western blotting	Protein	Antibody

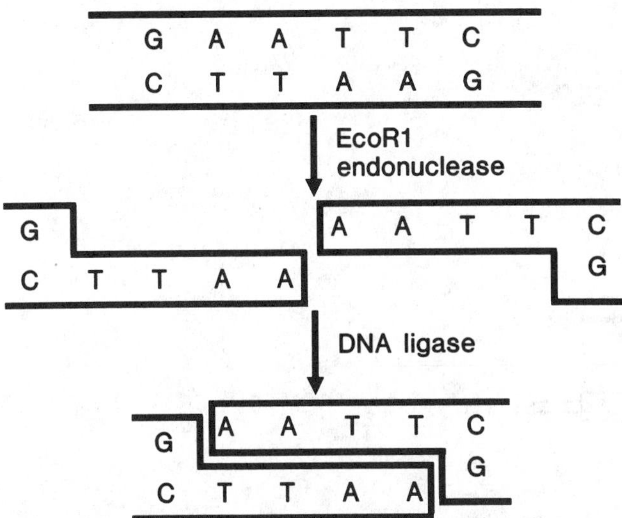

FIGURE 1-15 Restriction endonucleases recognize specific sequences and cut in a specific manner. The sequences recognized may be anywhere from 3 to 8 bp and may cut to give a blunt end or a staggered end ($EcoR_1$). Enzymes that provide staggered ends (cohesive or sticky ends) have unpaired bases which are easy to ligate together since they are complementary to each other as shown in this illustration. This feature is exploited in cloning or in the formation of any recombinant DNA molecule. For cloning purposes the fragment of DNA to be inserted is digested with the same restriction enzyme as is used to digest the DNA of the vector into which it will be inserted. Thus, the sticky ends of the DNA insert and the vector will be complementary and easy to ligate together in the presence of the enzyme DNA ligase as illustrated in Fig. 1-16. *(From Mares A Jr, Towbin J, Bies, RD, Roberts R: Molecular biology for the cardiologist. Curr Probl Cardiol 1992; 17: 9–72. Reproduced with permission from the publisher and authors.)*

to size has been overcome by the development of a technique referred to as yeast artificial chromosome (YAC),[39] which provides for DNA inserts up to 100,000 to 2,000,000 bp. This has markedly accelerated the cloning of large fragments of DNA. Cloning, as discussed, is performed to obtain multiple copies of DNA, and, unless specifically designed, the DNA is neither transcribed into protein nor translated into mRNA. If one desires to express a particular DNA fragment or gene, one must then select what is referred to as an expression vector. It is imperative to provide a promotor element that is appropriate for the host, and the gene must contain the appropriate 5′ untranslated region for binding to the ribosome as well as the appropriate 3′ region for translation and stability of the message. An example would be the expression of rt-PA in mammalian cells, whereby the protein is expressed and secreted to be harvested and commercially processed for use as a thrombolytic agent.

Development of Gene Libraries

Gene libraries are usually referred to as either genomic or cDNA. A genomic library refers to one made from nuclear DNA. A library is really a collection of DNA fragments that have been cloned in an appropriate vector and grown in a particular host, usually bacteria. A major difference between a genomic and a cDNA library is that a genomic library contains DNA fragments composed of introns and exons, whereas the cDNA library made from mRNA reflects only exons that have been transcribed to mRNA. Furthermore, the cDNA library is tissue specific by constructing it from the mRNA expressed in, for example, human cardiac tissue. A genomic library made from the human heart or any human tissue will obviously also have the genes for all other tissues. The libraries are often classified as complete or incomplete: in the case of the genomic library, whether it contains all of the human genes (the whole human genome) or only part of the genome; in the case of the cDNA library, completeness refers to whether it contains all or some proportion of the mRNA for that particular organ. The completeness often depends on the skill of the investigator and the total number of clones in the library since there must be severalfold more clones selected than there are genes. The collection of clones representing the library can be stored indefinitely and used as a renewable source for genomic or cDNA sequences. cDNA libraries of the whole heart and specific structures of the heart such as the Purkinje system are now available.[40] To isolate a particular gene or fragment of DNA or cDNA from a library requires a radioactive complementary cDNA probe.

Polymerase Chain Reaction

The polymerase chain reaction (PCR) has revolutionized the application of the techniques of molecular biology. This technique was not developed until 1985,[41,42] but its impact already has been felt throughout medicine and biotechnology. This procedure, conveniently and without the tedium of cloning, can provide 1,000,000 copies of a DNA fragment in 3 to 4 h and a billion copies within 24 h. PCR simply and ingeniously takes advantage of the natural DNA replication process. The sequence of the two ends of the DNA fragment desired to be amplified should be known, but short sequences of 15 to 30 bp are adequate, and fragments in between these sequences as large as 2 to 4 kb can be amplified. The sequence is used to make two oligonucleotides, referred to primers, with one for each end of the DNA fragment. One is made in the sense direction, and the other is made in the antisense direction (Fig. 1-17). The primers are used to prime the synthesis of complementary DNA strands and are designed such that the DNA between the primers is the fragment of interest to be amplified. If mRNA is to be amplified, it must be converted to a cDNA using the enzyme reverse transcriptase. The primers (oligonucleotides) are added in excess, together with the necessary bases for synthesis, the enzyme Taq DNA polymerase (catalyze DNA synthesis) and a sample containing the DNA to be amplified. There are three steps to each cycle: Initially, one must denature the DNA (separate the primers and the native DNA) into separate strands, which is done by increasing the temperature to 95°C. The temperature is then decreased to 50°C so the primers and the native DNA will reanneal to their complementary base sequences. The native DNA strands will bind not only to each other, but also the primers. The temperature is now increased to 65°C for synthesis of the new DNA fragments. Synthesis in the presence of Taql polymerase is initiated at the 5′ end and further nucleotides are added in the 5′ to 3′ direction to provide the desired double-stranded DNA fragment. Taql DNA

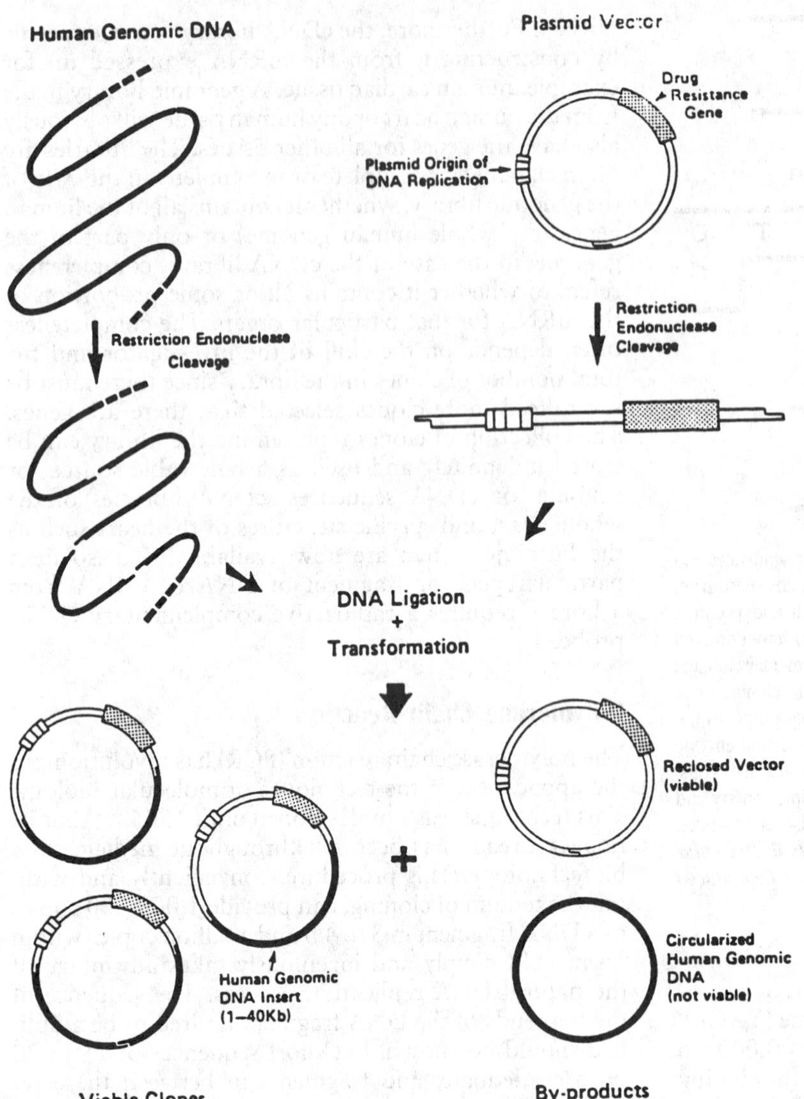

FIGURE 1-16 DNA cloning. The basic objective of cloning is to provide multiple copies of a DNA fragment of interest. The fundamental principles for in vitro cloning of specific DNA fragments are (1) the human genome DNA of interest is isolated after being digested by a restriction endonuclease, which is often referred to as the DNA insert; (2) a DNA vector is selected (shown on the right); the vector is a plasmid that has circular DNA and contains the necessary replication site and the reporter gene (drug resistance) subsequently to recognize which host has the insert. The vector and the DNA fragment to be inserted are digested with the same restriction endonuclease so that the ends are complementary for ligation; (3) DNA ligase ligates compatible insert and vector ends together; (4) host cells are transformed by incorporating vectors containing insert fragments and are identified by characteristics encoded by resident genes on the vector. Some of the clones will be viable and others not. *(From Mares A Jr, Towbin J, Bies RD, Roberts R: Molecular biology for the cardiologist. Curr Probl Cardiol 1992; 17: 9–72. Reproduced with permission of the publisher and authors.)*

polymerase, isolated from *thermus aquaticus*, is thermostable, which is of tremendous advantage in performing the PCR reaction. Since the high temperatures of up to 95°C do not destroy this polymerase, it negates the need to add DNA polymerase between each cycle. Furthermore, since Taq polymerase has an optimal activity temperature of around 70°C, one can significantly accelerate DNA synthesis. The cycle is then repeated and after about 30 cycles over 3 h one should have about 1,000,000 copies. There are many clinical applications for PCR. To make a diagnosis of viral myocarditis, for example, one can use PCR to amplify from a myocardial biopsy any specific viral RNA or DNA for which primers can be made. Viral RNA must first be converted to cDNA as noted before being amplified. The sensitivity of most conventional techniques is inadequate to detect molecules unless present in 50,000 to 100,000 copies per cell. In contrast only one copy of RNA or DNA is needed for PCR and in 3 to 4 h up to 1,000,000 copies can be generated and subsequently detected by most conventional techniques. PCR offers hereto unknown diagnostic sensitivity and specificity for cardiac disorders such as myocarditis, and, in patients undergoing cardiac transplantation, it may be used to enhance sensitivity for detecting infection or immunological rejection. Another application of PCR is to detect and amplify mutations associated with hereditary disorders using genomic DNA of any cell or cDNA of cardiac biopsies.

MOLECULAR BASIS OF CARDIAC CONTRACTION

Cardiac myocytes are large cells of up to 120 μm in length.[43] They are joined together in a syncytium. The sarcolemma surrounding the myocyte through the intercalated disk joins to adjacent cells and invaginates into the myofibril through the T-tubules. Cardiac muscle is composed of fibers, which in turn are composed of myofibrils. The myofibril has a periodicity imparted to it by the sarcomere, which is the working unit of contraction. The sarcomeres are joined in series with each other via the Z-lines. The sarcomere is composed primarily of myosin and actin, the thick and thin filaments, respectively. There are, however, four other proteins attached

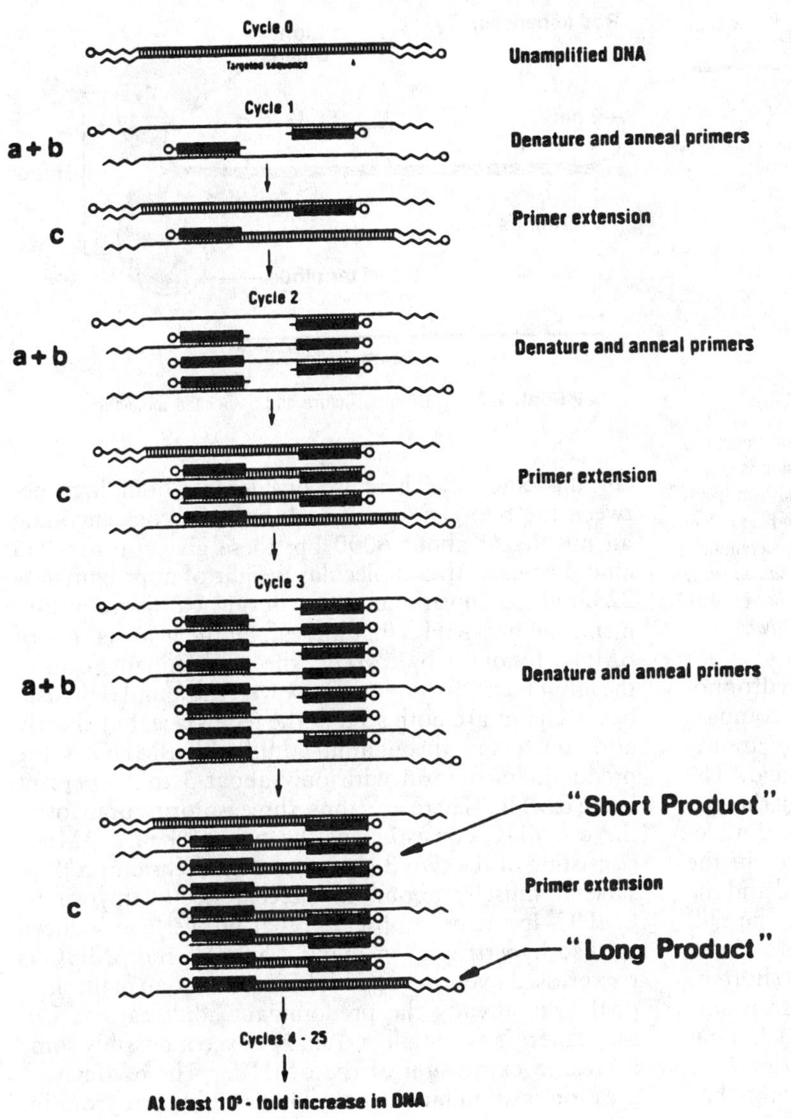

FIGURE 1-17 The polymerase chain reaction (PCR). Single copy segments of DNA may be amplified up to a millionfold by repetitive cycles of: (1) heat denaturing the target segment of DNA into two single-stranded templates; (2) annealing complementary primer sequences to the 5′ and 3′ ends of the single-stranded templates; and (3) synthesizing double-stranded DNA complementary to each strand by extension from the primer by a heat-stable DNA polymerase. This repetitive reaction increases the amount of target DNA logarithmically. *(From Mares A Jr, Towbin J, Bies RD, Roberts R: Molecular biology for the cardiologists. Curr Probl Cardiol 1992; 17: 9–72. Reproduced with permission of the publisher and authors.)*

to the actin filament: tropomyosin and troponins C, T, and I, and two myosin light chain molecules attached to the myosin heavy chains. The sarcomeres comprise about 50 percent of the mass of the cardiac myocyte and, depending on the state of contraction, vary from 1.6 to 2.2 μm in length as shown in Fig. 1-18. The individual proteins involved with the regulation of sarcomeric contraction including myosin, actin, troponin, and tropomyosin, together with the proteins involved with their assembly and those of the cardiac cytoskeleton will be discussed briefly (see also Chap. 5.)

The Contractile Proteins

Myosin

Myosin is present in muscle and nonmuscle cells of animals, plants, and many microorganisms. There are two forms of myosin termed Type I and Type II. Type II, found in muscle and nonmuscle cells, is by far the most extensively studied and contains a globular region that binds to actin and a long fibrous tail that aggregates with other myosin molecules to form the thick filaments of the sarcomere. The thick myosin filament is limited to the A-band of the sarcomere and is about 100 to 150 nm in diameter and 1.5 to 1.6 μm in length. Each thick filament of myosin consists of 300 to 400 molecules of myosin stacked longitudinally and laterally to each other by the terminal end of the tail at the M-line (Fig. 1-19). The Type 1 myosin has a molecular weight of 110,000, contains only the globular actin-binding region, lacks the fibrous tail, and is present only in nonmuscle cells and will not be discussed further. The myosin Type II molecule[44–46] has a molecular weight of about 500,000 and consists of two identical heavy chains, each with a molecular weight of 223,000, and two pairs of light chains of two different types: one with a molecular weight of 16,000 and the other 20,000 (Fig. 1-20). Each myosin heavy chain has a globular head formed by the amino terminus and a rodlike double-strand α-helical tail region of about 120 nm. Bound to the myosin head is the pair of myosin light chains. Each myosin heavy chain is an α-helical coil with 3.6 amino acids per turn. The two myosin heavy chains are coiled around each other to form a long, rigid, coiled tail; then they separate, and each amino terminus turns back on itself to give the bilobular myosin head. The two α-helical-coiled myosin

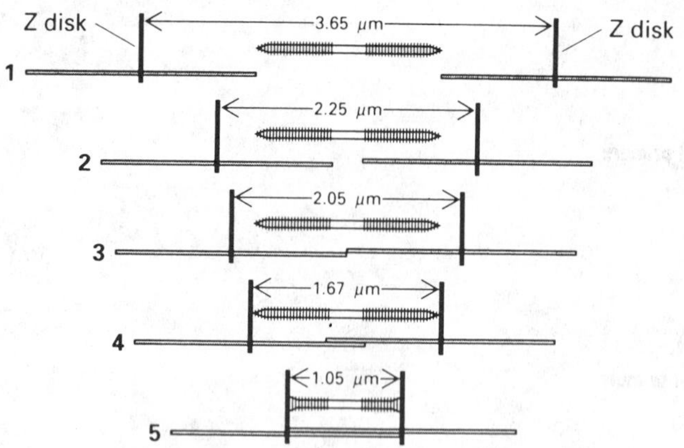

FIGURE 1-18 Relationship of sarcomere length and tension generated during isometric contraction of striated muscle. Maximum tension is generated at sarcomere lengths that allow maximum interaction of myosin heads and actin filaments (positions 2 and 3). If the sarcomere length is too short (positions 4 and 5), actin filaments overlap one another and prevent optimum interaction with myosin heads. [*From Darnell J, Lodish H, Baltimore D (eds): Molecular Cell Biology. New York, Scientific American Books, W.H. Freeman, 1990. Reproduced with permission from the publisher.*]

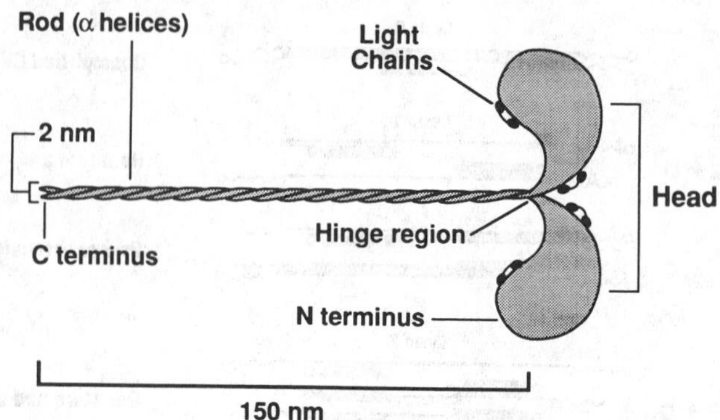

FIGURE 1-20 Myosin structure and associated molecules.

heavy chain molecules are bound together by hydrophobic residues (residues that repel H_2O). This is a common mechanism for many proteins.[47] In myosin there are hydrophobic side chains every seventh amino acid. The hydrophobic residues fit together while repelling the surrounding aqueous medium and stabilizing the double-stranded α-helix. There are two flexible hinges in the myosin molecule, one at the junction of the head and the tail, and the other in the proximal portion of the tail. These are crucial in its function as a motor protein to flex and move the actin filaments, and to induce shortening. Each myofibril of myosin in the sarcomere is surrounded by six actin filaments, and in turn, each actin filament is surrounded by two myosin filaments.

The molecular genetics of myosin heavy chains has been elucidated considerably in recent years.[48,49] Interest is intensifying due to the recent finding that hypertrophic cardiomyopathy may be due to a mutation in the βMHC gene. The heavy chain myosins are encoded by two genes, one for the βMHC and the other the αMHC[50] (Fig. 1-21). Both genes are located adjacent to each other on chromosome 14. There is considerable homology between the two genes, and each has 40 exons encoding an mRNA of about 6000 bp; these give rise to 1935 amino acids with a molecular weight of approximately 223,000. In lower mammals during cardiac development, the first MHC that appears in the heart is that of βMHC followed by αMHC, the predominant form in the adult heart. In humans, however, the α and β myosin heavy chains are both seen in the fetal stage, but shortly after birth and throughout adulthood, βMHC is the predominant myosin with only about 3 to 10 percent being αMHC. There are, thus, three isoforms of myosin: the α/αMHC consisting of the two α chains, βMHC consisting of the two β chains, and the hybrid of α/β. In skeletal muscle, about 15 percent of the myosin is βMHC. It has been observed that in overload-induced cardiac hypertrophy in many mammals the βMHC is reexpressed over that of αMHC. However, in man, since βMHC is already the predominant adult cardiac isoform, there is essentially no change except possibly some decreased expression of the αMHC.[51] The αMHC expression is stimulated by thyroxine in hyperthyroid-induced hypertrophy[52] (see also Chap. 6B).

Actin

The precise molecular structure of actin is yet to be fully determined, but overall it has a dumbbell shape with a

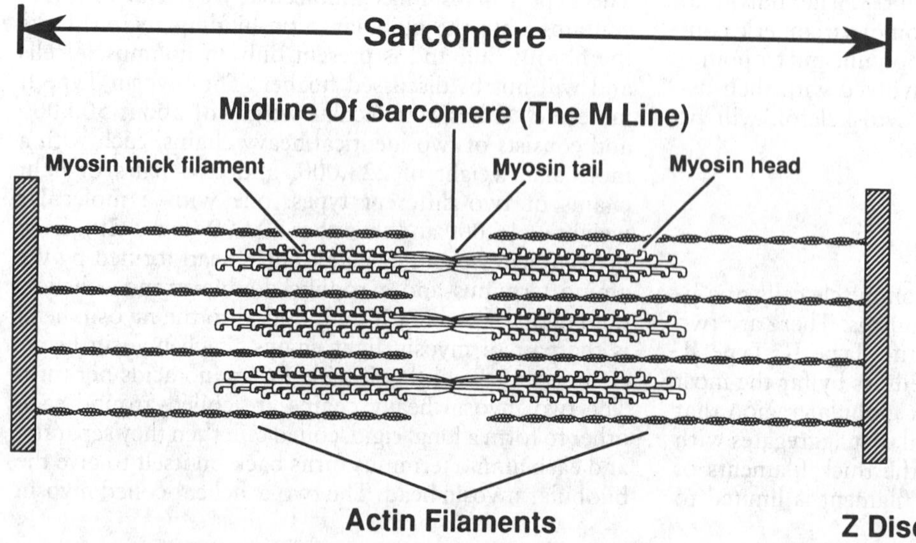

FIGURE 1-19 Sarcomere ultrastructure.

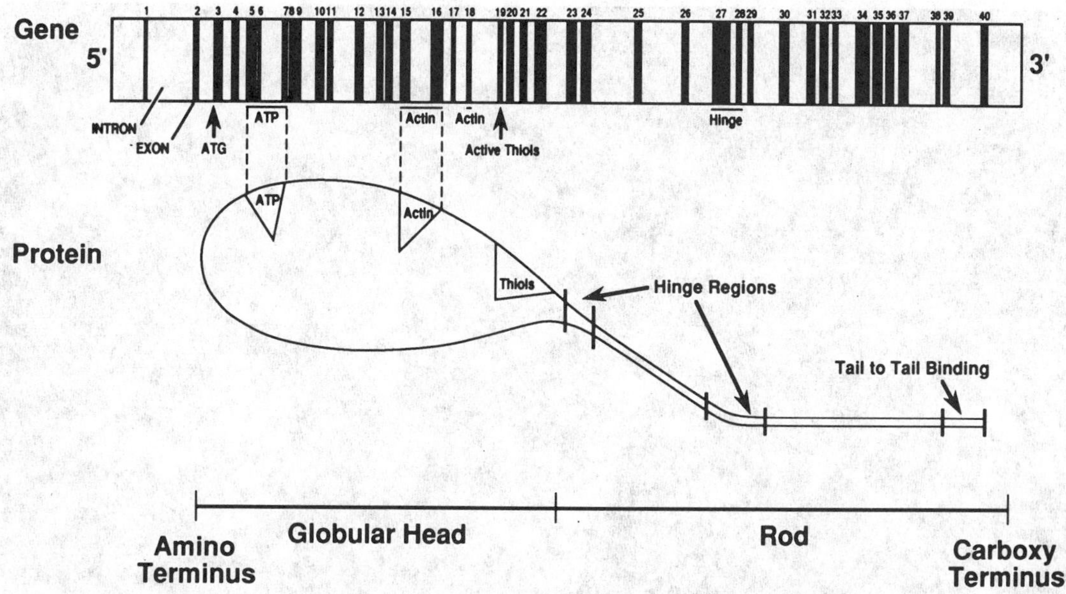

FIGURE 1-21 Structures of the βMHC and its gene. Illustrated here in the top rectangular bar are the 40 exons and the intervening introns of the gene for βMHC. Shown below is the βMHC protein and the recognized domains. The regions of the gene that encode for these functional domains are indicated by the arrows.

dimension of 6.7 × 4 × 4 nm.[53] Each actin subunit has a defined polarity, and the subunits always polymerize head to tail. Each molecule combines with another to form a double α-helix, consisting of two strands of about 1 μm in length and 50 nm in diameter. The individual monomer has a molecular weight of 42,000 often referred to as G-actin, and in its polymerized filamentous form is referred to as F-actin. The subunits of actin filaments, because of their defined polarity, all point in the same direction. Each monomer is roughly perpendicular to the helix axis and has major connections with, at least, two of its closer myosins. Polymerization of the globular actin monomers is induced by magnesium, potassium, or sodium in concentrations similar to those found in the cell cytosol. Polymerization of actin is accompanied by a large increase in the viscosity of the cytoplasm. Actin from diverse organisms can copolymerize, indicating that they have come from a common ancestral gene and are highly conserved during evolution. Since actin polymerizes at cellular concentration of potassium, it is very stable, and although it can easily depolymerize, it is almost always in a filamentous state.

There are six actin proteins expressed in the adult mammal, each the product of a separate gene: one expressed in skeletal muscle, another in heart muscle, two in smooth muscle and two others referred to as nonmuscle, or cytoplasmic, actins.[54] Actin appears to be a necessary component of the cytoskeleton of practically all cells. In the chick embryo, the initial actin expressed in the myocardium is that of smooth muscle followed by skeletal actin, which in turn is followed by cardiac actin—the adult form. It has recently been observed in the rat that pressure-overload-induced cardiac hypertrophy is associated with reappearance of fetal isoforms of the contractile proteins, and both skeletal actin and smooth muscle actin are re-expressed. The actin proteins differ from each other by only 7 percent in their amino acid sequences, and this difference is primarily in the amino terminus, which may have some subtle influence on actin polymerization. Otherwise, it is not certain that the amino acid differences have any functional consequence. For example, cardiac actin induced in a fibroblast will polymerize with the endogenous actins and appear to perform normally.

Tropomyosin and Troponin

Tropomyosin, like myosin, is a coil of two parallel α-helical polypeptides each with 284 amino acids and a molecular weight of 35,000.[55,56] This long stretched-out rodlike molecule is about 40 nm in length. Tropomyosin molecules polymerize head-to-tail to form filaments that lie in one of the grooves of the actin helix to give the actin molecule rigidity. Each tropomyosin molecule has seven actin-binding sites, which bind to seven actin monomers. In addition, bound to a specific site on each tropomyosin molecule are three troponin peptides called troponin-T, I, and C (Fig. 1-22). The presence of troponin and tropomyosin on the thin filaments in the absence of calcium inhibits the myosin ATPase activity by inhibiting the interaction of myosin with actin. Troponin-T has a molecular weight of 37,000, is also an elongated protein that binds along the C-terminal third of tropomyosin, and links both troponin-I and troponin-C to tropomyosin. Troponin-I with a molecular weight of 22,000 binds to actin as well as troponin-T. Troponin-I in concert with tropomyosin causes a small conformational change in the actin, so that it binds weakly to myosin heads but cannot activate the myosin ATPase. Troponin-C, the calcium-binding subunit, has a structure and function very similar to that of calmodulin. Occupation by calcium ions of all the calcium binding sites on troponin C releases the tropomyosin-troponin I inhibition of the actin-myosin ATPase activity, thus activating muscle contraction. This calcium binding triggers a slight movement or rotation of the tropomyosin helix toward the

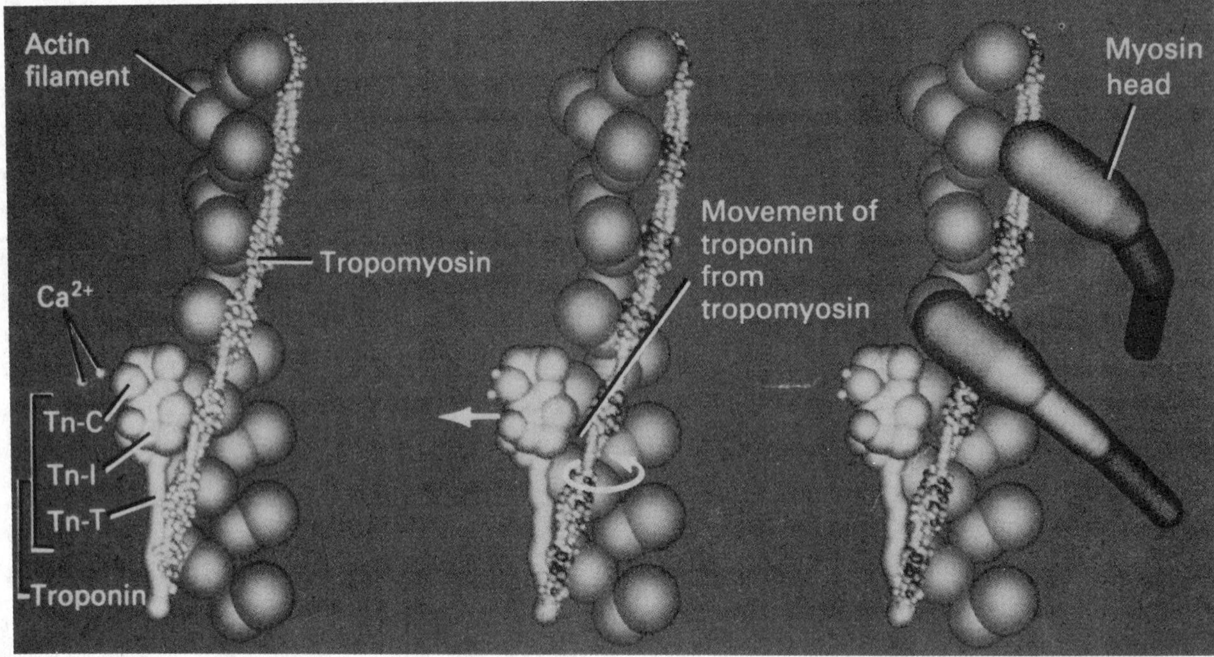

FIGURE 1-22 Effect of Ca^{2+} ions on tropomyosin and myosin binding to actin filaments. (a) In the "off" (resting) state, tropomyosin is bound to the outer domains of seven actin monomers along the helical actin filament. One troponin complex (without bound Ca^{2+}) is bound to each tropomyosin. (b) In the "on" (active state), troponin C (Tn-C) binds Ca^{2+} ions, causing TN-C and Tn-I to move away from tropomyosin. The freed tropomyosin rotates so as to bind to a slightly more inward position on the actin monomers. (c) Rotation of tropomyosin allows myosin heads to bind strongly to actin. *(From Phillips GN Jr., Filliers JP, Cohen C. J Mol Biol 1986;222:111. Reproduced with permission from the publisher. Photographs courtesy of Dr. C Cohen.)*

center of the actin filament. This shift of the tropomyosin exposes a region of the actin monomers to which the myosin heads bind in such a manner that myosin ATPase is activated. There are multiple isoforms of tropomyosin and troponin generated by alternative splicing of the mRNA[57,58] (see also Chap. 5).

Molecular Basis for Contraction and Relaxation

The proposed mechanism[59] whereby the actin filaments slide over the myosin filaments and induce shortening or contraction is illustrated in Fig. 1-23. Cardiac contraction and relaxation are regulated in part by calcium. Calcium released by sarcoplasmic calcium ATPase induces contraction by releasing calcium and relaxation by sequestering it. Hydrolysis of ATP at a rate of one molecule per myosin head is required for each cycle, as the actin filament moves a distance of about 7 nm. In the relaxed state, myosin is prohibited from binding to actin by the presence of tropomyosin and troponin, which blocks the receptor site for myosin. Myosin has minimal ATPase activity in the absence of actin; nevertheless, it does induce some hydrolysis of ATP to ADP and P_i. Systolic contraction is induced by calcium which, upon influx, binds to troponin C that induces a slight movement of tropomyosin that exposes the receptor site on actin for myosin. The resulting binding of actin to myosin increases the ATPase activity of myosin by about 200-fold which hydrolyzes the ATP to ADP. The ADP is released from the head of the myosin, which further enhances the binding of the myosin to actin. The head of the myosin, which is oriented at a 90° angle to the actin, flexes to a 45° angle and in so doing moves the actin filaments closer together. Subsequently, the calcium is again sequestered, and ATP binds to the myosin head, which inhibits binding to the actin, relaxes the sarcomere, and reinitiates diastole. Using high intensity X-ray from a synchrotron, it has been possible to follow the changes in muscle-diffraction patterns during muscle contractions. The increase in cytosolic calcium and tropomyosin movement occur 17 ms after a muscle is stimulated. The myosin head attaches to actin after about 25 ms and the tension is generated after about 40 ms (see also Chap. 5).

BIOLOGY OF THE CYTOSKELETAL PROTEINS

Cytoskeleton refers to the fibrous proteins that are present in the cytoplasm. The cytoskeletal fibers give the cell strength and rigidity. They also control movement within the cell. For example, the microtubules provide the tracks along which vesicles are transported by actin-binding molecules. These cytoskeletal proteins form three major classes subdivided according to their size into microfilaments,[60] microtubules,[61] and intermediate filaments.[62] The microfilaments are polymers of the protein subunit actin; the microtubules are polymers of the subunits of α and β tubulin and the intermediate filaments of five different rod-shaped protein subunits. The polymerization and depolymerization of these fibers are closely regulated by the cell.

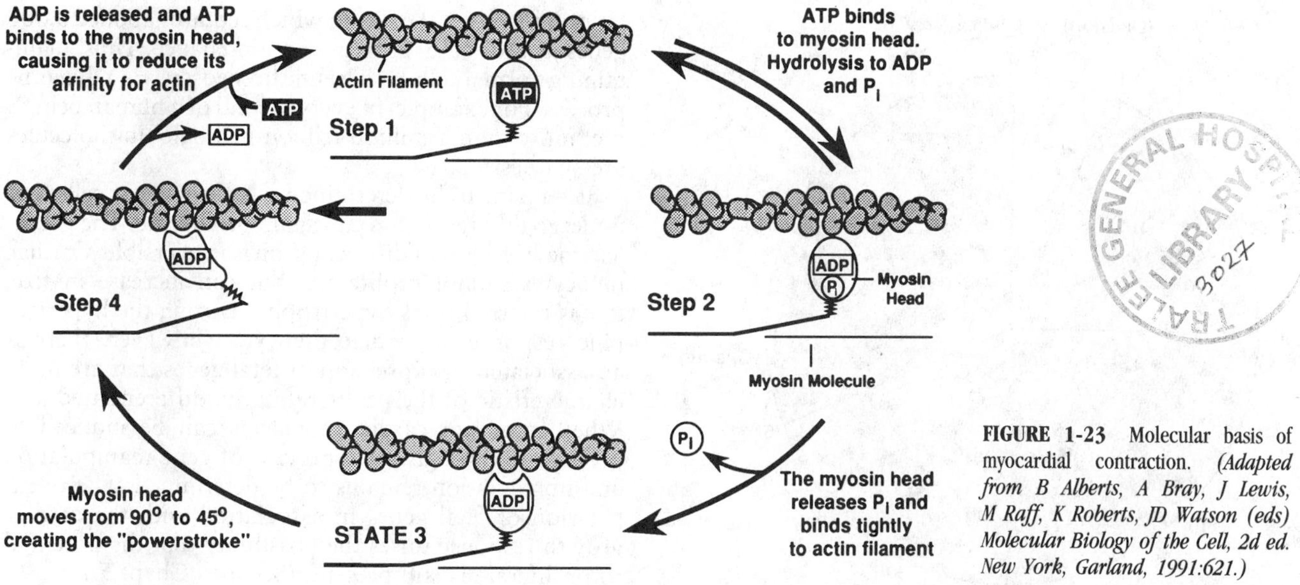

FIGURE 1-23 Molecular basis of myocardial contraction. *(Adapted from B Alberts, A Bray, J Lewis, M Raff, K Roberts, JD Watson (eds) Molecular Biology of the Cell, 2d ed. New York, Garland, 1991:621.)*

Microfilaments

In addition to the organized actin of the sarcomere, actin filaments are distributed throughout the cytoplasm of essentially all cells and serve to anchor many proteins crucial to cell survival. In addition, actin is associated with several other proteins that enable the actin filaments to perform their specific functions. The full normal function of actin and its associated proteins and their alteration during pathological states are not known. In the growth response of cardiac hypertrophy or the healing and remodeling following myocardial infarction, it is possible that these proteins play pivotal roles. *Titan,* which binds myosin to the Z line, is essential to the velocity and force developed by myosin-actin interaction, as is *nebulin,* which attaches actin to the Z line. Abnormalities related to these proteins, both acquired and inherited, are beginning to emerge. *Dystrophin* is the protein encoded by the gene responsible for Duchenne muscular dystrophy (DMD) and is known to be a subsarcolemmal protein with the function of anchoring actin to the plasma membrane. Elucidation of the mechanism by which defective dystrophin induces the well-recognized cardiomyopathy associated with DMD should provide information applicable to many cardiac disorders.[63,64] *Spectrin* has several isoforms critical to the cytoskeleton of the erythrocyte, and certain inherited abnormalities are known to induce anemia. Recently, a spectrin isoform specific to the heart was identified,[65] which also appears to be involved with the binding of actin to the plasma membrane.

Microtubules

With rare exceptions such as the erythrocyte, microtubules are found in the cytoplasm of all cells from the ameba to higher plants and animals. These fibers are about 24 nm in diameter, vary widely in length from a fraction of a micrometer to tens of micrometers. The microtubule wall is made up of globular subunits about 4 to 5 nm in diameter, and these subunits are arranged in 13 longitudinal rows encircling the hollow-appearing center. This basic design is present in practically all microtubules. Colchicine, which inhibits microtubule assembly, does so by binding to the tubulin. Microtubules are involved in movement and organization of cell organelles.

Intermediate Filaments

In contrast to actin and tubulin, which are widely distributed among cell types, the rather insoluble intermediate filaments are tissue and cell specific. Actin and tubulin are globular and the polymers they form are rather like beads on a string. In contrast, intermediate filament (IF) subunit proteins are extended molecules that form rope-like polymers. The IF proteins include desmin, vimentin, neurofilaments, glial fibrillary acid protein, and the keratins. In cardiac myocytes, desmin filaments connect the desmosomes from one muscle cell to the other and form the scaffold for both the Z-disk and the myofibrils. The desmin filament is responsible for the transmission of the stress and strain of the contractile force between cardiac myocytes.

MOLECULAR BASIS FOR CELLULAR GROWTH

Patterns of Growth

Understanding growth requires understanding its different stages; namely, developmental growth, cellular differentiation, normal constitutive protein synthesis of the different cells, and the growth response to certain stimuli such as exercise or injury. During early development in the fetal and embryonic stages, practically all cells proliferate as well as increase in size and are said to be in cell cycle (Fig. 1-24). Throughout this process certain cells drop out of cell cycle, cease proliferating, and undergo the process of differentiation. At birth or within weeks thereafter, certain cells of organs, such as the heart and brain, lose their ability to proliferate, and growth is

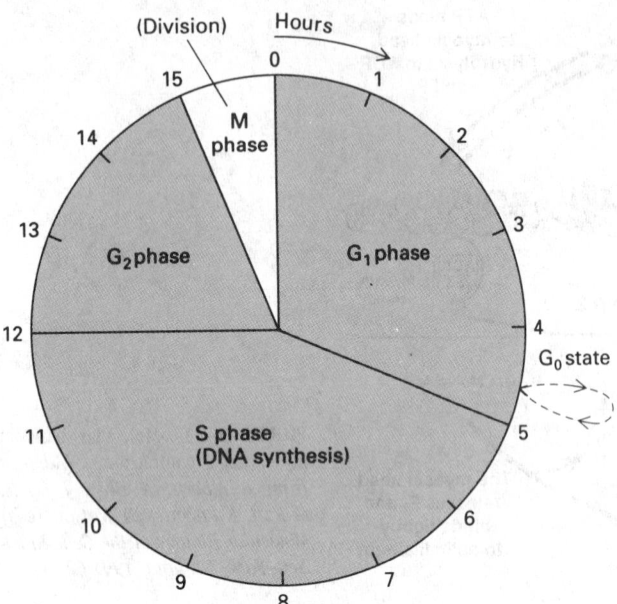

FIGURE 1-24 The cell cycle in a mammalian cell having a generation time of 16 h. The three phases spanning the first 15 h or so—the G_1 (first gap) phase, and S (synthetic) phase, and the G_2 (second gap) phase-make up the interphase, during which DNA and other cellular macromolecules are synthesized. The remaining hour is the M (mitotic) phase, during which the cell actually divides.

restricted to maintaining normal cell size or increasing cell size without an increase in number. Many of the genes expressed in embryonic development subsequently downregulate after birth. Conversely, genes that code for proteins serving specialized function in the differentiated cell may be inhibited in the proliferating, undifferentiated cell only to be expressed upon differentiation. For example, the muscle cell, upon differentiation, downregulates the gene that encodes for BB creatine kinase and upregulates the gene for MM creatine kinase. Similarly, upregulation occurs in the genes that encode for myosin, actin, and other sarcomeric proteins essential to perform the contractile activity of the cell. It is estimated that the human body has a total of 10^{14} cells of only 200 to 250 different types. The specialized functions are dependent upon the repertoire of genes expressed by a particular cell type.

In the adult organism, there are three ongoing dynamic growth responses: hyperplasia, constitutive "growth," and hypertrophy. In certain organs, such as the liver or skin, there are relatively undifferentiated cells that can proliferate and increase in number, a process referred to as proliferative growth, or hyperplasia. Subsequently, a proportion of these cells differentiate. The continuous synthesis of constitutive proteins that are necessary to maintain cell integrity without necessarily changing in size may be viewed in the broadest sense as growth.

Proteins are synthesized to replace those catabolized while maintaining the normal size, shape, and function of the cell. It is estimated that most of the proteins of the heart are replaced every five days. It is estimated that all of man's functions are determined by about 30,000 to 50,000 genes, and about 10,000 genes (proteins) are required to maintain basal cellular integrity of a particular organ, except the brain, which requires about 20,000 genes just for basal growth or maintenance. Thus, maintaining normal cellular baseline homeostasis is a dynamic process. For example, in every second of a human being's life, more than a million trillion hemoglobin molecules are synthesized.

It remains to be determined whether or not cells that undergo differentiation can again proliferate. The prevalent view holds that differentation is irreversible. Cardiac myocytes cannot proliferate, but can increase in size; this is referred to as hypertrophy. During the hypertrophic response of cardiac myocytes, however, there is an associated re-expression of fetal genes that are more characteristic of the proliferating, undifferentiated cell. Whether or not cardiac myocytes can be induced to proliferate through some process of gene manipulation and upregulation remains to be determined. The re-expression of fetal genes in association with the cardiac growth response raises the possibility that the potential to proliferate is still present. (See also Chap. 5.)

Receptor and Signalling Proteins Underlying the Growth Response

There are a number of extracellular membrane receptors involved in mediating or modulating growth responses: (1) channels, (2) G-protein coupled and (3) tyrosine kinase-containing receptors[66] (Fig. 1-25). There are two common, highly utilized intracellular transducing or signalling cascades referred to as the cyclic AMP system and the inositol triphosphate pathway. The channel receptors are distributed throughout the nervous system. Each receptor spans the lipid bilayer with an extracellular component and an intracellular cytoplasmic component. The receptors are named according to their ligands and include the acetylcholine, glycine, GABA, and glutamate receptors. These ligands bind to the receptor and induce a voltage-dependent channel opening in the membrane, which permits ions to cross the lipid bi-layer.

The G-protein coupled receptors are a widespread family of receptors consisting of well over 100 subtypes. They are referred to as G-protein receptors since they activate the guanine-nucleotide-binding proteins (GDP, GTP). These receptors are believed to have a common topology. The amino terminus of each receptor is outside of the cell, and the intracellular carboxyl terminus contains sites that can be phosphorylated. The core of the receptor consists of seven hydrophobic α-helices that span the membrane bi-layer and contain the binding sites for the ligand. The best recognized and characterized example of this kind of receptor is that of the adrenergic receptor (see Chap. 3). Receptor activation of the G-protein involves dissociating of GDP and the binding of GTP, which, in turn, activates one of the two signaling pathways. In the case of adenylate cyclase, protein kinase A or other cyclic-AMP-dependent protein kinase, will be activated. The inositol triphosphate pathway will activate phospholipase-C to generate IP-3 and diacylglycerol leading to activation of protein kinase C (see Chap. 2). There is also considerable evidence the G-proteins regulate potassium and calcium channel proteins in the brain and in skeletal and cardiac muscle.

The tyrosine-kinase receptors, so-named because of

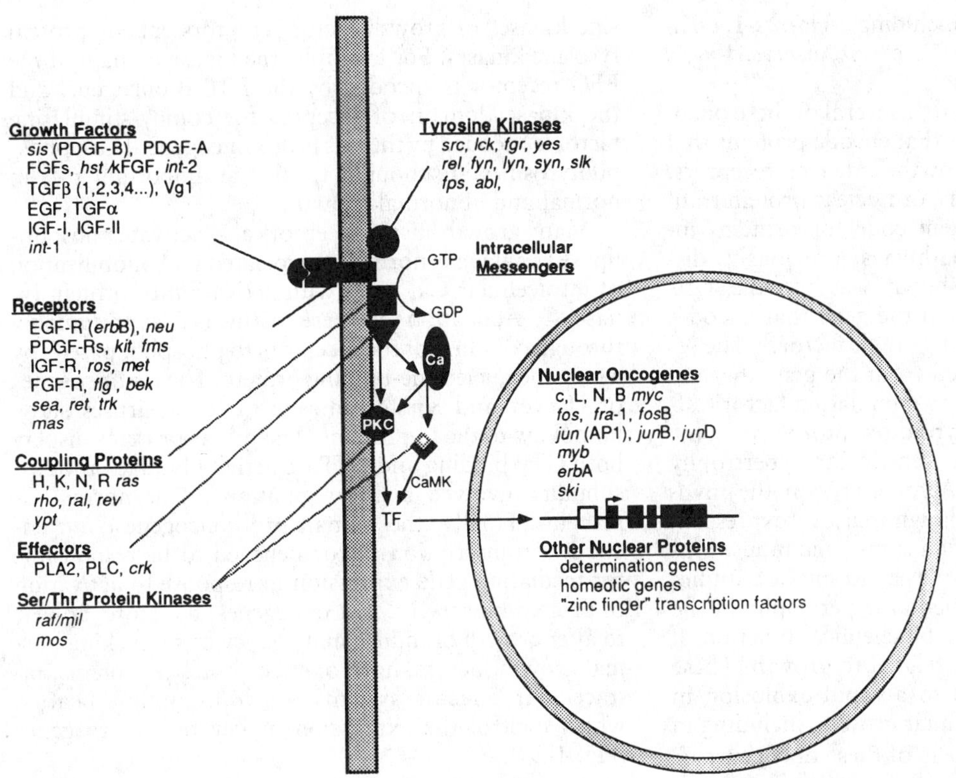

FIGURE 1-25 Illustration of the many proteins with varied functions for which oncogenes are known to encode. Oncogenes encode proteins that function as growth factors, receptors, coupling proteins, signaling proteins, as well as transcriptions factors.

their intrinsic tyrosine kinase activity,[67,68] have an extracellular domain, a transmembrane domain, and a cytoplasmic domain and are rather large proteins of about 1000 amino acids. The intracellular domain contains the tyrosine kinase activity. Typical ligands are the epidermal growth factor (EGF), the platelet-derived growth factor (PDGF), and insulin-like growth factor-1 (IGF-1). This group of receptors is of great interest because of their importance in cell growth and division. Well over a third of the oncogenes (to be described later) are thought to effect their responses on growth through this receptor pathway. Over 40 protein tyrosine kinases have now been identified; however, the mechanism by which the signals are relayed to the nucleus and effect gene expression is yet to be delineated fully.

Another class of receptors[69] involved with growth are intracellular localized either in the cytoplasm (i.e., progesterone) or on the nuclear membrane (i.e., thyroxine and estrogen). In these cases, lipophilic ligands rapidly penetrate the cell membrane and bind to their receptor, and the ligand-receptor complex activates or inhibits transcription of the corresponding gene. Several circulating hormones, including estrogen, progesterone, mineralcorticoids, glucocorticoids, thyroxine, aldosterone, and retinoic acid, utilize these receptors. There is also a group of protein kinases[70] in which serine or threonine is phosphorylated; it has been implicated in the growth response, but the signaling pathway and the mechanisms of altering gene expression or other target activities remain unknown.

Oncogenes—Definition and Background

A large body of our knowledge on growth and its regulation is derived from the study of oncogenes.[66] An oncogene is a gene whose abnormal expression or altered gene product will induce features of neoplastic growth in its host. Oncogenes were first discovered in association with viral-induced neoplasms. The oncogene was isolated from a retrovirus, which has as its nucleic acid RNA. The virus, an obligate parasite, enters the cell and, in the presence of the enzyme reverse transcriptase, transcribes its RNA into DNA, which then inserts itself into the cell's genome and replicates. These viruses are called retroviruses, and, since they possess reverse transcriptase, replication in the reverse direction (RNA to DNA) is possible. The first of these tumor-associated viruses to be discovered was the Rous sarcoma virus.[71] These viruses, upon injection into select animals, induced neoplasms and so were named oncogenes. It was soon discovered that genes analogous to those of the oncogenes are present in normal cells.[72–74] It has subsequently been shown that these oncogenes present in retroviruses are most likely derived from normal cellular genes. The normal cellular genes are referred to as proto-oncogenes, or cellular oncogenes (c-oncogene), and those of viruses as v-oncogenes. Several of the retroviruses and their respective oncogenes were isolated from human neoplasms; examples include c-*abl* from chronic myeloid leukemia and c-*myc* from Burkitt's lymphoma. The oncogenes code for proteins, some of which are well-known to mediate cellular growth and are almost identical to the products of their normal cellular counterpart. It is expected that there will be a cellular gene for every oncogene. The oncogenes capable of inducing malignancy represent a modified form of the normal cellular gene, most commonly due to structural mutation. Well over 50 protooncogenes have been recognized in the human genome, and their transformation to an oncogene and involvement in human cancer have been unquestionably documented in several cases, including c-Ha-*ras*-1, c-Ki-*ras*-2, N-*ras,* c-*erb*-B1, c-*erb*-B2, c-*myc,* n-*myc,* l-*myc,* and c-*abl.*[66]

Subsequent studies showed that several of these oncogenes were derived from genes that encode proteins that are known to mediate cell growth, either as receptors, intracellular signalling proteins, or nuclear protein transcription factors. Most of them code for proteins involved with the normal pathways previously discussed.[75,76] The first to be shown was for the v-*sis* oncogene which is derived from the gene that encodes the *B*-chain of platelet derived growth factor.[77] The V-*erb*-B was shown to be derived from the gene that encodes for the receptor for colony-stimulating factor (csf-1)[78] and V-*erb*-A[79] from the thyroid receptor gene. In the rat, pressure-overload-induced ventricular hypertrophy led to upregulation of mRNA for c-*myc* in the myocyte.[80,81] Jackson et al[82] have shown that overexpression of c-*myc* in the myocardium of a transgenic mouse was associated with cardiac hyperplasia. Results of studies in cell culture[83-85] and experimental hypertrophy in the intact rat also indicate that the biochemical function of the product of the gene c-*myc* related to growth. These and similar findings have led to a rapid explosion in research on oncogenes and cellular growth, including in the heart. Several of the products of these oncogenes or their normal cellular analogues affect cardiac growth through utilization of the biochemical pathways previously discussed. The interaction of the oncogenes with these pathways will be discussed in the next section (see also Chap. 6B.)

Growth Factors and Their Oncogenic Derivatives

Normal and pathologic growth are controlled by factors that are either stimulators or inhibitors.[86] Some of the growth factors are very analogous to endocrine hormones in that they are produced by one cell type, secreted into the blood, and circulate to act on receptors on cells at considerable distances. Several of the endocrine hormones, such as growth hormone, thyroxine, mineralocorticoids, and the glucocorticoids in some cases act as growth factors. Growth factors[87] such as TGFβ and the fibroblastic growth factors (FGF) produce paracrine or autocrine effects. Paracrine activity refers to effects of a secreted agent on adjacent cells. Autocrine activity refers to effects of an agent on the cell that produced it. In general, growth factors initiate their effects by binding to a membrane receptor that, in turn, activates intracellular secondary messengers; these activate nucleus transcription factors. These transcription, or transacting, factors regulate gene expression and subsequent protein synthesis. Regulation of protein synthesis may also result from altered rate of translation or stability of mRNA. Unlike the normal endocrine response, the growth response to hormones or growth factors occurs several hours after the initial stimulation and is more likely to occur if two or more growth factors have been activated (see also Chap. 6B.)

Some growth factor receptors, including those for EGF, insulin, IGF-1, PDGF, and colony stimulating factor (CSF-1), have intrinsic tyrosine kinase activity. Many oncogenes that have homologies with the intrinsic tyrosine kinases of growth factor receptors encode protein tyrosine kinases. For example, the kinase domain of the EFG receptor is encoded by the ERB-B oncogene, and the kinase domain of receptor for colony-stimulating factor is encoded by the fms proto-oncogene. Thus, phosphotyrosines are thought to play an important role in normal and abnormal growth.

Many growth-factor receptors also activate phospholipase C, which is normally associated with mobilization of intracellular Ca^{2+} and with activation of protein kinase C. Activation of these pathways is presumably through coupling of the receptors to phospholipase C by a guanine nucleotide-binding protein. The ras oncogenes of Harvey and Kirsten murine sarcoma viruses show homology to the G-proteins. The p^{21} ras proteins display both GTP binding and GTPase activity but lack the two subunits involved in the regulation of the normal G-proteins. Finally, the human protooncogene c-*jun* encodes a transcription factor believed to be responsible for mediating gene expression in response to activation of protein kinase-C. Most oncogenes, therefore, appear to alter growth or induce malignancy by mimicking normal growth factors, hormone receptors, G-proteins, intracellular effector systems, or transcription factors, which control the expression of key regulatory genes (Fig. 1-25).

Intracellular Ionic Changes of the Growth Response

The general molecular events associated with growth stimulation include a rapid ionic change in ion concentrations,[88,89] generally with increases of intracellular calcium and pH.[90-93] These events appear to be common to all growth factors and occur through multiple mechanisms. The increase in the pH may not be absolutely essential for the growth response; however, considerable evidence suggests that for DNA synthesis an increase in pH is essential. While the time scale varies, a representative temporal sequence[94] is reflected by that observed for protooncogene c-*fos:* transcription is initiated 10 to 15 min after stimulation; peaks at about 30 min; and returns to baseline in about 1½ h.[95] It is also of interest that, while the process of stimulating gene expression leads to synthesis of the specific gene product, the process in itself does not require protein synthesis.[66]

MOLECULAR BASIS FOR THE CARDIAC GROWTH RESPONSE

The growth response of the myocardium to injury, whether it be myocardial infarction, hypertension, or valvular disease, is a major determinant of morbidity and mortality. Growth is the major long term adaptive mechanism of the heart (see also Chap. 6B). The clinical and pathological features associated with cardiac hypertrophy have been described extensively.[96] Meerson[97] put forward the concept that early compensatory growth is beneficial while subsequent growth may become pathological and contribute to increased mortality. The mechanism underlying cardiac failure that occurs in association with prolonged cardiac hypertrophy remains to be elucidated, but a variety of postulates have been put forward: (1) The cardiac myocyte outgrows its blood supply; (2) the architecture of the cell is, including the organelle arrangement, altered, so that energy transport across the cytoplasm is deranged and inadequate; (3) the overall architecture and fiber orientation of the myocardium are altered such that adequate velocity and force cannot be generated; or (4) the muscle can no longer continue to increase in size in response to its needs. Despite the extensive literature characterizing hypertrophy, there has been very little knowledge regarding the molecular basis for the cardiac growth response. Application of the techniques of recombinant DNA promises to provide insights that will lead to beneficial manipulation of this response. The obvious questions to be answered include: (1) What are the stimuli that initiate the cell to activate the growth response? (2) What are the receptors that detect the stimuli? (3) What intracellular molecules mediate the response from the receptor to the nucleus? (4) How does that molecule interact with the DNA to promote or inhibit the growth response? (5) Are new proteins synthesized (phenotype), and is this synthesis adaptive, maladaptive, or just part of a triggered programmed response that is all or nothing? (6) Finally, can the process be modulated?

Cardiac myocytes are terminally differentiated and unable to proliferate. They are, therefore, similar to the differentiated skeletal myocyte, except skeletal muscle has undifferentiated satellite cells that can proliferate while the myocardium does not. The myocardium, however, as previously noted, participates in protein synthesis to compensate for protein catabolism and to maintain normal function, size, and shape. In response to cardiac injury of almost any type, there is an immediate adaptive growth response. Following myocardial infarction, even when 30 to 40 percent of the myocardium is destroyed, the normal surviving myocardium compensates by myocyte enlargement (hypertrophy as opposed to hyperplasia). Chronic cardiac failure, regardless of the etiology, is consistently associated with hypertrophy, which is a very dynamic process under the influence of several extracellular and intracellular factors. Modification of this maladaptive response is a major objective for therapeutic development.

Autocrine or Paracrine or Intracrine Mechanisms Mediate Cardiac Hypertrophy

Developmental growth of multiple organs during prepuberty and puberty is associated with orchestrated stimuli from a variety of hormones such as the growth hormone. This is in sharp contrast to the restricted organ growth observed in response to injury. For example, in aortic constriction, the left ventricle responds with increased mass, while the right ventricle is not affected. Hammond et al.[98] in 1979 proved conclusively that the growth stimulus was indeed localized to the affected organ. In these experiments, left ventricular hypertrophy was induced by aortic coarctation in the dog. Supernatants of the homogenized, hypertrophied left ventricle from dogs with aortic coarctation and normal dogs were used to perfuse a normal canine heart. Messenger RNA in that perfused heart was increased by extracts from the hypertrophied, but not the normal, myocardium, indicating the presence of a growth factor in the hypertrophied ventricle. These experiments did not shed light on the nature of the stimulus or the mechanism involved with gene regulation, but established the presence of a localized cellular stimulus acting through autocrine, paracrine, or intracrine mechanisms to induce cardiac hypertrophy. This was confirmed by Imamura et al.[99] in 1990; they showed that hypertrophy occurs in the left ventricle in response to aortic coarctation without growth in other chambers of the heart, while banding the pulmonary artery-induced hypertrophy of the right ventricle without involvement of the left ventricle. These investigators also observed an upregulation of the βMHC gene, indicated by increased mRNA and protein, and a downregulation of the αMHC gene. Circulating hormones, such as thyroxine and catecholamines, remained normal. Similarly, hypertrophy induced by volume overload, or myocardial infarction,[100] or other forms of injury are restricted to the cardiac chamber involved.

Cardiac Hypertrophy Is Associated with Reexpression of Fetal Proteins

As noted, cardiac myocytes do not increase in number after birth but do increase in size.[101,102] The best characterized system for muscle growth is that of skeletal muscle,[33,103–105] which upon differentiation drops out of cell cycle (Fig. 1-26). The genes for proliferation are downregulated, and genes specific for sarcomere function, such as myosin, are upregulated. In contrast, the cardiac myocyte, during its hypertrophic response to increase size, exhibits DNA synthesis (multiple nuclei)[106] and the reexpression of several fetal proteins otherwise expressed only in the undifferentiated cells.[107] The rational basis for the reexpression of fetal protein is not obvious. The response has been referred to as adaptive, maladaptive, or part of a triggered program response.[30] This response is most obvious in the rat in which there is a switch with hypertrophy from the predominant α-myosin heavy chain (αMHC) isoform to the embryonic βMHC isoform.[108,109] βMHC is known to be more efficient than αMHC since there is less myosin ATPase activity, and it uses less oxygen to do the same amount of work. Such dramatic changes do not occur, however, in the human ventricle where the βMHC is the predominant isoform in both embryo and adult, and the pattern is not altered significantly by hypertrophy. The atrial naturetic factor gene, however, is expressed in the hypertrophied human ventricle, as it is in the embryonic state, but it is not expressed in the normal adult ventricle.[110,111] The response of inducing the release of atrial naturetic factor from the ventricle, which has diuretic activity, could be adaptive in attenuating the retention of salt and water associated with cardiac failure. On the other hand, calcium ATPase, an enzyme essential to cardiac contractility, is decreased in both the hypertrophied rodent and the human ventricle.[112] It is well documented in the developing mammalian heart in utero that the initial actin gene expressed is that of smooth muscle, followed by that of skeletal, and finally cardiac muscle.[113] Smooth muscle and skeletal muscle actin are both reexpressed at

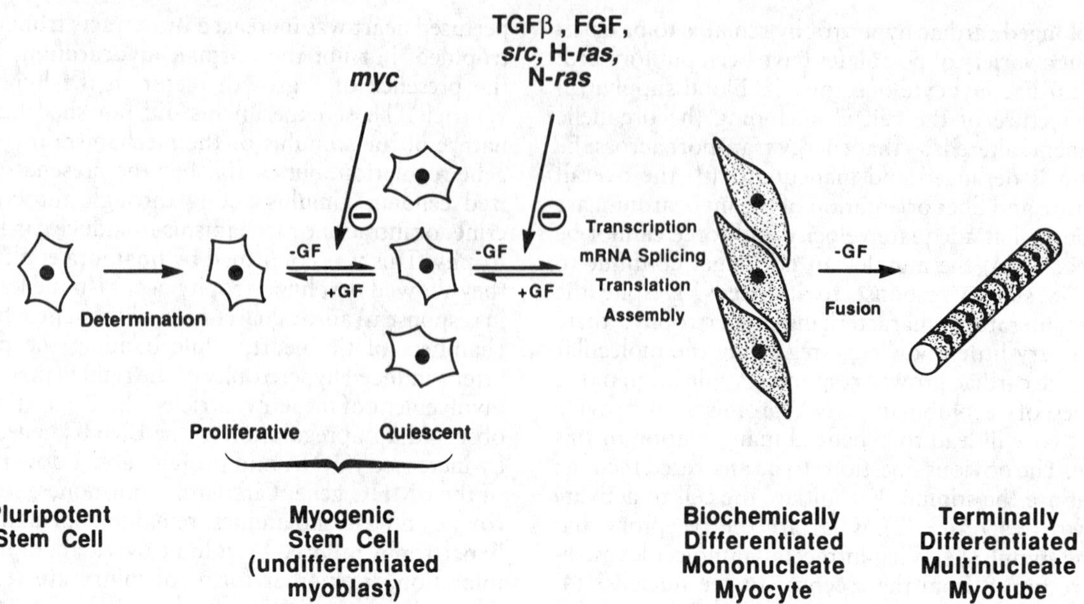

FIGURE 1-26 Development of a mature skeletal muscle cell from an undifferentiated stem cell, illustrating the various stages of differentiation and potential steps of control as exercised by growth factors and cellular oncogenes. The entry of the primitive cell into the myogenic pathway ("determination") does not, of itself, result in expression of muscle-specific genes. The affects of c-*myc* on muscle differentiation varies in relationship to the potential of the modified cell to sustain proliferation. In contrast, H-*ras* and N-*ras* genes, like inhibitory growth factors (GF) such as FGF and TGFβ, prevent the induction of muscle-specific genes even in quiescent myoblasts. Neither inhibitory growth factors nor activation of an inducible mutant ras gene can suppress the myogenic phenotype after fusion and "terminal" differentiation of a multinucleate myotube. *(From R Roberts, JA Towbin, T Parker, R Bles: A Primer of Molecular Biology. New York, Elsevier, 1992:158.)*

the level of a several-fold increase in the rodent during pressure-overload-induced cardiac hypertrophy.[114] Thus, the actin genes, during pathological hypertrophy, recapitulate ontogeny. The consequence of hypertrophy is initially a compensatory increase in myocardial function; however, the development of cardiac failure is often the ultimate outcome. The functional significance, if any, of the reexpression of fetal genes when the cardiac growth program is turned on in the adult heart is unknown. It is possible that the growth response can only be activated through expression of a family of genes. The master gene controlling expression of such a family could be triggered by a growth factor stimulated by pressure overload, this could result in a cascade of genes expressed, most of which are incidental rather than adaptive or maladaptive. For example, in skeletal muscle there is a master gene, myo-D,[115,116] which triggers the differentiation of mesenchymal cells in the skeletal muscle. When this occurs, a cascade of genes are downregulated and another cascade of genes upregulated. Myo-D is not expressed in cardiac muscle, and no such triggering factor has been found for cardiac myocyte differentiation.

Stimuli and the Receptors Mediating Cardiac Hypertrophy

Cardiac growth and hypertrophy are universal in man following a variety of stimuli, including pressure and volume overload, adrenergic stimulation secondary to pheochromocytoma, in association with myocarditis and myocardial infarction, and in other cardiomyopathies of diverse etiologies. Several other known factors are likely to also induce cardiac growth, such as angiotensin II[117] and endothelin.[118] The precise nature of the stimulus that activates cardiac growth and protein synthesis following pressure- or volume-induced hypertrophy remains to be elucidated. The mechanical stimulus, however, appears to be important and sufficient, since myocytes grown on membranes and subsequently stretched respond with increased mRNA levels and IP-3 turnover[119] as well as with upregulation of c-*myc* and c-*fos*[120] and increased calcium.[121] Thus, the pressure stimulus alone can induce the necessary signaling pathways for increased growth. In cultured, differentiated, primary cardiac myocytes, it has been demonstrated that α-adrenergic stimulation induces cardiac myocyte growth characterized by expression of fetal proteins similar to the in vivo response to pressure overload.[122] More recently, growth factors such as TGFβ and acidic and basic FGF have been shown in cultured primary rat myocytes to induce responses that were analogous to those observed following pressure overload induced hypertrophy in the intact animal.[33,123-125] Acidic FGF was associated with a hyperplastic response, while basic FGF was associated with increased protein synthesis analogous to hypertrophy. In contrast, TGFβ did not induce either a hyperplastic or hypertrophic response. All of the growth factors were associated with reexpression of fetal proteins; namely, an increase in βMHC and the reexpression of smooth and skeletal muscle actin, ventricular ANF, together with a decrease in αMHC and sarcoplasmic reticulum Ca^{2+} ATPase. Despite the homology of the two fibroblastic growth factors, they exhibited a significantly different pattern of fetal gene expression. The growth factors (FGF and TGFβ) are of great interest as increased expression of these factors in myocytes has been observed following experimental myocardial infarction in the rat.[126,127] Whether or not these factors play a role in compensatory growth following infarction remains to be determined.

The growth factor TGFβ and the fibroblastic growth factors are upregulated in early primordial cardiac tissue and are responsible for induction of cellular proliferation.[128,129] This is clearly an exciting area of research of great therapeutic potential. The similarity of response suggests a common mechanism for the various stimuli including pressure overload, volume overload, catecholamine, and the FGF and TGF1 growth factors. Hypertrophy induced by thyroxine,[52] however, is through a specific nuclear receptor and is somewhat different, in that αMHC rather than βMHC is upregulated, and the expression of the various fetal proteins characteristic of pressure overload or stimulation by the growth factors does not occur. Similarly, hypertrophy induced by exercise is not associated with reexpression of fetal proteins.[130]

Oncogenes as Signaling Proteins for Cardiac Hypertrophy

There is considerable evidence supporting a role for cellular protooncogenes in cardiac growth. During the development of the avian heart, virtually all cells contain the protooncogene c-*myc*. C-*myc* and v-*myc* genes are expressed at high levels in both embryonic and newborn hearts and are downregulated during cardiac maturation.[131] In neonatal rat myocytes in cell culture, differentiation into nonproliferating cardiac cells that occurs 5 to 10 days postbirth was associated with a downregulation of several protooncogenes, including c-*myc*, c-*fos*, and Ha-*ras*.[83-85] Coincident with myocyte differentiation is the expression of M creatine kinase over that of B creatine kinase. Induced persistent expression of c-*myc* in myocytes delayed but did not prevent cell differentiation, indicating c-*myc* was not sufficient to induce proliferation or abolish differentiation.[85] Persistent expression of Ha-*ras* oncogene prevented cell differentiation in cell culture.[84] Pressure-induced hypertrophy in the rat was associated with the reexpression of c-*myc*,[81] c-*jun*, *jun*-b, and c-*fos*.[118] C-*jun* and c-*fos* are bona fide transcription factors and were transiently expressed within hours of coarctation preceding the expression of fetal genes such as smooth muscle and skeletal muscle actin. This is of some note since it is now well documented that c-*fos* dimerizes with c- or *jun*-b to form a leucine zipper transcription factor.[30] As noted earlier, c-*myc* overexpressed in the transgenic mouse developed cardiac hyperplasia.[82] Expression of c-*myc* has also been documented in the hearts of hypertensive rats. Hypertrophy induced by TGF and fibroblastic growth factors is also associated with the upregulation of c-*fos* and *jun*-b.[33] Thyroxine, which induces hypertrophy through a nuclear receptor,[52] is encoded for by the erb A oncogene.[80]

Clues from Inherited Abnormalities of the Contractile Proteins

There is now great interest in the contractile proteins and cardiac hypertrophy in view of the finding of βMHC as a putative gene responsible for hypertrophic cardiomyopathy (see Chap. 90). In this disease, the primary defect is excessive growth, primarily of the ventricular septum. Studies have indicated that the gene responsible for this disease is located on chromosome 14[9,10] in the region of βMHC. Several mutations[132-134] have been shown to be present in the βMHC gene and would appear to be responsible for this disease. It was recently shown that a missense mutation in exon 13 of the β myosin heavy chain gene is expressed in the mRNA of cardiac tissue of an individual with HCM, but not in unaffected members of the family.[135,136] Studies are now ongoing to unravel further mutations and to determine how these mutations induce hypertrophic cardiomyopathy.

REFERENCES

1. Roberts R: The impact for molecular biology in cardiology. *Am J Physiol* 1991;261(suppl):8–14.
2. Roberts R: Integrated program for the training of cardiovascular fellows in molecular biology. In: Albertini A, Lenfant C, Paoletti R (eds): *Biotechnology in Clinical Medicine.* New York, Raven, 1987:99–105.
3. Katz AM: Molecular biology in cardiology, a paradigmatic shift (editorial). *J Mol Cell Cardiol* 1988;20:355–366.
4. Patterson SW, Piper H, Starling EH: The regulation of the heart beat. *J Physiol* 1914;48:465.
5. Meerson FZ: The myocardium in hyperfunction, hypertrophy, and heart failure. *Circ Res* 1963;25(suppl II):1–163.
6. Haudenschild CC, Grunwald J: Proliferative heterogeneity of vascular smooth muscle cells and its alteration by injury. *Exp Cell Res* 1985;157:364–370.
7. Grunwald J, Haudenschild CC: Intimal injury in vivo activates vascular smooth muscle cell migration and explant outgrowth in vitro. *Arteriosclerosis* 1984;4:183–188.
8. Califf RM, Ohman EM, Frid DJ, Fortin DF, Mark DB, Hlatky MA, et al: Restenosis: The clinical issues. In: *Textbook of Interventional Cardiology.* Philadelphia, Saunders, 1990:363–394.
9. Jarcho JA, McKenna W, Pare JAP, Solomon, SD, Holcombe RF, Dickie S, et al: Mapping a gene for familial hypertrophic cardiomyopathy to chromosome 14q1. *N Engl J Med* 1989;321:1372–1378.
10. Hejtmancik JF, Brink PA, Towbin J, Hill R, Brink L, Czernuszewicz GZ, et al: Localization of the gene for familial hypertrophic cardiomyopathy to chromosome 14q1 in a diverse American population. *Circulation* 1991;83:1592–1597.
11. Pennica D, Holmes WE, Kohr WJ, Harkins RN, Vehar GA, Ward CA, et al: Cloning and expression of human tissue-type plasminogen activator cDNA in E. coli. *Nature* 1983;301:214–221.
12. Larsen GR, Henson K, Blue Y: Variants of human tissue-type plasminogen activator. *J Biochem Chem* 1988;263:1023–1029.
13. Watson JD, Crick FHC: Molecular structure of nucleic acids: A structure for deoxyribose nucleic acid. *Nature* 1953;171:737–738.
14. Watson JD, Crick FHC: Genetic implications of the structure of deoxyribonucleic acid. *Nature* 1953;171:964–967.
15. Franklin RE, Gosling RG: Molecular configuration in sodium thymonucleate. *Nature* 1953;171:740–741.
16. Wilkins MHF, Stokes AR, Wilson HR: Molecular structure of deoxypentose nucleic acids. *Nature* 1953;171:738–740.
17. Schekman R, Weiner A, Kornberg A: Multienzyme systems of DNA replication. *Science* 1956;186:987–993.
18. Marmor J, Lane L: Strand separation and specific recombination in deoxyribonucleic acids: Biological studies. *Proc Natl Acad Sci USA 1960;46:453–461.*
19. Doty P, Marmor J, Eigner J, Schildkraut C: Strand separation and specific recombination in deoxyribonucleic acids: Physical chemical studies. *Proc Natl Acad Sci USA* 1960;46:461–476.
20. Leder P, Nirenberg M: RNA codewords and protein synthesis, II. Nucleotide sequence of a valine RNA codeword. *Proc Natl Acad Sci USA* 1964;52:420–427.
21. Nishimura S, Jones DS, Khorana HG: The in vitro synthesis

of a co-polypeptide containing two amino acids in alternating sequence dependent upon a DNA-like polymer containing two nucleotides in alternating sequence. *J Mol Biol* 1981;146:1–21.
22. Olivera BM, Hall ZW, Lehman IR: Enzymatic joining of polynucleotides. V. A DNA adenylate intermediate in the polynucleotide joining reaction. *Proc Natl Acad Sci USA* 1968;61:237–244.
23. Smith HO, Wilcox KW: A restriction enzyme from *Hemophilias influenzae*. I: Purification and general properties. *J Mol Biol* 1970;51:379–391.
24. Kelly TJ Jr., Smith HO: A restriction enzyme from *Hemophilias influenzae*. II: Base sequence of the recognition site. *J Mol Biol* 1970;51:393–409.
25. Baltimore D: Viral RNA-dependent DNA polymerase. *Nature* 1970;226:1209–1211.
26. Termin HM, Mizutani S: RNA-dependent DNA polymerase in virions of Rous sarcoma virus. *Nature* 1970;226:1211–1213.
27. Cohen S, Chang A, Boyer H, Helling R: Construction of biological functional bacterial plasmids in vitro. *Proc Natl Acad Sci USA* 1973;70:3240–3244.
28. Sanger F, Coulson AR: A rapid method for determining sequences in DNA by primed synthesis and DNA polymerase. *J Mol Biol* 1975;94:444–448.
29. Maxam AM, and Gilbert W: A new method of sequencing DNA. *Proc Natl Acad Sci USA* 1977;74:560–564.
30. Roberts R: Molecular biology of the cardiovascular system. In: Roberts R (ed): *Molecular Biology Series*. Hamden, CT, Blackwell, 1992:1–14.
31. Knight, SL: Molecular zippers in gene regulation. *Sci Am* 1991;264:54–64.
32. Brown D: The role of stable complexes that repress and activate eucaryotic genes. *Cell* 1984;37:359–365.
33. Schneider MD, Roberts R, Parker TG: Modulation of cardiac genes by mechanical stress. The oncogene signalling hypothesis. *Mol Biol Med* 1991;8:167–183.
34. Falvey E, Schibler U: How are the regulators regulated? *JASEB J* 1991;5:309–314.
35. Aaij C, Borst P: The gel electrophoresis of DNA. *Biochim Biophys Acta* 1972;269:192–200.
36. Sharp PA, Sugden B, Sambrook J: Detection of two restriction endonuclease activities in *Emophilus Parainfluenzae* using analytical agarose-ethidium bromide electrophoresis. *Biochemistry* 1973;12:3055–3062.
37. Southern EM: Detection of specific sequences among DNA fragments separated by gel electrophoresis. *J Mol Biol* 1975;98:503–517.
38. Sambrook J, Fritsch EF, Maniatis T: Analysis and cloning of eucaryltic genomic DNA. In: *Molecular Cloning: A Laboratory Manual*. New York, Cold Spring Harbor laboratory Press, 1989:9.14–9.23.
39. Schwarz DC, Cantro CR: Separation of yeast chromosome-sized DNAs by pulsed field gradient gel electrophoresis. *Nucleic Acids Res* 1984;37:67.
40. Cortez MD, Friedman DL, Shih H, Roberts R, Perryman B: A distinct MM creatine kinase isoform is present in human and canine myocardial purkinje fibers. *Circulation* 1989; 80(suppl II):II-1831.
41. Saiki RK, Scharf S, Faloona F, Mullis KB, Horn GT, Erlich HA, et al: Enzymatic amplification of β-globin genomic sequences and restriction site analysis of diagnosis of sickle cell anemia. *Science* 1985;230:1350–1354.
42. Saiki RK, Gelfand DH, Stoffel S, Scharf SJ, Higuchi R, Horn GT, et al: Primer-directed enzymatic amplification of DNA with a thermostable DNA polymerase. *Science* 1988;239:487–491.
43. Darnell J, Lodish H, Baltimore D: Actin, myosin, and intermediate filaments: Cell movements and cell shape. In: Darnell J, Lodish H, Baltimore D (eds): *Molecular Cell Biology* 2d ed., New York, W.H. Freeman, 1990.
44. Jaenicke T, Diederich KW, Haas W, Schleich J, Lichter P, Pfordt M, et al: The complete sequence of the human β-myosin heavy chain gene and a comparative analysis of its product. *Genomics* 1990;8:194–206.
45. Yamauchi-Takihara K, Sole MJ, Liew J, Ing D, Liew CC: Characterization of human cardiac myosin heavy chain genes. *Proc Natl Acad Sci USA* 1989;86:3504–3508.
46. Jandreski MS, Sole MJ, Liew CC: Sequence of cDNA encoding the syrian hamster cardiac β-myosin heavy chain. *Nucleic Acids Res* 1988;16:4734.
47. Warrick HM, Spudich JA: Myosin structure and function in cell motility. *Annu Rev Cell Biol* 1989;3:379–421.
48. Leinwand LA, Fournier REK, Nadal-Ginard B, Shows TB: Multigene family for sarcomeric myosin heavy chain in mouse and human DNA: Localization on a single chromosome. *Science* 1983;221:766–768.
49. Emerson CP, Bernstein SI: Molecular genetics of myosin. *Annu Rev Biochem* 1987;56:695–726.
50. Matsuoka R, Chambers A, Kimura M, Kanda N, Bruns G, Yoshida M, et al: Molecular cloning and chromosomal localization of a gene encoding for human cardiac myosin heavy chain. *Am J Med Genet* 1988;29:369–376.
51. Nadal-Ginard B, Mahdavi V: Molecular basis of cardiac performance. *J Clin Invest* 1989;84:1693–1700.
52. Izumo S, Nadal-Ginard B, Mahdavi V: All members of the MHC multigene family respond to thyroid hormone in a highly tissue-specific manner. *Science* 1986;231:597–600.
53. Amos LA: Structure of muscle filaments studied by electron microscopy. *Annu Rev Biophys Chem* 1985;14:291–313.
54. Chang KS, Zimmer WE Jr, Bergsma DJ, Dodgson JB, Schwartz RJ: Isolation and characterization of six different chicken actin genes. *Mol Cell Biol* 1984;4:2498–2508.
55. Payne MR, Rudnick SE: Regulation of vertebrate striated muscle contraction. *Trends Biochem Sci* 1989;14:357–360.
56. Zot AS, Potter JD: Structural aspects of troponin-tropomyosin regulation of skeletal muscle contraction. *Annu Rev Biophys* Chem 1987;16:535–559.
57. Andreadis A, Gallego ME, Nadal-Ginard B: Generation of protein isoform diversity by alternative splicing: Mechanistic and biological implications. *Annu Rev Cell Biol* 1987;3:207–242.
58. Breitbart RE, Andreadis A, Nadal-Ginard B: Alternative splicing: A ubiquitous mechanism for the generation of multiple protein isoforms from single genes. *Annu Rev Biochem* 1987;56:467–495.
59. Cooke R: The mechanism of muscle contraction. *CRC Crit Rev Biochem* 1986;21:53–118.
60. Pollard TD, Cooper JA: Actin and actin-binding proteins. A critical evaluation of mechanisms and functions. *Annu Rev Biochem* 1986;55:987–1035.
61. Darnell J, Lodish H, Baltimore D: Microtubules and cellular movements. In: Darnell J, Lodish H, Baltimore D (eds): *Molecular Cell* Biology, 2d ed. New York, W.H. Freeman, 1990.
62. Steinert PM, Roop DR: Molecular and cellular biology of intermediate filaments. *Annu Rev Biochem* 1988;57:593–626.
63. Bies RD, Friedman D, Roberts R, Perryman MB, Caskey CT: Expression and localization of dystrophin in human cardiac purkinje fibers. *Circulation* 1992;86:147–153.
64. Bies RD, Phelps SF, Cortez MD, Roberts R, Caskey CT, Chamberlain JS: Human and murine dystrophin mRNA transcripts are differentially expressed during skeletal muscle, heart, and brain development. *Nucleic Acids Res 1992;20:1725–1731.*
65. Vybiral T, Winkelmann JC, Roberts R, Joe E-H, Casey DL, Williams JK, Epstein HF: Human cardiac and skeletal muscle spectrins: Differential expression and localization. *Cell Motil Cytoskeleton* 1992;21:291–304.
66. Marshall CJ: Oncogenes and cell proliferation: An overview. In: Glover DM, Hames BD (eds): *Oncogenes*. New York, IRL Press, 1989:1–21.
67. Hunter T, Cooper JA: Protein-tyrosine kinases. *Annu Rev Biochem* 1985;54:897.
68. Foulkes JG, Rich-Rosner M: Tyrosine-specific protein kinases as mediators of growth control. In: Cohen P, Housley MD (eds): *Molecular Aspects of Cellular Regulation,* Vol 4. Amsterdam, Elsevier, 1985.
69. Connelley OM, Sullivan WP, Toft DO, Birnbaumer M, Cook RG, Maxwell BL, et al: Molecular cloning of chicken progesterone receptor. *Science* 1986;233:767–770.
70. Edelman AM, Blumenthal DK, Krebs EG: Protein serine/threonine kinases. *Annu Rev Biochem* 1987;56:567–613.
71. Bishop JM: Viral oncogenes. *Cell* 1985;42:23–38.
72. Macara IG: Oncogenes and cellular signal transduction. *Physiol Rev* 1989;69:797–820.
73. Schneider MD, Olson EN: Control of myogenic differentiation by cellular oncogenes. *Mol Neurobiol* 1988;2:1–39.
74. Mulvagh SL, Roberts R, Schneider MD: Cellular oncogenes in cardiovascular disease. *J Mol Cell Cardiol* 1988;20:657–662.

75. Bishop JM: Cellular oncogenes and retroviruses. *Annu Rev Biochem* 1983;52:301–354.
76. Varmus HE: The molecular genetics of cellular oncogenes. *Annu Rev Genet* 1984;18:553–612.
77. Waterfield MD, Scrace GT, Whittle N, Stroobant BP, Johnson A, Wasteson A, et al: PDGF is structurally related to the putative transforming protein P28[sis] of simian sarcoma virus. *Nature* 1983;304:35.
78. Downward J, Yarden Y, Mayes E, Scrace G, Totty N, Stockwell P, et al: Close similarity of EGF receptor and v-*erb*-B oncogene protein sequences. *Nature* 1984;307:521–527.
79. Sap J, Munoz A, Damm K, Goldberg Y, Ghysdael J, Leutz A, et al: The c-*erb*-A protein is a high-affinity receptor for thyroid hormone. *Nature* 1986;324:635–640.
80. Mulvagh SL, Michael LH, Perryman MB, Roberts R, Schneider MD: A hemodynamic load in vivo induces cardiac expression of the cellular oncogene, c-*myc*. *Biochem Biophys Res Commun* 1987;147:627–636.
81. Izumo S, Nadal-Ginard B, Mahdavi V: Proto-oncogene induction and reprogramming of cardiac gene expression produced by pressure overload. *Proc Natl Acad Sci USA* 1988;85:339–343.
82. Jackson T, Allard M, Sreenan C, Doss L, Bishop S, Swain JL: Increased expression of c-*myc* during cardiac development produces myocyte hyperplasia in transgenic mice. *Mol Cell Biol* 1990;10:3709–3716.
83. Schneider MD, Payne PA, Ueno H, Perryman MB, Roberts R: Dissociated expression of c-*myc* and a *fos*-related competence gene during cardiac myogenesis. *Mol Cell Biol* 1986;6:4140–4143.
84. Payne PA, Olson EN, Hsiau P, Roberts R, Perryman MB, Schneider MD: An activated c-Ha-*ras* allele blocks the induction of muscle-specific genes whose expression is contingent on mitogen withdrawal. *Proc Natl Acad Sci USA* 1987;84:8956–8960.
85. Schneider MD, Perryman MB, Payne PA, Spizz G, Roberts R, Olson EN: Autonomous *myc* expression in transfected muscle cells does not prevent myogenic differentiation. *Mol Cell Biol* 1987;7:1973–1977.
86. Rayter SI, Iwata KK, Michitsch RW, Sorvillo JM, Valenzuela DM, Foulkes JG: Biochemical functions of oncogenes. In: Glover DM, Hames BD (eds): *Oncogenes*. New York, IRL Press, 1989:113–189.
87. Roberts AR, Sporn MB: The transforming growth factor-betas. In: Sporn MB, Roberts AR (eds.): *Peptide Growth Factors and Their Receptors. Handbook of Experimental Pharmacology.* Heidelberg, Springer-Verlag, 1990:419–472.
88. Rozengurt E, Mendoza SA: Synergistic signals in mitogenesis: Role of ion fluxes, cyclic nucleotides and protein kinase C in Swiss 3T3 cells. *J Cell Sci* 1985;3(suppl):229–242.
89. Rozengurt E: Early signals in the mitogenic response. *Science* 1986;234:161–166.
90. Berridge MJ, Heslop JP, Irvine RF, Brown KD: Inositol triphosphate formation and calcium mobilization in response to platelet-derived growth factor. *Biochem J* 1984;222:195–201.
91. Vara F, Rozengurt E: Stimulation of Na^+/H^+ antoport activity by epidermal growth factor in insulin occurs without activation of protein kinase C. *Biochem Biophys Res Commun* 1985;130:646.
92. Besterman JM, Tyrey SJ, Cragoe EJ, Cuatrecasas P: Inhibition of epidermal growth factor-induced by amiloride and an analog: Evidence against a requirement of Na^+/H^+ exchange. *Proc Natl Acad Sci USA* 1984;81:6762–6766.
93. Puoysser J, Chambard JC, Franchi A, Paris S, Van Obberghen-Schilling E: Growth factor activation of the sodium $^+$-H^+ antiporter controls growth of fibroblast by regulating intra-cellular pH. *Cancer Cells* 1985;3:409–415.
94. Greenberg ME, Ziff EB: Stimulation of 3T3 cells induces transcription of the c-*fos* proto-oncogene. *Nature* 1984;311:433–438.
95. Linzer DIG, Anthans D: Growth-related changes in specific mRNAs of cultured mouse cells. *Proc Natl Acad Sci USA* 1983;80:4271–4275.
96. Roberts R, Towbin J, Parker TG, Bles R (eds): *A Primer of Molecular Biology*. New York, Elsevier Science, 1992.
97. Meerson FZ: *The Failing Heart: Adaptation and Maladaptation.* New York, Raven, 1983:51–52.
98. Hammond GL, Wieben E, Markert CL: Molecular signals for initiating protein synthesis in organ hypertrophy. *Proc Natl Acad Sci USA* 1979;76:2455–2459.
99. Imamura SI, Matsuoka R, Hiratsuka E, Kimura M, Nishikawa, T, Takao A: Local response to cardiac overload on myosin heavy chain gene expression and isozyme transition. *Circ Res* 1990;66:1067–1073.
100. Rubin SA, Correa M, Rabines A, Fishbein MC: Beta blockade alters myosin heavy chain gene expression after rat infarction. *Circulation* 1989;80:II–458.
101. Oberpriller JO, Oberpriller JC: Cell division in cardiac myocytes. In: Ferrans VF, Rosenquist G, Weinstein C (eds) *Cardiac Morphogenesis.* Elsevier Science, New York, 1985:12–22.
102. Olson EN, Caldwell KC, Gordon JI, Glaser L: Regulation of creatine phosphokinase expression during differentiation of BC_3H1 cells. *J Biol Chem* 1983;258:2644–2652.
103. Sejersen T, Suemegi J, Ringertz NR: Density-dependent arrest of DNA replication is accompanied by decreased levels of c-*myc* mRNA in myogenic but not in differentiation-defective myoblasts. *J Cell Physiol* 1985;125:465–470.
104. Stockdale FE: Myoblast commitment and the embryogenesis of skeletal muscle. In: Pearson ML, Epstein HE, (eds): *Muscle Development: Molecular and Cellular Control.* Cold Spring Harbor, New York, Cold Spring Harbor Laboratory, 1982:339–344.
105. Blau HM, Baltimore D: Differentiation requires continuous regulation. *J Cell Biol* 1991;112:781–783.
106. Clubb JR, Bishop FJ, Bishop SP: Formation of binucleated myocardial cells in the noenatal rat: An index for growth hypertrophy. *Lab Invest* 1984;50:571–577.
107. Parker TG, Packer SE, Schneider MD: Peptide growth factors can provoke "fetal" contractile protein gene expression in rat cardiac myocytes. *J Clin Invest* 1990;85:507–514.
108. Alpert NR, Gordon MS: Myofibrillar adenosine triphosphate activity in congestive heart failure. *Am J Physiol* 1962;202:940–946.
109. Katz AM: Cardiomyopathy of overload: A major determinant of prognosis in congestive heart failure. *N Engl J Med* 1990; 322:100–110.
110. Seidman CE, Wong DW, Jarcho JA, Bloch JD, Seidman JG: Cis-acting sequences that modulate atrial natriuretic factor gene expression. *Proc Natl Acad Sci USA* 1988;85:4104–4108.
111. Saito Y, Nakao K, Arai H, Nishimura K, Okumura K, Obata K, et al: Augmented expression of atrial natriuretic polypeptide gene in ventricle of human falling heart. *J Clin Invest* 1989;83:298–305.
112. Mercardier JJ, Lompre AM, Duc P, Boheler KR, Fraysse JB, Wisnewsky C, et al: Altered sarcoplasmic reticulum Ca^{2+}-ATPase gene expression in the human ventricle during end-stage heart failure. *J Clin Invest* 1990;85:305–309.
113. Ruzicka DL, Schwartz RJ: Sequential activation of a α-actin genes during avian cardiogenesis: Vascular smooth muscle α-actin gene transcripts mark the onset of cardiomyocyte differentiation. *J Cell Biol* 1988;107:2575–2586.
114. Black FM, Packer SE, Parker TG, Michael LH, Roberts R, Schwartz RJ, Schneider MD: The vascular smooth muscle α-actin gene is reactivated during cardiac hypertrophy provoked by load. *J Clin Invest* 1991;88:1581–1588.
115. Olson EN: MyoD family: A paradigm for development? *Genes Dev* 1990;4:1454–1461.
116. Davis RL, Weintraub H, Lassar AB: Expression of a single transfected cDNA converts fibroblasts to myoblasts. *Cell* 1987;51:987–1000.
117. Katoh Y, Komuro I, Shibasaki Y, Yamaguchi H, Yazaki Y: Angiotensin II induces hypertrophy and oncogene expression in cultured rat heart myocytes. *Circulation* 1986;80:II–450.
118. Shubeita HE, McDonough PM, Harris AN, Knowlton KU, Glembotski CG, Brown JH, Chien KR: Endothelin induction of inositol phospholipid hydrolysis, sarcomere assembly, and cardiac gene expression in ventricular myocytes: A paracrine mechanism for myocardial cell hypertrophy. *J Biol Chem* 1990;265:555–562.
119. Mann DL, Kent RL, Cooper G: Load regulation of the properties of adult feline cardiocytes: Growth induction by cellular deformation. *Circ Res* 1989;64:1079–1090.
120. Komuro I, Kaida T, Shibazaki Y, Kurabayashi M, Katch Y, Hoh E, et al: Stretching cardiac myocytes stimulates proto-oncogene expression. *J Biol Chem* 1990;265:3595–3598.

121. Marban E, Koretsune Y: Cell calcium, oncogenes, and hypertrophy. *Hypertension* 1990;15:652–658.
122. Bishopric N, Simpson PC, Ordahl CP: Induction of the skeletal α-actin gene in x_1-adrenoreceptor-mediated hypertrophy of rat cardiac myocytes. *J Clin Invest* 1987;80:1194–1199.
123. Parker TG, Packer SE, Schneider MD: Peptide growth factors can provoke "fetal" contractile protein gene expression in rat cardiac myocytes. *J Clin Invest* 1990;85:507–514.
124. Parker TG, Chow KL, Schwartz RJ, Schneider MD: Differential regulation of skeletal α-actin transcription in cardiac muscle by two fibroblast growth factors. *Proc Natl Acad Sci USA* 1990;87:7066–7070.
125. Parker TG, Chow KL, Schwartz RJ, Schneider MD: A proximal segment of the skeletal α-actin promoter, resembling the c-fos serum response element, is induced selectively in cardiac muscle by basic, but not acidic, fibroblast growth factor (Abstr). *Clin Res* 1991;39:191a.
126. Thompson NC, Bazoberry F, Speir EH, Casscells W, Ferrans VJ, Flanders KC, et al: Transforming growth factor beta-1 in acute myocardial infarction in rats. *Growth Factors* 1988;1:91–99.
127. Chiba M, Bazoberry F, Speir EH, Sasse J, Nesbitt CP, Baird A, et al: Role of basic fibroblast growth factor in angiogenesis, healing and hypertrophy after rat myocardial infarction (abstr). *Circulation* 1989;80:II-452.
128. Akhurst RJ, Lehnert SA, Faissner A, Duffle E: TGF beta in murine morphogenetic processes: The early embryo and cardiogenesis. *Development* 1990;108:645–656.
129. Lyons KM, Pelton RW, Hogan BLM: Organogenesis and pattern formation in the mouse: RNA distribution patterns suggest a role for bone morphogenic protein-2A (BMP-2A). *Development* 1990;109:833–844.
130. Morris GS, Baldwin KM, Lash JM, Hamlin RL, Sherman WM: Exercise alters cardiac myosin isozyme distribution in obese Zucker and Wistar rats. *J Appl Physiol* 1990;69:380–383.
131. Ueno H, Perryman MB, Roberts R, Schneider MD: Differentiation of cardiac myocytes following mitogen withdrawal exhibits three sequential stages of the ventricular growth response. *J Cell Biol* 1988;107:1911–1918.
132. Tanigawa G, Jarcho JA, Kass S, Solomon SD, Seidman CE: A molecular basis for familial hypertrophic cardiomyopathy: An alpha/beta cardiac myosin heavy chain hybrid gene. *Cell* 1990;62:991–998.
133. Geister-Lawrance AA, Kass S, Tanigawa G, Vosberg H-P, McKenna W, Seidman CE, Seidman JG. A molecular basis for familial hypertrophic cardiomyopathy: A beta-cardiac myosin heavy chain gene missense mutation. *Cell* 1990;62:999–1006.
134. Marian AJ, Yu Q-T, Mares A, Hill R, Roberts R, Perryman MB: Detection of a new mutation in the β-myosin heavy chain gene in an individual with hypertrophic cardiomyopathy. *J Clin Invest* 1992;90:2156–2165.
135. Perryman MB, Mares A Jr., Hejtmancik F, Gooch G, Roberts R: The β myosin heavy chain missence mutation in exon 13, a putative defect for HCM is present in only one of 39 families. *Circulation* 1991;84:II-418.
136. Perryman MB, Yu Q-T, Marian AJ, Mares A, Czernuszewicz G, Ifwegu J, Roberts R: Expression of a missense mutation in the mRNA for β myosin heavy chain in a myocardial biopsy from a patient with familial hypertrophic cardiomyopathy. *J Clin Invest* 1992;90:271–277.

Chapter 2

Cellular Biology of Blood Vessels

Kathy K. Griendling, Ph.D. ■ *R. Wayne Alexander, M.D., Ph.D.*

Knowledge of the biology of the vascular wall is essential to understanding the pathophysiology of atherosclerosis, vasospasm, and hypertension, as well as the rationale behind the development and application of new therapeutic strategies for vascular disease. As the major strategy for treating vascular disease shifts from treating secondary manifestations to treating the primary dysfunction, understanding the biologic basis of disease becomes of central importance. It is likely that much cardiovascular disease reflects dysfunctional endothelium. This chapter is designed to give an introduction to vascular biology with emphasis on the function of the endothelium.

STRUCTURE OF THE VESSEL WALL

Arteries consist of three layers: the innermost intima, the media, and the outermost adventitia. The intima is comprised of a single layer of endothelial cells embedded in an extracellular matrix. The media is separated from the intima by the internal elastic lamina, and consists of smooth muscle cells, elastic laminae, bundles of collagen fibers, and elastic fibrils, all embedded in an extracellular matrix. The adventitia is the most variable layer, containing dense fibroelastic tissue, nutrient vessels, and nerves.

The actual composition of each of these layers varies with the type of blood vessel. Large, conduit arteries are typically referred to as elastic arteries, because of their high ratio of elastic laminae to smooth muscle cells. Muscular arteries are generally smaller and have a prevalence of smooth muscle cells, while arterioles consist of only one to two layers of smooth muscle cells. The smallest vessels are the capillaries, made up of a single layer of endothelial cells that are occasionally apposed to pericytes—smooth muscle-like cells that serve a contractile function. The venous system has a similar architecture to that of the arterial system, the main difference being the orientation of the smooth muscle cells within the wall.

Physiologically, the two most important cell types in the vascular system are the endothelial cell and the vascular smooth muscle cell. The endothelial cell is generally oriented with the direction of blood flow parallel to the main axis of the vessel. Endothelial cells are held together by junctional complexes that regulate permeability and control cell-to-cell communication. The smooth muscle cell is a spindle-shaped cell whose orientation varies with the type of artery, but is generally helical in large, elastic arteries and concentric in muscular arteries. Vascular smooth muscle cells contain three types of filaments: thick (myosin), thin (actin), and intermediate. The proteins that form these filaments undergo phosphorylation exposure to certain vasoactive agonists, thus altering their orientation and interactions and supporting force development (see below). In normal arteries, the smooth muscle cells are primarily in the "contractile" phenotype described above. Under conditions where smooth muscle cells are proliferating, however—such as atherosclerotic plaques, intimal hyperplasia as a result of angioplasty, or placement in culture—these cells "modulate" morphologically and biochemically to a growth mode and lose their differential contractile features.

PHYSIOLOGY OF THE ENDOTHELIAL CELL

Normal endothelial cell function is crucial to homeostasis in the vascular system. As mentioned above, diseases such as atherosclerosis ultimately are manifestations of endothelial dysfunction. The endothelium has three major functions: as a metabolically active, secretory tissue; as an anticoagulant, antithrombotic surface; and as a barrier to indiscriminant passage of blood constituents into the arterial wall. The implications of these physiologic properties for vascular biology will be considered separately. In this subsection we shall discuss the processing of various substances by the endothelium.

Endothelial Cell Metabolism and Secretion

As discussed in more detail below, endothelial cells secrete vasoactive substances both into the lumen and ablumenally into the vessel wall. These molecules include prostacyclin, endothelial-derived relaxing factor (EDRF), and endothelial-derived hyperpolarizing factor (EDHF), which serve as vasodilators[1–3]; endothelin[4] and endothelial-derived contracting factor (EDCF), which act as vasoconstrictors; factor VIII antigen, von Willebrand's factor, and plasminogen activator, which are involved in the coagulation/fibrinolytic pathways; structural components of the extracellular matrix (collagen, elastin, glycosaminoglycans, fibronectin)[7,8]; and heparans and growth factors that regulate smooth muscle cell proliferation.[9–12] In addition, endothelial cells are able to clear and metabolically alter blood-borne and locally produced substances including plasma lipids and lipoproteins,[13] adenine nucleotides and nucleosides,[14] serotonin, catecholamines, bradykinin, and angiotensin I.[15]

Endothelial cells are involved in the metabolism of plasma lipids in several ways. Lipoprotein lipase, an enzyme that hydrolyzes triglycerides into constituent fatty acids, is bound to the endothelial cell surface by heparan sulfates.[16] The interaction of this enzyme with chylomicrons or very-low-density lipoprotein (VLDL) particles results in the release of free fatty acids, which can then cross the subendothelial space to the underlying smooth muscle or inflammatory cells in atherosclerosis. In addition, endothelial cells possess receptors for low density lipoprotein (LDL),[17] which regulate the transport and modification of LDL. Normally, LDL receptors are downregulated because receptor processing is inhibited in the nongrowing monolayer.[17] There are, however, two other pathways for uptake of LDL. First, LDL can be transported across the endothelium by an unknown, active, receptor-independent mechanism.[18] Second, modified, or oxidized LDL can be taken up by "scavenger" LDL receptors,[19] the expression of which is unaffected by the growth state of the endothelial cells. These cells also have the capacity to modify LDL,[20] thus enhancing its uptake and ultimately leading to an increase in cholesterol esters in the vessel wall and, importantly, facilitating LDL uptake by inflammatory cells in disease.

The Endothelial Cell and Thrombosis

Quiescent endothelial cells normally present an antithrombotic surface that resists platelet adhesion and does not activate coagulation. (For a more detailed discussion of thrombosis, see Chap. 7.) The continuity of the endothelium is essential to this function, and nonthrombogenicity has been attributed in part to the negative charge on the surface of these cells.[21] Endothelial cells are, however, capable of synthesizing and secreting prothrombotic factors, especially when stimulated with cytokines or other inflammatory agents. The endothelium thus represents a functional antithrombotic-thrombolytic/thrombotic balance (Fig. 2-1). Potent anticoagulants elaborated by the endothelium include prostacyclin, which inhibits platelet aggregation,[22] heparin-like molecules,[23] and thrombomodulin, which activates protein C.[24] In addition, antithrombin III binds to the surface-bound heparin-like molecules and serves as a clearance (via internalization) molecule for thrombin, as well as a thrombin inhibitor.[25] These cells also produce tissue plasminogen activator (TPA) and plasminogen activator inhibitor-I (PAI-I), and can bind plasminogen on their surface via fibronectin and thrombospondin.[26] The relative amounts of tPA and PAI-I can be up- or downregulated, respectively, by thrombin and other vasoactive substances to control clot lysis.

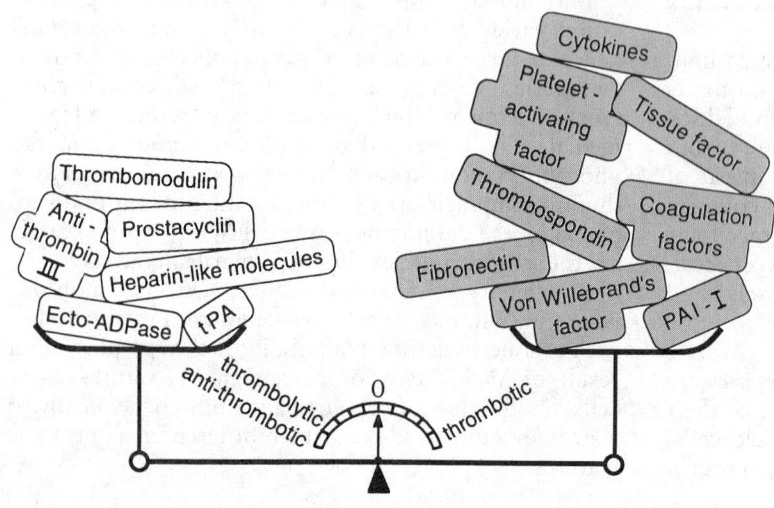

FIGURE 2-1 Hemostatic/thrombotic balance in endothelial cells. Endothelial cells express and secrete both prothrombotic and antithrombotic/thrombolytic molecules. Under normal conditions, endothelial cells present an antithrombotic surface. Upon stimulation with cytokines or other inflammatory agents, they synthesize and secrete prothrombotic factors. The hemostatic status of the endothelium is thus highly dependent upon the balance between these two opposing classes of compounds. Abbreviations: tPA = tissue plasminogen activator; PAI-I = plasminogen activator inhibitor-I. (Courtesy of Bernard Lassègue, Ph.D.)

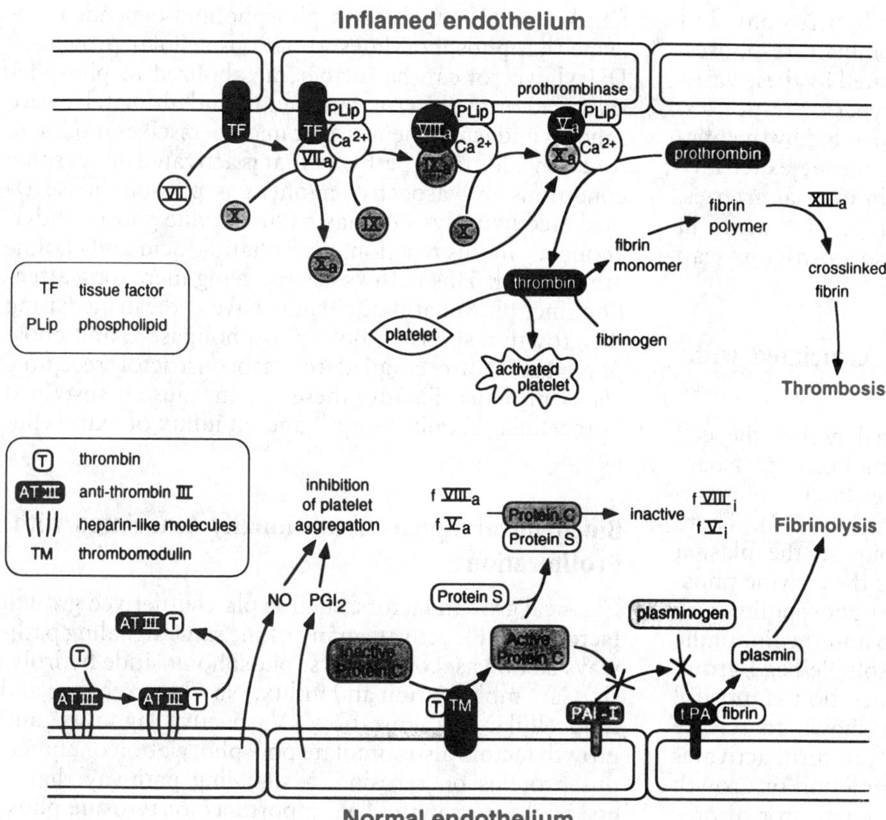

FIGURE 2-2 Pathways of thrombosis and thrombolysis. Under normal conditions, the endothelium is antithrombotic. Antithrombin III (ATIII) binds thrombin and serves to clear thrombin from the circulation. Prostacyclin (PGI_2) inhibits platelet aggregation, and thrombomodulin (TM) activates protein C, which inhibits plasminogen activator inhibitor-I (PAI-I) and interacts with protein S to inactivate activated factors V and VIII, thus limiting thrombosis. Since PAI-I inhibits the tissue plasminogen activator (tPA)-catalyzed conversion of plasminogen to plasmin, PAI-I inhibition leads to accumulation of plasmin and fibrinolysis. Upon stimulation with inflammatory cytokines, there is increased expression of tissue factor on the endothelial cell surface. Tissue factor participates in the activation of Factor X, which, in turn, promotes assembly of the prothrombinase complex, producing thrombin. Under these conditions, endothelial cells thus amplify the thrombotic response. (Courtesy of Bernard Lassègue, Ph.D.)

As alluded to earlier, the endothelium, under conditions of injury or inflammation, may become prothrombotic (Fig. 2-2). On stimulation with inflammatory cytokines, endothelial cells increase the surface expression of tissue factor[27] and leukocyte adhesion molecules,[28] and decrease the expression of thrombomodulin.[27] Thrombin itself stimulates further production of von Willebrand's factor,[29] which, along with thrombospondin and fibronectin, participates in the thrombotic response. Furthermore, endothelial cells can bind factor IX,[30] which, when tissue factor is expressed, can be activated by tissue factor-VIIa complex, leading to activation of factor X in the presence of factor VIII. Activated factor X (Xa) can then promote assembly of the prothrombinase complex. Thus, under inflammatory conditions, endothelial cells can amplify the prothrombotic response. All of the factors controlling the expression of pro- and antithrombotic/fibrinolytic molecules are not known, but it is clear that the endothelium functions as a major regulator of hemostasis.

Barrier Function and Endothelial Cell Permeability

There are three routes by which the endothelium selectively regulates the influx of plasma macromolecules into the arterial wall: intercellular tight junctions, vesicles and/or transendothelial channels, and the lipid phase of the endothelial membrane. These pathways enable the intact endothelium to serve as a barrier, preventing or impeding highly mitogenic, thrombotic, or vasoactive substances from coming into direct contact with the underlying vascular smooth muscle. Each route has both active and passive components, and the extent to which they are utilized depends to a certain degree on the location of the endothelial cells. Thus, capillaries and postcapillary venules respond to vasoactive agents, some of which (histamine, prostaglandins) are secreted by the endothelial cell itself, with increased flux through tight junctions.[31] The tight junctions found in arteries tend to be more occlusive, but may also be influenced by hypertension[32] and various agonists. Vesicular transport is mainly utilized by the cell to transfer water-soluble macromolecules from the luminal surface to the abluminal surface, but the permanence of such structures and whether they form transendothelial channels is a matter of debate. Lipid phase transport has been proposed as a mechanism whereby lipid-soluble molecules (e.g., free fatty acids) could be transferred to the abluminal surface of the endothelial cell.[33] These molecules could enter the outer leaflet of the membrane from the circulation and diffuse along the lipid bilayer to be released or bind to extracellular matrix components in the subintimal area. Thus, the endothelium has both passive and active roles in the control of vascular permeability by acting as a physical permeability barrier and by modulating the expression of cell-surface and secreted agonists and molecules that are capable of altering permeability.

PHYSIOLOGY OF THE VASCULAR SMOOTH MUSCLE CELL

The smooth muscle cell normally responds to hormonal stimulation with contraction or relaxation. However, in certain disease states, growth and/or hypertrophy and migration to the intima are the predominant responses. Some of the biochemical signals generated by these vasoactive agonists are similar for both types of responses, with the final physiological response dictated by the phenotype and environment of the cell, and the exact biochemical pathways activated. Thus, in normal arteries, growth factors can act as vasoconstrictors,[34] while in modulated smooth muscle cells, vasoconstrictors can stimulate hypertrophy or hyperplasia.[35]

Biochemical Signals Traditionally Associated with Contraction

Some of the earliest signals generated within the cell following stimulation with calcium-mobilizing vasoactive agonists involve hydrolysis of a specific class of membrane lipids, the phosphoinositides[36] (Fig. 2-3). There are three major inositol phospholipids in the plasma membrane that serve as substrates for the enzyme phospholipase C. Phospholipase C cleaves phospholipids to liberate the water-soluble head group and the lipophilic molecule, diacylglycerol. The water soluble head group that is most important for signal generation is inositol trisphosphate (IP_3), which has been shown to release Ca^{2+} from intracellular stores.[37] Ca^{2+}, in turn, activates a cascade of enzymes leading to contraction or growth (see below). Diacylglycerol is a potent activator of protein kinase C, a Ca^{2+}- and phospholipid-dependent enzyme that phosphorylates numerous cellular proteins.[38] Diacylglycerol can be further metabolized to phosphatidic acid or to glycerol, fatty acids, and ultimately, eicosanoids and leukotriences that may themselves modulate tone. An additional pathway that is activated under some conditions by vasoactive agonists is phospholipase D-mediated hydrolysis of plasma membrane phosphatidylcholine.[39] In this reaction, phosphatidic acid and choline are released. This pathway is receiving increasing attention since phosphatidic acid may have a role in mediating the growth response.[40] Both phospholipase C and phospholipase D are coupled to vasoconstrictor receptors via G proteins. Finally, these agents cause a sustained intracellular alkalinization[41] and an influx of extracellular Ca^{2+}.[42]

Biochemical Signals Traditionally Associated with Proliferation

Classical growth factors, such as platelet-derived growth factor (PDGF), activate many of the same signaling pathways as do vasoconstrictors: phosphoinositide hydrolysis, Ca^{2+} mobilization and influx, Na^+/H^+ exchange and intracellular alkalinization. Vasoactive agonists and growth factors also stimulate phosphorylation of numerous proteins on tyrosine, a signaling pathway that is essential for growth. The importance of tyrosine phos-

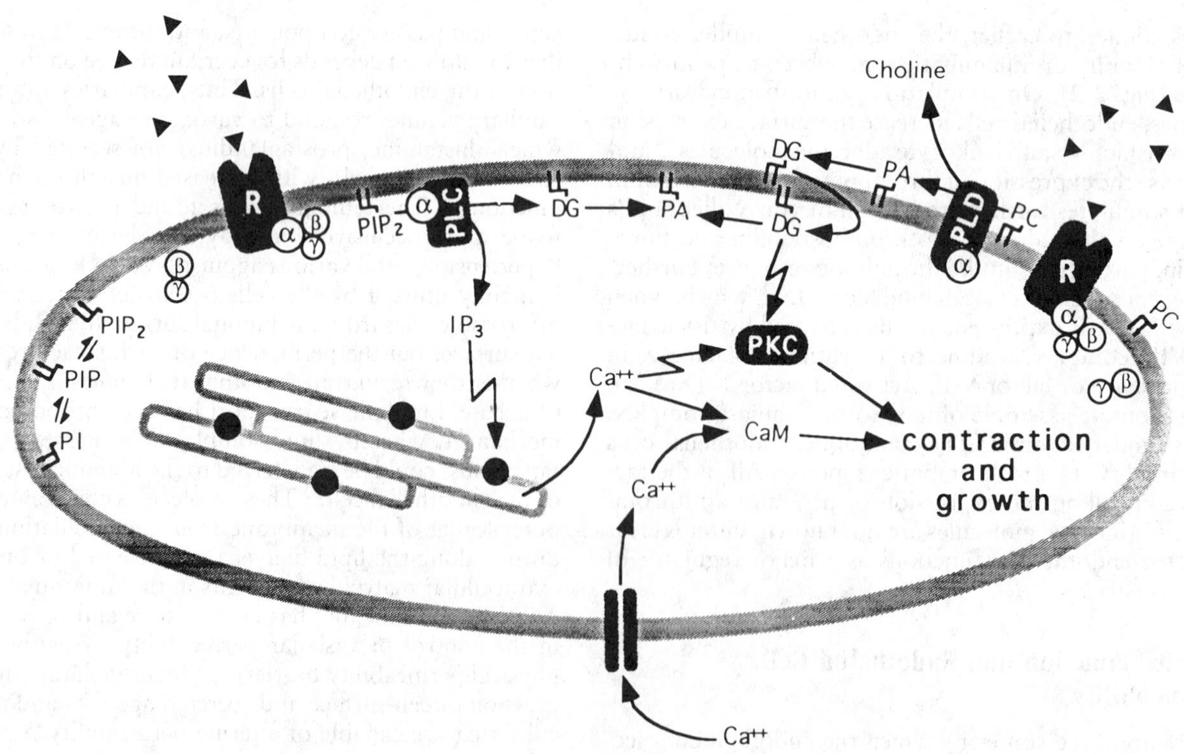

FIGURE 2-3 Signaling pathways in vascular smooth muscle. Vasoconstrictor agonists interact with specific receptors (R) on vascular smooth muscle. These receptors are linked to a G protein, which then couples to phospholipase C (PLC) or phospholipase D (PLD). PLC cleaves the inositol phospholipids to yield diacylglycerol (DG) and inositol phosphates, in particular, inositol trisphosphate (IP_3). IP_3 releases calcium from intracellular stores, activating calmodulin (CaM), while DG activates the Ca^{2+}- and phospholipid-dependent enzyme protein kinase C (PKC). PLD cleaves phosphatidycholine (PC) to release phosphatidic acid (PA) and choline. DG and PA can be interconverted, and in vascular smooth muscle, PLD-mediated PC hydrolysis is probably the main source of DG. The Ca^{2+}- and PKC-induced phosphorylation of various cellular proteins lead ultimately to contraction or growth. Abbreviations not given above: PI = phosphatidylinositol; PIP = phosphatidylinositol 4-phosphate; PIP_2 = phosphatidylinositol 4,5-bisphosphate. (Courtesy of Bernard Lassègue, Ph.D.)

phorylation in mediating the growth response is best shown by the observation that mutant PDGF receptors, which lack the normal, intrinsic tyrosine kinase domain, are incapable of mediating proliferation in response to PDGF.[43] In addition, a tyrosine kinase inhibitor, genestein, has been shown to inhibit growth.[44] There is also increasing evidence that tyrosine phosphatases are able to counteract the mitogenic effects of growth factors by inhibiting tyrosine phosphorylation of specific substrates.[45]

PDGF possibly has been the most extensively studied growth factor in terms of the biochemical signals involved in the tyrosine kinase pathway. A complex of substrates is postulated to become associated with activated growth factor receptor complexes and subsequently to activate a cascade of intracellular events leading to the final cellular response.[46] This complex is proposed to be comprised of phospholipase C-γ, phosphatidylinositol-3-kinase, GTPase-activating protein (GAP), and the protooncogene *c-raf*. Upon addition of PDGF to various cell types, the receptor dimerizes and auto-tyrosine phosphorylates, and each of the above proteins is phosphorylated on tyrosine, presumably leading, either directly or indirectly via association with the activated receptor, to their activation. At present, it is clear that the "signal transfer particle," as the activated receptor and its associated substrates has been called, or its components play a role in transduction of the growth signal, but the exact mechanism by which this occurs is not understood.

Contraction Cascade

Contractions induced by various vasoactive hormones differ not only in magnitude and time course, but also differ between vessels. In general, there is an initial, rapid component of force generation and a more sustained phase of contraction. Some agonists, such as angiotensin II, induce only a transient constriction of many vessels, while others, including norepinephrine and vasopressin, nearly always cause a sustained contraction. The initial phase of force development has been shown to depend on the formation of actin-myosin cross-bridges, but the mechanisms underlying the sustained phase of contraction are less clear.

Phasic contraction of smooth muscle is proposed to be regulated by a sliding-filament mechanism similar to that seen in skeletal muscle. Force generation is accomplished by attachment of the myosin heads (or cross-bridges) to actin filaments. This attachment catalyzes ATP hydrolysis to generate tension, and occurs in a cyclic manner for the duration of the stimulus. Smooth muscle has a relatively greater content of actin and a lower content of myosin than does skeletal muscle, and in contrast to skeletal muscle, the major site of calcium regulation of smooth muscle actomyosin is on the myosin molecule. Smooth muscle myosin consists of two large subunits, each with an M_r of 200 kDa, and two small subunits of 20 and 16 to 17 kDa, known as the myosin light chains. Force generation in smooth muscle is regulated by the phosphorylation/dephosphorylation of the 20-kDa protein (Fig. 2-4). Once phosphorylation occurs, actin-activated Mg^{2+}-ATPase activity is stimulated, resulting in cross-bridge cycling. Myosin light chain phosphorylation is mediated by an enzyme known as myosin light chain kinase (MLCK). This protein associates with calmodulin, a calcium-binding protein required for activation of numerous cytoplasmic enzymes. Thus, when Ca^{2+} increases within the cell in response to hormonal stimulation, Ca^{2+} binds to calmodulin, which, in turn, associates with MLCK, converting it from an inactive to an active form. MLCK then phosphorylates the myosin light chain, permitting actin activation of the Mg^{2+}-ATPase and resulting in cross-bridge formation. When the intracellular Ca^{2+} concentration drops below about 100 nM, Ca^{2+} dissociates from calmodulin, calmodulin detaches from MLCK, and MLCK becomes inactive. Myosin light chain phosphatase activity then predominates, myosin is dephosphorylated, and cross-bridge *cycling* ceases. However, during sustained contraction, the intracellular Ca^{2+} concentration is low, and energy consumption is reduced, suggesting the development of a latch-bridge, or of a low cycling state.[47] Alternatively, the sensitivity of the contractile apparatus to Ca^{2+} may be increased, a response posited to be regulated by protein kinase C.[48]

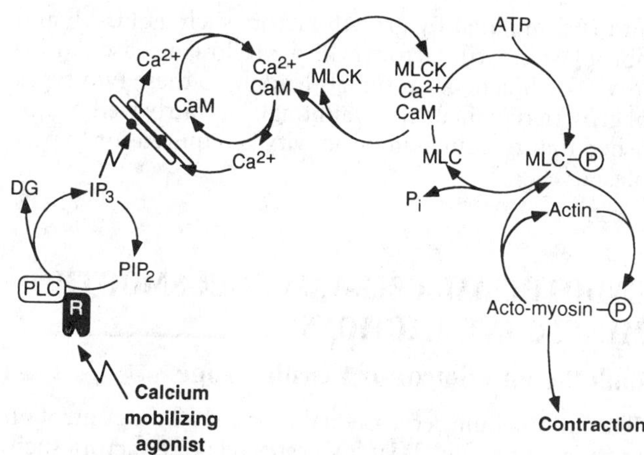

FIGURE 2-4 Contraction cascade. Activation of smooth muscle by a vasoconstrictor hormone leads to a cascade of biochemical signals, ultimately resulting in phosphorylation of actomyosin, cross-bridge formation, and force generation. The release of Ca^{2+} from intracellular stores is one of the major initiating events, since Ca^{2+} combines with calmodulin to activate myosin light chain kinase. This enzyme phosphorylates the myosin light chain, which is then able to interact with actin. Abbreviations: R = receptor; PLC = phospholipase C; DG = diacylglycerol; PIP_2 = phosphatidylinositol 4,5–bisphosphate; IP_3 = inositol trisphosphate; CaM = calmodulin; MLCK = myosin light chain kinase; MLC = myosin light chain; P = phosphate. (Courtesy of Bernard Lassègue, Ph.D.)

Growth

Vascular smooth muscle cell growth takes two forms: hypertrophy and hyperplasia. In general, hypertrophy appears to occur in response to long-term stimulation with vasoconstrictor-type agents, while hyperplasia occurs in response to the classical growth factors. Hypertrophy is characterized by an increase in smooth muscle cell mass due to increased protein synthesis, and has been shown to occur in response to angiotensin II[49] and thrombin,[50] as well as in large vessels during hypertension. Hyperplasia is characterized by cell replication, and is stimulated by growth factors such as PDGF and fibroblast growth factor (FGF)[51,53] following vascular injury. The biochemical signals leading to these two types of growth remain unclear, although it is fairly well-established that tyrosine kinase activity is required for hyperplasia.

ENDOTHELIAL CELL-VASCULAR SMOOTH MUSCLE INTERACTIONS

Endothelial Control of Vascular Tone

The endothelium serves a dual function in the control of vascular tone (Fig. 2-5). It secretes relaxing factors such as nitric oxide and adenosine, and constricting factors such as the endothelins. Vessel tone is thus dependent on the balance between these factors, as well as upon the ability of the smooth muscle cell to respond to them. The most important regulatory molecules are discussed separately.

Endothelium-Derived Relaxing Factor/Nitric Oxide

An endothelium-derived relaxing factor (EDRF) was first described by Furchgott and Zawadzki,[2] who observed that aortic rings dilated in response to acetylcholine only when the rings maintained an intact endothelium. EDRF is released from endothelial cells. The predominant form of EDRF, derived from L-arginine by the action of the enzyme nitric oxide synthase, is nitric oxide (NO), or a closely related nitroso compound.[53] This conclusion is based on the observation that both EDRF and NO activate guanylate cyclase, are inhibited by oxygen free radicals, methylene blue, and heme-containing proteins, and have a mechanism of action that is independent of prostaglandins generated by the cyclooxygenase pathway.[54] Like EDRF, NO is highly unstable and is rapidly oxidized to form nitrite and nitrate. NO easily crosses the smooth muscle cell membrane and binds to the heme moiety of the soluble guanylate cyclase, thereby enhancing the formation of cyclic GMP. Cyclic GMP, in turn, reduces intracellular Ca^{2+} concentrations leading to dephosphorylation of the myosin light chain and relaxation.[55] It should be noted that the drug nitroglycerin exerts its vasodilator effects by being converted to NO. Nitroglycerin thus is substituting for a natural product. Deficiency in release of active NO is an important contributing factor leading to vasospasm (see Chap. 56).

Many factors have been shown to regulate the release of EDRF/NO[56] by increasing intracellular Ca^{2+}. These include hormones such as acetylcholine, norepinephrine, bradykinin, thrombin, ATP, and vasopressin; the platelet-derived factors, serotonin and histamine; fatty acids; ionophores; and physical forces.

Prostacyclin

Prostacyclin, or PGI_2, is a prostanoid derived from the action of cyclooxygenase on arachidonic acid. It is released by the endothelium and relaxes vascular smooth muscle by increasing its intracellular content of cyclic AMP.[57] Prostacyclin is also platelet-suppressant and antithrombotic, and reduces the release of growth factors from endothelial cells and macrophages.[22] Among the agonists that stimulate prostacyclin synthesis are bradykinin (one of the most potent), substance P, PDGF and EGF, and adenine nucleotides,[22] while aspirin has been shown to inhibit it transiently. Therapeutically, the debate about the appropriate dose of aspirin in ischemic coronary syndrome revolves around finding a dose that will inhibit platelet function without inhibiting endothelial PGI_2 synthesis.

Adenosine and Related Compounds

Both adenine nucleosides (adenosine) and nucleotides (ADP, ATP) are released by the endothelium in response to such stimuli as thrombin[58] and flow.[59] Adenine nucleosides bind to P1 purinergic receptors that activate cyclic AMP leading to relaxation, while adenine nucleotides stimulate P2 receptors that are coupled to phosphoinosi-

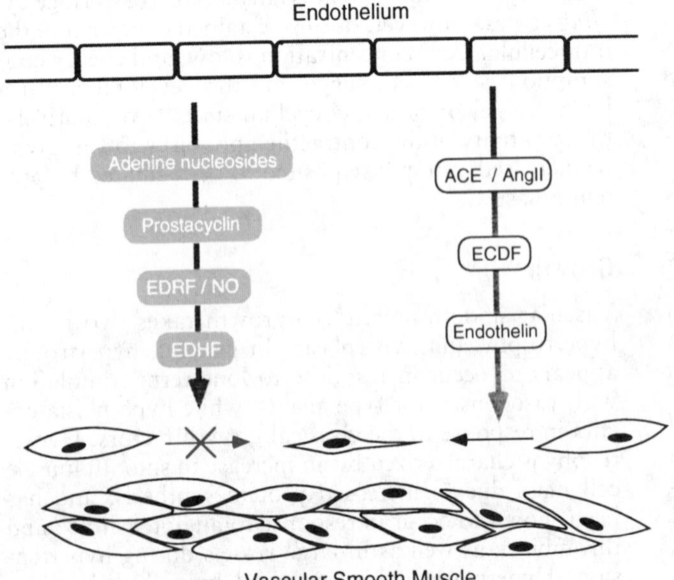

FIGURE 2-5 Endothelial control of vascular tone. Endothelial cells synthesize and secrete both vasodilator substances (colored boxes) and vasoconstrictor compounds (white boxes). Vessel tone is dependent on the balance between these factors, as well as on the ability of the smooth muscle cells to respond to them. Abbreviations: EDRF = endothelial-derived relaxing factor; NO = nitric oxide; EDHF = endothelial-derived hyperpolarizing factor; ACE = angiotensin-converting enzyme; AngII = angiotensin II; EDCF = endothelium-derived contracting factor. (Courtesy of Bernard Lassègue, Ph.D.)

tide hydrolysis. Stimulation of P2 receptors in endothelial cells results in an increase in intracellular Ca^{2+} and release of EDRF/prostacyclin,[60] while P2 receptors on vascular smooth muscle mediate contraction.[61] Thus, depending on the relative amounts of adenosine, ATP, and ADP in the vessel wall, and the presence of a functional endothelium, these compounds can have a net dilatory or constrictor effect on vascular smooth muscle. Additionally, the endothelium possesses an extracellular ectonucleotidase enzymatic system that mediates the conversion of ATP or ADP to adenosine, thereby regulating the local levels of these compounds.[14] These systems are important in determining the vascular response to ADP released from platelets at the site of thrombus formation.

Endothelin

The endothelins are a family of closely related peptides made and secreted by endothelial cells in some, but not all, vascular beds. They are among the most potent vasoconstrictors ever identified. The slow, sustained contraction induced by these compounds in smooth muscle appears to be the result of activation of the phosphoinositide/protein kinase C signaling pathway, as well as of opening voltage-dependent L-type calcium channels.[62] Endothelial cells themselves also have receptors for endothelin,[63] but their physiological role is unknown.

Angiotensin Converting Enzyme

Endothelial cells have been shown to synthesize and express at their surface angiotensin-converting enzyme (ACE),[64] the protein that converts angiotensin I to the potent vasoconstrictor angiotensin II and that degrades and inactivates bradykinin. ACE associated with the endothelial cell membrane serves to modify both locally produced or circulating angiotensin I and bradykinin, and hence contributes importantly to the regulation of vasomotor tone.

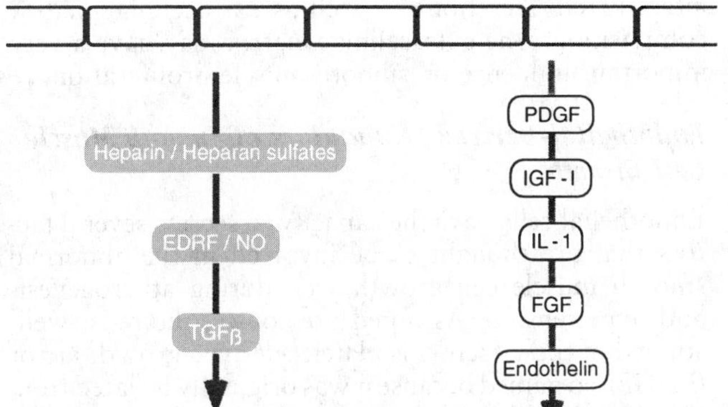

Endothelial Control of Vascular Growth

As with vascular tone, the endothelium also exerts a dual effect on vascular growth (Fig. 2-6). Both growth-promoting and growth-inhibitory factors are made and secreted by endothelial cells, making them pivotal in the control of smooth muscle responsiveness. Endothelial cells are involved in two types of vascular growth: angiogenesis and abnormal growth of smooth muscle during disease.

Angiogenesis

Angiogenesis in vivo occurs during normal wound healing and during the vascularization of solid tumors. It is a complex process involving degradation of the basement membrane, the migration and proliferation of endothelial cells, and tube formation. Several factors have been shown to stimulate angiogenesis, including fibroblast growth factor (FGF), vascular permeability factor (VPF), transforming growth factor-α (TGF-α), angiogenin, transforming growth factor-β (TGF-β), tumor necrosis factor-α (TNF-α)[65], and insulin-like growth factor I (IGF-I).[66] Their properties are summarized in Table 2-1. Some of these factors stimulate angiogenesis by inducing endothelial cell migration and proliferation (FGF, VPF); others appear to do so by stimulating endothelial cell differentiation (TGF-β, TNF-α) or by activating a secondary cell type to produce angiogenic factors (angiogenin, TGF-β, TNF-α). Angiogenesis may be negatively regulated by both naturally occurring and synthetic compounds. It can be inhibited by the combination of heparin and cortisone,[67] thrombospondin, platelet factor IV, and γ-interferon. Many of these agents bind to heparin, suggesting that they exert their growth-inhibitory effects by blocking the action of heparin-binding growth factors, such as FGF. It is likely that the control of angiogenesis rests on the maintenance of a balance between the stimulatory and inhibitory factors, the regulation of which is not yet fully understood.

FIGURE 2-6 Endothelial control of vascular growth. As with vasoactive substances, endothelial cells make and secrete both growth-promoting (white boxes) and growth-inhibitory (colored boxes) compounds. Under normal conditions, the net effect of the endothelium is growth-inhibitory. Abbreviations: EDRF = endothelial-derived relaxing factor; NO = nitric oxide; TGF = β-transforming growth factor-β; PDGF = platelet-derived growth factor; IGF-I = insulin-like growth factor I; IL-1 = interleukin 1; FGF = fibroblast growth factor. (Courtesy of Bernard Lassègue, Ph.D.)

TABLE 2-1
Angiogenic Stimulators and Inhibitors

	Angiogenesis	Origin	Release	Endothelial Cell Proliferation	Endothelial Cell Chemotaxis	Tubule Formation
FGF	+	Endothelial cells	Cell lysis	+ +	+ (EC)	+
VPF	+	Follicular cells, (neuroblastoma glioma)	Secreted	+ +		
TGF-α	+	Transformed fibroblasts, macrophages (adenocarcinoma cells)	Secreted	+ +		
Angiogenin	+	Lymphocytes, Liver	Secreted	0	−	
TGF-β	+	Endothelial cells	Secreted	—	− (EC) + (monocytes)	+
TNF-α	+	Activated macrophage tumor cells	Secreted	—	+	+
Angiostatic Steroids	−	Synthetic	—	—		
Thrombospondin	−	Platelets	Secreted	—		
Platelet Factor IV	−	Platelets	Secreted	—		
γ-interferon	−	Activated T-cells, macrophages	Secreted	−		

Endothelial-Derived Inhibitors of Smooth Muscle Cell Growth

Normally, smooth muscle cells are relatively refractory to growth stimuli, and are maintained in a quiescent, differentiated state. It has been proposed, based on at least two lines of evidence, that the endothelium is important in maintaining this smooth muscle phenotype. First, removal of the endothelium experimentally allows initiation of the mitogenic response, and second, regrowth of *normal* endothelium inhibits further proliferation.[68] One mechanism by which such a tonic inhibitory influence on smooth muscle cell growth could be effected is the secretion by endothelial cells of specific inhibitors of cell proliferation. Alternatively, the endothelium could be an effective barrier limiting access of blood-borne growth factors to vascular smooth muscle. Attention so far has focused on heparin and other glycosaminoglycans (including heparan sulfate) as possible candidates for endothelial-derived growth inhibitory factors. Heparin inhibits VSMC mitogenesis and migration in vivo and in vitro, and is able to reduce neointimal proliferation if administered during the first 3 days after vascular injury.[69] However, the inhibition is not complete, and it seems likely that other endothelial cell factors may be involved. Another possibility is EDRF (NO), which is usually associated with vascular relaxation. NO is released tonically from the endothelium of large arteries, which have a relatively minor role in the control of vascular tone, suggesting that it may have an additional function in these vessels. Studies on cultured VSMC have shown that pharmacologic agents such as sodium nitroprusside and 8-bromo-cyclic GMP, which mimic the effect of NO on vascular smooth muscle G kinase, can inhibit mitogenesis.[70] This raises the possibility that NO may have an important role in maintaining the normal artery in a state refractory to mitogens. Finally, endothelial cells have been shown to make and secrete TGF-β,[11] which is subsequently activated by smooth muscle cells. This growth factor inhibits smooth muscle growth directly,[71] and also alters PDGF secretion[72] as well as extracellular matrix composition. The extracellular matrix may have a very important influence on smooth muscle proliferation.

Endothelial-Derived Stimulators of Smooth Muscle Cell Growth

Endothelial cells have the capacity to secrete several factors that are thought to be involved in the abnormal smooth muscle cell growth seen during atherogenesis and hypertension. As noted previously, the most well-studied of these factors is platelet-derived growth factor (PDGF), so named because it was originally isolated from platelets. PDGF is a dimer composed of two distinct peptide chains (designated A and B chains), and can be produced as an AB heterodimer, or an AA or BB homodimer. Endothelial cells contain the mRNA for both peptides,[72] although the precise form in which PDGF is secreted is unclear. Release of PDGF from the endothelium is regulated by second messengers such as cAMP and activators of protein kinase C; other growth factors including TGF-β, FGF, and TNF; circulating factors; and locally produced factors such as thrombin.[72] A second growth factor made and secreted by endothelial cells is insulin-like growth factor I (IGF-I).[12] IGF-I is a progression factor that facilitates movement of cells through the cell cycle but, by itself, is not a particularly strong mitogen. In vitro, it enhances the mitogenic effect of PDGF on smooth muscle.[73] IGF-I production by endothelium has been shown to be regulated by PDGF and hydrostatic pressure, but its role in the control of vascular growth remains unclear.

Other factors made by the endothelium that are able to alter smooth muscle proliferation include interleukin-1 (IL-1), FGF, and endothelin. IL-1 is an inflammatory cytokine that has numerous vascular effects in addition to mitogenesis, including the stimulation of procoagulant activity,[74] induction of leukocyte adhesiveness (see below), and inhibition of contraction.[75] IL-1 regulates its own expression,[76] and, in addition, its production is regulation by TNF-α,[65] lipopolysaccharide, and γ-interferon.[76] As noted above, basic FGF has been detected in endothelial cells,[16] and has been shown to be a potent smooth muscle mitogen, particularly after denuding injury.[52] FGF does not contain the signal peptide that usually provides a mechanism for transporting proteins out of cells, and thus is thought not to be secreted by endothelial cells. It is, however, present and stored in the subendothelial matrix, and may be released on cell lysis or death.[77] FGF released from vascular smooth muscle cells may be particularly important in the growth response induced by injury to the arterial wall after balloon angioplasty. FGF bound to the matrix can be released by heparin and proteinases,[78] suggesting that the matrix may serve as a store for rapidly mobilizing this growth factor. Finally, the vasoconstrictor endothelin has also been shown under certain circumstances to act as a smooth muscle mitogen,[79] possibly by increasing PDGF-A chain secretion in the smooth muscle cells themselves.

Potential Signaling Mechanisms

The response of vascular smooth muscle cells to these growth factors depends on the balance of the hormonal and environmental influences to which the cells are subjected. For example, intact arteries are relatively unresponsive to FGF, only showing a proliferative response when the endothelium has been damaged or removed.[52] This raises the possibility that the cellular mechanism of action of factors secreted by the endothelial cells is to induce a protein or factor in smooth muscle cells that makes them refractory to mitogenic stimulation. One candidate for such a protein is a tyrosine phosphatase. As noted above, most growth factors activate a cascade of tyrosine kinases as an initial step in the mitogenic stimulus. The level of tyrosine in cellular proteins is also controlled by tyrosine phosphatases, enzymes that remove phosphates from tyrosine residues. Thus, in cells with very active tyrosine phosphatases, tyrosine kinases may be unable to induce a sustained phosphorylation of proteins on tyrosine, theoretically inhibiting the growth response. Evidence for such a mechanism of growth control is only now becoming available with the recent isolation and cloning of membrane-spanning and cytosolic tyrosine phosphatases.[80] It has been shown that somatostatins act as growth inhibitors in neoplastic cells through activation of a tyrosine phosphatase.[81] Furthermore, angiopeptin, a somatostatin analog, has been shown to inhibit neointimal proliferation after balloon injury,[82] suggesting that activators of tyrosine phosphatases may be important in growth control. Recently, TGF-β, one of the major growth inhibitors produced by endothelial cells, has been proposed to stimulate tyrosine phosphatase activity.[83] These observations raise the possibility that one of the mechanisms by which endothelial cells help to maintain smooth muscle quiescence is by the induction of tyrosine phosphatase activity in the smooth muscle cells.

ENDOTHELIAL CELL-LEUKOCYTE INTERACTIONS

Endothelial cells have recently been shown to participate actively in the development of inflammatory reactions. They are central to the recruitment of leukocytes to sites of inflammation by secreting chemotactic molecules and expressing adhesion molecules that interact with surface proteins on leukocytes.

Inflammatory cytokines increase synthesis of vasodilators by the endothelium, which causes increased blood flow to the injured area. Histamine, which is released at the site of vascular inflammation, also contracts endothelial cells in certain areas, thus increasing permeability.[84] Cytokines also stimulate endothelial secretion of leukocyte chemoattractant proteins (interleukin-8) and monocyte chemotactic protein (MCP-1), and expression of adhesion molecules such as intercellular adhesion molecules-1 and -2 (ICAM-1 and ICAM-2), endothelial-leukocyte adhesion molecule-1 (ELAM-1), vascular cell adhesion molecule-1 (VCAM-1), and GMP-140, which are important regulators of leukocyte accumulation on the vascular surface.[85] ELAM-1 and GMP-140 bind resting, but not activated, neutrophils; VCAM-1 binds to the VLA-4 antigen on monocytes and T-lymphocytes; and ICAM-1 and -2 bind to the LFA-1 integrin receptor on B-lymphocytes.[85] The expression of these molecules appears to be differentially regulated by cytokines, thrombin, and histamine,[85] so that their surface expression determines the type of leukocytes attached to the endothelial monolayer. It has been suggested that the sequential accumulation of different leukocyte classes at sites of inflammation can be explained by the differential induction of these endothelial cell adhesion molecules.[86] Leukocyte adhesion molecules and chemoattractant proteins are also likely to be important in atherogenesis (see below).

ENDOTHELIAL RESPONSES TO HEMODYNAMIC INFLUENCES

In addition to being influenced by the integration of circulating blood cells, vascular smooth muscle cells, and matrix, the endothelium responds to the physical forces of pressure, stretch, and shear stress imposed by the hemodynamics of the circulation. Flow-mediated, endothelium-dependent vasodilation has been described in many vascular beds,[87] and shear stress has been proposed to play a role in controlling endothelial cell proliferation.[88] Elevated pressure, stretch of the vessel wall, and shear stress have all been shown independently to affect endothelial cell morphology and/or function. Pressure alone appears to increase the production of IGF-I by endothelial cells in vitro, and to have a role in the generalized hypertrophy of the vessel wall that occurs during hypertension. Studies in cultured cells have shown that stretching endothelial cells leads to changes in cell shape, intracellular signal generation with an increase in calcium concentration, and proliferation.[88] Shear stress has numerous effects on endothelial cells. Initially, it was found that exposure of endothelial cell monolayers to elevated shear stresses in vitro caused them to align in the direction of flow. This reorientation was accompanied by changes in the cytoskeleton of the cells, including reorganization and alignment of the actin filaments and microtubules. Similar mechanisms presumably also account for the orientation of endothelial cells parallel to the longitudinal axis in areas of laminar flow in the arterial system. The function of endothelial cells is also altered by shear stress: a K^+ current is activated; secretion of vasoactive factors, including NO, endothelin, and prostacyclin[70] is increased; PDGF receptor expression is increased; uptake of LDL is elevated; and tissue plasminogen activator secretion is increased.[88]

The importance of these observations lies in the variation in hemodynamic forces throughout the circulation. High pressure, such as that which occurs in hypertension, causes changes in the morphology and function of the vessel wall.[89] In addition, the areas of the vasculature exposed to low shear stress (branch points and curvatures) exhibit a predilection to the formation of atherosclerotic lesions.[90] It is thus clear that the hemodynamic environment of the endothelium and underlying smooth muscle is a potentially powerful regulator of vascular function.

The mechanism(s) by which the endothelial cell can sense and transduce mechanical signals is unknown. Possibilities include a surface mechanoreceptor, a flow-sensitive ion channel, changes in cytoskeletal stress due to deformation, and flow-dependent gradients of bioactive substances along the surface of the cell.

ENDOTHELIAL DYSFUNCTION AND VASCULAR SMOOTH MUSCLE ABNORMALITY

In general, the normal endothelium is in an inhibitory mode—inhibiting contraction, thrombosis, white cell adhesion, and vascular smooth muscle growth (Figs. 2-1, 2-5, and 2-6.). Endothelial dysfunction is one of the important concepts that has developed in vascular biology over the last decade. Implicit in the term is the recognition that the fundamental or normal functions of the endothelium are not fixed, but are regulatable. Thus, the endothelium in a given area may lose its vasodilator prominence, become prothrombotic or less thrombolytic, begin to support leukocyte adherence (which may be a normal response in the inflammatory process), or stimulate rather than inhibit smooth muscle migration and proliferation. It is likely that endothelial dysfunction accounts ultimately for a large portion of all cardiovascular disease.

Atherosclerosis

Atherosclerosis is the prototypic disease characterized by endothelial dysfunction. Many of its cardinal features are directly explainable in this context. Thus, mononuclear and lymphocytic infiltration, hypercontractility, LDL modification and smooth muscle cell growth, and intimal migration are likely related to abnormalities of the endothelium induced by hyperlipidemia, hypertension, smoking, and unknown hereditary factors. The pathogenesis of atherosclerosis viewed as a disease of endothelial dysfunction is depicted in Fig. 2-7. (For a more detailed discussion, see Chap. 54.)

Clinically, endothelial dysfunction in atherosclerosis has primarily been defined by impairment of endothelial-dependent relaxation.[91] This defect, which likely accounts for the vasospastic tendency of diseased arteries, appears to be attributable to defective generation or delivery of active EDRF/NO.[92] Impairment of coronary endothelial-dependent vasodilator function occurs in patients with risk factors such as hypercholesterolemia prior to angiographically demonstrable coronary disease.[93] In hypercholesterolemic animals, Minor et al.[92] have found marked decreases in EDRF activity accompanied by increases in the release of NO metabolites. This apparent paradox is likely explained by the fact that the enhanced NO produced by the hypercholesterolemic endothelium is rapidly degraded to inactive metabolites of NO. Since the vasodilator defect in these animals could be corrected both in vivo and in vitro by administration of polyethylene glycol-linked superoxide dismutase (PEG-SOD),[94] an enzyme that inactivates intracellular superoxide radicals, it is probable that excessive oxygen free radicals produced by the endothelium as a consequence of the oxidative metabolic stress induced by hypercholesterolemia degrade NO and, thus, account for the decreased vasodilator activity.

A second manifestation of a dysfunctional endothelium that is apparent very early after initiation of cholesterol feeding in animals is the recruitment of monocytes and macrophages into the vessel wall.[95] This recruitment is likely the result of induction of VCAM-1 expression[96] as well as of secretion of MCP-1.[97] The molecular linkage between hyperlipidemia and MCP-1/adhesion molecule expression is unknown, but may reflect in part the metabolic (oxidative) stress imposed by this change in milieu. Inflammatory cytokines are also important mediators of adhesion molecule expression, and their production by the endothelium and inflammatory cells in the vessel wall may also contribute to adhesion molecule expression in both the early and late stages of the disease.

The intimal proliferation observed in atherosclerotic lesion formation results from migration and hyperplasia

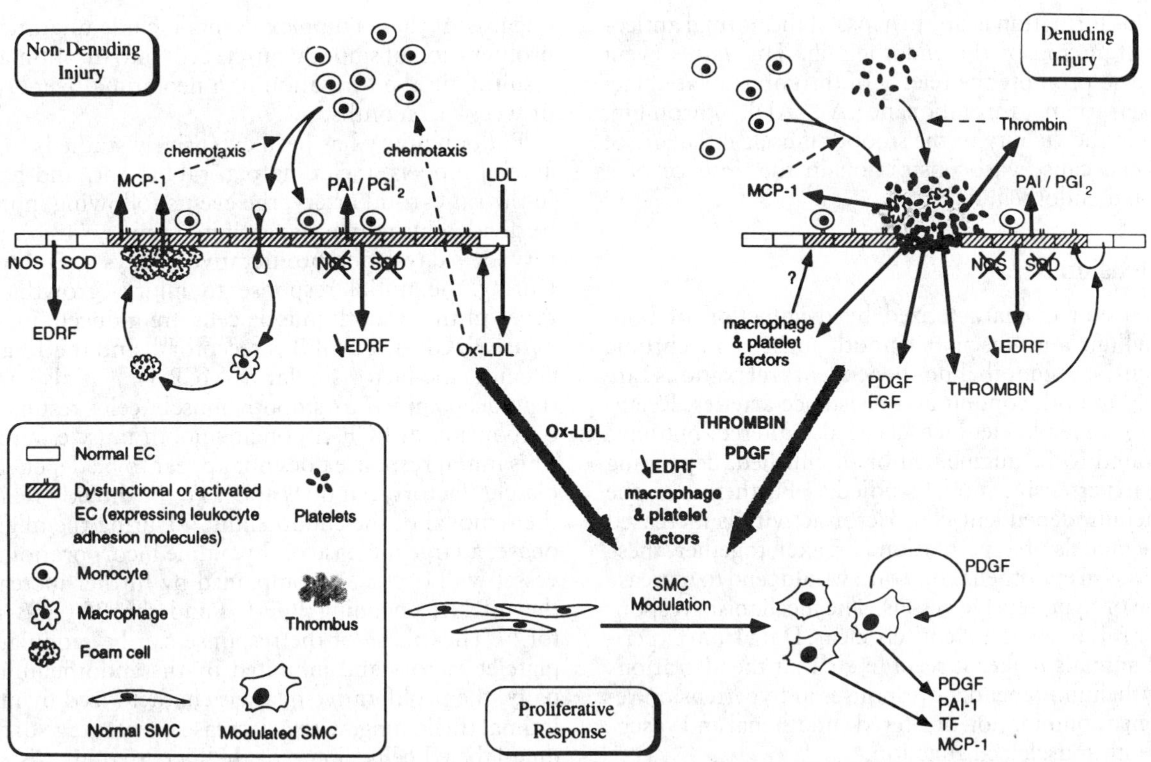

FIGURE 2-7 Theoretical initiating events in vascular lesion formation: *Nondenuding injury:* LDL enters the subendothelial space where it is converted to oxidized LDL (ox-LDL), which induces monocyte chemoattraction and endothelial dysfunction. Dysfunctional endothelial cells (EC) express cell adhesion molecules (ICAM, ELAM, and VCAM) leading to increased monocyte adhesion and movement into the vessel wall. Monocytes in the vessel wall differentiate into macrophages, take up lipids, and remain locally as foam cells, subsequently evolving into fatty streaks. The foam cells in the fatty streak and the overlying endothelium express monocyte chemotactic protein-1 (MCP-1), resulting in further enhanced monocyte chemoattraction and adhesion. Dysfunctional EC may synthesize less nitric oxide synthase (NOS) or superoxide dismutase (SOD, an enzyme that metabolizes oxygen radicals that have been shown to inactivate NO). This decreases endothelial-derived relaxing factor (EDRF) release/activity. The loss of EDRF together with the direct effects of ox-LDL, or growth factors secreted by the foam cells or endothelium, act on the quiescent contractile smooth muscle cells in the vessel wall, giving rise to the proliferative phenotype, with division and migration into the endothelium. *Denuding injury:* Loss of endothelium leads to platelet deposition, tissue factor-mediated activation of extrinsic coagulation to generate thrombin, cleavage of fibrinogen to fibrin, and the formation of thrombus. Thrombin gives rise to endothelial expression of adhesion molecules and consequent monocyte attachment, together with secretion of platelet granular constituents. Monocytes enter the thrombus and differentiate into phagocytic macrophages expressing tissue factor and MCP-1. This leads to further monocyte chemoattraction into the vessel wall. Smooth muscle cell proliferation is produced by (a) thrombin generation at the site of denuding injury; (b) platelet-derived growth factor (PDGF) or other growth factors released from platelets in the thrombus; (c) factors secreted by the macrophages ingesting the thrombus; and (d) the loss of EDRF activity caused by endothelial dysfunction. *Proliferative response:* Modulated smooth muscle cells (SMCs) proliferate and synthesize factors that promote plaque development. SMCs synthesize: (a) PDGF and other growth factors that cause self-perpetuating autocrine or paracrine stimulation of SMC proliferation; (b) tissue factor (TF) and plasminogen activator inhibitor-1 (PAI-1) that act locally to produce thrombin or inhibit fibrinolysis of the fibrin network used to facilitate cell migration; and (c) MCP-1 which increases monocyte chemoattraction into the lesion thereby leading to lesion development. (We thank Drs. Laurence Harker, Josiah Wilcox, and Bernard Lassègue for their creative and intellectual development of this figure.)

of vascular smooth muscle cells.[98] Proliferation has been attributed to growth factors such as PDGF, FGF, and IGF-I. Since these growth factors can be produced by the endothelium in vitro, it is very likely that the dysfunctional endothelium in atherosclerosis also produces growth factors while shifting from a growth-inhibitory to a growth-promoting mode. Furthermore, there is evidence that products of oxidative metabolism may also release growth factors.

The recent rapid advance in our understanding of vessel wall cell biology provides insight into the biologic mechanisms responsible for the pathogenesis of atherosclerosis. There is now a basis for developing a unifying concept of the disease that revolves around endothelial dysfunction mediated by changes in oxidative metabolism. Oxidative modification of LDL thus assumes a central role in atherogenesis (Fig. 2-7). The role of oxidized LDL is discussed more completely in Chap. 54, and the relationship of the cell biology of atherosclerosis to coronary ischemic syndrome is discussed in Chap. 56.

Vasospasm

When the endothelium becomes dysfunctional as in atherosclerosis, the underlying smooth muscle cells often become hyperreactive to certain vasoconstrictor stimuli, including serotonin and ergonovine.[99] Coronary spasm leading to myocardial infarction is one of the most clinically relevant problems arising from this phenomenon. Proposed mechanisms to account for this vasoconstrictor abnormality that can result in total occlusion include supersensitivity of the smooth muscle cells themselves to constrictor stimuli and loss of endothelial-dependent relaxing mechanisms. The increased tendency towards thrombus formation is due to a loss of the normal anticoagulant function of the endothelium. This latter event would also promote the release of thrombus-related factors (serotonin, thromboxane A_2, ADP, thrombin, PDGF) in the vicinity of the smooth muscle cells, any of which can cause vasoconstriction in the absence of a functional endothelium.[100]

Hypertension

Hypertension is characterized by dysfunction of both endothelium and vascular smooth muscle. In chronic hypertension, endothelium-dependent relaxations are impaired in both conduit and resistance arteries. Relaxations to some platelet factors are also altered, but have been found to be augmented or diminished, depending on the hypertensive model studied.[101] Furthermore, the endothelium-dependent constrictor activity is increased in some models of hypertension.[101] Taken together, these alterations in endothelial function would tend to increase the tone of hypertensive vessels. The mechanism responsible for this effect is not entirely clear. Data from experimental animals makes it seem likely that the alterations in endothelium-dependent responses in hypertension result from a combination of altered endothelial and vascular smooth muscle cell function.

Hypertension is also characterized by an increase in vessel wall mass. In the aortas of spontaneously hypertensive and Goldblatt hypertensive rats, this increase can be attributed to an increase in the size of the existing smooth muscle cells.[102,103] This hypertrophy is accompanied by an increase in ploidy; that is, an increased DNA content per cell.[102,103] In contrast, resistance vessels from these same animals appear to increase their mass by hyperplasia of the smooth muscle cells.[104] The stimuli responsible for these changes in the hypertensive vascular wall are unknown. Vascular remodelling appears to have two stages: (1) an initial, reversible intense vasoconstriction mediated by neural or endogenous signals, followed by (2) a remodeling of the vessel wall characterized by increased smooth muscle mass and narrowing of the vessel lumen. There is some evidence that this response is dependent on the presence of the endothelium.[89]

Restenosis

Restenosis is the development of a neointima that occurs following angioplasty, often leading to reocclusion of the initial lesion. The response of the arterial wall to the injury induced by angioplasty (removal of the endothelium and stretching of the vessel wall) involves several distinct events (Fig. 2-7). Removal of the endothelium not only alters the paracrine hormonal environment in which vascular smooth muscle cells exist, but it also exposes a thrombogenic surface to which platelets and other circulating factors can adhere, resulting in the formation of a thrombus. In addition, injury to the underlying smooth muscle may release factors such as FGF, which have mitogenic effects on the remaining smooth muscle cells. Finally, infiltration and subsequent activation of macrophages into the denuded vessel wall brings an additional set of hormonal influences to bear on the vascular smooth muscle. The pathophysiological consequences of these complex events include migration and proliferation of smooth muscle cells into the intimal area, resulting in the formation of a neointima over a period of weeks to months.

Balloon injury has been extensively studied in several animal models, including pig, rabbit, rat, and baboon. In the rat carotid artery, the events following injury can be divided into three stages: initial (injury–48 h), migratory (3–7 days), and proliferative (7 days to 3–4 weeks). During the initial response to injury, growth-related genes in the smooth muscle cells are induced, including c-*fos*, PDGF-A, PDGFB-β receptor[105] and the JE gene (a chemotactic factor similar to MCP-1).[106] It also appears that deep injury to smooth muscle cells results in an outpouring of FGF, a potent smooth muscle mitogen.[77] This initial response does not appear to be dependent on platelet factors, but does appear to be directly related to the removal of the endothelium.[68] During the migratory phase, a large increase of thymidine incorporation in the vessel wall occurs, accompanied by further increases in the mRNA encoding IGF-I[107] and the PDGF-β receptor.[105] This phase of the response can be modulated by platelet factors and inhibited by the endothelium.[68] Finally, the proliferative phase is characterized by marked intimal thickening, with a decreased percentage of thymidine-labeled cells. Some of the increased area is due to deposition of extracellular matrix, and the majority of the proliferative activity occurs at the luminal surface of the vessel. This proliferative phase seems ultimately to be inhibited by regrowth of normal functioning endothelium.

Thus, during the process of restenosis after angioplasty, both the loss of endothelium and the transformation of smooth muscle cells appear to contribute to neointimal formation. At least two lines of evidence implicate the endothelium as having a crucial role in the response of the vessel wall to injury. First, removal of the endothelium allows initiation of the mitogenic response, and second, regrowth of *normal* endothelium inhibits further proliferation. Furthermore, gentle denudation with a nylon loop, accompanied by rapid regeneration of endothelium, results in significantly less neointimal proliferation.[108] In addition, proliferating smooth muscle cells have characteristics distinct from the differentiated smooth muscle cells in the medial layer. Their cytoskeleton is similar to that found in cultured cells. It seems likely, therefore, that two of the most important causes of restenosis are the loss of endothelium-derived growth inhibitory factors, and the transformation of smooth muscle cells into a phenotype able to respond to platelet- and endothelial-derived factors with proliferation.

Gene Transfer

One of the most interesting and potentially promising new approaches to development of treatments for restenosis and abnormal vascular growth in atherosclerosis is gene therapy. Gene therapy can be defined as the introduction of genetically engineered genes into the somatic cells of patients to correct inherited or acquired disorders through the induction of in vivo synthesis of the missing or defective gene product. Gene therapy applied to cardiovascular pathology is still in its experimental stage, but several approaches have been successfully used in animal models of vascular disease. In some instances autologous endothelial or smooth muscle cells have been removed and cultured, transfected in vitro, and reintroduced into a denuded artery by means of a double balloon catheter.[109] A second method that has been tested involves direct genetic modification of vascular cells in vivo using a retroviral vector[110] or DNA liposomes.[111] Successful transfer of adenosine deaminase,[109] tPA,[112] β-galactosidase,[112] luciferase,[113] and class I MHC[111] has been accomplished in model systems, and has been used to study mechanism of proliferation[111] and to improve stent function by local delivery of thrombolytic molecules.[112] Gene transfer thus holds promise as a potential treatment for diverse vascular diseases.

REFERENCES

1. Moncada S, Vane JR: Arachidonic acid metabolites and the interaction between platelets and blood vessel walls. *N Engl J Med* 1979;300:1142–1147.
2. Furchgott RF, Zawadzki JV: The obligatory role of endothelial cells in the relaxation of arterial smooth muscle by acetylcholine. *Nature* 1980;288:373–376.
3. Taylor SG, Weston AH: Endothelium-derived hyperpolarizing factor: A new endogenous inhibitor from the vascular endothelium. *Trends Pharmacol Sci* 1988;9:272–274.
4. Yanagisawa Y, Kurihara H, Kimura S, Tomobe Y, Kobayashi M, Mitsui Y, et al: A novel potent vasoconstrictor peptide produced by vascular endothelial cells. *Nature* 1988;332:411–415.
5. Jaffe EA, Hoyer LW, Nachman RL: Synthesis of von Willebrand factor by cultured human endothelial cells. *Proc Nat Acad Sci USA* 1974;71:1906–1909.
6. Loskutoff DJ, Edgington TS: Synthesis of a fibrinolytic activator and inhibitor by endothelial cells. *Proc Nat Acad Sci USA* 1977;74:3903–3907.
7. Stenmark KR, Orton EC, Reeves JT, Voelkel NF, Crouch EC, Parks WC, et al: Vascular remodeling in neonatal pulmonary hypertension. *Chest* 1988;93 (Suppl 3):127S–133S.
8. Sato T, Arai K, Ishiharajima S, Asano G: Role of glycosaminoglycan and fibronectin in endothelial cell growth. *Exp Mol Pathol* 1987;47:202–210.
9. Castellot JJ Jr., Addonizio ML, Rosenberg R, Karnovsky MJ: Cultured endothelial cells produce a heparin-like inhibitor of smooth muscle cell growth. *J Cell Biol* 1981;90:372–379.
10. Zerwes HG, and Risau W: Polarized secretion of a platelet-derived growth factor-like chemotactic factor by endothelial cells in vitro. *J Cell Biol* 1987;105:2037–2041.
11. Hannan RL, Kourembanas S, Flanders KC, Rogel SJ, Roberts AB, Faller DV, et al: Endothelial cells synthesize basic fibroblast growth factor and transforming growth factor beta. *Growth Factors* 1988;1:7–17.
12. Delafontaine P, Bernstein KE, Alexander RW: Insulin-like growth factor I gene expression in vascular cells. *Hypertension* 1991;17:693–699.
13. Wang-Iverson P, DeRosa PM, Brown WV: Plasma lipoprotein interaction with endothelial cells. In: Ryan U (ed): *Endothelial Cells*. Boca Raton, FL, CRC Press, 1988:179–187.
14. Gordon EL, Pearson JD, Slakey LL: The hydrolysis of extracellular adenine nucleotides by cultured endothelial cells from pig aorta. *J Biol Chem* 1986;33:15496–15504.
15. Cary DA, Mendelsohn FA: Effect of forskolin, isoproterenol and IBMX on angiotensin converting enzyme and cyclic AMP production by cultured bovine endothelial cells. *Mol Cell Endocrin* 1987;53:103–109.
16. Shimada K, Gill PJ, Silbert JE, Douglas WHJ, Fanburg BL: Involvement of cell surface heparan sulfate in the binding of LPL to cultured bovine endothelial cells. *J Clin Invest* 1981;68:995–1002.
17. Vlodavsky I, Fielding PE, Johnson LK, Gospodarowicz D: Inhibition of low density lipoprotein uptake in confluent endothelial cell monolayers correlates with a restricted surface receptor redistribution. *J Cell Physiol* 1979;100:481–495.
18. Hashida R, Anamizu C, Kimura J, Ohkuma S, Yoshida Y, Takano T: Transcellular transport of lipoprotein through arterial endothelial cells in monolayer culture. *Cell Struct Funct* 1986;11:31–42.
19. Baker DP, Van Lenten BJ, Fogelman AM, Edwards PA, Kean C, Berliner JA: LDL, scavenger and beta-VLDL receptors on aortic endothelial cells. *Arteriosclerosis* 1984;4:248–255.
20. Morel DW, DiCorleto PE, Chisolm GM: Endothelial and smooth muscle cells alter low density lipoprotein in vitro by free radical oxidation. *Arteriosclerosis* 1984;4:357–364.
21. Danon D, Skutelsky E: Endothelial surface charge and its possible relationship to thrombogenesis. *Ann NY Acad Sci* 1976;275:47–63.
22. Gryglewski RJ, Botting RM, Vane JR: Mediators produced by the endothelial cell. *Hypertension* 1988;12:530–548.
23. Rosenberg RD, Rosenberg JS: Natural anticoagulant mechanisms. *J Clin Invest* 1984;74:1–6.
24. Esmon CT, Owen WG: Identification of an endothelial cofactor for thrombin-catalyzed activation of Protein C. *Proc Nat Acad Sci USA* 1981;78:2249–2252.
25. van Iwaarden F, Acton DS, Sixma JJ, Meijers JCM, de Groot PG, Bouma BN: Internalization of antithrombin III by cultured human endothelial cells and its subcellular localization. *J Lab Clin Med* 1989;113:717–726.
26. Podor TJ, Curriden SA, Loskutoff DJ: The fibrinolytic system of endothelial cells. In: Ryan US (ed): *Endothelial Cells*, vol I. Boca Raton, FL, CRC Press, 1988:127–148.
27. Schorer AE, Moldow CF: Production of tissue factor. In: Ryan US (ed): *Endothelial Cells*, vol I. Boca Raton, FL, CRC Press, 1988:85–105.
28. Whelan J, Ghersa P, Hooft-an-Huijsduijnen R, Gray J, Chandra G, Talabot F: An NF kappa B-like factor is essential but not sufficient for cytokine induction of endothelial leukocyte adhesion molecule 1 (ELAM-1) gene transcription. *Nucleic Acids Res* 1991;19:2645–2653.
29. Sporn LA, Marder VJ, Wagner DD: Von Willebrand Factor released from Weibel-Palade bodies binds more avidly to extracellular matrix than that secreted constitutively. *Blood* 1987;69:1531–1534.
30. Stern DM, Nawroth PP: Modulation of endothelial cell coagulant properties. In: Ryan US (ed): *Endothelial Cells*, vol I. Boca Raton, FL, CRC Press, 1988:149–165.
31. Svensjo E, Grega GJ: Evidence for endothelial cell-mediated regulation of macromolecular permeability by post-capillary venules. *Fed Proc* 1986;45:89–95.
32. Huttner I, Boutet M, Rona G, More RH: Studies on protein passage through arterial endothelium: III. Effect of blood pressure levels on the passage of fine structural protein tracers through rat arterial endothelium. *Lab Invest* 1973;29:536–546.
33. Scow RO, Blanchette-Mackie EJ, Smith LC: Role of capillary endothelium in the clearance of chylomicrons: A model for lipid transport from blood by lateral diffusion in cell membranes. *Circ Res* 1976;39:149–162.
34. Berk BC, Alexander RW, Brock TA, Gimbrone MA Jr, Webb RC: Vasoconstriction: A new activity for platelet-derived growth factor. *Science* 1986;232:87–90.
35. Owens GK: Control of hypertrophic vs. hyperplastic growth of vascular smooth muscle cells. *Am J Physiol* 1989;257:H1755–H1765.
36. Berridge MJ, Irvine RF: Inositol trisphosphate, a novel second messenger in cellular signal transduction. *Nature* 1984;312:315–321.
37. Yamamoto H, van Breeman C: Inositol 1,4,5–trisphosphate releases calcium from skinned cultured smooth muscle cells. *Biochem Biophys Res Commun* 1985;130:270–274.
38. Nishizuka Y: The role of protein kinase C in cell surface signal transduction and tumor promotion. *Nature* 1984;308:693–698.
39. Lassègue B, Alexander RW, Clark M, Griendling KK: Angiotensin II-induced phosphatidylcholine hydrolysis in cultured vascular smooth muscle cells: Regulation and localization. *Biochem J* 1991;276:19–25.
40. Moolenaar WH, Kruijer W, Tilly BC, Verlaan I, Bierman AJ, de Laat SW: Growth-factor-like action of phosphatidic acid. *Nature* 1986;323:171–173.
41. Berk BC, Aronow MS, Brock TA, Cragoe E Jr., Gimbrone MA Jr,

Alexander RW: Angiotensin II-stimulated Na+/H+ exchange in cultured vascular smooth muscle cells: Evidence for protein kinase C dependent and independent pathways. *J Biol Chem* 1987;262:5057–5064.

42. Brock TA, Alexander RW, Ekstein LS, Atkinson WJ, Gimbrone MA Jr.: Angiotensin increases cytosolic free calcium in cultured vascular smooth muscle cells. *Hypertension* 1985;7(Suppl 1): I-105–I-109.
43. Williams LT: Signal transduction by the platelet-derived growth factor receptor. *Science* 1989;243:1564–1570.
44. Clegg KB and Sambhi MP: Inhibition of epidermal growth factor-mediated DNA synthesis by a specific tyrosine kinase inhibitor in vascular smooth muscle cells of the spontaneously hypertensive rat. *J Hypertension* 1989;7(Suppl 6):S144–S145.
45. Liebow C, Reilly C, Serrano M, Schally AV: Somatostatin analogues inhibit growth of pancreatic cancer by stimulating tyrosine phosphatase. *Proc Natl Acad Sci USA* 1989;86:2003–2007.
46. Ullrich A, Schlessinger J: Signal transduction by receptors with tyrosine kinase activity. *Cell* 1990;81:203–212.
47. Dillon PF, Aksoy MO, Driska SP, Murphy RA: Myosin phosphorylation and the cross-bridge cycle in arterial smooth muscle. *Science* 1981;211:495–497.
48. Morgan KG: Role of calcium ion in maintenance of vascular smooth muscle tone. *Am J Cardiol* 1987;59:24A–28A.
49. Berk BC, Vekshtein V, Gordon HM, Tsuda T: Angiotensin II-stimulated protein synthesis in cultured vascular smooth muscle cells. *Hypertension* 1989;13:305–314.
50. Berk BC, Taubman MB, Griendling KK, Cragoe EJ Jr., Fenton JW II, Brock TA: Thrombin-stimulated events in cultured vascular smooth muscle cells. *Biochem J* 1991;274:799–805.
51. Golden MA, Au YPT, Kirkman Tr, Wilcox JN, Raines EW, Ross R, et al: Platelet-derived growth factor activity and mRNA expression in healing vascular grafts in baboons. *J Clin Invest* 1991;87:406–414.
52. Lindner V, Lappi DA, Baird A, Majack RA, Reidy MA: Role of basic fibroblast growth factor in vascular lesion formation. *Circ Res* 1991;68:106–113.
53. Myers PR, Minor RL, Guerra R Jr., Bates JN, Harrison DG: The vasorelaxant properties of the endothelium derived relaxing factor more closely resemble S-nitrosocysteine than nitric oxide. *Nature* 1990;345:161–163.
54. Ignarro LJ: Endothelium-derived nitric oxide: Actions and properties. *FASEB J* 1989;3:31–36.
55. Rapoport RM, Draznin MB, Murad F: Endothelium-dependent relaxation in rat aorta may be mediated through cyclic GMP-dependent protein phosphorylation. *Nature* 1983;306:174–176.
56. Furchgott RF, Vanhoutte PM: Endothelium-derived relaxing and contracting factors. *FASEB J* 1989;3:2007–2018.
57. Ito T, Ogawa K, Enomoto I, Hashimoto H, Kai I, Satake T: Comparison of the effects of PGI_2 and PGE_1 on coronary and systemic hemodynamics and coronary arterial cyclic nucleotide level in dogs. *Adv Prostaglandin Thromboxane Leukotriene Research* 1980;7:641–646.
58. Carwile LE, Ager A, Gordon JL: Effects of neutrophil elastase and other proteases on porcine aortic endothelial prostaglandin I_2 production, adenine nucleotide release, and responses to vasoactive agents. *J Clin Invest* 1984;74:1003–1010.
59. Milner P, Bodin P, Loesch A, Burnstock G: Rapid release of endothelin and ATP from isolated aortic endothelial cells exposed to increased flow. *Biochem Biophys Res Comm* 1990;170:649–656.
60. Pearson JD, Slakey LL, Gordon JL: Stimulation of prostaglandin production through purinoceptors on cultured porcine endothelial cells. *Biochem J* 1983;214:273–276.
61. O'Connor SE, Wood BE, Leff P: Characterization of P2x-receptors in rabbit isolated ear artery. *Br J Pharm* 1990;101:640–644.
62. Brock TA, Danthuluri NR: Cellular actions of endothelin in vascular smooth muscle. In: Ruybanyi G (ed): *Endothelin*. Oxford University Press, in press.
63. Ogawa Y, Nakao K, Arai H, Nakagawa O, Hosoda K, Suga S: Molecular cloning of a non-isopeptide-selective human endothelin receptor. *Biochem Biophys Res Comm* 1991;178:248–255.
64. Gumkowski F, Kaminska F, Kaminiski M, Morrissey LW, Auerbach R: Heterogeneity of mouse vascular endothelium: In vitro studies of lymphatic, large blood vessel and microvascular endothelial cells. *Blood Vessels* 1987;24:11–23.
65. Klagsbrun M, D'Amore PA: Regulators of angiogenesis. *Ann Rev. Physiol* 1991;53:217–239.
66. Hansson HA, Brandsten C, Lossing C, Petruson K: Transient expression of insulin-like growth factor I immunoreactivity by vascular cells during angiogenesis. *Exp Mol Path* 1989;50:125–138.
67. Folkman J, Langer R, Linhardt RJ, Haudenschild C, Taylor S: Angiogenesis inhibition and tumor regression caused by heparin or a heparin fragment in the presence of cortisone. *Science* 1983;221:719–725.
68. Clowes AW, Clowes MM, Fingerle J, Reidy MA: Regulation of smooth muscle cell growth in injured artery. *J Cardiovasc Pharm* 1989;14 (Suppl 6): 12–15.
69. Clowes AW, Clowes MM: Kinetics of cellular proliferation after arterial injury. IV. Heparin inhibits rat smooth muscle mitogenesis and migration *Circ Res* 1986;58:839–845.
70. Garg UC, Hassid A: Nitric oxide-generating vasodilators and 8-bromo-cyclic GMP inhibit mitogenesis and proliferation of cultured rat vascular smooth muscle cells. *J Clin Invest* 1989;83:1774–1777.
71. Owens GK, Geisterfer AA, Yang Y W-H, Komoriya A: Transforming growth factor β induced growth inhibition and cellular hypertrophy in cultured vascular smooth muscle cells. *J Cell Biol* 1988;107:771–780.
72. Kavanaugh WM, Harsh GR IV, Starksen NF, Rocco CM, Williams LT: Transcriptional regulation of the A and B chain genes of PDGF in microvascular endothelial cells. *J Biol Chem* 1988;263:8470–8472.
73. Clemmons DR: Exposure to platelet-derived growth factors modulates the porcine aortic smooth muscle cell response to somatomedin-C. *Endocrinology* 1985;117:77–83.
74. Bevilacqua MP, Gimbrone MA Jr.: Modulation of endothelial cell procoagulant and fibrinolytic activities by inflammatory mediators. In: Ryan US (ed): *Endothelial Cells*, vol I. Boca Raton, FL, CRC Press 1988:107–118.
75. Beasley D, Cohen RA, Levinsky NG: Interleukin 1 inhibits contraction of vascular smooth muscle. *J Clin Invest* 1989;83:331–335.
76. Schindler R, Ghezzi P, Dinarello CA: IL-1 induces IL-1 IV. Interferon-γ suppresses IL-1 but not lipopolysaccharide-induced transcription of IL-1. *J Immunol* 1990; 144:2216–2222.
77. Lindner V, Reidy MA: Proliferation of smooth muscle cells after vascular injury is inhibited by an antibody against basic fibroblast growth factor. *Proc Natl Acad Sci USA* 1991;88:3739–3743.
78. Bashkin P, Doctrow S, Klagsbrun M, Svahn CM, Folkman J, Vlodavsky I: Basic fibroblast growth factor binds to subendothelial extracellular matrix and is released by heparinase and heparin-like molecules. *Biochemistry* 1989;28:1737–1743.
79. Hirata Y, Takagi Y, Fukuda Y, Marumo F: Endothelin is a potent mitogen for rat vascular smooth muscle cells. *Atherosclerosis* 1989;78:225–228.
80. Hunter T: Protein-tyrosine phosphatases: The other side of the coin. *Cell* 1989;58:1013–1016.
81. Liebow C, Reilly C, Serrano M, Schally AV: Somatostatin analogues inhibit growth of pancreatic cancer by stimulating tyrosine phosphatase. *Proc Natl Acad Sci USA* 1989;86:2003–2007.
82. Conte JV, Foegh ML, Calcagno D, Wallace RB, Ramwell PW: Peptide inhibition of myointimal proliferation following angioplasty in rabbits. *Trans Proc* 1989;21:3686–3688.
83. Gruppuso PA, Mikumo R, Brautigan DL, Braun L: Growth arrest induced by transforming growth factor β1 is accompanied by protein phosphatase activation in human keratinocytes. *J Biol Chem* 1991;266:3444–3448.
84. Majno G, Shea SM, Leventhal M: Endothelial contraction induced by histamine-type mediators: an electron microscopic study. *J Cell Biol* 1969;42:647–672.
85. Pober JS, Cotran RS: What can be learned from the expression of endothelial adhesion molecules in tissues? *Lab Invest* 1991;64:301–305.
86. Pober JS, Cotran RS: The role of endothelial cells in inflammation. *Transplantation* 1990;50:537–544.
87. Marshall JJ, Kontos HA: Endothelium-derived relaxing factors: A perspective from in vivo data. *Hypertension* 1990;16:371–386.
88. Nerem RM, Girard PR: Hemodynamic influences on vascular endothelial biology. *Toxicol Path* 1990;18:572–582.
89. Schwartz SM, Majesky MW, Dilley RJ: Vascular remodeling in

hypertension and atherosclerosis. In: Laragh JH, Brenner BM, (ed): *Hypertension: Pathophysiology, Diagnosis and Management.* New York, Raven 1990:521–539.

90. Asakura T, Karino T: Flow patterns and spatial distribution of atherosclerotic lesions in human coronary arteries. *Circ Res* 1990;66:1045–1066.
91. Freiman PC, Mitchell GG, Heistad DD, Armstrong ML, Harrison DG: Atherosclerosis impairs endothelium-dependent vascular relaxation to acetylcholine and thrombin in primates. *Circ Res* 1986;58:783–789.
92. Minor RL, Myers PR, Guerra R, Bates JN, Harrison DG: Diet-induced atherosclerosis increases the release of nitrogen oxides from rabbit aorta. *J Clin Invest* 1990;86:2109–2116.
93. McLenachan JM, Williams JK, Fish RD, Ganz P, Selwyn AP: Loss of flow-mediated endothelium-dependent dilation occurs early in the development of atherosclerosis. *Circulation* 1991;84:1273–1278.
94. Mugge A, Elwell JH, Peterson TE, Heistad DD, Harrison DG: Chronic treatment with polyethylene-glycolated superoxide dismutase partially restores endothelium-dependent vascular relaxation in cholesterol-fed rabbits. *Circ Res* 1991; 69:1293–1300.
95. Hansson GK, Seifert PS, Olsson G, Bondjers G: Immunohistochemical detection of macrophages and T lymphocytes in atherosclerotic lesions of cholesterol-fed rabbits. *Arteriosclerosis Thrombosis* 1991;1:745–750.
96. Cybulsky MI, Gimbrone MA Jr: Endothelial expression of a mononuclear leukocyte adhesion molecule during atherogenesis. *Science* 1991;251:788–791.
97. Wang JM, Sica A, Peri G, Walter S, Padura IM, Libby P, et al: Expression of monocyte chemotactic protein and interleukin-8 by cytokine-activated human vascular smooth muscle cells. *Arteriosclerosis Thrombosis* 1991;11:1166–1174.
98. Ross R: The pathogenesis of atherosclerosis—an update. *N Engl J Med* 1986;314:488–500.
99. Vita JA, Treasure CB, Nabel EG, McLenachan JM, Fish RD, Yeung AC, et al: The coronary vasomotor response to acetylcholine relates to risk factors for coronary artery disease. *Circulation* 1990;81:491–497.
100. Rubanyi GM: Endothelium-derived relaxing and contracting factors. *J Cell Biochem* 1991;46:27–36.
101. Luscher TF, Vanhoutte PM: Endothelium-dependent contractions to acetylcholine in the aorta of the spontaneously hypertensive rat. *Hypertension* 1986;8:344–348.
102. Owens GK, Schwartz SM: Alterations in vascular smooth muscle mass in the spontaneously hypertensive rat. Role in cellular hypertrophy, hyperploidy and hyperplasia. *Circ Res* 1982;51:280–289.
103. Owens GK, Schwartz SM: Vascular smooth muscle cell hypertrophy and hyperploidy in the Goldblatt hypertensive rat. *Circ Res* 1983;53:491–501.
104. Halpern W, Warshaw DM, Mulvany MJ: Mechanical and morphological properties of arterial resistance vessels in young and old spontaneously hypertensive rats. *Circ Res* 1979;45:250–259.
105. Majesky MW, Reidy MA, Bowen-Pope DF, Hart CE, Wilcox JN, Schwartz SM: PDGF ligand and receptor gene expression during repair of arterial injury. *J Cell Biol* 1990;111:2149–2158.
106. Taubman MB, Rollins BJ, Poon M, Marmur J, Green RS, Berk BC, et al: JE mRNA accumulates rapidly in aortic injury and in platelet-derived growth factor-stimulated vascular smooth muscle cells. *Circ Res* 1992;70:314–325.
107. Cercek B, Fishbein MC, Forrester JS, Helfant RH, Fagin JA: Induction of insulin-like growth factor I messenger RNA in rat aorta after balloon denudation. *Circ Res* 1990;66:1755–1760.
108. Fingerle J, Au YP, Clowes AW, Reidy MA: Intimal lesion formation in rat carotid arteries after endothelial denudation in absence of medial injury. *Atherosclerosis* 1990;10:1082–1087.
109. Lynch CM, Clowes MM, Osborne WRA, Clowes AW, Miller AD: Long-term expression of human adenosine deaminase in vascular smooth muscle cells of rats: A model for gene therapy. *Proc Natl Acad Sci USA* 1992;89:1138–1142.
110. Nabel EG, Plautz G, Nabel GJ: Gene transfer into vascular cells. *J Am Coll Cardiol* 1991; 17:189B–194B.
111. Nabel EG: Direct gene transfer into the arterial wall. *J Vasc Surg* 1992;15:931–932.
112. Dichek DA, Neville RF, Zwiebel JA, Freeman SM, Leon MB, Anderson WF: Seeding of intravascular stents with genetically engineered endothelial cells. *Circulation* 1989;80:1347–1353.
113. Lim CS, Chapman GD, Gammon RS, Muhlestein JB, Bauman RP, Stack RS et al: Direct in vivo gene transfer into the coronary and peripheral vasculatures of the intact dog. *Circulation* 1991;83:2007–2011.

Chapter 3

Structure and Function of Cardiovascular Membranes, Channels, and Receptors

Gary L. Stiles, M.D.

Every living cell must have the ability to maintain a controlled intracellular environment. In order to accomplish this, a variety of substances such as ions, water, and proteins must be transported into or out of the cell as needed. In addition, cells must be responsive to environmental perturbations such as hormones, drugs, or other molecules even when these factors do not physically enter the cell. The structural entity that allows this to be accomplished is the plasma membrane. The plasma membrane effectively gives structure to the cells while selectively insulating the extracellular from the intracellular world. Although the plasma membrane can be thought of as a simple cellular envelope, it is anything but simple and inert.[1-4] The membrane is, in fact, a highly organized structure composed of lipids, proteins, and carbohydrates dynamically interacting and largely associated through noncovalent bonds. The general structure for a membrane is shown in Fig. 3-1 wherein there is a lipid bilayer in which charged portions of the lipids face the extracellular and intracellular spaces while hydrophobic (nonpolar) fatty acyl chains interact with each other.

As can be seen in Fig. 3-1, not only is there a very heterogeneous population of substances that constitute the membrane but also these molecules are arranged in an asymmetric distribution with certain substituents having a predilection for the extracellular surface (glycoproteins) whereas others are more frequently encountered on the cytoplasmic surface (phosphotidylserine).

Approximately 50 percent of the mass of the plasma membrane are lipids. The major type of lipid encountered are phospholipids that have a polar head group and two hydrophobic hydrocarbon tails. Phospholipids

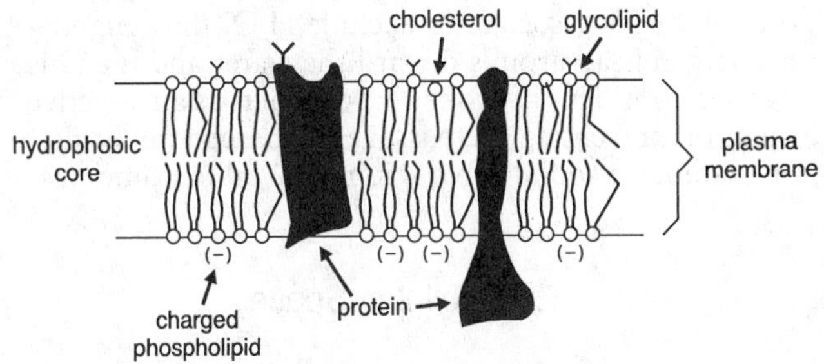

FIGURE 3-1 Schematic representation of plasma membrane. The polar head groups represented by small circles are arranged at the extracellular and intracellular surfaces. The lipid (fatty acid) chains face each other to form the hydrophobic core. The unsaturated fatty acid chains (containing double bonds) are represented by the "kinked" tails. The large proteins shown represent transmembrane proteins embedded in the lipid matrix. One of the proteins and several of the lipids (glycolipids) are represented as containing a carbohydrate substituent (γ). The charged phospholipids are shown on the intracellular surface.

themselves are a mixture of different compounds that vary in the length of the hydrocarbon tails, the degree of double-bond saturation in the tail, and the type of substituents in the polar head groups. Of particular importance in the functioning of the membrane is the degree of saturation or unsaturation in the fatty acid tails of the phospholipids. When the fatty acid chains are unsaturated, i.e., have double bonds between carbon atoms, the chain is kinked (as depicted in Fig. 3-1) and, hence, cannot be packed as tightly together, leading to a greater mobility or fluidity within the membranes. Theoretically at least, there may be an association between the diet content of saturated versus unsaturated fats and the composition of plasma membrane, which could ultimately provide a link between diet and how cells function and respond to stimuli. This may directly affect how the proteins can move or function within the lipid bilayer.[1-3]

Cholesterol is another major constituent of the membrane and tends to promote membrane rigidity rather than fluidity.[1,2,4] Cholesterol, which is a rigid heterocyclic compound, aligns itself in the membrane with its hydroxyl group near the polar head groups of the phospholipid and its hydrophobic tail interacting with the fatty acid tails within the lipid bilayer. Cholesterol's rigidity decreases the ability of fatty acid tails to move and thereby promotes membrane rigidity.

Glycolipids make up the last large class of lipids that comprise the lipid bilayer. These lipids contain carbohydrates in the form of oligosaccharides. The oligosaccharides are a very heterogeneous group of compounds that range from a single-sugar substituent to very complex gangliosides that contain multiple sugar residues terminating in sialic acid giving them an overall negative charge. As mentioned earlier, glycolipids are only found on the extracellular face where their glycan components are exposed to the extracellular environment. The function of this class of molecules remains speculative but may relate to cell-cell interaction or may act as specific cell surface receptors.

The very nature of lipid molecules makes them spontaneously form bilayers when exposed to a water environment. The association of lipids occurs when the hydrophobic tails associate to exclude H_2O, thus aligning the charged head groups toward the water and the tails toward a core. This hydrophobic core acts as an effective insulation preventing the passage of charged molecules. For example, a sodium (Na^+) ion is 10 billion times less likely to cross a lipid bilayer than is a water molecule. If the structure of the plasma membrane contained only lipids as described, then although it would be an effective barrier, it would by and large not allow for the transport of substances into or out of the cell or for the transduction of transmembrane signals.

To accomplish these specific functions, the lipid bilayer acts as a matrix to support proteins in the appropriate conformation to allow them to carry out their appointed tasks. Although there is a general scheme for the types of lipids found in plasma membranes, there is great diversity and disparity among the types of proteins embedded in the plasma membrane from cell to cell. There are, however, two general classes of proteins. The first is an integral membrane protein that either passes directly through the lipid bilayer (transmembrane protein) or is attached via a lipid side-chain interaction to the lipid bilayer. These proteins do not readily dissociate from the plasma membrane and can be released only through disruption of the membrane structure by detergents or organic solvents. The other class of proteins (peripheral or loosely associated) do penetrate the lipid bilayer but are more closely associated with integral membrane proteins by noncovalent associations and can be dissociated from the membrane without physically disrupting the membrane bilayer. That is to say, simple changes in the ionic strength of solutions in contact with the membrane may be able to dissociate the proteins from the membrane.

For the purposes of this chapter, the integral membrane proteins are most important. This class of proteins represents the major constituents of both membrane-bound receptors and ion channels. These integral membrane proteins can pass through the membrane once or multiple times. Proteins that span an odd number of times will obviously have their amino and carboxy termini on opposite sides of the lipid bilayer, while proteins that span an even number of times will have the carboxy and amino termini on the same side (see Fig. 3-2*A*).

Since these proteins must interact with the relatively aqueous (hydrophilic) cytosolic and extracellular spaces as well as the hydrophobic lipid bilayer, most proteins contain stretches of hydrophilic amino acids interspersed with hydrophobic domains. The hydrophobic domains are incorporated into the lipid bilayer so that the nonpolar regions of the amino acids interact with the fatty acid chains while the polar peptide bonds and polar side chains are grouped to shield themselves from the fatty

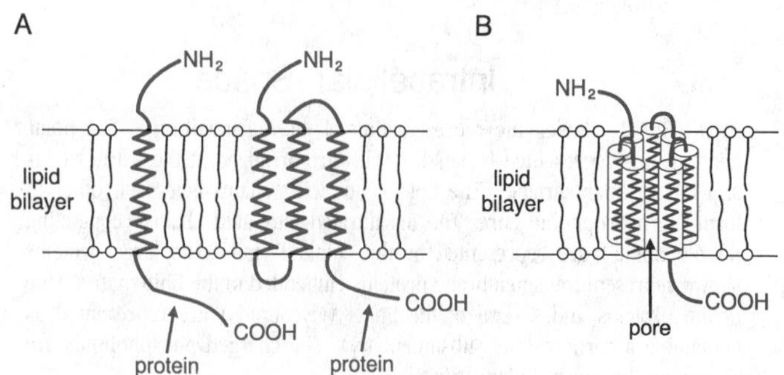

FIGURE 3-2 Arrangement of transmembrane proteins in lipid bilayer. *A*. Transmembrane proteins can traverse the lipid bilayer once or multiple times. The crooked lines represent stretches of hydrophobic amino acids usually 20 to 28 in number that constitute the transmembrane domain. For proteins that contain multiple transmembrane domains the hydrophobic domains are separated by hydrophilic domains represented by smooth lines. Although these proteins are shown with their amino terminus as extracellular, this is not always the case. *B*. When multiple transmembrane domains exist, they may arrange to form a bundle with a central core or pore. This arrangement is frequently seen in ion channels and receptors as described in text.

acids. As we shall see, when the proteins span the lipid bilayer multiple times, the transmembrane segments can arrange themselves in a bundle so as to create a hydrophilic core, pore, or channel and a hydrophobic perimeter to interact with the fatty acid chains (see Fig. 3-2*B*). This pore can be utilized as a site for interaction of ligands, hormones, or drugs to interact with the protein (receptor) or as a hydrated channel through which ions or other small molecules can pass into or out of the cell. As might be imagined, the orientation of the protein in the membrane is critical to its function. A significant proportion of integral membrane proteins have post-translational modifications including glycosylation (addition of sugars) or fatty acid acylation. The carbohydrate chains are always on the extracellular face of the cell while the lipid modifications can be attached to either face of the membrane. In some cases these modifications are absolutely required for function of the protein; in other cases the alterations have no apparent effect.

Membranes, as mentioned earlier, display a property known as fluidity, which permits proteins and lipids to have mobility in the lipid bilayer. This property allows distinct proteins to come together and interact to produce a functional coupling (lateral diffusion), e.g., receptors and guanine nucleotide binding proteins (G proteins) or the clustering of low-density lipoprotein receptors. The lipid bilayer cannot, however, be viewed as an unstructed liquid through which proteins float at random. Membranes, in fact, have discrete structural domains in which certain ion channels or enzymes are confined to specific areas and are not free to diffuse around the cell.[1]

ION CHANNELS

Few fields in science have witnessed a more rapid expansion in knowledge than that of ion channel structure and function. Ion channels function primarily to regulate the flow of ions across the cell membrane and thereby modulate the electrical potential of the cell.[5] It has long been recognized that channel proteins must in some way form a regulatable water-filled pore through which select ions can pass. Under the appropriate conditions a single channel can maintain a high degree of specificity toward a single type of ion yet allow more than a million of these ions to pass per second. Ion channels can be thought of as a passive conduit through which ions move down a concentration gradient. That is to say, energy in the form of adenosine triphosphate (ATP) is not expended during the ion movement. This is in contrast to an energy-dependent ion pump, which can move ions against a concentration gradient.[1]

Channels must inherently have the ability to open and close in response to the cells' need or appropriate stimuli. If the channel were to remain open, an ionic equilibrium would quickly be reached between the outside and inside of the cells and no ionic gradient or electrical potential across the membrane would be maintained. This would lead to cellular dysfunction and/or death.

The "gating" function of ion channels is intrinsic to the protein structure of the channel and can be regulated by several distinct signaling processes including mechanical stimulation of the channel such as stretch (mechanically gated channel), voltage changes across the membrane (voltage-gated channels), or the binding of hormones or drugs (ligand-gated channels).[6–13] This last class of channels can be regulated via external neurotransmitters such as acetylcholine, epinephrine, or adenosine.[7,10–13] These substances may interact directly with the channel protein (acetylcholine) or through distinct receptors, such as the β-adrenergic receptor (epinephrine) or A_1 adenosine receptor (adenosine), which in turn activate specific G proteins. The G proteins can then modulate channel activity either through direct intramembrane interactions or indirectly via a second-messenger system, such as adenosine 3′,5′-cyclic monophosphate (cAMP) or cyclic guanosine monophosphate (cGMP).[7,10–13] These channel subtypes should not be taken to be mutually exclusive since a voltage-sensitive channel may also have its function modulated by receptor-mediated G-protein interactions.

The fact that external stimuli can regulate channel pore opening and closing immediately begins to provide insight into the protein architecture of the channel. First, the protein must span the membrane to allow a pore to form. Second, the pore must have inherent properties that allow only specific ions to enter and traverse the pore. Third, the pore must have the ability to close and open (gate). Finally, the channel protein must have regulatory regions through which the appropriate signals can be imparted to the channel such as sites for G-protein interaction, sites that sense changes in voltage or sites for covalent modifications such as phosphorylation. See Fig. 3-3 for a schematic representation.

In addition to classification by regulatory mechanisms, channels are frequently categorized by their ion selectivity and whether they promote outward or inward currents. For example, in the outward current channel class, the K^+-selective channels are by far the most important and the most abundant in terms of different subtypes. This class of channels acts to hyperpolarize the cell and, therefore, frequently is responsible for repolarizing cells after the action potential created largely by the Na^+ channel (inward current) has depolarized the cell. As mentioned previously, the K^+ movement is down its concentration gradient and hence K^+ moves outward. The K^+ channels are highly regulated in the heart.[5,10] Acetylcholine acting through muscarinic receptors and adenosine acting via A_1 adenosine receptors activate a pertussis-toxin-sensitive G protein that subsequently activates a K^+ channel to promote hyperpolarization of the cell.[5,10] The effect of hyperpolarization on pacemaker and conducting system cells would be to decrease spontaneous depolarization and hence decrease chronotropy and to slow conduction. This is reasonable since it is well known that adenosine can slow heart rate and atrioventicular (AV) nodal conduction.[14] In extracardiac tissues such as neurons, muscarinic receptors acting through pertussis-toxin-insensitive G proteins can inhibit K^+ channels (M currents) through mechanisms distinct from those described above.[10] In addition, there are several other types of K^+ channels in the heart including the ATP depletion–dependent K^+ channel, the Na^+-dependent K^+ channels, and the delayed rectifying K^+ channels.[5] *Rectifying channels* are those that have a net current

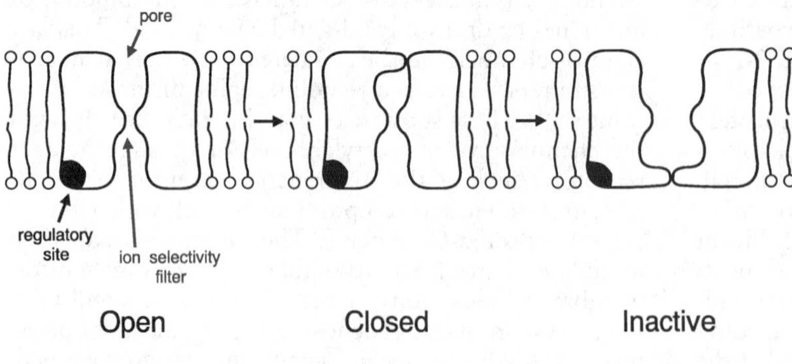

FIGURE 3-3 Schematic representation of a generic ion channel in lipid bilayer. The major functional features of an ion channel are depicted. These include a central pore, or "channel," through which ions can pass and a selectivity filter that permits only a specific ion to pass. The regulatory site represents a domain on the protein responsible for regulating the function (ability of ions to pass) of the channel. This could range from a phosphorylation site, an actual hormone binding site, or the site for interaction with G proteins. Three discrete states of the channel are shown—open, closed, or inactive.

usually in the outward direction that rectify or counteract the depolarized state. A delayed rectifying channel simply opens late in the depolarization process. This latter group of channels function primarily during the most depolarized states of the cell. In the heart, cAMP will increase the outward current thereby accelerating repolarization and shortening the action potential. There are a variety of additional outward rectifying K^+ channels that are modulated by time (A current channels) or Ca^{2+}—the Ca^{2+}-activated outward-rectifying K^+ channels. The great diversity of K^+ channels makes a detailed description of each type impossible in this chapter, and the reader is referred to the references.[5,6,8,15–17]

There are two main types of inward channels that promote depolarization of the cell with which we should be concerned, i.e., the Na^+ and Ca^{2+} channels. The calcium channels are primarily responsible for increasing intracellular Ca^{2+} leading to contraction of muscle.[5,6,18] There are three major classes of voltage-dependent Ca^{2+} channels, which have been designated L type, N type, and T type.[5] The channels can be differentiated by their sensitivity to the dehydropyridine class of Ca^{2+} channel blockers, by the membrane potential at which they are activated and inactivated, and by their gating and permeation characteristics. These channels are positively and negatively regulated by G-protein coupled receptors. For example, in the heart β-adrenergic receptors acting via the G_s protein promote the opening of Ca^{2+} channels. This effect can be mediated by two distinct pathways. The first is mediated by an enhanced level of intracellular cAMP, which activates protein kinase A leading to phosphorylation of the Ca^{2+} channels.[10]

The second involves the direct activation of the channel by activated G_s protein independent of cAMP. This is one of an exceedingly rare, if not unique, β-adrenergic receptor mediated effects that is a cAMP-independent mechanism. A number of receptors are capable of inhibiting the activity of Ca^{2+} channels via distinct mechanisms. Certain muscarinic (M2) receptors and A_1 adenosine receptors inhibit Ca^{2+} currents by suppressing cAMP levels following activation of inhibitory G_i proteins. In contrast, atrial natriuretic factor acting via its receptor can activate cGMP leading to an enhancement of a cyclic nucleotide phosphodiesterase that degrades cAMP.[5] This functionally produces the same effect as that mediated by the A_1 adenosine receptor described above but by a distinctly different mechanism. Receptors that activate protein kinase C may also inactivate Ca^{2+} channels.

The last class of channels to be described are the Na^+ channels. This channel is largely responsible for the rapid inward movement of Na^+ ions, which results in the rapid upstroke of the action potential. This channel will be used as a representative of the larger class of voltage-sensitive ion channels that undergo inactivation and includes K^+ channels (A channel) and dihydropyridine-sensitive Ca^{2+} channels since they all share structural and functional homologies.[6,18,19] The voltage-gated Na^+ channels are largely responsible for generating the action potential so critical in cardiac muscle and conducting tissue.[20] The action potential is a rapid transient self-propagating electrical current that traverses the membrane. The cell normally has a potential difference across the membrane of about −80 to −100 mV. A depolarization of the membrane, i.e., shift in the membrane potential to a less negative value, leads to the opening of voltage-gated Na^+ channels and an influx of Na^+ (down its concentration gradient) into the cell. This leads to a further depolarization that permits additional Na^+ to enter. This positive-feedback loop enhances the propagation of the depolarization wave. There must, however, be a mechanism to terminate this process since the cell obviously does not find itself in a situation where all Na^+ channels are open and no Na^+ gradient exists. The process that protects the cell against this possibility is called the *inactivation* state of the channel. This state of the channel is distinctly different from simple channel closure (Fig. 3-3). When "inactivated," the channel cannot reopen until the local membrane potential has returned to its resting negative value and the channel protein reassumes its closed configuration. The exact mechanism(s) responsible for this inactivation state and the process returning the protein to its closed state remains largely unknown.

Molecular studies undertaken in the past few years have revealed strong structural similarities among Na^+, K^+, and Ca^{2+} channels.[6,18,19] These channels may be a single-subunit protein complex or may contain multiple subunits.[6,18,19] There are homologous motifs within the primary subunit of each channel. For example, each channel has multiple membrane-spanning hydrophobic domains including a so-called S4 sequence in which positively charged basic amino acid residues, such as arginines, are located every third amino acid within this membrane domain. This specialized sequence may function as the voltage sensor.[6,18,19] In addition, there are multiple hydrophilic regions that traverse the membrane to form the aqueous pore through which the ions pass. The gating function is envisioned as a twisting or "screw-like" motion of the helices upward in the membrane resulting in the opening of the channel.[15,16]

Multiple Na^+ channels have now been cloned and/or purified.[6,21–23] Purification studies indicate that there is one large subunit (of over 1800 amino acids) and several smaller subunits.[6,19] The large subunit by itself can form functional Na^+ channels with many but not all of the properties expected of the native Na^+ channel. Within the large subunit there are multiple repeats of similar sequences.[6] Thus, the large protein is composed of four homologous domains linearly arranged in series. Within each of these domains lie multiple stretches of hydrophobic amino acids that likely represent the transmembrane spanning regions and a single so-called S4 sequence described above (see Fig. 3-4*A*).

In contrast to the Na^+ channel, the K^+ channel is much simpler and contains only one of the basic repeat units contained in the Na^+ channel (Fig. 3-4*B*). Multiple K^+ channels have been cloned and all have the basic single-subunit motif but differ in their amino and carboxy termini.[6,8] This suggests that the common or shared portions of these channels are responsible for the ion pore, the ion selectivity, and the voltage sensitivity mechanisms whereas the two ends may function to impart specific regulatory functions.

The Ca^{2+} channels are known to be multimeric having both large and small subunits. The large α_1 subunit has many of the structural features of the Na^+ channel, as shown in Fig. 3-4*A*, in that it has four homologous domains that contain multiple membrane-spanning regions and a single S4 sequence.[18,19,24]

The striking similarities among the channel structures suggest that nature has taken a relatively simple functional building block and then created variations on a theme in order to create diversity and specialization for different types of ion channels with defined functions.

RECEPTORS

Cell surface (transmembrane) receptors function to permit extracellular substances to regulate intracellular function or metabolism without necessarily having to enter the cell. A number of different types of receptors can initiate a transmembrane signal that ultimately modulates cellular function. In this chapter we shall focus only on the largest group—the G-protein coupled receptors, which utilize G proteins to act as the intermediary between a given receptor and the actual inhibition or activation of an effector system, such as adenylyl cyclase.[25–28] The other classes of receptors, which will not be discussed, include those that have intrinsic tyrosine kinase activity such as the receptor for epidermal growth factor or insulin,[29] those that transport the ligand itself

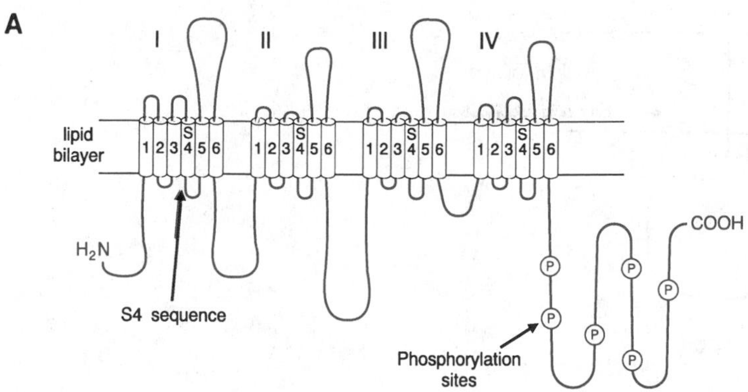

B

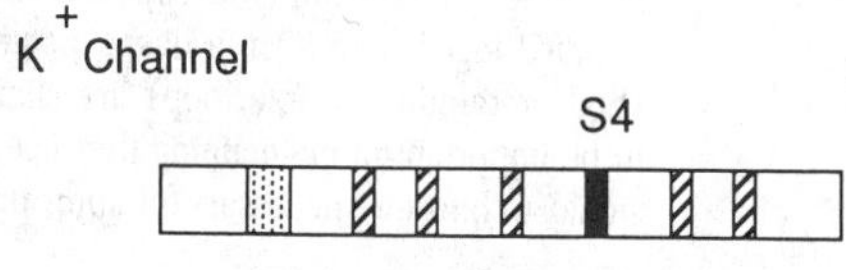

FIGURE 3-4 Structural characteristics of sodium channels. *A.* Schematic representation of Na^+ channel protein/membrane architecture. The large protein tranverses the membrane multiple times with both the amino and carboxyl termini on the intracellular side of the membrane. The transmembrane regions are grouped into four motifs each containing six transmembrane spans. Within each motif there is a specific span termed the S4 region that likely contains the voltage sensing region. Phosphorylation sites are shown on the carboxyl tail that help to regulate channel function. *B.* Comparison of a schematic representation of the Na^+ channel with its four motifs with that of a K^+ channel in which a single similar motif comprises the channel pore.

into the cell such as those for the low-density lipoprotein,[30] and the ion channels that themselves contain the receptor for their own ligand such as the nicotinic acetylcholine receptor.[7]

Receptor Structure

As alluded to in the previous section, there is a close functional association between ion channels and membrane receptors. In addition, there are structural similarities between the G-protein coupled receptors and ion channels. Recent years have witnessed the purification and cloning of a large number of these G-protein coupled receptors. This has provided an abundance of information of their structure, function and regulation.[28,31] The G-protein coupled receptors are part of a large ever-growing gene family of cell surface receptors that bind such diverse agonists (ligands) as adenosine, catecholamines, "light," odorants, acetylcholine, prostaglandins, angiotensin, vasoactive intestinal protein, and histamine.[25,31] The receptors for each of these endogenous substances are integral membrane proteins that contain seven transmembrane domains that likely associate to form a "bundle" with a central "pocket"—much like that described for ion channels (see Figs. 3-2*B* and 3-4*A*). Instead of forming an aqueous pore, however, the pocket forms the binding site for the ligand. Much like the ion pore, which has a selectivity filter that permits only selective ions to pass through the pore, the pocket determines the ligand specificity for each receptor. In addition, each receptor contains an extracellular amino terminal tail and three extracellular loops connecting the transmembrane domains. There are three intracellular loops and an intracellular carboxyl tail (see Fig. 3-5*A*).

All of these receptors are single-subunit proteins and each of the seven transmembrane domains contain 20 to 28 hydrophobic amino acids. These domains are likely arranged as an α helix, as shown in Fig. 3-5*B*. The extracellular and intracellular loops largely contain more hydrophilic amino acids that can interact with the aqueous environment. In pioneering work performed with rhodopsin and bacteriorhodopsin (one of the G-protein coupled receptors) high-resolution electron diffraction studies have established the validity of the seven-membrane spanning motif.[32,33] This work has permitted models for other G-protein coupled receptors to be proposed, as shown in Fig. 3-5*B*. There are currently many laboratories attempting to validate and understand the secondary and tertiary structure of these receptors.

The function of the extracellular domains is largely unknown, although it is clear that the amino terminus tail or extracellular loop II are the sites for glycosylation.[34] The role of glycosylation in the functioning of the receptor remains unclear.[34] The extracellular loops I and

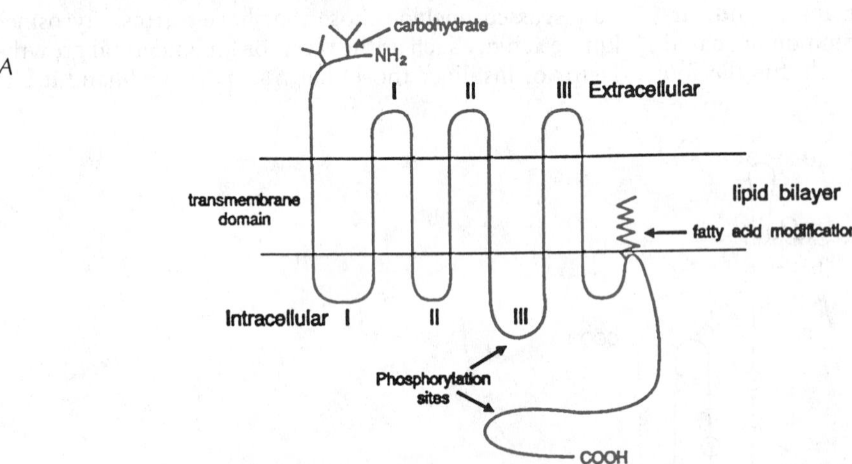

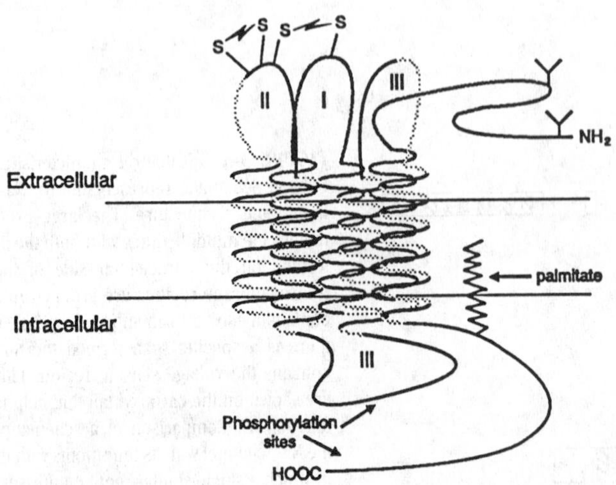

FIGURE 3-5 Receptor structure. *A*. Planar model of a prototypic G-protein coupled receptor and its arrangement in the lipid bilayer. These receptors have their amino terminus on the extracellular surface. Most receptors have carbohydrate modifications on the extracellular surface either on the amino terminus (as shown) or on the second extracellular loop. Sites for protein phosphorylation exist on the third intracellular loop and/or the carboxyl terminus. Phosphorylation of these sites likely results in less efficient coupling of the receptor to the effector system. Some receptors have lipid modifications that attach the protein to the lipid bilayer. *B*. Model of receptor with the transmembrane domains bundled together to form a ligand pocket. Disulfide bonds (both intraloop and interloop) are shown and are known to be important in maintaining the receptor's three-dimensional architecture necessary for appropriate ligand binding.

TABLE 3-1
G Proteins

G Proteins	Variants (α Subunit)	Effector	Response
G_s	4 (1 gene, 4 splices)	Adenylyl cyclase	+
		Ca^{2+} channel	+
G_i	3 (3 genes)	Adenylyl cyclase	−
		K^+ channel	+
		Na^+ channel	+
G_o	2 (? splice variants)	Ca^{2+} channel	−
		? K^+ channel	
		? Phospholipase C	
G_q	?	Phospholipase C	+
G_t	2	cGMP phosphodiesterase	+

II contain cysteine residues that likely form disulfide bonds, which are important in stabilizing the ligand binding pocket.[34,35]

As mentioned above, the transmembrane domains contain the ligand binding site and determine the pharmacologic specificity of the receptors. At present the exact regions (and amino acids) of the domains responsible for the ligand binding site for agonists and antagonists are largely unknown. For further details see Refs. 36 to 38.

The cytoplasmic regions, particularly loop III and the carboxyl tail, are important for receptor coupling to its G protein and contain sites for posttranslational modifications such as phosphorylation important for regulation of receptor function.[34] The functions of cytoplasmic loops I and II remain largely unknown.

Receptor Coupling

G-protein coupled receptors functionally interact with a wide variety of G proteins, which are heterotrimeric protein complexes consisting of α, β, and γ subunits.[39] The α subunits are likewise an ever-expanding superfamily of proteins that currently have more than 10 members, some of which are listed in Table 3-1,[25] the more common being α_s, which is responsible for activating adenylyl cyclase; α_i (three subtypes known), which inhibit adenylyl cyclase; α_o (two types), which may regulate K^+ channels, Ca^{2+} channels, and phospholipase C; and $\alpha_{Z(?P,X)}$, which is responsible for activating phospholipase C.

Each of the α subunits are capable of coupling to receptors and are multifunction proteins of about 40,000 daltons molecular weight. Within the α subunit resides a specific domain that allows it to interact with its attendant receptor, a site for interacting with the appropriate effector system, and a region that binds guanosine triphosphate (GTP) and then has the ability to hydrolyze GTP to inactive guanine nucleotide (GDP) (GTPase activity).[40]

A full understanding of receptor-mediated transmembrane signaling requires insight into how the three known components of a prototypic stimulatory adenylyl cyclase system interact.[25,26,34] For this system, the β-adrenergic receptor (β-AR), the stimulatory G_s protein, and the enzyme adenylyl cyclase are the three protein components. The β-AR acts as the recognition unit for a hormone—epinephrine (see Fig. 3-6). When an agonist such as epinephrine binds to the receptor in its appropriate pocket, it induces a conformational change in the receptor that allows it to functionally interact with its G protein, G_s, which in the basal (inactive) state is in its heterotrimeric state αβγ. In the basal state, GDP is bound to the α subunit. Under the influence of the agonist, an agonist-specific high-affinity receptor–G-protein complex forms and the G protein is induced to undergo a conformational change that promotes the exchange of GTP for GDP. This is the active guanine nucleotide. The binding of GTP likely results in the dissociation of the receptor from the G protein as well as the dissociation of the α-GTP from the βγ subunit. These reactions are all known to require the presence of Mg^{2+}. The activated α-GTP is then able to interact functionally with the catalytic unit of adenylyl cyclase, thereby activating it to convert ATP to cAMP.

The mechanism responsible for terminating this process is the hydrolysis of GTP to GDP + P_i. This GTPase activity resides within the α subunit itself.[25,39] When the GTP is hydrolyzed to GDP, α-GDP is no longer able to activate adenylyl cyclase and the α subunit reassociates with βγ allowing the complex to recycle back to interact with the receptor if an agonist is present to start the process again. If no agonist is present, the α-GDP(βγ) remains in its basal state.

An analogous process is likely responsible for G-protein mediated activation of ion channels, phospholipase C, phospholipase D and A, and the cGMP-phosphodiesterase. The exact mechanism by which inhibitory receptors, such as the A_1 adenosine or the α_2 adrenergic, act to suppress cAMP is still debated but most investigators believe that activation of the G_i protein by inhibitory receptors is analogous to that described above. Following the dissociation of α_i-GTP from βγ, however, the mechanism for inhibition of adenylyl cyclase becomes less clear. The most likely scenario is that following the release of βγ, the βγ may by the process of mass action promote the reassociation of α_s with βγ thereby inactivating α_s. Thus, G_i appears to inactivate G_s rather than directly inhibiting the catalytic unit. The other potential mechanism would be that activated α_i-GTP directly inhibits the catalytic unit itself.[25,39] In the final analysis

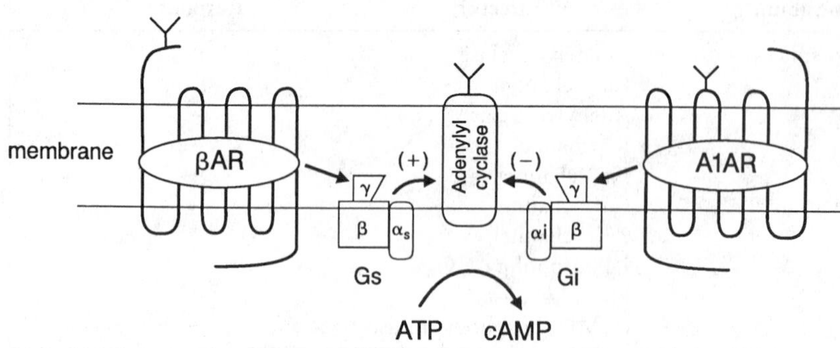

FIGURE 3-6 Typical hormone-sensitive adenylyl cyclase system. The β-adrenergic receptor (β-AR) is a typical stimulating receptor that interacts with the stimulatory G protein (G_s) shown in its heterotrimeric form with the α, β, γ subunits. The enzyme adenylyl cyclase is shown as a transmembrane protein (actually has multiple transmembrane domains) with a carbohydrate chain (γ) shown on its extracellular surface. The A_1 adenosine receptor (A_1-AR) is a typical inhibitory receptor that interacts with the inhibitory guanine nucleotide binding protein (G_i) to inhibit the enzyme adenylyl cyclase. Each receptor contains a carbohydrate chain (γ).

both mechanisms may be operative but under different conditions.

Receptor Function

The original concept of transmembrane signaling put forward by Sutherland's group[41] in 1967 was that a hormone activated a specific receptor, which in turn directly activated an effector. This model was constructed based on what was known about multisubunit enzymes. As the complexity of the signaling systems in terms of components, cofactors, and component interactions became apparent, more diverse pathways and interactions had to be expected and explained.

For example, traditionally receptor classes were defined by their relative affinities for specific agonists and antagonists. Thus, a distinct pharmacologic potency series defined a given receptor type or class. Evidence slowly accumulated that there appeared to be pharmacologic variations within receptor classes leading to the concept of receptor subtypes. With the recent application of the techniques of molecular biology to the field of receptor classification, we are only now beginning to appreciate the great diversity nature has to offer. For illustrative purposes we can again use adrenergic receptors as a model. Ahlquist,[42] in 1948, first demonstrated that catecholamines exerted their effects through two different receptors based on a pharmacologic profile. He termed these alpha and beta receptors. With the advent of radioligand binding studies and the synthesis of new ligands it became clear that each of these receptor types could be subdivided into β_1- and β_2-adrenergic and α_1- and α_2-adrenergic receptors by pharmacologic criteria. Now with molecular cloning techniques it is clear that there is a β_3 receptor found predominantly in fat tissues and that there are at least three subtypes of each of the α_1- and α_2-adrenergic receptors. Where this proliferation of receptor subtypes will end is not at all clear at the present time.

Not only has the number of receptor subtypes grown dramatically but so has the number of G proteins and effector systems to which each receptor may couple. Dogma has been that β-ARs always activate cAMP as their mechanism for cell signaling, and by implication the only effector system that the G_s protein could activate was adenylyl cyclase. Recent studies now clearly document that β-ARs acting via G_s can directly open Ca^{2+} channels without first activating adenylyl cyclase and cAMP.[25] Similarly, the A_1 adenosine receptor (A_1-AR), which was thought to produce its effect only via inhibition of adenylyl cyclase, is now known to also open K^+ channels.[25] Whether or not there are separate and distinct G_i-like proteins that mediate these two effects remains unproven. To further complicate matters, a single receptor subtype may well be capable of activating several different G proteins.[25]

As is evident from this brief discussion, our ability to find and study the components of the signaling apparatus has far outstripped our ability to define how each component interacts to maintain selectivity and specificity in a physiologically relevant manner. Much additional work will be necessary to better define the processes (pathways) involved between receptor activation and physiologic responses.

Receptor Regulation

G-protein coupled receptors have long been recognized to be dynamic entities capable of being regulated by pathophysiologic processes.[26,34,43–45] This regulation is now known to occur at multiple levels, i.e., transcriptional, translational, and posttranslational. In addition, it is clear that activation of certain G-protein coupled receptors can lead to alterations in the quantity and functionality of G proteins.[46–48] These multiple levels of regulation make possible a very fine "tuning" mechanism for controlling the transmembrane signal transduction process for either an enhancement or a diminuation of receptor signaling. The last decade has demonstrated that each of the components of hormone-sensitive adenylyl cyclase systems can be modified either quantitatively or functionally or both in a variety of model systems. Table 3-2 lists the known or possible modes of regulation. Obviously, not all of these changes occur in any one cell system or for any pathophysiologic perturbation.

TABLE 3-2
Modes of Receptor Signaling Regulation

I. Changes in receptor number
  a. Increase or decrease in transcriptional rate (mRNA)
  b. Alteration in translatability or stability of mRNA
  c. Alteration in protein half-life or stability
  d. Removal of receptor from membrane
II. Covalent alterations of receptor
  a. Phosphorylation
  b. Fatty acid acylation
III. Alterations in receptor-G protein coupling
IV. Changes in G protein quantity and/or functionality
V. ? Alterations in G protein–Effector interaction
VI. ? Alterations in effector unit quantity or functionality

There are now a large number of conditions known to modulate receptor signaling including agonist-induced desensitization, antagonist-induced sensitization, changes in steroid and thyroid hormone levels, cAMP changes, congestive heart failure (CHF), diabetes, and ischemia.[26,43,45] One of the physiologically and therapeutically important modes of regulation is the phenomenon of agonist-induced desensitization. Desensitization refers to the attenuation of responsiveness to an agonist in its continued presence—a phenomenon well appreciated in clinical medicine. At least two major mechanisms are responsible for agonist-mediated desensitization including regulation of receptor number on the cell surface and the ability of these receptors to interact with the appropriate G proteins to transmit a signal. These two final pathways for regulation can result from changes occurring at many different levels. In the β-AR system at least three different processes are involved with desensitization. The first is uncoupling of the receptor from its G_s protein, which is rapid (seconds to minutes). Second is sequestration of the receptor away from its normal cell surface membrane domain to a less accessible compartment. Third is down regulation, wherein there is an absolute decrease in the total cellular receptor population. Agonist-specific or homologous desensitization is usually defined as a decrease in adenylyl cyclase responsiveness to a single agonist after chronic exposure to that agonist. In contrast, heterologous desensitization occurs when the responsiveness of a number of receptor-mediated agonists or nonreceptor activators of adenylyl cyclase, such as guanine nucleotides or sodium fluoride, are decreased after an exposure to a single agonist.[34,49] These two processes may not be mutually exclusive, however, and heterologous desensitization may occur in addition to homologous desensitization, particularly if agonist exposure is prolonged.[34,49] Recent evidence links the phosphorylation of the receptor with the rapid uncoupling of the receptor from the effector units.

A major step forward in elucidating potential mechanisms involved in homologous desensitization was the discovery and characterization of a new receptor-specific kinase by Benovic et al.[50] This kinase has been called the β-AR kinase, although it is now known that it can phosphorylate other integral membrane receptors. This kinase is different and distinct from other kinases, such as the cAMP-dependent protein kinase or protein kinase C. The most interesting property of β-AR kinase is that it preferentially phosphorylates the agonist-occupied receptor rather than an antagonist or unoccupied receptor. This raises the prospect that in vivo phosphorylation of the agonist-occupied receptor may play a direct role in the desensitization process. There is compelling circumstantial evidence that this may be the case. First, the phosphorylated receptor under the appropriate in vitro conditions displays an 80 percent decrease in its ability to interact with G_s (uncoupled). Second, the time course for phosphorylation of the β-AR in intact cells parallels the time course of desensitization. Third, β-AR kinase displays wide tissue distribution. Finally, the sequestration of phosphorylated receptors into the cell is subsequently associated with their dephosphorylation and recycling back to the cell membrane.

Homologous desensitization is not thought to be a cAMP-mediated event, i.e., elevated concentrations of cAMP without receptor activation and consequent increased protein kinase A activity do not mimic catecholamine-induced desensitization.

In contrast, heterologous desensitization may involve multiple pathways that include both receptor protein changes as well as alterations in the other components of the adenylyl cyclase system. This form of desensitization usually results from a more prolonged exposure to agonists and the process proceeds at a slower rate. In contrast to homologous desensitization, heterologous desensitization can be directly induced by increases in cAMP concentrations in some systems.[49] Thus, administration of stable analogues of cAMP to cells can totally mimic the phenomenon of catecholamine-induced desensitization in some model systems. This suggests that activation of protein kinase A may be a mediator of some forms of desensitization.

The mechanism(s) responsible for sequestration of the receptor is much less clear and may not involve phosphorylation. The sequestration does appear to be agonist dependent and may involve a specific conformation of the receptor that initiates the translocation process. Where this sequestered region is and how the receptor stays there are also unknown.

Down regulation as mentioned above refers to the state wherein there is an actual decrease in the total cellular pool of receptors associated with a decreased agonist responsiveness. This down regulation appears to be a much slower process than is uncoupling and sequestration. There is at present an incomplete understanding of how down regulation occurs. When the quantity of any protein changes, there are always at least two possible mechanisms involved, including altered synthesis, altered degradation, or both. In the case of G-protein coupled receptors, both possibilities appear to be implicated. Evidence has recently been put forth to suggest that there is enhanced proteolysis of the receptor during desensitization.[34] In addition, altered synthesis of new messenger ribonucleic acid (mRNA) involving regulation of transcription likewise has been documented.[45] The cloning of the genes for G protein receptors has now permitted the evaluation of receptor regulation at the deoxyribonucleic acid (DNA)/RNA levels.[45]

Several groups have now documented that prolonged

exposure of cells to β-ARs, cAMP analogues, or forskolin (a diterpine that activates adenylyl cyclase) produces a down regulation of β-ARs that is accompanied by a significant decrease in β-AR mRNA levels.[45] A number of the above agents are known to increase cAMP and hence to activate protein kinase A. A logical assumption, therefore, is that the protein kinase A pathway must be involved in this pathway. The pathway leading to decreased transcription is likely independent of the well-known cAMP regulating motif (CRE) found in many promoter/enhancer regions of genes that act to increase transcription.[45] A mechanism for decreasing the quantity of mRNA is that of decreasing messenger stability and hence decreasing its half-life. A decreased half-life results in less time available for the mRNA to be translated. Evidence for just such a mechanism has now been described for the β-AR. When a smooth-muscle cell line was treated with agonist, the half-life of the β-AR mRNA was significantly decreased. Although the mechanism responsible for the change in stability is not known, the 3′-untranslated region of the β_2-AR mRNA contains sequences that have been found in other mRNAs that are short lived and highly regulated.[45]

Although agonist-induced receptor regulation has been highlighted here, for completeness the effect of endocrine modulation on receptor regulation should be briefly mentioned. Hormones, such as cortisol and thyroid hormone, have long been recognized to modulate receptor responsiveness.[26] The glucocorticoids increase β-AR number and epinephrine responsiveness in many cells. In addition, cotreatment of cells with glucocorticoids and catecholamines leads to a diminished desensitization compared to treatment with catecholamines alone.[45] This suggests that glucocorticoids might act by enhancing receptor synthesis or preventing down regulation. Recent studies have documented that glucocorticoids can directly increase the rate of β_2-AR gene transcription and that a rapid elevation of mRNA preceded an increase in the number of β-AR found at the cell surface.[45] Glucocorticoids are known to promote increases in gene transcription via a specific DNA motif in the enhancer/promoter region, which has been termed a glucocorticoid response element (GRE). This enhancer is a 15 base pair element that binds a specific glucocorticoid-protein complex.[45] A similar GRE has been identified in the β_2-AR gene, and this may explain the effect of glucocorticoid responsiveness of the β-AR.[45]

G-Protein Regulation

Not only are receptors capable of being regulated but so too are G proteins. This regulation of G proteins by G-protein coupled receptor activation remains enigmatic compared to what is known concerning receptor regulation. The earliest pathophysiologic condition known to modulate G-protein quantity was probably altered thyroid hormone levels.[26] The most common scenario is that hyperthyroidism is associated with an increased quantity of G_s while hypothyroidism is associated with a decrease in G_s.[26] This is, however, not found in all cell types studied. Chronic activation of G-protein receptors has been associated with modulation of G proteins.[47,48] An excellent example of this is the activation of the A_1 adenosine receptor (A_1-AR) in adipocytes. In this in vivo rat model, following long-term activation of the A_1-AR by agonists, there is a decrease in the ability of adenosine to mediate inhibition of adenylyl cyclase. This desensitization occurs concomitantly with a sensitization to the effects of agonists that stimulate adenylyl cyclase.[47,48] These changes are associated with a decreased quantity of the G_i proteins and an increased quantity of the G_s proteins.[47,48] These changes occur with no alteration in the quantity of the mRNAs for these proteins.[48] The mechanism for these changes remains speculative. The changes in the G proteins may well explain the phenotypic changes seen in cellular responsiveness following desensitization in this system.[47,48] Similar changes in G proteins have now been described for a variety of receptor systems.[5]

Receptor Signaling in the Heart

The heart has been the focus of a large number of studies on how pathophysiologic conditions may modify G-protein coupled receptor initiated transmembrane signaling. As described above, much has been learned concerning the regulation of receptors in model systems, but a detailed understanding of receptor systems in the heart has lagged behind. There are several reasons for the disparity in knowledge. First, there were no continuous cell lines of myocardial cells. Second, the number of receptors on myocardial cells is typically much lower (by a factor of 10 to 100) than on many other cells and tissues. Third, myocardial membranes have been labile and sensitive to proteinases, which renders them unresponsive to agonist-mediated effector activation. Even with these difficulties many pathophysiologic conditions are known to modulate receptors, G proteins, and responsiveness of adenylyl cyclase systems.[52,53] If we have learned anything about these systems, it has been that regulation is complex and multifactorial. Simply to count receptors or G proteins is not sufficient, and detailed studies of each of the components and their interactions is necessary to comprehend how a complex organ such as the heart is regulated. Even when much information is available, it is still not always clear whether the changes seen are cause or effect. An example of this occurs during CHF in the human heart. Many studies have documented that a number of alterations occur in the adenylyl cyclase system of the heart in CHF.[53] These include a decreased cAMP responsiveness to catecholamines, decreases in β-AR number, an uncoupling of β-ARs from G_s, and an increased quantity of the inhibitory G protein, G_i. All of these changes could help explain the decreased contractile responsiveness to catecholamines in CHF. On the other hand, a causal relationship between the changes in the receptor system and the decreased contractile response has not been documented. An equally plausible possibility is that the receptor system changes are a consequence of the high circulating catecholamines seen in end-stage CHF, which essentially induce a state of desensitization. These caveats are not mentioned to disparage the work thus far performed in CHF, but only to point out that much additional information is necessary before any definitive statement can be made relating to the role receptor signaling systems play in the pathophysiology

TABLE 3-3
Pathophysiology and Regulation of Receptor Components in the Heart

Disease/Intervention	Receptor Number	G-Protein Coupling	G-Protein Quantity/ Function
Congestive heart failure	β-AR (↓) A_1-AR (○)	↓ Coupling	↑ G_i; G_s (↓,○)
Hyperthyroidism	β-AR (↑)	↑ Coupling	?
Hypothyroidism	β-AR (↓)	?	?
Desensitization (catecholamines)	β-AR (↓)	↓ Coupling	No change
β -Blockers	β-AR (↑,○)	?	No change
Methylxanthines	A_1-AR (↑)	↑ Coupling	No change
Ischemia	β-AR (↑)	?	?

↓ = decrease, ↑ = increase, ○ = no change; β_1-AR = β-adrenergic receptor, A_1-AR = A_1 adenosine receptor.

of CHF. Table 3-3 is a partial listing of pathophysiologic conditions (treatments) known to regulate components of the G-protein coupled receptor system in the heart. (See also Chap. 25.)

SUMMARY

This chapter has attempted to highlight some of the recent advances in the areas of cell membrane structure, ion channels, and G-protein coupled receptors. A major aim has been to illustrate that these topics are not in any way distinct or separate topics but rather are intimately related structurally, functionally, and in how they are regulated. As our knowledge of these membrane components increases, we will better be able to understand cardiac pathophysiology and to develop rational therapeutic and preventive modalities to decrease morbidity and mortality associated with heart disease.

REFERENCES

1. Alberts B, Bray D, Lewis J, Raff M, Roberts K, Watson JD (eds): *Molecular Biology of the Cell*, 2d ed. New York, Garland, 1989.
2. Vouce DE, Vouce JE (eds): *Biochemistry of Lipids and Membranes*. Menlo Park, CA, Benjamin/Cummings, 1985.
3. Benga G, Tager JM: *Biomembranes: Basic and Medical Research*. New York, Springer-Verlag, 1988.
4. Jain M, Wagner R: *Introduction to Biological Membranes*. New York, Wiley, 1980.
5. Lewis DL, Lechleiter JD, Kim D, Nanavati C, Clapham DE: Intracellular regulation of ion channels in cell membranes. *Mayo Clin Proc* 1990; 65:1127–1143.
6. Jan LY, Jan YN: Voltage-sensitive ion channels. *Cell* 1989; 56:13–25.
7. Hartzell HC: Regulation of cardiac ion channels by catecholamines, acetylcholine and second messenger systems. *Prog Biophys Mol Biol* 1988; 52:165–247.
8. Rehm H, Tempel BL: Voltage-gated K^+ channels of the mammalian brain. *FASEB J* 1991; 5:164–170.
9. Krueger BK: Toward an understanding of structure and function of ion channels. *FASEB J* 1989; 3:1906–1914.
10. Brown AM, Birnbaumer L: Ionic channels and their regulation by G protein subunits. *Annu Rev Physiol* 1990; 52:197–213.
11. Numa S: A molecular view of neurotransmitter receptors and ionic channels. In: *The Harvey Lectures*, Series 83. New York, Alan R. Liss, 1989: 121–165.
12. Bolton TB, Beech DJ, Komori S, Prestwich SA: Voltage- and receptor gated channels. In: *Frontiers in Smooth Muscle Research*. New York, Alan R. Liss, 1990; 229–243.
13. Birnbaumer L, Codina J, Yatani A, Mattera R, Graf R, Olate J, et al: Molecular basis of regulation of ionic channels by G proteins. In: *Recent Progress in Hormone Research*, vol 45. New York, Academic, 1989: 121–208.
14. Belardinelli L, Linden J, Berne RM: The cardiac effects of adenosine. *Prog Cardiovasc Dis* 1989; 32:73–97.
15. Guy HR, Conti F: Pursuing the structure and function of voltage-gated channels. *Trends Neurosci* 1990; 13:201–206.
16. Montal M: Molecular anatomy and molecular design of channel proteins. *FASEB J* 1990; 4:2623–2635.
17. Agnew WS: A Rosetta stone for K channels. *Nature* 1988; 331:114–115.
18. Catterall WA: Excitation-contraction coupling in vertebrate skeletal muscle: A tale of two calcium channels. *Cell* 1991; 64:871–874.
19. Catterall WA: Structure and function of voltage-sensitive ion channels. *Science* 1988; 242:50–61.
20. Hille B: *Ionic Channels of Excitable Membranes*. Sunderland, MA, Sinauer, 1984.
21. Loughney K, Kreser R, Ganetzley B: Molecular analysis of the paralocus, a sodium channel in drosophila. *Cell* 1989; 58:1143–1154.
22. Kayano T, Noda M, Flockerzi V, Takahashi H, Numa S: Primary structure of rat brain sodium channel III deduced from the cDNA sequence. *FEBS Lett* 1988; 228:187–194.
23. Noda M, Ikeda T, Suzaki H, Takeshima H, Takahashi T, Kuno M, et al: Expression of functional sodium channels from cloned cDNA. *Nature* 1986; 322:826–828.
24. Froehner SC: New insights into the molecular structure of the dihydropyridine-sensitive calcium channel. *Trends Neurosci* 1988; 11:90–92.
25. Birnbaumer L, Abramowitz J, Yatani A, Okabe K, Mattera R, Graf R, et al: Roles of G proteins in coupling of receptors to ionic channels and other effector systems. *Biochem Mol Biol* 1990; 25:225–244.
26. Stiles GL, Caron MG, Lefkowitz RJ: The β-adrenergic receptor: Biochemical mechanisms of physiological regulation. *Physiol Rev* 1984; 64:661–743.
27. Parker EM, Ross EM: G protein-coupled receptors: Structure and function of signal-transducing proteins. In: *Current Topics in Membranes and Transport*, vol 36. New York, Academic, 1990: 131–144.
28. Caron MG: The guanine nucleotide regulatory protein-coupled receptors for nucleosides, nucleotides, amino acids and amine neurotransmitters. *Cell Biol* 1989; 1:159–166.
29. Carpenter G, Cohen S: Epidermal growth factor. *J Biol Chem* 1990; 265:7709–7712.
30. Brown MS, Goldstein JL: Lipoprotein receptors: Therapeutic implication. *J Hypertens* (Suppl) 1990; 8:533–535.

31. Dohlman HG, Caron MG, Lefkowitz RJ: A family of receptors coupled to guanine nucleotide regulatory proteins. *Biochemistry* 1987; 26:2657–2664.
32. Nathans J, Thomas D, Hogness DS: Molecular genetics of human color vision: The genes encoding blue, green, and red pigments. *Science* 1986; 232:193–202.
33. Henderson R, Unwin PNT: Three dimensional model of purple membrane obtained by electron microscopy. *Nature* 1975; 257:28–32.
34. Raymond JR, Hnatowich M, Lefkowitz RJ, Caron MG: Adrenergic receptors: Models for regulation of signal transduction processes. *Hypertension* 1990; 15:119–131.
35. Dohlman HG, Caron MG, DeBlasi A, Frielle T, Lefkowitz RJ: A role of extracellular disulfide bonded cysteines in the ligand binding function of the β_2-adrenergic receptor. *Biochemistry* 1990; 29:2335–2342.
36. Lefkowitz RJ, Caron MG: Adrenergic receptors: Models for receptors coupled to guanine nucleotide regulatory proteins. *J Biol Chem* 1988; 263:4993–4996.
37. Strader CD, Sigal IS, Dixon RAF: Structural basis of β-adrenergic receptor function. *FASEB J* 1989; 3:1825–1832.
38. Hibert MF, Trumpp-Kallmeyer S, Bruinvels A, Hoflack J: Three-dimensional models of neurotransmitter G-binding protein-coupled receptors. *Mol Pharmacol* 1991; 40:8–15.
39. Gilman AG: G proteins: Transducers of receptor-generated signals. *Annu Rev Biochem* 1987; 56:615–649.
40. Birnbaumer L: Transduction of receptor signal into modulation of effector activity by G proteins: The first 20 years or so. . . . *FASEB J* 1990; 4:3068–3078.
41. Robinson GA, Butcher RW, Sutherland EW: Adenylyl cyclase as an adrenergic receptor. *Ann NY Acad Sci* 1967; 139:703–723.
42. Ahlquist RP: A study of the adrenotropic receptors. *Am J Physiol* 1948; 153:585–600.
43. Stiles GL: Adenosine receptors and beyond: Molecular mechanisms of physiological regulation. *Clin Res* 1990; 38:10–18.
44. Sibley DR, Benovic JL, Caron MG, Lefkowitz RJ: Regulation of transmembrane signaling by receptor phosphorylation. *Cell* 1987; 48:913–922.
45. Collins S, Caron MG, Lefkowitz RJ: Regulation of adrenergic receptor responsiveness through modulation of receptor gene expression. *Annu Rev Physiol* 1991; 53:497–508.
46. Ramkumar V, Bumgarner JR, Jacobson KA, Stiles GL: Multiple components of the A_1 adenosine receptor-adenylate cyclase system are regulated in rat cerebral cortex by chronic caffeine ingestion. *J Clin Invest* 1988; 82:242–247.
47. Parsons WJ, Stiles GL: Heterologous desensitization of the inhibitory A_1 adenosine receptor-adenylate cyclase system in rat adipocytes: Regulation of both N_s and N_i. *J Biol Chem* 1987; 262:841–847.
48. Longabaugh JP, Didsbury J, Spiegel A, Stiles GL: Modification of the rat adipocyte A_1 adenosine receptor-adenylate cyclase system during chronic exposure to an A_1 adenosine receptor agonist: Alterations in the quantity of $G_{s\alpha}$ and $G_{i\alpha}$ are not associated with changes in their mRNAs. *Mol Pharmacol* 1989; 36:681–688.
49. Hausdorff WP, Caron MG, Lefkowitz RJ: Turning off the signal: Desensitization of β-adrenergic receptor function. *FASEB J* 1990; 4:2881–2889.
50. Benovic JL, DeBlasi A, Stone WC, Caron MG, Lefkowitz RJ: β-Adrenergic receptor kinase: Primary structure delineates a multigene family. *Science* 1989; 246:235–240.
51. Rich KA, Codina J, Floyd G, Sekura R, Hildebrandt JD, Iyengar, R: Glucagon-induced heterologous desensitization of the MDCK cell adenylyl cyclase. *J Biol Chem* 1984; 259:7893–7901.
52. Stiles GL, Lefkowitz, RJ: Cardiac adrenergic receptors. *Annu Rev Med* 1984; 35:149–164.
53. Stiles GL: Adrenergic receptor responsiveness and congestive heart failure. *Am J Cardiol* 1991; 67:13C–17C.

Chapter 4

Anatomy of the Heart

Bruce F. Waller, M.D. ■ Robert C. Schlant, M.D.

GROSS ANATOMY OF THE HEART AND BLOOD VESSELS

Andreas Vesalius (1514–1564) is considered the "father" of modern anatomy. Since his day, however, new observations have been made that provide an important framework for understanding cardiac physiology and pathophysiology, for examining the patient, and for interpreting noninvasive and invasive tests of the heart.[1-14]

The heart is situated in the middle mediastinum with its "long axis" oriented from the left upper abdominal quadrant to the right shoulder. The heart has a *base*, which is formed by the atria and great arteries, and an *apex*, which is formed by the junction of the ventricles and ventricular septum.

The sternum and costal cartilages of the third, fourth, and fifth ribs overlie the heart anteriorly. About two-thirds of the heart is left of the midline. The heart rests upon the diaphragm and is tilted forward and to the left so that the apex is anterior to the rest of the heart. The normal apex impulse can be palpated in the fourth or fifth intercostal space near the midclavicular line. The weight and size of the heart vary considerably depending on age, sex, body length, epicardial fat, and general nutrition. The average human adult heart averages approximately 325 ± 75 g in men and 275 ± 75 g in women.[10]

The borders of the normal cardiac silhouette in a frontal view are formed by the following structures (Fig. 4-1): The top of the cardiac silhouette is formed by the transverse and ascending aorta. The upper right margin is delineated by the superior vena cava. The right atrium provides the remaining right lateral cardiac border. Most of the inferior border is composed of right ventricle. The apex and the lower left lateral cardiac border consist of the left ventricle. The left atrial appendage perches atop the left ventricle and to the side of the pulmonary artery, interjecting on the cardiac border between the left ventricle and pulmonary outflow tract. The pulmonary outflow area forms the rest of the upper left border.

External Features

The atria are separated from the ventricles externally by the *coronary sulcus* [atrioventricular (AV) sulcus], which circles the heart between the atria and ventricles (Figs. 4-1 and 4-2). The right coronary artery, after leaving the aorta, travels in this sulcus between the right atrium and right ventricle until it descends on the posterior surface of the heart. Similarly, the left circumflex artery is found in the coronary sulcus between the left atrium and left ventricle until the artery ramifies posteriorly.

Externally, the two ventricles are delineated by interventricular sulci, which descend from the coronary sulcus toward the apex. Epicardial fat often obscures these landmarks (Fig. 4-2). The anterior interventricular sulcus contains the left anterior descending coronary artery and courses over the muscular ventricular septum between the right and left ventricles to the apex. It then turns around the apex and continues in the posterior interventricular sulcus on the diaphragmatic surface of the heart.

The posterior interventricular sulcus is the pathway for the posterior descending coronary artery, which is usually the terminal branch of the right coronary artery or, less frequently, of the left circumflex artery (Fig. 4-

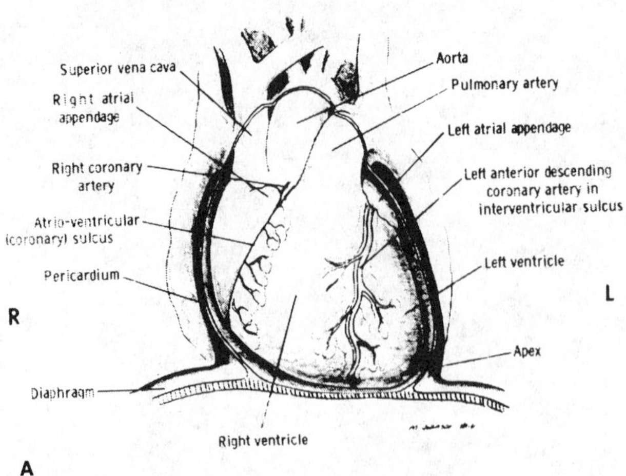

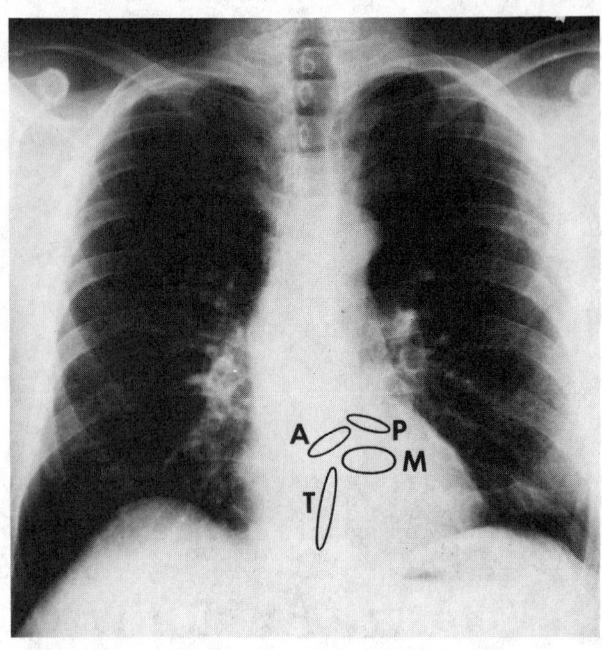

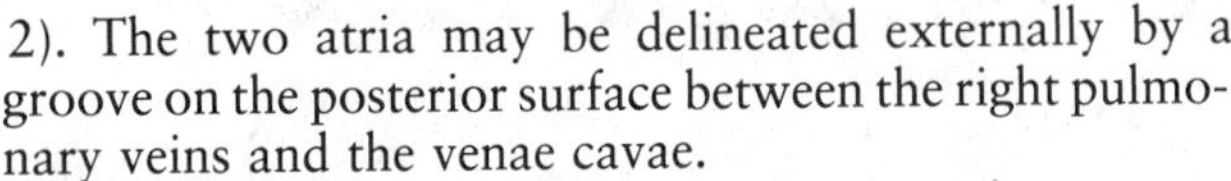

FIGURE 4-1 *A.* Diagram showing the normal relations of the pericardium, great vessels, ventricles, and atria as viewed in the frontal position. R = right; L = left. *B.* Frontal (AP) roentgenogram of the heart. The components that form the cardiac silhouette can be readily identified from *A*. A = aortic valve ring; P = pulmonary valve ring; M = mitral valve ring; T = tricuspid valve ring. (*Diagram by McClaren Johnson, Jr., M.D.*)

2). The two atria may be delineated externally by a groove on the posterior surface between the right pulmonary veins and the venae cavae.

The *crux* of the heart refers to the area on the posterior-basal surface where the coronary sulcus meets the posterior interventricular sulcus (Fig. 4-2). Internally at this junction, the atrial septum joins the ventricular septum. The coronary artery that crosses this area makes a sharp inward turn at the crux and provides a small artery to the nearby AV node. The area of the heart below the crux is referred to as the diaphragmatic, or inferior, surface of the heart. A transverse section through the heart is extremely helpful in demonstrating the relations of the cardiac chambers (Figs. 4-3 to 4-5). The ventricular and atrial septa are aligned obliquely 45° to the left of the midline with the planes of the septa directed approximately from right scapula to left nipple.[7] The entire right side of the heart is to the right of this plane, placing most of the right atrium anterior to the left atrium and most of the right ventricle anterior to the left ventricle.

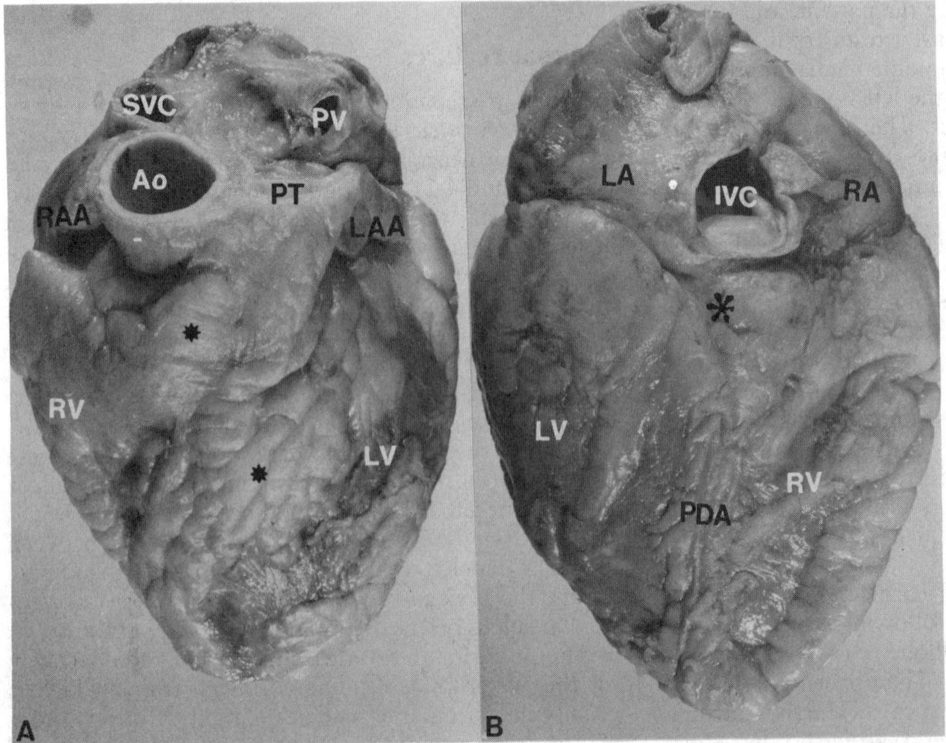

FIGURE 4-2 External views of the heart. *A.* Anterior surface showing epicardial fat*, which obscures the interventricular sulci containing the left anterior descending artery. Ao = aorta; LAA = left atrial appendage; LV = left ventricle; PT = pulmonary trunk; PV = pulmonary vein; RAA = right atrial appendage; RV = right ventricle; SVC = superior vena cava. *B.* Posterior surface of heart showing location of posterior descending artery (PDA), crux of the heart*, and inferior vena cava (IVC). LA = left atrium; RA = right atrium.

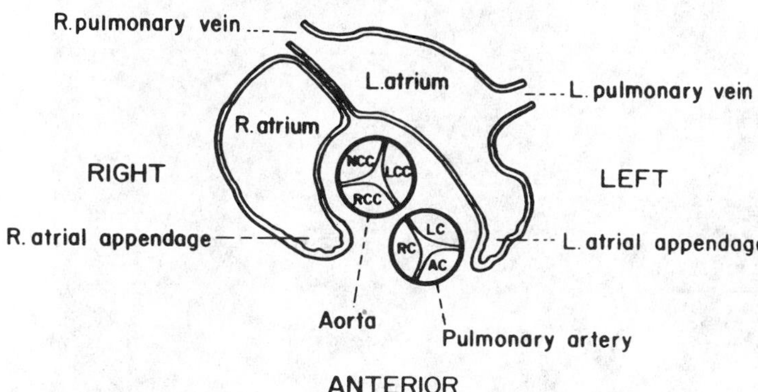

FIGURE 4-3 Schematic transverse section through the heart at approximately the level of the second intercostal space. The relation between the left and right atria and the interatrial septum is illustrated. The relative positions of the aortic and pulmonary valves and their cusps are shown. AC = anterior cusp; RC = right cusp; LC = left cusp of the pulmonary valve; LCC = left coronary cusp; RCC = right coronary cusp; NCC = noncoronary cusp of the aortic valve.

Fibrous Skeleton

A fibrous tissue framework affords a firm anchor for the attachments of the atrial and ventricular musculature as well as the valvular tissue (Figs. 4-6 and 4-7). At the center of the heart the central fibrous body (right fibrous trigone) fuses together the medial aspect of the mitral and tricuspid valve and the aortic root. The left fibrous trigone is formed by compact bundles of connective tissue that course from the central fibrous body to the left, posterior inferiorly and anteriorly. Continuations of fibroelastic tissue from the central fibrous body (right fibrous trigone) and the left fibrous trigone partially encircle the mitral and tricuspid valves. These rings of tissue are the mitral and tricuspid annuli, which serve as attachments for the mitral and tricuspid valves as well as for the atrial and ventricular muscle. In general, the fibrous skeleton is less well developed around the tricuspid valve. A triple scalloped line of heavy collagenous tissue extends anteriorly from the left and right fibrous trigones to provide a three-pointed, crownlike skeletal support for the aortic root and cusps. A substantial ligament of tissue, the conus ligament, passes from the right side of the aortic root to a similar arrangement of scalloped tissue that surrounds the pulmonic root.

An important extension of the fibrous skeleton, the membranous ventricular septum, extends inferiorly and anteriorly from the central fibrous body (right fibrous trigone).[7,9,15] This membranous septum is located at the summit of the muscular ventricular septum, where it provides support for the right coronary and noncoronary aortic cusps (Fig. 4-8). A portion of the membranous

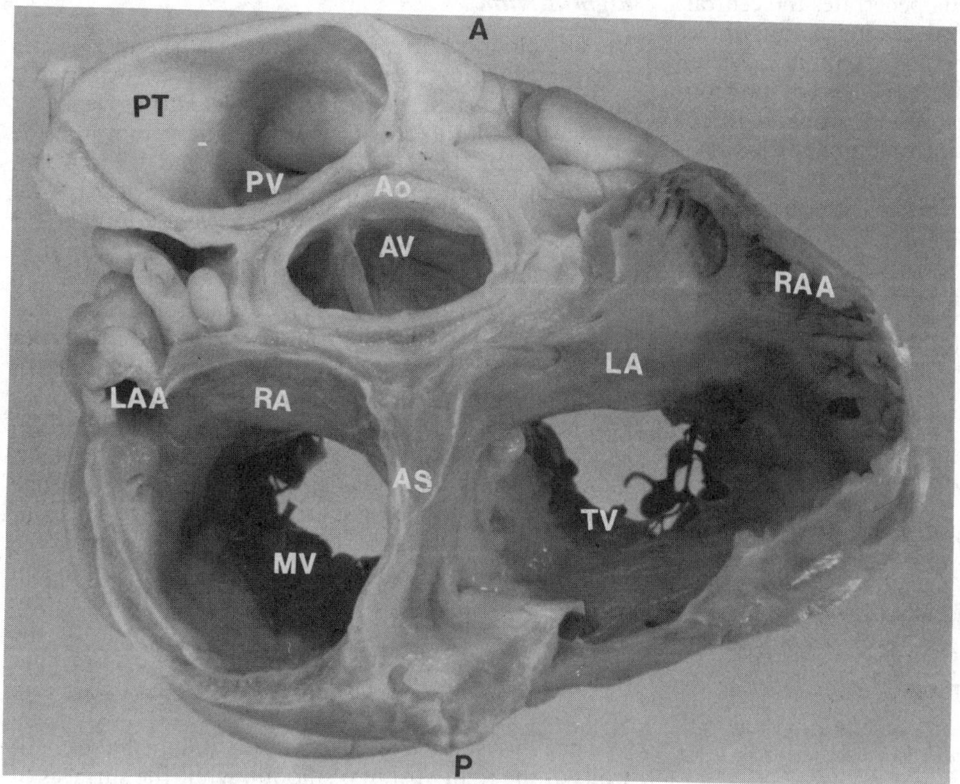

FIGURE 4-4 Transverse section through base of heart showing relationship of various chambers and great vessels. A = anterior; AO = aorta; AS = atrial septum; AV = aortic valve; LA = left atrium; LAA = left atrial appendage; MV = mitral valve; RA = right atrium; RAA = right atrial appendage; P = posterior; PT = pulmonary trunk; PV = pulmonic valve; TV = tricuspid valve. [*From BF Waller et al: Tomographic views of normal and abnormal hearts: The anatomic basis for various cardiac imaging techniques. Clin Cardiol 13:804(pt I), 877(pt II), 1990. Reproduced with permission from the publisher and authors.*]

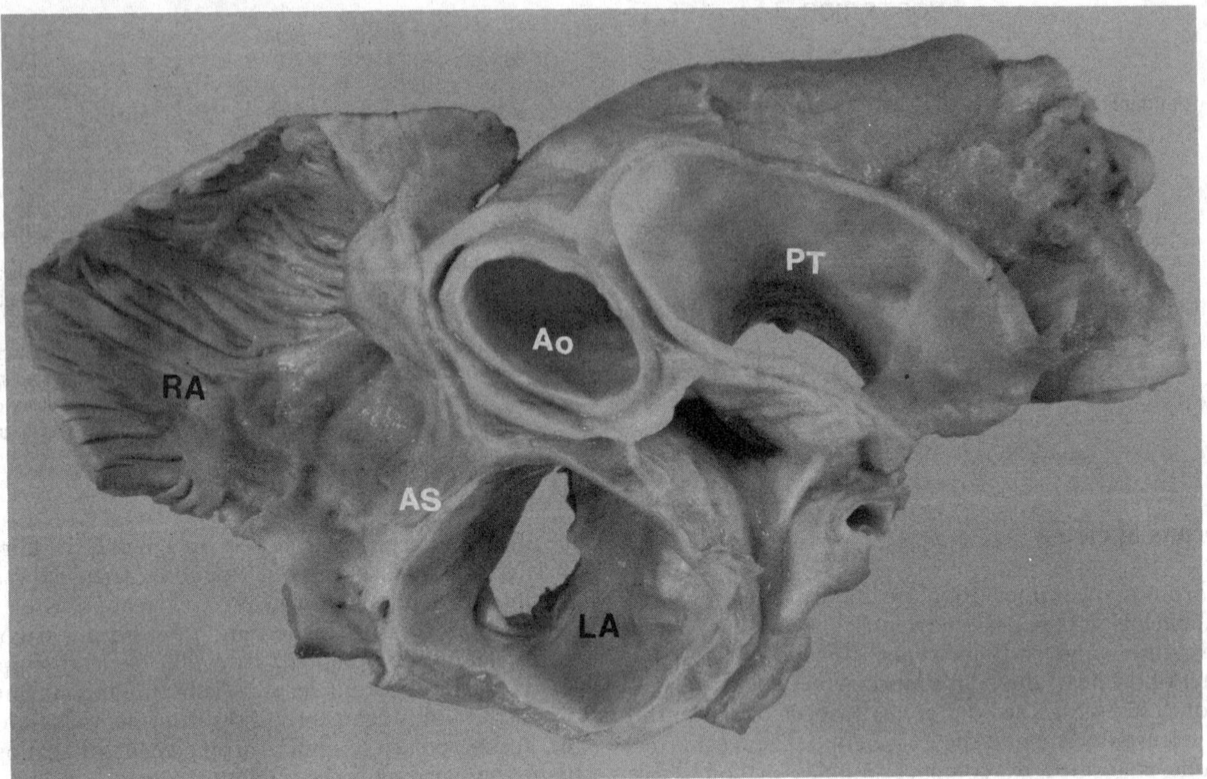

FIGURE 4-5 Basal view of heart showing relationship of great vessels and atria. The left atrium (LA) has a smooth endocardium while the right atrium (RA) is trabeculated. The aorta (Ao) is posterior to the pulmonary trunk (PT) but anterior to the atrial septum (AS). [*From BF Waller et al: Tomographic views of normal and abnormal hearts: The anatomic basis for various cardiac imaging techniques. Clin Cardiol 13:804(pt I), 877(pt II), 1990. Reproduced with permission from the publisher and authors.*]

ventricular septum extends slightly above the tricuspid valve, forming a small portion of the medial wall of the right atrium.[16] The bundle of His penetrates the central fibrous body and travels along the inferior margin of the membranous portion of the ventricular septum.[17] At the crest of the muscular septum, above the level of junction of the right coronary and posterior (noncoronary) aortic cusps, the His bundle separates into a left bundle branch and a right bundle branch. The left bundle subsequently subdivides into multiple branches that fan out as they spread to the left ventricle.

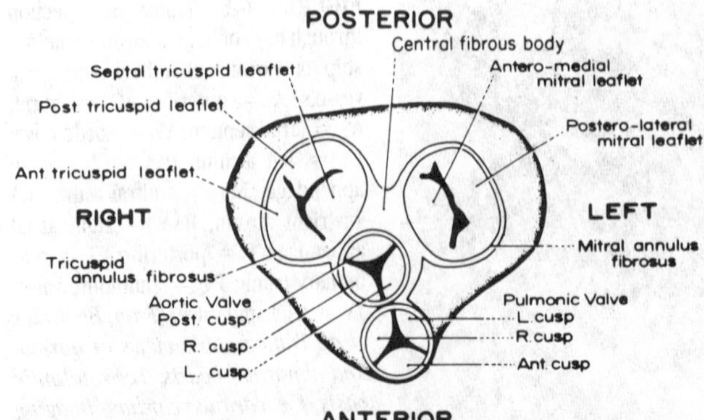

FIGURE 4-6 Schematic anterosuperior view of the heart with the atria removed. The components of the fibrous skeleton and the orientation of the leaflets of each valve are shown.

Cardiac Chambers

Right Atrium

Venous blood returns to the heart via the superior and inferior venae cavae into the right atrium, where it is stored during right ventricular systole. During ventricular diastole, blood flows from the right atrium into the right ventricle (Figs. 4-1, 4-2, 4-4, 4-7, and 4-9 to 4-11). The right atrium forms the right lateral cardiac border and is above, behind, and to the right of the right ventricle (Figs. 4-4 and 4-7). Most of the right atrium is to the right and anterior to the left atrium (Figs. 4-4 and 4-7). Anteromedially, the right atrial appendage protrudes from the right atrium and overlaps the aortic root (Figs. 4-1 and 4-2). On the posterior external surface of the right atrium a ridge, the *sulcus terminalis* (or terminal groove), extends vertically from the superior to the inferior vena cava. This corresponds to an internal muscular bundle, the crista terminalis, which runs along the edge of the entrance to the right atrial appendage to the front of the orifice of the superior vena cava and then to the right side of the inferior vena cava[7] (Figs. 4-9 to 4-11). The sinus node is usually located at the lateral margin of the junction of the superior vena cava with the right atrium and the atrial appendage, beneath or near the sulcus terminalis (terminal groove) (Figs. 4-1 and 4-2).

The inner surface of the posterior and medial (septal) walls of the right atrium is smooth, while the surfaces of

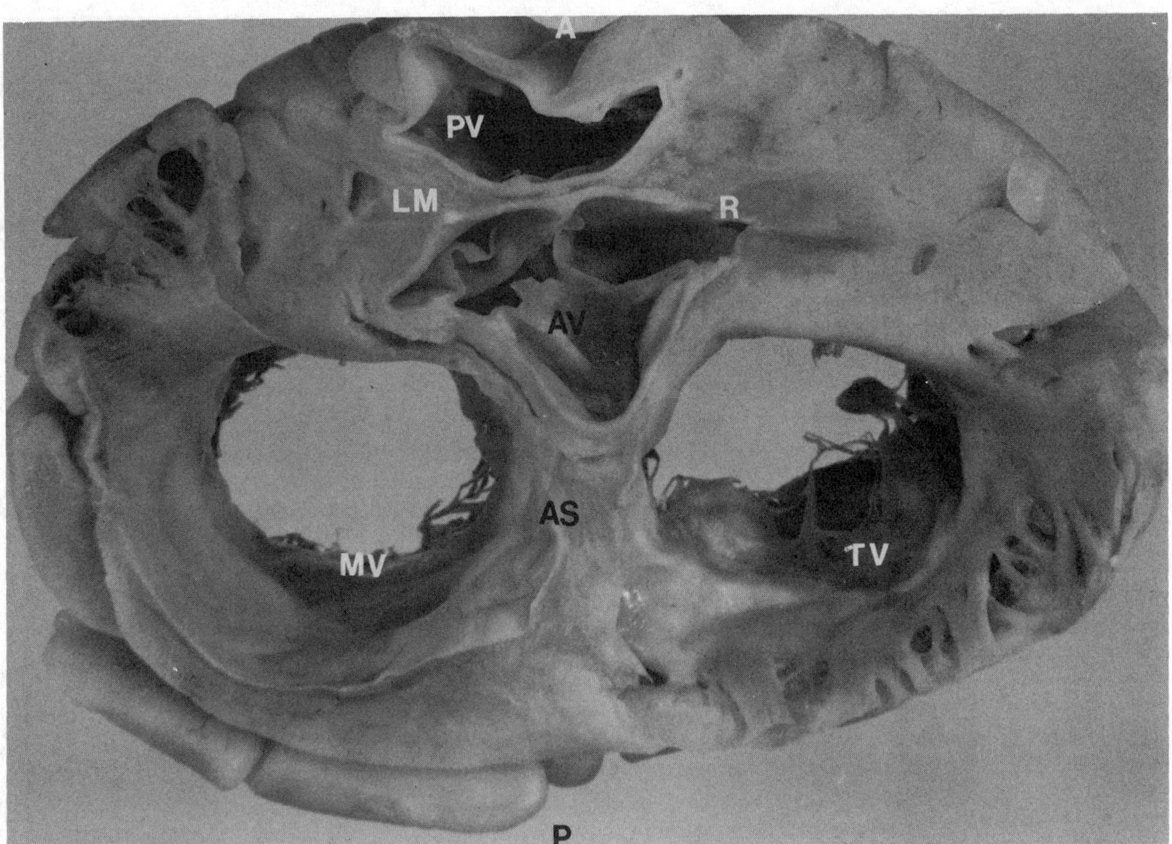

FIGURE 4-7 Cross-sectional view of heart showing aortic valve (AV), pulmonary trunk (PT), origin of the right (R) and left main (LM), coronary arteries, tricuspid (TV) and mitral (MV) valves, and atrial septum (AS). A = anterior; P = posterior. [*From BF Waller et al: Tomographic views of normal and abnormal hearts: The anatomic basis for various cardiac imaging techniques. Clin Cardiol 13:804(pt I), 877(pt II), 1990. Reproduced with permission from the publisher and authors.*]

the lateral wall and of the right atrial appendage are composed of parallel muscle bundles, the pectinate muscles[7] (Figs. 4-7 and 4-11). The right atrial wall measures almost 2 mm in thickness. The superior and inferior venae cavae enter the right atrium posteriorly and medially at its superior and inferior aspects. The orifice of the superior vena cava usually has no valve; the orifice of the inferior vena cava is flanked anteriorly by an inconstant, rudimentary valve, the *eustachian valve*, formed by a crescentic fold. The caval orifices may vary in shape and diameter depending upon the phase of respiration, the cardiac cycle, and the contraction or relaxation of surrounding muscular bands. The variation in the orifice may play some role in promoting venous return or preventing atrial reflux.

The medial wall of the right atrium includes the atrial septum and is also important because of its proximity to several structures[7] (Figs. 4-7 and 4-9 to 4-11). Anteriorly, the posterior (noncoronary) cusp and the right coronary cusp of the aortic root lean against the medial right atrium, forming a normal slight bulge known as the *torus aorticus*, which is a useful landmark during transseptal catheterization of the left side of the heart. The proximal right coronary artery is in the immediate vicinity as it enters the coronary sulcus. The proximity of the aortic root to the right atrium permits an aneurysm of the sinus of Valsalva to rupture into the right atrium.

The atrial septum (Figs. 4-3, 4-4, 4-7, and 4-9 to 4-11) is found in the posteroinferior portion of the medial wall of the right atrium and extends obliquely forward from right to left.[18] Near the center of the atrial septum there is a shallow depression, the *fossa ovalis*, which often has a prominent fold, or limbus, anteriorly. The ostium of the coronary sinus is located between the inferior vena cava and the tricuspid valve (Figs. 4-9 to 4-11). The orifice of the coronary sinus is guarded by a rudimentary flap of tissue, the Thebesian valve. The AV node is located in the lower atrial septum, anterior and medial to the coronary sinus, just above the septal leaflet of the tricuspid valve. The sinus and AV nodes, as well as the entire conducting pathways, are not grossly visible.

Right Ventricle

The right ventricle receives venous blood from the right atrium during ventricular diastole and propels blood into the pulmonary circulation during ventricular systole (Figs. 4-9 to 4-14). The right ventricle is normally the most anterior cardiac chamber, lying directly beneath the sternum (Figs. 4-1 and 4-2). Enlargement or hyperactivity of the right ventricle may often be detected by palpation of the sternum or the lower left sternal border. The right ventricle is partially below, in front of, and medial to the right atrium but anterior and to the right

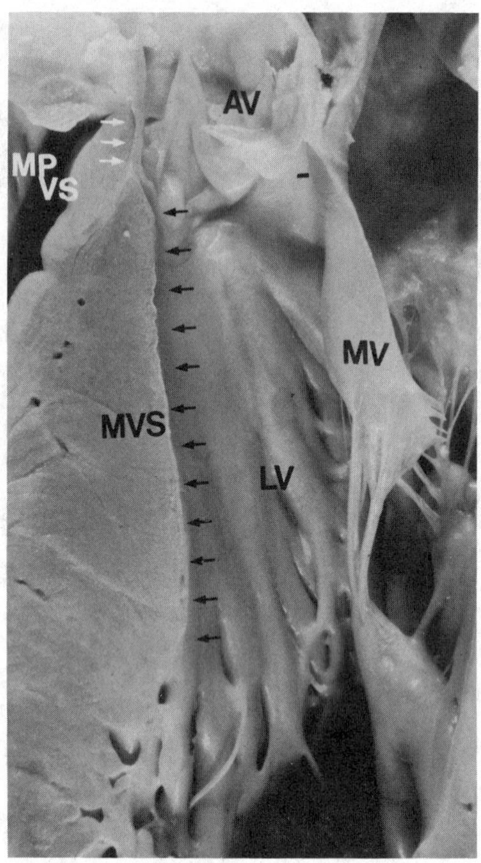

FIGURE 4-8 Specimen showing the muscular ventricular septum (MVS) (black arrows) and membranous portion of the ventricular septum (MPVS) (white arrows). LV = left ventricle; MV = mitral valve.

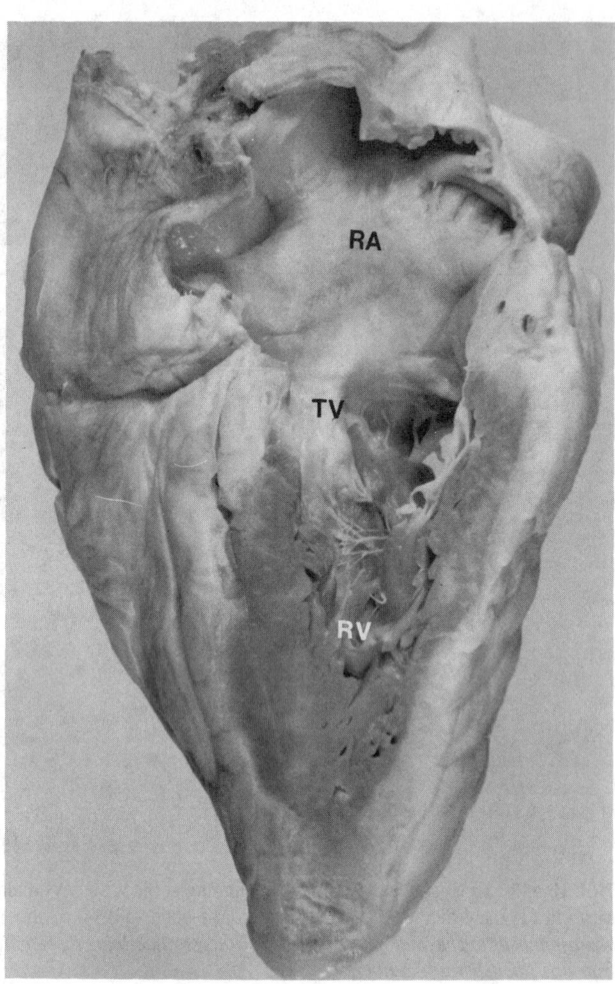

FIGURE 4-9 Long-axis view of right side of heart showing right ventricle (RV), right atrium (RA), and tricuspid valve (TV). The RV walls are heavily trabeculated. [*From BF Waller et al: Tomographic views of normal and abnormal hearts: The anatomic basis for various cardiac imaging techniques. Clin Cardiol 13:804(pt I), 877(pt II), 1990. Reproduced with permission from the publisher and authors.*]

of the left ventricle. Most of the entire inferior border of the frontal roentgenogram view of the heart consists of the right ventricle (Fig. 4-1).

The striking difference in configuration between the two ventricles is illustrated by a transverse section (Figs. 4-12 and 4-13). The left ventricular chamber is an ellipsoidal sphere surrounded by relatively thick (8 to 15 mm at autopsy) musculature, well suited to ejecting blood against the high resistance of the systemic vessels. The right ventricle, which normally contracts against very low resistance, has a crescent-shaped chamber and a thin outer wall, measuring 4 to 5 mm in thickness.[19] The anterior right ventricular wall curves over the ventricular septum, which normally bulges into the right ventricular cavity. Although the ventricular septum forms the medial wall of both ventricles, it seems to contribute predominantly to left ventricle function in normal subjects. The anterior and inferior walls of the right ventricular cavity are lined by muscle bundles, the *trabeculae carneae*, which often form ridges along the inner surface of the wall or cross from one wall to the other (Figs. 4-9 to 4-14). A rather constant muscle, the *moderator band*, crosses from the lower ventricular septum to the anterior wall, where it joins the anterior papillary muscle (Figs. 4-9 to 4-11). The right bundle branch, after traveling through the muscular ventricular septum, courses through the moderator muscle to the endocardium of the right ventricle.

Functionally, the right ventricle can be partitioned into an inflow tract, an outflow tract, and an apical trabecular component (body). The trabecular muscles in the apex of the right ventricle are much more coarse than those in the left ventricle. The inflow tract, consisting of the tricuspid valve and the trabecular muscles of the anterior and inferior walls, directs entering blood anteriorly, inferiorly, and to the left at an angle of 60° to the outflow tract[20] (Fig. 4-9). The smooth-walled outflow tract, also referred to as the *infundibulum*, forms the superior portion of the right ventricle. It is separated from the inflow tract by a thick muscle, the *crista supraventricularis*, which arches from the anterolateral wall over the anterior leaflet of the tricuspid valve to the septal (medial) wall, where it joins other constrictor bands of muscle that encircle the outflow tract[14,21] (Figs. 4-9 and 4-14). Blood entering the infundibulum is ejected superiorly and posteriorly into the pulmonary trunk.

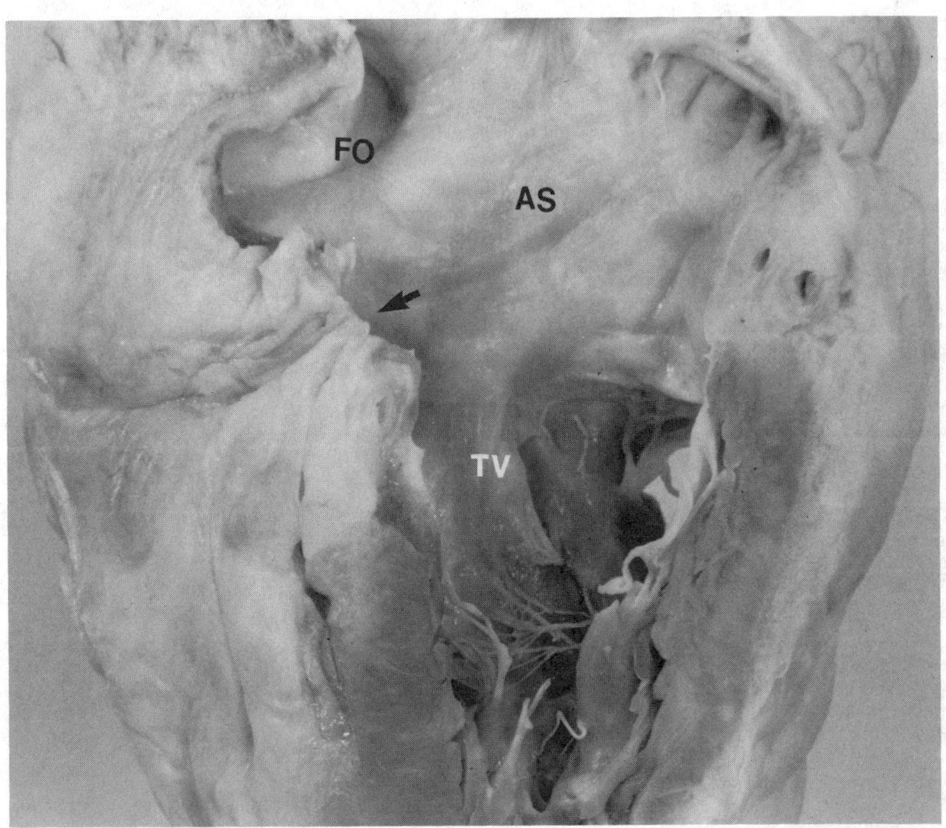

FIGURE 4-10 Closeup of right atrium showing atrial septum (AS), foramen ovale (FO), entrance to orific of coronary sinus (arrow), and tricuspid valve (TV).

Left Atrium

The left atrium receives blood from the pulmonary veins and serves as the reservoir during left ventricular systole and as a conduit during left ventricular filling. In addition, left atrial contraction provides a significant increment of blood to the left ventricle, stretching the ventricle and priming it for ventricular ejection. This is sometimes referred to as the "atrial kick" or atrial component of ventricular filling. (See Chap. 5.)

The left atrium is located superiorly, in the midline, and posterior to the other cardiac chambers (Figs. 4-3, 4-4, 4-7, 4-11, and 4-15). As a consequence of this posterior position, the left atrium is not normally seen in the frontal roentgenogram. The esophagus abuts directly on its posterior surface, while the aortic root impinges on its anterior wall. The right atrium is located to the right and anterior (Fig. 4-3). The left ventricle is to the left, anterior, and inferior. The posterior position of the left atrium makes it impossible to palpate externally unless it is massively dilated. With severe mitral regurgitation, however, expansion of the left atrium from the regurgitation and the ejection recoil of the anteriorly located ventricles may force the heart anteriorly, producing a late systolic sternal lift. The left atrium usually enlarges posteriorly and laterally in mitral stenosis or regurgitation, occasionally even reaching the right or left lateral chest wall.

The wall of the left atrium is 3 mm, slightly thicker than that of the right atrium. Two pulmonary veins enter posterolaterally on each side, conveying oxygenated blood from the lungs. Though there are no true valves at the junction of the pulmonary veins and the left atrium, "sleeves" of atrial muscle extend from the left atrial wall around the pulmonary veins for 1 or 2 cm and may exert a partial sphincter-like influence, tending to lessen reflux during atrial systole or mitral regurgitation (Figs. 4-11 and 4-15).

The endocardium of the left atrium is smooth and slightly opaque (Figs. 4-11 and 4-15). Pectinate muscles are present only in the left atrial appendage, which projects from the anterolateral left atrium, alongside the pulmonary artery. The atrial septum is smooth but may contain a central shallow area, corresponding to the fossa ovalis (Figs. 4-11 and 4-15).

Left Ventricle

The left ventricle receives blood from the left atrium during ventricular diastole and ejects blood into the systemic arterial circulation during ventricular systole (Figs. 4-11 to 4-13 and 4-15). The left ventricle is roughly bullet shaped with the blunt tip directed anteriorly, inferiorly, and to the left, where it contributes, with the lower ventricular septum, to the apex of the heart.[22] Although the left ventricle forms the lower left lateral cardiac border in the frontal roentgenogram, the major portion of its external surface is posterolateral (Fig. 4-1). The left ventricle is posterior and to the left of the right ventricle and inferior, anterior, and to the left of the left atrium. The left ventricular chamber is approximately an ellipsoidal sphere, surrounded by thick muscular walls measuring 8 to 15 mm, or approximately

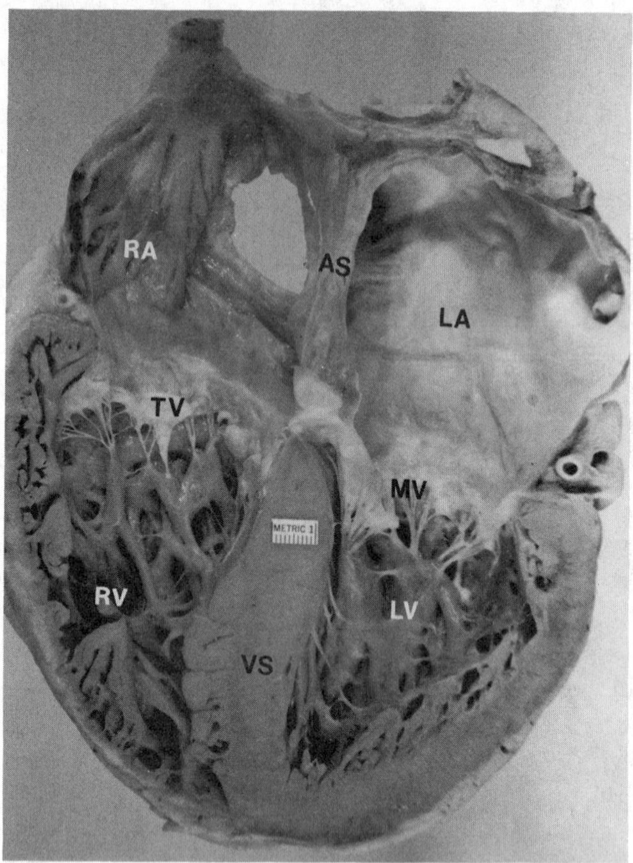

FIGURE 4-11 Four-chamber view of heart showing morphologic differences between the four chambers. The right atrium (RA) is more trabeculated than the left (LA), and the right ventricle (RV) is more heavily and coarsely trabeculated compared to the left ventricle (LV). AS = atrial septum; MV = mitral valve; TV = tricuspid valve; VS = ventricular septum. [*From BF Waller et al: Tomographic views of normal and abnormal hearts: The anatomic basis for various cardiac imaging techniques. Clin Cardiol 13:804(pt I), 877(pt II), 1990. Reproduced with permission from the publisher and authors.*]

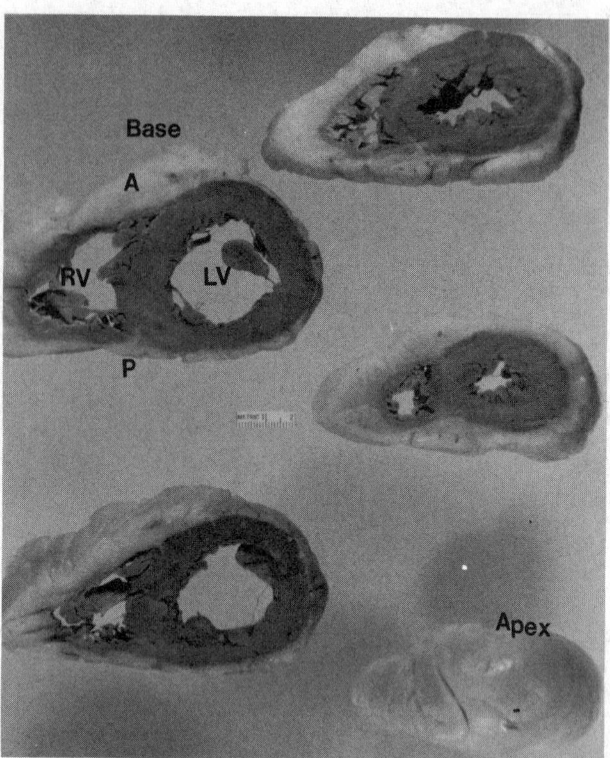

FIGURE 4-12 Family of ventricular slices from base to apex. A = anterior; LV = left ventricle; RV = right ventricle; P = posterior; VS = ventricular septum. The LV cavity is more "circular" shaped compared to the more "triangular" shaped RV cavity. [*From BF Waller et al: Tomographic views of normal and abnormal hearts: The anatomic basis for various cardiac imaging techniques. Clin Cardiol 13:804(pt I), 877(pt II), 1990. Reproduced with permission from the publisher and authors.*]

two to three times the thickness of the right ventricular wall. The tip of the left ventricular apex is often thin, sometimes measuring 2 mm or less. The medial wall of the left ventricle is the *ventricular septum*, which is shared with the right ventricle (Figs. 4-2, 4-11 to 4-13, and 4-15). The septum, which is roughly triangular in shape with the base of the triangle at the level of the aortic cusps, is entirely muscular except for the small membranous septum, located superiorly just below the right coronary and the posterior coronary cusps (Figs. 4-8, 4-11, and 4-15). The upper third of the septum is smooth endocardium. The remaining two-thirds of the septum and the remaining ventricular walls are ridged by interlacing muscles, the *trabeculae carneae*. The ventricular wall exclusive of the septum is often referred to as the free wall of the left ventricle.

The anteromedial leaflet of the mitral valve, which is the larger and more mobile of the two mitral leaflets, extends from the top of the posteromedial septum across the ventricular cavity to the anterolateral ventricular wall and separates the left ventricular cavity into an inflow and an outflow tract (Figs. 4-15 and 4-16). The funnel-shaped inflow tract, which is formed by the mitral annulus and by both mitral leaflets and their chordae tendineae, directs the entering atrial blood inferiorly, anteriorly, and to the left (Figs. 4-15 and 4-16). The outflow tract, surrounded by the inferior surface of the anteromedial mitral leaflet, the ventricular septum, and the left ventricular free wall, orients the blood flow from left ventricular apex to the right and superiorly at an angle of 90° to the inflow tract.[7] With the onset of ventricular systole, both mitral leaflets are propelled together and upward, converting the entire left ventricle into an expulsion chamber. The apical portion of the left ventricle is characterized by fine trabeculations.

Cardiac Valves

The heart contains four cardiac valves: two semilunar and two atrioventricular.[23] The two semilunar valves, aortic and pulmonic, guard the outlet orifice of their respective left and right ventricles. The two AV valves, mitral and tricuspid, guard the inlet orifice of their respective left and right ventricles. The four cardiac valves are surrounded by fibrous tissue forming partial or complete "rings" (valve annulus). These fibrous rings join to form the fibrous skeleton of the heart, to which also are attached atrial and ventricular myocardium. The area between the septal leaflet of the tricuspid valve, the ante-

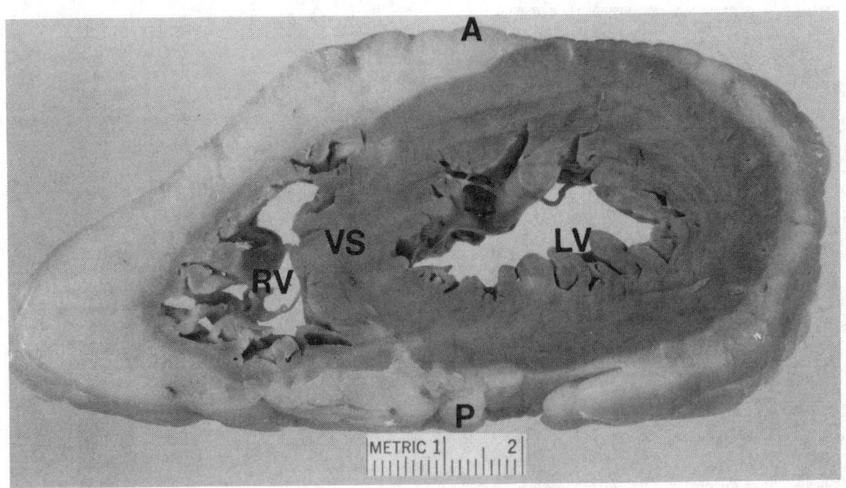

FIGURE 4-13 Closeup of ventricular slice seen in Fig. 4-12. This view corresponds to the short-axis echocardiographic views of the ventricular cavities. A = anterior; LV = left ventricle; RV = right ventricle; VS = ventricular septum. [*From BF Waller et al: Tomographic views of normal and abnormal hearts: The anatomic basis for various cardiac imaging techniques. Clin Cardiol 13:804(pt I), 877(pt II), 1990. Reproduced with permission from the publisher and authors.*]

rior leaflet of the mitral valve, and the posterior or noncoronary cusp of the aortic valve forms one part of the central fibrous body. The remaining portion is made up of fibrous tissue connecting the left aortic cusp and the anterior leaflet of the mitral valve.[23]

Histological Structure

Each cardiac valve has a central collagenous core, the fibrosa, which is continuous with the collagen of the cardiac skeleton and of the chordae tendineae. Both sides of the fibrosa are covered by loose fibroelastic tissue, usually containing mucopolysaccharides, and the entire valve is covered by endothelium. The endothelium and connective tissue of the AV valves are continuous with atrial and ventricular endocardium, and those of the semilunar valves are continuous with the aortic and pulmonary intima. Gross and Kugel[24] have proposed that the loose connective tissue on the atrial aspect of the AV valves be termed the *atrialis*, that on the ventricular surface of all four valves the *ventricularis*, and that on the aortic or pulmonary side of the semilunar valves the *arterialis*. Smooth and striated cardiac muscle may extend onto the proximal one-third of the atrialis in the AV valves and often contains blood vessels. The distal two-thirds of the normal AV valve and all the semilunar valve are avascular.[23–27]

Semilunar Valves

The semilunar aortic and pulmonary valves are similar in configuration, except the aortic cusps are slightly thicker.[23, 28–30] They are situated at the summit of the outflow tract of their corresponding ventricle, the pulmonary valve being anterior, superior, and slightly to the left of the aortic valve (Figs. 4-4, 4-6 to 4-8, and 4-14 to 4-19). Each valve is composed of the three fibrous cusps. The pulmonary valve differs from the aortic valve by having no discrete annulus or fibrous ring. The U-shaped convex lower edges of each cusp are attached to and

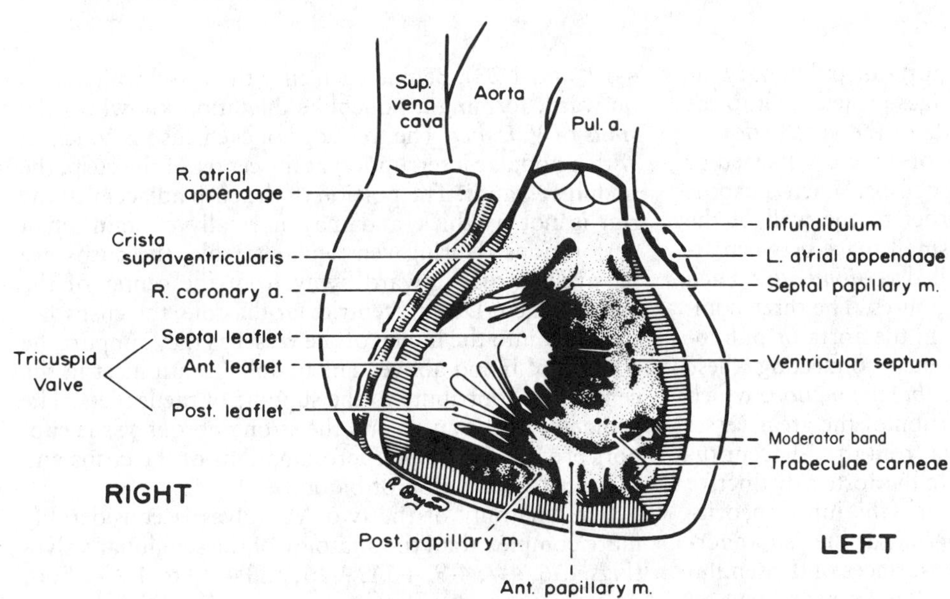

FIGURE 4-14 Schematic representation of a frontal view of the heart. The anterior right ventricular wall has been removed to demonstrate the orientation of the tricuspid leaflets and the papillary muscles. The anterior papillary muscle is sectioned. The trabeculated inflow portion of the right ventricle is contrasted with the smooth infundibular (outflow) area.

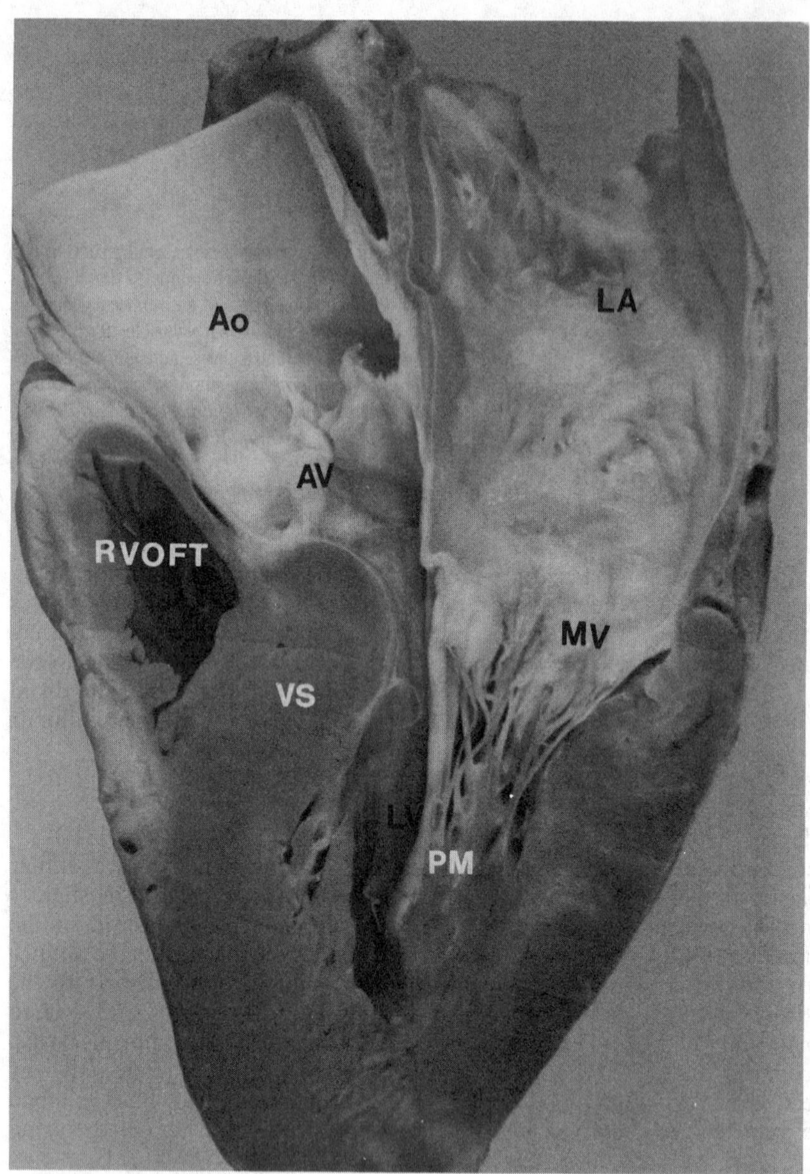

FIGURE 4-15 Long-axis view of left side of heart showing aorta (Ao), left atrium (LA), left ventricle (LV), mitral valve (MV), papillary muscle (PM) of mitral valve, aortic valve (AV), and right ventricular outflow tract (RVOFT). [*From BF Waller et al: Tomographic views of normal and abnormal hearts: The anatomic basis for various cardiac imaging techniques. Clin Cardiol 13:804(pt I), 877(pt II), 1990. Reproduced with permission from the publisher and authors.*]

suspended from the root of the aorta or pulmonary artery, with the upper free valve edges projecting into the lumen. The cusps circle the inside of the vessel root.[31]

Each semilunar valve consists of three equal-sized or nearly equal-sized semicircular cusps. Each cusp is attached by its semicircular border to the wall of the aorta or pulmonary trunk. The small space between attachments of adjacent cusps is called a *commissure*. Each semilunar valve has three commissures. The three commissures lie equally spaced around the aorta or pulmonary trunk, and the circumference connecting these points has been termed the *sinotubular junction*, which may also be described as the portion of the great vessel separating the sinuses of Valsalva from the adjacent tubular portion of the great artery. In the aorta a distinctive circumferential "hump" or line marks this junction, originally described by Leonardo da Vinci as the "supraaortic ridge." Each of the ventricular surfaces of the semilunar cusps has a small nodule [much more prominent on the aortic valve (*noduli Arantii*)] in the center of the free edge marking the contact sites of closure (Figs. 4-18, 4-19, and 4-23). Behind each cusp the vessel wall bulges outward, forming a pouchlike dilatation known as the *sinus of Valsalva*. The free edge of each cusp is concave, with a nodular interruption at the center of the cusp, the nodulus Arantii. The portion of the cusp adjacent to the rim is not as thick and may normally contain small perforations. During ventricular systole, the cusps are passively thrust upward away from the center of the aortic lumen. During ventricular diastole, the cusps fall passively into the lumen of the vessel as they support the column of blood above. The noduli Arantii meet in the center and contribute to the support of the leaflets. The geometry of the cusps and the strong fibrous tissue support provide excellent approximations of the cusps and prevent regurgitation of blood.

The anatomy of the two AV valves is considerably more complex than the anatomy of the semilunar valves (Figs. 4-6, 4-7, 4-9, 4-11, 4-15, and 4-20 to 4-23). Both AV valves consist of leaflets (two mitral and three tricuspid), chordae tendineae, papillary muscles (two or three, respectively), and valve annuli. The leaflets are demar-

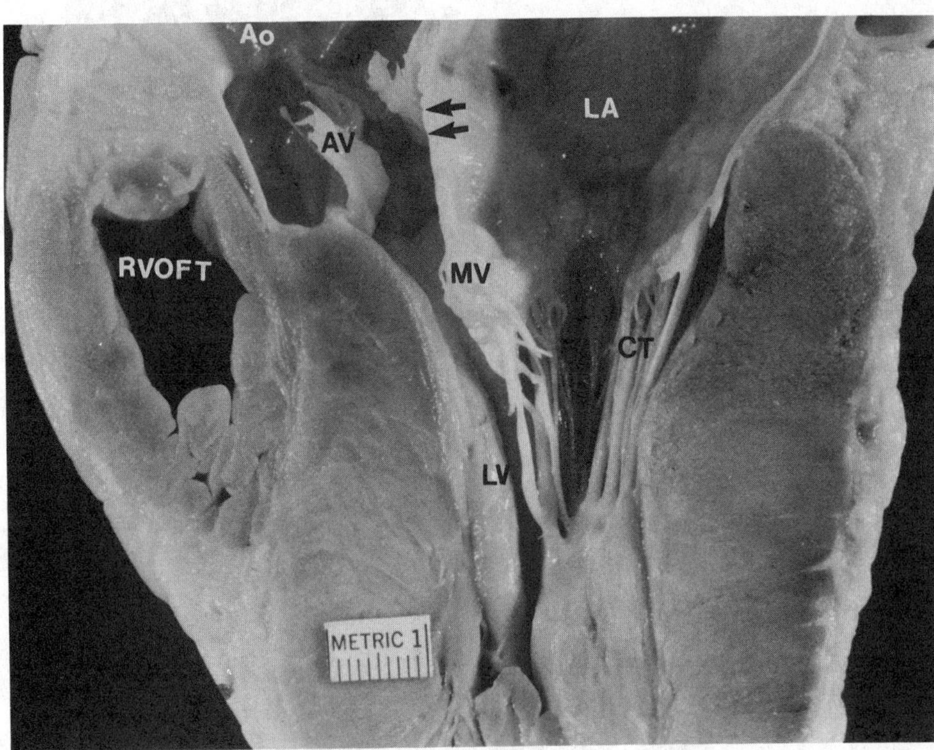

FIGURE 4-16 Long-axis view of left ventricle showing continuity of aortic (AV) and mitral (MV) valves (arrows) and chordae tendineae (CT) of MV. Ao = aorta; LA = left atrium; LV = left ventricle; RVOFT = right ventricular outflow tract.

cated by commissures located along the valve annular attachment. The anterior leaflet of each of the AV valves is the largest and is roughly semicircular in shape. The posterior mitral leaflet and the posterior and septal tricuspid leaflets have shorter annulus to free edge distances but longer basal attachments, compared to the respective anterior leaflet. Complex chordal structures arise from papillary muscles or directly from ventricular myocardium and insert onto the free edge and several millimeters from the margin on the ventricular surface. The annular structure of the mitral valve primarily surrounds the posterior leaflet, while the anterior leaflet does not have a

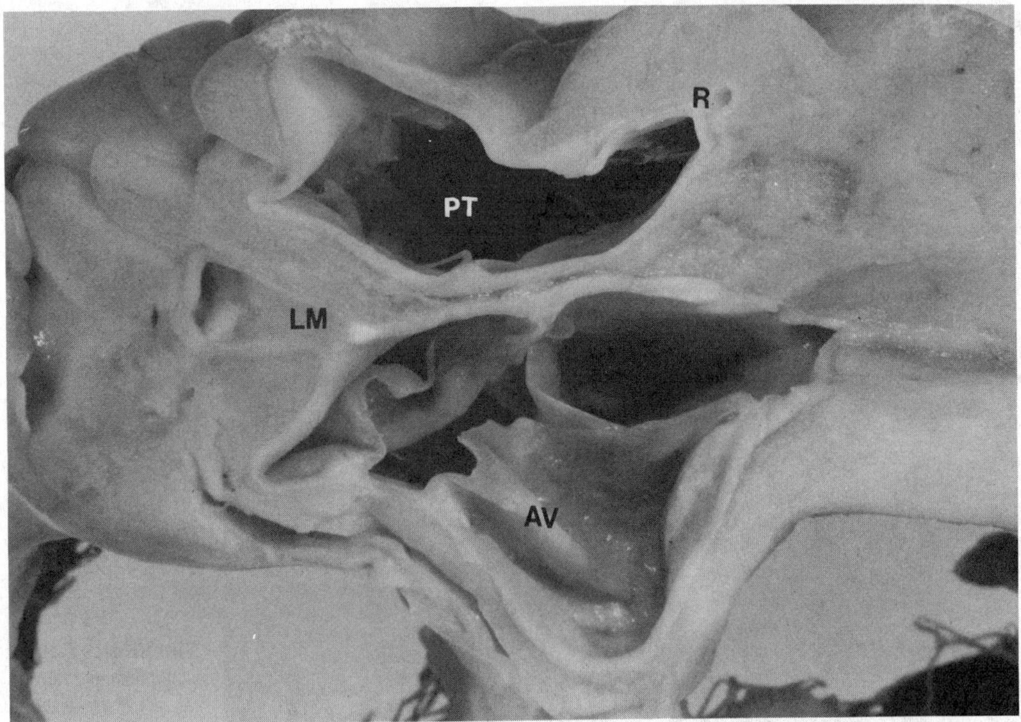

FIGURE 4-17 Short-axis view of three-cuspid aortic valve (AV) and pulmonary trunk (PT). L = left main coronary ostium; R = right coronary ostium. [*From BF Waller et al: Tomographic views of normal and abnormal hearts: The anatomic basis for various cardiac imaging techniques. Clin Cardiol 13:804(pt I), 877(pt II), 1990. Reproduced with permission from the publisher and authors.*]

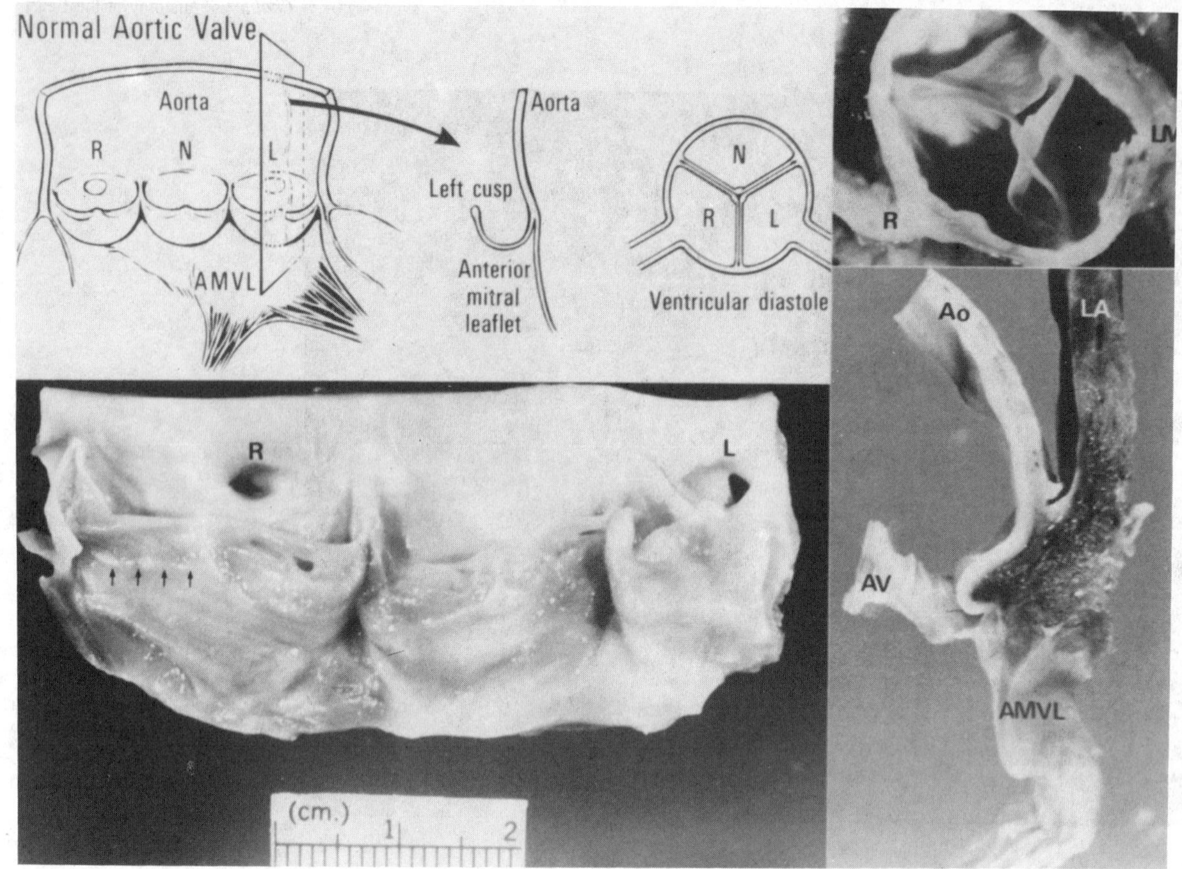

FIGURE 4-18 Morphology of the normal aortic valve. AMVL = anterior mitral valve leaflet; Ao = aorta; AV = aortic valve; LV = left main; N = noncoronary cusp; LA = left atrium; R = right; RC = right coronary artery. Arrows point to line of closure. Portion of aortic cusp above the line of closure is called the lunula. *(From BF Waller: Morphologic aspects of valvular heart disease: Part I. Curr Prob Cardiol IX:13, 1985. Reproduced with permission from the publisher and author.)*

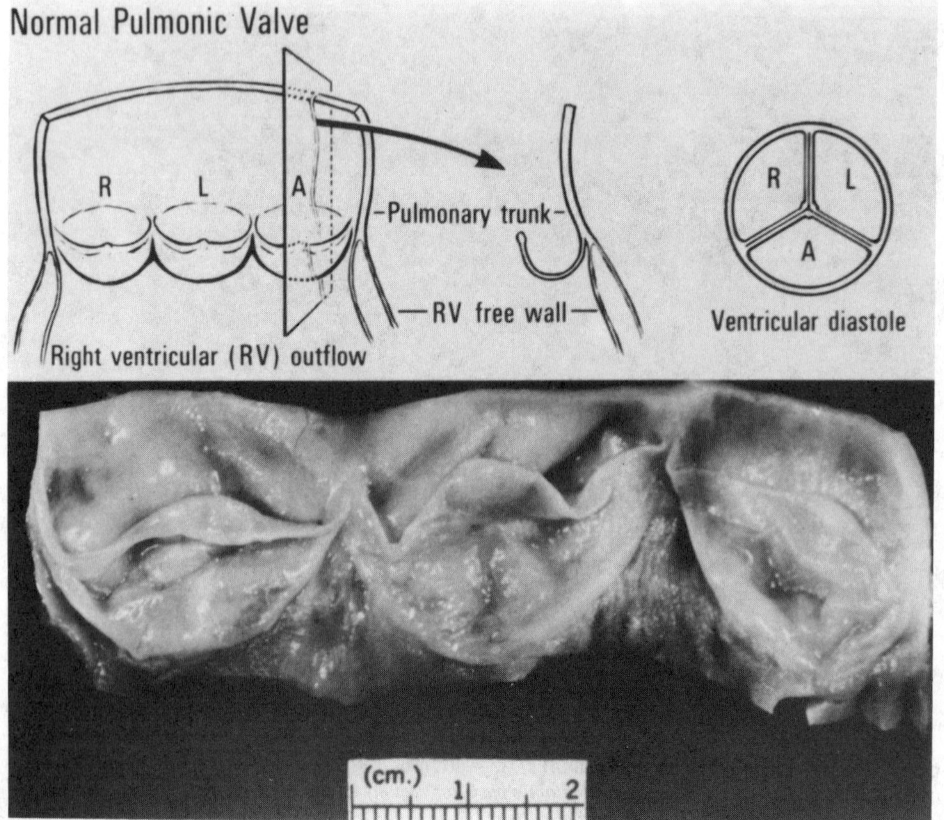

FIGURE 4-19 Morphology of the normal pulmonic valve. A = anterior; L = left; R = right. *(From BF Waller: Morphologic aspects of valvular heart disease: Part I. Curr Prob Cardiol IX:13, 1985. Reproduced with permission from the publisher and author.)*

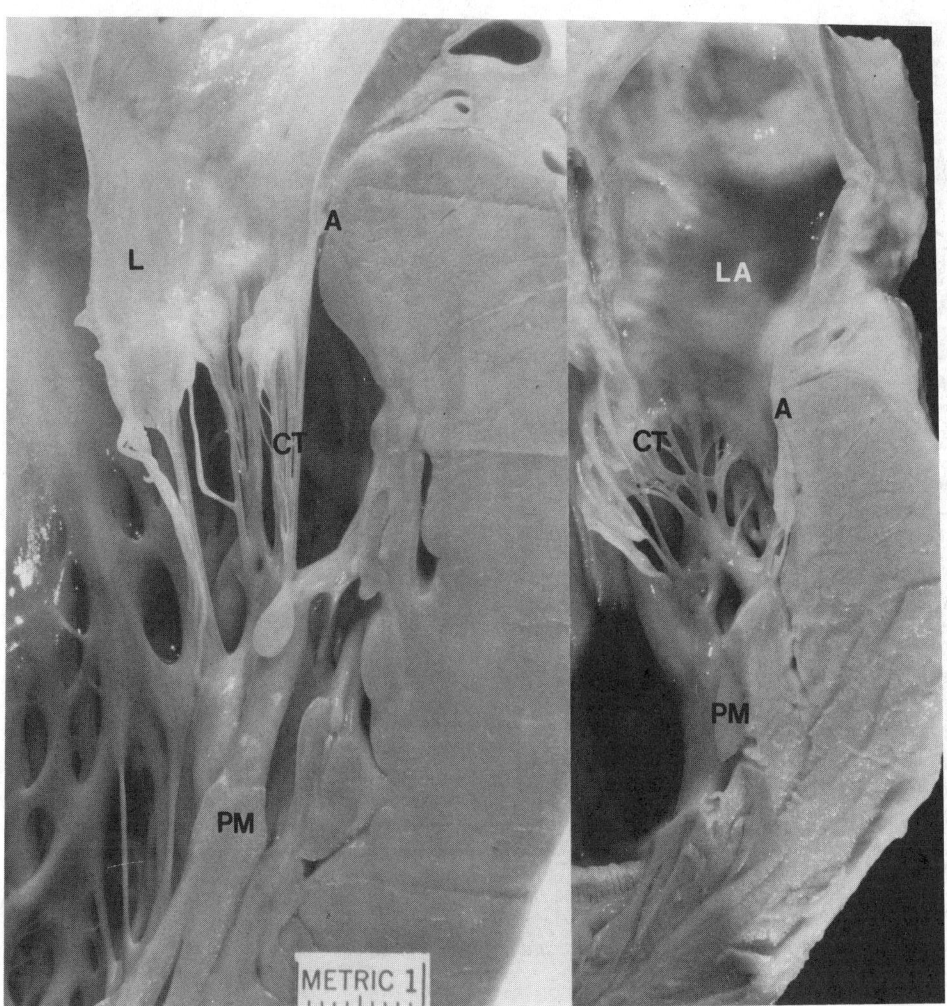

FIGURE 4-20 Mitral valve apparatus. *Left*: Chordae tendineae (CT); leaflet (L); annulus (A); papillary muscle (PM). *Right*: Left atrium (LA). Note the interchordal connections (arrows) and chordal connections from both anterior and posterior mitral leaflets to the posteromedial papillary muscle (right). [*From BF Waller et al: Tomographic views of normal and abnormal hearts: The anatomic basis for various cardiac imaging techniques. Clin Cardiol 13:804(pt I), 877(pt II), 1990. Reproduced with permission from the publisher and authors.*]

true annulus but is continuous with the wall of ascending aorta, aortic valve, and membranous ventricular septum. The annulus of the tricuspid is nearly circumferential, is larger than the mitral annulus, and lies at a lower level (i.e., more apical) than the mitral annulus. On the atrial surface of the AV valves, 0.5 to 1.0 cm from the free edge, is a line of nodular thickening (more prominent on the mitral valve), marking the contact points of closure.[23]

Specific Valve Structure

Aortic Valve

General The normal tricuspid aortic valve (Figs. 4-17 and 4-18) is a symmetric structure in which the orifice of the fully opened valve is central and the cusps are easily mobile and retract to the aortic commissures. When the valve is closed, all three cusps meet and overlap equally. The circumferential distances between each of the three commissures and the depth of the aortic valve sinus (from sinotubular junction to base of sinus) in a normally formed valve are similar (Fig. 4-18). Each of the ventricular surfaces of the aortic cusps has a small nodule in the center of the free edge that marks the closure contact site. A small rim of valve tissue above this nodule, known as the *lunula*, overlaps the neighboring cusp and serves as a supporting strut. Fenestrations of the lunula are quite common but are of no functional consequence. Fenestrations of the aortic valve lunula increase with age.[30]

The sinotubular junction, the aortic sinuses of Valsalva, the valve cusps and commissures, and the junction of aortic valve with the ventricular septum and anterior mitral valve leaflet make up the aortic valve complex. The narrowest circumference is at the lowermost portion of this complex, the junction with ventricular septum. This circumference (diameter), referred to as the *aortic ring*, is measured by surgeons to determine the size of an aortic prosthetic valve. Pathologists at necropsy, on the other hand, measure the circumference (8 to 10 cm) at the sinotubular junction, which more closely corresponds to the measurements made by the echocardiographers during life.

The three aortic valve cusps have been termed the left, right, and noncoronary (posterior) cusps, with each of the left and right sinuses of Valsalva giving rise to the left and right main epicardial coronary artery, respectively. Knowledge of the adjacent anatomic structures or chambers of the aortic valve is important in determining potential sites of left-to-right shunting. Rupture of the right and noncoronary sinuses of Valsalva may communicate with right-sided chambers (right ventricular outflow

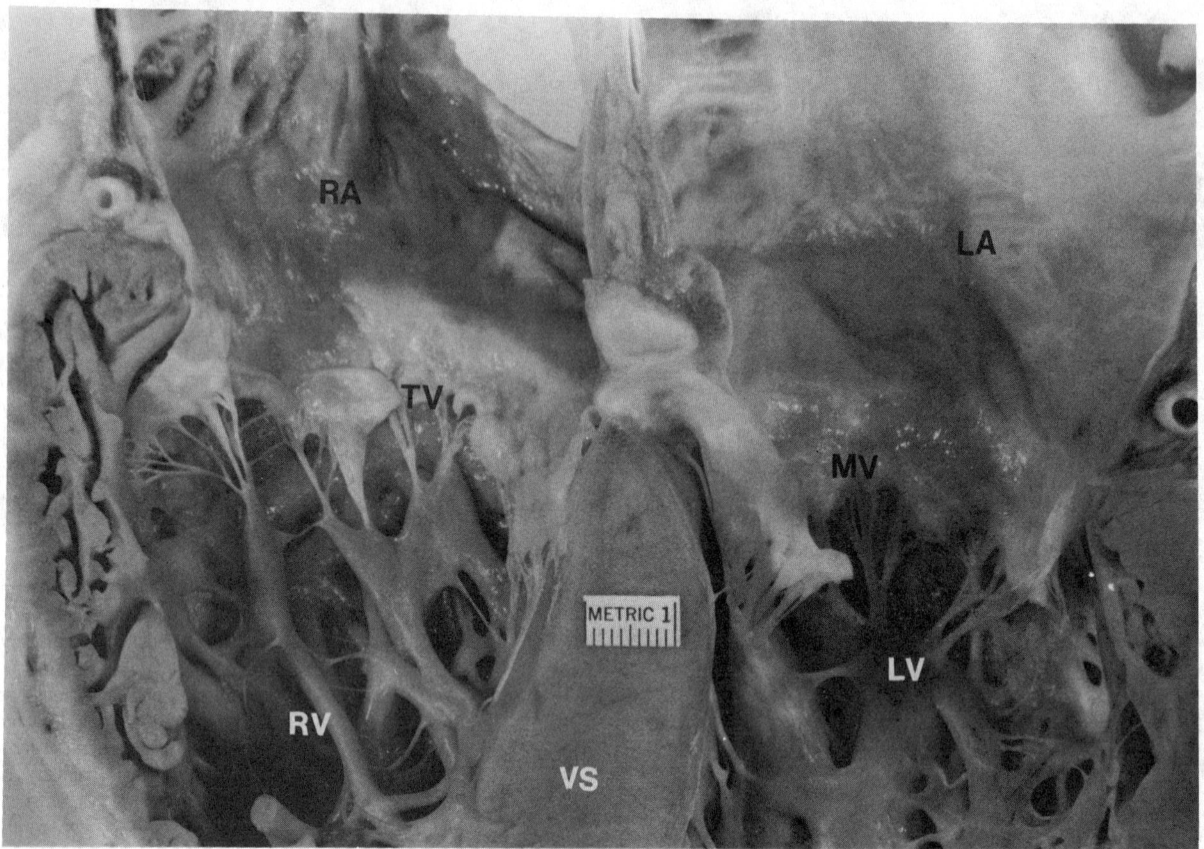

FIGURE 4-21 Four-chamber view showing mitral (MV) and tricuspid (TV) valves. The annulus of the tricuspid valve is more spiral than the annulus of the mitral valve (MV). LA = left atrium; LV = left ventricle; RA = right atrium; RV = right ventricle; VS = ventricular septum. [*From BF Waller et al: Tomographic views of normal and abnormal hearts: The anatomic basis for various cardiac imaging techniques. Clin Cardiol 13:804(pt I), 877(pt II), 1990. Reproduced with permission from the publisher and authors.*]

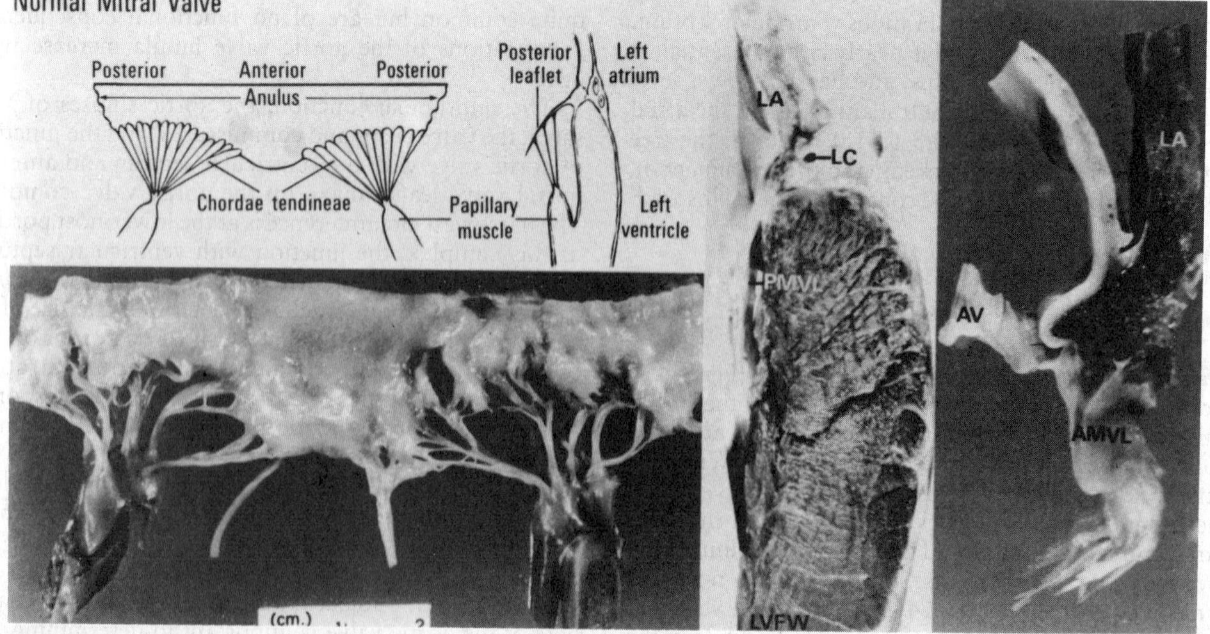

FIGURE 4-22 Morphology of the normal mitral valve. AMVL = anterior mitral valve leaflet; AV = aortic valve; LA = left atrium; LC = left circumflex coronary artery; LVFM = left ventricular free wall; PMVL = posterior mitral valve leaflet. (*From BF Waller: Morphologic aspects of valvular heart disease: Part I. Curr Prob Cardiol IX:13, 1985. Reproduced with permission from the publisher and author.*)

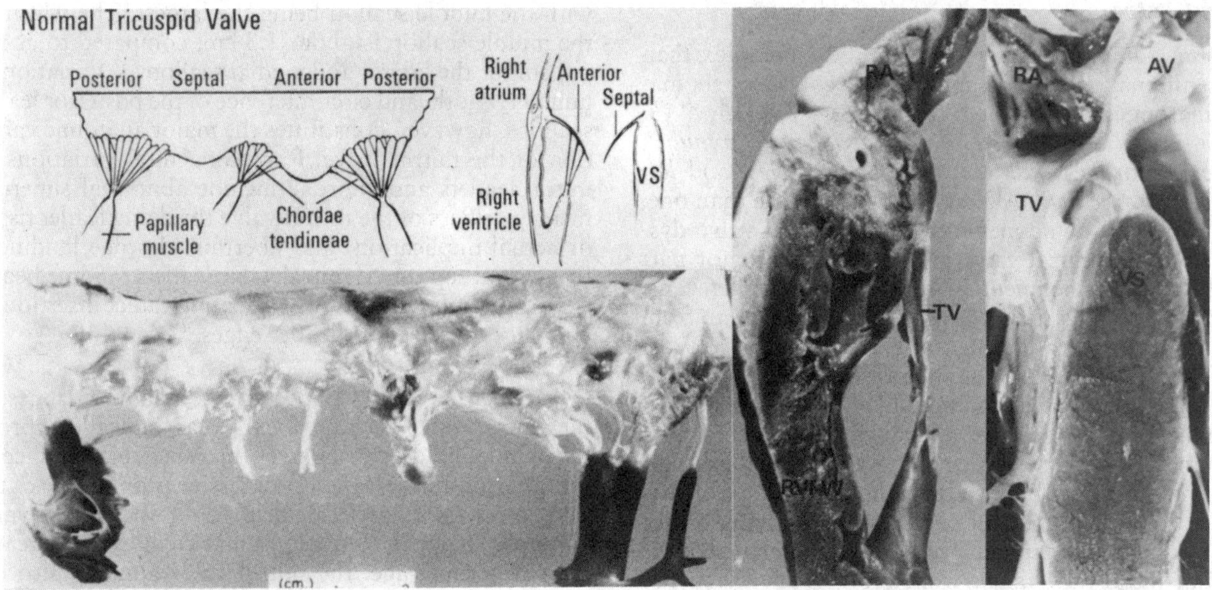

FIGURE 4-23 Morphology of the normal tricuspid valve. AV = aortic valve; RA = right atrium; RVFW = right ventricular free wall; TV = tricuspid valve; VS = ventricular septum. *(From BF Waller: Morphologic aspects of valvular heart disease: Part I. Curr Prob Cardiol IX:13, 1985. Reproduced with permission from the publisher and author.)*

tract, right atrium), while rupture of the left sinus of Valsalva generally communicates with left-sided chambers (left atrium or left ventricular outflow tract). Portions of the left and noncoronary cusp are continuous with the anterior leaflet of mitral valve.

Anatomic Variation The normal tricuspid aortic valve is a symmetric structure composed of three equal-sized cusps. Detailed measurements of commissural diameters and cuspal depth show that some tricuspid aortic valves have marked variation in these measurements.[31,32] The circumference between one set of commissures may be longer or shorter than in the remaining two sets of commissures, one sinus of Valsalva may be deeper or shallower than the remaining two sinuses, or the combination of these variables may occur in the same aortic valve. These variations in cusp size result in asymmetric lines of closure and may result in accelerated "wear and tear" (aging) of the valve structure. These congenitally malformed tricuspid valves may be the basis for some of the isolated aortic valve stenoses seen in patients over age 65 years.[31,32]

Age-Related Changes The normal cuspal markings become more prominent with age. The central cuspal nodules thicken and enlarge and the bases of the sinuses of Valsalva typically contain calcific deposits. The body of the aortic valve cusps also thickens, while the cusp lunula often thins and develops fenestrations. Commissures characteristically remain open with normal aging changes, and the sinuses of Valsalva dilate with increasing age.[33]

Pulmonic Valve

General Like the aortic valve, the normal tricuspid aortic valve is a symmetric structure (Figs. 4-7 and 4-19) in which the orifice of the fully opened valve is central and the cusps are easily mobile and retract to the pulmonary trunk attachments. The circumferential distances between each of the three commissures and the depth of the pulmonary valve sinus in a normally formed valve are similar. With the exception of adjacent anatomic connections and coronary ostia, the normal pulmonic and aortic valves are identical in design. The lines of cusp apposition and the central nodules are less prominent in pulmonic valves than in aortic valves, as might be expected from the lower right-sided ventricular pressures. With age, fenestrations of the cusp lunulae appear but, as in the aortic valve, have no functional significance. The three pulmonic valve cusps are named in relation to the aortic cusps—right, left, and anterior. The pulmonic valve annulus is about 1.5 cm above the level of the aortic valve annulus, but its circumference is similar (7 to 9 cm). The pulmonic valve is discontinuous with the tricuspid valve because of muscular structures of the right ventricular outflow tract.

Anatomic Variation As with the aortic valve, detailed measurements of commissural diameters and cuspal depth reveal variations. The long-term functional significance of these congenitally abnormal tricuspid pulmonic valves with asymmetric closure lines differs from that of the aortic valve in that acquired "senile" (old age) pulmonic stenosis does not occur. This difference presumably is due to the difference in right- and left-sided ventricular systolic pressures.

Age-Related Changes With increasing age, the pulmonic valve cusps thicken slightly, but far less than the aortic valve leaflets. Calcific deposits in the base of the pulmonic valve sinuses were not observed in 40 hearts from patients aged 90 to 103 years.[33]

Mitral Valve

General The mitral valve is much more complex than the semilunar valves. The mitral valve consist of six major anatomic components[34] (Figs. 4-6, 4-7, 4-15, 4-16, and 4-20 to 4-22): *posterior left atrial wall, annulus, leaflets, chordae tendineae, papillary muscles*, and *left ventricular free wall.* Alterations of one, more than one, or all of these components can cause mitral valve dysfunction. The mitral valve annulus forms a major part of the basal attachment of the posterior leaflet. This bundle of fibrous tissue separates left ventricular from left atrial myocardium and is located posterior to the posterior mitral leaflet. The anterior leaflet does not have a true annulus but is continuous with the wall of ascending aorta, aortic valve, and membranous ventricular septum. The valve measurement used by surgeons ("mitral ring") or that obtained by pathologists at autopsy is not really a measurement of the mitral annulus but of the mitral valve circumference. The circumference of the normal mitral valve ranges from 8 to 10.5 cm (mean, 9.4 cm).[34–36]

Unlike the other three cardiac valves, which each have three leaflets or cusps, the mitral valve consists of only two leaflets. The anterior leaflet has a much longer base to margin of closure width (2.3 cm) than the posterior leaflet (1.2 cm),[37] but the circumference (6 cm) of the posterior leaflet (annular attachment) is about twice that of the anterior leaflet (3 cm). Whereas the base-to-margin widths and circumferences of each mitral leaflet are different, the surface area of each leaflet is similar.[34,35] The total surface area of both leaflets is about two and one-half times that of the orifice area calculated using the mitral valve circumference.[38] The leaflets are connected to each other at junctions called commissures. In contradistinction to the semilunar commissures, which represent "spaces" between cusps, the commissures of the AV valves are "junctions" of continuous leaflet tissue.

The chordae tendineae of the mitral valve consist of primary, secondary, and tertiary chordae[34] that subdivide as they extend from papillary muscles to leaflets (Figs. 4-20 to 4-22). Some chordae tendineae from each papillary muscle attach to both anterior and posterior mitral leaflets. The spaces between the multiple chordal subdivisions function as secondary orifices between the left atrium and left ventricle.[34] The two left ventricular papillary muscles are termed anterolateral and posteromedial. The anterolateral papillary muscle is usually larger than the posteromedial. The major blood supply of the anterolateral muscle is the left anterior descending coronary artery, while the right coronary artery supplies the posteromedial muscle.[39] The left circumflex artery supplies blood to both papillary muscles. The apices of papillary muscles appear to be sensitive indicators of myocardial hypoxia, since blood supply to the papillary muscle must travel the full thickness of the left ventricular free wall and then retrogradely up the longer axis of the papillary muscle body.[40]

Anatomic Variations The posterior leaflet of the mitral valve shows considerable variation in its subdivision into one to three scallops—lateral, middle, and medial.[37] Virtually all posterior leaflets (96 percent) are triscalloped, with the middle scallop being the largest. The width of the middle scallop is about 1.3 cm, compared to about 1.0 cm for the lateral and medial scallops.[37] Variation in number, width, and circumference of the posterior leaflet scallops, however, constitutes the major anatomic variation of the mitral valve. Rare congenital variations of mitral leaflets and chordae include abnormal supernumerary orifices of the mitral valve (bridging leaflet tissue or actual duplication) and aberrant chordae tendineae from atrial septum to mitral valve leaflets.[41] Some hearts have "muscular chords" representing direct insertion of papillary muscles into leaflet edges.[36]

Age-Related Changes Expected age-related changes of the mitral valve include focal areas of leaflet fibrous thickening, lipid deposits over the ventricular surface of the anterior mitral leaflet, progressive prominence of the lines of closure, and calcification of the mitral valve annulus.[33] Since the left ventricular cavity size decreases with increasing age, the mitral valve annulus also decreases with age.[40] This latter change promotes further leaflet contact and increases leaflet fibrous changes. This change in ventricular cavity also creates ventriculo–leaflet area disproportion, so the segments of normal leaflet prolapse into the left atrium.[33]

Tricuspid Valve

General The tricuspid valve, like the mitral valve, is a complex structure made up of six major anatomic components: right atrial wall, annulus, three leaflets, chordae tendineae, papillary muscles, and right ventricular free wall. The three leaflets are termed anterior, posterior, and septal (Figs. 4-6, 4-7, 4-9 to 4-11, 4-14, and 4-23). The anterior leaflet is usually the largest, with a width of 2.2 cm. The septal leaflet and posterior leaflet measure about 1.5 cm and 2.0 cm in width, respectively.[42] The tricuspid annulus is a nearly circular fibrous structure, much less prominent than the mitral valve annulus but slightly larger in circumference (10 to 12.5 cm). The posterior leaflet makes up the largest portion of the annulus (7.5 cm), followed by the anterior (3.7 cm) and septal (3.6 cm) leaflets. The septal leaflet has a characteristic fold or indentation where its annulus passes from the posterior ventricular free wall to the membranous septum (Fig. 4-23). The chordae tendineae of the tricuspid valve are made up of five types: fan shaped, rough zone, basal, free edge, and deep[42] (Fig. 4-23). Of these, the free-edge and deep chordae are unique to the tricuspid valve.[42] The chordae arise from a single large anterior papillary muscle, double or multiple septal papillary muscles, and several small posterior papillary muscles. The papillary muscles are attached to the corresponding walls of the right ventricle.

Anatomic Variations The posterior leaflet of the tricuspid valve shows considerable variation in its subdivision into one to three scallops. The scallops are produced by small clefts marked by fan-shaped chordae. Rare congenital tricuspid valve anomalies include supernumerary orifices created by bridging leaflet tissue or actual valve duplication.[43, 44]

Age-Related Changes With increasing age, the tricuspid valve leaflet margins of closure become more prominent, and the leaflet acquires focal areas of fibrous thickening. Leaflet or annular calcification is rarely seen unless there is an abnormal calcium balance[45] or the patient has inborn metabolic abnormalities.[36]

Papillary Muscles

The papillary muscles of both ventricles are located below the commissures of the AV valves.[46] These muscles project from the trabeculae carneae and may be single, bifid, or occasionally a row of muscles arising from the ventricular wall. In the left ventricle the two groups of papillary muscles, located below the anterolateral and posteromedial commissures, arise from the junction of the apical and middle third of the ventricular wall (Figs. 4-8 to 4-11, 4-15, 4-16, 4-20, 4-21, and 4-24). In the right ventricle there are usually three papillary muscles (Figs. 4-10 and 4-11). The largest is the anterior papillary muscle, which is found below the commissure between the anterior and posterior leaflets, originating from the moderator band as well as from the anterolateral ventricular wall. The posterior papillary muscle lies beneath the junction of the posterior and septal leaflets. A small septal papillary muscle, originating from the wall of the infundibulum, tethers the anterior and septal leaflets high against the infundibular wall. At times this muscle is virtually absent, and the chordae tendineae arise from a small tendinous connection to the infundibulum. The septal leaflet of the tricuspid valve usually has extensive attachments to the ventricular septum. The papillary muscles, because of their relatively parallel alignment to the ventricular wall and their chordal attachments to two adjacent valve leaflets, pull the leaflets of the mitral valve and tricuspid valve together and downward at the onset of isovolumic ventricular contraction.

Chordae Tendineae

Strong cords of fibrous tissue, the chordae tendineae,[47] spring from the tip of each papillary muscle (Figs. 4-8, 4-11, 4-15, 4-16, 4-20, and 4-21). They often subdivide and interconnect before they attach to the two leaflets directly above. The chordae may attach directly into a fibrous band running along the free edge of the valves or they may become incorporated into the ventricular surface of the leaflet a few millimeters back from the edge. Additional chordae run directly from the ventricular wall into the undersurface of the posterolateral leaflet of the left ventricle and the septal and posterior leaflets of the right ventricle. The chordae tendineae, by their attachments to most of the free valvular border and by their numerous cross connections, allow the valve leaflets to balloon upward and against each other and evenly distribute the forces of ventricular systole. Dysfunction or rupture of a papillary muscle or rupture of a chorda tendinea may undermine the support of one or more valve leaflets, producing regurgitation.

Endocardium

Endocardium endothelium appears to share many, if not all, of the many functions of vascular endothelium described below. A newly found agent from endocardial endothelial cells that prolongs myocardial contraction has been provisionally referred to as "endocardin." The prolongation of contraction by endocardin can be overridden by stimulation of endothelium-derived relaxing factor (EDRF), which shortens the duration of contraction. (See Chaps. 2, 5, 25, and 56.)

Pericardium[48,49]

The heart is enclosed by the pericardium, the two surfaces of which can be visualized by considering the heart as a fist that is plunged into a large balloon or serous pericardium (Figs. 4-1 and 4-25). The surface of the balloon in intimate contact with the fist is analogous to the visceral pericardium or epicardium. This surface encases the heart, extending several centimeters onto each of the great vessels. It is then reflected back, as is the outer surface of the balloon, to form the parietal

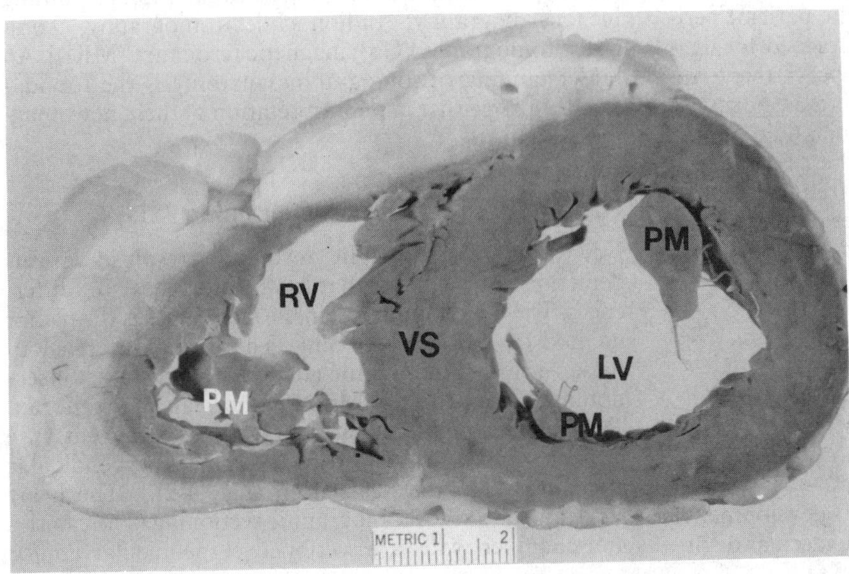

FIGURE 4-24 Short-axis view of ventricles showing papillary muscles (PM) of mitral valve (PM black) and tricuspid valve (PM white). LV = left ventricle; RV = right ventricle; VS = ventricular septum.

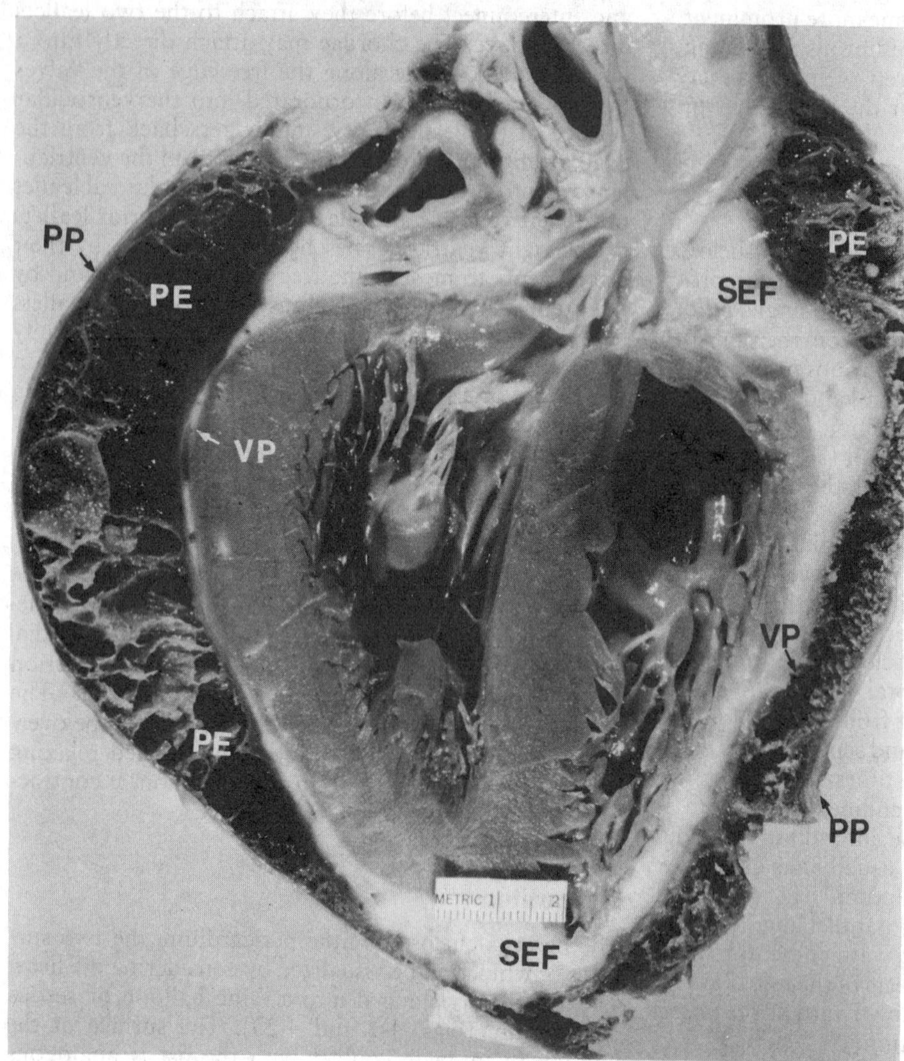

FIGURE 4-25 Fibrous pericardial effusion (PE) helps to delineate the two normal layers of the pericardial sac: visceral pericardium (VP) and parietal pericardium (PP). Subepicardial fat (SEF) is located just beneath the visceral layer of pericardium.

pericardium, which is fused to the fibrous pericardium to form the fibrous layer. The two pericardial surfaces are lined by smooth, glistening serous tissue and are separated by a thin layer of lubricating fluid, which allows the heart to move freely within the parietal pericardium. The parietal pericardium is attached by ligaments to the manubrium, the xiphoid process, the vertebral column, and the diaphragm. There is normally about 10 to 50 mL of thin, clear pericardial fluid, which moistens the contracting surfaces of the visceral and parietal pericardium. Four recesses are frequently present in images or examination of the pericardial space: the superior sinus, the transverse sinus, the postcaval recess, and the oblique sinus.[49]

TOMOGRAPHIC VIEWS OF NORMAL HEART: ANATOMIC BASIS FOR VARIOUS CARDIAC IMAGING TECHNIQUES

During the last several years, dramatic developments have taken place in the diagnosis of cardiovascular disorders in the area of cardiac imaging techniques.[13,14] From a previous era of imaging by silhouettes (chest roentgenography, fluoroscopy, angiocardiography), we have emerged into an era of imaging by tomographic scanning [echocardiography, radionuclide tomography, computed tomography (CT), magnetic resonance (MRI)]. An understanding of tomographic anatomy is the foundation for proper use and interpretation of these new imaging modalities.

Position of Heart and Tomographic Axis

New tomographic imaging techniques result in various depictions of the heart that have similarities and differences. The major similarity in the techniques is the planar method of cardiac sectioning. The major difference in these various tomographic techniques is the axis of sectioning relative to the position of the heart in the thorax. Two-dimensional echocardiographic imaging cuts the heart in transverse and longitudinal planes perpendicular and parallel to the heart itself (Fig. 4-26). The heart serves as the axis of tomographic sectioning. The cavities and chamber walls are sectioned perpendicular and/or

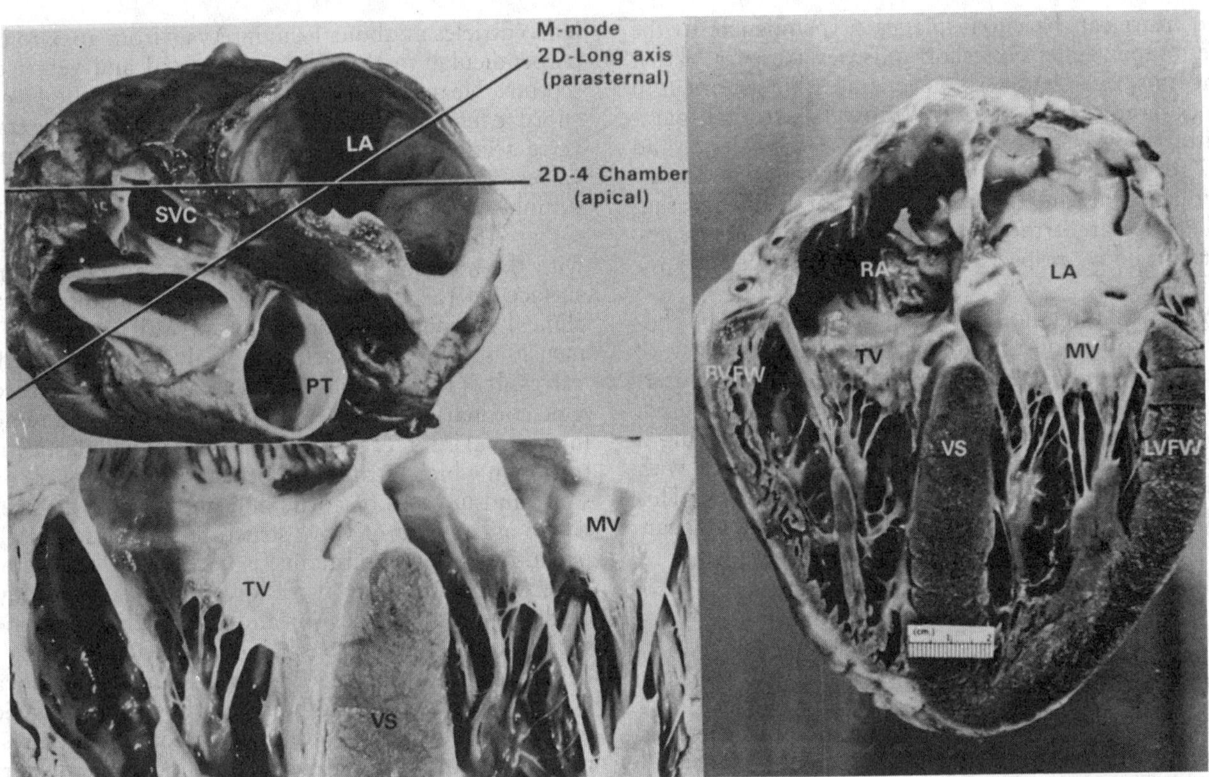

FIGURE 4-26 Composite showing method of cutting a heart and resultant tomographic views. *A.* Basal view of heart showing planes of base-apex sectioning in order to obtain two-dimensional long-axis and two-dimensional, four-chamber echocardiographic views. The parasternal long-axis view is also used to correlate images obtained from M-mode echocardiography. *B.* Closeup of four-chamber view showing atrioventricular valves [tricuspid (TV), mitral valve (MV)]. The annulus of the TV is located more apically than the MV annulus. VS = ventricular septum. *C.* Four-chamber view of heart. LA = left atrium; LVFM = left ventricular free wall; RA = right atrium; RVFM = right ventricular free wall. *(From BF Waller: Morphologic aspects of valvular heart disease: Part I. Curr Prob Cardiol IX:13, 1985. Reproduced with permission from the publisher and author.)*

parallel to their respective axis. In contrast, CT and MRI cut the thorax in transverse and longitudinal planes. The body serves as the axis of tomographic sectioning. The heart sits in an oblique position relative to the thorax: The atria are located posteriorly and only slightly superiorly; the cardiac apex is directed leftward, anteriorly, and somewhat inferiorly; and the atrial and ventricular septae and AV valves are directed anteriorly and somewhat inferiorly. Thus, the right atrium is a right lateral chamber, the left atrium is a midline posterior chamber, the right ventricle is an anterior chamber, and the left ventricle is a posterior chamber. Sectioning the heart in tomographic planes using the thorax as the axis of reference necessarily results in "distortions" of cardiac cavities, valve structures, and thickness of chamber walls. Oblique sectioning of the cavities and chamber walls may not provide precise anatomic correlates but produces truncated or inflated measurements. Technical changes in CT and MRI presently under development will permit tomographic cardiac sectioning using the heart as the axis of reference. In contrast to imaging modalities using the thorax as the axis of sectioning, echocardiography uses the heart as the axis of sectioning.

Thus, precise anatomic correlates can be made in terms of measurements of wall thickness and chamber sizes. Debate among pathologists and anatomists concerning the "proper anatomic orientation" and "display" of tomographic cardiac images[50–52] centers around the principle of reference axis. Arguments that depiction of the heart in an echocardiographic four-chamber view ("valentine shape") is "unconventional" and "nonanatomic" are based upon tomographic imaging that uses the body as the reference axis. When one uses the heart as the reference axis, however, the echocardiographic four-chamber view is quite conventional and anatomic.[4, 13, 14]

Preparation of Necropsy Heart and Methods of Cutting to Display Tomographic Anatomy

At necropsy, planar sectioning of the heart requires formalin fixation with or without perfusion for 12 to 24 h before cutting. If pressure fixation is not available, gentle "stuffing" of the atria with paper towels can help distend these chambers. The paper towels should not be placed through the AV valves as this will abnormally distort the valve leaflets. Adult as well as infant hearts can be sectioned in tomographic planes if prepared by the above described methods. Actual tomographic cutting of the heart can be done with the use of a large 12- to 16-in knife, which allows smooth, straight sectioning. Sectioning the heart in tomographic planes without formalin fixation will result in irregular rough cavity walls and distortions in the cardiac chambers.

Clinically, multiple cuts in different planes are obtained in each patient. Anatomically, multiple cuts in different planes are a more difficult task but can be obtained with the use of cyanoacrylate glue. The formalin fixed heart can be cut in planes perpendicular to the base-to-apex dimension (short-axis view) or parallel to it (long-axis, two-chamber, four-chamber views) or cut in planes parallel to the thorax (transverse, frontal, parasagittal views) (Figs. 4-4, 4-5, 4-7, 4-9 to 4-12, and 4-27 to 4-31). The short-axis, two-chamber, and four-chamber planes and the transverse, frontal, and parasagittal planes are orthogonal sets of images but use the heart or body, respectively, as the reference axis for sectioning.

A particular method of cutting a heart should be chosen so as to demonstrate the specific disease or lack of disease in each heart. Each necropsy specimen is different, and no "standard" or "universal" cut can be used. The traditional "flow of blood" method of cutting a heart appears to have lost its clinical relevance with respect to the new cardiac imaging techniques. This method is particularly poor for demonstrating myocardial or valvular anatomy or heart disease.

The Heart as the Reference Axis

Short-Axis Method

The short-axis method of sectioning the heart also has been referred to as the "bread loaf" or "ventricular slice" method (Figs. 4-4, 4-5, 4-7, 4-12, 4-13, and 4-31). The technique involves transverse sectioning of the right and left ventricles at about 1-cm intervals from apex to base perpendicular to the axis of the atrial and ventricular septum. Near the base of the heart (about the level of chordae tendineae–papillary muscle junction), the transverse sections may skip to the level of the semilunar valves and atria (Figs. 4-12, 4-13, and 4-31). The resulting sections produce a "family of slices" from apex to base (Figs. 4-12 and 4-13). These slices are oriented with the anterior surface on the top and the posterior surface on the bottom. The short-axis method allows clinical morphologic correlation of wall and cavity dimensions and cross-sectional analysis of the cardiac valves. It is the method of choice in cases of atherosclerotic coronary heart disease in which recent and remote myocardial infarcts are likely; in cases of neoplastic infiltration in which location of metastatic implants are possible; and in cases of aortic and mitral valve disease in which assessment of valve structure and value function (stenotic, purely regurgitant) is necessary. This method of sectioning the heart also allows classification of myocardial infarcts into location and size: anterior, posterior, septal, and/or lateral; basal, midventricular, apical, or base to apex; transmural or nontransmural (subendocardial, subepicardial). Another use of the short-axis view of the aortic valve and adjacent anatomic structures is recognition of the right and left main coronary arteries (Figs. 4-4, 4-5, and 4-7). The bifurcation of the left main into left anterior descending and left circumflex arteries

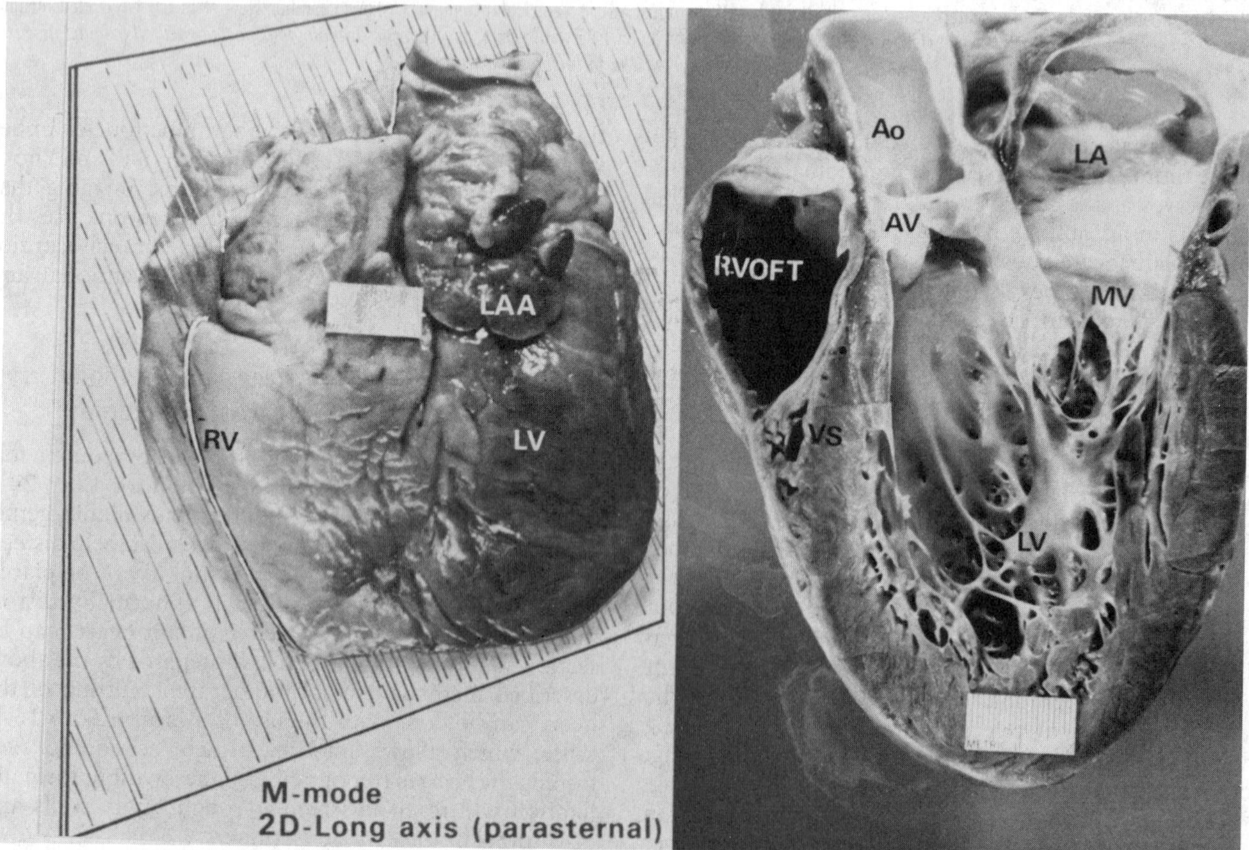

FIGURE 4-27 Tomographic sectioning of the heart from base to apex along the planar lines shown in Fig. 4-2 produces views that correlate with echocardiographic parasternal long-axis images. Ao = aorta; AV = aortic valve; LA = left atrium; LAA = left atrial appendage; LV = left ventricle; MV = mitral valve; RV = right ventricle; RVOFT = right ventricular outflow tract; VS = ventricular septum. *(From BF Waller: Morphologic aspects of valvular heart disease: Part I. Cur Prob Cardiol IX:13, 1985. Reproduced with permission from the publisher and author.)*

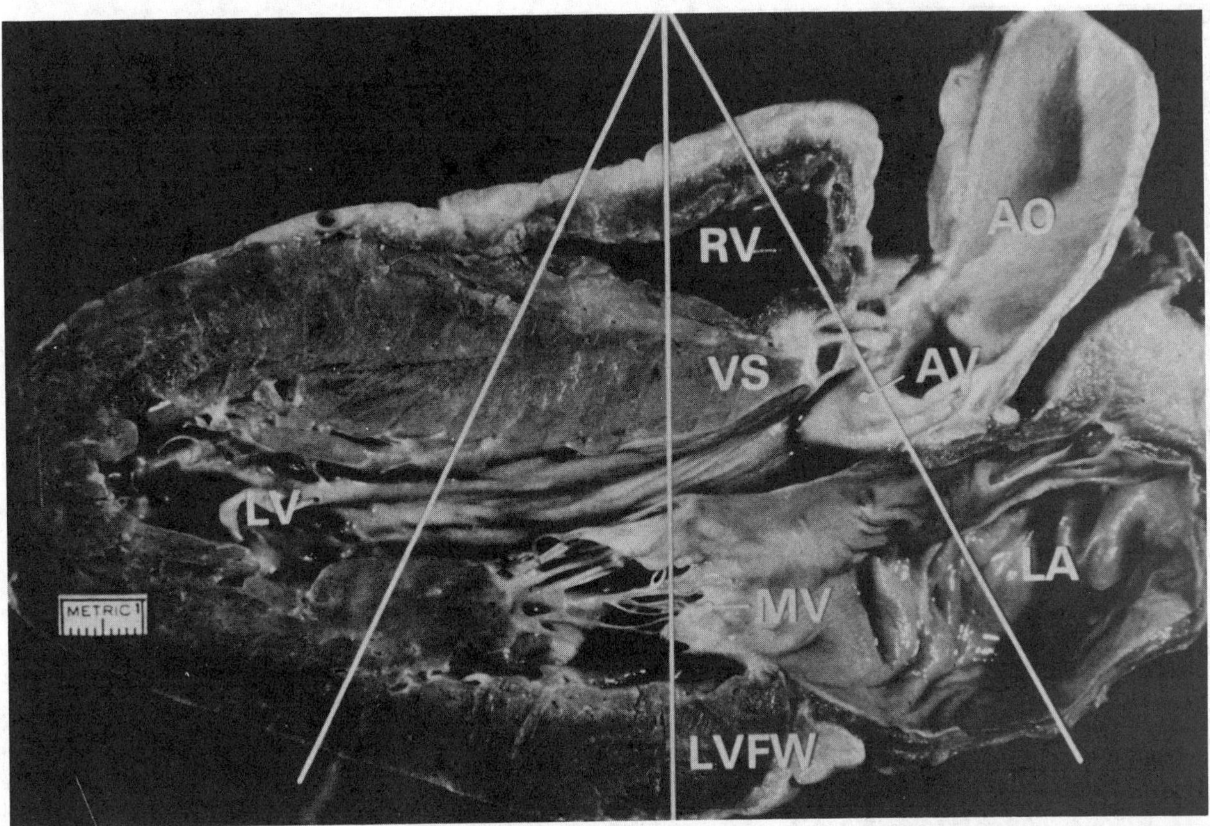

FIGURE 4-28 M-mode echocardiographic view showing "ice-pick" views of selected areas of the heart. One view displays the right ventricle (RV), aortic valve (AV), portions of aorta (Ao), and left atrium (LA). Another more apical view show the RV, ventricular septum (VS), left ventricular cavity (LV), and left ventricular free wall (LVFW). MV = mitral valve. [*From BF Waller et al: Tomographic views of normal and abnormal hearts: The anatomic basis for various cardiac imaging techniques. Clin Cardiol 13:804(pt I), 877(pt II), 1990. Reproduced with permission from the publisher and authors.*]

and proximal portions of these main arteries can often be identified with two-dimensional echocardiography. Anomalous origin of the right and left coronary ostia can also be recognized occasionally.

Two-Chamber Method

The two-chamber method involves sectioning the heart through the inflow tract of the left ventricle and inflow and a portion of the outflow tracts of the right ventricle. The plane of left ventricular sectioning is through the left ventricle and left atrium in an anteroposterior fashion and extending from base to apex. The two-chamber left ventricular plane discloses views of left atrium, anterior (septal), and posterior (mural) portions of the mitral valve leaflets, left ventricular cavity, and the anterior, apical, and posterior walls of the left ventricle. This view currently is used in assessment of the left ventricle in patients with atherosclerotic coronary heart disease. It provides another plane of sectioning for classification of left ventricular damage. A parallel cut on the right side of the heart discloses a similar view of the right ventricular inflow (right atrium, tricuspid valve, right ventricular body) but also discloses a portion of the right ventricular outflow tract. Although this particular tomographic view has been used less commonly in echocardiography, it would appear to be ideal in assessing right ventricular wall damage, intracavitary masses, and right ventricular outflow tract obstruction.

Four-Chamber Method

The four-chamber method involves sectioning the heart from base to apex in a right-to-left plane along the acute margins of right and left ventricles and corresponding walls of the atria (Figs. 4-11, 4-21, and 4-26). In the bisected specimen, portions of the tricuspid valve (posterior and septal leaflet), mitral valve (primarily posterior leaflet), AV valve annuli, chordae tendineae, papillary muscles, and each of the four cardiac chambers are visualized. In this view, it is readily apparent that the tricuspid valve annulus is located more apical than the mitral valve annulus. This anatomic finding is useful in identification of the right ventricle in complex congenital heart disease. Once the ventricle is identified, the AV valve follows concordantly. The corollary is also true in that if the AV valve can be morphologically identified, the ventricle follows concordantly (i.e., recognition of the tricuspid valve as the apical most AV valve also identifies the morphologic right ventricle). The four-chamber view is useful in cardiomyopathies for measurement of all four chambers and wall thickness and for identification of cavitary thrombus or tumor.

Long-Axis Method

The long-axis method of cutting or imaging the heart produces a unique left ventricular inflow/outflow tract view (Figs. 4-9, 4-10, 4-15, 4-16, 4-27, 4-28, and

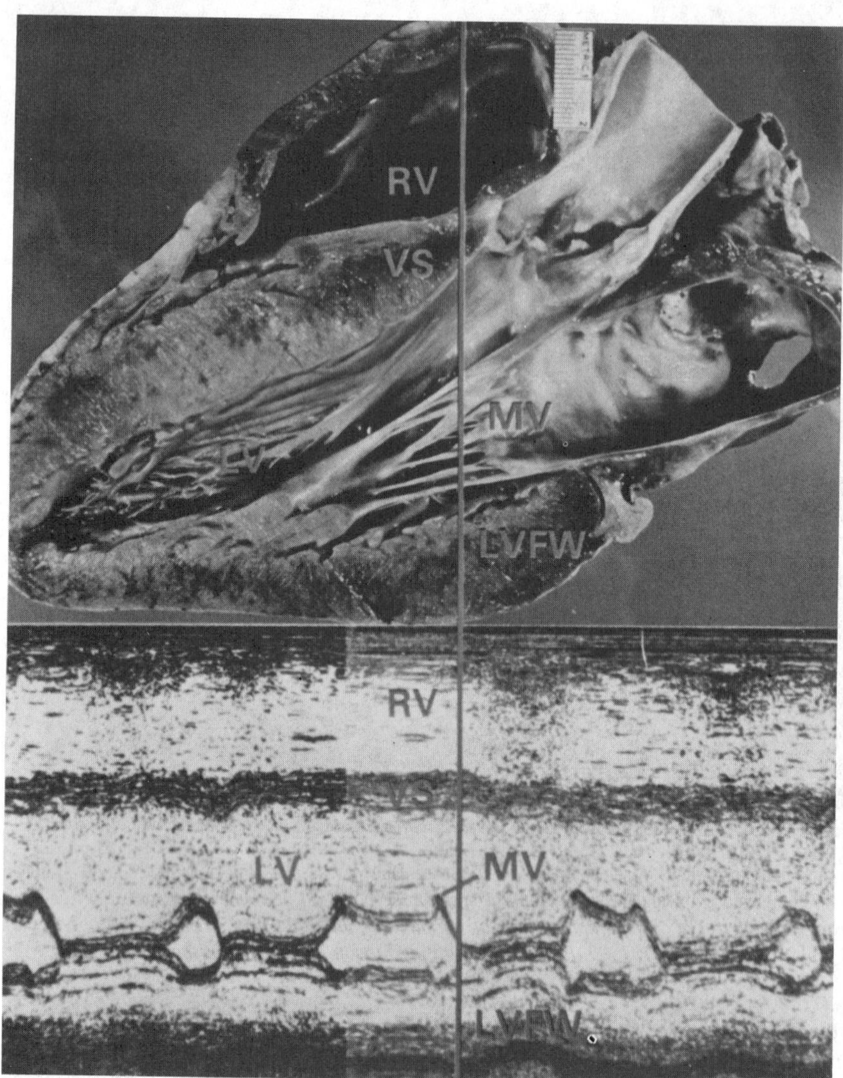

FIGURE 4-29 Parasternal long-axis view of heart with correlating M-mode echocardiogram. The ice-pick view through the midportion of the heart shows the right ventricle (RV) outflow tract, the ventricular septum (VS), left ventricular (LV) cavity, mitral valve (MV), and left ventricular free wall (LFVW). Systolic measurements on M-mode echocardiogram correspond to measurements on the formalin-fixed heart. [*From BF Waller et al: Tomographic views of normal and abnormal hearts: The anatomic basis for various cardiac imaging techniques. Clin Cardiol 13:804(pt I), 877(pt II), 1990. Reproduced with permission from the publisher and authors.*]

4-32). The left ventricular long-axis view is obtained by sectioning the heart in an anterolateral plane from base to apex. In this longitudinal plane, evaluation of the aortic and mitral valves, proximal portion of the ascending aorta (sinus portion and proximal tubular portion), left ventricular outflow, left ventricular and atrial walls, and chamber is possible. Also, a portion of right ventricular outflow tract just apical to the pulmonic valve is viewed on the left ventricular long-axis plane. The right-sided parallel longitudinal section views the right atrium, tricuspid valve, and body of the right ventricle. The left ventricular long-axis view is one of the "standard" two-dimensional echocardiographic views of the heart and thus is used for coronary, valvular, and myocardial heart disease. The long-axis left ventricular section also corresponds to the traditional M-mode echocardiographic image with "ice pick" views of the aorta and left atrium, left ventricular outflow tract and mitral valve, and proximal portion of the ventricular septum, left ventricular cavity, and left ventricular free wall. Anatomically, the left ventricular free wall imaged in this plane represents the lateral left ventricular free wall.

The Body (Thorax) as the Reference Axis

Tomographic sections of the heart obtained by use of the body as the reference axis result in cardiac images that differ from those described earlier. Three standard anatomic planes are generally used in CT and MRI: transverse (horizontal), frontal (coronal), and parasagittal (paramedian) (Figs. 4-33 and 4-34). Corresponding anatomic cardiac sections produced by these tomographic planes have been well illustrated in several anatomic atlases.[53–56]

Transverse (Horizontal) Method

Transverse tomographic planes of the thorax produce sections of the heart with truncated or expanded views of chambers and walls because of the oblique position of the heart within the thorax (Figs. 4-33 and 4-34). Some of the transverse views appear similar to the echocardiographic short-axis views. Transverse sectioning at the level of the great vessels provides an anatomic display of the pulmonary trunk and its bifurcation into the right

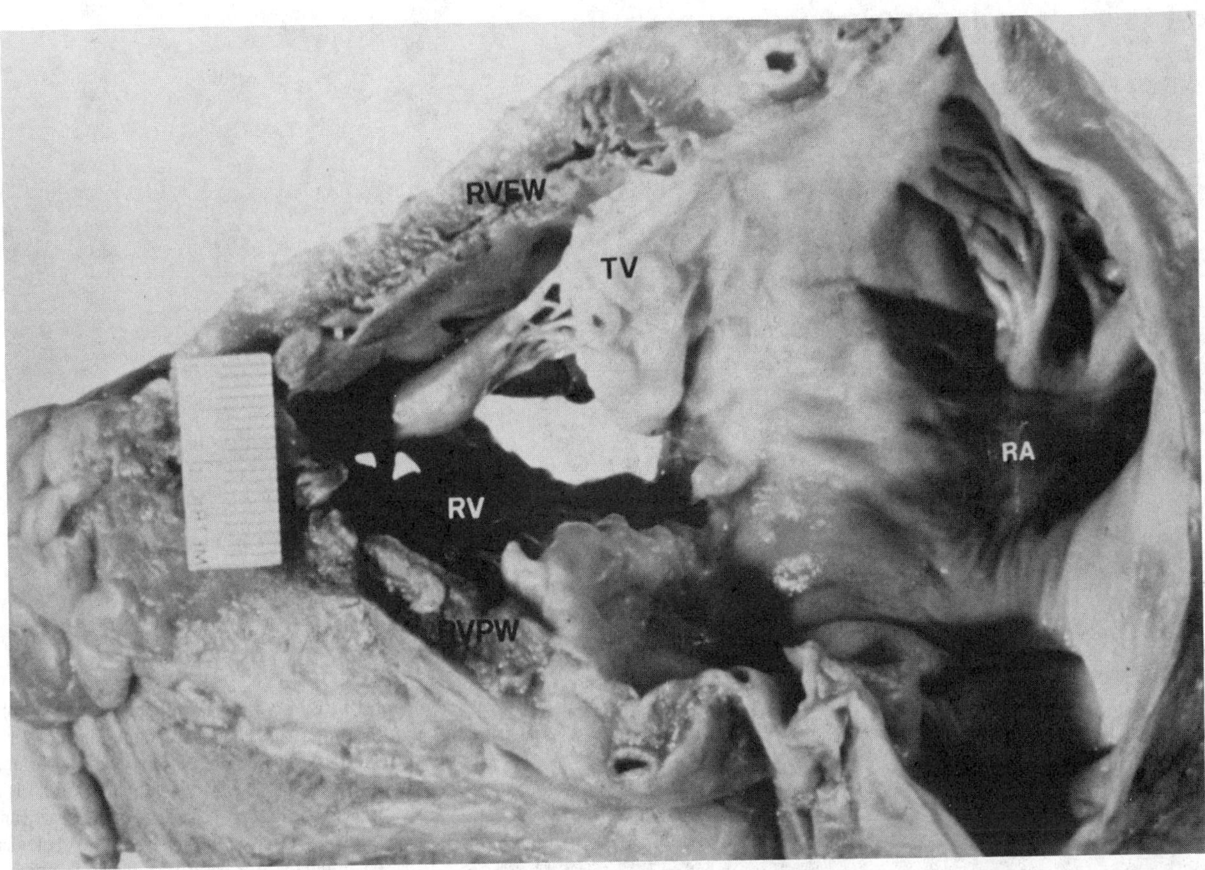

FIGURE 4-30 Tomographic cut of heart through right-sided structures as viewed by a parasternal long-axis, two-dimensional echocardiogram. RA = right atrium; RV = right ventricle; RVFW = right ventricular free wall (anterior); RVPW = right ventricular posterior wall; TV = tricuspid valve. [*From BF Waller et al: Tomographic views of normal and abnormal hearts: The anatomic basis for various cardiac imaging techniques. Clin Cardiol 13:804(pt I), 877(pt II), 1990. Reproduced with permission from the publisher and authors.*]

and left main pulmonary arteries and an adjacent cross section of the ascending aorta. Transverse sections taken of the heart "from the head to the feet" produce a family of oblique cross sections. One horizontal view produces a foreshortened four-chamber view that when viewed from the left, appears as a two-chamber echocardiographic cut and when viewed from the right appears as a truncated view of right ventricular inflow and an inflated view of the right atrium. Horizontal planes are useful in evaluation of patients with coronary and pericardial heart disease and in patients with diseases of the great vessels (dissection, aneurysm, mediastinal masses).

Frontal (Coronal) Method

Frontal tomographic planes of the body (thorax) produce the least familiar cardiac images compared with echocardiographic images. Sectioning the thorax from the anterior to the posterior (sternum to spine) results in cardiac sections that, at any one time, contain portions of left and right ventricles, aorta and pulmonary trunks, and left and right atria. These cardiac sections also cut the heart obliquely, preventing adequate assessment of chamber size and wall thickness or thinness. This method provides excellent views of the right ventricular outflow tract, pulmonary trunk, and pulmonary trunk bifurcation that are not available in the previously described tomographic cardiac sections. Also, the frontal plane is useful in evaluation of the aortopulmonary window and the vena cava.

Parasagittal (Paramedian) Method

Parasagittal tomographic planes of the body (thorax) produce another set of generally unfamiliar views of the heart. Planes of sectioning cut the heart in right-to-left fashion from shoulder to shoulder. Thus, the right-sided structures (vena cavae, right atrium, right ventricle) are viewed last. Some sections resemble the echocardiographic two-chamber views of the right and left sides. This method also cuts chambers and vessels in an oblique fashion that precludes adequate assessment of chamber size and wall thickness in most images. This method is excellent in anatomic evaluation of the aortic aneurysm, dissection, and coarctation.

In addition to conventional transverse, coronal, and sagittal imaging, oblique imaging planes are possible with MRI.[57–59] Oblique planes permit cuts of the heart along its long and short axes. The resultant cuts are analogous to the angiographic right and left anterior oblique views.

The newer cardiac imaging modalities (MRI, cine CT,

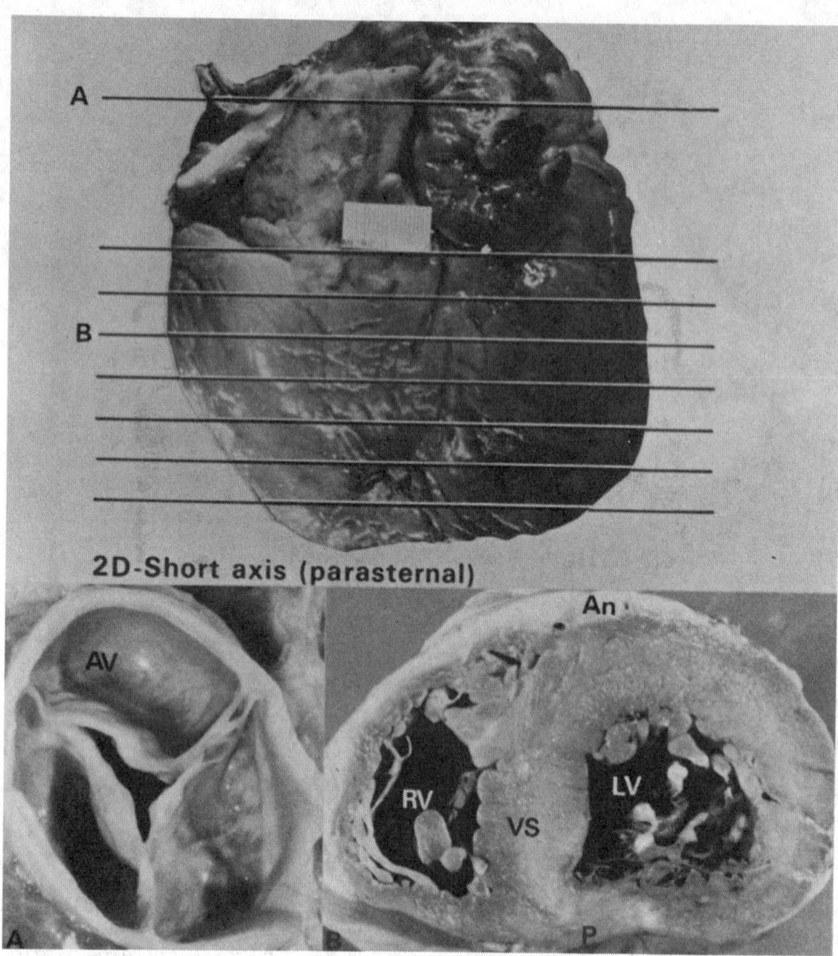

FIGURE 4-31 Tomographic sectioning of the heart in a "breadloaf" fashion produces a series of short-axis views of the left ventricle (LV) from apex to base. This "family of ventricular slices" is seen in Fig. 4-12. A very basal view of the heart (line *A*) produces a view of the aortic valve (AV) (*A*). Line *B* corresponds to a basal view of the ventricles (*B*) showing right ventricle (RV) and LV, anterior (An) and posterior (P) surfaces of the heart, and the ventricular septum (VS).

positron emission tomography) not only provide depiction of cardiac anatomy with the limitations mentioned above but also provide an excellent technique for characterization of myocardial tissue. Distinguishing ischemic and scarred myocardium, tumor and fat infiltration, and intracavitary tumor versus thrombus are useful morphologic data that cannot be assessed using present echocardiographic modalities.[58-60] (See Chap. 15.)

Scintigraphic Thallium Imaging

Scintigraphic thallium testing is a popular technique used in conjunction with exercise testing. Present methods of sectioning the heart produce images that closely resemble two-dimensional echocardiographic views yet are variants of the oblique and sagittal planes. The similarity of these images to that of the echocardiographic views results from using the heart primarily as the axis for imaging. (See Chap. 134.)

INNERVATION OF THE HEART

Although the sinus or SA (sinoatrial) node, AV (atrioventricular) node, and specialized conduction system of the heart possess the inherent ability for spontaneous, rhythmic initiation of the cardiac excitation impulse, the autonomic nervous system also influences the rate of spread of the excitation impulse, the depolarization and repolarization of the myocardium, and the contractility of both the atria and the ventricles.

The parasympathetic innervation of the heart originates in the medulla and passes through the right and left vagus nerves (Fig. 4-35). Two sets of cardiac nerves arise from each vagus nerve: the superior (superior and inferior cervical) cardiac nerves, which arise from the vagi in the neck, and the inferior (thoracic) cardiac nerves, which arise from either the vagus nerves or the recurrent branches of the vagi. The sympathetic innervation of the heart passes from the spinal cord to the upper four or five thoracic ganglia. Some fibers from the upper thoracic ganglia pass up the cervical sympathetic to the superior, middle, or inferior cervical ganglia. The superior (cervical), middle (cervical), and inferior (cervical) cardiac nerves originate from their respective ganglia and pass downward through the deep and superficial parts of the cardiac plexus to the heart. When the inferior cervical and first thoracic ganglia are fused together, the resulting ganglion is known as the *stellate ganglion*. Additional cardiac branches arise from the upper four or five thoracic ganglia and pass to the cardiac plexuses, which surround the root and arch of the aorta near the tracheal bifurcation. The cardiac and coronary plexuses are formed by cardiac branches from both the sympathetic and parasympathetic systems. Both sympathetic and parasympathetic fibers influence the SA node, the AV

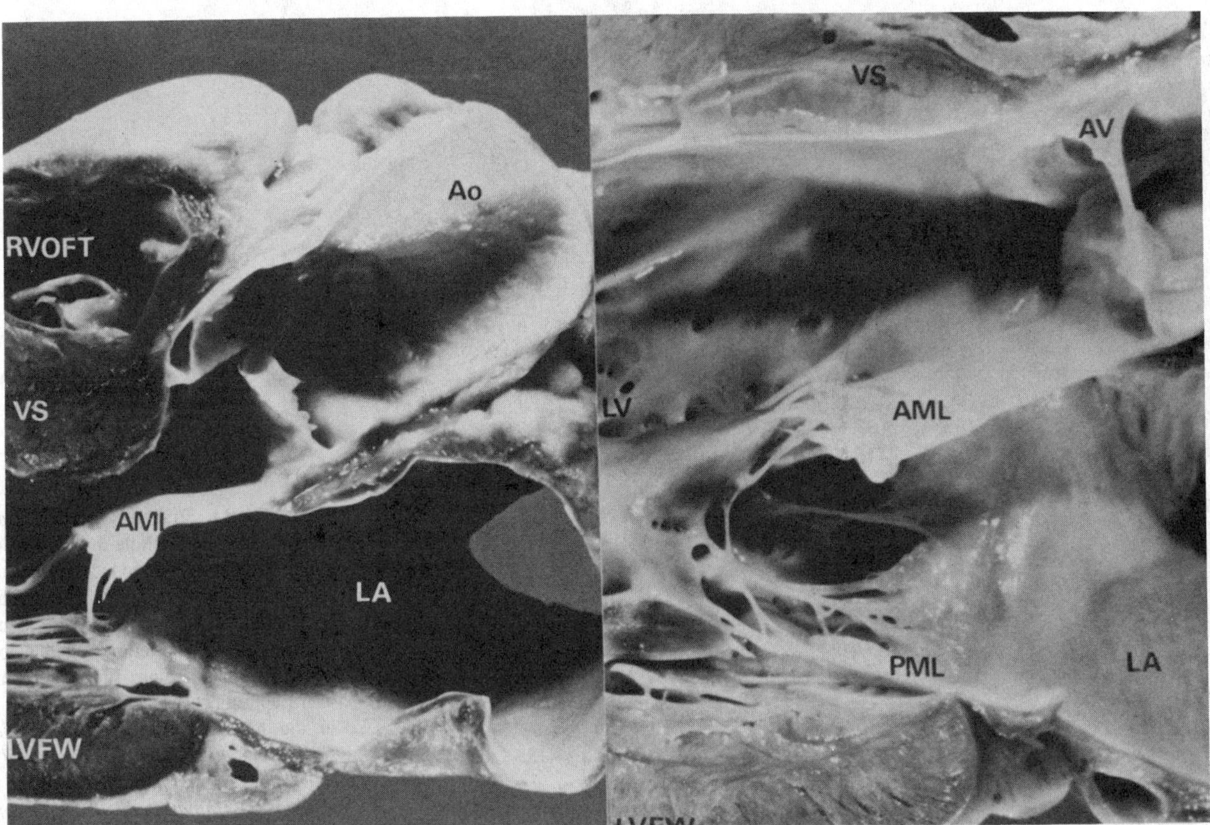

FIGURE 4-32 Parasternal long-axis view of the heart as viewed on a two-dimensional echocardiogram. *Left*: This view provides anatomic information about the basal ventricular septum (VS), left ventricular (LV) cavity, and aortic (AV) and mitral (MV) valves. AML = anterior mitral leaflet; Ao = aorta; LA = left atrium; LVFM = left ventricular free wall; RVOFT = right ventricular outflow tract. *Right*: Closeup view of LV outflow tract showing fibrous continuity of AV and AML. PML = posterior mitral leaflet. *(From BF Waller: Morphologic aspects of valvular heart disease: Part I. Curr Prob Cardiol IX:13, 1985. Reproduced with permission from the publisher and author.)*

node, and both the atrial and ventricular myocardium, although vagal fibers to the ventricles are rather sparse. Sympathetic fibers are dense to the epicardial coronary arteries and veins and are moderate to intramural vessels. Sympathetic stimulation to the heart is largely mediated by the release of norepinephrine. Cardiac parasympathetic impulses are transmitted by acetylcholine.

Afferent impulses from chemoreceptors and mechanoreceptors in the pericardium, connective tissue, adventitia, and walls of the heart pass by peripheral sensory

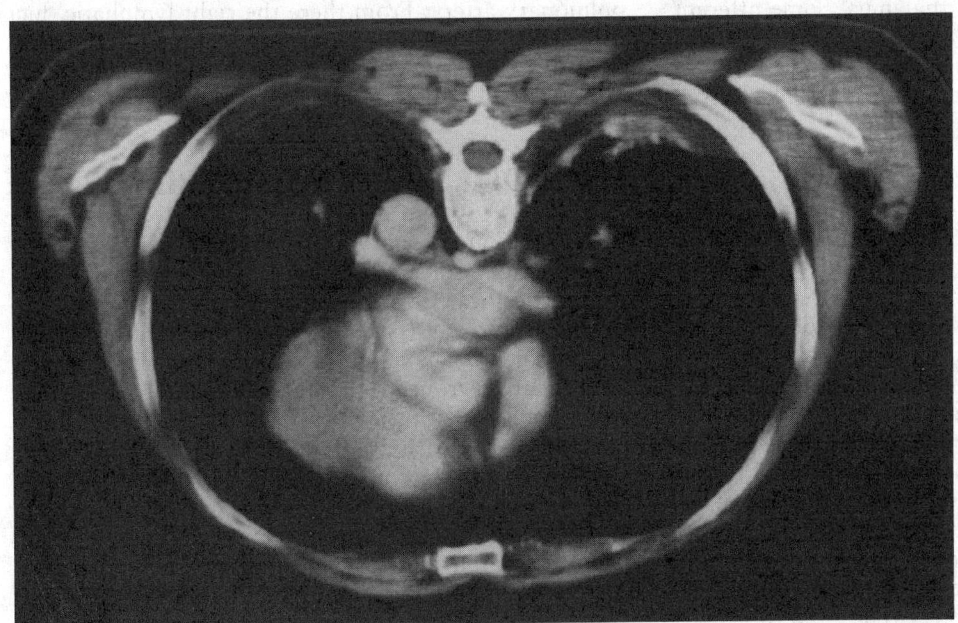

FIGURE 4-33 Transverse section of the heart from a CT scan. The perpendicular cut of the thorax creates oblique cuts of the heart. [*From BF Waller et al: Tomographic views of normal and abnormal hearts: The anatomic basis for various cardiac imaging techniques. Clin Cardiol 13:804(pt I), 877(pt II), 1990. Reproduced with permission of the publisher and authors.*]

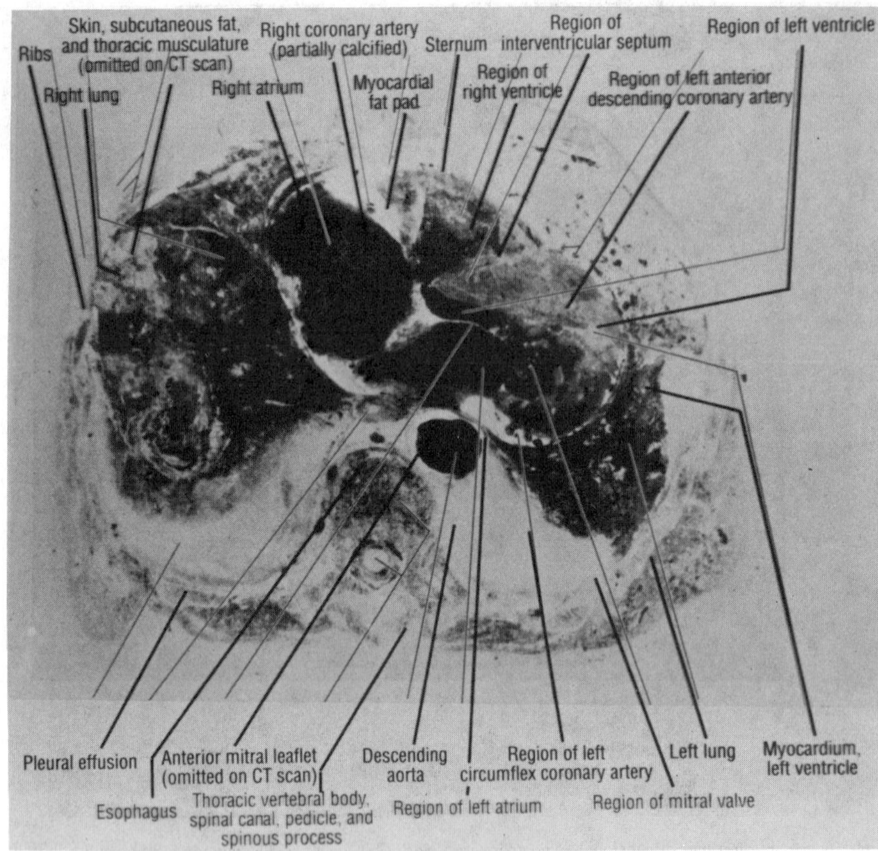

FIGURE 4-34 Transverse section of a human cadaver thorax. Note the perpendicular cut through the thorax produces truncated and expanded views of various cardiac structures. The anterior left ventricular wall is much thicker than the posterior wall due to the oblique cardiac section. The anterior mitral leaflet appears closer to the right atrium than to the left atrium in this cut. *(From G Gambarelli et al: Computerized Axial Tomography. An Anatomic Atlas of Serial Sections of the Human Body. Berlin, Springer-Verlag, 1977. Reproduced with permission from the publisher and author.)*

axons through sympathetic plexuses and through the lower two cervical and upper four thoracic sympathetic ganglia to thoracic dorsal ganglia, where the cell bodies of the neurons are located. The impulses are carried by the central axon of this neuron through the dorsal roots to the posterior gray column of the spinal cord, where the fibers synapse with the second-order neuron. From this neuron, fibers cross the median plane, ascend in the ventral spinothalamic tract, and terminate in the posteroventral nucleus of the thalamus. Some afferent vagal ganglia have been found in the left coronary artery system. Impulses passing through these neurons and ganglia are thought to be important in the Bezold-Jarisch reflex.

LYMPHATIC SYSTEM OF THE HEART

The lymphatic drainage of the heart flows from subendocardial vessels to an extensive capillary plexus lying throughout the subepicardium.[64,65] These capillaries converge in collecting lymphatic channels that run alongside the coronary vessels: a posterior interventricular trunk paralleling the posterior descending coronary artery up to the crux of the heart and then circling around to the right from posterior to anterior in the right coronary sulcus; an anterior interventricular trunk ascending from the apex to the base next to the left anterior descending coronary artery; and an obtuse marginal trunk running alongside the left circumflex artery (Fig. 4-36).

The two major left ventricular channels—the anterior interventricular trunk and the obtuse marginal trunk—join near the base of the pulmonary artery to form the left coronary channel. More often, the right coronary channel unites with the left coronary channel to become a main supracardiac channel, the principal cardiac lymphatic, which passes upward beneath the left atrial appendage, behind the pulmonary artery, to enter a pretracheal node between the arch of the aorta and the pulmonary artery. From there the right lymphatic duct runs cephalad in the mediastinum to drain into the junction of the internal jugular and right subclavian veins.

EPICARDIAL CORONARY ARTERIES

The epicardial coronary artery system[66] consists of the left and right coronary arteries, which normally arise from ostia located in the left and right sinuses of Valsalva, respectively (Figs. 4-37 and 4-38). In about 50 percent of humans a "third coronary artery" ("conus artery") arises from a separate ostium in the right sinus. Additional smaller ostia may be found in the right sinus, which give rise to multiple right ventricular branches. Up to five separate coronary ostia have been described (Fig. 4-39).[67]

The left main (LM) coronary artery ranges in length from 1 to 25 mm before bifurcating into the left anterior descending (LAD) and left circumflex (LC) branches.[68] The LAD coronary artery measures from 10 to 13 cm

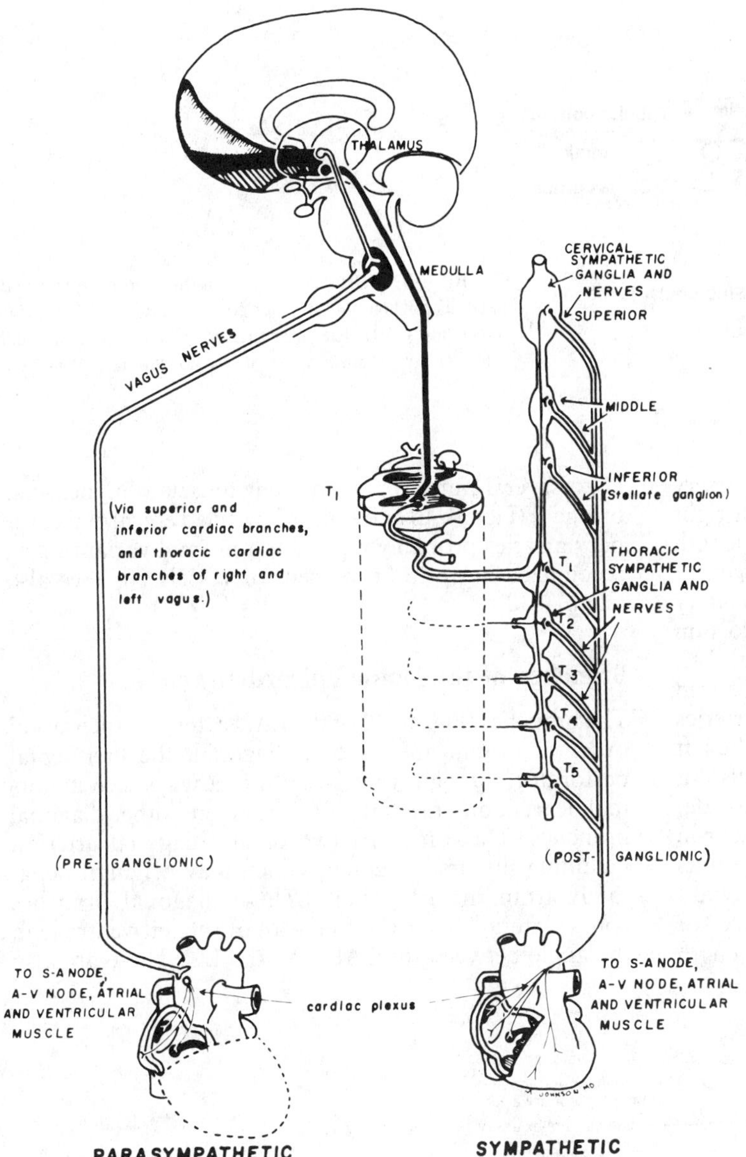

FIGURE 4-35 A simplified, diagrammatic representation of the efferent autonomic innervation of the heart. The parasympathetic and sympathetic nerves to the heart, many of which closely accompany each other in and through the various cardiac and coronary plexuses, have been separated for illustrative purposes. See text for details. *(Diagram by McClaren Johnson, Jr., M.D.)*

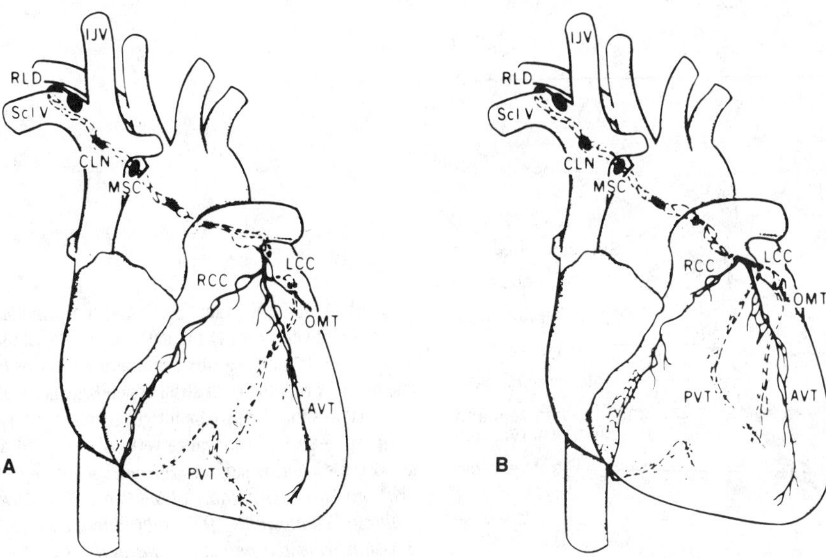

FIGURE 4-36 Diagrams of two different anatomic patterns (*A* and *B*) of lymphatic drainage channels of the heart. PVT = posterior interventricular trunk; RCC = right coronary channel; LCC = left coronary channel; AVT = anterior interventricular trunk; OMT = obtuse marginal trunk; MSC = main supracardiac channel; CLN = cardiac lymph node; RLD = right lymphatic duct; SciV = right subclavian vein; IJV = internal jugular vein. *(From M Feola, R Merklin, S Cho, et al: The terminal pathway of the lymphatic system of the human heart. Ann Thorac Surg 24:531, 1977. Reproduced with permission from the publisher and authors.)*

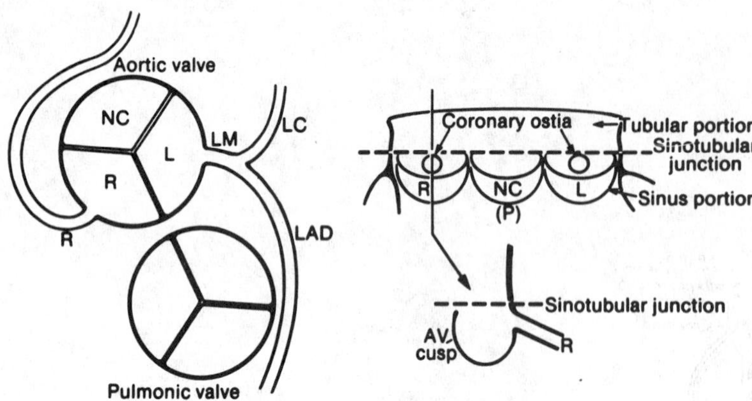

FIGURE 4-37 Diagram showing normal aortic origin and initial distribution of four major coronary arteries: left anterior descending (LAD), left circumflex (LC), left main (LM), and right (R). AV = aortic valve; NC = noncoronary; P = posterior.

in length, whereas the usual nondominant LC artery measures about 6 to 8 cm in length. The dominant right coronary artery (RCA) is about 12 to 14 cm in length before giving rise to the posterior descending artery (PDA). The luminal diameters of the major coronary arteries in adults range as follows: LM, 2.0 to 5.5 mm (mean 4 mm); LAD, 2.0 to 5.0 mm (mean 3.6 mm); LC, 1.5 to 5.5 mm (mean 3.0 mm); and RCA, 1.5 to 5.5 mm (mean 3.2 mm).[68] Although the LAD and LC arteries generally taper in diameter as each extends from the left main bifurcation, the RCA maintains a fairly constant diameter until just before the origin of its posterior descending branch. The subepicardial coronary arteries run on the surface of the heart embedded in various amounts of subepicardial fat. Portions of the epicardial coronary arteries may dip into the myocardium ("mural artery" or "tunneled artery") and be covered for a variable length (1 to several mm)[21] by ventricular muscle ("myocardial bridge") (Figs. 4-40 and 4-41). Tunneled epicardial coronary arteries probably represent a normal variant being recognized in up to 86 percent of vessels.[69, 70] (See also Chap. 138.)

Branches of the Major Epicardial Arteries

The branches (Fig. 4-38) of the LAD artery, in their usual order of origin, are the first diagonal, the first septal perforator, the right ventricular (not always seen in normal hearts), other septal perforators, and other diagonal branches. There may be two to six diagonal arteries, including the first diagonal, which may originate separately from the LM trunk. These diagonal branches course laterally over the free wall of the left ventricle in the angle between the LAD and the LC. There are also

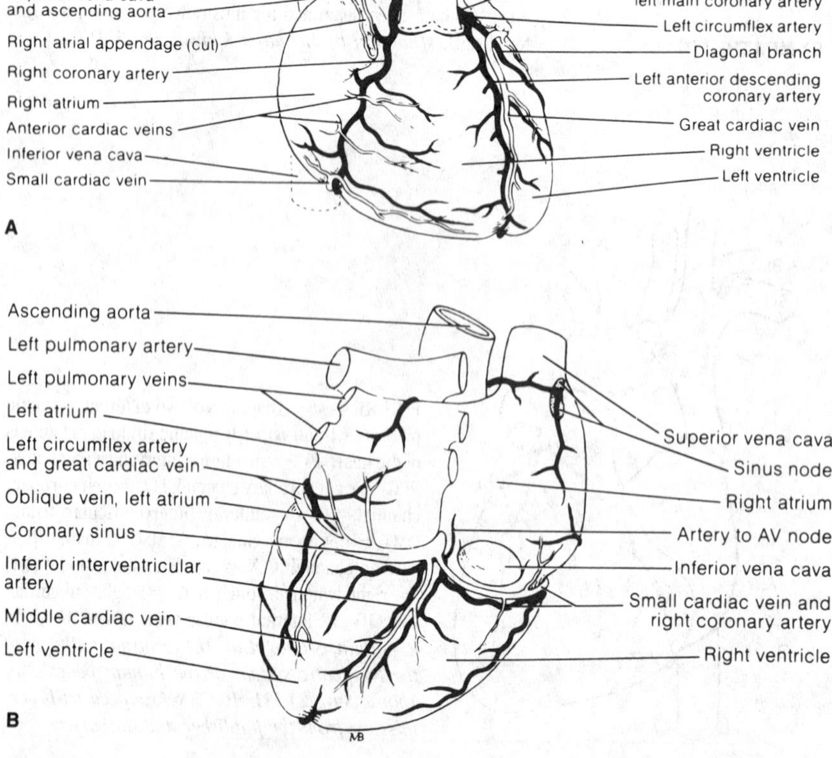

FIGURE 4-38 Diagram illustrating the principal arteries and veins on (*A*) the anterior surface of the heart and (*B*) the posterior and inferior surfaces of the heart. Part of the right atrial appendage has been resected to show the proximal right coronary artery. In *B* the heart is shown more vertically oriented to expose the inferior surface. *(From R Walmsley, H Watson: Clinical Anatomy of the Heart. New York, Churchill Livingstone, 1978. Reproduced with permission from the publisher and authors.)*

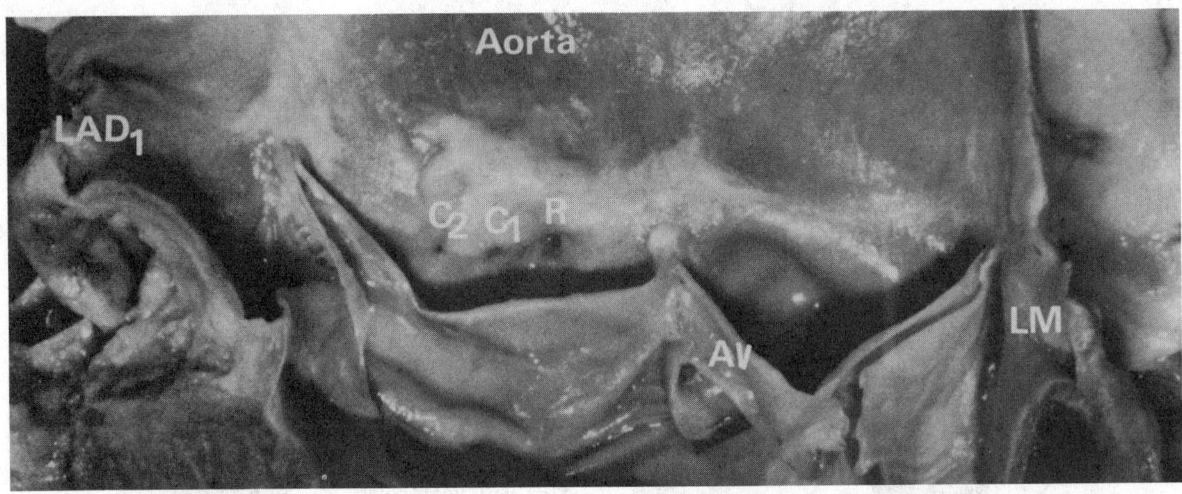

FIGURE 4-39 Photograph of ascending aorta showing five separate coronary ostia: duplicate left anterior descending (LAD_1), duplicate conal arteries (C_1, C_2), left main (LM), and right (R). AV = aortic valve. *(From BF Waller: Five coronary ostia: Duplicate left anterior descending and right conus coronary arteries. Am J Cardiol 52:137, 1983. Reproduced with permission from the publisher and author.)*

three to five septal branches, which leave the LAD artery at a right angle and plunge deeply into the ventricular septum (Fig. 4-43).

The branches of the LC are variable but may include the sinus node artery (40 to 50 percent), the left atrial circumflex branch, the anterolateral marginal, the distal circumflex, one or more posterolateral marginals, and the PDA (10 to 15 percent). The anterolateral marginal, which is usually the largest branch, is directed along the anterolateral wall toward the apex.

The branches of the RCA include the conus artery (which may originate from a separate ostia in the right coronary sinus in 40 to 50 percent of hearts) to the right ventricular outflow area, the artery to the sinus node (50 to 60 percent), several anterior right ventricular branches, right atrial branches, the acute marginal branch, the artery to the AV node and proximal bundle branches, the PDA, and terminal branches to the left ventricle and left atrium. When the sinus node artery originates from the RCA, it runs along the anterior right atrium to the superior vena cava, which it encircles in a clockwise or counterclockwise direction before it penetrates the sinus node.[71] In 40 to 50 percent of hearts, the sinus node artery originates from the proximal LC and crosses behind the aorta and in front of the left atrium to reach the superior vena cava.

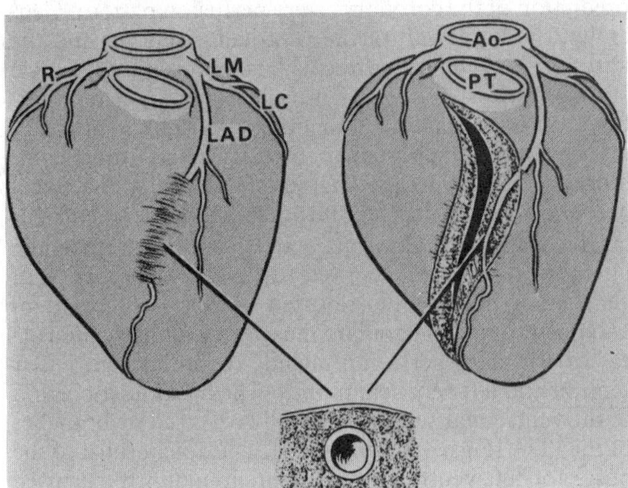

FIGURE 4-40 Diagram and photomicrograph showing tunneled epicardial coronary artery. *Left*: Middle portion of left anterior descending coronary artery (LAD) lies within ventricular myocardium. Ao = aorta; LC = left circumflex; LM = left main; PT = pulmonary trunk; R = right. (×100). *(From BF Waller: Anatomy, histology, and pathology of the major epicardial coronary arteries relevant to echocardiographic imaging techniques. J Am Soc Echo 2:232, 1989. Reproduced with permission from the publisher and author.)*

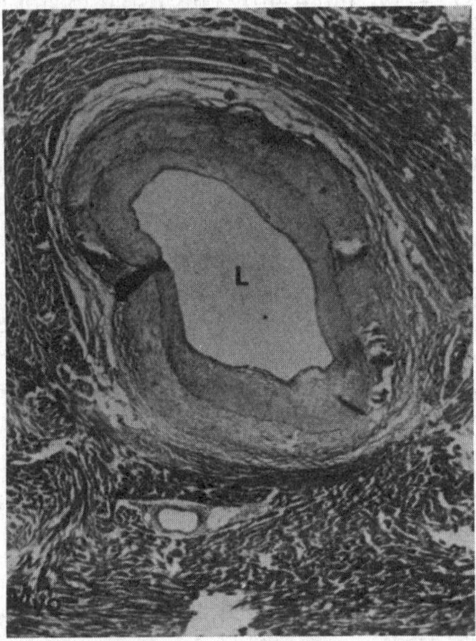

FIGURE 4-41 Tunneled left anterior descending coronary artery. The artery is surrounded by myocardium (Myo). L = lumen. *(From BF Waller: Anatomy, histology, and pathology of the major epicardial coronary arteries relevant to echocardiographic imaging techniques. J Am Soc Echo 2:232, 1989. Reproduced with permission from the publisher and author.)*

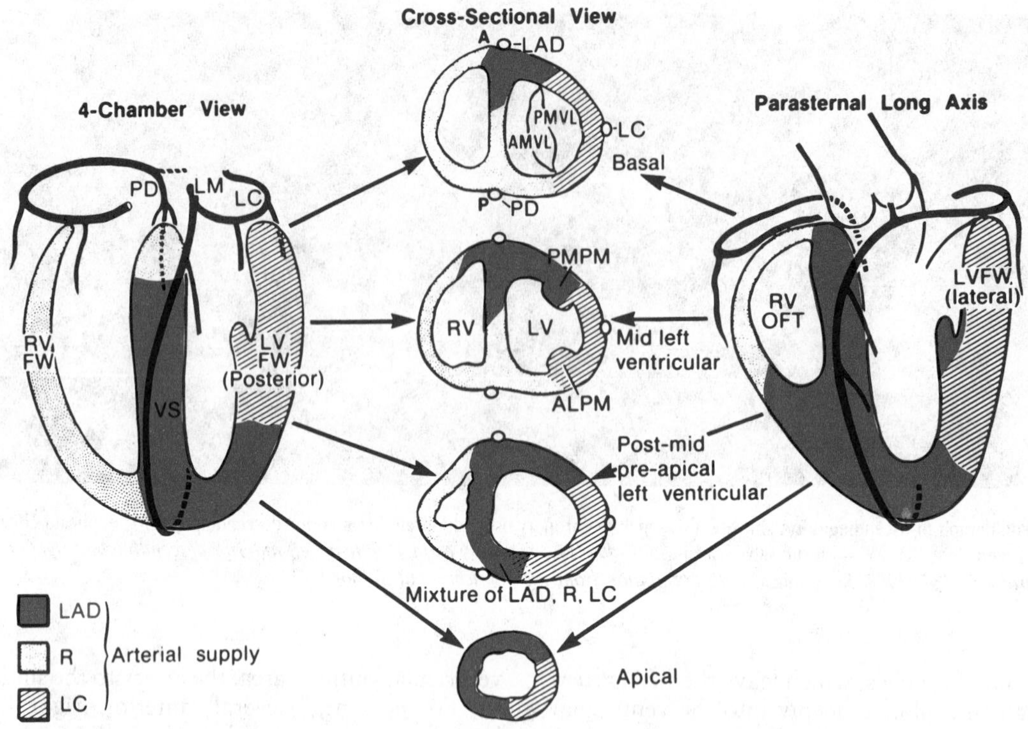

FIGURE 4-42 Diagram showing myocardial perfusion patterns of major epicardial coronary arteries as viewed from three tomographic cuts: four-chamber view, cross-sectional view, and parasternal long axis. A = anterior; ALPM = anterolateral papillary muscle; LC = left circumflex; LAD = left anterior descending; LM = left main; LV = left ventricle; LVFM = left ventricular free wall; P = posterior; PMPM = posteromedial papillary muscle; RV = right ventricle; RVFM = right ventricular free wall; RVOFT = right ventricular outflow tract. *(Modified from H Feigenbaum: Echocardiography. Philadelphia, Lea & Febiger, 1986: 462.)*

Coronary Ostia

The left and right coronary ostia arise normally within a sinus of Valsalva or at the junction of the sinus and tubular portions of aorta (sinotubular junction) (Figs. 4-37, 4-39, and 4-40). This ostial location allows maximal coronary filling during ventricular diastole. Occasionally, the right or left coronary ostium arises 1 cm or more above the sinotubular junction. This ostial dislocation has been termed high takeoff coronary artery. The record position for a high takeoff coronary artery is 2.5 cm above the sinotubular junction.[72] In addition to the normal variants of a separate conus ostium or several right ventricular branch ostia, certain congenital coronary artery anomalies give rise to a reduced number (single coronary artery), increased number (separate origin of the LAD, LC, or both) (Fig. 4-40), or altered shapes (acute angle takeoff, slitlike) or the coronary ostia. (See Chap. 97.)

Coronary Artery Distribution and Myocardial Supply

In the current era of reperfusion therapy for evolving acute myocardial infarction, it has become popular to refer to the "infarct artery" of the "ventricular myocardium at risk." These phrases indicate that there is a well-established relation between a given epicardial coronary artery and its myocardial supply. Although general statements can be made about the coronary distribution, the amount of myocardium supplied by a vessel is variable and is affected by collateral vessels, congenital variations, and other factors. Figure 4-42 shows a scheme whereby certain areas on various views of the two-dimensional echocardiogram can provide a reasonable prediction of the coronary artery perfusion pattern. Generally, the basal half of the ventricular septum and the anterior left ventricular free wall is perfused by the LAD coronary artery. A dominant right coronary artery perfuses anterior, lateral, and posterior right ventricular myocardium. The posterior coronary artery (most commonly arising from the RCA) supplies blood to the apical half of the ventricular septum and posterior left ventricular free wall. The LC coronary artery usually perfuses the lateral wall of the left ventricle (defined as that portion of ventricular myocardium located between anterolateral and posteromedial papillary muscles). Unappreciated areas of coronary perfusion include the basal ventricular septum and left ventricular apex. The basalmost portion of the ventricular septum is usually perfused by branches of the PDA (Figs. 4-42 and 4-43). The apical third of the posterior left ventricle may be predominantly perfused by the LAD artery as it wraps around the cardiac apex for variable lengths along the posterior left ventricle. At present it is believed that the LAD artery and its branches nourish the apical wall of the left ventricle, most of the right and left bundle branches, and the anterolateral papillary muscle of the left ventricle. When the PDA is provided by the circumflex artery, the entire septum is vascularized by the left coronary system.[73] The LAD

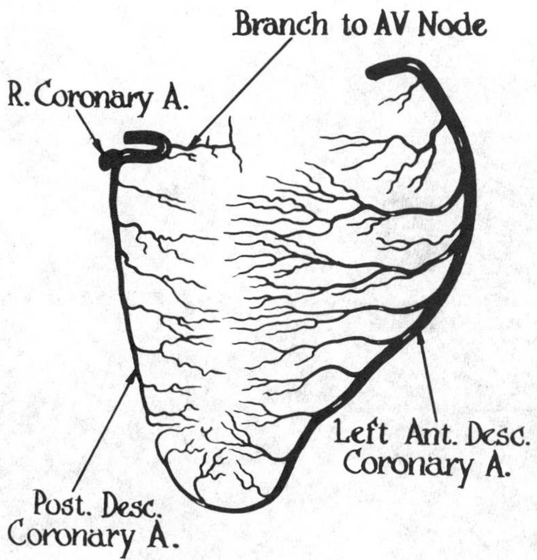

FIGURE 4-43 Drawing illustrating the normal blood supply of the human ventricular septum. *(From TN James, GE Burch: Blood supply of the human interventricular septum. Circulation 17:391, 1958. Reproduced with permission from the American Heart Association and the authors.)*

artery can also provide collateral circulation to the anterior right ventricle via the circle of Vieussens, to the posterior ventricular septum by the septal perforators, and to the PDA from the distal LAD artery or a diagonal branch.

Kogel's artery[74] arises from the proximal RCA or LC or, rarely, the LM; it courses posteriorly into the lower portion of the atrial septum and anastamoses with the AV node artery.

Histological Features of the Normal Coronary Artery

The basic organization of the coronary arterial wall is similar to all arteries in that three concentric layers can be distinguished (Figs. 4-44 and 4-45): an inner (luminal) layer, the intima (tunica intima, intimal layer); a medial layer; and an outer (external) layer, the adventitia (tunica adventitia, adventitial layer).

The intima consists of a lining layer of endothelial cells, a subendothelial layer containing connective tissue, and smooth-muscle cells. The endothelium provides a smooth luminal lining and a selective diffusion barrier between the blood and the other wall layers. The endothelial cells are oriented longitudinally relative to the artery and are attached by occluding junctions and gap lium was considered a simple, passive barrier modulating diffusion. In contrast, it is now known that endothelial (communicating) junctions. Until recently, the endothe- cells have a number of metabolic and endocrine functions that play a critical role both normally and in various disease states. Endothelium-derived relaxing factor, which is now thought to be nitric oxide produced from L-arginine, stimulates guanylate cyclase to produce vasodilating cyclic guanosine monophosphate. Endothelium-derived relaxing factor is an important modulator of subadjacent vascular smooth-muscle tone and of the vascular response to a number of vasoactive hormones (such as adenosine, acetylcholine, serotonin, and bradykinin) in both conduit and resistance vessels. The release of EDRF under the stimulus of increased shear stress plays an important role in the production of vasodilatation in some vascular beds during conditions of increased flow. (See also Chaps. 2, 5, and 56.) Some of the many other functions of the arterial endothelial cell include production of a potent vasoconstrictor peptide, *endothelin;* an antithrombotic agent (prostacyclin, PGI_2); a prothrombotic agent (factor VIII or von Willebrand's factor); a fibrinolytic agent (tissue plasminogen activator); an inflammatory mediator (interleukin-1); and important growth factors, including platelet-derived growth factor (PDGF) and fibroblast growth factor. It contains receptors for low-density lipoprotein, thrombin, and factor X.[75] The intimal layer is also the site of many of the pathological changes seen in elastic arteries, such as atherosclerosis. The intimal layer is separated from the medial layer by the internal elastic membrane (internal elastic lamina, elastic interna) which is a fenestrated sheet of elastic tissue (Figs. 4-44 and 4-45). The internal elastic membrane may be fragmented, duplicated, or focally lost with advancing age or intimal disease. (See Chap. 55.)

The media consists of multiple layers of smooth-muscle cells and connective tissue (elastic fibers, collagen, proteoglycans). The amount of elastic tissue is less and the number of smooth-muscle cells is greater in the epicardial coronary arteries compared with other elastic vessels.[68] The media consists of up to 40 layers of circumferentially or helically oriented smooth muscles. The normal media ranges in thickness from 125 to 350 μm (average 200 μm).[76] Medial thicknesses underlying diseased intima (atherosclerotic plaque) are considerably thinner, ranging from 16 to 190 μm (mean 80 μm).[76] The smooth-muscle cells are embedded in a glycoprotein mix that stains heavily with the periodic acid Schiff reac-

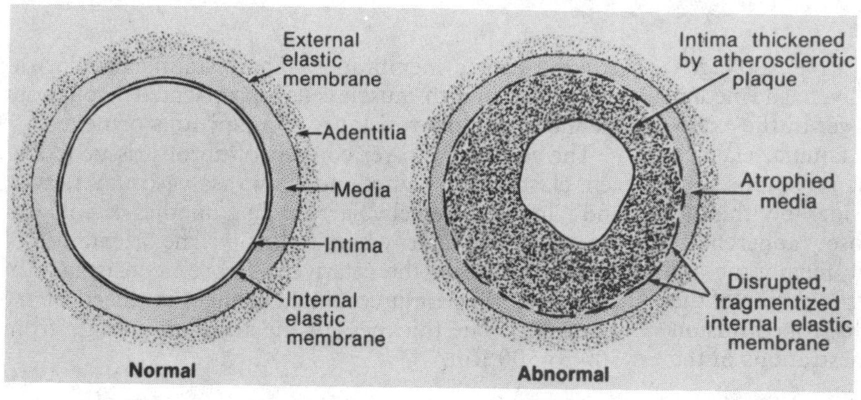

FIGURE 4-44 Diagram showing histologic structure of normal and diseased epicardial coronary artery. *(From BF Waller: Anatomy, histology, and pathology of the major epicardial coronary arteries relevant to echocardiographic imaging techniques. J Am Soc Echo 2:232, 1989. Reproduced with permission from the publisher and author.)*

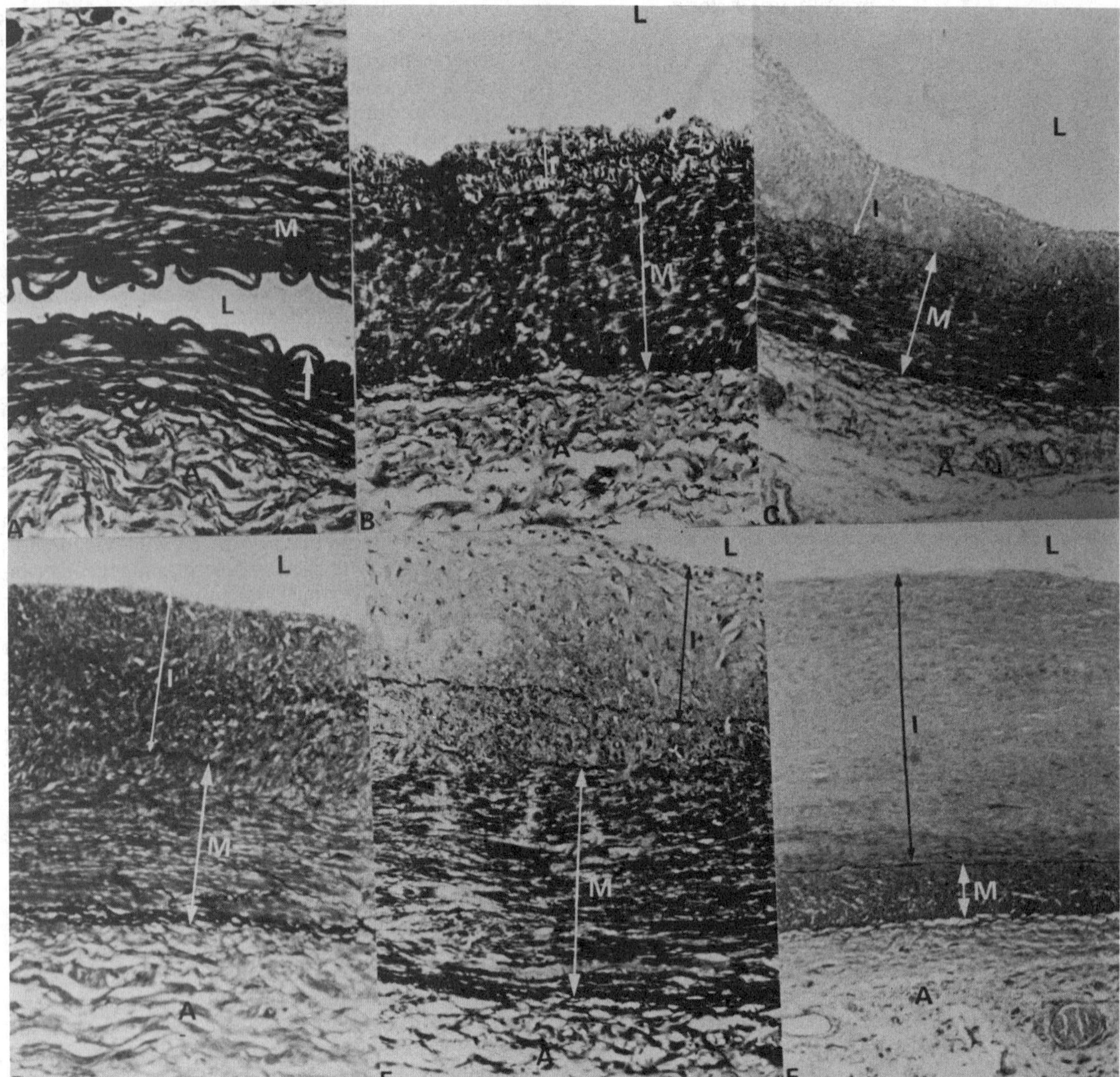

FIGURE 4-45 Composite of histologic sections of wall of various epicardial coronary arteries. *A*. One-day-old artery showing underdeveloped intima, wavy internal elastic membrane (arrow), and well-developed media (M). *B*. Teenage coronary artery showing further development of intima and media. *C–F*. Diseased epicardial coronary arteries showing varying degrees of intimal thickening by atherosclerotic plaque, fragmented or disrupted internal elastic membrane, and thinning of media. A = adventitia; L = coronary lumen. *(From BF Waller: Anatomy, histology, and pathology of the major epicardial coronary arteries relevant to echocardiographic imaging techniques. J Am Soc Echo 2:232, 1989. Reproduced with permission from the publisher and author.)*

tion [*para*-aminosalicylic acid (PAS) positive]. Collagen and elastic fibers are also present in this layer. The medial layer is separated from the adventitial layer by the external elastic membrane (external elastic lamina, elastica externa). The external elastic membrane is composed of interrupted layers of elastin and is considerably thinner than the internal elastic membrane. Closely adherent to the outer border of the external elastic membrane are unmyelinated nerve axons. The neural stimulation of the medial smooth muscles apparently results from diffusion of the neurotransmitter through the fenestrations of the external elastic membrane.[77] The resulting depolarization of the smooth-muscle cells is propagated throughout the media by low-resistance gap junctions or nexus.[77]

The adventitial layer consists of fibrous tissue (collagen, elastic fibers) surrounded by vasa vasorum, nerves, and lymphatic vessels. Surrounding bundles of collagen are oriented primarily longitudinally. The orientation of the collagen and the relatively "loose" consistency of the adventitia permit continual changes in the coronary diameter.[77] The thickness of the adventitia ranges from 300 to 500 μm.

Developmental and Aging Changes of the Epicardial Coronary Arteries

The epicardial coronary arteries normally undergo significant changes between the fetal state and old age (Fig. 4-46).[78,79] In fetal coronary arteries the intima is not well developed, consisting of a thin layer of elongated endothelial cells in close contact with the internal elastic membrane. The internal elastic membrane appears as a continuous tube (Fig. 4-46). The media in fetal coronary arteries is well developed, consisting of a layer of circular smooth-muscle cells and fine elastic fibers (Fig. 4-46). The adventitia is less well developed and consists of a thin layer of connective tissue.[78] Changes in various layers begin after birth and consist of splitting and fragmenting of the internal elastic membrane, proliferation of fibroblasts, and an increase in ground substance in the subendothelium. The medial smooth muscles alter their shape and position, presumably as a result of a reaction to hemodynamic changes after birth.[78] In the next several months smooth muscles appear between the split internal elastic membrane and form the "musculoelastic layer" between the intima and media. Intimal "cushions" of fibroblasts and elastic fibers occur focally along the intima. The external elastic membrane forms by 6 months. By 1 year the intima contains a collection of subendothelial collagen and elastic fibers and a musculoelastic layer that eventually is incorporated into the mature media. In normal human coronary arteries, the amount of smooth muscle and fibroelastic tissue in the intima is a function of age. The intima progressively thickens, so that by late adolescence it is as thick as the media; after adolescence the intima becomes thicker than the media.[79] In middle age the intima may become diseased and markedly thickened by atherosclerotic plaque. The underlying media thins and loses smooth-muscle cells. The internal elastic membrane fragmentizes, duplicates, or focally disappears. Degenerative changes such as calcium deposition take place in the intima (atherosclerotic plaque), but calcific deposits rarely involve the media (Mönckeberg's medial sclerosis).[80] In old age the coronary arteries become tortuous, the luminal diameter increases, the media thins, and calcific deposits increase.[81] (See also Chap. 55.)

THE CORONARY VEINS

An extensive intercommunicating network of veins provides venous drainage for the coronary circulation. Three venous drainage systems can be considered: the coronary sinus and its tributaries, the anterior right ventricular veins, and the Thebesian veins (Fig. 4-38).[82]

The coronary sinus, located in the posterior AV groove near the crux of the heart, receives venous blood from the great, middle, and small cardiac veins, the posterior veins of the left ventricle, and the left atrial oblique vein (of Marshall). The coronary sinus predominantly drains blood from the left ventricle. The anterior interventricular vein lies in the anterior interventricular sulcus, parallel to the left anterior descending coronary artery. It ascends to near the bifurcation of the left main coronary artery and then turns leftward to circle posteriorly under the left atrium in the left AV sulcus, where it is referred to as the great cardiac vein. Along its posterior course, the great cardiac vein receives venous blood from large marginal and posterior left ventricular branches and then becomes the coronary sinus near the posterior margin of the left atrium. The posterior interventricular vein (middle cardiac vein) arises near the posterior aspect of the cardiac apex and ascends in the posterior interventricular sulcus next to the posterior descending coronary artery and drains either into the right atrium directly or into the coronary sinus just before it empties into the right atrium. The oblique vein of Marshall runs along the posterior left atrium and joins the great cardiac vein at the point where the latter becomes the coronary sinus. The coronary sinus extends 2 to 3 cm within the posterior AV groove before it opens into the infero-posterior-medial aspect of the right atrium, between the orifice of the inferior vena cava and the septal tricuspid leaflet. A crescent-shaped, rudimentary valve, the Thebesian valve, can be seen at its entrance. The total distance from the bifurcation of the left coronary artery to the Thebesian valve is about 9 cm. About 85 percent of the coronary venous blood, including the drainage from the ventricular septum, the left ventricle, both atria, and some of the right ventricle, is carried by this elaborate system of veins. It is important to note that studies involving catheterization of the coronary sinus often require placing the tip of a catheter in the coronary sinus beyond the entrance of the posterior interventricular vein and other major veins draining the posterior left ventricle.

There are two to four anterior cardiac veins that originate in and drain the anterior right ventricular wall, travel superiorly to cross the right AV sulcus, and enter either directly into the right atrium anteriorly or into a collecting vein at the base of the right atrium. The small cardiac vein, which receives some branches from the right ventricle and the right atrium, winds around the right side of the heart in the AV sulcus and terminates either in the coronary sinus or the right atrium. The Thebesian veins are tiny venous outlets draining the myocardium directly into the cardiac chambers, primarily into the right atrium and right ventricle.

THE CONDUCTION SYSTEM OF THE HEART

The specialized tissues of the heart (neuromyocardial cells) that initiate and conduct the cardiac impulse consist of three major parts: (1) *sinus node* (sinu-atrial node, sinoatrial node, SA node, sinoauricular node, pacemaker, node of Keith-Flack); (2) *atrioventricular junctional area*, including the *atrioventricular node* (AV node, node of Tawara, node of Aschoff-Tawara, compact portion of atrioventricular junctional area) and the His bundle (penetrating bundle, AV bundle, common bundle); and (3) bundle branches (branching portion of AV bundle, bifurcation, ventricular conduction tissue) and terminal Purkinje fibers (Purkinje cells, peripheral conduction system, network of Purkinje) (Figs. 4-47 to 4-63). Controversy still exists about whether impulses

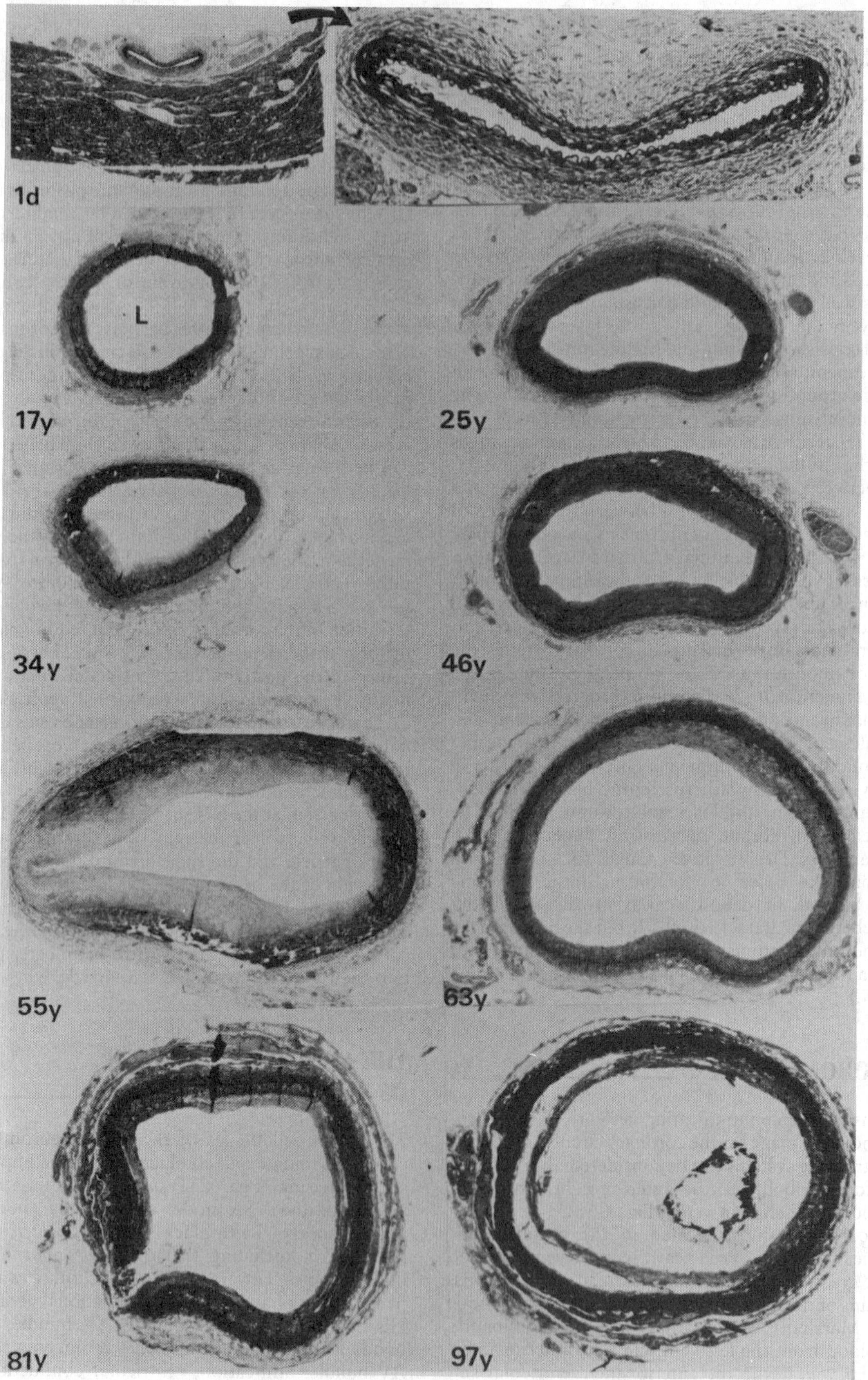

FIGURE 4-46 Photomicrographs of left anterior descending coronary artery from nine patients spanning nine decades of life. All arteries (except top right) are photographed at same magnification (×10). With advancing age, luminal diameter and cross-sectional area increase, intima thickens, and media thins. All arteries are from patients dying of noncardiac disease. D = day; y = year. *(From BF Waller: Anatomy, histology, and pathology of the major epicardial coronary arteries relevant to echocardiographic imaging techniques. J Am Soc Echo 2:232, 1989. Reproduced with permission from the publisher and author.)*

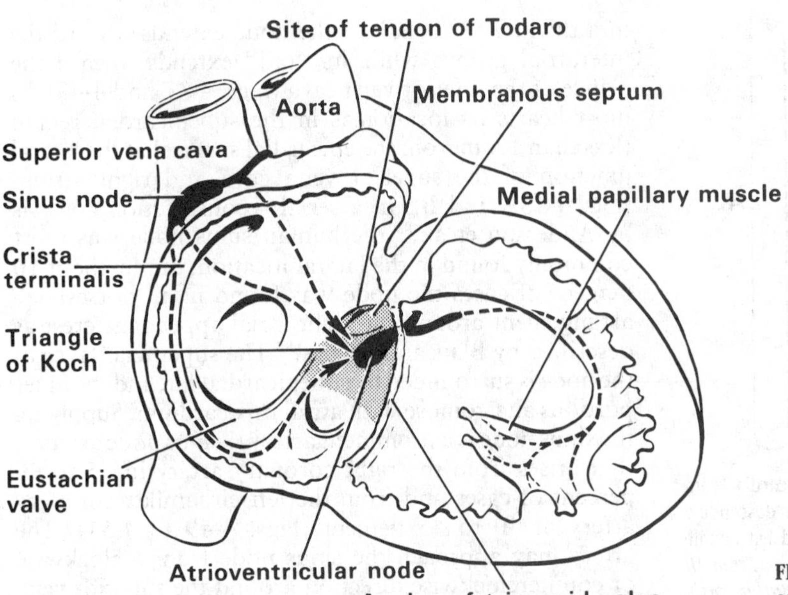

FIGURE 4-47 Diagram showing the anatomic landmarks of the cardiac conduction system.

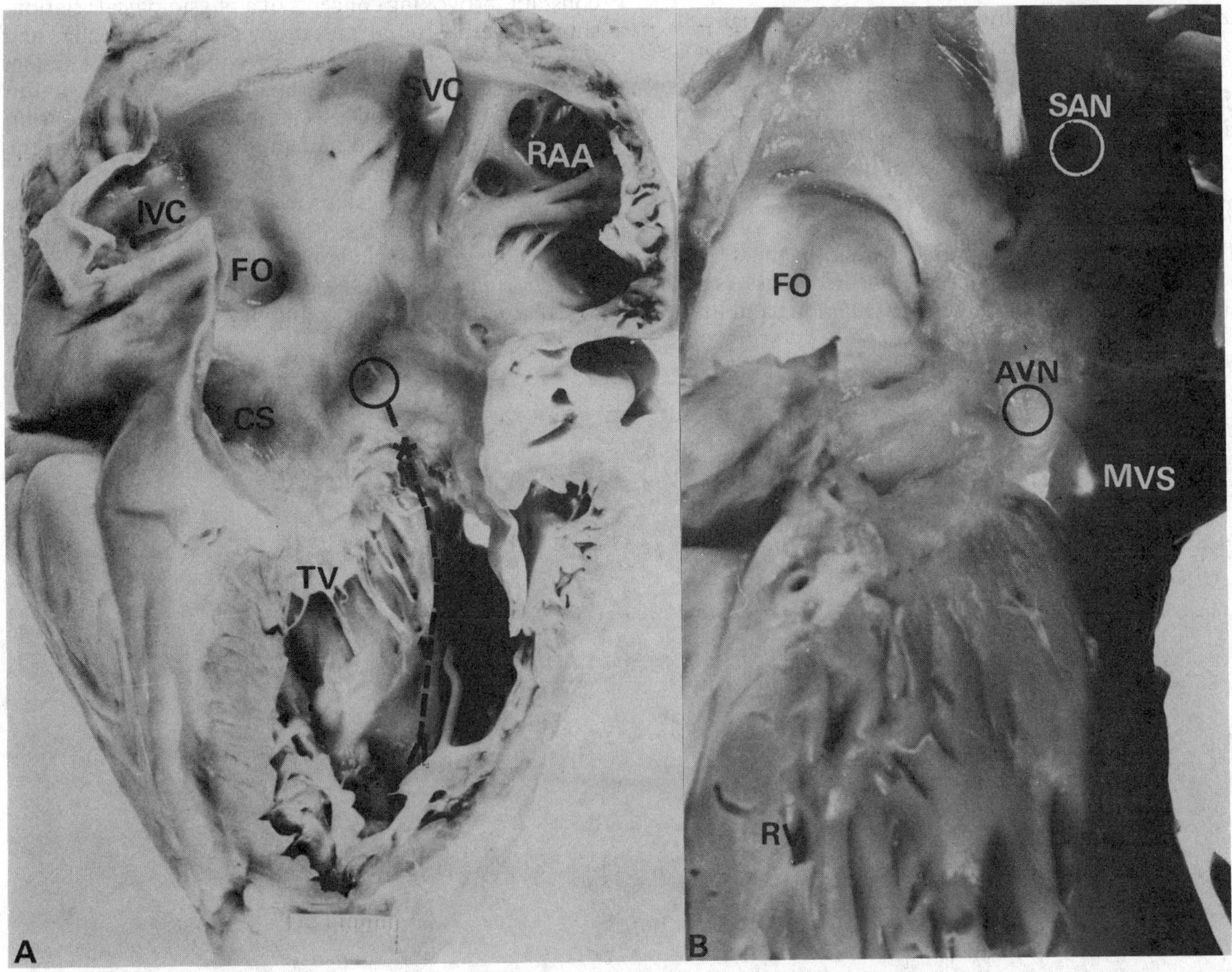

FIGURE 4-48 Photographs of heart showing anatomic landmarks of the cardiac conduction system. *A*. Tomographic cut of the right side of the heart showing the location of the atrioventricular node (circle) and right bundle branch (*- - -). CS = coronary sinus; FO = fossa ovale; IVC = inferior vena cava; RAA = right atrial appendage; SVC = superior vena cava; TV = tricuspid valve. *B*. Closeup of annulus of tricuspid valve showing approximate location of sinoatrial node (SAN) and atrioventricular node (AVN, circle). MVS = membranous ventricular septum; RV = right ventricle.

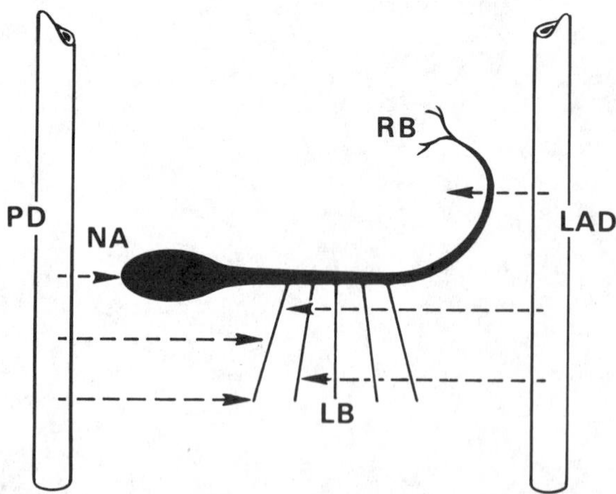

FIGURE 4-49 Diagram showing arterial blood supply of the cardiac conduction system. The nodal artery (NA) arises from the posterior descending artery (PD). The bulk of the arterial blood supply to right and left bundle branches comes from the left anterior descending artery (LAD). *(From MJ Davies: Pathology of Conducting Tissue of the Heart. London, Butterworth, 1979. Reproduced with permission from the publisher and author.)*

from the sinus node to the AV node travel over specialized conducting "pathways" ("specialized atrial cells") or over nonspecialized plain atrial myocardium. Because of this controversy, the internodal area has not been listed in the three-part structure of specialized conduction tissues. (See also Chaps. 34 and 35.)

Sinus Node

The sinus node, first reported by Keith and Flack in 1907,[83–85] is an oval-shaped, elongated mass (spindle shaped) measuring about 10 to 20 mm long and up to 5 mm thick. The "head" of the node extends toward the interatrial groove while its "tail" extends toward the orifice of the inferior vena cava (Figs. 4-47 and 4-48). In most hearts its location is in the subepicardial region (less than 1 mm from the epicardial surface) at the lateral junction of the superior vena cava and right atrium (Fig. 4-48*A* and *B*). In a serial reconstruction analysis by Anderson et al.,[86] the human sinus node was most commonly found in the lateral location, but in about 10 percent of cases the node was found in a "horseshoe" arrangement around the right atrial appendage crest as described by Blair and Davies.[87] The superficial layer of the node is surrounded by subepicardial fat, and the inner portions anastomose with atrial myocardium. Supplying the sinus node is a prominent artery ("sinus node artery") that arises from the right coronary artery in 55 to 60 percent of cases and from the left circumflex coronary artery in 40 to 45 percent (Figs. 4-49 to 4-51). The artery may approach the sinus node from a clockwise or counterclockwise direction around the superior vena caval–right atrial junction or completely encircle the atriocaval junction.[86] A dual blood supply to the sinus node is present in 11 percent of individuals.[89] The relationship of the artery to the node has been thought to be fairly constant, provoking concepts of a physiological relationship between arterial pulsation, arterial diameter, and sinus node discharge rate in a feedback control system ("servomechanism").[90] On the other hand, variation in arterial disposition suggests an inconsistent relationship between the artery and node and casts doubt upon the servomechanism concept.[86]

Histologically, the sinus node is easily recognized at low magnifications (Figs. 4-52 to 4-54). Specific cell types in the sinus node include *nodal cells, transitional cells,* and *atrial muscle cells.* Nodal cells (P cells) are small (3 to 10 μm), ovoid, pale standing, and poorly striated

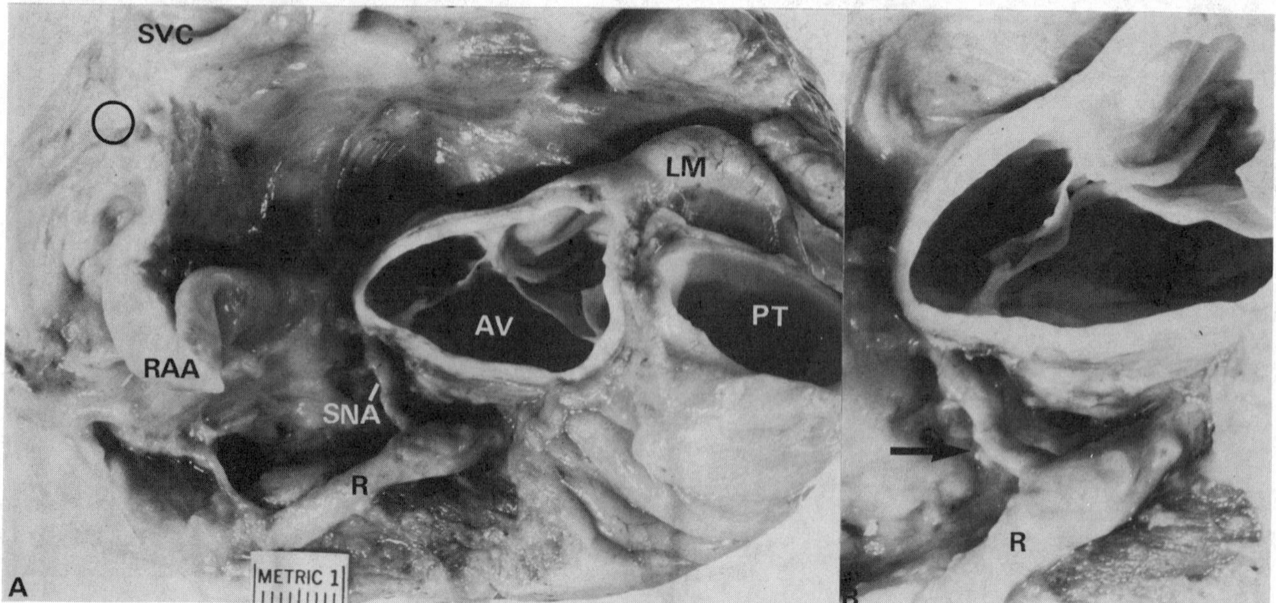

FIGURE 4-50 Photographs of heart showing origin of the sinus nodal artery (SNA). *A.* Sinus nodal artery arising as early branch of the right (R) coronary artery. Dark circle indicates approximate location of the sinus node (SN). PT = pulmonary trunk, RAA = right atrial appendage, SVC = superior vena cava. *B.* Closeup of right coronary artery.

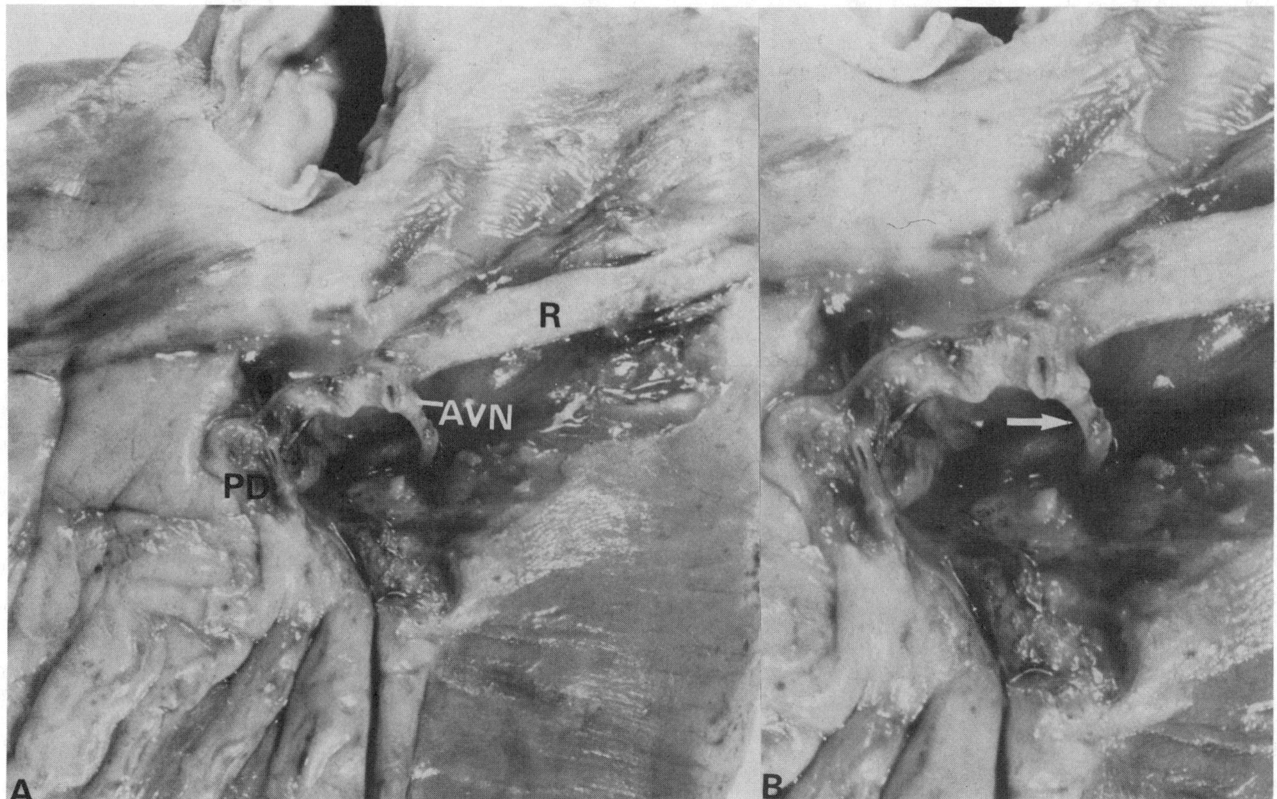

FIGURE 4-51 Photographs of posterior surface of the heart at the crux showing the origin of the atrioventricular nodal (AVN) artery from the right (R) coronary artery. *A*. The AVN artery arises near the origin of the posterior descending (PD) coronary artery. *B*. Closeup of origin of AVN artery (arrow).

compared to the general myocardial cells.[91] Although the nuclei are of normal size, the nodal cells contain fewer mitochondria compared to contractile cells. The nodal cells are grouped together in interconnecting fascicles placed in a background of fibrous matrix.[92] The interweaving fascicles of nodal cells surround the sinus nodal artery (body of node). Although contact between nodal cells was thought to occur by opposing cell membranes (a factor possibly correlating with the slow conduction within the sinus node), more recent studies suggest the presence and role of nexus connections.[93, 94] Nodal cells are thought to be the source of normal impulse formation in the sinus node.[95–97] Transitional cells (T cells) are elongated cells with characteristics intermediate between the packed nodal cells and the individual atrial myocardial cells.[92] The T cells are located at the margins of the node where the nodal cells become contiguous with atrial myocardium. T cells near nodal cells have simple intercellular connections, while more fully developed intercalated discs exist in T cells near atrial myocardium.[93] In some areas discrete fibrous septae form junctions that separate the node from atrial myocardium, and in other area projections of transitional cells ("tongues") extend for short distances into the working atrial myocardium[92] (Fig. 4-53). Since nodal cells make contact with each other or with T cells, the T cells may provide a "functional pathway" for distribution of the sinus impulses formed in the nodal cells to the rest of the atrial myocardium.[97] The third type of cell present in the sinus node is the working atrial myocardial cell. These cells also extend as projections or tongues into the nodal boundaries. James[97] has described large, clear cells ("Purkinje") at the margins of the sinus node, whereas Becker and colleagues[98] have not found these cells in infant hearts.

Marked differences are present between the histology of the sinus node in an infant and that in an adult.[99] In the infant sinus node, the nodal cells predominate relative to the fibrous matrix. In contrast, in the adult sinus node the fibrous tissue is predominant with the nodal cells scattered within the connective tissue.[99] Part of the increase in fibrosis is likely to be related to an imbalance between proliferating fibrous tissue and more static nodal cells.[92] Surrounding fat also increases with advancing age.

Internal Atrial Myocardium

As noted, the method of travel of the sinus impulse to the AV node remains controversial.[85, 100–110] Investigators agree that a certain population of atrial cells has different electrophysiological properties from other atrial cells. The controversy revolves around whether or not the population of atrial cells with "specialized" action potentials is involved in the orderly transmission of the sinus impulse within the atrium and whether or not these "specialized" cells can be distinguished histologically from "working" atrial myocardium.[92] James[105] and James and Sherf[111] have reviewed the original studies of Bachman,[112] Wenckebach,[113] and Thorel[100] and have supported the concept of three specific internodal tracts

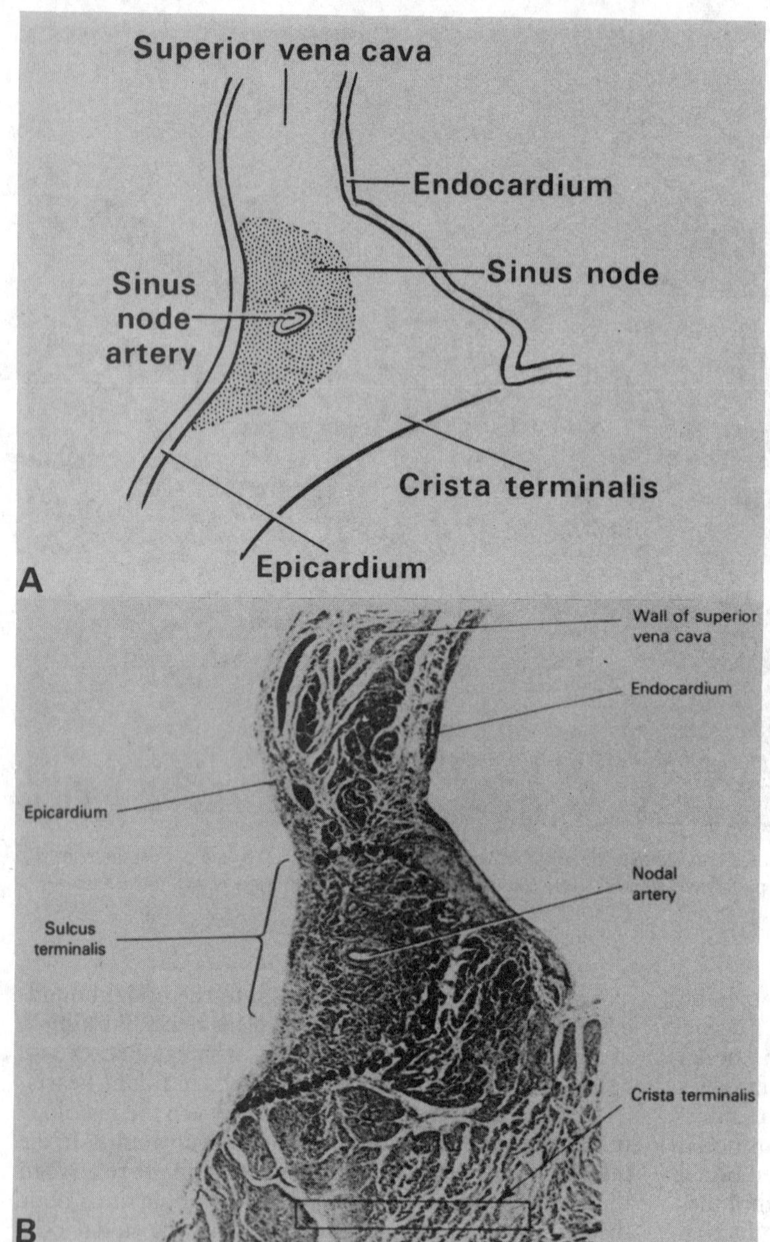

FIGURE 4-52 Diagram (*A*) and photomicrograph (*B*) of sinus node. *(B. From MJ Davies et al: The Conduction System of the Heart. London, Butterworth, 1983. Reproduced with permission from the publisher and authors.)*

between sinus and atrioventricular nodes: *anterior internodal tract* (Bachmann-James'), *middle internodal tract* (Wenckebach's), and *posterior internodal tract* (Thorel's). All three tracts anastomose with each other above the AV node. In these bundles are transitional cells and common atrial myocardial cells. Purkinje cells have been reported near the proximal and distal course of these fascicles,[114] whereas in the middle course common atrial myocardial cells are prevalent, making it difficult and uncertain to follow the fascicles anatomically. In contrast to the concept of specialized atrial "tracts," Janse and Anderson[110] favor the preferential transmission of the sinus node impulse by the shortest routes between the nodes over the thickest bundles of working atrial myocardium. These investigators also question the presence of Purkinje-like cells in the internodal atrial myocardium. Thus, the issue of atrial conduction pathways (?tracts) has not been settled,[115] but presently the evidence does not support the presence of specialized internodal tracts resembling the discrete histologically identifiable bundle branches in the ventricles.[116] Preferential internodal conduction in some parts of the atrium compared to other parts probably does exist and may be due to atrial myocardial fiber orientation, size, geometry, or other factors rather than specialized tracts located between the nodes.[86, 92, 93]

Interatrial Conduction

Bachmann's bundle appears to conduct the cardiac impulse preferentially from the right to the left atrium. This large muscle bundle (see earlier) begins along the anterior margin of the sinus node and travels posteriorly around the aorta to the left atrium. James[97] indicates that the middle and posterior internodal tracts may also extend fibers from the right atrium to the left atrium.

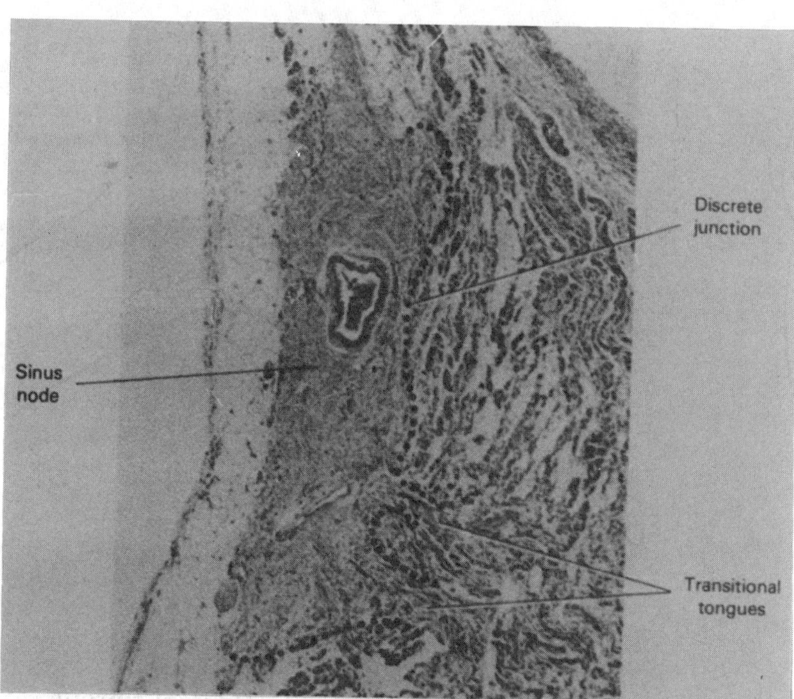

FIGURE 4-53 Photomicrographs of section of sinus node showing junction of sinus node and atrial myocardium and area of transitional cells. *(From MJ Davies et al: The Conduction System of the Heart. London, Butterworth, 1983. Reproduced with permission from the publisher and authors.)*

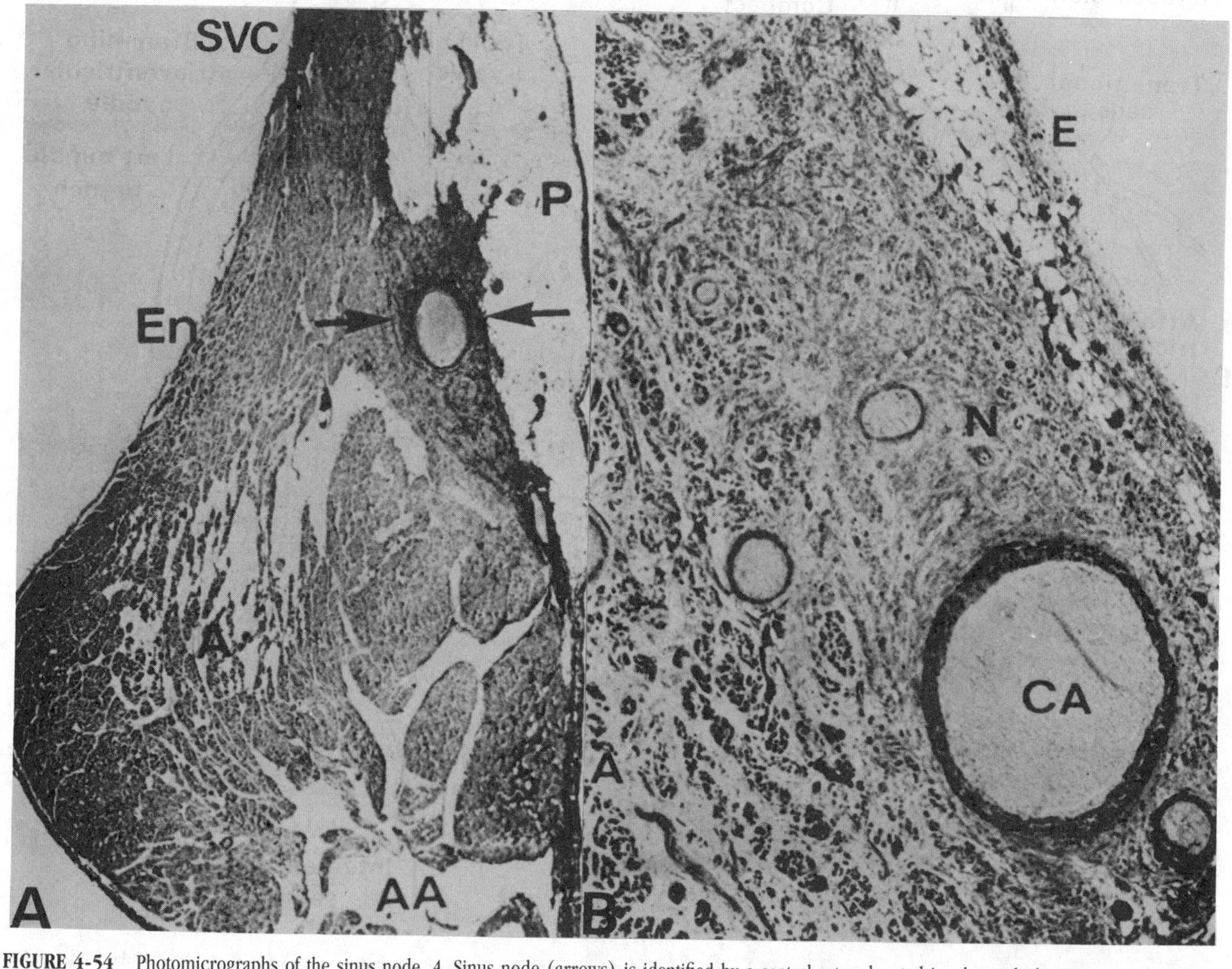

FIGURE 4-54 Photomicrographs of the sinus node. *A.* Sinus node (arrows) is identified by a central artery located just beneath the epicardial surface. A = right atrium; AA = atrial appendage; EN = endocardium; SVC = superior vena cava. *B.* Closeup of sinus node (N) showing a matrix of collagen and muscle fibers. A = atrium; CA = central artery; E = endocardium. *(From MJ Davies: Pathology of Conducting Tissue of the Heart. London, Butterworth, 1971. Reproduced with permission from the publisher and author.)*

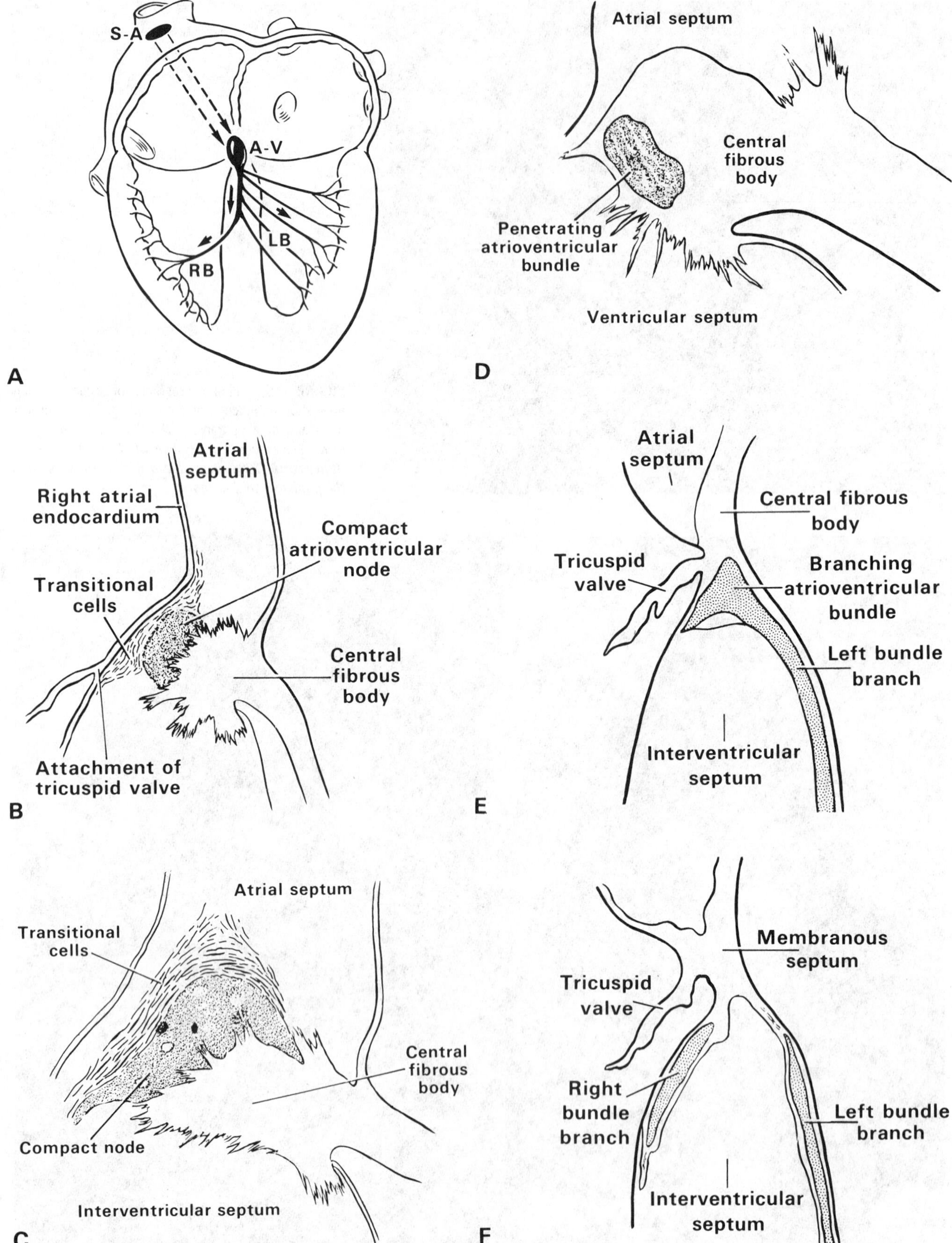

FIGURE 4-55 Diagrammatic composite showing the anatomy of the atrioventricular junctional area from the proximal area of atrioventricular node (*B*,*C*) to the penetrating bundle (*D*), branching atrioventricular bundle (*E*), to the distal area of the right (R) and left (L) bundle (B) branches (*F*). AV = atrioventricular node; SA = sinus node.

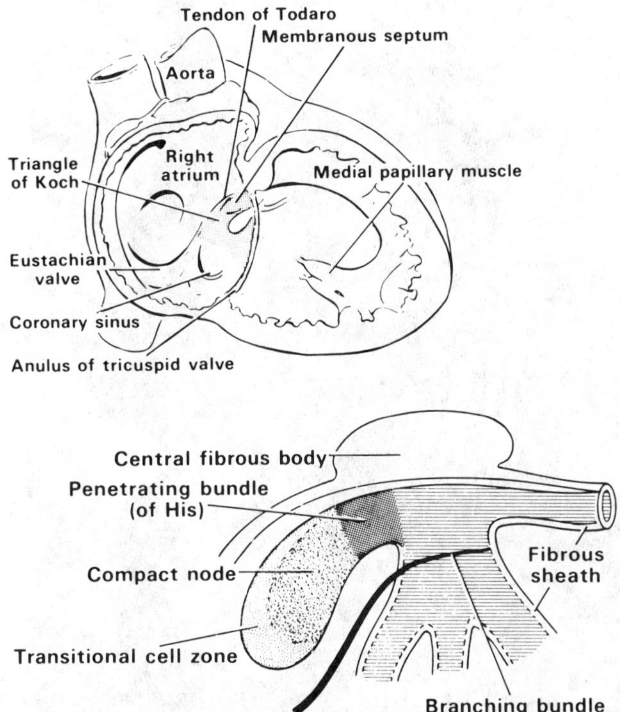

FIGURE 4-56 Diagram of the anatomy of the atrioventricular junction. *(From RH Anderson et al: Anatomicro-electrophysiological correlations in the conduction system—a review. Br Heart J 45:67, 1981. Reproduced with permission from the publisher and authors.)*

Atrioventricular Junctional Area

The normal AV junctional area can be divided into three distinct regions: *transitional cell zone*[117] ("nodal approaches"[118]), *atrioventricular node* (compact portion, Tawara's node[117]) and *penetrating portion* of the AV bundle (His bundle, common bundle) (Figs. 4-47 to 4-63). Some authors[92] include the branching AV bundle (bundle branches) as the fourth region.

Transitional Cell Zone (Nodal Approaches)

The connections by which the myocardium of the right atrium anastomoses with the AV node can be regarded as a "transitional" area between working and specialized cardiac muscle or as an "outer layer" of the AV node (Figs. 4-55 and 4-56). This outer zone concept was originally described by Tawara[117] in 1906 and recently reemphasized by Anderson and colleagues.[119] Rossi[120] indicates that the transitional zone is not a definite layer external to the compact AV node but is made up of thin separate fascicles. These junctional bundles have been subdivided into three main groups: anterior (superior), middle, and posterior (inferior).[105,121] James[84] described some fibers passing from the posterior internodal tract to the distal portion of the AV node (His bundle), which may provide an anatomic substrate for a bypass tract. Other investigators have been unable to confirm these findings, and the functional significance of these fibers has not been demonstrated.

Atrioventricular Node

The compact portion of the AV junction (AV node) seems to occupy a position in the middle of the heart but actually is an epicardial structure (Figs. 4-57 to 4-59). The node lies just beneath the right atrial posterior epicardium, anterior to the ostium of coronary sinus, and directly above the insertion of the septal leaflet of the tricuspid valve (Fig. 4-59). It is located at the apex of a triangle formed by the tricuspid annulus and the tendon of Todaro (*triangle of Koch*).[122] The tendon of Todaro, which originates in the central fibrous body, passes posteriorly through the atrial septum with the eustachian valve. The base of the triangle of Koch[122] is the ostium of the coronary sinus (Figs. 4-57 and 4-58). The atrial component of the junctional area is entirely contained in this triangle. The compact AV node becomes the penetrating bundle of His at the apex of the triangle of Koch and passes into the ventricular tissues below the point of attachment of the tendon of Todaro to the central fibrous body. Within the ventricles, the gross landmark of the AV junctional area is the *membranous septum* (Fig. 4-57). The branching and nonbranching bundles are located between the membranous and the muscular ventricular septum.

In the adult human, the AV node is a compact ovoid structure measuring about 1 × 3 × 5 mm. Histologically, the AV node is composed of a thick mesh of tiny pale cells, which anastomose with one another by short pluridirectional projections of their cytoplasm ("star cells").[120] These cells are interwoven with collagen and elastic fibers. At the electron microscopic level, James and Sherf[111] examined two human hearts and described four types of AV nodal cells: P cells, transitional cells, common myocardial cells, and Purkinje cells. The arterial supply to the AV node ("AV nodal artery") is a branch from the right coronary artery in 85 to 90 percent of human hearts and a branch of the left circumflex coronary artery in the remaining 10 to 15 percent[88] (Figs. 4-49 to 4-51). The innervation of the AV junction, though less prominent than that of the sinus node, is richly supplied by adrenergic and cholinergic fibers with regional differences relevant to function.[122, 123]

The Bundle of His (Penetrating Portion of the AV Bundle) The penetrating bundle (*His bundle*) is a continuation of the distal part of the AV node without any definite histocytological boundary (Fig. 4-60). The bundle of His is a cordal structure measuring 20 mm in length and up to 4 mm in diameter. Conventionally, the beginning of the common bundle is at a point where the specialized myocardial cells lose their network arrangement and form parallel strands just before entering into the membranous septum.[120] These changes are quite variable, but the differences in structure may be quite abrupt and distinct to allow a reliable histologic distinction. Proximal cells of the penetrating portion are heterogenous, resembling those of the compact node, whereas the distal cells of the common bundle are similar to cells in the proximal bundle branches. In general, the Hisian fibers have larger diameters and more parallel arrangement compared to the nodal structures.

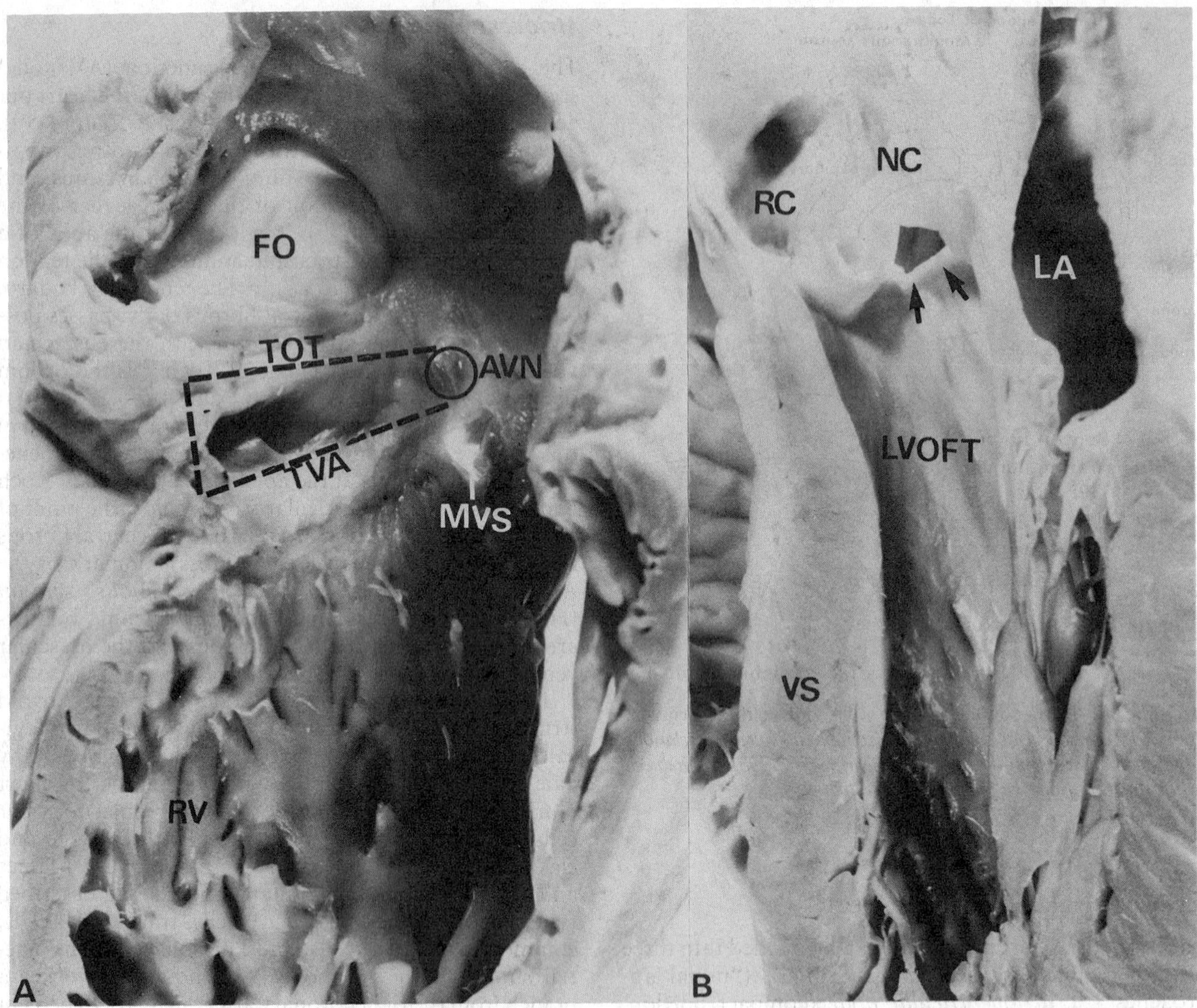

FIGURE 4-57 Photomicrographs of the heart showing anatomic landmarks of the atrioventricular node (AVN). *A*. Triangle of Koch (dashed lines) showing location of AVN. The membranous ventricular septum (MVS) has been excised. CS = coronary sinus; FO = fossa ovale; RV = right ventricle; TOT = tendon of Todaro; TVA = tricuspid valve annulus. *B*. View of left ventricular outflow tract (LVOFT) showing location of excised MVS (arrows) beneath the noncoronary (NC) cusp of aortic valve. LA = left atrium; RC = right coronary cusp; VS = ventricular septum.

The course of the common bundle has been subdivided anatomically into three portions: (1) *nonpenetrating* (proximal, distal to AV node), (2) *penetrating* (within the fibrous tissue of the central body and membranous septum, "tunneled segment"), and (3) *branching* (bifurcation at the crest of muscular ventricular septum).[120] The names "proximal," "middle," and "distal" tract of the AV common bundle have also been applied to these subdivisions. "Upper connections"[120] sometimes connect the common bundle with the crest of the ventricular septum (Fig. 4-63). These fibers were first described by Mahaim[124] in 1947 and are termed either Mahaim fibers or paraspecific fibers. These "bypass" fibers can be separated into "nodoventricular" and "fasciculoventricular" fibers and have been implicated as a substrate for preexcitation in adult hearts. These fibers may connect the node to the ventricular septum or connect various portions of the penetrating bundle to the septal crest. The presence of these fibers as islands of conduction tissue within the central fibrous body have been implicated in sudden infant death syndrome[125] and as a possible cause for circus rhythm circuits.[126] (See Chap. 35.) Arterial branches from both the left anterior and posterior descending coronary arteries supply the upper muscular ventricular septum, making this portion of the conduction system less subject to ischemic damage.[97] Nerve trunks are found along blood vessels, and small strands of beaded nerve fibers lie inside and near the bundle.[127]

Bifurcation and Bundle Branches

Anatomically, the bifurcation is the lowest part of the common bundle (Figs. 4-55 and 4-61 to 4-63). The bifurcation begins on the left side at about the point where the common bundle emerges from the central fibrous body while the right bundle divides at a more anterior point in the distal membranous septum.[120] Variations in the bifurcation site have potential clinicopathologic correlates including right- or left-sided His bundle bifurcation[128] and intraseptal bifurcation.[120]

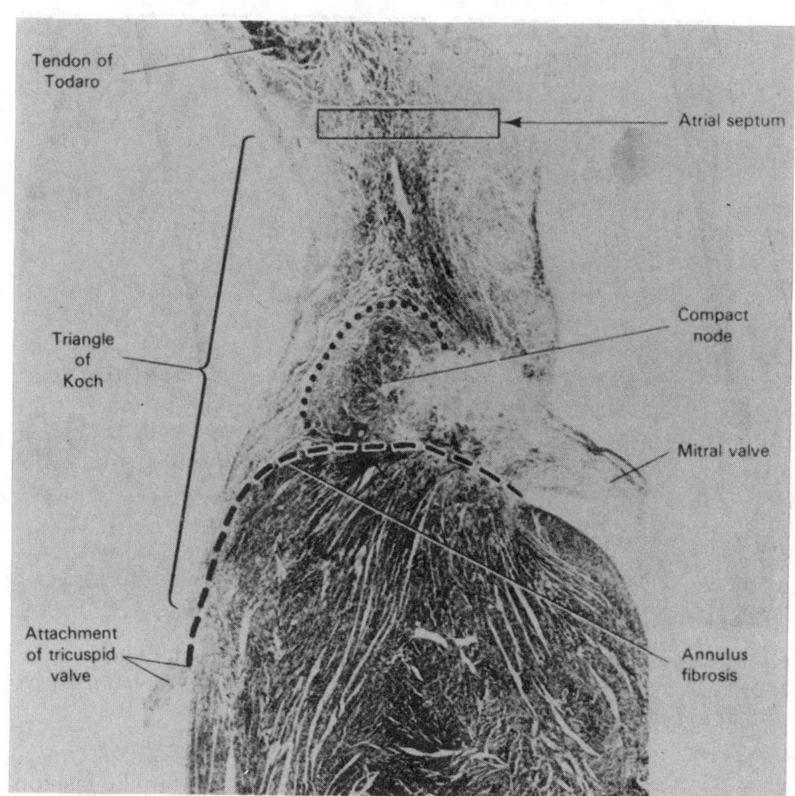

FIGURE 4-58 Photomicrograph showing the boundaries of the triangle of Koch and location of the atrioventricular node (compact node). *(From MJ Davies et al: The Conduction System of the Heart. London, Butterworth, 1983. Reproduced with permission from the publisher and authors.)*

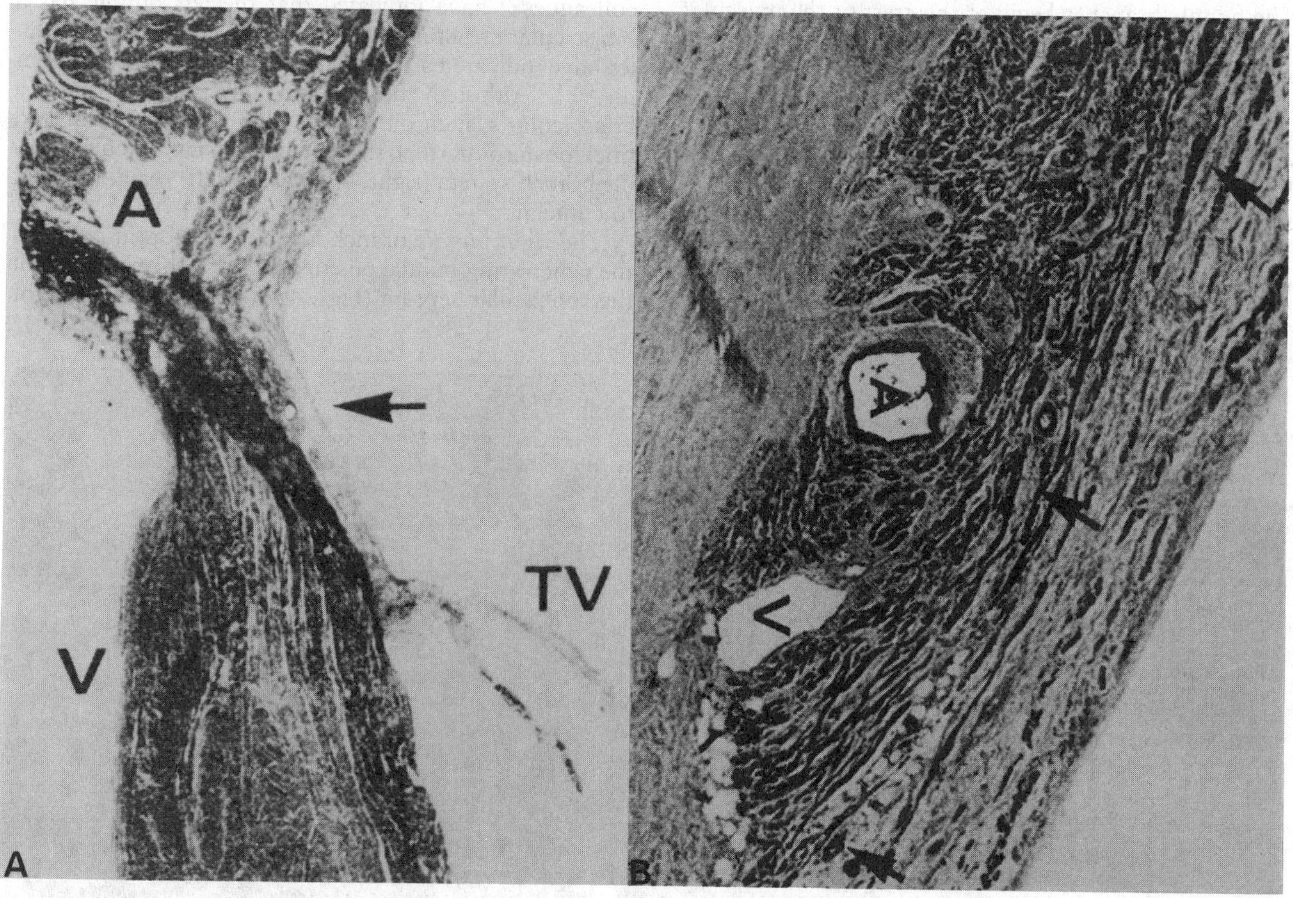

FIGURE 4-59 Photomicrographs of normal atrioventricular node (AVN). The AVN (arrow) is adjacent to the central fibrous body (CFB) and lies beneath the right atrial *A.* endocardium just above the insertion of the tricuspid valve (TV). V = left ventricle. *B.* Closeup of AVN (arrows) showing artery (A) and vein (V). *(From MJ Davies: Pathology of Conducting Tissue of the Heart. London, Butterworth, 1971. Reproduced with permission from the publisher and author.)*

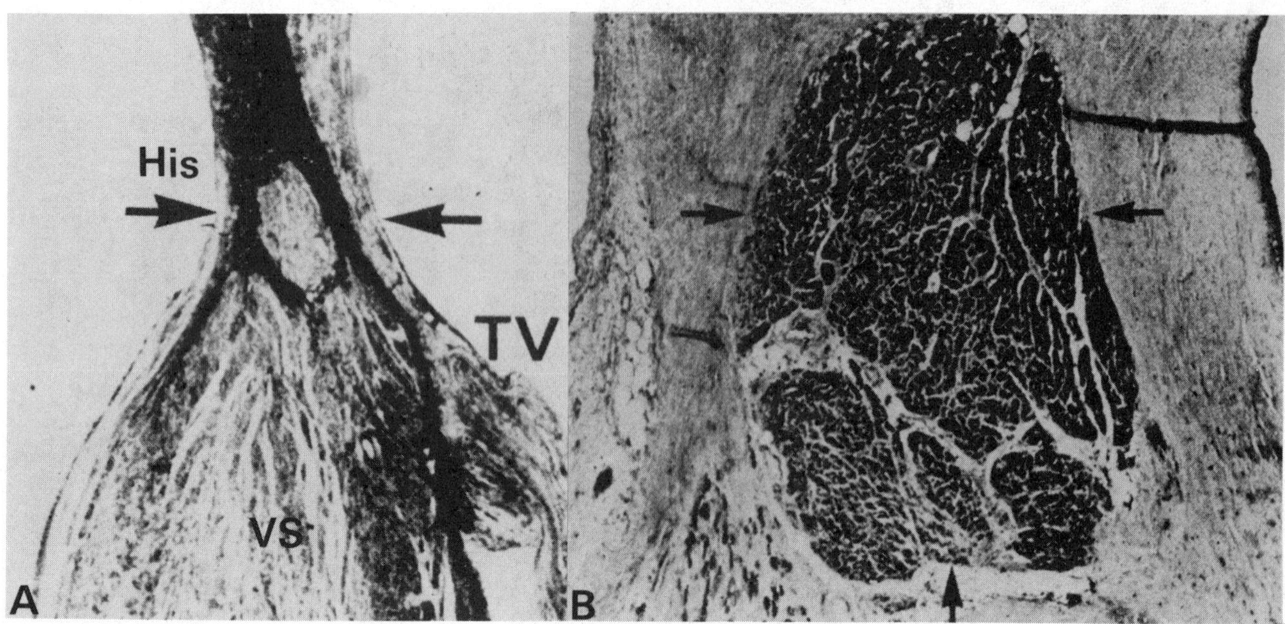

FIGURE 4-60 Photomicrographs of normal main bundle of His. *A*. Emerging from the central fibrous body is the main bundle of His (arrow). TV = tricuspid valve; VS = ventricular septum. *B*. Closeup of normal main bundle of His. *(From MJ Davies: Pathology of Conducting Tissue of the Heart. London, Butterworth, 1971. Reproduced with permission from the publisher and author.)*

Bundle Branches

The bundle branches begin at the crest of the muscular ventricular septum immediately distal to the membranous septum with fibers of the *left bundle* branch forming a cascade down the left ventricular septal surface beneath the noncoronary aortic cusp (Figs. 4-55, 4-61, and 4-62). The morphology of the left bundle branch has been a subject of debate. The initial left bundle fibers separate from the branching bundle as a continuous "fan" of cells along the left ventricular septum. The disagreement concerns the fashion in which the fan of cells divides as it passes into the left ventricle. Tawara[117] showed that the left bundle radiates in a fanlike fashion with three major divisions (Plate I, 4-1). Rosenbaum and colleagues[129] have indicated that the left bundle has a bifascicular structure. More recent reconstruction studies have indicated a trifascicular division of the left bundle.[128, 130] Although the anatomy may not conform to a bifascicular system on the left (thin anterosuperior and thick posteroinferior), the concept of a trifascicular bundle branch system (right, bifascicular left) remains useful to clinicians.[93]

The *right bundle* branch is the direct continuation of the penetrating bundle positioned along the right side of the ventricular septum (Figs. 4-55 and 4-61). The right

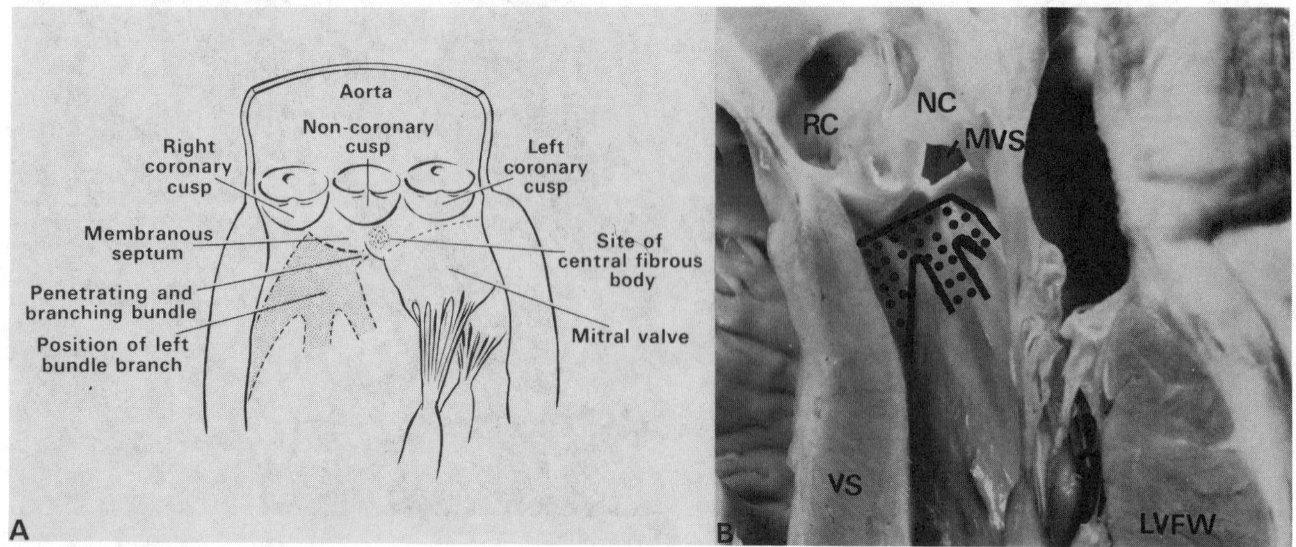

FIGURE 4-61 Anatomy of the left side of the heart showing landmarks of the conduction system. *A*. Diagram of conduction system. *B*. Photograph of heart showing excised membranous ventricular septum and location of left bundle branch. NC = noncoronary cusp; RC = right cusp of aortic valve; LVFW = left ventricular free wall; VS = ventricular septum.

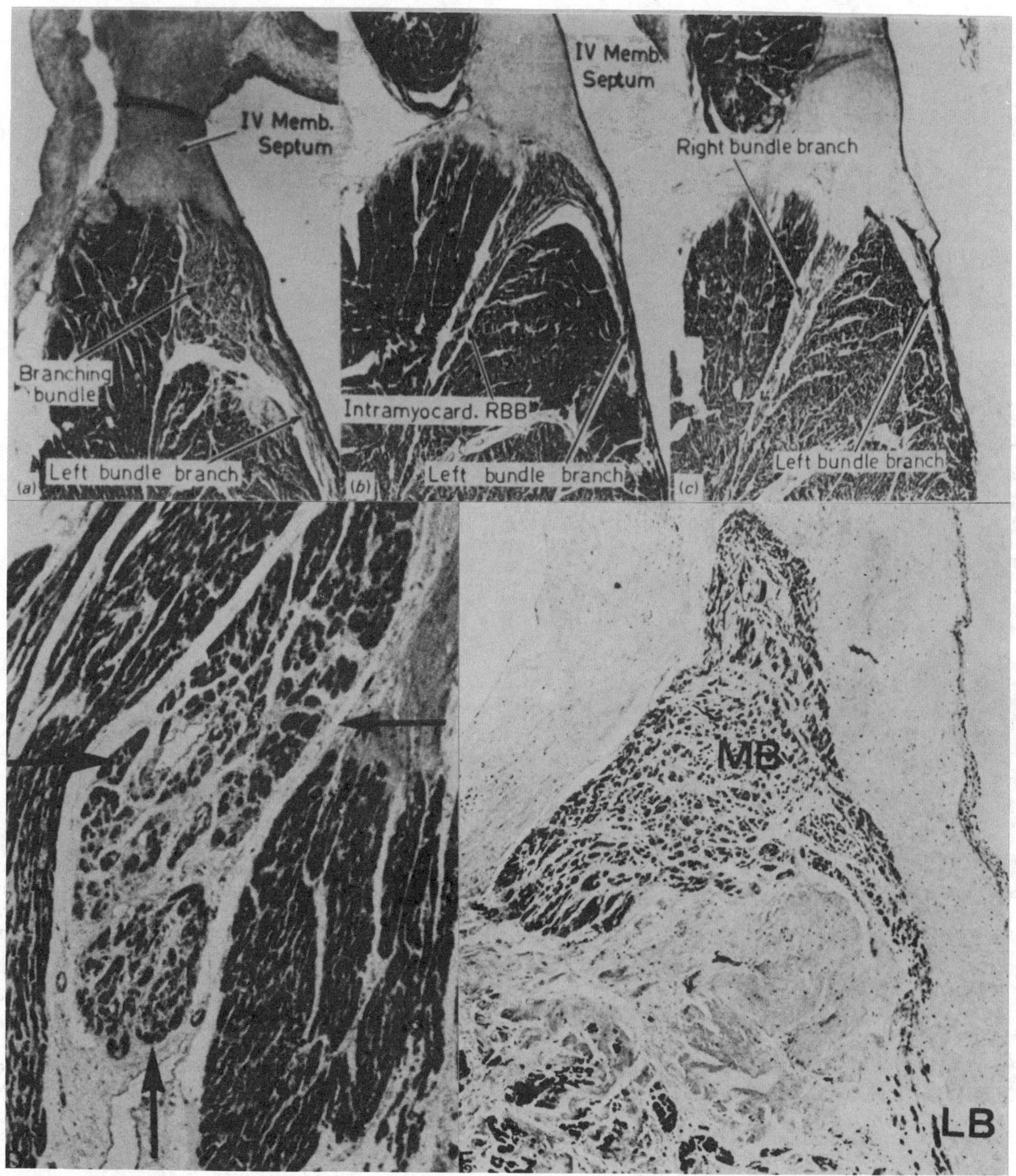

FIGURE 4-62 Photomicrographs of normal branching atrioventricular bundle and right (R) and left (L) bundle branches (BB). *A–C.* Series showing origin of branching bundle. *D–E.* Closeups showing origin of left bundle (LB) from main bundle (MB). *(A–C. From MJ Davies et al: The Conduction System of the Heart. London, Butterworth, 1983. D, E. From MJ Davies: Pathology of Conducting Tissue of the Heart. London, Butterworth, 1971. Reproduced with permission from the publisher and authors.)*

bundle becomes a subendocardial structure in the middle and lower thirds of the ventricular septum and can be seen grossly. In some hearts, the right bundle branch forms an obtuse angle with the His bundle.[128] It remains unbranched to the apex of the right ventricle.

The cells of the bundle branches are traditionally described as Purkinje cells (large and vacuolated). As in the His bundle, the proximal portions of the bundle branches have longitudinal strands of Purkinje-like cells. These cells have loosely arrayed mitochondria with few myofibrils. While the Purkinje fibers also exhibit side-to-side connections, the major intercellular connections are end to end through intercalated discs that may facilitate rapid longitudinal conduction.[97, 131] (See Chap. 34.)

The left bundle branch is supplied blood by both the left anterior descending and posterior descending (right)

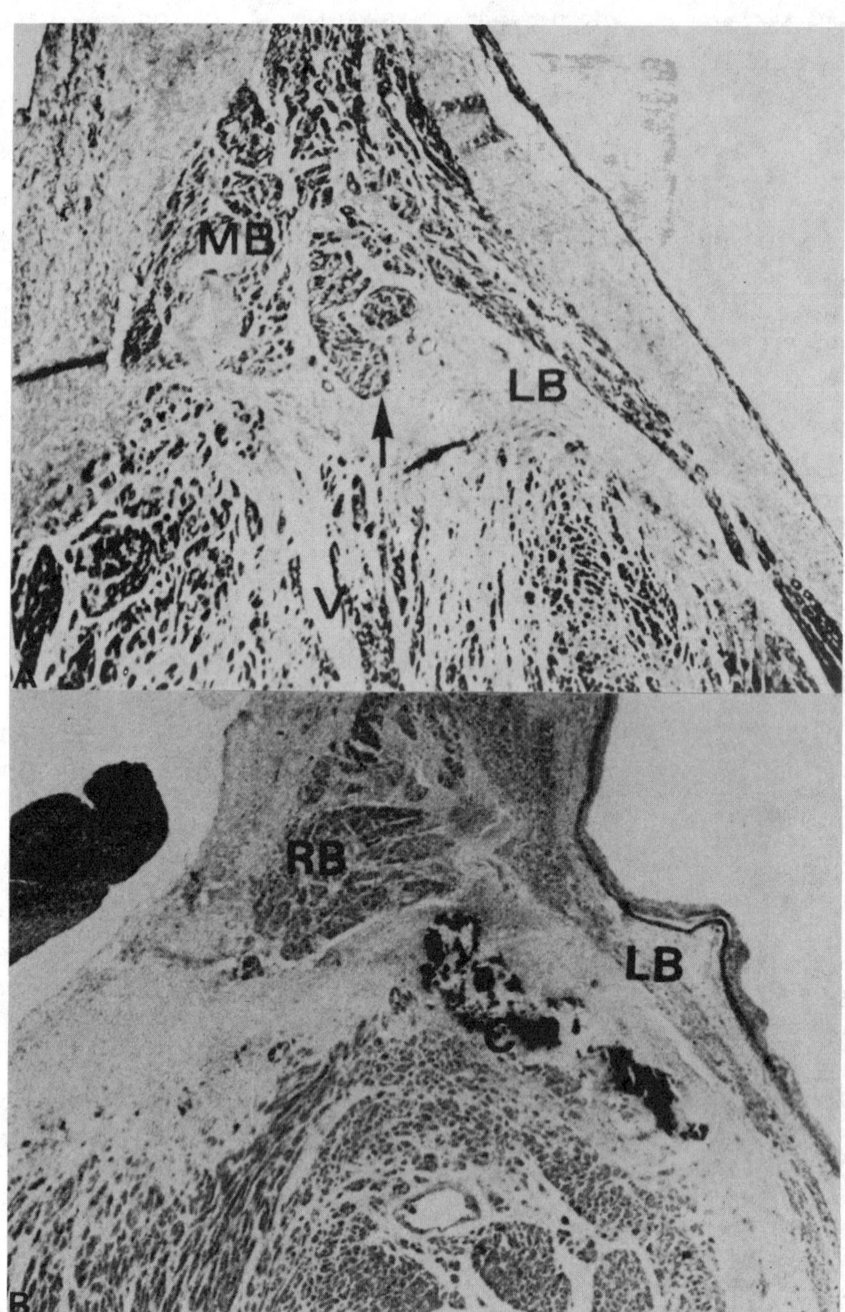

FIGURE 4-63 Variants of normal main bundle and branching bundles. *Top:* Closeup of main bundle (MB) and origin of left bundle (LB). A muscle strand (arrow) leaves the main bundle to enter the upper ventricular septum (V) bypassing the bundle branches. *Bottom:* Normal origin of left bundle (LB) showing calcium (C) as aging change in the crest of ventricular septum. RB = right bundle. *(From MJ Davies: Pathology of Conducting Tissue of the Heart. London, Butterworth, 1971. Reproduced with permission from the publisher and author.)*

coronary arteries (Figs. 4-49 to 4-51). The anterior and middle radiations of the left bundle branch are supplied mainly through septal perforations of the left anterior descending coronary artery. The right bundle branch is supplied from both right and left anterior descending coronary arterial systems.[132]

Terminal Purkinje Fibers

These fibers connect with the ends of the bundle branches to form interweaving networks on the endocardial surface of both ventricles. Practically, however, it is very difficult to trace the distal connections of the bundle branch system in humans. Purkinje fibers tend to be concentrated at papillary muscle tips rather than at the base of the ventricles. Purkinje fibers, which penetrate the subendocardium and myocardium at varying distances (species dependent), appear to be more resistant to ischemia than common myocardial fibers.[118]

ULTRASTRUCTURE OF THE MYOCARDIUM

The functions of the heart may be classified into the following three types: electrical, mechanical, and endocrine. Many myocardial cells are specialized for one of these functions. The myocardial cells concerned primarily with mechanical shortening are similar, although there are some differences between atrial and ventricular myocardium.[133] Several different types of cells have electrical or endocrine activity as a major function, and the structure of such cells is significantly different from that of contractile, or "working," myocardial cells.[84, 91, 105, 134]

Some special cells of the heart are particularly developed for the generation and very rapid conduction of an electrical impulse to the working cells.[105] There are four types of cells generally recognized in this system of impulse formation and rapid conduction: *P cells, transitional cells, ameboid cells*, and *Purkinje cells*. The P cells are numerous in the sinus node and are also present in the AV node and internodal pathways.[111] Transitional cells are found predominantly in the sinus node, the AV node, internodal pathways, and for considerable distances the atrial tissue adjacent to both nodes. Ameboid cells are found primarily in the eustachian ridge area. Purkinje cells are found at the margins of the sinus node; in the internodal pathways, which also contain intermingled transitional cells and ordinary working myocardial cells; adjacent to the AV node; and in the His bundle and its branches. The His bundle consists primarily of Purkinje cells, while the bundle branches consist of Purkinje cells intermingled with ordinary working cells.

The P cells are so named[91, 135] because of their pale appearance on microscopy and their resemblance to primitive myocardial cells and because they are thought to be the site of origin of the pacemaker impulse. They are usually ovoid or rounded, in contrast to the usual elongated shape of other myocardial cells. They measure 5 to 10 μm in greatest diameter and are the smallest type of myocardial cell.

Transitional cells are a heterogeneous group of cells that include all cells with a microscopic appearance intermediate between the P cells and the more complex working myocardial cells. They are more elongated than P cells but shorter and narrower than working myocardial cells.

Ameboid cells have been described[136, 137] in electron micrographs from the eustachian ridge. They may be elongated, triangular, oval, or nongeometric in shape. They have multilobular nuclei and pseudopodic prolongations that fill the spaces between neighboring cells and are often filled with a heavy concentration of electron-opaque granules that tend to give the cells a dark appearance. They have many mitrochondria and myofibrils. Although the exact function of the ameboid cells is unknown, they may act as an auxiliary pacemaker or may be a source of atrial natriuretic factor.

Purkinje cells are identified primarily on the basis of their ultrastructure. Purkinje cells tend to be both broader and shorter than working myocardial cells and measure from 10 to 30 μm in cross section and 20 to 50 μm in length.

Contractile or "working" myocardial cells are similar, whether they are from atrial or ventricular myocardium. They are characterized by hundreds of myofibrils in a special arrangement. Working myocardial cells are arranged longitudinally in series, with multiple cells forming a "fiber." Multiple fibers are generally arranged in parallel. Although cardiac muscle fibers have many lateral and end-to-side connections, the contractile cells are not a true anatomic syncytium. Intercalated disks at the terminal margins and junctions of contractile cells form a specialized transversely oriented cell boundary.[138] The myofibrils of working myocardial cells insert in the region of the intercalated disk. Contractile cells have many mitochondria and a nucleus, which tends to be centrally located and slightly elongated. These myocardial cells are about 10 to 20 μm in diameter and 50 to 100 μm in length.

Contractile cells contain an intricate sarcotubular system of tubules, vesicles, and cisternae.[139, 140] One component of this system consists of the periodic invagination of the sarcolemma by transversely oriented tubules known as the T system. Focal dilatations of the T-system tubules are seen in the area of the Z band, forming a cisternlike structure, the intermediary vesicle.[141] A second component of the sarcotubular system is the series of interconnecting longitudinal tubules that tend to be oriented parallel to the myofibrils, which they surround. Near the Z band, these tubules have local dilatations, lateral sacs, or terminal cisternae, which, together with the intermediary vesicle, form a triad. A triad consists of an intermediary vesicle from the T system and two lateral sacs from the longitudinal system. Although the three components of the triad are very close to each other, they probably are not in direct communication. The term subsarcolemma cisternae describes both the central (T-system) and peripheral (sarcolemma) sites of proximity. (See Chap. 5.)

Transverse tubules are arranged perpendicular to the long axis of the cell but branch longitudinally and can directly connect with other transverse tubules.[142, 143] In contrast, the internal longitudinal system (or sarcoplasmic reticulum) is a plexiform labyrinth of vesicles and tubules, some of which may also be transversely oriented.[144]

The sarcotubular system plays an important role in both electrical impulse conduction[145] and electromechanical coupling.[141] The impulse spreads rapidly on the surface of cells, down the transverse tubules, and stimulates the lateral sacs or vesicles and the entire sarcoplasmic reticulum to release large amounts of calcium around the contractile elements of the cell and initiate myocardial contraction.[146]

The myofibrils form longitudinally oriented strands of interdigitating myosin and actin filaments, which are the contractile elements of working, contractile myocardial cells (Figs. 4-64 and 4-65). The repeating morphologic and functional unit of contractile cells, the sarcomere, produces a regular band pattern of dark and light areas. The length of each sarcomere varies from 1.5 to 2.2 μm long.[147] The dark Z bands, where the intercalated disks are located, provide a boundary at the ends of the sarcomere to which the actin filaments are attached. These thin filaments of actin and some tropomyosin B project into the center of the sarcomere, where they interdigitate with the thick myosin filaments, which lie in the central part of the sarcomere. The thick filaments of myosin measure 1.5 μm and have small excresences produced by cross-bridges.[148] On microscopy, the

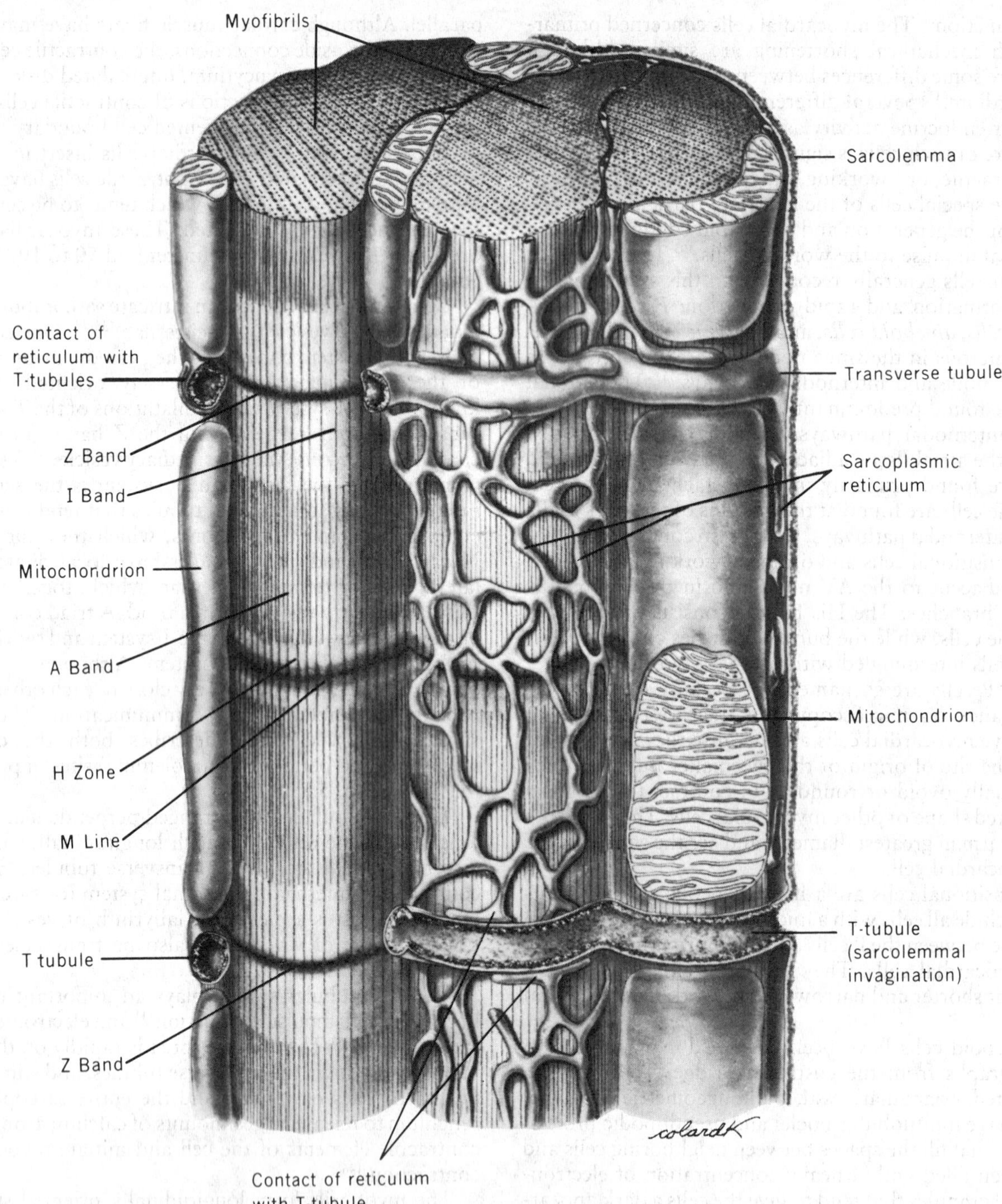

FIGURE 4-64 Schematic representation of myocardium. One sarcomere extends from one Z band to the other. Mitochondria, sarcoplasmic reticulum, and T tubules are also shown. *(From W Bloom, DW Fawcett: Textbook of Histology. Philadelphia, WB Saunders Company, 1969, and DW Fawcett, NC McNutt: Ultrastructure of the myocardium: I. Ventricular papillary muscle. J Cell Biol 42:1, 1969. Copyright and permission of the Rockefeller University Press. Modified and reproduced with permission from the publishers and authors.)*

dark and light zones of the sarcomere are produced by the periodic, interdigitating relations between the thin actin and the thick myosin filaments (Figs. 4-64 to 4-66). When the myofibrils are moderately stretched, the following pattern is seen: The I band consists of thin actin filaments attached to each side of the dark Z band. The A band is the wide dark area between two peripherally located I bands. The H zone is a lighter band of thick myosin filaments in the center of the A band. Crossing the center of the H zone is a thin dark line, the M line, consisting of the knoblike excrescences of the myosin filaments. The portions of the A band that extend in

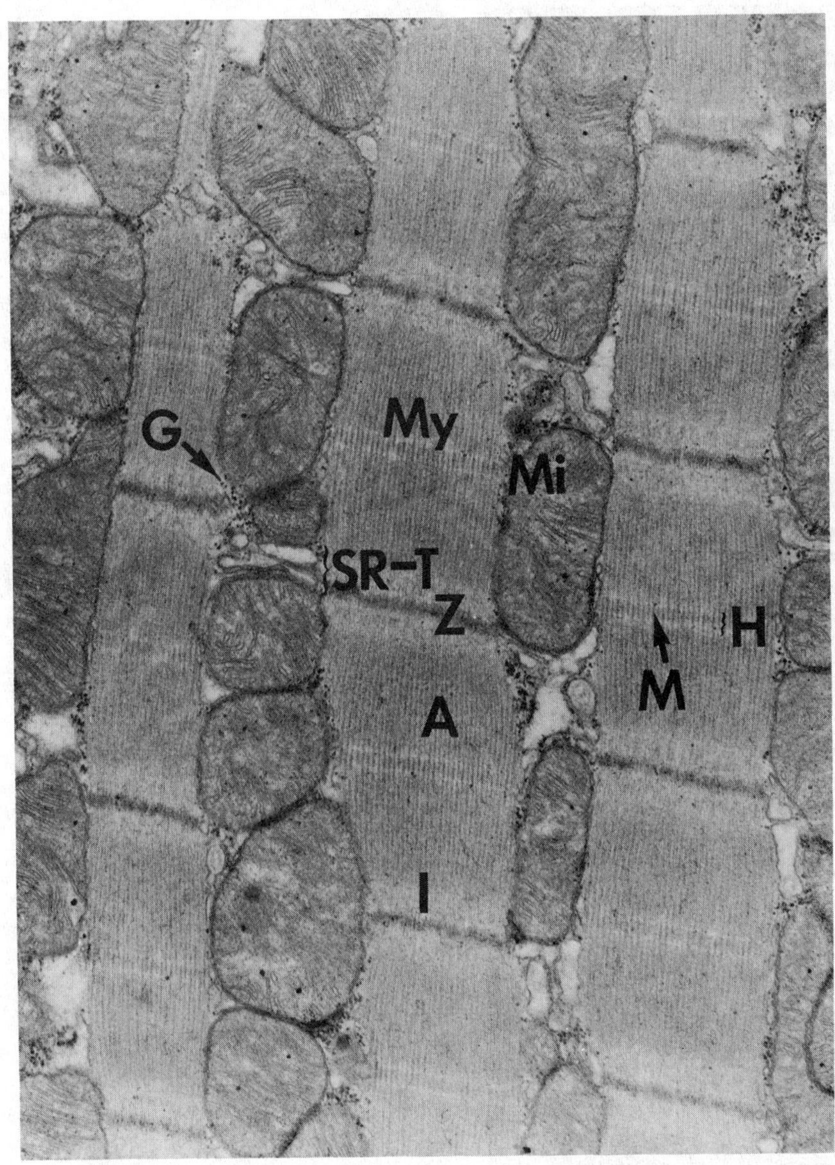

FIGURE 4-65 Electron micrograph of hamster myocardium, longitudinal section. Thick myosin and thin actin filaments are arranged into myofibrils (My) that exhibit the characteristic banding pattern. Mi = mitochondrion; G = glycogen particles; SR-T = elements of sarcoplasmic reticulum and T-tubule system; A = A band; Z = Z band; I = I band; M = M line; H = H zone. *(Courtesy of Claudia R. Adkison, Ph.D.)*

either direction from the H zone to each adjacent I band are darker than the H zone because they contain both thin actin and thick myosin filaments.

The appearance of a transverse section of myofibril depends upon the level of the sarcomere at which the cut is made. The H zone and M line area contain only thick myosin filaments arranged in a hexagonal pattern; the I band contains only evenly spaced thin actin filaments, except in the H zone; the A band shows the thick myosin and thin actin filaments arranged in a hexagonal pattern with six thin actin filaments surrounding each thick myosin filament (Fig. 4-67).

Each working myocardial cell contains hundreds of parallel myofibrils with rows of mitochondria between them (Figs. 4-64 to 4-66). The alignment of Z bands, I bands, and A bands of adjacent myofibrils is responsible for the typical cross striations seen on light microscopy.

Many studies have supported the application of Huxley and Hanson's "sliding filament hypothesis"[149–151] to both skeletal and myocardial muscle. In their theory, linkages between the actin and myosin pull or propel the actin filaments toward the center of the sarcomere. The two sets of filaments slide past each other, causing the muscle fiber to shorten. The myosin component for the linkage is heavy (H) meromyosin,[150] which combines with actin and also contains the adenosine triphosphatase (ATPase) necessary to split the ATP to provide the energy for contraction. When a myocardial cell is activated, the concentration of free intracellular Ca^{2+} combines with troponin and releases the actinmyosin inhibition, thereby permitting the actin and myosin fibers to slide and the muscle fiber to shorten. The mitochondria of working myocardial cells (Figs. 4-64 to 4-66) are cylindrically shaped and measure 2 by 0.5 μm. They have many infoldings, or cristae, which project inward from the membrane. Mitochondria are very numerous and comprise 25 to 50 percent of the total mass of myocardium.[147] (See also Chap. 5.)

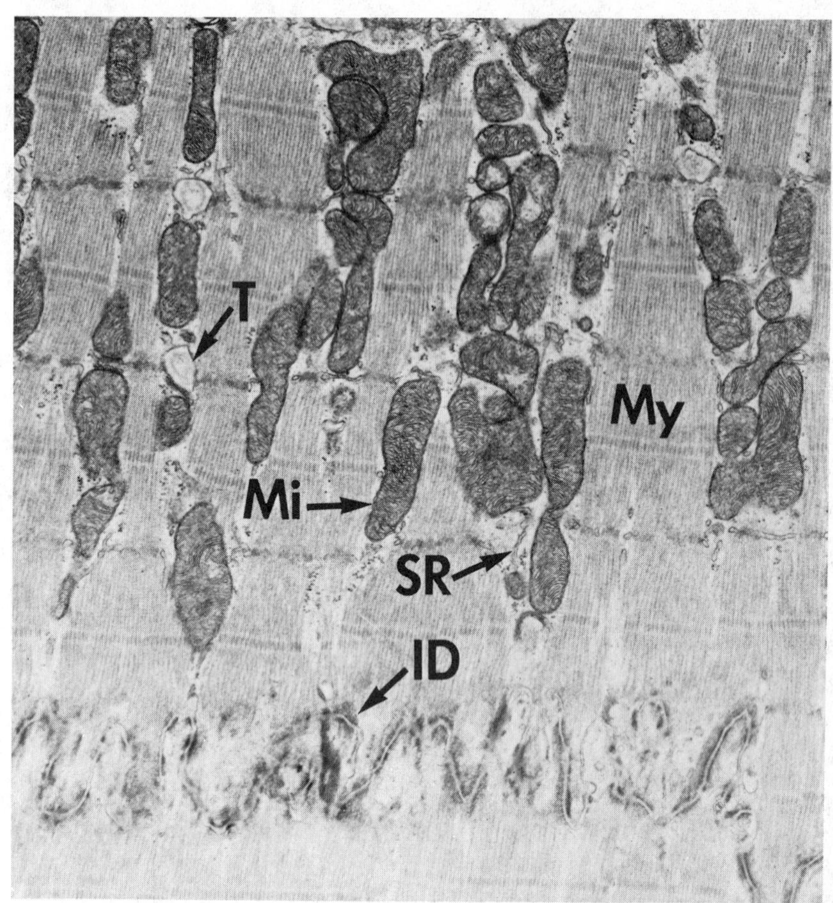

FIGURE 4-66 Electron micrograph of human myocardium, longitudinal section. Cytoplasm is packed with a regular array of myofibrils (My), showing the distinct banding pattern. Mitochondria (Mi) and elements of the sarcoplasmic reticulum (SR) and the T-tubule system (T) are arranged around the myofibrils. Portions of two cells are shown joined end to end at the intercalated disk (ID). *(Courtesy of Claudia R. Adkison, Ph.D.)*

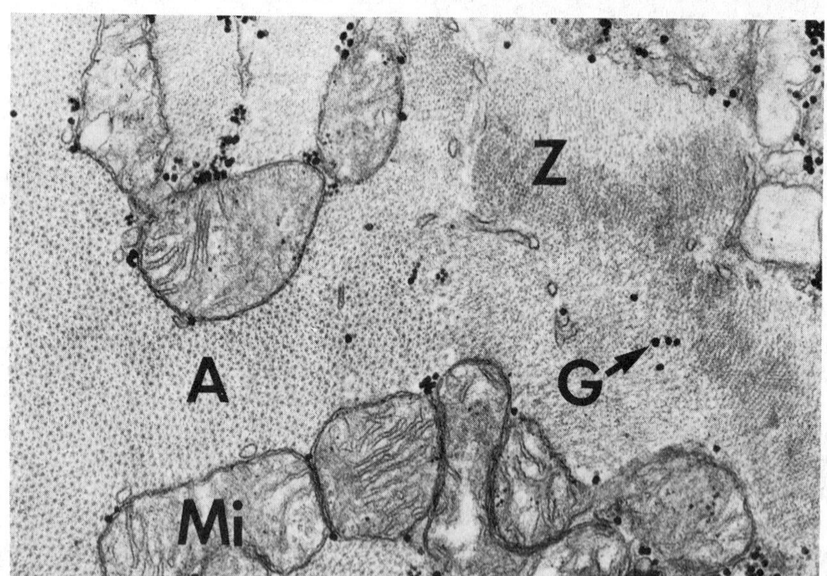

FIGURE 4-67 Electron micrograph of dog myocardium, cross section. Thin actin and thick myosin filaments form a hexagonal array in the A band (A) of a myofibril. Z = Z band; G = glycogen particles; Mi = mitochondrion. *(Courtesy of Claudia R. Adkison, Ph.D.)*

REFERENCES

1. Anderson RH, Wilcox BR, Becker AE: Anatomy of the normal heart. In: Hurst JW (ed): *Atlas of the Heart*. New York, McGraw-Hill and Gower Medical Publishing, 1988: 1–10.
2. Burton AC: The importance of the shape and size of the heart. *Am Heart J* 1957; 54:801–810.
3. Zimmerman J: The functional and surgical anatomy of the heart. *Ann R Coll Surg Engl* 1966; 39:348–366.
4. Waller BF: Anatomic basis for newer imaging techniques. *Am J Cardiac Imag* 1987; 1:311–322.
5. Davies MJ, Pomerance A, Lamb D: Techniques in examination and anatomy of the heart. In: Pomerance A, Davies MJ (eds): *The Pathology of the Heart*. Oxford, Blackwell Scientific Publications, 1975: 1–10.
6. McAlpine WA: *Heart and Coronary Arteries*. New York, Springer-Verlag, 1975: 1–50.
7. Walmsley R, Watson H: *Clinical Anatomy of the Heart*. New York, Churchill Livingstone, 1978: 1–24.

8. Nazarian GK, Julsrud PR, Ehman RL, Edwards WD: Correlation between magnetic resonance imaging of the heart and cardiac anatomy. *Mayo Clin Proc* 1987; 62:573–583.
9. Wilcox BR, Anderson RH: *Surgical Anatomy of the Heart.* New York, Raven, 1985: 1–9.6.
10. Edwards WD: Applied anatomy of the heart. In: Brandenburg RO, Fuster V, Giuliani ER, et al (eds): *Cardiology: Fundamentals and Practice.* Chicago, Year Book Medical Publishers, 1987: 47–112.
11. Scholz DG, Kitzman DW, Hagan PT, Ilstrup DM, Edwards WD: Age-related changes in normal human hearts during the first 10 decades of life. Part I (growth): A quantitative anatomic study of 200 specimens from subjects from birth to 19 years old. *Mayo Clin Proc* 1988; 63:126–136.
12. Anderson RH, Becker AE: *Cardiac Anatomy.* Gower Medical Publishing, London, 1980: 1–10.30.
13. Waller BF, Taliercio CP, Slack JD, Orr CM, Howard J, Smith ML: Tomographic views of normal and abnormal hearts: The anatomic basis for various cardiac imaging techniques. Part I. *Clin Cardiol* 1990; 13:804–812.
14. Waller BF, Taliercio CP, Slack JD, Orr CM, Howard J, Smith ML: Tomographic views of normal and abnormal hearts: The anatomic basis for various cardiac imaging techniques. Part II. *Clin Cardiol* 1990; 13:877–884.
15. Lev M, Bharati S: The fibrous skeleton of the heart. In: Hurst JW (ed): *Update IV: The Heart.* New York, McGraw-Hill, 1982: 7–14.
16. Rosenquist GC, Sweeney LJ: The membranous ventricular septum in the normal heart. *Johns Hopkins Med J* 1974; 135:9–16.
17. Titus JL: Normal anatomy of the human cardiac conduction system. *Mayo Clin Proc* 1973; 48:24–30.
18. Sweeney LF, Rosenquist GC: The normal anatomy of the atrial septum in the human heart. *Am Heart J* 1979; 98:194–199.
19. Prakash R: Determination of right ventricular wall thickness in systole and diastole: Echocardiographic and necropsy correlation in 32 patients. *Br Heart J* 1978; 40:1257–1261.
20. Grant RP, Downey FM, MacMahon H: The architecture of the right ventricular outflow tract in the normal heart and in the presence of ventricular septal defects. *Circulation* 1961; 24:223–235.
21. James TN: Anatomy of the crista supraventricularis: Its importance for understanding right ventricular function, right ventricular infarction and related conditions. *J Am Coll Cardiol* 1985; 6:1083–1095.
22. Kennedy JW, Baxley WA, Figley MM, Dodge HT, Blackmon JR: Quantitative angiocardiography: I. The normal left ventricle in man. *Circulation* 1966; 34:272–278.
23. Waller BF: Morphologic aspects of valvular heart disease: Part I. *Curr Prob Cardiol* 1985; IX:13–26.
24. Gross L, Kugel MA: Topographical anatomy and histology of the valves in the human heart. *Am J Pathol* 1931; 7:445–476.
25. Clark JA: An x-ray microscopic study of the blood supply to the valves of the human heart. *Br Heart J* 1965; 27:420–423.
26. Duran CMG, Gunning AJ: The vascularization of the heart valves: A comparative study. *Cardiovasc Res* 1968; 3:290–296.
27. Montiel MM: Muscular apparatus of the mitral valve in man and its involvement in left-sided cardiac hypertrophy. *Am J Cardiol* 1970; 26:341–344.
28. Zimmerman J: The functional and surgical anatomy of the aortic valve. *Isr J Med Sci* 1969; 5:862–868.
29. Merklin RJ: Position and orientation of the heart valves. *An M Anat* 1969; 125:375–380.
30. Davies MJ: *Pathology of Cardiac Valves.* London, Butterworth, 1980.
31. Vollebergh FEMG, Becker AE: Minor congenital variations of cusp size in tricuspid aortic valves: Possible link with isolated aortic stenosis. *Br Heart J* 1977; 39:1006–1011.
32. Roberts WC: The structure of the aortic valve in clinically isolated aortic stenosis—an autopsy study of 162 patients over 15 years of age. *Circulation* 1970; 42:91–97.
33. Waller BF, Roberts WC: Cardiovascular disease in the very elderly: Analysis of 40 necropsy patients aged 90 years and over. *Am J Cardiol* 1983; 51:403–421.
34. Perloff JK, Roberts WC: The mitral apparatus: Functional anatomy of mitral regurgitation. *Circulation* 1972; 46:227–239.
35. Waller BF, Morrow AG, Maron BJ, DelNegro AA, Kent KM, McGrath FJ, et al: Etiology of clinically isolated, severe, chronic, pure mitral regurgitation: Analysis of 97 patients over 30 years of age having mitral valve replacement. *Am Heart J* 1982; 104:276–288.
36. Roberts WC: Morphologic features of the normal and abnormal mitral valve. *Am J Cardiol* 1983; 51:1005–1028.
37. Ranganathan N, Lam JHC, Wigle ED, Silver MD: Morphology of the human mitral valve: II. The valve leaflets. *Circulation* 1970; 41:459–467.
38. Brock RC: The surgical and pathologic anatomy of the mitral valve. *Br Heart J* 1952; 14:489–513.
39. Estes EH Jr, Dalton FM, Entman ML: The anatomy and blood supply of the papillary muscles of the left ventricle. *Am Heart J* 1966; 71:356–362.
40. Roberts WC, Perloff JK: Mitral valve disease: A clinicopathologic survey of the conditions causing the mitral valve to function abnormally. *Ann Intern Med* 1972; 77:939–975.
41. Edwards BS, Edwards WD, Bambara JF, Van der Bel-Kahn J, Bove KE, Edwards JE: Anomalies of the left atrium and mitral valve: Cords, flaps and duplication of valves. *Arch Pathol Lab Med* 1983; 107:29–33.
42. Silver MD, Lam JHC, Ranganathan N, Wigle ED: Morphology of human tricuspid valve. *Circulation* 1971; 43:333–348.
43. Cascos AS, Rabago P, Sokolowski M: Duplication of the tricuspid valve. *Br Heart J* 1967; 29:943–946.
44. Elfenbein B, Paplanus SH: Duplication of the mitral and tricuspid valves. *Arch Pathol* 1968; 85:675–680.
45. Roberts WC, Waller BF: Effect of chronic hypercalcemia on the heart: An analysis of 18 necropsy patients. *Am J Cardiol* 1981; 71:371–384.
46. Estes EH Jr, Dalton FM, Entman ML, Dixon HB II, Hackel DB: The anatomy and blood supply of the papillary muscles of the left ventricle. *Am Heart J* 1966; 71:356–362.
47. Lam JHC, Ranganathan N, Wigle ED, Silver MD: Morphology of the human mitral valve: I. Chordae tendineae. *Circulation* 1970; 41:449–458.
48. Holt JP: The normal pericardium. *Am J Cardiol* 1970; 26:455–465.
49. Choe YH, Im J-G, Park JH, Ho MC, Kim CW: The anatomy of the pericardial space: A study in cadavers and patients. *Am J Radiol* 1987; 149:693–698.
50. Edwards WD, Tajik AJ, Seward JB: Standardized nomenclature and anatomic bases for regional tomographic analysis of the heart. *Mayo Clin Proc* 1981; 56:479–497.
51. Silverman NH, Hunter S, Anderson RH, Ho SY, Davies MJ, Sutherland GR: Anatomic basis for cross-sectional echocardiography. *Br Heart J* 1983; 50:421–431.
52. Edwards WD: Anatomic basis for tomographic analyses of the heart at autopsy. In: Waller BF (ed): *Cardiac Morphology.* Philadelphia, FA Davis, 1984: 485–506.
53. Carter BL, Morehead J, Wolpert SM, Hammerschlag SB, Griffiths HJ, Kahn PC: *Cross-sectional Anatomy, Computed Tomography and Ultrasound Correlation.* New York, Appleton-Century-Crofts, 1977: 1–60.
54. Bo WJ, Mechan I, Krueger WA: *Basic Atlas of Cross-sectional Anatomy.* Saunders, Philadelphia, 1980: 1–28.
55. Gambarelli J, Guerinel G, Chevrot L, Matteri M: *Computerized Axial Tomography. An Anatomic Atlas of Serial Sections of the Human Body.* Berlin, Springer-Verlag, 1977: 1–41.
56. Han MC, Kim CW: *Sectional Human Anatomy. Transverse, Sagittal and Coronal Sections Correlated with Computed Tomography and Magnetic Resonance Imaging.* Seoul, Ilchokok, 1985: 1–20.
57. Nazarian GK, Julsrud PR, Ehman RL, Edwards WD: Correlation between magnetic resonance imaging of the heart and cardiac anatomy. *Mayo Clin Proc* 1987; 62:573–583.
58. Higgins CB: New horizons in cardiac imaging. *Radiology* 1985; 156:577–588.
59. Higgins CB: Overview of MR of the heart—1986. *Am J Radiol* 1986; 146:907–914.
60. Higgins CB, Carlsson E, Lipton MJ: *CT of the Heart and Great Vessels.* Mount Kisco, NY, Futura, 1983: 1–48.
61. Mitchell GAG: *Cardiovascular Innervation.* Baltimore, Williams & Wilkins, 1956.
62. Janes RD, Brandys JC, Hopkins DA, Johnstone DE, Murphy DA, Armour JA: Anatomy of human extrinsic cardiac nerves and ganglia. *Am J Cardiol* 1986; 57:299–309.
63. Randall WC (ed): *Nervous Control of Cardiovascular Function.* New York, Oxford University Press, 1984.

64. Feola M, Merrlin R, Cho S, Brockman SK: The terminal pathway of the lymphatic system of the human heart. *Ann Thorac Surg* 1977; 24:531–536.
65. Miller AJ: *Lymphatics of the Heart*. New York, Raven, 1982.
66. Waller BF: Anatomy, histology, and pathology of the major epicardial coronary arteries relevant to echocardiographic imaging techniques. *J Am Soc Echo* 1989; 2:232–252.
67. Waller BF: Five coronary ostia: Duplicate left anterior descending and right conus coronary arteries. *Am J Cardiol* 1983; 52:137–146.
68. Baroldi G: Diseases of the coronary arteries. In: Silver MD (ed): *Cardiovascular Pathology*, vol 1. New York, Churchill Livingstone, 1983: 317–391.
69. Schulte MA, Waller BF, Hull MT, Pless JE: Origin of the left anterior descending coronary artery from the right aortic sinus with intramyocardial tunneling to the left side of the heart via the ventricular septum: A case against clinical and morphologic significance of myocardial bridging. *Am Heart J* 1985; 110:499–501.
70. Polacek P: Relation of myocardial bridges and loops on the coronary arteries to coronary occlusions. *Am Heart J* 1961; 61:44–52.
71. Anderson KR, Ho SY, Anderson RH: Location and vascular supply of sinus node in human heart. *Br Heart J* 1979; 41:28–32.
72. Spring DJ, Thomsen JH: Severe atherosclerosis in the "single coronary artery." Report of a previously undescribed pattern. *Am J Cardiol* 1973; 31:662–665.
73. James TN, Burch GE: Blood supply of the human interventricular septum. *Circulation* 1958; 17:391–396.
74. Kugel MA: Anatomical studies on the coronary arteries and their branches: I. Arteria anastomotica auricularis magna. *Am Heart J* 1927; 3:260–270.
75. Benditt EP, Schwartz SM: Blood vessels. In: Rubin E, Farber JL (eds): *Pathology*. Philadelphia, Lippincott, 1988: 454–65.
76. Waller BF: The eccentric coronary atherosclerotic plaque: Morphologic observations and clinical relevance. *Clin Cardiol* 1989; 12:14–20.
77. Fawcett DW: Blood and lymph vascular systems. In: Fawcett DW (ed); *A Textbook of Histology*. Philadelphia, Saunders, 1986: 367–381.
78. Neufeld HN, Schneeweiss A: *Coronary Artery Disease in Infants and Children*. Philadelphia, Lea & Febiger, 1983: 1–42.
79. Vlodaver Z, Edwards JE: Pathology of coronary atherosclerosis. *Prog Cardiovasc Dis* 1971; 14:256–274.
80. Mönckeberg JG: Uber die reine Mediaverkalkung der Extremitatenarterien und ihr Vorhalten zur Arterioskierwose. *Virchows Archiv [A]* 1903; 171:14–30.
81. Waller BF, Morgan R: The very elderly heart. *Cardiovasc Clin* 1987; 18:361–410.
82. James TN: *Anatomy of the Coronary Arteries*. New York, Hoeber Medical Division, Harper & Row, 1961: 1–77.
83. Keith A, Flack M: The form and nature of the muscular connections between the primary division of the vertebrate heart. *J Anat Physiol* 1907; 41:172–182.
84. James TN: Anatomy of the human sinus node. *Anat Rec* 1961; 141:109–139.
85. Lev M, Bharati S: Anatomy of the conduction system in normal and congenitally abnormal hearts. In: Roberts NK, Gelband H (eds): *Cardiac Arrhythmias in the Neonate, Infant and Child*. New York, Appleton-Century-Crofts, 1977: 29–53.
86. Anderson KR, Ho SY, Anderson RH: The location and vascular supply of the sinus node in the human heart. *Br Heart J* 1979; 41:28–32.
87. Blair DM, Davies F: Observations on the conducting system of the heart. *J Anat* 1935; 69:303–325.
88. James TN: *Anatomy of the Coronary Arteries*. New York, Harper & Row, 1961: 1–50.
89. Vieweg WVR, Alpert JS, Hagan AD: Origin of the sinoatrial node and atrioventricular node arteries in right, mixed and left inferior emphasis systems. *Cathet Cardiovasc Diag* 1975; 1:361–373.
90. James TN: The sinus node as a servomechanism. *Circ Res* 1973; 32:307–313.
91. James TN, Sherf L, Fine G, Morales AR: Comparative ultrastructure of the sinus node in man and dog. *Circulation* 1966; 34:139–163.
92. Davies MJ, Anderson RH, Becker AE: *The Conduction System of the Heart*. London, Butterworth, 1983: 1–200.
93. Zipes DP: Genesis of cardiac arrhythmias: Electrophysiological consideration. In: Braunwald E (ed): *Heart Disease. A Textbook of Cardiovascular Medicine*, 2d ed. Philadelphia, Saunders, 1984: 581–620.
94. Masson-Pevel M, Bleeker WK, Gas D: The plasma membrance of leading pacemaker cells in the rabbit sinus node: A qualitative and quantitative ultrastructural analysis. *Circ Res* 1979; 45:621–629.
95. Trautwein W, Uchizono K: Electron microscopic and electrophysiologic study of the pacemaker in the sinoatrial node of the rabbit heart. *Z Zellforsch Mikrosk Anat* 1963; 61:96–101.
96. Bleeker WK, Mackaay AJ, Masson-Pevet M, Bowman LN, Becker AE: Functional and morphological organization of the rabbit sinus node. *Circ Res* 1980; 46:11–21.
97. James TN: Anatomy of the conduction system of the heart. In: Hurst JW, Logue RB, Rackley CE, Schlant RC, Sonnenblick EH, Wallace AG, Wenger NK (eds): *The Heart*, 5th ed. New York, McGraw-Hill, 1982: 46–56.
98. Becker AE, Bowman LN, Janse MJ, Anderson RH: Functional anatomy of the cardiac conduction system. In: Harrison DC (ed): *Cardiac Arrhythmias: A Decade of Progress*. Boston, GK Hall, 1981.
99. Lev M: Aging changes in the human sinoatrial node. *J Gerontol* 1954; 9:1–10.
100. Thorel C: Verlaufige Mitteilung uber eine besondere Muskelverbindung Zwischen der Cava Superior und dem Hisschen Bundel. *Munchener Med Wochenschrift* 1909; 56:2159–2163.
101. Condorelli L: Uber die Bahnen der Reizleitung von Keith-Flackschen Knoten zeiden Vorhofen. *Zeits Gesam Exper Med* 1929; 68:493–497.
102. Franco PM: Recherches sur les faisceaux de connexion auriculaires dans les condition normales et pathologues. *Arch Mal Coeur* 1951; 44:287–292.
103. Osawa M: Histologic study on the conducting systems in the atrial portion of the dog's heart. 3. Specific pathways conducting between the sinus node and the tawara node. *Jpn Circ J* 1959; 23:1014–1019.
104. Robb JS, Petri R: Expansion of the atrioventricular system in the atria. In: Paes de Carvalho A (ed): *The specialized tissues of the Heart*. Amsterdam, Elsevier, 1961.
105. James TN: The connecting pathways between the sinus node and the A-V node and between the right and left atrium in the human heart. *Am Heart J* 1963; 66:498–508.
106. Meredith J, Titus JL: The anatomical atrial connections between sinus and AV node. *Circulation* 1968; 37:566–579.
107. Spach MS, King TD, Barr RC, Boaz DE, Marrow MN, Giddens SH: Electrical potential distribution surrounding the atria during depolarization and repolarization in the dog. *Circ Res* 1969; 24:857–873.
108. Truex RC: The sinoatrial node and its connections with the atrial tissues. In: Wellens HJJ, Lie KI, Janse MJ (eds): *The Conduction Systems of the Heart—Structure, Function and Clinical Implications*. Philadelphia, Lea & Febiger, 1976: 209–215.
109. Lev M, Bharati S: Lesions of the conduction system, and their functional significance. *Path Ann* 1974; 9:157–207.
110. Janse MJ, Anderson RH: Specialized internodal atrial pathways—fact of fiction. *Eur J Cardiol* 2:117–136.
111. James TN, Sherf L: Specialized tissue and preferential conduction in the atria of the heart. *Am J Cardiol* 1971; 28:414–427.
112. Bachman G: The interauricular time interval. *Am J Physiol* 1916; 41:309–320.
113. Wenckebach KF: Beitrangae zur Kenntnis der menschlichen Herztatigkeit. *Arch Anat Physiol* 1908; 3:53–58.
114. Isa L, Matturri, Rossi L: Contributo isto-citologico al riconoscimento delle connessioni internodali atriali. *G Ital Cardiol* 1976; 4:1024–1025.
115. Hoffman BF: Fine structure of the internodal pathways. *Am J Cardiol* 1979; 44:385–386.
116. Becker AE, Bouman LN, Janse MK, Anderson RH: Functional anatomy of the cardiac conduction system. In Harrison DC (ed): *Cardiac Arrhythmias: A Decade of Progress*. Boston, GK Hall, 1981: 1–18.
117. Tawara S: *Das Reizleitungssystem des Saugetierkerzens*. Jena, Gustav Fischer, 1906.
118. Hecht HH, Kossmann CE, Childers RW, Langendorf R, Ler M,

Rosen KM, et al: Atrioventricular and intraventricular conduction. Revised nomenclature and concepts. *Am J Cardiol* 1973; 31:232–244.

119. Anderson RH, Becker AE, Brechenmacher C, Davies MJ, Rossi L: The human atrioventricular junctional area. A morphological study of the AV node and bundle. *Eur J Cardiol* 1975; 3:11–25.
120. Rossi L: *Histopathology of Cardiac Arrhythmias*, 2d ed. Melano, Casa Editrice Ambrosiana, 1979: 1–75.
121. Becker AE, Anderson RH: Morphology of the human atrioventricular junctional area. In Wellens JHH, Lie KI, Janse MJ (eds): *The Conduction System of the Heart—Structure, Function and Clinical Implications*. New York, Lea & Febiger, 1976: 263–271.
122. Thaemert JC: Atrioventricular node innervation in ultrastructural three dimensions. *Am J Anat* 1970; 128:239–249.
123. Thaemert JC: Fine structure of the atrioventricular node in ultrastructural three dimensions. *Am J Anat* 1973; 136:43–65.
124. Mahaim I: Kent's fiber in the A-V paraspecific conduction through the upper connection of the bundle of His—Tawara. *Am Heart J* 1947; 33:651–653.
125. James TN: Sudden death in babies. New observations in the heart. *Am J Cardiol* 1968; 22:479–484.
126. James TN, Marshall ML: De Subitaneis Mortibus 18. Persistent fetal dispersion of the atrioventricular node and His bundle within the central fibrous body. *Circulation* 1976; 53:1026–1034.
127. Rossi L: *Sistema di Conduzione e Nervi nel Aiore dell'Uomo*. Milano, Casa Ed Ambrosiana, 1954: 1–66.
128. Massing GK, James TN: Anatomical configuration of the His bundle and bundle branches in the human heart. *Circulation* 1976; 53:609–621.
129. Rosenbaum MB, Elizari MV, Lazzari JO: *The Hemiblocks*. Tampa, FL, Tracings, 1970.
130. Demoulin JC, Kulbertus HE: Histopathological examination of concept of left hemiblock. *Br Heart J* 1972; 34:807–814.
131. Weidmann S: The diffusion of radiopotassium across intercalated disks of mammalian cardiac muscle. *J Physiol* 1966; 187:323–342.
132. Davies MJ: *Pathology of Conducting Tissue of the Heart*. London, Butterworth, 1971: 1–49.
133. Anderson RH, Becker AE, Tranum-Jensen J, Janse MJ: Anatomicro-electrophysiological correlations in the conduction system—a review. *Br Heart J* 1981; 45:67–82.
134. Sommer JR, Jennings RB: Ultrastructure of cardiac muscle. In: Fozzard HA, Haber E, Jennings RD, et al (eds): *The Heart and Cardiovascular System: Scientific Foundations*. New York, Raven, 1986: 61–75.
135. James TN, Sherf L: Ultrastructure of the human atrioventricular node. *Circulation* 1968; 37:1049–1070.
136. Sherf L, James TN: Fine structure of cells and their histological organization within internodal pathways of the heart: Clinical and electrocardiographic implications. *Am J Cardiol* 1979; 44:345–369.
137. Sherf L, James TN: Functional anatomy and ultrastructure of the internodal pathways. In: Little RC (ed): *Physiology of Atrial Pacemakers and Conductive Tissues*. New York, Futura, 1980: 67–72.
138. Sjostrand FS, Andersson-Cedergran E: Intercalated discs of heart muscle. In: Bourne GH (ed): *The Structure and Function of Muscle*. New York, Academic, 1960: 421–429.
139. Porter KR, Palade GE: Studies on the endoplastic reticulum: III. Its form and distribution in striated muscle cells. *J Biophys Biochem Cytol* 1957; 3:269–276.
140. Hoffman BF: Physiology of atrioventricular transmission. *Circulation* 1961; 24:506–517.
141. Essner E, Novikoff AB, Quintana N: Nucleoside phosphatase activities in rat cardiac muscle. *J Cell Biol* 1965; 25:201–215.
142. Fawcess DW, McNutt NS: The ultrastructure of the cat myocardium. I. Ventricular papillary muscle. *J Cell Biol* 1969; 42:1–45.
143. Forssmann WG, Giardier L: A study of the T system in rat heart. *J Cell Biol* 1970; 44:1–19.
144. Sommer JR, Johnson EA: A comparative study of Purkinje fibers and ventricular fibers. *J Cell Biol* 1968; 36:497–526.
145. Huxley AF, Taylor RE: Local activation of striated muscle fibers. *J Physiol* 1958; 144:426–441.
146. Huxley AF: The links between excitation and contraction. *Proc R Soc Lond Ser B* 1964; 160:486–488.
147. Braunwald E, Ross J Jr, Sonnenblick EH: Mechanisms of contraction of the normal and failing heart. *N Engl J Med* 1967; 277:794–800.
148. Hasselbach W: ATP driven active transport of Ca in the membranes of the sarcoplasmic reticulum. *Proc R Soc Lond Ser B* 1964; 160:501–504.
149. Huxley HE, Hanson J: Changes in the cross-striations of muscle during contraction and stretch and their structural interpretation. *Nature* 1954; 173:973–976.
150. Huxley HE: Structural arrangement and the contraction mechanism in striated muscle. *Proc R Soc Lond Ser B*, 1964; 160:442–448.
151. Huxley HE: Structural evidence concerning mechanism of contraction in striated muscle. In: Paul WM, Kay CM, Monckton G (eds): *Muscles*. Toronto, Pergamon 1965: 3–18.

Chapter 5

Normal Physiology of the Cardiovascular System

Robert C. Schlant, M.D. ■ Edmund H. Sonnenblick, M.D.

The cardiovascular system has the following three basic functions: (1) to transport oxygen and other nutrients to the cells of the body, (2) to remove metabolic waste products from the cells, and (3) to carry substances such as hormones from one part of the body to another. In addition, the heart and blood vessels themselves have important neurohumoral functions.

With every beat, the performance of the heart may be considered the net result of the following three major determinants: *preload, afterload,* and *contractility* (the inotropic state). The heart rate then determines the performance of the heart relative to time. Cardiac performance is further influenced by many factors, including the synchrony of ventricular contraction, atrial function, neural control, drugs, hormones and metabolic products, and pericardial properties. This chapter reviews myocardial excitation-contraction coupling, the fundamentals of muscle mechanics, the major factors influencing cardiac performance, the major mechanisms of cardiac reserve, the coronary circulation, the response to exercise, and the cardiac cycle. Detailed discussions are found in the general reference sources.[1–18] The evaluation of cardiac and myocardial function is further discussed in Chap. 23 and the pathophysiology of heart failure in Chap. 25.

MYOCARDIAL EXCITATION-CONTRACTION COUPLING

In recent years there has been a great increase in our understanding of the mechanisms by which the action potential stimulus initiates the contractile process in heart muscle. All studies have emphasized the central role in excitation-contraction coupling of the calcium ion (Ca^{2+}),[11,19–29] which has been known to be essential for myocardial contraction since the classic studies of Ringer.[30] The Ca^{2+} ion is now known to have two major roles in excitation-contraction: the initiation of contraction (trigger substance) and the regulation of the extent of myocardial contraction (regulating factor).

With the initiation of the action potential in ventricular myocardium (Fig. 5-1), there is a very rapid influx of Na^+ (or change in Na^+ *conductance*), which produces the rapid electrical spike and overshoot during phase zero of the action potential[31,32] (see Chap. 34). During the plateau phase of the action potential (phase 2), there is a slow inward flux of Ca^{2+} through slow channels in the myocardial cell membrane, or sarcolemma, into the intracellular fluid (sarcoplasm, or cytosol) and possibly into the sarcoplasmic reticulum.[33,34] There is evidence that some extracellular Ca^{2+} ions are temporarily bound to special sites on the sarcolemmal surface for one or more beats prior to being transported into the sarcoplasm by subsequent action potentials.[11,23] The action potential also spreads from the myocardial cell membrane down the extensive *transverse (T) tubular system,* which consists of sarcolemma invaginations, especially near the Z bands, that are in direct continuity with the extracellular or interstitial space (see Chap. 4 for anatomic details). During the passage of the action potential, the T system contributes qualitatively to intracellular Ca^{2+} in the same manner as the regular sarcolemma. The action potential descends the T system near the Z bands into *triadic*

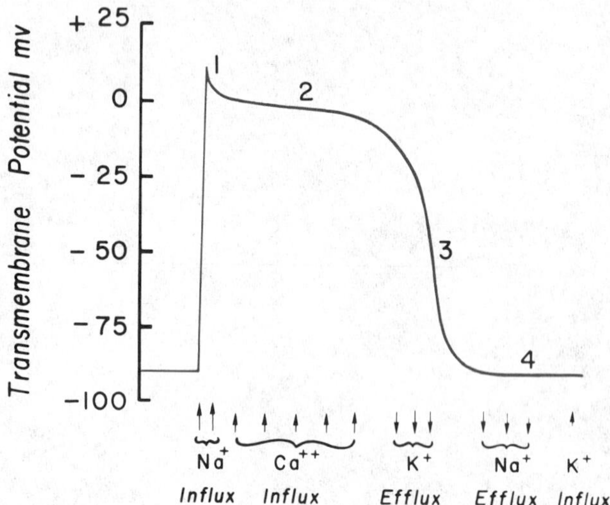

FIGURE 5-1 Schematic action potential of human ventricular myocardium together with probable electrolyte movements. The initial phase 0 spike and overshoot is related to a sudden influx of Na^+. This is followed by a slower, maintained influx of Ca^{2+} during the plateau phase 2. The phase of Ca^{2+} efflux is not well defined for human ventricular myocardium, but presumably it occurs during phase 4.

junctions, in which a single T-system tubule is in extremely close proximity to, but not in open communication with, two terminal *cisternae,* or extensions (lateral sacs), of the *sarcoplasmic reticulum (SR).*

The SR is an extensive system of intracellular tubules more or less floating in the sarcoplasma and surrounding the myofibrils. It has many branches near the transverse tubules and the surface membranes (sarcolemma) and invests every myofibril in the cell. While the SR is present in all mammalian cardiac cells, the T system is usually present where the cells are relatively large and serves to extend the surface membrane deep into the fiber. In small atrial fibers and cells of the conduction system, the T system is generally absent.

The mechanism by which the action potential depolarization "signal" is transferred from the sarcolemma and the T system to the intracellular sarcoplasmic reticulum is not precisely known, although it is probable that the relatively small initial transsarcolemmal calcium flux mediates this role (Fig. 5-2).[11,21,22,24–28,33,34] Once the sarcoplasmic reticulum is depolarized, however, the excitation spreads rapidly throughout the SR, and relatively large amounts of free Ca^{2+} are released from the SR into the sarcoplasm during the plateau phase of the action potential. The Ca^{2+} binds to a specific protein, troponin C (Tn C), which is part of a complex unit (tropomyosin-troponin) on the thin actin filament which normally inhibits actin and myosin from interacting. When Ca^{2+} is bound to this unit, this inhibition is removed and sites of actin can now interact with myosin, permitting the fibril to contract (Fig. 5-3). It appears probable that the Ca^{2+} is released particularly from the terminal cisternae (or *vesicles* or *lateral sacs*) of the SR (Fig. 5-4). In some species, mitochrondia can also release Ca^{2+} into the intracellular fluid, but it is doubtful that this mechanism normally contributes significantly to intracellular Ca^{2+} in human myocardium, although mitochondria may serve as a buffer under conditions of high cellular Ca^{2+} load.[35,36] Some Ca^{2+} may also be released from the sarcolemma surface or its glycocalyx coat.[11] Thus, a very low concentration of inward Ca^{2+} movement produced by the action potential is the initiating stimulus for the "calcium-triggered," "calcium-induced," or "regenerative" release of Ca^{2+} primarily from SR. Additional Ca^{2+} that enters through Ca^{2+} channels during the later portion of the plateau phase of the action potential, as well as Ca^{2+} that enters by the Na^+–Ca^{2+} exchanger, contributes to the continued regenerative release of Ca^{2+}. This late-entering Ca^{2+} may also be stored in the sarcoplasmic reticulum to provide Ca^{2+} for subsequent contractions.[11,21,22,24–29,33,37]

The increased sarcoplasmic "free," or "activating," Ca^{2+} diffuses to the myofibrils, where it binds to the Tn C subunit of the troponin-tropomyosin complex, which is located periodically along thin actin filaments. In the absence of Ca^{2+}, troponin works through tropomyosin, which courses along the actin filament, to prevent actin

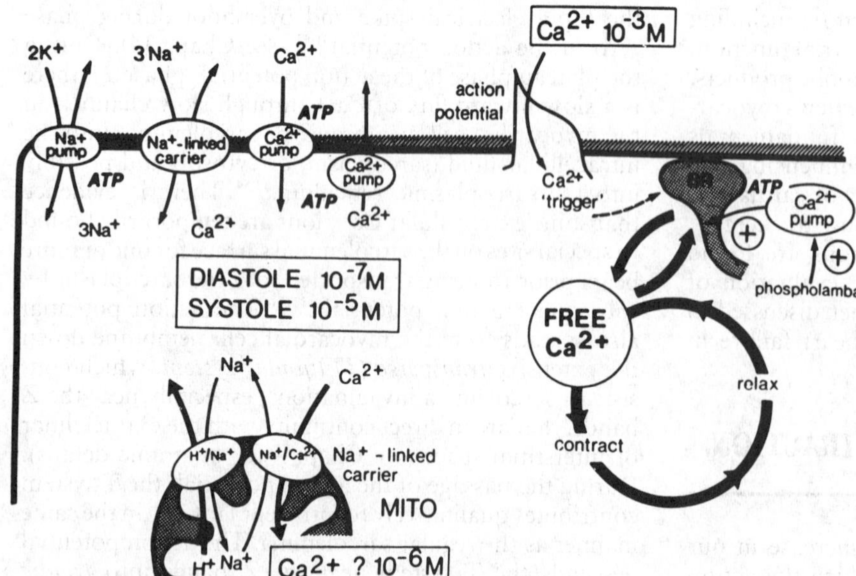

FIGURE 5-2 Calcium fluxes in the myocardium. Note the much higher extracellular (10^{-3} *M*) than intracellular value and a hypothetical mitochondrial value of about 10^{-6} *M*. The mitochondria could act as a buffer against excessive changes in the free cytosolic calcium concentration. MITO, mitochondria; SR, sarcoplasmic reticulum. *(From LH Opie: The Heart: Physiology and Metabolism. New York, Raven Press, 1991. Reproduced with permission from the publisher and author.)*

A Myocardial Contraction

Action Potential
↓
Depolarization of Sarcolemma and transverse "T" tubular system
↓
Influx of Ca^{2+}
↓
Calcium-induced Ca^{2+} Release from SR
↓
Increased binding of Ca^{2+} to troponin C
↓
Release of inhibition of actin and myosin
↓
Actin-myosin contraction

B Myocardial Relaxation

Increased SR uptake of Ca^{2+}
↓
Ca^{2+} efflux → Decreased sarcoplasmic Ca^{2+}
↓
Decreased Ca^{2+} binding to troponin C
↓
Increased troponin-tropomyosin complex inhibition of actin-myosin contraction
↓
Actin-myosin relaxation

FIGURE 5-3 Schematic diagram of the events that produce, *A*, myocardial excitation-contraction coupling and, *B*, myocardial relaxation. With depolarization of the cardiac cell membranes (sarcolemma and transverse T system), the Na^+ channels open, followed by the Ca^{2+} channels. The initial transsarcolemmal influx of Ca^{2+} triggers the release of Ca^{2+} from the sarcoplasmic reticulum (SR). Ca^{2+} in higher concentration then binds to troponin C; this produces conformational changes in whole troponin (troponin I–troponin C–troponin T complex) that relieves a troponin I interaction with actin, thereby allowing tropomyosin to roll back into the grooves of the F-actin superhelix and allowing the interaction of actin and myosin to produce contraction. The transsarcolemmal Ca^{2+} current has both a faster and a slower component. It is possible that the former may act to trigger the release of Ca^{2+} from the SR, whereas the slow component may cause the SR to accumulate calcium. Ca^{2+} influx may also occur by the Na^+-Ca^{2+} exchanger. Relaxation is initiated by an unknown stimulus that produces the active uptake of Ca^{2+} by the SR Ca^{2+} ATPase, which is under the control of phospholamban. The resulting lower concentration of cytoplasmic Ca^{2+} produces decreased Ca^{2+} binding to troponin C and relaxation. During relaxation, Ca^{2+} efflux may occur both by Ca^{2+} ATPase and by a Na^+ Ca^{2+} exchanger.

from interacting with myosin. There are three troponin (Tn) proteins: Tn C, which binds Ca^{2+}; Tn I, which affects tropomyosin so as to keep actin from associating with myosin; and Tn T, which attaches these units to tropomyosin. Once Ca^{2+} attaches to troponin C, a conformational change occurs in tropomyosin via Tn I that enhances the formation of crossbridges between myosin and actin, resulting in contraction.[11,14,21,22,24–29,33,38] This loss of inhibition, or "derepression," allows enzyme sites on myosin bridges to interact with actin so that the resultant actomyosin adenosine triphosphatase (ATPase), in the presence of bound adenosine triphosphate (ATP) and magnesium, allows bridge motion and myocardial contraction through the sliding filament mechanism. An increase in the free Ca^{2+} concentration from 5×10^{-7} to 6×10^{-6} *M* results in the production of approximately 90 percent of the maximum force. The fraction of myofibrillar Ca^{2+} bound by Tn C and necessary for activation is not exactly known, although about 22 μmol is needed by the myofibril for 50 percent activation and 90 μmol for maximal activation. The increased sarcoplasmic Ca^{2+} also influences myocardial metabolism by activating glycogen phosphorylase, which results in increased glycogenolysis. The energy for myocardial

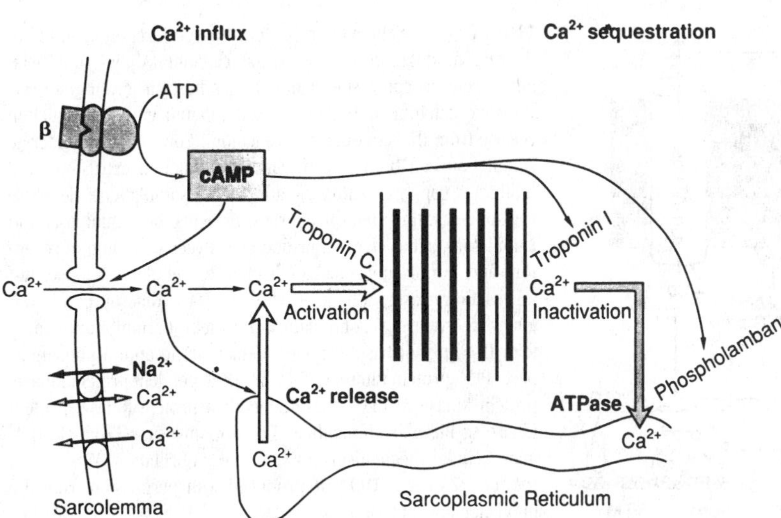

FIGURE 5-4 Effect of calcium ion cycling on activation and inactivation of contractile proteins. Calcium influx across the sarcolemma as well as calcium released from sarcoplasmic reticulum stores allow association and cross-linking of the myofibrillar proteins actin and myosin, with resultant cellular contraction. This rapid increase in intracellular calcium concentration is then countered by rapid sequestration of calcium into the sarcoplasmic reticulum by calcium ATPase. The decrease in intracellular calcium concentration allows "inactivation" of the actin myosin cross-bridges, with resultant cellular relaxation. Stimulation of sarcolemmal beta-adrenergic receptors increases the intracellular concentration of cyclic AMP (cAMP), which enhances activation and also facilitates inactivation, by phosphorylation of troponin I (which reduces contractile protein affinity for calcium) and of phospholamban (which augments calcium ATPase activity.) *(From RO Bonow, JE Udelson: Left ventricular diastolic dysfunction as a cause of congestive heart failure: Mechanisms and management. Ann Intern Med 117:502–510, 1992. Reproduced with permission from the publisher and authors.)*

contraction is obtained from molecules of magnesium ATP that are split by an ATPase site on the myosin filament heads during each interaction with actin (see Chap. 6A).

Relaxation is initiated by an unknown stimulus (or loss of inhibition) that produces an increased uptake of sarcoplasmic Ca^{2+}, predominantly by the SR, with removal of Ca^{2+} from Tn C. It is not certain exactly where or how this decrease in intracellular Ca^{2+} occurs in human myocardium.[28,39–44] It has been suggested that Ca^{2+} uptake occurs on the sarcoplasmic surface of the longitudinal tubules of the SR, directly back into the terminal cisternae of the SR and on the sarcolemma.[11,23] The route that would be taken by Ca^{2+} after being reabsorbed into longitudinal tubules at the SR is also uncertain.[28] It may be transported or diffused back to the terminal cisternae within the SR, and some may be diffused to the T system and to the interstitial space. Relaxation of the actin-myosin myofibrils occurs as the result of an inhibition produced by the troponin-tropomyosin complex in the presence of low intracellular Ca^{2+} (Figs. 5-3 and 5-4).

The primary transport system for the efflux of Ca^{2+} from myocardial cells appears to be the sodium-calcium exchanger, in which one calcium ion leaves the cell in exchange for three sodium ions, which are subsequently pumped out of the cell by the sodium-potassium ATPase in exchange for two potassium ions.[14] The ATP-dependent Ca^{2+} pump may also play a role.[45]

The velocity and the amount of tension developed by the actin-myosin myofilaments are directly related to the amount of Ca^{2+} available to inhibit troponin and induce contraction. It should also be noted that the Ca^{2+} that enters electrogenically during phase 2 (slow current) of the action potential indirectly modulates myocardial contractility by contributing significantly to the amount of intracellular calcium. When the heart rate is abruptly increased, there is an associated progressive increase or decrease in contractile force, known as the *Bowditch, staircase,* or *treppe phenomenon.* This effect is also associated with altered amounts of Ca^{2+} available for activation.[46] It is likely that many drugs (such as digitalis,[26,47–51] sympathomimetic amines,[37,51–55] calcium antagonists, xanthines, and phosphodiesterase inhibitors), as well as conditions such as an increase in heart rate,[56–59] paired pacing,[60] or postextrasystolic potentiation,[61] ultimately have their influence on myocardial contractility through their effect upon available intracellular Ca^{2+}.[11,24,26,52,62,63] The negative inotropic effect of acidosis upon myocardial contractility may also be related to a decrease in the quantity of Ca^{2+} released from the sarcoplasmic reticulum[64] (see also Chap. 28). An increase in the intracellular Na^+ concentration decreases the influx of Na^+ via the bidirectional Na^+-Ca^{2+} exchange system and thereby decreases the efflux of Ca^{2+}. The net result is an increase in intracellular Ca^{2+} and in contractility.[11,24,26,65] Figures 5-5 and 5-6 diagrammatically illustrate the major components that regulate calcium homeostasis in myocardial membranes and that directly influence myocardial contractility by their influence upon intracellular Ca^{2+}.

Digitalis, which binds to and inhibits membrane sodium-potassium ATPase and thereby inhibits the active extrusion of sodium that enters with each systole in exchange for potassium, produces much of its effect by increasing intracellular Na^+, which, through the Na^+-Ca^{2+} exchanger, results in an increased concentration of intracellular activator Ca^{2+} [26,43,49,50] (see Chaps. 25 and 27). Other conditions that increase intracellular Na^+ may also increase myocardial contractility.[26,65] Studies have also suggested that significant defects in the kinetics of intracellular calcium are present in the myocardium of patients with heart failure[46] (see Chap. 25).

FUNDAMENTAL MYOCARDIAL MUSCLE MECHANICS

The contraction of heart muscle is regulated by four distinct, although interrelated, factors:

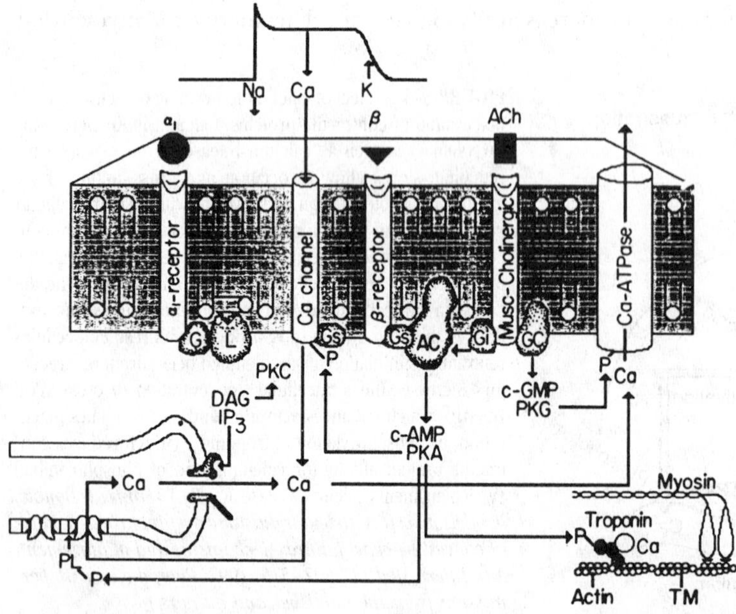

FIGURE 5-5 Schematic representation of adrenergic and cholinergic modulation of myocardial calcium. Alpha- and beta-adrenergic receptor stimulation acts synergistically to increase cytosolic calcium by both increased calcium entry and calcium release from the sarcoplasmic reticulum. Conversely, cholinergic stimulation can both directly (increase calcium extrusion) and indirectly (oppose action of adrenergic stimulation) decrease cytosolic calcium. Heterotrimeric G proteins, both inhibitory and stimulatory, act as signal transducers between activation of receptors and cytoplasmic changes leading to cellular response. AC, adenylate cyclase; ACh, acetylcholine; DAG, diacylglycerol; GC, guanylate cyclase; G_s, stimulatory G protein; G_i, inhibitory G protein; IP_3, inositol trisphosphate; L, membrane-bound phospholipase; PKC, protein kinase C; PKA, cAMP-dependent protein kinase, protein kinase A; PKG, cGMP-dependent protein kinase, protein kinase G; PL, phospholamban; TM, tropomyosin. (From GE Billman: Cellular mechanisms for ventricular fibrillation. *News Physiol Sci* 7:254–25, 1992. Reproduced with permission from the publisher and author.)

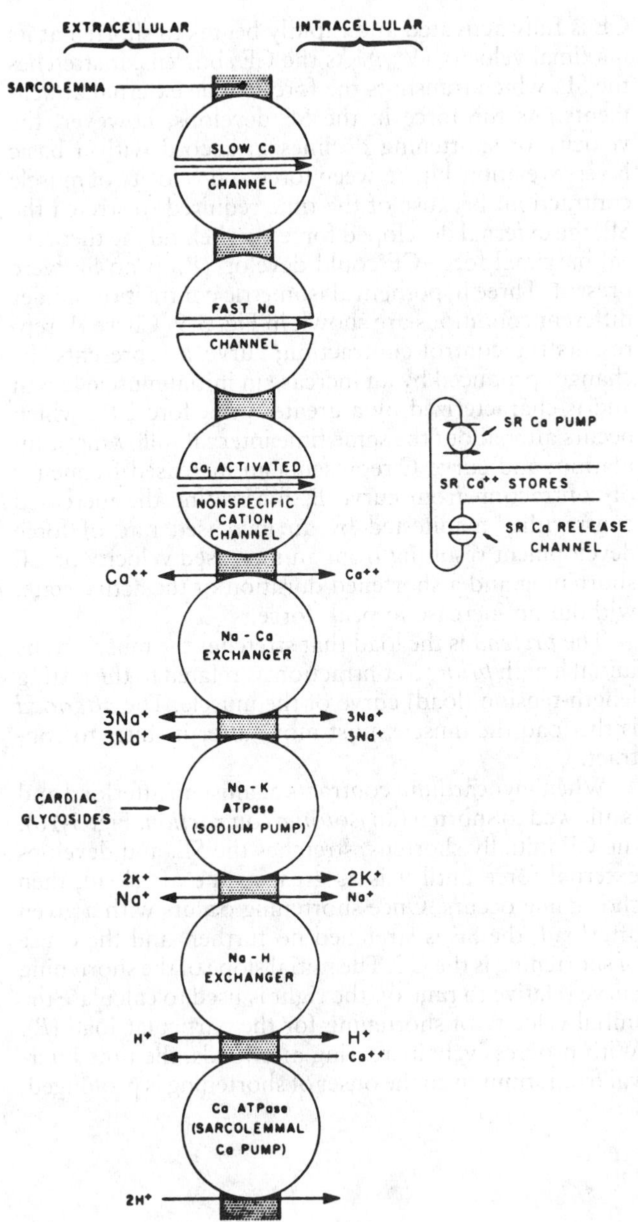

FIGURE 5-6 Selected components regulating cellular calcium homeostasis in myocardial membrane systems. (1) The slow calcium channel, a voltage-sensitive protein complex that carries the slow inward calcium current during phase 2 of the cardiac action potential, provides the pulse of intracellular calcium (Ca^{2+}) that triggers calcium-induced release of a much larger amount of activator calcium from stores in the sarcoplasmic reticulum (SR). The arrow indicates the principal direction of ion movement when the channel is activated. (2) The fast sodium channel, another voltage-sensitive structure, mediates the upstroke of the cardiac action potential; this depolarization event results in activation of the slow calcium channel. (3) A putative intracellular calcium-activated nonspecific cation channel, less well characterized than the preceding components (1 and 2), is thought to account for the transient depolarizing (and hence arrhythmogenic) inward current that occurs in response to toxic doses of cardiac glycosides. (4) The sodium-calcium exchanger is a membrane component that mediates the facilitated, bidirectional exchange of sodium for calcium across the sarcolemmal membrane. This process is sensitive to membrane potential because of the asymmetry of charge movement inherent in the stoichiometry of the process (three sodium ions for every calcium ion). (5) The Na-K-ATPase, or sodium pump—the cardiac glycoside-binding site—is located on the outward-facing surface of the alpha subunit of this enzyme, which mediates the active transport of sodium and potassium ions against their respective concentration gradients. (6) The sodium-hydrogen exchanger, an amiloride-sensitive protein, mediates the electroneutral exchange of sodium for hydrogen ions and helps to facilitate the accumulation of intracellular sodium (and hence intracellular calcium) in response to cardiac glycosides. (7) The sarcolemmal calcium pump has a relatively low-capacity but high-affinity ATP-dependent ion-transport protein that extrudes calcium from cardiac cells against a large electrochemical gradient and helps to maintain the low levels of intracellular calcium ions that prevail during diastole. To the right of the sarcolemmal membrane are represented (8) the sarcoplasmic reticulum ATP-dependent calcium pump that is responsible for diastolic relaxation by rapid sequestration of calcium at end systole, and (9) the ryanodine-sensitive sarcoplasmic reticulum calcium-release channel that accounts for calcium-induced release of most of the calcium that activates contractile proteins in mammalian myocardium. (*From TW Smith: Digitalis: Mechanisms of action and clinical use. N Engl J Med 318:358, 1988. Reproduced with permission from the publisher and author.*)

1. The *preload* (Starling's law of the heart), which is the passive load that establishes the initial muscle length of the cardiac fibers prior to contraction. Preload is described by the resting length-tension curve in isolated muscle. In the intact heart, this comprises the diastolic pressure-volume curve.
2. The *afterload,* which is the sum of all the loads against which the myocardial fibers must shorten during systole, including the aortic impedance, the arterial resistance, the peripheral vascular resistance, the end-diastolic pressure, acting through the Laplace relationship, and the mass of blood in the aorta and great arteries, as well as the viscosity of the blood.
3. The *contractility,* or *inotropic state* of the heart, which is reflected in the speed and shortening capacity of the myocardium at a given instantaneous load.
4. The *heart rate,* or frequency of contraction.

These four factors are interrelated in the intact organism and are not independent. As will be described, fiber length appears to influence primarily the number of active force-generating sites in the myocardium, whereas a change in the contractile state (or contractility) is related to a qualitative change in the force generated by the sites, that is, a change in their activations, with or without a change in their number.[66–70] Before discussing these mechanisms, however, a brief review of fundamental myocardial mechanics as described by force-velocity-length relationships is appropriate.[71] More detailed discussions are presented in specialized reviews.[10,71–93]

Hill[94,95] suggested a model for muscular contraction that has been exceedingly useful for understanding myocardial mechanics and predicting their changes under a number of different circumstances. In this model (Fig. 5-7), muscle contraction behaves as if there were a *contractile element* (CE), which is capable of developing force and of shortening; a *series elastic component* (SE), which is passively stretched by shortening the CE; and a *parallel elastic component* (PE), which supports resting tension but plays little role during contraction. The model does

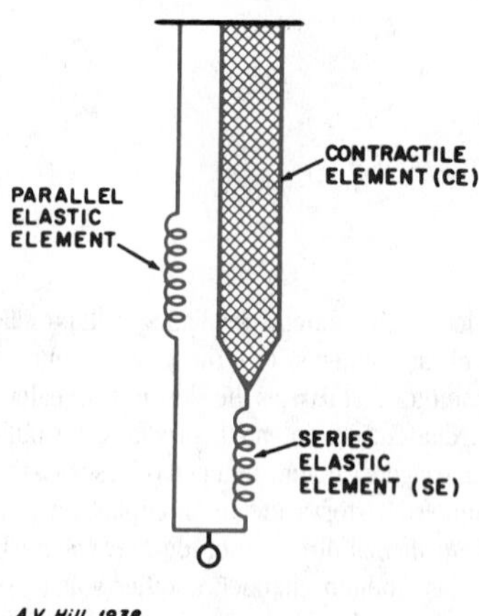

FIGURE 5-7 Hill's three-component model for muscle. See the text for details. (*From EH Sonnenblick: The Mechanics of Myocardial Contraction. In: SA Briller, HL Conn Jr, eds: The Myocardial Cell: Structure, Function, and Modification by Cardiac Drugs. Philadelphia, University of Pennsylvania Press, 1966, 173. Reproduced with permission from the publisher and author.*)

not denote specific anatomic sites of the components or, indeed, their arrangement. Rather, it describes how force and shortening are transferred from contractile sites to the external world, and anatomic reality is not implied. As such, it is a useful "working" model for understanding how isometric and isotonic contractions are related. In isolated muscle preparations, this SE is created by damaged elastic ends of the muscle; in the intact heart, the SE includes valves and elastic structures. For these reasons, when compared to skeletal muscle, the functional SE of heart muscle is four to five times as compliant.

After stimulation of a strip of heart muscle that is not allowed to shorten (*isometric contraction*, Fig. 5-8), the CE is fully activated and rapidly begins to shorten at its maximal velocity (V_{max}). As the CE shortens, it stretches the SE, which transmits the force to the external attachments. As the force in the SE develops, however, the velocity of shortening declines in accord with a basic inverse relationship between force and velocity of muscle contraction. Because of the time required to stretch the SE, the external developed force lags behind the theoretical maximal force CE could develop (P_0) if no SE were present. Three hypothetical isometric contractions under different conditions are shown in Fig. 5-9. Curve *A* represents the control contraction; curve *B* represents the changes produced by an increase in initial muscle length and is characterized by a greater peak force, P_0, which occurs after about the same time interval following stimulation; and curve *C* represents an increased frequency of contraction from curve *B*, illustrating the increased contractility manifested by an increased rate of force development resulting from an increased velocity of CE shortening and a shortened duration of the active state, without an increase in peak force.

The *preload* is the load that stretches the muscle to its initial length *prior* to contraction as related to the resting length-tension (load) curve of the muscle. The *afterload* is the load the muscle must move after it starts to contract.

When myocardium contracts against an afterload and is allowed to shorten (an *isotonic contraction*, Fig. 5-10), the CE initially shortens, stretches the SE, and develops external force until it is as great as the afterload; then shortening occurs. Once shortening occurs with a given afterload, the SE is stretched no further, and the cause of shortening is the CE. The initial slope of the shortening curve relative to time on the right is used to calculate the initial velocity of shortening for the particular load (*P*). With progressively increasing afterloads, the time interval from stimulus to the onset of shortening is prolonged,

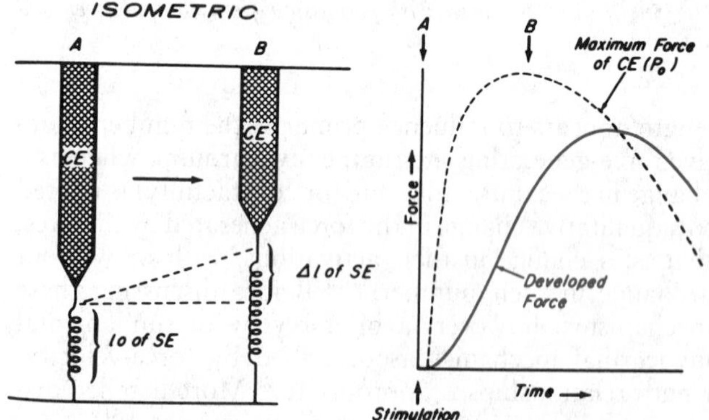

FIGURE 5-8 Schematic model of an isometric contraction of a strip of heart muscle. *Left:* The muscle model with a contractile element (CE) and a series elastic-component (SE). The initial length of the SE (L_0) increases by Δl between *A* and *B*. *Right:* The time course of development of external force together with the hypothetical instantaneous force of CE that it might develop if no SE attachments were present. Point *A*, the initial resting state; point *B*, some time during active activation. See the text for details. [*From EH Sonnenblick: The Mechanics of Myocardial Contraction. In: SA Briller, HL Conn Jr, eds: The Myocardial Cell: Structure, Function, and Modification by Cardiac Drugs. Philadelphia, University of Pennsylvania Press, 1966, 173. Reproduced with permission from the publisher and author.*]

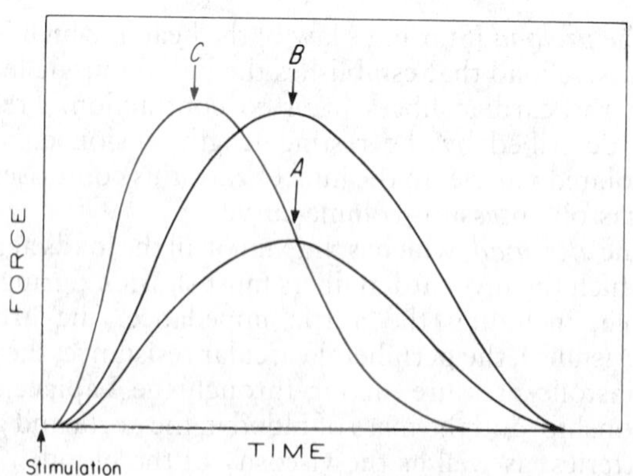

FIGURE 5-9 Hypothetical isometric force developed by three hypothetical contractions. *A.* Control. *B.* Increased initial muscle length. *C.* The muscle in curve *B* contracting more frequently. See the text for details. [*From EH Sonnenblick: The mechanics of myocardial contraction. In: SA Briller, HL Conn Jr, eds: The Myocardial Cell: Structure, Function, and Modification by Cardiac Drugs. Philadelphia, University of Pennsylvania Press, 1966, 173. Reproduced with permission from the publisher and author.*]

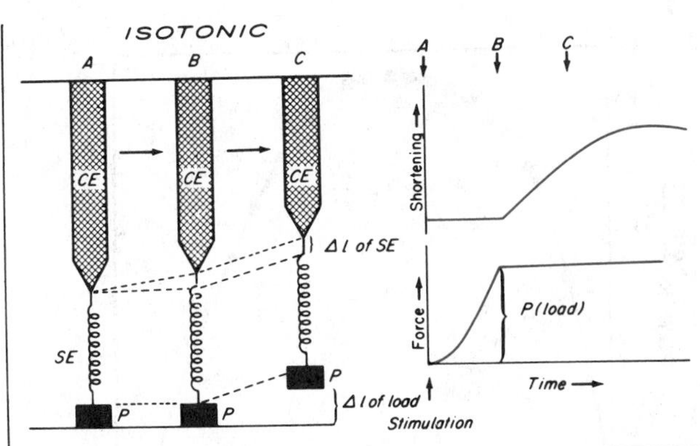

FIGURE 5-10 An afterloaded isotonic contraction of myocardium. On the left is the muscle model attached to a load *P*, which is supported when the muscle is at rest (*A*). This type of load *P* that is encountered by the CE only when the CE attempts to shorten is the afterload, whereas the small load used to stretch the system to its initial length is the preload. With stimulation of the system, the CE begins to shorten at maximum speed V_{max}. During the isometric portion of the contraction, between *A* and *B*, the CE shortens, the SE matches the load *P*, and the load starts to move. Once the load begins to move to point *B*, the SE remains constant in length, and shortening of the system reflects shortening of the CE alone. The curves on the right reflect force and shortening as functions of time after stimulation. The tangent to the slope of the curve of initial shortening is used to obtain the initial velocity of isotonic shortening for a given load. After plotting the initial velocity of shortening for different loads, one may extrapolate the curve to zero load to obtain the theoretic intrinsic or maximal velocity V_{max}. See Fig 5-12. (*From EH Sonnenblick: The mechanics of myocardial contraction. In: SA Briller, HL Conn Jr, eds: The Myocardial Cell: Structure, Function, and Modification by Cardiac Drugs. Philadelphia, University of Pennsylvania Press, 1966, 173. Reproduced with permission from the publisher and author.*)

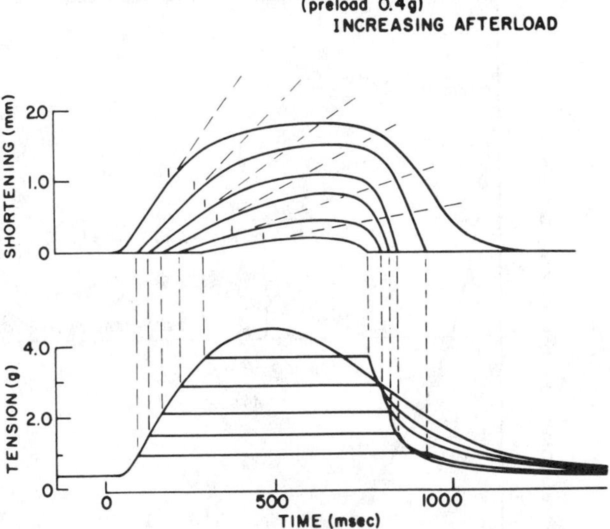

FIGURE 5-11 A series of superimposed tracings made from isolated papillary muscle that was arranged in such a manner that both initial isometric contraction and subsequent isotonic shortening are possible. *Below:* Serial isometric contraction at increasing afterloads (horizontal lines). *Above:* Successive isotonic shortening corresponding to the increasing afterloads in the lower tracing (*dashed lines*). The dashed lines on the upper tracing represent the initial velocity of shortening. As the afterload increases, the initial velocity of shortening decreases and the extent of shortening decreases, but the isometric relaxation phase increases. [*From EH Sonnenblick: The mechanics of myocardial contraction. In: SA Briller, HL Conn Jr, eds: The Myocardial Cell: Structure, Function, and Modification by Cardiac Drugs. Philadelphia, University of Pennsylvania Press, 1966, 173. Reproduced with permission from the publisher and author.*]

but the time to maximal shortening is unchanged (Fig. 5-11). In addition, the initial velocity of isotonic shortening for each load, which is obtained by drawing a tangent to the initial shortening slope, decreases with increasing loads. This basic curvilinear relationship is further illustrated in Figs. 5-12 and 5-13, in which the force-velocity relationships of isolated papillary muscles are plotted to illustrate the basic principle of a decrease in the initial velocity of shortening with increasing loads. As shown in Fig. 5-12, extrapolation of the curve to zero load yields the theoretic maximal velocity (V_{max}) of shortening of the contractile elements in the unloaded muscle. V_{max} in turn is altered by factors that modify the activation of the muscle, but not by a change in initial muscle length within physiological resting lengths.[2,71] Thus, it forms one index of the contractility of the myocardial fibers being examined.

PRELOAD: THE FRANK-STRAUB-WIGGERS-STARLING PRINCIPLE

In 1871, Bowditch[96] showed that if the condition of the heart muscle remains unaltered, contractions remain equal in strength, regardless of the strength of stimuli applied. This principle, which has become known as the *all-or-nothing law of the heart*, implied that cardiac muscle either does not contract at all or responds to the fullest extent, but that the magnitude of the all-or-none response is determined by the inherent "condition" of the muscle. In 1884, Howell and Donaldson[97] presented unequivocal evidence that the heart itself has intrinsic mechanisms by which its output is adjusted to the venous input. Using a heart-lung preparation, they found that increasing the venous return increased cardiac output and stroke as well as right atrial pressure. In 1895, Frank[98] published his classic studies on the dynamics of heart muscle. His object was to correlate the reactions of cardiac muscle with the responses of skeletal muscle, the force of contraction of which had been previously shown by Fick,[99] von Kries,[100] and Blix[101] to be related to the initial length and resting tension. Frank studied the frog atria and ventricles and showed that, within limits, stepwise increases in diastolic volume and pressure just before contraction—the *presystolic* or *end-diastolic* volume and pressure—determine the magnitude of the all-or-none response. His studies emphasized the dependence of the cardiac response on hemodynamic events immediately preceding excitation.

In 1914, Wiggers[102] demonstrated that the reactions established by Frank for the frog's ventricle also apply to the naturally beating right ventricle of dogs. He concluded that the rate of isometric pressure rise and the peak systolic pressure are determined by changes in the initial tension, as long as marked changes in inherent contractility are not simultaneously produced by experimental procedures. Also in 1914, Straub[103] and Starling

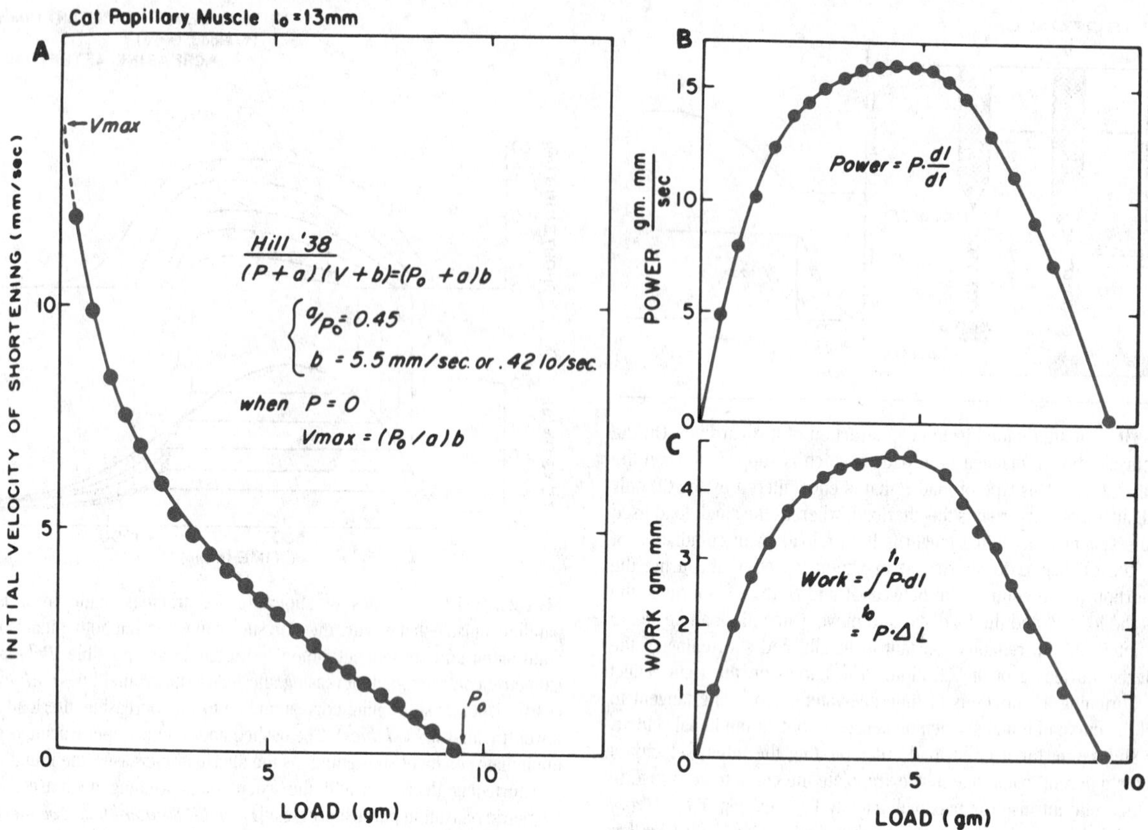

FIGURE 5-12 *A.* Force-velocity relationships of a papillary muscle, illustrating the decreasing initial velocity of shortening with increasing loads. The insert gives Hill's equation for muscular contraction with the derived constants. When the curve is extrapolated to zero load, one obtains the V_{max}, or the intrinsic velocity of shortening. When the load is increased to the point at which no shortening can occur (an isometric contraction), the maximum force is manifest (P_0 or intrinsic force). *B.* The load versus the power (force versus velocity of shortening). *C.* The load versus work (force or load versus displacement). Note that peak power and work are obtained at loads approximately 50 percent of the maximal force of contraction P_0 obtained during isometric conditions. Instantaneous force-velocity of shortening is measured at a constant time after stimulation by quick-release techniques. [*From EH Sonnenblick: The mechanics of muscle contraction. In SA Briller, HL Conn Jr, eds: The Myocardial Cell: Structure, Function, and Modification by Cardiac Drugs. Philadelphia, University of Pennsylvania Press, 1966, 173. Reproduced with permission from the publisher and author.*]

and associates[104,105] independently reported their studies of the effect of changes in initial tension and length on the response of isolated hearts. The studies of Starling and associates have received the greatest amount of attention in the English-speaking areas of the world; however, in deference to Frank, the general principle is often referred to as the *Frank-Starling law of the heart.*[106] On the basis of highly suggestive, but not quite conclusive, studies on the heart-lung preparation, Starling and associates concluded that "the mechanical energy set free on passage from the resting to the constricted state depends on the area of chemically active surfaces, i.e., on the length of the muscle fibers."

Wiggers[107] has pointed out that, although there is a general impression that the often-reproduced representation of the law by Starling and associates was based on data from their own experiments, the published curves were reproductions of graphs previously published by Blix and by Frank. Although it is not certain whether the responsiveness of the heart is fundamentally related to changes in presystolic pressure (initial tension) or to changes in volume (initial length), it is obvious that fiber length and resting tension are interrelated.

Wiggers[107] has emphasized the importance of other factors affecting the responsiveness of the myocardium and has stressed that the statement of the law of the heart, in which the energy of contraction is a function of the length of the muscle fiber, should be modified by the phrase "under equivalent states of responsiveness," or what one would call contractility today.[108] Sarnoff and Berglund[109,110] demonstrated this principle as a "family of curves" relating stroke work to left atrial pressure that exists for each ventricle and that many other factors, such as humoral agents, neural influences, and metabolic condition of the myocardium, determine which particular "curve" the ventricle is operating on at a given moment. The studies of Braunwald and associates[2,111,112] have shown the applicability of the law of the heart in both the normal and the diseased human heart.

As discussed below, changes in muscle length not only change the number of bridges that can be formed to develop force but also affect the amount of force produced by the same amount of Ca^{2+} activation.[66–69,72] Thus, although V_{max} is not altered by changing muscle length, the sensitivity of the contractile system to Ca^{2+} is length-dependent. In this sense, muscle length effects (preload) and contractility (inotropism) are interrelated.

Although pressure and volume (initial fiber length)

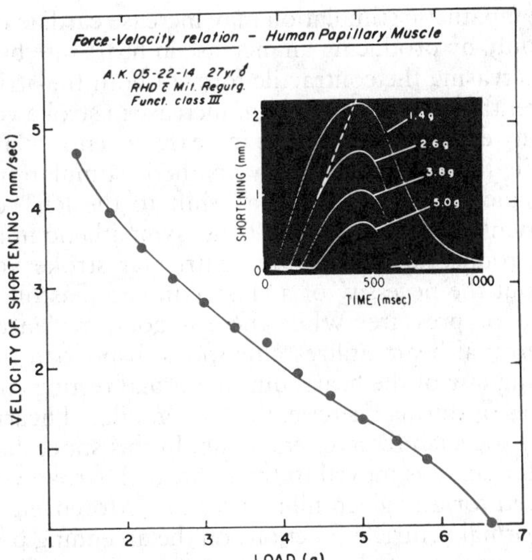

FIGURE 5-13 Relationship between the initial velocity of isotonic shortening and afterload of a human papillary muscle stimulated at a rate of 12 stimuli per minute. The preload was 1.4 g, with a muscle length of 15 mm. Note the significant decrease in initial velocity as the load increases. The insert shows four recordings with different afterloads; the decrease in rate of shortening with increasing afterload is apparent from the altered slopes of the length-time curves. *(From EH Sonnenblick, E Braunwald, AG Morrow: The contractile properties of human heart muscle: Studies on myocardial mechanics of surgically excised papillary muscles. J Clin Invest 44:966. 1965. Reproduced with permission from The American Society for Clinical Investigation and the author.)*

are related, the relationship may be altered under certain circumstances. *Distensibility* or *compliance* is the ratio of change in ventricular volume to change in ventricular diastolic pressure ($\Delta V/\Delta P$), while ventricular *stiffness* is the reciprocal, or the change in pressure for a given change in volume ($\Delta P/\Delta V$).[93,113-121] Steady-state compliance determined just before systolic contraction comprises only part of the determinants of ventricular filling. Early ventricular filling following closure of the aortic valves depends on rapidity of the ventricular relaxation with *elastic recoil* creating a gradient of rapid early ventricular filling. This active elastic recoil depends on a small end-systolic volume and helps early filling, especially during tachycardia. Late filling depends on diastolic compliance as well as completed ventricular relaxation. Defining changes in compliance is especially complex in certain pathological conditions. For example, with chronic volume overloads, the curve relating diastolic volume to pressure moves to the right so that there is greater volume for any given filling pressure and a greater volume at zero filling pressure (V_0). Nevertheless, at larger volumes, very small changes in volume may produce large diastolic pressure changes, consistent with increased wall stiffness. Thus, the curve is changed with increased compliance at small volumes and reduced compliance with large volumes. Such alterations reflect ventricular wall remodeling due to the volume overload (see Chap. 25).

Most of the recognized changes in static ventricular compliance occur chronically. Conditions that may change ventricular compliance include ventricular distension, resulting in increased compliance; ventricular hypertrophy, resulting in reduced compliance; fibrosis; infiltrative diseases; pericardial tamponade or constriction; lymphatic obstruction; engorgement of the coronary circulation; ventricular septal hypertrophy; or disease or dilatation of the contralateral ventricle (decreased compliance). Aging also is associated with an increase in ventricular stiffness or decreased compliance, reflecting age-dependent myocyte loss, fibrosis, and reactive hypertrophy.[122,123] Except in response to hypoxia, ischemia, acidosis, afterload, or tachycardia, significant acute changes in the pressure-volume relationship or in the relaxation and distensibility of ventricles probably do not occur, nor do many inotropic agents produce significant acute changes.[113,120,124] On the other hand, the rate of ventricular relaxation can be increased by late systolic loading or catecholamines.[125-127] There is some evidence that some calcium antagonists and other agents may favorably influence early relaxation and distensibility, particularly in the hypertrophied heart.[128-130] Marked tachycardia and asynchrony also influence relaxation and ventricular filling.[131,132] (See also Chap. 25.)

Ventricular distensibility is often significantly influenced by filling of the opposite ventricle, especially when filling pressures are acutely elevated with an intact pericardium.[133-139] Thus, the pressure-volume relationships of one ventricle can be immediately influenced by acute changes in the filling of the contralateral ventricle. At cardiac catheterization, it is possible to obtain reasonable estimations of ventricular end-diastolic and end-systolic volumes and very accurate measurements of end-diastolic pressure. As discussed in Chap. 25, the ventricular end-diastolic pressure may be elevated either by an altered compliance due to myocardial hypoxia, fibrosis, infiltrative processes, pericardial tamponade or constriction, failure, or by ventricular hypertrophy itself.[2,113-117,121,140,141] The term *lusitrophy* has been used to refer to the diastolic properties of myocardium and cardiac chambers.[142]

The Frank-Starling law of the heart is one of the major mechanisms by which the normal right and left ventricles maintain equal minute outputs even though their stroke outputs may vary considerably during normal respiration. Thus, if the right ventricle temporarily pumps more blood into the pulmonary circulation than the left ventricle pumps into the systemic circulation, the proper balance between the two pumps is soon achieved, since the venous return to the left atrium and ventricle causes the left ventricular end-diastolic fiber length to be greater, increasing left ventricular stroke output. In addition, a decreased left ventricular stroke output would eventually lead to decreased return of blood to the right atrium and ventricle, producing a decrease in right ventricular stroke output. By this mechanism the two ventricles, which function as two pumps in series, are able to balance their outputs and prevent pulmonary edema despite marked variations in stroke volumes.

A left ventricular "function curve" is shown in Fig. 5-14, in which left ventricular stroke volume is plotted as a function of left ventricular end-diastolic pressure. The initial ventricular function curves[109] utilized stroke work (stroke volume × blood pressure); however, stroke volume and derived stroke work are greatly dependent on the blood pressure, and thus the use of stroke volume

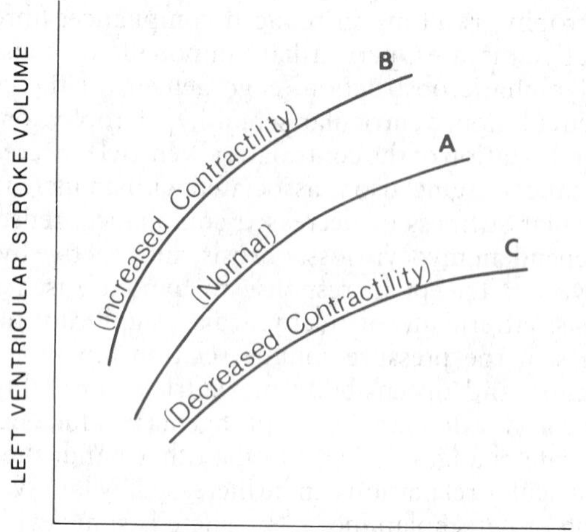

FIGURE 5-14 Relationship between left ventricular end-diastolic pressure and left ventricular stroke volume. *A.* The normal function. *B.* The shift to the left of the original curve associated with increased contractility, such as might result from sympathetic stimulation of the ventricle or the infusion of epinephrine or norepinephrine. *C.* A shift to the right of the original curve associated with decreased contractility, such as might result from ventricular failure from ischemia or myocardial depressant drugs. A ventricle functioning on a curve *C* might be restored to a curve *A* by the action of digitalis or inotropic drugs, such as norepinephrine or epinephrine. Similar but not identical curves are obtained when left ventricular stroke volume or cardiac output is plotted against left ventricular end-diastolic pressure or left atrial mean pressure. Function curves such as these may be obtained from both ventricles and both atria.

is more appropriate. Because end-diastolic fiber length and intraventricular pressure are normally related to each other, it is common in clinical situations to measure left ventricular end-diastolic pressure, since fiber length is difficult to determine in patients. In Fig. 5-14, curve *A* represents a hypothetical normal left ventricular function curve. Curve *B* represents a "shift to the left" of the function curve of the same ventricle under the influence of sympathetic stimulation or the infusion of epinephrine, norepinephrine, or other catecholamines. Curve C represents a "shift to the right" of curve *A*, such as might occur with myocardial depression from hypoxia, cardiodepressant drugs, or myocardial "failure." Note that under normal conditions (curve *A*), very slight changes in fiber length, which can be produced by small changes in filling pressure, are associated with significant increases in stroke volume. As mentioned above, this is one of the major mechanisms by which the two ventricles have balanced outputs over any period of time, even though their stroke outputs may vary considerably from beat to beat, particularly during the respiratory cycle. Cardiac output is increased by an increase in preload (i.e., the Frank-Starling relationship) in many conditions, including those associated with an increase in venous return and a decrease in peripheral vascular resistance, such as exercise, anemia, fever, pregnancy, or other forms of peripheral arteriovenous fistulas. Changes in external pressure on the body, such as those encountered in either space flight or immersion of the lower body in water, are associated with increased preload and increased intrathoracic blood volume.

Sympathetic stimulation may increase cardiac output not only by producing an increase in heart rate but also by increasing the contractile force of both the atria and the ventricles, with a resultant increase in stroke volume for any extent of filling. The increase in ventricular contractile force produced by sympathetic stimulation may be depicted graphically as a "shift to the left" of the ventricular function curve. Thus, sympathetic impulses can produce an increase in ventricular stroke volume without the necessity of a change in end-diastolic fiber length or pressure. While there is good evidence that the normal heart utilizes alterations in preload (or the Starling law of the heart) during normal resting circumstances or during exercise, the failing, dilated heart may have little such reserve remaining. In this state, the ventricular curve is moved to the right, with stroke volume reduced for any given filling pressure. Moreover, while the normal ventricle functions on the ascending portion of the curve, the failing ventricle functions on a flattened curve and an increase in falling pressure does not produce an increase in stroke volume. Thus, the hearts of patients with heart failure and cardiac dilatation operate near the top (L_{max}) of their force-length curve, where sarcomere lengths are about 2.2 mm after fixation (see Fig. 5-16) and are therefore unable to respond significantly to increased filling or stretch with a greater force of contraction. There is probably no true descending limb for a function curve, although changes in afterload reflecting the Laplace relationship and increased volume may produce an apparent descending limb.[143–146]

Figure 5-15 illustrates the interrelationships between ventricular end-diastolic volume, end-diastolic pressure, and stroke work. As indicated in Fig. 5-15*A*, the relationship between stoke volume and end-diastolic volume is nearly linear. On the other hand, the relationship between end-diastolic pressure and volume (Fig. 5-14*B*) is curvilinear, with a definite volume at zero pressure and a rather sharp increase in pressure above a certain volume. Figure 5-14C illustrates the familiar curvilinear relationship between ventricular end-diastolic pressure and stroke volume.

Ultrastructural Basis of Starling's Law

The length-tension relationship of a papillary muscle is shown in Fig. 5-16. The length of a myocardial sarcomere at which maximal force develops is approximately 2.2 μm after fixation, at which length the thin actin and thick myosin myofilaments are optimally overlapped to provide the greatest number of force-generating sites.[2,70,76,147–157] When the sarcomere is stretched beyond about 2.2 μm, the developed force decreases as the myofilaments become partially disengaged and fewer contractile sites are brought into play. In addition, actual damage to the myocardial cells and sarcomeres occurs when the fibers are excessively stretched.[145] In skeletal muscle, at a length of 3.65 μm, the actin and myosin myofilaments are completely disengaged, and developed tension drops to zero. These long sarcomeres are seen only in skeletal fibers, since cardiac sarcomeres and cells are too stiff to become that overstretched. While consistent with a "sliding-filament" mechanism, such longer sarcomere lengths at which force falls are not seen physi-

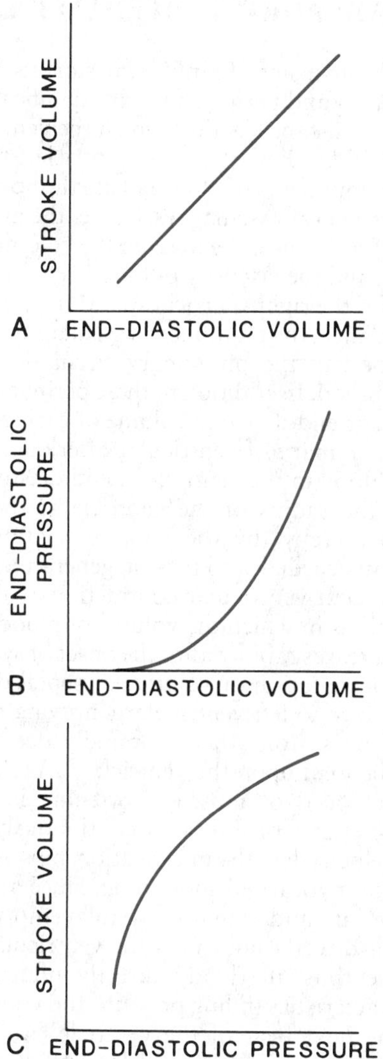

FIGURE 5-15 Illustration of the approximate interrelationships among stroke work, ventricular end-diastolic volume, and end-diastolic pressure. *A.* The relationship between stroke volume and end-diastolic volume is nearly linear. *B.* The relationship between end-diastolic pressure and end-diastolic volume is curvilinear, with a definite volume at zero pressure and a rather sharp increase in pressure above a certain volume. *C.* The familiar curvilinear relationship between stroke volume and ventricular end-diastolic pressure, similar to that shown in Fig. 5-12.

ologically. At sarcomere lengths less than 2.2 μm, the actin myofilaments first pass into the center of the sarcomere, and at 2.0 μm they bypass one another and developed tension decreases. The reason for the fall in force with shortening sarcomere length in this physiologic portion of the curve is not clear. Among the possible explanations are interference of the thin filaments, restoring forces, and/or a decrease in Ca^{2+} sensitivity of the sarcomere at short lengths.[69,158] As the papillary muscle in Fig. 5-16 is increasingly stretched, the resting tension increases, at first slowly and then more markedly. The *stiffness* of myocardial muscle can be defined as the slope of the curve relating the change in resting tension to the change in length. Relative to skeletal muscle, cardiac muscle is very stiff, with resting tension rising exponentially. If there is no resting tension, diastolic sarcomere length is about 1.95 μm. As sarcomeres reach 2.2 μm, resting tension is very great. Compressive forces occur in systole at shorter lengths, and this creates elastic recoil on relaxation.

A sarcomere length (after fixation) of 2.2 μm, which produces peak active tension (L_{max}), occurs in normal dogs at about the upper limit of normal left ventricular filling pressure (10 to 12 mmHg). At normal filling pressures, the sarcomere length in the midwall of the left ventricle varies from about 2.07 μm at end diastole to 1.8 μm at end systole.[150,151] Theoretically, the normal ventricle may have an ejection fraction of 55 percent with a shortening of individual sarcomere length of only 13 percent.[106,107] Endocardial sarcomeres must, of course, shorten more than epicardial sarcomeres. Theoretically, 50 percent of the normal stroke volume can be accounted for by the pistonlike effect produced by about 25 to 35 percent ventricular wall thickening[159]; thus, the ejection of blood from the ventricles results from the generation of intraventricular pressure that is produced by both shortening and thickening of individual myocardial sarcomeres.

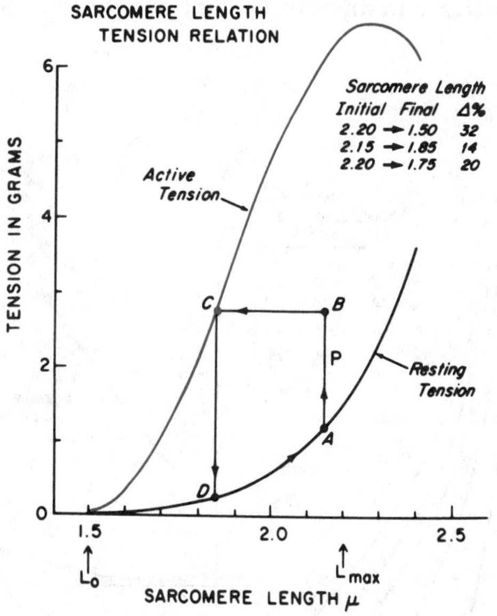

FIGURE 5-16 Relationship among papillary sarcomere length, resting tension, and developed or active tension. Note that active tension increases up to a sarcomere length of 2.2 μm (L_{max}) and then decreases. The resting tension increases markedly above a sarcomere length of 2.0 to 2.2 μm, which corresponds to an end-diastolic pressure of about 10 to 12 mmHg. The course of a normal contraction is shown in *ABCD.* Contraction starts at point *A* and develops a force equal to an imposed load *P,* reaching point *B.* The fiber then shortens until the active tension curve is reached at *C,* when relaxation occurs and returns the course to *D* at the end of systole. Normally, the ventricle functions on the ascending limb of the active tension curve at length below L_{max}, where greatest active tension develops, with sarcomere lengths between 1.8 and 2.2 μm. The descending limb of the length-active tension curve occurs at sarcomere lengths greater than L_{max}. There is normally moderate heterogeneity of sarcomere lengths in the heart, sarcomeres in the subendocardial layers tending to be longer and to shorten more than sarcomeres from the midwall or epicardium. In patients with marked ventricular dilatation, most of the dilatation is due to rearrangement and plastic "slippage" of the muscle fibers and myofibrils together with an increase in length of fibers due to synthesis of sarcomeres in series rather than to stretching of individual sarcomeres. (*From EH Sonnenblick, HM Spotnitz, D Spiro: Role of the sarcomere in ventricular function and the mechanism of heart failure. Circ Res 15(suppl 2):70, 1964. Reproduced with permission from the American Heart Association and the author.*)

Influences of Fiber Length and Heart Rate on Force-Velocity Relationships

The influence of increased initial fiber length on the force-velocity relationships of a papillary muscle is shown in Fig. 5-17. With increasing fiber length there is an increase in the maximal actively developed isometric force (P_0). In contrast, there is little or no change in the maximal velocity of shortening (V_{max}).[160] The increase in intrinsic force P_0 with unchanged V_{max} produced by increased initial muscle length appears related to an increased sarcomere sensitivity to intracellular Ca^{2+}.[66–68] The change in contractility associated with an increase in heart rate occurring in both atrial and ventricular muscle is shown by the *force-frequency relationship;* it is also termed the *Bowditch effect*, or *treppe*.[57–59,74,76,79,161,162] In many conditions associated with an increase in heart rate there is associated increased sympathetic stimulation of the myocardium, which activates adenylate cyclase, resulting in increased production of adenosine 3′,5′-monophosphate (cyclic AMP, or second messenger), which causes an increased influx of Ca^{2+} through slow calcium channels and an increase in myocardial contractility.

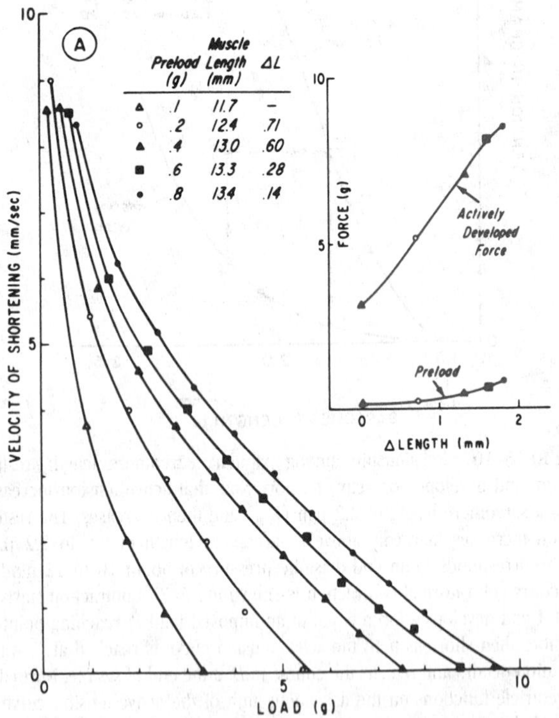

FIGURE 5-17 The effects of increasing initial muscle length on the force-velocity relationship. The initial velocity of shortening is plotted against preload, increases in which increase the initial length. In the insert, the maximal force developed is plotted against the change in muscle length. It is apparent that an increased muscle length produces little or no increase in V_{max}, the velocity of shortening at zero load obtained by extrapolation, but increases the actively developed maximal force P_0, which is produced under isometric conditions when the load is increased so much that no shortening can occur. (*From EH Sonnenblick: Series elastic and contractile elements in heart muscle: Changes in muscle length. Am J Physiol 207:1330, 1964. Reproduced with permission from the American Physiological Society and the author.*)

AFTERLOAD: AORTIC IMPEDANCE

It has been known since Frank's experiments[98] that ventricular ejection and performance are significantly influenced by the resistance against which the ventricles contract.[104,107,146,163–170] For the left ventricle, the major peripheral components of afterload are the aortic impedance, the peripheral vascular resistance, the arterial wall (or stiffness) resistance, the mass of the column of blood in the aorta, and the viscosity of blood. The corresponding factors for the right ventricle are the main pulmonary artery impedance, the pulmonary vascular resistance, the mass of blood in the pulmonary circulation, and the viscosity of blood. In addition to these peripheral factors, the preload, or end-diastolic volume of each ventricle, is a major determinant of ventricular afterload. Thus, the amount of blood in the ventricle at end diastole directly determines the radius of the ventricle at the onset of systole and thereby (by the Laplace relationship) the amount of myocardial wall tension generated during the onset of the next ventricular contraction.

In conditions in which the volume of blood in the left ventricle decreases rapidly after the onset of systole (such as mitral regurgitation or ventricular septal defect), the total impedance to left ventricular emptying rapidly decreases during systole, thereby rapidly decreasing significantly the load upon the ventricle.[168] As the load decreases, the speed of muscle shortening increases. In general, the effects of afterload continuously influence the force-velocity-length-time relationships throughout the course of myocardial shortening. Since afterload influences the rate and extent of systolic emptying of the ventricles, it directly influences the ventricular end-systolic volume; thus, afterload indirectly influences the diastolic characteristics (filling pressure and volume or preload) of the next beat of the ventricle. An additional influence of changes in afterload is manifested by an increase in ventricular performance several beats after aortic pressure is raised (the *Anrep effect* or homeometric autoregulation).[171] Some studies have indicated that this phenomenon may be due to recovery from transient subendocardial ischemia caused by the sudden change in arterial pressure.[172]

CONTRACTILITY AND THE INOTROPIC STATE

The third major mechanism by which myocardial function is altered is a change in the inotropic state (contractility) of the muscle independent of a change in preload (fiber length) or afterload.[2,16,68–91,173–179] The biochemical events that are responsible for increases in contractility, or inotropism, remain the subject of active investigation. Abbott and Mommaerts[180] and Sonnenblick and associates[2,57,69,71–81,160,178] have noted that an increase in the contractile state of a muscle is characterized by an increase in V_{max} with or without a change in P_0, the maximal force under isometric conditions at zero velocity. Acute alterations in contractility can also be evaluated by shifts in the linear relationship between end-systolic pressure and end-systolic volume of the ventricle. All of these changes reflect a change in the force-velocity-length relationships of the myocardium and thus the ventricle, as noted below. (See also Chap. 23.)[71,181–187]

An increase in heart rate increases the contractile state, as shown by an increase in the velocity of shortening at any level of tension and by changes in location of V_{max}, obtained by extrapolating to zero load, without a change in P_0. An increase in heart rate also increases the rate of relaxation, or negative dP/dt.[188] Strophanthidin and norepinephrine both produce a significant shift to the right in the force-velocity curves and an increase in both V_{max} and P_0 in association with a decrease in the time from stimulation to peak shortening.[75] Increased contractility can also be illustrated by ventricular function curves (Fig. 5-14); however, a "function curve" tends to be a less sensitive indicator of changes in the contractile state of isolated myocardium than a force-velocity curve. Thus, function curves, which relate end-diastolic pressure to stroke volume and stroke work, may show only small changes at a time when significant changes are apparent in the force-velocity curves.[79] The increased contractility produced by an increase in heart rate (the *force-frequency relationship* or the *Bowditch phenomenon*)[56–59,78,161,162,188] affects primarily the speed of contraction and is thus more readily shown by force-velocity curves than by ventricular function curves. On the other hand, the increased contractility produced by large amounts of norepinephrine or by large increases in heart rate may be apparent in both types of curves.

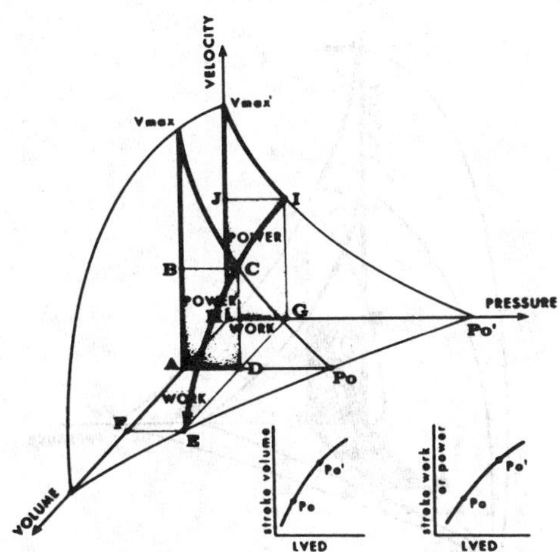

FIGURE 5-19 The effect of increasing preload (left ventricular end-diastolic pressure) on the force-velocity-volume relationship. Blood pressure remains the same. Maximum isometric force increases from P_0 to P'_0; work increases from *ADEF* to *HGEF*, while power increases from *ABCD* to *HGIJ*. This increase in the end-diastolic volume of the ventricle does not represent a change in the contractile state of the myocardium, since V_{max} is not changed. The insert in the lower right shows the predicted relations of stroke volume, stroke work, and stroke power to left ventricular end-diastolic pressure (LVED), reflecting changes in work and power areas from the three-dimensional diagram. [*From EH Sonnenblick: The mechanics of myocardial contraction. In: SA Briller, HL Conn Jr, eds: The Myocardial Cell: Structure, Function, and Modification by Cardiac Drugs. Philadelphia, University of Pennsylvania Press, 1966:173. Reproduced with permission from the publisher and author.*]

The complex interrelationships among *force, velocity,* and *length* of both isolated myocardium and intact ventricles can best be represented by a three-dimensional graph.[2,71,77,173,174] Figure 5-18 is a diagram of such a graph for a ventricle with the superimposed course of a single contraction; Fig. 5-19 illustrates the effect of increasing preload or initial muscle length; Fig. 5-20 illustrates the effects of an increased contractile state. This indicates that when contractility is augmented, the myocardium shortens faster at any given muscle length, for any given load and also shortens further or generates more force. It should be noted that myocardial contractility at any moment is best defined by the *surface* of the curved surface relating force, velocity, and length.[71]

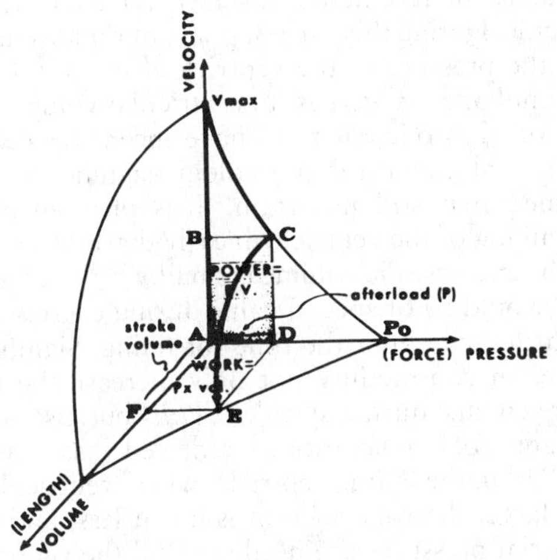

FIGURE 5-18 Force-velocity-length (force-velocity-volume) diagram of the intact ventricle. The force is the equivalent of load, which is the sum of preload (end-diastolic pressure) and afterload (aortic pressure). The length axis is derived from intraventricular volume. The superimposed dark line portrays the course of a single contraction. Starting at *A*, with activation, the CE velocity rises toward V_{max}. With CE shortening, force is built up and velocity of shortening decreases to *C*. This represents the isometric (isovolumic) phase of contraction. At *C*, the force equals the load, and shortening begins from *C* to *E*. During muscle shortening between *C* and *E*, velocity of shortening changes as a function of the decrease in muscle length that ensues. The shaded area on the force-velocity (vertical) plane represents calculated power (*ABCD*); the shaded area on the base represents work for a load *P* (*ADEF*). [*From EH Sonnenblick: The mechanics of myocardial contraction. In: SA Briller, HL Conn Jr, eds: The Myocardial Cell: Structure, Function, and Modification by Cardiac Drugs. Philadelphia, University of Pennsylvania Press, 1966: 173. Reproduced with permission from the publisher and author.*]

When sympathetic stimulation causes the heart to beat with increased contractility and at a faster rate, not only is the contraction more forceful and faster, but the relaxation and elastic recoil of the ventricular musculature ("diastolic suction") are also more rapid.[188–194] Both the more forceful contraction and the more vigorous relaxation tend to increase the stroke volume of the next beat, since the diastolic filling period is longer than it would otherwise be and since, with the more rapid elastic recoil, the ventricular pressure is lower earlier and more rapidly, and possibly absolutely. The increased emptying produced by increased contractility also means that the fiber length will be less at the beginning of the next diastole. This shorter length tends to increase the distensibility of the ventricle, augment rapid early filling, and allow greater filling at a lower filling pressure.

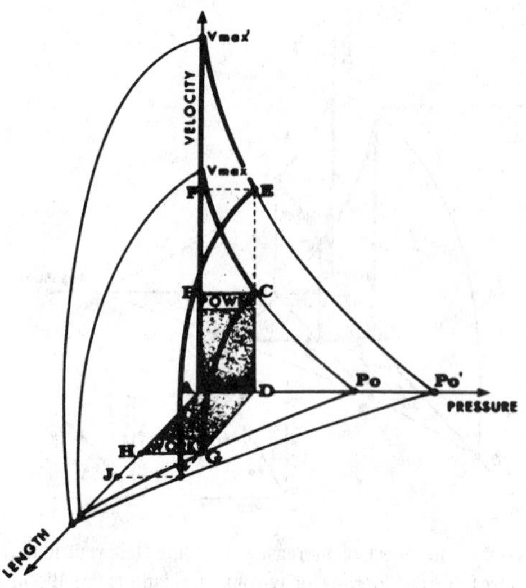

FIGURE 5-20 The effect of increasing the contractile state on the force-velocity-volume relation of the ventricle. Both V_{max} and P_0 are augmented, while the load (pressure) has been kept constant. Work and power are augmented. [*From EH Sonnenblick: The mechanics of myocardial contraction. In: SA Briller, HL Conn Jr, eds: The Myocardial Cell: Structure, Function, and Modification by Cardiac Drugs. Philadelphia, University of Pennsylvania Press, 1966:173. Reproduced with permission from the publisher and author.*]

HEART RATE

The fourth major determinant of cardiac function is the heart rate, or the frequency of cardiac contraction. This is probably the major mechanism by which most individuals increase their cardiac output during periods of modest increased demand or exercise. An increase in heart rate may also increase myocardial contractility and relaxation and improve diastolic performance; the systolic force-interval relationship is known as *treppe,* the *staircase phenomenon,* or the *Bowditch effect.*[56–59,78,79,161,162,188] This effect is much more apparent in an anesthetized animal or depressed heart than in the intact, conscious state.[2,161,195] Even in the intact individual, however, the duration of each systole decreases as the heart rate increases, within limits. The rate of relaxation also increases with an increase in heart rate. Nevertheless, since there are more systoles per minute, the total time per minute spent in systole increases. Presumably, the increase in heart rate results in the release of more Ca^{2+} from the stores within the myocardial cell, thus enhancing myofibrillar contraction. The "recuperative effect of a long pause" upon the strength of contraction is known as the *Woodworth phenomenon,* or as negative, or reverse, staircase phenomenon.[196,197]

OTHER FACTORS INFLUENCING VENTRICULAR FUNCTION AND CONTRACTILITY

Sequence of Ventricular Contraction

An additional concept of importance in the application of the law of the heart to the ventricle as a whole concerns the sequence of ventricular activation and contraction. Since the ventricular myocardial fibers contract sequentially, the strength of contraction of the later-contracting myocardial fibers theoretically is influenced by the strength, the rate, and the sequence of contraction of the fibers that contract earlier and that stretch the later-contracting fibers.[198–200] Since one aspect of increased contractility is a faster rate of contraction, an increased contractility of the initially contracting fibers may increase the end-diastolic fiber length of the myocardial fibers that have not yet begun to contract and thereby directly increase the force of contraction of those fibers that contract later. This phenomenon has been referred to as *idioventricular kick,*[201] in analogy with the increased ventricular filling and performance, the *atrial kick,* produced by atrial systole. An abnormal sequence of ventricular contraction or *dyssynergy* is also mechanically less efficient and relatively wasteful of energy, particularly if there are areas of akinesis or dyskinesis (see Chap. 57).

Ventricular Suction

Ventricular filling is enhanced by any increases in the pressure difference between the atrium and ventricle, whether produced by increased atrial pressure or by lower ventricular diastolic pressure. The latter phenomenon, which can be produced by increased elastic recoil and ventricular relaxation, is referred to as *diastolic suction.* One form is present normally during early diastole, immediately following opening of the atrioventricular (AV) valve, and its extent is inversely related to ventricular volume. During this earliest phase of rapid ventricular filling, the pressure in the ventricle *decreases* despite a rapid simultaneous *increase* in ventricular volume. Other forms of diastolic suction have been reviewed by Brecher,[202] although the physiologic significance of the phenomenon is still uncertain. This phenomenon enhances filling of the ventricle in early diastole, especially when the end-systolic volume is small.[193,203] Such a mechanisms would be of special value during exercise, when tachycardia may limit the time for filling. Significantly, increases in contractility not only increase the rate of pressure change during systole (dP/dt) but also increase the rate of relaxation, reflected as negative dP/dt.[188,194] In the failing ventricle, where ventricular volume is large, diastolic suction is much less, and higher mean atrial pressures are needed to fill the ventricle.

Atrial Function

The atria have two main functions: a transport, or pump, function and a reservoir function to contain blood available for rapid ventricular filling.[204–209] Like the ventricles, the atria respond to an increase in fiber length by an increased force of contraction. Increased atrial contractility characterized by a shift to the left of atrial function curves (or a shift to the right of their force-velocity curves) may be produced by increased sympathetic stimulation, by inotropic agents such as digitalis or catecholamines, or by decreased vagal stimulation. Each of these causes the atrium to pump a greater amount of blood forward into the ventricle, with a resultant increase in ventricular end-diastolic fiber length and pressure (the *atrial kick*), thereby causing the ventricle to increase its force of contraction. When the atrial transport function is lost (e.g., by atrial fibrillation) in a person with an otherwise normal heart, the normal circulatory reserve mechanisms are able to maintain the cardiac output at rest within normal limits, although the response of the cardiac output to strenuous exercise is usually diminished. In a patient with ventricular disease, however, where compliance of the ventricle may be reduced, producing diastolic dysfunction, the mean diastolic pressure may be elevated, producing pulmonary congestion, and even the resting cardiac output may be diminished significantly by this form of *atrial failure* (see Chap. 25).

The atria also produce atrial natriuretic peptides (ANPs) that have natriuretic and diuretic actions and relax intestinal smooth muscle.[210-219] Some ANPs also relax vascular muscle. It is probable that atrial distension triggers the release of ANP, leading to diuresis and natriuresis. ANPs also inhibit the production of aldosterone.[221] The importance of ANPs (or *atrial natriuretic factor*) in normal homeostasis, congestive heart failure, or essential hypertension remains under active investigation.

Nervous Control[13,54,222-228]

The nerve endings of sympathetic fibers, which lie between the myocardial fibers, synthesize norepinephrine and store it in granules. Both atria and ventricles contain β_1 and β_2 receptors, with the atria usually having somewhat more. Other studies have indicated that β_2 receptors are located especially in vascular smooth muscle or in the sinoatrial (SA) and AV nodes.[229] On stimulation, sympathetic fibers cause the local release of norepinephrine, which acts locally on beta receptors, which are present on the fiber surface, to enhance the activity of adenylate cyclase, which in turn catalyzes the conversion of ATP to cyclic AMP.[230] Cyclic AMP activates protein kinases that phosphorylate the slow calcium channel, increasing myocellular Ca^{2+} entry and myocardial contractility (inotropic effect)[54,55] (Fig. 5-5). At the same time, protein kinases phosphorylate a protein, *phospholamban,* which causes the sarcoplasmic reticulum to take up Ca^{2+} more rapidly, enhancing relaxation (lusitropic effect). Once nerve stimulation stops, the same nerve endings take up and store norepinephrine for reutilization. A small amount of the norepinephrine is also metabolized locally. Sympathetic nerve fibers reach the entire atria and ventricles, as well as the sinus or SA and AV nodes, while vagal fibers, which cause the local release of acetylcholine, influence predominantly the atrial musculature and SA and AV nodes. Some vagal innervation, however, has also been shown to reach the ventricles, and vagal stimulation can decrease ventricular contractility modestly.[231] Further, vagal stimulation reduces the extent of the inotropic response produced by the sympathetic stimulation.[231] In general, sympathetic stimulation increases atrial and ventricular contractility, increases heart rate, and speeds the spread of excitation through the AV node and, very slightly, through the ventricles. There is also evidence that the coronary vessels and heart muscle may produce neuropeptides that can influence coronary vascular resistance and myocardial contractility.[232,233]

Vagal stimulation generally exerts effects opposite to those of sympathetic stimulation on the sinus node of the atria. At any given instant, the effect of the nervous system on the heart is the net balance of these two opposing controls, which usually vary reciprocally. It is probable that the vagal parasympathetic stimulation, which is generally inhibitory, normally predominates in the conscious state and maintains the usual resting heart rate of about 65 to 75 beats per minute. The resting bradycardia of exercise training is due predominantly to a slowing of the intrinsic rate of the sinus node pacemaker due to enhanced vagal activity in association with a decrease in the adrenergic influence.[234] Neural reflexes, particularly from stretch receptors in the carotid sinus and aorta, form a major extrinsic control mechanism that influences myocardial performance directly and indirectly.[223-226] When carotid sinus stretch decreases, as with arterial hypotension, a reflex venoconstriction is produced by the sympathetic nervous system that increases venous return and thereby increases ventricular end-diastolic fiber length. Simultaneously, carotid sinus hypotension produces reflex arterial vasoconstriction, increasing peripheral vascular resistance and aortic impedance. In addition, carotid sinus hypotension elicits reflexes that increase atrial and ventricular contractility. Stimulation of the carotid sinus nerve, such as might occur with carotid sinus hypertension, produces opposite effects.

Cardiac Renin-Angiotensin System

There is good evidence of a cardiac renin-angiotensin system that produces active peptides with physiologic effects.[235-239]

Drugs and Hormones

Myocardial contractility is increased by increased activation of the myocardium that is mediated in one form or another by an enhanced availability of Ca^{2+} ions inside the cell.[11,24-28] Increased Ca^{2+} bathing the heart produces this action. Some of the major mechanisms that regulate myocardial cellular Ca^{2+} homeostasis are illustrated in Figs. 5-5 and 5-6. Catecholamines, including norepinephrine, epinephrine, and isoproterenol, act on β-adrenergic receptors on the myocardial cells, which activate a G protein as the signal transducer to activate adenylate cyclase, increasing the production of cyclic AMP, which in turn activates sarcolemmal protein kinases that phosphorylate the slow calcium channel, resulting in increased intracellular Ca^{2+}.[240] Protein kinases also phosphorylate phospholamban, which causes the sarcoplasmic reticulum to take up Ca^{2+} more rapidly, enhancing relaxation. These actions result in increased myocardial contractility and more rapid relaxation (see Fig. 25-11). Digitalis glycosides enhance contractility by inhibiting the Na^+K^+-ATPase in the cell surface membrane, thereby leaving larger amounts of Na^+ within the cell, decreasing the Na^+-Ca^{2+} exchange and resulting in an increased concentration of Ca^{2+} within the fiber (Figs.

5-5 and 5-6).[49,50] (See also Chaps. 25 and 27.) Contractility is also increased to some degree by corticosteroids, aldactone, angiotensin II, serotonin,[241] and glucagon.[242]

The physiologic role of other substances such as prostaglandins,[243] secretin,[244] neurotensin, endogenous opiates, enkephalins, and nucleotide and polypeptide systems such as kinekard, vasoactive intestinal polypeptide (VIP), and neuropeptide Y[232,245–247] in the regulation of myocardial contractility is unclear. Vascular endothelial cells release substances that may affect myocardial contractility, such as *endothelin,* which is also a potent vasoconstrictor.[248–258] Endocardial cells also appear to affect contractility.[259–263] The importance of these factors to myocardial contractility is unknown (see below). The actions of thyroxine on myocardial contractile functions are complex, but in general its effects are to increase rates of contraction and relaxation (see Chap. 102).

Myocardial contractility is decreased by hypoxia, ischemia, and by many drugs, including barbiturates, quinidine, procainamide, disopyramide, lidocaine, most beta blockers (Chap. 66), and calcium antagonists (Chap. 67). Acidosis also depresses myocardial contractility, particularly if the sympathoadrenal system function is impaired.[264] Morphine produces a very mild negative inotropic effect upon isolated myocardial strips, but in the conscious dog it can produce a beta-adrenergic-mediated increase in myocardial contractility and alpha-adrenergic-mediated coronary vasoconstriction.[265]

A number of neuropeptides have been shown to have significant effects on myocardial contractility and coronary vascular resistance.[232,245–247] Some of these occur in significant amounts in the heart and may play important roles in the normal regulation of myocardial contractility and coronary blood flow.

Anesthesia

General anesthesia from halothane or pentobarbital may depress myocardial contractility significantly. In addition, the reflex control mechanisms influencing heart rate may be significantly altered by anesthesia. For example, in the conscious state, the reflex bradycardia of acute hypertension is caused mainly by withdrawal of sympathetic stimulation, while under anesthesia, it is caused almost entirely by parasympathetic restraint.[195] In the intact conscious animal, the force-frequency relationship, or the Bowditch phenomenon, appears to influence myocardial contractility relatively little, whereas an increase in heart rate causes a much larger increase in contractility if the level of contractility is first depressed by generalized anesthesia.[195] Similarly, in anesthetized animals, the increase in heart rate produced by acute volume loading and presumed stimulation of low-pressure receptors in the atria (the *Bainbridge reflex*) is erratic; on the other hand, the reflex is consistently found in conscious animals and can be blocked by the combination of atropine and propranolol.[266] In contrast, the Anrep effect, or the positive inotropic effect of an acute increase in afterload, has been demonstrated in the anesthetized animal but is difficult to demonstrate in the conscious subject with a low spontaneous heart rate.[195]

Postextrasystolic Potentiation

When an extraventricular depolarization is imposed or occurs spontaneously between normal beats, the subsequent normal beat is potentiated. The extent of *postextrasystolic potentiation* is generally related to the closeness of the extra beat to the previous normal beat. The mechanism of this type of postextrasystolic potentiation is probably related to increased availability of calcium ions near the contractile sites of the actin and myosin myofilaments. Advantage has even been taken clinically of this phenomenon by placing an electrically induced extra beat close to the spontaneous beat and continuing it.[267–269] The clinical use of "paired electrical stimulation," which markedly increases myocardial contractility is limited by the danger of inducing ventricular fibrillation.

MECHANISMS OF CARDIAC RESERVE

Normal homeostatic mechanisms regulate cardiac output to meet the demands of the body, which can increase its cardiac output five- to sixfold during exercise. It is not possible to separate sharply those mechanisms by which the cardiovascular system is normally controlled and those mechanisms of *cardiac reserve* (Table 5-1) that the heart may utilize to meet increased demands on the normal heart and/or to maintain cardiac function in the presence of disease of the heart or circulatory system. Many of these homeostatic and regulatory mechanisms act synergistically in the intact organism; others, such as the sympathetic and parasympathetic nervous control of the heart, are in a state of constantly varying balance. Although the relative contributions of each mechanism in the experimental animal can be separated and quantified, in humans this is generally not possible. Indeed, the demonstration of mechanisms during physiologic experiments indicates only *potential* mechanisms of reserve or control, not what actually happens in the intact organism. Furthermore, since most of the mechanisms are interrelated and affect one another, the contribution of one mechanism depends on, and changes with, the contribution of the other mechanisms. In the following discussion, we shall consider some of these mechanisms from the standpoint of their use as forms of *cardiac reserve,* although many of the same mechanisms are utilized in the *normal circulatory regulation* (see also Chaps. 23 and 25).

The two basic mechanisms of cardiac reserve by which

TABLE 5-1

Mechanisms of Cardiac Reserve
Increased heart rate
Increased stroke volume
Increased oxygen extraction
Redistribution of blood flow
Anaerobic metabolism
Cardiac dilatation
Cardiac hypertrophy

the heart or any other pulsatile pump can increase its output in the face of increased demand (or attempt to maintain output in the presence of myocardial disease) are (1) change in rate and (2) change in stroke volume.

Heart Rate

A change in pulse rate is one of the simplest and most effective ways of increasing cardiac output in response to an increase in venous return. In individuals who are not trained athletes, under conditions of moderately increased demands, an increase in cardiac output occurs primarily by an increase in heart rate mediated by decreased parasympathetic (vagal) tone. An increase in heart rate by itself may mediate an increase in cardiac output about four- to fivefold in highly trained athletes. Above certain limits, however, cardiac output may actually begin to fall as heart rate rises. This rate is about 170 to 180 beats per minute for most normal young individuals but may be 200 to 220 in trained athletes or only 120 to 140 in older, untrained persons or in patients with heart disease. The decrease in cardiac output above a certain rate is due largely to the shortening of the time of diastole per minute, limiting both the time for adequate filling of the ventricles and for coronary blood flow, which occurs primarily during diastole in the left ventricle.

Although an increase in heart rate may produce a modest increase in myocardial contractility and a shortening in the absolute duration of each systole,[56–59,76–78,161,162,186] negative inotropic effects of tachycardia can become apparent above a certain rate.[59] The shape of the curve relating heart rate to contractility varies according to species and the conditions under which it is studied. Most changes in pulse rate with normal activities are effected by decrease in vagal inhibition and during more vigorous stress by the addition of sympathetic stimulation of the sinus node of the heart.[222–226]

Stroke Volume

In a normal individual in the recumbent position, the relation of left ventricular stroke volume (SV) to end-diastolic volume (EDV), termed the *ejection fraction,* is about 60 to 75 percent and tends to be linear. Since the curve relating EDV to filling pressure is curvilinear, when end-diastolic pressure is substituted for EDV, the curve relating SV to filling pressure is curved and, due to the exponential rise in filling pressure relative to volume, tends to flatten at high filling pressures (Fig. 5-15).[71] Increased contractility may increase the ejection fraction and the SV with a decreased end-systolic volume (ESV), with the EDV either decreasing or remaining the same. An increased SV can also be produced either by a primary increase in venous return, which utilizes preload reserve and increases the end-diastolic fiber length of the atria and ventricles, or by a decrease in afterload, which permits enhanced emptying of the ventricle.[170] In the early stages of heart failure, since there is often an increase in EDV and fiber length, which tends to maintain the SV, the ejection fraction is decreased. Indeed, a decrease in ejection fraction is a hallmark of ventricular failure. Since SV is load-dependent, the ejection fraction may be increased when impedance of ventricular emptying is reduced (e.g., mitral regurgitation) or reduced when impedance is high (e.g., aortic stenosis). (See Chaps. 23 and 25.)

Increased Oxygen Extraction

When the tissue requirements for oxygen increase or the supply of blood decreases, the tissues may, up to a point, extract more oxygen from the volume of blood passing through the tissue. The entry of oxygen into myocardial cells is facilitated by myoglobin, which has oxygen dissociation characteristics favorable to the diffusion of oxygen into the cells.[270] Increased oxygen extraction is a major reserve mechanism utilized by the tissues of the body acutely during extreme exertion or chronically when the cardiac output is diminished. This reserve mechanism is of less value to the myocardium, which even normally extracts about 75 percent of its arterial oxygen content.

Redistribution of Blood Flow[13,17,18,238,252,254,257,271–274]

The redistribution of cardiac output is a major mechanism of reserve for the body under conditions of increased demand, as during exercise or under conditions of diminished cardiac output. The general result is to maintain blood flow to the brain, the heart, and the tissues acutely requiring blood flow while sacrificing blood flow to tissues and organs not being utilized or less essential to immediate survival. The mechanisms by which this redistribution occurs are complex. Although the following explanation is over-simplified, redistribution may be considered the integrated response of two mechanisms: (1) a local autoregulation of the metabolically active tissue or organ, by which local changes in P_{O_2}, P_{CO_2}, pH, potassium ion (K^+) concentration, and other metabolic products and mechanical shear stress affect the endothelium of local blood vessels, reducing small vessel resistance and increasing blood flow (see below); and (2) an integrated response of the central nervous system, mediated by the sympathetic and parasympathetic nervous systems, producing vasodilation of the active or exercising organ and vasoconstriction of many other tissues and organs. In addition, there often appears to be a venoconstriction mediated by the sympathetic nervous system, which increases venous return to the heart and performs a type of internal transfusion or shifting of blood from the large venous reservoirs to the heart, arterial system, and active organs.

Anaerobic Metabolism

Many tissues, particularly skeletal muscle utilize anaerobic metabolism as a reserve mechanism, although the value of this mechanism for the myocardium is also quite limited. In a normal individual during moderate exercise, anaerobic metabolism may account for about 5 percent of the energy utilized; patients with heart failure may obtain 30 percent of their immediate total energy requirements by anaerobic metabolism during exercise.

Dilatation and Hypertrophy

Dilatation and hypertrophy are forms of compensatory reserve, although they are also swords of Damocles for the heart. Their effects in heart failure are discussed in Chaps. 23 and 25, and their significance in athletes is discussed in Chap. 114.

REGULATION OF REGIONAL BLOOD FLOW

The amount of blood flowing to an individual organ of the body is determined by the difference between the arterial and venous pressures in the vessels supplying the organ and by the vascular resistance of the organ. Although the arterial and venous pressures change in situations such as exercise, eating, or emotional stress, most of the alterations in the distribution of blood flow are the consequence of changes in vascular resistance of the organ.[5,13,17,18,238,252,254,257,271–280]

The major mechanisms by which decreases in organ vascular resistance are effected are an increase in caliber of the vessels and an opening of new vascular channels. Since most of the vascular resistance appears to be located at the level of the small arteries and arterioles, it is probable that most of the regulation occurs by changes in caliber of these vessels, although changes in the capillaries and veins may at times play an important role.

In a consideration of the local control of blood flow, several fundamental relationships and definitions should first be introduced.

The *resistance* to blood flow through a given portion of the circulation is usually expressed by the ratio of the mean pressure difference between two points in the vascular system to the mean amount of blood passing from one point to the other. It is usually calculated using mean pressures and flows, although most vascular flow is pulsatile. If it were possible to measure accurately instantaneous pressure differences and flows, it would be theoretically more proper to calculate vascular *impedance,* which is the ratio of pulsatile pressure to pulsatile flow and which varies with the frequency of the pulse. Vascular resistance may be expressed in various units: by *peripheral resistance units* (PRU), or pressure gradient (mmHg) per unit blood flow (mL/s); by Aperia's formula, to give results in absolute or metric (cgs, or centimeter-gram-second) units by multiplying PRU units by a conversion factor of 1332 to express resistance in terms of dynes · second per centimeter^5; or by the ratio of pressure gradient (mmHg) to blood flow (liters/min) to give *R units.* R units may be converted approximately to dynes · second per centimeter^5 by multiplying by 80.

Minor changes in calculated resistance are usually of no significance, not only because of possible errors in pressure or flow measurements, but also because changes in apparent resistance may result from the distending effect of inflow or exit pressures. Since resistance is the slope of the relationship of pressure to flow and this relationship is curvilinear, resistance can change merely by changing either pressure or blood flow. Moreover, if both are changing, the change in resistance is difficult or impossible to evaluate. In addition, alterations in the distending force may mask changes in the vascular bed. Because of such considerations and the nonlinear relationship between pressure and flow of most vascular beds, changes in calculated resistance cannot be equated simply with vasoconstriction or vasodilatation. This is particularly true if there are changes in both pressure and flow.

The relationship of the various factors affecting the resistance to fluid flow in rigid tubing is expressed by *Poiseuille's equation:*

$$\text{Fluid flow} = \frac{\pi(\text{pressure difference})(\text{radius})^4}{8(\text{vessel length})(\text{fluid viscosity})}$$

Since the experiments from which the equation was derived were performed in straight, rigid tubes with steady, streamlined flow of an ideal, viscous fluid, the relationship cannot be directly applied to the vascular system, in which the vessels are neither straight nor rigid, the blood is not a simple viscous fluid, and the flow is not always streamlined. Nevertheless, the predominant influence on flow is the radius of the vessel, which is raised to the *fourth* power in the above equation, is apparent. Of the other factors, changes in vessel length are thought to be ordinarily relatively unimportant; however, changes in viscosity related to changes in hematocrit, temperature, and serum protein levels are often of marked significance, particularly in small blood vessels. It should also be noted that in most vascular beds, most of the blood vessels are connected in parallel rather than in series. The total resistance of vessels connected in parallel is calculated by adding the *conductance* of each individual vessel ($1/R$, the reciprocal of the individual resistance) to obtain the total conductance of all the vessels (Fig. 5-21). Because of these relationships for vessels in parallel and in accordance with Poiseuille's laws, the resistance of four small tubes in parallel is four times as great as that of a single large tube of equal total cross-sectional area. Actually, it requires 16 small tubes with four times the total cross-sectional area to have a resistance as low as a single wide tube or vessel.

Since all normal blood vessels are distensible at least to some extent, it follows that increasing the *intraluminal*

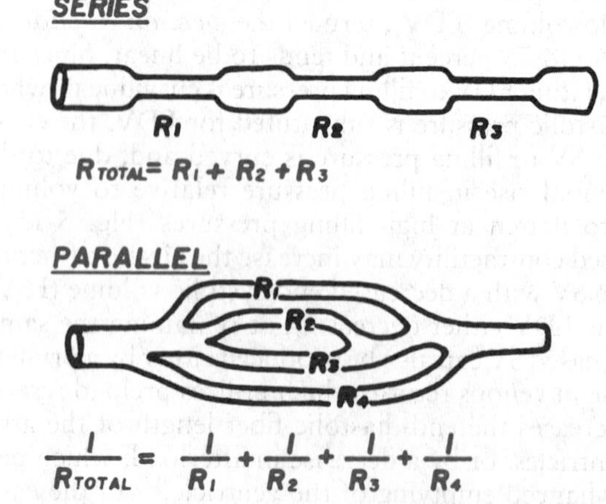

FIGURE 5-21. Comparison of the calculation of vascular resistance of vessels in series and in parallel. In most vascular beds, most of the blood vessels of the same size are connected in parallel.

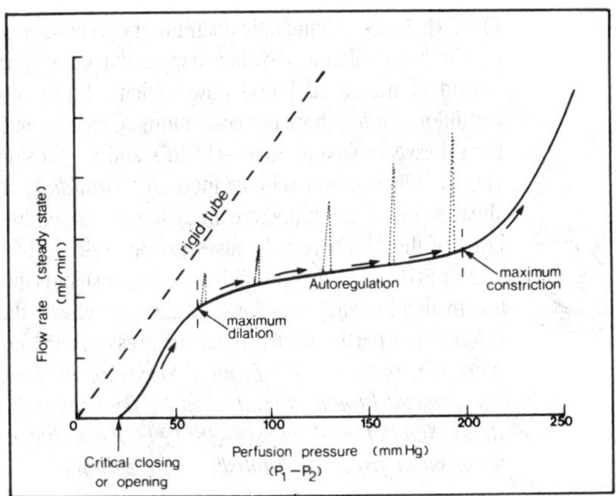

FIGURE 5-22 Effect of perfusion pressure on flow rate in a rigid tube perfused with a Newtonian fluid (---) and in a vascular bed (muscle) perfused with blood (—). Note the autoregulation of steady-state blood flow within certain limits of perfusion pressure in the circulation through muscle. The dotted lines represent the immediate increase in blood flow, which declines to the steady level when vascular smooth muscle reacts to stretch and washout of vasodilator metabolites. (*Figure modified by Dr. Badeer from HS Badeer: Cardiovascular Physiology: A Synopsis. Basel, Karger, 1984, 146. Reproduced with permission from the publisher and author.*)

pressure will increase the *transmural pressure* on the vessel wall and increase the diameter and radius of the vessel. This effect is seen in Fig. 5-22, which illustrates the pressure-flow curve of an isolated peripheral vascular bed. Flow is maintained relatively equally by autoregulation within a wide range of perfusion pressure. The pressure at about 20 mmHg, at which flow ceases entirely, has been sometimes referred to as the *critical closure pressure;* however, it is perhaps better referred to as the *critical flow pressure,* since it is unlikely that there is often complete anatomic closure of the vessels.

The amount of distension present in an individual blood vessel is dependent on the stiffness, or *tone,* of the vessel and on the *distending,* or *transmural, pressure,* that is, the difference between the intraluminal pressure, which tends to expand the vessel, and the external pressure, which tends to compress the vessel. The tone, or stiffness, of a blood vessel is determined by the geometry of the vessel and by the mechanical properties of the vessel wall. *Myogenic tone* refers to the contraction of vascular smooth muscle in response to stretch.[18,281–284] Such tone, which may be either maintained or rhythmic, is important in the local autoregulation of blood flow.

Important relationships between the distending pressure and the tension in the wall of a blood vessel are expressed in the following form of the *law of Laplace:*

$$\text{Wall tension} = \text{distending pressure} \times \frac{\text{vessel radius}}{2 \times \text{wall thickness}}$$

From this equation it is apparent that the tension in the wall of a blood vessel tending to expand it is greater either if the radius of the vessel is greater or if the blood vessel wall is thinner. Thus, veins with greater radii and thinner walls than their arterial counterparts have a greater wall tension than their arterial counterparts *at the same pressure.* As noted previously, the same considerations hold for the heart. The degree of stretching of the vessel wall produced by wall tension depends on the elastic stiffness of the vessel wall. The term *distensibility* is usually defined by the pressure-volume characteristics of a given vessel and is dependent on the above-mentioned factors, among others.

The regulation of vascular stiffness achieved by alterations in the physicochemical-mechanical properties of vascular smooth muscle is referred to as *vasomotion.* The major factors by which changes in vasomotion and changes in vessel caliber are accomplished are (1) metabolic, chemical, and hormonal substances carried in the blood and/or locally produced; (2) pressure (wall stretch);[283] (3) flow (shear stress);[285,286] and (4) the activity of fibers from the autonomic nervous system innervating the blood vessels and locally releasing norepinephrine or acetylcholine. The relative importance of these mechanisms varies markedly from one vascular bed to another and in different sizes of vessels in the same bed.[286] The relative importance is also significantly different at rest and during activity of the organ.

Most systemic arteries, and probably veins, respond to hypoxia and/or an increase in P_{CO_2} with vasodilatation.[268–271] The vasodilatation produced by hypoxia in many vascular beds is significantly augmented by an increase in K^+ concentration. Many substances are important in the local control of vasomotion, including endothelium-derived relaxing factor (EDRF), which is thought to be nitric oxide[280,287]; *endothelin,* a very potent vasoconstricting substance released by the endothelium[248–258,288]; prostaglandins[273,289]; lactic acid; histamine; neuropeptides and other vasoactive peptides; and unknown "metabolic products." The cerebral vessels are particularly sensitive to P_{CO_2} whereas the coronary vessels respond strikingly to changes in P_{O_2},[271,279,290–294] although qualitatively similar changes are found in most other systemic vessels. It is probable that the myocardial vasodilatation produced by hypoxia is ordinarily mediated by the metabolite adenosine rather than by a direct effect of lowered P_{O_2}, unless the hypoxia is extreme.[6,17,18,238,253,280,284] Local prostaglandins and neuropeptides released in the heart may also be important (see below).[232,244,289,290] In most organs, the effects of P_{O_2}, P_{CO_2}, K^+, prostaglandins, and metabolic products work synergistically with the autonomic nervous system to regulate regional blood flow.[283] In contrast to systemic vessels, the pulmonary vessels seem to respond in the opposite manner to changes in P_{CO_2}, pH, and P_{O_2}. Thus, alveolar hypoxia results in regional vasoconstriction of the pulmonary arterioles, which tends to decrease perfusion of poorly ventilated areas and to help maintain normal O_2 saturation of arterial blood. In addition to their regional effects, P_{O_2} and P_{CO_2} in the mixed venous blood returned to the heart appear to be involved in the control of the total output of the heart through poorly understood mechanisms.

Endothelial Control of Blood Vessels

The endothelium plays a very active role in the modulation arteriolar and arterial tone.[233,238,250–258,287,294–298] EDRF, one form of which is nitric oxide (NO) produced from L-arginine, stimulates guanylate cyclase to produce cyclic guanosine monophosphate (cyclic GMP), which produces relaxation of vascular smooth muscle by de-

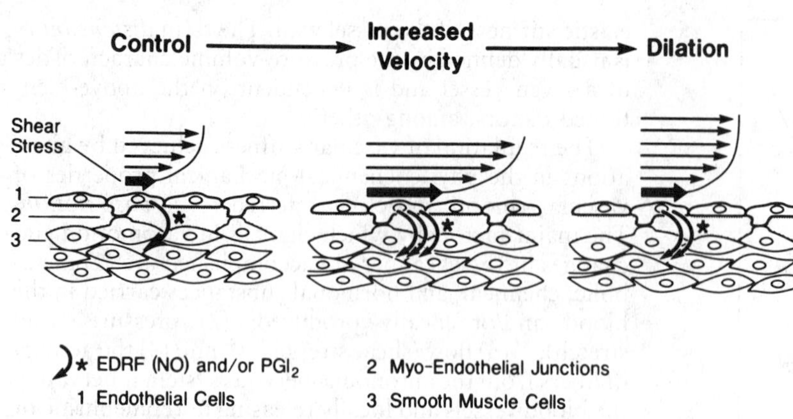

FIGURE 5-23 Schematic diagram of current concept of flow-induced dilation showing changes that occur during a period of increased blood flow velocity. Under control conditions (*left*), there is a continuous release of endothelium-derived relaxing factor (EDRF) and/or prostacyclin (PGI_2). When blood velocity increases (*middle*), rise in shear stress of the bloodstream acting on the endothelial layer of the blood vessel causes greater release of EDRF and/or PGI_2, as well as possibly vasodilator signals through the myoendothelial junctions, leading to vessel dilation (*right*) and partial return of shear stress toward control state. NO, nitric oxide. (*From V Smiesko, PC Johnson: The arterial lumen is controlled by flow-related shear stress. News Physiol Sci 8:34–38, 1993. Reproduced with permission from the publisher and authors.*)

creasing cytosolic free Ca^{2+}.[287] EDRF is an important modulator of the local vascular response to vasoactive substances such as acetylcholine, ATP, adenosine diphosphate (ADP), adenosine monophosphate AMP, substance P, histamine, serotonin, and bradykinin. In most vascular beds, the release of EDRF is stimulated by an increase in shear stress associated with an increase in the velocity of flow and thereby plays an important role in vasodilatation (Fig. 5-23).[252–254,257,280,285–286,294–304] EDRF may also help modulate the response to changes in oxygen tension.[250,257,287,297,299–301,305,306] Metabolic dilatation of distal arterioles can result in dilatation of upstream arterioles by both flow-dependent and myogenic mechanisms and can result in decreased vascular resistance and improved oxygen delivery (Fig. 5-24). The endothelium is often functionally impaired in atherosclerosis.[250,254,257,297,300,301,306–313]

The endothelium also forms prostacyclin (PGI_2) from arachidonic acid. PGI_2 inhibits platelet adherence to the endothelium[314] and also produces relaxation of vascular smooth muscle. Nitrates, sodium nitroprusside, adenosine, hydrogen ions, CO_2, and K^+ act directly on vascular smooth muscle cells, and their actions are not endothelium-mediated.

The endothelium can also release vasoconstricting substances. One of these is endothelin, which produces very strong vascular smooth muscle vasoconstriction by acting on an endothelin receptor to stimulate Ca^{2+} entry

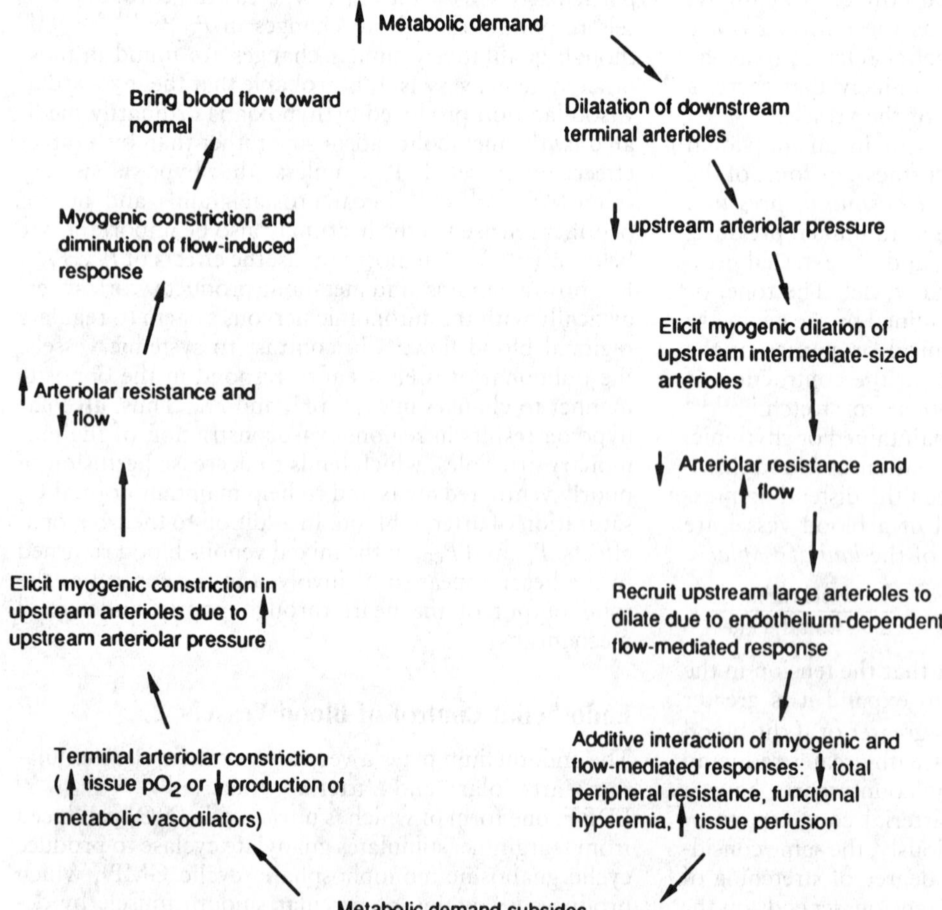

FIGURE 5-24 Integrative role of metabolic, myogenic, and flow-mediated regulation of coronary arteriolar tone during functional hyperemia. Note that metabolic dilatation of small arterioles can result in dilatation of upstream arterioles by flow-dependent and myogenic mechanisms that lessen overall vascular resistance and improve tissue oxygenation. (*From L Kuo, MJ Davis, WM Chilian: Endothelial modulation of arteriolar tone. NIPS 7:5–9, 1992. Reproduced with permission from the publisher and authors.*)

through the Ca^{2+} channel[249] and to stimulate the formation of IP_3,[248–251,255,256,258,288,315] which increases cytosolic calcium in vascular smooth muscle by stimulating the release of Ca^{2+} from intracellular sources. Many substances cause endothelin to be released, including vasopressor hormones, such as angiotensin II, epinephrine, and arginine vasopressin (AVP); coagulation products, such as thrombin; cytokines, such as interleukin-1; oxygen free radicals; and substances derived from aggregating platelets, such as transforming growth factor β (TGFB).[258] Endothelium can also synthesize endothelial-derived contracting factors (EDCF), which are not endothelin.

Plasma endothelin-1 concentration is increased in patients with unstable angina, acute myocardial infarction, heart failure, or renal insufficiency and in some patients with systemic arterial hypertension (see Chaps. 25 and 56). Impaired endothelial function in advanced heart failure leads to decreased vasodilatation of the vasculature in exercising skeletal muscles and to decreased capacity for exercise. The same deadaptation occurs with inactivity of muscle and is restored over time with muscle use (exercise). See Chaps. 2 and 56 for more detailed discussions of endothelial function.

Neural Control of Blood Vessels[3,13,18,225,226,272,275,276]

Three main types of nerve fibers are important in the control of blood vessels: (1) sympathetic vasoconstrictor fibers, (2) sympathetic vasodilator fibers, and (3) parasympathetic vasodilator fibers.

Sympathetic vasoconstrictor fibers are found in both arteries and veins throughout the body, but not in capillaries. These fibers appear to effect vasoconstriction by the release of norepinephrine at the nerve fiber endings, which acts on α_1-adrenergic receptors in vascular smooth muscle. Vasodilatation may be produced by inhibition of the discharge rate of these nerve fibers. These fibers are important in responding to local or regional stimuli of many types. During exercise, they also produce arterial vasoconstriction in nonworking muscles and venous vasoconstriction of capacitance vessels, thereby helping to restrict blood flow to those areas and to maintain blood flow to either vital beds or exercising muscle. In addition, these fibers are the major pathways for reflex changes in peripheral resistance secondary to changes in carotid sinus and aortic stretch receptors, as well as reflex changes from the carotid body chemoreceptors and from stretch receptors in the low-pressure areas of the intrathoracic vascular bed.[225] They are thought to be the principal mechanism by which impulses from the cortical and subcortical areas of the brain influence total and regional peripheral resistance. The effect of these nerve fibers on the coronary and cerebral blood vessels is ordinarily very slight, being overshadowed by the influence of P_{O_2} and P_{CO_2}, although the adrenergic vasoconstriction may limit the concomitant metabolic vasodilatation and may help maintain blood flow to the inner layer of the left ventricle during tachycardia.[271–274,316,317] The influence of sympathetic stimulation and coronary reflexes is considered in Chap. 57.

Sympathetic vasodilator fibers appear to be of importance in skeletal muscles, although it is possible that some cutaneous blood vessels and coronary vessels also receive this type of fiber. Probably these fibers are not normally active tonically and are not influenced significantly by the carotid sinus or aortic arch stretch receptors, but they may be important in increasing blood flow to active muscles during the initiation of exercise. The effector agent at the nerve fiber ending is thought to be acetylcholine.

Parasympathetic vasodilator fibers are restricted to the tongue and salivary glands and to the sacral area, particularly the erectile vessels of the genital organs. In the sacral area they subserve local regulation of blood flow through the release of acetylcholine. Parasympathetic stimulation of the salivary glands releases *kallikrein,* which acts on kininogen, a plasma α_2 globulin synthesized in the liver, to form lysyl-bradykinin, which is converted by an aminopeptidase to *bradykinin,* a substance with powerful vasodilating properties. This is the same enzyme that converts inactive angiotensin I to the active angiotensin II (see Chap. 30). The sweat glands of the skin, innervated by sympathetic cholinergic fibers, may also liberate a kallikrein, and a kallikrein precursor in plasma may be activated by certain physical and chemical factors. In addition, the release of kallikrein and the formation of kinins may contribute to the hypotension associated with endotoxin and anaphylactic shock, the dumping syndrome, and carcinoid syndrome.[318–320]

In general, vasoconstriction occurs as the result of increased activity of the sympathetic nervous system, which causes the local release of norepinephrine at the nerve fiber endings in blood vessels, whereas vasodilatation is produced by the inhibition of sympathetic vasoconstrictor impulses and/or by endothelial and metabolic vasoactive products and local environmental conditions (P_{O_2}, P_{CO_2}, pH, K^+, etc.; Fig. 5-25). Localized vasodilatation may also be produced in exercising muscle by sympathetic vasodilator fibers and in the sacral area and salivary glands by parasympathetic fibers. In some areas vasodilatation may be produced by the formation of neuropeptides and other polypeptides under autonomic nervous system influence.[238,245,247,318–320] Prostaglandins are also very important in local circulatory control.

The anatomic pathways by which the central nervous system helps to control cardiovascular function are still poorly defined. The mechanisms by which the nervous system is able to integrate impulses from all levels—the cortex and limbic system, reticular system, diencephalon, mesencephalon, medulla oblongata, spinal cord, and so on—and to synthesize these impulses in order to provide the organism with responses varying from the massive sympathetic discharge associated with shock to very discrete vasomotor changes are also not well delineated. Three major pools of spontaneously active neurons appear important in control of both the heart and the peripheral blood vessels: the *cardiovascular excitatory center* (pressor area), located in the rostrolateral portion of the medulla; the *cardiovascular inhibitory center* (depressor area), located in the mediocaudal portion of the medulla; and the *dorsal motor nucleus of the vagus nerve,* which exerts a cardiac inhibitory influence.[3] It is also apparent that impulses from high levels at times bypass lower integrative areas. There is also little information regarding the mechanisms of conditioning involving the autonomic nervous system.

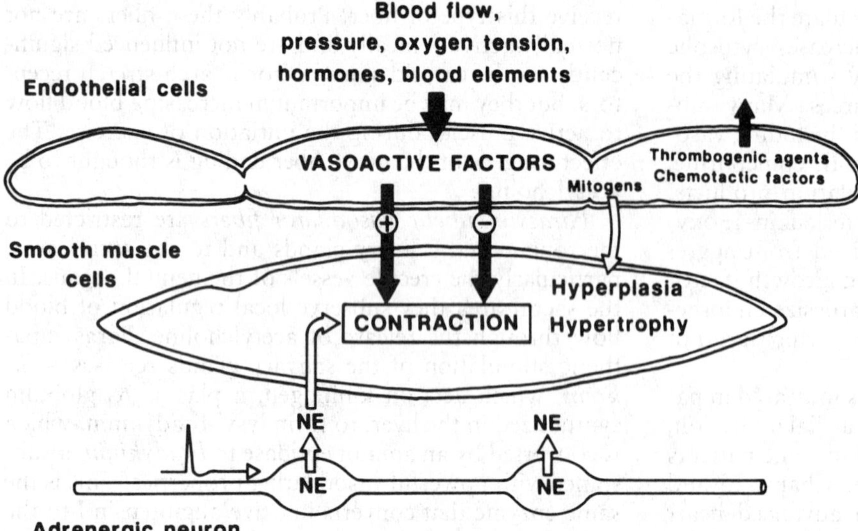

FIGURE 5-25 Schematic representing regulatory systems responsible for control of peripheral vascular tone. Adrenergic neurons, through release of norepinephrine (NE), regulate adjustments in tone relative to the activity of cardiopulmonary, baro-, and chemoreceptors. In response to changes in blood flow, oxygen tension, circulating levels of hormones, and substances released from blood elements (aggregating platelets and activated macrophages), the endothelium releases vasoactive substances that can either contract or relax the smooth muscle. Some vasoactive factors can also be mitogenic and inhibit platelet and macrophage adhesion or aggregation. (*From VM Miller: Interactions between neural and endothelial mechanisms in control vascular tone. News Physiol Sci 6:60–63, 1991. Reproduced with permission from the publisher and author.*)

MYOCARDIAL OXYGEN CONSUMPTION

The hemodynamic determinant of myocardial oxygen consumption ($M\dot{V}_{O_2}$) was related in 1907 by Barcroft and Dixon to external work, or the product of aortic pressure and flow.[321] In 1912, Rohde concluded that ventricular pressure and heart rate together determined myocardial oxygen consumption,[322] and in 1915 Evans and Matsuoka[323] reported a "relation between the tension set up on contraction and the metabolism of the contractile tissue." They noted that volume work was performed with less oxygen consumed than was an equal amount of pressure work and noted that the tension in the wall of the heart "varies roughly as the endocardiac pressure and as the square of the radius of the heart cavities," the now-familiar Laplace relationship. Subsequently, many studies have confirmed the importance of active intramyocardial tension or wall stress developed by the ventricle, or a related variable, as a major determinant of myocardial oxygen consumption.[324] Related variables have been correlated with $M\dot{V}_{O_2}$, including the product of pressure and heart rate, the product of integrated ventricular pressure and heart rate (the "tension-time index"),[325] developed wall tension, and contractile element work. Clearly, *wall tension* and *heart rate* are the major determinants of myocardial oxygen consumption.

The inotropic state (contractility, or the velocity of contraction) is the second major determinant of myocardial oxygen consumption.[324–327] The results of several earlier studies relating $M\dot{V}_{O_2}$ to ventricular end-diastolic fiber length or diastolic volume were probably related to changes in developed tension or velocity of contraction. Similarly, the net effect on myocardial oxygen consumption of various positive inotropic interventions, such as sympathetic nerve stimulation or excitement, paired electrical stimulation, or the infusion of digitalis glycosides, catecholamines, or calcium, depends to a large degree on the relative effects on the tension developed and on the contractile state.[324] Most of the increase in myocardial oxygen uptake produced by catecholamines is related to the hemodynamic alterations they induce, although large doses can increase oxygen uptake in the nonbeating heart by a small amount. The effect of digitalis and other positive intropic agents on $M\dot{V}_{O_2}$ depends on its relative effects on the contractile state of the heart, which it increases, causing $M\dot{V}_{O_2}$ to increase, and upon ventricular wall tension, which can decrease $M\dot{V}_{O_2}$ significantly if the heart radius decreases sufficiently.[324,327]

As shown in Table 5-2, the seven determinants of myocardial oxygen consumption can be classified as four major determinants and three minor determinants. The oxygen cost of electrical activation is probably less than 1 percent of the total $M\dot{V}_{O_2}$, and the costs for contractile-state activation and deactivation and for the maintenance of the active state are also small.[324,326] Clinically, relative myocardial oxygen requirements can be estimated by determining the product of systolic blood pressure and heart rate, the *tension-time index*,[325] or *pressure-time per minute*.[328] One may also factor the product of pressure and heart rate by the total duration of systole per minute.

Coronary flow and pressure affect oxygen consumption in the nonworking heart but have variable effects in the beating heart.[329] Alcohol stimulates the myocardial uptake of oxygen, whereas hypothermia markedly decreases oxygen consumption.

TABLE 5-2

Determinants of Myocardial Oxygen Consumption
Major determinants
Myocardial mass
Intramyocardial tension or wall stress (pressure × volume)
Inotropic state (contractility)
Heart rate
Minor determinants
External work (load × shortening)
Basal oxygen requirements
Activation energy

CORONARY CIRCULATION

The normal coronary circulation is able to provide oxygen to the heart under a wide range of conditions and is able to increase its flow five to six times the value at rest.[253,280,284,290–293,297,317,330–336] *Coronary vascular reserve* is the capacity of the coronary circulation to provide additional oxygenated blood to the myocardium. At rest, however, the coronary blood flow (CBF) is approximately 70 to 90 mL/100 g per min and the oxygen consumption of the heart approximately 8 to 10 mL/100 g per min.[290–294,330] Even at rest, however, the heart, which is normally aerobic (Chap. 6A), extracts and utilizes most of the oxygen contained in its blood supply. Consequently, the oxygen content of the blood in the coronary sinus is about 5 mL/100 mL blood, which corresponds to about 30 percent saturation and a P_{O_2} of 18 to 20 mmHg. As a result, relatively little additional oxygen can be made available to the heart by greater oxygen extraction, and any increase in demand for oxygen by the heart must be met by an increase in CBF. Thus, any increase in the myocardial oxygen requirement (Table 5-2) will normally result in a proportional increase in CBF. Coronary arteries diseased with atherosclerosis may fail to dilate normally under conditions of increased need and may actually narrow (see Chap. 57).

Physical Factors Influencing CBF

The arterial pressure gradient (aortic-left ventricular diastolic pressure) and the time spent in diastole are the major determinants of CBF. Excessively elevated diastolic pressure, however, does not result in unneeded perfusion because of autoregulation.[337] On the other hand, when the perfusion pressure is very low, the coronary circulation is maximally dilated, and CBF is linearly related to the perfusion pressure. In general, CBF is maintained throughout a fairly wide range of perfusion pressure by autoregulation via myogenic changes in coronary artery tone.[281,282,284,321] CBF may be decreased by factors decreasing effective coronary perfusion pressure, such as congenital anomalies of the coronary arteries or obstruction of a coronary artery by atherosclerosis, thrombosis, or vasoconstriction. In general, it is necessary to decrease the lumen, or cross-sectional area, of an epicardial coronary vessel by at least two-thirds to cause a significant decrease in resting coronary flow. CBF also varies with the length and character of the obstruction, and lesser degrees of obstruction can cause a significant obstruction under conditions that increase the need for coronary blood flow (see also Chap. 57).

During ventricular systole, the left ventricular intramyocardial pressure exceeds left ventricular cavitary pressure or aortic systolic pressure, and the penetrating coronary vessels in the wall of the left ventricle are markedly compressed, or "throttled," preventing forward blood flow and even producing retrograde flow.[338] In addition to the physical systolic compression of the vessels, CBF is impeded by increased shear caused by twisting of the coronary vessels during systole.[339] Thus, for all intents and purposes, the left ventricle receives the majority of its CBF during diastole. The right ventricle receives flow more nearly equally during both systole and diastole (Fig. 5-26). In patients with coronary artery disease or even with marked left ventricular hypertrophy, tachycardia can predispose to myocardial ischemia, not only by the direct increase in oxygen consumption, but by significantly limiting the amount of time occupied by diastole. Indeed, in the markedly hypertrophied left ventricle, coronary reserve is significantly reduced, although resting flow corrected for mass may be normal. Furthermore, as noted above, coronary vascular resistance may actually increase during conditions of stress, such as exercise, in patients with coronary atherosclerosis (see Chap. 57).

Tissue pressure and especially left ventricular diastolic pressure also influence and can decrease CBF, especially to the subendocardium of a "failing" left ventricle and particularly if arterial hypotension is also present. An elevation of outlet pressure in the coronary sinus or right atrium can also offer some impediment to coronary perfusion, although this is seldom a significant factor in the

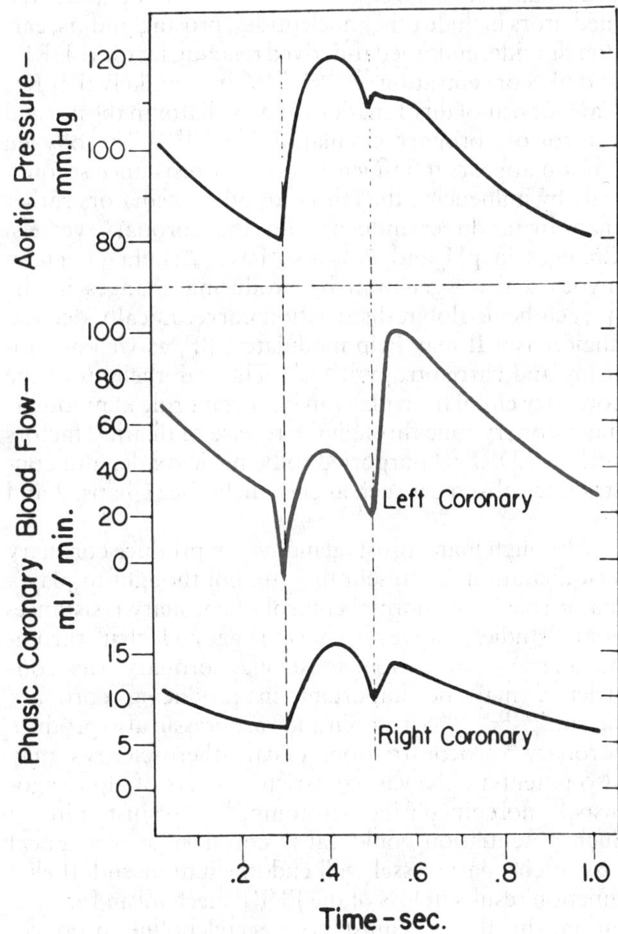

FIGURE 5-26 Comparison of phasic coronary blood flow in the left and right coronary arteries. Note the marked decrease in flow in the left coronary artery during left ventricular ejection. The decrease in blood flow to the left ventricle begins with the onset of left ventricular systole, shortly before the beginning of ejection of blood from the left ventricle, which is indicated by the first vertical line. (*From RM Berne, MN Levy: Cardiovascular Physiology, 6th ed. St. Louis, Mosby Year Book, 1992. Reproduced with permission from the publisher and authors.*)

absence of severe coronary artery disease. Blood viscosity is an additional factor that may contribute to a limitation of CBF, particularly in the presence of coronary artery disease. A myogenic mechanism, or Bayliss phenomenon, also contributes to the autoregulation of CBF.[281,282,284,321] Additional physical factors affecting the adequacy of CBF include the total myocardial mass and the diffusion distance of oxygen from coronary capillaries to the center of hypertrophied myocardial cells.

Metabolic Factors Influencing CBF

CBF normally increases linearly with increased myocardial oxygen requirements, and most of the increase in CBF is by coronary vasodilatation secondary to metabolic autoregulation (Table 3-2). Several mediators or metabolic vasodilators are responsible for the metabolic autoregulation of the coronary circulation. Adenosine, which is formed by dephosphorylation of AMP and which has strong coronary vasodilating properties, has most of the criteria for the physiological regulation of CBF and may play a major role in the metabolic control of coronary resistance.[284,290–294,332,333,339–342] Other potential mediators include other nucleotides, prostaglandins, carbon dioxide, endothelial-derived relaxing factor (EDRF), and pH concentration.[238,253,254,284,297] It is unlikely that K^+, Ca^{2+}, or osmolality functions as a mediator in the normal control of coronary circulation.[290–294,332,333] The oxygen tension appears to influence coronary resistance secondarily by influencing the release of other mediators rather than by a direct influence on the coronary vessels. Changes in pH and P_{CO_2} also have a slight effect on myocardial oxygenation by producing changes in the oxygen-hemoglobin dissociation curve. Locally derived angiotensin II may help modulate CBF, as well as inotropy and chronotropy.[235–237,239] The endothelium of the coronary circulation plays an important role in modulating coronary tone through the release of dilating factors such as EDRF,[233] purported to be nitric oxide, and constricting substances such as endothelin (see Chaps. 2 and 56).

Although many prostaglandins can produce coronary vasodilatation, at present they are not thought to play a major role in the normal control of coronary resistance. Some studies, however, have suggested that thromboxane A_2, an extremely strong coronary vasoconstrictor, may be important in producing coronary spasm.[332,333,342–346] Serotonin and vasopressin also produce coronary vasoconstriction. Local atherosclerosis may also potentiate the vasoconstrictor effects of alpha agonists,[347] norepinephrine, serotonin,[348–350] or histamine.[351] Such potentiation could cause coronary spasm. Focal loss of coronary vessel wall endothelium or endothelial function results in loss of the EDRF mechanism for dilatation. In this circumstance, acetylcholine produces paradoxical vasoconstriction in diseased coronary vessels[306–313,352] (see Chaps. 56 and 58).

Humoral Factors Influencing CBF

Catecholamines such as norepinephrine and epinephrine stimulate alpha receptors in the coronary vessels and produce direct coronary vasoconstriction but indirectly they produce coronary vasodilatation and an increase in CBF due to the marked increase in myocardial contractility and thus increased myocardial oxygen consumption.[238,353] The effects of dopamine on the coronary circulation vary markedly with the dose administered, but in general it produces mild coronary vasodilatation. Isoproterenol stimulates beta vasodilator receptors and produces an increase in coronary venous oxygen saturation in normal animals.[354]

Angiotensin II produces coronary vasoconstriction, although this effect is partially obscured by its other effects that increase myocardial oxygen consumption by increases in systemic pressure and left ventricular wall stress, heart rate, and myocardial contractility. It may also release prostaglandins E_2 and F, which produce coronary vasodilatation.[355,356]

High concentrations of vasopressin produce direct coronary vasoconstriction.[357–359] Coronary vascular tone is probably not significantly affected by changes in concentration of Na^+, K^+, Ca^{2+}, or Mg^{2+}, although studies have suggested that Ca^{2+} produces mild vasoconstriction; Mg^{2+} produces vasodilatation; Na^+ produces no effect; and K^+ produces a biphasic response, with small doses producing vasodilatation and large doses vasoconstriction.

Thyroid hormone produces coronary vasodilatation secondary to its effects on heart rate and myocardial contractility to increase myocardial oxygen consumption.[360,361] Adrenal steroids affect CBF and resistance secondarily by their tendency to produce systemic hypertension and left ventricular hypertrophy. Glucagon produces coronary vasodilatation that is secondary to an increase in heart rate and contractility. Beriberi is associated with increased CBF and decreased myocardial oxygen extraction,[362] perhaps as part of generalized arterial vasodilatation.

Adenosine and acetylcholine both produce marked coronary vasodilatation in normal vessels. As noted above, in patients with coronary atherosclerosis and endothelial dysfunction, acetylcholine may produce paradoxic coronary artery vasoconstriction.[306–313,352] (See also Chaps. 56 and 58.) Histamine produces coronary vasodilatation, both directly and indirectly, by its positive inotropic and chronotropic effects.[290] Serotonin also produces direct and, to a lesser degree, indirect coronary vasodilatation.

Polypeptides are also possibly important in the regulation of CBF.[290–294,318,339,340] Bradykinin increases CBF, possibly by the actions of prostaglandins.[363,364] Substance P produces moderate endothelium-dependent coronary vasodilatation, but its role in the normal regulation of CBF is unknown.[284,365–367] Vasoactive intestinal polypeptide (VIP) appears to produce both direct coronary vasodilatation (strong endothelium-dependent, weaker endothelium-independent) and indirect vasodilatation due to its positive inotropic effects.[247,367–370] Neuropeptide tyrosine Y (NPY), which is very widespread, coexists with norepinephrine in the peripheral nervous system, including nerves to coronary blood vessels. NPY may play a role in some instances of coronary spasm.[232,284,368] Calcitonin gene-related peptide (CGRP) produces endothelium-dependent coronary vasodilation. Its importance in the control of CBF in normal individuals or patients with disease is unknown.[284]

Many prostaglandins produce coronary vasodilatation, especially prostacyclin (PGI_2), which is synthesized by endothelial cells and which also inhibits platelet aggregation.[238,371] Thromboxane A_2 is a very strong coronary vasoconstrictor released from platelets that may be important in producing episodic, vasospastic, clinically significant decreases in coronary blood flow[320,342] (see Chap. 59).

Neural Factors Influencing CBF

Sympathetic Nerves

As described in Chap. 4, sympathetic nerves to the heart and coronary vessels arise from the three cervical and the first four thoracic sympathetic ganglia.[227] Sympathetic adrenergic fibers extensively innervate both the epicardial and the intramural arteries and veins. Large coronary vessels appear to have both α and β_2 receptors, while small vessels have predominantly β_2 receptors. The coronary vessels do not appear to have either β_1 adrenergic receptors, which appear to be limited to the myocardium, or sympathetic cholinergic fibers.[372]

Stimulation of cardiac sympathetic nerves produces a direct vasoconstriction of the coronary arteries. This vasoconstriction, however, is normally overwhelmed by vasodilatation secondary to the increase in myocardial metabolism produced by the sympathetic stimulation of heart rate and myocardial contractility.[227,317] Coronary vascular beta adrenergic receptors are not thought to contribute to the response to nerve stimulation.

Parasympathetic Nerves

Experimentally, stimulation of the vagus nerves produces some direct coronary vasodilatation that is mediated by the release of acetylcholine and can be blocked by atropine.[373] In the intact organism, however, vagal stimulation produces bradycardia and may decrease myocardial contractility, both of which decrease myocardial oxygen requirements and result in secondary coronary vasoconstriction. Acetylcholine inhibits adenylate cyclase by a guanine inhibitory protein and decreases myocardial cyclic AMP but augments cyclic GMP, both of which decrease myocardial contractility[227] (see Fig. 25-11). Since vagal fiber innervation of ventricular myocardium is relatively small, however, the effect on function is minor.

Coronary Reflexes

Although coronary vascular resistance is primarily determined by metabolic autoregulation, it is also modulated by the sympathetic nervous system in response to changes in arterial pressure that are sensed by baroreceptors in the carotid sinus.[3,5,8,164,222-225] Carotid chemoreceptors, which may be initiated by acidosis, hypoxemia, or hypercapnia, can also influence coronary resistance by a predominant vasodilator effect mediated by the vagi and perhaps by a lesser vasoconstrictor effect mediated by the sympathetic nerves and only apparent if the vagal reflex is blocked.[223,225,290,293] There is no convincing evidence, however, of a coronary-to-coronary reflex except following the intracoronary administration of veratridine, which is known to elicit the Bezold-Jarisch reflex, a coronary-to-periphery reflex producing hypotension and bradycardia.[228,330] There is evidence that reflex vasodilatation of some peripheral vascular beds as well as changes in heart rate and contractility may occur in some patients following coronary occlusion.[228,374] On the other hand, there is little substantial evidence of reflex vasoconstriction of coronary vessels from peripheral phenomena such as gastritis or cholecystitis. There is good evidence for a pulmonary inflation reflex that produces coronary vasodilatation in part mediated by a withdrawal of sympathetic tone.[375] The role of cardiac mechanoreceptors in the regulation of coronary blood flow is uncertain.[228,376]

Coronary Collateral Circulation

The stimuli and mechanisms for the development of coronary collateral circulation are not precisely known.[377-380] Hypoxia appears to play a major role. It has been postulated that hypoxia releases vasodilator metabolites that dilate preexisting microscopic collateral vessels without a smooth muscle component, increasing their pressure and tangential wall stress and damaging the vessel walls. This initial damage is then followed by reparative processes and the development of large-lumen, thick-walled collateral vessels with smooth muscle responsive to constrictive and dilating influences.[228,377-380] Fibroblast-stimulating factor increases coronary collateral flow into acutely ischemic areas and reduces resultant infarct size.[381] In human beings, the presence of coronary collateral circulation usually signifies the presence of significant coronary artery disease.[377-380] Once formed by hypoxia, collateral circulation may persist, although it may not be evident when primary flow sources are adequate.

Distribution of CBF

Current evidence indicates that the blood flow to the left ventricle is closely related to its oxygen demands. In experimental animals, this is also true within the left ventricle, where the left ventricular subendocardium at rest consumes 10 to 30 percent more oxygen per gram than the subepicardium and has a proportionately higher blood flow.[334,382-384] During tachycardia or other conditions that increase myocardial oxygen requirements and CBF of the experimental animal, however, CBF of experimental animals is more nearly equal in different layers of left ventricular myocardium. Estimates of CBF distribution in normal human beings, however, have suggested a fairly homogeneous distribution of coronary flow in the layers of the left ventricle at rest.[385] Most studies have indicated that the left ventricular subendocardium, which possesses a very dense vasculature, has a higher systolic intramyocardial pressure, calculated wall stress, and oxygen consumption than the subepicardium.[382,386] CBF to the left ventricular subendocardium is especially likely to be compromised by tachycardia, hypertrophy, an aged ventricle, or elevation of left ventricular diastolic pressure. The latter may be seen chronically in patients with hypertension, aortic stenosis, or hypertrophic cardiomyopathy[387] and may produce chronic diastolic dysfunction (see Chaps. 25 and 26). It may occur acutely secondary to myocardial ischemia with angina pectoris or myocardial infarction. In this situation, it may produce acute or even "flash" pulmonary edema.[388,389]

THE CARDIAC CYCLE

The successive mechanical events of the cardiac cycle may be described by a modification (Plate II, 5-1) of Wiggers' classic diagram, which divided the cardiac cycle into two *periods*, systole and diastole, and subdivided these periods into *phases* of cardiac activity.[390–392] In the following discussion, the cardiac cycle is divided according to events on the left side of the heart. Corresponding periods and phases may also be described for events on the right side of the heart, with some differences (see below). The echocardiogram is very useful for estimating changes in ventricular volume and for timing valvular events.[393,394]

The first phase of ventricular systole is *isovolumic (isovolumetric* or *isochoric) contraction.* This phase begins with the first detectable rise in left ventricular pressure after the *z point;* it is associated with the initial, mitral component (MC) of the first heart sound and the beginning of the isovolumic contraction (IC) wave of the apex cardiogram. The end of the isovolumic contraction phase and the beginning of the succeeding *rapid ventricular ejection* phase are indicated by the opening of the aortic valve (AO), a rise in aortic pressure, a decrease in ventricular volume, and the peak of the ejection E wave of the apex cardiogram. The onset and termination of the next phase of *reduced ventricular ejection* are less well defined; however, this phase may be said to begin when the shape of the ventricular volume curve indicates a significant decrease in the rate of ejection. This normally occurs prior to the peak systolic pressure in the left ventricle and aorta. The phase of reduced ejection lasts until the end of actual ventricular ejection and the beginning of diastole, which occurs just before the recording of the incisura on the aortic pressure tracing. The very brief initial phase of diastole preceding the incisura is referred to as *protodiastole* and represents the time required for the reversal of flow in the aorta and for closure of the aortic valve, which is responsible for the *incisura* of the aortic pressure tracing.

The beginning of the next phase of *isolvolumic relaxation* of the left ventricle is signified by the closure of the aortic valve, as indicated by the aortic component (AC) of the second heart sound and by an inward isovolumic relaxation (IR) wave of the apex cardiogram. Isovolumic relaxation lasts until the left ventricular pressure falls below the left atrial pressure and blood begins to flow from the atrium into the ventricle. Usually, the left ventricular pressure falls below the left atrial pressure tracing slightly *after* the peak of the left atrial *v* wave, since there is a slight fall in left atrial pressure caused by a decrease in the upward bulging of the atrioventricular (AV) valve structures during ventricular isovolumic relaxation. In a sense, this is the opposite of the mechanism thought to produce the *c* wave in the atria during early ventricular systole. Both isovolumic relaxation and the following phase of rapid ventricular filling are produced by elastic recoil and active relaxation of the ventricular myocardium.

The end of the isovolumic relaxation phase and the beginning of the *rapid ventricular filling phase* are indicated by an increase in the ventricular volume curve, and by the O point of the apex cardiogram, which coincides with the opening of the mitral valve (MO). If the mitral valve is diseased, the opening of the valve may be audible as an "opening snap" (OS). This rapid ventricular filling phase is associated with a continuation of the decrease in atrial pressure (the *y descent*) begun during isovolumic relaxation, a rapid increase in ventricular volume, and an outward rapid-filling wave (RFW) in the apex cardiogram.

The end of the rapid ventricular filling phase and the beginning of the *slow ventricular filling phase* are evidenced by a change in the slope of the ventricular volume curve, which indicates a change in the rate of ventricular filling. At times, the end of rapid ventricular filling is associated with low-frequency vibrations or a sound, termed the S_3 or *ventricular gallop*, which occurs very shortly before the nadir of the *y* descent of the atrial pressure tracing. On the apex cardiogram the end of the rapid ventricular filling phase (and the identification of S_3) is indicated at the moment when an abrupt change in slope occurs at the transition from the rapid-filling wave (RFW) to the slow-filling wave (SFW). This may be associated with a brief outward pulsation which is referred to as an *F wave*, or *peak*, on the apex cardiogram; frequently an S_3 is both visible and palpable (see Chap. 11).

During the phase of *slow ventricular filling*, or diastasis, the pressures in the left atrium and left ventricle slowly increase as the ventricle is passively filled until the next atrial systole produces the *a wave* in the left atrial pressure tracing. At times, an *h wave* is present in late diastasis prior to the *a* wave. Atrial contraction and the increased ventricular filling produced by atrial contraction (or "atrial kick") are reflected in an increase in ventricular pressure, an increase in ventricular volume, and an outward *a* wave of the apex cardiogram. Toward the peak or the second half of the atrial *a* wave there may be a sound (S_4), particularly if there is a vigorous atrial contraction and relaxation. After the *a* wave of atrial contraction and relaxation, there is a very brief period or point (*z* point) when the atrial and ventricular pressures are essentially equal in normal individuals. The next cardiac cycle begins when the next ventricular contraction causes a definite sharp rise in pressure from the *z* point.

As one would expect from the location of the sinus node, contraction of the right atrium and opening of the tricuspid valve occur slightly before the corresponding events on the left side of the heart (Plate II, 5-1; Plate III, 5-2). On the other hand, excitation and contraction of the left ventricle begins prior to contraction of the right ventricle, although the beginning of ejection of blood into the pulmonary artery slightly precedes ejection into the aorta, since the pressure in the right ventricle does not have to increase to such a high level before ejection begins (Plate II, 5-1). It is interesting to note that right ventricular ejection lasts beyond left ventricular ejection, producing the normal interval between the aortic component of the second heart sound (A_2) and the pulmonic component of the second heart sound (P_2). The shorter duration of left ventricular ejection is related to the greater contractile force of the left ventricle and to differences in the aorta and the pulmonary artery impedance and compression-chamber (*Windkessel*) characteristics.

During the brief phase of left ventricular isovolumic systole, the central aortic pressure pulse may show a slight positive wave that is produced by slight bulging of the aortic valve due to the rapidly increasing left ventricular pressure. During left ventricular ejection, the left ventricular pressure exceeds aortic pressure only during the early part of ejection and actually is slightly less than aortic pressure during most of systole.[395] It should also be noted that, although several components of the first and second heart sounds are referred to by the name of the valve commonly associated with the production of that sound, the sounds are not produced by the actual closure or striking together of the valve leaflets. *The sounds are more properly considered to be produced by the sudden acceleration and deceleration of blood with tensing of the entire valve structures, and vibrations of all cardiac structures.* Actually, there is evidence that the AV valves and the aortic valve may be closed physiologically at a slightly different time than when these sounds occur.[396–402] In most clinical situations, the two components of the first heart sound, the mitral (M) and the tricuspid (T) component, are produced by sudden acceleration-deceleration of blood, the valves, and cardiac structures in association with abrupt closure of the mitral and tricuspid valves, respectively.

The shape of an apex cardiogram recording varies significantly depending on the particular instrumentation used to record it. The drawing of a tracing shown in Plate II, 5-1 was obtained with a piezo crystal.

While ventricular pressure is traditionally expressed in relation to time (Plate II, 5-1), pressure can also be expressed in relation to ventricular volume in pressure-volume loops of individual heartbeats (see Fig. 26-5). Such loops are very useful in the evaluation of systolic and diastolic ventricular function and of myocardial contractility.[403] The slope of the line connecting the points at the end of systole (point C in Fig. 25-5) on different pressure-volume loops is called the *end-systolic elastance*, or Ees, reflecting the shortening capacity of the ventricle, (i.e., the end-systolic length-tension curve). As such, it has been used as one index of contractility.[183–187,403] (See Chaps. 23 and 25).

THE ARTERIAL PULSE

The arterial pressure pulse is produced by the ejection of blood from the left ventricle into the aorta and great vessels at a rate faster than its runoff into the peripheral circulation. In human beings, an average left ventricular stroke volume of 60 to 100 mL is ejected in about 0.25 s, and, of this volume, approximately two-thirds is ejected during the rapid-ejection phase. Although the peak rate of ejection of blood occurs prior to the peak pressure in the left ventricle or aorta, the pressure continues to rise in the aorta as long as blood is ejected into the aorta faster than it runs off into the peripheral arteries. Sometimes there is a slight notch in the central arterial pulse wave during or toward the end of the rapid-ejection phase. This is referred to as the *anacrotic notch*, or *shoulder*; it is accentuated in valvular aortic stenosis. At the end of ventricular ejection (and after the very brief phase of protodiastole), the aortic valve closes. In central aortic pressure tracings, this event is reflected by a sharp downward deflection, or *incisura*, on the descending limb of the pressure tracing and a gradual fall during diastole. At times, left ventricular isovolumic contraction causes a slight positive deflection in central arterial tracings just before the onset of the main arterial pulse wave.

As the arterial pressure pulse wave passes to the periphery, there are significant changes in its form (Fig. 5-27).[404] As the pulse moves away from the heart, the initial upstroke of the pulse becomes steeper, there is normally no anacrotic pause on the ascending limb, and the systolic maximum becomes peaked and increased in magnitude. The *dicrotic notch*, or *halt*, which corresponds to the incisura recorded more centrally, tends to occur later and lower and to be smoother in contour than the incisura. The positive wave that follows the dicrotic notch is referred to as the *dicrotic wave*; in many peripheral arteries this is normally more prominent than the slight upward deflection recorded centrally following the incisura. Although the systolic pressure may increase as the wave moves to the periphery, the diastolic and mean arterial pressures decrease slightly. The major factors responsible for these changes in the arterial pulse contour are (1) distortion of the components of the pulse waves as they travel peripherally, (2) different rates of transmission of various components of the pulse wave, (3) amplification or distortion of different components of the pulse by *standing* or *reflected waves*, (4) differences in elastic behavior and in caliber of the arteries, and (5) conversion of some kinetic energy to hydrostatic energy. Further details of the arterial pulse are discussed in Chap. 10.

THE VENOUS PULSE

The form of the venous pressure pulse[205,405] is determined by the rate of return of the blood from the peripheral tissues into the venous segment, the pressure-volume characteristics of the segment of the vein, the nature of the resistance to flow or distensibility offered by the right atrium and ventricle during the different phases of the cardiac cycle, and, to a slight degree, the tissues overlying the veins at the point of observation. Although the venous pressure pulse wave travels peripherally away from the heart, there is at the same time a venous flow of blood in the opposite direction toward the heart.

The *a* wave of the venous pressure pulse is related to contraction of the right atrium and is followed by the *z* point immediately preceding ventricular systole. In the jugular venous pulse, the *c* wave as usually recorded is predominantly produced by the systolic impulse in the

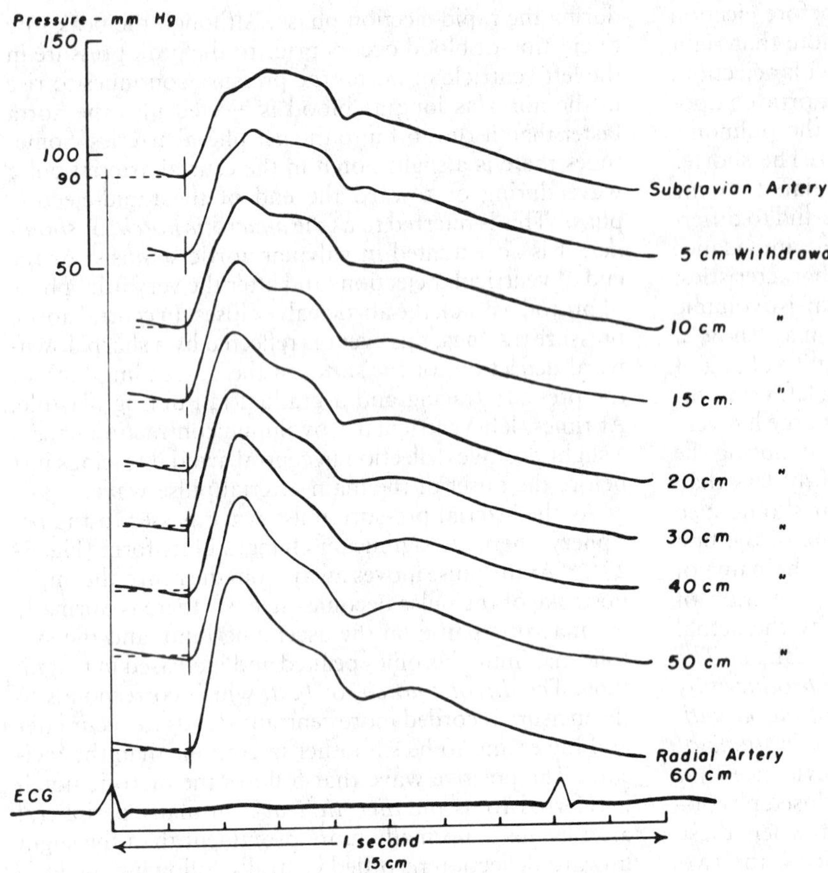

FIGURE 5-27 Pulse contours in a healthy 30-year-old man, showing transformation of pressure pulse in subclavian-radial system. Pressure pulses were recorded consecutively during withdrawal of the tip of an adrenal catheter from the subclavian artery near the aorta to the radial artery in the left arm. Onsets of pressure pulses are aligned for purposes of comparison. As the pulse wave moves peripherally, the initial wave steepens and increases in magnitude, the dome-shaped systolic maximum becomes peaked, and the dicrotic halt moves down and to the right and becomes slurred. Low-amplitude, central postdicrotic wave is not seen after catheter has been withdrawn 10 cm or more. Prominence of radial dicrotic wave is due, in part, to change in position of dicrotic halt. Horizontal broken line intersecting onset of each pulse contour is calibration reference point (90 mmHg). Interval of time from peak of R wave of electrocardiogram to onset of systolic upswing of each pulse wave is indicated by duration of each tracing to left side of short vertical lines, which mark onset of systole from each pulse. [*From HW Marshall, HF Helmbolz, EH Wood: Physiologic consequence of congenital heart disease. In: WF Hamilton, P Dow, eds: Handbook of Physiology, sec 2: Circulation, vol 1. Bethesda, MD, American Physiological Society, 1962, 417. Reproduced with permission from the publisher and authors.*]

adjacent carotid artery, with some contribution produced by right ventricular contraction and upward bulging of the tricuspid valve. In the early part of ventricular systole and following the brief *c* wave, there is a rapid inflow of blood to the right atrium, produced in part by descent of the tricuspid valve ring, which produces the normal negative venous wave during ventricular systole, the negative *x* wave, or *x descent* (or systolic collapse). The *x descent* is also produced by the ejection of blood from both ventricles, which decreases the intrapericardial pressure and therefore the pressure in both atria. As the venous inflow continues into the atria after the *x* descent, the pressure in the atria and in the veins builds up, producing the *v* wave during approximately the second half of ventricular systole. The peak of the right atrial *v* wave occurs shortly before or simultaneously with opening of the tricuspid valve and the beginning of the phase of right rapid ventricular filling. During early ventricular diastole, the rapid flow of blood from the great veins and right atrium into the right ventricle produces the negative *y* descent (or diastolic collapse) of the peripheral venous pulse wave. When recorded externally, the venous pulse wave is somewhat damped, and even when recorded directly, the waves are usually less steep in rise and descent than the corresponding waves of the atria. In part this is due to the damping effect of the large veins, which can accommodate markedly different volumes of blood without a marked change in pressure.

Clinically, venous pulse waves are particularly difficult to evaluate in the presence of tachycardia, obesity, or shock or during the administration of drugs that produce venoconstriction. Further details of the venous pulse are discussed in Chap. 10.

NORMAL PRESSURES AND FLOW RATES IN THE CARDIOVASCULAR SYSTEM[406–408]

In general, the pressure in the systemic arteries is about five to six times greater than in the pulmonary arteries, although the amount of blood flowing in each unit is essentially the same. The left ventricular output may be slightly greater than the right ventricular output, due to the small amount of bronchial artery flow that returns in the pulmonary veins and the drainage of a few thebesian veins into the left atrium and ventricle. In order to compare measurements between individuals of different sizes, measurements of flow and resistance are often expressed in terms of square meters of body surface area; that is, instead of comparing cardiac output in absolute number of liters per minute, the output of the heart is expressed as the *cardiac index*, or liters per minute per square meter of body surface area. There is still a need for additional data to establish the limits of "normal" for vascular pressures, flow, and resistance for normal individuals of all ages under conditions of rest, exercise, or emotional stress. Furthermore, some of the slight differences in normal values reported from different laboratories are related to the use of different methods of measurement or different baselines for measurement of

TABLE 5-3
Hemodynamic Values of Normal Recumbent Adults

Measurement	Mean	Range
Cardiac index, liters/min per/m²	3.4	2.8–4.2
Stroke index, mL/beat	47	30–65
Arteriovenous oxygen difference, mL per liter of blood	38	30–48
Arterial saturation, %	98	94–100
Pressure,* mmHg		
Brachial artery		
Systolic	130	90–140
Diastolic	70	60–90
Mean	85	70–105
Left ventricle		
Systolic	130	90–140
End-diastolic	7	4–12
Left atrium		
Maximum	13	6–20
Minimum	3	−2–+9
Mean	7	4–12
Pulmonary artery wedge (PC)		
Maximum	16	9–23
Minimum	6	1–12
Mean	9	6–15
Pulmonary artery		
Systolic	24	15–28
Diastolic	10	5–16
Mean	16	10–22
Right ventricle		
Systolic	24	15–28
End-diastolic	4	0–8
Right atrium		
Maximum	7	2–14
Minimum	2	−2–+6
Mean	4	−1–+8
Venae cavae		
Maximum	7	2–14
Minimum	5	0–8
Mean	6	1–10
End-diastolic volume		
Left ventricular, mL/m²	70	50–90
Resistance, dyn·s/cm⁵		
Total systemic	1150	900–1400
Systemic arteriolar	850	600–900
Total pulmonary	200	150–250
Pulmonary arteriolar	70	45–120

*Baseline for pressure measurements one-half of anteroposterior chest diameter. 1 mmHg = 133.332 Pascal (Pa) = 0.133 kPa.

pressure. Table 5-3 lists the mean and range of hemodynamic measurements for normal resting adults, and Table 5-4 gives the distribution of systemic blood flow and oxygen consumption in a hypothetical 70-kg normal resting male.

RESPONSE TO EXERCISE[2,5,76,409–421]

The mechanisms utilized to increase the cardiac output during dynamic exercise vary, depending on the age, condition, posture, and athletic training of the person. (See also Chap. 114). In particular, the relative contribution of heart rate and stroke volume has been the subject of considerable interest. In general, pulse rate may increase three-fold (or even five-fold in some highly trained athletes), whereas stroke volume increases considerably less.[422] With extreme increases in heart rate, stroke volume may even decline slightly. Most "normal" but untrained individuals in the supine position increase their cardiac output during mild to moderate dynamic exercise predominantly by an increase in pulse rate rather than by an increase in stroke volume. With the increase in ventricular contractility, end-diastolic volume tends to decrease with an increase in ejection fraction. With more extreme exercise, stroke volume increases about 10 to 15 percent in the supine position and by 30 to 100 percent in the upright position, despite a considerably shortened systolic ejection period. In individuals who are accustomed to physical exertion, there is an earlier and more marked increase in stroke volume in both positions, and stroke volume often doubles during extreme upright exercise. The increase in ejection fraction during supine exercise is often associated with an increase in end-diastolic volume in untrained subjects but with a decrease in end-systolic volume in well-trained individuals.[423] During upright exercise in some normal subjects, the increase in ejection fraction is associated with an increase in end-diastolic volume.[424] The ejection fraction may decrease rather than increase during upright exercise in apparently normal individuals over 65 years of age.[425]

Dynamic exercise results in increased sympathetic adrenergic nervous activity to the resistance vessels of the kidney and splanchnic area and to the uninvolved muscles, while increasing blood flow to the exercising muscles by sympathetic vasodilatation and by locally mediated vasodilatation resulting from increased metabolic activity. The increase in sympathetic nervous system activity is roughly proportional to the intensity of exercise. The arterial systolic blood pressure often increases 40 to 60 mmHg during moderate or severe exercise, although the mean arterial blood pressure increases much less. The diastolic pressure changes variably. Calculated total arterial resistance normally decreases considerably during exercise.

An increase in cardiac output is further moderated by an increase in venous return produced by the combination of vasodilatation of the exercising muscles and the increased mechanical activity of the skeletal muscles, which rhythmically compress the peripheral veins, and by the rhythmic increase and decrease of the pressure in the peritoneal and thoracic cavities. The latter is sometimes referred to as the *abdominothoracic pump*. Exercise also produces a decrease in the volume of blood in venous reservoirs, especially the splanchnic blood volume. The result of these shifts makes more blood available to the heart, arterial vessels, and exercising muscles. On the other hand, during prolonged exercise, plasma volume may decrease significantly, with a resultant increase in hematocrit.[426,427] An increase in venous return to the atria may also produce an increase in heart rate by the Bainbridge reflex; this is more apparent in patients with a low resting heart rate or with hypervolemia in

TABLE 5-4
Distribution of Systemic Blood Flow and Oxygen Consumption in a Normal Subject* at Rest in a Comfortable Environment

Circulation	Blood Flow, mL/min	Percentage of Total Flow	AV†O_2 Difference, mL/dL	O_2 Consumption mL/min	Percentage of Total Consumption
Splanchnic	1400	24	4.1	58	25
Renal	1100	19	1.3	16	7
Cerebral	750	13	6.3	46	20
Coronary	250	4	11.4	27	11
Skeletal muscle	1200	21	8.0	70	30
Skin	500	9	1.0	5	2
Other organs	600	10	3.0	12	5
Total	5800	100	4.0	234	100

*Weight, 70 kg; surface area, 1.7 m^2.
†AV = arteriovenous.
SOURCE: Wade OL, Bishop JM: *Cardiac Output and Regional Blood Flow.* Blackwell Scientific, Oxford, 1962. Reproduced with permission from the publisher and authors.

association with hemodilution. Isometric exercises of relatively mild degree may produce significant increases in blood pressure and pulse rate,[428–433] factors of considerable importance in patients with coronary artery disease (see Chaps. 57 and 58).

During exercise, there is a significant redistribution of the elevated cardiac output. During mild-to-moderate dynamic exercise, coronary blood flow and blood flow to the active skeletal muscles increases, and cerebral flow is maintained, whereas renal and splanchnic flows diminish. During more severe exercise, these changes are exaggerated, and flow to the resting skeletal muscles may decrease. During maximal exercise, cerebral flow may also decrease, in association with hyperventilation and respiratory alkalosis. Skin blood flow may decrease initially during exercise, but it increases with continued exercise and contributes to the elimination of body heat. Exercise at high altitude imposes special problems, including sustained stimulation of the sympathetic nervous system.[434]

In general, there is evidence of a generalized sympathetic discharge during exercise that in active muscles is overridden by local endothelial control, vasodilator metabolites, and changes in P_{O_2}, P_{CO_2}, pH, and K^+. In exercising skeletal muscles, there may be increased activity of sympathetic vasodilator fibers in addition to decreased vasoconstrictor activity. Venoconstriction during exercise tends to shift blood toward the central circulation and to the active skeletal muscles. Similar venoconstriction may occur in response to cold, emotion, hyperventilation, or norepinephrine. The plasma levels of both norepinephrine and epinephrine increase during dynamic exercise, but the level of norepinephrine is increased much less during isometric exercise.

REFERENCES

1. Hamilton WF, Dow P (eds): *Handbook of Physiology, sec. 2 Circulation.* Bethesda, MD, American Physiological Society, vols. 1–3, 1962–1965.
2. Braunwald E, Ross J Jr, Sonnenblick EH: *Mechanisms of Contraction of the Normal and Failing Heart,* 2d ed. Boston, Little, Brown, 1976.
3. Berne RM (ed): *Handbook of Physiology, sec. 2: The Cardiovascular System,* vol. 1: *The Heart.* Bethesda, MD, American Physiological Society, 1979.
4. Braunwald E, Ross J Jr: Control of cardiac performance. In: Berne RM (ed): *Handbook of Physiology, sec 2: The Cardiovascular System,* vol. 1: *The Heart.* Bethesda, MD, American Physiological Society, 1979: 533.
5. Shepherd JT, Abboud FM (eds): *Handbook of Physiology, sec 2: The Cardiovascular System,* vol III: *Peripheral Circulation and Organ Blood Flow,* parts 1 and 2. Bethesda, MD, American Physiological Society, 1983.
6. Renkin EM, Michel CC (eds): *Handbook of Physiology, sec. 2: The Cardiovascular System,* vol. IV: *Microcirculation,* Part 1. Bethesda, MD, American Physiological Society, 1984: 1–626.
7. Badeer HS: *Cardiovascular Physiology.* New York, Karger, 1984.
8. Sperelakis N: *Physiology and Pathophysiology of the Heart.* Boston, Martinus Nijhoff, 1984.
9. Nathan RD (ed): *Cardiac Muscle: The Regulation of Excitation and Contraction.* Orlando, Academic Press, 1986.
10. Rupp H: *The Regulation of Heart Function.* New York, Georg Thieme, 1986.
11. Langer GA (ed): *Calcium and the Heart.* New York, Raven, 1990: 1–387.
12. Chien S (ed): *Molecular Biology of the Cardiovascular System.* Philadelphia, Lea & Febiger, 1990: 1–262.
13. Zucker IH, Gilmore JP (eds): *Reflex Control of the Circulation.* Boca Raton, FL, CRC Press, 1991: 1–1053.
14. Opie LH: *The Heart: Physiology, Metabolism, Pharmacology, and Therapy.* Orlando, Grune & Stratton, 1984.
15. Fozzard HA, Haber E, Jennings RB, Katz AM, Morgan HE (eds): *The Heart and Cardiovascular System: Scientific Foundations,* 2d ed. New York, Raven, 1991:1–2193.
16. Katz AM: *Physiology of the Heart.* 2d ed. New York, Raven Press, 1992.
17. Berne RM, Levy MD: *Cardiovascular Physiology,* 6th ed. St. Louis, Mosby Year Book, 1992: 1–298.
18. Loscalzo J, Creager MA, Dzau VJ (eds): *Vascular Medicine.* Boston, Little, Brown, 1992: 1–1211.
19. Langer GA: Calcium at the sarcolemma. *J Mol Cell Cardiol* 1984; 16:147–153.
20. McDonald TF: Excitation-contraction coupling: Relationship of the slow inward current to contraction. In: Sperelakis N (ed): *The Physiology and Pathophysiology of the Heart.* Boston, Martinus Nijhoff, 1984: 187–198.
21. Fabiato A, Baumgarten CM: Methods for detecting calcium release from the sarcoplasmic reticulum of skinned cardiac cells and the relationships between calculated transsarcolemmal calcium movements and calcium release. In: Sperelakis N (ed): *The Physi-*

ology and Pathophysiology of the Heart. Boston, Martinus Nijhoff, 1984: 215–254.

22. Tada M, Shigekawa M, Nimura Y: Uptake of calcium by the sarcoplasmic reticulum and its regulation and functional consequences. In: Sperelakis N (ed): *The Physiology and Pathophysiology of the Heart.* Boston, Martinus Nijhoff, 1984: 255–277.
23. Pierce GN, Rich TL, Langer GA: Trans-sarcolemmal Ca^{2+} movements associated with contraction of the rabbit right ventricular wall. *Circ Res* 1987; 61:805–814.
24. Bers DM (ed): *Excitation-Contraction Coupling and Cardiac Contractile Force.* Boston, Kluwer, 1991: 1–258.
25. Ebashi S: Excitation-contraction and the mechanism of muscle contraction. *Annu Rev Physiol* 1991; 53:1–16.
26. Sheu S-S, Blaustein MP: Sodium/calcium exchange and control of cell calcium and contractility in cardiac and vascular smooth muscles. In: Fozzard HA, Haber E, Jennings RB, Katz AM, Morgan HE (eds): *The Heart and Cardiovascular System,* 2d ed. New York, Raven, 1991: 903–943.
27. Gibbons WR, Zygmunt AC: Excitation-contraction coupling in the heart. In: Fozzard HA, Haber E, Jennings RB, Katz AM, Morgan HE (eds): *The Heart and Cardiovascular System,* 2d ed. New York, Raven, 1991: 1249–1279.
28. Callewaert G: Excitation-contraction coupling in mammalian cardiac cells. *Cardiovasc Res* 1992; 26:923–932.
29. Langer GA: Calcium and the heart: exchange at the tissue, cell, and organelle levels. *FASEB J* 1992; 6:893–902.
30. Ringer S: A further contribution regarding the influence of the different constituents of the blood on the contraction of the heart. *J Physiol (Lond)* 1885; 4:29–42.
31. Coraboeuf E: Ionic basis of electrical activity in cardiac tissue. In: Levy MN, Vassale M (eds): *Excitation and Neutral Control of the Heart.* Baltimore, Williams & Wilkins, 1982: 1–35.
32. Glitsch HG: Characteristics of active sodium transport in intact cardiac cells. In: Levy MN, Vassale M (eds): *Excitation and Neural Control of the Heart.* Baltimore, Williams & Wilkins, 1982: 36.
33. Philipson KD, Bers DM, Nashimoto AY, Langer GA: Binding of Ca^{2+} and Na^{+} to sarceblemmal membranes: Relating to control of myocardial contractility. *Am J Physiol* 1980; 238: H373–378.
34. McDonald T: Excitation-contraction coupling: Relation of the slow inward current to contraction. *J Gen Physiol* 1985; 85:187.
35. Lehninger AL: Ca^{2+} transport by mitochondria and its possible role in the cardiac contraction-relaxation cycle. *Circ Res* 1974; 35(suppl 3):83–90.
36. Carafoli E, Tiozzo R, Lugli G, Crovetti F, Kratzing C: The release of calcium from heart mitochondria by sodium. *J Mol Cell Cardiol* 1974; 6:361–371.
37. Sperelakis N: The slow action potential and properties of the myocardial slow channels. *J Gen Physiol* 1985; 85:159.
38. Winegrad S: Regulation of cardiac contractile proteins. *Circ Res* 1984; 55:565–574.
39. Carofoli E: The homeostasis of calcium in heart cells. *J Mol Cell Cardiol* 1985; 17:203–212.
40. Carafoli E: The intracellular homeostasis of calcium: An overview. *Ann N Y Acad Sci* 1988; 551:147–157.
41. LePeuch CJ, Demaille JG: Covalent regulation of the cardiac sarcoplasmic reticulum calcium pump. Review article. *Cell Calcium* 1989; 10:397–400.
42. Schatzmann HJ: The calcium pump at the surface membrane and at the sarcoplasmic reticulum. *Annu Rev Physiol* 1989; 51:473–485.
43. Carafoli E: Calcium pump of the plasma membrane. *Physiol Rev* 1991; 71:129–153.
44. Missiaen L, Waytack F, Raeymaekers L, Demedt H, Droogmans G, Declerck I, et al: Ca^{2+} extrusion across plasma membrane and Ca^{2+} uptake by intracellular stores. *Pharmacol Ther* 1991; 50:191–232.
45. Caroni P, Carafoli E: The Ca^{++}-pumping ATPase of heart sarcolemma. *J Biol Chem* 1981; 256:3263–3270.
46. Siri FM, Kruoger J, Nordin C, Ming Z, Aronson RS: Depressed intracellular calcium transients and contractions in myocytes from hypertrophied and failing guinea pig hearts. *Am J Physiol* 1991; 26:H514–H540.
47. Barry WH, Biedert S, Miura DS, Smith TW: Changes in cellular Na, K, and Ca contents, monovalent cation transport rate, and contractile state during washout of cardiac glycosides from cultured chick heart cells. *Circ Res* 1981; 49:141–149.
48. Mullins LJ: The role of Na-Ca exchange in heart. In: Sperelakis N (ed): *The Physiology and Pathophysiology of the Heart.* Boston, Martinus Nijhoff, 1984: 199–214.
49. Eisner DA, Smith TW: The Na-K pump and its effectors in cardiac muscle. In: Fozzard HA, Haber E, Jennings RB, Katz AM, Morgan HE (eds): *The Heart and Cardiovascular System,* 2d ed. New York, Raven, 1991: 863–902.
50. Smith TW: Digitalis: Mechanisms of action and clinical use. *N Engl J Med* 1988; 318:358–365.
51. Hicks MJ, Shigekawa M, Katz AM: Mechanism by which cyclic adenosine 3′:5′-monophosphate-dependent protein kinase stimulates calcium transport in cardiac sarcoplasmic reticulum. *Circ Res* 1979; 44:384–391.
52. Sperelakis N: Cyclic AMP and phosphorylation in regulation of CA^{++} influx into myocardial cells and blockade by calcium antagonistic drugs. *Am Heart J* 1984; 107:347–357.
53. Colucci WS, Wright RF, Braunwald E: New positive inotropic agents in the treatment of congestive heart failure. *N Engl J Med* 1986; 314:290, 349–358.
54. Vatner SA: Sympathetic mechanisms regulating myocardial contractility in conscious animals. In: Fozzard HA, Haber E, Jennings RB, Katz AM, Morgan HE (eds): *The Heart and Cardiovascular System,* 2d ed. New York, Raven, 1991: 1709–1728.
55. Williamson JR, Monck JR: Second messengers of inositol lipid metabolism and Ca^{2+} signaling. In: Fozzard HA, Haber E, Jennings RB, Katz AM, Morgan HE (eds): *The Heart and Cardiovascular System,* 2d ed. New York, Raven, 1991: 1729–1744.
56. Koch-Weser J, Blinks JR: The influence of the interval between beats on myocardial contractility. *Pharmacol Rev* 1963; 15:601–652.
57. Covell JW, Ross J Jr, Taylor R, Sonnenblick EH, Braunwald E: Effects of increasing frequency of contraction on the force-velocity relation of left ventricle. *Cardiovasc Res* 1967; 1:2–8.
58. Arentzen CE, Rankin JS, Anderson PAW, Feezor MD, Anderson RW: Force-frequency characteristics of the left ventricle in the conscious dog. *Circ Res* 1978; 42:64–71.
59. Johnson EA: Force-interval relationship of cardiac muscle. In: Berne RM (ed): *Handbook of Physiology, sec 2: The Cardiovascular System,* vol 1: *The Heart.* Bethesda, MD, American Physiological Society, 1979: 475–496.
60. Braunwald E, Sonnenblick EH, Frommer PL, Ross J Jr: Paired electrical stimulation of the heart: Physiologic observations and clinical implications. *Adv Intern Med* 1967; 13:61–96.
61. Hoffman BF, Bindler E, Suckling EE: Postextrasystolic potentiation of contraction in cardiac muscle. *Am J Physiol* 1956; 185:95–102.
62. Braunwald E: Mechanisms of action of calcium channel blocking agents. *N Engl J Med* 307:1618–1627.
63. Watanabe AM, Lindemann JP: Mechanisms of adrenergic and cholinergic regulation of myocardial contractility. In: Sperelakis N (ed): *Physiology and Pathophysiology of the Heart.* Boston. Martinus Nijhoff, 1984: 377–404.
64. Fabiato A, Fabiato F: Effects of pH on the myofilaments and sarcoplasmic reticulum of skinned cells from cardiac and skeletal muscles. *J Physiol* 1978; 276:233–255.
65. Eisner DA, Lederer WJ, Vaughan-Jones RD: The quantitative relationship between twitch tension and intracellular sodium activity in sheep cardiac Purkinje fibers. *J Physiol (Lond)* 1984; 355:251–266.
66. Allen DG, Kentish JG: The cellular basis of the length-tension relation in cardiac muscle. *J Mol Cell Cardiol* 1985; 17:821–840.
67. Hoh JFY, Rossmanith GH, Kwan LJ, Hamilton AM: Adrenaline increases the rate of cycling of crossbridges in rat cardiac muscle as measured by pseudo-random binary noise-modulated perturbation analysis. *Circ Res* 1988;62:452–461.
68. LaKatta EG: Starling's law of the heart is explained by an intimate interaction of muscle length and myofilament calcium interaction. *J Am Coll Cardiol* 1987; 10:1157–1164.
69. Babu A, Sonnenblick EH, Gulati J: Molecular basis for the influence of muscle length on myocardial performance. 1988; 240:74–76.
70. Lakatta EG: Length modulation of muscle performance: Frank-Starling law of the heart. In: Fozzard HA, Haber E, Jennings RB, Katz AM, Morgan HE (eds): *The Heart and Cardiovascular System,* 2d ed. New York, Raven, 1991: 1325–1351.
71. Brutsaert DL, Sonnenblick EH: Cardiac muscle mechanics in the evaluation of myocardial contractility and pump function:

Problems, concepts and directions. *Prog Cardiovasc Dis* 1973; 16:337–361.
72. Sonnenblick EH: Implications of muscle mechanics in the heart. *Fed Proc* 1962; 21:975–990.
73. Sonnenblick EH: Instantaneous force-velocity-length determinants in the contraction of heart muscle. *Circ Res* 1965; 16:441.
74. Sonnenblick EH: Braunwald E, Morrow AG: The contractile properties of human heart muscle: Studies on myocardial mechanics of surgically excised papillary muscles. *J Clin Invest* 1965; 44:966-977.
75. Glick G, Sonnenblick EH, Braunwald E: Myocardial force-velocity relations studied in intact unanesthetized man. *J Clin Invest* 1965; 44:978–988.
76. Sonnenblick EH, Braunwald E, Williams JF Jr, Glick G: Effects of exercise on myocardial force-velocity relations in intact unanesthetized man: Relative roles of changes in heart rate, sympathetic activity, and ventricular dimensions. *J Clin Invest* 1965; 44:2051–2062.
77. Sonnenblick EH: The mechanics of myocardial contraction. In: Briller SA, Conn HL Jr (eds): *The Myocardial Cell: Structure, Function and Modification by Cardiac Drugs.* Philadelphia, University of Pennsylvania Press, 1966: 173–250.
78. Sonnenblick EH, Morrow AG, Williams JF Jr: Effects of heart rate on the dynamics of force development in the intact human ventricle. *Circulation* 1966; 33:945–951.
79. Covell JW, Ross J Jr, Sonnenblick EH, Braunwald E: Comparison of the force-velocity relation and the ventricular function curve as measures of the contractile state of the intact heart. *Circ Res* 1966; 19:364–372.
80. Braunwald E, Sonnenblick EH, Ross J Jr, Gault JH: Insights into cardiovascular physiology derived from muscle mechanics. *Am J Cardiol* 1967; 20:705–711.
81. Pool PE, Sonnenblick EH: Mechanochemistry of heart muscle: I. The isometric contraction. *J Gen Physiol* 1967; 50:951–965.
82. Gault JH, Ross J Jr, Braunwald E: Contractile state of the left ventricle in man: Instantaneous tension-velocity-length relations in patients with and without disease of the left ventricular myocardium. *Circ Res* 1968; 22:451–463.
83. Pool PE, Chandler BM, Seagren SC, Sonnenblick EH: Mechanochemistry of cardiac muscle: II. The isotonic contraction. *Circ Res* 1968; 22:465–472.
84. Barns JW, Covell JW, Ross J Jr: The mechanics of isotonic left ventricular contractions. *Am J Physiol* 1973; 224:725–732.
85. Langer GE, Brady AJ: *The Mammalian Myocardium.* New York, John Wiley, 1974.
86. Mahler F, Ross J Jr, O'Rourke RA, Covell JW: Effects of changes in preload, afterload and inotropic state on ejection and isovolumic phase measures of contractility in the conscious dog. *Am J Cardiol* 1975; 35:626–634.
87. Skelton CL, Sonnenblick EH: Physiology of cardiac muscle. In: Levine JH (ed): *Clinical Cardiovascular Physiology.* New York, Grune & Stratton, 1976: 57–120.
88. Jewell BR: A reexamination of the influence of muscle length on myocardial performance. *Circ Res* 1977; 40:221–230.
89. Alpert NR, Hamrell BB, Mulieri LA: Heart muscle mechanics. *Annu Rev Physiol* 1979; 41:521–537.
90. Brady AJ: Mechanical properties of cardiac fibers. In: Berne RM (ed): *Handbook of Physiology, sec 2: The Cardiovascular System,* vol 1: *The Heart.* Bethesda, MD, American Physiological Society, 1979: 461–474.
91. Strobeck JE, Sonnenblick EH: Myocardial contractile properties and ventricular performance. In: Fozzard HA, Haber E, Jennings RB, Katz AM, Morgan HE (eds): *The Heart and Cardiovascular System: Scientific Foundations.* New York, Raven Press, 1986: 31–49.
92. Shroff SG, Janick JS, Weber KT: Mechanical and energetic behavior of the intact left ventricle. In: Fozzard HA, Haber E, Jennings RB, Katz AM, Morgan HE (eds): *The Heart and Cardiovascular System,* 2d ed. New York, Raven, 1991: 129–150.
93. Grossman W, Lorell BH (eds): *Diastolic Relaxation of the Heart: Basic Research and Current Applications for Clinical Cardiology.* Boston, Martinus Nijhoff, 1988: 1–310.
94. Hill AV: The heat of shortening and the dynamic constants of muscle. *Proc R Soc London Ser B* 1938: 126: 136–195.
95. Hill AV: *First and Last Experiments in Muscle Mechanics.* Cambridge, University Press, 1970: 141.
96. Bowditch HP: Ueber die Eigenthumlichkeiten der Reizbarkeit, welche die Muskelfasern des Herzens zeigen. *Verh K Sachs Ges Wochenshr, Leipzig Math Phys Cl* 1871; 23:652.
97. Howell WH, Donaldson F Jr: Experiments upon the heart of the dog with reference to maximum volume of blood sent out by left ventricle in a single beat. *Philos Trans R Soc London Ser B* 1884; 175:139.
98. Frank O: Zur Dynamik des Herzmuskels. *Z Biol* 1895; 32:370; Chapman CB, Wasserman E (trans), *Am Heart J* 58:282–317, 467–478.
99. Fick A: Mechanische Arbeit und Warmeentwickelung bei der Muskeltatigheit, Leipzig, FA Brockhaus, 1882.
100. Kries J von: Untersuchungen zur Mechanik der quergestreiften Muskels. *Arch Physiol Leipzig* 1885; 67:348–374.
101. Blix M: Die Lange und die Spannung des Muskels. *Skand Arch Physiol* 1895; 5:173.
102. Wiggers CJ: Some factors controlling the shape of the pressure curve in the right ventricle. *Am J Physiol* 1914; 33:382–396.
103. Straub H: I. Dynamik des Saugetierherzens; II. Mitteilung Dynamik des Rechten Herzens. *Dtsch Arch Klin Med* 1914; 115:531–595, 116:409–436.
104. Patterson SW, Starling EH: On the mechanical factors which determine the output of the ventricles. *J Physiol* 1914; 48:357–379.
105. Patterson SW, Piper H, Starling EH: The regulation of the heart beat. *J Physiol* 1914; 48:465–513.
106. Starling EH: *The Linacre Lecture on the Law of the Heart.* London, Longman, Green, 1918.
107. Wiggers CJ: Determinants of cardiac performance. *Circulation* 1951; 4:485–495.
108. Strobeck JE, Krueger J, Sonnenblick EH: Load and time considerations in the force-length relations of cardiac muscle. *Fed Proc* 1980; 39:175–182.
109. Sarnoff SJ, Berglund E: Ventricular function: I. Starling's law of the heart studied by means of simultaneous right and left ventricular function curves in the dog. *Circulation* 1954; 9:706–718.
110. Sarnoff SJ: Myocardial contractility as described by ventricular function curves: Observations on Starling's law of the heart. *Physiol Rev* 1955; 35:107–122.
111. Braunwald E, Ross J Jr: Applicability of Starling's law of the heart to man. In: Evans Jr (guest ed): Symposium: Structure and function of heart muscle. *Circ Res* 1964; 15(suppl 2): 169–178.
112. Braunwald E: The control of ventricular function in man. *Br Heart J* 1965; 27:1–16.
113. Levine HJ: Compliance of the left ventricle. *Circulation* 1972; 46:423–426.
114. Gaasch WH, Cole JS, Quinones MA, Alexander JK: Dynamic determinants of left ventricular diastolic pressure-volume relations in man. *Circulation* 1975; 51:317–323.
115. Mirsky I: Assessment of passive elastic stiffness of cardiac muscle: Mathematical concepts, physiologic and clinical considerations, directions for future research. *Prog Cardiovasc Dis* 1976; 18:277–308.
116. Grossman W, McLaurin LP: Diastolic properties of the left ventricle. *Ann Intern Med* 1976; 84:316–326.
117. Gaasch WH, Levine HJ, Quinones MA, Alexander JK: Left ventricular compliance: Mechanisms and clinical implications. *Am J Cardiol* 1976; 38:645–653.
118. Nayler WG, Williams A: Relaxation in heart muscle: Some morphological and biochemical considerations. *Eur J Cardiol* 1978; 7(suppl):35–50.
119. Mirsky I: Elastic properties of the myocardium: A quantitative approach with physiological and clinical applications. In: Berne RM (ed): *Handbook of Physiology, sec 2: The Cardiovascular System,* vol 1: *The Heart.* Bethesda, MD, American Physiological Society, 1979; 497–531.
120. Smith V-E, Zile MR: Relaxation and diastolic properties of the heart. In: Fozzard HA, Haber E, Jennings RB, Katz AM, Morgan HE (eds): *The Heart and Cardiovascular System,* 2d ed. New York, Raven, 1991: 1353–1367.
121. Grossman W, Lorell BH (eds): *Diastolic Relaxation of the Heart: Basic Research and Current Applications for Clinical Cardiology.* Boston, Martinus Nijhoff, 1988.
122. Weisfeldt ML, Loeven WA, Shock NW: Resting and active mechanical properties of trabeculae carneae from aged male rats. *Am J Physiol* 1971; 220:1921–1927.
123. Olivetti G, Melissari M, Capasso JM, Anversa P: Cardiomyopa-

thy of the aging human heart: Myocyte loss and reactive cellular hypertrophy. *Circ Res* 1991; 68:1560–1568.

124. Nakamura Y, Wiegner AW, Bing OHL: Measurement of relaxation in isolated rat ventricular myocardium during hypoxia and reoxygenation. *Cardiovasc Res* 1986; 20:690–697.
125. Blaustein AS, Gaasch WH: Myocardial relaxation: VI. Effects of adrenergic tone and asynchrony on LV relaxation rate. *Am J Physiol* 1983; 244:H417–422.
126. Hori M, Inoue M, Kitakaze M, Tsujioka K, Ishida Y, Fukunami M: Loading sequence is a major determinant of afterload-dependent relaxation in intact canine heart. *Am J Physiol* 1985; 249:H747–754.
127. Gaasch WH, Ariel Y, McMahon TA: Dynamics of left ventricular diastolic filling abstr. *J Am Coll Cardiol* 1986; 7:243A.
128. Hanrath P, Mathey DG, Kremer P, Sonntag F, Bleifeld W: Effect of verapamil on left ventricular isovolumic relaxation time and regional left ventricular filling in hypertrophic cardiomyopathy. *Am J Cardiol* 1980; 45:1258–1264.
129. Lorell BH, Paulus WJ, Grossman W: Modification of abnormal left ventricular diastolic properties by nifedipine in patients with hypertrophic cardiomyopathy. *Circulation* 1982; 65:499–507.
130. Suwa M, Hirota Y, Kawamura K: Improvement in left ventricular diastolic function during intravenous and oral diltiazem therapy in patients with hypertrophic cardiomyopathy: An echocardiographic study. *Am J Cardiol* 1984; 54:1047–1053.
131. Bahler RC, Martin P: Effects of loading conditions and inotropic state on rapid filling phase of left ventricle. *Am J Physiol* 1985; 248:H523–533.
132. Heyndrickx GR, Vantrimpont PJ, Rousseau MF, Pouleur H: Effects of asynchrony on myocardial relaxation at rest and during exercise in conscious dogs. *Am J Physiol* 1988:254 (*Heart Circ Physiol* 23): H817–H822.
133. Taylor RR, Covell JW, Sonnenblick EH, Ross J Jr: The independence of ventricular distensibility in the filling of the opposite ventricle. *Am J Physiol* 1967; 213:711–718.
134. Bemis CE, Serur JR, Borkenhagen D, Sonnenblick EH, Urschel CW: Influence of right ventricular filling pressure on left ventricular pressure and dimension. *Circ Res* 1974; 34:498–504.
135. Shirato K, Shabetai R, Bhargava V, Franklin D, Ross J Jr: Alteration of the left ventricular diastolic pressure-segment length relation produced by the pericardium: Effects of cardiac distention and afterload reduction in conscious dogs. *Circulation* 1978; 57:1191–1198.
136. LeWinter MM, Pavelec R: Influence of the pericardium on left ventricular end-diastolic pressure-segment relations during early and late stages of experimental chronic volume overload in dogs. *Circ Res* 1981; 50:501–509.
137. Bhargava V, Shabetai R, Ross J Jr, Pavelec RS, Mason PA: Influence of the pericardium on left ventricular diastolic pressure-volume curves in dogs with sustained volume overload. *Am Heart J* 1983; 105:995–1001.
138. Hess OM, Bhargava V, Ross J Jr, Shabetai R: The role of the pericardium in interactions between the cardiac chambers. *Am Heart J* 1983; 106:1377–1383.
139. Little WC, Badke FR, O'Rourke RA: Effect of right ventricular pressure on the end-diastolic left ventricular pressure-volume relationship before and after chronic right ventricular pressure overload in dogs without pericardia. *Circ Res* 1984; 54:719–730.
140. Braunwald E, Ross J Jr: The ventricular end-diastolic pressure appraisal of its value in the recognition of ventricular failure in man. *Am J Med* 1963; 34:147–150.
141. DiDonna G, LeWinter M, Johnson A, Peterson K: Effects of left ventricular hypertrophy on diastolic wall stiffness. *Circulation* 1974; 50(suppl 3):45–49.
142. Smith VE, Katz AM: Inotropic and lusitropic abnormalities in the genesis of heart failure. *Eur Heart J* 1983; 4 (suppl A):7–17.
143. Katz AM: The descending limb of the Starling curve and the failing heart. *Circulation* 1965; 32:871–875.
144. Monroe RG, Gamble WJ, LaFarge CG, Kumar AE, Manasek FJ: Left ventricular performance at high end-diastolic pressures in isolated perfused dog hearts. *Circ Res* 1970; 26:85–99.
145. Ross J Jr, Sonnenblick EH, Taylor RR, Spotnitz HM, Spiro D: Diastolic geometry and sarcomere lengths in the chronically dilated canine left ventricle. *Circ Res* 1971; 28:49–61.
146. MacGregor DC, Covell JW, Mahler F, Dilley RB, Ross J Jr: Relations between afterload, stroke volume, and the descending limb of Starling's curve. *Am J Physiol* 1974; 227:884–890.
147. Sonnenblick EH, Spotnitz HM, Spiro D: Role of the sarcomere in ventricular function and the mechanism of heart failure. *Circ Res* 1964; 15(suppl 2):70–80.
148. Spiro D, Sonnenblick EH: The structural basis of the contractile process in heart muscle under physiological and pathological conditions. *Prog Cardiovasc Dis* 1965; 7:295–335.
149. Spiro D: The fine structure and contractile mechanism of heart muscle. In: Briller SA, Conn HL Jr (eds): *The Myocardial Cell: Structure, Function, and Modification by Cardiac Drugs.* Philadelphia, University of Pennsylvania Press, 1966: 13.
150. Ross J Jr, Sonnenblick EH, Covell JW, Kaiser G, Spiro D: Architecture of the heart in systole and diastole: Technique for rapid fixation and analysis of left ventricular geometry. *Circ Res* 1967; 21:409–421.
151. Sonnenblick EH, Ross J Jr, Covell JW, Spotnitz HM, Spiro D: The ultrastructure of the heart in systole and diastole: Changes in sarcomere length. *Circ Res* 1967; 21:423–431.
152. Sonnenblick EH, Ross J Jr: Some ultrastructural considerations in myocardial failure: Sarcomere overextension and length dispersion. In: Tanz RD, Kavaler F, Roberts J (eds): *Factors Influencing Myocardial Contractility.* New York, Academic Press, 1967: 43–48.
153. Leyton RA, Sonnenblick EH: The sarcomere as the basis of Starling's law of the heart in the left and right ventricles. In: Bajusz E, Jasmin G (eds): *Methods and Achievements in Experimental Pathology,* vol 5, Basel, S Karger AG, 1971: 22–59.
154. Yoran C, Covell JW, Ross J Jr: Structural basis for the ascending limb of left ventricular function. *Circ Res* 1973; 32:297–303.
155. Sonnenblick EH, Skelton CL: Reconsideration of the ultrastructural basis of cardiac length-tension relations. *Circ Res* 1974; 35:517–526.
156. Skelton CL, Sponitz WW, Feldman D, Serur JR, Mirsky I, Sonnenblick EH: Ultrastructural and functional correlates of acute cardiac distension. (abstr). *Clin Res* 1974; 22:304a.
157. Sommer JR, Jennings RB: Ultrastructure of cardiac muscle. In: Fozzard HA, Haber E, Jennings RB, Katz AM, Morgan HE (eds): *The Heart and Cardiovascular System: Scientific Foundations* 2d ed. New York, Raven Press, 1991:3–50.
158. Allen DG, Kurihara S: Calcium transients at different muscle length in rat ventricular muscle. *J Physiol (Lond)* 1979; 292:68P–69P.
159. Dodge HT, Frimer M, Stewart DK: Functional evaluation of the hypertrophied heart in man. *Circ Res* 1974; 35(suppl 2):122–127.
160. Sonnenblick EH: Series elastic and contractile elements in heart muscle: Changes in muscle length. *Am J Physiol* 1964; 207:1330–1338.
161. Higgins CB, Vatner SF, Franklin D, Braunwald E: Extent of regulation of the heart's contractile state in the conscious dog by alteration in the frequency of contraction. *J Clin Invest* 1973; 52:1187–1194.
162. Mahler F, Yoran C, Ross J Jr: Inotropic effect of tachycardia and poststimulation potentiation in the conscious dog. *Am J Physiol* 1974; 227:569–575.
163. Imperial ES, Levy MN, Zieske HJ Jr: Outflow resistance as an independent determinant of cardiac performance. *Circ Res* 1961; 9:1145–1155.
164. Sarnoff SJ, Mitchell JH: The control of the function of the heart. In: Hamilton WF, Dow P (eds): *Handbook of Physiology, sec 2: Circulation,* vol 1. Bethesda, MD, American Physiological Society, 1962: 489.
165. Sonnenblick EH, Downing SE: Afterload as a primary determinant of ventricular performance. *Am J Physiol* 1963; 204:604–610.
166. Levine HJ, Forwand SA, McIntyre KM, Schechter E: Effect of afterload on force-velocity relations and contractile element work in the intact dog heart. *Circ Res* 1966; 18:729–744.
167. Evans GL, Smulyan H, Eich RH: Role of peripheral resistance in the control of cardiac output. *Am J Cardiol* 1967; 20:216–221.
168. Urschel CW, Covell JW, Sonnenblick EH, Ross J Jr, Braunwald E: Myocardial mechanics in aortic and mitral valvular regurgitation: The concept of instantaneous impedance as a determinant of the performance of the heart. *J Clin Invest* 1968; 47:867–883.
169. Milnor WR: Arterial impedance as ventricular afterload. *Circ Res* 1975; 36:565–570.

170. Ross J Jr: Mechanisms of cardiac contraction. What roles for preload, afterload and inotropic state in heart failure? *Eur Heart J* 1983; 4(suppl A):19–28.
171. Von Anrep G: On the part played by suprarenals in the normal vascular reactions of the body. *J Physiol* 1912; 45:307–317.
172. Vatner SF, Monroe RG, McRitchie RJ: Effects of anesthesia tachycardia and autonomic blockade on Anrep effect in intact dogs. *Am J Physiol* 1974; 226:1450–1456.
173. Brutsaert DL, Sonnenblick EH: Force-velocity-length-time relations of the contractile elements in heart muscle of the cat. *Circ Res* 1969; 24:137–149.
174. Brutsaert DL, Claes VA, Sonnenblick EH: Effects of abrupt load alterations on force-velocity-length and time relations during isotonic contractions of heart muscle: Load clamping. *J Physiol* 1971; 216:319–330.
175. Noble MIM: Problems concerning the application of concepts of muscle mechanics to the determination of the contractile state of the heart. *Circulation* 1972; 45:252–255.
176. Peterson KL, Skloven D, Ludbrook P, Uther JB, Ross J Jr: Comparison of isovolumic and ejection phase indices of myocardial performance in man. *Circulation* 1974; 49:1088–1101.
177. Brady AJ: Mechanics of the myocardium. In: Langer GA, Brady AJ (eds): *The Mammalian Myocardium.* New York, John Wiley, 1974: 163–192.
178. Sonnenblick EH, Strobeck JE: Derived indices of ventricular and myocardial function. *N Engl J Med* 1977; 296:978–982.
179. Brady N: Contractile and mechanical properties of the myocardium. In: Sperelakis N (ed): *The Physiology and Pathophysiology of the Heart.* Boston, Martinus Nijhoff, 1984: 279–299.
180. Abbott BC, Mommaerts WFHM: A study of inotropic mechanisms in the papillary muscle preparation. *J Gen Physiol* 1959; 42:533–551.
181. Tanz RD, Kavaler F, Roberts J (eds): *Factors Influencing Myocardial Contractility.* New York, Academic Press, 1967.
182. Mehmel HC, Stocking B, Ruffmann K, von-Olshausen K, Schuler G, Kubler W: The linearity of the end-systolic pressure-volume relationship in man and its sensitivity for assessment of left ventricular function. *Circulation* 1981; 63:1216–1222.
183. Sagawa K: The end systolic pressure-volume relation of the ventricle: Definition, modifications and clinical use. *Circulation* 1981; 63:1223–1227.
184. McKay RG, Aroesty JM, Heller GV, Royal H, Parker JA, Silverman KJ, et al: Left ventricular pressure-volume diagrams and end-systolic pressure-volume relations in human beings. *J Am Coll Cardiol* 1984; 3:301–312.
185. Maughan WL, Sunagawa K, Burkhoff D, Sagawak K: Effect of arterial impedance changes on end-systolic pressure-volume relation. *Circ Res* 1984; 54:595–602.
186. Kaseda S, Tomoike H, Ogaa I, Ogata I, Nakamura M: End-systolic pressure-volume, pressure-length, and stress-strain relations in canine hearts. *Am J Physiol* 1985; 18:H648–654.
187. Lee J, Tajimi T, Widmann TF, Lee JD, Tajimi T, Widmann TF, Ross J Jr: Application of end-systolic pressure-volume and pressure-wall thickness relations in conscious dogs. *J Am Coll Cardiol* 1987; 9:136–146.
188. Freeman GL, Little WC, O'Rourke RA: Influence of heart rate on left ventricular performance in conscious dogs. *Circ Res* 1987; 61:455–464.
189. Parmley WW, Sonnenblick EH: Relation between mechanics of contraction and relaxation in mammalian cardiac muscle. *Am J Physiol* 1969; 216:1084–1091.
190. Cohn PF, Liedtke AJ, Serur J, Sonnenblick EH, Urschel CW: Maximal rate of pressure fall (negative *dP/dt*) during ventricular relaxation. *Cardiovasc Res* 1972; 6:263–267.
191. Weisfeldt ML, Scully HE, Frederiksen J, Rubenstein JJ, Pohost GM, Beierholm E, et al: Hemodynamic determinants of maximum negative *DP/DT* and the periods of diastole. *Am J Physiol* 1974; 227:613–621.
192. Strobeck JE, Bahler AS, Sonnenblick EH: Isotonic relaxation in cardiac muscle. *Am J Physiol* 1975; 229:646–651.
193. Brutsaert DL, Rademakers FE, Sys SU, Gillebert TC, Housmans PR: Analysis of relaxation in the evaluation of ventricular function of the heart. *Prog Cardiovasc Dis* 1985; 28:143–163.
194. Chemla D, Lecarpentier Y, Martin JL, Clerque R, Antonetti A, Hatt P: Relationship between inotropy and relaxation in rat myocardium. *Am J Physiol* 1986; 250:H1008–H1016.
195. Vatner SF, Braunwald E: Cardiovascular control mechanisms in the conscious state. *N Engl J Med* 1975; 293:970–976.
196. Woodworth RS: Maximal contraction, staircase contraction, refractory period, and compensatory pause of the heart. *Am J Physiol* 1902; 8:213–249.
197. Hajdu S: Mechanism of the Woodworth staircase phenomenon in heart and skeletal muscle. *Am J Physiol* 1969; 216:206–214.
198. Hawthorne EW: Instantaneous dimensional changes of the left ventricle in dogs. *Circ Res* 1961; 9:110.
199. Schlant RC, Dixon F, Elson SH, Rawls WJ, Williamson FR Jr: Modification of the law of the heart: Influence of early contracting areas. (abstract). *Circulation* 1964; 30 (suppl 3): 153.
200. Schlant RC, Rawls WJ, Dixon F, Elson S: An additional determinant of ventricular performance (abstract). *Clin Res* 1965; 13:62.
201. Schlant RC: Idoventricular kick (abstract). *Circulation* 1966; 34(suppl 3):209.
202. Brecher GA: Experimental evidence of ventricular diastolic suction. *Circ Res* 1956; 4:513–518.
203. Sonnenblick EH: The structural basis and importance of restoring forces and elastic recoil for the filling of the heart. *Eur Heart J* 1980; 1(suppl A): 107–110.
204. Mitchell JH, Gilmore JP, Sarnoff SJ: The transport function of the atrium: Factors influencing the relation between mean left atrial pressure and left ventricular end diastolic pressure. *Am J Cardiol* 1962; 9:237–247.
205. Brecher GA, Galletti PM: Functional anatomy of cardiac pumping. In: Hamilton WF, Dow P (eds): *Handbook of Physiology, sec 2: Circulation,* vol 2. Bethesda, MD, American Physiological Society, 1963: 759–798.
206. Braunwald E: Hemodynamic significance of atrial systole. *Am J Med* 1964; 37:778–779.
207. Burchell HB: A clinical appraisal of atrial transport function. *Lancet* 1964; 1:775.
208. Williams JF Jr, Sonnenblick EH, Braunwald E: Determinants of atrial contractile force in the intact heart. *Am J Physiol* 1965; 209:1061–1068.
209. Mitchell JH, Gupta DN, Payne RM: Influence of atrial systole on effective ventricular stroke volume. *Circ Res* 1965; 17:11–18.
210. Dietz JR: Release of natriuretic factor from rat heart-lung preparations by atrial distention. *Am J Physiol* 1984; 247:R1093–1096.
211. Debold AJ: Atrial natriuretic factor: A hormone produced by the heart. *Science* 1985; 230:767–770.
212. Yamaji T, Ishibashi M, Takaka F: Atrial natriuretic factor in human blood. *J Clin Invest* 1985; 76:1705–1709.
213. Tikkanen I, Fyhrquist F, Metsarinne K, Leidenius R: Plasma atrial natriuretic peptide in cardiac disease and during infusion in healthy volunteers. *Lancet* 1985; 2:66–69.
214. Espiner EA, Crozier IG, Nicholls MG, Cuneo R, Yondle TG, Ikram H: Cardiac secretion of atrial natriuretic peptide. *Lancet* 1985; 2: 398–399.
215. Ballermann BJ, Brenner BM: Role of atrial peptides in body fluid homeostasis. *Circ Res* 1986; 58:619–630.
216. Raine AE, Erne P, Burgisser E, Muller FB, Bolli P, Burkart F, et al: Atrial natriuretic peptide and atrial pressure in patients with congestive heart failure. *N Engl J Med* 1986; 315:533–537.
217. Mulrow PJ, Schrier R (eds): *Atrial Hormones and Other Natriuretic Factors.* Bethesda, MD, American Physiological Society, 1987: 1–178.
218. Genest J, Cantin M: Atrial natriuretic factor. *Circulation* 1987; 75(suppl 1): 118–124.
219. Wildey GM, Misono KS, Graham RM: Atrial natriuretic factor: Biosynthesis and mechanisms of action. In: Fozzard HA, Haber E, Jennings RB, Katz AM, Morgan HE (eds): *The Heart and Cardiovascular System,* 2d ed. New York, Raven, 1991: 1777–1796.
220. Currie MG, Geller DM, Cole BR, Boylan JG, Yu Seng W, Holmberg SW, et al: Bioactive cardiac substances: Potent vasorelaxant activity in mammalian atria. *Science* 1983; 221:71–73.
221. Atarashi K, Mulrow PJ, Franco-Saenz R, Snajdar R, Rapp J: Inhibition of aldosterone production by an atrial extract. *Science* 1984; 224:992–994.
222. Levy MN, Martin PJ: Neural control of the heart. In: Berne RM (ed): *Handbook of Physiology, sec 2: The Cardiovascular System* vol 1: *The Heart.* Bethesda, MD, American Physiological Society, 1979: 581–620.

223. Brown AM: Cardiac reflexes. In: Berne RM (ed): *Handbook of Physiology, sec 2: The Cardiovascular System,* vol 1: *The Heart.* Bethesda, MD, American Physiological Society, 1979: 677–689.
224. Korner PI: Central nervous control of autonomic cardiovascular function. In: Berne RM (ed): *Handbook of Physiology, sec 2: The Cardiovascular System,* vol 1: *The Heart.* Bethesda, MD, American Physiological Society, 1979: 691.
225. Mancia G, Mark AL: Arterial baroreceptors in humans. In: Shepherd JT, Abboud FM (eds): *Handbook of Physiology, sec 2: The Cardiovascular System,* vol III: *Peripheral Circulation and Organ Blood Flow,* part 2. Bethesda, MD, American Physiological Society, 1983: 755–793.
226. Randall WC (ed): *Nervous Control of Cardiovascular Function.* New York, Oxford University Press, 1984.
227. Armour JA: Anatomy and function of the intrathoracic neurons regulating the mammalian heart. In: Fozzard HA, Haber E, Jennings RB, Katz AM, Morgan HE (eds): *The Heart and Cardiovascular System,* 2d ed. New York, Raven, 1991: 1–37.
228. Hainsworth R: Reflexes from the heart. *Physiol Rev* 1991; 71:617–658.
229. Susanni EE, Vatner DE, Homcy CJ: The beta-adrenergic receptor/adenylyl cyclase system. In: Fozzard HA, Haber E, Jennings RB, Katz AM, Morgan HE (eds): *The Heart and Cardiovascular System,* 2d ed. New York, Raven, 1991: 1685–1708.
230. Sutherland EW: On the biological role of cyclic AMP. *JAMA* 1970; 214:1281–1288.
231. DeGeest H, Levy MN, Zieske H, et al: Depression of ventricular contractility by stimulation of the vagus nerves. *Circ Res* 1965; 17:222–235.
232. Franco-Cerecada A, Lundberg JM, Dahlof C: Neuropeptide Y and sympathetic control of heart contractility and coronary vascular tone. *Acta Physiol Scand* 1985; 124:361–365.
233. Bassenge E, Busse R: Endothelial modulation of coronary tone. *Prog Cardiovasc Dis* 1988; 30:349–380.
234. Badeer HS: Resting bradycardia of exercise training: A concept based on currently available data. In: Roy PE, Rona G (eds): *The Metabolism of Contraction,* vol 10: *Recent Advances in Studies on Cardiac Structure and Metabolism.* Baltimore, University Park Press, 1975: 553.
235. Dzau VJ, Re RN: Evidence for the existence of renin in the heart. *Circulation* 1987; 75:1134–1136.
236. Dzau VJ: Cardiac renin-angiotensin system: Molecular and functional aspects. *Am J Med* 1988; 84:22–27.
237. Lindpainter K, Ganten D: The cardiac renin-angiotensin system: An appraisal of present experimental and clinical evidence. *Circ Res* 1991; 68:905–921.
238. O'Rourke ST, Vanhoutte PM: Vascular pharmacology. In: Loscalzo J, Creager MA, Dzau VJ (eds): *Vascular Medicine: A Textbook of Vascular Biology and Diseases.* Boston, Little, Brown, 1992: 133–155.
239. Dostal DE, Baker KM: Evidence for a role of an intracardiac renin-angiotensin system in normal and failing hearts. *Trends Cardiovasc Med* 1993; 3:67–74.
240. Holmer SR, Homey CJ: G proteins in the heart: A redundant and diverse transmembrane signaling network. *Circulation* 1991; 84:1891–1902.
241. Saman S, Thandroyen F, Opie LH: Serotonin and the heart: Effects of ketanserin on myocardial function, heart rate, and arrhythmias. *J Cardiovasc Pharmacol* 1985; 7(suppl 7):S70–S75.
242. Zaritsky AL, Horowitz M, Chernow B: Glucagon antagonism of calcium channel blocker-induced myocardial dysfunction. *Crit Care Med* 1988; 16:246–251.
243. Dzau VJ, Packer M, Lilly LS, Swartz SL, Hollenberg NK, Williams GH: Prostaglandins in severe congestive heart failure: Relation to activation of the renin-angiotensin system and hyponatremia. *N Engl J Med* 1984; 310:347–352.
244. Gunnes P, Reikeras O: Distribution of the increased cardiac output secondary to the vasodilating and inotropic effects of secretin. *Scand J Clin Lab Invest* 1987; 47:383–388.
245. Gu J, Adrian TE, Tatemoto K, Polak JM, Allen JM, Bloom SR: Neuropeptide tyrosine (NPY): A major cardiac neuropeptide. *Lancet* 1983; 1:1008–1010.
246. Su C: Extracellular functions of nucleotides in heart and blood vessels. *Annu Rev Physiol* 1985; 47:665–676.
247. Franco-Cereceda A, Bengtsson L, Lundberg JM: Inotropic effects of calcitonin gene-related peptide, vasoactive intestinal polypeptide and somatostatin on the human right atrium in vitro. *Eur J Pharmacol* 1987; 134:69–76.
248. Marsden PA, Danthuluri NR, Brenner BM, Ballermann BJ, Brock TA: Endothelin action on vascular smooth muscle involves inositol triphosphate and calcium mobilization. *Biochem Biophys Res Commun* 1988; 158:86–93.
249. Goto K, Kasuya Y, Matsuki N, Takuwa Y, Kurihara H, Ishikawa T, et al: Endothelin activates the dihydropyridine-sensitive, voltage-dependent Ca^{2+} channel in vascular smooth muscle. *Proc Natl Acad Sci U S A* 1989; 86:3915–3918.
250. Lüscher TF, Yang Z, Diederich D, Bühler FR: Endothelium-derived vasoactive substances: Potential role in hypertension, atherosclerosis, and vascular occlusion. *J Cardiovasc Pharmacol* 1989; 14:563–569.
251. Vane JR, Botting R, Masaki T (eds): Endothelin. *J Cardiovasc Pharmacol* 1989; 13(suppl): S1–S231.
252. Vanhoutte, PM: Endothelium and control of vascular function. *Hypertension* 1989; 13:658–667.
253. Bassenge E, Heusch G: Endothelial and neuro-humoral control of coronary blood flow in health and disease. *Rev Physiol Biochem Pharmacol* 1990; 116:77–165.
254. Vane JR, Änggård EE, Botting RM: Regulatory functions of the vascular endothelium. *N Engl J Med* 1990; 323:27–36.
255. Masaki T, Kimura S, Yanagisawa M, Goto K: Molecular and cellular mechanisms of endothelin regulation: Implications for vascular function. *Circulation* 1991; 84:1457–1468.
256. Rubany GM, Botelho LHP: Endothelins. *FASEB J* 1991; 5:2713–2720.
257. Lerman A, Burnett JC Jr: Intact and altered endothelium in regulation of vasomotion. *Circulation* 1992; 86(suppl III): III-12–III-19.
258. Lüscher TF, Boulanger CM, Dohi Y, Yang Z: Endothelium-derived contracting factors. *Hypertension* 1992; 19:117–130.
259. Brutsaert DL, Meulemans AL, Sipido KR, Sys SU: Effects of damaging the endocardial surface on the mechanical performance of isolated cardiac muscle. *Circ Res* 1988; 62:358–366.
260. Brutsaert DL: The endocardium. *Annu Rev Physiol* 1989; 51:263–273.
261. Brutsaert DL: Role of endocardium in cardiac overloading and failure. *Eur Heart J* 1991; 11(suppl G): G-8–G-16.
262. Brutsaert DL, Andries LJ: The endocardial endothelium. *Am J Physiol* 1992; 263(*Heart Circ Physiol* 32):H985–H1002.
263. Henderson AH, Lewis MJ, Shah AM, Smith JA: Endothelium, endocardium, and cardiac contraction. *Cardiovasc Res* 1992; 26:305–308.
264. Rocamora JM, Downing SE: Preservation of ventricular function by adrenergic influences during metabolic acidosis in the cat. *Circ Res* 1969; 24:373–381.
265. Vatner SF, Marsh JD, Swain JD: Effects of morphine on coronary and left ventricular dynamics in conscious dogs. *J Clin Invest* 1975; 55:207–217.
266. Horwitz LD, Bishop VS: Effect of acute volume loading on heart rate in the conscious dog. *Circ Res* 1972; 30:316–332.
267. Frommer PL, Robinson BF, Braunwald E: Paired electrical stimulation: A comparison of the effects on performance of the failing and nonfailing heart. *Am J Cardiol* 1966; 18:738–774.
268. Cranefield PF, Hoffman BF: The physiologic basis and clinical implications of paired pulse stimulation of the heart. *Dis Chest* 1966; 49:561–567.
269. Braunwald E, Sonnenblick EH, Frommer PL, Ross J Jr: Paired electrical stimulation of the heart: Physiologic observations and clinical implications. *Adv Intern Med* 1967; 13:61–96.
270. Wittenberg JB: Myoglobulin-facilitated oxygen diffusion: Role of myoglobin in oxygen entry into muscle. *Physiol Rev* 1970; 50:559–636.
271. Korner PI: Control of blood flow to special vascular areas: Brain, kidney, muscle, skin, liver, and intestine. In: Guyton AC, Jones CE (eds): *Cardiovascular Physiology, Physiology,* ser I. vol 1, Baltimore, University Park Press, 1974: 123.
272. Zelis R (ed): *The Peripheral Circulations.* New York, Grune & Stratton, 1975.
273. Messina EJ, Weiner R, Kaley G: Prostaglandins and local circulatory control. *Fed Proc* 1976; 35:2367.
274. Abboud FM, Schmid PG, Heistad DD, Mark AL: Regulation of peripheral and coronary circulation. In: Levine HJ (ed): *Clinical*

Cardiovascular Physiology. New York, Grune & Stratton, 1976: 143–205.
275. Shepherd JT, Vanhoutte PM: *Veins and Their Control*. Philadelphia, WB Saunders, 1975: 269.
276. Abboud FM, Schmid PG, Heistad DD, Mark AL, Barnes RW: The venous system. In: Levine HJ (ed): *Clinical Cardiovascular Physiology*. New York, Grune & Stratton, 1976: 207–257.
277. Dobrin PB: Vascular mechanics. In: Shepherd JT, Abboud FM (eds): *Handbook of Physiology, sec 2: The Cardiovascular System*, vol III: *Peripheral Circulation and Organ Blood Flow*, part 2. Bethesda, MD, American Physiological Society, 1983: 65.
278. Zweifach BW, Lipocosky HH: Pressure-flow relations in blood and lymph microcirculation. In: Renkin EM, Michel CC (eds): *Handbook of Physiology, sec 2: The Cardiovascular System*, vol III: *Microcirculation*, part 1. Bethesda, MD, American Physiological Society, 1984: 251–307.
279. Rose CP, Goresky CA: Interactions between capillary exchange, cellular entry, and metabolic sequestration processes in the heart. In: Renkin EM, Michel CC (eds): *Handbook of Physiology, sec 2: The Cardiovascular System*, vol III: *Microcirculation*, part 1. Bethesda, MD, American Physiological Society, 1984: 781–798.
280. Parent R, Paré R, Lavallée M: Contribution of nitric oxide to dilation of resistance coronary vessels. *Am J Physiol* 1992; 262(*Heart Circ Physiol 31*):H10–H16.
281. Bevan JA: Vascular myogenic or stretch-dependent tone. *J Cardiovasc Pharmacol* 1985; 7(suppl 3):S129–S136.
282. Nichols WW, O'Rourke MF: *McDonald's Blood Flow in Arteries*. 3d ed. Philadelphia, Lea & Febiger, 1990: 1–456.
283. Davis MJ: Myogenic response gradient in an arteriolar network. In: Mulvany MJ, Aalkjaer C, Heagerty AM, Nyborg NCB, Strandgaard S (eds): *Resistance Arteries: Structure and Function*. Amsterdam, Elsevier, 1991: 51–55.
284. Olsson RA, Bunger R, Spaan, JAE: Coronary circulation. In: Fozzard HA, Haber E, Jennings RB, Katz AM, Morgan HE (eds): *The Heart and Cardiovascular System*, 2d ed. New York, Raven, 1991: 1393–1425.
285. Smiesko V, Lang DJ, Johnson PC: Dilator response of rat mesenteric arcading arterioles to increased blood flow velocity. *Am J Physiol* 1989; 257(*Heart Circ Physiol* 26):H1958–H1965.
286. Kuo L, Davis MJ, Chilian WM: Endothelium-dependent, flow-induced dilation of isolated coronary arterioles. *Am J Physiol* 1990; 259(*Heart Circ Physiol 28*):H1063–H1070.
287. Moncada S, Palmer RM, Higgs EA: Nitric oxide: physiology, pathophysiology, and pharmacology. *Pharmacol Rev* 1991; 43:109–142.
288. Simonson MS, Dunn MJ: Endothelin. Pathways of transmembrane signaling. *Hypertension* 1990; 15(suppl I):I-5–I-12.
289. Needleman P: The synthesis and function of prostaglandins in the heart. *Fed Proc* 1976; 35:2376–2381.
290. Marcus ML: *The Coronary Circulation in Health and Disease*. New York, McGraw-Hill, 1983.
291. Feigl EO: Coronary physiology. *Physiol Rev* 1983; 63:1–205.
292. Olsson RA, Bunger R, Spaan JAE: Coronary circulation. In: Fozzard HA, Haber E, Jennings RB, Katz AM, Morgan HE (eds): *The Heart and Cardiovascular System: Scientific Foundations*, 2d ed. New York, Raven Press, 1991:1393–1425.
293. Spaan JAE, Bruschke AVG, Gittenberger-DeGroot AC (eds): *Coronary Circulation*. Dordrecht, Martinus Nijhoff, 1987.
294. Busse R, Trogisch G, Bassenge E: The role of endothelium in the control of vascular tone. *Basic Res Cardiol* 1985; 80:475–490.
295. Vanhoutte PM, Miller VM, Houston DS: Modulation of vascular smooth muscle contraction by the endothelium. *Annu Rev Physiol* 1986; 48:307–320.
296. Vanhoutte PM: Endothelium-dependent contractions in arteries and veins. *Blood Vessels* 1987; 24:141–144.
297. Bassenge E, Busse R: Endothelial modulation of coronary tone. *Prog Cardiovasc Dis* 1988; 30:349–380.
298. Inoue T, Tomoike H, Hisano K, Nakamara M: Endothelium determines flow-dependent dilation of the epicardial coronary artery in dogs. *J Am Coll Cardiol* 1988; 11:187–191.
299. Rubanyi GM, Romero JC, Vanhoutte PM: Flow-induced release of endothelium-derived relaxing factor. *Am J Physiol* 1986; 250:H-1145–H-1149.
300. Vanhoutte PM, Shimokawa H: Endothelium-derived relaxing factor and coronary vasospasm. *Circulation* 1989; 80:1–8.
301. Henderson AH: Endothelium in control. *Br Heart J* 1991; 65:116–125.
302. Holtz J, Forstermann U, Pohl U, Giesler M, Bassonge E: Flow-dependent, endothelium-mediated dilatation of epicardial coronary arteries in conscious dogs: effects of cyclooxygenase inhibition. *J Cardiovasc Pharmacol* 1984; 6:1161–1169.
303. Pohl U, Holtz J, Busse R, Bassenge E: Crucial role of endothelium in vasodilator response to increased flow in vivo. *Hypertension* 1986; 8:37–44.
304. Kuo L, Davis MJ, Chilian WM: Endothelium-dependent flow-induced dilation of isolated coronary arterioles. *Am J Physiol* 1990; 259:H1063–H1070.
305. Dewey JG, Vanhoutte PM: Anoxia and endothelium-dependent reactivity in canine femoral artery. *J Physiol (Lond)* 1983; 335:65–74.
306. Yasue H, Horio Y, Nakamura N, Fujii H, Imoto N, Sonoda R, et al: Induction of coronary artery spasm by acetylcholine in patients with variant angina: Possible role of the parasympathetic nerve system in the pathogenesis of coronary artery spasm. *Circulation* 1986; 74:955–963.
307. Okumura K, Yasue H, Horio Y, Takaoka K, Matsuyama K, Fujii H, et al: Multivessel coronary spasm in patients with variant angina: A study with intracoronary injection of acetylcholine. *Circulation* 1988; 77:535–542.
308. Ludmer PL, Selwyn AP, Shook TL, Wayne R, Mudge GH, Alexander RW, et al: Paradoxical vasoconstriction induced by acetylcholine in atherosclerotic coronary arteries. *N Engl J Med* 1986; 315:1046–1051.
309. Yamamoto H, Bossaller C, Cartwright J Jr, Henry PD: Videomicroscopic demonstration of defective cholinergic arteriolar vasodilatation in atherosclerotic rabbit. *J Clin Invest* 1988; 81:1752–1758.
310. Cox DA, Vita JA, Treasure CB, Fish RD, Alexander RW, Ganz P, et al: Atherosclerosis impairs flow-mediated dilation of coronary arteries in humans. *Circulation* 1989; 80:458–465.
311. Yasue H, Matsuyama K, Matsuyama K, Okumura K, Morikami Y, Ogawa H: Responses of angiographically normal human coronary arteries to intracoronary injection of acetylcholine by age and segment: Possible role of early coronary atherosclerosis. *Circulation* 1990; 81:482–490.
312. Marshall JJ, Kontos HA: Endothelium-derived relaxing factors: A perspective from in vivo data. *Hypertension* 1990; 16:371–386.
313. Flavahan NA: Atherosclerosis or lipoprotein-induced endothelial dysfunction: Potential mechanisms underlying reduction in EDRF/nitric oxide activity. *Circulation* 1992; 85:1927–1938.
314. Ware JA, Heistad DD: Platelet-endothelium interactions. *N Engl J Med* 1993; 328:628–635.
315. Rubanyi GM, Vanhoutte PM: Hypoxia releases a vasoconstrictor substance from the canine vascular endothelium. *J Physiol (Lond)* 1985; 364:45–56.
316. Feigl EO: The paradox of adrenergic coronary vasoconstriction. *Circulation* 76:737–745.
317. Gutterman DG, Brody MJ, Marcus ML: Neural regulation of coronary blood flow. In: Fozzard HA, Haber E, Jennings RB, Katz AM, Morgan HE (eds): *The Heart and Cardiovascular System*, 2d ed. New York, Raven, 1991: 695–736.
318. Sander GE, Huggins CG: Vasoactive peptides. *Annu Rev Pharmacol* 1972; 12:227–264.
319. Oates JA, Fitzgerald GA, Branch RA, Jackson EK, Knapp HR, Roberts LJ: Clinical implications of prostaglandins and thromboxane A_2 formation. *N Engl J Med* 1988; 319:689–698.
320. Zusman RM: Eicosanoids: Prostaglandins, thromboxane, and prostacyclin. In: Fozzard HA, Haber E, Jennings RB, Katz AM, Morgan HE (eds): *The Heart and Cardiovascular System*, 2d ed. New York, Raven, 1991: 1797–1815.
321. Barcroft J, Dixon WE: The gaseous metabolism of the mammalian heart. *J Physiol* 1907; 35:182–204.
322. Rohde E: Uber den Einfluss der mechanischen Bedingungen auf die Tatigkeit und den Sauerstoffverbrauch des Warmbluterherzens. *Arch Exp Pathol Pharmakol* 1912; 68:401–420.
323. Evans CL, Matsuoka Y: The effect of various mechanical conditions on the gaseous metabolism and efficiency of the mammalian heart. *J Physiol* 1915; 49:378–405.
324. Sonnenblick EH, Skelton CL: Oxygen consumption of the heart: Physiological principles and clinical implications. *Mod Concepts Cardiovasc Dis* 1971; 40:9–16.
325. Sarnoff SJ, Braunwald E, Welch GH, Case RB, Stainsby WN, Macruz R: Hemodynamic determinants of oxygen consumption

of the heart with special reference to the tension-time index. *Am J Physiol* 1958; 192:148.

326. Sonnenblick EH, Ross J Jr, Covell JW, et al: Velocity of contraction as a determinant of myocardial oxygen consumption. *Am J Physiol* 1965; 209:919–927.
327. Covell JW, Braunwald E, Ross J Jr, Sonnenblick EH: Studies on digitalis: XVI. Effects on myocardial oxygen consumption. *J Clin Invest* 1966; 45:1535–1542.
328. Neill WA, Levine HJ, Wagman RJ, Gorlin R: Left ventricular oxygen utilization in intact dogs: Effect of systemic hemodynamic factors. *Circ Res* 1963; 12:163–169.
329. Gregg DE: Effect of coronary perfusion pressure or coronary flow on oxygen usage of the myocardium. *Circ Res* 1963; 13:497–500.
330. Berne RM, Rubio R: Coronary circulation. In: Berne RM (ed): *Handbook of Physiology, sec 2: The Cardiovascular System,* vol. 1: *The Heart.* Bethesda, MD, American Physiological Society, 1979: 873.
331. Rose CP, Goresky CA: Interactions between capillary exchange, cellular entry, and metabolic sequestration processes in the heart. In: Renkin EM, Michel CC (eds): *Handbook of Physiology, sec 2: The Cardiovascular System,* vol IV: *Microcirculation,* part 2. Bethesda, MD, American Physiological Society, 1984: 781–798.
332. Dole WP: Autoregulation of the coronary circulation. *Prog Cardiovasc Dis* 1987; 29:293–323.
333. Olsson RA, Bunger R: Metabolic control of coronary blood flow. *Prog Cardiovasc Dis* 1987; 29:369–387.
334. Hoffman JI: Transmural myocardial perfusion. *Prog Cardiovasc Dis* 1987; 29:429–464.
335. McHale PA, Dube GP, Greenfield JC Jr: Evidence for myogenic vasomotor activity in the coronary circulation. *Prog Cardiovasc Dis* 1987; 30:139–146.
336. Young MA, Knight DR, Vatner SF: Autonomic control of large coronary arteries and resistance vessels. *Prog Cardiovasc Dis* 1987; 30:211–234.
337. Hanley FL, Messina LM, Grattan MT, Hoffman IE: The effect of coronary inflow pressure on coronary vascular resistance in the isolated dog heart. *Circ Res* 1984; 54:760–772.
338. Wiggers CJ: The interplay of coronary vascular resistance and myocardial compression in regulating coronary flow. *Circ Res* 1954; 2:271–279.
339. Bache RJ, Dymek DJ: Local and regional regulation of coronary vascular tone. *Prog Cardiovasc Dis* 1981; 24:191–212.
340. Klocke FJ, Ellis AK: Control of coronary blood flow. *Annu Rev Med* 1980; 31:489–508.
341. Berne RM: The role of adenosine in the regulation of coronary blood flow. *Circ Res* 1980; 47:807–813.
342. Conti CR (ed): *Coronary Artery Spasm: Pathophysiology, Diagnosis and Treatment.* New York, Marcel Dekker, 1986: 1–347.
343. Folts JD, Crowell EB Jr, Rowe GG: Platelet aggregation in partially obstructed vessels and its elimination with aspirin. *Circulation* 1976; 54:365–370.
344. Kuzuya T, Tada M, Inoue M, Kodama K, Takeda H, Mishima M, et al: Increased levels of thromboxane A_2 in peripheral and coronary circulation in patients with angina pectoris (abstr.). *Am J Cardiol* 1980; 45:454.
345. Robertson RM, Robertson D, Roberts LJ, Maas RL, Fitzgerald GA, Friesinger GC, et al: Thromboxane A_2 in vasotonic angina pectoris. *N Engl J Med* 1981; 304:998–100.
346. Esumi K, Tada M, Kuzuya T, Ohmori M, Matsuda H, Inoue M, et al: Thromboxane A_2 and prostaglandin I_2 in canine circulation during transient myocardial ischemia (abstr.). *Circulation* 1981; 64(suppl 4):266.
347. Yokoyama M, Goldman M, Henry PD: Supersensitivity of atherosclerotic arteries to ergonovine is partially mediated by a serotonergic mechanism (abstr.). *Circulation* 1979; 60(suppl 2):100.
348. Heistad DD, Armstrong ML, Marcus ML, Marcus ML, Piegors DJ, Mark AL: Augmented responses to vasoconstrictor stimuli in hypercholesterolemic and atherosclerotic monkeys. *Circ Res* 1984; 54:711–718.
349. Mudge GH Jr, Goldberg S, Gunther S, Mann T, Grossman W: Comparison of metabolic and vasoconstrictor stimuli on coronary vascular resistance in man. *Circulation* 1979; 59:544–550.
350. Johannsen UJ, Mark AL, Marcus ML, Armstrong ML: Effects of dietary hyperlipoproteinemia on coronary vascular responsiveness in vivo (abstr.). *Circulation* 1980; 64(suppl 4):267.
351. Shimokawa H, Tomoike H, Nabeyama S, Yamamoto H, Araki H, Nakamura M, et al: Coronary artery spasm induced in atherosclerotic miniature swine. *Science* 1983; 221:560–562.
352. Harrison DG, Minor RL, Guerra R, Quillen JE, Selke FW: Endothelial dysfunction in atherosclerosis. In: Rubanyi GM (ed): *Cardiovascular Significance of Endothelium-Derived Vasoactive Factors.* Mt Kisco, NY, Futura, 1991: 263–280.
353. Vatner SF, Higgins CB, Braunwald E: Effects of norepinephrine on coronary circulation and left ventricular dynamics in the conscious dog. *Circ Res* 1974; 34:812–823.
354. Krasnow N, Rolett EL, Yurchak PM, Hood WB, Gorlin R: Isoproterenol and cardiovascular performance. *Am J Med* 1964; 37:514–525.
355. Dusting GJ, Moncada S, Vane JR: Prostaglandins, their intermediates and precursors: Cardiovascular actions and regulatory roles in normal and abnormal circulatory systems. *Prog Cardiovas Dis* 1979; 21:405–430.
356. Gunther S, Cannon PJ: Modulation of angiotensin II coronary vasoconstriction by cardiac prostaglandin synthesis. *Am J Physiol* 1980; 238:H895–901.
357. Nakano J: Cardiovascular actions of vasopressin. *Jpn Circ J* 1973; 37:363–381.
358. Nakano J: Cardiovascular responses to neurohypophysial hormones. In: Greep RO, Astwood EB (eds): *Handbook of Physiology, sec 7: Endocrinology,* vol 4. Bethesda, MD, American Physiological Society, 1974: 395–442.
359. Khayyal MA, Eng C, Franzen D, Breall JA, Kirk ES: Effects of vasopressin on the coronary circulation reserve and regulation during ischemia. *Am J Physiol* 1985; 248:H516–522.
360. Buccino RA, Spann JF Jr, Pool PE, Sonnenblick EH, Braunwald E: Influence of thyroid state on the intrinsic contractile properties and energy stores of the myocardium. *J Clin Invest* 1967; 46:1669–1682.
361. Skelton CL, Sonnenblick EH: Cardiovascular system. In: Werner SC, Ingbar SH (eds): *Hyperthyroidism.* New York, Harper & Row, 1978: 688.
362. Hackel DB, Kleinerman J: Effects of thiamin deficiency on myocardial metabolism in intact dogs. *Am Heart J* 1953; 46:1.
363. Needleman P, Marshall GR, Sobel BE: Hormone interactions in the isolated rabbit heart: Synthesis and coronary vasomotor effects of prostaglandins, angiotensin, and bradykinin. *Circ Res* 1975; 37:802–808.
364. Regoli D, Barabe J, Therialult B: Does indomethacin antagonize the effects of peptides and other agents on the coronary circulation of rabbit isolated hearts? *Can J Physiol Pharmacol* 1977; 55:307–310.
365. Losay J, Mroz EA, Treagear GW, Leeman SE, Gamble WJ: Action of substance P on the coronary blood flow in the isolated dog heart. In: von Euler US, Pernow B (eds): *Substance P.* New York, Raven Press, 1976.
366. Carretero OA, Scicli AG: The kallikrein-kinin system. In: Fozzard HA, Haber E, Jennings RB, Katz AM, Morgan HE (eds): *The Heart and Cardiovascular System.* 2d ed. New York, Raven, 1991: 1851–1874.
367. Brum JM, Bove AA, Vanhoutte PM: Participation of the endothelium in the vasodilator effects of vasoactive intestinal peptide and substance P in the coronary arteries (abstract). *Circulation* 1985; 72(suppl III):III-83.
368. Said SI: VIP: Overview, in Bloom SR (ed): *Gut Hormones.* Edinburgh, Churchill Livingstone, 1978: 465–469.
369. Rudehill A, Solleri A, Franco-Cereceda A, Lundberg JM: Neuropeptide Y (NPY) and the pig heart: Release and constrictor effects. *Peptides* 1987; 7:821–826.
370. DeNeef P, Robberecht P, Chatelain P, Chatelaim P, Waelbroeck M, Christophe J: The in vitro chronotropic and inotropic effects of vasoactive intestinal peptide (VIP) on the atria and ventricular papillary muscle from *Cy-anomologus* monkey heart. *Regul Pept* 1984; 8:237–244.
371. Needleman P, Kaley S: Cardiac and coronary prostaglandin synthesis and function. *N Engl J Med* 1978; 298:1122–1128.
372. Stiles GL, Lefkowitz RJ: Cardiac adrenergic receptors. *Annu Rev Med* 1984; 35:149–164.
373. Feigl EO: Parasympathetic control of coronary blood flow in dogs. *Circ Res* 1969; 25:509–519.
374. Hanley HG, Costin JC, Skinner NS Jr: Differential reflex adjustments in cutaneous and muscle vascular beds during experimental coronary artery occlusion. *Am J Cardiol* 1971; 27:513–521.
375. Vatner SF, McRitchie RJ: Interaction of the chemoreflex and the

pulmonary inflation reflex in the regulation of coronary circulation in conscious dogs. *Circ Res* 1975; 37:664–673.

376. Shepherd JT: Cardiac mechanoreceptors. In: Fozzard HA, Haber E, Jennings RB, Katz AM, Morgan HE (eds): *The Heart and Cardiovascular System,* 2d ed. New York, Raven, 1991: 1481–1504.
377. Schaper W: Collateral circulation. In: Schaper W (ed): *The Paraphysiology of Myocardial Perfusion.* Amsterdam, Elsevier/North-Holland, 1979: 1–276.
378. Schaper W, Bernotat-Danielowski S, Nienaber C, Schaper J: Collateral circulation. In: Fozzard HA, Haber E, Jennings RB, Katz AM, Morgan HE (eds): *The Heart and Cardiovascular System,* 2d ed. New York, Raven, 1991: 1427–1464.
379. Schaper W: *Collateral Circulation: Heart, Brain, Kidney, Limbs.* Norwell, MA, Kluwer Academic Publications, 1993.
380. Gregg DE, Patterson RE: Functional importance of the coronary collaterals. *N Engl J Med* 1980; 303:1404–1406.
381. Yanagisawa-Miwa A, Uchida Y, Nakamuru F, Tomara T, Kido H, Kamijo T, et al: Salvage of infarcted myocardium by angiogenic action of basic fibroblast growth factor. *Science* 1992; 25:1401–1403.
382. Hoffman JIE, Buckberg GD: Transmural variations in myocardial perfusion. In: Yu PN, Goodwin JF (eds): *Progress in Cardiology.* Philadelphia, Lea & Febiger, 1976: 37–89.
383. Hoffman JIE: Determinants and prediction of transmural myocardial perfusion. *Circulation* 1978; 58:381–391.
384. Wangler RD, Peters KG, Marcus ML, Tomanek RJ: Effects of duration and severity of arterial hypertension on cardiac hypertrophy and coronary vasodilator reserve. *Circ Res* 1982; 51:10–18.
385. Schelbert HR, Phelps ME, Hoffman EJ, Huang SC, Selin CE, Kuhl DE: Regional myocardial perfusion assessed with N-13 labeled ammonia and positron emission computerized axial tomography. *Am J Cardiol* 1979; 43:209–218.
386. Hoffman JIE: The effect of intramyocardial forces on the distribution of intramyocardial blood flow. *J Biomed Eng* 1979; 1:33–40.
387. Bache R: Effects of hypertrophy on the coronary circulation. *Prog Cardiovasc Dis* 1988; 30:403–440.
388. Lee FA, Cabin HS, Francis CK: The syndrome of flash pulmonary edema: Clinical definition and angiographic findings (abstract). *J Am Coll Cardiol* 1988; 11(suppl A):151A.
389. Schlant RC: "Flash" pulmonary edema. *Am Coll Cardiol Curr J Rev* 1992; 1:74–75.
390. Wiggers CJ: Studies on the consecutive phases of the cardiac cycle: I. The duration of the consecutive phases of the cardiac cycle and the criteria for their precise determination. *Am J Physiol* 1921; 56:415–438.
391. Wiggers CJ: Studies on the consecutive phases of the cardiac cycle: II. The laws governing the relative durations of ventricular systole and diastole. *Am J Physiol* 1921; 56:439–459.
392. Schlant RC: Events during cardiac cycle. In: Altman PL, Dittmer DS (eds): *Respiration and Circulation,* 2d ed. Bethesda, MD, Federation of American Society for Experimental Biological Proceedings, 1973: 304.
393. Laniado S, Yellin E, Kotler M, Levy L, Stadler J, Terdiman R: A study of the dynamic relations between the mitral valve echogram and phasic mitral flow. *Circulation* 1975; 51:104–113.
394. Laniado S, Yellin E, Terdiman R, Meytes I, Stadler J: Hemodynamic correlates of the normal aortic valve echogram: A study of sound, flow, and motion. *Circulation* 1976; 54:729–737.
395. Spencer MP, Greiss FC: Dynamics of ventricular ejection. *Circ Res* 1962; 10:274–279.
396. Grant C, Greene DG, Bunnell IL: The value-closing function of the right atrium: A study of pressures and atrial sounds in patients with heart block. *Am J Med* 1963; 34:325–328.
397. MacCanon DM, Arevalo F, Meyer EC: Direct detection and timing of aortic valve closure. *Circ Res* 1964; 14:387–391.
398. Piemme TE, Barnett GO, Dexter L: Relationship of heart sounds to acceleration of blood flow. *Circ Res* 1966;18:303–315.
399. Delman AJ: Hemodynamic correlations of cardiovascular sounds. *Annu Rev Med* 1967; 18:139–158.
400. Craige E, Fortuin NJ: Genesis of heart sounds and murmurs as demonstrated by echocardiography. In: Joyner CR (ed): *Ultrasound in the Diagnosis of Cardiovascular-Pulmonary Disease.* Chicago, Year Book Medical, 1974: 119–132.
401. Waider W, Craige E: First heart sound and ejection sounds: Echocardiographic and phonocardiographic correlation with valvular events. *Am J Cardiol* 1975; 35:346–356.
402. Chandraratna PAN, Lopez JM, Cohen LS: Echocardiographic observations on the mechanism of production of the second heart sound. *Circulation* 1975; 51:292–296.
403. Sagawa K, Maughan L, Suga H, Sunagawa K: *Cardiac Contraction and the Pressure-Volume Relationship.* New York, Oxford University Press, 1988: 1–480.
404. Marshall HW, Helmholz HF, Wood EH: Physiologic consequences of congenital heart disease. In: Hamilton WF, Dow P (eds): *Handbook of Physiology, sec 2: Circulation,* vol 1. Bethesda, MD, American Physiological Society, 1962: 417–487.
405. Mackay IFS: The true venous pulse wave, central and peripheral. *Am Heart J* 1967; 74:48–57.
406. Barratt-Boyes BG, Wood EH: Cardiac output and related measurements and pressure values in the right heart and associated vessels, together with an analysis of the hemodynamic response to the inhalation of high oxygen mixtures in healthy subjects. *J Lab Clin Med* 1958; 51:72–90.
407. Braunwald E, Brockenbrough EC, Fraham CJ, Ross J Jr: Left atrial and left ventricular pressures in subjects without cardiovascular disease. *Circulation* 1961; 24:267–269.
408. Wade OL, Bishop JM: *Cardiac Output and Regional Blood Flow,* Oxford, Blackwell Scientific, 1962.
409. Dexter L, Whittenberger JL, Haynes FW, Goodale WT, Gorlin R, Sawyer CG: Effect of exercise on circulatory dynamics of normal individuals. *J Appl Physiol* 1951; 3:439–453.
410. Barratt-Boyes BG, Wood EH: hemodynamic response of healthy subjects to exercise in the supine position while breathing oxygen. *J Appl Physiol* 1957; 11:129–135.
411. Wang Y, Marshall RJ, Shepherd JT: The effect of changes in posture and of graded exercise on stroke volume in man. *J Clin Invest* 1960; 39:1051–1061.
412. Epstein SE, Beiser GD, Stampfer M: Characterization of the circulatory response to maximal upright exercise in normal subjects and patients with heart disease. *Circulation* 1967; 35:1049.
413. Braunwald E, Sonnenblick EH, Ross J Jr, Glick G, Epstein SE: An analysis of the cardiac response to exercise. *Circ Res* 1967; 20(suppl 1): 1–58.
414. Chapman CB (ed): Physiology of muscular exercise. *Circ Res* 1967; 20(suppl 1): 1.
415. Bevegard BS, Shepherd JT: Regulation of the circulation during exercise in man. *Physiol Rev* 1967; 47:178–213.
416. Smith EE, Guyton AC, Manning RD, White RJ: Integrated mechanisms of cardiovascular response and control during exercise in the normal human. *Prog Cardiovasc Dis* 1976; 18:421–444.
417. Astrand PO, Rodahl K: *Textbook of Work Physiology: Physiological Bases of Exercises,* 3d ed. New York, McGraw-Hill, 1986.
418. Scheuer J, Tipton CM: Cardiovascular adaptations of physical training. *Annu Rev Physiol* 1977; 39:221–251.
419. Blomqvist CG, Saltin B: Cardiovascular adaptations to physical training. *Annu Rev Physiol* 1983; 45:169–189.
420. Brengelmann GL: Circulatory adjustments to exercise and heat stress. *Annu Rev Physiol* 1983; 45:191–212.
421. Schlant RC: Physiology of exercise. In: Fletcher GF (ed): *Exercise in the Practice of Medicine,* 2d ed. Mount Kisco, NY, Futura, 1988:1–47.
422. Upton MT, Rerych SK, Roeback JR Jr, Newman GE, Douglas JM Jr, Wallace AG, et al: Effect of brief and prolonged exercise on left ventricular function. *Am J Cardiol* 1980; 45:1154–1160.
423. Bar-Shlomo B-Z, Druck MN, Morch JE, Jablonsky G, Hilton JO, Feiglin DH, et al: Left ventricular function in trained and untrained healthy subjects. *Circulation* 1982; 65:484–488.
424. Kelbaek H, Gjorup T, Christensen WJ, Vestergaard B, Godtredsen J: Cardiac function and plasma catecholamines during upright exercise in healthy young subjects. *Int J Cardiol* 1986; 10:223–235.
425. Port S, Cobb FR, Coleman RE, Jones RH: Effect of age on the response of the left ventricular ejection fraction to exercise. *N Engl J Med* 1980; 303:1133–1137.
426. Astrand PO, Saltin B: Plasma and red cell volume after prolonged severe exercise. *J Appl Physiol* 1964; 19:819–832.
427. Lundvall J, Mellander S, Westling H, White T: Fluid transfer between blood and tissues during exercise. *Acta Physiol Scand* 1972; 85:258–269.

428. Lind AR, McNicol GW: Circulatory responses to sustained handgrip contractions performed during other exercise, both rhythmic and static. *J Physiol* 1967; 192:595–607.
429. Lind AR, McNicol GW: Cardiovascular responses to holding and carrying weights by hand and by shoulder harness. J Appl Physiol 1968; 25:261–267.
430. Nutter DO, Schlant RC, Hurst JW: Isometric exercise and the cardiovascular system. *Mod Concepts Cardiovasc Dis* 1972; 41:11–15.
431. Fisher ML, Nutter DO, Jacobs W, Schlant RC: Haemodynamic responses to isometric exercise (handgrip) in patients with heart disease. *Br Heart J* 1973; 35:422–432.
432. Martin CE, Shaver JA, Leon DF, Thompson ME, Reddy PS, Leonard JJ: Autonomic mechanism in hemodynamic responses to isometric exercise. *J Clin Invest* 1974; 54:104–115.
433. McCloskey DI, Streatfield KA: Muscular reflex stimuli to the cardiovascular system during isometric contractions of muscle groups of different mass. *J Physiol* 1975; 250:431–441.
434. Grover RF, Weil JV, Reeves JT: Cardiovascular adaptation to exercise at high altitude. *Exercise Sports Sci Rev* 1986; 14:269–302

Chapter 6A

The Physiological Chemistry of Energy Production in the Heart

E. Douglas Lewandowski, Ph.D. ■ *Joanne S. Ingwall, Ph.D.*

Adenosine triphosphate (ATP) is the high-energy phosphate-containing compound directly used for excitation-contraction in muscle cells. Cleavage of the terminal phosphate (the phosphoryl bond) by proteins called ATPases releases chemical energy that is converted into the work of contraction (myosin ATPase), ion movements (Na^+ and Ca^{2+} ATPases), and macromolecular synthesis. The reaction is

$$MgATP + H_2O \rightarrow MgADP + P_i + H^+ \quad (1)$$

Chemical energy that can be used to do work is called free energy. Although the free energy of ATP hydrolysis is high (−7.3 kcal/mol) compared to other high-energy phosphate-containing compounds, the concentration of ATP in the cytosol of cardiac myocytes is low. Adult mammalian ventricular tissue contains approximately 5 mmol per gram wet weight, which is equivalent to 8 to 10 mmol per liter of intracellular water or 30 to 35 nmol per milligram of cardiac protein. Indeed, this amount of ATP is sufficient to maintain pump function for only about 50 beats. Thus, the cell must continually resynthesize ATP to maintain normal pump function and cellular viability. The metabolic pathways that produce ATP in the heart are described in this chapter. Illustrative examples of how these pathways for ATP synthesis change in disease states are also given.

The distinction between the amount or concentration of ATP versus its *turnover rate* is central to our understanding of bioenergetics and the metabolic consequences of pathophysiological conditions (such as ischemia) on the control of metabolism. In the normal heart, ATP concentration remains constant but its rate of synthesis and degradation (turnover rate) varies. The energetics of changing cardiac work illustrates this principle. As the work load of the heart increases, oxygen consumption (a good index of ATP synthesis rate) proportionately increases; yet ATP content is essentially unchanged. Thus ATP turnover rate, but not its concentration, increases. This example also illustrates the important principle that ATP synthesis rate matches ATP utilization rate.

Another important principle essential for our understanding of bioenergetics is that the chemical reactions that use ATP are "driven" by high ratios of ATP to adenosine diphosphate (ADP) while ATP synthesis reactions are inhibited by high ATP/ADP ratios. Atkinson[1] introduced the expression the adenylate energy charge, defined as $\frac{(ATP + \frac{1}{2} ADP)}{(ATP + ADP + AMP)}$, to distinguish between utilizable ATP (the numerator) and the total adenine nucleotide pool (the denominator) (AMP = adenosine monophosphate). In well-perfused tissue the cystosolic ATP, ADP, and AMP concentrations are approximately 10 mM, 30μM, and 0.1μM, respectively, while during ischemia, ATP falls to below 1 mM and ADP and AMP increase 10-fold or more. Thus, the adenylate energy charge is close to 1 in healthy tissue and less than 0.9 in ischemic tissue.

Given the critical need to maintain both a constant and high level of ATP, it is not surprising that the cell uses many reactions and pathways to synthesize ATP.

The remarkable feature of intermediary metabolism is that constant ATP concentration is maintained by the integration of multiple pathways. De novo synthesis of the purine ring of ATP from formate, carbon dioxide, and amino acids occurs slowly. Indeed, repleting 40 percent of the ATP pool following 15 min of coronary artery occlusion in the dog heart takes more than 3 days.[2] Phosphorylation of preformed purine via salvage pathways is more rapid, occurring in minutes or hours instead of days. Examples are salvage of ADP via the adenylate kinase reaction (2ADP $\rightleftharpoons$ ATP + AMP) and phosphorylation of purine nucleobases (such as hypoxanthine) or nucleosides (such as inosine or adenosine) by enzymes located in myocytes and endothelial cells.

The major nonpurine high-energy phosphate-containing compound in the heart is phosphocreatine (PCr) (free energy = −10.3 kcal/mol). In the heart the PCr concentration is twice the ATP concentration. The transfer of the high-energy phosphate group between PCr and ATP is catalzyed by *creatine kinase:*

$$\text{PCr} + \text{MgADP} + \text{H}^+ \rightleftharpoons \text{creatine} + \text{MgATP} \quad (2)$$

The overall equilibrium position is far to the right. Using the nuclear magnetic resonance (NMR) technique of magnetization transfer, investigators have measured the unidirectional velocity of the creatine kinase reaction in vivo. Adenosine triphosphate synthesis via creatine kinase is 10 times faster than the net ATP synthesis rate estimated from the physiological index of oxygen consumption. In the anesthesized open chest rat heart, measured creatine kinase reaction velocity was about 5 m*M*/s.[3] Discoveries of the localization of the mitochondrial creatine kinase isoenzyme on the inner mitochondrial membrane[4] and some of the MM isoenzyme in the M band of the myofibril[5] have led to the hypothesis that creatine kinase "shuttles" chemical energy between sites of ATP production (mitochondria) and sites of ATP utilization (myofibrils and ion transport across membranes) (Fig. 6A-1). Although creatine kinase rapidly rephosphorylates ADP to maintain high levels of ATP and hence a high adenylate energy charge, PCr is also rapidly depleted (within 100 beats) if not resynthesized from ATP.

Many changes occur in the creatine kinase system in disease states, including isoenzyme shifts (typically increases in BB and MB creatine kinase), changes in total tissue activity (V_{max}) and depletion of the total creatine pool. Because creatine kinase reaction velocity is so rapid, decreases in V_{max} and/or substrate (guanidino) concentration reduce the capacity of the heart to maintain normal ATP content. Because ATP is consumed by cell functions, phosphate transfer will eventually cease without the continual generation of chemical energy. Such energy is generated by the breakdown of carbon-based fuels.

ATP Synthesis from Carbon-Based Fuels

Adenosine triphosphate is generated by the metabolic breakdown, or catabolism, of carbon-based fuels through two fundamental processes: (1) substrate-level phosphorylation and (2) the generation of reducing equivalents for oxidative energy production (Fig. 6A-1). An example of substrate level phosphorylation is the glycolytic production of ATP from glucose in the cytosol. The generation of reducing equivalents, from either glycolysis or the tricarboxylic acid (TCA) cycle, contributes to the production of ATP via the linkage between the respiratory chain and oxidative phosphorylation within the mitochondria. In the normal heart, oxidative production of ATP predominates over substrate level phosphorylation as the source of ATP for the energetic support of cell functions and contractile activity. However, changes in the functional state or pathophysiology of the heart can result in a shift toward substrate level phosphorylation as the primary mode of energy production, as in the oxygen-limited or ischemic heart. In either case, the fuels required for energy production must be made available to the myocyte from either intracellular stores or circulating plasma levels of carbohydrates, fats, amino acids, or ketone bodies.

These fuels are generally referred to as *substrates* to indicate that they are converted to other intermediates through a series of enzyme-catalyzed reactions (Fig. 6A-1). The normal heart preferentially utilizes fatty acids as the substrate for oxidative energy production, although nutritional, metabolic, and hormonal influences can induce a greater contribution from carbohydrates. Recent studies indicate that the contractile performance of postischemic, reperfused myocardium is improved in response to increased glucose metabolism.[6,7] Carbohydrates are also known to play a major role in supporting the energetics of the heart under the anaerobic conditions of hypoxia and ischemia. Starches and sugars can enter glycolysis as the monomeric sugars, glucose or fructose. Glycogen is a starch that is composed of polymerized glucose units and serves as an intracellular store of glucose. Less utilized directly as fuels are amino acids, which nonetheless are involved in the shuttling of carbon chains to and from the energy-yielding metabolic pathways. Ketones can also serve as substrates but normally contribute very little to the total percentage of oxidative energy production. Only during extreme circumstances, such as starvation and severe diabetic ketosis, are ketones likely to account for a significant amunt of the energy produced within myocardium. The regulation of intermediary pathways, which determine the production of energy from this menu of carbon-based fuels, is described in the following sections of this chapter.

GLUCOSE METABOLISM IN THE HEART

Uptake of glucose by the heart is controlled by the glucose transporter in the sarcolemmal membrane. No energy is required for this glucose transport, because the extracellular glucose concentration is much higher than the intracellular concentration. The transporter is stimulated by (1) increased demands for anaerobic glycolysis, as in hypoxia; (2) increased work performance; (3) high plasma glucose concentrations, as in the fed state following a high carbohydrate meal; and (4) the actions of the circulating hormone, insulin. The reverse situations of glycolytic inhibition, decreased cardiac work, fasting conditions, and uncontrolled diabetes mellitus all lead

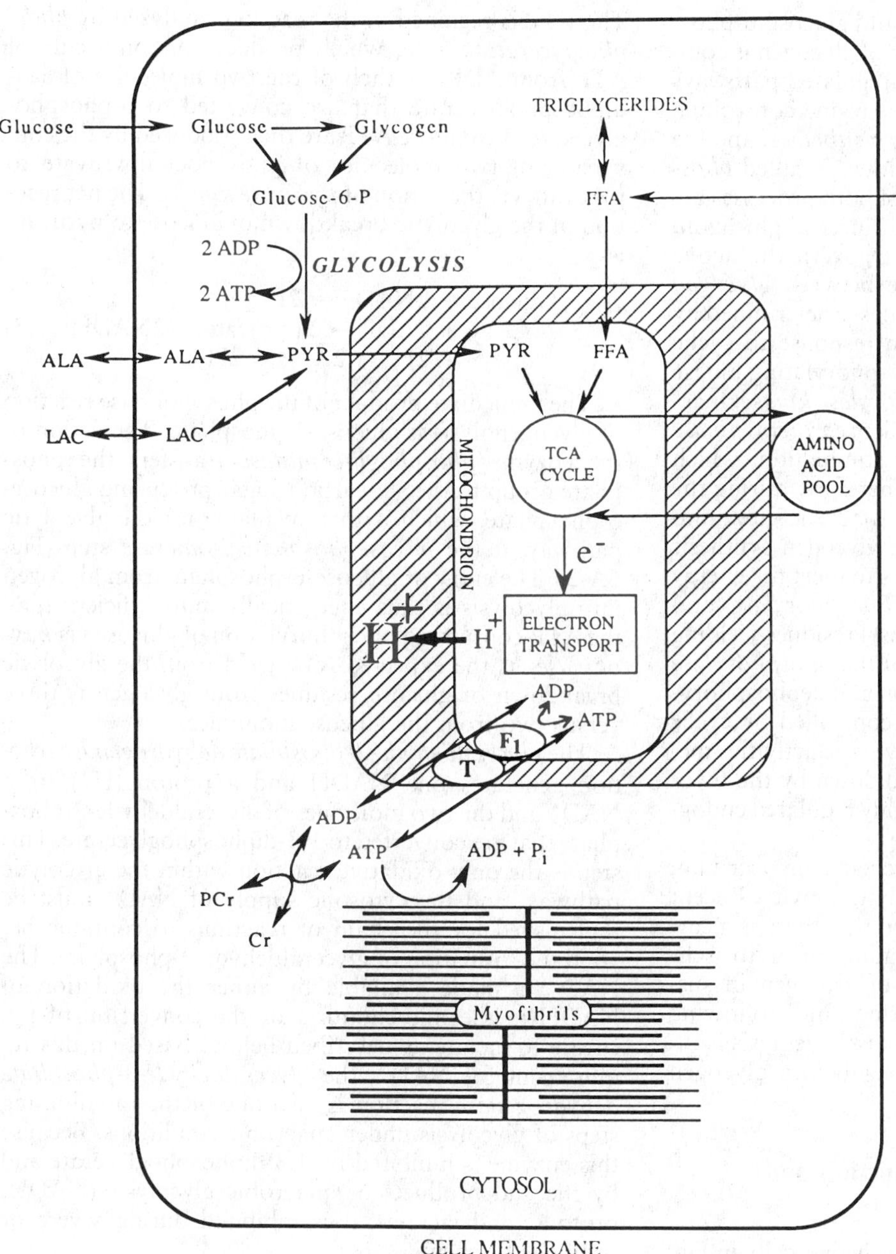

FIGURE 6A-1 Energy production from carbon-based fuels in the myocyte. Glucose uptake across the sarcolemmal membrane supplies both glycogen storage and substrate level energy production via glycolysis. Cytosolic metabolism of pyruvate (PYR) produces alanine (ALA) and lactate (LAC), which either leave the cell or are reconverted to pyruvate for oxidation within the mitochondria. Free fatty acids (FFAs) enter the cell by passive, facilitated diffusion across the sarcolemmal membrane and are either stored through triglyceride formation or transported into the mitochondria for oxidative metabolism. Both PYR and FFAs are metabolized to form two carbon, acetyl groups that enter oxidative metabolism within the tricarboxylic acid (TCA) cycle. The TCA cycle is also fueled by amino acids that are in exchange between the mitochondrial matrix and the cytosol. The oxidative production of reducing equivalents from the TCA cycle supplies electrons (e^-) to the electron transport chain, which generates a proton (H^+) gradient across the inner mitochondrial membrane. This proton gradient drives F_1 ATPase (F_1) converting ADP to ATP, which is coupled to the nucleotide translocase (T). The high-energy phosphoryl group of ATP supports the energy requirements of excitation-contraction coupling. Energy is also supplied by ATP and creatine (Cr). Energy-yielding processes are highlighted in blue.

to reduced activity of the glucose transporter and slow glucose entry into the myocyte, as will high levels of fatty acid oxidation by the myocyte. Thus, the first step of regulation in the utilization of glucose within the myocyte occurs at the level of the sarcolemmal membrane.

Once glucose enters the myocyte, the metabolism of this six-carbon sugar is directed toward either the pentose shunt, glycolytic breakdown into three-carbon (triose) units, or glycogen synthesis. Of the three metabolic pathways, the pentose shunt is the least involved in the production of energy, although the five-carbon pentose phosphates from this pathway can reenter glycolysis. The pentose shunt supplies carbon chains for the formation of adenine nucleotides, such as AMP and guanosine triphosphate (GTP), and also regenerates the cofactor $NADP^+$ (the oxidized form of nicotinamide–adenine dinucleatide phosphate). The process of glycolysis is the primary entry point for glucose into energy-yielding metabolism. This series of enzymatic reactions can occur in the heart under both aerobic conditions, with the ultimate oxidation of glucose, and under anaerobic conditions, when glycolysis serves as the primary source of ATP production. Glycogen synthesis allows the storage of glucose, and this process is regulated by a complex network of enzyme activation in response to metabolic and hormonal stimuli within the cell. The balance between glycogen synthesis, called *glycogenesis*, from glucose monomers and the degradation of glycogen stores, or *glycogenolysis*, to produce glucose-1-phosphate is discussed next.

Glycogen

Glucose is stored in the heart in the form of glycogen granules, a branched polysaccharide. The functional role of glycogen in heart muscle is to provide an energy source in the form of glucose-1-phosphate and glucose-6-phosphate for glycolysis. The metabolism of glycogen is complex, involving separate and highly regulated pathways for synthesis and degradation. The enzyme controlling glycogen synthesis is called *glycogen synthetase*, and the enzyme controlling glycogen breakdown is called *phosphorylase*. The regulatory enzymes of both processes are under hormonal control (by epinephrine and glucagon) by way of reciprocal reactions that govern the active state of each enzyme. The balance between *glycogen synthetase* and *phosphorylase* activities is determined by a *cascade* of enzymatic reactions in response to cyclic AMP activation of two different phosphorylating kinase enzymes, *protein kinase* and *phosphorylase kinase*. Inactivation by the cyclic AMP-dependent *protein kinase* occurs in response to β-adrenergic stimulation, which increases the level of cyclic AMP. Therefore, during the inotropic and chronotropic effects of β-adrenergic stimulation, the heart is able to shut off glycogen synthesis and mobilize available carbohydrates to meet the energy demands of increased cardiac work. *Phosphorylase* catalyzes the sequential removal of glycosyl residues yielding glucose-1-phosphate. The activity of the *phosphorylase* is also dependent on phosphorylation and dephosphorylation reactions that are indirectly controlled by cyclic AMP. The reciprocal control of enzymatic activities mediating glycogen synthesis and breakdown by the myocyte is evidence that glycogen is a highly regulated endogenous energy source.

Glycogen content is reduced in ischemic myocardium as a consequence of increased glycolytic activity. Recent experimental findings have suggested that there is a cardioprotective effect of glycogen loading prior to ischemia.[8] However, the effectiveness of glycogen in sustaining the cardiac function during and following ischemia remains controversial, because glycolysis is inhibited in ischemic heart tissue long before glycogen stores are completely depleted.[9]

Glycolytic Pathway: Energy Production and Regulation

The pathway of glycolysis is shown schematically in Fig. 6A-2. For purposes of energy accounting, this pathway can be separated into two distinct stages: (1) the ATP-requiring stage, which comprises the formation of glucose-6-phosphate from glucose and the subsequent production of fructose-1,6-bisphosphate, while consuming two molecules of ATP, and (2) the ATP-yielding stage, which comprises the formation of two triose units per six carbon sugars and ultimate formation of pyruvate, while yielding four molecules of ATP. Thus, the net energy yield of this pathway is two molecules of ATP.

As shown in Fig. 6A-2, the enzyme *hexokinase* catalyzes the transfer of a phosphate group from one molecule of ATP, forming ADP and converting glucose into glucose-6-phosphate. (Glucose-6-phosphate can also be generated from the end production of glycogen breakdown, glucose-1-phosphate, as described below.) Another molecule of ATP is consumed in the reaction catalyzed by the enzyme *phosphofructokinase*, which transfers the phosphate group from ATP to fructose-6-phosphate in producing fructose-1,6-bisphosophate. The ATP is regained in the reaction catalyzed by *phosphoglycerate kinase*, which produces one molecule of ATP from ADP for each of the two molecules of 1,3-diphosphoglycerate that are converted to 3-phosphoglycerate. Two more ATP are then produced by the conversion of two molecules of phosphoenolpyruvate to pyruvate via the action of *pyruvate kinase*. The net reaction of the glycolytic breakdown of glucose to pyruvate is

$$\begin{aligned}\text{Glucose} &+ 2\text{NAD}^+ + 2\text{P}_i \\ &+ 2\text{ADP} \rightarrow 2\text{ pyruvate} + 2\text{NADH} \\ &+ 2\text{H}^+ + 2\text{ATP} + 2\text{H}_2\text{O}\end{aligned} \qquad (3)$$

The immediate product of the phosphorylase reaction of glycogenolysis is glucose-1-phosphate. The action of the enzyme *phosphoglucomutase* transfers the phosphate group to the six-carbon sugar producing glucose-6-phosphate, which is then available for the glycolytic pathway at the *hexosephosphate isomerase* step (Fig. 6A-2). The entry of glucose-6-phosphate from glycogen into glycolysis is thus energetically more efficient than the ATP-consuming phosphorylation of glucose via *hexokinase*, as the expected ATP yield from the glycolytic breakdown of glucose residues from glycogen is three versus two from the glucose monomer.

The *glyceraldehyde-3-phosphate dehydrogenase* reaction generates one NADH and a proton (H^+) from NAD^+ and the two molecules of glyceraldehyde-3-phosphate that are converted to 1,3-diphosphoglycerate. This step is the only oxidative reaction within the glycolytic pathway, and the cytosolic supply of NAD^+ must be replenished for the chain of reactions to continue beyond the formation of glyceraldehyde-3-phosphate. The NAD^+ is made available by either the oxidation of NADH in the mitochondria or the conversion of pyruvate to lactate as described below. Based on this requirement for NAD^+, the *glyceraldehyde-3-phosphate dehydrogenase* reaction is also one of the rate-limiting steps of glycolysis under anaerobic conditions. Because this enzyme is inhibited by 1,3-diphosphoglycerate and by the end products of anaerobic glycolysis (NADH, protons, and lactate), it is inhibited during severe or prolonged ischemia.

Another enzyme of great importance in regulating glycolytic flux is *phosphofructokinase*, which is responsible for the conversion of fructose-6-phosphate to fructose-1,6-biphosphate. Unlike *glyceraldehyde-3-phosphate dehydrogenase*, which is dependent on the redox state and the ability of the heart to undergo oxidative metabolism, this enzyme is more responsive to the energetic state of the cytosol (the adenylate energy charge). The *phosphofructokinase* reaction is irreversible and determines the intracellular content of glucose-6-phosphate. When *phosphofructokinase* is activated by a fall in ATP or by elevated levels of ADP, AMP, and inorganic phosphate (causing a decrease in the adenylate energy charge), the resultant decrease in glucose-6-phosphate content stimulates glucose metabolism and the activity of the *hexokinase* enzyme. During such activation, the rate-limiting step in glycolysis then becomes the *glyceraldehyde-3-phosphate dehydrogenase* reaction. However, *phosphofructokinase* can also become rate limiting by an inhibitory response to high levels of ATP (high adenylate

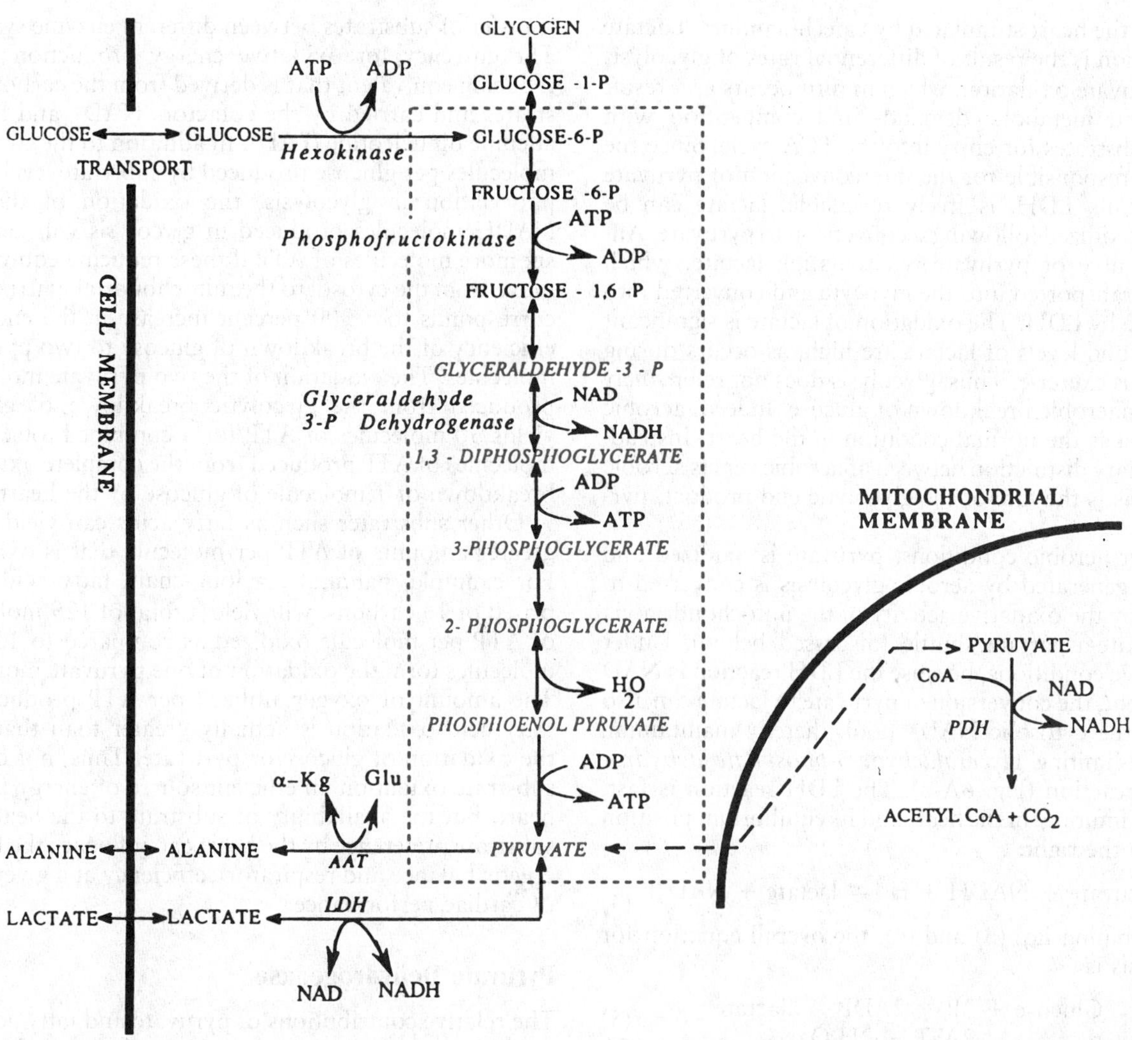

FIGURE 6A-2 Metabolism of glucose and pyruvate. The glycolytic pathway is indicated in the blue box. Two triose units are produced from each molecule of glucose and are highlighted in blue. Key enzymes of glucose metabolism are highlighted in blue. Pyruvate is the pivotal intermediate between nonoxidative metabolism in the cytosol via alanine aminotransferase (AAT) and lactate dehydrogenase (LDH) and the oxidative metabolism in the mitochondria via the action of the pyruvate dehydrogenase (PDH) enzyme complex. α-Kg, α-ketoglutarate; Glu, glutamate; CoA, coenzyme A.

energy charge) or the TCA cycle intermediate citrate. Therefore, while many enzymes are involved in the glycolytic pathway, the ability of the heart to regulate glycolytic flux in response to energetic state and oxidative metabolism is provided by the balance between the activity of these regulatory enzymes, *phosphofructokinase* and *glyceraldehyde-3-phosphate dehydrogenase*.

Glycolytic ATP production can partially support the energetic requirements of the hypoxic or ischemic heart. Increasing glycolytic metabolism in ischemic myocardium delays the progression of ischemic contracture and rigor formation, improving the chances that the functional state of the heart will be restored upon reperfusion.[10] A recent relevant experimental finding is that maintenance of the ischemic myocardium is influenced not only by the amount of glycolytic ATP produced but also by the rates of glycolytic flux and ATP production.[11] Part of these effects of glycolysis may not be attributed to ATP production alone but may also include an interrelationship between glycolytic flux and cation homeostatasis. This theoretical "functional compartmentation" is controversial, and precedents for the necessary physical compartment within the cytosol (such as protein–protein complex) have yet to be established.

Aerobic and Anaerobic Glycolysis

Under normal aerobic conditions in the myocardium, glycolysis proceeds in the cytosol as the breakdown of glucose to three-carbon units in the form of pyruvate. In aerobic glycolysis, pyruvate is converted to acetyl coenzyme A (CoA) via the action of pyruvate dehydrogenase in the mitochondria (Fig. 6A-2). In contrast, under anaerobic conditions such as hypoxia and ischemia, pyruvate oxidation is inhibited, pyruvate is converted to lactate in the cytosol via the *lactate dehydrogenase* (LDH) reaction, and lactate accumulates. The myocardial production of lactate is now well recognized as an indicator of anaerobic glycolysis subsequent to oxygen deprivation. It is important to emphasize, however, that some lactate is also produced under aerobic conditions. An example is the work load-dependent recruitment of glycolytic activity in the heart stimulated by catecholamines. Lactate production is the result of differential rates of glycolysis and pyruvate oxidation, which in turn occurs as a result of altered metabolic demands and competition with other substrates for entry into the TCA cycle. Since the enzyme responsible for the interconversion of pyruvate and lactate, LDH, is freely reversible, lactate can be rapidly oxidized following reconversion to pyruvate. Another source of pyruvate is circulating lactate, which can be transported into the myocyte and converted into pyruvate by LDH. The oxidation of lactate is significant when blood levels of lactate are high, as occurs during strenuous exercise. Thus, glycolysis does not refer *solely* to the anaerobic breakdown of glucose. Indeed, aerobic glycolysis is the normal condition in the heart. Instead, the primary distinction between anaerobic versus aerobic glycolysis is the fate of the glycolytic end product, pyruvate.

Under aerobic conditions, pyruvate is oxidized and NADH generated by aerobic glycolysis is converted to NAD^+ by the oxidative activity of the mitochondria via the malate-aspartate shuttle (discussed below). Under anaerobic conditions, because the LDH reaction is NAD dependent, the conversion of pyruvate to lactate can also restore the cytosolic NAD^+ pool, thereby maintaining the rate-limiting *glyceraldehyde-3-phosphate dehydrogenase* reaction (Fig. 6A-2). The LDH reaction is fast, not rate limiting, in the heart and its equilibrium position is far to the right:

$$\text{Pyruvate} + \text{NADH} + H^+ \rightleftharpoons \text{lactate} + NAD^+ \quad (4)$$

Combining Eq. (3) and (4), the overall equation for glycolysis is

$$\text{Glucose} + 2P_i + 2\text{ADP} \rightarrow 2\text{lactate} + 2\text{ATP} + 2H_2O \quad (5)$$

In either aerobic or anaerobic glycolysis, the complete pathway of glycolysis generates a net energy yield of two molecules of ATP per breakdown of one molecule of glucose. Glycolytic ATP supplements oxidative production of ATP, constituting 5 to 10 percent of the total ATP under aerobic conditions, but is the sole energy source in anaerobic conditions. The ATP that is produced independently of oxygen via the glycolytic breakdown of glucose is generated by substrate level phosphorylation. Although the fate of pyruvate is primarily to be converted to either acetyl-CoA or lactate, pyruvate also participates in the transamination reaction between pyruvate and glutamate to produce alanine and α-ketoglutarate.[10,12] Pyruvate is also a reactant, with carbon dioxide, in the $NADP^+$-dependent malic enzyme reaction, which produces malate used in the *citrate synthase* step of the TCA cycle,[13] as discussed below.

OXIDATIVE METABOLISM

The heart is a highly aerobic organ that derives over 90 percent of its energy production from the progressive oxidation of carbon-based fuels. Unlike glycolysis, which takes place in the cytosol, oxidative metabolism occurs in the mitochondria. The mitochondrial matrix is a dense protein environment allowing for rapid and efficient transfer of substrates between different enzyme systems. The currency for oxidative energy production is the reducing equivalent that is derived from the carbon substrates and carried by the cofactors NAD^+ and flavin–adenine dinucleotide (FAD). In addition to the two ATP molecules per glucose produced by substrate level phosphorylation in glycolysis, the oxidation of the two NADH molecules produced in glycolysis will generate six more molecules of ATP if these reducing equivalents move from the cytosol to the mitochondrial matrix. This corresponds to a 300 percent increase in the energetic efficiency of the breakdown of glucose to two pyruvate molecules. The oxidation of the two pyruvate molecules produced from the glycolytic breakdown of glucose yields 30 molecules of ATP for a combined total of 38 molecules of ATP produced from the complete oxidative breakdown of 1 molecule of glucose by the heart.

Other substrates such as fatty acids can yield much greater amounts of ATP per molecule that is oxidized. For example, palmitate, a long-chain fatty acid comprised of 16 carbons, will yield a total of 129 molecules of ATP per molecule oxidized as compared to 15 ATP molecules form the oxidation of one pyruvate molecule! The amount of oxygen utilized per ATP produced by fatty acid oxidation is actually greater than that with the oxidation of glucose or pyruvate. Thus, not only is substrate oxidation an efficient source of energy for the heart, but the availability of substrate to the heart and substrate preference by the heart can influence the bioenergetic balance and respiratory efficiency at a given level of cardiac performance.

Pyruvate Dehydrogenase

The relative contributions of pyruvate and fatty acids to oxidative metabolism are variable and are regulated by the activity of the *pyruvate dehydrogenase* (PDH), a large protein complex located in the inner mitochondrial membrane. The next reaction is to decarboxylate the three-carbon pyruvate to a two-carbon, acetyl group bonded to (CoA):

$$\text{Pyruvate} + \text{CoA-SH} + NAD^+ \rightarrow \text{acetyl-CoA} + CO_2 + \text{NADH} + H^+ \quad (6)$$

The PDH contains multiple phosphorylation sites that regulate its enzymatic activity. Phosphorylation of PDH by a *protein kinase* inactivates this enzyme in response to end product activation of the kinase by NADH and acetyl-CoA. The PDH is also phosphorylated to the inactive form by *PDH kinase* in response to NADH. The *PDH phosphatase* dephosphorylates PDH to the active form. The *PDH phosphatase* is inhibited by NADH and end products of oxidative metabolism. The sensitivity of the PDH kinase and phosphatase enzymes to the NADH/NAD ratio in the myocyte allows the formation of acetyl-CoA to be shut down during hypoxia or ischemia in the heart, allowing pyruvate to be converted to lactate via LDH to sustain anerobic glycolysis.

The extent of pyruvate oxidation is governed by the percentage of PDH enzyme that is in the active dephosphorylated state (PDHa). The inhibition of carbohydrate oxidation by fatty acid metabolism is mediated through PDH, as the increases in acetyl-CoA, TCA intermediates,

NADH, and ATP that are associated with fatty acid oxidation serve to increase *PDH phosphatase* activity and decrease *PDH kinase* activity. The active PDHa is also regulated by the intramitochondrial ratios of NADH/NAD and acetyl-CoA/CoA. The PDH activity is also responsive to changes in mitochondrial calcium levels, providing a physiological control of carbohydrate oxidation.

Experiments on the intact heart have demonstrated reduced pyruvate oxidation in the presence of the preferred, long-chain fatty acid substrate in the form of palmitate.[7] The level of active PDHa also appears to play a role in the recovery of contractile function in the postischemic, reperfused heart. During early, but not late, reperfusion, an unusually high percentage of PDH is in the phosphorylated inactive form.[14] The resultant, transient reduction in pyruvate oxidation during early reperfusion has been confirmed in intact heart preparations.[15] Evidence exists to support the notion that countering this transient depression of carbohydrate oxidation during early reperfusion is important in resetting the contractile state of the postischemic heart and ultimately improving contractile recovery from reversible ischemia.[6]

Fatty Acid Metabolism

Fats are available to the heart in the form of plasma triglycerides and free fatty acids. Triglycerides are composed of fatty acids that are bound to a three-carbon sugar, glycerol. Circulating free fatty acids are bound to plasma proteins, primarily albumin. As an energy source, these fats supply over twice as much energy per gram as carbohydrate or protein sources. Free fatty acids are more readily oxidized by the heart than triglycerides and are the predominant oxidative fuel for the heart. Triglycerides must first be broken down into the glycerol and fatty acid components before the fatty acids can be oxidized.

The uptake of fatty acid by the myocyte occurs by passive diffusion across the sarcolemmal membrane, facilitated by fatty acid carrier proteins. The rate of transport is dependent on the size of the gradient for plasma and myocyte fatty acid content. Thus, raising plasma fatty acid concentrations will increase the uptake by the myocytes. Once in the cytosol, the fatty acid must be activated to acyl-CoA prior to transport into the mitochondria for subsequent oxidation. Alternatively, acyl-CoA can be utilized for the formation of more complex lipids in the myocyte. This activation involves the formation of an active complex with CoA at the expense of two high-energy phosphate bonds (pyrophosphate) from ATP. The activated acyl-CoA in the cytosol is then converted to acyl-carnitine, which is transported into the mitochondria via the action of the acyl-carnitine transferases. This transfer is driven by the concentration differences in acyl-carnitine (high cytosolic levels) and acyl-CoA (high mitochondrial levels) across the mitochondrial membrane. The transferase reaction is mediated by two components of acyl-carnitine transferase: (1) *acyl-carnitine transferase I*, which is located on the cytosolic side of the inner mitochondrial membrane and transfers acyl-carnitine across the membrane, and (2) *acyl-carnitine transferase II*, which is located on the mitochondrial side of the inner mitochondrial membrane and converts acyl-carnitine back to acyl-CoA within the matrix.

The accumulation of these activated fatty acid esters in ischemic or hypoperfused myocardium is one of the deleterious events leading to the disruption of cell function. Elevation of acyl-carnitine in the cytosol inhibits the sodium-potassium pump, and high levels of serum fatty acids have been associated with arrhythmogenesis in man,[16,17] Elevated acyl-esters may also inhibit energy transfer between the cytosol and the mitochondria by inhibiting the *adenine nucleotide translocase*. In addition, free fatty acids within the cytosol exert a detergent-like action, disrupting the highly ordered membrane structure of the myocyte. Therefore, the very fuel that supports normal cardiac function can contribute to the disruption of myocyte function when oxidative metabolism is impaired in the presence of residual fatty acid content. The ischemic myocardium responds to the excess fatty acids by complexing them into less deleterious lipid complexes. The formation of such lipid droplets has been visualized in the areas surrounding ischemic myocardium.[18] In reperfused myocardium, oxidative metabolism of fatty acids in the mitochondria may contribute to oxygen wastage by uncoupling oxidative phosphorylation from the respiratory chain. Alleviating the oxidative burden of fatty acid metabolism in the postischemic heart by increasing carbohydrate utilization (i.e., glucose) improves the efficiency of oxygen utilization per unit of mechanical work performed by experimental heart preparations.[6]

β Oxidation

In the mitochondria, activated fatty acids are broken down by the multistep process of β oxidation into two carbon fragments for entry into the TCA cycle (Fig. 6A-3). The first of four steps in β oxidation is the oxidation of acyl-CoA by *acyl-CoA dehydrogenase*, forming enoyl CoA and reducing the cofactor FAD into $FADH_2$. The second step is the hydration of the enoyl-CoA by *enoyl CoA hydratase*, consuming a molecule of water and producing hydroxyacyl-CoA. The third step is another oxidation reaction catalyzed by *hydroxyacyl-CoA dehydrogenase* to form ketoacyl-CoA, reducing NAD^+ to NADH. The fourth step is the thiolytic cleavage of the ketoacyl CoA into acetyl-CoA and new acyl-CoA chain that has been shortened by two carbons. This last reaction of the *thiolase* enzyme utilizes an additional CoA to form the new acyl-CoA, which is again available for further breakdown via the four steps of β oxidation. In this one round of β oxidation, the reducing equivalents produced are available for oxidation via the respiratory chain and additional ATP synthesis. The process of β oxidation continues to break down the fatty acid chain into two-carbon acetyl-CoA units by the progressive cleavage of the chain at the β-carbon position, thus the name of this pathway. The action of β oxidation on odd-numbered fatty acids culminates in the formation of the activated three-carbon fatty acid, propionyl-CoA (from propionate). Propionyl-CoA can then enter oxidative metabolism by conversion to the TCA intermediate succinyl CoA.

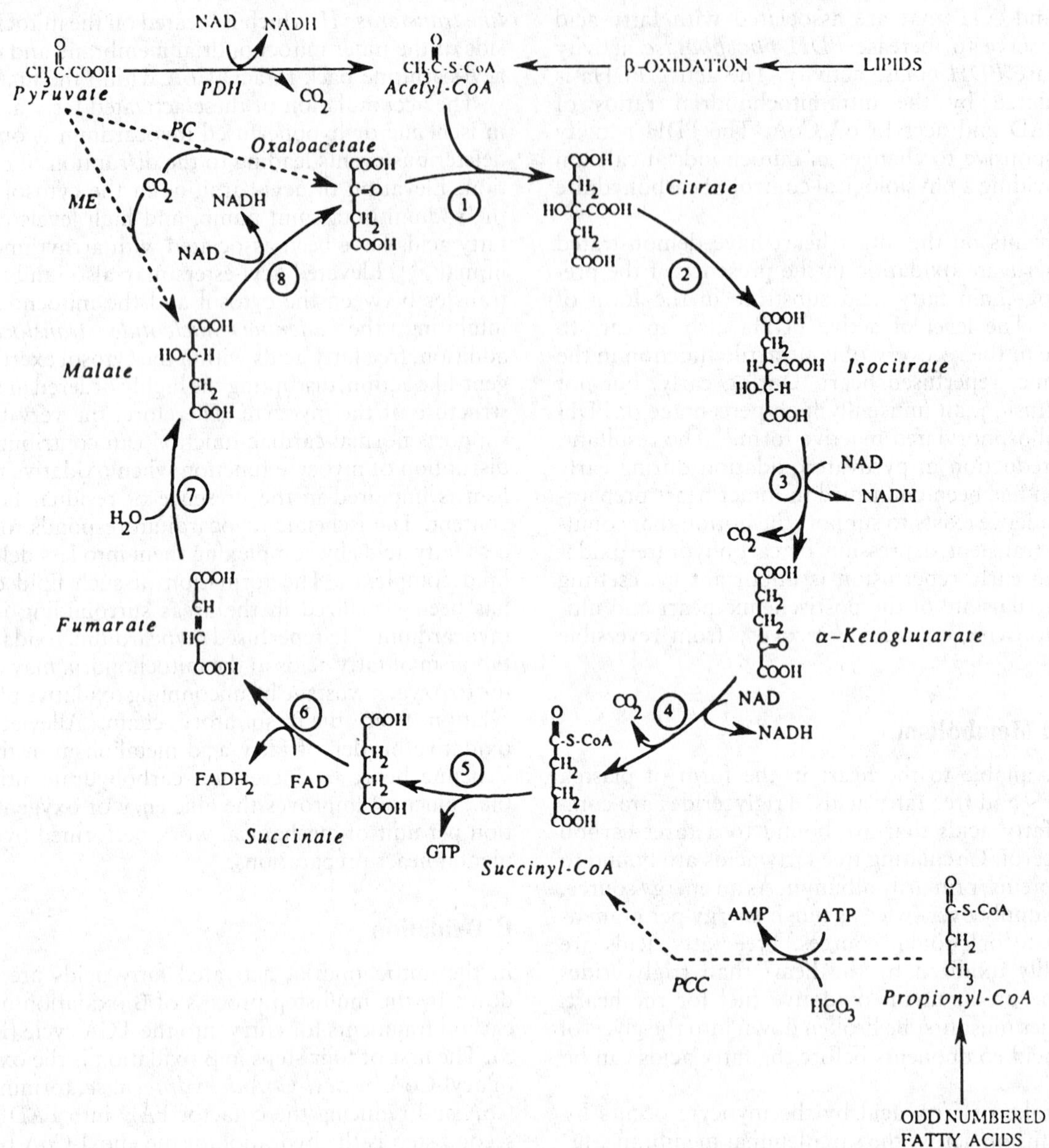

FIGURE 6A-3 Tricarboxylic acid (TCA) cycle. Numbered reactions within the TCA cycle are catalyzed by the following enzymes: 1, citrate synthase; 2, aconitase; 3, isocitrate dehydrogenase; 4, α-ketoglutarate dehydrogenase; 5, succinyl CoA synthase; 6, succinate dehydrogenase; 7, fumarase; 8, malate dehydrogenase. Energy-yielding products are highlighted in blue, as the formation of reducing equivalents or the high-energy phosphate bond of GTP. Other enzymatic reactions contributing to the formation of TCA cycle intermediates include the reactions of pyruvate dehydrogenase (PDH), pyruvate carboxylase (PC), $NADP^+$-dependent malic enzyme (ME), and propionyl CoA carboxylase (PCC).

Tricarboxylic Acid Cycle

The primary source of NADH from the oxidation of carbon-based substrates is the TCA cycle (Fig. 6A-3). This pathway is also commonly called the citric acid cycle or the Krebs cycle, in honor of Sir Hans Krebs of Oxford, who first described this cycle. The TCA cycle can be divided into two parts or spans. The first is from acetyl-CoA to succinyl-CoA and the second is from succinyl-CoA to oxaloacetate.

The net conversion of acetyl-CoA to CO_2 begins when the two-carbon acetyl-CoA units, from the breakdown of carbon-based substrates, enter the TCA cycle by a condensation reaction with the four-carbon organic acid oxaloacetate (Fig. 6A-3). This reaction is catalyzed by *citrate synthase* to produce the six-carbon organic acid citrate and can be rate limited by the availability of carbon substrate. The activity of *citrate synthase* is reduced by ATP, which provides a level of regulation by the energetic state of the heart. Successive dehydration and hydration reactions by *aconitase* interchange the positions of a hydrogen and a hydroxyl group within the citrate molecule, forming isocitrate. *Isocitrate dehydrogenase* catalyzes the oxidative decarboxylation of isocitrate to liberate carbon dioxide and produce the five-carbon α-ketoglutarate and NADH in the first step, yielding a reducing equivalent for the oxidative production of ATP. The production of α-ketoglutarate is under regulation through inhibition of the enzyme by NADH and stimulation by ADP. A second oxidative decarboxylation is catalyzed by *α-ketoglutarate dehydrogenase*, liberating another carbon dioxide from α-ketoglutarate and forming succinyl-CoA and a second reducing equivalent as NADH. For this reaction to proceed, CoA must be freely available as a reactant. Flux through the α-ketoglutarate dehydrogenase reaction is very sensitive to the availability of carbon substrate, and the enzyme activity is affected by the mitochondrial calcium level.[19] This reaction is also subject to feedback inhibition by the products succinyl-CoA and NADH.

The conversion of succinyl-CoA to succinate via the action of *succinyl-CoA synthase* is readily reversible. In the forward direction, the reaction is coupled to the phosphorylation of GDP to form GTP from the only substrate level phosphorylation reaction in the TCA cycle. This GTP can then donate the phosphate group to ADP to produce ATP. The four-carbon organic acid succinate is then oxidized by *succinate dehydrogenase* to form fumarate and reduce FAD to $FADH_2$. The two electrons that are donated to form $FADH_2$ are then directly transferred to the respiratory chain to generate oxidatively two molecules of ATP. The *fumarase* enzyme catalyzes the hydration of fumarate to produce malate. Malate is oxidized by *malate dehydrogenase* in the production of oxaloacetate, which generates reducing equivalents that are transferred to NAD^+ to form the reduced NADH. The NADH produced by this reaction is then also available for oxidation by the respiratory chain to yield three molecules of ATP. Coming full circle, oxaloacetate is then available as a reactant in the condensation reaction of an additional acetyl group by citrate synthase.

The energy yield from one "turn" of the TCA cycle, starting from the entry of acetyl-CoA, is 12 ATP molecules. One of these ATP molecules is produced by substrate level phosphorylation during the conversion of succinyl CoA to succinate, and the other 11 ATP molecules come from the oxidation of 3 NADH (3 ATP for each NADH) and 1 $FADH_2$ (2 ATP for each $FADH_2$). In the process, the carbon pool, which is distributed among all of the TCA cycle intermediate pools, is conserved within the cycle with the net reaction shown below:

$$\begin{aligned}\text{Acetyl CoA} &+ 3\text{NAD}^+ + \text{FAD} + \text{GDP}\\ &+ \text{P}_i + 2\text{H}_2\text{O} \rightarrow 2\text{CO}_2\\ &+ 3\text{NADH} + \text{FADH}_2 + \text{GTP}\\ &+ 3\text{H}^+ + \text{CoA}\end{aligned} \tag{7}$$

This pathway is often represented as a spinning loop that speeds up in response to metabolic indicators of increased oxidative energy demands, largely mediated by TCA cycle intermediate levels and the NADH/NAD ratio in the mitochondria. This pathway is not a closed loop, however, and points of entry in addition to acetyl-CoA at citrate synthase may occur, determined by the work load and pathophysiological state of the heart. The TCA cycle rate changes with substrate choice[20] and the rate of oxygen consumption, indicating a reciprocal relationship between the physiological demands of the heart and the metabolically controlled redox (reduction-oxidation) state of heart. Therefore, the activity and regulation of the TCA cycle are important links between the respiratory activity of the mitochondria and the functional state of the myocardium.

Since the entry of two carbon acetyl groups into the TCA cycle at citrate synthase is balanced by the liberation of two CO_2 molecules, other reactions must govern the regulation of the total carbon pool within the TCA intermediates. These reactions are responsible for the differences in the total TCA cycle intermediate pool that have been observed at different work loads or with different substrates. The reactions that contribute to the formation of the TCA cycle intermediate pools are anaplerotic (from the Greek meaning "to fill up") reactions, and opposing reactions contributing to net efflux of carbon from the TCA cycle are cataplerotic reactions. Anaplerosis includes the reactions of pyruvate and propionate carboxylation to the four-carbon organic acids and the transaminase reactions involving glutamate and aspartate or alanine (Fig. 6A-3). Cataplerotic reactions are less well defined in the heart but may involve the reverse reactions of anaplerosis. The balance between these two types of reactions regulates the TCA cycle intermediate pool size and is involved in both the feedback control of TCA cycle flux rates and transfer of metabolic signals between the mitochondrial compartment and the cytosol.

Metabolic disorders, such as diabetic or alcoholic ketosis, can lead to contractile failure of the heart subsequent to the "derailment" of the span between *citrate synthase* and *α-ketoglutarate dehydrogenase* from the span between *succinyl-CoA synthase* and *citrate synthase*.[21] As CoA is sequestered by the activation of ketones from the plasma, succinyl-CoA is formed. The carbon pool within this first span of the TCA cycle will then accumulate, starving the second span of its carbon pool. Unless anaplerotic sources of carbon are available in the form of pyruvate from carbohydrates or propionate from odd-numbered fatty acids to replenish the TCA intermediate pool within the second span, *citrate synthase* will become substrate starved and the cycle will grind to a halt. Alternatively, a redistribution of the TCA intermediate carbon pool will ensue, adjusting the TCA cycle rate via feedback inhibition, as described in the previous section. Such a redistribution of the total carbon pool between the intermediates of either span of the TCA cycle provides internal regulation of cycle flux and the capability to adjust the rate of oxidative substrates metabolism to the carbon flux through the multiple entry/exit points of the cycle. Thus, the TCA cycle is in communication with other intermediary pathways both within the mitochondria and in the cytosol, thereby maintaining a balance between the metabolic state of the heart and the physiological demand for oxidative energy production.

Malate-Aspartate Shuttle

One mechanism that provides metabolic communication between the mitochondrial matrix and the cytosol is the malate-aspartate shuttle (Fig. 6A-4). The primary function of this shuttle is the transport of reducing equivalents from cytosolic NADH to the mitochondria for oxidation and replenishing the cytosolic supply of NAD^+. In the process, NADH is oxidized to NAD^+ by the coupled reaction with oxaloacetate to produce malate in the cytosol. Malate is then carried into the mitochondria, indirectly transporting the reducing equivalents from cytosolic NADH. Mitochondrial oxidation of

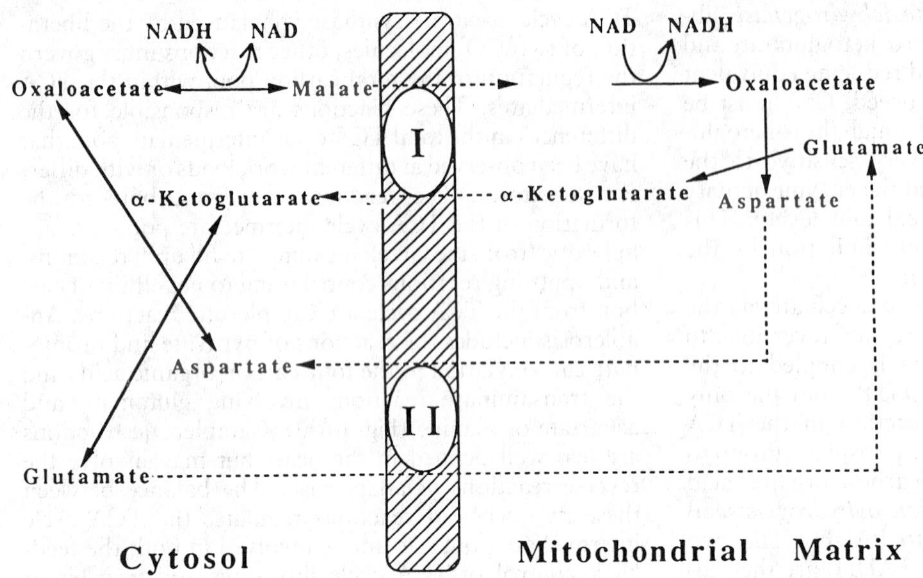

FIGURE 6A-4 Malate-aspartate shuttle. The NADH produced in the cytosolic compartment of the myocyte is oxidized to NAD^+ during conversion of oxaloacetate to malate. Malate crosses the mitochondrial membrane in exchange for α-ketoglutarate through the activity of the antiport carrier system (I). The malate and NAD^+ in the mitochondrial matrix are then reconverted to oxaloacetate and NADH. Oxaloacetate, which is impermeable to the mitochondrial membrane, is replenished in the cytosolic compartment by transamination between aspartate and α-ketoglutarate. The glutamate formed by this transamination is transported into the mitochondria via exchange for the outward transport of aspartate at the antiport carrier system (II). Thereby, steady-state levels of oxaloacetate are maintained in the cytosol, while net transfer of NADH into the mitochondria occurs.

malate to oxaloacetate reduces mitochondrial NAD^+ to NADH. The oxaloacetate reduced from the oxidation of transported malate is not permeable, so to complete the cycle, oxaloacetate undergoes transamination with glutamate to form matrix α-ketoglutarate and aspartate. An antiport carrier (I) catalyzes the transport of malate in exchange for α-ketoglutarate from the mitochondrial matrix to the cytosol. Another antiport carrier (II) transports aspartate out of the mitochondrial matrix and into the cytosol in exchange or glutamate. In the cytosol, the α-ketoglutarate and aspartate are involved in a transaminase reaction to produce glutamate and restore oxaloacetate. The net result of this complex shuttle system is the indirect transport of reducing equivalents by malate into the mitochondrial matrix with overall increases in mitochondrial NADH and cytosolic NAD^+. However, the shuttle also provides a mechanism, via the α-ketoglutarate-aspartate carrier, for the myocyte to accommodate transient changes in flux within the two spans of the TCA cycle as determined by *α-ketoglutarate dehydrogenase* activity. Additionally, the exchange of metabolites between the mitochondrial and cytosolic compartments by the action of this shuttle provides a mechanism for translating the levels of TCA intermediates (i.e., citrate) within the mitochondrial matrix to the cytosol for the regulation of glycolysis.

Oxidative Phosphorylation

In the heart, nearly all ATP synthesis occurs via oxidative phosphorylation in the inner mitochondrial membrane. Oxidative phosphorylation is the process whereby ATP is formed as electrons are transferred from NADH or $FADH_2$ (which were made by glycolysis in the cytosol or by fatty acid oxidation and the citric acid cycle in the mitochondrial matrix) to molecular O_2 by a series of electron carriers. The driving force of oxidative phosphorylation is derived from the high affinity of O_2 for electrons. Electrons are transferred from NADH to O_2 through a chain of three large protein complexes—*NADH-Q reductase, cytochrome reductase*, and *cytochrome oxidase*—interspersed with electron carriers coenzyme Q and cytochrome c. The $FADH_2$ enters at the level of coenzyme Q. The specific electron-carrying groups are the flavins, iron-sulfur clusters, hemes, and copper ions. The flow of electrons through these three complexes leads to the pumping of protons from the matrix to the cytosolic side of the inner mitochondrial membrane, creating a proton-motive force (Fig. 6A-1). The net reaction is

$$NADH + \tfrac{1}{2}O_2 + H^+ \rightarrow H_2O + NAD^+ \qquad (8)$$

The oxidation of NADH and $FADH_2$ is coupled to the phosphorylation of ADP to form ATP via the ATPase complex, also known as H^+-ATPase, F_0, F_1-ATPase, or ATP synthase. This ATPase is driven by the flow of protons back to the matrix. The ATP-synthesizing complex consists of the F_1 subunit, which is located on the matrix side and contains the catalytic site for ATP synthesis; the transmembrane F_0 subunit, which contains the proton channel; and the F_1 inhibitor protein, which is the stalk between the F_0 and F_1 subunits and regulates proton flow and ATP synthesis. Based on elegant ^{18}O exchange experiments, Boyer[22] showed that the role of the proton gradient is not to form ATP (since equal amounts of bound ATP and ADP are in equilibrium at the catalytic site) but rather to release ATP from the enzyme. The net reaction is

$$ADP^{3-} + Pi^{2-} + H^+ \rightarrow ATP^{4-} + H_2O \qquad (9)$$

Oxidation of each NADH yields three ATP and each $FADH_2$ yields two ATP.

The ATP and ADP are not permeable to the inner mitochondrial membrane. The coupled exchange of cytosolic ADP for mitochondrial ATP occurs via the ATP-ADP translocase. The result is a net transfer of one negative charge out of the matrix, decreasing the membrane potential. About 25 percent of the energy obtained from respiration is used to restore this membrane potential. In this way, electron transport is tightly coupled to phosphorylation and hence the high efficiency of ATP synthesis via oxidative phosphorylation (Fig. 6A-1). The net reaction for the complete oxidation of glucose in heart is

$$\text{Glucose} + 38\text{ADP} + 38\text{p}_i + 38\text{H}^+ + 6\text{O}_2 \rightarrow 6\text{CO}_2 + 38\text{ATP} + 42\text{H}_2\text{O} \quad (10)$$

Respiration is controlled by availability of NADH, O_2, ADP, and P_i. Based on experiments using isolated mitochondria, the notion that ADP is the most important regulator became widely accepted. Using ^{31}P NMR spectroscopy to measure ATP, PCr, and pH in vivo, one can now calculate cytosolic ADP concentrations with reasonable confidence. Coordinate changes in ADP and respiration rates can be shown in some,[23] but not all,[24,25] experimental conditions. Thus, regulators other than ADP must also function to regulate respiration *in vivo*. The choice is governed by the physiology and pathophysiology of the heart. The existence of multiple regulators minimizes fluctuations in ATP production and maintains high adenylate energy charge and a related expression, the phosphorylation potential, [ATP]/[ADP]/[P_i]. This is particularly important during ischemia and hypoxemia, when creatine kinase fails to maintain low levels of ADP and P_i and O_2 could be (but probably is not) limiting.

NEW METHODS FOR METABOLIC EVALUATION OF THE HEART

Metabolic support of contractile function is best understood in the intact beating heart. Metabolism is also an important component in evaluating the pathological state of tissue and may also provide an index of tissue viability. Unfortunately, traditional methods to study metabolism are not well suited to concurrent measurements of physiological function. This is due to the requirements of tissue sampling and to the inherent nature of biochemical assay of dilute enzymes. In short, the invasive nature of most metabolic analyses limits our understanding of the basic physiology of intact myocardium and the clinical evaluation of diseased hearts. Therefore, progress in cardiovascular science is greatly enhanced by new nondestructive methods that allow for repeated or continual metabolic evaluation of the same region of myocardium. Two methodologies fulfill the criteria of providing nondestructive, kinetic information: positron emission tomography (PET) (Chap. 137) and NMR spectroscopy (Chap. 136). Positron emission tomography provides information on the cardiac uptake and spatial distribution of positron-emitting nuclei in exogenous metabolic agents that can then be related to the pathophysiological state. Nuclear magnetic resonance spectroscopy is uniquely able to provide chemical information about the metabolism of specific molecules and pathways. The NMR-detectable nuclei include ^{31}P and ^{13}C, which allow for nondestructive, repetitive measurement of energy production, utilization, and turnover rate. Thus, NMR methods provide kinetic information of tissue biochemistry in intact myocardium by targeting specific metabolic reactions that may characterize pathophysiology. Specific examples follow.

Phosphorus-31 NMR spectroscopy provides measurement of tissue content of ATP, PCr, and P_i as well as intracellular pH. Using the tool of magnetization transfer, the velocity of the forward (or reverse) creatine kinase reaction has been measured in heart *in vivo* (Fig. 6A-5). Other examples of the ability of NMR to measure

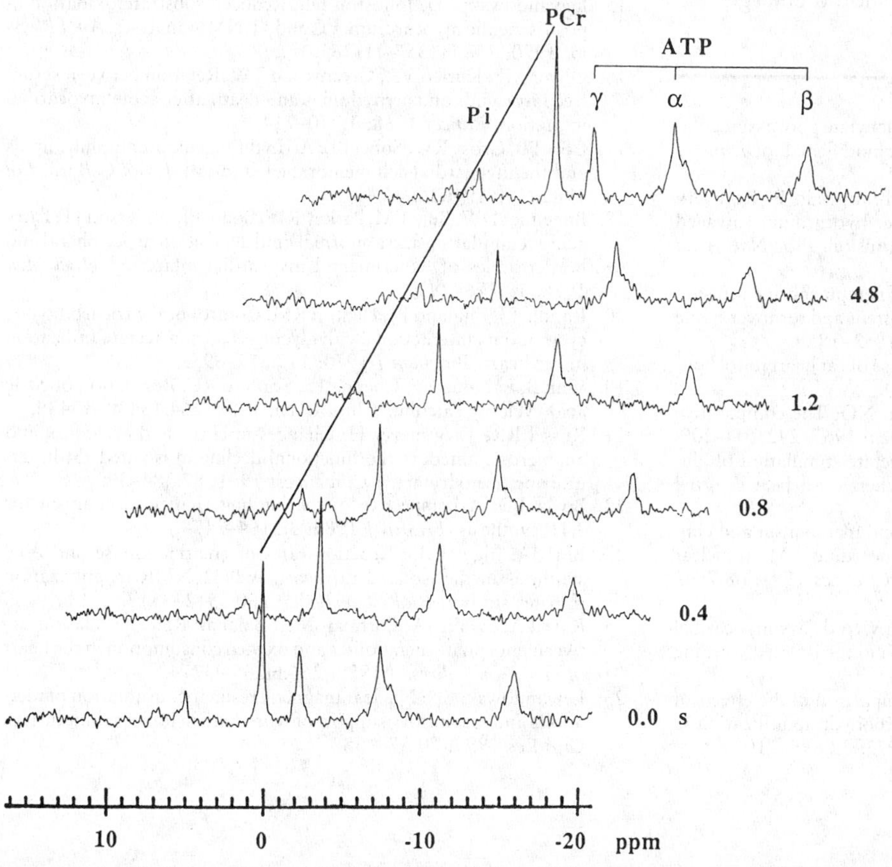

FIGURE 6A-5 Magnetization Transfer. Stacked plot of ^{31}P NMR spectra illustrating the magnetization transfer method used to measure flux through the creatine kinase reaction. The duration of saturation of the [γ-P] ATP signal (in seconds) is denoted to the right of each spectrum. The major resonances are assigned from left to right as inorganic phosphate (P_i), phosphocreatine (PCr), and γ-, α-, and β-phosphates of ATP. Values for the pseudo-first-order rate constant of the forward creatine kinase reaction PCr→[γ-P]ATP is calculated from the exponential decay of the PCr peak area and time of saturation of γ-ATP. Flux through the reaction is calculated by multiplying the pseudo-first-order rate constant and tissue PCr content. Each spectrum was obtained by signal averaging 40 scans of 90° read pulses following the saturation pulse interleaved in groups of 8 and separated by a constant delay of 7 s (including the saturation pulse time).

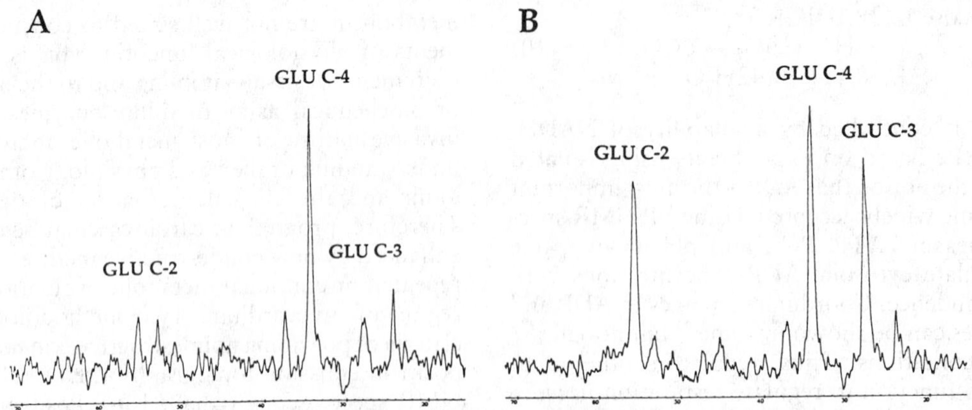

FIGURE 6A-6 Dynamic changes in NMR spectra from intact heart. Sequential, pre-steady-state ^{13}C NMR spectra from isolated rabbit heart oxidizing [2-^{13}C] acetate are shown. Spectrum *A* was acquired at the 3- to 6-min period of perfusion with ^{13}C-enriched substrate. Spectrum *B* was acquired at steady-state enrichment of glutamate during the 25- to 28-min period of perfusion with ^{13}C-enriched substrate. Note evolution of ^{13}C spectra from intact heart over time. Relative signal intensity of ^{13}C-labeled carbon positions within the tissue glutamate pool approaches steady-state isotopic enrichment at a rate determined by the work load and carbon flux through substrate oxidation. Each spectrum represents 3 min of signal acquisition. Carbon positions of glutamate (GLU) are labeled as indicated for the 2-, 4-, and 3-carbons.

whole-organ enzymology include net ATP synthesis using ^{31}P magnetization transfer and carbon-based substrate utilization using exogenous ^{13}C-labeled metabolites. Recently, ^{13}C NMR spectra obtained sequentially from intact hearts with different levels of cardiac performance and respiratory rates (Fig. 6A-6) show that turnover within the TCA cycle intermediate pool correlates with the energetic demand of contractile activity. Therefore, dynamic ^{13}C NMR analysis from intact hearts provides information uniquely related to carbon flux through oxidative pathways in the whole heart. By the use of new approaches such as these, new insights integrating biochemistry and physiology should emerge.

REFERENCES

1. Atkinson DE: The energy change of the adenylate pool as a regulatory parameter. Interaction with feedback modifiers. *Biochemistry* 1968; 7:4030–4034.
2. Kloner RA, DeBoer LWV, Ingwall JS, Braunwald E: Recovery from prolonged abnormalities of canine myocardium salvaged from ischemic necrosis by coronary reperfusion. *Proc Natl Acad Sci USA* 1981; 78:7152–7156.
3. Bittl JA, Balschi JA, Ingwall JS: Effects of nerepinephrine infusion on myocardial high-energy phosphate content and turnover in the living rat heart. *J Clin Invest* 1987; 79:1852–1859.
4. Jacobus WE, Lehringer AL: Creatine kinase of rat heart mitochondria. *J Biol Chem* 1973; 248:4803–4810.
5. Eppenburger HM, Dawson DM, Kaplan NO: The comparative enzymology of creatine kinase. *J Biol Chem* 1967; 242:204–209.
6. McViegh JJ, Lopaschuk GD: Dichloroacetate stimulation of glucose oxidation improves recovery of ischemic rat hearts. *Am J Physiol* 1990; 259:H1079–H1085.
7. Johnston DL, Lewandowski ED: Fatty acid metabolism and contractile function in the reperfused myocardium: Multinuclear NMR studies of isolated rabbit hearts. *Circ Res* 1991; 68:714–725.
8. Schneider CA, Taegtmeyer H: Fasting in vivo delays myocardial cell damage after brief periods of ischemia in the isolated working rat heart. *Circ Res* 1990; 6:1045–1050.
9. Rovetto MJ, Whitmer JT, Neely JR: Comparison of the effects of anoxia and whole heart ischemia on carbohydrate utilization in isolated working rat hearts. *Circ Res* 1973; 32:699–710.
10. Lewandowski ED, Johnston DL, Roberts R: Effects of inosine on glycolysis and contracture during myocardial ischemia. *Circ Res* 1991; 68(2):578–587.
11. Owen P, Dennis S, Opie LH: Glucose flux rate regulates onset of ischemic contracture in globally underperfused rat hearts. *Circ Res* 1990; 66:344–353.
12. Taegtmeyer H, Peterson MB, Ragavan VV, Ferguson AG, Lesch M: De novo alanine synthesis in isolated oxygen-deprived rabbit myocardium. *J Biol Chem* 1977; 252:5010–5018.
13. Russell RR, Taegtmeyer H: Pyruvate carboxylation prevents the decline in contractile function of rat hearts oxidizing acetoacetate. *Am J Physiol* 1991; 261:H1756–H1762.
14. Kobayashi K, Neely JR: Effects of ischemia and reperfusion on pyruvate dehydrogenase activity in isolated rat hearts. *J Mol Cell Cardiol* 1983; 15:359–367.
15. Lewandowski ED, Johnston DL: Reduced substrate oxidation in post-ischemic myocardium: ^{13}C and ^{31}P NMR analyses. *Am J Physiol* 1990; 258:H1357–H1365.
16. Oliver MF, Kurien VA, Greenwood TW: Relation between serum free fatty acids and arrhythmias and death after acute myocardial infarction. *Lancet* 1968; 1:710–714.
17. Corr PB, Gross RW, Sobel BE: Arrhythmogenic amphiphilic lipids and the myocardial cell membrane (editorial). *J Mol Cell Cardiol* 1982; 14:619–626.
18. Bilheimer DW, Buja LM, Parkey RW, Bonte FJ, Willerson JT: Fatty acid accumulation and abnormal lipid deposition in peripheral and border zones of experimental myocardial infarcts. *J Nucl Med* 1978; 19:276–283.
20. Randle PJ, England PJ, Denton RM: Control of the tricarboxylate cycle and its interactions with glycolysis during acetate utilization in rat heart. *Biochem J* 1970; 117:677–695.
19. Wan B, LaNoue KF, Cheung JY, Scaduto RC: Regulation of citric acid cycle by calcium. *J Biol Chem* 1989; 264:13430–13439.
21. Russel RR, Taegtmeyer H: Changes in citric acid cycle flux and anaplerosis antedate the functional decline in isolated rat hearts utilizing acetoacetate. *J Clin Invest* 1991; 87:384–390.
22. Boyer PD: A perspective of the binding change mechanism for ATP synthesis. *FASEB J* 1989; 3:2164–2178.
23. Bittl JA, Ingwall JS: Reaction rates of creatine kinase and ATP synthesis in the isolated rat heart: A P-31 NMR magnetization transfer study. *J Biol Chem* 1985; 260:3512–3517.
24. Katz LA, Swain JA, Portman MA, Balaban RS: The relation between phosphate metabolites and oxygen consumption in the heart *in vivo*. *Am J Physiol* 1989; 256:H265–H274.
25. Lewandowski ED: Nuclear magnetic resonance evaluation of metabolic and respiratory support of work load in intact rabbit hearts. *Circ Res* 1992; 70:576–582.

Chapter 6B

Molecular and Cellular Control of Cardiac Growth and Hypertrophy

Howard E. Morgan, M.D. ■ Kenneth M. Baker, M.D.

In Chap. 1 the receptors and signal proteins of the major pathways involved in regulating cardiac growth were discussed with emphasis on how they exert their control through transcription. Regulation of growth through these pathways is also implemented through translation (protein synthesis) and posttranslation and will be the emphasis in this chapter. Protein synthesis and degradation play a major role in regulating growth whether it be constitutive, in response to injury, mechanical overload, or other stimuli. Rapid cardiac growth usually follows an increased work load that is imposed on the heart as the result of hypertension, following myocardial infarction, or at birth.[1-3] Associated with increased work load in vivo, there are changes in plasma concentrations of substances such as adrenergic agonists, thyroxine, and angiotensin. A continuing question is whether the hypertrophy of cardiac muscle cells is due to direct effects of these neurotransmitters and hormones on cardiac growth through receptor binding or growth depends on mechanical deformation of the heart imposed directly by pressure overload. A corollary question is whether increased work load and associated stretching of the ventricular wall can generate intracellular signals that will result in net protein formation without the intervention of neurotransmitters, hormones, or growth factors. The mechanisms through which physical forces are converted to biochemical signals (mechanotransduction) have been shown to involve stretch-activated ion channels, adenylyl cyclase, Na^+-H^+ exchange, and activation of protein kinase C (Fig. 6B-1).[4] The same intracellular signaling mechanisms, cations, cyclic adenosine monophosphate (cAMP), diacylglycerol (DAG), protein kinase A (PKA), and protein kinase C (PKC) are involved in G-protein-linked pathways that include cell surface receptors for hormones and neurotransmitters (Fig. 6B-2).[5] In many instances, the signaling pathways involve phosphorylation of components of the complex of factors that catalyze protein synthesis through peptide chain initiation and elongation[6] as well as through deoxyribonucleic acid (DNA) transcription.[7] Phosphorylation causes both inhibition and activation of protein synthesis.[6] Inhibition of protein synthesis results primarily from modifications of the α subunit of the initiation factor eIF-2 or the elongation factor eEF-2. However, a large number of phosphoproteins have been identified including 13 initiation factor subunits, 3 of the 4 elongation factors, 3 ribosomal proteins, and a number of aminoacyl–transfer ribonucleic acid (tRNA) synthetases. Phosphorylation of eIF-2B, eIF-3, eIF-4B, eIF-4F, and ribosomal protein S6 correlates with activation of protein synthesis in vivo or in vitro.[6] These proteins are phosphorylated by PKC as well as by other protein kinases, some of which may be specific for the individual protein, for example S6 kinase. Protein kinase C has also been most closely linked with control of transcription.[7] Addition of phorbol esters, analogues of DAG, the physi-

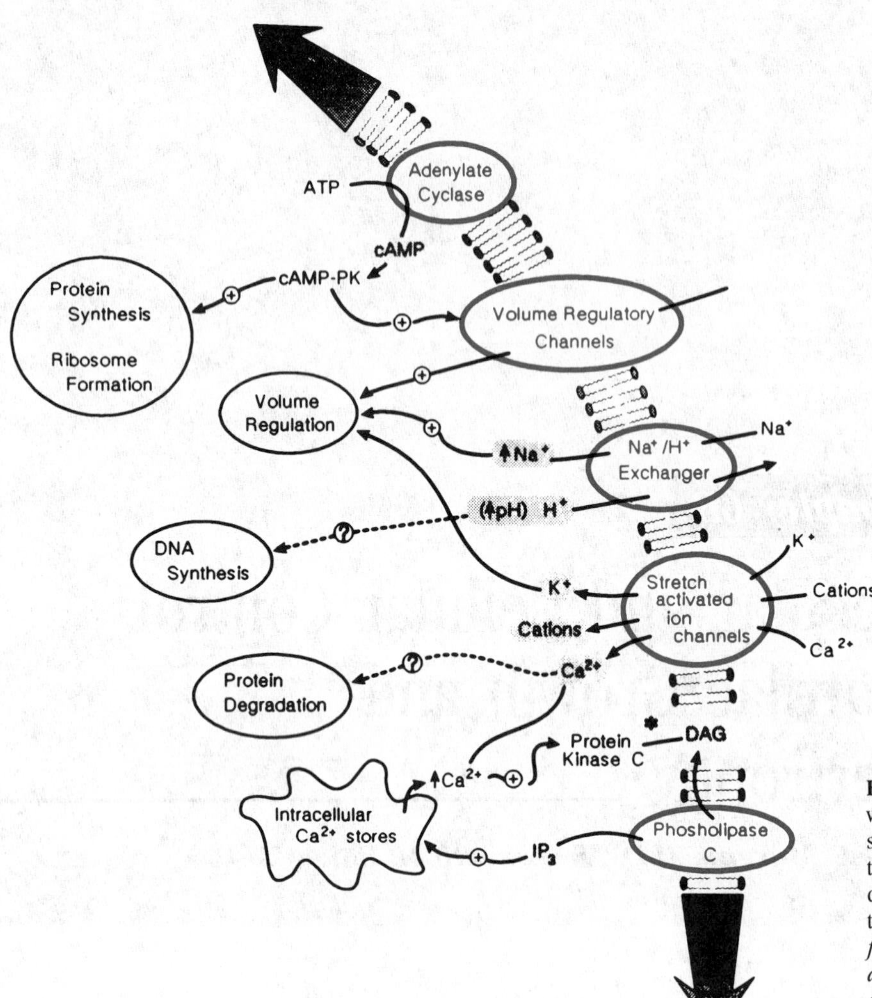

FIGURE 6B-1 Candidate mechanotransducers involved in alterations in cellular biochemistry in response to mechanical forces. Signals generated by these catalysts are indicated by shading. DAG, 1,2-diacylglycerol. Asterisk indicates activated state of protein kinase C. (*From PA Watson, Function follows form: generation of intracellular signals by cell deformation. FASEB J 5:2013–2109, 1991. Reproduced with permission from the publisher, editor, and author.*)

ological activator of PKC, stimulates growth of quiescent cardiac myocytes in culture and accelerates ribosomal DNA transcription.[8] Stimuli that increase growth of cultured cardiomyocytes, including norepinephrine, endothelin, angiotensin II, and contraction, activate PKC.[1,7] In addition to phosphorylation, binding of intracellular signaling compounds (e.g., cAMP) or hormones (e.g., thyroid hormone or glucocorticoids) to DNA binding proteins can regulate gene expression[1,7] (see Chap. 1).

In order to increase the rate of protein synthesis, the rate of the step that is slowest must be accelerated. In the case of cardiomyocytes, what limits the rate of protein synthesis? In regard to a specific protein, the limiting component is often the cytoplasmic concentration of its messenger RNA (mRNA). For global protein synthesis that is required for hypertrophy, mRNA availability does not appear to limit the rate.[1,3] In rat heart, approximately 90 percent of the ribosomal subunits are active in polysomes, which indicates that the rate of protein synthesis is not limited by mRNA availability. Instead, the rate of protein synthesis reflects the content of ribosomes and other components of the protein synthesis pathway.[3,9] The question then becomes what limits the rate of ribosome formation and what physiological stimuli accelerate this process? In addition, what factors sustain optimal rates of peptide chain initiation and elongation and provide the basis for limitation of the rate by the content of ribosomes. These questions are the focus of the remainder of this chapter.

REGULATION OF PROTEIN DEGRADATION AND THE EFFICIENCY OF PROTEIN SYNTHESIS

Hypertrophy and reduction in cardiac mass depend upon changes in the relative rates of synthesis and degradation of all heart proteins. The half-time for turnover of heart proteins and RNA varies from 1 h to several days.[3] The average half-life for a heart protein is 5 days. As a result, a nearly complete complement of new protein is synthesized about every 3 weeks; from this point of view, a person has essentially a "new heart" each month. The significance of the rapid turnover rate is that myofibrillar or enzymatic components of the heart can change in quantity or in type of isozyme over short time periods. Protein turnover in the heart is affected by mechanical activity, availability of hormones and growth factors, oxidative substrates, and oxygen. Decreased availability of these factors may perturb the protein balance of the heart.

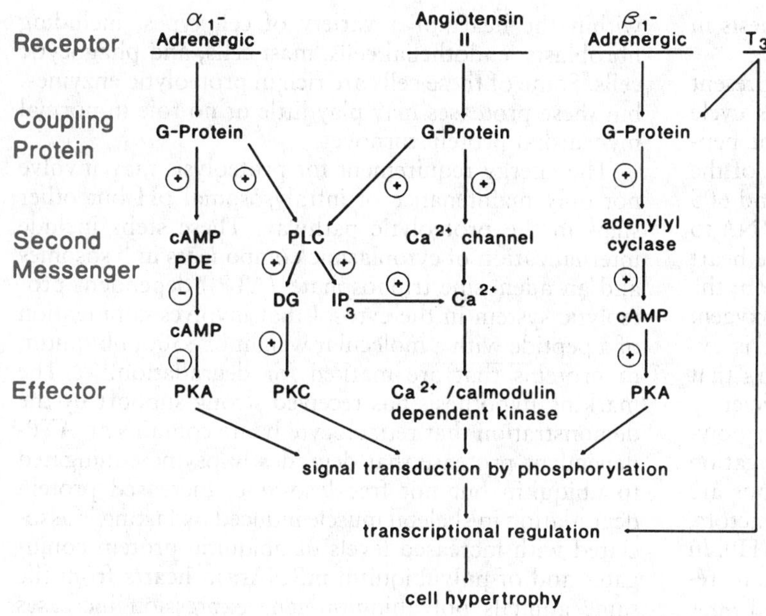

FIGURE 6B-2 Neural and endocrine pathways with possible coupling proteins, second messengers, and effector mechanisms for transcriptional regulation of cardiac cell hypertrophy. G proteins, guanine nucleotide binding proteins; cAMP, cyclic AMP; PDE, phosphodiesterase; PLC, phospholipase C; DG, diacylglycerol; IP_3, inositol triphosphate; PKC, protein kinase C; PKA, cAMP-dependent protein kinase. (*From HE Morgan, KM Baker: Cardiac hypertrophy. Circulation 83:13–25, 1991. Reproduced with permission from the publisher, editor, and author.*)

The pathway of protein synthesis is shown in Fig. 6B-3. Transport of amino acids into the intracellular pool is considered to be the first step in protein synthesis. On the other hand, extracellular availability of amino acids does not appear to restrain protein synthesis in the heart when normal plasma levels of amino acids are present.

The contents of amino acids within the intracellular pool are determined by (1) the rate of entry from the extracellular space; (2) the rate of exit from the cell; (3) rates of formation or destruction of the compound by transamination, oxidation, or other metabolic processes; and (4) rates of protein synthesis and degradation. As a result, intracellular levels of amino acids may fall even though protein synthesis is accelerated. These findings, in addition to the observation that 90 percent of the tRNA is in the aminoacyl form, indicate that steps later in the protein synthetic pathway, such as the content of

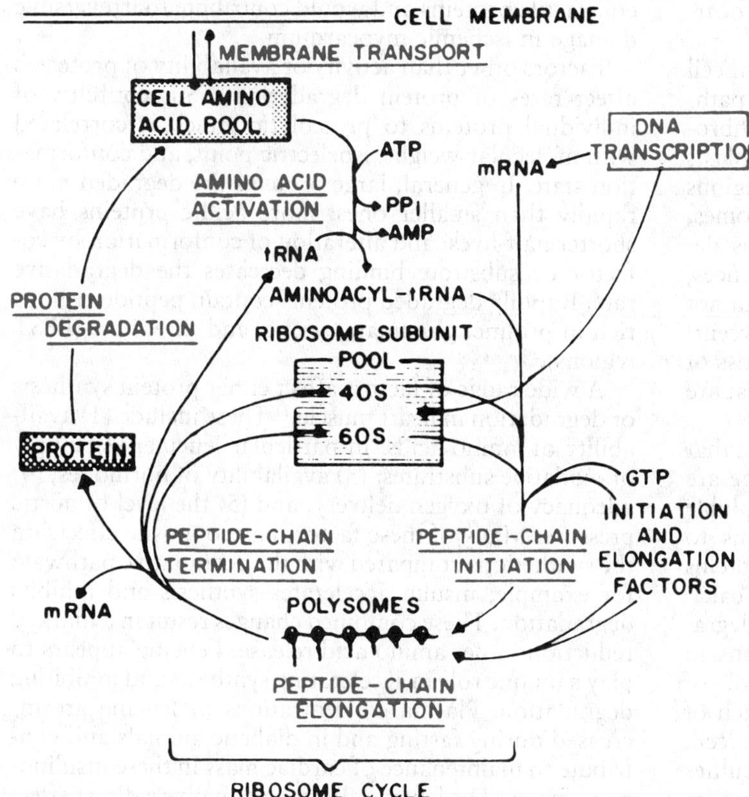

FIGURE 6B-3 Pathway of protein turnover. Amino acids are supplied to the intracellular pool by either membrane transport or protein degradation. Intracellular amino acids are activated to form aminoacyl derivatives by combination with tRNA. Polymerization of activated amino acids into protein is catalyzed by a series of ribosome-catalyzed reactions that make up the ribosome cycle. These reactions include initiation of peptide chains on the ribosomes and elongation and termination of chains. Peptide chain initiation refers to binding of mRNA and initiator tRNA (methionyl tRNA) to the small ribosomal subunit (40S), followed by the binding of the large subunit (60S). Both steps require GTP and initiation factors. Peptide chain elongation refers to successive addition of activated amino acids as determined by the code contained within mRNA. This process is dependent on elongation factors. When the protein is complete, the peptide chain and ribosomal subunits are released into the cytoplasm. Protein degradation refers to reactions catalyzed by proteases and results in the release of free amino acids into the intracellular pool. [*From HE Morgan, et al: Protein metabolism of the heart. In: RM Berne (ed): Handbook of Physiology, sec 2: The Cardiovascular System. Bethesda, MD, American Physiological Society, 1979. Reproduced with permission from the publisher, editor, and author.*]

ribosomes, are flux controlling for protein synthesis in vivo.

The heart contains a pool of ribosomes that is present as either subunits or polysomes. These particles cycle from the subunit pool into polysomes through the peptide chain initiation reactions. Initiation consists of the binding of mRNA, an initiator tRNA, and 40S and 60S subunits and is followed by translation of the mRNA to form a protein. Initiation of peptide chains in the heart is controlled by insulin, epinephrine, and glucagon; the availability of amino acids, fatty substrates, and oxygen; and the work loads and pH to which the heart is exposed.[2,3,10,11] As a result of the breadth of factors that regulate initiation, these reactions remain sufficiently rapid to keep most of the ribosomal subunits in polysomes and to shift the flux-generating step to elongation and termination of peptide chains. These reactions are limited by the supply of ribosomes, elongation factors, aminoacyl tRNA, and guanosine triphosphate (GTP). In anoxic or ischemic hearts, high-energy phosphate reserves are depleted, including the GTP levels, and rates of protein synthesis are inhibited at the level of these ribosome-catalyzed reactions. In normal situations, however, the supply of ribosomes is the major determinant of the rate.

The exact pathway by which proteins are degraded to free amino acids is not known, but lysosomes and cytoplasmic proteases appear to be involved.[3,12–14] Lysosomes contain a number of hydrolytic enzymes, including acid proteases that are capable of degrading protein to free amino acids. Lysosomal proteases have pH optima that are in the range of 2 to 4, a value much lower than the overall intracellular pH. One mechanism of the energy requirement of protein degradation appears to involve maintenance of low intralysosomal pH. Lysosomes often appear in the perinuclear region of myocardial cells and in the rows of mitochondria.

Fasting of animals or deprivation of serum from cell cultures has been used to examine the proteolytic pathway in heart, liver, skeletal muscle, and cultured fibroblasts.[14] An increased rate of proteolysis in fibroblasts involves targeting of proteins containing peptide regions similar to Lys-Phe-Glu-Arg-Gln (KFERQ) to lysosomes, and the cytosolic concentrations of these proteins decline. All tissues contain proteins with these sequences, but they disappear with fasting in heart and liver but not in skeletal muscle. The loss in heart weight (7 percent) during a 24-h fast appears to be due entirely to loss of proteins containing KFERQ-like peptide regions that are degraded in lysosomes.[14]

In addition to acid proteases, proteolytic enzymes that have pH optima in the neutral and alkaline range are present in the heart. These enzymes include two soluble Ca^{2+}-activated proteases[13,15] that degrade proteins to peptides and particulate proteases that degrade proteins to free amino acids. The physiological function of calcium-dependent proteases is unknown, and protein degradation in heart is not affected by wide variations in extracellular Ca^{2+}.[16] Similarly, the physiological role of the particulate proteases is in doubt, because much of the activity appears to be localized in a nonmuscle cell, the mast cell. This finding illustrates one of the difficulties in defining the proteolytic pathway, namely, the presence within the heart of a variety of cell types, including fibroblasts, endothelial cells, mast cells, and phagocytic cells. Some of these cells are rich in proteolytic enzymes, but these proteases may play little or no role in normal myocardial protein turnover.

The energy requirement for proteolysis may involve not only maintenance of intralysosomal pH but other steps in the proteolytic pathway. These steps include internalization of cytoplasmic components in lysosomes and an adenosine triphosphate–(ATP-) dependent proteolytic system in the cytosol that involves conjugation of a peptide with a molecular weight of 8500, ubiquitin, to proteins that are marked for degradation.[17,18] The marking hypothesis has received strong support by the demonstration that reticulocyte lysate contains an ATP-dependent protease that degrades lysosyme conjugated to ubiquitin but not free lysosyme. Increased protein degradation in skeletal muscle induced by fasting is associated with increased levels of ubiquitin-protein conjugates and of polyubiquitin mRNAs; in hearts from the same animals polyubiquitin-gene expression increases only slightly. These results do not support an important role for a nonlysosomal ATP-dependent proteolytic process in the loss of heart weight during fasting. In heart, the energy requirement appears to involve initial steps in the proteolytic pathway because factors that reduce levels of high-energy phosphates, such as anoxia and ischemia, prevent the loss of activity of a specific enzyme, S-adenosyl methionine decarboxylase, and do not lead to the accumulation of the products of proteolysis, peptides and free amino acids, within the heart. In regard to effects of reduced oxygen delivery on protein degradation in the heart, it is important that the initial step in the pathway be blocked. Otherwise, proteolysis would proceed and result in inactivation of enzymes and contractile proteins and would contribute to irreversible damage in ischemic myocardium.

Factors other than activity or availability of proteases affect rates of protein degradation.[19] Susceptibility of individual proteins to proteolytic attack is correlated with molecular weight, isoelectric point, and conformation state. In general, large proteins are degraded more rapidly than smaller ones; more acidic proteins have shorter half-lives; and alteration of conformation by cofactor or substrate binding decreases the degradative rate. Rapidly degraded proteins contain peptide regions rich in proline, glutamate, serine, and threonine (PEST regions).[20]

A wide range of factors affect either protein synthesis or degradation in heart muscle.[21] These include (1) availability of amino acids, in particular leucine; (2) supply of oxidative substrates; (3) availability of hormones; (4) adequacy of oxygen delivery; and (5) the level of aortic pressure. Many of these factors have opposite effects on the synthetic as compared with the degradative pathway; for example, insulin accelerates synthesis and inhibits degradation. These combined changes result in a marked reduction in net amino acid release. Leucine appears to play a unique role in accelerating synthesis and inhibiting degradation. Plasma concentrations of leucine are increased during fasting and in diabetic animals and contribute to maintenance of cardiac mass in these insulinopenic states. The leucine effect may involve a direct effect of the amino acid on enzymes in the pathway or may result indirectly through its oxidation.

Both protein synthesis and degradation are energy-requiring processes, and as a result, oxidizable substrate must be supplied to maintain energy levels for both processes. Glucose can serve as a satisfactory substrate for ATP synthesis but is unable to support control rates of protein synthesis or degradation. On the other hand, fatty acids and other similar substrates are able to support energy generation and maintain equal rates of protein synthesis and degradation and nitrogen balance.[21] Effects of these substrates appear to be important in insulin-deficient states, such as diabetes, in which plasma levels of fatty acids and ketone bodies are elevated.

Stretch of the ventricular wall maintains high efficiency of protein synthesis by affecting both peptide chain initiation and elongation.[21] The rate of protein synthesis is increased by raising the perfusion pressure of Langendorff heart preparations that are supplied glucose as oxidizable substrate. The effect of increasing aortic pressure from 60 to 120 mmHg is still present in hearts that are arrested with tetrodotoxin and have a drain in the ventricle. An increase in intraventricular pressure from 0 to 25 mmHg in arrested isolated rat hearts accelerates the rate of protein synthesis to the same extent as elevation of aortic pressure from 60 to 120 mmHg. These studies indicate that stretch of the ventricular wall is the mechanical parameter most closely linked to the acceleration of protein synthesis.

Increased cytosolic [Ca^{2+}], Na^+ uptake, and content of cAMP have been suggested to represent intracellular signals that link stretch to increased protein synthesis. The involvement of higher cytosolic [Ca^{2+}] was detected in skeletal muscle, but evidence to support this relationship could not be obtained in heart.[21] Stretch of ferret papillary muscle accelerates protein synthesis and Na^+ uptake, and both of these events are blocked by addition of streptomycin. Streptomycin does not block the increased rate of protein synthesis that follows, raising the perfusion pressure from 60 to 120 mmHg.[21] The latter observation does not support the proposed role of Na^+ influx as a transducer of growth. In rat heart increased content of cAMP may serve as the intracellular signal linking stretch to cardiac growth.[21] Elevation of aortic pressure increases cAMP content, the activity of the cAMP-dependent protein kinase, and the rate of protein synthesis. All of these changes are blocked by a muscarinic-cholinergic agonist, methacholine. As noted above, hypoosmotic swelling of avian erythrocytes and S49 lymphoma cells increases cellular cAMP, indicating that cellular deformation directly stimulates adenylyl cyclase and cAMP accumulation.[4] Inositol phosphates are also raised by stretching of the right atrium and ventricle, perhaps due to activation of phospholipase C.[21] If so, DAG content would also increase and lead to activation of PKC. Stretching of rat neonatal cardiomyocytes that are cultured on deformable dishes increases inositol phosphate levels, total cell RNA and mRNA levels for the protooncogene *c-fos* and skeletal α-actin.[22] These changes are inhibited by down regulation of PKC. Future work must define the molecular mechanism(s) of transcriptional control and cardiac growth.

REGULATION OF THE CAPACITY FOR PROTEIN SYNTHESIS

Capacity for protein synthesis reflects the quantities of ribosomes, peptide chain initiation and elongation factors, and tRNA and mRNA that are available to catalyze protein synthesis. Because the availability of mRNA, aminoacyl-tRNA, and initiation factors is sufficient to result in approximately 90 percent of all ribosomes being in the form of polysomes, the capacity for protein synthesis is determined by the quantity of ribosomes. In rat heart, the rate of protein synthesis is a linear function of RNA concentration, an index of ribosome content.[3] During hypertrophic growth of neonatal myocytes in culture, faster rates of RNA synthesis account for the increase in RNA content, and as a result, the rate of protein synthesis is accelerated.[23] The mechanism of accelerated ribosomal RNA synthesis in contracting as compared to quiescent myocytes is a faster rate of ribosomal DNA transcription, which has been observed in both cells and nuclei of contracting myocytes.[24] In newborn pig hearts whose left ventricle (LV) increases in size by 71 percent during the first 3 days of life, content of total RNA in the LV doubles, and rates of ribosome formation increase prior to an increase in rates of total protein synthesis.[25]

CONTROL MECHANISMS IN RAPID CARDIAC GROWTH

Hypertrophy of hearts in adult animals and rapid growth of the newborn hearts provide opportunities to explore the control mechanisms that are involved. In response to hypertension or following loss of heart muscle due to myocardial infarction, the ability of heart muscle cells to hypertrophy allows the heart to cope with the increased demand, but increased LV mass is associated with increased cardiovascular disease risk and, with the exception of age, is the most potent determinant of this risk.[26] As a result, reduction of load on the heart is the strategy of choice in adult animals. In newborn hearts, the physiological situation is entirely normal, but the LV grows rapidly and the right ventricle slowly, presumably as the result of increased aortic pressure and greater work load imposed on the LV from changes in the neonatal circulation at birth.[25] The rapid increase in LV size occurs during the first week of life.

Pressure-overload hypertrophy induced by aortic banding in animal models is associated with stretch of the ventricular wall and with changes in the release of neurotransmitters or plasma concentrations of hormones.[1] Because elevated arterial pressure and increased myocardial mass can be dissociated in hypertensive animals and humans, other growth stimuli may be involved, including α- and β-adrenergic agonists, thyroxine, and angiotensin II.[1]

Recent studies in the rat[27] and cat[28] have led to opposite conclusions regarding the importance of adrenergic agonists in growth. Zierhut and Zimmer[27] found that norepinephrine infusion increased LV mass, total RNA, and the RNA-to-DNA ratio. An α_1-adrenergic blocker, prazosin, and metropolol, a β_1 and β_2 blocker, each partially prevented the increase in LV mass, and together, the blockers totally prevented the increased size of the LV. Verapamil reversed the functional changes but did not prevent growth of the LV in response to norepinephrine infusion. This study supports a role for adrenergic agonists in growth. Conversely, Cooper et al.[28] studied the effects of pulmonary artery banding in a cat right ventricle in which a papillary muscle was unloaded by section of its tendon. The unloaded papillary muscle atrophied while the pressure-overloaded ventricle hypertrophied. The hypertrophy was not impaired by denervation of the heart or α- or β-adrenergic blockade. These findings do not support the hypothesis that adrenergic stimulation is required for growth of the heart.[28] Although infusions of isoproterenol clearly lead to cardiac hypertrophy, a direct effect of growth has not been established because of inability to control the hemodynamic parameters, occurrence of areas of myocardial necrosis, and metabolic changes.[1]

Angiotensin II (AII) also has direct and indirect effects on the heart.[1] The indirect effects lead to increased sympathetic outflow to the heart, vasoconstriction, and increased aldosterone synthesis and release. The direct effects are mediated by membrane receptors and include greater cardiac contractility and faster protein synthesis that may be linked to activation of phospholipase C, increased DAG and inositol phosphate contents, activation of PKC, and opening of L-type Ca^{2+} channels.[29] In rats with an abdominal aortic constriction, administration of enalapril, an angiotensin converting enzyme (ACE) inhibitor, prevents hypertrophy of the left ventricle, although cardiac afterload does not change.[30] Similarly, infusion of AII, but not saline, into rats for 7 days increases left ventricular weight. This increase is prevented by an AII receptor antagonist (DuP 753) but not by an ACE inhibitor or a vasodilator (hydralazine) that normalizes blood pressure.[31] These findings indicate that AII and pressure overload are directly involved in cardiac hypertrophy in vivo in adult animals.

In the heart of newborn pigs, the LV increases in size by 71 percent over the first 3 days of life while the right ventricle does not grow. Faster growth of the LV is accounted for by greater capacity of protein synthesis, as evidenced by greater RNA content.[25] When hearts from 2-day-old pigs are perfused in vitro, however, rates of ribosome formation and total protein synthesis are insensitive to addition of glucagon, 1-methyl-3-isobutylxanthine, or a combination of norepinephrine and propranolol.[32] These findings indicate that the newborn heart is maximally stimulated to grow by the combination of hemodynamic, neural, and endocrine perturbations at birth. To restrain LV growth, newborn pigs were treated with enalapril or DuP 753, an AII receptor antagonist. Treatment with either of the drugs decreases left ventricular growth by about 50 percent during the first 3 days of life. When hearts from 3-day-old pigs treated with enalapril are perfused in vitro, rates of ribosome formation and protein synthesis are reduced and account for the reduced rate of growth. These results indicate that AII plays a role, either directly or indirectly, in the rapid growth of the LV in the first few days of life.

CONCLUSIONS

Rapid cardiac growth in response to pressure overload in adult or newborn animals involves direct effects of (1) cell deformation and (2) receptor binding of neurotransmitters and hormones to generate intracellular signals that control the capacity and efficiency of protein synthesis. In vivo, the efficiency of peptide chain initiation is high because the pathway is saturated with substrates, such as amino acids, mRNA, and high-energy phosphates. Initiation of peptide chains is accelerated by insulin, epinephrine, glucagon, fatty substrates, stretch of the ventricular wall, and the pH to which the heart is exposed. As a result, the capacity for protein synthesis, as represented by the content of ribosomes, determines the rate of protein synthesis. The rate of ribosome formation is the major factor controlling ribosome content and is limited by the rate of ribosomal DNA transcription. Intracellular signaling pathways that involve protein kinase A and C regulate transcription, but the molecular mechanisms remain to be defined.

REFERENCES

1. Morgan HE, Baker KM: Cardiac hypertrophy: Mechanical, neural and endocrine dependence. *Circulation* 1991; 83:13–25.
2. Sugden PH, Fuller SJ: Regulation of protein turnover in skeletal and cardiac muscle. *Biochem J* 1991; 273:21–37.
3. Morgan HE, Rannels DE, McKee EE: Protein metabolism of the heart. In: Berne RM (ed): *Handbook of Physiology*, sec. 2: *The Cardiovascular System*. Bethesda, MD, American Physiological Society, 1979: 845–871.
4. Watson PA: Function follows form: Generation of intracellular signals by cell deformation. *FASEB J* 1991; 5:2013–2019.
5. Dohlman HG, Thorner J, Caron MG, Lefkowitz RJ: Model system for the study of seven-transmembrane-segment receptors. *Ann Rev Biochem* 1991; 60:653–688.
6. Hershey JWB: Translational control in mammalian cells. *Ann Rev Biochem* 1991; 60:717–755.
7. Chien KR, Knowlton KU, Zhu H, Chien S: Regulation of cardiac gene expression during myocardial growth and hypertrophy: Molecular studies of an adaptive response. *FASEB J* 1991; 5:3037–3046.
8. Allo SN, McDermott PJ, Carl LL, Morgan HE: Phorbol ester stimulation of protein kinase C activity and ribosomal DNA transcription: Role in hypertrophic growth of cultured cardiomyocytes. *J Biol Chem* 1991; 266:22003–22009.
9. Morgan HE, Gordon EE, Kira Y, Chua BHL, Russo LA, Peterson CJ, et al: Biochemical mechanisms of cardiac hypertrophy. *Ann Rev Physiol* 1987; 49:533–543.
10. Kent RL, Mann DL, Cooper G IV: Signals for cardiac hypertrophy in hypertension. *J Cardiovasc Pharm* 1991; 17(suppl 2):S7–S13.
11. Sugden PH, Fuller SJ: Correlations between cardiac protein synthesis rates, intracellular pH and the concentrations of creatine metabolites. *Biochem J* 1991; 273:339–346.
12. Benyon RJ, Bond JS: Catabolism of intracellular protein: Molecular aspects. *Am J Physiol* 1986; 251:C141–C152.
13. Bond JS, Butler PE: Intracellular proteases. *Ann Rev Biochem* 1987; 56:333–364.
14. Wing SS, Chiang HL, Goldberg AL, Dice JF: Proteins containing peptide sequences related to Lys-Phe-Glu-Arg-Gln are selectively depleted in liver and heart, but not skeletal muscle of fasted rats. *Biochem J* 1991; 275:165–169.
15. DeMartino GN, Croall DE: Calcium-dependent proteases: A prevalent proteolytic system of uncertain function. *News Physiol Sci* 1987; 2:82.
16. Gordon EE, Kira Y, Demers LM, Morgan HE: Aortic pressure as a determinant of cardiac protein degradation. *Am J Physiol* 1986; 250:C932–938.

17. Rechsteiner M: Ubiquitin-mediated pathways for intracellular proteolysis. *Ann Rev Cell Biol* 1987; 3:1–30.
18. Driscoll J, Goldberg AL: The proteasome (multicatalytic protease) is a component of the 1500-kDa proteolytic complex which degrades ubiquitin-conjugated proteins. *J Biol Chem* 1990; 265:4789–4792.
19. Dice JF: Molecular determinants of protein half-lives in eukaryotic cells. *FASEB J* 1987; 1:349–357.
20. Loetscher P, Pratt G, Rechsteiner M: The C terminus of mouse ornithine decarboxylase confers rapid degradation on dihydrofolate reductase. *J Biol Chem* 1991; 266:11213–11220.
21. Morgan HE, Chua BHL, Russo L: Protein synthesis and degradation. In: Fozzard HA, Haber E, Jennings RB, Katz AM, Morgan HE (eds): *The Heart and Cardiovascular System*. New York, Raven, 1991: 1505–1524.
22. Komuro I, Katoh Y, Kaida T, Shibazaki Y, Kurabayashi M, Hoh E, et al: Mechanical loading stimulates cell hypertrophy and specific gene expression in cultured rat cardiac myocytes. *J Biol Chem* 1991; 226:1265–1268.
23. McDermott PJ, Morgan HE: Contraction modulates the capacity for protein synthesis during growth of neonatal heart cells in culture. *Circ Res* 1989; 64:542–553.
24. McDermott PJ, Carl LL, Conner KJ, Allo SN: Transcriptional regulation of ribosomal RNA synthesis during growth of cardiac myocytes in culture. *J Biol Chem* 1991; 226:4409–4416.
25. Camacho JA, Peterson CJ, White GJ, Morgan HE: Accelerated ribosome formation and growth in neonatal pig hearts. *Am J Physiol* 1990; 258(*Cell Physiol* 27):C86–C91.
26. Levy D: Clinical significance of left ventricular hypertrophy: Insights from the Framingham study. *J Cardiovasc Pharm* 1991; 17(suppl 2):S1–S6.
27. Zierhut W, Zimmer HG: Significance of myocardial α- and β-adrenoceptors in catecholamine-induced cardiac hypertrophy. *Circ Res* 1989; 65:1417–1425.
28. Cooper G IV, Kent RL, Uboh CE, Thompson EW, Marino TA: Hemodynamic versus adrenergic control of cat right ventricular hypertrophy. *J Clin Invest* 1985; 75:1403–1414.
29. Baker KM, Booz GW, Dostal DE: Cardiac actions of angiotensin II: Role of an intracardiac renin-angiotensin system. *Ann Rev Physiol* 1992; 54:227–241.
30. Baker KM, Chernin MI, Wixson SK, Aceto JF: Renin-angiotensin system involvement in pressure overload cardiac hypertrophy in rats. *Am J Physiol* 1990; 259:H324–H332.
31. Dostal DE, Baker KM: Angiotensin II stimulation of left ventricular hypertrophy in adult rat heart: Mediation by the AT_1 receptor. *Am J Hypertens* 1992; 5:276–280.
32. Beinlich CJ, Baker KM, White GJ, Morgan HE: Control of growth in the neonatal pig heart. *Am J Physiol Suppl (Oct)* 1991; 261:3–7.
33. Beinlich CJ, White GJ, Baker KM, Morgan HE: Angiotensin II and left ventricular growth in newborn pig heart. *J Mol Cell Cardiol* 1991; 23:1031–1038.

Chapter 7

Thrombus Formation and Dissolution

Marschall S. Runge, M.D., Ph.D. ■ Laurence A. Harker, M.D.

The most common causes of death in the western world, acute myocardial infarction and stroke, result from vascular thrombosis. Recent advances in our understanding of the molecular mechanisms of thrombogenesis have given rise to new therapeutic approaches to its treatment and prevention. Moreover, there is renewed appreciation that coagulation proteases and regulatory proteins acting during thrombus formation may initiate vascular proliferative responses. In this chapter we shall (1) define the clinical problem of thrombogenesis for both arterial and venous thrombosis, (2) review the current clinical uses of thrombolytic and antithrombotic agents, (3) describe the recent advances in the development of naturally occurring and synthetic coagulation proteins and anticoagulants that may enable clinicians to treat thrombosis more effectively in the near future, and (4) analyze the evidence that initiation of intravascular thrombosis may be a critical component of the maladaptive proliferative response to arterial injury [e.g., the restenosis that follows percutaneous transluminal coronary angioplasty (PTCA)].

CLINICAL PROBLEM OF VASCULAR THROMBOSIS

Role of the Normal Vessel Wall in Preventing Thrombosis

The intact endothelium maintains blood fluidity by multiple mechanisms (Fig. 7-1).[1,2] The electronegative charge of the endothelial membrane prevents cell deposition on its surface.[3] The endothelium inhibits platelet aggregation by degrading adenosine diphosphate (ADP)[4] and inhibits platelet reactivity by synthesizing and secreting prostacyclin[5] and nitric oxide [endothelium-derived relaxing factor (EDRF)].[6,7] The endothelium also prevents fibrin deposition by increasing local concentrations of activated protein C, which downregulates thrombin generation[8,9] and promotes fibrinolysis by increasing production of tissue plasminogen activator (tPA) in response to thrombin.[10,11] Further prevention of vascular thrombosis results from the rapid inactivation of coagulation serine proteases by the following natural inhibitors: (1) endothelial heparan sulfate, (2) antithrombin III, (3) heparin cofactor II, (4) α-2-macroglobulin, and (5) α-1-antitrypsin (potent coagulation-protease inhibitors present on the endothelial cell surface) (see Harpel[12] for a review). Finally, activated prothrombotic molecules are diluted into flowing blood and then rapidly removed from the circulation by the tissue mononuclear phagocytic system. Thus, the presence of a normal, intact endothelium protects against pathological thrombus formation. (See Chaps. 2 and 56.)

Intravascular Thrombus Formation

Thrombus forms as a pathological consequence of interactions between blood hemostatic mechanisms and components of the injured vessel wall. *Thrombin* activates platelets by cleavage of a specific thrombin receptor.[13] Moreover, thrombin-stimulated platelet activation pro-

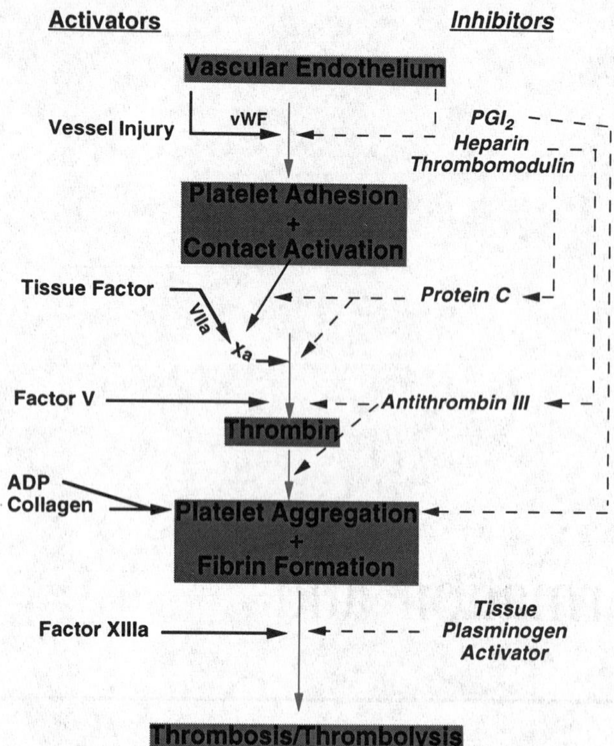

FIGURE 7-1 Naturally occurring activators and inhibitors of thrombosis. The process of hemostasis is shown by the vertical arrows, with key steps in shaded boxes. The solid horizontal arrows show the roles of thrombosis activators and other naturally occurring procoagulants in thrombosis. The dashed horizontal arrows show naturally occurring inhibitors of this process and their roles.

duces a marked positive-feedback mechanism for the activation of factors V and VIII. Thrombin converts fibrinogen into fibrin and facilitates fibrin crosslinking by activating factor XIII. Thus, once the thrombotic process begins, thrombin promotes progressively more rapid thrombus accretion by virtue of its interactions with platelets and fibrin. In addition, it appears that thrombin may play a central role in the vascular response to injury by interacting with a specific cell surface receptor present on platelets, vascular endothelial cells, and smooth-muscle cells.

Arterial and venous thrombosis differ in their genesis as well as in the approaches required for their prevention and treatment. Arterial thrombotic occlusion complicates atherosclerosis and causes acute myocardial or cerebral infarction. Initiation of arterial thrombosis most likely results from vascular injury, with exposure of highly thrombogenic components of the subendothelium and atherosclerotic plaque, primarily collagen and tissue factor, to high shear flow. The "arterial-type" thrombus that forms is rich in platelets but poor in fibrin and red cells ("white" thrombus; Fig. 7-2*A*), in contrast to venous thrombotic disease, which is generally characterized by the activation of coagulation factors in areas of blood stasis that result from vascular compression, dysfunction, or less commonly, damage. The "red" thrombus (Fig. 7-2*B*) seen in venous thromboembolic disease is rich in fibrin and red blood cells and relatively poor in platelets. Venous thrombi also differ from arterial thrombi in their ability to propagate and their potential for causing pulmonary embolism. Antiplatelet agents (e.g., aspirin) can effectively limit arterial thrombosis by interfering with platelet recruitment into the forming thrombus, but aspirin is much less effective in preventing venous thrombosis. Anticoagulants (e.g., heparin) inhibit the production or the activity of serine coagulation proteases, particularly thrombin, and are useful in treating venous thrombosis but less effective in the treatment of arterial thrombosis.[14] Fibrinolytic agents are useful for the treatment of patients with either arterial or venous thrombosis. They destroy a formed thrombus by degrading its fibrin network. It is becoming increasingly evident that in patients with coronary artery thrombosis and acute myocardial infarction, the administration of anticoagulants and/or antiplatelet agents enhances fibrinolysis and helps to prevent reformation of the thrombus. (See also Chap. 68.)

Arterial Thrombosis

Arterial thrombosis typically occurs after vascular injury. Atherosclerosis is usually present, and the actual injury may represent spontaneous rupture of an atherosclerotic plaque or may follow mechanical or thermal disruption of the atherosclerotic plaque (e.g., balloon

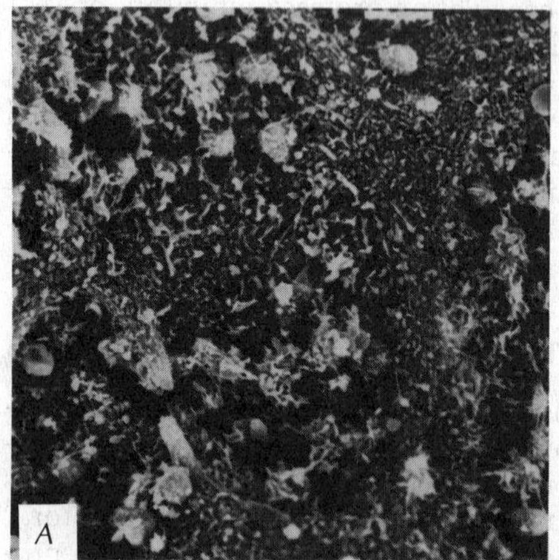

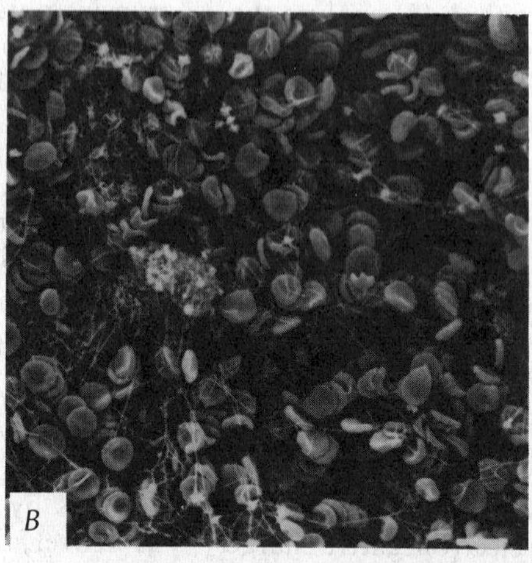

FIGURE 7-2 Comparison of platelet-rich and fibrin-rich thrombus morphology by scanning electron microscopy (800-fold magnification). *A.* Accumulation of deposited and fusing platelets at a thrombogenic site under arterial flow conditions. The relative sizes of the platelet masses are illustrated by the appearance of the occasional red cells. *B.* Appearance of fibrin strands entrapping red cells at sites of thrombus forming under venous flow conditions.

angioplasty, atherectomy, or laser therapy). Once the normal endothelium is injured, subendothelial structures (such as collagen, smooth-muscle cells, and connective tissue) and/or the contents of an atherosclerotic plaque are exposed to circulating blood and platelets. Platelets adhere to the subendothelium as a first step in both normal hemostasis and pathological thrombosis. This platelet adherence is mediated by the interaction of any of several platelet membrane glycoproteins with adhesive proteins present on subendothelial and connective tissue cells. Several specific proteins are thought to be important in the adhesion of platelets to the vessel wall. Von Willebrand factor (vWF) present on the platelet surface is important for platelet adhesion, particularly at high shear rate (i.e., in small vessels), although it also has detectable effects at lower shear rates.[15] The interaction of vWF with adhesion proteins appears to be necessary both for initiating the contact between platelets and the subendothelium and for optimal platelet adhesion.[16] Another adhesion protein that is important in the interaction of platelets with the subendothelium is fibronectin, which is also involved in platelet adhesion at low shear rates.[17]

Following adherence, platelets become activated and release their granule contents, particularly ADP. Platelets also generate thromboxane A_2 (TXA_2) and promote the production of thrombin. Thrombin, ADP, and TXA_2 independently induce platelets to express a functional fibrinogen receptor from the membrane GPIIb/IIIa heterodimer. Fibrinogen then forms the structural backbone of these platelet-rich thrombi. Serotonin, epinephrine, and platelet-activating factor are weaker agonists of platelet activation and probably require the presence of other stimulatory agents for maximal effectiveness.[18] (Platelet activation is discussed in more detail in Chap. 68.) In addition to the role of these granule proteins in platelet activation, there is accumulating evidence that other granule proteins, such as platelet-derived growth factor, may cause the induction of cell proliferation.[19,20] Finally, some molecules, like thrombin, appear to play roles in both thrombosis and cell proliferation.[20]

Venous Thrombosis

Static blood flow contributes to the pathogenesis of venous thrombosis. In general, thrombi in veins are found at sites of maximum stasis, such as in valve pockets.[21] At these sites, annular vortex flow prolongs residence time of blood cells and procoagulant material, thus increasing the likelihood of thrombosis.[22] It is therefore not surprising that the first episode of deep venous thrombosis (DVT) most frequently occurs in patients with prolonged inactivity. Similarly, in patients with a tendency toward DVT, prolonged immobilization of the legs (in an automobile or airplane seat) greatly increases the chance that a thrombus will form. A prothrombotic state is also a risk factor for the development of DVT, regardless of whether on a hereditary or on an acquired basis. There is also an increase in venous thrombosis in pregnancy and in the presence of some malignancies, which may be considered "acquired" prothrombotic states. Finally, "hypofibrinolysis," a decrease in endogenous tPA activity or an increase in the activity of plasminogen activator inhibitor 1 (PAI-1)[23] predisposes to venous thrombosis.

Hip surgery of any type deserves a special note.[24] Among hospitalized patients, hip surgery is probably the most common precipitant of venous thrombosis. In fact, venography shows that up to 30 percent of patients undergoing hip surgery have some degree of venous thrombosis (though this is most frequently not symptomatic). It is likely that the underlying mechanism is local mechanical damage to the femoral vein during the surgical procedure together with venous stasis. This would explain why thrombosis following hip surgery is less responsive to standard anticoagulant prophylaxis than are other venous thrombotic events associated with surgery.[25]

TREATMENT OF CORONARY ARTERY THROMBOSIS

The use of intravenous thrombolytic therapy has revolutionized the treatment of patients with acute myocardial infarction. The impact of thrombolytic therapy has only occurred in the last decade, however, long after it was first suggested that arterial thrombosis was the cause of acute myocardial infarction. Herrick[26] originally described patients with coronary thrombosis in 1912 and suggested that this was the most common cause of myocardial infarction. There was a great deal of debate about this until DeWood et al.[27] demonstrated that most patients had thrombotic occlusion of the infarct-related artery soon after acute myocardial infarction. In the interim, the development of coronary care units, bedside hemodynamic monitoring, coronary angiography, and pharmacologic advances (including the development and use of beta blockers, calcium channel blockers, nitroglycerin, and antiarrhythmic agents) reduced the mortality in hospitalized patients with acute myocardial infarction from approximately 20 to 30 percent to approximately 10 to 12 percent. Thrombolytic therapy has become an integral part of the management of acute myocardial infarction since the mid-1980s and has further reduced in-hospital mortality to 6 to 8 percent, except in elderly or other high-risk groups. (See also Chap. 60.)

In the United States, three thrombolytic agents are currently available for intravenous use: streptokinase (SK), tPA, and anisoylated plasminogen-streptokinase activator complex (APSAC). [Two other agents, single-chain urokinase-type plasminogen activator (scuPA) and urokinase (UK), have been used clinically in Europe.] The agents approved for use in the United States are generally considered "plasminogen activators" and vary somewhat in their biological and pharmacologic properties. (See Chap. 68 for a more detailed discussion.) Certainly all three agents are effective. The potential clinical significance of their different pharmacologic characteristics is responsible for literally hundreds of reports yearly. An understanding of the differences in their molecular structures and mechanisms of action is necessary to appreciate the potential and realized clinical differences of these agents.

Fibrin Formation and Platelet Activation

Fibrin is the end result of the interaction of two coagulation pathways, one intrinsic and one extrinsic (see Fig. 7-3). The convergence of these pathways results in cleavage of prothrombin to thrombin. Thrombin then cleaves fibrinogen to fibrin. The initial reaction in the intrinsic pathway is the activation of factor XI on the membrane surface. The initial reaction in the extrinsic pathway is the activation of factor VII on the membrane surface. The intrinsic and extrinsic pathways converge in the enzymatic activation of factor X, which also occurs on a membrane surface. Factor Xa is an integral component of the "ten-ase" complex that is assembled on the platelet membrane surface and consists of factor Xa and factor Va and Ca^{2+}. This ten-ase complex efficiently converts prothrombin to thrombin. Thrombin generation is further amplified by two cofactors, factors Va and VIIIa. Factors Va and VIIIa are subject to positive-feedback regulation by thrombin. Thus, the initial formation of thrombin is followed by a marked amplification in thrombin formation as a result of this positive-feedback system involving factors Va and VIIIa. Once formed, thrombin not only cleaves fibrinogen to form fibrin but also activates platelets.

Fibrinolysis involves the degradation of insoluble fibrin to soluble fibrin fragments. The rate-limiting step in this process is the conversion of inactive plasminogen into the active enzyme plasmin (see Fig. 7-4). Streptokinase, tPA, and APSAC are all efficient activators of plasminogen, although the precise molecular mechanism of activation differs. Tissue plasminogen activator is unique in that its catalytic efficiency is increased more than 1000-fold when it is bound to fibrin. It was initially thought that this property would result in fibrin-specific plasmin generation and safer and more efficient fibrinolysis. To date, this has not resulted in a major clinical improvement. (See also Chaps. 60 and 68.)

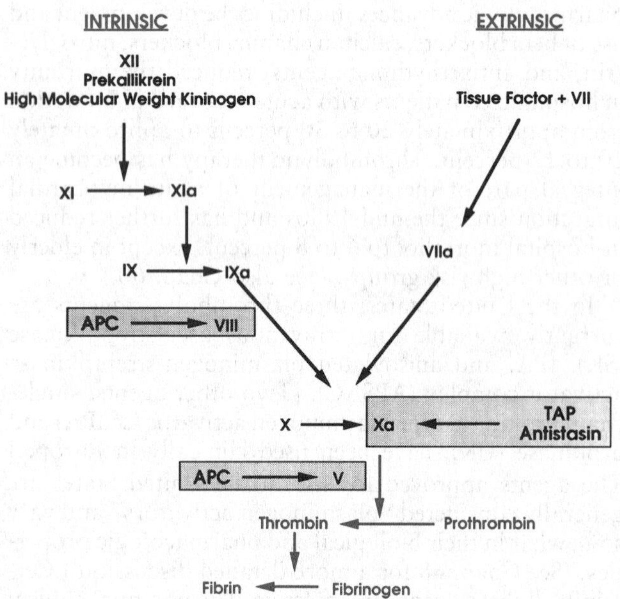

FIGURE 7-3 Intrinsic and extrinsic coagulation pathways. The essential proteins that comprise the intrinsic and extrinsic pathways are shown. The sites of action for the coagulation inhibitors, tick anticoagulant peptide (TAP), antistasin, and activated protein C (APC), are shaded. *(From MS Runge: The future of thrombolytic therapy. Heart Dis Stroke 1:39–42, 1992. Reproduced with permission from the publisher and author.)*

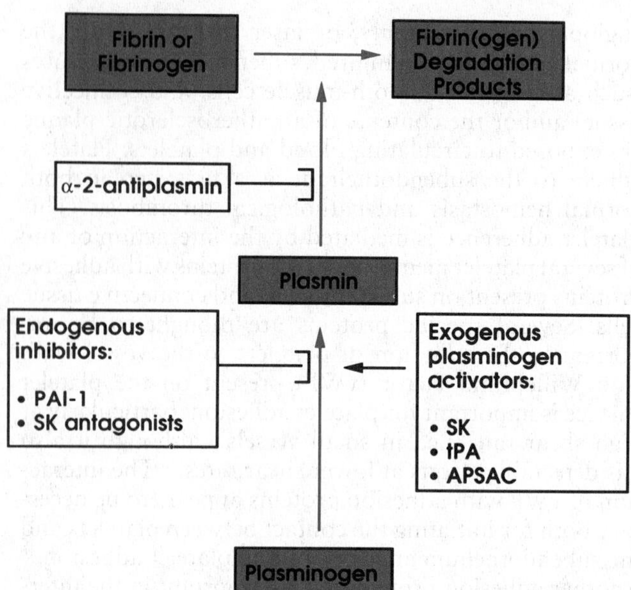

FIGURE 7-4 Essentials of fibrinolysis. Exogenously administered plasminogen activators convert plasminogen into plasmin. The principal inhibitors of this step are plasminogen activator inhibitor 1 (PAI-1), which inhibits tPA, and antistreptokinase antibodies (particularly in patients who have previously been treated with streptokinase), which can inhibit SK or APSAC. The α-2-antiplasmin is the principal inhibitor of plasmin. Plasmin degrades fibrin into fibrin degradation products, which are anticoagulants themselves. Plasmin is relatively nonspecific and can also degrade fibrinogen and other plasma proteins.

Thrombolytic Therapy

Surprisingly, the large multicenter clinical trials currently published[28–31a] have shown that although the three available agents differ considerably in their intrinsic properties, there is relatively little clinical difference among these agents as currently administered. (See Chap. 60.) Several possible explanations have been suggested. First, the naturally occurring plasminogen activators may lack clinical efficiency because they function best in situations where the amount of thrombus is small and readily accessible to blood flow (as in the subclinical thrombi that are likely lysed by endogenous plasminogen activators). Conversely, it is possible that the naturally occurring plasminogen activators require more intensive adjunctive anticoagulant and/or antiplatelet therapy because of their specificity, short duration of action, and rapid lytic effects. The nonspecific plasminogen activation by streptokinase certainly results in the generation of a lytic state and the production of fibrin degradation products, both of which lead to systemic anticoagulation and lessen the chance of rethrombosis. Of note, the recently presented results of the GUSTO trial[31a] showed that patients treated with tPA administered according to an accelerated dosing regimen with intravenous heparin therapy fared better than patients treated with streptokinase. The 30-day mortality in the tPA-treated group was 6.3 percent, while that in the SK-treated group was 7.3

percent, overall a 14 percent reduction in mortality (see Chap. 60).

The major clinical trials currently published have shown that:

- The fibrin-selective agents (tPA and scuPA) produce more rapid and more efficient initial recanalization of the infarct artery than the non-fibrin-selective agents.
- The overall rate of achieving patent infarct-related arteries by hospital discharge is similar for tPA, scuPA, SK, and APSAC, owing to a higher incidence of "early reocclusion" in patients treated with tPA or scuPA than in those treated with SK or APSAC. It is unclear whether this relates to the plasma half-life of the plasminogen activator or to the generation of a lytic state. (Both SK and APSAC have longer plasma half-lives and more of a tendency toward a lytic state than tPA.)
- Serious bleeding complications are uncommon but do not differ significantly among the three activators.
- Although serious allergic reactions occur with SK and APSAC, these are infrequent and tend to be easily treated or prevented by the preadministration of corticosteroids.

These large, multicenter, randomized clinical trials clearly show that the early administration of thrombolytic agents reduces mortality in patients with acute myocardial infarction. It is generally agreed that thrombolytic therapy would be more effective if (1) thrombi can be lysed more quickly, (2) the underlying substrate can be modified to decrease the frequency of reocclusion, and (3) untoward side effects such as systemic bleeding and allergic reactions can be eliminated or markedly reduced. (See Chaps. 60 and 69.)

The indications, contraindications, and specific regimens for the thrombolytic therapy of patients with acute myocardial infarction are discussed in Chaps. 60 and 69. It should be noted that many investigators feel that patients with residual evidence of a previous stroke or with other evidence of significant cerebrovascular disease should not receive thrombolytic therapy. The issue of treatment of patients with ongoing cerebral ischemia from a thrombotic stroke is currently being studied in clinical trials. A second problem relates to patients who previously received SK or APSAC, who frequently develop anti-SK antibodies that may be detectable for several years, and in whom a second treatment with either SK or APSAC can result in an anaphylactic reaction. This is relatively rare and can usually be prevented with preadministration of intravenous corticosteroids. Even if the anaphylactic reaction is prevented with corticosteroids, however, the presence of anti-SK antibodies can prevent effective thrombolysis by binding to and inhibiting the administered SK. Thus, it is advisable to consider tPA (or another intervention) in patients who have previously received SK or APSAC.

New Thrombolytic Agents on the Horizon

An enormous research effort has focused on improving the clinical properties of the available plasminogen activators. The goals are to increase the rate of recanalization, decrease the rate of rethrombosis, and improve safety by decreasing the tendency for intracranial (and systemic) bleeding.

One approach to improving the effectiveness of these agents has been to achieve fibrin-specific plasminogen activation by localizing the plasminogen activator to the area of the thrombus. Theoretically, this would allow efficient thrombolysis and limit the disruption of the hemostatic system. Molecular biology techniques have been used to alter specific properties of tPA and scuPA, with the goal of increasing clot specificity. The type of modifications made include (1) combinations of different portions of tPA and scuPA into a single molecule, (2) "targeting" the plasminogen activators to thrombi using a fibrin-specific or a platelet-specific monoclonal antibody, and (3) using variants found elsewhere in nature [a tPA-like molecule manyfold more fibrin-specific than human tPA has been purified from the saliva of the vampire bat (*Desmodus*)[32]]. Only one of these approaches, that of using recombinant hybrid molecules that combine a human plasminogen activator with a fibrin-specific antibody, appears to offer clinical promise.

A second approach has been to increase the plasma half-life of tPA or scuPA, since it is thought that the effectiveness of SK and APSAC therapy is at least in part due to their prolonged plasma half-life. The plasma half-life of tPA in humans is 4 to 6 min, while that of SK is about 25 min, and that of APSAC exceeds 45 min. Determinants of the half-life of tPA have been defined by examination of the molecular properties of tPA, and altered tPA molecules have been produced that have a markedly prolonged half-life (on the order of 60 min). In a canine model, a tPA mutant with a prolonged half-life produced more rapid clot lysis, and with less reocclusion, than did native tPA.[33]

A third approach being investigated is to modify tPA so that it is less responsive to the normally occurring inhibitors found in human plasma, which tend to be elevated in some patients with acute myocardial infarction. Altered forms of tPA that are resistant to inhibition are in the early stages of development. It is likely that tPA in human beings is rapidly inhibited by PAI-1, which is secreted by activated platelets. Madison et al.[34] described a mutant of tPA that is resistant to PAI-1 inhibition. The efficacy and safety of this tPA mutant is not yet known. (See also Chap. 69.)

An attractive alternative to changing the characteristics of a plasminogen activator is to coadminister a plasminogen activator with a very potent anticoagulant or a platelet aggregation inhibitor. As described above, the combination of heparin (to inhibit thrombin) or aspirin (to inhibit platelet aggregation) and tPA therapy in patients has clinically proven benefits.[35,36] Even more specific and potent antithrombin and antiplatelet agents have been identified and are in the early stages of clinical trials, which will help define the role of potent thrombin and platelet inhibition in the treatment of patients with acute myocardial infarction.

Immediate Angioplasty

Because the limitations of thrombolytic therapy and the exclusion criteria (Chap. 60) prevent administration of thrombolytic therapy to a significant number of patients presenting with acute myocardial infarction, a number of investigators have suggested that primary PTCA for acute myocardial infarction may be a reasonable alternative. Interest in this approach has been stimulated because of the success of primary PTCA in the treatment of patients with cardiogenic shock.[37,38] In addition, a number of trials have suggested that primary PTCA for acute myocardial infarction (in the absence of cardiogenic shock) is as effective as thrombolytic therapy[39–41]; however, the number of patients in these studies is small. Selected subgroups of patients who are ineligible for thrombolytic therapy but who have a potentially high mortality rate may benefit from primary PTCA.[42–44] (See Chaps. 60 and 70.)

Antiplatelet Therapy

Aspirin

Several different antiplatelet drugs have been used in animal studies and in humans. These include the nonsteroidal anti-inflammatory drugs (aspirin, indomethacin, phenylbutazone, etc.) and ticlopidine. Of these, aspirin is the antiplatelet agent most widely used.

Clinically, aspirin is a very effective antithrombotic agent. Aspirin (300 to 1500 mg daily) has been shown to be effective in reducing transient ischemic attacks (TIAs), stroke, and death in patients with transient cerebral ischemia.[45,46] Similarly, aspirin reduces the incidence of myocardial infarction and cardiac death in patients with unstable angina and prevents reinfarction and vascular death in patients who have suffered both remote and acute myocardial infarction.[30,47] Aspirin prevents the occlusion of aortocoronary saphenous vein bypass grafts[48] and arteriovenous shunts.[49] Aspirin may also be effective in the primary prevention of myocardial infarction, although the present results are controversial.[50–52] (See also Chaps. 62 and 68.)

Two important effects of aspirin are to abolish platelet production of thromboxane A_2 (TXA_2, a potent vasoconstrictor and platelet agonist) and endothelial cell synthesis of prostacyclin (PGI-2, a potent vasodilator and platelet antagonist). These effects result from the acetylation and inactivation of cyclooxygenase in platelets and endothelial cells.[53,54] The effect of aspirin is different on platelets and on endothelial cells because platelets do not synthesize cyclooxygenase, and therefore, the effect of aspirin persists for the life span of any exposed platelets. In contrast, endothelial cells resynthesize cyclooxygenase, and the effect of aspirin on endothelial cells is reversible over about 24 to 36 h.

There is debate about the optimal dose of aspirin in patients with cardio- or cerebrovascular disease. From a theoretical standpoint, it should be possible to select an aspirin dose that maintains endothelial cell synthesis of PGI-2 but abolishes platelet TXA_2 production, thus allowing normal vasodilation to occur but preventing platelet aggregation. In practice, it has not been possible to find such a dose. Even with very low doses (35 mg/day), PGI-2 production is markedly decreased.[55] With high doses, there is increased incidence of the dose-dependent side effects, such as gastrointestinal and cutaneous bleeding. Based on the comparable therapeutic effectiveness of doses ranging from 160 to 1500 mg daily in adults[46,56] and the dose-related increase in side effects,[46,57,58] the current general recommendation is to administer 325 mg aspirin orally once daily.

Dipyridamole

Dipyridamole increases cyclic adenosine monophosphate (AMP) by inhibiting phosphodiesterase activity.[59] Experimentally, dipyridamole has been shown to be an effective antithrombotic that acts synergistically with aspirin.[60] Currently, its clinical indication is limited to the prevention of systemic embolism in patients with prosthetic heart valves, and it is administered in combination with warfarin.[61] In the treatment of cerebrovascular disease and coronary thrombotic events or for the prevention of saphenous vein bypass graft thrombosis, dipyridamole is ineffective by itself and provides no additional benefit when given with aspirin. (See also Chap. 68.)

Ticlopidine

Ticlopidine inhibits platelets by an as-yet undefined mechanism. It does not affect phosphodiesterase, adenylcyclase, cyclooxygenase, or thromboxane synthetase activities. Ticlopidine may inhibit platelet aggregation and activation by binding to platelet surface receptors.[62] It is likely that the in vivo activity of ticlopidine is due to an active metabolite, since there is little activity in vitro. In thrombosis models, ticlopidine is a more potent antithrombotic than aspirin.[63] The long half-life of ticlopidine complicates its clinical use. The onset of action is slow (there is a delay of several days before the drug is fully effective) and the effect persists for several days after discontinuing treatment. Additionally, occasional idiosyncratic neutropenia and gastrointestinal side effects may occur during its use. Clinically, ticlopidine (250 mg twice a day) is effective in the secondary prevention of stroke: Recurrence of stroke and cardiovascular death is reduced by 30 percent compared to placebo.[64] In fact, in one study ticlopidine (250 mg twice daily) was 30 percent more effective than aspirin (650 mg twice daily) in preventing the occurrence of nonfatal stroke and death in patients with TIA.[65] Other indications of ticlopidine currently under study are in the treatment of peripheral vascular disease, in ischemic heart disease, and in surgery requiring cardiopulmonary bypass. (See also Chap. 68.)

Other Antiplatelet Agents

Several agents that inhibit platelet aggregation or activation are undergoing clinical and preclinical trials. These agents are discussed in detail in Chap. 68. Selected antithrombins and platelet inhibitors are also discussed below with respect to their potency in preventing rethrombosis. Five general categories of agents are being investigated at present: (1) inhibitors of TXA_2, (2) prostacyclin and its derivatives, (3) dietary *n*-3 fatty acids, (4) direct thrombin inhibitors, and (5) inhibitors of platelet aggregation.

Combined Approaches to Treatment of Rethrombosis

The ability to dissolve an initial thrombus has led to a new problem: rethrombosis. Both initial thrombosis and rethrombosis result in arterial occlusion, although by somewhat different mechanisms. These differences may have important implications for the development of therapeutic approaches. The initial thrombotic occlusion of a coronary artery results in the formation of "mixed thrombi," rich in both platelets and fibrin, whereas rethrombosis produces thrombi rich in platelets but low in fibrin.

In experimental models and in humans, the platelet-rich, fibrin-poor thrombi associated with rethrombosis do not respond to fibrinolytic therapy as well as the platelet- and fibrin-rich initial thrombi. Thus, most efforts to treat rethrombosis focus on blocking the process by inhibiting platelet aggregation and recruitment. Even with the clinically available antiplatelet and anticoagulant agents, aspirin and heparin,[30,66] however, rethrombosis after pharmacologic or mechanical treatment of arterial occlusion is common. The reported incidence of acute thrombosis after PTCA ranges from 2 to 10 percent.[67,68] (See also Chaps. 70 and 71.) The incidence of reocclusion after successful thrombolytic therapy for acute myocardial infarction is approximately 12 to 18 percent.[69,70] (See also Chap. 60.)

Because thrombin plays a central role in platelet activation and fibrin formation, its inhibition appears to be a particularly effective way to prevent unwanted thrombosis. Of the growing number of antithrombins under evaluation, heparin (see below) has been studied most intensively. Heparin reduces platelet deposition in experimental animals following balloon angioplasty[71,72] but does not completely prevent arterial thrombosis in doses used clinically. The low-molecular-weight heparins (which have increased anti–factor Xa activity compared to heparin) also fail to prevent arterial thrombosis. It is particularly important to coadminister intravenous heparin when tPA is used as the thrombolytic agent. (See Chaps. 60 and 69.) The relative failure of heparin to inhibit arterial thrombosis probably relates to inability of the heparin-antithrombin complex to inhibit clot bound thrombin. (See also Chap. 68.) On the other hand, clot bound thrombin can be effectively inhibited by *hirudin,* a naturally occurring anticoagulant found in the medicinal leech.[73] Hirudin is a potent antithrombin that binds directly to and inhibits thrombin. Hirudin has been shown to be more effective than heparin alone or than heparin plus aspirin in the reduction of platelet-thrombus deposition in an experimental angioplasty model.[72] Synthetic antithrombins that have been studied in animal models include the tripeptide D-phenylalanyl-L-prolyl-L-arginyl chloromethyl ketone (D-FPRCH $_2$Cl),[74] MD-805 (or argipidine),[75,76] and derivatives of the serine protease inhibitor, benzamidine.[77] All inhibit thrombin by mechanisms independent of antithrombin III and prevent platelet aggregation and thrombus formation in animal models. For all of these agents, however, effective antithrombotic doses result in impaired hemostasis and prolonged bleeding times. (See also Chap. 68.)

Two new approaches to inhibiting thrombin offer clinical promise. Both prevent the amplification of thrombin by intrinsic and extrinsic pathways (see Fig. 7-3). Activated protein C (APC), a physiological anticoagulant, enzymatically degrades factors Va and VIIIa, thus attenuating the normal amplification of thrombin. Modulation of coagulation by APC may allow sufficient thrombin to be generated to facilitate the formation of hemostatic plugs, thereby preventing hemorrhage, while preventing excessive amplification of thrombin and, hence, rethrombosis. Data in nonhuman primates support this hypothesis.[78] A similar approach has taken advantage of two recently described specific inhibitors of factor Xa: tick anticoagulant protein (TAP)[79] and antistasin.[80] These molecules downregulate the prothrombinase complex by impairing the activity of the ten-ase complex. The factor Xa inhibitors thus allow small amounts of thrombin to be generated but prevent amplification in a manner analogous to that of APC.

An alternative approach to preventing thrombosis is to block the "final common pathway," the binding of fibrinogen with its receptor on the platelet glycoprotein IIb/IIIa complex. Several inhibitors of fibrinogen–glycoprotein IIb/IIIa binding have been discovered or developed. These include monoclonal antibodies,[81,82] small synthetic peptides, and "natural" inhibitors found in the venom of vipers, such as trigramin,[83] echistatin,[84] bitistatin,[85] applaggin,[86] and kistrin.[87] All of these inhibitors prevent platelet aggregation, thrombus formation, and arterial occlusion in animal models. Like the direct thrombin inhibitors, however, therapeutic doses are most frequently associated with impaired hemostasis.[74]

TREATMENT OF VENOUS THROMBOSIS AND PULMONARY EMBOLISM

Development of Deep Venous Thrombosis and Pulmonary Embolism

Of the three general classes of antithrombotic agents (antiplatelet, anticoagulant, and fibrinolytic), anticoagulants with or without antiplatelet agents are most often used to treat patients with venous thrombosis.[88] Fibrinolytic agents, used primarily in arterial thrombosis, may also be indicated in the treatment of massive DVT or life-threatening pulmonary emboli. (See Chap. 100 for details of the management of patients with pulmonary embolism.)

Anticoagulants

Heparin

In clinical practice, standard unfractionated heparin is the most widely used antithrombotic agent.[14] Heparin is a heterodisperse mixture of polysaccharides of molecular weight ranging from 3000 to 40,000 daltons, averaging about 15,000 daltons. Heparin catalyzes bimolecular complex formation between plasma antithrombin III and serine-proteases of the coagulation pathway. The anticoagulant action of heparin primarily results from its inhibition of thrombin. At high concentrations, heparin induces thrombin inhibition through heparin cofactor II, another specific plasma antithrombin. (See also Chap. 68.)

Both antithrombotic efficacy and bleeding complications are dose dependent. Heparin monitoring by coagulation tests is critical, since the anticoagulant response to heparin varies greatly among different individuals and in the same individual at different times during the course of thromboembolic diseases.[89,90] The gold standard for determining therapeutic efficacy is the plasma heparin level. Because the activated partial thromboplastin time (APTT) correlates relatively well with plasma heparin levels, and since the APTT is quicker and less expensive to determine than plasma heparin levels, APTT is generally used to monitor therapy.[14,91] Monitoring of platelet count is also important since heparin-induced thrombocytopenia has been reported in about 1 to 5 percent of patients receiving therapeutic heparin.

Heparin may be administered by bolus, continuous intravenous injection, or subcutaneously. Subcutaneous administration is usually reserved for prophylaxis against venous thrombosis perioperatively, for medical patients at bed rest, or for the treatment of DVT during pregnancy because of the risk to the fetus of warfarin therapy. A recent review of more than 70 randomized trials in 16,000 patients indicates that the perioperative use of low-dose heparin (5000 IU twice daily) decreases the risk of pulmonary emboli by about half and the risk of DVT by about two-thirds in patients undergoing urologic, orthopedic, or general surgery.[92] Patients undergoing elective hip surgery, however, require adjusted subcutaneous heparin doses producing APTT values in the high normal range rather than fixed low doses.[14,93] (See also Chap. 100.)

Low-Molecular-Weight Heparins

Low molecular weight heparins (LMWHs) are prepared by fractionation of standard heparin. Several different preparations of LMWHs exist. Common features of all of these preparations are a relative increase in their ability to inhibit activated factor X (anti-Xa activity) and a relative decrease in their ability to inhibit thrombin, resulting in a decreased prolongation of the APTT at therapeutic antithrombotic doses. Thus, anti-Xa activity is generally used for laboratory monitoring. Experimentally, LMWHs have been shown to exhibit antithrombotic effects that are comparable to unfractionated heparin but without as much bleeding. This suggests that LMWHs might have a more favorable therapeutic ratio[94] in patients. To date, however, most clinical studies have failed to confirm an improved hemostatic safety for LMWHs.[95]

Vitamin K Antagonists: Warfarin

Vitamin K is necessary for gamma carboxylation of clotting factors II, VII, IX, and X and protein C and protein S. The carboxylated residues are necessary for calcium binding by these proteins, and calcium is essential for their activity. Vitamin K antagonists result in the production of biologically inactive coagulation proteins. Warfarin is the most widely used vitamin K antagonist, because of its rapid metabolism (half-life about 35 h) and good bioavailability.[96] The anticoagulant effect of vitamin K agonists is fully manifest 36 to 72 h after administration, when clotting factor activity is reduced to about 10 percent of normal. Individuals vary greatly in their response to vitamin K antagonists. The prothrombin time (PT) is generally used to monitor warfarin therapy. To standardize the PT, an international reference preparation of thromboplastin has been designated, and the observed PT ratio is now converted to an international normalized ratio (INR) using an international sensitivity index.[96–98] The high intensity regimen (to achieve an INR of 2.5 to 3.5) generally corresponds to standard laboratory PTs of 1.6 to 2.0 × control. Recently it has been demonstrated that moderate intensity anticoagulation producing an INR of 2.0 to 3.0 (PT approximately 1.3 to 1.6 × control) is as effective as the high intensity regimen (and causes fewer bleeding complications) in the prevention and treatment of venous thrombosis as well as in the prevention of systemic embolism in patients with acute myocardial infarction or atrial fibrillation. The higher therapeutic range (INR 2.5 to 3.5; PT approximately 1.6 to 2.0 × control) is recommended for patients with mechanical prosthetic valves or with recurrent systemic embolism.[98] (See Chaps. 68 and 100.)

New Anticoagulants

Many new thrombin inhibitors are being evaluated in clinical trials. It remains to be seen whether or not any of these agents will offer an improved ratio of therapeutic efficacy in comparison with the heparins or warfarin. In particular, APC and the factor Xa inhibitors appear to be the most promising. One additional anticoagulant that has been used for both arterial and venous thrombosis is dermatan sulfate. Unlike heparin, dermatan sulfate catalyzes the heparin cofactor II–thrombin interaction but has no action on antithrombin III–serine protease interactions. Dermatan sulfate has been shown to be antithrombotic without exhibiting antihemostatic effects.[99]

Fibrinolytic Therapy

Fibrinolytic therapy has several theoretical advantages over anticoagulants in the treatment of DVT and pulmonary embolism. These include (1) the preservation of native structures in the deep veins, (2) prevention of the postphlebitic syndrome,[100] and (3) the more rapid and complete lysis of thrombi. (See also Chap. 100.) Fibrinolytic agents are most effective in recently formed thrombi and less effective in old thrombi. Thus, in DVT and pulmonary embolism, fibrinolytic agents should be administered as soon as feasible after the onset of symptoms. (See Chap. 100 for further discussion of the fibrinolytic therapy of patients with pulmonary embolism.)

REFERENCES

1. Furie B, Furie BC: Molecular and cellular biology of blood coagulation. *N Engl J Med* 1992; 326:800–806.
2. Badimon L, Badimon JJ, Fuster V: Pathogenesis of thrombosis. In: Verstraete M, Fuster V (eds): *Thrombosis in Cardiovascular Disease,* Philadelphia, Saunders, 1992: 17–40.
3. Sawyer S, Srinivasan S: The role of electrochemical surface properties in thrombosis at vascular interfaces: Cumulative experience of studies in animals and man. *Bull NY Acad Med* 1972; 48:235–256.
4. Pearson JD, Carlton JS, Gordon JL: Metabolism of adenine nucleotides by ectoenzymes of vascular endothelial and smooth-muscle cells in culture. *Biochem J* 1980; 190:421–429.
5. Moncada S, Vane JR: Arachidonic acid metabolites and their interactions between platelets and blood vessel wall. *N Engl J Med* 1979; 300:1142–1147.
6. Moncada S, Palmer RMJ, Higgs EA: Prostacyclin and endothelium-derived relaxing factor: Biological interactions and significance. In: Verstraete M, Vermylen J, Lijnen R, and Arnout J (eds): *Thrombosis and Haemostasis 1987,* Leuven, Leuven University Press, 1987: 505–523.
7. Moncada S, Higgs EA: Prostaglandins in the pathogenesis and prevention of vascular disease. *Blood Rev* 1987; 1:141–145.
8. Lollar P, Owen WG: Clearance of thrombin from the circulation in rabbits by high-affinity binding sites on the endothelium: Possible role in the inactivation of thrombin by antithrombin III. *J Clin Invest* 1980; 66:1222–1230.
9. Esmon NL, Owen WG, Esmon CT: Isolation of a membrane-bound cofactor for thrombin-catalyzed activation of protein C. *J Biol Chem* 1982; 257:859–864.
10. Levin EG, Loskutoff DJ: Cultured bovine endothelial cells produce both urokinase and tissue-type plasminogen activators. *J Cell Biol* 1982; 94:631–636.
11. Levin EG, Marzec UM, Anderson J, Harker LA: Thrombin stimulates tissue plasminogen activator release from cultured human endothelial cells. *J Clin Invest* 1984; 74:1988–1995.
12. Harpel P: Blood proteolytic enzyme inhibitors: Their role in modulating blood coagulation and fibrinolytic pathways. In: Colman RW, Hirsh J, Marder VJ, Salzman EW (eds): *Hemostasis and Thrombosis: Basic Principles and Clinical Practice,* 2d ed. Philadelphia, Lippincott, 1987: 219–234.
13. Vu T-KH, Hung DT, Wheaton VI, Coughlin SR: Molecular cloning of a functional thrombin receptor reveals a novel proteolytic mechanism of receptor activation. *Cell* 1991; 64:1057–1068.
14. Hirsh J: Heparin. *N Engl J Med* 1991; 324:1565–1574.
15. Badimon L, Badimon JJ, Turitto VT, Fuster V: Role of von Willebrand factor in mediating platelet–vessel wall interaction at low shear rate: The importance of perfusion condition. *Blood* 1989; 73:961–967.
16. Fressinaud E, Baruch D, Girma JP, Sakariassen KS, Baumgartner HR, Meyer D: von Willebrand factor–mediated platelet adhesion to collagen involves platelet membrane glycoprotein IIb–IIIa as well as glycoprotein Ib. *J Lab Clin Med* 1988; 112:58–67.
17. Nievelstein PFEM, Sixma JJ: Glycoprotein IIb–IIIa and RGD(S) are not important for fibronectin-dependent platelet adhesion under flow conditions. *Blood* 1988; 72:82–88.
18. Holmsen H: Platelet secretion. In: Colman RW, Hirsh J, Marder VJ, Salzman EW (eds): *Hemostasis and Thrombosis: Basic Principles and Clinical Practice,* 2d ed. Philadelphia, Lippincott, 1987: 606–617.
19. Lindner V, Reidy MA: Proliferation of smooth muscle cells after vascular injury is inhibited by an antibody against basic fibroblast growth factor. *Proc Natl Acad Sci USA* 1991; 88:3739–3743.
20. Okazaki H, Majesky MW, Harker LA, Schwartz SM: Regulation of platelet-derived growth factor (PDGF) ligand and receptor gene expression by alpha-thrombin in vascular smooth muscle cells. *Circ Res* 1992; 71:1285–1293.
21. Sevitt S: The structure and growth of valve-pocket thrombi in femoral veins. *J Clin Pathol* 1974; 27:517–528.
22. Kareno T, Motoniya M: Flow through a venous valve and its implication for thrombus formation. *Thromb Res* 1984; 36:245–257.
23. Nilsson IM, Ljungner H, Tengborn L: Two different mechanisms in patients with venous thrombosis and defective fibrinolysis: Low concentration of plasminogen activator or increased concentration of plasminogen activator inhibitor. *Br Med J* 1985; 290:1453–1456.
24. Hirsh J: Prevention of venous thrombosis in patients undergoing major orthopaedic surgical procedures. *Acta Chir Scand Suppl* 1990; 556:30–35.
25. Thomas DP: Overview of venous thrombogenesis. *Semin Thromb Hemost* 1988; 14:1–8.
26. Herrick JB: Clinical features of sudden obstruction of the coronary arteries. *JAMA* 1912; 59:2015–2020.
27. DeWood MA, Spores J, Notske R, Mouser LT, Burroughs R, Golden MS, et al: Prevalence of total coronary occlusion during the early hours of transmural myocardial infarction. *N Engl J Med* 1980; 303:897–902.
28. Anglo-Scandinavian Study of Early Thrombolysis (ASSET): Trial of tissue plasminogen activator for mortality reduction in acute myocardial infarction. *Lancet* 1988; 2:525–530.
29. Gruppo Italiano per lo Studio della Streptochinasi nell' Infarcto miocardico, GISSI: Effectiveness of intravenous thrombolytic treatment in acute myocardial infarction. *Lancet* 1986; 1:397–401.

29a. GISSI: Long-term effects of intravenous thrombolysis in acute myocardial infarction. Final report of the GISSI study. *Lancet* 1987; 2:871–874.

29b. Gruppo Italiano per lo Studio della Sopravvivenza nell' Infarcto miocardico. GISSI-2: A factorial randomized trial of alteplase versus streptokinase and heparin versus no heparin among 12,490 patients with acute myocardial infarction. *Lancet* 1990; 336:65–71.

30. ISIS-2 (Second International Study of Infarct Survival) Collaborative Group: Randomised trial of intravenous streptokinase, oral aspirin, both, or neither among 17,187 cases of suspected acute myocardial infarction: ISIS-2. *Lancet* 1988; 2:349–360.

30a. The International Study Group: In-hospital and clinical course of 20,891 patients with suspected acute myocardial infarction randomized between alteplase and streptokinase with or without heparin. *Lancet* 1990; 336:71–75.

31. ISIS-3 (Third International Study of Infarct Survival) Collaborative Group: ISIS-3: A randomized comparison of streptokinase vs tissue plasminogen activator vs anistreplase and of aspirin plus heparin vs aspirin alone among 41,299 cases of suspected acute myocardial infarction. *Lancet* 1992; 339:753–770.

31a. Topel E, et al. for the GUSTO Investigators: *Global Utilization of Streptokinase and Tissue Plasminogen Activator for Occluded Coronary Arteries (GUSTO).* Findings presented at the annual meeting of the American Federation for Clinical Research, Washington, DC, April 30, 1993.

32. Gardell SJ, Duong LT, Diehl RE, York JD, Hare TR, Register RB, et al: Isolation, characterization and cDNA cloning of a vampire bat salivary plasminogen activator. *J Biol Chem* 1989; 264:17947–17952.
33. Jackson CV, Crowe VG, Craft TJ, Sundboom JL, Grinnell BW, Bobbitt JL, et al: Thrombolytic activity of a novel plasminogen activator, LY 210825, compared with recombinant tissue-type plasminogen activator in a canine model of coronary artery thrombosis. *Circulation* 1990; 82:930–940.
34. Madison EL, Goldsmith EJ, Gerard RD, Gething M-J, Sambrook JF: Serpin-resistant mutants of human tissue-type plasminogen activator. *Nature* 1989; 339:721–724.
35. Hsia J, Hamilton WP, Kleiman N, Roberts R, Chaitman BR, Ross AM: A comparison between heparin and low-dose aspirin as adjunctive therapy with tissue plasminogen activator for acute myocardial infarction. Heparin-Aspirin Reperfusion Trial (HART) Investigators. *N Engl J Med* 1990; 323:1433–1437.
36. Bleich SD, Nichols TC, Schumacher RR, Cooke DH, Tate DA, Teichman SL: Effect of heparin on coronary arterial patency after thrombolysis with tissue plasminogen activator in acute myocardial infarction. *Am J Cardiol* 1990; 66:1412–1417.
37. Lee L, Bates ER, Pitt B, Walton JA, Laufer N, O'Neill WW: Percutaneous transluminal coronary angioplasty improves survival in acute myocardial infarction complicated by cardiogenic shock. *Circulation* 1988; 78:1345–1351.
38. Verna E, Repetto S, Boscarini, M, Ghezzi I, Binaghi G: Emergency coronary angioplasty in patients with severe left ventricular dys-

function of cardiogenic shock after acute myocardial infarction. *Eur Heart J* 1989; 10:958–966.
39. Grines CL, Browne KF, Marco J, Rothbaum D, Stone GW, O'Keefe J, et al., for the Primary Angioplasty in Myocardial Infarction Study Group: A comparison of immediate angioplasty with thrombolytic therapy for acute myocardial infarction. *N Engl J Med* 1993; 328:673–679.
40. Zijlstra F, de Boer MJ, Hoorntje JCA, Reiffers S, Reiber JHC, Suryapranata H: A comparison of immediate coronary angioplasty with intravenous streptokinase in acute myocardial infarction. *N Engl J Med* 1993; 328:680–684.
41. Gibbons RJ, Holmes DR, Reeder GS, Bailey KR, Hopfenspirger MR, Gersh BJ, for the Mayo Coronary Care Unit and Catheterization Laboratory Groups: Immediate angioplasty compared with the administration of a thrombolytic agent followed by conservative treatment for myocardial infarction. *N Engl J Med* 1993; 328:685–691.
42. Kahn JK, O'Keefe JH, Rutherford BD, McConahay DR, Johnson WL, Giorgi LV, et al: Timing and mechanism of in-hospital and late death after primary coronary angioplasty during acute myocardial infarction. *Am J Cardiol* 1990; 66:1045–1048.
43. Kahn JK, Rutherford BD, McConahay DR, Johnson W, Giorgi LV, Ligon RW, et al: Usefulness of angioplasty during acute myocardial infarction in patients with prior coronary artery bypass grafting. *Am J Cardiol* 1990; 65:698–702.
44. Lee TC, Laramee LA, Rutherford BD, McConahay DR, Johnson WL Jr, Giorgi LV, et al: Emergency percutaneous transluminal coronary angioplasty for acute myocardial infarction in patients 70 years of age and older. *Am J Cardiol* 1990; 66:663–667.
45. The Canadian Cooperative Study Group: A randomized trial of aspirin and sulfinpyrazone in threatened stroke. *N Engl J Med* 1978; 299:53–59.
46. UK-TIA Study Group: The UK-TIA Aspirin Trial: Interim results. *Br Med J* 1987; 296:316–320.
47. Antiplatelet Trialists' Collaboration: Secondary prevention of vascular disease by prolonged antiplatelet treatment. *Br Med J* 1988; 296:320–331.
48. Goldman S, Copeland J, Moritz T, Henderson W, Zadina K, Ovitt T, et al: Improvement in early saphenous vein graft patency after coronary artery bypass surgery with antiplatelet therapy: Results of a Veterans Administration cooperative study. *Circulation* 1988; 77:1324–1332.
49. Harter HR, Burch JW, Majerus PW, Stanford N, Delmex JA, Anderson CB, et al: Prevention of thrombosis in patients on hemodialysis by low-dose aspirin. *N Engl J Med* 1979; 301:577–579.
50. The Steering Committee of the Physicians Health Study Research Group: Findings from the aspirin component of the ongoing Physicians' Health Study. *N Engl J Med* 1988; 318:262–264.
51. Peto R, Gray R, Collins R, Wheatley K, Hennekens C, Jamrozik K, et al: Randomised trial of prophylactic daily aspirin in British male doctors. *Br J Med* 1988; 296:313–316.
52. Hennekens CH, Peto R, Hutchinson GB, Doll R: An overview of the British and American aspirin studies. *N Engl J Med* 1988; 318:923–924.
53. Burch JW, Stanford PW: Inhibition of platelet prostaglandin synthetase by oral aspirin. *J Clin Invest* 1979; 61:314–319.
54. Majerus PW: Arachidonate metabolism in vascular disorders. *J Clin Invest* 1983; 72:1521–1525.
55. Kyrle PA, Eichler HG, Jager U, Lechner K: Inhibition of prostaglandin and thromboxane A2 generation by low-dose aspirin at the site of plug formation in man in vivo. *Circulation* 1987; 75:1025–1029.
56. Bousser MG, Eschwege E, Haguenau M, LeFaucconnier JM, Thibult N, Touboul D, et al: "AICLA" controlled trial of aspirin and dipyridamole in the secondary prevention of atherothrombotic cerebral ischemia. *Stroke* 1983; 14:5–14.
57. Levy M: Aspirin use in patients with major upper gastrointestinal bleeding and peptic ulcer disease. *N Engl J Med* 1974; 290:1158–1162.
58. Lewis HD, Davis JW, Archibald DG, Steinke WE, Smitherman TC, Doherty JE, et al: Protective effects of aspirin against acute myocardial infarction and death in men with unstable angina. *N Engl J Med* 1983; 309:396–403.
59. FitzGerald GA: Dipyridamole. *N Engl J Med* 1987; 316:1247–1257.
60. Hanson SR, Harker LA, Bjornsson TD: Effects of platelet-modifying drugs on arterial thromboembolism in baboons. Aspirin potentiates the antithrombotic actions of dipyridamole and sulfinpyrazone by mechanism(s) independent of platelet cyclooxygenase inhibition. *J Clin Invest* 1985; 75:1591–1599.
61. Chesebro JH, Fuster V, Elveback LR, McGoon DC, Pluth JR, Puga FJ, et al: Trial of combined warfarin plus dipyridamole or aspirin therapy in prosthetic heart valve replacement: Danger of aspirin compared with dipyridamole. *Am J Cardiol* 1983; 51:1537–1541.
62. Saltiel E, Ward A: Ticlopidine. A review of its pharmacodynamic and pharmacokinetic properties, and therapeutic efficacy in platelet-dependent disease states. *Drugs* 1987; 34:222–262.
63. Hanson SR, Harker LA: Baboon models of acute arterial thrombosis. *Thromb Haemostas* 1987; 58:801–805.
64. Gent M: The Canadian American Ticlopidine Study (CATS) in thromboembolic stroke (abstr). Book of Abstracts: Symposia, Oral and Poster Presentations 1988; XXII Congress of the International Society of Hematology, Milan, August 28–September 2, 1988: 75.
65. Hass WK: The Ticlopidine-Aspirin Study (TASS): Review and results (abstr). Book of Abstracts: Symposia, Oral and Poster Presentations 1988; XXII Congress of the International Society of Hematology, Milan, August 28–September 2, 1988: 75.
66. SCATI Group: Randomised controlled trial of subcutaneous calcium-heparin in acute myocardial infarction. *Lancet* 1989; II:182–186.
67. Holmes DR, Vlietstra RE, Smith HC, Vetrovec GW, Kent KM, Cowley MJ, et al: Restenosis after percutaneous transluminal coronary angioplasty (PTCA): A report from the PTCA registry of the National Heart, Lung and Blood Institute. *Am J Cardiol* 1984; 53:77C–81C.
68. Barnathan ES, Schwartz JS, Taylor L, Laskey WK, Kleaveland JP, Kussmaul WG, et al: Aspirin and dipyridamole in the prevention of acute coronary thrombosis complicating coronary angioplasty. *Circulation* 1987; 76:125–134.
69. Chesebro JH, Knatterud G, Roberts R, Borer J, Cohen LS, Dalen J, et al: Thrombolysis in Myocardial Infarction (TIMI) Trial, Phase 1: A comparison between intravenous tissue plasminogen activator and intravenous streptokinase. Clinical findings through hospital discharge. *Circulation* 1987; 76:142–154.
70. Topol EJ, Morris DC, Smalling RW, Schumacher RR, Taylor CR, Nishikawa A, et al: A multicenter, randomized, placebo-controlled trial of a new form of intravenous recombinant tissue-type plasminogen activator (activase) in acute myocardial infarction. *J Am Coll Cardiol* 1987; 9:1205–1213.
71. Heras M, Chesebro JH, Penny WJ, Bailey KR, Lam JYT, Holmes DR, et al: Importance of adequate heparin dosage in arterial angioplasty in a porcine model. *Circulation* 1988; 78:654–660.
72. Heras M, Chesebro JH, Penny WJ, Bailey KR, Badimon L, Fuster V: Effects of thrombin inhibition on the development of acute platelet-thrombus deposition during angioplasty in pigs. *Circulation* 1989; 79:657–665.
73. Weitz JI, Hudoba M, Massel D, Maraganore J, Hirsh J: Clot-bound thrombin is protected from inhibition by heparin-antithrombin III but is susceptible to inactivation by antithrombin III–independent inhibitors. *J Clin Invest* 1990; 86:385–391.
74. Hanson S, Harker L: Interruption of acute platelet-dependent thrombosis by the synthetic antithrombin D-phenylalanyl-L-prolyl-L-arginyl chloromethyl ketone. *Proc Natl Acad Sci USA* 1988; 85:3184–3188.
75. Eidt JF, Allison P, Noble S, Ashton J, Golino P, McNatt J, et al: Thrombin is an important mediator of platelet aggregation in stenosed canine coronary arteries with endothelial injury. *J Clin Invest* 1989; 84:18–27.
76. Jang I, Gold HK, Leinbach RC, McNary JE, Fallon JT, Collen D: Acceleration of reperfusion by combination of rt-PA and a selective thrombin inhibitor, argatroban (abstr). *Circulation* 1989; 80(suppl):II:217.
77. Sturzebecher J, Struzebecher U, Vieweg H, Wagner G, Hauptmann J, Markwardt F: Synthetic inhibitors of bovine factor Xa and thrombin comparison of their anticoagulant efficiency. *Thromb Res* 1989; 54:245–252.
78. Gruber A, Hanson SR, Kelly AB, Yan BS, Bang N, Griffin JH, et al: Inhibition of thrombus formation by activated recombinant protein C in a primate model of arterial thrombosis. *Circulation* 1990; 82:578–585.
79. Vlasuk G, Sipko G, Shebuski R: Specific factor Xa inhibition

enhances thrombolytic reperfusion and prevents acute reocclusion in the canine copper coil model of arterial thrombosis. *Circulation* 1990; 82(suppl):III-603.

80. Scarborough RM, Rose JW, Hsu MA, Fried VA, Phillips DR, Nannizzi L, et al: Characterization of a potent and GPIIb–IIIa specific platelet aggregation inhibitor from the venom of the southeastern pigmy rattlesnake (abstr). *Circulation* 1990; 82:III-370.
81. Gold HK, Coller BS, Yasuda T, Saito T, Fallon JT, Guerrero JL, et al: Rapid and sustained coronary artery recanalization with combined bolus injection of recombinant tissue-type plasminogen activator and monoclonal antiplatelet GPIIb/IIIa antibody in a canine preparation. *Circulation* 1988; 77:670–677.
82. Hanson SR, Pareti FI, Ruggeri ZM, Marzec UM, Kunicki TJ, Montgomery RR, et al: Effects of monoclonal antibodies against the platelet glycoprotein IIb/IIIa complex on thrombosis and hemostasis in the baboon. *J Clin Invest* 1988; 81:149–158.
83. Huang TF, Holt JC, Kirby EP, Niewiarowski S: Trigramin: Primary structure and its inhibition of von Willebrand factor binding to glycoprotein IIb/IIIa complex on human platelets. *Biochemistry* 1989; 28:661–666.
84. Gan Z-R, Gould RJ, Jacobs JW, Friedman PA, Polokoff MA: Echistatin: A potent platelet aggregation inhibitor from the venom of the viper, *Echis carinatus*. *J Biol Chem* 1988; 263:19827–19832.
85. Shebuski RJ, Ramjit DR, Bencen GH, Polokoff MA: Characterization and platelet inhibitory activity of bitistatin, a potent arginine–glycine–aspartic acid–containing peptide from the venom of the viper *Bitis arietans*. *J Biol Chem* 1989; 264:21550–21556.
86. Chao BH, Jakubowski JA, Savage B, Chow EP, Marzec UM, Harker LA, et al: *Agkistrodon piscivorus piscivorus* platelet aggregation inhibitor: A potent inhibitor of platelet activation. *Proc Natl Acad Sci USA* 1989; 86:8050–8054.
87. Dennis MS, Henzel WJ, Pitti RM, Lipari MT, Napier MA, Peisher TA, et al: Platelet glycoprotein IIb/IIIa protein antagonists from snake venoms: Evidence for a family of platelet aggregation inhibitors (abstr). *Blood* 1989; 74:129.
88. Hirsh J: Antithrombotic therapy in deep vein thrombosis and pulmonary embolism. *Am Heart J* 1992; 123:1115–1122.
89. Hirsh J, van Aken WG, Gallus AS, Dollery CT, Cade JF, Yung WL: Heparin kinetics in venous thrombosis and pulmonary embolism. *Circulation* 1976; 53:691–695.
90. Simon TL, Hyers TM, Gaston JP, Harker LA: Heparin pharmacokinetics: Increased requirements in pulmonary embolism. *Br J Haematol* 1978; 39:111–120.
91. Cruickshank MK, Levine MN, Hirsh J, Roberts R, Siguenza M: A standard heparin homogram for the management of heparin therapy. *Arch Int Med* 1991; 151:333–337.
92. Collins R, Scrimgeour A, Yusuf S, Peto R: Reduction in fatal pulmonary embolism and venous thrombosis by perioperative administration of subcutaneous heparin. *N Engl J Med* 1988; 318:1162–1173.
93. Leyvraz PF, Richard J, Bachman F, van Melle G, Treyvaud JM, Livio JJ, et al: Adjusted versus fixed-dose subcutaneous heparin in the prevention of deep-vein thrombosis after total hip replacement. *N Engl J Med* 1983; 309:954–958.
94. Hirsh J, Ofosu FA, Levine M: The development of low molecular weight heparins for clinical use. In: Verstraete M, Vermylen J, Lijnen R, Arnout J (eds): *Thrombosis and Haemostasis 1987*. Leuven, Leuven University Press, 1987: 325–348.
95. Hirsh J, Buchanan MR: Comparative effects of heparin and LMW heparin on hemostasis. *Thromb Res Suppl* 1991; 14:11–17.
96. Hirsh J: Oral anticoagulant drugs. *N Engl J Med* 1991; 324:1865–1875.
97. Poller L: Laboratory control of anticoagulant therapy. *Semin Thromb Hemost* 1986; 12:13–19.
98. Dalen JE, Hirsh J (eds): Third American College of Chest Physicians Consensus Conference on Antithrombotic Therapy. *Chest* 1992; 102(suppl):303S–549S.
99. Fernandez F, van Ryn J, Ofosu F, Hirsh J, Buchanan MR: The haemorrhagic and antithrombotic effects of dermatan sulphate. *Br J Haematol* 1986; 64:309–317.
100. Marder VJ, Sherry S: Thrombolytic therapy: Current status (2). *N Engl J Med* 1988; 318:1585–1595.

Chapter 8

Incidence, Prevalence, and Mortality of Cardiovascular Diseases

William B. Kannel, M.D., Ph.D. ■ *Thomas J. Thom, B.A.*

Life expectancy has never been higher in the United States than at present, largely as a result of the improved standard of living and quality of life. Accounting for most of the improvement over the past 25 years, however, has been the 49 percent decline in the age-corrected death rate for the cardiovascular diseases, suggesting the extent to which these leading causes of death are amenable to preventive and therapeutic management.

CARDIOVASCULAR DISEASES AS A MAJOR HEALTH HAZARD

General Morbidity and Mortality

During the past 25 years there have been major reductions in mortality rates for the various forms of cardiovascular disease in the United States.[1,2] Yet cardiovascular disease continues to be the most serious threat to life and health. One in every 3 men in the United States can expect to develop some major cardiovascular disease before reaching age 60; the odds for women are 1 in 10.[3] Coronary heart disease is a major cause of death beginning around age 40 in men and 65 in women.[4] The most common cardiovascular diseases are hypertension and heart disease, but a common underlying condition is atherosclerosis, which is clinically manifested as coronary heart disease (heart attack), cerebrovascular disease (stroke), and peripheral arterial disease. An estimated 8 percent of the population, 20 million persons, have some form of heart disease and 63 million, one-fourth of the population, have hypertension defined as a systolic blood pressure of 140 mmHg or greater or a diastolic pressure of 90 mmHg or greater or are on antihypertensive medication.[2,5] Almost one-third of persons with heart disease and 5 percent of those with hypertension are limited in their usual activity by the condition.[6] These diseases rank third and fourth, respectively, as chronic conditions causing limitation of activity. More than two-thirds of persons over age 65 have hypertension, as defined above, and nearly 30 percent have heart disease. Yet two-thirds of all persons with hypertension are under 65 and over 50 percent of all persons with heart disease are under 65 years of age. In 1989, there were an estimated 39 million days in short-stay hospitals and 56 million visits to physicians' offices for these diseases.[7,8] Heart disease and hypertension account for an estimated 455 million days of restricted activity, 184 million bed days, and 23 million work-loss days annually.[6,9]

Cardiovascular disease constitutes an expanding problem in the elderly, causing 70 percent of all deaths beyond age 75.[4] Coronary heart disease is the most common and most lethal cardiovascular event in both sexes, exacting a large toll in disability and quality of life in old age. Unrecognized myocardial infarctions are especially common and are as lethal as symptomatic infarctions.[10] Beyond age 65, women become as vulnerable to cardiovascular mortality as men.[4] The predisposing modifiable risk factors for coronary disease, stroke, peripheral arterial disease, and cardiac failure are similar in young and old and in men and women. These major established risk factors include hypertension, dyslipidemia, impaired glucose tolerance, physical indolence, and cigarette smoking. An attenuated risk ratio for some risk factors is offset by a greater incidence of cardiovascular disease in advanced age so that the attributable risk and the potential benefit of treatment rises with age.[11] In old age, cholesterol and low-density lipoproteins are considerably higher in women than in men. Some 10 million elderly persons and two women for every man will require investigation and treatment for elevated lipids by National Heart, Lung, and Blood Institute guidelines. Cardiovascular risk profiles composed of the major risk factors predict coronary heart disease as efficiently in the elderly as in the young. This and the fact that the decline in cardiovascular mortality has included the elderly suggest potential for intervention. Because of the preponderance of women in the elderly population, trials of the efficacy of correcting risk factors in general and lipids in particular should include women.

Cardiovascular diseases accounted for 43 percent of all deaths in 1991, a total of 923,000.[12] Largely because there are many more older women than older men in the U.S. population, the equivalent percentage is higher in women (48 percent) than in men (42 percent), and the number of deaths from cardiovascular diseases is greater in women than in men.[4] Of all cardiovascular disease deaths, 38 percent occurred "prematurely," i.e., before 75 years of age, the average life expectancy in 1989.[13] That compares to 62 percent in 1949.[14] Atherosclerosis, when manifested as coronary heart disease, cerebrovascular disease, or peripheral arterial disease, accounted for 72 percent of all deaths from the cardiovascular diseases in 1991.[12] Heart disease is the leading cause of death followed by cancer and then cerebrovascular diseases.[4] Death rates for cardiovascular disease are highest in black males, next highest in white males followed by black females, and lowest in white females. Prevalence and mortality from the cardiovascular diseases decrease with increasing family income and with increasing levels of education.[5,15]

Because cardiovascular disease accounts for 43 percent of the nation's mortality and much of the nation's morbidity, its cost to the nation's economy is by far the largest for any diagnostic group, an estimated $159 billion in 1990 according to the National Heart, Lung, and Blood Institute.[12] For cardiovascular disease patients that year, the nation spent $85 billion for hospital care, physician and other professional services, drugs, and nursing home care. This amounts to more than 1 percent of the nation's gross national product. The economy lost $74 billion in productivity due to illness ($17 billion) and premature death ($57 billion) attributed to these diseases. Included in the $57 billion is the discounted value of future productivity that would have occurred if those who died from cardiovascular diseases in 1990 had lived to normal life expectancy. It has also been estimated that the 5-year medical cost of a myocardial infarction (i.e., diagnostic and therapeutic services) is $51,211 in 1986 dollars.[16]

Although there are national data on hospitalized patients, national incidence and case fatality data for the cardiovascular diseases are nonexistent. Data from the Framingham (Massachusetts) Heart Study provide reliable estimates for 36 years of follow-up of a defined population sample of 5209 men and women aged 35 to 94. Average annual rates of first major cardiovascular events rose from 5 per 1000 men at ages 35 to 44 years to 59 per 1000 at ages 85 to 94 (Table 8-1). For women, comparable rates are achieved 10 years later in life, with the gap closing with advancing age. Coronary heart disease is the predominant cardiovascular event comprising more than one-half of all such events in men and women under age 75 (Table 8-2). But the proportions of cardiovascular events due to coronary heart disease decline with age as the proportions due to stroke and congestive

TABLE 8-1

Incidence of Major Cardiovascular Events: Framingham Study, 36-Year Follow-up*

	Cardiovascular Disease (All Types)		Coronary Heart Disease		Stroke and Transient Ischemic Attack		Congestive Heart Failure		Peripheral Arterial Disease	
Age	Men	Women	Men	Women	Men	Women	Men	Women	Men	Women
35–44	5	2	5	1	†	†	†	†	†	†
45–54	15	7	11	4	2	1	2	1	2	1
55–64	28	16	21	11	5	3	5	3	5	3
65–74	39	24	26	14	10	8	9	6	7	4
75–84	57	46	32	22	21	17	17	13	5	3
85–94	59	66	25	23	†	27	31	28	†	†
35–64‡	18	9	14	6	3	2	3	2	3	2
65–94‡	43	30	27	17	12	11	11	9	6	3

*Average annual incidence per 1000 persons free of specified disease.
†Results are omitted when fewer than five individuals experience an event.
‡Age-adjusted rates.
SOURCE: National Heart, Lung, and Blood Institute

TABLE 8-2

Percentage of First Cardiovascular Events by Type of Event, Framingham Study, 36-Year Follow-up

Age (years)	Cardiovascular Disease, *n* (All Types)		Coronary Heart Disease (%)		Stroke and Transient Ischemic Attack (%)		Congestive Heart Failure (%)		Peripheral Arterial Disease (%)	
	Men	Women	Men	Women	Men	Women	Men	Women	Men	Women
35–54	269	147	76.2	61.2	8.6	17.7	7.8	12.9	7.4	8.2
55–64	441	348	69.4	62.9	11.3	12.6	6.8	10.1	12.5	14.4
65–74	345	342	62.9	57.6	17.4	23.4	8.1	9.6	11.6	9.4
75–94	154	269	55.3	46.9	25.3	31.6	12.3	15.6	7.1	5.0

heart failure increase with age. Under age 75, there is a higher proportion of cardiovascular events due to coronary heart disease in men than in women and a higher proportion due to congestive heart failure in women than in men.

Secular and Historical Trends

The trend in mortality from the cardiovascular diseases as a group has been downward since about 1940, with long-term declines for the three subgroups, rheumatic, cerebrovascular, and hypertensive diseases, and a decline for coronary heart disease (CHD) since the mid-1960s (Fig. 8-1). The coronary decline antedates effective antithrombolytic and antihypertensive treatment. Prior to 1940 cardiovascular mortality increased and became the predominant cause of death because of control of infectious and parasitic diseases and an epidemic increase in fatal coronary attacks. Cardiovascular mortality declined just under 1 percent per year in the 1950s and 1960s.[2] The decline became more precipitous in the 1970s, with the rate falling 3 percent per year since then. Sixty-two percent of the decline between 1950 and 1989 occurred in the 17 years since 1972. For CHD, there has been over a 50 percent decline in the age-adjusted death rate since the peak in 1963; the current decline is about 3 to 4 percent per year. For stroke, the rate of decline since 1972 has exceeded 6 percent per year, but the annual rate of decline has lessened in recent years.

A striking feature of the recent decline in cardiovascular mortality has been its universal nature; i.e., it has declined in all races, both sexes, all age groups, and all geographic areas in the United States. However, greatest improvements have been noted in young adults and the higher socioeconomic subgroups, and there are geographic differences in the rate of decline.[2,17] The largest percentage declines are noted for hypertension and cerebrovascular diseases, and in recent years the largest absolute decline has been in CHD. Except for lung cancer and chronic obstructive pulmonary diseases, mortality from other natural causes has also been declining. But because cardiovascular diseases account for one-half of all deaths, declines in these diseases are largely responsible for the major improvement of average life expectancy, which by 1989 was 75.2 years.[13]

The decline in CHD mortality reverses the earlier epidemic rise persisting into the 1960s; it coincides with improvements in the major cardiovascular risk factors, more vigorous and effective treatment of the acute episode, and greater efforts at secondary prevention.[17–22] The decline in CHD mortality in the United States exceeds that observed in most countries.[23] Many Western countries only recently began experiencing a downward trend in CHD mortality, and the trend is still upward in countries of Eastern Europe.

The decline in cardiovascular mortality indicates that the major force of mortality is controllable. Whether attributable more to changes in disease-promoting lifestyle or to better medical care of those already afflicted, it is clear that cardiovascular disease is not an inevitable

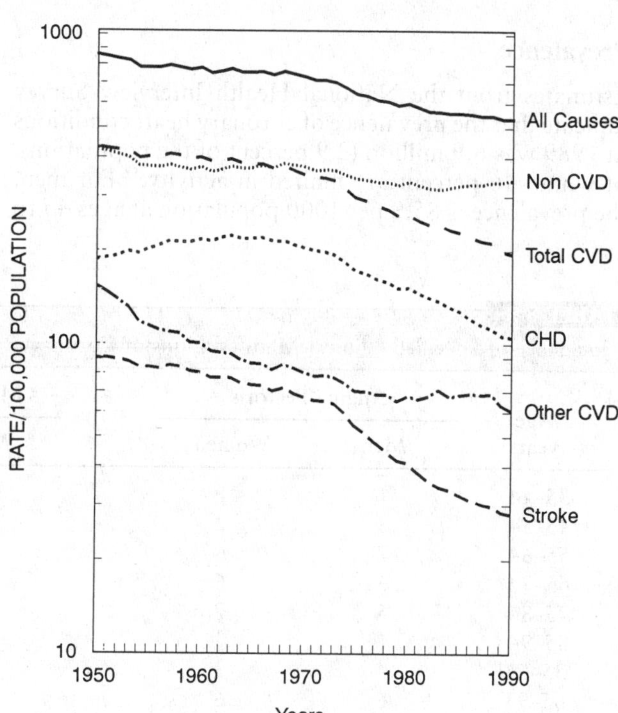

FIGURE 8-1 Age-adjusted U.S. death rates for selected causes, 1950–1990 (CVD = cardiovascular disease; CHD = coronary heart disease). *(From Vital Statistics of the United States, National Center for Health Statistics.)*

burden of aging or genetic makeup. Although causes of the decline in cardiovascular mortality are uncertain, the decline has been substantial, sustained, and real. The decline has coincided with increased efforts to achieve healthier living habits and with improvements in the ambient burden of cardiovascular risk factors.

Unfortunately, there are very few uniform statistics on trends in morbidity. This is important because reduction in mortality without a decline in the attack rate would indicate better medical care was responsible, while a reduction in both morbidity and mortality suggests environmental influences and/or preventive measures have improved. If reduction in mortality continues, the size of the elderly population will continue to increase over and above the increase related to demographic effects. Some studies, but not all, suggest that there have been declines in incidence of the cardiovascular diseases.[17-22]

CORONARY HEART DISEASE

Coronary heart disease kills and disables people in their most productive years and, according to the National Heart, Lung, and Blood Institute, accounted for $22 billion in medical care costs and $32 billion in indirect economic costs in 1989.[2] Coronary disease is the third most frequent cause of short-stay hospitalizations, exceeded only by childbirth and injuries.[7] Per-admission hospital costs for coronary disease are among the highest. Coronary heart disease is the leading cause of premature, permanent disability in the American labor force, accounting for 19 percent of disability allowances by the Social Security Administration.[24]

Prevalence

Estimates from the National Health Interview Survey indicate that the prevalence of coronary heart conditions in 1989 was 6.9 million (2.9 percent of the population), of whom 46 percent are limited in activity.[5,6] For men, the prevalence is 85.9 per 1000 population at ages 45 to 64 and 168.9 at 65 and over. For women, the corresponding estimates by age are 25.6 at 45 to 64 years and 113.0 at 65 and over, substantially lower than in men.

Incidence

Coronary heart disease causes about 800,000 new heart attacks each year and 450,000 recurrent attacks.[2] Incidence in women lags behind men by 10 years for total CHD and by 20 years for more serious clinical manifestations such as myocardial infarction and sudden death (Table 8-3). Male predominance is least striking for uncomplicated angina pectoris.

The first coronary presentation for women is more likely to be angina, whereas in men it is more likely to be myocardial infarction (Table 8-4). More angina in men occurs after infarction than before. Only 20 percent of coronary attacks are preceded by long-standing angina, fewer if the infarction is silent or unrecognized. Serious manifestations of coronary heart disease such as infarction or sudden death are rare in the premenopausal female. The incidence and severity of CHD increase with age in both sexes. There seems to be a more precipitous increase for women after the menopause, with CHD rates in postmenopausal women two to three times that of women the same age who remain premenopausal.[25] This applies whether the menopause is natural or surgical and, in the latter, whether the ovaries are removed or not. The sex ratio in incidence narrows progressively with advancing age.

Unrecognized myocardial infarctions are common, numbering at least one in four infarctions (Table 8-5). Half of the unrecognized infarctions are silent, and the rest are atypical so that neither the patient nor the physician entertains the possibility. More than half of these subjects eventually develop some overt clinical manifestations of CHD and hence come under medical care. Angina is less frequent in subjects with unrecognized infarction than in those with recognized symptomatic myocardial infarction, either before or after the infarction occurs. Despite the apparent mild nature of unrecognized infarction, the risk of subsequent mortality is

TABLE 8-3

Incidence of Specified Clinical Manifestations of Coronary Heart Disease: Framingham Study, 36-Year Follow-up*

Age (years)	Angina Pectoris		Myocardial Infarction		Sudden Death	
	Men	Women	Men	Women	Men	Women
35–44	1	<1	2	†	†	†
45–54	3	2	5	1	1	†
55–64	7	6	9	3	2	1
65–74	6	6	13	5	3	1
75–84	5	7	19	10	5	3
85–94	†	†	†	12	†	6
35–64‡	4	3	6	2	1	<1
65–94‡	6	6	14	7	3	2

* Average annual incidence rate per 1000 persons free of coronary heart disease.
† Results are omitted when fewer than five individuals experienced the event.
‡ Age adjusted.

TABLE 8-4

Percentage of First Events of Coronary Heart Disease by Type of Event, Framingham Study, 36-Year Follow-up

Age (years)	Coronary Heart Disease, *n* (All Types)		Myocardial Infarction* (%)		Angina Pectoris (%)		Coronary Insufficiency (%)		Sudden Death from Coronary Heart Disease (%)		Non–Sudden Death from Coronary Heart Disease (%)	
	Men	Women	Men	Women	Men	Women	Men	Women	Men	Women	Men	Women
35–54	212	84	43.9	29.8	34.9	58.3	8.0	4.8	9.4	4.8	3.8	2.4
55–64	339	245	44.5	26.9	40.7	57.1	3.2	7.3	8.8	5.7	2.7	2.9
65–74	252	222	50.8	36.0	29.8	46.8	4.0	7.2	11.9	7.2	3.6	2.7
75–94	102	141	58.8	47.5	18.6	28.4	3.9	4.3	13.7	17.0	4.9	2.8

*Recognized or unrecognized.

TABLE 8-5

Percentage of Unrecognized Myocardial Infarction: Framingham Study, 36-Year Follow-up

Age (years)	Total	Men	Women
35–94	36	33	38
35–64	33	27	48
65–94	40	42	37

nearly the same as with recognized infarction. Diabetic men and hypertensive persons of both sexes are particularly susceptible to silent or unrecognized infarctions.

Prognosis

After surviving the acute stage of a myocardial infarction morbidity and mortality is 2 to 9 times that of the general population (Table 8-6).[26] The rates of occurrence of reinfarction, sudden death, angina pectoris, cardiac failure, and stroke are all substantial. The relative and absolute risks of these events are as great in women as in men. Within 6 years following a recognized myocardial infarction, 23 percent of men and 31 percent of women will have a recurrent infarction, and 41 percent of men and 34 percent of women will develop angina. About 20 percent will be disabled with cardiac failure and 9 percent of men and 18 percent of women will have a stroke. Sudden death will be experienced by 13 percent of men and 6 percent of women. Prognosis is as bad, if not worse, following an unrecognized infarction (Table 8-6). Although about two-thirds of myocardial infarction patients do not make a complete recovery, 88 percent under age 65 are able to return to their usual occupations.[27]

Mortality

Coronary heart disease is the leading cause of death in American adults, accounting for more than one-fourth of the deaths in persons over age 35.[4] In 1989, there were 498,000 coronary deaths.[13] Mortality from this disease increases with age, but it is also a prominent cause of death in adults at the peak of their productive lives.

In a substantial number of CHD deaths, the progression from inapparent clinical disease to death is rather swift. Much of the premature mortality from CHD comes on with little warning in a population prone to this disease. Sudden, unexpected, out-of-hospital coronary deaths that occur too rapidly to allow arrival alive at the hospital account for more than one-half of all coronary fatalities. The proportion of coronary deaths that are sudden deaths is lower in women than in men and lower in elderly men than in the young (Table 8-7). However, the percentage of sudden coronary deaths that occur without prior CHD is much greater in women than in men and greater in younger than in older persons (Table 8-8). In 48 percent of men and 63 percent of women who died suddenly, there was no prior evidence of overt coronary disease.

About 80 percent of coronary mortality in persons under age 65 occurs during the initial coronary attack.[3] Thus, despite a higher risk of death with a prior coronary attack, most coronary deaths arise from the population still free of symptomatic CHD. After myocardial infarction, sudden deaths occur at four to six times the rate of the general population. Hence, primary prevention appears to offer more to society than secondary prevention. The first year following a recognized myocardial infarction is especially dangerous, with 27 percent of men and 44 percent of women succumbing (Table 8-9). Long-term survival following unrecognized myocardial infarction is only slightly better than for recognized infarctions, and survival is better for women than for men (Table 8-10). Following uncomplicated angina pectoris, the survival picture for men under age 65 is nearly the same as it is for recognized infarctions and is much worse than survival in women.

Coronary heart disease is either the leading cause or one of the leading causes of death in men and women and in every racial or ethnic group.[2] The death rate for CHD is four and a half times higher in men than in women at ages 25 to 34, but that ratio declines to one and a half by ages 75 to 84. The coronary death rate is twice as high in blacks than in whites at ages 25 to 34, and that difference disappears by age 75. Heart disease mortality is not quite as high among the Hispanic population as it is among blacks and whites.[28]

TABLE 8-6

Six-Year Prognosis Following Myocardial Infarction*: Framingham Study, 30-Year Follow-up

	Men		Women	
	Percent	Risk Ratio†	Percent	Risk Ratio†
Recognized				
Death	40	2.6	46	3.9
Sudden death	13	4.0	6	4.4
Myocardial infarction	23	2.8	31	8.5
Angina pectoris	41	6.2	34	5.7
Cardiac failure	17	4.2	23	7.7
Stroke/transient ischemic attack	9	2.7	18	5.1
Unrecognized				
Death	50	2.7	36	2.5
Sudden death	14	4.8	6	6.2
Myocardial infarction	19	2.0	24	4.8
Angina pectoris	19	2.7	26	4.9
Cardiac failure	27	5.8	18	5.3
Stroke/transient ischemic attack	16	4.3	12	2.6

*Surviving 30 days.
†Standardized morbidity and mortality ratios (times 0.01).

HYPERTENSION

Hypertension is the most prevalent cardiovascular disease, and it is one of the most powerful contributors to cardiovascular morbidity and mortality. It is the most important factor contributing to the 500,000 cases of stroke that occur each year and is a major factor in the estimated 1.25 million annual heart attacks.[2] Each year, about 32,000 deaths are classified with hypertensive disease as the underlying cause, and it is the main contributor to the 147,000 deaths from stroke, 42,000 deaths from cardiac failure, many of the 498,000 deaths from CHD, and many of the 22,000 deaths from kidney disease that occurred in 1989.[13]

Prevalence

Data from the National Health and Nutrition Examination Survey for 1976 to 1980 indicate a hypertension prevalence of 29.7 percent for persons 18 to 74 years of age in the United States.[29] For that estimate hypertension is defined as blood pressure equal to or greater than 140/90 mmHg. When persons below that level but on antihypertensive medication are included and data are extrapolated to 1989 for all ages, prevalence is about 63 million: one-fourth of the total population, one-third of the adult population.[2] Prevalence of mild hypertension, defined as a diastolic blood pressure of 90 to 104 mmHg, is about 25 million persons. Prevalence of isolated systolic hypertension, defined as systolic blood pressure over 160 mmHg and diastolic under 95 mmHg, is about 4 million persons, comprised mostly of older persons.

Percent prevalence increases with age and is highest among blacks and the elderly. Isolated systolic hypertension is a common and distinctly hazardous condition in the elderly. There is recent evidence from the Systemic Hypertension in the Elderly Program (SHEP) that treatment of this form of hypertension in the elderly is distinctly efficacious not only against stroke but against coronary disease as well.[30] This benefit accrued despite the use of a diuretic (clorthalidone). The benefit in the face of diuretic use may derive from the lower impact of

TABLE 8-7

Percentage of Coronary Heart Disease Deaths as Sudden Deaths: Framingham Study, 36-Year Follow-up

Age (years)	Total	Men	Women
35–94	41	45	33
35–64	49	52	39
65–94	36	40	32

TABLE 8-8

Percentage of Sudden Deaths without Prior Coronary Heart Disease: Framingham Study, 36-Year Follow-up

Age (years)	Total	Men	Women
35–94	52	48	63
35–64	50	50	83
65–94	49	45	57

TABLE 8-9

Percentage of Deaths within One Year Following Initial Cardiovascular Event: Framingham Study, 36-Year Follow-up

Age (years)	Recognized Myocardial Infarction		Stroke/Transient Ischemic Attack		Congestive Heart Failure	
	Men	Women	Men	Women	Men	Women
35–94	27	44	30	31	41	37
35–64	16	30	19	24	34	26
65–94	43	50	36	34	46	41

TABLE 8-10

Percentage of Deaths by Time Interval Following Initial Cardiovascular Event and Survival for 30 days: Framingham Study, 36-Year Follow-up

Interval length (years)	Angina Pectoris Uncomplicated		Recognized Myocardial Infarction		Unrecognized Myocardial Infarction		Stroke/ Transient Ischemic Attack		Intermittent Claudication		Congestive Heart Failure	
	Men	Women	Men	Women	Men	Women	Men	Women	Men	Women	Men	Women
Ages 35–74 years												
1–2	3	1	7	15	8	2	14	14	2	1	38	15
2–4	11	3	14	21	20	8	24	16	10	10	51	25
4–8	20	11	32	33	44	23	39	33	27	21	75	49
8–12	41	22	45	55	63	39	58	48	48	38	80	58
12–16	54	31	58	79	76	44	69	51	61	56	85	72
16–20	65	45	71	90	91	62	84	65	73	70	89	79
Ages 65–94 years												
1–2	4	5	24	22	18	23	24	25	3	1	46	38
2–4	10	19	43	49	40	46	38	35	13	9	65	54
4–8	27	35	67	68	63	62	62	61	45	30	86	80
8–12	59	47	80	79	84	74	76	75	64	60	92	90
12–16	85	69	90	89	90	84	88	90	82	79	98	95
16–20	—	81	—	—	96	91	—	95	94	92	—	97

side effects on lipids and glucose tolerance in the elderly or the lower dose of diuretics used in this trial than in former trials. Persons with hypertension face serious excess risks of cardiovascular sequelae, and since much of this excess risk is attributable to mild hypertension, there is need for intervention through preventive life-style modification, if not through drug treatment. Because of the higher prevalence of milder hypertension, almost 60 percent of the excess mortality attributable to hypertension comes from this blood pressure range. Risks of cardiovascular sequelae are proportional to the blood pressure level at any age, in either sex, whether the elevation is systolic or diastolic. Approximately one-half of the persons who suffer a first heart attack and two-thirds who suffer a first stroke have blood pressures above 160/95 mmHg.

Although in most affluent populations there is a rise in blood pressure with age in both sexes, this is not universal and it does not mean that blood pressure must inevitably rise with age or that in those whose pressures do rise it reflects a normal aging process. There is about a 20 mmHg systolic and 10 mmHg diastolic rise from age 30 to age 64. Systolic pressures continue to rise into the eighties in women and into the seventies in men. Diastolic pressures level off earlier and, in men, decline precipitously beyond age 55. The pressures start lower in young adult women and rise more steeply in middle age (50 and over), so that they equal those of men in the fifties and then progressively exceed those of men in later life; this crossover is observed for both systolic and diastolic pressures. In some populations in the world, blood pressure does not rise with age.

There have been apparent large improvements between 1960 to 1962 and 1976 to 1980 in the percentage of hypertensives (160/95 mmHg or greater or on medication) aware of it (from 48 to 71 percent), on antihypertensive medication (from 30 to 45 percent), and under control (from 12 to 23 percent) during that time.[29] "Under control" in this case means on antihypertensive medication and having blood pressures below 160/95 mmHg. These secular trends in blood pressure are difficult to interpret because of the increased use of antihypertensive therapy for milder degrees of hypertension.

Incidence

Longitudinal observation of blood pressures as people age reveals a different pattern than cross-sectional data. The reason for this difference is obscure. Diastolic pressures are essentially parallel in the sexes, with women's pressures consistently below those of men. Systolic pressures in women, initially lower than those in men, rise more steeply in women to converge at age 60 with those of men but never to exceed them. A progressive and disproportionate rise in systolic pressure with advancing age is presumed to result from loss of arterial elasticity. Blacks have higher blood pressures than whites in most Western cultures. The crossover in blood pressures in the sexes appears to occur 10 years earlier in blacks than in whites.

Mortality

Only 3 percent of cardiovascular deaths in 1989 were nominally attributed to hypertensive disease, a gross underestimate of its impact on mortality. Hypertensive disease mortality is largely due to atherosclerotic sequelae such as coronary disease, stroke, and cardiac failure. Renal failure due to necrotizing arteriolar disease is uncommon, and malignant hypertension is vanishing as a cause of death. In 1979 only 6 percent of deaths directly attributed to hypertension were ascribed to malignant hypertension. The marked downward trend in mortality attributed to hypertensive disease and stroke strongly suggests that mortality resulting from hypertension is on the decline.

Determinants

While genetic susceptibility plays a large role, this may be only permissive, requiring one or more environmental cofactors such as salt intake, alcohol, or weight gain to bring on hypertension. Of all the identifiable determinants of hypertension, weight gain and adiposity, particularly abdominal in distribution, seem to be predominant. New underlying causes of hypertension are discovered every decade, but the causes of the vast majority of cases remain undetermined. Of the identifiable causes, chronic renal diseases, renovascular disease, and hypertension induced by oral contraceptives head the list. Routine search for underlying causes not suggested by signs or symptoms is usually unrewarding and often counterproductive. Recent research suggests that insulin resistance occurring in association with obesity may play a fundamental role.[31]

STROKE

Prevalence

There are about 10 stroke patients per 1000 population in the United States, a total of 2.6 million persons according to the National Health Interview Survey of 1989.[5] An estimated 41 percent of stroke patients are limited in their usual activity because of this disease.[6] Prevalence rises in men from 14.6 per 1000 adults at 45 to 64 years to 77.5 for men ages 75 and over and from 15.9 to 79.6 in the respective age groups in women.[5] In the Framingham Study, the most common variety of stroke is atherothrombotic brain infarction, which accounts for 64 percent of all strokes (excluding transient ischemic attacks). Next most common are cerebral embolus, subarachnoid hemorrhage, and intracerebral hemorrhage. Intracerebral hemorrhage has apparently declined most in recent years.

Incidence

The chance of having a stroke before age 70 in the Framingham Study is 1 in 20 for either sex.[32] However, incidence rates vary depending on the age of the study sample, whether the sample is derived from the general population or from some select subgroup such as hospitalized patients, and whether recurrent strokes are included. Thirty-one percent of stroke survivors needed assistance in self-care, 20 percent required help in ambulation, and 71 percent had an impaired vocational capacity when examined an average of 7 years after their stroke.[33]

Cerebrovascular disease need not be a result of aging. Modifiable contributing factors offer the possibility of prevention by identifying stroke candidates for corrective measures. Stroke prevention requires early treatment of persons with hypertension, cardiac disorders, and transient cerebral ischemic attacks.

Mortality

Cerebrovascular disease, the third leading cause of death, was responsible for 214,000 deaths in 1973, but by 1989 the number had declined to 147,000.[13] This decline is remarkable because the population of older persons increased substantially during that time. The age-adjusted death rate declined by 55 percent over this period, although the rate of decline has diminished in recent years.[2] The rate of decline in mortality for stroke accelerated from a 1 percent per year decline in the 1940s and 1950s and a 2 percent per year decline in the 1960s to a 6 percent per year decline in the 1970s. But since 1980 the decline slowed to less than 4 percent per year. Yet this disease still accounts for 1 of every 14 deaths, and 46,000 of them occur prior to 75 years of age. Under age 65 the mortality rate is three times greater in the black than in the white population, largely as a result of the higher prevalence and increased severity of hypertension. The proportion of strokes that result in death within 1 year is about 31 percent, less if the stroke occurs before age 65 (Table 8-9). Long-term survivorship is poorer in men than in women; over two-thirds of the men with stroke die within 8 years (Table 8-10).

HEART FAILURE

Heart failure is the end stage of cardiac disease after the myocardium has used all its reserve and compensatory mechanisms. Once overt signs appear, half of the patients will be dead within 5 years despite modern medical management.[34] Heart failure is a tragic consequence of a variety of heart diseases, particularly hypertensive, coronary, rheumatic, and congenital heart disease. Risk of heart failure is increased two- to sixfold with coronary disease, angina conferring half the risk of myocardial infarct. The dominant cause is hypertension, which precedes failure in 75 percent of cases. Coronary heart disease, generally accompanied by hypertension, is responsible in 39 percent of cases.[35] Precursive rheumatic heart disease, noted in 21 percent of cases of cardiac failure, is also often accompanied by hypertension.

According to the National Heart, Lung, and Blood Institute, from 2 to 3 million Americans have heart failure and an estimated 400,000 new cases occur each year, and there are almost 700,000 hospitalizations annually.[2,7] Based on the Framingham Study, occurrence is equally as frequent in men and women and annual occurrence approaches 10 per 1000 population after 65 years of age (Table 8-1). Survivorship following diagnosis of heart failure is poorer in men than in women, but even in women only about 15 percent survive much longer than 8 to 12 years (Table 8-10). The outlook is not much better than for cancer. The case fatality rate for heart failure is high, with one in five dying. Sudden death is a common mode of exodus occurring at six to nine times the general population rate. Multiple-cause-of-death tabulations mentioned heart failure 200,000 times on death certificates in 1982 with over 85 percent designated as a secondary diagnosis.[36] With an increasing geriatric population, heart failure is a formidable problem. It is the leading *diagnosis-related group* in hospitalized patients over 65 years of age.[37]

Despite the availability of potent glycosides, diuretics, and antihypertensive agents, heart failure continues at a high incidence. Preventive management requires early detection and correction of impaired myocardial function, and treatments that do not potentiate or induce arrhythmia. Greater emphasis must be given to preventive measures instituted before the heart has exhausted its reserve and compensatory mechanisms. Since hypertension is such an important predisposing factor, early and sustained treatment would seem a key to the prevention of heart failure. If preventive programs are to be developed, identification of factors that predispose and influence the course of the disease is essential. Using ordinary office procedures, one can detect high-risk candidates for heart failure before there is an overt manifestation present.

There is little indication that the declines in death rates from heart disease in general and from CHD in particular in the United States have been accompanied by an improvement in the incidence of heart failure. Data from the Framingham Study indicate very little improvement in the ominous outlook following onset of congestive heart failure. Median survival of 652 incident cases of congestive heart failure was only 1.7 years in men and 3.2 years in women. Overall survival rates at 5 years were only 25 percent for men and 38 percent for women. Mortality increased with age in both sexes. Adjusting for age, no significant change in the prognosis of congestive heart failure was evident over the past four decades despite improvements in treatment. Thus, congestive heart failure remains a highly lethal condition with a better prognosis in women and younger victims. Advances in treatment of hypertension, myocardial ischemia, and valvular heart disease have not resulted in improvements in survival once heart failure ensues.

Mortality and hospital discharge rates for heart failure have failed to decline substantially since 1970 despite a marked decline in CHD mortality and marked improvement in hypertension control.[36] This cannot be readily explained. Some postulate that improved survival of cases of angina, myocardial infarction, and hypertensive heart disease may result in an increased prevalence of chronic heart disease and ultimately heart failure.[38] There is also uncertainty about the prevalence of underlying etiologies for congestive heart failure. Etiologies may have shifted in recent years from predominantly hypertension to CHD.[39] (See also Chap. 25.)

IDIOPATHIC CARDIOMYOPATHY

The causes of idiopathic dilated (congestive) and hypertrophic cardiomyopathy remain ill defined so that opportunities for preventing them are few. Reliable estimates of the prevalence and incidence of these disorders are unavailable because of the comparatively uncommon occurrence of these diseases in the general population. Examination of National Center for Health Statistics data from 1987 indicated 18,660 deaths assigned to cardiomyopathy. About 87 percent of these were coded as congestive or dilated cardiomyopathy.[40] Hypertrophic cardiomyopathy accounted for only 2 percent of cases in men and less than 6 percent in women. Alcoholic heart muscle disease (cardiomyopathy) appears to account for 8 percent. This condition appears to be 2.5 times as frequent in blacks as in whites.

In 1989 cardiomyopathy was responsible for 53,000 hospitalizations and 484,000 days of hospital care in the United States.[7] Mortality was highest in older persons, men, and blacks. Death rates rose sharply since 1970 for reasons that are unclear. This could be an artifact of changes in diagnostic criteria and death certification practices.

ARRHYTHMIAS

An arrhythmia is a disturbance of the cardiac impulse. It is a manifestation of most major cardiac diseases, a major cause of morbidity in rheumatic heart disease, and a contributor to half of the mortality from CHD. Many such victims die suddenly, without warning. Together with cardiac failure, arrhythmias are the final common pathways of heart disease.

Although the frequency of arrhythmias is not known, in 1989 there were an estimated 2.8 million hospital discharges with arrhythmias listed as one of the diagnoses.[7] In about one-fifth of these cases arrhythmia was the primary diagnosis. In 1989 there were an estimated 2 million physician office visits for this condition, larger than the number due to stroke. It is not known how many deaths are directly attributed to arrhythmias each year because it is the immediate cause, not the underlying cause, of much cardiac mortality.

The Framingham Study reported incidence rates for atrial fibrillation. In that population the chance of developing this condition was about 2 percent within 20 years.[41] About 70 percent of the cases evolved following development of overt cardiovascular disease. Cardiac failure and rheumatic heart disease were the most powerful precursors with the relative risks in excess of fivefold. Hypertensive cardiovascular disease was the most common prior cardiovascular disease, largely because of its great frequency in the general population. Neither hypertension alone or CHD was a significant precursor. Among the risk factors, only diabetes and left ventricular hypertrophy on electrocardiogram were significantly or substantially related to the occurrence of atrial fibrillation. Cardiovascular mortality was doubled by development of atrial fibrillation.

RHEUMATIC FEVER AND RHEUMATIC HEART DISEASE

Rheumatic fever is the chief cause of serious valvular heart disease. Acute rheumatic fever and subsequent rheumatic heart disease remain one of the important cardiovascular problems in the tropical and subtropical developing countries in South America, Africa, the Middle East, and Asia.[42] It occurs there with a frequency seen in the United States and Europe a century ago. Although preventable, this disease occurs because of overcrowding, the deceptive self-limited nature of symptoms in streptococcal pharyngitis, and the mild and often clinically inapparent nature of streptococcal infections. The availability of penicillin to treat these infections, living conditions that are less crowded than formerly, and evolution of different strains of streptococcus have made rheumatic fever uncommon in the United States, although incidence remains high in disadvantaged subgroups such as blacks, Puerto Ricans, Mexican-Americans, and American Indians.[42] Because this disease has not been eradicated in this country, there is need to define better the incidence and prevalence and the infective endocarditis that follows as well as better to define those at risk.

The estimated prevalence in 1989 of active rheumatic fever and chronic rheumatic heart disease is 1.7 million persons, 7 per 1000 persons of all ages, over 13 per 1000 above age 45.[5] About 15 percent of these persons are limited in activity because of the resulting chronic carditis.[6] Incidence, generally thought to be about 100,000 new cases per year, may be overestimated; there are no good national estimates. Occurrence is concentrated in the lower socioeconomic subgroups. Rheumatic fever is rare before age 3, occurring most frequently between 5 and 15 years of age, when streptococcal infections are most frequent. During epidemics of streptococcal pharyngitis, the rheumatic fever attack rate is 3 percent, whereas in endemic situations it is only 0.3 percent. Many of the 56,000 annual open heart operations on cardiac valves in 1989 were rheumatic heart disease patients.[7]

With decline in rheumatic fever in the United States, its clinical manifestations have also moderated so that carditis is detected in less than 20 percent of acutely affected patients.[43] Annual mortality has declined to about 6000 deaths per year, which reflects an 89 percent decline in the age-adjusted death rate from 1950 to 1989. But because the cardiac sequelae of rheumatic fever are still seen in adults and adequate treatment can reduce attacks by 90 percent, rheumatic fever and rheumatic heart disease are still the two most preventable serious cardiovascular disorders. It seems clear that at least part of the decline in rheumatic fever was due to prompt antistreptococcal treatment by physicians. However, the decline in rheumatic fever appears to have antedated the advent of antistreptococcal agents. We are currently unable to explain definitively the decline in rheumatic fever possibly because we do not fully understand its etiologic factors. (See also Chap. 78.)

In developing countries, rheumatic fever is the most frequent cause of heart disease in the 5- to 13-year-old group, causing 25 to 40 percent of all cardiovascular diseases and 33 to 50 percent of all hospital admissions.[44] The persistence of rheumatic fever both in the United States and abroad does not allow complacency.

OTHER VALVULAR DISEASE

In the two decades since mitral valve prolapse was described, the syndrome has changed from a curiosity to the most frequently diagnosed valvular deformity. The exact prevalence is not clear. It appears to occur in 6 to 10 percent of presumably normal young women[45] and is reported in about 4 percent of healthy young men.[46] Although the condition may become manifest at any age, it is reported most frequently in young women aged 14 to 30, where it may reach a prevalence exceeding 10 percent. Echocardiographic studies indicate that it may be even more common with 10 to 15 percent of the population possibly afflicted; however, many diagnosed by echocardiography exhibit neither clinical nor angiographic evidence of the syndrome. The fact that 6 to 10 percent of asymptomatic young women have this syndrome is prima facie evidence that it is generally a benign condition. The natural history is not well established. Few cases progress to a severe form, and the risk of sudden death appears to be less than originally thought. The major importance may be the threat of endocarditis, which must be rare, and arrhythmias, which may be common. (See also Chap. 80.)

CONGENITAL HEART DISEASE

The prevalence of congenital heart disease at birth as determined during the infant's brief stay in the hospital is likely to be underestimated, and recognition of specific lesions may be inaccurate. Most data are deficient for congenital heart disease diagnosed after the first week of life. Prevalence data based on autopsy findings are unreliable because they reflect a fraction of the deaths and relate only to fatal lesions. Most information comes from retrospective studies based extensively on referral practices.

Structural abnormalities of the heart or intrathoracic great vessels seem to affect 8 to 10 of every 1000 infants born alive in the United States. If bicuspid aortic valves and mitral valve prolapse manifested later in life are counted, the rate may well exceed 1 percent of live births. About 1 newborn per 1000 live births has a cardiac birth defect that cannot be managed medically or surgically. Most infants who previously would have died now survive to adult life because of improved treatment, but 5 to 6 per 1000 live births require frequent medical or surgical attention.

Except for the recent unexplained twofold increase in ventricular septal defects and the threefold increase in patent ductus arteriosus, the incidence of most congenital heart diseases has remained stable. Rubella vaccine has reduced rubella-caused congenital heart disease, and congenital heart defects associated with Down's syndrome are less common because older women are having fewer babies. Preventive strategies are impeded by lack of knowledge of the cause of most congenital heart disease, although we have learned that alcohol, trimethadione, and lithium can cause cardiac defects. The majority of congenital heart disease may involve complex genetic-environmental interactions that remain to be elucidated.

About 72 of each 1000 live births in the United States are premature, with the infants weighing less than 2500 g. Almost half of premature infants weighing less than 1750 g will maintain patency of their ductus arteriosus, possibly because their immature lungs do not properly metabolize prostaglandins that cause the ductus to remain open.[47] The growing number of teratogens identified appear to account for only 5 percent of all human malformations, and single mutant genes are said to be responsible for only 3 percent of cases.[48] (See also Chap. 96).

In all evaluations of mortality from congenital heart disease, death in infancy predominates at 1.3 to 2.8 per 1000 live births. Later mortality is more speculative, about 0.4 per 1000 live births over the subsequent 3 years. About 25 percent of infants with congenital heart disease have a malformation incompatible with life beyond the first year; possibly half of these can be treated surgically to improve the quality of life, if not to produce a cure. About 2.5 per 1000 live-born infants require specialized services for diagnosis and treatment of congenital heart disease shortly after birth, and another 2.5 per 1000 will need these resources later in childhood.

With the exception of bicuspid aortic valve in older patients, ventricular septal defect is the most common variety, accounting for 30 percent of congenital heart disease. Some 75 percent of congenital heart disease in infants and children is encompassed by eight defects: ventricular septal defect, pulmonary stenosis, patent ductus arteriosus, tetralogy of Fallot, aortic stenosis, coarctation of the aorta, and transposition of the great arteries. There is an excess of birth defects in blacks. The rate among siblings is 17 per 1000 compared to 2.6 per 1000 in the general population. (See also Chap. 97.)

PULMONARY THROMBOEMBOLISM

Estimates of mortality from pulmonary embolism vary widely, depending on the source and accuracy of data. It is probably directly responsible for 50,000 deaths annually in the United States. If untreated, recurrent episodes are frequent and more than 25 percent will be fatal. Mortality is probably underreported since two-thirds of cases found at autopsy were overlooked before death. More than 60 percent of fatalities occur within 1 h of onset; hence, pulmonary embolism is likely to be confused with sudden coronary death.

Among the white U.S. population, the age-adjusted death rate for pulmonary embolism decreased 12 percent in men and 20 percent in women between 1970 and 1978.[49] Despite protocol changes that increased the number of diagnoses coded and the introduction of prospective payment and diagnosis-related groups from 1983 to 1985, no increases in rates were noted from 1979 to 1985. The rate of hospital discharges with diagnosis of pulmonary embolism declined 15 to 45 percent, particularly in younger age groups, between 1979 and 1985.

Death rates and hospital rates for pulmonary embolism increase with age and are higher in men than in women and in blacks than in whites. Pulmonary embolism contributed to nearly 30,000 deaths in 1986 and was diagnosed 91,000 times in hospitals in 1989.[4,7]

The incidence of pulmonary embolism is even more uncertain than the mortality. Only 10 percent of cases occur in normal persons without predisposing factors such as chronic cardiopulmonary and malignant disease, estrogen therapy, orthopedic trauma, immobilization, operative procedures, obesity, pregnancy, or blood dyscrasias. The elderly are more vulnerable.

Postoperative pulmonary emboli alone produce 4000 to 8000 deaths annually. It is a major cause of death postpartum and in patients hospitalized for orthopedic conditions. Evidence from Britain suggests that the annual mortality from pulmonary embolism has been increasing for several decades despite anticoagulant drugs. More than 5 million persons over age 40 undergo major surgery each year in the United States; 1 or 2 of each 1000 will die postoperatively from pulmonary embolism. The recent advent of low-dose heparin prophylaxis may substantially reduce this risk.[50]

Epidemiologic surveys suggest that pulmonary thromboembolism causes 50,000 deaths annually in the United States, although only 1 in 10 emboli sustained is fatal. Taking this into account, it is estimated that there are 500,000 pulmonary embolus events annually. Routine autopsies find evidence of recent or old embolism in 25 to 30 percent.[51] When a special search is made, they are found in 60 percent of autopsies. It is estimated that pulmonary embolism is grossly underdiagnosed, since only 10 to 30 percent of autopsied cases with evidence of embolism had an antemortem diagnosis.

More than 95 percent of pulmonary emboli arise from deep venous thrombi in the legs (above the knee); the remaining arise from the right cardiac chambers or other veins. The majority of deaths occur suddenly and can be avoided only by prophylaxis. Patients who survive to reach the hospital for medical treatment generally have a good outlook with little morbidity and resolution of the emboli. (See also Chap. 100).

PREVENTIVE IMPLICATIONS

Examination of the incidence, prevalence, mortality, and natural history of cardiovascular disease suggests the need for a preventive approach. Further innovations in diagnosis and treatment for cardiovascular disease will undoubtedly improve the outlook of patients surviving the initial attack. But this can have only a limited impact because of the high initial mortality. When the heart or brain is infarcted, no therapy can be expected to restore full function. If the initial presentation is sudden death, therapy is unavailing. A preventive approach involving correction of predisposing factors in advance of the overt clinical expression of the disease can be expected to have the greater impact.

Coronary heart disease often strikes without warning: One in five coronary attacks presents as sudden death, and two-thirds of the deaths occur in the community too precipitously to be brought under medical attention.

While some strokes may give warning by transient ischemic attacks, most do not. Even when they do, intervention at that stage does not necessarily avoid a permanently damaging stroke or prolong life.

Heart valves damaged by rheumatic heart disease and infective endocarditis can be surgically repaired or replaced by prosthetic appliances; this approach often requires potentially dangerous anticoagulants to prevent emboli, and valve failure and hemolysis are distressingly common. Although such patients live longer, more comfortable lives than formerly, their survival does not approach that of patients with rheumatic fever kept from progressing to severe valve damage by antibiotic prophylaxis against recurrent disease.

Hypertension that progresses to target organ involvement is less manageable than if vigorously treated prior to such manifestations. The first sign of target organ involvement is too often a stroke, myocardial infarction, or sudden death. Half such cardiovascular catastrophes occur before evidence of organ involvement can be discovered on biennial examination.

Awaiting overt signs and symptoms of cardiovascular disease is no longer justified. In some respects, the occurrence of symptoms may be more properly regarded as a medical failure rather than as the initial indication for treatment.

A major impact on cardiovascular morbidity and mortality should derive from the practice of preventive medicine, from public health measures to alter life-style to one more favorable to cardiovascular health, and from health education to inform people of what they must do to protect their cardiovascular health.[17,52] Recent expansion and improvements have occurred in these measures conceivably contributing significantly to the dramatic 45 percent decline in cardiovascular mortality during the past two decades, which is responsible for 79 percent of the decline in overall mortality.

REFERENCES

1. National Center for Health Statistics: *Health, United States, 1990.* DHHS pub no (PHS) 91-1232. US Government Printing Office, 1991.
2. National Heart, Lung, and Blood Institute: *Morbidity and Mortality Chartbook on Cardiovascular, Lung, and Blood Diseases/1992.* US Dept of Health and Human Services, 1992.
3. Gordon T, Kannel WB: Premature mortality from coronary heart disease: The Framingham Study. *JAMA* 1971; 215:1617–1625.
4. National Center for Health Statistics: *Vital Statistics of the United States, 1988*, vol II, *Mortality*, pt A. US Government Printing Office, 1991.
5. National Center for Health Statistics, Adams PF, Benson V: Current estimates from the National Health Interview Survey, United States, 1989. *Vital and Health Statistics.* DHHS pub no (PHS) 90-1504. US Government Printing Office, 1990.
6. National Center for Health Statistics, Collins JG: Prevalence of selected chronic conditions, United States, 1986–88. *Vital and Health Statistics.* DHHS pub no (PHS) 93–1510. US Government Printing Office, 1993.
7. National Center for Health Statistics, Graves EJ: Detailed diagnoses and procedures, National Hospital Discharge Survey, 1989. *Vital and Health Statistics*, ser 13, no. 107, DHHS pub no. (PHS) 91-1768. US Government Printing Office, 1991.
8. National Center for Health Statistics, DeLozier JE, Gagnon RO: National ambulatory medical care survey: 1989 summary. *Advance Data from Vital and Health Statistics.* No. 128, DHHS pub no (PHS) 87-1250. US Government Printing Office, 1987.
9. National Center for Health Statistics, Wilder CS: Disability days United States, 1983. *Vital and Health Statistics.* DHHS pub no (PHS) 87-1586. US Government Printing Office, 1986.
10. Kannel WB, Cupples LA, Gagnon DR: Incidence, precursors and prognosis of unrecognized myocardial infarction. *Adv Cardiol* 1990; 37:202–214.
11. National Heart, Lung, and Blood Institute: Cholesterol and Heart Disease in Older Persons and Women: Review of an NHLBI Workshop. *Ann Epidemiol* 1992, vol 2, 161–176.
12. National Heart, Lung, and Blood Institute: *NHLBI Fact Book, Fiscal Year 1992.* US Dept of Health and Human Services, National Institutes of Health, February 1993.
13. National Center for Health Statistics: Annual summary of births, marriages, divorces, and deaths; United States, 1989. *Monthly Vital Statist Rep*, vol 38, no 13, August 30, 1990.
14. National Office of Vital Statistics: *Vital Statistics of the United States*, 1949, pt II, 1951.
15. Rogot E, Sorlie PD, Johnson NJ, Schmitt C: Second data book; a study of 1.3 million persons: By demographic, social, and economic factors: 1979–1985 follow-up: US National Longitudinal Mortality Study. US Dept of Health and Human Services, National Institutes of Health pub no 92-3297, 1992.
16. Wittels EH, Hay JW, Gotto AM: Medical costs of coronary artery disease in the United States. *Am J Cardiol* 1990; 65:432–440.
17. Thom TJ, Kannel WB: Factors in the decline of coronary disease mortality. In: Connor WE, Bristow JD (eds): *Coronary Heart Disease: Prevention, Complications, and Treatment.* Philadelphia, Lippincott, 1985:5–20.
18. Higgins MW, Luepker RV (eds): *Trends in Coronary Heart Disease Mortality: The Influence of Medical Care.* New York, Oxford University Press, 1988.
19. Higgins MW, Luepker RV: Trends and determinants of coronary heart disease mortality: International comparisons. *Int J Epidemiol* 1989; 18(suppl 1):51.
20. Sytkowski PA, Kannel WB, D'Agostino RB: Changes in risk factors and the decline in mortality from cardiovascular disease: The Framingham Study. *N Engl J Med* 1990; 322(23):1635–1641.
21. D'Agostino RB, Kannel WB, Belanger AJ, Sytkowski PA: Trends in CHD and risk factors at age 55–64 in the Framingham Study. *Int J Epidemiol* 1989; 18(3,suppl 1):567–572.
22. Burke GL, Sprafka JM, Folsom AR, Luepker RV, Norsted SW, Blackburn H: Trends in CHD mortality, morbidity and risk factor levels from 1960 to 1986: The Minnesota Heart Survey. *Int J Epidemiol* 1989; 18(3, suppl):573–581.
23. Uemura K, Pisa Z: Trends in cardiovascular disease mortality in industrialized countries since 1950. *World Health Stat Q* 1988; 41:155–177.

24. US Dept of Health and Human Services, Social Security Administration: *Characteristics of Social Security Disability Insurance Beneficiaries.* SSA pub no 13-11947, 1982.
25. Gordon T, Kannel WB, Hjortland MC, McNamara PM: Menopause and coronary heart disease. *Ann Intern Med* 1978; 89:157–161.
26. Cupples LA, D'Agostino RB: Survival following initial cardiovascular events: 30-Year follow-up Framingham Heart Study, section 35. In: Kannel WB, Wolf PA, Garrison RJ (eds): *The Framingham Study: An Epidemiological Investigation of Cardiovascular Disease.* Bethesda, MD, National Heart, Lung, and Blood Institute, National Institutes of Health pub no 88-2969, 1988.
27. Kannel WB: *The Natural History of Myocardial Infarction: The Framingham Study.* Leiden, Leiden University Press, 1973.
28. National Center for Health Statistics: Deaths of Hispanic origin, 15 reporting states, 1979–81. *Vital and Health Statistics,* ser 20. No 18, DHHS pub no (PHS) 91-1855. US Government Printing Office, December 1990.
29. National Center for Health Statistics, Drizd T, Dannenberg AL, Engel A: Blood pressure levels in persons 18–74 years of age in 1976–80, and trends in blood pressure from 1960 to 1980 in the United States. *Vital and Health Statistics.* DHHS pub no (PHS) 86-1684. US Government Printing Office, 1986.
30. SHEP Cooperative Working Group: Prevention of stroke by antihypertension drug treatment in older persons with isolated systolic hypertension: Final results of the Systolic Hypertension in the Elderly Program (SHEP). *JAMA* 1991; 265(24):3255–3264.
31. Reaven GM, Hoffman BB: A role for insulin, the aetiology and causes of hypertension? *Lancet* 1987; 2(8556):435–437.
32. Gresham GE, Fitzpatrick TE, Wolf PA, McNamara PM, Kannel WB, Dawber TR: Residual disability in survivors of stroke: The Framingham Study. *N Engl J Med* 1975; 293:954.
33. Kannel WB, Wolf PA, Dawber TR: An evaluation of the epidemiology of atherothrombotic brain infarction. *Milbank Mem Fund Q* 1975; 405–448.
34. Kannel WB, Belanger AJ: Epidemiology of heart failure. *Am Heart J* 1991; 121(3,pt 1):951–957.
35. Kannel WB, Castelli WP, McNamara PM, McKee PA, Feinleib M: Role of blood pressure in the development of congestive heart failure: The Framingham Study. *N Engl J Med* 1972; 287:781–787.
36. Gillum RF: Heart failure in the United States, 1970–1985. *Am Heart J* 1987; 113:1043–1045.
37. National Center for Health Statistics, Graves EJ: Diagnosis-related groups using data from the National Hospital Discharge Survey, United States, 1985. *Advance Data from Vital and Health Statistics.* No. 137, DHHS pub no (PHS) 87-125. US Government Printing Office, July 2, 1987.
38. Gillum RF, Folson AR, Blackburn H: The decline in coronary heart disease mortality: Old questions and new facts. *Am J Med* 1984; 76:1055–1065.
39. Turlink JR, Goldhaber SJ, Pfiffer MA: An overview of contemporary etiologies of congestive heart failure. *Am Heart J* 1991; 121:1852–1853.
40. Gillum RF: Idiopathic cardiomyopathy in the United States, 1970–1982. *Am Heart J* 1986; 111(4):752–755.
41. Kannel WB, Abbott RD, Savage DD, McNamara PM: Epidemiologic features of chronic atrial fibrillation: The Framingham Study. *N Engl J Med* 1982; 306:1018–1022.
42. Gillum RF: Trends in acute rheumatic fever and chronic rheumatic heart disease: A national perspective. *Am Heart J* 1986; 111(2): 430–432.
43. Persellin RH: Acute rheumatic fever: Changing manifestations. *Ann Intern Med* 1978; 89:1002–1004.
44. Markowitz M: Observations in the epidemiology and preventability of rheumatic fever in developing countries. *Clin Ther* 1981; 4:240–251.
45. Procacci PM, Savran SV, Schreiter SL, Bryson AL: Prevalence of clinical mitral valve prolapse in 1969 young women. *N Engl J Med* 1976; 294:1086–1088.
46. Sbarbaro JA, Mehlman DJ, Wu L, Brooks HL: A prospective study of mitral valvular prolapse in young men. *Chest* 1979; 75(5):555–559.
47. Department of Health, Education, and Welfare: *Proceedings of the Second Conference on the Epidemiology of Aging.* DHEW pub no 80-969, 1980.
48. Michaelson M: *Report on a Study of Congenital Cardiovascular Malformations—Etiology, Incidence, Natural History and Organization of Diagnostic and Therapeutic Services.* World Health Organization, Regional Office for Europe, 1979.
49. Gillum RF: Pulmonary embolism and thrombophlebitis in the United States, 1970–1985. *Am Heart J* 1987; 114:1262–1266.
50. Clagett GP, Anderson FA Jr, Levine MN, Salzman EW, Wheeler HB: Prevention of venous thromboembolism. *Chest* 1992; 102(suppl.):3915–4075.
51. Moser KM: Pulmonary thromboembolism. In: Wilson JD, Braunwald E, Isselbaecher KJ, Petersdorf RG, Martin JB, Fauci AS, et al: (eds): *Harrison's Principles of Natural Medicine,* 12th ed. New York, McGraw-Hill, 1991:1090–1096.
52. Havlik RJ, Feinleib M (eds.): *Proceedings of the Conference on Decline of Coronary Heart Disease Mortality.* Washington, National Institutes of Health, 1979.

PART II

General Evaluation of the Patient

SECTION A
History and Physical Examination

Chapter 9A

Introduction to the General Evaluation of the Patient

Robert A. O'Rourke, M.D.

In assessing patients with definite or suspected cardiac disease, one obtains important information from the history, physical examination, chest roentgenogram, electrocardiogram and other routine laboratory tests. In many patients this data base will provide the necessary background for making an accurate diagnosis and appropriate decisions concerning therapy. In other patients more information is necessary and additional, more technical, noninvasive cardiac tests such as echocardiography and/or radionuclide studies are needed. In certain patients the general assessment of the patient indicates the need for cardiac catheterization and contrast angiography, with or without additional noninvasive cardiac testing. For example, the proper approach to specific patients with symptomatic coronary artery disease may include both coronary arteriography and cardiac catheterization (anatomy and hemodynamics) as well as myocardial perfusion imaging with thallium-201 (extent of inducible ischemia).

It should be emphasized that *not all patients need every test* and that the skillful use of low technology including the history and general examination of the patient may preclude the need for additional studies or may be important in determining which of a wide variety of available sophisticated tests should be chosen for a particular patient. The purpose of this section (Chaps. 9A to 22) is to discuss the proper application of the history, physical examination, and frequently performed diagnostic and monitoring procedures in patients with cardiac disease and to delineate the differential diagnosis in patients who present with certain common cardiovascular symptoms.

The physician assessing patients with cardiovascular disease must be cognizant of the sensitivity, specificity, predictive value, and accuracy of the results of selected diagnostic tests (Table 9A-1).[1] *Sensitivity* indicates the frequency of a positive test result in a population of patients *with* a particular disease. *Specificity* indicates the frequency of a negative test result in a group of patients *without* a certain disease. The positive predictive value of a diagnostic test result defines the percentage of patients *with* a specific disease in a group of patients in whom the test results are positive. The negative predictive value indicates the percentage of patients *without* a certain disorder in a population of patients in whom the test results are negative. The overall diagnostic accuracy of a test is defined as the percentage of patients correctly classified by the test. *Bayes' theorem* states that the predictive value of a test result is predetermined by the incidence of the disease in the population being evaluated. The posttest likelihood of a particular disorder is equal to the pretest likelihood times the probability that the test result is a true one. Thus, a false positive diagnostic test result is most likely to occur when the test is applied to a member of a patient group in whom the particular disease is very uncommon. The posttest probability of disease can be calculated from the disease prevalence in a particular patient group and the sensitivity and specificity of the diagnostic test as indicated in Table 9A-1.[1]

TABLE 9A-1

Validity Measures of a Diagnostic Test*

Sensitivity: $\frac{TP}{TP + FN}$ Specificity: $\frac{TN}{TN + FP}$

Predictive Value of a Positive Test: $\frac{TP}{TP + FP}$

Predictive Value of a Negative Test: $\frac{TN}{TN + FN}$

Overall Diagnostic Accuracy: $\frac{TP + TN}{\text{Total number of tests}}$

Bayes' theorem:

Probability of disease presence with a positive test $= \frac{\text{sensitivity} \times \text{prevalence}}{(\text{sensitivity} \times \text{prevalence}) + [(1 - \text{specificity}) \times (1 - \text{prevalence})]}$

Probability of disease presence with a negative test $= \frac{(1 - \text{sensitivity}) \times \text{prevalence}}{(1 - \text{sensitivity} \times \text{prevalence})[\text{specificity} \times (1 - \text{prevalence})]}$

*True positive (TP) = Positive result in patient with disease; True negative (TN) = Negative result in patient *without* disease; False positive (FP) = Positive result in patient *without* disease; False negative (FN) = Negative result in patient with disease.

SOURCE: From Steingart RM, Scheuer J: Assessment of myocardial ischemia. In: Hurst JW, Schlant RC (eds): *The Heart,* 7th ed, New York, McGraw-Hill, 1990: 357.

In assessing the patient with cardiovascular disease, an orderly approach is a necessity (Table 9A-2). It is prudent to ascertain the etiology, abnormal anatomy, altered physiology, cardiac status, and prognosis of the cardiovascular disease as recommended in the guidelines set forth by the New York Heart Association.[2-4] As indicated in the guidelines, the *etiologic, anatomic,* and *physiological* diagnosis of cardiovascular disease relies on a careful analysis of the patient's history, an attentive physical examination, and, when indicated, a variety of laboratory studies.[2-4] Some of the latter do not evaluate specifically the cardiovascular system but often help delineate the patient's major problem.[2-4] Other tests, such as electrocardiography, echocardiography, cardiac nuclear studies, cardiac catheterization, and angiography are used to determine the cause of heart disease or to identify specific anatomic and physiologic abnormalities.[2-4] The *etiology* of cardiovascular disease should be determined by considering both structural and functional abnormalities. If two or more possible causes of heart disease are present, each should be mentioned.[2-4] *Anatomic* lesions of the cardiovascular system often are recognized clinically. Many times the presence of a structural lesion is suggested from recognizing the cause of the heart disease, identifying the resulting physiological abnormalities, or both.[2-4] When more than one anatomic abnormality exists, each should be included in the anatomic diagnosis. Some different *physiological* abnormalities often have similar clinical manifestations, and identifying the cause of the abnormality may depend upon knowledge of the etiologic or anatomic diagnoses. If more than one physiological abnormality is present, all should be included in the physiological diagnosis.[2-4]

TABLE 9A-2

New York Heart Association Classification of a Complete Diagnosis of Cardiovascular Disease*

Old (prior to 1973)[2]	New (after 1973)[3,4]
Etiology	Etiology
Anatomy	Anatomy
Physiology	Physiology
Functional Capacity*	Cardiac Status and Prognosis
Therapeutic	(Specific Recommendations)

*The old *Functional and Therapeutic Classifications* of the 6th edition in 1964 were replaced by the patient's overall *Cardiac Status and Prognosis* in the 7th edition in 1973.

SOURCE: Reproduced with permission from the New York Heart Association, Inc., and the publisher.[3,4]

A complete cardiac diagnosis should include one or more titles from each of the principal diagnostic categories of this nomenclature: etiologic, anatomic, physiological, and cardiac status and prognosis (Table 9A-2). The purpose of the classification, "Cardiac Status and Prognosis," is to assess the current cardiac state of the patient and to provide a prognosis of the patient's future status as modified by optimal therapy.[3-4] The cardiac status includes a total assessment of the etiologic, anatomic, and physiological diagnoses. The prognosis is based on an estimation of the likely effects of optimal current medical and surgical therapies. The classification of each patient should be reviewed frequently and revised as indicated. This appraisal should indicate to others the physician's opinion of the patient's status and prognosis without consideration of specific management. A recommendation for further diagnostic procedures, medical and surgical therapies, and limitation of physical activity should be detailed at the end of the classification.[1]

A functional classification based on symptoms is still needed in patients with angina pectoris or heart failure for determining the indications for certain forms of therapy, for evaluating the response to therapy, for judging

TABLE 9A-3
The Old New York Heart Association Functional Classification

Class 1	No symptoms with ordinary physical activity.
Class 2	Symptoms with ordinary activity. Slight limitation of activity.
Class 3	Symptoms with less than ordinary activity. Marked limitation of activity.
Class 4	Symptoms with any physical activity or even at rest.

SOURCE: Reproduced with permission from the New York Heart Association, Inc., and the publisher.[2]

the extent of disability, and for classifying patients who are included in clinical trials.[1] The Canadian Cardiovascular Society classification[5] commonly is used to describe the amount of effort required to produce angina pectoris (see Table 19-2). When such a classification is used it should be displayed after the term angina pectoris, which is located in the physiology category of the New York Heart Association classification of a "complete cardiovascular diagnosis." The grading of dyspnea and/or fatigue due to heart failure needs further clarification; however, in some circumstances it still is reasonable to use the old New York Heart Association classification (Table 9A-3).[2] For example, this classification of the extent of dyspnea and/or fatigue has been used frequently to classify patients with heart failure, and it is commonly employed in determining entry criteria for patients participating in clinical research trials.

REFERENCES

1. Hurst JW: The physician's approach to the patient: goals and cardiac appraisal. In: Hurst JW, Schlant RC (eds): *The Heart*, 7th ed. New York, McGraw-Hill, 1990: 115–121.
2. The Criteria Committee of the New York Heart Association: *Diseases of the Heart and Blood Vessels: Nomenclature and Criteria for Diagnosis*, 6th ed. New York, New York Heart Association/ Little, Brown and Company, 1964.
3. The Criteria Committee of the New York Heart Association: *Nomenclature and Criteria for Diagnosis of Diseases of the Heart and Great Vessels*, 8th ed. New York, New York Heart Association/ Little, Brown and Company, 1979.
4. The Criteria Committee of the New York Heart Association: *Nomenclature and Criteria for Diagnosis of Diseases of the Heart and Great Vessels*, 7th ed. New York, New York Heart Association/ Little, Brown and Company, 1973.
5. Campeau L: Letter to the editor. *Circulation* 1976; 54:522.

Chapter 9B

The History: Symptoms and Past Events Related to Cardiovascular Disease

J. Willis Hurst, M.D. ■ Douglas C. Morris, M.D.

The physician's interview with the patient has a dual purpose: to obtain important medical information and to establish a bond of trust between the patient and physician.

The purpose of this chapter is to emphasize the important technique of history taking[1-3] and to discuss briefly the symptoms caused by cardiovascular disease.

ERRORS MADE IN HISTORY TAKING

The Inhumane Interview

When the history-taking period is over, patients should realize that the physician knows a lot about them and cares about their well-being. When patients perceive that physicians give of themselves, they in turn trust the physicians.

Unfortunately, history taking does not always create a good doctor-patient relationship. In fact, the interview may establish adversary roles for the physician and the patient. The interview will fail if the interviewer is too hurried; demands precise answers and displays irritation when such are not given; shows disdain when the answers to questions are not known; insists on probing deeper into areas that are emotionally painful to the patient; fails to look up from the desk during the interview; receives multiple telephone calls during the interview; seems to treat dreaded diseases casually; gives nonverbal signals of personal unhappiness; and seems to be automated rather than understanding. Should any of these occur, the interview will be perceived by the patient as the most inhumane and cruel portion of the entire medical workup.

Today there is considerable discussion about the inhumaneness of medicine; it is usually blamed on machines and technology. Machines, however, are either used or misused by physicians and their helpers, who sometimes disturb patients by what they say. When the medical interview fails because of improper conversation, the physician will be unable to establish a relationship with the patient and the medical information will often be wrong because the patient tries to avoid the process of a cold interrogation.

The Flaw in Dealing with the Chief Complaint

Physicians are taught to ask patients to state their *chief complaint*. The patient's chief complaint may not lead the physician to identify the patient's most serious problem. The physician, however, must always deal with the patient's chief complaint; not to do so will lead to instant patient dissatisfaction because the patient perceives the chief complaint as the most serious one and feels that the physician is insensitive when it is ignored. The physician must not fail to identify symptoms other than the patient's chief complaint because they may be important and serious.

The Flaw in Dealing with the Present Illness

The historical details related to the chief complaint are labeled the *present illness*. Should the interviewer's mind be dominated by this lock-step sequence, he or she may not pursue all the patient's complaints. It is far better to ask patients to enumerate all their symptoms and to establish a present illness for each of the symptoms the physician judges to be significant.

Use and Abuse of Medical Questionnaires

A medical questionnaire is helpful when it is given to the patient well in advance of the interview. The patient can then record certain data more accurately because he or she will have time to think about the question, ask others about the question, and look up details about the question in personal papers. The abnormalities perceived by the patient should be probed, and related areas should be pursued by the physician. This approach, when properly implemented, should ensure that nothing important has been overlooked and permit more time for the physician to personalize the interview.

The medical questionnaire may be harmful if the physician allows it to act as a substitute for his or her interaction with the patient or fails to show the patient that it is a very important part of the medical record.

Failure to Interpret Properly the Past History

Physicians may make an error when they accept a past event as fact. We seem willing to accept a past history of rheumatic fever as fact but demand strict criteria for the current diagnosis of the disease. We seem willing to accept the past diagnosis of myocardial infarction when the basis of the belief may be hearsay evidence. The past history is very important, but at times it can mislead the physician.

Failure to Talk with the Family

It is important to obtain information from family members about the patient's symptoms and his or her reaction to the illness. Every experienced physician knows that the successful care of the patient is frequently determined by the physician's relationship with members of the patient's family. It is essential to establish a doctor-family relationship as well as a doctor-patient relationship.

Failure to Assess the Patient's Feelings

Good historians will know their patient's reaction to illness, feelings about disability, feelings about surgical intervention, and emotional reactions. Also, when the interview is over, the patient should perceive the physician as a knowledgeable and caring person.

Failure to Live Through a Day with the Patient

It is important for the physician to "live through" a day with the patient. This is accomplished by simply asking the patient to enumerate the activities of the day, beginning with getting up in the morning and ending with getting up 24 h later. When this is done, many new insights about the patient's life will be discovered.

PAST HISTORY

Although the past history is at times misleading, it may offer an important clue to the presence of disease. There may be a history of congenital heart disease in the family. The patient's mother may give a history of rubella during the first few months of pregnancy, which makes patent ductus, pulmonary valve stenosis, coarctation of the pulmonary arteries, and aortic septal defect more likely to be present. A definite history of rheumatic fever may be helpful in the effort to establish the cause of a heart murmur, whereas a negative history of rheumatic fever does not eliminate it as a cause of a heart murmur. As stated earlier, the physician must be cautious in accepting a vague history of rheumatic fever as being accurate because the diagnosis was formerly made with inadequate data. The history of hypertension in family members increases the chances that the cause of a patient's high blood pressure is essential hypertension. Coronary artery disease in young family members increases a patient's chances of having the disease. Old trauma may be responsible for constrictive pericarditis, a thoracic aortic aneurysm, or an arteriovenous fistula as well as other types of cardiac lesions. Drugs, including alcohol, may cause heart disease. Accordingly, a detailed history of the use of medication, addicting drugs, and alcohol is essential. A past history of pulmonary embolism, thrombophlebitis, or systemic embolism must not be overlooked.

A history of dental work, or some other diagnostic or therapeutic procedure, or recent infection should alert the physician to consider the possibility of infective endocarditis in a patient with valvular heart disease.

SYMPTOMS AS DIAGNOSTIC MARKERS: PREDICTIVE VALUE

Years ago our predecessors taught us that 70 percent of the diagnostic information was found in the medical history, 20 percent was found in the physical examination, and 10 percent was discovered as the result of laboratory procedures including the electrocardiogram and chest x-ray. We now realize that this assessment of the diagnostic value of the various techniques is not correct because it is the patient's disease that predetermines the techniques that are likely to reveal the abnormalities. For example, faint aortic regurgitation is usually identified by hearing the heart murmur with the stethoscope.

The proper way to view the various methods of data collection (history, physical examination, electrocardiogram and chest x-ray, and other laboratory data) is to recognize that all of these methods are needed to detect the presence and severity of cardiovascular disease. Which method or methods yield the proper diagnostic clue is predetermined by the type and severity of the disease process.

It must be remembered that serious heart disease can be present in patients with mild or no symptoms. Modern medicine requires that physicians understand the sensitivity, specificity, and predictive value of test results. Physicians, as a rule, apply these standards to laboratory test results but have not applied them to symptoms and physical signs. It is, in fact, as important to know the sensitivity, specificity, and predictive value of the response to a question or the presence or absence of a physical sign as it is to know the sensitivity, specificity, and predictive value of laboratory test results.

The physician must learn the predictive value of symptoms and determine whether or not the history obtained is sufficiently adequate to be used in the decision-making process about the patient. The physician then adds this information to the results (with their predictive values) obtained from the performance of the physical examination, the analysis of the electrocardiogram, and the interpretation of the chest x-ray and determines whether or not a definite decision can be made. If a definitive decision cannot be made, the physician then asks whether or not more information is needed. If the answer is yes, the physician determines which additional diagnostic procedure should be performed.

PRESENCE AND MAGNITUDE OF SYMPTOMS RELATED TO HEART DISEASE

If the absence of symptoms always signified the absence of heart disease, a physician would only have to ask, "How do you feel?" If the patient answered, "Fine," the physician could pronounce the patient well. The inadequacy of this approach is highlighted by the fact that many patients who experience sudden death or massive myocardial infarction had no warning symptom before the tragic event occurred. Patients with treacherous ventricular rhythm disturbances may not know that the abnormal rhythm is occurring. Patients with evidence of pulmonary congestion on the chest x-ray may not have dyspnea.

Patients may, however, have many symptoms as the result of minor disorders. For example, a patient with occasional premature ventricular contractions may feel each abnormal beat and be petrified with the fear of death. The patient with severe and terrifying angina pectoris due to coronary atherosclerosis may have only a high-grade obstruction of the midportion of the right coronary artery. Such a lesion is usually accompanied by a good long-term prognosis compared with the poor long-term prognosis of a patient with high-grade obstruction of the left main coronary artery.

Some patients deny the presence of symptoms, often at a deep psychological level, since they cannot face the reality of the problem, while others may willfully withhold information from the physician because they might lose their job if the truth were known. Other patients may, for personal gain, proclaim their symptoms as more severe than they really are.

Some patients whose symptoms are dependent on effort will have no symptoms because they do not do enough to produce them. Elderly patients, sedentary patients, and patients whose physical activity is limited by another illness fall into this category. Some patients with angina pectoris due to coronary atherosclerosis or dyspnea due to mitral stenosis may walk more slowly in order to avoid symptoms. In fact, physicians frequently advise such patients to do less walking in order to avoid symptoms. When the patient follows the physician's advice, the physician may conclude erroneously that the patient is "better" because he or she describes fewer symptoms.

Elderly patients with cerebral atrophy may not be able to recall symptoms and may become frustrated when the details of symptoms are pursued. Patients who are psychiatrically disturbed may be unable to perceive symptoms or to give a meaningful account of them.

SYMPTOMS ASSOCIATED WITH CARDIOVASCULAR DISEASE

Pain

The ability to evaluate pain is a direct index of the expertise of the physician. It is necessary for the physician to determine the location of the pain, the size of the painful area, the radiation of the pain, the quality of the pain, how long the pain has been present, how long each episode of pain lasts, the factors that produce the pain, and the factors that relieve the pain.

Chest Pain

Pain Due to Myocardial Ischemia The most common cause of myocardial ischemia is atherosclerotic coronary heart disease (see Chaps. 58 to 60). Other causes of myocardial ischemia include aortic stenosis and regurgitation (Chap. 79), cardiomyopathy (Chaps. 89 to 91), and rare forms of coronary artery disease, including coronary artery spasm (Chaps. 58, 59, and 64).

Chest pain, or discomfort, occurs when coronary atherosclerosis reaches a critical degree of severity and the lumen of the coronary arteries becomes sufficiently narrowed to produce myocardial ischemia. Myocardial ischemia may develop when coronary blood flow, which is adequate at rest, is not adequate when the myocardial oxygen demands on the heart are increased by physical effort or when spasm or thrombosis impedes coronary blood flow when the patient is at rest (Chaps. 56 to 59). Myocardial ischemia due to valve disease or cardiomyopathy signifies the severity of the conditions. (See Chaps. 79 and 89 to 91.)

The brief "pain" of myocardial ischemia is called angina pectoris. This serious disorder is discussed more fully in Chaps. 19, 58, and 59. Angina pectoris may be overlooked if the physician inquires only about pain. Many patients with angina pectoris deny a sensation of pain but complain of aching, a heavy feeling, chest pressure, chest tightness, indigestion in the chest, or a squeezing sensation in the chest.

Angina pectoris characteristically occurs during physical effort; it also occurs when the patient is at rest. It may occur just after the patient assumes the recumbent position or immediately after the patient gets up in the morning. It is precipitated by emotions, especially anger, and exposure to cold and may follow meals. The distress may occur when a combination of precipitating factors occurs.

The unpleasant sensation is usually located in the retrosternal region of the chest or across the anterior portion of the upper part of the chest. The discomfort usually affects an area about the size of a clenched fist. As pointed out by Dr. Samuel Levine, the patient frequently clenches his or her fist and places it on the region of the chest to indicate where the discomfort is located. It is useful to have the patient identify the size of the painful area by using a single finger to circumscribe the area.

The pain may radiate to the neck, jaw, hard palate, tongue, left arm, right arm, shoulder, elbow, wrist, upper portion of the back, or upper part of the abdomen. The discomfort may be more pronounced in these areas or, on rare occasion, may be felt only in one or more of the areas mentioned.

The discomfort that is labeled angina pectoris usually lasts for 1 to 3 min if the provoking cause is discontinued. Patients soon learn to stop walking or to slow their pace when they feel the discomfort. The angina pectoris provoked by anger may last longer than that caused by effort but rarely lasts longer than 10 min.

Angina pectoris may be aggravated by many other medical conditions, including emotional stress, obesity, anemia, and thyrotoxicosis. Angina pectoris is usually relieved promptly after nitroglycerin is placed under the tongue. Some patients relieve their angina pectoris by performing the Valsalva maneuver.

The electrocardiogram may be normal at rest and show ST-segment displacement only during an episode of angina.

The identification of angina pectoris is strengthened when the discomfort is reproducible and when a specified degree of effort produces the discomfort.

Some patients may answer all leading questions with affirmative responses. As pointed out by Dr. Samuel Levine, a more accurate response may be obtained if the physician asks, "I suppose the discomfort is worse when you walk *down hill* isn't it?" Should the patient counter with, "Oh no, it is worse when I walk up hill," the diagnosis of angina is likely because the patient answers negatively to a question that, at times, would lead some patients to answer affirmatively.

The subsets of myocardial ischemia include stable angina pectoris, unstable angina pectoris, Prinzmetal's angina (variant angina), syndrome X, postinfarction angina, angina equivalents, and prolonged myocardial ischemia with or without objective signs of myocardial infarction. They are discussed in detail in Chaps. 19 and 58 to 60.

Pain Due to Dissecting Aneurysm of the Aorta Acute aortic dissection, due to medial cystic necrosis of the aorta, is commonly associated with excruciating pain. (See Chaps. 19 and 123.) The pain is usually located in the anterior portion of the chest, lasts for hours, and is frequently of maximal intensity at the onset. The pain tends to radiate into the thoracic portion of the back more often than the pain of myocardial infarction. The pain may be felt predominantly or only in the back. The pain is not aggravated by deep breathing or turning. The pain may be located in the abdomen if the arteries of the abdominal viscera are involved. Occasionally, the pain seems to shift from one area of the chest to a lower portion of the chest as the dissection progresses. More than the usual amount of opiates may be needed to relieve the pain.

Pain Due to Aortic Aneurysm A thoracic aortic aneurysm due to atherosclerosis may rupture and produce chest pain (see Chaps. 19 and 123).

Pain Due to Acute Pericarditis The pain of acute pericarditis (Chaps. 19 and 92) is not related to effort; it is usually aggravated by deep inspiration. It is often described by the patient as feeling "sharp" or "cutting." The pain is usually located in the precordial area and may radiate to the upper portion of the shoulders or sides of the neck. The patient tends to avoid deep inspiration or even normal respiratory movements because of the intense aggravation of the discomfort associated with this activity. Turning the body from side to side may aggravate the pain, as may swallowing. Leaning forward may occasionally relieve the discomfort. The pain may occur only in the neck, shoulders, or interscapular area. The absence of a pericardial friction rub does not exclude pericarditis.

Pain Due to Pulmonary Emboli The majority of small pulmonary emboli (Chaps. 19 and 100) produce no chest pain. In fact, the patient may not identify any symptoms that are directly due to pulmonary emboli, which is why the majority of emboli are not diagnosed. The pain of pulmonary embolism may, at times, be similar to that of myocardial ischemia. Acute distressing dyspnea is the most common symptom related to pulmonary embolism. Pulmonary infarction may follow pulmonary embolism. The pain of pulmonary infarction is due to pleuritis, which is usually located in the lateral portion of the chest; it is aggravated by deep inspiration.

Pain Related to Pulmonary Hypertension The chest pain associated with pulmonary hypertension (Chaps. 19 and 99) may simulate angina pectoris and occurs, most often, in patients with mitral stenosis or Eisenmenger's syndrome. The pain has been thought to be due to dilatation of the pulmonary artery, but it is more likely due to right ventricular myocardial ischemia.

Chest Discomfort Due to Noncardiovascular Causes The most common cause of chest pain is not related to cardiovascular disease but is associated with *anxiety* (Chaps. 19 and 117 to 118). The discomfort is usually located in the left inframammary region and rarely radiates to other locations. The pain does not occur during effort but may occur after effort. It is not aggravated by breathing but is associated with other signs of anxiety such as periodic deep-sighing respiration, hyperventilation, sinus tachycardia, fatigue, and a fear of "closed-in" places. The discomfort may be characterized as a series of short sticks and stabs lasting no longer than it takes to snap one's fingers or it may be a dull ache lasting for hours to days at a time. This type of discomfort may be disabling to patients and may consume their every thought. The discomfort may also be located in the retrosternal area and anterior chest region. The discomfort may be so similar to myocardial ischemia that it is not possible to separate the two conditions without a coronary arteriogram. Some of these patients have mitral valve prolapse, but the symptoms described commonly occur in patients without mitral valve prolapse or any other recognizable disease.

Since angina pectoris and the discomfort associated with anxiety (or other causes) may coexist, great skill is needed by the physician to clarify such problems. The medical history commonly yields the major diagnostic clue that enables a physician to determine the coexistence of two different causes of chest discomfort.

Chest discomfort may also be caused by the shoulder-hand syndrome; esophageal rupture; esophageal spasm; esophageal reflux; acute esophageal impaction; a cafe coronary; stomach and duodenal disorders; gallbladder disease; diseases of the spine, shoulder girdle, pleura, lung, and mediastinum (including mediastinal emphysema); thrombophlebitis of the chest wall; herpes zoster; and other chest wall syndromes. The characteristics of the chest pain due to these conditions are discussed in Chaps. 19 and 58 to 60.

Pain in the Extremities

Intermittent claudication of the lower extremities due to peripheral atherosclerosis (Chap. 124) is frequently overlooked because the physician believes the discomfort should always be localized in the calf of the leg. Peripheral arterial vascular disease must also be considered when discomfort develops in the arch of the foot, calf of the leg, thighs, hips, or gluteal region during effort.

The symptom associated with acute arterial occlusion of the lower extremities due to an embolus may, at its onset, be no more than the sensation of hypesthesia (interpreted by the patient as "the leg going to sleep").

Intermittent claudication of the upper extremities and masseter muscles may occur. This symptom is usually due to a nonatherosclerotic cause of arterial disease such as arteritis.

The pain of Raynaud's disease may be noted in the fingers after exposure to cold. The patient may note pallor of the fingers prior to feeling pain. This symptom should lead the physician to inquire about dysphagia and look for the skin changes of progressive systemic sclerosis (scleroderma).

Pain and swelling of the lower extremity may be due to thrombophlebitis (Chap. 124).

Head Pain

The pain of myocardial ischemia may be felt in the jaw, hard palate, cheek, and rarely deep in the ear canals.

The pain of temporal arteritis is usually localized to the temporal region of the head. It may be associated with visual difficulty and polymyalgia rheumatica.

Migraine headache is vascular in origin and may be quite severe. Other clues include nausea, scotoma, and intolerance to light.

Hypertension does not usually produce headache, but severe headache may occur in patients with severe hypertension.

Pain in the Abdomen

The pain of expanding or rupturing atherosclerotic abdominal aneurysm is located in the midabdomen and lower portion of the back. This condition is discussed in Chap. 123.

Abdominal angina due to vascular disease of the mesenteric arteries is discussed in Chap. 123.

The pain of myocardial ischemia or pericarditis may be located in the upper portion of the abdomen.

The liver may become painful and tender as a result of heart failure. Liver discomfort may be aggravated by effort in such patients.

Joint Pain

Almost all forms of arthritis may be associated with heart disease. Rheumatic fever, rheumatoid arthritis, lupus erythematosus, psoriatic arthritis, ankylosing spondylitis, gonococcal arthritis, Reiter's disease, and Lyme arthritis may be associated with heart or pericardial disease.

Dyspnea (Difficult Breathing)

Dyspnea is a distressing symptom (Chap. 20). The patient complains of shortness of breath or that he or she "can't get enough air."

There are many causes of dyspnea. The investigation of dyspnea must include a search for the factors that precipitate and relieve it.

Obviously, an infant or small child does not complain of shortness of breath. Therefore, other clues to respiratory distress are required (Chap. 97). The rate of breathing is greatly increased in this age group when there is heart failure or acute lung disease. Unlike children the respiratory rate of adults with dyspnea due to chronic heart failure may not be greatly increased.

Chronic dyspnea can be caused by heart failure, pulmonary disease, sighing respiration associated with anxiety, obesity, poor physical fitness, pleural effusions, and effort asthma.

Acute dyspnea may occur with acute pulmonary edema, hyperventilation associated with anxiety, pneumothorax, pulmonary embolism, pneumonia, and airway obstruction.

Dyspnea on Effort

Dyspnea on effort is a common complaint. It is usually due to congestive heart failure, chronic pulmonary disease, or poor physical condition (Chaps. 20 and 26). It is necessary to establish the degree of activity required to produce dyspnea. This may be done by inquiring about the daily activity of each patient. It is also valuable to determine when the patient began to notice increasing dyspnea. For example, if the patient has only recently noted difficulty in climbing a hill, the dyspnea is more likely to be due to heart failure than to chronic lung disease. The dyspnea could be associated with chronic lung disease, but it would then be wise to look for recent complications such as pneumothorax, atelectasis, and pulmonary infection in order to explain the recent increase in symptoms.

Dyspnea related to effort may be the equivalent of angina pectoris in some patients with coronary atherosclerosis who develop transient global myocardial ischemia during effort.

Dyspnea and Wheezing

When a patient complains of wheezing associated with dyspnea, he or she may have lung disease or heart disease. If the symptoms have developed recently in an adult over the age of 40, the physician should search for other clues that indicate heart disease (Chaps. 20 and 26). When the wheezing is due to heart disease, the patient is said to have cardiac asthma. If there is a history of periodic wheezing and dyspnea since childhood, bronchial asthma and lung disease are more likely to be the cause. One must remember, however, that patients who have had bronchial asthma for many years may develop heart disease and heart failure. When this occurs, the heart failure may precipitate more bronchial asthma.

Wheezing on effort may be due to either heart failure or chronic lung disease. Wheezing due to bronchial asthma may become apparent because the effort evokes deeper respiratory excursions and, in some patients, the effort precipitates a special type of *effort asthma*.

Orthopnea

Orthopnea is a specific type of dyspnea (Chaps. 20 and 26). It implies that patients have less difficulty breathing in the sitting position than in the recumbent position. The patient relates that he or she places two or three pillows under the head in order to have a restful night. This symptom is often associated with congestive heart failure but may also be associated with severe chronic lung disease.

The fatigue associated with the effort of breathing seems to be less when the dyspnea is due to chronic pulmonary disease than when it is due to heart failure.

Paroxysmal Nocturnal Dyspnea

Paroxysmal nocturnal dyspnea is a very important variety of shortness of breath (see Chaps. 20 and 26). The predictive value of this symptom as a sign of heart failure is excellent but not perfect. Characteristically, the patient has little difficulty falling asleep in the recumbent position. A few hours later he or she is awakened from sleep with acute shortness of breath. The patient seeks relief by sitting on the side of the bed or in a chair and may go to an open window searching for air. After a time, the dyspnea subsides and the patient returns to the recumbent position. The patient may then sleep comfortably the remainder of the night.

Other causes for this unusual sequence of events include the hyperventilation syndrome due to anxiety, pulmonary emboli, and rarely, acute bronchial asthma or laryngeal stridor. The latter may be caused by esophageal reflux. The hyperventilation syndrome due to anxiety and bronchial asthma is not completely relieved by sitting up, and it would be unusual for pulmonary emboli to occur at the same hour for several nights in a row.

Acute Pulmonary Edema

Acute pulmonary edema is usually due to disease of the left ventricle or to mitral valve disease (Chaps. 20 and 26). The patient experiences the sudden development of dyspnea and cough and may produce frothy, blood-tinged sputum. The symptoms may occur without previous warning as in myocardial infarction or may be preceded by dyspnea on effort or cardiac asthma.

Cheyne-Stokes Breathing

Cheyne-Stokes breathing is characterized by periods of hyperpnea that alternate with periods of apnea. This type of breathing usually occurs in older patients with heart failure. Patients with Cheyne-Stokes respiration usually have cerebral vascular disease and abnormal left heart function. Patients with Cheyne-Stokes respiration rarely complain of dyspnea, perhaps because they are so sick. They are occasionally aware of acute shortness of breath during the hyperpneic phase of the cycle. Cheyne-Stokes respiration rarely occurs in children or in patients with cor pulmonale. Normal newborn babies, however, may exhibit a breathing pattern that is somewhat similar to Cheyne-Stokes respiration.

Sleep Apnea Syndrome

The type of breathing associated with the sleep apnea syndrome is characterized by episodes of snoring alternating with prolonged periods of apnea due to upper airway obstruction (Chaps. 20 and 104).

Dyspnea Due to Pulmonary Embolism

The sudden dyspnea of acute pulmonary embolism (Chaps. 20 and 100) may be profound and is usually the only symptom associated with this event. This condition should be suspected when sudden dyspnea occurs during the postsurgical or postpartum period or in a patient who has chronic heart failure.

Dyspnea Due to Anxiety

Dyspnea due to anxiety is a common cause of breathing difficulty. It is not caused by heart disease but may be mistaken by the patient and physician as being due to heart disease. A diagnostic error may be made when a patient with known heart disease has dyspnea due to anxiety. In such a case the dyspnea may be thought to be due to heart failure (Chaps. 20 and 117 to 118).

The shortness of breath associated with anxiety assumes two forms, either of which is disturbing to patients. Patients may feel as though the air "does no good" or "does not go down far enough" or may say they "can't get a good, satisfying breath." Normal breathing is interrupted by deep sighs. Some patients experience claustrophobia. Fatigue, palpitation, and precordial "aching" or "sticks and stabs" of chest discomfort may also be present. Patients may develop prolonged periods of hyperventilation that are frequently associated with numbness of the arms, hands, and lips, tetany, and unreal sensation. Such attacks are commonly referred to as "panic attacks."

Dyspnea due to anxiety may occur in patients who also have pulmonary disease or heart disease, thereby testing the diagnostic acumen of the physician.

Dyspnea Due to Hypoxia

The dyspnea associated with congenital heart disease (Chap. 97) and a right-to-left intracardiac shunt is related to hypoxia. When the dyspnea is related to effort and is due to a right-to-left shunt and decreased pulmonary blood flow, it is relieved when the young patient squats. Such episodes are common in patients with tetralogy of Fallot. Young children with this malformation may have hypoxic spells that are relieved when the mother pulls the child's legs under the child's buttock, thereby simulating the squatting position.

Severe anemia and methemoglobinemia may be the sole cause of dyspnea on effort and is a contributing factor in patients who have heart disease.

Dyspnea Due to Thyrotoxicosis

The dyspnea of thyrotoxicosis (Chap. 102) is due to associated myopathy and an increase in the body's need for oxygen.

The "Dyspnea" of Pregnancy and Acidosis

The full-term pregnant female may "huff and puff" with effort but has a curious reaction to the audible respiratory effort; she seems quite conscious of her labored breathing but is rarely alarmed by it. Accordingly, she is not truly dyspneic (Chap. 113).

Patients with compensatory hyperpnea associated with metabolic acidosis due to diabetes mellitus or uremia rarely complain of true dyspnea.

Cough

A dry, nonproductive cough may be related to the pulmonary congestion associated with heart failure (Chap. 26). It may occur with effort or at rest. Although dyspnea is usually present, cough may dominate the clinical picture.

The cough that accompanies acute pulmonary edema is often associated with frothy, pink-tinged sputum, whereas the sputum associated with chronic bronchitis is usually white and mucoid. The sputum accompanying pneumonia is often thick and yellow. The sputum associated with pulmonary infarct may be bloody, as may be the sputum associated with cancer of the lung or bronchiectasis.

Cough may be caused by angiotensin converting enzyme inhibitors, which are often prescribed for heart failure.

Hemoptysis (Coughing up Blood)

Posterior epistaxis associated with systemic hypertension may cause blood-streaked sputum, and localized disease of the nose may give a similar clinical picture. Patients who are receiving warfarin may have epistaxis that simulates hemoptysis. In most patients, however, epistaxis is obvious and is not confused with bloody sputum.

Alveolar Pulmonary Edema

Pink, frothy sputum is frequently associated with acute alveolar pulmonary edema secondary to left ventricular disease or mitral stenosis. Blood-streaked sputum may occur with acute pulmonary congestion when the classic findings of acute pulmonary edema are not fully developed. The bleeding is due to an abrupt increase in pulmonary venous pressure; the pulmonary capillaries rupture (Chap. 26).

Mitral Stenosis

Hemoptysis due to mitral stenosis (Chap. 80) is frequently induced by physical exercise, sexual intercourse, or excitement. It may be the first symptom of mitral stenosis and may occur during pregnancy. The bleeding results from pulmonary venous hypertension and is due to rupture of pulmonary or bronchopulmonary venules. Episodes of pulmonary hemorrhage of this type may subside as the veins adapt to the high pressure or as pulmonary arteriolar disease develops.

Pulmonary Infarction

When hemoptysis occurs in a patient with heart failure, it is wise to consider the possibility of pulmonary infarction (Chap. 100). The bloody sputum usually appears within a few hours to a day after the embolus and is due to necrosis and hemorrhage into the alveoli.

Aortic Aneurysms

An aortic aneurysm (Chap. 123) may rupture into the tracheobronchial tree and produce lethal hemoptysis. Aneurysms due to syphilis, atherosclerosis, and dissection may cause this catastropic event.

Other Causes of Hemoptysis

Other causes of hemoptysis include pulmonary tuberculosis pneumonia, bronchiectasis, bronchogenic carcinoma, primary pulmonary hemosiderosis, Osler-Rendu-Weber disease with a pulmonary arteriovenous aneurysm, and necrotic pulmonary arterial lesions due to periarteritis nodosa or lupus erythematosus.

Palpitation

The term *palpitation* is used to describe a disagreeable awareness of the heartbeat (Chap. 21). The patient may complain of a "pounding," "stopping," "jumping," or "racing" in the chest. A parent may observe an abnormal heart rhythm when looking at or feeling a child's precordium.

The sensitivity of the nervous system determines whether or not the patient complains of palpitations. The complaint is not directly related to the seriousness of the heart disease or to the type of arrhythmia.

When patients have a premature cardiac contraction, they feel the post-extrasystolic beat, which is associated with a large stroke volume. On rare occasions a patient may be aware of his or her heartbeat after digitalis medication has been given because of the increased force of myocardial contraction induced by the drug.

A patient may be aware of a cardiac arrhythmia by detecting an uncomfortable sensation in the neck. This is probably due to distension of the neck veins when the right atrium contracts against a closed tricuspid valve.

Patients may complain when the heartbeat is slow or fast and when the heartbeat is regular or irregular. The patient may be able to determine if the onset and offset of the rapid beat is abrupt or gradual. The patient may complain of forceful, regular heartbeats. Ectopic beats, atrial fibrillation, and other arrhythmias may be more troublesome to patients with aortic regurgitation because, in such cases, the variations of stroke output are so radically different from normal.

It is useful to ask if anyone counted the patient's pulse during an episode of tachycardia. The heart rate of 150 beats per minute suggests atrial flutter with 2:1 atrioventricular block or sinus tachycardia. A regular heart rate of 180 beats per minute may be due to supraventricular tachycardia or ventricular tachycardia.

The patient may give a history of increased urine output during an episode of supraventricular tachycardia.

Syncope

Cardiac syncope (Chap. 21) is defined as the transient loss of consciousness due to an inadequate cerebral blood flow secondary to an abrupt decrease in cardiac output. *Near syncope* may be applied to the clinical situation in which the patient feels dizzy and weak and tends to lose postural tone but does not lose consciousness.

Syncope may occur in many types of heart disease and circulatory disorders, including atherosclerotic coronary heart disease; aortic stenosis; aortic regurgitation; mitral stenosis; idiopathic hypertrophic cardiomyopathy; left atrial tumor; pulmonary embolism; primary pulmonary hypertension; pulmonary arteriolar disease secondary to left-to-right shunts (Eisenmenger's syndrome); pulmonary valve stenosis; tetralogy of Fallot; paroxysmal rapid heartbeat (atrial tachycardia and ventricular tachycardia); sinus arrest ("sick-sinus" syndrome); ventricular standstill or fibrillation related to atrioventricular block due to coronary atherosclerosis, Lev's disease, or Lenegre's disease (Adams-Stokes attacks); acute blood loss; etc. There are certain types of syncope that can be characterized as postural hypotension, carotid sinus syncope, cough syncope, micturition syncope, vagovagal syncope, and vasodepressor syncope. Bilateral carotid artery stenosis or vertebral artery obstruction may produce syncope. (See also Chap. 21.)

Worrisome Movements and Noises

Patients may hear or feel several worrisome cardiovascular events other than palpitation. The murmurs of ventricular septal defect, aortic valve stenosis, retroversion of an aortic valve cusp, rupture of the chordae tendineae of the mitral valve, retroversion of a porcine mitral valve, and arteriovenous fistula may be heard by the patient and family members. Some of these noises can even be heard at a considerable distance from the patient.

Patients and their family members may be disturbed by the uncontrollable movements of chorea associated with acute rheumatic fever.

Patients with severe tricuspid regurgitation may feel the expanding venous pulse in the neck. Some feel the pulse wave hit the ear, and others note that their collars are "too tight" with each ventricular systole. Expanding venous pulsations due to complete heart block or ventricular pacing may be felt in the neck when the right atrium contracts against a closed tricuspid valve. Patients with aortic regurgitation may complain that their heads "bob."

History of Swelling of the Legs, Weight Gain, or Enlarging Abdomen

Edema of the lower extremities may be found on physical examination although the patient may be unaware of its existence (Chap. 26). On the other hand, there may be a history of "swelling," and edema may be absent at the time of the examination. Although edema is not required to establish the diagnosis of heart failure, it is unfortunate that many physicians still demand the presence of at least some edema before seriously considering the diagnosis of congestive heart failure. Other subtle signs of heart failure are usually present long before the appearance of edema.

Considerable weight gain due to retention of extracellular fluid may occur without associated edema. This may, at times, be as much as 10 to 15 lb. On the other hand, there are numerous causes of edema other than congestive heart failure, and its presence is not diagnostic of congestive heart failure.

Local factors play a major role in determining the distribution of fluid in the body. Pulmonary edema due to mitral stenosis provides a good illustration of the importance of local factors. When ventricular diastole is shortened to a critical point in a patient with mitral stenosis, pulmonary edema develops because the right ventricle continues to pump more blood into the lungs than can pass the stenosed mitral valve. Under these circumstances there will be no weight gain or peripheral edema. The body fluid has simply been redistributed and it accumulates in the lungs. The patient with chronic congestive heart failure who has gained weight because of retention of sodium and water secondary to altered renal function may detect edema of the ankles and lower legs during the day and note that it diminishes during the night. The edema of the legs occurs because of local hydrostatic factors related to the upright position.

It is important to ascertain whether edema of the extremities preceded or followed dyspnea on effort. Although there are many exceptions, the edema due to poor function of the left ventricle, mitral stenosis, or cor pulmonale is usually preceded by dyspnea.

Edema may be due to hypoproteinemia such as occurs in nephrosis and starvation. As with heart failure, the edema may occur in the dependent portion of the body. Such edema usually occurs when the total blood protein is below 5 g/dL.

Edema of one leg is usually due to local factors in the same leg such as varicose veins, thrombophlebitis, or lymphedema. When there is bilateral leg edema due to heart failure, with more edema in one leg compared to the other, one can conclude that a local factor is also present in the leg exhibiting the most edema. Edema may shift from the extremities to the sacral region when a patient is confined to bed.

Periorbital edema is more common in children than in adults. Although this finding on history or physical examination may be due to renal disease, it also occurs in heart failure. It simply indicates that salt and water have been retained and that the tissue pressure around the eyes of the child is low when compared to other areas. Rare causes of periorbital edema include trichinosis and superior vena caval obstruction.

Ascites may be recognized by the patient as an increase in swelling of the abdomen. Ascites due to congestive heart failure is not common today and usually follows peripheral edema. A local factor, such as cirrhosis of the liver, is also likely to be present when ascites seems to be out of proportion to the peripheral edema in a patient with heart failure. Constrictive pericarditis and restrictive cardiomyopathy should also be considered in this setting (Chaps. 91 and 92). The child with heart failure forms ascites more readily than does the adult.

The calcium antagonist nifedipine may produce bilateral edema of the lower portion of the legs. Edema of the lower extremities may rarely occur in patients with thyrotoxicosis. (See also Table 22-1.)

Fatigue and Weakness

There are many causes of fatigue and weakness (Chap. 20), and therefore these symptoms are not specific for heart disease. The most common cause of these symptoms is anxiety and depression. Anemia, thyrotoxicosis, and other chronic disease states may be associated with fatigue and weakness. The least common cause is Addison's disease.

When a patient with heart disease is waterlogged or when there is pulmonary congestion due to heart disease, the patient is likely to complain of dyspnea. With modern diuretic therapy, this complaint may be supplanted by the feelings of fatigue and weakness. The actual physiological mechanism of the fatigue associated with heart failure is not known, but it is probably related to an inadequate cardiac output. The heart fails in its prime objective of nourishing all the tissues and organs of the body, including the skeletal muscles. Potassium depletion due to the use of diuretics is a common cause of weakness.

A patient may experience exhaustion related to effort as a manifestation of transient global myocardial ischemia due to atherosclerotic coronary heart disease (Chap. 20). Dyspnea and hypotension may also occur at the time such a patient detects the exhaustion. These complaints have been labeled as angina equivalents.

Finally, drugs such as beta blockers may produce fatigue and weakness (Chap. 125) and antihypertensive medication may produce postural hypotension and weakness.

Abnormal Skin Color

The patient or family members may detect cyanosis of the lips and relate the observation to the physician. Four grams of reduced hemoglobin per deciliter of blood is needed for cyanosis to occur, and arterial oxygen saturation must be about 85 percent or less for cyanosis to be detected. Cyanosis is unlikely when the hemoglobin is less than 33 percent of normal because reduced hemoglobin cannot be produced in an amount sufficient to cause the bluish color. When the hemoglobin is normal, about one-third of it must be in the reduced form for the bluish color to appear.

A bluish tint to the skin may not be due to congenital heart disease with a right-to-left shunt or to pulmonary disease; it may be due to argyria or methemoglobinemia.

When cyanosis occurs suddenly in a patient with chronic congestive heart failure, it should suggest the possibility of acute pulmonary embolism.

A patient or a family member may detect that the cyanosis is more intense in the feet than in the hands (Chap. 97). This suggests a right-to-left shunt through a patent ductus arteriosus in a patient with Eisenmenger physiology.

A history of flushing of the face and trunk, sometimes precipitated by alcohol, should lead one to search for the other signs and symptoms of carcinoid heart disease.

Jaundice may be detected by the patient or by a member of the family. As a rule, hepatic congestion due to heart failure will not produce jaundice. When jaundice does occur in a patient with heart failure, it is appropriate to consider pulmonary infarction in addition to the hepatic congestion or cirrhosis of the liver. Hemolysis of red blood cells may occur in patients with prosthetic valves and can produce jaundice. On rare occasions hemolytic anemia and jaundice may be caused by severe aortic valve stenosis.

Cardiomyopathy due to hemochromatosis should be considered in a patient with diabetes whose skin color has changed from normal to bronze.

Patients with cyanosis who are also icteric may have a slightly green color to their skin. This color may be seen in patients with cyanosis due to heart failure, tricuspid regurgitation, or stenosis and liver dysfunction.

A slatelike color of the skin of the hands and nose may develop in patients who take amiodarone for otherwise uncontrollable ventricular arrhythmias.

Recurrent Bronchitis and Pulmonary Infection

Recurrent coughing due to heart failure is often thought to be due to bronchitis, and patients with chronic bronchitis may cough more when heart failure ensues. Patients with increased pulmonary blood flow due to left-to-right shunts are subject to pulmonary infection. Patients with high pulmonary venous pressure are more prone to the development of pulmonary edema when they have viral pneumonitis than are patients with normal pulmonary venous pressure. This is especially true in patients with mitral stenosis.

Insomnia

The most common causes of insomnia are mental conflict, emotional disturbances, and depression. Heart failure, however, may also cause insomnia. The patient with Cheyne-Stokes respiration may sleep during the apneic phase and wake during the hyperpneic phase of the condition. Patients with pulmonary congestion due to heart failure may have insomnia before they detect nocturnal dyspnea.

Cerebral Symptoms

Patients may have dizziness, near syncope, and syncope, as discussed under "Syncope" earlier in this chapter.

Patients with decreased cardiac output secondary to heart failure may become mentally confused and disoriented. Such symptoms may also be due to hypoxia, to drugs that are invariably prescribed for such patients, or to renal or hepatic failure.

A completed stroke may be caused by a lacunar infarct, cerebral hemorrhage, cerebral arterial thrombosis, or a cerebral embolus (Chap. 122). A transient cerebral ischemic attack is commonly due to an embolus. The embolus may originate in an atheromatous ulcer in the carotid artery system or be related to infective endocarditis, a recent myocardial infarction, atrial fibrillation, or clots on a prosthetic valve or originate in the leg veins and pass through a patient's foramen ovale to the brain (Chap. 122).

The patient with cardiogenic shock or the patient with violent tachycardia who also has considerable intracranial or extracranial vascular disease may have such severe cerebral hypoxia that coma occurs. Hypoxic coma may follow cardiac resuscitation and occasionally occurs after cardiopulmonary bypass, which is used for cardiac surgery.

A cerebral abscess may occur in patients with congenital heart disease and a right-to-left shunt.

Hoarseness

Hoarseness is usually unrelated to cardiovascular disease. It can occur in patients with an aortic aneurysm that involves the left recurrent laryngeal nerve. Mitral stenosis may occasionally produce hoarseness, but this is rarely seen today because the condition is usually treated surgically before it produces such a symptom. The hoarseness in such patients is due to the pressure of a large pulmonary artery on the recurrent laryngeal nerve.

Pericardial effusion may be related to myxedema, which may be associated with a coarse, low-pitched voice.

Hoarseness and loss of voice may occur following the use of an endotracheal tube during cardiac surgery.

Epistaxis

Severe nosebleed may occur in patients with hypertension. This can, on rare occasions, be so severe as to place the life of the patient in danger from exsanguination. Epistaxis occurs with acute rheumatic fever, but rheumatic fever is unusual in the United States today. Trauma is the most common cause of nosebleed. Severe epistaxis may occur in patients who are also receiving the anticoagulant warfarin. (See also Chap. 22.)

Anorexia, Nausea, and Vomiting

Anorexia, nausea, and vomiting may be caused by digitalis. Patients with myocardial infarction may complain of nausea and exhibit vomiting, but opiates may, and often do, cause the symptoms in such patients. Patients with heart failure may have anorexia and nausea without any other apparent cause.

Indigestion

Many patients with angina pectoris due to coronary atherosclerosis erroneously attribute their symptoms to indigestion or heartburn, while patients with heartburn, esophageal reflux, and esophageal spasm may believe they have angina pectoris.

Hiccups

Hiccups may occasionally occur in patients with myocardial infarction and are common during the postoperative period after cardiac surgery.

Dysphagia

Dysphagia may occur in patients with progressive systemic sclerosis, an aortic arch anomaly, or an extremely large left atrium.

Weight Loss, Malnutrition, and Cachexia

Patients with long-standing heart failure may give a history of eating poorly, and this may be associated with weight loss. Therefore, calorie, protein, and vitamin malnutrition may occur.

Urinary Symptoms

Patients with chronic heart failure may note oliguria during the day and polyuria at night. Men with urinary tract obstruction due to enlargement of the prostate may have more difficulty voiding when heart failure ensues, and this in turn may make the heart failure worse. Polyuria may occur during supraventricular tachycardia.

Fever and Chills

Patients with rheumatic fever do not have chills unless aspirin has been used for treatment. Chills are common in patients with bacterial endocarditis (Chap. 94). Fever may accompany pericarditis. Myalgia, chills, and fever may, on rare occasions, be related to myocardial infarction, presumably because of some form of immunologic response to necrotic myocardial tissue.

It is important to inquire whether there has been any recent dental work (including cleaning) or other procedures in patients with heart murmurs and fever, because this may be a clue to the diagnosis of endocarditis.

Patients Who Say They Have Had a Heart Attack

Many patients state that they have had a heart attack because, to them, any abrupt incident thought to be related to the heart is considered to be a heart attack. This includes chest pain with or without proof of myocardial infarction, a cardiac arrhythmia, pulmonary edema, and hyperventilation. Accordingly, a physician should not automatically conclude that a patient actually had a previous myocardial infarction when the patient says he or she had a heart attack.

ACKNOWLEDGMENTS

Dr. Edward R. Dorney contributed to this chapter in previous editions of *The Heart*. Regrettably, Dr. Dorney died in 1990 prior to revision of this chapter. We also thank Dr. I. Sylvia Crawley for her contribution to this chapter in the previous editions of the book.

REFERENCES

1. Mackenzie J: *Principles of Diagnosis and Treatment in Heart Affections.* London, Oxford Medical Publications, 1916.
2. White PD: *Heart Disease.* New York, Macmillan, 1931.
3. Wood PD: *Diseases of the Heart and Circulation,* 2d ed. Philadelphia, Lippincott, 1957.

Chapter 10

General Examination of the Patient

Robert A. O'Rourke, M.D. ■ Mark E. Silverman, M.D. ■
Robert C. Schlant, M.D.

In certain patients with definite or suspected cardiovascular disease, general inspection will result in the detection of specific findings that indicate the presence of a syndrome or disease that can be associated with various types of cardiovascular abnormalities. Important clues from the general inspection of the patient that can lead to the etiologic diagnosis of congenital and acquired heart disease are detailed in this chapter. Since this discussion is organized according to the specific type of heart disease, many etiologies are mentioned several times and each disorder is italicized and its major manifestations described only the first time it is named.[1]

SYNDROMES ASSOCIATED WITH CONGENITAL HEART DISEASE

Congenital heart disease due to syndromes often associated with major cardiovascular manifestations may be divided into heritable disorders, connective tissue disorders, inborn areas of metabolism, chromosomal abnormalities, sporadic disorders, and teratogenic disorders. (See also Chaps. 95 to 98.) Occasionally, a particular syndrome falls into more than one category. In the first category, the *Ellis–van Creveld syndrome* is a heritable form of dwarfism characterized by short extremities, polydactyly, dysplastic teeth and nails, and multiple frenula binding the upper lid to the alveolar ridge (Fig. 10-1). Over half of the patients have heart disease, usually a large atrial septal defect or a single atrium.[2] The *thrombocytopenia–absent radius (TAR) syndrome* includes bilateral radial aplasia with the presence of the thumb and thrombocytopenia and may be associated at times with an ostium secundum atrial septal defect and/or tetralogy of Fallot.[3] The *Holt-Oram syndrome,* an autosomal dominant trait, combines an atrial septal defect or other congenital heart disease with an abnormal thumb (Fig. 10-2).[3] The thumb may be absent, hypoplastic, bifid, triphalangeal, or unusually long. *Laurence-Moon-Bardet-Biedl syndrome,* mental retardation, polydactyly, obesity, retinitis pigmentosa, and hypogonadism occur in association with congenital heart disease.[4]

Arteriovenous fistulas involving the lung, liver, and mucous membrane are associated with multiple telangiectasia in patients with the *Osler-Weber-Rendu syndrome.*[5] The *Cornelia de Lange syndrome* is characterized by bushy, confluent eyebrows, downward-slanting eyes, small mandible, low-set ears, hirsutism, long eyelashes, broad, flat upturned nose, severe growth and mental retardation, and a peculiar "chicken-wing" extremity with a single thumblike digit (Fig. 10-3).[3] A ventricular septal defect, patent ductus arteriosus, pulmonic stenosis, anomalous venous return, or atrial septal defect may be present.

There appears to be an increased incidence of congenital heart disease in children with a cleft palate or lip.[6] In the *Pierre Robin syndrome,* the cleft palate is associated with a hypoplastic mandible causing a "shrewlike" face (Fig. 10-4). A cleft palate, micrognathia, low-set ears, and truncus arteriosus may be present in the familial *third and fourth pharyngeal pouch syndromes.*[1]

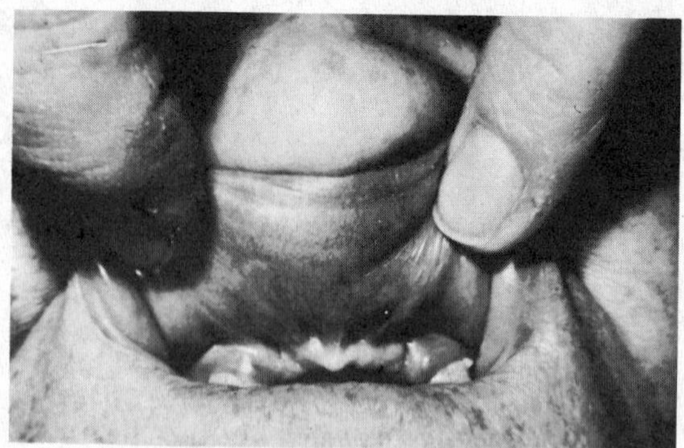

A

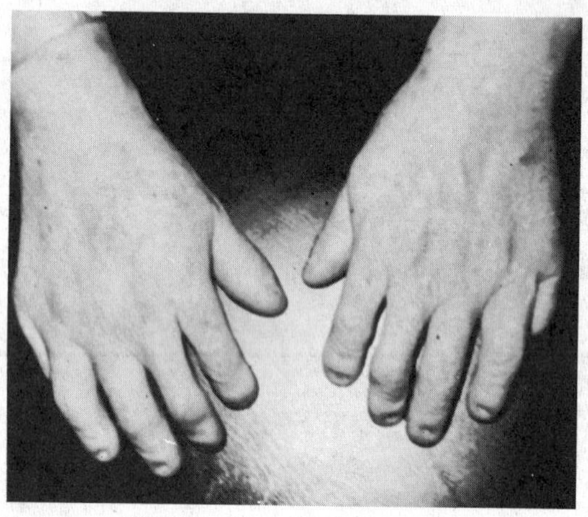

B

FIGURE 10-1 Ellis–van Creveld syndrome. *A.* Typical "lip tie" due to multiple frenulum. *B.* Polydactyly. This patient has a large atrial septal defect.

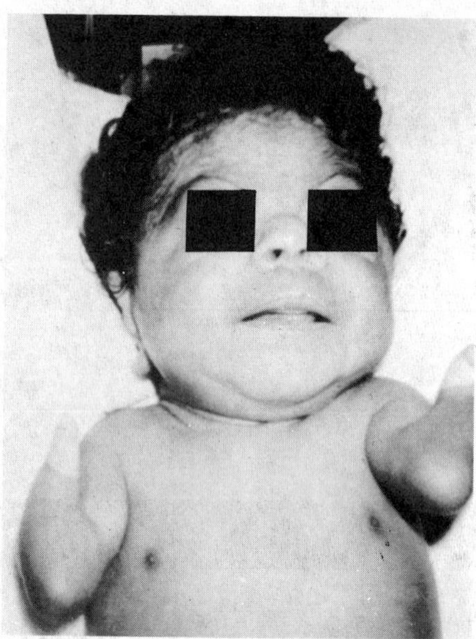

FIGURE 10-3 Cornelia de Lange's syndrome: low hairline, hirsutism, bushy eyebrows, phocomelia, and a single thumblike digit. May be associated with ventricular septal defect.

Of the connective tissue disorders, *cutis laxis* is a generalized disruption of elastic fibers with diminished skin resilience, frequent hernias, and pulmonary artery branch stenosis.[7] Patients with *Ehlers-Danlos syndrome* (Fig. 10-5*A* and *B*) have hyperextensible joints and hyperelastic and friable skin that often is associated with arterial dilation and rupture, aortic regurgitation, or mitral regurgitation, the latter usually due to mitral valve prolapse.[8,9] Patients with *osteogenous imperfecta* have

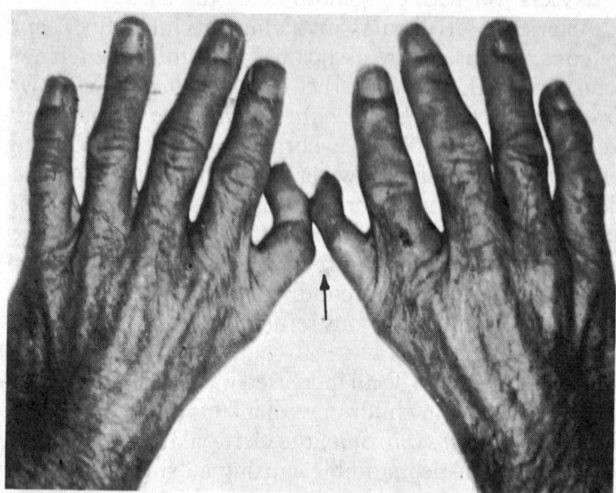

FIGURE 10-2 Holt-Oram syndrome: fingerized thumb (arrow) associated with an atrial septal defect.

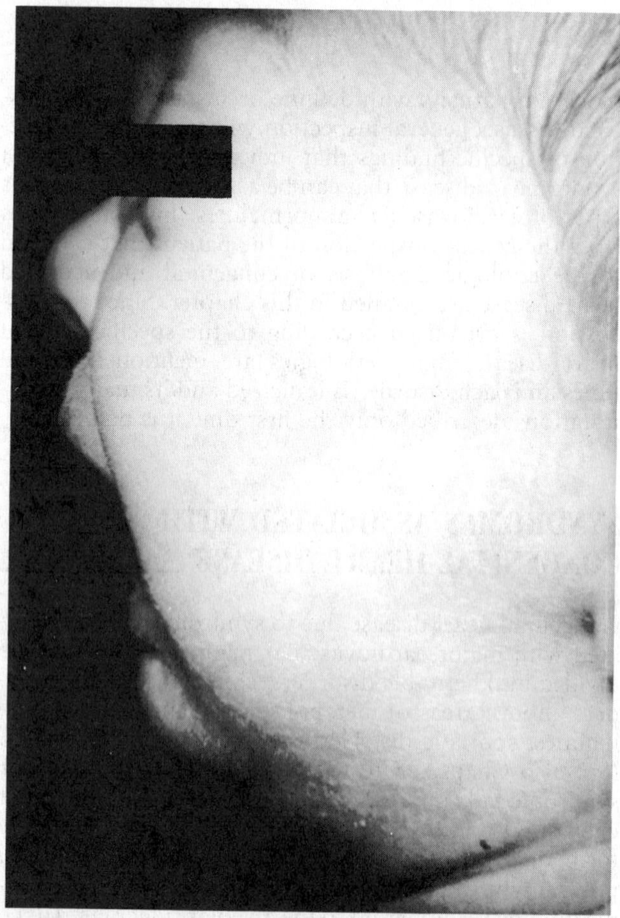

FIGURE 10-4 Pierre Robin syndrome: hypoplastic mandible associated with a ventricular septal defect.

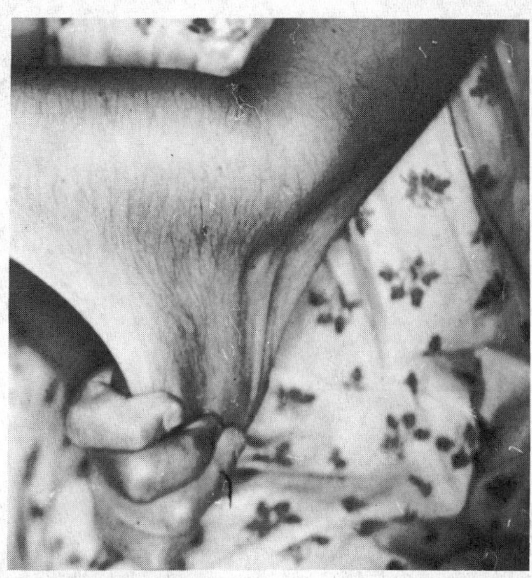

A

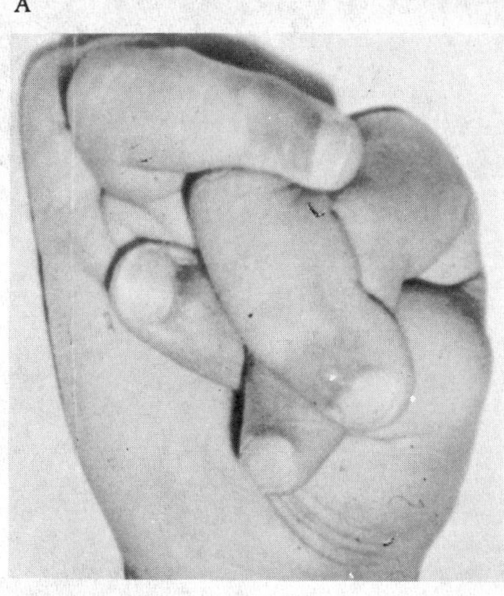

B

FIGURE 10-5 Ehlers-Danlos syndrome. *A.* Hyperextensible skin. *B.* Lax joints. Redundant chordae tendineae and arterial rupture may occur.

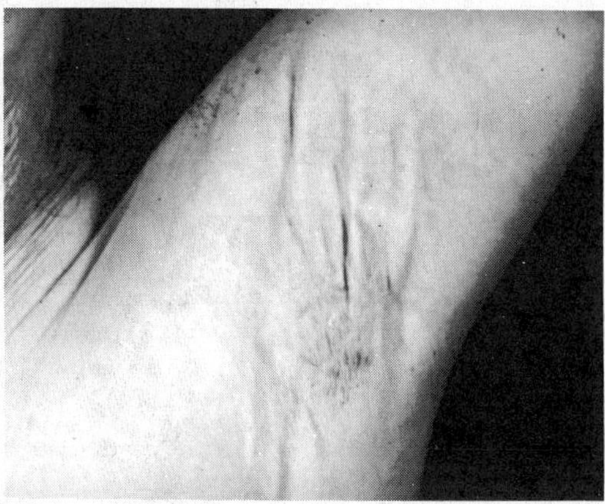

FIGURE 10-6 Pseudoxanthoma elasticum: grooved, skin in a typical location. Arterial calcification may occur.

brittle bones, blue sclera, and short legs and have an increased incidence of aortic regurgitation due to root dilatation and mitral regurgitation.[10] Patients with *pseudoxanthoma elasticum* have dermal elastic fiber degeneration, retinal angioid streaks, aortic regurgitation, and coronary artery disease (Fig. 10-6).[10]

Marfan's syndrome, an autosomal dominant trait, is suggested by certain skeletal features such as increased height, long fingers, narrow palms, lax joints, kyphoscoliosis, pectus excavatum or carinatum, elongated face, high arch palate, and flat feet (Fig. 10-7).[1,11] The legs are disproportionally long, resulting in an abnormal ratio of the upper segment to lower segment of at most 0.85. The arm span may exceed the height. When patients with Marfan's syndrome clench a hand around the flexed thumb, the thumb protrudes past the ulnar side of the hand.[11] They can also easily encircle their wrist by grasping it with the fifth finger and thumb of the other hand (Fig. 10-7*B*). Often the signs include bilateral subluxation of lens, severe myopia, and blue sclera (Fig. 10-7*D*). Subcutaneous tissue is sparse. Valvular disease is common, and patients with Marfan's syndrome may have mitral valve prolapse, minimal to severe mitral regurgitation, a dilated and often calcified mitral annulus, and eventual chordal rupture. Aortic regurgitation is a consequence of a dilated aortic root, prolapse of the aortic cusps, or aortic dissection. (See also Chaps. 79, 80, 96, and 123.)

Aortic regurgitation has also been described in patients with inborn errors of metabolism including *Morquio's syndrome* (mucopolysaccharidosis IV) and *Scheie's syndrome* (mucopolysaccharidosis V).[12] Patients with Morquio's syndrome are identified by short stature, short neck, barrel chest, broad mouth, short nose, widely spaced teeth, and cloudy cornea. In Scheie's syndrome, growth retardation, sternal protrusion, facial abnormalities, and cloudy cornea are present. In *Fabry's disease* angiokeratomas, which are purplish, pinpoint skin lesions, occur on the lips, trunk, and penis (Fig. 10-8). Mitral regurgitation is often associated with this sex-linked recessive disorder in which there is a genetic deficiency of the enzyme α-galactosidase A.[13]

Many chromosomal abnormalities have been associated with congenital heart disease. The well-recognized characteristics of *Down syndrome* (trisomy 21) include a small head, shallow orbits, epicanthal folds, low-set ears, widely spaced eyes (hypertelorism), Brushfield's spots of the iris, protruding tongue, transverse palmer creases, and mental retardation (Fig. 96-2). Congenital heart disease appears in 40 to 60 percent of patients, with a ventricular septal defect or endocardial cushion defect as the most frequent findings.[14] Less commonly, tetralogy of Fallot, secundum atrial septal defect, patent ductus arteriosus, and other abnormalities are present.[14,15] (See also Chaps. 96 and 97.)

Kleinfelter's syndrome is characterized by gynecomastia, small testicles, eunuchoid appearance, tall stature, and long extremities. Associated atrial septal defects have been described.[16]

Abnormalities involving chromosomes 1, 9, 11, and 22 have been described in association with congenital heart disease.[17] The findings with *chromosome 1 abnormalities* include peaked nose, micrognathia, and long tapering fingers. Children with *chromosome 9 abnor-*

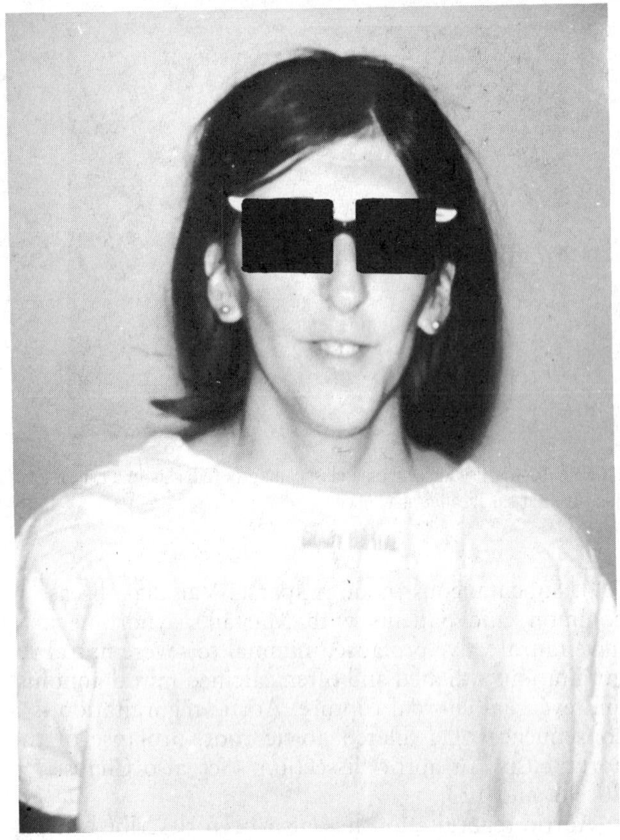

A

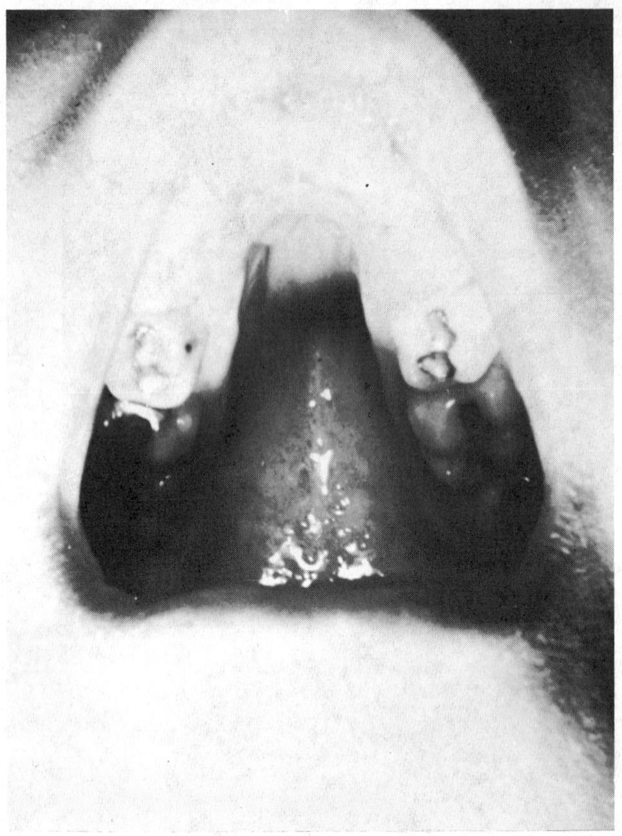

C

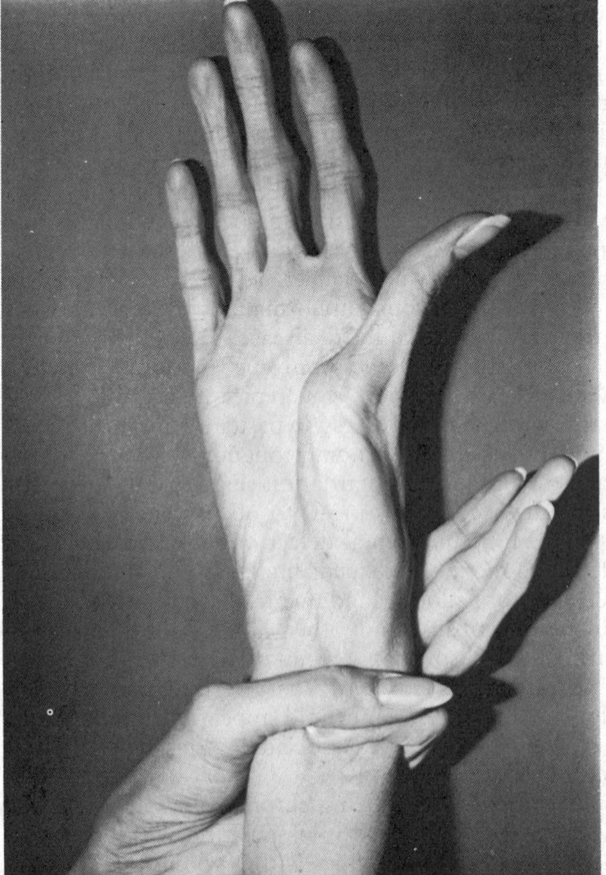

B

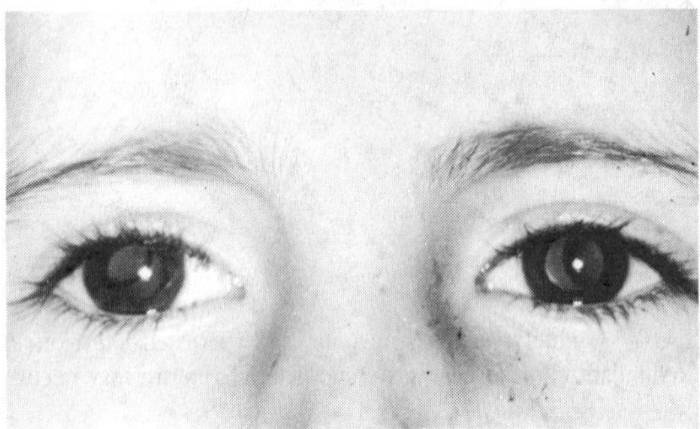

D

FIGURE 10-7 Marfan's syndrome. *A.* Long, narrow face. *B.* Arachnodactyly and positive wrist sign. *C.* High arched palate. *D.* Ectopia lentis associated with aortic aneurysm and severe aortic regurgitation in a teenage girl.

malities have prominent foreheads, hypertension, anteverted nostrils, long upper lip, a short neck, mental retardation, and external ear malformations. A *chromosome 11 abnormality* has similar features plus retraction of the lower lip. Psychomotor retardation, coloboma, hypertelorism (widely spread eyes), downward slanting of the eyes, and preauricular tags or fistulas are clues to a *chromosome 22 defect.*[1]

Congenital heart disease, primarily patent ductus arteriosus, has been associated with the *49 XXXXY syndrome.*[1] This unusual disorder should be suspected when a child has psychomotor retardation, hypoplastic genitals, prognathism, clinodactyly (inward curving of the fifth finger), and radioulnar synostoses.

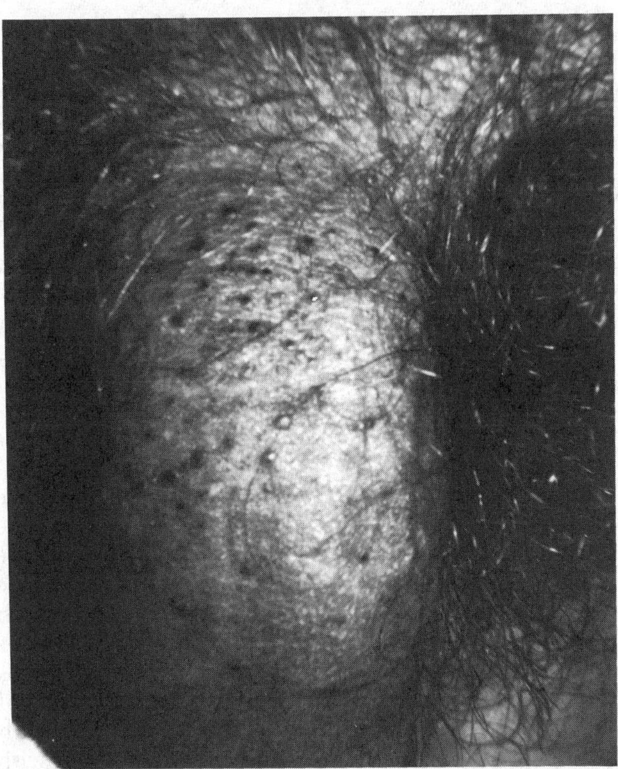

FIGURE 10-8 Fabry's disease: dark red angiokeratomas on the penis may be linked with coronary artery disease.

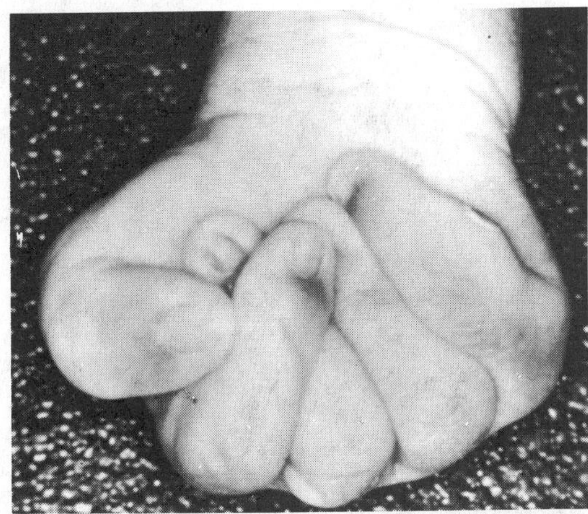

FIGURE 10-9 Trisomy 18 syndrome: tightly clenched fist with overlapping index and fifth fingers. A ventricular septal defect was present.

Congenital heart disease of varied types is common in *trisomy 13* and *trisomy 18 syndromes*.[1] In *trisomy 13 syndrome* the child has a cleft palate and lip; the ocular tissue and the nose may be missing. Polydactyly in combination with retroflexible thumbs, transverse creases, hyperconvex narrow nails, and flexion of the fingers and hands are characteristic of this syndrome. The features of the *trisomy 18 syndrome* are a small triangular mouth with receding chin, small mandible, webbed neck, and tightly clenched fists with the index finger overlapping the third finger and the fifth finger over the fourth (Fig. 10-9).

Low hairline, low-set ears, deafness, small jaw, and short, webbed neck are physical findings common to both *Turner's syndrome* and the *Klippel-Feil syndrome*. Turner's syndrome also includes short stature, broad chest with widely spaced nipples, epicanthal folds, widely spaced eyes (hypertelorism), pigmented moles, ptosis, clinodactyly, and a shortened fifth finger (Fig. 10-10).[18,19] Coarctation of the aorta, aortic stenosis, and hypertrophic cardiomyopathy are the usual cardiovascular considerations. The Klippel-Feil syndrome may cause facial asymmetry, cleft palate, torticollis, scoliosis, deafness, strabismus, and hydrocephaly. Ventricular septal defect is the most common associated cardiac disorder.[20]

There are many sporadic disorders associated with congenital heart disease. An imperforate anus may be associated with a cardiovascular malformation.[21] This may occur as an isolated finding or as a component of the *VATER association*,[22] the *asplenia syndrome*,[23] the *CHARGE syndrome*[24] (coloboma, heart disease, atresia choanae, retarded growth, genital hypoplasia, ear anomalies), or *cat's-eye pupil*[25] (a fissure of the iris and choroid associated with cardiac defect). The VATER association also includes vertebral defect, tracheoesophageal fistula, and radial and renal dysplasia.[22] A ventricular defect occurs in 80 percent of these patients. The asplenia syndrome has a high incidence of complex congenital heart

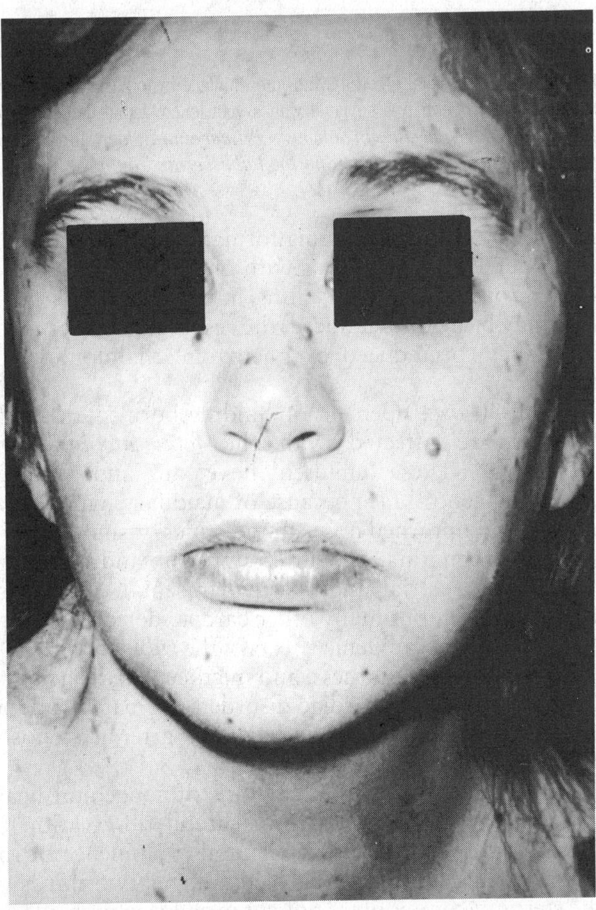

FIGURE 10-10 Turner's syndrome: epicanthal folds, pigmented moles, hypertelorism, and scars on the neck where webs have been removed may be associated with coarctation of the aorta.

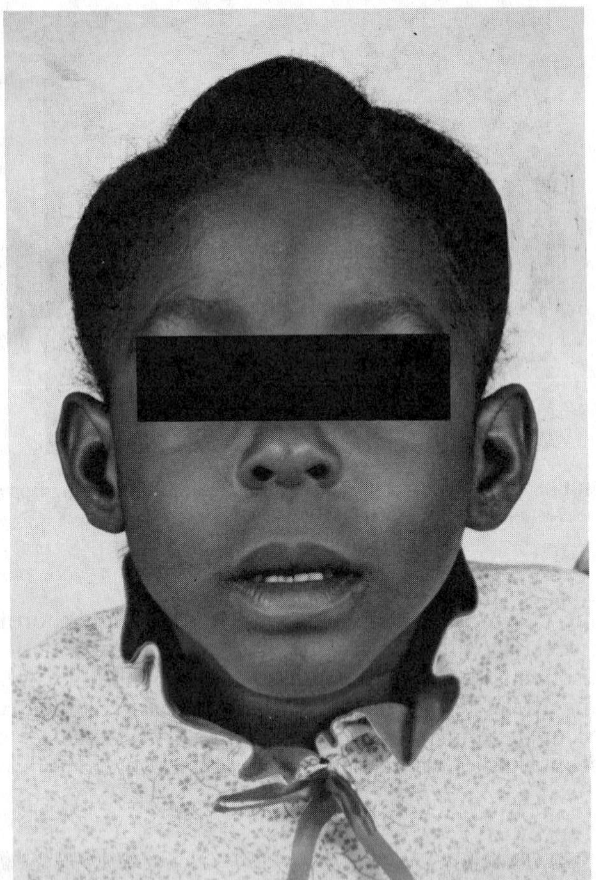

FIGURE 10-11 Fetal alcohol syndrome: midface hypoplasia, absent philtrum, and microcephaly associated with a ventricular septal defect. *(From ME Silverman: Visual clues to diagnosis. Primary Cardiology, August 1987. Reproduced with permission from the publisher and author.)*

disease.[23] Cardiovascular malformations are found in 15 to 25 percent of newborns with omphalocele.[26]

Teratogenic effects resulting in congenital heart disease may be alcohol induced, the result of rubella during pregnancy, or induced by phenytoin, thalidomide, or lithium.[27]

From 30 to 40 percent of children born to alcoholic mothers are affected with the *fetal alcohol syndrome.*[1,28,29] These children have an undeveloped-appearing central face because of maxillary hypoplasia, a small and upturned nose, an indistinct or smooth philtrum, micrognathia, and a thin upper lip and vermilion (Fig. 10-11). Atrial and ventricular septal defects are most common, but many other cardiac defects can also be found. The teratogenic effects of the *rubella syndrome* include cataracts, deafness, and microcephaly. The most frequent congenital cardiac disorders are patent ductus arteriosus, pulmonic valvular and/or arterial stenosis, and atrial septal defect.[30]

Important clues to the diagnosis of congenital heart disease may be obtained from careful observation of the thorax and extremities. Bilateral prominence of the anterior chest with bulging of the upper two-thirds of the sternum commonly is present in children with a large ventricular septal defect. A unilateral bulge at the fourth and fifth intercostal spaces at the lower left sternal border often is found in adults with ventricular septal defects.[31] A bulge in the area of the second and third intercostal space at the left sternal border may result from an underlying atrial septal defect. Scoliosis is commonly present in cyanotic congenital heart disease. Underdeveloped musculature of the lower extremities compared with the upper extremities occurs with coarctation of the aorta. Clubbing of the digits and cyanosis of the skin or nails suggest congenital heart disease with right to left shunting of blood (Plate IV, 10-1).

Specific forms of differential cyanosis often provide a clue to exact pathological anatomy.[32] Cyanosis of the fingers greater than the toes suggests complete transposition of the great vessels with preductal coarctation or complete interruption of the aortic arch, pulmonary hypertension, and a reverse shunt through a patent ductus arteriosus delivering oxygenated blood to the lower extremities (Plate IV, 10-2). In this anomaly, the presence of aortic coarctation can be distinguished from complete interruption of aortic arch.[1] Slightly less cyanosis of the left arm when compared with the right arm favors aortic coarctation; while intense symmetric cyanosis of both arms is seen with complete aortic interruption. Cyanosis and clubbing of the toes associated with pink finger nails of the right hand and minimal cyanosis and clubbing of the left hand are due to pulmonary hypertension with normally related great vessels and a reversed shunt with the patent ductus arteriosus bringing unoxygenated blood to the left arm and lower extremities (Plate V, 10-3). The same pattern results from interruption of the aortic arch and a patent ductus arteriosus delivering desaturated blood to the legs. If the right subclavian artery arises proximal to the aortic obstruction, then the right hand may be pink and the left hand cyanotic. However, when an anomalous right subclavian artery originates from the descending aorta, both hands are cyanotic. Red fingertips "tuft erythema" may signify a small, intermittent right to left shunt with only slight reduction in arterial oxygen saturation (Plate V, 10-4).

Anotia (congenital absence of the pinna) and facial paralysis may be signs of underlying ventricular septal defect and pulmonic stenosis.[33] The presence of any congenital somatic abnormality should always prompt a search for congenital heart disease. Extracardiac anomalies were found in 25 percent of infants seen during the first year for significant cardiac disease in one study.[34] The defects were commonly found in the musculoskeletal system and were associated with specific syndromes. (For further specific details concerning the clinical presentation of patients with congenital heart disease the reader is referred to Chaps. 95 to 98.)

DISORDERS AFFECTING THE VALVES

The cutaneous lesions of *infective endocarditis* (Chap. 94) include Osler's nodes, Janeway lesions, clubbing of the fingers (Plate V, 10-5), splinter hemorrhages of the nails, and petechiae.[35,36] *Osler's nodes* are reddish-purple, tender nodules typically found in the distal pad of the finger or toe (Fig. 10-12; Plate V, 10-6). By contrast, *Janeway lesions* are hemorrhagic but nontender and involve the palms or soles. Splinter hemorrhages are linear and black and affect the distal third of the fingernail.

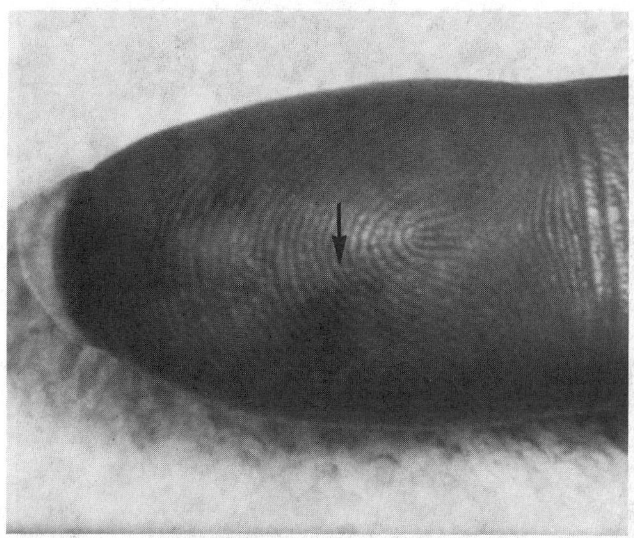

FIGURE 10-12 Bacterial endocarditis: valvular infection associated with a tender, purplish nodule (Osler's node) in the finger pad (arrow).

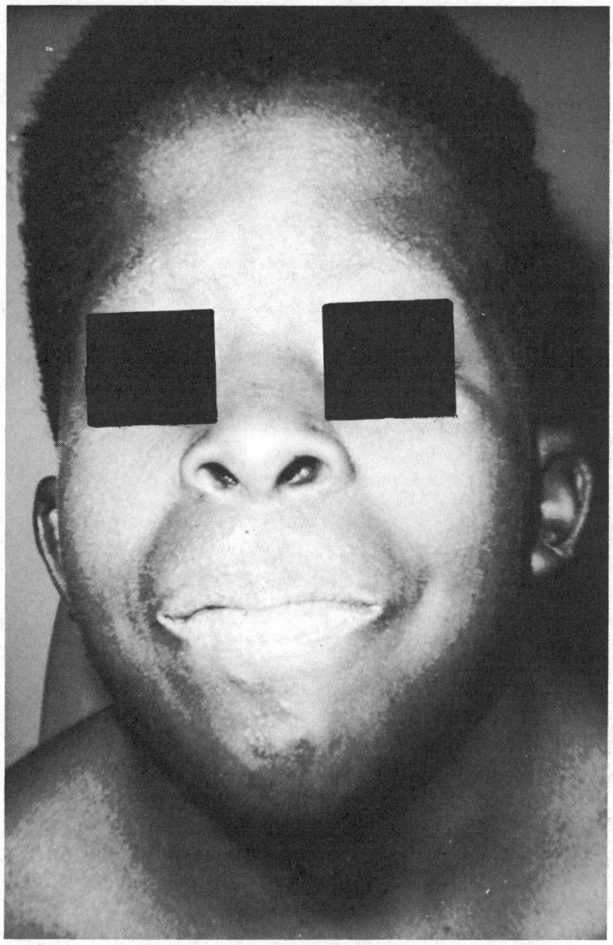

FIGURE 10-13 Noonan's syndrome: ptosis, hypertelorism, and low-set ears associated with valvular pulmonic stenosis.

They also are present in many unrelated diseases and may result from trauma in otherwise healthy people.

Certain features suggest primary valvular heart disease (Chaps. 78 to 82). The murmur of pulmonic stenosis may be part of Noonan's syndrome, Turner's syndrome (previously discussed), Rubinstein-Taybi syndrome, rubella syndrome (see above), the multiple lentigines syndrome, pulmonary valve dysplasia, or Watson's syndrome. In *Noonan's syndrome*[37] the characteristic findings include ptosis, low-set ears, downward-slanting eyes, webbed neck, hypertelorism, low posterior hairline, short stature, mental retardation, and normal chromosomes (Fig. 10-13). Broad toes and thumbs, a slanting forehead, a thin, beaked nose, and large, low-set ears are seen in *Rubinstein-Taybi* syndrome (Fig. 10-14).[38] Café au lait spots and mental retardation are linked to pulmonic valve stenosis in *Watson's syndrome.*[1]

The *multiple lentigines syndrome* is identified by the presence of multiple tan-to-brown macules varying in size from pinpoint to 5 cm in diameter (Fig. 10-15). These cutaneous lesions may affect the entire body but are most heavily concentrated on the neck and upper thorax. Other findings in this syndrome include hearing loss, short stature, hypertelorism, ptosis, prognathism, pectus excavatum or carinatum, kyphoscoliosis, café au lait spots, and other skeletal defects.[39]

The *carcinoid syndrome* may present as intense flushing of the face; a chronic cyanotic hue and telangiectasia may be present. Stenosis and/or regurgitation of the tricuspid and/or pulmonic valves often result when hepatic metastases are present.[40,41] When a patent ductus arteriosus, lung metastases, or a patent foramen ovale is present, the left-sided heart valves often are affected.[1]

In *progressive systemic sclerosis,* tightening of the skin on the fingers and then the hands, forearms, upper chest, and face is associated with hair loss and disappearance of subcutaneous tissue and skin creases (Fig. 10-16). Flexion contractures on the fingers may cause a clawlike hand deformity. Raynaud's phenomenon often is an early manifestation. Although valvular changes include thickening of the edges of the mitral, aortic, and tricuspid valves as well as thickening and shortening of the mitral chordae, the resulting valve disease rarely is significant.[1,42]

Joint disease associated with cardiac valvular disease is frequent with systemic lupus erythematosus, rheumatoid arthritis, rheumatic fever, polychondritis, ankylosing spondylitis, alkaptonuria, and Whipple's disease. In *systemic lupus erythematous,* the joint inflammation is usually symmetrical and nondeforming. Typical skin lesions include an erythematous, scaling eruption over the cheeks and bridge of the nose, circumscribed reddish-purple plaques, telangiectasia, and patchy hair loss (Fig. 10-17). Verrucous endocarditis may involve any of the four cardiac valves; however, severe valvular dysfunction is unusual. Valvular disease may be more common in patients with antiphospholipid antibodies.[43,44] (See also Chap. 103.)

In patients with *rheumatoid arthritis,* the metacarpophalangeal joints, proximal interphalangeal joints, wrists, metatarsophalangeal joints, shoulders, knees, ankles, and elbows are involved with inflammation and subsequent destruction. Advanced disease results in ulnar deviation of the fingers, flexion of the distal interphalangeal joints with hyperextension of the proximal interphalangeal joints producing a "swan-neck" deformity, and a Z-shaped configuration of the thumb.[1] Subluxa-

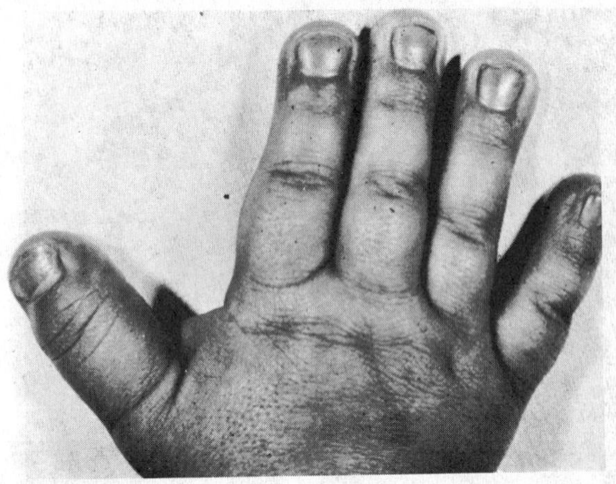

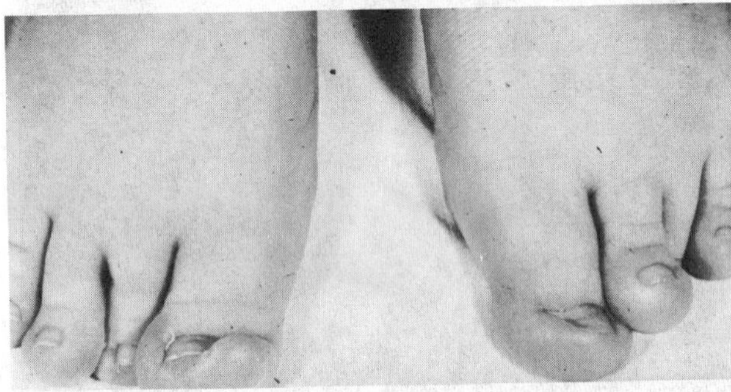

FIGURE 10-14 Rubinstein-Taybi syndrome may be associated with a variety of congenital heart defects. *(From ME Silverman, JW Hurst: The hand and the heart. Am J Cardiol 22:718, 1968. Reproduced with permission from the publisher and authors.)*

tion of the metacarpophalangeal joints with interosseal muscle wasting and thickening of the wrists are common. Granulomatous aortic or mitral valve disease with regurgitation is most common in patients who are seropositive and have subcutaneous nodules or classic rheumatoid deformities.[45] *Rheumatic fever,* often with cardiac involvement, should be suspected in patients with erythema marginatum, urticaria, and migratory polyarthritis involving the large joints. Subcutaneous nodules are less frequently found. Marked ulnar deviation at the metacarpophalangeal joints, suggesting rheumatoid arthritis, can be due to repeated attacks of rheumatic fever and is known as *Jaccoud's or post–rheumatic fever arthritis.*[46] In contrast to rheumatoid arthritis, the fingers can be moved freely into a correct alignment and x-rays of the hands are normal.

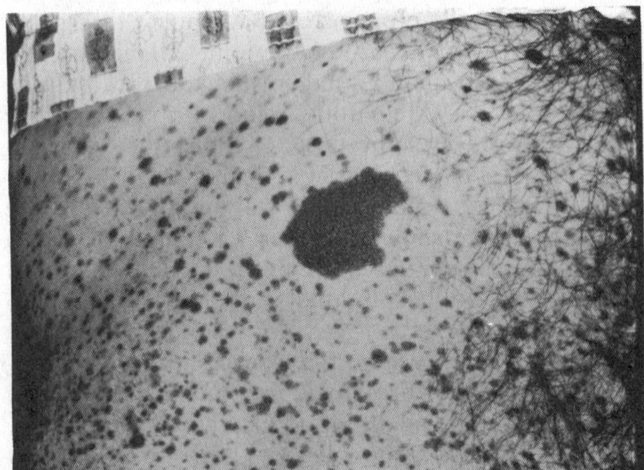

FIGURE 10-15 Multiple lentigines syndrome: dark brown macular lesions on the abdomen associated with hypertrophic subaortic stenosis. *(From ME Silverman: Visual clues to diagnosis. Primary Cardiology, October 1986. Reproduced with permission from the publisher and author.)*

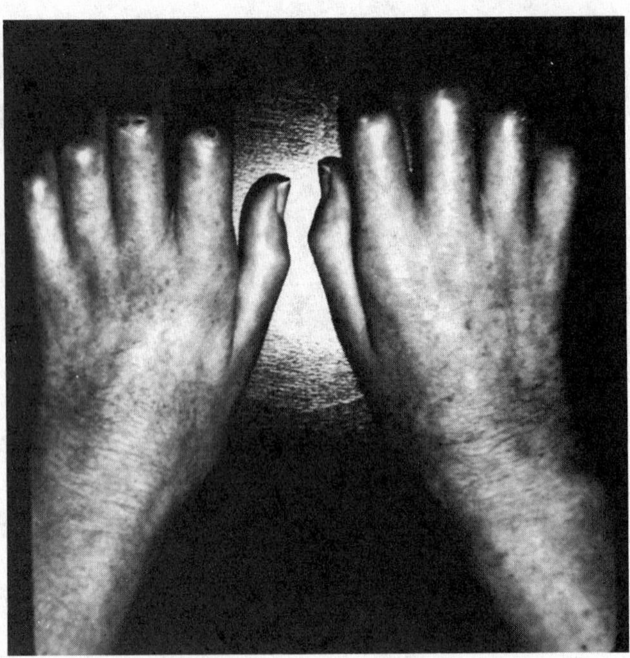

FIGURE 10-16 Scleroderma: clawlike hand deformity and shiny, tight skin may be linked with myocardial fibrosis.

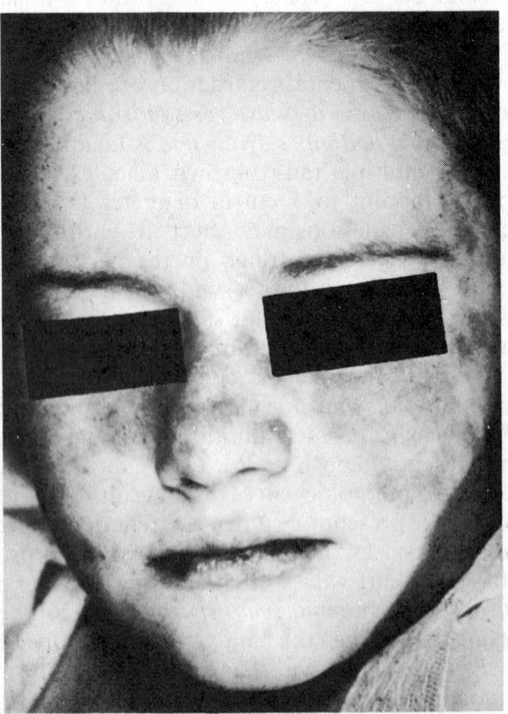

FIGURE 10-17 Systemic lupus erythematosus: butterfly rash associated with pericardial, myocardial, and endocardial disease.

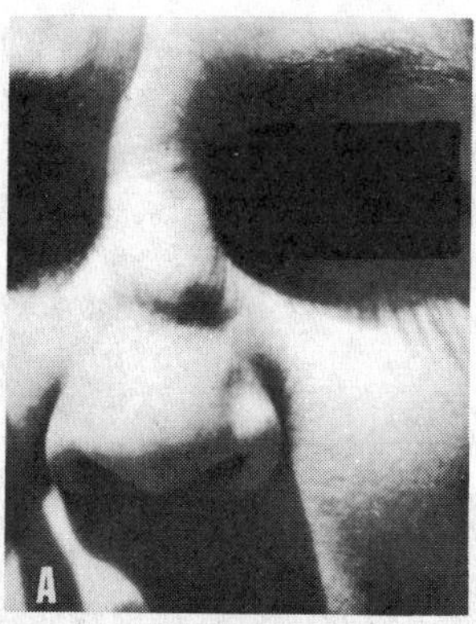
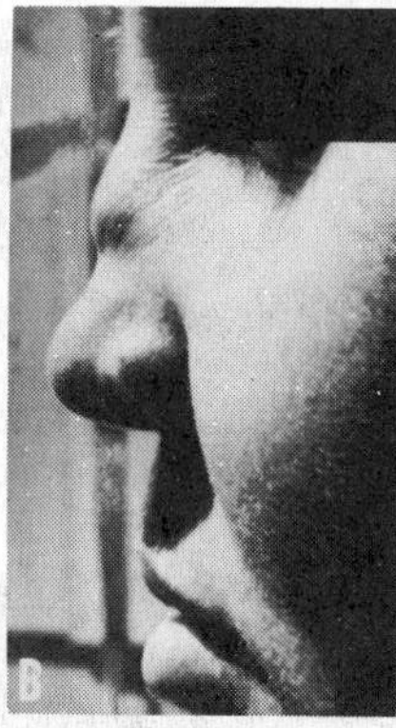

FIGURE 10-18 Polychondritis. *A, B.* Destruction of cartilage of nose, producing a "saddle nose" in association with aortic regurgitation. *(Courtesy of Dr. Warren Sarrell, Anniston, AL.)*

Polychondritis causes an inflammatory destruction of the cartilage of the face resulting in a saddle-shaped collapse of the nose or a cauliflower ear.[1] Aortic regurgitation, aortic aneurysm, and rarely aortic root dissection are associated (Fig. 10-18).[47,48]

Chronic synovitis involving the fibrocartilaginous joints of the spine occurs in patients with *ankylosing spondylitis.* The disease may be confined to the sacroiliac area or spread slowly upward. The patient with advanced disease is bent forward, is unable to stand upright, and must walk with a stiff and halting gait (Fig. 10-19). Aortic regurgitation, due to thickening and shortening of the aortic cusps from perivascular inflammation and fibrosis, occurs in up to 10 percent of patients.[49] Mitral regurgitation and complete heart block may also occur. *Cogan's syndrome,* consisting of ophthalmic inflammation and audiovestibular symptoms, is another cause of vasculitis involving the aortic root and leading to aortic regurgitation.[50]

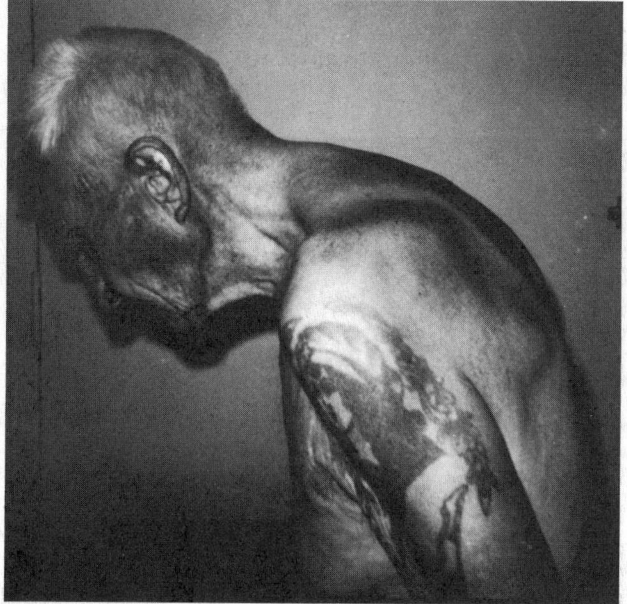

FIGURE 10-19 Ankylosing spondylitis: immobile, curved spine with forward jutting of head may be seen with AV block or aortic regurgitation. *(From ME Silverman: Visual clues to diagnosis. Primary Cardiology, June 1987. Reproduced with permission from the publisher, author, and patient.)*

Whipple's disease is suggested by the combination of polyarthritis, abdominal pain, and diarrhea. Aortic and mitral regurgitation and endocarditis are known complications.[51] Aortic or mitral valvulitis may also be due to an accumulation of homogentisic acid in *alkaptonuria.*

External signs of mitral valve prolapse (see also Chap. 80) include a straight thoracic spine, pectus excavatum, scoliosis, hypomastia, joint laxity, and various neuromuscular disorders. Systolic and rarely diastolic murmurs have been described with chest wall deformities due to *straight-back syndrome* and *pectus excavatum,* which may impinge on or displace the heart.

DISORDERS ASSOCIATED WITH CARDIOMYOPATHY

Hypertrophic cardiomyopathy (Chap. 90) has been associated with Friedreich's ataxia, Turner's syndrome, Noonan's syndrome,[52] Fabry's disease, neurofibromatosis, and the multiple lentigines syndrome. *Friedreich's ataxia* is a spinocerebellar degenerative disorder that results in a broad-based, lurching gait, impaired vibration, position, and joint sense, and incoordination. Kyphoscoliosis and pes cavus (high instep, retraction of the toes at the metatarsal-phalangeal joints, and hammer toes) are two important physical signs (Fig. 10-20). Concentric and asymmetric left ventricular hypertrophy and a dilated cardiomyopathy have each been described.[53]

Myocardial hypertrophy may be secondary to extreme *obesity or acromegaly.* With acromegaly, the broad forehead, thickened skin, and enlarged nose, lip, and tongue produce coarsened facial features (Fig. 10-21) while elongation of the mandible leads to prognathism and overbite. The large sausage-shaped fingers and spadelike configuration of the hands are typical.[54]

Cor pulmonale and right ventricular hypertrophy may be secondary to pulmonary hypertension caused by *kyphoscoliosis, restrictive lung disease,* progressive systemic sclerosis, *upper airway blockade* by enlarged tonsils[55] and adenoids, or the *sleep apnea syndrome* associated with extreme obesity.

Myocarditis (Chap. 88) occurs with systemic lupus erythematosus, rheumatic fever, Reiter's syndrome,[56] Kawasaki's disease,[57] Lyme arthritis,[58] and occasionally Whipple's disease.[59] *Reiter's syndrome* is characterized by conjunctivitis and hyperkeratotic coalescing lesions encrusted on the soles and palms, associated with arthritis and urethritis. *Kawasaki's disease* begins with fever, cervical adenopathy, and a strawberry tongue. Later, the palms and soles become indurated and purplish-red and then peel. A widespread erythematous rash may appear and then desquamate. *Lyme arthritis,* caused by the spirochete *Borrelia burgdorferi,* begins with an expanding erythematous rash with a bright red border (Fig. 10-22).[60] The center of the rash may clear, indurate, blister, or become necrotic. Multiple annular lesions may develop.

Diseases that cause myocardial fibrosis include dermatomyositis, Duchenne's muscular dystrophy, myotonic

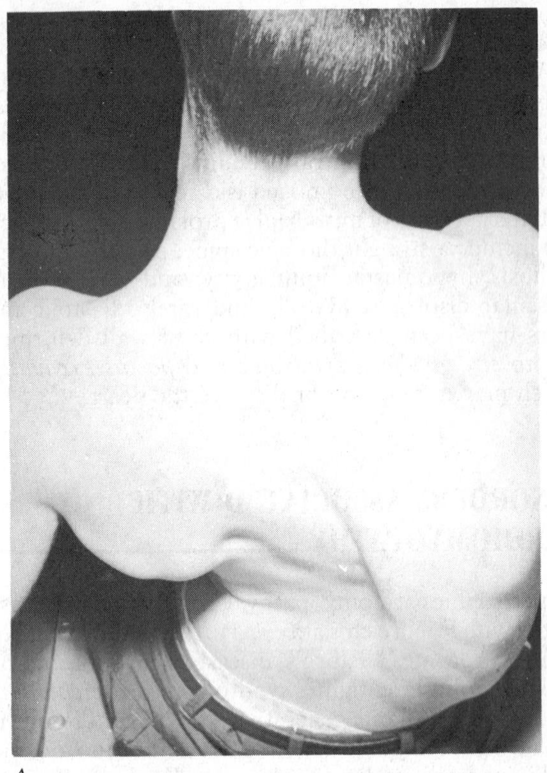

A

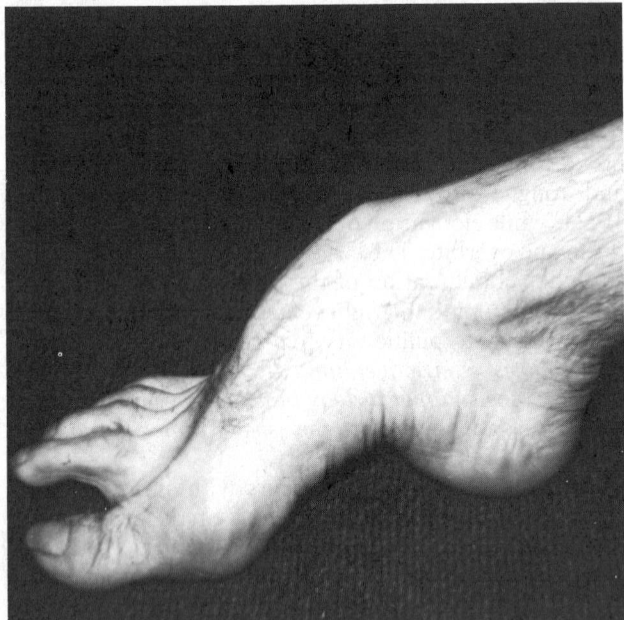

B

FIGURE 10-20 Friedreich's ataxia (photographs from different patients). *A.* Kyphoscoliosis. *B.* Pes cavus. Myocardial fibrosis and hypertrophy are often present. *(From ME Silverman: Visual clues to diagnosis. Primary Cardiology, June 1987. Reproduced with permission from the publisher and authors.)*

muscular dystrophy, Kearns-Sayre syndrome, Friedreich's ataxia,[61] sarcoidosis, and progressive systemic sclerosis. With *dermatomyositis*, an erythematous eruption and periorbital heliotropic discoloration affects the face (Plate V, 10-7) and a scaly, erythematous rash may cover

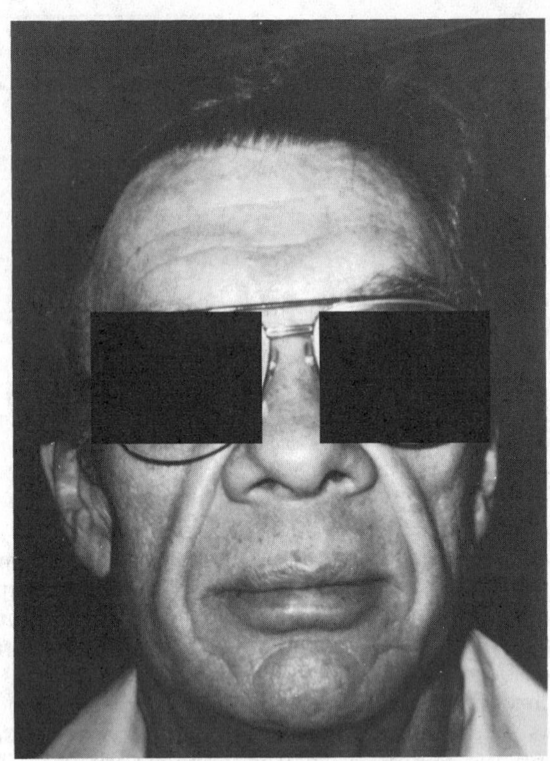

FIGURE 10-21 Acromegaly: coarse facial features, folds of skin, and prognathism are associated with myocardial hypertrophy and fibrosis. *(From ME Silverman: Visual clues to diagnosis. Primary Cardiology, February 1987. Reproduced with permission from the publisher, author, and patient.)*

the knuckles, sparing the interphalangeal region.[62] A waddling gait and pseudohypertrophic calves are characteristic of *Duchenne's muscular dystrophy*. The electrocardiogram (ECG) commonly is consistent with fibrosis of the posterior left ventricle.[63] In *myotonic dystrophica*, drooping eyelids, cataracts, a receding hairline, and a masklike expression are present.[64,65] The *Kerns-Sayre*

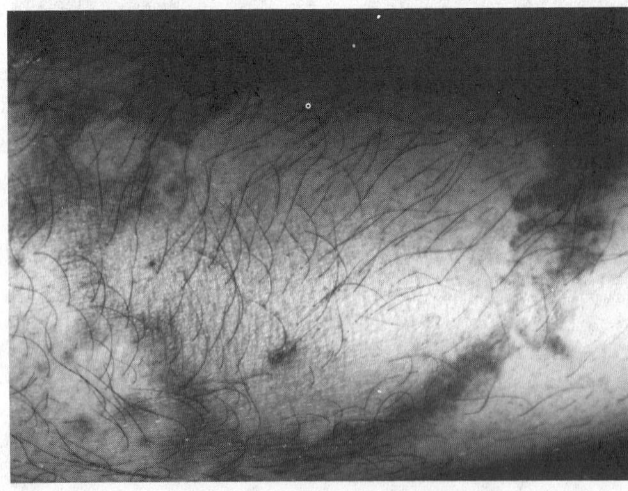

FIGURE 10-22 Lyme arthritis: annular expanding rash with a clear central area may be associated with pericarditis and AV block. *(From ME Silverman: Visual clues to diagnosis. Primary Cardiology, December 1986. Reproduced with permission from the publisher and author.)*

syndrome is a form of ocular muscular dystrophy in which external ophthalmoplegia, ptosis, and retinitis pigmentosa occur.[66,67] The skin manifestations of *sarcoidosis* include erythema nodosum, lupus pernio (a red or violet plaque with a predilection for the nose, cheeks, eyelids, and ears), and waxy translucent papules found on the cheeks, periorbital areas, ears, nasolabial folds, and elsewhere.[68,69] Uveitis, bilateral parotid gland enlargement, and arthritis often are present.

Isolated noncompaction of the left ventricular myocardium is characterized by numerous, prominent ventricular trabeculations, deep intertrabecular recesses, arrhythmias, and a distinctive facial dysmorphism.

Infiltrative diseases of the myocardium include Wilson's disease, Cori's disease, Fabry's disease, hemochromatosis, amyloidosis, glycogen storage disease, and sarcoidosis. (See also Chaps. 91 and 96.) *Wilson's disease* is an autosomal recessive disorder in which copper accumulates in tissues including the myocardium.[70] Arrhythmias, autonomic dysfunction, and cardiomyopathy have been reported. Kayser-Fleischer rings, usually golden-brown in color and circling the edge of the cornea, provide a major clue to the correct diagnosis. *Cori's disease* (type III glycogenosis) is suspected when a patient has xanthomas and a yellowish skin. In *hemochromatosis,* the skin has a bronze or slate-gray coloration; myocardial infiltration with iron deposits often cause a dilated or rarely a restrictive cardiomyopathy associated with arrhythmias and heart failure.[71] Macroglossia and waxy nodules of the skin and eyelids, which may hemorrhage when pinched, are clues to the diagnosis of *amyloidosis* (Fig. 10-23).[72] (See also Chap. 91.) Glycogen storage disease also enlarges the tongue.

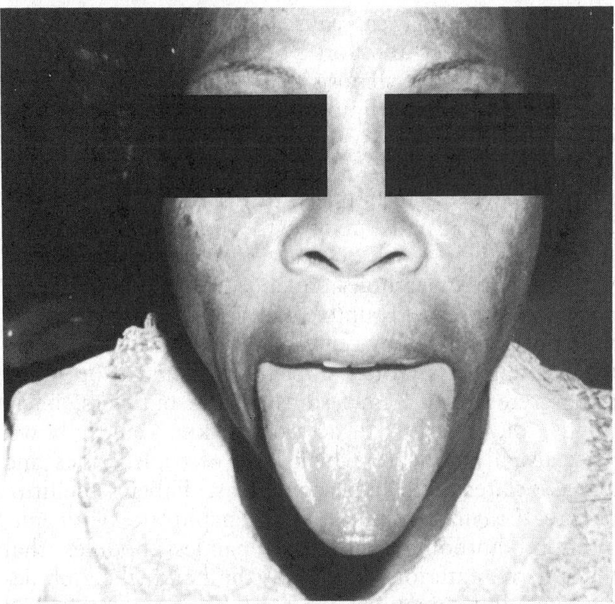

FIGURE 10-23 Amyloidosis: enlarged tongue may be a sign of an infiltrative cardiomyopathy. *(From ME Silverman: Visual clues to diagnosis. Primary Cardiology, November 1987. Reproduced with permission from the publisher, author, and patient.)*

DISORDERS ASSOCIATED WITH PERICARDIAL DISEASE

Pericarditis may be a result of Reiter's syndrome, Whipple's disease, Kawasaki's disease, systemic lupus erythematosus, rheumatoid arthritis,[73] rheumatic fever, dermatomyositis, hemochromatosis, Behçet's disease, Degos' disease, uremia, mulibrey nanism, polychondritis, hypothyroidism, or metastatic disease among others. (See also Chap. 92.) The components of *Behçet's disease* include erythema nodosum, superficial phlebitis, oral and genital ulcers, and iritis.[74,75] Patients with *Degos' disease* (malignant atrophic papulosis) present with painless, oval, cutaneous lesions that have a white center and surrounding erythema.[76] In this rapidly fatal disease occlusive fibrosis of small- and medium-size arteries produces pleuritis and pericarditis. In far-advanced renal disease, urochrome pigmentation of the skin and uremic frost are cutaneous manifestations.[77] The term *mulibrey nanism* describes a syndrome involving muscle, liver, brain, and eyes.[78] These patients have a triangular face, bulging forehead, low nasal bridge, growth retardation, pigmentary changes in the fundus, hemangiomas, and constrictive pericarditis.[1] Hypothyroidism, a cause of often-massive pericardial effusions, distorts the face with thickened skin, dry hair, puffy eyelids, and enlarged tongue.

DISORDERS CAUSING CONDUCTION SYSTEM DISEASE

Acquired causes of atrioventricular (AV) block or bundle branch block include sarcoidosis,[68] rheumatic fever, gout, Reiter's syndrome,[79,80] dermatomyositis, amyloidosis,[72] Kawasaki's disease,[57] ankylosing spondylitis, systemic lupus erythematosus,[81] and Lyme arthritis.[58] In *gout,* uric acid crystals may form nodules affecting the conduction system, and AV block may be an early cardiac manifestation of ankylosing spondylitis.[82]

Inherited or congenital disorders associated with conduction defects include systemic lupus erythematosus, Friedreich's ataxia, Kearns-Sayre syndrome, multiple lentigines syndrome, muscular dystrophy,[83] myotonic dystrophy, tuberous sclerosis, and Refsum's disease. Maternal lupus is an important cause of congenital complete AV block in the newborn.[84] In *Refsum's disease,* a lipidosis and genetically determined neuropathy characterized by high levels of phytanic acid, cerebellar ataxia, night blindness, deafness, ichthyosis, cataracts, and polyneuropathy have been associated with myocardial disease and conduction abnormalities.

DISORDERS AFFECTING THE VASCULAR SYSTEM

Aortic aneurysms and dissection (Chap. 123) are frequent cardiovascular complications of Marfan's and Ehlers-Danlos syndromes.[85] Aneurysms of other vessels and arterial rupture also may occur. A progressive looseness of skin, producing pendulous folds and droopy eyelids, can be due to *cutis laxa,* a generalized destruction of elastic tissue that can cause dilatation of the aorta or pulmonary artery and aortic rupture.[85]

Coronary artery stenosis from atherosclerosis can be associated with hyperlipidemia,[86] cerebrotendinous xanthomatoses, Werner's syndrome, uremia, progeria, acromegaly, and diabetes mellitus. *Hyperlipidemia* may be suspected when xanthomas or arcus senilis are present. Xanthelasma usually involve the upper eyelid. When they occur before age 50, there is a strong association with familial hypercholesterolemia and premature coronary artery disease. Eruptive xanthomata are recognized as papules with yellow centers surrounded by an erythematous halo. They often appear with sudden outbreak of discrete 1- to 4-cm lesions on the buttocks, back, thighs, and exterior surfaces of the knees and elbows. They usually indicate a high level of triglycerides and are associated with hyperlipidemias, diabetes mellitus, pancreatitis, myxedema, and the nephrotic syndrome. Tendon xanthomata are firm, painless nodules that thicken the exterior tendons of the hand, the Achilles tendons, and sometimes the tendons of the knees and elbows (Fig. 10-24). *Cerebrotendinous xanthomatoses* is a rare disorder in which tendon xanthomas, cataracts, dementia, ataxia, neuropathy, and accelerated atherosclerosis are present. Tuberous xanthomata are yellow to deep-orange papules erupting over the elbows, knees, buttocks, and heels. They may coalesce or be pedunculated and are a manifestation of hyperlipidemia, myxedema, and liver disease. Large, orange, lobulated tonsils are a finding in *Tangier disease,* in which there is deficiency of high-density lipoprotein.

In *Werner's syndrome,* the skin is tightly stretched over the underlying bones.[87,88] There is marked loss of subcutaneous tissue, and ulcerations occur over the legs. Severe coronary atherosclerosis often results in myocardial infarction at an early age. Physical findings in diabetes mellitus may include tight skin and necrobiosis diabeticorum, an atrophy of the skin of the lower extremities. *Progeria* is a rare disorder in which the face is small and prematurely aged, the eyes bulge, and the nose is beaked. Severe atherosclerosis with early myocardial infarction is a common cause of death in early life.[89,90] In some studies a diagonal earlobe crease and short tufts of ear-canal hair have been curiously associated with coronary atherosclerosis.[91,92]

Nonatherosclerotic arterial disease can be attributed to homocystinuria, pseudoxanthoma elasticum, Fabry's disease, Hurler's syndrome, Whipple's disease,[93] and scleroderma. *Homocystinuria,* a disorder of methionine metabolism, causes thrombosis of veins and intermediate-size arteries.[85] Patients resemble those with Marfan's syndrome because they have long extremities, pectus carinatum, and kyphoscoliosis. Pseudoxanthum elasticum has been associated with fibrosis of coronary arteries and calcification of peripheral arteries.[85] A glycosphingolipid is deposited in the arterial endothelium of patients with Fabry's disease and may result in angina pectoris or myocardial infarction. Patients with *Hurler's syndrome* have mental retardation; a large, boat-shaped head; a broad nose; large lips; small and widely spaced teeth; and a large protuberant tongue.[94] Glycosaminoglycan deposition in the coronary arteries is present. Myocardial fibrosis due to repeated coronary small-vessel spasm has been postulated to be a result from progressive systemic sclerosis.[42]

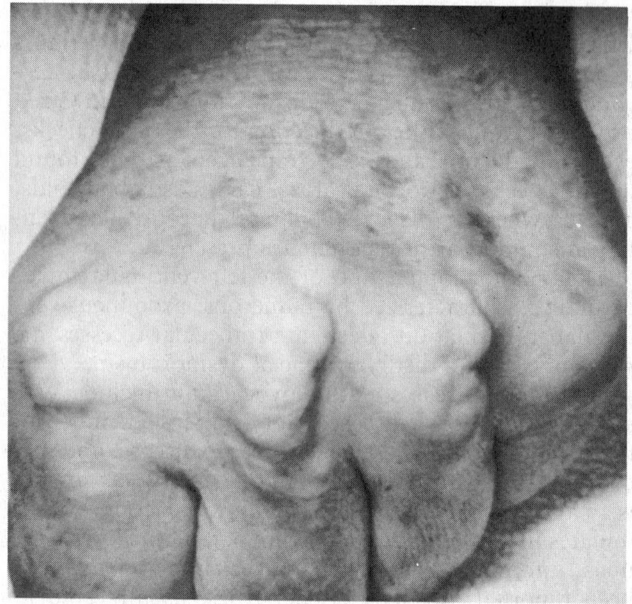

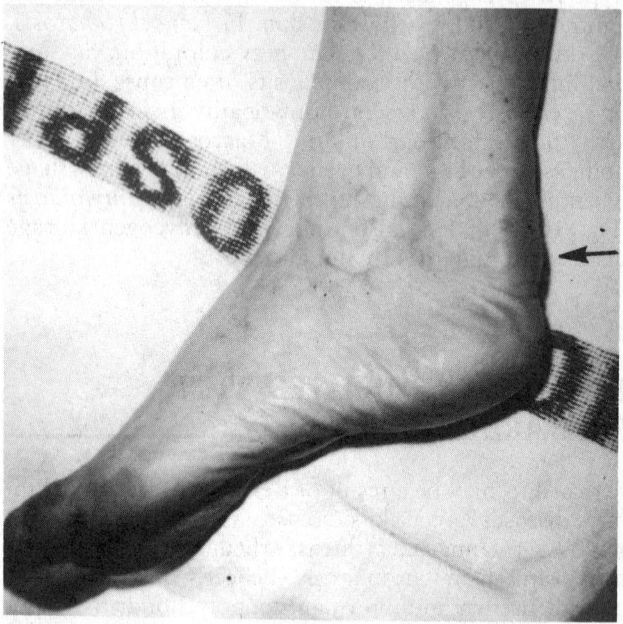

FIGURE 10-24 Hyperlipidemia: xanthomata. Associated with coronary artery disease. *A.* On the extensor tendons of the hand. *B.* On the Achilles tendon (arrow).

Vasculitis may be due to systemic lupus erythematosus, rheumatoid arthritis, Behçet's disease,[74] Kawasaki's disease,[57] and polyarteritis. Cutaneous infarction, nodules, petechiae, livedo reticularis, gangrenous digits, myocardial infarction, heart failure, and hypertension may be due to polyarteritis.[95]

Arteriovenous shunts may be found in extensive skin disease, hereditary hemorrhagic telangiectasia (HHT), and the Klippel-Trenaunay-Weber syndrome. *Kaposi's*

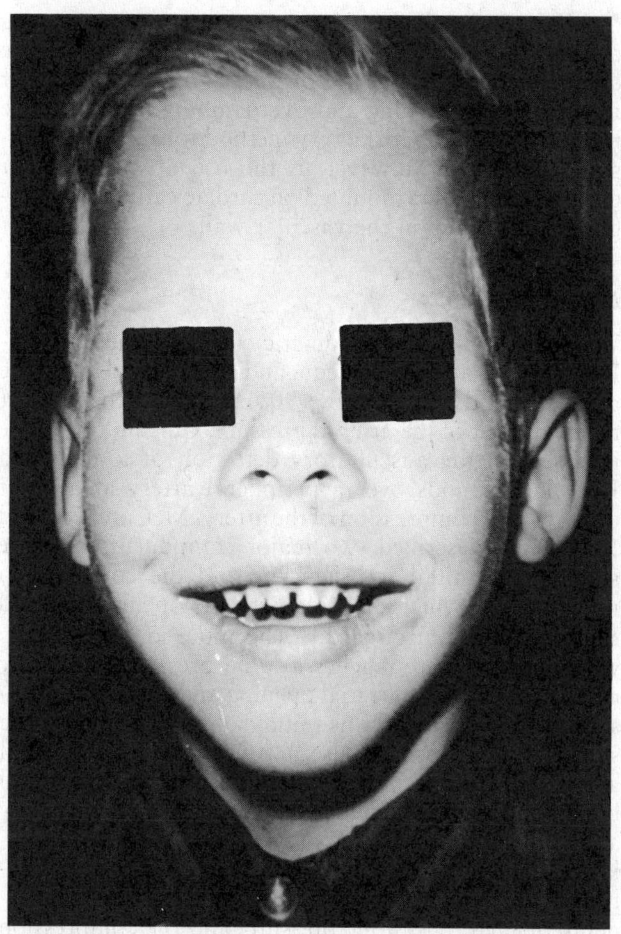

FIGURE 10-25 Supravalvular aortic stenosis: turned-up nose, broad cheeks, large mouth with peg-shaped teeth, and large ears.

sarcoma or exfoliative dermatitis due to psoriasis may divert the blood supply through shunts in the skin to produce high-output cardiac failure. Clues to underlying *arteriovenous fistula* as a cause of high-output failure include a barely discernible scar from a knife wound or a surgical incision. Telangiectasia of the fingertips, lips, and tongue and pulmonary and hepatic arteriovenous fistulas are components of *hereditary hemorrhagic telangiectasia.*[96] The triad of anomalies that *Klippel-Trenaunay-Weber syndrome* comprises are vascular nevus, large varices, and bony or soft-tissue hypertrophy.[97] Marked enlargement of a limb(s) and facial hemihypertrophy are features of this disorder in which part or all of the deep venous system is absent and arteriovenous malformation is often present. Hemangiomas of the skin may also indicate multinodular hemangiomatosis of the liver, a cause of high-output heart failure in infancy.

Stenosis of large arteries may occur with supravalvular aortic stenosis, rubella syndrome, Turner's syndrome, and neurofibromatosis. The face of a child with *supravalvular aortic stenosis* (William's syndrome) is almost diagnostic (Fig. 10-25). The head is small, with an elflike appearance; the cheeks are full and baggy and the mouth is large.[98] Thick lips and peg-shaped, widely spaced teeth are typical findings. The forehead is prominent and broad. Mental retardation is often present. The supravalvular aortic stenosis may be a localized ridge or a diffuse narrowing of the aorta beginning just above the sinuses of Valsalva. Pulmonic artery branch stenosis is frequently present. Coarctation of the aorta is a common cardiac lesion in Turner's syndrome and neurofibromatosis has been associated with renal artery stenosis.

Facial swelling and jugular venous distension may be early signs of *superior vena caval obstruction* from clot or tumor.

MISCELLANEOUS DISORDERS

Multiple lentigines, cutaneous myxomas, myxoid fibroadenomas of the breast, and various endocrine abnormalities are features of a recently described inherited disorder in which single or multiple cardiac myxoma occur.[99]

Telangiectasia of the tongue and lips may be associated with a pulmonary arteriovenous fistula (Plate V, 10-8 and 10-9).

A susceptibility to atrial fibrillation and atrial flutter has been documented in patients who have *facioscapulohumeral muscular dystrophy.*[100] Sinus node dysfunction, elbow contractures, and humeroperoneal weakness are *manifestations* of *Emery-Dreifuss muscular dystrophy.*

Single or multiple rhabdomyomas may develop within the myocardium and cause heart failure, valvular obstruction, or arrhythmias in patients with *tuberous sclerosis* (Plate V, 10-10).[101] The diagnosis is suggested by the presence of yellow-brown angiofibromas ("adenoma sebaceum") on the face, subungual fibromas around the fingernail, café au lait spots, and subcutaneous nodules.

MEASUREMENT OF ARTERIAL PRESSURE*

Noninvasive assessment of the arterial blood pressure using a pneumatic cuff is the most frequently used method for determining the status of the circulation and the interaction between the heart and arterial system. Blood pressure deviations from normal often provide important diagnostic information in patients with a variety of cardiac and noncardiac diseases.

Physical Determinants of the Arterial Pressure

The arterial blood pressure, a measure of the lateral force per unit area of vascular wall, is quantitated as millimeters of mercury or dynes per square centimeter. The determinants of the peak systolic blood pressure include the volume and velocity of left ventricular ejection, the peripheral arteriolar resistance, the distensibility of the arterial wall, the viscosity of the blood, and the end-diastolic volume in the arterial system. The subsequent diminution in pressure during diastole is in turn

*The portion of this chapter dealing with the measurement of systemic blood pressure appeared in the fifth and sixth editions of *The Heart.* It was written by Dr. Donald Nutter and is reproduced here, with slight modification, with the permission of Dr. Nutter.

influenced by blood viscosity, arterial distensibility, peripheral resistance to flow, and the length of the cardiac cycle.[102] Important physical factors affecting arterial distensibility include (1) the elastic modulus of the arterial wall, the ratio of stress (force acting to deform the wall) to strain (the proportional deformation produced), and (2) the geometry of the arterial wall, i.e., the internal radius *(r)* and wall thickness *(h)*, which govern wall tension *(T)* according to the modified Laplace equation $T = Pr/h$, where P is intravascular pressure. A decrease in elasticity or an increase in radius results in diminished distensibility and a greater rise in pressure per unit volume of blood.[102]

The mean arterial pressure is the product of the cardiac output and the total peripheral resistance, the latter often being increased by many mechanisms including alpha-adrenergic stimulation, the renin-angiotensin system, or other circulating hormonal or humoral factors.[103]

Methods for Measuring the Arterial Pressure

Direct Methods

In 1733 Stephen Hales recorded the arterial pressures in animals by cannulation and a blood-filled glass column.[104] Current techniques for the direct and continuous measurement of arterial pressure utilize the electromanometer, a transducer that converts mechanical energy into an electric signal suitable for amplification, display, and recording. The artery is cannulated with a saline-filled catheter or needle that mechanically couples the circulation to the arterial manometer. Pressures are recorded using atmospheric pressure as the "zero" reference level, and intravascular pressures are further referenced to the level of the heart by addition or subtraction of a gravitation factor. The gravitation factor is expressed by the formal pgh, where p is the density of blood (in grams per milliliter), g is the acceleration due to gravity (980 cm/s^2), and h is the transducer height (centimeters) above or below the horizontal plane of the heart.

The strain gauge manometer commonly is used for the precise and accurate measurement of the arterial pressure. However, error may originate in the catheter or coupling system, in which the properties of inertia, friction, and elasticity interact to produce damping of the frequency response. Systems may be overdamped or underdamped, both resulting in signal distortion. Nevertheless, the appropriate combination of an inelastic cardiac catheter and connecting tube filled with bubble-free fluid produces "critical" damping in which the system response is constant to some desirable frequency level and adequate for the clinical recording of intravascular pressures.[102]

Measurement errors also occur when an end-hole catheter is positioned axial to flow in a vessel and may become important during high arterial flow when kinetic energy may exceed 10 percent of the total fluid energy. The use of a side-hole catheter positioned in a large, patent artery allows measurement of the true arterial pressure. Also, pressure transients due to catheter whip can falsely elevate the measured arterial pressure.[102]

Miniature, self-flushing strain gauge manometers attached directly to an intravascular catheter or needle eliminate many of the problems related to transducer mounting and flushing and overdamping by connective tubing. The most satisfactory method for reducing measurement errors, however, is the use of intravascular electromanometers mounted on cardiac catheters or surgically implanted in the vascular wall.

Indirect Methods

The invention of the pneumatic cuff manometer (Riva-Rocci, 1896) and the subsequent discovery and use of the arterial sounds (Korotkoff, 1905) permitted the indirect measurement of the arterial pressure. Current technique is based on the auscultatory detection of low-pitched Korotkoff sounds over a peripheral artery at a point distal to cuff compression of the artery. McCutcheon and Rushmer[105] described two major components of these sounds: the initial transient (k_i) and the compression murmur (k_c), which coincide with the opening tap and rumble sounds of Rodbard.[106] The initial sound K_i occurs when cuff pressure reaches arterial pressure and likely results from abrupt arterial opening and vascular distension. The intensity of this initial sound depends on the slope of the pressure pulse and the level of the distal arterial pressure at the time of arterial opening, the sound being louder with vasodilatation and high-velocity flow and softer with arterial constriction or circulatory collapse. The initial transient probably is caused by oscillation of the arterial walls as the occluded segment is suddenly opened by systolic pressure, and the compression murmur is caused by a turbulent jet of flow distal to the partially compressed segment.

The Korotkoff sounds have been divided into five phases occurring in sequence as the occluding pressure declines. Phase I consists of clear tapping sounds (k_i) that occur when the cuff pressure has fallen to the arterial peak systolic level. These sounds are initially soft and gradually become louder as cuff pressure falls. Phase II consists of k_i sounds followed by swishing sounds or murmurs (k_c). Phase III is an augmentation of phase II sounds as an increased volume of blood passes through the partially compressed artery. Phase IV is signaled by the abrupt, distinct muffling of the sounds, resulting in a blowing quality that slowly diminishes in intensity. It is due to diminution and loss of component k_i as cuff pressure approaches arterial diastolic levels and reduction in component k_c as the flow period lengthens and velocity decreases. Phase V, complete cessation of sound, occurs when the artery is no longer compressed to an extent that produces turbulent flow. The cuff pressure at which sound disappears may be extremely low or nonexistent when high-flow velocities (e.g., from exercise, anemia, fever) already exist in the circulation. This indirect method slightly underestimates the true arterial pressure.

Proper technique is important for obtaining accurate measurements of blood pressure by the indirect method. The inflatable rubber bag within the compression cuff should have a width that is 20 percent greater than the limb diameter and a length adequate to encompass two-thirds the limb. The cuff should be applied snugly, with the inflatable bag positioned over the artery, at the level of the heart. Before auscultation the cuff is quickly inflated to a pressure 20 mmHg above the systolic, as indicated by obliteration of the radial pulse. The stethoscope is then applied lightly but firmly over the artery and auscultatory pressure is determined by noting the onset (peak systole) and behavior of the Korotkoff sounds as the cuff is deflated at a rate of 3 mmHg/s. When the sounds disappear, the bag should be rapidly decompressed and 1 or 2 min allowed to pass before repeat determinations are made. Whenever possible, the blood pressure should be taken when the subject is upright as well as supine. In the elderly, determination of the blood pressure in both arms is recommended. An American Heart Association report[107] recommends that the systolic pressure be recorded as the point at which the first tapping sound occurs for two consecutive beats (phase I) and that the diastolic pressure be recorded in adults as the point at which sounds become inaudible. In children and in adults with a hyperkinetic circulation, the diastolic pressure should be recorded as the point at which muffling of the sounds occurs (onset of phase IV). The arterial pressures at both the onset of muffling and the disappearance of sound should be recorded. The mean blood pressure can be estimated by the addition of one-third the pulse pressure (systolic pressure minus diastolic pressure) to the diastolic pressure.

This indirect method provides several potential sources of error due to improper equipment, inaccurate detection of the Korotkoff sounds, and observer techniques.[102] For example, a cuff with smaller than recommended width may result in falsely elevated arterial pressure measurements. The standard pneumatic cuff may often be unsatisfactory for pressure measurement in the arms or in the legs of very obese subjects.[108] The arterial pressure may be underestimated if the cuff is deflated too rapidly, particularly when bradycardia or an irregular rhythm is present or if inadequate inflation does not result in complete arterial occlusion. When the cuff is deflated too slowly or is immediately reinflated for multiple pressure determinations, the resultant venous congestion may artificially elevate the diastolic pressure and may falsely decrease the systolic pressure by decreasing the intensity of phase I or phase II sounds to an inaudible level. An erroneously low systolic pressure may also result from the failure to detect the presence of an auscultatory gap, a silent interval occasionally present just below the systolic pressure level.[102]

Studies correlating direct and indirect blood pressure measurements have been characterized by considerable variability between individual subjects but in general have shown a good correlation between indirect and direct measurements of blood pressure in the arm.[108] The observed trend has been for the indirect method to underestimate systolic pressure by several millimeters of mercury, to overestimate diastolic pressure by several millimeters of mercury when phase IV is used as an end point, and to slightly underestimate diastolic pressure in normal individuals when phase V is taken as the end point.

Home blood pressure recordings using manual or automatic inflation and deflation of the cuff and detection of Korotkoff sounds by a microphone, stethoscope, or ultrasonic transducer are being used with increasing frequency for the ambulatory assessment of patients with hypertension.[109–111] Ambulatory blood pressure devices are now available that meet the standards for automated devices of the Association for the Advancement of Medical Instrumentation.[112,113]

More recently, arterial tonometry has been used as a completely noninvasive method for monitoring the arterial pressure. This probe with a micromanometer in its tip operates on the principle of a piezo-resistive transducer of cantilever construction.[114]

Normal Arterial Pressure

Normal pressures have been defined on the basis of values included within two standard deviations of the mean of pressures obtained in a large population of apparently healthy individuals. The normal blood pressure range varies with age, sex, and socioracial grouping.[115] In the United States, the pressure increases rapidly during the first few days of life and then increases gradually, with a slightly greater increment in systolic than in diastolic values, throughout life. The pressure tends to be higher in western, industrialized societies than in Asian and African and technically underdeveloped societies.

With increasing age beyond maturity and into senescence, the aorta undergoes progressive dilation and elongation, with increasing stiffness of its walls.[116] As a result of this diminished vascular distensibility, there is an increase in systolic arterial pressure with less change in diastolic pressure.[117]

The normal blood pressure limits for adults (younger than 40 and of mixed sex and race) living in the United States are approximately 100 to 140 mmHg systolic and 60 to 90 mmHg diastolic. However, in an individual subject, baseline pressures above or below these levels do not define a pathological state, since the physiological range of normal for an individual may overlap with the statistical range of abnormality.[102] The systolic arterial pressure rises slowly and progressively in most Americans between ages 20 and 60 and more rapidly later, increasing by about 20 mmHg between ages 60 and 80.[118] Diastolic pressure usually rises very little after age 45.[119]

It has been demonstrated in mildly to moderately hypertensive persons that the blood pressure "casually" recorded by a physician is significantly higher than the average value of a series of intermittent indirect determinations or continuous direct recordings made during normal activity.[119] To estimate basal blood pressure, measurements have been obtained during sleep, when the subject first awakens in the morning while still recumbent, or after several hours of reclining.

Many factors contribute to variations in an individual's blood pressure during daily activities. These include (1) body posture; (2) state of muscular, cerebral, or gastrointestinal activity; (3) emotional or painful stimuli; (4) environmental factors such as temperature and noise level; and (5) the use of tobacco, coffee, and other drugs with direct or neurally mediated vasomotor properties.[102] Twenty-four-hour pressures, obtained from normal and hypertensive subjects with an automatic recorder, have shown considerable variability with activity and emotional stimuli.[120,121] The average diurnal pattern of blood pressure consists of an increase throughout the day and early evening and a significant, rapid decline to a low point during the early, deep stage of sleep.

With normal respiration the peak systolic blood pressure is greater during expiration by as much as 10 mmHg than during inspiration. An augmentation of this difference occurs in patients with pericardial tamponade (pulsus paradoxicus; see Chap. 92) and during hyperventilation.

Isotonic exercise in both the supine and upright positions produces a moderate increase in blood pressure (systolic pressure greater than mean greater than diastolic pressure). Sustained isometric muscular contractions produce an abrupt increase in systolic, mean, and diastolic blood pressure that is dependent on the strength of the contraction.[122]

Abnormal Arterial Pressure

Increased Pulse Pressure

An increase in arterial pulse pressure is commonly observed during routine blood pressure recordings. This usually results from an increase in stroke volume and ejection velocity, often associated with a decrease in peripheral resistance. Fever, anemia, hot weather, exercise, hyperthyroidism, or arteriovenous fistulas may produce this change. Several cardiac diseases, such as aortic regurgitation, patent ductus arteriosus, or truncus arteriosus, often result in a widened pulse pressure. An increased pulse pressure due to a large stroke volume may occur with complete heart block or marked sinus bradycardia.[102]

Atherosclerosis of the large arteries often reduces arterial compliance and with a normal or even decreased stroke volume results in an elevated systolic pressure. The systolic hypertension of the elderly does not necessarily represent a change in arteriolar resistance. Efforts to lower this type of systolic pressure elevation are often appropriate but can result in diminished peripheral perfusion. The increased pulse pressure associated with systemic arteriovenous fistulas is less common; a relative tachycardia may be the only clinical clue.

Reduced Pulse Pressure

A narrow pulse pressure is uncommon in normal subjects but may result from an increased peripheral resistance (increased circulating catecholamines in heart failure), decreased stroke volume (severe aortic stenosis), and/or markedly decreased intravascular volume (diabetic ketoacidosis).[102]

Unequal Pulse Pressures

The diagnostic importance of blood pressure differences between right and left arms has been enhanced in recent years by the recognition of supravalvular aortic stenosis[123] in children and the subclavian steal syndrome in adults. Most patients with the former have greater than 20 mmHg higher blood pressure in the right arm. The subclavian steal syndrome, often accompanied by symptoms of cerebrovascular insufficiency, usually results in a pronounced lowering or absence of brachial artery pressure in the ipsilateral extremity.[102]

A progressive increase in systolic pressure normally occurs as the point of measurement is moved peripherally from the central aorta, and the increment in systolic pressure is equivalent in the large arteries of the upper arm and the thigh. Direct recordings of femoral and brachial arterial pressures (systolic, diastolic, and mean) in adults[124] and children[125] and indirect measurement of popliteal and brachial pressures using appropriate pressure cuffs[126] have demonstrated that pressures are equal at these sites. A difference in arm and leg pressures may occur because of coarctation of the aorta or acquired disease such as aortic dissection, aortic arch syndrome, or the subclavian steal syndrome.[102]

Pulsus Alternans

Pulsus alternans may be detected by palpating a peripheral artery. The femoral artery is probably best for this purpose. One must, of course, be certain the heart rhythm is normal. The sphygmomanometer can also be used to identify the beat-to-beat variation in pressure that accompanies pulsus alternans.

Pulsus alternans is discussed later in this chapter. It occurs in patients with severe heart disease who exhibit impaired left ventricular contraction. It can occur for a few beats following supraventricular tachycardia in normal persons. It can also occur when the respiratory rate is half the pulse rate. This may be apparent when pulsus paradoxus is present in patients with cardiac tamponade.

Pulsus Paradoxus

A normal person may exhibit a 10- to 12-mmHg drop in systolic pressure during normal inspiration. A fall in pressure greater than this amount may be identified in patients with acute cardiac tamponade, constrictive pericarditis, severe obstructive lung disease, and restrictive cardiomyopathy.

It may be detected by inflating the blood pressure cuff above systolic pressure and then slowly releasing it. As the cuff pressure is gradually reduced, the blood pressure sounds become audible during expiration. The difference in pressure between the first audible sound heard on expiration and the pressure level at which the sounds are heard during all phases of respiration gives a measurement of magnitude of pulsus paradoxus.

The mechanism of pulsus paradoxus is discussed in Chap. 92.

THE ARTERIAL PULSE

Palpation of the arterial pulse is a basic and important element of the physical examination.[127,128] Any discussion of the arterial pulse must include recent advances in measurement of arterial hemodynamics, assessment of the arterial wave contour, and frequency analysis of the pressure pulse.[128–134]

Physical Determinants of the Arterial Pulse

Genesis of the Arterial Pulse

Pressure and blood flow measurements in the ascending aorta result from the interaction between the heart and arterial system. The rise in left ventricular pressure, on exceeding the aortic pressure, becomes the driving force for the movement of blood into the ascending aorta.[135,136] This driving force is dependent on the intrinsic contractility of ventricle muscle, the size and shape of the left ventricle, and the heart rate. It is opposed by several forces that impede the development of flow and are interrelated in a complex manner. Three major factors contributing to arterial impedance include (1) resistance, (2) inertia, and (3) compliance. Resistance is related to blood viscosity and the geometry of the vasculature; it opposes flow and is unaffected by changes in heart rate. Inertia is related to the mass of the blood, opposes the rate of change of arterial blood flow (i.e., acceleration), and is heart rate dependent. Compliance is related to the distensibility of the vascular walls, opposes changes in arterial blood volume, and is also heart rate dependent. The heart rate dependency of inertia and compliance introduces phase shifts between instantaneous pressure and flow in a pulsatile system.[135] Inertia and compliance are important determinants of the character of ventricular ejection, especially in early systole when flows and pressures are changing rapidly.

The arterial pulse wave begins with aortic valve opening and the onset of left ventricular ejection. Aortic pressure rises rapidly in early systole since the left ventricular stroke volume enters the aorta faster than it flows to distal sites. The rapid-rising portion of the arterial pressure curve is often termed the *anacrotic limb* (from Greek, "upbeat"). Studies in experimental animals and in patients indicate that peak proximal aortic flow velocity occurs slightly earlier than peak pressure.[130] After its peak, aortic pressure declines as ventricular ejection slows and peripheral blood flow continues. During isovolumic relaxation, a transient reversal of flow from the central arteries toward the ventricle just prior to aortic valve closure is associated with an incisura on the descending limb of the aortic pressure pulse. The subsequent smaller, secondary positive wave has been attributed to the elastic recoil of the aorta and aortic valve but is partially due to reflected waves from more distal arteries. Subsequently, aortic pressure decreases again as further "runoff" in the peripheral circulation occurs in diastole.

The proximal aortic pulse pressure is directly proportional to the ratio of stroke volume to arterial distensibility, but multiple factors influence this complex relationship.[137] Arterial distensibility diminishes as the distending arterial pressure increases. Accordingly, the pulse pressure for a constant stroke volume will be larger if the mean blood pressure is elevated. In addition, arterial distensibility varies inversely with the rate of rise of intraluminal pressure. When the systolic ejection rate increases, the stiffer arterial wall results in a greater pulse pressure. Finally, the arterial pulse pressure may be modified by reflected pressure waves and by the rate of blood flow from arterioles to veins.

Contour of the Arterial Pulse

Pulsatile changes in arterial diameter are virtually identical to the pressure pulse, with minor differences explained in terms of nonlinear elasticity and viscosity of the arterial wall. In 1939, Hamilton and Dow defined the pressure wave contour in different arteries in terms of wave reflection between the aortic valve and peripheral sites.[138] In their explanation, the arterial pulse bounded back and forth between the aortic valve and peripheral reflecting sites, setting up a system of "standing waves" in the aorta. The standing wave hypothesis is not completely accurate, however, since some attenuation to the wave in travel occurs and there is incomplete reflection of the wave.[139]

More precise information about the arterial pulse has been obtained from quantitative studies in which a regularly repeated pressure or flow wave is considered as a series of harmonics.[129,140] Each harmonic component has a definite modulus (amplitude) and a definite phase (delay) from a set point of reference. Given the modulus and phase of the different harmonics of the pulse, the original wave can be resynthesized, and corresponding components of waves recorded simultaneously can be compared. By measuring and correlating mean values of the waves, vascular resistance can be calculated and the resistance properties of vessels downstream can be interpreted. The corresponding frequency components of pressure and flow can be compared in order to determine vascular impedance, the relation of pressure to flow at frequencies which are multiples of the heart rate.[129]

Usually, there is a linear relation between pressure and flow at the same point in an artery and between pressure and pressure at different points in the arterial system. From impedance curves, it is possible to identify the factors responsible for the relation between pulsatile pressure and flow.[130,131,136,141] Furthermore, the coefficient of reflection in peripheral vessels can be calculated from the relation of resistance to the minimal and subsequent values of impedance modulus. The peripheral arterial pressure wave recorded is the summation of the incident (initial) and reflected waves. The systemic circulation has been represented by a simple asymmetric T-tube model which emphasizes the importance of wave reflection at two arteriolar reflecting sites in the upper and lower parts of the body.[129,132] An important patient study indicates major reflection sites at the aortic level of the renal arteries and at a point distal to the terminal abdominal aorta bifurcation.[133]

Peripheral Transmission of the Arterial Pulse

As the normal aortic pulse wave is transmitted peripherally, significant changes in its contour occur due to (1) distortion and damping of pulse wave components; (2) different rates of transmission of various components; (3) distortion or exaggeration by reflected, resonant, or standing waves; (4) conversion of kinetic energy into hydrostatic or potential energy; (5) differences in distensibility and caliber of the arteries; and (6) changes in the vessel wall due to age and/or disease.[142]

The arterial pressure pulse enters the proximal aorta and travels distally at a velocity many times faster than

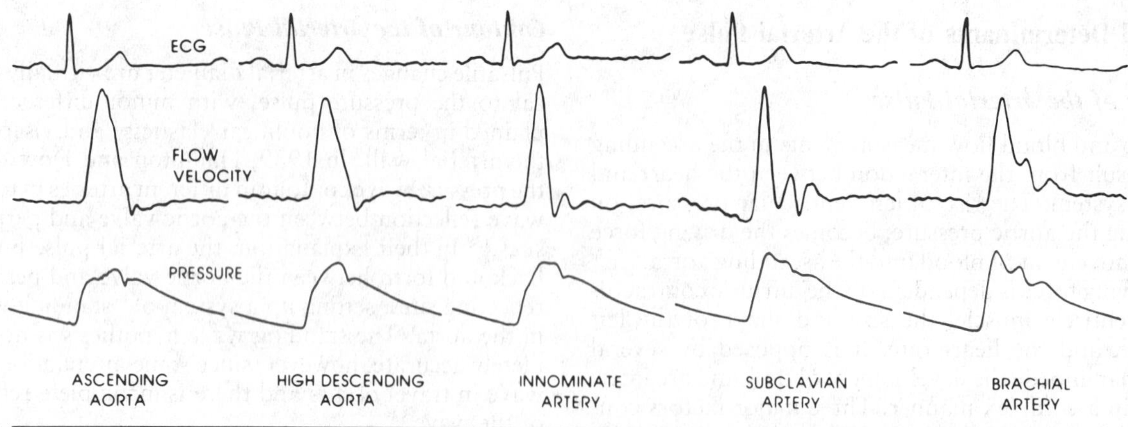

FIGURE 10-26 Simultaneous recording of ECG, catheter-tip flow velocity, and micromanometer pressure in a normal subject as the catheter is moved distally from the ascending aorta. [*From JH Stein (ed): Internal Medicine, 2d ed. Boston, Little, Brown and Company, 1987: 315. Used with permission from the publisher and author.*]

maximum blood flow. The pressure wave is accompanied by a traveling wave distending the arterial wall, the pulse wave velocity increasing as arterial wall distensibility diminishes.[137] This normally occurs distally, as the arteries branch into smaller channels and their walls become stiffer. With increasing age and with systemic hypertension, however, arterial wall distensibility diminishes and pulse wave velocity is correspondingly greater.[129,143,144]

The pulse wave arrives progressively later at more peripheral sites when timed from the QRS complex on the ECG. Representative time delays from the central aorta are as follows: carotid, 30 ms; brachial, 60 ms; radial, 80 ms; and femoral, 75 ms.

The arterial pulse wave undergoes a progressive change in shape during its transmission distally (Fig. 10-26). The pulse pressure and systolic amplitude increase, and the ascending limb of the pulse wave becomes steeper. The incisura of the central aorta pulse is gradually replaced by a smoother, somewhat later, dicrotic notch which occurs at lower pressure levels. The dicrotic notch and the following positive secondary or dicrotic wave probably result from the summation of the forward pulse wave and reflected waves from the peripheral vessels.

Examination of the Arterial Pulse

All major arterial pulses should be examined bilaterally both for patency and for waveform characteristics. The thickness and hardness of the arterial walls often can be assessed by "rolling" the vessel against underlying tissue. A pulse in the foot should not be considered absent unless examined with the foot in the dependent position. Otherwise, the arterial pulses usually are examined with the patient supine and with the trunk of the body slightly elevated.

The examiner uses tactile receptors in the tips of the fingers to sense movement of the arterial wall associated with the pressure pulse as it passes the site of palpation. Measurements in the proximal aorta show cyclic movement in both diameter and length proportional to the pulse pressure.[145] In more peripheral arteries with connective tissue attachments, however, the detectable movement is small and variable, with radial expansion by only about 2 percent of the end-diastolic cross-sectional area.[146]

The usual technique for palpating the arterial pulse is to press with the examining fingers until the maximum pulse is sensed. The pulse is felt as changing displacement superimposed on the "baseline" displacement produced by compressing the artery. The examiner should apply varying degrees of pressure while concentrating on the separate phases of the pulse wave. This method, referred to as *trisection,* is useful for assessing the upstroke, systolic peak, and diastolic slope of the arterial pulse.[142] Controversy exists as to how many fingers should be used to palpate the pulse, and the examiner should use whichever method he or she prefers, being careful not to perceive the examining fingertip pulse as well.

Palpation of the carotid artery is preferred for assessing cardiac performance, since the carotid pulse corresponds more closely to the central aortic pressure. In certain cardiac diseases (e.g., aortic regurgitation), however, the abnormalities detected in the carotid pulse are accentuated in the peripheral pulses. For determining the cardiac rate and rhythm, the radial pulse most often is used; but if it is irregular, cardiac auscultation often provides more reliable information. To evaluate the integrity of the peripheral arterial blood supply and to localize any lesions that exist, the arterial pulses in all four extremities should be examined and compared (Chap. 124).

Inspection of the carotid arterial and jugular venous pulsations should be performed at the same time. The carotid pulse usually is best examined with the sternocleidomastoid muscles relaxed and with the head rotated slightly toward the examiner. The carotid pulse may be timed from the first heart sound, which is heard slightly before the pulsation. The carotid pulse should be palpated in the lower half of the patient's neck in order to avoid carotid sinus compression. Occasionally, it is useful to palpate two arteries simultaneously (e.g., radial and femoral) to detect an apparent pulse wave delay such as occurs in patients with coarctation of the aorta.

The examination of arterial pulses in the abdomen

and upper and lower extremities should be performed carefully in all patients and compared using a scale such as 0 = complete absence of pulsation; 1+ = small or reduced pulsation; 2+ = normal or average pulsation; and 3+ = large or bounding pulsation. Furthermore, auscultation over the major arteries should be performed since an audible bruit may be a clue to partial occlusion or may (e.g., carotid) indicate transmission of a cardiac murmur.

Normal Arterial Pulse

The normal carotid pulse has a smooth, rapid upstroke or ascending limb to a smooth, dome-shaped summit (Fig. 10-27). Then a downstroke occurs which is somewhat less rapid than the upstroke. The dicrotic notch and secondary diastolic wave usually are not felt but may be palpable in some normal individuals or during fever, exercise, or excitement. The dicrotic notch usually occurs about 300 ms after the onset of the pulse wave when corrected for heart rate.

In arteries distal to the carotid, the pulse wave arrives later and has a steep initial wave that rises to a high peak pressure, whereas the diastolic pressure and the mean pressure are slightly lower. The systolic upstroke time (onset of pulse wave to its peak) tends to be shorter and the apparent left ventricular ejection time (onset of pulse wave to incisura) longer in more peripheral arterial pulses. In the brachial artery, the heart rate–corrected systolic upstroke time averages 120 ms (range, 90 to 160 ms) and the systolic ejection time about 320 ms (range, 280 to 360 ms).

Graphic recordings of the arterial pulses frequently show two positive deflections during systole, the first shoulder being referred to as the *percussion wave* and the second as the *tidal wave*. In the normal proximal aortic pulse the percussion wave is due to arrival of the impulse generated by left ventricular ejection, the tidal wave may represent its echo from the upper part of the body, and the dicrotic or diastolic wave is a reflection from the lower part of the body.[129] The contour of the distal pulses can be explained in similar terms with altered time relations between incident and reflected waves at different distances from peripheral reflecting sites.

With aging, there is a relative increase in the second (tidal) systolic wave and the height of the incisura relative to the first systolic wave.[118,131,141,147] The systolic upstroke time is longer, and the amplitude and duration of the diastolic wave tend to be less prominent.

Abnormal Arterial Pulses

In hypertension and arteriosclerosis, the pressure pulse amplitude is increased, the tidal wave is prominent, and the diastolic wave is absent. All features of the pulse can be explained by increased wave velocity.[118,131] Reflected waves return to the proximal aorta during late systole, augmenting the tidal wave and increasing systolic pressure.[118] With systemic hypotension, the pulse wave velocity is decreased and the later tidal and diastolic waves are further displaced from the percussion wave.

Impairment of the pulse of one or both carotid arteries usually is produced by atherosclerosis, but multiple other causes include thrombosis, embolus, arteritis, and diseases of the aortic arch. Kinking of the carotid or brachiocephalic artery is relatively frequent, particularly in hypertensive patients, and may simulate aneurysmal dilatation. Femoral pulses may be diminished in the child and young adult as a result of coarctation of the aorta. In most adults, however, the diminution of the femoral pulsation is caused by atherosclerosis of the abdominal aorta, aortic bifurcation, or ileofemoral arteries (Chap. 123).

Hyperkinetic Arterial Pulse

Large, bounding arterial pulses usually indicate the rapid ejection of an increased volume of blood from the left ventricle (Fig. 10-27*A*). Commonly, the arterial pulse pressure is increased and the peripheral arterial resistance is diminished. The hyperdynamic arterial pulse is sometimes referred to in terms that describe a particular component of the pulse wave. Thus, the water-hammer pulse, named after a Victorian toy, refers to an extremely

A. Hyperkinetic Pulse

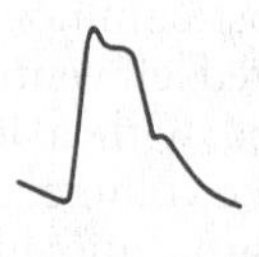

Normal

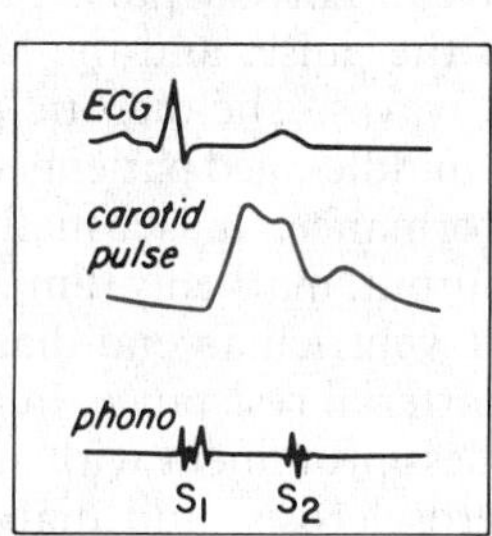

B. Bisferiens Pulse

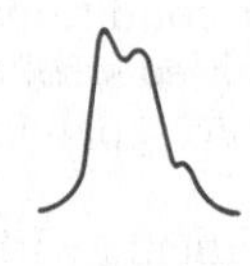

C. Hypokinetic Pulse

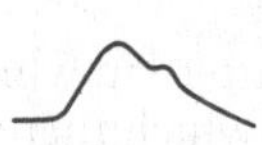

D. Parvus et Tardus Pulse

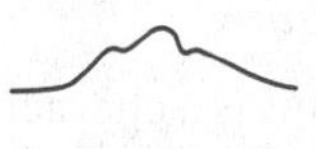

E. Dicrotic Pulse + Alternans

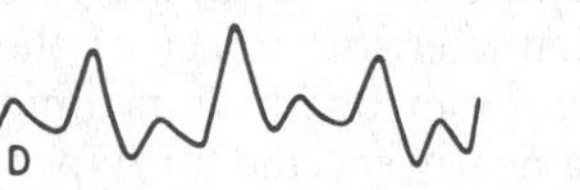

FIGURE 10-27 Schematic representation of the normal carotid arterial pulse, five types of abnormal pulses and pulsus alternans. ECG = electrocardiogram; phono = phonocardiogram; S_1, S_2 = first and second heart sounds; S = systolic; D = diastole.

rapid, forceful ascending limb of the arterial pulse wave.[148] By contrast, "collapsing pulse" refers to a quick, marked decrease in the arterial pulse wave following its peak. Hyperkinetic pulses often are more prominent in the brachial, radial, or femoral arteries than in the carotid artery. The term *Quincke pulse* refers to visible small pulsations in the nail bed of patients with hyperdynamic arterial pulses from any cause, including aortic regurgitation.

Hyperkinetic arterial pulses occur in normal subjects with a hyperkinetic circulation (e.g., exercise, fever), patients with cardiovascular diseases associated with increased stroke volume, and subjects with marked bradycardia and an extremely large stroke volume (e.g., athletes). A hyperdynamic arterial pulse also occurs in patients with an abnormally rapid runoff of blood from the arterial system (e.g., patent ductus arteriosus, arteriovenous fistulas). Patients on chronic hemodialysis often have hyperdynamic pulses produced by the combination of a surgical arteriovenous fistula, anemia, and hypertension.

In aortic regurgitation, the rapid-rising, bounding arterial pulse results from an increase in stroke volume and the rate of left ventricular ejection. The early systolic flow often produces palpable vibrations manifested as a thrill on the steep ascending limb. Later in systole, the rate of ventricular ejection and the arterial pulse wave decrease sharply, often resulting in systolic collapse.[136]

Bisferiens Arterial Pulse

The bisferiens (from Latin, "twice beating") pulse has a waveform characterized by two positive waves during systole (Fig. 10-27*B*). The pulse wave upstroke rises rapidly and forcefully, producing the first systolic peak (percussion wave). A brief decline in pressure is followed by a smaller and somewhat slower-rising positive pulse wave (tidal wave). Abnormalities of left ventricular ejection and reflected waves from peripheral arteries contribute to the prominence of the second systolic wave in the bisferiens pulse. The bisferiens pulse, usually felt in the carotid artery, is sometimes more easily palpable in a brachial or radial artery. A bisferiens pulse often occurs in patients with aortic regurgitation and in patients with combined aortic stenosis and severe aortic regurgitation.[149–152] It also occurs commonly in other conditions associated with the rapid ejection of an increased stroke volume from the left ventricle (e.g., exercise, fever, patent ductus arteriosus).

The bisferiens pulse often is present in patients with hypertrophic cardiomyopathy, many of whom have a pressure gradient in the left ventricular outflow tract.[153] In this syndrome, the midsystolic negative wave usually coincides with a marked decrease in the rate of left ventricular ejection. The second systolic wave, or tidal wave, most likely is produced by reflected waves from the periphery. The bisferiens pulse may be elicited by maneuvers that decrease the left ventricular size or increase its contractility. The most characteristic aspect of the arterial pulse in hypertrophic cardiomyopathy is its rapid rate of rise. A physical finding nearly specific for hypertrophic cardiomyopathy is a much smaller arterial pressure pulse in the cardiac cycle following a premature ventricular beat. (See also Chap. 90.)

Hypokinetic Arterial Pulse

A small, weak arterial pulse frequently is present in patients with a diminished stroke volume (Fig. 10-27*C*). Usually, the decreased stroke output is associated with decreased rate and duration of left ventricular ejection, and there is a narrow arterial pulse pressure despite an increased arterial resistance. Common causes include hypovolemia, left ventricular failure, and mitral or aortic valve stenosis.

Parvus et Tardus Pulse

Patients with moderate or severe valvular aortic stenosis often have an arterial pulse that is small and has a delayed systolic peak.[154,155] Occasionally, there may be a detectable shoulder on the upstroke of the carotid pulse, referred to as anacrotic (Fig. 10-27*D*).[156] Palpable coarse vibrations are often present as a systolic thrill over the slowly rising carotid pulse. The *parvus et tardus* pulse is much easier to detect in the carotid arteries than in more distal arteries.

Most middle-aged patients with uncomplicated severe aortic stenosis have a parvus et tardus pulse, but this pulse may also occur in relatively mild stenosis. Furthermore, an apparently normal arterial pulse is not unusual in elderly patients with severe aortic stenosis due to the decreased distensibility of the large arteries, which also alters the character of the arterial pulse.[119,157] Severe left ventricular failure often results in a small, weak pulse which may be difficult to distinguish from that of aortic stenosis.

Dicrotic Arterial Pulse

The dicrotic (from Greek, "double beating") pulse is a twice-peaked pulse with one peak in systole and the second in diastole, the latter due to an accentuated and palpable dicrotic wave that follows the second heart sound (Fig. 10-27*E*).[158] It is usually felt best in the carotids, although it may also be palpated over more peripheral arteries. Major abnormalities include a short systolic ejection phase, a low dicrotic notch, a large diastolic wave, a narrow pulse pressure, a diminished rate of rise of the pulse, and the lack of distinct percussion and tidal waves. The dicrotic pulse is most common in young or middle-aged patients with impaired left ventricular performance. It is usually associated with a low cardiac output, markedly diminished stroke volume, elevated left ventricular end-diastolic pressure, and high systemic arterial resistance. In general, the dicrotic wave becomes less prominent with age, hypertension, generalized atherosclerosis, and diabetes. Rarely, the dicrotic wave can be palpated in young febrile patients in whom none of the other abnormal features of the dicrotic pulse are present.

Pulsus Alternans

Pulsus alternans is a characteristic pulse pattern in which the beats occur at regular intervals but in which there is a regular attenuation of the systolic height of the pressure pulses (Fig. 10-27*E*).[159,160] Rarely, pulsus alternans is so marked that the weaker pulses are not felt at all. When pulsus alternans is noticed first after a premature beat, the extent of the difference in systolic pressure in alternating beats declines for several cycles until the pulse amplitude is again constant. The initiation of post-premature ventricular beat pulsus alternans is probably related to the increased duration of left ventricular filling after the premature beat, resulting in a greater end-diastolic volume and hence increased contractile force due to the Frank-Starling mechanism.[161]

Severe depression of left ventricular performance often results in sustained pulsus alternans. There is an alteration in aortic flow, systolic left ventricular pressure, aortic systolic pressure, left ventricular *dP/dt,* and left ventricular end-diastolic pressure. Sustained pulsus alternans likely is due to alteration of the contractile state of at least part of the myocardium, which may be caused by the failure of electromechanical coupling in some cells during the weaker contraction.[162] A subsequent stronger contraction would then represent contraction of all cells, some of which were potentiated.

Pulsus alternans may be better appreciated when palpating a distal artery that has a slightly wider pulse pressure than the carotid artery. It is often brought out or accentuated when the patient assumes the upright position, thus decreasing venous return. The patient's respiration should be held since the small changes in arterial pressure caused by normal respiration may obscure the recognition of pulsus alternans. Pulsus alternans can be confirmed by using a sphygmomanometer and is usually associated with a left ventricular third heart sound.

Pulsus Paradoxus

A paradoxical pulse (see also Chap. 92) is defined as a marked decrease in the pulse amplitude during normal quiet inspiration or a decrease in the systolic arterial pressure by more than 10 mmHg. The normal small decline in systolic blood pressure probably is produced predominantly by relative pooling of blood in the pulmonary vessels during inspiration and may also reflect the delayed transmission through the lungs of the preceding expiratory fall in venous pressure and right ventricular cardiac output.[142]

In patients with cardiac tamponade, fluid accumulation in the pericardium increases intrapericardial pressure, and the heart's filling capacity is reduced. During inspiration, the expected augmentation of venous return to the right side of the heart occurs despite the elevated intrapericardial pressure.[163] The diminished thoracic pressure also causes a pooling of blood in the pulmonary capillaries and diminishes pulmonary venous return to the left atrium. Since the high intrapericardial pressure limits flow to the heart and the total cardiac filling capacity is limited, the increase in right-sided heart volume with inspiration causes an obligatory decrease in left-sided heart filling. This, along with the pooling of blood in the pulmonary bed, produces a decline in left ventricular stroke volume and systolic blood pressure during inspiration.[164] Pulsus paradoxus is common with cardiac tamponade but infrequent with constrictive pericarditis. (See also Chap. 92.)

Different hemodynamic mechanisms contribute to the production of a paradoxical pulse in certain patients with superior vena cava obstruction, asthma, or obstructive airway disease and in some patients with pulmonary embolism, shock, or postthoracotomy.[142]

The extent of pulsus paradoxicus can be quantitated by cuff sphygmomanometry as the pressure difference between the first discernible Korotkoff sound on expiration and the pressure level at which Korotkoff sounds are audible during all phases of respiration.

Effects of Arrhythmias on the Arterial Pulse

Premature Ventricular Depolarizations

A premature ventricular depolarization may be associated with no pulse, a small-amplitude pulse, or a normal arterial pulse, depending on timing and whether or not the left ventricular pressure generated is able to open the aortic valve. The arterial pulse following a premature beat usually is greatly enhanced because of decreased aortic impedance, increased left ventricular filling, and augmented left ventricular contractility. At times, premature ventricular beats are so common as to produce an irregularly irregular pulse. Then, the presence of cannon *a* waves in the jugular venous pulse should alert one to the correct diagnosis.

Tachyarrhythmias

The ECG usually is needed for the definitive diagnosis of any abnormality of heart rate or rhythm. On the other hand, careful observation of the arterial and jugular venous pulses frequently leads to the correct diagnosis.

Most tachycardias associated with a regular pulse are of supraventricular origin. In sinus tachycardia the arterial pulse will gradually slow with carotid sinus pressure and then again gradually increase. Paroxysmal atrial tachycardia has an "all-or-none" response. Carotid sinus pressure will increase the block at the AV junction in patients with atrial flutter, the pulse rate slowing and subsequently returning to its original rate in a "jerky" fashion.

In patients with ventricular tachycardia and AV dissociation, the variation in the atrial-ventricular sequence of contraction and resulting pulse amplitude may often be detected by palpation.

An irregularly irregular pulse with a varying pulse pressure is usually the result of atrial fibrillation; however, multifocal atrial tachycardia is also a common cause of this finding in patients with severe chronic obstructive lung disease.

Bradyarrhythmias

An unusually slow heart rate frequently is associated with a decrease in the rate of rise and amplitude of the arterial pressure pulse. Complete heart block is readily diagnosed by the variability in the arterial pulse amplitude, the changing intensity of the first heart sound, and intermittent cannon *a* waves in the jugular venous pulse.

VENOUS PULSE

The evaluation of the venous pulse is an integral part of the physical examination since it reflects both the mean right atrial pressure and the hemodynamic events in the right atrium. Factors influencing the right atrial and central venous pressure (CVP) include the total blood volume, the distribution of blood volume, and right atrial contraction.

Venous blood returning from the systemic capillaries is nonpulsatile. Changes in volume flow created by skeletal muscles and respiratory pump are nonsynchronous with the pulsatile activity of the heart. Changes in flow and pressure caused by right atrial and ventricular filling, however, produce pulsations in the central veins that are transmitted toward the peripheral veins, opposite to the direction of blood flow. With the possible exception of the *c* wave, which is the combined result of carotid arterial impact and an upward movement of the tricuspid valve, the pulsations observed in the neck are produced by right atrial and ventricular activity.[165]

Examination of the Jugular Venous Pulse

The two main objectives of the bedside examination of the neck veins are the estimation of the CVP and the inspection of the waveform. Usually, the right internal jugular vein is superior for both purposes. In most normal subjects, the maximum pulsation of the internal jugular vein is observed when the trunk is inclined by less than 30°. In patients with an elevated venous pressure, it may be necessary to elevate the trunk further, sometimes to as much as 90°.[166] When the neck muscles are relaxed, shining a beam of light tangently across the skin overlying the internal jugular vein exposes its pulsations. Simultaneous palpation of the left carotid artery aids the examiner in deciding which pulsations are venous.

Measurements of Venous Pressure

The difference between venous distension and venous pressure elevation must be considered. Veins may be markedly dilated with minimal increase in pressure or may not be visibly distended despite a very high venous pressure. Venous pressure may be estimated by examining the veins in the dorsum of the hand. With the patient sitting or lying at a 30° elevation or greater, the arm is slowly and passively raised from a dependent position. When the venous pressure is normal, the veins collapse when the dorsum of the hand reaches the level of the sternal angle of Louis. Unfortunately, local venous obstruction or augmented peripheral venous constriction may diminish the accuracy of estimating CVP by this method.

The external or internal jugular veins may also be used to estimate venous pressure.[167] Because of its more direct route to the right atrium, the internal jugular vein is superior for the estimation of venous pressure and assessment of the venous waveform. The patient is examined at the optimum degree of trunk elevation for visualization of venous pulsations. The vertical distance from the top of the oscillating venous column to the level of the sternal angle is generally less than 3 cm (3 cm + 5 cm = 8 cm). Greatly elevated venous pressure may be missed by failing to elevate adequately the patient's head. It may be necessary to actually have the patient sit upright. If the "pulsating meniscus" is very high, pulsations may be inappropriate in the lower neck. When venous engorgement is marked, the patient's earlobe may pulsate and even the veins on the top of the head may be distended.

In patients suspected of right ventricular failure but having normal resting venous pressure, the abdominojugular (also known as hepatojugular) test is useful.[168] With the patient breathing normally, firm pressure is applied with the palm of the hand to the upper right quadrant of the abdomen for 10 or more s. The patient should be instructed to continue to breathe normally during the test. In most subjects the venous pressure is not altered significantly. In some normal patients there is a transient increase in jugular venous pressure with a *rapid return* to or near baseline in less than 10 s. The dysfunctioning right ventricle, however, is unable to accept the increment in blood volume due to enhanced venous return without a marked increase in its filling pressure, which is transmitted to the neck veins. In patients with right ventricular failure, which often results from left-sided heart failure, the venous pressure either rises rapidly and declines slowly during abdominal compression or remains elevated by 4 or more centimeters of blood until pressure is released (Fig. 10-28).[172] Ducas et al. also studied the abdominojugular test and attested to the accuracy of the test results.[169]

Analysis of Venous Waveforms

Again the patient's trunk should be inclined to whatever elevation is necessary to reveal the top of the oscillating venous column.[128,170] Having the patient take a slow, deep inspiration will increase the amplitude of the presystolic *a* wave while decreasing the mean right atrial pressure. This is a useful technique for identifying the site at which the pulsations will be best visualized. Simultaneous palpation of the left carotid artery aids the examiner in relating the venous pulsations to the timing of the cardiac cycle.

Normal Venous Pulse

The normal jugular venous pulse (JVP) reflects phasic pressure changes in the right atrium and consists of three positive waves and two negative troughs (Fig. 10-29). In considering this pulse, it is useful to refer to the events of the cardiac cycle. The positive presystolic *a* wave is produced by right atrial contraction and is the dominant wave in the JVP, particularly during inspiration.

During atrial relaxation, the venous pulse descends from the summit of the *a* wave. Depending on the PR interval, this descent may continue until a plateau (z point) is reached just prior to right ventricular systole. More often, the descent is interrupted by a second positive venous wave, the *c* wave, which is produced by bulging of the tricuspid valve into the right atrium during right ventricular isovolumic systole and by the impact of the carotid artery adjacent to the jugular vein.[171] Following the summit of the *c* wave, the JVP contour declines,

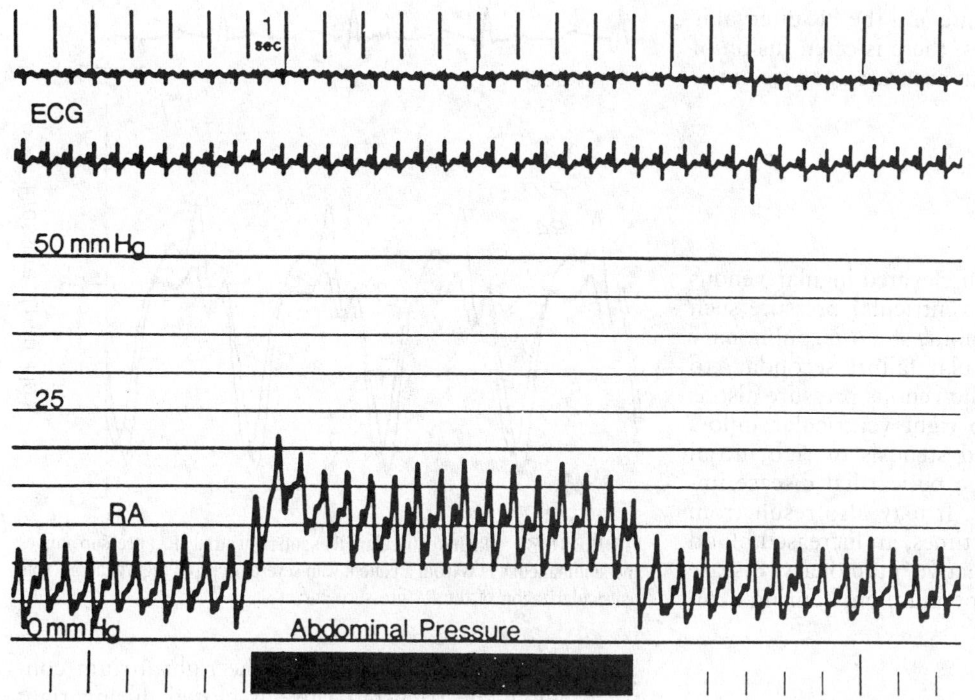

FIGURE 10-28 Elevation in right atrial (RA) pressure observed during abdominal pressure in patient with mild congestive heart failure. *(From GA Ewy: The abdominojugular test: Technique and hemodynamic correlates. Ann Intern Med 109:456, 1989. Used with permission from the publisher and author.)*

forming the normal negative systolic wave, the *x* wave. The *x* descent is due to a combination of atrial relaxation, the downward displacement of the tricuspid valve during right ventricular systole, and the ejection of blood from both ventricles.

The positive, late systolic *v* wave in the JVP results from the increase in blood volume in the venae cavae and right atrium during ventricular systole when the tricuspid valve is closed. After the peak of the *v* wave is reached, the right atrial pressure decreases because of the diminished bulging of the tricuspid valve into the right atrium and the decline in right ventricular pressure which follow tricuspid valve opening. The latter occurs at the peak of the *v* wave in the JVP. Following the summit of the *v* wave, there is a negative descending limb, referred to as the *y* descent or diastolic collapse, which is due to the tricuspid valve opening and the rapid inflow of blood into the right ventricle. The initial *y* descent corresponds to the right ventricular rapid-filling phase. The trough of the *y* wave occurs in early diastole and is followed by the ascending limb of the *y* wave, which is produced by continued diastolic inflow of blood into the right side of the heart. The velocity of this ascending pressure curve depends on the rate of venous return and the distensibility of the chambers of the right side of the heart. When diastole is long, the ascending limb of the *y* wave is often followed by a small, brief, positive wave, the *h* wave, which occurs just prior to the next *a* wave. At times, there is a plateau phase rather than a distinct *h* wave. With increasing heart rate, the *y* trough and *y* ascent are followed immediately by the next *a* wave. (See also Plate II, 5-1.)

Usually, there are three visible major positive waves *(a, c, v)* and two negative waves *(x, y)* when the pulse

A. Tricuspid Regurgitation

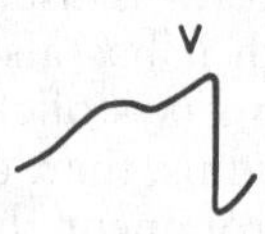

Normal

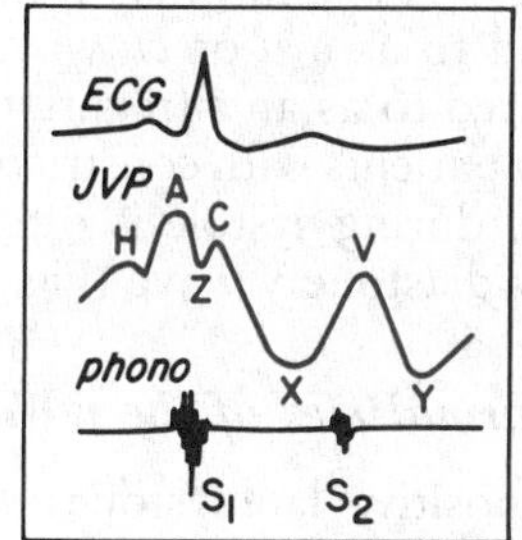

B. Tricuspid Stenosis

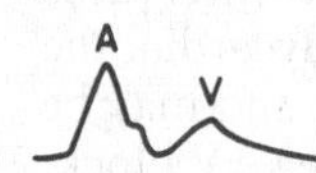

C. Constrictive Pericarditis

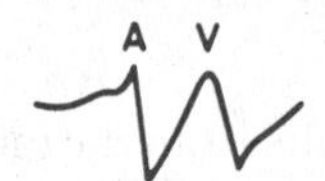

D. Atrial Septal Defect

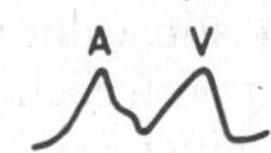

E. Atrial Fibrillation

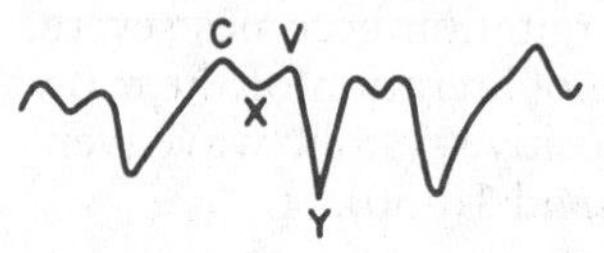

F. First Degree AV Block

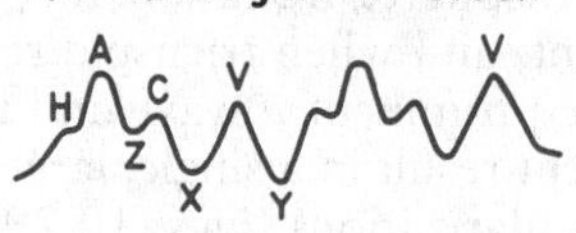

G. Complete AV Block

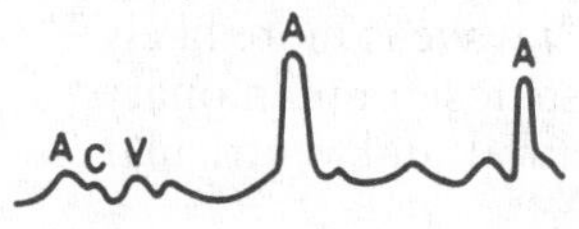

FIGURE 10-29 Schematic representation of the normal jugular venous pulse (JVP), four types of abnormal JVPs, and the JVPs in three arrhythmias. See text for definition of H, A, Z, C, X, V, and Y.

rate is below 90 beats per minute and the PR interval is normal. With faster heart rates, there is often fusion of some of the pulse waves, and an accurate analysis of the waveform is more difficult.

Abnormal Venous Pulse

Elevated Venous Pressure

The most common cause of an elevated jugular venous pressure is an increased right ventricular pressure such as occurs in patients with pulmonic stenosis, pulmonary hypertension, or right ventricular failure secondary to right ventricular infarction. The venous pressure also is elevated when obstruction to right ventricular inflow occurs, such as with tricuspid stenosis or right atrial myxoma, or when constrictive pericardial disease impedes right ventricular inflow. It may also result from vena cava obstruction and, at times, an increased blood volume. Patients with obstructive pulmonary disease may have an elevated venous pressure only during expiration.

Kussmaul's Sign

Normally there is an increase in the *a* wave of the JVP but a decrease in the mean jugular venous pressure during inspiration as a result of the increased filling of the right-sided chambers associated with the decline in intrathoracic pressure. An inspiratory increase in the venous pressure may occur in patients with severe constrictive pericarditis when the heart is unable to accept the increase in right ventricular volume without a marked increase in the filling pressure.[172] Although Kussmaul's sign was first described in patients with constrictive pericarditis, its most common cause is severe right-sided heart failure, regardless of etiology. The presence of Kussmaul's sign is also useful in the diagnosis of right ventricular infarction.[173] (See also Chap. 92.)

Abnormalities of the a Wave

The *a* wave in the JVP is absent when there is no effective atrial contraction, such as in atrial fibrillation (Fig. 10-29*E*). In certain other conditions, the *a* wave may not be apparent. In sinus tachycardia the *a* wave may fuse with the preceding *v* wave, particularly if the PR interval is prolonged. In some patients with sinus tachycardia, the *a* wave may occur during the *v* or *y* descent and may be small or absent. In the presence of first-degree AV block, a discrete *a* wave with ascending and descending limbs is often completed prior to the first heart sound and the *ac* interval is prolonged (Fig. 10-29*F*).

Large *a* waves are of considerable diagnostic value (Fig. 10-29*B*). When giant *a* waves are present with each beat, the right atrium is contracting against an increased resistance. This may result from obstruction at the tricuspid valve (tricuspid stenosis or atresia, right atrial myxoma) or conditions associated with increased resistance to right ventricular filling. A giant *a* wave is more likely to occur in patients with pulmonic stenosis or pulmonary hypertension in whom both the atrial and ventricular septa are intact.

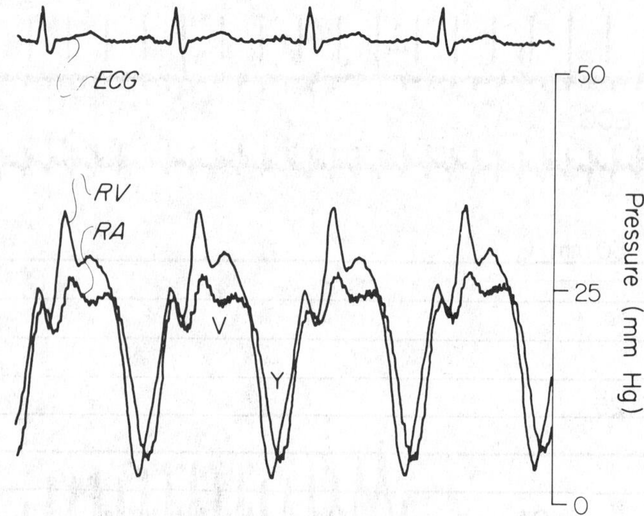

FIGURE 10-30 Right ventricular (RV) and right atrial (RA) pressure curves and simultaneous ECG from a patient with severe tricuspid regurgitation. Note ventricularization of the RA pressure curve.

Cannon *a* waves occur when the right atrium contracts while the tricuspid valve is closed during right ventricular systole. Cannon waves may occur either regularly or irregularly and are most common in the presence of arrhythmias (Fig. 10-29*G*).

Abnormalities of the x Wave

The most important alteration of the normally negative systolic collapse (*x* wave) of the JVP is its obliteration or even replacement by a positive wave. This is usually due to tricuspid regurgitation.[174,175] Although atrial relaxation may contribute to the normal *x* descent, the development of atrial fibrillation does not obliterate the *x* wave except in the presence of tricuspid regurgitation. Accordingly, the occurrence of a positive wave in the JVP during ventricular systole is strong evidence of tricuspid regurgitation (Figs. 10-29*A* and 10-30). Mild tricuspid regurgitation lessens and shortens the downward *x* wave as the regurgitation of blood into the right atrium produces a positive wave that diminishes the usual systolic fall in venous pressure. In some patients with moderate tricuspid regurgitation, there is a fairly distinct positive wave during ventricular systole between the *c* and *v* waves. This abnormal systolic waveform is usually referred to as a *v* or *cv* wave, although it has also been referred to as an *r* (regurgitant) or an *s* (systolic) wave.

In patients with constrictive pericarditis, the *x* descent wave during systole is often more prominent than the early diastolic *y* wave (Fig. 10-29*C*).

Abnormalities of the v Wave

The positive, late systolic *v* wave results from the increasing right atrial blood volume during ventricular systole when the tricuspid valve normally is closed. With mild tricuspid regurgitation, the *v* wave becomes more prominent, and when tricuspid regurgitation becomes severe, the prominent *v* wave and the obliteration of the *x* descent result in a single, large positive systolic wave (ventricularization) (Figs. 10-29*A* and 10-30).

Normally the *v* wave is lower in amplitude than the *a* wave in the JVP. In patients with an atrial septal defect, however, the higher left atrial pressure is transmitted to the right atrium and the *a* and *v* waves are often equal in the right atrium and the JVP (Fig. 10-29*D*).[176] In patients with constrictive pericarditis and sinus rhythm, the right atrial *a* and *v* waves may also be equal, but the venous pressure is increased, which is unusual with isolated atrial septal defect. In patients with constrictive pericarditis who are in atrial fibrillation, the *cv* wave is prominent and the *y* descent rapid.

Abnormalities of the y Trough

The *y* descent, or diastolic collapse, is produced mainly by the tricuspid valve opening and the rapid inflow of blood into the right ventricle. A rapid, deep *y* descent in early diastole occurs with severe tricuspid regurgitation (Fig. 10-29*A*). A venous pulse characterized by a sharp *y* descent, a deep *y* trough, and a rapid ascent to the baseline is seen in patients with constrictive pericarditis or with severe right-sided heart failure. A slow *y* descent in the JVP suggests an obstruction to right ventricular filling and may be the only abnormal finding in patients with tricuspid stenosis or right atrial myxoma (Fig. 10-29*B*). In both constrictive pericarditis and severe right-sided heart failure, the venous pressure is elevated with a sharp *y* dip in the JVP. (See also Chap. 92.) The presence of a large positive systolic venous wave favors the diagnosis of severe heart failure.

Effects of Arrhythmias of the Venous Pulse

Large *a* waves in the JVP during arrhythmias are present when the P wave (atrial contraction) occurs between the onset of the QRS complex and the termination of the T wave (Fig. 10-29*G*). Such cannon *a* waves may occur regularly in junctional rhythm. More commonly, they occur irregularly when AV dissociation accompanies premature ventricular beats, ventricular tachycardia, or complete heart block. The *a* wave is absent in patients with atrial fibrillation, and flutter *a* waves at a regular rate of 250 to 300 per minute frequently are observed in patients with atrial flutter and varying degrees of AV block. Patients with multifocal atrial tachycardia often have prominent and somewhat variable *a* waves in the JVP. In these patients, many of whom have pulmonary hypertension secondary to lung disease, the *a* waves are often very large.

INSPECTION AND PALPATION OF THE PRECORDIUM

Inspection and palpation of the cardiac pulsations on the anterior chest have been practiced by physicians since ancient times and have a solid scientific basis.[178–180] The results of precordial inspection and palpation have been correlated with noninvasive studies, hemodynamic data, and surgical and autopsy studies.[179,180] Currently, inspection and palpation of the precordium remain an important part of the cardiovascular examination.[181–184] Their usefulness depends on an understanding of cardiovascular physiology, the proficiency of the examiner and the ability to integrate findings with history, the information obtained by other portions of the physical examination, the ECG, chest roentgenogram, and other diagnostic tests.[180] Thoughtful inspection and palpation of the precordium form the foundation for accurate interpretation of the arterial and venous pulses, heart sounds, and murmurs.[179]

Precordial Pulsations Due to the Heartbeat

Precordial pulsations, reflecting underlying movement of the heart and great vessels, occur principally in seven areas of the anterior chest[179,180] (Fig. 10-31):

1. the sternoclavicular area,
2. the aortic area,
3. the pulmonic area,
4. the right ventricular (left parasternal) area,
5. the apical (left ventricular) area,
6. the epigastric area, and
7. ectopic (variable-location) areas.

This classification requires some qualification.[179] While the cardiac apex usually is occupied by the left ventricle, it sometimes consists of an enlarged right ventricle that displaces the left ventricle laterally and posterior. Occasionally, the cardiac position is abnormal due to dextroposition, dextroversion, dextrocardia, or other changes in intrathoracic structures. Although the cardiac apex impulse commonly is referred to as *point of maximal impulse* (PMI), the two terms are not necessarily synonymous since the maximal precordial pulsation may reflect an enlarged or hypertrophied right ventricle, a dilated aorta or pulmonary artery, or a left ventricular wall motion abnormality. Therefore, precordial pulsations should be described by their location, timing, contour, and duration.[179,180,184]

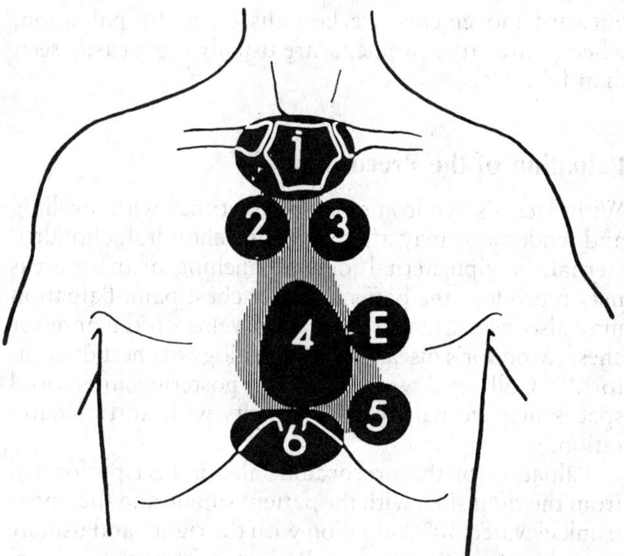

FIGURE 10-31 Seven areas to be examined for abnormal cardiovascular pulsations by inspection and palpation. *(From RC Schlant, JW Hurst: Examination of the Precordium: Inspection and Palpation. New York, American Heart Association, 1990: 1–28. Used with permission from the publisher and authors.)*

Inspection of the Precordium

The examiner should first inspect the thorax from the foot of the bed with the subject supine, the legs horizontal, and the head and trunk elevated to approximately 30°.[179] Important information often results. The patient may have a barrel-shaped chest with an increased anteroposterior diameter, a straight-back syndrome, pectus excavatum, pectus carinatum, kyphoscoliosis, or ankylosing spondylitis. Each may produce or be associated with cardiac abnormalities. Asymmetry of the thorax due to convex bulging of the precordium suggests the presence of heart disease since childhood. Exaggerated movements of the cardiac apex often can be detected from this observation point.

Next, the examiner should move to the patient's right side and observe the patient's chest tangentially, rather than from above. A light beam directed across the precordium may enhance subtle findings.[179,180] Precordial movements frequently can be more easily recognized if the tip of an applicator stick, tongue blade, or light pencil is held against the impulse as a fulcrum. Motion of the underlying chest wall is transmitted to the free end of the instrument and exaggerated, making the movements more obvious.[179,180]

In patients with an abnormally prominent apical impulse and in some thin, normal individuals, the apical impulse or apex beat can be seen. Presystolic apical motion associated with the atrial contribution to ventricular filling (a fourth heart sound) sometimes may be visualized as may the diastolic waveform due to rapid ventricular filling (a third heart sound). A late systolic bulge either at the apex or in an ectopic area, usually located either medial and superior or lateral to the apical impulse, may be observed in patients with a large dyskinetic ventricular aneurysm.[180]

It is important to inspect the entire anterior chest. When precordial pulsations are exaggerated, they become visible as well as palpable. However, in general, outward movements are best discerned by palpation, whereas inward movements are usually more easily seen than felt.[179,180]

Palpation of the Precordium

With Tietze's syndrome pain, sometimes with swelling and tenderness, may affect the costochondral, chondrosternal, or xiphisternal joints. Touching of these areas may reproduce the patient's exact chest pain. Palpation may also reveal tender superficial veins on the anterior chest (Mondor's disease), a rare etiology of chest discomfort.[180] Collateral vessels in the posterior intercostal spaces may be palpable in patients with aortic coarctation.[180]

Palpation of the precordium also is best performed from the right side, with the patient supine and the upper trunk elevated 30°. Palpation with the right hand usually provides more information. Patients with suspected cardiovascular disease should also be examined in the left lateral decubitus position, rotated 45 to 90°.[180,184,185] In this position, the normal left ventricular impulse may be displaced several centimeters leftward and may appear more prominent and sustained. The size of the apex impulse rather than its distance from the midsternal or midclavicular line determines its normality.[185] Often, the apex impulse and other palpable events such as a left ventricular rapid filling wave (S_3) or presystolic *a* wave (S_4) may be felt only in this position.[180,185]

The examiner should define the location and size of the cardiac apex impulse, characterize its contour, and identify any abnormal precordial pulsations. The palm of the hand, ventral surface of the proximal metacarpals, and fingers should all be used for the optimal appreciation of specific movements. The fingers appear to be particularly insensitive to relatively large amplitude, very low frequency movements.[187] This is consistent with the clinical observation that an examiner's hand occasionally can be visualized to move up and down with precordial motion, although the same movements are imperceptible by palpation alone.[179] By contrast, higher frequency events, such as the vibrations associated with abnormally loud aortic or pulmonic components of the second heart sound, are easily palpable, even though the amplitude of their movement is not readily visible.[179]

The pads of the fingers are most useful for detecting left ventricular and normal right ventricular motion while the palm and proximal metacarpals are best used for palpating larger, low-frequency movements such as the parasternal systolic lift of right ventricular hypertrophy.[179] Varying pressure with the hand is useful. High-frequency movements such as ejection sounds, valve closure sounds, and mitral opening snaps are more easily detected with the hand held firmly against the chest while low-frequency movements such as ventricular diastolic filling events are best recognized with light pressure with the fingertips.

Thrills are palpable vibrations from murmurs or bruits ordinarily associated with grade 4/6 murmurs or louder (Chap. 11). The location of a thrill often helps identify its origin. Thrills are most easily palpated with the fingertips or with firm pressure using either the palm of the hand or proximal metacarpals. Sometimes, thrills are felt better during a held-end expiration with moderate pressure applied from the right hand on top of the left hand, which is placed on the chest.[180] Occasionally, palpable murmurs are more readily detected with the right palm placed over the anterior chest and the left hand supporting the posterior thorax with equal force.[180]

To detect abnormal right ventricular motion, the heel of the hand should be placed over the lower half of the sternum with the patient's breath held at end expiration.[179] The parasternal lift due to right ventricular hypertrophy often is better visualized than actually felt. In patients with chronic obstructive pulmonary disease, subxyphoid and epigastric palpation with the patient's breath held at end inspiration is useful for assessing right ventricular motion.[180]

As indicated above, proper patient positioning is important. The location of the apex impulse usually is described in terms of its distance from the midsternal or midclavicular line and the intercostal space in which it is located. Although heart size commonly is estimated based on the size and location of the apex impulse with the patient supine, this is not always a reliable indicator of left ventricular end-diastolic volume.[185–187] The apex impulse is often faint or not palpable with the patient supine because of the distance of the ventricular apex from the chest wall. Palpation of the cardiac apex with the patient in the left lateral position, however, permits optimal assessment of the size (diameter) and contour of the systolic outward movement at the apex; diastolic movements are also best appreciated with the patient in this position.[185,188] Since the apex impulse may shift several centimeters laterally when the patient rotates to the left lateral position, the location of the apex impulse may be incorrect in this position. Palpation with coincident cardiac auscultation often is useful for identifying the systolic or diastolic timing of various precordial pulsations. Simultaneous palpation of the apical impulse and carotid pulse may be helpful in assessing the severity of aortic stenosis. An appreciable lag time between the onset of the apex impulse and carotid pulse usually indicates severe aortic stenosis.[189]

Physiology of Precordial Motion

Although only the apical impulse is palpable normally, a brief right ventricular systolic motion can be felt at the left sternal edge in asthenic individuals. With the onset of isovolumic left ventricular contraction there is anterior movement of the left ventricle toward the chest wall (Fig. 10-32).[179] Counterclockwise rotation of the left ventricle along its longitudinal axis occurs as the cardiac apex moves anteriorly and makes contact with the chest wall in early systole.[189–193] The maximal outward movement occurs coincident with or just after aortic valve opening. After rapid early ejection, the left ventricle moves away from the chest wall and the apex retracts during latter systole and returns to baseline well before the second heart sound.[179] The outward apex movement in early systole normally is palpable but the later systolic inward movement is only visible (Fig. 10-32). Palpable movements of the apex in diastole result from left ventricular filling. The early diastolic outward movement due to rapid ventricular filling (F wave) is occasionally palpable in normal children and young adults (Fig. 10-32). Late diastolic filling due to left atrial contraction (A wave) is not normally palpable. Precordial motion is modified by age, chest wall thickness, lung disease, and pleural or pericardial effusion.[179]

Area 1: Sternoclavicular Area Pulsations

The sternoclavicular area (Fig. 10-31) includes the right and left sternoclavicular joints, the manubrium, and the upper sternum. Usually, no pulsation is noted in this area. A slight, brief systolic pulsation of a sternoclavicular joint or the manubrium may be due to aortic regurgitation. Abnormal pulsations and movements in the sternoclavicular area are commonly produced by enlargement, dilatation, or diseases of the aorta, particularly aortic dissection, atherosclerotic aneurysm, or syphilitic aneurysm.[180] An abnormal pulsation of a sternoclavicular joint in patients with chest pain may be an early clue to diagnosis of aortic dissection.[194,195] A slight pulsation in the right sternoclavicular area may suggest a right-sided aortic arch in patients with cyanotic heart disease, particularly tetralogy of Fallot.[196] A kinked, tortuous right carotid artery or dilation and tortuosity of other brachiocephalic vessels may produce visible and palpable pulsations in the suprasternal notch or the supraclavicular areas.[180]

Area 2: Aortic Area Pulsations

Vibrations of the aortic component (A_2) of the second heart sound may be palpated when they are accentuated, as in arterial hypertension. With valvular aortic stenosis a systolic thrill is present frequently in the second and less commonly in the first and third right intercostal spaces near the sternum (Fig. 10-31). It often radiates upward toward the right side of the neck and to the suprasternal notch and right supraclavicular area. Less frequently, the thrill is palpable at the second or third left interspace next to the sternum or at the apex. A systolic thrill in the aortic area and in the right carotid artery can also occur in patients with pure aortic regurgitation. Abnormal systolic pulsations in the aortic area may be due to dilation of the ascending aorta due to aneurysm and/or chronic aortic regurgitation.

Area 3: Pulmonic Area Pulsations

Vibrations associated with a loud pulmonic component (Fig. 10-31) of S_2 are often palpable in patients with pulmonary hypertension from any cause. During simultaneous palpation of the carotid pulse, a palpable P_2 or A_2 coincides with the early downslope of the carotid pulse. A systolic thrill in the second and third left intercostal space near the sternum often occurs with pulmonic valve stenosis. The thrill often radiates toward the left side of the neck, in contrast to the thrill with aortic stenosis, which radiates upward and to the right.

Pulsations of a dilated pulmonary artery may be seen or felt in the second or third left intercostal space near the sternum.[197] In normal infants and children or anxious adults with thin chest walls, a slight, brief, early systolic pulsation may be present in this area. This pulsation is accentuated by conditions that cause an increased cardiac output (e.g., fever, pregnancy). Idiopathic dilatation of the pulmonary artery may also cause a palpable systolic impulse in the same area.[180]

The common causes of an accentuated and sustained systolic pulsation in the pulmonary artery area are pulmonary hypertension, increased pulmonary blood flow, or their combination. In general, pulmonary hypertension causes a relatively slow, sustained, and forceful pulmonary artery pulsation, while a large pulmonary blood flow (e.g., atrial septal defect) produces an extremely active, more vigorous but less sustained pulsation. Valvular pulmonary stenosis with poststenotic dilation of the pulmonary artery may be associated with a palpable, sustained pulsation in this area, often with a slow rise of the initial phase.[180]

Area 4: Left Parasternal–Right Ventricular or Tricuspid Area Pulsations

A systolic thrill in the third, fourth, or fifth intercostal space in the parasternal area to the left of the sternum (Fig. 10-31) is characteristic of ventricular septal defect,

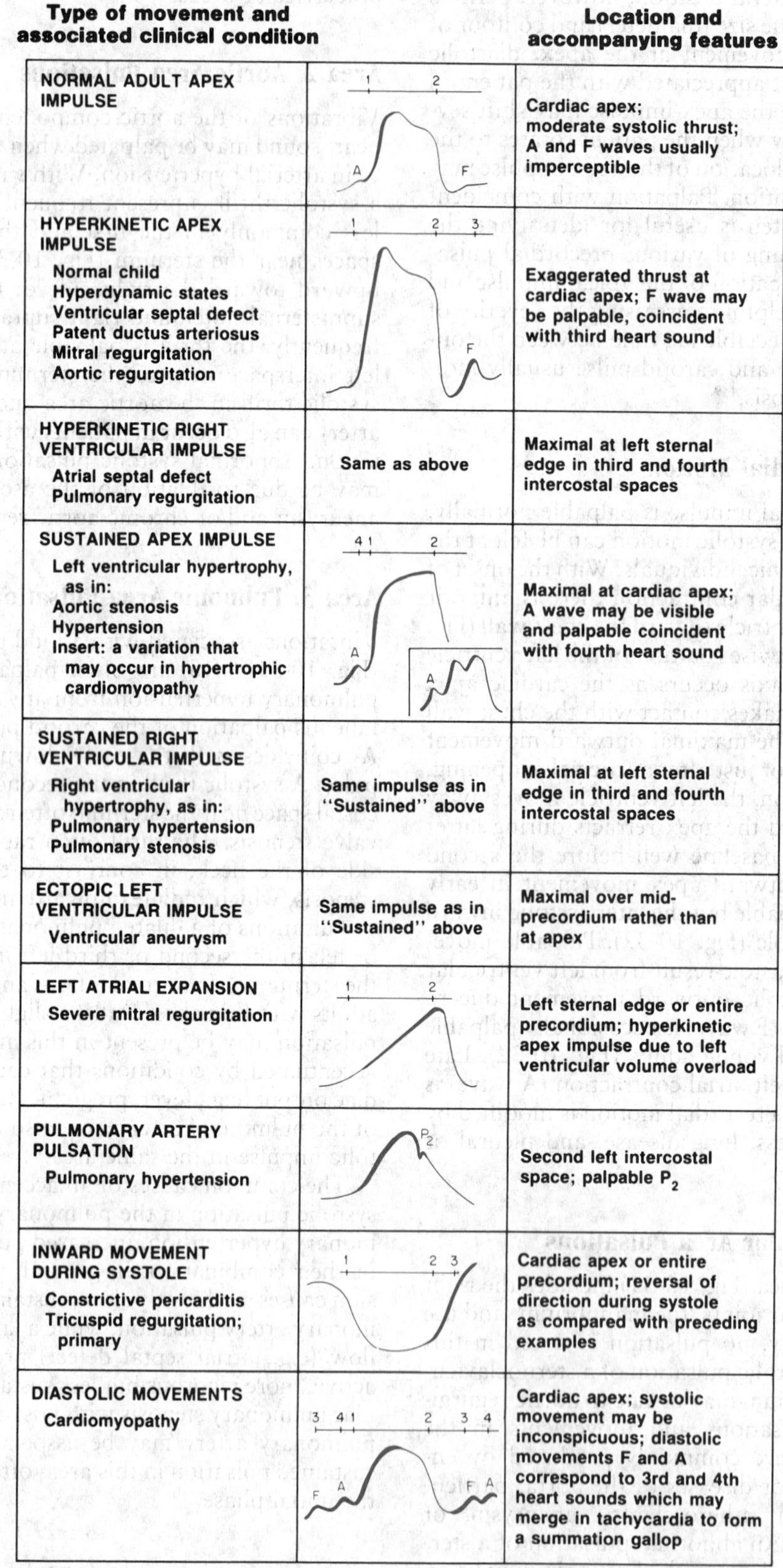

Graphic Representation
(palpable features in heavy line)

Type of movement and associated clinical condition		Location and accompanying features
NORMAL ADULT APEX IMPULSE	1 2 A F	Cardiac apex; moderate systolic thrust; A and F waves usually imperceptible
HYPERKINETIC APEX IMPULSE Normal child; Hyperdynamic states; Ventricular septal defect; Patent ductus arteriosus; Mitral regurgitation; Aortic regurgitation	1 2 3 F	Exaggerated thrust at cardiac apex; F wave may be palpable, coincident with third heart sound
HYPERKINETIC RIGHT VENTRICULAR IMPULSE Atrial septal defect; Pulmonary regurgitation	Same as above	Maximal at left sternal edge in third and fourth intercostal spaces
SUSTAINED APEX IMPULSE Left ventricular hypertrophy, as in: Aortic stenosis; Hypertension; Insert: a variation that may occur in hypertrophic cardiomyopathy	4 1 2 A A	Maximal at cardiac apex; A wave may be visible and palpable coincident with fourth heart sound
SUSTAINED RIGHT VENTRICULAR IMPULSE Right ventricular hypertrophy, as in: Pulmonary hypertension; Pulmonary stenosis	Same impulse as in "Sustained" above	Maximal at left sternal edge in third and fourth intercostal spaces
ECTOPIC LEFT VENTRICULAR IMPULSE Ventricular aneurysm	Same impulse as in "Sustained" above	Maximal over mid-precordium rather than at apex
LEFT ATRIAL EXPANSION Severe mitral regurgitation	1 2	Left sternal edge or entire precordium; hyperkinetic apex impulse due to left ventricular volume overload
PULMONARY ARTERY PULSATION Pulmonary hypertension	P_2	Second left intercostal space; palpable P_2
INWARD MOVEMENT DURING SYSTOLE Constrictive pericarditis; Tricuspid regurgitation; primary	1 2 3	Cardiac apex or entire precordium; reversal of direction during systole as compared with preceding examples
DIASTOLIC MOVEMENTS Cardiomyopathy	3 4 1 2 3 4 F A F A	Cardiac apex; systolic movement may be inconspicuous; diastolic movements F and A correspond to 3rd and 4th heart sounds which may merge in tachycardia to form a summation gallop

FIGURE 10-32 Graphic representation of apical movements in health and disease. Heavy line indicates palpable features. P_2, pulmonary component of second heart sound; A, atrial wave, corresponding to fourth heart sound (S_4) or atrial gallop; F, filling wave, corresponding to third heart sound (S_3) or ventricular gallop. [*From P Willis IV: Inspection and palpation of the precordium. In JW Hurst (ed): The Heart, 7th ed. New York, McGraw-Hill, 1990: 164. Reproduced with permission.*]

although tricuspid regurgitation can also produce a thrill here.

The lower left parasternal region normally retracts very slightly during systole, and right ventricular activity is not palpable. Slight, gentle outward pulsations of the lower sternum and left parasternal areas may be recorded in normal children and young adults, in thin adults with a small anterior-posterior thoracic diameter, or in patients with pectus excavatum. Sometimes, these pulsations can be palpated in the subxiphoid area. They are increased by hyperdynamic cardiac function.[180]

Abnormal pulsations of the sternal and left parasternal areas are most commonly due to right ventricular hypertrophy or dilation. The pulsation associated with right ventricular hypertension usually is more sustained throughout systole and tends to rise more gradually than the pulsation produced by a right ventricular volume load, which usually is more vigorous but often briefer.[198]

A predominant right ventricular pressure load occurs with pulmonic stenosis and pulmonary hypertension due to left ventricular failure, mitral valve disease, a left-to-right shunt, or pulmonary vascular disease. The sustained anterior precordial pulsation associated with isolated valvular pulmonic stenosis may not occur with tetralogy of Fallot because the thick right ventricle is not excessively dilated.[180] Atrial septal defect and ventricular septal defect are two congenital lesions frequently associated with a right ventricular volume load.[199]

Moderate or severe mitral regurgitation may produce an abnormal late systolic anterior left parasternal pulsation even in the absence of pulmonary hypertension.[200–202] This precordial lift is brisk, and its greatest force coincides with the accentuated V wave in the left atrial pressure wave. It likely is due to the large volume of blood regurgitated into the expanding left atrium, which is located centrally behind the right ventricle and anterior to the spine. While expansion of the left atrium may contribute somewhat to the anterior motion of the heart, it is likely that most of the anterior motion and force is the result of a jet or squid effect.

Conditions associated with a decrease in right ventricular compliance, such as right ventricular hypertrophy secondary to pulmonary hypertension, may be associated with a palpable "right-sided" S_4 in this area or, occasionally, in the epigastric area. Although a palpable S_3 in this area may reflect a large right ventricular volume load, it usually indicates right ventricular dysfunction or failure. Right ventricular S_3 and S_4 vibrations may be augmented during inspiration and may be attenuated or even disappear during expiration (Chap. 11).

Area 5: Apical Area Pulsations

As mentioned above, the apex impulse (Fig. 10-31) is not synonymous with maximum impulse or PMI. The location, size, and character (duration, contour or shape, amplitude, and apparent force) of the apex impulse should be determined.[180] The examiner should focus on one phase of the cardiac cycle at a time and correlate the findings with other cardiovascular events.

The normal apex (apical) impulse usually is located within 10 cm of the sternal midline, at or within the left midclavicular line in the fifth intercostal space when the patient is supine. It may be located lateral to the midclavicular line when associated with a high diaphragm, pregnancy, marked pectus excavatum, or other conditions which displace a normal heart to the left. The normal apex impulse is less than 3 cm in diameter and, in most instances, is considerably smaller.[185] The early systolic outward movement of the apical area (Fig. 10-32) begins at about the same time as that of the S_1, just before the upstroke of the carotid pulse. Peak outward motion normally occurs with or just after blood is ejected into the aorta; then the apex normally moves inward. The outward movement of the apical impulse is normally not excessively forceful and is felt only during the first third of systole.

The apex impulse may be hyperkinetic or hyperdynamic with increased amplitude in normal individuals who have a thin chest wall, a flat chest, or a depressed sternum. Lying on the left side may cause a normal apical impulse to move laterally and to have increased amplitude and duration[180,185]; however, it should still not exceed a diameter of greater than 3 cm.[185] A hyperdynamic apex impulse may also be found in anxious children, in patients with high cardiac output states, and in patients with a mild to moderate left ventricular volume load from mitral or aortic regurgitation.[180] The apex impulse is more sustained when mitral or aortic regurgitation is more severe or when left ventricular systolic function is decreased.[203,204] In general, a greatly sustained apex impulse indicates either marked left ventricular hypertrophy or depressed left ventricular systolic function, while left ventricular dilation displaces the apex impulse laterally and inferiorly.[180]

Concentric left ventricular hypertrophy without an increase in left ventricular cavity size may occur in systemic hypertension, valvular aortic stenosis, and hypertrophic cardiomyopathy. Characteristically, the apex impulse is not displaced but is both abnormally forceful and sustained.[205,206] An S_4 vibration may be palpable or visible or both.

Severe left ventricular dilation whether due to volume load or ventricular failure may displace the apex impulse laterally and inferiorly and cause marked increase in size. The duration of the apex impulse is more sustained in patients with left ventricular systolic dysfunction, particularly when associated with marked left ventricular dilation.

Important information about relative amounts of ventricular hypertrophy and dilatation often can be obtained from the apex impulse. Thus, in valvular aortic stenosis, with marked concentric left ventricular hypertrophy but little or no dilation, the apex impulse characteristically is small, forceful, and sustained but not displaced.[207] A presystolic S_4 is often palpable at the apex. By contrast, in severe aortic regurgitation with marked dilation of the left ventricle plus considerable eccentric hypertrophy, there is a diffuse apex impulse with increased force, duration, and amplitude that is displaced laterally and inferiorly.[180]

In some patients with acute myocardial infarction, a sustained apex impulse may simulate that due to left ventricular hypertrophy.[208–210] Those developing mitral regurgitation secondary to myocardial infarction (papillary muscle dysfunction) may manifest left ventricular dilation and hypertrophy by a displaced and sustained, forceful, large apex impulse.[180] A late systolic bulge at the cardiac apex may be due to a functional left ventricular aneurysm, occasionally resulting in a bifid apex impulse. In other patients, a late systolic bulge may be palpable in an ectopic area between the apex impulse and the left parasternal area.[180]

A bifid apex impulse during systole may also be due to marked left ventricular dilation and hypertrophy in patients with both aortic stenosis and regurgitation and in those with hypertrophic cardiomyopathy.[211] Infrequently, a faint systolic notch or vibration is palpable in the apex impulse of patients with mitral valve prolapse at the moment of a nonejection midsystolic click. Systolic retraction of the apical impulse usually indicates either constrictive pericarditis or severe tricuspid regurgitation with marked right ventricular dilation (Fig. 10-32).[212] An apical systolic thrill most commonly is produced by mitral regurgitation and often is diffuse, whereas a diastolic thrill is usually produced by mitral stenosis and is localized to a small, discrete area (Chap. 11).

Diastolic Events: Palpable Third and Fourth Heart Sounds

During early diastole, brief outward chest wall movement corresponding to a left ventricular rapid filling or a third heart sound (S_3) may occasionally be seen or felt, even if not audible with a stethoscope (Fig. 10-32). In children and young adults, the presence of an early diastolic ventricular filling sound (S_3) and movement is usually normal. On the other hand, the presence of such a movement or sound (Chap. 11) in a sedentary adult or a patient with heart disease usually indicates an elevated left ventricular diastolic pressure and volume, and likely ventricular decompensation, often with a decreased ejection fraction. Patients with acute myocardial infarction or transient myocardial ischemia during angina pectoris frequently develop a transient palpable and audible ventricular filling S_3, which reflects the acutely decreased ventricular compliance (Chap. 11). A palpable ventricular rapid filling wave (S_3) may be present in patients with left ventricular failure from any cause; however, hemodynamic systolic ventricular failure is often not always present when a ventricular filling wave or sound occurs in the presence of volume loading and dilation of the left ventricle, such as with mitral regurgitation or aortic regurgitation.

The presystolic left atrial contribution to the apical impulse (referred to as the atrial impulse or *a* wave) may be detected during late diastole, just prior to S_1 (Fig. 10-32). Usually, a palpable atrial impulse coincides with an audible fourth heart sound. A palpable S_4 usually is associated with an increased left ventricular end-diastolic pressure and decreased compliance (Chap. 11). In general, an S_4 is not normally palpable but may be felt at the apex with its associated S_4 in some normal adults if the PR interval is long and circulation is hyperdynamic.[180] In some patients with ischemic heart disease, a palpable apical S_4 may develop or become more prominent during an episode of angina pectoris or even during exertion without chest pain.[213] A palpable presystolic impulse, S_4, or both occur frequently in patients with acute myocardial infarction and also frequently is present in other conditions producing a decrease in left ventricular compliance and increased end-diastolic pressure.

In a patient with mitral valve disease, the presence of a palpable left-sided atrial impulse or S_4, a palpable left-sided ventricular filling sound or S_3, or an abnormally sustained apical impulse is evidence against the diagnosis of isolated important mitral stenosis and suggests the presence of coincident left ventricular disease.

A double, or bifid, apical impulse may be present in various circumstances, most commonly in the combination of an outward movement during ventricular systole and a second outward pulsation during diastole.[180] The diastolic impulse may occur either in early diastole (S_3) or in late diastole or presystole (S_4).

A bifid apical impulse with two systolic impulses may be present in patients with hypertrophic obstructive cardiomyopathy, complete left bundle branch block, or myocardial infarction. If these patients also develop a palpable impulse during either early (S_3) or late (S_4) diastole, a triple or trifid apical impulse may occur.[180] When such patients develop both a palpable S_3 and a palpable S_4, it occasionally is possible to see and feel a quadruple apical impulse.

Area 6: Epigastric Area Pulsations

Some normal and many hyperkinetic individuals have visible or palpable pulsations of the aorta in the epigastric area (Fig. 10-31). Abnormally large pulsations of the aorta may be due to an aortic aneurysm or aortic regurgitation. Hepatic movements may be identified in the epigastric area, particularly in patients with tricuspid regurgitation, tricuspid stenosis, or marked right ventricular dilatation, hypertrophy, and hyperactivity.

In some patients with pulmonary hypertension due to chronic lung disease, the detection of right ventricular hypertrophy by precordial palpation is difficult because the shape of the chest often conceals the enlarged right ventricle. To detect abnormal right ventricular pulsations in patients with emphysema, the palm of the right hand should be placed on the epigastric area and moved cephalad while gently sliding the fingers under the rib cage.[180] Aortic pulsations can be detected by the palmar surface of the fingers, and pulsations due to right ventricular hypertrophy can be felt in the fingertips.

Area 7: Ectopic Area Pulsations

Occasionally, cardiac pulsations are encountered in areas other than those previously described; that is, between the pulmonary and apical areas (Fig. 10-31). Ischemic heart disease is the most common cause of an ectopic systolic pulsation, which may occur transiently during an episode of angina pectoris. A similar paradoxical systolic outward movement may be detected after acute myocardial infarction and may persist; more commonly, it disappears within a few weeks. A persistent paradoxical ectopic pulsation may also be found in patients who develop a ventricular aneurysm after myocardial infarction.

Ectopic pulsations on the anterior chest wall can also be found in patients with cardiomyopathies of varying etiologies. In patients with severe mitral regurgitation and a giant left atrium that extends to the right, an ectopic systolic pulsation of the atrium may occasionally be felt in the right anterior or lateral chest or in the left axilla.[180]

Percussion Versus Inspection and Palpation of the Precordium

When performed by a skilled examiner, percussion of the heart can provide an estimate of cardiac size and shape. Percussion of the heart only gives information about the location of the borders of cardiac dullness, however, whereas precordial inspection and palpation provide both information about the location of the outer limits of cardiac pulsations and a determination of the size and character of the pulsations.

Although percussion has been used in the diagnosis of pericardial effusion, it has limited value when the results are objectively correlated with the diagnosis as determined by more sensitive and specific noninvasive and invasive testing.

PHYSICAL EXAMINATION OF THE CHEST, ABDOMEN, AND EXTREMITIES

Physical examination of the lung is a painless noninvasive technique, requiring only a stethoscope.[214,215] An abnormal examination often indicates the need for a chest roentgenogram. Wheezing and a pleural friction rub are detected only by the clinical evaluation. The pleural friction rub may be a clue to the diagnosis of pulmonary infarction. Pleural fluid due to heart failure is usually located in the right pleural space. When pleural fluid is localized predominated to the left, a cause other than or in addition to heart failure, such as a pulmonary infarction, should be considered.[215]

A pneumothorax may develop as a consequence of spontaneous mediastinal emphysema or be iatrogenic due to procedures.[215] Hyperresonance and diminished breath sounds may be due to pulmonary emphysema. Signs of pulmonary consolidation may be due to pneumonia or pulmonary infarction. Wheezing and rales may be due to bronchial disease. Heart failure may be associated with rales in the lung bases, wheezing, and pleural fluid. Importantly, heart failure frequently is *not* associated with rales and interstitial pulmonary edema usually does *not* produce rales.[215]

The diameter of the *abdominal* aorta should be determined in every patient (see also Chap. 123).[215] An abdominal aortic aneurysm may be missed if the examiner fails to assess the area above the umbilicus.

Specific abnormalities of the abdomen may be secondary to heart disease. A large and tender liver is common in patients with heart failure or constrictive pericarditis. Systolic hepatic pulsations are frequent in patients with tricuspid regurgitation. A palpable spleen is a common, but late, sign in patients with severe heart failure and is also often present in patients with infective endocarditis.

Although hepatic cirrhosis is the most common cause of ascites, it may occur with heart failure alone, although this has become less common with the use of diuretic therapy. Patients with severe tricuspid regurgitation, such as caused by infective endocarditis in drug addicts, may develop prominent systolic pulsation of the internal jugular veins in the neck; a large, moving, and pulsating liver; and ascites. Constrictive pericarditis should be considered when ascites are out of proportion to peripheral edema. In such patients the heart size is normal or only slightly enlarged, a pericardial "knock" is heard, and there is a rapid x and/or y descent in the internal jugular vein pulsation.[215] Restrictive cardiomyopathy can mimic constrictive pericarditis, but the heart is usually large in patients with restrictive cardiomyopathy. When there is an arteriovenous fistula in the abdomen, a continuous murmur may be heard over the abdomen. Fistulas due to trauma and surgery may occur.

A systolic bruit may be heard over the kidney areas and may signify renal artery stenosis, particularly in patients with systemic hypertension. A systolic bruit often is auscultated over the abdominal aorta, but its presence does not indicate the severity of disease of the aorta.[215]

Examination of the upper and lower *extremities* may provide important diagnostic information. (See also Chap. 124.) The clinical detection of arterial disease and thrombophlebitis is important.[2] Atherosclerosis of the peripheral arteries may produce intermittent claudication of the buttock, calf, thigh, or foot, with severe disease resulting in tissue damage of the toes. Peripheral atherosclerosis is an important risk factor for ischemic heart disease, and its presence increases the likelihood of coronary atherosclerosis. Thrombophlebitis often causes pain in the calf or thigh, or edema, and its presence should raise the consideration of pulmonary emboli as well. Edema is a late sign of heart failure, and its predictive value as a diagnostic sign is poor. It frequently involves the right leg prior to the left. Considerable heart failure and a resulting weight gain may be present without edema being present. Edema of the lower extremities may be secondary to local factors such as varicose veins or thrombophlebitis or the removal of veins at coronary artery bypass surgery. Under such circumstances, the edema often occurs in only one leg.

Edema may result from restrictive garments, and venous stasis often is secondary to a long trip in a car or airplane.[215] Edema may be due to salt and water retention in patients with primary renal disease. In the differential diagnosis of edema local factors should be considered first. If local factors can be excluded, the cause of the salt and water retention should be determined with an assessment for evidence of heart disease and other signs of heart failure or evidence of primary renal disease. Rarely, peripheral edema can be an early sign of lymphatic obstruction produced by metastatic disease in the pelvis or abdomen.

REFERENCES

1. Silverman ME: Inspection of the patient. In: Hurst JW (ed): *The Heart,* 7th ed. New York, McGraw-Hill, 1990: 135–149.
2. McKusick VA, Egeland JA, Eldridge R, Krusem DE: Dwarfism

in the Amish. I. The Ellis–van Creveld syndrome. *Bull Johns Hopkins Hosp* 1964; 115:306–330.
3. Lin AE, Perloff JK: Upper limb malformations associated with congenital heart disease. *Am J Cardiol* 1985; 55:1576–1583.
4. Holmes LB, Brennerhasset JB, Austin KF: A reappraisal of Kartagener's syndrome. *Am J Med Sci* 1968; 255:13–17.
5. Burckhardt D, Stalder GA, Ludin H, Bianchi L: Hyperdynamic state due to Osler-Weber-Rendu disease with intrahepatic arteriovenous fistulas. *Am Heart J* 1973; 85:797–805.
6. Shah CV, Pruyansky S, Harris WS: Cardiac malformations with facial clefts. *Am J Dis Child* 1970; 119:238–244.
7. Beighton P: The dominant and recessive forms of cutis laxa. *J Med Genet* 1972; 9:916–925.
8. Jaffe AS, Geltman EM, Rodey GE, Vitto J: A consistent manifestation of Type IV Ehlers-Danlos syndrome. The pathogenic role of the abnormal production of type III collagen. *Circulation* 1981; 64:121–125.
9. Cupo LN, Pyeritz RE, Olson JL, McPhee SJ, Hutchins GM, McKusick VA: Ehlers-Danlos syndrome with abnormal collagen fibrils, sinus of valsalva aneurysms, myocardial infarction, panacinar emphysema and cerebral heterotopia. *Am J Med* 1981; 71:1051–1058.
10. Hortop J, Tsipouras P, Hanley JA, Maron BJ, Shapiro JR: Cardiovascular involvement in osteogenesis imperfecta. *Circulation* 1986; 73:54–61.
11. Bruno L, Tredia S, Mangiavaechi M, Colombo V, Mozzota FG, Sirtori CR: Cardiac skeletal and ocular abnormalities in patients with Marfan's syndrome and their relatives. *Br Heart J* 1984; 51:220–230.
12. Schieken RM, Kerber RE, Iowasecu VV, Zellinger H: Cardiac manifestations of the mucopolysaccharidases. *Circulation* 1975; 52:700–705.
13. Goldman ME, Cantor R, Schwartz M, Baker M, Desnick RJ: Echocardiographic abnormalities and disease severity in Fabry's disease. *J Am Coll Cardiol* 1986; 7:1157–1161.
14. Tandon R, Edwards JE: Cardiac malformations associated with Down's syndrome. *Circulation* 1973; 47:1349–1355.
15. Goldhaber SZ, Rubin LI, Brown W, Robertson N, Stubblefield F, Sloss LT: Valvular heart disease (aortic regurgitation and mitral valve prolapse) among institutionalized adults with Down's syndrome. *Am J Cardiol* 1986; 57:278–281.
16. Rosenthal A: Cardiovascular malformations in Klinefelter's syndrome: Report of three cases. *J Pediatr* 1972; 80:471–473.
17. Lewandowski RC Jr, Yunis J: New chromosomal syndromes. *Am J Dis Child* 1975; 129:515–529.
18. Van der Hauwaert LG, Fryns JP, Dumoulin M, Logghe N: Cardiovascular malformations in Turner's and Noonan's syndrome. *Br Heart J* 1978; 40:500–509.
19. Subramaniam PN: Turner's syndrome and cardiovascular anomalies. *Am J Med Sci* 1989; 297:260–262.
20. Helmi C, Pruzansky S: Craniofacial and extracranial malformations in the Klippel-Feil syndrome. *Cleft Palate J* 1980; 17:65–88.
21. Greenwood RD, Rosenthal A, Nadas AS: Cardiovascular malformations associated with imperforate anus. *J Pediatr* 1975; 86:576–579.
22. Quan L, Smith DW: The VATER association. *J Pediatr* 1973; 82:104–107.
23. Freedom RM: The asplenia syndrome: A review of significant extracardiac structural abnormalities in 29 necropsied patients. *J Pediatr* 1972; 81:1130–1133.
24. Cyran SE, Martinez R, Daniels S, Dignan P, Kaplan S: Spectrum of congenital heart disease in CHARGE association. *J Pediatr* 1987; 110:576–578.
25. Ho CK, Kaufman RL, Podos SM: Ocular colobomata, cardiac defect, and other anomalies. *J Med Genet* 1975; 12:289–293.
26. Greenwood RD, Rosenthal A, Nadas AS: Cardiovascular malformations associated with omphalocele. *J Pediatr* 1974; 85:818–821.
27. Nora JI, Nora AH: Maternal transmission of congenital heart diseases. New recurrence risk figures and the questions of cytoplasmic inheritance and vulnerability to teratogens. *Am J Cardiol* 1987; 59:459–463.
28. Sandor GGS, Smith DF, McLeod PM: Cardiac malformations in the fetal alcohol syndrome. *J Pediatr* 1981; 98:771–773.
29. Ouellette EM, Rosett HL, Rosman MP, Weiner L: Adverse effects on offspring of maternal alcohol abuse during pregnancy. *N Engl J Med* 1977; 297:528–530.
30. Rowe RD: Maternal rubella and pulmonary artery stenosis. *J Pediatr* 1963; 32:180–185.
31. Arosemena E, Elliot LP, Eliot RS: Chest deformity in adults with congenital heart disease. *Am J Cardiol* 1967; 20:309–313.
32. Aziz K, Sanyal SK, Goldblatt E: Reversed differential cyanosis. *Br Heart J* 1968; 30:288–290.
33. Pearl W: Syndrome of anotia, facial paralysis, and congenital heart disease. *J Pediatr* 1984; 105:441–442.
34. Jaigesimi P, Antia AV: Extracardiac defects in children with congenital heart disease. *Br Heart J* 1979; 42:475–479.
35. Hermans PE: The clinical manifestations of infective endocarditis. *Mayo Clin Proc* 1982; 57:15–21.
36. Proudfit WL: Skin signs of infective endocarditis. *Am Heart J* 1983; 106:1451–1453.
37. Mendez HMM, Opitz JM: Noonan syndrome: A review. *Am J Med Genet* 1985; 21:493–506.
38. Gellis SS, Feingold M: Rubinstein-Taybi syndrome. *Am J Dis Child* 1971; 121:327–328.
39. St. John Sutton MG, Tajik AJ, Giuliana ER, Gordon H, Daniel WP: Hypertrophic obstruction cardiomyopathy and lentiginosis: A little known neural ectodermal syndrome. *Am J Cardiol* 1981; 47:214–217.
40. Callahan JA, Wrolewski EM, Reeder GS, Edwards WD, Seward JB, Tajik AS: Echocardiographic features of carcinoid heart disease. *Am J Cardiol* 1982; 50:762–768.
41. Himelman RB, Schiller NB: Clinical and echocardiographic comparison of patients with the carcinoid syndrome with and without carcinoid heart disease. *Am J Cardiol* 1989; 63:347–353.
42. Goldman AP, Kotler MN: Heart disease in scleroderma. *Am Heart J* 1985; 110:1043–1046.
43. O'Rourke RA: Antiphospholipid antibodies: A marker of lupus carditis. *Circulation* 1990; 82:636–638.
44. Nihoyannopoulos P, Gomez PM, Joshi J, Loizou S, Walport MJ, Oakley CM: Cardiac abnormalities in systemic lupus erythematosus. *Circulation* 1990; 82:369–375.
45. Nomier AM, Turner RA, Watts LE: Cardiac involvement in rheumatoid arthritis. *Arthritis Rheum* 1979; 22:561–564.
46. Bittle JA, Perloff JK: Chronic post-rheumatic fever arthropathy of Jaccoud. *Am Heart J* 1983; 105:515–517.
47. Michet CJ Jr, McKenna CH, Luthra HS, O'Fallon WM: Relapsing polychondritis. *Ann Intern Med* 1986; 104:74–78.
48. Bowness P, Hawley IC, Morris T, Dearden A, Walport MJ: Complete heart block and severe aortic incompetence in relapsing polychondritis. *Arthritis Rheum* 1991; 34:97–100.
49. Bergfeldt L, Edhag O, Rajs J: HLA-B27-associated heart disease. *Am J Med* 1984; 77:961–967.
50. Vollersten RS, McDonald TJ, Younge BR, Banks PM, Stanson AW, Ilstrup DM: Cogan's syndrome: Eighteen cases and a review of the literature. *Mayo Clin Proc* 1986; 61:344–361.
51. McAllister HA, Fenoglio JJ: Cardiac involvement in Whipple's disease. *Circulation* 1975; 52:152–156.
52. Doynama K, Hirose K, Fujiwara H: Asymmetric septal hypertrophy in a 41-year-old woman with Noonan's syndrome. *Chest* 1990; 97:1480–1481.
53. Child JS, Perloff JK, Bach PM, Wolfe AD, Perlman S, Kark RA: Cardiac involvement in Friedreich's ataxia: A clinical study of 75 patients. *J Am Coll Cardiol* 1986; 7:1370–1378.
54. Lie JT, Grossman SJ: Pathology of the heart in acromegaly: Anatomic findings in 27 autopsied patients. *Am Heart J* 1980; 100:41–52.
55. Sofer S, Weinhouse E, Tal A, Wanderman KL, Margulis G, Leiberman A: Cor pulmonale due to adenoidal or tonsillar hypertrophy or both in children. *Chest* 1988; 93:119–127.
56. Collins P: Aortic incompetence and active myocarditis in Reiter's disease. *Br J Vener Dis* 1972; 48:300–303.
57. Nakano H, Saito A, Ueda K, Nojima K: Clinical characteristics of myocardial infarction following Kawasaki disease. *J Pediatr* 1986; 108:198–203.
58. Olson LJ, Okafor EC, Clements IP: Cardiac involvement in Lyme disease: Manifestations and management. *Mayo Clin Proc* 1986; 61:745–749.
59. Southern JF, Moscicki RA, Magro C, Dickersin GR, Fallon JT, Bloch KJ: Lymphedema, lymphocytic myocarditis, and sarcoid-like granulomatosis. Manifestations of Whipple's disease. *JAMA* 1989; 261:1467–1470.
60. Cox J, Krajden M: Cardiovascular manifestations of Lyme disease. *Am Heart J* 1991; 122:1449–1455.
61. Giunta A, Maione S, Biagini R, Filla A, De-Michele G, Campa-

nella G: Noninvasive assessment of systolic and diastolic function in 50 patients with Friedreich's ataxia. *Cardiology* 1988; 75:321–327.
62. Stern R, Goldbold JH, Chess O, Kagen LJ: ECG abnormalities in polymyositis. *Arch Intern Med* 1984; 144:2185–2189.
63. Perloff JK: Cardiac rhythm and conduction in Duchenne's muscular dystrophy: A prospective study of 20 patients. *J Am Coll Cardiol* 1984; 3:1263–1268.
64. Perloff JK, Stevenson WG, Roberts NK, Cabeen Weiss J: Cardiac involvement in myotonic muscular dystrophy (Steinert's disease): A prospective study of 25 patients. *Am J Cardiol* 1984; 54:1074–1081.
65. Nguyen HH, Wolfe JT, Holmes DR, Edwards WD: Pathology of the cardiac conduction system in myotonic dystrophy. *J Am Coll Cardiol* 1988; 11:662–671.
66. Gallastegui J, Hariman RJ, Handler B, Lev M, Bharatis S: Cardiac involvement in the Kearns-Sayre syndrome. *Am J Cardiol* 1987; 60:385–388.
67. Schwartzkopff B, Frenzel H, Breithardt G, Deckert M, Losse B, Toyka KV, et al: Ultrastructural findings in endomyocardial biopsy of patients with Kerns-Sayre syndrome. *J Am Coll Cardiol* 1988; 12:1522–1528.
68. James DG, Williams WJ: *Sarcoidosis and Other Granulomatous Disorders.* Philadelphia, Saunders, 1985.
69. Winters S, Cohen M, Greenberg S, Stein B, Curwin J, Pe E, et al: Sustained ventricular tachycardia associated with sarcoidosis: Assessment of the underlying cardiac anatomy and the prospective utility of programmed ventricular stimulation, drug therapy and an implantable antitachycardia device. *J Am Coll Cardiol* 1991; 18:937–943.
70. Kuan P: Cardiac Wilson's disease. *Chest* 1987; 91:579–583.
71. Olson LJ, Edwards WD, McCall JT, Ilstrup DM, Gersh BJ: Cardiac iron deposition in idiopathic hemochromatosis: Histologic and analytic assessment of 14 hearts from autopsy. *J Am Coll Cardiol* 1987; 10:1239–1243.
72. Cueto-Garcia L, Reeder GS, Kyle RA, Wood DL, Seward JB. Naessens J, et al: Echocardiographic findings in systemic amy loidosis: Spectrum of cardiac involvement and relationship to survival. *J Am Coll Cardiol* 1985; 6:737–747.
73. Hara KS, Ballard DJ, Ilstrup DM, Connolly DC, Vollertsen RS: Rheumatoid pericarditis: Clinical features and survival. *Medicine* 1990; 69:81–91.
74. James DG, Thompson A: Recognition of the diverse cardiovascular manifestations in Behçet's disease. *Am Heart J* 1982; 103:457–458.
75. Di Eusanio G, Mazzola A, Gregorini R, Esposito G, Di Nardo W, Di Manici G, et al: Left ventricular aneurysm secondary to Behçet's disease. *Ann Thorac Surg* 1991; 51:131–135.
76. Pierce RN, Walker Smith GJ: Intrathoracic manifestations of Degos' disease (malignant atrophic papulosis). *Chest* 1978; 73:79–84.
77. Scharf S, Wexler J, Longnecker RE, Blaufox MD: Cardiovascular disease in patients on chronic hemodialytic therapy. *Prog Cardiovasc Dis* 1980; 22(5):343–356.
78. Turiteri L, Perheentupa J, Rapola J: The cardiopathy of mulibrey nanism: A new inherited syndrome. *Chest* 1974; 65:628–631.
79. Hassel D, Heinsimer J, Califf R, Benson A, Rice J, German L: Complete heart block in Reiter's syndrome. *Am J Cardiol* 1984; 53:967–968.
80. Deer T, Rosencrance JG, Chillag SA: Cardiac conduction manifestations of Reiter's syndrome. *South Med J* 1991; 84:799–800.
81. Borenstein DG, Fye WB, Arnett FC, Stevens MB: The myocarditis of systemic lupus erythematosus. *Ann Intern Med* 1978; 89:619–624.
82. Bergfeldt L, Edhag O, Vedin L, Vallin H: Ankylosing spondylitis: An important cause of severe disturbances of the cardiac conduction system. *Am J Med* 1982; 73:187–191.
83. Stevenson WG, Perloff JK, Weiss JN, Anderson TL: Facioscapulohumeral muscular dystrophy: Evidence for selective, genetic electrophysiologic cardiac involvement. *J Am Coll Cardiol* 1990; 15:292–299.
84. Vetter VL, Rashkind WJ: Congenital complete heart block and connective-tissue disease. *N Engl J Med* 1983; 309:236–238.
85. Bowen J, Boudoulas H, Wooley CF: Cardiovascular disease of connective tissue origin. *Am J Med* 1987; 82:481–488.
86. Sprecher DL, Schaefer EJ, Kent KM, Gregg RE, Zech LA, Hoeg JM: Cardiovascular features of homozygous familial hypercholesterolemia: Analysis of 16 patients. *Am J Cardiol* 1984; 54:20–30.
87. Cohen JI, Arnett EN, Kolodny AL, Roberts WC: Cardiovascular features of the Werner syndrome. *Am J Cardiol* 1987; 59:493–495.
88. Epstein CJ, Martin GM, Schultz AL, Motalsky AG: Werner's Syndrome: A review of its symptomatology, natural history, pathologic features, genetics, and relation to the natural aging process. *Medicine* 1966; 45:177–221.
89. Dyck JD, David TE, Burke B, Webb GD, Henderson MA, Fowler RS: Management of coronary artery disease in Hutchinson-Gilford syndrome. *J Pediatr* 1987; 111:407–410.
90. Badame AJ: Progeria. *Arch Dermatol* 1989; 125:540–544.
91. Elliott WJ: Ear lobe crease and coronary artery disease. *Am J Med* 1983; 75:1024–1032.
92. Elliott WJ, Karrison T: Increased all-cause and cardiac morbidity and mortality associated with the diagonal earlobe crease. *Am J Med* 1991; 91:247–254.
93. James TN, Bulkley BH: Abnormalities of the coronary arteries in Whipple's disease. *Am Heart J* 1983; 105:481–491.
94. Renteria VG, Ferrans VS, Roberts WC: The heart in Hurler syndrome: Gross histologic and ultrastructural observations in five necropsy cases. *Am J Cardiol* 1976; 38:487–501.
95. Przybojewski JZ: Polyarteritis nodosa in the adult: Report of a case with repeated myocardial infarction and a review of cardiac involvement. *S Afr Med J* 1981; 60:512–518.
96. Perry WH: Clinical spectrum of hereditary hemorrhagic telangiectasia (Osler-Weber-Rendu disease). *Am J Med* 1987; 82:989–997.
97. You CK, Rees J, Gillis DA, Steeves J: Klippel-Trenaunay syndrome: A review. *Can J Surg* 1983; 26:399–403.
98. Pagon RA, Bennett FC, LaVeek B, Stewart KB, Johnson J: Williams syndrome. *J Pediatr* 1987; 80:85–91.
99. Carney JA, Hruska LS, Beauchamp CD, Gordon H: Dominant inheritance of the complex of myxomas, spotty pigmentation, and endocrine overactivity. *Mayo Clin Proc* 1986; 61:165–172.
100. Hopkins LC, Jackson JA, Elsas LJ: Emery-Dreifuss humeroperoneal muscular dystrophy: An X-linked myopathy with unusual contractures and bradycardia. *Ann Neurol* 1981; 10:230–237.
101. Gibbs JL: The heart and tuberous sclerosis. *Br Heart J* 1985; 54:596–599.
102. Nutter DO: Measurements of the systolic blood pressure. In: Hurst JW (ed): *The Heart,* 5th ed. New York, McGraw-Hill, 1982.
103. Frohlich ED: Hypertension in the elderly. *Curr Probl Cardiol* 1988; 13(5):313–367.
104. Hales S: *Statistical Essays: Containing Haema-staticks; or, an Account of Some Hydraulick and Hydrostatical Experiments Made on the Blood and Blood-Vessels of Animals.* London, Innys W, Manby R, 1733.
105. McCutcheon EP, Rushmer RF: Korotkov sounds: An experimental critique. *Circ Res* 1967; 20:149–161.
106. Rodbard S: The components of the Korotkov sounds. *Am Heart J* 1967; 74:278–282.
107. Kirkendall WM, Feinleib M, Freis ED, Mark AL: AHA Committee Report: Recommendations of human blood pressure determination by sphygmomanometers. *Circulation* 1980; 62:1146A–1155A.
108. Neilsen PR, Janniche H: The accuracy of auscultatory measurement of arm blood pressure in very obese subjects. *Acta Med Scand* 1974; 196:403–409.
109. Hla KM, Feussner JR: Screening for pseudohypertension: A quantitative non-invasive approach. *Arch Intern Med* 1988; 148:673–676.
110. Krakoff LR, Eison H, Phillips RH, Leiman SJ, Lev S: Effect of ambulatory blood pressure monitoring on the diagnosis and cost of treatment for mild hypertension. *Am Heart J* 1988; 116:1152–1154.
111. Zachariah PK, Sheps SG, Ilstrup DM, Long CR, Bailey KR, Wiltgen CM: Blood pressure load: A better determinant of hypertension. *Mayo Clin Proc* 1988; 63:1085–1091.
112. Littler WA, Komsuoglar B: Which is the most accurate method of measuring blood pressure? *Am Heart J* 1989; 117:723–728.
113. Evans CE, Haynes RB, Goldsmith Ch, Hewson SA: Home blood pressure–measuring devices: A comparative study of accuracy. *J Hypertens* 1989; 7:133–142.

114. Kelly RP, Haywood C, Ganis J, Avolio A, O'Rourke M: Noninvasive registration of the arterial pressure waveform using high-fidelity applanation tonometry. *J Vasc Med Biol* 1989; 1(3):142–149.
115. Frohlich ED, Gifford RW, Hall WD: Hypertensive cardiovascular disease, in 18th Bethesda Conference Report: Cardiovascular disease in the elderly. *J Am Coll Cardiol* 1987; 10(suppl A):57A–59A.
116. LaKatta ED, Mitchell JH, Pomerance A, Rowe GG: Human aging: Changes in structure and function, in 18th Bethesda Conference Report: Cardiovascular disease in the elderly. *J Am Coll Cardiol* 1987; 10(suppl A):42–47.
117. O'Rourke MF: *Arterial Function in Health and Disease.* New York, Churchill Livingstone, 1982.
118. Wei JY, Gersh BJ: Heart disease in the elderly. *Curr Probl Cardiol* 1987; 12:1–65.
119. Kaplan NM: *Clinical Hypertension,* 5th ed. Baltimore, Williams & Wilkins, 1990.
120. Littler WA, Honour AJ, Pugsley DJ, Sleight P: Continuous recording of direct arterial pressure in unrestricted patients. *Circulation* 1975; 51:1101–1106.
121. Richardson DW, Honour AJ, Fenton DW, Scott FH, Pickering GW: Variation in arterial pressure throughout the day and night. *Clin Sci* 1964; 26:445–460.
122. Donald KW, Lind AR, McNicol GW, Humphreys PW, Taylor SH, Staunton HP: Cardiovascular responses to sustained contractions. *Circ Res* 1967; 20(suppl 1):15–30.
123. Wooley CF, Hosier DM, Booth RW, Molnar W, Sirak HD, Ryan JM: Supravalvular aortic stenosis. *Am J Med* 1961; 31:717–725.
124. Pascarelli EF, Bertrand CA: Comparison of blood pressure in the arms and legs. *N Engl J Med* 1964; 270:693–698.
125. Park MK, Guntheroth WG: Direct blood pressure measurements in brachial and femoral arteries in children. *Circulation* 1979; 41:231–237.
126. Felix WR, Hochbert HM, George MED, Schmalzback EL, Vaserberg R: Ultrasound measurement of arm and leg blood pressure. *JAMA* 1973; 226:1096–1099.
127. Crawford MH: Inspection and palpation of venous and arterial pulses. In: *Examination of the Heart; Part 2.* New York Am Heart Association, 1990.
128. O'Rourke MF, Kelly R, Avolio A: *The Arterial Pulse.* Philadelphia, Lea and Febiger, 1992.
129. O'Rourke MF: The arterial pulse in health and disease. *Am Heart J* 1971; 82(5):687–702.
130. Murgo JP, Westerhof N, Giolma JP, Altobelli SA: Aortic input impedance in normal man: Relationship to pressure wave shapes. *Circulation* 1980; 62:105–116.
131. O'Rourke MF: Pressure and flow waves in systemic arteries and the anatomic design of the arterial system. *J Appl Physiol* 1967; 23:139–149.
132. O'Rourke MF, Auido AP: Pulsatile flow and pressures in human systemic arteries: Studies in man and in a multibranched model of the human systemic arterial tree. *Circ Res* 1980; 46:363–372.
133. Murgo JP, Westerhof N, Giolma JO, Altobelli SA: Effects of exercise on aortic impedance and pressure wave shapes in normal man. *Circ Res* 1981; 48:334–343.
134. Latham RD, Westerhof N, Sipkema P, Rubal BJ, Reuderick P, Murgo JP: Regional wave travel and reflections along the human aorta: A study with six simultaneous micromanometer pressures. *Circulation* 1985; 72:1257–1269.
135. Murgo JP, Altobelli SA, Dorethy JF: Normal ventricular ejection dynamics in man during rest and exercise. *AHA Monograph* 1975; 46:92.
136. Westerhof N, Murgo JP, Sipkema P: Arterial impedance. In: Hwang NHC, Gross DR, Patel DJ (eds): *Quantitative Cardiovascular Studies.* Baltimore, University Park Press, 1979: 111–150.
137. Marx HJ, Yu PN: Clinical examination of the arterial pulse. *Prog Cardiovasc Dis* 1967; 10:207–235.
138. Hamilton WF, Dow P: An experimental study of the standing waves in the pulse propagated through the aorta. *Am J Physiol* 1939; 125:48.
139. McDonald DA, Taylor MG: The hydrodynamics of the arterial circulation. *Prog Biophys* 1959; 9:105–173.
140. McDonald DA: The relation of pulsatile pressure to flow in arteries. *J Physiol* 1955; 127:533–552.
141. O'Rourke MF, Taylor MG: Input impedance of the systemic circulation. *Circ Res* 1967; 20:365–380.
142. Schlant RC, Felner JM: The arterial pulse—clinical manifestations. *Curr Prob Cardiol* 1977; 2(5):1–50.
143. O'Rourke MF, Blazek JV, Morreels CL, Krovetz LJ: Pressure wave transmission along the human aorta. *Circ Res* 1968; 23:567–579.
144. Freis ED, Heath WC, Luchsinger PC, Snell RE: Changes in the carotid pulse which occurs with age and hypertension. *Am Heart J* 1966; 71:757–765.
145. Patel DJ, Greenfield JC, Dry DL: In vivo pressure length-radius relationships of certain blood vessels in man and dog. In: Attinger EO (ed): *Pulsatile Blood Flow.* New York, McGraw-Hill, 1964: Chap 17.
146. Stead EA, Greenfield JC: Pressures and pulses. *Physiol Phys* 1964; 2:1–6.
147. Freis ED, Kyle MC: Computer analysis of carotid and brachial pulse waves: Effects of age in normal subjects. *Am J Cardiol* 1968; 22:691–695.
148. Corrigan DJ: On permanent patency of the mouth of the aorta, or inadequacy of the aorta valves. *Edinburgh Med Surg* 1832; 37:225.
149. Clarke JM: On the pulsus bisferiens of aortic regurgitation. *Lancet* 1894; 2:1529–1541.
150. Broadbent W: Pulsus bisferiens. *Br Med J* 1899; 1:75.
151. Fleming PR: The mechanism of the pulsus bisferiens. *Br Heart J* 1951; 19:519–524.
152. Ikram H, Nixon PGF, Fox JA: The hemodynamic implications of the bisferiens pulse. *Br Heart J* 1964; 26:452–459.
153. Wigle ED: The arterial pressure pulse in muscular subaortic stenosis. *Br Heart J* 1963; 25:97–105.
154. Steell G: The pulse in aortic stenosis. *Lancet* 1894; 2:1206–1217.
155. Feil HS, Katz LN: The transformation of the central into the peripheral pulse in patients with aortic stenosis. *Am Heart J* 1926; 2:12–17.
156. Dow P: The development of the anacrotic and tardus pulse of aortic stenosis. *Am J Physiol* 1940; 131:432.
157. Rahimtoola SH, Cheitlin MD, Hutter AM: Valvular and congenital heart disease, in 18th Bethesda Conference Report: Cardiovascular disease in the elderly. *J Am Coll Cardiol* 1987; 10(suppl A):60–62.
158. Ewy GA, Rios JC, Marcus FI: The dicrotic arterial pulse. *Circulation* 1969; 39:655–661.
159. White PD: Alternation of the pulse: A common clinical condition. *Am J Med Sci* 1915; 150:82–96.
160. Cohn KE, Sandler H, Hancock EW: Mechanisms of pulsus alternans. *Circulation* 1967; 36:372–380.
161. Mitchell JH, Sarnoff SJ, Sonnenblick EH: The dynamics of pulsus alternans: Alternating end-diastolic fiber length as a causative factor. *J Clin Invest* 1963; 42:55–63.
162. Pace JB, Priola DV, Randall WC: Alternatives in cardiac synchrony and contractility during induced pulsus alternans. *Physiologist* 1966; 9:259.
163. Shabetai R, Fowler NO, Fenton JC, et al: Pulsus paradoxus. *J Clin Invest* 1965; 44:1882–1898.
164. Shabetai R, Fowler NO, Guntheroth WG: The hemodynamics of cardiac tamponade and constrictive pericarditis. *Am J Cardiol* 1970; 26:480–489.
165. Hurst JW, Schlant RC: Examination of the veins. In: Hurst JW (ed): *The Heart,* 4th ed. New York, McGraw-Hill, 1978: chap 15.
166. Fowler NO, Marshall WJ: Cardiac diagnosis from examination of arteries and veins. *Circulation* 1964; 30:272–283.
167. Ewy GA, Marcus FI: Bedside estimation of the venous pressure. *Heart Bull* 1968; 17:41.
168. Ewy GA: The abdominojugular test: Technique and hemodynamic correlates. *Ann Intern Med* 1989; 108:456–460.
169. Ducas J, Magder S, McGregor M: Validity of the hepatojugular reflux as a clinical test for congestive heart failure. *Am J Cardiol* 1983; 52(10):1299–1303.
170. Fowler NO: Inspection and palpation of venous and arterial pulses. In: *Examination of the Heart.* New York, American Heart Association, 1972: 1–41.
171. Wood P: *Diseases of the Heart and Circulation,* 2d ed. Philadelphia, Lippincott, 1957.
172. Kussmaul A: Uber Schwielige Mediastino-pericarditis und Den Parodoxen Pulse. *Berl Klin Wochenschr* 1873; 10:433.
173. Dell'Italia L, Starling MR, O'Rourke RA: Physical examination for exclusion of hemodynamically important right ventricular infarction. *Ann Intern Med* 1983; 99:608–612.

174. Messer AL, Hurst JW, Rappaport MB, Sprague HB: A study of the venous pulse in tricuspid valve disease. *Circulation* 1950; 1:388–393.
175. Meuller O, Shillingford J: Tricuspid incompetence. *Br Heart J* 1954; 16:195–207.
176. Dexter L: Arterial septal defect. *Br Heart J* 1956; 18:209–225.
177. Perloff JK, Harvey WP: Clinical recognition of tricuspid stenosis. *Circulation* 1960; 22:346–364.
178. Corvisart JN: *An Essay on the Organic Diseases and Lesions of the Heart and Great Vessels.* Translated from the French, with notes, by Jacob Gates. New York, Hafner Publishing, 1962.
179. Willis PW IV: Inspection and palpation of the precordium. In: Hurst JW (ed): *The Heart,* 7th ed. New York, McGraw-Hill, 1990: 163–169.
180. Schlant RC, Hurst JW: *Examination of the Precordium: Inspection and Palpation.* New York, American Heart Association 1990: 1–28.
181. Stapleton JF, Groves BM: Precordial palpation. *Am Heart J* 1971; 81:409–427.
182. Basta LL, Bettinger JJ: The cardiac impulse: A new look at an old art. *Am Heart J* 1979; 97:96–111.
183. Perloff JK: The physiòlogic mechanisms of cardiac and vascular physical signs. *J Am Coll Cardiol* 1983; 1:184–198.
184. Abrams J: Precordial motion in health and disease. *Mod Concepts Cardiovasc Dis* 1980; 49:55–60.
185. Eilen SD, Crawford MH, O'Rourke RA: Accuracy of precordial palpation for detecting increased left ventricular volume. *Ann Intern Med* 1983; 99:628–630.
186. Smith D, Craige E: Enhancement of tactile perception as employed in palpation. *Circulation* 1980; 62:1114–1118.
187. Corn RD, Cole JS: The cardiac apex impulse. *Ann Intern Med* 1971; 75:185.
188. Bethell HJN, Nixon PGF: Examination of the heart in supine and left lateral positions. *Br Heart J* 1973; 35:902–907.
189. Chun PKC, Dunn BE: Clinical care of severe aortic stenosis. *Arch Intern Med* 1982; 142:2284–2288.
190. Deliyannis A, Gillam PMS, Mounsey JPD, Steiner RE: The cardiac impulse and the motion of the heart. *Br Heart J* 1964; 26:396–411.
191. McDonald IG: The shape and movements of the human left ventricle during systole. *Am J Cardiol* 1970; 26:221–230.
192. Sutton GC, Prewitt TA, Craige E: Relationship between quantitated precordial movement and left ventricular function. *Circulation* 1970; 41:179–190.
193. Abrams J: *Essentials of Cardiac Physical Diagnosis.* Lea & Febiger, Philadelphia, 1987.
194. Logue RB, Sikes C: A new sign in dissecting aneurysm of aorta: Pulsation of a sternoclavicular joint. *JAMA* 1952; 148:1209–1212.
195. Lindsey J Jr, Hurst JW: Clinical features and prognosis in dissecting aneurysm of the aorta: A re-appraisal. *Circulation* 1967; 35:880–888.
196. Perloff JK: The movements of the heart—Observation, palpation, and percussion. In: *Physical Examination of the Heart and Circulation.* Philadelphia, Saunders, 1982: 130–170.
197. Burstin L: Determination of pressure in the pulmonary artery by external graphic recordings. *Br Heart J* 1967; 29:396–404.
198. Eddleman EE Jr, Thomas HD: The recognition and differentiation of right ventricular pressure and flow loads. A correlative study of kinetocardiograms, electrocardiograms, fluoroscopy, and cardiac catheterization data in patients with mitral stenosis, septal defect, pulmonic stenosis and isolated pulmonary hypertension. *Am J Cardiol* 1959; 4:652–661.
199. Nagle RE, Tamara FA: Left parasternal impulse in pulmonary stenosis and atrial septal defect. *Br Heart J* 1967; 29:735–741.
200. Ronon JA Jr, Steelman RB, DeLeon AC Jr, Waters TJ, Perloff JK, Harvey WP: The clinical diagnosis of acute severe mitral insufficiency. *Am J Cardiol* 1971; 27:284–290.
201. Sutton GC, Craige E, Grizzle JE: Quantitation of precordial movement. II. Mitral regurgitation. *Circulation* 1967; 35:483–491.
202. Basta LL, Wolfson P, Eckberg DL, Abboud FM: The value of left parasternal impulse recordings in the assessment of mitral regurgitation. *Circulation* 1973; 48:1055–1065.
203. Eddleman EE Jr: Kinetocardiographic findings in aortic insufficiency. *Am Heart J* 1957; 53:530–541.
204. Abrams J: Precardial palpation. I: Horwitz LD and Graves BM (eds) *Signs and Symptoms in Cardiology.* Philadelphia, Lippincott, 1985:156–177.
205. Nagle RE, Boicourt OW, Gillam PM, Mounsey JP: Cardiac impulse in hypertrophic obstructive cardiomyopathy. *Br Heart J* 1966; 28:419–425.
206. Rios JC, Massumi RA: Correlation between the apex cardiogram and left ventricular pressure. *Am J Cardiol* 1965; 15:647–655.
207. Tafur E, Cohen LS, Levine HD: The apex cardiogram in left ventricular outflow tract obstruction. *Circulation* 1964; 30:392–399.
208. Harvey WP: Some pertinent physical findings in the clinical evaluation of acute myocardial infarction. *Circulation* 1969; 39/40(suppl IV):IV-175–181.
209. Heikkila J, Luomanmaki K, Pyorala K: Serial observations on left ventricular dysfunction in acute myocardial infarction. 1. Gallop sounds, ventricular asynergy, and radiological signs. *Acta Med Scand* 1971; 190:89–104.
210. Lane FJ, Carroll JM, Levine HD, Gorlin R: The apexcardiogram in myocardial asynergy. *Circulation* 1968; 37:890–899.
211. Shah PM: Newer concepts in hypertrophic obstruction cardiomyopathy. II. *JAMA* 1979; 242:1771–1776.
212. Boicourt OW, Nagle RE, Mounsey JP: The clinical significance of systolic retraction of the apical impulse. *Br Heart J* 1965; 27:379–391.
213. Eddlemand EE Jr, Harrison TR: The kinetocardiogram in patients with ischemic heart disease. *Prog Cardiovasc Dis* 1963; 6:189–211.
214. Walker HK, Hall WD, Hurst JW: *Clinical Methods: The History, Physical, and Laboratory Examination,* 2d ed. Boston, Butterworths, 1980: 200, 628–648, 726, 740–775.
215. Hurst JW, Robinson PH: Physical examination of the chest, abdomen and extremities. In: Hurst JW, et al (eds): *The Heart,* 7th ed. New York, McGraw-Hill, 1990: 242–243.

Chapter 11

Auscultation of the Heart

James A. Shaver, M.D. ■ *Rosemarie Salerni, M.D.*

Since the invention of the stethoscope by Laënnec in 1826,[1] cardiac auscultation has played a key role in the evaluation of the patient with cardiovascular disease.[1] In the past four decades, tremendous technologic advances have been made in cardiac diagnosis. One of the important benefits of these new diagnostic techniques has been a better understanding of the relationship between intracardiac pressure, flow, and valve motion on one hand and the resultant sound phenomena on the other. The analysis of heart sounds and murmurs by phonocardiography together with information obtained by cardiac catheterization, angiography, echocardiography, and cardiac surgery have made cardiac auscultation a precise discipline based on firm physiologic principles. These very accurate methods of cardiac investigation have not made the stethoscope obsolete; on the contrary, they have given auscultation an even more important place in cardiac diagnosis.[2]

TECHNIQUES AND APPROACH TO AUSCULTATION

The Stethoscope

The physician must choose a stethoscope that fits the ears comfortably, has as short a segment of flexible tubing as possible, and is equipped with a diaphragm and a bell. Selection of the proper earpieces for comfort and the best transmission of sound is based on individual preference and is best evaluated by trial and error. A snug, comfortable fit depends on the size of the earpieces as well as the angle at which they enter the ear canal; the angulation of the rigid metal tubing must therefore be chosen to suit the comfort of the individual. The rubber tubing should be as short as feasible, and experience indicates that tubing about 12 in. long is the best compromise. Rapaport and Sprague[3] have shown that thick-walled tubing about $\frac{1}{8}$ in. in diameter is best suited to transmit sounds and murmurs.

The human ear is most sensitive to auditory vibrations that occur in the frequency range between 1000 and 4000 to 5000 Hz, and the sensitivity falls off sharply when the frequency of vibration is below 1000 Hz. This is particularly true of low-frequency sounds, which must be of considerably greater amplitude to reach the threshold of audibility than sounds of higher frequency. Most cardiovascular sounds and murmurs that are of diagnostic importance are between 30 and 1000 Hz, thereby placing the auscultator at considerable disadvantage.[4] Therefore, it is imperative that a stethoscope be equipped with both a diaphragm and a bell and that each of these pieces be applied to the chest wall with optimal pressure.

The diaphragm brings out the high frequencies and attenuates the lows. In order to do this properly, it should be fairly rigid. When the diaphragm is used to accentuate high-pitched sounds, it should be pressed very firmly against the skin. This technique will make high-frequency murmurs such as the faint diastolic blowing murmur of aortic valve regurgitation audible at the base when they would otherwise be missed. The bell accentuates the low-frequency sounds and filters out the high-pitched tones. Often, low-frequency sounds are more easily appreciated by palpation than by auscultation; in these situations, the stethoscope should be placed very lightly on the skin with just enough pressure to seal the edge at the point of maximal impulse. The bell can also be used as a filter. With very light pressure, the low-pitched sounds are accentuated; however, with firm pressure of the bell against the skin, the skin itself becomes a relatively tight diaphragm and the low-frequency sounds are suppressed. Although this technique can be very helpful, the stethoscope should always be equipped with a valve system that permits one to switch from the diaphragm to the bell with ease.

Examination of the Patient

The examination should take place in a quiet room that is well lighted and comfortably heated. The patient should be properly gowned, with adequate exposure to the waist. The examining table should be large enough so that the patient can be instructed to lie flat, sit up, or roll to one side with complete ease. Usually, the physician will examine from the right side, and it is equally important that the physician be comfortable as well as the patient.

Prior to auscultation, the clinician should take advantage of the information obtained from the history as well as from the examination of the arterial, venous, and cardiac pulsations. (See Chap. 10.) When abnormalities are found, their auscultatory counterparts should be diligently pursued. For example, prominent *a* waves in the jugular venous pulse should alert the clinician to search carefully for a low-pitched, right-sided fourth heart sound (S_4) or the subtle presystolic murmur of tricuspid stenosis, while large *v* waves that augment with inspiration should suggest tricuspid regurgitation. The presence of pulsus alternans should always demand a careful search for third and fourth heart sounds (S_3, S_4) as well as for the presence of functional mitral or tricuspid regurgitation often present in severe cardiac decompensation. A rapid, jerky rise of the carotid pulse may be the clue to the diagnosis of hypertrophic cardiomyopathy, which can be confirmed by manipulating the systolic murmur with maneuvers that change the pre- and afterloading conditions of the heart. Since every patient cannot be examined in every position or with complete evaluation by physiologic or pharmacologic interventions, the extent of the examination must be dictated by the patient's overall clinical presentation.

There are four primary areas of cardiac auscultation: (1) the primary and secondary aortic areas in the second right interspace and the third left interspace adjacent to the sternum, respectively; (2) the pulmonary area in the second left interspace; (3) the tricuspid area in the fourth and fifth interspaces adjacent to the left sternal border; and (4) the mitral area at the cardiac apex. However, this does not mean to imply that auscultatory events arising from each valve are heard only in their respective areas. The murmur of aortic stenosis in the elderly is often heard best (and at times only) at the apex, while the murmur of a flail posterior mitral leaflet may radiate to the base and simulate the murmur of aortic stenosis. Ejection sounds arising from the stenotic aortic valve are usually most prominent at the apex, while the opening snap of mitral stenosis is heard best midway between the tricuspid and mitral areas. The murmur of tricuspid regurgitation may be appreciated best at the classical mitral area if the right ventricle occupies the apex. Furthermore, cardiac auscultation should not be restricted to just these four areas. For example, the murmur of aortic regurgitation secondary to abnormalities of the aortic root may be heard best to the right of the sternum, while the murmur of tricuspid regurgitation in the emphysematous patient with pulmonary hypertension is best ausculted in the epigastrium. The continuous murmur of a patent ductus arteriosus is heard just below the left clavicle, while the murmur of large bronchial collaterals may be most prominent in the posterior thorax. Again, the patient's overall clinical presentation will guide the experienced clinician to the appropriate area to auscult.

During auscultation, one listens both specifically and selectively for heart sounds and then for murmurs, first during systole and then during diastole. As described by Levine and Harvey,[5] the physician should adopt a systematic way of listening: starting at the apex, then moving to the lower left sternal border, and progressing along the sternal border to the base of the heart. The patient should be lying on his or her back, and each area should be surveyed with both chest pieces. In each area examined, the physician listens specifically for the first heart sound (S_1), noting its intensity, constancy, presence of splitting, and variation with respiration. This is followed by selective listening to the second heart sound (S_2), noting the same characteristics. Then extra sounds are searched for and carefully listened to, first in systole, then in diastole, with mental notations as to their time of appearance, pitch, and other characteristics that may identify them as gallop sounds, ejection sounds, or valve opening sounds. Whether the examination is initiated at the base by listening to S_2 or at the apex listening to S_1 depends on the physician's preference. Of greater importance is that the examination be performed in a compulsive, systematic way, with the physician listening intently for one event at a time. Attention is then first turned to systole and then to diastole for the presence of murmurs. After this general survey, the physician listens selectively for certain sounds and murmurs. With the bell applied lightly to the skin at the apex, the patient is instructed to roll onto the left side and the clinician selectively "tunes in" to diastole and the low-frequency range. This allows the physician to determine the presence or absence of diastolic filling sounds or diastolic rumbles arising from the atrioventricular valves.

The examination is continued with the patient in the sitting position. While the patient leans slightly forward during quiet respiration, the clinician can optimally appreciate splitting of S_2. With the breath held in deep expiration, the physician examines the aortic and pulmonic areas with the diaphragm firmly pressed against the chest wall, selectively "tuning in" to the high-frequency range in an effort to hear the faint blowing diastolic murmur of aortic regurgitation or, if the clinical situation warrants, the presence of a pericardial friction rub. Sounds and murmurs such as these are discovered only when they are searched out carefully with intent listening and concentration. Otherwise, the examiner's attention is directed only to the medium- and high-pitched sounds and murmurs that are loud and obvious to the ear.

Auscultation of the heart should be considered a dynamic exercise. In addition to ausculting the patient in the left lateral decubitus position, he or she should, when possible, also be examined while standing, squatting, and during the Valsalva maneuver and following its release. This type of dynamic examination changes the pre- and afterloading conditions of the heart and may yield diagnostic information because of the typical response of heart sounds and murmurs to these maneuvers.

Once the attentive physician has heard an unusual sound or murmur, it will never be forgotten. An analogy can be made with the distinctiveness of the sounds emanating from a violin versus those from the piccolo. Once heard and defined, they will never be confused. Likewise, the whooping murmur of a prolapsed mitral valve, once heard, will never be confused with the rough systolic ejection murmur of aortic stenosis; nor will the high-frequency opening snap of a mobile mitral valve be confused with a loud summation gallop. Often, the experienced clinician can arrive at a definitive diagnosis by careful attention to the very specific characteristics of certain heart sounds and murmurs.

Phonocardiography

Modern phonocardiography is a graphic representation of the cardiovascular examination[6] and is used to demonstrate what we see, feel, and hear at the bedside. Although inferior to the actual cardiac examination at the bedside, it greatly complements the written word. It includes not only the recording of the auscultatory events of the precordium but also the recording of the carotid, venous, and apical precordial pulsations simultaneously with the electrocardiogram (ECG). This technique may enhance the accuracy of the cardiac examination because it allows precise timing of cardiac auscultatory events as well as accurate and quantitative reproduction of physiologic events of the cardiac cycle. It is an excellent teaching aid, particularly in terms of training the clinician's ear to the timing of closely sequenced sounds. However, the high-frequency events such as the soft murmur of aortic regurgitation are almost impossible to record. In that situation, the "tuned-in" ear is far superior. When phonocardiography is combined with echocardiography (phonoechocardiography), instantaneous valvular and ventricular wall motion can be correlated with sound and pressure events, further enhancing its diagnostic and teaching value.

HEART SOUNDS

Heart sounds are of two types: high-frequency transients associated with the abrupt terminal checking of valves that are closing or opening, and low-frequency sounds related to early and late diastolic filling events of the ventricles. Sounds related to closing and opening of the atrioventricular valves include mitral and tricuspid closing sounds (M_1, T_1), nonejection sounds, and the opening snaps; while sounds related to closing and opening of the semilunar valves include aortic and pulmonic closure sounds (A_2, P_2) and early valvular ejection sounds or clicks. Low-frequency sounds include the physiologic heart sound (S_3) and the pathologic S_3 gallop associated with early ventricular filling events and the presystolic atrial S_4 gallop associated with late diastolic events resulting from the atrial contribution to ventricular filling. With tachycardia these sounds may fuse, producing a summation gallop.

In recent years, sophisticated studies using phonoechocardiography, high-fidelity micromanometry, instantaneous flow and flow velocity measurements, and high-speed cineangiography have given us better understanding of the sound, pressure, flow, and motion correlates of these heart sounds.[7,8] These approaches will be emphasized in subsequent sections to provide a better understanding of both the mechanisms of production and the clinical relevance of these sounds in health and disease.

The First Heart Sound

The first heart sound (S_1) as recorded by high-resolution phonocardiography consists of four sequential components: (1) small low-frequency vibrations, usually inaudible, that coincide with the beginning of left ventricular contraction and felt to be muscular in origin; (2) a large high-frequency vibration, easily audible, related to mitral valve closure (M_1); (3) followed closely by a second high-frequency component related to tricuspid valve closure (T_1); and (4) small low-frequency vibrations that coincide with acceleration of blood into the great vessel (Fig. 11-1). The two major components audible at the bedside are the louder M_1 heard best at the apex followed by T_1

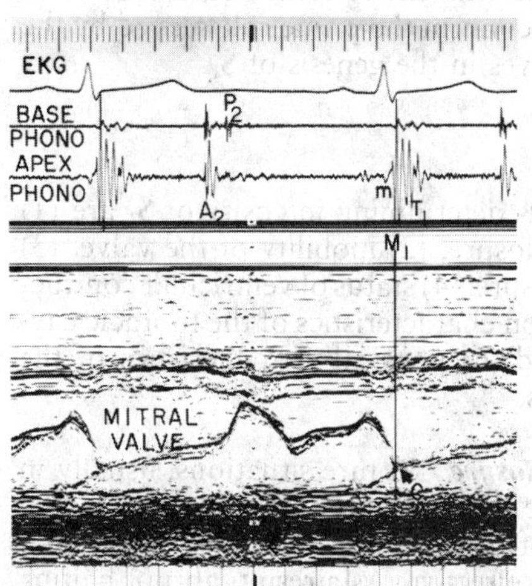

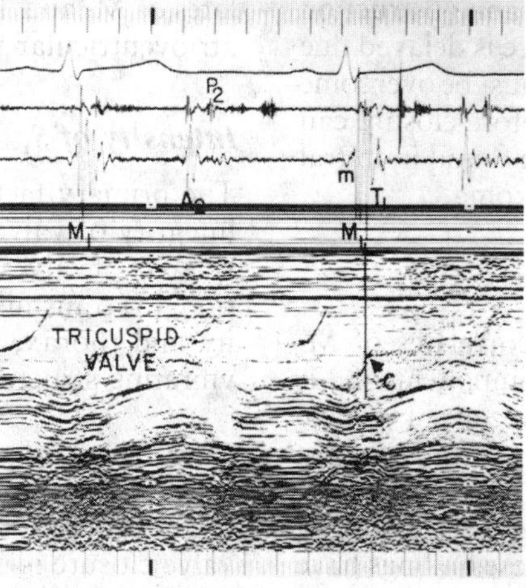

FIGURE 11-1 The apex phonocardiogram is recorded with the mitral valve echocardiogram (*left panel*) and tricuspid valve echocardiogram (*right panel*) in a normal subject. The mitral (M_1) and tricuspid (T_1) components of the first heart sound are coincident with the closure point (C) of the mitral and tricuspid valves, respectively. A small, low-frequency vibration (m) is seen prior to M_1, and a few low-frequency vibrations follow T_1 in early systole.

heard best at the left lower sternal border. They are separated by only 20 to 30 ms and at the apex are usually appreciated only as a single sound in the normal subject. Although controversy exists regarding the genesis of these two major components, several hemodynamic and phonoechocardiographic studies have supported the original observations of Dock[9] and Leatham[10] regarding the role played by the atrioventricular valves in generating these sounds.

Echocardiographic Correlates and Splitting of S_1

Several studies have shown that the first high-frequency component of S_1 coincides with the complete coaptation of the anterior and posterior leaflets of the mitral valve.[11–18] This sound is not due to the clapping together of the two delicate leaflets, but rather to the sudden deceleration of blood setting the entire cardiohemic system into vibration when the elastic limits of the closed, tensed valves are met.[19] It is unlikely that complete coaptation of the complex valve leaflets and final tensing are simultaneous; presumably it is the latter event that is associated with vibrations perceived as M_1. For practical purposes, however, the resolution of M-mode echocardiography is inadequate to distinguish between these two events, and M_1 and the C point of the mitral valve echocardiogram are considered to be coincident.[18] Similar echocardiographic correlates are more difficult to demonstrate for T_1 in the normal subject because it is often impossible to clearly identify the onset of T_1 as the two components of S_1 are often synchronous or narrowly split (Fig. 11-1). However, when T_1 is more widely separated from M_1, identical echocardiographic correlates have been demonstrated in patients with wide splitting of S_1 due to Ebstein's anomaly of the tricuspid valve.[7,20] This exaggerated T_1, or "sail sound," and its wide separation from M_1 has been a helpful sign in the diagnosis of this entity.[20] Wide splitting of S_1 with normal sequencing (M_1, T_1) is also present in right bundle branch block of the proximal type as well as in left ventricular pacing, ectopic beats, and idioventricular rhythms originating from the left ventricle due to a delayed contraction of the right ventricle.[21] In a similar manner, pacing from the right ventricle and ectopic beats and idioventricular rhythms originating from the right ventricle will produce reversed splitting of S_1 (T_1, M_1) due to delay in left ventricular contraction. Reversed splitting of S_1 may also be present in patients with hemodynamically significant obstruction of the mitral valve, as mitral valve closure is delayed due to the increased left atrial pressure that must be overcome by the rising left ventricular pressure before closure can occur.[22] Similar delay in M_1 may also be found in mitral obstruction secondary to left atrial myxoma.

Hemodynamic Correlates of S_1

In Fig. 11-2, the sound and pressure correlates of M_1 are shown. The first high-frequency component of M_1 coincides with the downstroke of the left atrial *c* wave and is delayed from the left ventricular–left atrial pressure crossover by 30 ms. Similar delays in M_1 following atrioventricular pressure crossover have been reported by other investigators.[23,24] In the past, these findings have

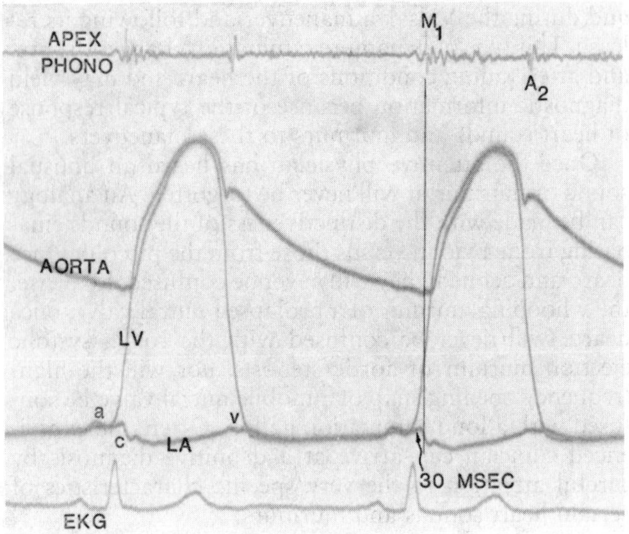

FIGURE 11-2 The apex phonocardiogram is displayed simultaneously with the cardiac cycle, as recorded by high-fidelity catheter-tipped micromanometers in the central aorta, left ventricle (LV), and left atrium (LA). The first high-frequency component of M_1 is coincident with the downstroke of the left atrial *c* wave and is separated from left ventricular–left atrial pressure crossover by an interval of 30 ms. (*From JA Shaver, et al: Normal and abnormal heart sounds in cardiac diagnosis. Part I: Systolic sounds, Curr Probl Cardiol 10(3):10, 1985. Reproduced with permission of the publisher and the authors.*)

caused considerable confusion regarding the origin of both M_1 and T_1, as it was assumed that these sounds occurred at atrioventricular pressure crossover. However, the elegant studies of Laniado et al.[12] recording both valve motion and phasic flow across the mitral valve simultaneously resolved this issue. This study clearly established that forward flow continued for a short period following left ventricular–left atrial pressure crossover due to the inertia of mitral flow, with M_1 occurring 20 to 40 ms later, coincidental with cessation of mitral flow and closure of the valve. An even greater delay between the occurrence of T_1 and right ventricular–right atrial pressure crossover has been shown by Mills and associates,[11] and the micromanometer study of O'Toole and associates[25] has shown that T_1 also coincides with the downstroke of the right atrial *c* wave. These hemodynamic data, together with the echocardiographic correlates of M_1 and T_1, confirm the prime role played by the atrioventricular valves in the genesis of S_1.

Intensity of S_1

The primary factors determining intensity of S_1 are (1) integrity of valve closure, (2) mobility of the valve, (3) velocity of valve closure, (4) status of ventricular contraction, (5) transmission characteristics of the thoracic cavity and thorax, and (6) physical characteristics of the vibrating structures.

Integrity of Valve Closure In rare situations, usually in the setting of severe mitral regurgitation, there is inadequate coaptation of the mitral leaflets to a degree that valve closure is not effective. As a result, abrupt halting

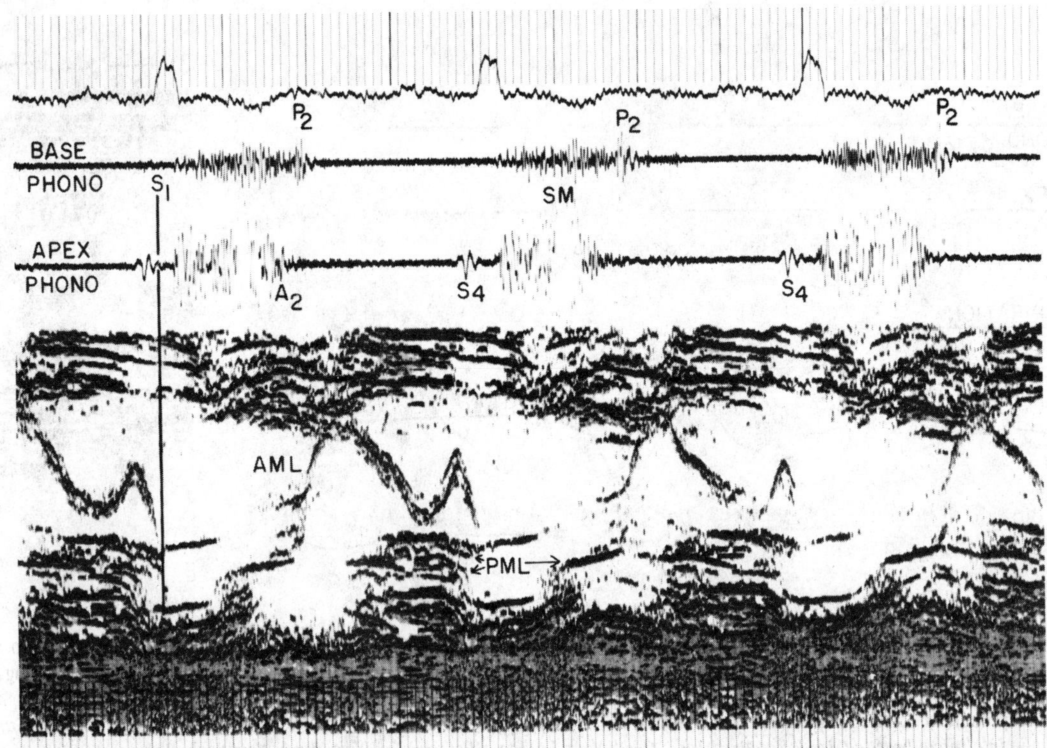

FIGURE 11-3 Base and apex phonocardiograms are recorded simultaneously with the mitral valve echocardiogram in a 62-year-old man who developed acute mitral regurgitation secondary to rupture of the chordae tendinae of a myxomatous valve. During diastole multiple echos arise from the flail posterior mitral leaflet (PML), and during early ventricular systole effective mitral valve closure does not occur, resulting in an inaudible low-frequency vibration on the apex phonocardiogram. During systole, there is separation of the anterior (AML) and posterior mitral leaflets, resulting in severe mitral regurgitation. The murmur has a crescendo-decrescendo contour simulating the murmur of aortic stenosis ending prior to A_2. Wide physiologic splitting of S_2 is present. The prominent S_4 present on the apex phonocardiogram was associated with an apical presystolic impulse. [*From JA Shaver: The physical examination in cardiac diagnosis. Cardiol Consult 6(3):3, 1985. Reproduced with permission of the publisher and the author.*]

of the retrograde blood column during early ventricular contraction does not occur, and S_1 may be markedly attenuated or absent. Such may be the case in severe mitral regurgitation due to a flail mitral leaflet, as shown in Fig. 11-3.[26]

Mobility of the Valve Severe calcific fixation of the mitral valve with complete immobilization will cause a markedly attenuated M_1. This is most commonly seen in the setting of longstanding mitral stenosis, as shown in Fig. 11-4.

Velocity of Valve Closure The velocity of valve closure is the most important factor affecting the intensity of S_1 and is determined by the timing of mitral valve closure in relation to the left ventricular pressure rise in early systole.[11,14,18,27–29] The relative timing of left atrial and left ventricular systole may vary this relationship, as shown in Fig. 11-5, in an anesthetized dog preparation using the technique of sequential atrioventricular pacing.[27] As the PR interval progressively decreased from 130 to 30 ms, there is a progressive increase in the intensity of M_1 and progressive delay in M_1 relative to the onset of left ventricular contraction. However, when left atrial and left ventricular systole occur almost simultaneously at a PR interval of 10 ms, S_1 again becomes soft. At short PR intervals (30 to 70 ms), the mitral valve leaflets are maximally separated by atrial contraction at the onset of left ventricular systole. With left ventricular contraction, the mitral valve closes at a high velocity with a large excursion. This results in a loud, late M_1 occurring on a steeper part of the left ventricular pressure curve when the retrograde blood column is suddenly decelerated at the moment the elastic limits of the mitral valve are met. At longer PR intervals, there is less separation of the mitral valve leaflets, which have already begun to close with atrial relaxation. When left ventricular systole begins, there is less excursion of the mitral valve until tensing occurs, and S_1 occurs earlier relative to the onset of left ventricular contraction at a lower left ventricular pressure. Thus, less force is applied to the mitral valve, its closing velocity is decreased, and less energy is generated when a column of retrograde blood is abruptly halted, resulting in a softer M_1. Although simultaneous motion of the mitral valve is not shown in Fig. 11-5, subsequent investigations using cineradiography and echocardiographic techniques to visualize the mitral valve during variations of the PR interval have further confirmed the relationship between the rate of mitral valve closure and the intensity of M_1.[14,24,30]

The clinical finding of marked variation in the intensity of S_1 in a patient with a slow heart rate will often alert the clinician at the bedside to the diagnosis of complete heart block with atrioventricular (AV) dissociation. Other conditions in which there are beat-to-beat variations in the intensity of S_1 include Möbitz type I heart

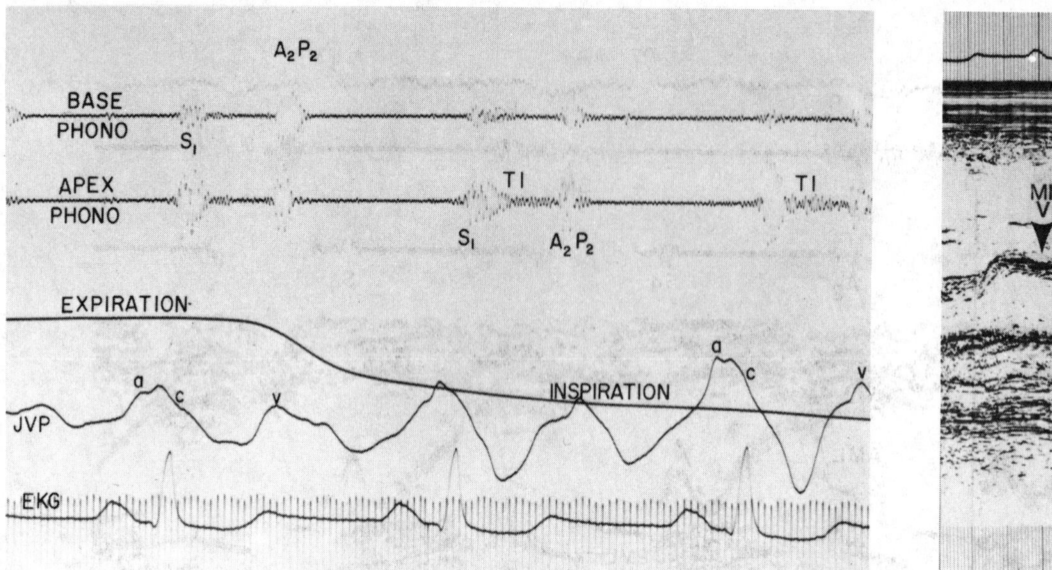

FIGURE 11-4 *Left panel:* Base and apex phonocardiograms are recorded simultaneously with the jugular venous pulse (JVP) and ECG in a patient with calcific fixation of a severely stenotic mitral valve (as shown in the right panel). S_1 is soft, and there is no evidence of an opening snap during early diastole or a diastolic rumble. Note that with inspiration, a functional tricuspid regurgitation murmur develops in the apex phonocardiogram, and the *a* wave on the JVP becomes more prominent. Cardiac catheterization confirmed severe mitral stenosis and pulmonary hypertension. [*From JA Shaver: Current uses of phonocardiography in clinical practice. In: E Rapaport (ed): Cardiology Update—Reviews for Physicians. New York, Elsevier, 1981, p 362. Reproduced originally in part (left panel) with permission of the publisher and authors; and from JA Shaver, et al: Normal and abnormal heart sounds in cardiac diagnosis. Part 1: Systolic sounds. Curr Probl Cardiol 10(3):20, 1985, p 20. Re-produced in total with permission of the publisher and the authors.*]

block and ventricular tachycardia with AV dissociation. Variations in the intensity of S_1 also occur with atrial fibrillation with both normal and stenotic atrioventricular valves. The loud S_1 occurs at short RR intervals, while a softer S_1 occurs at longer RR intervals when the valve leaflets have partially closed.[31] Mills and Craige[18] have shown an excellent correlation ($R = 0.90$) between the terminal closing rate of the anterior mitral leaflet and the amplitude of M_1 in patients with atrial fibrillation without mitral obstruction.

The position of the mitral valve at the onset of ventricular systole may be altered not only by the relative timing of atrial and ventricular systole but also by altering the rate of left ventricular filling during atrial systole. Leonard and associates[32] have shown that the timing and intensity of both S_1 and S_4 in hypertensive patients can be influenced by variations in venous return (Fig. 11-6). It is suggested that the mitral leaflets have a greater separation when venous return is decreased to the noncompliant hypertensive left ventricle because there is more effective atrial volume transport into a relatively underfilled ventricle. As shown in the right panel of Fig. 11-6, this results in a softer S_4 that migrates toward an increased S_1. When venous return is increased (center panel), the atrial contribution of ventricular filling is now operating on the steeper portion of the left ventricular pressure volume curve. The S_4 becomes louder and earlier, and S_1 is decreased in amplitude due to partial atriogenic closure of the mitral valve. This is the most likely explanation of a soft S_1 frequently noted in hypertensive patients with normal PR intervals.

Status of Ventricular Contraction The status of ventricular contractility is also an independent factor determining the amplitude of S_1.[27,28,30,33] In normal subjects, both exercise and catecholamine infusion have been shown to increase the amplitude of S_1, while administration of beta-blocking agents decreases it.[28,34] In both situations, the prime factor in altering the intensity of S_1 is the rate of pressure development in the ventricle. This increased rate of pressure development partially explains why S_1 is increased in patients with anemia, arteriovenous fistulas, pregnancy, anxiety, and fever.[35] It is also likely that these high-output states, often associated with tachycardia, result in wider separation of the AV valves at the onset of ventricular systole due to high flow through a shortened diastolic period. In a similar fashion, the loud T_1 in an atrial septal defect is due to high flow through the tricuspid valve, secondary to the left-to-right shunt at the atrial level. A decrease in the intensity of S_1 associated with a decrease in the rate of left ventricular pressure development is found in myxedema, cardiomyopathy, and acute myocardial infarction.[35,36] Beat-to-beat variation in the intensity of S_1 (auscultatory alternans) has also been found in patients with pulsus alternans, in whom beat-to-beat alteration in the rate of left ventricular pressure development occurs.[37]

Transmission Characteristics of the Thoracic Cavity and Chest Wall The degree of attenuation of heart sounds generated by the vibrating cardiohemic system is a function of both sound frequency and the distance of the heart from the chest wall. The higher frequency heart sounds are attenuated to a greater extent than are lower frequency sounds.[38] Conditions such as obesity, emphysema, or large pleural or pericardial effusions will decrease the intensity of all auscultatory events, while a thin-body habitus would tend to increase the intensity.

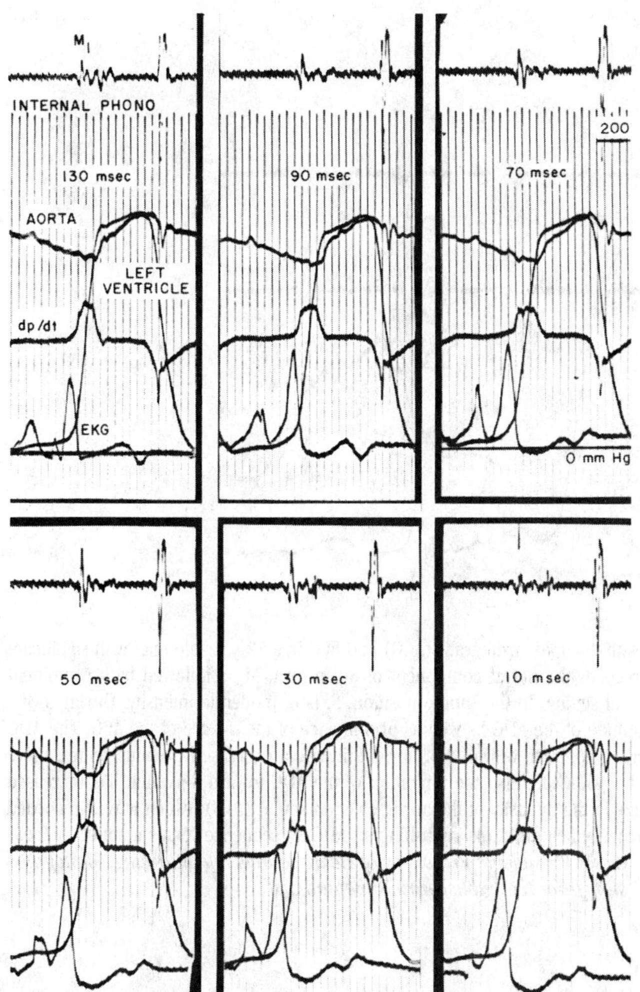

FIGURE 11-5 The effect of changing the PR interval on left ventricular sound and pressure events, as recorded by high-fidelity catheter-tipped micromanometers in an anesthetized dog preparation. The M_1 amplitude is markedly increased at the shorter PR intervals, while the maximum *dP/dt* is decreased. At the 10-ms PR interval, the M_1 amplitude is again decreased. Note that as the PR interval shortens, both M_1 and the notch on the *dP/dt* tracing occur later in systole and a plateau develops preceding the notch. (*From ME Stept, et al: Effect of altering P-R interval on the amplitude of the first heart sound in the anesthetized dog. Circ Res 25:259, 1969. Reproduced with permission from the American Heart Association, Inc., and the authors.*)

Physical Characteristics of the Vibrating Structures Alterations in the physical characteristics of the vibrating structures may also vary the intensity of S_1. Both myocardial infarction and ischemia induced by pacing have been shown to decrease the intensity of S_1 secondary to these alterations.[39,40]

S_1 *in Pathologic Conditions*

Careful attention to the intensity of S_1 is an extremely important aspect of cardiac auscultation, often giving clues to the proper diagnosis and the degree of abnormality of the involved structures. The following conditions are examples where alterations in the intensity of S_1 play a key role in the correct diagnosis.

S_1 in Mitral Stenosis A loud, late M_1 is the hallmark of hemodynamically significant mitral stenosis.[28,41,42] When M_1 is loud, it is associated with a loud opening snap, and the intensity of both M_1 and the opening snap correlate with valve motility (Fig. 11-7, left panel). When calcific fixation of the stenotic mitral valve occurs, M_1 is soft and the opening snap is absent (Fig. 11-4). The relationship between sound and pressure and echocardiographic mitral valve motion is shown in Fig. 11-8.[43] Significant scarring of the mitral valve is evident as a result of the rheumatic process. The increased left atrial pressure delays the time of pressure crossover between the left atrium and the left ventricle. As a result, M_1 occurs later and at a much higher than normal left ventricular pressure, at a time when there is a more rapid rate of development of left ventricular pressure. The presystolic gradient between the left atrium and left ventricle prevents preclosure of the mitral valve leaflets. As a result, the closure of the leaflet begins from a domed position within the left ventricular cavity and takes place over a much greater distance than normal following the onset of left ventricular contraction. Both of these factors increase the velocity of mitral valve closure and the momentum of blood directed toward the mitral valve leaflets, resulting in a loud M_1 when the elastic limits of the stenotic mitral valve are met. A similar mechanism is responsible for the booming S_1 with aftervibrations in left atrial myxoma (Fig. 11-7, center panel).[44,45]

S_1 in Mitral Valve Prolapse Tei and colleagues[26] have reported a loud M_1 heard over the apex in patients with nonrheumatic mitral regurgitation; this is indicative of holosystolic mitral valve prolapse (Fig. 11-7, right panel). Patients with the more common middle to late systolic prolapse have a normal S_1, while a soft or absent S_1 may indicate a flail mitral leaflet (Fig. 11-3). The increased amplitude of leaflet excursion with prolapse beyond the line of closure explains the loud M_1 associated with holosystolic prolapse. An alternate explanation may be a summation of a normal M_1 and an early nonejection click of valvular prolapse.

S_1 and Left Bundle Branch Block In left bundle branch block (LBBB), M_1 is decreased in intensity and is frequently delayed, at times resulting in reversal of sequence of S_1 (Fig. 11-9).[28,46–48] The reason for the delay and the decreased intensity of M_1 in this condition is multifactional, with different mechanisms operative in different patients depending on the degree of completeness of the LBBB, the site of block (proximal versus peripheral), and especially the status of left ventricular function.[49–51] The primary factors involved are (1) delay in onset of left ventricular contraction, (2) degree of left ventricular dysfunction, (3) presence of concomitant first-degree heart block, and (4) presence of a noncompliant left ventricle facilitating atriogenic preclosure of the mitral valve. It is likely that more than one factor is operative in most patients with LBBB, with one or two factors predominating.

S_1 in Acute Aortic Regurgitation One of the important auscultatory findings in acute aortic regurgitation is attenuation or absence of M_1, as shown in Fig. 11-10.[28,30,52,53] Severe regurgitation into a left ventricle that has not had time to adapt to the acute volume

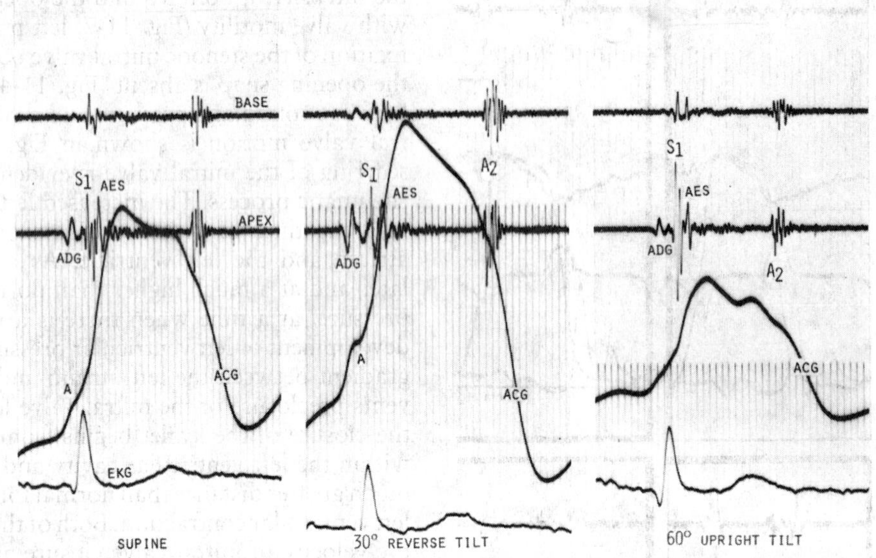

FIGURE 11-6 Base and apex phonocardiograms are recorded simultaneously with the apexcardiogram (ACG) and ECG in a 52-year-old man with significant systemic hypertension. In all three postures, an atrial diastolic gallop (ADG) precedes the mitral component of S_1. In turn, M_1 is followed by a prominent second component that is mostly likely an aortic root ejection sound in this clinical setting. In the supine position, S_1 is of moderate intensity. During a 30° reverse tilt with increased venous return, there is significant increase in the amplitude of the ADG as well as prominence of the *a* wave of the ACG. The ADG is also further separated from the mitral component of S_1, which is slightly softer. In contrast, with 60° of upright tilt and a decrease in venous return, there is a significant decrease in the intensity of the ADG and loss of the *a* wave on the ACG. Note also the migration of the ADG toward S_1, which has increased significantly in intensity. With these postural changes, there is no significant change in the intensity of the aortic ejection sound (AES), which is well recorded at the apex and at the base. These simple maneuvers at the bedside can be particularly helpful in distinguishing an ADG–S_1 sequence versus a split S_1. [*From JA Shaver, et al: Ejection sounds of left-sided origin. In: DF Leon, JA Shaver, (eds): Physiologic Principles of Heart Sounds and Murmurs, Monograph 46. Dallas, American Heart Association, 1975, p 31. Reproduced with permission from the publisher and the authors.*]

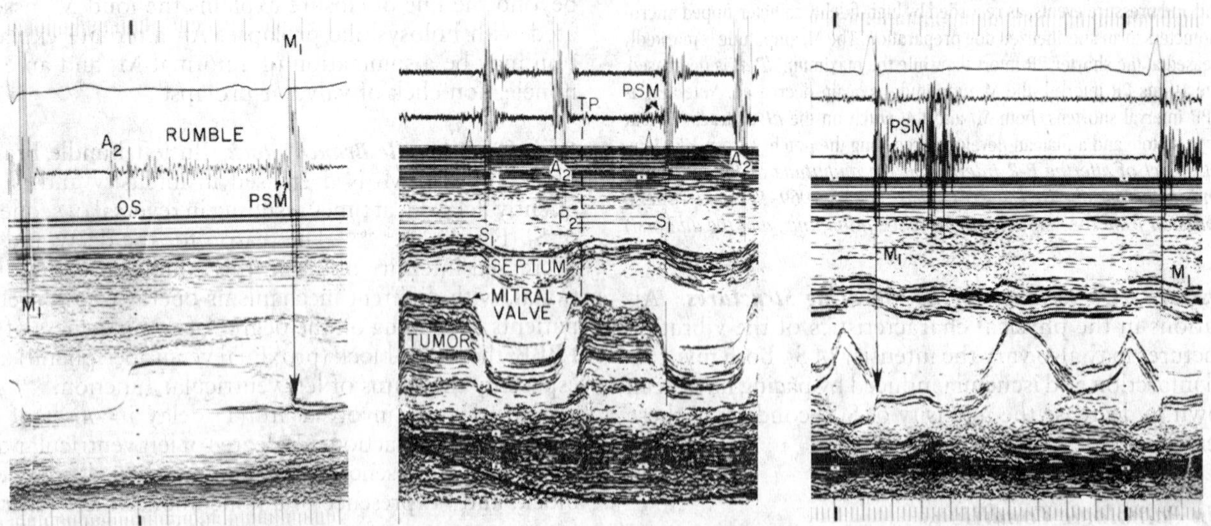

FIGURE 11-7 Simultaneous phonocardiograms are recorded with the mitral valve echocardiograms in three patients: mitral stenosis (*left panel*), left atrial myxoma (*center panel*), and prolapse of the mitral valve (*right panel*). In each condition, a loud M_1 is present and coincident with the closing point of the mitral valve echocardiogram. Common to each condition is wide separation of the mitral leaflets at the onset of left ventricular systole with high-velocity closure occurring over a large excursion. In the left panel a mobile stenotic valve is demonstrated, and a loud opening snap is coincident with the E point. In the center panel, an early diastolic tumor plop (TP) is coincident with the maximal excursion of the tumor during its rapid descent into the ventricle. Note the presystolic crescendo murmur (PSM) occurring during the rapid closure of the mitral valve in both mitral stenosis and left atrial myxoma. In the right panel, a pansystolic murmur (PSM) with late systolic accentuation is secondary to the prolapse of the mitral valve with late systolic hammocking. [*From JA Shaver: Current uses of phonocardiography in clinical practice. In: E Rapaport (ed): Cardiology Update—Reviews for Physicians. New York, Elsevier, 1981, p 370. Reproduced in part (center panel) with permission of the publisher and the author. Copyright 1981 by Elsevier Science Publishing Co., Inc.*]

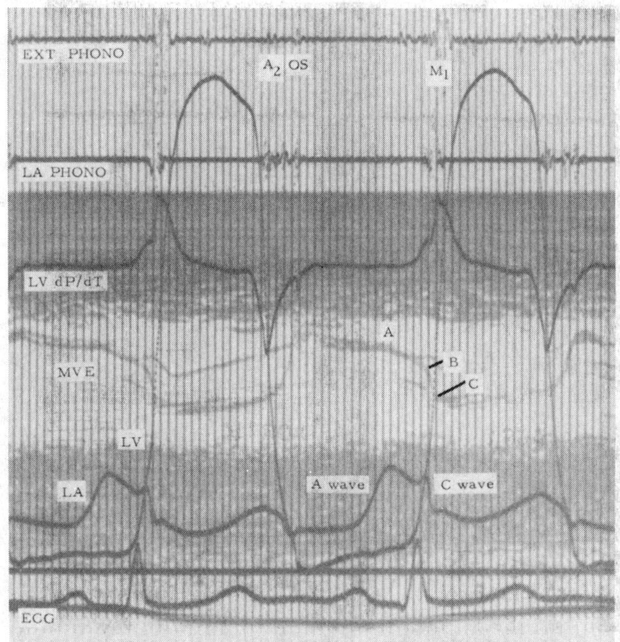

FIGURE 11-8 External sound, equisensitive left ventricular and left atrial pressures (catheter-tipped micromanometer), left ventricular *dP/dt*, and left atrial sound are recorded simultaneously with the mitral valve echocardiogram in a patient with hemodynamically significant mitral stenosis. A significant presystolic gradient is present due to atrial contraction, and the onset of the rapid closure of the mitral valve (B) is delayed until the left ventricular pressure exceeds left atrial pressure. This occurs 40 ms after the beginning of the left ventricular pressure rise at a time when left ventricular *dP/dt* is much higher than normal. Following left atrial–left ventricular pressure crossover, there is rapid ventriculogenic closure of the mitral valve (B-C), resulting in a very loud M_1 coincident with the C point of the mitral valve echocardiogram and the downstroke of the *c* wave of the left atrial pressure. A prominent opening snap is coincident with the E point of the mitral valve echocardiogram. Its separation from A_2 is determined by both the level of the left atrial pressure and the rate of left ventricular pressure decline. (*From JA Shaver, et al: Normal and abnormal heart sounds in cardiac diagnosis. Part 1: Systolic sounds. Curr Probl Cardiol 10(3):21, 1985. Reproduced with permission of the publisher and the authors.*)

overload causes a marked increase in the left ventricular end-diastolic pressure, resulting in premature closure of the normal mitral valve in middiastole. With the onset of left ventricular systole minimal valve excursion occurs, causing a marked reduction in the intensity of M_1.

Systolic Ejection Sounds

Ejection sounds are early systolic ejection events that can originate from either the left or the right side of the heart. These sounds have been classified as *valvular,* arising from deformed aortic or pulmonic valves, or as *vascular*, or root events caused by the forceful ejection of blood into the great vessels. Careful attention to the presence or absence of valvular ejection sounds is of great benefit in defining the level of right or left ventricular outflow tract obstruction while root ejection sounds give insight into abnormalities of the great vessels with or without systemic or pulmonary hypertension.

Aortic Valvular Ejection Sounds

Aortic valvular ejection sounds are found in nonstenotic congenital bicuspid valves and in the entire spectrum of mild to severe stenosis of the aortic valve. This sound introduces the typical ejection murmur of aortic stenosis, is widely transmitted, and is often heard best at the apex. As shown in the left panel of Fig. 11-11, the aortic valvular ejection sound is delayed 20 to 40 ms after the onset of pressure rise in the central aorta and is coincident with the sharp anacrotic notch on the upstroke of the aortic pressure curve. Simultaneous sound, pressure, and cineangiographic studies have shown that this sound is coincident with the maximal excursion of the domed valve when its elastic limits are met.[54–57] The abrupt deceleration of the oncoming column of blood sets the entire cardiohemic system into vibration, the lower frequency components being recorded as the anacrotic notch and the high-frequency components representing the valvular ejection sound. Inherent in this mechanism of sound production is the ability of the deformed valve to move. With severe calcific fixation of the valve, no excursion or pistonlike ascent of the deformed valve is possible; therefore, no sudden tensing of the valve leaflets or abrupt deceleration of the column of blood occurs. As shown in the right panel of Fig. 11-11, neither an anacrotic notch on the upstroke of the aortic pressure nor a valvular ejection sound is recorded in this situation.

Sound and motion correlates identical to those demonstrated by cineangiography have been found with phonoechocardiography, clearly showing the onset of the ejection sound to be coincident with the maximal opening of the valve (Fig. 11-12).[15,58] The intensity of the ejection sound correlates directly with the mobility of the valve, but there is no correlation between intensity and the severity of the obstruction. In mobile, nonstenotic bicuspid valves, the ejection sound is not only loud but also widely separated from S_1 due to the prolonged excursion of the mobile valve (Fig. 11-13, left panel).[59] The presence of an aortic valvular ejection sound is a valuable physical finding at the bedside; it not only defines the left ventricular outflow obstruction at the valvular level but also gives insight into the mobility of the valve (Fig. 11-13).

Pulmonary Valvular Ejection Sounds

Pulmonary valvular ejection sounds have identical sound and pressure correlates as aortic valvular ejection sounds.[60] Echocardiographic correlations have also shown that the onset of the pulmonary ejection sound occurs at the maximal excursion of the stenotic pulmonary valve.[15,58] In contrast to the aortic valvular ejection sounds and to most right-sided auscultatory events, the pulmonic sound or ejection click decreases in intensity or disappears with inspiration in mild to moderate stenosis. The hemodynamic mechanism responsible for this phenomenon[60–62] is shown in Fig. 11-14. The elegant phonoechocardiographic studies of Weyman and associates[63] and Mills and Craige[18] have documented this dynamic movement of the pulmonary valve with respiration. In very mild valvular pulmonic stenosis, respiratory varia-

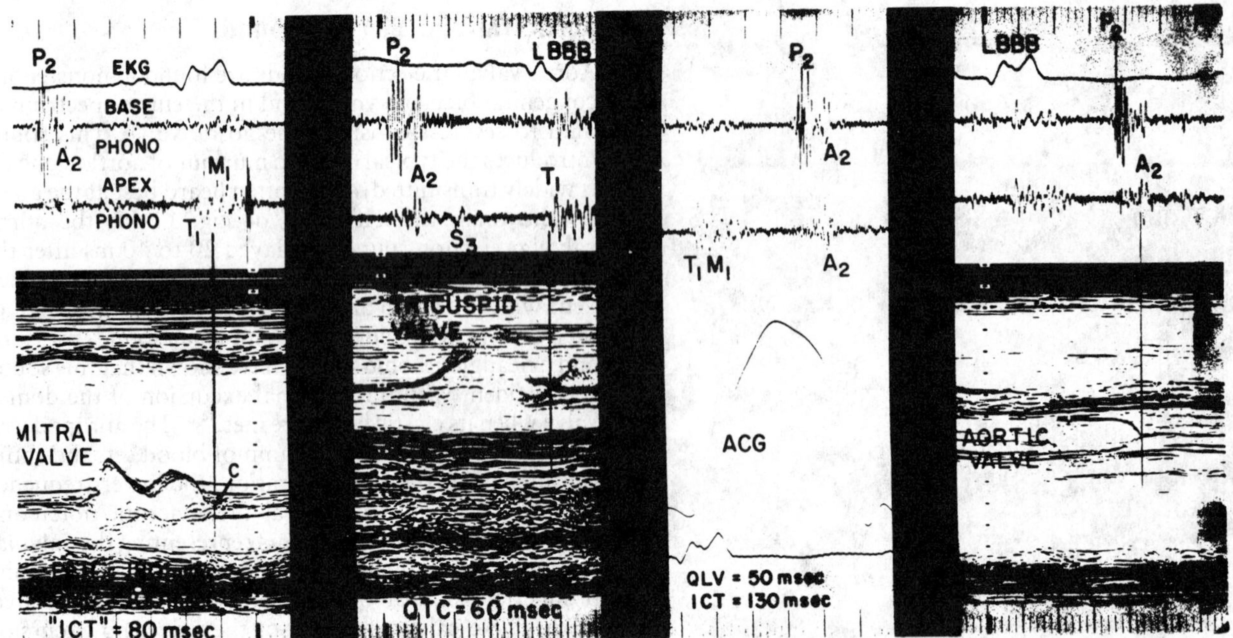

FIGURE 11-9 Base and apex phonocardiograms are recorded simultaneously with the mitral and tricuspid valve echocardiogram, the apexcardiogram (ACG), and the aortic valve echocardiogram in a patient with LBBB and significant left ventricular dysfunction. A markedly delayed M_1 is coincident with complete coaptation of the anterior and posterior leaflets of the mitral valve. The sequence of S_1 is reversed. The mitral valve echocardiogram shows significant atriogenic preclosure of the anterior and posterior leaflets and is followed by slow ventriculogenic closure of the valve, resulting in a soft M_1. In the next panel, T_1 is clearly shown to be coincident with the final closure point of the tricuspid valve and precedes M_1. Reversed splitting of S_2 is present and is confirmed by simultaneous recording of the aortic valve echocardiogram in the far right panel. In this patient with LBBB, the electromechanical interval (Q–left ventricular) was within normal limits, and the reversed splitting of S_1 and S_2 was due to severe left ventricular dysfunction with marked prolongation of isovolumic contraction time. (*From JA Shaver, et al: Effects of left bundle branch block on the events of the cardic cycle. Acta Cardiol 43:461–462, 1988. Reproduced with permission of the publisher and authors.*)

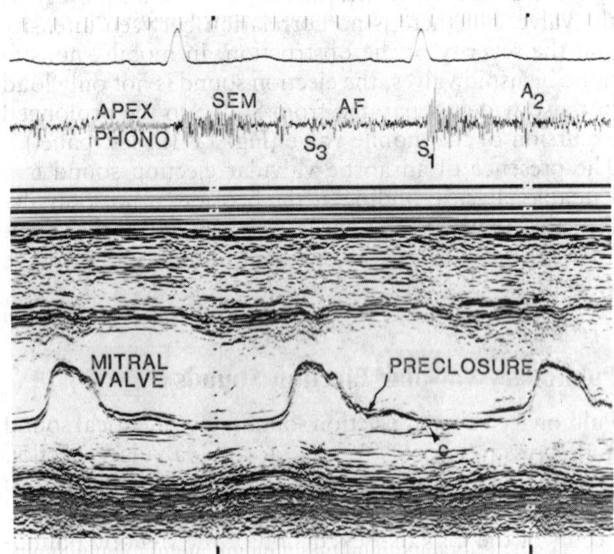

FIGURE 11-10 The apex phonocardiogram is recorded simultaneously with the mitral valve echocardiogram in a patient with acute aortic regurgitation. There is middiastolic preclosure of the mitral valve, and a very soft S_1 is recorded coincident with the terminal closing motion of the mitral valve following the onset of ventricular systole. A systolic ejection murmur (SEM) is present during systole, and an Austin Flint murmur (AF) is introduced by an S_3 gallop during early diastole. Note the absence of the presystolic component of the Austin Flint murmur. (*From JA Shaver, et al: Normal and abnormal heart sounds in cardiac diagnosis. Part I: Systolic sounds. Curr Probl Cardiol 10(3):25, 1985. Reproduced with permission of the publisher and the authors.*)

tion may be absent.[60] In very severe valvular obstruction, a vigorous atrial contraction can completely preopen the pulmonic valve in diastole, causing a crisp preejection sound.[64,65] In this situation, it has been shown that right ventricular pressure at the time of the atrial kick actually exceeds pulmonary artery end-diastolic pressure.[60] As the severity of the pulmonic stenosis increases, both the excursion of the deformed valve and the right ventricular isovolumic contraction time decrease. The net effect of both of these events is migration of the pulmonary ejection sound toward S_1.

Aortic Vascular Ejection Sounds

Ejection sounds originating from the aortic root are common in systemic hypertension in the setting of a tortuous sclerotic aortic root, a tight, noncompliant arterial tree, and forceful left ventricular ejection. They are coincident with the upstroke of the high-fidelity central aortic pressure and have been interpreted as an exaggeration of the ejection component of the normal S_1.[54,55] Echocardiographic correlations by Mills and associates,[58] however, have shown that this sound occurs at the moment of complete opening of the aortic valve and always on the pressure upstroke of the high-fidelity aortic pressure curve. These observations have led them to conclude that this sound probably originates from the valve leaflets. At the present time, these minor discrepancies regarding the

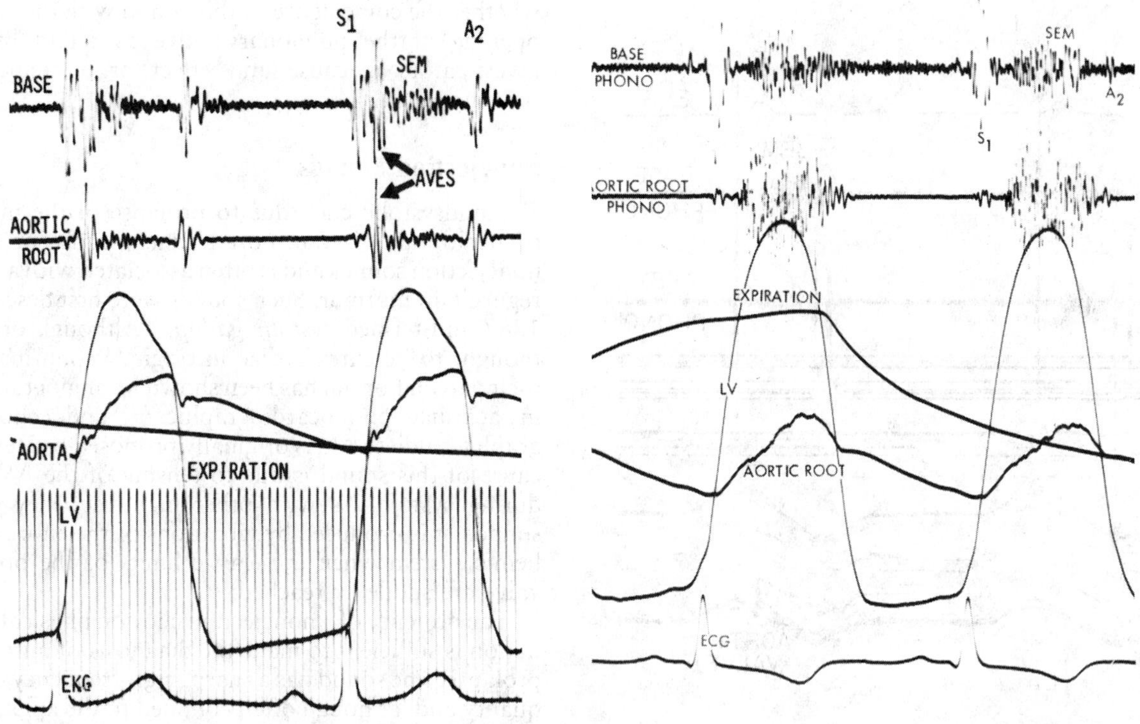

FIGURE 11-11 Base and aortic root phonocardiograms are recorded simultaneously with high-fidelity catheter-tipped micromanometers in the central aorta and left ventricle in a 23-year-old man with mild valvular aortic stenosis (*left panel*) and in an elderly patient with severe calcification of the aortic valve (*right panel*). In valvular aortic stenosis, the murmur is introduced by a loud aortic valvular ejection sound (AVES). The peak gradient across the aortic valve was less than 30 mmHg, and the systolic ejection murmur ends well before the prominent aortic closure sound. With calcific fixation of the aortic valve, a valvular ejection sound is not recorded on either the base or the aortic root phonocardiogram, nor is an anacrotic notch present on the upstroke of the central aortic pressure trace. Note also that the aortic closure sound is barely recordable at the base. [*From JA Shaver: Innocent murmurs. Hosp Med, April 1978, p 25. © 1978. Reproduced from Hospital Medicine in part (left panel) with permission of Hospital Publications, Inc. and the author; and from JA Shaver, et al: Ejection sounds of left-sided origin. In: DF Leon, JA Shaver (eds): Physiologic Principles of Heart Sounds and Murmurs, Monograph 46. Dallas, American Heart Association, 1975, p 33. Reproduced in part (right panel) with permission from the publisher and the authors.*]

exact mechanisms of production of this sound have not been resolved.

In contrast to the ejection sound of the stenotic aortic valve, these root sounds tend to be poorly transmitted from the aortic area and are not heard well at the apex. It may be difficult at times (if not impossible) to differentiate this sound from the tricuspid component of a widely split S_1, which is best heard at the fourth left parasternal area and often increases with inspiration. The bedside decision as to whether this is T_1 versus an ejection sound will often be dictated by the clinical situation. In either condition, it should be emphasized that the benign S_1 ejection sound or M_1-T_1 complex is frequently misinterpreted as a pathologic S_4-S_1 sequence. Factors that favor the presence of an S_4-S_1 complex are an associated palpable presystolic apical impulse, optimal audibility of the S_4 with the stethoscope bell applied lightly at the apex, and a change in the intensity of the S_4 with maneuvers that vary venous return (Fig. 11-6).

Pulmonary Vascular Ejection Sounds

Vascular or root ejection sounds may also arise from the pulmonary artery, and the common denominator is dilation of the pulmonary artery.[60] This dilation can be idiopathic or secondary to severe pulmonary hypertension. Although Leatham and Vogelpoel[66] have stated that this sound is louder during expiration, there is no consensus on this point. Unlike splitting of S_1, which is heard best at the mitral or tricuspid area, this sound is louder in the second and third left intercostal spaces.

Echocardiographic correlates of the pulmonary root ejection sound show it to be coincide with complete opening of the pulmonary valve, occurring during the upstroke of the high-fidelity pulmonary artery pressure recording.[58,67] This has led to the conclusion that these vascular ejection sounds may originate from semilunar valve cusps that have undergone changes in structure in response to increased pressure.[18] Other investigators have found that the pulmonary root ejection sounds in the setting of pulmonary hypertension coincide with the upstroke of the high-fidelity pulmonary artery pressure tracing, while in both idiopathic dilation of the pulmonary artery and atrial septal defect, this sound occurs during the upstroke of the pulmonary pressure tracing.[60] In each of these conditions, it has been suggested that this sound is related to sudden checking of the rapidly accelerating blood column by the "tight" or "loose" pulmonary artery when its elastic limits are met. At the present time, it is not possible to state with certainty

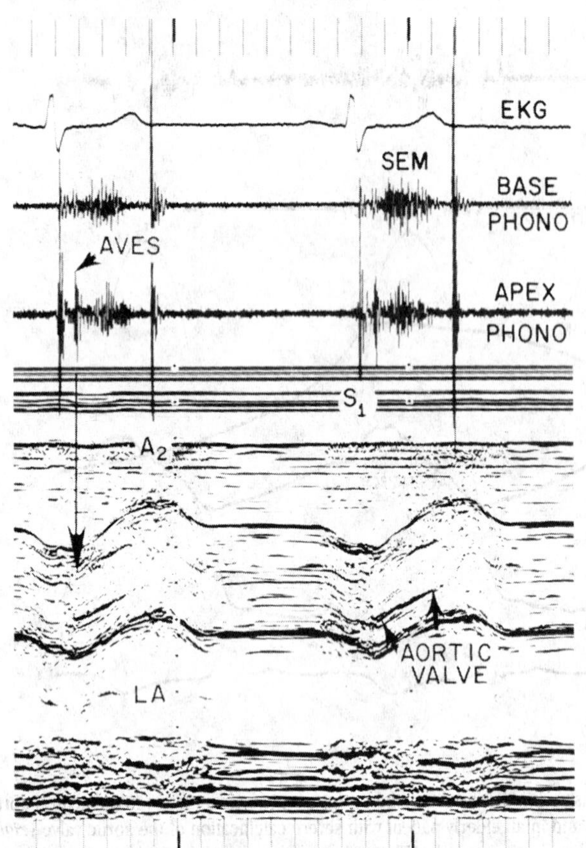

FIGURE 11-12 Base and apex phonocardiograms are recorded simultaneously with the aortic valve echocardiogram in a young man with valvular aortic stenosis. A prominent aortic valvular ejection sound (AVES) is recorded at the apex and is coincident with the maximal excursion of the aortic valve in early systole. It is followed by a crescendo-decrescendo systolic ejection murmur (SEM) that ends well before a loud A_2.

whether the coincidence of this sound with the maximal opening of the pulmonary valve as found by some investigators is cause and effect or a chance relationship.

Nonejection Sounds

The midsystolic click due to prolapse of the mitral or tricuspid valve is the most frequent cause of systolic nonejection sounds and is often associated with a systolic regurgitant murmur. Such sounds were first described in 1887 and termed *systolic gallop*.[68] Although originally thought to be extracardiac in origin,[69] confirmation of their valvular origin has been shown by angiographic,[70,71] intracardiac phonocardiographic,[72,73] and echocardiographic studies.[74–76] As originally proposed by Reid,[77] the cause of this sound is due to tensing of the AV valves during systole. As with other high-frequency cardiac sounds, it is produced by vibrations of the entire cardiohemic system when the elastic limits of the prolapsed valve are suddenly reached.

The presence of a nonejection click on physical examination is sufficient to make the diagnosis of mitral valve prolapse. The sound has a sharp, high-frequency clicking quality and, although often confined to the apex, can be transmitted widely on the precordium. It may be an isolated finding occurring most often in middle to late systole or there may be multiple clicks, presumably as a result of different areas of the large, redundant, scalloped mitral leaflets prolapsing at different times (Fig. 11-15). Numerous echocardiographic studies have shown the presence of the characteristic mid- to late systolic prolapse as well as holosystolic prolapse in patients with clicks. All of these patterns may be seen in the presence of an isolated systolic click, click and late systolic mur-

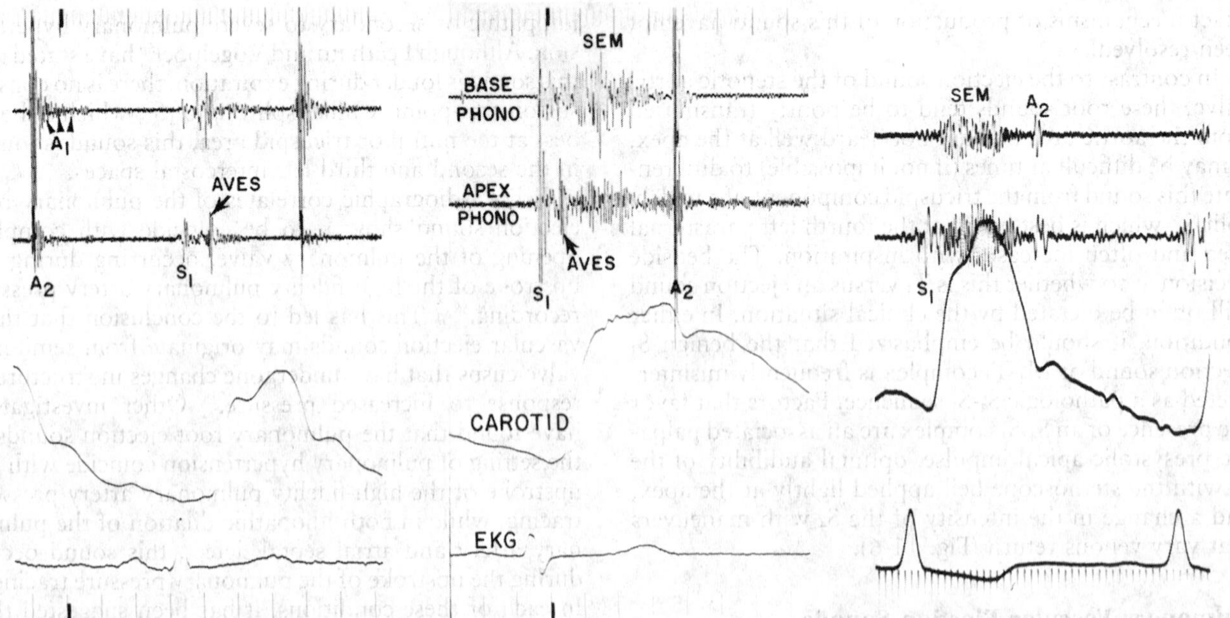

FIGURE 11-13 A prominent aortic valvular ejection sound (AVES) of a congenital nonstenotic and stenotic bicuspid aortic valve is shown on the left and center panels, respectively. On the right panel there is no evidence of a valvular ejection sound in a patient with severe fixed orifice subaortic stenosis. The valvular ejection sound of the nonstenotic bicuspid valve is widely separated from S_1 and unassociated with a subsequent murmur. The ejection sound of the stenotic bicuspid valve introduces the typical crescendo-decrescendo murmur of valvular aortic stenosis. In both conditions, A_2 is well preserved.

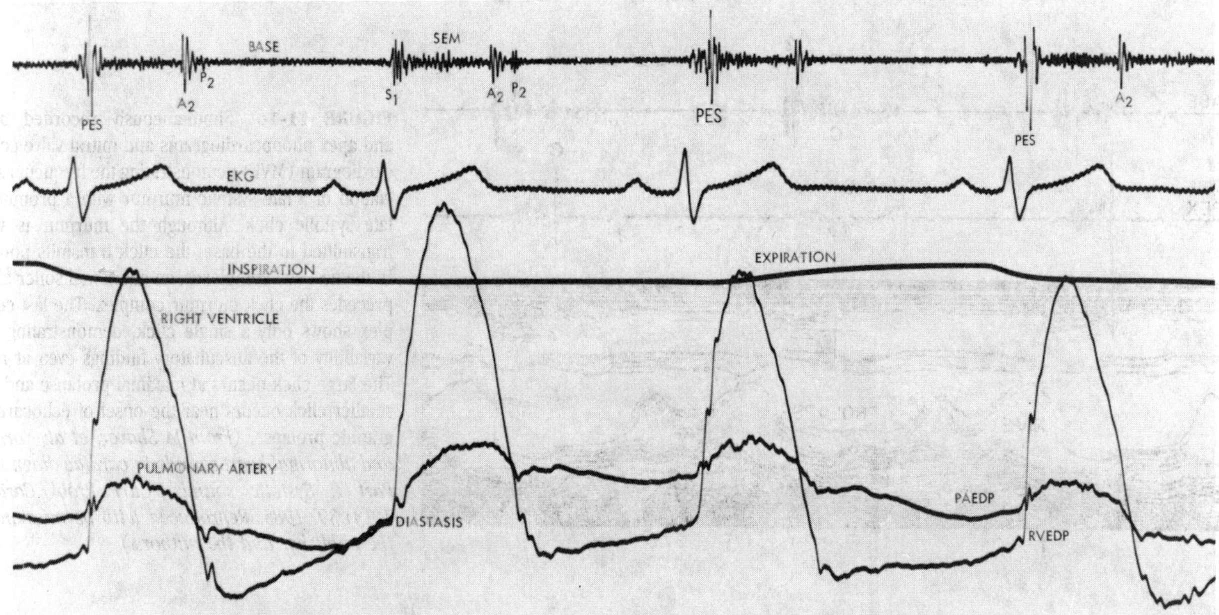

FIGURE 11-14 Simultaneous right ventricular and pulmonary artery pressures are recorded with the phonocardiogram showing the mechanism of the attenuation of the pulmonary valvular ejection sound (PES) during respiration in a patient with mild valvular pulmonic stenosis. In the second complex, the valvular ejection sound has disappeared and there is complete equalization of the diastolic pressures in the right ventricle and pulmonary artery. With equalization of pressure there is preopening of the deformed stenotic valve, and with the onset of right ventricular systole no further excursion of the domed valve is possible, and the ejection sound is absent. During expiration, the pulmonary artery diastolic pressure is significantly higher than the right ventricular end-diastolic pressure, and the prominent ejection sound is again recorded. Considerable variation of the ejection sound occurs during various phases of respiration and is caused by varying degrees of preopening of the valve. Note the tendency for the ejection sound to occur later during the expiratory phase. (*From PS Reddy, et al: Cardiac systolic murmurs: Pathophysiology and differential diagnosis. Prog Cardiovasc Dis 14:14, 1974. Reproduced in part with permission of the publisher and the authors.*)

mur, or the late systolic murmur alone. The click usually occurs at the time of maximum prolapse; the lack of exact correlation of maximal valvular prolapse and the auscultatory findings is the result of the M-mode echocardiographic technique, which allows visualization of only a small portion of the valve.

A feature of mitral valve prolapse is the variability of the auscultatory findings from examination to examination and even from beat to beat (Fig. 11-16). The timing of the click, or click and the late systolic murmur, vary considerably with changes in posture (Fig. 11-17).[78] In the upright posture, the heart becomes smaller due to decreased venous return, and the click moves earlier in systole. Angiographic studies have confirmed an earlier and greater degree of prolapse in the upright posture compared to the supine position.[79] Squatting, which

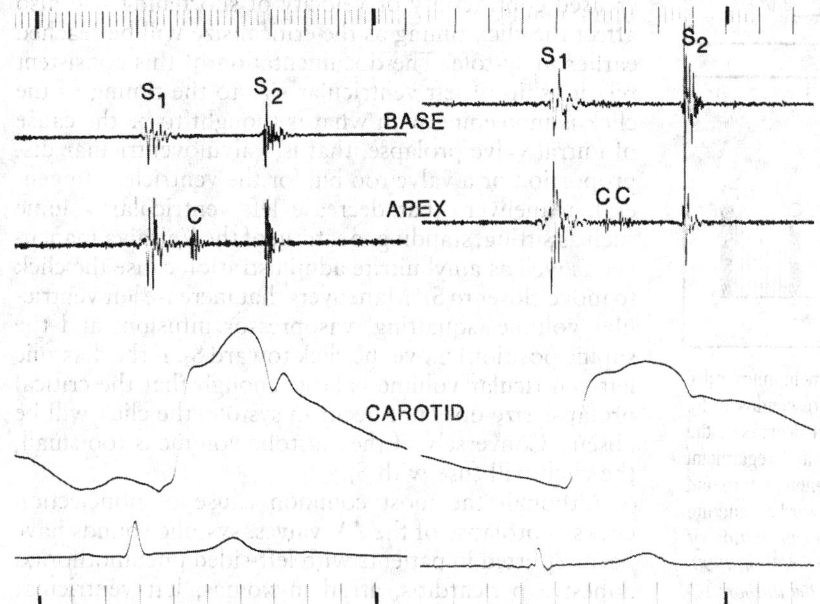

FIGURE 11-15 Base and apex phonocardiograms in two patients with nonejection clicks. The apex phonocardiogram shows an isolated systolic click (*left*). In the right panel are two close clicks 40 ms apart. On examination, multiple clicks may sound like a scratchy murmur rather than individual clicks. (*From JA Shaver, et al: Normal and abnormal heart sounds in cardiac diagnosis. Part I: Systolic sounds. Curr Probl Cardiol 10(3):38, 1985. Reproduced with permission of the publisher and the authors.*)

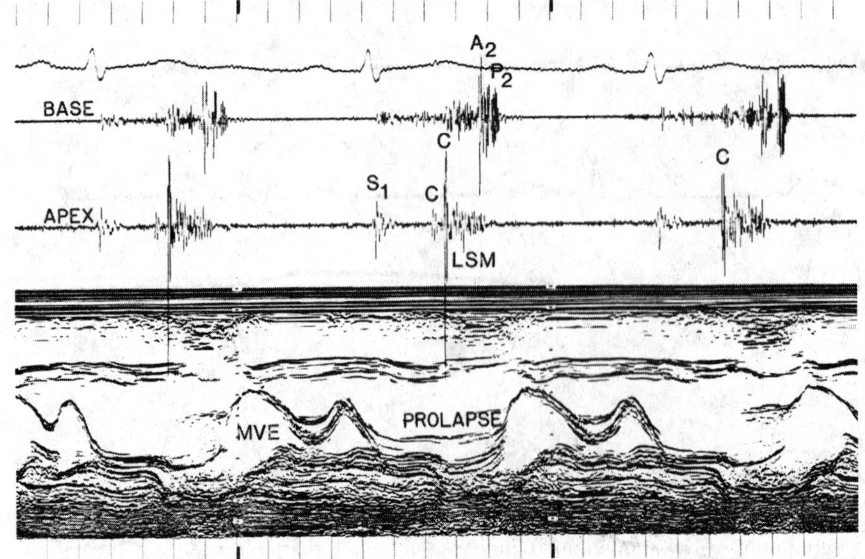

FIGURE 11-16 Simultaneously recorded base and apex phonocardiograms and mitral valve echocardiogram (MVE) demonstrating the frequent association of a late systolic murmur with a prominent late systolic click. Although the murmur is well transmitted to the base, the click transmits poorly. In the first two complexes, an additional softer click precedes the click murmur complex. The last complex shows only a single click, demonstrating the variability of the auscultatory findings even at rest. The large click occurs at maximal prolapse and the smaller click occurs near the onset of echocardiographic prolapse. *(From JA Shaver, et al: Normal and abnormal heart sounds in cardiac diagnosis. Part I: Systolic sounds. Curr Probl Cardiol 10(3):39, 1985. Reproduced with permission of the publisher and the authors.)*

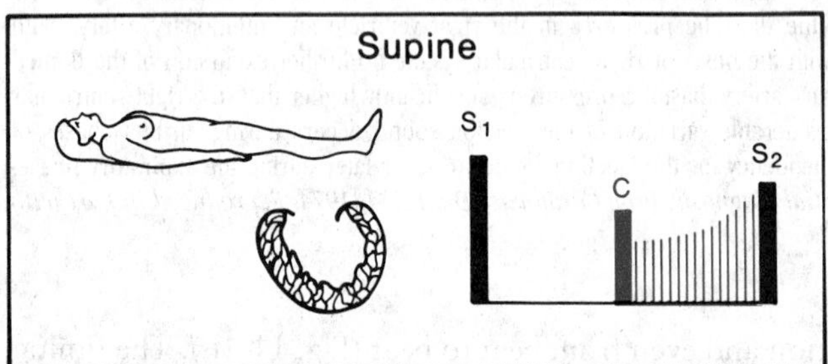

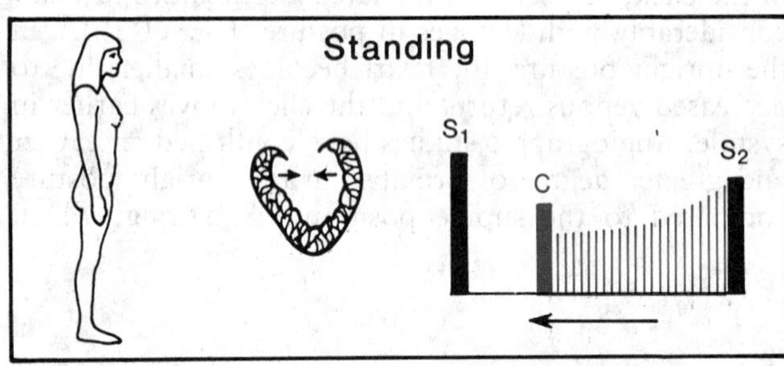

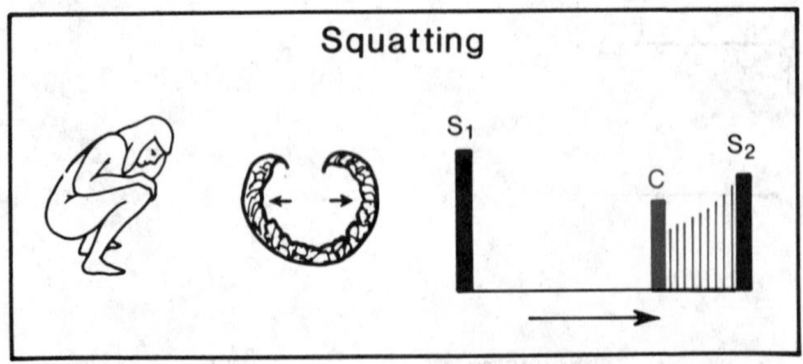

FIGURE 11-17 A midsystolic nonejection sound (C) occurs in mitral valve prolapse and is followed by a late systolic murmur that crescendos to S_2. With the assumption of the upright posture, venous return decreases, the heart becomes smaller, the C moves closer to S_1, and the mitral regurgitant murmur has an earlier onset. With prompt squatting, both venous return and afterload increase, the heart becomes larger, the C moves toward S_2, and the duration of the murmur shortens. *(From JA Shaver, et al: Examination of the Heart, Part IV, Auscultation, Dallas, American Heart Association, 1990, p 13. Reproduced with permission of the publisher and the authors.)*

causes an immediate increase in venous return and afterload, increases left ventricular volume, resulting in later prolapse and movement of the click toward S_2. At the bedside, these simple maneuvers are helpful in differentiating the nonejection click from early ejection sounds, a split S_2, or an S_3.

Other physiologic and pharmacologic maneuvers that vary the loading conditions of the heart also cause changes in the timing of the auscultatory event. Phonoechocardiographic correlations during the inhalation of amyl nitrite have confirmed the cause-and-effect relationship between the echocardiographically demonstrated prolapse and the timing of the click.[76] Mathey and associates[80] have demonstrated that echocardiographically determined left ventricular diameter was relatively constant at the time of the click during supine, upright, and amyl nitrite conditions, indicating that a critical size was necessary for prolapse to occur. Increased contractility or velocity of shortening will also affect the click timing as the critical size will be reached earlier in systole. The documentation of this consistent relationship of left ventricular size to the timing of the click is in keeping with what is thought to be the cause of mitral valve prolapse, that is, valvuloventricular disproportion or a valve too big for the ventricle.[81] In general, maneuvers that decrease left ventricular volume such as sitting, standing, or strain of the Valsalva maneuver as well as amyl nitrite administration cause the click to move closer to S_1. Maneuvers that increase left ventricular volume (squatting, vasopressor infusion, and the supine position) move the click toward S_2. If the diastolic left ventricular volume is large enough that the critical prolapse size does not occur in systole, the click will be absent. Conversely, if the diastolic volume is too small, the click will fuse with S_1.

Although the most common cause of nonejection clicks is prolapse of the AV valves, systolic sounds have been reported in patients with left-sided pneumothorax, adhesive pericarditis, atrial myxomas, left ventricular aneurysm, aneurysm of the membranous ventricular septum associated with a ventricular septal defect, and incompetent heterograft valves.[82–85] The presence of these conditions can usually be recognized by the clinical setting and by the absence of the typical changes in the timing of the click associated with physiologic and pharmacologic maneuvers.

The Second Heart Sound

Leatham[86] has emphasized the importance of the S_2 in the cardiac examination by labeling it the "key to auscultation of the heart." To appreciate the significance of the normal and the abnormal S_2, knowledge of its relationship to the hemodynamic events of the cardiac cycle is essential.[87–89] In Fig. 11-18, the two components of S_2 are recorded simultaneously with the cardiac cycle by high-fidelity catheter-tipped micromanometers. The A_2 and P_2 are coincident with the incisura of the aorta and pulmonary artery pressure trace, respectively, and terminate the left and right ventricular ejection periods. Right ventricular ejection begins prior to left ventricular ejection, has a longer duration, and terminates after left ventricular ejection, resulting in P_2 normally occurring after A_2 (plates II and III). Right and left ventricular systole are nearly equal in duration, and the pulmonary artery incisura is delayed relative to the aortic incisura, primarily due to a larger interval separating the pulmonary artery incisura from the right ventricular pressure, compared with the same left-sided event. This interval has been called the "hangout" interval, a purely descriptive term coined in our laboratory over 15 years ago. Its duration is felt to be a reflection of the impedance of the vascular bed into which the blood is being received.[90–92] Normally, it is less than 15 ms in the systemic circulation and only slightly prolongs the left ventricular ejection time. In the low-resistance, high-capacitance pulmonary bed, however, this interval is normally much greater than on the left, varying between 43 and 86 ms, and therefore contributes significantly to the duration of right ventricular ejection.[90] Awareness of this interval is essential for proper understanding of normal physiologic splitting and for the abnormal splitting seen in conditions where significant alterations in pulmonary vascular impedance have occurred.

Echocardiographic Correlations and Mechanism of Sound Production

In Fig. 11-19, the relationship between the aortic and pulmonary valve echocardiogram and A_2 and P_2 is shown. The first high-frequency component of both A_2 and P_2 is coincident with completion of closure of the aortic and pulmonic valve leaflets. Identical correlations have been found by other investigators.[93,94] As with sounds arising from the AV valves, A_2 and P_2 are not due to the clapping together of the valve leaflets but are produced by the sudden deceleration of retrograde flow of the blood column in the aorta and pulmonary artery when the elastic limits of the tensed leaflets are met. This abrupt deceleration of flow sets the cardiohemic system into vibration; the lower frequency vibrations are recorded as in the incisura of the great vessels, while the higher frequency components result in A_2 and P_2. This

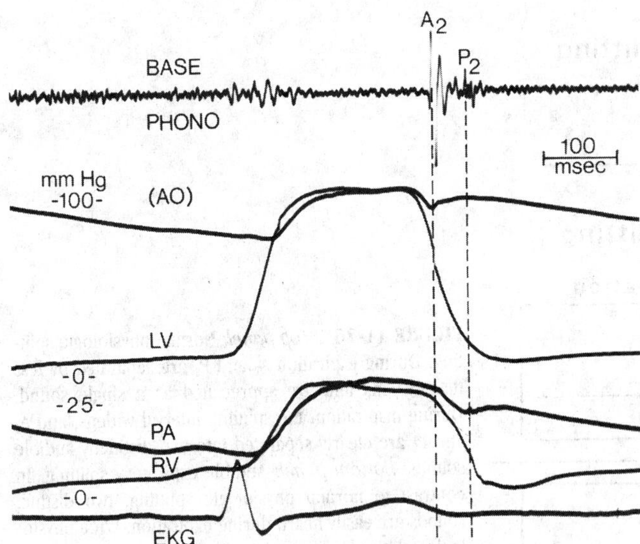

FIGURE 11-18 The cardiac cycle recorded by high-fidelity catheter-tipped micromanometers. The aortic (A_2) and pulmonic (P_2) closure sounds are coincident with the incisurae of their respective arterial traces. Although the left and right ventricular mechanical systole are nearly equal in duration, the right ventricular (RV) systolic ejection period terminates after left ventricular (LV) ejection because of an increased right-sided "hangout" interval. (*From JA Shaver, et al: The second heart sound: Newer concepts. Part 1: Normal and wide physiological splitting. Mod Concepts Cardiovasc Dis 46:7, 1977. Reproduced with permission from the American Heart Association, Inc., and the authors.*)

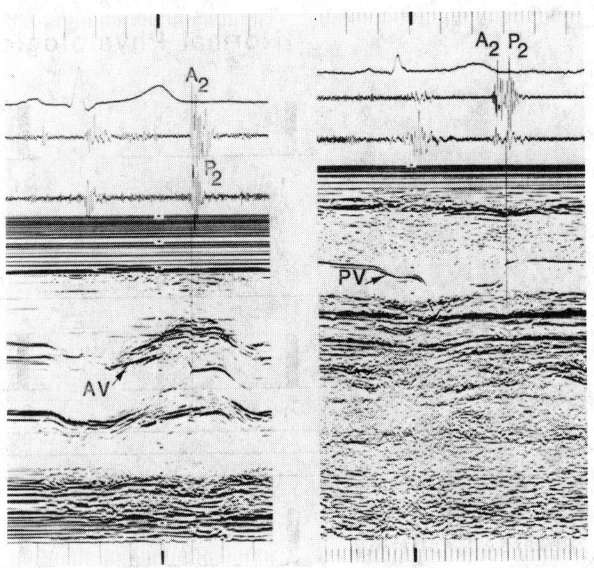

FIGURE 11-19 *Left panel:* The base and apex phonocardiograms are recorded simultaneously with the aortic valve echocardiogram. The first high-frequency component of A_2 is coincident with the completion of closure of the aortic valve. *Right panel:* Base and apex phonocardiograms are recorded with the pulmonary valve echocardiogram. The first high-frequency component of P_2 is coincident with the completion of closure of the pulmonic valve. (*From JA Shaver, et al: Normal and abnormal heart sounds in cardiac diagnosis. Part 1: Systolic sounds. Curr Probl Cardiol 10(3):43, 1985. Reproduced with permission of the publisher and the authors.*)

mechanism of sound production is consistent with Rushmer's[19] original observations as well as with several subsequent investigations.[90,95,96] In further support of this theory are additional observations showing that the amplitude of A_2 and P_2 is directly proportional to the rate of change of the diastolic pressure gradient that develops across the valves, that is, the driving force accelerating the blood mass retrograde into the base of the great vessels.[95,97] This pressure gradient is the result of both the level of the diastolic pressure in the great vessel and the rate of pressure decline in the ventricle and is consistent with the well-known clinical observation of increased intensity of A_2 and P_2 in systemic and pulmonary hypertension.

Normal Physiologic Splitting

Normally during expiration, A_2 and P_2 are separated by an interval of less than 30 ms and are heard by the clinician as a single sound.[98,99] During inspiration, both components become distinctly audible as the splitting interval widens, primarily due to a delayed P_2,[10,100] although an earlier A_2 contributes to a lesser degree (Fig. 11-20).[101-106] The traditional explanation of normal splitting was that the delayed P_2 during inspiration was secondary to increased venous return, prolonging the duration of right ventricular systole, while a concomitant decrease in venous return to the left heart shortened left ventricular systole.[107-109] More recent studies have shown that the delayed P_2 and early A_2 associated with inspiration are due to a complex interplay between dynamic changes in pulmonary vascular impedance and changes in systemic and pulmonary venous return.[106] The net effect of these changes is prolongation of right ventricular ejection and a concomitant decrease in left ventricular ejection that results in widening of the splitting interval during inspiration.

On auscultation, splitting of S_2 is usually best heard at the second or third left intercostal space; the normal P_2 is softer than A_2 and is rarely audible at the apex.[105] When P_2 is heard at the apex, either significant pulmonary hypertension is present or the apex is occupied by the right ventricle—a situation commonly seen in normotensive atrial septal defect. The absolute value of inspiratory splitting varies with age and the depth of respiration. In younger subjects, maximal splitting during inspiration averages 40 to 50 ms; with age this value decreases such that a single S_2 during both phases of respiration may be normal in subjects older than 40 years.[105,110-112]

Abnormal Splitting

All conditions in which abnormal splitting of S_2 exist can be identified at the bedside by the presence of audible expiratory splitting (more than 30 ms), that is, the ability to hear two distinct sounds during expiration (Fig. 11-20).[87,110] This finding must be present when the patient is auscultęd in both the supine and upright positions, as some normal subjects have audible expiratory splitting in the recumbent position that becomes single when the upright position is assumed.[110] There are three causes of audible expiratory splitting: (1) wide physiologic splitting primarily due to delayed P_2, (2) reversed splitting primarily due to delayed A_2, and (3) narrow physiologic splitting as seen in pulmonary hypertension, where A_2 and P_2

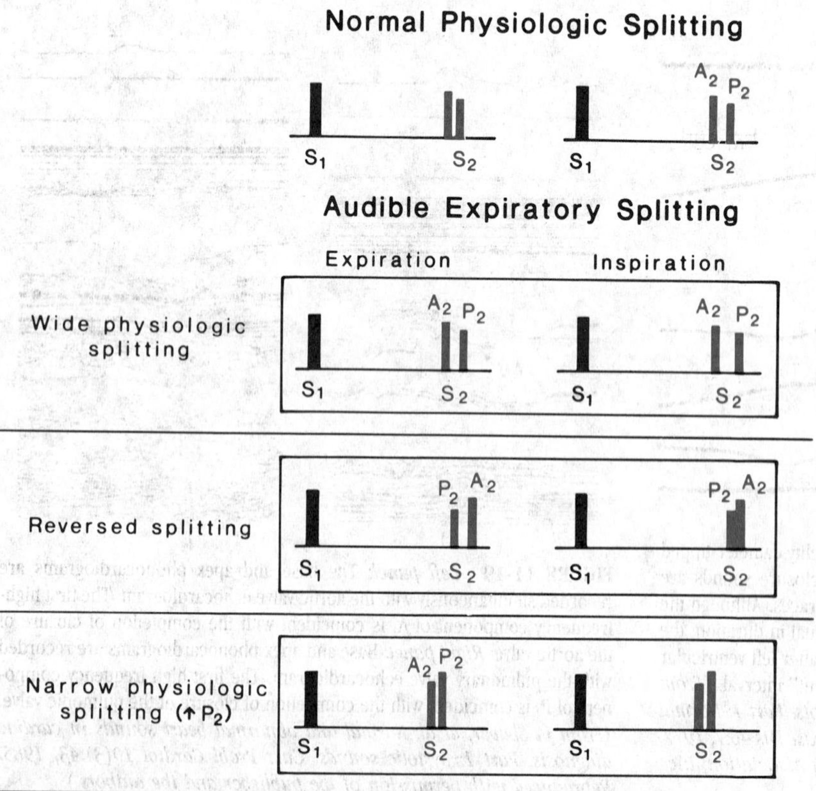

FIGURE 11-20 *Top panel:* Normal physiologic splitting. During expiration A_2 and P_2 are separated by less than 30 ms and are appreciated as a single sound. During inspiration, the splitting interval widens, and A_2 and P_2 are clearly separated into two distinctly audible sounds. *Bottom panel:* Audible expiratory splitting. In contrast to normal physiologic splitting, two distinct sounds are easily heard during expiration. Wide physiologic splitting is due to delay in P_2. Reversed splitting is due to delay in A_2, resulting in paradoxical movement; that is, with inspiration, P_2 moves toward A_2, and the splitting interval narrows. Narrow physiologic splitting is seen in pulmonary hypertension, and both A_2 and P_2 are heard during expiration at a narrow splitting interval due to an increased intensity and high-frequency composition of P_2. (*From JA Shaver, et al: Examination of the Heart. Part IV, Auscultation, Dallas, American Heart Association, 1990, p 17. Reproduced with permission of the publisher and the authors.*)

are heard as two distinct sounds during expiration at a narrow splitting interval. In Tables 11-1 and 11-2, the common causes of wide physiologic splitting and reversed splitting of S_2 are classified according to the abnormality of the cardiac cycle responsible for the altered timing of A_2 and P_2. In each table, the cardiac cycle has been divided into three phases (Fig. 11-18): (1) the electromechanical couple interval, the time from the onset of the Q wave to the rise of ventricular pressure; (2) ventricular mechanical systole, the sum of the isovolumic contraction time plus the ejection period minus the "hangout" interval (abnormalities of this interval exclude those conditions in which prolongation of the hangout interval is primarily responsible for the increased ejection time); and (3) hangout or impedance interval, the time between the incisura of the arterial trace and the ventricular pressure at the same level as the incisura (includes all conditions in which prolongation of this interval is primarily responsible for the increased ejection time).

Wide Physiologic Splitting of S_2 An example of wide physiologic splitting of S_2 due to delayed electrical activation of the right ventricle secondary to right bundle branch block is shown in Fig. 11-21. In Figs. 11-22 and 11-23, prolongation of right ventricular mechanical systole secondary to severe pulmonary hypertension and pulmonic stenosis is responsible for the delayed P_2. In Fig. 11-24, the classic wide, fixed splitting of S_2 found in atrial septal defect is demonstrated. A composite in Fig. 11-25 documents the role played by decreased impedance of the pulmonary vascular bed in the audible expiratory splitting found in atrial septal defect, idiopathic dilation of the pulmonary artery, and mild pulmonic stenosis with aneurysmal dilation of the pulmonary artery. In each case, there is a marked increase in the hangout interval as measured by high-fidelity pressure tracings. In Fig. 11-3, wide physiologic splitting secondary to a decreased left ventricular ejection time is shown in a patient with acute mitral regurgitation. For a more detailed analysis of each of the conditions producing wide physiologic splitting of S_2, the reader is referred to the references listed in Table 11-1.

TABLE 11-1

Wide Physiologic Splitting of the Second Heart Sound

Delayed pulmonic closure
- Delayed electrical activation of the right ventricle
  - Complete RBBB (proximal type)[21]
  - Left ventricular paced beats[21]
  - Left ventricular ectopic beats[21]
- Prolonged right ventricular mechanical systole
  - Acute massive pulmonary embolus[113,114]
  - Pulmonary hypertension with right heart failure[115,116]
  - Pulmonic stenosis with intact septum (moderate to severe)[64,117]
- Decreased impedance of the pulmonary vascular bed (increased "hangout")
  - Normotensive atrial septal defect[87,118]
  - Idiopathic dilation of the pulmonary artery[87,90]
  - Pulmonic stenosis (mild)[87,90]
  - Atrial septal defect, postoperative (70%)[7,98]
  - Unexplained AES in the normal[119]

Early aortic closure
- Shortened left ventricular mechanical systole (LVET)
  - Mitral regurgitation[87,98,100]
  - Ventricular septal defect[98]

RBBB = right bundle branch block; AES = audible expiratory splitting; LVET = left ventricular ejection time.

SOURCE: From Shaver JA, et al: The second heart sound: Newer concepts. Part 1: Normal and wide physiological splitting. *Mod Concepts Cardiovasc Dis* 1977; 46:9. Reproduced with permission from the American Heart Association, Inc. and the authors.

TABLE 11-2

Reversed Splitting of the Second Heart Sound

Delayed aortic closure
- Delayed electrical activation of the left ventricle
  - Complete LBBB (proximal type)[49,121,122]
  - Right ventricular paced beat[21]
  - Right ventricular ectopic beat[21]
- Prolonged left ventricular mechanical systole
  - Complete LBBB (peripheral type)[49,110,121,122]
  - Left ventricular outflow tract obstruction[89,121,123,124]
  - Hypertensive cardiovascular disease[126]
  - Arteriosclerotic heart disease
    - Chronic ischemic heart disease[127–129]
    - Angina pectoris[127–129]
- Decreased impedance of the systemic vascular bed (increased "hangout")
  - Poststenotic dilation of the aorta secondary to aortic stenosis or regurgitation[121,124,125]
  - Patent ductus arteriosus[121,130]

Early pulmonic closure
- Early electrical activation of the right ventricle
  - Wolff-Parkinson-White syndrome, type B[131,132]

LBBB = left bundle branch block.

SOURCE: From Shaver JA, et al: The second heart sound: Newer concepts. Part 2: Paradoxical splitting and narrow physiological splitting. *Mod Concepts Cardiovasc Dis* 1977; 46:13. Reproduced with permission from the American Heart Association, Inc. and the authors.

Reversed Splitting of S_2 Almost all cases of reversed splitting of S_2 are due to a delay in A_2. As a result, the sequence of closure sounds is reversed, with P_2 preceding A_2. At the bedside, this abnormality is recognized by paradoxical movement of A_2 and P_2 with respiration.[120] During inspiration, P_2 moves toward A_2 and the splitting interval narrows, whereas during expiration the two components separate, and audible expiratory splitting is present (Fig. 11-20). The presence of paradoxical splitting of S_2 almost always indicates significant underlying cardiovascular disease.

Both right ventricular ectopic and paced beats produce a delay in the onset of left ventricular contraction, resulting in reversed splitting of S_2.[21] The mechanism responsible is a delayed activation of the left ventricle, prolonging the Q to left ventricular pressure rise interval. The most common cause of reversed splitting is complete

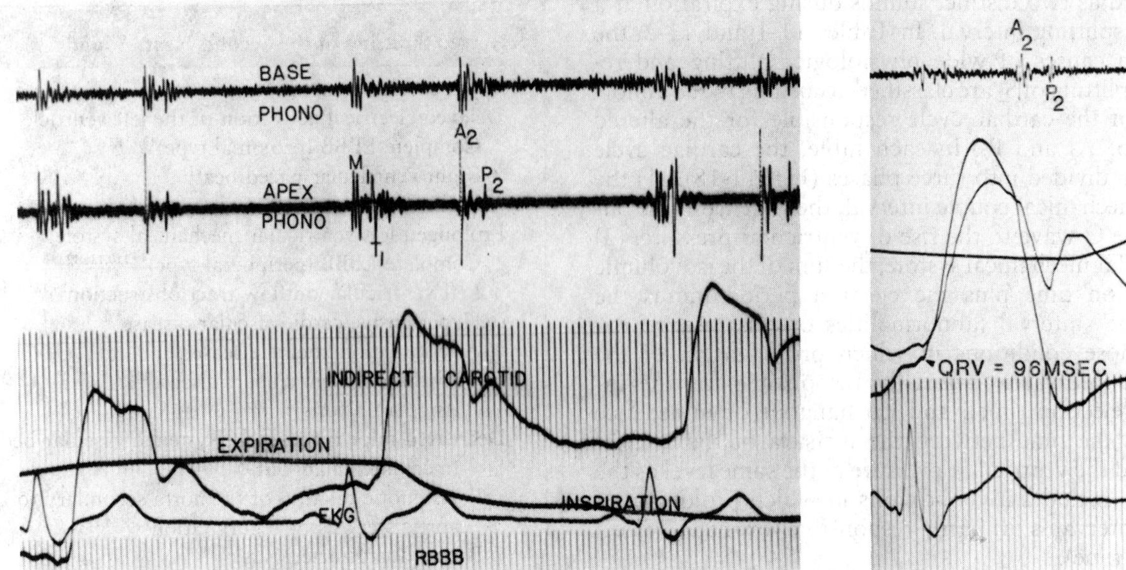

FIGURE 11-21 *Left panel:* Wide physiologic splitting of S_2 is seen in a patient with complete right bundle branch block. Audible expiratory splitting that widens normally with inspiration is present. Note also the wide splitting of the first heart sound into its mitral (M_1) and tricuspid (T_1) components, as recorded at the apex. *Right panel:* The base phonocardiogram is recorded simultaneously with high-fidelity catheters in the right ventricle and pulmonary artery during cardiac catheterization. There is marked prolongation of the Q to the onset of the right ventricular pressure rise of 96 ms, resulting in wide physiologic splitting of S_2. The delayed P_2 is secondary to the delayed activation of the right ventricle. [*From JA Shaver: Current uses of phonocardiography in clinical practice. In: E Rapaport (ed): Cardiology Update—Reviews for Physicians. New York, Elsevier, 1981, p 337. Reproduced originally in part (left panel) with permission of the publisher and author; and from JA Shaver, et al: Normal and abnormal heart sounds in cardiac diagnosis. Part 1: Systolic sounds. Curr Probl Cardiol 10(3):48, 1985. Reproduced in total with permission of the publisher and authors.*]

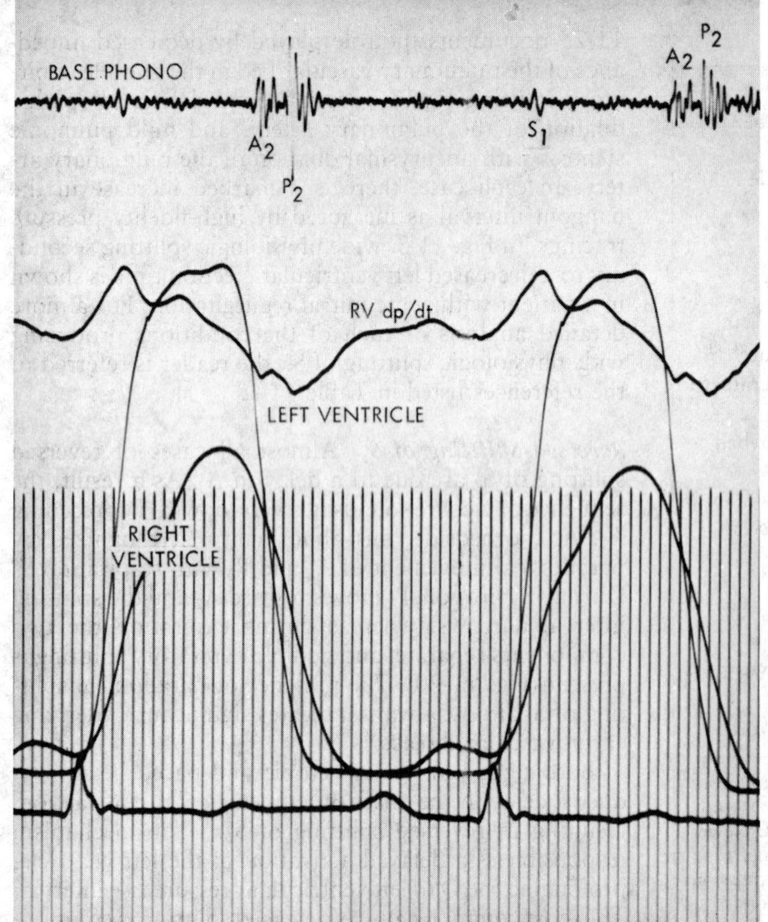

FIGURE 11-22 Simultaneous high-fidelity left and right ventricular pressures are recorded with the base phonocardiogram in a 35-year-old chronic drug abuser with severe pulmonary hypertension. Wide, fixed splitting of S_2 is recorded, and the intensity of P_2 is greater than that of A_2. Significant prologation of right ventricular systole is responsible for the delay in P_2, due primarily to prolongation of the right ventricular isovolumic contraction time. (*From Shaver JA, et al: Normal and abnormal heart sounds in cardiac diagnosis. Part I: Systolic sounds. Curr Probl Cardiol 10(3):50, 1985. Reproduced with permission of the publisher and authors.*)

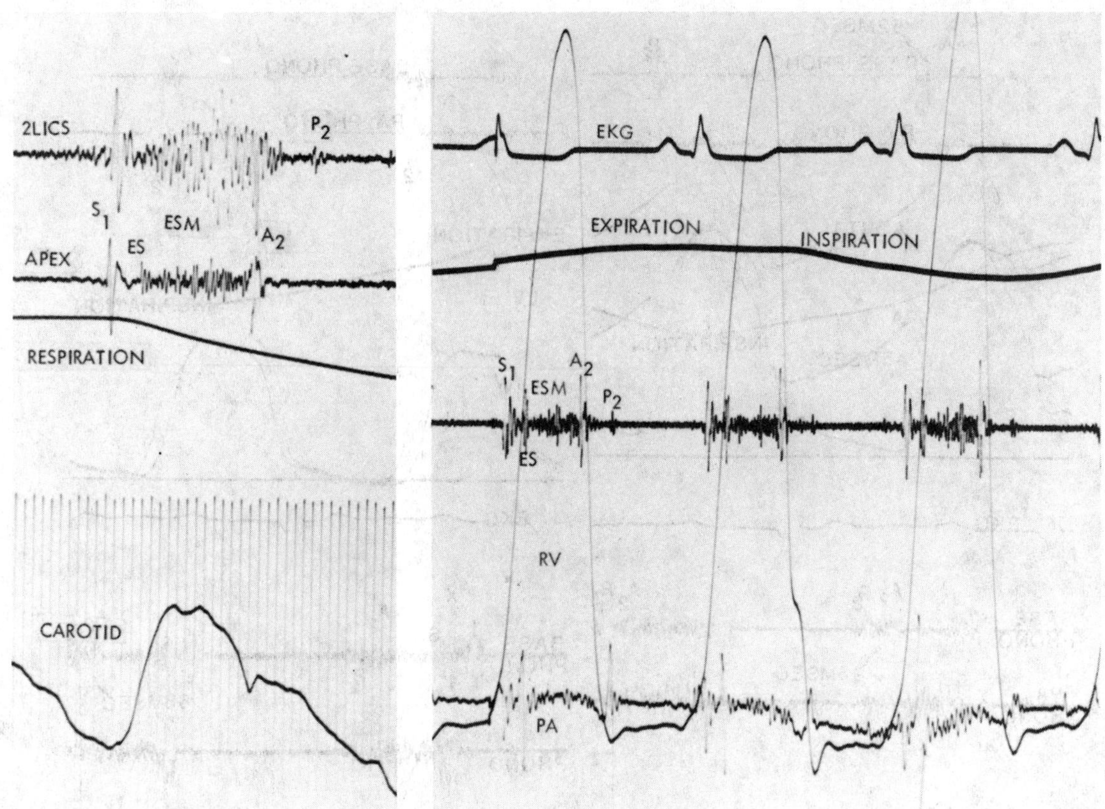

FIGURE 11-23 *Left panel:* The phonocardiogram of a patient with severe valvular pulmonic stenosis as recorded at the second left intercostal space (2LICS) and the apex. The long ejection murmur (ESM) has late systolic peaking and spills through A_2. There is a marked delay in P_2, which is very small in amplitude. *Right panel:* At cardiac catheterization, the markedly delayed P_2 is shown to be secondary to a very large systolic pressure gradient, and its decreased intensity is due to the low pulmonary artery pressure at the time of valve closure. The late peaking of the ejection murmur correlates with the maximal pressure gradient between the right ventricle and the pulmonary artery. *(From EI Curtiss et al: First and second heart sound. In: LD Horwitz (ed): Signs and Symptoms in Cardiology. Philadelphia, JB Lippincott, 1985, p 200. Reproduced with permission of the publisher and authors.)*

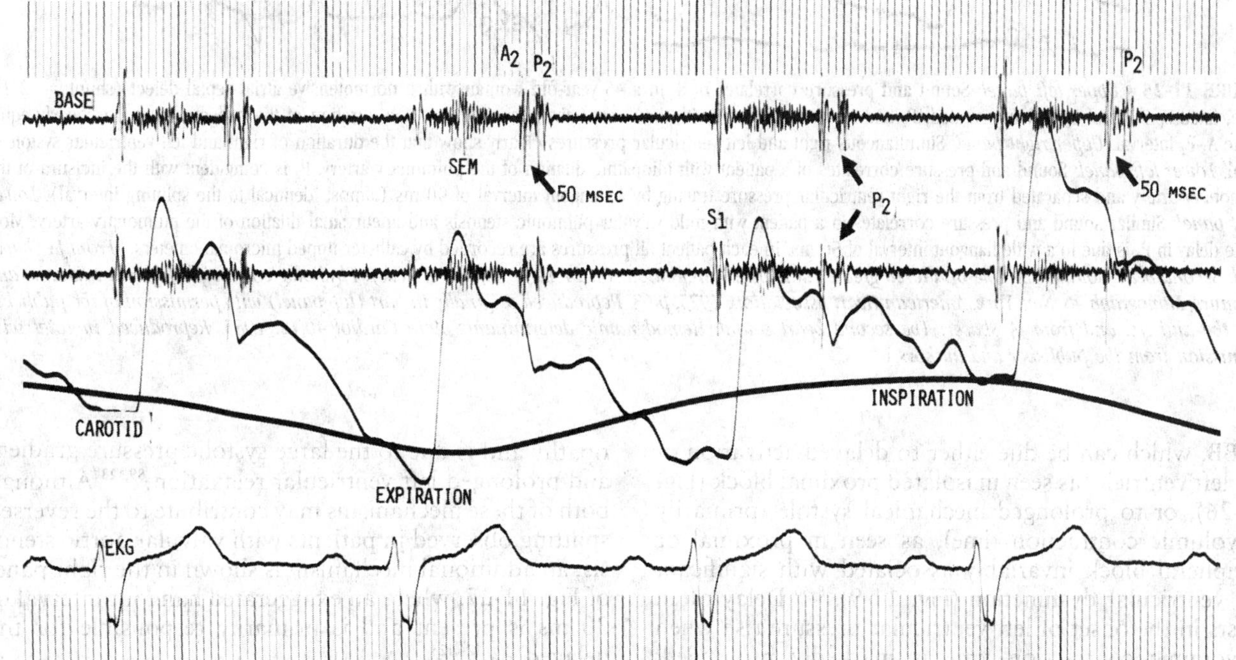

FIGURE 11-24 Simultaneous base and apex phonocardiograms are recorded together with the carotid pulse during quiet respiration in a young woman with a large atrial septal defect. Wide, fixed splitting of S_2 is present, and P_2 is easily recorded at the apex. A prominent systolic ejection murmur (SEM) is recorded at the base and is due to the large stroke volume across the right ventricular outflow tract. *(From JA Shaver: Innocent murmurs. Hosp Med, April 1978, p 15. © 1978. Reproduced with permission of Hospital Publications, Inc., and the author.)*

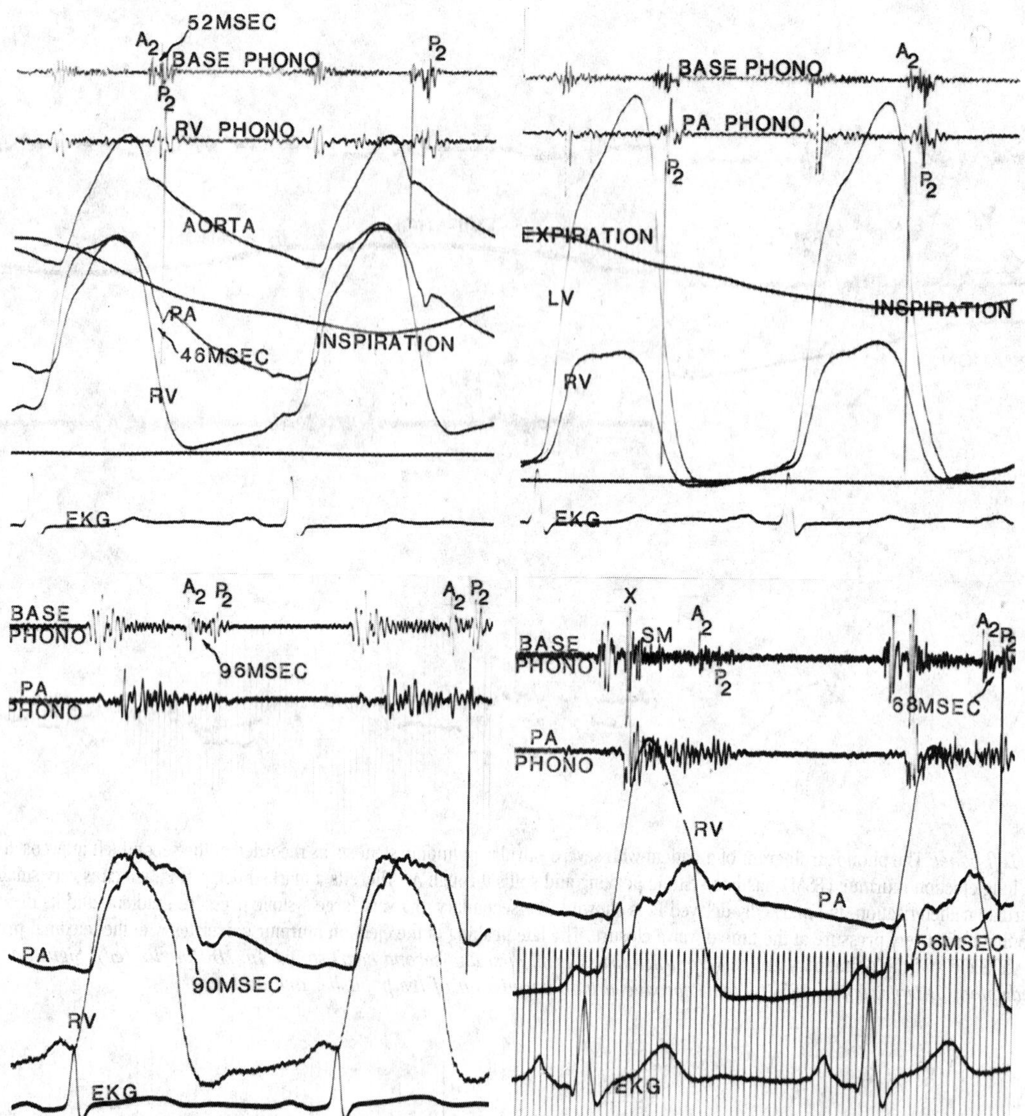

FIGURE 11-25 *Upper left panel:* Sound and pressure correlates of S_2 in a 45-year-old woman with a normotensive atrial septal defect (shunt = 2:1). Wide, fixed splitting of S_2 is demonstrated; P_2 and A_2 are coincident with their respective incisurae, and the duration of the hangout interval is nearly equal to the A_2-P_2 interval. *Upper right panel:* Simultaneous right and left ventricular pressures clearly show that the duration of right and left ventricular systole is equal. *Lower left panel:* Sound and pressure correlates of a patient with idiopathic dilation of the pulmonary artery. P_2 is coincident with the incisura of the pulmonary artery and separated from the right ventricular pressure tracing by a hangout interval of 90 ms (almost identical to the splitting interval). *Lower right panel:* Similar sound and pressure correlates in a patient with mild valvular pulmonic stenosis and aneurysmal dilation of the pulmonary artery. Most of the delay in P_2 is due to a wide hangout interval of 56 ms. In each patient all pressures are recorded by catheter-tipped micromanometers. [*From JA Shaver et al: Second heart sound: The role of altered greater and lesser circulation. In: DF Leon, JA Shaver (eds): Physiologic Principles of Heart Sounds and Murmurs, Monograph 46. New York, American Heart Association, 1975, p 63. Reproduced originally in part (top panel) with permission of the publisher and the authors; and from JA Shaver: The second heart sound; Hemodynamic determinants. Acta Cardiol 40:12, 1985. Reproduced in total with permission from the publisher and authors.*]

LBBB, which can be due either to delayed activation of the left ventricle, as seen in isolated proximal block (Fig. 11-26), or to prolonged mechanical systole (primarily isovolumic contraction time), as seen in proximal or peripheral block invariably associated with significant left ventricular dysfunction (Fig. 11-9).[48-50] Delay often exists in the onset of left ventricular pressure rise when isovolumic contraction time is markedly prolonged, since in most cases of LBBB varying degrees of both mechanisms are present, with one predominating.[121,122]

In the left panel of Fig. 11-27, reversed splitting of S_2 is demonstrated in a patient with hypertrophic cardiomyopathy and is due to the large systolic pressure gradient and prolonged left ventricular relaxation.[89,123] Although both of these mechanisms may contribute to the reversed splitting observed in patients with valvular aortic stenosis, an additional mechanism is shown in the right panel of Fig. 11-27, where an exaggerated hangout interval of 30 ms is present and is primarily responsible for the delayed A_2.[124,125]

In hypertensive cardiovascular disease, splitting is usually physiologic with the intensity of A_2 increased. However, rare instances of reversed splitting do occur. The elevation of blood pressure produced by intravenous

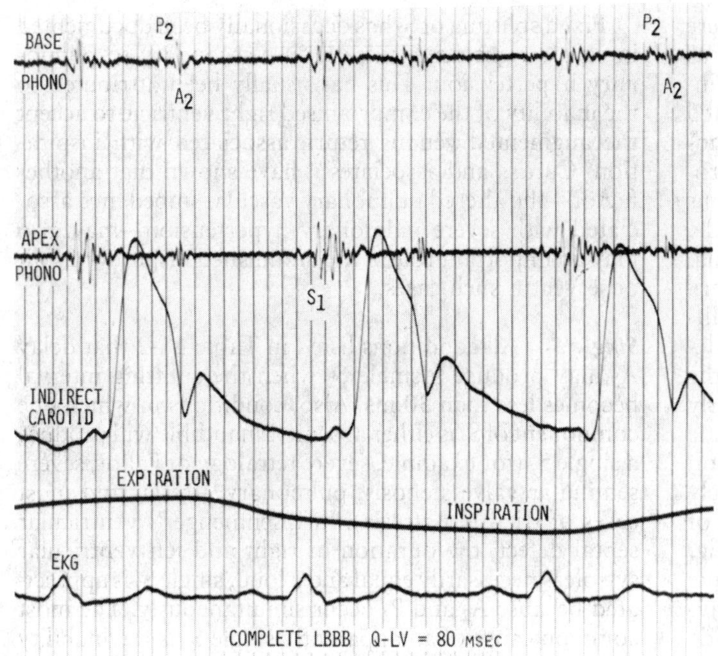

FIGURE 11-26 Reversed splitting of S_2 with paradoxical movement in a patient with complete left bundle branch block. A_2 is confirmed by the simultaneous indirect carotid pulse, and with inspiration there is slight narrowing of the splitting interval. At cardiac catheterization, a marked increase in the Q to left ventricular rise interval of 80 ms was documented and was primarily responsible for the delayed A_2. A slight increase in the isovolumic contraction time was also present. (*From JA Shaver, et al: Normal and abnormal heart sounds in cardiac diagnosis. Part I: Systolic sounds. Curr Probl Cardiol 10(3):56, 1985. Reproduced with permission of the publisher and the authors.*)

administration of methoxamine has been shown to produce reversed splitting in a normal subject due to prolongation of both left ventricular ejection time and the isovolumic contraction time in the face of an increased afterload.[126] Reversed splitting of S_2 has also been reported in ischemic heart disease and during episodes of angina pectoris.[127,128] The latter is extremely uncommon and has rarely been documented by phonocardiography. It is most likely due to a prolonged isovolumic contraction time of the ischemic left ventricle, although during angina it may also be due to an increase in systemic arterial pressure or transient LBBB.[129]

Decreased impedance in the systemic vascular bed can also contribute to the delayed A_2 seen in poststenotic dilation of the aorta, as shown in the right panel of Fig. 11-27. It also plays a role in the reversed splitting occasionally seen in both chronic aortic regurgitation and patent ductus arteriosus.[121,130] Reversed splitting of S_2 has also been reported in some cases of type B Wolff-Parkinson-White syndrome, where early activation of the right ventricle through an accessory pathway has caused P_2 to occur prematurely.[131,132]

Narrow Physiologic Splitting Narrow physiologic splitting of S_2 is a common finding in severe pulmonary hypertension, as shown in Fig. 11-20.[115,133] In contrast to the normal situation where only a single sound is heard during expiration, both A_2 and P_2 are easily heard, even though the splitting interval is less than 30 ms because of the increased intensity and high-frequency composi-

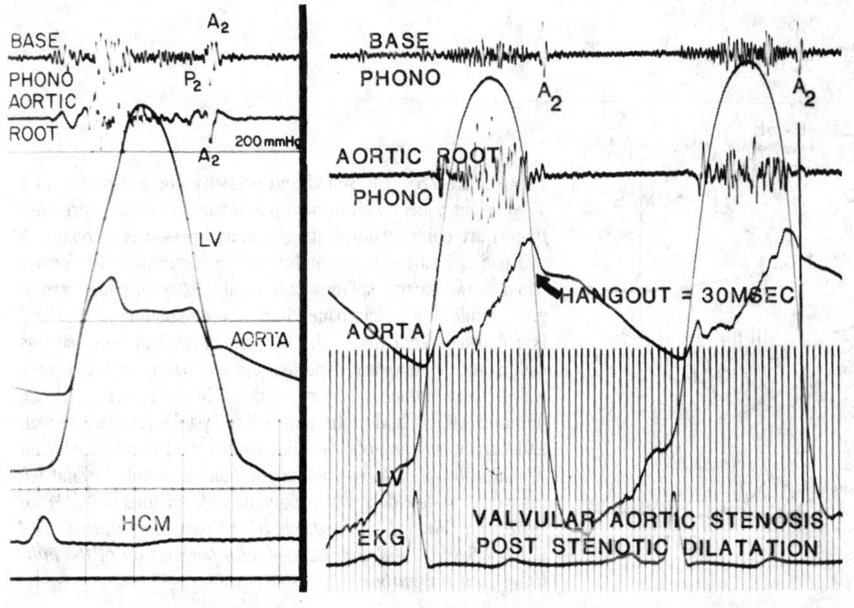

FIGURE 11-27 *Left panel:* External sound and aortic root sound are recorded simultaneously with pressures in the left ventricle and central aorta (catheter-tipped micromanometers) in a patient with hypertrophic cardiomyopathy. Reversed splitting of S_2 is present, and the delayed A_2 is due to the large systolic pressure gradient and the prolonged left ventricular relaxation. *Right panel:* Catheter-tipped micromanometers are recording pressures in the left ventricle and central aorta in a patient with valvular aortic stenosis having marked poststenotic dilation of the aorta; A_2 is coincident with the central aortic incisura and separated from the left ventricular pressure by a wide hangout interval of 30 ms. This interval is nearly twice as long as the normal left ventricular hangout interval, as shown in Figs. 11-2 and 11-18. (*From JA Shaver: The second heart sound: Hemodynamic determinants. Acta Cardiol 40:7, 1985. Reproduced with permission of the publisher and the author.*)

tion of P_2. Narrow splitting, although common in severe pulmonary hypertension, is not always the case, as shown in Fig. 11-22, where wide splitting with an increased amplitude of P_2 is present. It has been suggested by Shapiro and associates[116] that a wide split in pulmonary hypertension may indicate a more severely compromised ventricle than a normal split. Similar observations have also been made by Perloff,[115] who states that wide, persistent splitting becomes a useful sign of abnormal right ventricular performance in patients with primary pulmonary hypertension. In order to reconcile these different responses in S_2 when pulmonary hypertension develops, it is essential to appreciate that normally the duration of right and left ventricular systole is nearly equal and that a potential interval (the normally wide right-sided hangout interval) can be encroached upon as a process of pulmonary hypertension progressively decreases the capacitance and increases the resistance of the pulmonary vascular bed (Fig. 11-18).[88–91,121,134] In Fig. 11-28, the sound and pressure correlates of two patients with severe pulmonary hypertension are shown, one having narrow splitting of S_2 and the other having wide splitting of S_2. Common to both patients is marked narrowing of the normally wide right-sided hangout interval. In the center panel, the duration of right and left ventricular mechanical systole is nearly equal at the time of the pulmonary artery incisura, and the splitting interval is narrow. In contrast, the right panel shows that there has been a marked prolongation of right ventricular mechanical systole in the face of chronic pressure overload, and the net effect is a delayed P_2 resulting in wide splitting of S_2. Thus, a spectrum of the width of splitting may be seen in pulmonary hypertension, depending on the degree of selective prolongation of right ventricular systole, always in the setting of a narrow hangout interval. Furthermore, it is clear that varying degrees of splitting may be seen in the same patient during different stages of the disease process, producing the pulmonary hypertension. Similar hemodynamic correlates have been found in patients having hyperkinetic pulmonary hypertension secondary to large atrial septal defects.[91,118]

Fixed splitting of S_2 has occasionally been documented in severe right ventricular failure secondary to pulmonary hypertension. This has usually been attributed to the inability of the compromised right ventricle to accept the augmented venous return associated with inspiration. Curtiss and associates[106] have shown that another factor—the altered pulmonary vascular impedance associated with severe pulmonary hypertension—may also play an important role in the diminished inspiratory split observed in such cases.

Single S_2 All conditions listed in Table 11-2 that delay A_2 may produce a single S_2 when the splitting interval becomes less than 30 ms. Also, conditions in which one component of S_2 is either absent or inaudible will produce a single S_2 (for example, severe tetralogy of Fallot, severe semilunar valve stenosis, pulmonary atresia, and most cases of tricuspid atresia). In Eisenmenger's ventricular septal defect, the duration of right and left ventricular systole is necessarily equal and a loud, single S_2 is appreciated because A_2 and P_2 occur simultaneously. The most common cause of an apparently single S_2 is the inability to hear the fainter of the two components of the sound (usually P_2) because of emphysema, obesity, or respiratory noise. Another common cause of single S_2 is seen in individuals over age 50. Although this has been attributed to a delayed A_2,[112,130] a decreased inspiratory delay in P_2 has also been reported.[111] This latter finding has been shown to be due to a decreased right-sided hangout interval, most likely related to aging changes in the pulmonary vascular bed.[99]

Opening Snaps

Opening of the normal atrioventricular valve is almost always a silent event. However, with thickening and deformity of the leaflets, usually rheumatic in origin, a sound is generated in early diastole in a manner analogous to ejection sounds arising from deformed semilunar valves. The term *opening snap* was first used by Thayer[135] in 1908 to describe the high-frequency early diastolic

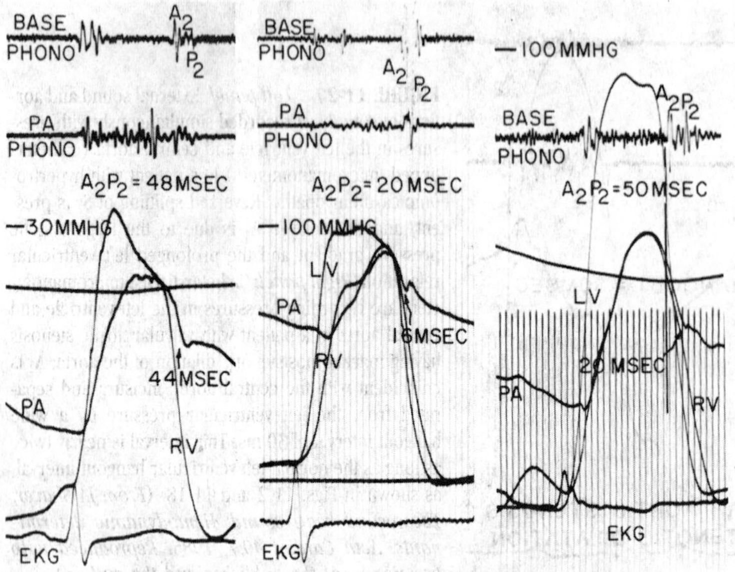

FIGURE 11-28 The sound and pressure correlates of S_2 in a 17-year-old patient with normal pulmonary artery pressure (*left panel*) are contrasted with the sound and pressure correlates of two patients having severe pulmonary hypertension. The center panel shows narrow splitting of S_2 on the external phonocardiogram, while in the right panel there is wide splitting of S_2. There is a marked reduction in the hangout interval in both patients with severe pulmonary hypertension compared to the patient with normal pulmonary artery pressure. In the center panel, the duration of left and right ventricular systole is nearly equal, and narrow splitting of S_2 results. In the right panel, significant prolongation of right ventricular mechanical systole beyond left ventricular systole delays P_2, producing wide splitting of S_2. (*From JA Shaver: Clinical implications of the hangout interval. Int J Cardiol 5:396, 1984. Reproduced with permission of the publisher and the author.*)

sound in mitral stenosis. Margolies and Wolferth[136] provided the first extensive description of the sound and its timing and proposed that the mechanism of production was a sudden stopping of the opening movement of the valve. They also recognized that the sound had been absent in those patients who, on autopsy, had markedly thickened and essentially immobile valves. This mechanism was confirmed by hemodynamic and angiographic studies that show sudden checking of the early diastolic descent of the funnel-shaped stenotic valve when its elastic limits were met.[42,137,138] Phonoechocardiography has given an even more precise correlation of the opening snap with the maximum opening motion of the anterior mitral leaflet (Fig. 11-7, left panel).[43,139]

The opening snap is a crisp, sharp sound that can be heard in the midprecordial location, usually best in the area from the left sternal border to just inside the apex. It may often be heard well at the base of the heart and is frequently not well heard at the maximal intensity of the diastolic murmur. The diastolic rumble generally follows the opening snap by a short interval. There is no variation in the intensity or timing of the mitral opening snap with respiration.

As with ejection sounds of valvular origin, the intensity of the mitral opening snap correlates well with the mobility of the valve. A loud opening snap is found in mobile stenotic valves with good excursions (Fig. 11-7, left panel), while the opening snap is absent with severe calcific fixation of the valve (Fig. 11-4; Fig. 11-29, center panel). The intensity of M_1 parallels the intensity of the opening snap; mobile valves having a loud opening snap have an accentuated M_1, and immobile valves having a decreased or absent opening snap have marked attenuation of M_1. Although the presence of valvular calcification decreases valve mobility and the audibility of the opening snap, the sound is actually found in 50 to 60 percent of patients with calcific valves. The mere presence of valvular calcium does not preclude some mobility of the valve leaflets and therefore an opening snap (Fig. 11-29, left panel).

The opening snap follows A_2 by an interval of 0.03 to 0.15 s. In patients with mild mitral stenosis the interval is usually long, whereas with more severe stenosis the A_2-opening snap (A_2-OS) interval is shorter. The A_2-OS interval in atrial fibrillation can vary with cycle length, as shown in Fig. 11-30. With a short preceding RR interval, the left atrium has not had time to empty, the left atrial pressure remains high, and the A_2-OS interval is short. With a longer preceding RR interval, the left atrial pressure falls, and the A_2-OS interval widens.

There have been a number of attempts to use the A_2-OS interval to predict the level of the left atrial pressure and severity of mitral stenosis.[140–142] The hemodynamics responsible for the timing of the opening snap are shown in Fig. 11-8. The opening snap occurs at the maximal mitral valve opening shortly after left ventricular–left atrial pressure crossovers. Factors that influence the timing of the opening snap relative to A_2 are (1) the rate of left ventricular pressure decline, (2) the level of the left ventricular pressure at the time of A_2, and (3) the level of the left atrial pressure. Increasing severity of mitral stenosis is usually accompanied by an increasing left atrial pressure and therefore a shortening of the A_2-OS interval. Because this interval is multifactorially determined, there is an imperfect correlation between the A_2-OS interval and the mitral valve area.[143,144]

Tricuspid valve stenosis can also produce an opening snap.[145–147] This sound is frequently not detected because the findings of coexisting mitral stenosis, which is almost invariably present, overshadow those of tricuspid stenosis. The maximum intensity of the tricuspid opening snap tends to be found closer to the left sternal border and,

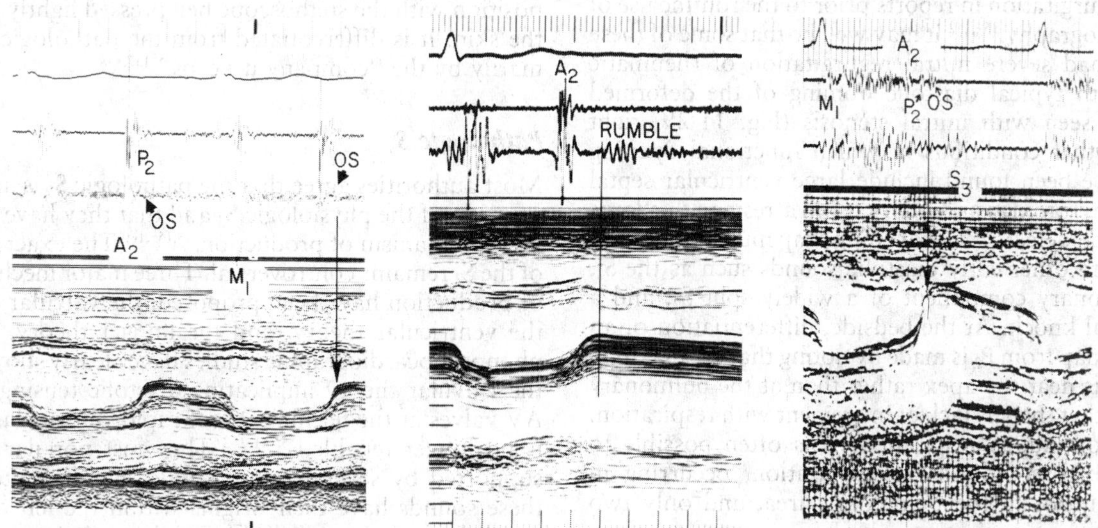

FIGURE 11-29 Base and apex phonocardiograms are recorded simultaneously with the mitral valve echocardiogram in three patients with chronic rheumatic mitral valve disease. In the left panel, a soft opening snap is coincident with the maximal opening of a thickened, relatively immobile, stenotic mitral valve. In the center panel, calcific fixation of a severely stenotic mitral valve is present, and an opening snap is absent. Note that the onset of the diastolic rumble begins after the maximal anterior excursion of the heavily calcified valve. In the right panel, an opening snap occurs at the maximal opening of the nonstenotic rheumatic valve. A holosystolic murmur of mitral regurgitation is present, and no gradient was found across the mitral valve at cardiac catheterization. A loud S_3 gallop follows the opening snap and occurs during the early E-F slope of the rheumatic mitral valve.

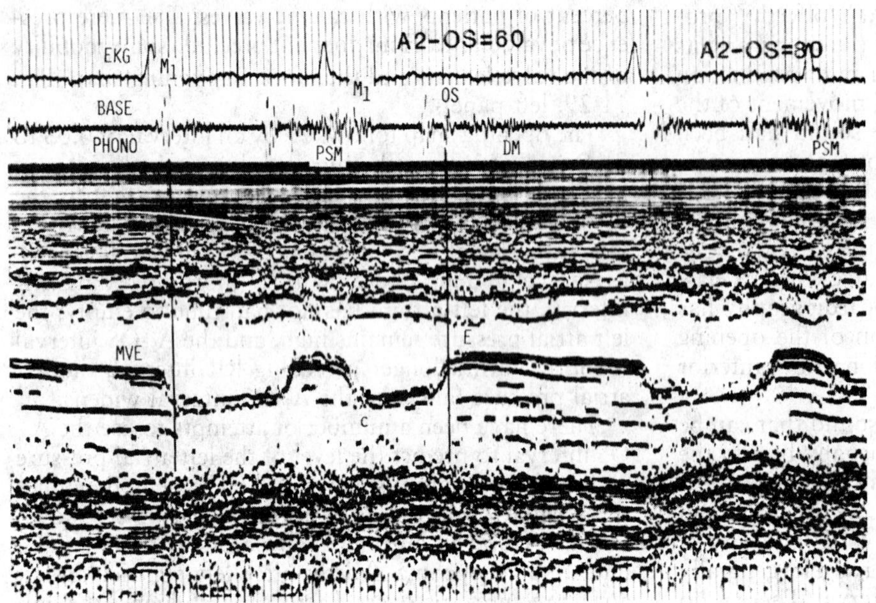

FIGURE 11-30 The base phonocardiogram is recorded with the mitral valve echocardiogram in a patient having mitral stenosis with atrial fibrillation and varying RR cycles. Following a short diastolic filling period, the A_2-OS interval in complex 2 is 60 ms. After a longer diastolic filling period, the A_2-OS interval in complex 3 is lengthened to 80 ms because of the decrease in left atrial pressure. The crescendo presystolic murmur (PSM) preceding complex 2 is caused by ventriculogenic closure of the stenotic mitral valve shortly after it has opened. The PSM is absent in complex 3 following a longer diastolic filling period. DM = diastolic murmur; E = maximal point of mitral valve opening. (*From PS Reddy, et al: Normal and abnormal heart sounds in cardiac diagnosis. Part 2. Diastolic sounds. Curr Probl Cardiol 10(3):12, 1985. Reproduced with permission of the publisher and the authors.*)

unlike the mitral snap, the intensity of the tricuspid snap increases with inspiration. When present, it generally follows the mitral opening snap.[146]

An early diastolic sound can also be caused by a right or left atrial myxoma.[44] Although the clinical findings of a left atrial myxoma may be similar to those of mitral stenosis, the echocardiographic picture is classic (Fig. 11-7, center panel). The tumor "plop" occurs at the maximal diastolic descent of the myxoma.

Although an opening snap is rarely found in patients with normal valves, it may be heard in situations where high flow exists across the AV valves.[148] An early diastolic sound is frequently present in large atrial septal defects,[149] coincident with maximal opening of the tricuspid valve.[150] Opening snaps have also been observed in severe mitral regurgitation in reports prior to the routine use of echocardiography.[151,152] It may well be that some of these patients had severe mitral regurgitation of rheumatic origin with typical diastolic doming of the deformed valve, as seen with mitral stenosis (Fig. 11-29, right panel). Other conditions in which functional opening snaps have been found include large ventricular septal defects, thyrotoxicosis, and tricuspid atresia with a large atrial septal defect.[148] The opening snap must be differentiated from other early diastolic sounds such as the S_3, the pulmonary component of a widely split S_2, and a pericardial knock. At the bedside, differentiation of an opening snap from P_2 is made by noting that the maximal intensity is near the apex rather than at the pulmonary area and that there is lack of movement with respiration. During continuous respiration, it is often possible to appreciate three sounds on inspiration, occurring in rapid sequence in the pulmonary area, and only two components on expiration.

The Third and Fourth Heart Sounds

The third and fourth heart sounds (S_3, S_4) are low-frequency events related to early and late diastolic filling of the ventricles (Fig. 11-31). When they are heard in disease states, they are called *gallop* sounds, and their presence gives valuable information to the clinician regarding the status of ventricular function and compliance.

The Third Heart Sound

Physiologic S_3 The physiologic S_3 is a benign finding commonly heard in children, adolescents, and young adults.[153,154] It is rarely present in the adult after age 40 and, when present, is often associated with a thin, esthenic body habitus.[155] This is a low-frequency sound that follows A_2 by 120 to 200 ms and occurs during the rapid filling wave of the apexcardiogram (Fig. 11-32, top panel).[156] It is best ausculted at the apex in the left lateral position with the stethoscope bell pressed lightly against the skin. It is differentiated from the pathologic S_3 primarily by the "company it keeps."[157,158]

Pathologic S_3

Most authorities agree that the pathologic S_3 is an exaggeration of the physiologic S_3 and that they have a common mechanism of production.[19,159,160] The exact genesis of the S_3 remains controversial. Three major mechanisms of production have been proposed: the valvular theory, the ventricular theory, and the impact theory. Recent phonoechocardiographic studies have clearly shown that the valvular theory implicating diastolic tensing of the AV valves at the termination of rapid ventricular filling is no longer tenable.[158,161–163] The most popular theory supported by several recent studies has indicated that these sounds have their origins within the left or right ventricle or their walls.[162–175] The dynamic interplay between the force of delivery of blood into the ventricle on one hand and the ability of the ventricle to accept this flow on the other hand is thought to be the important factor in the genesis of this sound. When there is appropriate interaction between these factors, the S_3 occurs when the ventricle suddenly reaches its elastic limits and abruptly decelerates the onrushing column of blood,

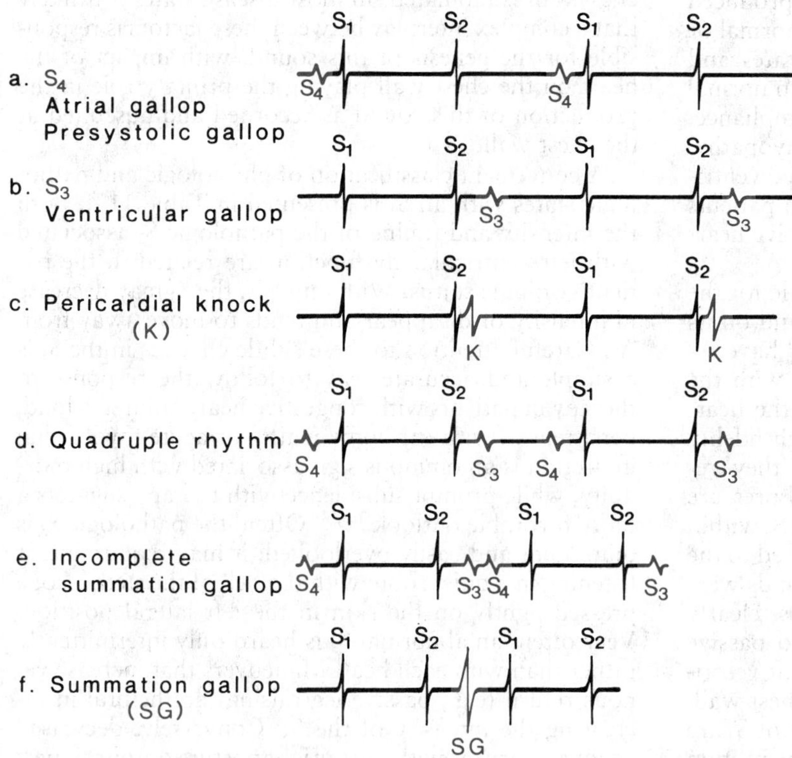

FIGURE 11-31 *A.* The S_4 occurs in presystole and is frequently called an atrial or presystolic gallop. *B.* The S_3 occurs during the rapid phase of ventricular filling. It is a normal finding and is commonly heard in children and young adults, disappearing with increasing age. When it is heard in the patient with cardiac disease, it is called a pathologic S_3 or ventricular gallop and usually indicates ventricular dysfunction or AV valvular incompetence. *C.* In constrictive pericarditis, a sound in early diastole, the pericardial knock (K) is heard earlier and is louder and higher pitched than the usual pathologic S_3. *D.* A quadruple rhythm results if both S_4 and S_3 are present. *E.* At faster heart rates, the S_3 and S_4 occur in rapid succession and may give the illusion of a middiastolic rumble. *F.* When the heart rate is sufficiently fast, the two rapid phases of ventricular filling reinforce each other, and a loud summation gallop (SG) may appear; this sound may be louder than either the S_3 or S_4 alone. *(From JA Shaver, et al: Examination of the Heart, Part IV, Auscultation, Dallas, American Heart Association, 1990, p 27. Reproduced with permission of the publisher and the authors.)*

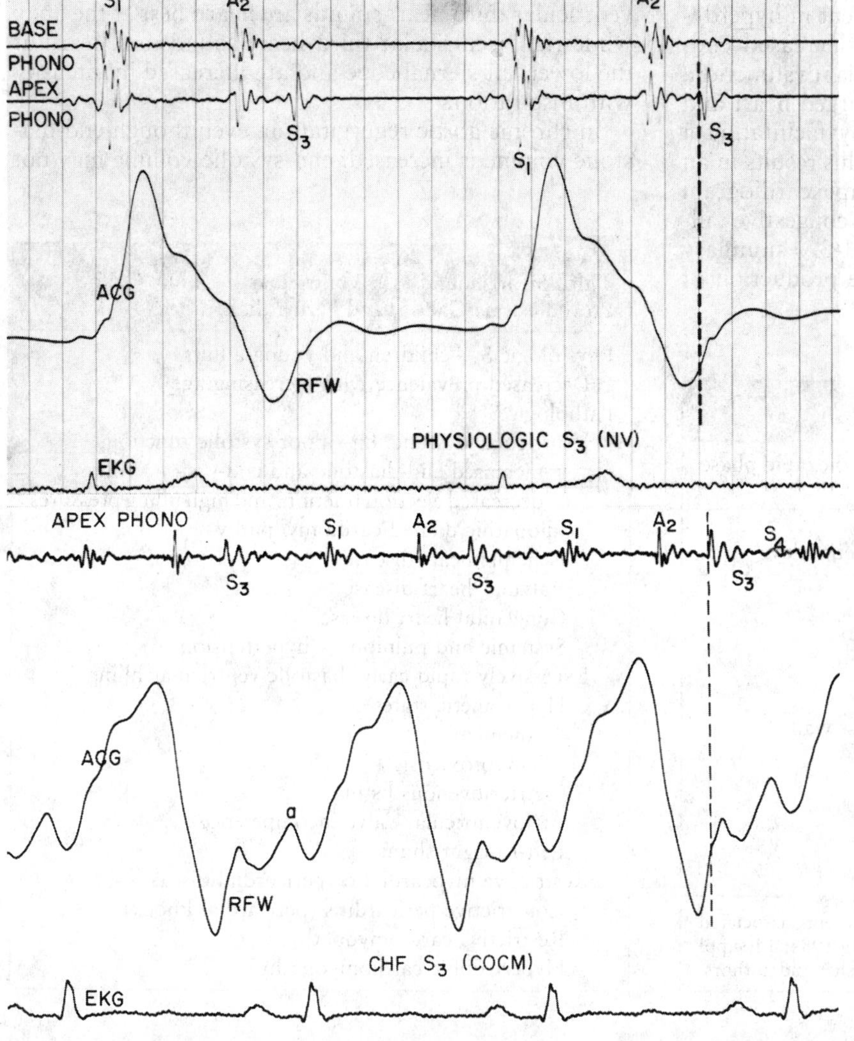

FIGURE 11-32 *Top panel:* A physiologic S_3 recorded in a 24-year-old woman without evidence of cardiovascular disease. The onset of the S_3 occurs during the rapid filling wave (RFW) of the ACG between the O and F points. The remainder of the cardiovascular examination was entirely within normal limits. *Bottom panel:* A very prominent S_3 gallop is recorded in a patient with severe congestive cardiomyopathy (COCM). On physical examination, there was a small-volume carotid pulse and marked engorgement of the neck veins with elevated venous pressure. The ACG shows a very prominent presystolic pulsation (*a*) and an extremely RFW is present. The onset of the S_3 occurs during the RFW of the ACG. The first heart sound is soft. *[From JA Shaver, et al: Early diastolic events associated with the physiologic and pathologic S_3. J Cardiography 14(suppl 5):30, 1984. Reproduced with permission of the publisher and the authors.]*

thereby setting the entire cardiohemic system into vibration. In keeping with this theory, an S_3 may be produced by excessive rapid filling into a ventricle with normal or increased compliance, as with high-output states and mitral regurgitation, or by a normal or less than normal rate of filling into a ventricle with decreased compliance, such as in patients with hypertrophic cardiomyopathy. Likewise, decreased rates of filling into overfilled ventricles with large end-systolic volumes, as seen in patients with poor left ventricular function and congestive heart failure, will produce this sound.[176,177]

Although this mechanism is likely responsible for the sound recorded within the ventricular cavity and on its epicardial surface, Reddy and associates[8,177–180] have reported convincing data that the sound heard with the stethoscope is due to the dynamic impact of the heart with the chest wall. Using equisensitive high-fidelity transducers with identical electronic filters, they recorded external and left ventricular sound and pressure simultaneously and consistently found that the S_3 within the left ventricle was softer or absent as compared to the external sound.[177] Furthermore, when both sounds were present, they often occurred at different times, clearly indicating that the external S_3 was not due to passive transmission of a sound originating from the left ventricle through the intervening structures to the chest wall. The force of the impact and resultant intensity of S_3 are dependent primarily on the size of the heart, the motion of the heart within the thorax, and the chest wall configuration. This theory explains the S_3 present in hyperdynamic states as well as those with an increased end-systolic volume secondary to left ventricular dysfunction. In the latter, the space between the enlarged heart and lateral chest wall is diminished, thereby facilitating a more forceful impact in early diastole. This results in an exaggerated rapid filling wave on the apexcardiogram and the prominent S_3 pathognomonic of congestive failure (Fig. 11-32, lower panel). In Table 11-3, a summary of the major factors responsible for the production of the S_3 as recorded within the left ventricle and on the chest wall is tabulated. In most disease states it is likely that a complex interplay between these factors is responsible for the genesis of this sound, with impact of the heart on the chest wall playing the primary role in the production of this sound as recorded and ausculted at the chest wall.

A convenient classification of physiologic and pathologic states with an S_3 is presented in Table 11-4. Both the intensity and timing of the pathologic S_3 associated with left ventricular dysfunction are related to the patient's volume status. With diuresis, the S_3 may decrease in intensity or disappear and tends to move away from A_2. Careful attention to these subtle changes in the S_3 is a simple and accurate way to follow the response to therapy in patients with congestive heart failure. A loud, persistent S_3 with cardiomyopathy or acute myocardial infarction is an ominous sign associated with high mortality, while prompt subsidence with therapy suggests a more favorable outlook.[165,181] Often, the pathologic S_3 is quite faint and easily overlooked; it may require intent listening in a quiet room with the bell of the stethoscope pressed lightly on the skin in the left lateral position. Very often, an abnormal S_3 is heard only intermittently rather than with each beat. Maneuvers that increase venous return (e.g., passive leg raising) are helpful in increasing the intensity of the S_3. Conversely, decreased venous return, as with the upright posture or tourniquets about the extremities, will decrease the intensity.[182] Left ventricular third heart sounds are heard best at the apex while right ventricular third heart sounds are heard at the lower left sternal edge and are increased in intensity with inspiration.

In chronic aortic regurgitation, even though end-diastolic volume is increased, end-systolic volume may not

TABLE 11-3

Hemodynamic Determinants of the S_3

Ability of the ventricle to accept flow during the rapid phase of diastolic filling
- Rate of relaxation of the ventricle
- End-systolic or residual volume of the ventricle
- Compliance of the relaxed ventricle
- Nonobstructed atrioventricular valve

Atrial pressure head
- Atrial blood volume
- Atrial compliance

Dynamic impact of the heart with the chest wall
- Architecture of the thorax
- Cardiac size
- Cardiac motion within the thorax
- Phase of respiration
- Position of the patient

SOURCE: From Shaver JA, et al: Early diastolic events associated with the physiologic and pathologic S_3. *J Cardiog* 1984; 14(suppl 5):45. Reproduced with permission of the publisher and authors.

TABLE 11-4

Third Heart Sound (S_3), Ventricular Diastolic Gallop, Protodiastolic Gallop, and Pericardial Knock

Physiologic S_3—children and young adults
- Decreased prevalence with increasing age

Pathologic S_3
- Ventricular dysfunction—poor systolic function, increased end-diastolic and end-systolic volume, decreased ejection fraction, and high filling pressures
  - Idiopathic dilated cardiomyopathy
  - Ischemic heart disease
  - Valvular heart disease
  - Congenital heart disease
  - Systemic and pulmonary hypertension
- Excessively rapid early diastolic ventricular filling
  - Hyperkinetic states
    - Anemia
    - Thyrotoxicosis
    - Arteriovenous fistula
  - Atrioventricular valve incompetence
  - Left-to-right shunts
- Restrictive myocardial or pericardial disease
  - Constrictive pericarditis (pericardial knock)
  - Restrictive cardiomyopathy
  - Hypertrophic cardiomyopathy?

be increased until left ventricular dysfunction develops. As left ventricular dysfunction develops, the ejection fraction decreases, resulting in an increased end-systolic volume, and a pathologic S_3 appears in these patients.[183] An S_3 is very common in acute aortic regurgitation and is usually followed by the middiastolic component of the Austin Flint rumble (Fig. 11-10).[52]

A pathologic S_3 resulting from excessive early diastolic filling is common in hyperkinetic states and AV valve regurgitation (Fig. 11-29, right panel) and often initiates a short flow rumble. It is often present in large left-to-right shunts due to high flow across the mitral valve with ventricular septal defect or patent ductus arteriosus and high flow across the tricuspid valve with atrial septal defect. The presence of this sound in these conditions does not imply congestive heart failure, and such patients may maintain normal myocardial contractility for years after the S_3 is detected.[184]

Pathologic third heart sounds are heard in both restrictive and hypertrophic cardiomyopathy. At times, they occur somewhat earlier after A_2 and may have durations that simulate a short diastolic rumble. In constrictive pericarditis, an early prominent sound of a somewhat higher frequency is heard—the pericardial knock. The evidence to date points to the simultaneous occurrence of the pericardial knock and the termination of rapid filling of the ventricles.[185] Whether this relationship is causal or coincidental is unclear. The apex cardiac pulsation may show systolic retraction followed by an exaggerated diastolic impulse. As shown in Fig. 11-33, this results in an apexcardiogram that is a mirror image of the normal, with the knock occurring at the peak of the diastolic impulse consistent with the impact theory

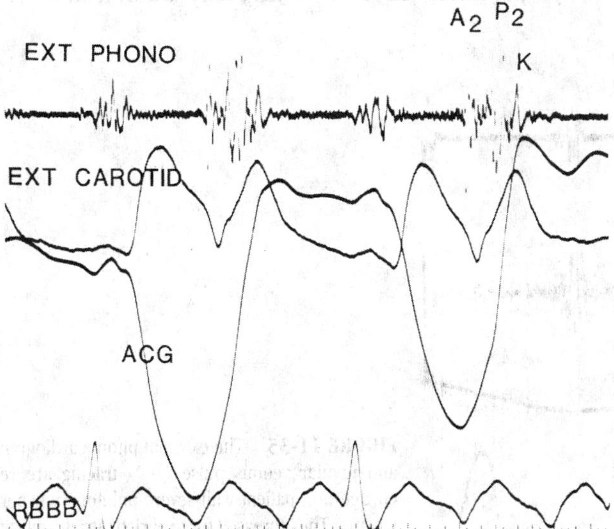

FIGURE 11-33 The ACG, external phonocardiogram, and external carotid pressure are recorded in a patient with chronic constrictive pericarditis, atrial flutter, and right bundle branch block (RBBB). Note the wide splitting of S_2 and the presence of a pericardial diastolic knock (K). The ACG shows systolic retraction and a prominent diastolic wave that peaks at the time of occurrence of the knock. [*From PS Reddy: Hemodynamics of constrictive pericarditis. In: PS Reddy et al (eds): Pericardial Disease. New York, Raven, 1982, p 291. Reproduced in part with permission of the publisher and the authors.*]

of Reddy.[8] The pericardial knock usually increases in intensity with inspiration and occurs near the nadir of the *y* descent of the jugular venous pulse (Fig. 11-34). Atrial fibrillation is commonly present in severe constrictive pericarditis, and at times the loud early knock may be confused with the opening snap of mitral stenosis. Careful attention to the classic contour of the jugular venous pulse in this condition will usually allow the correct diagnosis at the bedside.

The Fourth Heart Sound

Precordial vibrations resulting from atrial contraction are normally neither palpable nor audible. Under pathologic conditions, forceful atrial contraction generates a low-frequency sound (S_4) just prior to S_1 (also termed the *atrial diastolic gallop* or the *presystolic gallop*).

Atrial contraction must be present for production of an S_4. It is absent in atrial fibrillation and in other rhythms in which atrial contraction does not precede ventricular contraction. The S_4 follows the onset of the P wave of the ECG by approximately 70 ms. Audibility of the S_4 depends not only on its intensity and frequency but also on its separation from S_1. The degree of this separation is determined primarily by the PR interval, but it is also somewhat influenced by the PS_4 and the QS_1 interval. A loud S_1 may also mask the audibility of a preceding softer S_4.

The S_4 is best heard at the apex impulse with the patient turned in the left lateral position. It varies considerably with respiration, usually being heard best during expiration. Both the intensity and timing of the S_4 are closely related to the end-diastolic volume of the ventricle. Maneuvers that increase venous return increase the audibility by increasing the intensity of the sound and by causing it to occur earlier, thereby separating it further from S_1 (Fig. 11-6).[32] Decreased venous return does the opposite. Audible fourth heart sounds are usually accompanied by a palpable presystolic apical impulse in the absence of obesity, emphysema, etc., but occasionally palpable presystolic impulses are not audible. The S_4 generated by a forceful right atrial contraction is usually heard best at the lower left sternal border. Unlike the left-sided S_4, it tends to be accentuated with inspiration (Fig. 11-35). It is also accompanied by prominent *a* waves in the jugular venous pulse and is occasionally audible over the right jugular vein.[186]

As with the S_3, both the ventricular origin of this sound due to the abrupt deceleration of the atrial contribution to late diastolic filling[169] and the impact theory[8] have been proposed. It is likely that the former is responsible for the sounds recorded within the ventricular cavities or on their epicardial surfaces, while the latter mechanism is responsible for the S_4 ausculted at the chest wall.

Regardless of the exact mechanism of production, the presence of an S_4, particularly when associated with a palpable presystolic apical impulse, is an abnormal finding. Although considered to be a normal finding in older subjects by some investigators,[187] many other experienced cardiologists feel strongly that a definite S_4 in a middle-aged or older person is not likely to be a normal event.[186,188] The study of Reddy and associates[155] has shed light on this controversy, showing that the absolute in-

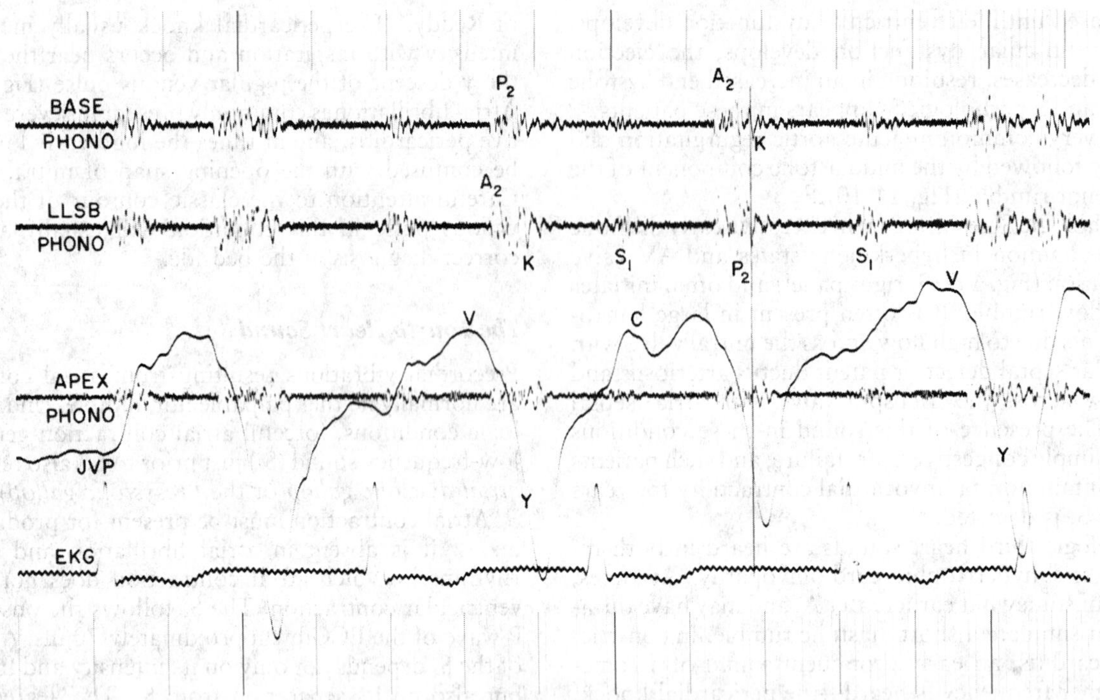

FIGURE 11-34 Phonocardiograms at the base, left sternal border, and apex are recorded with the jugular venous pulse in a patient with constrictive pericarditis and chronic atrial fibrillation. Wide splitting of S_2 is present and a relatively high-frequency sound, the pericardial knock (K), occurs near the nadir of the *y* descent of the jugular venous pulse (JVP). Note the increase in the intensity of the knock associated with the more prominent *y* descent during inspiration on the first complex.

tensity of S_4 does not decrease with age as does the absolute intensity of S_1, resulting in a relative increase in the intensity of S_4 compared to S_1. This relative change in intensity may well explain the increased frequency of recordable and audible fourth heart sounds in older subjects. Conditions such as obesity, emphysema, or barrel-chest deformity may hinder the clinical detection of both an S_4 and an apical presystolic impulse.

The common pathologic conditions in which S_4 is heard are listed in Table 11-5. A forceful atrial contraction into a hypertrophied noncompliant ventricle almost always produces an early and easily audible and re-

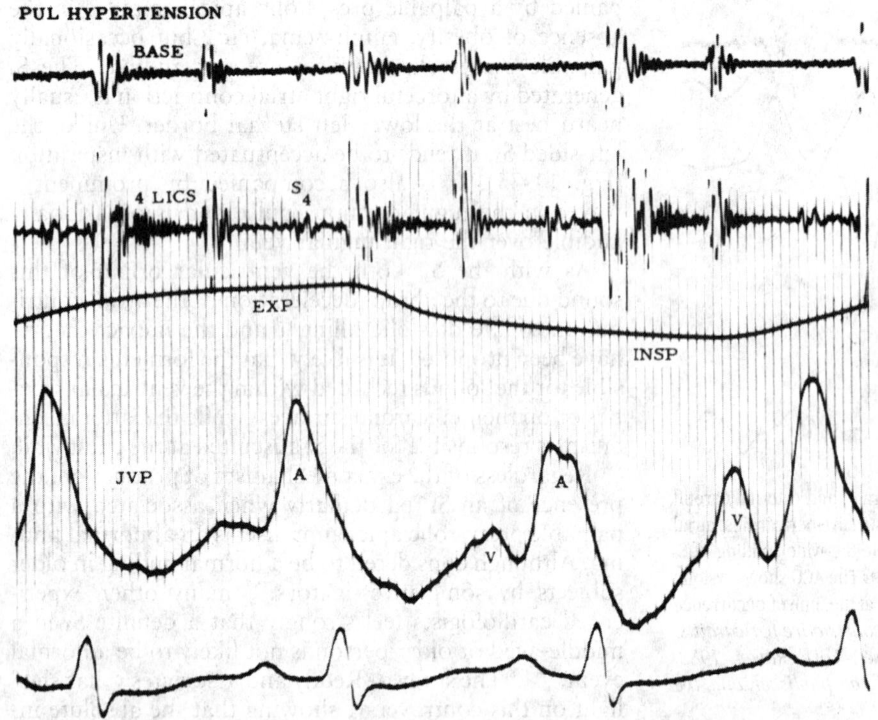

FIGURE 11-35 The external phonocardiogram and jugular venous pulse (JVP) tracing are recorded in a patient with severe pulmonary hypertension. The increased force of right atrial contraction is evident from the prominent *a* wave in the JVP. The S_4 is recorded in the fourth left intercostal space (4LICS) along the lower left sternal border. Note the increased amplitude of the S_4 with inspiration. [*From JA Shaver: Current uses of phonocardiography in clinical practice. In: E Rapaport (ed): Cardiology Update. New York, Elsevier, 1981, p 352. Reproduced with permission of the publisher and the author. Copyright 1981 by Elsevier Publishing Co., Inc.*]

TABLE 11-5

Fourth Heart Sound (S_4), Atrial Diastolic Gallop, and Presystolic Gallop

Physiologic—recordable, rarely audible
Pathologic
- Decreased ventricular compliance
  - Ventricular hypertrophy
    - Left or right ventricular outflow obstruction
    - Systemic or pulmonary hypertension
    - Hypertrophic cardiomyopathy
  - Ischemic heart disease
    - Angina pectoris
    - Acute myocardial infarction
    - Old myocardial infarction
    - Ventricular aneurysm
  - Idiopathic dilated cardiomyopathy
- Excessively rapid late diastolic filling secondary to vigorous atrial systole
  - Hyperkinetic states
    - Anemia
    - Thyrotoxicosis
    - Arteriovenous fistula
  - Acute atrioventricular valve incompetence
- Arrhythmias
  - Heart block

cordable S_4. The severe left ventricular hypertrophy present in systemic hypertension, severe valvular aortic stenosis, and hypertrophic cardiomyopathy is responsible for the loud S_4 recorded in Figs. 11-6, 11-36, and 11-37. In each case, the S_4 is associated with a prominent apical presystolic impulse and is widely separated from S_1. Although Goldblatt et al.[189] have reported that an S_4 in patients with aortic stenosis correlates with a peak systolic gradient of 70 mmHg or more and a left ventricular end-diastolic pressure of 13 mmHg or greater, Caulfield and associates[190] have modified this observation, stating that an S_4 is good evidence of significant aortic stenosis only in patients under age 40.

An audible S_4 with a palpable presystolic impulse is common in patients with ischemic heart disease during an acute episode of angina and in the early phases of transmural myocardial infarction. Its prevalence is also increased in patients with prior myocardial infarction. However, audible fourth heart sounds in patients with ischemic heart disease without prior infarction is quite uncommon.[8] In patients with left ventricular aneurysm or idiopathic or ischemic cardiomyopathy, abnormal fourth heart sounds are commonly present and often associated with an S_3, producing a quadruple rhythm. If tachycardia is present or if the PR interval is prolonged, S_3 and S_4 may fuse, giving rise to a loud summation gallop (Fig. 11-31).

Quadruple rhythms are common in hyperkinetic states where the S_3 is due to excessively rapid early diastolic filling and the S_4 results from a forceful atrial contraction into a volume-loaded ventricle. With varying degrees of tachycardia, incomplete summation may occur, simulating a diastolic rumble, or complete fusion may occur, generating a loud summation gallop (Fig. 11-31). In acute incompetence of the AV valve, vigorous atrial contraction into an acutely volume-loaded ventricle produces an S_4 associated with a presystolic apical impulse (Fig. 11-3).[191] At times it may be difficult to appreciate because of the masking effect of the loud systolic murmur. This contrasts with most patients with chronic mitral regurgitation, who do not have an S_4 but rather frequently have an S_3. (See also Chap. 80.)

Presystolic and isolated diastolic fourth heart sounds as well as summation gallops may be heard with varying degrees of heart block. First-degree heart block facilitates audibility of the S_4 because it further separates S_4 from S_1. In 2 : 1 heart block, an isolated S_4 may be heard in diastole and also a presystolic S_4 may be audible because

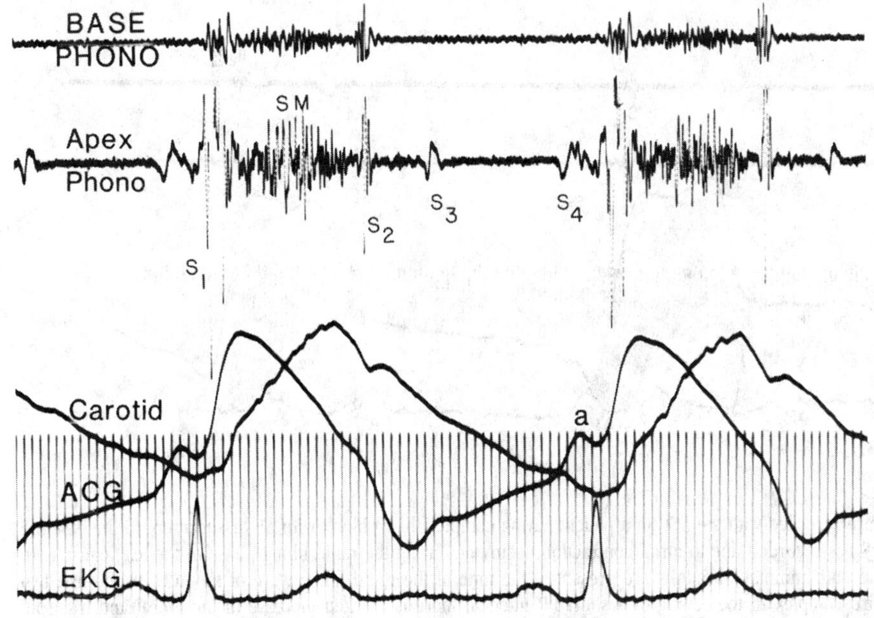

FIGURE 11-36 Atrial diastolic (ADG) and ventricular diastolic (VDG) gallops are recorded in an adult with severe calcific aortic stenosis. The ADG is associated with a prominent presystolic apical impulse (*a*) and the VDG occurs during the rapid filling wave of the ACG. The carotid pulse has a very slow rate of rise and a markedly prolonged left ventricular ejection time. The classic diamond-shaped systolic ejection murmur (SM) is present at the base and apex. Note the higher-frequency composition of the SM at the apex but preservation of the crescendo-decrescendo pattern. [*From JA Shaver: Current uses of phonocardiography in clinical practice. In: E Rapaport (ed): Cardiology Update—Reviews for Physicians. New York, Elsevier, 1981, p 356. Reproduced with permission of the publisher and author. Copyright 1981 by Elsevier Publishing Co., Inc.*]

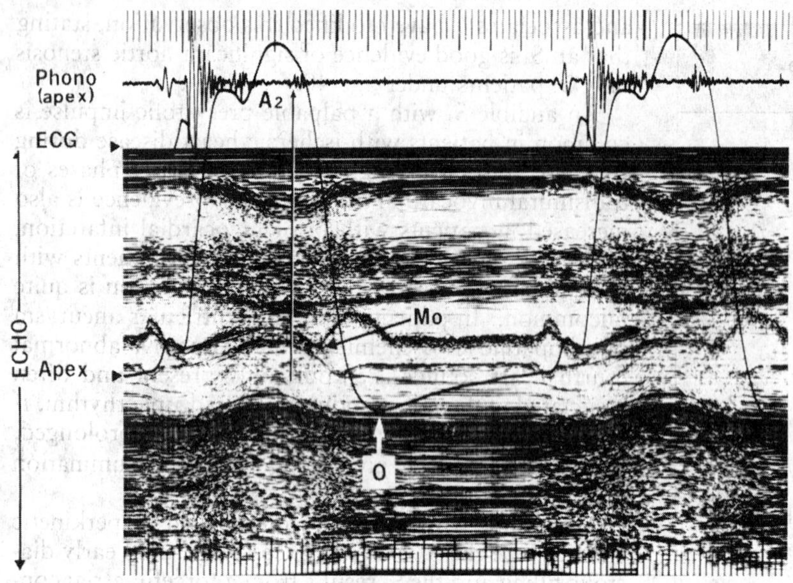

FIGURE 11-37 The apex phonocardiogram is recorded simultaneously with the ACG and mitral valve echocardiogram. A prominent S_4 is widely separated from S_1 and is coincident with the rapid upstroke of the *a* wave on the ACG. Asymmetrical septal hypertrophy is present, and the left ventricular cavity is small. At cardiac catheterization, no gradient was found across the left ventricular outflow tract. [*From RF Alvares, et al: Isovolumic relaxation period in hypertrophic cardiomyopathy. J Am Coll Cardiol 3(1):75, 1984. Reproduced with permission from the American College of Cardiology and the authors.*]

of the increase in diastolic volume. In complete heart block, S_4 may be heard randomly throughout diastole, and when it occurs simultaneously with rapid early ventricular filling, a loud summation gallop may occur (Fig. 11-38). Fourth heart sounds have also been reported in ventricular systole when atrial contraction occurred during systole in a patient with heart block. The occurrence of an S_4 when the mitral valve is closed excludes its ventricular origin due to either a pressure or volume change and is in keeping with the impact theory of S_4 sound production.[8]

Prosthetic Valve Sounds

The sounds produced by prosthetic valves are varied, depending on the type of valve, its position, and whether or not it is functioning normally. Mechanical valves produce opening and closing clicks that are easily audible and in many patients can be heard even without a stethoscope. Ball-in-cage valves such as the Starr–Edwards produce the loudest and most distinctive opening and closing clicks in any position as long as there is normal valve and ventricular function (Fig. 11-39).[192,193] In the aortic position, a crisp opening click occurs 0.06 to 0.07 s after S_1 and is coincident with maximal ball excursion as demonstrated by echocardiography.[194] The metallic ball of the Starr–Edwards valve also produces multiple early systolic clicks when the freely moving ball bounces against the cage during early systolic ejection.[193,195] These clicks occur during the harsh systolic ejection murmur. Absence or decrease in intensity of these clicks occur with valve obstruction or left ventricular dysfunction. A decrease in the intensity of the opening and closing clicks, which normally have an intensity ratio of more than 0.5, and the absence of the opening click are also indications of valve malfunction.[193,194]

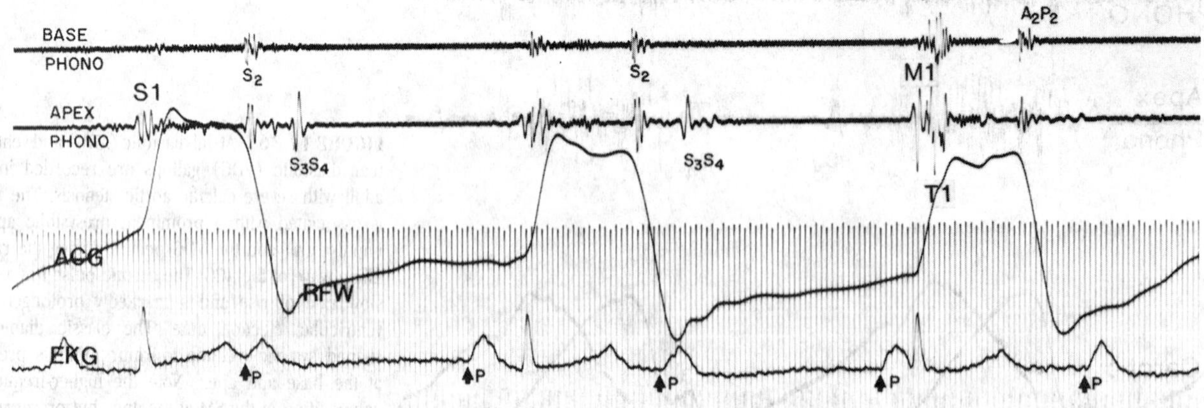

FIGURE 11-38 Base and apex phonocardiograms are recorded with the ACG in a patient having complete heart block with AV dissociation. In the first and second complexes a prominent summation gallop (S_3S_4) is recorded due to atrial contraction occurring during the rapid filling phase of the left ventricle. In the third complex, atrial contraction occurs later, and only minimal vibrations are present at the time of the rapid filling wave of the ACG. In the first two complexes, the intensity of S_1 is soft, while in the third complex in the setting of a short PR interval, there is marked increase in the mitral and tricuspid components of S_1.

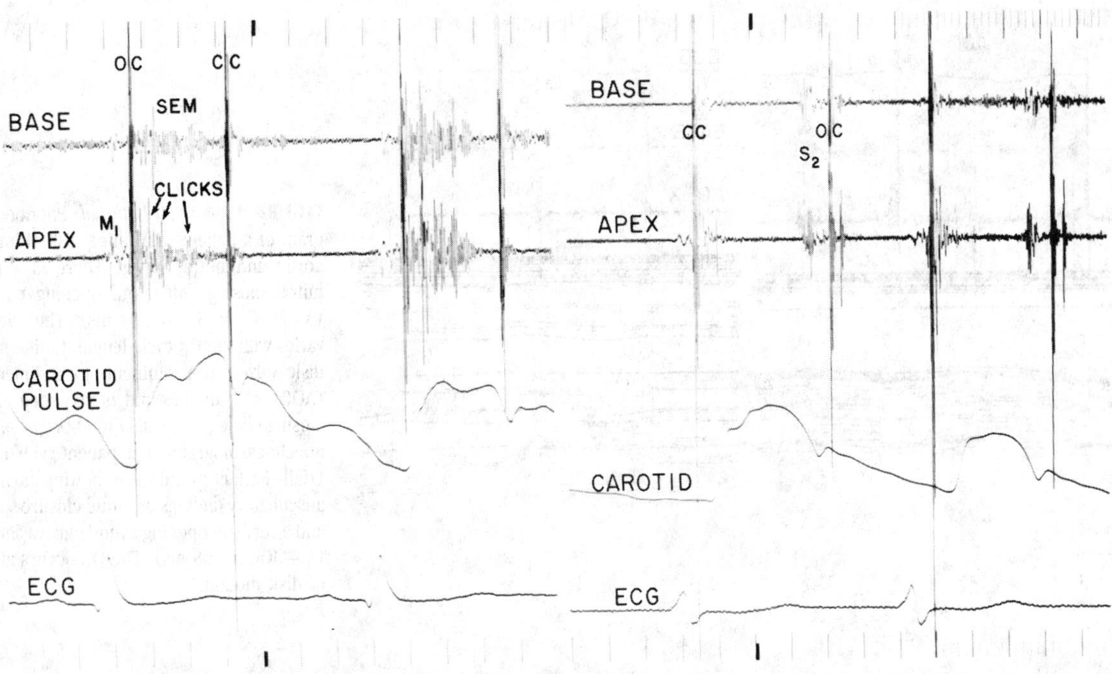

FIGURE 11-39 *Left panel:* Phonocardiogram of a patient with a Starr–Edwards aortic valve. A loud aortic closing click (CC) is present. A slightly softer aortic opening click (OC) follows a much softer S_1 (S_1–OC = 55 ms). A harsh ejection murmur with overlying systolic clicks is recorded (*arrows*). *Right panel:* Phonocardiogram of a patient with a Starr–Edwards mitral valve. There is a very loud mitral closing click (CC). A prominent opening click (OC) occurs 65 ms after aortic closure (A_2). A softer sound follows the OC and is due to the ball bouncing against the cage.

In the mitral position, a prominent opening click occurs 0.05 to 0.15 s after A_2.[196] Narrowing of this interval indicates an elevation of left atrial pressure, which may be due to either valvular obstruction or regurgitation. Interference with ball motion can also produce prolongation or significant beat-to-beat variation of this interval. A closing click is also prominent. Just as is seen with the normal S_1, there is variability in the intensity of the closing click, with the changing RR intervals of atrial fibrillation being louder with short RR intervals and softer with long. A decreased intensity with first-degree AV block also occurs due to partial atriogenic closure of the valve, thus reducing the ball excursion and therefore the click intensity. Although a decreased intensity of the valve clicks occurs with valve malfunction, the presence of normal ball motion on an echocardiogram suggests that a nonvalvular cause such as severe left ventricular dysfunction is responsible for the decreased intensity.[192]

The auscultatory findings of disk valve prostheses vary, depending upon the type of disk valve. Central occluder valves such as the Beall valve, which was used predominantly in the mitral and tricuspid positions, produce distinct, audible opening and closing sounds.[193,194] The more commonly used tilting disk valves do not ordinarily produce audible opening sounds in either the aortic or mitral position, although a soft opening sound can usually be demonstrated by phonocardiography (Fig. 11-40). Phonoechocardiography has shown that these sounds occur at the onset rather than at the maximal opening of the disk.[193,197] In the mitral position, the A_2-OS interval is 0.05 and 0.09 s; abbreviation of this interval occurs with valvular regurgitation or obstruction, both of which elevate the left atrial pressure. The aortic opening click usually follows S_1 by 0.04 s. The closing sounds of disk valves are distinct and easily heard in both aortic and mitral positions. Left ventricular dysfunction, first-degree AV block, or other arrhythmia that causes the disk to move to a partially closed position prior to the onset of ventricular contraction will result in a softer sound. This finding must be distinguished from malfunction caused by either fibrosis or thrombus disturbing the disk motion. Auscultation of the bileaflet St. Jude valve is similar to that of the tilting disk valve.[198]

The sounds produced by tissue prosthetic valves are more like normal heart sounds than the sounds from a mechanical valve (Fig. 11-41).[193,194] In the aortic position, an opening sound is usually not audible. In the mitral position, an opening sound is audible in about 50 percent of patients at an interval of 0.07 to 0.11 s after A_2.

Extracardiac Sounds

Pacemaker Sounds

High-frequency sounds of brief duration are occasionally present in patients with transvenous pacemakers located in the right ventricular apex. They are extracardiac in origin, occurring nearly synchronous (within 6 to 10 ms) with the pacemaker spike, and are due to stimulation of intercostal nerves adjacent to endocardial electrodes.[199] This stimulus results in contraction of the intercostal muscles, and frequently twitching of the muscle can be observed. The presence of these sounds should always suggest possible myocardial perforation by the endocardial lead, although this is not always present. Stimulation of the pectoral muscles as well as diaphragmatic stimulation has also been reported to produce these extracardiac sounds. They have also been observed in patients having transthoracically placed epicardial leads.

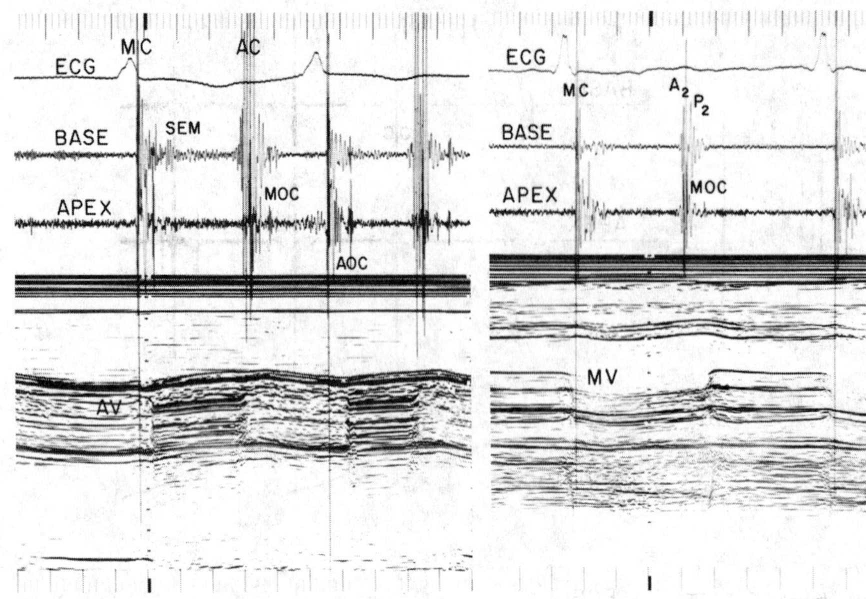

FIGURE 11-40 *Left panel:* Phonoechocardiogram of a patient with tilting disk (Bjork–Shiley) aortic and mitral valves. There is a prominent mitral closing (MC) and opening click (MOC) (A_2–MOC = 55 to 110 ms). The click interval varies with the RR cycle length. Unlike most tilting disk valves, a prominent aortic opening click (AOC) was audible and is recorded. The aortic closing click (AC) is also loud. *Right panel:* Phonoechocardiogram of a patient with tilting disk (Hall–Kaster) mitral valve showing the more usual auscultatory findings of a loud closure sound (MC) and a very soft opening sound that was not audible. (A_2–MOC = 65 ms). The OC occurs at the onset of disk motion.

Pericardial Friction Rub

Inflammation of the pericardial sac with or without fluid may cause a pericardial friction rub. These friction sounds are very high-pitched, leathery, and scratchy in nature. They seem close to the ear and are ausculted best with the patient leaning forward or in the knee-chest position, holding his or her breath after forced expiration. The pericardial rub may have three components during the intervals of the cardiac cycle when the heart has the greatest excursions within the pericardial sac—at the time of atrial systole, at the time of ventricular contraction, and during rapid early diastolic filling. The usual friction rub occurs during the first two intervals, although three-component rubs may be heard. Triple-component friction rubs are common in uremic pericarditis, particularly when the underlying cardiac disease is hypertension. In this situation, the heart is hyperkinetic due to both pressure and volume overload as well as to the anemia associated with renal failure. Pericardial friction rubs are very common in the acute phase of transmural myocardial infarction, although they often last for only a few hours. There is a common misconception that friction rubs are not heard when there is a large amount of fluid in the pericardial sac; this is not the case, because usually some portions of the visceral and parietal pericardial surfaces are in contact in spite of the large amount of fluid.[2] (See also Chap. 92.)

Occasionally, certain midsystolic (ejection) murmurs have a scratchy character and may be misinterpreted as friction rubs. This is particularly true of the short, scratchy pulmonic ejection murmur heard in hyperthyroidism (Means–Lerman sign).[200] Such scratchy sounds

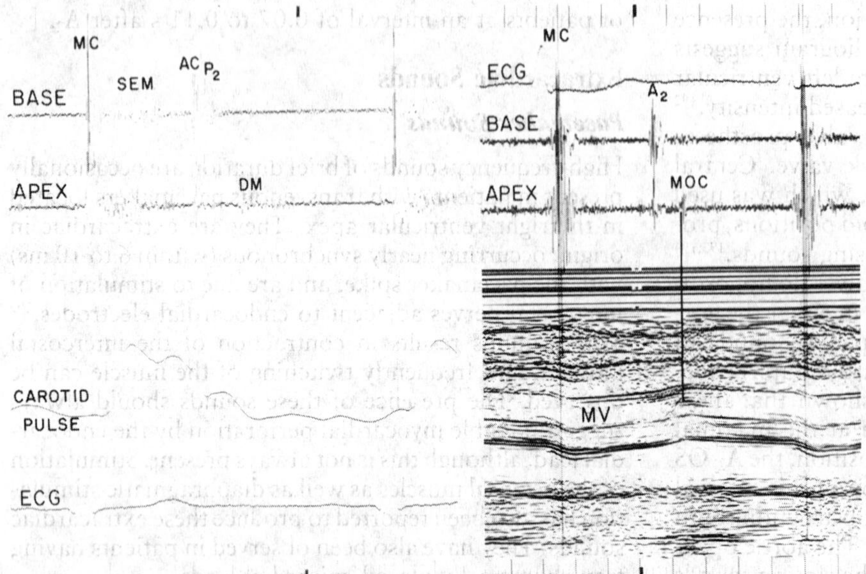

FIGURE 11-41 *Left panel:* Phonocardiogram of a patient with heterograft aortic and mitral valves. There is no distinct aortic or mitral opening click. Closing clicks of both valves are prominent. (AC = aortic closure; MC = mitral closure). There is a mitral middiastolic rumble at the apex (DM) and a systolic ejection murmur (SEM); both are frequently found with heterograft valves. *Right panel:* Phonoechocardiogram of a patient with the more typical auscultatory findings of a heterograft mitral valve. There is a prominent mitral closing sound (MC). A softer but still audible mitral opening sound (MOC) occurs just after maximum excursion of the valve leaflets. A_2–MOC = 90 ms. No diastolic rumble was recorded.

should not be considered to be a friction rub unless both systolic and diastolic components are heard.

Mediastinal Crunch: Hamman's Sign[201]

When air is present in the mediastinum, a series of scratchy sounds may occur, related indirectly to both heartbeat and respiratory excursion. These sounds occur most frequently during ventricular systole and in a random fashion. The diagnosis of mediastinal emphysema may be confirmed by crepitation in the neck secondary to subcutaneous air. Often, the patient is aware of the sound and may volunteer what position or phase of respiration will accentuate it. These crunching sounds due to air in the mediastinum are common following cardiac surgery.

HEART MURMURS

A *cardiac murmur* is defined as a relatively prolonged series of auditory vibrations of varying intensity (loudness), frequency (pitch), quality, configuration, and duration.[202] Although the exact physical principles that govern the production of murmurs have been debated for years, most authorities now agree that turbulence is the prime factor responsible for most murmurs.[19,203] Turbulence arises when blood velocity becomes critically high due to high flow, flow through an irregular or narrow area, or a combination of both. Leatham has attributed the production of murmurs to three main factors[204]: (1) high flow rate through normal or abnormal orifices, (2) forward flow through a constricted or irregular orifice or into a dilated vessel or chamber, and (3) backward or regurgitant flow through an incompetent valve, septal defect, or patent ductus arteriosus. Frequently, a combination of these factors is operative.

While the intensity of a systolic murmur is not always proportional to the hemodynamic disturbance, grading the loudness of a murmur from 1 to 6 as described by Freeman and Levine[205] is generally utilized. A grade 1 murmur is so faint that it can be heard only with special effort. A grade 2 murmur is faint but can be easily heard. A grade 3 murmur is moderately loud; a grade 4 murmur is very loud; and a grade 5 murmur is extremely loud and can be heard if only the edge of the stethoscope is in contact with the skin but cannot be heard if the stethoscope is removed from the skin. A grade 6 murmur is exceptionally loud and can be heard with the stethoscope just removed from contact with the chest. Experience has shown that systolic murmurs of grade 3 or more in intensity are usually hemodynamically significant. Systolic thrills are usually associated with murmurs of grade 4 or louder. As pointed out by Leatham, the intensity of the murmur varies directly with the velocity of blood flow across the area of murmur production. The velocity in turn is directly related to the pressure head that drives the blood across the murmur-producing area. For example, high velocity of flow through a small ventricular septal defect produces a loud murmur, whereas a large flow at low velocity through an atrial septal defect produces no murmur. The intensity of a murmur as ausculted at the chest wall is also determined by the transmission characteristics of the tissues intervening between the source of the murmur and the stethoscope. Obesity, emphysema, and the presence of significant pericardial or pleural effusion will decrease the intensity of a murmur, while a thin, esthenic body habitus will often accentuate it.

McKusick[206] has shown that the frequency of a murmur bears a direct relationship to the velocity of blood flow, as does the intensity of the murmur. The low-velocity flow resulting from a small pressure head across a stenotic mitral valve produces a low-pitched rumbling murmur, while the large diastolic pressure gradient across an incompetent aortic valve causes a high-pitched murmur. A recent study has further demonstrated that the dominant frequencies contained in heart murmurs due to stenotic lesions are directly related to the instantaneous jet velocities distal to the associated obstruction.[207] Occasionally, the frequency composition of the same systolic murmur may vary, depending on the area ausculted. For example, the systolic murmur of aortic stenosis frequently sounds higher pitched at the apex than at the base.[208] Some murmurs, such as the "cooing dove" regurgitant murmur of a ruptured or retroverted aortic cusp,[209] the systolic "whoop" or "honk" of mitral valve prolapse,[210] or the high-pitched systolic murmur of a degenerated bioprosthetic valve,[211] have a very distinctive musical quality. Recent data support the theory that such musical murmurs result from a uniform periodic vibration of a cardiac structure such as a valve leaflet or chordae tendineae that begins to resonate in response to turbulent energy.[212,213]

In addition to the intensity and frequency of murmurs, their timing should also be described. There is seldom any difficulty distinguishing between systole and diastole, since systole is considerably shorter at normal heart rates. However, at rapid heart rates, the durations of these two intervals approach each other. Under such circumstances, the examiner can usually time the murmur by simultaneous palpation of the right carotid artery or can rely on the fact that the second heart sound (S_2) is usually the louder sound at the base. Once S_2 is identified, murmurs can be properly located in the cardiac cycle as systolic or diastolic. If the murmur in question is at the apex, the proper timing can be ensured by the "inching" technique popularized by Harvey and Levine.[5] This consists of slowly moving the stethoscope down from the base to the apex while repeatedly fixing the cardiac cycle in mind, using S_2 as a reference point. With sinus tachycardia, carotid sinus pressure may temporarily slow the rate and make it possible to differentiate systole from diastole. If extra systoles are occurring and one listens carefully to identify the beat that follows a compensatory pause, the first subsequent sound will be the first heart sound (S_1). Continuous murmurs are heard throughout the cardiac cycle in systole and diastole and usually have their peak intensity around S_2.

The location and radiation of a murmur is multifactionally determined by its site of origin, intensity, and direction of blood flow as well as by the physical characteristics of the chest.[214] The duration and time intensity contour (*murmur "envelope"*) of a specific murmur is intimately related to the instantaneous pattern of blood flow velocity causing the murmur.

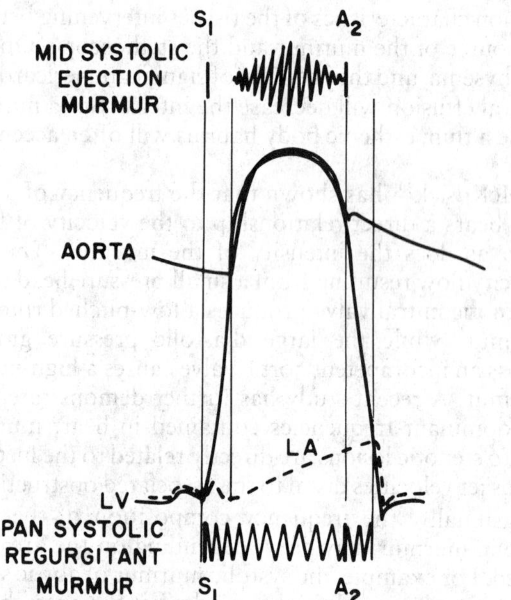

FIGURE 11-42 Diagrammatic representation of the midsystolic ejection murmur and pansystolic regurgitant murmur as related to left ventricular (LV), aortic, and left atrial (LA) pressures. The systolic ejection murmur occurs during the period of LV ejection; the onset of the murmur is separated from the first heart sound (S_1) by the period of isovolumic contraction, and the crescendo-decrescendo murmur terminates before aortic valve closure. The pansystolic murmur begins with and may replace S_1. This murmur continues up to and through the aortic closure sound (A_2), as LV pressure exceeds LA pressure during this time. (*From PS Reddy, et al: Cardiac systolic murmurs: Pathophysiology and differential diagnosis. Prog Cardiovasc Dis 14:19, 1971. Reproduced with permission from the publisher and the authors.*)

Systolic Murmurs

Systolic murmurs may be classified into two basic categories—ejection murmurs and regurgitant murmurs (Fig. 11-42). This simple classification, popularized by Leatham,[204] is most attractive because it has a physiologic as well as a descriptive basis. Systolic ejection murmurs are due to forward flow across the left or right ventricular outflow tract, while systolic regurgitant murmurs are due to retrograde flow from a high-pressure cardiac chamber to a low-pressure chamber.

Systolic Ejection Murmurs

The systolic ejection murmur begins shortly after the pressure in the left or right ventricle exceeds the aortic or pulmonic diastolic pressure sufficiently to open the aortic or pulmonic valve. As a result, there is a delay between the S_1, which occurs shortly after AV pressure crossover and the beginning of the murmur (Fig. 11-42). The murmur then waxes and wanes in a crescendo-decrescendo fashion often described as "diamond shaped" or "spindle shaped" in configuration. The murmur ends before the semilunar valve closure of the side from which it originates. The contour of the time-intensity pattern or "envelope" of the murmur corresponds to the contour of the flow velocity, and the murmur is heard when the sound produced during the peak turbulence exceeds the audible threshold.[215] Thus, not only is the overall intensity of the murmur proportional to the rate of ventricular ejection, but also its shape depends on the instantaneous flow velocity during the period of ejection. As can be seen in Fig. 11-43, during normal left ventricular ejection, a disproportionately large volume flow occurs in early systole. If velocity of flow exceeds the murmur threshold, a short midsystolic or "ejection" murmur results, and its envelope corresponds to the flow velocity pattern. If the stroke volume of the ventricle is increased, this pattern of ejection persists in an exaggerated fashion; the resultant murmur has a tendency to peak early in systole and fade out about halfway through the ejection phase. Such murmurs have been referred to as "kite shaped," and are common in high-output states or conditions such as aortic regurgitation or heart block, where stroke volume is high.

It should be pointed out that the flow characteristics of normal right ventricular ejection are somewhat different. Early ejection rates are not nearly as high and the flow curve peaks somewhat later, having a more rounded contour.[216] This flow pattern may well explain some of the long systolic ejection murmurs heard in atrial septal defects and the straight-back syndrome, where only min-

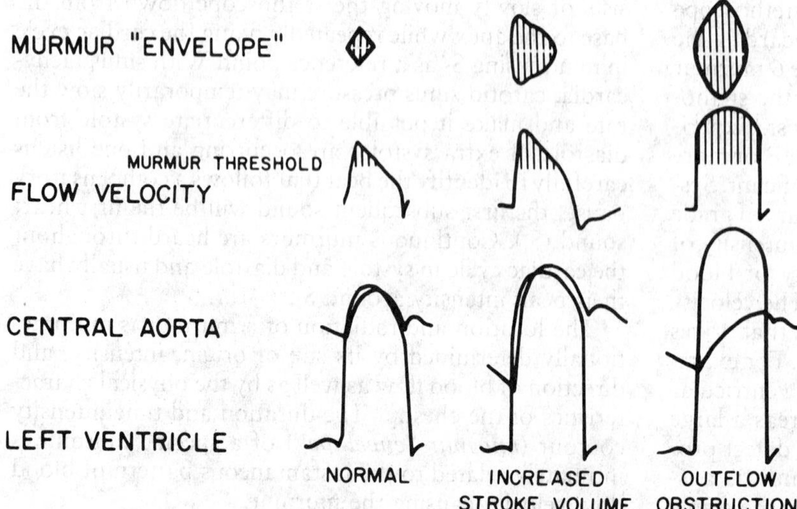

FIGURE 11-43 The simultaneous time-intensity course of the murmur "envelope," aortic flow velocity, and left ventricular (LV) and central aortic pressure. During normal LV ejection (*left panel*), peak flow velocity is early with two-thirds of the ventricular volume ejected during the first half of systole. The murmur threshold may be exceeded during the early peak flow and the corresponding murmur envelope inscribed. The center panel shows exaggeration of the normal pattern of LV ejection with a high stroke volume as in high-output states. With critical aortic stenosis (*right panel*), rapid early ejection is no longer possible; the flow velocity is increased and the contour becomes rounded and prolonged, producing the typical diamond-shaped murmur of aortic stenosis. (*Modified from PS Reddy, et al: Cardiac systolic murmurs: pathophysiology and differential diagnosis. Prog Cardiovasc Dis 14:4, 1971. Reproduced with permission of the publisher and the authors.*)

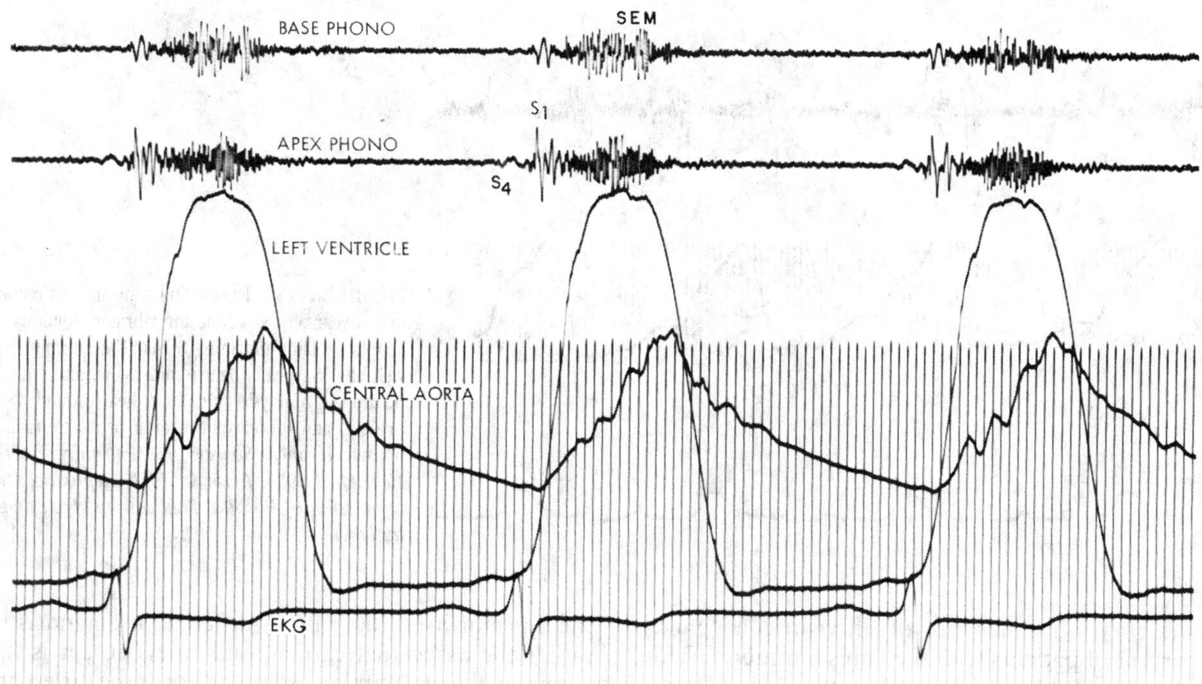

FIGURE 11-44 Base and apex phonocardiograms are recorded simultaneously with left ventricular (LV) and central aortic pressures in a patient with severe calcific aortic stenosis. A valvular ejection sound is absent, and A_2 is not recorded. The murmur is crescendo-decrescendo, and its contour correlates well with the instantaneous pressure gradient. Note that the murmur has a much higher frequency content on the apex phonocardiogram. A soft S_4 gallop is also recorded at the apex.

imal gradients are found across the right ventricular outflow tract.[217] With true valvular obstruction, rapid early ejection is no longer possible; the aortic flow velocity pattern becomes rounded, resulting in the more symmetrical murmur of aortic stenosis. In such cases, the instantaneous flow pattern is determined by the instantaneous pressure head with the resultant high correlation between the contour of the gradient and the murmur envelope (Fig. 11-44). If left or right ventricular obstruction is severe, systole is prolonged and the semilunar valve closure sound is delayed. The murmur, however, always stops before the closure sound of the side from which it originates, although it may envelop the closure sound of the opposite side of the circulation. Because of the high correlation between the shape of the murmur and its underlying flow velocity characteristics, during auscultation careful attention must be given to the shape and duration of the murmur as well as to its intensity.

The intensity of ejection murmurs closely parallels changes in cardiac output. Any condition that increases forward flow—such as exercise, anxiety, fever, or increased stroke volume associated with the long diastolic filling period after a premature beat—increases the intensity of the murmur. Likewise, conditions that decrease cardiac output—congestive heart failure, beta blockade, or other negative inotropic agents—will decrease the intensity of the ejection murmur. This intimate relationship to flow, particularly with beat-to-beat variations, will usually allow the clinician to differentiate a systolic ejection murmur from a systolic regurgitant murmur. Furthermore, the definitive diagnosis of the systolic murmur can often be made during auscultation by careful attention to the response of the murmur to various bedside maneuvers that alter the flow and loading conditions of the heart.[218] These maneuvers include respiration, the strain and release phases of the Valsalva maneuver, standing, squatting, passive leg elevation, isometric hand grip exercise, inhalation of amyl nitrite, and transient arterial occlusion.

Innocent Murmurs Innocent murmurs are always systolic ejection in nature and occur without evidence of physiologic or structural abnormalities in the cardiovascular system when peak flow velocity in early systole exceeds the murmur threshold.[219] These murmurs are almost always less than grade 3 in intensity and vary considerably from examination to examination and with body position and level of physical activity. They are not associated with a thrill or with radiation to the carotid arteries or axillae. They may arise from flow across either the normal left or right ventricular outflow tract and always end well before semilunar valve closure.

Innocent murmurs are found in approximately 30 to 50 percent of all children. In young children, especially ages 3 to 8, the vibratory systolic (Still's) murmur is common (Fig. 11-45).[220] It has a very distinctive quality described as "groaning," "croaking," "buzzing," or "twanging." It is heard best along the left sternal border at the third or fourth interspace and disappears by puberty. Considerable controversy exists as to the origin of the vibratory systolic murmur. One group of investigators has suggested that left ventricular bands, which cross the left ventricular outflow tract, could be responsible for the production of turbulence resulting in the vibratory

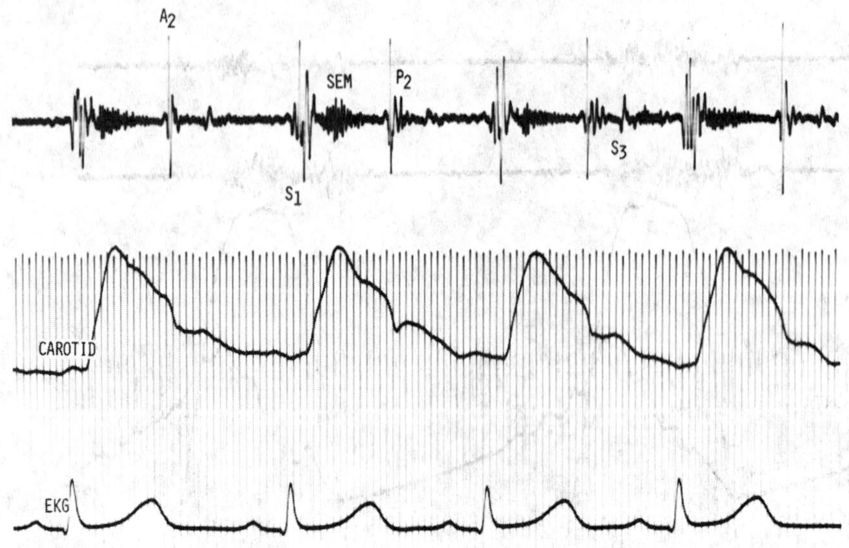

FIGURE 11-45 Typical Still's murmur as recorded in a 4-year-old boy. Note the vibratory quality of the systolic ejection murmur (SEM). The murmur begins well after S_1, peaks before midsystole, and ends well before A_2. A physiologic third heart sound (S_3) is present, and the carotid arterial pressure tracing is normal. (*From JA Shaver: Innocent murmurs. Hosp Med, April 1978, p 15. © 1978. Reproduced with permission of Hospital Publications, Inc., and the author.*)

murmur. They found this type of left ventricular bands in 76 percent of patients with the Still's murmur.[221] This finding was not confirmed in another study using Doppler and two-dimensional echocardiography.[222] In this report, it was suggested that the origin of the Still's murmur was related to the finding of a small ascending aortic diameter associated with a concomitant high aortic blood flow velocity. Regardless of the exact cause, most authorities agree that this murmur originates from flow across the left ventricular outflow tract.

Innocent systolic ejection murmurs have also been attributed to flow across the normal right ventricular outflow tract and have been termed innocent pulmonic systolic murmurs because the site of their maximal intensity is ausculted best in the pulmonary area at the second left interspace with radiation along the left sternal border. These are low to medium in pitch, with a blowing quality, and are common in children, adolescents, and young adults. However, Stein et al.,[223] using high-fidelity catheter-tipped micromanometers to record intracardiac sound and pressure in the aorta and pulmonary artery in adults with normal valves, invariably recorded the ejection murmur in the region of the aortic valve. They concluded that these murmurs, in spite of their precordial location, were aortic in origin.

In adults over age 50, innocent murmurs due to flow across the left ventricular outflow tract are often heard and may be of a higher frequency, with a musical quality, and frequently loudest at the apex. They may be associated with a tortuous, dilated sclerotic aortic root, often in the setting of systolic hypertension. Mild sclerosis of the aortic valve may also be present.

The preceding descriptive breakdown of innocent murmurs is based primarily on age, precordial location, and distinctive acoustic qualities. Since all of these murmurs are equally innocent and because there is considerable overlap among them in respect to origin, transmission, and frequency composition, they are best characterized as systolic ejection murmurs without associated abnormalities of the cardiovascular system. Since both innocent and pathologic ejection murmurs have the same mechanism of production, it is not the nature of the murmur itself that allows differential diagnosis but rather the associated cardiac findings. Thus, it is "the company the murmur keeps" that affords the differential diagnosis of the pathologic systolic ejection murmur from the innocent murmur (Fig. 11-46).[224]

For a murmur to be considered innocent, the examination of the cardiovascular system must disclose no abnormalities. Blood pressure and contour of the carotid, femoral, and brachial arteries should always be evaluated carefully. For example, a seemingly innocent murmur in the setting of hypertension, particularly in a younger patient, should always suggest the diagnosis of coarctation of the aorta, which can readily be diagnosed by palpation of weak or nearly absent femoral pulses and confirmed by taking the blood pressure in the lower extremities. There should be no elevation of the jugular venous pulse, and the contour of the jugular pulse should be normal, without exaggeration of either the *a* or *v* wave. Evidence of cardiac enlargement on physical examination should be absent, and the palpation of the apex in the left lateral position should show no evidence of a presystolic impulse, sustained systolic motion, or hyperdynamic circulation. On auscultation, normal physiologic splitting should be present. A physiologic S_3, as shown in Fig. 11-45, is often present in association with an innocent murmur in children and young adults but should not be heard after age 30. An S_4 is rarely heard in normal children and adults (younger than 50 years) and should always be considered to be abnormal when associated with a presystolic impulse. Systolic ejection sounds of valvular origin as well as midsystolic nonejection sounds should be absent, as they point to minor abnormalities of the semilunar and AV valves, respectively (Fig. 11-46). The remainder of the physical examination should show no evidence of a cardiac cause of pulmonary or systemic congestion. In almost all patients with innocent murmurs, the ECG and the cardiac silhouette on chest x-ray should be normal.

The supraclavicular arterial murmur or bruit is a common finding in normal individuals, particularly children and adolescents.[225] These murmurs are maximal in intensity above the clavicles and tend to be louder on the

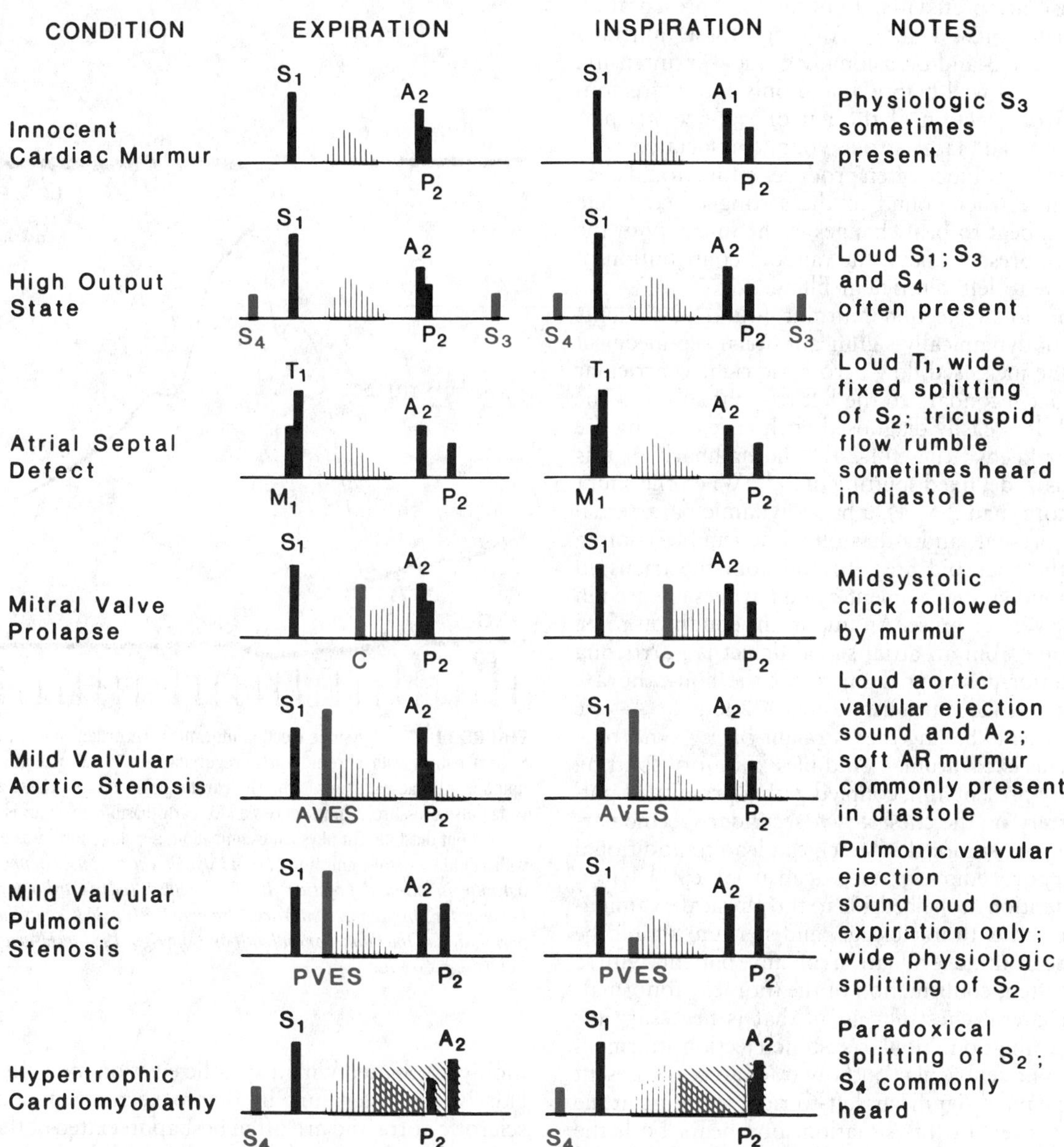

FIGURE 11-46 The differential diagnosis of the innocent murmur versus the Pathologic systolic murmur is made by "the company the murmur keeps." The innocent murmur must be found in the setting of an otherwise normal cardiovascular examination. C = midsystolic nonejection sound; AVES = aortic valvular ejection sound; PVES = pulmonary valvular ejection sound; AR = aortic regurgitation. (*From JA Shaver, et al: Examination of the Heart. Part IV, Auscultation, Dallas, American Heart Association, 1990, p 40. Reproduced with permission of the publisher and the authors.*)

right, although they are often heard bilaterally. The bruit begins shortly after S_1, is diamond shaped, and is of brief duration, usually occupying less than half of systole. Although the exact mechanism of production is unknown, it is related to peak flow velocity near the origin of the normal subclavian, innominate, or carotid artery. When particularly prominent, this murmur may transmit to the basal region of the heart and simulate a systolic ejection murmur. However, unlike the cardiac ejection murmur, the supraclavicular murmur is always louder above the clavicles than below them. Complete compression of the subclavian artery may cause the murmur to disappear completely, while partial compression may occasionally intensify it. Hyperextension of the shoulders is a simple bedside maneuver that may decrease the intensity of the murmur and cause it to disappear completely.[226] In the adult, the supraclavicular murmur must be distinguished from the murmur of true organic carotid obstruction, this latter murmur being longer, often extending through S_2, and frequently associated with a history suggestive of transient ischemic attacks.

Functional Systolic Ejection Murmurs Systolic ejection murmurs produced by high cardiac output states are functional and flow related but are excluded from the category of innocent murmurs because of their associated altered physiologic state.[219] These include the cardiac flow murmurs of thyrotoxicosis, pregnancy, anemia, fever, exercise, and peripheral arteriovenous fistula and are best interpreted in light of the total presentation of the patient (Fig. 11-46).[227] Although these murmurs are often grade 3 and occasionally grade 4 in intensity, they always end well before S_2 and only rarely are confused with obstruction of the left or right ventricular outflow tract. The large stroke volume associated with high-degree heart block often produces a functional ejection murmur; when found in the setting of complete heart block, beat-to-beat changes in the intensity of the murmur are present due to the random contribution of atrial systole to left ventricular filling.

The functional ejection murmur found in patients with a hemodynamically significant atrial septal defect is due to the increased flow across the right ventricular outflow tract secondary to the left-to-right shunt at the atrial level. It is easily diagnosed at the bedside "by the company it keeps" (Fig. 11-24). The hallmark of this condition is wide, fixed splitting of S_2.[149] When the shunt is large (more than 2.5 : 1), a hyperdynamic parasternal impulse is present, and a diastolic flow rumble is often heard in the tricuspid area. In addition, the tricuspid closure is loud, and prominent *a* and *v* waves are seen in the jugular venous pulse. An important condition to be differentiated from an atrial septal defect is narrowing of the anterior-posterior diameter of the bony thorax. Prominent systolic murmurs—often grade 3 or 4—are heard in patients having the "straight-back" syndrome and/or pectus excavatum.[228] Audible expiratory splitting is frequently present and, coupled with a prominent pulmonary artery on the chest x-ray (secondary to the narrow anterior-posterior diameter), can lead to additional unnecessary procedures to rule out an atrial septal defect. Careful attention at the bedside to the physical examination of the spine, thoracic cage, and sternum should be part of the routine evaluation of any patient with a murmur. Often, confirmation of the thoracic abnormality with a lateral chest film is all that is necessary for definitive evaluation. Similar systolic ejection murmurs from the right ventricular outflow tract are also present in patients having significant left-to-right shunting at the ventricular level. In this situation, one hears both the holosystolic murmur of the ventricular septal defect and the systolic ejection murmur, with the ejection components of the murmur appreciated best at the base.

Prominent systolic ejection murmurs are the rule in patients with significant aortic regurgitation secondary to the large forward stroke volume (Fig. 11-47). Although no significant left ventricular outflow gradient is found in these patients, the intensity of such murmurs may be grade 4 or 5, and occasionally they are associated with a thrill. However, they always end well before aortic closure and are clearly separated from the early regurgitant murmur. Such a murmur is rarely confused with significant valvular obstruction because of the peripheral findings of wide-open aortic regurgitation. When true valvular obstruction is present (mixed stenosis and regurgitation of the aortic valve), the longer systolic ejection murmur is often associated with a prominent thrill. Systolic ejection murmurs due to large right ventricular stroke volume are also seen in severe organic pulmonic valvular regurgitation.

Ventricular ejection into a dilated great vessel is commonly associated with a systolic ejection murmur. In the elderly, such murmurs are due to ejection into a dilated, sclerotic aorta and are often best appreciated at the apex. Frequently, degenerative changes of mild sclerosis of the aortic valve are also present, and the clinician is faced with a difficult decision as to whether true obstruction exists. The presence of significant calcification on fluoroscopic examination favors true obstruction and can be confirmed when a significant gradient is demonstrated by Doppler studies.

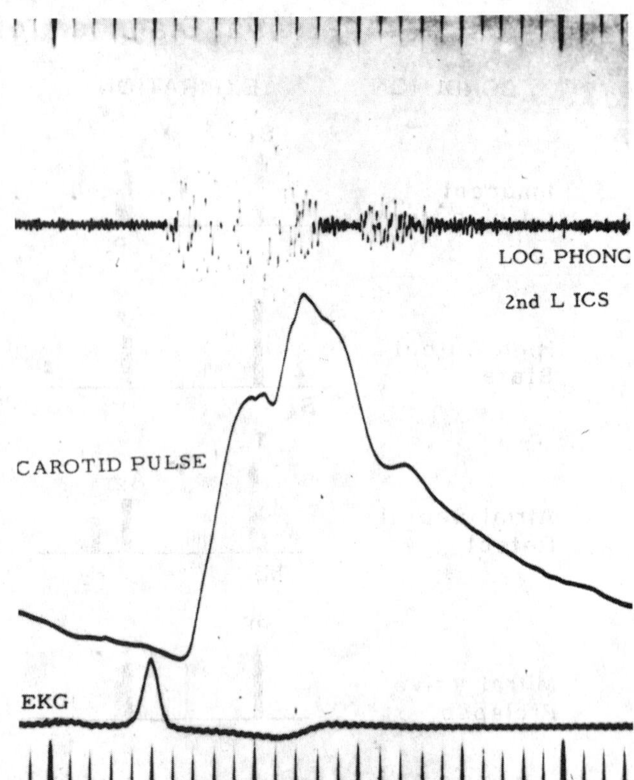

FIGURE 11-47 A systolic ejection murmur is recorded ending well before S_2 in a patient with chronic aortic regurgitation. No valvular gradient was found at cardiac catheterization. The carotid pulse is rapid rising and has a wide pulse pressure. A long decrescendo–early diastolic murmur is recorded throughout diastole. On physical examination, a systolic thrill was associated with a grade 5 systolic murmur. [*From J Shaver: Current uses of phonocardiography in clinical practice. In: E Rapaport (ed): Cardiology Update: Reviews for Physicians. New York, Elsevier, 1981, p 363. Reproduced with permission of the publisher and author. Copyright 1981 by Elsevier Science Publishing Co., Inc.*]

A systolic ejection murmur due to right ventricular ejection into a massively dilated pulmonary artery is present in idiopathic dilation of the pulmonary artery (Fig. 11-25),[66] which is often confused with an atrial septal defect due to the wide auditory expiratory splitting present in this condition. Also, the prominent pulmonary ejection sound may be confused with a loud tricuspid closure sound of a patient having an atrial septal defect. Careful clinical examination may not allow differentiation of these two conditions; however, the standard posterior-anterior and lateral chest x-ray will not show evidence of increased pulmonary flow, and the echocardiogram will easily demonstrate the large hyperdynamic right ventricle of the atrial septal defect not seen with isolated pulmonary artery dilation. Short systolic ejection murmurs frequently associated with a prominent late pulmonary ejection sound are also seen in dilated pulmonary arteries secondary to severe pulmonary hypertension of any cause.[66] They are identified by "the company they keep." Physical findings of severe pulmonary hypertension are always present, including a prominent parasternal impulse and increased intensity of the pulmonic component of S_2, which is well heard at the apex. Prominent *a* waves in the neck and the presence of a right-sided S_4 that increases with inspiration are present if the ventricular septum is intact (Fig. 11-35). If the pulmonary hypertension is associated with intracardiac shunting, cyanosis is frequently present. A high-pitched, early diastolic murmur of pulmonic regurgitation secondary to severe pulmonary hypertension is often present.

Left Ventricular Outflow Tract Murmurs Obstruction to left ventricular outflow may be congenital or acquired and may be located at the valvular, supravalvular, or subvalvular level. Stenosis is occasionally present at more than one level. In the clinical evaluation, one should attempt to define the severity and the level of obstruction. However, it is not the purpose of this chapter to give an exhaustive differential diagnosis of the various forms of left ventricular outflow obstruction; the reader is referred to three excellent articles reviewing this subject in detail.[229–231] For completeness, however, a summary of this differential diagnosis can be found in Table 11-6.

The murmur of fixed stenosis of the left ventricular outflow tract, regardless of the site, is crescendo-decrescendo, and its contour closely parallels the instantaneous pressure gradient (Fig. 11-44). As long as cardiac output is maintained, there is an excellent correlation between the intensity and length of the murmur with severity of obstruction, as shown in Figs. 11-11 and 11-44. Although there is a tendency toward late peaking of the murmur with increasing severity of the obstruction, this delayed peaking has not been found to correlate as well with the severity of valvular obstruction in aortic stenosis as it has in pulmonic stenosis.[232] The murmur of significant fixed left ventricular outflow tract obstruction is usually best heard at the second right and second and third left interspaces near the sternum. It radiates widely into the neck and along the great vessels. With radiation to the apex, particularly in the elderly patient, the high-frequency components of the murmur predominate and the apical murmur has a high pitch and often a musical quality (Figs. 11-36, 11-44).[208] This characteristic change in the pitch between the proximal and distal radiation of the murmur is a repeated source of confusion on

TABLE 11-6

Differential Diagnosis of Left Ventricular Outflow Obstruction

	Congenital Aortic Stenosis				
Parameter	Valvular	Subvalvular	Supravalvular	Acquired Aortic Stenosis	Hypertrophic "Obstructive" Cardiomyopathy
Physical appearance	Normal	Normal	Characteristic facies	Normal	Normal
Arterial pulse	Slow rise, sustained peak	Slow rise, sustained peak	Right brachial and carotid > left	Slow rise, sustained peak	Brisk rise, unsustained double peak
S_4 presystolic impulse	Yes	Yes	Yes	Yes	Yes
Left ventricular systolic impulse	Sustained, single	Sustained, single	Sustained, single	Sustained, single	Sustained, may be double
Aortic ejection sound	Typical ↓ with calcif.	Rare	Rare	Common ↓ with calcif.	Rare exception
Midsystolic ejection murmur; maximal site	First or second right interspace	First or second right interspace	First right interspace and over right carotid	First or second right interspace; apex in elderly	Apex, lower left sternal edge
Second sound splitting	Usually normal or single	Usually normal or single	Usually normal or single	Usually single or reversed	Usually reversed or single
Intensity of aortic closure	Normal or increased ↓ with calcif.	Normal or decreased	Normal or decreased	Decreased or absent with calcif.	Normal
Murmur of aortic regurgitation	Common	Common	Uncommon	Common	Rare exception

Calcif. = calcification.

SOURCE: Modified from Reddy PS, et al: Cardiac systolic murmurs; pathophysiology and differential diagnosis. *Prog Cardiovasc Dis* 1971; 14:6. Reproduced with permission of the publisher and authors.

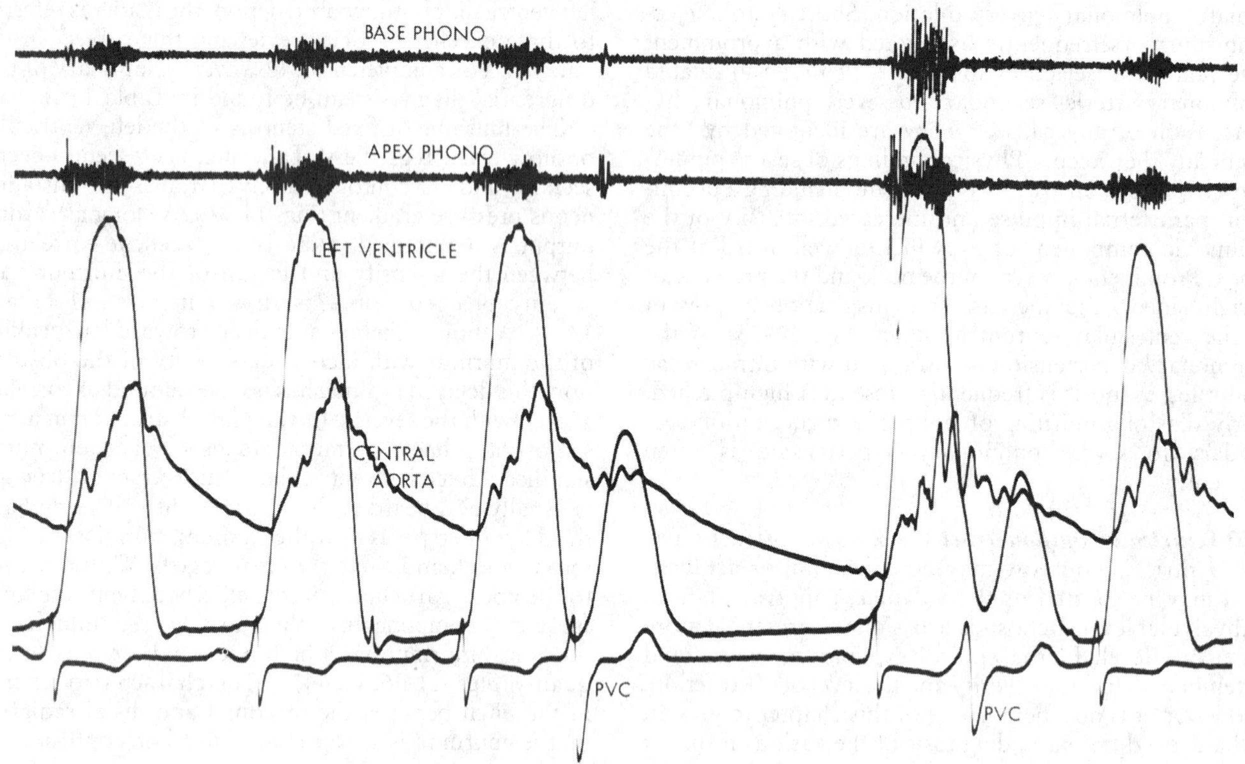

FIGURE 11-48 Effect of the long diastolic filling period following a premature ventricular contraction (PVC) on the intensity of the systolic ejection murmur (SEM) in the same patient as in Fig. 11-44. There is a marked increase in the intensity of the aortic stenosis murmur recorded at the base and at the apex. In spite of the higher frequency content of the apical murmur, this response clearly identifies this murmur as ejection in nature. [*From H Paley: Left ventricular outflow tract obstruction: Heart sounds and murmurs. In: DF Leon, JA Shaver (eds): Physiologic Principles of Heart Sounds and Murmurs, Monograph 46. Dallas, American Heart Association, 1975, p 112. Reproduced with permission from the publisher and the author.*]

auscultation. There is an almost overpowering urge to call it a separate murmur of mitral regurgitation; however, observations repeatedly demonstrate that this murmur, regardless of its timbre or harmonics, retains a diamond-shaped configuration whenever it is heard or recorded. Of help in confirming the ejection nature of such a high-pitched murmur is the relationship between the intensity of the systolic murmur and the length of preceding diastole as described by Henke and associates.[233] They noted that the murmur of aortic stenosis varied directly with the length of the preceding diastole; the longer the preceding ventricular filling period, the louder the systolic murmur (Fig. 11-48). In contrast, the apical murmur of mitral regurgitation is associated with little or no variation in intensity with varying cycle lengths. This observation is useful in patients with atrial fibrillation or frequent premature contractions and serves to identify whether an apical murmur is due to radiation of an ejection murmur or is an additional regurgitant murmur of mitral regurgitation. Beat-to-beat variations in the intensity of the murmur of aortic stenosis have been noted in both pulsus alternans[234] and AV dissociation,[235] again demonstrating the intimate relationship between beat-to-beat changes in stroke volume and the intensity of the systolic ejection murmur.

A loud early systolic valvular ejection sound or click is the hallmark of congenital valvular aortic stenosis, and its presence defines the obstruction at the valvular level (Fig. 11-12).[236] As discussed earlier in this chapter, its intensity correlates well with the motility of the valve, and there is no correlation with the severity of the obstruction. As shown in Fig. 11-11, it disappears when the valve becomes immobile due to calcific fixation and is absent in fixed subaortic stenosis (Fig. 11-13). With progressive increase in the severity of the outflow obstruction, the duration of left ventricular ejection is prolonged,[237,238] resulting in narrow, single, or reversed splitting of S_2. Reversed splitting of S_2 in aortic stenosis, in the absence of LBBB, is always associated with severe obstruction. (See also Chap. 79.)

Regardless of the site of obstruction, significant stenosis always results in left ventricular hypertrophy, with a decreased diastolic compliance. Clinically, this manifests as a presystolic apical pulsation on palpation and as an S_4 on auscultation (Fig. 11-36). In patients above age 12, the S_4 is generally associated with a left ventricular diastolic pressure above 11 mmHg and a left atrial *a*-wave peak of about 13 mmHg.[189] The relationship between the severity of obstruction and the presence of S_4 gallops is an indirect one, reflecting hypertrophy and decreased compliance of the left ventricle rather than obstruction per se. Because of the frequent coexistence of hypertensive or arteriosclerotic heart disease in the elderly patient with calcific aortic stenosis, the presence of an S_4 may be nonspecific and correlate poorly with the severity of obstruction.[190] The

S_3 gallops may also be heard in left ventricular outflow tract obstruction, particularly when decompensation occurs (Fig. 11-36).

The diagnosis of hemodynamically significant aortic stenosis in the elderly presents a particularly difficult problem.[239] The murmur is often of low intensity due to the decreased cardiac output and poor left ventricular function. An ejection sound or click is rarely present, due to calcific fixation of the valve leaflets, and S_2 is of low amplitude. The murmur is often loudest at the apex, has a high-frequency content, and may be difficult to define as ejection in nature because S_1 and A_2 may be poorly heard and therefore lost as landmarks defining the onset and end of mechanical systole. In most patients with severe aortic stenosis, no A_2 is heard and the murmur obliterates P_2. In the elderly the rate of rise of the carotid pulse may be nearly normal due to the hard, sclerotic vessels even with severe obstruction. As shown in Fig. 11-48, the response of the murmur following a premature ventricular contraction (PVC) may be very helpful in confirming the ejection nature of the murmur. Differentiation from the benign murmur of mild aortic sclerosis may be difficult and often necessitates confirmation of obstruction by echo-Doppler examination.[240] (See also Chap. 130.)

Right Ventricular Outflow Tract Obstruction Obstructions to right ventricular outflow are congenital anomalies and may be at the level of the valve, infundibulum, and proximal or distal branches of the pulmonary artery. Isolated infundibular pulmonic stenosis with an intact septum is rare and is usually associated with a large ventricular septal defect (tetralogy of Fallot). When the ventricular septum is intact, there is an excellent correlation between both the intensity and duration of the murmur and the severity of obstruction.[64,241] In Fig. 11-49, the auscultatory findings of progressively more severe valvular pulmonic stenosis with intact ventricular septum are contrasted with those found in tetralogy of Fallot with progressively more severe right ventricular outflow obstruction.[242,243] As with valvular aortic stenosis, an early systolic ejection sound defines the level of obstruction at the valve. In mild to moderate valvular obstruction, the intensity of this sound is markedly attenuated or may disappear with inspiration (Fig. 11-14).[62] In more severe valvular obstruction, this sound may fuse with S_1 or may actually present as a presystolic click when the pressure generated by a forceful right atrial contraction exceeds right ventricular end-diastolic pressure, causing doming of the stenotic valve in late diastole. Although obstruction to right ventricular outflow in tetralogy of Fallot is usually at the infundibular level, valvular stenosis may also be present. In this setting a pulmonary valvular ejection sound introduces a systolic murmur, and little variation in the intensity of the ejection sound is found with respiration.[244] (See also Chap. 97.)

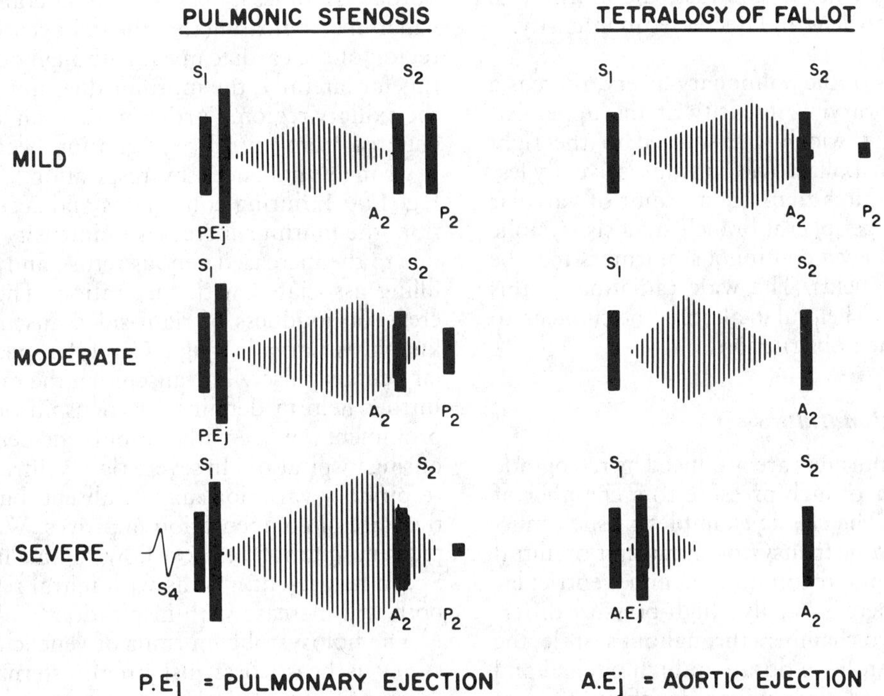

FIGURE 11-49 In valvular pulmonic stenosis with intact ventricular septum, right ventricular systolic ejection becomes progressively longer with increasing obstruction to flow. As a result, the murmur becomes louder and longer, enveloping the aortic closure sound. At the same time, pulmonic closure occurs later; splitting becomes wider but is more difficult to appreciate because the aortic closure sound is lost in the murmur, and the pulmonic closure sound becomes progressively softer due to the low pulmonary artery pressure. With increasing severity of pulmonic stenosis, the pulmonary ejection sound may fuse with S_1. In severe obstruction with concentric hypertrophy and decreased right ventricular compliance, an S_4 appears. In tetralogy of Fallot with increasing obstruction at the infundibular area, more and more right ventricular blood is shunted across a silent ventricular septal defect with less flow across the obstructed right ventricular outflow tract. With increasing obstruction, the murmur becomes shorter, earlier, and fainter. The pulmonic closure sound is absent in severe tetralogy of Fallot. The dilated aorta receives almost all of the cardiac output from both ventricular chambers, and there is an aortic ejection sound (AEj). (*From J Leonard et al: Examination of the heart series. Part four: Auscultation. Dallas, American Heart Association, 1974, p 45. Reproduced with permission from the publisher and the authors.*)

The classic late peaking of the systolic ejection murmur of severe pulmonic stenosis with intact ventricular septum is demonstrated in Fig. 11-23. Note that the late vibrations of the murmur completely envelop A_2, while P_2 is markedly delayed and decreases in intensity secondary to the low pulmonary artery closing pressure. In moderate to severe valvular pulmonic stenosis, an excellent correlation has been found between the A_2-P_2 interval and the right ventricular peak pressure.[64] When the ventricular septum is intact in severe right ventricular outflow obstruction, prominent *a* waves are present in the jugular venous pulse, in association with a right-sided S_4 that increases with inspiration. Neither of these findings is present in uncomplicated tetralogy of Fallot. Occasionally, in very severe pulmonic stenosis, a low-pitched, presystolic murmur may be present due to forward flow across the stenotic valve that has been prematurely opened by forceful right atrial contraction in late diastole.[64] Such patients are often cyanotic due to right-to-left shunting through a patent foramen ovale.

In isolated infundibular obstruction, a pulmonic ejection sound is usually not encountered[245] and the pulmonic closure (P_2) is usually not audible except in the mildest cases. The site of maximal intensity of the murmur is of little help in differentiating the site of obstruction. Both valvular pulmonic stenosis and isolated infundibular pulmonic stenosis with intact septum can be differentiated from tetralogy of Fallot by noting the marked intensification of the ejection murmur after the inhalation of amyl nitrite. In contrast, the murmur of tetralogy of Fallot shortens and decreases in intensity.[246] (See also Chap. 97.)

In branch stenosis of the pulmonary artery, there is a systolic murmur of varying intensity at the upper left sternal border that is widely transmitted to the right chest, back, and both axillae. The murmur is usually less harsh and of higher pitch than the murmur of valvular stenosis. With more peripheral branch stenosis, systolic ejection murmurs or even continuous murmurs may be heard over the lung fields. The wide radiation of this murmur is particularly helpful in alerting the clinician to this type of right-sided obstruction.

Systolic Regurgitant Murmurs

Systolic regurgitant murmurs are produced by retrograde flow from a chamber of high pressure to a chamber of lower pressure.[204,247] The classic examples of such murmurs are the holosystolic (pansystolic) murmur of mitral regurgitation, tricuspid regurgitation, and ventricular septal defect. Since there is usually a high-pressure differential between the two chambers throughout systole, the murmurs are holosystolic in duration, high pitched and blowing in quality, and plateaulike in configuration.

Holosystolic Regurgitant Murmurs The murmur of chronic mitral regurgitation is the prototype of the holosystolic regurgitant murmur, as shown in Figs. 11-42 and 11-50. It begins with or replaces S_1 and continues throughout systole in a plateaulike fashion beyond A_2, finally terminating when the left ventricular pressure drops to the level of the left atrial pressure during isovolumic relaxation.[152,248,249] In contrast to the systolic ejection murmur, there is little variation in its intensity with varying cycle lengths (Fig. 11-50).[250] It is heard best at the apex and radiates well into the axilla; only the loudest murmurs are associated with a thrill at the apex. There is little variation in its intensity with respiration, and it is frequently accompanied by a loud diastolic filling sound followed by a short rumble.[251] In this situation, the loud S_3 is not a manifestation of congestive failure but a reflection of hemodynamically significant mitral regurgitation. Likewise, the short rumble does not mean concomitant obstruction at the mitral valve but rather is secondary to extremely rapid early diastolic filling. As shown in Fig. 11-51, the intensity of the murmur is directly related to the pressure gradient between the left ventricle and the left atrium. With amyl nitrite, there is a dramatic decrease in the left ventricular–left atrial gradient and in the intensity of the murmur. The opposite response is seen with vasoconstrictive agents that increase the left ventricular–left atrial pressure gradient.

It should be emphasized that the diagnosis of hemodynamically significant mitral regurgitation is established by the presence of the holosystolic regurgitant murmur and loud S_3 associated with a short flow rumble. However, the etiology is determined by the clinical presentation and associated physical findings and is best confirmed by echocardiography.[252]

The classic holosystolic (pansystolic) murmur of tricuspid regurgitation in the setting of right ventricular pressure overload is best heard at the lower left sternal border.[2] At times it may be heard laterally to the midclavicular line, indicating that the right ventricle occupies the region of the cardiac apex. Although occasionally heard this far laterally, the murmur does not radiate well into the axillary region. Furthermore, it can usually be differentiated from mitral regurgitation because its intensity is strongly influenced by respiration.[253,254] As shown in Fig. 11-52, during continuous and accentuated respiration, the murmur increases in intensity with inspiration due to the increased venous return and right ventricular filling associated with inspiration. The inspiratory increase in loudness of right-sided auscultatory events is known as Carvallo's sign. Careful inspection of the jugular venous pulse while ausculting the murmur will be of further help in defining its tricuspid origin, showing a prominent *v* wave with a rapid *y* descent that augments during inspiration. In severe right ventricular failure, this respiratory variation may be absent, but it reappears as the state of compensation improves. With severe tricuspid regurgitation, a short flow rumble introduced by an S_3 can be present, just as with mitral regurgitation, and both will increase with inspiration.[255]

The holosystolic murmur of ventricular septal defect (VSD) is heard best just off the sternal border in the fourth, fifth, and sixth intercostal spaces and is usually accompanied by a forceful thrill.[256,257] The murmur does not radiate to the axilla as with mitral regurgitation and does not have the respiratory variation characteristic of tricuspid regurgitation. Wide physiologic splitting with an easily heard P_2 is usually present when the left-to-right shunt is hemodynamically significant. When the shunt is large, there is a left ventricular S_3 followed by a short flow rumble. The regurgitant murmur is due to high-velocity flow from the high-pressure left ventricle

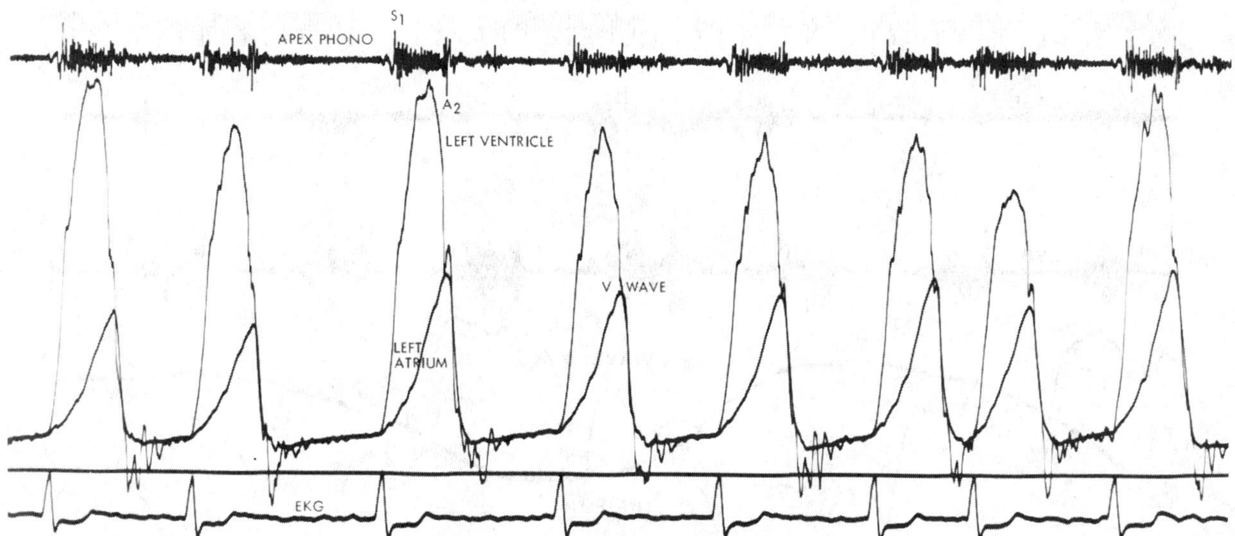

FIGURE 11-50 The apex phonocardiogram is recorded simultaneously with the left ventricular (LV) and left atrial (LA) pressures in a patient with chronic mitral regurgitation. The murmur is plateaulike in character, spilling through A_2 and having minimal variation in intensity with the varying cycle lengths of atrial fibrillation. This is in marked contrast to the post-PVC response of valvular aortic stenosis as shown in Fig. 11-48. [*From H Paley: Left ventricular outflow tract obstruction: Heart sounds and murmurs. In: DF Leon, JA Shaver (eds): Physiologic Principles of Heart Sounds and Murmurs, Monograph 46. Dallas, American Heart Association, 1975, p 112. Reproduced with permission from the publisher and the authors.*]

to the lower pressure right ventricle, and its intensity correlates poorly with the degree of left-to-right shunting. For example, a grade 5 murmur may be associated with a very high velocity flow through a small hemodynamically insignificant muscular VSD (Roger).[258] On the other hand, an equally loud murmur associated with a thrill may be present with a larger defect having massive left-to-right shunting. However, when the defect is very large and the right and left ventricular pressures are equal, no murmur may be produced across the defect; instead, the short pulmonary ejection murmur of severe pulmonary hypertension is present (Eisenmenger's VSD).[259] As shown in Fig. 11-53, the murmur of ventricular septal defect is very sensitive to vasoactive agents that alter vascular impedance, and a marked decrease in both the left ventricular–right ventricular pressure gradient and the intensity of the murmur are seen following the administration of amyl nitrite.

Early Systolic Regurgitant Murmurs Rarely, a regurgitant murmur confined to early systole is seen in the presence of a small ventricular septal defect. This murmur begins in the usual manner at the onset of ventricular systole and stops suddenly in early or midsystole.[260,261] The sudden cessation of the murmur is due to the fact that as ejection continues and ventricular size decreases,

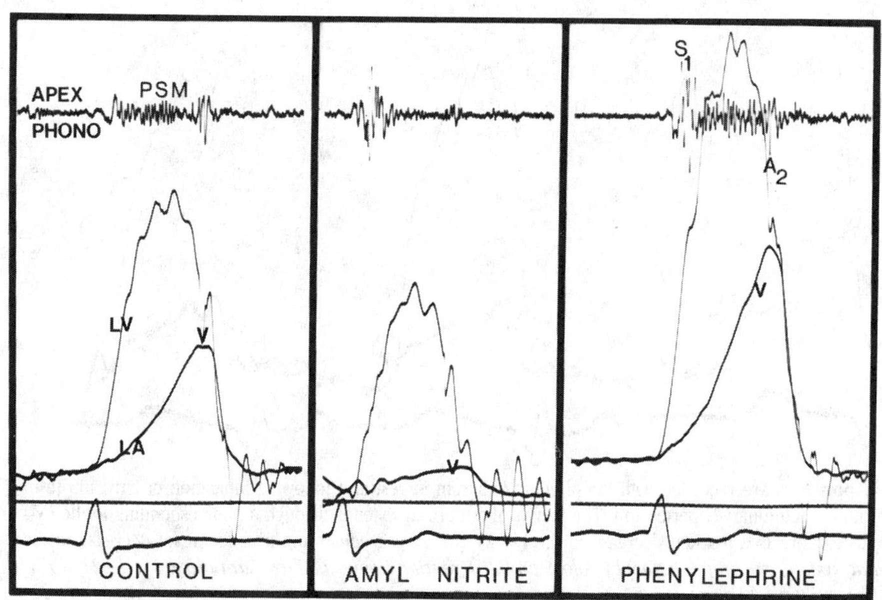

FIGURE 11-51 Simultaneous apex phonocardiogram. Left atrial (LA) and left ventricular (LV) pressures are recorded during the control state, the inhalation of amyl nitrite, and phenylephrine infusion in a patient with longstanding mitral regurgitation. During control observation, a significant LV–LA pressure gradient was associated with a pansystolic murmur (PSM) recorded at the apex. After inhalation of amyl nitrite, the peak LV pressure, the height of the *v* wave, and the LV–LA pressure gradient are decreased. Associated with this is a marked diminution in the intensity of the pansystolic murmur. In contrast, after the infusion of phenylephrine, all three pressure parameters as well as the intensity of the murmur are increased. [*From J Shaver: The physical examination in cardiac diagnosis. Cardiol Consult 6(3):8, 1985. Reproduced with permission of the publisher and the author.*]

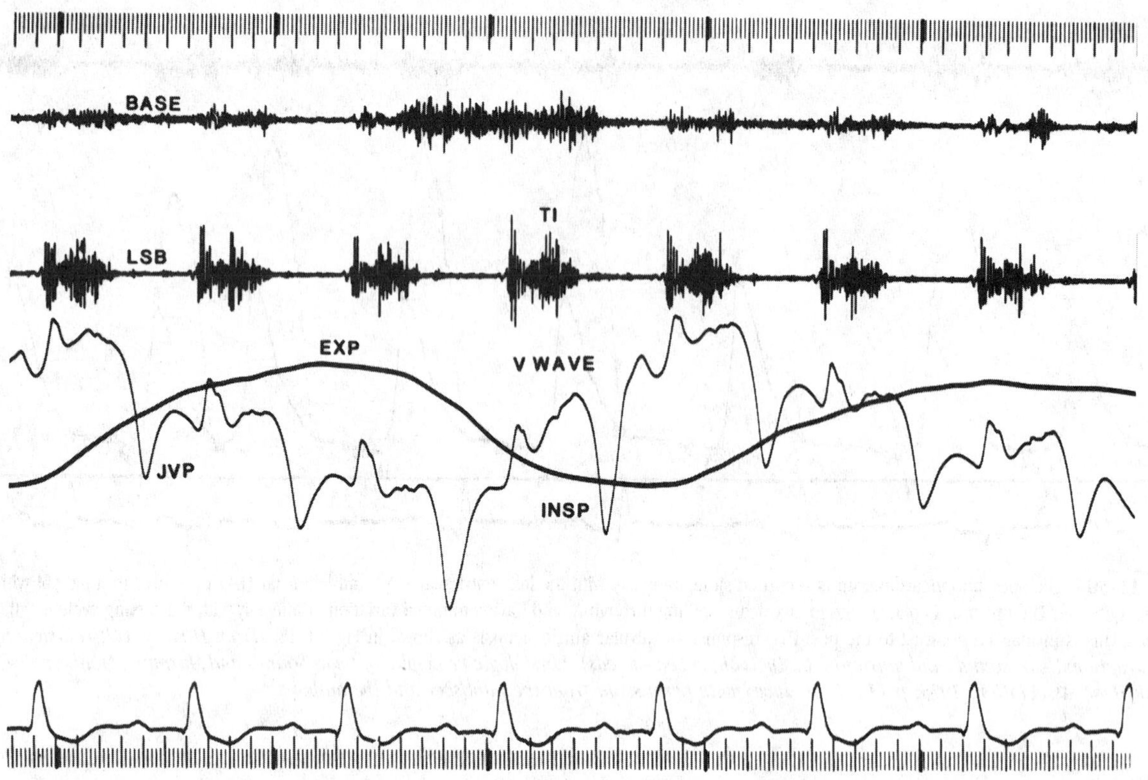

FIGURE 11-52 Phonocardiograms at the base and left sternal border (LSB) are recorded with the jugular venous pulse during exaggerated respiration in a patient with cor pulmonale. Augmentation of the pansystolic murmur at the left sternal border confirms its tricuspid origin. The jugular venous pulse shows prominent *v* waves having an increased pulse pressure and *y* descent during inspiration, characteristic of tricuspid regurgitation. [*From R Salerni, et al: Noninvasive graphic evaluation: Phonocardiography and echocardiography. In: WS Frankl, AN Brest (eds): Cardiovascular Clinics: Valvular Heart Disease—Comprehensive Evaluation and Management. Philadelphia: FA Davis, 1986, p 201. Reproduced with permission of the publisher and the authors.*]

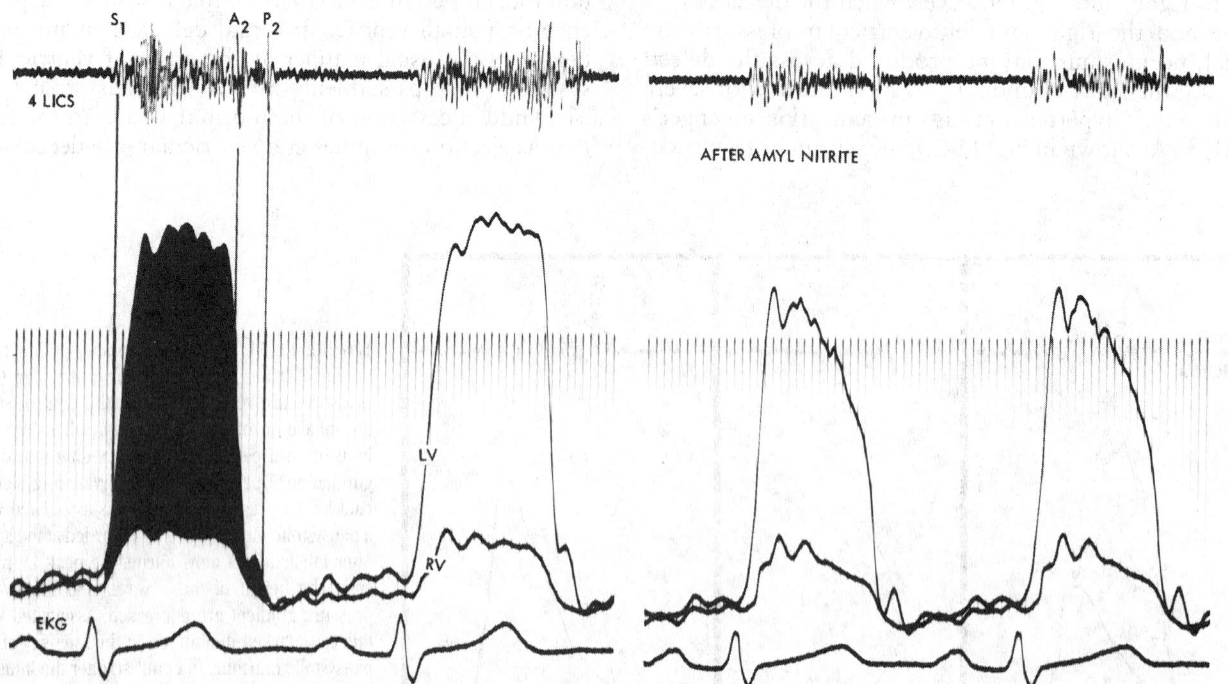

FIGURE 11-53 Right (RV) and left ventricular (LV) pressures are recorded with the phonocardiogram at rest and following inhalation of amyl nitrite in a 26-year-old woman with a ventricular septal defect without pulmonary hypertension. The pansystolic murmur extends through A_2, corresponding to the LV–RV pressure gradient. Following inhalation of amyl nitrite, there is a marked decrease in the LV–RV pressure gradient and a concomitant decrease in the intensity of the murmur. (*From PS Reddy, et al: Cardiac systolic murmurs; pathophysiology and differential diagnosis. Prog Cardiovasc Dis 14:21, 1971. Reproduced with permission of the publisher and the authors.*)

the small defect is sealed shut as the ventricular septum thickens during systole and the flow ceases. This murmur is important because it is characteristic of the type of ventricular septal defect that may disappear with age.

In contrast to the holosystolic murmur of chronic mitral regurgitation, acute severe mitral regurgitation may present as an early systolic murmur.[262–264] Common conditions producing acute mitral regurgitation include spontaneous rupture of the chordae tendineae of a myxomatous valve, acute or subacute bacterial endocarditis of the mitral valve, papillary muscle rupture or dysfunction secondary to acute myocardial infarction, and disruption of the mitral apparatus due to chest trauma.[265–268] In each of these conditions, large-volume flow regurgitates into a relatively normal left atrium that has not had the time to make the adaptive changes in compliance seen in chronic longstanding mitral regurgitation. As a result, an extremely high *v* wave is generated in the left atrium. This high *v* wave abolishes the left ventricular–left atrial gradient during the latter part of systole, resulting in termination of retrograde flow and abbreviation of the systolic murmur. As shown in Fig. 11-3, in a patient with acute mitral regurgitation secondary to spontaneous rupture of the chordae tendineae of a myxomatous valve, the murmur ends before A_2. Audible expiratory splitting with an accentuated P_2 is present at the base, and a loud S_4 is recorded at the apex. The presence of the S_4 associated with a prominent presystolic impulse on palpation is an important clue that indicates the acute nature of the mitral regurgitation and is rarely present in mitral regurgitation of a chronic nature.[191] The systolic murmur of acute mitral regurgitation may have classic radiation to the axilla and back, especially if it is due to prolapse of the anterior leaflet of the valve with flow directed over the posterior leaflet. When the murmur is loud, it may be conducted to the top of the head and to the sacrum along the spinal column. Occasionally, the murmur is conducted to the base of the heart and great vessels, simulating aortic stenosis.[269] The quick-rising carotid pulse with rapid falloff as well as the wide physiologic splitting of the second heart sound will readily allow differentiation from aortic stenosis.[270] (See also Chap. 80.)

The systolic murmur of organic tricuspid regurgitation is often unimpressive and presents as an early systolic murmur ending well before A_2, even in the presence of severe regurgitation.[271] In this condition, the right ventricular pressure is nearly normal, and massive regurgitation may be present with only a small pressure differential between the right ventricle and the right atrium (Fig. 11-54). The small pressure head results in a low-velocity flow, minimal turbulence, and a soft, abbreviated murmur. Occasionally, only minimal early systolic vibrations are heard, as demonstrated in Fig. 11-54. In most patients, large *v* waves are readily apparent in the jugular venous pulse (see also Chap. 10). The murmur retains the characteristic inspiratory augmentation seen in right-sided regurgitant murmurs and is frequently associated with an S_4 that increases in intensity with inspiration. A right-sided S_4 together with a prominent diastolic tricuspid flow rumble are the rule when the tricuspid regurgitation is acute, as in endocarditis of the tricuspid valve. After total excision of the tricuspid valve for infective endocarditis related to intravenous drug

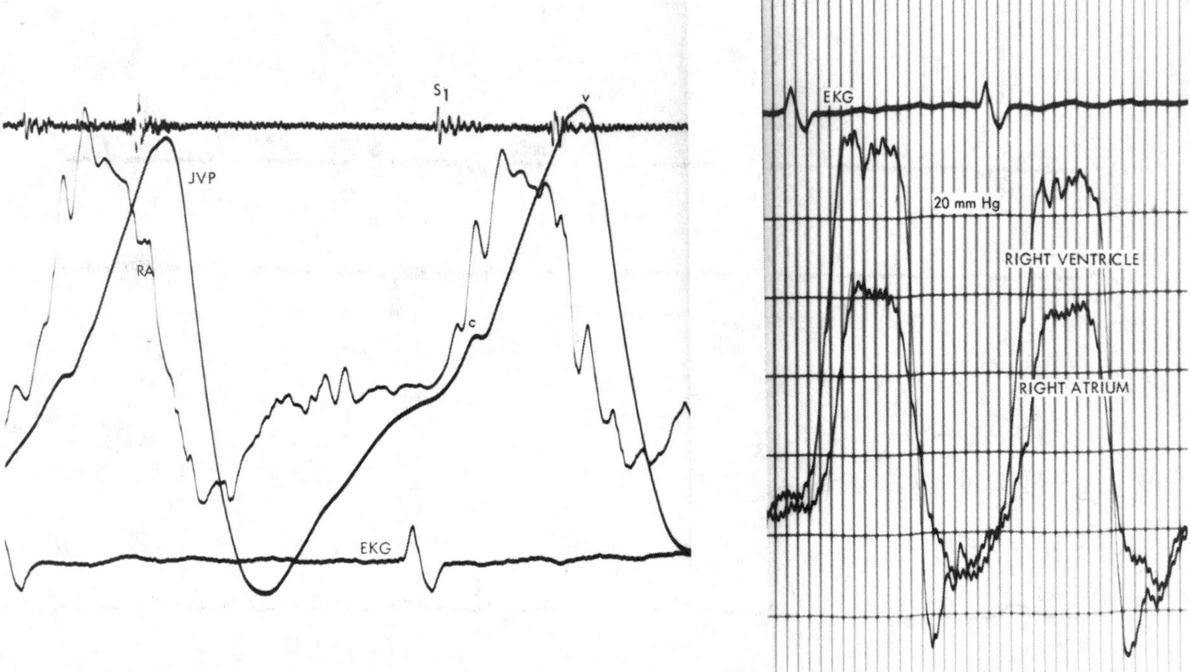

FIGURE 11-54 The phonocardiogram is recorded simultaneously with the jugular venous pulse and right atrial pressure in a patient with severe organic tricuspid regurgitation. Only minimal early systolic vibrations are recorded on the phonocardiogram, and a huge CV wave is present on the jugular venous pulse. In the right panel, simultaneous right ventricular and right atrial pressures are shown, demonstrating ventricularization of the right atrial pressure. There is a minimal pressure gradient across the tricuspid valve, resulting in low-velocity retrograde flow and absence of a significant murmur.

abuse, the systolic murmur is often very unimpressive or may be completely absent. Giant *v* waves in the neck are easily visible, however, and palpable venous thrills and a murmur at the base of the neck may be present secondary to rapid retrograde flow in the jugular system.[272] Other causes of organic tricuspid regurgitation include carcinoid heart disease, right ventricular infarction, chest trauma, and damage of the tricuspid valve during open heart surgery. (See also Chap. 81.)

Mid- and Late Systolic Regurgitant Murmurs Midsystolic murmurs can occur with mitral regurgitation due to papillary muscle dysfunction as originally described by Burch et al.[273] The timing of the murmur of papillary muscle dysfunction may also be late systolic and may be intermittent or constant. It occurs with ischemia or infarction of either the posterior medial or anterior lateral papillary muscle. Often these murmurs are transient, being provoked by episodes of ischemia.

Varying degrees of mitral valve prolapse are the most frequent cause of a late systolic murmur, and this entity is one of the most common causes of systolic murmurs seen in clinical practice. The murmur is best heard at the apex and often has a tendency to a late systolic crescendo. It is frequently introduced or accompanied by nonejection clicks. These clicks may be single or multiple, and they can occur independently without an accompanying systolic murmur (Fig. 11-15). As shown in Fig. 11-16, the click occurs near the time of maximal prolapse in midsystole, and the late systolic murmur continues up to and through A_2 due to prolapse of the posterior leaflet during the remainder of systole. In the past, the late systolic murmurs and mid- and late systolic clicks were considered to be innocent and thought to be extracardiac in origin—that is, pleural or pericardial.[274,275] Subsequent studies with intracardiac phonocardiography have localized these acoustic events to the mitral valve and subvalvular structures,[72,73] while left ventricular cineangiograms have demonstrated late systolic mitral regurgitation with billowing or prolapse of one or both leaflets into the left atrium.[70,71,276]

The timing and intensity of these murmurs vary with physiologic and pharmacologic maneuvers that alter the end-diastolic volume of the heart (Figs. 11-17 and 80-16). These murmurs are also sensitive to conditions that alter the peripheral vascular impedance as well as the inotropic state of the heart.[81] These variations in the timing and duration of the murmur can be most easily understood by considering mitral valve prolapse as a condition in which the valve is too big for the ventricle. This valvuloventricular disproportion manifests itself at a given geometric size and configuration during left ventricular contraction. Situations that decrease the end-diastolic volume of the heart, decrease peripheral vascular impedance, or increase the inotropic state allow the heart to reach this critical geometry sooner, resulting in an earlier onset of the click and a longer murmur. Increase in the size of the heart and peripheral vascular impedance and a decrease in the inotropic state will result in the opposite changes, with the click moving toward S_2 and the murmur becoming shorter. (See also Chap. 80.) These dynamic changes can best be appreciated at the bedside by examining the patient in the supine, left lateral, sitting, and standing positions as well as during prompt squatting. The effect of decreased venous return associated with the assumption of the upright posture is shown in Fig. 11-55 in a patient without a murmur in the supine position and emphasizes the importance of

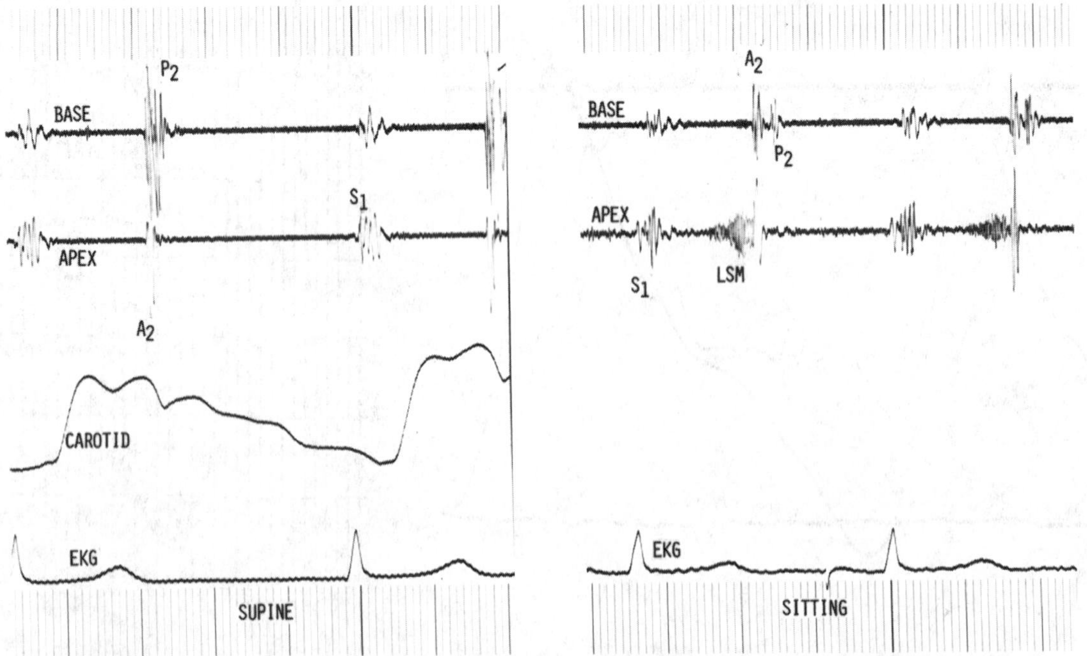

FIGURE 11-55 Base and apex phonocardiograms are recorded in the supine and sitting positions in a patient with late mitral valve prolapse. Note the absence of a late systolic murmur in the supine position. Upon assuming the sitting posture, a late systolic murmur is produced secondary to the decreased venous return. A nonejection click is not present in this patient. [*From RO Brandenburg, et al (eds): Cardiology. Fundamentals and Practice. Chicago: Year Book Medical Publishers, 1987, p 256. Reproduced with permission from the publisher and the authors.*]

examining the patient suspected of mitral valve prolapse in more than one posture. The inhalation of amyl nitrite is also very helpful at the bedside; the decreased end-diastolic volume of the ventricle secondary to the reflex tachycardia, coupled with the marked decrease in peripheral vascular impedance, causes the murmur to become earlier, longer, louder, and at times holosystolic. The click also migrates toward S_1. Late systolic murmurs may also originate from prolapse of the tricuspid valve.[255] (See also Chap. 80.)

Levine and Harvey[5] described a musical, apical systolic murmur that they called a "whoop" because it simulated the "whoop" of whooping cough. Rackley and associates[277] called a similar sound a "precordial honk" because it suggested to them the honking noise of a goose. These murmurs are loud, high pitched, musical, sonorous, and vibratory; are best heard at the apex in late systole; and are frequently intermittent. They may vary strikingly with respiration, from beat to beat, and from examination to examination. They are often preceded by clicks originally thought to be extracardiac in origin but confirmed by intracardiac phonocardiography to originate in the mitral valve.[73] They are associated with ballooning of the mitral valve or mitral regurgitation (or both),[210] and their unusual quality is secondary to the high-frequency vibrations of the mitral apparatus. The systolic whoop or honk together with late systolic murmurs with or without associated clicks are part of a continuum representing abnormalities of the mitral valve apparatus of varying etiologies. (See also Chap. 80.) Similar honking noises, with or without clicks, may arise from the tricuspid valve and also have been produced by transvenous pacemaker catheters situated across the valve. These murmurs are best auscultated at the fourth left intercostal space and have the typical inspiratory augmentation of tricuspid murmurs.

Murmur of Hypertrophic "Obstructive" Cardiomyopathy The classic cardiac findings of hypertrophic cardiomyopathy (HCM) with a left ventricular outflow gradient are demonstrated in Fig. 11-56, and the echocardiogram on the right gives insight into the mechanism of production of the systolic murmur. Most authorities now agree that systolic anterior motion (SAM) of the mitral apparatus impinges on the massively thickened septum, producing high-velocity flow in mid- and late systole, resulting in a midsystolic ejection murmur usually with its maximal intensity at the left sternal edge.[278] Varying degrees of mitral regurgitation may also be present during systole due to the distorted mitral apparatus. Frequently on auscultation the skilled clinician has difficulty deciding whether the systolic murmur found in HCM is ejection or regurgitant in nature.[279] The explanation for this confusion is readily understood by analysis of the intracardiac sound and pressure recordings shown in Fig. 11-57. A typical systolic ejection murmur is recorded from the catheter-tipped micromanometer in the left ventricular outflow tract, while a late systolic murmur of mitral regurgitation is recorded from the transseptal left atrial micromanometer. The onset of this latter murmur begins shortly after contact of the anterior mitral leaflet with the septum (SSC), as timed by simultaneous M-mode echocardiography of the mitral valve. Thus, the resulting external murmur recorded by the precordial phonocardiogram is the summation of both murmurs as transmitted to the chest wall.[61,280,281]

In patients with dynamic left ventricular outflow gradients, the intensity of both the systolic ejection murmur

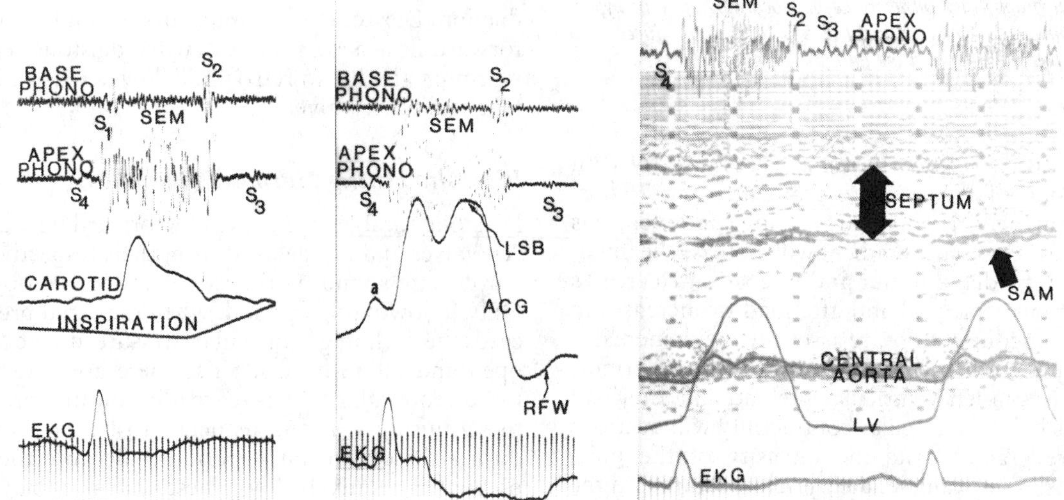

FIGURE 11-56 Simultaneous base and apex phonocardiograms are recorded with the carotid pulse and ACG in the left and center panels respectively in a 54-year-old man with hypertrophic cardiomyopathy. The carotid pulse rises rapidly and has a late systolic plateau and a prolonged ejection period. Prominent S_4 and S_3 are demonstrated and are associated with the *a* wave and the rapid filling wave (RFW), respectively, of the ACG. Note the late systolic bulge (LSB) on the ACG. S_2 is single. A loud grade 5 systolic ejection murmur is present and is of greatest intensity at the apex. In the right panel, the apical systolic murmur is recorded together with the M-mode echocardiogram. Simultaneous high-fidelity left ventricular and central aortic pressures are recorded by catheter-tipped micromanometers. Marked thickening of the interventricular septum and SAM of the mitral valve are present on the echocardiogram. A large systolic pressure gradient is demonstrated beginning shortly after the onset of the SAM. (*From JA Shaver, et al: Phonoechocardiography and intracardiac phonocardiography in hypertrophic cardiomyopathy. Postgrad Med J 62:538, 1986. Reproduced with permission of the publisher and the authors.*)

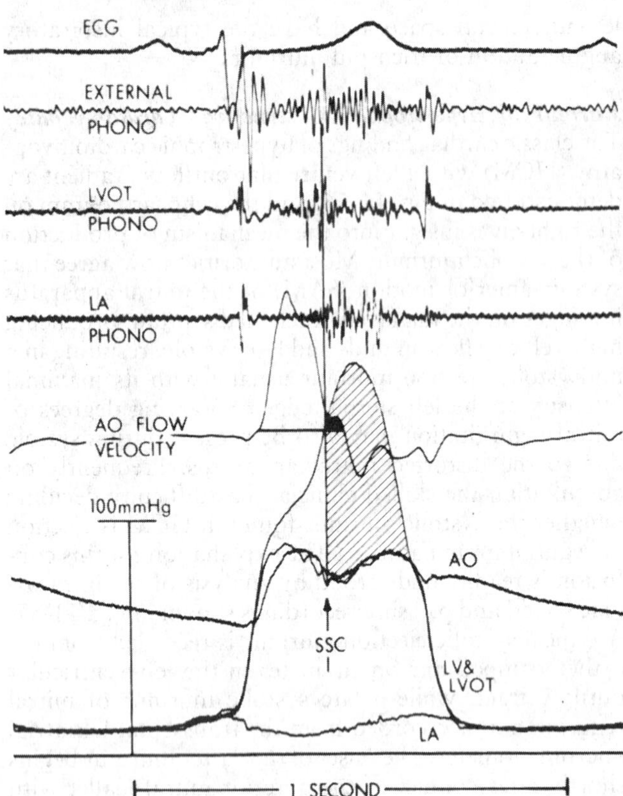

FIGURE 11-57 Catheter-tipped micromanometer pressures are recorded from the left atrium, left ventricle, left ventricular outflow tract (LVOT), and aorta, together with external sound and intracardiac sound recorded from micromanometers in the left atrium and LVOT in a patient with hypertrophic cardiomyopathy. Aortic flow velocity is recorded by a flow probe in the central aorta. The vertical line denotes the time of SAM-septal contact (SSC) as determined by simultaneous M-mode echocardiography of the mitral valve. Note that the majority of aortic flow occurs before SSC. A systolic ejection murmur is recorded from the LVOT, and a late systolic mitral regurgitant murmur is recorded from the left atrium. The external phonocardiogram represents the summation of these two murmurs. (*From JA Shaver, et al: Phonoechocardiography and intracardiac phonocardiography in hypertrophic cardiomyopathy. Postgrad Med J 62:539, 1986. Reproduced with permission of the publisher and the authors.*)

and the mitral regurgitant murmur varies directly with the magnitude of the pressure gradient.[278,279,282] Thus, physiologic maneuvers and pharmacologic interventions that increase the pressure gradient will increase the intensity of the precordial murmur and vice versa. Decreases in left ventricular preload and afterload or increases in left ventricular contractility are associated with increases in the pressure gradient and the intensity of the murmur, while increases in left ventricular preload and afterload or decreases in left ventricular contractility will decrease the pressure gradient and the intensity of the murmur.[61,278,282–284] For example, the upright posture and the strain phase of the Valsalva maneuver decrease venous return and left ventricular preload, and the murmur increases in intensity. Upon reclining or with prompt squatting, augmented venous return increases left ventricular preload and the murmur decreases in intensity. Vasoactive drugs such as amyl nitrite decrease blood pressure, and a marked increase in the intensity of the murmur occurs; whereas vasoconstrictive drugs such as phenylephrine increase the afterload, and the murmur is decreased or abolished (Fig. 11-58).[283] (See also Chap. 90.)

These responses to vasoactive drugs should be compared to the diametrically opposite responses shown in Fig. 11-51 in a patient with a holosystolic murmur of chronic mitral regurgitation. In patients with HCM, inotropic drugs such as digitalis and catecholamines increase the intensity of the murmur while beta blockade usually decreases it. The responses to these interventions are relatively specific for HCM, although occasionally patients with mitral valve prolapse behave similarly.[281] However, the clinical setting of this entity is usually easily differentiated from HCM; when this is not possible, echocardiography provides the definitive diagnosis.

In the absence of a left ventricular outflow gradient at rest or with provocation, the murmur of HCM is less impressive. Although a short ejection murmur is usually recorded due to rapid early left ventricular ejection, it is often softer and extends through less of systole than when a gradient is present (Fig. 11-37).[285] There is also little variation in the intensity with changes in preload, afterload, or contractility.

In HCM with and without a gradient across the left ventricular outflow tract, massive left ventricular hypertrophy is present, and a prominent presystolic impulse associated with a left ventricular S_4 is the rule when normal sinus rhythm is present (Figs. 11-37, 11-56). An S_3 is also a common finding in patients with HCM, and occasionally there is an early diastolic rumble that may mimic the diastolic murmur of mitral stenosis. Such rumbles are felt to be due to the increased impedance to left ventricular filling secondary to the decreased diastolic compliance of the left ventricle.[279] (See also Chap. 90.)

Diastolic Murmurs

Diastolic murmurs have two basic mechanisms of production. Diastolic filling murmurs or rumbles are due to forward flow across the AV, while diastolic regurgitant murmurs are due to retrograde flow across an incompetent semilunar valve.[286]

Diastolic Filling Murmurs (Rumbles)

Diastolic rumbles are caused by forward flow across the AV valves and are delayed from their respective semilunar closure sound by the isovolumic relaxation period. Only following this period, when the atrial pressure exceeds the declining ventricular pressure, do the AV valves open and filling begins. Since there are two phases of rapid ventricular filling—early diastole and presystole—these murmurs have a tendency to be most prominent during these two filling periods.[2] Because the velocity of flow is relatively low, these murmurs have a low-frequency content and are rumbling in character.

Diastolic Rumbles Due to Obstruction of the Atrioventricular Valve The murmur of mitral stenosis is heard best at the apex in the left lateral position, and its duration correlates well with the duration of the mitral diastolic gradient. Its intensity is related to the severity of the obstruction and to the flow across the valve.[287] As a

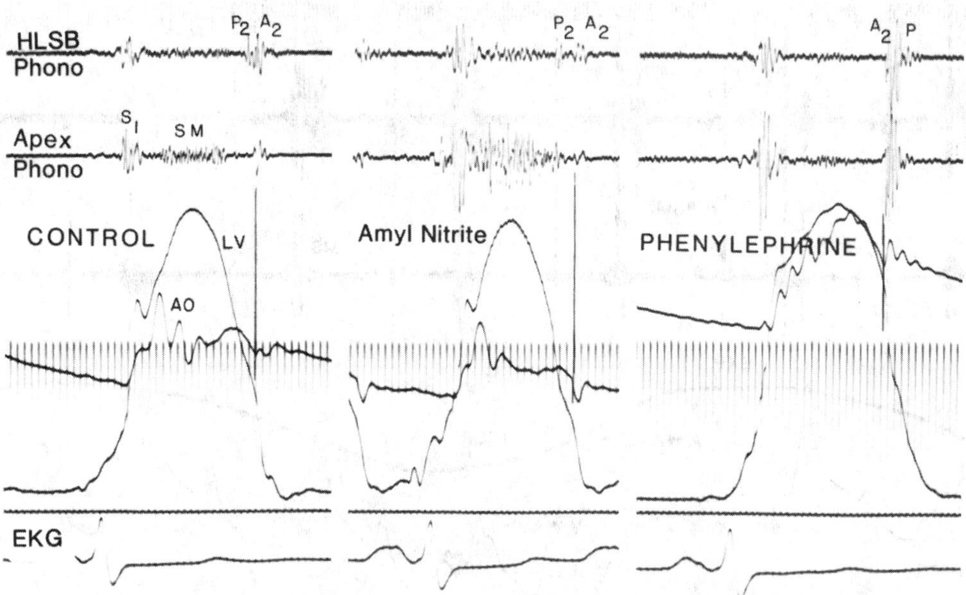

FIGURE 11-58 Simultaneous high left sternal border (HLSB) and apex phonocardiograms are recorded with left ventricular (LV) and central aortic pressure in the control state, following inhalation of amyl nitrite and the intravenous administration of phenylephrine in an 18-year-old woman with hypertrophic cardiomyopathy. In the control state, a large LV–aortic pressure gradient is present, and the duration of LV ejection is markedly prolonged, resulting in reversed splitting of S_2. A grade 3 systolic ejection murmur is recorded by the apex phonocardiogram during the pressure gradient. Following the administration of amyl nitrite, there is an increase in the LV–aortic pressure gradient and a marked increase in the intensity of the systolic murmur as recorded at the apex. Note that on the base phonocardiogram reversed splitting of S_2 persists, with an even greater delay in A_2. Following administration of phenylephrine, there is complete obliteration of the LV–aortic pressure gradient and almost total disappearance of the apical murmur. The contour of the central aortic pressure is normalized, and physiologic splitting of S_2 is now present. As compared to the control state, the inhalation of amyl nitrite and the infusion of phenylephrine result in no significant change in peak LV pressure; the increased gradient during inhalation of amyl nitrite was secondary to a decrease in aortic pressure. Contrast these responses to the administration of amyl nitrite and phenylephrine with those shown in Fig. 11-51—a patient with chronic mitral regurgitation. (*From PS Reddy, et al: Cardiac systolic murmurs: Pathophysiology and differential diagnosis. Prog Cardiovasc Dis 14:31, 1971. Reproduced in part with permission from the publisher and the authors.*)

result, there is poor correlation between the intensity of the murmur and the severity of the obstruction; for example, high flow across a mild obstruction may produce a loud rumble, while low flow across a severely stenotic valve may produce a very soft murmur or may be silent.[288]

When the stenotic mitral valve is mobile, the murmur is introduced by a prominent opening snap (OS) (Fig. 11-7, left panel). The duration of the interval between A_2 and the opening snap correlates well with the level of left atrial pressure; the shorter the A_2-OS interval, the higher the left atrial pressure, and vice versa.[140,144,147] The S_1 is also loud when the stenotic valve is mobile and is usually preceded by a crescendo murmur. Although originally attributed to increased flow secondary to left atrial systole, phonoechocardiographic studies by Criley et al.[289] have suggested that this short "presystolic" murmur is actually due to high-velocity antegrade flow through a progressively narrowing mitral orifice during very early (isovolumic) ventricular systole (Fig. 11-7, left panel). This mechanism may also be responsible for the brief crescendo presystolic murmur observed in patients with mitral stenosis in atrial fibrillation following a short cycle length (Fig. 11-30).[290] The exact physical principles causing the production of this crescendo murmur are still in question, as a study by Hada and associates[291] has not confirmed high-velocity flow by Doppler echocardiography during the rapid closing motion of the stenotic mitral valve. Regardless of the exact mechanism, these sounds are dependent on the presence of antegrade mitral flow at the time of very early ventricular contraction.[292]

Although the intensity of the diastolic rumble in mitral stenosis correlates poorly with the severity of obstruction, there is an excellent correlation of severity with the duration of the murmur. When sinus tachycardia or rapid atrial fibrillation is present, a rumble starting with an opening snap and continuing to S_1 may not be meaningful because of the short diastolic time. Carotid sinus pressure may be very helpful in temporarily slowing the heart rate, thereby allowing the clinician to uncover the potential length of the rumble. (See also Chap. 80.)

Obstruction of the mitral orifice can also be produced by a left atrial tumor. The diastolic murmur may be very similar to that produced by mitral stenosis, as shown in Fig. 11-7, center panel.[44] A loud tumor "plop" is present instead of the opening snap, and the presystolic crescendo murmur occurs as the protruding tumor mass returns rapidly through the mitral orifice into the left atrium during early ventricular systole. A systolic murmur of mitral regurgitation may also be present, and both murmurs may vary from examination to examination and with changes in body position.

The murmur of tricuspid stenosis is usually heard in the xiphoid area just off the sternal border. Since right atrial systole occurs earlier than left, the diastolic murmur of tricuspid stenosis may have a crescendo-decre-

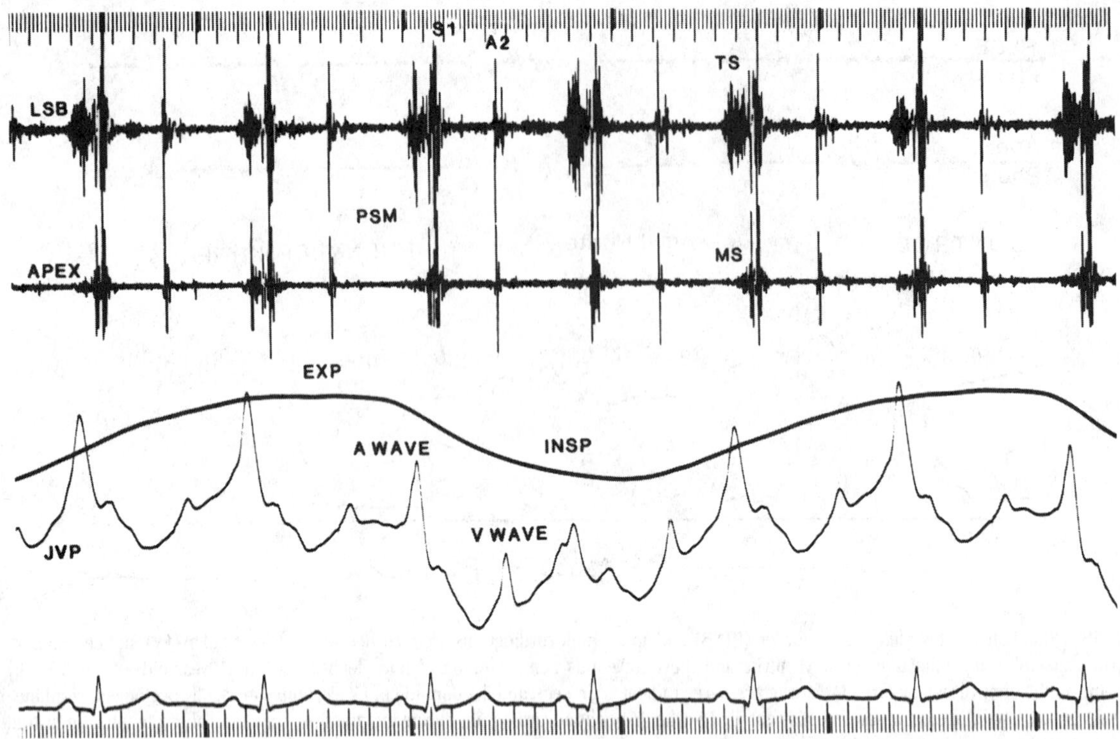

FIGURE 11-59 Phonocardiograms at the left sternal border (LSB) and apex are recorded together with the jugular venous pulse in a patient originally thought to have only mitral stenosis. The jugular venous pulse shows prominent *a* waves and the phonocardiogram at the LSB clearly shows inspiratory augmentation of a diamond-shaped presystolic murmur (TS) of tricuspid stenosis, in contrast to the apical mitral stenosis murmur (MS) that begins later and crescendos to S_1. [*From R Salerni, et al: Noninvasive graphic evaluation: Phonocardiography and echocardiography. In: WS Frankl, AN Brest (eds): Cardiovascular Clinics: Valvular Heart Disease—Comprehensive Evaluation and Management. Philadelphia, FA Davis, 1986, p 199. Reproduced with permission of the publisher and the authors.*]

scendo configuration (Fig. 11-59).[293] Even when the PR interval is normal, the presystolic accentuation of the diastolic rumble may terminate before S_1. Since tricuspid stenosis almost always occurs in the presence of mitral stenosis, this diastolic diamond-shaped murmur that augments during inspiration and the presence of large *a* waves in the jugular venous pulse are clues to this additional diagnosis.[294] When atrial fibrillation is present, the murmur is in middiastole and has the typical inspiratory augmentation. However, it is often very difficult to appreciate and must be carefully sought out, since both the presystolic murmur and large *a* waves alerting the clinician to this diagnosis are absent.[295] A tricuspid opening snap, which usually follows the mitral opening snap, may also be present and may initiate the murmur.[147]

Diastolic Rumbles Due to High Flow across the Atrioventricular Valves High-velocity flow across the normal or insufficient AV valve may result in short middiastolic rumbles often accompanied by an S_3 and should not be confused with murmurs produced by true obstruction of the AV valves. Such rumbles are common in both ventricular septal defect and patent ductus arteriosus due to the large flow across the mitral valve secondary to the left-to-right shunt.[296,297] Likewise, the left-to-right shunt in a large atrial septal defect often produces a tricuspid rumble.[149] Similar low-pitched rumbling murmurs may also be present in hyperkinetic states. Common to all these conditions is high-volume flow during the latter phase of the rapid filling period. Phonoechocardiography has shown that these murmurs occur during the rapid closing motion of the mitral valve, suggesting a functional "obstruction" during the period of rapid early diastolic filling.[298] Identical phonoechocardiographic correlates have also been shown with mitral and tricuspid regurgitation, where early diastolic filling is also extremely rapid. With tricuspid regurgitation, the early rumble will increase with inspiration, typical of right-sided murmurs across the tricuspid valve. During rapid atrial fibrillation, ventriculogenic closure of the normal mitral valve during the rapid filling phase of a short cardiac cycle may cause a "presystolic" murmur by a similar mechanism (Fig. 11-60).

Mitral valvulitis during an episode of acute rheumatic fever may cause a short diastolic rumble, the Carey Coombs murmur.[299] This rumble, especially in children or in the presence of fever and anemia, may be introduced by an S_3 rather than by an opening snap. This combination of an S_3 with a short rumble indicates that there is not enough obstruction to the valve to alter the characteristics of rapid early ventricular filling.

The Austin Flint murmur as originally described by Flint in 1862[300] consisted of an apical presystolic murmur observed in two patients with considerable aortic regurgitation and no evidence of mitral stenosis at autopsy. Since its original description, the timing of this murmur has been extended to include a middiastolic component (Fig. 11-61). It is heard best at the apex and has many

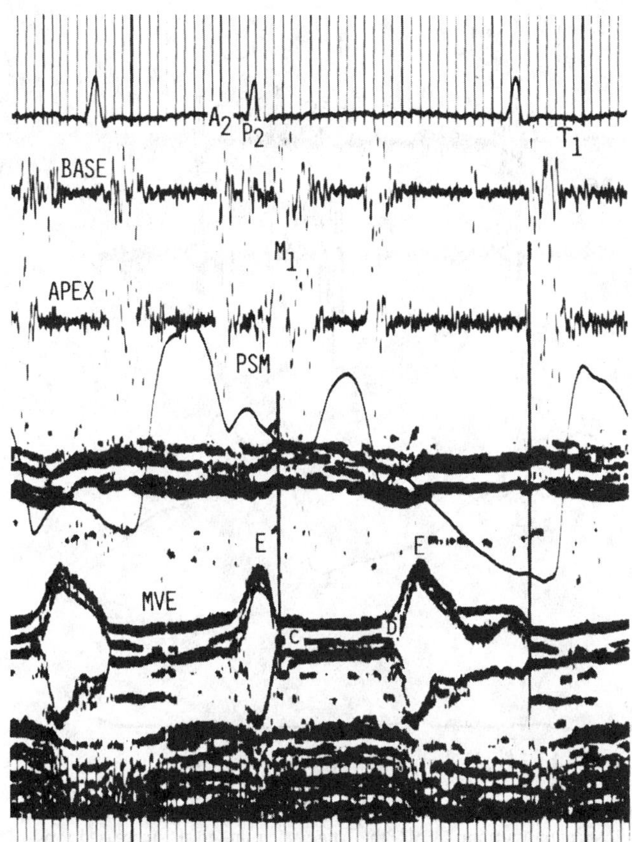

FIGURE 11-60 Phonoechocardiogram showing the mechanism of the presystolic murmur (PSM) in rapid atrial fibrillation without obstruction at the mitral valve. A rapidly closing normal mitral valve causes a crescendo murmur in complex 2. This finding is not present at longer cycle lengths. [*From R Salerni, et al: Noninvasive graphic evaluation: Phonocardiography and echocardiography. In: WS Frankl, AN Brest (eds): Cardiovascular Clinics: Valvular Heart Disease—Comprehensive Evaluation and Management. Philadelphia, FA Davis, 1986, p 178. Reproduced in part with permission of the publisher and the authors.*]

of the qualities of the murmur of mitral stenosis. However, it is introduced by an S_3 rather than by an opening snap, and S_1 is of normal or decreased amplitude.[301] Maneuvers or pharmacologic agents that increase the degree of aortic regurgitation, such as hand grip or vasoconstricting drugs, will increase the intensity of the rumble, while vasodilating agents such as amyl nitrite will decrease its intensity. In most cases of severe aortic regurgitation, particularly when the regurgitation is acute, the presystolic component of the Austin Flint murmur is lost (Fig. 11-10). In this situation, there is marked elevation of the left ventricular end-diastolic pressure (LVEDP), and the reverse pressure gradient between the left ventricle and left atrium causes premature closure of the mitral valve. (See also Chap. 79.)

A complete understanding of the origin of this murmur is still forthcoming, but most investigators agree that it is not secondary to late diastolic mitral regurgitation or isolated vibrations of the mitral leaflets. Elegant phonoechocardiographic studies have shown that the murmur is associated with the rapid closing motion of the mitral valve leaflets during middiastole and presystole; it is presumably due to antegrade flow across a closing orifice and to mechanisms similar to the flow rumble of AV valvular regurgitation and high-output states.[302,303] However, Austin Flint murmurs have been observed in the absence of rapid closing of the mitral valve, and Reddy et al.[304] have suggested that incomplete valve opening rather than excessively rapid closure rates may be the essential requirement for producing the increased mitral flow velocity. One echo-Doppler study has suggested that patients with an Austin Flint murmur usually have an aortic regurgitant jet aimed directly at the mitral valve, causing deformity and shuddering of the valve, in contrast to patients with equally severe regurgitation in whom the murmur is absent.[305] It is most likely that a combination of these factors is responsible for the turbulence that occurs across the mitral valve when the regurgitant jet collides with the antegrade flow through the mitral orifice and with the mitral leaflets. Right-sided Austin Flint murmurs of similar quality have been reported in association with severe pulmonic regurgitation associated with pulmonary hypertension.[306] It has not been reported in organic pulmonic regurgitation with normal pulmonary artery pressures.

Diastolic Regurgitant Murmurs

Holodiastolic Aortic Regurgitant Murmurs The early diastolic murmur of aortic regurgitation is blowing and high pitched in character and is often more difficult to record than to hear because of its high-frequency content. Since isovolumic relaxation of the left ventricle is very rapid, a large gradient quickly develops between the aortic and left ventricular diastolic pressures, and the murmur builds up to maximum intensity almost immediately after A_2.[2] As diastole progresses, the gradient between the two chambers slowly falls, and the murmur envelope closely parallels the pressure drop in a decrescendo fashion up to S_1 (Figs. 11-47, 11-61). When the aortic regurgitation is valvular in origin, the murmur is usually best heard at the third and fourth left parasternal areas. The finding that the murmur is heard best to the right of the sternum should alert the clinician to an aortic root etiology of the regurgitation.[307] It should be pointed out that this finding is helpful only if present, as aortic regurgitation secondary to dilation of the aortic root may have the usual radiation with peak intensity to the left of the sternum.[308] Although the frequency content of the murmur is in a range advantageous to the human ear, the amplitude of the vibrations may be quite small and the murmur quite faint. Therefore, the murmur may be overlooked if the examiner does not listen with the patient sitting up and leaning forward and does not listen with the diaphragm of the stethoscope firmly pressed against the chest wall. In addition, since the pitch of the murmur approaches that of respiratory sounds, one should listen while the patient holds his or her breath after deep expiration.

The degree of aortic regurgitation is directly proportional to the pressure head driving the flow in a retrograde fashion. Maneuvers or pharmacologic agents that increase or decrease the diastolic aortic–left ventricular pressure gradient will increase or decrease the intensity of the regurgitant murmur. Prompt squatting will often bring out a very faint aortic regurgitant blowing murmur

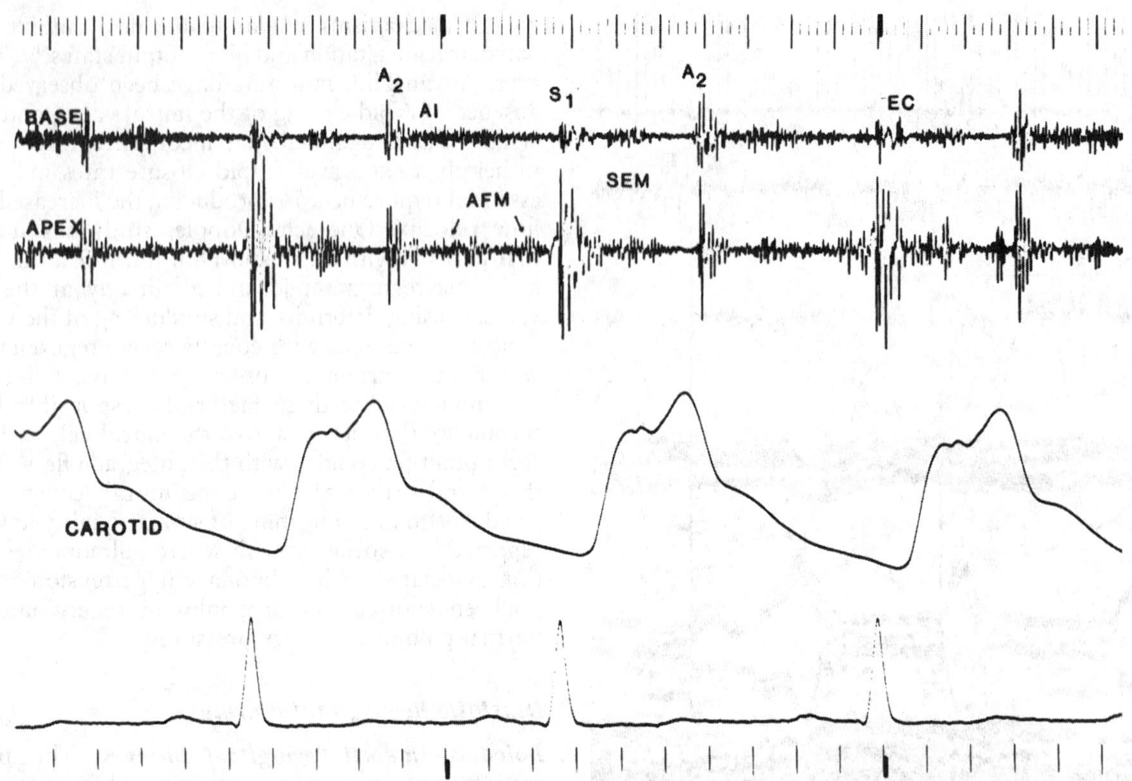

FIGURE 11-61 The early diastolic and presystolic component of the Austin Flint murmur (AFM) is recorded in a 26-year-old man with chronic aortic regurgitation. S_1 and S_2 are normal. A soft ejection click (EC) introduces a systolic ejection murmur (SEM), the latter being due to the increased forward stroke volume. The early diastolic murmur at the base (AI) begins with A_2 and extends through most of diastole. The carotid pulse is full with a wide pulse pressure. [*From R Salerni, et al: Noninvasive graphic evaluation: Phonocardiography and echocardiography. In: WS Frankl, AN Brest (eds): Cardiovascular Clinics: Valvular Heart Disease—Comprehensive Evaluation and Management. Philadelphia, FA Davis, 1986, p 193. Reproduced with permission of the publisher and the authors.*]

at the bedside, and inhalation of amyl nitrite will markedly decrease its intensity. It should be remembered that the murmur of mild aortic regurgitation often disappears during the latter stages of pregnancy due to the low peripheral vascular resistance. As shown in Fig. 11-47, pure aortic regurgitation without associated valvular stenosis may present with a prominent systolic ejection murmur as well as an Austin Flint rumble at the apex (Fig. 11-61). The carotid pulse is rapid rising and has a large volume. The A_2 is often diminished or even absent when the regurgitation is valvular in origin, due to inadequate coaptation and checking of the retrograde blood column by the deformed leaflets.[309]

The etiology of the aortic regurgitation usually cannot be determined by the quality of the murmur. An exception to this rule is the presence of a "cooing dove" or musical diastolic murmur, which usually denotes a rupture or retroversion of an aortic cusp. Such ruptures occur secondary to trauma, bacterial endocarditis, and occasionally in the presence of arteriosclerotic involvement of the aortic valve.[209] Retroversion and subsequent rupture of the aortic valve with a musical murmur is also a complication of syphilitic aortic regurgitation.[310] (See also Chap. 79.)

Abbreviated Aortic Diastolic Regurgitant Murmur The murmur of very mild aortic regurgitation may be abbreviated and end by middiastole. This is particularly true of the functional aortic regurgitant murmur of systemic arterial hypertension. As the volume of blood in the aorta decreases during diastole, the aortic ring becomes smaller and coupled with the decreasing aortic–left ventricular diastolic gradient, retrograde flow ceases, and the murmur disappears.

The murmur of aortic regurgitation may also be abbreviated if the aortic regurgitation is acute.[52] Acute regurgitation of blood into a ventricle that has not had time to adapt to a large-volume load results in marked elevation of the LVEDP and equilibration of the aortic and left ventricular diastolic pressures. With this, retrograde flow ceases and the murmur disappears in the latter part of diastole, as demonstrated in Fig. 11-62. In the syndrome of acute aortic regurgitation, there may be preclosure of the mitral valve resulting in a soft or absent S_1 as well as absence of the presystolic component of the Austin Flint murmur (Fig. 11-10). Common causes of this syndrome include aortic valve endocarditis, trauma, acute aortic dissection, and dehiscence of an aortic valve prosthesis.

Holodiastolic Pulmonary Regurgitant Murmur Pulmonic regurgitation is most commonly found in the setting of severe pulmonary hypertension and dilation of the pulmonary artery with inadequate coaptation of the leaflets of the pulmonic valve. The functional murmur of pulmonary regurgitation (Graham Steell murmur)[311] is similar

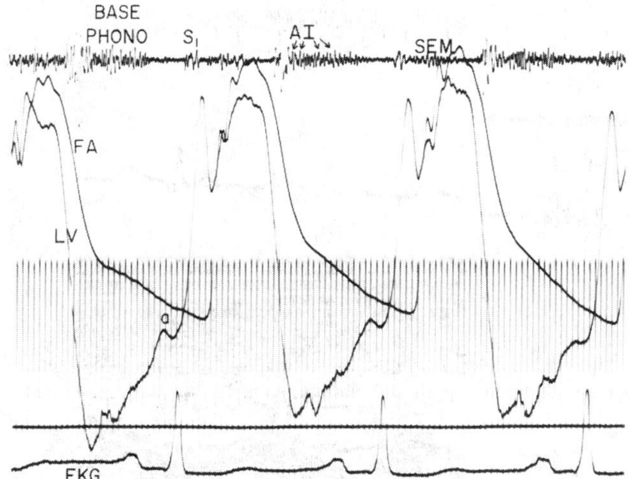

FIGURE 11-62 The base phonocardiogram is recorded simultaneously with the left ventricular and femoral artery pressures in a patient with acute aortic regurgitation, producing a number of atypical auscultatory findings as compared with chronic compensated aortic regurgitation. There is marked elevation of the LVEDP to 32 mmHg, with equilibration of the aortic and LVEDPs. With this equilibration of pressures, there is abbreviation of the aortic regurgitation murmur with a silent gap before S_1. The decreased intensity of S_1 is due to partial preclosure of the mitral valve secondary to the elevated LVEDP owing to regurgitant flow into a noncompliant left ventricle. [*From JA Shaver: Current uses of phonocardiography in clinical practice. In: E Rapaport (ed): Cardiology Update—Reviews for Physicians. New York, Elsevier, 1981, p 338. Reproduced with permission of the publisher and the author. Copyright 1981 by Elsevier Science Publishing Co., Inc.*]

in both frequency and contour to that of aortic regurgitation because the hemodynamics responsible for their production are identical. These murmurs cannot be differentiated by either their quality or location on the chest wall. Thus, the differential diagnosis is made by the "company the murmur keeps," and when associated with the peripheral signs of hemodynamically significant aortic regurgitation or with the findings of severe pulmonary hypertension, there is rarely a problem. However, when rheumatic mitral stenosis is the primary lesion, the semilunar regurgitant murmur may be secondary either to associated rheumatic aortic regurgitation or to the Graham Steell murmur if the pulmonary hypertension is severe. Careful investigation of the semilunar blowing murmur in the setting of mitral stenosis has shown that it is almost always due to aortic regurgitation, even when significant pulmonary hypertension is present.[312] More common causes of the Graham Steell murmur of functional pulmonary regurgitation are primary pulmonary hypertension and Eisenmenger's syndrome.

Early diastolic murmurs are occasionally heard in end-stage renal failure, particularly when there is concurrent anemia, hypertension, and fluid overload. In a study using Doppler echocardiography, Perez and associates[313] demonstrated that these murmurs are usually pulmonic in origin. They are often transient in nature and are related to fluid overload. Such murmurs are diminished by extracellular fluid removal and reflect correctable pulmonary hypertension.[313]

Delayed Pulmonary Regurgitant Murmur The murmur of organic pulmonary regurgitation is quite different in quality and duration, as compared to either aortic regurgitation or the Graham Steell murmur of pulmonary hypertension.[314] As shown in Fig. 11-63, the murmur is delayed from P_2 by a short interval and then builds up quickly to a crescendo followed by a decrescendo that ends well before S_1. In organic pulmonary regurgitation, the pulmonary artery pressure may be normal, and the diastolic gradient between the pulmonary artery and right ventricle may be very small, resulting in low-velocity retrograde flow and a lower pitched murmur. The murmur is heard only during the period of maximal gradient in early and middiastole, as the pulmonary artery pressure begins to equilibrate with the right ventricular end-diastolic pressure in the latter part of diastole. This type of murmur may be congenital or acquired as with pulmonary valve endocarditis, carcinoid syndrome, or surgical procedures on the pulmonic valve. It is often associated with a prominent systolic ejection murmur secondary to the large right ventricular stroke volume.

Continuous Murmurs

A continuous murmur is defined as one that begins in systole and extends through S_2 into part or all of diastole.[202] It need not occupy the entire cardiac cycle; therefore, a systolic murmur that extends into diastole without stopping at S_2 is considered to be continuous even if it fades completely before the subsequent S_1. A physiologic classification of continuous murmurs as described by Myers[315] is detailed in Table 11-7.

Continuous Murmurs Due to Rapid Blood Flow

High-velocity blood flow through veins and arteries may cause a continuous murmur. The cervical venous hum is a continuous murmur with diastolic accentuation and is easily heard in almost all children.[316] This murmur can also be heard in healthy adults and is present in nearly all women in the later stages of pregnancy. High cardiac output states such as thyrotoxicosis and anemia are also associated with easily heard venous hums. This murmur is usually poorly heard in the supine position, and its presence in this position in an adult strongly suggests a hyperdynamic circulatory state. Peak intensity is in the supraclavicular fossa just lateral to the sternocleidomastoid muscle, and it is usually more prominent on the right side. When the murmur is loud, it may radiate below the clavicles and occasionally can be confused with the continuous murmur of patent ductus arteriosus. However, this error should never be made because the cervical venous hum can easily be terminated by digital compression of the jugular venous pulse.

The mammary souffle is another example of a continuous murmur occurring in 10 to 15 percent of pregnant women during the second and third trimesters and in the early postpartum period, particularly in lactating women, and is heard between the second and sixth anterior intercostal spaces.[317] This murmur may be obliterated by firm pressure on the stethoscope or by digital pressure applied just lateral to the site of auscultation and should therefore not be confused with the continuous

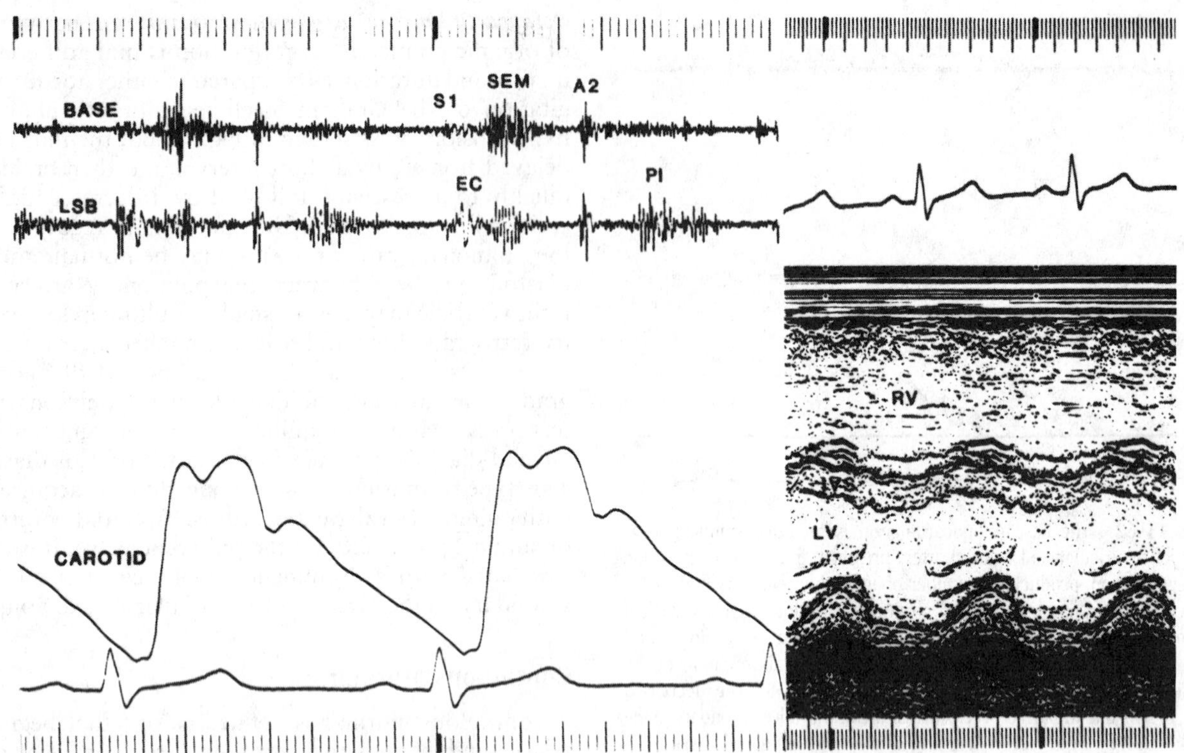

FIGURE 11-63 Phonocardiogram and echocardiogram of a 32-year-old man with organic pulmonary regurgitation. At the left sternal border (LSB), a middiastolic diamond-shaped murmur (PI) that is delayed from the soft P_2 is typical of organic pulmonic regurgitation. A prominent systolic ejection murmur is present due to the increased stroke volume across the right ventricular outflow tract. The echocardiogram shows a dilated right ventricle (RV) and a paradoxical septal motion of right ventricular volume overload. [*From R Salerni, et al: Noninvasive graphic evaluation: Phonocardiography and echocardiography. In: WS Frankl, AN Brest (eds): Cardiovascular Clinics: Valvular Heart Disease—Comprehensive Evaluation and Management. Philadelphia, FA Davis, 1986, p 206. Reproduced with permission of the publisher and the authors.*]

murmur of patent ductus arteriosus or with arteriovenous fistula.[318] The mammary souffle disappears after termination of lactation. Other causes of continuous murmurs due to rapid blood flow through arterial or venous channels are outlined in Table 11-7.

Continuous Murmurs Due to High-to-Low Pressure Shunts

A group of congenital cardiovascular anomalies has shunting from the high-pressure systemic (aortic) circulation to the low-pressure pulmonary arterial circulation, resulting in a large gradient between the two systems throughout the cardiac cycle. The murmur of patent ductus arteriosus is the classic example of this type of anomaly (Fig. 11-64). It is heard best in the left infraclavicular area and the second left intercostal space. The peak intensity of the murmur is at the time of S_2, after which it gradually wanes until it terminates before S_1.[319] The length of the murmur is determined by the difference in the vascular resistance between the greater and lesser circulation.[115] As the pulmonary vascular resistance increases, the diastolic pressure in the pulmonary artery approaches and finally reaches systemic levels, diminishing and finally abolishing diastolic flow and the diastolic portion of the murmur. With equilibration of aortic and pulmonary artery pressure, systolic flow across the shunt diminishes and finally disappears, leaving the ductus silent [Eisenmenger's patent ductus arteriosus (PDA)]. Surgically produced aortopulmonary connections (Blalock, Waterston, or Pott's shunts) as well as the murmur of aortic pulmonary window have identical qualities, and the effect of pulmonary hypertension on their length is analogous. (See also Chap. 97.)

It is important for the clinician to distinguish these types of continuous murmurs from to-fro murmurs. The latter is a combination of the systolic ejection murmur and a semilunar diastolic murmur. The classic example of a to-fro murmur is the murmur of aortic stenosis and regurgitation. The continuous murmur builds to a crescendo around S_2, whereas the to-fro murmur has two components. The midsystolic ejection component decrescendos and may disappear as it approaches S_2, leaving a silent period before the onset of the regurgitant murmur (Fig. 11-47).

Truncus arteriosus is a rare congenital anomaly and probably produces a continuous murmur only if there is coexisting pulmonary artery stenosis. In the presence of severe right ventricular outflow obstruction, bronchial collateral arteries can enlarge their normal precapillary anastomoses with pulmonary arteries, and the resultant aortic pulmonary fistula can produce a continuous murmur. This murmur can be heard in the same location as the patent ductus but radiates widely, especially over the posterior thorax. Large bronchial collateral arteries producing such continuous murmurs are more common with pulmonary atresia but also occur with tetralogy of Fallot.[320] Bronchial artery–pulmonary artery collaterals

TABLE 11-7

Physiologic Classification of Continuous Murmurs

A. Continuous murmurs due to rapid blood flow
  1. Venous hum
  2. Mammary souffle
  3. Hemiangioma
  4. Hyperthyroidism
  5. Acute alcoholic hepatitis
  6. Hyperemia of neoplasm (hepatoma renal cell carcinoma, Paget's disease)

B. Continous murmurs due to high-to-low pressure shunts
  1. Systemic artery to pulmonary artery (patent ductus arteriosus, aortopulmonary window, truncus arteriosus, pulmonary atresia, anomalous left coronary, bronchiectasis, sequestration of the lung)
  2. Systemic artery to right heart (ruptured sinus of Valsalva, coronary artery fistula)
  3. Left-to-right atrial shunting (Lutembacher's syndrome, mitral atresia plus atrial septal defect)
  4. Venovenous shunts (anomalous pulmonary veins, portosystemic shunts)
  5. Arteriovenous fistula (systemic or pulmonic)

C. Continuous murmurs secondary to localized arterial obstruction
  1. Coarctation of the aorta
  2. Branch pulmonary stenosis
  3. Carotid occlusion
  4. Ciliac mesenteric occlusion
  5. Renal occlusion
  6. Femoral occlusion
  7. Coronary occlusion

SOURCE: From Myers JD: The mechanisms and significances of continuous murmurs. In: Leon DF, Shaver JA (eds): *Physiologic Principles of Heart Sounds and Murmurs*, Monograph 46. New York, American Heart Association, 1975: 202. Reproduced with permission from the American Heart Association, Inc. and author.

sufficient to produce continuous murmurs are also found in far advanced bronchiectasis[321] and sequestration of the lung.

An anomalous left coronary artery arising from the pulmonary artery may cause a continuous murmur when the left-to-right shunt flow is large and is usually best heard at the left sternal border. In this condition, the origin of the right coronary artery is from the aorta, and the left-to-right shunt is from the high-pressure right coronary arterial bed through large arterial collaterals to the left coronary system, which empties into the low-pressure pulmonary artery. (See Chap. 97.)

Sinus of Valsalva aneurysms may cause continuous murmurs when they rupture into the right heart. In almost all cases, rupture occurs from the right and noncoronary sinuses into the right atrium or the right ventricle. The murmur is heard maximally at the lower sternal border or xiphoid over the area corresponding to the fistulous tract.[286] Diastolic accentuation of this murmur is an important sign to differentiate ruptured sinus from patent ductus arteriosus or arteriovenous fistula. Systolic suppression of the murmur is due to both mechanical narrowing of the fistulous tract during systolic contraction as well as the probable Venturi effect created by the rapid ejection of blood past the aortic origin of the fistula.[322] The continuous murmur may be very loud and occasionally can be heard from the foot of the bed.

Coronary artery fistulas usually empty into the right atrium or ventricle and cause a continuous murmur that is best heard to either the left or the right of the lower sternal area. Since the majority of coronary flow occurs during diastole, the diastolic component of the murmur is louder. When the coronary artery fistula empties into a high-pressure right ventricle, only a diastolic murmur may be heard because the pressure gradient across the shunt is reduced during systole.

Left-to-right shunting through an uncomplicated atrial septal defect produces no murmur audible on the chest wall because of the minimal pressure gradient and absence of turbulence. However, when mitral valve obstruction is present, as with Lutembacher's syndrome or mitral atresia, there is a high-pressure gradient between the left and right atria across the defect, and a continuous murmur may be present.[323] This murmur increases in intensity with inspiration and decreases with the Valsalva maneuver. Occasionally, a small atrial septal defect is produced following transseptal catheterization or balloon valvuloplasty for mitral stenosis, and a continuous murmur is produced due to high-velocity flow resulting from the large pressure gradient from left to right atrium. This is especially likely to occur if the mitral obstruction is not adequately relieved by the balloon valvuloplasty.

Total anomalous pulmonary venous drainage into a systemic vein may produce a continuous venous hum usually heard in the pulmonary area or the left infraclavicular area.[324] Frequently, a constriction at the junction of the anomalous venous conduit and the innominate vein or superior vena cava may cause augmentation of the murmur.

Arteriovenous fistulas between peripheral vessels produce a classic continuous murmur with systolic accentuation caused by shunting of a large volume of blood at rapid flow rates from a high-pressure artery into a low-pressure vein. These murmurs are best heard at the site of the fistula. Local compression of the veins may decrease the intensity of the murmur by raising venous pressure and reducing the arteriovenous pressure gradient. Complete obliteration of the fistula will terminate the murmur, and if the shunt is of considerable magnitude, a baroreceptor-mediated reflex bradycardia may occur (Branham's sign). Likewise, a reflex tachycardia will occur upon release of the obstruction. Pulmonary arteriovenous fistulas usually produce only a systolic murmur because the peripheral vascular resistance of the normal lung is very low, and the normally small diastolic pressure gradient from pulmonary artery to pulmonary vein is not significantly increased by the presence of the fistula.[315]

Continuous Murmur Secondary to Localized Arterial Obstruction

Localized stenosis of systemic or pulmonary arteries may produce a continuous murmur or bruit if the obstruction is critical and adequate collateral flow is not available.[325] Most partially obstructed arteries have only systolic mur-

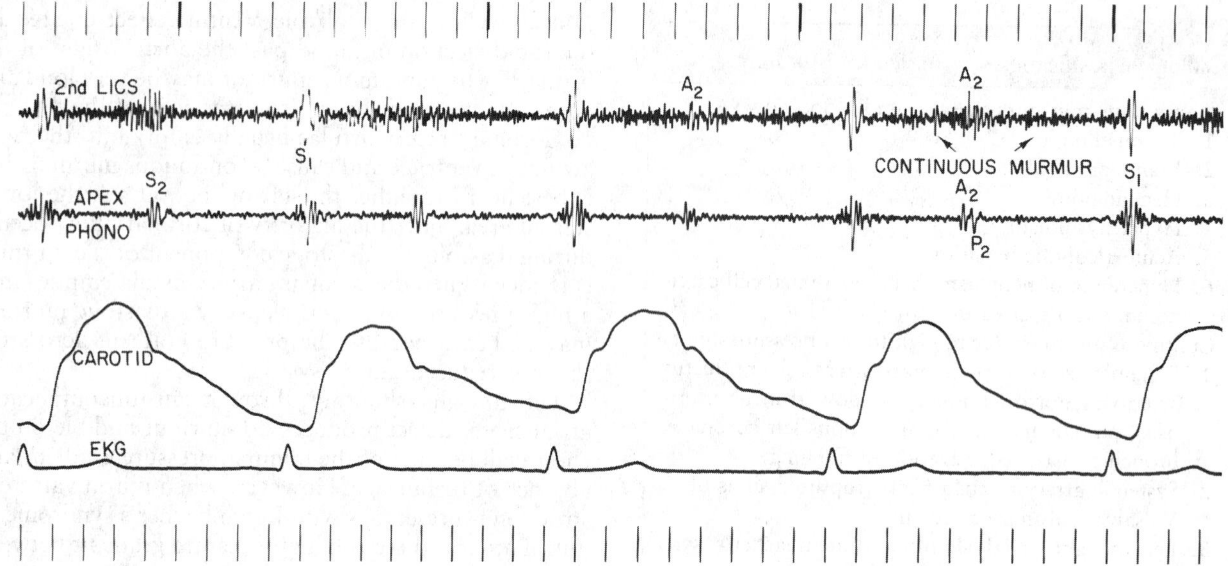

FIGURE 11-64 The classic contour of a continuous murmur of a large patent ductus arteriosus (PDA) as recorded at the second intercostal space. The murmur begins in systole, peaks at S_2, and continues in a decrescendo manner during diastolic runoff. The carotid pulse is prominent with a prolonged left ventricular ejection time. [*From JA Shaver: Current uses of phonocardiography in clinical practice. In: E Rapaport (ed): Cardiology Update—Reviews for Physicians. New York, Elsevier, 1981, p 366. Reproduced with permission of the publisher and the author. Copyright 1981 by Elsevier Science Publishing Co., Inc.*]

murs that are delayed relative to cardiac systole, depending upon the transit time of pulsatile flow from the heart to the site of obstruction. Edholm and associates[326] have shown that a considerable systolic pressure gradient exists across partial arterial obstructions but there is usually no diastolic gradient. This lack of diastolic gradient was explained by the fact that the collateral arteries around the obstruction deliver adequate flow such that the diastolic pressure on either side of the localized obstruction is essentially equal. Thus, a localized, partial arterial obstruction characteristically produces only a systolic murmur or bruit. If adequate collateral flow is not present however, a diastolic and a systolic pressure gradient is produced, and a continuous murmur with systolic accentuation is present. Depending on the degree of inadequacy of collaterals, the murmur is truly continuous when collateral circulation is essentially nonexistent or it extends only partially through diastole when collateral flow is somewhat compromised. Such is the case in severe coarctation of the aorta, where, in addition to the systolic and/or continuous murmurs heard over the thorax produced by rapid blood flow through the tortuous intercostal collaterals, a continuous murmur may be produced at the site of the coarctation.[327] This latter murmur is best heard over the back, midline between the scapulas. (See also Chap. 97.)

Continuous murmurs may also arise from branch pulmonary stenosis or partial obstruction of a major pulmonary artery occluded by a massive pulmonary embolus. Other common locations of continuous murmurs secondary to localized arterial obstructions are listed in Table 11-7. Common to all these murmurs is critical narrowing of the vessel with inadequate collateral flow, such that a continuous pressure gradient is produced throughout the cardiac cycle. Murmurs produced by obstruction of major coronary arteries are rarely loud enough to be transmitted to the chest wall. When audible, they produce only diastolic murmurs, even with inadequate collateral circulation.[328,329] This is because most coronary flow normally occurs during diastole due to the high wall tension in the left ventricle during systolic contraction. Inhalation of amyl nitrite is helpful in differentiating this murmur from that of mitral stenosis. The diastolic murmur of partial coronary obstruction decreases in intensity during inhalation of amyl nitrite, due to the decreased coronary perfusion pressure.[330] In contrast, the diastolic murmur of mitral stenosis increases in intensity secondary to the increased flow across the mitral valve.

REFERENCES

1. Laënnec RTH: *Traité de l'auscultation médiate,* 2d ed. Paris, Brosson et Chaude, 1826.
2. Shaver JA, Leonard JJ, Leon DF: *Examination of the Heart.* Part 4: *Auscultation of the Heart.* Dallas, American Heart Association, 1990.
3. Rapaport MB, Sprague HB: The effects of tubing bore on stethoscope efficiency. *Am Heart J* 1951; 42:605–609.
4. Butterworth JS, Chassin MR, McGrath R, et al: *Cardiac Auscultation.* New York, Grune & Stratton, 1960.
5. Levine SA, Harvey WP: *Clinical Auscultation of the Heart,* 2d ed. Philadelphia, Saunders, 1959.
6. Shaver JA: Current uses of phonocardiography in clinical practice. In: Rapaport E (ed): *Cardiology Update—Reviews for Physicians.* New York, Elsevier, 1981: 327–378.
7. Shaver JA, Salerni R, Reddy PS: Normal and abnormal heart sounds in cardiac diagnosis. Part I: Systolic sounds. *Curr Probl Cardiol* 10, March 1985.
8. Reddy PS, Salerni R, Shaver JA: Normal and abnormal heart sounds in cardiac diagnosis. Part II. Diastolic sounds. *Curr Probl Cardiol* 10, April 1985.
9. Dock W: Mode of production of the first heart sound. *Arch Intern Med* 1933; 51:737–746.

10. Leatham A: Splitting of the first and second heart sounds. *Lancet* 1954; 267:607–614.
11. Mills PG, Chamusco RF, Moos S, Craige E: Echophonocardiographic studies of the contribution of the atrioventricular valves to the first heart sound. *Circulation* 1976; 54:944–951.
12. Laniado S, Yellin EL, Miller H, Frater WM: Temporal relation of the first heart sound to closure of the mitral valve. *Circulation* 1973; 47:1006–1014.
13. Shah PM, Kramer DH, Gramiak R: Influence of the timing of atrial systole on mitral valve closure and on the first heart sound in man. *Am J Cardiol* 1970; 26:231–237.
14. Burggraf GW, Craige E: The first heart sound in complete heart block: Phono-echocardiographic correlations. *Circulation* 1974; 50:17–24.
15. Waider W, Craige E: First heart sound and ejection sounds: echocardiographic and phonocardiographic correlation with valvular events. *Am J Cardiol* 1975; 35:346–356.
16. Criley JM, Chambers RD, Blaufuss AH, Friedman NJ: Mitral stenosis: mechanico-acoustical events. In: Leon DF, Shaver JA (eds): *Physiologic Principles of Heart Sounds and Murmurs*, Monograph 46. New York, American Heart Association, 1975: 149–159.
17. Brooks N, Leech G, Leatham A: Factors responsible for normal splitting of first heart sound: High-speed echophonocardiographic study of valve movement. *Br Heart J* 1979; 42:695–702.
18. Mills P, Craige E: Echophonocardiography. *Prog Cardiovasc Dis* 1978; 20:337.
19. Rushmer RF: *Cardiovascular Dynamics,* 3d ed. Philadelphia, Saunders, 1970: 305.
20. Milner S, Meyer RA, Venables AW, Korfhagen J, Kaplan S: Mitral and tricuspid valve closure in congenital heart disease. *Circulation* 1976; 53:513–518.
21. Haber E, Leatham A: Splitting of heart sounds from ventricular asynchrony in bundle-branch block, ventricular ectopic beats, and artificial pacing. *Br Heart J* 1965; 27:691–696.
22. Hultgren HN, Leo TF: The tricuspid component of the first heart sound in mitral stenosis. *Circulation* 1958; 18:1012–1016.
23. DiBartolo G, Nunez-Dey D, Muiesan G, et al: Hemodynamic correlates of the first heart sound. *Am J Physiol* 1961; 201:888–892.
24. Wexler LF, Pohost GM, Rubenstein JJ, O'Keefe DD, Vezeridis MP, Daggett WM: The relationship of the first heart sound to mitral valve closure in dogs. *Circulation* 1982; 66:235–243.
25. O'Toole JD, Reddy PS, Curtiss EI, Griff FW, Shaver JA: The contribution of tricuspid valve closure to the first heart sound: An intracardiac micromanometer study. *Circulation* 1976; 53:752–758.
26. Tei C, Shah PM, Cherian G, Wong M, Ormiston JA: The correlates of an abnormal first heart sound in mitral valve prolapse syndromes. *N Engl J Med* 1982; 307:334–339.
27. Stept ME, Heid CE, Shaver JA, Leon DF, Leonard JJ: Effect of altering P-R interval on the amplitude of the first heart sound in the anesthetized dog. *Circ Res* 1969; 25:255–263.
28. Thompson ME, Shaver JA, Leon DF, Reddy PS, Leonard JJ: Pathodynamics of the first heart sound. In: Leon DF, Shaver JA (eds): *Physiologic Principles of Heart Sounds and Murmurs*, Monograph 46. New York, American Heart Association, 1975: 8–18.
29. Leech G, Brooks N, Green-Wilkinson A, Leatham A: Mechanisms of influence of P-R interval on loudness of first heart sound. *Br Heart J* 1980; 43:138–142.
30. Shah PM: Hemodynamic determinants of the first heart sound. In: Leon DF, Shaver JA (eds): *Physiologic Principles of Heart Sounds and Murmurs*, Monograph 46. New York, American Heart Association, 1975: 2–7.
31. Rytand DA: The variable loudness of the first heart sound in auricular fibrillation. *Am Heart J* 1949; 37:187–204.
32. Leonard JJ, Weissler AM, Warren JV: Observations on the mechanism of atrial gallop rhythm. *Circulation* 1958; 17:1007–1012.
33. Sakamoto T, Kusukawa R, MacCanon DM, Luisada AA: Hemodynamic determinants of the amplitude of the first heart sound. *Circ Res* 1965; 16:45–57.
34. Hume L, Reuben SR: The effects of exercise on the amplitude of the first heart sound in normal subjects. *Am Heart J* 1978; 95:4–11.
35. Delman AJ: Hemodynamic correlates of cardiovascular sounds. *Ann Rev Med* 1967; 18:139–158.
36. Stein PD, Sabbah HN, Barr I: Intensity of heart sounds in the evaluation of patients following myocardial infarction. *Chest* 1979; 75:679–684.
37. Sakamoto T, Kusukawa R, MacCanon DM, Luisada AA: First heart sound amplitude in experimentally induced alternans. *Dis Chest* 1966; 50:470–475.
38. Ravin A: *Auscultation of the Heart,* 2d ed. Chicago, Yearbook Medical Publishers, 1967.
39. Adolph RJ, Stephens JF, Tanaka K: The clinical value of frequency analysis of the first heart sound in myocardial infarction. *Circulation* 1970; 41:1003–1014.
40. Clarke WB, Austin SM, Shah PM, Griffen PM, Dove JT, McCullough J, et al: Spectral energy of the first heart sound in acute myocardial ischemia. *Circulation* 1978; 57:593–598.
41. Wooley CF, Klassen KP, Leighton RF, Goodwin MS, Ryan JM: Left atrial and left ventricular sound and pressure in mitral stenosis. *Circulation* 1968; 38:295–307.
42. Thompson ME, Shaver JA, Heidenreich FP, Leon DF, Leonard JJ: Sound, pressure and motion correlates in mitral stenosis. *Am J Med* 1970; 49:436–450.
43. Salerni R, Reddy PS, Sherman ME, O'Toole JD, Leon DF, Shaver JA: Pressure and sound correlates of the mitral valve echocardiogram in mitral stenosis. *Circulation* 1978; 58:119–125.
44. Nasser WK, Davis RH, Dillon JC, Tavel ME, Helmen CH, Feigenbaum H, et al: Atrial myxoma: II. Phonocardiographic, echocardiographic, hemodynamic and angiographic features in nine cases. *Am Heart J* 1972; 83:810–824.
45. Gershlick AH, Leech G, Mills PG, Leatham A: The loud first heart sound in left atrial myxoma. *Br Heart J* 1984; 52:403–407.
46. Burggraf GW: The first heart sound in left bundle branch block: An echophonocardiographic study. *Circulation* 1981; 63:429–435.
47. Hultgren HN, Craige E, Nakamura T, Fujii J, Bilisoly J: Left bundle branch block and mechanical events of the cardiac cycle. *Am J Cardiol* 1983; 52:755–762.
48. Grines CL, Bashore TM, Boudoulas H, Olson S, Shafer P, Wooley CF: Functional abnormalities in isolated left bundle branch block. The effect of interventricular asynchrony. *Circulation* 1989; 79:845–853.
49. Baragan J, Fernandez-Caamano F, Sozutek Y, Coblence B, Lenegre J: Chronic left complete bundle-branch block: Phonocardiographic and mechanocardiographic study of 30 cases. *Br Heart J* 1968; 30:196–202.
50. Shaver JA, Rahko PS, Grines CL, Boudoulas H, Wooley CF: Effect of left bundle branch block on the events of the cardiac cycle. *Acta Cardiol.* 1988; 4:459–467.
51. Rahko PS, Shaver JA, Salerni R: Reversed closure sequence of the mitral and tricuspid valves in congestive heart failure. *Circulation* 1986; 74(suppl II):1196.
52. Reddy PS, Leon DF, Krishnaswami V, O'Toole JD, Salerni R, Shaver JA: Syndrome of acute regurgitation. In: Leon DF, Shaver JA (eds): *Physiologic Principles of Heart Sounds and Murmurs*, Monograph 46. New York, American Heart Association, 1975: 166–174.
53. Meadows WR, VanPraagh S, Indreika M, Sharp JT: Premature mitral valve closure: A hemodynamic explanation for absence of the first sound in aortic insufficiency. *Circulation* 1963; 28:251–258.
54. Whittaker AV, Shaver JA, Gray S III, Leonard JJ: Sound-pressure correlates of the aortic ejection sound: An intracardiac sound study. *Circulation* 1969; 39:475–484.
55. Shaver JA, Griff FW, Leonard JJ: Ejection sounds of left-sided origin. In Leon DF, Shaver JA (eds): *Physiologic Principles of Heart Sounds and Murmurs*, Monograph 46. New York, American Heart Association, 1975: 27–34.
56. Ross RS, Criley JM: Cineangiocardiographic studies of the origin of cardiovascular physical signs. *Circulation* 1964; 30:255–261.
57. Epstein EJ, Criley JM, Raftery EB, Humphries JO, Ross R: Cineradiographic studies of the early systolic click in aortic valve stenosis. *Circulation* 1965; 31:842–853.
58. Mills PG, Brodie B, McLaurin L, Schall S, Craige E: Echocardiographic and hemodynamic relationships of ejection sounds. *Circulation* 1977; 56:430–436.
59. Leech G, Mills P, Leatham A: The diagnosis of a non-stenotic bicuspid aortic valve. *Br Heart J* 1978; 40:941–950.
60. Martin CE, Shaver JA, O'Toole JD, Leon DF, Reddy PS: Ejection sounds of right-sided origin. In Leon DF, Shaver JA (eds): *Physio-*

logical Principles of Heart Sounds and Murmurs, Monograph 46. New York, American Heart Association, 1975: 35–44.

61. Reddy PS, Shaver JA, Leonard JJ: Cardiac systolic murmurs: Pathophysiology and differential diagnosis. *Prog Cardiovasc Dis* 1971; 14:1–37.
62. Hultgren HN, Reeve R, Cohn K, McLeod R: The ejection click of valvular pulmonic stenosis. *Circulation* 1969; 40:631–639.
63. Weyman AE, Dillon JC, Feigenbaum H, Chang S: Echocardiographic patterns of pulmonary valve motion in valvular pulmonary stenosis. *Am J Cardiol* 1974; 34:644–651.
64. Leatham A, Weitzman D: Auscultatory and phonocardiographic signs of pulmonary stenosis. *Br Heart J* 1957; 19:303–317.
65. Flanigan WH, Shah PM: Echocardiographic correlate of presystolic pulmonary ejection sound in congenital valvular pulmonic stenosis. *Am Heart J* 1977; 94:633–636.
66. Leatham A, Vogelpoel L: The early systolic sound in dilatation of the pulmonary artery. *Br Heart J* 1954; 16:21–33.
67. Sakamoto T, Matsuhisa M, Hayashi T, Ichiyasu H: Echocardiogram and phonocardiogram related to the movement of the pulmonary valve. *Jpn Heart J* 1975; 16:107–117.
68. Cuffer B: Nouvelle recherches sur le bruit galop. *Arch Gen Med* 1887; 1:131, 301.
69. Gallavardin L: Nouvelle observation avec autopsie d'un pseudo-devoublement mitral. *Prat Med Fra* 1932; 13:19.
70. Barlow JB, Pocock WA, Marchand P, Denny M: The significance of late systolic murmurs. *Am Heart J* 1963; 66:443–452.
71. Criley JM, Lewis KB, Humphries JO, Ross RS: Prolapse of the mitral valve: Clinical and cine-angiocardiographic findings. *Br Heart J* 1966; 28:488–496.
72. Ronan JA, Perloff JK, Harvey WP: Systolic clicks and the late systolic murmur. *Am Heart J* 1965; 70:319–325.
73. Leon DF, Leonard JJ, Kroetz FW, Page WL, Shaver JA, Lancaster JF: Late systolic murmurs, clicks, and whoops arising from the mitral valve. *Am Heart J* 1966; 72:325–336.
74. Kerber RE, Isaeff DM, Hancock EW: Echocardiographic patterns in patients with the syndrome of systolic click and late systolic murmur. *N Engl J Med* 1971; 284:691–693.
75. Popp RL, Brown OR, Silverman JF, Harrison D: Echocardiographic abnormalities in the mitral valve prolapse syndrome. *Circulation* 1974; 49:428–433.
76. Winkle RA, Goodman DJ, Popp RL: Simultaneous echocardiographic phonocardiographic recordings at rest and during amyl nitrite administration in patients with mitral valve prolapse. *Circulation* 1975; 51:522–529.
77. Reid JVO: Mid-systolic clicks. *S Afr Med J* 1961; 35:353–355.
78. Fontana ME, Pence HL, Leighton RF, Wooley CF: The varying clinical spectrum of the systolic click–late systolic murmur syndrome: A postural auscultatory phenomenon. *Circulation* 1970; 41:807–816.
79. Fontana ME, Wooley CF, Leighton RF, Lewis R: Postural changes in left ventricular and mitral valvular dynamics in the systolic click–late systolic murmur syndrome. *Circulation* 1975; 51:165–173.
80. Mathey DG, Decoodt PR, Allen HN, Swan HJC: The determinants of onset of mitral valve prolapse in the systolic click–late systolic murmur syndrome. *Circulation* 1976; 53:872–878.
81. Fontana ME, Kissel GL, Criley JM: Functional anatomy of mitral valve prolapse. In: Leon DF, Shaver JA (eds): *Physiological Principles of Heart Sounds and Murmurs*, Monograph 46. New York, American Heart Association, 1975: 126–132.
82. Roelandt J, Willems J, van der Hauwaert LG, deGeest H: Clicks and sounds (whoops) in left-sided pneumothorax: Clinical and phonocardiographic study. *Dis Chest* 1969; 56:31–36.
83. Martin CE, Hufnagel CA, deLeon AC Jr: Calcified atrial myxoma: Diagnostic significance of the "systolic tumor sound" in a case presenting as tricuspid insufficiency. *Am Heart J* 1969; 78:245–250.
84. Pickering D, Keith JD: Systolic clicks with ventricular septal defects: A sign of aneurysm of ventricular septum? *Br Heart J* 1971; 33:538–539.
85. Killebrew E, Cohn K: Observations on murmurs originating from incompetent heterograft mitral valves. *Am Heart J* 1971; 81:490–493.
86. Leatham A: The second heart sound, key to auscultation of the heart. *Acta Cardiol* 1964; 19:395–416.
87. Shaver JA, O'Toole JD: The second heart sound: Newer concepts. Part I: Normal and wide physiologic splitting. *Mod Concepts Cardiovasc Dis* 1977; 46:7–12.
88. Shaver JA: Clinical implications of the hangout interval. *Int J Cardiol* 1984; 5:391–398.
89. Shaver JA: The second heart sound: Hemodynamic determinants. *Acta Cardiol* 1985; 40:7–18.
90. Shaver JA, Nadolny RA, O'Toole JD, Thompson ME, Reddy PS, Leon DF, et al: Sound pressure correlates of the second heart sound: An intracardiac sound study. *Circulation* 1974; 49:316–325.
91. Shaver JA, O'Toole JD, Curtiss EI, Thompson ME, Reddy PS, Leon DF: Second heart sound: Role of altered greater and lesser circulation. In: Leon DF, Shaver JA (eds): *Physiologic Principles of Heart Sounds and Murmurs*, Monograph 46. New York, American Heart Association, 1975: 58–67.
92. Curtiss EI, Reddy PS, O'Toole JD, Shaver JA: Alterations of right ventricular systolic time intervals by chronic pressure and volume overloading. *Circulation* 1976; 53:997–1003.
93. Craige E: Echocardiography in studies of the genesis of heart sounds and murmurs. In: Yu P (ed): *Progress in Cardiology*, Philadelphia, Lea & Febiger, 1975: 1–21.
94. Hirschfeld S, Liebman J, Borkat G, Bormuth C: Intracardiac pressure-sound correlates of echocardiographic aortic valve closure. *Circulation* 1977; 55:602–604.
95. Kusukawa R, Bruch DW, Sakamoto T, MacCanon DM, Luisada AA: Hemodynamic determinants of the amplitude of the second heart sound. *J Appl Physiol* 1966; 21:938–946.
96. Brough RD, Talley RC: Temporal relation of the second heart sound to aortic flow in various conditions. *Am J Cardiol* 1972; 30:237–241.
97. Stein PD, Sabbah HN, Anbe DT, Khaja F: Hemodynamic and anatomic determinants of relative differences in amplitude of the aortic and pulmonary components of the second heart sound. *Am J Cardiol* 1978; 42:539–544.
98. Adolph RJ: Second heart sound: Role of altered electromechanical events. In: Leon DF, Shaver JA (eds): *Physiologic Principles of Heart Sounds and Murmurs*, Monograph 46. New York, American Heart Association, 1975: 45–57.
99. Curtiss EI, Shaver JA, Reddy PS, O'Toole JD: Newer concepts in physiologic splitting of the second heart sound. In: Leon DF, Shaver JA (eds): *Physiologic Principles of Heart Sounds and Murmurs*, Monograph 46. New York, American Heart Association, 1975: 68–73.
100. Leatham A, Towers M: Splitting of the second heart sound in health. In: Proceedings of the Thirtieth Annual General Meeting of the British Cardiac Society (Glasgow, May 10, 1951). *Br Heart J* 1951; 13:575.
101. Boyer SH, Chisholm AW: Physiologic splitting of the second heart sound. *Circulation* 1958; 18:1010–1011.
102. Shafter HA: Splitting of the second heart sound. *Am J Cardiol* 1960; 6:1013–1022.
103. Castle RF, Jones KL: Mechanism of respiratory variations in splitting of the second heart sound. *Circulation* 1961; 24:180–184.
104. Aygen MM, Braunwald E: Splitting of the second heart sound in normal subjects and in patients with congenital heart disease. *Circulation* 1962; 25:328–345.
105. Harris A, Sutton G: Second heart sound in normal subjects. *Br Heart J* 1968; 30:739–742.
106. Curtiss EI, Matthews RG, Shaver JA: Mechanism of normal splitting of the second heart sound. *Circulation* 1975; 51:157–164.
107. Shuler RH, Ensor C, Gunning RE, Moss WG, Johnson V: The differential effects of respiration on the left and right ventricles. *Am J Physiol* 1942; 137:620–627.
108. Lauson HD, Bloomfield RA, Cournand A: Influence of the respiration on the circulation in man: With special reference to pressures in the right auricle, right ventricle, femoral artery and peripheral veins. *Am J Med* 1946; 1:315–335.
109. Brecher GA, Hubay CA: Pulmonary blood flow and venous return during spontaneous respiration. *Circ Res* 1955; 3:210–214.
110. Adolph RJ, Fowler NO: The second heart sound: A screening test for heart disease. *Mod Concepts Cardiovasc Dis* 1970; 39:91–96.
111. Shah PM, Slodki SJ: The Q-II interval: A study of the second heart sound in normal adults and in systemic hypertension. *Circulation* 1964; 29:551–561.
112. Slodki SJ, Hussain AT, Luisada AA: The Q-II interval: III. A study of the second heart sound in old age. *J Am Geriatr Soc* 1969; 17:673–679.

113. Logue RB, Cobbs BW, Dorney ER: The second heart sound in pulmonary embolism and pulmonary hypertension. *Trans Am Clin Climatol Assoc* 1966; 78:38–50.
114. Susmano A, Kefer J, Kumar LV: Abnormal pulmonic sound during acute massive pulmonary embolism. *Chest* 1978; 74:45–49.
115. Perloff JK: Auscultatory and phonocardiographic manifestations of pulmonary hypertension. *Prog Cardiovasc Dis* 1967; 9:303–338.
116. Shapiro S, Clark TJH, Goodwin JF: Delayed closure of the pulmonary valve in obliterative pulmonary hypertension. *Lancet* 1965; 2:1207–1211.
117. Vogelpoel L, Schrire V: Auscultatory and phonocardiographic assessment of pulmonary stenosis with intact ventricular septum. *Circulation* 1960; 22:55–72.
118. O'Toole JD, Reddy PS, Curtiss EI, Shaver JA: The mechanisms of splitting of the second heart sound in atrial septal defect. *Circulation* 1977; 56:1047–1053.
119. Ehlers KH, Engle MA, Farnsworth PB, Levin AR: Wide splitting of the second heart sound without demonstrable heart disease. *Am J Cardiol* 1969; 23:690–696.
120. Gray IR: Paradoxical splitting of the second heart sound. *Br Heart J* 1956; 18:21–28.
121. Shaver JA, O'Toole JD: The second heart sound: Newer concepts. Part 2: Paradoxical splitting and narrow physiological splitting. *Mod Concepts Cardiovasc Dis* 1977; 46:13–16.
122. Luisada AA, Kumar S, Pouget MJ: On the causes of the changes of the second heart sound in left bundle branch block. *Jpn Heart J* 1972; 13:281–294.
123. Alvares RF, Shaver JA, Gamble WH, Goodwin JF: The isovolumic relaxation period in hypertrophic cardiomyopathy. *J Am Coll Cardiol* 1984; 3:71–81.
124. Gamble WH, Shaver JA, Alvares RF, Salerni R, Reddy PS: A critical appraisal of diastolic time intervals as a measure of relaxation in left ventricular hypertrophy. *Circulation* 1983; 68:76–87.
125. Kumar S, Luisada AA: Mechanism of changes in the second heart sound in aortic stenosis. *Am J Cardiol* 1971; 28:162–167.
126. Shaver JA, Kroetz FW, Leonard JJ, Paley HW: Effect of steady-state increases in systemic arterial pressure on the duration of left ventricular ejection time. *J Clin Invest* 1968; 47:217–230.
127. Agnew T, Bucher H, McDonald L, Seymour J: Delayed closure of the aortic valve in ischaemic heart disease. *Br Heart J* 1967; 29:775–777.
128. Yurchak PM, Gorlin R: Paradoxical splitting of the second heart sound in coronary heart disease. *N Engl J Med* 1963; 269:741–743.
129. Martin CE, Shaver JA, Leonard JJ: Physical signs, apexcardiography, phonocardiography, and systolic time intervals in angina pectoris. *Circulation* 1972; 46:1098–1114.
130. Luisada AA: The second heart sound in normal and abnormal conditions. *Am J Cardiol* 1971; 28:150–161.
131. Zuberbuhler JR, Bauersfeld SR: Paradoxical splitting of the second heart sound in the Wolff-Parkinson-White syndrome. *Am Heart J* 1965; 70:595–602.
132. Ito M, Fujino T, Kanaya S, Imanishi S, Mashiba H: Phono-, echo-, and electrocardiographic correlation in the Wolff-Parkinson-White syndrome, with special reference to the split pattern of second heart sound. *Jpn Heart J* 1977; 18:329–339.
133. Wood P: Pulmonary hypertension. *Br Med Bull* 1952; 8:348–353.
134. Dell'Italia LJ, Walsh RA: Acute determinants of the hangout interval in the pulmonary circulation. *Am Heart J* 1988; 16:1289–1297.
135. Thayer WS: The early diastolic heart sound. *Trans Assoc Am Phys* 1908; 13:326–357.
136. Margolies A, Wolferth CC: The opening snap (claquement d'ouverture de la mitrale) in mitral stenosis: Its characteristics, mechanism of production and diagnostic importance. *Am Heart J* 1932; 7:443–470.
137. Ross RS, Criley JM, Morgan RH: Cineangiography in mitral valve disease. *Trans Assoc Am Phys* 1961; 74:271–279.
138. McCall BW, Price JL: Movement of the mitral cusps in relation to the first heart sound and opening snap in patients with mitral stenosis. *Br Heart J* 1967; 29:417–421.
139. Friedman NJ: Echocardiographic studies of mitral valve motion: Genesis of the opening snap in mitral stenosis. *Am Heart J* 1970; 80:177–187.
140. Wells B: The assessment of mitral stenosis by phonocardiography. *Br Heart J* 1954; 16:261–266.
141. Oriol A, Palmer WH, Nakhjavan F, McGregor M: Prediction of left atrial pressure from the second sound-opening snap interval. *Am J Cardiol* 1965; 16:184–188.
142. Bayer O, Loogen F, Wolter HH: The mitral opening snap in the quantitative diagnosis of mitral stenosis. *Am Heart J* 1956; 51:234–245.
143. Rackley CE, Craig RJ, McIntosh HD, Orgain E: Phonocardiographic discrepancies in the assessment of mitral stenosis. *Arch Intern Med* 1968; 121:50–53.
144. Rahko PS, Shaver JA, Salerni R, Gamble WH, Reddy PS: Echophonocardiographic estimates of pulmonary artery wedge pressure in mitral stenosis. *Am J Cardiol* 1985; 55:462–469.
145. Bousvaros GA, Stubington D: Some auscultatory and phonocardiographic features of tricuspid stenosis. *Circulation* 1964; 29:26–33.
146. Luisada AA, Slodke SJ, Krol B: Double (mitral and tricuspid) opening snap in patients with valvular lesions. *Am J Cardiol* 1965; 16:800–806.
147. Tavel ME: Opening snaps: Mitral and tricuspid. In: Leon DF, Shaver JA (eds): *Physiologic Principles of Heart Sounds and Murmurs*, Monograph 46. New York, American Heart Association, 1975: 85–91.
148. Millward DK, McLaurin LP, Craige E: Echocardiographic studies to explain opening snaps in presence of nonstenotic mitral valves. *Am J Cardiol* 1973; 31:64–70.
149. Leatham A, Gray I: Auscultatory and phonocardiographic signs of atrial septal defect. *Br Heart J* 1956; 18:193–208.
150. Tavel ME, Baugh D, Fisch C, Feigenbaum H: Opening snap of the tricuspid valve in atrial septal defect. *Am Heart J* 1970; 80:550–555.
151. Nixon PGF, Wooler GH, Radigan LR: The opening snap in mitral incompetence. *Br Heart J* 1960; 22:395–402.
152. Perloff JK, Harvey WP: Auscultatory and phonocardiographic manifestations of pure mitral regurgitation. *Prog Cardiovasc Dis* 1962; 5:172–194.
153. Sloan AW, Campbell FW, Henderson AS: Incidence of the physiological third heart sound. *Br Med J* 1952; 2:853–855.
154. Harvey WP, Stapleton J: Clinical aspects of gallop rhythm with particular reference to diastolic gallops. *Circulation* 1958; 18:1017–1024.
155. Reddy PS, Haidet K, Meno F: Relation of intensity of cardiac sounds to age. *Am J Cardiol* 1985; 55:1383–1388.
156. Tavel ME, Campbell RW, Feigenbaum H, Steinmetz EF: The apex cardiogram and its relationship to haemodynamic events with the left heart. *Br Heart J* 1965; 27:829–839.
157. Craige E: Gallop rhythm. *Prog Cardiovasc Dis* 1967; 10:246–260.
158. Shaver JA, Reddy PS, Alvares FR: Early diastolic events associated with the physiologic and pathologic S_3. *J Cardiol* 1984; 14(suppl V):30–46.
159. Warren JV, Leonard JJ, Weissler AM: Gallop rhythm. *Ann Intern Med* 1958; 48:580–596.
160. Nixon PGF: The genesis of the third heard sound. *Am Heart J* 1963; 65:712–714.
161. Dock W, Grandell F, Taubman F: The physiologic third heart sound: Its mechanism and relation to protodiastolic gallop. *Am Heart J* 1955; 50:449–464.
162. Shah PM, Jackson D: Third heart sound and summation gallop. In: Leon DF, Shaver JA (eds): *Physiologic Principles of Heart Sounds and Murmurs*, Monograph 46. New York, American Heart Association, 1975: 79–84.
163. Sakamoto T, Ichiyasu H, Hayashi T, Kawaratani H, Amano K, Hada Y: Genesis of the third heart sound. Phonoechocardiographic studies. *Jpn Heart J* 1976; 17:150–162.
164. Kuo PT, Schnabel TG Jr, Blakemore WS, Whereat A: Diastolic gallop sounds, the mechanism of production. *J Clin Invest* 1957; 36:1035–1042.
165. Shah PM, Gramiak R, Kramer DH, Yu P: Determinants of atrial (S_4) and ventricular (S_3) gallop sounds in primary myocardial disease. *N Engl J Med* 1968; 278:753–758.
166. Potain C: Du bruit de galop. *Gars d'Hop* 1880; 53:529.
167. Ozawa Y, Smith D, Craige E: Origin of the third heart sound. I. Studies in dogs. *Circulation* 1983; 67:393–398.
168. Ozawa Y, Smith D, Craige E: Origin of the third heart sound. II. Studies in human subjects. *Circulation* 1983; 67:399–404.
169. VandeWerf F, Minten J, Carmeliet P, DeGeest H, Kesteloot H:

The genesis of the third and fourth heart sounds. A pressure-flow study in dogs. *J Clin Invest* 1984; 73:1400–1407.
170. VandeWerf F, Boel A, Geboers J, Minten J, Willems J, DeGeest H, et al: Diastolic properties of the left ventricle in normal adults and in patients with third heart sounds. *Circulation* 1984; 69:1070–1078.
171. VandeWerf F, Geboers J, Kesteloot H, DeGeest H, Barrios L: The mechanism of disappearance of the physiologic third heart sound with age. *Circulation* 1986; 73:877–884.
172. Wilken MK, Meyers DG, Laski PA, Yi FP, Starke H: Mechanism of disappearance of S_3 with maturation. *Am J Cardiol* 1989; 64:1394–1396.
173. Vancheri F, Gibson D: Relation of third and fourth heart sounds to blood velocity during left ventricular filling. *Br Heart J* 1989; 61:144–148.
174. Lavine SJ, Arends D: Diastolic filling correlates of the third heart sound. *Am J Noninvas Cardiol* 1989; 3:51–57.
175. Pozzoli M, Febo O, Tramarin R, Pinna G, Cobelli F, Specchia G: Pulsed Doppler evaluation of left ventricular filling in subjects with pathologic and physiologic third heart sound. *Eur Heart J* 1990; 11:500–508.
176. Porter CM, Baxley WA, Eddleman EE Jr, Frimer M, Rackley CE: Left ventricular dimensions and dynamics of filling in patients with gallop heart sounds. *Am J Med* 1971; 50:721–727.
177. Reddy PS, Meno F, Curtiss EI, O'Toole JD: The genesis of gallop sounds: Investigation by quantitative phono- and apexcardiography. *Circulation* 1981; 63:922–933.
178. Gamble WH, Reddy PS: Preservation of the third heart sound in mitral stenosis. *N Engl J Med* 1983; 308:498–502.
179. Aubert AE, Denys BG, Meno F, Reddy PS: Investigation of genesis of gallop sounds in dogs by quantitative phonocardiography and digital frequency analysis. *Circulation* 1985; 71:987–993.
180. Shaver JA, Reddy PS, Alvares RF, Salerni R: Genesis of the physiologic third heart sound. *Am J Noninvas Cardiol* 1987; 1:39–55.
181. Riley C, Russell R, Rackley C: Left ventricular gallop sound and acute myocardial infarction. *Am Heart J* 1973; 86:598–602.
182. Leonard J, Weissler A, Warren J: Modification of ventricular gallop rhythm induced by pooling of blood in the extremities. *Br Heart J* 1958; 20:502–506.
183. Abdulla AM, Frank MJ, Erdin RA Jr, Canedo M: Clinical significance and hemodynamic correlates of the third heart sound gallop in aortic regurgitation. *Circulation* 1981; 64:464–471.
184. Stapleton JF: Third and fourth heart sounds. In: Horwitz LD, Groves BM (eds): *Signs and Symptoms in Cardiology*. Philadelphia, Lippincott, 1985: 214–226.
185. Tyberg TI, Goodyer AVN, Langou RA: Genesis of pericardial knock in constrictive pericarditis. *Am J Cardiol* 1980; 46:570–575.
186. Fowler NO, Adolph RJ: Fourth sound gallop or split first sound? *Am J Cardiol* 1972; 30:441–444.
187. Spodick DH, Quary-Pigotti VM: Fourth heart sound as a normal finding in older persons. *N Engl J Med* 1973; 288:140–141.
188. Tavel ME: The fourth heart sound: A premature requiem? *Circulation* 1974; 49:4–6.
189. Goldblatt A, Aygen MM, Braunwald E: Hemodynamic-phonocardiographic correlations of the fourth heart sound in aortic stenosis. *Circulation* 1962; 26:92–98.
190. Caulfield WH, deLeon AC, Perloff JK, Steelman RB: The clinical significance of the fourth heart sound in aortic stenosis. *Am J Cardiol* 1971; 28:179–182.
191. Cohen LS, Mason DT, Braunwald E: Significance of an atrial gallop sound in mitral regurgitation. *Circulation* 1967; 35:112–118.
192. Kotler MN, Segal BL, Parry WR: Echocardiographic and phonocardiographic evaluation of prosthetic heart valves. *Cardiovasc Clin* 1978; 9:187–207.
193. Smith ND, Raizada V, Abrams J: Auscultation of the normally functioning prosthetic valve. *Ann Intern Med* 1981; 95:594–598.
194. Kotler MN, Mintz GS, Panidis I, Morganroth J, Segal BL, Ross J: Noninvasive evaluation of normal and abnormal prosthetic valve function. *J Am Coll Cardiol* 1983; 1:151–173.
195. Simon EB, Kotler MN, Segal BL, Parry W: Clinical significance of multiple systolic clicks from Starr–Edwards prosthetic aortic valves. *Br Heart J* 1977; 39:645–650.
196. Hultgren HN, Hubis H: A phonocardiographic study of patients with the Starr-Edwards mitral valve prosthesis. *Am Heart J* 1965; 69:306–319.
197. Gibson TC, Starek PJK, Moos S, Craige E: Echocardiographic and phonocardiographic characteristics of the Lillehei-Kaster mitral valve prosthesis. *Circulation* 1974; 49:434–440.
198. DePace NL, Kotler MN, Mintz GS, Lichtenberg R, Coel IP, Segal BL: Echocardiographic and phonocardiographic assessment of the St. Jude cardiac valve prosthesis. *Chest* 1981; 80:272–277.
199. Harris A: Pacemaker "heart sound." *Br Heart J* 1967; 29:608–615.
200. Lerman J, Means JH: Cardiovascular symptomatology in exophthalmic goiter. *Am Heart J* 1932; 8:55–65.
201. Hamman L: Spontaneous mediastinal emphysema. *Bull Johns Hopkins Hosp* 1939; 64:1–21.
202. Soffer A, Feinstein A, Luisada AA, Perloff JK, Rosner S, Schlant R, et al: Glossary of cardiologic terms related to physical diagnosis and history. *Am J Cardiol* 1967; 20:285–286.
203. Stein PD: *A Physical and Physiological Basis for the Interpretation of Cardiac Auscultation: Evaluations Based Primarily on the Second Sound and Ejection Murmurs*. Mt. Kisco, NY, Futura Publishing Company, 1981.
204. Leatham A: Systolic murmurs. *Circulation* 1958; 17:601–611.
205. Freeman AR, Levine SA: Clinical significance of systolic murmurs: Study of 1000 consecutive "non-cardiac" cases. *Ann Intern Med* 1933; 6:1371–1385.
206. McKusick VA: *Cardiovascular Sound in Health and Disease*. Baltimore, Williams and Wilkins, 1958.
207. Donnerstein RL: Continuous spectral analysis of heart murmurs for evaluating stenotic cardiac lesions. *Am J Cardiol* 1989; 64:625–630.
208. Gallavardin L, Ravault P: Le souffle du rétrécissement aortique puet changer de timbre et devenir musical dans sa propagation apexienne. *Lyon Med* 1925; 135:523–529.
209. Gelfand D, Bellet S: The musical murmur of aortic insufficiency: Clinical manifestations; based on a study of 18 cases. *Am J Med Sci* 1951; 221:644–654.
210. Behar VS, Whalen RE, McIntosh HD: The ballooning mitral valve in patients with the "precordial honk" or "whoop." *Am J Cardiol* 1967; 20:789–795.
211. Sabbah HN, Magilligan DJ, Lakier JB, Stein PD: Hemodynamic determinants of the frequency and amplitude of a musical murmur produced by a regurgitant mitral bioprosthetic valve. *Am J Cardiol* 1982; 50:53–58.
212. Stein PD, Sabbah HN, Lakier JB: Origin and clinical relevance of musical murmurs. *Int J Cardiol* 1983; 4:103.
213. Pennestri F, Boccardi L, Minardi G, DiSegni M, Pucci E, Biasucci LM, et al: Doppler study of precordial musical murmurs. *Am J Cardiol* 1989; 63:1390–1394.
214. Rushmer RF, Morgan CL: Meaning of murmurs. *Am J Cardiol* 1968; 21:722–730.
215. Spencer MP, Greiss FC: Dynamics of ventricular ejection. *Circ Res* 1962; 10:274–279.
216. Franklin DL, VanCitters RL, Rushmer RF: Balance between right and left ventricular output. *Circ Res* 1962; 10:17–26.
217. Murgo JP, Altobelli SA, Dorethy JF, Logsdon JR, McGranahan GM: Normal ventricular ejection dynamics in man during rest and exercise. In: Leon DF, Shaver JA (eds): *Physiologic Principles of Heart Sounds and Murmurs*, Monograph 46. New York, American Heart Association, 1975: 92–101.
218. Lembo NJ, Dell'Italia LJ, Crawford MH, O'Rourke RA: Bedside diagnosis of systolic murmurs. *N Engl J Med* 1988; 318:1572–1578.
219. Tavel ME: Innocent murmurs. In: Leon DF, Shaver JA (eds): *Physiologic Principles of Heart Sounds and Murmurs*, Monograph 46. New York, American Heart Association, 1975: 102–106.
220. Still GF: *Common Disorders and Diseases of Childhood*, 1st ed. London, H. Frowde, 1909.
221. Darazs B, Hesdorfer CS, Butterworth AM, Ziady F: The possible etiology of the vibratory systolic murmur. *Clin Cardiol* 1987; 10:341–346.
222. Schwartz ML, Goldberg SJ, Wilson N, Allen HD, Mark GR: Relation of Still's murmur, small aortic diameter and high aortic velocity. *Am J Cardiol* 1986; 57:1344–1348.
223. Stein PD, Sabbah HN: Aortic origin of innocent murmurs. *Am J Cardiol* 1977; 39:665–671.
224. Shaver JA: Innocent murmurs. *Hosp Med* April 1978; 8–35.
225. Fowler NO, Marshall WJ: The supraclavicular arterial bruit. *Am Heart J* 1965; 69:410–418.
226. Nelson WP, Hall RJ: The innocent supraclavicular arterial

bruit—utility of shoulder maneuvers in its recognition. *N Engl J Med* 1968; 278:778.

227. Leonard JJ, Renfro NL, deGroot WJ, Page WL: The auscultatory diagnosis of the hyperkinetic state. In: Segal BL (ed): *The Theory and Practice of Auscultation.* Philadelphia, F.A. Davis, 1964: 180–190.
228. deLeon AC Jr: "Straight back" syndrome. In: Leon DF, Shaver JA (eds): *Physiologic Principles of Heart Sounds and Murmurs,* Monograph 46. New York, American Heart Association, 1975: 197–208.
229. Perloff JK: Clinical recognition of aortic stenosis. The physical signs and differential diagnosis of the various forms of obstruction to left ventricular outflow. *Prog Cardiovasc Dis* 1968; 10:323–352.
230. Vogel JH, Blount SG: Clinical evaluation in localizing levels of obstruction to outflow from left ventricle. *Am J Cardiol* 1965; 15:782–792.
231. Paley HW: Left ventricular outflow tract obstruction: Heart sounds and murmurs. In: Leon DF, Shaver JA (eds): *Physiologic Principles of Heart Sounds and Murmurs,* Monograph 46. New York, American Heart Association, 1975: 107–121.
232. Gamboa R, Hugenholtz PG, Nadas AS: Accuracy of the phonocardiogram in assessing severity of aortic and pulmonic stenosis. *Circulation* 1964; 30:35–46.
233. Henke RP, March HW, Hultgren HN: An aid to identification of the murmur of aortic stenosis. *Am Heart J* 1960; 60:354–363.
234. Tavel ME, Nasser WK: Murmur alternans in aortic stenosis. *Chest* 1970; 57:176–179.
235. Kroetz FW, Leonard JJ, Shaver JA, Leon DF, Lancaster JF, Beamer VL: The effect of atrial contraction on left ventricular performance in valvular aortic stenosis. *Circulation* 1967; 35:852–867.
236. Hancock EW: Differentiation of valvular and supravalvular stenosis. *Guys Hosp Rep* 1961; 110:1–30.
237. Bonner AJ, Sacks HN, Tavel ME: Assessing the severity of aortic stenosis by phonocardiography and external carotid pulse recordings. *Circulation* 1973; 48:247–252.
238. Kligfield P, Okin P: Effect of ventricular function on left ventricular ejection time in aortic stenosis. *Br Heart J* 1979; 42:438–441.
239. Thompson ME, Shaver JA: Aortic stenosis in the elderly. *Geriatrics* 1983; 38:50–65.
240. Aronow WS, Kronzon I: Correlation of prevalence and severity of valvular aortic stenosis determined by continuous-wave Doppler echocardiography with physical signs of aortic stenosis in patients aged 62 to 100 years with aortic systolic ejection murmurs. *Am J Cardiol* 1987; 60:399–401.
241. Vogelpoel L, Schrire V: Auscultatory and phonocardiographic assessment of pulmonary stenosis with intact ventricular septum. *Circulation* 1960; 22:55–72.
242. Vogelpoel L, Schrire V: Auscultatory and phonocardiographic assessment of Fallot's tetralogy. *Circulation* 1960; 22:73–89.
243. Zuberbuhler JR, Lenox CC, Neches WH, Park SC, Shaver JA: Auscultatory spectrum of the tetralogy of Fallot. In: Leon DF, Shaver JA (eds): *Physiologic Principles of Heart Sounds and Murmurs,* Monograph 46. New York, American Heart Association, 1975: 187–192.
244. Martin CE, Reddy PS, Leon DF, Shaver JA: Genesis, frequency and diagnostic significance of the ejection sound in adults with tetralogy of Fallot. *Br Heart J* 1973; 35:402–412.
245. Mills P, Wolfe C, Redwood D, Leech G, Craige E, Leatham A: Non-invasive diagnosis of subpulmonary outflow tract obstruction. *Br Heart J* 1980; 43:276–283.
246. Vogelpoel L, Schrire V, Nellen M, Swanepoel A: The value of amyl nitrite in the differentiation of Fallot's tetralogy and pulmonary stenosis with intact ventricular septum. *Am Heart J* 1959; 57:803–819.
247. Leatham A: Auscultation of the heart. *Lancet* 1958; 2:757–765.
248. O'Rourke RA, Crawford MH: Mitral valve regurgitation. *Curr Probl Cardiol* 1984; 9:1–52.
249. Brigden W, Leatham A: Mitral incompetence. *Br Heart J* 1953; 15:55–73.
250. Karliner JS, O'Rourke RA, Kearney DJ, Shabetai R: Hemodynamic explanation of why the murmur of mitral regurgitation is independent of cycle length. *Br Heart J* 1973; 35:397–401.
251. Nixon PGF: The third heart sound in mitral regurgitation. *Br Heart J* 1961; 23:677–689.
252. Burgess J, Clark R, Kamigaki M, Cohen K: Echocardiographic findings in different types of mitral regurgitation. *Circulation* 1973; 48:97–106.
253. Rivero Carvallo JM: Signo para el diagnostico de las insufficiencias tricuspideas. *Arch Inst Cardiol Mex* 1946; 16:531.
254. Leon DF, Leonard JJ, Lancaster JF, Kroetz FW, Shaver JA: Effect of respiration on pansystolic regurgitant murmurs as studied by biatrial intracardiac phonocardiography. *Am J Med* 1965; 39:429–441.
255. Wooley CF: The spectrum of tricuspid regurgitation. In: Leon DF, Shaver JA (eds): *Physiologic Principles of Heart Sounds and Murmurs,* Monograph 46. New York, American Heart Association, 1975: 139–148.
256. Leatham A, Segal BL: Auscultatory and phonocardiographic findings in ventricular septal defect with left-to-right shunt. *Circulation* 1962; 25:318–327.
257. Craige E: Phonocardiography in interventricular septal defects. *Am Heart J* 1960; 60:51–60.
258. Roger H: Recherches cliniques sur la communication congénitale des deux coeurs par inocclusion du septum interventriculaire. *Bull Acad Med (Paris)* 1879; 8:1074, 1189.
259. Wood P: The Eisenmenger syndrome or pulmonary hypertension with reversed central shunt. *Br Med J* September 1958; 701–709.
260. Vogelpoel L, Schrire V, Beck W, Nellen M, Swanepoel A: Atypical systolic murmur of minute ventricular septal defect and its recognition by amyl nitrite and phenylephrine. *Am Heart J* 1961; 62:101–118.
261. Leatham A: The spectrum of ventricular septal defect. In: Leon DF, Shaver JA (eds): *Physiologic Principles of Heart Sounds and Murmurs,* Monograph 46. New York, American Heart Association, 1975: 135–138.
262. Leonard JJ, Shaver JA: Acute mitral insufficiency. *Hosp Pract,* May 1985; 75–96.
263. Sutton GC, Craige E: Clinical signs of severe acute mitral regurgitation. *Am J Cardiol* 1967; 20:141–144.
264. Ronan JA Jr, Steelman RB, DeLeon AC, Waters TJ, Perloff JK, Harvey WP: The clinical diagnosis of acute severe mitral insufficiency. *Am J Cardiol* 1971; 27:284–290.
265. Roberts WC, Braunwald E, Morrow AG: Acute severe mitral regurgitation secondary to ruptured chordae tendineae. *Circulation* 1966; 33:58–70.
266. Morrow AG, Cohen LS, Roberts WC, Braunwald NS, Braunwald E: Severe mitral regurgitation following acute myocardial infarction and ruptured papillary muscle. *Circulation* 1968; 37–38(suppl 2):124–132.
267. Perloff JW, Roberts WC: The mitral apparatus: Functional anatomy of mitral regurgitation. *Circulation* 1972; 46:227–239.
268. DePace NL, Nestico PF, Morganroth J: Acute severe mitral regurgitation. Pathophysiology, clinical recognition, and management. *Am J Med* 1985; 78:293–306.
269. Shapiro HA, Weiss DR: Mitral insufficiency due to ruptured chordae tendineae. *N Engl J Med* 1959; 261:272–276.
270. Braunwald E: Mitral regurgitation. *N Engl J Med* 1969; 281:425–433.
271. Rios JC, Massumi RA, Breesmen WT, Sarin RK: Auscultatory features of acute tricuspid regurgitation. *Am J Cardiol* 1969; 23:4–11.
272. Amidi M, Irwin JM, Salerni R, Lavine SJ, Zuberbuhler JR, Shaver JA, et al: Venous systolic thrill and murmur in the neck: A consequence of severe tricuspid insufficiency. *J Am Coll Cardiol* 1986; 7:942–945.
273. Burch GE, DePasquale NP, Phillips HJ: Clinical manifestations of papillary muscle dysfunction. *Arch Intern Med* 1963; 112:158–163.
274. Humphries JO, McKusick VA: The differentiation of organic and innocent "systolic murmurs." *Prog Cardiovasc Dis* 1962; 5:152–171.
275. Reid JA, Humphries JO: Systolic clicks (so-called systolic gallops): A study of their clinical significance. *Bull Johns Hopkins Hosp* 1955; 97:177–181.
276. Barlow JB, Bosman CK, Pocock WA, Marchand P: Late systolic murmurs and non-ejection ("mid-late") systolic clicks. *Br Heart J* 1968; 30:203–217.
277. Rackley CE, Whalen RE, Floyd WL, Orgain ES, McIntosh HD: The precordial honk. *Am J Cardiol* 1966; 17:509–515.
278. Wigle ED, Sasson Z, Henderson MA, Ruddy TD, Fulop J, Rakowski H, et al: Hypertrophic cardiomyopathy. The importance of the site and the extent of hypertrophy. A review. *Prog Cardiovasc Dis* 1985; 28:1–83.

279. Shaver JA, Alvares RF, Reddy PS, Salerni R: Phonoechocardiography and intracardiac phonocardiography in hypertrophic cardiomyopathy. *Postgrad Med J* 1986; 62:537–543.
280. Murgo JP, Miller JW: Hemodynamic, angiographic and echocardiographic evidence against impeded ejection in hypertrophic cardiomyopathy. In: Goodwin JF (ed): *Heart Muscle Disease.* Lancaster, England, MIP Press Limited, 1985: 187–211.
281. Criley M, Siegel RJ: Has "obstructive" hindered our understanding of hypertrophic cardiomyopathy? *Circulation* 1985; 72:1148–1154.
282. Shah PM: Controversies in hypertrophic cardiomyopathy. *Curr Probl Cardiol* 1986; 11(10):563–613.
283. Braunwald E, Lambrew CT, Rockoff SD, Ross J, Morrow A: Idiopathic hypertrophic subaortic stenosis. I: A description of the disease based upon an analysis of 64 patients. *Circulation* 1964; 30(suppl 4):3–119.
284. Shaver JA, Salerni R, Curtiss EI, Follansbee WP: A clinical presentation and noninvasive evaluation of the patient with hypertrophic cardiomyopathy. In Shaver JA, Brest AN (eds): *Cardiomyopathies: Clinical Presentation, Differential Diagnosis, and Management. Cardiovascular Clinics.* Philadelphia, F.A. Davis, 1988: 149–192.
285. Murgo JP, Alter BR, Dorethy JF, Altobelli SA, McGranahan GM: Dynamics of left ventricular ejection in obstructive and nonobstructive hypertrophic cardiomyopathy. *J Clin Invest* 1980; 66:1369–1382.
286. Craige E, Millward DK: Diastolic and continuous murmurs. *Prog Cardiovasc Dis* 1971; 14:38–56.
287. Wood P: An appreciation of mitral stenosis. *Br Med J* 1954; 1:1051–1063.
288. Ueda H, Sakamoto T, Kawai N, Watanabe H, Uozumi Z, Okada R, et al: "Silent" mitral stenosis. Pathoanatomical basis of the absence of diastolic rumble. *Jpn Heart J* 1985; 6:206–219.
289. Criley JM, Chambers RD, Blaufuss AH, Friedman NJ: Mitral stenosis: Mechanico-acoustical events. In: Leon DF, Shaver JA (eds): *Physiologic Principles of Heart Sounds and Murmurs,* Monograph 46. New York, American Heart Association, 1975: 149–159.
290. Criley JM, Hermer AJ: The crescendo presystolic murmur of mitral stenosis with atrial fibrillation. *N Engl J Med* 1971; 285:1284–1287.
291. Hada Y, Amano K, Yamaguchi T, Takenaka K, Takahashi H, Takikawa R, et al: Noninvasive study of the presystolic component of the first heart sound in mitral stenosis. *J Am Coll Cardiol* 1986; 7:43–50.
292. Tavel ME: Presystolic murmur of mitral stenosis revisited. *J Am Coll Cardiol* 1986; 7:51–52.
293. Wooley CF, Fontana ME, Kilman JW, Ryan JM: Tricuspid sounds. Atrial systolic murmur, tricuspid opening snap, and right atrial pressure pulse. *Am J Med* 1985; 78:375–384.
294. Killip T III, Lukas DS: Tricuspid stenosis: Clinical features in 12 cases. *Am J Med* 1958; 24:836–852.
295. Sanders CA, Hawthorne JW, DeSanctis RW, Austen G: Tricuspid stenosis: A difficult diagnosis in the presence of atrial fibrillation. *Circulation* 1966; 33:26–33.
296. Craige E: Phonocardiography in interventricular septal defects. *Am Heart J* 1960; 60:51–60.
297. Ravin A, Darley W: Apical diastolic murmurs in PDA. *Ann Intern Med* 1950; 33:903–914.
298. Fortuin NJ, Craige E: Echocardiographic studies of genesis of mitral diastolic murmurs. *Br Heart J* 1973; 35:75–81.
299. Coombs CF: *Rheumatic Heart Disease.* New York, William Wood, 1924: 190.
300. Flint A: On cardiac murmurs. *Am J Med Sci* 1862; 44:29–54.
301. Segal JP, Harvey WP, Corrado MA: The Austin Flint murmur: Its differentiation from the murmur of rheumatic mitral stenosis. *Circulation* 1958; 18:1025–1033.
302. Fortuin NJ, Craige E: On the mechanism of the Austin Flint murmur. *Circulation* 1972; 45:558–570.
303. Craige E: The Austin Flint murmur. In: Leon DF, Shaver JA (eds): *Physiologic Principles of Heart Sounds and Murmurs,* Monograph 46. New York, American Heart Association, 1970: 160–165.
304. Reddy PS, Curtiss EI, Salerni R, O'Toole JD, Griff FW, Leon DF, et al: Sound pressure correlates of the Austin Flint murmur: An intracardiac sound study. *Circulation* 1976; 53:210–217.
305. Rahko PS: Doppler and echocardiographic characteristics of patients having an Austin Flint murmur. *Circulation* 1991; 83:1940–1950.
306. Green EW, Agruss NS, Adolph RJ: Right-sided Austin Flint murmur. *Am J Cardiol* 1973; 32:370–374.
307. Harvey WP, Corrado MA, Perloff JK: "Right-sided" murmurs of aortic insufficiency. *Am J Med Sci* 1963; 245:533–543.
308. Sakamoto T, Kawai N, Uozumi Z, Yamada T, Inove K, Chang SY, et al: The point of maximum intensity of aortic diastolic regurgitant murmur. *Jpn Heart J* 1968; 9:117–133.
309. Sabbah HN, Khaja F, Anbe DT, Stein PD: The aortic closure sound in pure aortic insufficiency. *Circulation* 1977; 56:859–863.
310. Stembridge VA, Hejtmancik MR, Herrmann GR: Unusual musical murmurs of anterior cusp aortic regurgitation. Report of 10 cases. *Am Heart J* 1954; 48:163–172.
311. Steell G: The murmur of high pressure in the pulmonary artery. *Med Chron* 1888; 9:182.
312. Runco V, Molnar W, Meckstroth CV, Ryan JM: The Graham Steell murmur versus aortic regurgitation in rheumatic heart disease. *Am J Med* 1961; 31:71–80.
313. Perez JE, Smith CA, Meltzer VN: Pulmonic valve insufficiency: A common cause of transient diastolic murmurs in renal failure. *Ann Intern Med* 1985; 103:497–502.
314. Runco V, Levin HS: The spectrum of pulmonic regurgitation. In: Leon DF, Shaver JA (eds): *Physiologic Principles of Heart Sounds and Murmurs,* Monograph 46. New York, American Heart Association, 1975: 175–182.
315. Myers JD: The mechanisms and significances of continuous murmurs. In: Leon DF, Shaver JA (eds): *Physiologic Principles of Heart Sounds and Murmurs,* Monograph 46. New York, American Heart Association, 1975: 201–208.
316. Fowler NO, Gause R: The cervical venous hum. *Am Heart J* 1964; 67:135–136.
317. Tabatznik B, Randall TW, Hersch C: The mammary souffle of pregnancy and lactation. *Circulation* 1960; 22:1069–1073.
318. Hurst JW, Staton J, Hubbard D: Precordial murmurs during pregnancy and lactation. *N Engl J Med* 1958; 259:515–517.
319. Gibson GA: Lecture on patent ductus arteriosus. *Edinburgh Med J* 1900; 8:1–10.
320. Ongley PA, Rahimtoola SH, Kincaid OW, Kirklin JW: Continuous murmurs in tetralogy of Fallot and pulmonary atresia with ventricular septal defect. *Am J Cardiol* 1966; 18:821–826.
321. Victor S, Lakshmikanthan C, Shankar G, Parameswaran PG, Sreenivasan H, Sadasivan CS: Continuous murmur as sequel of augmented collateral circulation in suppurative lung disease: Report of 3 cases. *Chest* 1972; 62:504–505.
322. Minkoff SM, Fort ML, Sharp JT: Rupture of an aneurysm of the sinus of Valsalva into the right atrium. *Am J Cardiol* 1967; 19:278–284.
323. Ross J Jr, Braunwald E, Mason DT, Braunwald NS, Morrow AG: Interatrial communication and left atrial hypertension. A cause of continuous murmur. *Circulation* 1963; 28:853–860.
324. Keith JD, Rowe RD, Vlad P, O'Hanley JH: Complete anomalous pulmonary venous drainage. *Am J Med* 1954; 16:23–38.
325. Myers JD, Murdaugh HV Jr, McIntosh HD, Blaisdell RK: Observations on continuous murmurs over partially obstructed arteries. *Arch Intern Med* 1956; 97:726–737.
326. Edholm OG, Howarth S, Sharpey-Schafer EP: Resting blood flow and blood pressure in limbs with arterial obstruction. *Clin Sci* 1951; 10:361–367.
327. Spencer MP, Johnston FR, Meredith JH: Origin and interpretation of murmurs in coarctation of aorta. *Am Heart J* 1958; 56:722–736.
328. Dock W, Zoneraich S: Diastolic murmur arising in stenosed coronary artery. *Am J Med* 1967; 42:617–619.
329. Sangster JF, Oakley CM: Diastolic murmur of coronary artery stenosis. *Br Heart J* 1973; 35:840–844.
330. Cheng TO: Diastolic murmur caused by coronary artery stenosis. *Ann Intern Med* 1970; 72:543–546.

Chapter 12

Examination of the Retina

W. Banks Anderson, Jr., M.D.

Inspection of the smaller vessels of the body is possible in only three areas: the retina, the conjunctiva, and the nail beds. Helmholtz's gift of the ophthalmoscope has made the retina by far the easiest and most rewarding of these observation sites. Viewing this two-dimensional vascular display is generally much easier, especially in the aged, if the pupils are dilated. One drop of tropicamide 1% ophthalmic solution (Mydriacyl) will dilate the pupils in 15 or 20 min. Care should be taken to make pulse and blood pressure determinations prior to instillation of such rapidly acting mydriatics as both the pulse and the blood pressure may increase after absorption of the drops. Although complications of mydriasis are rare, patients in whom the iris seems closely apposed to the cornea or those with a history of closed-angle glaucoma are best left undilated.

Examination of the retina should proceed methodically. Best pupillary dilatation is maintained if the optic disk is observed first. Look for evidence of edema and blurred margins and for cupping with sharp contours. Rule out neovascularization or the pallor of optic atrophy. Next scan along the superior temporal arcade, inspecting the arteries carefully for embolic plaques at each bifurcation. Note the arteriovenous crossings for evidence of obscuration of the vein and for pronounced nicking and banking of the vessels. The lower arcade and the nasal vessels may be inspected next. Avoid the macular area until all else has been viewed, as the pupil constricts most intensely when this area is illuminated. To find diabetic microaneurysms early, look just temporal to the fovea along the horizontal raphe. To discover cotton-wool infarcts, look circularly around the disk two disk diameters out. With such a plan in mind, the retina can be efficiently searched for evidence of cardiovascular disease. (See Table 12-1.)

An appreciation of the pathophysiological variations in retinal architecture is essential for recognizing its disease processes. The following sections describe morphologic changes helpful in assessing the cardiac patient.

RETINAL VESSEL CALIBER CHANGES

Caliber changes along the course of a single artery or vein are of much greater significance than are estimates of arteriovenous ratios or absolute vascular diameter (see Plate VI, 12-1). Estimates of the degree of tortuosity or straightening are also generally valueless, except in the situation where the veins are large, dark, and tortuous. This constellation of findings implies outflow obstruction, arterial inflow obstruction, hypoxia, or all three.[1] Such dark and dilated veins may occur in patients with

TABLE 12-1
Retinal Topography

Finding	Most Common Location
Arteriovenous crossings	Upper temporal quadrant
Cotton-wool spots	Around optic disk
Hard exudates	Between disk and fovea
Microaneurysms	Temporal to fovea
Emboli	Arterial bifurcations
Diabetic new vessels	Nerve head and arcades

large right-to-left shunts and in the leukemias and hyperviscosity syndromes.

Autonomic innervation of the retinal vessels does not exist.[2] Nevertheless the retinal vessels may change in caliber both acutely and chronically. Autoregulation of the retinal vessels does occur, and oxygen is the most active vasomotor substance. With hyperoxia there is rapid constriction of both the arteries and veins, while in hypoxia vasodilatation occurs.[3] Elevated carbon dioxide tension is also a retinal vasodilator.[4] Striking clinical examples of these combined effects are the vasodilatation (darkening of the blood column) and retinal and disk edema seen in patients with marked pulmonary insufficiency and right-sided cardiac failure[5] and in children with cyanotic congenital heart disease.[6] At the opposite extreme, the marked vasoconstrictor effect of oxygen may produce retinal vasoobliteration in immature infants with resulting retinopathy of prematurity.

Estimates of arteriovenous ratios are of little clinical utility.[7] Of much greater significance are variations in the caliber of a single vessel. These changes may take the form of focal narrowing, sometimes called *beading* or *spasm*. Beading is produced by an abnormal constriction that may be contiguous with an abnormally dilated segment. Usually seen in the venous system, where there is venous outflow obstruction, such beading is particularly common in diabetic retinopathy. Beading of the arteries is *not* generally associated with systemic disease but is seen in congenital conditions such as von Hippel's angiomatosis, Coat's disease, and Leber's miliary aneurysms.

Segmental narrowing or spasm of the retinal vessels has been much described in the older literature. Most descriptions of rapid waves of "spasm" were probably observations of patients with moving fibrin or platelet emboli. Narrowing of the retinal vessels has been observed in response to injections of norepinephrine and angiotensin.[8] Autoregulatory narrowing of the retinal vessels is a response to hypertension and upon occasion may be focal. This narrowing is chronic, and "spasm" is not an apt description.

VASCULAR WALL THICKENING

Normally only the blood column is visible when the retinal vessels are viewed. When changes in the walls do occur, they are most visible along the sides of the vessels since in this location the tangential line of sight presents a greater thickness to the viewer. Vessels at the disk often appear sheathed. This normal variant may be associated with a veil of tissue in front of the disk (Bergmeister's papilla). More peripheral retinal vessels become sheathed or cuffed in response to intraocular inflammation, vasculitis, or multiple sclerosis. Fatty exudate (hard exudate) may collect along venous walls (never arteries), particularly in diabetic exudative retinopathy. These deposits are not intrinsic to the wall itself. After venous obstructive disease of some duration, a white uniform line may develop along either side of the retinal veins in the involved area. Ballantyne[9] terms this *halo sheathing*, and Kennedy and Wise[10] have found it to consist of increased collagen deposition in the vessel wall.

ARTERIOSCLEROSIS

Should the retinal arterial circulation be considered arterial or arteriolar? If vessel size is the criterion, then *arteriole* might be proper. Nevertheless, Hogan and Feeney[11] have demonstrated smooth-muscle cells several layers thick in the media of the retinal arterial vessels both posteriorly and in the periphery. We will therefore use the terms *arteriosclerosis* and *artery* without respect to the size of the vessels. In arteriosclerosis the medial smooth muscle (which may hypertrophy in chronic hypertension) becomes hyalinized with the deposition of collagen. As the wall thickens, the vessel takes on a burnished coppery luster that with further thickening may transmute to silver. Obscuration of the venous blood column at arterial crossings is early evidence of this process. Even when the artery walls become so thick as to resemble "silver wires," flow can ordinarily still be demonstrated by fluorescein angiography. The intensity of the light reflex from these older vessels is increased, although the width of the vascular light reflex itself does not appear to be related to age or blood pressure.[12]

ARTERIOVENOUS COMPRESSION

Arteriovenous compression, or "nicking," has as its histological basis the sharing by the artery and vein of a common adventitial sheath at their crossings. Arteriosclerotic thickening impedes venous outflow at these locations with venous tortuosity, engorgement, and darkening of the blood column distal to the compression. Where the vein dives beneath the thick artery wall, sometimes "banking" to intersect at right angles, its blood column is obscured and it appears nicked.

ATHEROSCLEROSIS

Atherosclerosis, or fatty infiltration of the intima, was once thought not to occur in the retina. Clinicopathologic confirmation of retinal atherosclerosis has been obtained.[13] Retinal atheromata have a predilection for the bifurcations and bends within the first two branches of the central retinal artery, appearing as segments of irregular yellowish sheathing and having the crystalline knobbiness of a salted pretzel stick. On occasion the thickening may progress to the point where no blood column is visible, although total obstruction is rare.

COTTON-WOOL SPOTS

Cotton-wool spots are generally a sign of serious systemic disease. They may be seen in patients with severe hypertension, blood dyscrasias, collagen diseases, or hemorrhagic shock. Cotton-wool spots are also frequently seen in patients with acquired immunodeficiency syndrome (AIDS).[14] They are almost invariably found within three disk diameters of the optic disk and have a feathery, woolly character because of their anterior involvement of the nerve fiber layer (see Plate VI, 12-2).

Cotton-wool "exudates" are *not* exudates but consist of a cluster of cell-like swollen ends of fragmented axones (cytoid bodies) in an area of edematous retina. They are evanescent and will often disappear in a few weeks, leaving behind no observable trace of their presence. Ischemia is almost certainly the cause of these spots, which may occur secondary to occlusion of peripapillary capillaries or occlusion of a small artery or secondary to hypoxia. The presence of these cotton-wool spots is usually indicative of serious systemic disease.

HARD EXUDATES

Hard exudates are most probably edema residues. They occur in situations where the vessels become leaky, and as the more watery component of the extravasation is resorbed, the lipid residue forms hard, yellow, waxy deposits. They may surround the leaking vessel in a circinate ring or may accumulate in the macula, radiating from the fovea in the spokes of a macular "star." Histologically found deep in the retina, these exudates will disappear in some months if the source of the leakage is eliminated. These exudates indicate a loss of vascular wall integrity and are associated with hypertension, diabetes, venous outflow obstruction, and retinal angiomas. They are not ischemic in origin but indicate chronic fluid extravasation and retinal edema.

MICROANEURYSMS

Microaneurysms are not unique to diabetes but occur in many disease states, including retinal venous obstructive disease, sickle cell disease, the dysproteinemias, Behçet's disease, sarcoidosis, and other forms of uveitis. A common factor in all these conditions seems to be the presence of both retinal hypoxia and viable capillary endothelial cells. Microaneurysms are outpouchings in capillary walls that range in size from 20 to 100 μm. Commonly found adjacent to zones of capillary obliteration, or "dropout," it has been suggested that they represent abortive attempts at revascularization of a compromised capillary bed. (See Plate VI, 12-3.) Their etiology is, however, still unknown.

NEOVASCULARIZATION

Neovascularization also occurs in conditions where microaneurysms are found. The new vessels generally originate from capillaries or from the venous side of the circulation and are associated with greater or lesser degrees of fibrosis. In all cases, however, the new vessels are incorporated in an associated fibrous membrane. Some of the channels appear to function as shunts and, in cases of venous outflow obstruction, may serve to bypass the obstructed site. Other neovascular channels branch in a fanlike fashion toward an avascular zone or forward into the vitreous cavity, proliferating along a posterior hyaloid membrane. Such a rete mirabile does not appear to have any shunting function and is more suggestive of an attempt at revascularization of an unperfused tissue. Clinically the likelihood of blinding vitreous hemorrhage is greatly increased in the presence of such neovascularization.[15]

RETINAL VESSEL LEAKAGE

Normally the retinal vessels are permeable only to quite small molecules. This *blood-retina barrier* is analogous to the blood-brain barrier and is facilitated by the overlapping of the endothelial cells and the tight endothelial cell junctions in retinal vessels. Enclosed within the basement membrane of the capillary is an intramural pericyte whose investment may contribute to the relative impermeability of these vessels.

The sodium fluorescein molecule normally does not traverse this vascular barrier, and by fluorescein angiography abnormal sites of leakage can be conveniently defined. With this technique, neovascular channels are found to leak profusely, as do microaneurysms. In severe hypertension small areas of leakage may be seen along tiny arteries in the vicinity of cotton-wool spots.[16] Vessels damaged by emboli may leak, as do obstructed veins or inflamed vessels. Retinal edema and hard exudates are the consequences of this leakage.

RETINAL HEMORRHAGE

Hemorrhage into the retina indicates further breakdown in the integrity of the vascular wall. When the hemorrhage occurs in the inner retina, as in hypertension, it assumes a feathery flame shape as it is molded and dispersed by the nerve fibers coursing toward the disk. Deeper hemorrhages, such as those in diabetics, take on a more rounded dot or blot shape. Diabetic neovascularization may result in large hemorrhages beneath the retinal internal limiting membrane or into the vitreous, which obscures the underlying retina. In obstructions of the central retinal vein, the fundus may be splattered with blood as if a tomato had ruptured on the disk. (See Plate VI, 12-4.) Small hemorrhages are difficult to differentiate from microaneurysms, but hemorrhages usually fade within several weeks while microaneurysms may persist for months to years.

Hemorrhage may occur *beneath* the retina and usually originates not from the retinal vessels but from proliferation of a choroidal neovascular membrane growing through Bruch's membrane. These hemorrhages commonly occur beneath the macula and may destroy central vision. They have the appearance of a gray-black mass with a red fringe and have been mistaken for malignant melanomas of the choroid.

VASCULAR OCCLUSION

When the central artery or one of its branches is occluded, the nonperfused retinal area becomes cloudy in a matter of minutes. At the fovea where the retina is one cell layer thick and nourished by the choroid, the normal color and transparency persist. By contrast with the surrounding pallor, the fovea then has a cherry-red appearance. Occlusion at the capillary level is identified by the surrounding microaneurysms or adjacent cotton-wool spots. With fluorescein angiography such areas can be directly identified by their lack of perfusion.

Occlusion of the central retinal vein results in retinal edema and the "squashed tomato" hemorrhages noted above (Plate VI, 12-4). Occlusions of branches of the central vein produce edema and hemorrhage in the drained area. These branch vein occlusions always occur at arteriovenous crossings. Examination of the retina of the opposite eye of such patients will generally reveal significant arteriovenous compression. As collateral drainage channels develop, the edema and hemorrhagic retinopathy subside, leaving white-walled veins, neovascularization, and microaneurysms in the affected area. Hemorrhage into the vitreous may occur as a late complication from the neovascularization. There is a very high incidence of diabetes and hypertension in patients with venous obstructive disease,[17] and retinal and systemic arteriosclerosis is usually present.

OPTIC DISK EDEMA

Increased intracranial pressure, retinal venous outflow obstruction, inflammation, and ischemia are the four major causes of optic disk edema. The term *papilledema* is reserved by ophthalmologists and neurologists for the form of disk edema that is the result of increased intracranial pressure. It therefore has an etiologic connotation and is not used generally to mean optic disk edema. Patients with papilledema see well, while other forms of disk edema are associated with poor vision. *Papillitis* is the term applied to inflammatory disk edema. Patients with ischemic optic neuritis commonly have a pale, edematous disk with an altitudinal field effect. When associated with elevations of the sedimentation rate, such patients should be suspected of having giant-cell arteritis (temporal arteritis). If this diagnosis can be established, steroid therapy is indicated to prevent visual loss in the opposite eye.

RETINAL DYSTROPHY

In the equatorial periphery can be seen the irregular pigment clumps typical of *retinitis pigmentosa*, or "night blindness." Such pigment spicules in association with bilateral palsies of ocular movement occur in Kearns-Sayre syndrome. Affected patients develop progressive atrioventricular block, which in turn may cause sudden death. The syndrome is now known to be the result of abnormal mitochondrial deoxyribonucleic acid (DNA).[18]

OPTIC ATROPHY

In eyes with retinal dystrophy, or with the resolution of disk edema in papillitis, or ischemic optic neuritis, the disk will become flat and pale. Both pallor and impaired visual function are necessary for the diagnosis of optic atrophy since both the color and vascularity of the disk are highly variable. If the disk is atrophic and cupped with a shift of the vessels to the nasal side, glaucoma should be suspected. Optic atrophy without cupping may indicate intracranial tumor and should be investigated. It is unlikely that tumor has caused the atrophy if vision was once poor and has returned to near-normal levels. This is the situation often observed in patients with demyelinating disease.

EMBOLISM

Embolism from the heart and great vessels occurs more commonly than is generally appreciated. A sudden increase in tinnitus in one ear, a fleeting woozy sensation, a scintillating scotoma, a transient monocular visual loss all may be symptoms of embolic ischemia. This clinical suspicion may be confirmed by ophthalmoscopy. In Table 12-2 we have listed characteristics of retinal emboli of cardiovascular significance. Of these, platelet emboli are at once the most common and the most evanescent. Within minutes after vision has returned, platelet emboli have usually broken into fragments too small to identify ophthalmoscopically. Most other emboli persist for days or years and are more lasting evidence of an embolic episode. Hollenhorst cholesterol plaques may be identified at the same bifurcations for months to years after the embolic shower.

Platelet emboli, Hollenhorst plaques (Fig. 12-1), and calcium emboli are usually seen along the course of a

TABLE 12-2
Emboli of Cardiovascular Significance

Type	Appearance	Significance
Platelet	Dull pink to gray often with associated fibrin	Downstream vegetations, mural thrombi
Hollenhorst plaque	Glistening yellow-orange plaques at bifurcations	Downstream atheroma (containing cholesterol)
Calcium plaque	Glistening white plaques	Calcific aortic stenosis
Roth spot	Hemorrhage with gray-white center (Plate VII, 12-5)	Blood dyscrasia or septic embolus as in subacute bacterial endocarditis (SBE)
Fat embolus	Fuzzy-bordered gray-white spot without hemorrhage	Severe trauma with long-bone fractures; prognosis grave
Myxoma	Disk edema, retinal edema in arterial supply zone	Life-threatening atrial myxoma

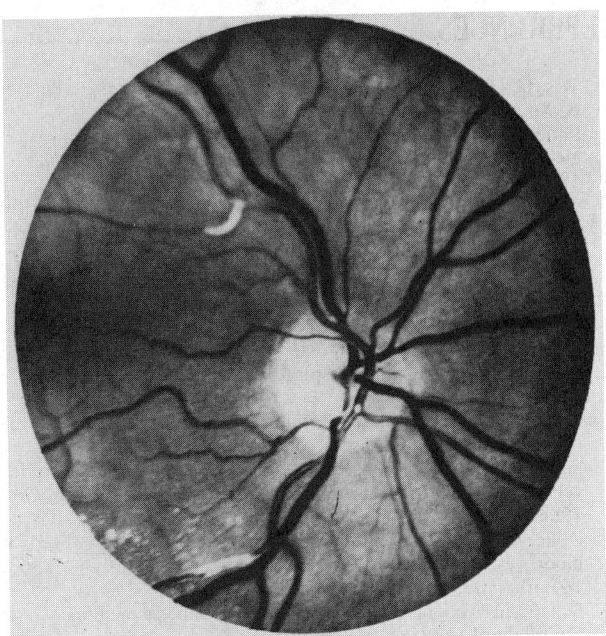

FIGURE 12-1 Retinal emboli often lodge at bifurcations, as in this patient with carotid atherosclerosis. Note that the embolic material often seems larger than the containing vessel, as in the embolus at the lower left edge of the photograph. Emboli may damage the vessel wall and cause leakage, as can be seen by the exudate deposited about the inferior embolus. Hollenhorst cholesterol plaques rarely completely obstruct arterial flow, and this patient maintained vision.

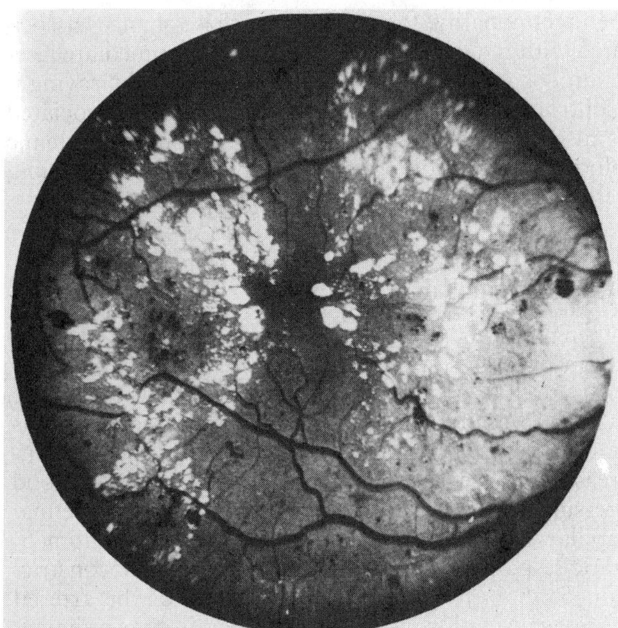

FIGURE 12-2 Exudative diabetic retinopathy, right eye, illustrating microaneurysms, dot and blot hemorrhages, and venous engorgement with extensive deposits of hard, yellow exudate.

retinal artery. Roth spots (see Plate VII, 12-5) and fat emboli may not appear to be intravascular and may not be associated with a vessel that is ophthalmoscopically visible.

Inspection of the retina may identify emboli that were deposited during cardiac catheterization or surgery. Valvular surgery is an especially likely source. In one series of 81 such patients, 12 percent were noted to have postoperative signs of retinal emboli.[19] The central retinal artery has been occluded by an embolus during cardiac catheterization.[20]

DISEASES

The eye is a major target for two extremely common diseases of cardiovascular significance: diabetes and hypertension. Blindness from the former now ranks as the second leading cause of acquired adult blindness in the United States, and these diabetic changes are commonly paralleled by severe renal and cardiac vasculopathy.

Diabetes

The average diabetic develops ophthalmoscopically visible retinal changes after 16 years of the disease. Focal loss of a portion of the capillary bed is followed by microaneurysm formation and vascular dilatation around the borders of the area of capillary dropout. (See Plate VI, 12-3.) Vascular leakage occurs with dot and blot hemorrhages and deposits of hard exudate (Fig. 12-2). New blood vessels develop along the vascular arcades and at the optic nerve head (Fig. 12-3). The proliferation of new blood vessels with their associated membranes often results in blinding hemorrhage into the vitreous cavity and tractional detachment of the retina.

The clinician must recognize early proliferative dia-

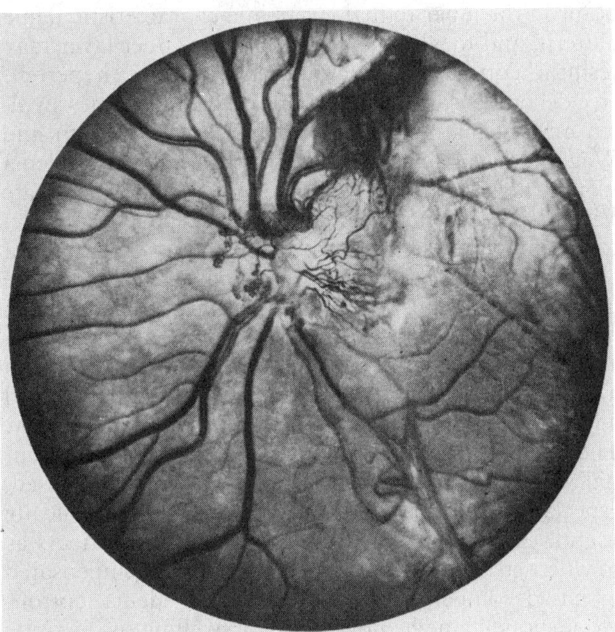

FIGURE 12-3 Proliferative diabetic retinopathy, left eye. There is extensive neovascularization of the disk with an associated small intravitreal hemorrhage that obscures the upper temporal vessels. Along the inferior termporal arcade is another area of neovascularization. These new vessels are incorporated in fibrous membranes that may tent up the vessels and cause traction detachments of the retina, as at the lower right edge of the photograph.

betic retinopathy, for not only are these changes associated with renal and cardiac disease, but immediate laser photocoagulation of the retina may be sight saving.[21] Control of the hypertension that is commonly associated is also of great importance, as elevations of systemic blood pressure compound the difficulty in controlling retinal vascular leakage. (See also Chap. 102.)

Systemic Arterial Hypertension

When the systemic blood pressure rises, the retinal circulation becomes especially vulnerable since its capillary pressure floor is determined by the intraocular pressure (about 16 mmHg) and not by the jugular or cavernous sinus pressure. The intraocular pressure does not increase in hypertension, and increases in systemic blood pressure would be directly reflected in increased retinal capillary perfusion pressure were it not for the homeostatic responses of the retinal vasculature. Vasoconstriction of the arterial tree and thickening of the arterial vessel walls with consequent reduction in lumen diameter are homeostatic responses to hypertension. (See Plate VI, 12-1 to 12-3; Plate VII, 12-6 to 12-8.) Arteriosclerotic narrowing of the vessels acts to insulate the capillary bed from the elevated arterial supply pressure. These arteriosclerotic changes are visible as narrowing, increases in central light reflexes, and copper and silver wiring of the arteries. (See Plate VII, 12-6.) If, however, increases in the systemic blood pressure are either very marked or very rapid, these homeostatic mechanisms are overwhelmed. The resulting decompensation of the capillary bed results in accumulations of fluid in the retina and optic nerve head. The aqueous portion of the fluid is more rapidly cleared than the lipid component, which accumulates as hard exudate. Hemorrhage may occur in the inner retinal layers in a characteristic flame pattern, and focal ischemia in the nerve fiber layer may result in cotton-wool microinfarcts. In severe hypertensive decompensation the optic nerve head becomes swollen and edematous. In the Scheie[22] and the Keith and Wagener[23] classifications, patients with disk edema would be assigned to the grade IV category. (See Plate VII, 12-6.) Patients with eclampsia or pheochromocytoma may have such marked and rapid elevations of capillary pressure that edema fluid floats the retina off the choroid, producing an exudative (nonrhegmatogenous) detachment of the retina.

Such retinal signs of capillary bed decompensation are usually paralleled by severe renal vasculopathy, and aggressive therapeutic efforts are indicated immediately. The likelihood that the patient suffers from a nonessential variety of hypertension is also markedly increased, especially if the patient is Caucasian.[24] It is clinically useful, therefore, to categorize hypertensive patients as to whether or not their retinal circulation is compensated or has decompensated with observable edema, cotton-wool spots, flame hemorrhages, or swelling of the optic disk.

REFERENCES

1. Wise GN, Dollery CT, Henkind P: *The Retinal Circulation.* Harper & Row, New York, 1971: 220–221.
2. Laties AM: Central retinal artery innervation: Absence of adrenergic innervation to the intraocular branches. *Arch Ophthalmol* 1967; 77:405–409.
3. Cusick PL, Benson OO, Boothby WM: Effect of anoxia and of high concentrations of oxygen on the retinal vessels. *Proc Mayo Clin* 1940; 15:500–502.
4. Frayser R, Hickam JB: Retinal vascular response to breathing increased carbon dioxide and oxygen concentrations. *Invest Ophthalmol* 1964; 3:427–431.
5. Stevens PM, Austen F, Knowles JH: Prognostic significance of papilledema in course of respiratory insufficiency. *JAMA* 1963; 183:161–164.
6. Petersen RA, Rosenthal A: Retinopathy and papilledema in cyanotic congenital heart disease. *Pediatrics* 1972; 49:243–249.
7. Stokoe NL, Turner RW: Normal retinal vascular pattern: Arteriovenous ratio as a measure of arterial caliber. *Br J Ophthalmol* 1966; 50:21–40.
8. Dollery CT, Hill DW, Hodge JV: The response of normal retinal blood vessels to angiotensin and noradrenaline. *J Physiol* 1963; 165:500–507.
9. Ballantyne AJ: The state of the retina in diabetes mellitus. *Trans Ophthalmol Soc UK* 1966; 66:503–543.
10. Kennedy JE, Wise GN: Retinochoroidal vascular anastomosis in uveitis. *Am J Ophthalmol* 1971; 71:1221–1225.
11. Hogan MJ, Feeney L: The ultrastructure of the retinal blood vessels. *J Ultrastruct Res* 1963; 9:10–28.
12. Brinchmann-Hansen O, Myhre K, Sandvik L: The light reflex in retinal vessels and its relations to age and systemic blood pressure. *Acta Ophthalmol* 1987; 65:206–212.
13. Brownstein S, Font RL, Alper MG: Atheromatous plaques of the retinal blood vessels: Histologic confirmation of ophthalmoscopically visible lesions. *Arch Ophthalmol* 1973; 90:49–52.
14. Rosenberg PR, Uliss AE, Friedland GH, Harris CA, Small CB, Klein, RS: Acquired immunodeficiency syndrome—ophthalmic manifestations in ambulatory patients. *Ophthalmology* 1983; 90:874–878.
15. The Diabetic Retinopathy Study Research Group: Four risk factors for severe visual loss in diabetic retinopathy. The third report from the diabetic retinopathy study. *Arch Ophthalmol* 1979; 97:654–655.
16. Hodge VJ, Dollery CT: Retinal soft exudates: A clinical study by color and fluorescence photography. *Q J Med* 1964; 33:117–131.
17. Quinlan PM, Elman MJ, Bhatt AK, Mardesich P, Enger C: The natural course of central retinal vein occlusion. *Am J Ophthal* 1990; 110:118–123.
18. Moraes CT, DiMauro S, Zeviani M, Lombes A, Shanske S, Miranda AF, et al: Mitochondrial DNA deletions in progressive external ophthalmoplegia and Kearns Sayre syndrome. *N Engl J Med* 1989; 320:1293–1299.
19. Pe'er J, Milgalter E, Matmoros N, Silberman S, Vidaurri L: Retinal emboli after open heart surgery (letter). *Arch Ophthalmol* 1989; 107:317.
20. Stefansson E, Coin T, Lewis WR, Belkin RN, Behar VS, Morris JJ, et al: Central retinal artery occlusion during cardiac catheterization. *Am J Ophthalmol* 1985; 99:586–589.
21. The Diabetic Retinopathy Study Research Group: Photocoagulation treatment in proliferative diabetic retinopathy. The second report of diabetic retinopathy study findings. *Ophthalmology* 1978; 85:82–106.
22. Scheie HG: Evaluation of ophthalmoscopic changes of hypertension and arteriolar sclerosis. *Arch Ophthalmol* 1953; 49:117–138.
23. Keith NM, Wagener HP, Barker NW: Some different types of essential hypertension: Their course and prognosis. *Am J Med Sci* 1939; 197:332–343.
24. Davis BA, Crook JE, Vestal RE, Oates JA: Prevalence of renovascular hypertension in patients with grade III or IV hypertensive retinopathy. *N Engl J Med* 1979; 301:1273–1276.

SECTION B

Frequently Performed Diagnostic and Monitoring Procedures

Chapter 13

The Resting Electrocardiogram

Agustin Castellanos, M.D. ■ *Kenneth M. Kessler, M.D.* ■ *Robert J. Myerburg, M.D.*

What is commonly called electrocardiogram (ECG) is the graph obtained when the electrical potentials of an electrical field originating in the heart are recorded at the body surface.[1-3] Emphasis should be placed on the fact that only potential differences in the field are registered since the ECG does not record *directly* the electrical activity of the heart itself. Classically, there are two major subdivisions of clinical electrocardiography[4]: (a) the analysis of arrhythmias (dealt with in Chap. 36) and (b) the study of the resting 12- (and occasionally more) lead ECG, which will be discussed in this chapter.

Although the ECG gives very useful clinical information, it only provides an approximation of the voltage produced by the source. Unfortunately, the ECG has not been able to achieve major *new* insights into its own basic theoretic limitations, which some have considered as the solutions of the "forward" problem and the "inverse" problem of electrocardiography.[1,2] Whereas the former seeks the description of a specific electrocardiographic pattern in response to a specific local or regional intracardiac change in electrical activity, the inverse problem seeks to predict the behavior of the cardiac generator from potentials recorded at the body surface.[1,2]

Despite these limitations, the ECG has many uses: It may serve as an independent marker of myocardial disease; it may reflect anatomic, hemodynamical, molecular, ionic, and drug-induced abnormalities of the heart; and it may provide information that is essential for the proper diagnosis and therapy of many cardiac[1] problems.[4] (See also Chap. 36.) In fact, it is the most commonly used laboratory procedure for the diagnosis of heart disease. While there are no complications related to the technique per se (by virtue of being a noninvasive procedure), underreading or misreading due to insufficient knowledge of pathological conditions, overreading due to inability to recognize technical errors, and most important, failure to correlate ECG findings with the clinical findings may result in iatrogenic heart disease. Every physician interpreting ECGs as well as those learning electrocardiographic interpretation should read the Guidelines for Electrocardiography of the American College of Cardiology, American Heart Association Task Force.[4] In fact, this also applies to paramedical personnel (nurses and technicians) having anything to do with ECGs.

VENTRICULAR DEPOLARIZATION AND REPOLARIZATION

Fluxes of ions across the cell membranes cause the differences in voltage between resting and activated myocardial cells. (See also Chap. 34.) To understand the somewhat complex study of the electrical forces produced by the heart as a whole at the body surface, it has been conventional to first discuss the electrical properties of a hypothetical muscle strip from the free wall of the left ventricle extending from endocardium to epicardium.[5-14]

In the resting or polarized state, the charges are at rest. A unipolar electrode facing the epicardial side of the strip, such as V_6, registers an isoelectric line.[5-13] If activation of this relatively large muscle strip starts in the endocardial side, it initiates the process called depolarization.[5-13] The *sequence* of this process is thus from endocardium to epicardium. Depolarization has been described as a moving wave *with the positive charges in front of* the negative charges. The previously mentioned lead V_6

overlying the epicardium of the left ventricle will record a positivity because it consistently faces positive charges throughout the entire depolarization sequence.[5-13] On the other hand, the *sequence* of ventricular repolarization is from epicardium to endocardium.[5-13] The *negative charges,* however, travel *in front* since repolarization tends to reestablish the resting, polarized state of the previously depolarized cells. As a consequence of the latter, V_6 will record a positive deflection (T wave) because it constantly faces positive charges throughout the entire repolarization sequence.

The earlier epicardial onset of repolarization has been attributed to the shorter duration of repolarization that epicardial cells have in comparison to endocardial cells. Thus, repolarization finishes at the epicardium while it still has not been completed at the endocardium. Hence, the *sequence* of repolarization is, as previously noted, from epicardium to endocardium. In contrast, in isolated (small) muscle strips the *sequence* of repolarization is from endocardium to epicardium (see "Ventricular Gradient" below).

ELECTROCARDIOGRAPHIC LEADS

To record an ECG an electric circuit between the heart and the electrocardiograph must be completed.[11] For this purpose, electrodes are placed on different parts of the body surface and are connected to the instrument by means of cables.[11] Thus, the whole system consists of an instrument, electrodes, cables, and leads.

Bipolar Standard Leads

An electrocardiographic lead can be defined as a pair of terminals with designated polarity, each of which is connected either directly or via a passive-active network to recording electrodes.

In 1913, Einthoven et al.[3] developed a method of studying the electrical activity of the heart by representing it graphically in a two-dimensional geometric figure, namely an equilateral triangle. While this is not strictly (mathematically) true, it has provided the clinician with a practical point with which to work. Of the many objections held against the theory, none has done away with it.[9,13] There are several simplifying assumptions upon which Einthoven's hypothesis is founded[3,13]:

- The body is a homogeneous volume conductor. Although the conductivity of the various tissues is not the same, the differences are not great enough to invalidate that the body can be considered as a homogeneous volume conductor.
- The sum of all the electric forces, or the mean of all the forces generated during the cardiac cycle, can be considered as originating in a dipole located in the electrical center of the heart.
- Electrodes placed on the right arm (RA), left arm (LA), and left leg (LL) are used to pick up the potential variations on these extremities. Standard (bipolar) leads (I, II, and III) are obtained by recording, respectively, the potential differences between LA and RA, LL and RA, and LL and LA. These leads record potential variations in the frontal plane only.
- Attachment between these limb electrodes, on the forearms and limbs, corresponds to a position in the root of the corresponding limb. For example, an electrode in the right forearm records the electrical activity that reaches the right shoulder. It should be pointed out that when the electrodes are placed proximally to the roots of the extremities, they lose their relatively "far" distance from the heart. Hence, Einthoven's equilateral theory does not hold. The latter is of importance to understand why leads placed proximally to the roots of the extremities, as those used for coronary care unit and Holter monitoring, by being only "equivalent" to the corresponding bipolar leads, are in some cases markedly different than the "true" standard bipolar leads.

Wilson Central Terminal

The sum of the potentials from RA, LA, and LL is equal to zero throughout the cardiac cycle with respect to any point at the body surface.[3,5,6,13] If leads are connected to electrodes at these points, their potential is zero with respect to any other electrode on the body surface. When this common point—Wilson's central terminal—is attached to the negative pole of the electrocardiographic machine through 5000-Ω resistors and an "exploring" electrode is connected to the positive pole, the potential variations recorded will be those of the latter only. A lead taken by this method is called a *unipolar* lead. Actually the central terminal is not zero because the right arm, left arm, and left leg are not equidistant from each other and from the heart; the body tissues vary in resistance; and the heart and the extremities do not lie in exactly the same plane in the body. The potential of the central terminal has been said to average around 0.3 mV.[9]

Unipolar Extremity Leads

Unipolar extremity leads were initially recorded by a system in which the central terminal of Wilson constituted the indifferent electrode and the exploring electrode was one of the three of the limb electrodes. It is important to understand that a lead is called indifferent if it approximates, for arbitrary sources in the heart, the potential existing at an infinite distance from these sources. Such leads were known as V_R, V_L, and V_F. At present, unipolar extremity leads are obtained by disconnecting the input to the central terminal of Wilson from the extremity being explored. This results in a one-and-a-half increase in their voltage. These *augmented* (a) extremity leads are the ones usually used for clinical electrocardiography and are labeled aV_R, aV_L, and aV_F.[5,9,13]

Unipolar Precordial Leads

The unipolar precordial ECG is obtained by placing the exploring electrode (connected to the positive pole of the electrocardiograph) on the classical six locations of the anterior and left portions of the chest.[5,6,13] The central terminal is used as the indifferent electrode. Unipolar leads made by this method are prefixed by the letter V (which stands for voltage) followed by subscript numbers 1 through 6, which indicate the corresponding chest sites. Precordial leads yield a positive deflection when facing positive charges and negative deflections when facing negative charges.[5,13] They do this according to what Wilson called the *solid-angle concept*.[5,13] A solid angle is merely an imaginary cone extending from the site in the chest throughout the heart. The precordial electrode is at its apex, and its base is at the opposite epicardial surface.[13] This concept is most important to understand precordial lead morphologies. For example, a lead displaying an old (Q-wave) infarction may show changes consistent with a new infarction. This occurs because the solid angle subtended by the corresponding lead explores more than the region generating the old scar.

Precordial leads record the electrical activity from the regions of the heart over which they are placed as well as from distant regions.[5] Thus, if V_2 is placed over (thereby facing) the right ventricle, part of the initial positive ventricular deflection reflects right ventricular activation, with the corresponding electrical forces moving toward the electrode.[13] Most portions of the terminal S wave represent activation of muscle other than the right ventricle (septum and free left ventricular wall), reflecting electric forces moving away from the electrode.[13] Lead V_2 is a right ventricular lead only because the electrode faces the right ventricle, not due to the fact that it just records the electrical activity of the right ventricle. For practical purposes, the peak of the r (or R) wave in this and all other precordial leads gives a rough estimate of the moment of arrival of excitation (intrinsicoid deflection) at the muscle underneath the electrode.[13] But this encompasses a considerable amount of muscle fibers (given by the solid-angle concept), in fact a greater amount than if the electrode is placed directly on the epicardial surface.[13] In the latter case, the moment of arrival of excitation at the electrode affects lesser number of fibers and is thus given by the intrinsic deflection.[13]

NORMAL ACTIVATION OF THE HEART: VENTRICULAR DEPOLARIZATION

After emerging from the sinus node, the cardiac impulse propagates throughout the atria in its journey toward the atrioventricular (AV) node. The *normal* P wave (resulting from activation of the myocardium of both atria) is a consequence of but does not directly represent sinus node activity. During sinus rhythm, the right atrium is activated before the left atrium.[6] This explains why high-fidelity recordings of the P waves of some normal persons show a small notch at the top. The latter simply reflects the normal asynchrony existing between both atria.[6] Because of the anatomic position of the sinus node, the sequence of atrial depolarization occurs in an inferior, leftward, and somewhat posterior direction. The normal P waves are always positive in leads I, II, aV_F, and V_3 to V_6 and negative in lead aV_R. According to the anatomic position of the heart, the P wave may be diphasic in V_1, III, and aV_L or negative in the latter lead. Atrial repolarization, also called T_a, is directly opposite in polarity to the P wave.[6,11] It is usually not seen because it coincides with the PR segment (not to be confused with the PR interval, as defined below) and QRS complex. Since the cardiac impulse reaches the AV node before the end of atrial depolarization, arrival of excitation at the AV node occurs at an undetermined moment (which can be roughly estimated by catheter recordings) within but before the end of the P wave.[14]

Activation of the ordinary ventricular muscle (onset of the QRS complex) starts as soon as the impulse emerging from the most distal ramifications of the bundle branches depolarizes a sufficiently large number of cells.[6,7,11] Therefore, the PR interval (used to estimate AV conduction time) includes conduction through the "true" AV structures (AV node, His bundle, bundle branches, and main divisions of the left bundle branch) as well as through those parts of the atria located between sinus and AV nodes.[8]

Conventional electrocardiographic theory holds that the onset of ventricular depolarization (given by the beginning of the normal q wave) reflects activation of the left side of the interventricular septum. This has been attributed to the fact that the left bundle system is shorter than the right bundle branch.[8,15] In addition, the large fanlike distribution of the ramifications of the fascicles of the left bundle branch on the left septal surface produces activation of a greater number of ordinary muscle cells per unit of time.[8,15] For this reason, the normal initial depolarization is oriented from left to right, therefore explaining the small q wave in lead V_6 and the small r wave in V_1. After the cardiac impulse descending through the right bundle branch reaches the right septal surface, the interventricular septum is activated in both directions. Septal activation is thereafter encompassed within or neutralized by free-wall activation. The most distal ramifications of both bundle branches (Purkinje fibers) form networks within the subendocardial regions of both ventricular walls. The latter are activated as soon as the multiple ramifications emerge from the Purkinje fibers.[15] The greater number of ordinary muscle fibers of the thicker left ventricular free wall explains why left ventricular free-wall events overpower those of the interventricular septum and right ventricular free wall.

ELECTRICAL AXIS

The electrical axis (EA) may be defined as a vector originating in the center of Einthoven's equilateral triangle.[3,13] A vector is a mathematical value expressed as an arrow that has magnitude, sense, and direction. On the other hand, scalar values only have magnitude. Moreover, a vector is a term for force, and since all electrocardiography deals with electrical forces, all electrocardiography can be considered vectorial. In practice, however, the term *vectorial* is used when referring to forces represented by arrows and loops rather than by complexes and waves.

When applied to the EA, the vector that represents it also gives the direction of the activation process as projected in the plane of the limb leads. Its length represents the manifest potential of the dipole in the center of the triangle. These general considerations apply either to the instantaneous EA (the vector indicating the direction of the impulse at the instant at which it is determined) as well as the mean EA (which is the resultant of all instantaneous electrical axes). Although the term EA can be used in reference to any of the major components of the ECG (P, T, or QRS), it is generally applied to the QRS.

There are many methods for determining the mean EA. The one recommended by electrocardiographers of the classical school consists of calculating the net areas enclosed by the QRS complex in leads I, II, and III.[3,6,7,12,13] The net area is the absolute sum of the positive and negative areas of the QRS complex in the corresponding lead. One of the drawbacks of this method is that the absolute values of the net area cannot be determined *accurately* by inspection. Since the absolute magnitude of the EA is not of fundamental clinical importance, it has been recommended that arbitrary units be used. When this is done, the results can be counterchecked by using Einthoven's law. For example, if in a given case, lead I is +4 units, lead II is +2 units, and lead III is −2 units, the calculation is accurate since the sum of leads I and III (+4 plus −2) must always equal lead II (+2). After having determined the net area, the results are plotted on the sides of the triangle, and perpendiculars are dropped from two or all three leads. The perpendiculars will meet at a point away from the center of the triangle. A line drawn from the latter to the former defines the mean EA.

A simpler, though less precise, method of calculating the quadrant (or parts of a quadrant) in which the EA is located consists of using the maximal QRS deflection in leads I and aV_F and, when necessary, lead II (Fig. 13-1). This method is inexact from the mathematical viewpoint but has the value of simplicity.[15,16]

Ventricular Repolarization

Although the depolarization process in the free left ventricular wall has been extensively studied, less known is how repolarization spreads throughout the interventricular septum and both ventricles.[12,13] This is probably related to the fact that in these structures repolarization is not a propagated process in the sense that depolarization is. It is for this reason that it is slower (takes longer time) and has a smaller voltage than depolarization. Moreover, it does not follow the same pathways.[12]

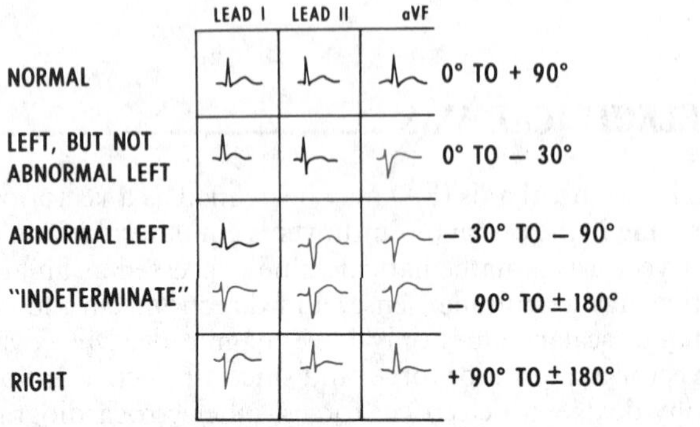

	LEAD I	LEAD II	aVF	
NORMAL				0° TO + 90°
LEFT, BUT NOT ABNORMAL LEFT				0° TO − 30°
ABNORMAL LEFT				− 30° TO − 90°
"INDETERMINATE"				− 90° TO ± 180°
RIGHT				+ 90° TO ± 180°

FIGURE 13-1 Determination of the quadrant, including parts of the left superior quadrant, in which the electrical axis can be located according to maximal ventricular deflections. The "indeterminate" quadrant is also called "right superior" and "northwest."

VENTRICULAR GRADIENT

The methods used to calculate the EA of the QRS complex can also be used to determine the T- and P-wave axis. The important relationship between the EA of the QRS complex and the T wave can be expressed by the *ventricular gradient.*[17] In contrast to what occurs in an epicardial-to-endocardial muscle strip (as previously mentioned), in the isolated muscle strip the *sequence* of ventricular depolarization occurs in the same direction as that of repolarization.[12] Although the QRS and T deflections have opposite polarity, the algebraic sum of QRS and T *areas* is zero. In the human heart, however, not only is the sequence different, but the pathways of ventricular depolarization and repolarization are not exactly the same.[12] Thus, the algebraic sum of QRS and T *areas* is no longer zero. Therefore, a gradient is said to exist. The ventricular gradient can be calculated by determining the electrical axis of the QRS and T (using *areas*) and then obtaining the resultant by the parallelogram method. Wilson considered that the ventricular gradient could be of help in determining between ischemic (symmetrical) T-wave inversion (primary changes) and T-wave changes due to abnormalities in depolarization such as bundle branch block, ventricular hypertrophy, ventricular pacing, and preexcitation syndromes (secondary changes).[12,13,17] In practice, calculation of the ventricular gradient is difficult and time consuming since it definitely has to be determined by areas and not maximal amplitude.

Challenges to Ventricular Gradient Concept: Electrotonic Modulation of T Waves and Cardiac Memory

According to Rosenbaum et al.,[18] the classical concept only applies to acute experiments and transient depolarization changes. These authors studied the prolonged depolarization occurring during long periods of ventricular stimulation and found two types of altered ventricular repolarization. One, corresponding to Wilson's classical theory, was transient and proportional in magnitude to the QRS complex but of opposite polarity. The other required a longer time (even days) to reach maximal effect as well as to disappear, becoming apparent only when normal activation recurred. The latter type was attributed to modulated electrotonic interactions occurring during cardiac activation in such a way that repolarization was accelerated at ventricular sites where depolarization begins and delayed in areas where depolarization terminates. T-wave changes occurring after the disappearance of prolonged depolarization showed accumulation and memory that persisted for days and weeks after the QRS complexes had again become narrow (see section on secondary ST-T-wave changes).[18] Evidence of electrotonic interaction operating under these circumstances has not been conclusively proven in the human heart.

ABNORMAL ST-SEGMENT CHANGES

In orthodox electrocardiographic language *injury* implies *abnormal* ST-segment changes, *necrosis* implies *abnormal* Q waves, and *ischemia* implies *symmetrical* T-wave inversion (or elevation).[5-7,9-13,16] Following conventional electrocardiographic theory, several authors consider that electrocardiographic "injury" occurs because the affected cells are unable to maintain their normal polarization during diastole.[5-7,12,16,19] Various hypotheses have been postulated to explain how this diastolic hypopolarization or generalized diastolic depolarization is manifested as abnormal ST-segment shifts in the surface ECG (Fig. 13-2).[20-22]

One hypothesis is based on the existence of a diastolic current of "injury." During the control (diastolic) period, both membrane resting potential and surface ECG baseline are at their normal level. At the onset of injury, the resting intracellular potential decreases (for example, from −90 to −70 mV) and the ECG baseline shifts

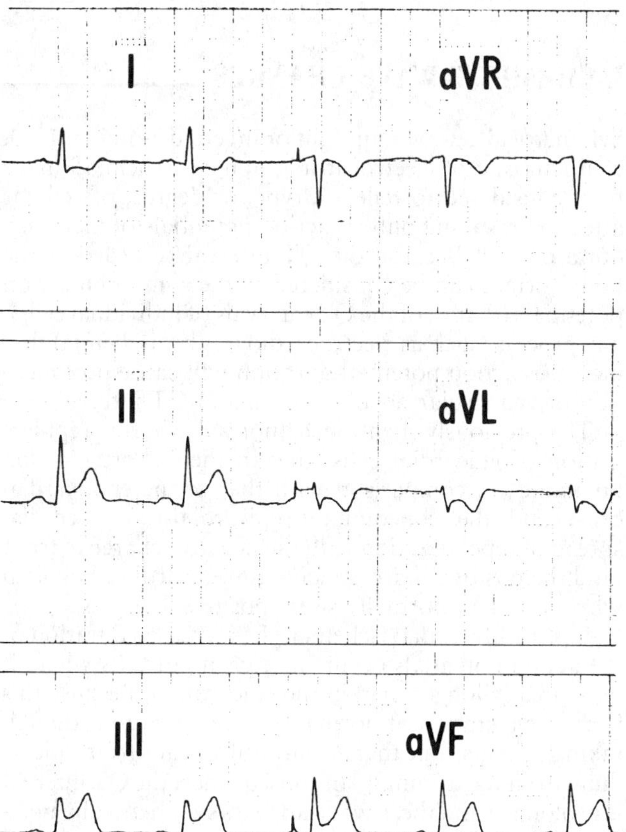

FIGURE 13-2 Acute inferior (diaphragmatic) myocardial infarction showing "indicative" ST-segment elevation in leads facing the inferior wall (II, III, and aV_F). Reciprocal changes are seen in the diametrically opposed leads (I and aV_L) located in the same (frontal) plane.

below its preinjury level. Because the injured cells leak negative ions, their *exterior* becomes relatively negative (or less positive) than that of the normal cells. Thus, a "current of injury" flows between the negative ("injured") zone and the positive (normal) region.[10] This produces a negative displacement of the surface electrocardiographic *baseline* in the leads facing the injured region.

In the surface ECG, depolarization (by virtue of the electrical negativization of the nonaffected area) practically reduces the potential difference between noninjured and injured regions. Therefore, the ST segment remains at the preinjury level, which is relatively *elevated* in reference to the injury baseline. Consequently, the ST-segment appears to be abnormally displaced above the latter. Note that the apparent presence of a systolic current of injury actually reflects disappearance of the diastolic current of injury. Finally, after the end of repolarization, the current of injury between injured and noninjured regions is reestablished and the ECG baseline is again depressed (as it was immediately before depolarization). Since the precise moment at which injury starts is not recorded in the surface ECG, the baseline that is almost invariably recorded is the postinjury baseline, which has been placed at an apparently adequate position by the recording instrument or by the ECG technician.[10]

It also has been shown that the abnormal ST-segment elevation in leads facing the affected zone does not merely represent the (passive) return of the baseline to its preinjury level but reflects a true, active, positive displacement.[10,20-23] Thus, when depolarization of both normal and injured regions has occurred, the surface of the normal cells will (on account of their greater initial polarization) be able to accumulate more negative ions. Hence, the normal regions become more negative than the injured regions, which are relatively more positive. In consequence, the ST segment becomes actively elevated above and beyond the preinjured baseline because of the relative potential difference existing at the end of depolarization. Most likely, injury reflects both disappearance of diastolic baseline shifts plus active ST elevation.[10,22]

According to the current-of-injury theory, this process results in ST-segment elevation when the injured muscle is located between normal muscle and the corresponding precordial electrode. On the other hand, ST-segment depression occurs when normal muscle is located between the injured tissue and the corresponding electrode.[10,12]

The precise moment at which ST-segment elevation due to acute myocardial infarction (MI) becomes irreversible has been greatly debated; several authors consider that this occurs at 6 months, others at 3 months, and some even at 2 weeks.[23] Mills et al.[24] found that patients with ST-segment elevation 2 weeks after an infarction also had ST-segment elevation at 6 months. In general, chronic ST-segment elevation indicates the existence of a large infarction, mainly anterior, usually with ventricular aneurysm.[23]

The mechanism of abnormal ST-segment elevation in anatomically defined ventricular aneurysms has not been fully established. Some authors consider that it results from the earlier repolarization of a ring of persistently viable (but nevertheless affected) tissue surrounding the aneurysm.[10] For other investigators, chronic ST-segment elevation reflects functional (echocardiographic) dyskinesia, thus not necessarily being due to a pathological ventricular aneurysm.[8,25]

Coronary artery disease is the most frequent cause of abnormal ST-segment changes. The latter, however, can also be due to epicardial injury due to pericarditis or subendocardial injury resulting from the effects of drugs.

ABNORMAL Q WAVES

Abnormal Q waves appearing several hours after total occlusion of a coronary artery result from the necrosis secondary to the decreased blood supply. The number of affected cells has to be large enough so as to produce changes reflected at the body surface. In general, the depth of the Q wave is proportional to wall thickness involvement.[7] Thus, in leads I and V_4 to V_6, a QS complex reflects transmural necrosis. The duration of the Q wave is proportional to the extent of the area of necrosis parallel to the epicardial surface.[7] If the latter starts in the subendocardium and extends toward (but not quite reaching) the epicardium, the corresponding leads will record QR or Qr complexes depending on the amount of living tissue located between dead tissue and recording electrode. Therefore, abnormal Q waves may occur in infarctions that are not completely transmural.[7] In this chapter, however, abnormal Q waves will be considered as reflecting transmural involvement.

In the course of the clinical entity known as acute MI, persisting Q waves are usually (but not invariably, as will be discussed subsequently) due to anatomic (lack of blood flow–related) necrosis. Abnormal Q waves can also occur transiently in unstable angina, Prinzmetal's angina, coronary artery spasm (without chest pain), and exercise-induced ischemia. This has been attributed to an intensity of cellular affectation ("injury") severe enough to produce a significant degree of hypopolarization (to, let us say, around -60 mV). Because the cells become electrically unexcitable (even though they are not anatomically, irreversibly necrotic),[7,8,15,16] abnormal Q waves occur. Spontaneous recanalization of an occluded vessel, spontaneous reversion of the ischemia, or spasm and interventions (pharmacologic or mechanical) that improve cellular metabolism and oxygenation can restore the normal polarization. If these cells become again excitable, the abnormal Q waves may disappear or vanish.[16,26]

Ischemic necrosis takes some hours to appear.[5] This contrasts with the accelerated occurrence of abnormal Q waves in the majority of patients with Q-wave MI after successful thrombolysis or following coronary artery angioplasty performed early in the course of the process. The genesis of these Q waves is not well understood.[26] Some authors consider them an expression of the acceleration of necrosis secondary to explosive cell swelling in already irreversibly injured tissue.[26] Because these Q waves also tend to disappear quickly, other authors consider that they reflect factors other than myocardial necrosis, such as reversal of regional dysmetabolism or the occurrence of transient interstitial ischemia or hemorrhage.[27]

Q waves that persist for more than 1 day may result from other causes than necrosis. Profound and prolonged ischemia can cause myocardial stunning with reversible functional, metabolic, ultrastructural, and electrophysiological abnormalities.[28] Thus, transient Q waves may be the electrocardiographic counterpart (electrical stunning) of the corresponding mechanical stunning.[26,29] It is possible for myocardial stunning to lag behind electrical recovery.[26]

Myocardial stunning should be differentiated from *myocardial hibernation.* The latter is a term used in reference to mechanical dysfunction of an ischemic area that is not transient but chronic.[30,31] Although the electrocardiographic counterpart of this type of mechanical dysfunction requires further studies, it is conceivable that (in some cases) the disappearance of chronic Q waves after coronary artery bypass surgery with improvement of wall motion abnormalities indicates that these Q waves were due not to cellular death but to cellular hibernation.[26] (See also Chaps. 57 to 60.)

Finally, abnormal Q waves need not be the end result of coronary artery disease since they may be seen after primary (due to infections or drugs) cellular necrosis (with angiographically normal coronary arteries) and in other pathological processes such as myocardial infiltration and certain types of interventricular septal hypertrophy.

ISCHEMIC T-WAVE CHANGES

Symmetrical T waves, upright or inverted as in Fig. 13-3, characteristic of electrocardiographic "ischemia," have been considered to reflect a type, or degree, of cellular affection resulting only in action potentials of increased duration.[7,10,16] Because the QT interval recorded at the body surface can be considered as the sum of all action potentials (that is, of the QT intervals of individual cells), any process (such as electrocardiographic ischemia) that increases action potential duration will cause prolongation of ventricular depolarization and QT interval.

The previously mentioned (normal) shorter repolarization of epicardial cells (due to their shorter action potentials, in comparison with that of the endocardial cells) and the concomitant epicardial-to-endocardial spread of repolarization with the negative charge in front (and the positive charges facing the epicardium) explain why V_5 and V_6 normally show positive T waves.[7,10]

In subendocardial ischemia, the increased duration of the action potentials occurs in a group of cells where it was already longer than in the epicardium. Because this is an exaggeration of normality, repolarization (though taking a longer time than usual) still spreads from epicardium to endocardium.[7,10] In consequence, the QT interval is prolonged and the T wave appears symmetrically positive. On the other hand, the increase in action potential duration that occurs in epicardial ischemia results not only in delayed repolarization (QT prolongation) but also in a change in the sequence of repolarization, which now starts at the earlier repolarized endocardium and

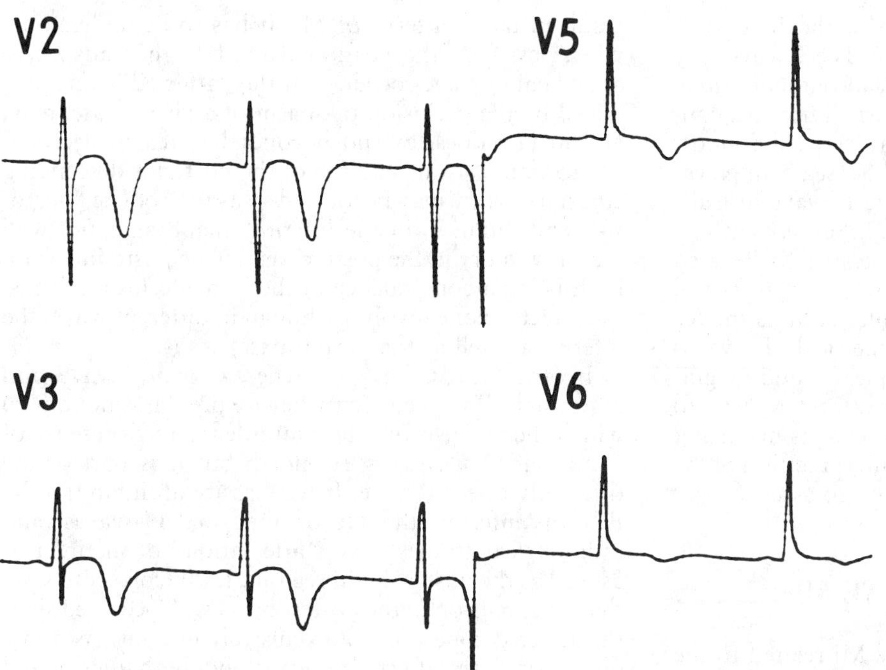

FIGURE 13-3 Electrocardiographic ischemia. Note symmetrical T-wave inversion in lead V_2.

then spreads toward the epicardium with the negative charges in front. The latter produces the characteristic symmetrical T-wave inversion.[7,10]

SECONDARY ST-T-WAVE CHANGES

Alterations in the sequence of ventricular depolarization (as those produced by bundle branch blocks, ventricular pacing, ectopic ventricular impulse formation, preexcitation syndromes, and ventricular hypertrophy) result in a change in the sequence of ventricular repolarization. The latter causes nonischemic T-wave inversions (secondary T-wave changes) in leads showing a predominantly positive QRS deflection.[6,10,12,17]

As mentioned in the section on ventricular gradients, the views of Rosenbaum and coworkers[18] are in conflict with Wilson's original concepts. An example is the type of ventricular repolarization changes (attributed to electrotonic modulation, memory, and accumulation) shown in Fig. 13-4. In intermittent chronic "complete" left bundle branch block (LBBB) when the ventricular complex becomes narrow, inverted T waves appear in leads (such as V_1 and V_2) where the S wave predominates (Fig. 13-4). In our opinion, the fact that changes in the ventricular activation sequence can produce what seems to be primary T-wave changes (that is, pseudoprimary repolarization abnormalities) capable of persisting long after cessation of the triggering factors has important clinical implications in intermittent bundle branch block, preexcitation syndromes, and posttachycardia syndrome and in patients with implanted pacemakers. Finally, ST-segment changes may occur during rapid supraventricular tachycardias in young patients without metabolic evidence of (physiological) ischemia.

CLASSIC PATTERN OF ACUTE Q-WAVE MI

This is said to occur in around 50 to 75 percent of patients with the clinical diagnosis of acute MI.[32] Obviously, these percentages will depend on whether stricter or looser criteria are used to diagnose MI.

The initial changes also depend on the moment at which the ECG is recorded, in reference to the moment

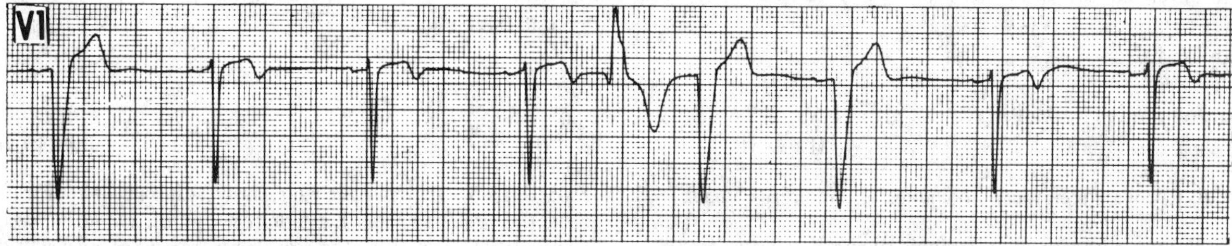

FIGURE 13-4 Tachycardia-dependent complete left bundle branch block. Pseudoprimary T-wave changes manifested as terminal T-wave inversion (when the left bundle branch block disappears) in leads showing a predominant negative (S-wave) deflection. The patient had "primary" conduction system disease with no other evidence of organic heart disease. The changes are those that correspond to the second type of secondary repolarization abnormalities described by Rosenbaum et al.[18]

of occurrence of the infarction. Thus, the first ECG change is usually an abnormal T wave. The T wave may be increased in magnitude, prolonged, and either positive or negative. A straightening of the normal upward concavity of the ST segment also has been reported. In most cases, the first ECG shows abnormal ST-segment elevation and an increase in the size of the R wave in leads exploring the affected area (Fig. 13-2). Subsequently, a Q wave appears, usually while the ST segment is elevated and generally before the T wave becomes negative. Thereafter the R wave becomes smaller and, as the ST segment returns to baseline, symmetrical T waves evolve.[6] The time of appearance, sequence, and magnitude of these changes, however, vary from patient to patient. It is as if each person has to serve as his or her own control, a factor that can make interpretation of the effects of specific interventions difficult to assess.[6]

LOCATION OF SITE OF Q-WAVE MI

Table 13-1 shows the location of the MI related to the leads in which abnormal Q waves appear according to the Criteria Committee of the New York Heart Association.[33] In addition, it depicts other processes, which, by also producing abnormal Q waves of different etiologies, result in false patterns of MI. It has to be understood, when classifying the location of an MI by the leads where abnormal Q waves occur, that the "affected" zone produced by the occlusion or spasm of a given vessel may, and in fact does, extend beyond the area of necrosis. For example, a single lesion of the posterior descending coronary artery may be located so as to produce "necrosis" and "injury" in the inferior (diaphragmatic) wall but only injury in the posterobasal (true posterior) wall, both being a consequence of the same occlusion. Thus, the affected zone involves (though in different ways) the inferior as well as the posterobasal walls.

In other words, the region where *normal* Q waves and abnormal ST-segment elevation are present is not one to which the necrosis or infarction (defined by presence of abnormal Q waves) is extended, but it is part of the originally affected zone. If we classify an infarction by ECG as inferior (the site of abnormal Q waves) and radionuclear studies show "affectation" of the inferior as well as the posterobasal regions, it is incorrect to state that an extension to the posterobasal wall occurred since the affected zone was not exclusively inferior. As previously stated, the affected zone includes both inferior and posterobasal (true posterior) walls in such a way that the former was necrotic and injured and the latter only injured.

TABLE 13-1

Electrocardiographic Location of Infarction Sites According to Leads Showing Abnormal Q Waves

Site	Leads	False Patterns
Inferior (diaphragmatic)	II, III, aV_F	WPW (PSAP), IHSS, PE
Inferolateral	II, III, aV_F, V_4–V_6	WPW (PSAP and LFWAP)
"True" posterior (posterobasal)	V_1 *	RVH, "atypical" incomplete RBBB
Inferoposterior	II, III, aV_F, V_1 *	WPW (PSAP and LFWAP), IHSS
Anteroseptal	V_1, V_2, V_3	LVH, chronic lung disease, LBBB
Anterolateral	I, II, aV_L, V_4–V_6	IHSS, ventricular septal defect
Extensive anterior	I, aV_L, V_1–V_6	
High anterolateral	I, aV_L	
Anterior (apical)	V_2–V_4	
High lateral	aV_L, "high" V_4–V_6	
Posterolateral	V_4–V_6, V_1	IHSS, WPW (LFWAP)

*Tall R wave, "reciprocal" to changes in "indicative" back lead.

NOTE: IHSS = idiopathic hypertrophic subaortic stenosis; LBBB = left bundle branch block; LFWAP = left free-wall accessory pathway; LVH = left ventricular hypertrophy; PE = pulmonary emphysema; PSAP = posteroseptal accessory pathway; WPW = Wolff-Parkinson-White syndrome.

RECIPROCAL ST-SEGMENT CHANGES

According to the theory of scalar leads, vectorial electrocardiography, as well as spatial vectorcardiography, in an inferior MI with abnormal Q waves and ST-segment elevation limited to this wall (that is, *without* "affectation" of the posterobasal, or true posterior, wall), the reciprocal ST-segment changes will occur in diametrically opposed leads located in the *same* plane. For example, "indicative" ST elevation in leads III and aV_F, which record the electrical activity of the inferior (posteroinferior, or diaphragmatic) wall, yields "reciprocal" ST-segment depression in leads I and aV_L because they face the superior (anterolateral) wall (Figs. 13-2 and 13-5,

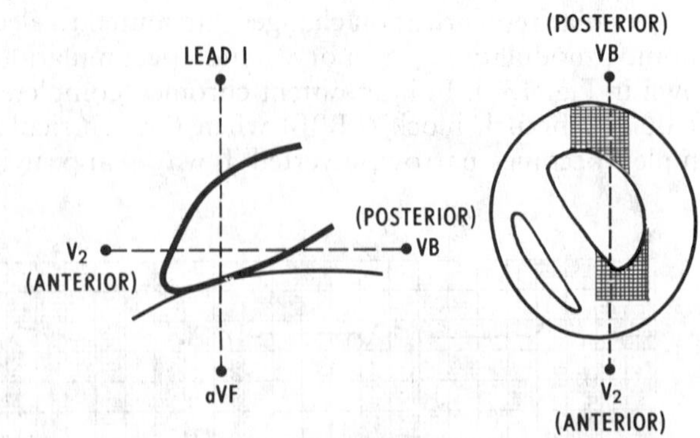

FIGURE 13-5 Diagrammatic representation explaining why, in a left lateral plane (left lateral x-ray view), anterior chest lead V_2 cannot be "reciprocal" to "inferior" lead aV_F (left). The right-sided schematic shows that ST-segment depression in anterior chest lead V_2 may reflect either anteroseptal wall subendocardial "injury" or posterobasal (true posterior) injury (transverse view from above corresponding to the electrovectorcardiographic horizontal plane). VB = unipolar chest lead (V) placed on the back of the thorax.

left).[11,34,35] For this reason, an inferior wall "injury" not affecting the posterobasal wall cannot produce "reciprocal" changes in a lead, such as V_2, which is located in a plane perpendicular to the frontal plane. The perpendicularity between vertical lead aV_F and horizontal lead V_2 can best be seen in a left sagittal plane where lead aV_F faces the inferior (diaphragmatic) wall and lead V_2 the anteroseptal and posterobasal walls (Fig. 13-5, left).

As a consequence of what was stated in a previous section, ST-segment depression in lead V_2 may reflect injury in the anterior subendocardial wall as well as injury in the posterobasal (or true posterior wall) (Fig. 13-5, right).[10] It should be emphasized that the ECG by itself cannot distinguish between these two possibilities.[10] The differential diagnosis can perhaps best be made by performing cardiac catheterization or radionuclear studies in the acute phase of the MI, when the ST changes are still present (Fig. 13-2). Another way is by analyzing ST-segment changes occurring during percutaneous transluminal coronary angioplasty in patients with proven single-vessel disease.[36]

NON-Q-WAVE MI

The "typical" pattern of non-Q-wave MI has been said to consist of abnormal ST-segment depression in all leads except aV_R, which shows ST-segment elevation (Fig. 13-6).[6] Classically, the abnormal repolarization changes persist for several days rather than disappearing in minutes or hours, as is the case with the transitory ST changes of the syndromes of coronary ischemia.[33] On the other hand, most cardiologists make the diagnosis of non-Q-wave MI when clinical, enzymatic, and, at times, radionuclear findings are associated with not only the previously mentioned repolarization changes but also the "ischemic" T-wave changes, nonspecific ST-T-wave changes, or rarely a normal ECG.

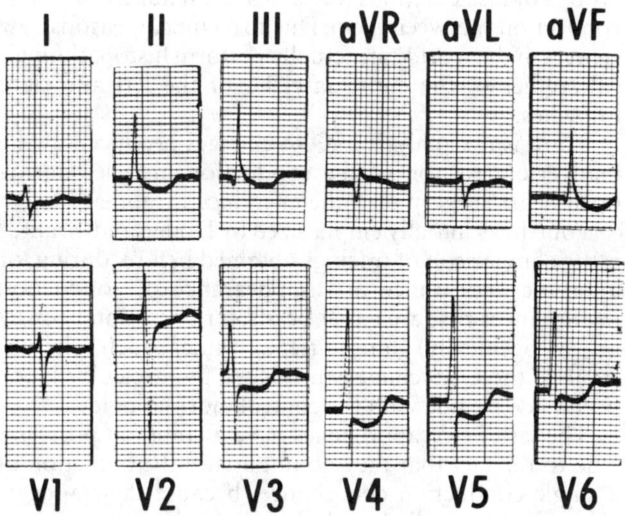

FIGURE 13-6 Classical subendocardial (non-Q-wave) infarction manifested by abnormal ST-segment depression in all leads except aV_R, which showed ST-segment elevation.

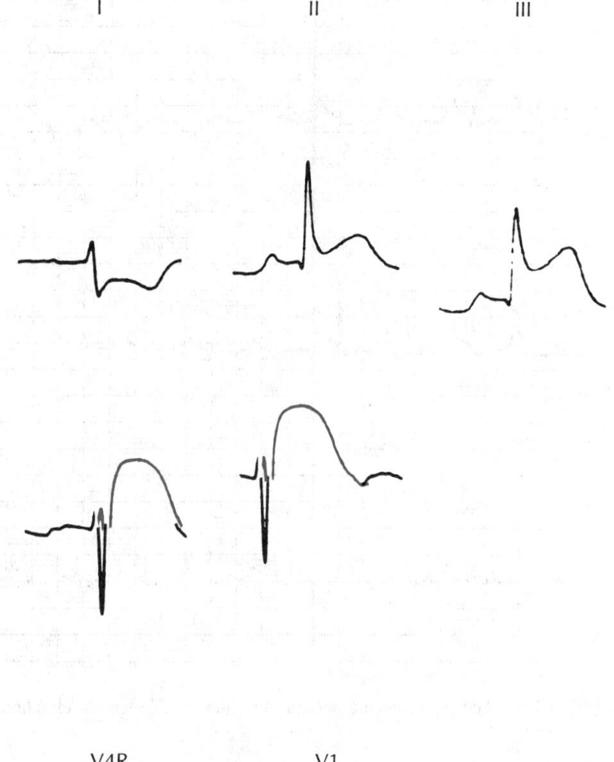

FIGURE 13-7 Acute inferior (diaphragmatic) MI with coexisting right ventricular infarction. Note ST-segment elevation in lead V_4R (and also in V_1). The ECG was taken 4 h after the onset of chest pain.

RIGHT VENTRICULAR MI

According to Braat et al.,[37] an ST-segment elevation of at least 1 mm in lead V_4R in patients with *acute inferior MI* had a sensitivity of 100 percent, a specificity of 87 percent, and a predictive accuracy of 92 percent for the diagnosis of right ventricular infarction (Fig. 13-7). These changes disappeared within 10 to 18 h after the onset of chest pain in 50 percent of their patients and after 72 h in the remaining patients.[37] Most authors agree that the electrocardiographic diagnosis of right ventricular infarction by the changes in V_4R has to be made within the initial 24 h. (See also Chap. 60.)

ATRIAL MI

Atrial infarction has been related to extensive ventricular MI.[38] In histopathological studies, important atheromatotic obstructions of the proximal portions of the right, left anterior descending, and circumflex coronary arteries are found.[38] Atrial infarction is suspected (but not proven) when an atrial arrhythmia develops in a patient with a large ventricular MI. Changes in morphology of the sinus P waves are also seen, but this finding is also nonspecific.[11,38] Other abnormalities, perhaps more diagnostic, are widespread PR-segment changes in the presence of an atrial arrhythmia, especially elevation of the PR segment in the left chest leads with reciprocal depression in the right chest leads or elevation in lead I with reciprocal depression in lead III.[11,39]

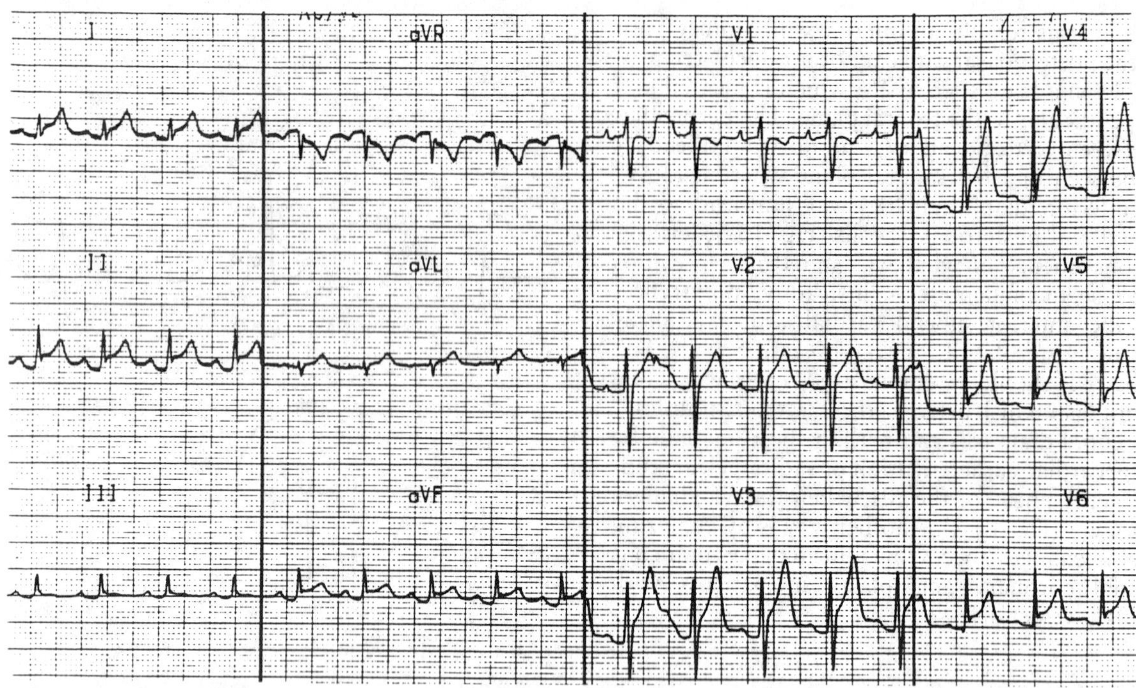

FIGURE 13-8 Acute nonspecific pericarditis showing ST-segment elevation in all leads except aV_R and V_1. (Compare with Fig. 13-6.)

PERICARDITIS

The electrocardiographic pattern of acute (generalized) pericarditis not due to MI is produced by the associated epicardial epimyocarditis, which in turn results in diffuse epicardial "injury."[6] The ST segments can be elevated in all leads except aV_R and, rarely, in V_1 (Fig. 13-8). Symmetrical T-wave inversion (due to epicardial "ischemia") usually develops after the ST segments have returned to the baseline (but can appear during the injury stage).[6] Neither reciprocal ST-segment changes nor abnormal Q waves are seen. In most cases of acute pericarditis, the PR segment is depressed in leads V_2 to V_6. Average electrocardiographic resolution occurs in close to 2 weeks.[11] The ECG pattern of acute pericarditis has to be differentiated from a normal variant occurring in some normal young persons that is often referred to incorrectly as early repolarization. The latter consists, in the left chest leads, of normal ST-segment elevation associated with usually large R waves that have small r′ deflections or notches starting *above* the baseline (Fig. 13-9).

FASCICULAR BLOCKS

Generalities

It seems appropriate to start this section by reviewing how our current knowledge regarding the fascicular blocks was obtained. For this purpose we should point out several ways of proving that a given QRS pattern is due to a specific type of conduction abnormality.[40]

First is extrapolation from animal experiments.[5,41–46] Unfortunately, the clinical recognition of left fascicular blocks was greatly delayed when applying information obtained from dogs, in whom bundle branch blocks and fascicular blocks result in changes different than in humans. The better correlation existing between humans and higher primate species such as the baboon has not been sufficiently explored, especially in investigations of right-sided fascicular blocks.

Second is ECG-pathological correlation.[47–56] There are also problems with this approach since a "lesion" in a site of the conduction system need not produce *persistent* ECG changes, and likewise, transient conduction disturbances may have a functional cause. Furthermore, studies of the most distal portions of the fascicles are not easy because the left branch fans out into what is usually considered to be three relatively broad, variably long groups of fasciculations (divisions) with numerous interconnections between them. Due to technical reasons, few centers in the world can actually perform histopathological studies of the entire fascicles of the left and right branches.

Third is the analysis of QRS changes produced by the inadvertent section of the conduction fascicles during open heart surgery or catheter-induced trauma.[57]

Fourth, as initially emphasized by Dodge and Grant,[58] is the comparison of tracings obtained before, during, or after the appearance or disappearance of conduction disturbances that are either persistent or (spontaneously or iatrogenically) intermittent. Under such circumstances, the QRS changes produced by fascicular block occur side by side with the control morphologies.[15,40,58,59]

The latter two approaches have a common problem. Due to the fact that they do not assure the induction of a single conduction disturbance (because their appearance is uncontrolled), what may be interpreted as a "pure" block of a given fascicle may be associated with an unidentified but electrocardiographically relevant conduction delay in another fascicle. The various criteria

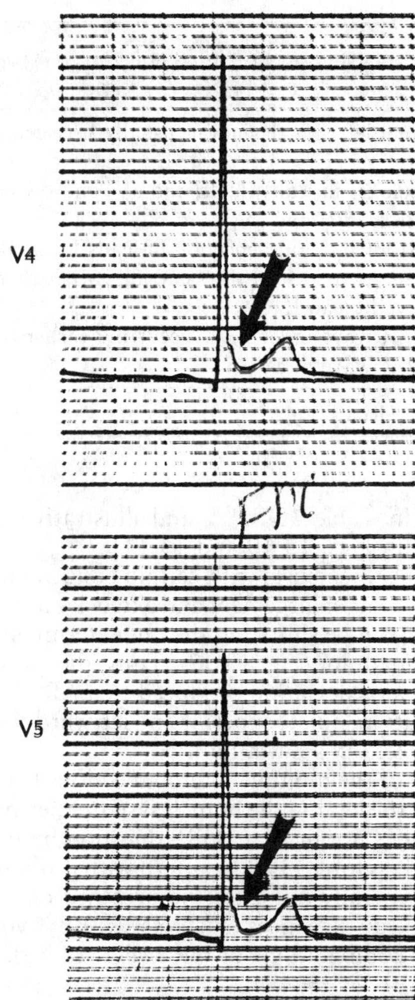

FIGURE 13-9 Normal variant ST elevation (not due to pericarditis) in a healthy 24-year-old male. Note large R waves with a notch (arrows) in its terminal part appearing as a small r′ wave starting a few millimeters above the baseline.

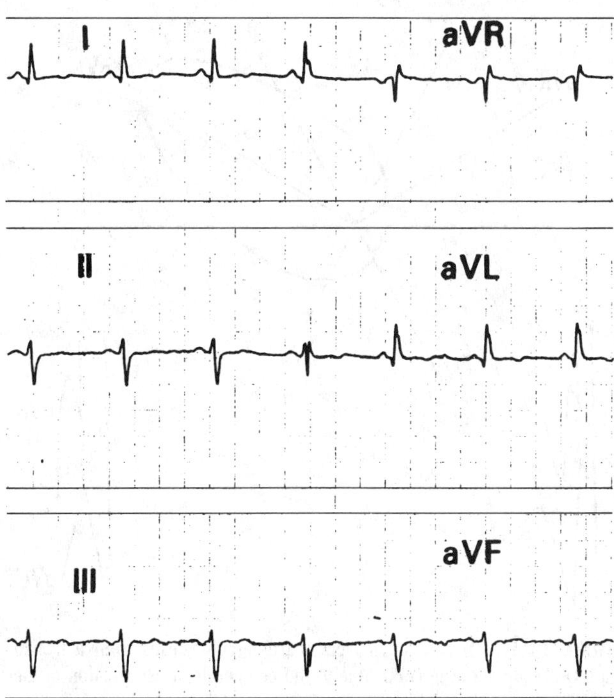

FIGURE 13-10 Left anterior fascicular block in a patient with primary conduction system disease.

proposed for diagnosis of fascicular blocks, though empirical, have been accepted for a very pragmatic reason: the need to interpret clinical ECGs. In reality, the sensitivity and specificity of these criteria require independent confirmation.[40,60] One can speculate that the latter may be provided by the newer methods of intraoperative mapping and refinements in the technique of phase imaging.

Left Anterior Fascicular Block

In left anterior fascicular block (LAFB), the posteroinferior regions of the left ventricular endocardium are activated abnormally before the anterosuperior left ventricular area.[8,15] After emerging from the posteroinferior division of the left bundle branch, the impulse first propagates in an inferior, rightward, and usually anterior direction for a short period of time. This orientation is responsible for the small q waves in leads I and aV_L and for the r waves in leads II, III, and aV_F (Fig. 13-10).

Occasionally, small q waves are not present in leads I and aV_L.[15] In the absence of MI, these initial QRS abnormalities have been attributed to "anatomic clockwise rotation of the heart" or to coexisting septal fibrosis or to incomplete LBBB.[15] The latter cannot explain a similar orientation of the initial vectors when LAFB is present with "complete" right bundle branch block (RBBB) because ventricular activation cannot be a function of the "completely" blocked right branch. In these cases, diffuse septal fibrosis or anatomic clockwise rotation appear more probable.[15] In pure LAFB, the general direction of the activation process (which determines the direction of the EA) occurs in a superior and leftward direction. Consequently, from the electrocardiographic viewpoint, the fascicles of the left branch behave more as if they were "superior" and "inferior" rather than "anterior" and "posterior" (Figs. 13-10 and 13-11). For this reason, the most significant abnormalities produced by left anterior and left posterior fascicular block (LPFB) (in the absence of complete RBBB) occur in the standard and unipolar extremity leads rather than in the precordial leads[15] (Figs. 13-10 and 13-11).

The degree of left axis deviation required for the diagnosis of complete LAFB has been a subject of debate and speculation.[8] It has been stated that if the EA lies between $-30°$ and $-60°$, LAFB is probably present, and if the EA is between $-60°$ and $-90°$, it is almost certainly present.[8] In our opinion, a cutoff of $-45°$ is a valid compromise. The analysis of QRS changes produced by atrial extrasystoles with aberration has shown that conduction delays through the left anterior fascicle can occur with less degree of left axis deviation. Incomplete LAFB, however, can only be diagnosed in these dynamic situations when the original (control) location of the EA is known. It should be remembered that LAFB is but one of the causes of left (superior and leftward) axis deviation (Table 13-2). Criteria for the diagnosis of pure LAFB are

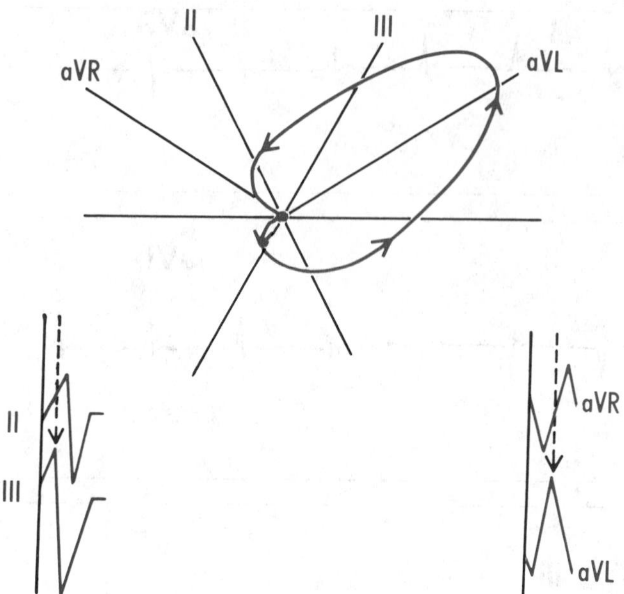

FIGURE 13-11 Derivation of electrocardiographic leads from a frontal plane QRS loop showing LAFB. Due to the counterclockwise rotation of the left superior loop, the peak of the R in aV_L preceded the peak of this deflection in aV_R (lower right). Furthermore, because the initial portion of the loop was inscribed on the positive half of the axis of lead III before it was inscribed in the positive half of the axis of lead II, the peak of the R in the former lead occurred before that in the latter lead. (*From A Castellanos, L Pina, L Zaman, et al: Recent advances in the diagnosis of fascicular blocks. Cardiol Clin 5:469–488, 1987. Reproduced with permission from the publisher and authors.*)

TABLE 13-2

Causes of Abnormal (−30° to −90°) Left Axis Deviation

Cause	Characteristic Features
1. Left anterior fascicular block	1. rS complexes in lead II with positive T waves
2. Extensive inferior wall MI	2. Qr complexes in lead II with ST-segment elevation and/or T-wave inversion
3. Extensive inferior wall MI with possible LAFB	3. QS pattern in leads II, III, and aV_F with ST-segment elevation and/or T-wave inversion
4. Wolff-Parkinson-White syndrome (posteroseptal accessory pathway)	4. Short PR interval; delta wave
5. Hyperkalemia	5. Wide QRS complexes; peaked T waves
6. Pulmonary emphysema	6. Low voltage; peaked P waves
7. Right ventricular apical pacing	7. Pacemaker spikes; predominantly negative ventricular deflections in V_1
8. Middle cardiac vein pacing	8. Pacemaker spikes; predominantly positive QRS deflections in V_1
9. Left coronary arteriography	9. Knowledge that dye was injected in left coronary artery

TABLE 13-3

Criteria for Diagnosis of Pure Left Anterior Fascicular Block

1. Abnormal left axis deviation (usually between −45° and −60°)
2. rS complexes in leads II, III, and aV_F and qR complexes in leads I and aV_L
3. Delayed intrinsicoid deflection in leads I and aV_L
4. Peak of r wave in lead III occurring earlier than peak of r wave in lead II
5. Peak of R wave in lead aV_L occurring earlier than peak of R wave in aV_R

SOURCE: Castellanos et al.[40]

presented in Table 13-3,[60–64] and illustrative examples are shown in Figs. 13-10 and 13-11.

When LAFB coexists with certain congenital types of right ventricular enlargement and extensive anterolateral MI, the EA can be shifted to the "undeterminate" (right superior) quadrant (Fig. 13-12). Thus, the constant feature of the axis deviation produced by LAFB is its *superior* orientation, not its superior and leftward orientation (abnormal left axis deviation).[40]

Because of the multiple interconnections between the fascicles of the left bundle branch system, the appearance of LAFB does not increase QRS duration by more than 0.025 s.[8] Therefore, a LAFB pattern with prolonged QRS duration generally indicates the presence of additional conduction disturbances such as RBBB, MI, "focal block," or combinations of these (Fig. 13-13).

Left Anterior Fascicular Block and Left Ventricular Hypertrophy

According to Rosenbaum et al.,[8,53,62,63] left ventricular hypertrophy (LVH) by itself does not produce *abnormal* left axis deviation. The left ventricular activation produced by LAFB, however, may lead to an increase in the voltage of the R wave in lead I and of the S wave in lead III, which can be capable of simulating a false pattern of LVH. Criteria for diagnosis of LVH coexisting with LAFB are discussed below.

Left Anterior Fascicular Block Coexisting with MI

The electrocardiographic changes imposed by MIs of different locations on the LAFB are shown in Fig. 13-14.

Focal Block

At this point, it is important to note that several names have been applied to the conduction disturbances occurring in the left-sided Purkinje-myocardial junctions, left septal surface, or free wall of the left ventricle: arborization block, diffuse (nonspecific) intraventricular block, periinfarction block, parietal block, etc.[8,64–71] Although some readers might disagree with what we consider (in keeping with Rosenbaum's concepts) to be "focal" block, they must nevertheless have a clear understanding of the concept that it implies.[5]

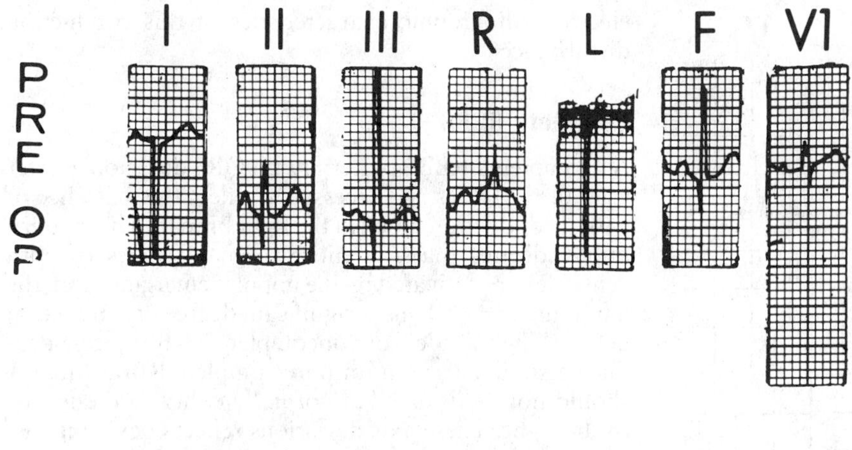

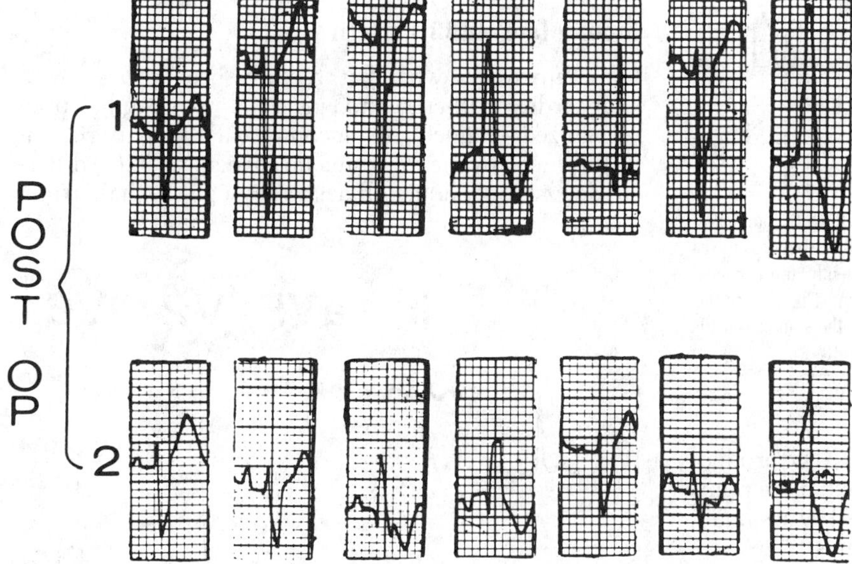

FIGURE 13-12 Transient postsurgical LAFB (with indeterminate axis) and persistent RBBB in a patient with tetralogy of Fallot (middle tracing). The top (control) tracing shows right axis deviation due to right ventricular hypertrophy with narrow QRS complexes. In the bottom tracing, recorded after disappearance of LAFB, right axis deviation due to right ventricular hypertrophy coexists with the persistent RBBB. (*From A Castellanos, L Pina, L Zaman, et al: Recent advances in the diagnosis of fascicular blocks. Cardiol Clin 5:469–488, 1987. Reproduced with permission from the publisher and authors.*)

These conduction disturbances have different electrogenetic mechanisms. Thus, the cellular "affectation" due to acute injury resulting from coronary artery disease, hyperkalemia, drugs, and intracoronary injections of contrast material occurs within (inside) the affected regions.[5,15,71] Focal blocks occurring in subacute or chronic MI after the appearance of abnormal Q waves (periinfarction block), as well as those occurring in the presence of diffuse myocardial fibrosis (of noncoronary etiology), are due to the circuitous and irregular activation of living cells surrounding areas of fibrotic tissue (Fig. 13-15).[5,64–71]

Left Posterior Fascicular Block

In pure LPFB, the impulse emerges from the unblocked anterosuperior division, thus producing small q waves in leads II, III, and aV_F.[8,15] Thereafter, the impulse moves through the electrically predominant left ventricle in an inferior and rightward direction, thus explaining the deep S waves in leads I and aV_L as well as the R waves in leads II, III, and aV_F.[8,15]

Radiologic studies of the human heart in situ have shown that the paraseptal regions of the posteroinferior (diaphragmatic) surface of the anatomic *left* ventricle are spatially located more to the *right* than certain (anterior) portions of the anatomic right ventricle.[15] Since the portions of the left ventricle that are spatially located to the right are less significant than those located superiorly, the degree of right axis deviation produced by pure LPFB is of lesser magnitude than that of left axis deviation produced by LAFB.[15] The hallmark of LPFB is, therefore, an "inferior" axis shift as much as "right" axis deviation (Figs. 13-16 to 13-18).

Because a similar sequence of ventricular activation can also occur in right ventricular hypertrophy, pleuropulmonary disease (acute or chronic), and extremely vertical anatomic heart positions due to a slender body build or chest wall deformities, it is evident that the diagnosis of "pure" LPFB cannot be made from the ECG alone. Additional clinical, radiologic, or pathological information is required for this purpose.[8,15,40,53]

The changes imposed in LPFB by MIs of different locations are depicted in Figs. 13-17 and 13-18 (third strip).

Left Fascicular Blocks Produced by Intra-His Bundle Lesions

Rosenbaum and coworkers[57] attributed surgically induced LAFB (coexisting with RBBB) to a lesion of the

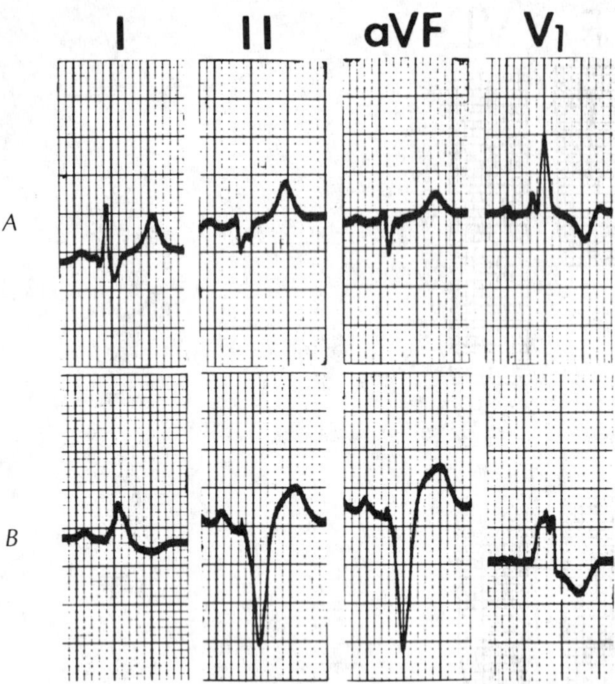

FIGURE 13-13 Left anterior fascicular block with wide QRS complexes. Whereas *A* shows LAFB with RBBB, in *B* these conduction disturbances coexist with diffuse septal and inferoposterior fibrosis. Consequently, the expected small q wave and the wide S wave in lead I are not present. This pattern has been called "masquerading" bundle branch block since the standard leads suggest LBBB while the chest leads are diagnostic of RBBB.

"pseudobifurcating" part of the His bundle. The production of LBBB and LPFB by catheters located in the right-sided cavities, however, cannot be explained by assuming direct affectation of these left-sided structures.[72,73] Nevertheless, they have been reported and attributed to the His bundle trauma produced by Swan-Ganz catheters.[72,73] In fact, certain clinical and experimental studies have shown that some bundle branch block patterns could be normalized by distal His bundle pacing.[74–77] Longitudinal dissociation of conduction within an usually diseased His bundle should be present for this to occur. There is, however, disagreement as to the mechanism involved, especially in regard to the predestination of fibers (within the His bundle) to specific right- or left-sided structures and to the role played by the transverse fibers connecting the various longitudinal strands.[73–77]

Left-Middle (Septal) Fascicular Blocks

This disorder has been anatomically demonstrated and associated with ischemic heart disease and fibrosis of the middle (septal) fascicle of the left branch.[48,55] While some authors consider that the right precordial leads show prominent R waves (similar to those found in true posterior, basal, myocardial infarction), others have described Q waves in leads V_1, V_2, and V_3.[78,79] It has also been considered that left-middle (septal) fascicular blocks are manifested by the absence of the expected q waves in leads V_5 and V_6 in electrocardiographic intermediate or horizontal hearts.[56] Such a diversity of diagnostic criteria shows that there are marked discrepancies regarding the electrocardiographic characteristics of this conduction disturbance.

Complete RBBB

A "complete" RBBB pattern (with QRS duration greater than 0.11 s) does not necessarily reflect the existence of a total conduction block in the right branch. This pattern only indicates that the entire or major parts of both ventricles are activated by the impulse emerging from the left branch.[15,80–82] Thus, a significant degree of conduction delay ("high-grade" or "incomplete" RBBB) can produce a similar pattern. In pure complete RBBB, the EA should not be deviated *abnormally* either to the left or to the right. These axis deviations reflect coexisting fascicular block or right ventricular hypertrophy.

Incomplete RBBB Pattern

For many years what has recently been proven with endocardial (catheter) and epicardial mapping has been recognized—namely, that incomplete RBBB patterns can be produced by the following mechanisms[80–92]: (1) different degrees of conduction delays through the main trunk

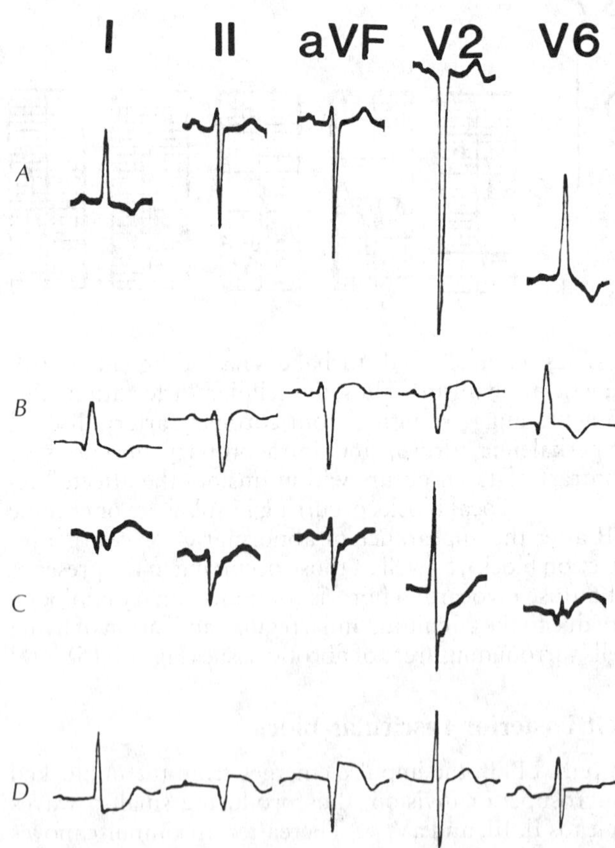

FIGURE 13-14 Diagnosis of LAFB associated with MI. Diagnostic feature given in parentheses. *A.* Left anterior fascicular block and anteroseptal MI (QS complex in right chest leads). *B.* Left anterior fascicular block and anterolateral MI (abnormal Q wave in leads I and V_6). *C.* Left anterior fascicular block and anterolateral MI with electrical axis in right superior ("indeterminate") quadrant (Q wave in leads I and V_6). *D.* Left anterior fascicular block and inferior wall MI (QS complexes and elevation of J point and ST segments in leads II and III).

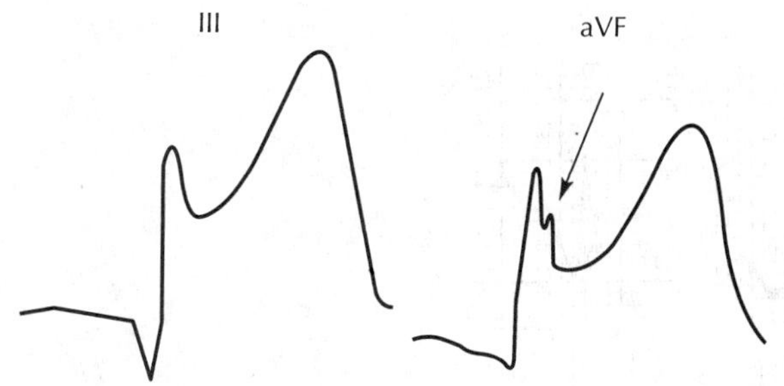

FIGURE 13-15 Left ventricular focal (inferior periinfarction) block (arrow).

of the right bundle branch (Fig. 13-19); (2) an increased conduction time through an elongated right bundle branch that is stretched because of a concomitant enlargement of the right septal surface (as in congenital volume overloading of the right ventricle); (3) a diffuse Purkinje-myocardial delay due to right ventricular stretch or dilatation; (4) surgical trauma or disease-related interruption of the major ramifications of the right branch ("distal" RBBB or "right fascicular blocks"); or (5) congenital variations of the distribution of the major distal ramifications resulting in a slight delay in activation of the crista supraventricularis.

Concealed RBBB

A conduction delay in the main trunk of the right bundle branch or in its major ramifications may be concealed (not manifested in the surface ECG) when there are coexisting (and of greater degree) conduction disturbances in the main left bundle branch, the anterosuperior division of the left bundle branch, and/or the free left ventricular wall.[15] A RBBB can also be concealed in some patients with Wolff-Parkinson-White syndrome if the ventricular insertion of the accessory pathway causes preexcitation of the right ventricular regions that would be activated late because of the RBBB.[93]

Complete LBBB

This conduction disturbance is characterized by wide (greater than 0.11 s) QRS complexes. The diagnostic criteria consist of prolongation of the QRS complexes (over 0.11 s) with neither a q nor an S wave in leads V_1 and in the *properly placed* V_6. A wide R wave with a notch on its top ("plateau") is seen in these leads. In hearts with an electrical (and anatomic) vertical position a small q wave may be seen in aV_L in the absence of MI. Right chest lead V_1 may or may not show an initial r wave, but the latter should be present ir lead V_2. Unfortunately, as mentioned in reference to complete RBBB, a complete LBBB morphology can be recorded in patients with high-degree (not necessarily complete) LBBB.

The direction of the electrical axis in patients showing QRS changes typical of complete LBBB has also been widely discussed.[15,16] In the majority of the human hearts, the site of exit from the right bundle branch does not seem to be at the lowermost right ventricular region (that called in pacemaker nomenclature the *right ventricular apex).*[15,16] If this were the case, all complete LBBBs would show (as when the right ventricular apex is paced) abnormal left axis deviation whereas the electrical axis in *uncomplicated* complete LBBB block usually is not located beyond −30°.

Complete LBBB with MI

Normally, in complete LBBB, the impulse emerges from the right bundle branch and propagates inferiorly, to the left and slightly anteriorly. This orientation of the initial forces tends to abolish previously present inferiorly and laterally located abnormal Q waves characteristic of inferior and lateral wall MIs.[15,94-96] If the infarction is antero-

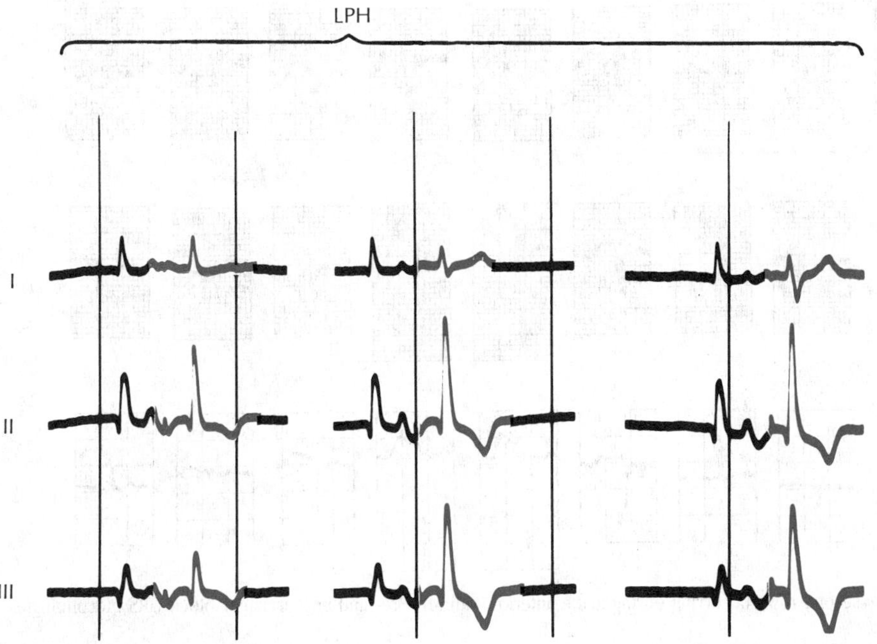

FIGURE 13-16 Premature atrial beats showing increasing degrees of (incomplete and complete) LPFB aberration. The first beats in all panels are escape beats with the same morphology as that of sinus beats. The second, aberrantly induced ventricular complexes show different degrees of right axis shift with an increase in size of the R waves in leads II and III. Note that the fundamental characteristic of LPFB was not right axis deviation (beyond +90°), but an inferior axis shift. (*From A Castellanos, RJ Myerburg: The Hemiblocks in Myocardial Infarction. New York, Appleton-Century-Crofts, 1976. Reproduced with permission from the publisher and authors.*)

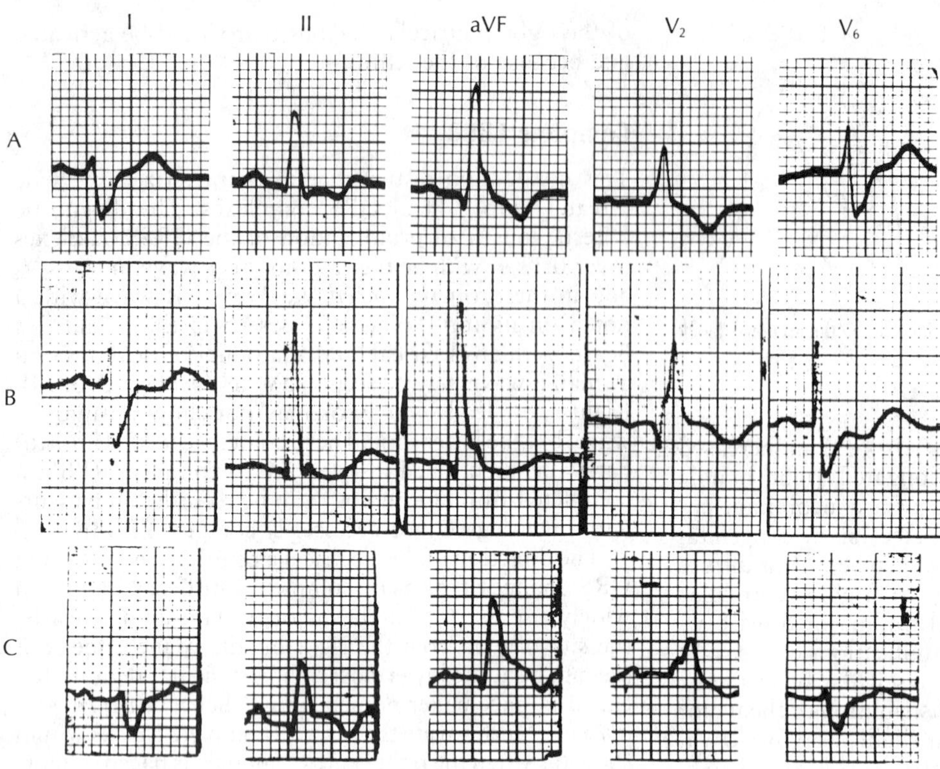

FIGURE 13-17 Left posterior fascicular block with RBBB. *A*. No MI. *B*. Anteroseptal MI (note q wave in V_2). *C*. Inferior MI (note ST-segment elevation and T-wave inversion in leads II and aV_F with slight ST-segment depression in lead I). The differences between *A* and *C* are not very marked since pure LPFB may produce an almost abnormal Q wave in the inferior leads. Conversely, this conduction disturbance, by producing an initial depolarization wave front oriented superiorly, is capable of decreasing the depth (thus normalizing) the abnormal Q-wave characteristic of inferior MI in leads II, III, and aV_F.

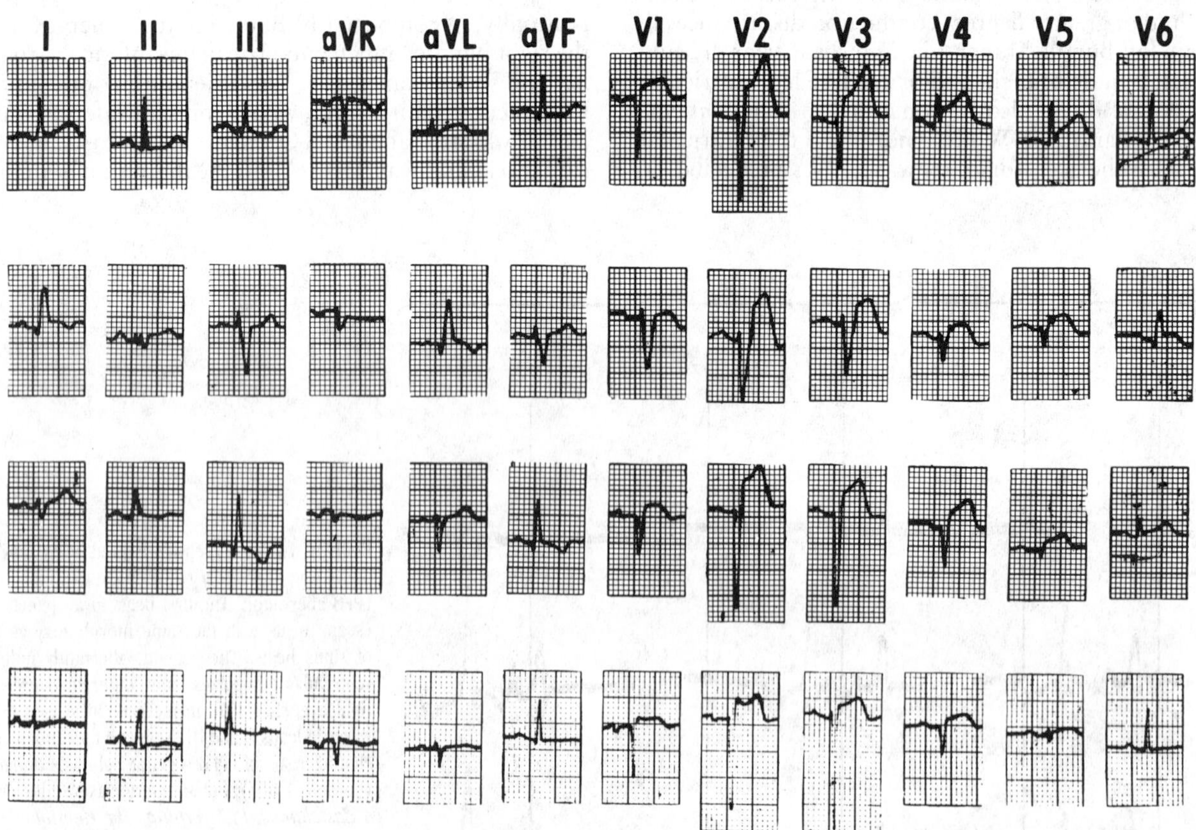

FIGURE 13-18 Pure LPFB (third row) and LAFB (second row) occurring during acute anterior wall MI. Pre- and postfascicular block QRS morphologies are shown in the top and bottom row, respectively.

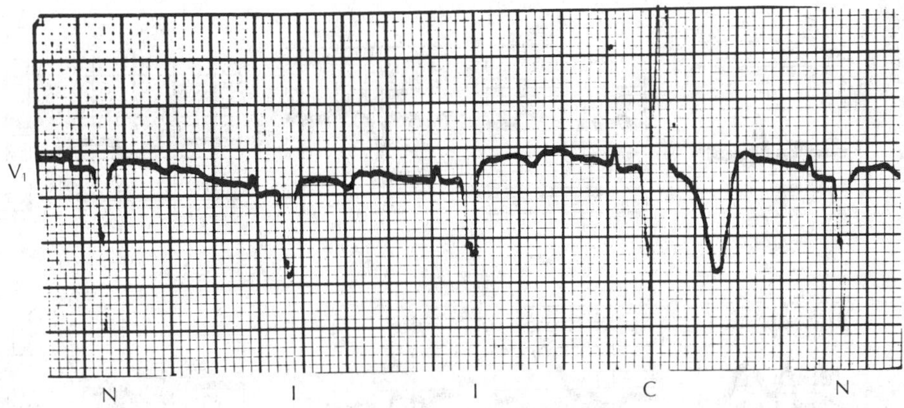

FIGURE 13-19 Possible 4 : 3 Wenckebach period in the right bundle branch (lead V_1). Because minor degrees of conduction delay through the right bundle branch produce a decrease in the depth of the S wave in lead V_1, it is conceivable for the first (and last) P waves to have been conducted normally through the right bundle branch. The second P wave could have been conducted with some delay, the third with a greater delay, whereas the fourth wave was completely blocked in the right bundle branch, thus ending the 4 : 3 Wenckebach sequence. (*A Castellanos, IL Pina, L Zaman, et al: Recent advances in the diagnosis of fascicular blocks. Cardiol Clin 5:469–488, 1987. Reproduced with permission from the publisher and authors.*)

septal, however, the impulse cannot propagate toward the left. Instead, the initial vectors point toward the free wall of the right ventricle because now the right ventricular free-wall forces are not neutralized by the normally preponderant septal and/or initial left ventricular free-wall forces. Thus, a small q wave will be recorded in leads (I, V_5, and V_6) where it is not normally recorded in complete LBBB (Fig. 13-20).

In a recent study, Wackers[96] showed that the most sensitive sign to detect acute MI was ST-segment elevation in leads facing the affected region (Fig. 13-21). Positive T waves in leads I, aV_L, V_5, and V_6 were not exclusively seen in patients with acute MI, since they were observed in a control group. The already discussed q wave and Cabrera's sign (notching of the ascending limb of the predominantly negative deflection in leads V_3 and V_4) were even less sensitive.[96]

Complete LBBB with LVH

This is discussed in the section dealing with LVH.

Incomplete LBBB Pattern

An incomplete LBBB pattern can be diagnosed in a heart with an electrically horizontal (or semihorizontal) heart position when leads I and V_6 show an R wave with a slurring in its upstroke (not on its top, as in complete LBBB).[6] Lead V_1 shows rS or QS complexes, and lead V_2 shows rS complexes. Although QRS duration usually ranges between 0.08 and 0.11 s, this pattern can be observed with QRS durations of 0.12 and 0.13 s. Not surprisingly, an incomplete LBBB pattern can be produced by various processes, including the following: (1) conduction delays in the main trunk of the left bundle branch, (2) conduction delays (of more or less equal degree) in the fascicles of the left bundle branch, (3) diffuse septal fibrosis, (4) small septal infarctions, (5) left ventricular enlargements (generally due to pressure overloading) in patients with congenital heart disease, and (6) combinations of all of the above.[15]

Wide QRS Complexes in Patients with Manifest Preexcitation Syndromes

The characteristic pattern of manifest Wolff-Parkinson-White syndrome consists of a short PR interval (reflecting faster than normal conduction through an accessory pathway of the Kent bundle type) preceding a wide QRS complex.[97] The latter usually shows an initial slurring (delta wave) followed by a terminal,[97] slender part. The

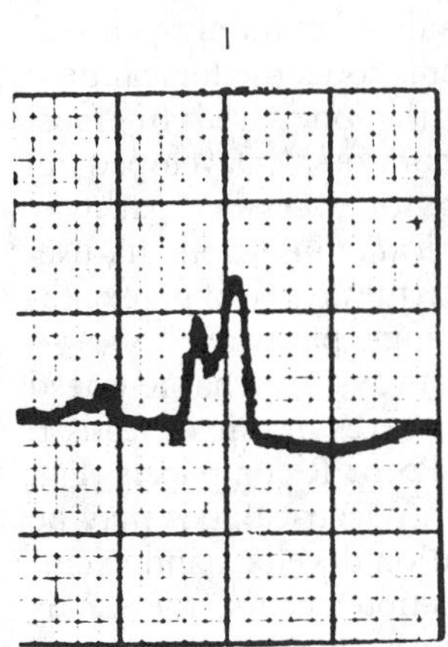

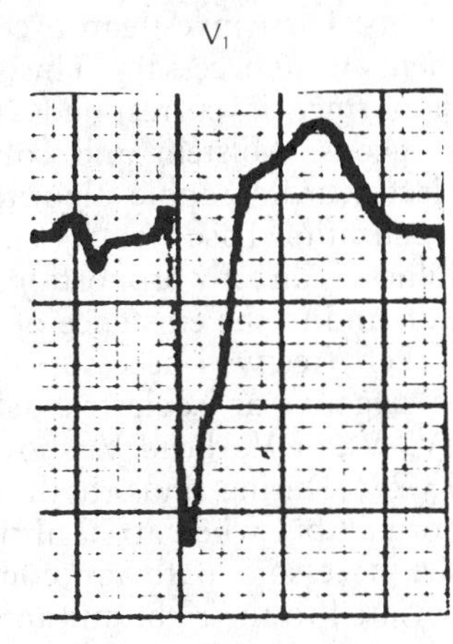

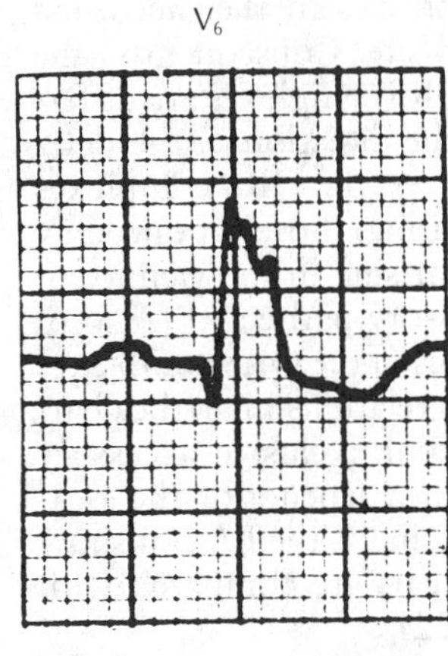

FIGURE 13-20 Complete LBBB with anteroseptal infarction. There is a small q wave in front of the otherwise typical wide ventricular complexes in leads I and V_6. A small r wave is present in V_1.

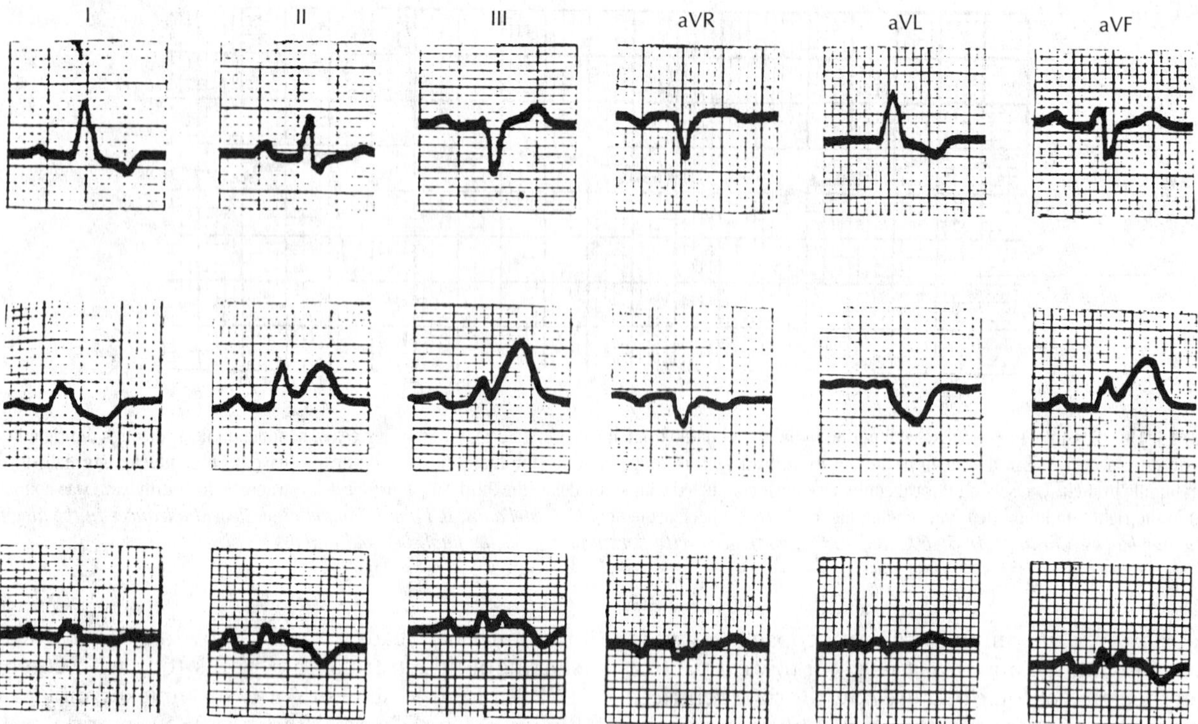

FIGURE 13-21 Complete LBBB (*top strip*) with an evolving acute inferior wall MI (*middle and bottom strips*). Note ST-T-wave changes.

classical ventricular complex is a fusion beat resulting from ventricular activation by two wave fronts. One, traversing the accessory pathway, produces the delta wave. The other, emerging from the normal AV pathway, is responsible for the terminal, more normal parts of the QRS complex.[98] The degree of preexcitation (amount of muscle activated through the accessory pathway) depends on many factors. Foremost among these are the distance between the sinus node and atrial insertion of accessory pathway and, more important, the differences in conduction time through the normal pathway and accessory pathway. Other things being equal, a patient with rapid (enhanced) AV nodal conduction will have a smaller delta wave than a patient with slow conduction through the AV node. Moreover, if there is total block at the AV node or His-Purkinje system, the impulse will be conducted exclusively via the accessory pathway bundle.[98] When this occurs, the QRS complexes are no longer fusion beats since the ventricles are then activated exclusively from the preexcited site. Consequently, the delta wave disappears and the QRS complexes are different than fusion beats, though the direction of the delta wave remains the same. Moreover, the QRS complexes are as wide as (and really simulating) those produced by artificial or spontaneous beats arising in the vicinity of the ventricular end of the accessory pathway.[98] Also of importance are the characteristics of the QRS complexes of beats without preexcitation in relationship to the characteristics of beats resulting from exclusive accessory pathway conduction (which in turn depends on the location of the pathway). Not surprisingly, the EA can show marked changes when fusion beats are compared with pure preexcited beats (Fig. 13-22).

In the past, to determine the location of the accessory pathway, the electrocardiographic classification of manifest Wolff-Parkinson-White syndrome proposed by F. F. Rosenbaum and coworkers[99] in 1945 was frequently used and misinterpreted. This classification is now of historical interest only.[98,100–105] Nevertheless, determining the anatomic position of the accessory pathway is presently of more clinical importance since the introduction of surgical and ablative techniques for symptomatic cases of Wolff-Parkinson-White syndrome. (See Chap. 43.) There are three major methods available for the anatomic localization of accessory pathways, namely, intraoperative mapping, catheter electrode techniques, and analysis of the 12-lead ECG. The latter is the least accurate, but the easiest, to use since it is noninvasive.

Milstein and coworkers[106] analyzed the direction of the delta wave and divided the mitral and tricuspid ring areas where the pathways are located into various segments. These investigators considered that only four segments were necessary. This seems to us the logical division since it corresponds to the one used by most surgeons. Milstein and collaborators[106] developed an electrocardiographic algorithm for accessory pathway localization based on its *ventricular* insertion. Its usefulness is directly proportional to the degree of preexcitation and to the existence of a single pathway.

Left free-wall accessory pathways are characterized by negative or isoelectric delta waves in one of leads I, aV_L, V_5, or V_6. Lead V_1 shows RS or R complexes (Fig. 13-22). During sinus rhythm, the electrical axis may be normal, but when atrial fibrillation develops and exclusive accessory pathway conduction occurs, the EA is deviated to the right and inferiorly (Fig. 13-22).

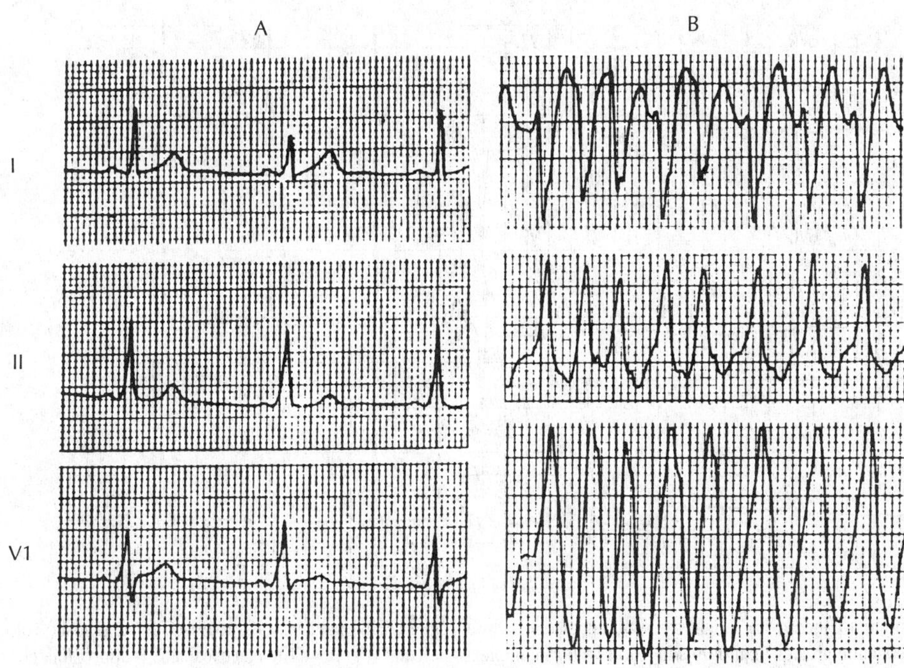

FIGURE 13-22 Wolff-Parkinson-White syndrome in a patient with a left free-wall accessory pathway. *A.* Sinus rhythm with fusion beats showing different degrees of preexcitation. *B.* Maximal preexcitation during atrial fibrillation. Note marked change in QRS duration and electrical axis.

Posteroseptal accessory pathways show negative or isoelectric delta waves in two of leads II, III, or aV_F and RS (or R) waves in V_1, V_2, or V_3 (Fig. 13-23). An Rs (or RS) wave in V_1 suggests a left paraseptal pathway; a QS complex in the same lead may correspond to a right paraseptal pathway.

Right free-wall accessory pathways display an LBBB pattern defined, for purposes of accessory pathway localization, by an R wave greater than 0.09 s in lead I and rS complexes in leads V_1 and V_2 with an electrical axis ranging between +30° to −60° (Fig. 13-24). The most rare right anteroseptal accessory pathways show an

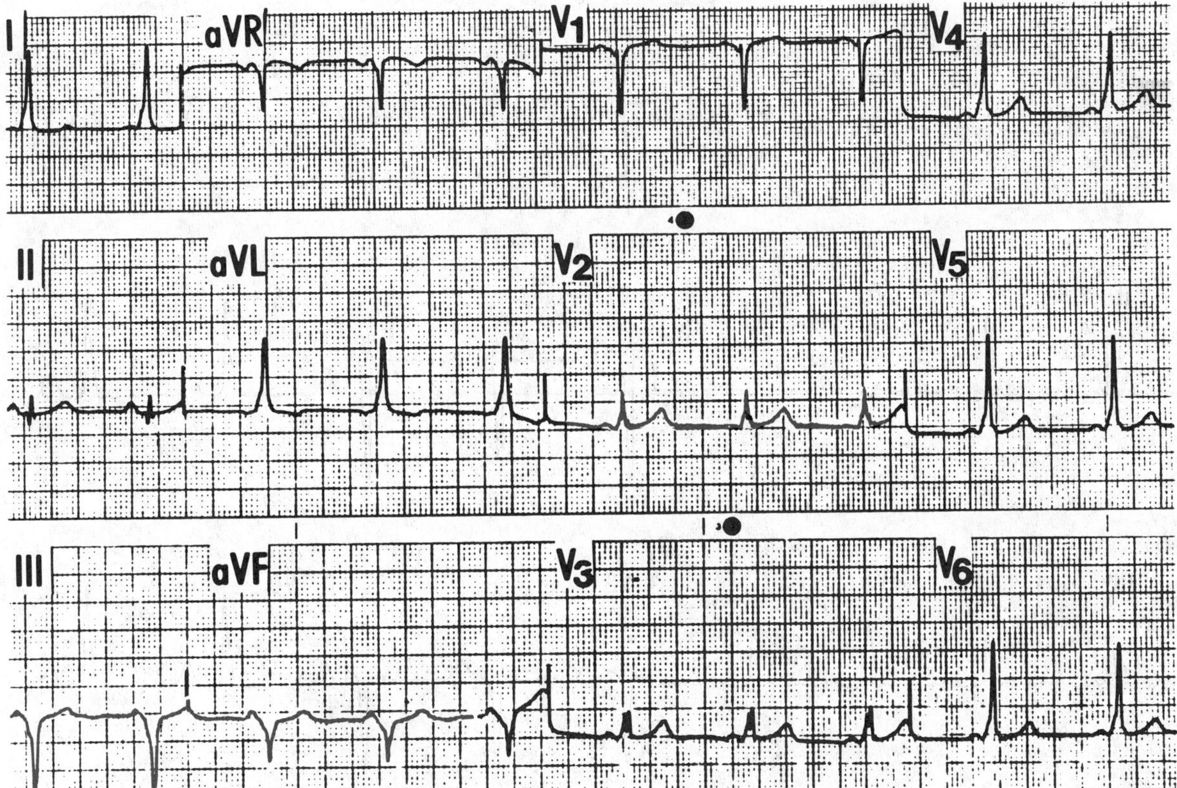

FIGURE 13-23 Wolff-Parkinson-White syndrome in a patient having a posteroseptal accessory pathway. Note short PR intervals with negative delta waves in III and aV_F. Lead V_2 shows all-positive QRS complexes.

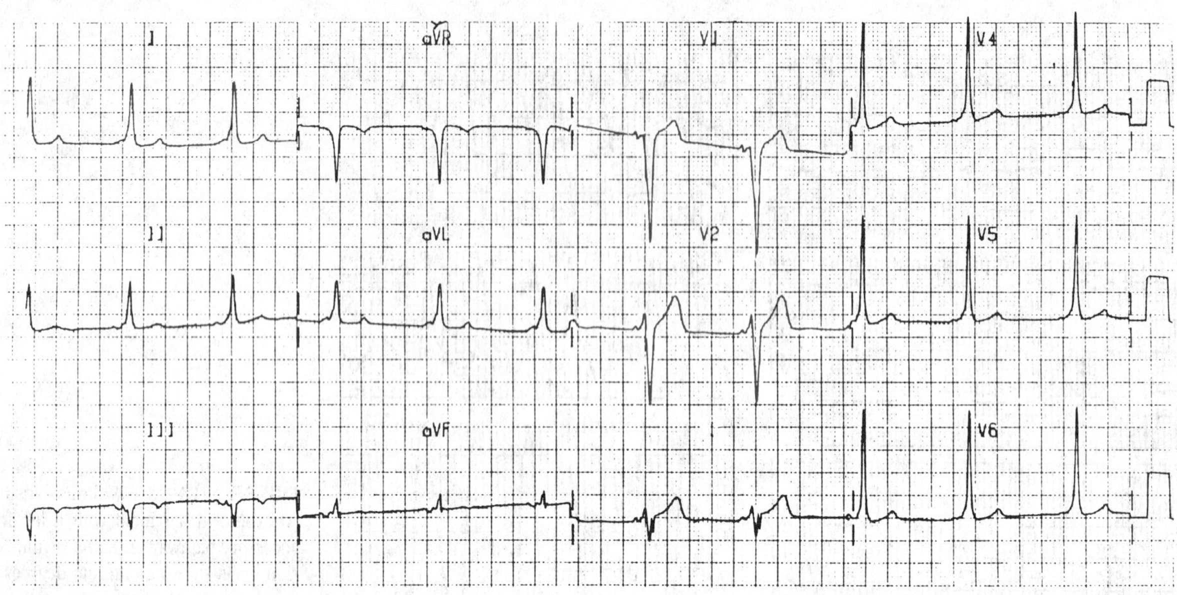

FIGURE 13-24 Wolff-Parkinson-White syndrome in a patient with a right free-wall accessory pathway. Note LBBB "pattern" characterized for diagnostic (of accessory pathway location) purposes by a QRS deflection greater than 0.09 s in lead I with rS complexes in leads V_1 and V_2. The electrical axis is approximately +15°.

LBBB pattern (as defined) with an electrical axis ranging between +30° and +120° (Fig. 13-25). A q wave may be present in lead aV_L but *not* in leads I or V_6.

Mixed patterns may result from the existence of two separate accessory pathways.

Nodoventricular (Mahaim) Fibers

During sinus rhythm, the surface ECG in patients having exclusively nodoventricular (Mahaim) fibers usually shows a normal PR interval without a distinct delta wave.[107] As a rule, the so-called classical pattern only

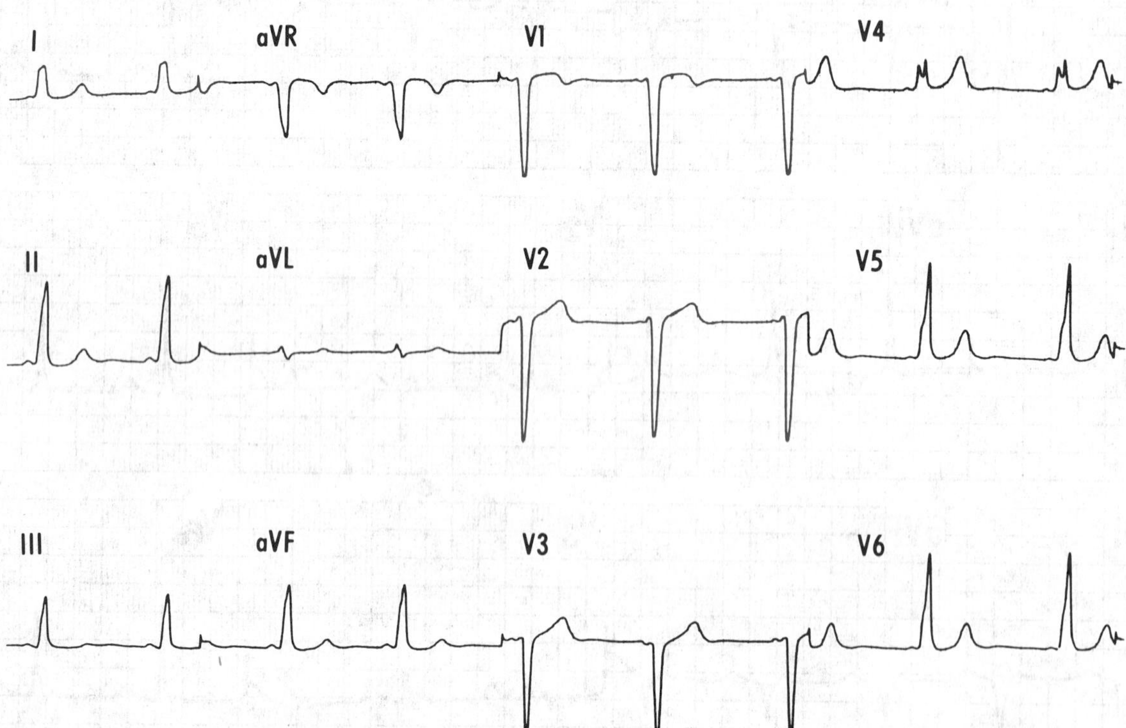

FIGURE 13-25 Wolff-Parkinson-White syndrome in a patient with a right anteroseptal accessory pathway. Note LBBB pattern (as defined in Fig. 13-24). The most important difference with Fig. 13-24, however, is that the electrical axis points more vertically, toward +60°, thereby being located within the range of the axis (+30° to +120°) reported for right anteroseptal accessory pathways.

appears during atrial pacing. According to data from intraoperative mapping, what had been usually considered to be Mahaim fiber conduction really represents anterograde propagation through a slowly conducting right free-wall accessory pathway.[108]

Wide QRS Complexes Produced by Ventricular Pacing from Different Sites

When determining the location of the stimulating electrodes, one should take special care not to consider that the distortion produced by large unipolar spikes constitutes parts of the pacing-induced QRS complexes. It is best *not* to describe the electrically produced ventricular beats as having an RBBB or LBBB morphology since what is relevant is the polarity of the properly positioned V_1 and V_2 electrodes and the direction of the EA (Fig. 13-26).[109,110] For example, endocardial or epicardial stimulation of the *anteriorly* located right ventricle at any site [apical (inferior), or mid/outflow tract (superior)] yields predominantly negative deflections in the right chest leads due to the *posterior* spread of activation (first and second vertical rows in Fig. 13-26). The reverse (positive deflections in V_1 and V_2) occurs when the epicardial stimulation of the superior and lateral portions of the posterior left ventricle by catheter electrodes in the distal coronary sinus or great and middle cardiac veins (or by implanted electrodes in the nearby muscle) results in *anteriorly* oriented forces (third and fourth vertical rows in Fig. 13-26). On the other hand, *superior* deviation of the electrical axis only indicates that a spatial (or cardiocephalic) *inferior* ventricular site has been stimulated, regardless of whether this site is the apical portion of the right ventricle or the inferior part of the left ventricle, the latter being paced through the middle cardiac vein (first and fourth vertical rows in Fig. 13-26). Conversely, an *inferior*, vertical axis is simply a consequence of pacing from a *superior* site, which can be the endocardium of the right ventricular outflow tract or the epicardium of the posterosuperior and lateral portions of the left ventricle (second and third vertical rows in Fig. 13-26).

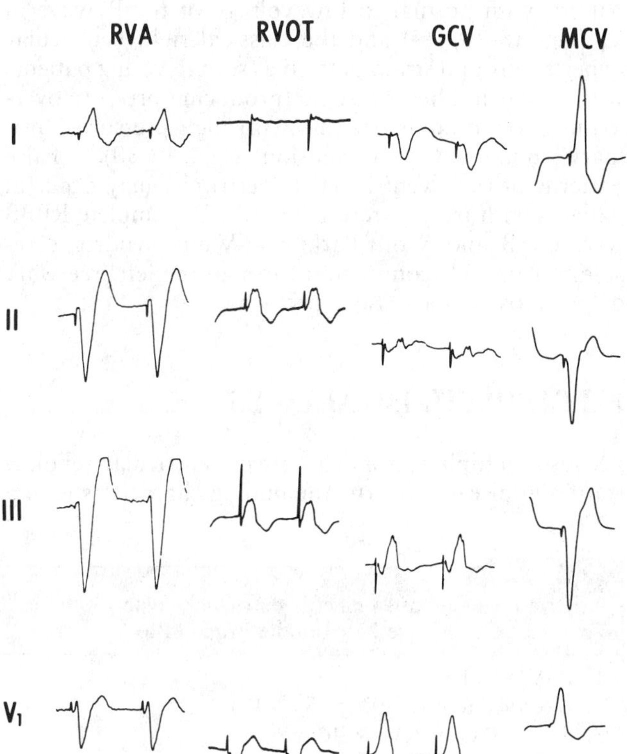

FIGURE 13-26 QRS changes (location of the electrical axis and polarity of lead V_1) produced by pacing from right ventricular apex (RVA), right ventricular outflow tract (RVOT), great cardiac vein (GCV), and middle cardiac vein (MCV).

LEFT ATRIAL HYPERTROPHY

Munuswamy et al.,[111] using M-mode echocardiography as the gold standard, evaluated the specificity and sensitivity of the most important clues for determining left atrial hypertrophy. These included (1) P-wave duration greater than 0.11 s and notched P wave with an interpeak interval in excess of 0.04 s and (2) negative phase of P in V_1 longer than 0.04 s and greater than 1 mm in lead V_1.

There are, however, problems when applying these criteria in a given ECG. For example, according to Josephson and Seides,[112] the mechanisms of prolonged duration of the P wave and of (posteriorly directed) terminal forces is delayed left atrial activation, not left atrial enlargement. In fact, most criteria mentioned above also apply for intraatrial block. Moreover, the previously mentioned findings in lead V_1[112] may reflect improper (high) placement of this lead, a common error made by ECG technicians. Generally, if the previously mentioned findings are found in patients with left ventricular enlargement or mitral stenosis, left atrial hypertrophy is most likely present, but in their absence, such findings most likely indicate an intraatrial conduction defect. In any case, the ECG pattern of left atrial hypertrophy results from a hypertrophy-induced intraatrial conduction delay.

LEFT VENTRICULAR HYPERTROPHY

As emphasized by Surawicz,[113] since the advent of other noninvasive techniques, there has been a changing role for the ECG in the diagnosis of ventricular hypertrophy. The ECG theory underlying the diagnosis of LVH has incorporated sound physical principles. Yet there are important limiting factors related to age, variable orientation of the heart in the chest, variable extracardiac factors, and the nonspecificity of each depolarization and repolarization abnormalities used in the diagnosis of LVH.[113] Necropsy studies have exposed the superiority of echocardiography (see Chap. 15) in respect to electrocardiography to detect LVH.[113] Echocardiography is also a better method for the serial follow-up of changes during progression or regression of LVH. In general, LVH increases the magnitude of left ventricular forces; tends to shift them posteriorly, to the left, and somewhat superiorly; prolongs left ventricular activation time; when significant, produces secondary ST-T-wave changes (the so-called left ventricular strain patterns); and is usually associated (again, when significant) with left atrial enlargement.[113]

As previously mentioned, however, many factors may decrease QRS voltage, while it is possible for other processes to increase intraventricular conduction time and to produce secondary ST-T-wave changes. Several criteria have been postulated to diagnose LVH in patients with narrow QRS complexes using necropsies as the gold standard (Tables 13-4 and 13-5).[114,115]

In addition, with echocardiography as the gold standard, several authors postulated electrocardiographic criteria for diagnosis of LVH in the presence of complete LBBB and LAFB (Tables 13-6 and 13-7).[116,117] It should be pointed out that the high sensitivity and specificity reported by Gertsch et al.[117] for diagnosis of LVH and LAFB have not been corroborated in preliminary studies performed in our department (unpublished observation; nevertheless indicated in Table 13-7).

TABLE 13-5

Point Score System of Romhilt and Estes for Diagnosis of Left Ventricular Hypertrophy

1. Amplitude, 3 points
   Any of the following:
   a. Largest R or S wave in the limb leads ≥ 20 mm
   b. S wave in V_1 or V_2 ≥ 30 mm
   c. R wave in V_5 or V_6 ≥ 30 mm
2. ST-T-segment changes (typical pattern of left ventricular strain with the ST-T-segment vector shifted in direction opposite to the mean QRS vector)
   Without digitalis, 3 points
   With digitalis, 1 point
3. Left atrial involvement, 3 points
   Terminal negativity of the P wave in V_1 is 1 mm or more in depth with a duration of 0.04 s or more
4. Left axis deviation: −30° or more, 2 points
5. QRS duration ≥ 0.09 s, 1 point
6. Intrinsicoid deflection in V_5, V_6 = 0.05 s, 1 point

SOURCE: Romhilt and Estes.[115]
NOTE: sensitivity, 54%; specificity, 97%.

PROCESSES PRODUCING OR LEADING TO RVH AND ENLARGEMENT

Right ventricular hypertrophy is manifest in the ECG only when the right ventricular forces predominate over those of the left ventricle. Since the latter has, roughly, three times more mass than the former, the right ventricle may double in size (when the left ventricle is normal) or triple its weight (when there is significant LVH) and still not result in the necessary requirements to pull the electrical forces anteriorly and to the right. For these reasons, right ventricular hypertrophy cannot be recognized easily in adult patients.

Despite these limitations, the ECG manifestations of right ventricular hypertrophy or enlargement can be subdivided into the following three main types[113]: (1) the posterior and rightward displacement of the QR forces associated with low voltage, as seen in patients with pulmonary emphysema (Fig. 13-27); (2) the incomplete RBBB pattern occurring in patients with chronic lung disease and some congenital cardiac malformation resulting in volume overloading of the right ventricle (Fig. 13-28); (3) the true posterior wall myocardial infarction pattern with normal to low voltage of the R wave in V_1 (Fig. 13-29); (4) and the classical right ventricular hypertrophy and strain pattern as seen in young patients with congenital heart disease (producing pressure overloading) or in adult patients with high pressure ("primary" pulmonary hypertension) (Fig. 13-30).[113] False patterns of right ventricular hypertrophy may occur in patients with true posterior (basal) MI, complete RBBB with LPFB and Wolff-Parkinson-White syndrome resulting from AV conduction through the left free wall, or posteroseptal accessory pathways.

TABLE 13-4

Voltage Criteria for Diagnosis of Left Ventricular Hypertrophy

	Sensitivity (%)	Specificity (%)
Limb lead criteria		
$R_1 + S_3 > 25$ mm	10.6	100
$RaV_L > 7.5$ mm	22.5	96.5
$RaV_L > 11$ mm	10.6	100
$RaV_F > 20$ mm	1.3	99.5
Precordial lead criteria		
$SV_1 + RV_5$ or $RV_6 > 35$ mm	42.5	95
SV_1 or $V_2 + RV_5$ or $RV_6 > 35$ mm	55.6	88.5
$SV_1 + RV_5$ or $RV_6 > 30$ mm	55.6	89.5
Greatest R + greatest S > 45 mm	45	93
RV_5 or $RV_6 > 26$ mm	25	98.5

SOURCE: Romhilt et al.[114]

ELECTROLYTE IMBALANCES

Because multiple factors can affect ventricular repolarization in diseased hearts, the finding characteristic of a

TABLE 13-6

Criteria for Diagnosis of Left Ventricular Hypertrophy in Presence of Complete Left Bundle Branch Block

1. RaV_L ≥ 11 mm
2. Electrical axis ≤ 40° (or $S_2 > R_1$)
3. $SV_1 + RV_5$ or RV_6 ≥ 40 mm
4. SV_2 ≥ 30 and SV_3 ≥ 25 mm

SOURCE: From Kafka et al.[16]
NOTE: sensitivity, 75%; specificity, 90%. Left ventricular hypertrophy diagnosed by echocardiography when left ventricular mass is ≥ 115 g/m².

TABLE 13-7

Criteria for Diagnosis of Left Ventricular Hypertrophy in Presence of Left Anterior Fascicular Block*

Study	ECG Criteria	Sensitivity (%)	Specificity (%)	Positive Predictive Value (%)	Negative Predictive Value (%)
Bozzi and Figini[117]	$SV_1 + (RV_5 + SV_5) \geq 25$ mm	69	92	90	73
Milliken[117]	$RaV_L \geq 13$ mm	35	92	82	56
Milliken[117]	SIII ≥ 15 mm	38	87	77	57
Gerstch et al.[117]	SIII + maximal sum of R+S in any single precordial lead	96	87	89	95
Reevaluated Gerstch criteria†		80	55	78	58

*Left ventricular hypertrophy diagnosed by echocardiography when left ventricular mass is ≥ 124 g/m².
†Unpublished observations performed in our department.
SOURCE: Gertsch et al.[117]

specific electrolyte abnormality may be modified, and even mimicked, by various pathological processes and the effects of certain drugs. In practice, the major problem with the electrocardiographic diagnosis of electrolyte imbalance is not the negative ECG with abnormal serum values, but the production of similar changes by other conditions in patients with normal serum values.[118]

Hyperkalemia

The initial effect of acute hyperkalemia is the appearance of peaked T waves with a narrow base (Fig. 13-31, left). The diagnosis of hyperkalemia is almost certain when the duration of the base is 0.20 s or less (with rates between 60 and 110 per minute).[118] As the degree of hyperkalemia increases, the QRS complex widens with the electrical axis usually being deviated abnormally to the left, and only rarely to the right (Fig. 13-31, right). In addition, the PR interval prolongs, and the P wave flattens until it disappears.[118] If untreated, death ensues either due to ventricular standstill or coarse slow ventricular fibrillation. Death can also result if wide QRS complexes occurring at fast rates are diagnosed as ventricular tachycardia and the patient is treated with antiarrhythmic drugs. On the other hand, Class IA and IC drugs as well as large doses of tricyclic antidepressants (especially when ingested for suicidal purposes) can also produce marked QRS widening. These processes, however, do not coexist with narrow-based, peaked T waves. Rarely, hyperkalemia produces (in the absence of coronary artery disease) a degree of ST-segment elevation in the right chest leads capable of suggesting anteroseptal myocar-

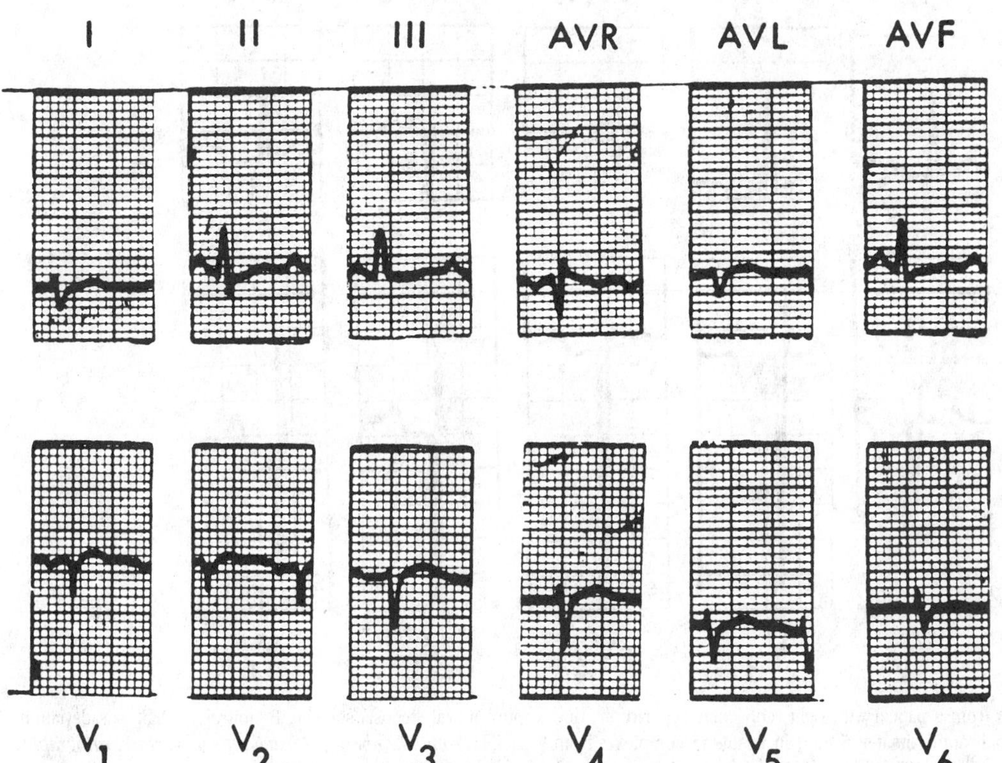

FIGURE 13-27 Electrocardiogram taken on a patient with pulmonary emphysema showing slight right axis deviation with small rS complexes in lead I, a vertical heart position, overall tendency to low voltage, and rS complexes in all chest leads. (*From L Lemberg, A Castellanos Jr: Vectorcardiography, 2d ed. New York, Appleton-Century-Crofts, 1975. Reproduced with permission from the publisher and authors.*)

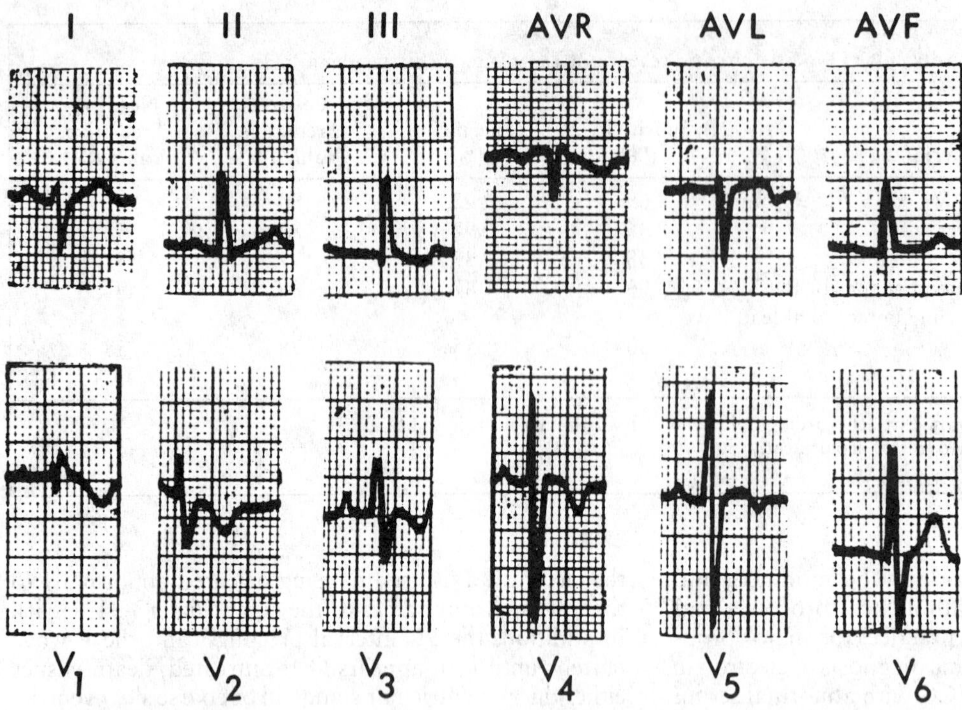

FIGURE 13-28 Electrocardiogram from a patient with right ventricular enlargement (volume overload in type) due to a small atrial septal defect (ostium secundum). Right axis deviation was associated with an incomplete RBBB pattern (rsR′ complexes in lead V_1). (*From L Lemberg, A Castellanos Jr: Vectorcardiography, 2d ed. New York, Appleton-Century-Crofts, 1975. Reproduced with permission from the publisher and authors.*)

dial injury. These constitute the "dialyzable currents of injury in potassium intoxication" reported by Levine et al.[119] (See also Chap. 37.)

Hypokalemia

The abnormal and delayed repolarization that occurs in hypokalemia is best expressed as QU, rather than QT, prolongation, since at times it can be difficult to differentiate between notching of the T wave and T- and U-wave fusion.[118] As the serum potassium falls, the ST segment becomes progressively more depressed and there is a gradual blending of T wave into what appears to be a tall U wave (Fig. 13-32, top).

An electrocardiographic pattern similar to that of hypokalemia can be produced by some antiarrhythmic

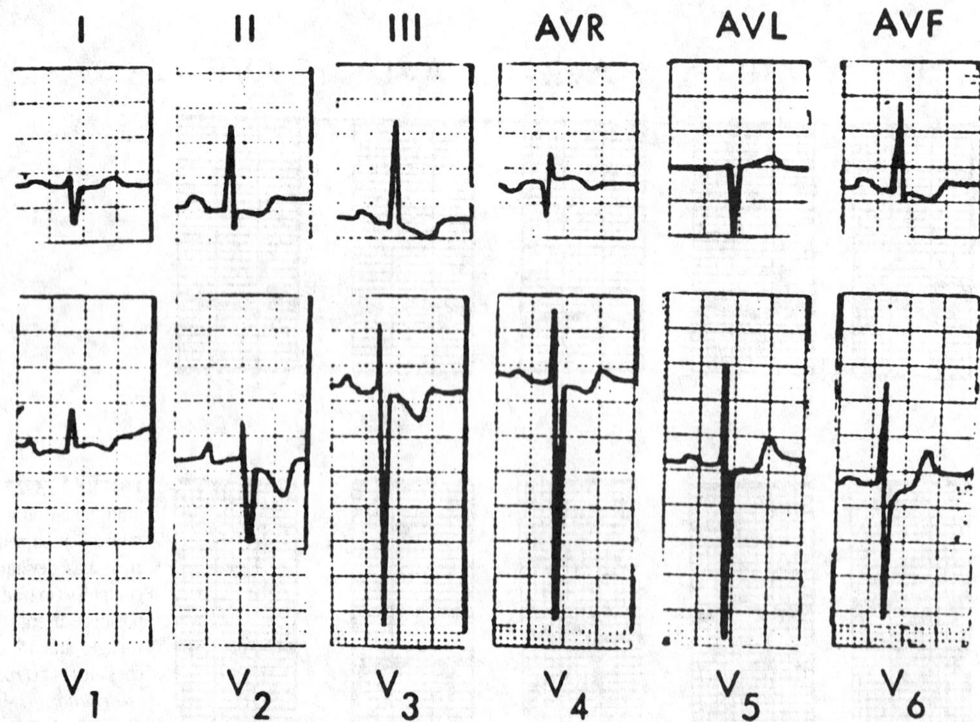

FIGURE 13-29 Electrocardiogram from a patient with right ventricular hypertrophy due to pure mitral stenosis showing P "mitrale," right axis deviation, an all-positive deflection (R wave of only approximately 5 mm) in V_1, and rS complexes from V_2 to V_6. (*From L Lemberg, A Castellanos Jr: Vectorcardiography, 2d ed. New York, Appleton-Century-Crofts, 1975. Reproduced with permission from the publisher and authors.*)

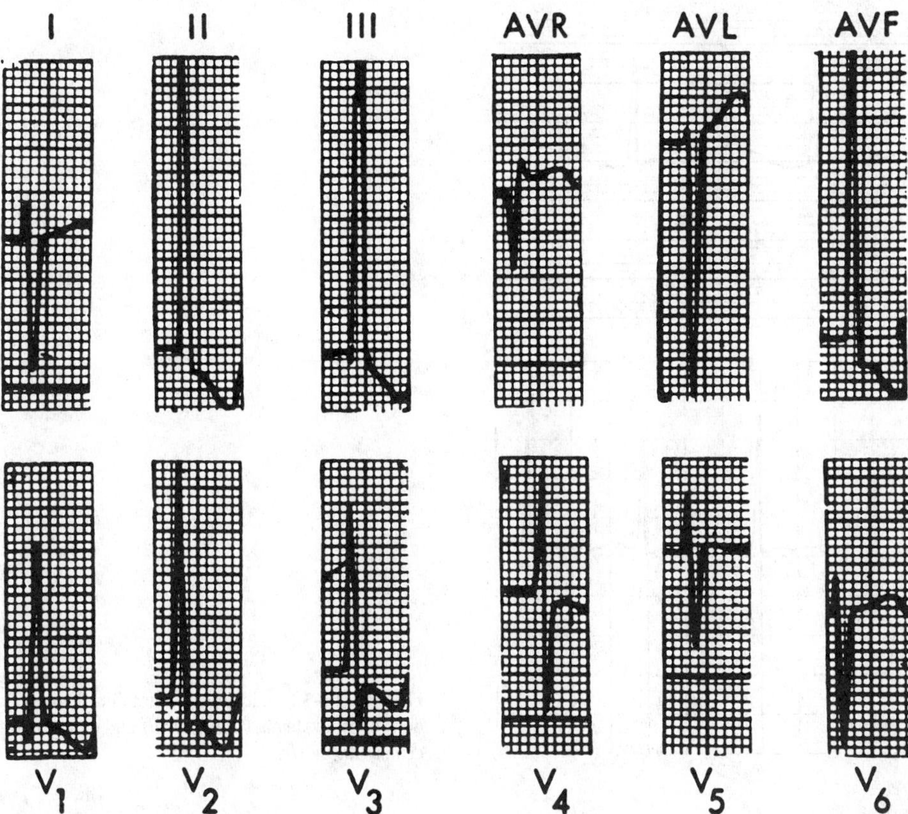

FIGURE 13-30 Electrocardiogram from a 17-year-old patient who had right ventricular enlargement (pressure overloading in type) due to severe pulmonic stenosis. Note extreme right axis deviation, overall high voltage, and qR complexes in lead V_1 *without* an incomplete RBBB pattern. (*From L Lemberg, A Castellanos Jr: Vectorcardiography, 2d ed. New York, Appleton-Century-Crofts, 1975. Reproduced with permission from the publisher and authors.*)

drugs, especially quinidine. These quinidine-induced repolarization changes may appear in patients receiving therapeutic doses who do not have elevated serum levels. Although at times these changes simply reflect that the patient is taking this drug, they should be viewed with extreme caution. When repolarization is greatly prolonged, however, they lead to multiform ventricular arrhythmias, including the so-called torsades de pointes. (See also Chap. 37.)

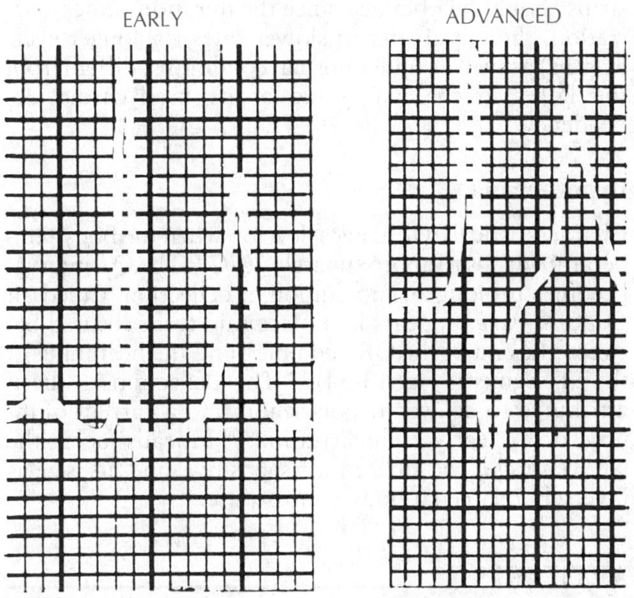

EARLY ADVANCED

FIGURE 13-31 Electrocardiographic manifestations of early hyperkalemia (narrow QRS complex with a peaked T wave having a very narrow base) and advanced hyperkalemia (absent P wave, wide QRS complex, and peaked T wave).

Hypomagnesemia

Hypomagnesemia does not produce QU prolongation unless the coexisting hypokalemia (with which it is almost invariably associated) is severe.[118] Long-standing and very marked magnesium deficiency lowers the amplitude of the T wave and depresses the ST segment.[118] It is difficult to differentiate between the changes produced by magnesium from those produced by potassium. For this reason it has been stated that hypomagnesia does not cause any changes in the ECG.[120] (See also Chap. 37.)

Hypermagnesemia

Similarly, in clinical tracings the effects of hypermagnesemia on the ECG are difficult to identify because the changes are dominated by calcium.[121] According to some authors, administration of intravenous magnesium to patients with normal ECGs may shorten the QT interval.[120] Other authors found no effects on ventricular refractoriness that are reflected by changes in the QT interval.[122] Intravenous magnesium given to patients with torsades de pointes controls the arrhythmia in a high percentage of patients without changing the prolonged QT interval significantly.[123] The calcium blocking activity of magnesium was suggested to be one of the mechanisms responsible for this antiarrhythmic activity.[121] (See also Chap. 37.)

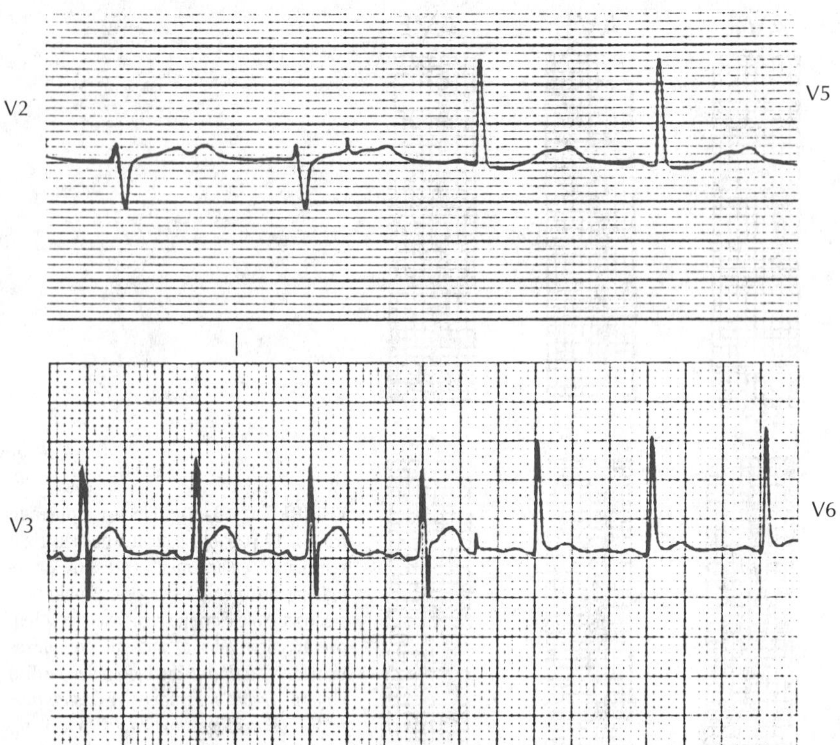

FIGURE 13-32 Electrocardiographic manifestations of hypokalemia (*upper strip*) and of hypercalcemia (*lower strip*).

Hypercalcemia

During sinus rhythm with normal rates the QT interval is short (Fig. 13-22, bottom). If factors known to modify the QT interval are not present, it has been said that a reasonably accepted correlation exists between the duration of the interval and serum calcium levels.[118] Occasionally, the ST segment is depressed and the T waves may become inverted in left and right chest leads. Digitalis also shortens the QT interval but produces its characteristic "effects" in leads where the R waves predominate. The classical upward concavity of the ST segment is seen in the left chest leads in patients with LVH and in V_1 and V_2 when there is right ventricular hypertrophy (with predominantly positive deflections in these leads). (See also Chap. 37.)

Hypocalcemia

The typical electrocardiographic pattern of hypocalcemia consists of QT prolongation at the expense of the ST segment.[118] The T wave is usually of normal width but can be narrow based if there is coexistent (moderate) hyperkalemia (Fig. 13-33). A very marked subendocardial ischemia (with the so-called hyperacute ST-T changes) can produce a similar pattern, but in those cases the T wave, though peaked, is not as narrow based. It has been said that hypocalcemia per se does not produce T-wave inversion. When present, the latter is usually a reflection of coexisting processes such as LVH and incomplete LBBB. An ECG pattern similar to that of hypocalcemia can be produced by some organic abnormalities of the central nervous system and by congenitally prolonged QT intervals such as the Jervell and Lange-Nielsen and Romano-Ward syndromes. (See next section.) (See also Chap. 37.)

DELAYED REPOLARIZATION SYNDROMES

Although it is not always easy to differentiate between prolonged QT and QU intervals, determining the existence of prolonged repolarization is not difficult, especially if intermediate (V_3 and V_4) chest leads are analyzed. For these reasons, it has been recommended that the single, more comprehensive, delayed depolarization syndrome be used (Table 13-8).[118,124–128] In these cases, long strips should be obtained since the duration of depolarization, though greater at slower rates (or longer cycle lengths) as well as under normal conditions, differs from the latter in the magnitude of its bradycardia dependency.

Hypothermia

Characteristic ECG changes develop when the body temperature drops to approximately 30°C.[11] The QT interval becomes prolonged. In addition, a deflection, called an *Osborn wave*, appears in a place said to be located between the end of the QRS complex and the beginning of the ST segment (Fig. 13-34).[129] This deflection has been attributed to delayed depolarization, to a current of injury, or to "early" repolarization.[130] In leads facing the left ventricle, the deflection is positive and its size is inversely related to body temperature.

ARTIFACTS

During the last few years the number and types of instruments used for noninvasive (nonelectrical) and invasive (electrical) study of cardiac functions have multiplied

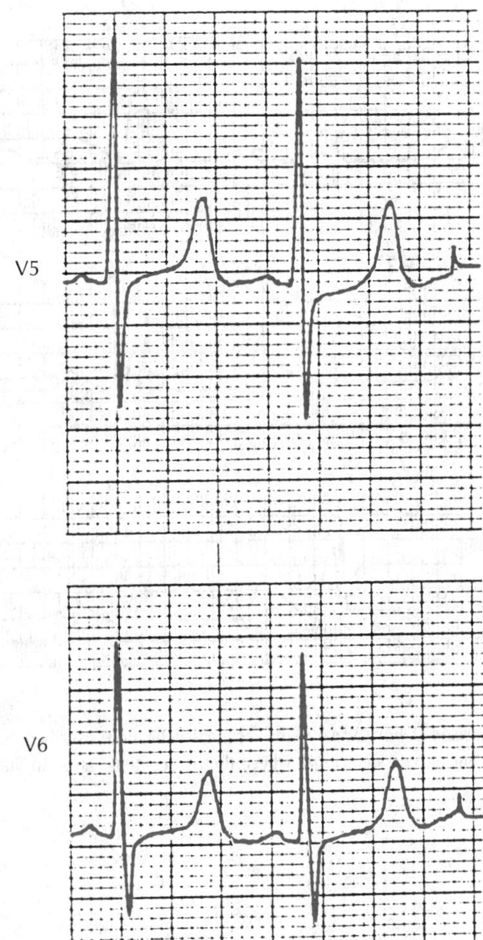

FIGURE 13-33 Electrocardiographic manifestations of hypocalcemia in a patient with coexisting hyperkalemia.

TABLE 13-8

Delayed Depolarization Syndromes (Prolonged QT and/or QU Intervals) Usually Bradycardia Dependent

1. Electrolyte disturbances
   a. Hypokalemia
   b. Hypocalcemia
   c. Hypomagnesemia
2. Drugs
   a. Class IA antiarrhythmic agents (quinidine, disopyramide, procainamide)
   b. Class III antiarrhythmic agents (amiodarone)
   c. Psychotropic drugs
3. Central nervous system diseases
   a. Subarachnoid hemorrhage
   b. Ruptured berry aneurysm
   c. Cryptococcal meningitis
4. Congenital syndromes
   a. Jervell and Lange-Nielsen syndrome
   b. Romano-Ward syndrome
5. Electrocardiographic ischemia
6. Arrhythmias
   a. Posttachycardia syndrome
   b. Cardiac arrest of any etiology
   c. Chronic idioventricular rhythms
7. Hypothermia

logarithmically. Naturally, physicians and hospital administrators have concentrated their attention on them. Technicians have been more interested in working in these more lucrative services. Such factors, and others, have downgraded the importance of 12-lead ECGs, relegating them to a tertiary role. Not surprisingly, the quality of technicians and of the ECG that they record have deteriorated in many centers. Optimal quality can only be achieved if the parties involved understand what is happening. The following are some of the artifacts commonly seen in current routine 12-lead ECGs.

Muscle Tremor and Alternating Current Interference

These are the most frequently encountered artifacts because some patients will continue to have disease processes producing tremor and because the amount of electronic equipment causing interference in a hospital environment has increased.

Improper Limb Lead Positioning

This has become not unusual after relaxation of quality control. It is more frequent in those institutions with inadequate standards for hiring technicians and with poor on-site training. Mixing up the cables from the electrocardiographic machine has gone beyond switching the right arm and left arm cables. Thus, various types of misplacement of only one cable are illustrated in Fig. 13-35. The method depicted in this illustration, based on the use of unipolar extremity leads only, is simpler than those incorporating the analysis of bipolar standard leads.[11] Not recognized in any textbook of electrocardiography is the uncontrovertible fact that in some centers even the "sanctity" of the attachment of the right leg (ground) cable to the right leg electrode has been violated (Fig. 13-36).[131] In our experience, this error is usually identified as improper cable attachment, but determination of the cables involved is usually not made correctly.[131]

Variations in Precordial Lead Placement

This is a problem more common now than when, in 1961, Simonson noted the considerable variation in chest lead placement in the same patients by different technicians and even by the same technician in several ECGs in the same patient.[132] This author found that in a controlled study, placement of the V_2 electrode varied 10 cm vertically and 8 cm horizontally in 103 healthy subjects.[132] Moreover, Kerwin et al.[133] found a rather large error in placement of chest electrodes (2 to 3 cm in both the horizontal and vertical directions) in repeated trials in the same patients by the same technicians. Perhaps the frequency of precordial lead misplacement is greater than that of somatic tremor.

Overshoot, Overdamping, and Running Down of the Standardization Battery

These problems, which can cause significant changes in QRS voltage and ST segments, may be enough to cause

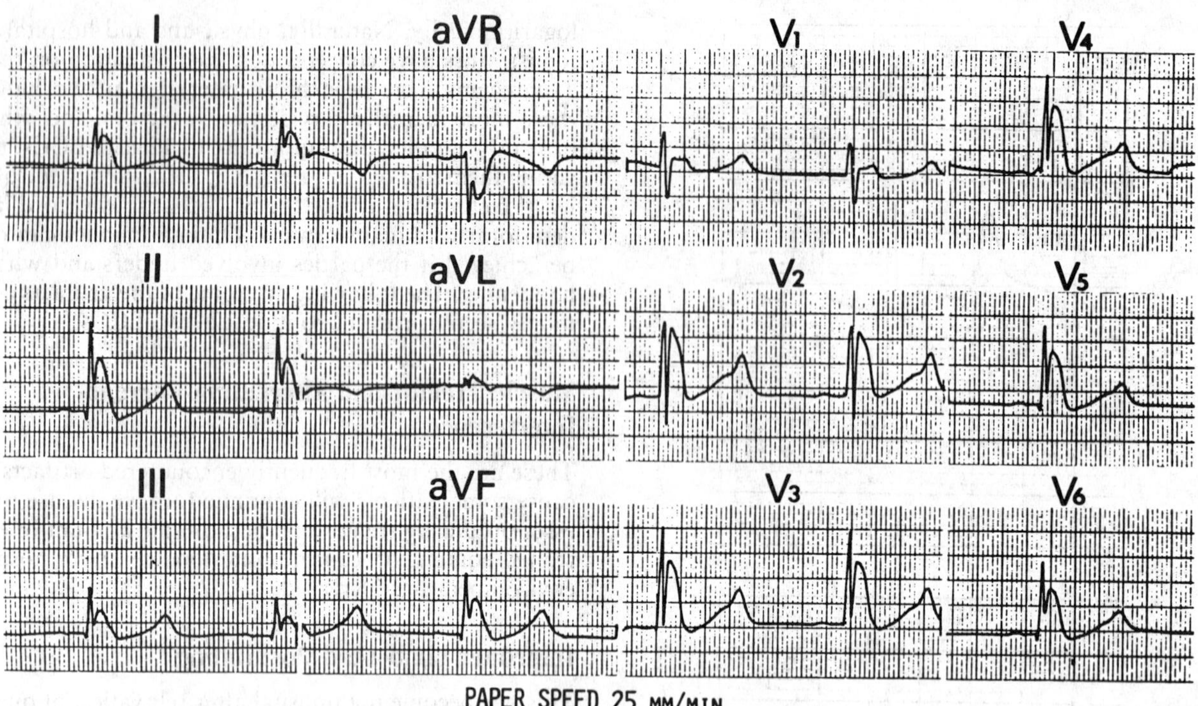

FIGURE 13-34 Electrocardiogram obtained from a patient with hypothermia. The characteristic Osborn wave is the terminal deflection inscribed between the slender part of the QRS complexes and the beginning of the ST segment. Note that it is not easy to determine where the ST segment starts. In addition, there is marked prolongation of the QT interval.

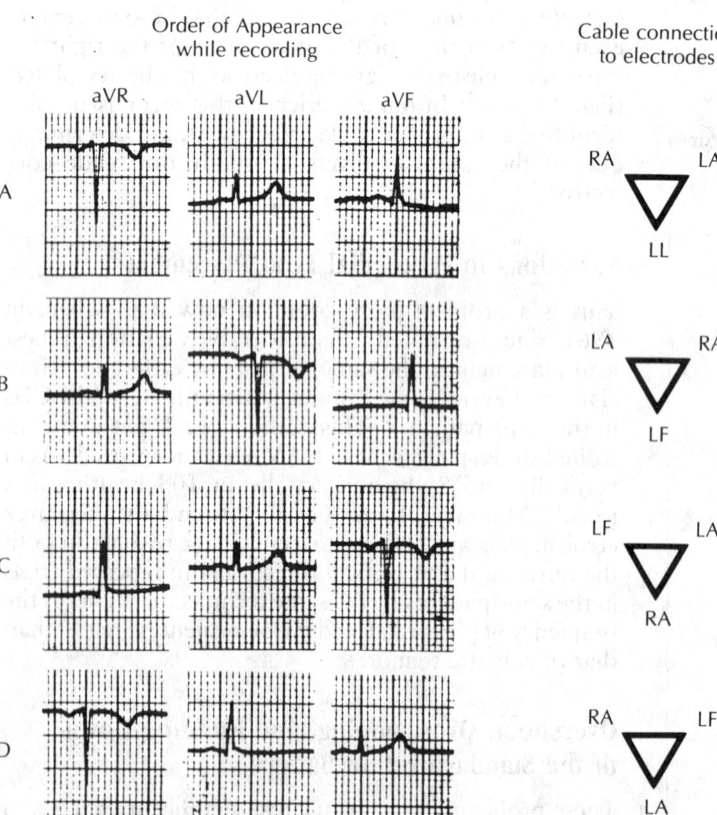

FIGURE 13-35 Identification of improper connections of a single *cable* from the electrocardiographic machine to the corresponding electrodes placed on the patient's limbs. Note that aV_R, aV_L, and aV_F invariably refer to *whatever morphology* is recorded when, while the ECG is being obtained, the corresponding knobs are turned in this order (regardless of whether the cables were properly or improperly attached). On the other hand, RA, LA, and LL (or LF) correspond to the *normal morphology* recorded by the cables so labeled. This method, based solely on the analysis of the unipolar extremity leads, is simpler than the method based on the study of the bipolar standard leads but is useful only when a single cable is misconnected. *A.* Normal. *B.* Since LA appears in aV_R and vice versa and RA appears in aV_L (with LF being in its normal position), the right arm and left arm cables must have been switched. *C.* Since LF appears in aV_R and RA appears in aV_F (with LA in its normal position), the right arm and left leg cables must have been switched. *D.* Since LA appears in aV_F and LF appears in aV_L (with RA in its normal position), the left arm and left leg cables must have been switched.

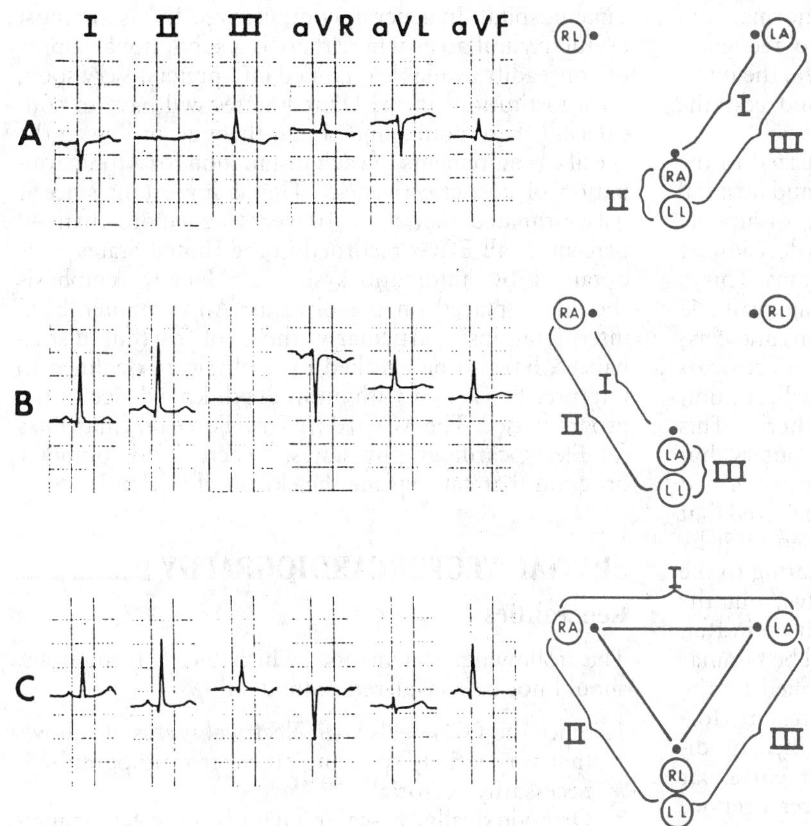

FIGURE 13-36 Identification of improper connections of the right leg (RL) (ground) cable. *C* can be regarded as almost equal to the control tracing since the RL (ground) and left leg (LL) cables were switched. The corresponding morphologies are not identical to the control morphologies since a very small difference in potential between both legs does exist. The latter is seen in *A*. Because the RL and RA cables were switched, lead II (RL, LL) records the difference in potential between both legs, which seems to be approximately 0.15 mV. The latter results in an almost straight line interrupted by a small blip. In addition, lead I represents the mirror image of normal lead III and lead III is the normal lead III. In *B*, where the LA and RL cables have been switched, lead III records almost a straight line. In addition, lead I is the normal lead II and lead II is the normal lead II. [*From A Castellanos, AN Saoudi, A Schwartz et al: Electrocardiographic patterns resulting from improper connection of the right leg (ground) cable. PACE 8:364–368, 1985. Reproduced with permission from the publisher and authors.*]

errors in the diagnosis of ventricular hypertrophy and coronary artery disease.

False Variations in Voltage

Garson noticed how, in several patients, ECGs taken weeks apart showed markedly different QRS voltages.[134] The latter were sometimes of enough magnitude to cause a pseudonormalization of a ventricular hypertrophy pattern. There had been no changes in hemodynamics, but different types of electrocardiographs were used. A study of this problem demonstrated that electrocardiographic data had a different voltage depending on whether they were recorded and displayed on an analog electrocardiograph or on a digital electrocardiograph. The potential importance of this study has to be emphasized, especially when information is input into a computer (see next section). Thus, if there is a statistically significant difference among ECGs, the serial comparisons must be done with the same machine. Moreover, criteria for voltage are only applicable to the type of instrument with which the data were gathered.

Wandering Baseline

Wandering baseline is usually due to unclean electrodes or electrodal sites.

How Should an ECG be Performed?

This question is appropriate in view of the many artifacts and technical (machine and human) problems occurring when ECGs are recorded. The Task Force of the American College of Cardiology (ACC)–American Heart Association (AHA) on Guidelines for Electrocardiography[4] have stated that the ECG should be performed and interpreted in accordance with the guidelines for optimal electrocardiography described in the ACC Tenth Bethesda Conference Report[135]; the guidelines for training described in the ACC Seventeenth Bethesda Conference Report on Cardiology Training[136]; the recommendations for standardization of leads and specifications for instruments in electrocardiography and vectorcardiography of the AHA[137]; and the recommendations for standardization and specifications for automated electrocardiography of the AHA.[138]

COMPUTER APPLICATIONS

It has been more than 30 years since the first attempts were made to apply computer technology to the interpretation of ECGs.[139] During this time, the field has progressed from initial attempts at the recognition of normal tracing to some of today's more sophisticated programs.[1,139–142] In general, computer systems for true analysis of ECGs have, as their main component, a program usually having the following four basic functions: (1) the measuring of electrocardiographic parameters, which includes an automatic wave front recognition section and a measurement section that extracts the wave fronts, a set of values, and control; (2) the interpretation of previously acquired information, responsible for the final statements generated by the program; (3) the identification of various rhythms, both normal and abnormal; and (4) the comparison with previous ECGs to recognize significant changes. Once a report is generated, the interpreter may simply correct (if necessary) and edit the computer interpretation.

A problem that is not sufficiently emphasized in the literature is the dilemma faced by physicians and hospital administrators who decide to computerize or update their ECG operation. This problem is the decision of selecting among the multiple available programs. This is so because substantial differences exist among available programs in regard to measurement definitions and classification criteria and terminology. As every electrocardiographer knows, there is a lack of standardized, universally agreed-on diagnostic terms and criteria. This problem, however, is not solely that of computers, but is related to all ECG interpretations, whether performed by individuals or machines. It has to be remembered that the program used depends on criteria imposed on it by human programmers. General guidelines relating to the selection of a program are not easy to give, but the interested reader may find pertinent information in Ref. 138. Physicians making the selections should be familiar with the diagnostic criteria employed (supplied by the manufacturers) and with the program's practical performance. The latter information can be obtained by directly communicating with other users. Of particular importance is knowledge of the manufacturer's service performance. Finally, the program selected has to be, at present, "tuned in" with the operational environment (community hospital or teaching institution, urban center or rural areas, etc.) in which it has to perform.

Once a program has been selected and is in use, it requires initial and periodic evaluation. The most practical method consists of accepting as standard constrained human observers, the constrained observers being given a set of measurements or criteria agreed upon before the evaluation. In academic centers, attempts to determine sensitivity and specificities should be made applying as standards electrocardiographically independent evidence, obtained using *more than one* of the currently available in vivo, noninvasive methods as well as (when possible) postmortem information.

Proper computerization has the following definite advantages:

1. Speed in providing reports with the resulting improved turnaround time.
2. Optimal utilization of emergency electrocardiographic services.
3. Reproducibility of measurements.
4. Improvements in quality control.
5. Possible decrease in physician's reading time and more consistency in interpretations.
6. Enhancement of the capacity to handle large volumes of ECGs.
7. Substantial improvement in record storage and retrieval with better comparison with previous tracings.

Computerized ECG programs also have to be evaluated using standard cost-effective methods. That is, the economics involved—initial investment, operational costs, payroll, overhead, and professional fees—have to be compared with those of the preexisting system in the same hospital. In general, computerized ECGs are most useful in rural areas where there is a suboptional supply of nonreadily available qualified interpreters. Very soon, most institutions in the United States will have to consider all these points and weigh them according to the specific requirements of each installation for a total evaluation of cost-effectiveness. This is important since it was estimated that even 10 years ago more than 40 percent of all ECGs recorded in the United States were obtained by automatic systems.[142] Finally, emphasis should be placed on the obvious: All computer ECG interpretations, particularly those of rhythm disturbances, have to be checked by a physician qualified to interpret ECGs and with an in-depth knowledge of the program used. The ACC/AHA Task Force on Guidelines for Electrocardiography states, "There is no computer program that can replace the skilled physician."[4]

SPATIAL VECTORCARDIOGRAPHY

Generalities

The following statements, which need reemphasis, should not be considered redundant:

1. Since the ECG deals with electrical forces, it follows that very strictly speaking all electrocardiography is necessarily vectorial.[81,143,144]
2. Orthodoxically, a scalar quantity only has magnitude, whereas a vector quantity has magnitude, direction, and sense.

When analyzing the vectorcardiogram (VCG), one should consider the activation of each muscle cell as producing an electrical force that can be represented by a vector depicting the spatial orientation and magnitude of this force.[143,145–147] During the spread of the activation process, innumerable electrical forces are generated. These multiple forces vary in magnitude and differ in direction. At any given moment, the resultant of these electrical forces can be represented by a spatial vector possessing magnitude, direction, and sense. This vector is referred to as an instantaneous vector and represents the resultant of *all* the forces of the heart acting at that particular moment. Immediately afterward, the wave of accession spreads to different areas of the myocardium, and the new instantaneous vector representing all the forces of the heart now occupies a different spatial position and has a different magnitude. This continues throughout the cardiac cycle, with the succeeding instantaneous vector occupying different spatial positions. At various times, the instantaneous vector may even have no appreciable magnitude. In the normal person, this corresponds to the PR segment, ST segment, and TP interval. If all manifest spatial vectors are diagrammatically represented as having a common point of origin, and if the distal points of the vectors are joined, a single spatial loop is formed for ventricular depolarization (QRS), ventricular repolarization (ST-T), and the atrial complex (P).

The VCG consists of four different loops. The electrical activity of the atria is recorded as a small loop designated the P loop; the depolarization of the ventricles is recorded as a large loop designated the QRS loop; while the repolarization of the ventricles is recorded as a smaller loop designated the ST-T loop. Finally, at high magnifications even a small U loop can also be recorded.

Electrovectorcardiography

The vectorial interpretation of the 12-lead ECG (electrovectorcardiography) has proven to be an important teaching tool. Strictly speaking, it is contradictory. Standard and unipolar extremity leads are truly vectorial (because of the "large" distance between electrodes and electrical center of the heart as given by the Einthoven theory). The same cannot be said about precordial leads because proximity effects render the truly vectorial concept unapplicable to them. Nevertheless, the latter is disregarded in electrovectorcardiographic interpretation.

Space: The Final Frontier

On the other hand, the theory of the truly spatial VCG is theoretically attractive. Because the heart is a tridimensional structure (located in space), its electrical activity should best be recorded by a spatial method. Indeed, space, as conceived by physicists through objects and their motion, has three dimensions, and positions are characterized by three numbers. The instant of an event is the fourth number. Four definite numbers correspond to every event; a definite event corresponds to any four numbers. Therefore, the world of events really forms a four-dimensional continuum. Unfortunately, judging by what is being published in the literature, the quest for finding an optimal method of visualizing the spatial loop has apparently been abandoned. Nevertheless, the spatial VCG is still of importance in children with congenital and acquired heart disease since in this population the criteria for pressure and volume overloading have proven value.[86] In our opinion, it is also of great value in categorizing the various types of intraventricular conduction defects.[146,147] While this may be attributed to the spatial technique per se, it can also be due to the use of instruments having a higher fidelity than routinely employed electrocardiographs. The VCG has also been found useful in detecting MI and certain types of right ventricular enlargement.

In practice, it has not been proven that the VCG gives more information than the routine 12-lead ECG, although some computer programs still use the Frank orthogonal leads X, Y, and Z. These programs thus constitute a 15-lead system. In addition, the time required to obtain a VCG is longer than the time required to record a 12-lead ECG. These are the main reasons for the logarithmic decrease in the use of spatial vectorcardiography during recent decades.

Other reasons are cost-effectiveness and the continuously increasing interest in other noninvasive methods of recording electrical activity (such as signal averaging and body surface mapping) or nonelectrical activity (such as echocardiography or magnetic resonance imaging, which looks at similar planes from *different* views).

To obtain the spatial VCG, electrodes are placed on the body surface in a way to record three leads whose planes are at right angles to each other. The true spatial VCG requires three corrected orthogonal leads with the following features[147,148]:

1. Mutual perpendicularity, with each lead being parallel to one of the rectilinear coordinate axes of the human body. Such axes are the horizontal, X (left-to-right and right-to-left) axis; the vertical, Y (inferosuperior or superoinferior) axis; and sagittal, Z (anteroposterior or posteroanterior) axis.
2. Equal amplitude from the vectorial viewpoint.
3. Retention of the same magnitude and direction for all points where cardiac electromotive forces are generated.

For example, even if two leads forming Einthoven's frontal plane were to be spatially correct, Einthoven's theory itself would make any electrodes placed for the purpose of obtaining the horizontal and sagittal planes (such as the tetrahedral system) spatially incorrect. The most used corrected spatial vectorcardiographic method in the world has been (and is) the one introduced by Frank.[148]

Since the spatial loop cannot be analyzed tridimensionally, it is customary to study its planar projections (Fig. 13-37). By proper attachment to the oscilloscope, the X and Y leads are used for the frontal plane, the X and Z leads for the horizontal plane, and the Z and Y leads for the sagittal plane (of which the right side has been the most popular).

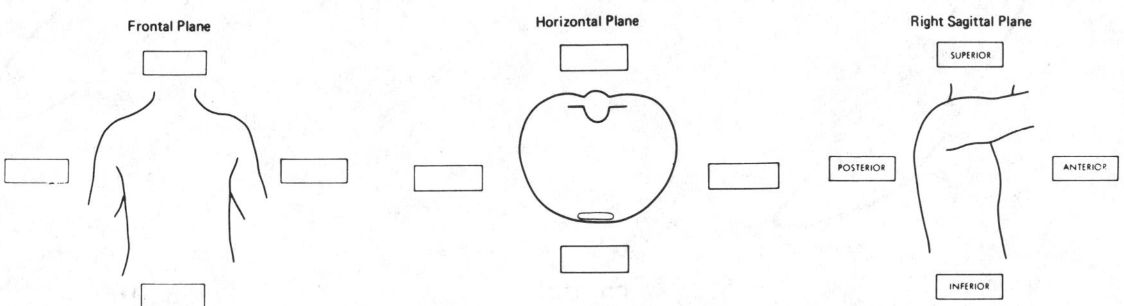

FIGURE 13-37 The spatial vectorcardiographic loops cannot be routinely analyzed in space with presently available techniques. Therefore, it is customary to study their projections in three planes seen as depicted in this figure. Note that (1) the frontal plane conforms to Einthoven's view of his equilateral triangle; (2) the horizontal plane is seen in such a way that the anterior surfaces of the heart and sternum are displayed in the inferior portions of the paper (in contrast to other noninvasive, nonelectrical methods); and (3) the sagittal plane is viewed from the right side of the patient. (*From L Lemberg, A Castellanos Jr: Vectorcardiography, 2d ed. New York, Appleton-Century-Crofts, 1975. Reproduced with permission from the publisher and authors.*)

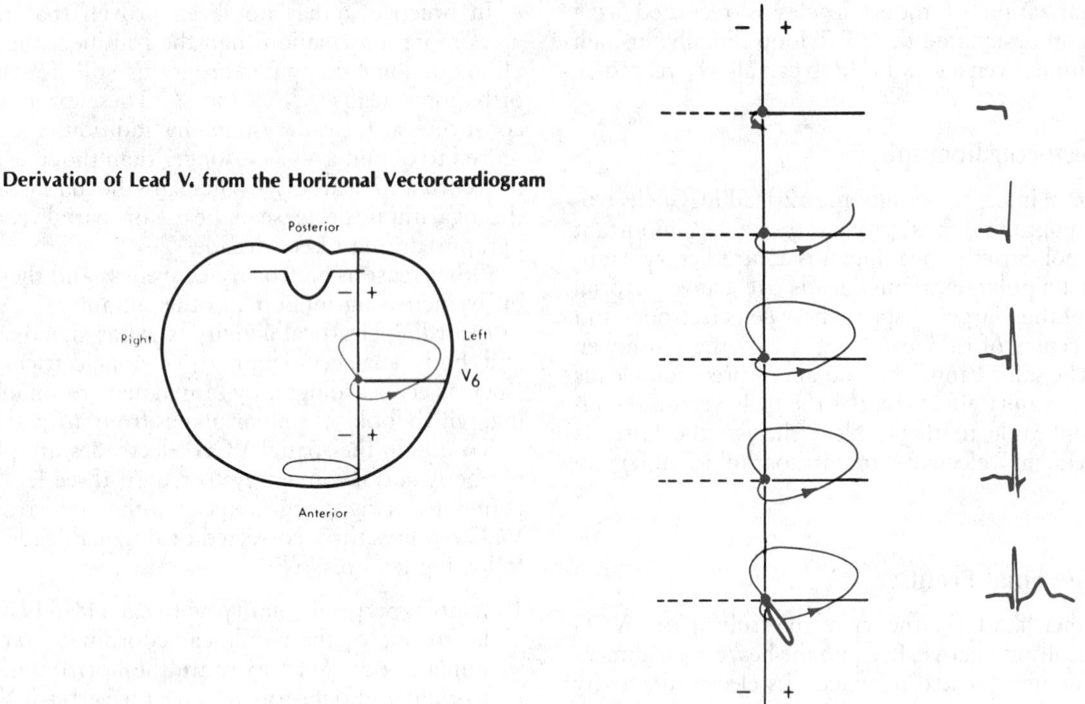

FIGURE 13-38 Method used to derive the morphology of a unipolar precordial lead (in this example lead V_6) from the horizontal plane QRS and ST-T loops. First (*left panel*), a line is drawn from the estimated location of the corresponding electrode to the point of origin of the loops. Thereafter, a perpendicular to this line passing from the point of origin is drawn. This divides the thorax into a negative area (for V_6) that is located beyond the perpendicular line and a positive area that is located between the perpendicular line and the electrode. Thus, in the top right schematic the small part of the loop located beyond the perpendicular line produces the small q wave in V_6. The other schematics show how progression of depolarization and repolarization produces parts of the QRS loop (and the entire ST-T loop), which are positive in lead V_6. The S wave occurs because the terminal part of the QRS loop is located beyond the perpendicular line. (*From L Lemberg, A Castellanos Jr: Vectorcardiography, 2d ed. New York, Appleton-Century-Crofts, 1975. Reproduced with permission from the publisher and authors.*)

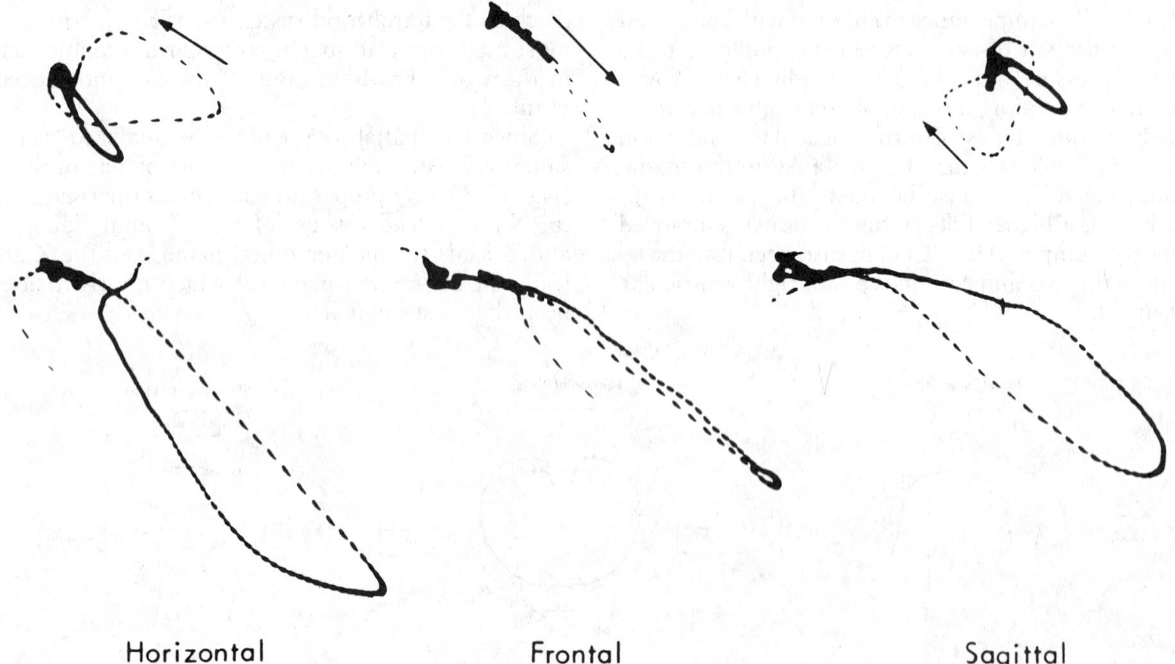

FIGURE 13-39 Planar projections of normal spatial VCG obtained with the Frank method. The ST-T loops are enlarged in the bottom view. In the horizontal plane, the QRS loop shows the expected, normal, counterclockwise (CCW) rotation (indicated by arrows). Although the narrow frontal plane QRS loop has clockwise (CW) rotation, in this plane either CCW, CW, or figure-eight rotations can be normal. In the right sagittal plane, the QRS loop displays its normal (CW) rotation. Enlargement of the ST-T loop clearly shows that its first half is inscribed more slowly. Therefore, the dashes (each representing 0.0025 s, or 25 ms) are closer together. Note that the rotation of the ST-T loop is similar to the rotation of the QRS loop in all planes. (*From L Lemberg, A Castellanos Jr: Vectorcardiography, 2d ed. New York, Appleton-Century-Crofts, 1975. Reproduced with permission of the publisher and authors.*)

Differences between Electrovectorcardiography and Spatial Vectorcardiography

In comparison with the ECG, the spatial VCG is another method of recording the electrical activity of the heart at the body surface. It is distinctly different than the various vectorial methods of ECG interpretation, such as those introduced by Sodi-Pallares et al.[7] and Grant.[34] In clinical practice and in teaching, both seem to be considered equal, but this is so only for pragmatic and didactic reasons. Although the spatial VCG and the ECG should each be studied as distinct methods, most electrocardiographers either memorize loop patterns or attempt to derive the leads with which they are familiar from the corresponding QRS loops.

Thus, bipolar standard and unipolar extremity leads are derived from the frontal plane more or less as when, in clinical ECG, they are derived from the electrical axis (in vectorcardiography the electrical axis is equated with the maximal QRS vector extending from the point of origin of the loop to its farthermost point). The unipolar precordial leads are derived from the horizontal plane loops (Fig. 13-38). Leads thus derived are different from the usual ECG leads. The latter, it was previously said, record electrical forces moving toward or away from them. But in the 12-lead ECG (especially when the precordial electrodes are misplaced) these forces can move spatially not only in a left-to-right and anterosuperior direction but also in an inferosuperior direction. On the other hand, the theory of spatial vectorcardiography states that the horizontal plane and unipolar leads just record left-to-right and anteroposterior forces. In spatial vectorcardiography, electrical forces oriented superiorly or inferiorly cannot be reflected in the horizontal plane, but only in the frontal and sagittal planes.

Most of the information contained in the sagittal plane is present in the frontal and horizontal planes. In practice, the sagittal plane is useful to act as a "judge" in cases of apparent discrepancy between the other two planes. For example, it serves to determine if a localized delay present in one of the two planes is "real" or is due to perpendicularity of vectors. It also serves for a better evaluation of the upward or downward direction of the initial 0.01- and 0.02-s vectors than the frontal plane. Normal QRS and ST-T loops obtained in the corresponding planes are depicted in Fig. 13-39.

REFERENCES

1. Macfarlane PW, Lawrie TDV (eds): *Comprehensive Electrocardiology. Theory and Practice in Health and Disease.* New York, Pergamon, 1989.
2. Myerburg RJ, Castellanos A: Resolution of nonspecific repolarization patterns from body surface signals: A new horizon of clinical electrocardiography. *J Am Coll Cardiol* 1989; 14:703–704.
3. Einthoven W, Fahr G, de Waart A: uber die Richtung und die manifeste Grosse der Pontetialschwankungen in menchlichen Herzen und uber den Einfluss der Herzlage auf die Form des Elecktrokardiogramms. *Arch Physiol* 1913; 150:275–315.
4. Task Force Report of the American College of Cardiology and the American Heart Association: ACC/AHA Guidelines for Electrocardiography. *Circulation* 1992; 19:473–481.
5. Johnston FD, Lepeschkin E (eds): *Selected Papers of Dr. Frank N. Wilson.* Ann Arbor, MI, Edwards Brothers, 1954.
6. Sodi-Pallares D, Calder RM: *New Bases of Electrocardiography.* St. Louis, CV Mosby, 1956: 169, 373.
7. Sodi-Pallares D, Medrano GA, Bisteni A, Ponce de Leon JJ: *Deductive and Polyparametric Electrocardiography.* Mexico, Inst Nac Cardiol Mexico, 1970: 36, 136.
8. Rosenbaum MB, Elizari MV, Lazzari JO: *The Hemiblocks.* Oldsmar, FL, Tampa Tracings, 1970.
9. Lipman BS, Massie E, Kleiger RE: *Clinical Scalar Electrocardiography,* 6th ed. Chicago, Year Book Medical Publishers, 1972: 210–215.
10. Schamroth L: *The Electrocardiology of Coronary Artery Disease,* 2d ed. Oxford, Blackwell Scientific, 1984.
11. Marriott HJL: *Practical Electrocardiography,* 8th ed. Baltimore, Williams & Wilkins, 1988.
12. Cabrera E, Gaxiola A: *Teoria y Practica de la Electrocardiografia,* 2d ed. Mexico, La Prensa Medica Mexicana, 1966.
13. Barker JM: *The Unipolar Electrocardiogram: A Clinical Interpretation.* New York, Appleton-Century-Crofts, 1952.
14. Lepeschkin E: *Modern Electrocardiography,* vol 1: *The P-Q-R-S-T-U Complex.* Baltimore, Williams & Wilkins, 1951.
15. Castellanos A, Myerburg RJ: *The Hemiblocks in Myocardial Infarction.* New York, Appleton-Century-Crofts, 1976.
16. Castellanos A Jr, Lemberg L: *A Programmed Introduction to the Electrical Axis and Action Potential.* Oldsmar, FL, Tampa Tracings, 1974: 34, 114.
17. Wilson FN, MacLeod AG, Barker PS, Johnston FD: The determination and significance of the areas of the ventricular deflections of the electrocardiogram. *Am Heart J* 1934; 10:46–61.
18. Rosenbaum MB, Blanco HH, Elizari MV, Lazzari JO, Vetulli HM: Electrotonic modulation of ventricular repolarization and cardiac memory. In: Rosenbaum MB, Elizari MV (eds): *Frontiers of Cardiac Electrophysiology.* Boston, Martinus Nijhoff, 1983: 67–99.
19. Bayley RH: An interpretation of injury and the ischemic effects of myocardial infarction in accordance with the laws which determine the flow of electric current in homogenous volume conductors and in accordance with relevant pathologic changes. *Am Heart J* 1942; 24:514–528.
20. Bruyneel KJJ: Use of moving epicardial electrodes in defining ST-segment changes after acute coronary occlusion in the baboon: Relation to primary ventricular fibrillation. *Am Heart J* 1975; 89:731–741.
21. Holland RP, Brooks H: TQ-ST segment mapping: Critical review and analysis of current concepts. *Am J Cardiol* 1977; 40:110–129.
22. Janse MJ: Electrophysiology and electrocardiology of acute myocardial ischemia. *Can J Cardiol* 1986; 2(suppl A):46A-52A (July).
23. Tzivoni D, Chenzbraun A: The significance of ST abnormalities in myocardial infarction. *Cardiol Clin* 1987; 5:419–426.
24. Mills RM, Young E, Gorlin R, Lesch M: Natural history of S-T segment elevation after acute myocardial infarction. *Am J Cardiol* 1975; 35:609–614.
25. Arvan S, Varat MA: Persistent ST-segment elevation and left ventricular wall abnormalities. A 2-dimensional echocardiographic study. *Am J Cardiol* 1984; 53:1542–1546.
26. Barold SS, Falkoff MD, Ong LS, Heinle RA: Significance of transient electrocardiographic Q waves in coronary artery disease. *Cardiol Clin* 1987; 5:367–380.
27. Timmis GC: Electrocardiographic effects of reperfusion. *Cardiol Clin* 1987; 5:427–446.
28. Braunwald E, Kloner RA: The stunned myocardium: Prolonged postischemic ventricular dysfunction. *Circulation* 1982; 66:1146–1149.
29. Bashour TT, Kabbani SS, Brewster HP, Wald SH, Hanna ES, Cheng TO: Transient Q waves and reversible cardiac failure during myocardial ischemia. Electrical and mechanical stunning of the heart. *Am Heart J* 1983; 106:780–783.
30. Rahimtoola SH: A perspective on the three large multicenter randomized clinical trials of coronary bypass surgery for chronic stable angina. *Circulation* 1985; 72(suppl 5):123–135.
31. Braunwald E, Rutherford JD: Reversible ischemic left ventricular dysfunction: Evidence for the "hibernating myocardium." *J Am Coll Cardiol* 1986; 8:1467–1470.
32. Abbott JA, Scheinman MM: Nondiagnostic electrocardiogram in patients with acute myocardial infarction: Clinical and anatomic correlations. *Am J Med* 1973; 55:608–613.
33. The Criteria Committee of the New York Heart Association: *Nomenclature and Criteria for Diagnosis of Diseases of the Heart*

and Great Vessels, 8th ed. Boston, Little, Brown and Company, 1979: 94.
34. Grant RP: Spatial vector electrocardiography: A method for calculating the spatial electrical vectors of the heart from conventional leads. *Circulation* 1950; 2:676–695.
35. Grant RP, Estes EH Jr: *Spatial Vector Electrocardiography*. New York, Blakiston, 1951.
36. Kracoff OH, Adelman AG, Marquis JF, Caspi A, Aldridge HE, Schwartz L: Twelve-lead electrocardiogram recording during percutaneous transluminal coronary angioplasty. Analysis of reciprocal changes. *J Electrocardiol* 1990; 23:191–198.
37. Braat SH, Brugrada P, den Dulk K, van Ommen V, Wellens HJJ: Value of lead V_4R for recognition of the infarct coronary artery in acute inferior myocardial infarction. *Am J Cardiol* 1984; 53:1538–1541.
38. Medrano GA, de Micheli A, Osornio A: Interatrial conduction and STa in experimental atrial damage. *J Electrocardiol* 1987; 20:357–363.
39. Liu CK, Greenspan G, Piccirillo RT: Atrial infarction of the heart. *Circulation* 1961; 23:331–338.
40. Castellanos A, Pina IL, Zaman L, Myerburg RJ: Recent advances in the diagnosis of fascicular blocks. *Cardiol Clin* 1987; 5:469–488.
41. Pruitt RD: Experimental bundle branch block. Fifty years ago. *Circulation* 1967; 36:625–627.
42. Pruitt RD, Watt TB Jr: On block of something less than a bundle branch or of something more. *Circulation* 1971; 43:775–777.
43. Rothberger CJ, Winterberg H: Experimentelle Beitrage zur Kenntnis der Reizleitungstorungen in den Kammern des Saugetierherzens. *Ges Exp Med* 1917; 5:264.
44. Watt TB Jr, Pruitt RD: Electrocardiographic findings associated with experimental arborization block in dogs. *Am Heart J* 1965; 69:642–654.
45. Watt TB Jr, Pruitt RD: Left posterior fascicular block in canine and primate hearts: An electrocardiographic study. *Circulation* 1969; 40:677–685.
46. Wilson FN, Johnston FD, Barker PS: Electrocardiograms of an unusual type in right bundle branch block. *Am Heart J* 1934; 9:472–479.
47. Davies MJ: *Pathology of Conducting Tissue of the Heart*. New York, Appleton-Century-Crofts, 1971.
48. Demoulin JC, Kulbertus HE: Histopathological examination of concept of left hemiblock. *Br Heart J* 1972; 34:807–814.
49. Grant RP: Left axis deviation. An electrocardiographic-pathologic correlation study. *Circulation* 1956; 14:233–249.
50. Kulbertus HE: Concept of left hemiblocks revisited: A histopathological and experimental study. *Adv Cardiol* 1975; 14:126–135.
51. Lenegre J: Contribution a l'etude des blocs de branch important notament les confortations electriques et histologiques. *Arch Mal Coeur* 1957; 50(suppl 1).
52. Massing GK, James TN: Anatomical configuration of the His bundle and bundle branches in the human heart. *Circulation* 1976; 53:609–621.
53. Rosenbaum MB, Elizari MV, Lazzari JO: *Los Hemibloqueos*. Buenos Aires, Ed Paidos, 1968.
54. Tawara S: Variations in the left bundle system. *Circulation* 1970; 41:782.
55. Uhley HN: Some controversy regarding the peripheral distribution of the conduction system. *Am J Cardiol* 1972; 30:919–920.
56. Uhley HN: The quadrifascicular nature of the peripheral conduction system. In: Dreifus LS, Likoff W (eds): *Cardiac Arrhythmias*. New York, Grune & Stratton, 1973: 743.
57. Rosenbaum MB, Corrado G, Oliveri R, Castellanos A, Elizari MV: Right bundle branch block with left anterior hemiblock surgically induced in tetralogy of Fallot. *Am J Cardiol* 1970; 26:12–19.
58. Dodge HT, Grant RP: Mechanisms of QRS complex prolongation in man. Right ventricular conduction defects. *Am J Med* 1956; 21:534–550.
59. Cohen SI, Lau SH, Stein E, Young MW, Damato AN: Variations of aberrant ventricular conduction in man: Evidence of isolated and combined block within the specialized conduction system. *Circulation* 1968; 38:899–916.
60. Miliken JA: Isolated and complicated left anterior fascicular block: A review of suggested electrocardiographic criteria. *J Electrocardiol* 1983; 16:199–211.
61. Warner RA, Hill NE, Mookerjee S, Smucyan H: Improved electrocardiographic criteria for the diagnosis of left anterior hemiblock. *Am J Cardiol* 1983; 51:723–726.
62. Rosenbaum MB, Elizari MV, Lazzari JO: The differential electrocardiographic manifestations of hemiblocks, bilateral bundle branch blocks and trifascicular blocks. In: Schlant RC, Hurst JW (eds): *Advances in Electrocardiography*. New York, Grune & Stratton, 1972: 145.
63. Rosenbaum MB, Elizari MV, Lazzari JO, Kretz A, Darvos HO: The clinical causes and mechanisms of intraventricular conduction disturbances. In: Schlant RC, Hurst JW (eds): *Advances in Electrocardiography*. New York, Grune & Stratton, 1972: 183–220.
64. Grant RP: Peri-infarction block. *Prog Cardiovasc Dis* 1959; 27:237–247.
65. Oppenheimer BS, Rothschild MA: Electrocardiographic changes associated with myocardial involvement: With special reference to prognosis. *JAMA* 1917; 69:429–431.
66. Castle CH, Keane WM: Electrocardiographic "peri-infarction block": A clinical and pathologic correlation. *Circulation* 1965; 31:403–408.
67. Corne RA, Parkin TW, Brandenburg RO, Brown AL Jr: Peri-infarction block: Postmyocardial-infarction intraventricular conduction disturbance. *Am Heart J* 1965; 69:150–153.
68. First SR, Bayley RH, Bedford DR: Peri-infarction block. *Circulation* 1950; 2:31–36.
69. Wilson FN, Herrmann GR: Bundle branch block and arborization block. *Arch Intern Med* 1920; 26:153–191.
70. Wilson FN, Hill IGW, Johnston FD: The form of electrocardiogram in experimental myocardial infarction. III. The later effects produced by ligation of the anterior descending branch of the left coronary artery. *Am Heart J* 1935; 10:903–915.
71. Castellanos A Jr: Diagnosis of left anterior hemiblock and left posterior hemiblock in the presence of inferior wall myocardial infarction. *Bull NY Acad Med* 1971; 47:923–930.
72. Jacobson LB, Scheinman M: Catheter-induced intra-Hisian and intrafascicular block during recording of His bundle electrograms. A report of two cases. *Circulation* 1974; 49:579–584.
73. Luck JC, Engel TR: Transient right bundle branch block with "Swan-Ganz" catheterization. *Am Heart J* 1976; 92:263–264.
74. Narula OS: Longitudinal dissociation in the His bundle. Bundle branch block due to asynchronous conduction within the His bundle in man. *Circulation* 1977; 56:996–1006.
75. El-Sherif N, Amat-y-Leon F, Schonfield C, Scherlag BJ, Rosen K, Lazzara R, et al: Normalization of bundle branch block patterns by distal His bundle pacing. Clinical experimental evidence of longitudinal dissociation in the pathologic His bundle. *Circulation* 1978; 57:473–483.
76. Scherlag BJ, El-Sherif N, Hope RR, Lazzara R: The significance of dissociation of conduction in the canine His bundle. Electrophysiological studies in vivo and in vitro. *J Electrocardiol* 1978; 4:343–354.
77. Scherlag BJ, El-Sherif N, Lazzara R: Bundle branch block due to His bundle lesions (abstr). *Am J Cardiol* 1974; 33:169.
78. Nakaya Y, Hiasa Y, Murayama Y, Lleda S, Nagao T, Niki T, et al: Prominent anterior QRS forces as a manifestation of left septal fascicular block. *J Electrocardiol* 1978; 11:39–46.
79. Gambetta M, Childers RW: Rate-dependent right precordial Q waves: "Septal focal block." *Am J Cardiol* 1973; 32:196–201.
80. Wilson FN, Herrmann GR: An experimental study of incomplete bundle branch block and of the refractory period of the heart of the dog. In: Johnston FD, Lepeschkin E, (eds): *Selected Papers of Dr. Frank N. Wilson*. Ann Arbor, MI, Edwards Brothers, 1954: 749–810.
81. Sodi-Pallares D, Bisteni A, Medrano GA: *Electrocardiografia y Vectorcardiografia Deductivas*. Mexico, La Prensa Medica Mexicana, 1964: 419.
82. Barker JM, Valencia F: The precordial electrocardiogram in incomplete right bundle branch block. In: Johnson FD, Lepeschkin E (eds): *Selected Papers of Dr. Frank N. Wilson*. Ann Arbor, MI, Edwards Brothers, 1954: 884–914.
83. Grishman A, Scherlis L: *Spatial Vectorcardiography*. Philadelphia, Saunders, 1952: 107.
84. Kossman CE, Berger AR, Rader B, Brumlik J, Briller SA, Donnelly JH: Intracardiac and intravascular potentials resulting from electrical activity of the normal human heart. *Circulation* 1950; 2:10–30.

85. Blount SG, Munyan EA Jr, Hoffman MS: Hypertrophy of the right ventricular outflow tract: A concept of the electrocardiographic findings in atrial septal defect. *Am J Med* 1957; 22:784–790.
86. Cabrera E, Gaxiola A: A critical re-evaluation of systolic and diastolic overloading patterns. *Prog Cardiovasc Dis* 1959; 2:219–236.
87. Moore EN, Hoffman BF, Patterson DF, Stuckey JH: Electrocardiographic changes due to delayed activation of the wall of the right ventricle. *Am Heart J* 1964; 68:347–361.
88. Fahr G: Some fundamental principles of electrocardiography. *Arch Intern Med* 1921; 26:126–130.
89. Punja MM, Schneebaum R, Cohen J: Bifascicular block induced by hyperkalemia. *J Electrocardiol* 1973; 6:71–75.
90. Sung RJ, Tamer DM, Agha AS, Castellanos A, Myerburg RJ, Gelband H: Etiology of the electrocardiographic pattern of "incomplete right bundle branch block" in atrial septal defect: An electrophysiologic study. *J Pediatr* 1975; 87:1182–1186.
91. Castellanos A, Ramirez AV, Mayorga-Cortes A, Pefkaros K, Rozanski JJ, Sprung C, et al: Left fascicular blocks during right-heart catheterization using the Swan-Ganz catheter. *Circulation* 1981; 64:1271–1276.
92. Pickoff AS, Wolff GS, Tamer D, Gelband H: Arrhythmias and conduction system disturbances in infants and children—Recent advances and contributions of intracardiac electrophysiology. In: Castellanos A, Brest AN (eds): *Cardiac Arrhythmia—Mechanisms and Management. Cardiovasc Clin* 1980; 11:203–219.
93. Garcia OL, Castellanos A, Sung RJ, Gelband H: Exposure of concealed right bundle branch block in Wolff-Parkinson-White type B by pacing from the vicinity of the A-V node. *Am Heart J* 1978; 96:662–668.
94. Sodeman WA, Johnston FD, Wilson FN: The Q1 deflection of the electrocardiogram in bundle branch block and axis deviation. *Am Heart J* 1944; 28:271–286.
95. Kindwall KE, Brown JP, Josephson ME: Predictive accuracy of criteria for chronic myocardial infarction in pacing-induced left bundle branch block. *Am J Cardiol* 1986; 57:1255–1260.
96. Wackers FJT: The diagnosis of myocardial infarction in the presence of left bundle branch block. *Cardiol Clin* 1987; 5:393–401.
97. Wolff L, Parkinson J, White PD: Bundle-branch block with short P-R interval in healthy young people prone to paroxysmal tachycardia. *Am Heart J* 1930; 5:685–704.
98. Castillo CA, Castellanos A Jr: His bundle recordings in patients with reciprocating tachycardias and Wolff-Parkinson-White syndrome. *Circulation* 1970; 42:271–285.
99. Rosenbaum FF, Hecht HH, Wilson FN, Johnston FD: The potential variations of the thorax and esophagus in anomalous atrioventricular excitation (Wolff-Parkinson-White syndrome). *Am Heart J* 1945; 29:281–326.
100. Wallace AG, Sealy WC, Gallagher JJ, Kasell J: Ventricular excitation in Wolff-Parkinson-White syndrome. In: Wellens HJJ, Lie KI, Janse MJ (eds): *The Conduction System of the Heart: Structure, Function and Clinical Implications.* Leiden, HE Stenfert Kroese BV, 1976: 613–630.
101. Befeler B, Castellanos A, Castillo CA, Agha AS, Vagueiro MC, Myerburg RJ: Arrival of excitation at the right ventricular apical endocardium in Wolff-Parkinson-White syndrome type B. *Circulation* 1973; 48:655–660.
102. Castillo CA, Castellanos A Jr, Befeler B, Myerburg RJ, Agha AS, Vagueiro MC: Arrival of excitation at right ventricular apical endocardium in Wolff-Parkinson-White syndrome Type A, with and without right bundle branch block. *Br Heart J* 1973; 35:594–600.
103. Castellanos A, Agha AS, Portillo B, Myerburg RJ: Usefulness of vectorcardiography combined with His bundle recordings and cardiac pacing in evaluation of the pre-excitation (Wolff-Parkinson-White) syndrome. *Am J Cardiol* 1972; 30:623–628.
104. Wellens HJJ: Contribution of cardiac pacing to our understanding of the Wolff-Parkinson-White syndrome. *Br Heart J* 1975; 37:231–241.
105. Gallagher JJ, Sealy WC, Kasell J, Wallace AG: Multiple accessory pathways in patients with the pre-excitation syndrome. *Circulation* 1976; 54:571–591.
106. Milstein S, Sharma AD, Guiraudon GM, Klein GJ: An algorithm for the electrocardiographic localization of accessory pathways in the Wolff-Parkinson-White syndrome. *PACE* 1987; 10:555–563.
107. Gallagher JJ, Smith WM, Kasell JH, Benson DW Jr, Sterba R, Grant AO: Role of Mahaim fibers in cardiac arrhythmias in man. *Circulation* 1971; 64:176–189.
108. Murdock CJ, Leitch JW, Klein GJ, Guiraudon GM, Yec R, Teo WS: Epicardial mapping in patients with "nodoventricular" accessory pathways. *Am J Cardiol* 1991; 68:208–214.
109. Castellanos A Jr, Ortiz JM, Pastis N, Castillo CA: The electrocardiogram in patients with pacemakers. *Prog Cardivasc Dis* 1970; 13:190–209.
110. Castellanos A Jr, Lemberg L, Salhanick L, Berkovits BV: Pacemaker vectorcardiography. *Am Heart J* 1968; 75:6–18.
111. Munuswamy K, Alpert MA, Martin RH, Whiting RB, Mechlin NJ: Sensitivity and specificity of commonly used electrocardiographic criteria for left atrial enlargement determined by M-mode echocardiography. *Am J Cardiol* 1984; 53:829–832.
112. Josephson ME, Seides SF (eds): *Clinical Cardiac Electrophysiology. Techniques and Interpretations.* Philadelphia, Lea & Febiger, 1979.
113. Surawicz B: Electrocardiographic diagnosis of chamber enlargement. *J Am Coll Cardiol* 1986; 8:711–724.
114. Romhilt DW, Bove KE, Norris RJ, Conyers E, Conradi S, Rowlands DT, et al: A critical appraisal of the electrocardiographic criteria for the diagnosis of left ventricular hypertrophy. *Circulation* 1969; 60:185–195.
115. Romhilt DW, Estes EH Jr: A point-score system for the ECG diagnosis of left ventricular hypertrophy. *Am Heart J* 1967; 75:752–758.
116. Kafka H, Burggraf GW, Milliken JA: Electrocardiographic diagnosis of left ventricular hypertrophy in the presence of left bundle branch block: An echocardiographic study. *Am J Cardiol* 1985; 55:103–106.
117. Gertsch M, Theler A, Foglia E: Electrocardiographic detection of left ventricular hypertrophy in the presence of left anterior fascicular block. *Am J Cardiol* 1988; 61:1089–1101.
118. Vander Ark CR, Ballantyne F III, Reynolds EW Jr: Electrolytes and the electrocardiogram. *Cardiovasc Clin* 1973; 5:269–294.
119. Levine HD, Wanzer SH, Merrill JP: Dialyzable currents of injury in potassium intoxication resembling acute myocardial infarction or pericarditis. *Circulation* 1956; 13:29–36.
120. Fisch C: Electrocardiography and vectorcardiography. In: Braunwald E. (ed): *Heart Disease.* Philadelphia, Saunders, 1988: 212.
121. Mosseri M, Porath A, Ovsyshcher I, Stone D: Electrocardiographic manifestations of combined hypercalcemia and hypermagnesemia. *J Electrocardiol* 1990; 23:235–241.
122. Kulick DL, Hong R, Ryzen E, Rude RK, Rubin JN, Elkayam U, et al: Electrophysiologic effects of intravenous magnesium in patients with normal conduction systems and no clinical evidence of significant cardiac disease. *Am Heart J* 1988; 115:367–373.
123. Tzivoni D, Keren A, Cohen AM, Loebel H, Zahavi I, Chenzbraun A, et al: Magnesium therapy for torsades de pointes. *Am J Cardiol* 1984; 53:528–530.
124. Schwartz PJ, Wolf S: QT interval prolongation as predictor of sudden death in patients with myocardial infarction. *Circulation* 1978; 57:1074–1077.
125. Burch GE: The EKG, the heart, the CNS, and autonomic nervous system. In: Schwartz PJ, Brown AM, Malliani A, et al (eds): *Neural Mechanisms in Cardiac Arrhythmias.* New York, Raven, 1978: 43–53.
126. James TN, Froggatt P, Atkinson WJ Jr, Lurie PR, McNamara DG, Miller WW, et al: De subitaneis mortibus: Observations on the pathophysiology of the long QT syndromes with special reference to the neuropathology of the heart. *Circulation* 1978; 57:1221–1231.
127. Schwartz PJ, Stone HL: Unilateral stellectomy and sudden death. In: Schwartz PJ, Brown AM, Malliani A, et al (eds): *Neural Mechanisms in Cardiac Arrhythmias.* New York, Raven, 1978: 107–122.
128. Myerburg RJ, Castellanos A: The diagnosis and management of patients with prolonged Q-T intervals. *Cardiology* 1979; 1:2–8.
129. Osborn JJ: Experimental hypothermia. Respiratory and blood pH changes in relation to cardiac function. Am J Physiol 1953; 175:389–398.
130. Santos EM, Kittle CF: Electrocardiographic changes in the dog during hypothermia. *Am Heart J* 1958; 55:415–420.
131. Castellanos A, Saoudi NC, Schwartz A, Sodi-Pallares D: Electrocardiographic patterns resulting from improper connections of the right leg (ground) cable. *PACE* 1985; 8:364–368.

132. Simonson E: *Differentiation between Normal and Abnormal in Electrocardiography*. St. Louis, CV Mosby, 1961: 262.
133. Kerwin AJ, McLean R, Tegelaar H: A method for the accurate placement of chest electrodes in the taking of serial electrocardiographic tracings. *Can Med Assoc J* 1960; 82:258–261.
134. Garson A Jr: Clinically significant differences between the "old" analog and the "new" digital electrocardiograms. *Am Heart J* 1987; 114:194–197.
135. Tenth Bethesda Conference of the American College of Cardiology: Optimal electrocardiography. *Am J Cardiol* 1978; 41:111–191.
136. Seventeenth Bethesda Conference of the American College of Cardiology: Adult cardiology training. *J Am Coll Cardiol* 1986; 7:1192–1218.
137. A.H.A. Committee Report: Recommendations for standardization of leads and of specifications for instruments in electrocardiography and vectorcardiography. Report of the Committee on Electrocardiography, American Heart Association. *Circulation* 1975; 52:11–31.
138. Bailey JJ, Berson AS, Garson A Jr, Horan LG, Macfarlane PW, Mortara DW, et al: Recommendations for standardization and specifications in automated electrocardiography: Bandwith and digital signal processing. A report for health professionals by an ad hoc writing group of the Committee on Electrocardiography and Cardiac Electrophysiology of the Council on Clinical Cardiology, American Heart Association. *Circulation* 1990; 81:730–739.
139. Taback L, Marden E, Mason HL, Pipberger HV: Digital recording of electrocardiographic data for analysis by a digital computer. *I.R.E. Trans Med Elect* 1959; 6:167–171.
140. Pipberger HV, Cornfeld J: What ECG computer program to choose for clinical application: The need for consumer protection. *Circulation* 1973; 47:918–920.
141. Laks MM, Ginzton L: Computerized electrocardiographic interpretation—A practical adjunct to the electrocardiographer. *Pract Cardiol* 1979; 5:127–144.
142. Proceedings of the Engineering Foundation Conference "Computerized interpretation of the electrocardiogram XII." *J Electrocardiol* 1987; 20(suppl):Preface.
143. Wilson FN, Johnston FD: The vectorcardiogram. *Am Heart J* 1938; 16:14–28.
144. Mann H: A method of analyzing the electrocardiogram. *Arch Intern Med* 1920; 25:238–294.
145. Massie E, Walsh TJ: *Clinical Vectorcardiography and Electrocardiography*. Chicago, Year Book Publishers, 1960.
146. Lemberg L, Castellanos A Jr: *Vectorcardiography*, 2d ed. New York, Appleton-Century-Crofts, 1975.
147. Chou TC, Helm RA, Kaplan S: *Clinical Vectorcardiography*, 2d ed. New York, Grune & Stratton, 1974.
148. Frank E: An accurate, clinically practical system for spatial vectorcardiography. *Circulation* 1956; 13:737–749.

Chapter 14

The Chest Roentgenogram and Cardiac Fluoroscopy

James T. T. Chen, M.D.

On November 8, 1895, Wilhelm Conrad Röntgen discovered x-rays and ushered in the new era of diagnostic roentgenology. With wavelengths only 1/10,000 those of visible light, x-rays can penetrate the human body to produce roentgenograms, thereby revolutionizing the field of medical diagnosis. Chest roentgenography in particular has since become a routine part of medical workup because of the invaluable information it can provide.

Familiarity with the altered anatomy and understanding of the underlying pathophysiology of a diseased heart are the keys to appropriate interpretation of its roentgen manifestations. The approach to the chest roentgenogram should be thorough and objective so that no clue is overlooked and no bias is incorporated in the process of radiographic analysis.[1,2] Rib notching (Fig. 14-1*A*), for example, is an important clue to the diagnosis of coarctation of the aorta.[6,7] To prevent occasional erroneous clinical information from misleading the radiographic interpretation, films should at first be read without any knowledge about the patient. A patient may be referred, for instance, because of "bronchial asthma" refractory to therapy, only to be found to actually suffer from cardiac asthma owing to critical mitral stenosis. In this circumstance, the classical radiographic manifestations of severe mitral stenosis should help clarify the confusion and prompt the change of patient management.

On other occasions, a secundum atrial septal defect may be misinterpreted as mitral stenosis because of similar physical signs. The split-second sound may be misinterpreted as the opening snap. The diastolic rumble owing to increased flow through a normal tricuspid valve may mimic the diastolic murmur of mitral stenosis. The

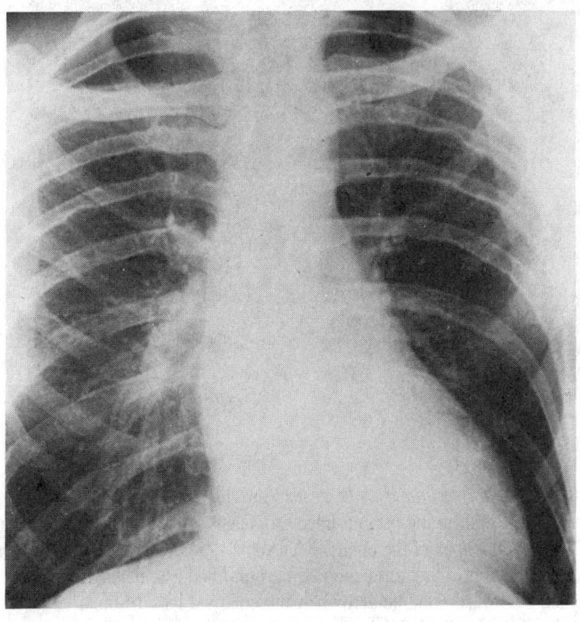

A

FIGURE 14-1 Practical application of four-view cardiac series. *A*. Posteroanterior view in a patient with coarctation of the aorta showing areas of rib notching bilaterally and left ventricular enlargement in the inferior and leftward direction.

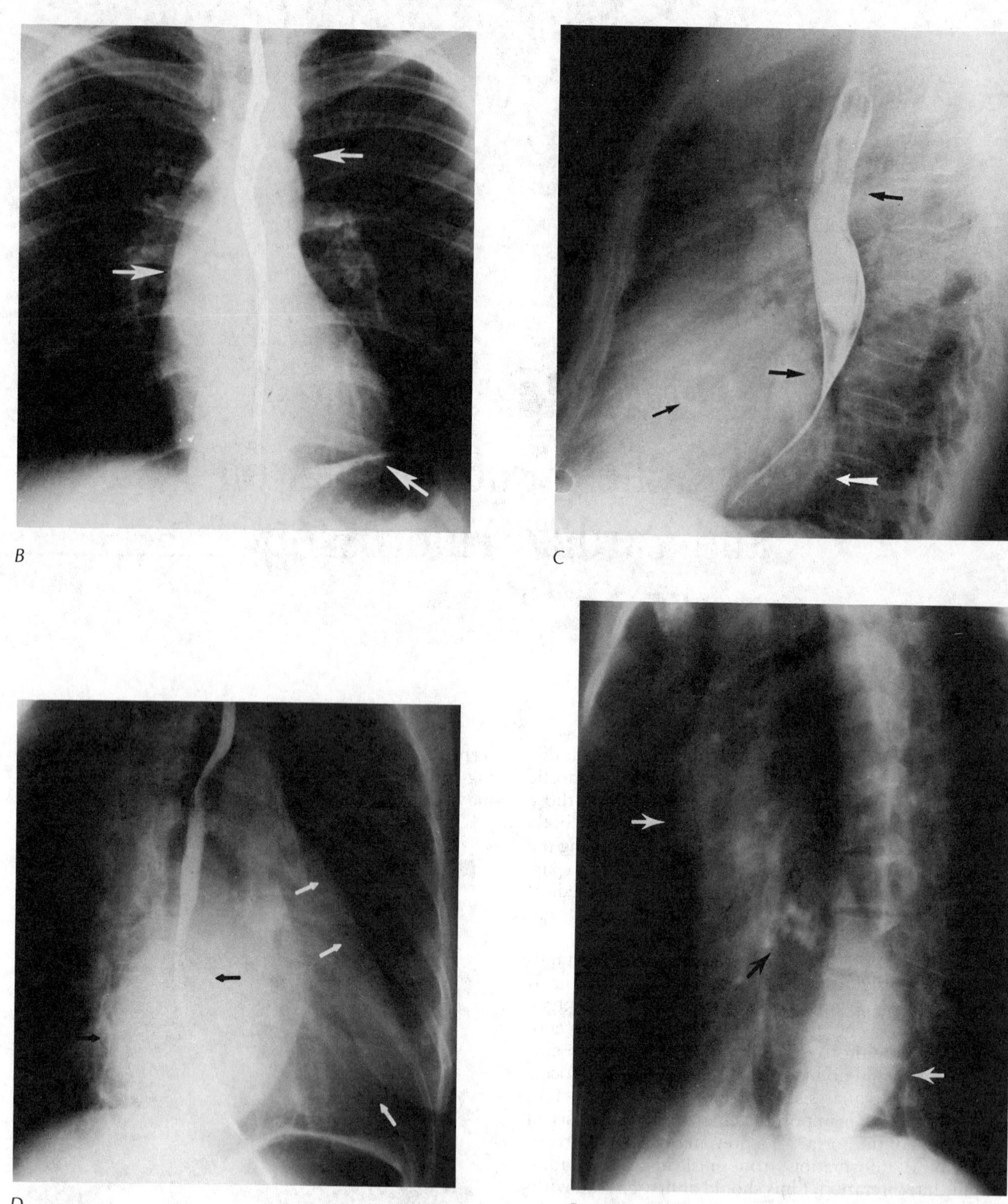

FIGURE 14-1 (*continued*) *B.* Posteroanterior view of another patient with coarctation of the aorta showing figure-three sign of the deformed descending aorta and E sign on the barium-filled esophagus. The upper arrow (on the patient's left) points to the level of coarctation. The lower arrow (on the patient's left) marks the apex of the enlarged left ventricle. The arrow on the patient's right indicates the dilated ascending aorta. *C.* Left lateral view of the third patient with coarctation of the aorta showing barium-filled esophagus to be pushed forward (upper arrow) by the poststenotic dilatation of the descending aorta and pushed backward (middle arrow) by the enlarged left atrium. The very large left ventricle (lower arrow) simply casts a shadow behind the esophagus without displacing it. The oblique arrow points to the calcium deposits in the stenotic bicuspid aortic valve. *D.* Right anterior oblique view of the same patient whose posteroanterior view is shown in Fig. 14-6*D*. Note the huge right atrium casting a triangular density (lower horizontal arrow) behind the esophagus without displacing it. The esophagus is deviated posteriorly by the enlarged left atrium (upper horizontal arrow). The upper oblique arrows indicate the direction of the enlarging pulmonary trunk and right ventricle. The lower oblique arrow points to the normal left ventricle with the undisturbed left costophrenic sulcus. *E.* Left anterior oblique view of a patient with valvular aortic stenosis. The dilated ascending aorta (upper white arrow) is found immediately above the flat anterior border of the normal right ventricle. The black arrow points to the calcified aortic valve. The lower white arrow marks the enlarged left ventricle.

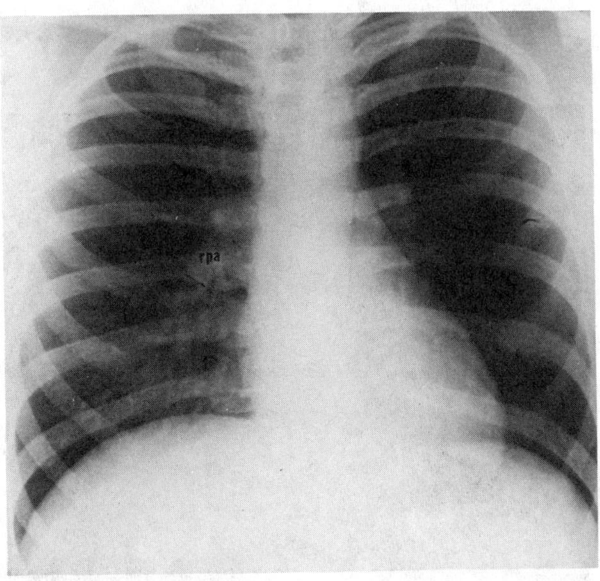

A

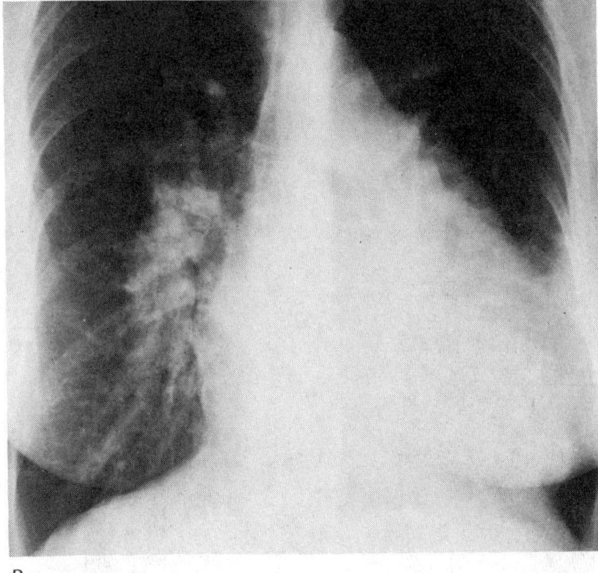

B

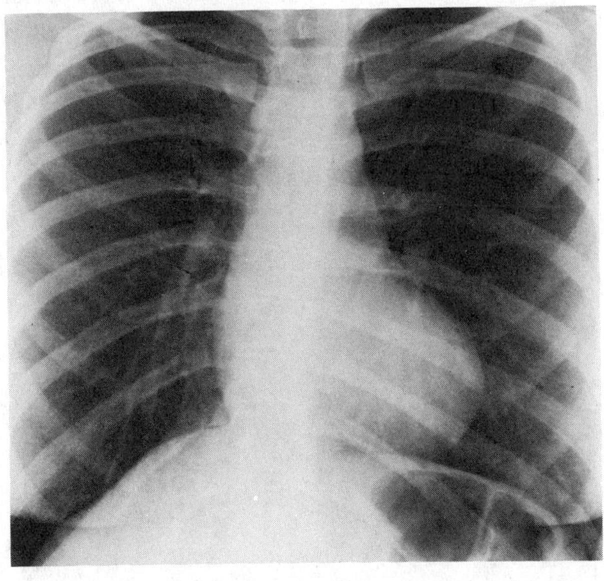

C

FIGURE 14-2 Roentgenographic assessment of the volume of pulmonary blood flow. *A.* Normal: There is caudalization of the pulmonary vascularity due to gravity. The right descending pulmonary artery (rpa) measures 13 mm in diameter in this young adult male patient. *B.* Increased: Patient with secundum atrial septal defect showing uniform increase in pulmonary vascularity bilaterally. The right descending pulmonary artery is markedly enlarged, measuring 27 mm. *C.* Decreased: Patient with tetralogy of Fallot showing a boot-shaped heart and uniform decrease in pulmonary vascularity. The right descending pulmonary artery is markedly decreased, measuring 6 mm.

x-ray signs, however, are quite different between the two entities (Figs. 14-2*B* and 14-3*A*).

The *final* radiologic conclusion, however, should be drawn only after correlating the x-ray findings with both clinical information and other laboratory parameters.

MAJOR STEPS OF ROENTGENOLOGIC EXAMINATION

Objective Analysis

Roentgenographic Examination for Anatomy

An Overview The first step is to survey the roentgenograms and look at the entire situation, searching particularly for noncardiac conditions that may reflect heart disease. For instance, a right-sided stomach with an absent inferior vena cava may direct our attention to the possibility of congenital interruption of inferior vena cava with azygos continuation[3,4] (Fig. 14-4). A narrowed anteroposterior diameter of the thorax may be the cause of an innocent murmur.[5]

Pulmonary Vasculature The lung may be likened to a mirror that faithfully reflects the underlying pathophysiology of the heart.[1,2,8–11] By careful evaluation of the pulmonary vasculature, one may narrow down the diagnostic possibility to a manageable level. For example, if uniform dilatation of all pulmonary vessels is present, the diagnosis of a left-to-right shunt (Fig. 14-2*B*) is preferred to a left-sided obstructive lesion. The latter typically shows a cephalad pulmonary blood flow pattern (Fig. 14-3*A*). More detailed analysis of the pulmonary vascularity will be given separately below.

Lung Parenchyma[9] When the right side of the heart fails, the lungs become unusually radiolucent because of decreased pulmonary blood flow. On the other hand, significant failure on the left side of the heart is characterized by the presence of pulmonary edema and a cephalad

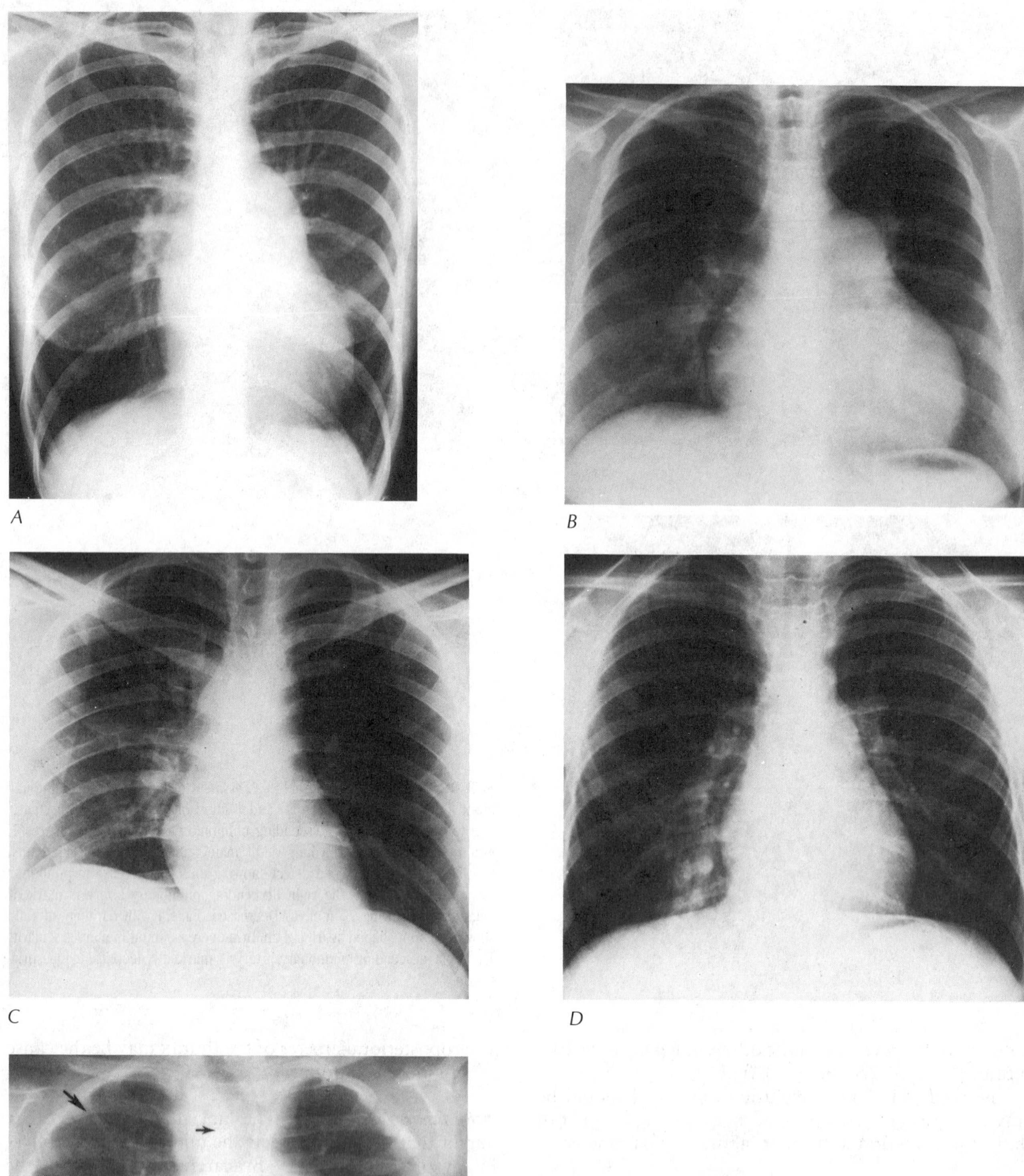

FIGURE 14-3 Abnormal pulmonary blood flow patterns. *A.* Cephalization: Patient with severe mitral stenosis showing dilatation of the upper vessels with constriction of the lower vessels. *B.* Centralization: Patient with primary pulmonary hypertension showing marked dilatation of the pulmonary trunk and the central segments of both pulmonary arteries with pruning of the peripheral branches. *C.* Lateralization: Patient with massive pulmonary embolism obstructing the left main pulmonary artery. Note the uneven distribution of blood flow between the two lungs in favor of the right. *D.* Localization: A cyanotic child showing localized vascular changes representing a large pulmonary arteriovenous fistula in the right lower lobe. *E.* Collateralization: A child with pseudotruncus arteriosus with cardiomegaly and a right aortic arch (small arrow). Note severe pulmonary oligemia with numerous small tortuous vessels (large arrow) in upper medial lung zones, representing bronchial arterial collaterals.

blood flow pattern (Fig. 14-5). Long-standing severe pulmonary venous hypertension may lead to hemosiderosis and/or ossification of the lung. When right-sided heart failure occurs as a result of severe left-sided heart failure, the preexisting pulmonary congestion will improve because of the decreased pulmonary blood flow (Fig. 14-5*B*).

Cardiac Size[10–13] A significantly enlarged heart is always abnormal, while mild cardiomegaly may reflect a higher than average cardiac output from a normal heart, as seen in athletes in active training. The cardiothoracic ratio remains the simplest and the most practical yardstick for the assessment of cardiac size.[1] The mean value for adults in deep inspiration is 44 percent. More accurate roentgen measurements of the cardiac size have been well documented[14,15] and are out of the scope of the present discussion. The nature of cardiomegaly can usually be determined by the specific roentgen appearance. As a rule, when the pulmonary blood flow pattern remains normal, cardiac lesions with volume overload tend to present a greater degree of cardiomegaly than lesions with pressure overload alone. For example, patients with aortic stenosis typically show features of left ventricular hypertrophy without dilation. On the other hand, the left ventricle both dilates and hypertrophies in the case of aortic regurgitation, producing a much larger heart even before congestive heart failure takes place. Both right-sided and left-sided heart failure can cause gross cardiac enlargement. The associated vascular abnormality in each case is, however, drastically different (see below under "Pulmonary Vascularity"). A heart smaller than average is encountered in patients with chronic obstructive pulmonary disease (Fig. 14-6*A*), Addison's disease, anorexia nervosa, and starvation. However, an abnormally small heart is difficult to define except in a retrospective fashion when the heart has returned to its normal capacity following successful therapy. For example, in patients with Addison's disease, the heart may become significantly larger following steroid therapy.

Cardiac Contour Any significant deviation from the normal cardiovascular contour may serve as a clue to the correct diagnosis. For instance, *coeur en sabot*, or a "boot-shaped heart" (Fig. 14-2C) is characteristic of tetralogy of Fallot. A bulge along the left cardiac border with a retrosternal double density is virtually diagnostic of left ventricular aneurysm (Fig. 14-7). A markedly widened right cardiac contour in association with a straightened left cardiac border is frequently seen in patients with severe mitral stenosis leading to tricuspid regurgitation (Fig. 14-6*D*).

Abnormal Densities Besides the familiar double density cast by an enlarged left atrium, other increased densities may be found within the confine of the heart, indicating a variety of dilated vascular structures, e.g., tortuous descending aorta, aortic aneurysm, coronary artery aneurysm, pulmonary varix, etc.[2] Furthermore, large cardiac calcifications are easily seen, particularly in the lateral and oblique views. If smaller calcific deposits are suspected, they should be promptly verified or ruled out by cardiac fluoroscopy. Any radiologically detectable calcification in the heart is of clinical importance. The heavier the calcification, the more significant it becomes (Fig. 14-1*E*). As a rule, the extent of valvular calcification is proportionate to the severity of the valve stenosis regardless of the other roentgen signs of the disease.[1,2]

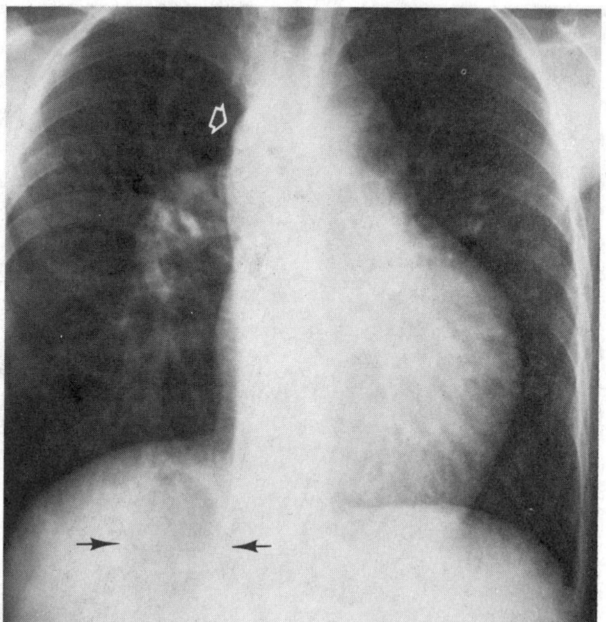

A

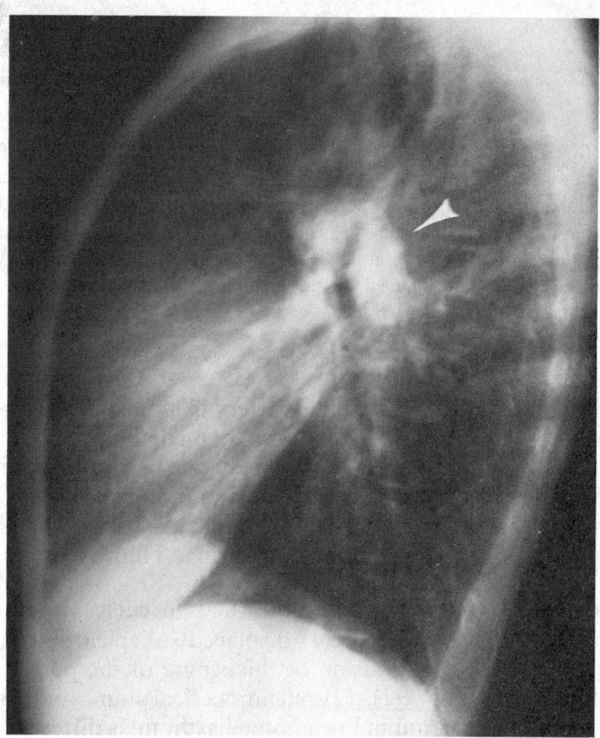

B

FIGURE 14-4 Patient with situs ambiguous, interruption of inferior vena cava, ventricular septal defect, and polysplenia. *A*. Posteroanterior view shows that the aortic arch and the heart are left sided and the stomach (lower arrows) is right sided. The azygos vein (upper arrow) is markedly enlarged. The heart is mildly enlarged and there is moderate increase in pulmonary vascularity. *B*. Lateral view shows an absent image of the inferior vena cava. The azygos arch (arrow) is markedly dilated.

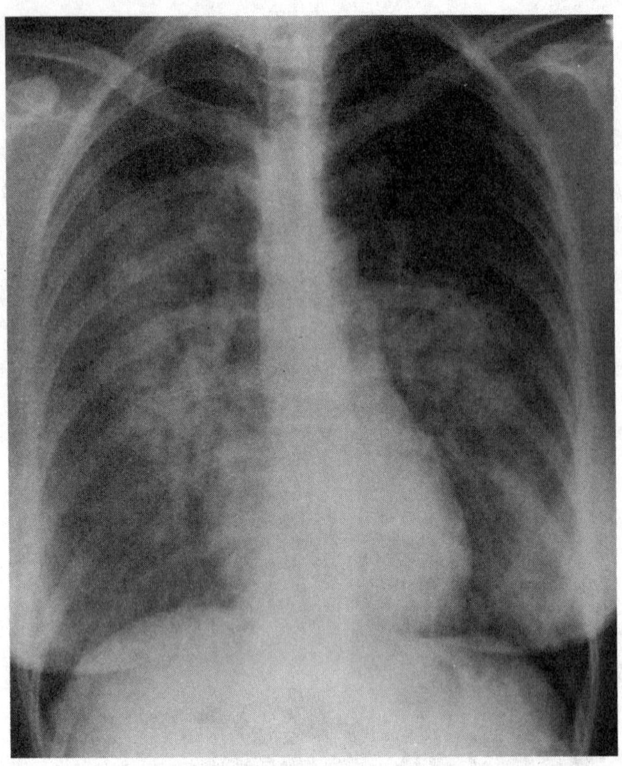

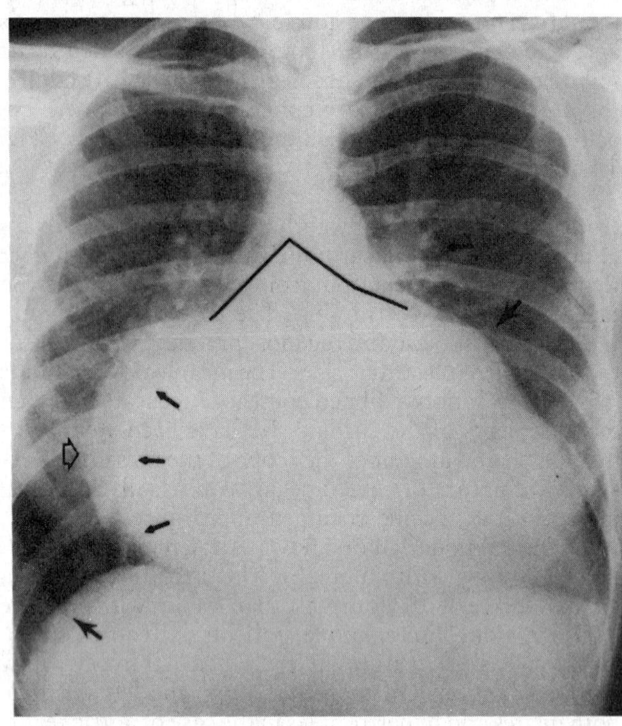

A B

FIGURE 14-5 Roentgen appearance of left-sided heart failure. *A*. Acute: Patient with acute mitral regurgitation due to rupture of chordae tendineae, showing "bat wings" appearance of severe alveolar type of pulmonary edema and a normal-sized heart. *B*. Chronic: Patient with severe rheumatic heart disease (severe mitral and tricuspid regurgitation and mild aortic regurgitation). This is a predominantly left-sided failure pattern. Note gross cardiomegaly with a striking cephalization of the pulmonary vascularity and interstitial pulmonary edema. The giant left atrium forms the right cardiac border (open arrow), makes its appendage bulge outward on the left side (upper large arrow), and splays the mainstem bronchi wide apart (solid lines). The huge right atrium forms a double density within the right cardiac border (3 small arrows). The upper small arrow marks the peribronchial cuffing of edema fluid. The lower large arrow points to multiple Kerley's B lines.

Calcification of the coronary artery is almost always of atherosclerotic nature. Mönckeberg medial calcification of the coronary system is extremely rare. A fluoroscopically detectable coronary calcification is correlated with major-vessel occlusion in 94 percent of patients with chest pain[16] (see below under "Cardiac Fluoroscopy").

Abnormal Lucencies The abnormal lucencies in and about the heart include (1) displaced subepicardial fat stripes caused by effusion or thickening of the pericardium (see Chap. 92), (2) pneumopericardium, and (3) pneumomediastinum. Pneumomediastinum is differentiated from pneumopericardium by the fact that the former shows a more superior extension of the air strip beyond the confine of the pericardium.

Cardiac Malpositions[3,4]

Dextrocardia By definition this is a mirror image of the heart and the abdominal viscera (situs inversus). A ninefold increase in the incidence of congenital cardiac defects is found in patients with dextrocardia (5 percent), as compared with that for the general population (0.6 to 0.8 percent). Also known is the tendency for these patients to have noncardiac lesions in Kartagener's triad: dextrocardia, sinusitis, and bronchiectasis.

Dextroversion Dextroversion represents an anomaly with situs solitus and a right-sided heart (the apex of the ventricles points to the right side and inferiorly). Roentgenographically, situs solitus is a certainty when both the aortic knob and the gastric air bubble are on the left side. Situs solitus also means that both the abdominal viscera and the atria are normal. Under these circumstances, if the ventricles fail to swing from their primitive right-sided position to their normal left-sided position, abnormal relationships between the ventricles and the rest of the cardiovascular structures are bound to occur.

The incidence of congenital cardiac defects was estimated at 98 percent in patients with dextroversion. Of these patients, over 80 percent had congenitally corrected transposition (or L-loop transposition) of the great arteries. The next commonly associated lesions were a combination of ventricular septal defect and pulmonary stenosis, a tetralogylike pathophysiology (Fig. 14-8). Therefore, from the statistical point of view, it is important to be able to differentiate dextroversion from dextrocardia, and this is readily accomplished on roentgen grounds alone. (See also Chap. 97.)

Levoversion This is a mirror image of dextroversion, consisting of a combination of situs inversus and a left-sided heart. The extremely high incidence of cyanotic congenital cardiac defects in patients with levoversion is comparable to that with dextroversion.

Cardiac Malpositions with Indeterminate Situs In this group, the patient's heart may be either left sided or right sided. The situs is ambiguous, with the roentgenogram showing aorticogastric bubble discordance. In other words, the aortic knob and the stomach are not on the same side, and therefore, the situs is unpredictable, though the left atrium tends to be on the side of the aorta. Under these circumstances, interruption of inferior vena cava with azygos continuation is almost always present (Fig. 14-4). The next most-commonly associated lesions are polysplenia and a left-to-right shunt, most frequently a ventricular septal defect. The only exception to the rule of indeterminate situs is an isolated right-sided aortic arch. (See Chaps. 95 to 97.)

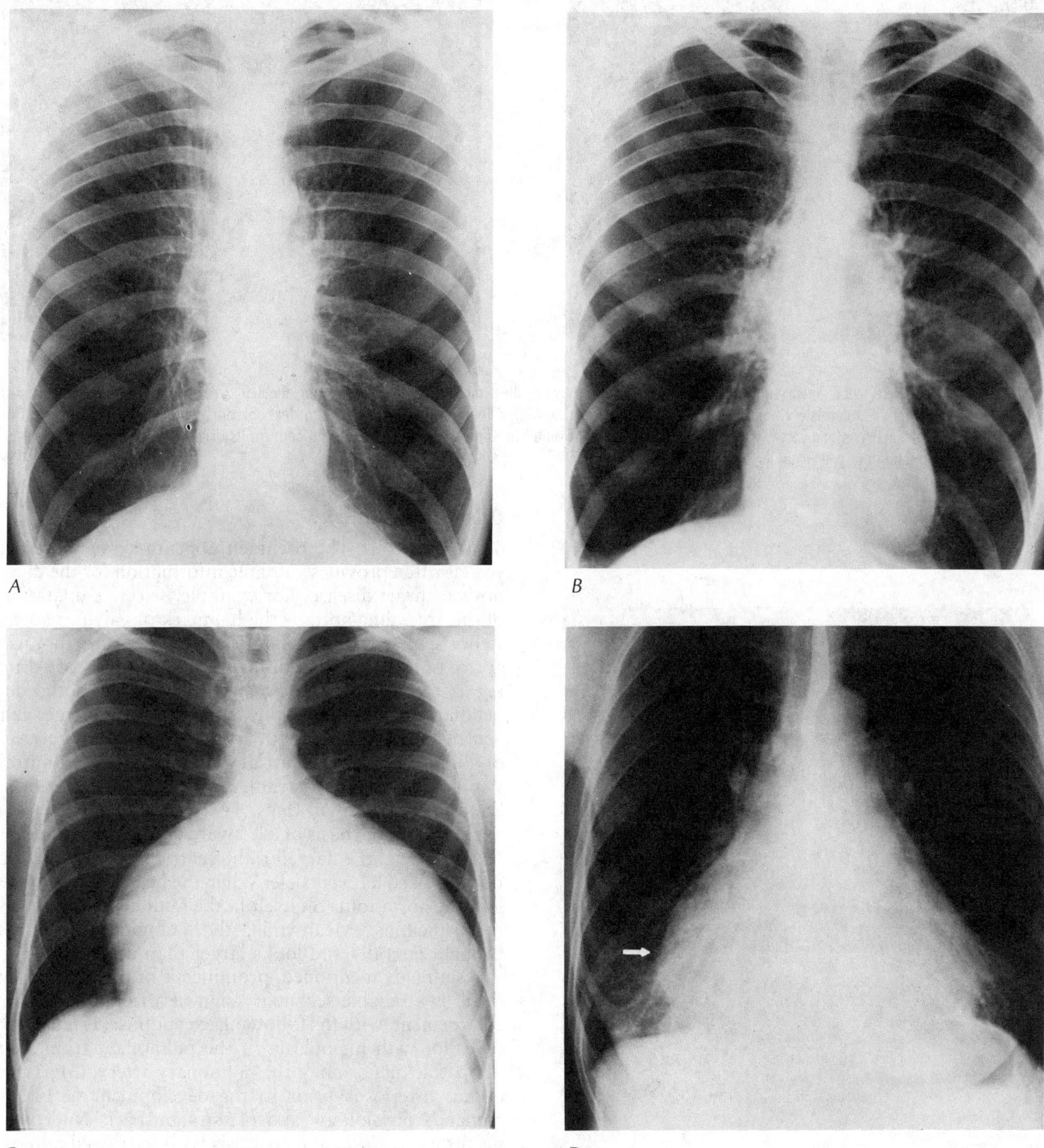

FIGURE 14-6 Roentgen appearance of right-sided heart failure. *A*. Patient with severe obstructive emphysema showing overaeration of the lungs, centralized flow pattern, and a small heart size. *B*. Three years later, the patient was in frank right-sided heart failure. Note that the heart got bigger as his emphysema got worse. The centralized flow pattern became more severe. *C*. Patient with Ebstein's anomaly showing gross cardiomegaly with severe decrease in pulmonary vascularity. The right cardiac border represents the huge right atrium, and the left cardiac border represents the giant right ventricle. *D*. Patient with rheumatic mitral stenosis showing a giant right atrium (arrow) representing severe functional tricuspid regurgitation secondary to unrelenting left-sided failure. The pulmonary venous congestion had improved following the onset of right-sided heart failure.

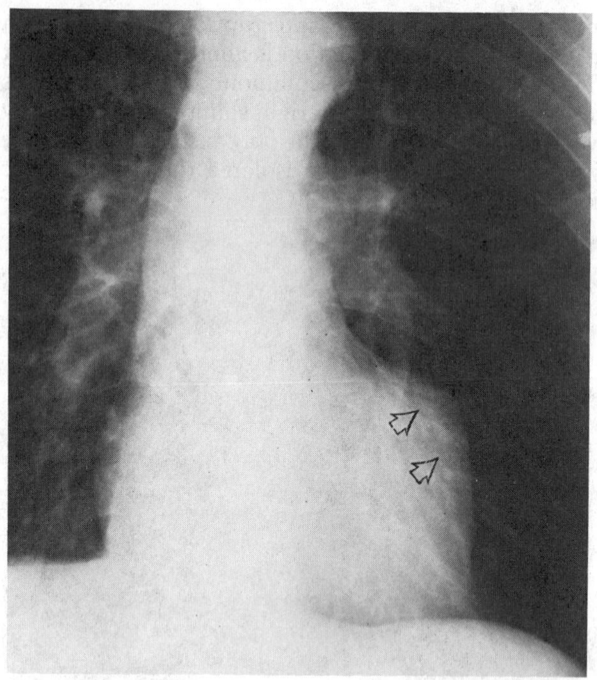

A

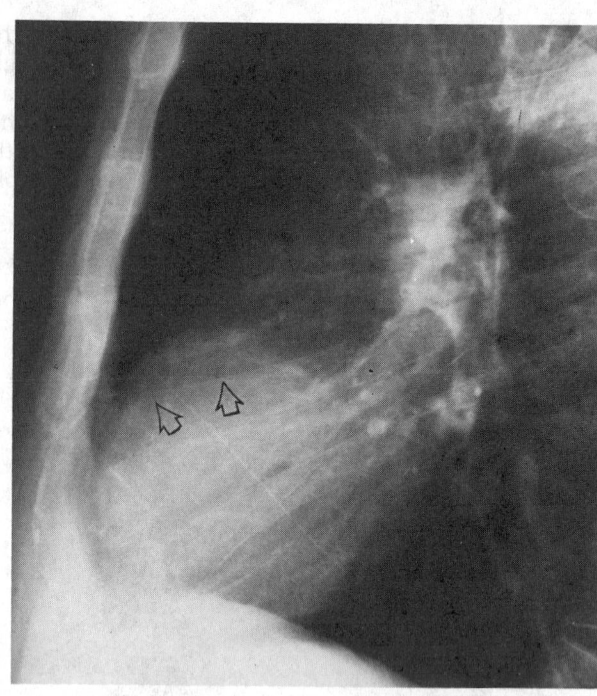

B

FIGURE 14-7 Left ventricular aneurysm. *A.* Posteroanterior view showing the typical bulge (arrows) along the left cardiac border representing a left ventricular aneursym of the anterolateral ventricular wall. *B.* Lateral view showing a double density with sharp borders anteriorly and superiorly (arrows). This is the left ventricular aneurysm that casts a shadow on the normal right ventricle. Fluoroscopically it is easy to confirm its origin and to separate it from the right ventricle by rotating the patient under direct vision.

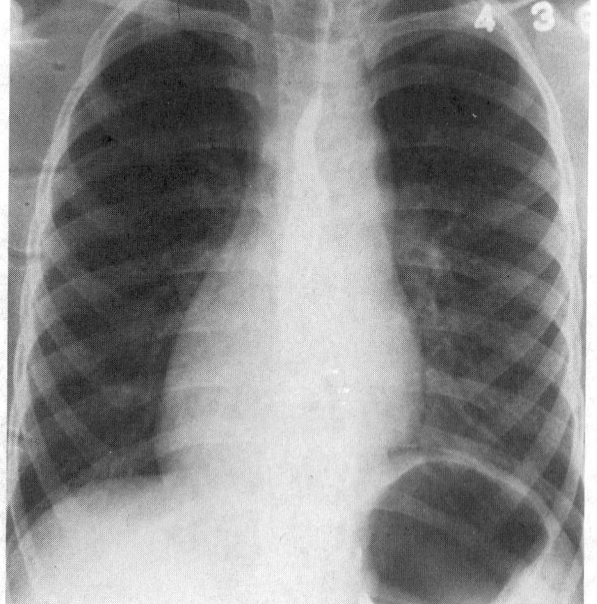

FIGURE 14-8 Posteroanterior view of a patient with dextroversion. Note that the aortic arch and the stomach air bubble are both on the left (situs solitus), and the apex of the ventricles is pointing to the right inferiorly. According to statistics and proved by cardiac catheterization, this patient had the typical combination of corrected transposition of great arteries, ventricular septal defect, and pulmonary stenosis. He was cyanotic. The pulmonary vascularity appears decreased.

Other Abnormalities

Great Vessels[1,12,13] The roentgen appearance of the great vessels often provides valuable information for the diagnosis of heart disease. For example, selective dilatation of the ascending aorta is the hallmark of valvular aortic stenosis; generalized dilatation of the entire thoracic aorta, on the other hand, favors the diagnosis of aortic regurgitation or systemic hypertension or both, depending on the size of the left ventricle. A larger left ventricle is associated with aortic regurgitation because of volume overload. In atrial septal defect and in mitral stenosis the pulmonary trunk is quite large and the aortic knob is usually small (Figs. 14-2*B* and 14-3*A*). This is explained on the basis of a leftward cardiac rotation that occurs when an enlarged right ventricle coexists with a normal-sized left ventricle. When the heart rotates to the left, the aorta folds on itself in the midline and becomes inconspicuous. Meanwhile, the pulmonary trunk is brought laterally and looks larger than it actually is.

As already mentioned, prominence of the pulmonary trunk is a reliable secondary sign of a right ventricular enlargement, with the following exceptions: (1) tetralogy of Fallot with hypoplasia of the pulmonary trunk, (2) idiopathic dilatation of the pulmonary artery, (3) patent ductus arteriosus prior to the development of Eisenmenger's physiology, and (4) straight-back syndrome, pectus excavatum, and scoliosis with narrowed anteroposterior diameter of the chest. Under the latter circumstances, the heart is compressed, displaced, and rotated to the left, giving rise to a falsely enlarged pulmonary artery.

In coarctation of the aorta, the engorged aortic knob and the poststenotic dilatation of the descending aorta cause an E sign on the barium-filled esophagus, outlining the site of coarctation[6] (Fig. 14-1*B*).

The abnormal size and distribution of both the pulmonary and the systemic veins are important clues to the presence of certain heart diseases, e.g., anomalous pulmonary venous connections and interruption of inferior vena cava with azygos continuation.

The significance of aortic arch anomalies will be discussed under the section on statistical guidance.

Mediastinal Structures[10,12,13,17,18] The mediastinal organs are frequently affected by the cardiovascular structures because of their close spatial interrelationships. An enlarged left atrium not only displaces the esophagus and the descending aorta but also elevates and compresses the left stem bronchus. A double aortic arch may compress both the trachea and the esophagus. On the other hand, malignant processes may invade the heart and great vessels, causing cardiac tamponade, or the superior vena cava syndrome, for example. More frequently than not, these mediastinal changes are evident on the chest roentgenogram and should be recognized promptly.

Pleura A right-sided pleural effusion is often present when the left side of the heart is failing. A bilateral hydrothorax, on the other hand, suggests bilateral heart failure or a noncardiac etiology of the effusion. Congestive heart failure is also known to be associated with a pseudotumor or "vanishing" tumor, representing interlobar collection of pleural fluid. As congestive heart failure improves, the "tumor" will disappear.

Bones and Joints Notching of the ribs has many origins. Basically any of the three major intercostal structures can enlarge, compress, and erode the lower borders of the ribs, producing areas of notching. They are intercostal arteries, veins, and nerves. Coarctation of the aorta[6] (Fig. 14-1*A*) represents the most common cause of rib notching due to dynamic dilatation and tortuosity of the arteries. Superior vena cava syndrome may cause a similar phenomenon of venous origin. Neurofibromatosis is known to produce rib notching by numerous intercostal neurofibromas.

Soft Tissues over the Chest Patients with renal failure may show severe edema in the soft tissues over the chest as part of the picture of general anasarca.

Extrathoracic Structures In Holt-Oram syndrome the upper extremity abnormalities may be evident in a chest roentgenogram or on other films in the patient's x-ray folder. A large arteriovenous malformation with curvilinear calcifications may be seen in the neck, thereby providing a clue as to the etiology of the patient's congestive heart failure. Radiographic evaluation of the patient's abdominal viscera is an integral part of the workup for cardiac malpositions.[3,4]

Fluoroscopic Observation for Dynamics

Cardiac fluoroscopy is a valuable adjunct to the chest roentgenogram.[1] Its advantages and limitations are detailed at the end of this chapter.

Comparison

To appreciate the acuteness or chronicity of the disease or its response to therapy, one must carefully compare the serial roentgenograms. As demonstrated in Fig. 14-6*B*, the heart might be considered neither enlarged nor failing if the baseline study made 3 years before (Fig. 14-6*A*) were not available for comparison (see below under "Heart Failure"). Similarly, a rapidly enlarging heart with a normal pulmonary vascularity is highly suggestive of pericardial effusion.

Statistical Guidance

Certain roentgenologic findings are by themselves diagnostic of a disease; other signs are indirectly suggestive of the diagnosis on the basis of statistics. Nevertheless, the latter can be quite useful by virtue of their high predictive value of a particular disease or a group of similar diseases. Therefore, one should always keep the statistical information in mind in the practice of cardiac roentgenology.

In addition to what has been mentioned under the section on cardiac malpositions, other anatomic settings may also provide useful statistical guidance for making a more precise radiographic diagnosis. Different types of aortic arch anomaly are good examples.

When a right-sided aortic arch is present, the incidence of congenital heart disease increases from 10- to 100-fold, depending on the anatomic details of the anomaly.[17,18] Of practical importance, there are only two types of right-sided aortic arch. The first has been called the *avian type*, implying a normal status for the birds but a seriously wrong one for human beings. The overwhelming majority of humans with this type would be born with cyanotic congenital heart disease. The second category may be called the *common type* because of a higher incidence of occurrence. Most patients with this type are physiologically normal, and their arch anomaly is usually discovered incidentally on routine chest x-rays or during a barium-meal study. The x-ray findings of the two types are similar in the posteroanterior view but are quite different in the lateral view (Fig. 14-9). The incidence of congenital heart disease in patients with a right-sided aortic arch[18] is shown in Table 14-1. In the presence of the avian type of right aortic arch the patient has only a 2 percent chance of being physiologically normal. The diagnosis of tetralogy of Fallot should be seriously considered under such conditions until proven otherwise.

Patients with a double aortic arch, on the other hand, rarely have congenital heart disease, though they tend to be symptomatic in infancy because of a compressing vascular ring.[17]

Clinical Correlation

The next step in the examination is to correlate the roentgenologic findings with the clinical information and other laboratory parameters for the final conclusion. It may become necessary at this point to reexamine the radiograph or to review the fluoroscopic observation or both. After detailed analysis of some finer points, a wrong impression may be corrected or a correct diagnosis reinforced.[1]

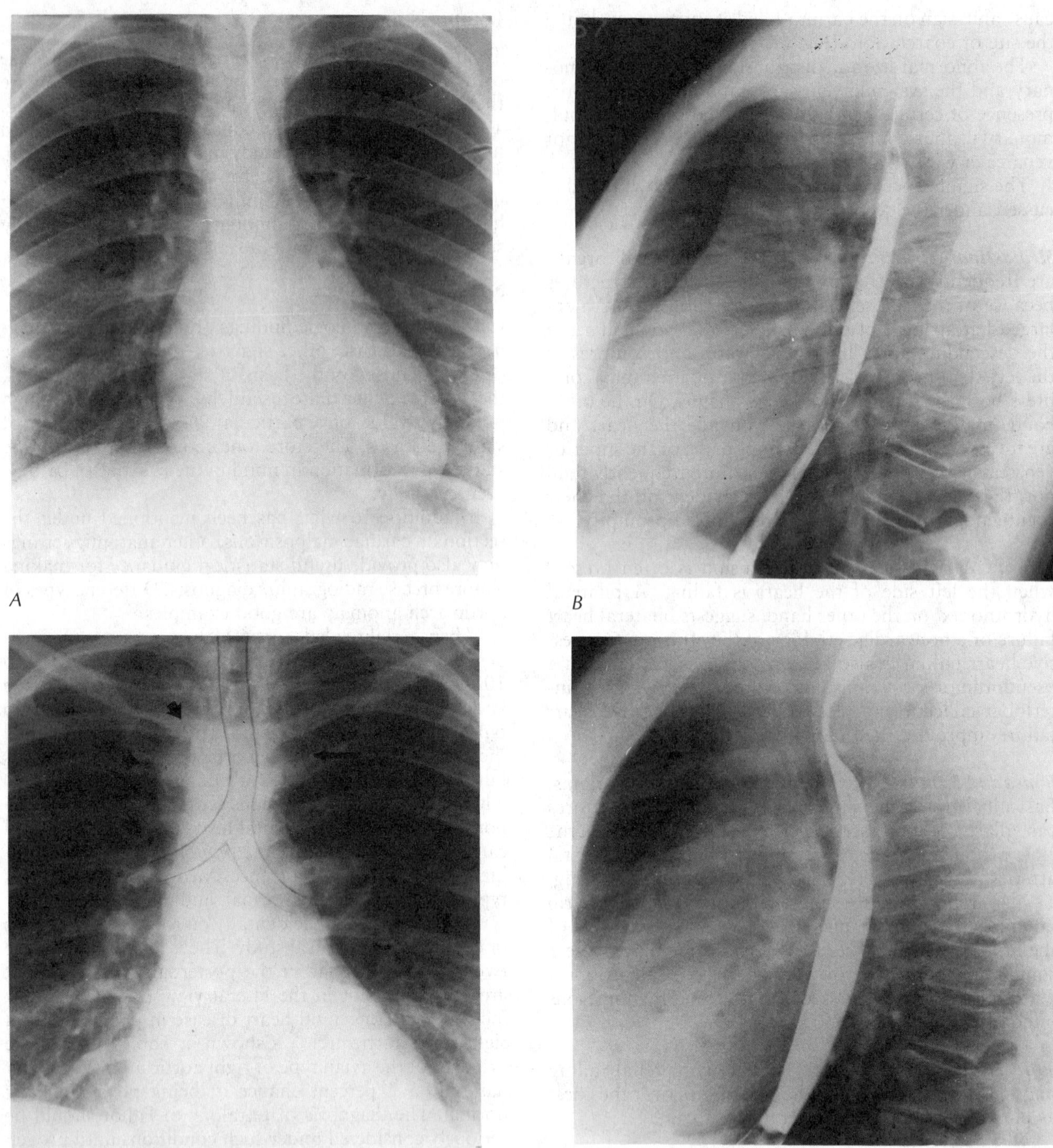

FIGURE 14-9 Statistical guidance focusing on the best diagnostic possibilities. *A.* Posteroanterior view of a patient with tetralogy of Fallot showing a right aortic arch, avian type. Note that the esophagus and trachea are deviated to the left. The cardiovascular structures are otherwise within normal limits. *B.* Lateral view of the same patient showing the aortic arch normally situated, in front of the trachea and esophagus. *C.* Posteroanterior view of a healthy man who was referred because of a "right superior mediastinal mass." Eventually this was proved to be a right aortic arch (short arrows) with an aberrant left subclavian artery (the common type). Note the large aortic diverticulum (long arrow) projected to the left of the midline. The margins of the trachea and main bronchi are traced with pencil. *D.* Lateral view of the same patient. Note the esophagus and the trachea, markedly displaced anteriorly by a huge aortic diverticulum from which arises the aberrant left subclavian artery.

PULMONARY VASCULARITY

Normal

The normal roentgen appearance of the pulmonary vasculature is typified by a caudad flow pattern because of gravity. The pressure differential between the apex and the base of the lung is approximately 22 mmHg in adults in upright position.[1,19] Therefore, more flow under higher distending pressure is expected in the lower lobe vessels than in the upper. Normally one sees very little vascu-

TABLE 14-1

Cardiac Defects Associated with Each Type of Right-Sided Aortic Arch

	Type of Anomaly	
	Avian	Common
Anatomic details	With mirror-image branching; the arch is anterior to the trachea	With aberrant left subclavian artery arising from a large aortic diverticulum that is posterior to the esophagus
Patients with cardiac defects, %	98	12
Type of defects, %		
Tetralogy of Fallot	90	71
Truncus arteriosus	2.5	
Transposition of great arteries	1.5	
Atrial septal defect and/or ventricular septal defect	0.5	21
Coarctation of aorta		7
Others	5.5	1

larity above the hilum, whereas more and larger vessels are found below the hilum. Since the pulmonary resistance is normal, all vessels taper gradually in a treelike manner from the hilum toward the periphery of the lung. The right descending pulmonary artery measures 10 to 15 mm in diameter in males and 9 to 14 mm in females (Fig. 14-2).[1,20]

Abnormal

Abnormal pulmonary vascularities can be classified into two categories, either in terms of volume or in terms of distribution.[1,9,11]

Abnormalities in Volume

In the evaluation of pulmonary vasculature the caliber of the vessels is more important than the length or the number. As long as the pulmonary blood flow pattern remains normal, with greater amount of flow to the bases than to the apices, the volume of the flow is proportional to the caliber of the pulmonary arteries (Fig. 14-2). In addition to measuring the right descending pulmonary artery, one may also assess the pulmonary blood volume by comparing the size of the pulmonary artery with that of the accompanying bronchus where they are viewed on end. Normally the two structures have approximately equal diameters.[1,21] When the artery-to-bronchus ratio is greater than unity, increased blood flow is suggested. Conversely, when the ratio is smaller than unity (Fig. 14-2C), decreased flow is likely.

Increased Pulmonary Blood Flow In the case of mild to moderate left-to-right shunts, for example, the vessels dilate in proportion to the increased flow with no significant change in pressure, resistance, or flow pattern. This phenomenon is also called *shunt vascularity* or *equalization*. The last expression is based on the fact that the distribution of blood flow tends to be equalized between the upper and lower lung zones; however, this change is not marked, and the lower lobes still receive a great deal more blood than the upper. Mild increase in pulmonary vascularity with slight cardiomegaly is commonly found in pregnant women and trained athletes with greater cardiac output and supernormal performance of the heart.

Decreased Pulmonary Blood Flow Patients with tetralogy of Fallot frequently show decreased pulmonary vascularity with smaller and shorter pulmonary arteries and more radiolucent lungs (Fig. 14-2C). Marked reduction in pulmonary blood flow is also encountered in patients with isolated right-sided heart failure without a right-to-left shunt (Fig. 14-6). This is attributed to the significant decrease in cardiac output from both ventricles.

Abnormalities in Distribution

An abnormal distribution of flow (or an abnormal flow pattern) always reflects a changed pulmonary vascular resistance, either locally or diffusely.

Cephalization In the presence of postcapillary pulmonary hypertension, physiological disturbances may begin when the total intravascular pressure exceeds the oncotic pressure of the blood. As a result, fluid leaks out of the vessels and collects in the interstitium before pouring into the alveoli.

Pulmonary edema interferes with gas exchange, resulting in a state of hypoxia. Hypoxia has a profound influence on the pulmonary vessels to constrict. Since there is a greater pressure increase in the lung bases than in the apices, the basilar vessels begin to constrict, forcing the blood to flow upward. This phenomenon actually represents a reversal of the normal blood flow pattern: redistribution or cephalization of the pulmonary vascularity. Cephalization occurs in any of three conditions: (1) left-sided obstructive lesions, e.g., mitral stenosis (Fig. 14-3*A*)[20] or aortic stenosis; (2) left ventricular failure, e.g., coronary heart disease or cardiomyopathies; and (3) severe mitral regurgitation even before pump failure of the left ventricle occurs. It should be emphasized that unless there is obvious constriction of the lower lobe vessels, the diagnosis of cephalization should not be made. Dilatation of the upper lobe vessels is of secondary importance and can be found without narrowing of the basilar vessels in a number of entities, most noticeably left-to-right shunts.

Centralization In the presence of precapillary pulmonary hypertension, the pulmonary trunk and central pulmonary arteries dilate, whereas the distal pulmonary arteries constrict in a concentric fashion from the periphery of the lung toward the hilum. This phenomenon is called centralization of the pulmonary vascularity. It occurs in patients with primary pulmonary hypertension (Fig. 14-3*B*), Eisenmenger's syndrome, or severe obstructive emphysema (Fig. 14-6*A* and *B*).

Lateralization Massive unilateral pulmonary embolism may cause a lateralized flow pattern. Since one major pulmonary artery is obstructed, the blood is forced to flow through the healthy lung only. The paucity of pulmonary vascularity in the diseased lung is termed *Westermark sign* (Fig. 14-3C).

Localization A localized abnormal flow pattern is exemplified by the arteriovenous fistula in a cyanotic child (Fig. 14-3*D*).

Collateralization Patients with markedly decreased pulmonary blood flow (severe tetralogy of Fallot, for example) tend to show numerous small and tortuous bronchial arterial collaterals in the upper medial lung zones near their origin from the descending aorta. The native pulmonary arteries are extremely small, though smooth and branching gracefully (Fig. 14-3*E*).[1]

Combined Abnormalities

In reality an abnormal pulmonary vascularity is, more frequently than not, a mixed type. There is a great variety of possible combinations, e.g., cephalization plus decreased flow in severe mitral stenosis (Fig. 14-3*A*) or centralization with increased flow in Eisenmenger's atrial septal defect.

Summary

Roentgen analysis of the pulmonary vasculature is accomplished in two steps. First, the volume of the pulmonary flow can be estimated by the degree of pulmonary arterial enlargement as long as the flow pattern remains normal. Second, the distribution of the pulmonary flow is assessed by the presence of an abnormal flow pattern. The volume and the distribution of pulmonary blood flow may change singly or in combination depending on the nature and the severity of the underlying heart disease.

Heart Failure

In addition to specific chamber enlargement, the pulmonary vasculature uniquely portrays the underlying pathophysiology of heart failure. In the chronic setting, decreased flow with increased pulmonary lucency is the hallmark of right-sided heart failure (Fig. 14-6); striking cephalization of the pulmonary vasculature is typical for left-sided decompensation (Figs. 14-3*A* and 14-5*B*).

Left-Sided

Acute Left-Sided Heart Failure The pulmonary vascular changes associated with acute left ventricular failure are usually not discernible for two reasons: (1) The resultant severe pulmonary edema obscures the pulmonary vasculature and (2) the redistribution of pulmonary blood flow secondary to acute left-sided heart failure is usually relatively mild. The combination of alveolar pulmonary edema and a normal-sized heart is the hallmark of acute left-sided heart failure (Fig. 14-5*A*),[9] most commonly seen in acute myocardial infarction. The edema fluid under this circumstance tends to distribute in a butterfly pattern.[22] The reason for this is poorly understood.

Chronic Left-Sided Heart Failure Chronic left-sided heart failure is characterized by striking cephalization of the pulmonary vasculature and interstitial pulmonary edema or fibrosis with multiple distinct Kerley's B lines (Fig. 14-5*B*). Pulmonary hemosiderosis, ossification, or both may result from long-standing severe postcapillary pulmonary hypertension.

Right-Sided

Acute Right-Sided Heart Failure Acute right-sided heart failure most commonly results from massive pulmonary embolism. The typical roentgen signs are rapidly developing centralization of the pulmonary vasculature and dilatation of the right-sided cardiac chambers and the venae cavae. In addition, the lungs may show localized or lateralized oligemia. Eventually, opacities in either or both lungs may develop as a result of pulmonary infarction.

Chronic Right-Sided Heart Failure Chronic right-sided heart failure has a number of causes. The common ones include congenital pulmonary stenosis, Ebstein's anomaly, severe chronic obstructive pulmonary disease, and recurrent pulmonary thromboembolic disease. Diffusely decreased pulmonary vascularity with unusually lucent lungs is seen in patients with right-sided heart failure without pulmonary hypertension (Fig. 14-6*C*). Centralized pulmonary flow pattern is encountered when the right-sided heart failure is secondary to precapillary pulmonary hypertension (Fig. 14-6*A* and *B*). Cephalized flow pattern with unusually lucent lungs is found in patients with right-sided heart failure secondary to severe left-sided heart failure (Fig. 14-6*D*). The degree of right-sided chamber enlargement is proportional to the severity of tricuspid insufficiency.

Combined

It is generally believed that right-sided heart failure is most often caused by severe left-sided heart failure. This is exemplified by patients with severe mitral stenosis leading to severe tricuspid regurgitation (Fig. 14-6*D*). Other examples of bilateral heart failure are cardiac tamponade and constrictive pericarditis, when both sides of the heart are affected (Fig. 14-10).

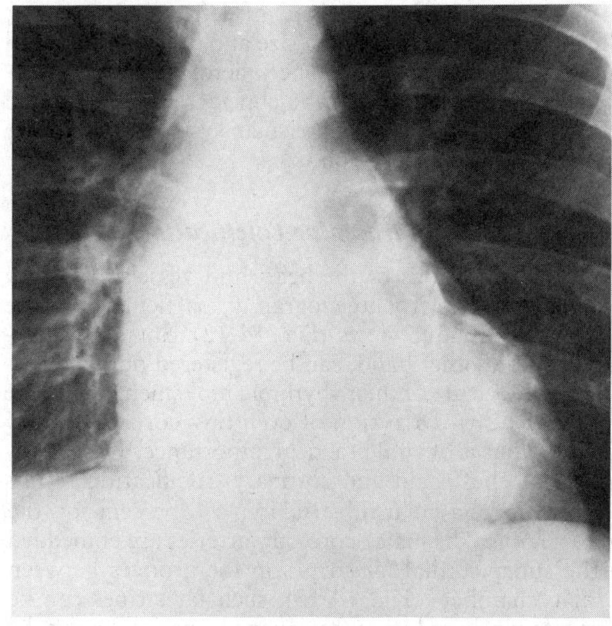

A

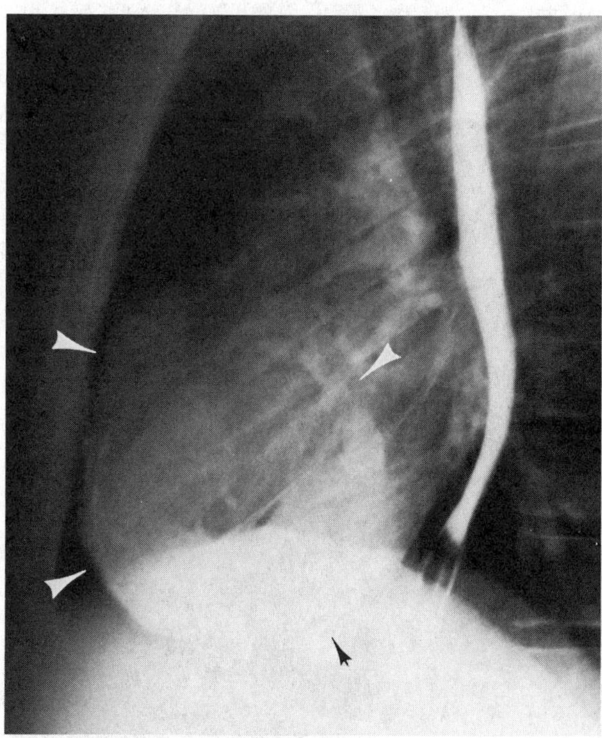

B

FIGURE 14-10 Patient with calcific constrictive pericarditis. Typically there is only mild postcapillary pulmonary hypertension due to left-sided constriction. Severe pulmonary venous congestion is prevented by the concurrent right-sided constriction. *A*. Posteroanterior view shows moderate cardiomegaly and mildly cephalad pulmonary blood flow pattern. *B*. Lateral view shows heavy calcification of the pericardium (arrows) and left atrial enlargement deviating the barium-filled esophagus.

CARDIAC FLUOROSCOPY

Cardiac roentgenography deals primarily with anatomic details by filming at short exposure times that stop the motion. *Cardiac fluoroscopy,* on the other hand, explores the dynamic features of the organ that are discernible only in motion.[23] The two techniques are mutually complementary.

Description[1,13]

A good-quality image intensifier is a prerequisite for the proper performance of cardiac fluoroscopy. The modern intensifier with the use of cesium iodide phosphors has increased the brightness of the fluoroscopic image by at least 10,000 times. Television viewing permits cone vision under dim light with better perception of detail. The attached videotape or videodisc recorder provides a means for instant playback as well as future analysis of the fluoroscopic observation.

The milliamperage and the kilovoltage of the fluoroscope should be adjusted according to the patient's size in different projections. The milliamperage ranges from 1.5 to 3.5 and the kilovoltage varies between 90 and 120. Too high a kilovoltage tends to reduce the contrast, and excessive milliamperage blurs off the margin of the image. The shortest fluoroscopic time and the smallest shutter opening are to be employed in order to reduce the dose of radiation to the minimal. The average examining time for this author is 3 min.

The patient is routinely examined in the erect position with four views. The patient should be asked to stop breathing during the brief moment of fluoroscopy. Barium meal is given only after a thorough search for cardiac calcifications is completed. Occasionally, a recumbent position is used for better visualization of small calcifications as well as for a critical evaluation of cardiac asynergy. The cardiac output increases and the heart rate decreases on assuming recumbency, thereby giving a truer and more representative picture of the left ventricular contractility. In obese patients, the thick layer of soft tissues over the thorax is compressed and pushed aside, thereby improving the fluoroscopic image significantly.

Results

When properly performed, cardiac fluoroscopy is quite useful in the following areas of investigation: (1) assessment of cardiovascular dynamics; (2) detection of small cardiovascular calcifications; (3) visualization of important anatomic landmarks, e.g., subepicardial fat stripes; (4) differentiation of cardiac from noncardiac disease; and (5) evaluation of cardiac valve prostheses, pacemakers, and radiopaque foreign bodies.

Precaution

Although no complication from modern fluoroscopy has been reported, both the patient and the examiner should be protected from excessive radiation. Even with an image intensifier, a routine cardiac fluoroscopy still involves more radiation than does two-view chest roentgenography. Therefore, the fluoroscopist should accomplish the task within the shortest possible period of time. Although all aspects of the heart are briefly surveyed, one should emphasize special areas of interest for each patient as suggested by the base-line radiographs. If coarctation of the aorta is suspected in a patient older than 40 years, for instance, particular attention should be paid to finding calcium in a stenotic bicuspid aortic valve.

Application

Assessment of Cardiovascular Dynamics[1,24–27]

The chest roentgenogram that is taken at random largely records the diastolic image of the heart. Fluoroscopy, on the other hand, provides a continuous vision of the pulsating organ through the entire cardiac cycle. On becoming familiar with the normal cardiovascular movements, the fluoroscopist will find that any deviation from the norm will be obvious.

The telltale x-ray signs of many cardiac lesions manifest themselves only in ventricular systole. Therefore, what may be missed on the film is often readily seen and diagnosed under the fluoroscope. For instance, left ventricular enlargement may be the only radiographic abnormality of severe aortic regurgitation in children or young adults. On fluoroscopy, however, the aorta is vigorously expanding in systole and rapidly collapsing in diastole. This dynamic alternation is characteristic of aortic regurgitation (Fig. 14-11). Other examples in the same vein include mild mitral regurgitation, mitral vale prolapse, left ventricular dyskinesia, and broad-based left ventricular aneurysm.

In valvular pulmonary stenosis, vigorous pulsation of the pulmonary trunk and its left branch is in bold contrast to the diminished pulsation of the right pulmonary artery.[26] Increased pulsation of diffusely enlarged pulmonary arteries is characteristic of left-to-right shunts. When marked discrepancy in size and pulsation is noted between the central and peripheral vessels, Eisenmenger's syndrome should be considered. Exaggerated left atrial expansion in ventricular systole is a reliable sign of mitral regurgitation.[27]

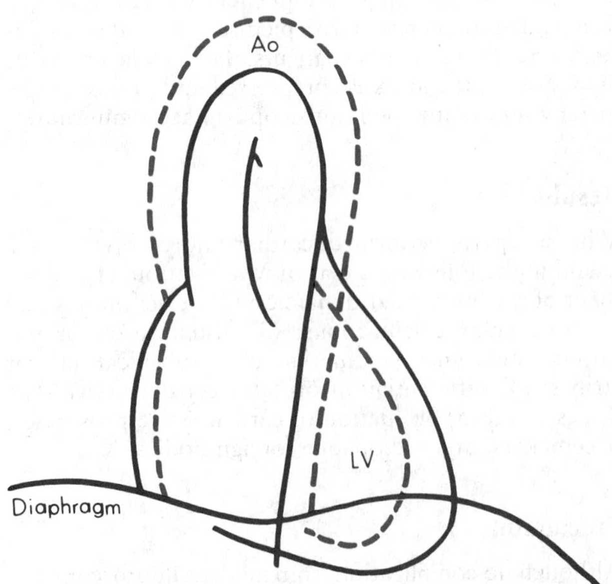

FIGURE 14-11 Schematic representation of dynamic changes of aortic regurgitation. Blue interrupted lines represent images in systole; solid lines, those in diastole.

Detection of Cardiovascular Calcifications[3,8]

Heavy calcifications of the heart and vessels are easily detected by chest roentgenography, particularly in the lateral and oblique views (Fig. 14-12). Small calcifications, on the other hand, can be registered only by fluoroscopy by virtue of their rhythmic movements from the pulsating heart. Detection of even tiny coronary artery calcifications is of vital practical importance. The combination of chest pain and coronary calcification results from major vascular obstruction 94 percent of the time.[16,28] Since the major coronary arteries are embedded in the subepicardial fat stripes in the grooves between cardiac chambers (Fig. 14-13), such fat stripes can be used effectively to locate the calcified arteries. Under the fluoroscope the fat stripes present as pulsating radiolucent (bright) lines, in contrast to the accompanying pulsating radiopaque (dark) lines of calcified coronary arteries. If the artery coincides with the fat line within the left atrioventricular groove (aL), it portrays the circumflex coronary artery. The right coronary artery is moving synchronously with the right atrioventricular groove (aR). The anterior descending artery coincides with the anterior interventricular groove (vA), as does the poste-

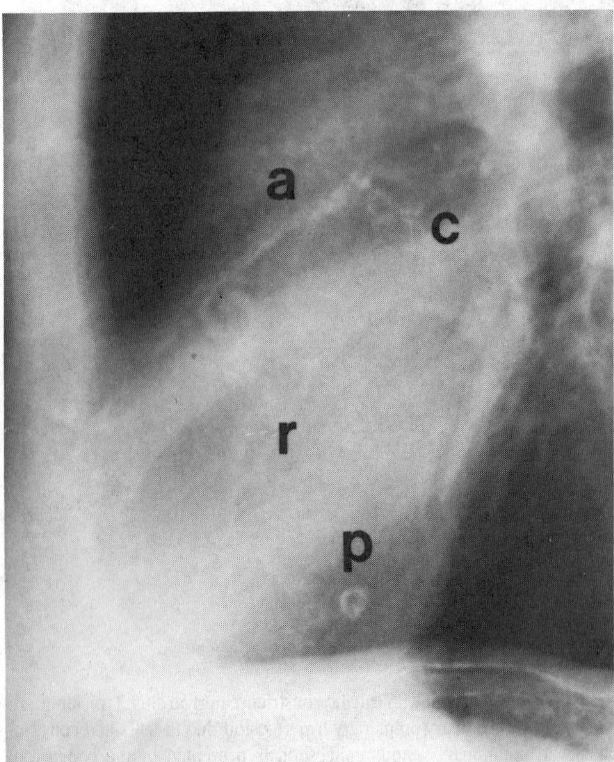

FIGURE 14-12 Lateral view shows heavy railroad-track-like calcification of all three major coronary arteries: r, right coronary artery; a, anterior descending; c, circumflex; p, posterior descending. Note the ringlike densities representing vessels viewed on end.

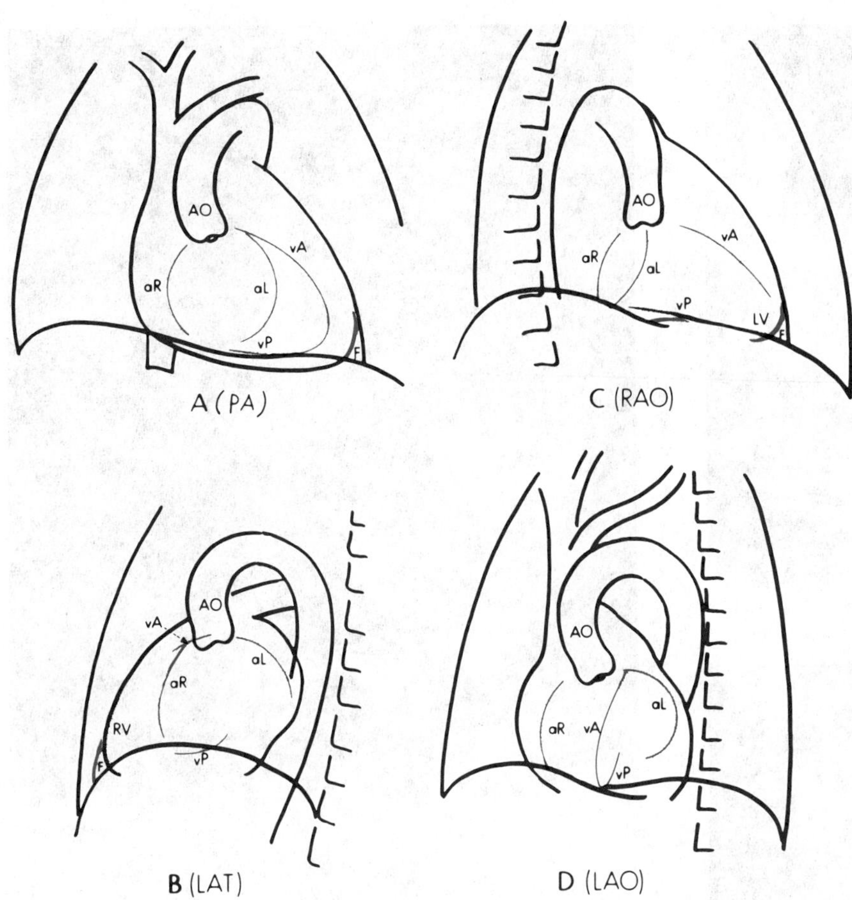

FIGURE 14-13 Schematic representation of the subepicardial fat stripes in relation to major coronary arteries. *A.* Posteroanterior view. *B.* Lateral view. *C.* Right anterior oblique view. *D.* Left anterior oblique view. Abbreviations: aL, left atrioventricular groove (circumflex); aR, right atrioventricular groove (right); vA, anterior interventricular groove (anterior descendings); vP, posterior interventricular groove (posterior descending); F, apical fat pad; AO, aorta; LV, left ventricle.

rior descending artery with the posterior interventricular groove (vP).

The lateral view is the best or the only view for the detection of a calcified right coronary artery. The left anterior oblique view at 20° to 30° is the most suitable for localizing the bifurcation of the left coronary artery. In this view, the left coronary artery is brought into relief between the hilar shadow anteriorly and the spinal column posteriorly. A ringlike density is frequently seen in this view, representing the end-on image of the calcified anterior descending artery. The right anterior oblique angle is used to view the calcified left main coronary artery. If both the anterior descending and the circumflex branches are also calcified, a Y-shaped density may be seen. The calcified cardiac valves, the myocardium, and the pericardium are easily confirmed by fluoroscopy.[1,24]

Visualization of Subepicardial Fat Stripes

The subepicardial fat lines are an important landmark in the diagnosis of heart disease. The *fat stripe* is a cushionlike structure separating the myocardium from the pericardium. Normally it is difficult to see the fat line because of the adjacent similar radiolucency of the air-filled lung. The in-between hairline density of the normal pericardium is delicate and also difficult to see except in the left lateral view (Fig. 14-14*A*). In the presence of pericardial effusion or thickening, the subepicardial fat line is displaced interiorly and becomes more visible because of the added background of water density (Fig. 14-14*B*). The subepicardial fat pulsates with the contracting myocardium within the immobile band of pericardial fluid. This is diagnostic of pericardial effusion.[29] In contrast, when pericardial thickening alone is present, the exterior border of the heart pulsates with the fat line. This, in turn, suggests the diagnosis of pericardial constriction.

Differentiation of Cardiac from Noncardiac Disease

When respiration is suspended, any structures that are moving are likely to be cardiovascular in nature. Conversely, noncardiac structures are immobile. This is exemplified by one bullet in the heart versus another in the chest wall. A pulmonary varix or an azygos vein collapses on Valsalva maneuver, with exaggerated pulsation following release of the breath. Enlarged nodes in these areas, on the other hand, will not change with such maneuver.

Evaluation of Valve Prostheses and Pacemakers

The normal movements of cardiac valve prostheses are parallel between the two phases of cardiac cycle. If a significant angle of tilt (more than 12°) is formed between the two phases, instability of the valve with associated insufficiency is nearly always present.[1,25,29,30]

The bileaflet St. Jude valve[31] has recently been used in both mitral and aortic positions. The valve is difficult to see radiographically (Fig. 14-15) but is readily detected

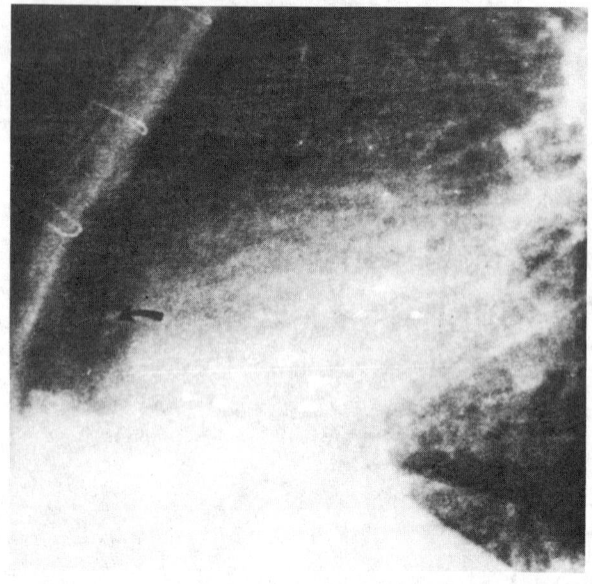

A

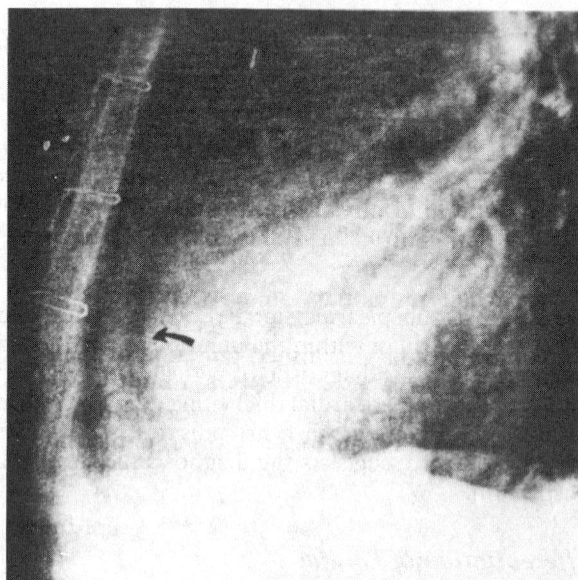

B

FIGURE 14-14 Subepicardial fat stripe in the diagnosis of pericardial effusion. *A.* Lateral view in a patient 3 weeks after coronary bypass procedure showing a normal pericardium as a hairline density (arrow) sandwiched between the subepicardial fat stripe interiorly and the mediastinal fat exteriorly. Also note the metallic sutures in the sternum and a surgical clip marking the origin of a venous graft in the ascending aorta. *B.* Lateral view of the same patient, who developed postpericardiotomy syndrome 5 weeks after operation. Note the subepicardial fat stripe (arrow) to be displaced interiorly by the widened pericardium. The fat stripe became more distinct in the presence of pericardial effusion.

under the fluoroscope.[1,31] When the leaflets move sluggishly, thrombotic stenosis of the valve should be suspected. Rarely one leaflet may dislodge and embolize distally, causing acute valvular insufficiency.[31]

The position of the pacemaker can be promptly determined under the fluoroscope and recorded on the film.[1,32] The subepicardial fat line overlies the myocardium and

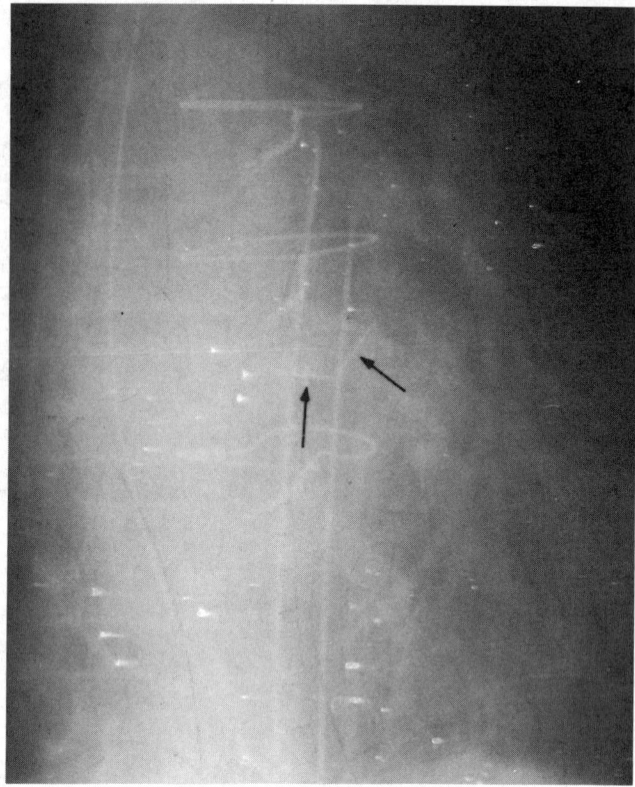

A

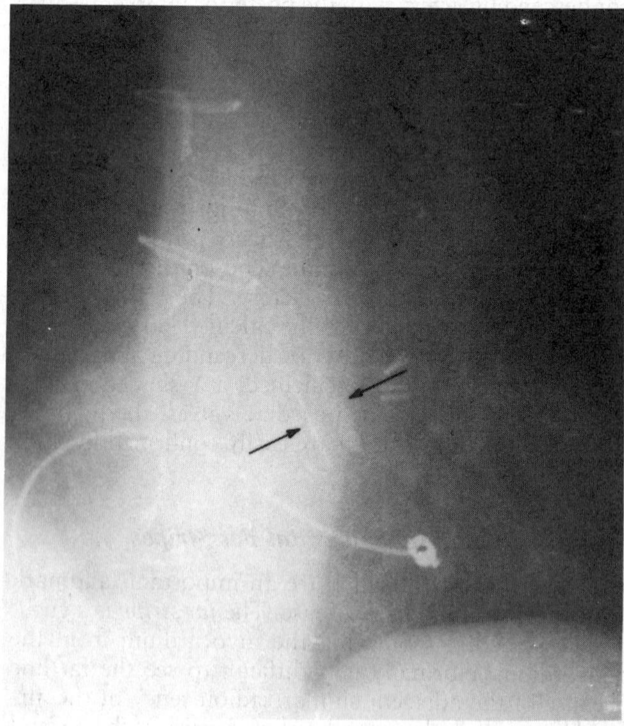

B

FIGURE 14-15 Status postmitral valve replacement with a St. Jude prosthesis. *A.* In systole the valve is closed and the two leaflets form a V-shaped density (arrows). *B.* In diastole, when the valve is open, the leaflets form a pair of parallel lines (arrows).

underlies the pericardium. If the pacing catheter is found within the fat stripe, it may have passed through the coronary sinus and entered one of the major cardiac veins. If the tip of the catheter is seen outside the fat stripe, it may have perforated the myocardium and thus be lying in the pericardium.[1,32] Although the wires and electrodes of a transmediastinal pacemaker may look normal on the films, minor breakage can only be appreciated in ventricular systole by aid of fluoroscopy.[32]

REFERENCES

1. Chen JTT: *Essentials of Cardiac Roentgenology.* Boston, Little, Brown and Company, 1987.
2. Chen JTT: The plain radiograph in the diagnosis of cardiovascular disease. In: Putman C (ed): Symposium on cardiopulmonary imaging. *Radiol Clin North Am* 1983; 21:609–621.
3. Elliott LP, Jue KL, Amplatz K: A roentgen classification of cardiac malpositions. *Invest Radiol* 1966; 1:17–28.
4. Elliott LP, Schiebler GL: *X-Ray Diagnosis of Congenital Cardiac Disease*, 2d ed. Springfield, Il, Charles C Thomas, 1979.
5. deLeon AC, Perloff JK, Twigg HL: The straight back syndrome: Clinical and cardiovascular manifestations. *Circulation* 1965; 32:193–203.
6. Figley M: Accessory roentgen signs of coarctation of the aorta. *Radiology* 1954; 62:671–686.
7. Juhl JH: *Essentials of Roentgen Interpretation*, 4th ed. Philadelphia, Harper & Row, 1981.
8. Edwards JE, Carey LS, Neufeld HN, Lester RG: *Congenital Heart Disease.* Philadelphia, Saunders, 1965.
9. Chen JTT, Capp MP, Johnsrude IS, Goodrich JK, Lester RG: Roentgen appearance of pulmonary vascularity in the diagnosis of heart disease. *Am J Roentgenol* 1971; 112:559–570.
10. Swischuck LE: *Plain Film Interpretation in Congenital Heart Disease*, 2d ed. Baltimore, Williams & Wilkins, 1979.
11. Milne ENC: Some new concepts of pulmonary blood flow and volume. *Radiol Clin North Am* 1978; 16:515–536.
12. Meszaros WT: *Cardiac Roentgenology.* Springfield, IL, Charles C Thomas, 1969.
13. Cooley RN: *Radiology of the Heart and Great Vessels*, 3d ed. Baltimore, Williams & Wilkins, 1978.
14. Keats TE: *Atlas of Roentgenographic Measurement*, 6th ed. St. Louis, Mosby-Year Book, 1990: 393–450.
15. Chickos PM, Figley MM, Fisher L: Correlation between chest film and angiographic assessment of left ventricular size. *Am J Roentgenol* 1977; 128:367–373.
16. Margolis JR, Chen JTT, Kong Y, Peter RH, Behar VS, Kisslo JA: The diagnostic and prognostic significance of coronary artery calcification. A report of 800 cases. *Radiology* 1980; 137:609–616.
17. Shuford WH, Sybers RG: *The Aortic Arch and Its Malformations.* Springfield, IL, Charles C Thomas, 1974.
18. Stewart JR, Kincaid OW, Titus JL: Right aortic arch: Plain film diagnosis and significance. *Am J Roentgenol* 1966; 97:377–389.
19. Fraser RG, Pare JAP: *Diagnosis of the Diseases of the Chest*, 2d ed. Philadelphia, Saunders, 1979: 97.
20. Chen JTT, Behar VS, Morris JJ, McIntosh HD, Lester RG: Correlation of roentgen findings with hemodynamic data in pure mitral stenosis. *Am J Roentgenol* 1968; 102:280–292.
21. Wojtowicz J: Some tomographic criteria for an evaluation of the pulmonary circulation. *Acta Radiol [Diagn] (Stockh)* 1964; 2:215.
22. Fleischner FG: The butterfly pattern of acute pulmonary edema. *Am J Cardiol* 1967; 20:39.
23. Jeffers K, Rees S (eds): *Clinical Cardiac Radiology,* 2d ed. London, Butterworths, 1980.
24. Chen JTT: Cardiac fluoroscopy. In: Kelley MJ (ed): *Symposium on Chest Radiography for the Cardiologist. Cardiol Clin* 1983; 1:565–573.
25. Chen JTT, McIntosh HD, Capp MP, Morris JJ Jr, Canent RV Jr, Lester RG: Intercalative angiocardiography: A method for recording cardiovascular dynamics on a single film. *Radiology* 1969; 93:499–506.
26. Chen JTT, Robinson AE, Goodrich JK, Lester RG: Uneven distribution of pulmonary blood flow between left and right lungs in isolated valvular pulmonary stenosis. *Am J Roentgenol* 1969; 107:343–350.
27. Chen JTT, Lester RG, Peter RH: Posterior wedging sign of mitral insufficiency. *Radiology* 1974; 113:451–453.
28. Bartel AG, Chen JTT, Peter RH, Behar VS, Kong Y, Lester RG: The significance of coronary calcification detected by fluoroscopy: A report of 360 patients. *Circulation* 1974; 49:1247–1253.
29. Jorgens J, Kundel R, Lieber A: The cinefluorographic approach to the diagnosis of pericardial effusion. *Am J Roentgenol* 1962; 87:911–916.
30. Gimenez JL, Soulen RL, Davila JC: Prosthetic valve detachment: Its roentgenographic recognition: Report of Cases. *Am J Roentgenol* 1968; 103:595–600.
31. Kotler MN, Panidis J, Mintz GS, Monaco O, Morris GC, Moschetto A: The role of noninvasive technique in the evaluation of the St. Jude cardiac prosthesis. In: DeBakey ME (ed): *Advances in Cardiac Valves: Clinical Perspectives.* New York, Yorke, 1983: 220.
32. Sorkin RP, Schuurmann BJ, Simon AB: Radiographic aspects of permanent cardiac pacemakers. *Radiology* 1976; 119:281–286.

Chapter 15

The Echocardiogram

Joel M. Felner, M.D. ■ *Randolph P. Martin, M.D.*

One of the most important noninvasive techniques for cardiovascular diagnosis that provides both reliable clinical information and patient safety is ultrasound. *Ultrasound* is defined as sound above the upper threshold of human hearing (20,000 Hz). Ultrasonics, the technology of high-frequency sound waves, deals with the transmission of these high-frequency waves through a medium. The high-frequency vibrations are created by striking an appropriate piezoelectric crystal with alternating electric current. A short burst or pulse of high-frequency, low-intensity sound is then emitted and directed through the human body to detect boundaries between structures of different acoustic impedance. This technique is termed *pulsed-reflected ultrasound.*

Ultrasound in the millions of cycles per second, or megaherz (MHz), range has become well established as a medical diagnostic tool primarily because of its biological safety (nonionizing radiation) and its ability to detect the position of both stationary and moving structures within the body. Ultrasound can not only determine the depth and position of echoes (reflected sonic waves) returned from the body but also accurately record the motion of structures over a period of time. Since the movement of patterns of the various cardiac components are related to function and have been found to change in pattern consistent with specific diseases, the heart and great vessels are ideally suited for ultrasonic examination. The transmission of pulsed-reflected ultrasound through the heart, with detection of the returning echoes detailing the position and movement of the cardiac acoustic interfaces, is termed *cardiac ultrasound* or *echocardiography.*

Cardiac ultrasound presently consists of three interrelated forms: M-mode echocardiography, two-dimensional echocardiography, and Doppler echocardiography and several different techniques: including transthoracic (precordial), transesophageal, and transabdominal, for fetal evaluation. Echocardiography is thus a multidimensional and multiplanar imaging modality. Motion or M-mode echocardiography, the original ultrasonic technique developed for cardiac examination, uses a narrow ultrasound beam to depict a one-dimensional slice of the target structure. Two-dimensional echocardiography is a system for recording a spatially correct image of the heart. Two-dimensional units scan the heart in an arclike motion, resulting in cross-sectional (tomographic) slices (planes) of cardiac structures. Doppler ultrasound tracks the direction and velocity of blood flow through the heart and great vessels. It is discussed in Chap. 130. Combining both two-dimensional echocardiography and Doppler echocardiography provides structural and functional information about cardiovascular structures. As such, echocardiography has become a multiplanar imaging modality.

Further details concerning transesophageal echocardiography are discussed in Chap. 131, stress echocardiography in Chap. 132, and intravascular echocardiography in Chap. 133.

The advantages of echocardiography over other noninvasive diagnostic tests are as follows:

1. It is biologically safe without any cumulative effects. As such, it can be used in children and in pregnant women.
2. It is a relatively painless procedure that can be perfomed without patient preparation.
3. The equipment is mobile and therefore can be moved

to any critical care areas, patient bedside, or even outpatient office settings.
4. A complete examination is relatively quick and takes anywhere from 15 to 60 min.
5. It can be performed serially.
6. It provides both anatomic (from two-dimensional imaging) as well as physiological (from Doppler) information about cardiac structure, function, and great-vessel anatomy.
7. It is a valuable screening device for early and accurate diagnosis leading to proper management.
8. It is useful for following serial changes over an extended period of time.

Information gleaned from this study can be used to pinpoint certain specific abnormalities and malfunctions and to furnish direction for diagnostic studies and treatment.

HISTORICAL PERSPECTIVES

Echo sounding, a technique used by certain birds and animals for distance perception, was first applied by human beings in the 1920s for depth recordings in oceanographic studies and submarine detection. The principles of diagnostic ultrasound have their roots in navy sonar, which uses sound impulses to detect objects and measure distance in water. The use of high-frequency ultrasonic waves as a diagnostic tool in medicine is a relatively recent development. In 1950, Keidel[1] was one of the first investigators to use ultrasound to examine the heart. It was not until the mid-1950s, however, that Edler and Hertz[2] pioneered the use of pulsed ultrasonic techniques in the description of certain aspects of cardiac anatomy. Echocardiography was popularized in the United States by Holmes and coworkers in 1957.[3] Initially, this technique was used for the assessment of mitral stenosis,[4] but more widespread interest followed its application in the diagnosis of pericardial effusion and the assessment of cardiac chamber size.[5,6]

A major development in the field of cardiac ultrasound was the introduction of two-dimensional echocardiography. The investigators most active in this area were Ebina et al.,[7] who developed ultrasound cardiotomography in the mid-1960s, and Bom et al.,[8] who developed the multielement cardiac scanner. This technique took a static image of cardiac anatomy and provided recognizable images of cardiac structure in real time.

The next significant milestone in the evolution of cardiac ultrasound was the addition of the pulsed Doppler device, initially investigated by Baker.[9] From the early days of pulse wave Doppler to the later developments of continuous wave Doppler, physiological information was added to functional/structural information provided by two-dimensional echocardiography.[10] Shortly after the maturation of Doppler echocardiography, transesophageal echocardiography, popularized by Hanrath et al. in Germany,[11] emerged as a milestone in the use of echocardiography. This technology allowed for assessment of unique cardiac anatomy in almost every patient as well as accounted for the movement of echocardiography into the operating room. Recent developments have included catheter-mounted transducers allowing for intracoronary and other intravascular ultrasound[12] (see Chap. 133). A recent evolutionary development in echocardiography is "digital" ultrasound, which has allowed for the digitization of ultrasound images leading to quantitative and semiquantitative analysis as well as tissue characterization.[10] The digitizing format allowed for the maturation of stress echocardiography including exercise or pharmacologic interventions.[13,14] (See Chap. 132.) Fetal echocardiography is also now being performed.[15]

BASIC PRINCIPLES OF ULTRASOUND

The ability to perform and interpret echocardiograms and to appreciate fully the capabilities, advantages, and limitations of this technique depends on an understanding of the basic principles of ultrasound.[16,17] M-mode and two-dimensional echocardiography are both based on the same fundamental ultrasonic principles. The basic circuitry of the pulsed-reflected ultrasound system causes the transducer, which contains one or more crystals with piezoelectric properties, to function as both a transmitter and a receiver of ultrasound. After the transducer is applied to the patient's skin over the area to be studied, a timer in the transmitter regulates the duration and frequency of the ultrasonic impulse. During the transmitting cycle the electronic circuit provides a very short burst or pulse (500 to 1500 pulses per second) of alternating current, causing the piezoelectric crystal to vibrate at a very high frequency. During the much longer receiving cycle, the same piezoelectric crystal detects the ultrasound vibrations and transforms them back into an electric signal that can be amplified and appropriately displayed and recorded. Any boundary or interface between materials having different acoustic impedances, or acoustic mismatch, will produce a sound reflection, or echo, back to the crystal. The difference between the M-mode and two-dimensional techniques is that the M-mode ultrasonic beam is aimed in one direction and therefore depicts only a single dimension of the target structure in an image that does not resemble cardiac structures, whereas the two-dimensional beam sweeps in an arc to yield a panoramic view of the heart that results in cross-sectional images that are anatomically recognizable.

Clinical echocardiography requires ultrahigh-frequency sound (2 to 7.5 MHz) so that it can be transmitted as a narrow beam and directed along a rather well-defined path through the soft tissues of the body. As the sound strikes a cardiac structure, a portion is reflected back to the receiver. Since the speed of sound in the body is known (approximately 1540 m/s), the time it takes for sound to travel to a cardiac structure and return to the receiver allows determination of the structure's distance from the transmitter.

The amount of ultrasound energy passing through the tissue is minimal, since the transducer acts as a transmitter less than 1 percent of the time and as a receiver more than 99 percent of the time. Tissue damage could be produced by very long exposure to high-energy ultrasound, because ultrasound excites molecules to move back and forth and to generate heat. Woodward et al.[18] have shown, however, that there is a wide margin of safety, despite much greater than normal exposure to sound vibrations, that is not likely to be reached in a routine clinical ultrasound study. There has been no validated case of human injury due to ultrasound in the exposure range used for diagnostic purposes.[19]

When an ultrasound pulse of sufficient energy travels through a medium and meets an acoustic interface, an echo of the sound wave may be produced. Sound waves lose energy or become attenuated when they pass through any medium. The strength of the echo returning to the transducer from the boundary, therefore, depends on several factors:

1. The degree of acoustic mismatch between the two media. Since echoes are generated only at interfaces of tissues with different acoustic impedances, no echoes are produced while the beam traverses a homogenous medium.
2. The absorption of the transmitted ultrasonic waves as they meet the interface.
3. The character of the interface (i.e., rough, smooth, calcified).
4. The resolution, penetration, and frequency of the ultrasound. *Resolution* is the ability to differentiate and recognize structures that are close to each other.[20] With the sound frequencies used clinically, two structures that are 1 to 2 mm apart within the heart can be differentiated. If two structures are not separated by at least this distance, they will appear as one on the oscilloscope face. *Penetration* is the ability to transmit sufficient ultrasonic energy into the chest to provide a satisfactory image. Both resolution and penetration are affected by the frequency of sound transmitted by the transducer. High-frequency sound (greater than 3.5 MHz) gives an excellent image at the expense of penetration, whereas low-frequency sound (1 to 3.5 MHz) penetrates better but has poorer resolving power. Therefore, for each patient examined the transducer chosen must balance the importance of resolution with the need for penetration.

The processed data from within the body can be displayed in three modes, A, B, and M, in order to present the clinical information in the most meaningful way. In A (amplitude) mode echoes are displayed as vertical spikes along the abscissa or horizontal axis. The distance between spikes (echoes) represents time required for echo return. The amplitude (height) of the spike corresponds to the relative intensity (strength) of the echo; its position along the horizontal axis indicates the depth of the structure. The A mode was the earliest presentation used in ultrasonic diagnosis and is currently used in echoencephalography and ophthalmology. It is not, by itself, suitable for use in echocardiography because it does not show motion. In the B (brightness) mode the horizontal baseline remains unchanged, but the echoes are now displayed as dots rather than spikes. The more intense the echo, the greater the brightness of the dot.

The M (motion) mode displays time and motion and is achieved by sweeping a B-mode display across the oscilloscope at a uniform speed. In this presentation the depth of an echo is shown along the vertical axis and the time is represented along the horizontal axis. The intensity of an echo is still proportional to its brightness, but the dots now appear as undulating lines. In effect, an M-mode recording is a continuous graph of the depth of the structures with respect to time. It provides an ideal means of following motion of cardiac structures.[21,22]

ULTRASONIC INSTRUMENTATION

The basic ultrasonic equipment in current use is an echocardiograph that consists of an oscilloscope, a transducer, and a photographic or video recorder. In a pulsed-echo system the echocardiograph transducer usually emits bursts of ultrasound energy for 1 μs; the echocardiograph transmits, receives, and electronically processes the data. These data, along with other physiological parameters such as the electrocardiogram (ECG) and respiratory cycle, are displayed on an oscilloscope monitor and fed into a physiological recorder.

The M-mode echocardiogram is obtained by using only one of the available crystals in the transducer housing to emit a single beam of sound. This produces a very narrow "ice-pick" image of cardiac structures, but the spatial resolution (1 to 2 mm along the axis of the sound beam) is the highest of any widely available, noninvasive cardiac diagnostic technique. Since this high-resolution image is obtained over a very short interval (it repeats its transmit-receive cycle about 1000 times per second), there is also a very high degree of temporal resolution. Therefore, if one is imaging a moving structure, its motion will be small compared to the interval of sampling by the M-mode ultrasound beam, and an accurate high-resolution representation of motion can be obtained (these motions include valve opening, closing, fluttering, and subtle wall motion abnormalities). Despite this high degree of axial and temporal resolution, there is no simultaneous field of view lateral to the transducer beam. The two-dimensional echocardiogram overcomes this shortcoming and has become the standard echocardiographic modality.

Two-dimensional instruments use a transducer containing one or more crystals that are mechanically rotated or electronically fired sequentially. This creates a fan-shaped, 60° to 90° image of the heart. Transmitting and receiving discrete beams through a 60° to 90° sector take substantially longer than pulsing a single M-mode beam (120 beams versus 1 individual beam are needed for an image). Therefore, building up a tomographic plane for two-dimensional images takes time and results in a limited frame rate—about 30 to 60 times per second rather than 1000 per second, as with M mode. These frame rates are fast enough to be integrated by the eye into a real-time presentation, but there is a substantial decrease in resolution. In addition, if the structure to be imaged is more than 16 cm from the transducer, the frame rate is reduced even further and resolution decreases even more.

Most modern ultrasound systems integrate M-mode and two-dimensional imaging in a convenient, easy-to-use, mobile unit. These units can display the two-dimensional image alone or simultaneously with an M-mode image, since one or two cursors are usually available to select from the two-dimensional sector the acoustic scan line(s) to be displayed in M mode. The availability of complementary and simultaneous M-mode displays, from known locations and orientations, has increased the sophistication and meaning of real-time M-mode studies by providing them with more accurate spatial orientation. A full range of adult, pediatric, and neonatal cardiac applications can be satisfied with most systems.

Recording Methods

Historically, ultrasound instruments have used either static frozen hard-copy pictures, strip-chart[23] recorders, video tape recording capabilities, or more recently, digital/computer manipulation of image/Doppler information. Modern-day instruments have replaced strip-chart recorders with video page printers and high-quality video recording instrumentation. Recent advances in digitizing and image manipulation have led to the integration of minicomputer systems within the ultrasound instruments, such that image manipulation, storage, and transfer will be readily available within the future.

Echocardiographic Controls

The controls on most machines can be grouped as follows: those affecting image size and position and those affecting image quality and intensity. The *depth control,* in centimeters, governs the maximum range of the ultrasonic field and hence the depth to which the beam travels as well as the size of the image of the cardiac structures. The *zoom control* enables a particular area of interest to be enlarged. The *position control* enables the operator to vary the position of the image on the oscilloscope, thus providing an area for recording other physiological parameters.

The majority of echocardiographic controls affect the image quality and intensity. Since ultrasound decreases in intensity as it travels through the body, echoes returning from the far field are weaker than those returning from the near field. If this normal attenuation were not corrected for before the image was displayed, the deeper structures would always appear less intense than the near-field structures even though the structures might be equivalent in size, mass, and reflectivity. To overcome this limitation, all echocardiographs have a circuit for suppressing near-field echoes and enhancing far-field echoes; it is referred to as *time gain compensation* (TGC). These controls (a series of levers or knobs) refine the image observed on the display screen by increasing or decreasing amplification of selected portions of the image. They must be adjusted for each patient and are frequently altered during the study.

An echocardiograph also has *power controls* (i.e., controls called the transmit, sensitivity, gain, reject, and damping controls) that uniformly decrease or amplify the intensity of the echoes as they are received. Increasing one of the power controls increases the amplitude of the ultrasonic waves transmitted into the tissue and results in a general brightening of the displayed image, enabling weaker reflective structures to come into view on the display. If the gain is too high, the brightness of the brightest structures may increase so much that weaker structures are difficult to distinguish. Approximately 30 different shades of gray can be obtained from the large variety of returning sound intensities, but overuse of the power controls can eliminate some of the subtle texture differences useful in diagnosis.

Most of the systems that are in use today generate two-dimensional echocardiograms in real time. Real-time systems currently available include the multiple-crystal scanner, designed by Bom[8]; the single-crystal mechanical scanner, designed by Griffith[24]; and the phased-array electronically steered scanner, adapted for cardiac imaging by von Ramm and Thurstone.[25] The basic requirement of these systems is that distance information (x axis) as well as height information (y axis) in the plane of the image can be displayed for echo targets semiquantitatively at image rates rapid enough to simulate real-time motion.

Two-Dimensional Scanners

Mechanical scanners may contain either a single crystal or a series of rotating crystals. The single-crystal mechanical scanners are similar to the M-mode units. The principal difference is that in two-dimensional systems the tranducer is not moved solely by hand; it is mounted on a head containing a motor and a drive assembly that mechanically oscillates the crystal(s). The crystal used is of about the same diameter as those used in conventional M-mode transducers, but the housing is larger and may vibrate. The mechanical scanners usually operate at a pulse repetition frequency of about 4000 per second, so that each frame contains about 133 lines when a frame rate of 30 per second is used. The quality of the individual frames, because of the high line density, is considerably better than that obtained with the multielement system. Mechanical scan heads, however, have identical focus in vertical and horizontal planes, thus necessitating changing scan heads to optimize image quality for the region of interest. The remainder of the ultrasonic system is identical to that used in M-mode echocardiography with the addition of a videotape recorder. These units are mobile and can be used for bedside examinations.

Electronic scanners contain multiple crystals and may be linear- or phased-array systems. The fixed-beam linear-array system developed by Bom uses a large transducer, usually 6 to 8 cm in length, that consists of 20 small ultrasonic elements.[8] The elements are fired rapidly and sequentially, and the end result is a virtually simultaneous firing of the individual elements. This forms a well-columned ultrasonic beam that is electronically swept along the length of the array and goes through the sequence rapidly (up to 60 times per second). The transducer is designed to image objects that lie just beneath each element. A linear scan of the heart produces a large rectangular image, so structures lying near the chest wall are displayed more completely than is possible with other scanners. Although it has not gained wide-spread acceptance, it is particularly advantageous in congenital heart disease, since right-side heart structures are well seen.[26] These units are small and allow portability to the bedside.

The *phased-array scanner* is the most advanced device for obtaining two-dimensional images of the heart.[25] This electronic device provides an image similar to that obtained with mechanical scanners, but it differs in the manner in which beam scanning is accomplished. The fan-shaped beam is electronically swept through the body tissue between 17 and 64 times per second. The applicator is small (2.5 mm in diameter), but the crystal is composed of 32 to 128 individual elements arranged linearly. A motor housing is not required, and there is no vibration. Free mobility and angulation of the transducer are possible. The scanning angle is adjustable and may be extended up to 90° for wide-angle viewing of a large portion of the heart. Frame rates up to 30 per second are utilitzed, and images are recorded on videotape.

In operation, the phased-array transducer is held stationary while the individual elements are excited sequentially, with a small delay interposed in the activation of individual crystals. This system is considerably more complex than mechanical sector scanners and therefore requires a computer or microprocessor for control of the individual elements. The phased-array principle can also be used to focus the beam and accomplishes it better than focusing done with acoustic lenses. The result is a marked improvement in the width of the beam and therefore of lateral resolution throughout the area of interest. In addition, the phased-array machines are the only instruments that can derive high-quality M-mode information from any angle on the sector scanner simultaneously with the real-time image. Conventional phased- or linear-array scanners, however, have fixed mechanical focus in the vertical plane and dynamic extended focus in the horizontal plane, resulting in an image that represents a relatively thick slice of tissue. To achieve superior focusing in both the vertical and horizontal directions, the *annular-phased-array transducer* was developed that results in a very thin tomographic slice and assures the highest resolution images. Phased-array systems are expensive, and some are rather large; some of them may not be transportable to the bedside, although the newest ones are mobile.

The Transducer

The selection of the appropriate transducer for the examination is of vital importance to the performance of a satisfactory echocardiogram. One of the most widely used transducers for adult echocardiography utilizes a piezoelectric crystal that emits sound signals with frequencies of 2.25 MHz and focuses the ultrasonic beam at a depth of 4 to 8 cm. This transducer is designed for maximum penetration. It is useful for scanning deep-seated (far-field) structures and examining patients of above-average body size. It permits an examination of 20 cm of tissue depth with a resolution of about 1 mm. In emphysematous patients or obese adults the desired effects of greater resolution must be compromised to achieve the necessary penetration. In such instances a transducer with a lower frequency response (e.g., 1.6 MHz) may be required.

The 3.5-MHz transducer, similar in design to the 2.25-MHz transducer, is especially useful for scanning patients of normal body size, since it offers an excellent combination of penetration and resolution. In young children and infants a smaller transducer is usually preferable, however, because penetration is much less important than resolution, since the heart is close to the transducer. The common transducers used in pediatric echocardiography have either 3.5 or 5 MHz of frequency, are 10 mm in diameter, and have short or medium focal length. For neonates and premature infants, a 5-MHz, 7-mm-diameter nonfocused transducer is especially useful when maximum resolution is desired.[27] The optimal choice of transducer for any sonographic study is, therefore, a balance between tissue penetration and resolution.

Digital Scan Converter

The addition of a digital scan converter to currently available ultrasound systems has resulted in major advances in image processing, display, and storage.[28] This device changes the ultrasound signal from analog to digital format. Digital data are then placed in the memory of a microprocessor, frame by frame, and can be read out in a real-time television format through a video recorder. In the absence of a digital scan converter some image degradation may occur when the unprocessed ultrasound data are fed through the television camera for the video image.

In addition to producing better image quality, the digital scan converter can manipulate measurements, store large amounts of data, and freeze the ultrasound image. The two-dimensional images, therefore, can be viewed as they are continuously updated on the screen in real time, can be frozen and recorded on videotape, or can be obtained as copies of individual freeze frames of real-time or videotaped images produced with a strip-chart recorder or Polaroid camera. The scan converter also allows a variety of pre- and postprocessing curves to be selected for additional image refining (e.g., curves for enhancing boundaries, for optimizing gray-scale presentation, and for studying tissue texture). *Postprocessing* can be applied to the real-time image or can be applied to the frozen images after digital storage, thus providing additional flexibility in adjusting image characteristics. Postprocessing can also affect videotaped material. Despite the advantages of the digital format over the standard analog format, recording of ultrasound signals on videotape may result in degradation of image quality with either technique. In some videotape systems only half of the scan lines displayed in real time are exhibited during stop-frame imaging.

Computer tomography with digital recording on floppy disks has allowed echocardiography to enhance its clinical potential. The advantages of storing individual pictures in a digital form are numerous, including savings in cost, storage, and editing as well as availability of automatic measurements and calibration. Most importantly, it permits the recording of a single cardiac cycle in a continuous loop that allows one to review a cardiac cycle for as long as necessary.

Other Features

Other features of the echocardiograph are an *alphanumeric keyboard, electronic calipers* (e.g., light pen or joystick), and an *electrocardiographic trigger,* which permits images to be frozen in preselected portions of the cardiac cycle (e.g., end systole and end diastole). These features provide considerable flexibility in documentation (e.g., recording patient identification, date, time, and tape number), making measurements on the frozen images (e.g., measuring the mitral valve orifice or determination of left ventricular volumes), and automatically displaying the calculated results.

TECHNIQUES FOR PERFORMING THE EXAMINATION

The acquisition of comprehensive and technically adequate echocardiographic studies requires a thorough knowledge of cardiac anatomy, physiology, and spatial orientation, since echocardiography requires immediate on-line interpretative evaluation. Unless the type and significance of abnormal structures, motion, and function are recognized, adequate views and complete anatomy will not be recorded and the study may not be adequate for diagnostic purposes. For these reasons, and so that the study can be directed along clinically relevant lines, certain information about the patient is necessary prior to the beginning of the examination. This includes height and weight (to determine body surface area), age, and cardiac findings. A complete echocardiographic examination, however, should be performed on all patients studied regardless of the clinical suspicions.

Echocardiograms should be performed and interpreted in accordance with the guidelines for optimal training set forth by the American Society of Echocardiography (ASE), the American College of Cardiology[29,30] (ACC), and the Society of Pediatric Echocardiography.[31] In addition, the uses of echocardiography in clinical cardiovascular practice should closely follow the recommendations set forth in the ACC/American Heart Association (AHA) guidelines for the clinical application of echocardiography.[32]

Both M-mode and two-dimensional echocardiographic examinations are performed with the patient in the supine position. This position serves to standardize the values for cardiac dimensions and also enables cardiac relations to be interpreted more consistently. Varying the position of the patient, however, may enhance the recording of the echoes from certain portions of the chest and should be a routine part of each study. Another position that is commonly employed is to have the patient lie in left lateral decubitus with the trunk raised about 30° to 45°. This enables the interventricular septum, and consequently the left ventricular, to be more accurately recorded, but it may distort right ventricular dimensions; interpretations may be erroneous if this is not appreciated. Therefore, we routinely examine the patient first in the supine position and then in the left lateral position. Pediatric patients frequently require sedation. For children aged 3 to 7 years, oral chloral hydrate in a dose of 50 to 100 mg/kg should be given about 30 min before the study.[33] Intramuscular phenobarbital, however, yields the best results in uncooperative patients. For infants we offer a sugar nipple or sugar water.[27]

The application of an electrocardiographic lead (usually II or III) is critical, not only for timing purposes and analyzing the echocardiogram but also because certain arrhythmias or conduction defects may cause motion abnormalities that may be confused with other cardiac abnormalities if the ECG is unknown.

We perform the echocardiographic examination from the patient's left side so that the transducer is at the long axis of the heart. When the patient is in a steep left lateral position, which is preferable for apical imaging, reaching across from the right side of the bed is much more difficult than working from the left, and if the patient is quite large or obese, it is harder to palpate and impossible to visualize the apex impulse. The direction from which the patient is approached, however, really does not matter as long as the examination is consistently performed and the scanning posture permits freedom of transducer movement, adequate room for reaching the controls, and an unimpeded view of the video screen.

The examination involves both hands. Usually the transducer is held in the left hand while the right hand is used to manipulate the controls of the echocardiograph and recorder. Alternatively, the left hand may be used as a stabilizing hand, with the forearm and hand resting on the patient, while the right hand is used to angulate and rotate the transducer as well as to operate the controls of the machine. Maintaining the transducer in a stable precordial position without excessive pressure or loss of image is critical; therefore, many echocardiographers rest the heel of the hand and some of the fingers on the patient's chest wall, whereas others prefer an arm rest to prevent the arm from becoming fatigued. A foot switch that manipulates the freeze-frame, strip-chart, and videotape controls is also extremely useful during two-dimensional scanning.

There must be airless contact between the transducer and the skin. Since the ultrasound beam is scattered in air, a liquid coupling medium (glycol based or water based) must be generously applied either over the area of the skin to be scanned or directly to the transducer head. Insufficient coupling medium can result in poor images. It is preferable to have the patient on a firm foam mattress approximately 8 in thick with a semicircular hole cut out on the left side. The patient is then positioned so that the cardiac apex is directly over this cutout, which facilitates apical imaging.

The examination is begun by placing the transducer on the skin overlying the precordium (precordial or transthoracic echocardiography) and moving it about in order to locate the best acoustic window. Since body size, structures, and organ positions vary considerably, the acoustic windows will be slightly different for each patient, making an initial search necessary. The best acoustic windows have little, if any, lung tissue or bony structures interposed between the skin and the heart, since both the air-tissue and the calcium-tissue interfaces almost totally reflect ultrasound, preventing it from reaching the deeper structures. This problem is not present in infants, since the ribs and sternum are cartilaginous. Once the desired image has been obtained, hold the transducer firmly over the area, being careful not to let the transducer slip.

Two-dimensional echocardiography has supplanted M-mode echocardiography as the standard imaging modality. Two-dimensional echocardiography overcomes many of the limitations of M-mode by providing a spatial orientation of the cardiac structures. Since these two imaging modalities are combined in the modern ultrasound system, the quality of the M-mode recording is significantly improved by employing simultaneous two-dimensional imaging to identify the precise location and direction of the M-mode cursor. This flexibility can provide more information about cardiac structures and function than either system could alone. Therefore, the M-mode and two-dimensional studies should be performed simultaneously or in sequence as part of the same echocardiographic examination, and measurements and interpretative information from both recordings should be incorporated into a single report. Nevertheless, since M-mode echocardiography is uniquely valuable because of its superior resolution, it will be discussed with an emphasis on the characteristic patterns.

Normal M-Mode Echocardiogram

The M-mode echocardiogram should usually be performed in conjunction with the two-dimensional study. The following discussion, however, will be focused solely on the M-mode examination, assuming that in many circumstances it is the only method available. Figure 15-1 is a schematic diagram of a cross section of the heart, showing how the ultrasonic beam can be swept in an arc between the cardiac apex and the base of the heart for structure identification. With the transducer at the third left intercostal space and angled toward the left hip, the ultrasonic beam traverses first the skin-transducer interface and then the chest wall, anterior right ventricular free wall, right ventricular cavity, interventricular septum, left ventricle, and posterior left ventricular wall. As the transducer tilts progressively cephalad, the posterior papillary muscles are imaged, then the mitral valve leaflets are traversed, and finally the aorta, aortic valve, and left atrial cavity are seen. In order to image the tricuspid and pulmonic valves, the ultrasound beam must angle between the right hip and left shoulder.

Figure 15-2 is a diagrammatic presentation of the M-mode scan as the transducer is swept from the cardiac apex toward the base of the heart. The letters correspond to the direction of the transducer in Fig. 15-1. These two illustrations demonstrate the relations of the heart valves and cardiac chambers to each other. For example, the left ventricle is about 2 to $2^1/_2$ times as large as the right ventricle, the aorta and left atrium are roughly equal in size, the septum is in continuity with the anterior aortic wall, and the anterior mitral leaflet is in continuity with the posterior aortic wall.

Begin the M-mode examination with a search for the mitral valve (Fig. 15-3). To understand the echocardiographic pattern produced by the anterior mitral leaflet, keep in mind that all motion is indicated relative to a fixed point on the anterior chest wall. The point of maximum excursion of the anterior leaflet is designated E, and the nadir of the initial diastolic closing valve is designated F. The middiastolic closing motion, referred to as the EF slope, represents the velocity of blood moving from the left atrium into the left ventricle. With atrial systole, blood is propelled through the mitral orifice and the leaflets reopen. The peak of this opening is designated A; with atrial relaxation, the valve begins to close again. Complete closure, point C, occurs following the onset of ventricular systole. The anterior mitral leaflet in diastole resembles the letter *M;* the mirror-image posterior leaflet resembles the letter *W.*

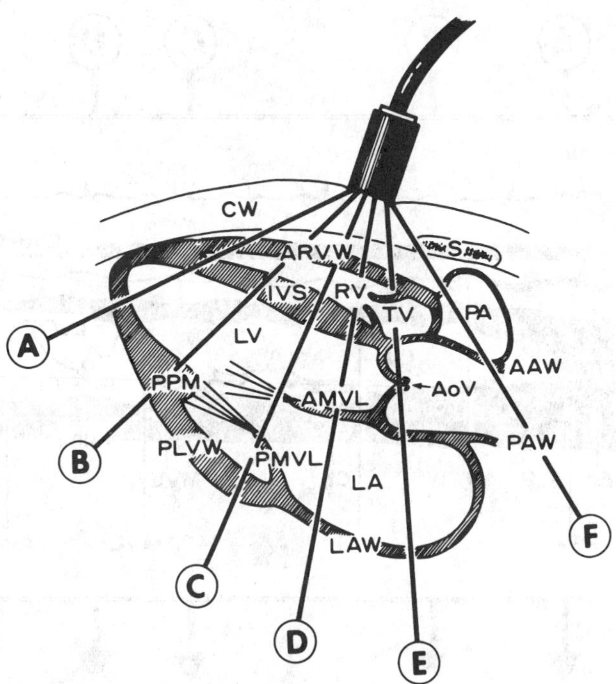

FIGURE 15-1 Cross section of the heart. Lines A through F show how the ultrasonic beam is swept in an arc between the apex and the base of the heart. With the transducer at A, the ultrasonic beam traverses the skin-transducer interface, chest wall (CW), anterior right ventricular wall (ARVW), right ventricle (RV), intraventricular septum (IVS), left ventricle (LV) at the apex, and posterior left ventricular wall (PLVW). As the transducer is tilted progressively cephalad, the following structures are imaged: at B, the left ventricle at the posterior papillary muscle (PPM); at C, anterior (AMVL) and posterior (PMVL) mitral valve leaflets; at D, anterior mitral leaflet at the junction of posterior left ventricular wall and left atrial wall (LAW); at E, tricuspid valve (TV), anterior (AAW) and posterior (PAW) aortic walls, aortic valve (AoV), and left atrium (LA); at F, pulmonary artery (PA). (*From JM Felner, RC Schlant: Echocardiography: A Teaching Atlas. New York, Grune & Stratton, 1976. Reproduced with permission from the publisher and authors.*).

The base-to-apex or apex-to-base scan should be obtained after identification of the mitral valve (Fig. 15-3). The anterior leaflet of the mitral valve smooths out in appearance and becomes the posterior wall of the aorta (anatomic posterior continuity); simultaneously the interventricular septum becomes the anterior wall of the aorta (anatomic anterior continuity). The two aortic walls will move parallel to each other (anteriorly in systole and posteriorly in diastole) and have a characteristic echo appearance. The leaflets of the aortic valve form a boxlike structure within the walls of the aorta (Fig. 15-3). The anterior (right coronary) and posterior (noncoronary) cusps can consistently be recorded, but the middle (left coronary) cusp, which is parallel to the ultrasound beam, is only occasionally seen. Posterior to the aorta is the left atrium. The left atrial posterior wall usually does not move at this level because it is attached to the mediastinum. The left ventricular cavity is bordered by the interventricular septum anteriorly and the

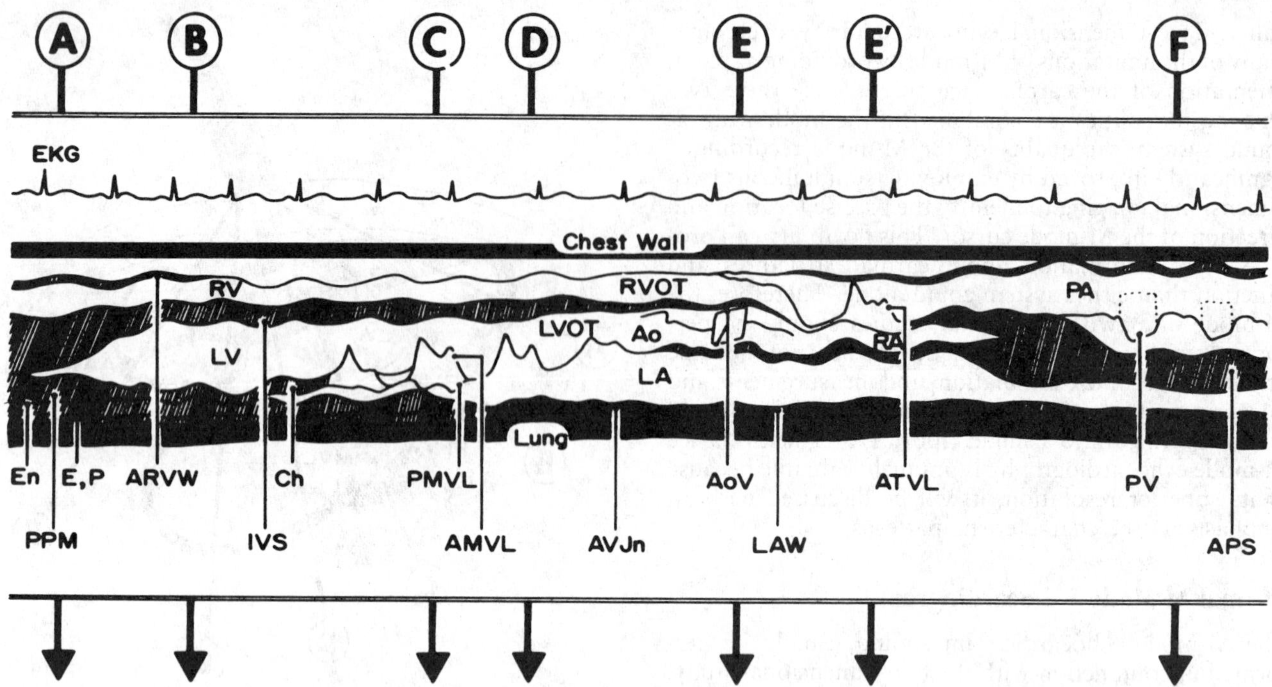

FIGURE 15-2 Representation of an M-mode echocardiographic recording as the ultrasonic beam is swept in an arc from the apex to the base of the heart. The arrows labeled A through F correspond approximately to the transducer positions in Fig. 15-1. An ECG is shown for timing. The ultrasound beam traverses the following structures: at A, the homogeneous, stationary echo of the chest wall (CW), anterior right ventricular wall (ARVW), right ventricle (RV), muscular portion of the interventricular septum (IVS), left ventricle (LV) at the level of the posterior papillary muscle (PPM), free left ventricular wall myocardium, consisting of endocardium (En) and epicardial (E) and pericardial (P) interface and lung; at B, left ventricle at the level of the chordae tendineae (Ch); at C, the right and left ventricles at the level of the anterior (AMVL) and posterior (PMVL) mitral valve leaflets; at D, the left ventricular outflow tract (LVOT) anterior to the mitral valve; at E, the right ventricular outflow tract (RVOT), ascending aorta (Ao), aortic valve (AoV), left atrium (LA), and left atrial wall (LAW); at E, the right ventricle, anterior tricuspid valve leaflet (ATVL), right atrium (RA), and left atrium; at F, the pulmonary artery (PA), pulmonic valve (PV), atriopulmonic sulcus (APS), and left atrium. (*From JM Felner, RC Schlant: Echocardiography: A Teaching Atlas. New York, Grune & Stratton, 1976. Reproduced with permission from the publisher and authors.*)

left ventricular free wall posteriorly. Both of these walls move, toward each other during systole and away from each other during diastole. A portion of the right ventricular cavity lies between the nonmoving chest wall and the septum; frequently the right ventricular free wall can be seen just beneath the chest wall echo.

Of the right-sided valves, only the anterior leaflet of the tricuspid valve and the posterior (left) pulmonic cusp can be recorded.

M-Mode Echocardiographic Measurements

The ASE has attempted to standardize the common M-mode measurements and has recommended that they be made by use of the *leading-edge* method.[34] That is, measurements from one structure to another should be made from the leading edge of the last echo produced by the anterior structure to the leading edge of the first echo produced by the posterior structure. It is also recom-

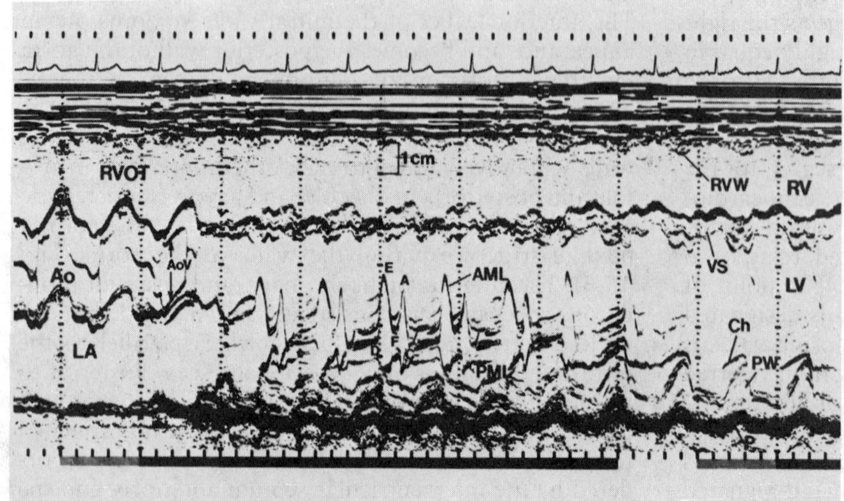

FIGURE 15-3 Normal M-mode echocardiographic base-to-apex scan. The leaflets of the boxlike aortic valve (AoV) open widely in systole, whereas in diastole they coapt and are midway between the anterior and posterior aortic walls. The aorta (Ao) and left atrium (LA) are equal in size. There are normal anterior continuity between the anterior aortic wall and the interventricular septum (VS) and normal posterior continuity between the posterior aortic wall and the anterior mitral leaflet (AML). The mitral valve has a characteristic M-shaped anterior leaflet and W-shaped posterior leaflet (PML). Onset of mitral valve opening is designated by the letter D, full opening of the anterior leaflet by E, middiastolic closure by F, atrial systole by A, and valve closure by C. RVW, right ventricular wall; RVOT, right ventricular outflow tract; Ch, chordae tendineae; LV, left ventricle.

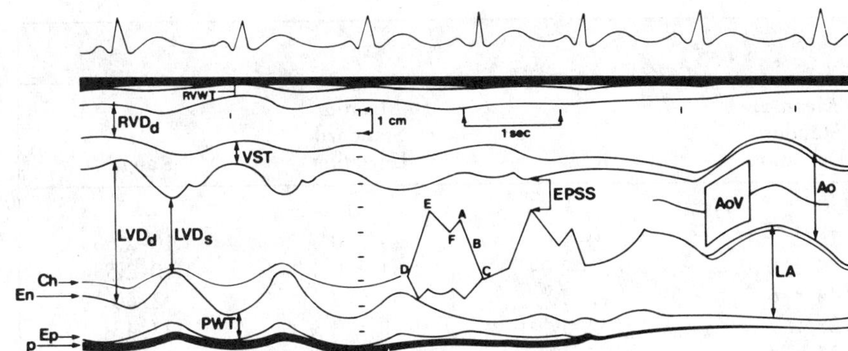

FIGURE 15-4 Schematic M-mode echocardiographic apex-to-base scan illustrating the location by determining intracardiac measurements. The anterior mitral leaflet is labeled A through F. See text for details. The mitral valve E point–ventricular septal separation (EPSS) is shown. RVWT, right ventricular wall thickness; RVD_d, right ventricular dimension, end-diastole; LVD_d left ventricular dimension, end diastole; LVD_s, left ventricular dimension, end systole; Ch, chordae tendineae; En, endocardium; Ep, epicardium; P, pericardium; VST, ventricular septal thickness; PWT, posterior wall thickness; AoV, aortic valve; Ao, aorta; LA, left atrium.

mended that all measurements be obtained by averaging five cardiac cycles recorded at end expiration, since inspiration causes an increase in right ventricular and a decrease in the left ventricular volume. The attempt to determine left ventricular dimensions from M-mode echocardiograms using the criteria advocated by the ASE has met with a diversity of opinion. There are data supporting their results from one group,[35] whereas another group believes that the recommendations are not clearly superior to other currently available techniques.[36]

The timing and locations of the various M-mode measurements, suggested by the ASE and supported by us, are shown in Fig. 15-4. Measurements should be made as follows:

1. The aortic root, the distance between the anterior edges of the two aortic walls, at end diastole.
2. The left atrium, the distance between the anterior portion of the posterior aortic wall and the anterior surface of the posterior left atrial wall, at end systole.
3. The left ventricle, the distance between the left side of the interventricular septum and the posterior left ventricular endocardium at the level of the chordae tendineae, except infants and young children, where it is best determined at the level of the mitral valve. Transducer position should be standard (i.e., perpendicular to the chest wall with very slight angulation),[37] since an abnormally low transducer placement may spuriously decrease left ventricular internal dimensions by producing a falsely thick septum. *End diastole* is defined as the onset of the QRS, and *end systole* is determined by the most posterior position of the septum. When septal motion is abnormal, the most anterior position of the posterior wall identifies end systole. Percent fractional shortening (percent delta D) of the left ventricle is determined as follows:

$$\frac{\text{End-diastolic dimension} - \text{End-systolic dimension}}{\text{End-diastolic dimension}} \times 100$$

4. The right ventricle, the distance between the anterior right ventricular free wall and the right side of the septum, at end diastole. The right ventricular dimension is subject to significant error because only a small portion of it is actually visualized and because the dimension varies depending on patient position and beam orientation.[21,22]
5. Septal wall thickness, the distance between the anterior right septal echo and the anterior left septal echo, at end diastole.
6. Posterior wall thickness, the distance between the anterior endocardial echo and the anterior surface of the epicardial echo, at end diastole.
7. The right ventricular free-wall thickness, the distance between the anterior epicardial and anterior endocardial surfaces, at end diastole.
8. The E point–septal separation (EPSS), the distance between the E point of the anterior mitral leaflet and the left margin of the ventricular septum, should not exceed 7 mm.[38]

Normal values for these M-mode echocardiographic measurements are shown in Table 15-1. These values, however, change during aging.[39] For example, increasing age correlates with increased aortic root diameter, left ventricular wall thickness, and left atrial size.

The Two-Dimensional Examination

There is almost a limitless number of possible cross-sectional (tomographic) planes through which the heart can be viewed or sliced.[23,40] This potential is highly advantageous, since the heart's position and architecture vary substantially from patient to patient. The ASE has attempted to standardize the two-dimensional examination by recommending a nomenclature for the various cardiac sections based on the position of the transducer (i.e., parasternal, apical, subcostal, and suprasternal) and the plane of cardiac anatomy being imaged (i.e., long-axis, short-axis, and four-chamber).[41]

The long-axis plane is the tomographic section that transects the heart parallel to the major axis of the left ventricle (Fig. 15-5). The short-axis plane is obtained by rotating the sector 90° and transecting the heart perpendicular to the plane of the long axis (Fig. 15-6). The four-chamber plane transects the heart approximately parallel to the dorsal and ventral surfaces of the body (Fig. 15-7). Each of these orthogonal planes, however, is actually a series or family of planes that can be generated by moving the transducer from side to side, from top to bottom, or clockwise to counterclockwise. For example, the long axis describes a family of planes parallel to the long axis of the heart and within 45° of the plane perpendicular to the dorsal and ventral surfaces of the body.

The ASE also recommends that an index mark be placed on every two-dimensional transducer in order to indicate the direction in which the ultrasound beam is being angled (Figs. 15-5 to 15-7).[41] Its main purpose, however, is to identify the portion of the image plane

TABLE 15-1
Normal Values

	Mean ± Standard Deviation	Range	Mean ± Standard Deviation	Range
No. of patients	25	—	50	—
Age, years	10 ± 3	4–18	24 ± 6	1.10–2.53
BSA, M^2	1.33 ± 0.38	0.72–2.04	1.81 ± .34	1.10–2.53
$LVID_d$, mm	44 ± 6	32–50	50 ± 3	42–60
$LVID_s$, mm	28 ± 7	32–50	50 ± 3	22–43
ΔD or FSLV	34 ± 4	25–42	33 ± 3	28–37
C_{cf} circ/s	1.09 ± 0.12	0.82–1.30	1.26 ± 0.3	0.95–1.60
Max_s PWV, mm/s	42 ± 10	32–55	60 ± 13	40–78
Max_d PWV, mm/s	137 ± 30	91–204	160 ± 48	110–280
IVS thickness, mm	8 ± 2	5–10	9 ± 1	7–12
IVS excursion, mm	7 ± 1	5–9	9 ± 1	7–12
PW_d thickness, mm	7 ± 2	4–9	9 ± 1	7–12
PW_s thickness, mm	12 ± 3	8–17	16 ± 2	13–20
Δ thickening PW	0.70 ± 0.25	0.41–0.95	0.50 ± 0.19	0.32–0.69
PW excursion	9 ± 2	7–14	11 ± 2	9–17
RVD_d supine, mm	—	—	15 ± 6	7–22
RVD_d left lateral, mm	—	—	20 ± 8	10–37
$Aorta_d$ mm	23 ± 4	15–27	28 ± 5	26–36
LAD_s mm	25 ± 5	20–31	27 ± 6	12–35

NOTE: BSA = Body surface area; $LVID_d$ = left ventricular internal diameter, end diastole; $LVID_s$ = left ventricular internal diameter, end systole; FSLV = fractional shortening of left ventricle; PWV = posterior wall velocity; IVS = interventricular septum; PW = posterior wall; RVD = right ventricular dimension; LAD = left atrial dimension.
SOURCE: JM Felner, RC Schlant: *Echocardiograpy: A Teaching Atlas.* New York, Grune & Stratton, 1976. Reproduced with permission from the publisher and authors.

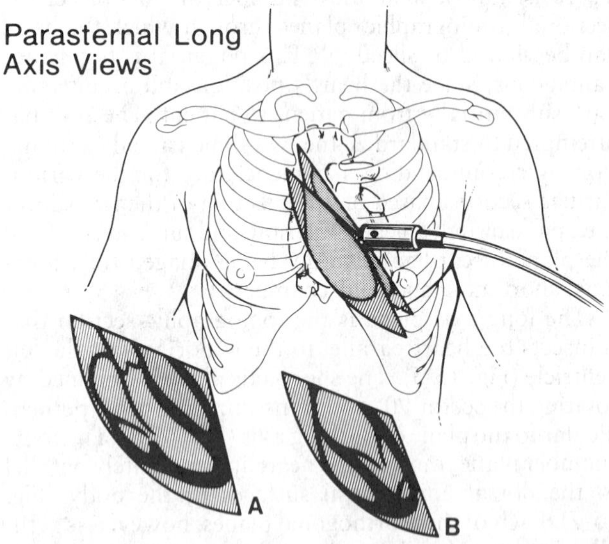

FIGURE 15-5 Anatomic reference drawing showing the position and inclination of the parasternal long-axis examining planes obtained with the transducer in the third intercostal space and the index mark (black dot) cephalad. *A.* Oriented with the sector beam between the right shoulder and left hip to show predominately structures of the left side of the heart. *B.* Oriented with the sector beam tilted medially and slightly inferiorly toward the right hip to show predominately structures of the right side of the heart. In real-time imaging, these two long-axis views are inverted and displayed as though the observer were viewing them from the patient's left side. (*The cardiac ultrasound examination—some commonly recorded views. Slightly modified and reproduced with permission from Hewlett-Packard.*)

that will appear on the right side of the display as the viewer faces the video screen. For example, if the index mark is pointing cephalad toward the right shoulder, in the direction of the aorta in a parasternal long-axis view, the aorta would appear on the right side of the video display. In addition, when the images are viewed on the screen, the signals returning from the structures located near the surface of the transducer should appear at the top of the screen in the narrowest part of the sector, while the structures located farthest from the transducer should appear at the bottom on the screen in the widest part of the sector wedge. If the equipment is provided with an image inversion switch, the operator can reverse the image; the structures near the surface (close to the transducer) will then appear at the bottom of the image and the more distant structures will appear at the top of display, without producing a change in the left-right orientation of the image. For best orientation, the transducer index mark should always be pointed either in the direction of the patient's head or to the patient's left side.

There are several techniques used in two-dimensional echocardiography that are not used in M-mode echocardiography. *Sliding* moves the transducer over the precordium, passing the sector into various positions within the heart. This maneuver is most helpful for evaluation of the size and shape of the heart and for preliminary estimation of the general direction of specific planes within the heart. *Angulation* extends the view of the

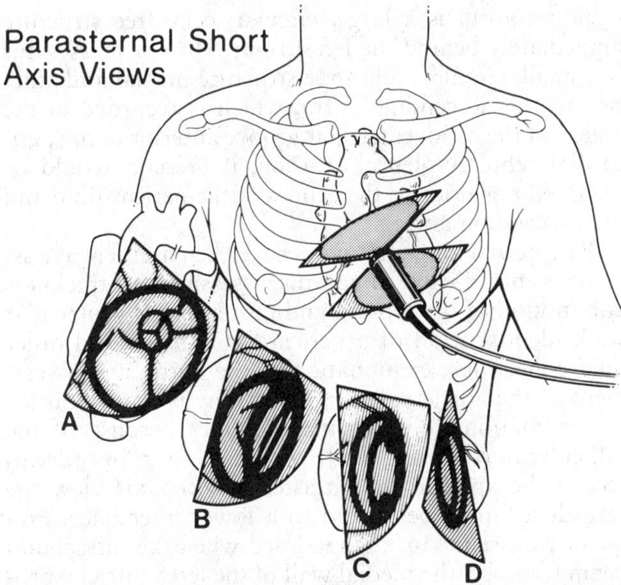

FIGURE 15-6 Anatomic reference drawing showing the position and inclination of some of the many parasternal short-axis examining planes obtained with the transducer in the third intercostal space and the index mark (black dot) to the patient's left. The short-axis planes shown are obtained by gradually tilting the transducer from base to apex. *A.* Aortic valve level. *B.* Mitral valve level. *C.* Papillary muscle level. *D.* Cardiac apex. In real-time imaging the apex image (*D*) is inverted. (*The cardiac ultrasound examination—some commonly recorded views. Slightly modified and reproduced with permission from Hewlett-Packard.*)

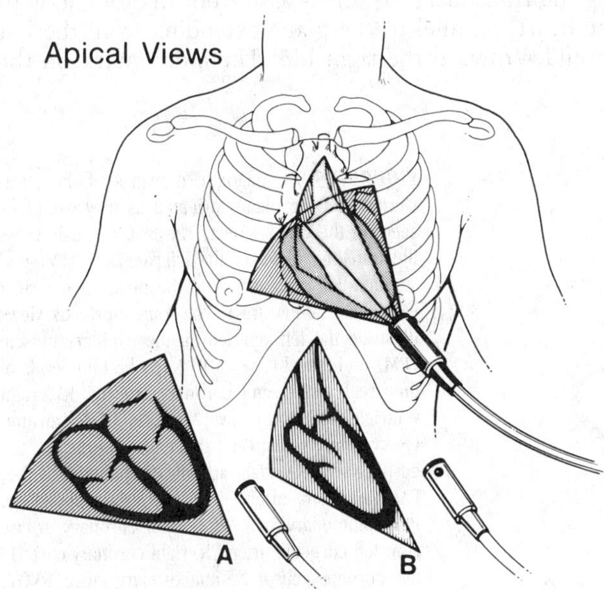

FIGURE 15-7 Anatomic reference drawing showing the position and inclination of two of the family of apical examining planes. *A.* Four-chamber view obtained with the index mark to the patient's left. *B.* Long-axis view obtained with the index mark cephalad. In real-time imaging the apical views are inverted and displayed as though the observer were looking down the heart. (*The cardiac ultrasound examination—some commonly recorded views. Slightly modified and reproduced with permission from Hewlett-Packard.*)

heart obtained by a particular sector and involves scanning the fan-shaped examination plane along its arc or width, thereby sequentially increasing the longitudinal extent of the area under study. *Tilting* displaces the sector in a direction perpendicular to its width and is useful for changing the plane of study and for development of three-dimensional spatial orientation of structures in a particular scanning plane. *Pivoting* is a rotational motion that changes the direction of the axis of the sector scan in relation to intracardiac structures. It is accomplished by rotating the transducer on its longitudinal axis while retaining a known target in the sector.

The two-dimensional examination begins with the patient usually positioned in the supine or left lateral position and the transducer (2.5, 3.5, or 5.0 MHz) placed at an acoustic window identical to that used for the M-mode examination. This examination, however, is usually performed using all four of the basic transducer positions: parasternal, apical, subcostal, and suprasternal (Fig. 15-8).[40] Recordability of parasternal views is highly influenced by body build and age. In normal children and young adults cardiac echoes are usually obtained from the second to fifth left intercostal spaces, but in elderly patients and in those with some degree of pulmonary emphysema the echocardiographic window shrinks in size so that only the lower intercostal spaces are usable. From this position the sector image of the heart along its long and short axes can be obtained. Additional transducer positions have also proved useful,

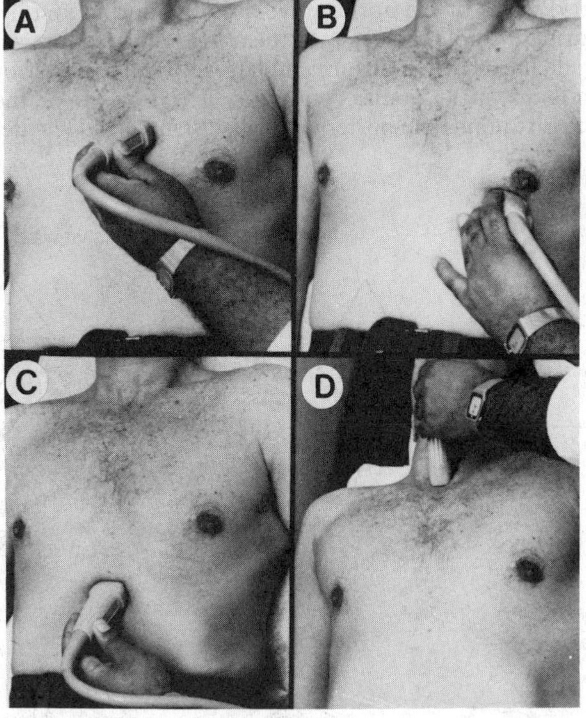

FIGURE 15-8 Commonly used transducer positions for the two-dimensional examination. *A.* Parasternal position at the third or fourth left intercostal space. *B.* Apical position directly over the palpable apex impulse. *C.* Subcostal position facilitated by flexing the patient's knees. *D.* Suprasternal notch position facilitated by placing a pillow behind the patient's neck and shoulders.

including imaging from the right side of the sternum and in the mid and low precordium.

The Tomographic Views

The *parasternal long-axis view* of the left ventricle extends from the right shoulder to the left hip. The index mark on the transducer points cephalad toward the right shoulder (Fig. 15-5). This plane is an excellent starting point, since it is comparable to the long-axis scan obtained from an M-mode examination and resembles an angiogram in the right anterior oblique projection. Therefore, most echocardiographers already appreciate the anatomy and motion of structures in this plane (Fig. 15-9). This two-dimensional image allows examination of the size and shape of the left ventricle, right ventricular outflow tract, left atrium, and aortic root, as well as examination of the motion of the mitral and aortic valves (Fig. 15-10). The point of the fan-shaped sector is occupied by the transducer artifact and the chest wall. In the middle of the sector almost the entire length of the left ventricle can be examined, although the cardiac apex is usually not seen in this view. The septum appears to become gradually thinner from the inferior (muscular) portion to the more superior (membranous) portion, where it is in anatomic continuity with the anterior wall of the aorta. Anterior to the aortic root and beneath the chest wall echo is the right ventricular outflow tract. The posterior wall of the aorta is in anatomic continuity with the large anterior mitral leaflet; the smaller posterior leaflet originates at the atrioventricular groove. Only the anterior (right coronary) and the posterior (noncoronary) cusps of the aortic valve are seen during systole. During diastole the cusps of the aortic valve coapt as a single line. The left atrium and left ventricular posterior walls are in anatomic continuity. The bottom of the sector contains the posterior cardiac structures. The descending aorta is a large, circular, echo-free structure immediately behind the left atrium. The coronary sinus is a small, circular, echo-free structure medial and anterior to the descending aorta, which is recorded in the region of the atrioventricular groove anterior to the pericardial echo. A pleural effusion, if present, would be recorded posterior to the echoes of the pericardium and the descending aorta.

Parasternal long-axis views have been useful in assessment of mitral valve apparatus, assessment of thickness and motion of the septum and posterior left ventricular wall, identification of a pericardial effusion and other fluid collections, examination of the aorta, and assessment of the aortic valve.[23,42] This view is not useful for the estimation of ventricular volumes because of the difficulty in recording the true cardiac apex. In order to record the apex in the parasternal long-axis view the transducer must be moved to a lower interspace. Frequently a pseudoapex is recorded when the ultrasound beam transects the medial wall of the left ventricle, producing a foreshortened image.

From the parasternal long-axis view of the left ventricle the transducer can be angled medially to image the long axis of the right ventricle and right atrium (Fig. 15-5). In this *right ventricular inflow tract view* the main orientation is through the right ventricle, tricuspid valve, and right atrium. The aorta has diasppeared, and only a small portion of the left ventricle and a portion of the membraneous septum are visualized (Fig. 15-9). The inflow portion of the right ventricle is bordered by the septum and anterior right ventricular wall. This view is useful for evaluating the tricuspid valve and for detecting right atrial masses.[23]

The *parasternal short-axis view* is obtained by rotating the transducer 90° clockwise from the long axis of the heart, parallel to the plane extending from the left shoulder toward the right hip. The index mark on the

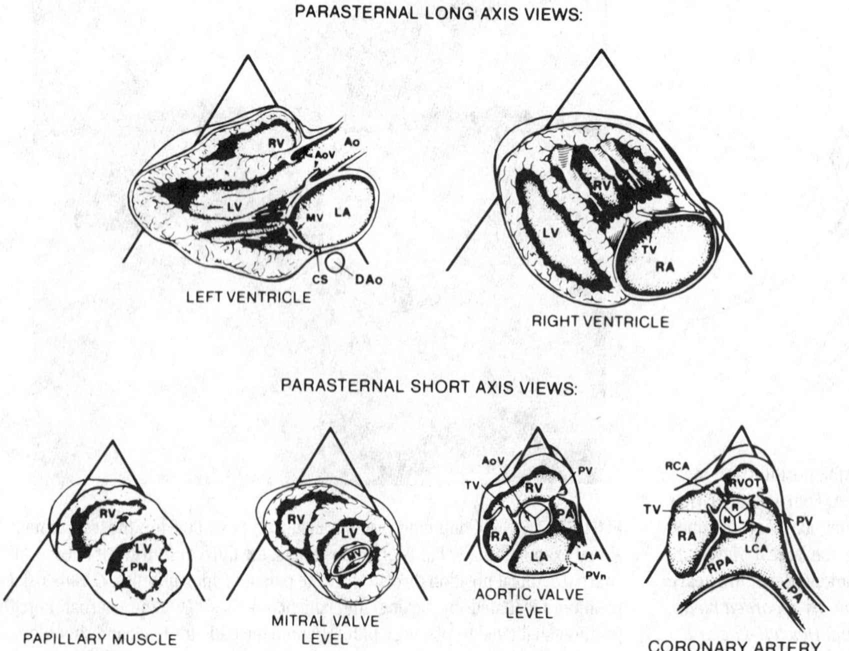

FIGURE 15-9 Anatomic drawings of the parasternal imaging planes oriented as they would be seen on the video screen. The two long-axis views illustrate the plane of the left ventricle (LV) and surrounding structures and the plane of the right ventricular inflow tract. The four short-axis views illustrate the left ventricle at the papillary muscle (PM) and mitral valve (MV) levels and the levels of the great vessels and coronary arteries. RV, right ventricle; AoV, aortic valve; Ao, aorta; LA, left atrium; CS, coronary sinus; DAo, descending aorta; TV, tricuspid valve; RA, right atrium; PV, pulmonic valve; PA, pulmonary artery; LAA, left atrial appendage; PVn, pulmonary vein; RCA, right coronary artery; LCA, left coronary artery; R, right coronary cusp; L, left coronary cusp; N, noncoronary cusp; RVOT, right ventricular outflow tract; RPA, right pulmonary artery; LPA, left pulmonary artery. [*From DJ Sahn, F. Anderson: Two-Dimensional Anatomy of the Heart: An Atlas for Echocardiographers. Copyright © 1982 John Wiley & Sons, New York. (Except figures in right upper and right lower portions of the illustration.) Adapted and reproduced with permission from John Wiley & Sons and the authors.*]

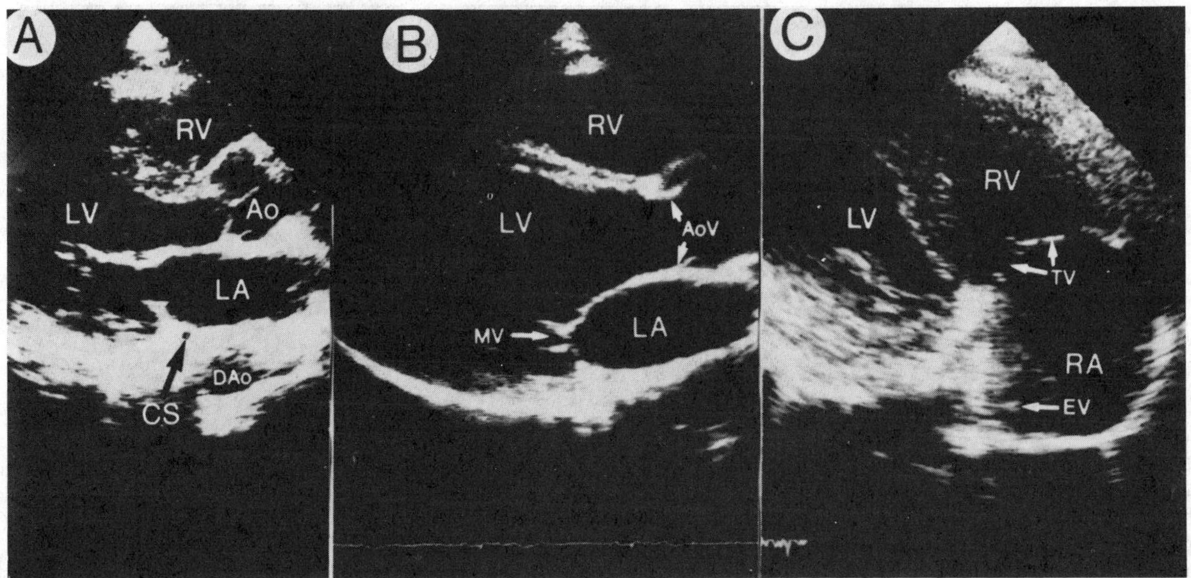

FIGURE 15-10 Two-dimensional parasternal long-axis views from a normal subject. *A.* Long-axis plane of the left ventricle (LV) in diastole. The aorta (Ao) and the left atrium (LA) are to the right of the sector image, and the apex of the left ventricle is to the left of the sector image. The outflow tract portion of the right ventricle (RV) appears anteriorly, at the top or narrowest part of the fan-shaped image; the posterior walls of the left ventricle and left atrium appear near the bottom or widest portion of the image. The coronary sinus (CS) and descending aorta (DAo) are the most posterior structures. *B.* Enlargement of view *A* in systole excludes the most posterior structures and shows that the leaflets of the aortic valve (AoV) open to the periphery and the leaflets of the mitral valve (MV) are closed. The left ventricle is two to three times the size of the right ventricle. *C.* Right ventricular inflow tract view shows the right atrium (RA), right ventricle, tricuspid valve (TV), and a small portion of the left ventricle.

transducer points to the patient's left side (Fig. 15-6). Short-axis views of the heart are unique to two-dimensional echocardiography—they are impossible to obtain with M-mode echocardiography or angiography. When the image plane is swept from the cardiac apex to the base of the heart, a series of short-axis planes at the levels of the true cardiac apex, papillary muscles, mitral valve orifice, and great arteries can be obtained (Figs. 15-6 and 15-9). Although these multiple short-axis views can often be recorded from the same parasternal interspace, it is frequently necessary to move the transducer into different locations over the left precordium to obtain all the short-axis images. For example, a more cephalad location (second interspace) may be advantageous in visualizing the great arteries, whereas a more caudad location (fourth or fifth interspace) is used to visualize the cardiac apex.[23,40,42]

Begin the short-axis examination with the transducer in the third interspace pointing directly posteriorly and locate the left ventricle and the papillary muscles as they project into the ventricular cavity (Fig. 15-11). The left ventricle will appear circular if the tomographic plane is truly perpendicular to the major axis of the heart. The posteromedial papillary muscle is located at 7 to 8 o'clock; the anterolateral papillary muscle is located at 3 to 4 o'clock. Pathological conditions of the papillary muscles, including hypertrophy, calcification, and rupture, can now be visualized; this is not possible with other techniques, including angiography. From the level of the papillary muscles, if the transducer is tilted inferiorly or moved to a lower interspace, the true left ventricular apex will be imaged in short axis. The size of the left ventricular cavity at this level is much smaller, and the trabeculations are more exaggerated. The right ventricular cavity is now quite small and will gradually disappear with further inferior angulation (Fig. 15-11).

From the papillary muscle level, tilt the transducer slightly cephalad to image the chordae tendineae and leaflets of the mitral valve in the center of the left ventricle (Fig. 15-11). At this level the right and left ventricular cavities are larger than they are at the papillary muscle level. The difference in size of the left ventricle during systole and diastole (Fig. 15-12), as well as the "fish mouth" appearance of the mitral valve as the leaflets open and close, can readily be appreciated. Short-axis views at the mitral valve level are useful for evaluation of regional wall motion, quantification of mitral orifice area, and observing various causes of mitral regurgitation. Portions of the right ventricle, tricuspid valve apparatus, ventricular septum, and left ventricular outflow tract are visualized anteriorly and to the left of the mitral valve. From this position, angling the transducer toward the right ventricle will more optimally record tricuspid valve motion.

As the transducer is tilted superiorly from the mitral valve area, the left ventricular outflow tract and then the great arteries at the base of the heart are sectioned transversely. The circular aorta containing the aortic valve is seen in the middle of the image (Figs. 15-6, 15-9, and 15-11). In diastole, the three aortic cusps usually form a Y configuration. Occasionally, the posterior junction, between the left and noncoronary cusps, is difficult to image because it is parallel to the plane of sound. When this occurs, only two of the three diastolic lines may be seen simultaneously, resulting in a V, rather than a Y, pattern. The anterior (right coronary) cusp is seen between the tricuspid and pulmonic valves. The left coronary cusp lies between the pulmonic valve and the left

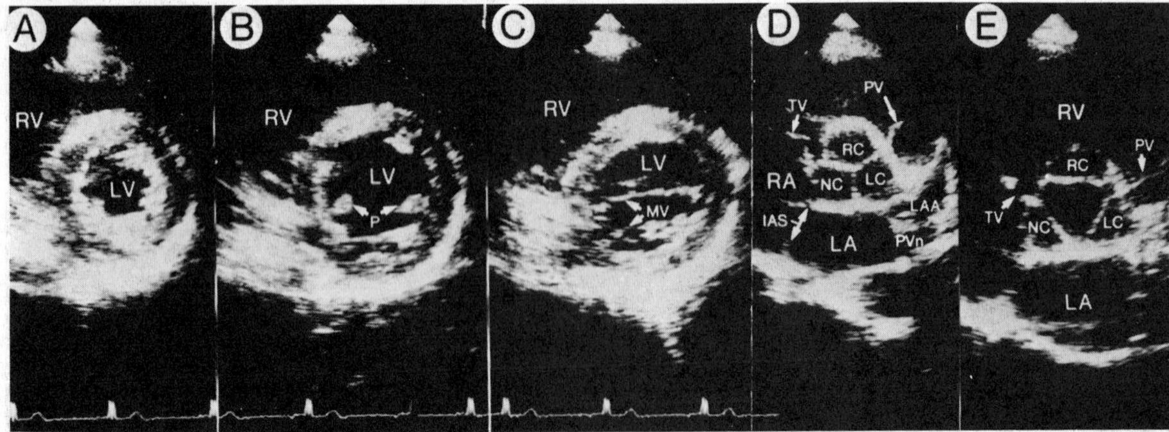

FIGURE 15-11 Two-dimensional parasternal short-axis views from a normal subject. *A.* The level of the cardiac apex shows a small, thick-walled left ventricle (LV) and only a very small portion of the right ventricle (RV). *B.* Left ventricle at the level of the papillary muscles (P). The right ventricle is larger and the left ventricular cavity is uniformly round and larger than at the apical level. *C.* Left ventricle, at the level of the partially opened mitral valve (MV), is larger than at the papillary muscle level. *D.* Diastolic frame at the base of the heart shows the closed aortic valve, with the right (RC), left (LC), and noncoronary (NC) cusps resembling the letter Y. The tricuspid (TV) and pulmonic (PV) valves are identified. *E.* Systolic frame at the same level as *D* shows the open aortic valve. IAS, interatrial septum; LA, left atrium; RA, right atrium; LAA, left atrial appendage; PVn, pulmonary vein.

atrium; the posterior (noncoronary) cusp lies between the left atrium and the tricuspid valve opposite the interatrial septum. The right ventricle appears sausage shaped in this view as it courses anteriorly around the aorta to reach the pulmonary artery. The pulmonic valve, at 2 o'clock on the aortic circle, separates the right ventricular outflow tract from the main pulmonary artery. The left atrial appendage, occasionally seen in this view, may be mistaken for a portion of the main pulmonary artery when the transducer beam is oriented so that a pulmonary vein is seen entering the left atrium. With slight medial angulation the septal and anterior tricuspid valve leaflets, at 10 o'clock on the aortic circle, form the transition between the right ventricle and the right atrium.

From the parasternal short-axis view at the base, tilting the transducer laterally toward the left shoulder identifies the pulmonary artery branches and a portion of the left main coronary artery, which originates at 4 o'clock on the aortic circle, just inferior to the pulmonic valve (Fig. 15-9). This tomographic plane affords an excellent view of the right ventricular outflow tract, pulmonic valve, main pulmonary artery, and bifurcation of right and left pulmonary arteries. Most of the left atrium is detected from this view, and portions of the tricuspid valve and right atrium are seen.

These two imaging planes at the base of the heart are best for evaluating the aortic valve, aortic root, and left atrium and are the primary views for assessing the rela-

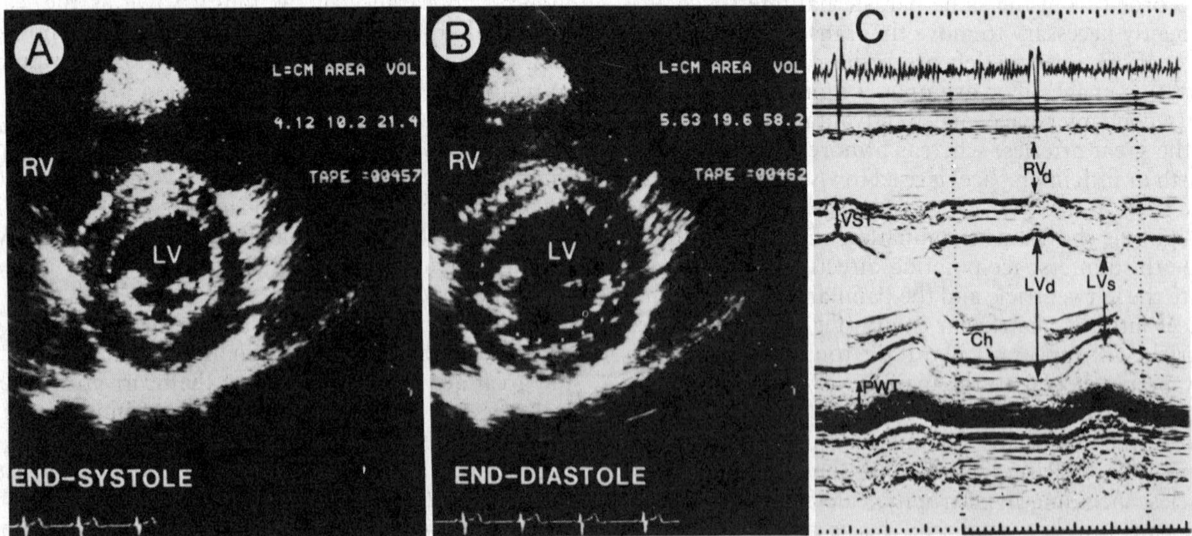

FIGURE 15-12 *A.* Two-dimensional parasternal short-axis view at end systole. *B.* Two-dimensional parasternal short-axis view at end diastole. *C.* A simultaneously obtained M-mode view of the left ventricle (LV) at the level of the chordae tendineae (Ch). The two-dimensional echograms demonstrate the method of calculating left ventricular volumes with a modern ultrasound system. The left ventricular endocardium is outlined (circular dots) permitting the on-line computer to calculate volume (VOL) shown at the upper right portion of the sector images. The ejection fraction is calculated to be 63 percent. RV, right ventricle, RV_d, right ventricle, end diastole; LV_d, left ventricle, end diastole; LV_s, left ventricle, end systole; VST, ventricular septal thickness; PWT, posterior wall thickness.

tive positions of the great vessels. In addition, the tricuspid and pulmonic valves can be analyzed and the diameter of the pulmonary artery and its branches can be determined. The origin of the coronary arteries can also be visualized.

The *apical views* are a family of planes obtained with the transducer positioned at the cardiac apex. The *apical four-chamber* view is the classic and most important of these.[23,42] To optimally obtain this view, turn the patient to a steeper left lateral position, place the transducer directly over the palpable apex impulse, and direct the beam toward the base of the heart (Fig. 15-7). The plane of the beam will be perpendicular to the septum while passing through the plane of the atrioventricular valves. The index mark is to the patient's left, so that the left ventricle is to the right and the right ventricle is to the left on the video screen.

The apical four-chamber view displays all four cardiac chambers, permits evaluation of the ventricular and atrial septa, and images the septal (medial) and anterior (lateral) leaflets of the tricuspid valve and the anterior (medial) and posterior (lateral) leaflets of the mitral valve (Figs. 15-13 and 15-14). A useful anatomic landmark is the central fibrous body (called the crux of the heart) where the interatrial and interventricular septa and atrioventricular valves meet. It appears as a high-intensity echo in the middle to posterior portion of the sector. Although side-by-side dimensions of the ventricles are obtainable, the left ventricle usually occupies more of the apical image than does the right ventricle, and the true right ventricular apex may not be imaged. The left ventricular free wall is the lateral wall and the right ventricular free wall is the anterior wall. The ventricles can be differentiated by the following: (1) the endocardial outline of the left ventricle is finer than that of the right ventricle; (2) the right ventricle has coarser trabeculations and has the moderator band near its apex; and (3) the septal tricuspid leaflet is anchored in a slightly more inferior (apical) position with reference to the anterior mitral leaflet. From this view, with slight cephalad angulation a portion of the aorta is seen at the junction formed by the interventricular septum, interatrial septum, anterior mitral leaflet, and septal tricuspid leaflet. This is then referred to as the *apical five-chamber view* (Fig. 15-14).

For total assessment of ventricular function and anatomy in patients with coronary artery disease the four-chamber view is essential.[23,43] It is the view best suited for examination of the left ventricular apex, where aneurysms and thrombi are usually located. This view is also useful for identifying the entry of the right and left inferior pulmonary veins into the left atrium and for showing the distribution of pericardial fluid. It is the best view for confirming the diagnosis of mitral valve prolapse (MVP). In patients with congenital heart disease this is also one of the most helpful views, since defects in the atrial and ventricular septa may be seen directly and the relation of the cardiac chambers to each other determined. The midportion of the interatrial septum is frequently not imaged, however, because (1) the region of the fossa ovalis is thin; (2) the sound beam is perpendicular to this portion of the septum; and (3) the distance from the transducer to this structure is great.[42]

When the transducer is rotated 90° counterclockwise from the apical four-chamber plane, the *apical long-axis view* is obtained. The plane of the beam is parallel to the

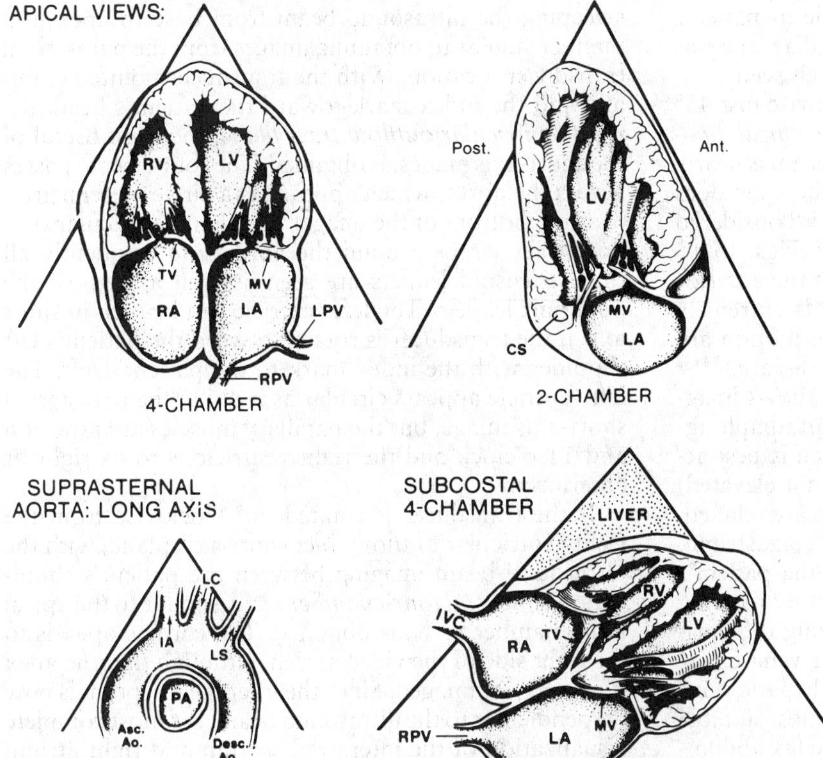

FIGURE 15-13 Anatomic drawings of some of the commonly obtained apical, suprasternal, and subcostal imaging planes oriented as they would be seen on the videoscreen. RV, right ventricle; LV, left ventricle; MV, mitral valve; RA, right atrium, LA, left atrium; LPV, left pulmonary view; RPV, right pulmonary vein; Post., posterior; Ant., anterior; CS, coronary sinus; Asc. Ao, ascending aorta; Desc. Ao. descending aorta; PA, pulmonary artery; IA, brachiocephalic artery; LC, left carotid artery; LS, left subclavian artery; IVC, inferior vena cava. *(From DJ Sahn: F. Anderson: Two-Dimensional Anatomy of the Heat: An Atlas for Echocardiographers. Copyright © 1982 John Wiley & Sons, New York. Adapted and reproduced with permission from John Wiley & Sons and the authors.)*

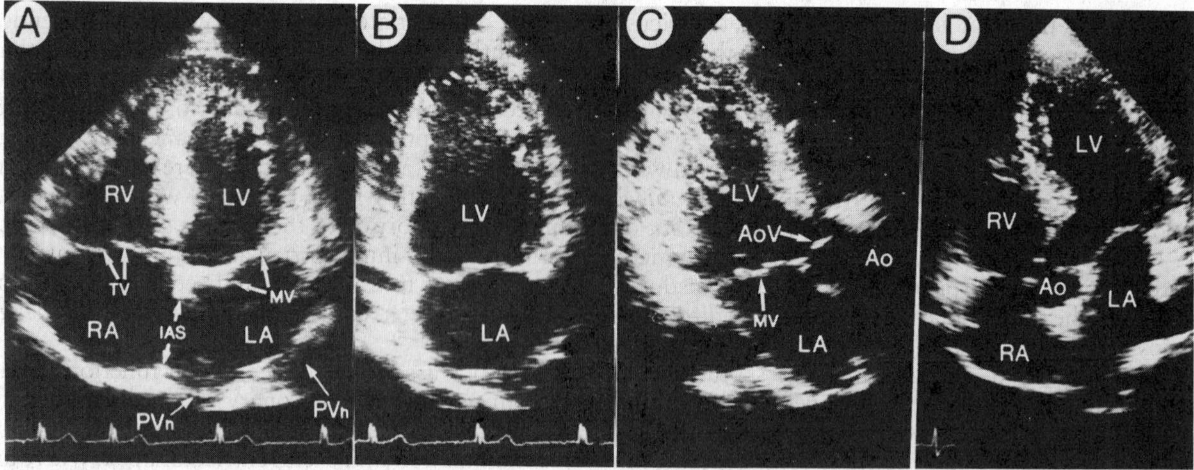

FIGURE 15-14 Family of two-dimensional apical views from a normal subject. *A.* Systolic frame of the four-chamber view shows the relations of the cardiac chambers, atrioventricular valves, and the interatrial and interventricular septa to each other. Note that the insertion of the tricuspid valve (TV) is inferior (more apical) to that of the mitral valve (MV) and that the common problem of partial drop-out of the midportion of the interatrial septum (IAS) is apparent. The entry of the pulmonary veins (PVn) into the left atrium (LA) is clearly seen. *B.* Systolic frame of the two-chamber view shows the left ventricle and left atrium with the closed mitral valve. *C.* Systolic frame of the long-axis view shows the aortic valve (AoV) and the proximal portion of the ascending aorta (Ao). The anterolateral and posteromedial walls of the left ventricle (LV) and the left atrium are also seen. The posteromedial papillary muscle, arising near the apex, may be seen in this view. *D.* Five-chamber view includes a portion of the aorta (Ao) seen at the junction formed by the cardiac septa and atrioventricular valves as well as the right (RA) and left atria and right (RV) and left ventricles.

ventricular septum and left ventricle, and therefore, the left atrium, left ventricular outflow tract, aortic valve, and proximal portion of the ascending aorta are imaged (Figs. 15-7 and 15-14). This view approximates the left ventricular silhouette seen on the right anterior oblique ventriculogram. In addition, it is quite similar to the image of the left ventricle in the parasternal long-axis view and may be an adequate substitute if a parasternal long-axis view is unobtainable. This view is particularly useful for examination of the left ventricle in patients with ischemic heart disease, since the cardiac apex as well as the septum and lateral walls are well seen.

If the transducer is rotated counterclockwise just 45° from the apical four-chamber image, the *apical two-chamber view* is obtained. The ultrasound beam is nearly parallel to the septum in this plane, but the view does not include the aorta or right ventricle and is considered to be a variant of the apical long-axis view (Figs. 15-13 and 15-14). Since this plane passes through the anterior and posterior left ventricular walls, it too is extremely useful for the evaluation of segmental wall motion abnormalities in patients with ischemic heart disease.[23,40,42]

The *subcostal* or *subxyphoid approach* allows imaging of the heart, great vessels, and several infradiaphragmatic structures (Fig. 15-15). This approach is best accomplished with the patient supine (head not elevated) with knees flexed so the abdominal muscles are relaxed. The transducer is placed in the upper epigastrium, pressed firmly back, and directed toward the patient's head with a little posterior and leftward tilt. By rotating the transducer inferiorly and rightward along the horizontal plane, one can visualize the inferior vena cava–right atrial junction and the drainage of the hepatic veins into the inferior vena cava (Fig. 15-15). The most suitable patient is thin, with a scaphoid abdomen and lax abdominal wall. This location provides a higher diagnostic yield in patients with chronic pulmonary disease because hyperinflation of the lungs and a low diaphragm usually preclude examination of the precordial and apical windows. Pulmonary emphysema may actually facilitate subcostal echocardiography by lowering the diaphragm, thereby bringing the heart closer to the transducer.

The subcostal approach allows images to be recorded from both short-axis and four-chamber planes (Fig. 15-15). A series of short-axis views can be recorded by sweeping the ultrasound beam from base to apex in a manner similar to obtaining images from the parasternal transducer location. With the transducer pointed cranially and the index mark toward the patient's head, the *right ventricular outflow tract plane,* the most useful of the short-axis planes, is obtained. The sound beam passes across the aorta, which appears as a circle or semicircle near the bottom of the image. The right ventricular outflow tract wraps around the aorta, and frequently all three tricuspid leaflets are seen as well as two of the pulmonic leaflets. The left ventricle can be seen in short axis if the transducer is rotated toward the patient's left shoulder with the index mark to the patient's left. The left ventricle appears circular as it did in the parasternal short-axis image, but the papillary muscles are now at 8 and 11 o'clock and the right ventricle is to its right or anteriorly.

If the transducer is rotated 90° clockwise from the right ventricular outflow tract short-axis plane, with the ultrasound beam imaging between the patient's shoulders, a *subcostal four-chamber view,* similar to the apical four-chamber view, is obtained. The cardiac apex is to the right side of the video screen, although the true apex is usually not imaged. Since the interatrial septum is now perpendicular to the ultrasound beam, the most complete visualization of the interatrial septum and right atrium is possible. The right and left superior pulmonary veins

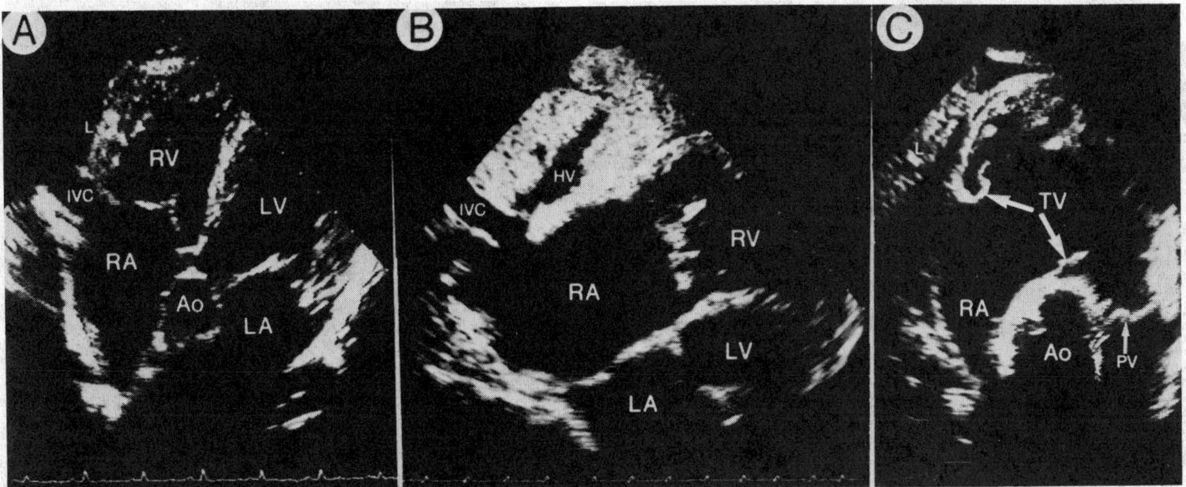

FIGURE 15-15 Two-dimensional subcostal views from a patient with chronic obstructive lung disease. The liver (L) is seen anteriorly in each frame. *A.* Five-chamber view, directed to include a portion of the inferior vena cava (IVC) at its junction with the right atrium (RA), shows the aorta (Ao) between the cardiac septa and atrioventricular valves in addition to the right and left (LA) atria and right (RV) and left (LV) ventricles. The cardiac apex is not seen in this view. *B.* Enlargement of the four-chamber view to best show the junction of the inferior vena cava (IVC) and the right atrium. The hepatic vein (HV) empties into the inferior vena cava. Complete imaging of the interatrial septum is appreciated in this view. *C.* Diastolic frame of the short-axis right ventricular outflow tract plane. The aorta (Ao) occupies the central portion of the image. Two of the open leaflets of the tricuspid valve (TV) and the closed pulmonic valve (PV) are identified. The pulmonic valve and pulmonary artery, often in the far field in this plane, may not be imaged as well as in the parasternal short-axis, but the subvalvular portion of the right ventricular outflow tract is more easily appreciated.

can be seen as they enter the left atrium; more of the left atrium is visualized in the subcostal four-chamber view than in the apical four-chamber view. The hepatic structures are usually interposed between the transducer and the right ventricular free wall anteriorly. With slight anterior angulation the aorta and left ventricular outflow tract are seen in a *subcostal five-chamber view*.

The subcostal view is most useful for evaluating the right ventricular free wall and the inferior vena cava and for the diagnosis of tricuspid regurgitation and atrial and ventricular septal defects. Positioning the right ventricular wall perpendicular to the M-mode cursor in the four-chamber view makes possible accurate recordings of right ventricular wall thickness. Since the ultrasonic beam is now perpendicular to the atrial septum, the entire length of the septum can be scanned for the presence and location of atrial septal defects.[44,45] It is also important to record the inferior vena cava in both four-chamber and short-axis views in order to assess its diameter and observe respiratory effects.[40,42] A special utility of this examining plane occurs in patients with a left pleural effusion, which complicates the ultrasonic diagnosis when the heart is viewed from the standard precordial positions.

The *suprasternal notch approach* visualizes mediastinal structures posterior to the sternum, including the ascending aorta, aortic arch, origin of the brachiocephalic vessels, and descending thoracic aorta (Fig. 15-13). Tomographic imaging from this transducer position, however, is more difficult than it is from any of the other locations. Therefore, make the patient as comfortable as possible by placing a pillow underneath the shoulders and upper back. This will extend the neck and facilitate manipulation of the transducer, which should be pressed firmly back in the groove just above the manubrium-sternum and clavicles (Fig. 15-8).

The *suprasternal long-axis view* images the ascending aorta, the transverse aorta with the origins of the major arterial branches (brachiocephalic innominate, left carotid, and left subclavian), and the descending aorta (Fig. 15-16). Proper transducer orientation with the index mark cephalad places the descending aorta on the right of the video screen. Posterior to the aortic arch, the right pulmonary artery is seen as a circle in short axis. The mainstem bronchus, being air filled, is a densely reflective structure between the aorta and the pulmonary artery. The left atrium is recorded posterior to the pulmonary artery. When the transducer is rotated 90° from this plane, the ascending aorta is seen in this *suprasternal short-axis view* as a circular, pulsating structure anteriorly, while the right pulmonary artery is imaged inferiorly in its long axis (Fig. 15-16). The superior vena cava–right atrial junction may be seen with slight anterior angulation. The right supraclavicular approach is an alternative plane that provides a view much like the suprasternal one (Fig. 15-16). It is used mainly for visualizing the motion of prosthetic aortic valves, particularly the Starr-Edwards ball valve, which is not well imaged from the precordium.

Echocardiographic examination from the suprasternal notch facilitates detection of aortic root abnormalities (e.g., saccular aneurysm, dissecting aneurysm, and coarctation), whereas elevation of the pulmonary artery and its branches may detect a patent ductus arteriosus.[33,40,42,46]

Two-Dimensional Echocardiographic Measurements

Two-dimensional echocardiographic measurements should be made using the leading-edge method.[47,48] Values for diastolic and systolic left ventricular diameters, systolic left atrial diameters, fractional shortening of the

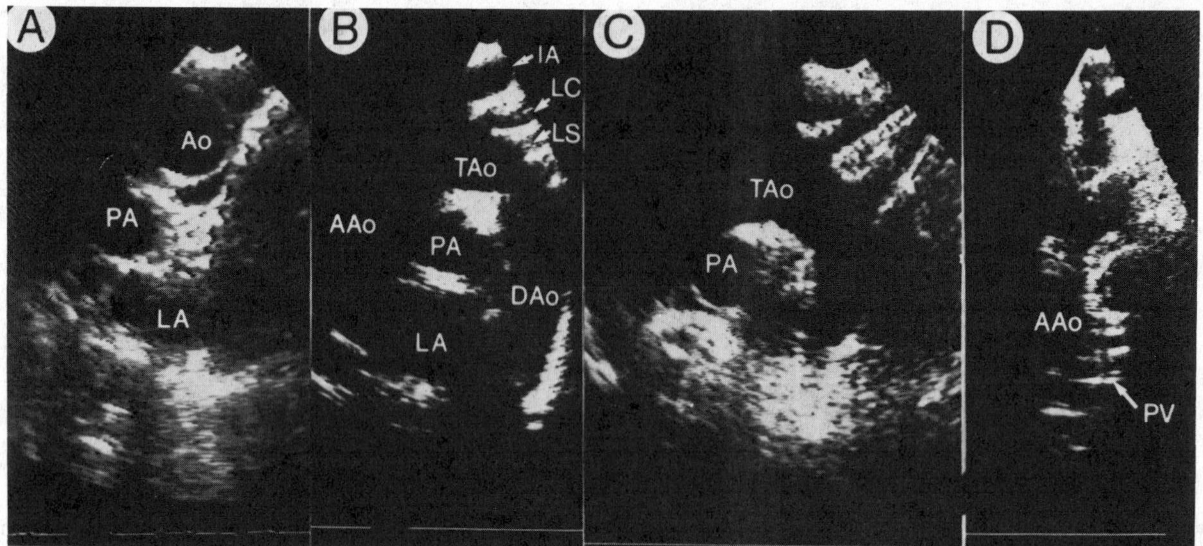

FIGURE 15-16 Two-dimensional suprasternal views of the great vessels from a normal subject. *A.* Short-axis plane shows the circular appearance of the transverse aorta (Ao). A portion of the long axis of the pulmonary artery (PA) is imaged beneath the aorta with the left atrium (LA) posterior to the pulmonary artery. In this view, with more medial angulation, the left and right brachiocephalic (innominate) veins may be seen entering the superior vena cava. *B.* Long-axis plane shows the ascending (AAo), transverse (TAo), and descending (DAo) aorta and the pulmonary artery, which appears to be circular because it is now seen in short-axis view. Arch vessels emerging from the transverse aorta are identified as the brachiocephalic (innominate) (IA), left common carotid (LC), and left subclavian (LS) arteries. *C.* Enlargement of view *B* to more clearly show the transverse aorta and arch vessels. *D.* Right supraclavicular transducer position enables one to rotate the imaging plane more anteriorly in order to image more of the ascending aorta and show its relation with the pulmonary artery and pulmonic valve (PV).

left ventricle, and left ventricular posterior and septal wall thicknesses are similar to those obtained with M-mode echocardiography.[40,47,48] The accepted echocardiographic views and locations for common two-dimensional measurements are shown in Fig. 15-17. Normal two-dimensional measurements for various intracardiac chambers and great vessels have been determined by several clinicians; a compilation of their findings is shown in Table 15-2.

The dimensions of the left ventricle and the thicknesses of both the interventricular septum and posterior wall are made at the level of the chordae tendineae in either the parasternal long-axis or short-axis views. The papillary muscles should not be included in assessment of wall thickness. Although M-mode echocardiography appears to be very sensitive for detection of true anatomic hypertrophy,[49] two-dimensional echocardiography is superior for quantitative assessment of left ventricular mass.[50] The shape and dimension of the left atrium varies in each tomographic view. The inferior-superior dimension is slightly greater than the anterior-posterior dimension in both the apical four-chamber and apical long-axis views.[40] The right ventricular and right atrial chambers are best evaluated from the apical four-chamber view.[51] The thickness of the right ventricular wall, however, is best determined from the subcostal four-chamber view by directing the M-mode cursor perpendicular to the right ventricular free wall.[52]

M-mode echocardiography has been useful for determining left ventricular volumes in patients with nonsegmental disease and has been easily quantitated, since it involves only making measurements on a strip-chart recording.[53–55] It is limited, however, since it is not spatially correct and has not been reliable in the presence of asynergy.[56,57] In addition, several assumptions must apply when M-mode dimensions are used to calculate left ventricular volumes: (1) the left ventricle approximates a prolate ellipse; (2) the major (long) axis of the left ventricle is twice the length of the minor (short) axis; and (3) the left ventricular wall motion sampled by the ultrasound beam is representative of the entire left ventricular chamber.[21] The reliability of quantitative two-dimensional echocardiography has been documented for both segmental and nonsegmental diseases. It thus appears superior to M-mode echocardiography for quantitative estimation of left ventricular volumes, because it directly measures all three hemiaxes, by imaging from apical as well as parasternal windows.[58–62]

Left ventricular volumes and left atrial volumes have been determined by two-dimensional echocardiography in a normal adult population and validated by angiography, radionuclide studies, and pathological measurements.[63–65] There are several ways of calculating left ventricular volumes, including the biplane area–length method, the single-plane ellipse method, and the modified Simpson rule.[40,48,62] The modified Simpson rule, originally developed for biplane angiography, appears to be a very reliable method, since it makes no assumptions about the geometry of the ventricles and is relatively unaffected by segmental wall motion abnormalities.[40,48,62] This method divides the left ventricle into slices of known thickness, and the volume of the left ventricle is then equal to the sum of the volumes of this series of slices. The major limitation of the Simpson rule method is the complexity of the calculations; therefore, computer assistance is necessary. There are several two-dimensional adaptations of Simpson's rule requiring different tomographic sections, including (1) apical four-chamber view

INTRACARDIAC DIMENSIONS

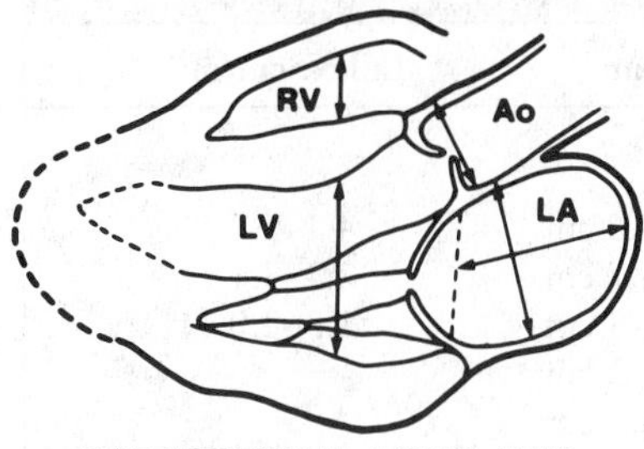

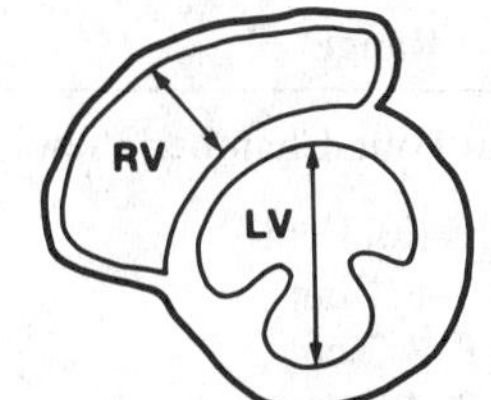

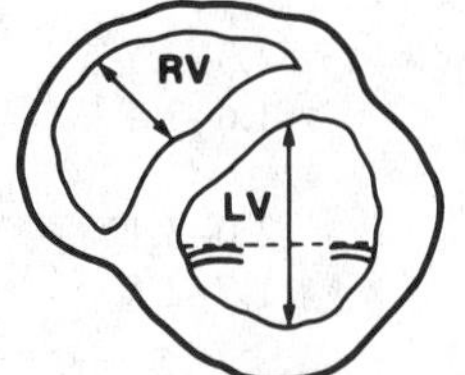

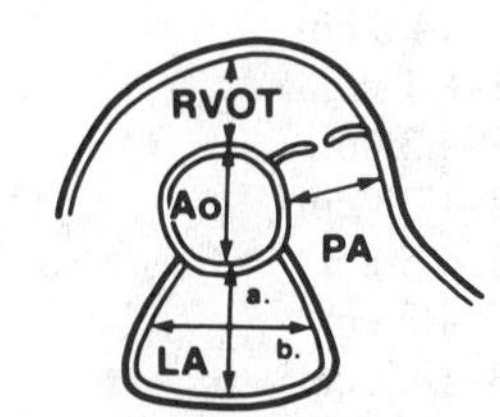

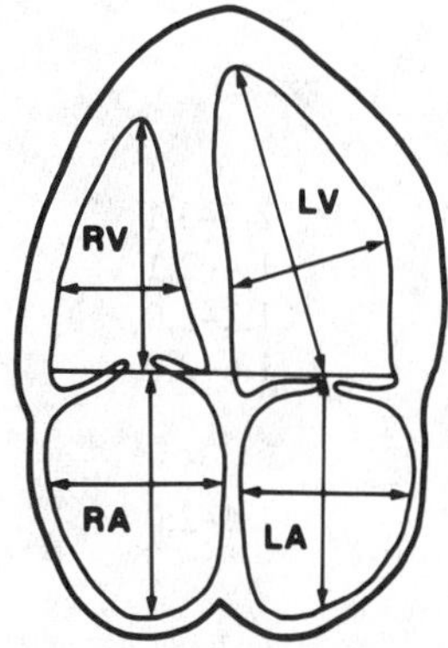

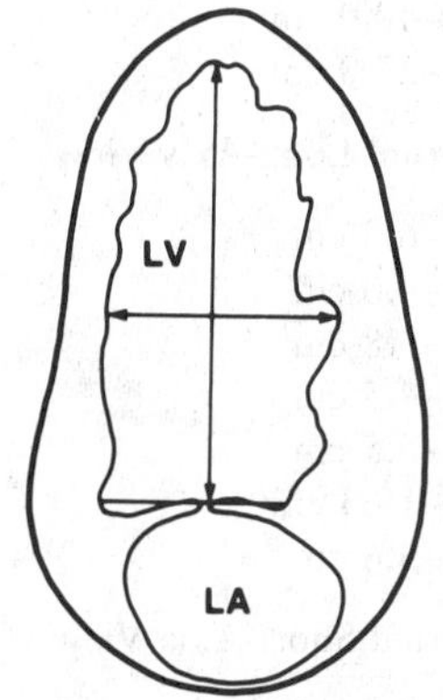

FIGURE 15-17 Some of the two-dimensional echocardiographic planes and locations for determining intracardiac dimensions. The left atrium (LA) is measured in both the anteroposterior (a) and inferolateral (b) dimensions, perpendicular to each other, from the parasternal long-axis, short-axis, and apical four-chamber views (as illustrated in the parasternal short-axis view). The right atrium (RA) is measured in the apical four-chamber view and also in the parasternal long-axis right ventricular inflow tract view, which is not shown. The major axis of each ventricle is measured in the four-chamber view from the atrioventricular plane to the apical endocardium. The left ventricular major axis is also measured in the two-chamber view. The minor axis of each ventricle is taken perpendicular to its major axis. This measurement may be taken at two-thirds of the length of the major axis (from the apical endocardium), as shown in the four-chamber view, or at the midpoint of the major axis, as shown in the two-chamber view. RV, right ventricle; LV, left ventricle; RVOT, right ventricular outflow tract; Ao, aorta; PA, pulmonary artery. (*From AE Weyman: Cross-Sectional Echocardiography. Philadelphia, Lea & Febiger, 1982, and I Schnittger, EP Gordon, PJ Fitzgerald, et al: Standardized intracardiac measurements of two-dimensional echocardiography. J Am Coll Cardiol 2:934, 1983. Drawn after studying multiple sources. Reproduced with permission from the publishers and authors.*)

and parasternal short-axis views at mitral and papillary muscle levels,[64] (2) apical four- and two-chamber views,[65] and (3) apical two-chamber view and parasternal short-axis view at the papillary muscle level.[62] The single apical plane analysis of Silverman et al. is especially useful when technical difficulties prevent adequate orthogonal long-axis views required by the Simpson rule algorithm.[63] Although there seems to be a consistent underestimation of left ventricular volumes using two-dimensional echocardiography as compared with volumes determined by angiography, these measurements have proved reliable when tested by interobserver and intraobserver methods.[62] Ejection fraction, however, correlates well with cineangiographic data, since two-dimensional echocardiography underestimates end-diastolic volume and end-systolic volume equally.[66,67] The Simpson rule method also permits accurate estimation of left ventricular mass. *Mass* is calculated as the product of the specific gravity of myocardium (1.05) and myocardial volume (i.e., the difference between total ventricular and intracavitary volumes).[68]

The determination of right ventricular volume is more difficult than that of left ventricular volume.[69] The left ventricle resembles a prolate ellipse (a convenient volumetric model), and the right ventricle has a complex shape, defying geometric description. The problem is compounded by irregular trabeculations, a separate infundibulum, and variations in shape with physiological conditions (e.g., respiration).

ADDITIONAL ECHOCARDIOGRAPHIC TECHNIQUES

Echophonocardiography

Echophonocardiography is the simultaneous recording of echocardiograms, usually M-mode data, and heart sounds on multichannel recorders.[70] Together with pulse tracings, the combination of echocardiography and phonocardiography increases the information available above that from both tests performed separately. Precise

TABLE 15-2
Cardiac Dimensions by Two-Dimensional Echocardiography

Cardiac Feature	Range	Mean	Index, cm/m^2
	Apical Four-Chamber View		
LV_a major	6.9–10.3 cm	8.6 cm	4.1–5.7
LV_d minor	3.3–6.1 cm	4.7 cm	2.2–3.1
LV_s minor	1.9–3.7 cm	2.8 cm	1.3–2.0
LV_d area	21.2–40.2 cm^2	31.2 cm^2	
LV_s area	8.0–21.1 cm^2	14.2 cm^2	
RV major	6.5–9.5 cm	8.0 cm	3.8–5.3
RV minor	2.2–4.4 cm	3.3–3.5 cm	1.0–2.8
RV_d area	12.0–22.2 cm^2	18.6–2.1 cm^2	
RV_s area	5.4–14.6 cm^2	9.9 cm^2	
LA major	4.1–6.1 cm	5.1 cm	2.3–3.5
LA minor	2.8–4.3 cm	3.5 cm	1.6–2.4
LA area	10.2–17.8 cm	14.7 cm^2	
RA major (inf-sup)	3.5–5.5 cm	4.3–4.5 cm	2.0–3.1
RA minor	2.5–4.9 cm	3.7 cm	1.7–2.5
RA area	11.3–16.7 cm^2	13.8–14 cm^2	
	Apical Two-Chamber View		
LV_d major	6.8–9.4 cm	8.0 cm^2	
LV_d minor	3.8–5.7 cm	4.6 cm^2	
LV_d area	19.4–48.0 cm^2	35.6 cm^2	
LV_s	8.9–27.0 cm	14.3 cm^2	
	Parasternal Long-Axis View		
LV_d	3.5–6.0 cm	4.8 cm	2.3–3.1
LV_s	2.1–4.0 cm	3.1 cm	1.4–2.1
RV	1.9–3.8 cm	2.8 cm	1.2–2.0
LA (A-P)	2.7–4.5 cm	3.6 cm	1.6–2.4
LA (S-I)	3.1–5.5 cm	4.4 cm	
LA area	9.0–19.3 cm^2	13.8 cm^2	
Ao	2.2–3.6 cm	2.9 cm	1.4–2.0
	Parasternal Short-Axis View		
Ao	2.3–3.7 cm	3.0–2.3 cm	1.6–2.4
RVOT	1.9–2.2 cm	2.7 cm	
RA	1.5–2.5 cm	1.9–2.2 cm	
LA	2.6–4.5 cm	3.6 cm	1.6–2.4
LA area	7.2–13.0 cm^2	10.8 cm^2	
LV_d (PM level)	3.5–5.8 cm	4.7 cm	2.2–3.1
LV_s (PM level)	2.2–4.0 cm	3.1 cm	1.4–2.2
LV_d area (PM level)	16.0–31.2 cm^2	22.2 cm^2	
LV_s area (PM level)	5.2–13.4 cm^2	8.5 cm^2	
LV_d (Ch. level)	3.5–6.2	4.8 cm	2.3–3.2
LV_s (Ch. level)	2.3–4.0 cm	3.2 cm	1.5–2.2
LV_d area (Ch. level)	16.4–32.3 cm^2	22.5 cm^2	
LV_s area (Ch. level)	6.1–16.8	10.7 cm^2	
	Subcostal View		
IVC diameter		1.8 cm	

SOURCE: The values shown in this table represent a compilation of data from three sources: I Schnittinger, EP Gordon, PJ Fitzgerald, et al: Standardized intracardiac measurements of two-dimensional echocardiography. *J Am Coll Cardiol* 5:934, 1983; M Triulzi, A Weyman: Normal cross-sectional measurements in adults. In: A Weyman (ed): *Echocardiography*. Philadelphia, Lea & Febiger, 1982: 497; AD Hagan, TG DiSessa, CM Bloor, et al: *Two-Dimensional Echocardiography: Clinical-Pathological Correlations in Adult and Congenital Heart Disease*. Boston, Little, Brown and Company, 1983: 553.

LV, left ventricle; LV_d, left ventricle, end diastole; LV_s, left ventricle, end systole; RV, right ventricle; RV_d, right ventricle, end diastole; RV_s, right ventricle, end systole; LA, left atrium; RA, right atrium; AO, aorta; RVOT, right ventricular outflow tract; PA, pulmonary artery; IVC, inferior vena cava.

timing of heart sounds and movements of cardiac structures with those heart sounds is possible through this combined technique. Research into the origin and significance of heart sounds and murmurs has been greatly advanced with this procedure. Clinically, it has greatly improved the noninvasive evaluation of prosthetic heart valves[71] and has proved useful in identifying the site of origin of systolic honks and murmurs.[72]

Systolic time intervals (STIs) can be derived from the M-mode echocardiogram.[21,73] Left-side STIs can be determined from either the aortic valve echocardiogram or a combination of the ECG, phonocardiogram, and carotid pulse tracing. Commonly determined intervals include the left ventricular ejection time and the preejection period. Right-side STIs can be derived only by imaging the pulmonic valve.[74]

Contrast Echocardiography

Contrast echocardiography has played an important role in the development of cardiac ultrasound. Initially, it was used to validate various structures by M-mode echocardiography.[75,76] More recently, contrast methods have been used with two-dimensional echocardiography to delineate structures not readily seen by M-mode examination (e.g., the superior and inferior venae cavae,[77] descending aorta, and coronary arteries[78]) as well as to evaluate intracardiac shunts,[79] regurgitant lesions,[80] and complex congenital heart problems.[81,82]

The contrast substance that has been used clinically consists of the microbubbles that occur with the injection of fluid into the intravascular system.[21,22] Almost any liquid contains expended microbubbles and will produce a contrast effect when injected. The addition of small amounts of gas to the liquid prior to injection will provide a maximal contrast effect. The contrast agents used most frequently are normal saline solution and indocyanine green dye. The latter substance has a very low surface tension, so that small bubbles stay suspended longer. Virtually any peripheral venous injection, even the handling of closed intravenous lines, will produce some echocardiographic contrast effect.[83] As the time from injection increases and the gases are gradually absorbed into the blood, the contrast effect diminishes. It further dwindles as the gas is absorbed during passage through the pulmonary and systemic capillary system, which acts as filters. The diameter of the pulmonary capillary bed is so small that contrast microbubbles capable of traversing this bed will dissolve owing to surface tension effects.[84] Therefore, contrast substance is not seen in the left side of the heart of normal subjects following the intravenous injections of fluids.

The actual performance of contrast echocardiography in the clinical setting is quite simple, and it can be employed either at the patient's bedside or in the echocardiographic laboratory. We use a three-way stop-cock attached to a scalp-vein intravenous line with two 10-mL syringes, each filled with 6 to 8 mL of saline solution, attached to the open ports of the stopcock. The saline solution becomes cloudy in appearance when vigorously injected back and forth between the two syringes, indicating that the amount of suspended air to be delivered is adequate. Then 6 mL of fluid from one syringe is injected rapidly and with extreme force into the vein. This procedure consistently produces an optimal contrast effect but obviously requires two individuals—one to perform the echocardiogram and the second to inject the bolus of fluid.

After the injection of saline solution and visualization of a satisfactory contrast effect, another contrast effect can often be obtained by raising the patient's arm over his or her head and then massaging the inner aspect of the upper arm toward the central circulation. This second contrast bolus, almost equal in intensity to the first, presumably is due to the release of residual contrast substance within the peripheral venous circulation. Echocardiographic contrast studies are best recorded during held respiration, although basic flow changes during respiration sometimes yield interesting physiological information. The Valsalva maneuver should be performed in patients suspected of having a small atrial septal defect or patent foramen ovale, since a momentary right-to-left shunt may be produced during the release phase.[84]

The widest use of contrast echocardiography is in the evaluation of blood flow patterns, specifically the demonstration of intracardiac shunting and valvular regurgitation. Once injected, echocardiographic contrast microbubbles flow with the blood and surface in markers that are easily imaged. Since these microbubbles do not pass through the lungs, the appearance of contrast echoes in a chamber of the left side of the heart following a peripheral venous injection confirms the presence of an abnormal right-to-left shunt. Two-dimensional echocardiography, however, must be used for accurate identification of the defect, because the precise site of a shunt cannot be visualized on the M-mode echocardiogram. The optimal imaging planes include the apical or subcostal four-chamber views, because either enables one to image the atria, ventricles, and interatrial and interventricular septa simultaneously. This has permitted the detection of even small numbers of microbubbles crossing a right-to-left shunt (Fig. 15-18).[85]

Most clinicians have found that contrast echocardiography is extremely sensitive and specific for evaluating patients with right-to-left shunts, since the diagnosis is confirmed if only a few microbubbles of the millions injected cross the defect.[79] Contrast echocardiography appears to be more sensitive than oximetry and at least as sensitive as dye dilution techniques in the detection of right-to-left shunts as small as 3 percent at the atrial, ventricular, or aortic levels. It is thus often sufficiently sensitive to disclose small right-to-left shunts in patients with a patent foramen ovale or surgically repaired atrial septal defects when other techniques show no such abnormalities.[85] When a large right-to-left shunt is suspected, it is best to limit the number of injections of contrast substance given. While undue effects of contrast substance administration are very rare, there are a few reported instances of central nervous system symptoms that have occurred in the setting of a large right-to-left shunt. In all cases, signs and symptoms were reversible.[86]

In addition to disclosing right-to-left shunts, contrast echocardiography can be extremely useful in demonstrating predominately left-to-right shunts using periph-

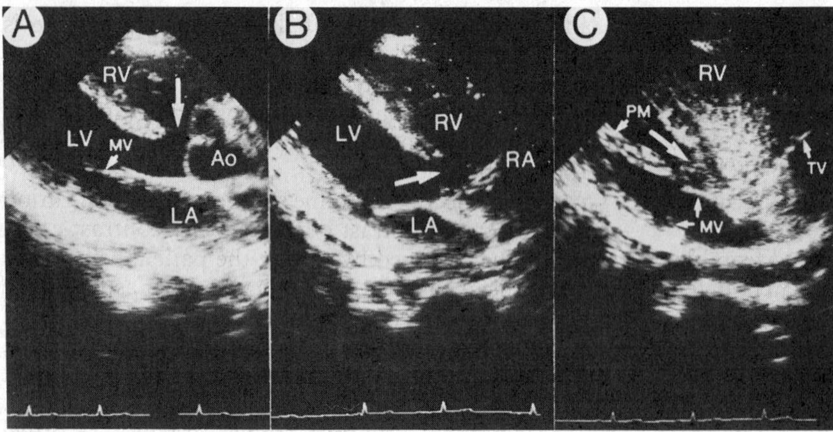

FIGURE 15-18 Two-dimensional echocardiogram from a patient with tetralogy of Fallot. *A.* Parasternal long-axis view demonstrates the aorta (Ao) overriding a large ventricular septal defect (arrow). *B.* Precordial four-chamber view shows the large ventricular septal defect (arrow). *C.* Same as view *B,* obtained during injection of aerated saline into an arm vein. Microbubbles, acting as contrast substance, virtually occlude the right atrium and right ventricle (RV), cross the ventricular septal defect (arrow), and enter the left ventricle (LV), MV, mitral valve; RA, right atrium; LA, left atrium; TV, tricuspid valve; PM, papillary muscle.

eral venous injections. It has been found that the majority of patients with predominately left-to-right shunts through an atrial septal defect also have small, transient right-to-left shunts. These transient right-to-left shunts can often be evoked by having the patient perform the Valsalva and/or Müller maneuvers, which alter intrathoracic and cardiac pressures sufficiently to cause some blood, and therefore contrast substance, to cross an atrial septal defect in a right-to-left direction.[84] In addition, a number of reports have demonstrated a *negative contrast effect* that is seen exclusively in patients with left-to-right shunts.[87] For example, if a left-to-right shunt exists at the atrial level, nonopacified blood from the left atrium will wash contrast microbubbles away from the interatrial area, yielding a contrast-free area or negative contrast effect.

Contrast echocardiography has proved to be of diagnostic value in the recognition of valvular regurgitation. From a noninvasive standpoint, the tricuspid valve is the only structure that can be conveniently assessed by this technique. When the inferior vena cava is imaged from the subcostal view in patients with a significant degree of tricuspid regurgitation, contrast substance may be observed to reflux into this vessel from the right atrium during systole following installation of the injectate into a peripheral vein.[88] The persistent reflux of large amounts of contrast substance into the inferior vena cava represents an accurate indication of tricuspid regurgitation, especially if the bubbles are seen to pass into the hepatic vein (Fig. 15-19).[80] This is an excellent technique for diagnosis of tricuspid regurgitation, despite the fact that transient, minor reflux of a few microbubbles into the inferior vena cava during atrial contraction may be observed in normal subjects. Analysis of the moment of appearance of the contrast substance bolus in the inferior vena cava, after an upper extremity vein injection, also aids in the diagnosis or exclusion of tricuspid regurgitation. If contrast microbubbles appear in the inferior vena cava in synchrony with the V wave of the atrial pressure curve, the diagnosis of tricuspid regurgitation can be made with a great degree of accuracy. Two-dimensional echocardiography has been used in this instance but may lead to a false-positive diagnosis because the timing of the appearance of contrast substance is less accurate than it is with M-mode recordings. Analysis of contrast echocardiograms should, therefore, include timing of appearance, pattern of opacification, duration of opacification (clearance time), intensity of contrast, and negative contrast effects.[89]

Doppler ultrasound has supplanted contrast echocardiography for the diagnosis of tricuspid regurgitation and shunt lesions. Development in contrast echocardiography, however, that will ensure its role in diagnosis include (1) quantitation of the contrast effect with specifically designed contrast agents whose gas content and size are controlled[90]; (2) specialized microbubbles capable of transit through the pulmonary vascular bed and thereby capable of opacification of the left side of the heart[91]; and (3) direct intracoronary injection of various contrast agents, including renograffin, peroxide, and sonicated albumin to delineate the coronary perfusion territory of individual coronary arteries. These injections result in formation of microbubbles and marked increase in myocardial brightness by echocardiography, which may determine the area at risk in coronary-prone patients.[92,93]

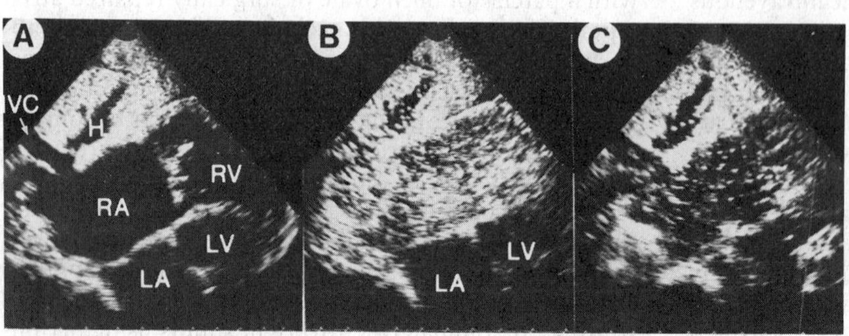

FIGURE 15-19 Two-dimensional subcostal four-chamber views, angled to show the junction between the inferior vena cava (IVC) and the right atrium (RA), the hepatic vein (H), and the right ventricle (RV), from a patient with severe tricuspid regurgitation. *A.* Prior to a peripheral intravenous injection of aerated saline solution. *B.* During the injection, microbubbles, acting as contrast substance, virtually occlude the inferior vena cava, hepatic vein, right atrium, and right ventricle. *C.* More than 30 s after the injection, microbubbles are still present in the hepatic vein, inferior vena cava, and right atrium. LA, left atrium; LV, left ventricle.

Exercise Echocardiography (See Chap. 132)

Supine (bicycle) or upright (treadmill) exercise has been used in conjunction with echocardiography during or immediately after the stress. The application of ultrasound to the study of exercise left ventricular dynamics was begun in the early 1970s.[94] In the 1980s exercise two-dimensional echocardiography assumed a clinical role in the evaluation and management of patients with ischemic disease, since it can (1) analyze both ventricles,[95] (2) accurately detect regional wall motion abnormalities, (3) determine the extent of regional myocardial thickening, and (4) measure global ejection fraction.[96,97]

The success in obtaining images of diagnostic quality with exercise two-dimensional echocardiography ranges between 71 and 100 percent but has depended on the modality of exercise, the position of the patient, the cardiac windows utilized, and the experience of the operator. Since ischemic regional wall motion abnormalities persist for several minutes following cessation of treadmill exercise, and since the left ventricle is adequately visualized in the first 30 to 60 s after exercise, echocardiography immediately after exercise gives excellent images because it avoids the technical problems of chest wall motion and hyperventilation.[95-100] If multiple left ventricular views are obtained in the first 5 min after exercise, success ranges from 85 to 100 percent. The apical window, with use of the four-chamber and two-chamber views, appears to be the best transducer position,[98,99] although the subcostal four-chamber view may also be useful.[100] The sensitivity of echocardiography is influenced by the prevalence of the disease as well as the population studied. However, its sensitivity varies between 66 and 93 percent with a specificity ranging between 69 and 100 percent.[95-99]

Contrast of exercise two-dimensional echocardiography with stress electrocardiography has been very successful. The addition of stress echo to an exercise ECG had led to a much higher degree of accuracy in diagnosis of coronary artery disease. Exercise echocardiography has proven to be a more accurate test than radionuclide multigated ventriculography in evaluating the ejection fraction response to exercise. Limited studies have compared exercise echocardiography to thallium scintigraphy, especially single-photon emission computed tomography (SPECT) thallium scintigraphy, but those studies have shown similar sensitivities and specificities.[95,100] Two-dimensional echocardiographic advantages over nuclide angiography include the following: (1) Analysis of beat-to-beat images of many cardiac cycles from multiple views gives inherently better resolution; (2) some areas of the heart are examined better with echocardiography than with radionuclide angiography; (3) there is a cost saving because two-dimensional echocardiography is less expensive than nuclear studies; (4) with echocardiography there is no need for intravenous injections or radiation hazard; (5) results are immediate, i.e., there is no time delay; and (6) two-dimensional echocardiography as well as Doppler echocardiography can easily be added to routine treadmill testing. The major limitation of two-dimensional echocardiography is the need for extensive observer interaction for reproducibility of measurements and observations. The interpretation of exercise echocardiograms has become simplified with the use of digital echocardiography and computer-assisted methods for image enhancement and endocardial border recognition. By digitalizing the echocardiographic recordings, individual cardiac cycles can be placed in a continuous (cine-) loop that virtually eliminates respiratory artifacts and permits rest and exercise recordings to be placed side by side for detailed comparison of wall motion.[101]

Pharmacologic and Physiological Interventions

Recent investigation has shown that pharmacologic stress echo may be extremely useful and as accurate as radionuclide pharmacologic stress testing. Dipyridamole echocardiography has been reported to have an overall specificity higher than that of exercise stress test (100 vs. 71 percent) and a similar overall sensitivity (74 vs. 69 percent).[97] Its reproducibility, however, has been somewhat questioned by multiple investigators. Recently, dobutamine stress echo has been used as well as adenosine stress echocardiography. The former appears quite promising in its diagnostic accuracy as well as safety.[13,14,102,103]

Pharmacologic and physiological interventions can influence left ventricular performance and valve motion while a patient is being monitored echocardiographically. Amyl nitrite can provoke systolic anterior motion of the mitral valve in patients with hypertrophic cardiomyopathy and systolic posterior motion of the mitral valve in patients with MVP.[104,105]

The Valsalva maneuver (forced expiration against a closed glottis) may help demonstrate the patency of the foramen ovale or detect a small atrial septal defect.[106]

Invasive Echocardiography

Although echocardiography is primarily a noninvasive technique, it has been used in a variety of invasive procedures, including (1) contrast echocardiography requiring an intravenous injection, (2) intracardiac echocardiography, (3) transesophageal echocardiography, and (4) intraoperative (epicardial) echocardiography, performed directly on the surface of the heart. (See Chap. 131.)

Contrast echocardiography has been used in the catheterization laboratory by injecting saline solution or indocyanine green through an intracardiac catheter with simultaneous echocardiography. Its major advantage is to obviate the need for cineangiography in young, critically ill patients, in pregnant women, in individuals allergic to iodine dye, and in patients not permitted a high osmotic load (e.g., uremic patients). Contrast echocardiography has also been used as a supplement to angiographic studies, especially in the neonate, since it helps provide a better control of the number and site of angiographic injections. When contrast medium is delivered to the left or right atrium through surgically placed pressure-monitor catheters, contrast echocardiographic studies in the postoperative period have proved useful in testing the effectiveness of surgical repair of anatomic and functional defects.[76] In many instances contrast echocardiography can be superior to standard angiography.[107]

Myocardial contrast echocardiography can assess myocardial perfusion by an in vivo technique of introducing contrast agents into the coronary circulation.[108–110] The echo texture of perfused myocardium is enhanced, while that of underperfused myocardium is unchanged. Contrast echocardiographic images can also provide an assessment of left ventricular function. These two features make this method suitable for study of ischemic heart disease.

Intracardiac echocardiography has also been used to obtain information on tissue characterization in studies in which a very high frequency two-dimensional echocardiographic transducer (10 to 40 MHz) is placed at the tip of an intracardiac catheter and the catheter is positioned against a myocardial wall.[111,112] Clear and detailed images of the coronary arteries have demonstrated atheroma, calcified plaques, and dissection after balloon angioplasty.

CLINICAL APPLICATION OF ECHOCARDIOGRAPHY

Echocardiography has numerous roles in the clinical evaluation of the patient with a cardiovascular problem and is now an integral part of the cardiovascular data base of many patients. It can definitively establish the diagnosis in a number of cardiovascular diseases (e.g., mitral stenosis and atrial myxoma) and is extremely useful in the differential diagnosis of a variety of cardiac symptoms, signs, and laboratory abnormalities including chest pain, heart murmurs, and the enlarged cardiac silhouette on chest x-ray. For instance, in patients with an enlarged cardiac silhouette on chest x-ray, echocardiography can separate those with pericardial effusion from those with true cardiomegaly, accurately identify the specific cardiac chamber enlarged, and distinguish cavitary dilatation from myocardial hypertrophy. In addition, it can aid in the therapy in several cardiac conditions (e.g., pericarditis, i.e., guided drainage of a pericardial effusion) and can provide prognostic information in the overall evaluation of a disease state (e.g., ischemic heart disease). Finally, it can be used as a screening test to exclude certain cardiovascular problems in patients with a family history of an inheritable cardiovascular disease or in competitive athletes. In order to describe accurately its many uses and indications, a thorough analysis of each application as to sensitivity, specificity, reproducibility, and quantitation would be necessary.

Two-dimensional echocardiography is the primary imaging modality because it is faster and easier to use

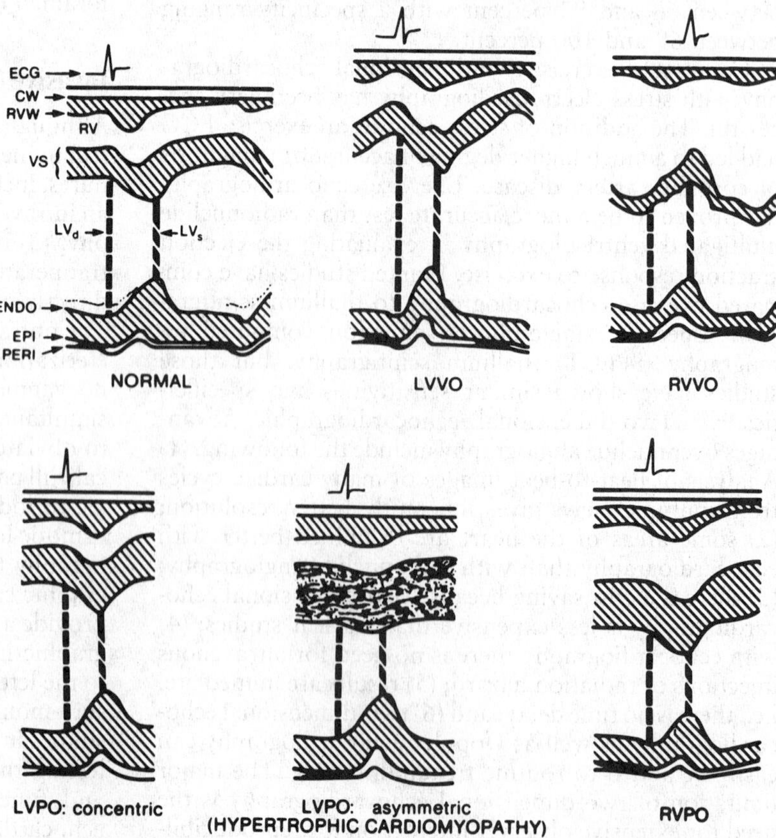

than M-mode echocardiography and is superior for most clinical applications. Since it provides a more comprehensive cardiac image and accurate spatial relationships of the cardiac structures, it is especially valuable in patients with segmental disease. M-mode recordings, however, yield a more convenient and accessible permanent record, give better detail and analysis of complex valve and wall motion patterns, and are more suitable for measuring cardiac chamber dimensions, wall thicknesses, and the slopes and amplitudes of the valve leaflets and myocardial walls. M-mode echocardiography also facilitates analysis of time relations with other simultaneously recorded physiological variables (e.g., ECGs, heart sounds, and pulse tracings). Since an understanding of the M-mode image is still essential for echocardiographic interpretation, a series of representative diagrams is shown in Figs. 15-20 to 15-22. In a modern, well-equipped diagnostic laboratory a comprehensive echocardiographic study should utilize both M-mode and two-dimensional recordings as well as Doppler ultrasound to provide information about cardiac anatomy and physiology for optimal patient care.[113-115]

Specific Cardiac Lesions

The diagnosis of *pericardial effusion* was one of the first medical uses for echocardiography,[5] and this technique is now considered the method of choice in patients with a suspected pericardial effusion.[116,117] The diagnosis is made when an echo-free space is seen between the visceral and parietal layers of the pericardium. A volume of fluid as small as 20 to 30 cc can be detected. The volume of fluid is best estimated semiquantitatively as follows: small, less than 100 cc; moderate, less than 500 cc; large, greater than 500 cc. M-mode echocardiography

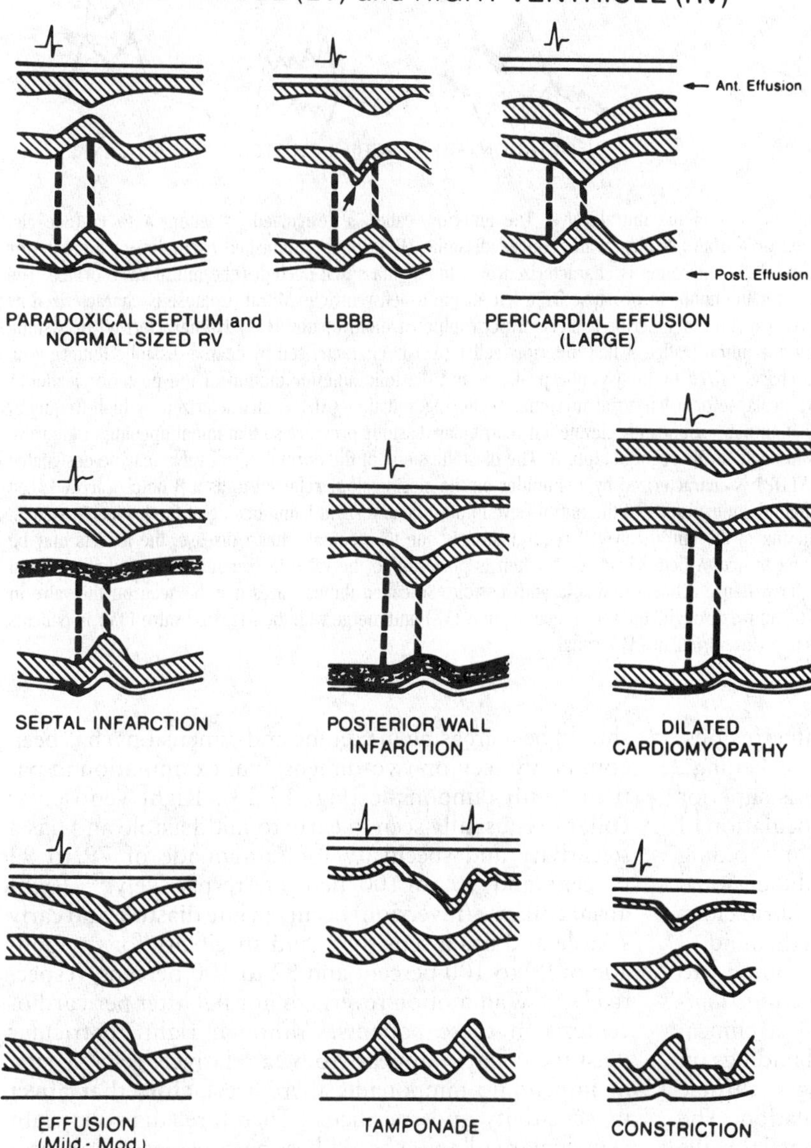

FIGURE 15-20 *A.* Schematic M-mode echocardiographic patterns of the left and right ventricles. The left ventricular dimensions at end diastole (LV_d) and end systole (LV_s) are identified by the broken vertical lines. A left ventricular volume overload (LVVO) lesion (e.g., aortic regurgitation and mitral regurgitation) is characterized by a dilated left ventricle and hyperdynamic ventricular septal (VS) and posterior wall motion. A right ventricular volume overload (RVVO) lesion (e.g., atrial septal defect and tricuspid regurgitation) is characterized by a dilated right ventricle (RV) and paradoxical septal motion. A left ventricular pressure overload (LVPO) lesion may have concentric hypertrophy (e.g., aortic stenosis and systemic arterial hypertension) or asymmetric septal hypertrophy (e.g., hypertrophic cardiomyopathy). Right ventricular hypertrophy is frequently present in both groups. A right ventricular pressure overload (RVPO) lesion (e.g., valvular pulmonic stenosis and tetralogy of Fallot) is characterized by right ventricular hypertrophy and asymmetric septal hypertrophy. CW, chest wall; RVW, right ventricular wall; Endo, endocardium; Epi, epicardium; Peri, pericardium. *B.* Paradoxical septal motion with a normal-sized right ventricle (RV) may be seen in patients with myocardial ischemia or infarction of the interventricular septum and patients after open heart surgery. Left bundle branch block (LBBB) is characterized by early posterior septal motion (arrow) followed by paradoxical septal motion. Pericardial effusions are classified as large if there is significant anterior and posterior fluid, moderate if there is significant posterior and small anterior fluid, and small (mild) if only posterior fluid is present. Myocardial infarction may demonstrate hypokinesis or akinesis of the septum or posterior wall with absence of systolic thickening. Congestive (dilated) cardiomyopathy is characterized by a dilated left ventricle with hypokinetic septal and posterior wall motion. Cardiac tamponade is characterized by anterior and posterior pericardial fluid with respiratory variation in chamber size and wall motion. Pericardial constriction is characterized by paradoxical septal motion and parallel movement of the epicardium and pericardium.

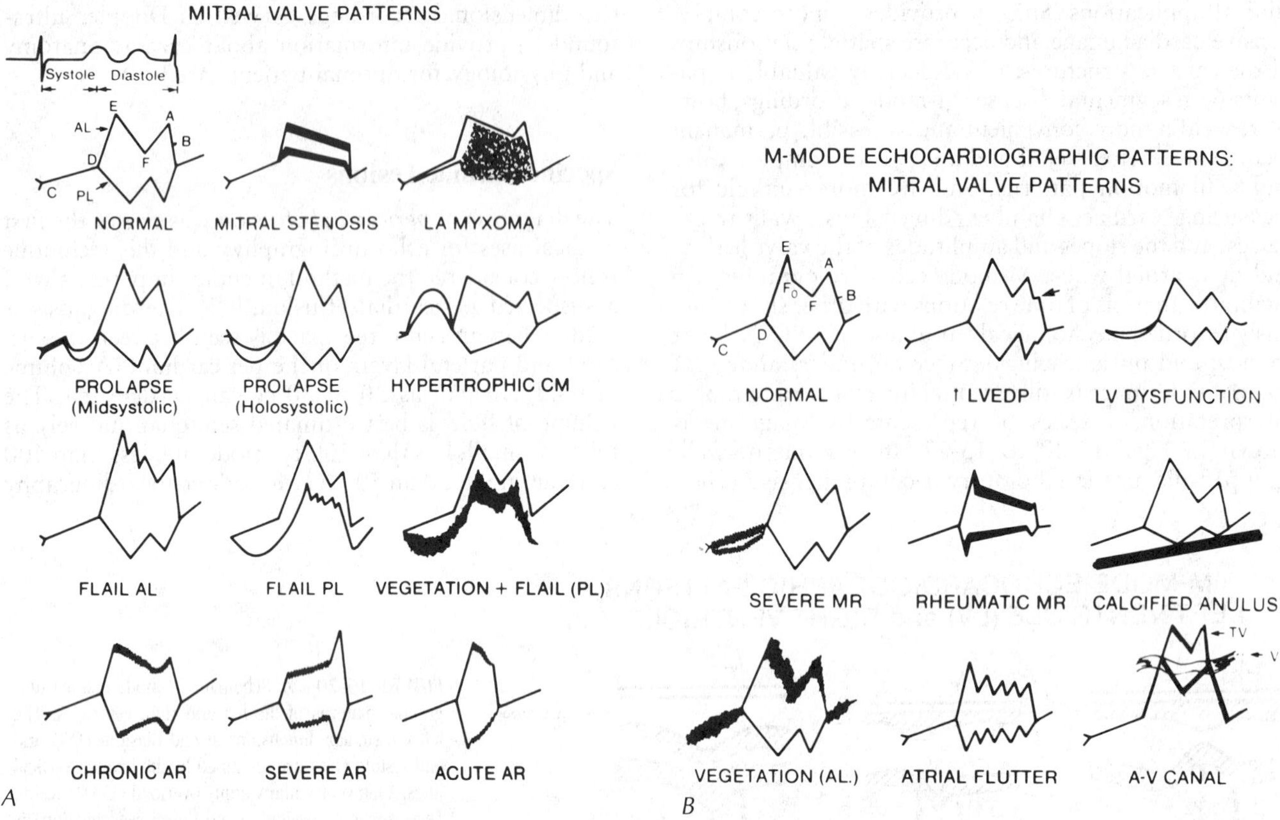

FIGURE 15-21 *A.* Schematic M-mode echocardiographic patterns of the mitral valve. The anterior leaflet is designated by letters A to F. (See Fig. 15-4.) Mitral stenosis is characterized by thickened (calcified or fibrotic) leaflets with reduced diastolic (EF) slope, diminished excursion of the anterior leaflet, and paradoxical motion of the posterior leaflet. Left atrial (LA) myxoma is characterized by a tumor mass that occludes the mitral valve orifice. The clear space in early diastole corresponds to the time required for the tumor to prolapse from left atrium to left ventricle. Mitral prolapse is characterized by either midsystolic or holosystolic posterior bowing of the posterior and/or anterior leaflets. Hypertrophic cardiomyopathy (CM) is characterized by systolic anterior motion and reduced diastolic (EF) slope of the anterior mitral leaflet. A flail anterior leaflet (AL) is characterized by coarse diastolic fluttering on the anterior leaflet, whereas a flail posterior leaflet (PL) is characterized by holosystolic prolapse and diastolic anterior motion of the posterior leaflet. A vegetation on a flail posterior leaflet may mimic mitral valve prolapse or a left atrial myxoma. Aortic regurgitation (AR) is characterized by high-frequency diastolic fluttering of the mitral leaflets. Severe aortic regurgitation may significantly elevate left ventricular diastolic pressure so that initial opening of the valve is absent or reduced, or the valve may close prematurely as in acute aortic regurgitation. *B.* The diastolic slope of the normal mitral valve may be designated EF or EF_0. Elevated left ventricular end-diastolic pressure (LVEDP) is characterized by a shoulder on the closing slope referred to as a B notch (arrow). Left ventricular (LV) dysfunction is characterized by a double-diamond configuration of the mitral valve in diastole and slight hammocking of the leaflets in systole. Mitral regurgitation (MR), if severe, may show systolic fluttering of the mitral valve. If regurgitation is due to rheumatic heart disease, the leaflets may be thickened and the anterior leaflet may have a "ski-slope" appearance. A dense band of calcium is posterior to the valve in patients with a calcified mitral annulus. Vegetations on the anterior leaflet (AL) appear as hazy, dense echoes in systole and diastole. So-called flutter waves may be seen on the valve in patients with atrial flutter. The anterior mitral leaflet appears to "move through" the ventricular septum (VS) and merge with the tricuspid valve (TV) in patients with partial (ostium primum atrial septal defect) or complete atrioventricular (AV) canal.

is superior in qualitative diagnosis (e.g., small effusions, constrictive hemodynamics, and pericardial thickening), whereas two-dimensional echocardiography is superior for assessing the amount, distribution, and loculation of pericardial fluid and is particularly useful in avoiding diagnostic pitfalls.[116–120] In addition, two-dimensional echocardiography can detect fibrous strands, fibrin clots, and tumor implants on the pericardium or in the fluid.[121] Two-dimensional echocardiography now appears to provide reliable criteria for the diagnosis of *cardiac tamponade.*[122,123] Although this is still primarily a clinical and hemodynamic bedside diagnosis, several findings on two-dimensional echocardiography can suggest cardiac compression from pericardial fluid accumulation. The collapse of the right ventricular and/or right atrial walls during diastolic filling (a time when the right ventricle should be increasing in volume and dimensions) has been commonly seen on two-dimensional examination in patients with tamponade (Fig. 15-23). Right ventricular collapse is usually seen in early to middiastole and has a sensitivity and specificity for tamponade of 79 to 92 percent and 90 to 100 percent, respectively.[122] Right atrial collapse (inversion) occurs in late diastole and early systole and has a sensitivity and specificity for tamponade of 90 to 100 percent and 82 to 100 percent, respectively.[124] Wall motion reverts to normal after pericardiocentesis in these patients. Although right ventricular diastolic collapse appears to be a relatively reliable sign of impending tamponade, there are factors that affect its sensitivity and specificity. Therefore, diastolic right ventricular collapse should best be considered only as a marker of the equalization of the right ventricular dia-

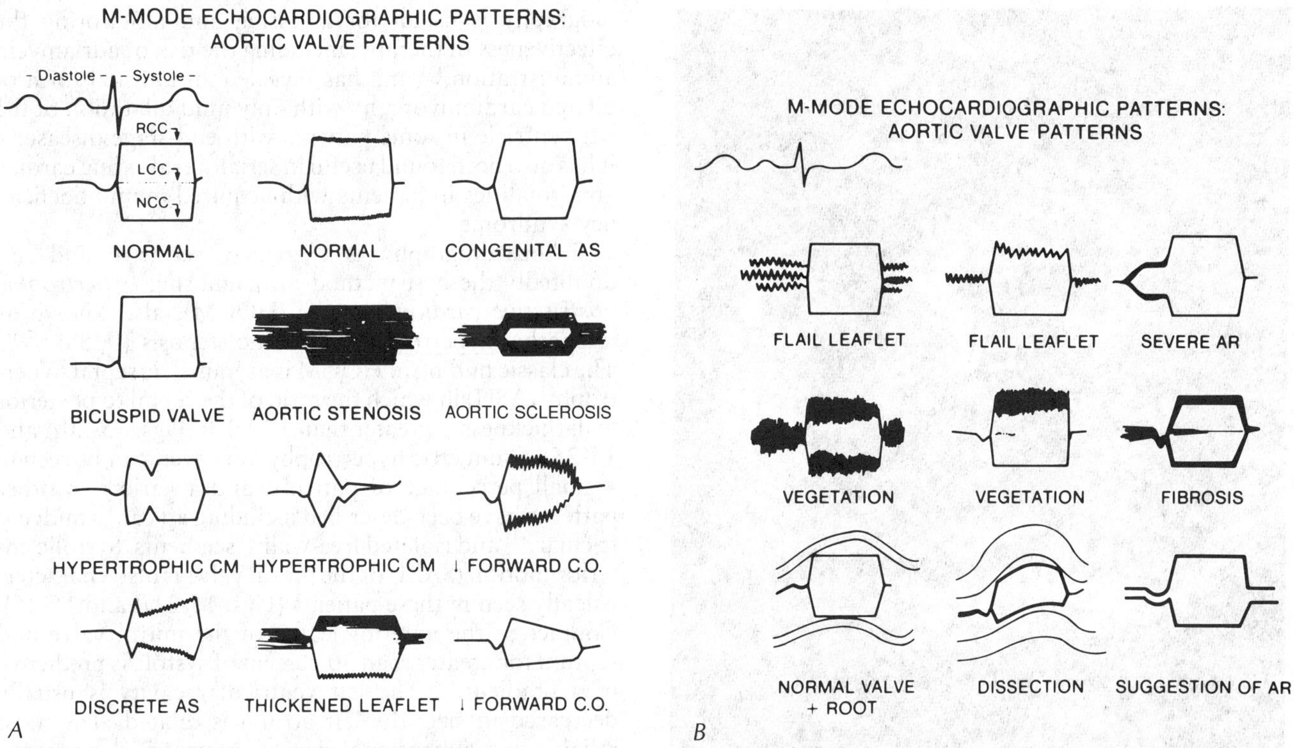

FIGURE 15-22 *A.* Schematic M-mode echocardiographic patterns of the aortic valve. The anterior or right coronary (RCC) and posterior or noncoronary (NCC) cusps are usually seen, but the middle or left coronary (LCC) cusp is parallel to the beam of sound and is not usually seen. The normal valve may occasionally exhibit high-frequency systolic vibrations. The valve may appear normal in patients with congenital aortic stenosis (AS), because the actual valve opening is out of the plane of the ultrasonic beam. A bicuspid aortic valve has eccentric diastolic closure. Calcific aortic stenosis, characterized by dense echoes (calcification) in systole and diastole and a reduced or absent valve orifice, must be differentiated from the thickened (fibrotic) leaflets of aortic valve sclerosis. Hypertrophic cardiomyopathy (CM) with obstruction has partial (notch) or complete midsystolic aortic valve closure, whereas discrete (membranous) subaortic stenosis has partial (notch) early systolic closure. Reduced forward cardiac output (CO), as seen with mitral regurgitation or left ventricular dysfunction, may show high-frequency systolic fluttering and gradual systolic closure. *B.* A flail aortic leaflet is characterized by coarse fluttering in systole and/or diastole. Premature opening of the aortic valve is evidence of elevated left ventricular diastolic pressure and is seen in severe aortic regurgitation (AR). Vegetations appear as dense, shaggy echoes on the leaflet(s) in systole and/or diastole. Separation of the leaflets in diastole of more than 3 mm is suggestive, but not diagnostic, of aortic regurgitation. The normal aorta is characterized by two parallel lines, each 1 to 3 mm thick, that move anteriorly in systole and posteriorly in diastole. The aortic leaflets normally open to the periphery of the aortic walls. Dissection of the aorta is characterized by a dilated aortic root (more than 42 mm), widened anterior or posterior (more than 9 mm) aortic walls, and thin aortic leaflets that open to the periphery of the inner lumen.

stolic and pericardial pressures. Its absence should not exclude tamponade, but in the setting of an otherwise normal right ventricle this absence makes the diagnosis of tamponade very unlikely. Plethora of the inferior vena cava (IVC) with blunted respiratory variation is a sensitive marker of a hemodynamically significant pericardial effusion because changes in the diameter of the wall of the IVC with inspiration closely reflect changes in the right ventricular filling pressure. The sign is defined as a decrease in inferior vena cava diameter by less than 50 percent after deep inspiration.[125]

Echocardiography is useful in defining the distribution of pericardial fluid and thus minimizing the hazards of pericardiocentesis.[126,127] The pericardiocentesis needle can be identified the scanning plane, and the position of the needle tip can be confirmed by contrast echocardiography so that the safest and most effective approach can be used for the procedure. The position of the needle or catheter should be monitored continuously during the procedure and it should be repositioned if necessary. Percutaneous pericardial biopsy, under two-dimensional echocardiographic guidance, has been introduced without complications reported to date.[128]

Constrictive pericarditis has relatively nonspecific echocardiographic findings. Pericardial thickening may be suggested by an increased echodensity, but measurements of pericardial thickness are not reliable.[129] In addition to pericardial thickening, other echocardiographic two-dimensional findings include rapid, early diastolic posterior motion of the left ventricular posterior wall; paradoxical motion and early and late diastolic notching and reduced systolic thickening of the ventricular septum; premature opening of the pulmonary valve; and lack of respiratory variation in the size of the inferior vena cava.[130] Pericardial tumors, presenting as epicardial nodules, and pericardial cysts may be detected by two-dimensional echocardiography.[131]

Echocardiography provides precise information about cardiac chamber enlargement and the extent of functional impairment. Determination of ventricular cavity dimensions, wall thickness, and systolic and diastolic function allows classification of the cardiomyopathies into three types: dilated, hypertrophic, and restrictive types. Echocardiography can thus accurately establish the morphologic diagnosis and assessment of the hemodynamic status of a patient with a cardiomyop-

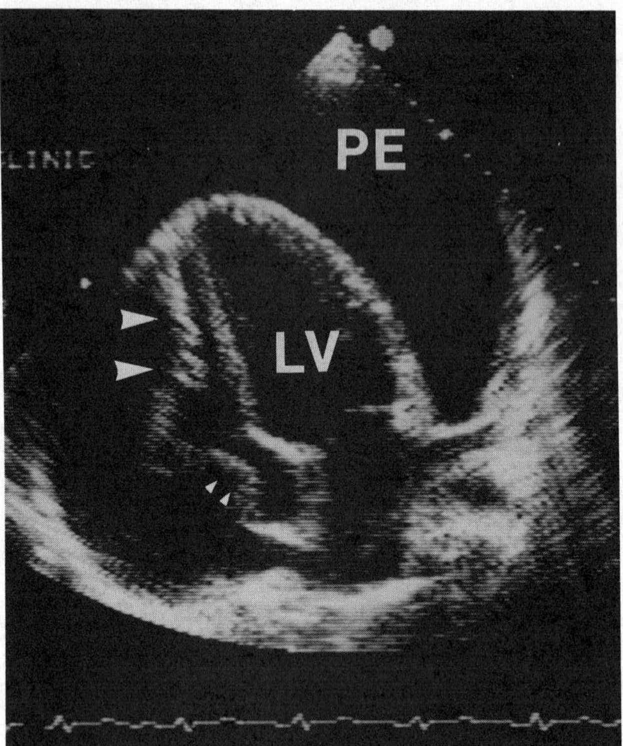

FIGURE 15-23 Two-dimensional apical four-chamber view from a patient with cardiac tamponade. This diastolic frame shows a large pericardial effusion (PE) that completely surrounds the heart. The right ventricular cavity is virtually nonexistent. There is both right ventricular wall collapse (large arrows) and right atrial wall collapse (small arrows) consistent with tamponade. LV, left ventricle.

athy.[132] (See also Chaps. 87 to 91.) *Idiopathic dilated cardiomyopathy* consists of dilatation of all four cardiac chambers, usually in a predictable, symmetrical pattern (Figs. 15-20*B* and 15-24).[133,134] Left ventricular systolic function is diminished, as evidenced by reduced septal and posterior wall motion, reduced delta D and ejection fraction. The cardiac valves are usually normal, but the excursion of the mitral and aortic valves is frequently diminished. Intracardiac thrombi may occasionally be identified and should always be searched for in each of the four cardiac chambers.[132] Two-dimensional echocardiography is useful for assessing and monitoring the effectiveness of therapy, including the risk of adriamycin administration,[135] and has revealed an unusual form of dilated cardiomyopathy with only mild dilatation of the left ventricle in some patients with end-stage disease.[136] It has also been found useful in serially evaluating cardiac abnormalities in patients with acquired immunodeficiency syndrome.[136a]

Echocardiography is extremely sensitive and undoubtedly the best method of diagnosing *hypertrophic obstructive cardiomyopathy* (HOCM), also known as idiopathic hypertrophic subaortic stenosis (IHSS).[137–141] The classic finding in HOCM is asymmetric septal hypertrophy (ASH) in which the ratio of the septal to posterior wall thickness is greater than 1.3 : 1.0 (Figs. 15-20*A* and 15-25). Symmetric hypertrophy, however, can be seen in a small percentage of patients, and a variety of other patterns have been described including apical,[139] midventricular,[142] and isolated free-wall[143] segments. Systolic anterior motion (SAM) of the mitral valve is also characteristically seen in these patients (Figs. 15-21*B* and 15-25). Contact of the anterior leaflet of the mitral valve and septum for greater than 30 percent of systole is predictive of a gradient.[144] The left ventricular cavity is usually decreased in size; the left atrium is dilated. The most reliable two-dimensional sign of left ventricular outflow tract obstruction in HOCM is midsystolic partial (notch) or complete closure of the aortic valve (Figs. 15-22*A* and 15-25).

Restrictive (infiltrative) cardiomyopathies have a multiplicity of etiologies and echocardiographically usually have ventricular wall hypertrophy with normal cavity size, dilated atria, normal or reduced systolic function, and reduced diastolic function. (See Chap. 91.) *Amyloidosis* is one of the most frequently encountered causes. The echocardiographic features of amyloidosis include concentric ventricular hypertrophy, normal or decreased left ventricular cavity size, and decreased left ventricular function both in systole and diastole. The valves and interatrial septum are thickened, and the hypertrophied left ventricular walls may have an abnormal glittering (or ground-glass) appearance[145,146] (Fig. 15-26). *Loeffler's endocarditis* also has well-delineated echocardiographic features, including fibrosis of the endocardium and subendocardium, concentric ventricular hypertro-

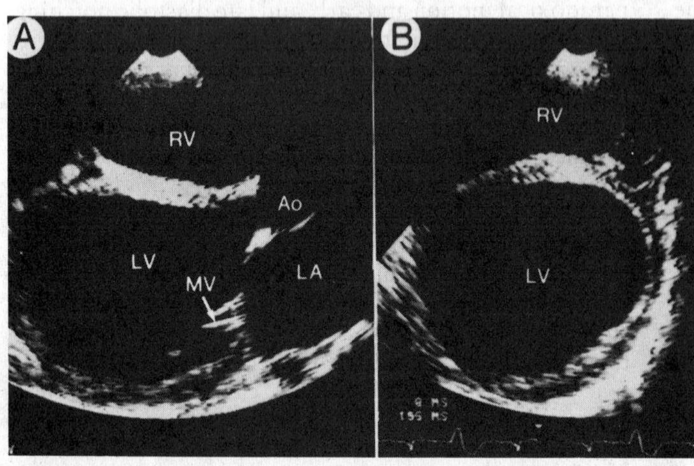

FIGURE 15-24 Two-dimensional echocardiogram from a patient with a congestive cardiomyopathy. *A.* Parasternal long-axis view shows a markedly dilated left ventricle (LV) and moderately dilated left atrium (LA) and right ventricle (RV). Although there appears to be a rounded apex, this is a foreshortened view and the true cardiac apex is not seen. In this end-systolic frame, the closed mitral valve (MV) is more than 30 mm from the septum, consistent with a markedly reduced ejection fraction. *B.* Parasternal short-axis view at end systole (identified by the electrocardiographic trigger at the bottom of the frame) shows that the septum and posterior wall appear thin in comparison with the dilated left ventricle.

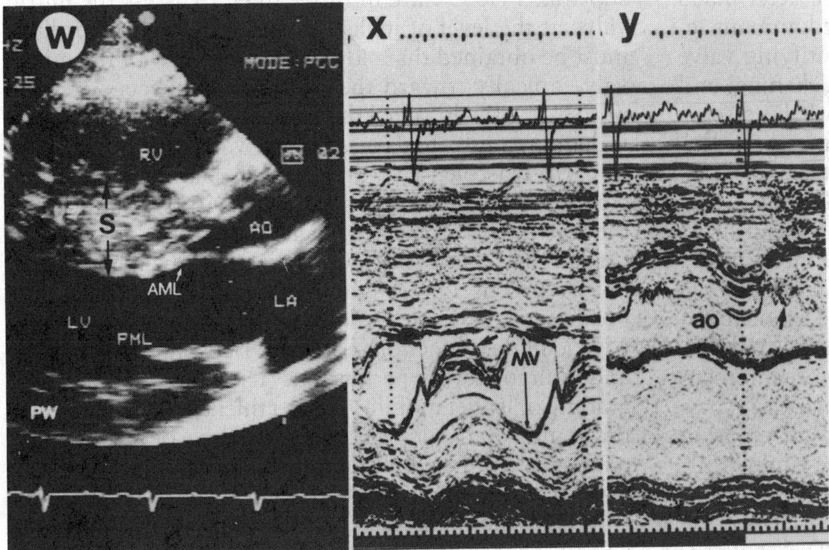

FIGURE 15-25 Echocardiogram from a patient with hypertrophic cardiomyopathy. *W.* Two-dimensional parasternal long-axis view in diastole demonstrates asymmetric septal hypertrophy. The thickness of the ventricular septal wall (S) is 30 mm and that of the posterior wall (PW) is 20 mm. Characteristic brightening of the septal echoes is evident. The left ventricular outflow tract between the anterior mitral leaflet (AML) and the septum is virtually obliterated. The left atrium (LA) is dilated. *X.* M-mode study at the level of the mitral valve shows systolic anterior motion (arrow) of the mitral valve and the mitral valve (MV) abuts against the intraventricular septum in diastole. *Y.* M-mode study at the level of the aorta shows premature closure (arrow) of the anterior aortic leaflet. PML, posterior mitral leaflet; Ao, aorta; RV, right ventricle.

phy, and high incidence of intraventricular thrombus.[147] Restrictive cardiomyopathies must be differentiated from other conditions that cause left ventricular hypertrophy, such as HOCM, systemic arterial hypertension, and aortic stenosis.

Echocardiography is an excellent technique for studying left ventricular structure and function. It is the noninvasive choice for evaluating the cardiac effects of hypertension.[35,148] It is more sensitive and specific for detecting the presence of hypertrophy and estimating left ventricular mass than electrocardiography or chest roentgenograms[149] and correlates accurately with necropsy data.[150] It is especially useful for patients with essential hypertension, with whom it is being used to (1) screen a large number of hypertensive individuals, (2) evaluate cardiac changes in population studies, and (3) assess regression of hypertrophy and mass after therapeutic intervention.[151]

Echocardiography is the noninvasive method of choice for the evaluation of valvular heart disease because of its unique ability to examine cardiac valve structure and motion. It has replaced cardiac catheterization as the definitive study for many types of valvular heart disease because it is of great value for determining both the causes and severity of valvular heart disease. In addition, it is excellent for deciphering organic murmurs in patients with cardiorespiratory symptoms. When evaluating a patient with suspected valvular heart disease, the

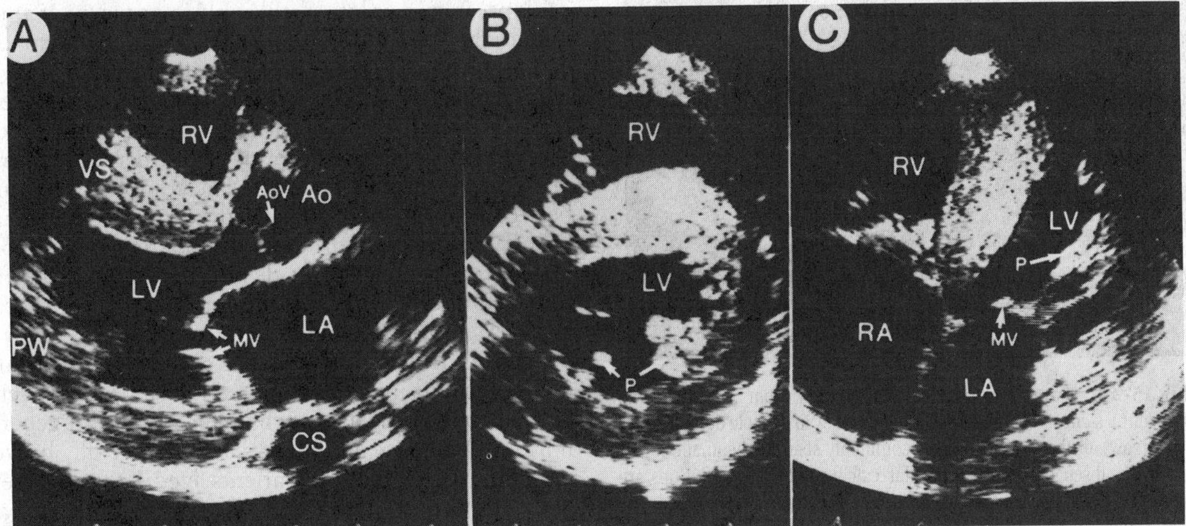

FIGURE 15-26 Two-dimensional echocardiogram from a patient with confirmed amyloid heart disease. *A.* Parasternal long-axis view in diastole shows right ventricular hypertrophy, concentric left ventricular hypertrophy, and bright reflectors of the interventricular septum (VS), characteristic of amyloid involvement of the myocardium. The left ventricular (LV) cavity is normal in size, but the left atrium is dilated. The mitral valve (MV) appears thickened. *B.* Short-axis view at the level of the hypertrophied papillary muscles (P) also shows right ventricular hypertrophy, concentric left ventricular hypertrophy, and a general increase in refractile pattern. *C.* Apical four-chamber view again shows the general increase in the refractile pattern of the septum and the hypertrophied papillary muscle (P) and chordae tendineae. The fact that the interatrial septum does not have significant dropout suggests that it, too, is hypertrophied. RV, right ventricle; CS, coronary sinus; PW, posterior wall; AoV, aortic valve; Ao, aorta; RA, right atrium.

following information is critical and can be determined by echocardiography: (1) defining the predominant lesion; (2) determining the etiology; (3) identifying valve morphology, including leaflet pliability, thickening, and calcification; (4) determining the severity of the disease process; (5) detecting coexisting abnormalities; (6) identifying complications; (7) evaluating ventricular function; and (8) reevaluating the patient after therapy. Criteria for valve stenosis and regurgitation for all four heart valves and specific indications for surgical intervention are emerging based on echocardiographic findings. The Doppler modality has greatly enhanced the echocardiographic diagnosis of the severity of valve abnormalities. The Doppler modality permits accurate measurement of pressure gradient and valve area calculation across stenotic valves as well as semiquantitative determination of the degree of valvular regurgitation. (See Chap. 130) Definitive surgery even without cardiac catheterization is now undertaken in some patients based solely on the accuracy of echocardiographic criteria.[152] Direct detection and quantitation of stenotic cardiac valves are virtually limited to the echocardiographic approach. In *mitral stenosis* leaflet motion is restricted, the orifice is reduced, and calcification is usually present (Figs. 15-21*A* and *B* and 15-27). This results in a fish-mouth-shaped parasternal short-axis appearance of the orifice. Echocardiography is the most sensitive and most specific noninvasive method for diagnosing mitral stenosis.[21,22,153] Published data have documented the usefulness of two-dimensional measurement of mitral valve area in patients with rheumatic mitral stenosis (Fig. 15-27).[154,155] Planimetry of the mitral valve orifice is performed from the parasternal short-axis view. Care must be taken to assess the mitral valve at the level of its leaflet tips; therefore, recordings must be obtained that slowly scan the body of the mitral valve apically toward the chordae tendineae. After the proper level is located, the image is slowly played until it demonstrates the largest mitral valve orifice size seen in early diastole. This area is then planimetered using computer-assisted area assessment. Direct planimetry of the valve area correlates well with those obtained at cardiac catheterization and surgery.[154] Echocardiography is also useful for confirming mitral stenosis in the presence of associated abnormalities such as left or right ventricular dysfunction, aortic or tricuspid valve disease, and pulmonary hypertension. The echocardiographic grading of leaflet mobility, leaflet thickening, subvalvular thickening, and calcification is predictive of the hemodynamic outcome of balloon mitral valvotomy.[156,157]

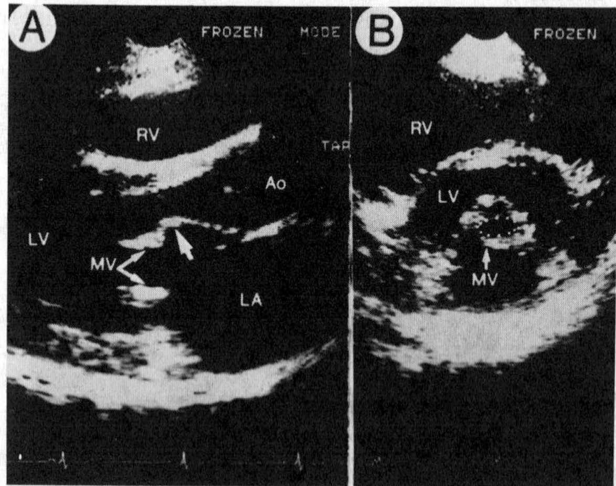

FIGURE 15-27 Two-dimensional echocardiogram from a patient with moderate mitral stenosis. *A* Parasternal long-axis view in diastole demonstrates doming (arrow) of the anterior leaflet, commonly seen in rheumatic mitral stenosis in the absence of marked valvular calcification. The leaflet tips are only moderately calcified, and the left atrium (LA) is moderately dilated. The extent of leaflet tip separation of the mitral valve (MV) is beneficial for identifying the true orifice in the parasternal short-axis plane and is also helpful as a rough guide to judge whether the parasternal short-axis image is precisely through the leaflet tips. *B*. Parasternal short-axis view through the tips of the mitral leaflets demonstrates the technique for determining mitral valve area. Planimetry of the valve area (dotted line) is performed at the onset of diastole when the orifice appears the largest; the valve orifice measures 1.2 cm.^{2} LV, left ventricle; RV, right ventricle; Ao, aorta.

Mitral regurgitation is frequently suggested by indirect signs including a left ventricular volume overload pattern characterized by a dilated, hypercontractile left ventricle, an increased ejection fraction or delta D, and systolic expansion of an enlarged left atrium (Fig. 15-20*A*).[158] The etiologic diagnoses, such as MVP, flail mitral leaflet, and calcified mitral annulus, are best determined by direct analysis of the motion and configuration of the mitral apparatus itself.[159,160]

Mitral valve prolapse can be considered the boon or bane of echocardiography (Fig. 15-21*A*). A very large number of patients are referred "to rule out" this condition, and substantial overdiagnosis seems to have become the rule. To provide better diagnostic definition of MVP, examine not only valve motion but also valve morphology.[161] Two-dimensional echocardiograms in patients with auscultatory and phonocardiographic evidence of MVP reveal a wide spectrum of valve types. Some valves are voluminous, thick, and redundant and prolapse regardless of the view (Fig. 15-28), whereas others are small, thin, and normal in appearance and prolapse in mid or late systole only in one view. It appears that diagnostic criteria using motion and morphology can separate patients with and without prolapse with a high degree of sensitivity and specificity and identify those at risk for complications. Patients with mild degrees of prolapse, however, may be difficult to differentiate from normal individuals. The complex relationship between the normal mitral valve and a saddle-shaped mitral annulus may produce an apparent bowing of the leaflets toward the atrial side of the annulus in the apical four-chamber view.[162] This finding was spuriously called prolapse in the past.[163] Mitral valve prolapse is now best defined as leaflet displacement above the plane of the mitral annulus in the parasternal long axis; displacement limited to the apical four-chamber view is, in general, a normal geometric finding.[164,165] Warth et al., however, noted that 34 percent of patients aged 10 to 18 meet the above criteria.[166] The morphology of the mitral leaflets has been shown to have prognostic importance in patients with prolapse. Those with thickened leaflets (>5 mm) have a higher incidence of endocarditis, severe regurgitation, and sudden death.[167,168] Mitral valve prolapse is occasionally associated with tricuspid valve prolapse and/or aortic valve prolapse.[169] In patients with a *flail mitral leaflet* the tip(s) of the valve, which remains

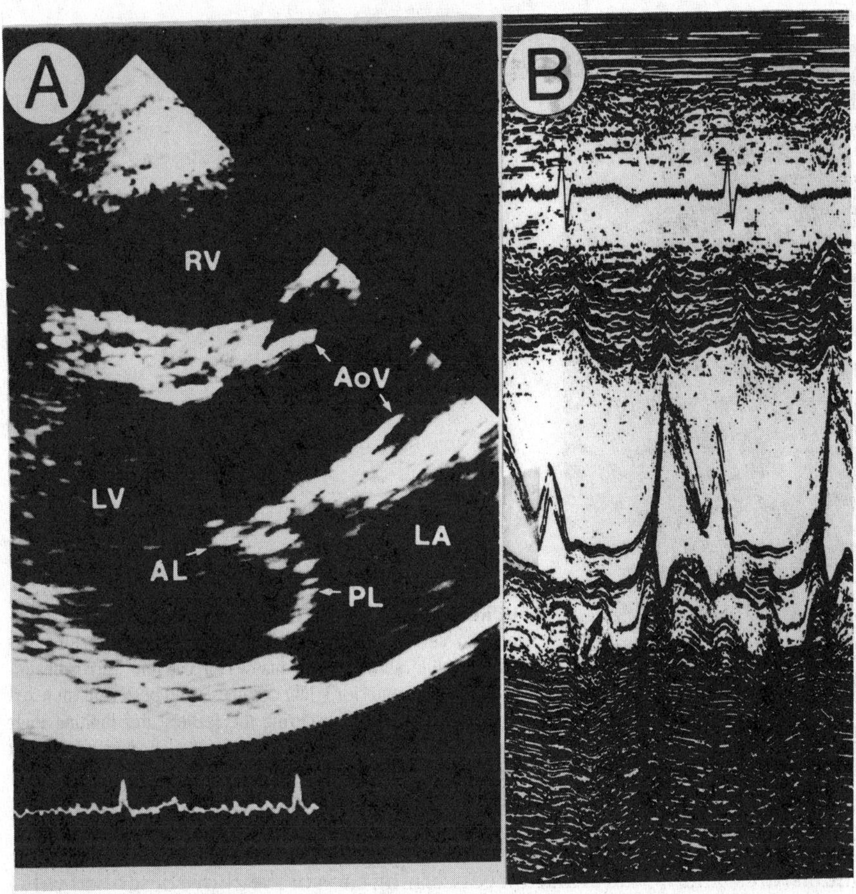

FIGURE 15-28 Echocardiogram from a patient with mitral valve prolapse. *A.* Parasternal long-axis view in systole shows the posterior leaflet (PL) of the mitral valve with superior displacement (bowing) into the left atrium (LA), i.e., arching posteriorly above the level of the atrioventricular groove and behind the normal coaptation point of the left atrium. *B.* M-mode study shows abrupt posterior displacement in midsystole (arrow) of the posterior mitral leaflet. There are multiple echoes arising in the area of the valve during systole as a result of the redundancy of the leaflets. These findings are characteristic of mitral valve prolapse. LV, left ventricle; AL, anterior leaflet of mitral valve; RV, right ventricle; AoV, aortic valve.

within the ventricle in prolapse, is displaced into the left atrium during systole.[170]

The sensitivity and specificity of ultrasound for identifying cardiac calcification are excellent. The echocardiographic pattern of *mitral annular calcification* is virtually diagnostic.[171] Echocardiography is more sensitive than chest roentgenography or fluoroscopy for detecting mitral annular calcification.

Aortic regurgitation produces high-frequency diastolic fluttering of the mitral leaflets and occasionally of the interventricular septum, best seen on M-mode examination. The left ventricle is dilated with the characteristic volume overload pattern.[172] M-mode echocardiography can frequently separate acute from chronic aortic regurgitation, since the former may show premature closure of the mitral valve, a sign of hemodynamically severe disease (Fig. 15-21*A*).[173] In the patient who has an apical diastolic rumbling murmur, echocardiography can determine the cause from among mitral stenosis, severe aortic regurgitation (Austin Flint murmur), left atrial myxoma, and severe mitral regurgitation.[21]

The aortic valve in patients with *valvular aortic stenosis* may show increased echogenicity (thickening or calcification) and reduced mobility of the leaflets (Figs. 15-22*A* and 15-29). Aortic stenosis is usually associated with concentric left ventricular hypertrophy and a dilated aortic root. Two-dimensional echocardiography is not as accurate in quantitating the aortic valve area as it is for the mitral valve area because the increased echogenicity of the cusps and irregular valve orifice make it difficult to accurately planimeter the aortic valve area. Two-dimensional echocardiography does have the ability to distinguish mild from severe aortic stenosis, which is often adequate for clinical purposes.[174,175] Severe stenosis can be excluded when the aortic cusps are separated by more than 12 mm. Cusp separation of less than 7 mm is only suggestive of severe stenosis, however. Problems in diagnosis occur in elderly patients, especially those with hypertension, who may show aortic leaflet thickening (fibrosis, sclerosis, or annular calcification). The Doppler modality provides the ability to noninvasively measure the peak and mean pressure gradients across the aortic valve and calculate the aortic valve area accurately and is much more valuable in determining the severity of aortic stenosis. (See Chap. 130.)

A *bicuspid aortic valve* is best diagnosed by two-dimensional visualization of the aortic valve, since this technique offers the advantage of being able to determine leaflet morphology, including systolic doming (seen best in the parasternal long-axis view), as well as cusp number (Fig. 15-30).[176] The sensitivity (78 percent) and specificity (96 percent) of the two-dimensional diagnosis of a bicuspid valve have been determined.[177] Analysis of the aortic valve can also establish the diagnosis of a flail aortic leaflet[178] and aortic valve prolapse[179] and detect the membrane of fixed subvalvular aortic stenosis.[180]

The echocardiogram plays an important role in the diagnosis of *tricuspid stenosis*.[181] The features of rheumatic tricuspid stenosis are identical to those of mitral stenosis, but it is not possible to directly measure the

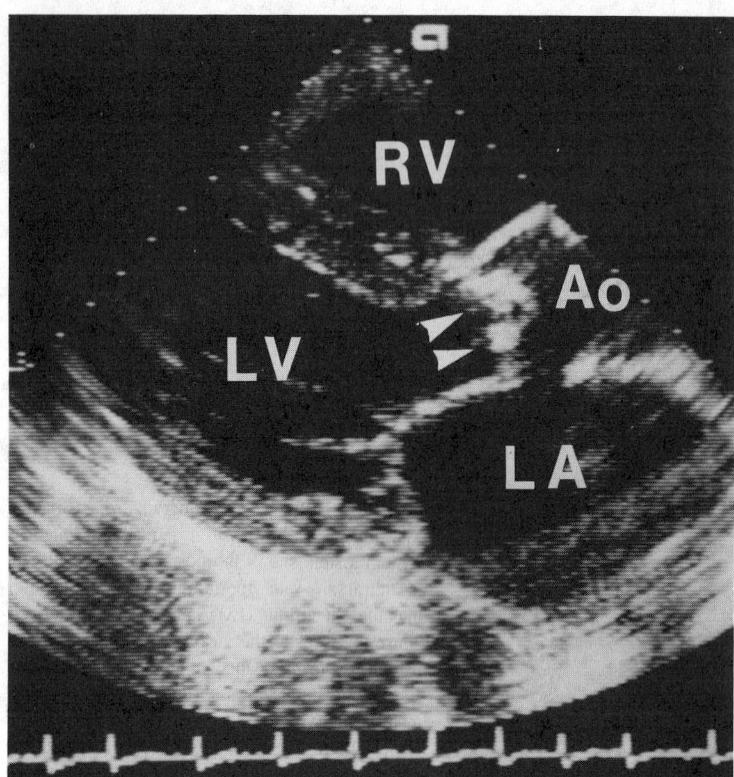

FIGURE 15-29 Two-dimensional echocardiogram from a patient with severe calcific aortic stenosis. Parasternal long-axis view in systole shows dense masses of calcium (arrowheads) representing the anterior (right coronary) and posterior (noncoronary) cusps virtually obscuring the leaflets and limiting their excursion. Ao, aorta; RV, right ventricle; LV, left ventricle; LA, left atrium.

tricuspid valve orifice. On the other hand, carcinoid tricuspid stenosis does not have fused commissures and coexistent mitral disease.[182]

The echocardiographic diagnosis of *valvular pulmonic stenosis* is defined by restricted cusp opening, systolic doming, and premature opening of the valve, frequently with a large *a* dip.[183] More precise quantitative information concerning each of the above described valvular lesions can be obtained noninvasively with Doppler ultrasound.

Echocardiographic assessment is the best noninvasive method for the evaluation of *prosthetic valves*. It is en-

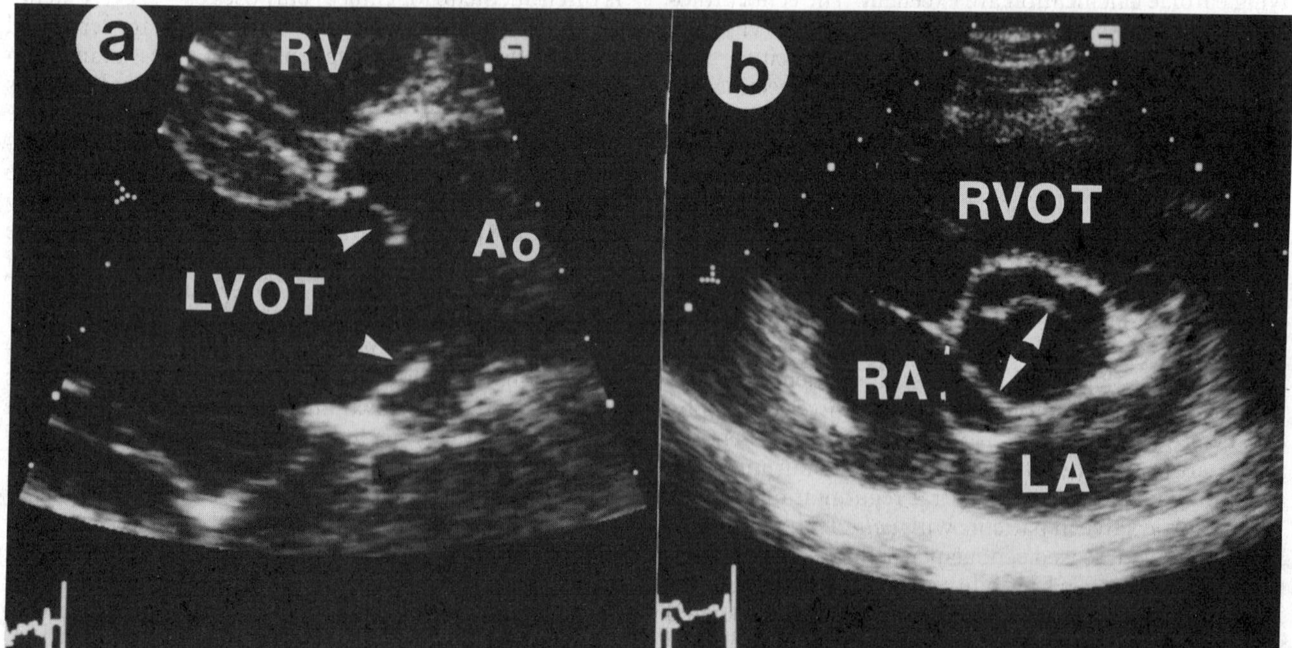

FIGURE 15-30 Two-dimensional echocardiogram from a patient with aortic stenosis due to a bicuspid aortic valve. *a*. Parasternal long-axis view shows systolic doming (bowing) of the anterior and posterior cusps of the aortic valve (arrowheads). *b*. Parasternal short-axis view at the level of the aorta shows only two cusps (arrowheads). Ao, aorta; LVOT, left ventricular outflow tract; RVOT, right ventricular outflow tract; RA, right atrium; LA, left atrium; RV, right ventricle.

hanced by the availability of a baseline study for comparison, and therefore a postimplantation study is recommended. (See also Chap. 83.) Mechanical prosthetic valves are difficult to evaluate because of the intense echogenicity of the mechanical elements that result in reverberations and attenuation (shadowing). Transesophageal echocardiography is therefore the procedure of choice, especially for the evaluation of mitral valve prostheses. (See Chap. 131.) Nevertheless, a variety of echophonocardiographic signs of dysfunction have been described[184] for transthoracic echocardiography including abnormalities of disk or ball motion and thrombus on struts, stents, or disks.[180] Bioprosthetic valves, however, can be evaluated more successfully because the leaflets can be identified routinely. Thickening, reduced mobility, vegetations, valve ring abscesses, and flail leaflets have been diagnosed. Torn cusps have been identified with a sensitivity of 82 percent and a specificity of 100 percent.[185,186] Echo-phonocardiographic studies have also proved useful in correlating valve clicks with disk or ball motion, especially in patients with more than one prosthesis. Evaluation of the severity of prosthetic valvular dysfunction is best determined by Doppler techniques. (See Chap. 130.)

Currently, echocardiography is the only technique available that can visualize a vegetation, except for cardiac surgery. *Infective vegetations* have been described on each of the four cardiac valves.[187–189] They appear as bright, mobile, echo-dense structures attached to the valve leaflets (Fig. 15-31). To be recognized echocardiographically, they must be greater than 2 mm in size and are generally irregular in shape and often move in a direction and speed different from the leaflet itself (Figs. 15-22*A* and 15-23*B*). The presence of a vegetation allows confirmation of the diagnosis and provides localization of involvement but does not determine whether the illness is acute or chronic. There is substantial controversy, however, as to its meaning when detected by echocardiography.[188] For instance, the mere presence of a vegetation is not, by itself, an indication for surgery; nor is its size. The actual size may be influenced by the presence of calcification that may spuriously give a larger appearance. Even the small, nonbacterial vegetations may be imaged.[190] Although there is evidence that vegetations larger than 1 cm are a risk for embolic events, the identification of such a mass is not by itself an indication for surgery.[191] The absence of a vegetation on echocardiography does not rule out endocarditis, since normal studies may be obtained with M mode in more than half of the patients with clinically diagnosed infective endocarditis. Two-dimensional echocardiography is much more sensitive, imaging vegetations in 70 to 85 percent of cases, especially right-sided vegetations.[192–194] Transesophageal echocardiography should improve the sensitivity for visualization of vegetations to nearly 90 percent.[191,193] (See Chaps. 94 and 131.) Echocardiography may also be useful in identifying vegetations in patients with culture-negative endocarditis.[195] Two-dimensional echocardiography not only can estimate vegetation size, shape, mobility, and location but also can detect many of the complications of endocarditis, such as leaflet destruction (e.g., ruptured chordae tendineae), shunt lesions, and valve ring abscesses as well as the hemodynamic consequences.[186] The risk of

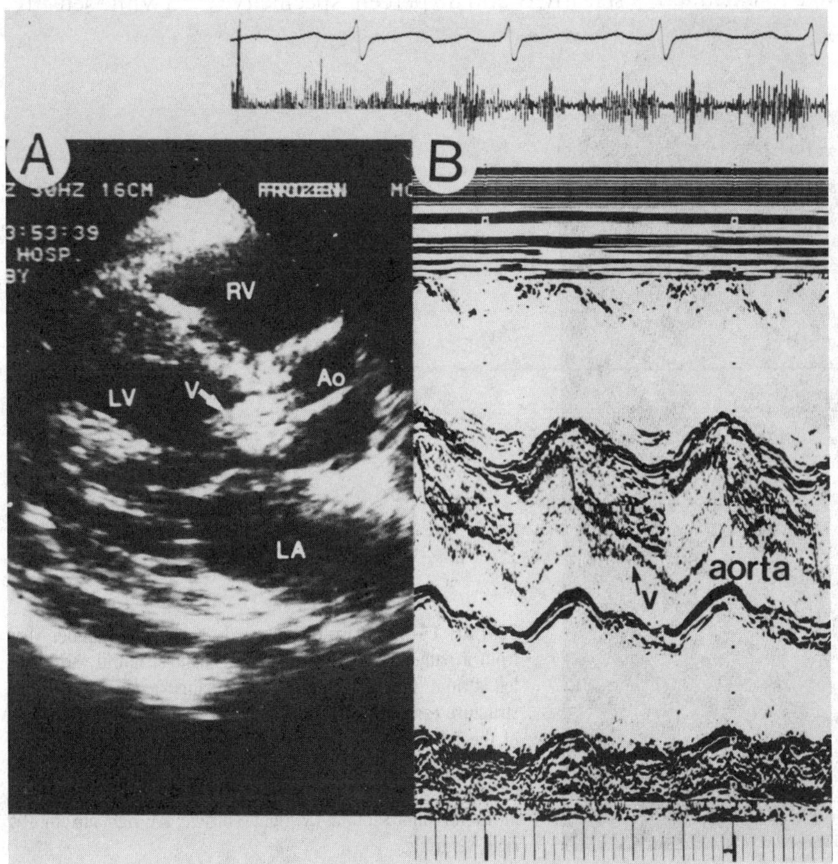

FIGURE 15-31 Echocardiogram from a patient with an aortic valve vegetation. *A.* Two-dimensional parasternal long-axis view shows a very dense, nodular structure (arrow v) that represents a large vegetation. This diastolic frame shows the vegetation projecting into the left ventricle (LV). *B.* M-mode study shows a shaggy, dense structure in diastole (arrow v) that represents the aortic valve vegetation. Ao, aorta; LA, left atrium; RV, right ventricle.

embolization appears to be greatest in patients with vegetative lesions at least 10 mm in diameter on two-dimensional echocardiography, especially if it is attached to the mitral valve.[191,194] If significant leaflet involvement is found, serial studies should be performed, since echocardiography is useful in assessing the extent of damage and the hemodynamic consequences. Serial echocardiograms, however, are not generally useful in assessing antibacterial therapy, since vegetations may persist for months to years after initial infection and bacteriologic cure.[21] A predischarge echocardiogram should be obtained to provide a baseline study, especially in drug-abuse patients, since recurrences are likely.

Prosthetic valve infective endocarditis is much more difficult to diagnose by transthoracic echocardiography because of the many image artifacts related to prosthetic material. The superior image quality of transesophageal echocardiography makes this technique more suitable, especially for evaluating mitral valve protheses. (See Chap. 131.)

Two-dimensional echocardiography has become the technique of choice for identifying *intracardiac masses,* since this method allows display of intracardiac structures in a spatial manner and visualizes areas of the heart that are not accessible by other noninvasive techniques (e.g., right atrium and left atrial appendage). Cardiac tumors, including atrial myxomas (Fig. 15-21*A*), sarcomas, and metastases as well as thromboembolic material have been identified in each of the cardiac chambers (Fig. 15-32).[131,196–202] Two-dimensional echocardiography is therefore useful for evaluating patients with *neurologic ischemic syndromes.* Patients with strokes should have an echocardiogram if there is a history of heart disease or if they are less than 45 years of age to exclude an intracardiac shunt lesion or MVP as a predisposing condition.[203]

Intracavitary left atrial thrombi are detected by two-dimensional echocardiography with a sensitivity of 70 to 90 percent and a specificity up to 98 percent.[203] Those that tend to form in the atrial appendage, however, are very difficult to image. In this location the sensitivity of two-dimensional echocardiography for detecting left atrial thrombi is reported to be 33 to 59 percent.[204] Transesophageal echocardiography is the modality of choice for suspected left atrial appendage thrombi. *Right atrial thrombi* may be mobile, serpentine structures prolapsing through the tricuspid valve and lacking any apparent attachment to the endocardium, fingerlike masses attached to the atrial wall or superimposed on a foreign body.[199] A "smokelike" pattern of swirling intracavitary echoes is indicative of low-flow regions of the heart.

Pathological intracardiac masses must be differentiated from normal cardiac anatomic variants, including the right atrial eustachian valve, right atrial Chiari network, left ventricular false tendon, and right ventricular moderator band as well as iatrogenic intracardiac masses such as the pacing wire or the Swan-Ganz catheter.

Transthoracic two-dimensional echocardiography can visualize certain portions of the thoracic aorta[205] and can be useful in the diagnosis of abnormalities such as dissecting aneurysm,[206,207] saccular aneurysm,[208] and coarctation of the aorta.[209] The echocardiographic features of *aortic dissection* include widening of the aorta to at lest 42 mm and demonstration of an intimal flap (Fig. 15-33). Parasternal long-axis and short-axis views as well as apical long-axis and suprasternal notch views are extremely important to attain the reported 100 percent sensitivity and 88 percent specificity.[210–212] While sensitiv-

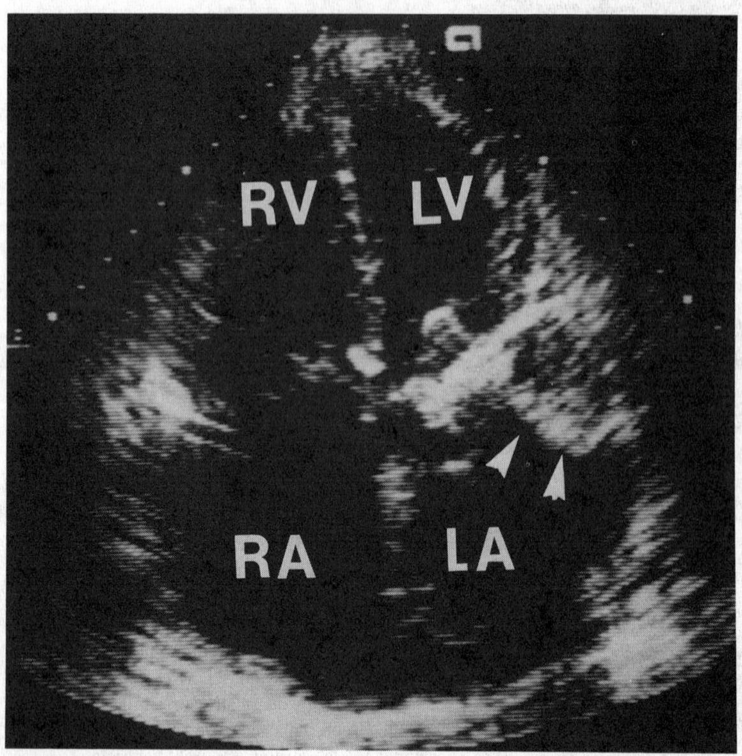

FIGURE 15-32 Two-dimensional apical four-chamber view from a patient with a prosthetic mechanical mitral valve. The left atrium (LA) is dilated and contains a dense echogenic structure (arrowheads) attached to the lateral wall in the region of the left atrial appendage that represents a large left atrial thrombus. A portion of the mitral valve prosthesis is seen projecting into the left ventricle (LV) and angling toward the intraventricular septum. LV, right ventricle; RA, right atrium; RV, right ventricle.

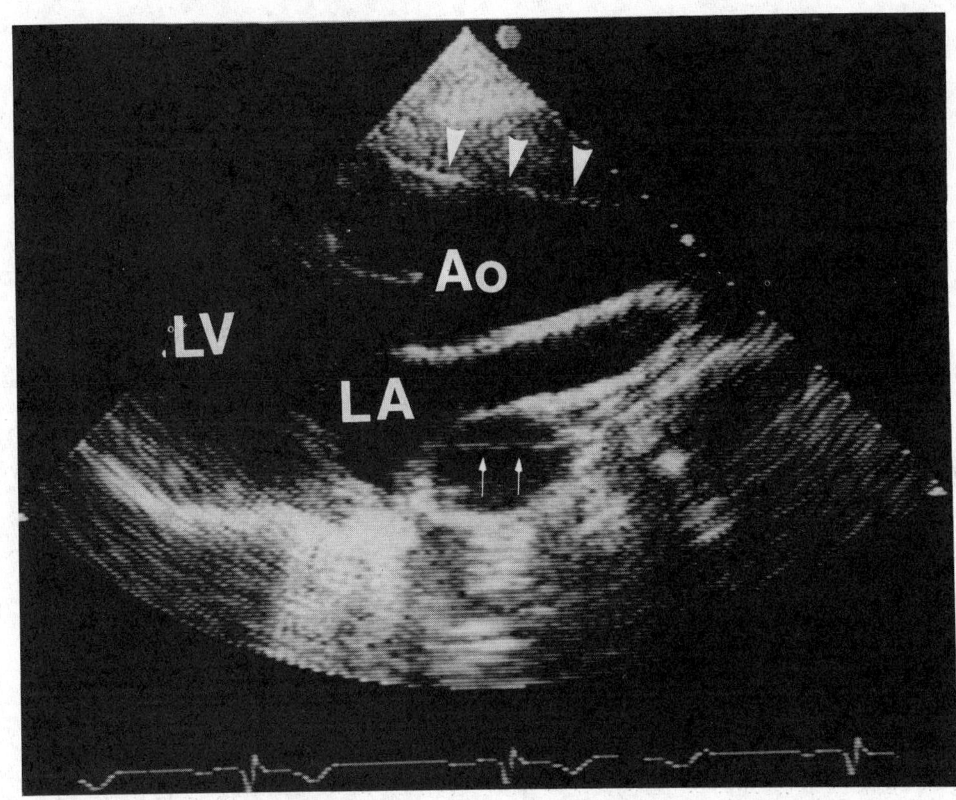

FIGURE 15-33 Two-dimensional parasternal echocardiogram from a patient with a Type I (proximal) dissection of the aorta. The ascending aorta (Ao) is dilated and contains a linear density (arrowheads) that represents the intimal flap, which separates the true and false lumen. The descending aorta is visible behind the left atrium (LA) and also contains the intimal flap (small arrows). LV, left ventricle.

ities and specificities for transthoracic echocardiographic detection of aortic dissection are reported to be high, most clinicians have recognized the inability of this test to diagnose accurately aortic dissections that are not true type I or type A dissections involving ascending aortic and aortic annulus. Transesophageal echocardiography, especially the biplane technique, has become the diagnostic modality of choice for aortic/thoracic aortic abnormalities. (See Chaps. 123 and 131.)

Two-dimensional echocardiography can evaluate both the superior and inferior vena cavae. A persistent left superior vena cava can be identified from the left supraclavicular fossa, whereas proximal inferior vena cava abnormalities (e.g., thrombus or tumor extension) can be imaged from the subcostal plane.[22]

Transesophageal echocardiography, however, is clearly the procedure of choice for evaluating abnormal conditions involving the aorta. (See Chap. 131.)

Echocardiography has been useful in patients with suspected *ischemic heart disease* for the differential diagnosis and evaluation of chest pain syndromes, determination of left ventricular performance, diagnosis, risk stratification, monitoring of serial changes in acute myocardial infarction and its complications, determining the prognosis, and planning therapy in chronic ischemic syndromes.[213,214] It can be used in the emergency room setting to detect a wall motion abnormality prior to the use of thrombolytic therapy and to aid in ruling out other chest pain syndromes, e.g., aortic dissection, MVP, aortic stenosis, and pericardial disease. The two-dimensional mode has become the principal echocardiographic technique in these patients,[215-222] but M-mode echocardiography is a useful adjunct because it can accurately record wall motion. M-mode echocardiography, however, cannot quantitate the amount of abnormally moving myocardium and cannot image all of the areas of the left ventricle (e.g., the apex and lateral wall). If images of suitable quality are obtained, it is possible with two-dimensional echocardiography to analyze ventricular wall motion on a regional basis and to apply quantitative descriptions to each segment of the myocardium.[213,216] A variety of methods have been used to divide the left and right ventricles anatomically.[42,45,50] One method of *regional analysis* and nomenclature that may be of considerable help in the evaluation of patients with suspected coronary artery disease is shown in Fig. 15-34. In patients with suspected ischemic heart disease all segments of the left ventricle must be evaluated systematically and related one to another in order to build a true three-dimensional image.[223]

Echocardiographic abnormalities occurring in patients with ischemic heart disease include changes in structure, such as thinning of the myocardial walls, and changes in wall motion (i.e., hypokinetic, akinetic, and dyskinetic changes). Visual assessment of the absence of systolic myocardial wall thickening or actual thinning of the wall are specific, but not sensitive, signs of the presence of myocardial infarction.[222-226] They are, however, more specific than are wall motion abnormalities, and they are especially useful when conduction abnormalities such as left bundle branch block are associated with the infarction. The simplest method of assessing wall motion is to note the differences between normal and abnormal adjacent segments.[227] Extensive regional wall motion abnormalities on two-dimensional echocardiography in patients with myocardial ischemia have predictive value and are useful in identifying high-risk patients.[219] Because of differences in views, however, it is often difficult to

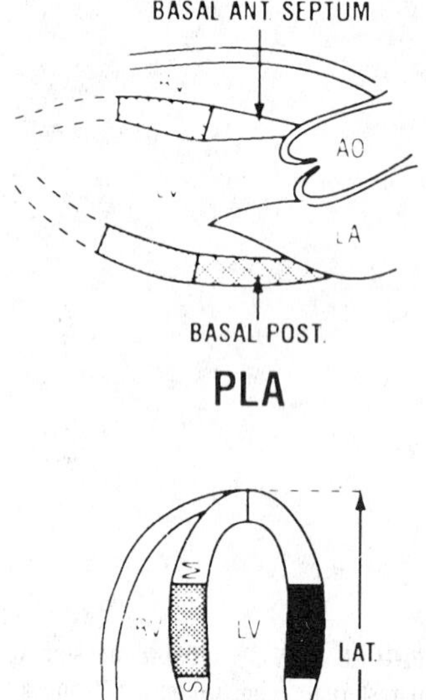

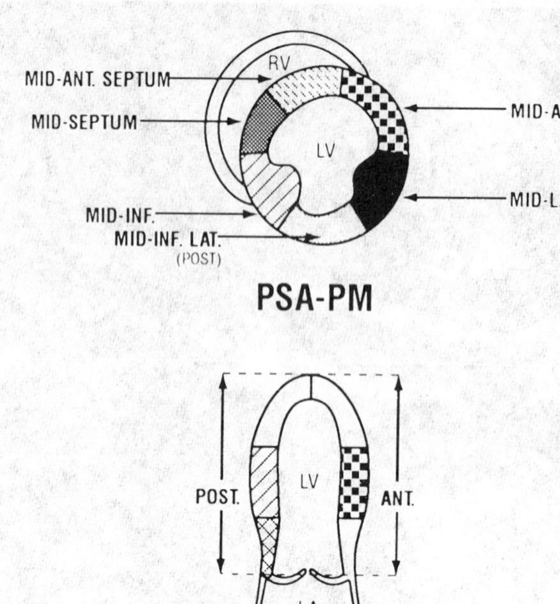

FIGURE 15-34 Regional analysis of the heart shows the four classic views used to determine the area of coronary artery involvement: PLA, parasternal long axis; PSA-PM, parasternal short axis at the papillary muscle level; 4C, apical four chamber; and 2C, apical two chamber. RV, right ventricle; LV, left ventricle; Ao, aorta; LA, left atrium; RA, right atrium; Ant, anterior; Post, posterior; Lat, lateral. (*From JM Felner: Echocardiography in coronary artery disease. In: Cardiovascular Disease and Chest Pain, vol 6, No. 2. New York, Cahners Publishing, 1990. Reproduced with permission.*)

make size comparisons between two-dimensional and angiographic assessments of wall motion abnormalities. Wall motion studies are extremely useful in excluding Q-wave (or transmural) myocardial infarction, since virtually all areas of transmural infarction will show akinesis or dyskinesis. Not all wall motion abnormalities are associated with demonstrable pathology, however, and non-Q-wave (or subendocardial) infarction may exist with an apparently normal echocardiogram. In patients with acute myocardial infarction, the ventricular wall motion abnormalities include not only the acutely infarcted segments but also previously infarcted segments and ischemic myocardium in adjacent zones. Furthermore, segmental wall motion abnormalities may also occur in patients with myocarditis, dilated cardiomyopathy,[228] and anorexia nervosa.[229]

Echocardiography also has prognostic value in patients with myocardial infarction, because it shows the relation and the extent of echocardiographic asynergy and the outcome of the infarction.[219,220] The extent of ischemic damage,[230] the presence of right ventricular infarction,[231] and certain complications such as left ventricular dysfunction,[232] aneurysm,[233] pseudoaneurysm,[234] left ventricular thrombi,[235] ventricular septal defect,[236] and papillary muscle rupture[237] can be accurately diagnosed by two-dimensional echocardiography. Two-dimensional echocardiography is excellent at diagnosing infarct expansion and differentiating it from infarct extension[238] as well as predicting left ventricular volume after infarction.[239] *Left ventricular aneurysms* are thin-walled dyskinetic segments readily detected by two-dimensional echocardiography. They are typically located at the apex and show systolic expansion while the rest of the functioning myocardium contracts inwardly and diastolic deformity[229] (Fig. 15-35).

Left ventricular thrombi are frequently seen (25 to 30 percent) in patients with acute anterior and apical myocardial infarctions, particularly within a left ventricular aneurysm.[240,241] These speckled-appearing intracavitary masses are found usually at the left ventricular apex but are virtually always in an area of decreased wall motion (Fig. 15-35). Appropriate use of the gain controls, together with multiple tomographic views, is very important if false-positive and false-negative results are to be prevented. Two-dimensional echocardiography has been reported to be the best method for detection of left ventricular thrombi associated with myocardial infarction, but age or activity cannot be accurately determined.[183,241,242] Sensitivity of two-dimensional echocardiography for the diagnosis of left ventricular thrombi ranges from 77 to 95 percent, whereas specificity is 88 to 95 percent.[232] Patients with echocardiographically demonstrated thrombus in the postinfarction period are at increased risk for embolism if the thrombus is protruding, pedunculated, or mobile.[243–245]

Transthoracic two-dimensional echocardiography is capable of directly visualizing the proximal portions of the coronary arteries.[246] Both the right and left coronary arteries have been identified but are difficult to image, since they are constantly moving in and out of the plane of examination. Left main coronary artery disease has been detected in some patients by two-dimensional echocardiography, but the sensitivity and specificity of the technique for this purpose have not been established.[247] In addition, patients with coronary artery disease may have high-intensity echoes, originating from the proximal portion of the left main coronary artery, that may be difficult to distinguish from surrounding structures. Transesophageal echocardiography is more useful for direct coronary artery visualization. (See Chap. 131.) The proximal identification of the coronary arteries may help detect congenital abnormalities (e.g., anomalous origin or fistula formation) or aneurysms that may develop as a complication of Kawasaki's disease.[248] This inflammatory pediatric disease should have serial echocardiographic evaluations since long-term abnormalities

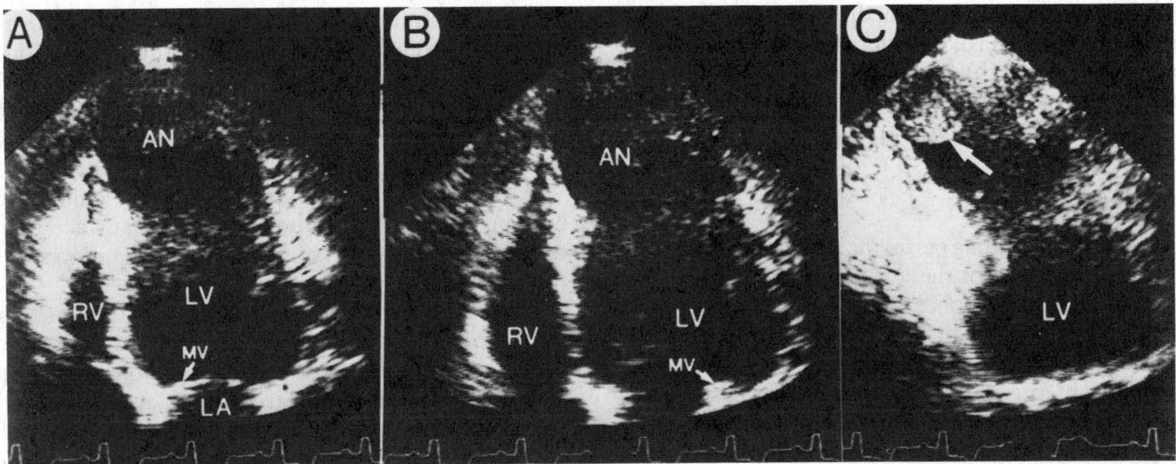

FIGURE 15-35 Two-dimensional echocardiogram from a patient with a recent anterior myocardial infarction. *A.* Systolic frame of the apical four-chamber view. *B.* Diastolic frame of the same view. Both show a large apical aneurysm (AN). The left ventricle (LV) is moderately dilated at its base, but there is extensive thinning of the apical wall. The aneurysm has a wide neck and fundus. *C.* Apical two-chamber view shows a round mass (arrow) partially filling the aneurysm as it extends from the surface of the akinetic wall, indicative of a mural thrombus. RV, right ventricle; LA, left atrium; MV, mitral valve.

of the coronary arteries occur after initial resolution and because therapeutic decisions may be affected.

The ability to image the cardiac structural relations and the lack of reliance on ionizing radiation have made echocardiography extremely useful in evaluating patients with congenital heart disease.[27,33,48,249,250] Valvular heart disease (e.g., bicuspid aortic valve and pulmonic stenosis), Ebsteins *anomaly* of the tricuspid valve, and great-vessel abnormalities (e.g., coarctation of the aorta) can be identified directly with two-dimensional echocardiography, and atrial and ventricular septal defects (Fig. 15-36) can be visualized directly and by contrast echocardiography.[251–253] Cyanotic heart lesions (e.g., tetralogy of Fallot and tricuspid atresia) also readily lend themselves to echocardiographic recognition.[21,22,27,33,42] Even complex congenital heart lesions have been detailed noninvasively using deductive two-dimensional echocardiography and accurate identification of the great arteries, atrioventricular and semilunar valves, interatrial and interventricular septa, and orientation of the ventricles.[254,255] In addition, Doppler ultrasound has been extremely useful in patients with congenital heart disease (Chap. 97). The appropriate use of ultrasound techniques has allowed some patients to undergo surgery without prior cardiac catheterization and angiography.

Fetal ultrasound is being used for prenatal care. Both transvaginal and transabdominal approaches at 10 to 12 and 16 to 18 weeks gestation, respectively, provide

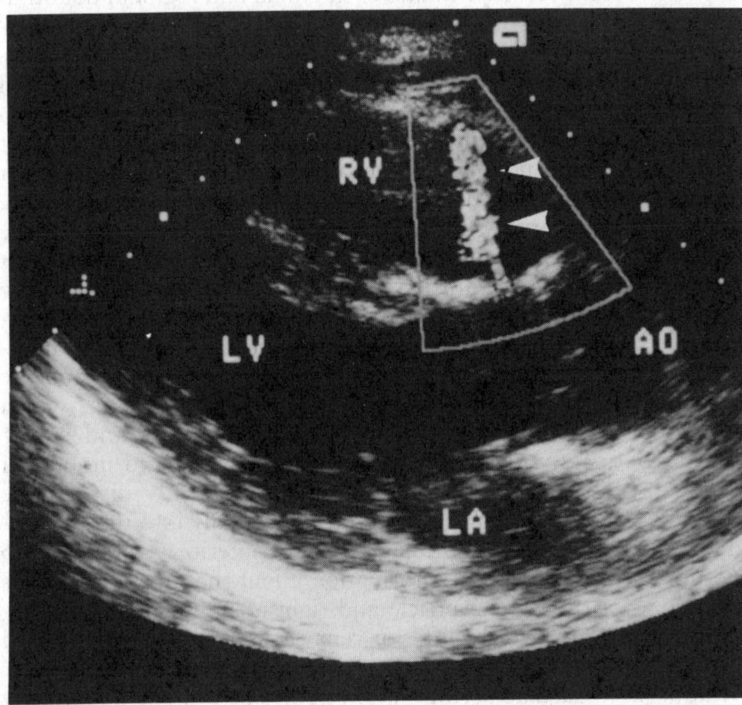

FIGURE 15-36 Parasternal long-axis view in systole of a color Doppler echocardiogram shown in black and white from a patient with a perimembranous ventricular septal defect. The jet of turbulent blood (arrows) is seen passing through the membranous septum into the right ventricle (RV). LV, left ventricle; Ao, aorta; LA, left atrium.

important information about cardiac anatomy and function in utero.[256] In utero, even fetuses with certain congenital lesions (e.g., hypoplastic left-sided heart syndrome and transposition of the great arteries) may now be diagnosed by echocardiography.[15,257]

Ventricular Function

The assessment of cardiac performance, especially global and regional function of the left ventricle, is one of the most valuable clinical applications of echocardiography. Cardiac chamber size can be accurately measured by both M-mode and two-dimensional echocardiography. Left ventricular internal dimensions at end systole and end diastole provide a reliable index of left ventricular chamber size, are subject to the least interobserver variability, and are the most reproducible (Figs. 15-12 and 15-20*A*).[258–262] Virtually all indexes of left ventricular pump performance have been derived from measurements of volume and pressure. The indexes derived from volume measurements, however, have proved to be of greatest clinical value.[258] Left ventricular volumes can be calculated by M mode but are not valid in asynergic ventricles.[56,259–261] Two-dimensional echocardiography offers considerable advantage over M mode for quantitating volumes because a variety of tomographic slices of the left ventricle can be analyzed. The correlations between volumes determined by angiography and by two-dimensional echocardiography in patients with and without asynergy have been excellent ($r = 0.8$ to 0.9).[58–62] Most laboratories measure left ventricular end-diastolic and end-systolic dimensions directly from M-mode studies rather than derive volumes because of the inconvenience and occasional inaccuracies of computerized methods.

Dynamic measurements of left ventricular function include (1) percent fractional shortening, (2) mean circumferential fiber shortening, (3) ejection fraction, (4) mitral E point–interventricular septal separation, (5) percent systolic wall thickening, and (6) wall motion analysis (i.e., hypokinesis, akinesis, dyskinesis). *Percent fractional shortening* of the left ventricle (percent delta D) is a valuable index of the overall left ventricular contractile state. This simple dimensional change, however, is valid only if regional contraction abnormalities are minimal or absent. Determination of mean circumferential fiber shortening (V_{CF}), calculated in the same manner as percent delta D except that ejection time is taken into consideration, is also a useful index of left ventricular performance but does not offer any practical advantages over percent delta D in characterizing left ventricular function. The *mitral E point–septal separation* (EPSS) has proved to be a sensitive and specific indicator of global left ventricular performance (Fig. 15-4).[38] The EPSS is independent of left ventricular size and is not influenced by regional wall motion abnormalities. *Ejection fraction* is the most useful single index of left ventricular function because it correlates best with the patient's clinical outcome.[66] M-mode ejection fraction, however, offers no advantage over the simpler percent delta D expression of contractility and may give spurious information in patients with segmental wall abnormalities. The ejection fraction derived from two-dimensional echocardiographic volumes, however, has been shown to have a more consistent relation to angiographic ejection fraction whether or not asynergy is present (Fig. 15-37). There are a variety of simple echocardiographic methods that provide rapid estimates of ejection fraction, including those of Quinones et al.[67] and Baran et al.[66]

A different index of global left ventricular function may be obtained with the endocardial surface mapping technique of Guyer et al.[263] that creates a planar map of the ventricle.

Two-dimensional echocardiography appears to be the ideal modality for analyzing left ventricular motion and determining regional contractile function, since virtually all segments of the myocardium are accessible with the variety of tomographic planes available.[264] Several specific views, however, apply particularly to wall motion analysis because they reproducibly outline left ventricular anatomy. These are the parasternal long-axis view, the parasternal short-axis view at both the mitral and papillary muscle levels, and the apical four-chamber and two-chamber views (Fig. 15-34). Analysis of regional endocardial wall motion (ie., hypokinesis, akinesis, and dyskinesis), as well as regional wall thickening, is necessary for discriminating between normal and ischemic or infarcted zones of myocardium. M-mode echocardiography is considerably restricted in analyzing regional left ventricular function, since it images only in the septal-posterolateral plane and is unreliable in the presence of asynergy. Nevertheless, because of its high resolution (1 to 2 mm), regional wall motion analysis, including amplitude and rate of motion from end diastole to peak systole and measurements of thickening of both the left side of the septum and the posterior wall, is even better than that obtained by radionuclide angiography.

The evaluation of right-sided cardiac chambers and function has not been reliable using M-mode echocardiography but has been greatly enhanced by two-dimensional echocardiography.[40,48,69] The unusual shape of the right ventricle makes even global and regional quantitative data difficult to obtain, but clinically useful qualitative information regarding right ventricular function, especially in patients with right ventricular infarction, can be provided. The right-sided structures are well seen in the parasternal long-axis right ventricular inflow tract view, since the anteroposterior dimension of the right ventricle and most of the right atrium are well visualized. Parasternal short-axis views of the left ventricle at the level of the chordae tendineae and parasternal short-axis views of the aortic root provide additional views of the right ventricle. The apical four-chamber view, however, appears to be the single most important view for evaluating the size and function of the right ventricle and the right atrium. Pulmonary arterial hypertension, which may cause right ventricular hypertrophy and subsequently dilatation, influences the shape and motion of the interventricular septum. It frequently distorts the septum, causing it to bulge abnormally into the left ventricle. Subcostal imaging of the inferior vena cava also provides useful information about the functional status of the right ventricle and right atrium. The respiratory collapse of the inferior vena caval diameter may be used to determine if the central venous pressure is elevated.[265]

Cardiac performance can also be evaluated indirectly

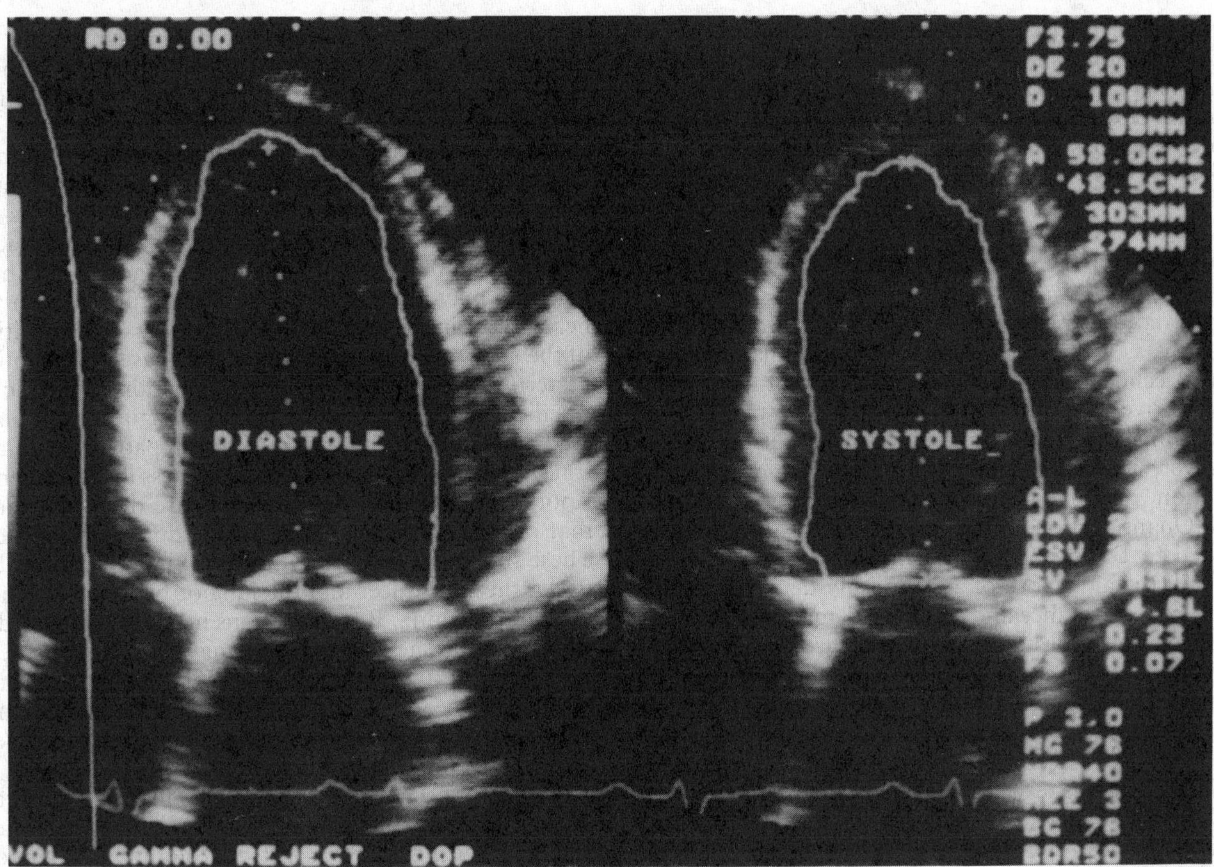

FIGURE 15-37 Two-dimensional apical two-chamber view shows a method for determining the left ventricular ejection fraction. The endocardium of the left ventricle is planimetered as shown at end diastole and end systole, respectively. From the left ventricular areas, the left ventricular volumes at end diastole (LVEDV) and end systole (LVESV) are calculated by standard formulas. The left ventricular ejection fraction is calculated as (LVEDV − LVESV)/LVEDV.

by analyzing the motion of the heart valves with M-mode echocardiography. Mitral valve analysis can relate hemodynamic information as follows: (1) Reduction in the diastolic (EF) slope suggests a reduced rate of left ventricular filling (Fig. 15-21*B*)[21,22]; (2) premature closure suggests elevated left ventricular diastolic pressure, especially in patients with acute aortic regurgitation (Fig. 15-21*A*)[173]; (3) increased EPSS inversely correlates with ejection fraction; (4) reduced E-point amplitude or delayed valve opening with an accentuated A wave suggests elevated left ventricular early diastolic pressure, especially in patients with severe chronic aortic regurgitation (Fig. 15-21*A*)[21,22]; and (5) a prominent shoulder (B notch) on the closing (AC) slope or a PR minus AC interval of less than 0.06 s suggests elevated left ventricular end-diastolic pressure (Fig.15-21*B*).[22] The rate of left atrial emptying (or left ventricular filling) is reflected by the slope of the posterior aortic root in early diastole. It is another useful indirect measurement of left ventricular function. A flat posterior aortic wall in early diastole suggests reduced left ventricular filling.[266]

The area of opening of the aortic valve and the pattern of leaflet motion provide qualitative information about left ventricular stroke volume.[21,22] Among structurally normal aortic valves, cusp separation is a function of initial forward left ventricular stroke volume, whereas the distance between cusps throughout systole and the time the cusps remain separated are affected by aortic flow volume, velocity, and heart rate. In low-output states or with significant mitral regurgitation, the aortic leaflets tend to open abruptly but close gradually throughout systole (early partial aortic valve closure) and, therefore, have a systolic pattern that more closely resembles a bullet than the usual parallelogram (Fig. 15-22*A*).[21] Premature opening of the aortic valve suggests markedly elevated left ventricular diastolic pressure, especially in patients with very severe aortic regurgitation (Fig. 15-22*B*).[267] Very early systolic partial closure (notch) is evidence of outflow tract obstruction in patients with discrete membranous subvalvular aortic stenosis, whereas early to midsystolic partial (notch) or complete closure is evidence of obstruction in patients with hypertrophic cardiomyopathy (Fig. 15-22*A*).[21,22]

Analysis of pulmonic valve motion may be useful in determining the hemodynamic status of the right side of the heart. Pulmonary arterial hypertension is suggested by a combination of reduced or absent *a* dip, midsystolic notch, flat EF slope, and/or abnormal right-sided systolic time intervals.[21,22] A midsystolic notch may suggest elevated pulmonary vascular resistance. An abnormally large *a* dip suggests valvular pulmonic stenosis, whereas coarse systolic fluttering suggests infundibular pulmonic stenosis. However, a normal *a* dip may be seen in patients with pulmonary hypertension complicated by right-sided heart failure, whereas an absent *a* dip may be seen in patients with valvular pulmonic stenosis and a fibrotic pulmonic valve. Tricuspid valve motion is also influenced by the functional status of the structures of the right side of the heart. For example, a prominent B notch on the tricuspid closing slope is evidence of elevated right ventricular end-diastolic pressure.[21,22]

LIMITATIONS OF ECHOCARDIOGRAPHY

As with all imaging procedures, echocardiography has strengths as well as weaknesses.[268–272] The major limitation of echocardiography has been lack of automated quantitative measurements, especially to two-dimensional imaging. This limitation is also its strength, however, since echocardiography allows a mental reconstruction of three-dimensional/tomographic information. Quantification that is automated has been widely applied to Doppler measurements, but echocardiography still remains more of a technically demanding skill as far as performance and clinically demanding as far as interpretation. One limitation of echocardiography is the inability to obtain complete diagnostic information in all patients. Delineation of total cardiac anatomic information may be achieved in only 80 to 90 percent of studies.[21,22,48] Recent advances in instrumentation and the use of multiple acoustic windows has improved, and some investigators believe that with higher frequencies complete studies can be obtained. Since ultrasound travels poorly through bone, lung, and thick-walled chests, ultrasound examination of the heart may be difficult in patients who have marked skeletal abnormalities such as pectus excavatum, patients with severe pulmonary disease (although subcostal windows often provide adequate information), and extremely obese patients.

M-mode echocardiography as an independent examination is rarely performed in North America. Obviously M mode, being an ice-pick view of the heart,[22] lacks spatial orientation of intracardiac structures and does not provide two-dimensional tomographic information. A major limitation of M-mode echocardiography is its inability to assess global LV function in the setting of marked regional wall motion abnormalities. Hence, the incorporation of M mode into the two-dimensional exam allows for this limitation of the M-mode technique to be bypassed.

A limitation of two-dimensional echocardiography, in addition to its somewhat qualitative analysis and lack of automated quantitative analysis, is the complexity of cardiac anatomic information provided by the two-dimensional imaging planes. For those not well versed in two-dimensional echocardiographic anatomy, initial views can be quite confusing. Improvement in standardization of views, as well as understanding of echocardiographic anatomy brought about by the use of transesophageal echo by many disciplines, has minimized this problem.

Misinterpretation of a cardiovascular study can be due to technical limitations. There is a real danger of mistaking artifacts or extraneous echos that result from the apparent or unexplained behavior of reflected ultrasound for evidence of cardiac disease.[271] It is possible for ultrasound to be reflected twice from a cardiac structure and appear on the echocardiographic tracing as an abnormal echo. These reverberatory or "phantom" echoes are the most common artifacts. They result from multiple reflections of acoustic energy and affect both the M-mode display and the two-dimensional images.[268] Careful measurement shows that these artifacts give the false impression of a second interface virtually twice as far from the transducer as the true echo (first interface), and their amplitude will be twice as large.[20,271,272] These reechoes may also occur between structures within the heart, resulting in an apparent deepening of the position of the structure and inversion of the phase of its motion pattern. Reverberations also occur within a fibrotic or calcified valve. This might partially explain the multilayered appearance of the mitral valve in patients with mitral stenosis and invalidates the thickness measurements. Another example of reverberations are the lung echoes that often obscure the entire image during inspiration. These shallow echoes are simply multiple reflections between the transducer and the lung or between the chest wall and the lung. Reverberations may also be recorded from intracardiac catheters, pacing wires, or prosthetic valves.[268,272] Ultrasound reflected from the plastic casing of the scan head of two-dimensional transducers tends to appear within the left ventricular image near its apex, thus mimicking a mural thrombus.

Artifactual echoes may also be produced by incorrect use of the echocardiographic controls.[271] Inappropriately high gain settings cause targets to "bloom" (i.e., appear larger and more distorted than their actual size and shape). This may result in valve orifices appearing reduced on two-dimensional echocardiographic studies when they are compared with the other targets. Other problems resulting from excessive gain include the following: (1) False-negative diagnoses because of obliteration of the echo-free space, as might be seen in the presence of a pericardial effusion. (2) Reduction in left ventricular cavity size by lengthening the trailing edge of the left-sided septal echo.[16,17] Since an interface is best displayed by the leading edge of its echo and not by its trailing edge, the use of high-gain settings to visualize the septum will lengthen the trailing edge of the left-sided septal echo. (3) Cloudlike noise in cardiac cavities, which may be misread as intracardiac thrombi. Artifacts can also be produced by inappropriate use of the near-gain compensation control and TGC control. The most common error introduced by incorrect use of these echocardiographic controls is the elimination of a portion of the echoes from the right side of the interventricular septum or even from the entire septum itself. This kind of artifact can be avoided by a judicious use of the TGC control, even if this results in unwanted echoes in the right ventricle.[269,270]

All transducers have beam patterns that contain "side-lobe" artifacts. These weaker beams of ultrasound energy are adjacent to the main beam and are generated from the edges of the individual transducer elements. They appear as an arclike, hazily bordered, lateral extension of a prominent echo-producing structure.[271,272] Characteristically, side-lobe artifacts produce extended echoes from strong reflecting surfaces such as pericardium, calcified valves, or prostheses and are depicted throughout the full sector image. Although these phantom echoes are generally weaker in intensity than those reflected from the main beam, they may occasionally be confused with true anatomic structure. Side-lobe artifacts can usually be diminished or eliminated by decreasing the gain settings or increasing the reject level of the ultrasound instruments.

One of the most serious limitations of the echocardiographic systems in current use is the width of the ultrasound beam, which determines lateral resolution.[22,39,40,271,272] Ultrasound energy cannot be accurately focused over the entire depth range of the beam but spreads over a finite angle. This causes some echoes to appear as if they are from structures in the central beam, whereas, in fact, they are echoes from structures off the main or display axis. These nonstructural spurious echoes are displayed at a site where there is no directly corresponding anatomic structure and may result in misinterpretation of clinical tracings. An echo from a target on the edge of the ultrasound beam may be displayed as if it were in the middle and will, therefore, not represent the true location of the target. The intensity of echoes from reflecting structures may vary widely, since they depend on several physical factors such as distance traveled, acoustic impedance, and angle of incidence of the sound beam. Thus, only structures that are relatively perpendicular to the ultrasonic beam will be accurately recorded, and target "dropout" results when the transducer-to-target relation is not maintained. Target dropout is quite common in two-dimensional echocardiography, because the multiple ultrasonic beams that are directed from the transducer are reflected from irregular cardiac targets, only some of which may be perpendicular to the interrogating beam.[42,271] Dropouts of the interventricular septum may falsely suggest the existence of an interventricular septal defect, whereas endocardial dropouts hamper the correct identification of the true ventricular wall contour in stop-frame images.

Two dimensional images are displayed on a cathode ray tube during the examination and are recorded on videotape, using a standard television camera or a digital scan converter, for a permanent record and subsequent analysis. This process may deteriorate image quality. In most systems only half of the scan lines, and thus only one-half of the information available during real-time study, is available for all off-line analyses. In addition, there is loss of information when the video format is displayed in stop-action. Furthermore, videotape remains a difficult, expensive, and cumbersome medium for data storage and retrieval. The television format itself can produce ghosts (persistent artifacts of structures that had appeared on the screen a moment before and had not quite faded away when the next image arrived).[40,271]

Electrical interference elsewhere in the building can also produce artifacts that appear as irregular, fine, linear markings on the tracing, with abrupt onset and cessation.[17,40,271] They should not be mistaken for the microbubbles produced by saline solution injections in contrast echocardiography or for swirling intracavitary blood in patients with low-cardiac-output syndromes.

Pitfalls may also be related to improper examination technique. When the transducer is at a higher than standard interspace, the anterior aortic wall is closer to the transducer than the septum is, and a false pattern of aortic-septal discontinuity may be recorded. A high transducer position can also give a pattern suggestive of MVP in normal subjects because the mitral leaflets move away from the transducer during systole when the base of the left ventricle moves toward the apex.

For most cardiac diseases clinical information is highly valuable for making intelligent echocardiographic conclusions. Professional interpretation of the ECG should not be separated from the individual conducting the study, an interpretation should be based only on what can be definitely identified. Making judgments from incomplete echoes or in the absence of electrocardiographic reference should be avoided.[269-271] As an example, paradoxical septal motion is not a specific abnormality and is seen in many conditions, such as right ventricular volume overload lesions and myocardial infarction and after open heart surgery or in the presence of left bundle branch block as shown by the ECG. Changing sensitivity and specificity of various echocardiographic criteria must also be known. For instance, asymmetric septal hypertrophy, once believed specific for hypertrophic cardiomyopathy, now is known to occur in newborns and in patients with systemic hypertension, aortic stenosis, pulmonary hypertension, and a variety of congenital heart diseases.

NEW APPLICATIONS AND THE FUTURE OF ECHOCARDIOGRAPHY

Several developments that have been perfected or are presently under investigation offer an exciting future for echocardiography. These include computerizing ("digitizing") the ultrasonic image, ultrasound tissue characterization, myocardial biopsy, intravascular ultrasound, myocardial perfusion imaging with contrast, and three-dimensional echocardiography. Most of the newer ultrasound equipment presently displays the echocardiographic images in a digital rather than analog format.[273] *Digital image processing* improves the image and allows for manipulation and evaluation of echoes by computer. Its main clinical uses include (1) ability to obtain quantitative information, (2) structure enhancement and identification that make regional wall motion abnormalities more apparent,[274] (3) three-dimensional reconstructing, and (4) detailed acoustic analysis of tissue.

Ultrasound tissue characterization is the study of using ultrasound to gain information about tissues beyond simply locating the positions of major cardiac structures and studying their motion patterns.[275-277] The variation in the amplitude of sound backscattered to the transducer from the myocardium appears to be related to muscle characteristics.[276,277] Clinical areas in which echocardiography has recognized alterations in cardiac tissue include the detection of fibrosis and calcification and the identification of myocardial scar.[278] Scarred areas of the myocardium, for example, are more echo intense and thinner than normal muscle. An alteration in the myocardial echoes has also been noted in patients with hypertrophic cardiomyopathy and amyloid heart disease.[279] Thus far, most of the observations using echocardiography for the analysis of tissue type have been qualitative in nature.

Conversion of the gray-scale image to color (so called B-color), which enhances the differences in the returning echoes and permits better identification of tissue types, has been performed, is commercially available, and may provide the impetus for further advancement in this area.[280] Less "echodense" tissue such as blood or fat displays darker shades of gray. Valve or scar tissue are displayed whiter and the myocardium is shown as varying levels of gray. The human eye, however, is more sensitive in distinguishing different shades of colors than shades of gray.[281] The color scale can be manipulated to emphasize higher or lower amplitudes, greatly enhancing the eye's perception of an image. For instance, apical ventricular thrombi are frequently difficult to differentiate from underlying myocardium by standard gray-scale compression. The B-color map may facilitate fine differentiation of fibrosed myocardium (denser, lighter shades) from thrombus (less dense, darker color). In addition, a redundant mitral valve may be imaged in B-color to resolve possible vegetations that may not be readily apparent by gray scale. The increasing use of computer analysis of echocardiographic data should help develop a quantative method for identifying subtle changes in acoustic properties, whether they be in color or various shades of gray. *Myocardial biopsy* under echocardiographic guidance to monitor heart transplant patients for episodes of rejection is now standard practice in our institution.

Intravascular ultrasound has been used to directly identify arterial vessel wall pathology by using extremely high frequency two-dimensional echocardiographic transducers mounted on vascular catheters.[12,282]

Myocardial perfusion imaging by contrast echocardiography employing intracoronary sonicated albumin can be used to evaluate left ventricular wall motion, investigate areas of ischemia, and detect reperfusion hyperemia.[283,284] When echo contrast is injected into a coronary artery, the myocardium supplied by that vessel "brightens" as the contrast travels into the myocardium.[285,286]

Reconstructed three-dimensional echocardiography may provide an enhanced appreciation for spatially oriented data. Several techniques are available for assessing the position and angle of the ultrasonic transducer, which is all that is necessary for the reconstruction of multiple two-dimensional images into a three-dimensional display.[284,287] Irrespective of how a three-dimensional echocardiogram is obtained, it theoretically should provide a more accurate spatial image of the heart and thus provide more accurate quantitative and qualitative information.

REFERENCES

1. Keidel WD: Über eine neue Methode zur Registrierung der Volumän-derungen des Herzens am Menschen. *Z Kreisl-Forsch* 1950; 39:257–271.
2. Edler I, Hertz CH: The use of ultrasonic reflectoscope for the continuous recording of movement of heart walls. *Kungl Fysiogr Sallski Fund Forhandl* 1954; 24:40–45.
3. Holmes JH, Howry DH, Posakony GJ, et al: Ultrasonic visualization of soft tissue structures in human body. *Trans Am Clin Climatol Assoc* 1955; 66:208–212.
4. Joyner CR, Reid JM, Bond, JP: Reflected ultrasound in the assessment of mitral valve disease. *Circulation* 1963; 27:503–509.
5. Feigenbaum H, Waldhausen JA, Hyde PP: Ultrasound diagnosis of pericardial effusion. *JAMA* 1965; 191:711–714.
6. Joyner CR, Jr, Reid JM: Application of ultrasound in cardiology and cardiovascular physiology. *Progr Cardiovasc Dis* 1963; 5:482–497.
7. Ebina T, Oka S, Tanaka M, et al: The ultrasonotomography of the heart and great vessels in living human subjects by means of ultrasonic reflection technique. *Jpn Heart J* 1967; 8:331–337.
8. Bom N, Lancee CT Jr, Van Zwieten G, Kloster FE, Roelandt J et al: Multiscan echocardiography: I. Technical description. *Circulation* 1973; 48:1066–1073.
9. Baker DW: Pulsed ultrasonic Doppler blood-flow sensing. *IEEE Trans Sonics Ultrasonics* 1970; SU-17(3).
10. Garcia E, Gueret P, Bennet M, et al: Digital image processing of two-dimensional echocardiograms: Identification of the endocardium. *Am J Cardiol* 1981; 48:479–486.
11. Hanrath P, Kremer P, Langenstein BA, Matsumoto M, Bleifeld W: Transosophageale Echokardiographie: Ein neues Verfahren zur dynamischen Ventrikelfunktions-analyse. *Dtsch Med Wochenschr* 1981; 106:523–525.
12. Pandian NG, Schwartz SL, Hsu TL, et al: Intracardiac echocardiography: Experimental observations on intracavitary imaging of cardiac structures with 20-MHz ultrasound catheters. *Echocardiography* 1991; 8:127–134.
13. Crouse LJ, Harbrecht JJ, Vacek JL, Rosamond TL, Kramer PH: Exercise echocardiography as a screening test for coronary artery disease and correlation with coronary arteriography. *Am J Cardiol* 1991; 67:1213–1218.
14. Distante A, Moscarelli E, Morales MA, Lattanzi F, et al: Pharmacologic methods instead of exercise for the assessment of coronary artery disease. *Echocardiography* 1991; 8:99–114.
15. Gidding SS, Huhta JC: Cardiac ultrasound: Its role in the recognition and management of fetal heart disease. *Echocardiography* 1991; 8:441–466.
16. Wells PNT: *Physical Principles of Ultrasonic Diagnosis*. London, Academic, 1969.
17. Hillard W: Basic physics of ultrasound. In: Schapira J, Charuzi Y, Davidson RM (eds): *Two-Dimensional Echocardiography*. Baltimore, Williams & Wilkins, 1982; 319.
18. Woodward B, Pond JB, Warwick R: How safe is diagnostic sonar? *Br J Radiol* 1970; 43:719–725.
19. Meltzer RS, Gramiak R: Safety considerations related to ultrasonic energy exposure during echocardiographic examinations. *Am J Cardiol* 1986; 58:1268–1269.
20. Roelandt J, van Dorp WC, Bom N, et al: Resolution problems in echocardiography: A source of interpretation error. *Am J Cardiol* 1976; 37:256–362.
21. Felner JM, Schlant RC: *Echocardiography: A Teaching Atlas*. New York, Grune & Stratton, 1976: 562.
22. Feigenbaum H: *Echocardiography*, 4th ed. Philadelphia, Lea & Febiger, 1986; 662.
23. Weyman AE: *Cross-Sectional Echocardiography*. Philadelphia, Lea & Febiger, 1982; 522.
24. Griffith JM, Henry WL: A sector scanner for real time two-dimensional echocardiography. *Circulation* 1974; 49:1147–1152.
25. von Ramm OT, Thurstone RL: Cardiac imaging using a phased array ultrasonic system: I. System design. *Circulation* 1976; 53:258–262.
26. Nishimura K, Hibi N, Fukui T, et al: Real-time observation of cardiac movement and structures in congenital and acquired heart disease employing high-speed ultrasonocardiotomography. *Am Heart J* 1976; 92:340–347.
27. Meyer, RA: *Pediatric Echocardiography*. Philadelphia, Lea & Febiger, 1977: 303.
28. Henry WL: Evaluation of left ventricular function using two-dimensional echocardiography. 1982; *Am J Cardiol* 49:319–327.
29. Pearlman AS, Gardin JM, Martin RP, et al: Guidelines for optimal physician training in echocardiography: Recommendations of the American Society of Echocardiography Committee for Physician Training in Echocardiography. *Am J Cardiol* 1987; 60:158–163.
30. Seventeenth Bethesda Conference: Adult cardiology training, November 1, 2, 1985, Bethesda, Maryland. *J. Am Coll Cardiol* 1986; 7:1191–1218.
31. Meyer RA, Hagler D, Huhta J, Smallhorn J, Snider R, Williams R: Guidelines for physician training in pediatric echocardiography: Recommendations of the Society of Pediatric Echocardiography

Committee on Physician Training. *Am J Cardiol* 1987; 60:164–165.

32. ACC/AHA guidelines: American College Cardiology/American Heart Assoc Task Force for the Clinical Application of Echocardiography *Circulation* 1990; 82:2323–2345.
33. Silverman NH, Snider AR: *Two-Dimensional Echocardiography in Congenital Heart Disease.* Norwalk, CT, Appleton-Century-Crofts, 1982.
34. Sahn D, DeMaria A, Kisslo J, Weyman AE: Recommendations regarding quantitation in M-mode echocardiography: Results of a survey of echocardiographic measurements. *Circulation* 1978; 58:1072–1083.
35. Friedman M, Roeske WR, Sahn DJ, et al: Accuracy of M-mode echocardiographic measurements of the left ventricle. *Am J Cardiol* 1982; 49:716–723.
36. Crawford MH, Grant D, O'Rourke RA, et al: Accuracy and reproducibility of new M-mode echocardiographic recommendations for measuring left ventricular dimensions. *Circulation* 1980; 61:137–143.
37. Popp R, Filly K, Brown OR, et al: Effect of transducer placement on echocardiographic measurement of left ventricular dimension. *Am J Cardiol* 1975; 35:537–541.
38. Massic BM, Schiller NB, Ratshin RA, et al: Mitral-septal separation: New echocardiographic index of left ventricular function. *Am J Cardiol* 1977; 39:1008–1016.
39. Henry WL, Gardin JM, Ware JH: Echocardiographic measurements in normal subjects from infancy to old age. *Circulation* 1980; 62:1054–1061.
40. Tajik AJ, Seward JB, Hagler DJ, et al: Two-dimensional real-time ultrasonic imaging of the heart and great vessels: Technique image orientation, structure, identification, and validation. *Mayo Clin Proc* 1978; 53:271–303.
41. Henry WL, DeMaria A, Gramiak R, et al: Report of the American Society of Echocardiography Committee on Nomenclature and Standards in Two-Dimensional Echocardiography. *Circulation* 1980; 62:212–217.
42. Sahn DJ, Anderson F: *Two-Dimensional Anatomy of the Heart. An Atlas for Echocardiographers.* New York, Wiley, 1982: 461.
43. Edwards WD, Tajik AJ, Seward JB: Standardized nomenclature and anatomic basis for regional tomographic analysis of the heart. *Mayo Clin Proc* 1981; 56:479–497.
44. Bierman FZ, Williams RG: Subxiphoid two-dimensional imaging of the interatrial septum in infants with congenital heart disease. *Circulation* 1979; 60:80–90.
45. Shub C, Dimopoulos IN, Seward JB, et al: Sensitivity of two-dimensional echocardiography in the direct visualization of atrial septal defect utilizing the subcostal approach: Experience with 154 patients. *J Am Coll Cardiol* 1983; 2:127–135.
46. Snider RA, Silverman NH: Suprasternal notch echocardiography: A two-dimensional technique for evaluating congenital heart disease. *Circulation* 1981; 63:165–173.
47. Schnittger I, Gordon EP, Fitzgerald PJ, et al: Standardized intracardiac measurements of two-dimensional echocardiography. *J Am Coll Cardiol* 1983; 2:934–938.
48. Hagan AD, DiSessa TG, Bloor CM, Culleja HB: *Two-Dimensional Echocardiography: Clinical-Pathological Correlations in Adult and Congenital Heart Disease.* Boston, Little, Brown, 1983: 568.
49. Woythaler JN, Singer SL, Kwan O, et al: Accuracy of echocardiography versus electrocardiography in detecting left ventricular hypertrophy: Comparison with postmortem mass measurements. *J Am Coll Cardiol* 1983; 2:305–311.
50. Reicheck N, Helak J, Plappert T, et al: Anatomic validation of left ventricular mass estimates from clinical two-dimensional echocardiography: Initial results. *Circulation* 1983; 67:348–352.
51. Bommer W, Weinert L, Neumann A, et al: Determination of right atrial and right ventricular size by two-dimensional echocardiography. *Circulation* 1979; 60:91–100.
52. Prakish R: Echocardiographic diagnosis of right ventricular hypertrophy: Correlation with ECG and necropsy findings in 248 patients. *Cathet Cardiovasc Diagn* 1981; 7:179–186.
53. Feigenbaum H, Popp RL, Wolfe SB, et al: Ultrasound measurements of the left ventricle: A correlative study with angiography. *Arch Intern Med* 1972; 129:461–467.
54. Belenkie I, Nutter DO, Clark DW, McCraw DB, Raizner AE: Assessment of left ventricular dimensions and functions by echocardiography. *Am J Cardiol* 1973; 31:755–762.
55. Murray JA, Johnston W, Reed J: Echocardiographic determination of left ventricular dimension, volumes and performance. *Am J Cardiol* 1972; 30:252–257.
56. Teichholz LE, Kruelen TH, Herman MV, Gorlin R: Problems in echocardiographic volume determinations: Echo-angiographic correlations in the presence or absence of asynergy. *Am J Cardiol* 1976; 37:7–12.
57. Abdulla AM, Frank MJ, Canedo ML, et al: Limitations of echocardiography in the assessment of left ventricular size and function in aortic regurgitation. *Circulation* 1980; 61:148–155.
58. Starling MR, Crawford MH, Sorensen SG, et al: Comparative accuracy of apical biplane cross-sectional echocardiography and gated equilibrium radionuclide angiography for estimating left ventricular size and performance. *Circulation* 1981; 63:1075–1081.
59. Erbel R, Schweizer P, Meyer J, et al: Left ventricular volume and ejection fraction determination by cross-sectional echocardiography in patients with coronary artery disease: A prospective study. *Clin Cardiol* 1980; 3:377–383.
60. Tortoledo FA, Quinones MA, Fernandez GC, et al: Quantification of left ventricular volumes by two-dimensional echocardiography: A simplified and accurate approach. *Circulation* 1983; 67:579–584.
61. Gordon EP, Schnittger I, Fitzgerald PJ, et al: Reproducibility of left ventricular volumes by two-dimensional echocardiography. *J Am Coll Cardiol* 1983; 2:506–513.
62. Wahr DW, Wang YS, Schiller NB: Left ventricular volumes determined by two-dimensional echocardiography in a normal adult population. *J Am Coll Cardiol* 1983; 1:863–868.
63. Gutman J, Wang YS, Wahr D, et al: Normal left atrial function determined by two-dimensional echocardiography. *Am J Cardiol* 1983; 51:336–340.
64. Folland ED, Parisi AF, Moynihan PF, et al: Assessment of left ventricular ejection fraction and volumes by real-time, two-dimensional echocardiography and radionuclide techniques. *Circulation* 1979; 60:760–766.
65. Silverman MH, Schiller NB: Apex echocardiography. *Circulation* 1978; 57:503–511.
66. Baran AO, Rogal GJ, Nanda NC: Ejection fraction determination without planimetry by two-dimensional echocardiography: A new method. *J Am Coll Cardiol* 1983; 1:1471–1478.
67. Quinones MA, Waggoner AD, Reduto LA, et al: A new simplified and accurate method for determining ejection fraction with two-dimensional echocardiography. *Circulation* 1981; 64:744–753.
68. Helak J, Reichek N: Quantitation of human left ventricular mass and volume by cross-sectional echocardiography: In vitro anatomic validation. *Circulation* 1981; 63:398–407.
69. Levine RA, Gibson TC, Aretz T, et al: Echocardiographic measurement of right ventricular volume. *Circulation* 1984; 69:497–505.
70. Mills P, Craige E: Echophonocardiography. *Prog Cardiovasc Dis* 1978; 20:337–351.
71. Felner JM, Miller DD: Echocardiographic characteristics of normally and abnormally functioning mechanical prosthetic heart valves. *Echocardiography* 1984; 1:261–310.
72. Felner JM, Harwood S, Mond H, et al: Systolic honks in young children. *Am J Cardiol* 1977; 40:206–211.
73. Stefadouros MA, Witham AC: Systolic time intervals by echocardiography. *Circulation* 1975; 51:114–117.
74. Hirschfeld S, Meyer RA, Schwartz DC, et al: Measurement of right and left ventricular systolic time intervals by echocardiography. *Circulation* 1975; 51:304–309.
75. Gramiak R, Shah PM, Kramer DH: Ultrasound cardiography: Contrast studies in anatomy and function. *Radiology* 1976; 92:939–948.
76. Tajik AJ, Seward JB: Contrast echocardiography. In: Kotler MN, Segal BL (eds): *Clinical Echocardiography,* and Brest AN (ed): *Cardiovascular Clinics.* Philadelphia, FA Davis, 1978: 317.
77. Wise NK, Myers S, Fraker TD, et al: Contrast M-mode ultrasonography of the inferior vena cava. 1981; *Circulation* 63:1100–1103.
78. Weyman A, Feigenbaum H, Dillon J, et al: Noninvasive visualization of the left main coronary artery by cross-sectional echocardiography. *Circulation* 1976; 54:169–174.
79. Valdes-Cruz LM, Sahn, DJ: Ultrasonic contrast studies for the detection of cardiac shunts. *J Am Coll Cardiol* 1984; 3:978–985.
80. DePace NL, Ross J, Iskandrian AS, et al: Tricuspid regurgitation:

Noninvasive techniques for determining causes and severity. *J Am Coll Cardiol* 1984; 3:1540–1550.
81. Seward JB, Tajik AJ, Hagler DJ: Peripheral venous contrast echocardiography. *Am J Cardiol* 1977; 39:202–212.
82. Truman AT, Syamasundar RP, Kulangara RJ: Use of contrast echocardiography in diagnosis of anomalous connection of right superior vena cava to left atrium. *Br. Heart J* 1980; 4:718–723.
83. Meltzer R, Tickner EG, Sahines TP, et al: The source of ultrasonic contrast effects. *JCU* 1980; 8:121–127.
84. DeMaria AN, Bommer W, Takeda P, et al: Value and limitations of contrast echocardiography in cardiac diagnosis. In: Fowler NO (ed), *Noninvasive Diagnostic Methods in Cardiology*. Philadelphia, FA Davis, 1983: 167.
85. Valdes-Cruz LM, Pieroni DR, Roland JMA, et al: Recognition of residual postoperative shunts by contrast echocardiographic techniques. *Circulation* 1977; 55:148–152.
86. Bommer WJ, Shah PN, Allen H, et al: The safety of contrast echocardiography: Report of the committee on contrast echocardiography in the American Society of Echocardiography. *J Am Coll Cardiol* 1984; 3:6–13.
87. Weyman AE, Wann LS, Caldwell RL, et al: Negative contrast echocardiography: A new method for detecting left-to-right shunts. *Circulation* 1979; 59:498–505.
88. Lieppe W, Behar VS, Scallion R, et al: Detection of tricuspid regurgitation with two-dimensional echocardiography and peripheral vein injections. *Circulation* 1978; 57:128–132.
89. Meltzer RS, Vered ZVI, Roelandt JOS, et al: Systematic analysis of contrast echocardiograms. *Am J Cardiol* 1983; 52:375–380.
90. Smith MD, Kwan OL, Reiser HJ, et al: Superior intensity and reproducibility of SHU-454, a new right heart contrast agent. *J Am Coll Cardiol* 1984; 3:992–998.
91. Ten Cate FJ, Feinstein S, Zwehl W, et al: Two-dimensional contrast echocardiography: II. Transpulmonary studies. *J Am Coll Cardiol* 1984; 3:21–27.
92. Maurer G, Ong K, Haendchen R, et al: Myocardial contrast two-dimensional echocardiography: Comparison of contrast disappearance rates in normal and underperfused myocardium. *Circulation* 1984; 69:418–429.
93. Shapiro JR, Reisner SA, Lichtenberg GS, Meltzer RS: IV contrast echocardiography with use of sonicated albumin in humans: Systolic disappearance of left ventricular contrast after transpulmonary transmission. *J Am Coll Cardiol* 1990; 16:1603–1607.
94. Kraunz RF, Kennedy JW: Ultrasonic determination of left ventricular wall motion in normal man: Studies at rest and after exercise. *Am Heart J* 1970; 79:36–43.
95. Maurer G, Nanda NC: Two-dimensional echocardiographic evaluation of exercise-induced left and right ventricular asynergy: Correlation with thallium scanning. *Am J Cardiol* 1981; 48:720–727.
96. Richards KL: Exercise echocardiography. *Am J Coll Cardiol* 1988; 11:1000–1001.
97. Applegate RJ, Dell'Italia LJ, Crawford MH: Usefulness of two-dimensional echocardiography during low-level exercise testing early after uncomplicated acute myocardial infarction. *Am J Cardiol* 1987; 60:10–14.
98. Morganroth J, Chen CC, David D, et al: Exercise cross-sectional echocardiographic diagnosis of coronary artery disease. *Am J Cardiol* 1981; 47:20–26.
99. Limacher MC, Quinones MA, Lawrence PR, et al: Detection of coronary artery disease with exercise two-dimensional echocardiography: Description of a clinically applicable method and comparison with radionuclide ventriculography. *Circulation* 1983; 67:1211–1218.
100. Crawford MH, Petru MA, Amon KW, et al: Comparative value of two-dimensional echocardiography and radionuclide angiography for quantitating changes in left ventricular performance during exercise limited by angina pectoris. *Am J Cardiol* 1984; 53:42–46.
101. Ryan T, Vasey CG, Presti CF, et al: Exercise echocardiography: Detection of coronary artery disease in patients with normal left ventricular wall motion at rest. *J Am Coll Cardiol* 1988; 11:993–999.
102. Sawada SG, Segar DS, Ryan T, et al: Echocardiographic detection of coronary artery disease during dobutamine infusion. *Circulation* 1991; 83:1605–1614.
103. Picano E, Lattanzi F, Masini M, et al: Comparison of high dose dipyridamole-echocardiography test and exercise two-dimensional echocardiography for diagnosis of coronary artery disease. *Am J Cardiol* 1987; 59:539–542.
104. Burggraf GW, Parker JD: Left ventricular volume changes after amyl nitrite and nitroglycerin in man as measured by ultrasound. *Circulation* 1974; 49:136–143.
105. Winkle RA, Goodman DJ, Popp RL: Simultaneous echocardiographic-phonocardiographic recordings at rest and during amyl nitrite administration in patients with mitral valve prolapse. *Circulation* 1975; 51:522–529.
106. Parisi AF, Harrington JJ, Askenazi J, et al: Echocardiographic evaluation of the valsalva maneuver in healthy subjects and patients with and without heart failure. *Circulation* 1976; 54:921–927.
107. Waldman JD, Rummerfield PS, Gilpin EA, et al: Radiation exposure to the child during cardiac catheterization. *Circulation* 1981; 64:158–163.
108. Reisner SA, Ong LS, Lichtenberg GS, et al: Myocardial perfusion imaging by contrast echocardiography with use of intracoronary sonicated albumin in humans. *J Am Coll Cardiol* 1989; 14:660–665.
109. Shapiro JR, Reisner SA, Meltzer RS: Prospects for transpulmonary contrast echocardiography. *J Am Coll Cardiol* 1989; 13:1629–1630.
110. Feinstein SB, Lang RM, Dick C, et al: Contrast echocardiography during coronary arteriography in humans: Perfusion and anatomic studies. *J Am Coll Cardiol* 1988; 11:59–65.
111. Glassman E, Kronzon I: Transvenous intracardiac echocardiography. *Am J Cardiol* 1981; 47:1255–1259.
112. Nissen SE, Gurley JC, Grines CL, et al: Intravascular ultrasound assessment of lumen size and wall morphology in normal subjects and in patients with coronary artery disease. *Circulation* 1991; 84:1087–1092.
113. Popp RL, Rubenson DS, Tucker CR, et al: Echocardiography: M-mode and two-dimensional methods. *Ann Intern Med* 1980; 93:844–853.
114. Kotler MN, Mintz GS, Segal BL, et al: Clinical uses of two-dimensional echocardiography. *Am J Cardiol* 1980; 45:1061–1082.
115. Bansal RC, Tajik AJ, Seward JB, Offord KP: Feasibility of detailed two-dimensional echocardiographic examination in adults: Prospective study of 200 patients. *Mayo Clin Proc* 1980; 55:291–308.
116. Horowitz MS, Schultz CS, Stinson EB, Harrison DC, Popp RL: Sensitivity and specificity of echocardiographic diagnosis of pericardial effusion. *Circulation* 1974; 50:239–247.
117. Martin RP, Rakowski H, French J, et al: Localization of pericardial effusion with wide angle phased-array echocardiography. *Am J Cardiol* 1978; 42:904–912.
118. Martin RP, Bowden R, Filly K: Intrapericardial abnormalities in patients with pericardial effusion: Findings by two-dimensional echocardiography. *Circulation* 1980; 61:568–572.
119. Schnittger I, Bowden RE, Abrams J, Popp RL: Echocardiography: Pericardial thickening and constrictive pericarditis. *Am J Cardiol* 1978; 42:388–345.
120. Tei C, Child JS, Tanaka H, et al: Atrial systolic notch on the interventricular septal echogram: An echocardiographic sign of constrictive pericarditis. *J Am Coll Cardiol* 1982; 1:907–912.
121. Chandraratna PAN, Aronow WS: Detection of pericardial metastases by cross-sectional echocardiography. *Circulation* 1981; 63:197–199.
122. Singh S, Wann S, Schuchard H, et al: Right ventricular and right atrial collapse in patients with cardiac tamponade—A combined echocardiographic and hemodynamic study. *Circulation* 1984; 70:966–971.
123. Gilliam LD, Guyer D, King ME, Marshall JE, Weyman AE: Hydrodynamic compression of the right atrium: A new echocardiographic sign of cardiac tamponade. *Circulation* 1983; 68:294–301.
124. Kronzon I, Cohen ML, Winer HG: Diastolic atrial compression: A sensitive echocardiographic sign of cardiac tamponade. *J Am Coll Cardiol* 1983; 2:770–775.
125. Himelman RB, Kircher B, Rockey DC, Schiller NB: Inferior vena cava plethora with blunted respiratory response: A sensitive echocardiographic sign of cardiac tamponade. *J Am Coll Cardiol* 1988; 12:1470–1477.
126. Chandraratna PAN, First J, Langevin E, et al: Clinical usefulness of echocardiographic contrast studies during pericardiocentesis. *Ann Intern Med* 1977; 87:199–203.

127. Callahan JA, Seward JB, Nishimura RA, et al: Two-dimensional echocardiographically guided pericardiocentesis: Experience in 117 consecutive patients. *Am J Cardiol* 1985; 55:476–479.
128. Cikes I: New echocardiographic possibilities in the etiological diagnosis and therapy of pericardial diseases. In: Hanrath P, Bleifeld W, Souquet J (eds): *Cardiovascular Diagnosis by Ultrasound. Transesophageal, Computerized, Contrast, Doppler Echocardiography.* The Hague, Martinus Nijhoff, 1982: 188.
129. Pandian NG, Skorton DJ, Kieso RA, Derber RE: Diagnosis of constrictive pericarditis by two-dimensional echocardiography: Studies in a new experimental model and in patients. *J Am Coll Cardiol* 1984; 4:1164–1173.
130. Nishimura RA, Connolly DC, Parker TW: Constrictive pericarditis: Assessment of current diagnostic procedures. *Mayo Clin Proc* 1985; 60:397–402.
131. Felner JM, Knopf W: Intracardiac and extracardiac masses diagnosed by two-dimensional echocardiography. *Echocardiography* 1985; 2:3–55.
132. Shah PM: Echocardiography in congestive or dilated cardiomyopathy. *J Am Soc Echo* 1988; 1:20–27.
133. Corya BC, Feigenbaum H, Rasmussen S, et al: Echocardiographic features of congestive cardiomyopathy compared with normal subjects and patients with coronary artery disease. *Circulation* 1974; 49:1153–1159.
134. Douglas PS, Morrow R, Ioli A, Reichek N: Left ventricular shape, afterload and survival in idiopathic dilated cardiomyopathy. *J Am Coll Cardiol* 1989; 13:311–315.
135. Ewy GA, Jones SE, Friedman MJ: Echocardiographic detection of adriamycin heart disease. *Proc Am Soc Clin Oncol* 1975; 16:228–231.
136. Keren A, Billingham ME, Popp RL: Features of mildly dilated congestive cardiomyopathy compared with idiopathic restrictive cardiomyopathy and typical dilated cardiomyopathy. *J Am Soc Echocardiogr* 1988; 1:78–87.
136a. Blanchard DB, Hagenhoff C, Chow LC, McCann HA, Kittrich HC: Reversibility of cardiac abnormalities in human immunodeficiency virus (HIV) infected individuals: A serial echocardiographic study. *J Am Coll Cardiol* 1991; 17:1270–1276.
137. Henry WI, Clark CE, Epstein SE: Asymmetric septal hypertrophy (ASH): Echocardiographic identification of the pathognomonic anatomic abnormality of IHSS. *Circulation* 1973; 47:225–233.
138. Martin RP, Rakowski H, French J, Popp RL: Idiopathic hypertrophic subaortic stenosis viewed by wide-angle, phased-array echocardiography. *Circulation* 1979; 59:1206–1217.
139. Maron BJ, Bonow RO, Seshagri TN, et al: Hypertrophic cardiomyopathy with ventricular septal hypertrophy localized to the apical region of the left ventricle. *Am J Cardiol* 1982; 49:1838–1848.
140. Rakowski H, Sasson Z, Wigle ED: Echocardiographic and Doppler assessment of hypertrophic cardiomyopathy. *J Am Soc Echo* 1988; 1:31–47.
141. Spirito P, Maron BJ: Relation between extent of left ventricular hypertrophy and age in hypertrophic cardiomyopathy. *J Am Coll Cardiol* 1989; 13:820–823.
142. Yamaguchi H, Ishimura T, Nishiyam S: Hypertrophic nonobstructive cardiomyopathy with giant negative T waves. *Am J Cardiol* 1979; 44:401–412.
143. Maron BJ, Gottchener JS, Bonow RC, Epstein SE: Hypertrophic cardiomyopathy with unusual locations of left ventricular hypertrophy undectable by M-mode echo cardiography: Identification by wide angle two-dimensional echocardiography. *Circulation* 1981; 63:409–418.
144. Gilbret BW, Pollick C, Adelman AG, Wigle ED: Hypertrophic cardiomyopathy: Subclassification by M-mode echocardiography. *Am J Cardiol* 1980; 54:861–872.
145. Siqueira-Filho AG, Cunha CLP, Tajik AJ, et al: M-mode and two-dimensional echocardiographic features in cardiac amyloidosis. *Circulation* 1981; 63:188–196.
146. Picano E, Pinamonti B, Ferdeghini EM, et al: Two-dimensional echocardiography in myocardial amyloidosis. *Echocardiography* 1991; 8:253–262.
147. Acquatella H, Schiller NB, Puigbo JJ, et al: Value of two dimensional echocardiography in endomyocardial disease with and without cosiphophilia. *Circulation* 1983; 67:1219–1226.
148. Pearson AC, Gudipati C, Nagelhort D, Sear J, Cohen JD, Labovitz AJ: Echocardiographic evaluation of cardiac structure and function in elderly subjects with isolated systolic hypertension. *J Am Coll Cardiol* 1991; 17:422–240.
149. Liebson PR, Savage DD: Echocardiography in hypertension: A review: I, Left ventricular wall mass, standardization and ventricular function. *Echocardiography* 1986; 3:181–188.
150. Devereux RB, Alonso DR, Lutas EM, et al: Echocardiographic assessment of left ventricular hypertrophy: Comparison to necropsy findings. *Am J Cardiol* 1986; 57:450–458.
151. Liebson PR, Savage DD: Echocardiography in hypertension: A review: II. Echocardiographic studies of the effects of antihypertensive agents on left ventricular wall mass and function. *Echocardiography* 1987; 4:215–249.
152. Kotlewski A, Kawanishi D, Rhamimtoola SH: Management of valvular heart disease: An illustrative cases approach. *Curr Probl Cardiol* 1991; 16:1–88.
153. Glover MU, Warren SE, Vieweg WVR, et al: M-mode and two-dimensional echocardiographic correlation with findings at catheterization and surgery in patients with mitral stenosis. *Am Heart J* 1983; 105:98–103.
154. Wann LS, Weyman AE, Feigenbaum H, et al: Determination of mitral valve area by cross-sectional echocardiography. *Ann Intern Med* 1978; 88:337–341.
155. Martin RP, Rakowski H, Kleiman JH, et al: Reliability and reproducibility of two-dimensional echocardiographic measurement of stenotic mitral valve orifice area. *Am J Cardiol* 1979; 43:560–568.
156. Herrmann HC, Wilkins GT, Abascal VM, Weyman AE, Block PC, Palacios IF: Percutaneous balloon mitral valvotomy for patients with mitral stenosis: Analysis of factors influencing early results. *J Thorac Cardiovasc Surg* 1988; 96:33–38.
157. Palacios IF, Block PC, Wilkins GT, Weyman AE: Follow-up of patients undergoing percutaneous mitral balloon valvotomy: Analysis of factors determining restenosis. *Circulation* 1989; 79:573–579.
158. Felner JM, Williams BR: Noninvasive evaluation of left ventricular overload and cardiac function. *Prac Cardiol* 1979; 5:158–196.
159. Mintz GS, Kotler MN, Segal BL, et al: Two-dimensional echocardiographic evaluation of patients with mitral insufficiency. *Am J Cardiol* 1979; 44:670–678.
160. Himelman RB, Kusumota F, Oken K, Lee E, Cahalan MK, Shah PM, Schiller NB: The flail mitral valve: Echocardiographic findings by precordial and transesophageal imaging and Doppler color flow mapping. *J Am Coll Cardiol* 1991; 17:272–279.
161. Felner JM: Echocardiographic evaluation of mitral valve prolapse. In: Miller DD (ed): *Cardiovascular Imaging Techniques.* Boston, Butterworths, 1987: 447–464.
162. Levine RA, Stathogiannis E, Newell JB, et al: Reconsideration of echocardiographic standards for mitral valve prolapse: Lack of association between leaflet displacement isolated to the apical four chamber view and independent echocardiographic evidence of abnormality. *J Am Coll Cardiol* 1988; 11:1010–1119.
163. Pini R, Greppi B, Roman MJ, Kramer-Fox R, Devereux RB: Time-motion reconstruction of mitral leaflet motion from two-dimensional echocardiography in mitral valve prolapse. *Am J Cardiol* 1991; 68:215–220.
164. Krivokapich J, Child JS, Dadourian BJ, Perloff JK: Reassessment of echocardiographic criteria for diagnosis of mitral valve prolapse. *Am J Cardiol* 1988; 61:131–135.
165. Perloff JK, Child JS: Mitral valve prolapse: Evolution and refinement of diagnostic techniques. *Circulation* 1989; 80:710–711.
166. Warth DC, King ME,Cohen JM, et al: Prevalence of mitral valve prolapse in normal children. *J Am Coll Cardiol* 1985; 5:1173–1177.
167. Marks AR, Choong CY, Sanfilippo AJ, Ferré M, Weyman AE: Identification of high-risk and low-risk subgroups of patients with mitral-valve prolapse. *N Engl J Med* 1989; 320:1031–1036.
168. Levine RA, Triulzi MO, Harrigan P, Weyman AE: The relationship of mitral annular shape to the diagnosis of mitral valve prolapse. *Circulation* 1987; 75:756–767.
169. Morganroth J, Jones RH, Chen CC, Naito N: Two-dimensional echocardiography in mitral, aortic and tricuspid valve prolapse. *Am J Cardiol* 1980; 46:1164–1177.
170. Mintz GS, Kotler MM, Parry WR, Segal BL: Statistical comparison of M-mode and two-dimensional echocardiographic diagnosis of flail mitral leaflets. *Am J Cardiol* 1980; 45:253–259.
171. D'Cruz I, Panetta F, Cohen H, Glick G: Submitral calcification or sclerosis in elderly patients: M-mode and two-dimensional

diagnosis and quantification of valvular aortic stenosis. *Circulation* 1980; 62:304–312.
175. Godley RW, Green D, Dillon JC, et al: Reliability of two-dimensional echocardiography in assessing the severity of valvular aortic stenosis. *Chest* 1981; 79:657–662.
176. Fowles RE, Martin RP, Abrams JM, et al: Two-dimensional echocardiographic features of bicuspid aortic valve. *Chest* 1979; 75:434–440.
177. Brandenburg RO, Tajik AJ, Edwards WD, et al: Accuracy of two-dimensional echocardiographic diagnosis of congenitally bicuspid aortic valve: Echocardiographic-anatomic correlation in 115 patients. *Am J Cardiol* 1983; 5:1469–1473.
178. Krivokapich J, Child JS, Skorton DJ: Flail aortic valve leaflets: M-mode and two-dimensional echocardiography. *Am Heart J* 1980; 99:425–431.
179. Mardelli TJ, Morganroth J, Naito M, et al: Cross-sectional echocardiograph detection of aortic valve prolapse. *Am Heart J* 1980; 101:295–300.
180. Wilcox WD, Seward JB, Hagler DJ, et al: Discrete subaortic stenosis: Two-dimensional echocardiographic features with angiographic and surgical correlation. *Mayo Clin Proc* 1980; 55:425–431.
181. Guyer DE, Gillam LD, Foale RA, et al: Comparison of the hemodynamic and echocardiographic diagnosis of rheumatic tricusp stenosis. *J Am Coll Cardiol* 1984; 3:1135–1144.
182. Howard RJ, Drobac M, Rider WD, et al: Carcinoid heart disease: Diagnosis by two-dimensional echocardiography. *Circulation* 1982; 66:1059–1065.
183. Weyman, AE, Hurwitz RA, Girod DA, et al: Cross-sectional echocardiographic visualization of the stenotic pulmonic valve. *Circulation* 1977; 56:769–774.
184. Felner JM, Miller DD: Echocardiographic characteristics of normally and abnormally functioning mechanical prosthetic heart valves. *Echocardiography* 1984; 1:261–310.
185. Alam, M, Lakie JB, Packard SD, et al: Echocardiographic evaluation of porcine bioprosthetic valves. *Am J Cardiol* 1983; 52:309–315.
186. Pollak S, Felner JM: Echocardiographic identification of prosthetic valve ring abscess. *J Am Coll Cardiol* 1986; 7:1167–1173.
187. Pratt C, Whitcomb C, Newmann A: Relationship of vegetations on echocardiograms to the clinical course in systemic emboli and bacterial vegetations (? endocarditis). *Am J Cardiol* 1980; 61:374.
188. Melvin ET, Berger M, Lutzker LG, et al: Noninvasive methods for detection of valve vegetations in infective endocarditis. *Am J Cardiol* 1981; 47:271–278.
189. Berger M, Delfin LA, Jelvehm M, et al: Two-dimensional echocardiography findings in right-sided infective endocarditis. *Circulation* 1980; 61:855–861.
190. Lopez JA, Ross RS, Fishbein MC, Siegel RJ: Nonbacterial thrombotic endocarditis: A review. *Am Heart J* 1987; 113:773–784.
191. Mugge A, Daniel WG, Frank G, Lichtlen PR: Echocardiography in infective endocarditis: Reassessment of prognostic implications of vegetation size determined by transthoracic and the transesophageal approach. *J Am Coll Cardiol* 1989; 14:631–638.
192. Robbins MJ, Soeiro R, Frishman WH, Strom JA: Right-sided valvular endocarditis: Etiology, diagnosis, and an approach to therapy. *Am Heart J* 1986; 111:128–135.
193. Shively BK, Gurule FT, Roldan CA, Leggett JH, Schiller NB: Diagnostic value of transesophageal compared with transthoracic echocardiography in infective endocarditis. *J Am Coll Cardiol* 1991; 18:391–397.
194. Jaffe WM, Morgan DE, Pearlman AS, Otto CM: Infective endocarditis, 1983–1988: Echocardiographic findings and factors influencing morbidity and mortality. *J Am Coll Cardiol* 1990; 15:1227–1233.
195. Rubenson DA, Tucker CR, Stinson EB, et al: The use of echocardiography in diagnosing culture-negative endocarditis. *Circulation* 1981; 64:641–646.
196. Ports TA, Cogan J, Schiller NB, et al: Echocardiography of left ventricular masses. *Circulation* 1978; 58:528–536.
197. DePace NL, Soulen RL, Kotler MN, et al: Two-dimensional echocardiographic detection of intraatrial masses. *Am J Cardiol* 1981; 48:954–960.
198. Stratton JR, Lighty GW Jr, Pearlman AS, et al: Detection of left ventricular thrombus by two-dimensional echocardiography: Sensitivity, specificity, and causes of uncertainty. *Circulation* 1982; 66:156–166.
199. Felner JM, Churchwell A, Murphy D: Right atrial thromboemboli: Clinical, echocardiographic and pathophysiologic manifestations. *J Am Coll Cardiol* 1984; 4:1041–1051.
200. Schweizer P, Bardos F, Erbel R, et al: Detection of left atrial thrombi by echocardiography. *Br Heart J* 1981; 45:148–152.
201. Herzog CA, Bass D, Kane M, et al: Two-dimensional echocardiographic imaging of left atrial appendage thrombi. *J Am Coll Cardiol* 1984; 3:1340–1344.
202. Keren A, Goldberg S, Gottlieb S, et al: Natural history of left ventricular thrombi: Their appearance and resolution in the posthospitalization period of acute myocardial infarction. *J Am Coll Cardiol* 1990; 15:790–800.
203. Meltzer RS, Tichner EG, Popp RL, Roelandt J: The source of echocardiographic contrast. In: Meltzer RS, Roelandt J, (eds): *Contrast Echocardiography*. The Hague, Martinus Nijhoff, 1982: 7–16.
204. Shrestha NK, Moreno FL, Narcisco FV, et al: Two-dimensional echocardiographic diagnosis of left atrial thrombus in rheumatic heart disease. *Circulation* 1983; 67:341–347.
205. Seward JB, Tajik AJ: Noninvasive visualization of the entire thoracic aorta: A new application of wide-angle two-dimensional sector echocardiography. *Am J Cardiol* 1979; 43:387.
206. Okumachi F, Yoshikawa J, Kato H, et al: Usefulness and limitations of two-dimensional echocardiography in the diagnosis of acute dissecting aneurysm of the aorta. *J Cardiog* 1981; 11:1169–1175.
207. Victor ME, Mintz GS, Kotler MN, et al: Two-dimensional echocardiographic diagnosis of aortic dissection. *Am J Cardiol* 1981; 48:1155–1159.
208. Iliceto S, Antonelli G, Biasco G, et al: Two-dimensional echocardiographic evaluation of aneurysms of the descending thoracic aorta. *Circulation* 1982; 66:1045–1049.
209. Weyman AE, Caldwell RL, Hurwitz RA, et al: Cross-sectional echocardiographic detection of aortic obstruction: 2. Coarctation of the aorta. *Circulation* 1978; 57:498–502.
210. Granato JE, Dee P, Gibson RS: Utility of two-dimensional echocardiography in suspected aortic dissection. *Am J Cardiol* 1985; 56:123–129.
211. Khandheria BK, Tajik AJ, Taylor CL, et al: Aortic dissection: Review of value and limitations of two-dimensional echocardiography in a six-year experience. *J Am Soc Echo* 1989; 2:17–24.
212. Erbel R, Daniel W, Visser C, et al: Echocardiography in diagnosis of aortic dissection. *Lancet* 1989; 1:457–461.
213. Morganroth J, Chen CC, David DD, et al: Echocardiographic detection of coronary artery disease: Detection of effects of ischemia on regional myocardial wall motion and visualization of left main coronary artery disease. *Am J Cardiol* 1980; 46:1178–1187.
214. Nishimura RA, Tajik AJ, Shub C, et al: Role of two-dimensional echocardiography in the prediction of in-hospital complications after acute myocardial infarction. *J Am Coll Cardiol* 1984; 4:1080–1087.
215. Parisi AF, Moynihan PF, Folland ED, et al: Quantitative detection of regional left ventricular contraction abnormalities by two-dimensional echocardiography: II. Accuracy in coronary artery disease. *Circulation* 1981; 63:761–767.
216. Gibson RS, Bishop HL, Stamm RB, et al: Value of early two-dimensional echocardiography in patients with acute myocardial infarction. *Am J Cardiol* 1982; 49:1110–1119.
217. Heger JJ, Weyman AE, Wann LS, et al: Cross-sectional echocardiography in acute myocardial infarction: Detection and localization of regional left ventricular asynergy. *Circulation* 1979; 60:531–538.
218. Horowitz RS, Morganroth J, Parrotto C, et al: Immediate diagnosis of acute myocardial infarction by two-dimensional echocardiography. *Circulation* 1982; 65:323–329.
219. Nishmura RA, Reeder GS, Miller JA, et al: Prognostic value of predischarge two-dimensional echocardiogram after acute myocardial infarction. *Am J Cardiol* 1984; 53:429–432.
220. Isaacsohn JL, Earle MG, Kemper AJ, Parisi AF: Postmyocardial infarction pain and infarct extension in the coronary care unit: Role of two-dimensional echocardiography. *J Am Coll Cardiol* 1988; 11:246–251.
221. Henschke CI, Risser TA, Sandor T, et al: Quantitative computer-assisted analysis of left ventricular wall thickening and motion

by two-Dimensional echocardiography in acute myocardial infarction. *Am J Cardiol* 1983; 52:960–964.

222. Likoff M, Reichek N, St. John-Sutton M, et al: Epicardial mapping of segmental myocardial function: An echocardiographic method applicable in man. *Circulation* 1982; 66:1050–1158.
223. Mann DL, Gillam LD, Weyman AE: Cross-sectional echocardiographic assessment of regional left ventricular performance and myocardial perfusion. *Prog Cardiovasc Dis* 1986; 29:1–52.
224. Pandian N, Kerber B: Two-dimensional echocardiography in experimental coronary stenosis: I. Sensitivity and specificity in detecting transient myocardial dyskinesis: comparison with somomicrometers. *Circulation* 1982; 66:597–602.
225. Armstrong WF: Echocardiography in coronary artery disease. *Prog Cardiovasc Dis* 1988; 30:267–288.
226. Nieminen M, Parisi A, O'Boyle JE, et al: Serial evaluation of myocardial thickening and thinning in acute experimental infarction: identification and quantification using two-dimensional echocardiography. *Circulation* 1982; 66:174–180.
227. Nixon JV, Brown CN, Smitherman TC: Identification of transient and persistent segmental wall motion abnormalities in patients with unstable angina by two-dimensional echocardiography. *Circulation* 1982; 65:1497–1503.
228. Pollick C, Cujec B, Parker S, Tator C: Left ventricular wall motion abnormalities in subarachnoid hemorrhage: An echocardiographic study. *J Am Coll Cardiol* 1988; 12:600–605.
229. Popp, RL: Echocardiogrpahy. *N Engl J Med* 1990; 323:101–109, 165–172.
230. Heger JJ, Weyman AE, Wann LS, Rogers EW, Dillon JC, Feigenbaun H: Cross-sectional echocardiographic analysis of the extent of left ventricular asynergy in acute myocardial infarction. *Circulation* 1980; 66:1113–1118.
231. D'Arcy BJ, Nanda NC: Two-dimensional echocardiographie features of right ventricular infarction. *Circulation* 1982; 65:167–173.
232. Pandian N, Koyanagi S, Skorton D, et al: Serial quantification of myocardial dyskinesis in acute myocardial infarction by two-dimensional echocardiography. *J Am Coll Cardiol* 1983; 1:619–628.
233. Visser CA, Kan G, David GK, et al: Echocardiographic-cineangiographic correlation in detecting left ventricular aneurysm: A prospective study of 422 patients. *Am J Cardiol* 1982; 50:337–347.
234. Catherwood E, Mintz GS, Kotler MN, et al: Two-dimensional echocardiogrpahic recognition of left ventricular pseudoaneurysm. *Circulation* 1980; 62:294–303.
235. Asinger RW, Mikell FL, Sharma B, et al: Observations on detecting left ventricular thrombus with two-dimensional echocardiography: Emphasis on avoidance of false positive diagnosis. *Am J Cardiol* 1981; 47:145–156.
236. Farcot JC, Boisante L, Rigaud M, et al: Two-dimensional echocardiographic visualization of ventricular septal rupture after acute myocardial infarction. *Am J Cardiol* 1980; 45:370–377.
237. Erbel R, Schweizer P, Bardos P, Meyer J: Two-dimensional echocardiographic diagnosis of papillary muscle rupture. *Chest* 1981; 79:595–601.
238. Erlebacher JA, Weiss JL, Weisfeldt ML, Bulkley BH: Early dilation of the infarcted segment in acute transmural myocardial infarction: Role of infarct expansion in acute left ventricular enlargement. *J Am Coll Cardiol* 1984; 4:201–208.
239. Abernethy M, Sharpe N, Smith H, Gamble G: Echocardiographic prediction of left ventricular volume after myocardial infarction. *J Am Coll Cardiol* 1991; 17:1527–1532.
240. Turpie, AGG, Robinson JG, Doyle DJ, et al: Comparison of high-dose with low-dose subcutaneous heparin to prevent left ventricular murals thrombosis in patients with acute transmural anterior myocardial infarction. *N Engl J Med* 1989; 320:352–357.
241. Reeder GS, Lengyel M, Tajik AJ, et al: Mural thrombus in left ventricular aneurysm: Incidence, role of angiography, and relation between anticoagulation and embolization. *Mayo Clin Proc* 1981; 56:77–83.
242. Weinreich DJ, Burke JF, Pauletto FJ: Left ventricular mural thrombi complicating acute myocardial infarction: Long term follow-up with serial echocardiography. *Ann Intern Med* 1984; 100:789–794.
243. Stratton JR, Nemanich JW, Johannessen KA, Resnick AD: Fate of left ventricular thrombi in patients with remote myocardial infarction or idiopathic cardiomyopathy. *Circulation* 1988; 78:1388–1393.
244. Johannessen KA, Nordrehaug JE, von der Lippe G: Left ventricular thrombosis and cerebrovascular accident in acute myocardial infarction. *Br Heart J* 1984; 51:553–556.
245. Kinney EL: The significance of left ventricular thrombi in patients with coronary heart disease: A retrospective analysis of pooled data. *Am Heart* 1985; 109:191–194.
246. Meyer RA: Echocardiography in assessing cardiac anatomy: Summary and discussion. *J Am Coll Cardiol* 1985; 5:44S–47S.
247. Rink LD, Feigenbaum H, Godley RW, et al: Echocardiographic detection of left main coronary artery obstruction. *Circulation* 1982; 65:719–724.
248. Yoshikawa J, Yanagihara K, Owaki T, et al: Cross-sectional echocardiographic diagnosis of coronary artery aneurysms in patients with mucocutaneous lymph node syndrome. *Circulation* 1979; 59:133–139.
249. Gutgesell HP: Echocardiographic assessment of cardiac function in infants and children. *J Am Coll Cardiol* 1985; 5:95S–103S.
250. Bierman FZ: Two-dimensional echocardiography in the older child. *J Am Coll Cardiol* 1985; 5:37S–43S.
251. Huhta JC, Gutgesell HP, Latson LA, Huffines FD: Two-dimensional echocardiographic assessment of the aorta in infants and children with congenital heart disease. *Circulation* 1984; 417–424.
252. Capelli H, Andrade JL, Somerrville J: Classification of the site of ventricular septal defect by two-dimensional echocardiography. *Am J Cardiol* 1983; 51:1474–1480.
253. Felner JM: Echocardiogrpahy: Acyanotic congential heart lesions. In: Kotler MN, Segal BL (eds): *Clinical Echocardiography, and Brest AN (ed): Cardiovascular Clinics*. Philadelphia, FA Davis, 1978: 251.
254. Solinger R, Elbl F, Minhas K: Deductive echocardiographic analysis in infants with congenital heart disease. *Circulation* 1974; 50:1072–1096.
255. Williams RG: Echocardiography in the neonate and young infant. *J Am Coll Cardiol* 1985; 5:30S–36S.
256. Schmidt KG, de Araujo LMD, Silverman NH: Evaluation of structural and functional abnormalities of the fetal heart by echocardiography. *Am J Cardiac Imaging* 1988; 2:57–76.
257. Copel JA, Pilu G, Green J, Hobbins JC, Leinman CS: Fetal echocardiographic screening for congenital heart disease: The importance of the four chamber view. *Am J Obstet Gynecol* 1987; 157:648–655.
258. Kreulen TM, Bove AA, McDonough MT, et al: The evaluation of left ventricular function in man: A comparison of methods. *Circulation* 1975; 51:677–688.
259. Popp RL, Alderman EI, Brown OR, et al: Sources of error in calculation of left ventricular volumes by echocardiography. *Am J Cardiol* 1973; 31:152–159.
260. Felner JM, Blumenstein BA, Schlant RC, et al: Sources of variability in echocardiographic measurements. *Am J Cardiol* 1980; 45:995–1004.
261. Felner JM: The value and limitations of echocardiography. In: Hurst JW (ed): *Update I: The Heart*. New York, McGraw-Hill, 1979: 47.
262. Force TL, Folland EL, Aebischer N, Sharma S, Parisi AF: Echocardiographic assessment of ventricular function. In: Marcus ML, Skorton DJ, Schelbert HR, Wolf GL (eds): *Cardiac Imaging—Principles and Practice*. Philadelphia, Saunders, 1990:374–402.
263. Guyer DE, Gibson TC, Gillan LD, et al: A new echocardiographic model for quantifying three-dimensional endocardial surface area. *J Am Coll Cardiol* 1986; 8:819–829.
264. Collins SM, Kerber RE, Skorton DJ: Quantitative analysis of left ventricular regional function by imaging methods. In: Miller DD, Burns RJ, Gill JB, Ruddy TD (eds): *Clinical Cardiac Imaging*. New York, McGraw-Hill, 1988: 233–259.
265. Simonson JS, Schiller NB: Sonospirometry: A new method for noninvasive estimation of mean right atrial pressure based on two-dimensional echographic measurements of the inferior vena cava during measured inspiration. *J Am Coll Cardiol* 1988; 11:557–564.
266. Dreslinski GR, Frohlich ED, Dunn FG, et al: Echocardiogrpahic diastolic ventricular abnormality in hypertensive heart disease: Atrial emptying index. *Am J Cardiol* 1981; 47:1087–1090.

267. Pietro DA, Parisi AF, Harrington JJ, et al: Premature opening of the aortic valve: An index of highly advanced aortic regurgitation. *JCU* 1978; 6:179–186.
268. Kotler MN, Segal BL, Mintz GS, et al: Pitfalls and limitations of M-mode echocardiogrpahy. *Am Heart J* 1977; 94:227–237.
269. Felner JM: Common errors made in echocardiography. *Med Times* 1979; 107:93–104.
270. O'Rourke RA, Crawford MH: How to avoid errors in use of echocardiography. *Cardiovasc Med* 1979; 4:1079–1086.
271. Roelandt J Lubse J: Limitations and pitfalls of M-mode and two-dimensional echocardiography. In: Roelandt J (ed): *The Practice of M-Mode and Two-Dimensional Echocardiography.* The Hague, Martinus Nijhoff, 1983: 53.
272. Latson LA, Cheathan JP, Gutgesell HP: Resolution and accuracy in two-dimensional echocardiography. *Am J Cardiol* 1981; 48:106–110.
273. Buda AJ, Delp EJ, Meyer CR, et al: Automatic computer processing of digital two-dimensional echocardiograms. *Am J Cardiol* 1983; 52:384–389.
274. Collins SM, Skorton DJ, Geiser EA, et al: Computer-assisted edge detection in two-dimensional echocardiography: Comparison with anatomic data. *Am J Cardiol* 1984; 53:1380–1387.
275. Skorton DJ, Collins SM, Nichols J, et al: Quantitative texture analysis in two-dimensional echocardiography: Application to the diagnosis of experimental myocardial contusion. *Circulation* 1983; 68:217–223.
276. Milunski MR, Mohr GA, Perez JE, et al: Ultrasonic tissue characterization with integrated backscatter: Acute myocardial ischemia, reperfusion, and stunned myocardium in patients. *Circulation* 1989; 80:491–503.
277. McPherson DD: Tissue characterization by ultrasound: What is possible now? What will be possible? *Echocardiography* 1991; 8:77–92.
278. Cohen RD, Mottley JG, Miller JG, et al: Detection of ischemic myocardium in vivo through the chest wall by quantitative ultrasonic tissue characterization. *Am J Cardiol* 1982; 50:838–843.
279. Fraker TD Jr, Nelson AD, Arthur JA, et al: Altered acoustic reflectance on two-dimensional echocardiography as an early predictor of myocardial infarct size. *Am J Cardiol* 1984; 53:1699–1702.
280. Bhandair AK, Nanda NC: Myocardial texture characterization by two-dimensional echocardiography. *Am J Cardiol* 1983; 51:817–825.
281. Thorell LG, Smith WJ: Using computer color effectively. Englewood Cliffs, NJ, Prentice-Hall, 1990:203.
282. Roelandt J, Gussenhoven WJ, Serruys PW, Tuccillo B, VanEgmond FC, Urk HV, et al: Clinical applications of intravascular echography. In Dagianti A, Feigenbaum H (eds): *Echocardiography 1990.* Excerpta Medica Internatl Cong Series. Amsterdam, Elsevier, 1990.
283. Armstrong WF, Gage SW: Evaluation of reperfusion hyperemia with myocardial contrast echocardiography. *J Am Soc Echocardiogr* 1988; 1:322–332.
284. Vandenberg BF: Myocardial perfusion and contrast echocardiography: Review and new perspectives. *Echocardiography* 1991; 8:65–76.
285. Sheikh KH, Smith SW, VonRamm O, Kisslo J: Real-time three-dimensional echocardiography: Feasibility and initial use. *Echocardiography* 1991 8:119–126.
286. Kaul S: Assessment of coronary blood flow reserve during myocardial contrast echocardiography. In *Echocardiography 1990.* Excerpta Medica Intl Cong Series. - Amsterdam, Elsevier, 1990.
287. Geiser EA, Ariet M, Conetta DA, et al: Dynamic three-dimensional reconstruction of the human left ventricle in vivo: Technique and initial observation in patients. *Am Heart J* 1982; 103:1056–1065.

Chapter 16

The Exercise Test

Gerald F. Fletcher, M.D. ■ Robert C. Schlant, M.D.

Exercise testing elicits the body's reaction to measured increases in acute exercise. The changes in heart rate, blood pressure, respiration, and perceived level of exertion provide data that permit quantitative estimation of cardiovascular conditioning and function. These data also correlate with more general aspects of conditioning such as flexibility and musculoskeletal strength. In addition to "numerical" data, exercise tests provide an opportunity to observe a person during exercise. By monitoring heart rate and blood pressure and continually observing the electrocardiogram (ECG), one can detect alterations in the hemodynamic response and ischemic-type ECG ST segment depression, and can detect and classify disturbances in cardiac rhythm and conduction associated with exercise.

THE CARDIOVASCULAR RESPONSE TO EXERCISE

Exercise, a common physiological stress, can elicit cardiovascular abnormalities not present at rest and can be used to assess function of the cardiovascular system. Exercise is only one of the many stresses to which human beings are exposed; therefore, it is frequently more appropriate to refer to an "exercise" test and not a "stress" test. Two types of muscular contraction (activity) can be used as an exercise test of the cardiovascular system: isometric (static) or isotonic (dynamic).[1] *Isometric (static) exercise,* defined as a constant muscular contraction without movement (e.g., handgrip), provokes more pressure than volume load on the left ventricle in relation to the body's ability to supply oxygen. The cardiovascular response to isometric exercise, however, is difficult to grade since the response to activation of a small muscle group is similar to the response to a large muscle group. In addition, cardiac output is not increased as much as resistance. *Isotonic (dynamic) exercise,* defined as muscular contraction of larger muscle groups resulting in movement, primarily provides a volume load to the left ventricle, and the cardiovascular response is proportional to the degree of the exercise.

Maximum Oxygen Uptake

When dynamic exercise begins, oxygen uptake by the lungs quickly increases. After several minutes, oxygen uptake usually remains relatively stable (steady state) at each intensity of exercise. During the steady state, heart rate (HR), cardiac output, blood pressure, and pulmonary ventilation are maintained at reasonably constant levels.[1]

Maximal oxygen consumption ($\dot{V}_{O_2max}$) is the greatest amount of oxygen a person can utilize while performing dynamic exercise involving large components of total muscle mass[2] and represents the amount of oxygen transported and used in cellular metabolism. It is convenient to express oxygen uptake in multiples of sitting/resting requirements. The metabolic equivalent (MET) is a unit of sitting/resting oxygen uptake [3.5 ml O_2 per kilogram of body weight per minute (mL kg^{-1} min^{-1})]. Rather than determining each person's true resting oxygen uptake, one MET is designated as this average. $\dot{V}_{O_2max}$ is significantly related to age, gender, exercise habits, heredity, and clinical cardiovascular status.

Maximum values of $\dot{V}_{O_2max}$ occur between ages 15 and 30 years and decrease progressively with age. At age 60, mean $\dot{V}_{O_2max}$ in men is approximately three-fourths that at age 20. Individuals with a sedentary lifestyle have a 9 percent reduction per decade versus less than five percent per decade in those with an active lifestyle. Up to age 12 to 16, there is no significant difference in $\dot{V}_{O_2max}$ among children. At age 12 to 14, however, a decrease is observed in girls. The reduced $\dot{V}_{O_2max}$ in women is related to less muscle mass, lower hemoglobin and blood volume, and smaller stroke volume than men.

Physical activity level has an important influence on $\dot{V}_{O_2max}$. After three weeks of bed rest, there is a 25 percent decrease in $\dot{V}_{O_2max}$ in healthy men. In moderately active young men, $\dot{V}_{O_2max}$ is about 12 METs, whereas individuals performing aerobic training such as distance running can have a $\dot{V}_{O_2max}$ as high as 18 to 24 METs (60–85 mL kg^{-1} min^{-1}). There appears to be a natural variation in $\dot{V}_{O_2max}$ related to genetic factors; in addition, $\dot{V}_{O_2max}$ is affected by the degree of impairment caused by intrinsic cardiovascular disease.

It is difficult to predict $\dot{V}_{O_2max}$ accurately based on exercise habits and age. Table 16-1 lists average levels of METs for various activities and the prognostic value of different levels of METs.

Maximum $\dot{V}_{O_2}$ is equal to maximum cardiac output times maximum arteriovenous oxygen ($a\dot{V}_{O_2}$) difference. Since cardiac output is equal to the product of stroke volume and HR, $\dot{V}_{O_2}$ is directly related to HR. The maximum $a\dot{V}_{O_2}$ difference during exercise has a physiological limit of 15 to 17 mL/dL; therefore, if maximum effort is achieved, $\dot{V}_{O_2max}$ can be used to estimate maximum cardiac output.

Myocardial Oxygen Uptake

Myocardial oxygen uptake (M_{O_2}) is determined by intramyocardial wall tension [left ventricular (LV) systolic pressure times end-diastolic volume, divided by LV wall thickness], contractility, and HR. Other, less important, factors include the external work performed by the heart, energy necessary for activation, and the basal metabolism of the myocardium. (See also Chap. 5.)

Accurate measurement of M_{O_2} requires cardiac catheterization; however, M_{O_2} can be estimated during exercise testing by the product of HR and systolic blood pressure, called the *rate pressure product*. In general, there is a linear relation between M_{O_2} and coronary blood flow. During exercise, coronary blood flow increases as much as fivefold above the resting value. A patient with obstructive coronary disease, however, may not have enough coronary blood flow to supply the metabolic demands of the myocardium during vigorous exercise, and as a consequence, myocardial ischemia occurs. (See also Chap. 57.)

TABLE 16-1

Clinically Significant Metabolic Equivalents (METs) for Maximum Exercise

1 MET	Resting
2 METs	Level walking at 2 mph
4 METs	Level walking at 4 mph
<5 METs	Poor prognosis; usual limit immediately after myocardial infarction; peak cost of basic activities of daily living
10 METs	Prognosis with medical therapy as good as coronary artery bypass surgery
13 METs	Excellent prognosis regardless of other exercise responses
18 METs	Elite endurance athletes
20 METs	World class athletes

MET = metabolic equivalent, or a unit of sitting resting oxygen uptake. 1 MET = 3.5 mL kg^{-1} min^{-1} oxygen uptake.

SOURCE: From Fletcher GF, Froelicher, VF, Hartley LH, Haskell WL, Pollock ML: Exercise standards: A statement for health professionals from the American Heart Association. *Circulation* 1990; 82:2286–2322. Reproduced with permission from the publisher and the authors.

RESPONSE TO DYNAMIC EXERCISE

The response to dynamic exercise consists of a complex series of cardiovascular adjustments to provide active muscles with blood appropriate for metabolic needs, to dissipate heat generated by active muscles, and to maintain blood supply to essential organs such as the brain and heart.

As cardiac output increases with dynamic exercise, vascular resistance decreases in active muscles but increases in tissues that do not function during exercise.[4] Since flow to active muscles increases much more than arterial pressure, there is a significant decrease in vascular resistance.

Heart Rate Response

An increase in HR due to a decrease in vagal outflow is an immediate response of the cardiovascular system to exercise. This is rapidly followed by an increase in sympathetic outflow to the heart and systemic blood vessels, which also contributes to the increase in HR. During dynamic exercise, HR increases linearly with work load and V_{O_2}. During low levels of exercise and at a constant work rate, HR will reach a steady state within several minutes; however, as work load increases, the time to stabilize progressively lengthens.

Heart rate response is influenced by several factors including age, sex, subject motivation, body habitus, and type of exercise. There is a decline in mean maximum HR with age,[5] which seems related to intrinsic cardiac changes rather than neural influences (see Chap. 115). Dynamic exercise increases HR more than isometric exercise, and an accentuated HR response is observed after bed rest. Other factors that influence HR include body position, general state of health, blood volume, and environment.

Arterial Blood Pressure Response

Systolic blood pressure increases with dynamic work as a result of increasing cardiac output, while diastolic pressure usually remains about the same or decreases slightly. An inadequate rise in systolic blood pressure (20 to 30 mmHg or less) can result from aortic outflow obstruction, left ventricular dysfunction, or myocardial ischemia. Patients who develop hypotension during exercise frequently have severe heart disease; patients with aortic valvular disease can also exhibit a drop in systolic blood pressure. Changes of blood pressure are strongly influenced by changes in peripheral resistance.

After maximum exercise, there is normally a decrease in systolic blood pressure, usually reaching resting levels in 6 min, then often remaining lower than pre-exercise levels for several hours. In some patients with coronary artery disease (CAD), higher levels of systolic blood pressure, at times even exceeding peak exercise values, may develop in the recovery phase. When exercise is terminated abruptly, some healthy persons have precipitous drops in systolic blood pressure due to venous pooling. Figure 16-1 shows the physiological response to submaximum and maximum treadmill exercise based on tests of more than 700 apparently healthy men aged 25 to 54. Maximum rate-pressure product ranges from a 10th percentile value of 25,000 to a 90th percentile value of 40,000.

The arterial blood supply to the myocardium and to other muscles and organs is usually adequate for the maximal perfusion requirement of which the organ is capable. If obstructive disease is present within a coronary artery, only minimal reduction in maximal blood flow will take place until the degree of arterial obstruction becomes quite advanced.[65] (See Chap. 5.) If the subject engages only in sedentary behavior, it is possible for an advanced degree of coronary arterial obstruction to develop without clinically significant underperfusion of the myocardium. The predictive importance of exertional myocardial ischemia is related to the intensity of cardiac activity at which the ischemia became apparent.[7] For example, if there is no evidence of ischemia at 75 percent of maximum exercise, but there is such evidence at 90 to 100 percent of maximal exercise, it would likely be associated with a less severe degree of coronary obstruction than if the ischemia had been detectable at only 25 to 50 percent of maximal exercise.

TESTING PROCEDURES

Exercise testing of patients should be conducted only by well-trained personnel with a basic knowledge of exercise physiology. In general, only physicians and other health professionals (especially nurses) familiar with normal and abnormal responses during exercise and qualified in Advanced Cardiac Life Support have the cognitive skills needed to perform exercise tests on patients competently.[8] Equipment, medications, and personnel trained to provide cardiopulmonary resuscitation (CPR) must be readily available. Although exercise testing of patients is considered safe, there are reports of acute myocardial infarction and death related to the procedure. Several surveys confirm that up to 10 myocardial infarctions or deaths, or both, can be expected per 10,000 tests. The risk is greater in postmyocardial infarction patients and in those being evaluated for malignant ventricular arrhythmias. Table 16-2 lists three classes of complications secondary to exercise tests.

Good clinical judgment is imperative in determining indications for and contraindications to exercise testing.[9] Table 16-3 lists the general indications for exercise testing, and Table 16-4 lists absolute and relative contraindi-

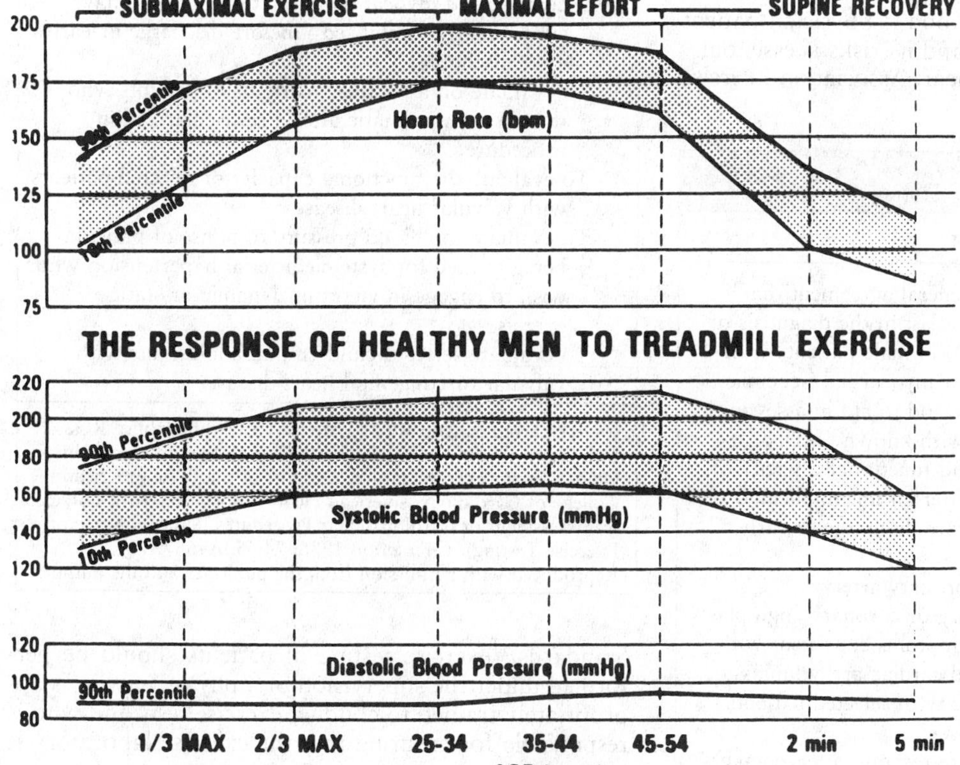

FIGURE 16-1 Normal response to progressive treadmill protocol in healthy subjects. (*From Froelicher VF: Exercise and the Heart: Clinical Concepts. Chicago, Year Book Medical Publishers, 1987. Reproduced with permission from the publisher and the author.*)

TABLE 16-2

Complications Secondary to Exercise Tests

Cardiac
Bradyarrhythmias Sinus Atrioventricular junctional Ventricular Atrioventricular block Asystole Sudden death (ventricular tachycardia/fibrillation) Myocardial infarction Congestive heart failure Hypotension and shock
Noncardiac
Musculoskeletal trauma
Ill-Defined and Miscellaneous
Severe fatigue, dizziness, fainting, general malaise, body aches, delayed ill feelings, and fatigue sometimes persisting for days

SOURCE: From Fletcher GF, Froelicher VF, Hartley LH, Haskell WL, Pollock ML: Exercise standards: A statement for health professionals from the American Heart Association. *Circulation* 1990; 82:2286–2322. Reproduced with permission from the publisher and the authors.

cations to exercise testing. Whereas absolute contraindications are quite definitive, in selected cases with relative contraindications, even submaximum testing may provide valuable information. The physician should be certain that the subject understands the procedure and acknowledges the risks. Good physician-patient communication about testing and its risks is essential.

As stated in the American Heart Association Exercise Standards,[9] exercise testing of patients should be performed under the supervision of a physician who is appropriately trained to conduct exercise tests and who is responsible for ensuring that the exercise laboratory is properly equipped and that the testing personnel are

TABLE 16-3

General Indications for Exercise Testing

Class I
Conditions for which there is general agreement that exercise testing is justified to assist in the diagnosis of coronary artery disease (CAD) in male patients with symptoms that are atypical for myocardial ischemia To assess functional capacity and to aid in assessing the prognosis of patients with known CAD To evaluate the prognosis and functional capacity of patients with CAD soon after an uncomplicated myocardial infarction (before discharge or early after discharge) To evaluate patients after coronary artery revascularization by surgery or coronary angioplasty To evaluate patients with symptoms consistent with recurrent, exercise-induced cardiac arrhythmias To evaluate functional capacity of selected patients with congenital heart disease To evaluate patients with rate-responsive pacemakers

TABLE 16-3

General Indications for Exercise Testing *(continued)*

Class II
Conditions for which exercise testing is frequently performed but in which there is a divergence of opinion with respect to its value and appropriateness To evaluate asymptomatic male patients over the age of 40 with special occupations (pilots, air traffic controllers, fire fighters, police officers, critical process operators, bus or truck drivers, and railroad engineers) To evaluate asymptomatic males over the age of 40 with two or more risk factors for CAD To evaluate sedentary male patients > 40 years who plan to enter a vigorous exercise program To assist in the diagnosis of CAD in women with a history of typical or atypical angina pectoris To assist in the diagnosis of CAD in patients who are taking digitalis or who have complete right bundle branch block To evaluate the functional capacity and response to therapy with cardiovascular drugs in patients with CAD or heart failure To evaluate patients with variant angina To follow-up serially (at 1-year intervals or longer) patients with known CAD To evaluate patients with a class I indication who have base-line ECG changes or coexisting medical problems that limit the value of the test (In some of these patients, exercise testing may still yield clinically useful information, such as duration of exercise, blood pressure response, and production of chest discomfort.) To evaluate patients who have sustained a complicated myocardial infarction but who have subsequently "stabilized" (before discharge or early after discharge) To evaluate on a routine, yearly basis patients who remain asymptomatic after a revascularization procedure To evaluate the functional capacity of selected patients with valvular heart disease To evaluate the blood pressure response of patients being treated for systemic arterial hypertension who wish to engage in vigorous dynamic or static exercise To evaluate selected children and adolescents with valvular or congenital heart disease

SOURCE: From Schlant RC, Blomqvist CG, Brandenburg RO, DeBusk R, Ellestad MH, Fletcher GF, et al: Special report. In: Guidelines for exercise tesing. A report of the Joint American College of Cardiology/American Heart Association Task Force on Assessment of Cardiovascular Procedures (Subcommittee on Exercise Testing). *Circulation* 1986; 74:653A–667A. Reproduced with permission from the publisher and the authors.

TABLE 16-4

Absolute and Relative Contraindications to Exercise Testing

Absolute	Relative*
Acute myocardial infarction or recent change on resting ECG	Less serious noncardiac disorder
Active unstable angina	Significant arterial or pulmonary hypertension
Serious cardiac arrhythmias	Tachyarrhythmias or bradyarrhythmias
Acute pericarditis	Moderate valvular or myocardial heart disease
Endocarditis	Drug effect or electrolyte abnormalities
Severe aortic stenosis	Left main coronary obstruction or its equivalent
Severe left ventricular dysfunction	Hypertrophic cardiomyopathy
Acute pulmonary embolus or pulmonary infarction	Psychiatric disease
Acute or serious noncardiac disorder	
Severe physical handicap or disability	

*Under certain circumstances and with appropriate precautions, relative contraindications can be superceded.

SOURCE: From Schlant RC, Blomqvist CG, Brandenburg RO, DeBusk R, Ellestad MH, Fletcher GF, et al: Special report. In: Guidelines for exercise testing. A report of the Joint American College of Cardiology/American Heart Association Task Force on Assessment of Cardiovascular Procedures (Subcommittee on Exercise Testing). *Circulation* 1986; 74:653A–667A. Reproduced with permission from the publisher and the authors.

appropriately trained. The level or degree of supervision needed during a test is determined by the clinical state of the patient being tested. Supervision must be designated by the physician or physician's staff, who ask pertinent questions about the patient's medical history, perform a brief physical examination, and review the standard 12-lead ECG performed immediately before testing. The physician should interpret data derived from testing, suggest further evaluation or therapy, and aid in providing effective and timely advanced CPR when necessary. A defibrillator and appropriate medications should be immediately available. Table 16-5 details safety measures for exercise testing.

The degree of supervision of an exercise test can range from assigning monitoring of the test to a properly trained nonphysician (i.e., nurse or exercise specialist) for testing apparently healthy younger persons (less than 40 years old) or assigning patients with stable chest discomfort syndromes to the physician who directly monitors blood pressure and the patient's status throughout exercise and recovery. The latter is the ideal for testing patients for diagnostic or prognostic purposes and is a requirement for testing all patients at increased risk for

TABLE 16-5

Safety Measures for Exercise Testing

1. Definite plan of emergency action, including the duties of each member of the team. In addition to direct patient care, the plan should include notification of appropriate individuals and providng other necessities for patient transfer.
2. Prompt admission to a coronary care unit.
3. All members of team trained in cardiopulmonary resuscitation.
4. Defibrillator within cable reach of treadmill, turned on and charged (200 J) during test. Full tube of electrode paste on top of unit.
5. Emergency drug kit.
6. Intravenous solutions, administration sets, needles and syringes.
7. Oropharyngeal airways, laryngoscope, endotracheal tubes, ventilation bag, and suction machine.
8. Equipment for the administration of oxygen.

SOURCE: From Fletcher GF (ed): *Exercise in the Practice of Medicine,* 2d ed. Mt. Kisco, NY, Futura, 1988. Reproduced with permission from the publisher and the author.

an exercise-induced complication. A physician should be immediately available during all exercise tests on patients.

Patient Preparation

Preparations for exercise testing include the following:

- The patient should be instructed not to eat or smoke for 2 to 3 h before the test and to dress appropriately for exercise. No strenuous physical efforts should be performed for at least 12 h before testing.
- Cessation of medications may, at times, be considered since some drugs interfere with exercise responses, complicating interpretation of exercise testing. There are, however, no formal guidelines for tapering medications, but rebound phenomena may occur rarely with discontinuance of beta blockers. Therefore, most patients are tested on their medications. Specific questioning is important to determine which drugs have been taken so the physician can be aware of possible electrolyte abnormalities and other effects.
- A brief history and physical examination should be done to rule out contraindications to testing or to detect important clinical signs such as murmurs, gallop sounds, pulmonary bronchospasm, or rales. Patients with a history of increasing or unstable angina or uncontrolled heart failure should not have exercise testing until their condition stabilizes. A cardiac physical examination should indicate which patients have valvular or congenital heart disease, particularly adult patients with severe aortic stenosis, who generally should not undergo exercise testing.
- A detailed explanation of the testing procedure should be given, outlining risks and possible complications. The patient should be told how to perform

the exercise test, and the testing procedure should be demonstrated.

- A standard resting 12-lead ECG should be obtained since it may differ from the resting pre-exercise ECG. This is essential, particularly in patients with known heart disease, since an abnormality or a change may contraindicate testing. Recording the ECG before starting the exercise test and after hyperventilation at another time may be helpful in detecting false-positive (indeterminate) ECG changes, particularly in women.
- Standing EG and blood pressure should be recorded to determine vasoregulatory abnormalities, particularly ST depression.

Electrocardiographic Recording

The most important aspect of the electrode-amplifier-recording system is the interface between the electrodes and the skin. Removing the superficial layer of skin significantly lowers resistance, decreasing the signal-to-noise ratio. The areas for electrode application are first shaved (if necessary) and then rubbed with an alcohol-saturated gauze. After the skin dries, it is marked with a "felt-tip" pen and rubbed with a fine sandpaper or other rough material to reduce skin resistance.

Many electrode systems are available for performing exercise testing; silver plate or silver chloride crystal pellets are preferred since they have the lowest offset voltage. The electrodes should have a metal interface that is sunken, creating a column to be filled with either an electrolyte solution or a saturated sponge. Connecting cables between the electrodes and recorder should be light, flexible, and properly shielded. Cables generally have a life span of a year or so, depending on use. Cables can eventually become a source of both noise and electrical discontinuity, requiring replacement.

Bipolar lead systems are advantageous in recording ECG changes during exercise. The relatively short placement time, freedom from motion artifacts, and the ease with which noise problems can be located are all factors that favor their use. The usual positive reference is one electrode placed in the same position as the positive reference for V_5 (the fifth intercostal space at the midclavicular line) and the negative reference at Wilson's central terminal. Figure 16-2 illustrates negative electrode placement for most bipolar lead systems. CM_5 is the most sensitive for ST segment changes. CC_5 excludes the vertical component included in CM_5 and decreases influence of atrial repolarization (T_a), reducing false-positive responses.[10]

Since a standard 12-lead ECG with electrodes placed on the limbs cannot be effectively obtained during exercise, other electrode placements have been used. Differences can be minimized by placing the arm electrodes as close to the shoulders as possible, and the leg electrodes below the umbilicus. Any modification of lead placement should be recorded on the tracing.

The lateral precordial leads (V_4 through V_6) are capable of detecting 90 percent of all ECG ST depression observed in multiple lead systems. A more extensive lead system, however, is preferred in certain patients with a high prevalence of previous myocardial infarction or symptoms suggesting coronary artery spasm. ST depression in five leads or more usually predicts multivessel disease. A three-lead system (V_2, II, and V_5) is usually adequate for localizing ischemia related to spasm and is also helpful for characterization of arrhythmias.

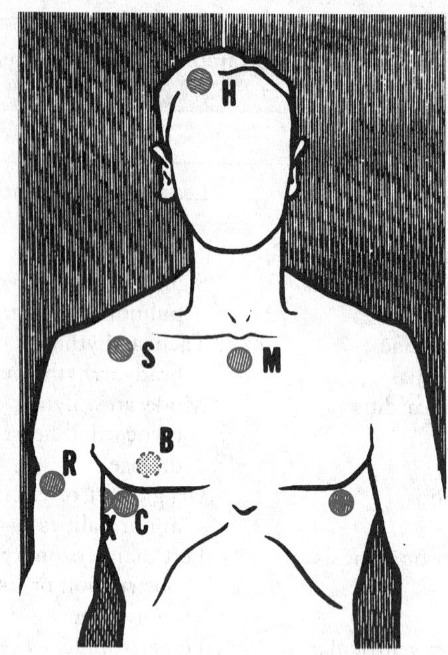

FIGURE 16-2 Negative electrode placement for most bipolar lead systems. B, on back, subscapular; M, top of manubrium; X, midaxillary line, fifth intercostal level; C, anterior axillary line, fifth intercostal level; H, above shoulders (neck or above); S, right clavicular edge; R, right arm; +, positive electrode placement for C_5 bipolar electrodes. (*From Froelicher VF: Exercise and the Heart: Clinical Concepts. Chicago Year Book Medical Publishers, 1987. Reproduced with permission from the publisher and the author.*)

There are various recorders designed to provide high-quality ECG data during exercise. Many use microprocessors to generate average waveforms and make ECG measurements; however, computer processing is not completely reliable because of software limitations in handling noise and inadequacy of the available algorithms. The physician must, therefore, compare the raw analog data with computer-generated output to validate its accuracy.

EQUIPMENT AND PROTOCOLS

Figure 16-3 illustrates the relation of METs to stages in the commonly used testing protocols. Numerous devices have been used to provide dynamic exercise for testing; however, the treadmill and the cycle ergometer remain the most commonly used dynamic exercise testing devices.

The treadmill should have front and side rails for patients to steady themselves; however, patients should not tightly grasp the front or side rails as this decreases V_{O_2} and work while increasing exercise time and muscle artifact. Most patients can walk without aid of the hand rails; however, older and poorly coordinated subjects may need such support. It is helpful if patients take their hands off the rails and place one or two fingers on the

TABLE III

FUNCTIONAL CLASS	CLINICAL STATUS	O_2 COST ml/kg/min	METS	BICYCLE ERGOMETER	TREADMILL PROTOCOLS															METS
					BRUCE		KATTUS		BALKE-WARE	ELLESTAD		USAFSAM		"SLOW" USAFSAM		McHENRY		STANFORD		
				1 WATT = 6 KPDS	3 MIN STAGES MPH	%GR	MPH	%GR	% GRADE AT 3.3 MPH 1-MIN STAGES	3/2/3 MIN STAGES MPH	%GR	MPH	%GR	MPH	%GR	MPH	%GR	% GRADE AT 3 MPH	% GRADE AT 2 MPH	
					5.5	20														
NORMAL AND I	HEALTHY, DEPENDENT ON AGE, ACTIVITY	56.0	16		5.0	18				6	15									16
		52.5	15	FOR 70 KG BODY WEIGHT KPDS								3.3	25							15
		49.0	14	1500			4	22	26 25 24 23 22 21 20 19 18 17 16 15 14 13 12 11 10 9 8 7 6 5 4 3 2 1	5	15									14
		45.5	13		4.2	16						3.3	20			3.3	21			13
		42.0	12	1350			4	18								3.3	18	22.5		12
	SEDENTARY HEALTHY	38.5	11	1200			4	14		5	10	3.3	15			3.3	15	20.0		11
		35.0	10	1050	3.4	14								2	25			17.5		10
		31.5	9				4	10						2	20			15.0		9
		28.0	8	900						4	10	3.3	10			3.3	12	12.5		8
	LIMITED	24.5	7	750	2.5	12	3	10		3	10			2	15			10.0	17.5	7
II	SYMPTOMATIC	21.0	6	600								3.3	5	2	10	3.3	9	7.5	14	6
		17.5	5	450	1.7	10	2	10		1.7	10					3.3	6	5.0	10.5	5
III		14.0	4	300	1.7	5						3.3	0	2	5			2.5	7	4
		10.5	3													2.0	3	0.0	3.5	3
		7.0	2	150	1.7	0						2.0	0	2	0					2
IV		3.5	1																	1

Aerobic cost of exercise protocols. This figure shows the predicted aerobic cost of the stages of many of the currently used treadmill protocols. Total exercise time is not as important a value as is the estimated oxygen consumption value of the protocol stage or workload reached.
MPH = miles per hour; %GR = percent grade; KPDS = kiloponds.

FIGURE 16-3 Treadmill protocols with approximate oxygen uptakes. (*From Froelicher VF: Exercise and the Heart: Clinical Concepts. Chicago Year Book Medical Publishers, 1987. Reproduced with permission from the publisher and the author.*)

rails to maintain balance after they are accustomed to walking on the treadmill. The treadmill should have both variable speed and grade capability and must be accurately calibrated.

Mechanical or electrically braked cycles are calibrated in kiloponds (kpm) or watts and are capable of varying the force to the pedaling speed (rate-independent ergometers). This permits more precise power output control since it is common for uncooperative or fatigued patients to decrease their pedaling speed. The highest values of V_{O_2} and HR are obtained with pedaling speeds of 60 to 80 rpm. One watt is equivalent to approximately 6 kpm and since exercise on a cycle ergometer is nonweight-bearing, kiloponds or watts can be converted to oxygen uptake in mL/min. METs are obtained by dividing V_{O_2} in mL/min by the product of body weight in kg $\times$ 3.5. The cycle ergometer is usually less expensive and occupies less space than a treadmill. Upper body motion is usually reduced, making it easier to obtain blood pressure measurements and to record the ECG; however, care must be taken to prevent isometric exercise of the arms.

There is a considerable difference between the body's response to acute exercise in the supine and erect positions. In healthy persons during supine cycle exercise, stroke volume and end-diastolic volume change relatively little, perhaps 10 to 20 percent, from volumes at rest, whereas during cycle exercise in the erect position, stroke volume increases (and may double during severe exercise) and then plateaus during mild work. In patients with intrinsic cardiac abnormalities, left ventricular filling pressure is more likely to increase during exercise in the supine than in the erect position. When patients with angina pectoris perform identical submaximum cycle work in the supine and erect positions, HR is higher in the supine position. Maximum work performed, however, is lower in the supine position, and angina develops at a lower rate pressure product. ST changes are more frequent during exercise in the upright position; however, ST-segment changes are usually greater during exercise in the supine position because of the greater left ventricular (LV) volume.

Protocols for clinical exercise testing should include an initial low load (warm-up), progressive uninterrupted exercise with an adequate duration in each level, and a recovery period. For cycle ergometry, the initial power output is usually 10 or 25 W (150 kpm/min), usually followed by increases of 25 W every 2 or 3 min until symptomatic or objective end-points are reached. If arm ergometry is substituted for cycle leg ergometry, a similar protocol may be used, except that initial power output and incremental increases are lower. Two-minute stages are most popular with arm ergometry.[11,12]

Several different treadmill protocols are in use, the most popular of which is the Bruce. The advantages of the Bruce protocol include a seventh or final stage, which cannot be completed by most individuals, and its use in many published studies, which provides extensive data for comparison. Its disadvantages include large increments in work load that make estimation of $\dot{V}_{O_2max}$ less accurate. In addition, the fourth stage can be either run or walked, probably resulting in different oxygen costs. Some subjects are forced to stop prematurely because of musculoskeletal difficulties or inability to tolerate the high work load increments. An initial zero and one half stages (1.7 mph at 0 percent, then 5 percent grade) may be used for some patients. Many exercise testing laboratories currently use Balke-type protocols (i.e., Naughton, Stanford, McHenry) with even MET levels for stage advances. Regardless of technique used, the optimum exercise testing protocol should last 6 to 12 min and should be adjusted to the type of patient being tested. Performance can be estimated with the oxygen cost of maximum work load or power output achieved rather than

TABLE 16-6
Schedule of Treadmill Exercise for the GXT

Stage Number	Time per Stage (min)	Elapsed Time at End of Stage	Speed		Treadmill Slope	
			km/h	(mph)	Grade, %	Elevation (degrees)
Zero*	3	3†	2.7	1.7	0 (level)	0 (level)
One-half*	3	3†	2.7	1.7	5	2.8
First	3	3	2.7	1.7	10	5.7
Second	3	6	4.0	2.5	12	6.8
Third	3	9	5.5	3.4	14	8.0
Fourth	3	12	6.8	4.2	16	9.0
Fifth	3	15	8.0	5.0	18	10.0
Sixth	3	18	8.9	5.5	20	11.0
Seventh	3	21	9.6	6.0	22	12.4

*Begin with stage zero or stage one-half if appearance and demeanor of subject suggest that walking capacity is severely limited.
†Exercise time in these preliminary stages is not counted when tabulating functional capacity.
GXT = graded exercise test.

SOURCE: From Fletcher GF (ed): *Exercise in the Practice of Medicine*, 2d ed. Mt. Kisco, NY, Futura, 1988. Reproduced with permission from the publisher and the author.

by total treadmill time if subjects do not use hand rails for support. This allows comparison of performance in different protocols.

Since there is strong evidence that the level of exercise required to produce ischemia is the most important part of the exercise test result, the question arises of how the exercise test work load shall be selected. There is overwhelming agreement on use of a progressively increasing exercise protocol beginning with a stage low enough to be tolerated by the "weakest" candidate for testing and ending with a stage sufficiently difficult to challenge the "fittest" candidate. Each stage should be long enough in duration for the subject to reach or closely approach steady state, and the work increments from one stage to the next should be small enough to permit the desired degree of precision in estimating work capacity.[13] The Bruce treadmill protocol is widely used (Table 16–6). Typical work output requirements for each stage in terms of oxygen consumption have been determined, and the range of stages is adequate both for sedentary individuals and athletes.[15] To increase applicability, two easier stages may be added below Stage 1 in order to accommodate virtually all ambulatory individuals.[15] In order for measurements of treadmill performance, exercise time, or rate-pressure response to be directly related to the actual cardiac work involved, the subject must have reached or closely approached "steady state." This implies that if the subject continued to exercise at this same intensity, cardiac output HR, and other indices would stay essentially the same until the point of fatigue. Steady state attainment requires at least 3 min, and perhaps longer on the treadmill, and exercise times shorter than this will not yield a reliable reflection of cardiovascular capacity.

Rather than assign a certain stage of exercise protocol as a goal for an individual (whether based on age, history of exercise participation, or level of condition), it is preferable to require the subject to exercise progressively through the protocol until it becomes excessively uncomfortable or impossible to continue, i.e., to an end-point of exhaustion unless other terminating end-points occur. As discussed below, there are several means of determining whether or not the subject makes a good effort so that the exercise time is a true representation of physical capacity. The most obvious criterion is HR, which can be predicted with about 90 percent accuracy.[17,18] Failure to attain an exercise tachycardia reasonably close to a predicted maximum may not provide an adequate indication of the degree of effort (Table 16-7).

SUBMAXIMUM VERSUS MAXIMUM EXERCISE TESTING

In some cases, testing is terminated when the patient reaches 90 percent of predicted maximum HR for age and level of training. The designated target HR, however, may be maximal for some subjects, beyond the limit of others, but submaximal for others. A test is considered maximal when the patient appears to give a true maximum effort (point of bodily exhaustion) or when other clinical end-points are reached.

Perceived Exertion

The subjective rating of exertion is a good indicator of relative fatigue and is used to quantify effort. Rather than using HR alone to clinically determine intensity of exercise, the 6 to 20 point Borg scale of perceived exertion[19] is useful (Table 16–8). Although there is some variation among patients in their actual rating of fatigue, individual patients rate consistently from test to test. Thus, the Borg scale can assist the clinician in judging the degree of fatigue with testing and in correlating the level of fatigue during testing with that experienced during daily activities.

TABLE 16-7

Predicted Exercise Heart Rate: Men/Women

Age	30	35	40	45	50	55	60	65
Maximal predicted heart rate								
(M)	193	191	189	187	184	182	180	178
(W)	190	185	181	177	172	168	163	159
80% of maximal predicted heart rate (HRi = .80)								
(M)	154	153	151	150	147	146	144	142
(W)	152	148	145	142	138	134	130	127

SOURCE: From Fletcher GF (ed): *Exercise in the Practice of Medicine,* 2d ed. Mt. Kisco, NY, Futura, 1988. Reproduced with permission from the publisher and the author.

Indications for Terminating Exercise Testing

Indications for discontinuing an exercise test include absolute and relative indications (Table 16-9).

Postexercise Period

Some abnormal responses occur only in recovery after exercise. For maximum sensitivity, patients should be supine in the postexercise period. Monitoring of blood pressure and ECG should continue for at least 6 to 8 min after exercise. An abnormal ECG response occurring only in the recovery period is not unusual; these responses are likely not false-positive unless they occur late in recovery. Mechanical dysfunction and electrophysiological abnormalities in the ischemic ventricle after exercise can persist from minutes to hours.

TABLE 16-8

Borg Scale for Rating Perceived Exertion

15-grade scale		10-grade scale	
6		0	Nothing
7	Very, very light	0.5	Very, very weak (just noticeable)
8		1	Very weak
9	Very light	2	Weak (light)
10		3	Moderate
11	Fairly light	4	Somewhat strong
12		5	Strong (heavy)
13	Somewhat hard	6	
14		7	Very strong
15	Hard	8	
16		9	
17	Very hard	10	Very, very strong (almost maximum)
18			
19	Very, very hard	°	Maximum
20			

SOURCE: From Pollock ML, Wilmore JH: *Exercise in Health and Disease: Evaluation and Prescription for Prevention and Rehabilitation,* 2d ed. Philadelphia, Saunders, 1990: 290. Reproduced with permission from the publisher and authors.

INTERPRETATION

Clinical Responses

Classical ischemic chest discomfort induced by the exercise test is strongly predictive of CAD and is even more predictive in the presence of ST depression. The patient's general appearance is also helpful. A decrease in skin temperature, cool perspiration, and peripheral cyanosis during exercise may indicate poor tissue perfusion due to inadequate cardiac output with secondary vasoconstriction, and higher work loads are not encouraged. Neurological manifestations such as light-headedness or vertigo can also indicate inadequate cardiac output.

TABLE 16-9

Indications for Terminating Exercise Testing

Absolute indications
Drop in systolic blood pressure (persistently below base line) despite an increase in work load
Onset of new or increasing anginal chest discomfort
Central nervous system symptoms (ataxia, dizziness, or near-syncope)
Evidence of poor peripheral perfusion (cyanosis or pallor)
Serious arrhythmias (i.e., high-grade ventricular, such as multiform complexes, triplets, and runs)
Technical difficulties in monitoring the ECG or systolic blood pressure
Patient's request to stop
Relative indications
ST or QRS changes such as excessive (≥ 3–4 mm) ST displacement, junctional depression, or marked QRS axis shift
Increasing chest discomfort
Fatigue, shortness of breath, wheezing, leg cramps, or intermittent claudication
General appearance (see discussion)
Less serious arrhythmias, including supraventricular tachycardias
Development of bundle branch block that cannot be distinguished from ventricular tachycardia

Physical Examination

Cardiac examination immediately after exercise can provide information about ventricular function. A precordial bulge or gallop rhythm can result from LV dysfunction. A mitral regurgitant murmur suggests papillary muscle dysfunction related to transient ischemia.

Exercise or Functional Capacity

The maximal oxygen consumption (V_{O_2max}) is the best index of maximal exercise capacity. A decrease in maximum cardiac output may be a consequence of CAD, and exercise may be limited by either anginal pain or an acute reduction in LV output. An increase in LV diastolic filling pressure and increasing pulmonary artery pressure will also limit exercise. A mean exercise capacity of 10 METs has been observed in nonathletic middle-aged healthy men. If patients with CAD reach 13 METs, their prognosis is good, regardless of other exercise test responses. As expected, patients with an exercise capacity of less than 5 METs have a higher mortality during follow-up than patients with higher capacities.

A normal exercise capacity does not exclude severe cardiac impairment. Mechanisms proposed to explain a normal exercise performance in such patients include increased peripheral oxygen extraction, preservation of chronotropic reserve, ability to tolerate elevated pulmonary wedge pressures without dyspnea, and increased levels of plasma norepinephrine at rest and during exercise.[3]

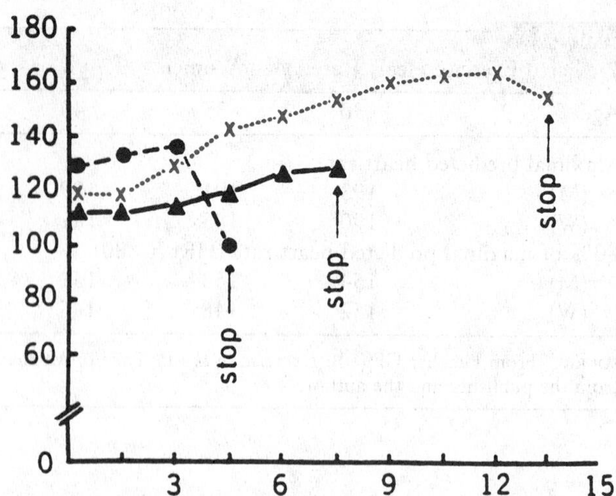

FIGURE 16-4 x = Normal response. Subject able to exercise 13½ min, drops blood pressure at peak of normal exercise capacity. ● = Abnormal. Subject increases systolic pressure initially, but pressure drops early in exercise before normal exercise capacity is reached. ▲ = Abnormal. Subject fails to raise systolic pressure to 130 mmHg or higher, even though exercise duration may be nearly normal. (*From Fletcher GF (ed): Exercise in the Practice of Medicine, 2d ed. Mt. Kisco, NY, Futura, 1988. Reproduced with permission from the publisher and the author.*)

HEMODYNAMIC RESPONSE

Blood pressure is a function of cardiac output and peripheral resistance. Although some normal subjects have a transient drop in systolic blood pressure at maximum exercise, this finding is frequently associated with severe CAD and ischemic dysfunction of the myocardium. Exercise-induced hypotension also identifies patients at increased risk for ventricular fibrillation in the exercise laboratory. Figure 16-4 illustrates normal and abnormal systolic blood pressure responses to exercise tests.

A relatively rapid HR during submaximum exercise or recovery could be due to vasoregulatory asthenia, decreased vascular volume or peripheral resistance, prolonged bed rest, anemia, or metabolic disorders and, therefore, may not reflect intrinsic cardiac disease. This finding is also relatively frequent in patients soon after myocardial infarction or coronary artery surgery. A relatively low HR at any point during submaximum exercise may be due to lack of training or drugs such as beta blockers. Conditions that affect the sinus node can also attenuate the normal response of HR during exercise testing. Table 16-7 shows predicted exercise HR in normals.

ECG Responses in Subjects with Normal Resting Electrocardiograms

During exercise, the P-wave vector tends to become more vertical and the P wave magnitude increases in the inferior leads. The PR segment (interval) shortens and slopes downward in the inferior leads. The change, which has been attributed to atrial repolarization (T_a wave), may cause false-positive or indeterminate ST depression in the inferior leads. Changes in R-wave amplitude are noted near maximum effort with a decrease in the R wave in the lateral leads (V_5) at maximum exercise and 1 min into recovery. In the lateral and vertical leads (V_5 and aVF), the S wave becomes greater in depth, showing a greater deflection at maximum exercise, and then gradually returning to resting values in recovery.

The J-junction is depressed in the lateral leads at maximum exercise, then gradually returns to pre-exercise values in recovery. A dramatic increase in J-junctional depression may be observed in all leads and may be greatest at 1 min into recovery. Subjects with resting J-junction elevation may develop an isoelectric J-junction with exercise as a normal finding. These changes revert in recovery. The normal ST segment vector response to both tachycardia and exercise is a shift rightward and upward in the frontal plane; however, there appears to be considerable biological variation in the degree of this shift. A gradual decrease in T wave amplitude is observed in all leads during early exercise. At maximum exercise the T wave begins to increase, and at 1-min recovery the amplitude is equivalent to resting values in the lateral leads.[3]

Abnormal Responses

The ST-segment level is measured relative to the PR segment since the U-P segment usually is unclear during exercise. ST elevation is measured as the deviation from the base-line ST level. If the base-line ST segment is depressed, the deviation from that level to the level during exercise or recovery is measured. The point for measuring the ST level is the J-junction; points 60 or 80 ms beyond this are usually used when the ST-segment slope is horizontal or downsloping. Considering a rapidly upsloping ST depression to be abnormal increases test sensitivity but decreases specificity. Various ST scores have been recommended, but none have been validated as superior to standard "visual" measurements. Exercise-induced myocardial ischemia can result in one of three ST-segment changes on the surface ECG: depression, elevation, and normalization.

ST-segment depression is the most common manifestation of exercise-induced myocardial ischemia. It usually reflects diffuse subendocardial ischemia, with vector direction determined largely by the area of ischemia and the placement of the heart in the thoracic cavity. The standard criterion for this abnormal response is horizontal or downsloping ST-segment depression of 0.10 mV (1.0 mm) or more for 80 ms in, at least, three consecutive "isoelectric" or level complexes. As shown in Fig. 16-5, however, other criteria have been considered. Downsloping (divergent) ST-segment depression usually reflects more ischemia than horizontal depression. In the presence of base-line abnormalities (especially in patients on digitalis), exercise-induced ST-segment depression is less specific for ischemia. Factors related to the probability and severity of CAD include the degree, time of appearance, duration, persistence in recovery, and number of leads with ST segment depression. The lower the work load and the double product at which the ST change occurs, the worse the prognosis and the more likely the presence of multivessel CAD.

ST elevation must be judged by whether or not it occurs in the presence of Q waves from a previous myocardial infarction. ST-segment elevation is more frequently observed in anterior leads (V_1 and V_2) with Q waves.[20]

Previous myocardial infarction is the most frequent cause of ST-segment elevation during exercise and seems to be related to dyskinetic areas or ventricular aneurysms. Approximately 50 percent of patients with recent anterior and 15 percent with inferior myocardial infarction exhibit this finding during exercise.[20] Patients with elevation usually have a lower left ventricular ejection fraction (LVEF) than those without such ST-segment elevation in leads with abnormal Q waves from prior myocardial infarction. These changes may result in reciprocal ST depression simulating ischemia in other leads. The development of both ST-segment elevation and depression during the same test may indicate multivessel coronary artery disease (CAD).

In patients without previous myocardial infarction (absence of Q waves on the resting ECG), ST-segment elevation during exercise frequently reflects severe transient ischemia resulting from significant proximal CAD or spasm.

In patients with variant angina, ST-segment elevation usually occurs during spontaneous anginal episodes, frequently at rest. During exercise, ST-segment elevation has been reported in about 30 percent of these patients and a reversible thallium-201 perfusion defect usually corresponds to the site of ST elevation. Another manifestation of ischemia may be the normalization of an ST segment. ECG abnormalities at rest, including T-wave inversion and ST-segment depression, may return to normal during attacks of angina and during exercise in some patients with myocardial ischemia. This can also be observed in subjects with a "persistent juvenile pattern" on the resting ECG.[3]

The R-wave amplitude may increase during exercise in certain subjects with cardiac disease; however, exercise-induced changes in R-wave amplitude have not improved diagnostic accuracy despite use of several lead systems, clinical subsets of patients, and different criteria for an abnormal response.

In normals, a gradual decrease in T-wave amplitude is observed in all leads during early exercise although the T wave begins to increase with maximum exercise. At 1-min recovery, T-wave amplitude usually returns to resting values. U-wave inversion may be associated with LV hypertrophy, CAD, and aortic and mitral regurgitation. Exercise-induced U wave inversion in patients with a normal resting ECG appears to be a marker of myocardial ischemia and suggests left anterior descending CAD. U-wave changes may, however, be difficult to assess during exercise, which increases HR and increases the proximity of the T and P waves.

Plasma potassium increases with maximal exercise testing and increases more after training in subjects on atenolol and propranolol therapy.[21] In addition (in sedentary individuals), both plasma potassium and magnesium increase significantly with maximal exercise, and these increases are unaffected by atenolol and propranolol blockade. To the contrary, propranolol, but not aten-

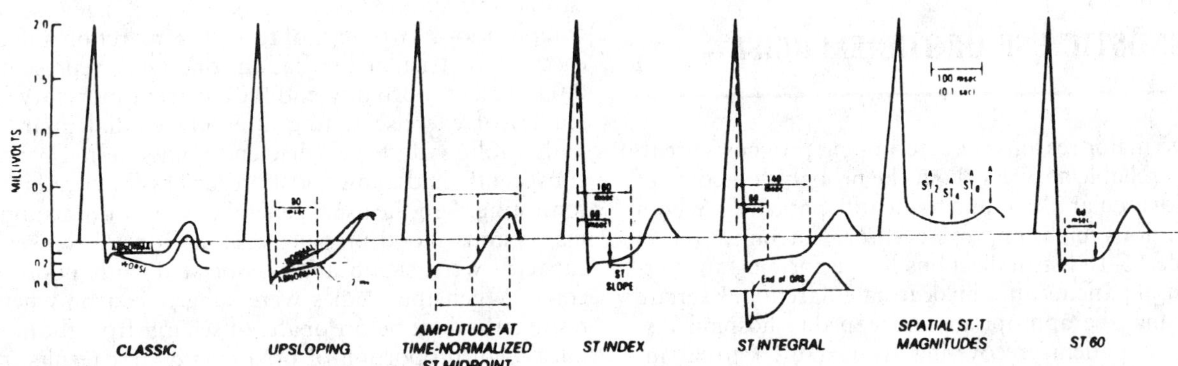

FIGURE 16-5 Types of abnormal ST responses. (*From Froelicher VF: Exercise and the Heart: Clinical Concepts. Chicago Year Book Medical Publishers, 1987. Reproduced with permission from the publisher and the author.*)

olol and placebo, prolongs the time of return to base line of potassium (compared to magnesium) after the acute exercise.[22] Such changes must be considered with exercise testing because of electrolyte effects on S-7, T, and U waves.

Exercise tests can be performed with radionuclide imaging to further evaluate myocardial perfusion. (See Chap. 134.) Echocardiographic images (Chap. 132) and Doppler flow measurements (Chap. 130) can also be made during and after exercise, and LV EF, wall motion, and valvular function can be assessed with these techniques.

DIAGNOSTIC VALUE OF THE EXERCISE TEST

Sensitivity and Specificity

Sensitivity and specificity are terms used to define how effectively a test detects disease. Sensitivity is the percentage of those with a disease who will have an abnormal test. Specificity is the percentage of those without the disease who will have a normal test. This may be affected by drugs, base-line ECG patterns, and whether a test is submaximal or maximal. Sensitivity and specificity are inversely related; when sensitivity is the highest, specificity is lowest, and vice versa.

If the population studied has a greater prevalence of disease, the test will have a higher sensitivity. (See also Chap. 9A.) For instance, the exercise test has a higher sensitivity in individuals with triple-vessel CAD than in those with single-vessel disease. A test can also have a lower specificity if it is used in individuals who are more likely to give false-positive (indeterminate) results, such as women or individuals with mitral valve prolapse.

Sensitivity and specificity of exercise-induced ST-segment depression can be demonstrated by comparing the results of exercise testing and coronary angiography.[23] In these studies, the exercise test with 0.1 mV horizontal or downsloping ST segment depression has approximately 84 percent specificity for angiographically significant CAD; that is, 84 percent of those without significant angiographic disease had a normal exercise test. These studies had a mean 66 percent sensitivity of exercise testing for significant angiographic CAD, with a range from 40 percent for one-vessel disease to 90 percent for three-vessel disease.

PROGNOSTIC USE OF THE EXERCISE TEST

The two major reasons for determining prognosis are to provide reliable answers about the probable outcome of a cardiovascular illness and to identify patients in whom interventions might improve eventual outcome.

Table 16-10 lists indications for performing an exercise test in patients after myocardial infarction. Exercise testing may be appropriate and expedite hospital discharge of patients recovering from a myocardial infarction. Ventricular arrhythmias not present at rest may be provoked during exercise and the patient's reaction to exercise at the time of discharge from the hospital can be assessed. An exercise test before discharge is important for providing guidelines for activity at home, reassurance of physical status, determination of risk of complications, and to provide a basis for advising the patient to resume or increase activity level and return to work.

TABLE 16-10

Purposes of Exercise Testing in Patients After Myocardial Infarction

Predischarge submaximum test
Setting safe exercise levels (exercise prescription)
Optimizing discharge
Altering medical therapy
Triaging for intensity of follow-up
Assuring, encouraging patient (first step in rehabilitation)
Reassuring spouse
Recognizing exercise-induced ischemia and arrhythmias
Maximum test for return to normal activities
Determining limitations (including exercise prescription)
Prognostication
Reassuring employers
Determining levels of disability
Triaging for invasive studies
Selecting medications

SOURCE: From Fletcher GF, Froelicher VF, Hartley LH, Haskell WL, Pollock ML: Exercise standards: A statement for health professionals from the American Heart Association. *Circulation* 1990; 82:2286–2322. Reproduced with permission from the publisher and the authors.

Some investigators perform exercise tests using symptom- or sign-limited end-points 2 or 3 weeks after myocardial infarction. In many, a submaximum limited test is quite appropriate. A HR limit of 130 to 140 beats per minute and a MET level of 5 to 7 is arbitrarily used, and a Borg perceived exertion level in the rage of 13 to 15 can be used as a test end-point, particularly for patients receiving beta blockers. A maximum test is probably more appropriate 3 or more weeks after myocardial infarction, when the patient is more often ready to resume full activities. (See also Chap. 60.)

One review of numerous predischarge and postmyocardial infarction exercise tests reported a few serious complications: two cases of recurrent infarction and two cases of ventricular fibrillation, one fatal, representing 0.05 percent morbidity and 0.02 percent mortality.[24] In studies of exercise testing after myocardial infarction with a follow-up for cardiac end-points, tested patients consistently had a lower risk, regardless of criteria used for testing.[24] Of the usual general criteria, only an abnormal systolic blood pressure response or a low exercise capacity were significantly associated with poor outcome. When the studies were subgrouped by whether testing was done before or after discharge from the hospital, a high proportion of predischarge test results indicated poor outcome. Submaximum testing resulted in the highest proportion of positive associations and the highest risk ratios, and abnormal responses at higher work loads were not as predictive as those at lower work loads.[24]

Studies using exercise testing of patients with stable CAD have provided data to predict angiographic findings, cardiac events in those with silent ischemia, or improved survival with coronary artery bypass surgery (CABS).

Exercise testing has been used to predict left main or triple-vessel coronary artery disease, or both, with varying results.[25]

Exertional Hypotension

In most studies, exercise-induced hypotension indicates a poor prognosis, and has a predictive value of 50 percent for left main/triple-vessel disease.[26] Exercise-induced hypotension can occur in patients with CAD, valvular heart disease, or cardiomyopathy. Occasionally, however, subjects without clinically significant heart disease will exhibit exercise-induced hypotension during exercise related to antihypertensive therapy or prolonged strenuous exercise.

Cardiac Events in Patients with Silent Ischemia

The prognostic implication of asymptomatic ("silent") ischemia detected during exercise testing is controversial. It has been suggested that those with silent ischemia are at greater risk for cardiac death; however, in three large studies of patients with a high prevalence of CAD who underwent exercise testing, those with ST-segment depression, with or without angina during testing, had similar prognoses.[27] Ischemia is asymptomatic in approximately 60 percent of patients with CAD and ischemic ST-segment depression, and silent ischemia occurring with treadmill testing does not appear to confer an increased risk for death relative to patients experiencing angina with signs of ischemia. Table 16–11 itemizes exercise testing findings associated with a poor prognosis in patients with CAD, and Table 16–12 shows data from eight studies in the prediction of cardiac events.[28–35] (See Chap. 58.)

In patients with CAD, exercise-induced ventricular arrhythmias are not an independent risk factor for subsequent mortality or coronary events. Some studies, however, suggest that these arrhythmias may add independent prognostic information to thallium-201, ST-segment, and HR changes,[36,37] and are associated with severe CAD and wall motion abnormalities. In selected subjects with CAD, exercise testing may be of considerable value in the evaluation of drug therapy of ventricular arrhythmias.

One study suggests that patients with multi-vessel CAD, cardiomegaly, exercise capacity of less than 5 METs, or a maximum systolic blood pressure of less than 130 mmHg do better if treated with surgery.[38] In another trial, patients who had an exercise test response of 1.5 mm of ST segment depression showed enhanced survival with surgery, which also improved survival in patients with base-line ST-segment depression or claudication.[39] In another study,[40] the benefit of surgery was greatest in patients with 1 mm ST-segment depression at less than 5 METs.

In several studies that evaluated graft occlusion and recurrence of symptoms, exercise-induced ST depression did not predict prognosis after CABS. An exercise capacity of 9 METs or more, however, indicates a good prognosis, regardless of other responses.[41]

Exercise testing may be of value in the routine (6 to 12 month) follow-up of patients who have undergone PTCA, especially in the evaluation of chest discomfort and detection of restenosis. Testing is of particular benefit in patients in cardiac rehabilitation programs (Chap. 63). It may be especially helpful in the patient with symptoms suggestive of ischemia or the patient whose progress in rehabilitation is limited.

There is substantial support for the use of exercise testing as the first noninvasive procedure after the history, physical examination, and resting ECG in the prognostic evaluation of patients with CAD. Exercise testing accomplishes both purposes of prognostic testing by providing information about the patient's clinical status and in helping provide recommendations for proper management. Exercise testing also helps select patients who should undergo further evaluation such as radionuclear studies and coronary angiography. Since the exercise test can be performed as an outpatient procedure and provides valuable information about activity levels, response to therapy, and disability, it is a reasonable first choice for prognostic assessment. Because of its widespread availability, the exercise test can have an enormous impact on cost-effective delivery of cardiovascular care. The exercise test is not usually recommended for

TABLE 16-11

Exercise Test Parameters Associated with Poor Prognosis and/or Increased Severity of CAD

Duration of symptom-limiting exercise
Failure to complete Stage II of Bruce protocol or equivalent work load ($\leq$ 6.5 METs*) with other protocols
Exercise heart rate (HR) at onset of limiting symptoms
Failure to attain HR $\geq$ 120/min (off beta blockers)
Time of onset, magnitude, morphology, and postexercise duration of abnormal horizontal or downsloping ST segment depression
Onset at HR < 120/min or $\leq$ 6.5 METs
Magnitude $\geq$ 2.0 mm
Postexercise duration $\geq$ 6 min
Presence in multiple leads
Systolic BP response during or following progressive exercise
Sustained decrease of > 10 mm Hg or flat BP response ($\leq$ 130 mmHg) during progressive exercise
Other potentially important determinants
Exercise-induced ST segment elevation in leads other than aVR
Angina pectoris during exercise
Exercise-induced U wave inversion
Exercise-induced ventricular tachycardia

* Energy expenditure at rest, equivalent to an oxygen uptake of approximately 3.5 mL O_2 per kilogram body weight per minute.

SOURCE: Reproduced with permission from Schlant et al.[9]

TABLE 16-12

Population Descriptors Including Clinical Variables, Exercise Testing, and Coronary Angiography from Studies of Multivariate Prediction of Cardiac Events

	LBVAMC	VACABS	CASS	Duke	Italian	German	Seattle	Buenos Aires
Years Entered	1984–1990	1970–1974	1974–1979	1969–1981	1976–1979	1975–1978	1971–1974	1972–1982
Population Size	592	245	4,083	2,842	1,083	1,034	733	180
Exercise Test								
% with 1mm ST Depression	58	72	44	35	—	—	—	65
Cardiac Cath Findings								
3V Left Main Disease (%)	21	68	23	27	20	45	12	44
Follow-Up								
Years	5	7	5	5	5.5	5	3.5	6
Annual CV Mortality (%)	2.7	NA	1.0	—	1.54	—	—	4.6
Independent Predictors of Mortality	CHF Q Waves <5 METs	E-I PVCs Max HR >140 bpm >2mm ST Depression	CHF Treadmill Stage ST Depression	ST Depression Angina Index Treadmill Time	Q Wave Prior MI Effort Ischemia Poor Ex Capacity	Ex Capacity Angina MHR	CHF Maximal DP Maximal SBP Angina Frequency Resting ST Depression	Max SBP <130 ST Elevation <4 METs

*LBVAMC, Long Beach Veterans Administration Medical Center; VACABS, Veterans Administration Coronary Artery Bypass Study; CASS, Coronary Artery Surgical Study; U vessel; CV, cardiovascular; CHF, congestive heart failure; METs, metabolic equivalents; E-I exercise induced; PVC, premature ventricular contractions; MI, myocardial infarction; Ex, exercise; MHR, maximal heart rate; DP, diastolis pressure; SBP, systolic blood pressure.

SOURCE: Reproduced with permission from references 28–35.

screening apparently healthy persons without risk factors since it has a high rate of false-positive results.[42,43]

OTHER USES OF THE EXERCISE TEST

Exercise testing has been used in patients with valvular heart disease to evaluate exercise-induced symptoms, to quantify disability, and to evaluate the response to medical and surgical therapy.[44] It has also been used to identify concurrent CAD; however, there is a high prevalence of false-positive responses because of frequently seen base-line ECG abnormalities and LV hypertrophy.

In selected patients with valvular heart disease exercise, testing may be useful to determine when surgery is indicated. (See Chaps. 79 and 80.) Effort syncope in patients with aortic stenosis[45,46] is an important symptom. Most guidelines for exercise testing list moderate to severe aortic stenosis as a contraindication for testing because of concerns about syncope and cardiac arrest. Therefore, exercise testing of patients with aortic stenosis should be restricted to subjects with mild to moderate gradients. Four proposed mechanisms for exercise-induced syncope in patients with aortic stenosis include carotid hyperactivity, LV failure, arrhythmias, and LV baroreceptor stimulation. Exercise testing, however, is relatively safe in both the pediatric and adult patient with mild to moderate aortic stenosis when performed very carefully and with experienced supervision. Attention should focus on the patient's symptoms, minute-by-minute response of blood pressure, slowing HR, and both ventricular and atrial arrhythmias. In the presence of an abnormal blood pressure response, the patient with aortic stenosis should take at least a 2-min cool-down walk at a lower stage of exertion to avoid acute LV volume overload, which may occur when the patient assumes the supine position. (See Chap. 79.)

Patients with aortic regurgitation[47] usually maintain a normal exercise capacity for a longer time than those with aortic stenosis, as volume work load of the myocardium requires less oxygen than pressure work. During exercise, there is a decrease in diastolic duration and regurgitant volume and a decrease in peripheral vascular resistance favoring forward output. As the myocardium fails, both LVEF and stroke volume decrease with an increase in both end-diastolic and end-systolic ventricular diameter. Exercise testing is useful for monitoring selected patients with aortic regurgitation, using appearance of ST-segment depression, a reduction of HR response to each work load, and decrease in $\dot{V}_{O_2max}$ as markers for decreasing LV function. (See Chap. 79.)

Patients with mitral stenosis[48] may have either a normal or excessive increase in HR during exercise. As stroke volume cannot be increased, the usual increase in cardiac output is less and may eventually fall during exercise, frequently accompanied by exercise-induced hypotension. The increase in HR and right ventricular pressure results in an increase in right ventricular myocardial oxygen demand. In patients with mitral stenosis, chest discomfort and ST-segment depression during exercise may occur either due to CAD or secondary to pulmonary hypertension. ST depression during exercise is attributed both to a decrease in coronary perfusion secondary to tachycardia and a fall in cardiac output and to an increase in myocardial oxygen demand secondary to right ventricular overload. The shortening of diastole associated with tachycardia and the increase in pulmonary blood flow associated with exercise increase left atrial pressure and may cause pulmonary congestion. (See Chap. 80.)

Patients with mild to moderate mitral regurgitation[49] maintain normal cardiac output during exercise. Blood pressure, HR, and ECG responses are usually also normal. When transient mitral regurgitation occurs suddenly during exercise as a result of ischemic papillary muscle dysfunction, however, a flat response in systolic blood pressure can occur. Patients with severe mitral regurgitation usually have decreased cardiac output and limited exercise capacity. ST-segment depression during exercise is infrequent in these patients; however, a hypotensive response can develop, and arrhythmias are frequent. (See Chap. 80.)

Several mechanisms have been suggested to explain the ST depression noted in some patients with mitral valve prolapse,[50] including regional ischemia of the papillary muscle, CAD, compression of the anterior descending artery, coronary spasm, and primary cardiomyopathy. ECG ST changes can be normalized by propranolol or other nonselective beta blockers, improving the specificity of the exercise test. (See Chap. 80.)

An exercise test is often used to evaluate the safety of an exercise training program and to formulate an exercise prescription. In general, an exercise test is useful for a sedentary individual who at the age of 40 decides to enter an exercise program of a higher intensity than walking at 50 to 60 percent of maximum HR reserve. Testing should also be done in younger individuals with coronary risk factors or a strong family history of CAD. It is preferable to determine an individual's maximum HR rather than give a predicted value for maximal HR to be attained during training, because of the wide scatter of maximum HR when plotted against age. An exercise test can be used in adult exercise or cardiac rehabilitation programs to safely advance an individual to a higher intensity. An improvement in exercise capacity on an exercise test can also be an effective incentive to continue the program and to encourage risk factor modification.

Exercise testing is used to determine the degree of impairment and disability of patients with various forms of heart disease. Patients who "exaggerate" their symptoms or who have a psychological impairment can often be identified. $\dot{V}_{O_2max}$ is the best noninvasive measurement of the exercise capacity of the cardiovascular system. Inability to reach 5 METs (below 18 mL kg^{-1} min^{-1}) without signs or symptoms is a criterion of disability used by the Social Security administration. The determination of a patient's exercise capacity affords an objective measurement of the degree of cardiac impairment.[51] (See also Chap. 142.)

The results of exercise testing do not add significantly to the risk stratification provided by the resting ECG in patients without known CAD who are candidates for major elective noncardiac surgery.[52] Therefore, exercise testing is not routinely recommended before major elective noncardiac surgery under general anesthesia. (See also Chap. 139.) The efficacy of angioplasty or surgery for peripheral vascular disease can be assessed by exercise testing.[53]

DRUGS AND EXERCISE TESTING

Beta Blockers

Maximum HR and systolic blood pressure product during exercise may be reduced by beta blockers. Patients with angina who receive beta blockers may have a greater exercise capacity with less ST-segment depression and less angina if the drugs prevent their reaching the ischemic rate pressure product. In some individuals, however, angina disappears, but ST depression occurs if the ischemic product can still be reached. (See also Chap. 66.)

Vasodilators

Vasodilators can increase exercise capacity in patients with angina or heart failure, or both.[54] To date, however, there is no good data that long-acting nitrates increase exercise capacity in patients with angina when they are tested after chronic administration.

Angiotensin-Converting Enzyme Inhibitors

Angiotensin-converting enzyme inhibitors decrease blood pressure both at rest and during exercise and can increase exercise capacity in patients with chronic heart failure.

Calcium Antagonists

Calcium antagonists have multiple hemodynamic effects. They can delay time to ischemia, improve exercise capacity, and delay ST segment depression until higher work loads. Heart rate and systolic blood pressure are decreased for a given level of exercise. (See also Chap. 67.)

Digitalis

ST-segment depression can be induced or accentuated during exercise in individuals who are taking digitalis, including both normal subjects and patients with CAD.[55] Profound ST-segment depression (> 2 mm more) compared to base line usually indicates ischemia, even in patients who are taking digitalis. Exercise-induced ST-segment depression related to digitalis has been said to persist for 2 or more weeks after digoxin is discontinued.

Other Drugs

Quinidine can cause prolongation of phase 2 of the ventricular action potential, decreasing the repolarization gradient during the ST segment and thus decreasing the magnitude of ST depression. A decrease of 20 beats per minute in maximum exercise HR has been reported in patients taking amiodarone. Amiodarone also increases duration of the QRS complex during exercise. Diuretics can cause hypokalemia, producing muscle fatigue, ventricular ectopy, and (rarely) ST-segment depression with exercise.

SPECIAL CASES OF EXERCISE TESTING INTERPRETATION

The difference in the predictive accuracy of exercise testing between men and women can be explained in part by the difference in prevalence of CAD[56]; however, the specificity of exercise testing is also lower in women. Several mechanisms have been suggested to explain the high false-positive (indeterminate) rate of ST depression in women, including estrogens and resting ST-T abnormalities. Since estrogens have a similar chemical structure to digitalis, it has been suggested that they may be partially responsible for the high prevalence of false-positive exercise test results in women.

Although exercise testing may detect labile hypertensives or individuals who will eventually become hypertensive, there is little valid support for this hypothesis.[57,58] Hypertensive patients frequently have ECG abnormalities (LV hypertrophy) and myocardial hypertrophy, both of which may result in false-positive ST responses.

Exercise testing has been used in patients with idiopathic dilated cardiomyopathy to determine exercise capacity, pulmonary response to LV dysfunction, grade of ventricular ectopy, and effectiveness of treatment.[59] Patients with LV dysfunction usually have reduced exercise capacity due to an inadequate increase in cardiac output during exercise, which limits V_{O_2max} and exercise tolerance. Initially, stroke volume may increase normally during upright exercise despite a decrease in LVEF; however, if there is limited chronotropic reserve with increasing exercise, the stroke volume and cardiac output cannot continue to meet the increase demands. A few patients may have normal exercise tolerance despite severe LV dysfunction. Several peripheral compensatory mechanisms have been proposed to explain the poor correlation between LV function and exercise capacity. (See also Chap. 89.)

Exercise may result in sudden death due to arrhythmias in hypertrophic cardiomyopathy.[60,61] Chest discomfort, an abnormal resting ECG, and exercise-induced ST-segment depression are frequent. In this condition, exercise testing under very careful supervision may be helpful to demonstrate the level at which significant events occur, such as the presence or severity of arrhythmias, myocardial ischemia, murmurs indicating obstruction in LV outflow, and presyncopal manifestations. (See Chap. 90.)

Intracardiac conduction blocks can either develop or resolve during exercise. Rate-dependent intraventricular blocks that occur during exercise often precede the appearance of chronic blocks present at rest.[62–64] The diagnosis of ischemia from the exercise ECG is not usually reliable when there is left bundle branch block, which can be associated with a marked degree of ST segment depression with exercise in addition to that found at rest. Left bundle branch block occurring with HR below 125 beats per minute in patients with typical angina is frequently associated with CAD. The presence of intraventricular blocks and their disappearance during exercise are rare. Rarely, patients with left bundle branch block develop a normal QRS pattern during exercise. Pre-existing right bundle branch block[65–69] does not influence interpretation of the exercise test except in the anterior (V_{1-2}) precordial leads; however, sensitivity of exercise testing in these patients is uncertain.

In addition to left or right bundle branch block, left anterior or posterior hemiblock and bifascicular block (a combination of right bundle branch block and either left anterior or posterior hemiblock) may be induced by exercise. The presence of such blocks is primarily a rate-related phenomenon occurring as the sinus rate increases beyond a critical point. Intraventricular block during exercise may be difficult to distinguish from ventricular tachycardia.

First-degree atrioventricular (AV) block occasionally occurs at the end of exercise or during the recovery phase. Medications or conditions that may produce prolonged AV conduction time (e.g., digitalis, propranolol, myocarditis) may predispose the individual to lengthening of the PR interval.

Second-degree AV block—Wenckebach (Mobitz type I) AV block—during exercise is rare. The clinical significance of exercise-induced Mobitz II AV block is not known but may also be a rate-related phenomenon, appearing as the sinus rate is accelerated beyond a critical level. It has been seen in patients with CAD.

Complete AV block at rest is a relative contraindication to exercise testing, but with very careful supervision, exercise testing may be performed in selected patients. Exercise testing can also be performed in patients with congenital complete AV block, provided there are no coexisting significant congenital anomalies.

Rarely, patients develop long periods of sinus arrest and sinoventricular conduction immediately after exercise. This usually occurs in patients with severe myocardial ischemia.

Exercise may provoke, abolish, or not affect anomalous AV conduction in individuals with known preexcitation such as Wolff-Parkinson-White syndrome (WPW).[70] Exercise usually does not abolish anomalous AV conduction; when it does occur, these individuals are thought to be in less danger of exercise-induced ventricular tachycardia. With anomalous AV conduction (such as WPW), significant ST depression can be observed during exercise testing and may not be due to ischemia but rather a false-positive (indeterminate) change. In general, there is a low prevalence of tachyarrhythmias during or after exercise in WPW patients. (See also Chap. 36.)

Exercise may induce cardiac arrhythmias under several conditions, especially diuretic and digitalis therapy.[71–73] The recent ingestion of alcohol or caffeine may also exacerbate exercise-induced arrhythmias. Since exercise increases myocardial oxygen demand, the presence of CAD can predispose some patients to arrhythmias during exercise. It appears that subendocardial ischemia (ST depression) is not as arrhythmogenic as transmural ischemia (ST elevation). Exercise-induced arrhythmias are generated by enhanced sympathetic tone and catecholamines, increased myocardial oxygen demand, or both. The immediate postexercise period is particularly of concern because of high catecholamine levels in combination with generalized vasodilation. The combination of peripheral arteriolar dilation induced by exercise and reduced cardiac output from diminished venous return secondary to the sudden termination of muscular activity may lead to a reduction in coronary perfusion while HR is elevated. The associated increased sympathetic tone may stimulate ectopic Purkinje pacemaker activity in the myocardium by accelerating phase 4 of the action potential, provoking spontaneous discharge and leading to increased automaticity.

Exercise can suppress cardiac arrhythmias present in patients at rest. This phenomenon has been attributed to the overdrive suppression of the ectopic impulse formation by sinus tachycardia induced by exercise-vagal withdrawal and increased sympathetic stimulation. (See also Chap. 35.)

Ectopic ventricular contractions are the most frequent typed cardiac arrhythmia that develops during exercise, followed by supraventricular arrhythmias. Their prevalence is directly related to age and cardiac abnormalities. In general, ectopic ventricular contractions are of concern in patients with a family history of cardiomyopathy, valvular heart disease, or known severe ischemia.

Sinus arrhythmias with periods of sinus bradycardia and wandering atrial pacemaker are relatively common during exercise and the immediate recovery phase. Atrial ectopy can occur in either normal or diseased hearts. Exercise-induced transient atrial fibrillation and flutter occur in less than 1 percent of individuals who undergo exercise testing.[74] These arrhythmias may be induced by exercise in both healthy individuals and patients with rheumatic heart disease, hyperthyroidism, WPW syndrome, or cardiomyopathy. Paroxysmal AV junctional tachycardia is rarely observed during exercise. Exercise-induced supraventricular arrhythmias alone are usually not related to CAD but are more often related to pulmonary disease, recent alcohol ingestion, or excessive caffeine.

REFERENCES

1. Rowell LB: *Human Circulation. Regulation During Physical Stress.* New York, Oxford University Press, 1986.
2. Cohn JN (ed): Quantitative exercise testing for the cardiac patient: The value of monitoring gas exchange: Introduction. *Circulation* 1987; 76(Suppl. VI):VI-1–VI-2.
3. Fletcher GF, Froelicher VF, Hartley LH, Haskell WL, Pollock ML: Exercise standards: A statement for health professionals from the American Heart Association. *Circulation* 1990; 82:2286–2322.
4. Higginbotham MB: Cardiac performance during submaximal and maximal exercise in healthy persons. *Heart Failure* 1988; 4:68–76.
5. Londeree BR, Moeschberger ML: Influence of age and other factors on maximal heart rate. *J Cardiac Rehabil* 1984; 4:44–49.
6. Gould KL, Lipscomb K: Effects of coronary stenoses on coronary flow reserve and resistance. *Am J Cardiol* 1974; 34:48–55.
7. Froelicher VF Jr: The detection of asymptomatic coronary artery disease. *Ann Rev Med* 1977; 28:1–12.
8. ACP/ACC/AHA Task Force on Exercise Testing. *JACC* 1990; 16(5):1061–1065.
9. Schlant RC, Blomqvist CG, Brandenburg RO, DeBusk R, Ellestad MH, Fletcher GF, et al: Special report. In: Guidelines for exercise testing. A report of the Joint American College of Cardiology/American Heart Association Task force on Assessment of Cardiovascular Procedures (Subcommittee on Exercise Testing). *Circulation* 1986; 74:653A–667A.
10. Becker RC, Alpert JS: Electrocardiographic ST segment depression in coronary heart disease. *Am Heart J* 1988; 115:862–868.
11. Franklin BA: Exercise testing, training and arm ergometry. *Sports Med* 1985; 2:100–119.
12. Balady GJ, Weiner DA, McCabe CH, Ryan TJ: Value of arm exercise testing in detecting coronary artery disease. *Am J Cardiol* 1985; 55:37–39.
13. Dalke B, Ware RW: An experimental study of "physical fitness" of Air Force personnel. *US Armed Forces Med J* 1959; 10:675–688.
14. Fletcher GF (ed): *Exercise in the Practice of Medicine,* 2d ed. Mt. Kisco, NY, Futura, 1988.
15. Bruce RA, Blackmon JR, Jones JW, Strait G: Exercising testing in adult normal subjects and cardiac patients. *Pediatrics* 1963; 32(Suppl):742–756.
16. Sheffield LT, Roitman D: Stress testing methodology. *Prog Cardiovasc Dis* 1976; 19:33–49.
17. Lester FM, Sheffield LT, Reeves TJ: Electrocardiographic changes in clinically normal older men following near maximal and maximal exercise. *Circulation* 1967; 36:5–14.
18. Sheffield LT, Maloof JA, Sawyer JA, Roitman D: Maximal heart rate and treadmill performance of healthy women in relation to age. *Circulation* 1978; 57:79–84.
19. Borg G: Psycho-physical bases of perceived exertion. *Med Sci Sports Exerc* 1982; 14:377–381.
20. Bruce RA, Fisher LD, Pettinger M, Weiner DA, Chaitman BR: ST segment elevation with exercise: A marker for poor ventricular function and poor prognosis. *Circulation* 1988; 77:897–905.
21. Fletcher GF, Fletcher BJ, Sweeney ME: Effects of exercise testing, training and beta blockade on serum potassium in normal subjects. *Am J Cardiol* 1990; 65:1242–1245.
22. Fletcher GF, Sweeney ME, Fletcher BJ: Blood magnesium and potassium alterations with maximal treadmill exercise testing: Effects of beta-adrenergic blockade. *Am Heart J* 1991; 121:105–110.
23. Gianrossi R, Detrano R, Mulvihill D, Lehmann K, Dubach P, Colombo A, et al: Exercise-induced ST depression in the diagnosis of coronary artery disease: A meta-analysis. *Circulation* 1989; 80:87–98.
24. Froelicher VF, Perdue S, Pewen W, Risch M: Application of meta-analysis using an electronic spread sheet to exercise testing in patients after myocardial infarction. *Am J Med* 1987; 83:1045–1054.
25. Lee TH, Cook EF, Goldman L: Prospective evaluation of a clinical and exercise-test model for the prediction of left main coronary artery disease. *Med Decis Making* 1986; 6:136–144.
26. Dubach P, Froelicher VF, Klein J, Oakes D, Grover-McKay M, Friis R: Exercise-induced hypotension in a male population: Criteria, causes, and prognosis. *Circulation* 1988; 78:1380–1387.
27. Dagenais GR, Rouleau JR, Hochart P, Magrina J, Cantin B, Dumesnil JG: Survival with painless strongly positive exercise electrocardiogram. *Am J Cardiol* 1988; 62:892–895.
28. Klein J, Froelicher VF, Detrano R, Dubach P, Yen R: Does the rest electrocardiogram after myocardial infarction determine the predictive value of exercise-induced ST depression? A two year follow-up study in a Veteran population. *J Am Coll Cardiol* 1989; 14:305–311.
29. Krone RJ, Dwyer EM, Greenberg H, Miller JP, Gillespie JA: Risk stratification in patients with first non-Q wave infarction: Limited value of the early low level exercise test after uncomplicated infarcts. *J Am Coll Cardiol* 1989; 14:31–37.
30. Hammermeister KE, DeRouen TA, Dodge HT: Variables predictive of survival in patients with coronary disease. Selection by univariate and multivariate analyses from the clinical, electrocardiographic, exercise, arteriographic, and quantitative angiographic evaluation. *Circulation* 1979; 59:421–430.
31. Mark DB, Hlatky MA, Harrell FE, Lee KL, Califf RM, Pryor DB: Exercise treadmill score for predicting prognosis in coronary artery disease. *Ann Intern Med* 1987; 106:793–800.

32. Brunelli C, Cristofani R, L'Abbate A, for the ODI Study Group: Long-term survival in medically treated patients with ischemic heart disease and prognostic importance of clinical and electrocardiographic data. (The Italian CNR Multicenter Prospective Study ODI). *Eur Heart J* 1989; 10:292–303.
33. Weiner DA, Ryan T, McCabe CH, Chaitman BR, Sheffield LT, Ferguson JC, et al: Prognostic importance of a clinical profile and exercise test in medically treated patients with coronary artery disease. *J Am Coll Cardiol* 1984; 3:772–779.
34. Gohlke H, Samek L, Betz P, Roskamm H: Exercise testing provides additional prognostic information in angiographically defined subgroups of patients with coronary artery disease. *Circulation* 1983; 68:979–985.
35. Peduzzi P, Hultgren H, Thomsen J, Angell W: Prognostic value of baseline exercise tests. *Progress Cardiovasc Dis* 1986; 28:285–292.
36. Kaul S, Lilly DR, Gascho JA, Watson DD, Gibson RS, Oliner CA, et al: Prognostic utility of the exercise thallium-201 test in ambulatory patients with chest pain: Comparison with cardiac catheterization. *Circulation* 1988; 77:745–758.
37. Marieb M, Beller G, Gibson R, Lerman B, Sanjiv K: Clinical relevancy of exercise-induced ventricular arrhythmias in suspected coronary artery disease. *Am J Cardiol* 1990; 66:172–178.
38. Bruce RA, Fisher LD, Hossack KF: Validation of exercise enhanced risk assessment of coronary heart disease events: Longitudinal changes in incidence in Seattle community practice. *J Am Coll Cardiol* 1985; 5:875–881.
39. European Coronary Surgery Study Group: Long-term results of prospective randomized study of coronary artery bypass surgery in stable angina pectoris. *Lancet* 1982; 2:1173–1180.
40. Weiner DA, Ryan TJ, McCabe CH, Chaitman BR, Sheffield LT, Fisher LD, et al: The role of exercise testing in identifying patients with improved survival after coronary bypass surgery. *J Am Coll Cardiol* 1986; 8:741–748.
41. Dubach P, Froelicher V, Klein J, Detrano R: Use of the exercise test to predict prognosis after coronary artery bypass grafting. *Am J Cardiol* 1989; 63:530–533.
42. McHenry PL, O'Donnell J, Morris SN, Jordan JJ: The abnormal exercise electrocardiogram in apparently healthy men: A predictor of angina pectoris as an initial coronary event during long-term follow-up. *Circulation* 1984; 70:547–551.
43. Sox HC Jr, Littenberg B, Garber AM: The role of exercise testing in screening for coronary artery disease [comments]. *Ann Intern Med* 1989; 110:456–469.
44. Hochreiter C, Borer JS: Exercise testing in patients with aortic and mitral valve disease: Current applications. *Cardiovasc Clin* 1983; 13:291–300.
45. Areskog NH: Exercise testing in the evaluation of patients with valvular aortic stenosis. *Clin Physiol* 1984; 4:201–208.
46. Atwood JE, Kawanishi S, Myers J, Froelicher VF: Exercise testing in patients with aortic stenosis. *Chest* 1988; 93:1083–1087.
47. Misra M, Thakur R, Bhandari K, Puri VK: Value of the treadmill exercise test in asymptomatic and minimally symptomatic patients with chronic severe aortic regurgitation. *Int J Cardiol* 1987; 15:309–316.
48. Vacek JL, Valentin-Stone P, Wolfe M, Davis WR: The value of standardized exercise testing in the noninvasive evaluation of mitral stenosis. *Am J Med Sci* 1986; 292:335–343.
49. Weber KT, Janicki JS, McElroy PA: Cardiopulmonary exercise testing in the evaluation of mitral and aortic valve incompetence. *Herz* 1986; 11:88–96.
50. Broustet JP, Douard H, Mora B: Exercise testing in arrhythmias of idiopathic mitral valve prolapse. *Eur Heart J* 1987; 8(Suppl D):37–42.
51. Lee TH, Shammash JB, Ribeiro JP, Hartley LH, Sherwood J, Goldman L: Estimation of maximum oxygen uptake from clinical data: Performance of the Specific Activity Scale. *Am Heart J* 1988; 115:203–204.
52. Carliner NH, Fisher ML, Plotnick GD, Garbart H, Rapoport A, Kelemen MH, et al: Routine preoperative exercise testing in patients undergoing major noncardiac surgery. *Am J Cardiol* 1985; 56:51–58.
53. McPhail N, Calvin JE, Shariatmadar A, Barber GG, Scobie TK: The use of preoperative exercise testing to predict cardiac complications after arterial reconstruction. *J Vasc Surg* 1988; 7:60–68.
54. Sullivan M, Savvides M, Abouantoun S, Madsen EB, Froelicher V: Failure of transdermal nitroglycerin to improve exercise capacity in patients with angina pectoris. *J Am Coll Cardiol* 1985; 5:1220–1223.
55. Sullivan M, Atwood JE, Myers J, Feuer J, Hall P, Kellerman B, et al: Increased exercise capacity after digoxin administration in patients with heart failures. *J Am Coll Cardiol* 1989; 13:1138–1143.
56. Guiteras P, Chaitman BR, Waters DD, Bourassa MG, Scholl JM, Ferguson RJ, et al: Diagnostic accuracy of exercise ECG lead systems in clinical subsets of women. *Circulation* 1982; 65:1465–1474.
57. Exercise hypertension: A symposium issue. *Herz* 1987; 12:76–149.
58. Liao Y, Emidy LA, Gosch FC, Stamler R, Stamler J: Cardiovascular responses to exercise of participants in a trial on the primary prevention of hypertension. *J Hypertens* 1987; 5:317–321.
59. Wilson JR, Fink LI, Ferraro N, Dunkman WB, Jones RA: Use of maximal bicycle performance in patients with congestive heart failure secondary to coronary artery disease or to idiopathic dilated cardiomyopathy. *Am J Cardiol* 1986; 15:601–606.
60. Losse B, Kuhn H, Loogen F, Schulte HD: Exercise performance in hypertrophic cardiomyopathies. *Eur Heart J* 1983; 4(Suppl F):197–208.
61. Savage DD, Seides SF, Maron BJ, Myers DJ, Epstein SE: Prevalence of arrhythmias during 24-hour electrocardiographic monitoring and exercise testing in patients with obstructive and nonobstructive hypertrophic cardiomyopathy. *Circulation* 1979; 59:866–875.
62. Heinsimer JA, Irwin JM, Basnight LL: Influence of underlying coronary artery disease on the natural history and prognosis of exercise-induced left bundle branch block. *Am J Cardiol* 1987; 60:1065–1067.
63. Vasey C, O'Donnell J, Morris SN, McHenry P: Exercise-induced left bundle branch block and its relation to coronary artery disease. *Am J Cardiol* 1985; 56:892–895.
64. Whinnery JE, Froelicher VF Jr, Stewart AJ, Longo MR Jr, Triebwasser JH, Lancaster MC: The electrocardiographic response to maximal treadmill exercise in asymptomatic men with left bundle branch block. *Am Heart J* 1977; 94:316–324.
65. Williams MA, Esterbrooks DJ, Nair CK, Sailors MM, Sketch MH: Clinical significance of exercise-induced bundle branch block. *Am J Cardiol* 1988; 61:346–348.
66. Wayne VS, Bishop RL, Cook L, Spodick D: Exercise-induced bundle branch block. *Am J Cardiol* 1983; 52:283–286.
67. Whinnery JE, Froelicher VF: Exercise testing in right bundle branch block (letter). *Chest* 1977; 72:684–685.
68. Whinnery JE, Froelicher VF Jr, Longo MR Jr, Triebwasser JH: The electrocardiographic response to maximal treadmill exercise of asymptomatic men with right bundle branch block. *Chest* 1977; 71:335–340.
69. Whinnery JE, Froelicher VF: Acquired bundle branch block and its response to exercise testing in asymptomatic air crewmen: A review with case reports. *Aviat Space Environ Med* 1976; 46:69–78.
70. Sharma AD, Yee R, Guiraudon G, Klein GJ: Sensitivity and specificity of invasive and noninvasive testing for risk of sudden death in Wolff-Parkinson-White syndrome. *J Am Coll Cardiol* 1987; 10:373–381.
71. Allen BJ, Casey TP, Brodsky MA, Luckett CR, Henry WL: Exercise testing in patients with life-threatening ventricular tachyarrhythmias: Results and correlation with clinical and arrhythmia factors. *Am Heart J* 1988; 116:997–1002.
72. Ryan M, Lown B, Horn H: Comparison of ventricular ectopic activity during 24-hour monitoring and exercise testing in patients with coronary heart disease. *N Engl J Med* 1975; 292:224–229.
73. Sami M, Chaitman B, Fisher L, Holmes D, Fray D, Alderman E: Significance of exercise-induced ventricular arrhythmia in stable coronary artery disease: A coronary artery surgery study project. *Am J Cardiol* 1984; 54:1182–1188.
74. Atwood JE, Myers J, Sullivan M, Forbes S, Friis R, Pewen W, et al: Maximal exercise testing and gas exchange in patients with chronic atrial fibrillation. *J Am Coll Cardiol* 1988; 11:508–513.
75. Froelicher VF: *Exercise and the Heart: Clinical Concepts.* Chicago, Year Book Medical Publishers, Inc., 1987.

Chapter 17

Techniques of Evaluating Pulmonary Function in Patients with Cardiac Disease

Eric G. Honig, M.D.

Pulmonary diseases may have adverse effects on cardiac function, and cardiac diseases may be manifested in alterations of pulmonary function. Cardiac enlargement may impinge on the tracheobronchial tree, causing lobar or segmental obstruction and atelectasis. Increased pulmonary venous pressure from left ventricular failure or mitral valve disease alters lung compliance, and increased lung water from pulmonary edema may decrease airflow as well. Increased pulmonary blood flow from left-to-right shunts have a similar mechanical effect on the lung and may alter gas-exchanging properties of the lung. Cardiac medications may cause airway reactivity or parenchymal pulmonary disease. Heart disease may affect the feedback loop controlling respiration leading to unstable respiratory rhythms. A decreased cardiac output may have disproportionate effects on respiratory muscle function.[1] Lung disease, in turn, may produce pulmonary hypertension and right ventricular dysfunction. Hypoxemia contributes to arrhythmogenesis. Poor pulmonary status adds to the risk of cardiac surgery. Heart or lung disease may lead to symptoms of dyspnea, decreased exercise tolerance, orthopnea, or cough. Tests of pulmonary function assist in determining to what degree symptomatology may be caused by pulmonary rather than cardiac disease and the degree to which known heart disease has compromised the respiratory system. While pulmonary function tests may reflect cardiac dysfunction, they cannot substitute for direct evaluation of cardiac physiology in patients with heart disease.

SPIROMETRY

Spirometry is the primary measure of pulmonary function. The spirometric maneuver consists of a full inhalation to total lung capacity followed by forced exhalation back down to residual volume. The spirogram plots volume as the dependent variable versus time while the flow-volume loop displays volume against its time differential, flow. The spirogram is best suited to analyzing late airflow events, while the flow-volume loop better displays events early in the forced expiration. The modern spirometer is usually attached to a computer that records and calculates time and volume data. Most systems today simultaneously display a flow-volume loop along with the volume-time trace for each expiratory effort.

Forced vital capacity (FVC) is defined as the total amount of air that can be breathed out in a single forced exhalation. The term FEV_1 is the amount breathed out in 1 s, FEV_3 that in 3 s. Both are normalized to the forced vital capacity as FEV_1/FVC and FEV_3/FVC. Flow over the middle of the vital capacity is described either by the FEF_{25-75}, the average flow from 25 to 75 percent vital capacity, or the $FEF_{200-1200}$, the average flow over 1 liter volume beginning from 200 mL below total lung capacity.[2] Midflow measurements are extremely sensitive indices of airflow limitation but are rarely significant in isolation.[3]

The expiratory limb of the flow-volume loop reflects intrathoracic physiology. The upper third of the flow volume loop is effort dependent, while the lower two-thirds is considered relatively effort independent and largely reflects the geometry of the distal airways. The peak expiratory flow rate (PEFR) is the chief index of effort-dependent flow while the instantaneous flow at 50 percent vital capacity ($\dot{V}_{max\ 50}$) is the most commonly used measurement of the effort-independent portion of the curve.[4]

Normal

The normal spirogram is characterized by a rapid initial slope of airflow with at least 75 percent of the vital capacity breath exhaled in the first second and 95 percent in the first 3 s. Because normal airways have completely emptied by this time, there is little further volume change after the first 3 s and the normal spirogram reaches a plateau.

The normal flow-volume loop reaches a rapid early peak with flows declining as lung volume decreases with continued exhalation. The expiratory limb of the flow-volume loop is nearly linear in its descent.

Obstruction

Obstruction is characterized by an increase in the time constant of exhalation and prolongation of the time needed to empty the airways. The obstructive spirogram will show a decreased initial slope and appreciable volume change still occurring after 3 s exhalation. Marked prolongation of expiration in severe obstruction may be accompanied by airway closure, trapping gas in the lung and reducing the vital capacity. A failure of the spirogram to reach a normal plateau indicates obstructive air trapping may be present.

The FEV_1 and FEV_3 as well as FEV_1/FVC and FEV_3/FVC will be reduced in clinically significant obstructive disease, and the vital capacity may be decreased when obstructive air trapping is present. An FEV_1 below 70 percent predicted has been found to carry 82 percent sensitivity and 98 percent specificity for obstructive disease.[5]

Obstruction is seen in the MEFV loop as concavity of the expiratory limb toward the volume axis. The more severe the obstruction, the higher the lung volume at which concavity will be observed. Usually, both the PEFR and $\dot{V}_{50}$ will be reduced.

Restriction

Restrictive disease is seen on the spirogram as compression of the volume axis. In pure restriction, airflow remains normal. There is a brisk upstroke of the spirogram and the tracing terminates in a normal plateau. Vital capacity, FEV_1, and FEV_3 will all be reduced while FEV_1/FVC and FEV_3/FVC are normal.

The flow-volume loop shows compression on the volume axis so that the loop resembles a vertically elongated bean. With preserved airflows, no concavity should be seen in the descending limb of the flow-volume loop.

In many restrictive lung disorders, coexisting airway disease may be present and the spirogram and flow-volume loops may show features of both processes.

An FVC of less than 80 percent predicted with an FEV_1 above 70 percent predicted is 82 percent specific and 93 percent sensitive for restrictive disease.[6]

Clinical Application

Spirometry is an important part of the evaluation of patients with dyspnea of unexplained etiology and in the assessment of pulmonary hypertension. (See Chap. 99.) Spirometry does not appear to be helpful in the evaluation of pulmonary amiodarone toxicity,[7] but it can be useful in the assessment of patients with cough due to angiotensin converting enzyme inhibitors or wheezing caused by beta blockers. Declines in spirometric performance may be sensitive early indicators of lung rejection in heart-lung transplants.[8] Vital capacity declines with severity of mitral stenosis and other forms of pulmonary venous hypertension, but pulmonary function is not sufficiently precise to supplant more direct methods of cardiac assessment. (See Chap. 80.) Available data do not permit a definitive assessment of the value of spirometry or other pulmonary function studies in the preoperative evaluation of patients for cardiac surgery.[9] Nonetheless, arterial blood gases and spirometry are suggested as "prudent" for patients with a history of tobacco use and dyspnea who are about to undergo cardiac surgery.[10]

INHALATION CHALLENGE

One of the defining characteristics of the asthmatic state is bronchial hyperresponsiveness leading to episodic cough, wheezing, or dyspnea. Asthmatic patients may show normal spirometry on pulmonary function testing. In order to document airways hyperreactivity, an inhalation challenge may be indicated.

Method

Methacholine Cl, a muscarinic cholinergic agent, is the most common stimulus employed, but histamine, carbachol, cold air, and exercise have all been used for bronchial challenges. Normal saline has been used to elicit nonspecific bronchial hyperresponsiveness. A challenge protocol measures baseline pulmonary function followed by inhalation of logarithmically increasing doses of the challenge stimulus with spirometry and measurement of lung volumes, airways conductance (sG_{aw}), and airways resistance (R_{aw}) at each challenge concentration. Bronchospasm will produce significant decreases in FVC, airflow, and sG_{aw} or increases in functional residual capacity (FRC) and R_{aw}. Results of a bronchial inhalation challenge are reported as the dose of challenge agent (PD) at which a clinically meaningful change is seen, $PD_{xxparam}$, where xx is the percentage change in the pulmonary parameter tested. The most commonly used expression is PD_{20FEV1}, a 20 percent decrease in FEV_1. Challenge data are plotted with log dose as the independent variable and the measured parameter as the dependent variable. The lower the PD, the greater the airway reactivity.[11,12]

Clinical Application

Bronchial inhalation challenge testing is indicated in the assessment of dyspnea, cough, or wheeze where intermittent airflow obstruction is suspected but not evident on simple spirometry. Bronchial hyperresponsiveness is characteristic of heart-lung transplants due to denervation hypersensitivity of the transplanted lung. Further increases in reactivity may indicate lung rejection even before spirometric abnormalities become evident. Bronchial hyperreactivity is also seen in the setting of pulmonary venous hypertension as "cardiac asthma." Cardiac asthma probably results from narrowing of airways by a peribronchial cuff of edema fluid as well as from activation or irritant receptors. It is largely reversible with correction of the underlying cardiac condition.[13]

LUNG VOLUMES

Lung volumes reflect a physiological balance between forces acting to increase the size of the lungs and thorax and those acting to reduce the volume of the lungs and thorax.

Method

Lung volumes can be measured by gas dilution (helium), gas washout (nitrogen), or planimetry of the chest roentgenogram but are most commonly determined by body plethysmography. Nitrogen washout is the most physiological approach and gives further information about the uniformity of distribution of ventilation, but its utility is limited by the reliability of available nitrogen analyzers. Helium dilution depends on the complete mixing of inspired helium in the lung over a period of 3 to 5 min. The result may be artifactually reduced by airways obstruction and poor penetration of inspired gas to obstructed lung or noncommunicating airspaces such as bullae. Body plethysmography is quick and convenient but may represent an overestimate in the presence of obstructive lung disease.

Clinical Application

Lung volumes are used to follow restrictive processes, assess obstructive air trapping and hyperinflation, and aid in the differential diagnosis of a decreased vital capacity. Lung volume measurements should be part of the assessment of patients with pulmonary hypertension looking for a restrictive pulmonary process. Uniformly low volumes suggest parenchymal restriction. A decreased total lung capacity (TLC) and normal FRC with an increased or normal residual volume (RV) are characteristic of congestive heart failure. A decreased inspiratory capacity with a preserved residual volume suggests neuromuscular disease while a decreased expiratory reserve volume is commonly seen in obesity.[14]

D_LCO

The carbon monoxide diffusing capacity (D_LCO) is often thought of as specific for uptake of CO across alveolar capillary membrane, but the test in fact reflects the entire gas exchange pathway from the mouth to red cell uptake of CO. The D_LCO is partitioned in parallel between membrane diffusion (D_m) and RBC uptake (θV_c). A low D_LCO may reflect anemia, decreased CO affinity by the erythrocyte, a decreased pulmonary capillary blood volume (θV_c), interstitial lung disease, an alveolar filling process, a reduction in the number of functioning alveoli, airways disease (D_m), or any combination of these.[15]

Method

Two methods are commonly used to measure D_LCO: single breath and steady state. The single-breath test (D_LCOsb) consists of a 10-s breath-hold of a total lung capacity inspiration of 2900 ppm CO mixed in 10 percent helium and air. Inspired and expired concentrations of He and CO are measured and the logarithmic disappearance rate of CO, which has a slope of D_L/VA, is calculated. Lung volume (VA) is determined by single-breath dilution of helium and multiplied by the disappearance slope to yield D_LCOsb.[16]

The steady-state measurement (D_LCOss) defines D_LCO as CO uptake/driving gradient. The driving gradient is defined as alveolar CO concentration and is estimated by the end-tidal CO concentration. The estimate is valid unless the distribution of ventilation is uneven, as in obstructive lung diseases where D_LCOss is biased low. The vulnerability of D_LCOss to inhomogeneity in ventilation may be reduced by measuring the steady-state D_LCO under exercise conditions. D_LCOsb is normally higher than D_LCOss at rest, and the two methods are not interchangeable. The two methods yield closer results when D_LCOss is measured in exercise.[17]

Clinical Application

A 15 to 20 percent fall in D_LCO has been shown to be 100 percent sensitive and 89 percent specific in the detection of pulmonary amiodarone toxicity, and a low-baseline D_LCO may indicate a subgroup at slightly increased risk for amiodarone toxicity. Patients with low-baseline pulmonary function will be more impaired by amiodarone toxicity, but the data cannot be used to justify avoiding the drug in patients with abnormal baseline pulmonary function. It would appear reasonable to obtain baseline pulmonary function studies including D_LCO at a point of clinical stability prior to initiating amiodarone and obtaining repeat assessments if the clinical picture is suggestive of toxicity. If the D_LCO remains at least 80 percent of baseline, the drug may be safely continued.[18,19]

The D_LCO is also useful in the evaluation of patients with pulmonary hypertension and for dyspneic patients in whom restrictive lung disease is being considered. D_LCO is reduced in emphysema but not in asthmatic patients.

POLYSOMNOGRAPHY

Polysomnography (PSG) is employed for definitive diagnosis of sleep-disordered breathing or excessive daytime somnolence.

Method

A PSG consists of continuous recording of airflow, respiratory effort, measured as rib cage and abdominal movements or directly as esophageal pressure, oxygen saturation, electrocardiography, electroencephalography for sleep staging, electrooculography to identify rapid eye movement sleep, and electromyography of selected upper airway muscles. The PSG is best carried out overnight for at least 8 h.[20] Shorter 4 to 5 h daytime nap studies have 88 percent sensitivity and 100 percent specificity for the diagnosis of sleep apnea compared with all-night studies but fail to accurately reflect sleep profile or oxygen desaturation.[21]

Sleep-disordered events are defined as a 50 percent or greater reduction of airflow for at least 10 s and classified as central or obstructive on the basis of inspiratory effort. The data are expressed as events per hour, the respiratory disturbance index (RDI) or apnea-hypopnea index (AHI), with 15 per hour as an upper limit of normal. The oxygen saturation profile and presence of arrhythmias are reported as a function of sleep stage. The efficiency of sleep and the frequency of electroencephalogram (EEG) arousals are noted.[22]

Clinical Application

A subgroup of patients with the clinical features of sleep apnea syndrome have been found on closer investigation to have Cheyne-Stokes respiration either alone or in association with central or obstructive apneas. Frank congestive heart failure or organic heart disease is a common underlying cause. Unlike typical sleep apnea, Cheyne-Stokes-associated hypersomnolence shows a good clinical response to theophylline.[23] Polysomnography or all-night oximetry may be helpful in detecting significant nocturnal oxygen desaturations in the evaluation of patients with cor pulmonale or pulmonary hypertension. A high prevalence of sleep apnea in patients awaiting transplant for ischemic cardiomyopathy suggests that polysomnography may have a role in this population as well.

RESPIRATORY MUSCLE FUNCTION

The diaphragm is the chief muscle of respiration. It is assisted in its function by the strap muscles of the neck, the trapezius, the intercostals, and the abdominal musculature. Although skeletal muscles, the respiratory muscles are similar to the myocardium in that they function throughout the patient's lifetime without significant rest or pause. Respiratory muscle weakness may be a cause of dyspnea or prolong ventilator dependence in the patient with mixed cardiac and respiratory failure.

Methods

Respiratory muscle function is assessed indirectly by ventilatory output and directly by respiratory forces or by measurement of transdiaphragmatic pressure. Maximum voluntary ventilation (MVV) is measured spirometrically. A patient is asked to breathe as deeply and as rapidly as possible. Exhaled volume is measured for 10 to 12 s and the result extrapolated to 60 s. MVV is not specific for muscle function, since it will also be reduced by obstructive or restrictive lung disease. The MVV is usually about 35 times the FEV_1. A disproportionately low MVV is suggestive either of respiratory muscle weakness or poor patient effort.

Maximal inspiratory and expiratory forces are a more direct evaluation of respiratory muscle strength. For the measurement, a mouthpiece is connected to a manometer. The patient is instructed to exhale fully to residual volume. At RV, the mouthpiece is occluded and the patient is instructed to inspire forcefully. The sustained maximal negative pressure is considered to be the maximal inspiratory force. The maximal expiratory force is measured from a maximal occluded expiratory effort from total lung capacity. Predicted normals for maximal expiratory forces are based on age and gender. Lower limits of normal inspiratory forces are 50 cmH_2O for females and 75 cmH_2O for males. Expiratory forces should be 95 cmH_2O for females and 140 cmH_2O for males. Maximal forces are critically dependent both on patient co-operation and the volume at which the measurement was made. Artifactual reductions will be seen if forces are determined below TLC or above RV.[24]

Diaphragmatic function can be assessed by the transdiaphragmatic pressure, P_{di}, defined as the difference between pleural pressure and intraabdominal pressure ($P_{abd} - P_{pl}$). Pleural pressure is measured from an esophageal balloon, while intraabdominal pressure is determined from a gastric balloon. Measurement of P_{di} has been simplified by the introduction of modified nasogastric tubes with dual measuring ports.

Clinical Application

Patients with congestive heart failure appear to have weakness of the diaphragm and respiratory muscles out of proportion to more generalized skeletal muscle weakness probably caused by reduced perfusion of the respiratory muscles. Since congestive failure leads to increased lung stiffness, elastic work of breathing is increased. The combination of increased elastic work and decreased diaphragmatic strength and endurance may lead to respiratory failure or prolonged ventilator dependence in combined respiratory and cardiac failure.[25]

There is a high incidence of diaphragm dysfunction associated with cardiac surgery attributable either to inadvertent crush injury of the phrenic nerve(s) or cold injury due to cardioplegic cooling.[26]

EXERCISE TESTING

The cardiac exercise tolerance test is well suited to the detection of cardiac ischemia (see Chap. 16). The addition of measurement of ventilation and expired oxygen and carbon dioxide concentrations allows a more global evaluation of work capacity and limits to exercise capacity. Cardiopulmonary exercise testing has become more widely available with the development of rapid-response O_2 and CO_2 analyzers and on-line calculation of gas exchange variables.

Method

Primary measurements in the cardiopulmonary exercise protocol are heart rate, blood pressure, minute ventilation, oxygen saturation, and the expired concentrations of CO_2 and O_2. Oxygen uptake ($\dot{V}_{O_2}$) and CO_2 output ($\dot{V}_{CO_2}$) are calculated from the expired gas concentrations and minute volume. Maximal oxygen uptake, ($\dot{V}_2$max) is defined by a plateau in $\dot{V}_{O_2}$ at increasing work levels. The anaerobic threshold typically occurs at 60 to 70 percent of $\dot{V}_{O_2}$max and is identified by an increase in $\dot{V}_{CO_2}$ or minute ventilation in response to the development of lactic acidemia. The O_2 pulse is defined as $\dot{V}_{O_2}$ per heart rate and reflects cardiac stroke volume. The dyspnea index is defined as the highest respiratory minute volume divided by the patient's MVV and indicates the patient's ventilatory reserve. Most cardiopulmonary exercise laboratories utilize 1 to 3 electrocardiographic leads for cardiac monitoring, but 12 leads are used when the likelihood of coronary artery disease is high.

After baseline spirometry and electrocardiography, patients are placed on a treadmill or cycle ergometer and exercised at increasing levels of work until $\dot{V}_{O_2}$max is reached. Work levels are calculated so that the patient reaches $\dot{V}_{O_2}$max within 8 to 12 min of exercise.

In cardiac disease, $\dot{V}_{O_2}$max will be measurable but below normal. Anaerobic threshold will be reached, oxygen saturation will be maintained, and the highest minute ventilation will be below 50 percent of MVV. Oxygen pulse is decreased. In pulmonary disease, $\dot{V}_{O_2}$max and the anaerobic threshold are typically not reached, desaturation may be seen, and MVV is closely approximated. Oxygen pulse is normal. Obesity or physical deconditioning is characterized by a normal $\dot{V}_{O_2}$max reached at a relatively low external work load.[27–29]

The addition of invasive measurements such as arterial blood gas sampling or right-sided heart catheterization may allow even more detailed delineation of the patient's pathophysiology.

Clinical Application

Cardiopulmonary exercise testing may be helpful in the differential diagnosis of dyspnea, in the evaluation of pulmonary hypertension, and in the determination of work capacity for the adjudication of disability. The results of cardiopulmonary exercise testing show good correlation with New York Heart Association functional classification in congestive heart failure and valvular heart disease.

REFERENCES

1. Remetz MS, Cleman MW, Cabin HS: Pulmonary and pleural complications of cardiac disease. *Clin Chest Med* 1989; 10:545–592.
2. Morris AH, Kanner RE, Crapo RO, Gardner RM: *Clinical Pulmonary Function Testing. A Manual of Uniform Laboratory Procedures*, 2nd ed. Salt Lake City, Intermountain Thoracic Society, 1984.
3. Stanescu DC, Rodenstein DO, Hoeven C, Robert A: "Sensitive tests" are poor predictors of the decline in forced expiratory volume in 1 second in middle-aged smokers. *Am Rev Respir Dis* 1987; 135:585–590.
4. Hyatt RE, Black LF: The flow-volume curve: A current perspective. *Am Rev Respir Dis* 1973; 107:191–199.
5. Gilbert R, Auchincloss JH Jr: The interpretation of the spirogram: How accurate is it for "obstruction"? *Arch Intern Med* 1985; 145:1635–1639.
6. Gilbert R, Auchincloss JH Jr: What is a "restrictive" defect? *Arch Intern Med* 1986; 146:1779–1781.
7. Magro SA, Lawrence EC, Wheeler SH, Krafcheck J, Lin H-T, Wyndham CRC: Amiodarone pulmonary toxicity: Prospective evaluation of serial pulmonary function tests. *J Am Coll Cardiol* 1988; 12:781–788.
8. Otulana BA, Higgenbottam T, Scott J, Clelland C, Igboaka G, Wallwork J: Lung function associated with histologically diagnosed acute lung rejection and pulmonary infection in heart-lung transplant recipients. *Am Rev Respir Dis* 1990; 142:329–332.
9. Zibrak JD, O'Donnell CR, Marton K: Indications for pulmonary function testing. *Ann Intern Med* 1990; 112:763–771.
10. Ameican College of Physicians: Preoperative pulmonary function testing. *Ann Intern Med* 1990; 112:793–794.
11. Braman SS, Corrao WM: Bronchoprovocation testing. *Clin Chest Med* 1989; 10:165–176.
12. Chai H, Farr RS, Froehlich LA, Matthison DA, McLean JA, Rosenthal RR, et al: Standardization of bronchial inhalation challenge procedures. *J Allergy Clin Immunol* 1975; 56:323–327.
13. Pison C, Malo JL, Rouleau JL, Chalaoui J, Ghazzo H, Malo J: Bronchial hyperresponsiveness to inhaled methacholine in subjects with chronic left heart failure at a time of exacerbation and after increasing diuretic therapy. *Chest* 1989; 96:230–235.
14. Ries AL: Measurement of lung volumes. *Clin Chest Med* 1989; 10:177–186.
15. Ayers LN, Ginsberg ML, Fein J, Wasserman K: Diffusing capacity, specific diffusing capacity and interpretation of diffusion defects. *West J Med* 1975; 123:255–264.
16. Crapo RO, Gardner RM (chair): Single breath carbon monoxide diffusing capacity (transfer factor): Recommendations for a standard technique. *Am Rev Respir Dis* 1987; 136:1299–1307.
17. Crapo RO, Forster RE: Carbon monoxide diffusing capacity. *Clin Chest Med* 1989; 10:187–198.
18. Kennedy JI Jr: Clinical aspects of amiodarone pulmonary toxicity. *Clin Chest Med* 1990; 11:119–129.
19. Dusman RE, Stanton MS, Miles WM, Klein LS, Zipes DP, Fineberg NS, et al: Clinical features of amiodarone-induced pulmonary toxicity. *Circulation* 1990; 82:51–59.
20. Phillipson EA, Remmers JE (chair): Indications and standards for cardiopulmonary sleep studies. *Am Rev Respir Dis* 1989; 139:559–568.
21. Sériès F, Cormier Y, LaForge J: Validity of diurnal sleep recording in the diagnosis of sleep apnea syndrome. *Am Rev Respir Dis* 1991; 143:947–949.
22. Funsten AW, Surratt PM: Evaluation of respiratory disorders during sleep. *Clin Chest Med* 1989; 10:265–276.
23. Dowdell WT, Javaheri S, McGinnis W: Cheyne-Stokes respiration presenting as sleep apnea syndrome. Clinical and polysomnographic features. *Am Rev Respir Dis* 1990; 141:871–879.

24. Celli BR: Clinical and physiologic evaluation of respiratory muscle function. *Clin Chest Med* 1989; 10:199–214.
25. Hammond MD, Bauer KA, Sharp JT, Rocha RD: Respiratory muscle strength in congestive heart failure. *Chest* 1989; 98:1091–1094.
26. Markland ON, Moorthy SS, Mahomet Y, King RD, Brown JW: Postoperative phrenic nerve palsy in patients with open heart surgery. *Ann Thorac Surg* 1985; 39:689–693.
27. Wasserman K, Hansen JE, Sue DY, Whipp BJ: *Principles of Exercise Testing and Interpretation*. Philadelphia, Lea & Febiger, 1987.
28. Neuberg GW, Friedman SH, Weiss MB, Herman MV: Cardiopulmonary exercise testing. The clinical value of gas exchange data. *Arch Intern Med* 1988; 148:2221–2226.
29. McElroy PA, Janicki JS, Weber KT: Cardiopulmonary exercise testing in congestive heart failure. *Am J Cardiol* 1988; 62:35A–40A.

Chapter 18

Hemodynamic Monitoring in Critical Care Units

Kanu Chatterjee, M.B., F.R.C.P.

Assessment of the severity of cardiovascular dysfunction, the mechanism of functional derangement and the response of cardiac function to therapeutic interventions, is frequently necessary for the appropriate management of critically ill patients. Although clinical evaluation, including electrocardiographic and radiologic investigations, should be performed in all patients with suspected cardiovascular dysfunction, these traditional approaches are not adequate to determine the precise mechanism of derangement of cardiac function in most critically ill patients. Furthermore, rapid changes in hemodynamic abnormalities, occurring spontaneously or during therapeutic intervention, cannot be ascertained by clinical evaluation alone.[1] With the advent of transthoracic and transesophageal echocardiography and radionuclide scintigraphy, it has been possible to assess the mechanism and severity of cardiovascular dysfunction even in critically ill patients. Presently, however, these techniques cannot be applied for continuous monitoring of cardiac function, which is necessary for the appropriate management of such patients. Since the introduction of flow-directed balloon-tipped flotation catheters, it has been possible to measure central hemodynamics and cardiac output by right-sided heart catheterization at the bedside, even in critically ill patients.[2,3] Hemodynamic monitoring can be applied to diagnose and understand cardiopulmonary pathophysiology as well as to assess the severity of hemodynamic abnormalities and response to therapeutic interventions. Thus, hemodynamic monitoring has become widely and frequently used by physicians from multiple medical specialties, including cardiologists, intensive care specialists, and anesthesiologists.

PROCEDURAL AND PHYSIOLOGICAL CONSIDERATIONS

Arterial Pressure Monitoring

Hemodynamic monitoring may include measuring arterial, right atrial, pulmonary artery, and pulmonary capillary wedge pressures and the determination of cardiac output. It is desirable to monitor intraarterial pressure directly by cannulation of an accessible peripheral artery. Arterial cannulation also allows repeated blood gas determinations. In patients with chronic heart failure and in those who are not in severe low-output state, intraarterial pressure monitoring may not be required. Most frequently, a radial artery is cannulated for monitoring intraarterial pressure. In patients with cardiogenic shock or when there is clinical evidence of marked peripheral vasoconstriction, it is sometimes desirable to monitor central arterial pressure by cannulation of a femoral artery. In the presence of extreme peripheral vasoconstriction from endogenous or exogenous catecholamine stimulation central arterial pressure may be considerably higher than the peripheral arterial pressure.

Another indication for monitoring intraarterial pressure pulse is for balloon inflation (dicrotic notch) and deflation (before the onset of upstroke) during the use of intraaortic balloon counterpulsation. In central aortic pressure pulse, aortic valve closure coincides with the incisura that occurs 20 to 40 ms before the dicrotic notch of the peripheral arterial pulse. This time delay for the onset of dicrotic notch in peripheral arterial pulse wave should be considered for the proper timing of balloon inflation. (See Chap. 31.)

CENTRAL HEMODYNAMICS

Right-sided heart catheterization with the use of balloon flotation catheters can be performed by appropriately trained physicians although extensive special training in cardiac catheterization laboratories is not required. Presently, triple-lumen catheters that allow measurement of right atrial, pulmonary arterial, and pulmonary capillary wedge pressures and cardiac output by thermodilution techniques are most frequently used in critical care units. Normally, pulmonary capillary wedge pressure does not exceed 15 mmHg, and right atrial pressure is usually less than 7 mmHg. In the presence of normal left and right ventricular function, there is a good correlation between changes in right atrial and in pulmonary capillary wedge pressures. In the presence of altered right or left ventricular function, however, this relationship is no longer preserved and the assessment of right and left ventricular function requires measurement of both right atrial and pulmonary capillary wedge pressures. These differences in right and left ventricular filling pressures result from the differences in right and left ventricular compliance.

Relating changes in right atrial and pulmonary capillary wedge pressures to changes in stroke work, stroke volume, or cardiac output allows construction of right and left ventricular function curves. (See Chaps. 23 and 25.) The true ventricular filling pressure, however, is the transmural pressure, which is the difference between ventricular diastolic and extramural pressures. Normally, extramural pressure (pericardial and mediastinal pressures) is negative, and measured left ventricular and right ventricular diastolic pressure represents left and right ventricular filling pressures. In clinical circumstances where there is considerable increase in extramural pressure, however, such as in patients with cardiac tamponade, measured right and left ventricular diastolic pressures (right atrial and pulmonary capillary wedge pressures) do not represent their true filling pressures.

Pulmonary capillary wedge pressure is higher than left ventricular diastolic pressure in patients with mitral valve obstruction. Decreased left ventricular compliance, resulting from hypertrophy, ischemia, or infiltrative disease, can result in an elevated left ventricular end-diastolic pressure that is produced by a vigorous atrial contraction ("kick") and that may be higher, for a very brief period, than the mean pulmonary capillary wedge pressure.

In patients with chronic obstructive pulmonary disease or patients who are being mechanically ventilated with positive end-expiratory pressure (PEEP), differences between pulmonary capillary wedge pressure and left atrial pressure are frequently observed. In most clinical situations, however, mean pulmonary capillary wedge pressure correlates well with mean left atrial and left ventricular diastolic pressures. Normally the difference between pulmonary artery end-diastolic pressure and mean pulmonary capillary wedge pressure does not exceed 5 mmHg, and pulmonary artery diastolic pressure can be used to estimate mean pulmonary artery capillary wedge pressures. When pulmonary vascular resistance is elevated, however, this difference increases. In patients with precapillary pulmonary hypertension and elevated pulmonary vascular resistance, pulmonary artery end-diastolic pressure cannot be used to represent pulmonary capillary wedge pressure.

MONITORING CARDIAC OUTPUT

With technical advances and the availability of the bedside computers, on-line repeated cardiac output measurements by thermodilution techniques are now routinely practiced in critical care and are usually performed by nursing personnel. The validity and expected precision of cardiac output measurements by thermodilution techniques have been established.[3,4] The variability of cardiac output measurements by thermodilution is between 2 and 4 percent. In patients with severe tricuspid regurgitation, the variability in cardiac output measurements by thermodilution techniques may be higher than usual because of unpredictable mixing of the cold indicator. Even in patients with tricuspid regurgitation and pulmonary hypertension, however, reproducible cardiac output measurements can usually be achieved by thermodilution techniques if the catheter position is proper and if proper techniques of delivery of cold indicator are practiced.

Determination of cardiac output is critical not only for the diagnosis and management of heart failure and shock syndromes but also to assess the prognosis.[5] When the cardiac index at rest exceeds 2.2 liters/min per m^2, the prognosis is usually favorable from the cardiovascular standpoint. A cardiac index between 1.8 and 2.2 liters/min per m^2 is borderline and barely adequate to meet the metabolic demand of severely ill patients. A cardiac index considerably less than 1.7 liters/min per m^2 is associated with a very poor prognosis unless that "low-output state" is promptly corrected by appropriate therapeutic interventions.

Right-sided heart catheterization allows determination of mixed venous oxygen saturation, and with the knowledge of arterial saturation, overall oxygen extraction can be estimated. Simultaneous determination of cardiac output permits estimation of both oxygen delivery and oxygen consumption. Inadequate oxygen delivery to meet the metabolic demand in acutely ill patients, as in high-risk postsurgical patients, is associated with an unfavorable prognosis.

Multipurpose Catheters

In addition to measurements of intracardiac pressures and cardiac output, multipurpose balloon flotation electrode catheters can be used for recording intracardiac electrograms that can be useful for the differential diagnosis of complex ventricular arrhythmias.[6] Although multipurpose electrode catheters were conceived originally to allow temporary atrial, ventricular, or atrioventricular sequential pacing, these catheters should not be used for pacing purposes because reliable pacing is usually not achieved. The multipurpose *right ventricular port catheter* can be used for temporary right ventricular pacing or for monitoring right ventricular pressure. Multipurpose *fiber-optic* catheters allow the monitoring of mixed venous oxygen saturation, which is sometimes useful to assess oxygen consumption and cardiac output.

The balloon flotation catheters are usually inserted percutaneously via internal jugular or subclavian veins. Antecubital or femoral veins should be used infrequently. The latter site should not be considered when prolonged hemodynamic monitoring is anticipated because of an increased incidence of catheter sepsis. For the proper placement of the balloon flotation catheters, fluoroscopy is usually not required; however, in patients with a markedly dilated right atrium and right ventricle, fluoroscopy may be useful for rapid placement of the catheter while avoiding complications such as catheter knotting and coiling. In patients with a dilated right atrium and right ventricle, the use of "guidewire" balloon flotation catheters is preferable for rapid catheter placement.

DIAGNOSTIC CONSIDERATIONS

Hypotension and *low output state*, pulmonary congestion, and hypoxia are frequently encountered clinical problems in intensive care units. These clinical syndromes are not produced by single or similar cardiovascular abnormalities, and the determination of central hemodynamics frequently defines the underlying pathophysiological mechanisms. The clinical conditions commonly encountered in critical care units and their hemodynamic characteristics are summarized in Table 18-1.[7]

TABLE 18-1

Hemodynamic Characteristics of Clinical Conditions Found in Critical Care Units

Hemodynamic Status	RAP	PAWP	PADP	PADP-PAWP	RAP = PAWP	Disproportionate Elevation of RAP	CO	PVR	SVR
Hypovolemic shock	Low	Low	Normal	Normal	Absent	Absent	Low	Normal	Normal or high
Predominant LV with or without shock	Normal or high	High	High	Normal	Absent	Absent	Low	Normal or high	Usually high
Primary RV failure	High	Normal or high	Normal or high	Normal or increased	Depends on etiology; usually present in RV infarct	Present	Low	Normal or elevated	Usually normal
Secondary RV failure	High	Normal or high	High	Increased	Usually absent	Present	Low	High	Normal or high
Cardiac tamponade	High	High	High	Normal	Present	Present	Low	Normal	High or normal
Acute, severe mitral regurgitation	Usually high, may be normal	High peaked *v* wave	High	Usually normal	Absent	Absent	Low	Normal or high	High or normal
Acute ventricular septal defect	Usually high	High	High	Usually normal	Absent	Usually absent	Low	Normal or high	High or normal
Septic shock	Usually low	Usually low or may be high	Normal or high	Normal or increased	Absent	Absent	High or normal	Normal or high	Low or normal
Adult respiratory distress syndrome	Normal or high	Normal	Normal or high	Usually increased	Absent	May be present	Depends on etiology	High or normal	Depends on etiology

RAP = right atrial pressure; PAWP = pulmonary artery wedge pressure; PADP = pulmonary artery diastolic pressure; PADP-PAWP = pulmonary artery diastolic and wedge pressure gradient; RAP = PAWP = equalization of diastolic pressures; CO = cardiac output; PVR = pulmonary vascular resistance; SVR = systemic vascular resistance; RV = right ventricular; LV = left ventricular.
SOURCE: WW Parmley, K Chatterjee.[7]

HYPOVOLEMIC SHOCK

Decreased cardiac output and hypotension in hypovolemic shock result from decreased right and left ventricular preloads. In the absence of altered ventricular compliance and of any changes in extramural pressures, right atrial and pulmonary capillary wedge pressures are less than normal. The upper limits of normal right atrial and pulmonary capillary wedge pressures are 7 and 15 mmHg, respectively. In hypovolemic shock, however, both right atrial and pulmonary capillary wedge pressures are much lower. For the hemodynamic diagnosis of hypovolemic shock it is necessary to establish that both right and left ventricular filling pressure are inadequate.

SEVERE LEFT VENTRICULAR FAILURE AND CARDIOGENIC SHOCK

The hemodynamic profile of patients with left ventricular failure is characterized by elevation of pulmonary capillary wedge pressure and, usually, reduction in cardiac index. With increasing severity of left ventricular failure, there is a progressive rise in pulmonary capillary wedge pressure. (See also Chap. 49.)

Right atrial pressure may remain normal, which suggests relatively normal right ventricular function. Elevated right atrial pressure may result from concomitant right ventricular failure due to significant pulmonary hypertension. In patients with chronic left ventricular failure, pulmonary vascular resistance may occasionally be increased; with a substantial increase in pulmonary vascular resistance the gradient between pulmonary artery end-diastolic pressure and mean pulmonary capillary wedge pressure increases (>5 mmHg). In patients with predominant left ventricular failure with secondary right ventricular failure, the ratio of mean right atrial to mean pulmonary capillary wedge pressure is usually less than 0.8. The magnitude of reduction in cardiac output is related to the severity of left ventricular failure, and in patients with cardiogenic shock, cardiac index is very low, usually less than 1.7 liters/min per m^2. (See Chap. 49.) It needs to be emphasized that the hemodynamic profile does not allow the diagnosis of the underlying mechanism of left ventricular failure. Both diastolic and systolic left ventricular dysfunction can be associated with similar hemodynamic abnormalities, and it is therefore desirable to assess the left ventricular ejection fraction. If the left ventricular ejection fraction is normal or near normal, one can assume that diastolic dysfunction is the principal mechanism for the hemodynamic abnormalities. In critical care, echo Doppler evaluation is a useful adjunctive investigation to assess left ventricular and right ventricular systolic function as well as to exclude significant valvular heart disease, which may also produce similar hemodynamic abnormalities. (See also Chaps. 15 and 130.)

Cardiogenic shock is a clinical syndrome characterized by hypotension (systolic blood pressure 90 mmHg or less) and clinical evidence of hypoperfusion such as oliguria, cold, clammy skin, and mental obtundation. (See Chap. 49.) This clinical syndrome most frequently is caused by severe acute or chronic left ventricular dysfunction. The hemodynamic abnormalities are similar to those associated with left ventricular failure without cardiogenic shock, except that the arterial pressure is always lower and the cardiac index is significantly reduced.

RIGHT VENTRICULAR FAILURE

Acute right ventricular failure can result from right ventricular myocardial infarction, acute massive pulmonary embolism, and acute severe tricuspid and pulmonary regurgitation. Postcapillary pulmonary hypertension and precapillary pulmonary hypertension are the most frequent causes of chronic right ventricular failure. (See Chap. 26.) Chronic primary right ventricular failure is encountered infrequently in adults. Chronic severe tricuspid regurgitation, secondary to chronic cor pulmonale, bacterial endocarditis, Epstein's anomaly, severe right ventricular dysplasia such as Uhl's syndrome, and carcinoid heart disease, may cause severe and predominant right ventricular failure. The usual hemodynamic abnormality of predominant right ventricular failure is a disproportionate elevation of right atrial pressure, compared to the changes in pulmonary wedge pressure; the ratio of right-atrial pressure to pulmonary capillary wedge pressure usually exceeds 0.8. In general, in patients with primary right ventricular failure, pulmonary artery pressure and pulmonary vascular resistance are normal or modestly elevated. In secondary right ventricular failure, pulmonary artery pressure and pulmonary vascular resistance are significantly elevated. In precapillary pulmonary arterial hypertension, pulmonary capillary wedge pressure is normal and pulmonary artery diastolic pressure is higher than mean pulmonary capillary wedge pressure by more than 5 mmHg.

In severe tricuspid regurgitation, the right atrial pressure is elevated and there is ventricularization of the right atrial pressure (Fig. 18-1). In severe tricuspid regurgitation, mean right atrial pressure may also be similar to mean pulmonary capillary wedge pressure (equalization of the diastolic pressures). Also, in right ventricular myocardial infarction, equalization of the right atrial and pulmonary capillary wedge pressure may occur. This equalization of the right and left ventricular diastolic pressures appears to result from increased intrapericardial pressure and a constraining effect of intact pericardium.[8] These hemodynamic abnormalities are very similar to those observed in constrictive pericarditis. (See Chap. 92.) Indeed, dip and plateau (square root sign) can be observed in the right ventricular pressure waveform in right ventricular myocardial infarction. In right ventricular myocardial infarction, the pulmonary artery pressure waveform is frequently distorted and a smooth upstroke, dicrotic notch or dicrotic waves may not be easily recognized. Right ventricular systolic pressure and peak pulmonary artery pressure are usually normal, and there is no abnormal gradient between pulmonary artery diastolic pressure and mean pulmonary capillary wedge pressure. Some elevation of pulmonary artery pressure,

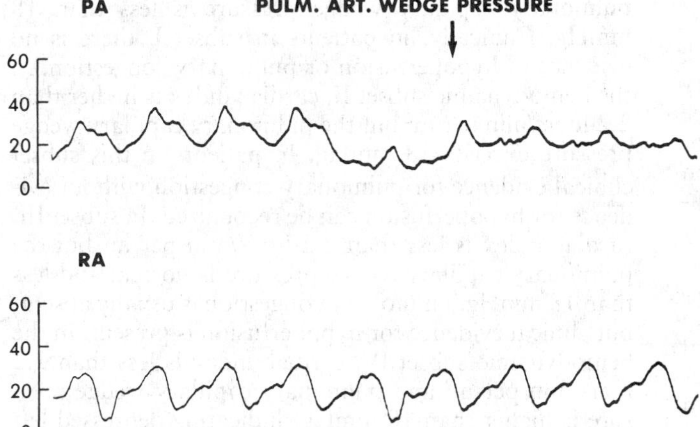

FIGURE 18-1 Right atrial (RA) and pulmonary artery wedge pressure (Pulm. Art. Wedge Pressure) in a patient with severe tricuspid regurgitation. Right atrial pressure tracing demonstrates "ventricularization," indicating severe tricuspid regurgitation. Mean pulmonary capillary wedge pressure and mean right atrial pressure were similar. [*Published with permission from K Chatterjee: Bedside hemodynamic monitoring. In: WW Parmley, K Chatterjee (eds): Cardiology, vol I. Philadelphia, JB Lippincott Company, 1987, Chap 55.*]

however, may occur if there is a substantial increase in mean pulmonary capillary wedge pressure due to increased pericardial pressure or due to preexisting left ventricular failure. It is apparent that equalization of the diastolic pressures can be observed in a number of clinical conditions, including cardiac tamponade, constrictive pericarditis, early stages of restrictive cardiomyopathy, acute right ventricular infarction, and severe tricuspid regurgitation. Bedside hemodynamic monitoring alone is not adequate for the differential diagnosis of these various conditions, and ancillary investigations are necessary to establish the diagnosis.

MITRAL REGURGITATION

In severe acute or subacute mitral regurgitation, the magnitude of the *v* wave (regurgitant wave) is markedly increased and a tall peaked *v* wave is frequently seen. (See Chap. 80.) It should be emphasized that a tall peaked giant *v* wave (height of the *v* wave exceeding the mean capillary wedge pressure by 10 mmHg or more) can also be seen in the absence of mitral regurgitation, as in patients with ventricular septal defect, aortic valve disease, and chronic coronary artery disease.[9] In the absence of significant dilatation of left atrium, the increased volume load into the left atrium will cause a substantial increase in the magnitude of the systolic *v* wave that may be similar to the changes observed in severe mitral regurgitation. Although the onset and the peak of the *v* wave in mitral regurgitation (regurgitant wave) is much earlier than normal and usually closely follows the QRS complex of the electrocardiogram, the timing of the onset of the *v* wave in mitral regurgitation is difficult to determine at the bedside. Thus, mitral regurgitation should not be diagnosed at the bedside from the changes in the pulmonary capillary wedge pressure wave form alone, and other investigations, particularly echo Doppler studies (see Chaps. 15 and 130), should be considered to confirm the diagnosis. In acute and subacute severe mitral regurgitation, a reflected *v* wave can occasionally be recognized in the pulmonary artery pressure waveform (Fig. 18-2). The reflected *v* wave tends to occur before the dicrotic notch of the pulmonary artery pressure tracing,[10] and this abnormality, when recognized, almost always indicates the presence of significant mitral regurgitation. It is important to note that chronic severe mitral regurgitation may exist without any substantial increase in mean pulmonary capillary wedge pressure or in the magnitude of *v* wave. This lack of change in mean pulmonary capillary wedge pressure and magnitude of *v* wave, despite severe mitral regurgitation, is observed when the left atrium is markedly enlarged. (See also Chaps. 80 and 138.)

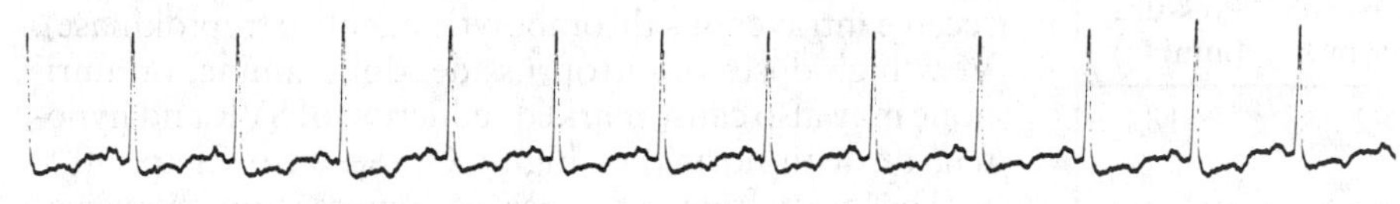

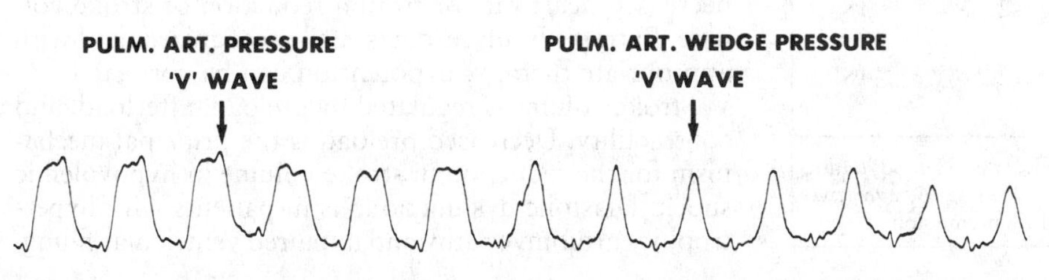

FIGURE 18-2 A tall peak *v* wave in the pulmonary artery wedge pressure tracing and a reflected *v* wave in the pulmonary artery pressure tracing in a patient with severe mitral regurgitation. [*Published with permission from K Chatterjee: Bedside hemodynamic monitoring. In: WW Parmley, K Chatterjee (eds): Cardiology, vol I. Philadelphia, JB Lippincott Company, 1987, Chap 55.*]

Ventricular Septal Defect

Because of left-to-right shunt at the ventricular level, there is a step-up in the oxygen saturation of pulmonary arterial blood compared to that in the right atrium. (See Chaps. 97 and 138.) In patients with severe acute or subacute mitral regurgitation, higher oxygen saturation may rarely be observed in blood drawn from distal pulmonary arterial branches than from proximal pulmonary artery or right ventricular samples. Thus, when pulmonary artery blood samples are drawn for the diagnosis of left-to-right shunt, it is desirable to check that the tip of the balloon flotation catheter is placed in the proximal pulmonary artery branches. Left-to-right shunt increases pulmonary blood flow, and cardiac output determined by thermodilution technique represents pulmonary blood flow, which is much higher than the systemic output. In patients with clinical features of low output state in whom the thermodilution cardiac output is high, it is desirable to exclude left-to-right shunt by other appropriate investigations. From measurements of pulmonary arterial, right atrial, and systemic arterial oxygen saturations, it is possible to estimate the relative pulmonary and systemic blood flows. Transthoracic and transesophageal echocardiography are useful for the diagnosis of mitral regurgitation and determining the anatomic location of ventricular septal defects. (See Chaps. 15 and 131.) Right heart catheterization, however, is required to assess the severity of hemodynamic abnormalities.

HEMODYNAMIC SUBSETS OF ACUTE MYOCARDIAL INFARCTION

The variable hemodynamic abnormalities resulting from acute myocardial infarction are related to the location and extent of the myocardial ischemic injury and to specific complications. (See Chap. 60.) Based on hemodynamic changes four subsets with distinctly different prognoses[11,12] have been proposed (Table 18-2). In subset I, cardiac index is higher than 2.2 liters/min per m^2 and pulmonary capillary wedge pressure is less than 18 mmHg. Clinically, in patients in subset I, there is no evidence of hypoperfusion or pulmonary congestion. In the hemodynamic subset II, cardiac index is higher than 2.2 liters/min per m^2 but the pulmonary capillary wedge pressure exceeds 18 mmHg. In patients in this subset clinical evidence for pulmonary congestion without evidence for hypoperfusion can be recognized. In subset III, cardiac index is less than 2.2 liters/min per m^2 but the pulmonary capillary wedge pressure is normal and less than 18 mmHg. Pulmonary congestion is usually absent, but clinical evidence for hypoperfusion is present. In the hemodynamic subset IV, cardiac index is less than 2.2 liters/min per m^2 and pulmonary capillary wedge pressure is higher than 18 mmHg, indicating depressed left ventricular pump performance. Clinical evidence for pulmonary congestion and hypoperfusion is recognized in patients in subset IV. The prognosis of patients in subset I, as expected, is most favorable and that of patients in subset IV is worst.

In clinical practice it is not always necessary to determine the hemodynamic subsets as there is a reasonable correlation between clinical subsets and the hemodynamic changes. In patients without evidence of hypoperfusion or pulmonary congestion or in patients who promptly recover from pulmonary congestion, hemodynamic monitoring is not required. On the other hand, for those patients who have persistent pulmonary congestion or evidence of hypoperfusion, determination of hemodynamics provides useful diagnostic information and facilitates appropriate therapeutic interventions.

TABLE 18-2
Prognosis Based on Hemodynamic Changes

Subset	Clinical Signs	Cardiac Index (liters/min per m^2)	Pulmonary Artery Wedge Pressure (mmHg)
I	No pulmonary congestion No hypoperfusion	>2.2	≤18
II	Pulmonary congestion No hypoperfusion	>2.2	>18
III	No pulmonary congestion Hypoperfusion	≤2.2	≤18
IV	Pulmonary congestion Hypoperfusion	≤2.2	>18

From Forrester JS, Diamond G, Chatterjee K, et al: Hemodynamic therapy of myocardial infarction. *N Engl J Med* 1976; 295 (two parts): 1356–1362, 1404–1413. Reprinted by permission.

HEMODYNAMIC DIFFERENTIAL DIAGNOSIS OF HYPOTENSION

Hypotension is a common clinical problem in critical care units. Appropriate therapy depends on the precise diagnosis of the mechanism of hypotension. (See Chap. 49.) Blood pressure is the product of cardiac output (CO) and systemic vascular resistance (SVR). Thus, hypotension can result from decreased CO or decreased SVR. Inappropriately reduced SVR as the cause of hypotension occurs most frequently in patients with septic shock, in which CO characteristically is high or normal. Right atrial pressure and pulmonary capillary wedge pressure may be low, normal, or slightly elevated. A similar hemodynamic profile may be observed in some patients who receive intravenous thrombolytic agents (streptokinase). Very high doses of nitroprusside, dobutamine, or amrinone may also cause marked reduction of SVR and hypotension with normal or high CO. (See also Chap. 30.)

The most frequent cause of hypotension, however, is decreased CO. A reduction in CO can result from decreased heart rate or from a reduction of stroke volume. Extreme bradycardia is easily recognized, and with appropriate therapy, hypotension can be corrected.

Stroke volume is regulated by preload, afterload, and contractility. Decreased preload is the principal mechanism for the reduction in stroke volume in hypovolemic shock. Diastolic dysfunction, as in patients with hypertrophic cardiomyopathy and impaired ventricular filling, may also be associated with decreased CO. Decreased preload in these patients, however, is not associated with decreased pulmonary capillary wedge pressure. Decreased CO due to decreased left ventricular preload is also the principal mechanism of hypotension in cardiac tamponade, constrictive pericarditis, and restrictive cardiomyopathy. Noninvasive investigations, particularly echocardiography, are necessary for the diagnosis of these clinical conditions. Increased afterload is associated with decreased stroke volume since an inverse relation exists between left ventricular afterload and stroke volume. Clinical conditions in which increased afterload is the principal mechanism for reduced stroke volume are infrequent. In patients with severe aortic valve stenosis, however, marked increase in left ventricular outflow resistance may decrease stroke volume sufficiently to reduce CO and produce hypotension. In elderly patients who present with low-output state and hypotension, it is desirable to exclude significant aortic valve stenosis that may not be clinically obvious. In general, bedside hemodynamic monitoring is not adequate to assess changes in ventricular afterload, except that calculated systemic vascular resistance is higher than normal. Impaired contractile function is the most frequent cause of decreased stroke volume. Contractile function, however, cannot be assessed by conventional bedside hemodynamic monitoring, and impaired contractile function is often assumed by the exclusion of other mechanisms for decreased stroke volume (decreased preload, increased afterload, mechanical defects). It is, however, feasible to apply bedside hemodynamic monitoring in conjunction with noninvasive investigations such as echocardiography for the differential diagnosis of the mechanism of hypotension and to develop a rational therapeutic approach.

HEMODYNAMIC MONITORING DURING THERAPEUTIC INTERVENTIONS

Hemodynamic monitoring is useful to assess response to therapy in critically ill patients. During intravenous fluid therapy in patients with hypovolemic shock, changes in CO and right atrial and pulmonary capillary wedge pressure help to determine the optimal filling pressures for the maximal increase in CO. In patients with acute myocardial infarction, the optimal filling pressure (pulmonary capillary wedge pressure) is usually between 14 and 18 mmHg.[13] In some patients with hemodynamic features of hypovolemic shock, intravenous fluid therapy does not increase CO appreciably despite maintaining adequate filling pressures. In these patients significant pump dysfunction should be suspected, and the treatment approach can be modified according to the hemodynamic response to addition of vasodilators or inotropic agents. During management of pump failure, choice of vasodilators can be made based on hemodynamic objectives such as decreasing systemic resistance and pulmonary capillary wedge pressures. Nitroglycerin is often more effective than sodium nitroprusside in reducing pulmonary capillary wedge pressure. Sodium nitroprusside, on the other hand, has greater potential to increase CO than nitroglycerin. The choice of inotropic agents and vasopressors should also be based on an individual patient's hemodynamic profile and objectives of therapy. To increase CO in the absence of hypotension, dobutamine and amrinone, which do not usually increase mean arterial pressure, can be used. For correction of hypotension, dopamine, epinephrine, norepinephrine, or neosynephrine are preferable. (See Chaps. 30 and 49). In hypotensive patients with coronary artery disease, intraaortic balloon counterpulsation therapy is useful to maintain coronary artery perfusion pressure. (See Chap. 31.) Hemodynamic monitoring is often necessary for appropriate selection of both individual drugs and combinations of vasoactive and inotropic drugs for management of pump failure and hypotension. The hemodynamic guidelines are summarized in Fig. 18-3.

Adult respiratory distress syndrome is a serious complication and requires aggressive therapy. For the diagnosis, as well as for determination of appropriate volume status of these patients, hemodynamic monitoring is useful. It has been suggested that in patients with adult respiratory distress syndrome, pulmonary capillary wedge pressure should be kept at a lower level to reduce permeability and thus pulmonary edema.

For the management of hypotension and the low-output state in patients after cardiac surgery or in patients with known cardiovascular abnormalities undergoing noncardiac surgery, hemodynamic monitoring is frequently employed. The therapeutic approaches in these patients are similar to those outlined above.

Shoemaker and colleagues[14–17] have reported that a normal $\dot{V}_{O_2}$ may not be adequate in critically ill patients after noncardiac surgery. It was reported that a $\dot{V}_{O_2}$ of greater than 600 mL/min per m^2 was associated with decreased mortality rates in these patients. A cardiac index of at least 4.5 liters/min per m^2 is associated with an improved prognosis. The therapeutic strategies involve administration of an adequate amount of intravenous fluid to maintain optimal left ventricular filling pressure, usually 15 mmHg or greater, and the use of vasodilators and inotropic agents, such as dobutamine, to optimize the increase in CO. Although conclusive evidence is lacking that such therapeutic interventions are universally successful in improving the prognosis of postoperative patients or patients with septic shock, these therapeutic manipulations with pharmacologic agents require hemodynamic monitoring.

RISKS AND BENEFITS

The complications related to hemodynamic monitoring are rather infrequent if proper precautions are undertaken and the recommended guidelines are followed.[18,19] Nonsustained ventricular and atrial arrhythmias and local infections and inflammations, however, are relatively common (15 to 40 percent). Pneumothorax, sustained arrhythmias, and important pulmonary complications occur in 3 to 4 percent of patients, usually those who are critically ill. The severity of the illness of the patient requiring hemodynamic monitoring and the experience, expertise, and knowledge of hemodynamic monitoring

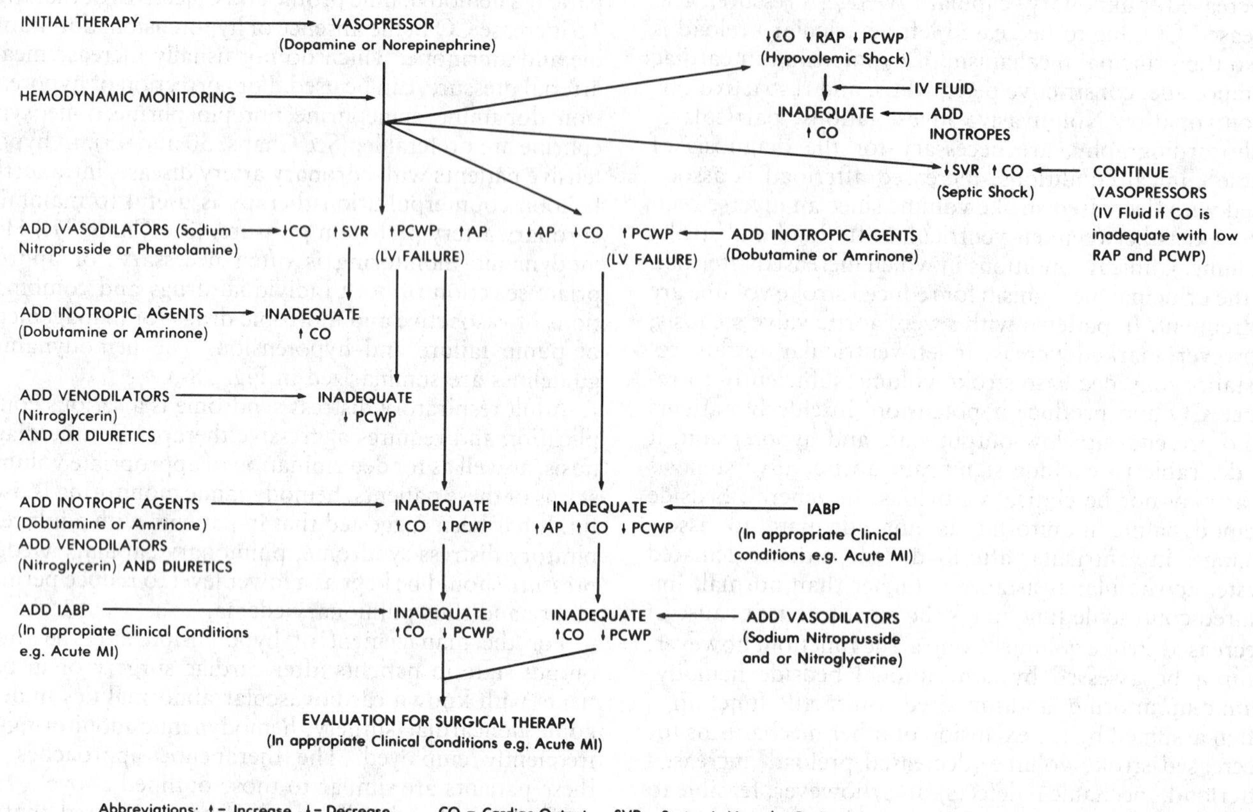

FIGURE 18-3 Therapeutic approach for hypotension based on hemodynamic changes. [*Published with permission from K Chatterjee: Bedside hemodynamic monitoring. In: WW Parmley, K Chatterjee (eds): Cardiology, vol I. Philadelphia, Lippincott, 1987, Chap 55.*]

of the individuals performing catheter insertion and determination of hemodynamics are major determinants of the rate of complications.

During insertion of the catheter, the most serious potential complications are sustained ventricular tachycardia, advanced atrioventricular block, or pneumothorax. Sustained ventricular tachycardia that requires treatment occurs in up to 3 percent of patients. The risk of serious arrhythmias is higher in unstable patients with electrolyte imbalance, acidosis, or myocardial ischemia. The prophylactic use of lidocaine in these higher risk patients may reduce the incidence of this complication. Even when life-threatening arrhythmias develop during hemodynamic monitoring, however, death from this complication is extremely rare because it almost always responds to treatment. In a recent prospective study advanced ventricular arrhythmias developed in 13 percent of patients, and the longest was a run of seven consecutive premature ventricular contractions.[20] In patients with preexisting left bundle branch block, transient interruption of conduction via the right bundle branch may occur during insertion of a balloon flotation catheter, which may result in complete atrioventricular block and ventricular asystole. Previous insertion of a pacing catheter or the use of a pacing port pulmonary artery catheter, however, can prevent this complication.

The reported incidence of pneumothorax during insertion of balloon flotation catheters via subclavian veins varies between 1 and 6 percent.[21-24] The use of internal jugular vein, however, has reduced considerably the incidence of pneumothorax to less than about 0.1 percent.[25]

Although earlier reports indicated an incidence of pulmonary infarction as high as 7.2 percent,[26] recent studies have reported a much lower incidence (0 to 1.3 percent).[27,28] Use of continuous flush with a heparin solution and more careful monitoring of pulmonary arterial waveforms are probably important reasons for the decrease in this complication.

The incidence of local thrombus formation around the catheter in the right side of the heart and in the internal jugular or subclavian vein has been reported in a number of studies.[29-31] In one autopsy study, a mural thrombus in the chambers of the right side of the heart was detected in one-third of patients. The incidence of pulmonary emboli, however, was no greater for patients with mural thrombi than for patients without mural thrombi. Recently, the reported incidence of these complications has been less, perhaps related to the use of heparin bonding on catheters. The thrombotic complications can also be minimized by reducing the time that the catheter is left in place.

Pulmonary artery rupture or perforation, a potentially

fatal complication, occurs in about 0.1 to 0.2 percent of patients.[27,32,33] Pulmonary arterial hypertension and recent cardiopulmonary bypass have been reported to be the risk factors for this complication. In patients undergoing cardiopulmonary bypass, it has been recommended that the catheter should be pulled before bypass and refloated to the pulmonary artery after bypass. The balloon should be inflated slowly with continuous pressure monitoring. In a prospective study, no cases of pulmonary artery rupture were reported in 1400 patients who had pulmonary artery catheterization for cardiac surgery.[25]

Septicemia related to hemodynamic monitoring tends to occur more frequently in patients requiring prolonged hemodynamic monitoring. In earlier studies, the incidence of septicemia during hemodynamic monitoring was reported in up to 2 percent of patients.[34,35] In recent years, however, the incidence of catheter-related sepsis has declined (0 to 1 percent).[25,36,37] The risk of catheter-related sepsis rises significantly if the catheter is left in place for more than 72 to 96 h. A number of recommendations have been proposed to reduce the risk of sepsis related to hemodynamic monitoring. These include the use of a sterile sleeve, antibiotic bonding to the catheter, and changing of the line with a guidewire. The value of these measures for reducing catheter-related infections requires prospective evaluation. It is apparent that improved catheter design and insertion technique, adherence to the recommended guidelines for catheter insertion and hemodynamic monitoring, and better care during hemodynamic monitoring and greater awareness of the potential complications have reduced significantly the incidence of minor and major complications of bedside catheterization of the right side of the heart. Nevertheless, bedside pulmonary artery catheterization should be considered to be an invasive procedure, and the risk of a serious complication always exists. Thus, one should always consider the relative risk and benefit of hemodynamic monitoring in an individual patient before bedside pulmonary artery catheterization is performed.[19,38]

Retrospective studies have indicated that pulmonary artery catheterization in patients with acute myocardial infarction complicated by heart failure, hypotension, or shock may be associated with a higher mortality than patients who do not undergo bedside hemodynamic monitoring.[39] A few randomized, prospective control trials of catheterizations of the right side of the heart in critically ill patients have also indicated that such catheterization with balloon flotation catheters may be associated with a higher mortality in critically ill patients.[40] It should be emphasized, however, that right-sided heart catheterization is a diagnostic, not a therapeutic, intervention. When appropriately performed and used, it is seldom associated with serious complications. As noted above, the fatalities resulting directly from right-sided heart catheterization are extremely rare. Recent studies suggest that often one cannot reliably diagnose the various pathophysiological conditions clinically or with the use of noninvasive investigative techniques with sufficient reliability to be useful for practical management of various cardiovascular abnormalities, such as hypotension and low-output syndrome in coronary care units and in postsurgical intensive care units.[19] In critically ill patients without acute myocardial infarction, clinical assessment of pulmonary artery wedge pressure and CO are frequently inaccurate.[1] In a prospective study comparing clinical diagnosis and hemodynamic data, it was reported that correct prediction of approximate CO was 71 percent, and for pulmonary artery wedge pressure it was only 62 percent.[41] Other investigators also reported that physical examination and a review of the chest radiograph identified the correct hemodynamic profile in only a minority of patients. The percentage of accurate prediction was low, ranging from 42 percent for pulmonary artery wedge pressure to 44 percent for CO.[1] Thus, it is apparent that clinical assessment and noninvasive investigations may not be adequate to predict the hemodynamic profile of many patients requiring prompt and aggressive therapeutic interventions. From the presently available data, it appears that right-sided heart catheterization provides hemodynamic information that can be used to select or change therapy.[42] The changes involved initiation or discontinuation of vasoactive and inotropic drugs, changing the rate of fluid administration or changing both fluid and drug therapy. Thus, bedside hemodynamic monitoring, if properly performed and with appropriate care, is useful in the management of critically ill patients. Hemodynamics monitoring with right-sided heart catheterization, however, should not be considered until there is a clear clinical indication.

REFERENCES

1. Connors AF Jr, McCaffree DR, Gray BA: Evaluation of right-heart catheterization in the critically ill patient without acute myocardial infarction. *N Eng J Med* 1983; 308:263–267.
2. Swan HJC, Ganz W, Forrester J, Marcus H, Diamond G, Chonette D: Catheterization of the heart in man with the use of a flow-directed balloon tipped catheter. *N Engl J Med* 1970; 283:447–451.
3. Forrester JS, Ganz W, Diamond G, Marcus H, Diamond G, Chonette D: Thermodilution cardiac output determination with a single flow directed catheter for cardiac monitoring. *Am Heart J* 1972; 83:306–311.
4. Ganz W, Donoso R, Marcus HS, Forrester JS, Swan HJC: A new technique for measurement of cardiac output by thermodilution in man. *Am J Cardiol* 1971; 27:392–396.
5. Swan HJC, Ganz W: Hemodynamic measurements in clinical practice: A decade in review. *J Am Coll Cardiol* 1983; 1:103–113.
6. Chatterjee K, Swan HJC, Ganz W, Gray R, Loebel H, Forrester JS, et al: Use of balloon-tipped flotation electrode catheter for cardiac monitoring. *Am J Cardiol* 1975; 36:56–61.
7. Chatterjee K: Bedside hemodynamic monitoring. In: Parmley WW, Chatterjee K (eds): *Cardiology*, vol I. Philadelphia, Lippincott, 1987: Chap. 55.
8. Goldstein JA, Vlahakes GJ, Verrier ED, Schiller NB, Botvinick E, Tyberg JV, et al: The role of right ventricular systolic dysfunction and elevated intrapericardial pressure in the genesis of low output in experimental right ventricular infarction. *Circulation* 1982; 65:513–522.
9. Fuchs RM, Henser RR, Yin FCP, Brinker JA: Limitations of pulmonary wedge V waves in diagnosing mitral regurgitation. *Am J Cardiol* 1982; 49:849–854.
10. Grose R, Strain J, Cohen MV: Pulmonary artery 'V' waves in mitral regurgitation: Clinical and experimental observations. *Circulation* 1984; 69:214–222.
11. Forrester JS, Diamond G, Chatterjee K, Swan HJ: Hemodynamic therapy of myocardial infarction (first of two parts). *N Engl J Med* 1976; 295:1356–1362.
12. Forrester JS, Diamond G, Chatterjee K, Swan HJ: Hemodynamic therapy of myocardial infarction (second of two parts). *N Engl J Med* 1976; 295:1404–1413.

13. Crexells C, Chatterjee K, Forrester JS, Dikshit K, Swan HJ: Optimal level of left heart filling pressures in acute myocardial infarction. *N Engl J Med* 1973; 289:1263–1266.
14. Shoemaker WC: A new approach to physiology, monitoring, and therapy of shock states. *World J Surg* 1987; 11:133–146.
15. Shoemaker WC: Circulatory mechanisms of shock and their mediators. *Crit Care Med* 1987; 15:787–794.
16. Shoemaker WC, Bland RD, Appel PL: Therapy of critically ill postoperative patients based on outcome prediction and prospective clinical trials. *Surg Clin North Am* 1985; 65:811–33.
17. Shoemaker WC, Appel PL, Kram HB, Waxman K, Lee T-S: Prospective trial of supranormal values of survivors as therapeutic goals in high-risk surgical patients. *Chest* 1988; 94:1176–1186.
18. Friesinger GC II, Williams SV: Clinical competence in hemodynamic monitoring. A statement for physicians from the ACP/ACC/AHA task force on clinical privileges in cardiology. *J Am Coll Cardiol* 1990; 15:1460–1464.
19. Matthay MA, Chatterjee K: Bedside catheterization of the pulmonary artery: Risks compared with benefits. *Ann Intern Med* 1988; 109:826–834.
20. Iberti TJ, Benjamin E, Gruppi L, Raskin JM: Ventricular arrhythmias during pulmonary artery catheterization in the intensive care unit. *Am J Med* 1985; 78:451–454.
21. Bernard RW, Stahl WM: Subclavian vein catheterization: A prospective study I. Noninfectious complications. *Ann Surg* 1971; 173:184–190.
22. Feliciano DV, Mattox KL, Graham JM, Beall AC Jr, Jordan GL Jr: Major complications of percutaneous subclavian vein catheters. *Am J Surg* 1979; 138:869–874.
23. Herbst CA: Indications for and management of subclavian catheters. *Ann Surg* 1978; 113:1421–1425.
24. Sznajder JI, Zveibil FR, Bitterman H, Weiner P, Bursztein S: Central vein catheterization. Failure and complication rates by three percutaneous approaches. *Ann Intern Med* 1986; 146:259–261.
25. Damen J, Bolton D: A prospective analysis of 1400 pulmonary artery catheterizations in patients undergoing cardiac surgery. *Acta Anaesthesiol Scand* 1986; 30:386–392.
26. Foote GD, Schabel SI, Hodges M: Pulmonary complications of the flow-directed balloon-tipped catheter. *N Engl J Med* 1974; 290:927–931.
27. Boyd KD, Thomas SJ, Gold J, Boyd AD: A prospective study of complications of pulmonary artery catheterizations in 500 consecutive patients. *Chest* 1983; 84:245–249.
28. Sise MJ, Hollingsworth P, Brimm JE, Petters RM, Virgilio RW, Shackford SR: Complications of the flow-directed pulmonary artery catheter: A prospective analysis of 219 patients. *Crit Care Med* 1981; 9:315–318.
29. Chastre J, Cornud F, Bouchama A, Viau F, Benacerraf R, Gilbert C: Thrombosis as a complication of pulmonary-artery catheterization via the internal jugular vein. *N Engl J Med* 1982; 306:278–281.
30. Rowley KM, Clubb KS, Smith GJ, Cabin HS: Right-sided infective endocarditis as a consequence of flow-directed pulmonary artery catheterization. *N Engl J Med* 1984; 311:1152–1156.
31. Connors AF Jr, Castele RJ, Farhat NZ, Tomashefski JF Jr: Complications of right heart catheterization. *Chest* 1985; 88:567–572.
32. McDaniel DD, Stone JG, Faltas AN, Khambatta HJ, Thys DM, Antunes AM, et al: Catheter-induced pulmonary artery hemorrhage: Diagnosis and management in cardiac operations. *J Thorac Cardiovasc Surg* 1981; 82:1–4.
33. Shah KB, Rao TL, Laughlin S, El-Etr A. A review of pulmonary artery catheterizations in 6245 patients. *Anesthesiology* 1984; 61:271–275.
34. Elliot CG, Zimmerman GA, Clemmer TP: Complications of pulmonary artery catheterization in the care of critically ill patients. *Chest* 1979; 76:647–652.
35. Prachar H, Dittel M, Jobst C, Kiss E, Machacek E, Nobis H, et al: Bacterial contamination of pulmonary artery catheters. *Intens Care Med* 1978; 4:79–82.
36. Michel L, Marsh HM, McMichan JC, Southorn PA, Brewer NS: Infection of pulmonary artery catheters in critically ill patients. *JAMA* 1981; 245:1032–1036.
37. Pinilla JC, Ross DF, Martin T, Crumb H: Study of the incidence of intravascular catheter infection and associated septicemia in critically ill patients. *Crit Care Med* 1983; 11:21–25.
38. Chatterjee K, Matthay M: Right-heart catheterization is a diagnostic procedure not a therapeutic intervention. *J Intens Care Med* 1991; 6:101–104.
39. Gore JM, Goldberg RJ, Spodick DH, Alpert JS, Dalen JE: A community-wide assessment of the use of pulmonary artery catheters in patients with acute myocardial infarction. *Chest* 1987; 92:721–727.
40. Guyatt G, Girotti M, Todd T, Hewson J, MacFarlane G, McIntyre R: A randomized control trial of right-heart catheterization in critically ill patients. *J Intens Care Med* 1991; 6:91–95.
41. Bayliss J, Norell M, Ryan A, Thurston M, Sutton LK: Bedside hemodynamic monitoring: Experience in a general hospital. *Br Med J [Clin Res]* 1983; 287:187–190.
42. Steingrub JS, Celoria G, Vickers-Lahti M, Teres D, Bria W: Therapeutic impact of pulmonary artery catheterization in a medical/surgical ICU. *Chest* 1991; 99:1451–1455.

PART III

The Major Cardiovascular Symptoms

Chapter 19

Chest Pain

Robert A. O'Rourke, M.D.

INTRODUCTION

Chest pain or chest discomfort is the foremost manifestation of myocardial ischemia and results from a disparity between myocardial oxygen demand and coronary blood flow in patients with coronary artery disease. The most common causes of myocardial ischemia are coronary atherosclerosis, coronary vasoconstriction, and/or coronary artery thrombosis, the latter occurring particularly in patients with acute coronary syndromes such as acute myocardial infarction and unstable angina (Chaps. 59 and 60).

It is now recognized that an increase in myocardial oxygen demand (MV_{O_2}) or demand ischemia, a decrease or inadequate blood flow (supply ischemia), or their combination may be responsible for anginal chest pain. The determinants of the myocardial oxygen demand include the ventricular wall stress, inotropic state, and heart rate. Thus, increases in afterload, preload, contractility, and heart rate often precipitate angina, and chronic exertional angina is commonly attributed to an increase in myocardial oxygen demand. However, flow-limiting narrowing of the coronary artery lumen by a complicated plaque with thrombus and/or vasoconstriction without an increment in oxygen demand often causes angina due to acute myocardial ischemia. This likely is the most common mechanism(s) for unstable angina (including variant angina) and acute myocardial infarction (Chaps. 56 to 60).

The responsible mechanism for cardiac pain is not clearly understood.[1] Nonmedullated small sympathetic nerve fibers that parallel the coronary arteries are thought to provide the afferent sensory pathway for angina and enter the spinal cord in the C8-T4 segments.[2] Impulses are transmitted to corresponding spinal ganglia and then through the spinal cord to the thalamus and cerebral cortex. Angina pectoris, like other pain of visceral origin, often is poorly localized and commonly is referred to the corresponding segmental dermatomes.

The differential diagnosis of chest pain is extensive. In addition to angina pectoris and myocardial infarction, other cardiovascular diseases, gastrointestinal diseases, psychogenic disease, neuromuscular disease, and diseases of the pulmonary system must be considered (Table 19-1). An accurate interpretation of the etiology of chest discomfort and its significance in individual patients is critically dependent on a carefully taken history (Chap. 9B). Important clinically relevant information may be missed if the overenthusiastic use of noninvasive and/or invasive diagnostic methods replaces rather than augments direct physician-patient communication.

In the differential diagnosis of chest discomfort, several historical features are important.[3] These include the quality of the chest discomfort; the site and radiation of the chest pain; the size of the area of discomfort; the time of the first episode of pain; the frequency of painful episodes; factors precipitating chest discomfort; action by the patient during an episode; and the factors relieving the chest discomfort.[3] Also important is the presence or absence of associated symptoms that often provide a clue to the correct etiology.

ANGINA PECTORIS AND MYOCARDIAL INFARCTION

Angina Pectoris

The original subjective description by William Heberden of his own angina in the late 18th century has not been surpassed.[4] He wrote:

TABLE 19-1

Differential Diagnosis of Chest Pain

1. Angina pectoris/myocardial infarction
2. Other cardiovascular causes
   a. Likely ischemic in origin
      (1) Aortic stenosis
      (2) Hypertrophic cardiomyopathy
      (3) Severe systemic hypertension
      (4) Severe right ventricular hypertension
      (5) Aortic regurgitation
      (6) Severe anemia/hypoxia
   b. Nonischemic in origin
      (1) Aortic dissection
      (2) Pericarditis
      (3) Mitral valve prolapse
3. Gastrointestinal
   a. Esophageal spasm
   b. Esophageal reflux
   c. Esophageal rupture
   d. Peptic ulcer disease
4. Psychogenic
   a. Anxiety
   b. Depression
   c. Cardiac psychosis
   d. Self-gain
5. Neuromusculoskeletal
   a. Thoracic outlet syndrome
   b. Degenerative joint disease of cervical/thoracic spine
   c. Costochondritis (Tietze's syndrome)
   d. Herpes zoster
   e. Chest wall pain and tenderness
6. Pulmonary
   a. Pulmonary embolus with or without pulmonary infarction
   b. Pneumothorax
   c. Pneumonia with pleural involvement
7. Pleurisy

> **"But there is a disorder of the breast marked with strong and peculiar symptoms, considerable for the kind of danger belonging to it and not extremely rare, which deserves to be mentioned more at length. The seat of it and sense of strangling and anxiety with which it is attended, make it not improperly called angina pectoris. They who are afflicted with it are seized while they are walking (more especially if it be up a hill and soon after eating) with a painful and most disagreeable sensation in the breast, which seems as if would extinguish life if it were to increase or to continue; but the moment they stand still, all this uneasiness vanishes."**

Angina pectoris is defined as chest pain or discomfort of cardiac origin that usually results from a temporary imbalance between myocardial oxygen supply and myocardial oxygen demand. It may occur only with exertion or spontaneously at rest; various subtypes are defined in Chaps. 9 and 46. The *quality* of the chest discomfort is usually described as "tightness," "pressure," "burning," "heavy," "aching," "strangling," or "compression."[5–8] Usually the patient is able to describe a deep rather than a superficial origin of the pain. Since the qualitative description of the pain is greatly influenced by the patient's intelligence, education, and social/cultural background, other characteristics of the chest discomfort are often extremely important in appropriately evaluating the symptoms. The most important of these are the *precipitating factors* for the onset of pain, its *mode* of *onset* and duration, its *pattern of disappearance*, and its *location*. Classically, the discomfort is induced by exercise, emotion, eating, or cold weather. A recognizable pattern of reproducibility of chest pain by certain activities is an important characteristic of angina, and the patient should be questioned specifically along these lines. Often, patients develop pain with exertion after meals, and there is greater tendency for arm work (e.g., showering, lifting, or carrying), which involves a greater element of isometric exercise rather than isotonic leg exercise, to produce distress.[5–8] Chest pain occurring only after exercise has been concluded or at the end of the day rarely is due to myocardial ischemia. Occasionally, angina will dissipate despite continued exercise (the walk-through phenomenon) or will not occur when a second exercise effort is undertaken which previously produced chest discomfort (warm-up phenomenon). Both circumstances may be attributed to the opening of functioning coronary arterial collaterals during the initial myocardial ischemia. Pain is more likely to occur when the patient is outdoors, especially when the temperature is extremely high or low and when the patient is walking uphill against the wind. Angina commonly occurs after the patient has eaten a heavy meal or when the patient is excited, angry, or tense. Hot or cold showers or baths, particularly after moderate to severe exercise, may precipitate pain as may brisk toweling afterwards. The sensory effects of temperature cause reflex autonomic changes in blood pressure and heart rate. Cold showers increase blood pressure and heart rate while hot showers cause an augmented cardiac output in response to vasodilation.[5–8] The chest pain during any type of activity often is made worse by the use of tobacco.[9] Carbon monoxide, a combustion product in cigarette smoke, may combine with hemoglobin and shift the hemoglobin-oxygen dissociation curve to the left, thereby diminishing tissue oxygen delivery. Also, the absorption of nicotine in cigarette smoke through the lungs or mucous membranes increases heart rate, systolic arterial pressure, and cardiac output through the release of endogenous catecholamines. All of the hemodynamic changes resulting from the use of nicotine increase the myocardial oxygen demand.[5–9]

Angina pectoris characteristically has a crescendo pattern at onset and "builds up." Pains, often described as "shooting" or "stabbing" that reach their maximum intensity virtually instantaneously often are not angina but are of musculoskeletal or neural origin. Angina usually is relieved within 5 to 15 min by rest, with or without the use of vasodilator drugs such as nitroglycerin, although nitroglycerin characteristically hastens relief. Failure to obtain relief with rest and/or nitroglycerin suggests another cause of pain or actual impending myocardial infarction. The reproducible relief of chest pain in an appropriate time frame (1 to 5 or 10 min) can be strong evidence favoring ischemia. A trial of nitroglycerin can be a useful diagnostic strategy. Patients with angina pectoris usually are classified functionally from Class I to Class IV (Table 19-2) depending on the amount of activity necessary to induce chest pain. Recommendations for limitation of physical exertion frequently are prescribed in accordance with functional capacity. The morbidity and mortality of patients with chronic ischemic heart disease is related inversely though roughly to the workload necessary to produce angina.

Localizing the *site* of chest discomfort provides additional information in determining its cause. Anginal pain is ordinarily retrosternal or felt slightly to left of the midline, beside or partly under the sternum. It rarely is isolated to the cardiac apex in the inframammary region. A pain that originates entirely outside the thorax and epigastrium or begins elsewhere and subsequently radiates through the chest often is not due to myocardial ischemia although pain beginning in typical angina radiation points such as arms are an exception as noted below. The chest pain of myocardial ischemia tends to *radiate* bilaterally across the chest into the arms (left more than right), and into the neck and lower jaw. Occasionally radiation to the back or occiput is noted. Angina usually does not radiate into the upper jaw, the lower back or below the umbilicus and is rarely felt in the abdomen alone. In the arms, the pain passes down the ulnar and volar surface to the wrist and then only into the ulnar fingers, never into the thumb or down the outer (extensor) surface of the arm which have a different dermatome pattern.[2-8] Pain may occasionally be felt only in the arm or may start in the arm and radiate to the chest. Attention to the patient's gestures that are utilized in characterizing and localizing the site of pain may be useful in determining its etiology. One or two clenched fists held by the patient over the sternal area (Levine's sign) is much more indicative of ischemic pain than is a finger pointed to a small circumscribed area in the left inframammary region.[2-8] The latter more likely represents chest pain of psychogenic origin.

As indicated above, the *duration* of chest pain may also be a useful differentiating feature. Angina pectoris rarely lasts less than 1 min or more than 15 min in the absence of myocardial infarction or persistent arrhythmias. Most patients with angina report prompt *relief* in less than 5 min after cessation of activity or with the use of sublingual nitroglycerin. Delayed relief of chest pain by sublingual nitroglycerin with its continuation for over 15 to 20 min is inconsistent with the rapid onset of action of the drug (less than 2 min) and may be ascribed to a placebo effect. Since nitrates are generalized smooth muscle relaxants, pain due to diffuse esophageal spasm or biliary colic may also be relieved by these same agents.[5-8] Similarly, they can be precipitated by smooth muscle constrictors such as ergonovine. Carotid sinus massage by the physician frequently will relieve anginal chest pain because of the reflex production of a relative bradycardia and a decrease in systolic blood pressure, thus reducing myocardial oxygen demand.[10] Carotid sinus massage should be performed only in the absence of extracranial occlusive cerebrovascular disease as manifested by carotid bruits and/or decreased carotid arterial pulsations and with careful auscultatory monitoring of the heart rate. The Valsalva maneuver may also relieve angina pain by decreasing myocardial wall tension as a result of the reduced venous return and left ventricular volume accompanying the increase in intrathoracic pressure. *Associated symptoms*, such as nausea, vomiting, faintness, fatigue, or diaphoresis, often accompany severe episodes of myocardial ischemia. Severe myocardial ischemia often produces severe dyspnea due to a marked increase in left ventricular diastolic filling pressure, sometimes producing an "angina equivalent" in the absence of chest discomfort.

No consideration of myocardial ischemia as a likely cause of chest discomfort is complete without carefully considering the chest pain in the context of known *risk factors* for coronary artery disease.[5-8] Established independent coronary risk factors include increasing age, male sex, hypercholesterolemia, cigarette smoking, diabetes, hypertension, and family history of premature coronary artery disease. A history of coronary artery disease at an early age in a first degree relative is an especially powerful predictor of the disease in a patient with chest pain.[1]

Angina pectoris should be considered as a symptom and not as a specific disease. Coronary arteriographic studies have demonstrated that more than 90 percent of patients with chest pain precipitated by exercise and relieved by rest have angiographic evidence of significant coronary disease.[5-8] However, other diseases may be associated with classic angina pectoris (see below). Any disorder condition which causes a transit disparity between myocardial oxygen demand and coronary blood

TABLE 19-2

Canadian Cardiovascular Society Functional Classification of Angina Pectoris

I. Ordinary physical activity, such as walking and climbing stairs, does not cause angina. Angina results from strenuous or rapid or prolonged exertion at work or recreation.

II. Slight limitation of ordinary activity. Walking or climbing stairs rapidly, walking uphill, walking or stair climbing after meals, in cold, in wind, or when under emotional stress, or only during the few hours after awakening. Walking more than two blocks on the level and climbing more than one flight of ordinary stairs at a normal pace and under normal conditions.

III. Marked limitations of ordinary physical activity. Walking one to two blocks on the level and climbing more than one flight under normal conditions.

IV. Inability to carry on any physical activity without discomfort—anginal syndrome *may be* present at rest.

SOURCE: Modified from Campeau L: Letter to the editor. *Circulation* 1976; 54:522. Reproduced with permission from the American Heart Association Inc. and the author.

flow may result in myocardial ischemia, particularly involving the subendocardium.[5–8]

Several reports have described certain patients with typical exertional chest discomfort and arteriographically normal coronary arteries.[11–15] These patients are more likely to be females, have fewer coronary risk factors, and, less commonly, have more relief of pain by sublingual nitroglycerin than patients with occlusive coronary artery disease. Although the underlying cause of this condition remains unsettled, the life expectancy of these patients appears no different from an age and sex-matched population without chest discomfort.

There is some evidence that abnormal small coronary artery function may cause limited coronary flow responses to stress or pharmacologic vasodilators in a subset of patients with anginal chest pain despite angiographically normal coronary arteries ("microvascular angina").[16–23] In the past, investigators arguing for or against the existence of this syndrome have often used the term "syndrome X" to describe their patient cohort. The term was first used by Kemp in a 1973[24] editorial response to an article by Arbogast and Bourassa,[25] in which patients with chest pain and angiographically normal coronary arteries were called "group X." These patients were selected because of ST segment depression during rapid atrial pacing.

Syndrome X appears to include a heterogenous group of patients with a wide spectrum of chest pain and a variety of vascular and smooth muscle hypersensitive constrictor responses. Multiple research studies continue in an effort to explain syndrome X.[26–34] However, a satisfactory explanation for chest pain in many patients with angiographically normal or nearly normal coronary arteries remains elusive. (See also Chap. 58.)

Although a history of characteristic angina with exertion is highly predictive of underlying coronary atherosclerosis, the specific features of the history differ from this idealized description in many patients with symptomatic ischemic heart disease. The physician must balance a high degree of suspicion stimulated by the high incidence and seriousness of myocardial ischemia with a unwillingness to make a premature and mistaken diagnosis of clinical coronary artery disease with its substantial impact on the psychic and socioeconomic aspects of the patient's future life.[5–8] Bayes' theorem stating that the predictive value of a test result is predetermined by the prevalence of the disease in the patient population being studied should be considered carefully.[35] Obviously, the likelihood of documenting severe coronary artery disease by arteriography differs in a 40-year-old menstruating female with no risk factors and atypical chest pain at rest from that in a 70-year-old man with hypertension, hypercholesterolemia, a positive family history, and classic exercise-induced chest discomfort of myocardial ischemia. The pretest likelihood of disease is low in the first patient and high in the second.

Some patients with coronary artery disease experience *angina at rest* as a complication or an isolated clinical manifestation of ischemic heart disease.[5–8] Myocardial ischemic pain at rest more likely results from an acute reduction in myocardial oxygen supply than from an increase in myocardial oxygen demand. Possible causative factors include isolated coronary artery spasm or embolism, coronary artery spasm superimposed on coronary atherosclerosis, and coronary thrombosis with spontaneous thrombolysis.[36–39] However, in patients with progressive coronary atherosclerosis, ischemic rest pain may also result from intermittent arrhythmias, that increase myocardial oxygen demand and/or decrease diastolic coronary blood flow, or from labile hypertension with its increased wall stress. Chest pain at rest may occur only as nocturnal angina. In addition to the above mechanism, nocturnal angina, also known as angina decubitus, may be produced by the increase in wall stress and, thus, MV_{O_2} secondary to redistribution of the intravascular blood volume in the recumbent position. Nocturnal angina may also be contributed to by the relative hypercapnia and acidosis that occurs during sleep. Nocturnal angina also has been accompanied by concomitant rapid eye movement sleep patterns on the electroencephalogram, that may result from augmented sympathetic discharge increasing MV_{O_2} and/or coronary constriction.[5–8] (See also Chap. 59.)

Despite the more malignant natural history observed in many patients with *rest angina*, the predictive value of the history alone is not as accurate as with exertional angina. The quality of pain is usually similar to that of exertional angina, but the discomfort may be more severe and its duration longer. In addition, angina at rest is commonly associated with nausea, vomiting, and/or diaphoresis. The onset of shortness of breath during or after the beginning of chest discomfort suggests that the pain is due to extensive myocardial ischemia and usually results from an acute elevation of left ventricular filling pressures secondary to the development of a large, transiently ischemic myocardial segment.[5–8] Such patients commonly are found to have multivessel occlusive coronary artery disease on arteriography. Syncope occasionally is associated with chest pain secondary to coronary artery spasm and may result from transient bradyarrhythmias such as complete heart block produced by ischemia of the specialized conduction system. A cyclic recurrence at the same time each day is an interesting but incompletely understood characteristic in some patients with pain resulting from coronary artery spasm.[5–8] (See Chap. 59.)

The physical examination of the patient during an episode of angina may reveal clues to the diagnosis, but often is normal in patients with no prior myocardial infarction (Table 19-3). During an episode, the systolic and diastolic blood pressures are often significantly elevated; or occasionally hypotension results when the ischemia is extensive. A mild tachycardia is often present,

TABLE 19-3

Clinical Findings during Chest Pain Due to Myocardial Ischemia

Increase or marked decrease in systolic blood pressure
Relative tachycardia or bradyarrhythmia
Palpable left ventricular asynergy
New S4 or S3
Reversed splitting of S2
Murmur of papillary muscle dysfunction
Bibasilar pulmonary rales

but bradyarrhythmias may also occur.[5–8] The presence of a new fourth or third heart sound, reverse splitting of S2, the murmur of mitral regurgitation, bibasilar pulmonary rales, palpable ventricular asynergy, or pulsus alternans suggest a cardiac cause for the patient's chest pain.[5–8]

The resting electrocardiogram (ECG) is normal in 25 to 50 percent of patients with stable angina. Evidence of prior myocardial infarction or ST–T wave changes of ischemia enhance suspicion that chest pain may represent angina. An ECG during chest pain reveals ischemic changes in apoproximately half of those with a normal resting electrocardiogram. The usefulness and cost of other noninvasive and invasive tests for determining whether or not rest or exercise-induced chest discomfort is due to myocardial ischemia from coronary artery disease should be carefully considered for each patient. (See also Chaps. 58 to 60.)

Myocardial Infarction

Chest pain or discomfort resulting from myocardial infarction is qualitatively similar to angina at rest. The differentiation between the pain resulting from ischemia and that due to myocardial necrosis is usually impossible to ascertain from the history alone.[5–8] Pain associated with transmural Q wave infarction usually is more severe and longer lasting than anginal pain and is often associated with nausea, vomiting, and diaphoresis. In addition, myocardial infarction is frequently accompanied by symptoms of sustained left ventricular dysfunction (dyspnea, orthopnea) and evidence of autonomic nervous system hyperactivity (tachycardia, diaphoresis, bradycardia).[5–8] However, painless or atypical presentations of myocardial infarction occur in up to 30 percent of patients, particularly in diabetic patients and the elderly. Thus, determination of serial serum enzymes and isoenzymes providing evidence of myocardial necrosis and serial ECGs indicating myocardial injury are necessary to establish the diagnosis in most patients. (See Chap. 60.)

CHEST PAIN DUE TO OTHER CARDIAC DISEASES

Ischemic Chest Pain Not Due to Coronary Atherosclerosis

There are two groups of cardiovascular diseases causing chest pain that is not due to coronary atherosclerosis (Table 19-1). The first group consists of cardiac diseases causing myocardial ischemia-related angina in the absence of coronary artery disease; ischemia is due to hemodynamic changes associated with an inadequate myocardial oxygen supply in relation to a normal or increased myocardial oxygen demand. Among these are left ventricular outflow obstruction secondary to *aortic valve stenosis* (Chap. 79), *hypertrophic cardiomyopathy* (Chap. 90), and *systemic arterial hypertension* (Chap. 76) in which left ventricular systolic pressure and left ventricular wall tension are greatly increased, and/or left ventricular hypertrophy is present.[5–8,40–42] Chest pain due to myocardial ischemia also occurs with severe *aortic regurgitation* (Chap. 79): The large ventricular volume load and increased ventricular dimensions result in increased myocardial oxygen demand, and the reduced diastolic perfusion pressure of the coronary arteries results in a relatively inadequate coronary blood flow.[5–8] Occasionally, very severe *anemia* or *hypoxia* may also produce myocardial ischemia by inadequate oxygen blood supply even in the absence of associated coronary artery disease.[43] In addition, severe *right ventricular systolic hypertension*, as often occurs with pulmonic stenosis or pulmonary hypertension, may cause exertional angina presumably on the basis of right ventricular subendocardial ischemia.[44]

Nonischemic Chest Pain

A second group of cardiac diseases causing chest pain that is not usually due to myocardial ischemia includes *pericarditis* (Chap. 92), *aortic dissection* (Chap. 123), and *mitral valve prolapse* (Chap. 80).

Pericarditis is a relatively common cause of chest pain.[45,46] The chest pain of pericarditis is most often sharp and penetrating in quality, and patients often obtain relief by sitting up and bending forward (Chap. 92). The cardinal diagnostic feature of pericardial pain is its frequent worsening by changes in body position, during deep inspiration, and occasionally when swallowing.[5–8] Radiation of the chest discomfort may involve the shoulders, upper back, and neck because of irritation of the diaphragmatic pleura, which is innervated through the phrenic nerve by fibers originating in cervical sympathetic ganglia C3 to C5. The visceral pericardium is virtually insensitive to pain and pain fibers originating in the parietal pericardium innervate only its diaphragmatic surface. Therefore, the chest discomfort associated with pericarditis is due predominately to parietal pleural irritation. This is the likely reason why pain is more prominent in viral or bacterial pericarditis than in noninfectious pericarditis, such as that caused by uremia and lupus. Occasionally, the pain of acute benign, presumptive viral, pericarditis may mimic that observed in acute myocardial infarction. Importantly, the most common cause of pericarditis in middle-aged or older people is acute myocardial infarction. The pericarditis usually occurs several days after the myocardial necrosis and must be distinguished from recurrent infarction or ischemia. Pericarditis may also be a cause of chest pain after cardiac surgery and may be a complication of aortic direction with leakage into the pericardium. Thus, the correct diagnosis depends on a careful analysis of the history, physical finding of an audible rub (Chap. 11), ECG (Chap. 13), and noninvasive diagnostic techniques such as echocardiography (Chap. 15), computed automated tomography (Chap. 135), and nuclear magnetic resonance imaging (Chap. 136). Rarely, patients with acute benign pericarditis may experience chest pain that is synchronous with each heartbeat.

Aortic dissection (Chap. 123) may be misdiagnosed on initial presentation as an acute myocardial infarction; indeed, myocardial infarction is a recognized complication of aortic dissection. However, the pain with dissection usually is of sudden onset as compared to the pain of myocardial ischemia, which builds intensity with time.[47]

Patients frequently characterize the pain as excruciating, the most severe discomfort that they have ever experienced, and as having a tearing quality. The discomfort may radiate widely into the neck, back, flanks, legs, and may migrate depending on the location and progression of the aortic dissection and the amount of arterial luminal compression.[5-8] Neurologic symptoms and signs may occur when dissection involves the cerebral arteries. With the exception of patients with Marfan's syndrome or idiopathic cystic medial necrosis, the majority of patients with aortic dissection will have a history of longstanding systemic arterial hypertension or evidence of it on physical examination (e.g., retinal arterial changes (Chap. 12), electrocardiography (Chap. 13), chest radiography (Chap. 14), or echocardiography (left ventricular hypertrophy) (see Chap. 15).

Mitral valve prolapse patients often present with atypical chest pain. In many, the pain appears to be psychogenic in origin. In some, the chest discomfort actually represents palpitation due to premature ventricular contractions. In most patients with mitral valve prolapse, myocardial perfusion imaging after exercise demonstrates no evidence of myocardial ischemia. (See Chapter 80.)

PSYCHOGENIC CAUSES OF CHEST PAIN

Psychogenic chest discomfort is a common type of recurrent chest pain that may be difficult to separate from angina pectoris, particularly when it occurs in patients with multiple risk factors for coronary artery disease or in otherwise asymptomatic patients with well-documented coronary artery disease.[5-8] The most common psychogenic cause of chest discomfort is *anxiety*.[48,49] (See also Chap. 118.) Although anxiety can coexist with, and often aggravate, chest pain due to myocardial ischemia, several characteristics of the pain help to differentiate these two conditions. Psychogenic chest pain often is described as sharp or stabbing, commonly is localized to the left inframammary area, and usually is sharply circumscribed. Terms such as stabbing or lightening-like may be used to describe extremely short (less than 1 min) episodes of pain. At times, the pain may persist for many hours or several days, in contrast to myocardial ischemia pain, that characteristically persists for shorter periods of time. Patients often note psychogenic pain after not doing activity or in the evening after work. Also, nonvocal communication, such as a flat or worried facial expression, retarded motor activity, and hand wringing may indicate underlying depression.[5-8] Observation of the patient during pain that occurs spontaneously or during exercise testing often provides insight into a potential psychogenic etiology. The pain often is atypical, the patient's emotional response inappropriate, and no other evidence for myocardial ischemia is apparent.[5-8] Patients with anxiety often have multiple complaints such as breathlessness, giddiness, and palpitation. Associated symptoms, such as air hunger, circumoral paresthesias, globus hystericus, and multiple somatic complaints may suggest a neurasthenic personality and/or hyperventilation syndrome. It is often worthwhile to determine if voluntary forced hyperventilation in the presence of the physician will reproduce the chest pain complaint with fidelity.[5-8] Many patients with mitral valve prolapse have atypical chest discomfort and often complain of chronic fatigue as well. A careful physical examination may disclose the presence of a midsystolic click and/or late systolic murmur, indicating that the atypical chest pain may be related to the mitral valve prolapse leaflet syndrome that some believe is specifically associated with atypical chest pain in certain patients (Chap. 80).

CHEST PAIN DUE TO GASTROINTESTINAL DISEASE

Pain originating in the gastrointestinal tract, particularly that of esophageal origin, is commonly confused with ischemic chest pain.[50] Diffuse esophageal spasm, a neuromuscular motor disorder of the esophagus characterized by chest pain, is the extracardiac condition that is most frequently confused with angina pectoris.[51-55] Esophageal spasm may occur in any age group but is more common in individuals in the fifth decade. The pain is usually retrosternal, may be burning, squeezing, or aching in quality, and often radiates to the back, arms, and jaw. It usually begins during or after a meal and can last minutes or hours. In some patients the pain may be precipitated or exacerbated by exercise, and relief may be obtained with nitroglycerin, which also relaxes esophageal smooth muscle. A useful feature in the differentiation of *diffuse esophageal spasm* from ischemic chest discomfort is its frequent association with pain as a result of swallowing, dysphagia, and the regurgitation of gastric contents. Episodes of pain are frequently precipitated either by extremely hot or cold drinks, or an emotional upset. The diagnosis of diffuse esophageal spasm is based on the history, the exclusion of cardiac and musculoskeletal causes of chest pain, and on the demonstration of abnormal esophageal motility on cineesophagrams or by esophageal manometry.[51-55]

Reflux esophagitis results from mucosal irritation produced by failure of the lower esophageal sphincter to prevent regurgitation of highly acidic gastric contents into the distal esophagus.[56-60] The pain is usually epigastric or retrosternal, is burning in quality, and frequently is precipitated by the recumbent position or by bending over. The "heartburn" and regurgitation often occur after meals or ingestion of coffee or after postural changes. Patients often are awakened by chest discomfort due to acid reflux which occurs in the recumbent position. Many of these patients are obese and report relief of discomfort from food, antacids, and/or elevation of the head of the bed.[5-8] Dysphagia may result from stricture formation secondary to long-standing esophageal reflux. The diagnosis is suggested by a history of "heartburn" in relation to meals and posture and by relief with antacids. The upper GI series may demonstrate hiatal hernia, but this does not establish the diagnosis of esophagitis or esophageal reflux. Esophagoscopy and esophageal biopsy may demonstrate mucosal lesions and are useful for assessing the severity of inflammation and for excluding malignancy. Sphincter incompetence may be documented by the use of esophageal manometry.[50] Esophageal acid perfusion testing (Bernstein test) will often provoke the patient's characteristic symptoms;

and distal esophageal pH monitoring will detect gastroesophageal reflux.

Acute esophageal rupture, a serious and often rapidly lethal event, causes severe retrosternal pain secondary to the chemical mediastinitis produced by acidic gastric contents.[5–8,50] Spontaneous rupture usually results from a prolonged bout of vomiting or retching after a heavy meal. Rupture is a recognized iatrogenic complication of esophageal instrumentation. The pain varies in location depending on the site and position. The diagnosis is based on symptoms and signs of mediastinal air following vomiting or esophageal instrumentation.

Although peptic ulcer disease and biliary colic are less commonly confused with chest pain of cardiac origin, myocardial ischemic pain may occasionally be described as burning in character and located near the epigastrium. Also, patients with coronary artery disease commonly receive aspirin therapy, which increases the risk of peptic ulcer disease.

NEUROMUSCULAR-SKELETAL CAUSES OF CHEST DISCOMFORT

Diseases involving the neuromuscular-skeletal systems may cause pain affecting dermatome patterns similar to those occurring with angina pectoris.[5–8] The *thoracic outlet syndromes*, in which various neural and vascular structures are compressed, may produce symptoms that are sometimes confused with cardiac chest pain. Although compression of the neurovascular bundle by a cervical rib or the scalenus anterior muscle may cause discomfort radiating to the head and neck, the shoulder region, or the axilla, most patients experience pain in the upper extremity resulting from somatic nerve compression, usually in the distribution of the ulnar nerve.[5–8] The presence of associated paresthesias, the presence of pain unrelated to physical exercise, the worsening of discomfort, and its aggravation by certain body positions are useful differentiating characteristics. The diagnosis of thoracic outlet syndrome can be confirmed in many patients by careful physical and neurologic examination.

Tietze's syndrome, or *idiopathic costochondritis*, is an occasional cause of anterior chest wall pain that is aggravated by movement and deep breathing.[61] The reproduction of the chest pain syndrome by direct pressure over the involved costochondral junction and/or the relief of pain after local infiltration with lidocaine are helpful diagnostic maneuvers.[62] *Degenerative arthritis* of the cervical and thoracic vertebrae may cause bandlike pain confined to the chest, neck, or back that often radiates to the arms.[63] Radiologic evidence of degenerative changes involving the cervical and thoracic vertebrae is often found in asymptomatic elderly patients. The production or exacerbation of pain by various postures, movement, sneezing, or coughing is more useful in the diagnosis of chest discomfort due to vertebral disease.[5–8]

The preeruptive stage of *herpes zoster* may be characterized by bandlike chest pain over one or more dermatomes. The advanced age of the patient, additional symptoms of malaise, headache and fever, the presence of hyperesthesia of the involved area on physical examination, and the eventual eruption of typical lesions 4 or 5 days after the onset of symptoms will result in the correct diagnosis. *Chest wall pain* and tenderness may occur for unknown reasons.[64] The discomfort may be reproduced by pressure over the painful area and by movements of the thorax such as bending, twisting, or turning. The variable duration of the pain and the absence of relief by nitroglycerin distinguish it from angina.

PULMONARY CAUSES OF CHEST PAIN

The syndrome of acute massive *pulmonary embolism* with its associated acute pulmonary hypertension and low cardiac output may occasionally simulate acute myocardial infarction, since myocardial ischemia may be present in both conditions.[65] The quality of chest pain may be identical to that observed in patients with nonradiating ischemic chest pain or may be pleuritic as described below. However, the associated signs of severe dyspnea, tachypnea, and intense cyanosis, accompanied by profound anxiety and agitation, favor the diagnosis of pulmonary embolism.[5–8] The physical examination often reveals evidence of pulmonary hypertension, tricuspid regurgitation, and acute right heart failure (Chap. 100).

The clinical setting may suggest the diagnosis because of the known increased likelihood of pulmonary embolism in the postpartum or postoperative state, during long trips, in patients with congestive heart failure and peripheral edema, and in those with deep vein thrombophlebitis.[5–8] Measurements of arterial blood gases, abnormal pulmonary-perfusion ventilation scans and if needed pulmonary arteriography will establish the correct diagnosis.[5–8]

Other pulmonary conditions associated with chest discomfort, such as pneumothorax, are rarely confused with ischemic chest pain because of additional characteristic clinical features.[5–8] *Spontaneous pneumothorax* usually occurs in young, otherwise healthy males in the third and fourth decades. The clinical presentation usually is characterized by the abrupt onset of agonizing unilateral pleuritic chest pain associated with severe shortness of breath. The plain or expiratory chest film provides the definitive diagnosis. Chest pain associated with *pneumonias* of various etiologies, as well as pulmonary infarctions as a consequence of pulmonary embolus, may result from pleural irritation. The discomfort is sharp, varies acutely with breathing, and is frequently accompanied by a reduced inspiratory effort. Associated signs of pulmonary parenchymal infection or infarction, such as fever, cough, and sputum production, or hemoptysis usually indicate the underlying diagnosis.

LIMITATIONS OF THE HISTORY IN ESTABLISHING THE CAUSES OF CHEST PAIN

Although a carefully obtained history is usually valuable for identifying the responsible causes of chest pain or in limiting the differential diagnosis, it occasionally is either not very beneficial or is frankly misleading. These limitations result from the variable skill of different physicians in obtaining a correct history or from the inability of the patient to delineate accurately the symptom complex because of educational, social, or cultural reasons.[3,5–8] Also, patients often minimize or deny symptoms for psychological reasons or for practical reasons such as maintaining job security. By contrast, some patients may exaggerate or fabricate symptoms in order to obtain disability compensation or other secondary gain.[5–8]

The history alone is not a very sensitive tool for the detection of ischemic heart disease. Angina is a relatively late event following hemodynamic or electrocardiographic changes or may not even develop in the myocardial "ischemic cascade."[66,67] "Silent" or asymptomatic myocardial ischemia is a frequently recognized and documented event of considerable clinical importance (Chap. 58).

REFERENCES

1. Malliani AM: The elusive link between transient myocardial ischemia and pain. *Circulation* 1986; 73:201–204.
2. Sampson JJ, Cheitlin M: Pathophysiology and differential diagnosis of cardiac pain. *Prog Cardiovasc Dis* 1971; 13:507–531.
3. Hurst JW: Atherosclerotic Coronary Heart Disease. In: Hurst JW, Schlant RC (eds): *The Heart*, 7th ed. New York, McGraw-Hill, 1990:965–968.
4. Heberden W: Some accounts of a disorder of the breast. *Med Trans* 1772; 2:59.
5. Walsh RA, O'Rourke RA: History and differential diagnosis of acute myocardial infarction. In: Karliner JS, Gregoratos G (eds): *Coronary Care*. New York, Churchill Livingstone, 1981:169–188.
6. Levine HJ: Difficult problems in the diagnosis of chest pain. *Am Heart J* 1980; 100:108–118.
7. Walsh RA, O'Rourke RA: Chest pain. In: Stein JH (ed): *Internal Medicine*, 3d ed. Boston, Little, Brown & Co., 1990: 60–64.
8. Christie LG Jr, Conti CR: Systematic approach to evaluation of angina-like chest pain: Pathophysiology and clinical testing with emphasis on objective documentation of myocardial ischemia. *Am Heart J* 1981; 102:897–912.
9. Oram S, Souton E: Tobacco angina. *Quart J Med* 1963; 32:115–120.
10. Levine SA: Carotid sinus massage. A new diagnostic test for angina pectoris. *JAMA* 1962; 182:1332–1356.
11. Epstein SE, Talbot TL: Dynamic coronary tone in precipitation, exacerbation and relief of angina pectoris. *Am J Cardiol* 1981; 48:797–803.
12. Proudfit WL, Shirey ED, Sones FM Jr: Selective cine coronary arteriography: Correlation with clinical findings in 1000 patients. *Circulation* 1966; 33:901–910.
13. Ockene IS, Shay MJ, Alpert JS, Weiner BH, Dalen JE: Unexplained chest pain in patients with normal coronary arteriograms. *N Engl J Med* 1980; 303:1249–1258.
14. Braschke AVG, Proudfit WL, Sones FM: Clinical course of patients with normal, and slightly or moderately abnormal coronary arteriograms. A follow-up study on 500 patients. *Circulation* 1973; 47:936–945.
15. Waxler EB, Kimbiris D, Dreifus LS: The fate of women with normal coronary arteriograms and chest pain resembling angina pectoris. *Am J Cardiol* 1971; 28:25–32.
16. Cannon RO: Microvascular angina: cardiovascular investigations regarding pathophysiology and management. *Med Clin N Am* 1991; 75:1097–1118.
17. Cannon RO III, Cattau EL Jr, Yakshe PN, Maher K, Schenke WH, Benjamin SB, et al: Coronary flow reserve, esophageal motility, and chest pain in patients with angiographically normal coronary arteries. *Am J Med* 1990; 88:217–222.
18. Panza JA, Epstein S, Quyyumi AA: Circadian variation in vascular tone and its relation to α-sympathetic vasoconstrictor activity. *N Engl J Med* 1991; 325:986–990.
19. Crake T, Canepa-Anson R, Shapiro L, Poole-Wilson PA: Continuous recording of coronary sinus oxygen saturation during atrial pacing in patients with coronary artery disease or with syndrome X. *Br Heart J* 1988; 59:31–38.
20. Miwa K, Fujita M, Ejiri M, Sasayama S: Comparative sensitivity of intracoronary injection of acetylcholine for the induction of coronary spasm in patients with various types of angina pectoris. *Am Heart J* 1990; 120:544–550.
21. Cannon RO III, Schenke WH, Quyyumi A, Bonow RO, Epstein SE: Comparison of exercise testing with studies of coronary flow reserve in patients with microvascular angina. *Circulation* 1991; 83(Suppl III):III-77–III-81.
22. Kaski JC, Tousoulis D, Galassi AR, McFadden E, Pereira WI, Crea P, et al: Epicardial coronary artery tone and reactivity in patients with normal coronary arteriograms and reduced coronary flow reserve (syndrome X). *J Am Coll Cardiol* 1991; 18:50–54.
23. Cannon RO III, Peden DB, Berkebile C, Schenke WH, Kaliner MA, Epstein SE: Airway hyperresponsiveness in patients with microvascular angina: evidence for a diffuse disorder of smooth muscle responsiveness. *Circulation* 1990; 82:2011–2017.
24. Kemp HG: Left ventricular function in patients with the anginal syndrome and normal coronary arteries. *Am J Cardiol* 1973; 32:375–376.
25. Abrogast R, Bourassa MG: Myocardial function during atrial pacing in patients with angina pectoris and normal coronary arteriograms. *Am J Cardiol* 1973; 32:257–263.
26. Attilio M: Syndrome X: still an appropriate name. *J Am Coll Cardiol* 1991; 17:1471–1472.
27. Levy RD, Cunningham D, Shapiro LM, Wright C, Mockus L, Fox KM: Diurnal variation in left ventricular function: a study of patients with myocardial ischaemia, syndrome X, and of normal controls. *Br Heart J* 1987; 57:148–153.
28. Turiel M, Galassi AR, Glazier JJ, Kaski JC, Maseri A: Pain threshold and tolerance in women with syndrome X and women with stable angina pectoris. *Am J Cardiol* 1987; 60:503–507.
29. Spinelli L, Ferro G, Genovese A, Ginquegrana G, Spadafora M, Condorelli M: Exercise-induced impairment of diastolic time in patients with X syndrome. *Am Heart J* 1990; 119:829–833.
30. Kern MJ: Extracting the coronary artery from syndrome X: Is epicardial vasomotion physiologic in patients with normal coronary arteriograms and reduced coronary flow reserve? *J Am Coll Cardiol* 1991; 18:55–56.
31. Opherk DO, Schuler G, Wetterauer K, Mathey J, Schwarz F, Kubler W: Four-year follow-up study in patients with angina pectoris and normal coronary arteriograms ("Syndrome X"). *Circulation* 1989; 80:1610–1616.
32. Galassi AR, Kaski JC, Pupita G, Margarita V, Crea F, Maseri A: Lack of evidence for alpha-adrenergic receptor-mediated mechanisms in the genesis of ischemia in syndrome X. *Am J Cardiol* 1989; 64:264–269.
33. Epstein SE, Cannon RO III, Bonow RO: Exercise testing in patients with microvascular angina. *Circulation* 1991; 83(Suppl III):III-73–III-76.
34. Cannon RO III, Quyyumi AA, Schenke WH, Fananapazir L, Tucker EE, Gaughan AM et al: Abnormal cardiac sensitivity in patients with chest pain and normal coronary arteries. *J Am Coll Cardiol* 1990; 16:1359–1366.
35. Diamond GA, Forrester JS: Analysis of probability as an aid in the clinical diagnosis of coronary artery disease. *N Engl J Med* 1979; 300:1350–1358.
36. Maseri A, Klassen GA, Lesch M (eds): *Primary and Secondary Angina Pectoris*. New York, Grune & Stratton, 1978.
37. Hillis DL, Braunwald E: Medical progress: coronary-artery spasm. *N Engl J Med* 1978; 229:695–702.
38. Prinzmetal M, et al: Angina pectoris. 1. A variant form of angina pectoris. *Am J Med* 1959; 26:375–388.
39. Herrick JB: Clinical features of sudden obstruction of the coronary arteries. *JAMA* 1912; 59:2015–2020.
40. Wood P: Aortic stenosis. *Am J Cardiol* 1958; 1:553–571.
41. Pasternac A, Noble J, Streulens Y, Elie R, Herschke C, Bourassa MG: Pathophysiology of chest pain in patients with cardiomyopathies and normal coronary arteries. *Circulation* 1982; 65:778–789.
42. Ouzts HG, Turner JL, Douglas JS Jr, Hurst JW: Prolonged chest pain suggesting myocardial infarction in patients with hypertrophic cardiomyopathy. In: Hurst JW (ed): *The Heart*, Update III. New York, McGraw-Hill Book Company, 1980: 139.

43. Pickering GW, Wayne EJ: Observations on angina pectoris and intermittence claudication in anemia. *Clin Sci* 1933; 1:305–309.
44. Ross RS, Babe BM: Right ventricular hypertension as a cause of angina. *Circulation* 1960; 22:801–802.
45. Barnes AR, Burchell HB: Acute pericarditis simulating myocardial infarction. *Am Heart J* 1942; 23:247–268.
46. Spodick DH: Pitfalls in the recognition of pericarditis. In: Hurst JW (ed): *Clinical Essays on the Heart*. Vol. 5. New York, McGraw-Hill Book Company, 1985.
47. Eagle KA, DeSanctis RW: Dissecting aortic aneurysm. *Curr Prob Cardiol* 1989; 14:227–278.
48. Cohen ME, White PD, Johnson RE: Neurocirculatory asthenia, anxiety necrosis or the effect syndrome. *Arch Intern Med* 1948; 81:260–281.
49. Katon W, Hall ML, Russo J, Cormier L, Hollifield M, Vitaliano PP: Chest pain: relationship of psychiatric illness to coronary arteriographic results. *Am J Med* 1988; 84:1–9.
50. Mellow MH: A gastroenterologist's view of chest pain. *Curr Prob Cardiol* 1983; 9:1–36.
51. Cassella RR, Ellis FH, Brown AL: Diffuse spasm of the esophagus. Fine structure of esophageal smooth muscle and nerve. *JAMA* 1965; 191:379–382.
52. Castell DO: The spectrum of esophageal motility disorders. *Gastroenterology* 1979; 76:639–640.
53. Gillis M, Nicks R, Skyring A: Clinical, manometric and pathogenic studies in diffuse esophageal spasm. *Br Heart J* 1967; 2:527.
54. Creamer B, Denoghue FE, Code CF: Pattern of esophageal motility in diffuse spasm. *Gastroenterology* 1958; 34:782–796.
55. Ferguson SC, Hodges K, Hersh T, Jinch H: Esophageal manometry in patients with chest pain and normal arteriograms. *Am J Gastroenterol* 1981; 75:124–129.
56. Richter JE, Castell DO: Gastroesophageal reflux: pathogenesis, diagnosis and therapy. *Ann Intern Med* 1982; 97:93–103.
57. Johnson LF, DeMeeter TR: Twenty-four hours pH monitoring of the distal esophagus: a quantitative measure of gastrointestinal reflux. *Am J Gastroenterol* 1974; 62:325–332.
58. Bernstein LM, Grain RC, Pacini R: Differentiation of esophageal pain from angina pectoris: role of esophageal acid perfusion test. *Medicine* 1962; 41:145–162.
59. Beng LJ, Hookin LA, Marguies S, Donner MW, Cauthorne RJ, Hendrix TR: A comparison of clinical measurements of gastroesophageal reflux. *Gastroenterology* 1972; 62:1–5.
60. Atkinson M: Monitoring esophageal pH. *Gut* 1987; 28:509–514.
61. Tietze A: Uber eine eigenartige Haufung on Fallen mit. Dystrophic der Ripenknorpel. *Berl Klin Wehr* 1921; 58:829.
62. Wolf E, Stern S: Costosternal syndrome. Its frequency and importance in differential diagnosis of coronary heart disease. *Arch Intern Med* 1976; 136:189–191.
63. Gunther L, Sampson JJ. The radicular syndrome in hypertrophic osteoarthritis of the spine, root pain and its differentiation from the heart pain. *JAMA* 1929; 93:514–519.
64. Epstein SE, Gerber LN, Boren JS: Chest wall syndrome. A common cause of unexpected pain. *JAMA* 1979; 241:2793–2797.
65. Bettmann MA, Salzman EW: Current concepts in the diagnosis of pulmonary embolism. *Mod Conc Cardiovasc Dis* 1984; 53:1–6.
66. Nesto RW, Kowalchuk GJ: The ischemic cascade: Temporal sequence of hemodynamic, electrocardiographic and symptomatic expressions of ischemia. *Am J Cardiol* 1987; 57:23C–30C.
67. Berman DS, Rozanski A, Knoebel SB: The detection of silent ischemia: Cautions and precautions. *Circulation* 1987; 75:101–105.

Chapter 20

Dyspnea and Fatigue

R. Wayne Alexander, M.D., Ph.D.

Dyspnea and fatigue are the most common symptoms of a number of cardiovascular diseases that are associated with abnormal ventricular function and/or decreased oxygen delivery to the periphery. Fatigue is the most common symptom limiting exercise in congestive heart failure while normal persons and, for example, patients with mitral stenosis appear to be limited equally by dyspnea and fatigue.[1]

FATIGUE

The term fatigue is rather nonspecific as commonly used. Patients may use this term to refer to the malaise associated with, for example, the systemic symptoms associated with an infection. Fatigue has been used to describe the premonitory symptoms of malaise or exhaustion that have been described as precursors of myocardial infarction or sudden death.[2–4] In a prospective study of risk factors for myocardial infarction exhaustion, over the relatively short term, was a less powerful predictor than age, smoking, or cholesterol but was more powerful than hypertension.[5] The data do not lend themselves to mechanistic interpretation but do confirm the importance of the symptom of fatigue as a risk factor for myocardial infarction that should be evaluated during routine history taking. It is possible that the general malaise that may be an antecedent to myocardial infarction may reflect the inflammatory nature of atherosclerosis in its active stages (see Chap. 56) and thus might be analogous to the systemic symptoms seen in other inflammatory diseases.

Fatigue is also used to describe the feeling of tiredness or weakness in skeletal muscle that may limit exercise in normal people as well as in those with disease. In cardiovascular disease the symptom refers to relatively premature exercise-limiting muscle weakness. Unusual fatigue at low levels of exertion is characteristic of any cardiac disease with decreased myocardial reserve and limited capability to increase cardiac output appropriately. In the particular case of congestive heart failure hypoperfusion of large muscle groups during exercise has been demonstrated and would presumably result in the early onset of anaerobic metabolism.[6–8] It is likely that the biochemical consequences of these metabolic changes are associated with the development of neural signals that are interpreted by the patient as fatigue. Recent work, however, has suggested that about 25 percent of patients with congestive heart failure have relatively normal skeletal muscle blood flow yet also exhibit fatigue with exercise.[9] This fatigue correlates with the development of lactate production by the muscle groups. It was concluded that this substantial group of patients exhibits skeletal muscle dysfunction. The implications are as yet unclear but suggest that cardiac rehabilitation programs might be particularly beneficial in this subgroup if these patients could be identified quickly and reliably. Muscle dysfunction might occur through disuse as there is increasing evidence that patients with heart failure decrease their activity markedly and do not usually approach even their limited exercise capacity during daily living.[10]

DYSPNEA

Dyspnea or the feeling of breathlessness occurs when there is higher demand for ventilation than can be met by comfortable breathing. It is frequently described as air hunger or as having to breathe too much or as not being able to breathe enough. Everyone, during vigorous exercise, has experienced the sensation, which is unpleasant but not painful in the usual sense.

It has frequently been assumed that dyspnea referred to a single sensation or symptom. It has become clear that "dyspnea" is used to denote a number of sensations that patients may describe as shortness of breath or breathlessness. Studies in normal volunteers in whom dyspnea was induced by a variety of maneuvers showed that the subjects chose a number of different descriptors from a designated list to characterize their sensations.[11] Cluster analysis revealed the grouping of descriptors indicating the ability to appreciate different sensations of breathlessness. An association was found between certain descriptors and the stimuli inducing dyspnea. These findings were consistent with the interpretation that in normal subjects dyspnea represents a number of different stimuli and thus is not explainable by a single physiological mechanism.

A similar approach has been used to study the sensations associated with breathlessness in patients with a spectrum of diseases causing dyspnea including congestive heart failure, chronic obstructive pulmonary disease, asthma, pulmonary hypertension, chest wall and neuromuscular disease, interstitial lung disease, and pregnancy.[12] Natural groupings of the same descriptors used in normal persons[11] were found in the patients indicating that they could distinguish different sensations of breathlessness. Furthermore, there was an association between descriptor groups and specific dyspnea causing conditions. These data indicate that there are different types of dyspnea in patients with a variety of cardiorespiratory abnormalities and suggest that the symptoms may be mediated by several mechanisms.

Pathophysiological Mechanisms of Dyspnea

There are a number of physiological mechanisms that have been described in both clinical and experimental settings to be associated with increased ventilatory drive. Excessive stimulation of these could be associated with dyspnea.[13] Ventilatory stimuli can result from increased pressures in the right atrium, right ventricle, pulmonary artery, and left atrium. These are sensed by mechanoreceptors. Similarly hypoxia, hypercapnia, and acidosis can result in stimulation of chemoreceptors in the carotid bodies or central nervous system (CNS). Mechanical stimuli have been found to be very important in the control of the ventilatory drive and these mechanisms may be particularly important in many clinical circumstances. The stimuli result from mechanoreceptors in muscle and lung. Psychogenic stimuli from the cerebral cortex may be important in hyperventilation associated with some psychoneuroses.

There has recently been a great deal of interest in the role of mechanoreceptors in the respiratory muscles and diaphragm in eliciting ventilatory drive and thus contributing to dyspnea. Proprioceptive signals from the respiratory muscles and diaphragm resulting from "length-tension inappropriateness" when there is excessive work of breathing contributes to dyspnea.[14–15] The length-tension inappropriateness theory was based on observations during loaded breathing and during breath-holding suggesting an important role for signals from the respiratory muscles. Thus, if at the break point during breath-holding, a rebreathing movement is performed that results in change in length of the respiratory muscles breath-holding time is prolonged and the discomfort is decreased although Pa_{CO_2} continues to increase and Pa_{O_2} falls.[16] The length-tension inappropriateness theory of Campbell and Howell proposed that, normally, there is an appropriate relationship between the displacement in muscle length and the tension developed by respiratory muscles. They suggested that increased respiratory load is detected because the volume displacement is less than that anticipated by muscle proprioceptor fibers. Breath holding then is an extreme example of "length-tension inappropriateness." The ability to prolong breath-holding beyond the break point during the rebreathing maneuver was thought to be attributed to shortening of the respiratory muscles and thus leading to an improved relationship between length and tension. Blocking of respiratory muscle contraction by curare, which would leave afferent nerve responses intact, markedly prolonged the time to discomfort with breath holding. The effect of muscular paralysis induced by D-tubocurarine on the duration and sensation of breath-holding during hypercapnia also has been assessed.[17,18] It was concluded that an important part of the distress from breath-holding and hypercapnia is due to stimuli rising in the respiratory muscles. A number of studies has suggested that the signals may arise from the diaphragm rather than from the intercostal muscles.[14]

It is likely that chemoreceptor drive sensitivity to hypercarbia also contributes to breathlessness.[14] High level quadriplegics totally dependent on mechanical ventilation can detect 10 mmHg increase in inspired CO_2.[19] The relative contributions of respiratory muscles and chemoreceptor stimulus to hypoxic or hypercarbic drive have not been resolved.[14]

Pulmonary receptors contribute to ventilatory drive especially in lung diseases. Upper airway mucosa receptors apparently play little role. On the other hand, receptors in the pulmonary parenchyma that have their afferent fibers traveling through the vagus nerve are important in ventilatory drive.

The role of vascular mechanoreceptors has been central to much of the thinking about control of ventilatory drive especially in congestive heart failure. There is compelling evidence for the existence of receptors in the sites previously mentioned that will stimulate ventilation.[13] Part of the conventional wisdom in clinical practice is that the dyspnea and ventilatory drive in congestive heart failure comes from increased pulmonary capillary wedge pressures. As will be seen below recent data cast doubt on this supposition.

Clinical Manifestations of Dyspnea

Dyspnea occurring during the usual activities of daily life is one of the most common manifestations of cardiac or pulmonary disease. The appreciation of breathlessness is usually dependent on the level of activity involved in

TABLE 20-1

Differential Diagnosis of Acute Dyspnea

Anxiety/hyperventilation
Asthma
Chest trauma
Pneumothorax
Fractured ribs
Pulmonary contusion
Pulmonary edema
Pulmonary embolism
Spontaneous pneumothorax

SOURCE: From Mahler.[20] Reprinted with permission of publisher and author.

a given patient's lifestyle.[20] Sedentary patients may reach an advanced state of cardiorespiratory compromise before experiencing dyspnea. On the other hand an athlete may experience unusual dyspnea with mild dysfunction. Distinguishing cardiac causes of dyspnea—most commonly congestive heart failure—from pulmonary causes, in fact, can sometimes be a major clinical problem. The differential diagnoses for the causes of acute and chronic dyspnea are shown in Tables 20-1 and 20-2.

Approach to the Evaluation of Chronic Dyspnea

History

A detailed history is essential in assessing chronic dyspnea and in attempting to distinguish between potential cardiac or pulmonic causes or to determine that the etiology might be marked deconditioning or even psychogenic. In many ways the approach is similar to that for evaluating chest pain. The frequency, duration, severity, precipitating events, and exercise threshold should be determined. Whether or not the dyspnea is associated with chest pain, exertion, wheezing, cough, anxiety, or sputum production should be established.

Physical Examination

A detailed physical examination should be performed to assess the cardiovascular and respiratory systems as outlined in Chaps. 10 and 11.

Laboratory Evaluation

Laboratory evaluation of chronic dyspnea should be guided by the history and physical examination. A chest x-ray is indicated in most patients and will provide information on heart size, specific chamber enlargement, pulmonary vascularity, and the presence of pulmonary edema, pleural effusion, pneumothorax, chest wall abnormalities, or evidence of pulmonary parenchymal disease. Distinguishing among various potential causes of dyspnea may require pulmonary function measurements and/or exercise testing. The pathophysiology of various disorders causing dyspnea and tests designed to identify them are summarized in Table 20-3.

TABLE 20-2

Differential Diagnosis of Chronic Dyspnea

Cardiovascular
Decreased cardiac output
Cardiomyopathy
Dilated
Hypertrophic
Infiltrative
Ischemic
Valvular disease
Pericardial disease
Congenital disease
Increased pulmonary venous pressure
Diastolic dysfunction
Hypertrophic disease
Ischemia
Mitral stenosis
Pulmonary venous occlusive disease
Right-to-left shunt
Respiratory
Airway disease
Upper airway obstruction
Asthma
Chronic bronchitis
Emphysema
Cystic fibrosis
Parenchymal lung disease
Interstitial lung disease
Malignancy—primary or metastatic
Pneumonia
Pulmonary vascular disease
Arteriovenous malformations
Intravascular obstruction
Vasculitis
Venous occlusive disease
Pleural disease
Effusion
Fibrosis
Malignancy
Chest wall disease
Deformities (e.g., kyphoscoliosis)
Abdominal "loading" (e.g., ascites, pregnancy, obesity)
Respiratory muscle disease
Neuromuscular disorders (e.g., myasthenia gravis, polio)
Phrenic nerve dysfunction
Weakness
Anemia
Anxiety/Psychological
Deconditioning

SOURCE: Modified from Mahler.[20] Reprinted with permission of publisher and author.

DYSPNEA IN CHRONIC CONGESTIVE HEART FAILURE

Although fatigue is the most common symptom in congestive heart failure, dyspnea occurs during daily living.

TABLE 20-3

Causes of Dyspnea, Pathophysiology, and Discriminating Clinical Measurements

Disorder	Pathophysiology	Discriminating Measurements
Anemia	O_2 carrying capacity	HB, ↓ $\dot{V}_{O_{2max}}$; ↓ AT
Cardiac		
Coronary artery	Ischemia	ECG changes; BP changes: $\dot{V}_{O_{2max}}$; ↓ AT; ↓ O_2-pulse
Valvular	Limited cardiac output	
Myopathy	Limited cardiac output	
Deconditioning	Detraining	↓ $\dot{V}_{O_{2max}}$; ↓ AT; ↓ O_2-pulse
Malingering	Hyper- and hypoventilation	Breathing pattern; Pa_{CO_2}
Obesity	↑ work to move body weight; if severe, respiratory restriction	↑ $\dot{V}_{O_2}$—work relationship; ↓ $\dot{V}_{O_{2max}}$
Pulmonary		
Airway obstruction	Diminished ventilatory capacity V/Q mismatching	↑ $\dot{V}_{Emax}$/MVV; expiratory flow limitation;
Interstitial disease	V/Q mismatching Diffusion impairment during exercise	↑ V_D/V_T; O_2 desaturation; ↓ $\dot{V}_{O_{2max}}$ ↑ O_2 desaturation during exercise; ↓ V_T and respiratory frequency; ↓ $\dot{V}_{O_{2max}}$
Pulmonary vascular	Physiological V_D	↑ V_D/V_T; O_2 desaturation during exercise ↑ $\dot{V}_E/\dot{V}_{O_2}$, ↓ $\dot{V}_{O_{2max}}$
Psychogenic	Hyperventilation with regular respiratory rate	Breathing pattern; Pa_{CO_2}

NOTE: Hb = hemoglobin value; $\dot{V}_{O_{2max}}$ = maximal oxygen consumption; AT = anaerobic threshold; ECG = electrocardiogram; BP = blood pressure; Pa_{CO_2} = arterial carbon dioxide tension; $\dot{V}_{Emax}$ = maximal exercise ventilation; MVV = maximal voluntary ventilation; V_D = dead space volume; V_T = tidal volume.
SOURCE: Adapted from Wasserman K, Whipp BJ: Exercise physiology in health and disease. *Am Rev Respir Dis* 1975; 112:219–249, with permission.

Dyspnea may occur with both isotonic and isometric exercise and extensive aerobic exercise is not necessary for it to be induced. As noted, the traditional view has been that increased pulmonary capillary wedge pressure was an important contributor to dyspnea in congestive heart failure. While this is probably true to some significant extent in acute pulmonary edema, recent work has failed to substantiate this view in the case of chronic ambulatory heart failure.[21,22] In fact, poor correlation exists between pulmonary capillary wedge pressure and the feeling of dyspnea (Fig. 20-1). Similarly, there is no evidence of sufficient changes in arterial blood gases

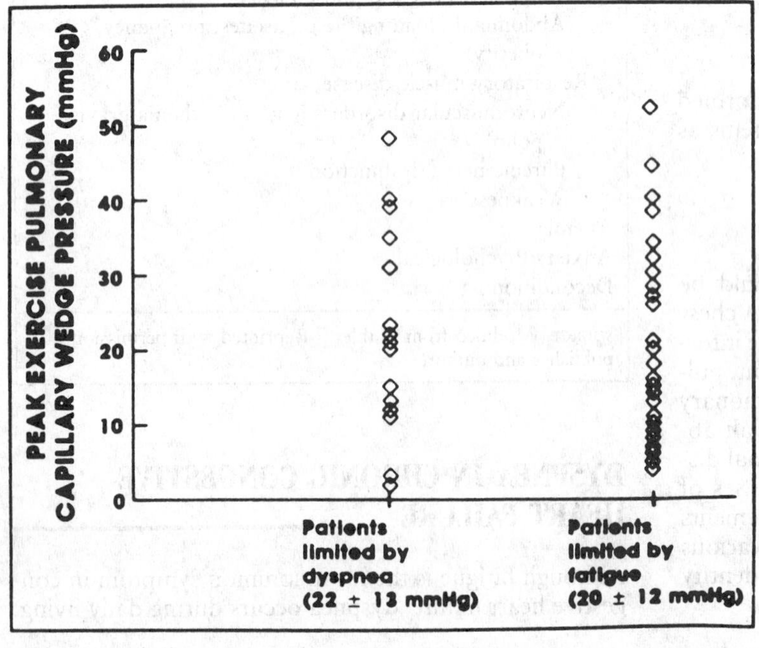

FIGURE 20-1 Peak exercise pulmonary capillary wedge pressure in patients limited to dyspnea versus those limited by fatigue. (From Sullivan et al.[21] Reprinted with permission of publisher, editor, and author.)

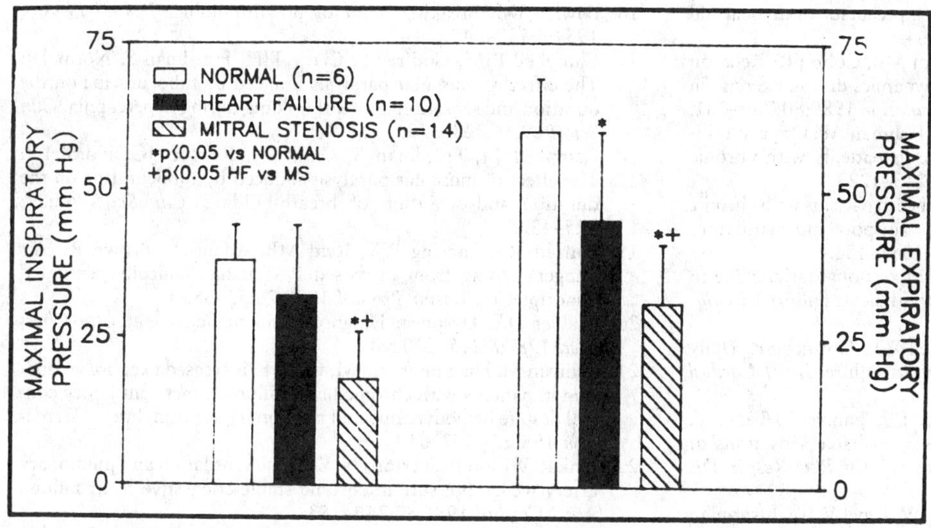

FIGURE 20-2 Maximal inspiratory and expiratory pressures in normal, heart failure, and mitral stenosis subjects. (From Mancine et al.[1] Reprinted with permission of publisher, editor, and author.)

during exercise in patients with heart failure to account for dyspnea by stimulation of arterial chemoreceptors.[21] Recent evidence suggests that ventilatory abnormalities may be centrally important in contributing to ventilatory drive in chronic congestive heart failure.[21] Although ventilatory control mechanisms regulated by, for example, CO_2 are normal in patients with congestive heart failure, there are demonstrable abnormalities in pulmonary mechanics. The most striking change was an increase in physiological dead space, which most likely was due to ventilation-perfusion abnormalities associated with decreased perfusion and dynamic ventilation-perfusion mismatch.[23] This change alone would require excessive ventilation during exercise to maintain normal blood gas values. In addition, congestive heart failure is associated with restrictive pulmonary changes and diffusion defects.[24] Obstructive defects are less common in chronic heart failure than in acute heart failure. Recent work has suggested that respiratory muscles may be a major source of the stimulus for breathlessness in chronic congestive heart failure.[1] There was evidence of respiratory muscle weakness (Fig. 20-2) and of correlation between maximal inspiratory and expiratory pressure with feelings of dyspnea. Furthermore, near-infrared spectroscopy has been used to demonstrate progressive respiratory muscle deoxygenation during exercise in patients with chronic congestive heart failure.[25] This deoxygenation probably results from the increased work of breathing in combination with hypoperfusion due to inadequate cardiac output. The feeling of dyspnea likely results from neural impulses generated in atrophic, underperfused and metabolically abnormal respiratory muscles.[1]

Special Types of Dyspnea in Congestive Heart Failure

Orthopnea

This term refers to the dyspnea that occurs in the supine but not in the upright position. It is characteristic of heart failure although it may occur in patients with lung disease or with weakness or paralysis of the diaphragm. In heart failure it is thought to result from the shift of blood volume from the periphery to the pulmonary circulation. Since pulmonary venous pressures are already elevated, mild pulmonary edema may develop and pulmonary mechanoreceptors are thought to be stimulated.

Paroxysmal Nocturnal Dyspnea

This symptom complex in a patient with congestive heart failure manifests as a sudden awakening from sleep with marked dyspnea that may take 5 to 15 min to clear after assuming the upright posture. The mechanisms are thought to be similar to those for orthopnea. Paroxysmal nocturnal dyspnea, like orthopnea, can occur in heart diseases of diverse etiologies ranging from dilated cardiomyopathy to valvular and coronary artery disease.

DYSPNEA IN OTHER CARDIOVASCULAR DISEASES

The mechanism of dyspnea in cardiovascular diseases other than congestive heart failure has not been studied extensively. It is likely that the mechanisms defined for chronic congestive heart failure also apply to the conditions listed in Table 20-2 that are characterized by limited abilities to increase cardiac output in response to exercise.

REFERENCES

1. Mancini DM, LaManca J, Henson D: The relation of respiratory muscle function to dyspnea in patients with heart failure. *Heart Failure* 1992;8:183–189.
2. Kuller LH: Prodromata of sudden death and myocardial infarction. *Adv Cardiol* 1978;25:61–72.
3. Rissanen V, Romo M, Siltanen P: Premonitory symptoms and stress factors preceding sudden death from ischaemic heart disease. *Acta Med Scand* 1978;204:389–396.
4. Alonzo AA, Simon AB, Feinleib M: Prodromata of myocardial infarction and sudden death. *Circulation* 1975;52:1056–1062.

5. Appels A, Mulder P: Excess fatigue as a precursor of myocardial infarction. *Eur Heart J* 1988;9:758–764.
6. Sullivan MJ, Knight JD, Higgenbotham MB, Cobb FR: Relation between central and peripheral hemodynamics during exercise in patients with chronic heart failure. *Circulation* 1989;80:769–781.
7. Weber KT, Kinasewitz GT, Janicki JS, Fishman AP: Oxygen utilization and ventilation during exercise in patients with chronic cardiac failure. *Circulation* 1982;65:1213–1223.
8. Wilson JR, Ferraro N: Exercise intolerance in patients with chronic left heart failure: Relation to oxygen transport and ventilatory abnormalities. *Am J Cardiol* 1983;51:1358–1363.
9. Wilson JR, Mancini D, Dunkman WB: Exertional fatigue due to skeletal muscle dysfunction in patients with heart failure. *Circulation* 1993;87:470–475.
10. Oka RK, Stotts NA, Dae MW, Haskell WL, Gortner SR: Daily physical activity levels in congestive heart failure. *Am J Cardiol* 1993;71:921–925.
11. Simon PM, Schwartzstein RM, Weiss JW, Lahive K, Fencl V, Techtsoonian M, Weinberger SE: Distinguishable sensations of breathless induced in normal volunteers. *Am Rev Respir Dis* 1989;140:1021–1027.
12. Simon PM, Schwartzstein RM, Weiss JW, Fencl V, Teghtsoonian M, Weinberger SE: Distinguishable types of dyspnea in patients with shortness of breath. *Am Rev Respir Dis* 1990;142:1009–1014.
13. Wasserman K, Casaburi R: Dyspnea: Physiological and pathological mechanisms. *Annu Rev Med* 1988;39:503–515.
14. Tobin MJ: Dyspnea: Pathophysiologic basis, clinical presentation and management. *Arch Int Med* 1990;150:1604–1613.
15. Campbell EJM, Howell JBL: The sensation of breathlessness. *Br Med Bull* 1963;18:36–40.
16. Fowler WS: Breaking point of breath-holding. *J Appl Physiol* 1954;6:539–545.
17. Campbell EJM, Godfrey S, Clark TJH, Freedman S, Normal J: The effect of muscular paralysis induced by tubocurarine on the duration and sensation of breathholding during hypercapnia. *Clin Sci* 1969;36:323–328.
18. Campbell EJ, Freedman S, Clark TJ, Robson JG, Normal J: The effect of muscular paralysis induced by tubocurarine on the duration and sensation of breath-holding. *Clin Sci* 1967;32:425–432.
19. Banzett RB, Lansing RW, Reid MB, Adams L, Brown R: 'Air hunger' arising from increased P_{CO_2} in mechanically ventilated quadriplegics. *Respir Physiol* 1989;76:53–68.
20. Mahler DA: Dyspnea: Diagnosis and management. *Clin Chest Med* 1987;8:215–230.
21. Sullivan M, Higginbotham M, Cobb F: Increased exercise ventilation in patients with chronic heart failure: Intact ventilatory control despite hemodynamic and pulmonary abnormalities. *Circulation* 1988;77:552–559.
22. Fink L, Wilson JR, Ferraro N: Exercise ventilation and pulmonary artery wedge pressure in chronic stable congestive heart failure. *Am J Cardiol* 1986;57:249–253.
23. Sullivan MJ: Exertional dyspnea and ventilatory control mechanisms in chronic heart failure. *Heart Failure* 1992;8:190–201.
24. Wright RS, Levine MS, Bellamy PE, Simmons MS, Batra P, Stevenson LW, et al: Ventilatory and diffusion abnormalities in potential heart transplant recipients. *Chest* 1990;98:816–820.
25. Mancini D, Ferraro N, Nazarro D, Chance B, Wilson JR: Respiratory muscle deoxygenation during exercise in patients with heart failure demonstrated with near-infrared spectroscopy. *J Am Coll Cardiol* 1991;18:492–498.

Chapter 21

Syncope, Presyncope, Palpitations, and Sudden Death

Bernardo Stein, M.D. ■ *Robert Roberts, M.D.*

INTRODUCTION

Physicians are frequently asked to evaluate patients with palpitations, "irregular" heart beating, dizziness, weakness, light-headedness, or frank syncope with disturbance of consciousness. The main tasks of the physician are to understand the nature of the event, establish the etiology, and either reassure the patient regarding the benign nature of the disorder or recommend further work-up and treatment. More specifically, the clinician must attempt to separate benign episodes (i.e., isolated ectopic beats in patients with no organic heart disease) from potentially life-threatening events (i.e., ventricular tachycardia in patients with myocardial dysfunction). It is the purpose of this chapter to review briefly the clinical approach to patients with palpitations, near syncope, syncope, and sudden cardiac death. A more detailed discussion on the subject can be found in Chaps. 50, 51, and 52.

Palpitations

Palpitation is a common symptom defined as an unpleasant awareness of the heartbeat. (See also Chap. 9B.) It may be caused by a variety of abnormalities of the cardiac rhythm: ectopic beats, compensatory pauses, atrial or ventricular tachycardia, hyperkinetic states, increased stroke volume, or sudden onset of bradycardia or heart block. Patients are commonly more aware of the postextrasystolic beat, which is associated with an increased stroke volume, than of the premature beat. Palpitations of abrupt onset and termination are usually due to paroxysmal supraventricular tachycardia, atrial flutter, or fibrillation, whereas slow onset and cessation may represent sinus tachycardia. Rapid, irregular, and chaotic heart beating suggests atrial fibrillation or multifocal atrial tachycardia. The pulse rate and regularity during the palpitation may offer some clues: 100 to 140 beats per minute suggests sinus tachycardia; 150 beats per minute suggests atrial flutter; more than 160 beats per minute suggests paroxysmal supraventricular tachycardia. An episode that is aborted by performing the Valsalva maneuver is compatible with supraventricular reentrant tachycardia.

An essential feature in the evaluation is to establish the presence or absence of organic heart disease. Palpitations in young, healthy individuals are rarely clinically significant, whereas those occurring in patients with heart disease may represent ventricular tachycardia, and thus directly influence prognosis.

The physical examination, chest x-ray, and, in selected cases, the echocardiogram, are helpful in detecting the presence of structural heart disease. The 12-lead electrocardiogram (ECG) may be entirely normal or disclose the presence of previous myocardial infarction, left ventricular hypertrophy, or conduction abnormalities. (See Chaps. 13, 35, and 36.) If the symptoms are isolated, mild, and there is no evidence of underlying heart disease, further work-up is generally unnecessary, and the patient should be reassured. In patients with heart disease or associated symptoms (dyspnea, chest pain, dizziness), further work up is usually indicated. Commonly used noninvasive tests include an ambulatory electrocardiographic recording, a self-activated event recorder, or transmission of the ECG signal transtelephonically to the clinic or the physician's office. (See Chap. 45.)

The need for additional tests depends on the nature of the suspected or proved organic heart disease. Echocardiography (Chap. 15) is an excellent tool for the detection and evaluation of valvular and myocardial disease. Radionuclide (Chap. 134) or angiographic ventriculograms (Chap. 138) provide information regarding global and regional myocardial function. Stress testing (Chap. 16) and/or coronary angiography (Chap. 138) are useful in the detection and evaluation of the severity of coronary stenoses in patients suspected of having ischemic heart disease. Electrophysiologic studies employing programmed cardiac stimulation (Chap. 46) are extremely informative. These are invasive and expensive procedures, however, and should be used selectively in patients with suspected ventricular tachyarrhythmias or severe conduction abnormalities.

Near Syncope and Syncope

Syncope refers to a sudden transient loss of consciousness, generally accompanied by inability to maintain postural tone (Chap. 50). Near syncope (or presyncope) is characterized by a transient episode of weakness, lightheadedness, faintness, awareness of surroundings but inability to interact, but does not result in complete loss of consciousness. Syncope is a fairly common disorder, accounting for about 1 percent of hospital admissions and 3 percent of emergency room visits. The pathophysiological mechanism is a transient reduction in cerebral blood flow and oxygenation.

Whereas syncope may represent a benign disorder with good prognosis in some patients, it may be a manifestation of a serious underlying cardiac or neurologic abnormality in others. Therefore, the physician should appropriately evaluate every patient presenting with syncope. The causes of syncope are multiple and depend, in part, on whether the population studied is derived predominantly from the intensive care and cardiology in-service departments, or from the emergency room and outpatient clinics. In general, cardiac disorders account for syncope in approximately 20 percent of cases (Table 21–1).[1,2,3,4,5] Vasodepressor syncope accounts for 30 percent of syncopal episodes and is the most common, identified cause of fainting. Other etiologies include neurologic disorders such as seizures, orthostatic hypotension, drugs and alcohol, metabolic, carotid sinus hypersensitivity, and psychogenic (Table 21–2). After initial workup, the cause of syncope remains unexplained in about one-third of patients. One study[6] suggests that electrophysiological studies and head-up tilt testing may identify the underlying cause of syncope in up to 74 percent of patients referred for unexplained syncope. (See Chap. 50.)

The history (Chap. 9B) remains the cornerstone of the evaluation of patients with syncope. Similar to the evaluation of patients with seizures, information from witnesses, when available, is invaluable. Because of the many causes of syncope (Tables 50-1, 50-2, and 50-4), the interviewer should attempt to obtain information regarding the course and duration of syncope, the position of the patient before fainting, the presence of premonitory symptoms, the presence of precipitating events or activities (fear, pain, head turning, swallowing, coughing, urinating, defecating, prolonged standing, etc.), associated signs during syncope (seizure activity, pallor, sweating), and the status during the recovery period. Information regarding the intake of medications, and drug and alcohol ingestion is essential. A social, psychological, and family history may also be valuable.

As noted, the most common type of syncope is the vasodepressor syncope. It is commonly precipitated by the sight of blood, pain, anxiety, fatigue, hunger, or a specific environmental setting such as being in a warm and crowded room. Premonitory symptoms include pallor, diaphoresis, nausea, and visual blurring. Loss of consciousness and postural tone follows rapidly, but consciousness is quickly restored in the recumbent position. Postsyncopal findings include persistent pallor, nausea, weakness, and diaphoresis. The main pathogenic mechanism is a profound reduction in total peripheral vascular resistance, unaccompanied by an increase in cardiac output. (See Chap. 50.)

TABLE 21-1
Major Causes of Cardiac Syncope

- Disturbances in cardiac rhythm
  - Sick sinus syndrome
  - AV block
    - AV node disease
    - His-Purkinje disease
  - Paroxysmal supraventricular arrhythmias
    - Atrial fibrillation
    - Atrial flutter
    - Atrial tachycardia
    - Preexcitation syndromes or enhanced AV nodal conduction
  - Ventricular tachyarrhythmias
    - Ventricular tachycardia
    - Paroxysmal ventricular fibrillation
    - Long QT syndrome (congenital or acquired)
  - Pacemaker-induced
    - Pacemaker malfunction
    - Pacemaker syndrome
    - Pacemaker-mediated tachycardia
- Obstruction to cardiac output
  - Right heart
    - Pulmonic stenosis
    - Pulmonary embolism
    - Pulmonary hypertension (primary or secondary)
    - Tetralogy of Fallot
    - Cardiac tamponade
  - Left heart
    - Aortic stenosis
    - Mitral stenosis
    - Hypertrophic obstructive cardiomyopathy
    - Left atrial myxoma
- Neurocardiogenic syncope (activation of ventricular mechanoreceptors)

NOTE: AV = atrioventricular.

TABLE 21-2

Causes of Syncope Not Associated with Cardiac Disease

Causes
Vasodepressor syncope
Orthostatic hypotension
Volume depletion
Autonomic dysfunction
Drug-induced
Carotid sinus syncope
Cardioinhibitory type
Vasodepressor type
Cerebrovascular disease
Situational
Micturition syncope
Defecation syncope
Cough syncope
Swallow syncope
Neuralgias
Glossopharyngeal
Trigeminal
Metabolic
Hypoglycemia
Hypoadrenalism
Other causes
Seizure disorders
Migraine attacks
Psychogenic
Syncope of unknown etiology

A fainting episode preceeded by light-headedness, weakness, palpitations, nausea, or diaphoresis, that occurs in the upright position and is followed by a prompt recovery without confusion suggests a cardiac arrhythmia. Exertional syncope is characteristic of patients with right or left ventricular outflow obstruction, as seen in aortic and pulmonic stenosis, hypertrophic cardiomyopathy, and severe pulmonary hypertension. Occasionally, syncope is associated with focal motor activity; less often, it can cause generalized seizure activity.

A clear distinction between syncope and a seizure disorder may occasionally be difficult. Seizures commonly occur abruptly without warning, or are preceded by a characteristic aura. An epileptic seizure can occur with the patients supine or recumbent, and follows a consistent pattern of motor or autonomic activity. It also runs an identical course each time. In contrast, the course of syncope is variable and may be aborted if the patient assumes the recumbent position. During the seizure, an apneic phase is followed by labored breathing, whereas in syncope, breathing is fast and shallow. Convulsive movements, tongue biting, loss of bladder and bowel function, and postictal confusion, sleepiness, and amnesia are characteristic of a seizure. Cardiac syncope that results in cerebral hypoxia may also be associated with seizure activity, convulsions, and loss of sphincter control.

Important aspects of the physical examination include an accurate measurement of the blood pressure and pulse in the supine, sitting, and standing positions. Often, it is useful to monitor the blood pressure while the patient stands for several minutes. A drop in the systolic pressure of 20 mmHg or more may be significant, particularly in the elderly and in those with cerebrovascular disease. Examination may reveal evidence of trauma. Particularly important aspects of the examination include the presence of murmurs suggestive of aortic, mitral, or pulmonic stenosis; third heart sound and apical enlargement or displacement suggestive of left ventricular dysfunction; and accentuated pulmonic component of the second heart sound and right ventricular heave suggestive of pulmonary hypertension. Carotid arterial bruits support the diagnosis of cerebrovascular disease. A complete neurologic examination is essential. When carotid sinus syncope is suspected, manual stimulation of the carotid sinuses under electrocardiographic and blood pressure monitoring should be part of the initial evaluation, provided that no significant carotid disease is present. (See Chap. 50.)

Laboratory tests are usually not helpful in discerning the cause of syncope. Occasionally, a low hematocrit is found in a patient with unsuspected gastrointestinal bleeding who presents with orthostatic syncope. Severe hypoglycemia may occur either in diabetic patients treated with oral hypoglycemic agents or insulin, or in those with insulinoma. Hyperkalemia may be the diagnostic clue in the rare patient with adrenocortical insufficiency.

The 12-lead ECG (Chap. 13) and rhythm strip are essential in every patient with syncope. The presence of severe sinus bradycardia, slow junctional rhythm, bifascicular or trifascicular block, or high grade atrioventricular block suggest that a bradyarrhythmia is perhaps the cause of syncope. In many patients with organic heart disease and conduction abnormalities, however, the etiology of syncope is not a bradyarrhythmia but ventricular tachycardia. Other helpful findings in the ECG are the presence of supraventricular arrhythmias in conjunction with preexcitation syndromes, repetitive ventricular ectopy, Q waves or ST segment shifts suggestive of ischemic heart disease, a prominent U wave from hypokalemia, or a long QT interval that may predispose to polymorphic ventricular tachycardia.

The chest x-ray is commonly entirely normal but may be abnormal in the presence of valvular heart disease or heart failure (Chap. 14). An echocardiogram is beneficial in patients with suspected right or left ventricular outflow obstruction, such as pulmonic or aortic valve stenosis or hypertrophic obstructive cardiomyopathy (Chap. 15). An assessment of left ventricular regional and global function is important when ventricular tachycardia is being considered as the cause of syncope. Echocardiography is also helpful in the rare patients in whom an intracavitary mass (i.e., atrial myxoma) is suspected. In addition, right ventricular overload, pulmonic insufficiency, or abnormal pulmonic valve motion may point toward the presence of pulmonary hypertension.

The appropriate work-up of patients with syncope is clearly dependent on the suspected etiology. Exercise testing (Chap. 16) may be useful in patients with coronary disease and in those suspected of having exercise-induced arrhythmias. Cardiac catheterization (Chap. 138) may be indicated in patients in whom myocardial ischemia is suspected to cause ventricular arrhythmias and syncope. Electroencephalography and computed tomography of the head should be reserved to patients suspected of having a seizure disorder or in whom the exam discloses a focal neurologic deficit. (See also Chap. 122.)

Most patients in whom an arrhythmic cause of syncope is suspected should be admitted to the hospital. Continuous ECG monitoring, which is the most widely used test for suspected arrhythmic syncope, may yield important information regarding the presence of brady- or tachyarrhythmias. However, a diagnosis of certainty is only reached when syncope occurs during the period of monitoring. This may be particularly difficult in patients with infrequent episodes. The sensitivity of 24-h ambulatory ECG monitoring to detect a clinically significant arrhythmia is about 50 to 60 percent in patients suspected of having an arrhythmic syncope, but less than 20 percent in unselected patients with a history of syncope. In cases of infrequent, non-life-threatening arrhythmias, patient-activated transtelephonic ECG recording may be very useful. In certain patients, this may be the only way of establishing a temporal relationship between the patient's symptoms and an arrhythmic event. (See Chap. 45.)

Another noninvasive tool for the evaluation of patients with syncope is the signal-averaged ECG (Chap. 47).[7] In patients with ischemic heart disease, the presence of high-frequency, low-amplitude signals in the terminal portion of the ECG (late potentials) suggests that a substrate for reentrant ventricular arrhythmias exists, whereas the absence of late potentials identifies patients with a low incidence of inducible ventricular tachycardia. Some centers use the signal-averaged ECG as a screening test for ventricular tachycardia in selecting patients for electrophysiological studies. The precise role and value of this test in patients with or without coronary disease is being defined and validated.

When the suspicion for an arrhythmic cause of syncope remains high despite a negative noninvasive evaluation, invasive electrophysiological studies (Chap. 46) are recommended. In the presence of organic heart disease, the yield of electrophysiological testing may be as high as 75 percent, whereas in patients with structurally normal hearts, the yield is significantly lower (less than 20 percent).[8] Therefore, invasive electrophysiological evaluation is recommended in patients with organic heart disease and syncope thought to be secondary to arrhythmias in whom noninvasive evaluation has been negative. It should be kept in mind that identification of abnormalities during electrophysiological testing does not mean they are the cause of syncope; clinical correlation is always necessary.

Another test that may be useful in the evaluation of syncope of unknown origin is the head-up tilt test.[6,9] (See Chap. 50.) This test is particularly useful in patients with recurrent syncope and no underlying organic heart disease. An abnormal response consists of the development of bradycardia, peripheral vasodilatation, arterial hypotension, and syncope occurring during the upright position. This paradoxical response has been termed "neurocardiogenic syncope" and is thought to be due to activation of ventricular mechanoreceptors leading to increased efferent vagal outflow and withdrawal of sympathetic tone. In susceptible individuals, bradycardia and hypotension during head-up tilt can be provoked by an infusion of isoproterenol.[10] In selected patients, tilt testing has an adequate sensitivity (70 percent) and specificity (80 percent).

Sudden Cardiac Death

It is commonly defined as unexpected cardiac death without preceding symptoms or with symptoms of less than 1 h in duration. The majority of episodes occur outside the hospital or physician's office. Four out of five patients who die suddenly have underlying coronary disease, and thus it is predominantly a disease of males. In one-fourth of patients, sudden death may be the first manifestation of heart disease. (See Chap. 51.)

The few available reports of the rhythm disturbance at the onset of sudden cardiac arrest have commonly shown the presence of ventricular fibrillation, often preceded by a short run of ventricular tachycardia. Only rarely have asystole or profound bradycardia been recorded. Sudden onset of electromechanical dissociation can occur in patients with myocardial ischemia. Pathological studies[11,12] have shown the presence of coronary thrombi overlying ruptured atherosclerotic plaques, and intramyocardial platelet aggregates resulting presumably from distal embolization of platelet thrombi in a substantial number of victims of ischemic sudden death. (See Chap. 55.)

An essential component of the evaluation of patients who survive an episode of cardiac arrest consists of identifying the underlying cardiac disorder as well as the precipitating arrhythmia since the rate of recurrence can be as high as 30 percent in the first year. In the absence of structural heart disease or conduction abnormalities, sudden death is very uncommon.

Patients who survive an episode of sudden death should be placed on continuous ECG monitoring in an intensive care setting. This may disclose the presence of repetitive ventricular ectopy, sustained or nonsustained ventricular arrhythmias, or severe bradycardia or conduction abnormalities. Acute myocardial infarction must be excluded; metabolic abnormalities that may predispose to arrhythmias, and which require immediate correction include hypokalemia, hypomagnesemia, and acidosis. Identification and withdrawal of medications with proarrhythmic potential, particularly antiarrhythmic drugs or digitalis, is important.

As mentioned above, 75 percent of sudden cardiac deaths are due to coronary atherosclerotic disease. Therefore, coronary angiography and left ventriculography (Chap. 138) are usually recommended. Other less common causes of sudden death unrelated to coronary disease include cardiomyopathies [dilated (Chap. 89) or hypertrophic (Chap. 90)], valvular disease [aortic stenosis (Chap. 79), mitral valve prolapse (Chap. 80)], or primary electrical abnormalities [atrioventricular block, congenital or acquired long QT syndrome, and ventricular preexcitation (Chaps. 13, 35, 36)]. Echocardiography (Chaps. 15 and 130) is very useful in the evaluation of patients with myocardial or valvular disorders.

The approach to the patient with sudden cardiac arrest should be individualized. A thorough cardiac evaluation should be directed to the identification and management of factors such as ischemia, heart failure, valvular disease, and primary electrical abnormalities. Most victims should have complete electrophysiological studies (Chap. 46). In about three-fourths of patients, a ventricular tachyarrhythmia can be induced by programmed electrical stimulation.[13] Suppression of inducible ventricular tachycardia with drugs or surgery portends a good prognosis. In contrast, patients in whom a ventricular arrhythmia is still inducible despite therapy have a recurrence rate as high as 40 percent. The increased utilization of various surgical (Chap. 44) and catheter ablative (Chap. 43) techniques for arrhythmias, and the advent of implantable defibrillators (Chap. 42) have made electrophysiological studies invaluable in the management of patients with sudden death (Chap. 51).

REFERENCES

1. Silverstein MD, Singer DE, Mulley A, Thibault GE, Barnett GO: Patients with syncope admitted to medical intensive care units. *JAMA* 1982; 248:1185–1189.
2. Day SC, Cook FF, Funkenstein H, Goldman L: Evaluation and outcome of emergency room patients with transient loss of consciousness. *Am J Med* 1982; 73:15–23.
3. Kapoor W, Karpf M, Wieand S, Peterson J, Levey G: A prospective evaluation and follow-up of patients with syncope. *N Engl J Med* 1983; 309:197–204.
4. Martin GJ, Adams SL, Martin HG, Mathews J, Zull D, Scanlon PJ: Prospective evaluation of syncope. *Ann Emerg Med* 1984; 13: 499–504.
5. Eagle KA, Black HR, Cook EF, Goldman L: Evaluation of prognostic classifications for patients with syncope. *Am J Med* 1985; 79:455–460.
6. Sra JS, Anderson AJ, Sheikh SH, Avitall B, Tchou PJ, Troup PJ, et al: Unexplained syncope evaluated by electrophysiologic studies and head-up tilt testing. *Ann Intern Med* 1991; 114:1013–1019.
7. Winters SL, Stewart D, Gomes JA: Signal averaging of the surface QRS complex predicts inducibility of ventricular tachycardia in patients with syncope of unknown origin: a prospective study. *J Am Coll Cardiol* 1987; 10:775–781.
8. Krol RB, Morady F, Flaker GC, DiCarlo LA, Baerman JM, Hewett J, et al: Electrophysiologic testing in patients with unexplained syncope: clinical and noninvasive predictors of outcome. *J Am Coll Cardiol* 1987; 10:358–363.
9. Grubb BP, Temesy-Armos P, Hahn H, Elliott L: Utility of upright tilt-table testing in the evaluation and management of syncope of unknown origin. *Am J Med* 1991; 90:6–10.
10. Almquist A, Goldenberg IF, Milstein S, Chen M-Y, Chen X, Hansen R, et al: Provocation of bradycardia and hypotension by isoproterenol and upright posture in patients with unexplained syncope. *N Engl J Med* 1989; 320:346–351.
11. Davies MJ, Thomas A: Thrombosis and acute coronary lesions in sudden cardiac ischemic death. *N Engl J Med* 1984; 310:1137–1140.
12. Davies MJ, Thomas AC, Knapman PA, Hangartner JR: Intramyocardial platelet aggregation in patients with unstable angina suffering sudden ischemic cardiac death. *Circulation* 1986; 73:418–427.
13. Wilber DJ, Garan H, Finkelstein D, Kelly E, Newell J, McGovern B, et al: Out-of-hospital cardiac arrest. Use of electrophysiologic testing in the prediction of a long-term outcome. *N Engl J Med* 1988; 318:19–24.

Chapter 22

Miscellaneous Cardiovascular Symptoms and Signs

Robert C. Schlant, M.D. ■ Edmund H. Sonnenblick, M.D.

This chapter and Chaps. 19 to 21 review selected common cardiovascular symptoms and signs. More extensive discussions are given in referenced chapters.

Cerebral vascular attacks or episodes refer to changes in cerebral function caused by an alteration in cerebral perfusion to a portion or all of the brain. Transient ischemic attack (TIA) refers to an abrupt onset of an episode of motor or sensory deficit that lasts longer than a few minutes but less than 24 h before complete recovery. Disability that persists more than 24 h but that resolves within 3 weeks is referred to as a *reversible ischemic neurologic disability* (RIND). (See Chap. 122.)

The alteration in cerebral perfusion in a TIA may be caused by an occlusion produced by a thrombus, an embolus, arterial dissection, vasospasm, or an acute decrease in perfusion pressure. In some patients, secondary cerebral hemorrhage may occur subsequent to initial obstruction of the vessel with focal infarction and may be detected by computerized tomographic (CT) imaging of the brain. Potential cardiovascular sources of cerebral emboli include thrombi from pulmonary venoocclusive disease; left atrial thrombi (especially in patients with atrial fibrillation or mitral valve disease); left atrial myxoma (Chap. 111); mitral valve prolapse (Chap. 80); mitral annular calcification (Chap. 122); left ventricular thrombi (especially in patients with prior myocardial infarction); nonbacterial thrombotic (marantic) endocarditis; mitral or aortic valve vegetations in patients with bacterial endocarditis (Chap. 94); calcific aortic stenosis (Chap. 79); prosthetic heart valves (Chap. 83); and atherosclerotic debris, cholesterol emboli, or small thrombi from atherosclerosis involving the ascending aorta, subclavian artery, carotid arteries or intracranial branches of the carotid arteries (Chaps. 122 to 124). Fat emboli from fractures of large bones may pass through the lungs and reach the brain (see Chap. 100). Paradoxic emboli may originate in systemic veins or the right atrium and pass to the systemic and cerebral circulation in patients with either a congenital heart defect with a right-to-left shunt such as Tetralogy of Fallot (see also Chap. 97) or a probe-patent foramen ovale that becomes transiently open due to an increase in right atrial pressure and volume. The latter may occur more frequently than is generally recognized. Patients with very high hematocrits, usually over 65 percent, or with a hypercoagulable state such as the antiphospholipid antibody syndrome (Chap. 103) may sustain a cerebral thrombus in either an arterial or a venous cerebral vessel.

In some patients, cerebral vascular perfusion pressure may be acutely decreased and produce syncope (Chap. 50) or, less often, focal or generalized seizure activity. This hypoperfusion may be related to a cardiac arrhythmia (Chap. 36), an acute decrease in cardiac output, severe heart failure or cardiogenic shock (Chap. 49), hypovolemia from any cause or excess systemic vasodilatation (Chaps. 21 and 50). Such episodes may be seen more commonly in patients with moderate obstructions in their internal carotid arteries that only become flow-limited during modest hypotension. Aortic dissection (Chap. 123) can involve the subclavian or carotid arteries and produce cerebral symptoms (Chap. 122).

Systemic arterial hypertension can cause rupture of

both congenital arterial microaneurysms in the cerebral circulation and apparently normal small vessels in the brain or meninges (Chap. 122). During cardiac catheterization (Chap. 138) air or thrombi can cause cerebral vascular accidents. Air embolization is a particular hazard of open heart surgery.

HEADACHE

Severe headache may be a prodrome to a subarachnoid hemorrhage, in which case the headache may be caused by an initial very slight bleed (Chap. 122). Patients with systemic arterial hypertension (SAH) may present with headache, although in a patient with moderate hypertension, there is a poor correlation between the level of blood pressure and the patient's perception of headache. On the other hand, headache is the most frequent presenting symptom of patients with severe or "malignant" hypertension. (See also Chaps. 76 and 77). Classically, the headache in patients with SAH is occipital or frontal in location although more often it is generalized.

EPISTAXIS

Epistaxis occasionally occurs in patients with SAH, particularly if the blood pressure is markedly increased, usually with a systolic pressure over 220 mmHg and/or a diastolic pressure more than 120 mmHg. More commonly, epistaxis is related to mechanical trauma, particularly in association with low humidity. Epistaxis, at times severe, used to be a more frequent and severe symptom of acute rheumatic fever (Chap. 78). Other causes of epistaxis include aplastic anemia, polycythemia vera, von Willebrand's disease, macroglobulinemia, and hereditary hemorrhagic telangiectasia.

EMBOLIC PHENOMENA

Arterial embolic phenomena may occur to any downstream organ from any of the sources noted above in the discussion of cerebral vascular attacks. Both the aorta and any artery can be the source of downstream embolic atherosclerotic debris, cholesterol, and thrombotic material. Most systemic emboli are probably either not recognized clinically or cause only momentary discomfort and are therefore ignored by the patient. This is commonly due to lysis of the embolus with reperfusion of the circulation involved.

Some of the more frequently recognized arterial emboli include the coronary arteries, where a coronary embolus may cause a myocardial infarction (Chap. 60) and the retinal artery, where an embolus, which sometimes can be seen on retinal examination (Fig. 12-1), can cause transient visual field defects. Emboli from left-sided endocarditis (Chap. 94) can cause sudden severe pain in a finger-tip and are probably etiologically related to both Osler's nodes (Plate V, 10-6 and Fig. 10-12) and Janeway lesions (Chap. 10). Splenic embolic can produce splenic infarction, which can cause sudden pain that is sometimes pleuritic in character. Emboli to the gastrointestinal tract can not only cause transient discomfort but can also produce fatal intestinal gangrene. Downstream emboli from atheromatous disease of the abdominal aorta can produce pain of the feet or toes, at times also leading to gangrene. Fat emboli from fractures of marrow-containing bones may pass through the pulmonary

TABLE 22-1

Some Causes of Edema

1. Congestive heart failure
2. Cirrhosis of the liver
3. Renal disease
   - A. Nephrotic syndrome
   - B. Glomerulonephritis
   - C. Diabetic glomerulosclerosis
   - D. Hypersensitivity reactions
   - E. Acute tubular necrosis
   - F. Chronic renal failure
4. Nutritional deficiencies
   - A. Starvation
   - B. Kwashiorkor
   - C. Beri-beri heart disease
5. Hormonal
   - A. Hypothyroidism
   - B. Pregnancy
   - C. Exogenous hyperadrenocortism
   - D. Administration of estrogen
   - E. Pre-menstrual
6. Mechanical
   - A. Posture
   - B. Immobility
   - C. Venous valvular insufficiency
   - D. Venous or lymphatic obstruction
     - *1* Malignancy
     - *2* Mechanical or inflammatory obstruction or destruction of channels
       - a. External compression by stockings or clothing
       - b. Thrombophlebitis
       - c. Chronic lymphangitis
       - d. Resection of regional lymph nodes
       - e. Filiariasis
   - E. Marked obesity
7. Increased capillary permeability
   - A. Damage to capillary endothelium
     - *1* Inflammatory edema
   - B. Allergic, hypersensitivity reactions
   - C. Chemical, thermal, mechanical injury
8. Vasodilators
   - A. Nifedipine
   - B. Minoxidil
9. Hypoalbuminemia
   - A. Severe nutritional deficiency
   - B. Severe, chronic liver disease
   - C. Protein-losing enteropathy
   - D. Congenital hypoalbuminemia
10. Idiopathic cyclic edema
11. Administration of excess fluids

circulation and produce emboli not only to the brain but also to the skin, where they may produce petechiae especially of the anterior and lateral chest, and to the kidney, where they can result in fatty material detectable in the urine (Chap. 100). Embolization from mechanical heart valves in some series has occurred at a rate of about 1 percent per year despite apparently adequate anticoagulation (Chaps. 79 to 84).

CLAUDICATION

Claudication, which literally means limping, is now used to refer not only to limping but also to discomfort in the distal or proximal lower extremity associated with exertion. The discomfort or pain, which most commonly is experienced in the calf and is often described as aching or cramping in character, is brought on by effort and relieved by rest. Occasionally, patients experience marked exertional weakness but only minimal discomfort. The claudication should be characterized by the distance or duration of walking before the onset of symptoms. In general, claudication is a sign of peripheral vascular disease (Chap. 124). In patients with lower aortic obstructive disease, discomfort or weakness may be felt in the buttocks or thigh while in patients with iliac disease, it is often localized to the calf.

EDEMA

Edema is one of the primary signs of heart failure from any cause. In most patients with heart failure, edema is associated with sodium and water retention and an increased blood volume. In many patients there is also an associated increase in systemic venous pressure (see Chap. 10). The location of the edema depends on the average position of the patient during the day and night. Accordingly, edema is most often found around the ankles and lower leg. More severe edema involves the upper legs and in males the scrotum and penis. *Anasarca* refers to massive generalized edema, which can involve the face and upper extremities as well as ascites. Occasionally, edema may only occur as a pleural effusion, which is often more on the right side than the left, or as ascites.

Edema can also result from many causes including acute or chronic renal insufficiency; chronic venous insufficiency, especially when combined with prolonged dependency of the legs; chronic lymphatic obstruction from chronic infectious diseases such as elephantiasis or from tumor involvement of pelvic lymph nodes; and marked hypoalbuminemia. When saphenous veins are used for coronary artery bypass surgery, mild edema is commonly experienced for a few months but tends to improve with time. Table 22-1 lists some of the common causes of edema.

PART IV

Heart Failure

SECTION A
Basic and Clinical Aspects

Chapter 23

Assessment of Cardiac Function and Myocardial Contractility

John Ross, Jr., M.D.

In evaluating the patient with cardiac dysfunction, a high index of suspicion about the underlying pathophysiological process after careful clinical examination and routine tests will aid greatly in the selection of additional procedures (if any) that may be needed to establish a diagnosis or to direct therapy. Before discussing the use of special tests and their application to selected clinical problems, it will be useful to consider first some general concepts about overall failure of the heart, myocardial failure, and the effects of altered loading conditions on cardiac function.

IS HEART FAILURE PRESENT OR NOT?

Failure of the heart as a *pump (overall heart failure)* is not synonymous with *myocardial failure.*

Overall Heart Failure

Ideally, we would like to have at least two measures that will determine the effects of heart failure on the tissues of the body: (1) the amount of blood pumped per minute relative to body surface area (the cardiac index) and (2) the pressures behind the pumping chambers (ventricular "filling pressures," reflected either by the mean atrial or the ventricular end-diastolic pressures) both at rest and during stress.

In clinical terms, failure of the right side of the heart at rest is evidenced by the presence of an elevated right-sided filling pressure (mean venous pressure 8 cmH_2O or greater) in the resting state, which may be associated with signs of congestion (peripheral edema, hepatomegaly, ascites). Left-sided heart failure at rest is evidenced by the presence of an abnormally elevated filling pressure on the left side of the heart sufficient to cause pulmonary venous congestion on the chest roentgenogram and may be associated with pulmonary rales or pleural effusion. A low cardiac index (2.4 liters/min per m^2 or less) would provide supportive evidence of overall heart failure at rest.

Further identification of overall heart failure is provided by inability of the left side of the heart to produce a normal increase in cardiac output with exercise with a reduction of maximum oxygen uptake (V_{O_2}).[1] Such impaired exercise responses are often associated with an abnormal increase in the right- or left-sided filling pressures or both during exercise. The finding of impaired functional capacity, reflected by a reduced maximal oxygen consumption determined noninvasively during exercise, also signifies overall heart failure since this measure correlates with the cardiac output and indicates that *cardiac reserve* is impaired.[2] However, it has been shown that some patients with poor left ventricular function at rest (ejection fraction below 30 percent) can exhibit good exercise capacity and oxygen uptake during a graded treadmill exercise test and vice versa.[2] Therefore, the presence of *abnormal ventricular function at rest does not necessarily indicate that overall heart failure is present, nor does the absence of overall cardiac failure necessarily mean that ventricular function is normal.* (See also Chap. 25.)

The above descriptions of overall heart failure say nothing about the *cause* of the failure, and with such a broad description heart failure may be due to such diverse etiologies as generalized myocardial disease, mitral stenosis, chronic pulmonary disease, or constrictive pericarditis. Nevertheless, such descriptions provide a starting point for the identification of right- and left-sided heart failure or both, from which one may proceed to determine whether or not signs of overall heart failure are due to myocardial disease, mechanical factors, or both. Regardless of cause, the manifestations of heart failure may be aggravated by other conditions such as fever, anemia, dysrhythmia, fluid overload, or metabolic disorders.

Myocardial Failure

Depression of myocardial function (reduced myocardial contractility or inotropic state) constitutes *one cause* of overall heart failure. Myocardial failure has been described using various frameworks.[3] It can be defined as the inability of each unit of muscle in the ventricle to shorten a normal distance at a normal velocity against a normal level of systolic load (afterload); it can also be described as the inability of the left ventricle to develop pressure or tension to a normal level and at a normal rate during isovolumetric contraction. The direct causes of most forms of myocardial failure remain unknown, but a few can be identified, such as acute depression of contractility produced by myocarditis, certain drugs, acidosis, or ischemia; chronic depression of contractility can be caused by scarring or patchy myofibrillar loss or damage to muscle cells caused by inflammation and other processes.

Most commonly, the clinical problem is to determine whether or not *basal myocardial contractility is depressed* in hearts of greatly differing sizes or in the same heart at different points in time under different loading conditions (for example, in serial studies after cardiac valve replacement).[4] To compare one heart with another, it is necessary to "normalize," or to correct for a given initial heart size. Therefore, when used to detect depressed contractility, systolic function is usually expressed as percentage change of the diastolic volume produced by systole (the ejection fraction), as discussed subsequently.

Ideally, systolic loading on the ventricles (afterload) should also be known and expressed in normalized terms, since the afterload affects wall shortening. Systolic pressure in the aorta or the left ventricle is often used to provide an index of afterload, but a variation of the Laplace equation should be applied if possible to define force per unit of cross-sectional area of the ventricular wall (wall stress). Thus, it is generally recognized that a large, thin-walled ventricle maintaining a normal systolic pressure in the resting state is carrying a higher than normal systolic wall stress, whereas a ventricle that is concentrically hypertrophied may be creating a very high systolic pressure but carrying a normal level of systolic wall stress.

Under some circumstances, excessive cardiac loading conditions alone can produce failure of the heart as a pump, as in aortic stenosis, even though myocardial contractility is not depressed.[4] Under other circumstances, favorable loading conditions and/or compensatory events may *mask* the presence of depressed myocardial contractility, as in mitral regurgitation.[4] In addition, impaired cardiac filling due to a variety of causes, i.e., diastolic dysfunction, can produce changes in overall cardiac performance without impaired myocardial systolic function. Finally, severe segmental contraction disorders can coexist with areas of supranormal regional contraction to yield normal overall cardiac function.

These general categories of *dissociation* between cardiac pump function and myocardial contractility are summarized in Table 23-1.

Heart Failure without Myocardial Failure

Mechanical Overload and Afterload Mismatch

The level of contractility or inotropic state of the myocardium significantly affects the behavior of the heart. It is useful to distinguish *cardiac performance* from *myocardial contractility* per se, since performance is also importantly influenced by the interplay between the preload and the afterload. In making this distinction, however, it is important to recognize that changes in resting fiber length can directly affect contractility—so-called length-dependent activation.[5] Examples of how cardiac performance can be greatly impaired by mechanical overload are severe acute hypertension or sudden aortic regurgitation, which can quickly lead to left ventricular pump failure without myocardial depression (Table 23-1); this situation can be described within a framework termed *afterload mismatch with limited preload reserve.*[6] Afterload mismatch can be simply defined as inability of

TABLE 23-1

Dissociations between Pump Function and Myocardial Function

Overall Heart Failure without Myocardial Failure
Acute mechanical overload
Acute cor pulmonale
Malignant hypertension
Acute volume overload (valvular regurgitation)
Chronic severe overload
High cardiac output states (Paget's disease, beriberi)
Valvular and congenital heart disease
Impaired cardiac filling
Pericardial restriction
Restrictive myocardial disease
Mechanical obstruction (mitral and tricuspid stenosis, tumor)
Tachycardias
Low cardiac output due to heart block or bradycardia
Myocardial Failure without Overall Heart Failure
Systolic unloading of the ventricle
Mitral regurgitation
Vasodilator drugs
Compensated myocardial failure
Segmental contraction disorders
Transient myocardial ischemia
Myocardial infarction

the ventricle operating at any stable level of inotropic state to maintain a normal forward stroke volume against the prevailing systolic load.

Afterload mismatch tends to occur when preload reserve is unavailable and the ventricle is therefore unable to compensate for altered afterload (Table 23-2). Thus, when the normal heart is pushed to the limit of its preload reserve, a further increase in afterload (as by acute hypertension, which leads to augmentation of systolic wall stress) can produce a reduction in wall shortening and in the forward stroke volume of the left ventricle (Fig. 23-1).[7] This situation resembles that in the normal heart under experimental circumstances where the preload is controlled and held constant and only the afterload is varied; there is an *inverse* relation between the systolic pressure and the stroke volume.[7] Similarly, in the failing heart, when preload reserve is fully utilized, if aortic pressure is increased, the ventricle cannot compensate and stroke volume falls,[8] yielding an apparent descending limb of function due to afterload mismatch (Fig. 23-1). That is, the failing ventricle behaves *as if its preload were fixed,* and any increase in systolic pressure induces afterload mismatch. Afterload mismatch can also occur in the normal heart when a vasopressor drug is administered and the venous return is inadequate to allow the ventricle to maintain stroke volume[9]; reflex venodilation or other peripheral regulatory factors may be responsible for such responses, which in the normal or failing heart can lead to displacement of the function curve relating stroke volume to end-diastolic volume upward or downward by decreases or increases in afterload, respectively, rather than by changes in myocardial contractility.[9] Finally, afterload mismatch can occur even without intervention when the failing ventricle is unable to deliver a normal stroke volume at the prevailing level of normal aortic pressure.[4,6] Thus, under conditions in which the reserve provided by increasing preload is limited or unavailable, the *stroke volume becomes inversely related to the afterload.* An apparent "descending limb" of ventricular function under these conditions is undoubtedly due primarily to excess afterload (afterload mismatch) rather than to sarcomere overstretch.[4–6]

These principles are illustrated in Fig. 23-1 using two different schemes for describing cardiac function (ventricular function curves and pressure-volume loops with end-systolic pressure-volume relations). Of course, all of these responses, which reflect alterations in ventricular performance due to induced changes in loading, can be altered by inducing changes in the inotropic state. In

TABLE 23-2

Factors Causing Limited Preload Reserve That Predispose to Afterload Mismatch

Peripheral	Cardiac
Venous return held constant experimentally	Acute volume loading to limit of ventricular filling
Venous return limited by peripheral factors	Chronic cardiac dilation
	Increased impedance to cardiac filling

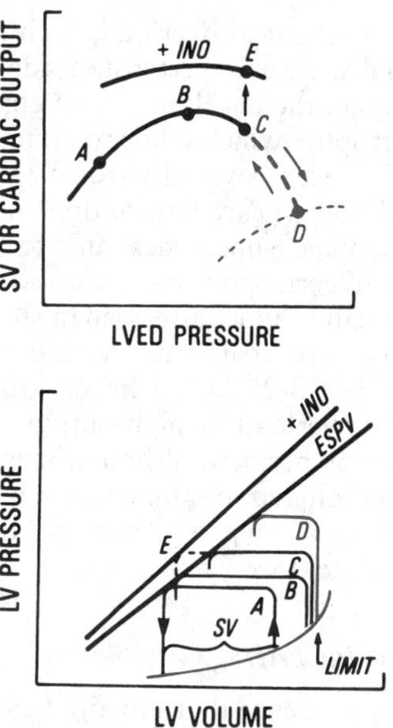

FIGURE 23-1 Two different frameworks for describing ventricular function and the effects of afterload mismatch and alterations in contractility. *Upper panel:* Relation between left ventricular end-diastolic (LVED) pressure and stroke volume (SV) or cardiac output in the presence of mild depression of ventricular function but with considerable preload reserve. Points *A* to *B* show the effects of a volume load: the stroke volume and cardiac output increase. Points *B* to *C* show the response to a small dose of a vasopressor, such as angiotensin II or phenylephrine, and points *C* to *D* show the effect of a high dose of vasopressor: a marked increase in left ventricular systolic pressure and an apparent descending limb of cardiac function [increased LVED pressure with decreased stroke volume, as the LV reaches the limit of preload reserve (heavy dashed line to point *D*)]. Reduction of the aortic pressure (correction of afterload mismatch) would move the ventricle back to point *C*. Point *D* may also be seen as operation of the ventricle on a downwardly displaced "cardiac output curve," the curve being displaced by the effects of increased resistance to ventricular ejection. Also seen are the effects of a positive inotropic drug (+INO), administered at point *C*, which shifts the function curve upward allowing the delivery of a larger stroke volume or cardiac output from the same LVED pressure (point *E*). *Lower panel:* Diagram of the same responses in another framework: left ventricular (LV) pressure-volume loops and the linear end-systolic pressure-volume relation (ESPV).[7] The curved lower line represents the diastolic pressure-volume relation. Beat *A* is a control contraction (corresponding to point *A* in upper diagram), showing the counterclockwise loop during LV isovolumetric contraction, ejection, and isovolumetric relaxation, and the stroke volume (SV) is indicated. With volume loading there is a mild pressure increase as the ventricle moves to beat *B*. With infusion of a vasopressor in low dose, the ventricle moves to point *C* and continues to reach the linear ESPV relation at end ejection; the stroke volume drops slightly (point *C*). With a marked pressor stress (beat *D*), the ventricle reaches the limit of its preload reserve; it cannot compensate for the increased systolic pressure and the stroke volume drops markedly (beat *D*, corresponding to point *D* in panel above). This response is due to afterload mismatch, and *not* to change in myocardial contractility. The effect of a positive inotropic agent (+INO) to shift the linear end-systolic pressure-volume relation upward and to the left is shown, and the stroke volume increases (beat *E* compared to beat *C*).

acute overall heart failure due to *afterload mismatch* (apparent descending limb, point D, Fig. 23-1), reduction of the overload by vasodilator therapy or by replacement of a defective valve with a prosthesis should promptly reverse the pump failure since myocardial contractility is basically intact.[6] Augmentation of the inotropic state with a positive inotropic drug will further improve ventricular performance (Fig. 23-1, point *E*).

In *chronic* mechanical overload, such as that due to valvular heart disease or hypertension, adaptations occur primarily through the development of concentric or eccentric hypertrophy, which tends to compensate for the overload and prevent overall cardiac failure. In most of these conditions, heart failure does not occur until myocardial damage supervenes due to long-standing overload and hypertrophy. As discussed subsequently, aortic stenosis can produce afterload mismatch and heart failure *without* irreversible depression of myocardial contractility (Fig. 23-2). Less is known about heart failure due to the overload of high-output states, such as Paget's disease or beriberi, although it is likely that in these conditions altered sodium balance with fluid retention can lead to a congested state in the absence of myocardial failure. (See Chap. 24.)

Impaired Cardiac Filling

There is ample evidence that impaired cardiac filling of various types can lead to heart failure (Table 23-1).

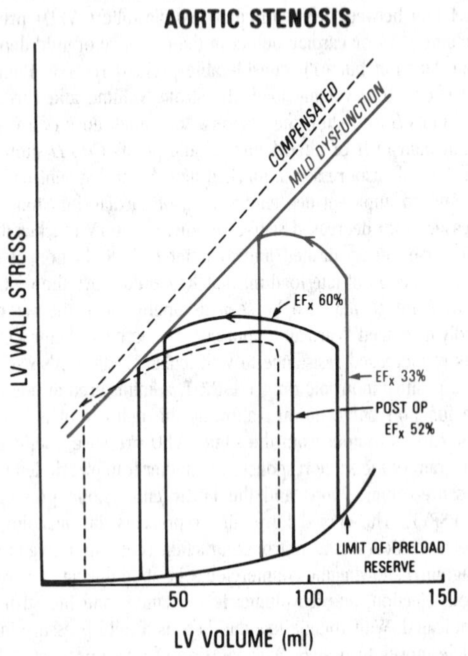

FIGURE 23-2 Diagrammatic examples of left ventricular (LV) function in valvular aortic stenosis. Loops of LV volume versus wall stress are shown during single contractions. The curved relation between diastolic LV volume and wall stress is also shown, along with the linear end-systolic wall stress–volume relation. In compensated aortic stenosis (dashed lines), the LV volume and the LV wall stress–volume loop are normal, with a fall of wall stress during ejection and a normal level of systolic wall stress despite elevated systolic pressure, due to concentric LV hypertrophy (see text). With development of mild depression of myocardial contractility, the linear end-systolic relation is shifted somewhat to the right, the left ventricle enlarges to encroach on its preload reserve, and the wall stress rises somewhat during ejection, although the ejection fraction (EF_X) is well maintained at 60 percent. With further progression of critical stenosis, the ventricle reaches the limit of its preload reserve, the wall stress rises markedly during ejection as the ventricle is unable to unload itself, and the stroke volume drops sharply (EF_X = 33 percent). This response is due to afterload mismatch, not to further depression of myocardial contractility. Following aortic valve replacement, there is persistence of mild depression of myocardial contractility, but the afterload mismatch is corrected and the ejection fraction returns to near normal postoperatively (EF_X = 52 percent).

Pericardial Restraint It has been well documented that decreased forward cardiac output and elevation of cardiac filling pressures are often associated with normal systolic function in chronic constrictive pericarditis and in acute cardiac tamponade.[10] There is also experimental evidence that acute volume overload, as by overtransfusion, can cause elevated cardiac filling pressures and impaired filling of the left side of the heart due to limitation of pericardial expansion as the right side of the heart overfills.[10] This response is associated with elevation of the *intrapericardial pressures,* with *apparent* depression of the ventricular function curve. It also leads to a shift upward of the entire diastolic pressure-volume relation of the left and right ventricles, due to changes of intrapericardial pressure, and the shift can be corrected by bleeding or by the use of a vasodilator such as nitroprusside.[10] Such responses may explain acute shifts downward of the left ventricular diastolic pressure-volume relation observed clinically with vasodilators,[11] and elevated intrapericardial pressures could play a role in producing the high filling pressures in severe acute heart failure. (See Chaps. 25 and 92.)

Diastolic Myocardial Dysfunction Ventricular relaxation (an active process of Ca^{2+} reuptake that is also influenced by loading conditions and nonuniformity[12]), when abnormally slow, primarily affects early ventricular filling, reflected on the Doppler tracing by reduction of peak early mitral inflow velocity, often with a compensatory increase in the late velocity during atrial contraction.[13] Increased ventricular chamber stiffness (reduced compliance) also diminishes peak early inflow velocity, but it also reduces peak late velocity during atrial contraction due to the increased impedance to atrial emptying.[13] Impaired relaxation shifts the early portion of the ventricular diastolic pressure-volume curve upward, associated with a decreased maximum rate of left ventricular pressure fall during isovolumetric relaxation, as occurs in acute regional ischemia of the left ventricle induced by exercise.[14] On the other hand, increased chamber stiffness typically steepens and displaces the entire ventricular diastolic pressure-volume curve upward, as in severe left ventricular hypertrophy or chronic coronary heart disease.[13] Noninvasive techniques may allow differentiation between myocardial restrictive and pericardial constrictive disease, but sometimes cardiac catheterization is required.[15] (See also Chap. 25.)

Restrictive disease of the ventricular chambers, such as in amyloidosis, can lead to elevated diastolic ventricular and atrial pressures often with normal systolic contractile function of the myocardium.[15]

Mechanical Obstruction to Ventricular Filling Mitral and tricuspid valve stenosis, cor triatriatum, fibrosing mediastinitis, and intraatrial clots or tumors can cause impaired ventricular filling and lead to pulmonary or systemic venous hypertension.

Arrhythmias Very rapid ventricular and atrial tachyarrhythmias, including atrial fibrillation, can cause marked reduction of the diastolic ventricular filling time per minute along with inappropriate timing or loss of atrial systole, which can lead to elevated cardiac filling pres-

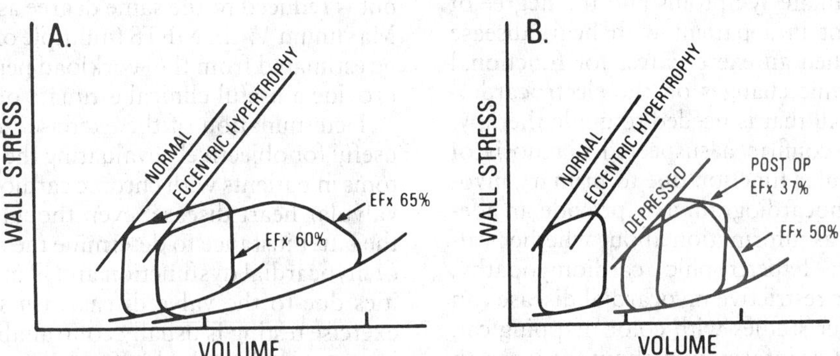

FIGURE 23-3 Diagrammatic examples of left ventricular (LV) function in mitral regurgitation. *A.* Volume overload hypertrophy (eccentric hypertrophy) causes displacement to the right of the curved diastolic pressure-volume relation and the linear end-systolic volume–wall stress relation, and the loop of a single LV contraction (volume versus wall stress) shows delivery of a very large total stroke volume. Because of the low-impedance leak into the left atrium, the ejection fraction is maintained at high-normal level (EF_X = 65 percent). *B.* The development of markedly depressed myocardial contractility shifts the linear end-systolic volume–wall stress relation downward and to the right. In this setting, prior to mitral valve replacement, the ventricle can still maintain a relatively low mean systolic wall stress, wall stress being reduced in particular early and late during ejection because of the regurgitant leak; therefore the total stroke volume remains high and ejection fraction is only mildly reduced (EF_X = 50 percent). Following mitral valve replacement, despite some reduction in end-diastolic volume in this example, the LV must now eject entirely into the aorta with its high impedance of the aorta, the wall stress early and late during ejection rises, and the ejection fraction falls (postoperative EF_X = 37 percent). This postoperative response, the opposite of that in the patient with aortic stenosis (Fig. 23-2), is again due to altered systolic loading conditions rather than a change in myocardial contractility produced by the operation. *(From J Ross Jr: Left ventricular function and the timing of surgical treatment of valvular heart disease. Ann Intern Med 94:498, 1981. Modified and reproduced with permission from the publisher and author.)*

sures and a fall in cardiac output. Also, marked bradyarrhythmias can impair the cardiac output.

All of these conditions, which impair or limit cardiac filling in diastole (Table 23-1), can produce signs of overall heart failure despite relatively normal systolic function of the ventricular myocardium, that is, a dissociation between cardiac pump function and myocardial contractility.

Myocardial Failure without Heart Failure

As might be anticipated, the converse of afterload mismatch can occur when the preload is adequate but the afterload or wall stress on the myocardial fibers is abnormally low. This may occur in mitral regurgitation, in which the low-impedance leak into the left atrium early in systole may result in maintenance of a normal ejection fraction until late in the clinical course, when depression of myocardial contractility has already occurred.[16] Thus, favorable loading conditions can mask depressed contractility, which, under normal loading conditions, would produce a low ejection fraction (Fig. 23-3).

Favorable loading conditions can be produced by treatment of the failing heart with a vasodilator drug that lowers the afterload during ejection[17] (Table 23-1). Experimental studies indicate that in acute heart failure, favorable effects of a vasodilator such as nitroprusside on the cardiac output result from both decreased afterload and peripheral circulatory effects. In this setting, left ventricular unloading by nitroprusside produces a large shift of blood volume from the distended central circulation to the peripheral bed, which is sufficient to counterbalance the peripheral pooling of blood due to the drug's dilating action on the veins. This shift of blood volume allows the venous return to increase and, when coupled with reduced resistance to ventricular ejection and afterload, which shift the ventricular function curve upward, leads to an increase in the output of the failing heart by the vasodilator.[18] Overall heart failure may thereby be relieved, despite severe persistent depression of myocardial contractility.

WHICH SPECIAL PROCEDURE SHOULD BE SELECTED?

Special diagnostic procedures to identify and quantify cardiac dysfunction or myocardial failure must be selected with careful regard to the question being asked as well as the overall safety, usefulness, and cost of each procedure (Table 23-3). For example, if the question can be answered by an extremely safe, noninvasive procedure such as echocardiography or treadmill exercise testing, there is little reason to use a more expensive procedure

TABLE 23-3

Potential Steps in Assessing Ventricular Dysfunction
Exercise capacity
Echocardiography
Two dimensional, M mode for ventricular size; ejection phase indexes; Doppler studies
Radionuclide angiography for ejection fraction
Magnetic resonance imaging
Balloon catheterization of right side of the heart
Cardiac output, filling pressures, systemic vascular resistance
Formal cardiac catheterization
Hemodynamic variables; quantitative ventriculography; ejection fraction (isovolumic phase indexes); coronary arteriography

that requires intravenous injection of a radioisotope. If the problem is to evaluate symptoms and the degree of functional impairment in a patient with heart disease of known etiology, then an exercise test for functional capacity or for ischemic changes on the electrocardiogram (ECG) may be all that is needed to guide therapy. If the problem is to confirm a suspected diagnosis of depressed left ventricular function due to primary myocardial disease, an echocardiogram may provide an adequate answer as well as information about whether valvular heart disease, hypertrophic cardiomyopathy, pericardial disease, or restrictive myocardial disease can be implicated. Doppler studies with color mapping can also provide quantitative information about the location and severity of valve lesions. If, for technical reasons, the echocardiogram is not conclusive for evaluating the degree of left ventricular dysfunction, a radionuclide angiographic determination of the ejection fraction provides an appropriate next step. Particularly if one needs to assess the level of global left ventricular dysfunction in coronary artery disease when regional wall motion abnormalities are present or suspected, the nongeometric technique of radionuclide ventriculography is a more reliable first step; also, the noninvasive tomographic technique of magnetic resonance imaging of the ventricle is becoming available in some centers for assessing global ventricular function and wall motion.[19]

If such noninvasive tests do not provide a diagnosis that is sufficiently accurate to allow effective medical or surgical therapy, then cardiac catheterization is usually indicated. In the presence of acute, severe heart failure with or without hypotension and sometimes in severe chronic heart failure, right-sided heart catheterization with pulmonary artery wedge pressure measurement in the intensive care setting may be highly useful, both in the diagnosis of causative factors and in guiding the responses to acute therapy.

Assessment of Overall Heart Failure

In evaluating symptoms of severe dyspnea, orthopnea, or edema, special procedures are usually not required for identifying the presence of right- or left-sided heart failure at rest. Knowledge of the cardiac output is generally not required, and filling pressures can be estimated from the venous pressure and chest radiograph.

Exercise Capacity

By the use of a treadmill or bicycle ergometer, exercise capacity can be determined from the maximum workload that the patient is able to carry out. The V_{O_2} when the patient performs a truly maximum effort is the best indicator of overall cardiac function, since it equals the product of the maximum cardiac output and the maximum arteriovenous O_2 difference. Noninvasive measurement of respiratory gas exchange during exercise has provided a useful approach for characterizing cardiac functional class based on the maximum V_{O_2}; class A (normal) exceeds 20 ml/min per kg; class B is 16 to 20 ml/min per kg; class C is 10 to 15 ml/min per kg; and class D is below 10 ml/min per kg.[20] In class D patients, for example, there is an inability to increase the stroke volume during exercise, although the resting cardiac output is reduced to the same degree as in class C patients.[20] Maximum V_{O_2} in METS (multiple of resting V_{O_2}) can also be estimated from the workload performed, and this can provide a useful clinical estimate of functional capacity.

Determination of the exercise capacity can be highly useful for objectively evaluating the significance of symptoms in patients with chronic cardiomyopathy or chronic valvular heart disease, even though it is not possible in the latter instance to determine the relative contributions of myocardial dysfunction and hemodynamic abnormalities due to the valve disease. (In severe aortic stenosis exercise testing is usually contraindicated.) Exercise testing can also be valuable for following responses to various forms of treatment, such as vasodilator therapy in chronic heart failure, or for reaching decisions concerning cardiac transplantation.[20]

The response to exercise is determined primarily by the exercise cardiac output, but many other factors, including adaptations in the skeletal muscles and the peripheral vascular bed, cardiovascular reflexes, motivation, and drug therapy, are also operative. It is therefore not surprising that good functional capacity has been reported in some individuals who have markedly impaired left ventricular function at rest, and vice versa.[2,21] For example, Franciosa et al.[21] reported some patients with ejection fractions of only 25 percent who were able to exercise for 17 min and others with normal ejection fractions who had exercise times of less than 5 min. (See also Chap. 16.)

Right-Sided Heart Catheterization

Catheterization of the pulmonary artery by the Swan-Ganz technique (Chap. 18) may be useful for evaluation and management of severe overall heart failure in certain clinical settings. This approach is frequently employed for evaluating severe heart failure in acute myocardial infarction,[22] particularly when complicated by hypotension (Chap. 18). For example, exclusion of relative hypovolemia as a cause of hypotension and low cardiac output together with a test of left ventricular function can be performed by using a small volume load (200- to 300-ml dextrose infusion) and measuring the response of the cardiac output, stroke volume, or stroke work index relative to the accompanying rise in pulmonary artery wedge pressure. A flat or descending relation indicates that left ventricular function is severely depressed with maximum use of the preload reserve. Catheterization of the right side of the heart in the intensive care unit is also sometimes indicated to quantitate chronic refractory heart failure, and it may be invaluable for selecting an appropriate vasodilator and monitoring its initial hemodynamic effects.[22]

Assessment of Myocardial Failure

The most common cause of ventricular dysfunction is depressed systolic contraction due to reduced myocardial fiber shortening. The first step is the *detection* of such an abnormality; then further steps may be needed to define its cause (e.g., overload due to valvular disease or primary myocardial failure). In chronic disease, such an abnormality is almost always accompanied by diastolic enlargement of the ventricle. Less commonly, systolic function is preserved and diastolic dysfunction (increased myocardial stiffness, pericardial disease) is responsible for high filling pressures. Often, the basic problem is to distinguish reduced ventricular performance due to mechanical abnormalities from that due to myocardial failure. Several measures of ventricular function, obtained by a variety of methods, can be used for this purpose.

Contractility Indexes

For evaluating *basal contractility* in many types of heart disease it is *not* necessary to rely on hemodynamic indexes of contractility that are independent of preload and afterload. In effect, when preload reserve has been fully utilized, depressed myocardial contractility will result in an "afterload mismatch" in the resting state, which will be expressed by inability of the ventricle to maintain normal performance *per unit* of its circumference or volume. In this setting, the afterload (wall stress) may be somewhat increased (and further contribute to impaired performance), but this increase occurs *because* depressed myocardial function has produced chamber enlargement. Therefore, measurement of normalized ejecting performance will effectively detect depressed myocardial contractility.

In the resting state, the so-called ejection phase indexes based on measurements of the left ventricular chamber size are perhaps the *most useful and practical* means of detecting depressed myocardial function. Such indexes include the percentage of the end-diastolic volume that is ejected (the *ejection fraction,* for which 55 percent is the lower limit of normal), the percentage shortening of the ventricular end-diastolic diameter (the *fractional shortening,* for which the lower limit of normal is 28 percent), and the mean velocity of internal diameter or circumferential fiber (CF) shortening, the *mean* V_{CF} (lower limit of normal is 1.2 circumferences per second). The ejection fraction is most commonly employed, and a reduced value measured in the resting state usually can detect depressed basal ventricular contractility. Like all of the "ejection phase" measures it is particularly sensitive to *changes in afterload* and under some conditions may not reflect depressed basal myocardial contractility when the level of afterload is *low* or *high*. The ejection phase indexes effectively separate normal patients from patients with clear-cut left ventricular myocardial disease.[23] The ejection phase measures have the advantage that they can be determined noninvasively by echocardiography or radionuclide angiography, and good agreement with measurements made from angiograms has been found.

Analyses of right ventricular function have been limited, primarily because of the complex shape of this chamber and the difficulty of computing right ventricular volumes angiographically. However, radionuclide techniques (nongeometric) have permitted assessment of the left and right ventricular ejection fractions at rest and during stress. At rest, the lower limit of normal of the right ventricular ejection fraction is approximately 40 to 43 percent.[24]

In chronic, compensated valvular heart disease or chronic hypertension, the left ventricular wall undergoes hypertrophy of the volume or pressure overload type, so that the mean systolic wall stress is often maintained at relatively normal or only mildly elevated levels.[25] In sudden aortic or mitral regurgitation, in acute hypertension, or with long-standing severe hypertension, the ejection phase measures may become unreliable for evaluating myocardial contractility, since a reduced ejection fraction can be due to afterload mismatch (Table 23-1). Alternatively, the systolic unloading of the left ventricle in chronic mitral regurgitation may yield a normal or near normal ejection fraction even when myocardial contractility is depressed (Fig. 23-3).[16] Under such circumstances, *limitations* of the ejection phase measures for identifying impaired myocardial contractility *must be recognized.* If measurement of the degree of depression of myocardial contractility or lack thereof is desired, normalized ventricular performance can be examined at the operating level of systolic *wall stress* and compared with the performance of the normal ventricle at a comparable level of wall stress.

Calculation of wall stress remains largely a research technique,[25,26] although it can be done in simple terms noninvasively using echocardiography.[27] On the other hand, it is rarely necessary to determine wall stress for effective clinical management if one keeps in mind the above caveats about loading conditions. Several techniques have been described for assessing myocardial contractility under abnormal loading conditions using analysis of wall stress. Some involve determining the inverse relation between afterload and a normalized measure of systolic function (such as velocity or stroke volume) over a range of loading conditions in the normal heart and then comparing the function of the heart in question with the normal relationship.[6] One such approach used clinically compares a given value of end-systolic wall stress and fractional shortening to a plot of the normal inverse relationship measured in a large group of normal subjects (Fig. 23-4).[28] Also, the linear relationship between left ventricular end-systolic volume and end-systolic wall stress (E_{max}) produced by acutely changing loading conditions with nitroprusside, phenylephrine, or angiotensin has been used to define normal and depressed contractility (see Fig. 23-2).[26,29–31]

Noninvasive Methods

Echocardiography (two-dimensional and M-mode) is the most common method employed for assessing global and regional myocardial function; it also allows identification of mechanical cardiac disorders and provides clues to impaired filling. Diastolic dysfunction is signaled by abnormal Doppler indexes, as described earlier, reduced E-F slope of the mitral valve on echo and by left atrial enlargement. Chamber enlargement can be confirmed (left ventricular end-diastolic size is increased if the dimension is over 5.6 cm or 3.2 cm/m^2 body surface area). All of the above-mentioned ejection phase indexes of contractility can be calculated, including fractional shortening and ejection fraction, together with chamber wall thickness, left ventricular end-diastolic volume, an myocardial mass (Chap. 15).

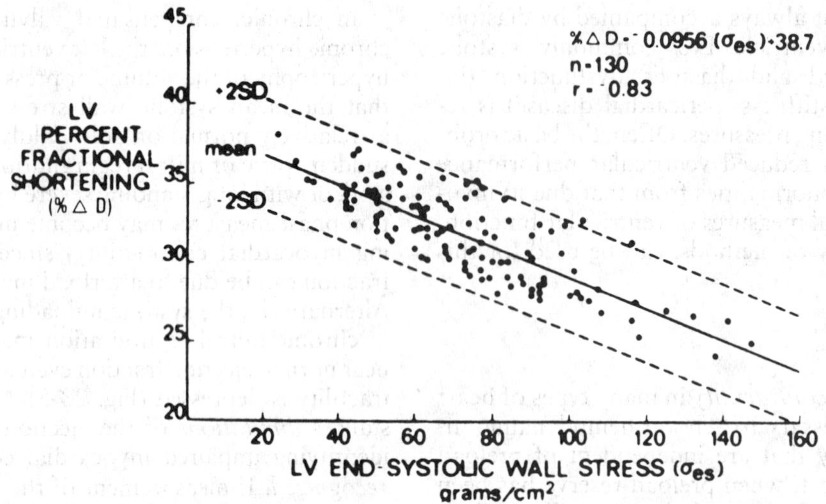

FIGURE 23-4 Example of one approach, employed by Borow et al.,[28] for defining basal myocardial contractility when systolic loading conditions are abnormal. Shown are the relations between left ventricular (LV) fractional shortening (percentage change of LV internal diameter, *D*, determined by echocardiography) over a range of LV end-systolic wall stress values. The LV systolic pressure and wall stress were varied in these normal patients by graded infusions of phenylephrine to produce the linear regression shown (standard deviations indicated). Using such a plot, a patient with normal end-systolic wall stress (70 g/cm^2, for example) in the resting state could be characterized as having myocardial failure if the fractional shortening were below approximately 30 percent. Alternatively, in a patient with aortic stenosis in whom the end-systolic wall stress is elevated (120 g/cm^2), fractional shortening might be below 25 percent, but this reduction is due to afterload mismatch rather than to depressed myocardial contractility (see also Fig. 23-1). (*From RM Borow, LH Greene, W Grossman, E Braunwald: Left ventricular end-systolic stress-shortening and stress-length relations in humans. Am J Cardiol 50:1301, 1982. Reproduced with permission from the publisher and author.*)

Radionuclide angiography (Chap. 134) is particularly suitable for determining the ejection fraction of the ventricles,[32] and it correlates well with angiography. Measurements of absolute ventricular volumes and diastolic filling rates have also been reported.[33] Radionuclide ventriculography is a reliable approach for obtaining serial ejection fraction values when needed (as in following a patient under treatment with adriamycin). This approach is valuable when technically adequate echo studies cannot be obtained, as for example in chronic obstructive pulmonary disease, or when assessment of global function independent of ventricular geometry and regional wall motion is needed in the presence of coronary heart disease, as in the predischarge assessment of a patient following acute myocardial infarction. An abnormal response (less than 5 percent increase) in the left or right ventricular ejection fraction during exercise occurs during regional myocardial ischemia in patients with coronary heart disease, but it may not be specific for ischemia.[32]

Cardiac Catheterization and Angiography

In the evaluation of cardiac and myocardial dysfunction, because of expense and some risk to the patient (Chap. 138), formal cardiac catheterization and coronary arteri-raphy are undertaken only when a precise diagnosis is cal to the selection of appropriate medical or surgical y and when that diagnosis cannot be achieved by sive techniques.

ve ventriculography using single or biplane left raphic studies to calculate the ejection frac- ejection phase measures (Chap. 138) has the standard for accurately quantifying of left ventricular size and function.[34] Chamber enlargement can be identified, the upper limit of normal of left ventricular end-diastolic volume being 110 ml/m^2 body surface area (2 SD).[35] High-fidelity pressure measurements together with volume and wall thickness calculations have also been used, largely as research tools, to study systolic wall stress,[36] diastolic filling rates,[37] diastolic stress-strain abnormalities,[38] and "isovolumic-phase indexes" of contractility.[39] Calculation of E_{max} as a load-independent measure of contractility (the slope of the relation between end-systolic pressure and end-systolic volume determined at two or more points by changing loading conditions) also remains largely a research tool, particularly for assessing chronic changes in myocardial contractility.[29–31] The simplest isovolumic index is the peak rate of rise of pressure (*dP/dt*) of the left ventricle; when it is reduced below about 1400 mmHg/s, myocardial contractility is usually depressed. This measure is affected by other factors, particularly the preload. In the author's view, various contractile indexes derived from isovolumic systole are generally less reliable than ejection phase indexes such as the ejection fraction in the individual patient.

Myocardial Biopsy

When cardiac catheterization studies fail to reveal a specific cause for unexplained severe cardiac failure, myocardial biopsy (Chap. 33) can sometimes reveal evidence of an unsuspected infiltrative cardiomyopathy, microvascular disease, or evidence of inflammation. In the past the diagnostic yield of such myocardial biopsies was relatively low, but more recently, using electron microscopy and special staining techniques, a considerable number of patients with unexplained congestive heart failure have shown evidence of inflammation and some have responded to immunosuppressive therapy.[40]

HOW SHOULD SPECIAL PROCEDURES BE USED TO SOLVE SPECIFIC CLINICAL PROBLEMS?

Recognition of Mechanical Factors Sufficient to Cause Heart Failure

In assessing the patient who has clinical signs of acute or chronic overall heart failure, it is important at the outset to consider the possibility that *mechanical factors* rather than myocardial depression are primarily responsible (Table 23-1). Impaired cardiac filling due to pericardial disease, myocardial disease, or other cause should be carefully excluded, as discussed subsequently in the section on myocardial disease. In some patients, a mechanical cause for secondary heart failure may be relatively obvious, as in severe systemic hypertension, coarctation of the aorta, arteriovenous fistula due to trauma or other cause, or other high-output states such as hyperthyroidism (see Table 23-1). In those settings, extensive evaluation of the associated cardiac dysfunction may not be necessary, since treatment of the primary disorder will correct the cardiac problem. In other patients, a congenital defect or acquired valvular lesion capable of producing an excessive flow or pressure load on one or both ventricles may be suspected. If mechanical overload is present, it is then necessary to establish whether or not there is a *sufficiently severe* mechanical overload to cause secondary myocardial dysfunction.

Once the presence of a significant mechanical problem is established, it is usually possible to exclude or detect the presence of associated depressed myocardial contractility by noninvasive methods. The most useful screening approach is echocardiography, in which direct measurements of the left-sided chamber dimensions, and sometimes right ventricular size, are made. The left or right ventricular ejection fraction also can be determined by radionuclide angiography. In the presence of chronic volume overload, the finding of normal systolic contractile function by echocardiography or a normal radionuclide ejection fraction, despite the presence of a moderately increased ventricular end-diastolic dimension, usually indicates the absence of significant depression of myocardial contractility. An important exception occurs in chronic mitral regurgitation, as discussed further in the section on myocardial function in valvular heart disease that follows. If coronary artery disease and regional wall motion abnormalities coexist with valvular heart disease, the M-mode echocardiogram can be unreliable and calculation of left ventricular volume by two-dimensional echocardiography may be feasible or the ejection fraction may be determined by the radionuclide technique.

In heart failure due to sudden, severe volume overload (consequent to infective endocarditis of the aortic or mitral valves, ruptured chordae tendineae, infarction of a papillary muscle, or ruptured interventricular septum), noninvasive studies should be performed and may provide clues to the mechanical cause of the heart failure as well as to the presence of severe ventricular dysfunction. Echocardiographic studies may allow the identification of a flail mitral valve leaflet, ventricular septal defect, or vegetations on the aortic, mitral, or tricuspid valves (Chap. 15); when coupled with pulsed color Doppler studies, the location of regurgitant leaks or ventricular septal rupture can be identified (Chap. 130). Diastolic fluttering of the anterior mitral valve leaflet may be noted in aortic valve regurgitation, and with acute severe aortic regurgitation preclosure of the mitral valve in middiastole may be identified (Chap. 15).

The echocardiogram or radionuclide ventriculogram will also allow identification of the reduction in fractional shortening and ejection fraction of the left ventricle that usually accompanies severe acute overload. This is often due primarily to full utilization of the preload reserve with acute afterload mismatch rather than to significant depression of myocardial contractility[6] and can occur with acute pressure overload (e.g., uncontrolled hypertension) as well as sudden volume overload (e.g., sudden aortic regurgitation). In the further diagnosis and treatment of heart failure due to sudden cardiac overload in the intensive care setting, the insertion of a balloon catheter usually is advisable to measure the wedge pressure, cardiac output, and vascular resistance, to search for a left-to-right shunt, and to guide vasodilator and other therapy.

Before one considers surgical treatment, full cardiac catheterization should usually be performed to ascertain the severity of the mechanical lesion and the state of the left ventricle and to examine the coronary arteries.[41]

Recognition of Myocardial Failure in Chronic Valvular Heart Disease

Valvular lesions that overload the left ventricle (aortic stenosis, aortic regurgitation, and mitral regurgitation) can, over time, produce severe left ventricular hypertrophy, which eventually is associated with myocardial fibrosis or other subcellular changes and left ventricular dysfunction.[42] Such dysfunction may persist even after surgical correction of the valve defect; patients with chronic valvular heart disease must therefore be carefully managed to avoid irreversible left ventricular dysfunction.[43] The types of special studies on the left ventricle and the frequency with which they should be performed vary somewhat among the three valvular lesions.

Valvular Aortic Stenosis

The adult with clinical features of significant aortic stenosis who develops symptoms of left ventricular dysfunction, syncope, or angina pectoris and in whom echocardiographic studies, including Doppler assessment of the aortic flow velocity (Chap. 130), suggest significant stenosis should have cardiac catheterization performed promptly (Chap. 79). Cardiac catheterization should document whether or not the aortic valve narrowing is significant (valve orifice area less than 0.75 cm^2 or 0.6 cm/m^2 body surface area are approximate guidelines)[43] and whether or not there is depressed left ventricular function. In male patients over age 35 years and females over age 40 years, coronary angiography is usually indicated to search for significant coronary atherosclerosis.[41] Generally, if the stenosis is severe and symptoms are present, operation is undertaken, since the outlook with medical therapy is poor.[44] (See also Chap. 79.) The adult patient who does not have significant symptoms, following initial evaluation including echocardiography with Doppler study, can be followed by clinical examination and watched closely for onset of symptoms, although if the Doppler studies suggest a particularly high aortic valve gradient, cardiac catheterization and consideration of operation may be appropriate in some individuals. (See Chap. 79.)

If left ventricular function is found to be moderately depressed preoperatively, ventricular function tends to return toward normal during the first 6 months postoperatively,[45–47] and hypertrophy regresses. Even in patients with severely depressed ventricular function preoperatively, the average ejection fraction can return to near normal or normal, although in a few patients it remains depressed.[46] These findings suggest that mechanical overload per se (*afterload mismatch*), rather than irreversibly depressed myocardial contractility, is often responsible for the reduced left ventricular function preoperatively.[43] The development of some dilation of the left ventricular chamber at end diastole, with relative thinning of the ventricular wall and reduced fractional shortening, may be due to increasing severity of critical aortic stenosis as well as to early left ventricular decompensation with utilization of the preload reserve. Further progression of the critical aortic stenosis will then result in afterload mismatch with a fall in the ejection fraction (Fig. 23-2).[43] In some patients, marked hypertrophy may result in impaired ventricular filling because of reduced ventricular compliance, so that the preload reserve is not fully utilized.[6] Aortic valve replacement allows the ventricle to eject more normally, with marked improvement of the ejection fraction in many instances (correction of afterload mismatch) (Fig. 23-2).

The current criteria for surgical treatment, based on the development of significant symptoms rather than the development of left ventricular dysfunction, remain appropriate. Thus, clinical results showing marked improvement of functional status at about 3 years after operation tend to be independent of the pre- and postoperative ejection fractions in patients with aortic stenosis, although most late deaths do tend to occur in patients with low pressure gradients.[48] Therefore, operation for aortic stenosis need not be considered *solely* to protect the left ventricle from irreversible myocardial damage. In addition, the data suggest that even in the patient with severe left ventricular dysfunction and an ejection fraction as low as 12 to 15 percent, operation should *not be denied,* since ventricular function frequently will improve postoperatively.[43] Nevertheless, operation should be carried out before patients develop severe ventricular dysfunction with cardiac enlargement and class III or IV symptoms, since even though symptoms improve, operative mortality is somewhat higher and 10-year survival is markedly reduced.[48] (See also Chap. 79.)

Aortic Regurgitation

In the adult patient with clinically severe aortic regurgitation (Chap. 79) and symptoms of left ventricular dysfunction or angina pectoris, it is generally advisable to proceed directly with cardiac catheterization, including coronary angiography when indicated, and consideration of surgical treatment. Such studies will characterize the severity of the regurgitation, the status of left ventricular function, and the presence or absence of associated coronary artery disease. Initial echocardiographic or radionuclide studies in such individuals may help to confirm the need for catheterization studies (see below).

In the patient without symptoms who has severe aortic regurgitation (regurgitant fraction over 40 percent or angiographic grade III or IV) and whose heart size is increased on the chest roentgenogram and by physical examination, a baseline echocardiogram should be obtained for measurement of the left ventricular dimensions. If moderate enlargement of the left ventricle (end-diastolic dimension less than 70 mm) with normal fractional shortening and calculated ejection fraction is found and the patient remains asymptomatic, serial echocardiographic studies about every 1 to 2 years can be recommended. In patients without symptoms, if left ventricular enlargement is more marked and systolic function is near the lower limit of normal (ejection fraction 45 to 50 percent), echocardiographic follow-up every 6 months to 1 year should be advised, since recent studies suggest that the proper timing of surgery can be identified. Bonow et al.[49] have shown in late follow-up studies from 3 to 7 years in patients who have undergone aortic valve replacement for aortic regurgitation that many patients who show improvement in left ventricular function early postoperatively show continued improvement at late study. If both left ventricular function and exercise capacity were impaired preoperatively, however, or left ventricular dysfunction (ejection fraction below 45 percent) had persisted preoperatively for more than $1\frac{1}{2}$ years, little postoperative improvement occurred.[49] Most of the few patients with a preoperative ejection fraction below 30 percent failed to show improvement in left ventricular function postoperatively.[49] Therefore, there should be close follow-up of patients whose ventricular function is close to the lower limit of normal with operation advised, even in the absence of significant symptoms, if the left ventricular ejection fraction falls below 45 percent, since the onset of depressed ventricular function has been reported to occur nearly simultaneously with the onset of symptoms[50] and operative results in this setting are highly satisfactory.[50] (See Chap. 79.)

When there is normal or only moderate depression of left ventricular function, by 6 months to 1 year after aortic valve replacement the heart size has diminished, hypertrophy has regressed, and left ventricular function has returned toward normal.[51] This sequence most likely reflects correction of afterload mismatch by the operation,[43] since the high systolic aortic pressure and volume overload preoperatively in aortic regurgitation make the systolic wall stress elevated (and higher than in mitral regurgitation).[52] In support of this view, other studies showing that early improvement in the ejection fraction at 2 years after valve replacement for aortic regurgitation can be explained entirely by lowered end-systolic wall stress postoperatively[53] (correction of afterload mismatch),[4] with some patients exhibiting persistent depression of contractility[53]; nevertheless, all patients exhibited improved functional class.[54] It would clearly be desirable to avoid persistent left ventricular dysfunction and potentially increased late mortality, and there is a growing tendency to consider earlier operation,[55] particularly if there is evidence of progressive left ventricular dysfunction,[43,49] as discussed above. (See Chap. 79.)

Mitral Regurgitation

In the patient with moderate chronic mitral regurgitation (Chap. 80), if the patient has limiting symptoms of left ventricular failure that are refractory to medical treatment and echocardiographic studies support the presence of severe regurgitation, cardiac catheterization should usually be performed to confirm the severity of the regurgitation, assess its etiology, evaluate the degree of left ventricular dysfunction, and examine whether or not associated disease of other valves or the coronary arteries[41] is contributory. In such patients, provided that left ventricular function is not severely depressed, replacement or surgical repair of the mitral valve is usually undertaken.

In the relatively asymptomatic patient with severe mitral regurgitation, the possibility of developing "silent" irreversible myocardial dysfunction poses an important problem.[43] As discussed earlier, mitral regurgitation places relatively favorable systolic loading conditions on the left ventricle, and eccentric hypertrophy coupled with the low-impedance leak early and late in systole yields a high normal ejection fraction when contractility is not reduced (Fig. 23-3*A*).[56] Even when myocardial contractility becomes severely depressed, a relatively normal ejection fraction can be maintained (Fig. 23-3*B*), although mean V_{CF} is sometimes reduced.[56] Thus, if significant cardiomegaly is seen on the chest roentgenogram or found on physical examination in such patients, a baseline echocardiographic study (or radionuclide ventriculogram) should be obtained to assess left ventricular performance.

In contrast to aortic regurgitation, studies before and after mitral valve replacement indicate that left ventricular function falls to some degree following operation in most patients, even though it may remain within the normal range postoperatively.[16,57] Moreover, when cardiomegaly remains only moderate, there is a progressive reduction in ventricular size and mass after valve replacement.[16,58] When there is a marked increase in left ventricular end-diastolic and particularly end-systolic dimensions preoperatively, with the fractional shortening and ejection fraction at low-normal or mildly depressed levels, ventricular function usually deteriorates further at 6 months to 1 year following mitral valve replacement, and ventricular hypertrophy and dilation fail to regress.[16,58] The marked fall in the ejection fraction following mitral valve replacement in these patients suggests that the ejection fraction was maintained at an artificially high value preoperatively, masking depression of myocardial function (Fig. 23-3*B*).[43] Following correction of the low-impedance leak, some of which occurs at low wall stress *early* in systole even though peak and mean wall stress values may be elevated,[36] the depression of ventricular function becomes manifest (presumably since all of ventricular ejection is now into the aorta with its high impedance) and the ejection fraction falls, reflecting afterload mismatch induced by relief of the regurgitant leak (Fig. 23-3*B*).

In the follow-up of the patient with severe mitral regurgitation who has few or no symptoms but who has cardiomegaly, serial echocardiographic studies should be performed annually. If on initial or serial studies the left ventricular end-diastolic diameter approaches 8.0 cm and the end-systolic diameter exceeds 5.0 cm (2.6 cm/m^2 body surface area) and, in addition, the fractional shortening approaches 30 percent[57] or the calculated ejection fraction falls below 55 percent, cardiac catheterization should be undertaken to confirm that the mitral regurgitation is severe (regurgitant fraction over 40 percent or angiographic grade III or IV), to study the coronary arteries if indicated (see earlier discussion), and to assess the status of left ventricular function.[43,58] Transesophageal echocardiography[59] may provide information as to the etiology of the mitral regurgitation (valve prolapse, rheumatic disease, chordal rupture) and thereby aid in determining whether or not mitral valve repair is feasible. If the echocardiographic findings are confirmed at cardiac catheterization, operative intervention to prevent further deterioration of myocardial function should then be considered.[43]

In contrast to aortic valve disease, since severe further deterioration of ventricular function appears to occur postoperatively in patients with significantly depressed left ventricular function, operation should be undertaken with caution if the ejection fraction is reduced below 40 percent. Nevertheless, if such patients survive operation, it appears that they often show improved functional status for many years despite ejection fraction values postoperatively of 30 to 40 percent.[56]

In patients with mitral regurgitation in whom mitral valve repair is feasible, such as those with mitral prolapse, initial studies suggest a more favorable postoperative course,[60] and further studies are needed to assess whether or not left ventricular function is less depressed postoperatively than in patients who have mitral valve replacement. (See also Chap. 80.)

Recognition of Myocardial Failure following Heart Surgery

Signs of left or right ventricular failure in the early or late postoperative period after aortic or mitral valve replacement can be due to irreversible myocardial disease existing preoperatively. Occasionally, the failure is due to intraoperative myocardial infarction or damage due to inadequate myocardial preservation of the hypertrophied heart, although the advent of hypothermic cardioplegia has made these complications less common. Heart failure in this setting can also be due to a paravalvular leak causing severe regurgitation or to prosthetic valve dysfunction due to clotting or fibrosis producing obstruction or regurgitation.

It is very important to identify a mechanical cause of the heart failure so that reoperation can be considered. In the postoperative setting, however, physical findings are often not definitive; for example, a severe paravalvular leak around a prosthetic mitral valve can occur with little or no systolic murmur.[61] Echocardiography or radionuclide ventriculography are useful for detecting severe left ventricular dysfunction or cardiac compression, and pulsed and color Doppler studies may point to a prosthetic valve abnormality (Chaps. 15 and 130). To definitively establish the cause of postoperative heart failure, it is often advisable to proceed with diagnostic cardiac catheterization and ventriculography together with coronary arteriography.

Recognition and Evaluation of Primary Myocardial Disease

In suspected myocardial disease, the initial goal should be to establish by the simplest possible methods whether or not myocardial dysfunction is present. The physiological pattern of the disease and its cause should then be sought, although information obtained by invasive studies may *not* be necessary to decide on appropriate treatment.

Is Myocardial Disease Present?

The most useful initial screening test is echocardiography. If such studies are technically unsatisfactory or inconclusive, a radionuclide angiogram can be performed to detect a depressed ejection fraction of either the left or right ventricle.

If the left ventricular end-diastolic chamber diameter is increased on the echocardiogram without a significant increase in wall thickness and the fractional shortening or calculated ejection fraction is reduced, it is likely that a cardiomyopathy (or myocarditis) of the dilated type is present (Chap. 89); the right ventricular internal diameter may also be increased in this condition. This diagnosis is particularly likely in the absence of a heart murmur, hypertension, prior myocardial infarction, or other cause for secondary ventricular enlargement and dysfunction. (See Chap. 89.)

In some endurance-trained athletes, the internal chamber diameter of the right or left ventricle or both may be abnormally large and associated with electrocardiographic evidence of ventricular hypertrophy. On the other hand, measures of systolic contractile function by echocardiography (fractional shortening, calculated ejection fraction, and V_{CF}) are normal in such individuals.[62] (See Chap. 114.)

If the echocardiogram shows an abnormally thickened left ventricular wall but the end-diastolic chamber diameter and systolic function are normal, hypertrophic cardiomyopathy is likely, provided hypertension and aortic stenosis are absent (Chap. 90). The echocardiogram will usually allow further differentiation into the symmetrical or asymmetrical type of hypertrophy, and if systolic anterior motion of the mitral valve is associated with a heart murmur, hypertrophic obstruction to left ventricular outflow should be considered. (See Chap. 90.)

If there is a significantly reduced ejection fraction slope of an otherwise normal mitral valve, decreased initial filling velocity on Doppler studies, together with significant left atrial enlargement, a restrictive pathophysiology is suggested. Such patients may have normal end-diastolic ventricular dimensions, with normal or depressed ventricular function.[15] A granular sparkling appearance with other features may suggest amyloidosis.[63] The diagnostic value of this finding has subsequently been found to be less than previously thought. (See Chap. 91.) Echocardiography may detect a thickened pericardium or pericardial effusion, valvular abnormalities, or unexpected wall motion disorders. The use of x-ray computed tomography[64] (Chap. 135) or magnetic resonance imaging[65] (Chap. 136) has been useful in excluding or confirming the presence of a thickened pericardium.[19] In some patients with cardiomyopathy, radionuclide angiography during exercise can demonstrate an abnormal decrease of or a failure to increase the ejection fraction, even when coronary heart disease is absent. Thus, for simply establishing the presence or absence of significant myocardial disease, cardiac catheterization is rarely necessary.

When Should Cardiac Catheterization Be Done?

Whenever the patient with myocardial disease is refractory to therapy or there is a deteriorating clinical course, as complete a pathophysiological diagnosis as possible should be reached by cardiac catheterization. When diagnostic cardiac catheterization is undertaken, right- and left-sided heart catheterization, left ventriculography, and coronary arteriography[41] should generally be done since even if a specific etiology is not identified, such studies often assist in management. In some patients, endomyocardial biopsy of either the right or the left ventricle may be performed to search for a tissue diagnosis, as discussed earlier.

One major goal of the cardiac catheterization study is to exclude the presence of surgically treatable disease, such as unsuspected congenital heart disease with a left-to-right shunt (atrial septal defect and anomalous venous connection are often missed clinically), unexpectedly severe valvular aortic stenosis or mitral regurgitation, a severe obstructive component of hypertrophic cardiomyopathy, constrictive pericarditis, or a significant contribution from unsuspected coronary atherosclerosis (see next section).

Another major goal is to establish the pathophysiological pattern of the myocardial disease in order to allow more rational selection of therapy. Basically, there are three patterns: congestive, hypertrophic, and restrictive (or several of these patterns may coexist) (Chaps. 89, 90, and 91). The congestive type is most common, and the pure restrictive type is quite rare. A restrictive pattern can be mimicked by constrictive pericarditis, and that condition should be carefully excluded (Chaps. 91 and 92). Selective ventriculography and analysis of pressure tracings from the right and left ventricles and atria will generally establish whether the disorder is primarily due to congestive cardiomyopathy with dilation of the chambers, wall thinning, and reduced systolic function or to restrictive disease. In restrictive disease, the chamber size and systolic function may be normal, although this is not always the case[15]; there may be a thickened left ventricular wall; and there is evidence of reduced ventricular diastolic compliance with impaired filling of the left ventricle.[37] Characteristically, there is an early diastolic dip followed by a rapid rise and then a plateau of pressure during diastasis, a prominent *a* wave with an elevated end-diastolic pressure, and a delayed *y* descent on the pulmonary artery wedge pressure or left atrial tracing indicating impaired atrial emptying into the diseased ventricle.[15,37] The right ventricle may also exhibit these phenomena. These features resemble constrictive pericarditis (Chap. 92), although typically in restrictive disease the right- and left-sided diastolic pressures do not equilibrate. In congestive cardiomyopathy, the above features generally are absent, although the ventricular end-diastolic pressure is usually elevated, and the early diastolic pressure is also high.

Thus, the dominant physiological pattern, congestive or restrictive, can usually be identified. Which pattern is present carries important implications for therapy since vigorous use of diuretics and positive inotropic stimuli are appropriate for the congestive pattern, whereas such therapy in the patient with restrictive pathophysiology can lead to decreased ventricular filling pressures and volumes with further impairment of the filling of the stiffened ventricle and a reduction of cardiac output. Likewise, afterload reduction therapy by vasodilators is more appropriate in the congestive setting, since in restrictive cardiomyopathy ventricular systolic emptying may already be near maximum, and dilating properties of these agents on the veins may also lead to reduced diastolic filling. (See Chaps. 91 and 92.)

The restrictive type of pathophysiology may blend with that due to outflow tract obstruction in hypertrophic cardiomyopathy, and surgical relief by myomectomy of a severe resting outflow gradient identified at cardiac catheterization may become necessary in occasional patients who are refractory to medical therapy.[66] (See Chap. 90.)

Coronary arteriography should accompany diagnostic studies to exclude the possibility of silent ischemia in the patient with cardiomyopathy.[41] Ischemic heart muscle disease ("cardiomyopathy") sometimes cannot be distinguished from other types of cardiomyopathy without such studies.

There are some settings in which limited cardiac catheterization should be considered. In the patient with established myocardial disease associated with severe heart failure that is refractory to treatment, if vasodilator therapy is being considered, it may be advisable to undertake balloon catheterization of the right side of the heart in order to characterize the hemodynamic setting.[22] Moreover, serial measurements following single oral doses of the proposed therapeutic regimen can allow selection of the most appropriate drugs.[17] Alternatively, the finding of an unexpectedly low cardiac filling pressure with a normal cardiac output, together with lack of response to a therapeutic test of vasodilators, may contraindicate the use of chronic vasodilator therapy.

Recognition and Evaluation of Ischemic Myocardial Dysfunction

The left ventricular ejection fraction determined noninvasively by radionuclide ventriculography, by 2-D echocardiography, or by intravenous digital or direct cine left ventriculography is highly useful in detecting global depression of cardiac function due to myocardial ischemia or infarction in patients with coronary artery disease. Since ischemic heart disease typically produces regional contraction abnormalities,[67] a normal left ventricular ejection fraction does not imply the absence of myocardial dysfunction. Thus, regional hypokinesia or even dyskinesia in one region can lead to compensatory hyperfunction in a normal region, with maintenance of a normal global ejection fraction.[67] Quantitative cine left ventriculography during cardiac catheterization is frequently used to precisely measure regional wall motion, as, for example, when studying the reversibility of ischemic dysfunction after therapeutic interventions such as thrombolysis in acute myocardial infarction.[68] Noninvasive approaches are also available for assessing regional wall motion abnormalities, including 2-D echocardiography for endocardial motion or regional systolic wall thickening (Chap. 15), assessing regional ejection fraction by radionuclide ventriculography (Chap. 134), or intravenous digital contrast angiography.[69]

Left Ventricular Function in Chronic Coronary Heart Disease

In patients with chronic coronary heart disease, the level of *global* left ventricular function has been found to be more important than the number of diseased coronary arteries in assessing mortality trends.[70] Thus, a depressed ejection fraction significantly reduces life expectancy regardless of the number of coronary vessels involved by significant stenoses, and it predicts a reduction in life expectancy even when one or two coronary arteries are diseased, a setting that has only a minor effect on annual mortality rate in the absence of depressed left ventricular function.[70] In some studies coronary bypass surgery has been found to improve life expectancy compared to medical treatment only in patients with left main disease or those with three-vessel disease who have a depressed ejection fraction.[71-73] There is other evidence, however, that in patients with significant symptoms coronary bypass surgery may improve survival in those with three-vessel disease even when left ventricular function is normal.[74] (See also Chaps. 58–61 and 73.)

Ventricular Function after Myocardial Infarction The ejection fraction has found increasing application in risk stratification following acute myocardial infarction, along with a number of variables including age, prior history of myocardial infarction, persistent ischemic pain, congestive heart failure in the hospital, and exercise-induced ischemia or limited exercise capacity near the time of hospital discharge. The presence of such prognostic indicators often leads to coronary angiography to determine whether or not myocardial revascularization by surgery or coronary angioplasty should be performed in an effort to reduce the increased risk.[41]

The level of the left ventricular ejection fraction, often determined by radionuclide angiography, is an independent determinant of mortality during the first 1 or 2 years following acute myocardial infarction,[75-77] and it has been used alone or in combination with several other variables for risk stratification after acute myocardial infarction. An ejection fraction below 45 percent close to the time of hospital discharge provides both optimum sensitivity and specificity for identifying patients at increased risk,[77] but does not have high predictive accuracy in identifying patients who will die, since a relatively large number of patients having a low ejection fraction will survive 1 year.[76,77] Nevertheless, the *sensitivity* of a reduced ejection fraction (<45 percent) for predicting 1-

year mortality (the percentage of patients who die who have a low ejection fraction) is relatively good (approximately 60 to 65 percent), and the sensitivity for sudden death is somewhat higher (over 70 percent, with 30 percent of deaths missed).[77] In another study, an ejection fraction of 40 percent was used as the breakpoint with similar sensitivity for defining sudden death (about 65 percent of the deaths were identified).[76]

The usefulness of the ejection fraction in prognosis after myocardial infarction can be considerably enhanced if clinical variables indicative of heart failure in the hospital are also considered. For example, in one multicenter study if two of four variables [ejection fraction below 40 percent, ventricular ectopic depolarizations at least 10 per hour, rales greater than bibasilar, and former New York Heart Association (NYHA) Class II to IV] were present (19 percent of the population), 2-year mortality ranged from about 8 to 22 percent.[75] In our data base, when two out of three variables (pulmonary congestion on x-ray examination, pulmonary rales, and S_3 gallop) were present during hospitalization or if the roentgenogram alone was positive, there was a three- to fourfold enhancement of the usefulness of a depressed ejection fraction for predicting 1-year mortality compared to use of the ejection fraction alone; in the absence of these variables, the ejection fraction lost a considerable degree of its predictive ability for 1-year mortality.[78]

Ischemic Heart Muscle Disease (Cardiomyopathy) In the patient with a clinical diagnosis of cardiomyopathy, the clinical symptoms and the electrocardiogram may not suggest prior myocardial infarction or recurrent ischemia, yet coronary heart disease may be the underlying process.[79-81] In some patients, attacks of dyspnea without pain or atypical pain may reflect recurrent myocardial ischemia or subendocardial infarction, and "silent" or painless myocardial ischemia is being recognized with increasing frequency.[82] The finding of coronary artery calcification on image intensification fluoroscopy may be very helpful in suggesting the diagnosis, and among a group of younger patients with heart muscle disease those shown on coronary arteriography to have an ischemic type showed calcification of either two or three coronary arteries.[79] Thallium perfusion imaging during and after exercise may also indicate the presence of myocardial scar at rest or show transient exercise-induced perfusion defects, and a fall in the radionuclide ejection fraction with exercise has been reported to be more indicative of ischemic heart muscle disease than of idiopathic dilated cardiomyopathy. Generally, however, if this diagnosis is suspected, cardiac catheterization with coronary arteriography will be required to fully characterize the degree of coronary atherosclerosis. In the more typical patient with ischemic heart muscle disease or "ischemic cardiomyopathy" a clear history of several previous myocardial infarctions and angina pectoris is obtained. Such patients should usually undergo cardiac catheterization as well, even if heart failure without angina pectoris is the presenting picture, since myocardial revascularization can result in improvement of dyspnea and heart failure or transient attacks of myocardial ischemia in some patients with ischemic heart muscle disease. Also, recent studies have indicated that patients with coronary heart disease and ejection fraction below 25 percent (usually with schematic symptoms) appear to show improved life expectancy following coronary artery bypass surgery.[83] (See also Chaps. 58–61 and 73.)

Reversibility of Myocardial Dysfunction Prolonged periods of partial ischemia lasting several hours, although followed by myocardial stunning, can be completely reversible with reperfusion.[84] During such conditions of low coronary flow, contraction is reduced in proportion to the reduction of regional myocardial blood flow, a condition that has been termed *perfusion-contraction matching*.[85] Such reversibility of contractile dysfunction (either complete or partial) has been demonstrated after coronary bypass surgery or balloon angioplasty in patients with unstable angina pectoris[86] and following thrombolysis in patients with acute myocardial infarction.[87,88]

Reversibility of contractile dysfunction has also been demonstrated to occur in some patients with chronic, stable coronary heart disease (without acute ischemia) after balloon angioplasty[89] or coronary bypass surgery.[90] This type of chronic dysfunction may represent either stunning, consequent to repeated episodes of ischemia, or the occurrence of very prolonged low-flow perfusion-contraction matching or both,[85] and the latter has been termed *myocardial hibernation*.[91] The detection of such poorly contracting but viable regions is important in patients with coronary artery disease and left ventricular dysfunction in whom revascularization might be beneficial, and it has been accomplished with combined flow (N^{13} ammonia) and metabolic imaging (F^{18} deoxyglucose) using positron emission tomography[92] and more recently by the thallium reinjection technique.[93] (See also Chaps. 57–60 and 134.)

Ventricular Aneurysm Sometimes heart failure or low cardiac output due to a left ventricular aneurysm is suggested by the ECG or the chest roentgenogram, and 2-D echocardiography has proved reliable in detecting the presence of an aneurysm (Chap. 15). If a ventricular aneurysm is seriously suspected in a patient who has significant symptoms due to heart failure, cardiac catheterization should be carried out to define the extent of the aneurysm and to assess the degree of coronary artery disease prior to considering corrective operation (Chap. 74).

REFERENCES

1. Weber KT, Janicki JS, McElroy PA: Determination of aerobic capacity and the severity of chronic cardiac and circulatory failure. *Circulation* 1987; 76(suppl VI):VI40–45.
2. Benge W, Litchfield RL, Marcus ML: Exercise capacity in patients with severe left ventricular dysfunction. *Circulation* 1980; 61:955–959.
3. Ross J Jr, Covell JW: Frameworks for analysis of ventricular and circulatory function: Integrated responses. In: West JB (ed): *Best and Taylor's Physiological Basis of Medical Practice*, 12th ed. Baltimore, Williams & Wilkins, 1991: 291.
4. Ross J: Cardiac function and myocardial contractility: A perspective. *J Am Coll Cardiol* 1983; 1:52–62.
5. LaKatta EG: Starling's law of the heart is explained by an intimate interaction of muscle length and myofilament calcium activation. *J Am Cardiol* 1987; 10:1157–1164.

6. Ross J Jr: Afterload mismatch and preload reserve: A conceptual framework for the analysis of ventricular function. *Prog Cardiovasc Dis* 1976; 18:255–264.
7. MacGregor DC, Covell JW, Mahler F, Dilley RB, Ross R Jr: Relations between afterload, stroke volume, and descending limb of starling's curve. *Am J Physiol* 1974; 227:884–90.
8. Ross J Jr, Braunwald E: The study of left ventricular function in man by increasing resistance to ventricular ejection with angiotensin. *Circulation* 1964; 29:739–49.
9. Lee JD, Tajimi T, Patritti J, Ross J Jr: Preload reserve and mechanisms of afterload mismatch in the normal conscious dog. *Am J Physiol* 1986; 19:H464–473.
10. Shabetai, R: *The Pericardium.* New York, Grune and Stratton, 1981.
11. Alderman EL, Glantz SA: Acute hemodynamic interventions shift the diastolic pressure-volume curve in man. *Circulation* 1976; 54:662–671.
12. Brutsaert DL, Rademakers FE, Sys SU: Triple control of relaxation: Implications in cardiac disease. *Circulation* 1984; 69:190–196.
13. Stoddard MF, Pearson AC, Kern MJ, Ratcliff J, Mrosek DG, Labovitz AJ: Left ventricular diastolic function: Comparison of pulsed Doppler echocardiographic and hemodynamic indices in subjects with and without coronary heart disease. *J Am Coll Cardiol* 1989; 13:327–336.
14. Miyazaki S, Guth BD, Miura T, Indolfi C, Schulz R, Ross J Jr: Changes of left ventricular diastolic function in exercising dogs without and with ischemia. *Circulation* 1990; 81(3):1058–1070.
15. Vaitkus PT, Kussmaul WG: Constrictive pericarditis versus restrictive cardiomyopathy: A reappraisal and update of diagnostic criteria. *Am Heart J* 1991; 122:1431–1441.
16. Schuler G, Peterson K, Johnson A, Francis G, Dennish G, Utley J, et al: Temporal response of left ventricular performance to mitral valve surgery. *Circulation* 1979; 59:1218–1231.
17. Chatterjee K, Parmley WW: Vasodilator therapy for acute myocardial infarction and chronic congestive heart failure. *J Am Coll Cardiol* 1983; 1:133–153.
18. Pouleur H, Covell JW, Ross J Jr: Effects of nitroprusside on venous return and central blood volume in the absence and presence of acute heart failure. *Circulation* 1980; 61:328–337.
19. Higgins CB, Lanzer P, Stark D, Botvinick E, Schiller NB, Lipton MJ, et al: Assessment of cardiac anatomy using nuclear magnetic resonance imaging. *J Am Coll Cardiol* 1985; 5:775–815.
20. Weber KT, Kinasewitz GT, Janicki JS, Fishman AP: Oxygen utilization and ventilation during exercise in patients with chronic cardiac failure. *Circulation* 1982; 65:1213–1223.
21. Franciosa JA, Park M, Levine TB: Lack of correlation between exercise capacity and indexes of resting left ventricular performance in heart failure. *Am J Cardiol* 1981; 47:33–39.
22. Swan HJC, Ganz W: Hemodynamic measurements in clinical practice: A decade in review. *J Am Coll Cardiol* 1983; 1:103–113.
23. Peterson KL, Sklovan D, Ludbrook P, Uther JB, Ross J Jr: Comparison of isovolumetric and ejection phase indices of myocardial performance in man. *Circulation* 1974; 49:1088–1101.
24. Berger HJ, Johnstone DE, Sands JM, Gottschalk A, Zaret BL: Response of right ventricular ejection fraction to upright bicycle exercise in coronary artery disease. *Circulation* 1979; 60:1292–1299.
25. Grossman W, Jones D, McLaurin LP: Wall stress and patterns of hypertrophy in the human left ventricle. *J Clin Invest* 1975; 56:56–64.
26. Lee J, Tajimi T, Widman TF, Ross J Jr: Application of end-systolic pressure-volume and pressure-wall thickness relations in conscious dogs. *J Am Coll Cardiol* 1987; 9:136–146.
27. Takahashi M, Sasayama S, Kawai C, Kotoure H: Contractile performance of the hypertrophied ventricle in patients with systemic hypertension. *Circulation* 1980; 62:116–126.
28. Borow KM, Green LH, Grossman W, Braunwald E: Left ventricular end-systolic stress-shortening and stress-length relations in humans. *Am J Cardiol* 1982; 50:1301–1308.
29. Mehmel HC, Stockins B, Ruffmann K, von Olshausen K, Schuler G, Kubler W: The linearity of the end-systolic pressure-volume relationship in man and its sensitivity for assessment of left ventricular function. *Circulation* 1981; 63:1216–1222.
30. McKay RG, Aroesty JM, Heller GV, Royal HD, Warren SE, Grossman W: Assessment of the end-systolic pressure-volume relationship in human beings with the use of a time-varying elastance model. *Circulation* 1986; 74:97–104.
31. Kass DA, Maughan WC: From "E_{max}" to pressure-volume relations: A broader view. *Circulation* 1988; 77:1203–1211.
32. Pitt B, Kalff V, Rabinovitch MA, Buda AJ, Colfen HT, Vogel RA: Impact of radionuclide techniques on evaluation of patients with ischemic heart disease. *J Am Coll Cardiol* 1983; 1:63–72.
33. Starling MR, Dell'Italia LJ, Walsh RA, Little WC, Benedetto AR, Nusynowitz ML: Accurate estimates of absolute left ventricular volumes from equilibrium radionuclide angiographic count data using a simple geometric attenuation correction. *J Am Coll Cardiol* 1984; 3:789–798.
34. Dodge HT, Sheehan FH: A quantitative contrast angiography for assessment of ventricular performance in heart disease. *J Am Coll Cardiol* 1983; 1:73–81.
35. Kennedy JW, Baxley WA, Figley MM, Dodge HT, Blackman JR: Quantitative angiocardiography: I. The normal left ventricle in man. *Circulation* 1966; 34:272–278.
36. Corin WJ, Monrad ES, Murakami T, Nonogi-Ho, Hess OM, Krayenbuehl HP: The relationship of afterload to ejection performance in chronic mitral regurgitation. *Circulation* 1987; 76:59–67.
37. Tyberg TL, Goodyer AVN, Hurst VW III, Alexander J, Langou RA: Left ventricular filling in differentiating restrictive amyloid cardiomyopathy and constrictive pericarditis. *Am J Cardiol* 1981; 47:791–796.
38. Peterson KL, Tsuji J, Johnson A, DiDonna J, LeWinter M: Diastolic left ventricular pressure-volume and stress-strain relations in patients with valvular aortic stenosis and left ventricular hypertrophy. *Circulation* 1978; 58:77–89.
39. Mahler F, Ross JP Jr, O'Rourke RA, Cavell JW: Effects of changes in preload, afterload and inotropic state on ejection and isovolumic phase measures of contractility in the conscious dog. *Am J Cardiol* 1975; 35:626–634.
40. Mason JW, O'Connell JB: Clinical merit of endomyocardial biopsy. *Circulation* 1989; 79:971–979.
41. Ross J Jr, Brandenburg R, Dinsmore R, Friesinger GC II, Holtgren HH, and the Subcommittee on Coronary Angiography: Guidelines for coronary angiography: A report of the American College of Cardiology/American Heart Association Task Force on Assessment of diagnostic and therapeutic cardiovascular procedures (Subcommittee on Coronary Angiography). *J Am Coll Cardiol* 1987; 10:935–950, 1987; and *Circulation* 1987; 76:963A–977A.
42. Schwarz F, Schaper J, Kittstein D, Flameng W, Walter P, Schaper W: Reduced volume fraction of myofibrils in myocardium of patients with decompensated pressure overload. *Circulation* 1981; 63:1299–1303.
43. Ross J Jr: Afterload mismatch in aortic and mitral valve disease: Implications for surgical therapy. *J Am Coll Cardiol* 1985; 5:811–826.
44. Frank S, Johnson A, Ross J Jr: Natural history of valvular aortic stenosis. *Br Heart J* 1973; 35:41–46.
45. Kennedy JW, Doces J, Stewart DK: Left ventricular function before and following aortic valve replacement. *Circulation* 1977; 56:944–950.
46. Smith N, McAnulty JH, Rahimtoola SH: Severe aortic stenosis with impaired left ventricular function and clinical heart failure, results of valve replacement. *Circulation* 1978; 58:255–264.
47. Rediker DE, Boucher CA, Block PC, Akins CW, Buckley MJ, Fifer MA: Degree of reversibility of left ventricular systolic dysfunction after aortic valve replacement for isolated aortic valve stenosis. *Am J Cardiol* 1987; 60:112–118.
48. Lund O, Jensen FT: Functional status and left ventricular performance late after valve replacement for aortic stenosis. Relation to preoperative data. *Eur Heart J* 1988; 9:1234–1243.
49. Bonow RO, Dodd JT, Maron BJ, O'Gara PT, White GG, McIntosh CL, et al: Long-term serial changes in left ventricular function and reversal of ventricular dilatation after valve replacement for chronic aortic regurgitation. *Circulation* 1988; 78:1108–1120.
50. Bonow RO, Rosing DR, McIntosh CL, Jones M, Maron BJ, Lan KK: The natural history of asymptomatic patients with aortic regurgitation and normal left ventricular function. *Circulation* 1983; 68:509–517.
51. Schuler G, Peterson KL, Johnson AD, Francis G, Ashburn W, Dennish G, et al: Serial non-invasive assessment of left ventricular hypertrophy and function after surgical correction of aortic regurgitation. *Am J Cardiol* 1979; 44:585–594.
52. Wisenbaugh T, Spann JF, Carabello BA: Differences in myocardial performance and load between patients with similar amounts of

chronic aortic versus chronic mitral regurgitation. *J Am Coll Cardiol* 1984; 3:916–923.
53. Taniguchi K, Nakano S, Kawashima Y, Sakai K, Kawamoto T, Sakaki S, et al: Left ventricular ejection performance, wall stress, and contractile state in aortic regurgitation before and after aortic valve replacement. *Circulation* 1990; 82:798–807.
54. Taniguchi K, Nakano S, Matsuda H, Shimazaki Y, Sakai K, Kawemoto T, et al: Timing of operation for aortic regurgitation: Relation to postoperative contractile state. *Ann Thorac Surg* 1990; 50:779–785.
55. Turina J, Turina M, Rothlin M, Krayenbuehl HP: Improved late survival in patients with chronic aortic regurgitation by earlier operation. *Circulation* 1984; 70(suppl I):I147–156.
56. Eckberg DL, Gault JH, Bouchard RL, Karliner JS, Ross J Jr: Mechanics of left ventricular contraction in chronic severe mitral regurgitation. *Circulation* 1973; 47:1252–1259.
57. Phillips HR, Levine RH, Carter JE, Boucher CA, Osbakken MD, Okada RD, et al: Mitral valve replacement for isolated mitral regurgitation: Analysis of clinical course and late postoperative left ventricular function. *Am J Cardiol* 1981; 48:647–654.
58. Zile MR, Gaasch WH, Carroll JD, Levine HJ: Chronic mitral regurgitation: Predictive value of preoperative echocardiographic indexes of left ventricular function and wall stress. *J Am Coll Cardiol* 1984; 3:235–242.
59. Matsuzaki M, Toma Y, Kusukawa R: Clinical applications of transesophageal echocardiography. *Circulation* 1990; 82:709–722.
60. Galloway AC, Colvin SB, Baumann FG, Hartz S, Spencer FC: Current concepts of mitral valve reconstruction for mitral insufficiency. *Circulation* 1988; 78:1087–1098.
61. Rockoff SD, Ross J Jr, Oldham EH, Mason DT, Morrow AG, Braunwald E: Ventriculo-atrial regurgitation following prosthetic replacement of mitral valve. *Am J Cardiol* 1966; 17:817–824.
62. Gilbert CA, Nutter DO, Felner JM, Perkins JV, Heymsfield SB, Schlant RC: Echocardiographic study of cardiac dimensions and function in the endurance-trained athlete. *Am J Cardiol* 1977; 40:528–533.
63. Siquera-Filho AG, Cunha CLP, Tajik AJ, Seward JB, Schattenberg TT, Giuliani ER: M-mode and two-dimensional echocardiographic features in cardiac amyloidosis. *Circulation* 1980; 63:188–196.
64. Isner JM, Carter BL, Bankoff MS, Pastore JO, Ramaswasny K, McAdam KP, et al: Differentiation of constrictive pericarditis from restrictive cardiomyopathy by computed tomographic imaging. *Am Heart J* 1983; 105:1019–1025.
65. Soulen RL, Stark DD, Higgins CB: Magnetic resonance imaging of constrictive pericardial disease. *Am J Cardiol* 1985; 55:480–484.
66. Maron BJ, Bonow RO, Cannon RO III, Leon BG, Epstein SE: Hypertrophic cardiomyopathy. Interrelations of clinical manifestations, pathophysiology, and therapy. *N Engl J Med* 1987; 316:844–852.
67. Ross J Jr: Perspective: Assessment of ischemic regional myocardial dysfunction and its reversibility. *Circulation* 1986; 74:1186–1190.
68. Dodge HT, Sheehan FH, Mathey DG, Brown BG, Kennedy JW: Usefulness of coronary artery bypass graft surgery or percutaneous transluminal angioplasty after thrombolytic therapy. *Circulation* 1985; 72:V-39–45.
69. Chappuis FP, Widmann TF, Nicod P, Peterson KL: Densitometric regional ejection fraction: A new three-dimensional index of regional left ventricular function. Comparison with geometric methods. *J Am Coll Cardiol* 1988; 11:72–82.
70. Mock MB, Ringqvist I, Fisher LD, Davis KB, Chaitman BR, Kouchoukos NT, et al: Survival of medically treated patients in the coronary artery surgery study (CASS) registry. *Circulation* 1982; 66:562–568.
71. Takaro T, Hultgren H, Lipton M, Thomsen J, Takaro T: V.A. cooperative randomized study for coronary arterial occlusive disease II. Left main disease. *Circulation* 1976; 54(suppl III):III107–117.
72. Murphy M, Hultgren H, Detre K, et al: Treatment of chronic stable angina. A preliminary report of survival data of the randomized Veterans Administration cooperative study. *N Engl J Med* 1977; 297:621–627.
73. CASS principal investigations and their associates: Coronary artery surgery study (CASS): A randomized trial of coronary artery bypass surgery. *Circulation* 1983; 68:939–950.
74. European Coronary Surgery Study Group: Long-term results of prospective randomized study of coronary artery bypass surgery in stable angina pectoris. *Lancet* 1982; 2:1173–1180.
75. Moss AJ, Bigger TJ, Case RB, Gillespie JA, Goldstein RE, Greenberg HM, et al: The multicenter postinfarction research group: Risk stratification and survival after myocardial infarction. *N Engl J Med* 1983; 309:331–336.
76. Mukharji J, Rude RE, Poole WK, Gustafson N, Thomas LJ, Strauss HW, et al: Risk factors for sudden death after acute myocardial infarction: Two-year follow up. *Am J Cardiol* 1984; 54:31–36.
77. Ahnve S, Gilpin E, Henning H, Curtis G, Collins D, Ross R Jr: Limitations and advantages of the ejection fraction for defining high risk after acute myocardial infarction. *Am J Cardiol* 1986; 58:872–878.
78. Nicod P, Gilpin E, Dittrich H, Chappuis F, Ahnve S, Engler R, et al: Influence on prognosis and morbidity of left ventricular ejection fraction with and without signs of left ventricular failure after acute myocardial infarction. *J Am Coll Cardiol* 1988; 61:1165–1171.
79. Johnson AD, Laiken SL, Shabetai R: Noninvasive diagnosis of ischemic cardiomyopathy by fluoroscopic detection of coronary artery calcification. *Am Heart J* 1978; 96:521–524.
80. Burch GE, Giles TD, Colclough HL: Ischemic cardiomyopathy. *Am Heart J* 1970; 79:291–292.
81. Dash H, Johnson RA, Dinsmore RE, Francis CK, Harthorne JW: Cardiomyopathic syndrome due to coronary artery disease: I. Relation to angiographic extent of coronary disease and to remote myocardial infarction. *Br Heart J* 1977; 39:733–739.
82. Chierchia S, Lazzari M, Freedman B, Brunelli C, Maseri A: Impairment of myocardial perfusion and function during painless myocardial ischemia. *J Am Coll Cardiol* 1983; 1:924–930.
83. Alderman EL, Fisher LD, Litwin P, Kaiser GC, Myers WO, Maynard C, et al: Results of coronary artery surgery in patients with poor left ventricular function (CASS). *Circulation* 1983; 68:785–795.
84. Matsuzaki M, Gallagher KP, Kemper WS, White F, Ross J Jr: Sustained regional dysfunction produced by prolonged coronary stenosis: Gradual recovery after reperfusion. *Circulation* 1983; 68:170–182.
85. Ross J Jr: Myocardial perfusion-contraction matching circulation: Implications for coronary heart disease and hibernation. *Circulation* 1990; 83:1076–1083.
86. Renkin J, Wijns W, Ladha Z, Col J: Reversal of segmental hypokinesis by coronary angioplasty in patients with unstable angina, persistent T wave inversion and left anterior descending stenosis. *Circulation* 1990; 82:913–921.
87. White HD, Norris RM, Brown MA, Takayama M, Maslowski, A, Bass NM, et al: Effect of intravenous streptokinase on left ventricular function and early survival after acute myocardial infarction. *N Engl J Med* 1987; 317:850–855.
88. Martin GV, Sheehan FH, Stadius M, Maynard C, Davis KB, Ritchie JL, et al: Intravenous streptokinase for acute myocardial infarction: Effects on global and regional systolic function. *Circulation* 1988; 78:258–275.
89. van den Berg EK Jr, Popma JJ, Dehmer GJ, Snow FR, Lewis SA, Vetrovec GW, et al: Reversible segmental left ventricular dysfunction after coronary angioplasty. *Circulation* 1990; 81:1210–1216.
90. Dilsizian V, Bonow RO, Cannon RO III, Tracy CM, Vitale AF, McIntosh CL, et al: The effect of coronary artery bypass grafting on left ventricular systolic function at rest: Evidence for preoperative subclinical myocardial ischemia. *Am J Cardiol* 1988; 61:1248–1254.
91. Rahimtoola SH: A perspective on the three large multicenter randomized clinical trials of coronary bypass surgery for chronic stable angina. *Circulation* 1985; 72(suppl V):V-123–135.
92. Tillisch J, Brunken R, Marshall R, Schwaiges M, Mandelkern M, Phelps M: Reversibility of cardiac wall-motion abnormalities predicted by positron-tomography. *N Engl J Med* 1986; 314:884–888.
93. Bonow RO, Dilsizian V, Cuocolo A, Bacharach SL: Identification of viable myocardium in patients with chronic coronary artery disease and left ventricular dysfunction: Comparison of thallium scintigraphy with reinjection and PET imaging with ^{18}F-fluorodeoxyglucose. *Circulation* 1991; 83:26–37.

Chapter 24

High-Cardiac-Output States

Noble O. Fowler, M.D.

In 1947 Burwell and Dexter[1] first demonstrated by the direct Fick method that cardiac output was increased in a patient with acute beriberi and congestive heart failure.

The disorders discussed in this chapter are those in which the resting cardiac output is increased in adult humans beyond the normal range (4 to 8 liters/min or a cardiac index of 2.3 to 3.9 liters/min per m^2). High-cardiac-output states are also known as hyperdynamic or hyperkinetic conditions.

High-cardiac-output states are important for several reasons. Recognition of their physical signs may be a clue to a systemic disease, e.g., hyperthyroidism or systemic arteriovenous fistula. Many of the high-cardiac-output states are curable conditions. The high-cardiac-output states provide information regarding the mechanisms that control cardiac output. The high-cardiac-output states may cause congestive heart failure that is refractory to conventional therapy and may aggravate preexisting heart disease. Finally, the high-cardiac-output states are usually associated with decreased peripheral vascular resistance, and the use of vasodilator therapy for congestive heart failure caused by them may aggravate the problem.

Cardiac output is the product of heart rate and cardiac stroke volume. Increased cardiac output at rest usually results from a combination of a moderate increase in both stroke volume and heart rate. Cardiac stroke volume is controlled by three major factors[2] (Table 24-1).

Increases in resting cardiac output usually result from changes in either cardiac loading conditions or cardiac contractility. The increased cardiac output of the hyperdynamic states usually does not result from increased cardiac contractility alone but usually involves changes in loading conditions. Right ventricular preload is estimated from right atrial or right ventricular end-diastolic pressure, while left ventricular preload is estimated from left ventricular end-diastolic pressure or pulmonary arterial wedge pressure. These values are seldom increased in the high-cardiac-output states unless congestive heart failure has supervened. However, pressure measurements may give a poor estimate of preload, because of alterations in ventricular compliance. For example, with increased ventricular compliance ventricular end-diastolic volume (and thus preload) may be increased even though the left ventricular end-diastolic pressure is normal.

Reduced left ventricular afterload is a major mechanism in many human hyperdynamic states. Left ventricular afterload is defined as the tension per unit of left ventricular wall acting on the muscle fibers after the onset of systolic shortening. Reduced left ventricular afterload may occur when there is peripheral shunting of blood (systemic arteriovenous fistula), central shunting (patent

TABLE 24-1

Physiological Mechanisms of Increased Cardiac Stroke Volume

1. Increased ventricular preload (blood volume, venous compliance, systemic arteriovenous fistula)
2. Decreased systemic arteriolar resistance
   a. Geometric; e.g., systemic arteriovenous fistula, metabolic, pregnancy, drugs such as hydralazine, angiotensin-converting enzyme inhibitors
   b. Rheologic; e.g., anemia
3. Increased cardiac contractility
   a. B_1 sympathetic stimulation
   b. Humoral factors; e.g., serotonin, thyroxin
   c. Drugs; e.g., amrinone, terbutaline, isoproterenol

ductus arteriosus), peripheral vasodilatation (hyperthyroidism), or reduced blood viscosity (anemia).

The cardiac output (CO) (direct Fick method) is calculated by dividing oxygen consumption by arteriovenous oxygen difference as follows:

$$\text{CO (liters/min)} = \frac{O_2 \text{ consumption}}{\text{systemic arterial blood } O_2 \text{ content } (Sa_{O2}) - \text{pulmonary arterial blood } O_2 \text{ content } (PA_{O_2})}$$

A normal cardiac index (CI) calculation is exemplified as follows:

$$\text{CI} = \frac{138 \text{ (normal } O_2 \text{ consumption/mL per min per m}^2)}{195\ (Sa_{O2}, \text{mL/liter}) - 150\ (PA_{O_2}, \text{mL/liter})}$$

$$= \frac{138}{45} = 3.1 \text{ liters/min per m}^2$$

In the high-cardiac-output states, usually the arteriovenous oxygen difference is less than the average normal value of 45 mL/liter or 4.5 mL per 100 mL of blood; this is due to an increase in the O_2 saturation of mixed venous blood in the presence of a normal systemic arterial blood oxygen saturation. The normal pulmonary arterial mixed venous blood oxygen saturation is 75 ± 5%. (See also Chap. 138.)

PHYSICAL FINDINGS IN THE HYPERDYNAMIC STATES

Heart Rate

The heart rate at rest is usually slightly increased and in the range of 85 to 105 beats per minute. Anemic patients with hyperdynamic states usually have a resting heart rate below 100 beats per minute unless there is acute blood loss.[3] In hyperthyroidism, the heart rate is seldom above 110 beats per minute unless there is severe thyrotoxicosis bordering on thyroid storm or complicating atrial fibrillation.

Systemic Veins

A cervical venous hum is commonly heard over the internal jugular veins, more often on the right. This continuous murmur with diastolic accentuation is a normal finding in children in the sitting position. When a cervical venous hum is readily heard in an adult, however, especially in the recumbent posture, a hyperdynamic state is suggested.

Systemic Arteries

The pulse pressure typically is wide, due to an increased stroke volume, with a decrease of diastolic pressure and an increase of systolic blood pressure. Pistol-shot sounds and Duroziez's murmur may be heard over the femoral arteries. A systolic bruit may be heard over the carotid arteries. In the absence of aortic regurgitation or patent ductus arteriosus, these signs are highly suggestive of an elevated left ventricular stroke volume owing to a hyperdynamic state.

Precordial Auscultation

The increased rate of ventricular ejection commonly produces turbulence, thus causing a midsystolic murmur in the second and third left intercostal spaces, which may stimulate valvular stenosis. The innocent vibratory Still's murmur, which usually disappears by the age of 30, may reappear in young adults. In patients with anemia, decreased blood viscosity may contribute to increased turbulence of blood flow. An increased rate of ventricular filling may produce a third heart sound at the cardiac apex. An apical fourth heart sound is common in hyperthyroidism if there is sinus rhythm. Although diastolic aortic murmurs have been described in patients with severe anemia or thyrotoxicosis, these are rare in the absence of associated aortic valvular disease or chronic uremia and systemic arterial hypertension.

Systemic and Pulmonary Congestion in the Hyperdynamic States

Patients with high-cardiac-output states may develop pulmonary or systemic congestion with elevated pulmonary capillary wedge pressure or right atrial pressure even in the absence of underlying heart disease. The cardiac output, although lower than before the onset of congestion, may remain above normal. Although it has been suggested that these patients be designated by the term *noncardiac circulatory congestion*, this discussion will use the more common label of congestive failure for these patients. (See also Chap. 25.)

HYPERTHYROIDISM (THYROTOXICOSIS)

Abnormal Physiology

Hyperthyroidism usually increases cardiac output. The increased total body oxygen consumption (usually 25 to 75 percent above normal) raises the cardiac output to supply metabolic needs; often there is an increase in cardiac output beyond this requirement with a decrease in arteriovenous oxygen difference. Peripheral vascular resistance is decreased, tending to increase cardiac output. Tachycardia also increases the output of the heart while cardiac stroke volume is maintained or increased.[4] Several factors are involved. Animal studies show that T_3 increases myosin V_1 and decreases myosin V_3 isoenzymes. This augments myosin adenosinetriphosphatase (ATPase) activity, increasing the velocity of cardiac contraction. Relaxation velocity is also increased, due to more efficient pumping of calcium ATPase by the sarcoplasmic reticulum.[5] The number of myocardial β-adrenergic receptors is increased and there is increased sensitivity to circulating epinephrine and norepinephrine.[5a] This tends to augment cardiac stroke volume. Studies of patients with hyperthyroidism have demonstrated that β-sympathetic receptor blockade reduced heart rate and lengthened the circulation time, while oxygen consumption remained elevated.[6] (See also Chap. 102.)

Clinical Manifestations

Most patients with hyperthyroidism have evidence of increased cardiac output without congestive heart failure. Many patients who have congestive heart failure with thyrotoxicosis have underlying heart disease, but in some, cardiac function returns to normal once the hyperthyroidism has been treated. In patients under the age of 35, one occasionally observes cardiac decompensation without evident additional heart disease.[4] Most patients with thyrotoxicosis demonstrate the usual physical findings of stare; exophthalmos; enlarged and firm thyroid gland with or without nodule formation; fine tremor of the outstretched hands; warm, moist skin of salmon hue; and tachycardia. In older patients thyrotoxicosis may be masked; the eye signs may be minimal or absent, and thyroid enlargement and tachycardia may be inconspicuous. There is often a loud cervical venous hum. Continuous murmurs over the thyroid gland in thyrotoxic patients are usually caused by a cervical venous hum rather than by dilated arteries within the gland. In thyrotoxicosis without heart failure, the cardiac rhythm is usually normal; approximately 10 percent of patients have atrial fibrillation, which is often paroxysmal. Atrial fibrillation is found more often in patients with heart failure.

Systolic blood pressure is usually increased with a modest decrease of diastolic pressure. The heart is usually of normal size, unless there is complicating heart disease or congestive heart failure. The first heart sound is often increased in intensity and may at times suggest an incorrect diagnosis of mitral stenosis. Both presystolic (S_4) and diastolic (S_3) apical gallop sounds are common.[7] Atrial fibrillation without obvious cause, increased arterial pulse pressure, and an unusually alert patient with congestive heart failure suggest hyperthyroidism. Studies for hyperthyroidism should be made in patients with unexplained atrial fibrillation or atrial flutter, especially when the ventricular rate fails to decrease with usual amounts of digitalis. Persistent unexplained sinus tachycardia, especially in elderly patients, also should suggest the possibility of thyrotoxicosis.

Catheterization

Hemodynamic studies reveal an increase of the resting cardiac output and usually increase of cardiac stroke volume in association with a decreased arteriovenous oxygen difference. The right atrial pressure is normal in the absence of congestive heart failure. When heart failure develops, the cardiac output is lower than before but usually remains above the normal range.

Noninvasive Studies

One echocardiographic study reported increased left ventricular end-diastolic volume and ejection fraction in hyperthyroid patients,[8] and another found no change in left ventricular end-diastolic dimension or end-systolic wall stress after treatment of thyrotoxic patients.[9] The latter authors concluded that the hyperkinesia of human thyrotoxicosis was due to augmented contractility rather than altered loading or chronotropic conditions.[9]

Seven young hyperthyroid subjects were studied before and after successful therapy.[10] Resting left ventricular ejection fractions were normal in both settings. Left ventricular ejection fraction did not show the normal increase with exercise of 5 percent or more in four of the seven but did show a normal increase later when the patients were euthyroid. Thus, in otherwise normal persons, the left ventricular ejection fraction was not increased at rest, but some patients had an impairment of the normal increase with exercise.

Diagnosis

The diagnosis of thyrotoxicosis is made by demonstrating a raised plasma total (protein-bound and unbound) thyroxine (total T_4), together with a raised radioactive triiodothyronine uptake (rT_3U). It is necessary to obtain both tests, since the total T_4 may be elevated by increased levels of thyroxine-binding globulin in the absence of thyroid dysfunction, as, for example, in pregnancy and during estrogen administration (including oral contraceptives). It is more satisfactory to measure free T_3 and T_4 directly by radioimmunoassay. These values may be misleadingly low in patients with a systemic illness. An elevated free T_4 indicates thyrotoxicosis unless the patient has one of the conditions that produce euthyroid hyperthyroxinemia. Free T_4 may also be increased with thyroiditis and following amiodarone therapy. Hyperthyroidism may occur in 1 to 2 percent of patients receiving amiodarone. In rare instances, the total plasma triiodothyronine (T_3) is elevated in the presence of a normal total T_4 and free T_4 (T_3 toxicosis). In borderline cases, the response of thyroid-stimulating hormone (TSH) to intravenous thyrotropin releasing hormone or the T_3 TSH suppression test may be useful. (See also Chap. 102.)

Management

Patients under the age of 25 years may be treated with subtotal thyroidectomy preceded by preparation with methimazole and Lugol's solution. A 1984 survey reported that the majority of thyroidologists preferred initial treatment with antithyroid drugs in young women and antithyroid drugs or radioiodine in young men.[11] In older patients, and especially in those with congestive heart failure or recurrent thyrotoxicosis after surgical treatment, the oral administration of radioactive iodine is usually preferred. In patients with a history of heart failure, oral antithyroid drugs, e.g., propylthiouracil, should be given before radioiodine treatment.[12] Beta-adrenergic antagonists frequently will improve the symptoms. These agents decrease the heart rate and cardiac output in thyrotoxic patients and are useful until the effects of thyroidectomy or radioactive iodine can be assessed. There is, however, some risk of a deleterious effect upon left ventricular function. In patients with hyperthyroidism and congestive failure, propranolol should be used only with caution. Initial treatment with digitalis and diuretics is recommended.[12] Certainly a major issue in any patient with hyperthyroidism and congestive heart failure is whether the hyperthyroidism is the major contributing factor or whether there is associated, serious underlying heart disease. Normal or relatively normal left ventricular function by echocardiogram could be reassuring in this regard. (See also Chap. 102.)

BERIBERI HEART DISEASE

Abnormal Physiology

Beriberi heart disease is due to thiamine deficiency, usually for 3 months or more. It is rare in the United States today. Blankenhorn[13] collected 12 cases from 1940 to 1948 at the Cincinnati General Hospital, and Akbarian and associates[14] reported four instances from the Boston City Hospital. Twenty-three cases in nonalcoholics were reported from Japan in 1980.[15] These patients, mostly teenagers, had a diet low in thiamine and high in polished rice, noodles, and soft drinks. Recently 15 cases with high-output heart failure were reported in South African black males who had consumed large amounts of Zulu beer.[16] Eight other patients had heart failure with metabolic acidosis and low cardiac output (shoshin beriberi). Two of these eight developed a hyperdynamic state as blood pressure improved with treatment.[16] In the Gambia, there was an outbreak of 140 cases of beriberi in 1988, attributed to the use of imported milled rice instead of native rice.[17]

The mechanisms of increased cardiac output in beriberi are obscure. Some patients with beriberi have lesions of the sympathetic nuclei[14] that may decrease peripheral arterial resistance, thus increasing cardiac work and leading to congestive failure.

Clinical Manifestations

Physical Examination

In Blankenhorn's study,[13] patients with beriberi heart disease were usually chronic alcoholics with either peripheral neuritis or pellagra. Biventricular congestive failure is usually present with elevation of systemic venous pressure, pulmonary rales, edema, and hepatic engorgement. Characteristically, there are widening of the arterial pulse pressure and bounding peripheral arterial pulses. Pistol-shot sounds may be heard over the peripheral arteries. The heart is usually dilated, and an apical S_3 is characteristically present.

Special Laboratory Studies: Catheterization

Right atrial and pulmonary wedge pressures are elevated, cardiac index is increased, and arteriovenous oxygen difference is decreased.[1,14] These abnormalities may return to normal after treatment with thiamine. Left ventricular ejection fraction may be normal or decreased. In a case report, the cardiac index (Fick method) was 8.0 liters; the left ventricular ejection fraction was 75 percent at rest and fell with exercise.[18] Sixteen days after thiamine therapy was begun, the cardiac index was 4.0 liters (thermodilution) and the ejection fraction rose with exercise. Figure 24-1 shows hemodynamic data from nine young patients with cardiac beriberi who were studied by Kawai et al.[15]

Diagnosis

The criteria for the diagnosis are a history of a thiamine-deficient diet for 3 months or longer, absence of another cause of heart disease, elevation of systemic venous pressure, edema, enlarged heart, minor electrocardiographic changes, evidence of peripheral neuritis or pellagra, and a response to thiamine with a decrease in heart size or autopsy findings consistent with the diagnosis.[13] Blood thiamine levels can be measured. Erythrocyte transketolase values may be low,[15] and their rise following thiamine treatment confirms the diagnosis.

Management

These patients should be treated with bed rest. Thiamine may be given parenterally in doses of 50 mg daily. Akbarian and associates[14] showed that ouabain might be beneficial. Sodium restriction and diuretics are of some value.

ANEMIA

Abnormal Physiology

A hyperdynamic state is typically found in chronic iron deficiency anemia when blood oxygen transport capacity falls to approximately one-half the normal value but may not be seen with recent blood loss or hemoglobinopathy. Cardiac output is usually not increased until the hemoglobin is below 7 g/dL of blood.[19] Experimentally, lesser degrees of anemia result only in a decreased exercise capacity and a reduced maximum cardiac output at maximum exercise.[20]

The elevated cardiac output of anemia is likely due to some increase in cardiac contractility, but the most important factor is a decrease in peripheral vascular resistance. β-adrenergic blockade does not prevent the increase of cardiac output with anemia. In patients with chronic anemia, there may be a humoral, noncatecholamine positive inotropic factor that might contribute to increased contractility.[21] The decrease in systemic vascular resistance is due to peripheral vasodilation and microvascular arteriovenous shunts; decreased blood viscosity may also be important. Experimentally, anemia increases the cardiac output less when blood viscosity is not allowed to fall.[22]

Clinical Manifestations

Most patients who develop congestive heart failure with anemia have underlying heart disease.[3] Rarely, congestive heart failure may occur from very severe anemia alone. This is unlikely unless the hemoglobin is below 5 g/dL of blood. When anemia results from sickle cell disease or from thalassemia, cardiac enlargement may occur with lesser degrees of anemia. In sickle cell anemia this may reflect myocardial microvascular disease and an altered oxyhemoglobin dissociation curve. Dyspnea, dependent edema, and reduction in vital capacity may all result from anemia alone without added congestive heart failure.

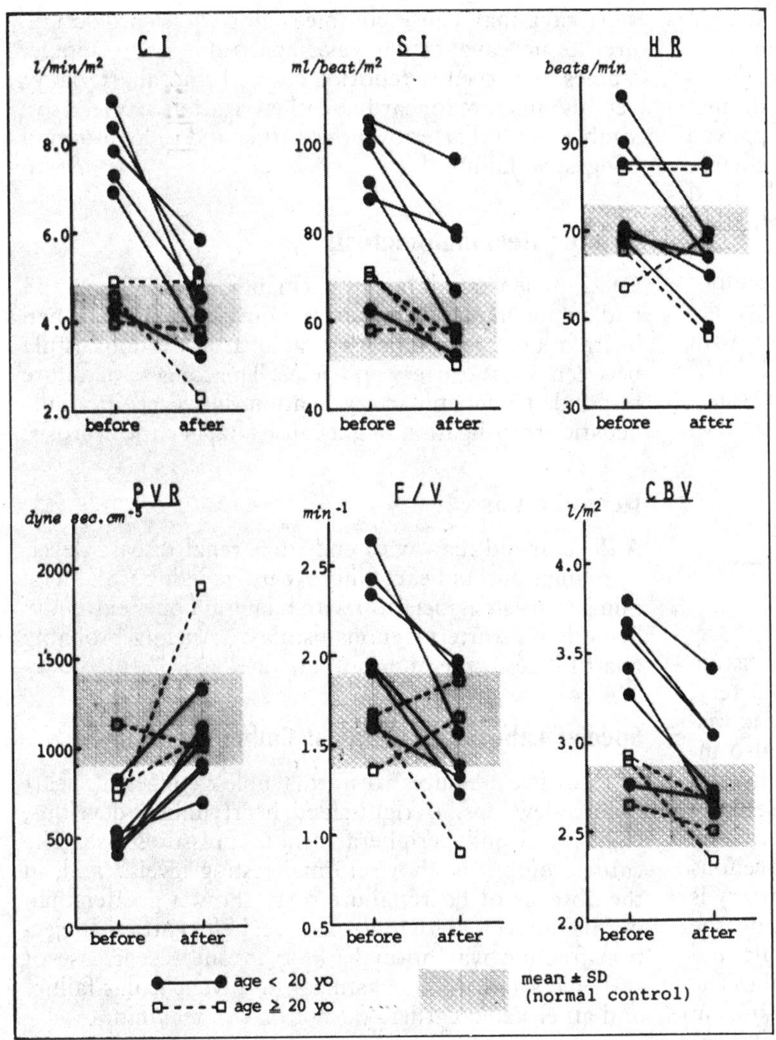

FIGURE 24-1 Changes of hemodynamic parameters before and after treatment in patients under and above 20 years of age. CI, cardiac index; SI, stroke index; HR, heart rate; PVR, peripheral vascular resistance; FV, blood turnover rate; CBV, circulatory blood volume. (*From C Kawai, A Wakabayashi, T Matsumura, et al: Reappearance of beriberi heart disease in Japan. Am J Med 69:383, 1980. Reproduced with permission from the publisher and the author.*)

The characteristic cardiovascular findings of chronic anemia have been described above.

Patients with sickle cell anemia may display a wider variety of cardiac murmurs. A diastolic apical murmur may suggest mitral stenosis, and as a rule the diagnosis of mitral stenosis should be made with great caution in patients with sickle cell anemia, usually after confirmation by echocardiogram. In children with sickle cell anemia, systolic murmurs are almost invariably present.[23] Most commonly, these are loudest in the second left intercostal space. A prominent third heart sound is common. There is a tendency to expiratory splitting of the second heart sound,[23] and the auscultatory findings of atrial septal defect may be simulated. In sickle cell anemia, cor pulmonale may develop because of pulmonary arterial thrombosis, but this complication is uncommon. A 1982 review was able to document only six cases of cor pulmonale related to sickle hemoglobinopathy.[24]

Catheterization and Noninvasive Studies

With severe anemia, there is an increase of resting cardiac output; cardiac stroke volume is usually increased.[25] With mild anemia (average hemoglobin 9.4 g) the cardiac output was normal at rest, but with exercise it rose more than normally.[25] In patients with anemia who develop congestive failure, the cardiac output may fall from the peak value but still remain above the normal resting value.[25] When studied by echocardiography, patients with sickle cell anemia have increased left ventricular systolic and diastolic dimensions; evidence of ventricular dysfunction may or may not be found.[26] A Doppler echocardiographic study of 30 patients with sickle cell anemia and normal systolic function showed abnormal diastolic filling patterns in 17.[27] Fifty-five percent of 40 adults with sickle cell anemia had left atrial dilation and 48 percent left ventricular dilation.[28] Only 10 percent had left ventricular hypertrophy and only 5 percent had severe pulmonary hypertension (PVR $>$ 400 dyne $\cdot$ s $\cdot$ cm^{-5}). In chronic iron-deficiency anemia, systolic time intervals were generally normal when blood hemoglobin was above 7 g/dL. In severe anemia without heart failure, the preejection period (PEP) was decreased and the left ventricular ejection time (LVET) was increased, indicating increased contractility. With severe anemia and heart failure, the PEP-LVET ratio was increased.[29]

Management

The treatment of anemia depends on the underlying cause. Digitalis is of uncertain value in congestive heart failure accompanied by severe anemia.[28] Bed rest, sodium restriction, and diuretics may be desirable. The anemia generally should be corrected gradually. In chronic anemia,[30] expansion of plasma volume tends to correct total blood volume almost to normal. The correction of anemia, for example, by transfusing large volumes of packed red blood cells too rapidly may cause pulmonary edema, especially in the elderly. Slow infusions of packed red blood cells should be performed with careful evaluation of the patient for dyspnea and auscultation of the lungs for evidence of pulmonary edema. Monitoring pulmonary wedge pressure with the Swan-Ganz flow-directed catheter may be desirable in occasional patients with cardiac enlargement or previous congestive heart failure. It may be necessary to employ diuretics simultaneously with transfusion to prevent a dangerous rise of pulmonary wedge pressure.

SYSTEMIC ARTERIOVENOUS FISTULA

Abnormal Physiology

As a rule, cardiac output is increased only with a fistula that involves a major artery: aorta, subclavian artery, femoral artery, common carotid artery, or the iliac vessels. Multiple small arteriovenous fistulas may also increase cardiac output. Pulmonary arteriovenous fistulas involve the low-resistance lesser circulation and seldom, if ever, lead to increased cardiac output, cardiac enlargement, or congestive heart failure. With an arteriovenous fistula, arterialized blood from a high-pressure artery is shunted into a low-pressure vein, thus decreasing the arterial blood flow to the tissue beyond the fistula and increasing the venous pressure distal to the fistula. The venous pressure proximal to the fistula and pressures in the right side of the heart are usually normal unless there is congestive heart failure. The heart rate and stroke volume increase secondary to the low systemic vascular resistance. The diastolic blood pressure is decreased, and the cardiac output is increased. Obliteration of the arteriovenous fistula by compression results in a fall in cardiac output. The plasma volume tends to be elevated in patients with systemic arteriovenous fistulas.

Physical Findings

An increased systemic arterial pulse pressure in the absence of aortic regurgitation suggests the possibility of a systemic arteriovenous fistula. If the patient has had an injury or a surgical operation, careful auscultation should be carried out over the site in order to look for the typical continuous murmur of arteriovenous fistula. Manual compression of the fistula tends to produce slowing of the heart (Branham's sign). Hereditary hemorrhagic telangiectasia may be complicated by hepatic arteriovenous fistulas with hepatomegaly and with thrill or audible bruit over the liver. There may be a hyperdynamic state with or without heart failure.[31] Patients with large arteriovenous fistulas may develop congestive heart failure rapidly or years later. One of our patients developed congestive heart failure 7 years following a gunshot wound involving the internal iliac artery and vein. Rupture of an abdominal aortic aneurysm into the inferior vena cava may cause curable high-output cardiac failure.[32] Aortocaval fistula was diagnosed by echo Doppler studies in a recently reported case.[33] Femoral arterial or venous puncture for cardiac catheterization may lead to a sizable femoral arteriovenous fistula and to high-output congestive failure.[34]

Hepatic Hemangiomatosis

Of 27 patients with hepatic hemangioendothelioma, 23 had cutaneous capillary hemangiomas and all but 2 had heart failure.[35] This lesion acts as an arteriovenous fistula between hepatic artery and veins. The congestive failure responds to hepatic artery ligation; however, in adults hepatic artery ligation might cause fatal hepatic necrosis.

Hemodialysis

A 26-year-old man with end-stage renal disease developed high-output heart failure (cardiac index 5.89 liters/min per m^2) in association with bilateral upper extremity hemodialysis arteriovenous fistulas.[36] Anemia probably contributed to the high-output state.

Special Laboratory Studies: Catheterization

Intracardiac pressures are normal unless congestive heart failure develops. If right-sided heart failure develops, right atrial and peripheral venous pressures rise. The cardiac output is above normal resting levels[37] and, in the absence of heart failure, may show a greater than normal increase with mild exercise. Left ventricular ejection fraction was normal (0.64) in one recent case of systemic arteriovenous fistula with biventricular failure and an elevated cardiac output of 16 liters/min.[38]

A 57-year-old man was hospitalized because of congestive heart failure for 4 years. Twenty-two years earlier he had sustained a gunshot wound producing a right subclavian arteriovenous fistula. Cardiac catheterization results shown in Table 24-2 were consistent with biventricular failure. Both right atrial and pulmonary wedge pressures were above normal. The cardiac index was well above the normal range of 3.1 ± 0.4 liters/min per m^2 and was associated with a narrow arteriovenous oxygen difference. Venous blood proximal to the fistula showed a step up in oxygen content of 3.4 volumes per

TABLE 24-2
Systemic Arteriovenous Fistula

	Rest	Exercise
Pressures, mmHg		
Right atrium	7	
Pulmonary artery	56/18(31)	64/28(43)
Pulmonary wedge	24	
Systemic arterial O_2 saturation, percent of capacity	92.5	94.4
Arteriovenous O_2 difference, mL/dL	3.3	4.4
O_2 consumption, mL/min	246	386
Cardiac index, liters/min per m^2	4.1	5.1

deciliter of blood. With exercise, there was a relatively normal increase of total cardiac output from 7.6 to 8.8 liters/min with an exercise-induced increment of oxygen consumption of 140 mL/min. Such response of cardiac output to exercise would be very unusual for patients with "low-output" heart failure.

Diagnosis and Treatment

If the characteristic continuous murmur with systolic accentuation is found in an area of trauma or surgical operation, no further studies should be required to establish the diagnosis. When there is doubt, arteriography may be employed. The systemic arteriovenous fistula may become infected so that there is endarteritis. This complication in turn may lead to infective endocarditis, most often involving the aortic valve. The treatment of a systemic arteriovenous fistula, when it is large enough to produce increased arterial pulse pressure, cardiac enlargement, or congestive heart failure, should be surgical repair. Details of surgical treatment are described in a recent article.[39]

HEPATIC DISEASE

Resting cardiac output may be increased in patients with liver disease, especially in those with cirrhosis or infectious hepatitis.[40] The mechanism is uncertain but has been attributed to increased blood volume, intrahepatic arteriovenous shunts, mesenteric arteriovenous shunts, and defects in inactivation of a circulating vasodilator.[41] Congestive heart failure may develop,[40] but most patients in this group probably die of hepatic failure before heart failure can develop. An echocardiographic study of 14 patients with liver cirrhosis found significant increases in cardiac index, left ventricular diastolic diameter, and mean velocity of left ventricular wall contraction.[41] Thirty patients with liver cirrhosis and 20 with surgical portasystemic shunts were studied by echocardiography.[42] Both groups had an increase in left ventricular end-diastolic volume index, which was significantly greater in the portasystemic shunt group than in the cirrhosis group. End-systolic volume index was not significantly increased, but stroke volume was significantly greater in both groups than in normal controls. Stroke volume was significantly greater in the group with shunts than in those with only cirrhosis. A study of 73 patients 6 months to 19 years old undergoing liver transplantation disclosed that 82 percent had an elevated cardiac output.[43] By echocardiography, 12 of 13 studied after liver transplantation had reduction of left ventricular end-diastolic dimension and 35 percent had a reduction of cardiac index.

PAGET'S DISEASE OF BONE

Paget's disease may increase systemic arterial pulse pressure and cardiac output. The increased cardiac output is presumably related to multiple, small systemic arteriovenous fistulas in the bones involved by this disorder, especially in the lower extremities. In one study, however, no evidence of increased arteriovenous shunting in the lower extremities was found using labeled microspheres.[43a] Cor pulmonale, aortic stenosis, and atrioventricular (AV) block may occasionally occur. Lequime and Denolin[44] found evidence of increased blood flow to limbs involved by Paget's disease, but an increase of resting cardiac output was unusual in their study. In patients with extensive bone involvement the cardiac output showed a greater than normal increase with exercise. The cardiac index could be correlated roughly with the percentage of skeletal involvement (Fig. 24-2). An echocardiographic study found that patients with greater than 15 percent skeletal involvement had increased right and left ventricular dimensions.[45] Those with less than 15 percent skeletal involvement did not differ from controls. Four of seven patients with more extensive skeletal involvement had increased resting cardiac output. Calcitonin therapy may decrease the elevated cardiac output.

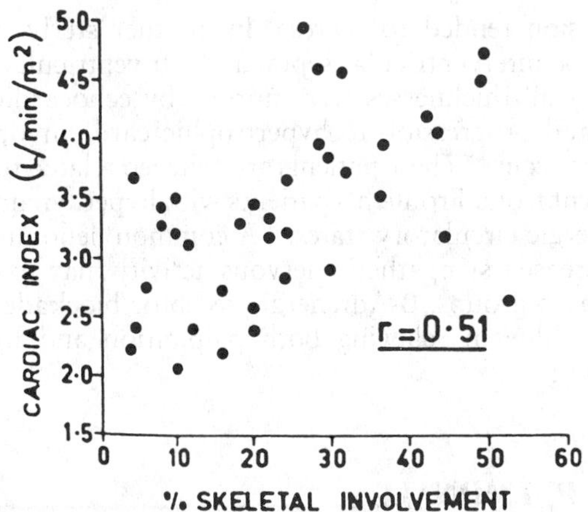

FIGURE 24-2 Scatter plot showing correlation between cardiac index and percentage of skeletal involvement in Paget's disease of bone. (*From JW Henley, RS Croxson, HK Ibbertson: The cardiovascular system in Paget's disease of bone and the response to therapy with calcitonin and diphosphonate. Aust NZ J Med 9:390, 1979. Reproduced with permission from the publisher and the author.*)

HYPERKINETIC HEART SYNDROME

Gorlin[46] described 24 patients with a hyperkinetic syndrome of unknown cause found principally in young and early middle-aged patients. These patients came to clinical attention because of dyspnea, chest discomfort, labile hypertension, and the presence of systolic murmurs. Most patients had an increased cardiac output at rest. Other patients did not, but they did have an increased rate of ventricular ejection. Heart failure developed in some patients observed for as long as 16 years. Electrocardiograms usually showed evidence of left ventricular enlargement. Systolic ejection sounds were common. Ejection and apical holosystolic murmurs were found. Nineteen were followed for 11 to 25 years.[47] Only two of nine reexamined were found to have a hyperkinetic heart on reexamination; in most patients electrocardiogram (ECG) abnormalities and systolic hypertension tended to regress. In another study of 14 patients, interventricular septal and left ventricular posterior wall thicknesses were normal by echocardiography, and progression to hypertrophic cardiomyopathy did not occur.[48] These patients are believed related to, but different from, Frohlich's patients with hyperdynamic β-adrenergic circulatory states.[49] A common denominator of increased sympathetic nervous activity may exist in these two groups. β-Adrenergic receptor blockade may be of value in relieving both palpitation and hypertension.[49]

COR PULMONALE

The resting cardiac output may be above normal in a minority of patients with chronic cor pulmonale associated with chronic obstructive airway disease. A study of 50 patients with chronic obstructive airway disease found an increased cardiac index (≥4.0 liters/min per m^2) in only two, and these had severe hypoxia and hypercapnia.[50] In our study, the cardiac output was on the average higher during heart failure than in patients with hypertensive or coronary artery disease accompanied by congestive heart failure.[51] (See also Chap. 101.)

POLYOSTOTIC FIBROUS DYSPLASIA (ALBRIGHT'S SYNDROME)

In polyostotic fibrous dysplasia the cardiac output may be increased. The cardiac index was 3.9 liters/min per m^2 or greater in five of six patients studied by McIntosh and associates.[52] Biopsy material from involved bones showed numerous thin-walled sinusoidal capillaries. The authors postulated that the lesions of polyostotic fibrous dysplasia act as minute arteriovenous fistulas, thus increasing cardiac output by lowering peripheral resistance.

CARCINOID SYNDROME

The resting cardiac output may be increased in patients with metastatic carcinoid tumors.[53] The patients may have a lowered arteriovenous oxygen difference and decreased peripheral vascular resistance. Serotonin, known to be elaborated by carcinoid tumors, increases myocardial contractility by direct action and is also a vasodilator. It seems likely that the increased cardiac output combined with tricuspid or pulmonary valve deformity, often found in patients with the carcinoid syndrome, may explain the high incidence of heart failure in this disease.

WARM AND HUMID ENVIRONMENT

Burch and associates[54] studied 10 subjects in New Orleans during the summers of 1957 and 1958. The mean of their cardiac outputs when in an air-conditioned ward was 4.0 liters/min. When the subjects were exposed to environmental conditions with the room temperature of 30.5 to 33.3°C (87 to 92°F) and relative humidity of 58 to 93 percent, the mean cardiac output rose 43 percent to 5.7 liters/min. Calculated ventricular work rose in some subjects, suggesting that air conditioning may reduce the work load of the heart in some patients with heart disease. Short periods of exposure to dry heat apparently had little effect on cardiac output. In another study, eight Marine recruits with heat stroke were evaluated.[55] Seven of the eight had increased cardiac index (>5.0 liters/min per m^2) that persisted after body temperature returned to normal. Systemic vascular resistance was decreased and central venous pressure tended to be increased. When whole-body hyperthermia was used to treat malignant neoplasms, a body temperature of 41.8°C (107.1°F) was associated with doubling of cardiac output.[56]

COLD ENVIRONMENT

In healthy young men exposed to 5°C ambient temperature, cardiac output and total body oxygen consumption were increased.[57] Since the arteriovenous oxygen difference was also increased, the rise of cardiac output can be explained by the increased metabolic demands of the tissues.

RENAL DISEASE

An increase of resting cardiac index not explained by fever or anemia may be found in patients with acute renal failure associated with tubular necrosis. With chronic renal failure and anemia, the cardiac output is also usually increased.[58] The cardiac output usually returns to normal when the anemia is corrected. Patients undergoing hemodialysis for the treatment of uremia tend to have an elevated cardiac output. An echocardiographic study of 23 men undergoing hemodialysis for 6 months or more showed an elevated stroke volume with a decreased ejection fraction.[59] In addition to anemia, the arteriovenous shunt used for dialysis and a uremic hypermetabolic state may contribute to the elevated cardiac output. The cardiac output in severe chronic renal disease was found to be highest at hemoglobin values of 6 to 7 g/dL blood and to decrease either above or below that value.[60] (See also Chap. 108.)

POLYCYTHEMIA VERA

The cardiac output and cardiac stroke index may be increased in patients with polycythemia vera.[61] The mechanism of increased cardiac output is uncertain but appears to be correlated with the degree of hypervolemia. Right atrial and pulmonary wedge pressures are not increased.

PREGNANCY

During normal pregnancy the cardiac output increases progressively until the seventh or eighth month. The increase averages 30 to 50 percent. Since systemic blood pressure tends to fall slightly, total peripheral resistance is considerably decreased. Cardiac output, stroke volume, systolic ejection fraction, and left ventricular end-diastolic dimension are still elevated 48 h postpartum but fall significantly by 2 weeks postpartum.[62] An echocardiographic study reported an increase in left atrial size, left ventricular mass, and stroke volume without a change in left ventricular dimensions.[63] The increased cardiac output is not entirely explained by increased maternal oxygen consumption or by increased uterine blood flow, and steroid hormone effects upon cardiac and vascular compliance may be important. (See also Chap. 113.)

Seven women were studied at 37 weeks gestation and at 12 weeks postpartum.[64] Cardiac output at rest at 37 weeks gestation (6.8 ± 1.6 liters/min) were significantly greater than at 12 weeks postpartum (4.3 ± 0.5 liters/min). Heart rate (86 ± 9 beats per minute) was also greater during pregnancy than postpartum (70 ± 8 beats per minute), while arteriovenous O_2 difference was significantly less during pregnancy (3.5 ± 0.4 mL/dL vs. 4.3 ± 0.6 mL/dL). Increases of cardiac output and stroke volume with exercise were significantly greater during pregnancy.

Cardiac outputs were compared in 14 patients with peripartum cardiomyopathy and 12 with dilated cardiomyopathy unrelated to pregnancy.[65] The mean cardiac index in the peripartum group (3.34 ± 1.36 liters/min per m^2) was significantly higher than in the dilated cardiomyopathy group (2.24 ± 0.72 liters/min per m^2). In three patients with peripartum cardiomyopathy, the resting cardiac index was above the normal range of 4.5 liters/min per m^2.

CERTAIN CUTANEOUS DISEASES

A significant increase in the resting cardiac output may occur in patients with "erythrodermic" skin disease. It is believed that increased blood flow to the skin might be at least partly responsible for the elevated cardiac output. Hecht and coworkers[66] found high resting cardiac output in psoriasis and in exfoliative dermatitis and also demonstrated a hyperdynamic state in patients with Kaposi's sarcoma.

OBESITY

In extreme obesity, the cardiac output tends to be increased, but only in proportion to the increased weight and oxygen consumption. The arteriovenous oxygen difference is not decreased.[67] Obese subjects (≥150 percent ideal body weight) were found to have increased cardiac output, stroke volume, and total blood volume and decreased peripheral resistance.[68] Cardiac stroke volume may be more greatly increased in visceral than in subcutaneous obesity.[69] (See also Chap. 104.)

SYSTEMIC ARTERIAL HYPERTENSION

The resting cardiac index has been found to be elevated in some patients with labile hypertension or borderline blood pressure elevation. The cardiac output tends to be higher in those patients with early, labile hypertension than in those with established hypertension. An increased cardiac output, however, may be found in some patients with severe hypertension.[70] (See also Chap. 75.)

DRUGS THAT TEND TO CAUSE A HIGH CARDIAC OUTPUT

The cardiac output may be raised by certain drugs that have a positive cardiac inotropic effect (isoproterenol, dopamine, epinephrine) and by certain vasodilators (nitrates, calcium channel blocking agents, hydralazine, angiotensin-converting enzyme inhibitors). In patients treated for congestive heart failure the cardiac output might even rise above normal levels with hydralazine therapy. In some patients the clinical signs of a hyperdynamic state can be found. A hyperkinetic circulation has been also observed with captopril therapy for congestive heart failure.[71] Interleukin-2, used in treating some advanced neoplasms, may have a vasodilator effect and may increase cardiac output.[72]

SEPTIC SHOCK

A study of 41 patients in septic shock found a decreased cardiac index in 5; cardiac index was moderately increased in 31 (3.5 to 7.0 liters/min per m^2); and in 5 there was an extreme hyperdynamic state (cardiac index >7.0 liters/min per m^2).[73] Extreme vasodilation was thought to be the mechanism. A panel discussion reported a consistent increase in cardiac index and a decrease in systemic vascular resistance in septic shock. Both ventricles were dilated with a decreased ejection fraction. Some degree of tachycardia was present. These values showed a return toward normal by 24 h in survivors.[74]

MISCELLANEOUS

Three patients with increased cardiac output and congestive heart failure associated with multiple myeloma have been described.[75] Anemia did not appear to be responsible for the increased cardiac output, and the presence of an unidentified vasodilator substance was postulated. High-output congestive heart failure was described in another patient with multiple myeloma.[76] Correction of anemia did not resolve the high-output state, which was attributed to massive arteriovenous shunting in the pelvis. High cardiac output, pulmonary congestion, and decreased systemic vascular resistance were described in two patients with acute adrenocortical insufficiency.[77] These findings should be confirmed.

REFERENCES

1. Burwell CS, Dexter L: Beri-beri heart disease. *Trans Assoc Am Phys* 1947; 60:59–64.
2. Braunwald E: On the difference between the heart's output and its contractile state (editorial). *Circulation* 1971; 43:171–174.
3. Varat MA, Adolph RJ, Fowler NO: Cardiovascular effects of anemia. *Am Heart J* 1972; 83:415–426.
4. Graettinger JS, Muenster JJ, Selverstone LA, Campbell JA: A correlation of clinical and hemodynamic studies in patients with hyperthyroidism with and without congestive heart failure. *J Clin Invest* 1959; 38:1316–1327.
5. Dillmann WH: Biochemical basis of thyroid hormone action in the heart. *Am J Med* 1990; 88:626–630.
5a. Williams LT, Lefkowitz RJ: Thyroid hormone regulation of β-adrenergic receptor number. *J Biol Chem* 1977; 252:2787–2789.
6. Grossman W, Robin NI, Johnson LW, Brooks HL, Selenkow HA, Dexter L: The enhanced myocardial contractility of thyrotoxicosis. Role of the beta adrenergic receptor. *Ann Intern Med* 1971; 74:869–874.
7. Leonard JJ, deGroot WJ: The thyroid state and the cardiovascular system. *Mod Concepts Cardiovasc Dis* 1969; 38:23–27.
8. Merillon JP, Passa P, Chastre J, Wolf A, Gourgon R: Left ventricular function and hyperthyroidism. *Br Heart J* 1981; 46:137–143.
9. Feldman T, Borow KM, Sarne DH, Neumann A, Lang RM: Myocardial mechanics in hyperthyroidism: Importance of left ventricular loading conditions, heart rate and contractile state. *J Am Coll Cardiol* 1986; 7:967–974.
10. Smallridge RC, Goldman MH, Raines K, Jones S, Van Nostrand O: Rest and exercise left ventricular ejection fraction before and after therapy in young adults with hyperthyroidism and hypothyroidism. *Am J Cardiol* 1987; 60:929–931.
11. Dunn JT: Choice of therapy in young adults with hyperthyroidism of Graves' disease. *Ann Intern Med* 1984; 100:891–893.
12. Blonde L, Skelton CL: Hyperthyroidism and cardiovascular disease: Concepts and management. *Cardiovasc Med* 1978; 3:1145–1158.
13. Blankenhorn MA: Effect of vitamin deficiency on the heart and circulation. *Circulation* 1955; 11:288–291.
14. Akbarian M, Yankopoulos NA, Abelmann WH: Hemodynamic studies in beriberi heart disease. *Am J Med* 1966; 41:197–212.
15. Kawai C, Wakabayashi A, Matsumura T, Yui Y: Reappearance of beriberi heart disease in Japan. *Am J Med* 1980; 69:383–386.
16. Naidoo DP: Beriberi heart disease in Durban. A retrospective study. *S Afr Med J*, 1987; 72:241–244.
17. Tang CM, Wells JC, Rolfe M, Cham K: Outbreak of beri-beri in the Gambia. *Lancet* 1989; 2:206–207.
18. Webster MWI, Ikram H: Myocardial function in alcoholic cardiac beriberi. *Int J Cardiol* 1987; 17:213–215.
19. Brannon ES, Merrill AJ, Warren JV, Stead EA Jr: The cardiac output in patients with chronic anemia as measured by the techniques of right atrial catheterization. *J Clin Invest* 1945; 24:332–336.
20. Celsing F, Nystrom J, Pihlstedt P, Werner B, Ekblom B: Effect of long-term anemia and retransfusion on central circulation during exercise. *J Appl Physiol* 1986; 61:1358–1362.
21. Florenzano F, Diaz G, Regonesi C, Escobar E: Left ventricular function in chronic anemia: Evidence of noncatecholamine positive inotropic factor in the serum. *Am J Cardiol* 1984; 54:638–645.
22. Fowler NO, Holmes JC: Blood viscosity and cardiac output in acute experimental anemia. *J Appl Physiol* 1975; 39:453–456.
23. Shubin H, Kaufman R, Shapiro M, Levinson DC: Cardiovascular findings in children with sickle cell anemia. *Am J Cardiol* 1960; 6:875–885.
24. Collins FS, Orringer EP: Pulmonary hypertension in the sickle hemoglobinopathies. *Am J Med* 1982; 73:814–821.
25. Graettinger JS, Parsons RL, Campbell JA: A correlation of clinical and hemodynamic studies in patients with mild and severe anemia with and without congestive failure. *Ann Intern Med* 1963; 58:617–626.
26. Chung EE, Dianzumba SB, Morais P, Sergeant GR: Cardiac performance in children with homozygous sickle cell disease. *J Am Coll Cardiol* 1987; 9:1038–1042.
27. Lewis JF, Maron BJ, Castro O, Moosa YA: Left ventricular diastolic filling abnormalities identified by Doppler echocardiography in asymptomatic patients with sickle cell anemia. *J Am Coll Cardiol* 1991; 17:1473–1478.
28. Simmons BE, Santhanam V, Castaner A, Rao KRP, Sachdev N, Cooper R: Sickle cell heart disease. Two-dimensional echo and Doppler ultrasonographic findings in the hearts of adult patients with sickle cell anemia. *Arch Intern Med* 1988; 148:1526–1528.
29. Abdullah AK, Siddiqui MA, Tajuddin M: Systolic time intervals in chronic anemia. *Am Heart J* 1977; 94:287–291.
30. Duke M, Herbert VD, Abelmann WH: Hemodynamic effects of blood transfusion on chronic anemia. *N Engl J Med* 1964; 271:975–980.
31. Peery WH: Clinical spectrum of hereditary hemorrhagic telangiectasia (Osler-Weber-Rendu disease). *Am J Med* 1987; 82:989–997.
32. Gordon JB, Newman KD, Marsh JD: Angina pectoris as the initial manifestation of an aortocaval fistula. *Am J Med* 1986; 80:514–516.
33. Daxini BV, Desai AG, Sharma S: Echo-Doppler diagnosis of aortocaval fistula following blunt trauma to abdomen. *Am Heart J* 1989; 118:843–844.
34. Kron J, Sutherland D, Rosch J, Morton MJ, McAnulty JH: Arteriovenous fistula: A rare complication of arterial puncture for cardiac catheterization. *Am J Cardiol* 1985; 55:1445–1446.
35. deLorimier AA, Simpson EB, Baum RS, Carlsson E: Hepatic artery ligation for hepatic hemangiomatosis. *N Engl J Med* 1967; 277:333–337.
36. Ingram CW, Satler LF, Rackley CE: Progressive heart failure secondary to a high output state. *Chest* 1987; 92:1117–1118.
37. Muenster JJ, Graettinger JS, Campbell AJ: Correlation of clinical and hemodynamic findings in patients with systemic arteriovenous fistulas. *Circulation* 1959; 20:1079–1086.
38. Johnson RA, Boucher CA: Normal left ventricular ejection fraction in systemic arteriovenous fistula. *Chest* 1981; 79:607–609.
39. Adolph RJ: Acquired peripheral arteriovenous fistula. In: Hurst JW (ed): *Current Therapy in Cardiovascular Disease*, 3d ed. Philadelphia, BC Decker, 1991: 409–412.
40. Murray JF, Dawson AM, Sherlock S: Circulatory changes in chronic liver disease. *Am J Med* 1958; 24:358–367.
41. Lewis BS, Tur-Kaspa R, Lewis N, Gotsman MS, Eliakim M: Left ventricular function in liver cirrhosis: An echocardiographic study. *Isr J Med Sci* 1980; 16:489–495.
42. Keller H, Bezjak V, Stegaru B, Buss J, Holm E, Heene DL: Ventricular function in cirrhosis and portasystemic shunt: A two-dimensional echocardiographic study. *Hepatology* 1988; 8:658–662.
43. Park SC, Beerman LB, Gartner JC, Zitelli BJ, Malatack JJ, Fricker FJ, et al: Echocardiographic findings before and after liver transplantation. *Am J Cardiol* 1985; 55:1373–1378.
43a. Rhodes BA, Greyson ND, Hamilton CR Jr, White RI Jr, Giargiana FA Jr, Wagner HN Jr: Absence of anatomic arteriovenous shunts in Paget's disease of bone. *N Engl J Med* 1972; 287:686–689.
44. Lequime J, Denolin H: Circulatory dynamics in osteitis deformans. *Circulation*, 1955; 12:215–219.
45. Arnalich F, Plaza I, Sobrino JA, Oliver J, Barbado J, Pena JM, et al: Cardiac size and function in Paget's disease of bone. *Int J Cardiol* 1984; 5:491–505.
46. Gorlin R: The hyperkinetic heart syndrome. *JAMA* 1962; 182:823–829.
47. Gillum RF, Teichholz LE, Herman MV, Gorlin R: The idiopathic hyperkinetic heart syndrome: Clinical course and long-term prognosis. *Am Heart J* 1981; 102:728–734.
48. Fiorentini C, Olivari MT, Moruzzi P, Guazzi, MD: Long-term follow-up of the primary hyperkinetic heart syndrome. *Am J Med* 1981; 71:221–227.
49. Frohlich ED: Beta adrenergic blockade in the circulatory regulation of hyperkinetic states. *Am J Cardiol* 1971; 27:195–199.
50. Burrows B, Kettel LJ, Niden AH, Rabinowitz M, Diener CF: Patterns of cardiovascular dysfunction in chronic obstructive lung disease. *N Engl J Med* 1972; 286:912–918.

51. Fowler NO, Westcott RN, Scott RC, Hess E: The cardiac output in chronic cor pulmonale. *Circulation* 1952; 6:888–893.
52. McIntosh HD, Miller DE, Gleason WL, Goldner JL: The circulatory dynamics of polyostotic fibrous dysplasia. *Am J Med* 1962; 32:393–403.
53. Schwaber JR, Lukas DS: Hyperkinemia and cardiac failure in the carcinoid syndrome. *Am J Med* 1962; 32:846–853.
54. Burch GE, dePasquale N, Hyman A, DeGraff AC: Influence of tropical weather on cardiac output, work, and power of right and left ventricles of man resting in hospital. *AMA Arch Intern Med* 1959; 104:553–560.
55. O'Donnell TF Jr, Clowes GHA Jr: The circulatory abnormalities of heat stroke. *N Engl J Med* 1972; 287:734–737.
56. Bull JM, Lees D, Schuette W, Whang-Peng J, Smith R, Bynum G, et al: Whole body hyperthermia. A phase-1 trial of a potential adjuvant to chemotherapy. *Ann Intern Med* 1979; 90:317–323.
57. Raven PB, Niki I, Dahms TE, Horvath SM: Compensatory cardiovascular responses during environmental cold stress, 5°C. *J Appl Physiol* 1970; 29:417–421.
58. Neff MS, Kim KE, Persoff M, Onesti G, Swartz C: Hemodynamics of uremic anemia. *Circulation* 1971; 43:876–883.
59. Cohen JL, Barooah B, Segal KR, Batuman V: Two-dimensional echocardiographic findings in patients on hemodialysis for more than six months. *Am J Cardiol* 1987; 60:743–745.
60. Hampl H, Schafer GE, Kessel M: Haemodynamic state in severe chronic renal failure. Pathophysiological aspects of cardiovascular function and the importance of bicarbonate dialysis. *Nephron* 1985; 39:102–111.
61. Cobb LA, Kramer RJ, Finch CA: Circulatory effects of chronic hypervolemia in polycythemia vera. *J Clin Invest* 1960; 39:1722–1728.
62. Robson SC, Dunlop W, Hunter S: Haemodynamic changes during the early puerperium. *Br Med J* 1987; 294:1065.
63. Vered Z, Poler SM, Gibson P, Wlody D, Perez JE: Noninvasive detection of the morphologic and hemodynamic changes during normal pregnancy. *Clin Cardiol* 1991; 14:327–334.
64. Pivarnik JM, Lee W, Clark SL, Cotton DB, Spillman HT, Miller JF: Cardiac output responses of primigravid women during exercise determined by the direct Fick technique. *Obstet Gynecol* 1990; 75:954–959.
65. Marin-Neto JA, Maciel BC, Urbanetz LLT, Gallo L Jr, Almeida-Filho OC, Amorim DS: High output failure in patients with peripartum cardiomyopathy: A comparative study with dilated cardiomyopathy. *Am Heart J* 1991; 121(1-pt 1):134–140.
66. Hecht HH and (by invitation) Candiolo BM, Malkinson FD, Nair KG, Saqueton AC: On cardio-cutaneous syndromes. *Trans Assoc Am Phys* 1967; 80:91–96.
67. Bray GA: Obesity and the heart. *Mod Concepts Cardiovasc Dis* 1987; 56:67–71.
68. Messerli FH, Sundgaard-Riise K, Reisin E, Dreslinski G, Dunn FG, Frohlich E: Disparate cardiovascular effects of obesity and arterial hypertension. *Am J Med* 1983; 74:808–812.
69. Nakajima T, Fujioka S, Tokunaga K, Matsuzawa Y, Tarui S: Correlation of intra-abdominal fat accumulation and left ventricular performance in obesity. *Am J Cardiol* 1989; 64:369–373.
70. Ibrahim MM, Tarazi RC, Dustan HP: Hyperkinetic heart in severe hypertension: A separate clinical hemodynamic entity. *Am J Cardiol* 1975; 35:667–674.
71. Fouad FM, Salcedo EE, Saragoca M, Bravo EL, Tarazi RC: Hyperkinetic circulation associated with captopril therapy for congestive heart failure (editorial). *N Engl J Med* 1981; 305:405–406.
72. Isner JM, Dietz WA: Cardiovascular consequences of recombinant DNA technology: Interleukin-2 (editorial). *Ann Intern Med* 1988; 109:933–935.
73. Baumgartner JD, Vaney C, Perret C: An extreme form of the hyperdynamic syndrome in septic shock. *Intens Care Med* 1984; 10:245–249.
74. Parillo JE, Parker MM, Natanson C, Suffredini AF, Danner RL, Cunnion RE, et al: Septic shock in humans. *Ann Intern Med* 1990; 113:227–241.
75. McBride W, Jackman JD Jr, Gammon RS, Willerson JT: High-output cardiac failure in patients with multiple myeloma. *N Engl J Med* 1988; 319:1651–1653.
76. Sanchez FW, Chuang VP, Skolkin MD: Transcatheter treatment of myelomatous AV shunting causing high-output failure. *Cardiovasc Intervent Radiol* 1986; 9:219–221.
77. Dorin RI, Kearns PJ: High output circulatory failure in acute adrenal insufficiency. *Crit Care Med* 1988; 16:296–297.

Chapter 25

Pathophysiology of Heart Failure

Robert C. Schlant, M.D. ■ Edmund H. Sonnenblick, M.D.

DEFINITIONS

The subject of heart failure requires a number of definitions to denote pathology, hemodynamic alterations, and clinical symptoms. The following definitions and classification (Table 25-1) are presented with the realization that future research will allow a much more precise analysis and classification of types of heart failure based on differences in their biochemistry and biophysics.[1–10] More detailed discussions are presented in later sections.

Circulatory Failure

Circulatory failure is a general term that refers to an inadequacy of the cardiovascular system in performing its basic functions of providing nutrition to the cells of the body and removing metabolic products from the cells. It may be caused primarily by either cardiac or noncardiac (peripheral) conditions. Noncardiac conditions that can cause circulatory failure include inadequate blood volume, decreased venous return, increased capacity of the vascular system, peripheral vascular abnormalities or disease, and inadequate oxyhemoglobin.

Circulatory overload or *congestion* is a general term referring to excess blood volume from either cardiac or noncardiac causes.[1] *Noncardiac circulatory overload* may be divided into two categories: (1) those conditions in which the primary defect appears to be an increase in blood volume, as may occur with the accumulation of excess salt and water due to salt-retaining steroids, excess blood or fluid administration, acute glomerulonephritis, oliguria, or anuria; and (2) those conditions in which the primary defect appears to be an increased venous return and/or decreased peripheral resistance, as may occur with arteriovenous fistulas, beriberi, cirrhosis, severe anemia, and so on, and in which the increase in blood volume is secondary. Many patients with noncardiac circulatory overload eventually develop secondary "high-output" heart failure (see Chap. 24).

Heart Failure

Heart failure exists when the heart is unable to pump sufficient blood to meet the metabolic needs of the body at normal filling pressures, provided the venous return to the heart is normal.

Congestive heart failure describes a syndrome with complex and variable symptoms and signs, including

TABLE 25-1

Classification of Circulatory Failure and Circulatory Overload

Circulatory failure
Heart (cardiac) failure
Noncardiac (peripheral) circulatory failure
Decreased return of blood to heart, inadequate blood volume
Increased capacity of vascular bed
Peripheral vascular abnormalities or disease
Inadequate oxyhemoglobin
Circulatory congestion
Cardiac circulatory overload
Heart (cardiac) failure
Noncardiac circulatory overload
Increase in blood volume
Increase in venous return and/or decrease in peripheral vascular resistance

dyspnea and increased fatigability, tachypnea, tachycardia, pulmonary rales, cardiomegaly, ventricular gallop sounds, and peripheral edema. In most patients, congestive heart failure and abnormal circulatory congestion occur as a result of both heart failure and subsequent changes in the peripheral circulation accompanied by activation of the sympathetic nervous system and the renin-angiotensin system. In most patients with clinical congestive heart failure due to mechanical or myocardial abnormalities, the heart (pump) failure is preceded by periods of *myocardial* dysfunction during which cardiac *pump* function and cardiac output (at least while at rest) may be maintained by compensatory mechanisms, including myocardial hypertrophy and ventricular dilatation. Initially the cardiac output fails to increase or may even decline during exercise or stress, and ultimately it is decreased even at rest. These changes are characterized by an increase in peripheral vascular resistance (PVR) at rest and a failure of the PVR to decrease with increased metabolic needs.

When intravascular circulatory congestion is present for any length of time with elevation of left ventricular diastolic and pulmonary venous pressures, increased transudation of fluid from the capillaries into the interstitial spaces occurs. Pulmonary edema develops in the pulmonary circulation if the rate of transudation exceeds the rate of lymphatic drainage. Initially, the edema may be detected by x-ray examination, and later audible rales may be detected on physical examination. In the systemic venous system, venous congestion may be visible and may result in the development of dependent peripheral edema and hepatomegaly. In the majority of patients, congestive heart failure develops chronically and is associated with the retention of sodium and water by the kidneys.

Acute heart failure can develop during acute ischemia of the ventricle, following a myocardial infarction of the left ventricle, following tachycardia, or following the rupture of a cardiac valve or structure. An acute shift of blood from the systemic circulation to the pulmonary circulation may occur before the retention of significant sodium or water. The term *congestive heart failure* should not be used unless there is congestion of cardiac origin. When the cause of the pulmonary or peripheral congestion is not clear, however, it is usually preferable to describe the symptoms or signs, which are nonspecific, and to avoid improperly diagnosing heart failure.

As mentioned above, *heart failure* or *cardiac failure* may be defined as that condition in which the heart is no longer able to pump an adequate supply of blood for the metabolic needs of the body at normal filling pressures of the ventricles, provided there is adequate venous return to the heart. Generally, systolic ventricular dysfunction is characterized by a decrease in stroke volume (SV), with a concomitant increase in end-diastolic volume (EDV) and a normal or somewhat reduced SV, resulting in a decrease in ejection fraction (EF). This relationship of SV to EDV is demonstrated by the Frank-Starling relationship (Fig. 5-14). The increase in EDV is associated with an increase in end-diastolic ventricular pressure (EDP) in consonance with the resting pressure-volume curve. As will be discussed, the filling pressures may be further elevated for a given end-diastolic volume by a thickened (hypertrophied) or fibrotic wall or may be decreased by chronic overdistension. In addition to this primary systolic or "pump" failure, there is often (but not always) an abnormally high diastolic pressure within the ventricle.

In patients with mild heart failure, the ventricular EDP and the cardiac output may be normal at rest, but the ventricular end-diastolic pressure may become elevated to abnormal levels during stress, such as exercise or an increase in afterload. The increase in cardiac output relative to the increase in oxygen consumption is also decreased (see below and Chap. 23). In patients with more severe systolic ventricular failure, both the early diastolic and the end-diastolic pressures may be elevated even at rest. The elevated left ventricular diastolic pressure is reflected in an elevation of pulmonary venous and capillary pressures and in dyspnea, which results from changes in pulmonary compliance due to pulmonary congestion and edema. It is also apparent that before one reaches this stage of clinical heart failure, the body has utilized many compensatory mechanisms after the onset of the initial abnormality or stress and that these compensatory mechanisms eventually have failed to maintain the needs for cardiac output (see below).

Since the fundamental characteristic of heart failure is an inability of the heart as a pump to supply adequately the demands of the body at normal filling pressures, it is apparent that this term could be applicable in a very general sense whenever the demands for increased cardiac output are not met as a result of cardiac limitations. This implies that any heart would eventually "fail" if the demands were increased sufficiently. In fact, this might rarely occur in persons with apparently normal hearts during extreme exertion. In most individuals, however, exertion is stopped prior to heart failure by fatigue or breathlessness, although these symptoms might be related to a limitation of cardiac output.

The causes of overall heart pump failure may be classified into three main categories: (1) failure primarily related to work overloads or mechanical abnormalities, (2) failure primarily related to primary myocardial abnormalities, and (3) failure related to abnormal cardiac rhythm or conduction disturbances (Table 25-2). Myocardial infarction may also be included as a special type of work overload. During the acute infarction, the EF falls as the EDV is increased to sustain SV, and this fall in EF is approximately proportional to the amount of myocardium lost. With time, the EF tends to remain at this reduced level. With healing of the infarction, this akinetic area does not contribute to ventricular emptying and may even contribute to the load. Thus, the entire load falls on the remaining nonischemic myocardium. This load is further increased by the increased diastolic volume, which causes wall tension to be increased for any given pressure and the nonischemic myocardium to hypertrophy in proportion to the amount of myocardium that is lost. Heart failure may ensue months or years later as a so-called *ischemic cardiomyopathy* that results from ventricular dilatation and reactive hypertrophy, termed *ventricular remodeling*, even in the absence of wall ischemia (see Chap. 61). Although heart failure is usually considered to be due to ventricular failure, atrial failure (see below) can contribute significantly.

TABLE 25-2
General Causes of Overall Heart Pump Failure

Mechanical abnormalities
Increased pressure load
Central (aortic stenosis, etc.)
Peripheral (systemic arterial hypertension, etc.)
Increased volume load (valvular regurgitation, shunts, increased venous return, etc.)
Obstruction to ventricular filling (mitral or tricuspid stenosis)
Pericardial constriction, tamponade
Endocardial or myocardial restriction
Ventricular aneurysm
Ventricular dyssynergy
Myocardial (muscular) abnormalities or loss of myocytes
Primary abnormalities or loss of myocytes
Cardiomyopathy
Neuromuscular disorders
Myocarditis
Metabolic (diabetes mellitus, etc.)
Toxic (alcohol, cobalt, etc.)
Presbycardia
Secondary myocardial abnormalities or loss of myocytes
Dysdynamic (secondary to mechanical abnormalities)
Ischemia (coronary heart disease)
Metabolic
Inflammation
Infiltrative diseases
Systemic diseases
Chronic obstructive lung disease
Myocardial depression due to drugs
Altered cardiac rhythm or conduction disturbances
Standstill
Fibrillation
Extreme tachycardia or bradycardia
Chronic tachycardia
Electrical asynchrony, conduction disturbances

There are several causes of both "primary" and "secondary" myocardial failure (Table 25-2). Myocardial failure is said to be *primary* when it is caused by (1) idiopathic cardiomyopathy (dilated, hypertrophic, or restrictive; (Chaps. 87–91); (2) cardiomyopathy due to a primary neuromuscular disease, such as Friedreich's ataxia, myotonic dystrophy, or Duchenne's muscular dystrophy (Chap. 96); (3) myocarditis (Chap. 88); (4) metabolic deficiencies that may affect the myocardium, such as diabetes mellitus, beriberi, and possibly hyper- or hypothyroidism (Chap. 102); (5) toxic effects of radiation, electricity, or chemicals, such as alcohol or cobalt (Chaps. 105 and 110); or (6) the process of aging, where myocytes are lost diffusely and progressively with reactive hypertrophy and focal fibrosis (Chap. 115).

Myocardial failure is said to be *secondary* (Table 25-2) when it is produced by (1) "dysdynamic" myocardial failure (see below); (2) myocardial ischemia, which may produce either an acute, "dysdynamic" myocardial failure or chronic, static failure due to a specific heart muscle disease with loss of myocytes and myocardial fibrosis, as noted above (Chaps. 57 and 61), (3) metabolic disorders, such as acromegaly, hypoparathyroidism, pheochromocytoma, and occasionally thyroid disease, or toxins (Chaps. 102, 110); (4) myocardial inflammation (Chap. 88); (5) myocardial infiltrative disorders and restrictive cardiomyopathies (Chap. 91); (6) systemic diseases (Chaps. 102–108); (7) acute or chronic lung disease (Chaps. 99–101); or (8) depression due to drugs, such as adriamycin (Chap. 110). The distinction between primary and secondary myocardial failure is frequently difficult and occasionally arbitrary. For example, in diabetes mellitus, heart muscle disease or cardiomyopathy may develop, most commonly associated with hypertension and diffuse myocyte loss. This loss may be due to microvascular spasm and focal ischemia.

The cause of left ventricular systolic dysfunction in patients with chronic obstructive lung disease is unknown, although the combination of hypoxia and hypercapnia may be important. Left ventricular diastolic dysfunction in such patients is, in part, secondary to the pronounced right ventricular hypertrophy and dilatation with secondary elevation of left ventricular diastolic pressure due to ventricular interdependence. The latter phenomenon is also important in the pathophysiology of acute pulmonary edema occasionally encountered in patients with acute pulmonary embolus.

Dysdynamic myocardial failure is a general term used to refer to the common forms of secondary myocardial failure that commonly develop after a period of increased ventricular preload or afterload. In response to an increased load, myocytes hypertrophy in accord with the Laplace relationship, as discussed below. When this adaptation is inadequate, ventricular dilatation ensues. These changes, together with any myocyte loss and resultant fibrosis, are termed *ventricular remodeling;* myocardial failure is a late stage in the process. Dysdynamic failure is frequently associated with hypokinesis, akinesis, and dyskinesis. The term *dysdynamic* (i.e., with impaired force or power) *myocardial failure* implied that the *systolic* mechanical performance, or myocardial contractility per unit mass, is significantly decreased; initially, however, the overall cardiac (pump) function may be maintained by the compensatory mechanisms noted above, and the cardiac output at rest may not be abnormally decreased.

In general, patients' symptoms are related to congestive heart failure, whereas patient survival is related to myocardial failure (Fig. 25-1).

Myocardial Failure

Myocardial dysfunction may be used to denote performance that is reduced, while *myocardial failure* refers to a more markedly decreased performance of the myocardium. When used in reference to myocardium, *function* has usually referred to systolic or shortening function, although there may also be diastolic abnormalities in the presence of minimal or no significant systolic abnormalities. In many patients with moderate or more marked myocardial dysfunction or myocardial failure, the decreased myocardial function can be detected by studies of overall cardiac pump function, whereas milder dys-

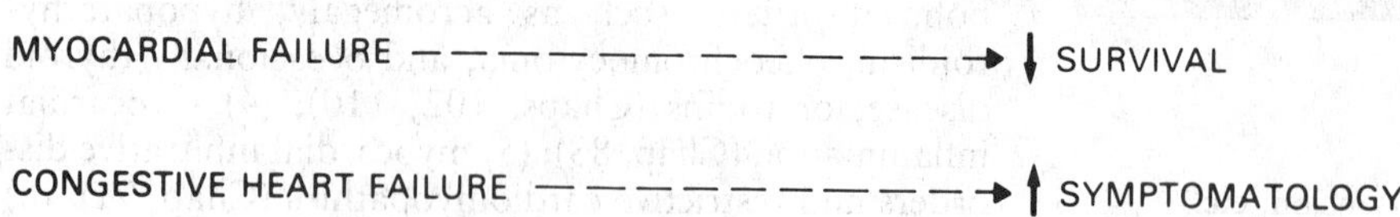

FIGURE 25-1 In general, the survival of patients with heart failure is related to the degree of myocardial failure, whereas their symptoms are related more to congestive heart failure and its compensatory mechanisms. See text for details.

function in other patients may be detected only by more specific and sensitive indices of myocardial contractility (see Chap. 23). In many patients with myocardial dysfunction or even myocardial failure, the overall cardiac pump function (and cardiac output at rest) may be maintained reasonably well by compensatory mechanisms such as increased ventricular filling or preload with dilatation and/or cardiac hypertrophy.

Myocardial failure may develop from many causes (Table 25-3). It may evolve from pressure overloads in which myocytes hypertrophy to meet the load. Hypertrophied cells contract and relax more slowly[11] and may be subject to metabolic limitations. When age-related myocyte loss is added, particularly in association with a late decrease in myocyte contractile activity, failure ensues with ventricular dilatation. Loss of myocytes—whether segmental, as in acute myocardial infarction, or diffuse, as in myocarditis—leads to reactive hypertrophy

TABLE 25-3

Possible Mechanisms of Myocardial Failure
Loss of myocytes
Hypertrophy of remaining myocytes
Energy production and utilization
Oxygen and energy supply
Substrate utilization and energy storage
Inadequate mitochondria mass and function
Ventricular remodeling
Contractile proteins
Abnormal myofibrillar or myosin ATPase
Abnormal myocardial proteins
Defective protein synthesis
Nonuniformity of contraction and function
Activation of contractile elements
Membrane $Na^+ - K^+$ – ATPase defects
Abnormal sarcoplasmic reticulum function
Abnormal CA^{2+} release
Abnormal CA^{2+} uptake
Abnormal myocardial receptor function
Down-regulation of beta adrenoreceptors
Decreased β_1 receptors
Decreased G_s protein
Increased G_1 protein
Autonomic nervous system
Abnormal myocardial norepinephrine function or kinetics
Abnormal baroreceptor function
Increased myocardial fibroblast growth and collagen synthesis
Aging changes, presbycardia
Sustained tachycardia
Miscellaneous

in remaining myocytes. As compensatory hypertrophy becomes more marked in some disease states, the unit contractility of the myocardium often declines. This is especially likely to occur in response to pressure overload, as in systemic hypertension or aortic stenosis, but also ensues when myocytes are lost.

Ultimately, the myocardial failure (plus mechanical abnormalities that may be present) often leads to a decrease in systolic pump function that is sufficient to produce overall pump or heart failure. In most patients, significant dysfunction and failure of the myocardium occurs before heart (pump) dysfunction or failure and the clinical syndrome of congestive heart failure become apparent (see Chap. 23).

Although both systolic and diastolic dysfunction or failure are present in the majority of patients with heart failure, and contraction and relaxation of the ventricle are coupled in patients with and without heart failure,[12] it is useful to consider separately the systolic and the diastolic properties of the myocardium and of the ventricle.[13] Thus, some patients may have marked *systolic ventricular dysfunction* or *failure* at a time when they do not have significant, if any, elevation of ventricular diastolic pressures. On the other hand, some patients have marked elevation of left ventricular diastolic pressure and pulmonary congestion (*diastolic dysfunction of the ventricle*) at a time when the systolic or pumping function of the ventricle, as characterized by a normal (≥50 percent) EF, is well maintained. The latter situation is especially likely to occur in some patients with hypertrophic cardiomyopathy, systemic hypertension, or aortic stenosis. In these patients the elevated ventricular diastolic pressure may be present due to a combination of the effects of ventricular hypertrophy and myocardial diastolic dysfunction at a time when the systolic function or cardiac output may be normal or even slightly elevated. In patients with severe pressure overload hypertrophy, the duration of contraction is prolonged and relaxation is delayed.[11] As a result, systole occupies a greater proportion of time. This effect is amplified by tachycardia, which may produce a high filling pressure for any given diastolic volume (i.e., diastolic dysfunction) despite well-maintained contractile force and EF. Acute, transient diastolic dysfunction may also occur in patients with coronary artery disease, with or without angina pectoris.[14–20] In general, most, but not all, patients with acute diastolic failure of the myocardium also have some systolic abnormalities of contraction.

High-Output Failure

Some patients with high-output states or primary noncardiac circulatory overload may develop pulmonary congestion and edema secondary to an abnormal elevation of ventricular diastolic pressure at a time when the total cardiac output (systolic, or pump, function) and EF of the left ventricle is normal or even increased (see Chap. 24). The latter syndrome can also occur in conditions associated with an increase in blood volume from the accumulation of excess salt and water due to salt-retaining steroids, excess blood or fluid administration, acute glomerulonephritis, oliguria, or anuria. In other patients, it may occur with an abnormally increased venous return and/or decreased peripheral resistance, as might occur in patients with arteriovenous fistulas, beriberi, hyperthyroidism, cirrhosis, severe anemia, and so on. Under such conditions, the chronic volume and/or pressure load on the ventricle may eventually produce myocardial and ventricular systolic (pump) dysfunction or failure. Ultimately, this can result in the reduction of cardiac output to abnormally low levels. Indeed, some part of this diastolic dysfunction results from systolic dysfunction. When symptoms of pulmonary congestion or pulmonary edema secondary to elevated diastolic pressure occur while the cardiac output is still normal or elevated, the syndrome is sometimes referred to as *high-output failure* (see Chap. 24).

Forward and Backward Failure

Forward failure and *backward failure* are expressions that have been used historically with somewhat different meanings. In oversimplified terms, *forward failure* was used to imply that most of the patient's symptoms and signs resulted from a low cardiac output, with easy fatigability, weakness, mental confusion, or even shock. *Backward failure* was used to imply that most of the patient's symptoms and signs resulted from elevation of venous pressure behind the failing ventricle or ventricles. This elevation of venous pressure was usually thought to be caused by the inability of the ventricle to empty itself properly or by obstruction of ventricular filling (mitral or tricuspid stenosis). The two expressions were also used in reference to concepts of the pathogenesis of the retention of salt and water. Even though the expressions are oversimplifications in this regard, they still have limited usefulness as clinical descriptors of clinical symptom-sign complexes. Thus, when the symptoms and signs are predominantly related to pulmonary or systemic venous congestion, backward failure may be said to exist. Conversely, if the symptoms are due to a marked decrease in cardiac output, forward cardiac failure, which is often acute, may be said to exist. It is likely that the terms will be used less frequently in the future.

"Left-" and "Right-Heart" Failure

"Left-heart" (left-sided) failure and *"right-heart" (right-sided) failure* are clinical terms for conditions in which the primary impairment is of the left side of the heart or of the right side of the heart, respectively. Since both sides of the heart are in a circuit, it is apparent that one side cannot pump significantly more blood than the other side for any length of time in the absence of abnormal shunts, communications, or regurgitation. Furthermore, experimentally produced failure of one ventricle may produce significant hemodynamic and biochemical abnormalities of the other ventricle, even without the usual hemodynamic manifestations of ventricular failure. Abnormal function of the left ventricle is not only reflected onto the right ventricle from augmented pulmonary pressures but may also affect the right ventricle via the shared septum and the phenomenon of ventricular interdependence, or interaction (see below). Altered elastic recoil of the left ventricle in diastole may also affect the right ventricle. Accordingly, even though the pumping ability of one ventricle may be primarily impaired, the output of the contralateral ventricle is secondarily decreased; the biochemistry and hemodynamics of the contralateral ventricle can also be abnormal even in "pure" one-sided failure.

Right-sided heart failure commonly follows left-sided heart failure. In most situations, the expression *left-sided heart failure* is clinically used in reference to symptoms and signs of elevated pressure and congestion in the pulmonary veins and capillaries, whereas *right-sided heart failure* is used in reference to symptoms and signs of elevated pressures and congestion in the systemic veins and capillaries. Actually, significant amounts of sodium and water retention, with subsequent peripheral edema formation, may occur with pure left-sided heart failure without hemodynamic evidence of right-sided heart failure. As noted previously, an increase in the diastolic pressure in either ventricle can increase the diastolic pressure or decrease the distensibility of the contralateral ventricle, especially if the pericardium is intact.

Compensated Heart Failure

Compensated heart failure is that condition in which the symptoms of heart failure are relieved by therapy, although the EDV and EDP often remain elevated and the EF remains reduced. As noted below, the usual "compensatory" mechanisms include increase sympathetic adrenergic stimulation of the heart, activation of the renal renin-angiotensin system, neurohumoral activation with increased vasoconstriction, fluid retention by the kidney with increased venous return and increased ventricular preload, and cardiac dilatation and hypertrophy. Clinically, myocardial compensation and a decrease in congestion may be produced by improved ventricular performance, and a decrease in congestion may be produced by digitalis glycosides, diuretics, or vasodilator drugs. The term *compensated heart failure* is frequently used in reference to patients with congestive heart failure whose symptoms and signs of pulmonary or peripheral congestion are relieved by diuretic therapy. In many such patients, reduced myocardial function and cardiac output persist, although symptoms are relieved by an improvement in peripheral circulation and the reduction in edema and congestion.

Atrial Failure

Although isolated atrial failure rarely, if ever, produces failure of the normal heart, the development of atrial fibrillation or flutter can precipitate heart failure in patients with compensated heart failure, especially when marked ventricular hypertrophy or diastolic dysfunction is present and when an "atrial kick" is important in maintaining cardiac output (see below). In the presence of severe hypertrophy of the left ventricle, the left atrium may play an important role in augmenting late diastolic filling and thus reducing mean filling pressures.

Stages of Heart Failure

Heart failure is a progressive disease, both in terms of cardiac function and the development of congestive heart failure. Later, the peripheral circulatory changes may become the dominant factor in the development of congestive heart failure and the evolution of symptoms (see below).

BASIC MECHANISMS OF MYOCARDIAL FAILURE

The basic biochemical and biophysical mechanisms of myocardial failure remain a very active area of investigation. It is likely that no single mechanism is present in all cases but, rather, that various mechanisms (Table 25-3) may contribute to myocardial failure under various circumstances. Moreover, many adaptive processes have been identified within the process of cardiac hypertrophy and heart failure. It is not clear which of these processes are central and primarily responsible for the progression of the disease and which are secondary. It should be emphasized that the following is an oversimplification of very complex processes, and the reader may want to consult more detailed references in this rapidly developing field.

Energy Production and Utilization

Oxygen and Energy Supply

Most patients with heart failure have a normal coronary blood flow at rest and a normal or elevated myocardial oxygen consumption per 100 g of tissue.[21] The total amount of oxygen consumed by the heart may be significantly increased because of the increased total mass, the increase in myocardial systolic wall tension due to the Laplace relationship in patients with heart failure, and perhaps some wasted contractile energy. This increase may result in the extraction of a greater amount of oxygen from each unit of coronary blood flow and a widening of the coronary arteriovenous oxygen difference. Many patients with heart failure are able to increase coronary blood flow during exercise; however, some patients with a dilated ventricle that increases in diameter during exercise may have a further widening of the coronary arteriovenous oxygen difference during exercise (Chaps. 5 and 23). In the presence of severe left ventricular hypertrophy, coronary blood flow is normal per unit mass of myocardium. On the other hand, the capacity of the coronary vascular bed to dilate during reactive hyperemia, which is normally four- to fivefold, is reduced. Nevertheless, no primary deficit in coronary blood flow or oxygen delivery has been demonstrated in heart failure associated with hypertrophy, except in the presence of obstructive coronary disease.

Substrate Utilization and Energy Storage

Although the myocardial uptake of fatty acids and glucose per 100 g of myocardium is normal in heart failure,[21] there is conflicting evidence on whether or not there is a primary decrease in energy liberation by mitochondrial oxidative phosphorylation.[4,5,21–25a] Although reductions in stores of myocardial high-energy phosphate, creatine phosphate (CP), and/or adenosine triphosphate (ATP) have often been found in heart failure, these changes are usually thought to be secondary and to be the consequence of the failure rather than the primary cause of the failure.[4,5,21–27] There also may be reduced levels of creatine kinase and changes in the isoenzymes of creatine kinase in heart failure (see Chap. 6A).[28–30]

Mitochondria Mass and Function

A significant decrease in the mass of mitochondria relative to the mass of myofibrils occurs in experimental cardiac hypertrophy.[31–34] It is possible that this is one of the limitations of severe hypertrophy. Defects in mitochondrial oxidative phosphorylation and in mitochondrial calcium metabolism may also be associated with myocardial failure.[21–25a,35–37] Except in circumstances where coronary flow is limited, such as with large vessel obstructive disease (Chap. 57) or purported microvascular obstructive or vasospastic disease, a primary role of energy limitation in the evolution of heart failure has yet to be demonstrated.[38] It is possible that it may play a role during periods of higher metabolic demand, such as tachycardia.[39]

Ventricular Remodeling

As noted in Chap. 5, when myocardial sarcomeres function at lengths up to the L_{max} at about 2.2 μm, they operate on the *ascending limb* of the length-tension curve and develop more active tension with increasing length (the Frank-Starling relationship). When the muscle strips and sarcomeres are stretched beyond the length at which maximal active tension is developed (L_{max}), however, the amount of active tension decreases and the sarcomeres are said to be operating on the *descending limb* of the length-tension curve[3,4,39a–47] (Fig. 5-16). The existence of a descending limb of cardiac function for the intact ventricle is highly unlikely, however, and much of the apparent decrease in function in some experimental studies was probably due to an increase in afterload associated with fluid overloading, the Laplace relationship of increased tension with increased ventricular volume, or to mitral regurgitation produced by ventricular dilatation.[44–46] At one time it was thought that sarcomere "overstretch" might be responsible for the decreased myocardial contractility with ventricular dilatation and heart failure. Subsequent studies showed, however, that acute volume loading is associated with an increase in left ventricular midwall mean sarcomere length to about L_{max} (2.2 to 2.4 μm after fixation) but not beyond. With chronic volume loading, there is additional recruitment of subendocardial and subepicardial sarcomere length to L_{max} but no sarcomere overstretch.[39a–41,47]

Other changes that contribute to the marked ventricular dilatation that is frequently present with volume overload include the synthesis of sarcomeres in series with preexisting sarcomeres, "slippage" of myofibrils and myocardial fibers, and rearrangement of myocardial fibers along cleavage planes of the left ventricle.[3,4,39a–44,47] Thus, although overstretch of sarcomeres may rarely be present very transiently, it does not appear to be an important primary mechanism of chronic heart failure. The effects of ventricular dilatation upon the law of Laplace have been noted above. Nonuniformity of myocardial contraction and functional mitral regurgitation also contribute to pump (heart) failure.[11,48]

Contractile Proteins

Myofibrillar and myosin adenosine triphosphatase (ATPase) are decreased as hypertrophy occurs, both in patients and in experimental animals with heart failure.[22,49–58] This correlates with a reduction in the velocity of shortening of the myocardium associated with hypertrophy. At the same time, the duration of contraction is prolonged and relaxation slowed, although the force of contraction is maintained. Thus, these changes may be viewed as an adaptation to load and not a cause of systolic failure. Slowed relaxation, however, can contribute to diastolic dysfunction.

In small animals, the decrease in myosin ATPase is associated with increased synthesis of slower V3 isoenzymes of myosin and a decrease in the faster V1 component. In humans, V3 is normally the entire component,[59] and the decreased ATPase activity may result from other alterations, perhaps in the troponin-tropomyosin system.

Heart failure in idiopathic dilated cardiomyopathy may be related to a decrease in levels of gene expression for phospholamban, a regulatory protein associated with the CA^{2+}—ATPase of the sarcoplasmic reticulum,[60] or for the proteolytic breakdown of a myosin light chain (LC2).[61] In other patients with heart failure due to idiopathic dilated cardiomyopathy or coronary artery disease, decreased expression of the human sarcoplasmic reticular Ca^{2+}—ATPase gene has been noted.[62–64]

Activation of Contractile Elements

Sarcolemma ATPase and Activating Ca^{2+}

Heart failure may also be associated with defects in the activity of the membrane transport enzyme Na^+-K^+-ATPase or the sarcolemmal transport of Ca^{2+},[4,65–67] although the role of these changes in the pathogenesis of myocardial failure is less definite.[22] In humans, in whom the V_3 isoenzyme system predominates, changes in the enzyme systems of the sarcolemmal and sarcoplasmic reticulum (SR) may be central to the slowing of contraction seen in hypertrophy and heart failure.

Sarcoplasmic Reticulum Function

There is substantial evidence of defects in both Ca^{2+} release and Ca^{2+} uptake by SR, which is accomplished by a Ca^{2+}-Mg^{2+}-dependent ATPase under the influence of phospholamban or by mitochondria in many types of clinical or experimental hypertrophy and heart failure.[6,9,22,35,68–90] These abnormalities of calcium metabolism appear to be of primary importance in some types of failure, whereas they may be secondary in other types. Intracellular acidosis decreases the affinity of troponin-C for Ca^{2+} and may contribute to some forms of heart failure, especially those associated with ischemia.[91] Patients with coronary artery disease may also have transient episodes of abnormal diastolic relaxation of the myocardium with acute changes in diastolic compliance that can produce an acute "stiff heart syndrome" and pulmonary edema.[14,20] These episodes, which may occur with or without angina pectoris, are thought to be caused by abnormalities of the intracellular uptake of Ca^{2+} by SR.[15–20] The amount of activator Ca^{2+} available for contraction can also be reduced by alterations in either intracellular Na^+ or K^+.[4,73,74,86,92]

The significance of abnormalities in the release of Ca^{2+} from SR in chronic myocardial failure is uncertain. As noted in Chap. 5, calcium release from SR is triggered by the increase of Ca^{2+} associated with the slow Ca^{2+} current of the action potential. It is also possible that Ca^{2+} release from the SR may be induced in the myocardium by inositol triphosphate or guanosine triphosphate, although this has not been well documented, especially in larger mammals. Most abnormalities of myocardial activation have been demonstrated only in the very late stages of the heart failure process. Thus, alterations in these systems may be the result of heart failure rather than its primary cause.

Myocardial Receptor Function

Myocardial beta-adrenergic receptor density and the production of "second-messenger" cAMP are decreased in heart failure due to down-regulation,[93–107] whereby the receptor remains but is not on the membrane surface. This may be the result of increased circulating catecholamines that are not buffered (i.e., removed from receptor sites) by dysfunctional sympathetic nerve terminals. Indeed, in severe heart failure, norepinephrine stores in sympathetic nerve endings are depleted, and these nerves neither synthesize, store, nor normally release catecholamines. Thus, the failing myocardium becomes functionally denervated, leaving exposed β_1-receptors. In the nonfailing human ventricular myocardium, the total beta-receptor density is approximately 90 fmol/mg, with the β_1 and β_2 proportions 80 and 20 percent, respectively. Most of the decrease in total beta-receptor density in failing myocardium is from a selective decrease in β_1 receptors.[93,97,108–112a] As a consequence, β_2-receptors constitute about 40 percent of the total beta-receptors in the failing human myocardium. The decrease in β_1-receptor density and beta-adrenoreceptor down-regulation probably account for much of the decrease in inotropic potential under the influence of beta-adrenergic receptors.

Although β_2-receptor density is relatively well preserved, the maximal adenylate cyclase response is decreased about 30 to 35 percent.[98] The H_2-histamine, the A_1 adenosine, and the α_1-receptor pathways appear to be relatively normal in heart failure.[113–116] There is evidence that the vasoactive intestinal peptide (VIP) receptors appear to be decreased in heart failure but to have increased receptor affinity, with a supersensitive dose-responsive curve.

Heart failure is associated with altered levels of G proteins (guanine nucleotide-binding regulatory proteins), which couple receptors to effector enzymes and which either stimulate or inhibit adenylate cyclase.[111,116b–125] Thus, there is evidence of a decrease in stimulatory guanyl nucleotide-binding protein (Gs)[111,117,126] and of an increase in inhibitory guanyl nucleotide-binding protein (G_i).[124,125,127–129] In terms of the changes in G_s and G_i, there are potentially important differences between patients with heart failure due to coronary artery disease and patients with failure due to idiopathic dilated cardiomyopathy.[125] Adenylate cyclase activity may also be decreased in heart failure.[104,130]

Autonomic Nervous System

In congestive heart failure, there are defects both in cardiac sympathetic neurotransmitters and in the cardiac parasympathetic control system.[5,93,131–154] These changes are not thought to be primary causes of the myocardial failure, although they may contribute significantly to its progression. The myocardial concentration of norepinephrine (NE) is significantly decreased (see "Compensatory Mechanisms" below).

Connective Tissue

Collagen and connective tissue increase during the process of hypertrophy and also following the loss of myocytes.[155–164] These changes in the cardiac skeleton, which have been termed *interstial heart disease,*[161] can contribute to the alterations of both diastolic and systolic function in the failing myocardium.[25,163] It may be significant that connective tissue hypertrophy regresses more slowly than myocyte hypertrophy in experimental studies of hypertrophy due to pressure loading. In addition, the collagen of the hypertrophied, pressure-overloaded myocardium apparently differs from that of normal myocardium. It is difficult, however, to separate alterations of loading due to increased fibrous tissue from those reflecting myocyte loss. The increase in fibrillar collagen not only increases myocardial stiffness but may also predispose to abnormal electrical dispersion.[160] Quantitative and qualitative changes in the connective tissue framework of the heart probably play a significant role in the ventricular remodeling process associated with various types of congestive heart failure and require further definition.

Senile Cardiomyopathy, Presbycardia, or Senile Heart Disease

With aging, many organs have diminished function, and the heart is no exception. In some elderly individuals, involutional changes of the myocardium may be associated with decreased elasticity of the skeleton of the heart and with mild fibrotic changes of the valves. In rats, myocytes appear to be lost as a process of aging, and the same process occurs in humans.[165] Thus, reactive hypertrophy may occur in the aged from the loss of cells and also as a consequence of the systolic hypertension resulting from decreased compliance of the aging aorta (see Chap. 115). The chemical basis of these aging changes and of the associated brown pigmentation of the heart is not known. This condition, known as *presbycardia, senile heart disease,* or *senile cardiomyopathy,* probably only rarely produces heart failure by itself; however, it does decrease the contractility, the rate of relaxation, and the adaptive reserve capacity of the heart.[166–171] Accordingly, patients with this condition more readily develop heart failure in the presence of other forms of heart disease or occasionally even from the increased demands of fever, moderate anemia, excess tachycardia, mild hyperthyroidism, excess fluid administration, myocardial ischemia, or a relatively small myocardial infarction. Aged myocardium has also been shown to have a diminished inotropic response to catecholamines[172,172a] (see Chap. 115).

Sustained Tachycardia

Experimentally, right ventricular pacing of dogs and pigs, usually at rates of about 240 to 260 beats per minute, produces a syndrome of heart failure after a few weeks that is similar to heart failure from idiopathic dilated cardiomyopathy in human beings and that may be reversible.[173–195] Clinically, sustained tachycardia can produce heart failure, especially in older patients or patients with marked ventricular hypertrophy.

Miscellaneous Mechanisms

Several other factors occur in heart failure that may contribute secondarily to myocardial heart failure. These factors include an increase in free radical production,[196] myocardial interstitial edema,[197] and direct toxic effects on myocardial cells from NE[198] and angiotensin II.[199]

COMPENSATORY MECHANISMS IN HEART FAILURE

Many of the adjustments and adaptations to heart failure are similar to the homeostatic mechanisms utilized by the body in response to circulatory failure from any cause, such as acute blood loss and acute myocardial infarction. Many of these neurohumoral compensatory mechanisms (Table 25-4) are also utilized by normal subjects during exercise or during periods of increased stress (see Chap. 5). In human beings with heart failure, it is often impossible to separate the many complex mechanisms of adjustment, many of which affect and modify one another. In patients with mild heart failure, these compensatory mechanisms are often able to restore to normal or near normal the arterial blood pressure, the organ perfusion, and the cardiac output at rest and at times during moderate exercise. When the failure is mild, no symptoms or clinically apparent organ dysfunction may result from these "compensatory" mechanisms. Eventually, however, many of the symptoms, signs, and organ dysfunction (and even death) that occur in patients with heart failure result from some of these same adaptive mechanisms (Fig. 25-2; see also Chaps. 9A and 23).

TABLE 25-4
Compensatory Mechanisms in Heart Failure

Autonomic nervous system
  Heart
    Increased heart rate
    Increased myocardial contractile stimulation
    Increased rate of relaxation
  Peripheral circulation
    Arterial vasoconstriction (increased afterload)
    Venous vasoconstriction (increased preload)
Kideny (renin-angiotensin-aldosterone)
  Arterial vasoconstriction (increased afterload)
  Venous vasoconstriction (increased preload)
  Sodium and water retention (increased preload and afterload)
  Increased myocardial contractile stimulation
Endothelin 1 (increased preload and afterload)
Arginine vasopressin (increased preload and afterload)
Atrial natriuretic peptides (decreased afterload)
Prostaglandins
Peptides
Frank-Starling law of the heart
  Increased end-diastolic fiber length, volume, and pressure (increased preload)
Hypertrophy
Peripheral oxygen delivery
    Redistribution of cardiac output
    Altered oxygen-hemoglobin dissociation
    Increased oxygen extraction by tissues
Anaerobic metabolism

Autonomic Nervous System

One of the more important acute adjustments to heart failure is a reflex increase in autonomic sympathetic excitation of the heart and most arteries and veins.[4,131,132,200–206] Generalized arterial vasoconstriction and an increase in venous tone are produced by the increased sympathetic activity, in combination with increased plasma concentrations of NE,[207] angiotensin II,[6] vasopressin,[141,208,209] endothelin-1,[210–216] neuropeptide Y,[217–220] and tumor necrosis factor[221–223] together with reduced endothelial-dependent vasodilatation[223–227] and reduced calcitonin gene-related peptide (CGRP).[228] Plasma aldosterone levels are frequently elevated.[229,230] Table 25-5 summarizes the neurohumoral changes that may occur in heart failure. The increased platelet activity reported in patients with heart failure[230a,230b] may result from these changes.

The increased sympathetic adrenergic stimulation of the heart is associated with an inhibition of cardiac parasympathetic activity.[132] An acute increase in sympathetic impulses to the heart normally stimulates the local release of NE and thereby produces beta stimulation with an increase in heart rate and an increase in myocardial contractility. NE also increases the rate of ventricular relaxation, which further contributes to increased ventricular filling. In addition, the generalized increased sympathetic activity and the release of NE from the adrenal medulla and the peripheral blood vessels contribute to increasing myocardial contractility.

Patients with chronic congestive heart failure have a significant decrease in the myocardial concentration of NE.[3,4,137,231,232] This is associated with decreased activity of myocardial tyrosine hydroxylase, which is the rate-limiting enzyme in the synthesis of NE.[138] It is of interest to note that, when right ventricular hypertrophy and failure are experimentally produced, the myocardial NE concentration is decreased in both the right and the left ventricle.[139] In experimental chronic heart failure, there is a decrease in the amount of myocardial NE released per nerve impulse as well as defects in the synthesis, uptake, and binding of NE.[137] On the other hand, net myocardial NE release may be markedly increased in patients with early heart failure,[233,234] perhaps related to a defective reuptake mechanism at the nerve endings for

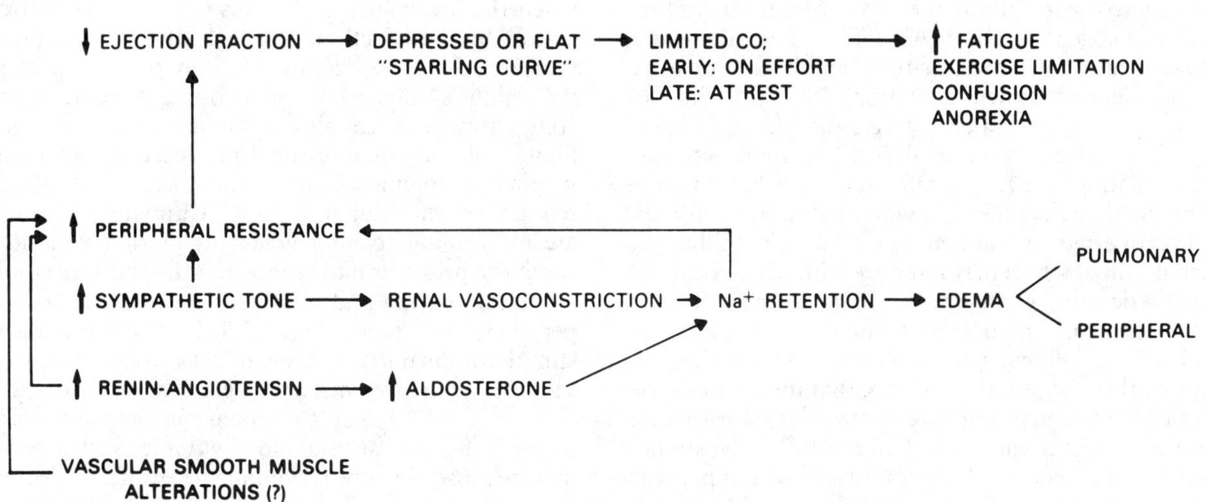

FIGURE 25-2 Schema of events in congestive heart failure leading to symptoms. Note that fatigue and other symptoms of limited cardiac output are primarily related to a decreased ejection fraction, whereas peripheral and pulmonary edema are related to Na^+ and water retention from increased sympathetic tone and increased renin-angiotensin-aldosterone. See text for details.

TABLE 25-5
Neurohumoral Changes in Heart Failure

Changes that increase vascular systemic resistance
Increased sympathetic nervous system activity (increased norepinephrine, epinephrine)
Increased endothelin
Increased arginine vasopressin
Increased renin and angiotensin II
Increased aldosterone
Increased neuropeptide Y
Increased tumor necrosis factor
Reduced endothelial-dependent vasodilatation
Reduced calcintonin gene-related peptide
Reduced parasympathetic nervous system activity
Impaired baroreceptor activity
Increased vasoconstrictor prostaglandins, kinines
Changes that decrease systemic vascular resistance
Increased atrial natriuretic peptide
Increased dopamine
Increased vasodilator prostaglandins (PGI_2, PGE_2)
Increased vasodilator peptides, (e.g., bradykinin, kalliden)

NOTE: Changes in individual patients vary significantly and changes may not always be present.

locally released NE.[235,236] In general, the arterial concentrations of NE and dopamine in patients with moderate to severe congestive heart failure are elevated at rest and increase more than normally during mild or moderate exercise.[237-240] This elevation of NE appears to be due predominantly to an increased synthesis in the peripheral vasculature and the adrenal medulla.[207] There is, however, a blunted response of plasma NE release during a 60 percent upright tilt.[241] The high plasma levels of NE and angiotensin II may potentiate the hypertrophic response of the remaining myocytes. Plasma epinephrine concentrations are only inconsistently increased in patients with heart failure.[239] Increased serum norepinephrine levels may also produce myocellular damage per se and further the progression of heart failure.[198]

Although the myocardial synthesis of NE is impaired in congestive heart failure, the myocardium can still respond to exogenous NE.[139] As noted above, there is a decreased catecholamine sensitivity and beta-adrenergic receptor density (down-regulation) in failing human hearts.[93,232,242] In general, however, the failing heart is responsive and may even be dependent upon extracardiac circulating NE. As a result, congestive heart failure is sometimes made somewhat worse by the acute administration of drugs such as beta blockers, guanethidine, or reserpine, all of which may interfere with the myocardial sympathetic adrenergic system. In many patients this effect is generally modest and often does not prevent their use (e.g., following acute myocardial infarction). In addition, there is growing evidence that the cautious use of beta blockers may improve ventricular performance in selected patients with heart failure.[243-255] A few studies have found no benefit[256-259] or found a benefit in patients with dilated cardiomyopathy but no benefit in heart failure due to coronary artery disease[249] (see Chap. 26).

In general, however, the defective synthesis and the depletion of myocardial NE do not appear to be major, primary causes of myocardial failure, although they may be important contributing mechanisms. Patients with chronic congestive heart failure may also have a significant depression of the normal parasympathetic nervous control of the heart.[133]

In patients with heart failure, the complex reflex actions of the autonomic nervous system and the local autoregulatory mechanisms tend to preserve circulation to the brain and heart while decreasing blood flow to the skin, skeletal muscles, splanchnic organs, and kidneys.[260-262] The increased sympathetic adrenergic stimulation of the peripheral arteries and the increased concentrations of circulating NE, angiotensin II, endothelin-1, and vasopressin contribute to arteriolar vasoconstriction, the maintenance of arterial pressure, and an increase in venous tone, which help to maintain venous return and ventricular filling and to support cardiac performance by Starling's law of the heart.[203] The arterial and arteriolar resistance of patients with congestive heart failure may also be increased by an increased sodium and water content, which increases their "stiffness."[263] The generalized increase in sympathetic nervous system activity also appears to play a facilitative role in sodium and water retention in heart failure.[261]

The increased systemic arteriolar vasoconstriction associated with heart failure is an example of a compensatory mechanism that probably evolved in response to an inadequate cardiac output from other causes, such as traumatic hemorrhage or an inadequate blood volume. In such an acute situation, the reflex maintains arterial pressure and perfusion of the brain and heart. On the other hand, in the patient with chronic heart failure, the compensatory increase in arteriolar resistance may actually make it more difficult for the failing heart to eject blood. One of the major cornerstones of the modern therapy of heart failure is the reduction of peripheral vascular resistance by converting enzyme inhibitors and other vasodilator drugs (see below and Chaps. 26, 30).

The Kidney in Heart Failure

The compensatory, homeostatic adjustments that occur when the heart fails tend to restore normal ventricular systolic pump function, although often at the price of increased diastolic pressures in the involved ventricle and the venous system filling the involved ventricle. A major compensatory mechanism is the increase in ventricular filling volume and pressures produced by an increase in plasma volume as the result of salt and water retention by the kidneys.[200-202,264] Ultimately, the mechanisms leading to an increase in plasma volume and capillary pressure may contribute to the formation of interstitial edema and may also contribute to increased peripheral resistance (Fig. 25-3).[265] The mechanism or stimuli for the initial changes in the kidneys that produce salt and water retention in heart failure are still not clear.[261,264,266-269] Possible mechanisms include a decrease in the "effective" arterial blood volume. Such a decrease may be sensed by arterial volume receptors, by decreased distending pressure in the carotid sinus and other cardiothoracic mechanoreceptors in the great arteries and veins, or by sensors in the thorax, kidneys, atria, and possibly the ventricles, liver, and central nervous sys-

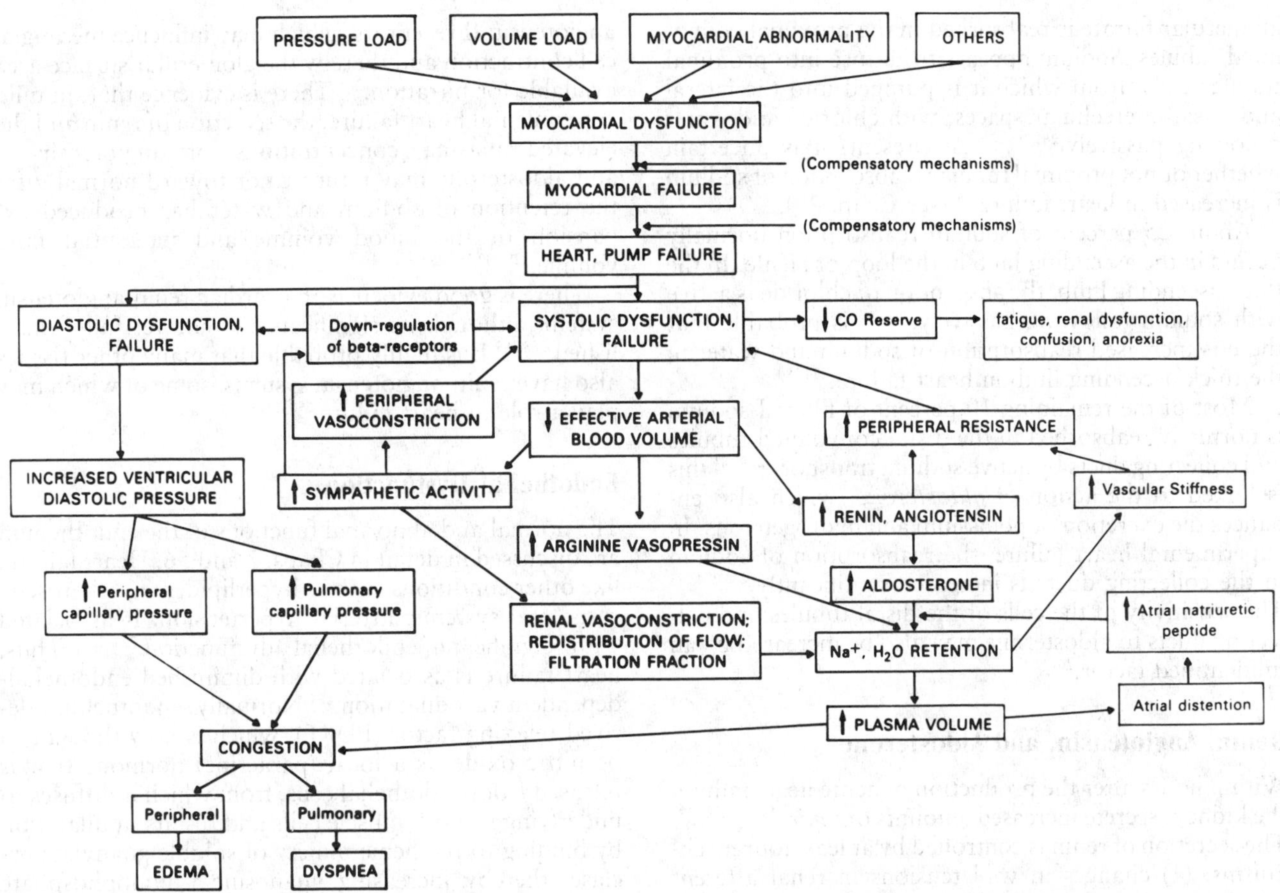

FIGURE 25-3 Schema of the sequence of events in heart failure. An increased load or myocardial abnormality leads to myocardial failure and eventually to heart failure. This results in increased sympathetic activity, increased levels of renin-angiotensin-aldosterone, pulmonary and peripheral congestion and edema, and decreased cardiac output reserve. Endothelial dysfunction also occurs, with decreased endothelial-dependent vasodilatation and with increased plasma levels of endothelin 1, a very strong vasoconstrictor. See text for details.

tem.[261,270–272] Increased renal venous pressure or decreased arterial perfusion pressure may also contribute to sodium retention by the kidneys.

During the phase of edema formation, patients with heart failure have a significantly delayed ability to excrete a load of either sodium chloride or water. In patients with very mild heart failure, if normal renal perfusion is restored by the expansion of blood volume, the handling of additional small amounts of sodium may return toward normal; however, patients with severe failure remain unable to excrete solute and water normally despite a marked expansion of blood volume and interstial fluid volume.

The renal vasoconstriction of patients with congestive heart failure is thought to result primarily from increased activity of both the sympathetic nervous system and the renin-angiotensin system.[203,264,268,269,273] Local redistribution of renal blood flow is also important. Prostaglandins and vasoactive peptides, especially neuropeptides and other endothelial products, may also be involved. In addition to a reduction in total renal blood flow, there is a redistribution of flow that produces a greater reduction of flow in the outer renal cortex with a relative maintenance of perfusion in the juxtamedullary areas.[261,264,269,274]

Patients with mild heart failure may have a normal glomerular filtration rate despite a reduced renal blood flow. This is the result of an increased filtration fraction due to marked vasoconstriction of efferent renal arterioles and decreased hydrostatic pressure in the peritubular capillaries.[275,276] In patients with more severe heart failure, total renal blood flow is even more decreased, and the glomerular filtration rate may be significantly decreased even though the filtration fraction may increase further. In this situation, "prerenal azotemia" is often present with an increase in the blood urea concentration.

The sympathetic nervous system, which can be activated by lowering of the arterial blood pressure or by direct stimulation of the renal nerves, plays a facilitative role in the renal retention of sodium and water in heart failure. An increase in renal venous pressure may also contribute to the retention of sodium and water. The increased tubular reabsorption of sodium and water in heart failure is aided by the marked redistribution of renal blood flow described above.[261,266,274] In addition, the uptake of fluid from the interstitium into the peritubular capillaries is enhanced by the efferent renal arteriolar vasoconstriction, which increases colloid osmatic pressure in the peritubular capillaries. These hemodynamic mechanisms work synergistically to increase sodium and water reabsorption.[261,277,278]

Patients with heart failure have significantly decreased excretion rates of sodium chloride due to increased tubular reabsorption, even when the glomerular filtration rate is normal. Normally, about 60 to 70 percent of the glomerular filtrate is reabsorbed in the proximal convoluted tubules. Sodium appears to diffuse into proximal tubular cells, from which it is pumped into the lateral and basal intercellular spaces, with chloride and water following passively.[261,266,279] At present, it is uncertain whether or not proximal tubular reabsorption of sodium is increased in heart failure[266] (see Chap. 29).

About 25 percent of sodium reabsorption normally occurs in the ascending limb in the loop of Henle. In the thick ascending limb, the absorption of chloride is active with sodium following passively.[261] It is probable that there is increased reabsorption of sodium and water in the thick ascending limb in heart failure.[274,280]

Most of the remaining 10 percent of filtered sodium is normally reabsorbed in the distal convoluted tubules and collecting ducts by active sodium transport,[274,281] this is linked to the action of *aldosterone,* which also enhances the excretion of potassium and hydrogen ions. In experimental heart failure, the reabsorption of sodium in the collecting ducts is increased significantly.[266,274,279] The sensitivity of the cells of the distal tubules and collecting ducts to aldosterone may also be increased by an unidentified factor.[261]

Renin, Angiotensin, and Aldosterone

Within hours after the production of acute heart failure, the kidneys secrete increased amounts of *renin.*[203,267,282,283] The secretion of renin is controlled by at least four mechanisms: (1) changes in wall tensions in renal afferent arterioles, (2) a macula densa receptor that detects changes in the rate at which sodium and/or chloride reaches the distal tubule, (3) a negative feedback effect from the elevated plasma levels of angiotensin II, and (4) the central nervous system, which influences renin secretion by the renal nerves, adrenal medulla, and the posterior pituitary gland.[284] Carotid sinus or atrial distension may also influence renin secretion.[266,267,272,284,285] In general, decreased renal perfusion pressure, decreased renal blood flow, and decreased sodium load at the distal tubule result in the release of renin. It is uncertain whether or not the increased levels of arginine vasopressin (AVP) often present in heart failure influence renin release.[285]

Renin acts upon angiotensinogen, which is produced mainly in the liver, to produce angiotensin I, which is converted to *angiotensin II.*[282,283] Angiotensin II has strong arterial vasoconstrictor properties and contributes to the increase in peripheral vascular resistance and the maintenance of blood pressure in heart failure when "effective" filling of the arterial circulation decreases.[261,286] Angiotensin II further constricts renal efferent arterioles; in the brain, it stimulates thirst; while in the adrenal gland, it stimulates secretion of *aldosterone,* which very strongly promotes the reabsorption of sodium and the excretion of potassium in the distal tubules and collecting ducts of the kidney. Plasma concentrations of both angiotensin II and aldosterone are usually elevated in patients with congestive heart failure. Angiotensin II also has some direct, albeit minor, inotropic properties and may augment the release of NE from nerve endings. It also appears to augment myocardial hypertrophy directly. Glomerular mesangial cells appear to have angiotensin II receptors, which may influence mesangial cell contraction and thereby the glomerular surface area available for filtration.[287] There is evidence that, in mild experimental heart failure, the secretion of renin and the elevated plasma concentrations of angiotensin II and aldosterone may return to or toward normal after the retention of sodium and water has produced expansion of the blood volume and interstitial fluid volume.[229,230,261,282]

There is good evidence of a cardiac renin-angiotensin system, although its significance is not yet fully established.[288,289] It is highly probable that many other tissues also have renin-angiotensin systems, some of which may play a role in heart failure.[290–291a]

Endothelial Dysfunction

The normal and abnormal functions of the endothelium are discussed in detail in Chaps. 2 and 56. Heart failure, like other conditions such as hyperlipidemia, atherosclerosis, and systemic arterial hypertension, is associated with significant endothelial dysfunction.[224–227] Thus, heart failure is associated with diminished endothelial-dependent vasodilatation.[224] Normally, endothelium-derived relaxing factor (EDRF), which is now thought to be nitric oxide, is a local (paracrine) hormone that is released from endothelial cells, from which it diffuses to underlying smooth muscle cells and results in dilatation by binding to the heme moiety of soluble guanylate cyclase, thereby increasing guanosine-5-monophosphate (cGMP) production.[292,293]

One of the more important physiologic stimulants of EDRF release is the longitudinal shear force on endothelial cells produced by changes in flow rate. The endothelium also releases endothelin-1, which is one of the most potent vasoconstrictor substances known. Patients with heart failure have increased circulating levels of endothelin-1.[210–216] It has also been suggested that the endocardial endothelium is capable of influencing the duration of cardiac contraction.[294–296] The importance of the latter phenomenon in human heart failure is unknown. (See also Chaps. 2 and 56.)

Arginine Vasopressin

In severe heart failure secretion of pituitary antidiuretic hormone or AVP is increased, particularly in patients with hyponatremia.[141,209,297–301] Although AVP may contribute to the decreased ability of some patients to secrete a water load, it appears not to play a major primary role in edema formation.[261,302] AVP is also a strong vasoconstrictor and contributes to the increase in systemic vascular resistance in heart failure.

Atrial Natriuretic Peptide (Factor)

The plasma concentration of atrial natriuretic peptide or factor (ANP or ANF) is increased in heart failure.[303–313] This should produce a natriuresis by its direct renal action, particularly since atrial natriuretic factor also decreases the production of aldosterone.[314] As noted above, however, it appears that the homeostatic control of circulatory blood volume by this mechanism is inadequate to overcome the stronger forces tending to retain sodium and water in heart failure.

The importance of ANP in the pathogenesis of the syndrome of congestive heart failure is unclear.[315-317] Atrial natriuretic factor also inhibits the production of aldosterone, renin, and AVP.[314,317,318] Many patients with heart failure do have increased plasma concentrations of ANP,[303-313] presumably released secondary to atrial distension, but their natriuretic and vasodilator properties are overwhelmed by the stronger factors producing retention of salt and water and vasoconstriction.

ANPs are made and stored in specialized atrial cells, from which they are released by the stimulus of atrial distension. Some may also be released by ventricular myocytes. They have both a natriuretic and a diuretic effect, and some relax vascular smooth muscle and/or intestinal smooth muscle.[314,315] Their role, if any, in heart failure is not clear.[266,283,314,319] Patients with severe heart failure may have down-regulation of the ANP receptors coupled to guanylate cyclase in their pulmonary vasculature.[320]

Prostaglandins

The kidneys synthesize prostaglandins PGE_2 and PGF_{2a} in the interstitial and collecting duct cells of the medulla. These substances are released into the renal interstitial fluid and renal venous blood and are metabolized in both the renal cortex and the lungs. Prostacyclin (PGI_2) and PGE_2 can be synthesized by renal vascular and smooth-muscle cells.[321] Their role in the maintenance of normal sodium balance or in heart failure is still unclear.[261,322] They may help maintain glomerular filtration in the presence of marked efferent arteriolar vasoconstriction.[323] PGI_2 and PGE_2 may stimulate the release of renin.[322,324]

Some patients with heart failure have increased levels of the metabolites of vasodilator prostaglandins, which may oppose the vasoconstriction produced by the renin-angiotensin-aldosterone system.[322-324] Those patients with heart failure, in whom the vasodilating effects of prostaglandins are important in opposing the many vasoconstricting influences, are susceptible to a worsening of their clinical condition when they are given agents that inhibit prostaglandin synthesis, such as indomethacin.[322-324] The negative inotropic effects of furosemide noted experimentally appear to be prostaglandin-mediated.[325]

Peptides

The vasodilator peptides bradykinin and kalliden, which are formed by the kallikrein-kinin system, may be involved in the intrarenal distribution of blood flow and the excretion of sodium,[325a,326] but their importance in heart failure is also unknown. The neuropeptide tyrosin (NPY), a 36-amino acid peptide, may be important in the control of myocardial contractility and the regulation of myocardial perfusion.[327] Increased plasma levels of neuropeptide Y[217-220] and substance P[219] have been found in some patients with heart failure.

Frank-Starling Law of the Heart

When the ventricle fails acutely, the Frank-Starling law of the heart is immediately brought into play. When the normally filled ventricle fails to eject a normal quantity of blood during one beat, its end-systolic volume increases. Consequently, this increased volume remains and is added to the blood entering the ventricle during the next diastole. The net result is an increased end-diastolic volume for the next beat. This increased "preload" produces an increased stroke volume during the next contraction in accordance with the Frank-Starling law of the heart. This increase in contractile force is related to an increase in sarcomere length that produces increased contractile bridge formation for a given amount of Ca^{2+} released into the myocyte[327a-333] (see Chap. 5).

Over a period of time, the ventricle may be able to maintain normal or nearly normal stroke volume and work at an increased end-diastolic fiber length and volume (Fig. 25-4). In many patients with a chronic increase in preload, as may be produced by aortic or mitral regurgitation, the ventricle dilates markedly and increases its end-diastolic volume strikingly without an increase in diastolic pressure. This reflects a shift in the passive pressure-volume curve to the right as a result of remodeling of the wall of the ventricle. As ventricular failure progresses, the increase in stroke volume (SV) associated with an increase in end-diastolic volume or end-diastolic pressure (EDP) is reduced. Due to the increased stiffness of the ventricle as volume is increased, any further increase in EDP produces very little increase in diastolic

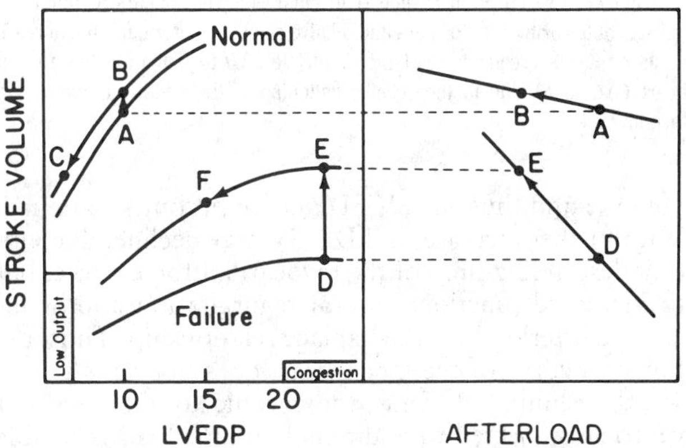

FIGURE 25-4 Relationship between stroke volume and left ventricular end-diastolic pressure (LVEDP) (*left*) and afterload (*right*). Normally, the ventricle operates on a sharply rising Frank-Starling curve with an LVEDP less than 12 mmHg (point *A*), where small changes in filling pressure yield large changes in stroke volume. Further, stroke volume is largely independent of the afterload. When failure occurs, ventricular function is characterized by a shift of the curve relating stroke volume to LVEDP to the right and downward. Low output may ensue if the curve is sufficiently depressed, while pulmonary congestion occurs as the LVEDP is increased. At the same time, since this failing ventricle is now highly afterload-dependent (point *D*), small changes in afterload produce large changes in stroke volume.

When afterload is reduced in the normal circulation (point *A* to point *B*, *right*) stroke volume rises very slightly. If venodilatation occurs at the same time, stroke volume falls to point *C* (*left*). The net result is a decrease in stroke volume. On the contrary, when afterload is reduced in the presence of severe ventricular failure, stroke volume is increased (point *D* to point *E*, *right*). Since the Frank-Starling curve is relatively flattened, a simultaneous decrease in venous tone leads to a decrease in LVEDP with only a small decrease in stroke volume (point *E* to point *F*, *left*). The net result of these opposing consequences may mean an increase in stroke volume. These results are observed clinically when nitroprusside is administered as an "unloading" agent for treating the failing ventricle.

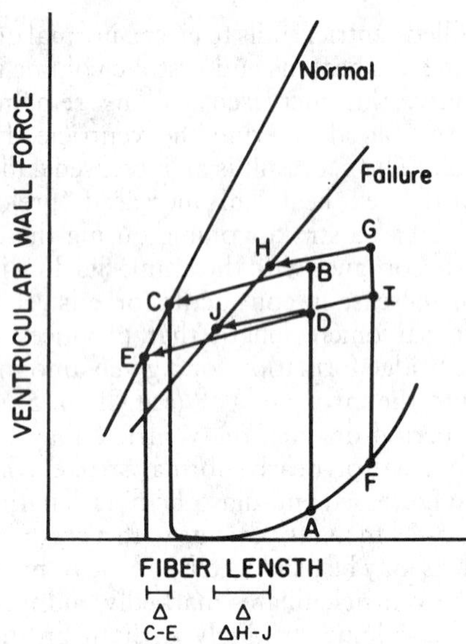

FIGURE 25-5 Relationship between ventricular wall force and fiber length. Hypothetical contractile cycles have been portrayed for the normal and failing ventricle. In the normal heart, contraction starts at point *A*, wall force rises until the aortic valve is opened (point *B*), *the ventricle empties* (point *B* to *C*), and relaxation ensues. When arterial pressure (afterload) is reduced (e.g., to point *D*), ejection starts at point *D* and proceeds to point *E*.

In the presence of ventricular failure, the fiber length in diastole is increased, and ventricular contraction starts at point *F*. With systolic contraction, ventricular wall force rises to point *G*, and with ventricular emptying, fiber length decreases to point *H*. When the afterload is decreased, wall force only needs to reach point *I* when ventricular emptying occurs to point *J*.

It is noteworthy that, for the same relative change in afterload, the increase in shortening is greater in the failing ventricle (Δ*H* to *J*) than in the normal heart (Δ*C* to *E*) due to the relative flattening of the systolic curve in the former case.

volume, and thus the SV-EDP curve becomes flattened. With further increases in EDP, SV may decline, due, not to a descending limb of the myocardial force curve, but to increased functional mitral regurgitation and/or increased afterload via the Laplace relationship. Thus, the function curve of the intact heart does not have a "descending limb."[45,46] Thus, the chronically dilatated left ventricle subjected to additional volume load is unable to utilize the Frank-Starling mechanism to a significant degree[39–41,47] (Fig. 25-4).

In patients with congestive heart failure the retention of salt and water by the kidneys increases effective blood volume, which tends to increase ventricular filling volume and to return stroke output toward normal. This mechanism may return stroke output tot normal or near normal, but at the expense of increased venous pressure in the pulmonary venous or the systemic venous systems. In some patients this increased filling pressure is necessary for a reasonable cardiac output. Such patients may develop symptoms of decreased cardiac output if the ventricular filling pressure is excessively decreased by diuretics. This need for a high filling pressure is particularly likely to occur in patients with pericardial constriction, aortic stenosis, restrictive cardiomyopathy, or hypertrophic cardiomyopathy (see Chaps. 79 and 90–92).

Another characteristic of the dilated, failing heart is that it becomes less influenced by preload and more afterload-dependent (Figs. 25-4 and 25-5). The normal heart can sustain large changes in systolic loading or afterload with relatively little change in cardiac output and with only minor changes in diastolic volume. When myocardial failure is present and the diastolic volume is increased and the heart is dilated, however, any further increase in afterload may lead to a substantial decrease in stroke volume. Alternatively, a decrease in afterload may substantially increase the cardiac output (Fig. 25-4).

Hypertrophy of the Heart

Hypertrophy is one of the major adaptations of the heart to chronically increased stress, but it may itself contribute to the progression of heart failure. Experimentally, there is metabolic evidence of hypertrophy within a few hours after an increase in cardiac work.[7,156,157,334] Hyperplasia, or an actual increase in the total number of myocardial cells, is generally thought to occur in human beings only if the increased stress occurs within the first few months of life. Recent evidence, however, suggests that hyperplasia can also occur later in life under conditions of excessive loading or myocyte loss.[335,336] Cardiac hypertrophy is associated with a significant increase in the number and/or size of sarcomeres within each myocardial cell. In general, chronic pressure loads tend to result in thicker myocardial cells with replication of sarcomeres in parallel, whereas chronic volume loads result in longer and somewhat thicker individual myocardial cells with replication of sarcomeres both in series and in parallel.[335,337–342] In addition, significant hyperplasia can occur in myocardial interstitial cells, which outnumber myocytes three to one in the normal adult myocardium (see below).[158–164]

Two classic types of left ventricular hypertrophy are recognized: concentric and eccentric. In pure *concentric hypertrophy* of the left ventricle, there is an increase in the thickness of the ventricular wall, but the ventricular chamber does not increase in diameter. In some instances, the ventricular chamber may actually decrease in size. Myocytes increase in diameter rather than in length. This type of hypertrophy is classically present in patients with isolated valvular aortic stenosis. In experimental models of pressure overload hypertrophy, capillary growth is less than the increase in muscle mass.[343–347] In pure *eccentric hypertrophy,* the thickness of the left ventricular wall and the internal diameter of the ventricle increase proportionately. This may be seen in normal growth, in endurance athletes, or in patients with volume overload of the left ventricle, as in isolated mitral regurgitation.[337–339,348] In these circumstances, myocytes elongate as well as thicken. As noted previously, *reactive hypertrophy* can occur in response to loss of myocytes from those remaining after myocardial infarction.[342,349]

Although the stimulus for myocardial hypertrophy is unknown,[7,156,157,328,329,350–352] it has been suggested that an increase in systolic wall tension of the ventricle in conditions associated with increased afterload stimulates the synthesis of sarcomeres in parallel to existing sarcomeres and thereby produces concentric hypertrophy[337–339] (see also Chap. 6B). Conversely, it has been suggested that an increase in diastolic wall tension under conditions of increased preload primarily stimulates the synthesis of sarcomeres in series with preexisting sarcomeres and produces eccentric hypertrophy. In so-called compensated hypertrophy, the increase in wall thickness is such that the tension in the wall is maintained in a normal range. It should be emphasized that hypertrophy of the remaining myocytes is very common in heart failure and that the increased stress on the remaining myocytes may result in their early loss and initiate a vicious cycle with even greater stress upon the surviving myocytes.[165,341,342,349,353]

As noted above, there is evidence that in some species there may be differences in the myosin present at various ages and synthesized in response to a stimulus to hypertrophy; these differences are more marked in atrial myosin.[59,350,354–356] In some species, such as the rat and the rabbit, the myosin synthesized in response to pressure loading may have more V_3 myosin than does that synthesized in response to volume loading.[357]

It is significant that the increase in individual myocardial cell length produced by the increase in the number of sarcomeres in patients with chronically dilated hearts is not adequate to explain the increase in heart size frequently encountered. In such patients, there is also myocardial "slippage" or rearrangement at the level of myofibrils, myocardial fibers, and muscle bundles. There may also be a significant increase in the amount of interstitial tissue.[4,41,43,159–164,337,358]

In general, most studies have indicated that the compensatory hypertrophy in many patients with chronic pressure or volume overload can be sufficient to return the calculated systolic wall tension to normal, although diastolic wall stress may remain abnormal in patients with volume overload (see Chap. 23).[4,6,47,337–339,359–363] Uncompensated failure is commonly characterized by an increase in systolic wall tension despite the compensatory hypertrophy. Many factors, including growth hormone, thyroid hormone, cortisol, angiotensin, and increased sympathetic stimulation of the heart, contribute to the development of cardiac hypertrophy in response to stress (see Chap. 6B).[363]

Hypertrophy is a natural adaptation to a systolic overload of the ventricle. Reactive hypertrophy occurs when myocardium is lost, such as following a myocardial infarction or with a cardiomyopathy. Moreover, as the hypertrophy increases, the tension per cell in the wall is reduced toward normal. As myocardial hypertrophy occurs, physiologic and biochemical alterations ensue. The rate of contraction of the myocardium decreases, the time to attain peak tension is delayed, and relaxation is slowed. Nevertheless, if enough time is available for contraction, peak force and shortening are maintained. As noted above, in some species, these physiologic alterations have a correlate in biochemical changes wherein, with hypertrophy, a slower myosin isoenzyme (V_3) is synthesized instead of the faster isoenzyme (V_1).[350,351,354,355,357] The same alteration in myosin tends to occur as a function of aging itself. With aging, however, myocytes are also lost, and the effects of aging and hypertrophy are additive. In addition, other enzyme systems that are associated with the control of activating Ca^{2+} for the heart are also slowed. In human beings, the latter changes appear to be major biochemical alterations in heart failure (see above).

Effect of Cardiac Hypertrophy on Diastolic Compliance

The diastolic compliance, or distensibility, of ventricles of patients with concentric hypertrophy due to pressure overload is typically much less than that of patients with eccentric hypertrophy due to volume overload in the absence of severe myocardial failure. Elastic recoil and the rate of relaxation may also be impaired. Thus, the extremely thick hypertrophied ventricle of a patient with concentric hypertrophy from aortic stenosis, systemic arterial hypertension, or hypertrophic cardiomyopathy may require a high left ventricular EDP for normal filling due to the hypertrophy itself.[364–369] In such patients, an elevation of ventricular diastolic pressure is not necessarily associated with systolic myocardial failure (Fig. 25-6).

These alterations form the substrate for "diastolic ventricular dysfunction," which is characterized by an elevated ventricular filling pressure with a normal SV and end-diastolic volume and thus a normal (50 to 75 percent) EF. Hypertrophy and delayed left ventricular relaxation may limit the time for diastolic filling and elevate filling pressure, producing pulmonary congestion, pulmonary edema, and the clinical picture of diastolic heart failure. This is amplified by tachycardia and a salt load.[63,364–376] Figure 25-7 illustrates the major parameters of diastolic dysfunction evaluated by noninvasive studies. Early left ventricular filling has multiple determinants in addition to muscle inactivation, such as elastic recoil forces viscoelastic effects, left ventricular filling pressure and left atrial pressure, left ventricular stiffness, ventricular interaction (interdependence), and pericardial constraint.[377,378] Obesity can be associated with impaired diastolic function even in normotensive subjects.[379]

In contrast, many patients with eccentric hypertrophy from mitral or aortic regurgitation may have markedly increased end-diastolic volumes with relatively normal diastolic pressures, often in the presence of significant myocardial and ventricular systolic dysfunction. These findings limit the value of ventricular EDP as an index of left ventricular performance, especially if the diastolic pressure is not correlated with other data (see Chap. 25).[380–388] Nevertheless, an elevated EDP is one of the hallmarks of left ventricular dysfunction.[63,369,371–376,389–391]

Left ventricular diastolic pressure-volume relationships may be significantly influenced by the phenomenon of ventricular interaction (interdependence) and by elevated right ventricular pressure and volume, particularly if the pericardium is intact.[377,392–398a]

The acute decrease in left ventricular distensibility produced by ischemia or hypoxia is greater in ventricles with chronic pressure overload hypertrophy than in normal ventricles.[399] The effects of myocardial ischemia upon ventricular systolic and diastolic function are discussed in more detail in Chap. 58. Left ventricular distensibility is frequently a contributing factor to left ventricular diastolic dysfunction. Factors influencing ventricular distensibility include alterations in the composition and geometry of the left ventricle, pericardial constraint, and coronary turgor from blood in the coronary circulation.[158,159,400–402] Figure 25-8 illustrates the important dif-

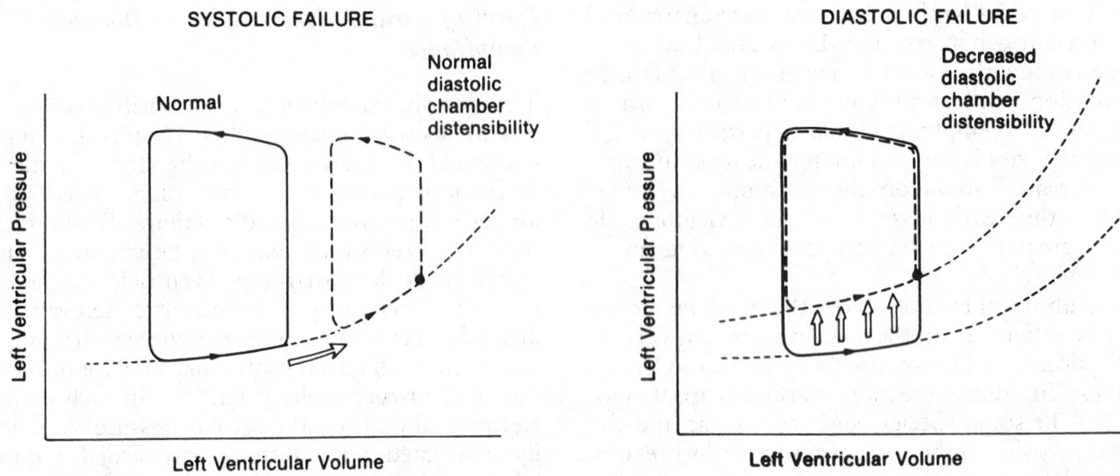

FIGURE 25-6 The left panel shows a schematized left ventricular pressure-volume loop from a patient with primary systolic failure. A normal left ventricular pressure-volume loop (*solid loop*) is shown on the left portion of the curve, and the transition to systolic failure (*dashed loop*) is shown on the right. Systolic failure is manifested as an increase in left ventricular end-systolic volume and as a reduction in the extent of shortening (stroke volume). LVEDP is increased because left ventricular volume is increased. As indicated by the arrow, the diastolic portion of the pressure-volume loop has simply shifted to the right along the same diastolic pressure-volume relationship. No change in the distensibility of the left ventricle has occurred. The right panel shows a left ventricular pressure-volume loop from a patient with primary diastolic failure (*dashed loop*). Note that the LVEDP is the same as that in the patient with primary systolic failure, as denoted by the • on the pressure-volume loops. However, in the right panel, this is related to an upward shift of the left ventricular diastolic pressure-volume relationship (*arrows*). This indicates a decrease in left ventricular diastolic distensibility such that a higher diastolic pressure is required to achieve the same diastolic volume. In this patient, no change in end-diastolic volume or systolic shortening has occurred. (*From BH Lorell: Left ventricular diastolic pressure-volume relations: Understanding and managing congestive heart failure. Heart Failure 4:206–223, 1988. Reproduced with permission from the publisher and author.*)

ference between diastolic distensibility and altered compliance. The possible mechanisms of impaired relaxation in ventricular hypertrophy include increased wall thickness, increased wall stress (afterload mismatch), fibrosis, and impaired myocardial relaxation from subendocardial ischemia or diastolic calcium overload intrinsic to hypertrophy.[364,367,369] Normally, the pressure in the left ventricle rapidly falls below the pressure in the left atrium and accelerates the flow of blood into the left ventricle.[401,403] This phenomenon of "ventricular suction" is frequently markedly impaired in patients with left ventricular failure. The term *lusitrophy* has been used to refer to the diastolic relaxation and compliance properties of the ventricles.[81]

Effects of Experimental Cardiac Hypertrophy on Indices of Myocardial Contractility

The evaluation of contractility may depend on the particular index used and the setting in which it is employed.[404] When the heart is experimentally caused to become hypertrophied by increasing ventricular preload (volume overload), the myocardial contractility per unit mass is usually not decreased initially but only later with severe pump failure.[4,47,405] In contrast, with the development of hypertrophy that is experimentally produced by increased ventricular afterload (pressure overload), namely, the experimental hypertrophy of aortic or pulmonic stenosis, contractile behavior is altered but cannot be said to be depressed. Thus, the speed of contraction is slowed and the duration of contraction is prolonged in association with slowed relaxation. Force development and shortening capacity, however, remain normal. Only in late failure does contractile force decline.[4,139,406,407] It has also been found that this altered contractility may be reversible if the experimental hypertrophy is reversed by unbanding before the onset of failure.[408] Other studies of pressure-induced hypertrophy have found that myocardial contractility per unit mass may also return to normal if the elevated pressure load is maintained for 24 weeks,[409] whereas other investigators have found normal ventricular function at rest in animals with stable hypertrophy from either volume or pressure overload.[410]

Overall, it appears that alterations in myocardial contractility with associated experimental cardiac hypertrophy are extremely variable and depend on the inciting stimulus, the experimental design and species studied, the particular index of contractility utilized, and when the ventricle is studied.[11,406–410] For example, left ventricular hypertrophy induced by high-altitude hypoxia is not associated with a decrease in the indexes of contractility, whereas there is a decrease in the indexes in experimental chronic coarctation of the aorta.[411] Some of these discrepancies among experimental studies may also depend on the acuteness and severity of the overload or preload, the extent of resultant hypertrophy, and the age of the individual when it occurs (see Chap. 23).

Heart Rate

The normal heart responds to an increase in heart rate by a positive inotropic effect, which is known as *frequency treppe* or the *Bowditch effect*.[412] In the failing heart, however, an increase in heart rate may produce a reduced or even a reversal of the normally positive force-frequency effect (*reversed* or *negative treppe*).[412a–414]

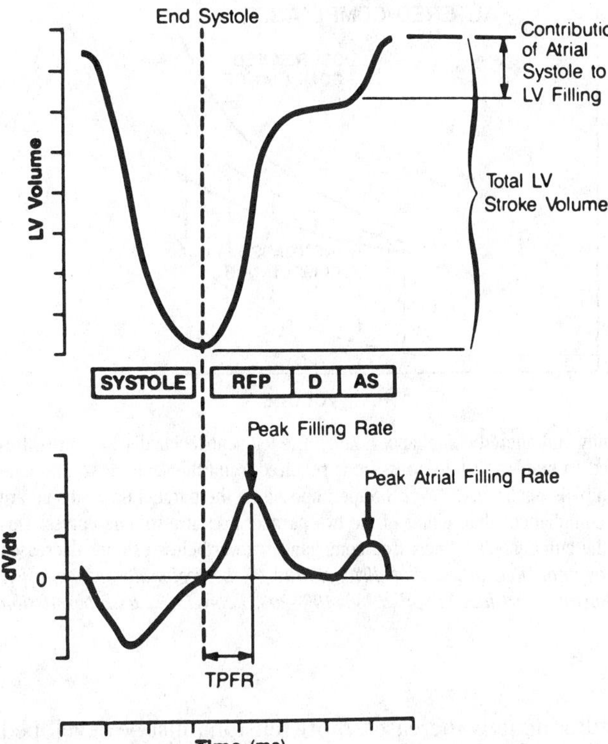

FIGURE 25-7 Idealized plot of left ventricular volume versus time (*top*) and the rate of change of volume (*dv/dt*) versus time (*bottom*), such as might be obtained from contrast or radionuclide ventriculographic studies. The representative cardiac cycle begins at end diastole. Subsequent events as depicted by the bars in the center of the figure are (1) systole, during which left ventricular volume decreases to a minimum and *dv/dt* reaches its maximum and (2) diastole, the beginning of which is signaled by the opening of the mitral valve and the onset of left ventricular filling. Diastole has three distinct phases in normal individuals: (1) the rapid filling phase (RFP), during which the left ventricle fills rapidly but passively and the peak filling rate occurs; (2) diastasis (D), during which relatively little left ventricular volume change occurs; and (3) atrial systole (AS), in which active atrial contraction fills the left ventricle to its end-diastolic volume. The diastolic parameters that have been derived from such analysis are the peak filling rate, the time to peak filling rate (TPFR), the percent contribution of atrial systole, and the first third filling fraction. *(From AJ Labovitz, AC Pearson: Evaluation of left ventricular diastolic function: Clinical relevance and recent Doppler echocardiographic insights. Am Heart J, 114:836–849, 1987. Reproduced with permission from the publisher and authors.)*

Peripheral Oxygen Delivery

Redistribution of Blood Flow

Patients with heart failure redistribute their diminished cardiac output. In general, perfusion of the brain and heart is maintained at the expense of circulation to the kidney, splanchnic area, and skin. The peripheral tissues in heart failure extract more oxygen per unit of blood flow, and this produces an increase in the arteriovenous oxygen difference of the whole body. This “venous oxygen reserve” is potentially less useful to the myocardium, which even normally extracts about 65 to 75 percent of the oxygen coming to it (see Chap. 5) or to the brain.

Oxygen-Hemoglobin Dissociation

The usual decrease in blood flow to the peripheral tissues in heart failure is associated with a progressive decline in the affinity of hemoglobin for oxygen, which is caused by an increase in 2,3-diphosphoglycerate (DPG).[415] This change in affinity for oxygen, which is reflected in a rightward shift in the oxygen-hemoglobin dissociation curve, facilitates the release of oxygen in the peripheral capillaries of underperfused tissues.

Anaerobic Metabolism

Some tissues utilize anaerobic metabolism during transient periods of increased stress, such as exercise. Unfortunately, this reserve mechanism is of limited value to the myocardium (see Chap. 6A) or the brain.

Peripheral Vascular Resistance

Patients with heart failure have an increase in peripheral vascular resistance due to multiple mechanisms, including increased sympathetic adrenergic vasoconstrictor activity and increased plasma concentrations of NE, angiotensin II, endothelin-1, and AVP. In addition, the sodium and water retention in heart failure tends to make the arterioles “stiff” from an increased content of sodium and water. An increase in tissue turgor can compress blood vessels and contribute to the increased peripheral vascular resistance at rest, as well as to the important failure of the peripheral vascular resistance to decrease normally during exertion. In the later stages of heart failure, hypertrophy of arteriolar smooth muscle may also limit normal metabolically mediated vasodilation.

In the early stages of heart failure, cardiac output and arterial vascular resistance are generally normal, despite marked reductions in EF. When symptoms develop, cardiac output may be somewhat reduced at rest, while peripheral vascular resistance is elevated; nevertheless, resistance can decrease markedly with reactive hyperemia and during exercise cardiac output may increase three- to fourfold with concomitant falls in vascular resistance. In patients with late, highly symptomatic failure, a further, important abnormality develops in the peripheral arterial circulation. At this stage, cardiac output is reduced at rest with an increased peripheral vascular resistance. During exercise, metabolically mediated arterial vascular dilatation is impaired, and blood flow to the exercising organ does not increase. Hence, there is little increase in cardiac output, and exercise performance becomes limited due to lack of skeletal muscle blood flow. This abnormality of dilatation may result from a reduction of the release by the vascular endothelium of EDRF (nitric oxide), which normally mediates dilatation. This abnormality is partially reversible with increased exercise training[415a,416,416a] or with long-term drug therapy for heart failure.[417]

THE LAW OF LAPLACE

The law of Laplace and the effects of ventricular dilatation on the mechanics and energetics of myocardial contraction are important factors in heart failure. On first

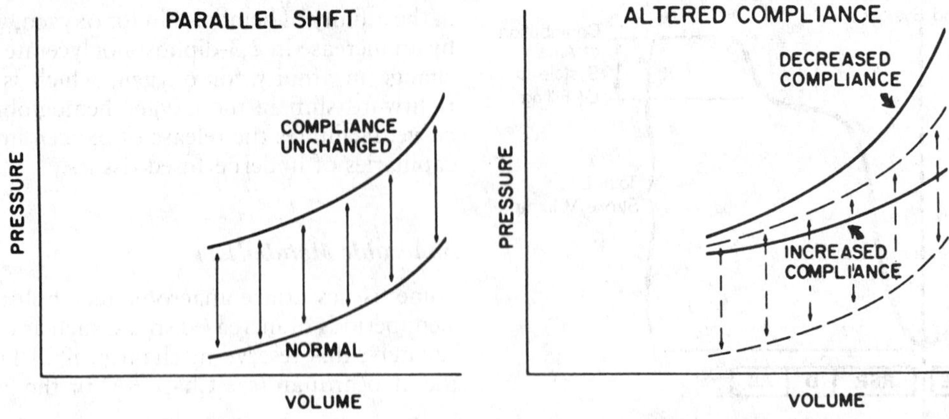

FIGURE 25-8 Schematic illustration of the difference between diastolic distensibility and altered compliance. (*Left*) The left ventricular diastolic pressure-volume relationship has undergone a parallel upward shift. Distensibility is decreased (a higher diastolic pressure is required to fill the ventricle to the same chamber volume), although compliance (the slope of the pressure-volume relationship) is unchanged. (*Right*) Superimposed on the parallel upward shift are curves whose slopes are steeper (decreased compliance) or less steep (increased compliance) than either of the two parallel pressure-volume curves. This illustrates the importance of distinguishing distensibility from compliance, because the curve labeled "increased compliance" nevertheless exhibits decreased distensibility compared to the normal pressure-volume relationship. *(From W Grossman: Relaxation and distensibility of the regionally ischemic left ventricle. In: W Grossman, BH Lorell (eds): Diastolic Relaxation of the Heart. Boston, Martinus Nijhoff, 1988: 193–203. Reproduced with permission from the publisher and authors.)*

thought, it might seem that ventricular dilatation is advantageous. With an increased end-diastolic ventricular volume and sarcomere length, each sarcomere would have to shorten less to eject a given volume of blood, and each myocardial fiber would be able to perform more work by virtue of greater preload (the Frank-Starling law of the heart). These seeming advantages, however, are negated by other consequences of dilatation. The more important of these is the need for the myocardial fibers in the wall of a dilatated ventricle to develop greater tension in order to produce a given pressure within the ventricle. In general, ventricular myocardial wall tension is calculated by employing the law of Laplace, which actually applies to a distensible membrane with a spherical or cylindrical shape, and by assuming that the ventricle has a spherical cavity. Figure 25-9 illustrates three definitions of contractile tension in the ventricular myocardium. In general, calculations of myocardial tension should usually be expressed in terms of force per unit of cross-section area (formula shown on right in Fig. 25-9).[359] By all three formulas, it is apparent that, as the radius acutely increases, more tension must be developed by each fiber to produce or maintain a given intraventricular pressure. In formula 3, an increased thickness of the ventricular wall tends to decrease the required systolic tension per cross-sectional area.

The law of Laplace expresses an additional disadvantage of the dilated ventricle. In a normal ventricle, the decrease in average radius of the ventricle during ejection is relatively large; consequently, the effect of this decrease in diameter on instantaneous wall tension is normally greater than the opposite effect of the increasing pressure in the ventricle. As a result, the myocardial fiber tension, or force, may actually *decrease* soon after the beginning of ejection from a normal-sized ventricle, and the tension is usually less at the moment of peak systolic pressure in the ventricle than at the beginning of ejection. On the other hand, if the ventricle is markedly dilated and the contractility, and thus the shortening capacity, of the myocardial fibers is reduced, both the relative and the absolute decrease in average radius is much less during the ejection of an equal volume. In a markedly dilated

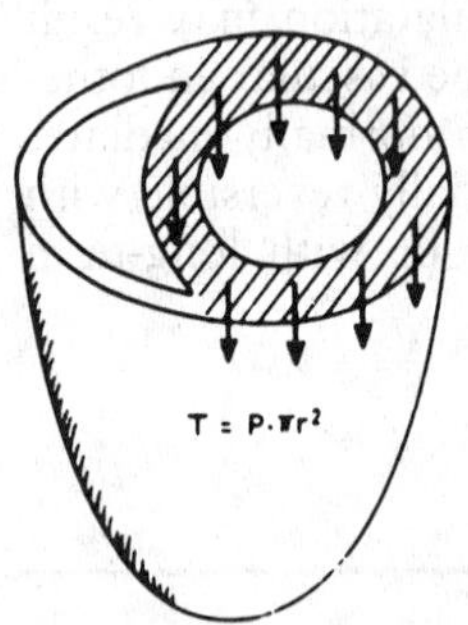

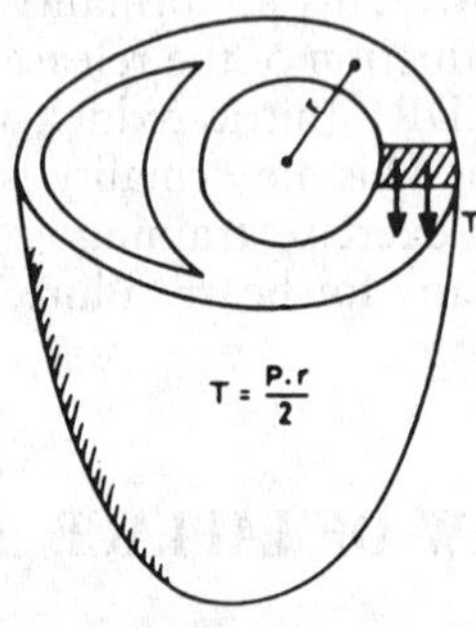

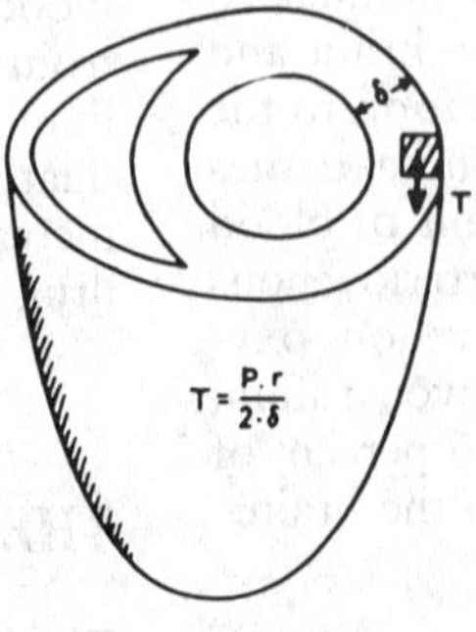

FIGURE 25-9 Three definitions of contractile force in the myocardium and the formulas based on the law of Laplace used to calculate each. *T*, contractile tangential tension or force in the wall of the ventricle; *P*, transmural pressure across the wall of the ventricle; *r*, average radius of the ventricle, assuming it to be spherical; δ, ventricular wall thickness. *(From HS Badeer: Contractile tension in the myocardium. Am Heart J 66:432, 1963. Reprinted with permission from the publisher and author.)*

ventricle, therefore, the average tension in the myocardial fibers may continue to increase from the beginning of ejection up to the peak systolic pressure.[359,418–420] In a sense, this is an additional type of "afterload" encountered during ejection by ventricles that are significantly dilated by increased "preload." A further disadvantage of dilatation is that the increased force, or tension, in the myocardial fibers required to develop a given pressure inside a dilated ventricle results in a decrease in the *rate* of myocardial fiber shortening (see Chap. 5), further limiting the ability of the ventricle to eject blood.[4,39,40,359,404,421,422] In mitral regurgitation, the early reduction in afterload (impedance) produced by the relatively rapid emptying of the left ventricle first into the low-pressure left atrium in early systole and then into the aorta helps to maintain left ventricular function for many years.[2,423] When the ventricle dilates and left atrial pressure is high, the unloading effect of rapid emptying is lost, thus adding to decompensation.

HEART FAILURE DUE TO PRESSURE OVERLOAD AND VOLUME OVERLOAD

Most types of congenital and acquired heart disease result in mechanical stress on the heart and myocardium. The two most common general types of mechanical cardiac stress are that resulting from an increased resistance to ventricular emptying of increased afterload (e.g., aortic stenosis, systemic hypertension, etc.) and that resulting from an increased preload or increased ventricular filling (e.g., aortic or mitral regurgitation, ventricular septal defect, etc.). The hemodynamics of several other specific types of mechanical abnormalities are described in more detail elsewhere: mitral stenosis (Chap. 80), pericardial tamponade or constriction (Chap. 92), endocardial restriction (Chap. 91), and the several varieties of ventricular dysynergy and aneurysm (Chap. 60). Figure 25-10 diagrams the progression from myocardial damage to left ventricular dysfunction to congestive heart failure.

In some patients with severe acute mechanical abnormalities, such as the acute rupture of a mitral chordae tendineae or an aortic valve leaflet, the overall capacity of the heart as a pump may be unable to meet the massive overload, although contractility of the myocardium may initially be normal. Similarly, some chronic mechanical abnormalities by themselves can prevent the heart from pumping an adequate amount of blood even without the development of myocardial failure. In most patients with a chronic pressure or volume load on the left ventricle, however, the development of either clinical congestive heart failure or pump failure is associated with the development of myocardial systolic dysfunction and eventually myocardial failure. This may be referred to as "dysdynamic" systolic dysfunction or failure. In this sense, heart failure, with its adaptations of hypertrophy and dilatation, *leads* to decreased myocardial contractility. As noted previously, some patients with marked hypertrophy from hypertrophic cardiomyopathy, systemic hypertension, or aortic stenosis may develop diastolic dysfunction or failure with pulmonary congestion before the development of systolic failure of the ventricle.

Myocardial Compensatory Mechanisms in Heart Failure Due to Increased Afterload (Pressure Overload)

The basic reaction of isolated myocardium to an increased afterload is to contract more forcefully but more slowly. In addition, when the heart of an experimental animal is acutely subjected to increased afterload, there is metabolic evidence of hypertrophy within a few hours.[156,157,327–329] The biochemical signal is unknown but may be related to a chronic increase in systolic wall tension (see Chaps. 1 and 6B).[157,328,337,338] As noted previously, the classic type of cardiac hypertrophy associated with aortic stenosis is *concentric hypertrophy,* in which there is marked thickening of the left ventricular wall (including the ventricular septum) but there is no increase in the size of the left ventricular cavity, which may even get smaller. Increased afterload effects myocardial thickening by replication of sarcomeres in parallel.[334] Although the contractility of the myocardium subjected to pressure overload may be decreased per unit mass later in the process (see above), overall ventricular compensation is maintained by the increase in myocardial mass. Systolic wall tension is generally returned to normal by the concentric hypertrophy and the spherical shape, although diastolic wall stress remains elevated.[4,7,23,328,334,337,359–361] During this phase of adaptive hyperfunction, function of the left ventricle is compensated, although the reserve may be reduced. Eventually, however, systolic, in addition to diastolic, myocardial dysfunction occurs and myocardial failure develops. Left ventricular diastolic volume increases, in association with cardiac pump dysfunction and failure, or "hyperadaptation" of Meerson.[327–329,411] Some of the possible structural and biochemical mechanisms responsible for myocardial failure are discussed above. An important consideration is diffuse loss of the hypertrophic myocytes with focal repair fibrosis. This loss results in an even greater load for the remaining myocytes.

In aortic stenosis there may be special difficulties with the delivery of adequate amounts of oxygen to the myocardial cells, particularly in the endocardium. Some of the factors responsible for inadequate oxygen delivery in aortic stenosis (and other conditions associated with marked concentric hypertrophy, such as hypertrophic cardiomyopathy and systemic hypertension) include the elevated myocardial oxygen requirements and the very high intramyocardial pressure, which throttles systolic coronary blood flow even more than usual, especially with tachycardia.[424–427] An elevated ventricular diastolic pressure, which may be necessary to fill the hypertrophied ventricle, will further impede diastolic coronary blood flow to the endocardium (see Chap. 5).[428] In addition, the growth of capillaries may be relatively less than the growth of myocytes, and the diffusion distance from myocardial capillaries to the center of the hypertrophied myocardial cells may be significantly increased.[429] Thus, there is a reduction in the relative increase in coronary blood flow during reactive hyperemia, which can be lim-

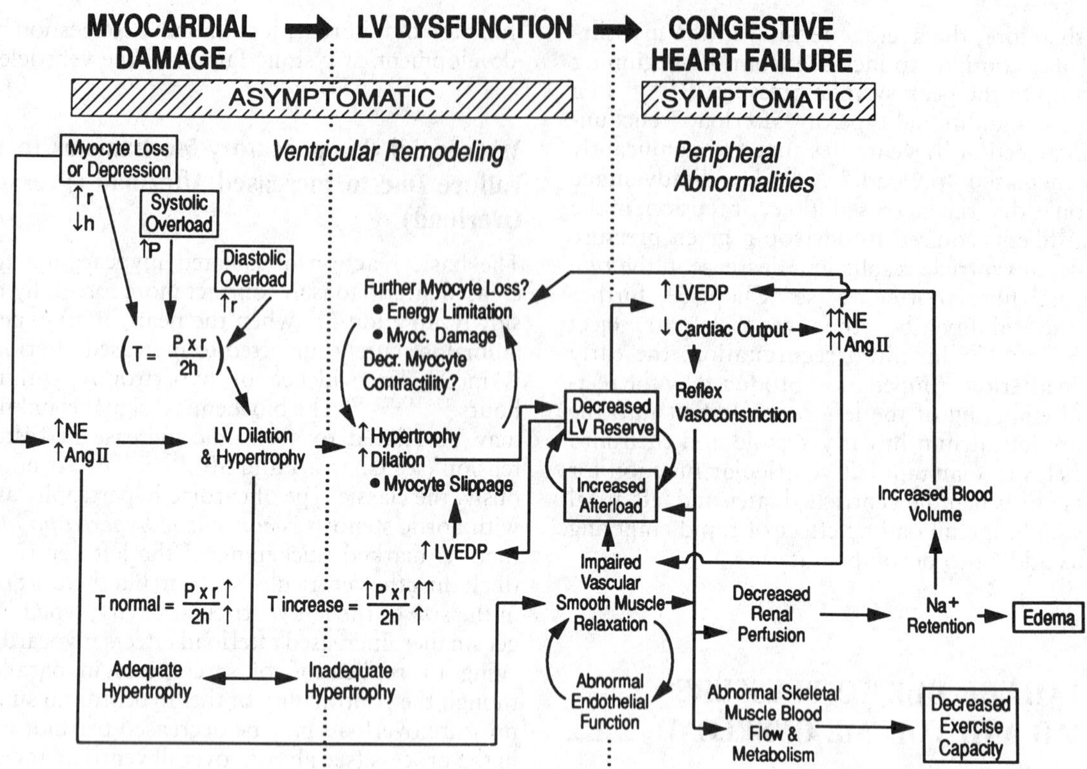

FIGURE 25-10 Evolution of myocardial damage to left ventricular function and ultimate congestive heart failure. The syndrome of congestive heart failure is the end result of processes that evolve in response to initial myocardial damage and/or cardiac overloads. The *initiating event* may be myocyte loss, either segmental, as with acute myocardial infarction, or diffuse, as with idiopathic cardiomyopathies and myocarditis; systolic overload, such as hypertension or aortic stenosis; or diastolic overload, such as mitral regurgitation or aortic regurgitation. Major loss of myocytes may also stimulate the renin-angiotensin and adrenergic systems, which may contribute to ventricular and vascular remodeling. All of these overloads create an increased workload for the heart, as characterized by Laplace relationship, where tension (t) is equal to the product of pressure (p) times the ventricular radius (r) over 2 times the wall of thickness (h). The initial adaptations to these overloads, termed *ventricular remodeling,* are an increase in both myocyte length and diameter as well as an increase in ventricular volume to maintain adequate stroke volume and hence cardiac output. If hypertrophy is adequate to normalize the tension load, a relatively steady state may be maintained. Myocytes continue to be lost as a function of aging per se, however, and this tends to lead to further myocyte hypertrophy and cardiac dilatation. Moreover, the aging process may be amplified by hypertrophy. Should there be a sudden increase in end-diastolic pressure within the ventricle, an added factor of relative myocyte slippage within the wall tends to occur, which may lead to a further decrease in myocytes across the ventricular wall, further increasing ventricular wall tension. This may create a downward spiral in which progressive cell loss leads to further ventricular remodeling and continued ventricular dilatation.

As noted above, the entire process of ventricular remodeling may occur asymptomatically, and myocardial damage progresses to left ventricular dysfunction, which is characterized by an increasing diastolic volume and thus a reduced ventricular ejection fraction. Symptoms associated with *congestive heart failure* occur when decreased left ventricular reserve limits cardiac output response to exercise. As the process of heart failure evolves, abnormalities of endothelial function in the peripheral arterioles lead to reduced ability of the peripheral vasculature to dilate in response to metabolic need. As these abnormalities occur, abnormal skeletal muscle blood flow occurs in response to exercise and decreased exercise tolerance. In addition, decreased renal perfusion leads to further activation of the renin-angiotensin-aldosterone system (RAAS), with increased aldosterone secretion and sodium retention. The combination of these two events leads to decreased exercise capacity and peripheral edema, important components of the symptom complex of congestive heart failure. Decreased cardiac performance promotes neurohumoral responses characterized by activation of the sympathetic nervous system and the renin-angiotensin-aldosterone system, leading to peripheral vasoconstriction and sodium accumulation. These factors feed back to increase the ventricular remodeling process and to amplify cardiac damage. Thus, initial myocardial damage progresses to ventricular dysfunction and ultimately to congestive heart failure. It is important to note that the myocardial damage and left ventricular dysfunction are often asymptomatic, and by the time symptomatic heart failure ensues, the disease process is far advanced. *(From LeJemtel TH, Sonnenblick EH: Heart failure and maladaptive processes: Introduction. Circulation 1993; 87(Suppl. VII):VII-1–VII-4. Reproduced with permission from the American Heart Association and the authors.)*

iting during periods of stress. Patients with marked concentric hypertrophy from aortic stenosis or other causes frequently have an elevation of left ventricular diastolic filling pressure (and a decreased rate of left ventricular relaxation and decreased left ventricular compliance or distensibility) due to the hypertrophy itself rather than to cardiac failure (see "Hemodynamic Characteristics of Heart Failure" below).[360,361,363,365–388]

Myocardial Compensatory Mechanisms in Patients with Increased Left Ventricular Preload (Volume Overload)

With increased left ventricular preload (volume overload), *eccentric hypertrophy* develops, and the ventricular chamber and the left ventricular wall increase in size proportionately.[156,157,327–329,334,337–339] It has been suggested that this type of hypertrophy is produced by a chronic increase in diastolic wall stress and is associated with the synthesis of additional sarcomeres, predominantly in series.[339] Since increased preload also increases systolic wall stress and afterload by the law of Laplace, some replication or sarcomeres in parallel also occur and help to normalize systolic stress.

When the ventricle is subjected acutely to an increased preload, the ventricle dilates and functions on a higher portion of the "ascending limb" of its length-tension function curve, with the sarcomere length ultimately increasing to about 2.2 μm in the midwall of the left ventricle. This length approximates L_{max}, the sarcomere length at which the maximal performance is achieved on the sarcomere length-tension function curve.[41–43] In experimental animals subjected to chronic left ventricular volume loading, the left ventricle continues to work on the ascending limb of a function curve. When the ventricle is subjected to increased preload, however, there does not appear to be any additional increase in sarcomere length in the midwall of the left ventricle beyond about 2.2 μm, although there is some additional recruitment in sarcomere length up to about 2.2 μm in the left ventricular endocardial and epicardial area.[39–47] At this point, sarcomeres are very stiff, and any further increase in diastolic volume produces a very large increase in diastolic pressure. Normally, the functioning sarcomere lengths are somewhat less in the endocardium and the epicardium than in the midwall of the left ventricle.[39] The marked ventricular dilatation of chronic volume loading is produced by several mechanisms, including an increase in individual sarcomere length, the synthesis of new sarcomeres in series and parallel with previous sarcomeres so that the myocytes are longer, "slippage" between and within myofibrils and fibers, and the rearrangement of myocardial fibers along the normal cleavage planes of the ventricle.[4,39–46,334,411] Taken together, these changes have been termed *ventricular remodeling.*

The performance of the ventricle with mitral regurgitation is aided by the fact that during systole the left ventricle is emptied relatively rapidly by regurgitation into the left atrium and by aortic ejection. This rapid decrease in the mean left ventricular diameter has the effect of rapidly decreasing the systolic wall tension and afterload (impedance) and thus increasing the velocity of contraction.[47,404,430] The diastolic capacity of the ventricle with chronically increased volume loads is often markedly increased so that it may accommodate a large volume without excess elevation of diastolic pressure,[47,327] although any additional volume loading may produce a precipitous elevation of diastolic pressure, indicative of reduced compliance.[431] When the myocardial contractility eventually becomes markedly decreased in patients with chronic volume overload, the many compensatory mechanisms, including ventricular dilatation and hypertrophy, are no longer able to maintain normal compensation. Functional mitral regurgitation commonly occurs at this point, and overall heart pump function fails.

Figure 25-11 shows the hypothetical changes in myocardial contractility and pump function following the onset of an abnormality such as increased cardiac stress or injury. Note that overall cardiac (pump) function may be reasonably maintained by the many adaptive and compensatory mechanisms until the myocardial failure is moderately severe.

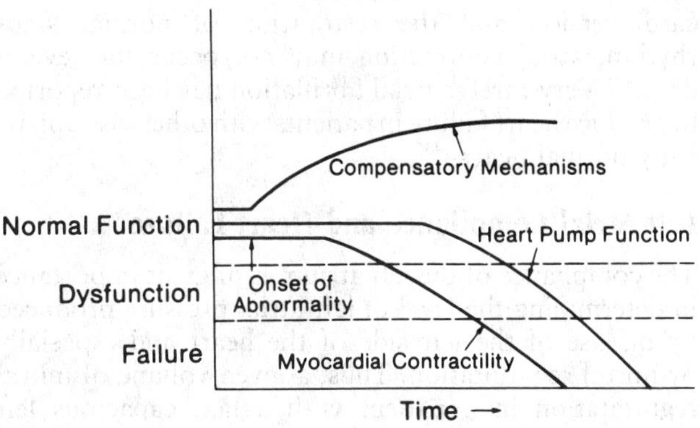

FIGURE 25-11 Hypothetical curves or compensatory mechanisms, overall cardiac or ventricular pump performance, and myocardial contractility following the onset of a significant stress, such as an increase in ventricular preload or ventricular afterload. Three levels of overall cardiac pump function and myocardial function (contractility) are shown; normal; dysfunction, or slightly to moderately decreased function; and failure, or markedly decreased function. In general, myocardial function or contractility decreases significantly prior to a decrease in overall cardiac pump function due to the compensatory mechanisms. Some studies have suggested that myocardial contractility may be decreased very early when hypertrophy occurs due to an increase in afterload. See text for discussion.

ATRIAL FAILURE AND HEART FAILURE[432,433]

The atria normally function as pumps and reservoirs.[458,459] In addition, the atria are the source of atrial natriuretic peptides.[304,305,313,317] Normally, the atria contribute approximately 15 to 20 percent of ventricular filling, but the relative contribution increases markedly with tachycardia. In normal individuals or patients with mild heart disease, loss of the atrial pumping function may result in no change in cardiac output at rest, although the response to exercise may be diminished. On the other hand, in patients with heart disease and limited cardiac reserve, atrial fibrillation or atrial flutter can produce *atrial failure* with severe detrimental effects on ventricular filling and on the pump function of the heart. This is particularly likely in patients with moderate or marked concentric cardiac hypertrophy from aortic stenosis, hypertrophic cardiomyopathy, or systemic arterial hypertension, where the stiffness of the ventricle is already increased.

The more common forms of atrial failure are due to arrhythmia (e.g., atrial fibrillation), mechanical abnormalities (e.g., mitral or tricuspid stenosis), or "dysdynamic" failure of the atrial myocardium. In some patients with compensated heart disease, congestive heart failure may be precipitated by the onset of atrial fibrillation, at times even when the ventricular response rate is controlled by digitalis. In these patients the restoration of normal sinus rhythm may result in a marked improvement in their hemodynamics, presumably by restoration of the normal "booster-pump" function of the atria. It is interesting to note that, in some patients following cardioversion and the restoration of normal sinus rhythm, atrial contraction may not occur for several days.[434] Very rarely, atrial fibrillation has been reported to produce heart failure in patients with otherwise apparently normal hearts.[435]

Left Atrial Compliance and Heart Failure

The compliance of the left atrium is of great importance in determining the level of left atrial pressure produced by disease of the left side of the heart and especially by mitral regurgitation. Thus, a given volume of mitral regurgitation in a patient with a lax, capacious left atrium, as is common in severe mitral regurgitation of long duration, may produce only slight elevation of left atrial pressure, whereas the same volume regurgitated into a smaller left atrium with less distensibility, as occurs with acute mitral regurgitation due to chordae tendineae rupture, produces marked elevation of left atrial pressure and severe pulmonary congestion (see Chap. 80).[47,436]

HEMODYNAMIC CHARACTERISTICS OF HEART FAILURE

The major hemodynamic alterations and several of the major compensatory mechanisms produced by myocardial and subsequent pump failure are diagrammatically shown in Fig. 25-12. Also indicated are the sites of action of major therapeutic interventions.

As described in Chaps. 5 and 23, the systolic performance of the intact heart should generally be assessed at two levels. The first type of analysis is an evaluation of the overall *cardiac pump function* as indicated by the relationship between stroke work (or cardiac output) and ventricular end-diastolic volume (or pressure). Ideally, these or other systolic indexes of pump performance are measured at rest and again during exercise or after induced changes in preload or afterload in order to construct a "function curve," although this is seldom done clinically. The second type of assessment is of systolic *myocardial function (myocardial contractility* or *inotropic state)*. Although decreases in myocardial contractility can sometimes be inferred from studies of overall cardiac function (i.e., when the cardiac output and SV are significantly decreased despite a markedly increased end-diastolic ventricular volume greater than 110 mL/m² and the presence of normal afterload and heart rate), more specific and more sensitive quantitative evidence of changes in myocardial contractility in patients is obtained from other special types of analyses. These include the following: (1) *isovolumic phase indexes* utilizing the rate of rise of ventricular pressure (*dP/dt*) or a derivative, (2) *ejection phase indexes* of contractility utilizing cir-

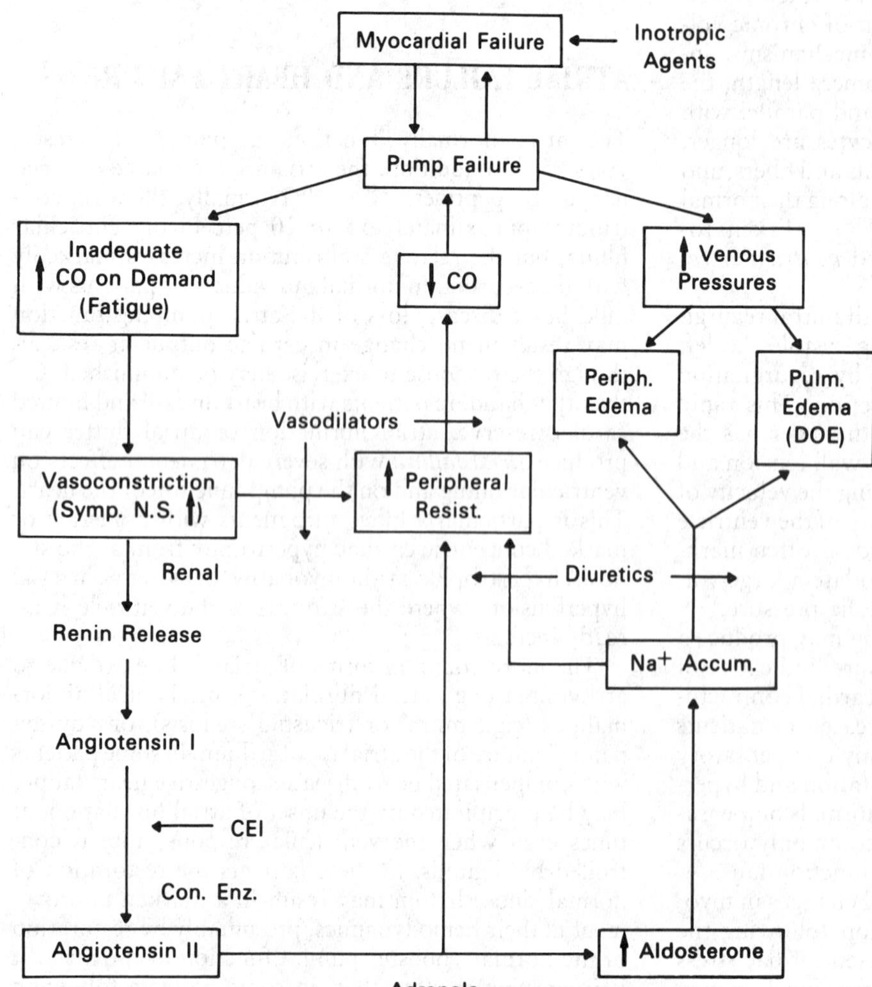

FIGURE 25-12 Schematic diagram of the major hemodynamic alterations and several of the major compensatory mechanisms that result from the development of myocardial failure and pump (heart) failure. Also shown are the sites of action of major therapeutic interventions: administration of inotropic agents, diuretics, converting enzyme inhibitors (CEI), and vasodilators.

cumferential fiber shortening rate (V_{cf}), and (3) *end-systolic indexes,* including analysis of ventricular end-systolic pressure or wall stress-volume relationships.[437] The techniques used clinically for evaluation of cardiac function and myocardial contractility are reviewed in Chap. 23.

Changes in the Contralateral Ventricle

The diastolic filling pressures of one ventricle affect the other across the common ventricular septum. Thus, elevated right ventricular filling pressure may produce an increase in left ventricular filling pressure (i.e., a "reversed" Bernheim effect).[396,438,441] These effects are much more apparent with an intact pericardium, which can substantially affect the left ventricular diastolic pressure-volume relationships.[441] In general, whenever there is moderate or marked ventricular hypertrophy of one ventricle, the diastolic pressure-volume relationships of the opposite ventricle may be altered.[377,392–398,442] This ventricular interdependence, or interaction, may occur chronically or acutely, as in patients with acute pulmonary embolus. In addition, in experimental heart failure models the contralateral left ventricle may have decreased NE concentration,[139,443] decreased myofibrillar adenosine triphosphatase activity,[50] and increased amounts of collagen.[155]

Secondary (Functional) Mitral or Tricuspid Regurgitation

"Functional" mitral valve regurgitation may develop secondary to left ventricular dilatation, and a similar form of tricuspid regurgitation occurs secondary to right ventricular dilatation. This may be a very major hemodynamic deficit in heart failure. In both instances the regurgitation is principally the result of failure of the papillary muscles and chordae tendineae of the dilatated ventricle to anchor or constrain the atrioventricular valve leaflets. A secondary mechanism, which is presented in chronic lesions, is dilatation of the valve annulus and failure of the valve annulus to constrict properly during systole. If the regurgitation is moderate or severe, the atrial pressure tracings may have a large regurgitant R wave ("giant *v* wave"). Heart failure is frequently associated with changes in left ventricular shape manifested by increased sphericity.[444–447] Functional mitral regurgitation may be more likely with a spherical left ventricle.[446,447]

Pulsus Alternans

Pulsus alternans may occur in patients with very severe heart failure, particularly from aortic stenosis. It may be associated with an alteration of end-diastolic volume or fiber length, with or without an alteration of EDP. In other patients, pulsus alternans may occur in the absence of alternation of either end-diastolic volume or pressure.[448–450] The latter cases appear to be associated with an isolated alteration of myocardial contractility. Pulsus alternans is probably related to a defect in the Ca^{2+} release-binding systems involved in excitation-contraction coupling. It may occur briefly in some apparently normal hearts during or following marked tachycardia.

Pulmonary Circulation in Heart Failure

In moderate or severe left ventricular failure, elevated left ventricular diastolic pressure is reflected in an elevation of left atrial, pulmonary capillary, and pulmonary artery diastolic pressures. Initially, the pulmonary artery pressure and right ventricular systolic pressure are abnormally elevated only during exercise, although later they may be chronically elevated to systemic levels at rest, particularly in patients with mitral valve disease (see Chap. 80). In the absence of significant pulmonary vascular disease or tachycardia, the pulmonary artery diastolic pressure can be used as a reasonably good reflection of mean left atrial pressure.

Right Ventricle in Heart Failure

Right ventricular dilatation and failure, with a decreased EF and rate of ejection, most often occur secondary to left ventricular failure, perhaps as a result of the pressure load created by elevated pulmonary pressures, but also from interactions across the ventricular septum that vitiate diastolic elastic recoil and may also slow emptying. There may also be secondary biochemical changes in the right ventricular myocardium (Fig. 25-13).[4,50,139,155,443] Right ventricular failure may be reflected in a decreased right ventricular SV and EF, despite an abnormal elevation of the right ventricular end-diastolic volume and pressure, the mean right atrial pressure, and the mean systemic venous pressure. If the failure is mild, these abnormalities may be absent at rest but apparent during exercise. Failure of the right ventricle may also be associated with development of right ventricular pulsus alternans, auscultatory alternans, and a right ventricular diastolic gallop (S_3) sound. The sequence of severe right ventricular failure secondary to left ventricular failure is frequently associated with the development of tricuspid regurgitation or occasionally with the development of functional pulmonary regurgitation due to dilatation of the pulmonary valve ring. Severe pulmonary regurgitation can produce an equalization of the pulmonary artery and right ventricular pressures during mid- or late diastole, although this rarely occurs with functional pulmonary regurgitation. Secondary, or so-called functional, tricuspid regurgitation is caused by the inability of the papillary muscles and chordae tendineae of the dilatated right ventricle to anchor and to maintain adequate closure of the tricuspid valve. Dilatation, or overstretch, of the tricuspid valve ring also contributes to the regurgitation when right ventricular dilatation is severe and chronic. Tricuspid regurgitation may produce large regurgitant R waves during systole in the right atrium and systemic veins (see Chap. 10). Clinically, the development of marked right ventricular failure in association with tricuspid regurgitation in a patient with severe left-sided heart failure may, very rarely, be associated with a significant decrease in the clinical symptoms of pulmonary congestion. More often, however, it is associated with a worsening of the pulmonary congestion.

Effects of Exercise in Patients with Heart Failure

During exercise in the supine position, the normal ventricle increases its cardiac output predominantly by an in-

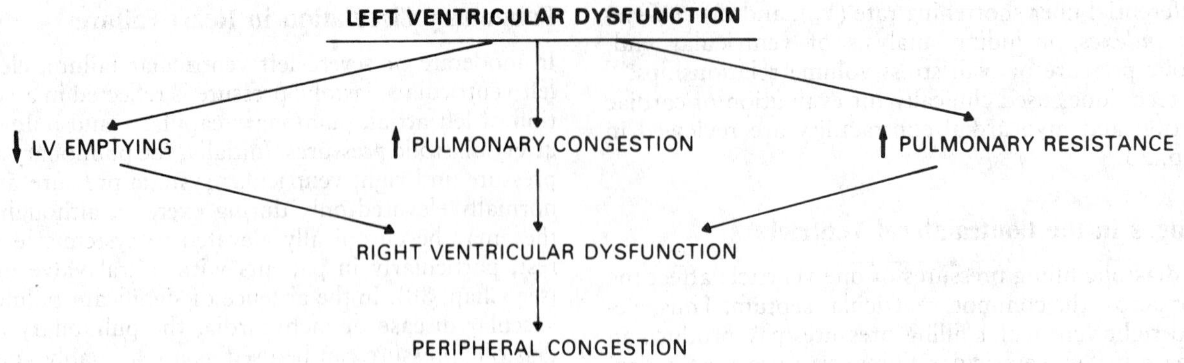

FIGURE 25-13 Relationship of left ventricular (LV) dysfunction to right ventricular dysfunction. See text for details.

crease in rate, although SV may increase 10 to 20 percent.[451] The increased SV occurs from an unchanged or slightly smaller end-diastolic volume and a decreased end-systolic volume;[452,453] consequently, the EF and SV may increase. The ventricular EDP normally stays the same or slightly decreases, whereas the systolic ejection period shortens and the mean systolic ejection rate and the rate of relaxation increase.[451–464] In contrast, during exercise in the upright position, SV may double,[465,466] and during maximal exercise the end-diastolic volume may increase.[4] The calculated efficiency (ratio of external work to oxygen consumed by the heart) increases during exercise in normal individuals, perhaps in part as the result of the decreased average ventricular radius throughout systole.

Conversely, in patients with heart failure due to dysdynamic myocardial failure, exercise may result in the following changes: an elevation of the EDP above 12 mmHg, only a slight increase or an actual decrease in SV despite an increased end-diastolic volume, a decreased EF,[467] an increased end-systolic volume, and a prolonged preejection phase.[4,449,454,467] The calculated ventricular efficiency decreases as the result of no increase (or an actual decrease) in SV despite an increased ventricular end-diastolic volume. The latter increases the mean radius of the ventricle and, by the Laplace relationship, increases the sarcomere tension necessary to produce a given intraventricular pressure. Not only does the increased tension required by the dilated ventricle increase the myocardial oxygen consumption ($M\dot{V}_{O2}$), it also decreases the velocity of shortening, further limiting the performance of the ventricle.[4,334,359,360,418–421,468] Exercise may also increase functional atrioventricular valvular regurgitation (see Chap. 23).

In patients with heart failure during dynamic exercise, the cardiac output either does not increase or does not increase adequately relative to the increased oxygen requirements of the body. One of the mechanisms for this is a failure of the peripheral vascular resistance to decrease normally during exertion.[469] Usually, the increase in blood flow to exercising limbs is less than normal in clinical heart failure, while there are marked decreases in the already diminished flow to skin, kidneys, and splanchnic organs. Coronary flow usually increases, whereas cerebral flow remains unchanged.[262] The excessive increase in venous tone and central venous pressure during exercise in heart failure may be in part related to a reflex with the afferent limb in the exercising muscle and the efferent limb in the sympathetic nervous system.[461] In addition, the plasma concentration of NE, which is often increased in moderate or severe congestive heart failure, is further increased. High plasma concentrations of angiotensin II, endothelin-1, and AVP may also contribute to the increase in arterial and venous tone. In general, exercise capacity in heart failure appears to be more closely related to the diastolic filling pattern of the left ventricle than to indices of left ventricular systolic function.[470]

The fact that the peripheral blood vessels of patients with heart failure have increased sodium and water content and are relatively stiff and relatively unresponsive to local metabolic vasodilator influences during exercise may have a protective influence in some patients with severe mitral stenosis. For example, if cardiac output did not increase or even decreased during extensive exercise, vasodilatation of large skeletal muscle groups could produce an excess fall in the mean arterial pressure. On the other hand, the increased stiffness tends to maintain arteriolar resistance and systemic blood pressure, although at the expense of increased total impedance to left ventricular emptying.

Effects of Heart Failure on the Peripheral Circulation

As noted above, in heart failure, there is evidence of a generalized state of arteriolar constriction and venoconstriction, resulting in an elevation of total peripheral vascular resistance and an increase in venous tone (i.e., the venous bed is less distensible than normal).[260] These changes tend to reduce cardiac output at rest as well as organ blood flow during exercise. They are mediated in part by sympathetic vasoconstrictor impulses, related to the generalized increase in sympathetic activity of the body, and perhaps by mechanical alterations in the distensibility of the resistance (arteriolar) vessels with increased "stiffness" due to increased sodium and water content.[260,263] In addition, the concentrations of NE, endothelin 1, angiotensin II, and AVP are elevated and contribute to both arterial vasoconstriction and the increase in venous tone.[207,286] Arteriolar smooth muscle hypertrophy may also occur in heart failure when endothelial dilator function in resistance vessels becomes abnormal. The mechanisms for these changes require further definition. Increased extravascular fluid or edema can also increase tissue pressure and external pressure on the systemic arterioles and veins. An increased plasma concentration of vasoconstrictor peptides or prostaglandins may also contribute to an increase in vascular tone. In some active organs with high oxygen requirements, these vasoconstrictor tendencies may be partially overridden by local metabolic vasodilators or local changes in adenosine, P_{O2}, P_{CO2}, pH, or K^+. In general, however, the usual markedly increased blood flow to exercising muscles is significantly attenuated.

Increased muscle fatigue in patients with heart failure is related not only to decreased blood flow during exertion but also to intrinsic changes in the skeletal muscles, including fiber atrophy and significant ultrastructure abnormalities that reflect a depressed oxidative capacity.[471–476] Altered skeletal muscle metabolism has been demonstrated by magnetic resonance spectroscopy.[472a,473,477] It is of interest that many patients appear to have a favorable training response.[478–482]

In heart failure associated with a diminished cardiac output, there is a significant redistribution of blood flow that in part resembles the normal redistribution occurring during exercise (Chap. 5).[262] Thus, in heart failure, the renal and skin blood flows are disproportionately reduced early, whereas the decreases in blood flow to the cerebral, splanchnic, and skeletal muscle areas are approximately proportional to the decrease in total cardiac output until the failure is severe. Coronary blood flow per 100 g of tissue tends to remain normal or nearly normal in most patients in heart failure. The decreased skin circulation contributes to the heat intolerance and even mild temperature elevations in heart failure, while the decreased flow to the brain and kidneys contributes significantly to the deranged functions of these organs.

As noted above, the increased sympathetic impulses to the kidney and the high blood levels of NE and angiotensin II produce a redistribution of intrarenal blood flow and lead to further retention of sodium and water.

In addition to a redistribution of blood flow in heart failure, the tissues extract more oxygen per unit of blood flow and utilize anaerobic metabolism to a greater extent than normal, particularly during acute exertion. The increased oxygen extraction results in a widening of the arteriovenous oxygen differences for most organs and for the body as a whole. The pulmonary arteriovenous oxygen difference, which indicates the average of the whole body, is one of the better parameters for judging the adequacy of the heart as a pump to provide oxygen to the tissues.

TABLE 25-6
Therapy for Heart Failure

Abnormality	Therapy
Preload	Salt restriction
	Diuretics
	Venous vasodilators
Afterload	Arterial vasodilators
	Angiotensin-converting enzyme inhibitors
	Angiotensin II-receptor blockers
Contractility	Inotropic agents
	Beta blockers (?)
Heart rate and rhythm	Pacemaker
	Antiarrhythmic agents, devices
	Beta blockers (?)

Baroreceptor Function

Heart failure is associated with significant impairment of baroreceptor reflexes that control both sympathetic and parasympathetic nervous system activity to the systemic arteries and veins and to the heart.[136,140,142–154,270,483–485]

PHYSIOLOGICAL BASIS OF THERAPY FOR HEART FAILURE

As discussed in Chap. 26, appropriate therapy and anticipated benefits depend on the phase of the disease. Early, a specific diagnosis is sought to treat as the primary damaging factor or factors, whether it is systolic overload, volume abnormalities, or ischemic myocardium. A fundamental aim is to prevent further myocyte loss. Once ventricular dysfunction is present, one seeks to limit the adaptive mechanisms that may become damaging, such as progressive ventricular dilatation (remodeling), while controlling salt and water accumulation. To prevent progression, it is important to prevent both further myocyte loss and continued dilatation. Late in the course of failure, while one still seeks these effects, major symptomatic improvement is gained by increasing peripheral organ perfusion and improving skeletal muscle performance.

It is useful in selecting the therapy for a patient with heart failure to consider each determinant of myocardial performance separately (Table 25-6). In general, an excessive increase in preload is treated with either diuretics or venous vasodilators. The relative increase in afterload associated with heart failure is treated with arterial vasodilators, compounds that inhibit the conversion of angiotensin I to angiotensin II, or compounds that block angiotensin II receptors (Chap. 30), while the excess sodium retention with peripheral or pulmonary edema or circulatory congestion is treated with diuretics (see Chap. 29). Figure 25-14 illustrates schematically the major mechanisms of action of vasodilator therapy in heart failure. Some of the benefits of therapy with angiotensin-converting enzyme (ACE) inhibitors in patients with mild to moderate heart failure or with left ventricular dysfunction without overt heart failure may be due to the effects of ACE inhibitors on tissue renin-angiotensin system activity (see also Chap. 26).

Myocardial systolic failure is present in most patients with systolic pump (heart) failure, either as a primary or as a secondary event. Direct therapy for a decrease in myocardial contractility includes the administration of digitalis (see Fig. 5-4) and other inotropic agents (Chap. 28) in addition to therapy to decrease afterload.[486,487] Figure 25-15 illustrates the mechanisms by which many inotropic agents increase myocardial contractility (see

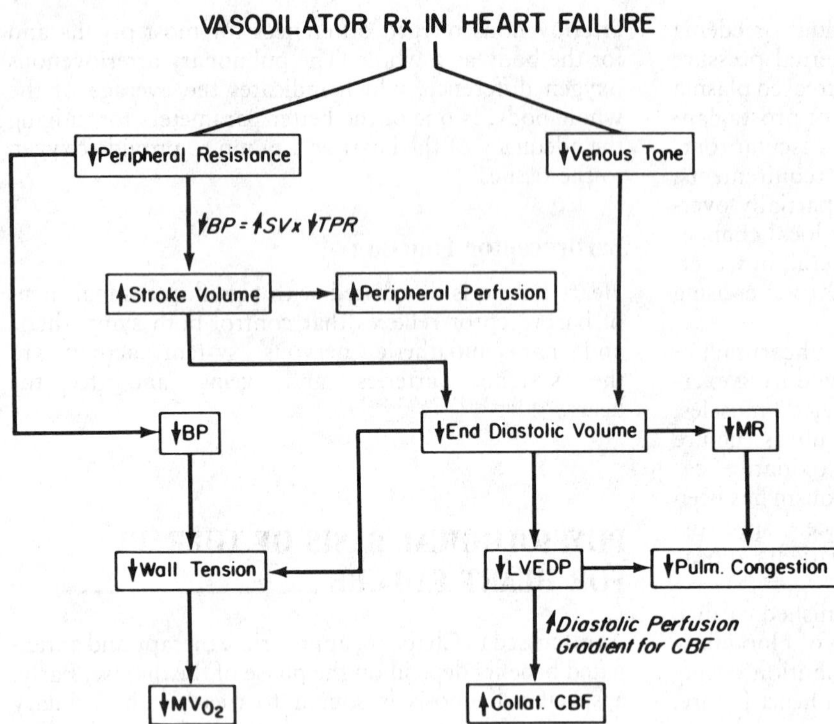

FIGURE 25-14 Schematic diagram of the major actions of vasodilator therapy in heart failure. The decrease in arterial resistance (decreased afterload) leads to an increase in stroke volume and improved peripheral perfusion. The decrease in arterial pressure combined with a decrease in end-diastolic volume (resulting from the decrease in venous tone) decreases systolic wall tension and myocardial oxygen requirements. The left ventricular end-diastolic volume is decreased as a result of both the improved stroke volume and the decreased venous return. It produces a decrease in LVEDP. This reduction may significantly improve coronary blood flow (CBF) and collateral blood flow to the left ventricle, particularly the subendocardium.

also Chaps. 27 and 28). Theoretically, inotropic agents used to treat mild myocardial failure might hasten the progression of the disease.[488] Improvement in central pump function permits progressive rehabilitation of the patient, which over several weeks is associated with a return toward normal of endothelial-dependent vascular vasodilatation and improved peripheral muscle blood flow during exercise. This permits increased exercise performance and, in terms of the inhibition of the renin-angiotensin system, improved quality of life. Digitalis may also have significant sympathoinhibitory actions in patients with heart failure.[489] (See Chap. 26 for further details of the treatment of heart failure.)

Diastolic dysfunction is treated acutely by the restoration, if necessary, of atrial contraction, the cautious use of diuretics to decrease pulmonary congestion, and the avoidance of myocardial ischemia and tachycardia. Chronically, the aim of therapy is to induce regression of the left ventricular hypertrophy.

PULMONARY FUNCTION AND PULMONARY EDEMA IN CONGESTIVE HEART FAILURE

Pulmonary Function in Congestive Heart Failure

The ventilatory functions of the lungs are frequently impaired due to pulmonary congestion from left ventricular failure or mechanical obstruction at the mitral valve.[490–492] The amount of intrathoracic space available for ventilation may be decreased by fluid in the interstitial, perivascular, and alveolar spaces; by hydrothorax; or, in some patients, by an increase in pulmonary blood volume.[493] The increased amount of fluid and congestion in the lungs decreases the compliance (increases the stiffness) of the lungs and increases the work and oxygen cost of breathing. Alveolar fluid decreases pulmonary compliance by altering the normal surface tension characteristics, while pericapillary thickening and interstitial edema interfere with alveolar-capillary diffusion of oxygen. The respiratory muscles, which have an increased workload because of the decreased pulmonary compliance, may suffer from relative ischemia and, rarely, may produce pain difficult to distinguish from pain of myocardial origin. As heart failure becomes severe, the oxygen consumption of the work of breathing becomes an increasing part of overall oxygen consumption and may ultimately become an overwhelming burden.[494]

Many patients with moderate pulmonary congestion have compensatory hyperventilation with respiratory alkalosis, although some patients with severe pulmonary edema can have metabolic and respiratory acidosis.[495] Pulmonary congestion alters many pulmonary function tests, and it is often difficult to distinguish by such tests between dyspnea due to cardiac causes and dyspnea due to pulmonary causes. In clear-cut instances, however, such a separation is often possible (see Chaps. 17 and 23).[491,492]

Pulmonary Edema[496–500]

General

The hydrostatic pressure in the pulmonary capillaries is normally 7 to 12 mmHg at rest in the supine position. When this pressure exceeds plasma oncotic pressure, which is normally 25 to 30 mmHg, net transudation of

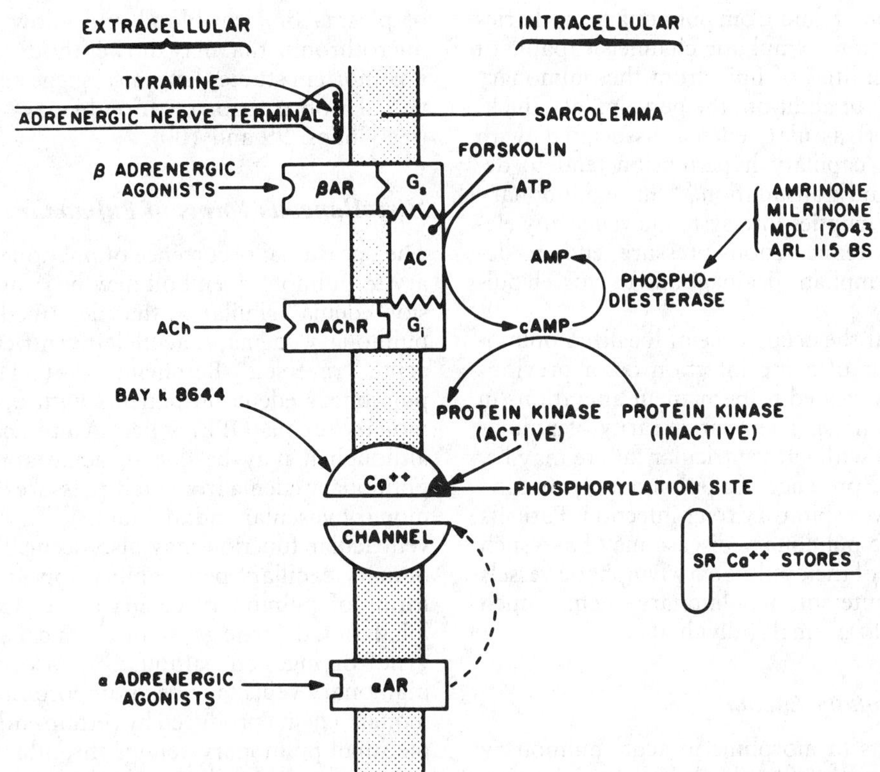

FIGURE 25-15 Diagram illustrating the sites of action of several positive inotropic agents. Circulating catecholamines, catecholamines released from adrenergic nerve terminals, and exogenous sympathomimetic drugs act on beta-adrenergic and alpha-adrenergic receptors (β-AR and α-AR, respectively). Stimulation of beta-adrenergic receptors causes activation of adenylate cyclase (AC), resulting in increased cyclic-AMP (cAMP) production, which in turn causes an increase in calcium influx through slow calcium channels, presumably due to the activation of protein kinases that phosphorylate the slow calcium channel. The mechanism by which stimulation of alpha-adrenergic receptors causes an increase in myocardial contractility is not fully understood, but it may also involve an action on the slow calcium channel. Tyramine acts on adrenergic nerve terminals to release catecholamines, which then act on adrenergic receptors. Calcium-channel agonists (e.g., the drug Bay k 8644) act directly on the calcium channel to increase calcium influx. Intracellular cAMP id degraded by phosphodiesterases, and inhibition of cardiac phosphodiesterases therefore results in an increase in intracellular cAMP levels. Several of the newer positive inotropic agents appear to act largely by this mechanism. cAMP can also be increased independently of beta-adrenergic receptors by direct stimulation of adenylate cyclase with forskolin. ACh, acetylcholine; G_I, quanine nucleotide inhibitory subunit; G_S, quanine nucleotide stimulatory subunit; mAChR, muscarinic ACh receptor; SR, sarcoplasmic reticulum. *(From WS Colucci, RF Wright, E Braunwald: New positive inotropic agents in the treatment of congestive heart failure. N Engl J Med 314:290, 1986. Reproduced with permission from the publisher and author.)*

fluid from the pulmonary capillaries occurs. Pulmonary edema occurs when this rate of transudation exceeds the rate of lymphatic drainage from the tissues. If the plasma oncotic pressure is low due to a decreased serum protein concentration, transudation of fluid across the pulmonary capillaries occurs at even lower pressure.[501] There is little evidence that altered capillary permeability due to central nervous system influences or hypoxia is ordinarily an important factor in the production of pulmonary edema in most patients, although changes in capillary permeability can be important in some specialized forms of pulmonary edema due to the "capillary leak syndrome"[502] or in some patients with virus infections of the respiratory tract. The major factor in cardiac pulmonary edema is the pulmonary capillary pressure.[492] The pulmonary capillaries have a significant "reserve" compared to systemic capillaries, since the pulmonary capillary pressure can ordinarily increase by 10 to 20 mmHg before significant transudation occurs.

An important consideration in the pulmonary circulation is the normal increase in hydrostatic pressure in both the arteries and veins in the dependent areas of the lungs. This increased pressure accounts, in part, for the initial appearance of pulmonary edema in the lower lobes in many patients with congestive failure. In normal persons in the upright position, relatively little pulmonary blood flow goes to the upper areas of the lungs. In patients with severe mitral stenosis or in severe left ventricular failure, however, the relative blood flow to the upper lobes may be equal or even exceed that to the lower lobes. It is uncertain whether this change in distribution of pulmonary blood flow is caused by local vasoconstriction produced by alveolar hypoxia, by a reactive hypertrophy and increased vascular tone of small arteries in the lower lobes secondary to the elevation of pulmonary arterial pressure, or by reflexes from the left atrium or pulmonary veins. Patients with marked elevation of left atrial pressure for long periods of time may often withstand elevations of pulmonary capillary pressure reasonably well, whereas the same level of pulmonary capillary pressure can produce severe, fulminating pulmonary edema in 5 to 10 min in a patient whose pulmonary circulation is not accustomed to these high pressure levels. The explanation for this difference may be that patients with chronic transudation of fluid from pulmonary capillaries often develop capacious lymphatic channels capable of removing large quantities of fluid from the pulmonary interstitial spaces.[503] In addition, the pericapillary thickening and the perivascular edema associated with chronic pulmonary capillary hypertension tend to decrease the rate of fluid transudation.[504] Since pulmonary lymphatic drainage empties into systemic veins, any elevation of central systemic venous pressure tends to decrease pulmonary lymphatic drainage and to worsen pulmonary edema.

It is probable that the occurrence of localized pulmonary edema in areas of acute infection or of previous infection is partially related to permanent alterations in local lymphatic drainage. The relative rarity of pulmonary rales in infants with left ventricular failure may be, in part, related to the presence of a pulmonary lymphatic system unscarred by respiratory tract infection. Patients with severe, chronic pulmonary disease may have such marked destruction of their pulmonary lymphatic vessels that they develop interstitial pulmonary edema much more readily than do normal individuals.

Morphine in Pulmonary Edema

The beneficial effects of morphine in acute pulmonary edema are in part produced by decreased arterial resistance and pressure secondary to a reduction of centrally mediated sympathetic neural tone, which decreases ventricular afterload; by a decrease in venous return, perhaps aided by depression of the respiratory pump; and by "pharmacologic phlebotomy" resulting from an increase in the capacity of the peripheral vascular beds with perfusion of unperfused areas and venous pooling.[505,506]

Noncardiac Pulmonary Edema

High-Altitude Pulmonary Edema

High-altitude pulmonary edema (HAPE) is apparently associated with marked pulmonary artery hypertension and pulmonary arteriolar vasoconstriction but with normal pulmonary artery wedge ("pulmonary capillary") pressure.[507–513] The mechanism of pulmonary edema in this rare syndrome is uncertain, although it is possible that the development of HAPE is related to an unusually marked, nonuniform vasoconstriction of the terminal pulmonary arterioles in response to decreased partial pressure of oxygen in the alveoli. As a consequence, there is excessive blood flow in the other areas of the lung, and the capillary bed may be relatively "unprotected" from the high pulmonary arterial pressure. An additional factor that may be important is the presence of preterminal arterioles, which are short, nonmuscular vessels that arise at right angles from small and medium-sized pulmonary arteries, bypass the pulmonary arterioles, and empty directly into the venous side of the pulmonary capillary bed.[514] These arterioles may be important in transmitting the strikingly elevated pulmonary artery pressure directly to the capillary bed in subjects with HAPE. Acute pulmonary hypertension may also damage the arterial walls and lead to direct transarterial leakage of plasma or even blood and allow the formation of microthrombi that may shower the distal capillary bed.[507] Postmortem studies have also suggested that pulmonary vascular obstruction by thrombi may occur in some cases (see Chaps. 99 and 100).

Miscellaneous Forms of Pulmonary Edema

The occasional occurrence of pulmonary edema secondary to pulmonary emboli may be related to "overperfusion edema" similar to that described for high-altitude pulmonary edema,[515] acute left ventricular failure, or an acute "reversed" Bernheim effect. The mechanism of pulmonary edema in patients with opiate-induced pulmonary edema (OPE) or heroin intoxication is uncertain, although it may be due to acute apnea with hypoxic pulmonary edema from high-pressure damage to the pulmonary vascular endothelium.[507,516] Acute depression of ventricular function may also occur.[517] Changes in pulmonary capillary permeability appear to occur in some forms of pulmonary edema associated with infection, inhalation of toxic gases, or chemicals, such as ethchlorvynol or ingested paraquat.[507] Vasoconstriction of the pulmonary veins may be an important factor in the pulmonary edema produced by certain endotoxins.[518] Multiple small pulmonary venous thrombi may also produce acute pulmonary edema. Neurogenic pulmonary edema appears to be associated with intensive elevations in systemic arterial and venous pressures and pulmonary arterial, capillary, and venous pressures. The abrupt elevation of pulmonary vascular pressure and volume may damage the vascular endothelium, altering reactivity and permeability and allowing pulmonary edema to develop.[507,519]

MORTALITY IN HEART FAILURE

The prognosis of patients with heart failure is generally poor; and in several series 50 percent of the patients with severe symptoms died within 12 months. In less severe heart failure, mortality approaches 50 percent in 3 to 4 years.[521–523] The primary factor determining prognosis is the left ventricular function, as reflected in the EF. Other factors that have been shown to have prognostic value include functional classification; electrolyte abnormalities such as hyponatremia; elevated levels of plasma catecholamines, angiotensin II, aldosterone, and atrial natriuretic factor; poor exercise tolerance; presence of atrial fibrillation; and coronary artery disease as the etiology of the heart failure.[524,525] Many patients with heart failure, perhaps 30 to 40 percent, die suddenly, presumably from ventricular arrhythmias. Moreover, increasing heart failure is associated with an increased incidence of ventricular arrhythmias, which may be decreased by aggressive, successful therapy for heart failure or by the prevention of hypokalemia or hypomagnesemia. Figure 25-16 diagrammatically illustrates the potential sequence of events in cardiac pump failure from initiating causes to myocardial failure to decreased survival. In patients surviving myocardial infarction, the prognosis is strongly related

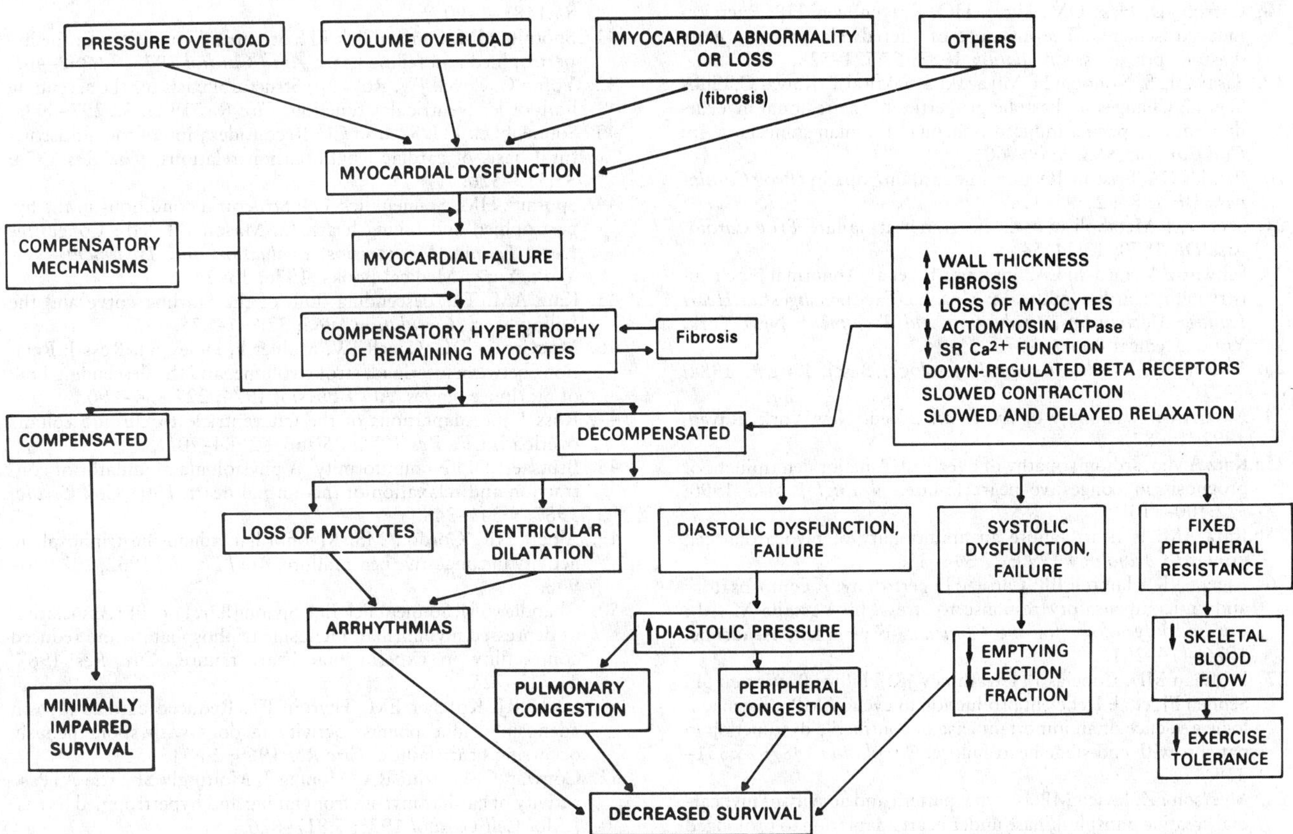

FIGURE 25-16 Sequence of events in cardiac pump failure from the initial load, myocardial damage, or loss progressing to myocardial failure and compensatory hypertrophy of the remaining myocytes. The decompensation of the myocardial and cardiac function due to a variety of causes may be manifested by systolic or diastolic dysfunction, further loss of myocytes, and ventricular dilatation, all of which contribute to decreased survival. The relatively fixed peripheral resistance contributes to the decreased exercise tolerance. See text for details.

to the left ventricular EF, in addition to the amount of myocardium that becomes ischemic during stress and the amount of ventricular ectopy (see Chaps. 23, 26, 60, 61, and 63).

REFERENCES

1. Eichna LW: Circulatory congestion and heart failure. *Circulation* 1960; 68:864–882.
2. Schlant RC, Nutter DO: Heart failure in valvular heart disease. *Medicine* 1971; 50:421–451.
3. Mason DT (ed): *Congestive Heart Failure: Mechanisms, Evaluation and Treatment.* New York, Yorke Medical Books, 1976: 1–448.
4. Braunwald E, Ross J Jr, Sonnenblick EH: *Mechanisms of Contraction of the Normal and Failing Heart,* 2d ed. Boston, Little, Brown, 1976: 1–417.
5. Weber KT, Janicki JS: The heart as a muscle-pump system and the concept of heart failure. *Am Heart J* 1979; 98:371–384.
6. Braunwald E, Mock MB, Watson J (eds): *Congestive Heart Failure: Current Research and Clinical Applications.* New York, Grune & Stratton, 1982: 1–384.
7. Alpert NR (ed): *Myocardial Hypertrophy and Failure: Perspectives in Cardiovascular Research,* vol. 7. New York, Raven, 1983: 1–682.
8. Levine HJ, Gaasch WH: *The Ventricle: Basic and Clinical Aspects.* Boston, Martinus Nijhoff, 1985: 1–345.
9. Rupp H: *Regulation of Heart Function: Basic Concepts and Clinical Applications.* Stuttgart, Thieme, 1986: 1–446.
10. Fozzard HA, Haber E, Jennings RB, Katz AM, Morgan HE (eds): *The Heart and Cardiovascular System: Scientific Foundations,* 2d ed. New York, Raven, 1991.
11. Skelton CL, Sonnenblick EH: Heterogeneity of contractile function in cardiac hypertrophy. *Circ Res* 1974; 35(suppl 2):83–96.
12. Eichhorn EJ, Willard JE, Alvarez L, Kim AS, Glamann DB, Risser RC, et al: Are contraction and relaxation coupled in patients with and without congestive heart failure? *Circulation* 1992; 85:2132–2139.
13. Mirsky I, Pfeffer JM, Pfeffer MA: Mechanical properties of normal and hypertrophied myocardium: Is there a relationship between diastolic and systolic function. In: Alpert NR (ed): *Perspectives in Cardiovascular Research,* vol 7. New York, Raven, 1983: 39–52.
14. Dodek A, Kassebaum DG, Bristow JD: Pulmonary edema in coronary-artery disease without cardiomegaly. *N Engl J Med* 1972; 286:1347–1350.
15. McLaurin LP, Rolett EL, Grossman W: Impaired left ventricular relaxation during pacing-induced ischemia. *Am J Cardiol* 1973; 32:751–757.
16. Barry WH, Brooker JZ, Alderman EL, Harrison DC: Changes in diastolic stiffness and tone of the left ventricle during angina pectoris. *Circulation* 1974; 49:255–263.
16a. Mann T, Brodie BR, Grossman W, McLaurin LP: Effect of angina on the left ventricular diastolic pressure-volume relationship. *Circulation* 1977; 55:761–766.
17. Bourdillon PD, Lorell BH, Mirsky I, Paulus WJ, Wynne J, Grossman W: Increased regional myocardial stiffness of the left ventri-

cle during pacing-induced angina in man. *Circulation* 1983; 67:316–323.
18. Carroll JD, Hess OM, Hirzel HO, Krayenbuehl HP: Exercise-induced ischemia: The influence of altered relaxation on early diastolic pressures. *Circulation* 1983; 67:521–528.
19. Sasayama S, Nonoogi H, Miyazaki S, Sakurai T, Kawai C, Eihos S, et al: Changes in diastolic properties of the regional myocardium during pacing-induced ischemia in human subjects. *J Am Coll Cardiol* 1985; 5:599–606.
20. Pantley GA, Bristow JD: Ischemic cardiomyopathy. *Prog Cardiovasc Dis* 1984; 27:95–114.
21. Scheuer J: Metabolism of the heart in heart failure. *Prog Cardiovasc Dis* 1970; 13:24–54.
22. Schwartz A, Sordahl LA, Entman ML, et al: Abnormal biochemistry in myocardial failure. In: Mason DT (ed): *Congestive Heart Failure: Mechanisms, Evaluation and Treatment.* New York, Yorke Medical Books, 1976: 25–44.
23. Badeer HS: *Cardiovascular Physiology.* Basel, Karger, 1984: 1–276.
24. Katz AM: *Physiology of the Heart* 2d ed. New York, Raven, 1992: 1–687.
25a. Katz AM: Cardiomyopathy of overload: A major determinant of prognosis in congestive heart failure. *N Engl J Med* 1990: 322:100–110
25b. Katz AM: Is heart failure an abnormality of myocardial cell growth? *Cardiology* 1990; 77:346–356.
26. Alpert NR, Hamrell BB: Cardiac hypertrophy: A compensatory and anticompensatory response to stress. In: Vassalle M (ed): *Cardiac Physiology for the Clinician.* New York, Academic, 1976: 174–201.
27. Feldman MD, Copelas L, Gwathmey JK, Phillips P, Warren SE, Schoen FJ, et al: Deficient production of cyclic AMP: Pharmacologic evidence of an important case of contractile dysfunction in patients with end-stage heart failure. *Circulation* 1987; 75:331–339.
28. Meerson FZ, Javich MP: Isozyme pattern and activity of myocardial creatine phosphokinase under heart adaptation to prolonged overload. *Basic Res Cardiol* 1982; 77:349–358.
29. Sievers R, Parmley WW, James T, Wikman-Coffelt J: Energy levels at systole and diastole in normal hamster hearts vs. myopathic hamster hearts. *Circ Res* 1983; 53:759–766.
30. Ingwall JS, Kramer MF, Fifer MA, Lovell BH, Shemin R, Grossman W, et al: The creatine kinase system in normal and diseased human myocardium. *N Engl J Med* 1985; 313:1050–1054.
31. Page E, McCallister LP: Quantitative electron microscopic description of heart muscle cells. *Am J Cardiol* 1973; 31:172–181.
32. Goldstein MA, Sordahl LA, Schwartz A: Ultrastructural analysis of left ventricular hypertrophy in rabbits. *J Mol Cell Cardiol* 1974; 6:265–273.
33. Rabinowitz M, Zak R: Mitochondria and cardiac hypertrophy. *Circ Res* 1975; 36:367–376.
34. Anversa P, Ricci R, Olivetti G: Quantitative structural analysis of the myocardium during physiologic growth and induced cardiac hypertrophy: A review. *J Am Coll Cardiol* 1986; 7:1140–1149.
35. Lentz RW, Harrison CE Jr, Dewey JD, Barnhorst DA, Danielson GK, Pluth JR: Functional evaluation of cardiac sarcoplasmic reticulum and mitochondria in human pathologic states. *J Mol Cell Cardiol* 1978; 10:3–30.
36. Unverfeth DV, Lee SW, Wallick ET: Human myocardial adenosine triphosphatase activities in health and heart failure. *Am Heart J* 1988; 115:139–146.
37. Schulze K, Becker BF, Schultheiss HP: Antibodies to the ADP/ATP carrier, an autoantigen in myocarditis and dilated cardiomyopathy, penetrate into myocardial cells and disturb energy metabolism in vivo. *Circ Res* 1989; 64:179–192.
38. Schever J: Metabolic factors in myocardial failure. *Circulation* 1993; 87(suppl VII): VII-54–VII-57.
39. Markiewicz W, Wu S, Sievers R, Parmley WW, Higgins CB, James TL, et al: Influence of heart rate on metabolic and hemodynamic parameters in the Syrian hamster cardiomyopathy. *Am Heart J* 1987; 114:362–368.
39a. Ross J Jr, Sonnenblick EH, Taylor RR, Spotnitz HM, Covell J: Diastolic geometry and sarcomere lengths in the chronically dilated left ventricle. *Circ Res* 1971; 28:49–61.
40. Spotnitz HM, Leyton RA, Kelly DT, Beiser GD, Pierce JE, Epstein SE, et al: Overstretched sarcomere in subacute volume-pressure loading of dog right ventricle (abstr.). *Circulation* 1972; 46(suppl 2):44.
41. Charney RH, Takahashi S, Zhao M, Sonnenblick EH, Eng C: Collagen loss in the stunned myocardium. *Circulation* 1992; 85:1483–1490.
41a. Spotnitz HM, Sonnenblick EH: Structural conditions in the hypertrophied and failing heart. *Am J Cardiol* 1973; 32:398–406.
42. Yoran C, Covell JW, Ross J Jr: Structural basis for the ascending limb of left ventricular function. *Circ Res* 1973; 32:297–303.
43. Sonnenblick EH, Skelton CL: Reconsideration of the ultrastructural basis of cardiac length-tension relations. *Circ Res* 1974; 35:517–526.
44. Spotnitz HM, Sonnenblick EH: Structural conditions in the hypertrophied and failing heart. In: Mason DT (ed): *Congestive Heart Failure: Mechanisms, Evaluation and Treatment.* New York, Yorke Medical Books, 1976: 13–24.
45. Katz AM: The descending limb of the Starling curve and the failing heart. *Circulation* 1965; 32:871–875.
46. MacGregor DC, Covell JW, Mahler F, Dilley RJ, Ross J: Relations between afterload, stroke volume, and the descending limb of Starling's curves. *Am J Physiol* 1974; 227:884–890.
47. Ross J Jr: Adaptations of the left ventricle to chronic volume overload. *Circ Res* 1974; 35(suppl 2):64–70.
48. Brutsaert DL: Nonuniformity: A physiologic modulator of contraction and relaxation of the normal heart. *J Am Coll Cardiol* 1987; 9:341–348.
49. Alpert NR, Gordon MS: Myofibrillar adenosine triphosphate activity in congestive heart failure. *Am J Physiol* 1962; 202:940–946.
50. Chandler BM, Sonnenblick EH, Spann JF Jr, Pool PE: Association of depressed myofibrillar adenosine triphosphatase and reduced contractility in experimental heart failure. *Circ Res* 1967; 21:717–725.
51. Luchi RJ, Kritcher EM, Thyrum PT: Reduced cardiac myosin adenosine-triphosphatase activity in dogs with spontaneously occurring heart failure. *Circ Res* 1969; 24:513–519.
52. Conway G, Heazlitt RA, Montag J, Mattingly SF: The ATPase activity of cardiac myosin from failing and hypertrophied hearts. *J Mol Cell Cardiol* 1975; 7:817–826.
53. Wikman-Coffelt J, McPherson J, Salel AF, Kamiyama T, Mason DT: Mechanism of impaired contractile protein function in aortic stenosis: Alterations in myosin ATPase activity in the chronically pressure overload canine left ventricle (absrt.). *Am J Cardiol* 1975; 35:177.
54. Wikman-Coffelt J, Walsh R, Fenner C, Kamiyama T, Salel A, Mason DT: Effects of severe hemodynamic pressure overload on the properties of canine left ventricular myosin: Mechanisms by which myosin ATPase activity is lowered during chronic increased hemodynamic stress. *J Moll Cell Cardiol* 1976; 8:263–270.
55. Wikman-Coffelt J, Mason DT: Mechanism of decreased contractility in chronic hemodynamic overload. In: Mason DT (ed): *Advances in Heart Diseases,* vol. 1. New York, Grune & Stratton, 1977: 491–504.
56. Leclercq JF, Swynghedauw B: Myofibrillar ATPase, DNA, and hydroxyproline content of human hypertrophied heart. *Eur J Clin Invest* 1976; 6:27–33.
57. Cummins P: Contractile proteins in muscle disease. *J Muscl Res Cell Motil* 1983; 4:5–24.
58. Pagani ED, Alonsi AA, Grant AM, Older TM, Dziuban SW, Allen PD: Changes in myofibrillar content and Mg-ATPase activity in ventricular tissues from patients with heart failure caused by coronary artery disease, cardiomyopathy, or mitral valve insufficiency. *Circ Res* 1988; 63:380–385.
59. Gorza L, Mercadier JJ, Schwartz K, Thornell LE, Sartore S, Schiaffino S: Myosin types in the human heart: An immunofluorescence study of normal and hypertrophied atrial and ventricular myocardium. *Circ Res* 1984; 54:694–702.
60. Feldman AM, Ray PE, Silan CM, Mercer JA, Minobe W, Bristow MR: Selective gene expression in failing human heart: Quantification of steady-state levels of messenger RNA in endomyocardial biopsies using the polymerase chain reaction. *Circulation* 1991; 83:1866–1872.
61. Margossian SS, White HD, Caulfield JB, Norton P, Taylor S, Slayter HS: Light chain 2 profile and activity of human ventricular myosin during dilated cardiomyopathy: Identification of a causal agent for impaired myocardial function. *Circulation* 1992; 85:1720–1733.
62. Mercadier JJ, Lompre A-M, Duc P, Boheler KR, Fraysse J-B, Wisnewsky C, et al: Altered sarcoplasmic reticulum Ca^{++}-AT-

Pase gene expression in the human left ventricle during endstage heart failure. *J Clin Invest* 1990; 85:305–309.
63. Grossman W: Diastolic dysfunction in congestive heart failure. *N Engl J Med* 1991; 325:1557–1564.
64. Arai M, Alpert NR, MacLennan DH, Barton P, Periasamy M: Alterations in sarcoplasmic reticulum gene expression in human heart failure: A possible mechanism for alterations in systolic and diastolic properties of the failing myocardium. *Circ Res* 1993; 72:463–469.
65. Mead RJ, Peterson MB, Welty JD: Sarcolemmal and sarcoplasmic reticular ATPase activities in the failing canine heart. *Circ Res* 1971; 29:14–20.
66. Dubois-Randé JL, Comoy E, Merlet P, Benvenuti C, Carville C, Hittinger L, et al: Relationship among neuropeptide Y, catecholamines and haemodynamics in congestive heart failure. *Eur Heart J* 1992; 13:1233–1238.
67. Beller GA, Conroy J, Smith TW: Ischemia-induced alterations in myocardial (Na^+ and K^+) ATPase and cardiac glycoside binding. *J Clin Invest* 1976; 57:341–350.
68. Dzau VJ, Packer M, Lilly LS, Swartz SL, Hollenberg NK, Williams GH: Prostaglandins in severe heart failure: Relation to activation of the renin-angiotensin system and hyponatremia. *N Engl J Med* 1984; 310:347–352.
69. Suko J, Vogel JH: Chidsey CA: Intracellular calcium and myocardial contractility: III. Reduced calcium intake and ATPase of the sarcoplasmic reticular fraction prepared from chronically failing calf hearts. *Circ Res* 1970; 27:235–247.
70. Sulakhe PV, Dhalla NS: Excitation-contraction coupling in heart: VII. Calcium accumulation in subcellular particles in congestive heart failure. *J Clin Invest* 1971; 50:1019–1027.
71. Sordahl LA, McCollum WB, Wood WG, Schwartz A: Mitochondria and sarcoplasmic reticulum function in cardiac hypertrophy and failure. *Am J Physiol* 1973; 224:497–502.
72. Ito Y, Suko J, Chidsey CA: Intracellular calcium and myocardial contractility: V. Calcium uptake of sarcoplasmic reticulum fraction in hypertrophied and failing rabbit hearts. *J Moll Cell Cardiol* 1974; 6:237–247.
73. Reuter H: Exchange of calcium ions in the mammalian myocardium: Mechanisms and physiological significance. *Circ Res* 1974; 34:599–605.
74. Katz AM: Congestive heart failure: Role of altered myocardial cellular control. *N Engl J Med* 1975; 293:1184–1191.
75. Dhalla NS, Das PK, Sharma GP: Subcellular basis on cardiac contractile failure. *J Mol Cell Cardiol* 1978; 10:363–385.
76. Factor SM, Sonnenblick EH: Pathogenesis of clinical and experimental congestive cardiomyopathies: Recent Concepts. *Prog Cardiovasc Dis* 1985; 27:395–420.
77. Staley NA, Noren GR, Einzig S: Early alterations in the function of sarcoplasmic reticulum in a naturally occurring model of congestive cardiomyopathy. *Cardiovasc Res* 1981; 15:276–281.
78. Dhalla NS, Alto LE, Heyliger CE, Pierce GN, Panagia V, Singal PK: Sarcoplasmic reticular Ca^{2+}-pump adaptation in cardiac hypertrophy due to pressure overload in pigs. *Eur Heart J* 1984; 5(suppl F):323–328.
79. Fein FS, Sonnenblick EH: Diabetic cardiomyopathy. *Prog Cardiovasc Dis* 1985; 4:255–270.
79a. Fizel A, Turcani M, Fizelova A, Maasovad D, Simko F: Calcium transport by intracellular membrane structures in the myocardium of hypertrophied and failing hearts. *Cor Vasa* 1986; 28:373–383.
80. Dhalla NS, Pierce GN, Panagia V, Singal PK, Beamish RE: Calcium movements in relation to heart function. *Basic Res Cardiol* 1982; 77:117–139.
81. Smith VE, Katz AM: Inotropic and lusitropic abnormalities in the genesis of heart failure. *Eur Heart J* 1983; 4(suppl A): 7–17.
82. Limas CJ, Olivari M, Goldenberg IF, Levine TB, Benditt DG, Simon A: Calcium uptake by cardiac sarcoplasmic reticulum in human dilated cardiomyopathy.
83. Gwathmey JK, Copelas L, MacKinnon R, Schoen FJ, Feldman MD, Grossman W, et al: Abnormal intracellular calcium handling in myocardium from patients with end-stage heart failure. *Circ Res* 1987; 61:70–76.
84. Movsesian MA, Bristow MR, Krall J: Ca^{2+} uptake by cardiac sarcoplasmic reticulum from patients with idiopathic dilated cardiomyopathy. *Circ Res* 1989; 65:1141–1144.
85. Morgan JP, Erny RE, Allen PD, Grossman W, Gwathmey JK: Abnormal intracellular calcium handling: A major cause of systolic and diastolic dysfunction in ventricular myocardium from patients with heart failure. *Circulation* 1990; 81:III21–III32.
86. Langer GA (ed): *Calcium and the Heart.* New York, Raven, 1990: 1–387.
87. Morgan JP: Abnormal intracellular modulation of calcium as a major cause of cardiac contractile dysfunction. *N Engl J Med* 1991; 325:625–632.
88. Siri FM, Krueger J, Nordin C, Ming Z, Aronson R: Depressed intracellular calcium transients and contraction in myocytes from hypertrophied and failing guinea pig hearts. *Am J Physiol* 1991; 261(*Heart Circ Physiol* 30):H514–H530.
89. Beuckelmann DJ, Näbauer M, Erdmann E: Intracellular calcium handling in isolated ventricular myocytes from patients with terminal heart failure. *Circulation* 1992; 85:1046–1055.
90. Hasenfuss G, Mulieri LA, Leavitt BJ, Allen PD, Haeberle JR, Alpert NR: Alteration of contractile function and excitation-contraction coupling in dilated cardiomyopathy. *Circ Res* 1992; 70:1225–1232.
91. Katz AM, Hecht HH: The early pump failure of the ischemic heart. *Am J Med* 1969; 47:497–502.
92. Van Winkle WB, Schwartz A: Ions and ionotropy. *Annu Rev Physiol* 1976; 38:247–272.
93. Bristow MR, Ginsburg R, Minobe W, Cubicciotti RS, Sageman WS, Lurie K, et al: Decreased catecholamine sensitivity and β-adrenergic-receptor density in failing human hearts. *N Engl J Med* 1982; 307:205–211.
94. Bristow MR, Kantrowitz NE, Ginsburg R, Fowler MB: β-adrenergic function in heart muscle disease and heart failure. *J Mol Cell Cardiol* 1985; 17(suppl 2):41–52.
95. Vatner DE, Vatner SF, Fuzii AM, Homcy CJ: Loss of high affinity cardiac beta-adrenergic receptors in dogs with heart failure. *J Clin Invest* 1985; 76:2259–2264.
96. Fowler MB, Laser JA, Hopkins GL, Minobe W, Bristow MR: Assessment of the beta-adrenergic receptor pathway in the intact failing human heart: Progressive β-receptor down-regulation and specific pharmacologic subsensitivity to agonist response. *Circulation* 1986; 74:1290–1302.
97. Bristow MR, Ginsburg R, Umans V, Fowler M, Minobe W, Rasmussen R, et al: β_1 and β_2-adrenergic receptor subpopulations in normal and failing human ventricular myocardium: Coupling of both receptor subtypes to muscle contraction and selective β_1 receptor down-regulation in heart failure. *Circ Res* 1986; 59:297–309.
98. Bristow MR, Ginsburg R, Gilbert EM, Hershberger RE: Heterogeneous regulatory changes in cell surface membrane receptors coupled to a positive inotropic response in the failing human heart. *Basic Res Cardiol* 1987; 82(suppl 2):369–376.
99. Colucci WS, Leatherman GF, Ludmer PL, Gauthier DF: Beta-adrenergic inotropic responsiveness of patients with heart failure: Studies with intracoronary dobutamine infusion. *Circ Res* 1987; 61(suppl I):I82–I86.
100. Bohm M, Beukelmann D, Brown L, Feiler G, Lorenz B, Nabaver M, et al: Reduction of beta-adrenoreceptor density and evaluation of positive inotropic responses in isolated, diseased human myocardium. *Eur Heart J* 1988; 9:844–852.
101. Feldman MD, Copelas L, Gwathmey JK, Phillips P, Warren SE, Schoen FJ, et al: Deficient production of cyclic AMP: Pharmacologic evidence of an important cause of contractile dysfunction in patients with end-stage heart failure. *Circulation* 1987; 75:331–339.
102. Bristow MR, Port JD, Hershberger RE, Gilbert EM, Feldman AM: The β-adrenergic receptor-adenylate cyclase complex as a target for therapeutic intervention in heart failure. *Eur Heart J* 1989; 10(suppl B):45–54.
103. Denniss AR, Marsh J, Quigg RJ, Gordon JB, Colucci WS: Beta-adrenergic receptor number and adenylate cyclase function in denervated transplanted and cardiomyopathic human hearts. *Circulation* 1989; 79:1028–1034.
104. Feldman AM: The receptor-G protein-adenylate cyclase complex in heart failure. In: Rapaport E (ed): *Cardiology Update: Reviews for Physicians.* New York, Elsevier, 1990: 213–233.
105. Stiles GL: Adrenergic receptor responsiveness and congestive heart failure. *Am J Cardiol* 1991; 67:13C–17C.
106. Bogaert MG, Fraeyman N: Receptor function in heart failure. *Am J Med* 1991; 90(suppl 5B):S-10–S-13.
107. Bristow MR, Minobe W, Rasmussen R, Larrabee P, Skerl L, Klein JW, et al: β-adrenergic neuroeffector abnormalities in the

failing human heart are produced by local rather than systemic mechanisms. *J Clin Invest* 1992; 89:803–815.

108. Brodde OE, Schüler S, Kretsch R, Brinkmann M, Borst HG, Hetzer R, et al: Regional distribution of β-adrenoceptors in the human heart: Coexistence of functional β_1- and β_2- adrenoceptors in both atria and ventricles in severe congestive cardiomyopathy. *J Cardiovasc Pharmacol* 1986; 8:1235–1242.
109. Boehm M, Benckelmann D, Brown L, Feiler G, Lorenz B, Näbauer M, et al: Reduction of beta-adrenoceptor density and evaluation of positive inotropic responses in isolated diseased human myocardium. *Eur Heart J* 1988; 9:844–852.
110. Brodde OE, Zerkowski HR, Borst HG, Maier W, Michel MC: Drug- and disease-induced changes of human cardiac β_1- and β_2-adrenoceptors. *Eur Heart J* 1989; 10(suppl B):38–44.
111. Gopalakrishnan M, Triggle DJ: The regulation of receptors, ion channels, and G proteins in congestive heart failure. *Cardiovasc Drug Rev* 1990; 8:255–302.
112. Steinfath M, Lavicky J, Schmitz W, Scholz H, Döring V, Kalmár P: Regional distribution of β_1- and β_2-adrenoceptors in the failing and nonfailing human heart. *Eur J Clin Pharmacol* 1992; 42:607–612.
112a. Homcy CJ, Vatner SF, Vatner DE: β-Adrenergic receptor regulation in the heart in pathophysiologic states: Abnormal adrenergic responsiveness in cardiac disease. *Annu Rev Physiol* 1991; 53:137–139.
113. Baumann G, Mercader D, Busch U, Felix SB, Loher J, Ludwig L, et al: Effects of the H_2-receptor agonist impromidine in human myocardium from patients with heart failure due to mitral and aortic valve disease. *J Cardiovasc Pharmacol* 1983; 5:618–625.
114. Bristow MR, Ginsburg R, Harrison DC: Histamine and the human heart: The other receptor system. *Am J Cardiol* 1982; 49:249–251.
115. Hershberger RE, Bristow MR: The A_1 adenosine receptor pathway in failing and nonfailing human heart. *Circulation* 1987; 76(suppl 4):433.
116. Bristow MR, Minobe W, Rasmussen R: Differential regulation of alpha and beta-adrenergic receptor in the failing human heart (abstr.). *Circulation* 1985; 72(suppl 2):329.
116a. Fedida D, Braun AP, Giles WR: α_1-Adrenoceptors in myocardium: Functional aspects and transmembrane signaling mechanisms. *Physiol Rev* 1993; 73:469–487.
116b. Horn EM, Corwin ST, Steinberg SF, Chow YK, Neuberg GW, Cannon PJ, et al: Reduced lymphocyte stimulatory guanine nucleotide regulatory protein and β-adrenergic receptors in congestive heart failure and reversal with angiotensin converting enzyme inhibitor therapy. *Circulation* 1988; 78:1373–1379.
117. Horn EM, Chow YK, Neuberg GW, Corwin SJ, Powers ER, Bilezikian JP, et al: The guanine nucleotide regulatory protein Ns is reduced in congestive heart failure. (Abstr.) *Circulation* 1986; 74(suppl II):II-198.
118. Bilezikian JP, Steinberg SF, Horn EM, Robinson RB, Rosen MR: G protein-adrenergic interactions in the heart. *Mol Cell Biochem* 1988; 82:5–11.
119. Majerus PW, Connolly TM, Deckmyn H, Ross TS, Bross TE, Ishii H, et al: The metabolism of phosphoinositide-derived messenger molecules. *Science* 1986; 234:1519–1526.
120. Kikkawa U, Nishizuka Y: The role of protein kinase C in transmembrane signaling. *Annu Rev Cell Biol* 1986; 2:149–178.
121. Hunter T: A thousand and one protein kinases. *Cell* 1987; 50:823–829.
122. Feldman AM, Cates AE, Baumgartner W, Baughman KL, Van Dop C: Alterations of the M_r 40,000 pertussin toxin substrate (AG_1) in human heart failure. *Circulation* 1987; 76(suppl 4):IV–432.
122a. Feldman AM: Modulation of adrenergic receptors and G-transduction proteins in failing human ventricular myocardium. *Circulation* 1993; 83(suppl IV):IV-27–IV-34.
123. Feldman AM, Cates AE, Veazey WB, Hershberger RE, Bristow MR, Baughman KL: Increase of the 40,000-mol wt pertussis toxin substrate (G protein) in the failing human heart. *J Clin Invest* 1988; 82:189–197.
124. Feldman AM: Experimental issues in assessment of G protein function in cardiac disease. *Circulation* 1991; 84:1852–1861.
125. Feldman AM: Alterations of the β-adrenergic signaling pathway in cardiac failure and its role in pathophysiology and treatment. *Curr Opinion Cardiol* 1992; 7:367–373.
126. Longabaugh J, Vatner D, Vatner S, Homey C: Decreased stimulatory guanosine triphosphate binding protein in dogs with pressure-overload left ventricular failure. *J Clin Invest* 1988; 81:420–424.
127. Neumann J, Scholz H, Döring V, Schmitz W, Meyerinck L, Kalmar P: Increase in myocardial G_i-proteins in heart failure. *Lancet* 1988; 2:936–937.
128. Boehm M, Gierschik P, Jacobs KH, Pieske B, Schnabel P, Ungerer M, et al: Increase of G_i in human hearts with dilated but not ischemic cardiomyopathy. *Circulation* 1990; 82:1249–1265.
129. Bristow MR, Hershberger RE, Port JD, Sandoval A, Rasmussen R, Cates AE, et al: β-Adrenergic pathways in nonfailing and failing human ventricular myocardium. *Circulation* 1990; 82(suppl I):I-12–I-25.
130. Bristow M, Ginsburg R, Strosberg A, Montgomery W, Minobe W: Pharmacology and inotropic potential of forskolin in the human heart. *J Clin Invest* 1984; 74:212–223.
131. Korner PI: Integrative neural cardiovascular control. *Physiol Rev* 1971; 51:312–367.
132. Higgins CB, Vatner SF, Braunwald E: Parasympathetic control of the heart. *Pharmacol Rev* 1973; 25:119–155.
133. Eckberg DL, Drabinsky M, Braunwald E: Defective cardiac parasympathetic control in patients with heart disease. *N Engl J Med* 1971; 285:877–883.
134. Rutenberg HL, Spann JF Jr: Alterations of cardiac sympathetic neurotransmitter activity in congestive heart failure. *Am J Cardiol* 1973; 32:472–480.
135. Braunwald E: Regulation of the circulation. *N Engl J Med* 1974; 290:1420–1425.
136. Goldstein RE, Beiser GD, Stampfer M, Epstein SE: Impairment of autonomically mediated heart rate control in patients with cardiac dysfunction. *Circ Res* 1975; 36:571–578.
137. Rutenberg HL, Spann JF Jr: Alterations of cardiac sympathetic neurotransmitter activity in congestive heart failure. In: Mason DT (ed): *Congestive Heart Failure: Mechanisms, Evaluation and Treatment*. New York, Yorke Medical Books, 1976: 85–95.
138. Pool PE, Covell JW, Levitt M, Gibb J, Braunwald E: Reduction of cardiac tyrosine hydroxylase activity in experimental congestive heart failure: Its role in the depletion of cardiac norepinephrine stores. *Circ Res* 1967; 20:349–353.
139. Spann JF Jr, Buccino RA, Sonnenblick EH, Braunwald E: Contractile state of cardiac muscle obtained from cats with experimentally produced ventricular hypertrophy and heart failure. *Circ Res* 1967; 21:341–354.
140. White CW: Abnormalities in baroreflex control of heart rate in canine failure. *Am J Physiol* 1981; 240:H793–H799.
141. Goldsmith SR, Francis GS, Cowley AW Jr, Levine TB, Cohn JN: Increased plasma arginine vasopressin levels in patients with congestive heart failure. *J Am Coll Cardiol* 1983; I:1385–1390.
142. Kubo SH, Cody RJ: Circulatory autoregulation in chronic congestive heart failure: Responses to head-up tilt in 41 patients. *Am J Cardiol* 1983; 52:512–518.
143. Levine TB, Francis GS, Goldsmith SR, Cohn JN: The neurohumoral and hemodynamic responses to orthostatic tile in patients with congestive heart failure. *Circulation* 1983; 67:1070–1075.
144. Ferguson DW, Abboud FM, Mark AL: Selective impairment of baroreflex-mediated vasoconstrictor responses in patients with ventricular dysfunction. *Circulation* 1984; 69:451–460.
145. Hirsh AT, Dzau J, Creager MA: Baroreceptor function in congestive heart failure: Effect of neurohormonal activity and regional vascular resistance. *Circulation* 1987; 75(suppl IV):36–48.
146. Vatner DE, Lee DL, Schwarz K, Longabaugh JP, Fuji AM, Vatner SF, et al: Impaired cardiac muscarinic receptor function in dogs with heart failure. *J Clin Invest* 1988; 81:1836–1842.
147. Ellenbogen KA, Mohanty PK, Szentpetery S, Thames MD: Arterial baroreflex abnormalities in heart failure. *Circulation* 1989; 79:51–58.
148. Mohanty PK, Arrowood JA, Ellenbogen KA, Thames MD: Neurohumoral and hemodynamic effects of lower body negative pressure in patients with congestive heart failure. *Am Heart J* 1989; 118:78–85.
149. Sopher SM, Smith ML, Eckberg DL, Fritsch JM, Dibner-Dunlap ME: Autonomic pathophysiology in heart failure: Carotid baroreceptor-cardiac reflexes. *Am J Physiol* 1990; 259(*Heart Circ Physiol* 28):H689–H696.
150. Ferguson DW, Berg WJ, Roach PJ, Oren RM, Mark AL, Kempf JS: Effects of heart failure on baroreflex control of sympathetic neural activity. *Am J Cardiol* 1992; 69:523–531.

151. Dibner-Dunlap ME, Thames MD: Control of sympathetic nerve activity by vagal mechanoreflexes is blunted in heart failure. *Circulation* 1992; 86:1929–1934.
152. Goldsmith SR, Hasking GJ: Dissociation of sympathetic responses to baroreceptor loading and unloading in compensated congestive heart failure secondary to ischemic or nonischemic dilated cardiomyopathy. *Am J Cardiol* 1992; 69:646–649.
153. Creager MA: Baroreceptor reflex function in congestive heart failure. *Am J Cardiol* 1992; 69:10G–16G.
154. Mancia G, Seravalle G, Giannattasio C, Bossi M, Preti L, Cattaneo BM, et al: Reflex cardiovascular control in congestive heart failure. *Am J Cardiol* 1992; 69:17G–23G.
155. Buccino RA, Harris E, Spann JF Jr, Sonnenblick EH: Response of myocardial connective tissue to development of myocardial connective tissue to development of experimental hypertrophy. *Am J Physiol* 1969; 216:425–428.
156. Alpert NR (ed): *Cardiac Hypertrophy*. New York, Academic, 1971: 1–223.
157. Zak R (ed): *Growth of the Heart in Health and Disease*. New York, Raven, 1984: 1–463.
158. Weber KT, Clark WA, Janicki JS, Shroff SG: Physiologic versus pathologic hypertrophy and the pressure-overloaded myocardium. *J Cardiovasc Pharmacol* 1987; 10(suppl 6):537–550.
159. Weber KT, Janicki JS, Shroff SG, Pick R, Abrahams C, Chen RM, et al: Collagen compartment remodeling in the pressure overloaded left ventricle. *J Appl Cardiol* 1988; 3:37–46.
160. Weber KT, Janicki JS, Shroff SG, Pick R, Chen RM, Bashey RI: Collagen remodeling of the pressure-overloaded hypertrophied nonhuman primate myocardium. *Circ Res* 1988; 62:757–765.
161a. Weber KT: Cardiac interstitium in health and disease: The fibrillar collagen network. *J Am Coll Cardiol* 1989; 13:1637–1652.
161b. Zhao M, Zhang H, Robinson TF, Factor SM, Sonnenblick EH, Eng C: Profound structural alterations of the extracellular collagen matrix in post-ischemic dysfunctional but viable myocardium. *J Am Coll Cardiol* 1987; 10:1322–1334.
162. Weber KT, Pick R, Silver MA, Moe GW, Janicki JS, Zucker IH, et al: Fibrillar collagen and remodeling of dilated canine left ventricle. *Circulation* 1990; 82:1387–1401.
163. Weber KT, Brilla CG: Pathological hypertrophy and cardiac interstitium: Fibrosis and renin-angiotensin-aldosterone system. *Circulation* 1991; 83:1849–1865.
164. Weber KT, Brilla CG, Janicki JS: Myocardial fibrosis: Functional significance and regulatory factors. *Cardiovasc Res* 1993; 27:341–348.
165. Olivetti G, Melissari M, Capasso JM, Anversa P: Cardiomyopathy of the aging human heart: Myocyte loss and reactive cellular hypertrophy. *Circ Res* 1991; 68:1560–1568.
166. Dock W: How some hearts age. *JAMA* 1966; 195:442–444.
167. Burch G, Giles T: Senile cardiomyopathy. *J Chronic Dis* 1971; 24:1–3.
168. Dock W: Cardiomyopathies of the senescent and senile. In: Burch GE (ed): *Cardiomyopathy*. Philadelphia, F A Davis, 1972: 361–373.
169. Miller TR, Grossman SJ, Schectman KB, Biello DR, Ludbrook PA, Ehsani AA: Left ventricular diastolic filling and its association with age. *Am J Cardiol* 1986; 58:531–535.
170. Bryg RJ, Williams GA, Labovitz AJ: Effect of aging on left ventricular diastolic filling in normal subjects. *Am J Cardiol* 1987; 59:971–974.
171. Lie JT, Hammond PI: Pathology of the senescent heart: Anatomic observations on 237 autopsy studies of patients 90 to 105 years old. *Mayo Clin Proc* 1988; 63:552–564.
172. Lakatta EG, Gerstenblith G, Angell CS, Shock NW, Weisfeldt ML: Diminished inotropic response of aged myocardium to catecholamines. *Circ Res* 1975; 36:262–269.
172a. Lakatta EG: Cardiovascular regulatory mechanisms in advanced age. *Physiol Rev* 1933; 73:413–467.
173. Whipple GH, Sheffield LT, Woodman EG, Theophilis C, Friedman S: Reversible congestive heart failure due to chronic rapid stimulation of the normal heart. *Proc N Engl Cardiovasc Soc* 1962; 20:39–40.
174. Coleman HN III, Taylor RR, Pool PE, Whipple GH, Covell JW, Ross J Jr, et al: Congestive heart failure following chronic tachycardia. *Am Heart J* 1971; 81:790–798.
175. Riegger AJG, Liebau G: The renin-angiotensin-aldosterone system: Antidiuretic hormone and sympathetic nerve activity in an experimental model of congestive heart failure in the dog. *Clin Sci* 1982; 62:465–469.
176. Armstrong PW, Stopps TP, Ford SE, DeBold AJ: Rapid ventricular pacing in the dog: Pathophysiologic studies of heart failure. *Circulation* 1986; 74:1075–1084.
177. Packer DL, Bardy GH, Worley SJ, Smith MS, Cobb FR, Coleman RE, et al: Tachycardia-induced cardiomyopathy: A reversible form of left ventricular dysfunction. *Am J Cardiol* 1986; 57:563–570.
178. Wilson JR, Douglas P, Hickey WF, Lanoce V, Ferraro N, Muhammad A, et al: Experimental congestive heart failure produced by rapid ventricular pacing in the dog: Cardiac effects. *Circulation* 1987; 75:857–867.
179. Damiano RJ, Tripp HF, Asano T, Small KW, Jones RH, Lowe JE: Left ventricular dysfunction and dilatation resulting from chronic supraventricular tachycardia. *J Thorac Cardiovasc Surg* 1987; 94:135–143.
180. Riegger GA, Elsner D, Kromer EP, Daffner C: Atrial natriuretic peptide in congestive heart failure in the dog: Plasma levels, cyclic guanosine monophosphate, ultrastructure of atrial myoendocrine cells, and hemodynamic, hormonal, and renal effects. *Circulation* 1988; 77:398–406.
181. Moe GW, Stopps TP, Howard RJ, Armstrong PW: Early recovery from heart failure: Insights into the pathogenesis of experimental chronic pacing-induced heart failure. *J Lab Clin Med* 1988; 112:426–432.
182. Moe GW, Stopps TP, Angus C, Forster C, De Bold AJ, Armstrong PW: Alterations in serum sodium in relation to atrial natriuretic factor and other neuroendocrine variables in experimental pacing-induced heart failure. *J Am Coll Cardiol* 1989; 13:173–179.
183. Morgan DE, Tomlinson CW, Qayumi AK, Toleikis PM, McConville B, Jamieson WRE: Evaluation of ventricular contractility indexes in the dog with left ventricular dysfunction induced by rapid atrial pacing. *J Am Coll Cardiol* 1989; 14:489–495.
184. Vaitkus PT, Curtis M, Marchlinski FE, Mancini DM: Incessant atrial tachycardia and heart failure. *Heart Failure* 1990; 6:183–188.
185. Spinale FG, Hendrick DA, Crawford FA, Smith AC, Hamada Y, Carabello BA: Chronic supraventricular tachycardia causes ventricular dysfunction and subendocardial injury in swine. *Am J Physiol* 1990; 259:H218–H229.
186. Calderone A, Bouvier M, Li K, Juneau C, de Champlain J, Rouleau JL: Dysfunction of the β- and α-adrenergic systems in a model of congestive heart failure: The pacing-overdrive dog. *Circ Res* 1991; 69:332–342.
187. Tomita M, Spinale FG, Crawford FA, Zile MR: Changes in left ventricular volume, mass, and function during development and regression of supraventricular tachycardia-induced cardiomyopathy: Disparity between recovery of systolic versus diastolic function. *Circulation* 1991; 83:635–644.
188. Shannon RP, Komamura K, Stambler BS, Bigaud M, Manders WT, Vatner SF: Alterations in myocardial contractility in conscious dogs with dilated cardiomyopathy. *Am J Physiol* 1991; 260:H1903–H1911.
189. Spinale FG, Pearce AP, Crawford FA, Schulte BA: Ventricular function and NA^+, K^+-ATPase activity and distribution with chronic supraventricular tachycardia. *Cardiovasc Res* 1991; 25:138–144.
190. Spinale FG, Tomita M, Zellner JL, Cook JC, Crawford FA, Zile MR: Collagen remodeling and changes in LV function during development and recovery from supraventricular tachycardia. *Am J Physiol* 1991; 261:H308–H318.
191. Spinale FG, Zellner JL, Tomita M, Tempel GE, Crawford FA, Zile MR: Reduced myocardial blood flow and altered capillary structure occur with chronic supraventricular tachycardia induced cardiomyopathy. *Am J Physiol* 1991; 261:H140–H148.
192. Zellner JL, Spinale FG, Eble DK, Hewett KW, Crawford FA Jr: Alterations in myocyte shape and basement membrane attachment with tachycardia-induced heart failure. *Circ Res* 1991; 69:590–600.
193. Moe GW, Angus C, Howard RJ, Parker TG, Armstrong PW: Evaluation of indices of left ventricular contractility and relaxation in evolving canine experimental heart failure. *Cardiovasc Res* 1992; 26:362–366.
194. Spinale FG, Fulbright M, Mukherjee R, Tanaka R, Hu J, Craw-

ford FA, et al: Relation between ventricular and myocyte function with tachycardia-induced cardiomyopathy. *Circulation Res* 1992; 71:174–187.
195. Juneau C, Calderone A, Rouleau J-L: Myocardial β-adrenergic and mechanical properties in pacing-induced heart failure in dogs. *Am J Physiol* 1992; 262(*Heart Circ Physiol* 31):H1458–H1467.
196. Belch JJF, Budges AB, Scott N, Chopra M: Oxygen free radicals and congestive heart failure. *Br Heart J* 1991; 65:245–248.
197. Laine GA, Allen SJ: Left ventricular myocardial edema: Lymph flow, interstitial fibrosis, and cardiac function. *Circ Res* 1991; 68:1713–1721.
198. Mann DL, Kent RL, Parsons B, Cooper G: Adrenergic effects on the biology of the adult mammalian cardiocyte. *Circulation* 1992; 85:790–804.
199. Tan LB, Jalil JE, Pick R, Janicki JS, Weber KT: Cardiac myocyte necrosis induced by angiotensin II. *Circ Res* 1991; 69:1185–1195.
200. Dzau VJ, Hollenberg NK, Williams GH: Neurohumoral mechanisms in heart failure: Role in pathogenesis, therapy and drug tolerance. *Fed Proc* 1983; 42:3162–3169.
201. Francis GS: Neurohumoral mechanisms involved in congestive heart failure. *Am J Cardiol* 1985; 55(suppl A):A15–A21.
202. Cody RJ: Neurohormonal influences in the pathogenesis of congestive heart failure. In: Weber K (ed): *Heart Failure Cardiology Clinics*. Philadelphia, Saunders, 1989; 7:73–86.
203. Forfar JC: Neuroendocrine activation in congestive heart failure. *Am J Cardiol* 1991; 67(suppl C):3C–15C.
204. Zucker IH: Baro and cardiac reflex abnormalities in chronic heart failure. In: Zucker IH, Gilmore JP(eds): *Reflex Control of the Circulation*. Boca Raton, FL, CRC Press, 1991: 849–873.
205. Katz AM: Heart failure. In: Fozzard HA, Haber E, Jennings RB, Katz AM, Morgan HE (eds): *The Heart and Cardiovascular System*. Scientific Foundations, 2d ed. New York, Raven, 1991: 333–353.
206. Alton M, Cody RJ: Neurohormonal mechanisms in congestive heart failure. *Curr Opin Cardiol* 1992; 7:374–380.
207. Thomas JA, Marks BH: Plasma norepinephrine in congestive heart failure. *Am J Cardiol* 1978; 41:233–243.
208. Creager MA, Faxon DP, Cutler SS, Kohlman O, Ryan TJ, Gavras H: Contribution of vasopressin to vasoconstriction in patients with congestive heart failure: Comparison with the renin-angiotensin system and the sympathetic nervous system. *J Am Coll Cardiol* 1986; 7:758–765.
209. Manthey J, Dietz R, Opherk D, Osterziel KJ, Leinberger H, Kübler W: Baroreceptor-mediated release of vasopressin in patients with chronic congestive heart failure and defective sympathetic responsiveness. *Am J Cardiol* 1992; 70:224–228.
210. Margulies KB, Hildebrand FL, Lerman A, Perrella MP, Burnett JC Jr: Increased endothelin in experimental heart failure. *Circulation* 1990; 82:2226–2230.
211. Cavero PG, Miller WL, Heublein DM, Margulies KB, Burnett JC Jr: Endothelin in experimental congestive heart failure in the anesthetized dog. *Am J Physiol* 1990; 259:F312–F317.
211a. Cody RJ, Haas GJ, Binkley PF, Caper Q, Kelley R: Plasma endothelin correlates with the extent of pulmonary hypertension in patients with chronic congestive heart failure. *Circulation* 1992; 58:504–509.
212. Rodeheffer RJ, Lerman A, Heublein DM, Burnett JC Jr: Increased plasma concentrations of endothelin in congestive heart failure in humans. *Mayo Clin Proc* 1992; 67:719–724.
213. Lerman A, Kubo SH, Tschumperlin LK, Burnett JC Jr: Plasma endothelin concentrations in humans with end-stage heart failure and after heart transplantation. *J Am Coll Cardiol* 1992; 20:849–853.
214. Cody RJ: The potential role of endothelin as a vasoconstrictor substance in congestive heart failure. *Eur Heart J* 1992; 13:1573–1578.
215. Stewart DJ, Cernacek P, Costello KB, Rouleau JL: Elevated endothelin-1 in heart failure and loss of normal response to postural change. *Circulation* 1992; 85:510–517.
216. McMurray JJ, Ray SG, Abdullah I, Dargie HJ, Morton JJ: Plasma endothelin in chronic heart failure. *Circulation* 1992; 85:1374–1379.
217. Maisel AS, Scott NA, Motulsky HJ, Michel MC, Boublik JH, Rivier JE, et al: Elevation of plasma neuropeptide Y levels in congestive heart failure. *Am J Med* 1989; 86:43–48.
218. Hulting J, Sollevia A, Ullman B, Franco-Cereceda A, Lundberg JM: Plasma neuropeptide Y on admission to a coronary care unit: Raised levels in patients with left heart failure. *Cardiovasc Res* 1990; 24:102–108.
219. Edvinsson L, Ekman R, Hedner P, Valdemarsson S: Congestive heart failure: Involvement of perivascular peptides reflecting activity in sympathetic, parasympathetic and afferent fibres. *Eur J Clin Invest* 1990; 20:85–90.
220. Valdemarsson S, Edvinsson L, Edman R, Hedner P, Sjöholm A: Increased plasma level of substance P in patients with severe congestive heart failure treated with ACE inhibitors. *J Int Med* 1991; 230:325–331.
220a. Dhalla NS, Singh JN, Fedelesova M, Balasubramanian V, McNamara DB: Biochemical basis of heart function: XII. Sodium-potassium stimulated adenosine triphosphatase activity in the perfused rat heart made to fail by substrate-lack. *Cardiovasc Res* 1974; 8:227–236.
221. Levine B, Kalman J, Mayer L, Fillit HM, Packer M: Elevated circulating levels of tumor necrosis factor in severe chronic heart failure. *N Engl J Med* 1990; 323:236–241.
222. McMurray J, Abdullah I, Dargie HJ, Shapiro D: Increased concentrations of tumour necrosis factor in "cachectic" patients with severe chronic heart failure. *Br Heart J* 1991; 66:356–358.
223. Han JJ, Leeper-Woodford SK, Drenning DH, Bechard D, Quigg R, Salyer J, et al: Circulating tumor necrosis factor and endothelial-derived relaxing factor in severe heart failure (abstr.). *J Am Coll Cardiol* 1992; 19:207A.
224. Kubo SH, Rector TS, Williams RE, Heifritz SM, Bank AJ: Endothelium-dependent vasodilation is attenuated in patients with heart failure. *Circulation* 1991; 84:1589–1596.
225. Drexler H, Lu W: Endothelial dysfunction of hindquarter resistance vessels in experimental heart failure. *Am J Physiol* 1992; 262 (*Heart Circ Physiol* 31):H1640–H1645.
226. Drexler H, Hayoz D, Münzel T, Hornig B, Just H, Brunner HR, et al: Endothelial function in chronic congestive heart failure. *Am J Cardiol* 1992; 69:1596–1601.
227. Katz SD, Biasucci L, Sabba C, Strom JA, Jondeau G, Galvao M, et al: Impaired endothelium-mediated vasodilation in the peripheral vasculature of patients with congestive heart failure. *J Am Coll Cardiol* 1992; 19:918–925.
228. Taquet H, Komajda M, Grenier O, Belas F, Landault C, Carayon A, et al: Plasma calcitonin gene-related peptide decreases in chronic congestive heart failure. *Eur Heart J* 1992; 13:1473–1476.
229. Anand IS, Ferrari R, Kalra GS, Wahi PL, Poole-Wilson PA, Harris PC: Edema of cardiac origin: Studies of body water and sodium, renal function, hemodynamic indexes and plasma hormones in untreated congestive cardiac failure. *Circulation* 1989; 80:299–305.
230. Weber KT, Villarreal D: Aldosterone and antialdosterone therapy in congestive heart failure. *Am J Cardiol* 1993; 71(suppl A):3A–11A.
230a. Mehta J, Mehta P: Platelet function studies in heart disease: Enhanced platelet aggregate formation in congestive heart failure. *Circulation* 1979; 60:497–503.
230b. Jafri SM, Ozawa T, Mammen E, Levine TB, Johnson C, Goldstein S: Platelet function, thrombin and fibrinolytic activity in patients with heart failure. *Eur Heart J* 1993; 14:205–212.
231. Chidsey CA, Braunwald E, Morrow AG, Mason DT: Myocardial norepinephrine concentration in man. *N Engl J Med* 1963; 269:653–658.
232. Bristow MR: The adrenergic nervous system in heart failure. *N Engl J Med* 1984; 311:850–851.
233. Swedberg K, Viquerat C, Rouleau J-L: Comparison of myocardial catecholamine balance in chronic congestive heart failure and in angina pectoris without failure. *Am J Cardiol* 1984; 54:783–786.
234. Hasking GJ, Esler MD, Jennings GL, Barton D, Johns JA, Korner PI: Norepinephrine spillover to plasma in patients with congestive heart failure: Evidence of increased overall and cardiorenal sympathetic nervous activity. *Circulation* 1986; 73:615–621.
235. Lund DD, Schmid PG, Johansen J, Roskoski R Jr: Biochemical indices of cholinergic and adrenergic automatic innervation in dog heart: Disparate alterations in chronic right heart failure. *J Mol Cell Cardiol* 14:419–425.
236. Rose CP, Burgess JH, Cousineau D: Tracer norepinephrine kinetics in coronary circulation of patients with heart failure secondary

to chronic pressure and volume overload. *J Clin Invest* 1985; 76:1740–1747.
237. Chidsey CA, Harrison C, Braunwald E: Augmentation of the plasma norepinephrine response to exercise in patients with congestive heart failure. *N Engl J Med* 1962; 267:650–654.
238. Minami M, Yasuda H, Yamazaki N, Kojima S, Nishijima H, Matsumura N, et al: Plasma norepinephrine concentration and plasma dopamine-beta-hydroxylase activity in patients with congestive heart failure. *Circulation* 1964; 67:1324–1329.
239. Francis GS, Goldsmith SR, Ziesche S, Cohn JN: Response of plasma norepinephrine and epinephrine to dynamic exercise in patients with congestive heart failure. *Am J Cardiol* 1982; 49:1152–1156.
240. Hasking GJ, Esler MD, Jennings GL, Dewar E, Lambert G: Norepinephrine spillover to plasma during steady-state supine bicycle exercise: Comparison of patients with congestive heart failure and normal subjects. *Circulation* 1988; 78:516–521.
241. Levine TB, Francis GS, Goldsmith SR, Cohn JN: The neurohumoral and hemodynamic response to orthostatic tilt in patients with congestive heart failure. *Circulation* 1983; 67:1070–1075.
242. Bristow MR: Myocardial beta-adrenergic receptor down regulation in heart failure. *Int J Cardiol* 1984; 5:648–652.
243. Waagstein F, Hjalmarson A, Varnaysclas E, Wallentin I: Effect of chronic β-adrenergic receptor blockade in congestive cardiomyopathy. *Br Heart J* 1975; 37:1022–1036.
244. Swedberg K, Waagstein F, Hjalmarson A, Wallentin I: Prolongation of survival in congestive cardiomyopathy in β-receptor blockade. *Lancet* 1979; 1:1374–1376.
245. Anderson JL, Lutz JR, Gilbert EM, Sorensen SG, Yanowitz FG, Menlove RL, et al: A randomized trial of low-dose beta-blockade therapy for idiopathic dilated cardiomyopathy. *Am J Cardiol* 1985; 55:471–475.
246. Engelmeier RS, O'Connell JB, Walsh R, Rad N, Scanlon PJ, Funnar R: Improvement in symptoms and exercise tolerance by metoprolol in patients with dilated cardiomyopathy: A double-blind, randomized, placebo-controlled trial. *Circulation* 1985; 72:536–546.
247. Heilbrunn SM, Shah P, Bristow MR, Valantine HA, Ginsburg R, Fowler MB: Increased beta-receptor density and improved hemodynamic response to catecholamine stimulation during long-term metoprolol therapy in heart failure from dilated cardiomyopathy. *Circulation* 1989; 79:483–490.
248. Eichhorn EJ, Bedotto JB, Malloy CR, Hatfield BA, Deitchman D, Brown M, et al: Effect of β-adrenergic blockade on myocardial function and energetics in congestive heart failure: Improvements in hemodynamic, contractile, and diastolic performance with bucindolol. *Circulation* 1990; 82:473–483.
249. Anderson JL, Gilbert EM, O'Connell JB, Renlund D, Yanowitz F, Murray M, et al: Long-term (2 year) beneficial effects of beta-adrenergic blockade with bucindolol in patients with idiopathic dilated cardiomyopathy. *J Am Coll Cardiol* 1991; 17:1373–1381.
250. Andersson B, Blomström-Lundqvist C, Hedner T, Waagstein F: Exercise hemodynamics and myocardial metabolism during long-term beta-adrenergic blockade in severe heart failure. *J Am Coll Cardiol* 1991; 18:1059–1066.
251. Eichhorn EJ: The paradox of β-adrenergic blockade for the management of congestive heart failure. *Am J Med* 1992; 92:527–538.
252. Bristow MR: Pathophysiologic and pharmacologic rationales for clinical management of chronic heart failure with beta-blocking agents. *Am J Cardiol* 1993; 71(suppl C):12C–22C.
253. Swedberg K: Initial experience with beta blockers in dilated cardiomyopathy. *Am J Cardiol* 1993; 71(suppl C):30C–38C.
254. Fowler MB: Controlled trials with beta blockers in heart failure: Metoprolol as the prototype. *Am J Cardiol* 1993; 71(suppl C):45C–53C.
255. Ikram H, Fitzpatrick D, Crozier IG: Therapeutic controversies with use of beta-adrenoceptor blockade in heart failure. *Am J Cardiol* 1993; 71(suppl C):54C–60C.
256. Ikram H, Fitzpatrick D: Double-blind trial of chronic oral beta-blockade in congestive cardiomyopathy. *Lancet* 1981; 2:490–493.
257. Ikram H, Fitzpatrick MA: Beta-blockade for dilated cardiomyopathy: The evidence against therapeutic benefit. *Eur Heart J* 1983; 4(suppl A):179–180.
258. Currie PJ, Kelly MJ, McKenzie A, Harper RW, Lim YL, Federman J, et al: Oral beta-adrenergic blockade with metoprolol in chronic severe dilated cardiomyopathy. *J Am Coll Cardiol* 1984; 3:203–209.
259. Brinkley PF, Lewe RF, Lima JJ, Al-Awwa A, Unverferth DV, Leier CV: Hemodynamic-inotropic response to beta-blockers with intrinsic sympathomimetic activity in patients with congestive cardiomyopathy. *Circulation* 1986; 74:1390–1398.
260. Vanhoutte PM: Adjustments in the peripheral circulation in chronic heart failure. *Eur Heart J* 1983; 4(suppl A):67–83.
261. Cannon P, Martinez-Maldonado M: The pathogenesis of cardiac edema. *Semin Nephrol* 1983; 3:211–224.
262. Leier CV: Regional blood flow in human congestive heart failure. *Am Heart J* 1992; 124:726–738.
263. Zelis R, Delea CS, Coleman HN, Mason DT: Arterial sodium content in experimental congestive heart failure. *Circulation* 1970; 41:213–216.
264. Raine AEG: Renal abnormalities in congestive heart failure. In: Fozzard HA, Haber E, Jennings RB, Katz AM, Morgan HE (eds): *The Heart and Cardiovascular System.* Scientific Foundations, 2d ed. New York, Raven, 1991: 1379–1391.
265. Casley-Smith JR: Mechanisms in the formation of lymph. In: Guyton AC, Halls JE (eds): *Cardiovascular Physiology IV, International Review of Physiology,* vol 26. Baltimore, University Park Press, 1982: 147–187.
266. deWardener H: The control of sodium excretion. In: Orloff J, Berliner RW (eds): *Handbook of Physiology,* sec 8, *Renal Physiology.* Bethesda, MD, American Physiological Society, 1973: 677–720.
267. Laragh JH, Scaley JE: The renin-angiotensin-aldosterone hormonal system and regulation of sodium, potassium, and blood pressure homeostasis. In: Orloff J, Berliner RW (eds): *Handbook of Physiology,* sec 8, *Renal Physiology.* Bethesda, MD, American Physiological Society, 1973: 831.
268. Hall JE: Regulation of renal hemodynamics. In: Guyton AC, Halls JE (eds): *Cardiovascular Physiology IV, International Review of Physiology,* vol 26. Baltimore, University Park Press, 1982: 243–321.
269. Schrier RW: Pathogenesis of sodium and water retention in high-output and low-output cardiac failure, nephrotic syndrome, cirrhosis, and pregnancy. *N Engl J Med* 1988; 319:1127–1134.
270. Bishop VS, Malliani A, Thoren P: Cardiac mechanoreceptors. In: Shepherd JT, Abboud FM (eds): *Handbook of Physiology.* Bethesda, MD, American Physiological Society, 1983: 497–556.
271. Peterson TV: Cardiac reflexes and control of renal function in primates. In: Zucker IH, Gilmore JP (eds): *Reflex Control of the Circulation.* Boca Raton FL, CRC Press, 1991: 313–358.
272. Shepherd JT: Cardiac mechanoreceptors. In: Fozzard HA, Haber E, Jennings RB, Katz AM, Morgan HE (eds): *The Heart and Cardiovascular System.* Scientific Foundations, 2d ed. New York, Raven, 1991: 148–1504.
273. Hasking GJ, Esler MD, Jennings GL, Burton D, Korner PI: Norepinephrine spillover to plasma in patients with congestive heart failure: Evidence of increased overall and cardiorenal sympathetic nervous activity. *Circulation* 1986; 73:615–621.
274. Stein JH, Boinjarern S, Wilson CB, Ferris TF: Alterations in intrarenal blood flow distribution. *Circ Res* 1973; (suppl):61–72.
275. Warren JV, Stead EA Jr: Fluid dynamics in chronic congestive heart failure. *Arch Intern Med* 1944; 73:138–147.
276. Merrill AJ: Edema and decreased renal blood flow in patients with chronic congestive heart failure: Evidence of forward failure as the primary case of edema. *J Clin Invest* 1946; 25:389–400.
277. Brenner BM, Troy JL, Daugharty TM: Quantitative importance of changes in post-glomerular colloid osmotic pressure in mediating glomerular tubular balance in the rat. *J Clin Invest* 1973; 52:190–197.
278. Ichikawa I, Brenner BM: Importance of efferent arteriolar vascular tone in regulation of proximal tubule fluid reabsorption and glomerulotubular balance in the rat. *J Clin Invest* 1980; 65:1192–1201.
279. deWardener HE: Mechanisms influencing urinary sodium excretion. In: Dickinson CJ, Marks J (eds): *Developments in Cardiovascular Medicine.* Baltimore, University Park Press, 1978: 179–190.
280. Mandin H: Cardiac edema in dogs: I. Proximal tubular and renal function (abstr.). *Kidney Int* 1976; 10:591.

281. Skorecki KL, Brenner BM: Body fluid homeostasis in man. *Am J Med* 1981; 70:77–88.
282. Dzau VJ, Collucci WS, Hollenberg NK, Williams GH: Relation of the renin-angiotensin-aldosterone system to clinical state in congestive heart failure. *Circulation* 1981; 63:645–651.
283. Dzau VJ, Pratt RE: Renin-angiotensin system. In: Fozzard HA, Haber E, Jennings JB, Katz AM, Morgan HE (eds): *The Heart and Cardiovascular System* 2d ed. New York, Raven, 1991: 1817–1849.
284. Linden RJ: Neurocirculatory control of sodium and water excretion. In: Dickinson CJ, Marks J (eds): *Developments in Cardiovascular Medicine.* Baltimore, University Park Press, 1978: 191–203.
285. Kiowski W, Julius S: Renin response in stimulation of cardiopulmonary mechanoreceptors in man. *J Clin Invest* 1978; 62:656–663.
286. Curtiss C, Cohn JN, Vrobel T, Franciosa JA: Role of the renin-angiotensin system in the systemic vasoconstriction of chronic congestive heart failure. *Circulation* 1978; 58:763–770.
287. Ausiello DA, Kreisberg JI, Roy C, Karnovsky MJ: Contraction of cultured rat glomerular cells of apparent mesangial origin after stimulation with angiotensin II and arginine vasopressin. *J Clin Invest* 1980; 65:754–760.
288. Dzau VJ: Cardiac renin-angiotensin system: Molecular and functional aspects. *Am J Med* 1988; 84(suppl 3A):22–27.
289. Lindpainter K, Ganten D: The cardiac renin-angiotensin system: An appraisal of present experimental and clinical evidence. *Circ Res* 1991; 68:905–921.
290. Dzau VJ, Hirsch AT: Emerging role of the tissue renin-angiotensin systems in congestive heart failure. *Eur Heart J* 1990; 11(suppl B):65–71.
291. Dzau VJ: Tissue renin-angiotensin system in myocardial hypertrophy and failure. *Arch Intern Med* 1993; 153:937–942.
291a. Lee MA, Böhm M, Paul M, Ganten D: Tissue renin-angiotensin systems. Their role in cardiovascular disease. *Circulation* 1993; 87(suppl IV):IV-7–IV-13.
292. Ignarro LJ: Biological actions and properties of endothelium-derived nitric oxide formed and released from artery and vein. *Circ Res* 1989; 65:1–21.
293. Moncada S, Palmer RMJ, Higgs EA: Nitric oxide: physiology, pathophysiology and pharmacology. *Pharmacol Rev* 1991; 43:109–142.
294. Brutsaert DL: The endocardium. *Annu Rev Physiol* 1989; 51:263–273.
295. Brutsaert DL: Role of endocardium in cardiac overloading and failure. *Eur Heart J* 1991; 11(suppl G):8–16.
296. Smith JA, Shah AM, Lewis MJ: Factors released from endocardium of the ferret and pig modulate myocardial contraction. *J Physiol* 1991; 439:1–14.
297. Cohn JN, Levine TB, Francis GS, Goldsmith S: Neurohumoral control mechanisms in congestive heart failure. *Am Heart J* 1981; 102:509–514.
298. Riegger GAJ, Liebau G, Kochsie K: Antidiuretic hormone in congestive heart failure. *Am J Med* 1982; 72:49–52.
299. Preibisz JJ, Sealey JE, Laragh JH: Plasma and platelet vasopressin in essential hypertension and congestive heart failure. *Hypertension* 1983; 5(suppl 1):1-129–1-138.
300. Pruszczynski W, Vahanian A, Ardaillou R, Acar J: Role of antidiuretic hormone in impaired water excretion of patients with congestive heart failure. *J Clin Endocrinol Metab* 1984; 58:599–605.
301. Share L: Role of vasopressin in cardiovascular regulation. *Physiol Rev* 1988; 68:1248–1284.
302. Cowley AW Jr: Vasopressin and cardiovascular regulation. In: Guyton AC, Halls JE (eds): *Cardiovascular Physiology IV, International Review of Physiology,* vol 26. Baltimore, University Park Press, 1982: 189–248.
303. Nakaoka H, Imataka K, Amano M, Fujii J, Ishibashi M, Yamaji T: Plasma levels of atrial natriuretic factor in patients with congestive heart failure. *N Engl J Med* 1985; 313:892–893.
304. Cody RJ, Atlas SA, Laragh JH, Kubo SH, Covitt AB, Ryman KS: Atrial natriuretic factor in normal subjects and heart failure patients: Plasma levels and renal, hormonal, and hemodynamic responses to peptide infusion. *J Clin Invest* 1986; 78:1362–1374.
305. Raine AEG, Erne P, Burgisser E, Muller FB, Bolli P, Burkart F: Atrial natriuretic peptide and atrial pressure in patients with congestive heart failure. *N Engl J Med* 1986; 315:553–557.
306. Ogawa K, Ito T, Hashimoto H, Ito Y, Ohno O, Tsuboi H, et al: Plasma atrial natriuretic factor in congestive heart failure. *Lancet* 1986; 1:106.
307. Burnett JC, Kao PC, Hu DC, Heser DW, Heublein D: Atrial natriuretic peptide elevation in congestive heart failure in the human. *Science* 1986; 231:1145–1147.
308. Bates ER, Shenker Y, Grekin RJ: The relationship between plasma levels of immunoreactive atrial natriuretic hormone and hemodynamic function in man. *Circulation* 1986; 73:1155–1161.
308a. Raine AEG, Erne P, Bürgisser E, Müller FB, Bolli P, Burkart F, et al: Atrial natriuretic peptide and atrial pressure in patients with congestive heart failure. *N Engl J Med* 1986; 315:533–537.
309. Pettersson A, Hedner J, Hedner T, Held P, Swedberg K, Towle AC: Increased plasma levels of atrial natriuretic peptide in patients with congestive heart failure. *Eur Heart J* 1986; 7:693–696.
310. Tsutamoto T, Bito K, Kinoshita M: Plasma atrial natriuretic polypeptide as an index of left ventricular end-diastolic pressure in patients with chronic left-sided heart failure. *Am Heart J* 1989; 117:599–606.
311. Donckier JE, De Coster PM, Vanoverschelde J-L, Brichant C, Cauwe F, Installe E, et al: Atrial natriuretic factor, cardiac volumes and filling pressures during exercise in congestive heart failure. *Eur Heart J* 1991; 12:322–327.
312. Nicholls DP, Riley M, Elborn JS, Stanford CF, Shaw C, McKillop JM, et al: Regulatory peptides in the plasma of patients with chronic cardiac failure at rest and during exercise. *Eur Heart J* 1992; 13:1399–1404.
313. Abraham WT, Hensen J, Kim JK, Dürr J, Lesnefsky EJ, Groves BM, et al: Atrial natriuretic peptide and urinary cyclic guanosine monophosphate in patients with chronic heart failure. *J Am Soc Nephrol* 1992; 2:1697–1703.
314. Atarashi K, Mulrow PJ, Franco-Saenz R, Mulrow PJ, Snajclar RM, Rapp JP: Inhibition of aldosterone production by an atrial extract. *Science* 1984; 224:992–994.
315. de Bold AJ, Borenstein HB, Veress AT, Sonnenberg H: A rapid and potent natriuretic response to intravenous injection of atrial myocardial extract in rats. *Life Sci* 1981; 28:89–94.
316. Ballerman BJ, Brenner BM: Role of atrial peptides in body fluid homeostasis. *Circ Res* 1986; 58:619–623.
317. Maack T, Marion DN, Camargo MJF, Kleinert HO, Laragh JH, Jaughan EO Jr: Effects of auriculin (atrial natriuretic factor) on blood pressure, renal function, and the renin-aldosterone system in dogs. *Am J Med* 1984; 77:1069–1071.
317a. Wildey GM, Misono KS, Graham RM: Atrial natriuretic factor: Biosynthesis and mechanisms of action. In: Fozzard HA, Haber E, Jennings RB, Katz AM, Morgan HE (eds): *The Heart and Cardiovascular System.* Scientific Foundations, 2d ed. New York, Raven, 1991: 1777–1796.
318. Samson WK: Atrial natriuretic factor inhibits dehydration and hemorrhage-induced vasopressin release. *Neuroendocrinology* 1985; 40:277–279.
319. Buckalew VM, Nelson DB: Natriuretic and sodium transport inhibitory activity in plasma of volume expanded dogs. *Kidney Int* 1974; 5:12–22.
320. Tsutamoto T, Kanamori T, Wada A, Kinoshita M: Uncoupling of atrial natriuretic peptide extraction and cyclic guanosine monophosphate production in the pulmonary circulation in patients with severe heart failure. *J Am Coll Cardiol* 1992; 20:541–546.
321. Levenson DJ, Simmons CE Jr, Brenner BM: Arachidonic acid metabolism, prostaglandins and the kidney. *Am J Med* 1982; 72:354–374.
322. Zusman RM: Eicosanoids: prostaglandins, thromboxane and prostacyclin. In: Fozzard HA, Haber E, Jennings JB, Katz AM, Morgan HE (eds): *The Heart and Cardiovascular System.* 2d ed. New York: Raven, 1991: 1797–1815.
323. Schor N, Ichikawa I, Brenner BM: Glomerular adaptations to chronic dietary salt restriction or excess. *Am J Physiol* 1980; 238:F428–F436.
324. Dzau VJ, Packer M, Lilly LS, Swartz SL, Hollenberg NK, Williams GH: Prostaglandins in severe congestive heart failure: Relation to activation of the renin-angiotensin system and hyponatremia. *N Engl J Med* 1984; 310:347–352.
325. Feldman AM, Levine MA, Gerstenblith G, Kaufman KO, Baughman KL: Negative inotropic effects of furosemide in the isolated

rabbit heart: A prostaglandin-mediated event. *J Cardiovasc Pharmacol* 1987; 9:493–499.

325a. Margolius HS, Horwitz D, Pisano JJ, Keiser HR; Relationships among urinary kallikrein, mineralocorticoids and human hypertensive disease. *Fed Proc* 1976; 35:203–206.

326. Carretero OA, Scicli AG: The kallikrein-kinin system. In: Fozzard HA, Haber E, Jennings RB, Katz AM, Morgan HE (eds): *The Heart and Cardiovascular System.* Scientific Foundations, 2d ed. New York, Raven, 1991: 1851–1874.

327. Gu J, Adrian TE, Tatemoto K, Bloom SR: Neuropeptide tyrosine (NPY): A major cardiac neuropeptide. *Lancet* 1983; 1008–1010.

327a. Meerson FZ, Javitz MP, Breger AM, Lerman MI: The mechanism of the heart's adaptation to prolonged load and dynamics of RNA synthesis in the myocardium. *Basic Res Cardiol* 1974; 484–499.

328. Allen DG, Kentish JG: The cellular basis of the length-tension relation in cardiac muscle. *J Mol Cell Cardiol* 1985; 17:821–840.

328a. Meerson FZ: Development of modern components of the mechanism of cardiac hypertrophy. *Circ Res* 1974; 35(suppl 2)11:58–63.

329. Meerson FZ, Katz AM (ed): *The Failing Heart: Adaptation and Deadaptation.* New York, Raven, 1983:1–323.

329a. LaKatta EG: Length modulation of muscle performance: Frank-Starling Law of the Heart. In: Fozzard HA, Haber E, Jennings RB, Katz AM, Morgan HE (eds): *The Heart and Cardiovascular System: Scientific Foundation.* 2d ed. New York, Raven Press, 1991: 1325–1351.

330. LaKatta EG: Starling's law of the heart is explained by an intimate interaction of muscle length and myofilament calcium activation. *J Am Coll Cardiol* 1987; 10:1157–1164.

331. Babu A, Sonnenblick E, Gulati J: Molecular basis for the influence of muscle length on myocardial performance. *Science* 1988; 240:74–76.

332. Hofmann PA, Fuchs F: Bound calcium and force development in skinned cardiac muscle bundles: Effect of sarcomere length. *J Mol Cell Cardiol* 1988; 20:667–677.

333. Hoh JF, Rossmanith GH, Kwan LJ, Hamilton AM: Adrenaline increases the rate of cycling of crossbridges in rat cardiac muscle as measured by pseudo-random binary noise-modulated perturbation analysis. *Circ Res* 1988; 62:452–461.

334. Grossman W, Carabello BA, Gunther S, Fifer MA: Ventricular wall stress and the development of cardiac hypertrophy and failure. In: Alpert NR (ed): *Perspectives in Cardiovascular Research,* vol 7. New York, Raven, 1983: 1–18.

335. Anversa P, Ricci R, Olivetti G: Quantitative structural analysis of the myocardium during physiological growth induced cardiac hypertrophy: A review. *J Am Coll Cardiol* 1986; 7:1140–1149.

336. Anversa P, Capasso JM, Olivetti G, and Sonnenblick EH: Cellular basis of ventricular remodeling in hypertensive cardiomyopathy. *Am J Hypertens* 1992; 5:758–770.

337. Linzbach AJ: Heart failure from the point of view of quantitative anatomy. *Am J Cardiol* 1960; 5:370–382.

338. Badeer HS: Biological significance of cardiac hypertrophy. *Am J Cardiol* 1964; 14:133–138.

339. Grossman W, Jones D, McLaurin LP: Wall stress and patterns of hypertrophy in the human left ventricle. *J Clin Invest* 1975; 56:56–64.

340. Marino TA, Kent RL, Uboh CI, Fernandez E, Thompson EW, Cooper G: Structural analysis of pressure versus volume overload hypertrophy of cat right ventricle. *Am J Physiol* 1985; 18:H371–H379.

341. Olivetti G, Ricci R, Lagrasta C, Maniga E, Sonnenblick EH, Anversa P: Cellular basis of wall remodeling in long-term pressure overload-induced right ventricular hypertrophy in rats. *Circ Res* 1988; 63:648–657.

342. Olivetti G, Capasso JM, Meggs LG, Sonnenblick EH, Anversa P: Cellular basis of ventricular remodelling after myocardial infarction in rats. *Circ Res* 1991; 68:856–869.

343. Breisch EA, Houser SR, Carey RA, Spann JF, Bove AA: Myocardial blood flow and capillary density in chronic pressure overload of the feline left ventricle. *Cardiovasc Res* 1980; 14:469–475.

344. Anversa P, Ricci R, Olivetti G: Quantitative structural analysis of the myocardium during physiologic growth and induced cardiac hypertrophy: A review. *J Am Coll Cardiol* 1986; 7:1140–1149.

345. Tomanek RJ, Palmer PJ, Peiffer GL, Schreiber KL, Eastham CL, Marcus ML: Morphometry of canine coronary arteries, arterioles, and capillaries during hypertension and left ventricular hypertrophy. *Circ Res* 1986; 58:38–46.

346. Anversa P, Beghi C, Kikkawa Y, Olivetti G: Myocardial infarction in rats: Infarct size, myocyte hypertrophy, and capillary growth. *Circ Res* 1986; 58:26–37.

347. Bache RJ: Effects of hypertrophy on the coronary circulation. *Prog Cardiovasc Dis* 1988; 31:403–440.

348. Schaper J: Hypertrophy in the human heart: Evaluation by qualitative and quantitative light and electron microscopy. In: Alpert NR (ed): *Perspectives in Cardiovascular Research,* vol 7. New York, Raven, 1983: 177–196.

349. Anversa P, Sonnenblick EH: Ischemic cardiomyopathy: Pathophysiologic mechanisms. *Prog Cardiovasc Dis* 1990; 33:49–70.

350. Jacob R, Kissling G, Rupp H, Vogt M: Functional significance of contractile proteins in cardiac hypertrophy and failure. *J Cardiovasc Pharmacol* 1987; 10(suppl 6):S2–S12.

351. Swynghedauw B, Schwartz K, Lecarpentier Y, Clapier-Ventura R, Perennec J, Waldenstron A, et al: Species-specificity of the isomyosin shift in cardiac overload. *J Appl Cardiol* 1988; 3:133–143.

352. Kitsis RN, Scheuer J: Correlations and dissociations between myosin isoenzymes and cardiac function. *J Appl Cardiol* 1988:327–335.

353. Anversa P, Palackal T, Sonnenblick EH, Olivetti G, Meggs LG, Capasso J: Myocyte cell loss and myocytecellular hyperplasia in the hypertrophied aging rat heart. *Circ Res* 1990; 67:871–885.

354. Jacob R, Ebrecht G, Kissling G, Rupp H, Takeda N: Functional consequences of cardiac myosin isoenzyme redistribution. In: Rupp H (ed): *Regulation of Heart Function: Basic Concepts and Clinical Applications.* New York, Thieme, 1986: 305–326.

355. Mercadier J-J, Lompre A-M, Wisnewsky C, Samuel JL, Bereovici J, Swynghedann B, et al: Myosin isoenzymatic changes in several models of rat cardiac hypertrophy. *Circ Res* 1981; 49:525–532.

356. Horowits R, Winegrad S: cAMP regulation of myosin ATPase activity in the maturing rat heart. *Circ Res* 1987; 61:914–924.

357. Cummins P, Lambert SJ: Myosin transitions in the bovine and human heart: A developmental and anatomical study of heavy and light chain subunits in the atrium and ventricle. *Circ Res* 1986; 58:846–858.

358. Olivetti G, Capasso JM, Sonnenblick EH, Anversa P: Side-to-side slippage of myocytes participates in ventricular wall remodeling acutely after myocardial infarction in rats. *Circ Res* 1990; 67:23–34.

359. Badeer HS: Contractile tension in the myocardium. *Am Heart J* 1963; 66:432–434.

360. Hood WP Jr, Rackley CE, Rolett EL: Wall stress in the normal and hypertrophied human left ventricle. *Am J Cardiol* 1968; 22:550–558.

361. Grossman W, McLaurin LP, Moos SP, Stefadouros M, Young DT: Wall thickness and diastolic properties of the left ventricle. *Circulation* 1974; 49:129–135.

362. Sasayama S, Ross J Jr, Franklin D, Bloor CM, Bishop S, Dilley RB: Adaptations of the left ventricle to chronic pressure overload. *Circ Res* 1976; 38:172–178.

363. Cohen J: Role of endocrine factors in the pathogenesis of cardiac hypertrophy. *Circ Res* 1974; 35(suppl II):II-49–II-57.

364. Lorell BH, Grossman W: Cardiac hypertrophy: The consequences for diastole. *J Am Coll Cardiol* 1987; 9:1189–1193.

365. Shapiro LM, Gibson DG: Patterns of diastolic dysfunction in left ventricular hypertrophy. *Br Heart J* 1988; 59:438–451.

366. Harizi RC, Bianco JA, Alpert JS: Diastolic function of the heart in clinical cardiology. *Arch Intern Med* 1988; 148:99–109.

367. Grossman W, Lorell BH (eds): *Diastolic Relaxation of the Heart: Basic Research and Applications for Clinical Cardiology.* Boston, Martinus Nijhoff, 1988: 1–310.

368. Gaasch WH, LeWinter MM (eds): *Left Ventricular Diastolic Dysfunction and Heart Failure.* Philadelphia, Lea & Febiger, 1993.

369. Perreault CL, Williams CP, Morgan JP: Cytoplasmic calcium modulation and systolic versus diastolic dysfunction in myocardial hypertrophy and failure. *Circulation* 1993; 87(suppl VII): VII-31–VII-37.

370. Dougherty AH, Naccarelli GV, Gray EL, Hicks CH, Goldstein RA: Congestive heart failure with normal systolic function. *Am J Cardiol* 1984; 54:778–782.

371. Soufer R, Wohlgelernter D, Vita NA, Amuchestegui M, Sostman HD, Berger HL, et al: Intact systolic left ventricular function in

clinical congestive heart failure. *Am J Cardiol* 1985; 55:1032–1036.
372. Kessler KM: Heart failure with normal systolic function: Update of prevalence, differential diagnosis, prognosis, and therapy. *Arch Intern Med* 1988; 148:2109–2111.
373. Grossman W: Diastolic dysfunction and congestive heart failure. *Circulation* 1990; 81(suppl III):III-1–III-7.
374. Yellin EL, Nikolic S, Frater RWM: Left ventricular filling dynamics and diastolic function. *Prog Cardiovasc Dis* 1990; 32:247–271.
375. Stauffer J-C, Gaasch WH: Recognition and treatment of left ventricular diastolic dysfunction. *Prog Cardiovasc Dis* 1990; 32:319–332.
376. Gaasch WH: Congestive heart failure in patients with normal left ventricular systolic function: A manifestation of diastolic dysfunction. *Herz* 1991; 16:22–32.
377. Glantz SA, Misbach GA, Moores WY, Mathey DG, LeKven J, Stowe DF: The pericardium substantially affects the left ventricular diastolic pressure-volume relationship in the dog. *Circ Res* 1978; 42:433–441.
378. Gilbert JC, Glantz SA: Determinants of left ventricular filling and of the diastolic pressure-volume relation. *Circ Res* 1989; 64:827–852.
379. Scaglione R, Dichiara MA, Indovina A, Lipari R, Ganguzza A, Parrinello G, et al: Left ventricular diastolic and systolic function in normotensive obese subjects: Influence of degree and duration of obesity. *Eur Heart J* 1992; 13:738–742.
380. Braunwald E, Ross J Jr: The ventricular end-diastolic pressure: Appraisal of its value in the recognition of ventricular failure in man. *Am J Med* 1963; 34:147–150.
381. Rackley CE, Hood WP Jr, Rolett EL, Young DT: Left ventricular end-diastolic pressure in chronic heart disease. *Am J Med* 1970; 48:310–319.
382. Levine HJ: Compliance of the left ventricle. *Circulation* 1972; 46:423–426.
383. Covell JW, Ross J Jr: Nature and significance of alterations in myocardial compliance. *Am J Cardiol* 1973; 32:449–455.
384. Grossman W, McLaurin LP: Diastolic properties of the left ventricle. *Ann Intern Med* 1976; 84:316–326.
385. Gaasch WH, Levine HJ, Quinones MA, Alexander JK: Left ventricular compliance: Mechanisms and clinical implications. *Am J Cardiol* 1976; 38:645–653.
386. Wisneski JA, Bristow JD: Left ventricular stiffness. *Annu Rev Med* 1978; 29:475–483.
387. Grossman W, Barry WH: Diastolic pressure-volume relations in the diseased heart. *Fed Proc* 1980; 39:148–155.
388. Lewis BS, Gotsman MS: Current concepts of ventricular relaxation and compliance. *Am Heart J* 1980; 99:101–112.
389. Gaasch WH, Levine HJ, Quinones MA, Alexander JK: Left ventricular compliance: Mechanisms and clinical implications. *Am J Cardiol* 1976; 38:645–653.
390. Gaasch WH, Zile MR: Evaluation of myocardial function in cardiomyopathic states. *Prog Cardiovasc Dis* 1984; 27:115–132.
391. Bonow RO, Udelson JE: Left ventricular diastolic dysfunction as a cause of congestive heart failure. *Ann Intern Med* 1992; 117:502–510.
392. Hefner LL, Coghlan CH, Jones WB: Distensibility of the dog left ventricle. *Am J Physiol* 1961; 201:97–101.
393. Janicki JS, Weber KT: The pericardium and ventricular interaction, distensibility, and function. *Am J Physiol* 1980; 238:H494–H503.
394. Bove A, Santamore W: Ventricular interdependence. *Prog Cardiovasc Dis* 1981; 23:365–388.
395. Maruyama Y, Ashikawa K, Isoyama S, Kanatsuka H, Ino-Oka E, Takishima T: Mechanical interactions between four heart chambers with and without the pericardium in canine hearts. *Circ Res* 1982; 50:86–100.
396. Little WC, Badke FR, O'Rourke RA: Effect of right ventricular pressure on the end-diastolic left ventricular pressure-volume relationship before and after chronic right ventricular pressure overload in dogs without pericardia. *Circ Res* 1984; 54:719–730.
397. Santamore WP, Constantinescu M, Vinten-Johansen J, Johnston WE, Little WC: Alterations in left ventricular compliance due to changes in right ventricular volume, pressure and compliance. *Cardiovasc Res* 1988; 22:768–776.
397a. Santamore WP, Shaffer T, Hughes D: A theoretical and experimental model of ventricular interdependence. *Basic Res Cardiol* 1986; 81:529–538.
398. Janicki JS: Influence of the pericardium and ventricular interdependence on left ventricular diastolic and systolic function in patients with heart failure. *Circulation* 1990; 82(2 suppl):III-15–III-20.
398a. Hoit BD, Dalton N, Bhargava V, Shabetai R: Pericardial influences on right and left ventricular filling dynamics. *Circ Res* 1991; 68:197–208.
399. Lorell BH, Wexler LF, Momomura S, Weinberg E, Apstein CS: The influence of pressure overload left ventricular hypertrophy on diastolic properties during hypoxia in isovolumically contracting rat hearts. *Circ Res* 1986; 58:653–663.
400. Grossman W, McLaurin LP, Moos SP, Stefadouras MA, Young DT: Wall thickness and diastolic properties of the left ventricle. *Circulation* 1974; 49:129–135.
401. Thiedemann KU, Holubarsch CH, Medugorac I, Jacob R: Connective tissue content and myocardial stiffness in pressure overload hypertrophy: A combined study of morphologic, morphometric, biochemical and mechanical parameters. *Basic Res Cardiol* 1983; 78;140–155.
402. Lorell BH: Significance of diastolic dysfunction of the heart. *Annu Rev Med* 1991; 42:411–436.
403. Cheng CP, Freeman GL, Santamore WP, Constantinescu MS, Little WC: Effect of loading conditions, contractile state, and heart rate on early diastolic left ventricular filling in conscious dogs. *Circ Res* 1990; 66:814–823.
404. Brutsaert DL, Sonnenblick EH: Cardiac muscle mechanics in the evaluation of myocardial contractility and pump function: Problems, concepts and directions. *Prog Cardiovasc Dis* 1973; 16:337–361.
405. Taylor RR, Hopkins BE: Left ventricular response to experimentally induced chronic aortic regurgitation. *Cardiovasc Res* 1972; 6:404–414.
406. Spann JF Jr, Covell JW, Eckberg DL, Sonnenblick EH, Ross J Jr, Braunwald E: Contractile performance of the hypertrophied and chronically failing cat ventricle. *Am J Physiol* 1972; 223:1150–1157.
407. Spann JF: Contractile and pump function of the pressure-overloaded heart. In: Alpert NR (ed): *Perspectives in Cardiovascular Research*, vol 7. New York, Raven, 1983: 19–38.
408. Cooper G IV, Satava RM, Harrison CE, Coleman HN 3d: Normal myocardial function and energetics after reversing pressure-overload hypertrophy. *Am J Physiol* 1974; 226:1158–1165.
409. Williams JF Jr, Potter RD: Normal contractile state of hypertrophied myocardium following pulmonary artery constriction in the cat. *J Clin Invest* 1974; 54:1266–1272.
410. Malik AB, Abe T, O'Kane HO, Geha AS: Cardiac performance in ventricular hypertrophy induced by pressure and volume overloading. *J Appl Physiol* 1974; 37:867–874.
411. Meerson FZ, Kapelko VI: The contractile function of the myocardium in two types of cardiac adaptation to a chronic load. *Cardiology* 1972; 57;183–199.
412. Noble MIM, Seed WA (eds): *The Interval-Force Relationship of the Heart: Bowditch Revisited.* Cambridge & Cambridge University Press, 1992: 1–368.
412a. Buckley NM, Penefsky ZJ, Litwak RS: Comparative force-frequency relationships in human and other mammalian ventricular myocardium. *Pfluegers Arch* 1972; 332:259–270.
413. Feldman MD, Gwathmey JK, Phillips P, Schoen F, Morgan JP: Reversal of the force-frequency relationship in working myocardium from patients with end-stage heart failure. *J Appl Cardiol* 1988; 3:273–283.
414. Mulieri LA, Hasenfuss G, Leavitt B, Allen PD, Alpert NR: Altered myocardial force-frequency relation in human heart failure. *Circulation* 1992; 85:1743–1750.
415. Valeri CR, Fortier NL: Red-cell 2,3-diphosphoglycerate and creatine levels in patients with red-cell mass deficiency or with cardiopulmonary insufficiency. *N Engl J Med* 1969; 281:1452–1455.
416. Coats AJS, Adamopoulos S, Radaelli A, McCance A, Meyer TE, Bernardi L, et al: Controlled trial of physical training in chronic heart failure: Exercise performance, hemodynamics, ventilation, and autonomic function. *Circulation* 1992; 85:2119–2131.
416a. Uren NG, Lipkin DP: Exercise training as therapy for chronic heart failure. *Br Heart J* 1992; 67:430–433.
417. Lindsay DC, Jiang C, Brunotte F, Adamopoulos S, Coats AJS,

Rajagopalan B, et al: Impairment of endothelium dependent responses in a rat model of chronic heart failure: Effects of an exercise training protocol. *Cardiovasc Res* 1992; 26: 694–697.

418. Mancini DM, LeJemtel TH, Factor S, Sonnenblick EH: Central and peripheral components of cardiac failure. *Am J Med* 1986; 80(suppl 2B):2–13.
419. Burch GE, Ray CT, Cronvich JA: Certain mechanical peculiarities of the human cardiac pump in normal and diseased states. *Circulation* 1952; 5:504–513.
420. Burch GE: Theoretic considerations of the time course of pressure developed and volume ejected by the normal and dilated left ventricle during systole. *Am Heart J* 1955; 50:352–355.
421. Burch GE, DePasquale NP, Cronvich JA: Influence of ventricular size on the relationship between contractile and manifest tension. *Am Heart J* 1965; 69:624–628.
422. Mason DT, Spann JF Jr, Zelis R, Amsterdam EA: Alterations of hemodynamics and myocardial mechanics in patients with congestive heart failure: Pathophysiologic mechanisms and assessment of cardiac function and ventricular contractility. *Prog Cardiovasc Dis* 1970; 12:507–557.
423. Winegrad S: Mechanism of contraction in cardiac muscle. In: Guyton AC, Halls JE (eds): *Cardiovascular Physiology IV, International Review of Physiology,* vol 26. Baltimore, University Park Press, 1982: 87–117.
424. Urschel CW, Covell JW, Sonnenblick EH, Ross J Jr, Braunwald E: Myocardial mechanics in aortic and mitral valvular regurgitation: The concept of instantaneous impedance as a determinant of the performance of the intact heart. *J Clin Invest* 1968; 47:867–883.
425. Vincent WR, Buckberg GD, Hoffman JIE: Left ventricular subendocardial ischemia in severe valvular and supravalvular aortic stenosis: A common mechanism. *Circulation* 1974; 49:326–333.
426. Brazier JR, Buckberg GD: Effects of tachycardia on the adequacy of subendocardial oxygen delivery in experimental aortic stenosis. *Am Heart J* 1975; 90:222–230.
427. Downey JM, Kirk ES: Inhibition of coronary blood flow by a vascular waterfall mechanism. *Circ Res* 1975; 36:753–760.
428. Brazier J, Cooper N, Buckberg G: The adequacy of subendocardial oxygen delivery: The interaction of determinants of flow, arterial oxygen content, and myocardial oxygen need. *Circulation* 1974; 49:968–977.
429. Honig CR, Bourdeau-Martini J: Extravascular component of oxygen transport in normal and hypertrophied hearts with special reference to oxygen therapy. *Circ Res* 1974; 35(suppl II): II-97–II-103.
430. Eckberg DL, Gault JH, Bouchard RL, Karliner JS, Ross J Jr: Mechanics of left ventricular contraction in chronic severe mitral regurgitation. *Circulation* 1973; 47:1252–1259.
431. McCullagh WH, Covell JW, Ross J Jr: Left ventricular dilatation and diastolic compliance changes during chronic volume overload. *Circulation* 1972; 45:943–951.
432. Mitchell JH, Gilmore JP, Sarnoff SJ: The transport function of the atrium: Factors influencing the relation between mean left atrial pressure and left ventricular end diastolic pressure. *Am J Cardiol* 1962; 9:237–247.
433. Braunwald E: Hemodynamic significance of atrial systole. *Am J Med* 1964; 37:665–669.
434. Ikram H, Nixon PGF, Arcan T: Left atrial function after electrical conversion to sinus rhythm. *Br Heart J* 1968; 30:80–83.
435. Brill IC, Rosenbaum EE, Flanery JR: Congestive failure due to auricular fibrillation in an otherwise normal heart. *JAMA* 1960; 173:784–785.
436. Suga H: Importance of atrial compliance in cardiac performance. *Circ Res* 1974; 35:39–43.
437. Borow KM, Green LH, Grossman W, Braunwald E: Left ventricular end-systolic stress-shortening and stress-length relations in humans: Normal values and sensitivity to inotropic state. *Am J Cardiol* 1982; 50:1301–1308.
438. Taylor RR, Covell JW, Sonnenblick EH, Ross J Jr: Dependence of ventricular distensibility on filling of the opposite ventricle. *Am J Physiol* 1967; 213:711–718.
439. Kelly DT, Spotnitz HM, Beiser GD, Pierce JE, Epstein SE: Effects of chronic right ventricular volume and pressure loading on left ventricular performance. *Circulation* 1971; 44:403–412.
440. Bemis CE, Serur JR, Borkenhagen D, Sonnenblick EH: Influence of right ventricular filling pressure on left ventricular pressure and dimension. *Circ Res* 1974; 34:498–504.
441. Glantz SA, Misbach GA, Moores WY, Mathey DG, Lekuen J, Stowe DF: The pericardium substantially affects the left ventricular diastolic pressure-volume relationship in the dog. *Circ Res* 1978; 42:433–441.
442. Little WC, Badke FR, O'Rourke RA: Effect of right ventricular pressure on the end-diastolic left ventricular pressure-volume relationship before and after chronic right ventricular pressure overload in dogs without pericardia. *Circ Res* 1984; 54:719–730.
443. Chidsey CA, Kaiser GA, Sonnenblick EH, Spann JF, Braunwald E: Cardiac norepinephrine stores in experimental heart failure in the dog. *J Clin Invest* 1964; 43:2386–2393.
444. Burton AC: The importance of the shape and size of the heart. *Am Heart J* 1957; 54:801–809.
445. Kono T, Sabbah HN, Stein PD, Brymer JF, Khaja F: Left ventricular shape as a determinant of functional mitral regurgitation in patients with severe heart failure secondary to either coronary artery disease or idiopathic dilated cardiomyopathy. *Am J Cardiol* 1991; 68:355–359.
446. Sabbah HN, Kono T, Stein PD, Mancini GBJ, Goldstein S: Left ventricular shape changes during the course of evolving heart failure. *Am J Physiol* 1992; 263 (*Heart Circ Physiol* 32):H266–H270.
447. Sabbah HN, Kono T, Rosman H, Jafri S, Stein PD, Goldstein S: Left ventricular shape: A factor in the etiology of functional mitral regurgitation in heart failure. *Am Heart J* 1992; 123:961–966.
448. Mitchell JH, Sarnoff SJ, Sonnenblick EH: The dynamics of pulsus alternans: Alternating end-diastolic fiber length as a causative factor. *J Clin Invest* 1963; 42:55–63.
449. Hada Y, Wolfe C, Craige E: Pulsus alternans determined by biventricular simultaneous systolic time intervals. *Circulation* 1982; 65:617–626.
450. Hess OM, Surber EP, Ritter M, Krayenbuehl HP: Pulsus alternans: Its influence on systolic and diastolic function in aortic valve disease. *J Am Coll Cardiol* 1984; 4:1–7.
451. Braunwald E, Goldblatt A, Harrison DC, Glick EP, Mason DT: Studies on cardiac dimensions in intact, unanesthetized man: III. Effects of muscular exercise. *Circ Res* 1963; 13:460–467.
452. Gorlin R, Cohen LS, Elliott WC, Klein MD, Lane FJ: Effect of supine exercise on left ventricular volume and oxygen consumption in man. *Circulation* 1965; 32:361–371.
453. Braunwald E: The control of ventricular function in man. *Br Heart J* 1965; 27:1–16.
454. Chapman CB (ed): Physiology of muscular exercise. *Circ Res* 1967; 20(suppl I):I-1–I-226.
455. Bevegard BS, Shepherd JT: Regulation of the circulation during exercise in man. *Physiol Rev* 1967; 47:178–213.
456. Horwitz LD, Atkins JM, Leshin SJ: Role of the Frank-Starling mechanism in exercise. *Circ Res* 1972; 31:868–875.
457. Vatner SF, Pagani M: Cardiovascular adjustments to exercise: Hemodynamics and mechanisms. *Prog Cardiovasc Dis* 1976; 19:91–108.
458. Bertrand ME, Carre AG, Ginestet AP, Lefebvre JM, Desplanaque LA, Lekieffre JP: Maximal exercise in normal subjects. *Eur J Cardiol* 1977; 516:481–491.
459. Astrand P-O, Rodahl K: *Textbook of Work Physiology: Physiological Basis of Exercise,* 3d ed. New York, McGraw-Hill, 1986.
460. Christensen NJ, Galbo H: Sympathetic nervous activity during exercise. *Annu Rev Physiol* 1983; 45:139–153.
461. Ludbrook J: Reflex control of blood pressure during exercise. *Annu Rev Physiol* 1983; 45:155–168.
462. Brengelmann GL: Circulatory adjustments to exercise and heat stress. *Annu Rev Physiol* 1983; 45:191–212.
463. Mitchell JH, Kaufman MP, Iwamoto GA: The exercise pressor reflex: Its cardiovascular effects, afferent mechanisms, and central pathways. *Annu Rev Physiol* 1983; 45:229–242.
464. Schlant RC: Physiology of exercise. In: Fletcher GF (ed): *Exercise in the Practice of Medicine,* 2d ed. Mount Kisco, NY: Futura, 1988: 1–47.
465. Epstein SE, Robinson BF, Kahler RL, Braunwald E: Effects of beta-adrenergic blockade on the cardiac response to maximal and submaximal exercise in man. *J Clin Invest* 1965; 44:1745–1753.
466. Robinson BF, Epstein SE, Kahler RL, Braunwald E: Circulatory

effects of acute expansion of blood volume: Studies during maximal exercise and at rest. *Circ Res* 1966; 19:26–32.

467. Bristow JD, Kloster FE, Farrehi C, Brodeur MT, Lewis RP, Griswold HE: The effects of supine exercise on left ventricular volume in heart disease. *Am Heart J* 1966; 71:319–329.
468. Skelton CL, Sonnenblick EH: Physiology of cardiac muscle. In: Levine HJ (ed): *Clinical Cardiovascular Physiology.* New York, Grune & Stratton, 1976: 57–120.
469. Zelis R, Nellis SH, Longhurst J, Lee G, Mason DT: Abnormalities in the regional circulations accompanying congestive heart failure. *Prog Cardiovasc Dis* 1975; 18:181–199.
470. Davies SW, Fussell AL, Jordan SL, Poole-Wilson PA, Lipkin DP: Abnormal diastolic filling patterns in chronic heart failure-relationship to exercise capacity. *Eur Heart J* 1992; 13:749–757.
471. Wiener DH, Fink LI, Maris J, Jones RA, Chance B, Wilson JR: Abnormal skeletal muscle bioenergetics during exercise in patients with heart failure: Role of reduced muscle blood flow. *Circulation* 1986; 73:1127–1136.
472. Massie BM, Conway M, Yonge R, Frostick S, Ledingham J, Sleight P, et al: Skeletal muscle metabolism in patients with congestive heart failure: Relation to clinical severity and blood flow. *Circulation* 1987; 76:1009–1019.

472a. Massie BM, Conway M, Yonge R, Frostick S, Sleight P, Ledingham J, et al: ^{31}P nuclear magnetic resonance evidence of abnormal skeletal muscle metabolism in patients with congestive heart failure. *Am J Cardiol* 1987; 60:309–315.

473. Massie BM, Conway M, Rajagopalan B, Yonge R, Frostick S, Ledingham J, et al: Skeletal muscle metabolism during exercise under ischemic conditions in congestive heart failure: Evidence for abnormalities unrelated to blood flow. *Circulation* 1988; 78:320–326.
474. Sullivan MJ, Green HJ, Cobb FR: Altered skeletal muscle metabolic response to exercise in chronic heart failure: Relation to skeletal muscle aerobic enzyme activity. *Circulation* 1991; 84:1597–1607.
475. Minotti JR, Christoph I, Oka R, Weiner MW, Wells L, Massie BM: Impaired skeletal muscle function in patients with congestive heart failure: Relationship to systemic exercise performance. *J Clin Invest* 1991; 88:2077–2082.
476. Minotti JR, Pillay P, Chang L, Wells L, Massie BM: Neurophysiological assessment of skeletal muscle fatigue in patients with congestive heart failure. *Circulation* 1992; 86:903–908.
477. Wilson JR, Fink L, Maris J, Ferraro N, Power-Vanwart J, Eleff S, et al: Evaluation of energy metabolism in skeletal muscle of patients with heart failure with gated phosphorus-31 nuclear magnetic resonance. *Circulation* 1985; 71:57–62.
478. Clausen JP: Circulatory adjustments to dynamic exercise and effect of physical training in normal subjects and in patients with coronary artery disease. *Prog Cardiovasc Dis* 1976; 18:459–495.
479. Sullivan MJ, Higginbotham MB, Cobb FR: Exercise training in patients with severe left ventricular dysfunction: Hemodynamic and metabolic effects. *Circulation* 1988; 78:506–515.
480. Sullivan MJ, Higginbotham MB, Cobb FR: Exercise training in patients with chronic heart failure delays ventilatory anaerobic threshold and improves submaximal exercise performance. *Circulation* 1989; 79:324–329.
481. Dubach P, Froelicher VF: Cardiac rehabilitation for heart failure patients. *Cardiology* 1989; 76:368–373.
482. Drexler H, Riede U, Münzel T, König H, Funke E, Just H: Alterations of skeletal muscle in chronic heart failure. *Circulation* 1992; 85:1751–1759.
483. Goldsmith SR, Francis GS, Levine TB, Cohn JN: Regional blood flow responses to orthostasis in patients with congestive heart failure. *J Am Coll Cardiol* 1983; 1:1391–1395.
484. Nolan J, Flapan AD, Capewell S, MacDonald TM, Neilson JMM, Ewing DJ: Decreased cardiac parasympathetic activity in chronic heart failure and its relation to left ventricular function. *Br Heart J* 1992; 67:482–485.
485. Zucker IH, Gilmore JP (eds): *Reflex Control of the Circulation.* Boca Raton, FL, CRC Press, 1991: 1–1053.
486. Colucci WS, Wright RF, Braunwald E: New positive inotropic agents in the treatment of congestive heart failure: Mechanisms of action and recent clinical developments. *N Engl J Med* 1986; 314:349–358.
487. Weber KT, Gill SK, Janicki JS, Maskin CS, Jain MC: Newer positive inotropic agents in the treatment of chronic cardiac failure: Current status and future directions. *Drugs* 1987; 33:503–519.
488. LeJemtel TH, Sonnenblick EH: Should the failing heart be stimulated? *N Engl J Med* 1984; 310:1384–1385.
489. Ferguson DW, Berg WJ, Sanders JS, Roach PJ, Kempf JS, Kienzle MG: Sympathoinhibitory responses to digitalis glycosides in heart failure patients: Direct evidence from sympathetic neural recordings. *Circulation* 1989; 80:65–77.
490. Fishman AP, Renkin EM (eds): *Pulmonary Edema.* Bethesda, MD, American Physiology Society, 1979:1–261.
491. Murray JF, Nadel JA (eds): *Textbook of Respiratory Medicine.* Philadelphia, Saunders, 1988.
492. Rapaport E: Dyspnea: Pathophysiology and differential diagnosis. *Prog Cardiovasc Dis* 1971; 13:532.
493. Luepker R, Liander B, Korsgren M, Varnauskas E: Pulmonary intervascular and extravascular fluid volumes in exercising cardiac patients. *Circulation* 1971; 44:626–637.
494. Myers J, Salleh A, Buchanan N, Smith D, Neutel J, Bowes E, et al: Ventilatory mechanisms of exercise intolerance in chronic heart failure. *Am Heart J* 1992; 124:710–718.
495. Aberman A, Fulop M: The metabolic and respiratory acidosis of acute pulmonary edema. *Ann Intern Med* 1972; 76:173–184.
496. Lee G de J: Pulmonary oedema. In: Yu PN, Goodwin JF (eds): *Progress in Cardiology,* vol 1. Philadelphia, Lea & Febiger, 1972: 261.
497. Fishman AP: Pulmonary edema: The water-exchanging function of the lung. *Circulation* 1972; 46:390–408.
498. Robin ED, Cross CE, Zelis R: Pulmonary edema. *N Engl J Med* 1973; 288:292–304.
499. Staub NC: Pulmonary edema. *Physiol Rev* 1974; 54:678–811.
500. Schreiner BF, Yu PN: Pulmonary circulation and edema: Anatomic and physiologic considerations. In: Levine HJ (ed): *Clinical Cardiovascular Physiology.* New York, Grune & Stratton, 1976: 635–706.
501. Gaar KA Jr, Taylor AE, Owens LJ, Guyton AC: Development of pulmonary edema. *Am J Physiol* 1967; 213:79–82.
502. Robin ED, Carey LC, Grenvik A, Glauser F, Gaudio R: Capillary leak syndrome with pulmonary edema. *Arch Intern Med* 1972; 130:66–71.
503. Uhley HN, Leeds SE, Sampson JJ, Friedman M: Right duct lymph flow in experimental heart failure following acute elevation of left atrial pressure. *Circ Res* 1967; 20:306–310.
504. Davies SW, Bailey J, Keegan J, Balcon R, Rudd RM, Lipkin DP: Reduced pulmonary microvascular permeability in severe chronic left heart failure. *Am Heart J* 1992; 124:137–142.
505. Zelis R, Mansour EJ, Capone RJ, Mason DT: The cardiovascular effects of morphine: The peripheral capacitance and resistance vessels in human subjects. *J Clin Invest* 1974; 54:1247–1258.
506. Vismara LA, Learman DM, Zelis R: Effects of morphine on venous tone in patients with acute pulmonary edema. *Circulation* 1976; 54:335–337.
507. Overland ES, Severinghaus JW: Noncardiac pulmonary edema. *Annu Rev Med* 1978; 23:307–326.
508. Hultgren HN, Grover RF: Circulation adaptation to high altitude. *Annu Rev Med* 1968; 19:119–152.
509. Roy SB, Guleria JS, Khanna PK, Manchanda SC, Pande JN, Subba PS: Haemodynamic studies in high altitude pulmonary oedema. *Br Heart J* 1969; 31:52–58.
510. Viswanathan R, Jain SK, Subramanian S: Pulmonary edema of high altitude: III. Pathogenesis. *Am Rev Resp Dis* 1969; 100:342–349.
511. Vogel JHK (ed): Hypoxia, high altitude and the heart. *Advances in Cardiology,* vol 5. Basel, S Karger, 1970.
512. Severinghaus JW: Transarterial leakage: A possible mechanism of high altitude pulmonary edema. In: Porter R, Knight J (eds): *High Altitude Physiology: Cardiac and Pulmonary Aspects,* London, Churchill Livingstone, 1971: 61–77.
513. Kleiner JP, Nelson WP: High altitude pulmonary edema: A rare disease? *JAMA* 1975; 234:491–495.
514. Recavarren S: The preterminal arterioles in the pulmonary circulation of high altitude natives. *Circulation* 1966; 33:177–180.
515. Hultgren HN, Robinson MC, Wuerflein RD: Over-perfusion pulmonary edema. *Circulation* 1966; 34(suppl 3):132–138.
516. Duberstein JL, Kaufman DM: A clinical study of an epidemic of heroin intoxication and heroin-induced pulmonary edema. *Am J Med* 1971; 51:704–714.
517. Paranthaman SK, Khan F: Acute cardiomyopathy with recurrent pulmonary edema and hypotension following heroin overdosage. *Chest* 1976; 69:117–119.

518. Kuida H, Hinshaw LB, Bilbert RP, Gilbert RP, Visscher MB: Effect of gram-negative endotoxin on pulmonary circulation. *Am J Physiol* 1958; 192:335–344.
519. Theodore J, Robin ED: Pathogenesis of neurogenic pulmonary edema. *Lancet* 1975; 2:749–751.
520. Packer M (ed): Physiologic determinants of survival in congestive heart failure. *Circulation* 1987; 75 (suppl IV):IV-1–IV-3.
521. McKee PA, Castelli WP, McNamara PM, Kannel WB: The natural history of congestive heart failure: The Framingham Study. *N Engl J Med* 1971; 285:1441–1446.
522. Kannel WB, Savage D, Castelli WP: Cardiac failure in the Framingham Study: Twenty-year follow-up. In: Braunwald E, Mock MB, Watson JT (eds): *Congestive Heart Failure: Current Research and Clinical Applications.* New York, Grune & Stratton, 1982: 15–30.
523. Rector TS, Cohn JN: Chronic heart failure: Incidence, prognosis, and the effects of medical interventions. In: Kapoor AS, Singh BN (eds): *Prognosis and Risk Assessment in Cardiovascular Disease.* New York, Churchill Livingstone, 1993: 283–289.
524. Cohn JN, Levine TB, Olivari MT, Garberg V, Lura D, Francis GS, et al: Plasma norepinephrine as a guide to prognosis in patients with chronic congestive heart failure. *N Engl J Med* 1984; 311:819–823.
525. Swedberg K, Eneroth P, Kjekshus J, Wilhelmsen L: Hormones regulating cardiovascular function in patients with severe congestive heart failure and their relations to mortality. *Circulation* 1990; 82:1730–1736.

Chapter 26

Diagnosis and Therapy of Heart Failure

Jay N. Cohn, M.D. ■ Edmund H. Sonnenblick, M.D.

Congestive heart failure is a clinical syndrome resulting from a primary abnormality in the function of the heart as a pump, and its diagnosis and ultimate therapy depend on an understanding of the underlying pathophysiology. This pathophysiology involves a wide variety of initial cardiac events as well as vascular and neurohormonal compensatory responses that contribute not only to the clinical syndrome but also to its progression and premature mortality. Primary cardiac overloads (e.g., hypertension or valve disease) or loss of myocardium (e.g., myocardial infarction) elicit adaptive myocardial changes including hypertrophy and ventricular dilation. These adaptations may result in myocardial dysfunction that, if extensive enough, produces ventricular dysfunction which ultimately eventuates in the syndrome of congestive heart failure. Thus, etiology of the heart disease forms only one part of the physiologic derangement. The evaluation and treatment of the overt clinical syndrome involves consideration of not only the initial cause of the cardiac dysfunction but also the evolving compensatory process (see Chap. 25).

TERMINOLOGY

In this chapter terminology will be used that requires precise definition. These terms include the following:

1. *Left ventricular dysfunction*: an abnormality of systolic or diastolic performance of the left ventricle such that either the contractile force is impaired and ventricular emptying reduced or the diastolic relaxation and filling are impaired, or both.
   a. *Systolic dysfunction*: an impairment of the contraction of the left ventricle such that the stroke volume is reduced for any given end-diastolic volume or filling pressure. In general, the end-diastolic volume is increased significantly while the stroke volume is reduced. Thus, the ratio of stroke volume (SV) to end-diastolic volume—the ejection fraction (EF)—is reduced. This may involve either or both ventricles.
   b. *Diastolic dysfunction*: a state in which ventricular filling rate and the extent of filling are reduced or in which a normal extent of filling is associated with an inappropriate rise in ventricular diastolic pressure. Normal systolic emptying (EF) may be maintained.
2. *Heart failure*: a clinical syndrome in which symptoms are associated with abnormalities in systolic or diastolic function. These symptoms may include fatigue, exercise limitation, dyspnea on exertion, orthopnea, or paroxysmal nocturnal dyspnea. (See also Chap. 25.)
3. *Congestive heart failure*: a clinical syndrome in which symptoms of cardiac dysfunction as noted under heart failure are accompanied by signs or symptoms of congestion, including peripheral edema or pulmonary congestion.
4. *Impedance*: the total force opposing left ventricular ejection and composed primarily of arterial compliance, arteriolar resistance, and inertance.

5. *Systemic vascular resistance*: the calculation resulting from the division of the mean systemic arterial pressure, minus the mean systemic venous pressure, by the cardiac output and representing the sum of the resistance to flow of all parallel vascular channels in the systemic circulatory system.
6. *Ventricular remodeling*: an adaptive process in which the ventricle is reshaped by structural changes resulting in increased chamber volume and increased myocardial mass. This involves myocyte hypertrophy with cell widening and elongation as well as myocyte rearrangements in the ventricular wall. Interstitial growth also is characteristic of the process.

ETIOLOGY OF HEART FAILURE

In general, heart failure begins with either an abnormality of coronary blood flow (ischemia and infarction), ventricular overloads whether from pressure (systemic arterial hypertension, aortic stenosis) or volume (mitral regurgitation or shunt lesions), or unexplained myocyte loss and depression (cardiomyopathies, viral myocarditis, toxins). It may also evolve from incessant arrhythmias (sustained tachycardia). Less commonly, the syndrome of congestive failure can result from external factors that limit ventricular filling (constrictive pericarditis).

The general pathophysiology of heart failure is further discussed in Chaps. 23 and 25. Some of the specific conditions that may cause heart failure with particular characteristics include the high output states (Chap. 24), coronary heart disease (Chaps. 58 to 61), systemic arterial hypertension (Chap. 75), aortic valvular disease (Chap. 79), mitral valve disease (Chap. 80), pulmonary and tricuspid valve disease (Chap. 81), multivalvular heart disease (Chap. 82), artificial heart valve disease (Chap. 83), myocarditis and secondary cardiomyopathies (Chap. 88), idiopathic dilated cardiomyopathy (Chap. 89), hypertrophic cardiomyopathy (Chap. 90), restrictive cardiomyopathy (Chap. 91), pericardial disease (Chap. 92), infective endocarditis (Chap. 94), genetic abnormalities (Chap. 96), congenital heart disease (Chaps. 97 and 98), pulmonary hypertension (Chap. 99), pulmonary embolism (Chap. 100), chronic cor pulmonale (Chap. 101), endocrine disease (Chap. 102), connective tissue disease (Chap. 103), obesity (Chap. 104), alcohol (Chap. 105), syphilis (Chap. 106), AIDS (Chap. 107), kidney disease (Chap. 108), noncardiac drugs, poisons, electricity, and radiation (Chap. 110), neoplasms (Chap. 111), trauma (Chap. 112), cerebrovascular disease (Chap. 122), and diseases of the aorta (Chap. 123).

Ischemic Heart Disease

Both systolic and diastolic dysfunction are early manifestations of myocardial iscehmia, since even modest reductions of blood flow may deprive the myocardium of adequate nutrition for generation of muscle contraction and muscle relaxation.[1] In humans the induction of ischemia, through either decreased coronary blood flow or increased oxygen need not met by increased blood flow, results in a rapid loss of contraction in the region involved. If blood flow is restored to the region before necrosis ensues, contractile activity does not return for hours or even days. This persistent loss of contractile activity for hours or days despite return of blood flow and the absence of necrosis is termed *stunning* and may contribute to ventricular dysfunction and symptoms of heart failure (see also Chap. 57).[2] Severe stunning may also produce persistent segmental dilatation of the ventricle by damaging connective tissue connections between cells, a form of remodeling.[3] Another concept, "hibernating" myocardium, refers to myocardium with a contractile dysfunction resulting from a chronic inadequacy of blood flow without histologic evidence of myocardial infarction.[4] Myocardial infarction results in a loss of functioning myocardium in the region served by the occluded coronary vessel. If the loss of coronary flow is incomplete, perhaps due to collateral blood flow, only a subendocardial infarction may result. Nevertheless, this leaves a larger load for the myocardium remaining in the region. The scar resulting from myocardial infarction may further contribute to left ventricular dysfunction by restricting filling or by creating an aneurysm.[5] With large infarctions, compensatory ventricular dilation occurs and reactive hypertrophy occurs in the remaining well-perfused myocardium. With large increases in diastolic filling pressures, "myocyte slippage" occurs and leads to further loads on the ventricular wall. These compensatory processes of myocyte hypertrophy, dilatation, and changes in wall conformation comprise *ventricular remodeling*.[6] Mitral regurgitation may also develop, secondary to either left ventricular dilatation or papillary muscle dysfunction. (See also Chaps. 25, 57, and 60.)

Thus, although the regional dysfunction or scar formation associated with coronary artery disease initially is confined to an area in the distribution of the involved coronary artery, this process often progresses to a dilated ventricle with global impairment of contractile function (hypokinesis). This chamber enlargement, or ventricular remodeling, may occur over days, weeks, months, or years and eventuate in a marked impairment of systolic function. In other instances, however, the regional dysfunction may persist and the ventricle may remain normal in size for many years. The reason why some ventricles remodel and others do not is not clear, but size of the initial infarct appears to be at least one important factor in this process. Some of this remodeling may result from an initial expansion of the infarct zone,[7] particularly with large infarcts involving the anterior wall of the left ventricle. The magnitude of systolic load placed on the left ventricle may contribute to the remodeling process by increasing systolic wall stress while the augmented diastolic pressure produces marked increases in diastolic wall stress. Hypertrophy is an almost invariable accompaniment of the remodeling process in patients with primary ischemic disease of the myocardium. This hypertrophy may, in part, represent a reactive process to normalize wall stress induced by dilatation of the chamber dimension.[8] Neurohumoral factors may also contribute to the ventricular hypertrophy.[9] (See Chap. 6B.) With these considerations in mind, therapy of ischemic processes is directed both to the ischemic event as well as to the ventricular remodeling it induces.

Nonischemic Disease

In a patient with epicardial coronary arteries that angiographically appear to be normal or nearly normal and with no other apparent disease, a dilated, poorly contracting left ventricle is usually diagnosed as idiopathic dilated cardiomyopathy (Chap. 89). Nonetheless, even in this clinical situation ischemia cannot be excluded as an important etiologic factor. Small vessel disease that can influence regional or global perfusion may not be demonstrable by angiographic techniques.[10] Furthermore, regional ischemia from epicardial or intramyocardial coronary disease is not always accompanied by chest pain, and even in the absence of structure or functional changes in the coronary arteries, subendocardial ischemia can result from the compressive force of a high left ventricular diastolic pressure.[11]

A primary disease affecting the myocyte and its contractile process appears to be the cause of most cases of idiopathic dilated cardiomyopathy. (See Chap. 89.) In general, idiopathic dilated cardiomyopathy is characterized by focal diffuse myocyte loss, replacement fibrosis, and reactive hypertrophy of remaining myocytes.[12] A variety of etiologic agents has been implicated (Tables 87-3 and 88-1), and the process can be multifactorial (see Chap. 88 and 89). In most instances the etiology of cardiomyopathy or heart muscle disease of unknown caused cannot be determined by histological examination. Aside from systemic arterial hypertension and coronary artery atherosclerosis, viruses,[13] alcohol,[14] and diabetes[15] may represent the most prevalent factors contributing to heart muscle myocardial dysfunction in North America. Diabetes may also be associated with large and small vessel obstructive disease.[16] (See also Chap. 102.)

Of particular interest are the changes in the myocardium that occur with aging; these changes might contribute to the prevalence of the syndrome of heart failure in the elderly in which diffuse loss of myocytes, increased fibrosis, and reactive hypertrophy of remaining myocytes have been demonstrated.[17,18] Perhaps due to these changes, aging appears to have an effect predominantly on diastolic rather than systolic function and thus may contribute to symptomatology because of impaired relaxation of the ventricle and a higher than normal filling pressure at a normal end-diastolic volume[19] (see below and Chap. 115). The poorly contracting ventricle in the syndrome of heart failure in the elderly also tends to remodel by dilatation and reactive hypertrophy. This remodeling process may occur quite early in the disease or may be delayed until the disease is quite advanced. As this progresses, the remodeling of the ventricle, often with superimposed mitral regurgitation, creates further abnormal loading of the ventricle via the Laplace relation. (See Chap. 5.) Regardless of mechanism, this ventricular dilatation is characterized by a fall in ejection fraction which appears to be a harbinger of morbidity and mortality.[20]

In the past, hypertension has been one of the most common cofactors in the development of heart failure.[21] In many populations the increasingly effective therapy has greatly reduced the incidence of hypertension as a primary cause of heart failure.[22] Nonetheless, even mild to moderate elevations of blood pressure may place a poorly tolerated load on the damaged left ventricle and thus may be an important cofactor in heart failure from other etiologies. Furthermore, hypertension is an important risk factor for the development of coronary disease[23] (see Chap. 62), and the presence of hypertension may be a marker for the coronary disease population.

PATHOPHYSIOLOGY

Ventricular Function

The myocardial abnormalities described above ultimately result in hemodynamic derangement of ventricular function. As the capacity for force development and shortening by the ventricular wall is lost, a compensatory increase in diastolic ventricular volume occurs. Thus, stroke volume is only maintained by an increase in diastolic volume and pressure. Moreover, the relation of stroke volume to end-diastolic pressure is not only depressed but flattened at higher filling pressures. Should marked ventricular hypertrophy without myocyte loss occur, such as with systemic arterial hypertension, prolonged systole, and delayed or incomplete diastolic relaxation of the ventricle, along with thicker ventricular wall, may elevate the end-diastolic filling pressures even with normal volumes, producing diastolic dysfunction. Alternatively, with chronic dilation of the ventricle, the pressure-volume curve may move to the right, and the end-diastolic pressure be actually less than expected for the increase in volume. (See also Chap. 25.)

In the early stages of left ventricular dysfunction, the hemodynamic abnormalities may be confined to exercise, when the increase in stroke volume demanded by exercise may be inadequate and/or accompanied by an abnormally brisk increase in left ventricular filling pressure. This reflects a shift downward and to the right of the Frank-Starling curve (i.e., a lower stroke volume for any given filling pressure) (Chap. 25). The left ventricle normally is capable of adjusting its work output to match an increasing aortic impedance over a wide physiological range[24] (Chap. 23). The dysfunctional left ventricle loses this ability and its performance becomes progressively more impaired as the impedance is increased.[25] (See also Chap. 25.) Thus, the failing left ventricle becomes very sensitive to impedance or afterload and, because of its depressed and flattened Frank-Starling curve, becomes quite insensitive to preload. This important physiological shift from a preload-dependent and afterload-independent ventricle in the normal individual to a preload-independent and afterload-dependent ventricle in the setting of heart failure has important therapeutic implications.

In most patients with heart failure some degree of diastolic dysfunction accompanies systolic dysfunction. The left ventricular diastolic dysfunction, or reduced diastolic ventricular compliance, implies that the left ventricle is stiffer than normal and therefore responds to a small increment in volume with a prominent increase in diastolic filling pressure that is transmitted backward into the pulmonary vasculature.[19] Diastolic dysfunction without apparent systolic dysfunction may be a cause of heart failure as characterized by pulmonary congestion and edema in a significant percentage of patients, particularly in the elderly and in those with a history of hypertension.[26] In general, diastolic dysfunction accompanies left ventricular hypertrophy, in which the myocardium characteristically contracts and relaxes more slowly and the time for diastolic ventricular filling becomes shorter. The thickened ventricular wall also requires higher filling pressures for the same volume of ventricular filling. With tachycardia and/or the loss of the atrial kick, as occurs with atrial fibrillation or flutter, diastolic filling pressure may rise enough to produce pulmonary edema, although systolic ventricular emptying may still be normal. Later, when the EF falls with systolic failure, diastolic dysfunction may still be an important factor. Some of the factors that influence left ventricular (LV) diastolic chamber distensibility are listed in Table 26-1. The syndrome of diastolic dysfunction or failure appears to have a better prognosis than heart failure associated with systolic dysfunction.[26]

In some patients with a reduced EF, the diastolic pressure-volume curve may also be shifted to the right so there is a greater diastolic volume than normal for any given filling pressure. At higher volumes, however, the slope of the pressure-volume curve changes, the wall becomes stiffer, and even the small increments in volume may lead to inordinate increases in filling pressure and vice versa. This phenomenon may be related to an increase in collagen in the interstitium of the myocardium.[27] (See also Chap. 23.)

TABLE 26-1

Factors that Influence Left Ventricular (LV) Diastolic Chamber Distensibility

Factors extrinsic to the LV chamber
- Pericardial restraint
- Right ventricular loading
- Coronary vascular turgor (erectile effect)
- Extrinsic compression by tumor, pleural pressure, etc.

Factors intrinsic to LV chamber
- Passive elasticity of LV wall (stiffness or compliance when myocytes are completely relaxed)
  - Thickness of LV wall
  - Composition of LV wall (muscle, fibrosis, edema, amyloid, hemosiderin) including both endocardium and myocardium
  - Temperature, osmolality
- Active elasticity of LV wall due to residual cross-bridge activation (cycling and/or latch state) through part or all of diastole:
  - Slow relaxation affecting early diastole only
  - Incomplete relaxation affecting early, mid-, and end-diastolic distensibility
  - Diastolic tone, contracture, or rigor
- Elastic recoil (diastolic suction)
- Viscoelasticity (stress relaxation, creep)

SOURCE: Grossman W: Evaluation of systolic and diastolic function of the myocardium. In Grossman W, Baim DS (eds): *Cardiac Catheterization, Angiography, and Intervention*, 4th ed. Philadelphia, Lea and Febiger, 1991: 319–339. Reproduced with permission from the publisher and editors.

A major consequence of the remodeling process in the left ventricle that results in an increase in end-diastolic volume is a reduction in left ventricular EF in patients with systolic heart failure. This remodeling involves elongation of myocytes as well as slippage of adjacent layers of myocytes to produce a larger chamber circumference.[28] When the chamber is enlarged, less shortening of the fiber is required to eject a normal stroke volume. On the other hand, more tension in the wall is required to generate the same pressure. Therefore, some of the apparent systolic functional abnormality in heart failure may be the *result* of chamber dilation and not the *cause* of dilation. (See also Chap. 25.)

Neurohormonal Activation

Neurohormonal systems are activated in the setting of left ventricular dysfunction, regardless of etiology. Activation of the sympathetic nervous system is manifested by elevated plasma norepinephrine levels,[29] increased spillover into the bloodstream of norepinephrine released into the synaptic cleft,[30] and evidence for increased sympathetic nerve traffic.[31] (See also Chap. 25.) This increased nervous system activity may be related to afferent signals to increase sympathetic discharge as well as to attenuation of the response of receptors that normally inhibit the sympathetic nervous system.[32] The status of sympathetic nerves in the heart is more complex. As heart failure proceeds, cardiac sympathetic nerves become dysfunctional and may lose their capacity to synthesize, store, and release norepinephrine.[33] Uptake of norepinephrine from the clefts where it acts on β_1 receptors may also be reduced, thus exposing the myocytes to continued catecholamine stimulation.[34]

The *renin-angiotensin system* also becomes activated in heart failure,[24,35] presumably through intrarenal mechanisms stimulated by changes either in pressure or changes in sodium load in the macula densa.[36] *Arginine vasopressin*, or antidiuretic hormone, also is increased in many patients with heart failure, probably through nonosmotic mechanisms stimulating the release of this hormone from the posterior pituitary.[37] *Atrial natriuretic peptide*, a hormone released from the atrium and perhaps also in abnormal states from the ventricle, circulates in higher than normal levels in patients with heart failure, presumably because of activation through stretch of the atrium or ventricles.[38] The physiological role of this hormone in the setting of heart failure has not been thoroughly demonstrated. There is also evidence for increased circulating or tissue levels of other hormonal systems, including *endothelin*,[39] a potent vasoconstrictor released by the endothelium. Impaired release of other tissue hormones has been demonstrated including *endothelial-derived relaxing factor (EDRF)*, or nitric oxide, which is a potent vasorelaxing material.[40] There is considerable evidence that at least some of these neurohormonal systems contribute to the symptomatology or progression of the heart failure syndrome, but the precise role of each hormone in this process remains to be elucidated (see Chap. 25). Many of the factors circulating or in the tissue in apparently increased concentrations are substances that also contribute to vascular smooth muscle or myocyte growth and hypertrophy. There is growing evidence that the mitogenic effect of these hormones may play a key role in the progression of the syndrome both in the myocardium and in the peripheral vasculature.[41] Indeed, in severe failure, some of the limitations of exercise performance may be due to reduced metabolically induced arteriolar vasodilation in exercising skeletal muscles.[42]

Peripheral Vasculature

An increase in systemic vascular resistance and a reduction of arterial and venous compliance are hallmarks of the syndrome of heart failure[43,44] and probably reflect constriction of vascular smooth muscle due to a number of possible mechanisms. Many of the hormonal systems activated are potent vasoconstrictors that probably contribute to the heightened vascular tone in this syndrome. The reduction or absence of vasodilator substances such as EDRF also may contribute to this heightened tone. No single mechanism apparently predominates, since a number of therapeutic interventions that interfere with different neurohormonal mechanisms may elicit vasodilation, but compensatory mechanisms often adjust the vascular tone despite continued inhibition of a single hormonal mechanism. The peripheral vasoconstriction in heart failure not only may contribute to the symptomatology of the disease by impairing blood flow to regional vascular beds both at rest and during exercise but also may contribute to the heightened impedance that places a systolic load on the left ventricle. The possible role of this vasoconstriction in the progression of the syndrome of heart failure will be considered in discussions of the management of the syndrome. The walls of the arterioles may also be swollen in heart failure, and in the case of systemic arterial hypertension, there may be significant medial hypertrophy.

CLINICAL MANIFESTATIONS OF HEART FAILURE

The four major clinical manifestations of heart failure are left ventricular dysfunction, exercise intolerance, congestion or edema, and ventricular arrhythmias.[45] Each of these may be documented clinically, and improvement in these abnormalities may serve as a therapeutic goal in the treatment of heart failure. Heart failure is characterized by an abnormality of left ventricular function accompanied by reduced capacity to exercise. As discussed below, a reduced EF may not be accompanied by severe impairment of exercise performance. Alternatively, in patients with diastolic ventricular dysfunction and a normal EF, dyspnea on exertion may limit exercise performance.

The most convenient way to assess the function of the left ventricle clinically is by imaging the chamber in diastole and systole, either by radionuclide methods (Chap. 134) or by echocardiography (Chap. 15). Radionuclide angiography provides a useful quantitation of left ventricular EF and thus may be used to quantitate the severity of the left ventricular disease and its progression. Echocardiography provides a more useful description of wall motion in several planes and thus allows for better description of the regional and global nature of the ventricular dysfunction. It also allows an assessment of ventricular wall thickness and dimensions from which diastolic and systolic volumes can be calculated. Estimation of end-diastolic volume, especially as it changes with time, is an important marker of the course of heart failure. The EF is a less sensitive measure of this. Furthermore, Doppler examination provides some clue to the rates of diastolic filling function of the left ventricle.[46] Doppler examination (Chap. 130) also allows quantitation of the severity of regurgitation through the aortic, mitral, and tricuspid valves; this may be important information in defining the mechanism of the left ventricular dysfunction. Valvular gradients can also be assessed accurately.[47] In evaluating left ventricular function it is sometimes useful to challenge the left ventricle in order to determine its functional capacity. Exercise is the most useful stress, and the change in EF with exercise may be an important diagnostic tool in an effort to detect the presence of significant coronary disease, which usually attenuates the normal increase in EF during exercise.[48] (See also Chap. 23.)

Exercise tolerance is often evaluated subjectively by historical information gained from the patient. A more precise way to quantitate exercise capacity is by the performance of an exercise test, which can be performed safely to maximal tolerated exercise in patients with heart failure.[49] This formal exercise testing often provides more information than one can obtain by history because it may well represent the most exercise a patient with heart failure has performed in recent months. Failure to complete even a modest work load in patients with heart failure may reflect the severity of abnormality of the heart failure syndrome but also may be importantly related to deconditioning of peripheral muscles from self-imposed inactivity.[50] (See Chap. 16.) The separation of disease from deconditioning is a problem that can be considerably resolved by performing gas exchange measurements during an exercise test. Newer methodology provides breath-by-breath analysis of expired O_2 and CO_2 for the calculation of oxygen consumption (V_{O_2}) and the onset of anaerobic metabolism during a progressive exercise test.[51] From this, a maximum oxygen consumption V_{O_2max}) can be determined. In apparently asymptomatic patients with considerable ventricular dysfunction, a modest reduction in V_{O_2max} may be demonstrated even though substantial levels of exercise as required by normal activities can be sustained. In later stages of heart failure, V_{O_2max} is poorly related to ejection fraction since a major component of the limitation of exercise then resides in peripheral mechanisms contributing to abnormal skeletal muscle flow and metabolism.

Pulmonary congestion or peripheral edema is often the reason the patient seeks medical help. Pulmonary congestion may be manifest as dyspnea on exertion, orthopnea, paroxysmal nocturnal dyspnea, or even acute pulmonary edema. (See also Chap. 20.) Peripheral edema is manifested by ankle swelling, weight gain, or abdominal bloating. Although sodium retention is a common manifestation of the heart failure syndrome, it is clear that exertional intolerance and disability may exist in some patients in the absence of overt congestion. This noncongestive heart failure is more difficult to recognize clinically and is often misdiagnosed. Even in the absence of edema, however, patients who exhibit exercise intolerance often have elevated pulmonary capillary wedge pressures which may relate to the exertional dyspnea.

Asymptomatic ventricular premature beats and runs of nonsustained ventricular tachycardia are common in patients with left ventricular dysfunction.[52] In the majority of instances these ventricular arrhythmias are not detected by the patient and are only noted by monitoring the electrocardiogram (ECG). The significance of these arrhythmias remains somewhat controversial. Sudden death is a common terminal even in patients with heart failure, and it is therefore intuitive to assume that these ventricular arrhythmias related in some way to the ventricular fibrillation that may be the immediate cause of death.[53] In most studies the presence of complex ventricular arrhythmias, including runs of nonsustained ventricular tachycardia, carries an adverse effect on survival.[54] Because these arrhythmias also become more severe as the left ventricle becomes more dysfunctional, it is important to separate the independent role of the arrhythmias from the ventricular dysfunction in influencing the course of the syndrome. In studies in which this has been carefully analyzed, it appears that ventricular arrhythmias do contribute independently, but only modestly, to the risk of dying from heart failure.[55]

CLINICAL DIAGNOSIS

The clinical diagnosis of heart failure depends on a careful history, a well-focused physical examination, and the performance of tests to document and quantitate the abnormalities.

History

The patient with early symptoms of heart failure may present with complaints of exertional dyspnea or fatigue, unusual tiredness, ankle edema at the end of the day, or modest orthopnea. Symptoms may only become manifest during periods of increased activity or following a more than normal salt intake. The distinction between exertional myocardial ischemia and exertional symptoms of heart failure is often difficult. In heart failure associated with or caused by coronary disease, left ventricular dysfunction is often a manifestation of ischemia and thus angina and dyspnea may coexist. Exercise-induced increases in myocardial oxygen consumption may produce transient segmental loss of contractile function (stunning) with resultant ventricular failure and even severe transient mitral regurgitation. Even in the absence of critical coronary stenoses, however, the left ventricular dysfunction associated with exercise in a patient with heart failure results in an increase in left ventricular diastolic pressure that may impair subendocardial perfusion and result in ischemia which may further aggravate the heart failure syndrome. Thus, ischemia and heart failure frequently coexist; in the former case intervention may be aimed primarily at restoring coronary perfusion or reducing myocardial oxygen requirements, whereas in the latter case intervention should emphasize treatment of the left ventricular failure.

Physical Diagnosis

Function of the left ventricle can be well assessed at the bedside by a careful physical examination. With the patient lying in the left lateral position, the left ventricular apical impulse can usually be felt and characterized on the basis of its forcefulness and size and how sustained it is during systole. A dilated left ventricle will result in a large, more diffuse apical impulse, whereas the hypertrophied ventricle results in a forceful but more localized impulse that is sustained through most of systole. (See Chap. 10.) A murmur of mitral regurgitation also is best sought in this left lateral position. Similarly, the presence of an S3 or S4 gallop often can be best appreciated by careful auscultation in the area of the left ventricular apex with the patient in the left lateral position. The finding of hypertrophied or dilated left ventricle does not, of course, make the diagnosis of heart failure but merely focuses attention on the function of the left ventricle. (See also Chaps. 9A to 11.) Pulsus alternans is virtually pathognomonic of left ventricular failure, but it is not present in most patients with heart failure.

An elevated venous pressure in the setting of ventricular function abnormalities suggests the diagnosis of heart failure. The central venous pressure is best assessed with the patient supine and the upper torso elevated to a sufficient degree to provide a manometer in which the venous pulse may be visible above the clavicle and below the ear. The deep venous pulse (from the internal jugular vein) in the neck should then be carefully visualized, and the level of the top of this pulse measured above either the angle of Louis or the level of the right atrium, which can be taken as the midaxillary line at the level of the nipple (Chap. 10). In patients with a normal jugular venous pressure at rest, right upper quadrant pressure can then be exerted while the central venous pressure is observed. A sustained increase in the jugular venous pressure while normal respiration and abdominal pressure are maintained (positive hepatojugular reflux) is a sign of impaired right ventricular performance. An elevated central venous pressure is a manifestation of right ventricular dysfunction. If the left atrial pressure (or pulmonary capillary pressure) is also elevated, there may be pulmonary rales or symptomatic orthopnea and radiologic evidence of pulmonary congestion or cephalization of pulmonary vascular markings (Chap. 14). Frequently, however, an elevated left atrial pressure may be asymptomatic and not accompanied by any overt signs. Right ventricular failure, which most often occurs as a consequence of left ventricular failure, is characterized by elevated venous filling pressures, hepatomegaly, and peripheral edema, occasionally with reduced or absent signs of pulmonary congestion. On rare occasions, orthopnea and paroxysmal nocturnal edema may also tend to disappear as right ventricular failure progresses.

Laboratory Tests

The upright chest film is a standard part of the workup of a patient with suspected heart failure (Chap. 14), but the size of the cardiac silhouette is not a sensitive guide to the size of the left ventricle, especially with mild disease. In one study, an abnormal increase in cardiothoracic ratio on the 6-ft (2-m) posteroanterior (PA) chest film was observed in no more than 50 percent of patients with clinical congestive heart failure.[56] When cardiomegaly is present and is accompanied by signs of congestion, including cephalization of pulmonary vascular markings, peripheral edema, or pleural effusions, the diagnosis of heart failure is nearly established. In addition, however, the chest x-ray provides information about the right ventricle and the atria that is not available from other tests. Because of this additional information in the chest x-ray, the cardiothoracic ratio has been found to be a predictor of mortality that on multivariate analysis is independent of left ventricular systolic function measured by radionuclide angiography.[57] Currently, echocardiography provides an excellent method for evaluating cardiac function (see Chap. 15). From transthoracic two-dimensional echos, right and left ventricular and atrial dimensions as well as wall thickness and motion may be determined and end-diastolic and end-systolic volumes calculated. Moreover, valvular motion and gradients can be determined with Doppler techniques (Chap. 130). As noted above, measurement of end-diastolic dimensions over time may provide important information as to the course of the disease.

Imaging the left ventricle by radionuclide angiography (Chap. 134) or ventriculography (Chap. 138) provides the most precise measure of chamber size and function, especially in patients in whom excellent echocardiographic images cannot be obtained. An end-diastolic chamber dimension can be calculated, and the ejection fraction can be quantitated. The EF from either these or echocardiographic measurements provides an acceptable means of quantifying systolic performance of the left ventricle since a value below 50 percent may be assumed to represent systolic left ventricular dysfunction. Diastolic dysfunction is diagnosed when the patient demonstrates symptoms of congestive heart failure and pulmonary congestion despite an ejection fraction greater than 50 percent. However, this figure is somewhat arbitrary. Table 26-2 lists some of the conditions that may cause heart failure in patients with normal systolic function.

An exercise test, particularly with measurement of gas exchange, can provide a useful quantitative index to the functional impairment in the patient with heart failure. A peak oxygen consumption <25 mL/kg per min (approximately 7 METs) or the appearance of symptoms of dyspnea or fatigue at work levels below those noted in healthy individuals is confirmatory evidence that the cardiac dysfunction is leading to symptoms. (See also Chap. 16.)

Ambulatory electrocardiographic (Holter) monitoring (see Chap. 45) is occasionally indicated in patients with heart failure because of asymptomatic ventricular premature beats and nonsustained ventricular tachycardia. Monitoring of the ECG for intervals up to 24 h provides quantitation of the ventricular arrhythmias and may provide some additional information regarding prognosis.[55] As noted in the section on treatment, however, therapy aimed at suppressing arrhythmias has not been found to be an effective strategy; nevertheless, it may still be useful to perform ambulatory ECG monitoring in selected patients as a guide to the severity of ventricular arrhythmias. Successful therapy to improve the performance of the heart may be accompanied by reduction of the frequency of arrhythmias. The cost effectiveness of ambulatory ECG monitoring in patients with heart failure has not been established.

Measurement of plasma hormone levels as a guide to the severity of heart failure has been a useful research technique but it is not necessarily applicable to clinical practice. High levels of plasma norepinephrine and plasma atrial natriuretic peptide have prognostic significance in heart failure,[58,59] and the reduction of circulating levels of these hormones might be construed to represent an improvement in the syndrome. A high plasma renin activity may be a marker for responsiveness to therapy with converting enzyme inhibitors. Although activation of these hormone systems indicates a more severe syndrome with a poorer prognosis and a more favorable

TABLE 26-2

Some Conditions that May Be Associated with Heart Failure and Normal Left Ventricular Systolic Performance

- Impaired ventricular relaxation
  - Left ventricular hypertrophy
    - Systemic arterial hypertension
    - Aortic stenosis
    - Hypertrophic cardiomyopathy
  - Myocardial ischemia
    - Coronary artery disease
    - Tachycardia
  - Aging
  - Ventricular asynchrony
- Increased myocardial stiffness
  - Myocardial infiltration
    - Amyloidosis
    - Hemochromatosis
  - Idiopathic restrictive cardiomyopathy
  - Interstitial fibrosis
  - Endomyocardial fibrosis
- Pericardial disease
  - Constriction
  - Tamponade
  - Effusive/constrictive
- Ventricular interaction
  - Acute pulmonary embolism
  - Right ventricular volume overload
  - Right ventricular infarction
  - Acute tricuspid regurgitation
- Mitral stenosis*
- Mitral regurgitation*
- Pulmonary venoocclusive disease*
- Chronic cor pulmonale*

* Conditions that may cause heart failure with normal left ventricular systolic function that are not due primarily to left ventricular diastolic dysfunction.

SOURCE: Adapted from Shah PM, Pai RG: Diastolic heart failure. *Curr Probl Cardiol* 1992; 17:783–868; and Bonow RO, Udelson JE: Left ventricular diastolic dysfunction as a cause of congestive heart failure. *Ann Intern Med* 1992; 117:502–510.

long-term response to converting enzyme inhibitor therapy, it is not necessary in clinical practice to measure hormone levels.

Cardiac catheterization provides the most precise measurements of cardiac dysfunction. Quantitation of pulmonary capillary wedge pressure, left ventricular EF, and the status of the coronary arteries determined by coronary angiography can all be useful measures in documenting the presence of heart failure, its etiology and prognosis, and its response to therapy. When it is important to identify a possible role for coronary disease in the etiology of heart failure, to quantitate the severity of valvular disease, or to quantitate the severity of hemodynamic derangement, cardiac catheterization may be a useful technique in this patient population (see Chap. 132). In general, however, most patients with heart failure do not require cardiac catheterization.

TREATMENT

The first responsibility of treatment is to correct or stabilize any primary abnormality or overload that can be identified. Thus, ischemia is controlled by medical or surgical intervention (Chap. 58), hypertension is rigorously treated (Chap. 77), and primary valve abnormalities (Chaps. 79 to 82) are evaluated for the possibility of repair.

Nonpharmacologic Therapy

Changes in diet and life-style are important parts of the management of heart failure. Salt restriction (2 g sodium or 5 g NaCl per day) is mandatory intervention in patients with signs or symptoms of congestion. Weight loss is an appropriate strategy in the overweight patient. In patients with coronary disease, risk factor reduction to slow the progression of atherosclerotic disease is an important part of management (see Chap. 62). Therefore, restriction of dietary saturated fat and cholesterol should be practiced by such patients. Smoking should be interdicted in all patients with heart failure, because of both its possible role in progression of coronary disease and the possibility of a smoking-induced sudden death.

Provision of an exercise prescription may be an important component of the management of heart failure (see Chap. 16). Whereas in the past many patients with heart failure were told to lead a sedentary existence, it is now common practice to urge patients with heart failure to continue to exercise up to their symptomatic limits. Exercise increases peak exercise capacity, which is reduced by inactivity, and may well improve the quality of life in patients with heart failure. Since there is as yet no firm evidence that chronic dynamic exercise is harmful or that it promotes progression of the disease, it seems appropriate to urge moderate exercise conditioning in most patients with heart failure. This exercise should be dynamic not isometric, however, since the latter exercise increases arterial pressure and left ventricular loading and may facilitate left ventricular remodeling and reduce ventricular performance.

It is also important in patients with heart failure to withdraw drugs that may adversely affect the performance of the heart. Alcohol should be interdicted or taken only in small amounts. Agents with negative inotropic effects probably should be avoided except where there may be a therapeutic benefit that warrants their use. For example, following acute myocardial infarction, beta-blocker therapy reduces mortality even in patients with reduced ejection fraction.[60] Accordingly, this therapy is advised but with appropriate monitoring. (See also Chap. 60.)

Pharmacologic Therapy

Diuretics

Impaired renal sodium excretory capacity commonly complicates both systolic and diastolic heart failure. The cause of sodium retention is apparently multifactorial and involves both hemodynamic and neurohormonal contributions. Patients who exhibit signs or symptoms of congestion, including pulmonary vascular engorgement, peripheral edema, or an increase in central venous pressure, usually require diuretic therapy in addition to dietary restriction of sodium. Despite the symptomatic benefits that result from diuretic therapy, however, diuretics may also induce some unwanted effects. (See also Chap. 29.) A drop in cardiac filling pressure may in some individuals result in a fall in cardiac output that could aggravate the fatigue of heart failure. Activation of the renin-angiotensin system and of the sympathetic nervous system in response to the diuresis may aggravate peripheral vasoconstriction, which can further increase the impedance load on the left ventricle. Potassium loss may precipitate ventricular arrhythmias, particularly in patients who are receiving concomitant digitalis therapy. Magnesium loss in response to diuretic therapy has also been identified as a potential risk factor for sudden death.

Initiation of diuretic therapy should be accompanied by a therapeutic goal. If symptoms of orthopnea or dyspnea on exertion are the indications for diuretic therapy, the relief of these symptoms is an appropriate target. If pedal edema is the problem, therapy should be aimed at relieving it. An elevated central venous pressure may be an indication for diuretic therapy even in the absence of symptoms; thus normalization of the central venous pressure would be an appropriate target for therapy. It is critical when initiating diuretic therapy to utilize the minimum dose of the drugs that can achieve the desired goal without inducing adverse side effects.

Intermittent diuretic therapy may be adequate for patients who have only mild sodium retention. In these cases a dose of a thiazide diuretic or of furosemide administered once or twice weekly may be effective in maintaining the patient edema-free with normal venous pressure. When continuous therapy is necessary and renal function is good, a thiazide diuretic administered once daily may be adequate to achieve the desired therapeutic goal, at times in combination with an intermittent loop diuretic (e.g., furosemide). Since, as discussed below, many patients requiring diuretic therapy for heart failure should be on concomitant angiotensin-converting enzyme (ACE) inhibitor therapy, potassium supplementation or potassium-retaining diuretics should only be administered if the serum potassium falls.

In patients with moderate to severe heart failure the use of a loop diuretic is generally required to maintain sodium balance. Under these circumstances, furosemide, bumetanide, or ethacrynic acid may be administered once or twice daily with titration of the dose to achieve the desired therapeutic goal. A dose of 40 to 80 mg furosemide administered once or twice daily is usually adequate in most patients with heart failure (see Chap. 29).

When fluid retention is recalcitrant, especially if renal function is moderately impaired, the use of a combination of diuretic agents is more effective than a single drug. Whenever doses of more than 100 mg/day of furosemide are necessary to control congestion, the addition of a more proximally acting diuretic can greatly augment the response to the loop diuretic. Metolazone is a particularly effective drug for that purpose and may be administered in a dose of 2.5 to 5 mg, usually given approximately 1 h before the oral dose of furosemide. This combination can produce a massive diuresis in some individuals, with considerable potassium loss. Therefore, close monitoring of potassium and supplementation with potassium chloride, when necessary, is of vital importance.

Enlistment of the patient in dosage adjustments of diuretic therapy is an appropriate strategy. Morning body weight can serve as a sensitive guide to the status of fluid retention. Once an ideal morning body weight has been established by relief of symptoms and normalization of central venous pressure, that weight can be used as a guide to needed adjustments of diuretic therapy. One strategy is to maintain a fixed daily dose of furosemide and to add metolazone intermittently as needed to maintain a predetermined morning weight. This strategy is often effective in preventing progressive fluid retention that leads to repeated hospitalizations. Although blood urea nitrogen may increase after the diuresis induced by metolazone, a modest increase in prerenal azotemia should not be a deterrent to continuation of this regimen. Patients with severe heart failure often exhibit chronic prerenal azotemia in response to diuretic therapy; however, prerenal azotemia usually has no long-term adverse effects and may be necessary for relief of symptoms.

Vasodilator Drugs

Increased impedance to left ventricular outflow and augmented venous tone are largely unwanted physiologic responses to heart failure and can contribute to further deterioration of left ventricular function. Therefore, drugs that relax the systemic vasculature and/or reduce venous tone may improve the performance of the left ventricle and relieve symptoms. The increase in left ventricular filling pressure that complicates heart failure is in part the product of a shift of blood from the peripheral venous system into the central venous system in response to venoconstriction accompanying heart failure. Thus, drugs that relax the venous vascular smooth muscle can redistribute the blood volume and reduce cardiac filling pressures, with a concomitant relief of symptoms of congestion. Moreover, such agents, by reducing the cardiac filling pressures, may help to reduce the progressive ventricular dilatation (remodeling) that produces further myocardial dysfunction as well as functional mitral regurgitation.

All vasodilator drugs appear to have an acute favorable hemodynamic effect in patients with heart failure, but the long-term benefits of these drugs in terms of symptoms or the progression of the disease appear to vary. Sodium nitroprusside is a potent, intravenously administered smooth-muscle dilator that relaxes both arterial and venous vasculature and results in a striking increase in cardiac output and reduction in cardiac filling pressure in patients with heart failure.[61] This therapy, which is markedly effective in patients with severe pump failure, usually requires continuous monitoring since arterial hypotension may complicate its use. Intravenous nitroglycerin produces venodilatation with much less effect on arterial vascular resistance. Thus in heart failure, nitrates produce a fall in both right and left ventricular filling pressures with little change in cardiac output or arterial pressure.[62] At higher doses, however, arterial hypotension may also ensue and limit further increase in dosage. Conversely, hydralazine reduces arterial resistance and increases cardiac output with little effect on the venous bed to reduce ventricular filling pressures.[63]

In order to replicate this hemodynamic effect chronically, oral drugs have been utilized with the therapeutic goal of relieving symptoms and improving exercise tolerance. The long-acting nitrates, which replicate the venous and some of the large arterial effects of sodium nitroprusside, may produce a profound reduction in the elevated cardiac filling pressure in patients with heart failure. Since these drugs do not have as much effect on the arteriolar vasculature as nitroprusside, they do not augment the cardiac output as much. Hydralazine, which has potent arteriolar dilating effects, works synergistically with nitrates to increase cardiac output. Thus, hydralazine and isosorbide dinitrate augment cardiac output and reduce filling pressure.[64] A chronic regimen of hydralazine and isosorbide dinitrate when added to a regimen of digoxin and diuretic therapy has been demonstrated to improve exercise tolerance and prolong life in patients with heart failure.[65] Current formulations of these drugs require their administration three or four times daily in order to maintain the hemodynamic benefit. Isosorbide dinitrate has usually been given in doses of 20 to 60 mg three or four times daily and hydralazine in divided doses of 200 to 300 mg daily. The major side effect of this therapy has been headache, which usually abates with chronic therapy. Some patients, however, are unable to tolerate these drugs because of symptomatic side effects, and alternative therapy must be sought. Since nitrate tolerance has been a concern during chronic nitrate therapy, it is prudent to administer the last evening dose of isosorbide dinitrate at least 10 h before the first morning dose in order to provide a drug-free interval.

The ACE inhibitors were introduced into the therapy of heart failure as vasodilator drugs because of their known action in inhibiting the effect of angiotensin II on blood vessels (Chap. 30). Although their vasodilator effect is an important pharmacologic action, it is likely that their beneficial effect in the syndrome of heart failure relates also to other actions that will be considered in a subsequent section. The evidence that therapy with ACE inhibitors can reduce mortality in patients with all degrees of symptomatic heart failure[66,67] has made their use a standard part of the regimen for the treatment of heart failure in most patients. (See also Chap. 25.)

Studies have also explored the use of ACE inhibitors in patients with left ventricular dysfunction not necessarily accompanied by symptoms of heart failure. In the Studies of Left Ventricular Dysfunction (SOLVD) trial, over 4000 patients with an EF <35 percent in the absence of heart failure symptoms were randomly assigned to receive placebo or enalapril therapy.[68] A trend for a reduction in total mortality in the enalapril-treated group did not reach statistical significance, but a striking delay in the onset of overt congestive heart failure and in the need for hospitalization was noted in the active treatment group. In the Survival and Ventricular Enlargement (SAVE) Trial, over 2000 patients from 3 to 16 days after an acute myocardial infarction and with an EF <40 percent were randomly assigned to receive placebo or captopril therapy.[69] The captopril-treated group exhibited a statistically significantly reduced mortality during follow-up.

Initiation of therapy with an ACE inhibitor in patients with heart failure must be done cautiously because of the possibility of a hypotensive reaction in some patients, especially those who have strong diuretic therapy and may have a decreased effective blood volume. This hypotension is generally well tolerated, however, and in the absence of significant orthostasis should not limit drug use. Sensitivity to the first dose of an ACE inhibitor usually relates to the level of activation of the renin-angiotensin system. Although a plasma renin activity measurement might provide that assessment, it is usually impractical and unnecessary to make this before initiating therapy. A serum sodium concentration may serve as a surrogate for plasma renin activity and provide a guide to the caution with which these drugs should be initiated.[70] A serum sodium level below 135 meq/liter is suggestive of heightened plasma renin activity and of an increased risk of a greater hypotensive response to the first dose. In patients who exhibit this degree of hyponatremia, very small doses of AC inhibitors should be administered initially with monitoring of blood pressure in a protective environment. In other patients, less caution is necessary. Since diuretics may induce a state of relative hypovolemia that can sensitize the circulation to an ACE inhibitor, it may be prudent to withhold diuretics for 24 h before initiating ACE inhibitor therapy.

An appropriate initial dose of an ACE inhibitor in a stable patient is the administration of 12.5 mg captopril or 2.5 mg enalapril. Captopril is generally administered three times daily and enalapril twice daily in patients with heart failure. Within 1 to 2 days after initiating this low-dose therapy, the dose may be increased if it has been well tolerated. For the management of heart failure the dose of captopril is approximately 75 to 150 mg daily and that of enalapril is 20 mg daily in divided doses. Since these dosing regimens have been demonstrated to have a favorable long-term effect in heart failure, it is imprudent to utilize lower doses unless the patient demonstrates intolerance. The major side effects of ACE inhibitor therapy are hypotension and azotemia; however, a modest persistent increase in creatinine is expected and poses no problem. Although most patients tolerate a moderate fall in blood pressure without symptoms, if the patient develops orthostatic dizziness or the serum levels of creatinine or blood urea nitrogen more than double, a reduction in dose of either the ACE inhibitor or, if appropriate, the diuretic agent being utilized concomitantly is mandated. Since inhibition of angiotensin II also inhibits adrenal aldosterone release, renal K^+ loss is reduced and hyperkalemia can occur, especially if oral potassium supplements are continued. A less serious, but sometimes troublesome, side effect of ACE inhibitor therapy is the development of cough. This symptom, which may relate to kinin production, appears not to be dose-related and may occur in some individuals in response to any ACE inhibitor. When cough begins to have an adverse effect on quality of life, it may be necessary to discontinue the drug and seek alternative therapy. Since hydralazine and isosorbide dinitrate in combination rarely produce hypotension or azotemia and do not cause cough, these drugs may be an appropriate alternative in patients who cannot tolerate converting enzyme inhibitor therapy.

A number of other vasodilator drugs have been utilized in heart failure, and new agents are currently in clinical testing. Alpha blockers have a favorable hemodynamic effect in heart failure but have not yet been demonstrated to exert a favorable clinical response on either symptoms or survival.[65] Therefore, these agents should not be viewed as preferred therapy at the present time. Minoxidil is a potent vasodilator drug which also exerts markedly favorable hemodynamic effects in heart failure but may result in sodium retention that can aggravate the symptoms of heart failure. Preliminary trials have not demonstrated favorable long-term effects of this drug.[71] Flosequinan, a new arterial and venous vasodilator, was withdrawn by the manufacturer after long-term studies suggested that its use might be associated with increased mortality.

Inotropic Drugs

Positive inotropic agents increase contractile force of the myocardium and have been considered a rational therapeutic approach to systolic heart failure. The arrhythmogenic potential of these agents, however, has raised questions relative to safety over longer periods of time, but digitalis glycosides have remained a popular and well-tolerated drug in the management of heart failure. Indeed, recent trials have provided support for the effectiveness of digoxin in relieving symptoms, increasing EF, and improving exercise tolerance in patients with heart failure even in normal sinus rhythm.[72,72a] The mechanism of action of digoxin may not be related exclusively to its positive inotropic effect but may also include neurohormonal inhibition related to activation of baroreceptor mechanisms.[73] In patients with atrial fibrillation digitalis glycosides are very useful in controlling heart rate.

One concern about the safety of digoxin administration in heart failure has been the risk of ventricular arrhythmias and sudden death. Ongoing clinical trials are addressing the long-term safety of digoxin in patients with heart failure. Until these studies are completed, it is appropriate to administer digoxin to patients who have moderate or severe systolic dysfunction in the presence of symptoms of heart failure. A dose of 0.25 mg daily is safe in most patients but should be reduced to 0.125 mg daily in older individuals, very small individuals, or those with mild renal insufficiency. Digoxin blood levels may be obtained when any question arises as to the adequacy and safety of the given dose of the drug. In the presence of atrial fibrillation, heart rate control is generally adequate to assess dose levels.

Other oral inotropic drugs have been under study for years with the aim of replacing or supplementing digoxin in an effort to increase contractile force of the ventricular myocardium in patients with heart failure. Although many agents have been demonstrated to have a favorable acute hemodynamic effect, the safety of most of these drugs has been brought into question in controlled clinical trials. Milrinone, a phosphodiesterase inhibitor which augments cyclic AMP levels to produce increased contractility of the heart as well as arterial and venous dilatation, was found to shorten survival in patients with very severe heart failure, possibly because of an arrhythmogenic effect of the drug.[74] This detrimental effect was not observed in less sick patients, and the relations to dose and interactions with digitalis glycosides are uncertain. Other agents that work through the beta-adrenergic receptor system have also been found to have an adverse effect on survival.[75] At present, none of these agents have been approved for clinical use although many remain in clinical investigation. Early studies with a unique new inotropic agent, vesnarinone, have suggested a favorable effect on survival.[76]

In severe acute heart failure the intravenous use of inotropic agents to augment cardiac performance is standard practice. The intravenous infusion of dobutamine can effect a striking increase in cardiac output,[77] particularly when administered in combination with sodium nitroprusside.[78] Other catecholamines have also been used in these circumstances together with low-dose dopamine to augment renal blood flow. Intravenous amrinone and milrinone (see Chap. 28) also increase cardiac output and lower filling pressures, the latter to an even greater extent than catecholamines.[79] Moreover, since dobutamine stimulates cyclic AMP while amrinone and milrinone, which are phosphodiesterase inhibitors, inhibit its breakdown, the combination of these agents is more potent than either alone. Although beta receptor down regulation in response to chronic stimulation with catecholamines has been demonstrated,[80] most studies suggest that a sustained benefit of these drugs is often maintained for several weeks. In an attempt to utilize this pharmacologic mechanism chronically, some physicians have employed intravenous infusion of dobutamine on an outpatient basis either continuously or intermittently through indwelling catheters.[81] The safety of this approach to management has not been proved, but anecdotal reports suggest that under carefully controlled situations it might be effective in improving symptoms and restoring otherwise bedridden patients to an ambulatory state.

Diastolic heart failure needs different therapy because decreased contractility is not the primary problem. In this circumstance, therapy is directed to cautious diuresis and slowing of the heart rate with restitution of sinus rhythm; in general, inotropic agents are not helpful in this situation and might even be detrimental with severe hypertrophy. (See also Chap. 25.)

Neurohormonal Inhibition

The evidence that activation of a variety of neuroendocrine mechanisms accompanies the syndrome of heart failure has led to speculation that this activation has an adverse effect on the long-term outcome of the syndrome. Not only may this neurohormonal activation cause redistribution of blood flow and vasoconstriction that may aggravate the symptoms of heart failure, but a number of neurohormonal mechanisms have been implicated in the myocardial remodeling and vascular remodeling associated with the syndrome.[41] It is therefore possible that the long-term progression of heart failure is related at least in part to these neurohormonal mechanisms.

Two groups of agents have been utilized to inhibit the progression of the syndrome. Most data are available on the ACE inhibitors, which appear to inhibit progression of left ventricular dysfunction and reduce mortality rate in the syndrome.[66-69] Although the beneficial mechanism of action of ACE inhibitors may be in part through their vasodilator effect in reducing impedance to left ventricular outflow, it is likely that some of the benefits relate to inhibition of neurohormonal mechanisms, including a reduction in circulating and tissue levels of angiotensin II and a reduction in norepinephrine.[82] Inhibition of myocardial hypertrophy and remodeling and vascular hypertrophy are also potential mechanisms for ACE inhibitor efficacy. (See also Chap. 25.)

Beta blockers have been utilized in the management of heart failure since early studies from Sweden claimed remarkable long-term benefits.[83,84] Although these agents would be expected to exhibit negative inotropic effect on left ventricular function, particularly in patients whose contractility is dependent on sympathetic nervous system activation, long-term favorable effects raise the possibility that this benefit results from other mechanisms. Long-term, carefully controlled trials have not yet been completed, and therefore the use of these agents in the management of heart failure must be viewed as experimental. Indeed, the mechanism of their potential beneficial effect is not understood. During initiation of therapy with beta blockers an aggravation of symptoms of heart failure and a deterioration of left ventricular function may be observed.[85] Therefore, it is usually advocated to begin this therapy at very low doses with careful titration up to a desirable level. Metoprolol is the drug most commonly employed for this purpose, but newer beta blockers that also possess vasodilator and inotropic actions might minimize the adverse hemodynamic effects when therapy is instituted.

Antiarrhythmic Therapy

Nearly half the cardiovascular deaths observed in patients with heart failure occur suddenly in a setting consistent with an arrhythmic terminal event.[86] Since ventricular arrhythmias, often asymptomatic nonsustained ventricular tachycardia, are commonly observed in patients with heart failure, it is natural to assume that the ventricular arrhythmias detected on ambulatory ECG monitoring bear some relationship to the subsequent sudden death. In carefully analyzed trials, ventricular arrhythmias recorded on ambulatory ECG monitors have on multivariate analysis been a modest independent predictor of mortality in patients with heart failure. Thus, although the severity of the symptoms of heart failure and the severity of left ventricular dysfunction are more powerful predictors of mortality, the presence of ventricular arrhythmias appears to have some independent influence. Therefore, attempts to suppress ventricular arrhythmias have been a high priority in interventional studies.

The strategy favoring ventricular arrhythmia suppression suffered a severe blow with the Cardiac Arrhythmia Suppression Trial (CAST) study, which demonstrated that effective suppression of premature beats with type 1C antiarrhythmic agents was associated with shortened life expectancy in patients with left ventricular dysfunction following myocardial infarction.[87] As a result of this trial it would currently be imprudent for physicians to prescribe such drugs in asymptomatic patients following myocardial infarction. When symptoms of ventricular arrhythmias, particularly syncopal episodes, are present, however, attempts to suppress the arrhythmia may be appropriate even in view of the risk; but in these patients other pharmacologic agents or implanted defibrillators may be a more effective strategy. Studies with amiodarone as an antiarrhythmic agent are currently in progress to determine if this drug can favorably affect survival without an unacceptable incidence of adverse effects.[88] (See also Chaps. 36, 42, and 60.)

Since some drugs that favorably influence left ventricular dysfunction and reduce mortality in heart failure appear to reduce mortality both from pump failure and from sudden death, it is hoped that a favorable impact on the syndrome of heart failure would also reduce the risk of sudden death. Further studies are required to demonstrate that pharmacologic intervention to improve ventricular function will be effective in reducing ventricular arrhythmias.

As noted above, an acute exacerbation of symptoms may occur with diastolic dysfunction during tachycardia or with atrial flutter or fibrillation; in this situation, rapid control of the heart rate and restoration of sinus rhythm is essential.

Anticoagulant Therapy

Thromboembolic events occur in patients with heart failure either because of stasis induced by inactivity and reduced regional blood flow or because of a hypercoagulable state produced by the syndrome. In patients with left ventricular mural thrombi on akinetic or dyskinetic segments of the left ventricular myocardium, anticoagulation often is employed in an effort to reduce the risk of systemic embolization (Chap. 60). In other patients, lower extremity venous thrombosis may result in pulmonary embolism (Chap. 100). In recent trials, the risk of clinically apparent thromboembolic events in patients with heart failure has been about 2.5 per 100 patient-years.[89,90] This low event rate combined with the evidence that few patients with heart failure appear to die of thromboembolic events has raised the question whether or not routine anticoagulation is appropriate in this patient population. In the absence of atrial fibrillation and in patients who are fairly active, there appears to be no strong indication for anticoagulation unless a previous thromboembolic event has occurred. The decision to anticoagulate depends on the physician's judgment of the risk of thromboembolism versus the risk of anticoagulation in an individual patient.

Invasive Approaches

Coronary Reperfusion

In patients with heart failure it is often difficult to assess the contribution of myocardial underperfusion to the left ventricular dysfunction. In the absence of chest pain or ECG changes of ischemia, the presence of coronary disease alone in a patient with a dilated left ventricle is not an adequate indication for surgical or interventional reperfusion. The most persuasive evidence supporting attempts to reperfuse the coronary circulation is the occurrence of repeated episodes of acute left heart failure associated with pulmonary edema even in the absence of chest pain. When these episodes occur in the absence of preceding dietary indiscretion or weight gain, the possibility of "flash" or acute ischemic left ventricular diastolic dysfunction must be seriously considered.[91,92] Under these circumstances coronary angiography to search for a treatable stenosis is often indicated. Additional studies to determine whether or not myocardium is viable may also be necessary.

When ischemia is more obvious by virtue of acute myocardial infarction, unstable angina, or suspicious ECG changes, the presence of left ventricular systolic dysfunction should not be a deterrent to coronary revascularization. Indeed, patients with left ventricular dysfunction and three vessel coronary disease often benefit most from coronary artery bypass surgery.[93–95] (See Chap. 73.) Aneurysmectomy, often combined with coronary artery bypass surgery, may significantly improve left ventricular performance in selected patients.[96] In selected high-risk patients, coronary angioplasty can effectively reperfuse critically stenotic arteries and also ideally improve the function of the left ventricle. (See also Chap. 70.)

Valvular Heart Disease

Mitral and tricuspid regurgitation often occur as functional complications of the dilated ventricular chambers in patients with heart failure. Medical rather than surgical attempts to reduce the degree of valvular regurgitation are usually preferred in this setting. Vasodilator drugs and diuretic therapy may strikingly reduce the degree of mitral and tricuspid regurgitation by reducing chamber size. Surgical approaches to functional mitral regurgitation, especially in very dilated ventricles, are associated with very high risk and usually very limited benefit. (See also Chaps. 79 to 86.)

Heart Transplantation

The most effective therapy for severe heart failure has been transplantation (Chap. 32). Because of the limitation of donor supply, this procedure has been available for only a minority of patients who develop intractable symptoms of heart failure. Criteria for eligibility for transplantation vary from center to center but usually favor patients below the age of 55 or 60 who do not have severe coexistent disease. Two-year mortality after heart transplantation has in recent years been reduced to <10 percent, and excellent long-term survival is possible although the development of coronary vascular disease is a limiting factor in some patients and may require a second heart transplantation. Indeed, long-term survival (>5 to 10 years) has been limited by the secondary development of large and small vessel obstructive disease (see also Chap. 32).

Mechanical Assistance

Short-term mechanical assistance in an attempt to tide a patient over an acute cardiac episode or to serve as a bridge to transplantation has been employed in a number of centers in the past decade. Considerable effort has been expended on the development of a totally implanted artificial heart that could substitute for heart transplants. Development of these devices is still proceeding, and an operational model may be available after the year 2000. (See also Chap. 31.)

Identification of Patients at Risk for Heart Failure

Most intervention trials in patients with heart failure have been conducted in symptomatic individuals who have moderate to severe left ventricular systolic dysfunction. Once this syndrome has developed the mortality is quite high, averaging more than 10 percent per year. In an effort to intervene earlier, recent studies have sought to initiate therapy prior to the development of symptoms of heart failure. Subjects in the SOLVD and SAVE trials were selected on the basis of reduced left ventricular EF even in the absence of symptoms.[68,69] In both these trials the administration of an ACE inhibitor (captopril or enalapril) was associated with a reduction of morbid events, an apparent slowing of the progression of left ventricular dysfunction, and a trend toward a reduction in mortality. These studies have raised the possibility that earlier intervention in heart failure might be an appropriate strategy.

Even in these studies, however, left ventricular systolic dysfunction already existed at the time of randomization. It is possible that the identification of patients at risk who have not yet developed systolic dysfunction might provide a population in whom intervention could affect long-term survival even more favorably. At the present time, however, it is premature to consider such an approach.

REFERENCES

1. Katz AM: Cellular mechanisms in congestive heart failure. *Am J Cardiol* 1988; 62:3A–8A.
2. Bolli R: Mechanisms of myocardial stunning. *Circulation* 1990; 82:723–738.
3. Zhao M, Zhang H, Robinson TF, Factor SM, Sonnenblick EH, Eng C: Profound structural alterations of the extracellular collagen matrix in post-ischemic "stunned" but viable myocardium. *J Am Coll Cardiol* 1987; 10:1322–1334.
4. Braunwald E, Rutherford JD: Reversible ischemic left ventricular dysfunction: Evidence for the "hibernating myocardium." *J Am Coll Cardiol* 1986; 8:1467–1470.
5. McKay RG, Pfeffer MA, Pasternak RC, Markis JE, Come PC, Nakao S, et al: Left ventricular remodeling after myocardial infarction: A corollary to infarct expansion. *Circulation* 1986; 74:693–702.
6. Pfeffer MA, Braunwald E: Ventricular remodeling after myocardial infarction. Experimental observations and clinical complications. *Circulation* 1990; 81:1161–1172.
7. Hutchins GM, Bulkley BH: Infarct expansion versus infarct extension: Two different complications of acute myocardial infarction. *Am J Cardiol* 1978; 41:1127–1132.
8. Grossman W: Cardiac hypertrophy. Useful adaptation or pathological process. *Am J Med* 1980; 69:576–584.
9. Laks M: Norepinephrine—the producer of myocardial cellular hypertrophy and/or necrosis and/or fibrosis. *Am Heart J* 1977; 94:394.
10. Factor SM, Sonnenblick EH: Hypothesis: Is congestive cardiomyopathy caused by a hypertensive myocardial microcirculation (microvascular spasm)? *Am J Cardiol* 1982; 50:1149–1152.
11. Salisbury PF, Cross CE, Rieban PA: Acute ischemia of inner layers of ventricular wall. *Am Heart J* 1963; 66:650–656.
12. Sonnenblick EH, LeJemtel TH, Eng C, Zhao M, Hochman J, Capasso M, et al: A role for ACE inhibitors in modulating ventricular remodelling and altering the course of ventricular dysfunction and resultant heart failure in ischemia and myocardial infarction. In: MacGregor GA, Sever PS, Caldwell D, Hollenberg NK (eds): *Current Advances in ACE Inhibition 2*. New York, Churchill-Livingstone, 1991: 38–42.
13. Peters NS, Poole-Wilson PA: Myocarditis—continuing clinical and pathologic confusion. *Am Heart J* 1991; 121:942–947.
14. Diamond I: Alcoholic myopathy and cardiomyopathy (editorial). *N Engl J Med* 1989; 72:458.
15. Fein FS, Sonnenblick EH: Diabetic cardiomyopathy. *Prog Cardiovasc Disc* 1985; 27:255–270.
16. Sunni S, Bishop SP, Kent SP, Geer JC: Diabetic cardiomyopathy. *Arch Pathol Lab Med* 1986; 110:375–381.
17. Wei JY: Age and the cardiovascular system. *N Engl J Med* 1992; 327:1735–1739.
18. Olivetti G, Melissari M, Capasso JM, Anversa P: Cardiomyopathy of the aging human heart: Myocyte loss and reactive cellular hypertrophy. *Circ Res* 1991; 68:1560–1568.
19. Gaasch WH, Levine HJ, Quinones MA, Alexander JK: Left ventricular compliance: Mechanisms and clinical implications. *Am J Cardiol* 1976; 38:645–653.
20. White HD, Norris RM, Brown MA, Brandt PW, Whitlock RM, Wild CJ: Left ventricular end-systolic volume is the major determinant of survival after recovery from myocardial infarction. *Circulation* 1987; 76:44–51.
21. McKee PA, Castelli WP, McNamara PM, Kannel WB: The natural history of congestive heart failure: The Framingham Study. *N Engl J Med* 1971; 285:1441–1446.
22. Kaplan NM: *Clinical Hypertension*, 5th ed. Baltimore, Williams and Wilkins, 1990.
23. Levy D, Wilson PWF, Anderson KM, Castelli WP: Stratifying the patient at risk from coronary disease: New insights from the Framingham Heart Study. *Am Heart J* 1990; 119:712–717.
24. Wilcken DEL, Charlier AA, Hoffman JIER, Guz A: Effect of alterations in aortic impedance on the performance of the ventricles. *Circ Res* 1964; 14:283–293.
25. Cohn JN: Vasodilator therapy for heart failure: The influence of impedance on left ventricular performance. *Circulation* 1973; 48:5–8.
26. Cohn JN, Johnson G: Heart failure with normal ejection fraction: The V-HeFT Study. *Circulation* 1990; 81:III-48–III-53.
27. Weber KT, Brilla CG: Pathological hypertrophy and cardiac interstitium. Fibrosis and renin-angiotensin-aldosterone system. *Circulation* 1991; 83:1849–1865.
28. Anversa P, Capasso JM, Puntillo E, Sonnenblick EH, Olivetti G: Structural mechanisms of the myocardial response to infarction.

In: Jacob R, Seipel L, Zucker IH (eds): *Cardiac Dilatation: Pathogenesis, Morphology, Hemodynamic and Energetic Consequences*. New York, Gustav Fischer, 1990:36–90.

29. Levine TB, Francis GS, Goldsmith SR, Simon A, Cohn JN: Activity of the sympathetic nervous system and renin-angiotensin system assessed by plasma hormone levels and their relationship to hemodynamic abnormalities in congestive heart failure. *Am J Cardiol* 1982; 49:1659–1666.
30. Hasking GJ, Esler MD, Jennings GL, Burton D, Johnson JA, Korner PI: Norepinephrine spillover to plasma in patients with congestive heart failure: Evidence of increased overall and cardiorenal sympathetic nervous activity. *Circulation* 1986; 73:615–621.
31. Sole MJ: Alterations in sympathetic and parasympathetic neurotransmitter activity. In: Braunwald E, Mock MG, Watson J (eds): *Congestive Heart Failure: Current Research and Clinical Applications*. New York, Grune & Stratton, 1982:101.
32. Goldstein RE, Beiser GD, Stampfer M, Epstein SE: Impairment of autonomically mediated heart rate control in patients with cardiac dysfunction. *Circ Res* 1975; 36:571–578.
33. Spann JF, Sonnenblick EH, Cooper T, Chidsey CA, Willman VL, Braunwald E: Cardiac norepinephrine stores and the contractile state of heart muscle. *Circ Res* 1966; 19:317–325.
34. Francis GS, Goldsmith SR, Levine TB, Olivari MT, Cohn JN: The neurohumoral axis in congestive heart failure. *Ann Intern Med* 1984; 101:370–376.
35. Levine TB, Francis GS, Goldsmith SR, Simon A, Cohn JN: Activity of the sympathetic nervous system and renin-angiotensin system assessed by plasma hormone levels and their relation to hemodynamic abnormalities in congestive heart failure. *Am J Cardiol* 1982; 49:1659–1666.
36. Olivari MT, Levine TB, Cohn JN: Evidence for a direct renal stimulating effect of prostaglandin E_2 on renin release in patients with congestive heart failure. *Circulation* 1986; 74:1203–1207.
37. Goldsmith SR, Francis GS, Cowley AW, Levine TB, Cohn JN: Increased plasma arginine vasopressin in patients with congestive heart failure. *J Am Coll Cardiol* 1983; 1:1385–1390.
38. Cody RJ, Atlas SA, Laragh JH, Kubo SH, Covit AB, Ryman KS, et al: Atrial natriuretic factor in normal subjects and heart failure patients: Plasma levels and renal hormonal and hemodynamic responses to peptide infusion. *J Clin Invest* 1986; 78:1362–1374.
39. Prasad K, Lee P, Kalra J: Influence of endothelin on cardiovascular function, oxygen-free radicals, and blood chemistry. *Am Heart J* 1991; 121:178–187.
40. Kubo SH, Rector TS, Bank AJ, Williams RE, Heifetz SM: Endothelium dependent vasodilation is attenuated in patients with heart failure. *Circulation* 1991; 84:1589–1596.
41. Francis GS, Cohn JN: Heart failure: Mechanisms of cardiac and vascular dysfunction and the rationale for pharmacologic intervention. Reviews. *FASEB* 1990; 4:3068–3075.
42. Mancini D, LeJemtel TH, Factor S, Sonnenblick EH: The central and peripheral components of heart failure. *Am J Med* 1966; 80(suppl 2B):2B–13B.
43. Finkelstein SM, Cohn JN, Collins RV, Carlyle PF, Shelley W: Vascular hemodynamic impedance in congestive heart failure. *Am J Cardiol* 1985; 55:423–427.
44. Wood JE: The mechanism of the increased venous pressure with exercise in congestive heart failure. *J Clin Invest* 1972; 4:2020–2024.
45. Cohn JN: Current therapy of the failing heart. *Circulation* 1988; 78:1099–1107.
46. Feigenbaum H: *Echocardiography*, 4th ed. Philadelphia, Lea & Febiger, 1986:211.
47. Stamm RB, Martin RP: Quantification of pressure gradients across stenotic valves by Doppler ultrasound. *J Am Coll Cardiol* 1983; 2:707–718.
48. Gardin JM, Kozlowski J, Dabestani A, Murphy M, Kusnick C, Allfie A, et al: Studies of Doppler aortic blood flow velocity during supine bicycle exercise. *Am J Cardiol* 1986; 57:327–332.
49. Tristani FE, Hughes VC, Archibald DG, Sheldahl LM, Cohn JN: Safety of graded symptom-limited exercise testing in patients with congestive heart failure. *Circulation* 1987; 76:VI-54–VI-58.
50. Holloszy JO: Adaptations of muscular tissue to training. *Prog Cardiovasc Dis* 1976; 18:445–458.
51. Wasserman K, McIlroy MB: Detecting the threshold of anaerobic metabolism in cardiac patients during exercise. *Am J Cardiol* 1964; 14:844–852.
52. Francis GS: Development of arrhythmias in the patient with congestive heart failure: Pathophysiology, prevalence, and prognosis. *Am J Cardiol* 1986; 57:3B–7B.
53. Cohn JN, Rector TS: Prognosis of congestive heart failure and predictors of mortality. *Am J Cardiol* 1988; 62:25A–30A.
54. Gradman A, Deedwania P, Cody R, Massie B, Packer M, Pitt B, et al, for the Captopril-Digoxin Study Group: Predictors of total mortality and sudden death in mild to moderate heart failure. *J Am Coll Cardiol* 1989; 14:564–570.
55. Goldman S, Johnson G, Cohn JN, Cintron G, Smith R, Francis G, for the V-HeFT VA Cooperative Studies Group: Mechanism of death in heart failure: The Vasodilator-Heart Failure Trials. *Circulation* 1993; 87(suppl VI):VI-24–VI-31.
56. Cohn JN, Archibald DG, Francis GS, Ziesche S, Franciosa JA, Harston WE, et al: Veterans Administration Cooperative Study on vasodilator therapy of heart failure: Influence of prerandomization variables on the reduction of mortality by treatment with hydralazine and isosorbide dinitrate. *Circulation* 1987; 75(suppl IV): IV-49–IV-54.
57. Cohn JN, Johnson GR, Shabetai R, Loeb H, Tristani F, Rector T, et al: Ejection fraction, peak exercise oxygen consumption, cardiothoracic ratio, ventricular arrhythmias and plasma norepinephrine as determinants of prognosis in heart failure. *Circulation* 1993; 87(suppl VI):VI-5–VI-16.
58. Cohn JN, Levine TB, Olivari MT, Garberg V, Lura D, Francis GS, et al: Plasma norepinephrine as a guide to prognosis in patients with chronic congestive heart failure. *N Engl J Med* 1984; 311:819–823.
59. Gottlieb SB, Kukin ML, Ahern D, Packer M: Prognostic importance of atrial natriuretic peptide in patients with chronic heart failure. *J Am Coll Cardiol* 1989; 13:1534–1539.
60. Beta-Blocker Heart Attack Trial Research Group: A randomized trial of propranolol in patients with acute myocardial infarction. I. Mortality results. *JAMA* 1982; 247:1707–1714.
61. Guiha NH, Cohn JN, Mikulic E, Franciosa JA, Limas CJ: Treatment of refractory heart failure with infusion of nitroprusside. *N Engl J Med* 1974; 291:587–592.
62. Franciosa JA, Mikulic E, Cohn JN, Jose E, Fabie A: Hemodynamic effects of orally administered isosorbide dinitrate in patients with congestive heart failure. *Circulation* 1974; 50:1020–1024.
63. Franciosa JA, Pierpont G, Cohn JN: Hemodynamic improvement after oral hydralazine in left ventricular failure: A comparison with nitroprusside infusion in 16 patients. *Ann Intern Med* 1977; 86:388–393.
64. Pierpont GL, Cohn JN, Franciosa JA: Combined oral hydralazine-nitrate therapy in left ventricular failure. Hemodynamic equivalency to sodium nitroprusside. *Chest* 1978; 73:8–13.
65. Cohn JN, Archibald DG, Ziesche S, Franciosa JA, Harston WE, Tristani FE, et al: Effect of vasodilator therapy on mortality in chronic congestive heart failure. Results of a Veterans Administration Cooperative Study (V-HeFT). *N Engl J Med* 1986; 314:1547–1552.
66. The SOLVD Investigators: Effect of enalapril on survival in patients with reduced left ventricular ejection fractions and congestive heart failure. *N Engl J Med* 1991; 325:293–302.
67. Cohn JN, Johnson G, Ziesche S, Cobb F, Francis G, Tristani F, et al: A comparison of enalapril with hydralazine-isosorbide dinitrate in the treatment of chronic congestive heart failure. *N Engl J Med* 1991; 325:303–310.
68. The SOLVD Investigators: Effect of enalapril on mortality and the development of heart failure in asymptomatic patients with reduced left ventricular ejection fractions. *N Engl J Med* 1992; 327:685–691.
69. Pfeffer MA, Braunwald E, Moyé LA, Basta L, Brown EJ, Cuddy TE, et al. The effect of captopril on mortality and morbidity in patients with left ventricular dysfunction following myocardial infarction: Results of the survival and ventricular enlargement (SAVE) trial. *N Engl J Med* 1992; 327:669–677.
70. Levine TB, Franciosa JA, Vrobel T, Cohn JN: Hyponatraemia as a marker for high renin heart failure. *Br Heart J* 1982; 47:161–166.
71. Franciosa JA, Jordan RA, Wilen MM, Reddy CL: Minoxidil in patients with chronic left heart failure: Contrasting hemodynamic and clinical effects in a controlled trial. *Circulation* 1984; 70:63–68.
72. Captopril Digoxin Multicenter Research Group: Comparative effects of therapy with captopril and digoxin in patients with mild to moderate heart failure. *JAMA* 1988; 259:539–544.

72a. Packer M, Gheorghiade M, Young JB, Costantini PJ, Adams KF, Cody RJ, et al: Withdrawal of digoxin from patients with chronic heart failure treated with angiotensin-converting-enzyme inhibitors. *N Engl J Med* 1993; 329:1–7.
73. Ferguson DW, Berg WJ, Sanders JS, Roach PJ, Kempf JS, Kienzle MG: Sympathoinhibitory responses to digitalis glycosides in heart failure patients: Direct evidence from sympathetic neural recordings. *Circulation* 1989; 80:65–77.
74. Packer M, Francis GS, Abrams J, Cobb FR, Eichhorn EJ, Giles TD, et al: Oral milrinone increases the risk of sudden death in severe chronic heart failure: The PROMISE Trial. *Circulation* 1991; 84:II-310.
75. The German and Austrian Xamoterol Study Group: Double-blind placebo-controlled comparison of digoxin and xamoterol in chronic heart failure. *Lancet* 1988; 1:489–493.
76. Feldman AM, Bristow MR, Parmley WW, Carson PE, Pepine CJ, Gilbert E, et al: Effects of vesnarinone on morbidity and mortality in patients with heart failure. *N Engl J Med* 1993; 329:149–155.
77. Akhtar N, Mikulic E, Cohn JN, Chaudhry MH: Hemodynamic effect of dobutamine in patients with severe heart failure. *Am J Cardiol* 1975; 36:202–205.
78. Mikulic E, Cohn JN, Franciosa JA: Comparative hemodynamic effects of inotropic and vasodilator drugs in severe heart failure. *Circulation* 1977; 56:528–533.
79. Gage J, Rutman H, Lucido D, LeJemtel TH: Additive effects of dobutamine and amrinone on myocardial contractility and ventricular performance in patients with severe heart failure. *Circulation* 1986; 74:367–373.
80. Bristow M, Ginsburg R, Minobe W, Cubicciotti RS, Sageman WS, Lurie K, et al: Decreased catecholamine sensitivity and beta adrenergic receptor density in failing human hearts. *N Engl J Med* 1982; 307:205–211.
81. Stecy P, Gunnar RM: Is intermittent dobutamine infusion useful in the treatment of patients with refractory congestive heart failure? In: Cheilin M (ed): *Cardiology Clinics, Dilemmas in Clinical Cardiology*. Philadelphia, Davis, 1990:277–289.
82. Francis GS, Cohn JN, Johnson G, Rector TS, Goldman S, Simon A, for the V-HeFT VA Cooperative Studies Group: Plasma norepinephrine, plasma renin activity, and congestive heart failure: Relations to survival and the effects of therapy in V-HeFT II. *Circulation* 1993; 87(suppl VI):VI-40–VI-48.
83. Waagstein F, Hjalmarson A, Varnauskas E, Wallentin I: Effect of chronic beta-adrenergic receptor blockade in congestive cardiomyopathy. *Br Heart* J 1975; 137:1022–1036.
84. Swedberg K, Hjalmarson A, Waagstein F, Wallentin I: Beneficial effects of long term beta-blockade in congestive cardiomyopathy. *Br Heart J* 1980; 44:117–133.
85. Waagstein F, Caidahl K, Wallentin I, Bergh CH, Hjalmarson A: Long-term β-blockade in dilated cardiomyopathy: Effects of short- and long-term metoprolol treatment followed by withdrawal and readministration of metoprolol. *Circulation* 1989; 80:551–563.
86. Franciosa JA, Wilen M, Ziesche S, Cohn JN: Survival in men with severe chronic left ventricular failure due to either coronary heart disease or idiopathic dilated cardiomyopathy. *Am J Cardiol* 1983; 51:831–836.
87. The Cardiac Arrhythmia Suppression Trial (CAST) Investigators: Preliminary report: Effect of encainide and flecainide on mortality in a randomized trial of arrhythmia suppression after myocardial infarction. *N Engl J Med* 1989; 321:406–412.
88. Cleland JGF, Cargie HJ, Findlay IN, et al: Clinical, hemodynamic and antiarrhythmic effects of long-term treatment with amidarone of patients in heart failure. *Br Heart J* 1987; 57:436.
89. Dunkman WB, Johnson GR, Carson PE, Bhat G, Farrell L, Cohn JN: Incidence of thromboembolic events in congestive heart failure. *Circulation* 1993; 87(suppl VI):VI-94–VI-101.
90. Cohn JN, Benedict CR, LeJemtel TH, Grover J, Shindler DM, Shelton B, et al: Risk of thromboembolism in left ventricular dysfunction: SOLVD (abstr). *Circulation* 1992; 86(suppl I): I-252.
91. Lee FA, Cabin CK: The syndrome of flash pulmonary edema: Clinical definition and angiographic findings (abstr). *J Am Coll Cardiol* 1988; 11(suppl A):151A.
92. Schlant RC: "Flash" pulmonary edema. *ACC Current Journal Review* 1992; 1:74–75.
93. Bounous EP, Mark DB, Pollock BG, Hlatky MA, Harrell FE Jr, Lee KL, et al: Surgical survival benefits for coronary disease patients with left ventricular dysfunction. *Circulation* 1988; 78 (suppl I)I-151–I-157.
94. Vigilante GJ, Weintraub WS, Klein LW, Schneider RM, Seelaus PA, Parr GVS: Improved survival with coronary by-pass surgery in patients with three-vessel coronary disease and abnormal left ventricular function. Matched case-control study in patients with potentially operable disease. *Am J Med* 1987; 82:697–702.
95. Kron IL, Flanagan TL, Blackbourne LH, Schroeder RA, Nolan SP: Coronary revascularization rather than cardiac transplantation for chronic ischemic cardiomyopathy. *Am Surg* 1989; 210:348–352.
96. Barrett-Boyes BG, White HD, Agnew TM, Pemberton JR, Wild CJ: The results of surgical treatment of left ventricular aneurysms: An assessment of risk factors affecting early and late mortality. *J Thorac Cardiovasc Surg* 1984; 87:87–98.

SECTION B

Drugs and Procedures Used to Treat Patients with Heart Failure

Chapter 27

Digitalis

Frank I. Marcus, M.D.

The publication of William Withering's book entitled *An Account of the Foxglove and Some of Its Medical Uses*[1] in 1785 laid the foundation for the scientific use of digitalis, still one of the most commonly prescribed cardiovascular drugs.

Digitalis is a term used to designate the entire class of cardiac glycosides. The cardiac glycosides are one of the most important and widely used groups of drugs in clinical medicine. Cardiac glycosides of medicinal importance are obtained from the plants *Digitalis pururea* (digitoxin, gitalin) and *D. lanata* [digoxin, lanatoside-C (Cedilanid), deslanoside (Cedilanid-D), acetyldigitoxin (Acylanid), and digitoxin].

CHEMISTRY

Cardiac glycosides have a characteristic ring structure known as an aglycone or genin coupled with one to four sugar molecules (Fig. 27-1). The aglycone portion of the glycoside consists of a steroid nucleus and a five- or six-membered α,β-unsaturated lactone ring at the C_{17} position of the steroid nucleus. A beta-oriented hydroxyl substitution is usually present at the C_3 and C_{14} positions. The sugar portion of the glycoside is attached to the steroid nucleus, usually through a hydroxyl group at the C_3 position. The most commonly used cardiac glycoside, digoxin, differs from digitoxin only by the presence of a C_{12} hydroxyl group.

STRUCTURE-ACTIVITY RELATIONS

Molecular requirements for potent cardiac effects include the unsaturated lactone ring, the C_{14} hydroxyl group, and the spatial (*cis*) configuration of the C-D ring structures containing carbons 8 through 17 (Fig. 27-1).[2] The particular *cis* configuration differentiates this steroid ring structure from those of endogenous steroids from mammalian species. Saturation of the lactone ring yields the dihydro derivative, a much less potent glycoside. Increasing the number of hydroxyl groups on the aglycone increases polarity and decreases lipid solubility and absorption. The number of sugars influences the pharmacokinetics more than it alters the potency. The lower the number of sugars attached to the genin of digitoxin (and presumably digoxin), the greater is the metabolism to water soluble metabolites and the shorter the half-life.[3–5] In general, the more lipid soluble cardiac glycosides, such as digitoxin, are metabolized prior to excretion while the more polar cardiac glycosides, such as digoxin, deslanoside, and lantoside-C, are excreted primarily by the renal route, mostly in unchanged form.

PHARMACOKINETICS

The pharmacokinetics of the two most widely used cardiac glycosides, digitoxin and digoxin, are summarized in Table 27-1.[6–16] In comparison with digitoxin, digoxin is less bound to plasma proteins, has a nearly 10-fold larger volume of distribution, and has a half-life four times as rapid as digitoxin.

Cardiac glycosides are widely distributed in body tissues. The highest concentrations are found in the kidney, followed by cardiac muscle.[17] The concentration of digoxin in skeletal muscle is less than in cardiac muscle, but since skeletal muscle represents approximately 40 percent of the total body weight, digoxin is distributed

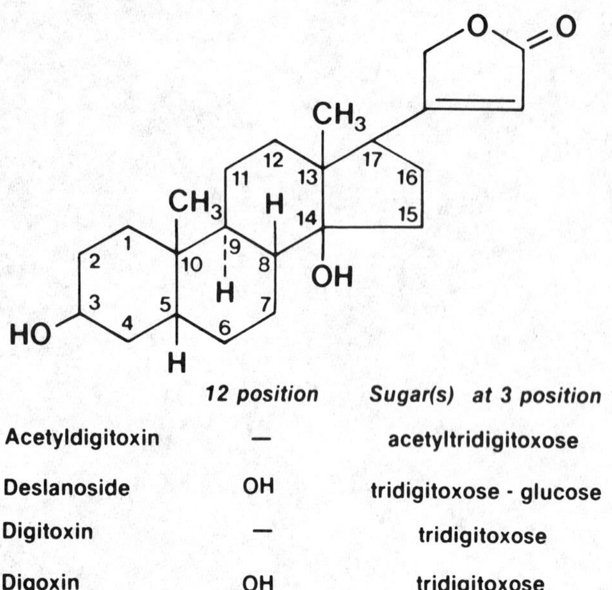

FIGURE 27-1 Comparative structures of cardiac glycosides. The aglycone is pictured. Digitoxose sugar has the molecular structure $C_6H_{10}O_3$.

principally to this tissue. About 60 percent of digoxin is excreted in the urine.[18] Until recently it was thought that digoxin was excreted primarily in unchanged form, but a variety of metabolites have now been identified, particularly the dihydro derivatives of digoxin.[19,20] Only about 15 percent of digitoxin is excreted unchanged in the urine, although an equal amount is excreted unchanged in the feces.

SPECIAL CONSIDERATIONS OF DIGOXIN PHARMACOKINETICS

An understanding of the potential variabilities in digoxin pharmacokinetics is important because these alterations may mandate a change in digoxin dosage.

Digoxin Bioavailability

Digoxin is unstable in acidic solutions. Significant hydrolysis of digoxin occurs if the intragastric pH is below 2, particularly if there is delayed gastric emptying time.[21] This observation may not be clinically important since the hydrolytic products recovered in the urine of patients with gastric hyperacidity are similar in patients without known gastric or duodenal ulcers.[22] Digoxin may be extensively metabolized in the gut to dihydro derivatives, as has been found in approximately 1 of every 10 subjects studied.[23] This biotransformation may account for resistance to therapy and unusually high digoxin requirements.[20] These patients are also susceptible to drug toxicity since abrupt changes in gut flora, such as occur with antibiotic treatment, may markedly enhance digoxin absorption.[24] The use of a highly bioavailable preparation such as an encapsulated liquid concentrate of digoxin minimizes this metabolic inactivation.[25] Patients with malabsorption syndromes due to short bowel syndrome or jejunoileal bypass do not have a significant decrease in absorption of digoxin from tablets.[26,27]

Infants and Children

Infants have been found to absorb digoxin in solution similarly to adults.[28] Binding of digoxin to several tissues, however, appears to be more extensive in infants than in adults, as exemplified by a larger volume of distribution. Thus, infants over 2 months of age and children may require larger doses (10 μg/kg per day) than adults (3 to 4 μg/kg per day) to achieve similar serum concentrations of digoxin. In infants (except neonates) the elimination half-life of digoxin is shorter than in adults. Infants and children also appear to tolerate higher serum concentrations of digoxin without development of tachyarrhythmias, although they may develop atrioventricular (AV) dissociation or heart block at these higher serum concentrations. The need for higher levels, however, has not been established on a pharmacodynamic basis.[29] Traditionally, digoxin is administered every 12 h to infants and children. A recent study indicated that the mean serum digoxin concentration was not different when the drug was given once daily, despite differences in trough and peak levels.[30] These changes were not associated with increased symptoms or signs associated with cardiac failure or digoxin toxic effects.

Elderly Patients

The alterations of digoxin pharmacokinetics in the elderly are in the reverse direction from those in the in-

TABLE 27-1
Pharmacokinetics of Digoxin and Digitoxin in Humans with Normal Renal Function*

Glycoside	Absolute Bioavailability (%)	Plasma Protein Binding (%)	Volume of Distribution (liters/kg)	Biological Half-Life (days)
Digoxin				
Tablet	60 (50–80)	25 (20–30)	5 (4–8)	1.7 (1.1–1.9)
Elixir	70 (60–80)	25 (20–30)	5 (4–8)	1.7 (1.1–1.9)
Capsules†	85 (80–100)	25 (20–30)	5 (4–8)	1.7 (1.1–1.9)
Digitoxin	90 (80–100)	93 (80–97)	0.46 (0.4–0.65)	7.0 (5–10)

* Data from normal subjects and patients. Numbers in parentheses are ranges.
† Lanoxicaps, Burroughs Wellcome Co.

fant.[31–33] There is a decrease in the apparent volume of distribution, principally due to a decrease in skeletal mass, and a decrease in the renal clearance of digoxin due to aging. These account for the well-known observation that the loading and maintenance doses of digoxin need to be decreased in the elderly. The prolongation of the half-life of digoxin in the elderly to approximately 73 h from a mean of 51 h in young subjects most likely reflects the age-related reduction in the renal filtration and secretion of digoxin.[31]

Obesity

The kinetics of digoxin is little altered in the obese individual since the concentration of digoxin in fatty tissue is quite low.[34,35] Thus, the dosage of digoxin should be calculated on the basis of lean body mass rather than on total body weight.

Renal Failure

Impaired kidney function is the most important condition that influences digoxin pharmacokinetics. Since digoxin is excreted primarily by the kidneys,[36] patients with renal failure have a decrease in digoxin clearance, with consequent increase in half-life, and thus require a smaller dose.[37–39] The increased fecal elimination of digoxin observed in anephric and other patients with renal failure does not compensate for its diminished renal excretion.[38] Digoxin metabolites accumulate in dialysis patients. Gault[40] found that an average of 22 percent of the immunoreactivity in a serum digoxin assay was due to metabolites in dialysis patients compared with 8 percent in other patients ($p < .001$). The metabolites are probably cardioinactive. Thus, cardioactivity tends to be lower than is suggested by the immunoassay results. There is a 35 to 50 percent decrease in the apparent volume distribution of digoxin in subjects with severe renal insufficiency.[41] The reason is not clear since the binding of digoxin to skeletal muscle is not decreased.[42] Possible explanations include reduction of tissue mass or reduced digoxin binding to organs other than skeletal muscle.[43] Whatever the explanation, a smaller than usual loading dose should be given to patients with severe renal insufficiency because of the decrease in volume of distribution.[41,44]

Hepatic Failure

The pharmacokinetics of digoxin are not significantly altered in patients with acute hepatitis[45] or in patients with chronic liver disease due to alcoholic cirrhosis.[46]

Pregnancy

It is not clear whether or not serum levels of digoxin are altered during pregnancy. Rogers et al.[47] found that levels in five pregnant patients were lower at delivery than 1 month later. On the other hand, Luxford and Kellaway[48] observed a significantly higher digoxin level in the third trimester compared to the postpartum period in 16 women who were maintained on the same dose of digoxin during this interval. This latter observation is puzzling since they found an increase in creatinine clearance and in the renal clearance and the 24-h excretion of digoxin during pregnancy relative to the postpartum period.[48] An increased absorption of digoxin during pregnancy was postulated.

Paired cord and maternal blood samples obtained at parturition show lower digoxin levels in cord blood.[49] This is of interest because of the occasional need to treat fetal supraventricular tachycardia with digoxin. Thus, higher maternal serum digoxin concentrations may be needed to obtain a therapeutic effect in the fetus. Daily maintenance doses of digoxin of 0.125 to 0.5 mg given to the mother, however, have treated successfully fetal supraventricular tachycardia.[50]

Although the concentration of digoxin in breast milk is approximately equal to the unbound plasma digoxin concentration, the quantity of digoxin ingested daily by infants is estimated to be between $\frac{1}{100}$ and $\frac{1}{20}$ of the recommended maintenance dose.[51] Therefore, breast feeding may safely be permitted in lactating mothers receiving digoxin therapy.

Hypothyroidism and Hyperthyroidism

After intravenous digoxin, serum levels are lower in hyperthyroid and higher in hypothyroid patients as compared to euthyroid patients for unexplained reasons.[52] There was no statistical difference in the excretion of a single dose of tritiated digoxin among hypothyroid or euthyroid patients. In studies in dogs with altered thyroid function there was no difference in the tissue concentration when the serum level differences were greatest. In addition, no differences were found in absorption or excretion after oral administration. Extensive subsequent studies by others of the pharmacokinetics of digoxin in altered thyroid states have not provided mechanistic insights into the original observations.[53–55] Since it is not clear whether end-organ sensitivity to digoxin is altered in hyper- or hypothyroidism, it seems reasonable to maintain serum digoxin concentration within the normal therapeutic range.

PHARMACOLOGIC EFFECTS

Withering[1] emphasized the diuretic action of digitalis, since this desirable effect was readily measurable. It was established only relatively recently that the primary therapeutic effect of digitalis in heart failure is due to its positive inotropic actions.[56] Over the past 50 years hundreds of investigators have attempted to clarify the mechanisms of action of digitalis, especially more recently at the subcellular level.[57–59] We now have a clear understanding of the effects of digitalis in humans. Digitalis acts by several mechanisms including an inotropic effect in both the normal and abnormal myocardium, an enhancement of the vagal and a diminution of the sympathetic effects on the heart, and finally, direct arterial vasoconstriction.

Inotropic Effect

Digitalis enhances contractility by increasing the availability of activated calcium to the contractile proteins in heart cells during excitation-contraction coupling by binding to and inhibiting Na^+,K^+-activated membrane ATPase.[60] The inhibition of Na^+,K^+-ATPase increases intracellular Na^+, which is exchanged for extracellular calcium. The net result of the increase in intracellular calcium is enhanced myocardial contractility. (See also Chaps. 5 and 28.)

Parasympathetic Activity

Digitalis increases the sensitivity of the arterial baroreceptor reflex so that afferent signals are augmented, resulting in an increase of vagal and a decrease in sympathetic efferent activity.[61] Digitalis also acts in the central vagal nuclei and nodose ganglia to enhance efferent signals.[62] Digitalis alters the electrical excitability of the efferent vagal fibers and impulse transmission in autonomic ganglia.[63] Finally, there is evidence that digitalis may increase the sensitivity of cardiac fibers to the actions of acetylcholine.[64] These parasympathomimetic effects are primarily responsible for the therapeutic efficacy of digitalis in the treatment of supraventricular arrhythmias.[65] In selected patients, the frequency of symptomatic angina and total duration of ischemia during 24 h may be decreased by the effect of digitalis in restoring cardiopulmonary reflexes.[66] There is evidence that ischemic ventricular myocardium can generate a powerful depressive reflex that may contribute to the resolution of myocardial ischemia by reducing myocardial oxygen consumption and coronary vascular tone. By restoring this reflex responsiveness in patients, particularly those with prior inferior myocardial infarction, ischemic episodes can be shortened. This provides a rationale for the benefit of digitalis as an antianginal drug in these patients.

Sympathetic Activity

Digitalis, through sensitization of baroreceptor reflexes, causes some decrease in efferent sympathetic activity, contributing to the decrease in sinus rate and prolongation of the AV nodal refractory period.[67] Digitalis-induced sympathetic inhibition may play a more important role in congestive heart failure than has been previously recognized. Thus, the increase in cardiac output and concomitant decrease in systemic vascular resistance following intravenous digoxin administration to patients with dilated cardiomyopathy is related to sympathetic withdrawal with preservation of parasympathetic tone, as indicated by spectral analysis of heart rate variability.[68] In addition, direct recordings of sympathetic nerve activity after digoxin administration show a marked and rapid attenuation of activity in patients with heart failure that precede the hemodynamic effects.[69] Evidence that the sympathetic effect is specific for digitalis and is not solely related to the increased contractility was suggested by the finding that administration of dobutamine with similar inotropic effects does not attenuate sympathetic nerve activity to muscle.

Direct Vasoconstrictor Effects

Digoxin induces contractions in isolated human arteries and veins that are not diminished by adrenoceptor blockade but are abolished by a calcium antagonist.[70] A neurogenic vasoconstrictor effect of digitalis on coronary vascular resistance has also been reported.[71] The vasoconstrictor effect of digitalis can result in an increase in systemic as well as pulmonary resistance,[72] which can worsen failure, particularly when given as a bolus.[73,74] In patients with ischemic heart disease without heart failure, there is a small, variable increase in systemic vascular resistance in response to intravenous digoxin.[75] The increase in the vasoconstrictor effect, which is rapid in onset, may precede the peak inotropic effect.[76]

Electrophysiological Effects

The influences of digitalis on the electrophysiological properties of the heart are complex. The effects vary with dose, type of cardiac tissue involved, and autonomic activity. There are direct effects on the transmembrane action potentials produced by the inhibition of Na^+,K^+-ATPase (sodium pump).[77] The most important properties relevant to the treatment of supraventricular arrhythmias are indirect and dependent upon vagal and antiadrenergic neural mechanisms. The electrophysiological effects of digitalis vary according to the animal species studied. These effects are summarized in Table 27-2.

Sinoatrial Node

In mammalian species, administration of therapeutic doses of digitalis causes little chronotopic effect on the sinoatrial (SA) node.[62,78–81] Administration of digoxin, 0.8 mg intravenously, to normal subjects causes only a slight decrease in the basal heart rate from 75 to 68 beats per minute.[82]Administration of digitalis to patients with ventricular failure often results in slowing of the sinus rate, which is largely explained by the fact that digitalis improves ventricular performance and results in a decrease in sympathetic tone. Digitalis can be administered to most patients with sinus bradycardia or asymptomatic sinus pauses without further decreasing sinus rate or accentuating the posttachycardia pauses.[83–85] The patient with "sick-sinus" syndrome, however, may have a lengthening of sinus node recovery time and SA conduction time[82,86] and an accentuation of symptoms due to secondary pauses after digitalis administration. If digitalis therapy is indicated for heart failure in patients symptomatic with sick-sinus syndrome, an electrophysiological study is usually indicated. The finding of a corrected sinus node recovery time of over 1000 ms has been found to be predictive of further lengthening of pauses in some, but not all, patients.[87] Twenty-four ambulatory electrocardiogram (ECG) recordings also should be done before and after digitalis administration in patients with sick-sinus syndrome.

Atrium

The electrophysiological effects of digitalis on atrial tissue are highly variable and are influenced by an interplay between drug concentration and the level of autonomic tone. In most intact animal studies, therapeutic concentrations of digitalis appear to have a predominant vagal

TABLE 27-2

Electrophysiological Effect of Digitalis on Cardiac Tissue

	Automaticity	Excitability	Conduction Velocity	Effective Refractory Period	Delayed After Depolarization
Sinoatrial node					
Therapeutic	↔ (or ↓)	–	↓*	–	–
Toxic	↔ or ↑ (↑)	–	↓↓*	–	–
Atrial muscle					
Therapeutic	↔	↔	↔ (↑)	↔ (↓†)	–
Toxic	↑	↓	↔ or ↓ (↓)	↑	+
Atrioventricular node					
Therapeutic	↔	–	↓	↑	–
Toxic	↑	–	↓↓	↑↑	–
Purkinje fibers					
Therapeutic	↔	↑	↔ or ↓	↔ or ↑ (↑)	–
Toxic	↑	↓	↓	↓	+
Ventricular muscle					
Therapeutic	↔	Variable	↔ or ↓	↓	–
Toxic	↑	↓	↓	↓	+
Accessory pathway					
Therapeutic	–	–	↑	↔ or ↓	–
Toxic	–	–	↑	↓	–

NOTE: Phrase or symbol inside parentheses indicates observations made only in animal studies. + = present; – = absent or not applicable; ↑ = increase; ↓ = decrease; ↔ = no effect; ↑↑ = markedly increased; ↓↓ = markedly decreased.
* Sinoatrial conduction.
† Increase after atropine.

action that results in shortening of the atrial effective refractory period and acceleration of conduction.[77,88,89] After denervation or atropine, digitalis increases atrial effective refractory period and slows conduction.[88,89] Therapeutic doses of cardiac glycosides have been shown to have no change[90,91] or to cause an increase in atrial refractory periods in humans.[82,92] Atrial conduction velocity, as measured by the P-A interval, has also been found to be increased[80] or show no change[93] following digitalis administration. These conflicting findings have been partially clarified by studies in which a time-dependent, biphasic electrophysiological response to methyldigoxin was found in the human right atrium.[94] There was initial prolongation of the action potential, which was maximal at 20 min after infusion and was associated with an increase in atrial effective refractoriness and vulnerability to atrial tachyarrhythmia induction. During the later phase (30 to 40 min) of infusion, atrial action potential shortened with a decrease in effective refractoriness and vulnerability to tachyarrhythmias. Atropine reduced the magnitude of both early and late components of the biphasic action potential response to digitalis. These observations of a time-dependent effect on atrial tachycardia induction are important when electrophysiological testing is performed for the evaluation of digitalis effect on supraventricular tachyarrhythmias.

Atrioventricular Node

Digitalis causes a prolongation of conduction and refractory periods of the AV node.[92] These effects are predominantly due to the vagal and antiadrenergic influence of digitalis.[67,79] Ouabain increases the effective refractory periods of both the fast and slow AV nodal pathways in the anterograde direction,[90] whereas the effects of digitalis on retrograde conduction in the AV node and the refractory period of AV conduction are variable.[81]

Purkinje Fibers and Ventricular Muscle

In therapeutic concentrations, there are few neural (indirect) effects of digitalis on Purkinje fibers and ventricular muscle.[95,96] Digitalis shortens the effective refractory period in the ventricle.[91]

Accessory Pathway

In human studies, there is a variable effect of digitalis on the anterograde effective refractory period of the accessory path in Wolff-Parkinson-White syndrome.[97,98] Jedeikin et al.[99] found that digitalis shortened this interval by more than 40 ms in nearly 40 percent of children. The retrograde effective refractory period of the accessory pathway is generally not affected by digitalis.[98,100]

USE OF DIGITALIS

Digitalis has two major uses. One is for the treatment of congestive heart failure and the other is for the treatment as well as the prevention of supraventricular arrhythmias. At present, the trend is not to rely completely on digitalis for the treatment of acute congestive heart failure since there are more potent inotropic drugs available for parenteral use. For the treatment of acute or chronic heart failure, diuretics may be administered intravenously or orally and can effectively relieve symptoms and signs of heart failure. Moreover, vasodilating drugs such as the angiotensin enzyme converting (ACE) inhibitors, or hydralazine and nitrates, are effective in relieving symptoms of congestive heart failure as well as increasing exercise tolerance. Digitalis, however, has many advantages as a drug for the treatment of chronic congestive heart failure. It is an inotropic drug that can be given orally once a day, has excellent short- and long-term tolerance, does not exhibit tachyphylaxis, and is inexpensive. It remains to be determined whether treatment for chronic congestive heart failure should be initiated with digitalis, diuretics, or vasodilators alone or in combination. In the United States the most common practice is to start therapy for congestive heart failure with digitalis in combination with diuretics. Angiotensin enzyme converting inhibitors are usually prescribed since they have been shown to reduce mortality rates when added to therapy with digoxin and diuretics in patients with severe congestive heart failure.[101] (See also Chap. 26.)

For the acute treatment of paroxysmal supraventricular tachycardia digitalis has been replaced to a large extent by adenosine, the calcium channel blocking drugs, verapamil and diltiazem, and beta blocking drugs. Digitalis is still the drug of choice for treatment of this condition in the patient who is also receiving beta blocking drugs or who has known sick-sinus syndrome, since the calcium channel blocking drugs may result in asystole or marked bradycardia after conversion. Digitalis has an advantage in treating paroxysmal supraventricular tachycardia in the presence of congestive heart failure since calcium channel blocking drugs such as verapamil as well as the beta blocking drugs decrease cardiac contractility.

Left Ventricular Failure in Patients with Acute Myocardial Infarction

Digitalis has minimal and unpredictable effects in patients with heart failure due to acute myocardial infarction,[102] and other drugs are preferable. When ouabain was compared with furosemide in patients with myocardial infarction who had an increase in pulmonary arterial pressure, furosemide caused a greater decrease in PA diastolic pressures than ouabain. Cardiac output was not markedly decreased with furosemide.[103] A comparison of dobutamine and digoxin in patients with acute myocardial infarction and cardiac failure showed that dobutamine markedly increased cardiac output, decreased filling pressure, and relieved pulmonary congestion, whereas digoxin did not affect either preload or afterload.[104] Thus, an intravenous inotropic drug alone or with a diuretic is the usual preferred treatment for patients with acute myocardial infarction who have congestive heart failure. An alternate therapy is the combination of digoxin and an afterload reducing agent such as nitroprusside. When nitroprusside is used alone in patients with congestive heart failure complicating acute myocardial infarction, there is a decrease in the wedge pressure as well as an increase in cardiac output. The addition of digoxin further increases cardiac output and decreases systemic vascular resistance.[105] (See also Chap. 60.)

Right-Sided Heart Failure Due to Cor Pulmonale

Digitalis has not been shown to be beneficial in patients with isolated cor pulmonale,[106,107] but patients with cor pulmonale who also have left-sided heart failure may be benefited by digitalis. Determination of radionuclide left and right ventricular ejection fraction may be helpful in clarifying the presence or absence of left-sided heart failure. Not only is digitalis not beneficial in patients with right-sided heart failure due to cor pulmonale but it may be especially hazardous, since such patients may have increased sensitivity to digitalis intoxication even in the absence of hypokalemia.[108] (See also Chaps. 99 and 101.)

Heart Failure Due to Left-to-Right Shunt in Infants and Children

There is a serious question as to whether or not the majority of infants and children with left-to-right shunt due to a ventricular septal defect or patent ductus arteriosus are benefited by digitalis.[29,109–111] There are also no controlled trials that document the efficacy of digitalis for infants with left-to-right shunts who may have normal left ventricular contractility and whose symptoms of heart failure may be due to circulatory overload.[112] In lambs with surgically created ventricular septal defect, digoxin slowed the heart rate and increased the stroke volume but did not alter systemic flow index or pulmonary flow index.[113]

Maintenance Digitalis and Chronic Heart Failure

Despite 200 years of digitalis use, the proper therapeutic role of digitalis in congestive heart failure with sinus rhythm is still controversial. It is firmly established that digoxin has a long-term inotropic effect in patients with normal sinus rhythm.[114] This effect is manifest by an increase in ejection fraction and cardiac output but no change in systemic vascular resistance.[115–117] It would be anticipated that these favorable changes would be accompanied by an increase in exercise duration in patients with congestive heart failure, and this has been documented in some[118,119] but not all studies.[120] There are two studies specifically designed to assess left ventricular performance during exercise in patients with congestive heart failure.[121,122] In one study, Sullivan et al.[121] showed an increase in ventilatory oxygen uptake with digoxin during submaximal and at maximal exercise, while the other study by Fleg et al.[122] showed an increase in ventricular performance (higher ejection fraction and systolic blood pressure at maximal effort) with digoxin. In patients with congestive heart failure, the combination of digitalis and vasodilators enhances cardiac performance in comparison with vasodilators alone.[123] A recent study involved 178 patients in New York Heart Association functional class II or III and normal sinus rhythm and impaired left ventricular systolic function (ejection fraction of 35 percent or less) on chronic therapy with digoxin, diuretics and ACE inhibitors.[124] In 93 patients switched to placebo in place of digoxin, worsening of failure with increased symptoms, decreased exercise tolerance and quality of life occurred in 23 patients, compared to only 4 of 85 patients who continued to receive digoxin. The clinical deterioration was often delayed by many weeks. Deterioration of function following withdrawal of digoxin has also been noted in other, smaller studies.[125–128] It can be concluded that a significant number of patients with chronic left-sided systolic heart failure deteriorate clinically and hemodynamically after digitalis withdrawal despite continuation of diuretic and ACE inhibitor therapy. As yet, it is unclear how to identify accurately patients in whom digitalis can be safely withdrawn. If the reason for initial digitalization was acute heart failure associated with myocardial infarction, pneumonia, or heart failure associated with surgery and signs of congestive heart failure have not recurred, it would seem reasonable to stop digitalis. One must be alert to the fact that an appreciable number of patients who have signs and symptoms of heart failure may have circulatory failure because of diastolic dysfunction, and digitalis is not likely to benefit these patients. These individuals may be identified by having a normal left ventricular ejection fraction in the presence of congestive heart failure. (See also Chaps. 25 and 26.)

Possible Enhanced Mortality in Patients on Chronic Digitalis Therapy after Myocardial Infarction

Until recently it has been assumed that the benefits of digitalis in chronic congestive heart failure outweigh its possible harmful effects. The controversy concerning the potential harmful effects of digitalis has been heightened by several reports that indicate that there may be an increase in mortality associated with digitalis treatment in the early months following an acute myocardial infarction.[129–131] The reported increase in mortality was present even after adjustment for major cardiac covariates such as left ventricular ejection fraction and ventricular ectopic beat frequency.[131] Other investigators have not been able to document an increase in mortality associated with digitalis either after myocardial infarction or in patients with chronic coronary artery disease.[132–135] The possible increased mortality associated with digitalis after infarction should cause the physician to evaluate carefully the need for digitalis therapy, particularly within the first year after myocardial infarction. One possible mechanism to explain enhanced mortality after myocardial infarction associated with therapeutic digoxin serum concentrations is an enhanced susceptibility to the development of ischemia-related lethal arrhythmias.[136]

TREATMENT OF ARRHYTHMIAS

Paroxysmal Supraventricular Tachycardia

Most paroxysmal supraventricular tachycardias (PSVTs) are due to reentry involving the AV node. By its modification of the critical relation between conduction time and refractory period of the slow and fast pathways in the AV node, digitalis can terminate paroxysmal AV nodal reentrant tachycardias.[90,137] Digitalis alone or in combination with beta blockers or calcium channel-blocking agents is useful in preventing PSVT. Prior to therapy with digitalis for PSVT, digitalis intoxication should be excluded as a cause of the arrhythmia, especially when it is associated with AV block. (See also Chap. 36.)

Atrial Fibrillation or Flutter

Digitalis is commonly used to treat atrial fibrillation or flutter with a rapid ventricular rate. Digitalis can decrease ventricular rate both at rest and during moderate exercise by increased concealed conduction into the AV node and prolonged refractoriness of the AV node.[138–140] Frequently there is an exaggerated ventricular rate response to moderate or maximal exertion despite therapeutic serum levels of digoxin.[141] Although it has been observed that serum digoxin levels decrease during exercise, the inadequate ventricular rate control with exertion is probably not due to displacement of digoxin from target organs. Addition of calcium channel- or beta-blocking agents may be useful when the ventricular rate is difficult to control by digitalis alone. The efficacy of digoxin has not been found to be different from placebo in conversion of recent-onset atrial fibrillation in patients without heart failure.[142] Nor is digoxin alone effective in preventing recurrence of atrial fibrillation in most patients with paroxysmal atrial fibrillation[143]: In fact, digoxin administration may result in longer duration of the episodes of atrial fibrillation. (See also Chap. 36.)

Multifocal Atrial Tachycardia

Digitalis is generally not effective in either abolishing this rhythm or slowing the ventricular response. In addition, since this arrhythmia is usually associated with severe obstructive pulmonary disease, a condition in which there is increased sensitivity to digitalis toxicity, the use of digitalis should be avoided in the treatment of multifocal atrial tachycardia unless there is concomitant congestive heart failure.[144] (See also Chap. 101.)

Ventricular Ectopy

The result of the use of digitalis in treatment of ventricular dysrhythmias is not impressive,[145] and it may cause confusion if there is suspicion of digitalis intoxication manifested by enhanced ventricular ectopy, ventricular tachycardia, and ventricular fibrillation. However, Lown et al.[146] reported that the frequency and grade of ventricular premature beats were reduced in 46 percent of patients receiving acetylstrophanthidin, unchanged in 26 percent, and increased in 28 percent. The antiarrhythmic action of acetylstrophanthidin does not appear to be related to its positive inotropic action.[147] Other observers[148,149] have found that digoxin was ineffective in suppressing complex ventricular ectopy and that the reduction in frequency of ectopy was found primarily in patients with normal ejection fractions. There is a general agreement that digitalis should not be withheld in patients with congestive heart failure and ventricular ectopy not due to digitalis intoxication. Interest in the use of digoxin to treat ventricular arrhythmias may be revived by a recent case report of the successful treatment of exercise-induced ventricular tachycardia. This arrhythmia had the characteristics of triggered activity and could reproducibly be terminated with adenosine.[150] (See also Chap. 36.)

Wolff-Parkinson-White Syndrome

Digitalis is being used infrequently in adult patients with Wolff-Parkinson-White syndrome who have narrow QRS paroxysmal circus movement tachycardia. In this type of tachycardia the anterograde conduction occurs by the AV node and the impulse returns to the atrium by way of the accessory pathway. Dhingra et al.[98] found that sustained tachycardia was still inducible in 89 percent of the 19 patients after the administration of intravenous ouabain. This suggests that digitalis alone may be of benefit only in a minority of patients who have this type of tachycardia. Combination therapy with type I drugs, such as procainamide or quinidine, or propranolol may be more effective in preventing recurrent tachycardia.[151] Digitalis may be hazardous in patients with the Wolff-Parkinson-White syndrome since it can increase the ventricular response via the accessory pathway and may result in ventricular fibrillation and sudden death.[152] Sellers et al.[99] found that treatment with digitalis was temporally related to the onset of ventricular fibrillation in 9 of 21 patients. Each of these patients had short RR intervals (220 ms or less) during atrial fibrillation in the control state. For this reason, it is suggested that digitalis not be used in patients with Wolff-Parkinson-White syndrome. If it must be used, an electrophysiological study should be performed before institution of long-term therapy. (See also Chap. 36.)

CHOICE OF DIGITALIS PREPARATION AND DOSING

Digoxin is the only cardiac glycoside in common use in the United States at this time. Ouabain is no longer available commercially. A loading dose of digoxin is usually not necessary unless there is urgency in achieving digitalis effect. In the absence of a loading dose, steady-state serum and tissue concentrations are achieved in 5 to 7 days. The usual oral maintenance dose is 0.25 mg. Generally, half that amount is prescribed for the elderly or for patients with severe renal insufficiency. In some patients, particularly those who have a large lean body mass, the dose may be 0.5 mg. The average oral loading dose of digoxin ranges from 1.25 to 1.5 mg given in divided doses over a 24-h period. The usual oral maintenance dose of digoxin in the encapsulated gel form of digoxin (Lanoxicaps), which has enhanced bioavailability, ranges between 0.1 to 0.4 mg/day. The oral loading dose for Lanoxicaps is 0.8 to 1.2 mg. Intravenous doses of digoxin are approximately 70 percent of the oral dose recommended for the tablet.

Digitilization with digitoxin is usually started with a loading dose since it would require approximately 1 month to achieve a steady state. The loading dose ranges from 0.8 to 1.2 mg in 24 h given in divided doses. The maintenance dose is usually 0.1 to 0.15 mg of digitoxin daily. The dose for the intravenous drug is the same as that for oral administration.

DRUG INTERACTIONS WITH DIGITALIS

The recognition that the serum levels of digoxin or digitoxin can be altered by coadministration of other medicines is of great importance.[153,154] There are two broad classifications of interactions that involve disposition of digoxin: (1) those due to drugs that alter the absorption of digoxin and (2) those due to drugs that primarily interfere with digoxin elimination. Interactions of the first type usually decrease digoxin serum concentration to a modest degree. The second type of interaction can cause a marked increase in serum concentration of digoxin and can result in digoxin toxicity. Interactions with digoxin are listed in Table 27-3.[155,177] (See also Chap. 109.) In many instances, the pharmacokinetic mechanisms of the interactions have been defined, but there is still uncertainty regarding the hemodynamics or electrophysiological effect of the alterations in digoxin serum levels as a result of drug interactions. Quantitation of the concentration of cardiac glycosides in the heart may not resolve the question because most of the cardiac glycoside in the heart muscle is nonspecifically bound to membrane lipids and other sites where it does not exert a pharmacologic effect. It is extremely difficult to relate the serum concentration of cardiac glycosides to receptor binding of the digitalis glycosides in heart muscle. Until further investigations clarify the clinical significance of serum levels as altered by concomitantly administered drugs, we should assume that digoxin serum concentrations reflect the intensity of the action of digoxin and strive to keep the serum levels within the accepted therapeutic range.

DIGITALIS TOXICITY

The incidence and mortality of digitalis intoxication appears to have decreased markedly over the past 20 years in hospitalized patients.[178] It is likely that a better knowledge of digoxin pharmacokinetics as well as an increase in the use of serum digoxin levels has contributed to the declining incidence of toxicity. The signs and symptoms of digitalis toxicity are well known. Among the more common manifestations are anorexia, nausea, fatigue, dizziness, and visual disturbances. Although these symptoms are not specific, their onset or exacerbation should raise the suspicion of digitalis toxicity. Risk factors for the development of digitalis toxicity are old age and elevated blood urea nitrogen and creatinine levels.[178] Patients can readily become confused when they are taking multiple drugs for treatment of congestive heart failure. Inadvertently they may take a daily dose of digitalis several times greater than has been prescribed. Other frequent causes of toxicity are drugs concomitantly prescribed that raise serum digoxin levels (Table 27-3) as well as diuretic-induced hypokalemia. Worsening heart failure may result in a decrease in renal function with

TABLE 27-3
Pharmacokinetic Interactions with Digoxin

Interfering Drugs	Mean Magnitude* of Interaction (%)	Mechanism of Interaction	Comments	Reference
Drugs That Alter Digoxin Absorption or Bioavailability				
Antacids; bran	−25	Unknown; ? absorption of digoxin	Give digoxin 1–2 h before antacid or bran	155, 156
Kaolin-pectin (Kaopectate)	−20–30	Absorption of digoxin	Give digoxin 1–2 h before kaolin-pectin	155
Cholestyramine (Questran)	−30	Physical binding to resin	Avoid by dosing cholestyramine bid, 8 h from digoxin administration	157
Metoclopramide (Reglan)	−25	↓ bioavailability by ↑ intestinal motility	(?) Administer digoxin as elixir or as Lanoxicaps	158, 159
Propantheline (Pro-Banthine)	−25	↑ bioavailability by ↓ intestinal motility	(?) Administer digoxin as elixir or as Lanoxicaps	157
Sulfasalazine (Azulfidine)	−20	↓ bioavailability		160
Erythromycin or tetracycline†	+43–150	↑ bioavailability due to inactivation of gut flora	Measure serum digoxin with coadministration of these antibiotics with digoxin	23, 24
Neomycin	−28	↓ bioavailability	Measure serum digoxin levels	161
Cancer chemotherapy	−50	↓ bioavailability due to damage to intestinal mucosa	Measure serum digoxin levels	162
Drugs That Interfere with Elimination of Digoxin				
Amiodarone (Cordarone)	+100	(?)↓ in renal and ↓ total body clearance of digoxin; inhibits uptake into hepatocies	↓ digoxin dose by $\frac{1}{2}$	163–167
Indomethacin‡	+50	↓ glomerular filtration	↓ dose of digoxin by $\frac{1}{4}$ to $\frac{1}{2}$	168
Propafenone (Rhythmol)	+20–80	↓ nonrenal clearance of digoxin	↓ dose of digoxin by $\frac{1}{4}$ to $\frac{1}{2}$	169
Quinidine	+100	(?) ↑ absorption ↓ volume of distribution ↓ renal and total body clearance of digoxin	↓ digoxin dose by $\frac{1}{2}$	170–173
Quinine	+75	↓ biliary clearance of digoxin	↓ digoxin dosage by $\frac{1}{2}$	174–175
Verapamil	+75	↓ renal and total body clearance of digoxin	↓ digoxin dose by $\frac{1}{2}$	160, 161

*Alteration in digoxin bioavailability or serum digoxin concentration. For single-dose studies, the magnitude of the anticipated change in serum digoxin concentration was estimated from pharmacokinetic data, particularly the change in total body clearance.
†Expected to occur in 10% of patients, those who have substantial conversion of digoxin to dihydro derivatives in the gut.
‡Interaction only in premature infants.

consequent decrease in renal and extrarenal excretion of digoxin with resultant digoxin accumulation. Under these circumstances the half-life of digoxin can approach that of digitoxin.

The therapeutic serum concentration of digoxin in adults is 1.0 to 2.0 ng/mL. Digoxin serum levels are frequently helpful in confirming the clinical suspicion of digitalis toxicity, especially if the serum digoxin level is greater than 3.0 ng/mL. A review of 43 reports showed that intoxicated patients had a mean serum digoxin concentration of 3.3 ng/mL.[179] If a serum digoxin level is less than 1.5 ng/mL in a patient who does not have hypokalemia and who is suspected of digoxin toxicity, the clinician must search for another explanation for the patient's symptoms since digitalis intoxication is unlikely. If the serum digoxin level is less than 1.0 ng/mL in a normokalemic patient, digitalis toxicity is sufficiently rare so as to exclude this diagnosis.

Electrocardiographic manifestations of digitalis toxicity are protean, are not diagnostic of this condition, and depend in part upon the age of the patient and the state of the myocardium. For example, accentuation of the vagal effects of digitalis are more commonly seen in young healthy individuals with digitalis overdose. In contrast, digitalis-intoxicated patients with advanced cardiac disease may develop ventricular ectopy at doses and blood levels below those required to produce AV conduction disturbances in patients without intrinsic cardiac disease.[180]

In a hospital population, accentuation of the vagal effects of digitalis is responsible for the majority of digitalis toxic arrhythmias. These include atrioventricular block, unexplained sinus bradycardia, junctional rhythm, and atrial fibrillation with a ventricular response below 50 per minute.[178]

The arrhythmogenic effects of digitalis are complex and have not been fully elucidated in humans. Possible mechanisms include delayed afterpotentials, enhanced diastolic depolarization, and reentry that appears to be due to intracellular calcium overload.[181–183] The magnitude of delayed afterpotentials and susceptibility to triggered activity may be enhanced in the presence of ischemia at cardiac glycoside concentrations that have no toxic effect in the absence of ischemia.[184]

Digitalis-induced arrhythmias may be best understood by considering those manifestations that are due predominantly to excessive parasympathomimetic effects on the heart and those that are related to enhanced ectopy. Manifestations of enhanced vagal effect include sinus bradycardia or SA exit block and AV nodal block often of the Wenckebach type. Examples of digitalis-induced ectopy include atrial premature beats, junctional tachycardia, and ventricular ectopic activity. Death may be due to digitalis-induced ventricular tachycardia and/or ventricular fibrillation. Ectopy may be combined with signs of excessive vagal effects to produce the ECG patterns of atrial tachycardia with AV block or junctional tachycardia with AV block. (See also Chap. 36.)

Therapy of digitalis toxicity will depend upon numerous factors including the time of the last dose ingested, the total amount of digitalis taken, the state of health of the patient, and the nature of the electrocardiographic manifestations of toxicity. For example, temporary discontinuation of digoxin is sufficient if the last dose of digoxin was taken longer than 6 h before examination, the dose was not massive, and the ECG manifestations are primarily vagal with an adequate ventricular response to maintain circulation. On the other hand, a temporary pacemaker must be inserted if there is inadequate circulation due to severe bradycardia or complete heart block. Correction of hypokalemia in addition to stopping the drug may be all that is needed to control digitalis-induced tachyarrhythmia, but potassium should be given very cautiously if there is AV block. Digitalis-induced atrial, junctional, or ventricular tachycardia should be treated by antiarrhythmia drugs. Lidocaine is effective, particularly in diminishing the severity and frequency of digitalis-induced ventricular ectopy. Procainamide may also be used. Diphenylhydantoin may be given intravenously in 100-mg doses every 5 min until the arrhythmia is abolished, until 1000 mg is administered, or until drowsiness, nystagmus, vertigo, or nausea occurs.[185] Diphenylhydantoin has been used successfully not only to suppress atrial and ventricular ectopy induced by digitalis but also to restore AV conduction. Quinidine should be avoided since it may displace digoxin from its binding sites to raise serum digoxin levels and will decrease both the renal and nonrenal excretion of digoxin. Beta-adrenergic blocking drugs should generally be avoided in treatment of digitalis toxicity. Anecdotal case reports indicate that amiodarone,[186] bretylium,[187] and intravenous magnesium[188,189] can suppress life-threatening ventricular arrhythmias due to digitalis intoxication. The fact that only vagal manifestations of toxicity are present in a patient who has ingested a massive amount of digitalis does not permit complacency, and preparations must be made to immediately rid the body of nonabsorbed digoxin as well as to administer digoxin antibodies to reverse anticipated lethal toxicity.

Therapy of massive overdose with digitalis has been revolutionized by the extraordinary success obtained with the administration of digoxin-specific sheep Fab fragments.[190] Recent reports of large-scale clinical studies[191,192] were preceded by a substantial body of experimental evidence accumulated over a decade showing that digitalis-specific antibodies are effective in reversing toxic effects of cardiac glycosides.[193] This approach is based on the ability to form a digoxin protein conjugate that, when injected into rabbits or sheep, induces highly specific antibodies. The affinity for digoxin is up to 50 times higher than that for digitoxin. The digoxin-specific antibodies bind and neutralize not only digoxin but also the major cardioactive metabolites of digoxin. The digoxin antibody globulin can be split into two Fab fragments and one Fc fragment by enzymatic digestion with papaine. The haptein-binding capacity of the Fab fragments is fully preserved, and the smaller molecular size of the Fab fragments may enable more rapid diffusion to cellular digoxin binding sites than complete antibody molecules. Following intravenous administration, specific Fab fragments bind to digoxin and rapidly accelerate the removal of digoxin from cellular membranes. This causes a marked increase in serum digoxin concentration; however, the digoxin is bound and therefore is pharmacologically inactive. Due to the smaller molecular weight, Fab fragments pass glomerular membranes and are excreted with a half-life of 16 to 20 h. Thus, the Fab fragments are capable of rapidly reversing digoxin-induced toxicity, and the glycoside is eliminated by the renal route, much of it in the protein bound form.[194] Administration of digoxin-specific Fab fragments is also effective in the treatment of toxicity due to digitoxin[195] as well as oleander.[196]

The safety and efficacy of the digoxin-specific Fab antibody fragments were demonstrated by the 150 cases reported by Antman and colleagues.[191] Of the 148 patients in whom a clinical response could be evaluated, 80 percent showed resolution of all signs and symptoms of digitalis toxicity and 10 percent improved. There were 15 patients (10 percent) who failed to respond to Fab; of these, 5 were moribund at the time of treatment (1 also received an inadequate dose of Fab), 4 were considered in retrospect not to be suffering from digitalis toxicity, and 1 was a true nonresponder. Adverse events included the rapid development of hypokalemia due to reversal of digitalis-induced block of the Na-K-ATPase system and exacerbation of heart failure. Although allergic reactions were not identified in this study in response to Fab treatment, there have been allergic reactions to Fab in 0.8 percent of patients subsequently reported.[192] None of these reactions have been of the anaphylactoid type, and the majority have occurred in patients with a history of allergy to antibiotics.

On the basis of the favorable experience in the treatment of digoxin toxicity with Fab, it would appear reasonable to extend this treatment to selected patients who have digitalis toxicity but do not have life-threatening arrhythmias. The major concern in using the Fab fragments for these less severely intoxicated patients is that immunogenicity is a potential problem, particularly if the patient requires a second administration of the antibody fragments.

Special consideration needs to be given to the patient intoxicated with digoxin who has renal failure.[197] Fab fragments are excreted renally. In humans with normal renal function the elimination half-life of Fab fragments is 15 to 20 h, whereas in patients with renal failure the half-life of the Fab fragments may be 330 h.[197] In patients with renal failure, the antigen-antibody combination may dissociate causing renewed intoxication. After the administration of Fab to patients with renal insufficiency, plasmapheresis can remove the antigen-antibody complexes, thus minimizing the later return of toxicity.[198]

There are two problems inherent in the measurement of serum digoxin concentration after administration of Fab fragments. The first is that Fab fragments may interfere with the immunoassay of digoxin.[199] The other is that assay of serum digoxin may measure both the free digoxin as well as digoxin that is bound to Fab and is therefore not biologically active. The Fab competes with the antibodies of the assay system for digoxin, disturbing the competition of antigen and tracer for antibody binding sites. When radioimmunoassay or fluorescence polarization immunoassay are used to measure digoxin in samples containing Fab, accurate results cannot be obtained. This problem can be obviated by separating the Fab fragments by boiling the Fab containing serum for 1 h, centrifuging the denatured pellet, and assaying the supernate.[200] Accurate assay of the free digoxin concentration can be quickly and accurately measured in samples containing Fab fragments by fluorescence polarization assay of the protein-free ultrafiltrate, which is obtained within minutes by centrifuging the serum through a protein-retaining membrane. Using the free digoxin level in conjunction with clinical data, one may administer additional Fab fragments if necessary.

Ancillary treatment for recent massive ingestion of digoxin and digitoxin toxicity includes the oral administration of activated charcoal with an initial dose of 50 to 100 g. It is not certain whether or not repeated doses are necessary. Activated charcoal enhances the rate of drug diffusion from the body into the gastrointestinal tract by efficiently absorbing the drug from gastrointestinal fluid. Activated charcoal may almost totally inhibit the absorption of digoxin ingested concomitantly[201] and can decrease the absorption of digoxin even when given 1 to 4 h after the glycoside.[202,203] In normal subjects digoxin clearance increased an average of 47 percent when activated charcoal was given at the same time as digoxin was infused intravenously.[204] Charcoal dosing was repeated on multiple occasions over the next 40 h. The mean half-life of elimination was shortened from 36.5 $\pm$ 11.8 to 21.5 $\pm$ 6.5 h. Charcoal was even more effective in enhancing digitoxin elimination in renal failure.[205] Activated charcoal has been shown to decrease the half-life of digitoxin in several patients who have taken an overdose of this medication.[206] The commonly recommended doses of activated charcoal for children is 15 to 30 g initially followed by 15 g every 3 to 4 h if needed. The adult dose is 30 to 100 g initially followed by 30 g every 3 to 4 h if needed.[207] The first dose of activated charcoal is usually given with a cathartic to prevent constipation and to prevent subsequent desorption of the compound from the charcoal that occurs with prolonged gastrointestinal residence. A new "superactive" charcoal has been developed that has greater potential for drug absorption than traditional activated charcoal.[207]

Cholestyramine has been advocated for the treatment of both digitoxin toxicity since it binds these glycosides and prevents reabsorption. Although cholestyramine has been reported to decrease the half-life of both digoxin and digitoxin after an overdose with these drugs, the decrease in half-life is variable.[208,209] Cholestyramine may be used as an adjunct, particularly for non-life-threatening overdose with the cardiac glycosides.[210] Although colestipol has many similarities to cholestyramine, it may not be effective in preventing the absorption of digoxin.[201]

The efficacy of removing digoxin or digitoxin by hemoperfusion is controversial. Theoretically this procedure should be more effective for removing an overdose of digitoxin since the plasma concentrations of digitoxin are 10-fold higher than digoxin due to a smaller volume of distribution and a smaller tissue bound fraction of the body load. Hemoperfusion has been used to successfully treat a patient with massive digitoxin overdose[211]; however, it is minimally effective, if at all, for digoxin.[212] Hemoperfusion has not been uniformly successful to treat digoxin poisoning.[213] If this method is used at all, hemoperfusion with XAD-4 resin appears to be more efficient than with charcoal hemoperfusion.[214]

REFERENCES

1. Withering W: *An Account of the Foxglove and Some of its Medical Uses: With Practical Remarks on Dropsy, and Other Diseases.* Birmingham, printed by M Swinney; for GGJ and J Robinson, Paternoster-Row, London, 1785.
2. American Hospital Formulary Service: Current drug therapy: Cardiac glycosides. *Am J Hosp Pharm* 1978; 35:1495–1507.
3. Gierke KD, Graves PE, Perrier D, Marcus FI, Mayersohn M, Goldman S: Metabolism and rate of elimination of digoxigenin bisdigitoxoside in dogs before and during chronic azotemia. *J Pharmacol Exp Ther* 1981; 212:448–451.
4. Graves PE, Fenster PE, MacFarland RT, Marcus FI, Perrier D: Kinetics of digitoxin and the bis and monodigitoxosides of digitoxigenin in normal subjects. *Clin Pharmacol Ther* 1984; 36:601–606.
5. Graves PE, Fenster PE, MacFarland RT, Marcus FI, Perrier D: Kinetics of digitoxin and the bis and monodigitoxosides of digitoxigenin in renal insufficiency. *Clin Pharmacol Ther* 1984; 36:607–612.

6. Lukas DS, DeMartino AG: Binding of digitoxin and some related cardenolides to human plasma protein. *J Clin Invest* 1969; 48:1041–1053.
7. Lukas DS: Some aspects of distribution and disposition of digitoxin in man. *Ann NY Acad Sci* 1971; 179:338–361.
8. Reuning RH, Sams RA, Notari RE: Role of pharmacokinetics in drug dosage adjustment. I. Pharmacological effect, kinetics and apparent volume of distribution of digoxin. *J Clin Pharmacol* 1973; 13:127–141.
9. Huffman DH, Manion CV, Azarnoff DL: Inter-subject variation in absorption of digoxin in normal volunteers. *J Pharm Sci* 1975; 64:433–437.
10. Rakin SW, Grupp G: A two-compartment open model for digoxin pharmacokinetics in patients receiving a wide range of digoxin doses. *Acta Cardiol* 1975; 30:343–351.
11. Marcus FI, Dickerson J, Pippins S, Stafford M, Bressler R: Digoxin bioavailability: Formulations and rates of infusion. *Clin Pharmacol Ther* 1976; 20:253–260.
12. Wettrell G, Andersson KE: Cardiovascular drugs II: Digoxin. *Ther Drug Monit* 1986; 8:129–139.
13. Perrier D, Mayersohn M, Marcus FI: Clinical pharmacokinetics of digitoxin. *Clin Pharmacokinet* 1977; 2:292–311.
14. Storstein L: Protein binding of cardiac glycosides in disease states. *Clin Pharmacokinet* 1977; 2:220–233.
15. Ochs R, Greenblatt DJ, Bodem G, Harmatz JS: Dose-independent pharmacokinetics of digoxin in humans. *Am Heart J* 1978; 96:507–511.
16. Doherty JE, Marcus FI, Binnion PF: A multicenter evaluation of absolute bioavailability of digoxin dosage forms. *Curr Ther Res* 1984; 35:301–306.
17. Doherty JE, Perkins WH, Flanigan WJ: The distribution and concentration of tritiated digoxin in human tissues. *Ann Intern Med* 1967; 66:116–124.
18. Marcus FI, Burkhalter L, Cuccia C, Pavlovich J, Kapadia GG: Administration of tritiated digoxin with and without a loading dose. A metabolic study. *Circulation* 1966; 34:865–874.
19. Gault MH, Longerich LL, Loo JCK, Ko PTH, Fine A: Digoxin biotransformation. *Clin Pharmacol Ther* 1984; 35:74–82.
20. Peters U, Falk L, Kalman SM: Digoxin metabolism in patients. *Arch Intern Med* 1978; 138:1074–1076.
21. Gault H, Kalra J, Ahmed M, Kepkay D, Longerich L, Barrowman J: Influence of gastric pH on digoxin biotransformation. II. Extractable urinary metabolites. *Clin Pharmacol Ther* 1981; 29:181–190.
22. Magnusson JO, Bergdahl B, Gustafsson S: Urinary excretion of digoxin and its metabolites in hyperacidic patients and in patients during coronary care. *Arzneim Forsch/Drug Res* 1984; 34:85–89.
23. Lindenbaum J, Rund DG, Butler VP Jr, Tse-Eng D, Saha JR: Inactivation of digoxin by the gut flora: Reversal by antibiotic therapy. *N Engl J Med* 1981; 305:789–794.
24. Norregaard-Hansen K, Klitgaard NA, Pedersen KE: The significance of the enterohepatic circulation on the metabolism of digoxin in patients with the ability of intestinal conversion of the drug. *Acta Med Scand* 1986; 220:89–92.
25. Rund DG, Lindenbaum J, Dobkin JF, Butler VP Jr, Saha JR: Decreased digoxin cardioinactive-reduced metabolites after administration as an encapsulated liquid concentrate. *Clin Pharmacol Ther* 1983; 34:738–743.
26. Marcus FI, Quinn EJ, Horton H, Jacobs S, Pippin S, Stafford M: The effect of jejunoileal bypass on the pharmacokinetics of digoxin in man. *Circulation* 1977; 55:537–541.
27. Heizer WD, Pittman AW, Hammond JE, Fitch DD, Bustrack JA, Hull JH: Absorption of digoxin from tablets and capsules in subjects with malabsorption syndromes DICP. *Ann Pharmacother* 1989; 23:764–769.
28. Wettrell G, Anderson KE: Clinical pharmacokinetics of digoxin in infants. *Clin Pharmacokinet* 1977; 2:17–31.
29. Redington AN, Carvalho JS, Shinebourne EA: Does digoxin have a place in the treatment of the child with congenital heart disease? *Cardiovasc Drugs Ther* 1989; 3:21–24.
30. Zalzstein E, Koren G, Levy M, Bentur Y, Macleod S, Freedom R: Once-daily vs twice daily dosing of digoxin in the pediatric age group. *J Pediatr* 1990; 116:137–139.
31. Ewy GA, Kapadia GG, Yao L, Lullin M, Marcus FI: Digoxin metabolism in the elderly. *Circulation* 1969; 39:449–453.
32. Cusak B, Kelly J, O'Malley K, Noel J, Lavan J, Horgan J: Digoxin in the elderly: Pharmacokinetic consequence of old age. *Clin Pharmacol Ther* 1979; 25:772–776.
33. Reid J, Kennedy RD, Caird FI: Digoxin kinetics in the elderly: *Age Aging* 1983; 12:29–37.
34. Ewy GA, Groves BM, Ball MS, Nimmo L, Jackson B: Digoxin metabolism in obesity. *Circulation* 1971; 44:810–814.
35. Abernathy DR, Greenblatt DJ, Smith TW: Digoxin disposition in obesity: Clinical pharmacokinetic investigation. *Am Heart J* 1981; 102:740–744.
36. Bloom PM, Nelp WB: Relationship of the excretion of tritiated digoxin to renal function. *Am J Med Sci* 1966; 251:133–144.
37. Doherty JE, Perkins WH, Wilson MC: Studies with tritiated digoxin in renal failure. *Am J Med* 1964; 37:536–544.
38. Marcus FI, Peterson A, Salel A, Scully J, Kapadia GG: The metabolism of tritiated digoxin in renal insufficiency in dogs and man. *J Pharmacol Exp Ther* 1966; 152:372–382.
39. Doherty JE, Flanigan WJ, Perkins WH, Ackerman GL: Studies with tritiated digoxin in anephric human subjects. *Circulation* 1967; 35:298–303.
40. Gault MH: Digitalis and renal failure. *Int J Artif Org* 1988; 11:141–143.
41. Aronson JK, Grahame-Smith EG: Altered distribution of digoxin in renal failure—a cause of digoxin toxicity? *Br J Clin Pharmacol* 1976; 3:1045–1051.
42. Jogestrand T, Ericsson F: Skeletal muscle digoxin binding in patients with renal failure. *Br J Clin Pharmacol* 1983; 16:109–111.
43. Jusko WJ, Weintraub M: Myocardial distribution of digoxin and renal function. *Clin Pharmacol Ther* 1974; 16:449–454.
44. Gault MH, Churchill DN, Kalra J: Loading dose of digoxin in renal failure. *Br J Clin Pharmacol* 1980; 9:593–597.
45. Zilly W, Richter E, Rietbrock N: Pharmacokinetics and metabolism of digoxin- and β-methyl-digoxin-12α^{3}H in patients with acute hepatitis. *Clin Pharmacol Ther* 1975; 7:303–309.
46. Marcus FI, Kapadia GG: The metabolism of tritiated digoxin in cirrhotic patients. *Gastroenterology* 1964; 47:517–524.
47. Rogers MC, Willerson JT, Goldblatt A, Smith TW: Serum digoxin concentration in the human fetus, neonate and infant. *N Engl J Med* 1972; 287:1010–1013.
48. Luxford AME, Kellaway GSM: Pharmacokinetics of digoxin in pregnancy. *Eur J Clin Pharmacol* 1983; 25:117–121.
49. Chan V, Jse TF, Wong V: Transfer of digoxin across the placenta and into breast milk. *Br J Obstet Gynecol* 1978; 85:605–609.
50. King CR, Mattioli L, Goertz KK, Snodgrass W: Successful treatment of fetal supraventricular tachycardia with maternal digoxin therapy. *Chest* 1984; 85:573–575.
51. Loughlan PM: Digoxin excretion in breast milk. *J Pediatr* 1978; 92:1019–1020.
52. Doherty JE, Perkins WH: Digoxin metabolism in hypo- and hyperthyroidism. *Ann Intern Med* 1966; 64:489–507.
53. Shenfield GM, Thompson J, Horn DB: Plasma and urinary digoxin in thyroid dysfunction. *Eur J Clin Pharmacol* 1977; 12:437–443.
54. Lawrence JR, Sumner DJ, Kalk WJ, Ratcliff WA, Whiting B, Gray K, et al: Digoxin kinetics in patients with thyroid dysfunction. *Clin Pharmacol Ther* 1977; 22:7–13.
55. Eichelbaum M: Drug metabolism in thyroid disease. *Clin Pharmacokinet* 1976; 1:339–350.
56. Gold H, Cattell M: Mechanism of digitalis action in abolishing heart failure. *Arch Intern Med* 1940; 65:263–278.
57. Repke K, Portius HJ: Uber die identitat der lonenpumpen-ATPase in der bel Zellmembran des Herzmuskels mit einem Digitalis-Rezeptorenzym. *Experientia* 1963; 19:452–458.
58. Fozzard HA, Sheets MF: Cellular mechanism of action of cardiac glycosides. *J Am Coll Cardiol* 1985; 5:10A–15A.
59. Katz AM: Effects of digitalis on cell biochemistry: Sodium pump inhibition. *J Am Coll Cardiol* 1985; 5:16A–21A.
60. Smith TW: Digitalis: Mechanisms of action and clinical use. *N Engl J Med* 1988; 318:358–365.
61. Pace DG, Gillis RA: Neuroexcitatory effects of digoxin in the cat. *J Pharmacol Exp Ther* 1976; 199:583–619.
62. Chai CY, Wang HH, Hoffman BF, Wang SC: Mechanisms of bradycardia induced by digitalis substances. *Am J Physiol* 1967; 212:26–34.
63. Ten Eick RD, Hoffman BF: The effect of digitalis on the excitability of autonomic nerves. *J Pharmacol Exp Ther* 1969; 169:95–108.

64. Toda M, West TC: The action of ouabain on the function of the atrioventricular node in rabbits. *J Pharmacol Exp Ther* 1969; 169:287–297.
65. Watanabe AK: Digitalis and the autonomic nervous system. *J Am Coll Cardiol* 1985; 5:35A–42A.
66. Trimalco B, Cierchia S, Lembo G, DeLuca N, Ricciardelli B, Condorelli G, et al: Prolonged duration of myocardial ischemia in patients with coronary heart disease and impaired cardiopulmonary receptor sensitivity. *Circulation* 1990; 81:1792–1802.
67. Ten Eick RD, Hoffman BF: Chronotropic effect of cardiac glycosides in cats, dogs and rabbits. *Circ Res* 1969; 25:365–378.
68. Binkley PF, Nunziata E, Cody RJ: Digoxin mediated reduction of sympathetic tone contributes to vasodilation in dilated cardiomyopathy (abstr). *Circulation* 1990; 82(suppl III):316.
69. Ferguson DW, Berg WJ, Sanders JS, Roach PJ, Kempf JS, Kienzle MG: Sympathoinhibitory responses to digitalis glycosides in heart failure patients. *Circulation* 1989; 80:65–77.
70. Mikkelsen E, Andersson KE, Lederballe Pedersen O: Effects of digoxin on isolated human peripheral arteries and veins. *Acta Pharmacol Toxicol* 1979; 45:249–256.
71. Hamlin NP, Willerson JT, Garan H, Powell WJ Jr: The neurogenic vasoconstrictor effect of digitalis on coronary vascular resistance. *J Clin Invest* 1974; 53:288–296.
72. Mikkelsen E: Effects of digoxin on isolated human pulmonary vessels. *Acta Pharmacol Toxicol* 1979; 45:139–144.
73. Haustein KO, Assmann I, Fiehring H: Problems of rapid digitalization in severe congestive heart failure. *Eur J Cardiol* 1980; 11:135–146.
74. DeMots H, Rahimtoola SH, McAnulty JH, Porter GA: Effects of ouabain on coronary and systemic vascular resistance and myocardial oxygen consumption in patients without heart failure. *Am J Cardiol* 1978; 41:88–93.
75. Powell AC, Horowitz JD, Hasin Y, Louis WJ: Relationship between systemic and coronary vascular responses to digoxin and concurrent drug therapy with verapamil/beta-adrenoreceptor antagonists in humans. *Clin Exper Pharmacol Physiol* 1990; 17:453–462.
76. Powell AC, Horowitz JD, Hasin Y, Syrjanen ML, Horomidis S, Louis WJ: Acute myocardial uptake of digoxin in humans: Correlation with hemodynamic and electrocardiographic effects. *J Am Coll Cardiol* 1990; 15:1238–1247.
77. Rosen MR, Wit AL, Hoffman BF: Electrophysiology and pharmacology of cardiac arrhythmias IV. Cardiac antiarrhythmic and toxic effects of digitalis. *Am Heart J* 1975; 89:391–399.
78. Toda N, West TC: Influence of ouabain on cholinergic responses in the sinoatrial node. *J Pharmacol Exp Ther* 1966; 53: 104–113.
79. Mendez C, Aceves J, Mendez R: Inhibition of adrenergic cardiac acceleration by cardiac glycosides. *J Pharmacol Exp Ther* 1961; 131:191–198.
80. Dhingra RC, Amet-Y-Leon F, Wyndham C, Wu D, Denes P, Rosen K: The electrophysiological effects of ouabain on sinus node and atrium in man. *J Clin Invest* 1975; 56:555–562.
81. Kugler JD, Garson A Jr, Gillette PG: Electrophysiologic effect of digitalis on sinoatrial nodal function in children. *Am J Cardiol* 1979; 44:1344–1348.
82. Bolognesi R, Benedini G, Ferrari R, Visioli O: Inhibitory effect of acute and chronic administration of digitalis on the sick sinus node. *Eur Heart J* 1986; 7:334–340.
83. Engel TR, Schaal SF: Digitalis in the sick sinus syndrome. *Circulation* 1973; 48:1201–1207.
84. Vera Z, Miller RR, McMillin D, Mason DT: Effects of digitalis on sinus nodal function in patients with sick sinus syndrome. *Am J Cardiol* 1978; 41:318–323.
85. Reiffel JA, Bigger JT, Cramer M: Effects of digoxin on sinus nodal function before and after vagal blockade in patients with sinus nodal dysfunction. *Am J Cardiol* 1979; 43:983–994.
86. Adornato E, Polimeni RM, Monea P, Travia G: Effetti della digitale sui parametri di funzione sinusale nella sindrome del seno malato. *G Ital Cardiol* 1984; 14:395–400.
87. Perrot G, Houppe JP, Ethevenot G, Cherrier F, Faivre G: Actions des digitaliques sur le noeud sinusal pathologique. *Arch Mal Coeur* 1983; 6:259–268.
88. Mendez C, Mendez R: The action of cardiac glycosides on the refractory period of heart tissues. *J Pharmacol Exp Ther* 1953; 107:24–36.
89. Mendez C, Mendez R: The action of cardiac glycosides on the excitability and conduction velocity of the mammalian atrium. *J Pharmacol Exp Ther* 1957; 121:402–413.
90. Wu D, Wyndham C, Amat-Y-Leon F, Denes P, Dhingra R, Rosen K: The effects of ouabain on induction of atrioventricular nodal re-entrant paroxysmal supraventricular tachycardia. *Circulation* 1975; 52:201–207.
91. Gomes JAD, Dhatt MS, Akhtar M, Carambas CR, Rubenson DS, Damato AN: Effects of digitalis on ventricular myocardial and His-Purkinje refractoriness and reentry in man. *Am J Cardiol* 1978; 42:931–938.
92. Schaal SF, Sugimoto T, Wallace AG, Sealy WC: Effects of digitalis on the functional refractory period of the AV node: Studies in awake dogs with and without cardiac denervation. *Cardiovasc Res* 1968; 4:356–359.
93. Engel TR, Gonzales ADC: Effects of digitalis on atrial vulnerability. *Am J Cardiol* 1978; 42:570–576.
94. Hayward RP, Hamer J, Taggart P, Emanuel R: Observations on the biphasic nature of digitalis electrophysiological actions in the human right atrium. *Cardiovasc Res* 1983; 17:533–546.
95. Hoffman BF, Singer DH: Effects of digitalis on electrical activity of cardiac fibers. *Prog Cardiovasc Dis* 1964; 7:226–260.
96. Rosen MR, Gelband H, Hoffman BF: Correlation between effects of ouabain in the canine electrocardiogram and trans-membrane potentials of isolated Purkinje fibers. *Circulation* 1973; 47:65–71.
97. Wellens HJJ, Durrer D: Effect of digitalis on atrioventricular conduction and circus-movement tachycardias in patients with Wolff-Parkinson-White syndrome. *Circulation* 1973; 47:1229–1233.
98. Dhingra RC, Palileo EV, Strasberg B, Swiryn C, Bauernfeind R, Wyndham C, et al: Electrophysiologic effects of ouabain in patients with preexcitation and circus movement tachycardia. *Am J Cardiol* 1981; 47:139–144.
99. Jedeikin R, Gillette P, Zinner A: Effect of ouabain on the antegrade effective refractory period of accessory atrioventricular connections in children (abstr). *Circulation* 1982; 66(II): 171.
100. Sellers TD Jr, Bashore TM, Gallagher JJ: Digitalis in the preexcitation syndrome. Analysis during atrial fibrillation. *Circulation* 1977; 56:260–267.
101. Consensus Trial Study Group: Effects of enalapril on mortality in severe congestive heart failure: Results of the Cooperative North Scandinavian Enalapril Survival Study (Consensus). *N Engl J Med* 1987; 316:1429–1435.
102. Hodges M, Friesinger GC, Riggins RCK, Dagenais GR: Effects of intravenously administered digoxin on mild left ventricular failure in acute myocardial infarction in man. *Am J Cardiol* 1972; 29:749–756.
103. Sjogren A: Left heart failure in acute myocardial infarction. *Acta Med Scand* 1970; 510:1–87.
104. Goldstein RA, Passamani ER, Roberts R: A comparison of digoxin and dobutamine in patients with acute infarction and cardiac failure. *N Engl J Med* 1980; 303:846–850.
105. Raabe DS: Combined therapy with digoxin and nitroprusside in heart failure complicating acute myocardial infarction. *Am J Cardiol* 1979; 43:990–994.
106. Mathur PN, Powles P, Pugsley SO, McEwan MP, Campbell EJM: Effect of digoxin on right ventricular function in severe chronic airflow obstruction. *Ann Intern Med* 1981; 95:283–288.
107. Mathur PN, Powles ACP, Pugsley SO, McEwan MP, Campbell EJM: Effect of long-term administration of digoxin on exercise performance in chronic airflow obstruction. *Eur J Respir Dis* 1985; 66:273–283.
108. Baum GI, Dick MM, Shotz S, Gumpel RC: Digitalis toxicity in chronic cor pulmonale. *S Med J* 1956; 49:1037–1042.
109. Berman W Jr, Dubynsky O, Whitman V, Friedman Z, Maisels MJ, Musselman J: Digoxin therapy in low-birth-weight infants with patent ductus arteriosus. *J Pediatr* 1978; 93:652–655.
110. Berman W Jr, Yabek SM, Dillon T, Niland C, Corlew S, Christensen D: Effects of digoxin in infants with a congested circulatory state due to a ventricular septal defect. *N Engl J Med* 1983; 308:363–366.
111. Lundell BPW, Boreus LO: Digoxin therapy and left ventricular performance in premature infants with patent ductus arteriosus. *Acta Pediatr Scand* 1983; 72:339–343.
112. White RD, Lietman PS: Commentary: A reappraisal of digitalis

for infants with left-to-right shunts and "heart failure." *J Pediatr* 1978; 92:867–870.
113. Boucek MM, Chang R, Synhorst DP: Hemodynamic consequences of inotropic support with digoxin or amrinone in lambs with ventricular septal defect. *Pediatr Res* 1985; 19:887–891.
114. Braunwald E: Effects of digitalis on the normal and the failing heart. *J Am Coll Cardiol* 1985; 5:51A–59A.
115. Kurogane K, Fujitani K, Fukuzaki H: Hemodynamic effects of digoxin on congestive heart failure in old myocardial infarction, dilated cardiomyopathy, acute myocardial infarction and mitral stenosis. *Jpn Heart J* 1985; 26:155–165.
116. Ribner HS, Plucinski DA, Hsieh Am, Bresnahan D, Molteni A, Askenazi J, et al: Acute effects of digoxin on total systemic vascular resistance in congestive heart failure due to dilated cardiomyopathy: A hemodynamic-hormonal study. *Am J Cardiol* 1985; 56:896–904.
117. Gheorghiade M, St Clair J, St Clair C, Beller GA: Hemodynamic effects of intravenous digoxin in patients with severe heart failure initially treated with diuretics and vasodilators. *J Am Coll Cardiol* 1987; 9:849–857.
118. Beaune J: For the Enalapril versus Digoxin French Multicenter Group. Comparison of enalapril versus digoxin for congestive heart failure. *Am J Cardiol* 1989; 63:22D–25D.
119. DiBianco R, Shabetai R, Kostuk W, Moran J, Schlant RC, Wright R: A comparison of milrinone, digoxin and their combination in the treatment of patients with chronic heart failure. *N Engl J Med* 1989; 320:677–683.
120. Captopril-Digoxin Multicenter Research Group: Comparative effects of therapy with captopril and digoxin in patients with mild to moderate heart failure. *JAMA* 1988; 259:539–544.
121. Sullivan M, Atwood JE, Myers J, Feuer J, Hall P, Kellerman B, et al: Increased exercise capacity after digoxin administration in patients with heart failure. *J Am Coll Cardiol* 1989; 13:1138–1143.
122. Fleg JL, Rothfeld B, Gottleib SH: Effect of maintenance digoxin therapy in aerobic performance and exercise left ventricular function in mild to moderate heart failure due to coronary artery disease: A randomized, placebo-controlled, crossover trial. *J Am Coll Cardiol* 1991; 17:743–751.
123. Ribner HS, Zucker MJ, Stasior C, Talentoski D, Standicki R, Lesch M: Vasodilators as first-line therapy for congestive heart failure: A comparative hemodynamic study of hydralazine, digoxin, and their combination. *Am Heart J* 1987; 114:91–95.
124. Packer M, Gheorghiade M, Young JB, Costantini PJ, Adams KF, Cody RJ, et al: Withdrawal of digoxin from patients with chronic heart failure treated with angiotensin-converting-enzyme inhibitors. *J Engl J Med* 1993; 329:1–7.
125. Dobbs SM, Kenyon WI, Dobbs RJ: Maintenance digoxin after an episode of heart failure: Placebo-controlled trial in outpatients. *Br Med J* 1977; 1:749–752.
126. Arnold SB, Byrd RC, Meister W, Melmon K, Cheitlin MD, Bristow JD, et al: Long-term digitalis therapy improves left ventricular function in heart failure. *N Engl J Med* 1980; 303:1443–1448.
127. Lee DC, Johnson RA, Bingham JB, Leahy M, Dinsmore RE, Goroll AH, et al: Heart failure in outpatients: A randomized trial of digoxin vs placebo. *N Engl J Med* 1982; 306:699–705.
128. Guyatt GH, Sullivan MJJ, Fallen EL, Tihal H, Rideout E, Halcrow S, et al: A controlled trial of digoxin in congestive heart failure. *Am J Cardiol* 1988; 61:371–375.
129. Moss AJ, Davis HT, Conard DL, Townsend M, Taylor DW, DeCamilla JJ, et al: Digitalis-associated cardiac mortality after myocardial infarction. *Circulation* 1981; 64:1150–1156.
130. Bigger JT Jr, Fleiss JL, Rolnitzky LM, Merab JP, Ferrick KJ: Effects of digitalis treatment on survival after acute myocardial infarction. *Am J Cardiol* 1985; 55:623–630.
131. Digitalis Subcommittee of the Multicenter Post-infarction Research Group: The mortality risk associated with digitalis treatment after myocardial infarction. *Cardiovasc Drug Ther* 1987; 1:125–132.
132. Madsen EB, Gilpin E, Henning H, Ahorre S, Le Winter M, Mazur J, et al: Prognostic importance of digitalis after acute myocardial infarction. *J Am Coll Cardiol* 1984; 3:681–689.
133. Ryan TJ, Bailey KR, McCabe CH, Luk S, Fisher LD, Mock MB, et al: The effects of digitalis on survival in high-risk patients with coronary artery disease: The Coronary Artery Surgery Study (CASS). *Circulation* 1983; 67:735–742.
134. Byington R, Goldstein S: Association of digitalis therapy with mortality in survivors of acute myocardial infarction: Observations in the beta-blocker heart attack trial. *J Am Coll Cardiol* 1985; 6:976–982.
135. Muller JE, Turi ZG, Stone PH, Rude RE, Raabe DS, Jaffe AS, et al: Digoxin therapy and mortality after myocardial infarction. *N Engl J Med* 1986; 314:265–271.
136. Lynch JJ, Montgomery DG, Lucchesi BR: Facilitation of lethal ventricular arrhythmias by therapeutic digoxin in conscious post infarction dogs. *Am Heart J* 1986; 111:883–890.
137. Wellens HJJ, Duren DR, Liem KL, Lie KI: Effect of digitalis in patients with paroxysmal atrioventricular nodal tachycardia. *Circulation* 1975; 52:779–788.
138. Redfors A: Digoxin dosage and ventricular rate at rest and exercise in patients with atrial fibrillation. *Acta Med Scand* 1971; 190:321–333.
139. Aberg H, Strom G, Werner I: The effect of digitalis on the heart rate during exercise in patients with atrial fibrillation. *Acta Med Scand* 1972; 191:441–445.
140. Meijler FL: An "account" of digitalis and atrial fibrillation. *J Am Coll Cardiol* 1985; 5:60A–68A.
141. Botker HE, Toft P, Klitgaard NA, Simonsen EE: Influence of physical exercise on serum digoxin concentration and heart rate in patients with atrial fibrillation. *Br Heart J* 1991; 65:337–341.
142. Falk RH, Knowlton AA, Bernard SA, Gotlieb NE, Battinelli NJ: Digoxin for converting recent-onset atrial fibrillation to sinus rhythm. *Ann Intern Med* 1987; 106:503–506.
143. Rawles JM, Metcalfe MJ, Jennings K: Time of occurrence, duration and ventricular rate of paroxysmal atrial fibrillation: The effect of digoxin. *Br Heart J* 1990; 63:225–227.
144. Wang K, Goldfarb BL, Gobel FL, Richman HG: Multifocal atrial tachycardia. *Arch Intern Med* 1977; 137:161–164.
145. DeMey C, Snoeck J: Review of the use of digitalis glycosides in ventricular dysrhythmias. *Acta Cardiol* 1980; 35:153–163.
146. Lown B, Graboys TB, Podrid PJ, Cohen BH, Stockman M, Gaughan CE: Effect of a digitalis drug on ventricular premature beats. *N Engl J Med* 1977; 296:301–306.
147. Podrid P, Lown B, Zielonka J, Holman BL: Effects of acetylstrophanthidin on left ventricular function and ventricular arrhythmias. *Am Heart J* 1984; 107:882–887.
148. Blumberg J, Hayes JG, Stevens M, Sullivan G, Killip T: Digitalis in treatment of ventricular extrasystoles in the otherwise normal heart (abstr). *Circulation* 1973; 48:18.
149. Gradman AH, Bergen H, Cunningham M, Harbison M, Zaret B: Effects of oral digoxin on ventricular ectopy and its relation to left ventricular function. *Am J Cardiol* 1983; 51:765–769.
150. Cook JR, Kirchhoffer JB, Fitzgerald JF: Treatment of a patient with an adenosine-sensitive ventricular tachycardia using digoxin. *J Cardiovasc Electrophysiol* 1991; 2:367–372.
151. Wu D, Amat-Y-Leon F, Simpson RJ, Latif P, Wyndham CRC, Denes P, et al: Electrophysiological studies with multiple drugs in patients with atrioventricular reentrant tachycardia utilizing an extranodal pathway. *Circulation* 1977; 56:727–736.
152. Dreifus LS, Haiat R, Watanabe Y, Arriaga J, Reitman N: Ventricular fibrillation: A possible mechanism of sudden death in patients with Wolff-Parkinson-White syndrome. *Circulation* 1971; 43:520–527.
153. Marcus FI: Pharmacokinetic interactions between digoxin and other drugs. *J Am Coll Cardiol* 1985; 5:82A–90A.
154. Rodin S, Johnson BF: Pharmacokinetic interactions with digoxin. *Clin Pharmacokinet* 1988; 15:227–244.
155. Brown DD, Juhl RP: Decreased bioavailability of digoxin due to antacids and kaolin-pectin. *N Engl J Med* 1976; 295:1034–1037.
156. Woods MN, Ingelfinger JA: The lack of effect of bran on digoxin absorption. *Clin Pharmacol Ther* 1979; 26:21–23.
157. Brown DD, Schmid J, Long RA, Hull JH: A steady-state evaluation of the effects of propantheline bromide and cholestyramine on the bioavailability of digoxin when administered as tablets or capsules. *J Clin Pharmacol* 1985; 25:360–364.
158. Johnson BF, Bustrack JA, Urbach DR, Hull JH, Marwaha R: Effect of metoclopramide on digoxin absorption from tablets and capsules. *Clin Pharmacol Ther* 1984; 36:724–730.
159. Kirch W, Janisch HD, Santos SR, Duhrsen U, Dylewicz P, Ohnhaus EE: Effect of cisapride and metoclopramide on digoxin bioavailability. *Eur J Drug Metab Pharmacokinet* 1986; 11:249–250.

160. Juhl RP, Summers RW, Guillory JK, Blaug SM, Cheng FH, et al: Effect of sulfasalizine on digoxin bioavailability. *Clin Pharmacol Ther* 1976; 20:387–394.
161. Lindenbaum J, Maulitz RM, Butler VP Jr: Inhibition of digoxin absorption by neomycin. *Gastroenterology* 1976; 71:399–404.
162. Bjornsson TD, Huang AT, Roth P, Jacob DS, Christenson R: Effects of high-dose cancer chemotherapy on the absorption of digoxin in two different formulations. *Clin Pharmacol Ther* 1986; 39:25–28.
163. Moysey JO, Jaggarao NSV, Grundy EN, Chamberlaind DA: Amiodarone increases plasma digoxin concentrations. *Br Med J* 1981; 282:272–273.
164. Fenster PE, White NW Jr, Hanson CD: Pharmacokinetic evaluation of the digoxin-amiodarone interaction. *J Am Coll Cardiol* 1985; 5:108–112.
165. Nademanee K, Kannan R, Hendrickson J, Burnam M, Kary I, Singh B: Amiodarone-digoxin interaction: Clinical significance, time course of development, potential pharmacokinetic mechanisms and therapeutic implications. *J Am Coll Cardiol* 1984; 4:111–116.
166. Robinson K, Johnston A, Walker S, Mulrow JP, McKenna WJ, Holt DW: The digoxin-amiodarone interaction. *Cardiovasc Drugs and Ther* 1989; 3:25–28.
167. Lambert C, Lamontagne D, Hottlet H, Du Souich P: Amiodarone-digoxin interaction in rats. *Drug Metab Disposition* 1989; 17:704–708.
168. Koren G: Interaction between digoxin and commonly coadministered drugs in children. *Pediatrics* 1985; 75:1032–1037.
169. Nolan PE Jr, Marcus FI, Erstad BL, Hoyer GL, Furman C, Kirsten EB: Effects of coadministration of propafenone on the pharmacokinetics of digoxin in healthy volunteer subjects. *J Clin Pharmacol* 1989; 29:46–52.
170. Ejvinsson G: Effect of quinidine on plasma concentrations of digoxin. *Br Med J* 1978; 1:279–280.
171. Hager WD, Fenster PE, Mayersohn M, Perrier D, Graves P, Marcus FI, et al: Digoxin-quinidine interaction. *N Engl J Med* 1979; 300:1238–1241.
172. Hager WD, Mayersohn M, Graves PE: Digoxin bioavailability during quinidine administration. *Clin Pharmacol Ther* 1981; 30:594–598.
173. Pedersen KE, Christiansen BD, Klitgaard NA, Nielsen-Kudsk F: Effect of quinidine of digoxin bioavailability. *Eur J Clin Pharmacol* 1983; 24:41–47.
174. Pedersen KE, Madsen JL, Klitgaard NA, Kjaer K, Hvidt S: Effect of quinine on plasma digoxin concentration and renal digoxin clearance. *Acta Med Scand* 1985; 218:229–232.
175. Hedman A, Angelin B, Arvidsson A, Dahlquist R, Nilsson B: Interactions in the renal and biliary elimination of digoxin "Stereoselective difference between quinine and quinidine." *Clin Pharmacol Ther* 1990; 47:20–26.
176. Klein HO, Lang R, DiSegni E, Kaplinsky E: Verapamil-digoxin interaction. *N Engl J Med* 1980; 303:160.
177. Pedersen KE, Dorph-Pedersen A, Hvidt S, Klitgaard NA, Nielsen-Kudsk F: Digoxin-verapamil interaction. *Clin Pharmacol Ther* 1981; 30:311–316.
178. Maydyoon H, Battilana G, Rosman H, Goldstein S, Gheorghiade M: The evolving pattern of digoxin intoxication: Observations at a large urban hospital from 1980–1988. *Am Heart J* 1990; 120:1189–1194.
179. Lee TH, Smith TW: Serum digoxin concentration and diagnosis of digitalis toxicity: Current concepts. *Clin Pharmacokinet* 1983; 8:279–285.
180. Smith TW, Willerson JT: Suicidal and accidental digoxin ingestion: Report of 5 cases with serum digoxin level correlations. *Circulation* 1971; 44:29–36.
181. Smith TW, Antman EM, Friedman PL, Blatt CM, Marsh JD: Digitalis glycosides: Mechanisms and manifestations of toxicity. *Prog Cardiovasc Dis* 1984; 26:413–485, 495–540; 27:21–56.
182. Rosen MR: Cellular electrophysiology of digitalis toxicity. *J Am Coll Cardiol* 1985; 5:22A–34A.
183. Gorgels APM, De Wit B, Beekman HDM, Dassen WRM, Wellens HJJ: Triggered activity induced by pacing during digitalis intoxication: Observations during programmed electrical stimulation in the conscious dog with chronic complete atrioventricular block. *PACE* 1987; 10:1309–1320.
184. Hariman RJ, Zeiler RH, Gough WB, El-Sherif N: Enhancement of triggered activity in ischemic Purkinje fibers by ouabain: A mechanism of increased susceptibility to digitalis toxicity by myocardial infarction. *J Am Coll Cardiol* 1985; 5:672–679.
185. Bigger TJ, Schmidt DH, Kutt H: Relationship between the plasma level of diphenylhydantoin sodium and its cardiac antiarrhythmic effects. *Circulation* 1968; 38:363–374.
186. Nicholls DP, Murtagh JG, Holt DW: Use of amiodarone and digoxin specific Fab antibodies in digoxin overdosage. *Br Heart J* 1985; 53:462–464.
187. Vincent JL, Dufaye P, Berre J, Kahn RJ: Bretylium in severe ventricular arrhythmias associated with digitalis intoxication. *Am J Emerg Med* 1984; 2:504–506.
188. French JH, Thomas RG, Siskind AP, Brodsky M, Iseri LT: Magnesium therapy in massive digoxin intoxication. *Ann Emerg Med* 1984; 13:562–565.
189. Reisdorff EJ, Clark MR, Walters BL: Acute digitalis poisoning: The role of intravenous magnesium sulfate. *J Emerg Med* 1986; 4:463–469.
190. Smith TW, Butler VP Jr, Haber E, Fozzard H, Marcus FI, Bremner F, et al: Treatment of life-threatening digitalis intoxication with digoxin-specific Fab antibody fragments. *N Engl J Med* 1982; 307:1357–1362.
191. Antman EM, Wenger TL, Butler VP Jr, Haber E, Smith TW: Treatment of 150 cases of life-threatening digitalis intoxication with digoxin-specific Fab antibody fragments. *Circulation* 1990; 81:1744–1752.
192. Hickey AR, Wenger TL, Carpenter VP, Tilson HH, Hlatky MA, Furberg CD, et al: Digoxin immune Fab therapy in the management of digitalis intoxication: Safety and efficacy results of an observational surveillance study. *J Am Coll Cardiol* 1991; 17:590–598.
193. Butler VP Jr, Watson JF, Schmidt DH, Gardner JD, Mandel WJ, Skelton CL: Reversal of the pharmacological and toxic effect of cardiac glycosides by specific antibodies. *Pharmacol Rev* 1973; 25:239–248.
194. Butler VP Jr, Schmidt DH, Smith TW, Haber E, Raynor BD, Demartini P: Effects of sheep digoxin-specific antibodies and their Fab fragments on digoxin pharmacokinetics in dogs. *J Clin Invest* 1977; 59:345–359.
195. Baud F, Bismuth C, Pontal PG, Scherrmann JM, Smith TW: Time course of antidigoxin Fab fragment and plasma digoxin concentrations in an acute digitalis intoxication. *J Toxicol Clin Toxicol* 1982/1983; 19:857–860.
196. Shumaik GM, Wu AW, Ping AC: Oleander poisoning: Treatment of digoxin-specific Fab antibody fragments. *Ann Emerg Med* 1988; 17:732–735.
197. Nuwayhid NF, Johnson GF: Digoxin elimination in a functionally anephric patient after digoxin-specific Fab fragment therapy. *Ther Drug Monit* 1989; 11:680–685.
198. Rabetoy GM, Price CA, Findlay JWA, Sailstad JM: Treatment of digoxin toxicity in a renal failure patient with digoxin specific antibody fragments and plasma plasmapheresis. *Am J Nephrol* 1990; 10:518–521.
199. Rainey RM: Effects of digoxin immune Fab (ovine) on digoxin immunoassays. *Am J Clin Pathol* 1989; 92:779–786.
200. Horsting MJ, Raisys VA, Opheim KE: Drug-specific Fab therapy in drug overdose. *Arch Pathol Lab Med* 1987; 111:693–697.
201. Neuvonen PJ, Kivisto K, Hirvisalo EL: Effects of resins and activated charcoal on the absorption of digoxin, carbamazepine and frusemide. *Br J Clin Pharmacol* 1988; 25:229–233.
202. Neuvonen PJ, Elfving SM, Elonon E: Reduction of absorption of digoxin, phenytoin and aspirin by activated charcoal in man. *Eur J Clin Pharmacol* 1978; 13:213–218.
203. Reissell P, Manninen V: Effect of administration of activated charcoal and fibre on absorption, excretion and steady state blood levels of digoxin and digitoxin. Evidence of intestinal secretion of the glycosides. *Acta Med Scand* 1982; 668(suppl):88–90.
204. Lalonde RL, Deshpande R, Hamilton PP, McLean WM, Greenway DC: Acceleration of digoxin clearance by activated charcoal. *Clin Pharmacol Ther* 1985; 37:367–371.
205. Park GD, Goldberg MJ, Spector R, Johnson GF, Feldman RD, Quee CK, et al: The effects of activated charcoal on digoxin and digitoxin clearance. *Drug Intell Clin Pharm* 1985; 19:937–941.
206. Pond S, Jacobs M, Marks J, Garner J, Goldschlager N, Hansen P: Treatment of digitoxin overdose with oral activated charcoal. *Lancet* 1981; 2:1177–1178.
207. Katona BG, Siegel EG, Cluxton RJ Jr: The new black magic:

Activated charcoal and new therapeutic uses. *J Emerg Med* 1987; 5:9–18.

208. Baciewitz AM, Isaacson ML, Lipscomb GL: Cholestyramine resin in the treatment of digitoxin toxicity. *Drug Intell Clin Pharm* 1983; 17:57–59.
209. Fresard F, Balant L, Noble J, Garcia B, Muller AF: Cholestyramine et intoxication á la digoxin: Efficacité therapeutique? *Schweiz Med Wschr* 1979; 109:431–436.
210. Henderson RP, Solomon CP: Use of cholestyramine in the treatment of digoxin intoxication. *Arch Intern Med* 1988; 148:745–746.
211. Gilfrich HJ, Kasper W, Meinertz T, Okonek S, Bork R: Treatment of massive digitoxin overdose by charcoal hemoperfusion and cholestyramine. *Lancet* 1978; 1:505.
212. Gilfrich HJ, Okonek S, Manns M, Schuster CJ: Digoxin and digitoxin elimination in man by charcoal hemoperfusion. *Klin Wochenschr* 1978; 56:1179–1183.
213. Bismuth C, Wattel F, Gosselin B, Lambert H, Genestal M, Galliot M: L'hemoperfusion sur charbon active enrobe experience des centres antipoisons francais: 60 intoxications. *Nouv Presse Med* 1979; 8:1235–1238.
214. Hoy WE, Gibson TP, Rivero AJ, Jain VK, Talley TT, Bayer RM, et al: XAD-4 resin hemoperfusion for digitoxic patients with renal failure. *Kidney Int* 1983; 23:79–82.

Chapter 28

Nonglycosidic Cardioactive Agents

Thierry H. LeJemtel, M.D. ■ *Edmund H. Sonnenblick, M.D.*

The therapy of acute and chronic heart failure and, more precisely, the role of positive inotropic agents have evolved greatly over the past few years.[1] When acute heart failure occurs in the setting of an acute myocardial infarction, early restoration of adequate myocardial perfusion by pharmacologic or mechanical revascularization is the primary mainstay of therapy in that it seeks to preserve myocardium. Positive inotropic agents represent a temporary measure to enhance ventricular performance and to sustain adequate cardiac output and blood pressure for the survival of vital organs. The assumption is made that ventricular contractility is recoverable, at least to some extent. Nevertheless, by itself, it may not alter the dismal prognosis of severe heart failure complicating an acute myocardial infarction. With regard to chronic congestive heart failure (CHF), substantial benefits of long-term angiotensin converting enzyme (ACE) inhibition have been documented on symptoms and mortality.[2–6] (See also Chap. 26.) In view of the benefits of ACE inhibitors, positive inotropic agents now appear indicated in most patients with mild heart failure when ACE inhibitors, other vasodilators such as nitrates, and potent diuretics no longer adequately control the symptoms. The treatment of heart failure is more fully discussed in Chap. 26. To reserve the use of nonglycosidic positive inotropic agents to late stages of CHF is justified as their safety is, to a large extent, unknown. Prolonged administration of specific phosphodiesterase (PDE) inhibitors to patients with CHF in functional classes III and IV of the New York Heart Association (NYHA) is accompanied by an increased mortality when compared to placebo.[7] The value of prolonged therapy with cardiac glycosides is currently being investigated. Some have even questioned the safety of all positive inotropic agents, including cardiac glycosides.[8] (See also Chap. 27.)

While the safety of inotropic agents is investigated, however, the need for therapeutic modalities other than nonspecific vasodilatation, ACE inhibition, diuretics, and digitalization is becoming more important. Patients who, prior to the thrombolytic era, would not have survived a large myocardial infarction, are now seen many years later with severe left ventricular dysfunction that most probably results from repeated, small myocardial infarctions. In addition, patients with chronic CHF whose lives have been prolonged by ACE inhibitors are more frequently hospitalized with clinical syndromes compatible with low cardiac output. In patients whose cardiac afterload has been optimally matched to depressed left ventricular performance by pharmacologic means, enhancement of myocardial contractility appears to remain the only therapeutic possibility.

REGULATION OF THE CONTRACTILE PROCESS AND POSSIBLE SITES OF ACTION OF POSITIVE INOTROPIC AGENTS

The rapidity of action of inotropic agents makes it unlikely that their effects could be mediated through structural changes in the contractile process or alteration of myosin adenosinetriphosphatase (ATPase) activity.[9] Increased delivery of activating Ca^{2+} to the contractile apparatus and/or increased affinity of the contractile apparatus for Ca^{2+} are therefore likely to mediate their positive inotropic actions. Although most of the Ca^{2+} that enters the cell during the plateau phase of the action potential is stored in the subsarcolemmal cisternae of the sarcoplasmic reticulum, a small portion triggers the release of Ca^{2+} from the intracellular stores into the cytosol to activate the contractile apparatus.[10] (See also Chap. 5.) Once the level of Ca^{2+} into the cytosol falls below the resting level following reuptake and storage of Ca^{2+} by sarcoplasmic reticulum and activation of the Na^{+}/Ca^{2+} exchange system, relaxation occurs. Control of the cytoplasmic Ca^{2+}, which plays a major role in the regulation of the contractile process, can be influenced through several mechanisms by the different nondigitalis, cardiotonic agents presently available. The precise events leading to the increase in cytoplasmic Ca^{2+}, which represents the final common pathway of action of most cardiotonic agents, will be reviewed separately for each class of these agents. The extent to which they may also modify the affinity of the contractility apparatus for Ca^{2+} will also be discussed.

For relaxation, intracellular Ca^{2+} must be reduced, presumably by sequestration into the sarcoplasmic reticulum and, to a lesser extent, extrusion from the cell. In heart failure, this mechanism appears abnormal.[11-13] Mechanisms that augment Ca^{2+} in cardiac myocytes are likely also to alter the excitation-contraction coupling of vascular smooth muscle, as discussed for specific agents.

CLASSIFICATION OF NONDIGITALIS CARDIOTONIC AGENTS

Nondigitalis cardiotonic agents can be classified into two major groups. The first includes the catecholamines (norepinephrine, dopamine) and their derivatives (such as dobutamine and isoproterenol) (Fig. 28-1). (See also Chap. 30.) These are only available for parenteral use, a feature that considerably limits their extended application. Other artificially synthesized catecholamines (such as aramine) act, to some extent, by releasing catecholamines from endogenous stores. The experimental oral catecholamine derivatives (pirbuterol and prenalterol) do not have demonstrated therapeutic value for the treatment of chronic CHF, because of excess β_2-receptor stimulation, leading to tachycardia, tachyphylaxis, ventricular arrhythmias, and adverse peripheral circulatory responses.[14]

The second group of nondigitalis cardiotonic agents is characterized by inhibition of myocardial cellular PDE (Type III). Their positive inotropic action may not be due entirely to PDE inhibition, however, as some agents, such as pimobendan, can sensitize myofibrils to Ca^{2+}.[15,16] These newer inotropic agents, which are orally active, also produce direct peripheral arterial and venous vasodilation, which in certain instances may be the predominant factor in improving cardiac performance. Thus, PDE III inhibition, which leads to increased cyclic adenosine 3′,5′-monophosphate (cAMP) levels in the cell, produces both enhanced contractility in the heart and vasodilatation in the peripheral circulation.[17] The prototype of these inotropic agents is amrinone; more recently developed agents include milrinone (Primacor), indolidan, enoximone, and pimobendan.[18]

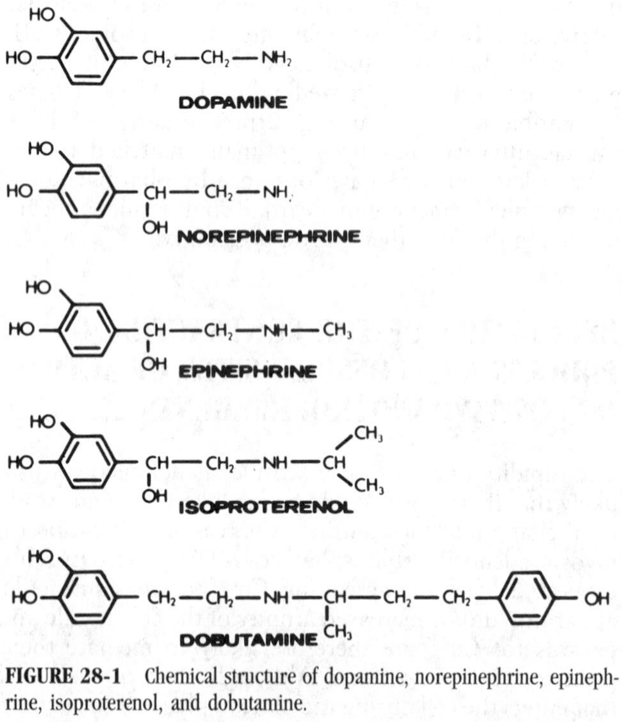

FIGURE 28-1 Chemical structure of dopamine, norepinephrine, epinephrine, isoproterenol, and dobutamine.

Catecholamines and Their Derivatives

Dopamine, a naturally occurring precursor of norepinephrine, and norepinephrine itself may be used to increase myocardial contractility. Both dopamine in high doses and norepinephrine constrict the peripheral arterioles, however, thus limiting their use. Dobutamine, which is a synthesized catecholamine derivative without vasoconstrictive activity, has become the most widely used parenteral inotropic agent.[19] (See also Chap. 30.)

Biochemistry, Regulation of Intracellular Calcium, and Pharmacokinetics

The endogenous catecholamines include dopamine, norepinephrine, epinephrine, and their derivatives. Norepinephrine is synthesized and stored in granules in sympathetic nerve endings and released with nerve stimulation, diffusing then to receptors located on the cell surface. More specifically, activation of the β-adrenoreceptor increases the levels of cAMP in the myocardial cells; this in turn activates cAMP-dependent protein kinase. The resulting phosphorylation of proteins in the sarcolemma, sarcoplasmic reticulum, and thin filaments increases calcium influx across the sarcolemma and the rate of calcium uptake into the sarcoplasmic reticulum and decreases myofibrillar calcium sensitivity. The overall effects of these changes are an increased rate and extent of shortening, along with an enhanced rate of relaxation. The half-life of endogenous catecholamines in the human plasma is brief, on the order of minutes (Figs. 5-5, 5-6).

Most inactivation of norepinephrine normally takes place from reuptake into the sympathetic nerve endings. Norepinephrine is also inactivated by two enzymes, catechol *O*-methyltransferase (COMT) and monoamine oxidase (MAO), and the products are mostly excreted in the urine. The former mechanism in the heart is severely compromised in CHF,[20] although the adrenergic receptors on the cardiac cells remain active. Dobutamine has a half-life of 2 min and is metabolized to inactive glucuronide conjugates and 3-O-methyl-dobutamine in the liver. These metabolites are mostly excreted in the urine.

Pharmacologic Actions

Endogenous catecholamines and dobutamine have different physiological actions that result from their relative specificity for α and β adrenoceptors.[21] Alpha receptors include α_1 receptors that are postsynaptic and are located either in the vascular smooth muscle or in the myocardium. The smooth-muscle α_1 receptors are responsible for vasoconstriction; the myocardial α_1 in humans mediates relatively weak positive inotropic and negative chronotropic responses. The α_2 adrenoreceptors are mostly presynaptic and responsible for decreasing norepinephrine release in the peripheral nerve terminals and decreasing sympathetic outflow in the central nervous system.[22] In addition, α_2-adrenergic receptors may be located in the smooth muscle and may be responsible for vasoconstriction in some vascular beds.[23] (See also Chap. 3.)

β-Adrenergic receptors include β_1 receptors located in the myocardium and responsible for positive inotropic, chronotropic, and dromotropic responses. They respond preferentially to neuronally released norepinephrine. The β_2 adrenoreceptors are located in the smooth muscle and mediate vasodilatation. The β_2 receptors may, however, also be located in the sinoatrial node and be responsible for positive chronotropy.[24] They respond preferentially to circulating norepinephrine released from the adrenal medulla and to exogenous catecholamines. In addition, there are specific dopaminergic receptors in the mesenteric and renal vascular bed that are responsible for arterial vasodilatation.[25] (See also Chap. 30.) The physiological actions of the endogenous catecholamines and their derivatives are thus determined by their specificity for the α_1-, β_1-, and β_2-adrenergic receptors (Table 28-1).

Dobutamine

The synthesis of dobutamine resulted from systemic modifications to the chemical structure of isoproterenol. In the intact dog dobutamine produces a potent positive inotropic action with little change of heart rate or vascular resistance.[26] It is generally accepted that the positive inotropic action of dobutamine is mediated through direct stimulation of β_1-adrenergic receptors in the myocardium, which in turn increases cAMP.[19] In addition, unlike dopamine, it does not stimulate the heart indirectly by releasing norepinephrine from the nerve endings. The relative lack of positive chronotropic effect of dobutamine is, however, not well understood. Either the chronotropic response to catecholamine may be mediated not by β_1 but by β_2 adrenoreceptors, which are only partially activated by dobutamine, or some of the positive inotropic action of dobutamine may result from stimulation of an α_1 myocardial receptor.[27] In the isolated rabbit papillary muscle, stimulation of the α adrenoreceptor increases substantially the force of contraction, although it does not alter calcium transient in the myocardial cell. Such disparity is consistent with an increase in myofibrillar sensitivity to Ca^{2+}.[28] Whether or not a similar mechanism occurs in human myocardium is controversial.

Independent of its exact mechanism of action, dobutamine is presently the cardiotonic agent that exerts the most potent inotropic action while producing limited undesirable effects on heart rate and blood pressure. In the setting of acute myocardial infarction complicated by severe left ventricular dysfunction refractory to appropriate vasodilators and diuretics, dobutamine is the cardiotonic of choice unless severe hypotension is present.[19] (See also Chaps. 30 and 60.) If systemic arterial pressure is substantially reduced, stimulation of β_2 adrenoreceptors may be detrimental and administration of high doses of dopamine or of norepinephrine may be required to maintain adequate blood pressure through α_1 vasoconstriction. Since dobutamine reduces left ventricular filling pressure while improving cardiac output, it tends to decrease heart size. This tends to offset the effect of augmented myocardial contractility upon myocardial oxygen requirements. In addition, dobutamine improves coronary perfusion by increasing diastolic perfusion time, as a result of a reduction in heart rate mediated by withdrawal of sympathetic tone. Dobutamine also increases the pressure gradient that drives blood flow into the ischemic tissue by reducing left ventricular diastolic pressure without affecting aortic diastolic pressure.

Administration of dobutamine to patients with acute myocardial infarction and left ventricular dysfunction is safe and most often improves cardiac performance without overtly worsening myocardial ischemia.[29] (See also Chap. 60.) The rate of infusion of dobutamine should start at 2 μg/kg per min and be titrated up to obtain optimal cardiac output while reducing left ventricular filling pressure to near normal value if these

TABLE 28-1
Receptor Activity of Sympathomimetic Amines

	α_{-1}	β_1	β_2	Dopaminergic
Norepinephrine	++++	++++	0	0
Epinephrine	++++	++++	++	0
Dopamine	++++	++	+	++++
Isoproterenol	0	++++	++++	0
Dobutamine	+++	++++	++	0

measurements are available. If they are not available, heart rate and blood pressure should be closely monitored to prevent tachycardia and major changes in blood pressure. The most serious side effect of dobutamine is the precipitation of ventricular arrhythmias that may necessitate drug dose reduction or even discontinuation.

In chronic CHF, administration of dobutamine is useful either during acute decompensation precipitated by a concomitant illness or for intermittent inotropic support that may require short-term hospitalization or be carried out on an outpatient basis with a small portable infusion pump.[30] Although patients with severe CHF have a decreased density and affinity of myocardial β-adrenergic receptors for catecholamines,[31] the majority of patients experience a hemodynamic and clinical improvement following administration of dobutamine. One usually has to increase the rate of infusion over time to maintain hemodynamic benefits similar to that initially observed. The reasons for the attenuation of the peak hemodynamic effects during long-term administration of dobutamine are poorly understood. The down regulation of the β adrenoreceptor in the failing human myocardium mostly affects β_1 receptors; the number and sensitivity of β_2 receptors are only minimally decreased.[32,33] Thus, activation of β_2 adrenoreceptor may be responsible for a substantial portion of the positive inotropic actions of dobutamine. The fate of the β_2 receptors and their coupling with adenylate cyclase during long-term administration of dobutamine are unknown. The mechanisms of the relatively prolonged clinical benefits of dobutamine after discontinuation of the infusion are most probably related to long-lasting effects on the peripheral circulation rather than on the myocardium. Concomitant infusion of dopamine at doses of 2 μg/kg per min or less may be useful to obtain dopaminergic renal arterial vasodilatation, to increase renal blood flow, and thus to promote sodium excretion.

Nondigitalis Noncatecholamine Cardiotonic Agents

Amrinone (Inocor) is the prototype of a new class of cardiotonic agents that do not act through the cellular mechanisms attributed to digitalis or catecholamines but are specific PDE Type III inhibitors, resulting in increasing levels of cAMP in the myocardium and peripheral smooth muscle (Fig. 28-2). Other cardiotonic agents in this class include milrinone, enoximone, and pimobendan.[18,34] At the present time, only the parenteral forms of amrinone and milrinone have been approved by the Federal Drug Administration (FDA) for use in CHF. The PDE activity appears more selective within the cardiac cell than that produced by papaverine and theophylline. Such selectivity may contribute to the relatively greater inotropic action of amrinone when compared to some other PDE inhibitors. The positive inotropic action of some of these cardiotonic agents may also result from increased sensitivity of contractile proteins for Ca^{2+}, a phenomenon documented with theophylline.[35] Of therapeutic interest, the positive inotropic action of these new agents may vary with the level of cAMP present in the cardiac cell and may therefore be more apparent after β_1-adrenergic stimulation, as during physical exercise or administration of exogenous catecholamines.[36,37]

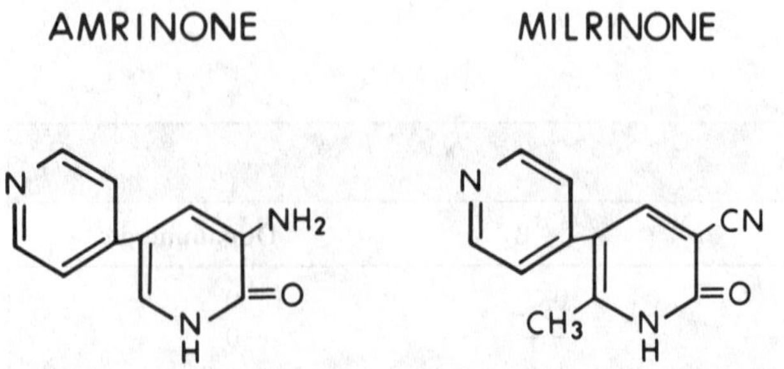

AMRINONE MILRINONE

FIGURE 28-2 Chemical structure of amrinone [5-amino (3,4′-bipyridine)-6(1*H*)-one] and milrinone [1,6-dihydro-2-methyl-6-oxo(3,4′-bipyridine)-5-carbonitrate].

Independent of their positive inotropic actions, these specific PDE inhibitors exert direct arteriolar and venous vasodilating properties that result from increasing levels of cAMP in the vascular smooth muscle. The exact mechanisms responsible for cAMP-induced vasorelaxation are incompletely understood. They may be mediated by cAMP-induced phosphorylation of purified myosin light-chain kinase, which renders it less sensitive to activation by calcium and calmodulin. Alternatively, cAMP-dependent protein kinase may increase Na^+-K^+-ATPase activity and thus facilitate extrusion of calcium through Na^+-Ca^+ exchange. A direct vasodilator effect of specific type III PDE inhibition occurs in patients with chronic CHF treated with milrinone.[38] Of importance, the dose response of the positive inotropic and vasodilating actions is probably different for each agent. For some agents, the direct vasodilating properties are present even at low doses; for others, the dilating properties are only observed at high doses. The direct vasodilator effect of specific PDE inhibitors may be somewhat attenuated by cardiac glycosides.[39]

Pharmacologic Actions

In vitro preparations of amrinone cause a dose-dependent increase in papillary muscle developed tension.[40] In anesthetized and unanesthetized dogs, amrinone increases cardiac contractile force and rate of left ventricular pressure rise, although it produces only small changes in heart rate or blood pressure.[40] Amrinone does not alter the action potential of driven or spontaneously beating canine Purkinje fibers; however, it shortens the functional refractory period and the conduction time of the canine atrioventricular node.[41] In experimental models of heart failure, amrinone increases cardiac output and reduces left ventricular filling pressures with minimal changes in heart rate or blood pressure.[42] These hemodynamic improvements are accompanied by an unchanged or decreased myocardial oxygen consumption.[42] In healthy dogs, amrinone enhances regional blood flow to the kidneys, spleen, and liver. In humans in heart failure, PDE III inhibition by milrinone reduces left ventricular filling pressure to a greater extent than does dobutamine for the same increase in cardiac output, and this reduction contributes to a decrease in myocardial oxygen consumption per minute with the former; with the latter, myocardial oxygen consumption tends to rise.[43]

Pharmacokinetics

In patients with CHF, the half-life of amrinone usually ranges from 5 to 8 h with considerable patient variation from 3 to 13 h. Amrinone is metabolized via conjugative pathways. Up to 40 percent of amrinone is excreted unchanged in the urine. In contrast, preliminary information indicates that the half-life of milrinone is shorter, on the order of 2 h.

Therapy with amrinone should be initiated with an intravenous bolus at a dose ranging from 0.75 to 3 mg/kg and followed by a continuous infusion at a rate ranging from 4 to 10 μg/kg per min. In patients with severe renal insufficiency, this rate of infusion should be subsequently decreased to prevent toxic plasma levels of amrinone and adverse potential reactions such as ventricular arrhythmias and hypotension.

Milrinone (Primacor) has pharmacologic actions and pharmacokinetics similar to amrinone[44] but may be less likely to produce thrombocytopenia and is less costly. It is about 20 times more potent than amrinone. The loading dose is 20 μg/kg administered intravenously slowly over 10 min. The standard maintenance dose is an infusion of 0.50 μg/kg per min (range 0.375 to 0.75 μg/kg per min) with a total daily dose of 0.77 mg/kg (range 0.59 to 1.13 mg/kg).

USE IN CONGESTIVE HEART FAILURE

Nonglycosidic cardioactive agents are only presently available for temporary use in parenteral form. Intravenous dobutamine, amrinone, and milrinone have been approved for temporary inotropic support by the FDA. Milrinone has the advantage over amrinone of having fewer side effects. In particular, thrombocytopenia does not appear to complicate prolonged use of milrinone. Milrinone and amrinone both increase cardiac output and reduce left ventricular pressure consistently, without producing overt changes in systemic arterial pressure or heart rate in patients with severe CHF.[45,46] The primary mechanism of the improvement in left ventricular performance appears to be due to the potent arteriolar and venodilating effects of milrinone and amrinone; the contribution of their positive inotropic effects is most often modest and variable from patient to patient. Of interest, the positive inotropic effects of dobutamine and amrinone are additive, and concomitant administration of amrinone at the recommended loading dose of 1.5 mg/kg and infusion rate of 5 to 60 μg/kg per min and dobutamine starting at a dose of 2 μg/kg per min with titration by increments of 1 μg/kg per min results in the optimal pharmacologic improvement in left ventricular performance in patients with decompensated CHF or acute heart failure.[36] Not only does the combined administration of amrinone and dobutamine exert greater hemodynamic benefits than that produced by either drug alone, but the combination appears to be better tolerated than higher doses of dobutamine in the range of 15 to 20 μg/kg per min. Moreover, the combined administration of amrinone and dobutamine should result in a lower metabolic cost on the myocardium, due to the potent venodilator effects of amrinone or milrinone to lower filling pressures. Moreover, β-adrenergic stimulation alone may increase myocardial oxygen requirements to a greater extent than specific PDE inhibition due to this action.

Long-term PDE inhibition with orally administered milrinone has been shown to have a detrimental impact on survival in patients with CHF in functional classes III and IV.[7] The increased mortality appears to be due, in part, to the proarrhythmic effect of PDE inhibitors. Whether or not the detrimental effect of milrinone on survival results from excessive doses of milrinone and perhaps of digoxin in patients hemodynamically unstable with deteriorating renal function is currently unclear. The negative experience with milrinone, however, should not decrease interest for the prolonged use of a nonglycosidic cardioactive agent for the treatment of chronic CHF refractory to ACE inhibition. As demonstrated by trials of ACE inhibitors on mortality, patients with CHF continue to deteriorate and eventually die of ventricular failure. Since only an extremely small number of these patients are candidates for cardiac transplantation, the development of safe, positive inotropic agents remains a very promising therapeutic approach.[47]

Vesnarinone (OPC-8212, ARKIN-Z) has been recently found to produce a decrease in mortality of approximately 50 percent in a study of 477 patients who were randomized to vesnarinone (60 mg/day, $n = 239$) or placebo ($n = 238$) and followed for 6 months.[48] A small percentage of patients developed neutropenia, usually within the first 16 weeks of therapy, that regressed when the agent was discontinued. The full mechanisms of action of this compound are not yet known, although it appears to affect myocyte Na^+ and K^+ channels in addition to producing very mild inhibition of PDE.

REFERENCES

1. Maskin CS, LeJemtel TH, Kugler J, Sonnenblick EH: Inotropic therapy in the management of congestive heart failure. *Cardiovasc Rev Rep* 1992; 13:8–23.
2. The CONSENSUS Trial Study Group: Effects of enalapril on mortality in severe congestive heart failure. Results of the Cooperative North Scandinavian Enalapril Survival Study (CONSENSUS). *N Engl J Med* 1987; 316:1429–1435.
3. The SOLVD Investigators: Effect of enalapril on survival in patients with reduced left ventricular ejection fractions and congestive heart failure. *N Engl J Med* 1991; 325:293–302.
4. Cohn JN, Johnson G, Ziesche S, Cobb F, Francis G, Tristani F, et al: A comparison of enalapril with hydralazine–isosorbide dinitrate in the treatment of chronic congestive heart failure. *N Engl J Med* 1991; 325:303–310.
5. Pfeffer MA, Braunwald E, Moye LA, Basta L, Brown Jr EJ, Cuddy TE, et al: Effect of captopril on mortality and morbidity in patients with left ventricular dysfunction after myocardial infarction. *N Engl J Med* 1992; 327:669–677.
6. The SOLVD Investigators: Effect of enalapril on mortality and the development of heart failure in asymptomatic patients with reduced left ventricular ejection fractions. *N Engl J Med* 1992; 327:685–691.
7. Packer M, Carver JR, Rodeheffer RJ, Ivanhoe RJ, Di Bianco R, Zeldis SM, et al, for the PROMISE Study Research Group: Effect of oral milrinone on mortality in severe chronic heart failure. *N Engl J Med* 1991; 325:1468–1475.
8. Katz AM: Potential deleterious effects of inotropic agents in the therapy of chronic heart failure. *Circulation* 1986; 73(suppl III): III-184–190.

9. Scheuer J, Bhan AK: Cardiac contractile proteins. Adenosine triphosphatase activity and physiological function. *Circ Res* 1979; 45:1–12.
10. Fabiato A, Fabiato F: Calcium and cardiac excitation-contraction coupling. *Annu Rev Physiol* 1979; 41:473–484.
11. Gwathmey JK, Copelas L, MacKinnon R, Schoen FJ, Feldman MD, Grossman W, et al: Abnormal intracellular calcium handling in myocardium from patients with end-stage heart failure. *Circ Res* 1987; 61:70–76.
12. D'Agnolo A, Luciani GB, Mazzucco A, Gallucci V, Salviati G: Contractile properties and Ca^{2+} release activity of the sarcoplasmic reticulum in dilated cardiomyopathy. *Circulation* 1992; 85:518–525.
13. Beuckelmann DJ, Nabauer M, Erdmann E: Intracellular calcium handling in isolated ventricular myocytes from patients with terminal heart failure. *Circulation* 1992; 85:1046–1055.
14. Weber KT, Andrews V, Janicki JS, Likoff M, Reichek N: Pirbuterol, an oral beta-adrenergic receptor agonist in the treatment of chronic cardiac failure. *Circulation* 1982; 62:1262–1667.
15. Ruegg JL: Effects of new inotropic agents on Ca^{++} sensitivity of contractile proteins. *Circulation* 1986; 73(suppl 3):78–84.
16. Bohm M, Morano I, Pieske B, Ruegg JC, Wankerl M, Zimmermann R, et al: Contribution of cAMP-phosphodiesterase inhibition and sensitization of the contractile proteins for calcium to the inotropic effect of pimobendan in the failing human myocardium. *Circ Res* 1991; 68:689–701.
17. Hardman JG: Cyclic nucleotides and regulation of vascular smooth muscle. *J Cardiovasc Pharmacol* 1984; 6:S639–S645.
18. Colucci WS, Wright RF, Braunwald E: New positive inotropic agents in the treatment of congestive heart failure. *N Engl J Med* 1986; 314:349–358.
19. Sonnenblick EH, Frishman WH, LeJemtel TH: Dobutamine: A new synthetic cardioactive sympathetic amine. *N Engl J Med* 1979; 300:17–22.
20. Chidsey CA, Braunwald E, Morrow AG: Catecholamine excretion and cardiac stores of norepinephrine in congestive heart failure. *Am J Med* 1965; 39:442–451.
21. Ahlquist RP: A study of the adrenotropic receptors. *Am J Physiol* 1948; 153:586–600.
22. Langer SZ: Presynaptic receptors and their role in the regulation of transmitter release: Sixth Gaddum Memorial Lecture. *Br J Pharmacol* 1977; 60:481–497.
23. Hoffman BB, Lefkowitz RJ: Alpha-adrenergic receptor subtypes. *N Engl J Med* 1980; 302:1390–1396.
24. Carlsson EC, Dahlof CG, Hedberg A, Persson H, Tangstrand B: Differentiation of cardiac chronotropic and inotropic effects of β-adrenoceptor agonists. *Naunyn Schmiedebergs Arch Pharmacol* 1977; 300:101–105.
25. Goldberg LI: Cardiovascular and renal actions of dopamine. Potential clinical applications. *Pharmacol Rev* 1972; 24:1–29.
26. Tuttle RR, Mills J: Dobutamine: Development of a new catecholamine to selectively increase cardiac contractility. *Circ Res* 1975; 36:185–196.
27. Williams RS, Bishop T: Selectivity of dobutamine for adrenergic receptor subtypes: In vitro analysis by radioligand binding. *J Clin Invest* 1981; 67:1703–1711.
28. Endoh M, Blinks JR: Actions of sympathomimetic amines on the Ca^{2+} transients and contractions of rabbit myocardium: Reciprocal changes in myofibrillar responsiveness to Ca^{2+} mediated through α- and β-adrenoreceptors. *Circ Res* 1988; 62:247–265.
29. Keung E, Siskind SJ, Sonnenblick EH, Ribner HS, Schwartz WJ, LeJemtel TH: Dobutamine therapy for acute myocardial infarction. *JAMA* 1981; 245:144–146.
30. Applefeld M, Newman KA, Grove WR, Sutton FJ, Roffman DS, Reed WP, et al: Intermittent, continuous outpatient dobutamine infusion in the management of congestive heart failure. *Am J Cardiol* 1983; 51:455–458.
31. Bristow WR, Ginsburg R, Minobe W, Cubbicciotti RS, Sageman WS, Lurie K, et al: Decreased catecholamine sensitivity and β-adrenergic receptor density in failing human hearts. *N Engl J Med* 1982; 307:205–211.
32. Bristow MR, Ginsburg R, Umans V, Fowler M, Minobe W, Rasmussen R, et al: β_1- and β_2-adrenergic receptor subpopulations in non-failing and failing human ventricular myocardium: Coupling of both receptor subtypes to muscle contraction and selective β_1-receptor down regulation in heart failure. *Circ Res* 1986; 59:297–309.
33. Bristow MR, Anderson FL, Port JD, Skerl L, Herschberger RE, Larrabee P, et al: Differences in β-adrenergic neuroeffector mechanisms in ischemic versus idiopathic dilated cardiomyopathy. *Circulation* 1991; 84:1024–1039.
34. Katz SD, Kubo SH, Jessup M, Brozena S, Troha JM, Wahl J, et al: A multicenter, randomized, double-blind, placebo-controlled trial of pimobendan, a new cardiotonic and vasodilator agent, in patients with severe congestive heart failure. *Am Heart J* 1992; 123:95–102.
35. Fabiato A: Effects of cyclic AMP and phosphodiesterase inhibitors on the contractile activation and the Ca^{2+} transient detected with aequorin in skinned cardiac cells from rat and rabbit ventricles. *J Gen Physiol* 1981; 78:15A–16A.
36. Gage J, Rutman H, Lucido D, LeJemtel TH: Additive effects of dobutamine and amrinone on myocardial contractility and ventricular performance in patients with severe heart failure. *Circulation* 1986; 74:367–373.
37. Guimond J, Matuschak G, Meyers F, Keating D: Augmentation of cardiac function in end-stage heart failure by combined use of dobutamine and amrinone. *Chest* 1986; 90:302–304.
38. Cody R, Muller FB, Kubo SH, Rutman H, Leonard D: Identification of the direct vasodilator effect of milrinone with an isolated limb preparation in patients with chronic congestive heart failure. *Circulation* 1986; 73:124–129.
39. Jondeau G, Klapholz M, Katz SD, Maher M, Galvao M, Levato P, et al: Control of arteriolar resistance in heart failure: Partial attenuation of specific phosphodiesterase inhibitor-mediated vasodilation by digitalis glycosides. *Circulation* 1992; 84:54–60.
40. Alousi AA, Farah AE, Lesher GY, Opalka CJ: Cardiotonic activity of amrinone-WIN 40680 5-amino-3′4′-bipyridin-6(1*H*)-one. *Circ Res* 1979; 45:666–677.
41. Nusrat A, Tepper D, Hertzberg J, Sonnenblick EH, Aronson RS: Effects of amrinone on atrioventricular conduction in the intact canine heart. *J Clin Pharmacol* 1983; 23:257–265.
42. Jentzer JH, LeJemtel TH, Sonnenblick EH, Kirk ES: Beneficial effect of amrinone on myocardial oxygen consumption during acute left ventricular failure in dogs. *Am J Cardiol* 1981; 48:75–83.
43. Grose R, Strain J, Greenberg M, LeJemtel TH. Systemic and coronary effects of intravenous milrinone and dobutamine in congestive heart failure. *J Am Coll Cardiol* 1986; 7:1107–1113.
44. Anderson JL, Baim DS, Fein SA, Goldstein RA, LeJemtel TH, Likoff MJ: Efficacy and safety of sustained (48 hour) intravenous infusions of milrinone in patients with severe congestive heart failure: A multicenter study. *J Am Coll Cardiol* 1987; 9:711–722.
45. Benotti JR, Grossman W, Braunwald E, Carabello BA: Effects of amrinone on myocardial energy metabolism and hemodynamics in patients with severe congestive heart failure due to coronary artery disease. *Circulation* 1980; 62:28–34.
46. LeJemtel TH, Maskin CS, Mancini D, Sinoway L, Feld H, Chadwick B: Systemic and regional hemodynamic effects of captopril and milrinone administered alone and concomitantly in patients with heart failure. *Circulation* 1985; 12:364–369.
47. Yuen J, Sonnenblick EH, LeJemtel TH: Principles of inotropic therapy in heart failure. In: Singh BN, Dzau VJ, Vanhoutte P, Woosley RL (eds): *Cardiovascular Pharmacology and Therapeutics.* New York, Churchill Livingstone, in press.
48. Feldman AM, Bristow MR, Parmley WW, Carson PE, Pepine CJ, Gilbert EM, et al: Effects of vesnarinone on morbidity and mortality in patients with heart failure. *N Engl J Med* 1993; 329:149–155.

Chapter 29

Diuretics

Juha P. Kokko, M.D., Ph.D.

Diuretics increase excretion of salt and water. While the primary clinical indication for their use is to decrease extracellular fluid volume, they have other uses not strictly related to their diuretic properties. This chapter will deal initially with understanding the nephrological sites affected and the molecular mechanism(s) of action of the various diuretics. The second part discusses the use and complications of the five major specific diuretic families. Finally, the clinical circumstances of special interest to the cardiologist will be emphasized. These include use in congestive heart failure and use as prophylaxis to prevent nephrotoxicity during radiocontrast infusions.

SITES AND MOLECULAR MECHANISM OF DIURETIC ACTION

Figure 29-1 shows schematically the various segments of the mammalian nephron and summarizes the principal transport mechanisms existing across these sites. The figure also contains an inset of the various families of diuretics with associated numbers that indicate those nephron segments where they exert their major effect.

Proximal Convoluted Tubule

The proximal convoluted tubule reabsorbs some two-thirds of the glomerular filtrate.[1] Since it is highly permeable to water,[2–7] the net fluid reabsorption across this segment occurs isoosmotically.[8–13] This reabsorption is complicated and occurs by both active and passive mechanisms. The proximal convoluted tubule reabsorbs most of the filtered glucose,[14–18] amino acids,[19–24] and other organic constituents as well as most of the bicarbonate.[14,25–31] With the reabsorption of the organic solutes and sodium bicarbonate early in the tubule, the remaining constituents are changed so that passive transport processes then contribute in a major way to net fluid reabsorption.[32]

One of the primary active transport processes contributing to the net fluid reabsorption across the proximal convoluted tubule is that of reabsorption of sodium bicarbonate by carbonic anhydrase–dependent mechanisms.[33–37] This explains the fact that net reabsorption of salt and fluid in the proximal convoluted tubule can be inhibited to a major extent by carbonic anhydrase inhibitors, such as acetazolamide (Diamox).[34,36] Similarly, since this segment is highly permeable to water and not permeable to solutes such as mannitol, it also is the primary site of action where tubular fluid reabsorption is inhibited by osmotic diuretics such as mannitol. It should be appreciated, however, that inhibition of proximal fluid tubule reabsorption has relatively small effect on net fluid homeostasis since nephron segments distal to the proximal tubule have tremendous unused capacity to reabsorb more salt and water if greater amounts are delivered to them. As a result, diuretics that have their major effect across the proximal tubule are weak diuretics.

Pars Recta

The pars recta is the straight component of the proximal tubule and also is highly permeable to water.[38,39] Thus, net fluid reabsorption across this segment, as is the case with the proximal convoluted segment, occurs isoosmotically. Since its capacity to reabsorb salt and water is

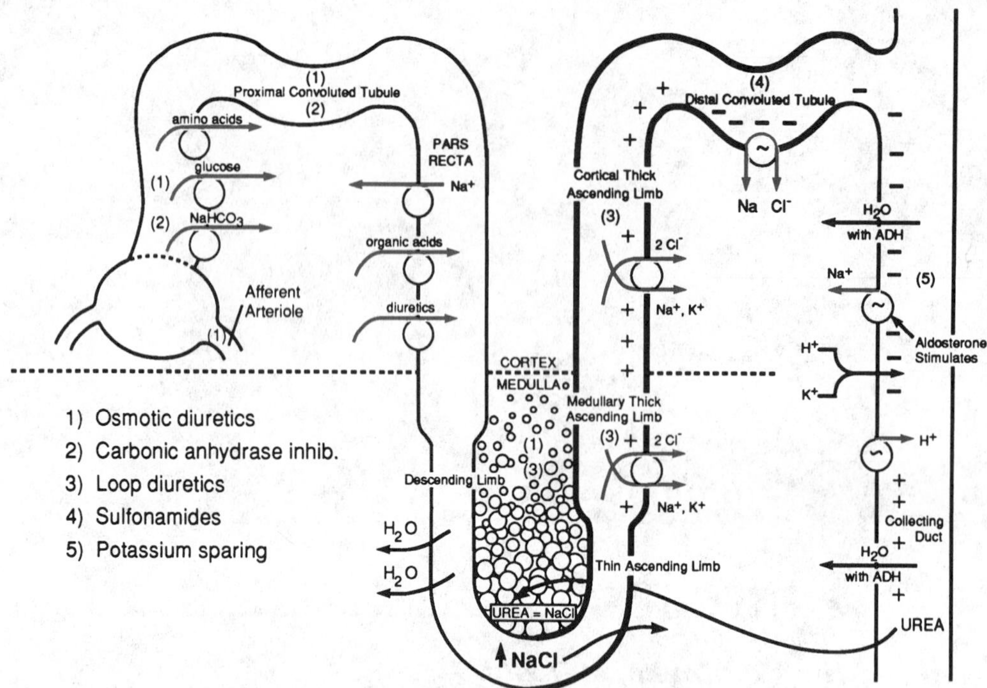

FIGURE 29-1 Major transport processes along the various segments of the mammalian nephron. The numbers refer to the respective site of action of the various diuretics. Blue lines represent active transport processes.

roughly a third of that of the proximal convoluted tubule,[40,41] inhibition of net salt and fluid reabsorption across the pars recta is clinically insignificant.

The pars recta is functionally important for the organic anion transport mechanism since it secretes many organic anions and cations including diuretics.[42–44] These secretory processes are important since all diuretics except spironolactone have their major effect from the urinary side of the tubule. It should be noted that diuretics are not filtered to a significant degree since they are carried in plasma by various nonfilterable proteins and that these secretory processes are critically important in obtaining clinically significant urinary concentrations of diuretics. The exact molecular mechanism of diuretic secretion has not been established, but membrane interactive processes on luminal as well as basolateral membranes play a role. Since organic anions and cations compete respectively with diuretics that are organic acids (thiazides, loop diuretics, acetazolamide) or organic bases (amiloride and triamterene) for secretory sites, it is not surprising that in clinical circumstances such as uremia and organic acidosis there is a lower concentration of organic acid diuretic in the urine for any given concentration of diuretic in the blood.[45–47] The urinary concentration of diuretics (determined by the pars recta) correlates more closely to the degree of induced natriuresis than do their blood concentrations.[48]

Descending Limb of Henle

Various lengths of descending limbs of Henle (DLH) descend toward the papillary tip into a normally progressively hypertonic environment (Fig. 29-1). Since all lengths of DLH are highly water permeable,[49–51] a significant amount of the fluid delivered to them from the proximal tubule is reabsorbed as a consequence of osmotic equilibration.[49] This segment does not possess any active transport processes to be inhibited by diuretics.[49] If loop diuretics obliterate the papillary hypertonicity by inhibiting active transport in segments generating this papillary hypertonicity, net water reabsorption will decrease significantly across the DLH. Indeed, a significant component of the increased *water* diuresis caused by diuretics is the result of decreased water reabsorption across the thin DLH.

Thin Ascending Limb of Henle

While the thin ascending limb of Henle is important for the countercurrent multiplication system, it does not have a major role in diuretic action since it is water impermeable and does not actively transport solutes transepithelially.[52–55]

Thick Ascending Limb of Henle

Both the cortical and the medullary thick ascending limb of Henle have important roles in diuretic function. The cortical thick ascending limb forms dilute urine while the function of the medullary thick ascending limb is to generate surroundings allowing formation of concentrated urine. Salt transport mechanisms are similar in both segments and are affected similarly by loop diuretics. Figure 29-2 summarizes schematically a secondary active chloride transport mechanism in these segments. Chloride is transported across epithelium against an electrochemical gradient,[56,57] but transport is dependent on the energy generated by the sodium potassium adenosinetriphosphatase (ATPase) on the blood side. Thus,

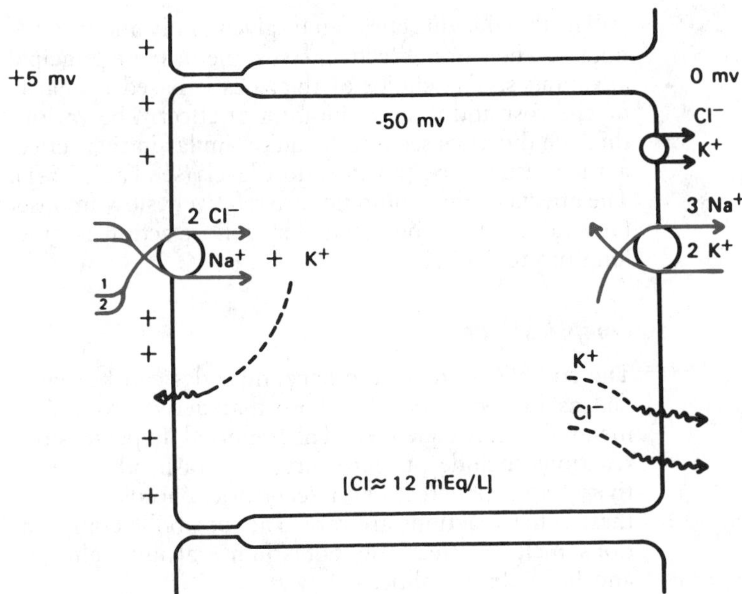

FIGURE 29-2 Cellular model of secondary active chloride transport across the thick ascending limb of Henle. The left side of the figure represents the luminal side with lumen positive +5 mV potential, the middle section is intracellular cytoplasm with −50 mV potential, while the right side of the figure is blood side at 0 mV potential. In this model, there are four ionic binding sites on the cotransport protein existing on the luminal surface. These binding sites must be occupied by sodium, potassium, and 2 chloride ions before translocation of these ions can take place from the luminal side into the intracellular space. The lumen positive potential occurs in a large part by potassium back diffusing into the lumen; it is this lumen positive potential difference that is responsible for a significant amount of passive sodium transport by paracellular routes. The loop diuretics compete for occupancy and act as a pseudosubstrate for one of the chloride transport sites, thus preventing the normal transport of chloride across this segment. Blue lines indicate membrane interactive transport processes.

active chloride transport is considered secondary.[58] In this model, the lumen positive potential difference (largely created by back diffusion of potassium into the lumen)[59] creates an electrochemical driving force for passive reabsorption of sodium through paracellular routes.[56,57] Thus, sodium is reabsorbed transcellularly and paracellularly while all chloride transport appears to be transcellular.[60]

The loop diuretics act lumenally to inhibit the Na-K-2Cl cotransporter, thus decreasing the lumen positive potential difference toward zero.[61–67] The mechanism is competitive inhibition of the chloride binding sites as a pseudosubstrate,[68,69] thus preventing the translocation of the electrolytes from the urinary side into the cell.

The thick ascending limb of Henle transports not only sodium and chloride by cotransporter but also divalent cations due to diffusion down the electrochemical gradient. While active calcium and magnesium transport mechanisms may exist in these segments, significant amounts of the cations are reabsorbed due to lumen positive potential differences.[70] Thus, loop diuretics that inhibit the lumen positive potential difference cause increased urinary loss of magnesium[71] as well as calcium.[72]

Distal Convoluted Tubule

The primary importance of the distal convoluted tubule in diuretic action is a luminal surface neutral sodium chloride transport mechanism[73,74] that is inhibited by thiazides.[73–77]

The process by which salt transport occurs out of the distal convoluted tubule is depicted in Fig. 29-1. Since this segment is impermeable to water with or without antidiuretic hormone,[78] it follows that it is also a diluting segment. Thus, thiazide diuretics inhibit the formation of dilute urine. This is the basis of thiazide-induced hyponatremia.[79] While some hydrogen and potassium secretion occurs, the capacity for transport of these ions is lower than that in the collecting duct.[80]

The Collecting Duct

The collecting duct traverses the cortex, outer medulla, and papilla, expressing functional differences in each area. However, the cortical collecting duct is the most important physiologically in the final urinary excretion of salt and acid-base in that it can be modified by the potassium-sparing diuretics. The cortical collecting tubule is composed of three primarily different types of cells that are depicted in Fig. 29-3.[81] The principal cell is involved with salt transport while the alpha and beta intercalated cells are involved with acid-base transport.

Aldosterone is the main determinant of the net transport of sodium across the principal cell.[78] In this cell, sodium gains access from lumen to intracellular space by traversing through sodium channels down electrochemical gradients.[82–87] The primary movement of sodium from lumen to cell creates a luminal electronegativity. Once the sodium is in the cell, it is pumped out by the peritubular sodium potassium ATPase whose activity is modulated by aldosterone levels.[88–95] Thus, increasing the sodium potassium ATPase activity by aldosterone increases net transport of sodium across this cell and creates a more lumen negative potential difference that favors passive secretion of hydrogen and potassium.

The primary effects of those diuretics affecting the collecting duct are upon the principal cell. Three different types of diuretics affect this segment. Amiloride and triamterene decrease the conductance of sodium channels and inhibit sodium reabsorption by that mechanism.[87,96] Spirolactones inhibit sodium reabsorption by competitive inhibition of the mineralocorticoid action.[97] Each of these compounds not only inhibits sodium reabsorption, but also secondarily decreases the generation of lumen negative potential difference and therefore is potassium sparing. These diuretics do not have clinically significant effects on salt and acid-base homeostasis across the more distal outer medullary or papillary collecting duct segments.

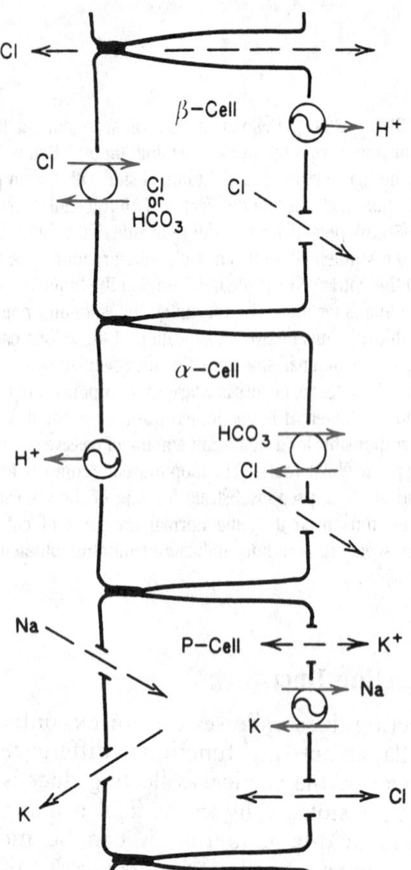

FIGURE 29-3 Schematics of the three cell types existing in the mammalian cortical collecting tubules. In each case the lumen is on the left side of the figure while the right side represents the blood side. The top two cells represent the two types of intercalated cells that are responsible for bicarbonate secretion (beta cell) and that are involved with acid secretion (alpha cell). The bottom cell summarizes the primary transport processes of the principal cell, which is responsible for salt transport and is the target organ for aldosterone. It is this cell that is primarily affected by the potassium-sparing diuretics. Blue lines indicate membrane interactive transport processes (*From V Schuster, J Stokes: Am J Physiol 22:F203–F212, 1987. Reproduced with permission from the publisher and the author.*)

DIURETIC FAMILIES

Benzothiazides

Mechanism of Action

While the thiazide diuretics were initially developed as inhibitors of carbonic anhydrase, studies in animals and humans led to the conclusion that their primary effect is to inhibit the function of the cortical diluting segment,[98–101] with no effect on sodium chloride transport in the medullary thick ascending limb of Henle.

The cortical diluting segment, however, includes epithelia of the cortical thick ascending limb of Henle, distal convoluted tubule, connecting tubule, and early segments of the cortical collecting duct. While there may be some species differences with respect to the exact site of action, thiazides appear to inhibit the electroneutral sodium-dependent chloride transport mechanism on the luminal side. The exact molecular mechanism of this inhibition is unknown.

The thiazide diuretics can be given orally and intravenously. Their oral effectiveness is one of their principal advantages. The choice of thiazides is based primarily on the cost and desired duration of effect. The various thiazide diuretics seem to be quite similar in their effect at their respective equivalent dose levels (see Table 29-1). The effects of these diuretics are relatively slow in onset (around 30 min), but their duration of action is quite long (up to 24 h).

Complications

The complications of the benzothiazides can be classified as idiosyncratic and those that derive from their metabolic consequences. The reported hypersensitive reactions include purpura, urticaria, rash, photosensitivity, and pancreatitis. Except for photosensitivity, these other reactions are rare. The metabolic complications include effects on potassium, calcium, glucose, and lipid abnormalities.

Hypokalemia The kaliuresis induced by thiazides results from increased delivery of sodium chloride to the potassium secretory segments of the nephron distal to the connecting segments. The resultant kaliuresis is highly dependent on the patient's aldosterone level. The higher the aldosterone level, the greater the potassium secretion.[102,103] While kaliuresis is an accepted consequence of thiazide therapy and drops in serum potassium of 0.4 to 0.8 meq/liter are not uncommon, significant total-body potassium deficiency (greater than 10 percent) is less common.[104–109] Approximately 20 to 30 percent of patients receiving normal doses of thiazides become hypokalemic to levels below 3.5 meq/liter and total potassium deficient to amounts greater than 10 percent of total-body potassium stores. It is interesting that the incidence of hypokalemia appears to be greater with thiazides than with loop diuretics, even though loop diuretics cause a higher fractional excretion of potassium.[108] This is because thiazides have a more prolonged effect. The shorter acting loop diuretics will have a longer nondiuretic compensatory period when the kidney can readjust to potassium deficits by increasing potassium reabsorption. It appears that those patients at the highest risk for developing potassium deficiency are those with the highest aldosterone levels, especially if coupled with a decreased potassium intake.

Thiazide-induced hypokalemia is causally associated with a number of untoward clinically significant side effects, including decreased insulin release (abnormal carbohydrate tolerance),[110–112] increased incidence of arrhythmias, both with and without digitalis,[113–120] decreased blood pressure with increased incidence of postural hypotension,[121–125] and potentiation of rhabdomyolysis.[126–130] Thus, potassium repletion should be considered in patients receiving thiazides, but by no means should this be a routine practice.[109,131] There are significant differences of opinion as to when to treat asymptomatic hypokalemia; however, it seems prudent that if patients are diabetic, have congestive heart failure, or are receiving digitalis, they should not be allowed to become total-body potassium deficient and their serum potassium should be kept at levels above 3.5 meq/liter.

TABLE 29-1
Oral Diuretic Agents

Generic Name	Trade Name	Usual Daily Dosage (mg)	Onset of Action (h)	Peak Effect (h)	Duration of Action (h)
Thiazide and related diuretics					
Bendroflumethiazide	Naturetin	2.5–15	2	4	6–12
Benzthiazide	Aquatag, Exna, Marazide	50–200	2	4–6	6–12
Chlorothiazide	Diuril, Diachlor, Diurigen	500–2000	1–2	4	6–12
Chlorthalidone	Hygroton, Hylidone	25–100	2	2–6	24–72
Cyclothiazide	Anhydron	2	Within 6	7–12	18–24
Hydrochlorothiazide	Esidrix, HydroDIURIL	25–100	2	4–6	6–12
Hydroflumethiazide	Diucardin, Saluron	50–200	2	4	6–12
Indapamide	Lozol	2.5–5	1–2	Within 2	Up to 36
Methylclothiazide	Enduron, Ethon	2.5–5	2	4–6	24
Metolazone	Diulo, Zaroxolyn	2.5–5	1	2	12–24
Polythiazide	Renese	2–4	2	6	24–48
Quinethazone	Hydromox	50–100	2	6	18–24
Trichlormethiazide	Metahydrin, Naqua	2–4	2	6	24
Loop diuretics					
Bumetanide	Bumex	0.5–2	0.5–1	1–2	4–6
Ethacrynic acid	Edecrin	50–100	Within 0.5	2	6–8
Furosemide	Lasix	29–80	Within 1	1–2	6–8
Potassium-sparing diuretics					
Amiloride	Midamor	5–20	2	6–10	24
Spironolactone	Aldactone	25–200	24–48	48–72	48–72
Triamterene	Dyrenium	200–300	2–4	6–8	12–16
Combination diuretics					
Amiloride and hydrochlorothiazide	Moduretic	5–10(A) 50–100(H)	See individual agents above	See individual agents above	See individual agents above
Spironolactone and hydrochlorothiazide	Aldactazide, Alazide	25–200(S) 25–200(H)	See individual agents above	See individual agents above	See individual agents above
Triamterene and hydrochlorothiazide	Maxide, Dyazide	37.5–100(T) 25–50(H)	See individual agents above	See individual agents above	See individual agents above

Compiled by Clyde Buchanan from Facts and Comparisons Drug Information, 1992.

Furthermore, patients who are at risk for developing arrhythmias, whether on digitalis or not, should also receive therapy to prevent potassium from falling below 3.5 meq/liter.[109,131] It has also been suggested that patients who are hospitalized with acute myocardial infarction have a mortality that increases if their serum potassium levels fall below 3.5 meq/liter.

Patients who are symptomatic from a decreased potassium concentration should be supplemented with potassium chloride.[109,131] There are numerous potassium supplements that are preferable to potassium-sparing diuretics since renal potassium regulatory processes are left unaltered with such supplementation.[132] In patients who refuse to take potassium supplements, it may be necessary to utilize a combination of potassium-sparing diuretics with thiazides.

Hyperglycemia Glucose intolerance may be associated with thiazides. Both in vitro and in vivo studies now suggest that the major reason is decreased beta-cell sensitivity to glucose during thiazide-induced hypokalemia with a fall of greater than approximately 1.0 meq/liter.[110–112] If potassium deficiency is prevented, glucose intolerance is not noted.[112]

Hyperuricemia Hyperuricemia is common in thiazide-treated patients, primarily due to circulatory volume contraction.[133,134] Volume contraction can cause proximal tubule reabsorption of all solutes including uric acid. The hyperuricemia with thiazides is usually mild (1 to 2 mg/dL) and of no clinical significance except in those patients with gout.[132] In nongouty patients the diuretic-induced hyperuricemia requires no therapy if uric acid levels are below 15 mg/dL.[135] The hyperuricemia usually responds rapidly to expansion of the effective arterial blood volume and discontinuation of thiazide diuretics. Probenecid can be given to lower uric acid if thiazides are needed in gouty patients.

Hypercalcemia Thiazides cause a 40 to 50 percent reduction in urine excretion of calcium.[136–138] The hypocalciuria is due to a direct thiazide effect to increase calcium reabsorption by the early portion of the distal tubule.[73] The reciprocal result of hypocalciuria, however, is a mild degree of hypercalcemia. Acutely, the rise may be 0.5 to 1.5 mg/dL, but with chronic use the expected rise in total serum calcium is often less than 0.2 mg/dL.[139,140] Clearly these changes are of no clinical significance unless they are superimposed on underlying hypercalcemia.

Hyperlipidemia Thiazide diuretics can increase total serum cholesterol by up to 10 percent.[141–147] Thiazides increase triglycerides, very low density lipoprotein (VLDL), and low-density lipoprotein (LDL) cholesterol by unknown mechanisms. Any changes in high-density lipoprotein (HDL) cholesterol are quite small or nonexistent.[148,149] Although controversial, some feel that even modest increases in cholesterol concentration can increase the rate of progression of atherosclerosis. In patients with hyperlipidemia or established atherosclerotic vascular disease, it is prudent to choose diuretics that do not induce hyperlipidemia.

Advantages

Thiazides have the advantages of being relatively inexpensive, orally active, and effective over an extended period.

Disadvantages

The primary disadvantages of thiazides are their relatively frequent metabolic side effects and their lower potency than loop diuretics in inducing salt and water excretion.

Use

Thiazides are indicated in those clinical states where mild diuresis is desired if no contraindications exist.[150] Low doses of thiazides are especially useful as antihypertensives. The antihypertensive effects can be obtained at such low doses that the expected adverse biochemical effects can be minimized.[151] Thiazide diuretics are not effective and are often contraindicated in chronic renal failure.

Loop Diuretics

The loop diuretics act by inhibiting transport of salt in the thick ascending limb of Henle. The three major diuretics in this group are furosemide, ethacrynic acid, and bumetanide. A number of newer loop diuretics are currently being developed but appear to have similar effects in clinically equivalent doses.

Mechanism of Action

As noted, the loop diuretics compete with chloride for occupancy of the luminal Na-K-2Cl cotransporter in the thick ascending limb of Henle (Fig. 29-2) and thus inhibit the translocation of sodium chloride from the luminal side to intracellular space.[152] In in vitro studies, the inhibition of salt transport across this segment occurs almost instantaneously, and once the diuretic is removed from the luminal fluid, the reabsorptive rate of chloride rapidly returns toward normal.[62,64,66,68] Since both the cortical and medullary thick ascending limbs of Henle are affected, it follows that both the diluting and concentrating capacities of the kidney are decreased. In vivo, these diuretics generally have a very rapid onset of action within minutes when given intravenously and within 30 min when given orally. They have a short duration of action of not more than 4 h. As noted, the loop diuretics are secreted into the urine by the pars recta by mechanisms that compete with endogenous organic acids.[45–47] Thus, under circumstances of organic acidosis, especially in the setting of chronic uremia, these diuretics have to be administered at higher than normal levels to achieve the same desired urinary concentration (see Table 29-2). Intravenous furosemide also produces venous vasodilatation, which may be beneficial in acute heart failure.

Complications Of Loop Diuretic Therapy

Loop diuretics as a group are quite well tolerated. Complications or adverse reactions generally can be classified into those due to hypersensitivity reactions to the drugs and those due to inhibition of the Na-K-2Cl cotransport mechanism. Hypersensitivity reactions are unpredictable and primarily dermatological with rare episodes of necrotizing angiitis, photosensitivity, exfoliative dermatitis, and pruritus. Rarely, hematologic reactions have been reported with thrombocytopenia and generalized suppression of the bone marrow. The predictable complications of loop diuretics are due to inhibition of the Na-K-2Cl cotransport mechanism. With this inhibition, there is an increased delivery of sodium and fluid to the cortical collecting tubule, resulting in increased kaliuresis. Usually, the fall in serum potassium concentration with loop diuretics is modest—0.3 to 0.4 meq/liter.[104,105,107,108,153] Only approximately 10 percent of patients develop hypokalemia of less than 3.5 meq/liter.[154,155] This degree of hypokalemia is less than that seen with thiazides—20 to 30 percent. The lower incidence of hypokalemia with the loop diuretics is due to their short duration of action. If the loop diuretics are combined with a chlorthalidone or other diuretic with a longer duration of action, the incidence of hypokalemia is increased significantly.[156,157]

Hypomagnesemia occurs with the loop diuretics since they inhibit magnesium reabsorption across the thick ascending limb of Henle and increase urinary magnesium excretion[158–161]; however, symptomatic hypomagnesemia is relatively rare except in the setting of chronic alcoholism or after prolonged use of the diuretics. Ventricular ectopy may occur as a consequence of decreased serum magnesium concentration, and magnesium deficiency should be corrected in patients with ventricular ec-

TABLE 29-2

Titration to Define a Single Effective Dose of Loop Diuretic in Patients with Chronic Renal Insufficiency

Creatinine clearance (mL/min)	20–50	<20
Starting dose		
Furosemide	40 mg IV	80 mg IV
Furosemide	80 mg PO	160 mg PO
Bumetanide	1 mg IV or PO	4 mg IV or PO
Ceiling dose		
Furosemide	120–160 mg IV	160–200 mg IV
Furosemide	240–320 mg PO	320–400 mg PO
Bumetanide	4–6 mg IV or PO	8–10 mg IV or PO

SOURCE: DC Brater.[48]

topy.[162,163] In some patients it is difficult to correct potassium deficiency until magnesium deficiency is corrected.

Metabolic alkalosis may occur with loop diuretics but is usually mild and of no clinical significance.[132] Hyperuricemia and hypoglycemia have also been reported with loop diuretics but less commonly than with the longer acting thiazide diuretics where the degree of hypokalemia may be greater. The mechanism of these metabolic abnormalities is similar to those induced by the thiazide diuretics discussed above.

One of the unique complications of loop diuretics has been ototoxicity. Ototoxicity has been reported with all the loop diuretics but was much more common in the past when very high doses were utilized.[164–168] Indeed, if cochlear function was checked before and after normal doses of loop diuretics by audiometry, no adverse effects were noted in a small study.[169] If the loop diuretics are given at high concentrations or if they are given with aminoglycosides or other ototoxic drugs, it is prudent to decrease or discontinue them if patients complain of buzzing in their ears or decreased hearing acuity. In most circumstances, ototoxicity is reversible, but irreversible ototoxicity has been reported.

Advantages

The advantages of the loop diuretics are their potency and rapid onset of action. They also exert their effect in most clinical states with metabolic abnormalities; however, increased doses must be given during organic acidosis.

Disadvantages

The two primary disadvantages of loop diuretics are cost and short duration of action. They should be discontinued if idiosyncratic reactions occur and should be discontinued or their dose reduced if major metabolic consequences occur.

Use

The loop diuretics can be used alone in essentially all instances where diuresis is indicated. They also are indicated in the first-line defense against hypercalcemia since these diuretics induce rapid calciuria.[158,159,170,171] This effect is due to inhibition of calcium reabsorption by the thick ascending limb of Henle, as noted.[172]

Potassium-Sparing Diuretics

As noted previously, spironolactone, amiloride, and triampterene cause natriuresis and antikaliuresis through effects across the cortical collecting tubule. As a group, these drugs induce a relatively mild natriuresis, and often the primary indication for their use is to produce potassium retention. The principal, but not sole, reason for the antikaliuresis is inhibition of the normally negative transepithelial potential difference across the cortical collecting tubule, which is the primary driving force for potassium secretion.[82–87] These diuretics have a relatively slow onset of action, especially the aldosterone receptor inhibitors. Transepithelial effects are not expressed until 3 or 4 h after administration in experimental studies, and it is usual for the maximal clinical effects of spirolactones to be seen only after several days. The effects of amiloride and triampterene are seen somewhat earlier, and their duration of action is in the intermediate range of 8 to 16 h.

Complications

A potential complication of the potassium-sparing diuretics is life-threatening hyperkalemia. In one study[173] hyperkalemia occurred in 8.6 percent of hospitalized patients receiving spironolactone. Life-threatening hyperkalemia has been reported in patients who have received these diuretics in a setting of renal insufficiency and diabetes, especially with the coadministration of potassium supplements.[174–178] Physicians should follow carefully the serum potassium concentration, especially in the initial phases of potassium-sparing diuretic use and should avoid the concurrent administration of potassium supplements and angiotensin converting enzyme (ACE) inhibitors. In addition, concurrent use of beta blockers and noninflammatory agents with potassium-sparing diuretics should be approached with some caution.[179]

Since the potassium-sparing diuretics also inhibit hydrogen ion secretion, one might expect that metabolic acidosis would be a common complication of their use. However, clinical experience has shown that metabolic acidosis is a relatively rare complication.[132]

A unique complication of spironolactone is gynecomastia.[180,181] The mechanism is not clear. This side effect has not been reported with sodium channel blockers. Various hypersensitivity reactions have been seen with the sodium channel blockers, and in some patients, nonspecific gastrointestinal symptoms such as nausea and anorexia occur.

Advantages

The primary advantage of this group of diuretics is to conserve potassium in patients with an intolerance to potassium supplementation or in whom potassium supplementation is not practical. Spironolactone is especially useful in those clinical states, such as cirrhosis, that are characterized by high concentrations of circulating aldosterone.

Disadvantages

The principal disadvantage of this group of diuretics is their lack of diuretic potency.

Use

The primary use of potassium-sparing diuretics is in the setting where potassium retention is desired. They also may be used as adjunct agents to potentiate other diuretics. Spironolactone is often indicated in patients with secondary aldosteronism as in cirrhosis and ascites.

Carbonic Anhydrase Inhibitors

Mechanism of Action

The principal diuretic effect of carbonic anhydrase inhibitors is the result of inhibition of carbonic anhydrase–mediated fluid reabsorption across the proximal convoluted tubule.[31-36] They also affect carbonic anhydrase–mediated processes in the distal tubule, but their primary diuretic effect (in contrast to the effect on hydrogen secretion) is through their effects on the proximal tubule. As a consequence, there is increased bicarbonate excretion and free-water formation. Because of a decrease in hydrogen ion excretion and an increase in delivery of bicarbonate to the collecting tubule, there is increased loss of potassium across the cortical collecting tubule. The onset of effect of carbonic anhydrase inhibitor occurs within minutes if given intravenously or within 30 min if given orally. The maximum effect occurs in several hours; the duration of action is 8 to 12 h.

Complications

Carbonic anhydrase inhibitors are remarkably nontoxic in both animals and in man. If acetazolamide is given at doses greater than 1 g per day, patients may complain of drowsiness and occasional numbness and tingling of fingers. At more clinically appropriate doses, however, this group of diuretics is well tolerated.

Carbonic anhydrase inhibitors have predictable metabolic complications. Metabolic acidosis is a necessary side effect since their primary effect is to increase excretion of bicarbonate; however, bicarbonate concentrations generally do not fall below 18 to 20 meq/liter,[182,183] and if more severe acidosis is demonstrated, other causes besides carbonic anhydrase inhibitors should be sought.[184,185] Since these diuretics increase distal delivery of non-reabsorbable bicarbonate, it is not surprising that kaliuresis is a common phenomenon and frank hypokalemia may occur, especially in the setting of increased aldosterone levels. Patients who are on maintenance levels of high doses of carbonic anhydrase inhibitors should have their serum potassium monitored.

Advantages

Carbonic anhydrase inhibitors generally are not used for their diuretic effects. In metabolic alkalosis they may have the advantage of promoting increased excretion of bicarbonate.

Disadvantages

Carbonic anhydrase inhibitors as a group are relatively ineffective diuretics.

Use

A primary use of carbonic anhydrase inhibitors is to alkalinize urine. This is especially useful when it is desirable to increase the excretion of those overdose drugs or toxins that are more soluble in alkaline urine. Carbonic anhydrase inhibitors may also increase excretion of endogenous compounds such as uric acid. Some use carbonic anhydrase inhibitors and volume expansion in the treatment of hematopoietic disorders in which high uric acid excretion rates are anticipated. They may also be useful in decreasing metabolic alkalosis, for example, in patients being weaned from a respirator.

Osmotic Diuretics

Mechanism of Action

Mannitol is the prototype osmotic diuretic. Under normal physiological conditions, mannitol has beneficial effects both on renal plasma flow and on the tubules causing decreased absorption of filtrate. The increase in renal plasma flow occurs as a consequence of at least three factors: increased plasma volume, increased release of atrial natriuretic peptide, and decreased resistance to renal plasma flow.[186-191] With increased renal plasma flow and with a decrease in the glomerular oncotic pressure caused by mannitol, there is a resultant increase in glomerular filtration rate.[190] Once this glomerular filtrate reaches the proximal tubule, there is a nonspecific inhibition of the proximal tubule reabsorption due to the osmotic effects of mannitol.[186] The onset of action of mannitol is immediate and its duration of action is only as long as the mannitol is still in circulation.

Complications

There are no specific complications associated with osmotic diuretics with the exception of increased blood volume.

Advantages

Mannitol is the most effective diuretic in restoring glomerular filtration rate during transient hypotension.[191,192]

Disadvantages

Mannitol must be given intravenously. Another disadvantage is that if it does not increase glomerular filtration rate, there is a danger of overexpansion of the blood volume with hyponatremia. Pulmonary edema can be produced or worsened.

Use

Osmotic diuretics are useful in many clinical settings with transiently decreased renal plasma flow. A decrease in renal plasma flow may occur during the induction phases of anesthesia or during the use of radiocontrast materials.[191] The dose of mannitol is 25 to 50 g as a single intravenous bolus in a 20 percent solution. If the urine flow does not increase within 10 min, further doses of mannitol are contraindicated. In those patients who respond favorably, a continuous infusion of a 10 to 15 percent solution may be started and continued as long as deemed necessary.

USE OF DIURETICS IN SPECIFIC CIRCUMSTANCES

Congestive Heart Failure

The primary reason for salt and water retention in acute congestive heart failure is the activation of the renin-angiotensin-aldosterone axis in a setting of low cardiac output with decreased blood flow to the kidney (Fig. 29-4).[193] Not only does the decrease in effective arterial blood volume increase proximal tubule reabsorption of salt and water, but sodium reabsorption is further increased by aldosterone-dependent mechanisms across the cortical collecting tubule.[88–95] Thus the therapeutic approaches to increasing natriuresis are fourfold: use of diuretics to increase salt excretion; use of ACE inhibitors to reduce afterload and increase renal blood flow; reduce salt and water intake; and increase cardiac output by inotropic agents. (See Chaps. 25 and 26.)

Generally speaking, the loop diuretics are most effective in moderate or severe congestive heart failure. They have the advantage of being potent natriuretic agents and being effective in patients with a wide variety of electrolyte abnormalities. Satisfactory diuresis can usually be obtained in patients with normal renal function with furosemide, 40 mg intravenously twice a day; ethacrynic acid, 50 mg intravenously twice a day; or bumetanide, 1 mg twice a day intravenously. If renal disease is present, the maximum necessary intravenous doses should be increased as summarized in Table 29-1.[48] If adequate diuresis is not achieved by the loop diuretics, a more proximally acting diuretic, such as metalazone, or a more distally acting diuretic, such as a potassium-sparing diuretic, can be added. Since the combination of metalazone and loop diuretics can lead to life-threatening hypokalemia, it is important to monitor carefully the serum potassium concentrations.[156,157]

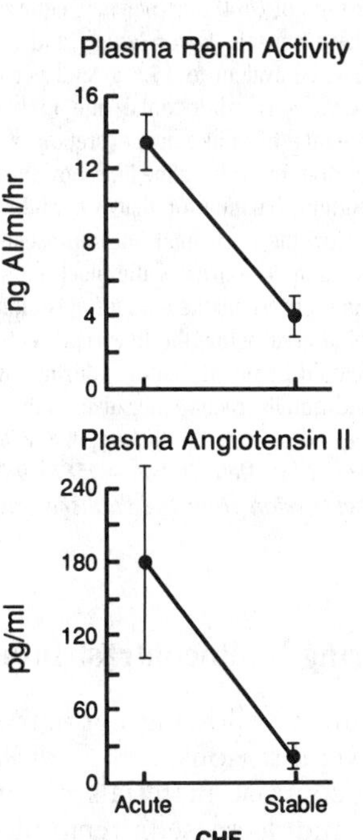

FIGURE 29-4 This figure demonstrates that in acute congestive heart failure, the renin-angiotensin system is activated (*left*) and that values return to normal once stabilization of congestive heart failure occurs (*right*). (*From VJ Dzau, WS Colucci, NK Hollenberg, et al: Circulation 63:645–651, 1981. Reproduced with permission from the publisher and the author.*)

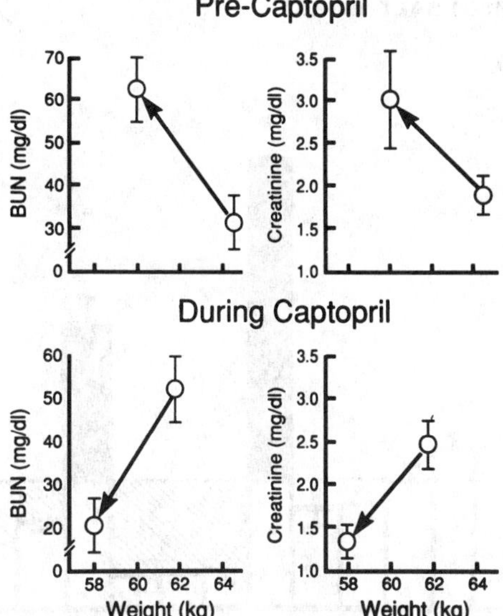

FIGURE 29-5 Studies in congestive heart failure patients that demonstrate the frequent finding whereby blood urea nitrogen (BUN) and creatinine increase with diuretics without the use of captopril, whereas with the additional use of captopril the BUN and creatinine can decrease with diuretics together with a reduction of edema and reduction of circulatory volume. (*From VJ Dzau, WS Colucci, GH Williams, et al: N Engl J Med, 302:1373–1379, 1980. Reproduced with permission from the publisher and the author.*)

One of the recent advances in the treatment of congestive heart failure is the appreciation of the importance of inhibiting the renin-angiotensin system.[194–197] Cardiologists are very aware that further forced decreases in effective arterial blood volume by diuretics in the setting of prerenal azotemia can worsen the degree of azotemia.[194] This adverse outcome can often be prevented with the simultaneous use of ACE inhibitors.[194] While the initial studies were conducted with captopril, similar beneficial effects on renal function in congestive heart failure have been seen with other ACE inhibitors.[198] Improved cardiac and renal function have been shown with the use of the combination of ACE inhibitors and diuretics both acutely (Fig. 29-5)[194] and chronically.[196,198,199] When ACE inhibitors are used in congestive heart failure and in the setting of presumed high angiotensin levels, it is prudent that an initial low dose is first used to be certain that an untoward hypotensive episode does not occur.[200] The potential for an inappropriate large decrease in blood pressure is more likely in patients who acutely or subacutely have elevated angiotensin levels than in patients who are in a steady state with elevated angiotensin levels, for example, those patients with high renin hypertension.

As noted in Chap. 26, salt restriction is a key component of treatment of congestive heart failure even with the use of diuretics and ACE inhibitors. Indeed, well-controlled studies have demonstrated that with a high sodium intake, loop diuretics given once a day fail to achieve a negative sodium balance.[201,202] The reason is

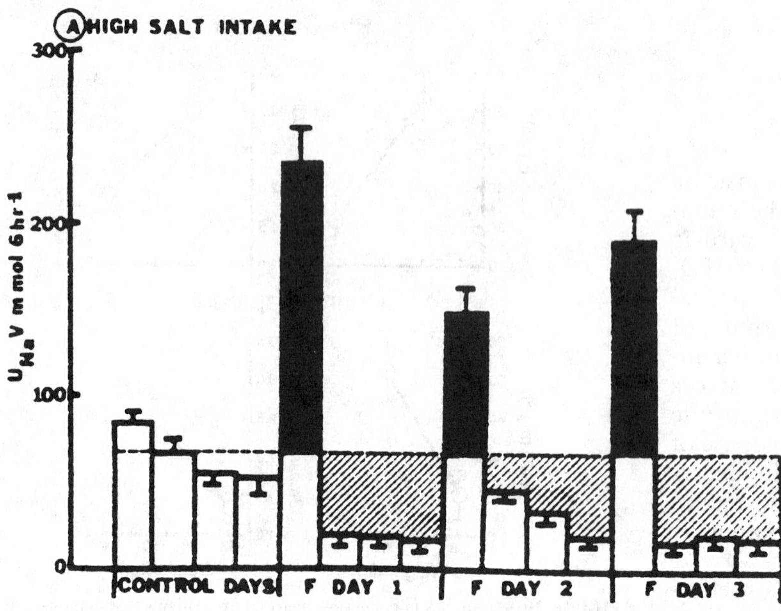

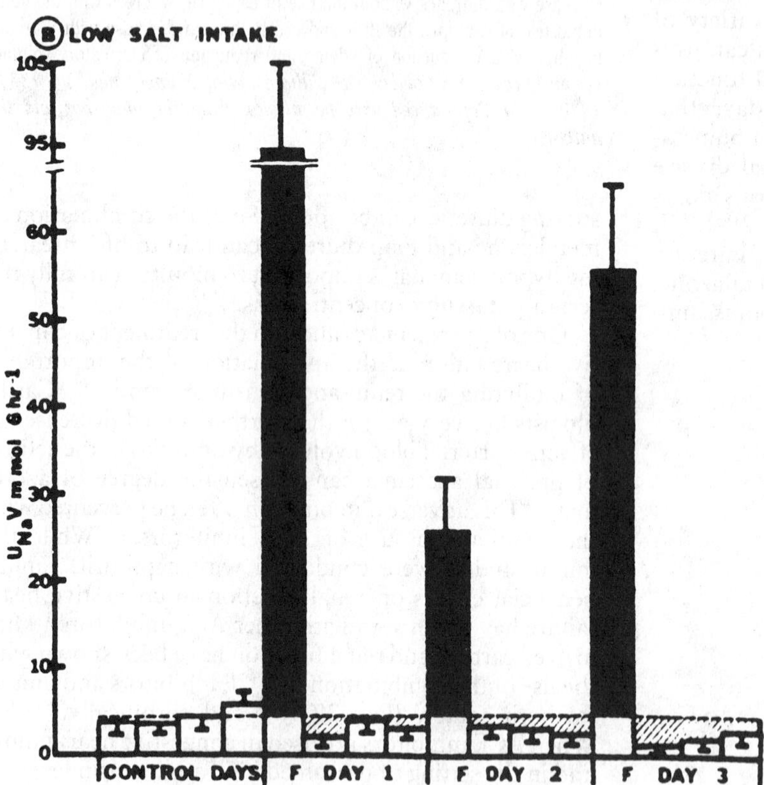

FIGURE 29-6 Mean 6-h balance studies of six normal subjects given 40 mg of furosemide on sodium intakes of 20 mmol (460 mg) per day, equivalent to 1.2 g NaCl per day (low salt, *lower panel*) and 270 mmol (6.2 g) per day, equivalent to 15.8 g NaCl per day (high salt, *upper panel*). The horizontal line in both panels represents balance of intake and excretion of sodium for that time period. Bars above the line show the magnitude of negative sodium balance for that 6 h while the distance of a bar below the horizontal line represents positive retention of sodium. The area of the black bars above the horizontal line represents the amount of sodium excretion, while the blue area below the line represents sodium retention. It should be noted that only during low salt intake do these individuals receive negative sodium balance for a 24-h period. (*From CS Wilcox, WE Mitch, RA Kelly, et al: J Lab Clin Med 102:450–458, 1983. Reproduced with permission from the publisher and the author.*)

that even though there is an impressive natriuresis for 3 h after the furosemide administration, there is a compensatory increase in sodium reabsorption in the remaining 24-h period that exactly matches the earlier losses, Fig. 29-6.[201] Thus, it is essential to limit the sodium intake to ensure negative sodium balances. Balance studies on normal humans have demonstrated that significant negative sodium balance can be predictably obtained with loop diuretics if sodium intake is limited to 20 meq/day (equivalent to 460 mg sodium or 1.2 g sodium chloride per day).

Diuretics during Radiocontrast Infusion

Acute renal failure following coronary angiography is not rare for several reasons[191,203–211]: direct tubular toxicity from radiocontrast materials,[212] intrarenal tubular obstruction,[213] and decrease in renal blood flow.[191,214–216] Radiocontrast-induced nephropathy is more common in individuals who have underlying renal disease and in those who have effective arterial blood volume contraction, such as in congestive heart failure.[210,217] In animal studies the decrease in renal blood flow after infusion of radiocontrast material may, in part, be due to increases in plasma and urinary concentrations of endothelin, a vasoconstrictor peptide.[218–220] Such a mechanism could contribute to radiocontrast-induced decrease in renal blood flow in humans.

In a recent study, 20 consecutive patients with chronic renal failure received mannitol for 2 h before and during cardiac catheterization in which diatrizoate was used.[191] Direct measurements of renal blood flow were made with thermodilution catheters in the left renal vein. In this study, the expected decrease in renal blood flow was not seen, and indeed renal blood flow increased in the diabetic subgroup of patients after receiving mannitol.[191] While these studies did demonstrate that mannitol can prevent a decrease in renal plasma flow, they also demonstrated a mean rise in serum creatinine of 0.2 mg/dL with mannitol, with a number of patients having a rise higher than 0.5 mg/dL. While this small study cannot be used to estimate the frequency of radiocontrast-induced nephropathy, it does show that the renal vasoconstrictive effect of radiocontrast infusion may be prevented by mannitol. It may therefore be prudent to suggest that selected patients be placed on mannitol diuresis prior to and during the cardiac catheterization. In the study cited[191] patients were infused with 15 percent mannitol mixed in 0.45 percent saline at the rate of 100 mL/h for 2 h before and during the cardiac catheterization. The use of other diuretics in the setting of expected acute renal failure in humans has not been as convincing as the results with mannitol.[221]

REFERENCES

1. Maddox DA, Gennari JF: The early proximal tubule: A high-capacity delivery-responsive reabsorptive site. *Am J Physiol* 1987; 252:F573–F584.
2. Ullrich KJ, Rumrich G, Fuchs G: Wasserpermeabilitat und transtubularer Wasserfluss corticaler Nephronabschnitte bei verschiedenen Diuresezustanden. *Pflugers Arch* 1964; 280:99–119.
3. Stolte H, Brecht JP, Wiederholt M, Hierholzer K: Einfluss von Adrenalektomie und Glucocorticoiden auf die Wasser-permeabilitat Cortikaler Nephronabschnitte der Rattenniere. *Pflugers Arch* 1968; 299:99–127.
4. Kokko JP, Burg MB, Orloff J: Characterization of NaCl and water transport in the renal proximal tubule. *J Clin Invest* 1971; 50:69–76.
5. Preisig PA, Berry CA: Evidence for transcellular osmotic water flow in rat proximal tubules. *Am J Physiol* 1985; 249:F124–F131.
6. DiBona GF: Effect of magnesium on water permeability of the rat nephron. *Am J Physiol* 1972; 223:1324–1326.
7. Green R, Giebisch G: Reflection coefficients and water permeability in rat proximal tubule. *Am J Physiol* 1989; 257:F658–F668.
8. Fromter EE, Rumrich G, Ullrich KJ: Phenomenological description of Na, Cl, and HCO_3 absorption from proximal tubules in the rat kidney. *Pflugers Arch* 1973; 343:189–220.
9. Green R, Giebisch G: Luminal hypotonicity: A driving force for fluid absorption from the proximal tubule. *Am J Physiol* 1984; 246:F167–F174.
10. Hierholzer K, Kawamura S, Seldin DW, Kokko JP, Jacobson HR: Reflection coefficients of various substrates across superficial and juxtamedullary proximal convoluted segments of rabbit nephrons. *Miner Electrolyte Metab* 1980; 3:172–180.
11. Jacobson HR, Kokko JP: Intrinsic differences in various segments of the proximal convoluted tubule. *J Clin Invest* 1976; 57:818–825.
12. Whittembury G, Oken DE, Windhager EE, Solomon AK: Single proximal tubules of Necturus kidney. IV. Dependence of H_2O movement on osmotic gradients. *Am J Physiol* 1959; 197:1121–1127.
13. Whittembury G, Paz-Aliaga A, Broudi A, Carpi-Medina P, Gonzales E, Linares H: Pathways for volume flow and volume regulation in leaky epithelia. *Pflugers Arch* 1985; 405:S17–S22.
14. Walker AM, Bott PA, Oliver J, MacDowell MC: The collection and analysis of fluid from single nephrons of the mammalian kidney. *Am J Physiol* 1941; 134:580–595.
15. Frohnert PP, Hohmann B, Zweibel R, Baumann K: Free flow micropuncture studies of glucose transport in the rat nephron. *Pflugers Arch* 1970; 315:66–85.
16. Barfuss DA, Schafer JA: Differences in active and passive glucose transport along the proximal tubule. *Am J Physiol* 1981; 240:F322–F332.
17. McKeown JW, Brazy PC, Dennis VW: Intrarenal heterogeneity for fluid, phosphate, and glucose absorption in the rabbit. *Am J Physiol* 1979; 237:F312–F318.
18. Tune BM, Burg MB: Glucose transport by proximal renal tubules. *Am J Physiol* 1971; 221:580–585.
19. Lingard J, Rumrich G, Young JA: Reabsorption of L-glutamine and L-histidine from various regions of the rat proximal convolution studied by stationary microperfusion: Evidence that the proximal convolution is not homogeneous. *Pflugers Arch* 1973; 342:1–12.
20. Bergeron M, Morel F: Amino acid transport in rat renal tubules. *Am J Physiol* 1969; 216:1139–1149.
21. Wright LA, Nicholson TF: The proximal tubular handling of amino acids and other ninhydrin-positive substances. *Can J Physiol Pharmacol* 1966; 44:183–193.
22. Eisenbach GM, Weise M, Stolte H: Amino acid reabsorption in the rat nephron. *Pflugers Arch* 1975; 357:63–76.
23. Silbernagl S: Tubular reabsorption of L-glutamine studied by free-flow micropuncture and microperfusion of rat kidney. *Int J Biochem* 1980; 12:9–16.
24. Lingard J, Rumrich G, Young JA: Kinetics of L-histidine transport in the proximal convolution of the rat nephron studied using the stationary microperfusion technique. *Pflugers Arch* 1973; 342:13–28.
25. Liu F-Y, Cogan MG: Axial heterogeneity in the rat proximal convoluted tubule. I. Bicarbonate, chloride, and water transport. *Am J Physiol* 1984; 247:F816–F821.
26. Liu F-Y, Cogan MG: Axial heterogeneity of bicarbonate, chloride and water transport in the rat proximal convoluted tubule. *J Clin Invest* 1986; 78:1547–1557.
27. Maddox DA, Atherton LJ, Deen WM, Gennari FJ: Proximal HCO_3 reabsorption and the determinants of tubular and capillary PCO_2 in the rat. *Am J Physiol* 1984; 247:F73–F81.
28. Maddox DA, Gennari FJ: Load dependence of HCO_3 and H_2O reabsorption in the early proximal tubule of the Munich-Wistar rat. *Am J Physiol* 1985; 248:F113–F121.
29. Maddox DA, Gennari FJ: Load dependence of proximal tubular bicarbonate reabsorption in chronic metabolic alkalosis in the rat. *J Clin Invest* 1986; 77:709–716.
30. Maddox DA, Horn JF, Famiano FC, Gennari FJ: Load dependence of proximal tubular fluid and bicarbonate reabsorption in the remnant kidney of the Munich-Wistar rat. *J Clin Invest* 1986; 77:1639–1649.
31. Jacobson HR: Effects of CO_2 and acetazolamide on bicarbonate and fluid reabsorption in rabbit proximal tubules. *Am J Physiol* 1981; 240:F54–F62.
32. Neumann KH, Rector FC: Mechanism of NaCl and water reabsorption in the proximal convoluted tubule of the rat kidney. *J Clin Invest* 1976; 58:1110–1118.
33. Rector FC, Carter NW, Seldin DW: The mechanism of bicarbonate reabsorption in the proximal and distal tubules of the kidney. *J Clin Invest* 1965: 44:278–290.
34. Lucci MS, Tinker JP, Weiner IM, DuBose TD: Function of proximal tubule carbonic anhydrase defined by selective inhibition. *Am J Physiol* 1983; 245:F443–F449.
35. Rector FC: Sodium, bicarbonate, and chloride absorption by the proximal tubule. *Am J Physiol* 1983; 244:F461–F471.
36. Cogan MG, Maddox DA, Warnock DG, Lin ET, Rector FC: Effect of acetazolamide on bicarbonate reabsorption in the proximal tubule of the rat. *Am J Physiol* 1979; 237:F447–F454.
37. Aronson PS: Mechanisms of active H^+ secretion in the proximal tubule. *Am J Physiol* 1983; 245:F647–F659.

38. Schafer JA, Patlak CS, Troutman SL, Andreoli TE: Volume absorption in the pars recta. II. Hydraulic conductivity coefficient. *Am J Physiol* 1978; 234:F340–F348.
39. Schafer JA: Mechanisms coupling the absorption of solute and water in the proximal nephron. *Kidney Int* 1984; 25:708–716.
40. Kawamura S, Imai M, Seldin DW, Kokko JP: Characteristics of salt and water transport in superficial and juxtamedullary straight segments of proximal tubules. *J Clinical Invest* 1975; 55:1269–1277.
41. Schafter JA, Troutman SL, Andreoli TE: Volume reabsorption, transepithelial potential differences and ionic permeability properties in mammalian superficial proximal straight tubules. *J Gen Physiol* 1974; 64:582–607.
42. Weiner IM: Organic acids and bases and uric acid. In: Seldin DW, Giebisch G (eds): *The Kidney: Physiology and Pathophysiology*. New York, Raven, 1985: 1703–1724.
43. Wright SH, Wunz TM: Amiloride transport in rabbit renal brush-border membrane vesicles. *Am J Physiol* 1989; 256:F462–F468.
44. Dantzler WH, Wright SH, Chatsudthipong V, Brokl OH: Basolateral tetraethylammonium transport in intact tubules: Specificity and transstimulation. *Am J Physiol* 1991; 261:F386–F392.
45. Rose HJ, O'Malley K, Pruitt AW: Depression of renal clearance of furosemide in man by azotemia. *Clin Pharmacol Ther* 1976; 21:141–146.
46. Rose HJ, Pruitt AW, Dayton PG, McNay JL: Relationship of urinary furosemide excretion rate to natriuretic effect in experimental azotemia. *J Pharmacol Exp Ther* 1976; 199:490–497.
47. Rose HJ, Pruitt AW, McNay JL: Effect of experimental azotemia on renal clearance of furosemide in the dog. *J Pharmacol Exp Ther* 1976; 196:238–248.
48. Brater DC: Use of diuretics in chronic renal insufficiency and nephrotic syndrome. *Semin Nephrol* 1988; 8:333–341.
49. Kokko JP: Sodium chloride and water transport in the descending limb of Henle. *J Clin Invest* 1970; 49:1838–1846.
50. Imai M, Hayashi M, Araki M: Functional heterogeneity of the descending limbs of Henle's loop. I. Internephron heterogeneity in the hamster kidney. *Pflugers Arch* 1984; 402:385–392.
51. Imai M, Taniguchi J, Yoshitomi K: Transition of permeability properties along the descending limb of long-loop nephron. *Am J Physiol* 1988; 254:F323–F328.
52. Imai M, Kokko JP: Sodium, chloride, urea, and water transport in the thin ascending limb of Henle. *J Clin Invest* 1974; 53:393–402.
53. Morgan T, Berliner RW: Permeability of the loop of Henle, vasa recta, and collecting duct to water, urea, and sodium. *Am J Physiol* 1968; 215:108–115.
54. Imai M: Function of the thin ascending limbs of Henle of rats and hamsters perfused in vitro. *Am J Physiol* 1977; 232:F201–F209.
55. Kondo Y, Imai M: Effect of glutaraldehyde on renal tubular function. II. Selective inhibition of Cl^- transport in the hamster thin ascending limb of Henle's loop. *Pflugers Arch* 1987; 408:484–490.
56. Burg M, Green N: Function of the thick ascending limb of Henle's loop. *Am J Physiol* 1973; 224:659–668.
57. Rocha AS, Kokko JP: Sodium chloride and water transport in the medullary thick ascending limb of Henle. Evidence for active chloride transport. *J Clin Invest* 1973; 52:612–623.
58. Kedem O: Criteria of active transport. In: Kleinzeller A, Kityk A (eds): *Membrane Transport and Metabolism*. Prague, Czechoslovak Academy of Sciences, 1961: 87–93.
59. Greger R, Schlatter E: Properties of the lumen membrane of the cortical thick ascending limb of Henle's loop of rabbit kidney. *Pflugers Arch* 1983; 396:315–324.
60. Hebert SC, Andreoli TE: Control of NaCl transport in the thick ascending limb. *Am J Physiol* 1984; 246:F745–F756.
61. Burg M, Green N: Effect of ethacrynic acid on the thick ascending limb of Henle's loop. *Kidney Int* 1973; 4:301–308.
62. Burg M, Stoner L, Cardinal J, Green N: Furosemide effect on isolated perfused tubules. *Am J Physiol* 1973; 225:119–224.
63. Greger R: Coupled transport of Na^+ and Cl^- in the thick ascending limb of Henle's loop of rabbit nephron. *Scand J Audiol* 1981; 14:1–15.
64. Greger R, Schlatter E: Cellular mechanism of the action of loop diuretics on the thick ascending limb of Henle's loop. *Kli Wochenschr* 1983; 61:1019–1027.
65. Kokko JP: Membrane characteristics governing salt and water transport in the loop of Henle. *Fed Proc* 1974; 33:25–30.
66. Imai M: Effect of bumetanide and furosemide on the thick ascending limb of Henle's loop of rabbits and rats perfused in vitro. *Eur J Pharmacol* 1977; 41:409–416.
67. Wangemann P, Wittner M, DiStefano A, Englert HC, Lang HJ, Schlatter E, et al: Cl^- channel blockers in the thick ascending limb of the loop of Henle. *Pflugers Arch* 1986; 407:S128–S141.
68. Greven J: Studies on the renal receptors of loop diuretics. *Clin Exp Hyper Theory Pract* 1983; A5:193–208.
69. Greven J: The pharmacological basis of the action of loop diuretics. In: Puschett JB, Greenberg A (eds): *Diuretics II*. New York, Elsevier Science, 1986: 173–181.
70. Quamme GA: Control of magnesium transport in the thick ascending limb. *Am J Physiol* 1989; 256:F197–F210.
71. Quamme GA: Effect of furosemide on calcium and magnesium transport in the rat nephron. *Am J Physiol* 1981; 241:F340–F347.
72. Suki WN, Rouse D, Ng RCK, Kokko JP: Calcium transport in the thick ascending limb of Henle. Heterogeneity of function in the medullary and cortical segments. *J Clin Invest* 1980; 66:1004–1009.
73. Costanzo LS, Windhager EE: Calcium and sodium transport by the distal convoluted tubule of the rat. *Am J Physiol* 1978; 235:F493–F506.
74. Shimizu T, Yoshitomi K, Nakamura M, Imai M: Site and mechanism of action of trichlormethiazide in rabbit distal nephron segments perfused in vitro. *J Clin Invest* 1988; 82:721–730.
75. Stokes J, Lee I, D'Amico M: Sodium chloride absorption by the urinary bladder of the winter flounder. A thiazide-sensitive, electrically neutral transport system. *J Clin Invest* 1984; 74: 7–16.
76. Ellison DH, Velazquez H, Wright FS: Thiazide-sensitive sodium chloride cotransport in early distal tubule. *Am J Physiol* 1987; 253:F546–F554.
77. Kunau RT, Weller DR, Webb HL: Clarification of the site of action of chlorothiazide in the rat nephron. *J Clin Invest* 1975: 56:401–407.
78. Gross JB, Imai M, Kokko JP: A functional comparison of the cortical collecting tubule and the distal convoluted tubule. *J Clin Invest* 1975; 55:1284–1294.
79. Ashraf N, Locksley R, Arieff A: Thiazide-induced hyponatremia associated with death or neurologic damage in outpatients. *Am J Med* 1981; 70:1163–1168.
80. Lucci MS, Pucacco LR, Carter NW, DuBose TD: Evaluation of bicarbonate transport in rat distal tubule: Effects of acid-base status. *Am J Physiol* 1982; 243:F335–F341.
81. Schuster VL, Stokes JB: Chloride transport by the cortical and outer medullary collecting duct. *Am J Physiol* 1987; 253:F203–F212.
82. Koeppen BM, Biagi BA, Giebisch G: Intracellular microelectrode characterization of the rabbit cortical collecting duct. *Am J Physiol* 1983; 244:F35–F47.
83. O'Neil RG, Helman SI: Transport characteristics of renal collecting tubules: Influences of DOCA and diet. *Am J Physiol* 1977; 233:F544–F558.
84. O'Neil RG, Sansom SC: Characterization of apical cell membrane Na^+ and K^+ conductances of cortical collecting duct using microelectrode techniques. *Am J Physiol* 1984; 247:F14–F24.
85. O'Neil RG, Sansom SC: Electrophysiological properties of cellular and paracellular conductive pathways of the rabbit cortical collecting duct. *J Membr Biol* 1984; 82:281–295.
86. Palmer LG, Frindt G: Amiloride-sensitive Na channels from the apical membrane of the rat cortical collecting tubule. *Proc Natl Acad Sci USA* 1986; 83:2767–2770.
87. Ling BN, Hinton CF, Eaton DC: Amiloride-sensitive sodium channels in rabbit cortical collecting tubule primary cultures. *Am J Physiol* 1991; 261:F933–F944.
88. Doucet A, Morel F, Katz AI: Microdetermination of Na-K-ATPase in single tubules: Its application for the localization of physiologic processes in the nephron. *Int J Biochem* 1980; 12:47–52.
89. El Mernissi G, Chabardes D, Doucet A, Hus-Citharel A, Imbert-Teboul M, Le Bouffiant F, et al: Changes in tubular basolateral membrane markers after chronic DOCA treatment. *Am J Physiol* 1983; 245:F100–F109.
90. Garg LC, Knepper MA, Burg MB: Mineralocorticoid effects on

Na-K-ATPase in individual nephron segments. *Am J Physiol* 1981; 240:F536–F544.

91. Horster M, Schmid H, Schimidt V: Aldosterone in vitro restores nephron Na-K-ATPase of distal segments from adrenalectomized rabbits. *Pflugers Arch* 1980; 384:203–206.
92. LeHir M, Kaissling B, Dubach UC: Distal tubular segments of the rabbit kidney after adaptation to altered Na- and K-intake. II. Changes in Na-K-ATPase activity. *Cell Tissue Res* 1982; 224:493–504.
93. Mujais SK, Chekal MA, Jones WJ, Hayslett JP, Katz AI: Regulation of renal Na-K-ATPase in the rat. *J Clin Invest* 1984; 73: 13–19.
94. O'Neil RG, Hayhurst RA: Sodium-dependent modulation of the renal Na-K-ATPase: Influence of mineralocorticoids on the cortical collecting duct. *J Membr Biol* 1985; 85:169–179.
95. Petty KJ, Kokko JP, Marver D: Secondary effect of aldosterone on Na-K-ATPase activity in the rabbit cortical collecting tubule. *J Clin Invest* 1981; 68:1514–1521.
96. Helman SI, Kizer NL: Apical sodium ion channels of tight epithelia as viewed from the perspective of noise analysis. *Cur Top Membr Transport* 1990; 37:117–155.
97. Fanestil DD: Mechanism of action of aldosterone blockers. *Semin Nephrol* 1988; 8:240–263.
98. Early LE, Kahn M, Orloff J: The effects of infusions of chlorothiazide on urinary dilution and concentration in the dog. *J Clin Invest* 1961; 40:857–866.
99. Suki W, Rector FC, Seldin DW: The site of action of furosemide and other sulfonamide diuretics in the dog. *J Clin Invest* 1965; 44:1458–1469.
100. Seldin DW, Eknoyan G, Suki WN, Rector FC: Localization of diuretic action from the pattern of water and electrolyte excretion. *Ann NY Acad Sci* 1966; 139:328–343.
101. Velazquez H, Wright FS: Effect of diuretic drugs on Na, Cl, and K transport by rat renal distal tubule. *Am J Physiol* 1986; 250:F1013–F1023.
102. Schwartz GJ, Burg MB: Mineralocorticoid effects on cation transport by cortical collecting tubules in vitro. *Am J Physiol* 1978; 235:576–585.
103. Field MJ, Stanton BA, Giebisch G: Differential acute effects of aldosterone, dexamethasone, and hyperkalemia on distal tubule potassium secretion in the rat kidney. *J Clin Invest* 1984; 74:1792–1802.
104. Finnerty FA, Maxwell MH, Kuhn J, Moser M: Long-term effects of furosemide and hydrochlorothiazide in patients with essential hypertension. *Angiology* 1977; 28:125–133.
105. Morgan DB, Davidson C: Hypokalemia and diuretics: An analysis of publications. *Br Med J* 1980; 280:905–908.
106. Multicenter Cooperative Study Group: Multiclinic comparison of amiloride, hydrochlorothiazide, and hydrochlorothiazide plus amiloride in essential hypertension. *Arch Intern Med* 1981; 141:482–486.
107. Araoye MA, Chang MY, Khatri IM, Freise D: Furosemide compared with hydrochlorothiazide. *JAMA* 1978; 240:1863–1866.
108. Anderson J, Godfrey BE, Hill DM, Munro-Faure AD, Sheldon J: A comparison of the effects of hydrochlorothiazide and furosemide in the treatment of hypertensive patients. *Q J Med* 1971; 15:541–560.
109. Schnaper HW, Freis ED, Friedman RG, Garland WT, Hall WD, Hollifield J, et al: Potassium restoration in hypertensive patients made hypokalemic by hydrochlorothiazide. *Arch Intern Med* 1989; 149:2677–2681.
110. Gorden P: Glucose intolerance with hypokalemia. *Diabetes* 1973; 22:544–551.
111. Sagild U, Andersen V, Andreasen PB: Glucose tolerance and insulin responsiveness in experimental potassium depletion. *Acta Med Scand* 1961; 169:243–251.
112. Helderman JH, Elahi D, Andersen DK, Raizes GS, Tobin JD, Schocken D, et al: Prevention of the glucose intolerance of thiazide diuretics by maintenance of body potassium. *Diabetes* 1983; 32:106–111.
113. Dyckner T, Helmers C, Lundman T, Wester PO: Initial serum potassium level in relation to early complications and prognosis in patients with acute myocardial infarction. *Acta Med Scand* 1975; 197:207–210.
114. Dyckner T, Helmers C, Wester PO: Cardiac dysrhythmias in patients with acute myocardial infarction: Relation to serum potassium level and prior diuretic therapy. *Acta Med Scand* 1984; 216:127–132.
115. Solomon RJ, Cole AG: Importance of potassium in patients with acute myocardial infarction. *Acta Med Scand* 1981; 647(suppl):87–93.
116. Nordrehaug JE, von der Lippe G: Hypokalemia and ventricular fibrillation in acute myocardial infarction. *Br Heart J* 1983; 50:525–529.
117. Johansson BW, Dziamski R: Malignant arrhythmias in acute myocardial infarction: Relationship to serum potassium and effect of selective and nonselective beta-blockade. *Drugs* 1984; 28(suppl 1):77-85.
118. Steiness E, Olesen KH: Cardiac arrhythmias induced by hypokalemia and potassium loss during maintenance digoxin therapy. *Br Heart J* 1976; 38:167–172.
119. Jelliffe RW: Effect of serum potassium level upon risk of digitalis toxicity. *Ann Intern Med* 1973; 78:821.
120. Seller RH: The role of magnesium in digitalis toxicity. *Am Heart J* 1971; 82:551–556.
121. Tannen RL: Potassium and blood pressure control. *Ann Intern Med* 1983; 98:773–780.
122. Paller MS, Linas SL: Hemodynamic effects of alterations in potassium. *Hypertension* 1982; 4(suppl):111-20–111-26.
123. Paller MS, Douglas JG, Linas SL: Mechanism of decreased vascular reactivity to angiotensin II in conscious, potassium-deficient rats. *J Clin Invest* 1984; 73:74–79.
124. Linas SL, Dickmann D: Mechanism of the decreased renal blood flow in the potassium-depleted conscious rat. *Kidney Int* 1982; 21:757–764.
125. Abbrecht PH: Cardiovascular effects of chronic potassium deficiency in the dog. *Am J Physiol* 1972; 223:555-560.
126. Knochel JP, Schlein EM: On the mechanism of rhabdomyolysis in potassium depletion. *J Clin Invest* 1972; 51:1750–1758.
127. Dominic JA, Koch M, Guthrie CP, Gallas JH: Primary aldosteronism presenting as myoglobinuric acute renal failure. *Arch Intern Med* 1978; 138:1433–1434.
128. Nadel SM, Jackson JW, Ploth DW: Hypokalemic rhabdomyolysis and acute renal failure: Occurrence following total parenteral nutrition. *JAMA* 1979; 241:2294–2296.
129. Bierbach H, Bohl J, Goldner HJ, Majdandzic J: Hypokalemic rhabdomyolysis associated with Barter's syndrome. *Klin Wochenschr* 1983; 61:183–186.
130. Patterson RE, Haut MJ, Montgomery CA, Lowensohn HS, McQuilken CT, Djuh YY, et al: Natural history of potassium-deficiency myopathy in the dog: Role of adrenocorticosteroid in rhabdomyolysis. *J Lab Clin Med* 1983; 102: 565–576.
131. Kaplan NM, Carnegie A, Raskin P, Heller JA, Simmons M: Potassium supplementation in hypertensive patients with diuretic-induced hypokalemia. *N Engl J Med* 1985; 12:746–749.
132. Nader PC, Thompson JR, Alpern RJ: Complications of diuretic use. *Semin Nephrol* 1988; 8:365–387.
133. Suki WN, Hull AR, Rector FC: Mechanism of the effect of thiazide diuretics on calcium and uric acid. *J Clin Invest* 1967; 46:1121.
134. Manuel MA, Steele TH: Changes in renal urate handling after prolonged thiazide treatment. *Am J Med* 1974; 57:741–746.
135. Langford HG, Blaufox MD, Borhani NO, Curb JD, Molteni A, Schneider KA, et al: Is thiazide-produced uric acid elevation harmful? *Arch Intern Med* 1987; 147:645–649.
136. Brickman AS, Massry SG, Coburn JW: Changes in serum and urinary calcium during treatment with hydrochlorothiazide: Studies on mechanisms. *J Clin Invest* 1972; 51:945–954.
137. Seitz H, Jaworski ZF: Effect of hydrochlorothiazide on serum and urinary calcium and urinary citrate. *Can Med Assoc J* 1964; 90:414–420.
138. Duarte CG, Winnacker JL, Becker KL, Pace A: Thiazide-induced hypercalcemia. *N Engl J Med* 1971; 284:828–830.
139. Yendt ER, Guay GF, Garcia DA: The use of thiazides in the prevention of renal calculi. *Can Med Assoc J* 1970; 102: 614–620.
140. Ljunghall S, Backman U, Danielson BG, Fellström B, Johansson G, Wikström B: Calcium and magnesium metabolism during long-term treatment with thiazides. *Scand J Urol Nephrol* 1981; 15:257–262.
141. Ames RP, Hill P: Antihypertensive therapy and the risk of coronary heart disease. *J Cardiol Pharm* 1982; 4:206–212.

142. Boehringer K, Weidmann P, Mordasini R, Schiffl H, Bachmann C, Riesen W: Menopause-dependent plasma lipoprotein alterations in diuretic-treated women. *Ann Intern Med* 1982; 97:206–209.
143. Gluck Z, Weidmann P, Mordasini R, et al: Increased serum low-density lipoprotein cholesterol in men treated short term with the diuretic chlorthalidone. *Metabolism* 1980; 29:240–245.
144. Grimm RH, Leon AS, Hunninghake DB, Lenz K, Hannan P, Blackburn H: Effects of thiazide diuretics on plasma lipids and lipoproteins in mildly hypertensive patients. *Ann Intern Med* 1981; 94:7–11.
145. Ames RP, Hill P: Elevation of serum lipid levels during diuretic therapy of hypertension. *Am J Med* 1976; 61:748–757.
146. Chrysant SG, Neller GK, Dillard B, et al: Effects of diuretics on lipid metabolism in patients with essential hypertension. *Angiology* 1976; 27:707–711.
147. Goldman AI, Steele BW, Schnaper HW, Fitz AE, Frohlich ED, Perry HM Jr: Serum lipoprotein levels during chlorthalidone therapy. A Veteran Administration–National Heart, Lung, and Blood Institute Cooperative Study on Antihypertensive Therapy: Mild Hypertension. *JAMA* 1980; 244:1691–1695.
148. Lasser NL, Grandits G, Caggiula AW, Cutler JA, Grimm RH Jr, Kuller LH, et al: Effects of antihypertensive therapy of plasma lipids and lipoproteins in the multiple risk factor intervention trial. *Am J Med* 1984; 76:52–66.
149. Middeke M, Weisweiler P, Schwandt P, et al: Serum lipoproteins during antihypertensive therapy with beta blockers and diuretics: A controlled long-term comparative trial. *Clin Cardiol* 1987; 10:94–98.
150. Black HR: Metabolic considerations in the choice of therapy for the patient with hypertension. *Am Heart J* 1991; 121:707–715.
151. Carlsen JE, Kober L, Torp-Pedersen C, Johansen P: Relation between dose of bendrofluazide, antihypertensive effect, and adverse biochemical effects. *Br Med J* 1990; 300:975–978.
152. Kinne R: Molecular properties of the sodium-potassium-chloride cotransport system in the kidney. In: Puschett JB, Greenberg A (eds): *Diuretics II: Chemistry, Pharmacology, and Clinical Applications.* New York, Elsevier Science, 1987: 138–144.
153. Dargie HJ, Boddy K, Kennedy AC, King PC, Read PR, Ward DM: Total body potassium and long term furosemide therapy: Is potassium supplementation necessary? *Br Med J* 1974; 4:316–319.
154. Manner RJ, Brechbill DO, Dewitt K: Prevalence of hypokalemia in diuretic therapy. *Clin Med* 1972; 79:15–18.
155. Licht JH, Haley RJ, Pugh B, Lewis SB: Diuretic regimens in essential hypertension: a comparison of hypokalemia effects, BP control, and cost. *Arch Intern Med* 1983; 143:1694–1699.
156. Black WD, Shiner PT, Roman J: Severe electrolyte disturbances associated with metolazone and furosemide. *South Med J* 1978; 71:380–385.
157. Epstein M, Lepp BA, Hoffman DS, Levinson R: Potentiation of furosemide by metolazone in refractory edema. *Curr Ther Res* 1977; 21:656–667.
158. Eknoyan G, Suki WN, Martinez-Maldonado M: Effect of diuretics on urinary excretion of phosphate, calcium, and magnesium in thyroparathyroidectomized dogs. *J Lab Clin Med* 1970; 76:257–266.
159. Davies DL, Lant AF, Millard NR, Smith AJ, Ward JW: Renal action, therapeutic use, and pharmacokinetics of the diuretic bumetanide. *Clin Pharm Ther* 1974; 15:141–155.
160. Shareghi GR, Agus ZS: Magnesium transport in the cortical thick ascending limb of Henle's loop of the rabbit. *J Clin Invest* 1982; 69:759–769.
161. Quamme GA: Effect of furosemide on calcium and magnesium transport in the rat nephron. *Am J Physiol* 1981; 241:340–347.
162. Hollifield JW: Potassium and magnesium abnormalities: Diuretics and arrhythmias in hypertension. *Am J Med* 1984; 77:28–32.
163. Dyckner T, Wester PO: Ventricular extrasystoles and intracellular electrolytes before and after potassium and magnesium infusions in patients on diuretic treatment. *Am Heart J* 1979; 97:12–18.
164. Rybak LP: Pathophysiology of furosemide ototoxicity. *J Otolaryngol* 1982; 11:127–133.
165. Meriwether WD, Mangi RJ, Serpick AA: Deafness following standard intravenous dose of ethacrynic acid. *JAMA* 1971; 216:795–798.
166. David DS, Hitzig P: Diuretics and ototoxicity. *N Engl J Med* 1971; 284:1328–1329.
167. Schwartz GH, David DS, Riggio RR, Stenzel KH, Rubin AL: Ototoxicity induced by furosemide. *N Engl J Med* 1970; 282:1413–1414.
168. Lloyd-Mostyn RH, Lord IJ: Ototoxicity of intravenous furosemide. *Lancet* 1971; 2:1156–1157.
169. Clasen W, Kindler J, Khartabil T, Imm S, Frisch J, Sieberth HG: Torasemide versus furosemide in patients with advanced chronic renal failure–Effect on saliuresis, renin-aldosterone-system and cochlear function. In: Puschett JB, Greenberg A (eds): *Diuretics II: Chemistry, Pharmacology, and Clinical Applications.* New York, Elsevier Science, 1987:53–57.
170. Suki WN, Yium JJ, Von Minden M, Saller-Hebert C, Eknoyan G, Martinez-Maldonado M: Acute treatment of hypercalcemia with furosemide. *N Engl J Med* 1970; 283:836–840.
171. Gadbow PA, Hanson TJ, Popovtzer MM, Schrier RW: Furosemide-induced reduction in ionized calcium in hypoparathyroid patients. *Ann Intern Med* 1977; 85:579–581.
172. Bourdeau JE, Buss SL, Vurek GG: Inhibition of calcium absorption in the cortical thick ascending limb of henle's loop by furosemide. *J Pharm Exp Ther* 1982; 221: 815–819.
173. Greenblatt DJ, Koch-Wester J: Adverse reactions to spironolactone. A report from the Boston collaborative drug surveillance program. *JAMA* 1973; 225:40–43.
174. McNay JL, Oran E: Possible predisposition of diabetic patients to hyperkalemia following administration of potassium-retaining diuretic, amiloride (MK 870). *Metabolism* 1970; 19:58–70.
175. Crosley AP, Ronquillo LM, Strickland WH, et al: Triamterene, a new natriuretic agent. *Ann Intern Med* 1962; 56:241–251.
176. Whiting GFM, McLaran CJ, Bochner F: Severe hyperkalemia with Moduretic. *Med J Aust* 1979; 1:409.
177. Cohen AB: Hyperkalemia effects of triamterene. *Ann Intern Med* 1966; 65:521–527.
178. Walker BR, Capuzzi DM, Alexander F, Familiar RG, Hoppe RC: Hyperkalemia after triamterene in diabetic patients. *Clin Pharm Ther* 1972; 13:643–651.
179. Ponce SP, Jennings AE, Madias NE, Harrington JT: Drug-induced hyperkalemia. *Medicine* 1985; 64:357–370.
180. Rose LI, Underwood RH, Newmark SR, Kisch ES, Williams GH: Pathophysiology of spironolactone-induced gynecomastia. *Ann Intern Med* 1977; 87:398–403.
181. Huffman DH, Kampmann JP, Hignite CE, Azarnoff DL: Gynecomastia induced in normal males by spironolactone. *Clin Pharmacol Ther* 1978; 24:465–473.
182. Counihan TB, Evans BM, Milne MD: Observations on the pharmacology of the carbonic anhydrase inhibitor "Diamox." *Clin Sci* 954; 13:583–598.
183. Epstein DL: Carbonic anhydrase inhibitor side effects. Serum chemical analysis. *Arch Ophthalmol* 1977; 95:1378–1382.
184. Siklos P, Henderson RG: Severe acidosis from acetazolamide in a diabetic patient. *Curr Med Res Opin* 1979; 6:284–286.
185. O'Sullivan PJ, Crowley JG, Muldowney FP: A case of acetazolamide induced (Diamox) acidotic coma in polycystic renal disease. *J Irish Med Assoc* 1967; 60:382–384.
186. Seely JF, Dirks JH: Micropuncture study of hypertonic mannitol diuresis in the proximal and distal tubule of the dog kidney. *J Clin Invest* 1969; 48:2330–2340.
187. Blantz RC, Israelit AH, Rector FC, Seldin DW: Relation of distal tubular NaCl delivery and glomerular hydrostatis pressure. *Kidney Int* 1972; 2:22–32.
188. Goldberg AH, Lilienfield LS: Effects of hypertonic mannitol on renal vascular resistance. *Proc Soc Exp Biol Med* 1965; 119: 635–642.
189. Flores J, DiBona DR, Beck CH, Leaf A: The role of all swelling in ischemic renal damage and the protective effect of hypertonic solute. *J Clin Invest* 1972; 51:118–226.
190. Blantz RC: Effect of mannitol on glomerular ultrafiltration in the hydropenic rat. *J Clin Invest* 1974; 54:1135–1143.
191. Kurnik BRC, Weisberg LS, Cuttler IM, Kurnik PB: Effects of atrial natriuretic peptide versus mannitol on renal blood flow during radiocontrast infusion in chronic renal failure. *J Lab Clin Med* 1990; 116:27–35.
192. Morris CR, Alexander EA, Bruns FJ, Levinsky MG: Restoration and maintenance of glomerular filtration by mannitol during hypofusion of the kidney. *J Clin Invest* 1972; 51:1555–1564.
193. Dzau VJ, Colucci WS, Hollenberg NK, Williams GH: Relation

of the renin-angiotensin-aldosterone system to clinical state in congestive heart failure. *Circulation* 1981; 63:645–651.
194. Dzau VJ, Colucci WS, Williams GH, Curfman G, Meggs L, Hollenberg NK: Sustained effectiveness of converting-enzyme inhibition in patients with severe congestive heart failure. *N Engl J Med* 1980; 302:1373–1379.
195. Ader R, Chatterjee K, Ports T, Brundage B, Hiramatsu B, Parmley W: Immediate and sustained hemodynamic and clinical improvement in chronic heart failure by an oral angiotensin-converting enzyme inhibitor. *Circulation* 1980; 61:931–937.
196. Captopril Multicenter Research Group: A placebo-controlled trial of captopril in refractory congestive heart failure. *J Am Coll Cardiol* 1983; 2:755–763.
197. Odemuyiwa O, Gilmartin J, Kenny D, Hall RJC: Captopril and the diuretic requirements in moderate and severe chronic heart failure. *Eur Heart J* 1989; 10:586–590.
198. SOLVD Investigators: Effect of enalapril on survival in patients with reduced left ventricular ejection fractions and congestive heart failure. *N Engl J Med* 1991; 325:293–302.
199. Davis R, Ribner HS, Keung B, Sonnenblick EH, LeJemtel TH: Treatment of chronic congestive heart failure with captopril, an oral inhibitor of angiotensin-converting enzyme. *N Engl J Med* 1979; 102:117–121.
200. Kokko JP: The role of the kidney in acute congestive heart failure: Treatment. *Cardiovasc Rev Rep* 1987; 8:60–63.
201. Wilcox CS, Mitch WE, Kelly RA, Skorecki K, Meyer TW, Friedman PA, et al: Response of the kidney to furosemide. I. Effects of salt intake and renal compensation. *J Lab Clin Med* 1983; 102:450–458.
202. Kelly RA, Wilcox CS, Mitch WE, Meyer TW, Souney PF, Rayment CM, et al: Response of the kidney to furosemide. II. Effect of captopril on sodium balance. *Kidney Int* 1983; 24:233–239.
203. D'Elia JA, Gleason RE, Alday M, Malarick C, Godley K, Warram J, et al: Nephrotoxicity from angiographic contrast material. *Am J Med* 1982; 72:719–725.
204. Eisenberg RL, Bank WO, Hedgcock MW: Renal failure after major angiography. *Am J Med* 1980; 68: 43–46.
205. Hou SH, Bushinsky DA, Wish JB, Cohen JJ, Harrington JT: Hospital acquired renal insufficiency: A prospective study. *Am J Med* 1983; 74:243–247.
206. Weinrauch LA, Healy RW, Leland OS, Goldstein HH, Kassissieh SD, Libertino JA, et al. Coronary angiography and acute renal failure in diabetic azotemic nephropathy. *Ann Intern Med* 1977; 86:56–59.
207. Martin-Paredero V, Dixon SM, Baker JD, Takiff H, Gomes AS, Busuttil RW, et al: Risk of renal failure after major angiography. *Arch Surg* 1983; 118:1417–1420.
208. Kumar S, Hull J, Lathi S, Cohen AJ, Pletka PG: Low incidence of renal failure after angiography. *Arch Intern Med* 1981; 141:1268–1270.
209. Gomes AS, Baker JD, Martin-Paredero V, Dixon SM, Takiff H, Machleder HI, et al: Acute renal dysfunction after major arteriography. *Am J Radiol* 1985; 145:1249–1253.
210. Taliercio CP, Vlietstra RE, Fisher LD, Burnett JC: Risks for renal dysfunction with cardiac angiography. *Ann Intern Med* 1986; 104:501–504.
211. Schwab SJ, Hlatky MA, Pieper KS, Davidson CJ, Morris KG, Skelton TN, et al: Contrast nephrotoxicity: A randomized controlled trial of a nonionic and an ionic radiographic contrast agent. *N Engl J Med* 1989; 320:149–153.
212. Humes HD, Hunt DA, White MD: Direct toxic effect of the radiocontrast agent diatrizoate on renal proximal tubule cells. *Am J Physiol* 1987; 252:F246–F255.
213. Zager RA, Timmerman TP, Merola AJ: Effects of immediate blood flow enhancement on the post ischemic kidney: Functional, morphologic and biochemical assessments. *J Lab Clin Med* 1985; 106:360–368.
214. Aperia A, Broberger O, Ekengren K: Renal hemodynamics during selective renal angiography. *Invest Radiol* 1968; 3:389–396.
215. Talner LB, Davidson AJ: Effect of contrast media on renal extraction of PAH. *Invest Radiol* 1968; 3:301–309.
216. Norby LH, DiBona GF: The renal vascular effects of meglumine diatrizoate. *J Pharm Exp Ther* 1975; 193:932–940.
217. Margulies KB, Hildebrand FL, Lerman A, Perella MA, Burnett JC: Increased endothelin in experimental heart failure. *Circulation* 1990; 82:2226–2230.
218. Margulies KB, McKinley LJ, Cavero PG, Burnett JC: Induction and prevention of radiocontrast-induced nephropathy in dogs with heart failure. *Kidney Int* 1990; 38:1101–1108.
219. Talner LB, Davidson AJ: Renal hemodynamic effects of contrast media. *Invest Radiol* 1968; 3:310–317.
220. Margulies KB, Hildebrand FL, Heublein DM, Burnett JC: Radiocontrast increases plasma and urinary endothelin. *J Am Soc Nephrol* 1991; 2:1041–1045.
221. Rudnick MR, Goldfarb S, Murphy MJ: Mannitol and other prophylactic regimens in contrast media–induced acute renal failure. *Coron Art Dis* 1991; 2:1047–1052.

Chapter 30

Drugs Used to Control Vascular Resistance and Capacitance

Jay N. Cohn, M.D.

The traditional role in medicine for vasoactive drugs that alter vascular resistance and capacitance has been to influence arterial pressure. Thus, vasodilator drugs that reduce systemic vascular resistance have been used as a rational approach to the treatment of hypertension, and vasoconstrictor drugs that increase systemic vascular resistance have, at least in the past, been advocated for the treatment of hypotensive states. Although variable venous capacitance effects of these drugs have been known to result in differing acute hemodynamic responses, the importance of these capacitive effects in the use of these agents has not traditionally been emphasized.

The demand for more selectivity in the choice of drug therapy for specific vascular syndromes had led in recent years to more attention to the regional vascular effects of these drugs. In myocardial ischemic syndromes, it has become important to understand effects of drugs on the large coronary arteries, the coronary arterioles, and the collateral channels as well as on the systemic arteries and veins to gain insight into antianginal effectiveness. The specific action of drugs on the pulmonary circulation has taken on importance not only because of growing interest in the interactions between the right and left ventricles but also because of therapeutic attempts to use vasoactive drugs to counteract pulmonary hypertension. Effects of drugs on the renal, splanchnic, and skeletal muscle circulations have become important as we become more sophisticated in our approach to hypertension, shock, and heart failure.

A further development in recent years has been an emphasis on the role of peripheral vascular factors in influencing the performance of the heart and its metabolic requirements. This newly awakened recognition of the importance of the vascular component of the cardiovascular system has led to the need for studying the effects of vasoactive drugs on the arterial and venous beds and for carefully assessing the left ventricular response to these drugs.[1] Only through an understanding of the pharmacologic actions of these drugs is it possible to employ rational vasoactive therapy in managing hypertension, angina pectoris, and heart failure.

HEMODYNAMIC EFFECTS OF VASODILATORS

Role of Preload Changes in Cardiac Performance

The importance of preload (end-diastolic myocardial fiber length) in controlling stroke volume from the left ventricle has long been recognized from the classical Frank-Starling curves.[2] (See also Chap. 5.) Several factors of particular importance when considering preload effects in the setting of heart disease must be considered:

- In the presence of myocardial disease the left ventricle may lose much of its sensitivity to preload, such that augmentation of preload may not result in much rise in stroke volume. A true descending limb of the Frank-Starling curve probably does not exist, however.[3] (See Chap. 25.)

- The dilated left ventricular chamber is not necessarily operating at a heightened preload, since much of the dilatation may reflect slippage of fibers rather than increased fiber length.[4]
- Changes in compliance of the ventricle may alter the relationship between diastolic pressure and volume and thus render change in filling pressure an unreliable guide to change in end-diastolic fiber length or preload.[5]
- Myocardial oxygen consumption is directly related to wall stress, which is a function of pressure and chamber diameter. Therefore, dilatation of the chamber should result in an increase in myocardial oxygen consumption. If the ventricle is operating on a flattened Frank-Starling curve, the increased oxygen consumption will not be accompanied by much increase in cardiac output (reduced external efficiency).[6]

Acute changes in ventricular preload may result from changes in vascular capacitance. Right ventricular preload is dependent on systemic venous capacitance as well as intravascular volume. Left ventricular preload is dependent on the capacitance of the pulmonary vascular bed as well as the output from the right ventricle. Interaction through the interventricular septum also may result in a direct effect on left ventricular compliance of changes in right ventricular filling.[7] (See also Chaps. 5 and 25.)

Role of Impedance Changes in Cardiac Performance

Although the normal left ventricle is able to maintain its performance in the face of a fairly wide range of outflow resistance (impedance), the damaged myocardium often loses this ability and ventricular performance becomes inversely related to impedance.[8] Thus, the impaired ventricle is characterized by reduced response to preload changes and heightened response to impedance changes.

In assessing the effects of drugs that alter impedance, one must give consideration to the following:

- Arteriolar resistance and arterial compliance are the major variables that influence impedance.[9] Afterload, or ventricular wall stress during ejection, is influenced by impedance, by the ventricular pressure generated by the force of ventricular contraction against a given impedance, by the end-diastolic chamber diameter, and by the shortening (stroke volume) during ejection. Vasoactive drugs may thus directly alter impedance but only secondarily influence afterload.
- Since increased impedance may decrease cardiac output in the presence of myocardial disease and at the same time result in increased pressure and volume and consequently increased myocardial oxygen consumption, the net effect of an increase in impedance is a decrease in cardiac efficiency.[10]
- Since vascular resistance and compliance are exquisitely sensitive to neurohumoral factors, changes induced by vasoactive drugs may be counteracted or magnified by reflex changes in activity of the sympathetic nervous system or the renin-angiotensin system.[11]
- Regional differences in effects of drugs on vascular tone influence peripheral distribution of blood flow. Cardiac output will respond to a change in total impedance, but the effects on flow to specific vascular beds relate to local vascular changes.[12]

Effects on Intravascular Volume

In addition to controlling resistance and capacitance, drugs that influence vascular tone influence the intravascular volume by altering capillary pressure, which determines the rate of capillary filtration. Since capillary pressure is influenced by the balance between precapillary arteriolar and postcapillary venular resistance, a drug that relaxes the venules would tend to lower capillary pressure and increase plasma volume, whereas one that lowered arteriolar resistance might increase capillary pressure and reduce plasma volume.[13] Changes in vascular volume become important, particularly when a therapeutic intervention is discontinued or during chronic administration of a drug. The concomitant use of diuretics with many vasoactive drugs will, of course, independently affect the intravascular volume.

DRUGS THAT DIRECTLY RELAX VASCULAR SMOOTH MUSCLE

A number of drugs that have been used to treat hypertension, angina pectoris, and congestive heart failure exert an effect on vascular smooth muscle that appears not to be dependent on receptor mechanisms. Some may depend for their effect on stimulation of cyclic guanosine monophosphate (GMP),[14] and with others the mode of action is not entirely clear.

Nitrates

Nitroglycerin and the various nitrates have been in use for the treatment of cardiac disease for more than 100 years. These agents have a profound venodilating effect that even in low doses results in an increase in vascular capacitance.[15] Although their effect on large-vessel compliance is more difficult to quantitate, considerable data indicate that even in relatively low doses these drugs increase the caliber and compliance of large-conductance muscular arteries.[16] A reduction in arteriolar resistance appears to occur in some vascular beds but may be dependent on high doses of the drug and may be a relatively transient effect of the nitrates.[17] Evidence also exists that nitrates have a relaxing effect on collateral vascular channels, particularly coronary collateral vessels, and this action may contribute to their beneficial effect in patients with angina pectoris.[18] The nitrates also appear to have a direct dilating effect on the pulmonary vasculature and therefore result in a lowering of pulmonary vascular resistance. The relative dilator effect of nitrates on various regional vascular beds is not entirely established, but it appears likely that the drugs have a prominent action on the cutaneous and skeletal muscle beds with a lesser effect on the visceral organs.[19]

Because of the diverse vascular actions of these agents, they have found a place in the management of a variety of cardiovascular diseases. *Nitroglycerin* (glyceryl trinitrate) serves as the drug of choice to treat anginal attacks because of the rapid onset and magnitude of action after sublingual administration. The remarkable effectiveness of nitroglycerin in angina pectoris is dependent on several actions of the drug, including a relaxing effect on stenotic coronary arteries, a reduction of blood pressure, and an increase in vascular capacitance, with a consequent reduction of ventricular volume. An increase in collateral flow to ischemic myocardium may be of special benefit when present.[20]

The organic nitrates appear to act through the formation of nitric oxide, which also appears to be the endogenous vasodilator released by the endothelium.[21] Endothelial release of nitric oxide appears to be impaired in hypertension, atherosclerosis, and heart failure.[21] Therefore, in some clinical situations organic nitrates may serve to replace deficient endogenous vasodilation.

The major issues with the nitrates in recent years have been related to the relative efficacy and pharmacokinetics of various formulations, the efficacy of chronic administration, and the possibility of tolerance to the drug (Table 30-1). Sublingual administration of nitroglycerin is clearly effective, and it is now well established that oral administration of the nitrates, particularly *isosorbide dinitrate,* produces a measurable hemodynamic response.[22] After absorption from the oral mucosa or gut, it is converted in the liver to active mononitrate metabolites.

Considerable variability exists in the dosage requirement for a vascular action after oral administration; isosorbide dinitrate doses of 20, 40, or 60 mg orally given at 4 to 6 h may be necessary to produce a sustained hemodynamic effect. *Isosorbide-5-mononitrate*, the longer-acting metabolite of *isosorbide dinitrate*, may be given 20 mg at 8 a.m. and 3 p.m. to produce similar effects.[23] Cutaneous administration of nitrates has long been utilized in ointment preparations that have been used for the treatment of angina.[24] Patches of nitroglycerine in matrix form for skin absorption are also widely used.[25] Some evidence suggests that absorption from these transdermal preparations is relatively modest and that large applications are necessary to produce hemodynamic effects comparable to what can be achieved with oral administration of nitrates.[26]

An unresolved issue is the appropriate dosing schedule for nitrate administration. Oral nitrates administered every 8 h or four times a day with an 8-h nighttime interval have been demonstrated to be effective in the treatment of heart failure. On the other hand, continuous administration of oral nitrates and, particularly, continuous transdermal administration may induce tolerance to the antianginal effects of the drug. Therefore, the current recommendation for chronic nitrate therapy of myocardial ischemia is to give oral nitrates on an eccentric dosing schedule (two daily doses of isosorbide-5-mononitrate or isosorbide dinitrate by midafternoon)[27] or to use transdermal preparations that are removed for at least 10 h at night.[28] There is reason to suspect that sensitivity and tolerance to the large arterial, arteriolar, and venous effects may not have the same time course. Therefore, appropriate dosing regimens for one clinical indication may not necessarily apply to other clinical indications.

Sodium Nitroprusside

Sodium nitroprusside is a potent smooth-muscle dilator that must be administered intravenously (see Table 30-2). The cellular mechanism of action of nitroprusside is very similar to that of the nitrates involving the formation of nitric oxide and cyclic GMP stimulation.[29] Intravenous titration of nitroprusside can produce progressively increasing arteriolar dilation and therefore progressive reduction of systemic vascular resistance. This arteriolar dilation is accomplished in concert with considerable venodilation and an increase in vascular capacitance. The net result of infusion of sodium nitroprusside is a dose-dependent reduction of arterial pressure in patients with hypertension and a dose-dependent decrease of impedance in patients with congestive heart failure. The drug has been of particular value for acute

TABLE 30-1

Effect of Commonly Used Nitrates

Drug	Route of Administration	Dosage	Onset of Effect	Duration of Effect	Reliability of Effect
Nitroglycerin (Nitrostat; Susadrin)	Sublingual	0.3–0.6 mg	30 s	15–30 min	High
Nitroglycerin (Nitrostat SR; Nitro-Bid)	Oral	2.5–19.5 mg	1h	2–4 h	Low
Nitroglycerin (Nitro-Bid; Nitrodisc; Nitro-Dur; Nitrol ointment; Transderm)	Transdermal	1–2 in (ointment) 10–60 cm^2 (patches)	1 h	6–14 h	Medium
Nitroglycerin (Tridil)	Intravenous	10–200 μg/min	Immediate	—	High
Isosorbide dinitrate (Isordil; Sorbitrate; Dilatrate)	Sublingual	2.5–10 mg	5 min	1–2 h	High
Isosorbide dinitrate (Isordil; Sorbitrate; Dilatrate)	Oral	10–60 mg	30 min	4–6 h	High
Isosorbide-5-mononitrate (ISMO)	Oral	10–20 mg	30 min	8–12 h	High

TABLE 30-2
Effect of Direct-Acting Vasodilators

Drug	Route of Administration	Dosage	Onset of Effect	Duration of Effect	Large Arteries	Arterioles	Veins
Sodium nitroprusside (Nipride)	Intravenous	25–400 μg/min	Immediate	—	+	+++	+++
Nitroglycerin (Tridil)	Intravenous	10–200 μg/min	Immediate	—	++	+	+++
Isosorbide dinitrate (Isordil; Sorbitrate, Isobid; Isotrate; Sorate, Sorbide; Dilatrate)	Oral	20–60 mg	30 min	4–6 h	++	+	+++
Hydralazine (Apresoline)	Oral	50–100 mg	30 min	6–12 h	0	+++	±
Minoxidil (Loniten)	Oral	10–30 mg	30 min	8–12 h	0	+++	0
Diazoxide (Hyperstat)	Intravenous bolus	100–300 mg	Immediate	4–12 h	0	+++	±

See Chapter 67 and Tables 67-1 to 67-14 for calcium antagonists. See also Chapter 77.

short-term management of unstable patients in whom adjustment of pressure and/or cardiac output is essential to maintaining clinical integrity. It frequently is used to control arterial pressure in aortic dissection, in hypertensive crisis, or in the postoperative cardiac patient, to produce hypotension during surgery and to augment left ventricular performance in acute myocardial infarction or severe congestive heart failure. (See also Chaps. 26 and 77.)

The regional vascular effects of nitroprusside may be of importance in its use. Cerebral blood flow increases,[30] and the drug has a pulmonary vasodilator effect,[31] but the systemic vasodilator effect does not favor the renal or splanchnic beds. Some experimental studies have suggested that myocardial ischemia may be aggravated by nitroprusside because of a coronary "steal" phenomenon,[32] but there is clinical evidence for efficacy of nitroprusside in myocardial ischemia.[33] In a carefully controlled multicenter study of acute myocardial infarction, early intervention with nitroprusside appeared to have a deleterious effect on mortality, whereas late intervention, when the goal was to improve persistently depressed cardiac function, had a beneficial effect.[34] Therefore, caution in administration of nitroprusside during the first 8 h after the onset of acute myocardial infarction is justified. Nitroglycerin is probably the preferred vasodilator in this clinical situation.

During titration of nitroprusside infusion, it is imperative that blood pressure be monitored closely and that infusion rate be carefully titrated. A wide variation in effective doses is noted, with some patients responding to doses as small as 20 to 40 μg/min, whereas others require as much as 600 to 800 μg/min. Toxicity of nitroprusside may be noted during prolonged administration of large doses of the drug, which may result in accumulation of thiocyanate that may lead to central toxicity.[35]

Hydralazine

Hydralazine exerts a dose-dependent arteriolar dilation that is effective in lowering systemic vascular resistance in patients with hypertension[36] and reducing impedance to left ventricular ejection in patients with heart failure[37] (Table 30-3). Reflex cardiac stimulation with tachycardia is common in hypertensive patients but is less often observed in patients with heart failure. Hydralazine exerts little, if any, effect on venous capacitance, and therefore an increase in cardiac output is not counterbalanced by much decrease in ventricular filling.[37]

Dosage levels of oral hydralazine are restricted by side effects, which include nonspecific musculoskeletal symptoms and occasionally a full-blown syndrome of systemic lupus erythematosus.[38] Toxicity from high-dose hydralazine is particularly prominent in individuals who are genetically slow acetylators and therefore tend to accumulate higher concentrations of the nonmetabolized drug in the blood. Angina may be precipitated by hydralazine, presumably in large part because of tachycardia, but also possibly related to coronary vascular effects precipitating maldistribution of flow in the myocardium or to a direct effect to increase myocardial contractility.[39]

For treatment of hypertension the dose of hydralazine generally is kept below 300 mg daily to avoid side effects. It usually is preferable to administer hydralazine in conjunction with a diuretic and/or a beta-adrenoceptor blocker to minimize the reflex tachycardia and reflex increase in cardiac output. In patients with congestive heart failure similar doses of hydralazine may be employed, although in some instances considerably higher doses may be necessary. Reflex tachycardia is attenuated in heart failure,[40] and therefore it usually is not necessary to inhibit this response. For most clinical indications it is probably possible to administer hydralazine on a twice-daily schedule. (See also Chap. 77.)

TABLE 30-3
Effect of Drugs That Inhibit Neurohumoral Vasoconstriction

Drug	Route of Administration	Dosage	Onset of Effect	Duration of Effect	Myocardial Contractility	Plasma Norepinephrine	Plasma Renin Activity
Clonidine (Catapres)	Oral	0.1–0.3 mg	1 h	6–12 h	=	=	–
Guanabenz (Wytensin)	Oral	8–24 mg	1 h	6–12 h	=	=	–
Methyldopa (Aldomet)	Oral	250–1000 mg	2–4 h	6–12 h	–	–	±
Reserpine (Serpasil)	Oral	0.1–0.5 mg	2–4 h	12–24 h	–	0	0
Propranolol (Inderal)	Oral	20–80 mg	30 min	4–8 h	=	+	=
Labetalol (Normodyne; Trandate)	Oral	200–800 mg	1 h	6–12 h	=	+	±
Guanethidine (Ismelin)	Oral	10–50 mg	1 h	24 h	–	+	±
Phentolamine (Regitine)	Intravenous	1–5 mg/min	Immediate	—	+	++	+
Prazosin (Minipress)	Oral	2–10 mg	30 min	4–8 h	0	±	+
Terazosin (Hytrin)	Oral	5–20 mg	2 h	12–24 h	0	±	+
Captopril (Capoten)	Oral	12.5–50 mg	30 min	4–8 h	0	–	++
Enalapril (MK421)	Oral	5–20 mg	1 h	12–24 h	0	–	++
Lisinopril (Zestril)	Oral	10–40 mg	2 h	24 h	0	–	++

Hydralazine–Isosorbide Dinitrate Combination

The vasodilator drugs hydralazine and isosorbide dinitrate, when used together, provide effects on arterial conductance vessels, arteriolar resistance vessels, and venous capacitance vessels. This combination has been studied extensively in patients with heart failure, in whom it produces a striking reduction in the elevated cardiac filling pressures and a prominent increase in stroke volume and cardiac output. In the Veterans Administration trial of vasodilators in heart failure (V-HeFT), the combination of 75 mg hydralazine and 40 mg isosorbide dinitrate administered four times daily to patients already treated with digoxin and diuretics led to a significant reduction of long-term mortality in patients with symptomatic heart failure.[41] Headache was a common side effect of the therapy, but most patients were able to be maintained on these drugs for the average 2.3 years of follow-up in the trial. In V-HeFT II the effect of the hydralazine–isosorbide dinitrate combination was compared to that of enalapril in patients with heart failure. The vasodilator combination produced a greater improvement in peak exercise performance and a greater improvement in left ventricular systolic performance than enalapril; however, the survival benefits of enalapril exceeded those of hydralazine and isosorbide dinitrate.[42]

Minoxidil

Minoxidil is an arteriolar dilator similar to hydralazine but apparently more potent (see Table 30-2). The drug may be administered twice daily and in higher doses may produce a profound dilator effect that is effective in lowering blood pressures in severe hypertension resistant to other interventions.[43] Reflex cardiac stimulation and sodium retention, possibly because of the arteriolar dilating effect of the drug or possibly because of a direct antinatriuretic effect on the kidney, are the major complicating hemodynamic effects of minoxidil.[44] Stimulation of lanugal hair growth over the face, extremities, and trunk is a common side effect of minoxidil and makes the drug less well tolerated by female patients. (See also Chap. 77.)

Diazoxide

Diazoxide is a nondiuretic thiazide derivative that exerts a potent arteriolar dilator effect when given intravenously (see Table 30-2). Its only place in cardiovascular therapy has been for acute management of hypertensive crisis, in which blood pressure lowering can be achieved quite rapidly and often can be maintained by continuous infusion or subsequent bolus injections. Sodium retention and hyperglycemia are common side effects of the drug, and these complications limit its use. For acute management of severe hypertension, sodium nitroprusside is more reliable and more easily titrated with fewer side effects.

CALCIUM ANTAGONISTS

In recent years a number of vasodilator drugs have been identified that appear to have in common inhibition of transmembrane calcium transport across slow channels in both cardiac muscle and vascular smooth muscle (see Chap. 67). These drugs also appear to inhibit intracellular calcium release that in some vascular tissue plays an important role in increasing cytosol calcium concentration to stimulate muscle contraction.[45] Many of the drugs in this family of compounds are still undergoing investigation and are not yet available for general clinical use.

Three classes of calcium antagonists are available for clinical use. Verapamil, a phenylalkylamine, exerts potent electrophysiological and negative inotropic effects as well as modest vasodilator actions. Diltiazem, a benzothiazepine, also has electrophysiological actions that make it effective, like verapamil, in the management of supraventricular arrhythmias. Both of these classes of calcium antagonists are effective in the treatment of hypertension and angina.

The dihydropyridines are a group of calcium antagonists that exert a range of cardiac and vascular effects but do not affect the cardiac conduction system. All are vasodilators, but the site and magnitude of the dilation varies among the different compounds. Furthermore, the drugs appear to differ considerably in the ratio of vasodilator to negative inotropic action so that some compounds appear to be devoid of cardiac effects at doses that produce prominent vasodilation. The original dihydropyridine, nifedipine, has now been joined in the marketplace by nicardipine, isradipine, felodipine, nimodipine, and amlodipine; it is likely that other dihydropyridines will follow this group.

The calcium antagonists in general relax the large-conductance arteries and the arterioles[46] but have fewer venous capacitance effects than the nitrates and some other vasodilators. (See also Chap. 67.) Considerable individual differences exist in the responsiveness of various vascular beds to individual calcium antagonists. Some of these agents, such as nisoldipine and nifedipine, may produce considerable arteriolar dilatation in the coronary bed and cause an increase in coronary blood flow.[47,48] Others have a less profound arteriolar dilator effect. Some experimental agents appear to have selective actions favoring the renal bed and the cerebral bed, whereas others appear to have a more prominent effect on the skeletal muscle vascular bed.[49,50] The pulmonary vasculature appears to be particularly responsive to at least some of the calcium antagonists but less responsive to others.[51] (See Chap. 99.)

Early clinical studies with calcium antagonists were devoted primarily to their use in angina pectoris. In myocardial ischemia these drugs exert a number of actions that appear to have a favorable effect on myocardial perfusion: (1) they increase large-conductance coronary artery caliber and therefore may reduce the severity of coronary stenoses; (2) they alter the resistance of coronary arterioles and coronary collateral channels and thus may augment myocardial perfusion in areas of ischemia; (3) they appear to inhibit reactive hyperemia in the coronary vascular bed, and this inhibition of inappropriate vasodilation may have favorable effects on the intramyocardial distribution of blood flow; (4) they reduce systemic vascular resistance, which may improve ventricular and myocardial oxygen consumption; (5) they may produce a modest reduction of myocardial preload and thus further reduce myocardial oxygen consumption; and (6) they may reduce exercise-induced blood pressure increase and tachycardia, the major determinants of myocardial oxygen consumption.

In recent years these drugs have also been employed for the management of hypertension in both the systemic and pulmonary vascular beds.[52,53] (See also Chap. 99.) Verapamil, diltiazem, and the dihydropyridines have been demonstrated in controlled experiments to be effective when used as monotherapy in the treatment of patients with systemic arterial hypertension. (See Chap. 77.) These agents appear to be particularly attractive because of the evidence for sustained effectiveness and the absence of severe side effects. Preliminary studies also have been carried out using drugs in this class in the management of subarachnoid hemorrhage, Raynaud's syndrome, migraine headache, etc.

Although interactions between calcium antagonists and other cardiovascular drugs have not been exhaustively studied, concern has been expressed for a possible additive negative inotropic effect of certain calcium antagonists and beta-adrenoceptor blockers. Caution thus must be exercised in the concomitant use of verapamil or diltiazem and beta blockers.[54] This caution does not appear to apply as strongly to the combined use of dihydropyridines with beta blockers. An interaction with digitalis also has been described with verapamil. It is therefore necessary to observe carefully for signs of digitalis toxicity when calcium antagonist therapy is initiated in the patient already receiving digitalis glycosides. (See Chap. 67.)

SYMPATHETIC VASOCONSTRICTOR INHIBITORS

Maintenance of tone in vascular smooth muscle in arteries, arterioles, and veins is dependent at least in part on sympathetic vasoconstrictor activity mediated largely through alpha-adrenoceptor stimulation (see Table 30-3). Inhibition of this sympathetic vasoconstriction will result in a reduction in systemic vascular resistance, redistribution of peripheral blood flow, and an increase in venous capacitance. Sympathetic blockade also tends to produce orthostatic hypotension. Inhibition may be accomplished at numerous sites along the course of the sympathetic vasoconstrictor apparatus.

Central Inhibition

Stimulation of central $alpha_2$ receptors results in a decreased sympathetic outflow and reduced sympathetic vasoconstrictor activity. This mechanism appears to account for the antihypertensive activity of *clonidine*.[55] *Guanabenz* and *guanfacine* are also available for this purpose.[56] These agents have an effect on both arterial and venous responses and thus increase systemic capacitance as well as lower vascular resistance. They also reduce sympathetic drive to the heart and therefore reduce heart rate and myocardial contractility. The negative inotropic effect of these drugs may limit their usefulness as vasodilator agents for the treatment of heart failure.[57] (See also Chap. 77.)

Other antihypertensive drugs also may exert a central inhibiting effect on sympathetic discharge. The action of *methyldopa*[58] and *reserpine*[59] may at least in part be related to central inhibition, and a central action has even been implicated in the antihypertensive effect of beta-adrenoceptor blockers[60] (see Table 30-3).

Tolerance has not been a problem with these centrally acting agents, but side effects of drowsiness, lethargy, and orthostatic dizziness are frequent enough with some of the drugs to warrant a search for alternate agents in many patients with hypertension. (See also Chap. 77.)

Ganglionic Blockade

Drugs that block sympathetic ganglia may be very effective in inhibiting sympathetic vasoconstriction, but the side effects of these drugs have practically eliminated them from clinical practice. Side effects of concomitant vagal blockade (constipation, urinary retention) and uncontrollable orthostatic hypotension are the most prominent complications of therapy.

Inhibition of Peripheral Norepinephrine Release

Guanethidine (see Table 30-3), *guanadrel, bethanidine,* and *bretylium* all inhibit postganglionic release of norepinephrine (NE) and thus reduce vascular tone and lower blood pressure. Since their action is accentuated when sympathetic tone is high, these agents all may produce orthostatic hypotension. Bethanidine and bretylium have an additional antiarrhythmic effect that has been useful in preventing and treating ventricular tachycardia/fibrillation.[61] (See Chap. 36.) Guanethidine is an attractive antihypertensive agent because of its potency and its once-a-day dosage. Guanadrel exerts similar effects but is shorter acting. Tolerance does not develop to these agents, and when combined with a diuretic, they are capable of normalizing standing pressure in the most severe hypertensives. However, side effects of orthostatic hypotension and diarrhea often occur when attempts are made to increase the dose to normalize supine pressure; consequently these drugs are now reserved for unusual special circumstances when the better tolerated agents prove ineffective.

Alpha-Adrenoceptor Blockers

Inhibition of sympathetic-mediated vasoconstriction by interference with the postganglionic alpha receptor has always appeared to be a rational approach to therapy of states in which the systemic vascular resistance is high. Early use of alpha-adrenoreceptor blockers was limited because the available agents, *phentolamine* (see Table 30-3) and *dibenzyline,* were poorly tolerated in clinical practice because of orthostatic hypotension and reflex tachycardia.[62] The introduction of *prazosin* (see Table 30-3) made it possible to utilize alpha-blocker therapy on a more chronic basis. The major difference between prazosin and the previously available alpha blockers appears to be related to the selectivity of effect on vascular alpha receptors. Whereas phentolamine and dibenzyline exert their action relatively nonselectively on both presynaptic and postsynaptic alpha receptors, prazosin's action is more highly localized to the postsynaptic alpha receptor.[63] This postsynaptic receptor, commonly referred to as the alpha$_1$ receptor, is the major mediator of sympathetic vasoconstriction of vascular smooth muscle. The presynaptic alpha$_2$ receptor appears to have a major effect on presynaptic release of NE.[64] Therefore alpha$_2$ stimulation tends to suppress NE release and alpha$_2$ blockade tends to enhance NE release. Therapeutic success with prazosin has therefore been attributed to the absence of inhibition of alpha$_2$ receptors and therefore the absence of enhanced NE release that might otherwise result in reflex tachycardia. Although prazosin may produce severe orthostatic hypotension after the first dose, this effect appears to wane with continued therapy.[65] The reason for tolerance to the orthostatic effects of prazosin has not been well explained, although it raises the possibility of some tolerance developing to the alpha$_1$-receptor blocking action of the drug. Longer acting alpha$_1$ blockers, terazosin and dexazosin, have recently become available for hypertension. These agents have been particularly advocated for use in hypertension and congestive heart failure. Recent studies suggest that these drugs also may be effective in relieving prostatic obstruction because of their inhibitor action on alpha$_1$ receptors in the prostate.

Although prazosin was formerly widely used for vasodilator therapy of heart failure, either tolerance to the hemodynamic effect of this drug or lack of a favorable effect of alpha$_1$ blockade has limited its usefulness in heart failure. The V-HeFT did not reveal a favorable effect of prazosin on mortality or exercise performance in patients with heart failure.[41] Therefore, this drug probably should not now be viewed as the vasodilator agent of choice for heart failure. Hydralazine plus isosorbide dinitrate or angiotensin converting enzyme inhibitors (ACEIs) are appropriate drugs for that purpose. (See also Chap. 26.)

Labetalol, an antihypertensive beta-adrenoceptor blocker, also exerts alpha-adrenoceptor blocking activity.[66] The alpha blocking activity appears to contribute to the blood pressure lowering effect and may also contribute to an orthostatic hypotensive effect of the drug.

Since sympathetic tone plays an important role not only on the arterial resistance vessels but also on the venous capacitance vessels, it would be anticipated that alpha-adrenoceptor blockers would increase capacitance and reduce cardiac preload as well as reduce peripheral arteriolar resistance. This appears to be the case with most of the alpha-adrenoceptor blockers that have been studied. The action of these alpha-adrenoceptor blockers on the renal vasculature and on renal tubular function is controversial. A sodium-retaining effect of alpha-adrenoceptor blockade, perhaps related to reduction of perfusion pressure, has been reported. On the other hand, data suggest that alpha$_2$ receptors may have a direct effect on renal tubular sodium reabsorption and may therefore have an independent effect on renal sodium handling.[67] These effects should become clearer as additional studies are carried out with some of the newer alpha-adrenoceptor blockers.

CONVERTING ENZYME INHIBITORS

Since angiotensin II is a potent constrictor of arteriolar resistance vessels, the development of ACEIs provided an attractive means of inhibiting vasoconstriction by inhibiting the production of the vasoactive octapeptide angiotensin II from the decapeptide angiotensin I (see Table 30-3).[68] The actions of *captopril, enalapril, lisinopril, quinapril, ramipril,* and *fosinopril* appear to be at least in large part related to their ability to inhibit production of angiotensin II; therefore, these drugs have a vasodilator effect that lowers systemic vascular resistance and have in addition a natriuretic effect by inhibition of aldosterone secretion.[69] The effects of ACEIs (see Table 30-3) in lowering blood pressure in patients with essential hypertension, and particularly in patients with renovascular hypertension, and in lowering systemic vascular resistance and improving left ventricular performance in patients with congestive heart failure have now been well established.[70,71] Other actions of ACEIs also cannot be disregarded. Inhibition of degradation of bradykinin may lead to increased levels of circulating bradykinin, which could also contribute to a vasodilator effect.[72] Since angiotensin II is an important stimulator of presynaptic NE release,[73] inhibition of production of angiotensin II also may reduce sympathetic vasomotor tone.[74] Central actions of angiotensin also may be important in influencing vascular resistance and salt and water balance; these actions may also be influenced by converting enzyme inhibition.[75,76] (See also Chap. 77.)

A variety of drugs with ACEI activity are now undergoing clinical investigation for use in hypertension, heart failure, and renal failure. The major differences between these drugs appear to be related to pharmacokinetics and molecular structure, although it is possible that they will prove to have differing effects on the tissue renin-angiotensin system in various organs. Some (e.g., enalapril) are pro-drugs that become active only after metabolism. Others (e.g., lisinopril) have a long duration of effect but are not pro-drugs. Some (e.g., captopril) have a sulfhydryl group as part of their structure, whereas others (e.g., enalapril, lisinopril) do not. The structure of these compounds may influence their side effects, their stimulation of kinins or prostaglandins, the tissue specificity of their effects, or their action on other biological systems, including free-radical formation.

The doses of ACEIs necessary for therapy of heart failure are based on blood pressure measurement, but the optimal dose needed for treatment of heart failure is controversial. Some early studies have been carried out with high doses (e.g., 300 mg daily captopril) whereas the drugs often are used in quite low doses in clinical practice. Careful dose-response studies on efficacy in heart failure have not been carried out, but it would be prudent for physicians to attempt to use doses proved effective in carefully controlled trials (100 to 150 mg daily captopril, 20 mg daily enalapril).

VASOCONSTRICTOR DRUGS

The use of vasoconstrictor agents for cardiovascular disorders has fallen into relative disrepute for several reasons: (1) Increases in vascular resistance may impair left ventricular output when the left ventricle is abnormal. Since an abnormality in left ventricular performance is common in shock and hypotensive states, administration of a vasoconstrictor drug may aggravate a flow deficiency in these syndromes even though it may at least temporarily support arterial pressure. (2) Vasoconstrictor drugs tend to redistribute peripheral blood flow away from vascular beds that are most sensitive to the vasoconstrictor effect of the administered agent. Since the renal bed may be particularly responsive to certain of these agents, a reduction of renal blood flow, often an undesirable effect, may accompany the systemic administration of many of these agents. (3) Tolerance to the vasoconstrictor effect of drugs may develop within a short period of time and may make it particularly difficult to maintain the vascular tone desired.

Despite these theoretical disadvantages, however, there are certain clinical situations in which support of arterial pressure is so critically important that an agent that reliably raises blood pressure by increasing vascular tone may have a place in emergency therapy. The coronary vascular bed and cerebral vascular bed are particularly sensitive to perfusion pressure, and the need for an adequate perfusion pressure is enhanced in the presence of stenotic lesions in the proximal coronary and cerebral vascular beds. Therefore, in circumstances when evidence of myocardial or cerebral ischemia is reduced, prompt restoration of blood pressure may be of great importance. Use of agents for this purpose is generally only temporary and can be replaced by more physiological approaches to the circulatory disturbances as soon as the mechanism of the abnormality can be identified.

Sympathetic Agonists

Drugs that stimulate alpha adrenoceptors may produce both arterial and venous constriction and thus raise systemic vascular resistance and increase cardiac filling. Administration of these drugs generally also increases capillary pressure and results in intravascular depletion of plasma volume.[13] The major difference among these agents relates to their action on the heart. Drugs such as NE and *metaraminol* exert beta-agonistic as well as alpha-agonistic effects; the cardiac effect tends to support cardiac output in the face of peripheral vasoconstriction. In contrast, agents such as *phenylephrine* and *methoxamine* exert little direct positive inotropic effect, and therefore their actions are predominantly confined to peripheral constriction. These agents tend to raise blood pressure but at the expense of a reduction of cardiac output and considerable cardiac slowing. *Ephedrine* and the ephedrine-like analogues produce alpha constriction and beta cardiac stimulation but also produce beta vasodilatation in the skeletal muscle. Administration of ephedrine results in a variable effect on blood pressure, accompanied by considerable cardiac stimulation. Redistribution of blood flow away from vascular beds heavily endowed with alpha receptors, such as the renal bed, accompany the hemodynamic response to these agents.[77] *Dopamine,* which is the immediate precursor of NE, increases myocardial contractility by directly stimulating beta adrenoreceptors and by causing the release of NE from nerve endings in the heart. In lower doses (<2 μg/kg per min), however, it predominantly stimulates both dopamine DA_1 receptors to produce direct vasodilatation in renal, mesenteric, coronary, and cerebral vascular beds and dopamine DA_2 receptors to inhibit NE release. Intermediate doses (2 to 5 μg/kg per min) produce an increase in myocardial contractility and cardiac output with unchanged or decreased peripheral vascular resistance. Larger doses (>5 to 10 μg/kg per min) produce an increase in peripheral resistance and a decrease in renal blood flow due to stimulation of both $alpha_1$ and serotonin receptors. (See also Chap. 28.)

Angiotensin Analogues

Angiotensin is a potent vasoconstrictor that at one time was used clinically for support of blood pressure in hypotensive states.[78] The angiotensin amide previously marketed has been withdrawn from the market and is no longer available for clinical use. Angiotensin has a modest inotropic effect by virtue of augmented NE release and direct positive inotropic action, but it also has a potent renal vasoconstrictor effect. There appears to be no clinical indication for the administration of angiotensin at the present time.

Vasopressin Analogues

Polypeptides of the *vasopressin* series are potent vasoconstrictor agents that exert an action on both the arterial and the venous bed. Some analogues have been developed that are essentially devoid of antidiuretic hormone properties and exert almost an exclusive action on the vasculature.[79] These agents are particularly effective on the coronary bed and have been used diagnostically to induce coronary spasm in susceptible individuals with atypical angina.[80] These agents also have a selective action on the mesenteric vascular bed and therefore have been used to control variceal bleeding by reduction of portal vein pressure.[81] Although the effectiveness of these agents in lowering portal pressure has been established, some question remains as to whether or not this vasoconstrictor effect persists during sustained administration and whether or not the portal pressure reduction can therefore be maintained. The action of these drugs on venous return and cardiac output appears to be somewhat species dependent, and the mechanism of the reduction of cardiac output is not entirely understood.

REFERENCES

1. Cohn JN: Vasodilator symposium. Introduction: Marriage of the heart and the peripheral circulation. *Prog Cardiovasc Dis* 1981; 24(3):189–190.
2. Sarnoff SJ, Berglund E: Ventricular function. I. Starling's law of the heart studied by means of simultaneous right and left ventricular function curves in the dog. *Circulation* 1954; 9:706–718.
3. Katz AM: The descending limb of the Starling curve and the failing heart. *Circulation* 1965; 32:871–875.
4. Linzbach AJ: Heart failure from the point of view of quantitative anatomy. *Am J Cardiol* 1960; 5:370–382.
5. Gaasch WH, Levine HJ, Quinones MA, Alexander JK: Left ventricular compliance: Mechanisms and clinical implications. *Am J Cardiol* 1976; 38:645–653.
6. Sonnenblick EH, Skelton CL: Myocardial energetics: Basic principles and clinical implications. *N Engl J Med* 1971; 285:668–675.
7. Ludbrook PA, Byrne JD, McKnight RC: Influence of right ventricular hemodynamics in left ventricular diastolic pressure-volume relations in man. *Circulation* 1979; 59:21–31.
8. Cohn JN: Vasodilator therapy for heart failure: The influence of impedance on left ventricular performance. *Circulation* 1973; 48:5–8.
9. Milnor WR: Arterial impedance as ventricular afterload. *Circ Res* 1975; 36:565–570.
10. Cohn JN, Mashiro I, Levine TB, Mehta J: Role of vasoconstrictor mechanisms in the control of left ventricular performance of the normal and damaged heart. *Am J Cardiol* 1979; 44:1019–1022.
11. Moskowitz RM, Cohn JN: Hemodynamic effects of oxdralazine and hydralazine in hypertension. *Clin Pharmacol Ther* 1980; 27:773–778.
12. Cohn JN, Tristani FE, Khatri M: Systemic vasoconstrictor and renal vasodilator effects of PLV-2 in man. *Circulation* 1968; 38:151–157.
13. Cohn JN: Relationship of plasma volume changes to resistance and capacitance vessel effects of sympathomimetic amines and angiotensin in man. *Clin Sci* 1966; 30:267–278.
14. Schultz G, Schultz KD, Bohme E, Krege VAW: The possible role of cyclic GMP in the actions of hormones and drugs on smooth muscle tone: Effects of exogenous cyclic GMP derivatives. *Adv Pharmacol Ther* 1978; 3:113.
15. Wilkins RW, Haynes FW, Weiss S: The role of the venous system in the circulatory collapse induced by sodium nitrite. *J Clin Invest* 1937; 85:85–91.
16. Brown BG, Bolson E, Peterson RB, Pierce CD, Dodge HT: The mechanisms of nitroglycerin action: Stenosis vasodilation as a major component of the drug response. *Circulation* 1981; 64:1089–1097.
17. Mason DJ, Braunwald EB: The effects of nitroglycerin and amyl nitrite on arteriolar and venous tone in the human forearm. *Circulation* 1965; 32:755–766.
18. Fam WM, McGregor M: Effect of coronary vasodilator drugs on retrograde flow in areas of chronic myocardial ischemia. *Circ Res* 1964; 15:355–365.
19. Vatner SF, Pagani M, Rutherford JD, Millard RW, Manders WT: Effects of nitroglycerin on cardiac function and regional blood flow distribution in conscious dogs. *Am J Physiol* 1978; 3:H244–H252.
20. McGregor M: The nitrates and myocardial ischemia. *Circulation* 1982; 66:689–692.
21. Vanhoutte PM: Endothelium-derived vasoactive factors. *Hypertens Ann* 1990; 3–20.
22. Franciosa JA, Mikulic E, Cohn JN, Jose E, Fabie A: Hemodynamic effects of orally administered isosorbide dinitrate in patients with congestive heart failure. *Circulation* 1974; 50:1020–1024.
23. Chasseaud LF, Dawn WH, Grundy RK: Concentrations of the vasodilator isosorbide dinitrate and its metabolites in the blood of human subjects. *Eur J Clin Pharmacol* 1975; 8:157–160.
24. Davis JA, Wiesel BH, Epstein SE: The treatment of angina pectoris with nitroglycerin ointment. *Am J Med Sci* 1955; 230:259–263.
25. Olivari MT, Cohn JN: Cutaneous administration of nitroglycerin: A review. *Pharmacotherapy* 1983; 3:149–157.
26. Olivari MT, Carlyle PF, Levine TB, Cohn JN: Hemodynamic and hormonal response to transdermal nitroglycerin in normal subjects and in patients with congestive heart failure. *J Am Coll Cardiol* 1983; 2:872–878.
27. Elkayam U: Tolerance to organic nitrates: Evidence, mechanisms, clinical relevance, and strategies for prevention. *Ann Intern Med* 1991; 114:667–677.
28. Rudolph W, Blasini R, Kraus F: Clinical efficacy of nitrates in the treatment of exertional angina pectoris. *Herz* 1982; 7:286–291.
29. Cohn JN, Burke LP: Diagnosis and treatment—drugs five years later: Nitroprusside. *Ann Intern Med* 1979; 91:752–757.
30. Ivankovich AD, Miletich DJ, Albrecht RF, Zaked B: Sodium nitroprusside and cerebral blood flow in the anesthetized and unanesthetized goat. *Anesthesiology* 1976; 44:21–27.
31. Pace JB: Pulmonary vascular response to sodium nitroprusside in anesthetized dogs. *Anesth Analg* 1978; 57:551–557.
32. Chiariello M, Gold HK, Leinbach RC, Davis MA, Maroko PR: Comparison between the effects of nitroprusside and nitroglycerin on ischemic injury during acute myocardial infarction. *Circulation* 1976; 54:766–773.

33. Awan NA, Miller RR, Vera Z, DeMaria AN, Amsterdam EA, Mason DT: Reduction of ST segment elevation with infusion of nitroprusside in patients with acute myocardial infarction. *Am J Cardiol* 1876; 38:435–439.
34. Cohn JN, Franciosa JA, Francis GS, Archibald D, Tristani F, Fletcher R, et al: Effect of short-term infusion of sodium nitroprusside on mortality rate in acute myocardial infarction complicated by left ventricular failure. *N Engl J Med* 1982; 306:1129–1135.
35. McDowall DG, Keaney NP, Turner JM, Lane JR, Okuder Y: The toxicity of sodium nitroprusside. *Br J Anaesth* 1974; 46:327–332.
36. Freis ED, Rose JC, Higgins TF, Finnerty FA, Kelley RT, Partenope EA: The hemodynamic effects of hypotensive drugs in man. IV. 1-Hydrazinopthalazine. *Circulation* 1953; 8:199–204.
37. Franciosa JA, Pierpont G, Cohn JN: Hemodynamic improvement after oral hydralazine in left ventricular failure: A comparison with nitroprusside infusion in 16 patients. *Ann Intern Med* 1977; 86:388–393.
38. Perry HM Jr: Late toxicity to hydralazine resembling systemic lupus erythematosus or rheumatoid arthritis. *Am J Med* 1973; 54:58–72.
39. Khatri I, Uemura N, Notargiacomo A, Freis ED: Direct and reflex cardiac stimulating effects of hydralazine. *Am J Cardiol* 1977; 40:38–42.
40. Levine TB, Francis GS, Goldsmith SR, Cohn JN: The neurohumoral and hemodynamic response to orthostatic tilt in patients with congestive heart failure. *Circulation* 1983; 67:1070–1075.
41. Cohn JN, Archibald DG, Ziesche S, Franciosa JA, Harston WE, Tristani FE, et al: Effect of vasodilator therapy on mortality in chronic congestive heart failure: Results of a Veterans Administration Cooperative Study (V-HeFT). *N Engl J Med* 1986; 314:1547–1552.
42. Cohn JN, Johnson G, Ziesche S, Cobb F, Francis G, Tristani, F, et al: A comparison of enalapril with hydralazine-isosorbide dinitrate in the treatment of chronic congestive heart failure. *N Engl J Med* 1991; 325:303–310.
43. DuCharme DW, Freyburger WA, Graham BE, Carlson RG: Pharmacologic properties of minoxidil: A new hypotensive agent. *J Pharmacol Exp Ther* 1973; 184:662–670.
44. Koch-Weser J: Vasodilator drugs in the treatment of hypertension. *Arch Intern Med* 1974; 133:1017–1027.
45. Katz AM, Messineo FC, Herbette L: Ion channels in membranes. *Circulation* 1982; 65(1):2.
46. Fleckenstein A: Specific pharmacology of cardium in myocardium, cardiac pacemakers and vascular smooth muscle. *Annu Rev Pharmacol Taxicol* 1977; 17:149–166.
47. Henry PD, Shuchleib LJ, Borda LJ, Roberts R, Williamson JR, Sobel BE: Effects of nifedipine on myocardial perfusion and ischemic injury in dogs. *Circ Res* 1978; 43:372–380.
48. Warltier DC, Meils CM, Gross GJ, Brooks HL: Blood flow in normal and ischemic myocardium after verapamil, diltiazem, nisuldipine—A new dihydropyridine calcium antagonist. *J Pharmacol Exp Ther* 1981; 218:296–302.
49. Shimizu K, Ohta T, Toda N: Evidence for greater susceptibility of isolated dog cerebral arteries to calcium antagonists than peripheral arteries. *Stroke* 1980; 11:261–266.
50. Kazda S, Garthoff B, Knorr A: Nitrendipine and other calcium entry blockers (calcium antagonists) in hypertension. *Fed Proc* 1983; 42:196–200.
51. Young TE, Lundquist LJ, Chesler E, Weir EK: Comparative effects of nifedipine, verapamil and diltiazem as pulmonary hypertensives in the anesthetized dog. (Abstr.) *Am J Cardiol* 1982; 49:942.
52. Olivari MT, Bartorelli C, Polese A, Fiorentini C, Moruzzi AS, Guazzi MD: Treatment of hypertension with nifedipine, a calcium antagonist agent. *Circulation* 1979; 59:1056–1062.
53. Olivari MT, Levine TB, Weir EK, Cohn JN: Hemodynamic effects of nifedipine at rest and during exercise in primary pulmonary hypertension. *Chest* 1984; 86:14–19.
54. Singh B, Ellrodt G, Peter CT: Verapamil: A review of its pharmacological properties and therapeutic uses. *Drugs* 1978; 15:169–197.
55. Raftos J, Bauer GE, Lewis RG, Stokes GS, Mitchell AS, Young AA: Clonidine in the treatment of severe hypertension. *Med J Aust* 1973; 1:786–793.
56. Baum T, Shropshire AT: Studies on the centrally mediated hypotensive activity of guanabenz. *Eur J Pharmacol* 1976; 37:31–34.
57. Giles TD, Iteld BJ, Mautner RK, Ragnoni PA, Dillenkoffer RL: Short-term effects of intravenous clonidine in congestive heart failure. *Clin Pharmacol Ther* 1981; 30:724–728.
58. Henning M: Studies on the mode of action of α-methyldopa. *Acta Physiol Scand* 1969; 75(suppl 322):1–37.
59. Shore PA: Transport and storage of biogenic amines. *Annu Rev Pharmacol* 1972; 12:209–226.
60. Tackett RL, Webb JG, Privitera PJ: Cerebroventricular propranolol elevates cerebrospinal fluid norepinephrine and lowers blood pressure. *Science* 1981; 213:911–913.
61. Bacaner MB, Benditt DG: Antiarrhythmic, antifibrillatory, and hemodynamic actions of bethanidine sulfate: An orally effective analog of bretylium for suppression of ventricular tachyarrhythmias. *Am J Cardiol* 1982; 50:728–734.
62. Richards DA, Woodings EP, Prichard BNC: Circulatory and alpha-adrenoceptor blocking effects of phentolamine. *Br J Clin Pharmacol* 1978; 5:507–513.
63. Doxey JC, Smith CFC, Walker JM: Selectivity of blocking agents for pre- and postsynaptic α-adrenoceptors. *Br J Pharmacol* 1977; 60:91–96.
64. Constantine JE, Weeks RA, McShane WK: Prazosin and presynaptic α-receptors in the cardioaccelerator nerve of the dog. *Eur J Pharmacol* 1978; 50:51–60.
65. Moulds RFW, Jauernig RA: Mechanism of prazosin collapse. *Lancet* 1977; 1:200–201.
66. Mehta J, Cohn JN: Hemodynamic effects of labetalol, an alpha and beta adrenergic blocking agent, in hypertensive subjects. *Circulation* 1977; 55:370–375.
67. Bosanac P, Dubb J, Walker B, Goldberg M, Agus ZS: Renal effects of guanabenz: A new antihypertensive. *J Clin Pharmacol* 1976; 16:631–636.
68. Cushman DW, Cheung HS, Sabo EF, Ondetti MA: Design of new antihypertensive drugs: Potent and specific inhibitors of angiotensin-converting enzyme. *Prog Cardiovasc Dis* 1978; 21:176–182.
69. Bravo EL, Tarazi RC: Converting enzyme inhibition with an orally active compound in hypertensive man. *Hypertension* 1979; 1:39–46.
70. Brunner HR, Gavias H, Waeber B, Kershaw GR, Turini GA, Vukovich RA, et al: Oral angiotensin-converting enzyme inhibitor in long-term treatment of hypertensive patients. *Ann Intern Med* 1979; 90:19–23.
71. Captopril Multicenter Research Group: A placebo-controlled trial of captopril in refractory chronic congestive heart failure. *J Am Coll Cardiol* 1983; 2(4):755–763.
72. McCaa RE, Hall JE, McCaa CS: The effects of angiotensin I-converting enzyme inhibitors on arterial blood pressure and urinary sodium excretion: Role for the renal-serum-angiotensin and kallikrein-kinin systems. *Circ Res* 1978; 43:I32–I39.
73. Zimmerman BG, Gomer SK, Lioa JC: Action of angiotensin on vascular adrenergic nerve endings: Facilitation of norepinephrine release. *Fed Proc* 1972; 31:1344–1357.
74. Antonaccio MJ, Kerwin L: Pre- and postjunctional inhibition of vascular sympathetic function by captopril in SHR: Implication of vascular angiotensin II in hypertension and antihypertensive actions of captopril. *Hypertension* 1981; 3:I54–I62.
75. Share L: Interrelations between vasopressin and renin-angiotensin system. *Fed Proc* 1979; 38:2267–2271.
76. Johnson AK, Mann JFE, Rosher W: Plasma angiotensin II concentrations and experimentally induced thirst. *Am J Physiol* 1981; 240:R229–R234.
77. Goodyer AVN, Jaeger CA: Renal response to non-shocking hemorrhage: Role of the autonomic nervous system and of the renal circulation. *Am J Physiol* 1955; 180:69–74.
78. Cohn JN, Luria MH: Studies in clinical shock and hypotension. II. Hemodynamic effects of norepinephrine and angiotensin. *J Clin Invest* 1965; 44:1494–1504.
79. Cohn JN, Tristani FE, Khatri IM: Systemic vasoconstrictor and renal vasodilator effects of PLV-2 in man. *Circulation* 1968; 38:151–157.
80. Conti CR, Curry RC, Christie LG, Pepine CJ: Clinical use of provocative pharmacoangiography in patients with chest pain. *Adv Cardiol* 1979; 26:44–54.
81. Shaldon S, Dolle W, Guevara L: Effect of pitressin on the splanchnic circulation in man. *Circulation* 1961; 24:797–807.

Chapter 31

The Percutaneous Intraaortic Balloon Pump and Ventricular Assist Devices

Joseph M. Craver, M.D. ■ *Mark W. Connolly, M.D.*

PERCUTANEOUS INTRAAORTIC BALLOON PUMP

The intraaortic balloon pump (IABP) is the most widely used form of mechanical circulatory assist. A nonocclusive balloon catheter device positioned in the descending thoracic aorta causes diastolic pressure augmentation by balloon inflation in diastole and afterload reduction by deflation during ventricular systole. This system for counterpulsation was first described by Mouloupoulos et al. in 1962.[1]

Since balloon counterpulsation permits the elevation of diastolic aortic pressure and augmentation of coronary blood flow while reducing the load against which the systolic heart must pump, it has been employed in the following circumstances:

1. It has been used in cardiogenic shock to try to maintain viable perfusion pressure in the patient whose heart is highly damaged, but in whom recovery is still possible.
2. It has been used as an adjunct to the therapy of the intermediate syndromes in which the balance between ischemia and infarction has not been established in the presence of impending myocardial infarction. In such a circumstance, where vasodilators and perhaps beta blockers have already been utilized, counterpulsation has been of added use in further reducing oxygen needs of the heart while augmenting coronary perfusion. Indeed, in some institutions this is a therapy of choice in order to stabilize the patient prior to further therapy.
3. It has been used in the postoperative period to aid ventricular performance so that the patient can be weaned from bypass. As improvements in bypass technique have occurred and less cardiac damage has followed the use of hypothermia and cardiac arrest, the need for this type of support in the postoperative period has been reduced.
4. It has been used effectively in supporting patients prior to emergency coronary bypass surgery when percutaneous coronary angioplasty fails and is complicated by refractory myocardial ischemia.[2]
5. It has been used to support patients awaiting cardiac transplantation who have chronic heart failure that has poorly responded or is refractory to pharmacologic therapy.

Hemodynamic Effects

Balloon counterpulsation offers both diastolic and systolic advantages. By inflating during diastole, the balloon displaces a volume of blood equal to its own volume, thereby raising aortic diastolic pressure and augmenting coronary perfusion, which occurs primarily during diastole. In systole, balloon deflation is made to occur just prior to the next aortic valve opening and abruptly reduces aortic pressure, thereby allowing the left ventricle to eject against a greatly reduced arterial impedance. This may lead to decreased systolic and diastolic ventricular volumes. Myocardial pressure work, and therefore myocardial oxygen consumption, is reduced.[3,4] If ventricular function is complicated by mitral regurgitation or by ventricular septal defect (e.g., after acute myocardial infarction), the reduced ventricular volumes and pressure improve hemodynamic function by reducing the regurgitant flow or left-to-right shunt, respectively.[5-7]

Technique

The Intraaortic Balloon

Significant advances have been made in the design and manufacture of the intraaortic balloon and catheter. First, an additional lumen has been incorporated into the catheter, through which can be passed a flexible guidewire over which balloon catheter insertion can be directed. This second lumen is also available to monitor central aortic pressure after insertion is completed and the wire removed. Second, reduction in the diameter of the catheter despite incorporation of the second lumen has enabled a balloon 40 mL in volume to be wrapped around the central catheter and yet maintain an overall unit diameter that can be inserted through a no. 11.5 French sheath.

There are presently six IABP systems: Model 700 (Aries), System 90 and 90-Transport (Datascope), K-2000 and KAAT transportable (Kontron), and Model 3000 (Mansfield [formerly S.M.E.C.]). Each company manufactures a variety of balloon catheters for percutaneous and/or surgical insertion. With the correct adaptors, balloon catheters from one company may be used with another's console. Balloons manufactured for percutaneous insertion incorporate a single-chambered 40 mL or 30 mL balloon mounted on a double-lumen catheter. Catheter size is 9.0 French for the 40 mL and 8.5 French for the 30 mL balloon.

Testing

Testing continues in an effort to reduce the catheter size without a decrease in efficiency, but smaller catheters may require a decrease in displacement volume as well. The technique of insertion without using a sheath is intended to reduce the area the system takes up in the femoral artery, but it has not gained widespread acceptance due to difficulty of insertion.

Balloons available for surgical insertion vary widely among the manufacturers. Balloons for surgical insertion are available in a range of sizes with volume displacement from 10 to 40 mL, with custom-made sizes on request (Datascope). Surgical insertion balloons are available in volume displacements of 20, 30, and 40 mL, with catheters sized down to 8.5 French (Kontron) from 6 to 60 mL in volume displacement (Mansfield). All are single-chamber and mounted on single-lumen catheters. Some balloons are manufactured from polyurethane (Datascope, Mansfield); others use (Kontron) Cardiothane-51. All have low-thrombogenic surface properties and excellent durability. All systems now inflate the balloons with helium.

Balloon Insertion

Insertion of the IABP balloon catheter is accomplished by one of three routes: (1) retrograde insertion through a sheath placed in the femoral artery by the Seldinger technique,[3,8,9] (2) insertion via a side arm graft sewn to the femoral artery, or (3) insertion through a graft attached to the ascending aorta.

Retrograde insertion of the IABP balloon catheter through a sheath in the femoral artery is the most commonly used method at this time and is applicable and practical under local anesthesia in virtually any location in which electrocardiogram (ECG) and arterial monitoring are possible. Once the ECG and arterial monitoring devices are functioning, the patient's groins are bilaterally prepared and draped. The common femoral artery having the strongest palpable pulse is selected. The technique is applied by percutaneously cannulating the femoral artery with a flexible guidewire then passed through the cannula well up into the lower abdominal aorta. The arterial puncture is enlarged by passing progressively larger arterial dilators over the wire until a no. 10 French sheath can be introduced into the artery. The length of the balloon catheter to be inserted is measured by placing the balloon tip at the angle of Louis and marking with a ligature the location on the catheter at which it would exit the femoral artery. The single-chambered balloon is prefolded at the factory. It is removed from its package after application of negative pressure to hold this prewrapped condition. The balloon is inserted through the sheath, usually over a guidewire, and passed into the thoracic aorta to the premeasured distance. Once the balloon is inserted, a one-way valve holding the vacuum is removed, and the balloon unwraps. It can then be connected to the pump console and counterpulsation can begin. Once the system is in place the balloon catheter must be securely fastened to the leg by separate heavy suture. Correct position is checked by portable chest x-ray or fluoroscopy, and any adjustment is made.

Modification of this technique for balloon insertion has been helpful when the patient is still on cardiopulmonary bypass, when femoral pulses are absent, or when percutaneous femoral cannulation is felt to be hazardous. In these situations surgically exposing the common femoral artery enables the operator to cannulate that artery under direct vision. Direct visualization during cannulation may avoid tangential arterial laceration, subintimal insertion, or excessive hematoma formation, which may lead to unsuccessful arterial cannulation.[10]

Prior to the development and refinement of a balloon catheter that could be inserted by the Seldinger technique, extensive experience was attained in inserting the balloon via a side arm graft sewn to the femoral artery. This technique is still employed in many centers and can be applied also under local anesthesia wherever ECG and arterial monitoring are possible. After both groins are prepared and draped, a 5-cm segment of common femoral artery just above the origin of the deep femoral artery is exposed and isolated between cotton vascular tapes, which are later used as tourniquets. Formerly the largest possible size of balloon (20, 30, or 40 mL) was selected, based on the size of the femoral artery. Now the 40 mL balloon used in the percutaneous technique is often selected for all vessels, since its total catheter diameter is smaller than that of even the former 20-mL surgical balloon catheter. Development is continuing into even smaller balloon catheters for use in extremely small femoral vessels. The balloon catheter is then passed through a 10-cm length of 10-mm woven Dacron graft, which is later sewn to the femoral artery. The balloon length to be inserted is measured as above. The patient is heparinized 3 min before the artery is opened. The femoral artery is occluded by using both vascular tourniquets and then is opened 1 cm. A flexible guidewire is inserted proximally into the aorta, and then the deflated, wrapped balloon catheter is inserted over the guidewire into the aorta until the length marked with the ligature is reached. The proximal vascular tourniquet is again tightened, the balloon is unwrapped, and counterpulsation can begin. The Dacron graft is sutured to the femoral arteriotomy. Heavy silk ligatures are tied around the graft and catheter to prevent bleeding. The tourniquets are then released and blood flow restored to the leg. The balloon catheter is separately secured to the leg with heavy suture. The wound is then checked for hemostasis, irrigated, and closed in layers over the graft and insertion site. Balloon position is checked as noted above.

The employment of a flexible wire passed into the aorta, over which the double-lumen balloon catheter can be passed during insertion, has been a major improvement in the ease, safety, and success of balloon insertion. With young patients in whom femoral blood flow is excellent, employment of the guidewire may not be necessary. On the other hand, in the elderly population and in all patients with aortoiliac obstructive disease utilization of the guidewire can reduce problems associated with balloon passage that may be related not only to obstructive atheroma in these vessels but also to the extreme tortuosity that can be present even when flow is not impaired.

Should obstruction be encountered in the aortoiliac vessels that prevents passage either of the guidewire or of the balloon catheter over the guidewire with reasonable pressure, the opposite femoral artery should be tried. If balloon passage meets obstruction in this second site as well, the femoral route is abandoned. Forcing the balloon past a vascular obstruction greatly increases the risk of major vascular complications and embolization.

The majority of intraoperative balloon insertions are performed during or after an open heart surgical procedure.[11,12] General anesthesia makes it easier to expose higher segments of the iliac artery system should obstructive atheroma be encountered in the femoral area. Also, having the heart and great vessels exposed for the cardiac surgical procedure provides an opportunity to attach the graft to the ascending aorta for anterograde balloon insertion should retrograde passage prove impossible.[13]

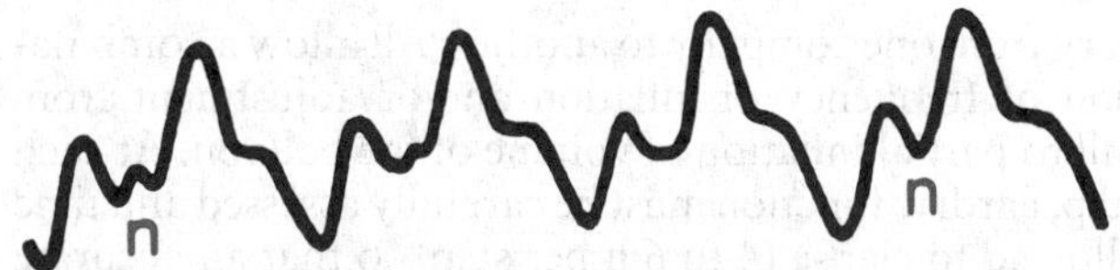

FIGURE 31-1 Timing of balloon inflation is adjusted to obliterate the dicrotic notch (n) on radial artery pressure curve.

Timing of Intraaortic Balloon Pump

Proper timing is essential if counterpulsation is to provide effective ventricular assist. The initial timing of IABP is done with the balloon at half volume and in the 1:2 mode. This enables one to see an unaugmented beat compared with a balloon-augmented beat. Ideally, the balloon should inflate immediately after aortic valve closure. If one is recording a central aortic pressure, this can be established accurately. If, however, a radial artery pressure trace is utilized, there will be a 50-ms delay in the waveform propagation. Therefore, balloon inflation is set to occur just before the dicrotic notch on the radial arterial pressure curve. As the proper timing interval for inflation is reached, one sees the obliteration of the dicrotic notch and a maximal height of the diastolic augmented peak (Fig. 31-1).

Adjustment of the deflation timing is equally important, in order to provide the maximum length of diastolic augmented interval and the greatest reduction in arterial impedance. Again, use of the 1:2 mode allows one to look at normal and augmented diastolic curves. By moving the deflation point closer to the ensuing systole, one seeks to achieve a waveform in which the end-diastolic dip is 10 to 15 mm below the level of the unaugmented diastolic level. Also one often sees a reduction in the height of the systolic peak that follows the augmented diastolic interval, when it is compared with the peak following an unaugmented beat (Fig. 31-2).

Weaning

IABP is continued in the 1:1 mode with the balloon at full volume until the patient's ventricular function appears satisfactorily restored and the need for the inotropic infusion has decreased. Weaning from IABP can then be accomplished over 6 to 12 h by systematic stepwise reductions of the assist mode.[14] Weaning choices

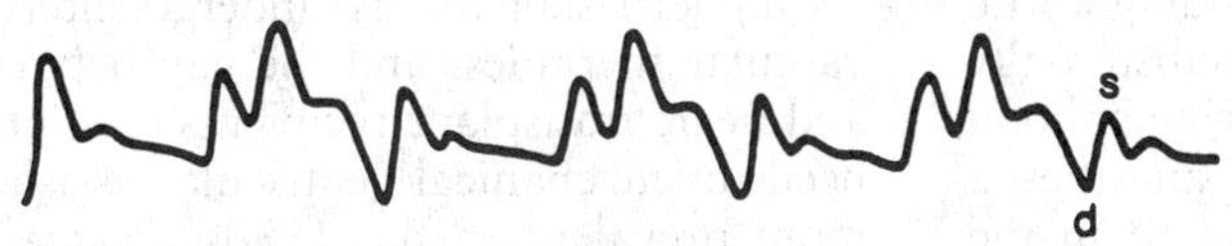

FIGURE 31-2 Timing of balloon deflation is adjusted to provide an end-augmentation diastolic dip (d) of 10 to 15 mmHg and to maximize reduction of ensuing ventricular systole (s).

vary from one company to another. All allow a combination of frequency of inflation and/or adjustment from full to partial inflation of volume of the balloon. At each step, cardiac function must be carefully assessed and time allowed to elapse (4 to 6 h per step) so that an accurate hemodynamic response is observed before further reduction in IABP assist is made. Measurements of cardiac index, arterial gas tensions, urine output, and pulmonary capillary wedge pressure along with careful clinical assessment of the patient's well-being serve as guides for further weaning or reinstitution of IABP assist. When hemodynamic independence of IABP assist is established, with the patient on minimal assist for 4 to 6 h, the balloon may be removed.

Balloon Removal

The procedure for balloon removal can be performed under local anesthesia in the intensive care unit. Removal of balloons inserted surgically is accomplished by re-exposing the femoral insertion site. If the balloon was inserted through a sheath the deflated balloon is withdrawn to the level of the sheath, then the sheath and balloon are removed simultaneously, while the femoral artery distal to the insertion site is temporarily occluded. This allows any thrombus that may be present in the artery, around the catheter or sheath or on the balloon itself, to exit via the insertion arteriotomy rather than to embolize distally in the artery. A careful prophylactic proximal and distal catheter embolectomy reduces retention of clot in the artery. Repair of the site can usually be performed with a few simple vascular sutures; rarely a vein patch repair may be needed if the artery is severely atherosclerotic. If a side arm graft was employed, the removal procedure is the same, with the graft usually being cut off near the insertion site and oversewn. Removal of the graft and primary arterial repair or vein patch repair of the anastomotic site can be done but usually are unnecessary.

Percutaneously inserted balloons are removed by similar techniques, simply by withdrawing the deflated balloon catheter to the level of the sheath and then removing both together while applying firm pressure to the femoral area just distal to the insertion site. Firm pressure just distal to the percutaneous insertion site is felt to reduce distal embolization of any clot or debris that may accompany balloon removal. Any such material egresses from the artery with the balloon catheter. After the balloon is removed, firm pressure over the femoral insertion site for 30 min to 1 h is essential, as is a normal coagulation profile, to avoid major groin hematoma. It may be that routine surgical removal and prophylactic proximal and distal catheter embolectomy may prove to be advisable on removal of percutaneously inserted balloons as well.[15]

When the balloon is inserted via an ascending aortic graft, usually the graft has been tunneled substernally into the epigastric subcutaneous tissue, allowing balloon removal by a similar procedure under local anesthesia. The end of the graft is then oversewn, buried in the wound, and allowed to clot. If the balloon cannot be removed or if a short graft has been used, reopening of the sternotomy is necessary.

Complications

Complications occur in approximately 5 to 35 percent of balloon insertions.[12,16–23] Ischemia of the extremity distal to the femoral insertion site is the most common complication of IABP and may be more frequent when the percutaneous insertion technique is employed.[20] Early removal of the catheter with thrombectomy is effective in most cases. Crossover grafts from the opposite femoral artery to a site distal to balloon insertion have been used as an alternative to removing the balloon when assist is still required.[19] Progressive ischemia requiring amputation of toes, the foot, or the lower leg has occurred in 1 to 2 percent of cases.[12,14–19]

Wound infection of the groin insertion site is the second most common complication, occurring in 3 to 4 percent of patients. These infections usually present themselves several days after the balloon has been removed and heal with topical care and systemic antibiotics. Deep infection requiring removal of the graft remnant is less frequent.[15–18]

Dissection or perforation of aortic, iliac, renal, or mesenteric vessels has been observed in 2 to 4 percent of patients and is usually suspected to stem from "difficult" balloon insertions.[12,18,20] Localized dissection or emboli are also thought responsible for the occasional case of spinal cord injury or small bowel or renal infarction (1 percent). Balloon insertion via the ascending aorta has been suggested to reduce the problem of dissection[13,15]; however, cannulation of visceral arteries with bowel infarction has been reported with this route.[21]

Thrombus formation on the balloon catheter with peripheral or visceral embolization has been reported.[7] Minidose heparin or infusion of low-molecular-weight dextran can prevent this but may cause bleeding complications.

Inability to pass the balloon catheter has been an important limitation of this technique in the past. Data regarding the frequency of this limitation are generally not available.[17] Utilization of the flexible guidewire to negotiate tortuous iliac vessels and obstructive atheromatous plaques in the femoral techniques and use of the ascending aorta as a site for insertion may reduce the incidence of nonpassage.

Balloon failure due to perforation is an increasing risk as balloon membranes are made thinner to accommodate smaller catheter sizes and as catheters are made more flexible. At first sign of balloon perforation—blood in the helium tubing—the balloon must be removed. A delay may prevent uncomplicated removal as the balloon fills with blood.

VENTRICULAR ASSIST DEVICES

As higher-risk patients undergo interventional cardiovascular therapies, and the gap between donor organs and heart transplant recipients continues to widen, the need for mechanical ventricular assistance will become more prevalent in the 1990s. Postcardiotomy cardiogenic shock refractory to pharmacological agents and intraaortic balloon pumping is estimated to occur in 1 percent of adult cardiac surgical cases.[24] This amounts to approximately 20,000 to 30,000 patients a year unable to be weaned from cardiopulmonary bypass. With available donor hearts leveling off at just over 3,000 per year in the United States, the United Network of Organ Sharing reports that 25 percent of potential recipients die waiting for a donor organ. Furthermore, the recipient waiting time for donor hearts continues to increase. Hence, the number of potential candidates for temporary and permanent mechanical circulatory assistance for end-stage heart failure will increase. Economic constraints will be the limiting factor in the use of these circulatory-assist devices.

Since the report of the first successful use of a ventricular assist device (VAD) in 1965,[25] technology has greatly progressed. A number of various devices are clinically in use today. Presently, in the United States, temporary VADs are approved for (1) *recovery* support in postcardiotomy, post-infarction or post-transplantation "stunned" myocardium; or for (2) *bridging* support in transplant or retransplant recipients in life-threatening heart failure. Permanent long-term support devices for refractory heart failure in patients not candidates for transplantation have not been clinically successful long-term. Technologic advances in blood-surface thromboresistant materials and implantable power sources are necessary before a permanent total artificial heart becomes clinically available.

Indications and Patient Selection

Patients in severe cardiogenic shock refractory to pharmacologic management and intraaortic balloon pumping are potential candidates for ventricular assistance. Hemodynamic monitoring with a Swan-Ganz arterial catheter and a left atrial line in postcardiotomy patients is necessary for decision making. Potential VAD candidates are patients with a cardiac index less than 1.8 liters/min/m^2, pulmonary capillary wedge or left atrial pressure (LAP) greater than 20 mmHg, right atrial pressure less than 15 mmHg, systolic arterial pressure less than 90 mmHg, and systemic vascular resistance greater than 2000 dynes·s/cm^5, representing severe *left* ventricular failure. Isolated *right* ventricular failure is present when the central venous pressure (CVP) exceeds 20 mmHg in the presence of relatively lower left-sided pressures (<15 mmHg) with a low cardiac index, low arterial pressure, and elevated systemic vascular resistance. *Biventricular* failure occurs when right- and left-side pressures are both significantly elevated (CVP and LAP > 20 mmHg). The differentiation between how much the right and left ventricle contributes to the shock state can be difficult. Intelligent decision-making determines the need for univentricular or biventricular assist-device insertion. Oliguria (< 20 mL/h) and metabolic acidosis support the hemodynamic criteria for VAD insertion (Table 31-1).

Patient selection is the most crucial factor in determining long-term survival with mechanical ventricular assistance.[25] In postcardiotomy patients, age greater than 70 years, renal failure and biventricular failure are predictors of poor outcome after VAD implantation.[26] Since transplant recipients have already undergone strict multisystem criteria for acceptance, they are usually better candidates for VAD implantation. End-organ dysfunction secondary to chronic low-out syndrome is frequently reversible with VAD support in transplant candidates with severe heart failure. The presence of infection, creatinine greater than 5 mg/dL, and respiratory failure predict negative outcomes with VAD bridging support in transplant recipients.[25,26] Primary cerebrovascular disease, presence of malignancy, peripheral vascular disease, chronic obstructive pulmonary disease, liver failure, blood dyscrasias, and presence of infection are other exclusion criteria.

TABLE 31-1

Hemodynamic Criteria for VAD Insertion

Cardiac index	< 1.8 liters/min per m^2
Systolic arterial pressure	< 90 mmHg
Systemic vascular resistance	> 2000 dynes·s/cm^5
Left atrial pressure	> 20 mmHg (LV failure)
Central venous pressure	> 20 mmHg (RV failure)
Oliguria or anuria	Urine output < 20 mL/h
Metabolic acidosis	

NOTE: VAD, ventricular-assist drive; LV, left ventricle; RV, right ventricle.

Predicting the reversibility of multiorgan failure secondary to cardiogenic shock after insertion of VAD can be difficult. Presently, there are no pre-VAD insertion criteria that accurately predict reversibility of multiorgan dysfunction. Therefore, careful pre-insertion patient selection and institutional VAD experience are necessary for successful patient outcomes.

Available Devices

The available devices are categorized *functionally* by the ventricle assisted (right, left, or biventricular), *mechanically* by the type of blood flow produced (pulsatile or nonpulsatile), by *position* (fully implanted or paracorporeal, heterotopic or orthotopic), or by *intended use* (temporary recovery of stunned myocardium or permanent long-term support). In paracorporeal or tethered VAD, the patient must be connected to external tubes or wires brought out through the skin, inhibiting the patient's postinsertion functional ability for rehabilitation. A fully implanted VAD allows the patient to be relatively free of external connections, allowing for more patient mobility and rehabilitation after insertion. Heterotopic or "piggy-back" VAD are the most commonly used today. Totally implantable or orthotopic devices (total artificial heart) have had limited use in recovery of stunned myocardium or bridging to transplantation. Permanent orthotopic devices are presently being developed and investigated for long-term use. The four types of VADs in present clinical use are external centrifugal pumps, external pulsatile devices, implantable left ventricular devices, and the paracorporeal Hemopump (Johnson & Johnson, Warren, NJ).

External Centrifugal Bypass Assist Devices

External centrifugal bypass pumps, including roller pumps, are readily available in any hospital performing open heart surgery. They are relatively inexpensive, simple to use, and do not require FDA approval. These devices are most commonly used for postcardiotomy cardiogenic shock, although many successes have been reported for bridge to transplantation.[28]

Cannulae are placed in the left atrium and aorta (LV bypass support) or in right atrium and pulmonary artery (RV bypass support), brought out through the chest, and connected to an external (roller or centrifugal) bypass pump. This system provides nonpulsatile flow rates from 2 to 6 liters/min. Centrifugal vortex pumps consist of magnetically driven, impeller rotator blades that propel blood from the inlet cannula to the outlet cannula, bypassing the support ventricle and providing arterial flow. The centrifugal VAD's most commonly used today are the Bio-Medicus, Inc. (Minneapolis, MN) and Sarns, Inc./3M (Ann Arbor, MI). After surgical bleeding has stopped, heparin infusion maintaining activated partial thromboplastin time (aPTT) at $1\frac{1}{2}$ to 2 times normal is recommended to prevent thromboembolic complications. Drive heads are frequently inspected for thrombus formation and should be changed regularly every 2 to 7 days to prevent embolic complications.

These devices are useful for short periods (5–7 days) of right, left, or biventricular ventricular support. If used for longer support, nonpulsatile perfusion may lead to multiorgan failure and significant damage to blood elements, producing complement activation, hemolysis, and thrombocytopenia. Significant perioperative bleeding, massive blood component transfusions, sepsis, and thromboembolic complications are frequent postoperative complications.

Experience with nonpulsatile VAD support for postcardiotomy cardiogenic shock patients has demonstrated a 20 to 35 percent hospital discharge rate[27,29,30] with an 86 percent 2-year patient survival in NYHA Class I or II.[27] Centrifugal VAD outcomes used for bridging to transplantation have been significantly better than postcardiotomy results, reaching 60 to 75 percent hospital discharge rates.[27]

External Pulsatile Ventricular Assist Devices

The external pulsatile VAD systems consist of pneumatically driven pumping chambers placed externally outside the body and connected to the heart chambers through cannulas brought in through the chest wall. Cannulae are placed in the right atrium (inflow) and pulmonary artery (outflow) for right ventricular support; and left atrium or ventricle (inflow) and aorta (outflow) for left ventricular assistance. The pumping chambers consist of polyurethane polymer thromboresistent diaphragms compressed by pulses of air delivered from the pneumatic, semi-portable, computer-controlled drive console. Prosthetic valves placed in the artificial chamber ensure one-way direction of pulsatile flow up to 6.5 liters/min.

The drive console has basically three different trigger modes of operation: asynchronous (fixed rate), external synchronous (ECG triggered), or volume-regulated. The commonly used volume mode or "full-to-empty" mode varies the pumping rate according to changes in the chamber's preload volume to maximize device output.

The Thoratec VAD system (Thoratec Laboratories, Inc., Berkley, CA), the Symbion Acute VAD (Symbion, Inc., Salt Lake City, UT), and the Abiomed BVS System 5000 (Abiomed, Inc., Danvers, MA) are the currently available external devices. All three can be used for right, left or biventricular support.

Farrar et al.[31] reported on the multi-institutional use of the Thoratec VAD system in 72 heart transplant recipients. Fifty-eight (81 percent) patients received biventricular support and fourteen patients left ventricular support only. Fifty-four underwent transplantation after a mean of 14.3 days of support (range 8 h to 81 days). Hospital 1- and 2-year survival rates (78 percent and 75 percent, respectively) were comparable to conventional nonbridged transplant patients.

Success has also been reported with its use as a temporary support device in postcardiotomy cardiogenic shock patients.[32]

Implantable Left Ventricular Assist Devices

Two implantable left ventricular assist devices (LVAD) for bridging to transplantation undergoing clinical evaluation under the Food and Drug Administration investigational device exemption are the Novacor LVAD (Novacor, Inc., Oakland, CA) and the Heartmate IP LVAD (Thermo Cardiosystems, Inc., Woburn, MA). Both systems consist of pusher-plate diaphragm chambers with bioprosthetic valves. The pumping chamber is implanted within the abdominal wall connected to external portable console through a percutaneous driveline. Asynchronous, ECG-triggered, and volume modes are available to maximize device output and patient support. The implantable pumping chamber and portable console allows for patient ambulation, exercise, and rehabilitation necessary to improving long-term results.

The Novacor LVAD is *electromechanically* driven. Inflow to the device is through left ventricular apical cannulation and outflow to a dacron graft sutured to the ascending aorta. Blood is pumped in parallel to the native heart at flow rates up to 9 liters/min.

The Heartmate LVAD is *pneumatically* driven. Inflow and outflow cannulation is similar to the Novacor LVAD. Textured polyurethane surfaces are used on the pusher-plate diaphragm. These textured surfaces promote pseudointimal lining formation on the diaphragm surface, which is felt to decrease thromboembolic complications. Most patients are anticoagulated long-term with warfarin regardless of type of device inserted.

Thermo Cardiosystems is currently testing a rechargeable internal battery source, and Novacor a totally implantable controller and power supply to further increase patient mobility.

Frazier et al.[33] recently reported the use of the Thermo Cardiosystems LVAD in 34 transplant recipients supported from 1 to 324 days. Sixty-five percent underwent transplantation and eighty percent were discharged from the hospital. Thromboembolic complications were rare. Similar results have been reported with the Novacor LVAD.[34]

Hemopump Left Ventricular Assist Device

The Hemopump (Nimbus, Inc., Rancho Cordova, CA) provides left ventricular assistance by pumping blood from the left ventricle into the aorta through a continuous flow catheter with an internal spiral vane cable rotating at 25,000 rpm. The intravascular catheter is inserted into the left ventricle from a graft sewn end-to-side to the femoral artery. Significant improvement in hemodynamics has been demonstrated after insertion in severe cardiogenic shock patients.[35] Disadvantages and complications are inability to insert through small, diseased femoral arteries, hemolysis, thrombocytopenia, ventricular arrhythmias, and thromboembolism. Experimentation and device design changes are being investigated until further clinical trials are resumed.

Total Artificial Heart

The Jarvik-7 Total Artificial Heart (Symbion, Inc., Tempe, AZ) has received much publicity in the past. Although still used clinically in a few centers as a bridge to transplant, it is no longer approved by the FDA for long-term orthotopic device insertion. New developments in power source supply, thromboresistance, and infection-resistant surfaces are necessary until a clinically useful, long-term device becomes available.

Summary

Relatively safe and reliable ventricular-assist devices have been successfully used for myocardial recovery in postcardiotomy cardiogenic shock and for bridging to transplantation (25 percent and 50 percent salvage rates, respectively). Patient selection, device selection, and timing of insertion before irreversible organ failure ensues remain at the forefront of successful outcomes. Thromboembolism, infection, and bleeding are significant device-related complications.

REFERENCES

1. Mouloupoulos SD, Topaz S, Kolff WJ: Diastolic balloon pumping (with carbon dioxide) in the aorta: Mechanical assistance to the failing circulation. *Am Heart J* 1962; 63:669–675.
2. Murphy DA, Craver JM, Jones EL, Curling PE, Guyton RA, King SB: Surgical management of acute myocardial ischemia following percutaneous transluminal coronary angioplasty: Role of the intraaortic balloon pump. *J Thorac Cardiovasc Surgery* 1984; 87:332–339.
3. Weber KT, Janicki JS: Intra-aortic balloon counterpulsation: A review of physiologic principles, clinical results, and device safety. *Ann Thorac Surg* 1974; 17:602–636.
4. Braunwald E, Covell JW, Maroko PR, Ross J Jr: Effects of drugs and of counterpulsation on myocardial oxygen consumption: Observation on the ischemic heart. *Circulation* 1969;40(suppl 4):220–228.
5. Buckley MJ, Leinbach RC, Kastor JA, Laird JD, Kantrowitz AR, Madras PN: Hemodynamic evaluation of intra-aortic balloon pumping in man. *Circulation* 1970; 41(suppl 2):130–136.
6. Phillips PA, Bregman D: Intra-operative application of intra-aortic balloon counterpulsation determined by clinical monitoring of the endocardial viability ratio. *Ann Thorac Surg* 1977; 23:45–51.
7. Dunkman WB, Leinbach RC, Buckley MJ, Mundth ED, Kantrowitz AR, Austen WG: Clinical and hemodynamic results of intraaortic balloon pumping and surgery for cardiogenic shock. *Circulation* 1972; 46:465–477.
8. Seldinger SI: Catheter replacement of the needle in percutaneous arteriography: A new technique. *Acta Radiol (Stockh)* 1953; 39:368–376.
9. Bregman D, Casarella WJ: Percutaneous intra-aortic balloon pumping: Initial clinical experience. *Ann Thorac Surg* 1980; 29:153–155.
10. Shahian DM, Neptune WB, Ellis FH: Intraaortic balloon pump morbidity: A comparative analysis of risk factors between percutaneous and surgical techniques. *Ann Thorac Surg* 1983; 36:644–653.
11. Buckley MJ, Craver JM, Gold HK, Mundth ED, Daggett WM, Austen WG: Intra-aortic balloon pump assist for cardiogenic shock after cardiopulmonary bypass. *Circulation* 1973; 46/47(suppl 3):90–94.
12. Craver JM, Kaplan JA, Jones EL, Kopchak J, Hatcher CR: What role should the intraaortic balloon pump have in cardiac surgery? *Surgery* 1979; 189:769–776.
13. Gueldner GL, Lawrence GH: Intra-aortic balloon assist through cannulation of the ascending aorta. *Ann Thorac Surg* 1975; 19:88–91.
14. Kaplan JA, Craver JM: Assisted circulation, In: Kaplan JA (ed), *Cardiac Anesthesia*. New York, Grune & Stratton, 1979:441–469.
15. Goldberg MJ, Kantrowitz A, Rubenfire M, Goodman G, Freed PS, et al: Intra-aortic balloon pump insertion: A randomized study comparing percutaneous and surgical techniques. *J Am Coll Cardiol* 1987; 9:515–523.
16. Creswell LL, Rosenbloom M, Cox JL, Ferguson TB Sr, Kouchoukos NT, Spray TL: Intraaortic balloon counterpulsation: Patterns of usage and outcome in cardiac surgery patients. *Ann Thorac Surg* 1992; 54:11–20.
17. Macoviak J, Stephenson LW, Edmunds LH Jr, Harken A, MacVaugh H: The intraaortic balloon pump: An analysis of five years' experience. *Ann Thorac Surg* 1980; 29:451–480.
18. Balooki H: *Clinical Application of the Intra-aortic Balloon Pump*. Mount Kisco, NY, Futura, 1977:1–490.
19. Lefemine AA, Kosowsky B, Madoff I, Black H, Lewis M: Results and complications of intra-aortic balloon pumping in surgical and medical patients. *Am J Cardiol* 1977; 40:416–420.
20. McEnany MT, Kay HR, Buckley MJ, Daggett WM, Erdman AJ, Mundth ED: Clinical experience with intra-aortic balloon pump support in 728 patients. *Circulation* 1978; 58(suppl 1):124–132.
21. Alpert J, Parsonnet V, Goldenkranz RJ, Bhaktan EK, Brief DK, Brenee BJ: Limb ischemia during intra-aortic balloon pumping: Indications for femoro-femoral cross-over graft. *J Thorac Cardiovasc Surg* 1980; 79:729–734.
22. Biddle TL, Stewart S, Stuart ID: Dissection of aorta complicating in intra-aortic balloon counterpulsation. *Am Heart J* 1976; 92:781–784.
23. Miller JF, Dodson TF, Salam AA, Smith RB: Vascular complications following intra-aortic balloon pump insertion. *Am Surg* 1992; 58:232–238.
24. Pennock JL, Pierce WS, Wisman CB, Bull AP, Waldenhausen JA: Survival and complications following ventricular assist pumping for cardiogenic shock. *Ann Surg* 1983; 198:469–478.
25. Spencer FC, Eiseman UG, Trinkle JK: Assisted circulation for cardiac failure following intracardiac surgery with cardiopulmonary bypass. *J Thorac Cardiovasc Surg* 1965; 45:56–59.
26. Pennington DG, McBridge LR, Swartz MT: Use of the Pierce-Donachy ventricular assist device in patients with cardiogenic shock after cardiac operations. *Ann Thorac Surg* 1989; 47:130–135.
27. Pae WE, Miller CA, Matthews Y, Pierce WS: Ventricular assist devices for postcardiotomy cardiogenic shock. *J Thorac Cardiovasc Surg* 1992; 104:541–553.
28. Miller CA, Pae WE, Pierce WS: Combined registry for clinical use of mechanical ventricular assist pumps and total artificial heart conjunction with heart transplantation. *J Heart Transplant* 1990; 9:453–458.
29. Killen DA, Piehler JM, Borkon AM, Reed WA: Bio-Medicus ventricular assist device for salvage of cardiac surgical patients. *Ann Thorac Surg* 1991; 52:230–235.
30. Curtis JJ, Walls JT, Schmaltz R, Boley TM, Nawarawong W, Landreneau RJ: Experience with the Sarns centrifugal pump in postcardiotomy ventricular failure. *J Thorac Cardiovasc Surg* 1992; 104:554–560.
31. Farrar DJ, Lawson JH, Litwak P, Cederwall G: Thoratec VAD system as a bridge to heart transplantation. *J Heart Transplant* 1990; 9:415–423.
32. Ruzevich SA, Kanter KR, Pennington DG, Swartz MT, McBride

LR, Termuhlen DF: Long-term follow-up study of survivors of postcardiotomy circulatory support. *Trans Am Soc Artif Intern Organs* 1988; 34:116–124.

33. Frazier OH, Rose EA, Macmanus Q, Burton Na, Lefrak EA, Poirer VL, et al: Multicenter clinical evaluation of the Heartmate 1000 IP left ventricular assist device. *Ann Thorac Surg* 1992; 53:1080–1090.

34. McCarthy PM, Portner PM, Tobler HG, Starnes FA, Ramasamy N, Oyer PE: Clinical experience with the Novacor ventricular assist system. *J Thorac Cardiovasc Surg* 1991; 102:578–587.

35. Wampler RK, Frazier OH, Lansing AM, Smalling RW, Nicklas JM, Phillips SJ, et al: Treatment of cardiogenic shock with the Hemopump left ventricular assist device. *Ann Thorac Surg* 1991; 52:506–513.

Chapter 32

Cardiac Transplantation

Sharon A. Hunt, M.D. ■ *John S. Schroeder, M.D.*
Margaret E. Billingham, M.D.

Although a number of advances in therapy for failing myocardium have saved or at least prolonged the lives of many patients with previously terminal myocardial dysfunction, there remains a sizable number of young patients who are fated to die or be severely disabled because of irreversible myocardial disease. In patients with such end-stage disease, biologic replacement of the heart has come to be a standard therapy and is currently widely accepted as a modality for prolonging life and improving its quality in carefully selected patients. As technological and engineering advances occur, mechanical replacement of the heart may well become a very competitive or complementary modality for treatment of such patients, but biologic replacement or transplantation is the current standard of therapy.

Interest in developing the surgical techniques to interpose a functioning heart into a recipient's circulation dates back at least to the early part of the twentieth century. In 1905 Alexis Carrel[1] first described heterotopic transplantation of a functioning donor heart into the neck of a dog. The heart in this model functioned in sequence with the recipient's heart in the circulation and was not actually capable of supporting the circulation. It was not until the 1950s that Demikhov[2] in Russia reported a series of technical advances in canine models in which a donor heart was placed in a heterotopic but intrathoracic position and the recipient heart excluded from the circulation so that the transplanted heart assumed the total burden of the circulation. In 1960 Lower and Shumway[3] described a technique for orthotopic transplantation of the canine heart that was elegant in its simplicity and remains the basis of standard clinical surgical transplant technique worldwide in the 1990s.

While these surgical techniques provided quite adequate anatomic and mechanical support and continuity of the circulation, they did not take into account the biologic phenomenon of immunologic rejection of a solid organ graft. This biologic phenomenon was simultaneously being encountered in the related field of kidney transplantation. Developments in the field of medical suppression of immune system reactivity led to the marriage of surgical and medical technology that is today known as organ transplantation. Clinical kidney transplantation first flourished in the mid 1960s.[4] The first human heart allograft procedure was performed in South Africa in 1967,[5] followed shortly by the first U.S. transplant by Shumway at Stanford in 1968 and then by a flurry of transplant activity in many centers for several years. This initial enthusiasm subsided as it became evident that postoperative survival was limited by a variety of complex medical complications including opportunistic infections and graft rejection. Most major centers discontinued performing heart transplantation in the early 1970s, and it was not until introduction of cyclosporine-based immunosuppression at Stanford in 1980 and demonstration of the attendant improvement in survival rates[6] that the procedure reemerged as widely accepted therapy for end-stage heart disease. In the 1990s most tertiary care centers provide programs for heart transplantation and most medical care payers in the United States, including the federal government, provide coverage for such care.

Cardiopulmonary transplantation was introduced at Stanford in 1981,[7] and subsequent experience with heart/lung and with both single- and double-lung transplantation in many centers has proven these procedures to be valid therapy for a wide variety of primary lung diseases and end-stage cardiopulmonary disorders.[8]

RECIPIENT SELECTION

As is the case with any surgical procedure, careful selection of patients for heart transplantation results in optimum postoperative survival rates. In contrast, however, to the quality-of-life or prolongation-of-life issues involved in decisions regarding more conventional heart surgery, decisions regarding candidacy for heart transplantation must take into consideration a limited donor supply, and therefore selecting recipients can be most difficult. Major guidelines for selection have been developed and are intended to provide the maximum benefit from a limited resource, namely that of donor organs. Selection criteria are in a state of change worldwide, and criteria for acceptance at one center may not match exactly those at another center. Nevertheless, some basic or general criteria can be described that are universally accepted and are summarized in Table 32-1. They include the most basic criterion: the existence of end-stage cardiac disease irremediable by other more conventional forms of medical or surgical therapy. The term *end stage* is, of course, difficult to define exactly, but in general, it refers to cardiac disease associated with New York Heart Association (NYHA) Functional Class IV symptomatic status and a clinically estimated probability of survival of less than 6 months. The definition of *more conventional* forms of therapy has certainly changed over the last several decades. Medical therapy with vasodilators and newer antiarrhythmic agents and devices, as well as surgical therapy for arrhythmias and formerly "inoperable" coronary disease, has at least delayed and in some patients avoided the need to resort to total cardiac replacement.

Age limits for cardiac transplant recipients are a second criterion for acceptance; these limits have been expanded considerably in both directions over the past several years. In the early years of experience with cardiac transplantation, older patients experienced very inferior survival rates and the upper limit of eligibility was set at age 50. Since the advent of cyclosporine-based immunosuppression in 1980, it has become apparent that survival rates are no longer inferior in older age groups. In the most recent year in which such data were analyzed in the Registry of the International Society for Heart Transplantation, the 30-day mortality rates according to age were identical (at 10 percent) for all ages between 10 and 69.[9] Reports from several centers have also attested to the excellence of both early and late postoperative survival rates in older patients.[10-13] Based on such data most centers have now advanced the official age of acceptability to 55, and many accept patients up to age 60. The lower age limits for transplantation eligibility have also been expanded recently with a number of major centers embarking on programs involving neonates and young children.

TABLE 32-1
Medical Criteria for Acceptance as Cardiac Transplant Recipient

Class IV cardiac disease
Not amenable to other surgical or medical therapy
Clinically estimated survival below 6 to 12 months
Age below 55 years
Absence of irreversible pulmonary hypertension
Absence of other systemic disease limiting survival
Absence of unresolved pulmonary infarcts

Potential cardiac transplant recipients are also screened for the existence of any other systemic disease that is likely separately to limit their survival. The coexistence of an active malignancy and the potentially increased tendency for its advancement in the presence of immunosuppression is one obvious problem, and such patients are routinely excluded. How to deal with a patient with end-stage heart disease and a remote history of malignancy is a more difficult problem. Edwards et al.[14] reported a small group of patients with a prior history of malignancy who were considered to have been cured of their malignant disease and were otherwise candidates for cardiac transplantation. Seven such patients had undergone transplantation; six had a remote history of lymphoproliferative disease, and one had had adenocarcinoma of the colon. Only the patient with colon cancer has had a recurrence of malignancy in follow-up averaging over 2 years. Thus, cautious acceptance of such patients may be justified.

The coexistence of one other major systemic disease, insulin-requiring diabetes, has been considered to be a contraindication to cardiac transplantation in otherwise acceptable patients. The rationale for this has been the well-known increase in incidence of early peripheral and cerebrovascular disease and nephropathy in these patients as well as their generally poor ability for wound healing and the difficulty of diabetic control during the period of constantly varying steroid doses early postoperatively. As steroid requirements have become lower, there has been discussion about relaxing this requirement to allow inclusion of stable (as opposed to "brittle") insulin-requiring diabetics, and in recent years several reports have attested to the safety and efficacy of heart transplantation in very carefully selected diabetic patients.[15-17] Human immunodeficiency virus (HIV) positivity is generally considered an absolute contraindication to heart transplantation due to the markedly poorer survival seen in other organ transplant recipients in this situation.

Other comorbid conditions must be considered on an individual basis, but irreversible organ dysfunction such as emphysema, severe peripheral vascular disease, and hepatic or renal dysfunction out of proportion to that predictable as a consequence of severe congestive heart failure are strong relative contraindications. The presence of an active infection is an (often temporary) absolute contraindication to transplantation because of the mandatory posttransplant institution of immunosuppression.

It was found early in the years of clinical experience with heart transplantation that a normal donor right ventricle is unable to increase its external work load acutely to overcome an elevated pulmonary vascular resistance (PVR). Because of this, patients who have end-stage heart disease with an elevated PVR may experience acute right-sided heart failure and cardiogenic shock after transplantation of a normal heart. This problem is a major cause of intraoperative deaths, and this fact has led to the setting of an upper limit of 4 Wood units of PVR (approximately 320 dynes-s/cm^5) (PAm-PAWm/CO) as the cutoff point or fourth criterion for suitability for cardiac transplantation. In recent years the concept of reactivity of the pulmonary vasculature and potential reversibility of elevated PVR has gained acceptance. Because of this, solidus potential candidates with PVR greater than 4 Wood units (320 dynes-s/cm^5) at baseline are usually subjected to pharmacologic maneuvers during hemodynamic monitoring using nitroprusside and/or prostaglandin E_1 to determine whether or not the elevated PVR is reversible; such patients are accepted as candidates for transplantation if the PVR can be reduced to acceptable levels while systemic arterial pressure remains adequate.

The last criterion that is accepted by most centers is the absence of unresolved pulmonary infarction. Pulmonary infarcts due to emboli from the dilated right ventricle, leg or pelvic veins, are common complications in patients with biventricular congestive heart failure awaiting transplantation in spite of systemic anticoagulation. Experience has shown that pulmonary infarcts have a high probability of becoming pulmonary abscesses after institution of immunosuppression. For this reason, waiting recipients who sustain pulmonary infarction usually are removed temporarily from the waiting list until the infarct resolves radiographically. Unfortunately, such resolution can be quite slow in this severely ill group of patients, and many never survive to return to the waiting list.

Based on these criteria, a group of patients is selected who are believed to have the best chance of benefitting from the operation and the attendant substantial commitment of medical resources. The type of underlying heart disease in the adult population selected for the procedure is nearly evenly split between idiopathic cardiomyopathy and ischemic disease, and in the pediatric population there is a higher percentage with congenital heart disease according to data from the International Society for Heart and Lung Transplantation (ISHLT) registry (Fig. 32-1).[18]

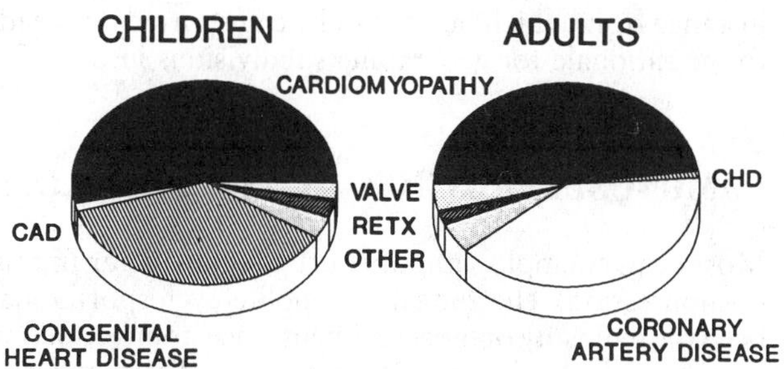

FIGURE 32-1 Etiology of underlying heart disease in transplant recipients. CAD = coronary artery disease; CHD = congenital heart disease; RETX = repeat transplantation. (*From JM Kriett, MP Kaye: J Heart Lung Transpl* 10:*491-498, 1991. Reproduced with permission.*)

DONOR SELECTION

Acceptance of the concept of brain death, both legally and medically, has been central to the emergence of organ transplantation (and particularly transplantation of unpaired organs such as the heart) in the modern era. The mandatory warm ischemic time involved if cardiopulmonary death were the only accepted criterion of death would make heart transplantation impossible. Acceptance of the concept of irreversible brain death has been a perhaps surprisingly recent phenomenon.

In 1970 Kansas became the first state in the United States to pass legislation recognizing the legal concept of brain death. Several states followed suit, and the medical and legal criteria for brain death have been refined over the years. The most recent and widely accepted set of guidelines was set out in the President's Commission Report in 1980.[19] It has been estimated that only 15 to 20 percent of persons who qualify as brain dead and have usable or transplantable organs become organ donors in the United States.[20] The reasons for this are complex and include public unawareness of the potential to donate organs as well as reticence among medical staff to make the request for donation. Efforts are being made in many areas to improve the percentage of organs from potential donors recovered for transplantation, but even with much higher recovery rates, heart transplantation will likely be a donor-limited field for the foreseeable future.

To be considered suitable donors for cardiac transplantation, brain-dead individuals must meet certain minimum criteria. Age criteria vary in different programs, but most cardiac donors have been under age 40. The donor should obviously not have had any significant cardiac disease, malignant disease, or acute chronic infection. Risk factors for cardiovascular disease such as diabetes or severe hypertension or hypercholesterolemia are relative exclusion factors. Donors are routinely screened serologically for HIV and for hepatitis B and C. Baseline serology for a number of other infectious diseases such as cytomegalovirus (CMV) is obtained in many programs but is usually not used prospectively in donor–recipient matching. If there is any suspicion of cardiac disease in the donor, appropriate diagnostic studies (including echocardiograms, cardiac catheterization, and coronary angiography) to assure the normalcy of the potential cardiac graft are pursued.

Once a potential donor is identified, the procurement process is initiated by contacting and referring to the local organ procurement organization (OPO), which has a registry of waiting recipients and coordinates equitable distribution of donor organs within a geographic area. Donor–recipient matching is fairly straightforward and requires ABO blood group compatibility as well as overall body size comparability with ±20 percent body weight considered to be an acceptable discrepancy. Human leukocyte antigen (HLA) matching is not attempted prospectively because of the difficulty in obtaining HLA typing promptly as well as the relatively small numbers of donors and recipients, which severely limits choices.

Most donor hearts currently are "harvested" or removed from the donor by a transplant donor team from a transplant center and transported back to the center for implantation. A cold ischemic time of 4 h in adults is generally considered safe; this requirement limits the distance from which hearts can be transported and leads to the rationale for geographic subdivisions into OPOs.

IMMUNOSUPPRESSION

Most centers employ multiple-drug regimens for immunosuppression. The fungal metabolite cyclosporine has been the mainstay of most regimens since its introduction into clinical practice over 10 years ago.[21] The number of drugs used and the timing of their administration varies from institution to institution, but several general principles are adhered to in the design of regimens.

The first principle is that immune reactivity and the tendency to graft rejection are highest early after graft implantation and decrease with time, although they likely never disappear entirely. Thus, most regimens employ the highest levels of immunosuppression immediately after surgery and decrease later, eventually settling on the lowest maintenance levels of suppression compatible with preventing recurrent graft rejection. The second principle is reminiscent of that originated in oncology chemotherapy regimens, that is, using low doses of several drugs without overlapping toxicities in preference to higher (and more toxic) doses of fewer drugs whenever feasible. As newer immunosuppressive agents and modalities are developed, the possible array of drug regimens can be expected to multiply accordingly, but these principles will likely remain.

The currently available immunosuppressive agents commonly used can be listed briefly. They include corticosteroids, azathioprine, cyclosporine, antithymocyte globulin (ATG), and OKT 3 monoclonal antibody preparation. A number of others are under investigation, and this list can be expected to increase over the coming 5 years. Table 32-2 outlines the current protocol used at Stanford University Medical Center for heart transplant recipients as an example of a typical cardiac transplant immunosuppressive regimen. Similar protocols are employed at most other transplant centers. Patients are begun on a relatively high dose of steroids and tolerable doses of cyclosporine and azathioprine initially. An initial 14-day prophylactic course of OKT3 is currently used and has recently replaced the routine use of equine ATG for this purpose. The intensity of immunosuppression is then tapered and is subsequently augmented only to treat graft rejection episodes.

TABLE 32-2

Stanford Cardiac Transplantation: Current Immunosuppressive Protocol

Stanford Cardiac Transplantation: Current Immunosuppressive Protocol
Cyclosporine
Loading dose 2–8 mg/kg 2–3 h preoperatively
Target serum level first month, 150–250 ng/mL
Target serum level thereafter, 100–200 ng/mL
Steroids
Methylprednisolone, 500 mg IV intraoperatively
Methylprednisolone, 125 mg IV q 8 h three times
Prednisone, beginning 0.6 mg/kg per day, tapering
Azathioprine
Loading dose, 4 mg/kg PO preoperatively
Maintenance dose, 1–2 mg/kg per day prn, white blood count above 4000
OKT3
5 mg IV daily 14 times beginning postoperatively on day 1

COMPLICATIONS

Rejection

In the first year following cardiac transplantation, the major cause of death is either acute rejection or infection. These two entities should be considered together, as insufficient immunosuppression will result in acute rejection whereas overtreatment with immunosuppression will result in infection. Acute rejection in cyclosporine-treated patients does not manifest itself clinically until rejection is end stage, at which point it is very severe and difficult to reverse. For this reason, patients are routinely monitored for acute rejection with serial endomyocardial biopsies. The endomyocardial biopsy has prevailed as the single most useful and accurate means of detecting acute rejection since it was first introduced into the cardiac transplantation program in 1973 at Stanford University.[22] Since then, many attempts have been made to use a noninvasive method to detect acute rejection. These efforts have been accelerated recently because of the recent need to manage neonates and very young children in whom the biopsy is a more hazardous and difficult procedure. Thus far, however, none of the techniques investigated has had the sensitivity and specificity to replace the biopsy.

Endomyocardial biopsy technique has been described and reported in depth in the literature.[23,24] (See Chap. 33.) The approach can vary, but in most cases the biopsy is performed percutaneously from the right internal jugular vein with pieces of tissue being retrieved from the right ventricular septum. In order to rule out acute rejection, a minimum of three to four good pieces (9 French bioptome size in adults) should be obtained to reduce the sampling error to an acceptable level. Even with three to four samples, a false-negative rate of 2 to 4 percent may result.[25] Biopsy specimens should be fixed immediately in 10 percent buffered formalin for light microscopy, and tissue can be frozen for immunohistochemical studies if required. Electron microscopy is usually not required, except for research purposes. After adequate fixation, the tissue is processed in the usual manner to provide thin well-stained (hematoxylin and eosin as well as Masson's trichrome) tissue specimens for review. It is recommended that the paraffin block be sampled at multiple levels.

Pathology of Acute Rejection

Gross Pathology

The rejected heart at autopsy or explantation is usually larger and heavier than normal. The heart is stiff and noncompliant and holds its shape. The outer surface may show a fibrinous pericarditis, and the heart in general is edematous and a dark plum color due to hemorrhage. The opened endocardial surface of the myocardium shows a distinct tinctorial difference between the darker red rejected donor heart myocardium and the light tan of the recipient myocardium, which can be compared along the atrial suture line. There are numerous subendocardial hemorrhages, and the trabeculae are swollen and prominent. Even the valves may be turgid and show some swelling. The interstitial edema and hemorrhage may impart an "amyloid quality" to the consistency and feel of the heart.

Microscopic Pathology

Hyperacute Rejection Fortunately such rejection does not occur often, but when it does, it is due usually to existence of ABO blood group incompatibility between the donor and the recipient. Hyperacute rejection manifests itself either immediately or within a few hours following transplantation. The heart will assume a darker red color due to the global interstitial hemorrhage that occurs from capillary breakdown. On histopathological examination, a hyperacutely rejected heart shows only interstitial edema and hemorrhage. If the heart is supported on cardiopulmonary bypass or other means until another donor heart is located, neutrophils will sometimes be admixed with the hemorrhage in the interstitium. Hyperacutely rejected hearts do not function and the recipient does not survive.

Acute Rejection and Grading of Acute Rejection Since the advent of cyclosporine for general use in 1981, there have come to be over 200 centers around the world performing cardiac transplants or combined cardiopulmonary transplants. It is inevitable, therefore, that many different grading systems for acute rejection have emerged.[26–28] Although different transplant centers may continue to use their preferred grading system, it has become necessary for the sake of comparing results from different centers as well as for multicenter trials that a uniform and standardized grading system be used. The ISHT now requires the use of the recently agreed-upon standardized system for all publications and trials.[29] For this reason, the new standardized grading system (Table 32-3) is used in this chapter. Use of the grading system requires an adequacy of sample with at least four pieces of myocardium, 50 percent of which must be evaluable myocardium (not biopsy site or scar). If a smaller bioptome (7-F or smaller) is used, then at least six pieces of myocardium are required. In this system, mild acute rejection is subdivided, with Grade 1A representing a focal perivascular or interstitial infiltrate that causes no myocyte damage. Several pieces of the biopsy may be involved. Grade 1B represents a more diffuse interstitial infiltrate that still does not cause any myocyte damage. Several pieces of tissue may be involved. Moderate acute rejection is represented by Grade 2, which is one focus of inflammatory infiltrate, which is sharply demarcated and is associated with myocyte damage. Grade 2 represents a solitary focus, and other biopsy pieces should be free of rejection or have a lesser grade. Grade 3A represents a multifocal moderate acute rejection that may be spread into several of the pieces. These infiltrates are associated with myocyte damage. Grade 3B is a more severe diffuse inflammatory process involving several of the pieces, if not all of them, and with significant myocyte damage (Fig. 32-2). This grade is often a borderline severe acute rejection. Severe acute rejection is represented by Grade 4, which is a diffuse polymorphous inflammatory infiltrate that may include neutrophils and eosinophils and in which there is frequently interstitial hemorrhage from vascular breakdown. Previous heavy immunosuppressive treatment or humoral rejection may result in more edema and hemorrhage than inflammatory infiltrate in severe acute rejection. Resolving or resolved acute rejection is denoted by a lesser grade on the biopsy than was noted on the prior biopsy.

Additional classifications using the new standardized grading system include reporting an inadequate biopsy, humoral rejection (positive immunofluorescence with vasculitis), or the so-called Quilty effect (an infiltrate usually confined to the endocardial surface only, which may or may not be associated with acute rejection).[29]

Pitfalls of Diagnosis of Acute Rejection

Not all inflammatory infiltrates in an endomyocardial biopsy necessarily represent acute rejection. In the first few weeks following cardiac transplantation, endomyocardial biopsies often show features of ischemia or ischemic damage to the myocardium, which is later replaced by granulation tissue. These changes are due to cold

TABLE 32-3

Standardized Cardiac Biopsy Grading

Grade	"New" Nomenclature	"Old" Nomenclature
0	No rejection	No rejection
1	A = Focal (perivascular or interstitial) infiltrate without necrosis B = Diffuse but sparse infiltrate without necrosis	Mild rejection
2	One focus only with aggressive infiltration and/or focal myocyte damage	"Focal" moderate rejection
3	A = Multifocal aggressive infiltrates and/or myocyte damage B = Diffuse inflammatory process with necrosis	"Low" moderate rejection "Borderline/severe"
4	Diffuse aggressive polymorphous ± infiltrate, ± edema, ± hemorrhage, ± vasculitis, with necrosis	"Severe acute" rejection

"Resolving" rejection denoted by a lesser grade.
"Resolved" rejection denoted by grade 0.
SOURCE: Reproduced with permission from *J Heart Lung Transpl.* 1990; 9:588.

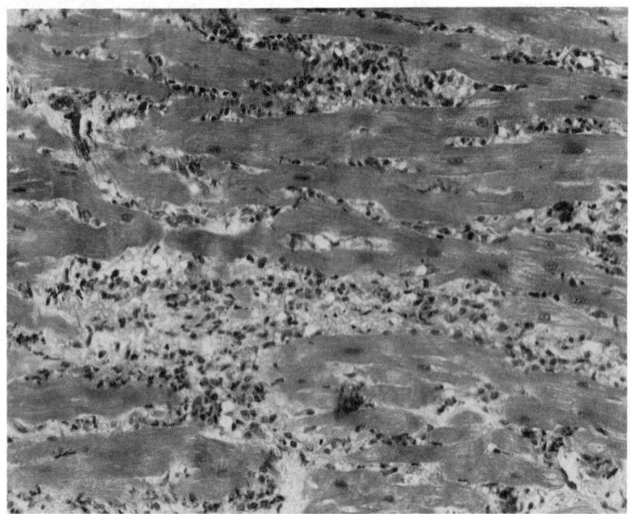

FIGURE 32-2 Endomyocardial biopsy showing acute rejection with myocyte replacement. H&E, ×100

ischemic time of the donor and may be exacerbated by a reperfusion syndrome following cardiac transplantation. There may also be small focal infiltrates of inflammatory cells as a result of using pressor agents either to support the donor prior to transplantation or to support the newly transplanted recipient. These infiltrates should not be confused with acute rejection. Infection, which is common in the immunosuppressed host, may also mimic or be confused with acute rejection. Inflammatory infiltrates due to infection, however, usually contain mixed inflammatory infiltrate (eosinophils and neutrophils as well as lymphocytes) and organisms may be found. Detailed descriptions of the above entities can be found in more extensive pathology papers.[18,30] Another pitfall causing confusion in biopsy interpretation is the occasional existence of granulation tissue due to residual inflammation from previous biopsy sites; however, usually other associated features make distinction from acute rejection possible.

In general, most patients can be monitored routinely with endomyocardial biopsy on a weekly basis for the first month following transplantation and then at monthly intervals for 6 months and then every 3 months or as required. In this way, severe acute rejection is seldom seen since most rejection episodes can be discovered and treated before they become severe. Biopsies are always done to assess the adequacy of a course of antirejection therapy.

Treatment for a rejection episode consists of augmentation of immune suppression. In the early postoperative period this usually is given as a 3-day pulse of intravenous corticosteroids. Subsequently, oral steroid pulses are commonly given. For resistant rejection, treatment or retreatment with lympholytic agents such as OKT3 is commonly used. For rejection refractory to such standard therapy, the use of total lymphoid irradiation (TLI)[31,32] or photophoresis[33] has offered some hope. Both are currently considered to be experimental therapy. Retransplantation remains the "ultimate" therapy for intractable rejection.

Infection

Infectious complications occurring as a consequence of chronic immunosuppression are the most frequent cause of death and morbidity in the posttransplant period. A wide variety of opportunistic organisms that are unusual as causes of clinical disease in the nonimmunocompromised population cause serious infections in organ transplant recipients. The lungs are the most commonly infected organs followed by the central nervous system. The clinical approach to such infectious complications includes a high level of vigilance for them and a very aggressive approach to prompt diagnosis and therapy.

Malignancy

All regimens of chronic immunosuppression are known to be accompanied by a subsequent increase in the incidence of lymphoproliferative malignancy, and organ transplant recipients have proved no exception.[33,34] The incidence of such malignancy in heart transplant recipients does not appear to be any higher than in other allograft recipients. There is increasing evidence that some of these malignancies may in fact be related to or subsequent to opportunistic infection with the Epstein-Barr (EB) virus.[35,36] They frequently occur in unusual extranodal locations and sometimes respond to reduction of immunosuppression.[37] According to the most recent registry report, malignancy accounts for 5 percent of deaths after heart transplantation.[38]

Graft Coronary Artery Disease

The above-described problems were all anticipated problems, given the nonspecific nature of currently available immunosuppression. The frequent development of diffuse and sometimes rapidly progressive graft epicardial coronary artery disease was not an anticipated sequela of cardiac transplantation but has in fact been found to occur to some extent in up to 40 percent of patients by 5 years posttransplant.[39–41]

Accelerated graft coronary disease in long-term cardiac allograft survivors is sometimes referred to as "chronic rejection," but this is a confusing term and probably should not be used unless or until the immunologic basis of the process is more clearly proven. Graft coronary disease may occur quite rapidly following cardiac transplantation in both children and adults. The pathologic findings include a concentric and longitudinal intimal proliferation, often with an intact elastica and not affecting the media of the vessel. Unlike "naturally occurring" atherosclerosis, asymmetric plaques, calcification, and atheromatous grumous material is seldom found except in long-term survivors over 10 years.[42] Also different from naturally occurring atherosclerosis are the fact that the entire vessel is often affected including the coronary artery branches and the small penetrating intramyocardial branches. It is of interest, although not surprising, that graft coronary disease may also occur in combined heart-lung transplants.[43]

Because it tends to affect the entire vessel and branches, graft coronary disease is not often amenable to atherectomy, angioplasty, or bypass surgery. Graft atherosclerosis is the leading cause of death, and complications after the first postoperative year and a better understanding of its underlying causes and development of prevention strategies are perhaps the most important areas of research in the field of cardiac transplantation.

DRUG-RELATED PROBLEMS

In addition to the above-described complications, a number of problems can and do occur in cardiac transplant recipients that are related specifically to the drugs used in the immunosuppressive regimen.

Cyclosporine

This agent has rather potent toxicity,[44] and much of what has been written and learned about its clinical use has been devoted to discovering ways of using it that minimize its toxicity. Table 32-4 lists the major unwanted or toxic side effects associated with the use of cyclosporine. Its inherent nephrotoxicity is by far the most important of these. Nephrotoxicity can be minimized, but not avoided, by careful monitoring of blood levels of the drug. A second and very important side effect associated with the use of cyclosporine is the frequent development of often severe arterial hypertension.[45] The exact mechanism of this hypertension has not been elucidated and is not apparently linked to the nephrotoxicity of cyclosporine. To date, no particular drug or class of drugs has been found to be uniformly efficacious, and many patients require multidrug antihypertensive regimens.

Prednisone

Chronic corticosteroid use is associated with perhaps the most formidable list of complications, including osteoporosis, glucose intolerance, skin fragility, cataract formation, and Cushingoid body habitus. Of these, the painful sequelae of osteoporosis with vertebral compression fractures and avascular necrosis of the hip and other weight-bearing joints are the most common causes of disability in late postoperative cardiac transplant recipients. For this reason, every effort is made to minimize and, when possible, eliminate the use of chronic maintenance corticosteroids in patient regimens.

Azathioprine

This agent was the mainstay of immunosuppressive regimens prior to the introduction of cyclosporine and has been reintroduced into the regimen in most programs in an effort to permit use of lower doses of cyclosporine and prednisone by adding an agent without overlapping toxicity. Its main toxic effect is that of dose-related bone marrow suppression, an effect that can easily be regulated by careful monitoring of peripheral blood counts.

TABLE 32-4

Cyclosporine Side Effects
Renal dysfunction
Hypertension
Headache
Hirsutism
Tremor

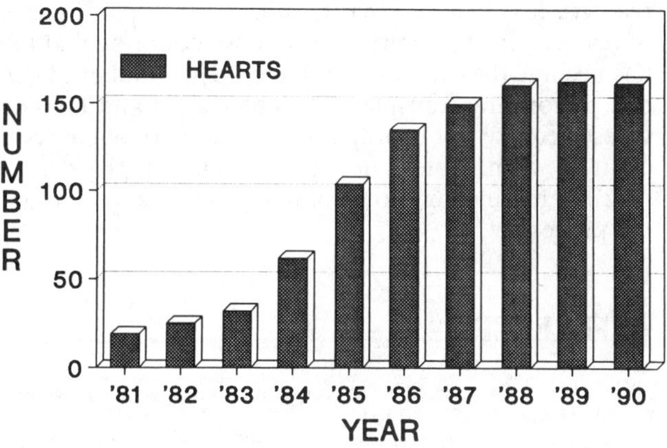

FIGURE 32-3 Number of centers reporting transplant procedures by year. (*Reproduced with permission* from JM Kriett, MP Kaye.[46])

RESULTS

The most recent ISHLT Registry data document a total of 16,687 heart transplant procedures performed worldwide as of January 1, 1991, the vast majority within the past 5 years.[46] Postoperative 1-year survival rates have increased from the 40 percent range in the early 1970s to the 60 percent range after the introduction of the endomyocardial biopsy and other advances in the mid-1970s to the 80 to 90 percent range after the introduction of cyclosporine-based immunosuppression in the early 1980s. The number of centers performing heart transplantation has increased concomitantly (and presumably because of the improved survival rates) since 1980, as shown in Fig. 32-3, as have the total number of transplant procedures per year, as shown in Fig. 32-4. Both numbers have plateaued in recent years, but for differing

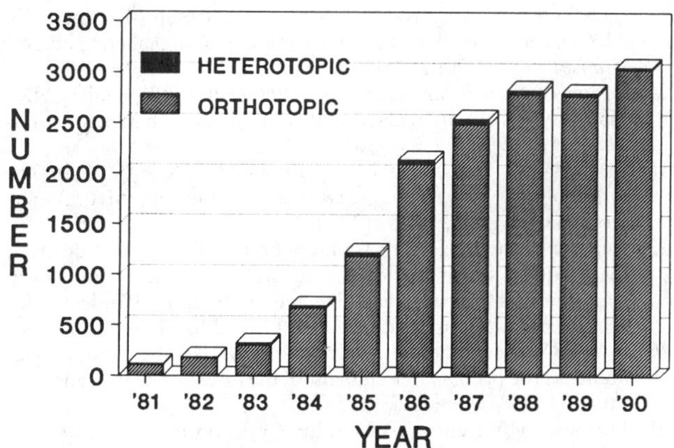

FIGURE 32-4 Numbers of heart transplant procedures by year. (*Reproduced with permission* from JM Kriett, MP Kaye.[46])

reasons. It is believed that number of transplant procedures per year has plateaued because donor availability has become the rate-limiting factor. The number of centers performing transplants has plateaued and may decrease because of the propensity of third-party payers to contract with centers doing a volume of procedures, possibly forcing very low volume programs to abandon the procedure.

REFERENCES

1. Carrel A, Gutterie CC: The transplantation of veins and organs. *Am J Med* 1905; 13:1101.
2. Demikhov VP: *Experimental Transplantation of Vital Organs.* Basil Hargh (translator). New York, Consultants' Bureau, 1962: 129.
3. Lower RR, Shumway NE: Studies on the orthotopic homotransplantation of the canine heart. *Surg Forum* 1960; 11:19.
4. Starzl TE, Marchioro RL, Waddell WR: The reversal of rejection in human renal homografts with subsequent development of homograft tolerance. *Surg Gynecol Obstet* 1963; 117:385–95.
5. Barnard CN: The operation. *S Afr Med J* 1967; 41:1274.
6. Oyer PE, Stinson EB, Jamieson SW, Hunt SA, Billingham M, Scott W, et al: Cyclosporin A in cardiac allografting: A preliminary experience. *Transpl Proc* 1983; 15:1247–1252.
7. Reitz BA, Wallwork JL, Hunt SA, Pennock JL, Billingham ME, Oyer PE, et al: Heart-lung transplantation—successful therapy for patients with pulmonary vascular disease. *N Engl J Med* 1982; 306:557–564.
8. Kriett JM, Kaye MP: The registry of the International Society for Heart Transplantation: Seventh official report—1990. *J Heart Transpl* 1990; 9:323–330.
9. Heck CF, Shumway SJ, Kaye MP: The registry of the International Society for Heart Transplantation: Sixth official report, 1989. *J Heart Transpl* 1989; 8:271–276.
10. Aravot DJ, Banner NR, Khaghani A, Fitzgerald M, Radley-Smith R, Mitchell AG, et al: Cardiac transplantation in the seventh decade of life. *Am J Cardiol* 1989; 63:90–93.
11. Olivari MT, Antolick A, Kaye MP, Jamieson SW, Ring WS: Heart transplantation in elderly patients. *J Heart Transpl* 1988; 7:258–264.
12. Miller LW, Vitale-Naedel N, Pennington G, McBride L, Kanter KR: Heart transplantation in patients over age fifty-five years. *J Heart Transpl* 1988; 7:254–257.
13. Carrier M, Emery RW, Riley JE, Levinson MM, Copeland JG: Cardiac transplantation in patients over 50 years of age. *J Am Coll Cardiol* 1986; 8:285–288.
14. Edwards BS, Hunt SA, Fowler MB, Valantine HA, Stinson EB, Schroeder JS: Cardiac transplantation in patients with preexisting malignant disease. *Am J Cardiol* 1990; 65:501–504.
15. Rhenman MJ, Rhenman B, Icenogle T, Christensen R, Copeland J: Diabetes and heart transplantation. *J Heart Transpl* 1988; 7:356–358.
16. Badellino MM, Cavarocchi B, Narins M, Jessup M, Alpern JB, McClurken JB, et al: Cardiac transplantation in diabetic patients. *Transpl Proc* 1990; 22:2384–2388.
17. Ladowski JS, Kormos RL, Uretsky BP, Griffith BP, Armitage JM, Hardesty RL: Heart transplantation in diabetic patients. *Transplantation* 1990; 49:303–305.
18. Billingham ME: Cardiac Transplantation. In: Sale GE (ed): *The Pathology of Organ Transplantation.* Stoneham, MA, Butterworth Heinemann, 1990: 133–152.
19. Reports of the medical consultants on the diagnosis of death to the President's Commission for the Study of Ethical Problems in Medicine and Biomedical and Behavioral Research: Guidelines for the determination of death. *JAMA* 1981; 246:2184–2186.
20. Evans RW, Mannines DL, Garrison LP, Maier MA: Donor availability as the primary determinant of the future of heart transplantation. *JAMA* 1986; 255:1892–98.
21. European Multicentre Trial Group: Cyclosporine in cadaveric renal transplantation: One year followup of a multicentre trial. *Lancet* 1983; 2:986–989.
22. Caves PK, Stinson EB, Graham AF, Billingham ME, Grehl TM, Shumway NE: Percutaneous transvenous endomyocardial biopsy. *JAMA* 1973; 225:228–291.
23. Mason JW: Techniques for right and left ventricular endomyocardial biopsy. *Am J Cardiol* 1978; 41:887–892.
24. Tilkian AG, Daily EK: Endomyocardial biopsy. In: Tilkian AG, and Daily EK (eds): *Cardiovascular Procedures.* St. Louis, MO, CV Mosby, 1986: 180–203.
25. Spiegelhalter DJ, Stovin PGI: An analysis of repeated biopsies following cardiac transplantation. *Statist Med* 1983; 2:33–40.
26. Billingham ME: The post-surgical heart: The pathology of cardiac transplantation. *Am J Cardiovasc Path* 1988; 1(3):319–334.
27. Kemnitz J, Cohnert T, Schafers HJ, Helmke M, Wahlers T, Hermann G, et al: A classification of cardiac allograft rejection. *Am J Surg Path* 1987; 11(7):503–515.
28. McAllister HA, Schnee MJ, Radovancevic B, Frazier H: A system for grading cardiac allograft rejection. *Texas Heart Inst J* 1986; 13:1–2.
29. Billingham ME, Cary NRB, Hammond ME, Kemnitz J, Marboe C, McAllister HA, et al: A working formulation for the standardization of nomenclature in the diagnosis of heart and lung rejection: Heart rejection study group. *J Heart Transpl* 1990; 9:587–592.
30. Yousem SA, Tazelaar HD: Combined heart-lung transplantation. In: Sale GE (ed): *The Pathology of Organ Transplantation.* Stoneham, MA, Butterworth Heinemann, 1990: 153–178.
31. Levin B, Bohannan L, Warvariv V, Bry W, Collins G: Total lymphoid irradiation (TLI) in the cyclosporine era—use of TLI in resistant cardiac allograft rejection. *Transpl Proc* 1989; 21:1793–1795.
32. Hunt SA, Strober S, Hoppe RT: Total lymphoid irradiation for treatment of intractable cardiac allograft rejection. *J Heart Lung Transpl* 1991; 10:211–216.
33. Costanzo-Nordin MR, Hubbel EA, O'Sullivan EJ, Johnson MR, Mullen GM, Heroux A, et al: Successful treatment of heart transplant rejection with photopheresis. *Transplantation,* 1992; 53:808–815.
34. Penn I: The price of immunotherapy. *Curr Prob Surg* 1981; 81:681–751.
35. Penn I: Cancers after cyclosporine therapy. *Transpl Proc* 1988; 20:276–279.
36. Hanto DW, Frizzera G, Gaul-Peczalska J, Purtilo DT, Klein G, Simmons RL, et al: The Epstein-Barr virus (EBV) in the pathogenesis of post-transplant lymphoma. *Transpl Proc* 1981; 8:756–760.
37. Young L, Alfieri C, Hennessy K, Evans H, O'Hara C, Anderson KC, et al: Expression of Epstein-Barr virus transformation-associated genes in tissues of patients with EBV lymphoproliferative disease. N *Engl J Med* 1989; 321:1080–1085.
38. Starzl TE, Porter FA, Iwatsuki S, Rosenthal JT, Shaw BW, Atchison RW, et al: Reversibility of lymphoma and lymphoproliferative lesions developing under cyclosporine-steroid therapy. *Lancet* 1984; 1:583–587.
39. Uretsky BF, Murali S, Reddy PS, Robin B, Lee A, Griffith BP, et al: Development of coronary artery disease in cardiac transplant patients receiving immunosuppressive therapy with cyclosporine and prednisone. *Circulation* 1987; 74:827–833.
40. Gao SZ, Schroeder JS, Alderman EL, Hunt SA, Valantine HA, Wiederhold V, et al: Prevalence of accelerated coronary artery disease in heart transplant survivors. *Circulation* 1989; 80(suppl III):III100–105.
41. Schroeder JS, Hunt SA: Cardiac transplantation: Where are we? (editorial). *N Engl J Med* 1986; 315:961–92.
42. Pucci AM, Forbes C, Billingham ME: Pathologic features in long-term cardiac allografts. *J Heart Transpl* 1990; 9:339–345.
43. Billingham ME: Cardiac transplant atherosclerosis. *Transpl Proc* 1987; XIX (suppl 5):19–25.
44. Myers BD, Ross J, Newton L, Luetscher J, Perlroth M: Cyclosporine-associated chronic nephropathy. *N Engl J Med* 1984; 311:699–705.
45. Thompson ME, Shapiro AP, Johnsen AM, Reeves R, Itzkoff J, Gindrereau E, et al: New onset of hypertension following cardiac transplantation: A preliminary report and analysis. *Transpl Proc* 1983; 15 (suppl I):2573–2577.
46. Kriett JM, Kaye MP: The registry of the international society for heart and lung transplantation: Eighth official report, 1991. *J Heart Lung Transpl* 1991; 10:491–498.

Chapter 33

The Technique of Myocardial Biopsy

Jerre F. Lutz, M.D.

Until the 1970s, the etiologic classification of diseases affecting the myocardium was based primarily on clinical and hemodynamic findings. The need to obtain biopsy specimens from orthotopically transplanted canine hearts resulted in the development of modern endomyocardial biopsy techniques and the long-awaited correlation between histological and physiological findings with resultant therapeutic implications. Presently, endomyocardial biopsy is indicated for the detection of cardiac allograft rejection or suspected myocarditis, for the monitoring of antineoplastic drug toxicity, and for the diagnosis of heart muscle disease due to conditions such as amyloidosis, sarcoidosis, or hemochromatosis.[1-3] Contraindications to the technique include bleeding dyscrasias, anticoagulant therapy, and mural thrombi.

DESCRIPTION

The Konno Method

The Konno myocardial bioptome, first described in 1962,[4] consists of a 100-cm catheter with a drive wire operated by a thumb ring that pushes and pulls the distal jaws open or closed. A cutdown technique using the basilic or saphenous vein or brachial artery is required to insert the broad biopsy head. There are multiple small parts, and although the outer jaw diameter is either 2.5 or 3.5 mm, there is a poor mechanical advantage often resulting in inadequate tissue samples. The shaft is rigid and entry into ventricles can be difficult. Problems with operation of the drive wire mechanism have also been reported.[5] This method is most frequently used in Japan and the Far East.

King's Method

In 1974, Brooksby and coworkers[6] and Richardson[7] used a modified Olympus fiberoptic bronchoscopy biopsy forceps inserted percutaneously through a no. 8 French long sheath into either an artery or a vein to perform right or left ventricular biopsy. The jaws are only 1.8 mm in diameter, resulting in small biopsy specimens, though the success rate is higher than with the Konno bioptome.[5] This method is most frequently used in the United Kingdom.

The Stanford Method

The no. 9 French 50-cm Stanford bioptome (Fig. 33-1) was designed by Caves et al.[8] in 1973 specifically for right ventricular septal biopsy following percutaneous insertion through a no. 9 French short sheath from the right internal jugular vein. The three main parts of the bioptome are the handle (modified by Mason[9] to be spring loaded, thus varying the cutting force), a flexible spiral wire catheter covered with Kynar tubing attached to one end of the handle, and a stiff, flexible wire that passes through the outer catheter and attaches to the other end of the handle. Opening and closing the handle controls the movement of the jaws welded to the distal end of the catheter and wire. Only one jaw is movable, but the span when open is 2.5 mm. The edges are sharp

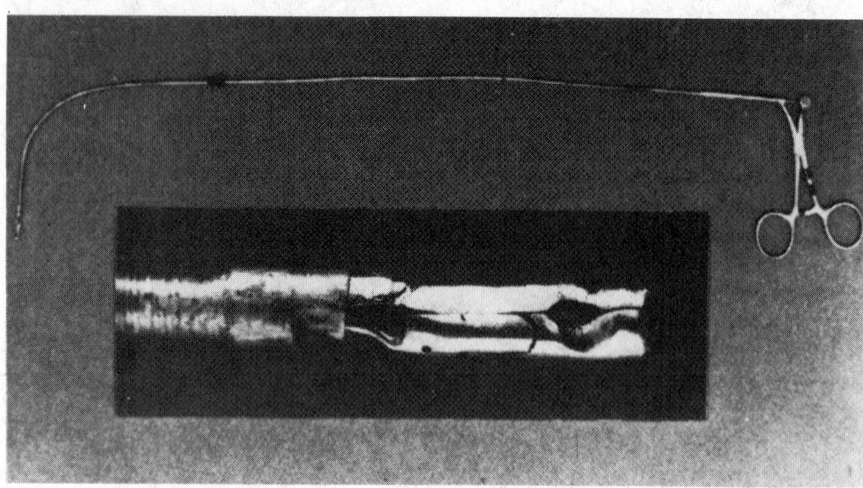

FIGURE 33-1 Stanford endomyocardial bioptome. (*From JW Mason: Techniques for right and left ventricular biopsy. Am J Cardiol 41:887–892, 1978. Reproduced with permission from the publisher and author.*)

enough to cut rather than avulse fragments of myocardium. Just prior to insertion, the catheter is bent at a right angle 7 cm from the distal tip and dipped into cold water to preserve the molded shape. Once inserted into the sheath, the catheter straightens to a 30° angle, ideal for crossing the tricuspid valve. This is the method most frequently used in the United States. Cooper and associates[10] have described a similar percutaneous technique using the supraclavicular approach for right ventricular biopsy in patients with heterotopic heart transplants. A long sheath remains in the right ventricle during the procedure to facilitate repetitive passes of the biopsy forceps.

Disposable Bioptome Technique

A no. 6 French disposable bioptome with two movable jaws can be inserted percutaneously via either venous or arterial access. Right ventricular biopsy using the disposable bioptome is performed through a multipurpose curved sheath introduced from the femoral vein across the tricuspid valve over a 125-cm multipurpose catheter. Left ventricular biopsy is performed by using a long straight sheath introduced into the left ventricle from the femoral artery over a pigtail catheter. Disposable biopsy forceps utilize either a 1.8- or 2.5-mm jaw diameter. Intravenous heparin is administered during left ventricular biopsy to prevent systemic emboli.[2] Lew and coworkers[11] have gently shaped the distal 7 to 10 cm of the disposable bioptome into a 60° to 90° curve for placement across the tricuspid valve via the internal jugular approach. Lurie and collaborators[12,13] have described techniques for attaining biopsy specimens in pediatric patients by using no. 4 and no. 5.5 French disposable biopsy catheters through the venous, arterial, and transseptal techniques.

ATTAINING BIOPSY SPECIMENS

Regardless of the technique, the patient's rhythm is monitored by an electrocardiogram and the passage of the forceps is monitored by fluoroscopy and/or two-dimensional echocardiography. Once the guiding sheath or bioptome is positioned across the tricuspid, mitral, or aortic valve (depending on the technique), the bioptome is advanced to the ventricular wall with jaws open to prevent perforation. In the correct fluoroscopic position for a right ventricular biopsy, the biopsy forceps is positioned well past the left border of the vertebral column and below the shadow of the left hemidiaphragm[5] (Fig. 33-2). Two-dimensional echocardiographic visualization has been useful in both visualizing the forceps and determining biopsy sites. The forceps should be aimed for the interventricular septum at the apex since this wall is relatively thicker than the free wall.[14] Mortensen and Egeblad[15] described good echocardiographic visualization in left ventricular (100 percent) but not right ventricular (18 percent) biopsies, whereas Pierard and associates[16] described good echocardiographic visualization in 100 percent of patients undergoing right ventricular biopsies. In left ventricular biopsies, the posterobasal segment of the ventricle is to be avoided.[17]

HANDLING OF BIOPSY SPECIMENS

Three to five biopsy specimens are attained. Mason[9] has described the Stanford protocol in which the first specimen is preserved in 10 percent buffered formalin and submitted for light microscopy. Serial sections are stained with hematoxylin-eosin, Masson's trichrome stain (for fibrosis), Congo red (for amyloid), and Prussian blue (for hemochromatosis). A second specimen is preserved in 2.5 percent glutaraldehyde for electron microscopy. The third specimen is flash frozen in isopentane and dry ice for immunofluorescent staining studies. Specimens can be placed directly into Earle's media for viral culture. Specimens should be teased from the biopsy forceps and excessive handling should be avoided.

RESULTS

Since the principal goal of endomyocardial biopsy is to attain material useful in the diagnosis and management

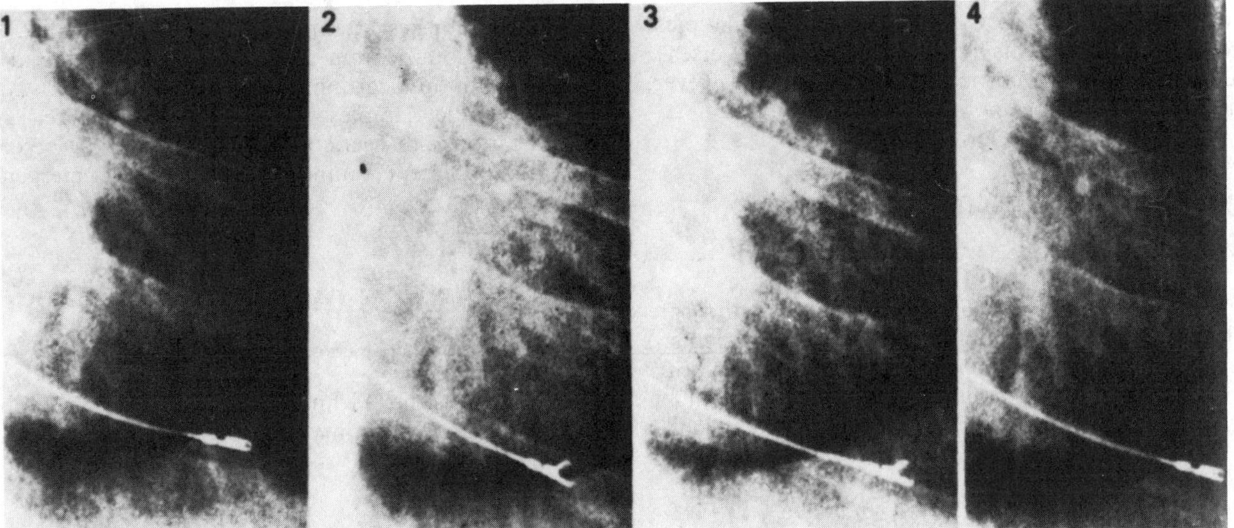

FIGURE 33-2 Fluoroscopic appearance of a right ventricular endomyocardial biopsy performed from the right internal jugular vein using the Stanford bioptome. *Panel 1:* Forceps across tricuspid valve. *Panel 2:* Jaws of forceps are open and slightly removed from ventricular wall. *Panel 3:* Jaws advanced open into ventricular wall. *Panel 4:* Jaws closed and biopsy specimen removed. A slight tug is sensed by the operator. (*Reproduced with permission from RE Fowles, JW Mason: Endomyocardial biopsy. Ann Intern Med 97:885–894, 1982.*)

of myocardial disorders,[18] one measure of success must be the frequency of attaining adequate material. Of the first 85 patients reported by Caves and coworkers,[8] diagnostic biopsy material was attained from all. Fowles and Mason[14] reported a 98 percent technical success in over 4000 biopsied cases. Cooper and collaborators[10] reported 96 percent success in patients with heterotopic heart transplants. Lew and coworkers[11] reported a 100 percent success rate in attaining material from more than 600 patients (85 percent outpatients) using the disposable bioptome.

Caves and associates[18] also reported good correlation between biopsy results and clinically apparent rejection in patients with orthotropic cardiac transplants (Fig. 33-3); moreover, biopsy-proven rejection often antedated clinically evident rejection by 2 to 4 days. Table 33-1 shows the noninfectious conditions in which material diagnostic of specific etiologies can presently be attained. Fowles and Mason[2] point out that the biopsy is not specific in the diagnosis of hypertrophied or dilated cardiomyopathy since there are no pathognomonic, histological, or biochemical features using current methods.

Specific diagnoses made by myocardial biopsy include cardiac allograft rejection, myocarditis, amyloidosis, sarcoidosis, hemochromatosis, glycogen storage disease, and eosinophilic infiltration of the endocardium. Infectious processes affecting the myocardium, including Chagas' disease and Lyme carditis can easily be diagnosed.[3] At Emory University, posttransplant biopsy specimens containing cytomegalovirus inclusion bodies and toxoplasmosis have led to specific diagnosis and therapy. An abnormal right ventricular biopsy demonstrating increased adipose and fibrous tissue may often be seen in patients with arrhythmogenic right ventricular dysplasia.[19] Open biopsies of donor hearts just prior to transplant to assess ischemic injury and left ventricular biopsy at the time of valve surgery to predict prognosis are research applications that may influence clinical treatment in the future.

The sensitivity of biopsy results must vary with the type of disease process studied. Although most pathological processes affect both ventricles, left ventricular biopsy is preferable in hypertrophic cardiomyopathy, certain forms of endomyocardial fibrosis, progressive systemic sclerosis involving only the left ventricle, and left ventricular radiation damage.[5] Olsen[20] has pointed out that good sensitivity can be attained if the process is diffuse or if the lesion (asymmetrical hypertrophy, tumors, or endocardial fibrosis) from which the specimen will be made can be localized. Thus, infiltrative cardiomyopathies such as amyloidosis (Fig. 33-4), sarcoid heart disease, and hemochromatosis can be readily diagnosed

TABLE 33-1

Disorders Specifically Diagnosed by Biopsy
Anthracycline cardiotoxicity
Carcinoid heart disease
Cardiac allograft rejection
Cardiac amyloidosis
Cardiac hemochromatosis
Cardiac sarcoidosis
Cardiac tumors
Endocardial fibroelastosis
Endocardial fibrosis
Fabry's disease of the heart
Glycogen storage diseases
Irradiation fibrosis of the heart
Myocarditis

SOURCE: From JA Laser, RE Fowles, JW Mason: Endomyocardial biopsy. *Cardiovasc Clin* 15:141–163, 1985. Reproduced with permission from the publisher and author.

by endomyocardial biopsy. The identification of a typical sarcoid granuloma is diagnostic of sarcoid heart disease and an indication for corticosteroid therapy[21]; however, a negative biopsy does not exclude the disorder.

ADVANTAGES OVER OTHER TECHNIQUES

Endomyocardial biopsy has become an easy and safe technique acceptable to both physicians and patients.[18] Previous to the development of this technique, myocardial biopsy was attained either by thoracotomy[22] or by percutaneous techniques resembling left ventricular puncture. Biopsies attained by Vim-Silverman needles were 1 cm long, 1 mm thick, and often composed of pericardium, myocardium, and endocardium.[14] Conversely, tissue samples were often inadequate. The complication rate was comparatively high (10 percent overall, 8 percent tamponade, 4 percent emergency thoracotomy).[23]

DISADVANTAGES OVER OTHER TECHNIQUES

Compared to other techniques, endomyocardial biopsy has great diagnostic utility with low morbidity. Problems

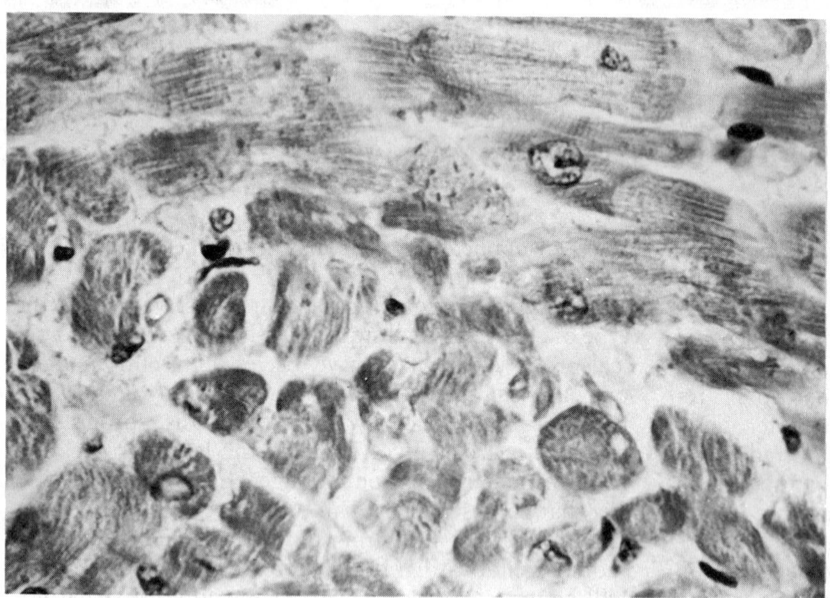

A

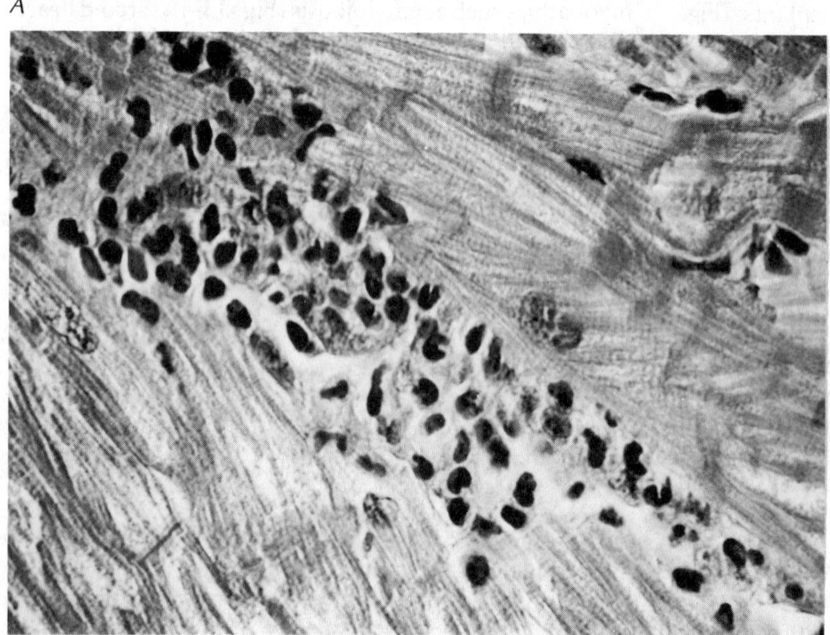

B

FIGURE 33-3 Allograft endomyocardial biopsies. *A*. A normal allograft biopsy shows myocytes in both longitudinal and cross sections (H&E × 400). *B*. Mild acute rejection is characterized by a discrete perivascular aggregate of small lymphocytes without myocyte injury (H&E × 400).

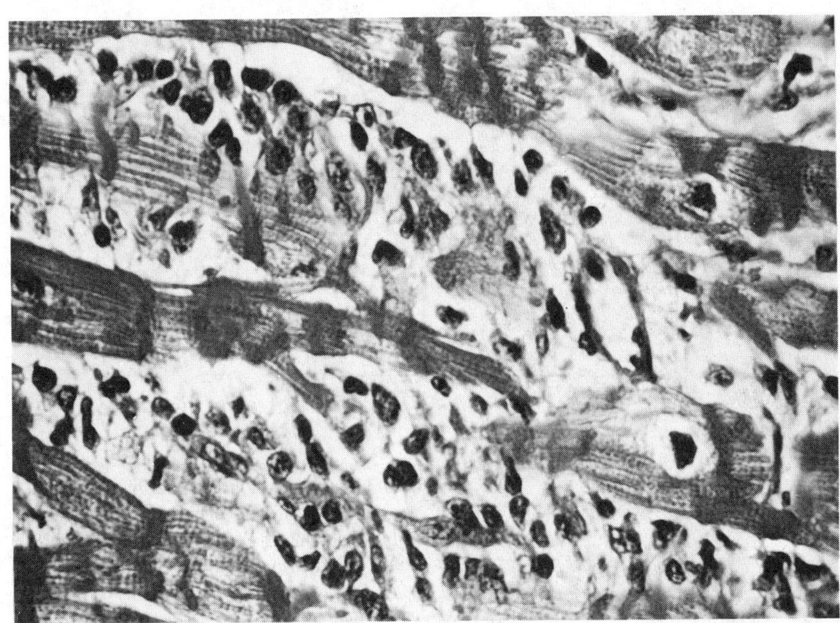

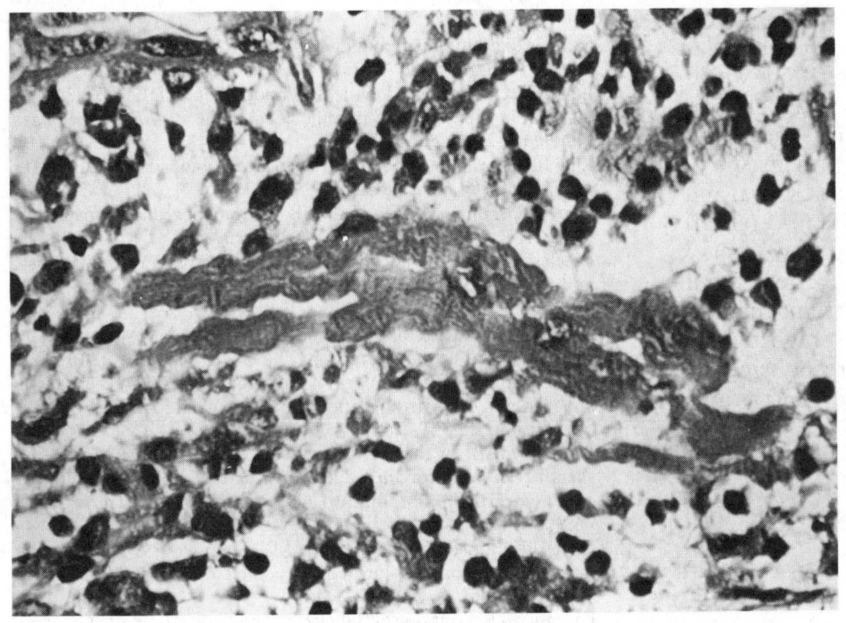

FIGURE 33-3 *(continued)* *C.* In moderate acute rejection, scattered foci of myocardium are slightly edematous and infiltrated by enlarged activated lymphocytes. A few myocytes show early damage with frayed cytoplasmic borders and loss of normal internal structure (H&E × 400). *D.* Severe acute rejection is characterized by marked diffuse edema and an intense inflammatory infiltrate of numerous segmented neutrophils as well as enlarged lymphocytes. Myocyte damage is extensive with frank myocyte necrosis (H&E × 400). (*Illustration courtesy of Gary Hertzler, M.D., Department of Pathology, Emory University School of Medicine, Atlanta, Georgia.*)

can arise, however, because of variability due to small sample size and intraobserver variation in pathological interpretation. Myocarditis and cardiomyopathy may not involve all muscle uniformly, thereby predisposing to sampling error. Vasculitis may not be evident on right ventricular biopsy since small vessels are relatively sparse compared to left ventricular tissue.[24] Old biopsy sites are characterized by extensive granulation tissue and can be mistaken for extensive subendocardial fibrosis.

Shanes and collaborators[25] reported a significant variability in the interpretation of fibrosis, hypertrophy, nuclear changes, abnormal lymphocyte counts, and diagnostic criteria for myocarditis when biopsies from 16 patients were submitted to seven different pathologists.

COMPLICATIONS

Chest discomfort during biopsy is unusual[20]; palpitations and discomfort at the bioptome insertion site are not unexpected. In the first 85 cases, Caves and coworkers[8] had one pneumothorax (related to the internal jugular approach) and one episode of atrial fibrillation. Fowles and Mason[2] reported tamponade in 0.14 percent of more than 4000 biopsies (none requiring thoracotomy). Additional complications included atrial fibrillation (three), pneumothorax (three), uncomplicated air embolus (six), transient recurrent laryngeal paresis (two), and Horner's syndrome (one). No patients died. Mason[9] also points out that in biopsy from the femoral approach, right

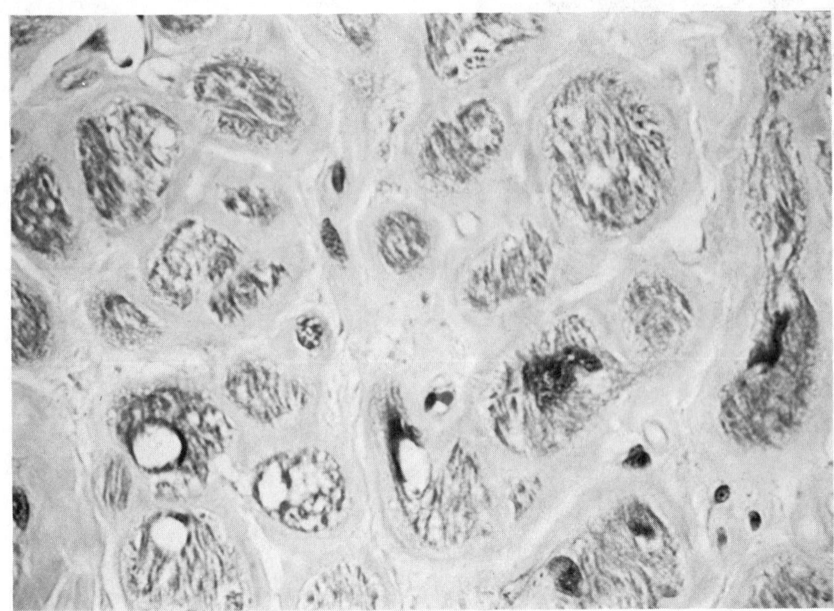

FIGURE 33-4 An endomyocardial biopsy demonstrates interstitial amyloid deposition. The amyloid forms thick pale rings around the myocytes (M) (H&E × 400). (*Illustration courtesy of Gary Hertzler, M.D., Department of Pathology, Emory University School of Medicine, Atlanta, Georgia.*)

bundle branch block is more likely because of the relatively higher position of the biopsy catheter. In a world survey of endomyocardial biopsy results, Sekiguchi and Take[26] reported perforation (0.42 percent) and death (0.03 percent) to be rare events in 6739 patients.

With regards to specific biopsy techniques, Kawai and Mutsumori[27] reported six systemic emboli (all cerebral) in 188 left ventricular biopsies. Lew and coworkers[11] reported that the carotid artery was inadvertently but uneventfully entered in 11 of 600 cases of internal jugular vein cannulation. Cooper and associates reported an overall complication rate of less than 1 percent using the supraclavicular approach in heterotropic heart transplant patients.[10]

Mason[9] clearly summarized matters when he stated that "the safety and success of the techniques for right and left heart biopsy described depend on meticulous attention to methodologic detail."

REFERENCES

1. Fenoglio JJ Jr, Ursell PC, Kellogg CF, Drusin RE, Weiss MB: Diagnosis and classification of myocarditis by endomyocardial biopsy. *N Engl J Med* 1983; 308:12–19.
2. Fowles RE, Mason JW: Endomyocardial biopsy. *Ann Intern Med* 1982; 97:885–894.
3. Dec GW: Current indications for endomyocardial biopsy. *Prim Cardiol* 1991; 17:34–46.
4. Sakakibara S, Konno S: Endomyocardial biopsy. *JN Heart J* 1962; 3:537–543.
5. Laser JA, Fowles RE, Mason JW: Endomyocardial biopsy. *Cardiovasc Clin* 1985; 15:141–163.
6. Brooksby IAB, Jenkins BS, Coltart DJ, Webb-Peploe MM: Left ventricular endomyocardial biopsy. *Lancet* 1974; 2:1222–1225.
7. Richardson PJ: King's endomyocardial bioptome. *Lancet* 1974; 1:660–661.
8. Caves PK, Schulz WP, Dong E, Stinson EB, Shumway N: New instrument for transvenous cardiac biopsy. *Am J Cardiol* 1974; 33:264–267.
9. Mason JW: Techniques for right and left ventricular biopsy. *Am J Cardiol* 1978; 41:887–892.
10. Cooper DKC, Fraser RC, Rose AG, Azenberg O, Oldfield GS, Hassoulas J, et al: Technique, complications and clinical value of endocardial biopsy in patients with heterotopic heart transplants. *Thorax* 1982; 37:727–731.
11. Lew BT, Olivari MT, Levine TB: Endomyocardial biopsy with a disposable bioptome: A modified technique. *Cathet Cardiovasc Diagn* 1987; 13:211–213.
12. Luri PR: Revision of pediatric endocardial biopsy technique. *Am J Cardiol* 1987; 60:368–370.
13. Lurie PR, Fujita M, Nuestein HB: Endomyocardial biopsy technique. *Am J Cardiol* 1978; 42:453–457.
14. Fowles RE, Mason JW: Role of cardiac biopsy in the diagnosis and management of cardiac disease. *Prog Cardiovasc Dis* 1984; 27(3):153–172.
15. Mortensen SA, Egeblad H: Endomyocardial biopsy guided by cross-sectional echocardiography. *Br Heart J* 1983; 50:246–251.
16. Piérard L, El Allaf D, D'orio V, Demoulin JC, Carlier J: Two-dimensional echocardiographic guiding of endocardial biopsy. *Chest* 1984; 85:759–762.
17. Brooksby IAB, Swanton RH, Jenkins BS, Webb-Peploe MM: Long sheath technique for introduction of catheter tip manometer of endomyocardial bioptome into left or right heart. *Br Heart J* 1974; 36:908–912.
18. Caves PK, Stinson EB, Billingham ME, Shumway N: Transvenous intracardiac biopsy using a new catheter forceps. *Heart Lung* 1975; 4:69–73.
19. Fontalivan F, Fontaine G, Fillette F, Aouate P, Chomette G, Grosgogeat F: Nosologic frontiers of arrhythmogenic dysplasia, quantitative variations of normal adipose tissue of the right ventricle. *Arch Mal Couer Vaiss* 1991; 84:33–83.
20. Olsen EGJ: Endomyocardial biopsy. *Br Heart J* 1978; 40:95–98.
21. Unverferth DV, Baker PB: Value of endomyocardial biopsy. *Am J Med* 1986; 80:22–32.
22. Weinberg M, Fell EH, Lynfield J: Diagnostic biopsy of the pericardium and myocardium. *AMA Arch Surg* 1958; 76:825–829.
23. Shirey EK, Hawk WA, Mukerji D, Effler DB: Percutaneous myocardial biopsy of the left ventricle. *Circulation* 1972; 46:112–122.
24. Melvin KR, Mason JW: Endomyocardial biopsy: Its history, techniques and current indications. *Can Med Assoc J* 1982; 126:1381–1386.
25. Shanes JG, Ghali J, Billingham ME, Ferrans VJ, Fenoglio JJ, Edwards WD, et al: Interobserver variability in the pathologic interpretation of endomyocardial biopsy results. *Circulation* 1987; 75:401–405.
26. Sekiguchi M, Take M: World survey of catheter biopsy of the heart. In: Sekiguchi M, Olson EGJ (eds): *Cardiomyopathy: Clinical, Pathological and Theoretical Aspects*. Baltimore, University Park Press, University of Tokyo Press, Tokyo, 1980: 217–225.
27. Kawai C, Mutsumori A: Myocardial biopsy. *Ann Rev Med* 1980; 31:139–157.

PART V

Disorders of Rhythm or Conduction

SECTION A

Electrophysiology, Diagnosis, and Management

Chapter 34

The Electrical Activity of the Heart

J. Thomas Bigger, Jr., M.D.

CARDIAC ELECTROPHYSIOLOGY

Along with nerve, skeletal muscle, and smooth muscle, heart muscle is one of the excitable tissues of the body. It shares many bioelectrical properties with other excitable tissues but has unique electrical features as well. The electrical activity of the heart is responsible for coordinating the sequence of cardiac activation and contraction. Understanding the normal electrocardiogram (ECG) requires a substantial knowledge of normal cardiac electrophysiology. Understanding cardiac arrhythmias requires knowledge of the electrical abnormalities that are their cause.

In this chapter, I will review briefly the basic principles of bioelectricity, some important aspects of excitable cardiac cell membranes, the ionic composition of cardiac cells, membrane ionic channels, cardiac action potentials, the normal sequence of activation in the heart, and some of the electrical abnormalities that cause cardiac arrhythmias. The mechanisms of cardiac arrhythmias and conduction disturbances are discussed in greater detail in Chap. 35.

Bioelectricity

Bioelectricity is the result of charge in tissue, usually as a result of positively or negatively charged ions.[1] A mole of ions contains 96,486 coulombs of charge (1 Faraday). Bulk physiological solutions, e.g., the extracellular fluid, usually are well-balanced electrically, containing an equal number of positively and negatively charged ions. Current is the flow of charge in some direction. Current flowing across a cell membrane is assumed to cross at a 90° angle to the cell surface and may be described as the amount of charge passing a point, e.g., the cell surface, per unit time, $i = dq/dt$. The ampere (A), which equals one coulomb per second, is the unit of current. Most currents in heart muscle range in amplitude from microamps (μA) to picoamps (pA), i.e., 1×10^{-6} A to 1×10^{-12} A. By convention, transmembrane current flow is designated as *negative* when positively charged ions move into the cell and as *positive* when positively charged ions move out of the cell. The total transmembrane current I_m is the sum of all ionic currents flowing at the instant when measurements are made. The electrical force that causes charges or ions to move is called voltage (V). The relationship between current and voltage is governed by Ohm's law:

$$V = IR$$

where V = voltage, I = current, and R = resistance. One ohm (Ω) is the amount of resistance that requires 1 V of force to cause 1 A of current flow. The interstitial and extracellular fluids have low resistance while the cell membrane has a high resistance. Membrane behavior often is described in terms of conductance (g), which is the inverse of resistance and is measured in siemens. Membrane conductance for an ion depends on membrane permeability to the ion and on the ion concentration. The conductance for an ion such as K^+ would be zero if K^+ were absent from the extracellular and intracellular fluid even though the membrane had a high permeability for K^+. The sarcolemma is a phospholipid bilayer and has substantial capacitance (C), i.e., ability to store charge. The amount of charge (q) stored on the membrane is proportional to the capacitance of the membrane and the voltage difference across the membrane:

$$q = CV$$

The Sarcolemma

The sarcolemma of cardiac cells is comprised of a phospholipid bilayer with its associated membrane glycoproteins.[2] The phospholipids are arranged so that their hydrophobic fatty acyl chains are in the membrane core while their polar head groups lie at the inner and outer surfaces of the membrane (Fig. 34-1). Cholesterol is found in the hydrophobic core of the membrane and probably contributes to its physical stability. The hydrophobic bilayer is about 50 Å, is very resistant to ion movement, and is an excellent capacitor. Proteins can be *extrinsic*, adsorbed to the membrane surface, or *intrinsic*, either embedded into one leaflet of the phospholipid bilayer or spanning the entire membrane to make contact with both extra- and intracellular fluid. Intrinsic proteins tend to fold or coil so that their apolar amino acids are on the surface of the protein in the lipid bilayer of the membrane. The lipid bilayer of the membrane is fluid so that the membrane has been likened to a collection of protein icebergs floating in a lipid sea.[2] Despite their relatively small fractional volume, proteins may comprise as much as half the membrane mass. The extrinsic proteins often are glycosylated and provide structural support to the sarcolemma. The intrinsic proteins serve as receptors, ion channels, and pumps.

Ionic Channels

Ionic channels are components of the membranes that permit movement of ions across the hydrophobic barrier of the cell membrane. The channels are thought to be membrane-spanning proteins that contain water so that hydrated ions can cross the membrane (Fig. 34-1). The channels have a selectivity filter that makes them selective to certain ions, e.g., a Na^+ channel preferentially conducts Na^+ ions and is less permeable to K^+ or Ca^{2+} ions.[1] Also, channels have gating mechanisms, i.e., they may be open or closed. Depending on the chemicals (agonists) in the channel or the transmembrane voltage field, the degree to which the channel is open may vary. The voltage dependence of channel opening can be explained by rearrangement of the charged portions of channel proteins according to the transmembrane charge field. Once open, channels have characteristic open times, e.g., about 1 ms for Na^+ channels and more than 100 ms for Ca^{2+} channels. Each channel seems to operate independently, i.e., the probability that a channel will be open or closed is not influenced by the state of neighboring channels. The number of channels per unit area of membrane has been measured for some channels. The membrane density of Na^+ channels has been measured using the binding of radioactive channel-specific agonists such as tetrodotoxin (TTX).[3] Only one TTX molecule binds to each Na^+ channel, and the binding has high affinity and specificity. Also, the number of Na^+ channels has been estimated using the opening-closing behavior in patch clamp studies.[4] These methods agree rather closely and suggest that the density of Na^+ channels in heart muscle, 5 to 10 per μ^2, is much less than that for squid giant axon, which is 200 to 500 per μ^2. The intensity of ionic current during activation usually is normalized to a unit area of membrane. Thus, the intensity of current will be proportional to the density of channels, i.e., number of channels per unit area of membrane. (See also Chap. 3.)

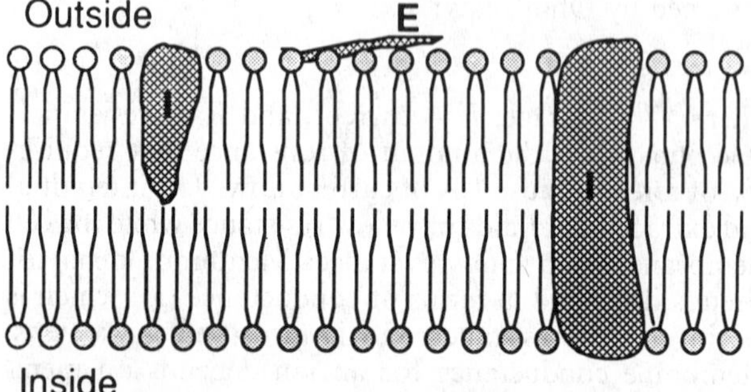

FIGURE 34-1 The myocardial cell membrane is composed of a lipid bilayer in which the polar heads of the phospholipid molecules face the extracellular or the intracellular fluid while the fatty acid tails face the core of the bilayer. Proteins can be intrinsic (I) or extrinsic (E).

Resting Transmembrane Voltage

Cardiac cells have a large transmembrane voltage difference during diastole, about −60 to −90 mV relative to the extracellular fluid potential. This resting transmembrane voltage or potential is an important factor in the electrical behavior of the cell, e.g., determining the action potential, and also in regulating transmembrane ion transport. In normal cardiac muscle, the resting transmembrane concentration gradients for ions such as K^+ and Na^+ are established by active ionic pumping and the membrane conductance for these ions. Typical normal values for electrolyte concentrations in myocardial cells are as follows:

$$[\mathrm{Na}]_o = 140\ \mathrm{m}M/\mathrm{liter} \qquad [\mathrm{Na}]_i = 25\ \mathrm{m}M/\mathrm{liter}$$

$$[\mathrm{K}]_o = 4.0\ \mathrm{m}M/\mathrm{liter} \qquad [\mathrm{K}]_i = 150\ \mathrm{m}M/\mathrm{liter}$$

$$\mathrm{gNa/gK} = 0.01 \text{ to } 0.07$$

where $[\ ]_o$ and $[\ ]_i$ refer to ionic concentrations outside and inside the cell. If there were no voltage gradient across the membrane, the movement of an ion such as K^+ would be determined only by the concentration gradient across the membrane and the permeability of the membrane to the ion.[5] Under these conditions, K^+ would diffuse out of the cell until the concentrations equalized across the sarcolemma. However, fixed negative charges inside the cell, presumably proteins and polypeptides too large to diffuse out of the cell, attract K^+ ions and impair their outward movement. When the chemical and electrical forces acting on an ion are equal and opposite, the system is in equilibrium and no net ion flux occurs.[5] The V_m at which electrochemical equilibrium occurs is called the equilibrium voltage or equilibrium potential.

According to the Nernst equation, the potassium equilibrium potential (V_K), i.e., the transmembrane voltage that would exist if the ionic concentrations given above were present and the membrane were permeable only to K^+, is given by

$$V_K = \frac{RT}{F} \ln \frac{[K]_o}{[K]_i} = -97 \text{ mV}$$

and the sodium equilibrium potential (V_{Na}) by

$$V_{Na} = \frac{RT}{F} \ln \frac{[Na]_o}{[Na]_i} = +46 \text{ mV}$$

where R is the universal gas constant, T is the absolute temperature, and F is the Faraday.[5] The Nernst equation states that for a given ratio of concentration (more properly the activity) of an ion across the semipermeable cell membrane, a transmembrane voltage exists that will maintain the concentration ratio constant. If the resting transmembrane voltage (resting V_m) were determined only by these two ions, then

$$V_m = \frac{RT}{F} \ln \frac{[K]_o + gNa/gK[Na]_o}{[K]_i + gNa/gK[Na]_i} = -90 \text{ mV}$$

Over a wide range of ionic concentrations, gNa/gK of the resting cell remains low and resting V_m is determined primarily by extracellular and intracellular K^+ concentrations. Raising $[K]_o$ from 3.8 to 6.0 m*M*/liter would decrease resting V_m from −90 to −80 mV even though gNa/gK remained constant. Under certain conditions, however, gNa/gK itself changes, producing changes in resting V_m. At very low values of $[K]_o$ (<0.5 m*M*/liter) or when cardiac muscle is stretched, g K decreases markedly. This increase in gNa/gK causes resting V_m to become less negative than the ionic concentration (activity) gradients would otherwise dictate. Purkinje fibers have a higher resting gNa than other cardiac myocytes, so that lowering K^+ has a dramatic effect on resting V_m (Fig. 34-2). Because of the decrease in gK as $[K]_o$ decreases below normal, resting V_m has the same value (about −60 mV) at $[K]_o$ = 1.0 m*M* and $[K]_o$ = 13.5 m*M*.[6,7] Despite the similarity of resting V_m, however, the response of cells to stimuli will be strikingly different at these two $[K]_o$. Ordinarily atrial and ventricular cells depolarize less than Purkinje fibers when $[K]_o$ is reduced because their resting gNa is lower.

The Na^+ Pump

There is a significant resting Na^+ influx in cardiac cells.[8] If Na^+ ions were not extruded by the cell, the resting potential would decrease as Na^+ accumulated. Extrusion of Na^+ from the cell requires energy because both electrical and chemical gradients oppose removal of Na^+. The energy for Na^+ pumping is provided by the alpha subunit of membrane-associated Na-K-adenosinetriphosphatase (ATPase) that extrudes three Na^+ and pumps in two K^+ for each molecule of ATP that is hydrolyzed.[9] This enzyme is stimulated by catecholamines and inhibited by digitalis glycosides. The activity of the Na^+ pump is electrogenic, i.e., more positive charge is pumped out than in (a 3 : 2 Na^+-K^+ ratio).[9] Under resting conditions, the pump current makes some contribution to resting V_m. Under conditions of increased Na^+ entry, e.g., increased heart rate, pump current will contribute more to diastolic V_m, driving it to more negative values.

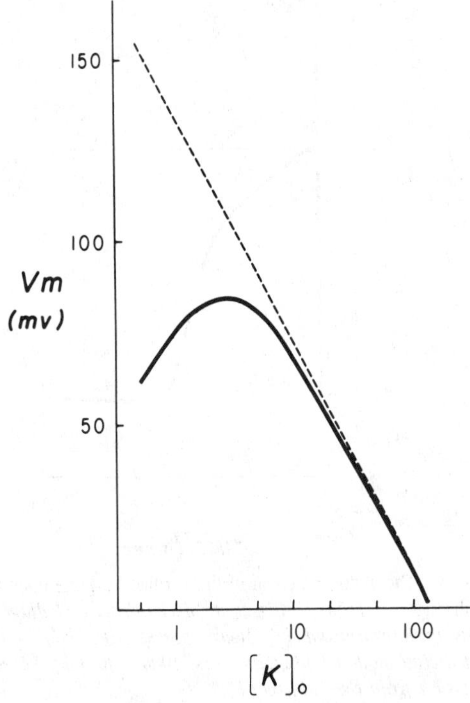

FIGURE 34-2 The resting transmembrane voltage of myocardial cells is determined by $[K]_o$. The dotted line shows the theoretical steady-state relationship between transmembrane voltage in the cardiac Purkinje fiber and $[K]_o$ from the Nernst equation using $[K]_i$ = 150 m*M* and the values of $[K]_o$ shown on the *x* axis. Note that in the physiological range of $[K]_o$, V_m departs significantly from theoretical values. When K is decreased below 2.5, the cell depolarizes markedly; V_m is about −60 mV, and $[K]_o$ is either 1.0 or 13.5 m*M*. [*From JT Bigger Jr: Mechanisms and diagnosis of arrhythmias. In: E Braunwald (ed): Heart Disease: A Textbook of Cardiovascular Medicine. Philadelphia, Saunders, 1980, 630–690. Reproduced with permission from the publisher.*]

THE CARDIAC ACTION POTENTIAL

Like other excitable cells, cardiac muscle cells produce an action potential when activated, i.e., a sudden regenerative depolarization of V_m, followed by a complex voltage-time course back to the resting V_m. Of all the excitable cells, cardiac cells have the longest action potential; their repolarization is the slowest. The cardiac Purkinje fiber action potential has five phases: 0, rapid depolarization; 1, immediate rapid repolarization; 2, slow repolarization or plateau; 3, rapid repolarization; and 4, the diastolic interval (Fig. 34-3). Other cardiac cell types have distinctive action potential contours that differ markedly from that of the Purkinje fiber (Fig. 34-4). To simplify the classification of cardiac action potentials, they can be thought of as belonging to one of two major groups, fast or slow action potentials (Fig. 34-5 and Table 34-1).

Fast Action Potentials and Fast Conduction

Most cardiac cells, such as ordinary or specialized atrial fibers, Purkinje fibers, and ventricular muscle cells, have

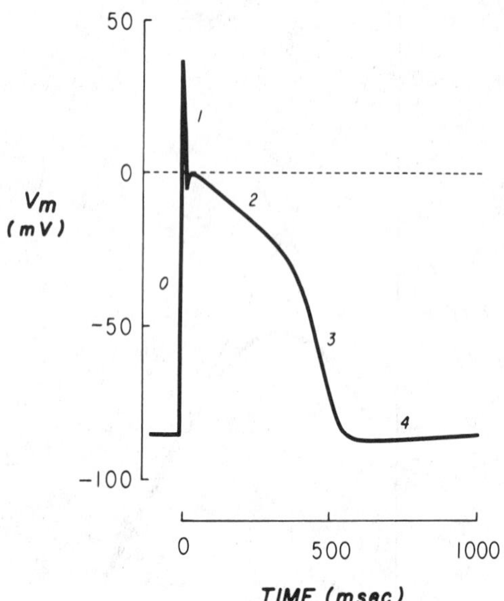

FIGURE 34-3 The action potential of the cardiac Purkinje fiber has five phases, 0 through 4. [*From JT Bigger Jr: Mechanisms and diagnosis of arrhythmias. In: E Braunwald (ed): Heart Disease: A Textbook of Cardiovascular Medicine. Philadelphia, Saunders, 1980, 630–690. Reproduced with permission from the publisher.*]

fast action potentials. These cells have high resting V_m and, when activated, generate a fast-rising, large-amplitude phase 0.[4] This type of phase 0 is associated with very rapid conduction. Cells with fast action potentials tend to have complex and highly developed intercellular connections.[10] The large surface area of complex cellular junctions provide a low-resistance pathway for current flow between cells. Coupling between adjacent cells is most highly developed in Purkinje fibers, and conduction is most rapid in these fibers.

Fast action potentials in the heart are generated by an inward rush of Na^+ through an ionic channel that is selectively permeable to Na^+ ions when the cell activates[5] (Fig. 34-6). The fast channel activates (opens) when V_m is rapidly brought from its resting value of -90 mV to the threshold voltage, about -75 mV. The Na^+ channel activates quickly, inactivates quickly (time constant 0.5 to 2 ms), and has a very high value for maximum ionic conductance when fully activated. The Na^+ channel is only open for 1 to 2 ms, but the inward Na^+ current is intense during that moment. The main modulator of Na^+ channel conductance is the value of V_m at the time of activation.[11] As resting V_m decreases and becomes less and less negative, the Na^+ channel will inactivate more and more so that the inward Na^+ current during activation becomes less and less intense. The weaker the Na^+ current, the smaller the amplitude and rate of rise of phase 0 and the slower impulse conduction will be. At a resting V_m of about -60 mV, the Na^+ channel is totally inactivated and no response can be elicited even with very strong stimuli. When the Na^+ channel activates from a normal resting V_m, the intense inward Na^+ current will carry V_m to very positive values ($+30$ mV), where the channel inactivates rapidly and will remain inactivated and incapable of responding to stimuli until the cell repolarizes. As the cell repolarizes, the Na^+ channel

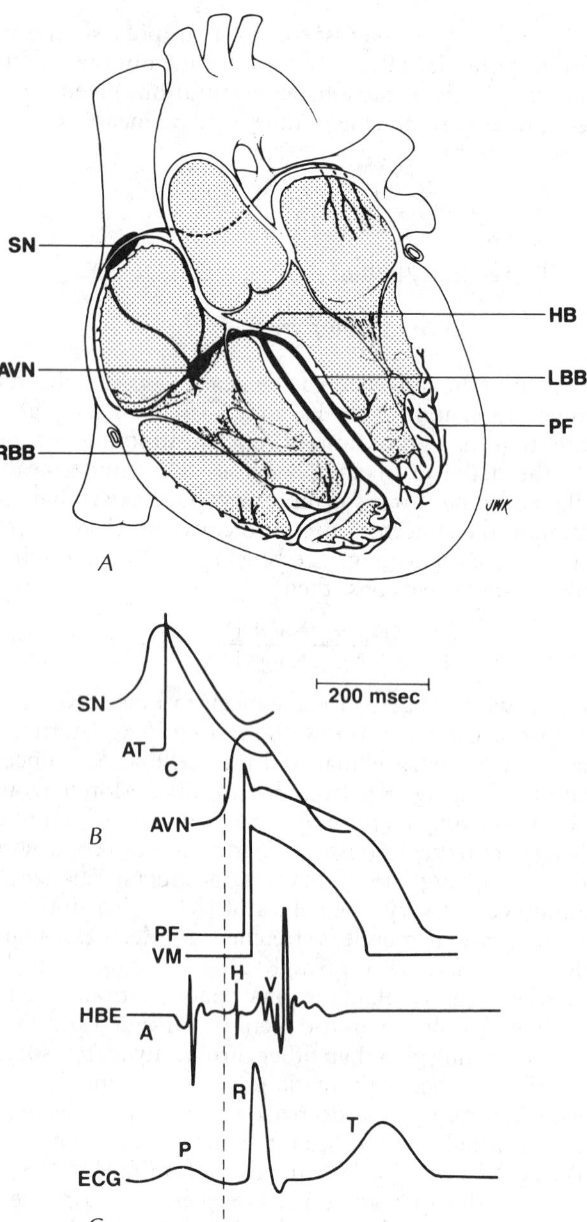

FIGURE 34-4 The anatomy and characteristic action potentials of the specialized impulse generating and conducting system of the heart. *A*. Diagram of the conduction system of the heart. SN = sinoatrial node; AVN = atrial ventricular node; HB = bundle of His; RBB = right bundle branch; LBB = left bundle branch block; PF = Purkinje fiber. *B*. Typical action potentials from the sinus node (SN), atrium (AT), atrial ventricular node (AVN), Purkinje fiber (PF), and ventricular muscle (VM). *C*. Relationship of action potentials in the His bundle electrocardiogram (HBE) to depolarization of the sites shown in *B* and to the electrocardiogram. Depolarization of the lower atrial septum (A), bundle of His (H), and ventricular septum (V) is recorded in the bipolar His bundle electrocardiogram. The H reflection partitions the PR interval into two subintervals, the AH interval, representing atrial ventricular nodal conduction, and the HV interval, which measures conduction in the His-Purkinje system.

reactivates progressively and reaches its maximum at V_m near -90 mV. Reactivation is a process that occurs with two time constants: most of the process has a time constant of a few milliseconds while the remainder has a time constant of 20 to 50 ms. When the cell has repolarized to -65 mV or so, it can be activated again; however,

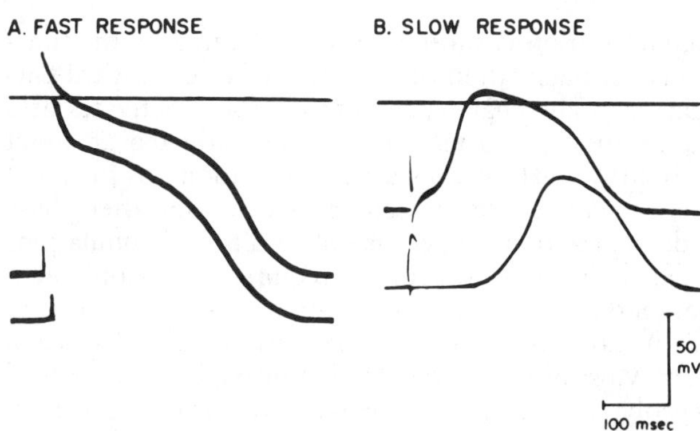

FIGURE 34-5 Fast and slow cardiac action potentials. *A.* Two fast response Purkinje fiber action potentials are recorded. The brief interval between the upstrokes of these action potentials indicates the rapid conduction velocity between the two recording sites. *B.* Two slow responses are shown with recording electrodes the same distance apart as in *A.* The long time interval between the upstrokes of these action potentials indicates the very slow conduction of the slow response. (*From AL Wit, MR Rosen, BF Hoffman: Electrophysiology and pharmacology of cardiac arrhythmias: II. Relationship of normal and abnormal electrical activity of cardiac fibers to the genesis of arrhythmias. Am Heart J 88:515–524, 1974. Reproduced with permission from the publisher and the author.*)

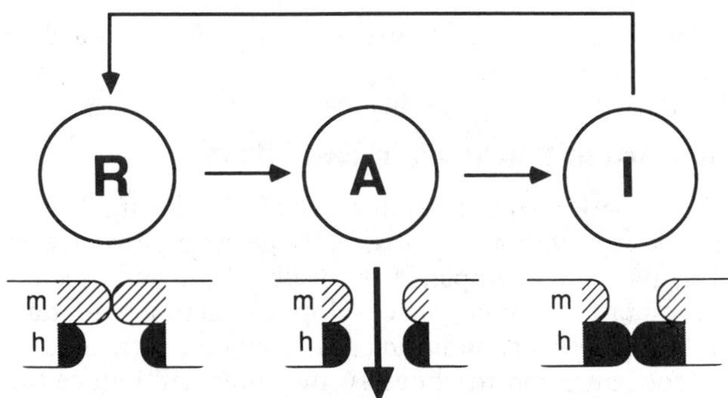

FIGURE 34-6 The sodium channel can exist in three states: (1) resting (R); (2) active or open (A); and (3) inactivated (I). The reactivation of sodium Na^+ channels is governed by the Hodgkin-Huxley voltage-dependent rate constant *m*. The bottom row of the diagram illustrates the sodium channel with its *m* and *h* gates. At normal resting transmembrane voltages the *h* gate is wide open but the *m* gate is closed. When the sodium channel activates, the *m* gate opens quickly. Shortly thereafter, the *h* gates close, inactivating the channel.

stimulation at this low value of V_m gives rise to a very low amplitude, slow-rising action potential. As repolarization proceeds from −65 to −85 mV, responses to premature stimulation will yield action potentials with larger amplitudes and faster depolarization rates. As soon as the maximum diastolic voltage is reached, the responses to premature stimulation will be near maximum.

This voltage-dependent responsiveness of fast action potentials is an important factor in arrhythmogenesis and operates in abnormal parts of the heart where cells are depolarized, for instance, by local hyperkalemia, by stretch injury, or during premature activation. The Na^+ channel is blocked by TTX and by many antiarrhythmic drugs with class I action, but not by Ca^{2+} channel-blocking drugs. The binding of TTX or antiarrhythmic drugs with class I action depends on the V_m and on the state of the channel, that is, whether it is resting, activated, or inactivated.

TABLE 34-1
Comparison of Slow and Fast Action Potentials

Electrophysiological Characteristics	Slow Potential	Fast Potential
Resting potential	−40 to −70 mV	−75 to −90 mV
Action potential amplitude	40–80 mV	90–120 mV
Phase 0 V_m	1–10 V/s	200–800 V/s
Overshoot	0–15 mV	10–30 mV
Conduction velocity	0.01–0.1 m/s	0.5–3.0 m/s
Threshold voltage	−50 to −30 mV	−75 to −65 mV
Depolarizing current carried by	Ca^{2+}, (Na^+)	Na^+
Ionic current activates	Slow (0.5 ms)	Fast (10–20 ms)
Ionic current inactivates	Slow (0.5 ms)	Fast (50–100 ms)
Channel blocked by	Mn^{2+}, La^{3+}, class IV antiarrhythmics	Tetrodotoxin, class I antiarrhythmics

Slow Action Potentials and Slow Conduction

The action potentials of sinus node P cells and atrioventricular (AV) nodal N cells are very characteristic and quite similar. These cells have a low maximum diastolic value of V_m and a small amplitude and relatively slow rising upstroke, i.e., phase 0, when they are activated (Fig. 34-5). These features of phase 0 in slow action potentials are associated with very slow conduction.[12] so, there are anatomic reasons for the slow conduction in the sinus node and AV node. The cell-to-cell connections between sinus node P cells or AV node N cells and their neighbors are sparse and primitive, contributing to the slow spread of excitation in these structures.[13,14]

The ionic basis for slow potentials is an ionic channel that, when activated, is selectively permeable to calcium (Ca^{2+}) and, to a lesser extent, to sodium (Na^+) ions.[15,16] The channel that carries slow inward current activates at rather positive values of V_m, such as −40 to −50 mV. The slow or L-type Ca^{2+} channel activates (opens) slowly, inactivates slowly (time constant 50 to 100 ms), and has a low value for maximum ionic conductance when fully activated (Table 34-1). The conductance of the channel is regulated to some extent by resting V_m and $[Ca]_i$ and is increased substantially by catecholamines. The L-type Ca^{2+} channel can be blocked by manganese or lanthanum or by drugs such as verapamil, diltiazem, or nifedipine.[17]

Slow-response action potentials propagate so slowly that some have questioned whether they actually propagate.[12] The slow propagation in the sinus and AV nodes permits reentrant excitation to occur in very small areas despite the long refractory period found in cardiac muscle.

Slow Action Potentials in Fast Fibers

Under abnormal circumstances, fibers that normally give rise to fast action potentials can develop slow action potentials. For example, Purkinje fibers, the prime example of a fast fiber type, can develop slow action potentials under a variety of conditions. Increasing the extracellular K^+ concentration to about 16 meq/liter will reduce the resting V_m of a Purkinje fiber to about -50 mV and inactivate the Na^+ channel. If catecholamines are applied to inactivated Purkinje fibers, the threshold for the Ca^{2+} channel will shift in a negative direction and the maximum inward Ca^{2+} current obtained during activation will increase.[18] Under these circumstances, electrical stimulation of the Purkinje fiber will evoke a slow action potential. These slow responses are unaffected by Na^+ channel-blocking agents such as TTX but are abolished by Ca^{2+} channel-blocking agents (Table 34-1). Action potentials of acutely ischemic cells resemble the slow responses that occur in high-K^+, high-catecholamine conditions. Under these conditions, the slow depolarization probably is caused by depressed Na^+channel action potentials. Ischemic slow action potentials are abolished by selective Na^+ channel blockers such as TTX[19] but not by Ca^{2+} channel blockers.[20] Purkinje fibers can generate "slow" action potentials during a variety of abnormal conditions via a variety of ionic mechanisms.

Repolarization of Cardiac Action Potentials and Refractoriness

One of the most striking attributes of the cardiac action potential is its long plateau; V_m remains more positive than -50 mV for several hundred milliseconds. This contrasts with the brief action potentials of peripheral nerves and skeletal muscle fibers which typically last for less than 5 ms. The long plateau provides adequate Ca^{2+} for contraction and prevents very rapid heart rates. Several ionic mechanisms are known to contribute to the long plateau. First, K^+ channels in Purkinje fibers show inward-going rectification positive to -50 mV so that the outward repolarizing currents carried by K^+ decrease during the plateau of the action potential.[5,21] Second, the cell tends to be held at plateau voltage by inward current carried by Na^+ and Ca^{2+}. There is a small component of I_{Na} that inactivates slowly and contributes to the inward current flowing during the plateau. The slow or secondary inward current (i_{Ca-L}) normally is triggered by the depolarization caused by phase 0 of the action potential (fast Na^+ inward current). The time constant for inactivating i_{Ca-L} is much longer (50 to 100 ms) than for inactivating i_{Na} (1 to 2 ms). Thus, i_{Ca-L} contributes depolarizing current for several hundred milliseconds during the action potential plateau. During the plateau, the small inward and small outward currents are almost perfectly balanced so that V_m changes very little for 200 to 400 ms. Phase 3 of the action potential (rapid repolarization) is due to inactivation of i_{Ca-L} and activation of i_K, an outward current.[5,21] As the slow channel inactivates, i_{Ca-L} decreases and the cell tends to repolarize. Repolarization is substantially accelerated by the time-dependent activation of a relatively large outward current, i_K.[22] The channel responsible for i_K activates at a V_m of about -50 mV and is fully activated at about $+20$ mV. The time constant for activation i_K is such that this current reaches its peak about 300 ms after phase 0 depolarization. Experimental results and simulations indicate that activation of i_K is required for action potential repolarization, i.e., inactivation of i_{Ca-L} alone is usually insufficient to cause repolarization in the absence of i_K.[5,22] Most of the charge flowing through the i_K channel is probably K^+. On the other hand, the reversal potential for i_K is -70 mV, which indicates that this channel is not strictly selective for K^+. As i_K carries V_m in a negative direction, inward rectification of other K^+ channels decreases and other outward (repolarizing) K^+ currents are recruited. The K^+ accumulation in narrow extracellular clefts may play a role in repolarization and certainly complicates attempts to study repolarizing K^+ currents in multicellular preparations with voltage clamp techniques.

Refractoriness

The recovery from refractoriness in cells with fast action potentials parallels repolarization and reflects primarily the instantaneous value of V_m and the reactivation of the Na^+ channel. Normal regulatory changes that decrease action potential duration in cardiac cells with fast action potentials, e.g., faster heart rates, also will shorten refractoriness. This effect is greater, in absolute terms, in Purkinje fibers than in ordinary ventricular muscle cells. Under abnormal conditions or under the influence of drugs that act on the Na^+ channel, recovery from refractoriness may lag repolarization. The recovery from refractoriness in cells with slow action potentials, e.g., sinus node or AV node cells, has a much longer time constant than in cells with fast action potentials. In these cells, refractoriness often is present for a significant time after full repolarization is achieved. Also, rapid heart rates may prolong rather than shorten refractoriness in cells with slow action potentials.[23]

INITIATION AND PROPAGATION OF THE CARDIAC IMPULSE

The normal heartbeat is governed by a specialized system that spontaneously generates and distributes each impulse through the heart in a coordinated way (Fig. 34-4). Normally the sinus node initiates the cardiac impulse while the His-Purkinje system serves as a backup should sinus node pacemaking fail or AV block occur. Normally, spontaneous impulse generation is much faster in the sinus node (60 to 100 per min) than in the His-Purkinje system (35 to 50 per min) placing the sinus node in control of cardiac rhythm. The cardiac impulse is generated in a small cluster of sinus node P cells that constitute the primary pacemaker for the heart and then spreads slowly through the sinus node and perinodal fibers to reach specialized atrial tracts and ordinary atrial muscle.[13] The specialized atrial tracts transmit the cardiac impulse rapidly from the sinus node to the AV node via the anterior, middle, and posterior internodal tracts and to the left atrium via Bachmann's bundle.[24,25]

The existence of specialized internodal tracts is still vigorously contested by some anatomists who often can find no histological structures to correspond to the function. There is, however, physiological evidence for specialized internodal tracts. Internodal conduction can be demonstrated in atria so depolarized by K^+ that ordinary atrial muscle is rendered inexcitable. This experiment takes advantage of the K^+-resistant properties of specialized conducting tissues. The only normal pathway for the cardiac impulse to conduct from atrium to ventricles is the AV node. As the cardiac impulse enters the AV node, it slows dramatically, accounting for most of the PR interval in the body surface ECG. When the impulse emerges from the AV node into the His bundle, conduction speeds dramatically and the spread of excitation through the bundle branches and peripheral Purkinje fiber network occurs with great rapidity in the normal heart. The action potential duration and refractoriness in the Purkinje system increases as a function of distance from the AV node to reach a maximum value about 2 to 3 mm from the Purkinje fiber–ventricular muscle junction. This area of longest refractoriness seems to exert a "gating" function. Ordinary ventricular muscle is activated almost simultaneously over much of its endocardial surface via the extensive subendocardial Purkinje fiber network. Activation of ventricular muscle spreads from endocardium to epicardium to complete the cardiac excitation cycle.

It is important to note that none of the events in the specialized impulse generating and conducting system can be recorded in the standard 12-lead ECG because the mass of these tissues is too small to generate electrical signals large enough to project on the body surface. Thus, during ECG analysis, the events in the sinus node, atrial specialized tracts, AV node, and His-Purkinje system must be inferred from the events that are recorded, the depolarization of the ordinary atrial and ventricular myocardium. Many of the events in the specialized conducting system can be recorded during clinical electrophysiological studies by placing electrodes on a catheter in contact with the structure of interest, e.g., the bundle of His.

Anisotropy

Propagation of the cardiac impulse in tissues composed of cells with fast action potentials shows variation in speed. Cablelike structures without extensive branches, such as the His bundle, bundle branches, or Purkinje fibers, conduct faster and with a greater safety factor than tissues with extensive three-dimensional branching, e.g., ordinary atrial or ventricular muscle, where the current sink is greater.[26] Also, spread of excitation is faster along the long axis of myocardial fiber bundles than transversely.[27]

Automaticity in Heart Muscle

Certain cells in the normal heart are capable of repetitive spontaneous self-excitation: the sinus node P cells and Purkinje fibers in the ventricles. There are other cells, e.g., atrial specialized fibers, that are not usually automatic but can become so under abnormal conditions.

Sinus Node

The sinus node P cell is an automatic cell that spontaneously generates slow potentials. When the P cell repolarizes after an action potential, it never rests at a stable value of V_m. Instead, V_m reaches a maximum negative value at the end of repolarization, and then slow spontaneous diastolic (phase 4) depolarization begins. When V_m reaches a critical value, the threshold voltage, an action potential ensues. The normal automatic process in the sinus node is finely modulated by the parasympathetic and sympathetic nervous systems. It is known that the parasympathetic neurotransmitter, acetylcholine, will cause hyperpolarization and a decrease in the slope of phase 4 depolarization in sinus node P cells. This effect is explained by an increase in the membrane K^+ conductance caused by acetylcholine.[5] Presumably, V_m is less negative than the K^+ equilibrium potential, V_K, so that the cell hyperpolarizes when K^+ conductance increases. The changes in ionic currents as a function of time that account for spontaneous phase 4 depolarization in P cells are controversial at the present time. The net inward current responsible for phase 4 depolarization increases steadily as a function of time and could be due to a decrease in I_K with a steady inward current or a time-dependent increase in inward current with a steady I_K. An inward current, carried by Na^+ through a relatively nonspecific cationic channel, I_f has been implicated in the pacemaker activity of the sinus node,[28] but there are many details about the normal automatic process that are yet to be defined.

His-Purkinje System

Cells from the junction of the AV node and His bundle to the most peripheral Purkinje fiber twigs are capable of automaticity. Under special experimental circumstances, AV nodal N cells can become automatic. When AV block occurs, a focus in the His bundle usually assumes the pacemaker function for the heart and fires regularly at a rate between 35 and 50 per minute. In diseased hearts, the pacemaker in the His-Purkinje system may be slower and located more distally. During sinus rhythm with intact AV conduction, pacemaking activity in the His-Purkinje system is supressed by the faster sinus node pacemaker. The cells of the His-Purkinje system are depolarized by the propagating sinus impulse before spontaneous diastolic depolarization reaches threshold. In addition, overdriving the His-Purkinje system by sinus rhythm or electrical pacing decreases the slope of phase 4 depolarization; this phenomenon is called overdrive suppression.[29]

One of the important mechanisms of overdrive suppression is "pump current." When cardiac cells are rhythmically activated, Na^+ enters the cell during each action potential. As cardiac rate becomes more rapid, the inward Na^+ flux becomes larger, and $[Na]_i$ increases. Even a small increase in $[Na]_i$ will increase the rate of Na^+-K^+ pumping in order to maintain normal transmembrane electrolyte gradients.[9] Exchange of Na^+ for K^+ is not electroneutral under these circumstances but electrogenic, i.e., when the pump is active, some 3 Na^+ are extruded for 2 K^+ entering the cell. This excess of positive-charge (Na^+) movement out of the cell is responsible for the pump current that hyperpolarizes the cell and counteracts phase 4 depolarization.[9]

Ionic Basis for Normal Pacemaker Activity in Cardiac Purkinje Fibers

The ionic basis for pacemaker activity in cardiac Purkinje fibers is still uncertain. Early studies showed that slope conductance fell as Purkinje fibers spontaneously depolarized.[30] Also, increasing extracellular K^+ from 2.7 to 5.4 m*M* caused a decrease of phase 4 depolarization and automatic firing finally ceased.[31] A voltage clamp applied at the onset of phase 4 depolarization to hold V_m at the maximum diastolic voltage showed a decrease in net inward current as a function of time.[32] Further voltage clamp experiments suggested that phase 4 depolarization was due to a current carried by K^+, called i_{K_2} that decayed with time in the presence of a steady inward Na^+ current.[5,33] Still later voltage clamp experiments showed that the pacemaker current was dependent on Na^+ and was blocked by low concentrations of Cs^+.[34,35] Additional evidence suggested that previous measurements of the reversal potential for i_{K_2} had been in error because of K^+ depletion in the intercellular clefts of Purkinje fibers during hyperpolarizing pulses.[34] DiFrancesco[34,35] showed that pacemaker current reversed near −20 mV and is carried by I_f. The apparent decrease in membrane slope conductance measured by Weidmann probably was due to inward rectification of K^+ channels as membrane depolarization proceeded. Although Na^+ carries the pacemaker current, the channel for I_f does not have voltage-dependent properties like the channel for I_{Na}; its reversal potential is −20 mV (i.e., far from the Na^+ equilibrium voltage), and it is not blocked by TTX.

MECHANISMS OF CARDIAC ARRHYTHMIAS

A classification of arrhythmia mechanisms is given in Table 34-2. Arrhythmias are categorized as due to abnormal impulse formation, abnormal impulse propagation, or combined abnormalities of impulse formation and propagation. Abnormalities of impulse formation include abnormalities of automaticity and early or delayed afterdepolarizations with triggered activity. Abnormalities of impulse propagation include conduction block and reentry of the cardiac impulse. Combinations of abnormalities of impulse formation and propagation can produce complex arrhythmias. In addition to the general mechanism of an arrhythmia, it is useful to know which cardiac tissues participate in the arrhythmia and the ionic mechanisms and structural abnormalities that promote the arrhythmia. When all of this information is available, strategies for management are usually suggested. (See also Chap. 35.)

TABLE 34-2

Mechanisms Responsible for Cardiac Arrhythmias
Abnormalities of impulse generation
Alterations of normal automaticity
Abnormal automaticity
Triggered activity
Early afterdepolarizations
Delayed afterdepolarizations
Abnormalities of impulse conduction
Slowing of conduction and block
Unidirectional block and reentry
Ordered reentry
Random reentry
Combined abnormalities of impulse generation and conduction
Conduction slowed by phase 4 depolarization
Parasystole

Altered Normal Automaticity

Alterations of the normal automatic mechanism can produce conduction abnormalities or arrhythmias. The normal sinus node pacemaker may fail in disease states or be excessively rapid under the influence of sympathetic activity. Pacemakers in the His-Purkinje system may control cardiac rhythm as escape pacemakers or when sympathetic activity is increased. The first situation occurs when sinus bradycardia or AV block reduces propagation of supraventricular impulses to a rate lower than the intrinsic rate of His-Purkinje pacemakers. Also, abnormal conditions, e.g., ischemia or drug treatment (sympathomimetic drugs or phosphodiesterase inhibitors), can lead to an increase in the rate of firing of pacemakers in the His-Purkinje system.

Abnormal Automaticity

Under abnormal conditions cells may become automatic due to abnormal mechanisms. For the first few days after experimental myocardial infarction, depolarized Purkinje fibers on the endocardial surface of the infarct become automatic at greatly reduced values of maximum diastolic V_m. At these reduced voltages, the phasic current that is associated with normal pacemaker activity is fully activated and, therefore, is probably not involved in the spontaneous firing.[5,34,35] The ionic mechanism of this form of automaticity is unknown.

Afterdepolarizations and Triggered Activity

Recently, there has been much interest in afterdepolarizations and triggered activity as a cause of cardiac arrhythmias. Afterdepolarizations are secondary depolarizations that occur after repolarization has begun. Triggered activity is single or repetitive firing of a cell or group of cells initiated by an afterdepolarization. Triggered activity is not a form of automaticity; triggered activity itself is not self-excitatory but rather depends on a preceding action potential and afterdepolarization to initiate the process. Two primary forms of afterdepolarizations, early and delayed, can initiate triggered activity.

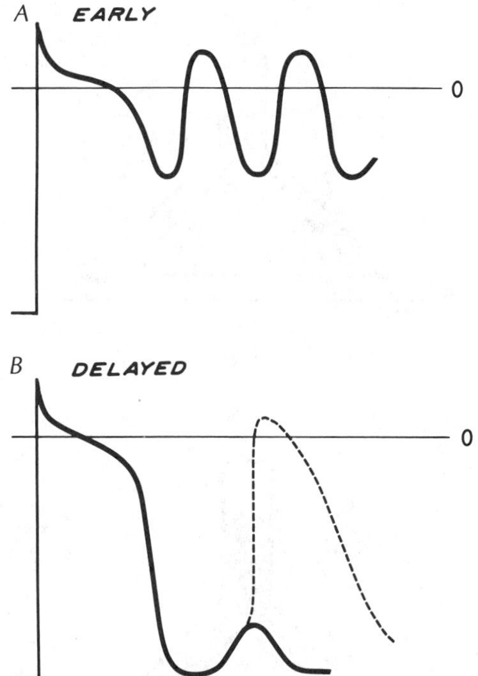

FIGURE 34-7 Afterdepolarizations and triggered activity. *A*. Early afterdepolarizations. Repolarization of the Purkinje fiber is interrupted by two secondary depolarizations before the fiber is fully repolarized. Such activity can be responsible for the clinical arrhythmia torsades de pointes. *B*. Delayed afterdepolarizations. After full repolarization of the Purkinje fiber a secondary depolarization occurred. The dashed line shows that if the afterdepolarization reaches threshold voltage, a propagating response can occur. [*From JT Bigger Jr: Electrophysiology for the clinician. Eur Heart J 5(suppl B):1–9, 1984. Reproduced with permission from the publisher.*]

Early Afterdepolarizations

Early afterdepolarizations are depolarizations that occur before the cell fully repolarizes (Fig. 34-7). They often arise from the plateau of the action potential but can occur during the rapid phase of repolarization. Early afterdepolarizations can occur in almost any type of heart cell, but they have been studied most extensively in cardiac Purkinje fibers and ventricular muscle cells.[36] Early afterdepolarizations often occur under conditions that cause striking delays in repolarization of heart cells, e.g., hypokalemia, slow heart rate, and drug toxicity. Early afterdepolarizations can trigger sustained rapid firing in Purkinje fibers. Since the Purkinje fiber action potential is much longer than those in adjacent ventricular muscle, ventricular muscle is likely to respond to early afterdepolarizations in the adjacent Purkinje fibers. The torsades de pointes form of ventricular tachycardia is very common clinically when patients have the same conditions that are known to produce early afterdepolarizations experimentally—hypokalemia, slow heart rate, or long QT produced by drugs. Often these factors occur together, e.g., diuretic-induced hypokalemia in patients taking quinidine. Thus, torsades de pointes may be the ECG counterpart of triggered activity initiated by early afterdepolarizations. This hypothesis needs further investigation. Treatments that shorten action potential duration are beneficial for experimental early afterdepolarizations caused by decreased extracellular K^+ concentration. Rapid pacing, increasing extracellular K^+ concentration, and drugs that increase K^+ conductance all tend to abolish early afterdepolarizations and triggered activity. All of these approaches share a common property: They increase K^+ conductance in heart muscle.

Delayed Afterdepolarizations

Delayed afterdepolarizations are small depolarizations (about 10 mV) that occur after the cell has repolarized (Fig. 34-7), usually soon after maximum diastolic voltage is reached. This behavior is present under normal conditions in a few cell types (cells in the coronary sinus[37] and in the AV valves[38]) and can be seen in many cell types under abnormal conditions. Delayed afterdepolarizations usually are too small to reach the threshold voltage, but their amplitude varies dynamically with change in heart rate or firing pattern. As heart rate increases or stimulation becomes more premature, the delayed afterdepolarization becomes larger and larger; if threshold voltage is reached, a run of rapid firing or triggered activity may be provoked (Fig. 34-8). Factors known to increase the amplitude of delayed afterdepolarizations include rapid pacing, premature activation, increased $[Ca]_o$, increased catecholamine concentrations, and digitalis toxicity.[39,40] Triggered activity initiated by delayed afterdepolarizations is *not* a form of automaticity; it requires the previous action potential and delayed afterdepolarization as the initiating events.[9] Although triggered activity is not self-initiating, it can be self-perpetuating.[12]

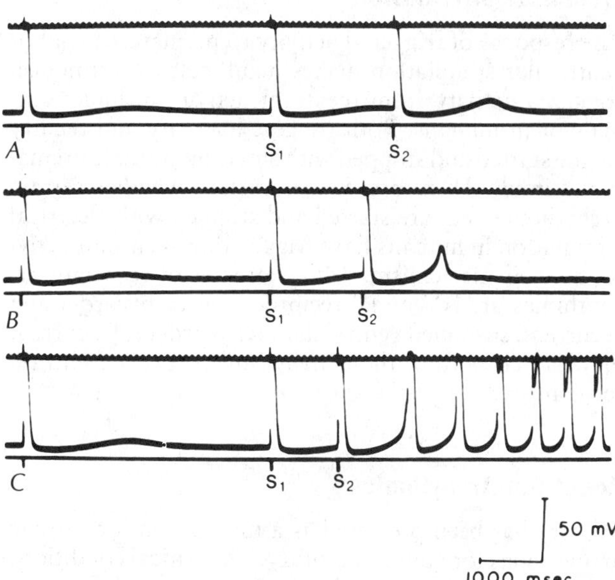

FIGURE 34-8 Afterdepolarizations and triggered activity in a coronary sinus cell from a dog. The fiber is stimulated at a regular cycle length of 4000 ms (S_1) and stimulated prematurely every eighth cycle (S_2). *A*. At a S_1S_2 interval of 2000 ms, the afterdepolarization is small and occurs about 1500 ms after the response to S_2. *B*. At a S_1S_2 of 4300 ms, afterdepolarization is larger and occurs about 900 ms after the response to the stimulus. *C*. At a S_1S_2 of 1000 ms, the afterdepolarization reaches threshold and causes a sustained run of triggered activity. Note the progressive decrease in cycle length at the beginning of triggered activity. (*From AL Wit, PF Cranefield. Reproduced with permission from the American Heart Association and the author.*)

Digitalis Toxicity and Triggered Activity

Although delayed afterdepolarizations do not normally occur in cardiac Purkinje fibers, they can develop during digitalis toxicity.[40] An abnormal current called "transient inward current" can develop in digitalis-intoxicated Purkinje fibers as a result of the following sequence of events. Digitalis binds to the portion of the Na-K-ATPase that is on the external surface of the sarcolemmal membrane. As a result, Na^+ pumping decreases and $[Na]_i$ increases. Then, cytosolic $[Ca]_i$ increases as a result of Na^+-Ca^{2+} exchange and leads to a phasic release of Ca^{2+} from internal stores in the sarcoplasmic reticulum.[41] Phasic increases in $[Ca]_i$ play an important role in generating the transient inward current.[40] A large increase in $[Ca]_o$ occurs after the upstroke of the action potential and subsides after about 100 ms. When afterdepolarizations are caused by digitalis toxicity, they are associated by a delayed second increase in $[Ca]_o$ that occurs simultaneously with the afterdepolarizations. The ion(s) responsible for transient inward current have not been identified and the current does not show typical Hodgkin-Huxley kinetics. Currently Na^+ seems to be the carrier, but the channel seems clearly different from the one carrying i_{Ca-L} or I_{Na}. Some of the digitalis-induced ventricular tachycardias in dogs and humans have characteristics that are compatible with triggered activity. Digitalis toxic arrhythmias are the most convincing example of human arrhythmias that may be caused by delayed afterdepolarizations and triggered activity.

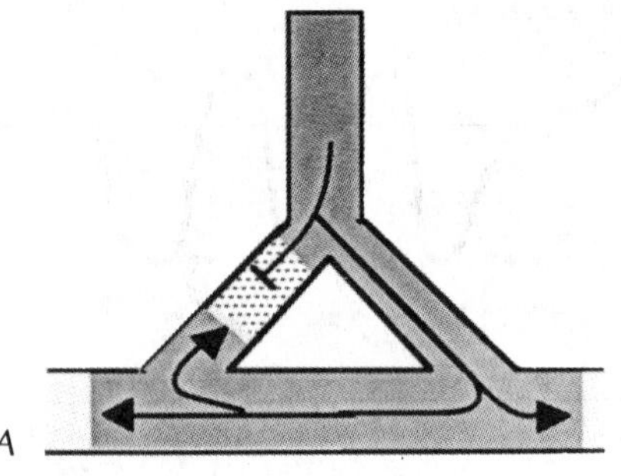

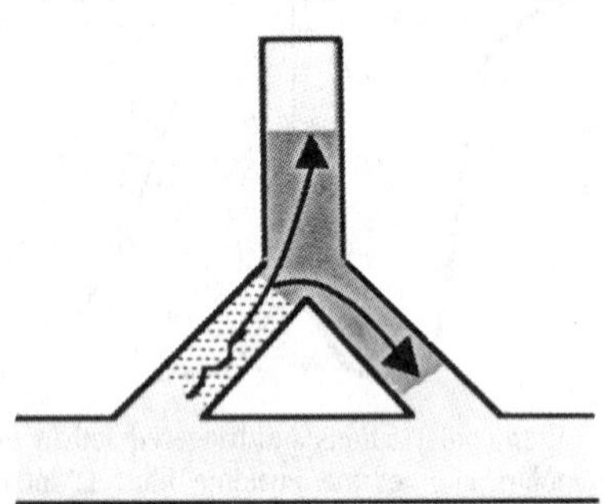

FIGURE 34-9 The Schmitt-Erlanger model of reentry. The diagram portrays a loop of cardiac fibers that could represent branches of Purkinje fibers terminating on ventricular muscle or a loop in the Purkinje fiber syncytium on the endocardium. The light stipple represents repolarized tissue with normal excitability. The dark stipple represents depolarized, refractory tissue. The dashed lines in the left branch indicate an area of persistently depolarized, relatively refractory tissue. *A*. Antegrade conduction blocks in the depolarized area in the left branch. *B*. Retrograde conduction in the left branch is slow but successful, permitting the impulse to reenter the right branch.

Premature Stimulation

The response of triggered activity to premature atrial or ventricular stimulation makes it difficult to distinguish triggered activity from reentrant activity in intact animals or in humans. Both triggered activity and reentry can be started and stopped with single or multiple premature stimuli. Therefore, it is uncertain whether certain arrhythmias that are started and stopped with electrical stimulation in humans have triggered or reentrant activity as their mechanism. Two examples of reentrant arrhythmias are AV nodal reciprocating tachycardia and recurrent, sustained ventricular tachycardia. The current view is that both of these arrhythmias have a reentrant mechanism.

Reentrant Arrhythmias

Reentry has been proposed as a mechanism for cardiac arrhythmias for almost a century. The critical conditions that permit reentry are slow conduction and one-way block in some portion of a circuit (Fig. 34-9). The one-way block may be permanent or dynamic. The exceedingly long refractory period of heart muscle tends to prevent reentry. Unless an impulse circulates for a very long time, cells in the circuit will still be refractory when the impulse returns to the site of one-way block. Slow responses and very depressed fast responses, however, can propagate slowly enough to permit reentry to occur even in fairly small circuits.[42] Application of KCl to localized zones of Purkinje fibers causes a number of phenomena that may be relevant to naturally occurring reentrant ventricular arrhythmias. Conduction delay or block is usually asymmetrical in a segment of Purkinje fiber depolarized by K^+, even though the geometry of the preparation is extremely simple—a single, thin, cablelike strand. This asymmetry makes unidirectional block easy to produce. Impulses entering a depolarized zone in a linear strand may reflect back to reexcite the portion of fiber from which they originally came, whether or not they successfully conduct through the depolarized zone (Fig. 34-9). In preparations with more complex geometries such as Y- or T-shaped networks, the behavior of the circuits becomes more complicated. Propagation across a T-shaped depolarized zone may occur only when impulses from two branches arrive at about the same time; this phenomenon is called *summation*. Conversely, propagation across a depolarized zone may be successful when impulses arrive from either branch separately but not when they arrive at the same time; this phenomenon is called *inhibition*. Summation and inhibition can cause a wide variety of electrophysiological behavior patterns in the complex networks of Purkinje fibers in mammalian hearts. Local areas of slow conduction can produce continuous reentrant rhythms in ringlike Purkinje networks without including ventricular muscle as an essential portion of the pathway. In experimental infarction, reentry can occur in a pathway that is confined to ventricular muscle. Thus, ventricular reentry can occur in either the Purkinje network or ventricular muscle alone or the reentrant path may include both of these cell types and their junctions.

Anomalous AV Connections

The most convincing example of a reentrant arrhythmia in humans is the AV reciprocating tachycardia seen in the preexcitation syndromes. Patients with preexcitation syndrome, the Wolff-Parkinson-White (WPW) syndrome, are born with one or more anomalous AV connections that cause a short PR interval and wide QRS complex due to eccentric and premature activation of the ventricles during sinus rhythm. During sinus rhythm, AV conduction of sinus impulses in the WPW syndrome uses both the AV node and the anomalous AV connection. The additional AV pathway promotes reentrant supraventricular tachycardia (AV reciprocating tachycardia). The common form of AV reciprocating tachycardia in the WPW syndrome often begins when a premature atrial impulse blocks the anomalous AV connection but conducts very slowly through the AV node (Fig. 34-10). The delay in the AV node is long enough for the anomalous AV connection to recover before the impulse reaches its ventricular end. The circulating impulse then reenters the atrium to complete the first cycle of sustained tachycardia. The eccentric position of many anomalous connections favors reentry. The excitation wave front that enters the ventricles via the AV node may take 100 ms or more to reach the ventricular insertion of an eccentric anomalous connection. Also, the diversity of electrophysiological properties of the tissues that comprise the reentrant circuit increases the likelihood that premature impulses will initiate reentrant tachycardia. Elaborate clinical electrophysiological mapping studies in the catheterization laboratory or operating room can determine the tachycardia pathway precisely. The evidence for reentry provided by excitation mapping is very strong. When the anomalous connection is divided, it becomes impossible to initiate the tachycardia. This is conclusive evidence for reentry.

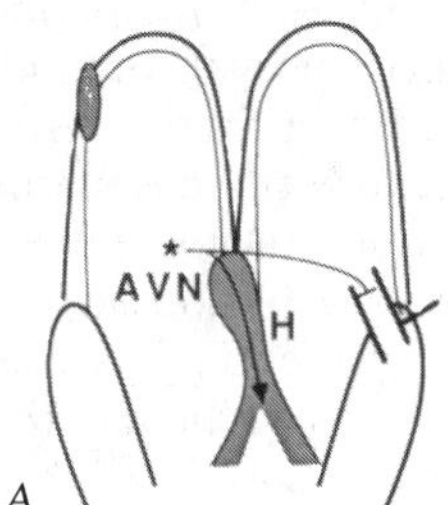

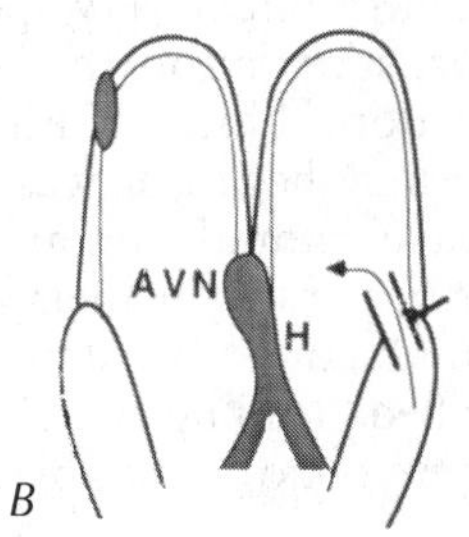

FIGURE 34-10 The onset of AV reentrant tachycardia in the Wolff-Parkinson-White syndrome. The diagram shows an anomalous AV connection between the left atrium and ventricle. *A.* An atrial premature depolarization (∗) blocks the anomalous AV connection but conducts slowly through the AV node. *B.* Retrograde conduction via the anomalous AV connection initiates AV reentrant tachycardia. SAN = sinoatrial node; AP = acessory pathway; H = His bundle; AVN = AV node.

Excitable Gap and Entrainment of Ventricular Tachycardia

The examples of reentry we have discussed above have an "excitable gap" in the reentry circuit. Most of the tissues in the circuit fully recover during a cycle of the AV reciprocating tachycardia in the WPW syndrome. One-way block is required in order to start the reentrant rhythm. The critical factor in sustaining these reentrant tachycardias, however, is very slow conduction restricted to a relatively small part of the circuit, e.g., the AV node in the case of AV reciprocating tachycardia in the WPW syndrome. The model suggested by Schmitt and Erlanger also assumes an excitable gap (Fig. 34-9). The presence of an excitable gap in the reentry circuit makes it possible for critically timed paced impulses to engage the circuit and alter the behavior of the reentrant tachycardia.[43,44] If a premature impulse arrives at a portion of the circuit that is at the end of the relative refractory period, the impulse can enter the circuit and propagate in both directions (Fig. 34-11). As the premature impulse propagates in the "retrograde" limb, it collides with the oncoming circulating wave front of the tachycardia and both wave fronts are extinguished. The premature impulse, however, may propagate in the "antegrade" direction and successfully traverse the entire reentry circuit. In this case, the tachycardia will be reset but will not be terminated. In a similar way, the first cycle of a train of stimuli can encounter a portion of the reentry circuit at the end of its relative refractory period and successfully complete

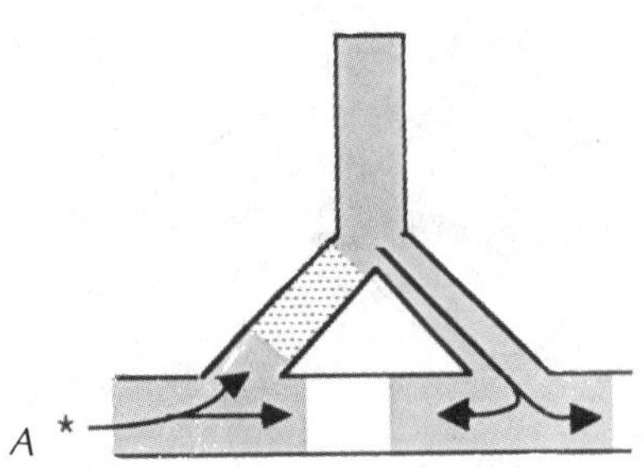

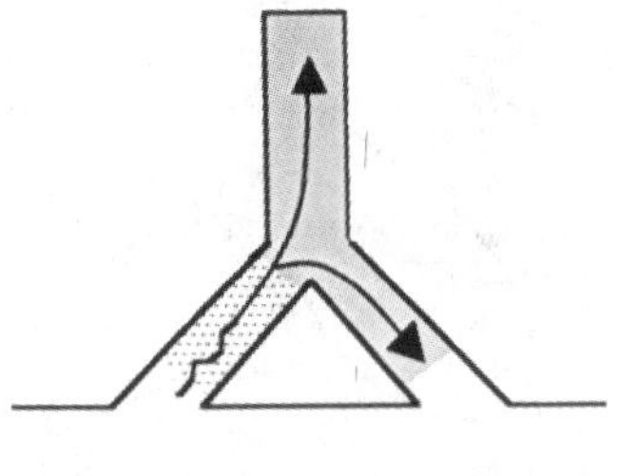

FIGURE 34-11 Entrainment of ventricular tachycardia. *A.* A critically-timed paced impulse (∗) propagates into a reentrant circuit that is responsible for ventricular tachycardia. The paced impulse collides with the tachycardia impulse. *B.* The paced impulse conducts retrograde in the left branch of the circuit through an area of slow conduction. The paced impulse finds the right branch recovered and is able to propagate around the circuit. The capture will "advance" the tachycardia and, if pacing is continued, the tachycardia can follow the pacing rate until pacing is stopped.

the circuit in the antegrade direction. If the second paced impulse is timed so that it blocks the retrograde wave front created by the first paced impulse but propagates successfully in the antegrade direction, the tachycardia will be "entrained" to the pacing rate.[44] At the faster pacing rate, there will be a less excitable gap. The tachycardia may follow the pacing rate until pacing is discontinued when the original tachycardia will resume its original rate. Instead of entraining the reentrant tachycardia, premature stimulation may terminate it. A premature impulse timed so that it blocks the tachycardia wave front in the retrograde limb but fails to propagate in the antegrade direction will terminate the tachycardia.

Static and Dynamic Block and Reentry

Experimentally, reentrant ventricular tachycardia can be initiated in subacute and chronically infarcted ventricles. A portion of the block is *static* due to barriers created by infarcted tissues and cell-to-cell uncoupling.[45] During the healing phase of myocardial infarction, part of the block can be *dynamic* due to the abnormal behavior of ischemically damaged but surviving cells in the epicardial rim overlying the infarcted zone.[45,46] In reentry due to dynamic block, the ventricular excitation wave front enters the ischemic zone to encounter an arc of refractoriness (dynamic block) that acts as a barrier to conduction (Fig. 34-12). The excitation wave front moves slowly in both directions around the arc of refractoriness and along its backside until it reaches a point near the center of the arc that has recovered from refractoriness where it conducts through the arc in the direction from whence it came. The impulse can then excite the normal ventricular muscle proximal to the abnormal tissue that has long since recovered and can cause a ventricular premature depolarization (VPD). If the wave front recirculates about the arc of refractoriness continuously, ventricular tachycardia will result. During the tachycardia, the lines of functional block are parallel to the fiber direction. A different activation pattern emerges when ventricular fibrillation is produced by premature stimulation of an acutely infarcting heart. Multiple independent wave fronts coexist on the epicardium along with multiple and shifting areas of dynamic block. The wave fronts can block, collide and extinguish, or summate. Also, the wave fronts lack a stable, repeating anatomic pathway but rather shift their position from cycle to cycle.[47]

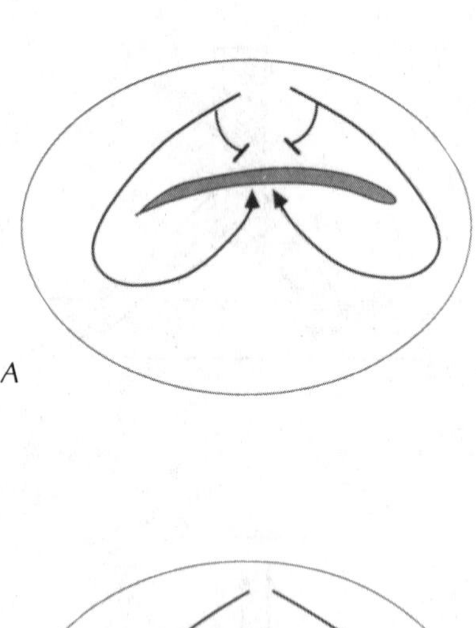

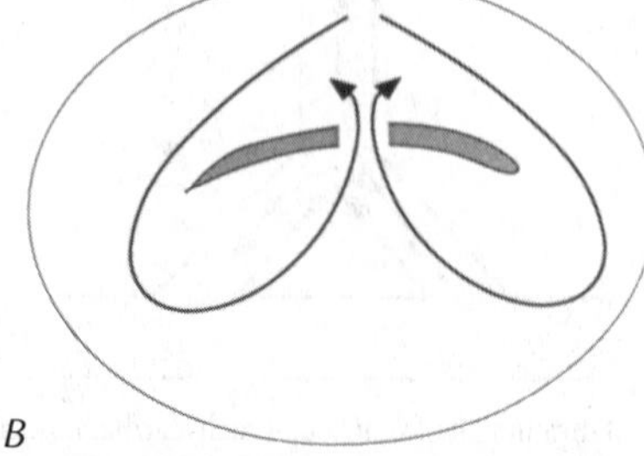

FIGURE 34-12 Reentry due to dynamic block in the epicardium of an ischemic area. *A.* A sinus impulse propagating into the ischemic area encounters an arc of block due to refractoriness. The impulse conducts slowly around the ends of the arc. *B.* As the impulse conducts around the arc of block, excitability recovers in the center of the arc, permitting the impulse to conduct across the arc in the direction from which it came.

Reentry Due to Anisotropy in Healed Infarcts

As the infarct heals, fibrosis separates the surviving muscle bundles in the epicardium over the infarct reducing the side-to-side connections.[47] Measurements of conduction on the epicardium over healed infarcts show marked anisotropy of conduction—conduction velocity is about four times as rapid in a direction parallel to the fiber orientation as in the transverse direction.[48] Critically timed premature impulses can cause block of the impulse in the longitudinal direction with slow spread in the direction tangential and transverse to the epicardial fiber orientation. Reentry may occur along the long axis of fiber orientation, and ventricular tachycardia can result. It is notable that premature stimuli are more likely to block in the long axis of fiber bundles, i.e., in the direction of more rapid conduction. This experimental result has been found by several investigators in atrium and ventricle.[27]

Leading Circle Reentry

Allessie et al.[49] demonstrated an extreme example of dynamic block as a critical factor in reentry. They showed that a small piece of atrial tissue that contained no natural barriers and no areas of slow conduction due to nodal tissue or pathological conditions could sustain reentry under very special circumstances. With premature stimulation, they were able to get one cycle of unidirectional block to initiate a rapid reentrant rhythm. After reentry began, it was sustained because the circulating wave front always arrived at the tissues ahead of it at a critical time in their relative refractory period so that conduction was slowed. This type of reentry has been called "leading circle" reentry to emphasize the fact that there is no "excitable gap" in the circuit.

Arrhythmias Due to Current of Injury

Janse and colleagues[47,50] have suggested that in experimental myocardial infarction a current of injury can flow across inexcitable boundaries. This current can be strong enough to excite adjacent ventricular muscle or Purkinje fibers. This mechanism might operate for brief periods of time after acute ischemic or mechanical injury to produce premature activation of the myocardium near the infarcting tissue.

Antiarrhythmic Drugs

Recently, a new classification of antiarrhythmic drugs has been proposed that is based upon arrhythmogenic mechanisms.[51]

REFERENCES

1. Fozzard HA, Arnsdorf MF: Cardiac electrophysiology. In: Fozzard HA, Haber E, Jennings RB, et al (eds): *The Heart and Cardiovascular System: Scientific Foundations,* 2d ed. New York, Raven, 1991: 63–98.
2. Katz AM: Membrane structure. In: Fozzard HA, Haber E, Jennings RB, et al (eds): *The Heart and Cardiovascular System: Scientific Foundations,* 2d ed. New York, Raven, 1991: 51–62.
3. Rogart R: Sodium channels in nerve and muscle membrane. *Ann Rev Physiol* 1981; 43:711–725.
4. Neher E, Stevens CF: Conductance fluctuations and ionic pores in membranes. *Ann Rev Biophys Bioeng* 1977; 6:345–381.
5. Noble D: *Initiation of the Heartbeat.* London, Oxford University Press, 1979.
6. Carmeliet EE: *Chloride and Potassium Permeability in Cardiac Purkinje Fibers.* Brussels, Presses Academiques Européenes, 1961.
7. Haas HG, Glitsch HG, Kern R: Kalium-fluxe und membran-potential am Froschvorhof in abhangigkeit von der kalium-aussenkonzentration. *Pflugers Arch* 1966; 288:43–64.
8. Bosteels S, Carmeliet EE: Estimation of intracellular Na concentration and transmembrane Na flux in cardiac Purkinje fibers. *Pflugers Arch* 1972; 336:35–47.
9. Eisner DA: The Na-K pump in cardiac muscle. In: Fozzard HA, Haber E, Jennings RB, et al (eds): *The Heart and Cardiovascular System: Scientific Foundations.* New York, Raven, 1986: 489–507.
10. Sommer JR, Johnson EA: Cardiac muscle: A comparative study of Purkinje fibers and ventricular fibers. *J Cell Biol* 1968; 36:497–526.
11. Weidmann S: The effect of the cardiac membrane potential on the rapid availability of the sodium-carrying system. *J Physiol* 1955; 127:213–224
12. Cranefield PF: *The Conduction of the Cardiac Impulse: The Slow Response and Cardiac Arrhythmias.* Mt. Kisco, NY, Futura Publishing, 1975.
13. James TN, Sherf L, Fine G, Morales AR: Comparative ultrastructure of the sinus node in man and dog. *Circulation* 1966; 34:139–163.
14. James TN, Sherf L: Ultrastructure of the human atrioventricular node. *Circulation* 1968; 37:1049–1070.
15. Reuter H: Divalent cations as charge carriers in excitable membranes. *Prog Biophys* 1973; 26:1–43.
16. Vitek M, Trautwein W: Slow inward current and action potential in cardiac Purkinje fibers. *Pflugers Arch* 1971; 323:204–218.
17. Hagiwara S, Nakajima S: Differences in Na and Ca spikes as examined by application of tetrodotoxin, procaine and manganese ions. *J Gen Physiol* 1966; 49:793–806.
18. Carmeliet E, Vereecke J: Adrenaline and the plateau phase of the cardiac action potential: Importance of Ca^{++}, Na^{+} and K^{+} conductance. *Pflugers Arch* 1969; 313:300–315.
19. Lazzara R, Hope RR, El-Sherif N, Scherlag BJ: Effects of lidocaine on hypoxic and ischemic cardiac cells. *Am J Cardiol* 1978; 41:872–879.
20. El-Sherif N, Lazzara R: Reentrant ventricular arrhythmias in the late myocardial infarction period: 7. Effect of verapamil and D600 and the role of the "slow channel." *Circulation* 1979; 60:605–615.
21. Trautwein W: Membrane currents in cardiac muscle fibers. *Physiol Rev* 1973; 53:793–835.
22. McAllister RE, Noble D, Tsien RW: Reconstruction of the electrical activity of cardiac Purkinje fibers. *J Physiol* 1975; 251:1–59.
23. Hoffman BF, Cranefield PF: *Electrophysiology of the Heart.* New York, McGraw-Hill, 1960.
24. James TN: The connecting pathways between the sinus node and the AV node and between the right and left atrium in the human heart. *Am Heart J* 1963; 66:498–508.
25. James TN, Sherf L: Specialized tissues and preferential conduction in the atria of the heart. *Am J Cardiol* 1971; 28:414–427.
26. Goldstein SS, Rall W: Changes in action potential shape and velocity for changing core conductor geometry. *Biophys J* 1974; 14:731–757.
27. Spach MS, Miller WT, Dolber PC, Kootsey JM, Sommer JR, Mosher CE Jr: The functional role of structural complexities in the propagation of depolarization in the atrium of the dog: Cardiac conduction disturbances due to discontinuities of effective axial resistivity. *Circ Res* 1982; 50:175–191.
28. Brown HF: Electrophysiology of the sino-atrial node. *Physiol Rev* 1982; 62:505.
29. Vassalle M: Electrogenic suppression of automaticity in sheep and dog Purkinje fibers. *Circ Res* 1970; 27:361–377.
30. Weidmann S: Effect of current flow on the membrane potential of cardiac muscle. *J Physiol* 1951; 115:227–236.
31. Vassalle M: Cardiac pacemaker potentials at different extra- and intracellular K concentrations. *Am J Physiol* 1965; 208:770–775.
32. Vassalle M: An analysis of cardiac pacemaker potential by means of a voltage clamp technique. *Am J Physiol* 1966; 210:1335–1341.
33. Noble D, Tsien RW: The kinetics and rectifier properties of the slow potassium current in cardiac Purkinje fibres. *J Physiol* 1968; 195:185–214.
34. DiFrancesco D: A new interpretation of the pacemaker current in calf Purkinje fibres. *J Physiol* 1981; 314:359–376.
35. DiFrancesco D: A study of the ionic nature of the pacemaker current in calf Purkinje fibres. *J Physiol* 1981; 314:377–393.
36. Hauswirth O, Noble D, Tsien RW: The mechanisms of oscillatory activity at low membrane potentials in cardiac Purkinje fibres. *J Physiol* 1969; 200:255–265.
37. Wit AL, Cranefield PF: Triggered and automatic activity in the canine coronary sinus. *Circ Res* 1977; 41:435–445.
38. Wit AL, Cranefield PF: Triggered activity in cardiac muscle fibers of the simian mitral valve. *Circ Res* 1976; 38:85–98.
39. Ferrier GR, Saunders JH, Mendez C: A cellular mechanism for the generation of ventricular arrhythmias by acetylstrophanthidin. *Circ Res* 1973; 32:600–609.
40. Kass RS, Tsien RW, Weingart R: Ionic basis of transient inward current induced by strophanthidin in cardiac Purkinje fibers. *J Physiol* 1978; 281:209–226.
41. Wier WG, Hess P: Excitation-contraction coupling in cardiac Purkinje fibers: Effects of cardiotonic steroids on the intracellular $[Ca^{2+}]$ transient, membrane potential, and contraction. *J Gen Physiol* 1984; 83:395–415.
42. Cranefield PF, Wit AL, Hoffman BF: Conduction of the cardiac impulse: III. Characteristics of very slow conduction. *J Gen Physiol* 1971; 59:227–246.
43. Janse MJ, Van Capelle FJL, Freud GE, Durrer D: Circus movement within the AV node as a basis for supraventricular tachycardia as shown by multiple microelectrode recording in the isolated rabbit heart. *Circ Res* 1971; 28:403–414.
44. MacLean WAH, Plumb VJ, Waldo AL: Transient entrainment and interruption of ventricular tachycardia. *Pace* 1981; 4:358–366.
45. El-Sherif N, Smith RA, Evans K: Canine ventricular arrhythmias in the late myocardial infarction period: 8. Epicardial mapping and reentrant circuits. *Circ Res* 1981; 49:255–265.
46. Wit AL, Allessie MA, Bonke FIM, Lammers W, Smeets J, Fenoglio JJ Jr: Electrophysiologic mapping to determine the mechanism of experimental ventricular tachycardia initiated by premature impulses. Experimental approach and initial results demonstrating reentrant excitation. *Am J Cardiol* 1982; 49:166–185.
47. Janse MJ, Van Capelle FJL, Morsink H, Kléber AG, Wilms-Schopman F, Cardinal R, et al: Flow of "injury current" and patterns of excitation during early ventricular arrhythmias in acute regional

myocardial ischemia in isolated porcine and canine hearts: Evidence for two different arrhythmogenic mechanisms. *Circ Res* 1980; 47:151–165.

48. Gardner PI, Ursell PC, Pham TD, Fenoglio JJ Jr, Wit AL: Experimental chronic ventricular tachycardia: Anatomic and electrophysiologic substrates. In: Josephson ME, Wellens HJJ (eds): *Tachycardias: Mechanisms, Diagnosis and Treatment.* Philadelphia, Lea & Febiger, 1981: 29–60.
49. Allessie MA, Bonke FIM, Schopman FJG: Circus movement in rabbit atrial muscle as a mechanism of tachycardia: III. The "leading circle" concept: A new model of circus movement in cardiac tissue without the involvement of an anatomical obstacle. *Circ Res* 1977; 41:9–18.
50. Janse MJ, Van Capelle FJL: Electrotonic interactions across an inexcitable region as a cause of ectopic activity in acute regional myocardial ischemia. *Circ Res* 1982; 50:527–537.
51. Task Force of the Working Group on Arrhythmias of the European Society of Cardiology: The Sicilian gambit. A new approach to the classification of antiarrhythmic drugs based on arrhythmogenic mechanisms. *Circulation* 1991; 84:1831–1851.

Chapter 35

Mechanisms of Cardiac Arrhythmias and Conduction Disturbances

Albert L. Waldo, M.D. ■ *Andrew L. Wit, Ph.D.*

OVERVIEW OF MECHANISMS OF CARDIAC ARRHYTHMIAS AND CONDUCTION DISTURBANCES

Introduction

Due to increasing availability of sophisticated electrophysiological techniques for the study of cardiac tissues, both in vivo and in vitro, and the ability to study arrhythmias and conduction disturbances in both experimental models and in patients, our knowledge of the mechanisms of arrhythmias and conduction disturbances has increased greatly in recent times. While much is now known, much remains to be understood.

Arrhythmias are due to normal or abnormal impulse generation, abnormal impulse conduction, or a combination of simultaneous abnormalities of impulse generation and conduction.[1] In this chapter we first provide an overview of these mechanisms and identify the clinical arrhythmias with which they are thought to be associated. Then we provide a detailed discussion of these mechanisms as they are currently understood.

Causes of Arrhythmias

Normal or Abnormal Impulse Initiation

Automatic Rhythms *Normal Mechanism* Cardiac cells normally capable of developing spontaneous diastolic (phase 4) depolarization are said to be pacemaker cells. When pacemaker cells manifest spontaneous diastolic depolarization (Fig. 35-1), and thereby are responsible for generating the cardiac rhythm, the rhythm is said to be an automatic rhythm. Normally, the dominant pacemaker of the heart is in the sinus node, which, in adults, fires at a rate of 60 to 100 beats per minute. Cells capable of developing spontaneous diastolic depolarization (i.e., of manifesting automaticity) also are normally found in the specialized fibers in the atria, in the atrioventricular (AV) junction, and in the His-Purkinje system. The normal rate of impulse formation in adults by these ectopic pacemakers is 40 to 60 beats per minute in the AV junction (the AV node and His bundle). Normal rates of more distally located ectopic pacemakers are uncertain, but are probably 20 to 40 beats per minute

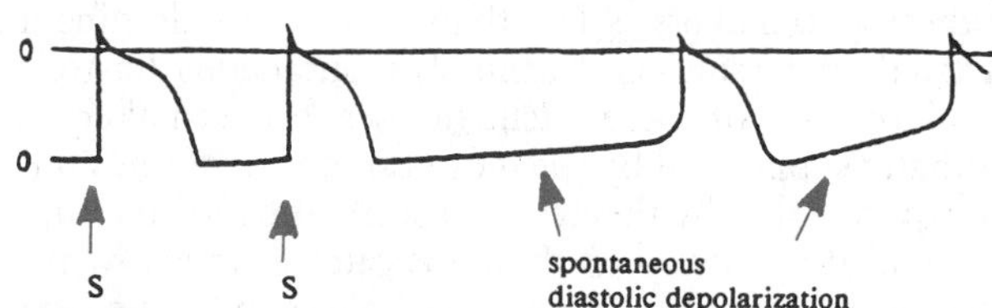

FIGURE 35-1 Arrhythmias may be caused by normal automaticity. Transmembrane potential recorded from a Purkinje fiber stimulated at a regular rate is shown. When the stimulus is turned off, spontaneous diastolic depolarization develops to cause automatic firing.

TABLE 35-1
Types of Tachycardias and Their Selected Characteristics and Documented or Presumed Mechanism

Tachycardia	Mechanism	Location	Rate Range	AV or VA Conduction
Sinus tachycardia	Automatic	Sinus node	≥100 bpm	1:1
Sinus node reentry	Reentry	Sinus node and right atrium	?110–180 bpm	1:1 or variable
Atrial fibrillation	Reentry	Atria	260–450 bpm, usually >300 bpm	Variable
Atrial flutter	Reentry	Right atrium	240–350 bpm, usually 300 ± 20 bpm	2:1 or variable
Atrial tachycardia	Reentry	Atria	150–240 bpm	1:1, 2:1, or variable
	Automatic	Atria	?	?
	Triggered (DADs) 2° to digitalis toxicity	Atria	150–240 bpm	1:1, 2:1, or variable
AV nodal reentry tachycardia	Reentry	AV node	120–250 bpm, usually 150–220 bpm	1:1
AV reentry (WPW or concealed accessory AV connection)	Reentry	Circuit includes accessory AV connection, atria, AV node, His, Purkinje system, ventricles	140–250 bpm, usually 150–220 bpm	1:1
Accelerated AV junctional tachycardia	Automatic or ? triggered	AV junction (AV node and His bundle)	61–200 bpm, usually 80–130 bpm	1:1 or variable
Accelerated idioventricular rhythm	Abnormal automaticity	Purkinje fibers	>60–? bpm	Variable, 1:1, or AV dissociation
Ventricular tachycardia	Reentry	Ventricles	120–300 bpm, usually 140–240 bpm	AV dissociation, variable, or 1:1
	Automatic (rare)	Ventricles	?	Variable, 1:1, or AV dissociation
Bundle branch reentrant tachycardia	Reentry	Bundle branches and ventricular septum	160–250 bpm, usually 195–240 bpm	AV dissociation, variable, or 1:1
Right ventricular outflow tract tachycardia	? Triggered (DADs)	Right ventricular outflow tract	120–220 bpm	AV dissociation, variable, or 1:1
Torsades de pointes	? Triggered (EADs)	Ventricles	>200 bpm	AV dissociation

DAD, delayed after depolarization; WPW, Wolff-Parkinson-White; EAD, early afterdepolarization; bpm, beats per minute.

in the bundle branches. These ectopic (i.e., nonsinus) pacemakers are also called latent or escape pacemakers for two related reasons: (1) the normal intrinsic rate of these pacemakers is less than that of the dominant pacemaker, the sinus node; and (2) spontaneous diastolic depolarization of these latent or escape pacemakers is normally suppressed by the more rapid rate of the sinus node pacemaker by the active process of overdrive suppression. It is only when the sinus rate slows below the intrinsic rate of these ectopic pacemakers that "the next one in line" warms up and fires. (See also Chap. 34.)

Arrhythmias of the sinus node An arrhythmia occurs when the sinus node pacemaker fires at a rate greater than 100 beats per minute (sinus tachycardia) (Table 35-1) or at a rate less than 60 beats per minute (sinus bradycardia) and is still the dominant pacemaker of the heart. A sinus tachycardia is usually an appropriate response to a precipitating factor (e.g., exercise, fever, hypotension, etc.), although, on occasion, it may be inappropriate, as in the presence of a sympathetic dysautonomia (inappropriate sinus tachycardia). On the other hand, sinus bradycardia more often reflects an abnormality not only of the sinus node pacemakers (they are too slow) but also of the latent or escape pacemakers (when the sinus rate slows abnormally, they do not escape). Sinus bradycardia may be due to an intrinsic abnormality of pacemaker cells, a parasympathetic dysautonomia (inappropriate sinus bradycardia), or an extrinsic factor such as suppression of automaticity by drug therapy (e.g., a beta blocker, a Ca^{2+} channel blocker, or an antiarrhythmic agent). For some patients, sinus bradycardia, particularly when only present at rest, may simply reflect a normal response to increased vagal tone, as in the well-trained athlete. Marked beat-to-beat variations in cycle length of the sinus rhythm, due virtually always to the influence of vagal tone on the pacemaker cells of the sinus node, is also considered an arrhythmia (sinus arrhythmia), even if the overall sinus rate is normal.

Ectopic automatic rhythms These arrhythmias occur when the site of the dominant pacemaker shifts to a site other than the sinus node (Table 35-1). The site of impulse initiation may shift from the sinus node to an ectopic (latent or escape) pacemaker if (1) the intrinsic rate of the sinus node decreases, e.g., when pacemaker dysfunction is limited to the sinus node; (2) the intrinsic rate of the ectopic (latent or escape) pacemaker increases, e.g., due to enhanced automaticity of latent pacemakers; or (3) the normal sinus impulse is prevented from being the dominant pacemaker of the heart, either because of sinus node exit block or sinoatrial block (i.e., the impulse cannot exit from the sinus node to excite the atria and subsequently the ventricles) or AV block (i.e., the impulse cannot excite the ventricles because of conduction block in the specialized AV conduction system, i.e., the AV node, His bundle, or both bundle branches. (See also Chaps. 34 and 36.)

Abnormal Mechanism Typically, normal working atrial and ventricular myocardial cells do not develop automaticity. Thus, when they manifest normal transmembrane potentials, no evidence of spontaneous diastolic (phase 4) depolarization is present. Under certain conditions, however, these cardiac muscle fibers, as well as specialized atrial and ventricular fibers, can develop an abnormal type of automatic firing. This occurs when the cell is relatively depolarized such that maximum diastolic potential is reduced to levels much lower than normal, usually by intrinsic cardiac disease. When this occurs, spontaneous diastolic (phase 4) depolarization may occur (Fig. 35-2). Such abnormal automaticity is caused by a pacemaker current that is different from the pacemaker current of normally automatic cells. The transmembrane action potentials associated with abnormal automaticity may be of the slow response type; i.e., the transmembrane action potential upstroke may depend on the slow inward (L-type) Ca^{2+} current because of inactivation of Na^{+} channels at the reduced level of membrane potential. Arrhythmias caused by abnormal automaticity will not be evident unless the rate of the abnormal focus is greater than that of the dominant automatic pacemaker (usually the sinus node) of the heart. Accelerated idioventricular rhythms after myocardial infarction may sometimes be caused by abnormal automaticity in Purkinje cells in the ischemic region. (See also Chap. 60.)

Triggered Rhythms These arrhythmias are caused by afterdepolarizations (Table 35-1).

Early afterdepolarizations (*EADs*) occur during repolarization of a transmembrane action potential that

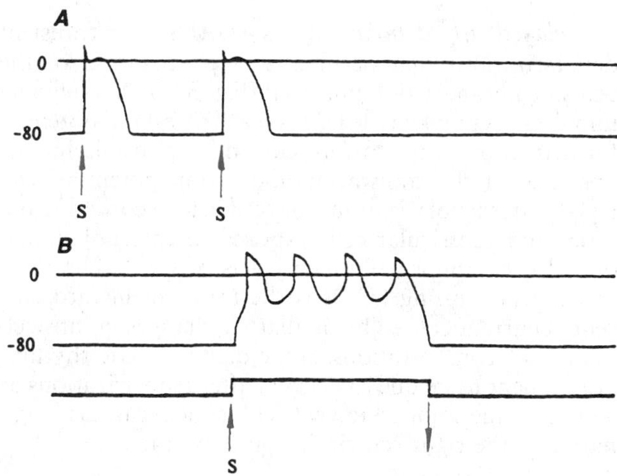

FIGURE 35-2 Arrhythmias may be caused by abnormal automaticity. Figure shows how abnormal automaticity may develop in a ventricular muscle fiber. *A.* Transmembrane potentials recorded from a muscle fiber with a normal resting potential are shown. When the fiber is not stimulated, phase 4 depolarization and automatic firing do not occur (compare with Fig. 35-1). *B.* At arrow, the membrane potential is reduced to −50 mV by a current pulse passed through a microelectrode. Automatic firing occurs at this low level of membrane potential. In the heart, certain abnormal states may cause similar decrease in membrane potential.

has been initiated from a normal level of membrane potential. They appear as a change in a membrane potential in a positive direction relative to the membrane potential expected during normal repolarization (Fig. 35-3*A* and *B*). Repetitive depolarizations may originate from the low level of membrane potential that occurs during the afterdepolarization. A clinical example of a triggered rhythm thought to be due to EADs is torsades de pointes associated with a toxic response to type IA or type III antiarrhythmic agents.

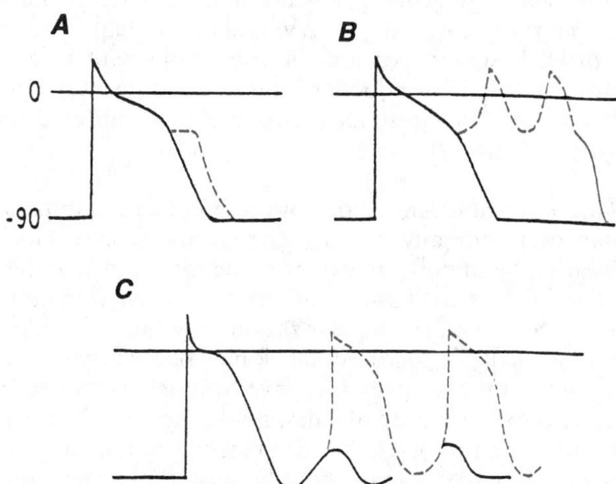

FIGURE 35-3 Triggered activity is caused by afterdepolarizations. *A.* Solid trace shows the normal transmembrane potential from a Purkinje fiber. The dashed trace shows an EAD that is subthreshold. *B.* Early afterdepolarization reached the threshold for the slow inward current, causing repetitive firing during the plateau of the Purkinje fiber action potential. *C.* Solid trace shows a transmembrane action potential followed by a subthreshold DAD. The dashed trace shows the triggered action potentials that occur when the afterdepolarization reaches threshold potential.

Delayed afterdepolarizations (*DADs*) are transient depolarizations that occur after repolarization of the transmembrane action potential (Fig. 35-3C). Triggered impulses occur when the DADs reach threshold potential for activation of the inward current responsible for the upstroke of the transmembrane action potential. Delayed afterdepolarizations have been recorded from atrial and ventricular cells exposed to catecholamines, digitalis, or abnormally high levels of Ca^{2+}. The ionic mechanism causing DADs is the transient inward current, a current caused by oscillatory changes in intracellular Ca^{2+} concentrations. Some digitalis toxic rhythms are thought to be due to delayed afterdepolarizations as well as some idiopathic ventricular tachycardias originating in the right ventricular outflow tract.

Abnormal Impulse Conduction

Prolongation of Conduction Time Prolongation of conduction time of the cardiac impulse may occur anywhere in the heart. It may result from slow conduction and be generalized, as in response to a type IC antiarrhythmic agent, or the slow conduction may be localized to a portion of the heart, e.g., a portion of the specialized AV conduction system or in ventricular myocardium injured by a myocardial infarction. Prolongation of conduction time resulting from slow conduction may also occur as a normal response of cardiac tissue, as in prolongation of AV nodal conduction time associated with a propagated premature beat. In addition to slow conduction, prolongation of conduction time may also occur when the cardiac impulse takes longer than normal to get from one place to another even though conduction velocity of the impulse along the route is normal. An example of the latter is found in patients with an endocardial cushion defect in which the sinus impulse takes an abnormally long time to reach the AV node. This occurs because the location of the ostium primum defect forces the activation wave front generated by the sinus impulse to take a longer route to reach the AV node.[2] As shall be seen shortly, however, perhaps the most important role of prolongation of conduction time is in the genesis and maintenance of most tachycardias due to ordered reentry.

Block of Conduction Block of the propagating impulse may occur for any number of reasons. It may block because the impulse arrives at tissue that is inexcitable, either because the tissue is still in its effective refractory period after a recent depolarization or because the tissue is abnormally depolarized. Block may occur because the strength of the propagating wave front is insufficient to excite the tissue ahead of it despite the fact that the tissue ahead of it is fully excitable (decremental conduction and block). Block also may occur because the propagating impulse encounters tissue intrinsically unable to conduct the cardiac impulse, e.g., scar tissue associated with a prior myocardial infarction or surgical incision.

If conduction block of the cardiac impulse occurs, disturbances of cardiac rhythm may occur in several different ways. If the sinus impulse fails to propagate to the right atrium (sinus node exit block or sinoatrial block), normally an ectopic (latent or escape) pacemaker will emerge and assume the role of cardiac pacemaker. If propagation of the cardiac impulse is impaired in the specialized AV conduction system so that the ventricles are not activated at a sufficiently rapid rate, an ectopic pacemaker (latent or escape) distal to the site of block will often emerge and assume the role of cardiac pacemaker. When either sinoatrial or AV block occurs, however, under some circumstances, an ectopic pacemaker may not emerge quickly enough and/or at a clinically adequate rate. Thus, either a period of asystole or marked bradycardia or both may occur. If either or both happen, the clinical problem may be quite serious and even life threatening. Block may also occur in one of the bundle branches, causing either left bundle branch block or right bundle branch block. Bundle branch block per se is rarely a clinical problem of any consequence except when the block occurs simultaneously in both bundle branches.

Unidirectional Block and Reentry During normal sinus rhythm, the conducted impulse from the sinus node pacemaker dies out after orderly and sequential activation of the atria, the specialized AV conduction system, and the ventricles, because the impulse is prevented from reactivating the myocardium by the refractoriness of the tissue that has just been activated. The heart then must wait for a new impulse from the sinus node pacemaker for each subsequent activation. The phenomenon of reentry occurs when the propagating impulse does not die out, but rather continues to propagate and reactivate the heart because the activation wave front continuously encounters excitable cardiac tissue. Almost all clinically important tachyarrhythmias are due to reentry (Table 35-1).

For reentry to occur, several conditions must be met. First, there must exist a substrate in the cardiac tissue capable of supporting reentry, i.e., a region in the heart with the appropriate electrical properties in which reentry can occur. Second, the excitation wave front must encounter unidirectional block. Third, the activation wave front must be able to circulate around a central area of block. Figure 35-4 (*A*, *B*, and *C*) illustrates a simple example of reentry in a loop of excitable tissue, as actually first demonstrated by Mayer in 1906 in the excitable ring of a jelly fish.[3] The center of the loop is a hole, and this serves as a central area of block around which the reentrant wave front can circulate. If the loop of excitable tissue is stimulated at a single point, two wave fronts of excitation circulate in the ring (Fig. 35-4*A*). Since the wave fronts collide, they die out. If block of one of the circulating wave fronts occurs, however, an excitation wave front can circulate in only one direction around the loop; i.e., unidirectional block of the stimulated wave front has occurred (Fig. 35-4*B*). If either conduction of the nonblocked impulse around the loop is slow enough (e.g., because of a region or regions of slow conduction) or, in the presence of normal conduction, the loop is long enough so that by the time the circulating wave front has returned to its site of origin, this latter region has recovered excitability, the wave front can then reexcite (i.e., reenter) tissue it has previously excited and continue to circulate (Fig. 35-4*C*). If the region of previous block remains unexcitable, then

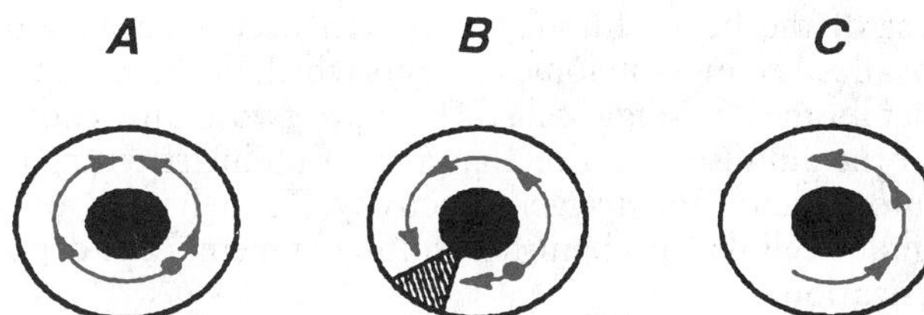

FIGURE 35-4 Schematic representation of reentry in a ring of excitable tissue. *A.* Ring was stimulated in the area indicated by the black dot. Impulses propagated away from the point of stimulation in both directions and collided; no reentry occurred. *B.* Cross-hatched area was compressed while the ring was stimulated, again at the black dot. The impulse propagated around the ring in only one direction, having been blocked in the other direction by an area of compression. Then immediately after stimulation the compression was relieved. *C.* Circulating impulse is shown returning to its point of origin and then continuing around the ring. Identical reentry would occur if the cross-hatched area was a region of unidirectional conduction block with block in the right-to-left direction.

bidirectional block at this site has prevented reentry. Since the block is unidirectional, reentry occurs.

In the presence of myocardium manifesting unidirectional block and a central inexcitable area around which an excitation wave front can circulate, as long as the wavelength (the product of the conduction velocity of the circulating wave front and the effective refractory period of the tissue of the reentrant circuit) of the circulating wave front is shorter than the length of the pathway in which it is traveling, the wave front will continue to circulate. The result is classical circus movement or reentrant excitation. Thus, an area of slow conduction is not an absolute requisite for reentrant excitation to occur. Reentry can occur at normal conduction velocities if the path length is sufficiently long; however, most reentrant circuits require the presence of an area of slow conduction. This is because in most circumstances, despite the presence of unidirectional block, the length of the potential reentrant circuit is too short so that without the presence of an area or areas of slow conduction, the nonblocked wave front would otherwise travel around the circuit so quickly that it would arrive at the point of origin of the wave front (the stimulus site in Fig. 35-4) before this site has repolarized sufficiently to become excitable again. In fact, presumably for this very reason, an area (or areas) of slow conduction is (are) part of the reentrant circuit for virtually all clinical reentrant rhythms.

Reentrant circuits may be located almost anywhere in the heart, and they can assume many sizes and shapes. Reentry in which the circulating wave front continuously reenters over the same stable pathway to generate the reentrant rhythm is called ordered reentry.[1] The circuit is usually comprised of a well-defined anatomic pathway, an anatomic circuit. One such example is the reentrant circuit in AV reentrant tachycardia (atrium, AV node, His-Purkinje system, ventricle, accessory AV connection). Functional circuits, which depend on cellular electrophysiological properties rather than anatomy, can also cause ordered reentry if the electrophysiological properties crucial for reentry are confined to a specific location and reentry only occurs in that location. Ordered reentry can also involve a combination of anatomic and functional pathways. Examples of ordered reentry include atrial flutter, most monomorphic ventricular tachycardias, AV nodal reentrant tachycardia, AV reentrant tachycardia involving an accessory AV connection, and sinus node reentrant tachycardia (Table 35-1). (See also Chap. 36.)

During random reentry,[1] propagation occurs in reentrant pathways that continuously change their size and location with time. For this to occur, circuits must, at least to a significant degree, be functional. Random reentry need not depend on any special electrophysiological abnormality in the heart, although electrophysiological abnormalities may also lead to random reentry. Examples of random reentry are atrial fibrillation and ventricular fibrillation (Table 35-1).

Reflection The term *reflection* has been used to describe a form of reentry in a linear bundle in which two excitable regions are separated by an area of depressed conduction.[4] During reflection, excitation occurs slowly in one direction along the bundle and is followed by continued propagation and excitation occurring in the opposite direction. One form of reflection may, in fact, be microreentry based on a functional longitudinal dissociation within the depressed segment.[5-7] How this might occur is diagrammed in Fig. 35-5. The diagram at the top of the figure depicts two adjacent fibers in a bundle. The entire shaded area is depressed (reduced membrane potential and slow action potential upstrokes), the darker area in the upper fiber indicating more severe depression than the lighter area in the lower fiber. Unidirectional conduction block occurs in the more severely depressed region. Arrows labeled I show the impulse entering the two fibers from the left end. Conduction of the impulse

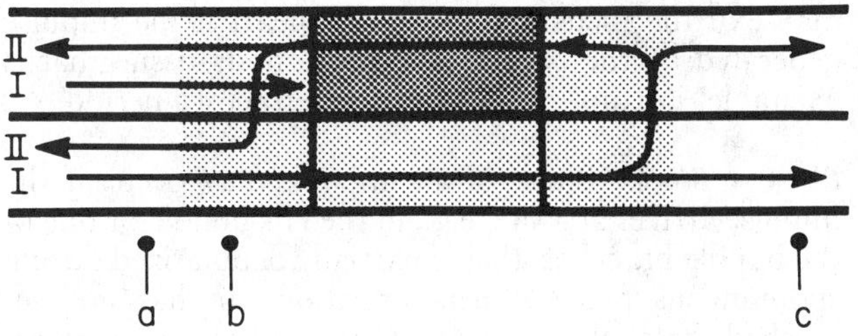

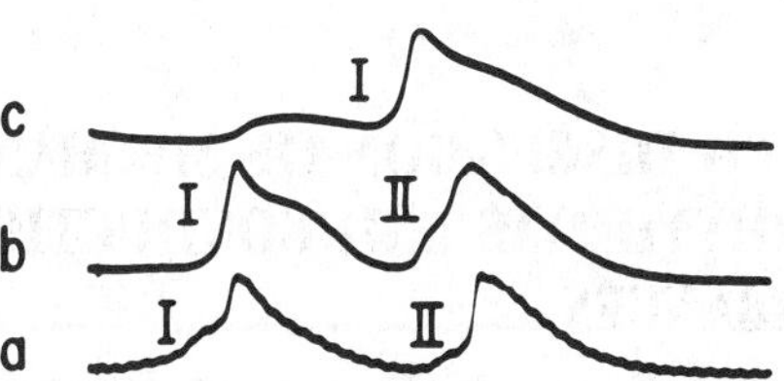

FIGURE 35-5 Diagram of reflection based on microreentry. *Top:* Schematic representation of two adjacent myocardial fibers. The shaded region indicates an area of depressed conduction. Arrows show the pattern of activation: Arrow I is a wave front conducting in an antegrade direction, and arrow II is a reflected wave front conducting in a retrograde direction. Action potentials shown below were recorded at sites *a*, *b*, and *c* on the diagram. (*Modified from Wit AL, Bigger JT Jr: Circulation 52:III96–115, 1975. Reproduced with permission from the publisher and authors.*)

(I) blocks in the fiber at the top, in the severely depressed region, but continues in the fiber at the bottom, which is not as depressed. The impulse conducts transversely from the bottom fiber to the top fiber once past the region of severe depression. It then conducts retrogradely through this severely depressed region in the top bundle. Arrows labeled II show the reflected impulse returning to reexcite the left end of the bundle. Action potentials that were recorded from sites *a*, *b*, and *c* in the bottom fiber are shown below: Action potentials labeled I were recorded as the impulse conducted from left to right; action potentials labeled II were recorded as the impulse conducted from right to left, returning to its origin. It is thought such reentry may occur in the His bundle or one of the bundle branches.

Simultaneous Abnormalities of Impulse Generation and Conduction

Parasystole At times, an ectopic pacemaker may be connected to the remainder of the heart through tissue(s) in which there is unidirectional block. The unidirectional block prevents the dominant rhythm, usually a sinus rhythm, from entering the region where the ectopic pacemaker is located. As a result, the ectopic pacemaker is not suppressed by the dominant rhythm of the heart. At the same time, because the block is unidirectional, impulses generated by the ectopic pacemaker can be conducted out to other regions of the heart provided they are not refractory, causing premature beats or even a tachycardia. This kind of rhythm is called *parasystole*. Thus, parasystole is a rhythm due to impulse generation (presumed to be due to an ectopic pacemaker, but it could be due to any mechanism) in a protected focus. The focus is protected because there is entrance block into the focus (due to unidirectional block). An impulse may exit the focus and excite the heart if the impulse generated by the parasystolic focus finds tissue that is excitable, i.e., not in the effective refractory period.

Phase 4 Block Block of an impulse may occur if the impulse arrives at a site, e.g., in the His bundle or one of the bundle branches, that is partially depolarized during spontaneous phase 4 depolarization but has not yet reached threshold. This spontaneous diastolic depolarization can sufficiently depolarize the tissue so that the fast Na^+ channels are inactivated enough to cause failure of propagation.[8]

DETAILED DISCUSSION OF MECHANISMS OF ARRHYTHMIAS AND CONDUCTION DISTURBANCES

Arrhythmias Caused by Impulse Initiation

Introduction

The term *impulse initiation* is used to indicate that an electrical impulse can arise in a single cell or group of closely coupled cells through depolarization of the cell membrane and, once initiated, can spread through the rest of the heart. Impulse initiation occurs because of localized changes in ionic currents which flow across the membranes of single cells. There are two major causes for the impulse initiation that may result in arrhythmias: automaticity and triggered activity. Each has its own unique cellular mechanism resulting in membrane depolarization.

Automaticity

It is convenient to subdivide automaticity into two kinds: normal and abnormal. Normal automaticity is found in the primary pacemaker of the heart, the sinus node, as well as in certain subsidiary or latent pacemakers which can become the pacemaker under conditions that are described later. Impulse initiation is a normal property of these latent pacemakers. On the other hand, abnormal automaticity, whether the result of experimental interventions or disease, only occurs in cardiac cells when major abnormal changes occur in their transmembrane potentials, in particular, in steady-state depolarization of the membrane potential. This property of abnormal automaticity is not confined to any specific latent pacemaker cell type but may occur almost anywhere in the heart.

Normal Automaticity: Pacemaker Mechanisms The normal site of impulse initiation is the sinus node. The cause of normal automaticity in the sinus node is a spontaneous decline in the transmembrane potential during diastole, referred to as the pacemaker potential or phase 4 or diastolic depolarization (the terms are interchangeable). Diastolic depolarization is that part of the sinus node membrane potential labeled dd in the top panel (*A*) of Fig. 35-6. When the depolarization reaches threshold potential (dashed line labeled TP), the upstroke of the spontaneous action potential is initiated. This fall in membrane potential during phase 4 reflects a gradual shift in the balance between inward and outward membrane currents in the direction of net inward (depolarizing) current.

Studies have been done to elucidate and characterize the membrane currents that cause diastolic (phase 4) depolarization in the sinus node using voltage-clamp techniques in small tissue preparations and in single dissociated sinus node cells. The cause of the pacemaker potential is still controversial. There is some evidence that diastolic depolarization results from the turning on of an inward current, called i_f, that is activated after repolarization of the sinus node actions potential. The net inward i_f current is carried by Na^+.[9] From the voltage-clamp studies, it is known that the i_f channels are inactivated at positive membrane potentials, begin to activate after hyperpolarization to around −40 mV, and are fully activated after hyperpolarization to around −100 mV.[10–12] Since the maximum diastolic potential of the sinus node pacemaker cells is between −60 and −70 mV, the i_f current is turned on during repolarization to this level, although it is not fully activated at the maximum diastolic potential. Activation of the i_f conductance also has a time dependency, and therefore, the inward current continues to increase after complete repolarization, causing the progressive fall in the membrane poten-

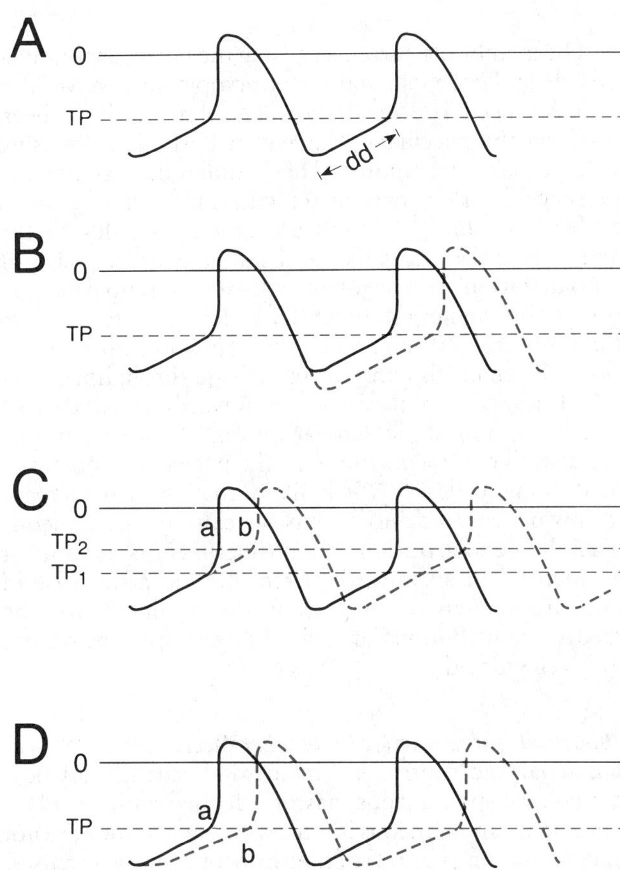

FIGURE 35-6 Diagrams of sinus node action potentials illustrating normal automaticity caused by spontaneous diastolic depolarization and the factors that change the rate of impulse initiation. *A.* Typical sinus node action potential with spontaneous diastolic depolarization (dd). *B.* Change in the rate when the maximum diastolic potential is shifted to a more negative level (from *a* to *b*). *C.* Change in rate caused by change in threshold potential to a less negative level (from TP1 to TP2). *D.* Change in rate that occurs when the slope of phase 4 depolarization is decreased (from *a* to *b*). (*Modified after Wit AL, Janes MJ: The Ventricular Arrhythmias of Ischemia and Infarction. The Electrophysiological Mechanisms. Mt. Kisco, NY, Futura Publishing, 1992. Reproduced with permission from the publisher and authors.*)

tial during phase 4. Important roles for other membrane currents, including the potassium current i_K and the T and L Ca^{2+} currents causing spontaneous diastolic depolarization, have also been proposed.[13–21] Therefore, there may be no single pacemaker current in the sinus node, but rather a number of currents may contribute to the occurrence of automaticity.[17]

The intrinsic rate at which sinus node pacemaker cells initiate impulses is determined by the interplay of three factors[22]: (a) the maximum diastolic potential; (b) the threshold potential; and (c) the rate or slope of phase 4 depolarization. Factor (c) is related to the properties of the pacemaker current(s). A change in any one of these factors will alter the time required for phase 4 depolarization to carry the membrane potential from its maximum diastolic level to threshold and thereby alter the rate of impulse initiation. For example, if the maximum diastolic potential increases (becomes more negative) going from solid trace *a* to dashed trace *b* in Fig. 35-6*B*, spontaneous depolarization to threshold potential will take longer and the rate of impulse initiation will fall. Conversely, a decrease in the maximum diastolic potential will tend to increase the rate of impulse initiation (going from trace *b* to trace *a*). Similarly, changes in threshold potential or changes in the slope of phase 4 depolarization will alter the rate of impulse initiation. In Fig. 35-6*C*, a change in threshold potential from TP1 to the less negative TP2 causes spontaneous diastolic depolarization to proceed for a longer time (dashed action potential trace) before an impulse is initiated, slowing the rate. In Fig. 35-6*D*, a decrease in the slope of spontaneous diastolic depolarization from *a* to *b* also results in a longer interval between action potentials (dashed trace) because of the longer time required for membrane potential to reach the threshold potential. In Fig. 35-6*C* and *D*, changes of threshold potential or slope of diastolic depolarization in the opposite direction would speed up the rate.

The alterations in the rate of impulse initiation in the sinus node resulting from the factors discussed above may lead to arrhythmias. They are often the result of the actions of the autonomic nervous system on the sinus node. Parasympathetic stimulation and the resultant release of acetylcholine hyperpolarize the membrane potential through stimulation of muscarinic receptors and activation of a K current (Fig. 35-6*B*).[23,24] Acetylcholine also decreases inward Ca^{2+} current and the i_f pacemaker current.[25] A combination of these effects slows the rate. Sympathetic stimulation and norepinephrine release increase the slope of diastolic depolarization and therefore sinus rate by increasing L-type Ca^{2+} current[26] and by increasing activation of the inward i_f current at the completion of action potential repolarization.[11,12,27] These effects are mediated through β_1-receptor stimulation.

In addition to the sinus node, cells with pacemaking capability in the normal heart are located in some parts of the atria and ventricles, although they are not pacemakers while the sinus node is functioning normally. These are latent or subsidiary pacemakers. Since spontaneous diastolic depolarization is a normal property, the automaticity generated by these cells is classified as normal. In the atria, cells with well-polarized membrane potentials (resting potentials of around −80 mV) and action potentials characterized by fast upstrokes, a plateau phase of repolarization and spontaneous diastolic depolarization, are located along the crista terminalis (Fig. 35-7*A*).[28] Subsidiary atrial pacemakers with somewhat lower maximum diastolic potentials (−75 to −70 mV) and prominent phase 4 depolarization are located at the junction of the inferior right atrium and inferior vena cava, near or on the Eustachian ridge (a remnant of the Eustachian valve of the inferior vena cava) (Fig. 35-7*B*).[29–31] Other potential atrial pacemakers are at the orifice of the coronary sinus (Fig. 35-7C)[32] and in the atrial muscle that extends into the tricuspid and mitral valves (Fig. 35-7*D*).[33–35] Action potentials of cells in the valves have slow upstrokes that are probably caused to a significant extent by L-type Ca^{2+} current. In the AV junction, AV nodal cells possess the intrinsic property of automaticity (Fig. 35-7*E*)[36] although there is still some uncertainty as to the exact location of these pacemakers in the node.[37] The intrinsic rate of the atrial pacemakers is greater than that of AV junctional pacemakers.[38] Both atrial and AV junctional subsidiary pacemakers are

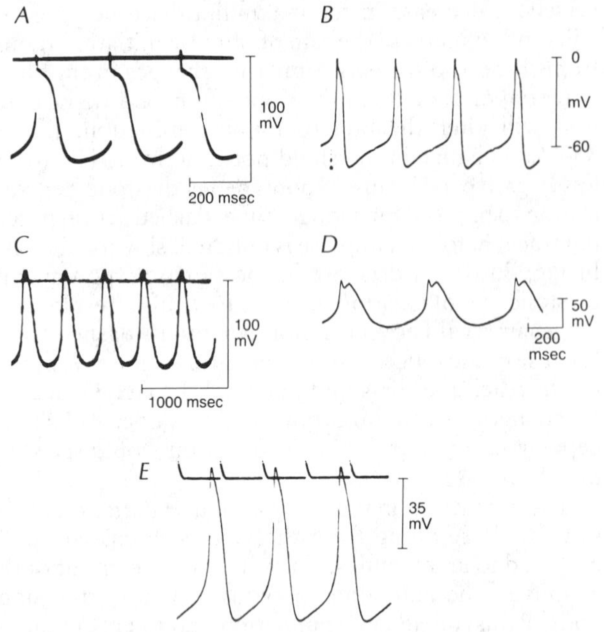

FIGURE 35-7 Transmembrane potentials recorded in isolated superfused preparations from some subsidiary pacemaker cells with the property of normal automaticity. Spontaneous diastolic depolarization that developed in the absence of overdrive suppression is shown in each panel. *A.* Atrial fiber in crista terminalis in the presence of isoproterenol. *B.* Atrial fiber in the inferior right atrium. *C.* Atrial fiber in ostium of coronary sinus in the presence of norepinephrine. *D.* Atrial fiber in stretched mitral valve leaflet. *E.* Atrioventricular nodal fiber of the rabbit heart after the AV node was separated from the atrium. (*From Wit AL, Janse MJ: The Ventricular Arrhythmias of Ischemia and Infarction. The Electrophysiological Mechanisms. Mt. Kisco, NY, Futura Publishing, 1992. Reproduced with permission from the publisher and authors.*)

under autonomic control, with the sympathetics enhancing pacemaker activity through B_1-adrenergic stimulation and the parasympathetics inhibiting pacemaker activity through muscarinic receptor stimulation.[39–42] In the ventricles, latent or subsidiary pacemakers are found in the His-Purkinje system, where Purkinje fibers have the property of spontaneous diastolic depolarization (Fig. 35-8).[22,43] The intrinsic Purkinje fiber pacemaker rate in general is less than the rate of atrial and AV junctional pacemakers and decreases from the His bundle to the distal Purkinje branches.[44] The spontaneous diastolic depolarization in this region is also under similar autonomic control. As in the atria, sympathetic activation enhances automaticity,[45] while parasympathetic activation can reduce it, mostly through inhibition of sympathetic influences.[46,47]

The membrane currents causing the normal spontaneous diastolic depolarization at ectopic sites have also been studied. The most thorough analyses have been done on the pacemaker current in Purkinje cells using voltage-clamp techniques. These studies have shown the presence of an i_f pacemaker current, as in the sinus node.[27,48,49] The i_f channels are deactivated during the action potential upstroke and initial plateau phase of repolarization but begin to activate as repolarization brings the membrane potential to levels more negative than about -60 mV. Since the activation kinetics are slow, the channels continue to activate throughout diastole, leading to an increasing net inward current carried by Na^+ and diastolic depolarization.[48,49] Other currents are also likely to contribute to the pacemaker potential in Purkinje cells.[27,50–52] It is likely that the net increase in inward current during diastole causing spontaneous diastolic depolarization in Purkinje fibers is a result of an increase in an inward current (i_f) and a decrease in outward current (i_{K_1} and i_K). In the coming years, the relative contributions of each of these currents are sure to be elucidated.

Abnormal Automaticity: Pacemaker Mechanisms Working atrial and ventricular myocardial cells do not normally have spontaneous diastolic depolarization and do not initiate spontaneous impulses even when they are not excited for long periods of time by propagating impulses. When the resting potentials of working atrial or ventricular myocardial cells are reduced sufficiently, however, spontaneous diastolic depolarization may occur and cause repetitive impulse initiation, a phenomenon called depolarization-induced automaticity or abnormal automaticity. The level of membrane potential at which abnormal automaticity occurs is often in a range between -70 and -30 mV.[53] Likewise, cells in the Purkinje system, which are normally automatic at high levels of membrane potential, also show abnormal automaticity when the membrane potential is reduced.[4,54] As discussed before, the i_f channels which participate in normal pacemaker activity in Purkinje fibers have a gating mechanism controlling channel opening and closing that is dependent on the transmembrane voltage. At membrane potentials that are positive to about -60 mV, such as after the upstroke and during the early phases of repolarization, the channels are closed. In response to the negative potentials that occur after complete repolarization, the channels reopen, generating the inward pacemaker current.[48,49] For this reason, when the steady-state membrane potential of Purkinje fibers is reduced to around

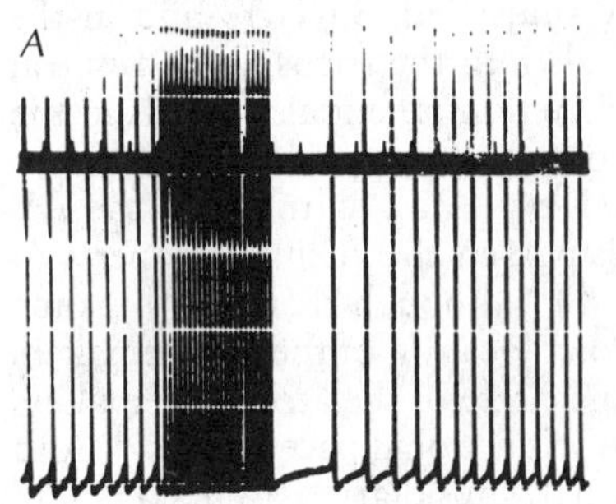

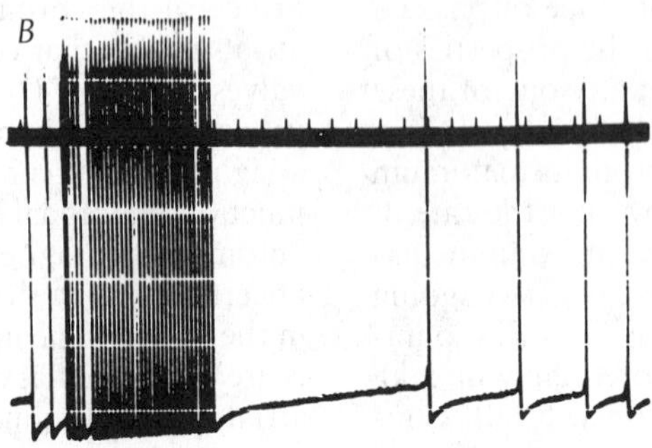

FIGURE 35-8 Overdrive suppression of normal automaticity in a canine Purkinje fiber. The action potentials are displayed at a slow oscilloscopic sweep speed so the time course of repolarization cannot be seen. Note the warmup of the spontaneous pacemaker following termination of pacing. (*From Cranefield PF: The Conduction of the Cardiac Impulse. The Slow Response and Cardiac Arrhythmia. Mt. Kisco, NY, Futura Publishing, 1975. Reproduced with permission from the publisher and author.*)

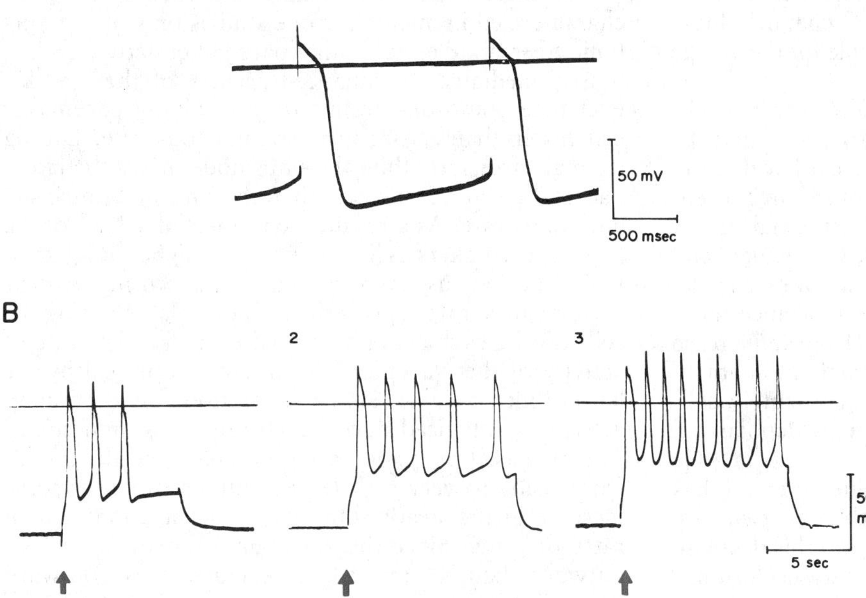

FIGURE 35-9 Normal and abnormal automaticity in a canine Purkinje fiber. *A.* Transmembrane potential recording from a Purkinje fiber with a normal maximum diastolic potential of −85 mV and spontaneous diastolic depolarization. *B.* Abnormal automaticity that occurred when membrane potential was decreased: (1) fiber was depolarized (at the arrow) to a membrane potential of −45 mV by injecting a long-lasting current pulse through a microelectrode; (2) membrane potential was reduced to −40 mV (at the arrow); (3) membrane potential was reduced to −30 mV (at the arrow). (*Reproduced from Wit AL, Friedman PF: Arch Int Med 1975; 135:459. Reproduced with permission from the publisher and author.*)

−60 mV or less, as may sometimes occur in ischemic regions of the heart, these normal pacemaker channels are not functional, and automaticity is not caused by the normal pacemaker mechanism. It can, however, be caused by an "abnormal" mechanism (described below). In Fig. 35-9, the transmembrane potential recorded from a spontaneously firing Purkinje fiber with normal automaticity is shown in panel *A*, and abnormal automatic activity occurring while the membrane potential was depolarized to progressively lower membrane potentials is shown in panel *B*: 1, 2, and 3. The abnormal automatic rate increased as membrane potential became more positive. This is a general characteristic of abnormal automaticity in atrial and ventricular cells as well.

A low level of membrane potential is not the only criterion for defining abnormal automaticity. If this was so, the automaticity of the sinus node would have to be considered abnormal. Therefore, an important distinction between abnormal and normal automaticity is that the membrane potentials of fibers showing the abnormal type of activity are reduced from their own normal level. For this reason, we do not classify automaticity in the AV node or valves, where membrane potential is normally low, to be abnormal automaticity.

A likely cause of automaticity at depolarized membrane potentials in ventricular muscle is activation and deactivation of the delayed rectifier K current.[55,56] The conductance of this K channel is activated during the normal action potential plateau, and the outward current that flows through it contributes to repolarization. The channel then deactivates during diastole. No significant outward current flows through this channel at normal diastolic potentials, since the resting potential lies near the reversal potential and the driving force is negligible.[56] When the membrane potential is depolarized, however, an outward current flows through this channel, which is activated at the depolarized membrane potentials. This current hyperpolarizes the membrane potential. As the channel then deactivates at the hyperpolarized potentials, spontaneous diastolic depolarization occurs. If either Na or Ca channels have been reactivated since the preceding action potential, the spontaneous depolarization caused by K-channel deactivation may lead to an upstroke caused by current flowing through one of these channels (depending on the level of the membrane potential).[56] A similar mechanism might cause abnormal automaticity in partially depolarized Purkinje fibers. Experiments on depolarized human atrial myocardium from dilated atria indicate that Ca^{2+}-dependent processes may also contribute to abnormal pacemaker activity at low membrane potentials.[57,58] It was proposed that intracellular Ca^{2+} released from the sarcoplasmic reticulum controls membrane permeability to an inward current during diastole that leads to spontaneous diastolic depolarization and abnormal automaticity. The mechanism may be similar to the one causing the transient inward current responsible for DADs (see the section on triggered activity). An increase in intracellular Ca^{2+} is also expected to cause an inward Na^+ current through Na^+-Ca^{2+} exchange.

In summary, therefore, several different mechanisms probably cause abnormal automaticity, including activation and deactivation of K^+ currents, Ca^{2+}-dependent activation of an inward current, inward Ca^{2+} currents and even some contribution by the pacemaker current i_f. It has not yet been determined which of the above mechanisms are operative in the different pathological conditions in which abnormal automaticity may occur.

The upstrokes of the spontaneously occurring action potentials generated by abnormal automaticity may be caused by either Na^+ or Ca^{2+} inward currents or, possibly, a mixture of the two. In the range of diastolic potentials between approximately −70 and −50 mV, repetitive activity is dependent on extracellular Na^+ concentration and can be decreased or abolished by the Na^+ channel blockers lidocaine and tetrodotoxin, indicating that the Na^+ inward current is involved. In a diastolic potential range of approximately −50 to −30 mV, repetitive activity depends on extracellular Ca^{2+} concentration and is reduced by the Ca^{2+} channel blockers, Mn^{2+} and verapamil, indicating a role for the L-type Ca^{2+} inward current.[4,59]

The decrease in membrane potential of cardiac cells required for abnormal automaticity to occur may be induced by a variety of factors related to cardiac disease. Although an increase in extracellular potassium concentration can reduce membrane potential, normal or abnormal automaticity in working atrial, ventricular, and Purkinje fibers usually does not occur when $[K]_o$ is elevated because of the increase in K^+ conductance (and, hence, net outward current) that results from an increase in $[K]^+_o$.[60,61] This argues against abnormal automaticity being responsible for arrhythmias arising in acutely ischemic myocardium, where cells are partially depolarized by increased extracellular K^+.[62–64] A decrease in $[K]_i$, which also causes a decreased membrane potential, has been shown to occur in the Purkinje fibers that survive on the endocardial surface of infarcts, and this decrease persists for at least 24 h after the coronary occlusion.[65] The reduction in $[K]_i$ contributes to the low membrane potential[66] and the accompanying abnormal automaticity.[67,68] Isolated preparations of diseased atrial and ventricular myocardium from human hearts superfused with Tyrode's solution show phase 4 depolarization and abnormal automaticity at membrane potentials in the range of -50 to -60 mV.[69–71] It has been proposed that a decrease in membrane potassium conductance is an important cause of the low membrane potentials in the atrial fibers.[70]

Suppression of Normal and Abnormal Automatic Subsidiary Pacemakers During sinus rhythm in the normal heart, the intrinsic rate of impulse initiation due to automaticity of cells in the sinus node is higher than that of the other potentially automatic cells, and the latent pacemakers are excited by propagated impulses from the sinus node before they can depolarize spontaneously to threshold potential. Not only are latent pacemakers prevented from initiating an impulse because they are depolarized before they have a chance to fire, but also the diastolic (phase 4) depolarization of the latent pacemaker cells with the property of normal automaticity is actually inhibited because they are repeatedly depolarized by the impulses from the sinus node.[72,73] This inhibition can be demonstrated by suddenly stopping the sinus node, e.g., by vagal stimulation (vagal stimulation also inhibits subsidiary pacemakers in the atria and AV junction) or in the tissue bath following termination of overdrive pacing (Fig. 35-8). Impulses then usually arise from a subsidiary pacemaker in the ventricular Purkinje system, but that impulse initiation is generally preceded by a long period of quiescence.[74,75] Impulse initiation by the Purkinje fiber pacemaker then begins at a low rate and only gradually speeds up to a final steady rate that is, however, still slower than the original sinus rhythm. The quiescent period following abolition of the sinus rhythm reflects the inhibitory influence exerted on the subsidiary pacemaker by the dominant sinus node pacemaker. This inhibition is called overdrive suppression. Similarly, the sinus node also overdrive suppresses subsidiary atrial pacemakers.[76]

The mechanism of overdrive suppression has been characterized in microelectrode studies on isolated Purkinje fiber bundles exhibiting pacemaker activity.[72] It is mostly mediated by enhanced activity of the Na^+-K^+ exchange pump that results from driving a pacemaker cell faster than its intrinsic spontaneous rate. During normal cardiac rhythm, the sinus node drives the latent pacemakers at a faster rate than their normal (intrinsic) automatic rate. As a result, the intracellular Na^+ of the latent pacemakers is increased to a higher level than would be the case were the pacemakers firing at their own intrinsic rate. This is the result of Na^+ entering the cells during each action potential upstroke. The rate of activity of the Na^+ pump is largely determined by the level of intracellular Na^+ concentration,[77] so that pump activity is enhanced during high rates of stimulation.[72] The increased pump activity prevents intracellular Na^+ from rising to very high levels, although there is some increase in the steady-state Na^+ concentration at high rates of firing. Since the Na^+ pump moves more Na^+ outward than K^+ inward, it generates a net outward (hyperpolarizing) current across the cell membrane.[78] When subsidiary pacemaker cells are driven faster than their intrinsic rate by the sinus node, the enhanced outward pump current hyperpolarizes the membrane potential and suppresses spontaneous impulse initiation in these cells, which, as described before, is dependent on the net inward current. When the dominant (overdrive) pacemaker is stopped, this suppression continues because the Na^+ pump continues to generate the outward current as it reduces the intracellular Na^+ levels toward normal. The continued Na^+ pump–generated outward current is responsible for the period of quiescence, which lasts until the intracellular Na^+ concentration, and hence the pump current, becomes small enough to allow subsidiary pacemaker cells to depolarize spontaneously to threshold. Intracellular Na^+ concentration decreases during the quiescent period because Na^+ is constantly being pumped out of the cell and little is entering.[59] Intracellular Na^+ and pump current continue to decline even after spontaneous firing begins because of the slow rate, causing a gradual increase in the discharge rate of the subsidiary pacemaker. The higher the overdrive rate, or the longer the duration of overdrive, the greater the enhancement of pump activity, so that the period of quiescence following the cessation of overdrive is directly related to the rate and duration of overdrive.[72]

The sinus node itself also can be overdrive suppressed if it is driven at a rate more rapid than its intrinsic rate. Thus, there may be a quiescent period after termination of either overdrive pacing or a rapid ectopic arrhythmia before the sinus rhythm resumes.[79–82] When overdrive suppression of the normal sinus node occurs, however, it is of lesser magnitude than that of subsidiary pacemakers overdriven at comparable rates.[29,79] The sinus node action potential upstroke is largely dependent on slow inward current carried by Ca^{2+} through the L-type Ca^{2+} channels, and far less Na^+ enters the fiber during the upstroke than in latent pacemaker cells such as Purkinje fibers. As a result, the activity of the Na^+ pump is probably not increased to the same extent in sinus node cells after a period of overdrive, and therefore, there is less overdrive suppression caused by enhanced Na^+ pump current. The relative resistance of the normal sinus node to overdrive suppression may be important in enabling it to remain as the dominant pacemaker even when its rhythm is transiently perturbed by external influences (such as transient shifts of the pacemaker to an ectopic site). The diseased sinus node, however, may be much more easily overdrive suppressed.[83]

There is an important distinction between the effects of the dominant sinus pacemaker on the two kinds of automaticity, as abnormal automaticity is not overdrive suppressed to the same extent as the normal automaticity that occurs at high levels of membrane potential.[84–86] The amount of suppression of spontaneous diastolic depolarization causing abnormal automaticity by overdrive is directly related to the level of membrane potential at which the automatic rhythm occurs.[85,86] For example, Purkinje fibers showing automaticity at moderately depolarized membrane potentials of −60 to −70 mV still manifest some overdrive suppression, although less than those fibers with automaticity at −90 mV. Automaticity in Purkinje fibers with membrane potentials less than −60 mV is only slightly suppressed by overdrive, if at all. These differences in the effects of overdrive may be related to the reduction in the amount of Na^+ entering the cell as membrane potential decreases, as we described for overdrive of the sinus node. At low levels of membrane potential, Na^+ channels are inactivated, decreasing the fast inward Na^+ current, and therefore, there is a reduction in the amount of Na^+ entering the cells during overdrive and the degree of stimulation of the sodium-potassium pump.[87]

In addition to overdrive suppression being of paramount importance for maintenance of normal rhythm, the characteristic response of automatic pacemakers to overdrive, as discussed in the previous paragraphs, is often useful for identifying mechanisms of arrhythmias in the in situ heart, where arrhythmia mechanisms cannot usually be identified by recording transmembrane potentials because of the technical difficulties. Not all mechanisms of arrhythmogenesis respond in the same way to overdrive as automatic pacemakers, and the differences in response can sometimes be used to distinguish among mechanisms. These differences are described in detail later in this chapter.

In addition to overdrive suppression, another mechanism that may suppress subsidiary pacemakers is the electrotonic interaction between the pacemaker cells and nonpacemaker cells in the surrounding myocardium.[88] This mechanism may be particularly important in preventing AV nodal automaticity[89,90] or automaticity in the distal Purkinje system where the pacemaking Purkinje fibers are in contact with nonpacemaking working ventricular muscle.[88,91,92]

Arrhythmias Caused by Automaticity Arrhythmias caused by either normal or abnormal automaticity of cardiac fibers may occur for several different reasons. Such arrhythmias might result simply from an alteration in the rate of impulse initiation by the normal sinus node pacemaker without a shift of impulse origin to a subsidiary pacemaker at an ectopic site. Sinus bradycardia and tachycardia are such arrhythmias. The cellular mechanisms that can change the rate of impulse initiation in the sinus node are described in Fig. 35-6. During alterations in sinus rate, there may be shifts of the pacemaker site within the sinus node.[22,93]

A shift in the site of impulse initiation to one of the regions where either normal or abnormal subsidiary pacemakers are located also results in arrhythmias. This would be expected to happen when any of the following occurs: (a) the rate at which the sinus node activates subsidiary pacemakers falls considerably below the intrinsic rate of the subsidiary pacemakers; (b) inhibitory electrotonic influences between nonpacemaker and pacemaker cells are interrupted; or (c) impulse initiation in subsidiary pacemakers is enhanced.

The rate at which the sinus node activates subsidiary pacemakers may be decreased in a number of situations. Impulse initiation by the sinus node may be slowed or inhibited altogether by heightened activity in the parasympathetic nervous system[94] or as a result of sinus node disease.[95] Alternatively, there may be block of impulse conduction from the sinus node to the atria or block of conduction from the atria to the ventricles. A latent pacemaker might also be protected from being overdriven by the sinus node if it is surrounded by a region in which impulses of sinus origin block (entrance block) prior to reaching the pacemaker cells. Such block, however, must be unidirectional so that activity from the pacemaker can propagate into surrounding myocardium whenever the surrounding regions are excitable. Some possible mechanisms for unidirectional block are discussed later in this chapter. The protected pacemaker is said to be a parasystolic focus.[96] In general, under these conditions such a protected focus of automaticity can fire at its own intrinsic frequency. Electronic current flow from surrounding regions may also influence the cycle length of a protected focus, either prolonging or abbreviating it, depending on whether the surrounding activity occurs during the early or late stage of diastolic depolarization.[97–99] Under any of the above conditions (sinus slowing, sinoatrial or AV block, parasystolic focus) there may be "escape" of a subsidiary pacemaker.

There is a natural hierarchy of intrinsic rates of subsidiary pacemakers having normal automaticity, with atrial pacemakers having faster intrinsic rates than AV junctional pacemakers, and AV junctional pacemakers having faster rates than ventricular pacemakers.[44,73] Once overdrive suppression is removed by sinus node inhibition, the pacemaker with the fastest rate becomes the site of impulse origin.[73] Sometimes mechanisms that are responsible for the suppression of impulse initiation in the sinus node also suppress pacemaker activity in the atria. The most prevalent atrial pacemaker site in experimental studies in which the sinus node is damaged or removed is at the junction of the inferior vena cava and posterior wall of the right atrium.[29,100–102] These atrial pacemakers may cause atrial arrhythmias if the sinus node or its arterial supply is damaged.[103]

Ectopic impulse initiation may occur in the AV junction. In fact, an AV junctional pacemaker may become the dominant rhythm in the absence of normal sinus node function. Atrioventricular junctional pacemakers may be located either in the AV node or His bundle. These different sites have somewhat different properties, including their intrinsic rate (faster in the node than in the His bundle) and response to autonomic nerve activity (parasympathetic activity suppresses AV nodal pacemakers to a greater extent than His bundle pacemakers). Atrioventricular junctional rhythms may occur during AV block, since the site of block is often proximal to the AV junctional pacemaker location.[37] If AV junctional pacemakers are also suppressed or if the site of disease causing AV block is in the His bundle or bundle branches, subsidiary pacemaker location is in the His-Purkinje system. The His bundle at the proximal end of the conducting system has a faster intrinsic rate than the more distally located Purkinje fibers.[44] The electrocardiogram (ECG) during idioventricular rhythm in patients with complete heart block is often characterized by a wide, aberrant QRS complex, suggesting impulse initiation in the distal Purkinje system.[104] In acute myocardial ischemia, particularly when occurring in the inferior wall, parasympathetic activity may be enhanced, depressing sinus rate or AV conduction or both.[105] Ectopic impulse initiation then may arise in the ventricular specialized conducting system.[106]

Any event which decreases intercellular coupling between latent subsidiary pacemaker cells and surrounding nonpacemaker cells may remove the inhibitory influence of electrotonic current flow on the latent pacemakers and allow them to fire at their intrinsic rate.[88] Coupling might be reduced by fibrosis which can separate myocardial fibers. For example, fibrosis in the atrial aspect of the AV junctional region that results in heart block might release nodal pacemakers from electrotonic suppression by surrounding atrial cells and permit them to become the dominant pacemakers driving the ventricles. Uncoupling might also be caused by factors that increase the intracellular Ca^{2+},[107] since elevated intracellular Ca^{2+} levels decrease coupling between myocardial cells. This might result, for example, from treatment with digitalis,[108] which inhibits Na^+ extrusion and thus increases Ca^{2+} levels in the cell.[109] In myocardial infarction, Purkinje fiber pacemakers may be uncoupled from damaged ventricular muscle cells, allowing the Purkinje fibers to fire at their normal intrinsic rates. Some inhibition of the sinus node is still necessary for the site of impulse initiation to shift to an ectopic site that is no longer inhibited because of uncoupling from surrounding cells, since, as explained above, the intrinsic firing rate of subsidiary pacemakers is still slower than the sinus node.

Subsidiary pacemaker activity also may be enhanced, causing impulse initiation to shift to ectopic sites even when sinus node function is normal. One cause may be enhanced sympathetic nerve activity. Norepinephrine released locally from sympathetic nerves steepens the slope of diastolic depolarization of latent pacemaker cells[22,32,33,110,111] and diminishes the inhibitory effects of overdrive.[112] The increase in slope of spontaneous diastolic depolarization may result from effects of norepinephrine on the i_f current, as described before, as well as from an increase in inward Ca^{2+} current in those cells in which this current participates in pacemaker activity. Localized effects on subsidiary pacemakers may occur in the absence of sinus node stimulation.[113] Therefore, sympathetic stimulation may enable membrane potential of ectopic pacemakers to reach threshold before they are activated by an impulse from the sinus node, resulting in ectopic premature impulses or automatic rhythms. There is evidence that in the subacute phase of myocardial ischemia, increased activity of the sympathetic nervous system may enhance automaticity of Purkinje fibers, enabling them to escape from sinus node domination.

Enhanced subsidiary pacemaker activity also may not require sympathetic stimulation. The flow of current between partially depolarized myocardium and normally polarized latent pacemaker cells might enhance automaticity.[114] This mechanism has been proposed to be a cause of some of the ectopic beats that arise at the borders of ischemic areas in the ventricle.[92] Inhibition of the electrogenic sodium-potassium pump results in a net increase in inward current during diastole because of the decrease in outward current normally generated by the pump and, therefore, may increase automaticity in subsidiary pacemakers sufficiently to cause arrhythmias. This might occur after adenosine triphosphate (ATP) is depleted during prolonged hypoxia or ischemia or in the presence of toxic amounts of digitalis.[115,116] A decrease in the extracellular potassium level also enhances normal automaticity,[74] as does acute stretch.[117] Stretch can induce rapid automatic rates in Purkinje fibers with normal maximum diastolic potentials.[118,119] Stretch of the ventricles can also induce arrhythmias in the intact heart,[120] although the site of origin of the ectopic impulses has not yet been localized. Stretch of the Purkinje system might occur in akinetic areas after acute ischemia or in ventricular aneurysms in hearts with healed infarcts.

At normal sinus rates, there may be little overdrive suppression of pacemakers with abnormal automaticity. As a result of the lack of overdrive suppression, even transient sinus pauses or occasional long sinus cycle lengths may permit an ectopic focus with a slower rate than the sinus node to capture the heart for one or more beats. On the other hand, ectopic pacemakers with normal automaticity would probably be quiescent during relatively short, transient sinus pauses because they are overdrive suppressed. It is also possible that the depolarized level of membrane potential at which abnormal automaticity occurs might cause entrance block into the focus and prevent it from being overdriven by the sinus node, even when impulses initiated in the focus could leave it (unidirectional block).[121] This would lead to parasystole, an example of an arrhythmia caused by a combination of an abnormality of impulse conduction and initiation. All these features of abnormal automaticity are evident in the Purkinje fibers that survive in regions of transmural myocardial infarction and cause ventricular arrhythmias during the subacute phase.[67]

The firing rate of an abnormally automatic focus might also be enhanced above that of the sinus node, leading to arrhythmias in the absence of sinus node suppression or conduction block between the focus and surrounding myocardium. The automatic rate is a direct function of the level of membrane potential—the greater the depolarization, the faster the rate.[4,54,56,122,123] Experimental studies have shown firing rates in muscle and Purkinje fibers of 150 to 200 per minute at membrane potentials less than -50 mV, and these rates should be sufficiently rapid to enable these pacemakers sometimes to control the rhythm of the heart. Catecholamines also increase the rate of firing caused by abnormal automaticity[124] and, therefore, may contribute to a shift in the pacemaker site from the sinus node to a region with abnormal automaticity. Among those clinical arrhythmias that are likely to be caused by abnormal automaticity is accelerated idioventricular rhythm after myocardial infarction. (See also Chap. 60.)

Triggered Activity

Triggered activity is a term used to describe impulse initiation in cardiac fibers that is dependent on afterdepolarizations.[125–127] Afterdepolarizations are oscillations in membrane potential that follow the upstroke of an action potential. There are two kinds of afterdepolarizations that may cause triggered activity. One occurs early, i.e., during repolarization of the action potential (EADs), and the other is delayed until repolarization is complete or nearly complete (DADs). When either kind of afterdepolarization is large enough to reach the threshold potential for activation of a regenerative inward current, action potentials result that are referred to as "triggered." Therefore, a key characteristic of triggered activity, discriminating it from automaticity, is that for triggered activity to occur, at least one action potential must precede it (the trigger). Automatic rhythms can arise de novo in the absence of any prior electrical activity, such as following long periods of quiescence, whereas triggered activity cannot.[4,127]

Triggered activity will cause arrhythmias when the site of impulse initiation shifts from the sinus node to the triggered focus. In order for this to occur, the rate of triggered impulses should be faster than the sinus rate, either transiently or persistently. This might result when firing of the sinus node is slowed or inhibited, when there is block of sinus impulses, or when the rate of triggered activity is faster than normal sinus node impulse initiation. The factors causing the shift in the site of impulse initiation should be very similar to those we described in our discussion of automaticity.

Delayed Afterdepolarizations and Triggered Activity Figure 35-10 shows an example of a DAD recorded with a microelectrode in a superfused preparation of atrial muscle exposed to catecholamines. The DAD is an oscillation in membrane potential that occurs after repolarization of the action potential (indicated in the figure by the unfilled arrow). The DAD is caused by events occurring during the action potential that will be described later. Figure 35-10*A* also shows that a DAD may be preceded by an afterhyperpolarization (black arrow), in which case the membrane potential transiently becomes more negative after the action potential than it was just before it. Afterhyperpolarizations, however, do not always precede DADs. The transient nature of the DAD clearly distinguishes it from normal spontaneous diastolic (pacemaker) depolarization, during which the membrane potential declines almost monotonically until the next action potential occurs (compare Fig. 35-10*A* with Fig. 35-6).

In addition to microelectrode recordings such as the one shown in Fig. 35-10*A*, DADs can also be identified using techniques for recording extracellular potentials.[128,129] A major problem that exists when this technique is used in situ to locate DADs in the heart, however, is discriminating the extracellular voltage deflections caused by afterdepolarizations from deflections that are a result of the motion of the heart, since movement alone can mimic DADs in extracellular recordings.[130] A second important problem is a possible difficulty in locating focal sites at which afterdepolarizations and triggered activity may be originating. Nevertheless, extracellular electrodes have been used to demonstrate what appear to be DADs occurring in the in situ heart.[131,132]

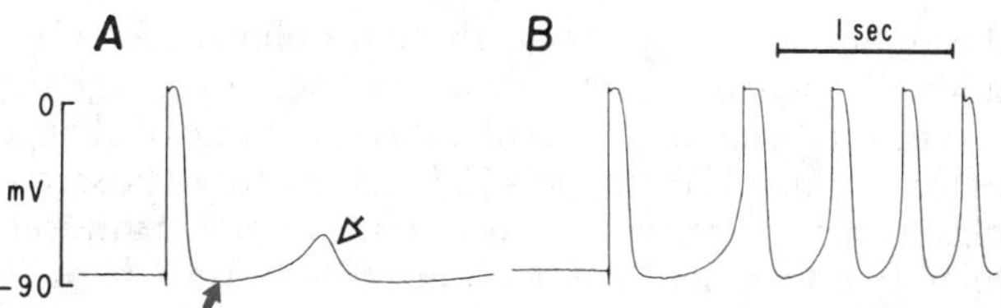

FIGURE 35-10 An example of a DAD (white arrow) recorded with a microelectrode from an atrial fiber in the canine coronary sinus. The black arrow indicates an afterhyperpolarization. *B.* The onset of triggered activity is shown. [*From Wit AL, Rosen MR: In: McFarlane PW, Veitch Lawrie TD (eds): Comprehensive Electrocardiology. Theory and Practice in Health and Disease, vol 2. New York, Pergamon, 1989: 801–841. Reproduced with permission from the publisher and author.*]

A triggered impulse is initiated when a DAD depolarizes the membrane potential to the threshold potential for activation of the inward current responsible for the upstroke of the action potential. Triggered impulses are shown in Fig. 35-10*B*. Afterdepolarizations do not always reach threshold, so that triggerable fibers may sometimes be stimulated at a regular rate without becoming rhythmically active, e.g., the stimulated action potential in Fig. 35-10*A*. Probably the most important influence that causes subthreshold DADs to reach threshold is a decrease in the cycle length (an increase in the rate) at which action potentials occur. Therefore, arrhythmias triggered by DADs can be expected to be initiated by either a spontaneous or a pacing-induced increase in the heart rate.

A triggered action potential is also followed by an afterdepolarization that may or may not reach threshold. When it does not reach threshold, only one triggered action impulse occurs. Quite often, the first triggered action potential is followed by a short or long "train" of additional triggered action potentials, each arising from the afterdepolarization caused by the previous action potential (Fig. 35-10*B*). The merging of the rising phase of the afterdepolarization with the upstroke of the action potential during triggered activity may be smooth, and as a result, the fiber may show phase 4 depolarization that is indistinguishable from the phase 4 depolarization seen during automatic activity.

Causes of Delayed Afterdepolarizations and Triggered Activity Delayed afterdepolarizations usually occur under a variety of conditions in which there is an increase in Ca^{2+} in the myoplasm and the sarcoplasmic reticulum above normal levels (sometimes referred to as *Ca overload*). Abnormalities in the sequestration and release of Ca^{2+} by the sarcoplasmic reticulum also may contribute to their occurrence. On depolarization of the membrane during an action potential, the intracellular free Ca^{2+} normally increases, primarily by Ca^{2+} influx through the L-type Ca^{2+} channels. Initially, this rapid rate of change of intracellular Ca^{2+} triggers Ca^{2+} release from the sarcoplasmic reticulum, which causes a further rise in intracellular free Ca^{2+} and contraction.[133] (See also Chaps. 5 and 34.) Repolarization then induces synchronous Ca^{2+} uptake by the sarcoplasmic reticulum in the cell and relaxation. If intracellular Ca^{2+} is very high or if catecholamines or cyclic adenosine monophosphate (AMP) are present, both of which enhance Ca^{2+} uptake by the sarcoplasmic reticulum, the Ca^{2+} in the sarcoplasmic reticulum may rise during repolarization to a critical level, at which a secondary spontaneous and synchronous release of Ca^{2+} from the sarcoplasmic reticulum occurs after the action potential and relaxation of contraction.[133] This secondary release of Ca^{2+} generates an aftercontraction as well as the transient inward (TI) current and the afterdepolarization. The TI current is an oscillatory membrane current that is distinct from the pacemaker currents.[134–141] After one or several afterdepolarizations, myoplasmic Ca^{2+} may decrease because Na^+-Ca^{2+} exchange extrudes Ca^{2+} from the cell, and membrane potential stops oscillating.

The exact mechanism by which the secondary rise in myoplasmic Ca^{2+} after repolarization causes the TI current is unclear and is still a source of controversy. Two possibilities are being actively considered. The first is that the Ca^{2+} released from the sarcoplasmic reticulum after repolarization acts on the sarcolemma to increase its conductance to ions (mainly Na^+) that flow into the cell down a concentration gradient through membrane channels. The second mechanism proposed for the origin of the TI current is that the rise in Ca^{2+} causes the TI current through an electrogenic (rheogenic) exchange of Ca^{2+} for Na^+. According to this hypothesis, the transient rise in myoplasmic Ca^{2+} that is released from the sarcoplasmic reticulum after the action potential is expected to result in "transport" of Ca^{2+} out of the cell across the sarcolemma by the Na^+-Ca^{2+} exchanger. Such an efflux is coupled to a Na^+ influx. If more than two Na^+ ions are exchanged for each Ca^{2+} ion, a net inward current occurs.[142–144]

The most widely recognized cause of DAD-dependent triggered activity is digitalis toxicity.[115,116,145–150] Afterdepolarizations caused by digitalis may sometimes reach threshold to cause triggered action potentials, particularly if the rate of stimulation is sufficiently rapid. Ventricular arrhythmias (repetitive responses) caused by digitalis in the heart in situ can also be initiated by pacing at rapid rates.[151] As toxicity progresses, the duration of the trains of repetitive responses induced by pacing increases.[152–154] We assume that these arrhythmias are caused by DADs. In addition, spontaneously occurring accelerated ventricular rhythms and ventricular tachycardia that occur during digitalis toxicity are likely to be caused by DADs.

Cardiac glycosides cause DADs by inhibiting the Na^+-K^+ pump. In toxic amounts, this effect results in a measurable increase in intracellular Na^+.[155,156] An increase in intracellular Na^+ in turn causes an increase in intracellular Ca^{2+}.[157] When intracellular Na^+ is increased, the concentration-dependent driving force for Na^+ across the sarcolemma is decreased, which in turn, diminishes Ca^{2+} extrusion from the cell by Na^+-Ca^{2+} exchange. Hence, there is a net inward Ca^{2+} movement.[43,158,159]

Catecholamines are probably the next most widely recognized cause of DADs. Delayed afterdepolarizations and triggered activity caused by catecholamines have been recorded with microelectrodes in atrial fibers of the mitral valve,[160] atrial fibers lining the coronary sinus,[32] atrial fibers in the inferior right atrium,[30] and atrial fibers from hearts with cardiomyopathy.[161] The DADs in Fig. 35-10 were caused by catecholamines in atrial fibers of the canine coronary sinus. Infusion of catecholamines through a catheter into the coronary sinus in the dog causes atrial tachycardia that has all the characteristics of triggered activity,[162] and therefore, some naturally occurring atrial tachycardias caused by triggered activity are probably induced by the sympathetic nervous system. Ventricular muscle and Purkinje fibers can also develop DADs in the presence of catecholamines.[163,164] Sympathetic stimulation may therefore also cause triggered ventricular arrhythmias, possibly some of the ventricular arrhythmias that accompany exercise[165] and some ventricular arrhythmias during ischemia and infarction.[166,167]

Catecholamines may cause DADs by increasing the slow inward L-type Ca^{2+} current through stimulation of beta-adrenergic receptors.[168,169] The net effect is an increase in trans-sarcolemmal Ca^{2+} entry into cardiac cells. In addition to increasing the inward Ca^{2+} current, catecholamines enhance uptake of Ca^{2+} by the sarcoplasmic reticulum leading to increased Ca^{2+} stored in the sarcoplasmic reticulum and the subsequent release of an increased amount of Ca^{2+} from the sarcoplasmic reticulum during the twitch.[133,170,171] The increased Ca^{2+} in the sarcoplasmic reticulum induced by catecholamines also may lead to the occurrence of DADs.

Delayed afterdepolarizations and triggered activity may also occur in the absence of pharmacologic agents, catecholamines, or an increase in extracellular Ca^{2+}. Triggerable fibers have been found in the upper pectinate muscles bordering the crista terminalis in the rabbit heart, in branches of the sinoatrial ring bundle or in transitional fibers between the ring bundle and ordinary pectinate muscle,[172] in apparently normal fibers in human atrial myocardium,[173] in human atrial fibers with very low membrane potentials (below −60 mV) and slow response action potentials,[69,70,173] in rat ventricular muscle that is hypertrophic secondary to renovascular hypertension (7.2 to 12.0 m*M*),[174] and in ventricular myocardium from diabetic rats.[175]

Properties of Delayed Afterdepolarizations The TI current that causes DADs is maximal at around −60 mV and diminishes at more positive and more negative membrane potentials.[137,139,176] As a result of the dependence of the TI current on the level of membrane potential, the amplitude of DADs and, therefore, the possibility of triggered activity are influenced by the level of membrane potential at which the action potentials occur. In the digitalis toxic Purkinje system, there is a "window" of membrane voltage for maximum diastolic potential, which is approximately between −75 and −80 mV, at which the amplitude of DADs tends to be greatest.[177,178] When DADs occur at the membrane potentials that favor a maximum amplitude, any intervention that hyperpolarizes or depolarizes the membrane tends to reduce their magnitude and to suppress any rhythms the afterdepolarizations might induce. Similarly, when there are no DADs in the presence of digitalis and the membrane potential is at a voltage less than or greater than the window, interventions that bring membrane potential into this voltage range often induce DADs. A similar dependence on membrane potential has been shown for DADs in atrial fibers of the coronary sinus[179] and in Purkinje fibers from infarcts.[180,181]

Delayed afterdepolarizations are influenced by the action potential duration, with longer action potential durations favoring the occurrence of DADs.[179] When action potential duration is longer, more Ca^{2+} is able to enter the cell. Drugs like quinidine, which prolong action potential duration, may increase DAD amplitude,[182] while drugs like lidocaine, which shorten action potential duration, may decrease DAD amplitude.[183]

The amplitude of DADs is dependent on the number of action potentials that precede them; i.e., after a period of quiescence, the initiation of a single action potential may be followed by either no afterdepolarization or only a small one. With continued stimulation, the afterdepolarizations increase in amplitude, and triggered activity may eventually occur.[32,116,146,160,184] The amplitude of DADs and their coupling interval to the previous action potentials are also dependent upon the cycle length at which action potentials are occurring, and triggered activity can be induced by a critical decrease in the drive cycle length.[116,146,160,167,172,174,175] This is illustrated by the effects of the stimulus cycle length on the amplitude of DADs recorded from an atrial fiber in the canine coronary sinus, shown in Fig. 35-11. The transmembrane potentials at the left were recorded when the stimulus cycle length was 2000 ms; the afterdepolarization amplitude following the last stimulated impulse is 5 mV. In the center, the stimulus cycle length was 1500 ms, and afterdepolarization amplitude after the last stimulated impulse is 15 mV. At the right, at a stimulus cycle length of 1200 ms, afterdepolarization amplitude reached 20 mV after the third stimulated action potential before triggered activity was initiated. Digitalis-induced DADs occur either singly or as two or more "damped" oscillations following the action potential.[116,146] When two or more afterdepolarizations are present, their relationship to the drive cycle length is complex. As drive cycle length decreases, the amplitude of the first afterdepolarization increases, reaching a peak at a cycle length of about 500 ms, and triggered activity may occur. If it does not, at shorter drive cycle lengths the magnitude of this first afterdepolarization decreases. The second DAD, however, continues to increase in magnitude as drive cycle length shortens further and may eventually reach threshold and induce triggered activity.

A decrease in the length of even a single drive cycle (i.e., a premature impulse) also results in an increase in the amplitude of the DAD that follows the premature cycle. The premature coupling interval at which triggered activity occurs is also dependent on the basic drive cycle length. As the basic drive cycle length decreases, the premature coupling interval needed to induce triggered activity increases.[185]

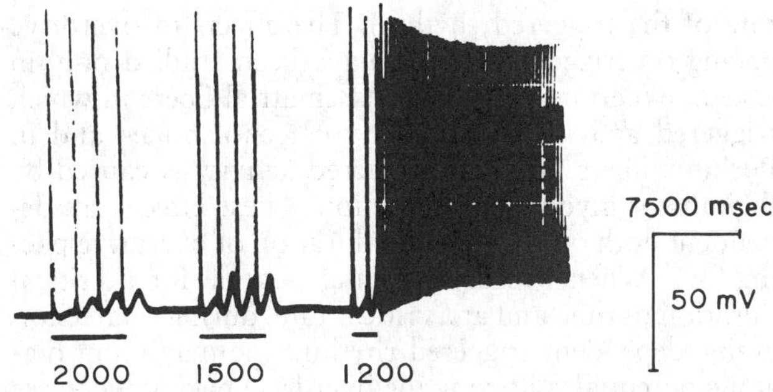

FIGURE 35-11 Effects of stimulation rate on DADs and triggered activity. Transmembrane action potentials were recorded from an atrial fiber in the canine coronary sinus superfused with Tyrode's solution containing norepinephrine. The stimulus cycle lengths and the periods of stimulation are indicated by the black bars. Sustained triggered activity occurred following stimulation at a cycle length of 1200 ms. The rate of triggered activity is so rapid that the individual action potentials cannot be seen at the slow oscilloscopic sweep speed. (*From Wit AL, Cranefield PF: Triggered and automatic activity in the canine coronary sinus. Circ Res 41:435, 1977. Reproduced with permission from the publisher and author.*)

Decreasing the drive cycle length, in addition to increasing amplitude, also tends to decrease the coupling interval of DADs to the action potential upstroke or terminal phase of repolarization by increasing the rate of depolarization of the afterdepolarization.[32,116,146,172] As a result, there is a direct relationship between the drive cycle length at which triggered impulses are initiated and the coupling interval between the first triggered impulse and the last stimulated impulse that induced them; i.e., as the drive cycle length is reduced, the first triggered impulse occurs earlier with respect to the last driven action potential. This characteristic property forms the basis for one of the indirect ways that triggered activity induced by a decrease in the drive cycle length in the whole heart is sometimes distinguishable from reentrant activity induced by a decrease in the drive cycle length, since the relationship for reentrant impulses initiated by rapid stimulation is often the opposite; i.e., as drive cycle length is reduced, the first reentrant impulse occurs later with respect to the last driven action potential (described in more detail later in the chapter). The increased time during which the membrane is in the depolarized state at shorter stimulation cycle lengths or after premature impulses increases Ca^{2+} in the myoplasm and the sarcoplasmic reticulum, thereby increasing the TI current responsible for the increased afterdepolarization amplitude and causing the current to reach its maximum amplitude more rapidly, decreasing the coupling interval of triggered impulses. The repetitive depolarizations can increase intracellular Ca^{2+} because of repeated activation of the inward Ca^{2+} current that flows through L-type Ca^{2+} channels.

We have discussed how triggered activity caused by DADs is initiated by stimulation. These characteristics may be of use in identifying triggered activity in the in situ heart (described later). Also of importance in identifying triggered arrhythmias in situ are the effects of electrical stimulation on established triggered activity.

In general, triggered activity is markedly influenced by overdrive pacing (i.e., pacing at a rate faster than the rate of the triggered rhythm). The effects of overdrive pacing on triggered activity have been studied only in several experimental situations: in atrial fibers in which triggered activity is caused by catecholamines and in Purkinje fibers in which triggered activity is caused by digitalis or myocardial infarction. These effects are dependent both on the rate and duration of overdrive pacing.[186,187] When overdrive pacing is done for a critical duration of time and at a critical rate, during a catecholamine-dependent triggered rhythm, the maximum diastolic potential following the overdrive pacing increases to levels more negative than before, and during the increase in membrane potential, the rate of triggered activity slows until the triggered rhythm stops. When triggered activity stops after a period of overdrive pacing at a moderate rate, some 10 to 50 impulses may occur after termination of the overdrive pacing before termination of the triggered activity occurs. The increase in maximum diastolic potential and the slowing and termination of triggered activity following a period of overdrive pacing are caused by an enhanced activity of the electrogenic Na^+ pump.[186] During a period of overdrive pacing, there is a transient increase in intracellular Na^+ because the increased number of action potentials stimulates the pump to generate increased outward current.[72,188]

In digitalis toxic Purkinje fibers, overdrive pacing can also terminate triggered activity, and this effect is dependent on the overdrive pacing cycle length but not on the overdrive pacing duration.[185,189] Termination occurs more frequently at more rapid overdrive pacing rates and may not be immediate; i.e., several triggered impulses may continue to occur after stimulation is stopped before triggered activity stops.[185] When overdrive pacing is not rapid enough to terminate the triggered rhythm, it can cause overdrive acceleration. Termination by overdrive pacing is not accompanied by hyperpolarization of the maximum diastolic potential and is probably not caused by increased Na-K pump activity, since the pump is partially inhibited by digitalis. The exact mechanism for termination has not been elucidated.

Premature stimuli may also terminate triggered rhythms, as shown in digitalis toxic Purkinje fibers,[185] Purkinje fibers in myocardial infarcts,[190] or atrial fibers exposed to catecholamines,[160,187] although termination is much less frequent than by overdrive pacing.[189] It has not been demonstrated that the premature impulse must occur at a critical point in the cycle length of triggered activity.

Early Afterdepolarizations and Triggered Activity Early afterdepolarizations are manifested as a sudden change in the time course of repolarization of an action potential such that membrane potential does not follow the trajectory characteristic of normal repolarization but suddenly shifts in a depolarizing direction. This is illustrated in the example of an EAD recorded with an intracellular microelectrode in a superfused Purkinje fiber shown in Fig. 35-12. The normal time course of repolarization of the action potential is shown in panel *A*. The arrow in panel *B* shows the deviation in membrane potential that constitutes the EAD. Early afterdepolarizations may appear at the plateau level of membrane potential, which is usually more positive than −60 mV, as in Fig. 35-12*B*, or they may appear later during phase 3 of repolarization. In Fig. 35-13*B*, trace 1 shows the normal time course of repolarization of a Purkinje fiber action potential, while trace 2 shows a deviation from this normal time course late during phase 3, which is the EAD. Early afterdepolarizations occurring late in repolarization occur at membrane potentials more negative than −60 mV in atrial, ventricular, or Purkinje cells that have normal resting potentials. Normally, a net outward membrane current shifts membrane potential progressively in a negative direction during repolarization of the action potential. An EAD occurs when, for some reason,

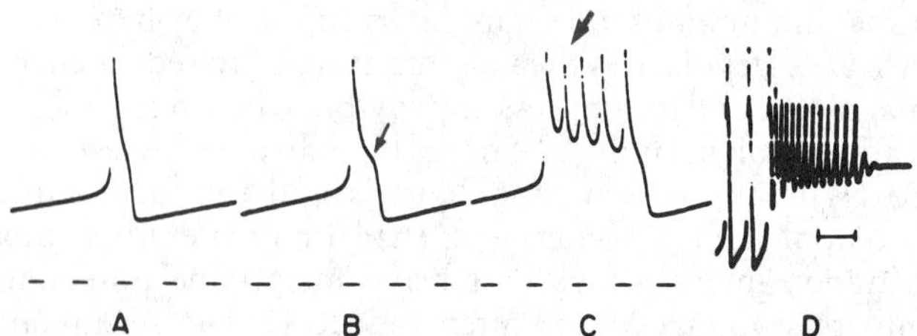

FIGURE 35-12 Early afterdepolarizations and triggered activity during repolarization in a Purkinje fiber. *A.* Transmembrane potential with normal repolarization of a spontaneously active Purkinje fiber. *B.* Early afterdepolarization (arrow) occurring during the plateau phase of the action potential. *C.* Triggered action potentials (arrow) during the plateau. *D.* Arrest of repolarization at a low level of membrane potential after a period of triggered activity. (*From Cranefield PF: Action potentials, afterpotentials and arrhythmias. Circ Res 41:415–425, 1977. Reproduced with permission from the publisher and author.*)

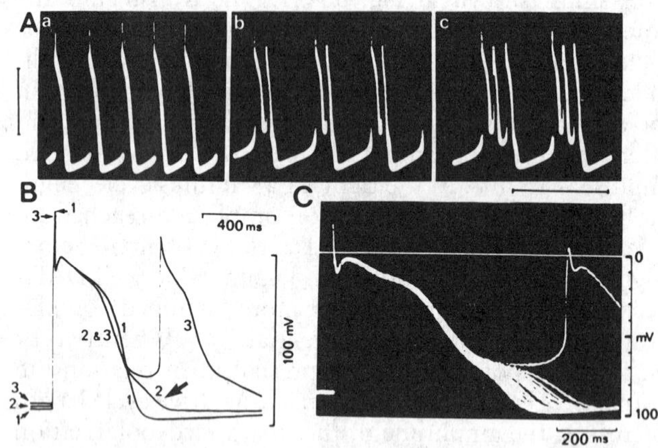

FIGURE 35-13 Early afterdepolarizations and triggered activity during late repolarization in a Purkinje fiber. *A.* Three panels are shown, *a, b,* and *c:* (*a*) a spontaneously firing Purkinje fiber with prominent phase 4 depolarization; (*b*) occurrence of a single triggered action potential caused by an EAD, occurring during repolarization of each spontaneous action potential; (*c*) occurrence of two triggered action potentials caused by an EAD, occurring during repolarization of each spontaneous action potential. *B.* Development of an EAD and a triggered action potential in three superimposed traces: (1) normal Purkinje fiber action potential; (2) alteration in the time course of late repolarization leading to the occurrence of an EAD (arrow); (3) further alteration in late repolarization, leading to a triggered action potential. *C.* Superimposed traces recorded from a Purkinje fiber in the course of developing EADs and a triggered action potential. [*From Coulombe et al: In Zipes DP, Jalife J (eds): Cardiac Electrophysiology and Arrhythmias. New York, Grune & Stratton, 1985: 43–49. Reproduced with permission from the publisher and author.*]

the current-voltage relationship is altered to cause outward current during repolarization to approach or attain 0, at least transiently. Such a shift can be caused by any factors that either decrease outward current, mostly carried by K^+, or increase inward current, carried by Na^+ or Ca^{2+}. If the change in the current-voltage relationship results in a region of net inward current during the plateau range of membrane potentials,[191] it could lead to a secondary depolarization (a triggered action potential) during the plateau or phase 3 by activating a regenerative inward current. Under certain conditions, EADs can lead to "second upstrokes"[4,126] or action potentials; when an EAD is large enough, the decrease in membrane potential leads to an increase in net inward (depolarizing) current, and a second action potential occurs prior to complete repolarization of the first, as shown in panel C (arrow) of Fig. 35-12 and by trace 3 in panel *B* of Fig. 35-13. The second action potential occurring during repolarization is triggered in the sense that it is evoked by an EAD, which in turn is induced by the preceding action potential. The second action potential may also be followed by other action potentials, all occurring at the low level of membrane potential characteristic of the plateau (Fig. 35-12C) or at the higher level of membrane potential of later phase 3 (Fig. 35-13, panels *Ab, Ac,* and *B*). Without the initiating action potential, there could be no triggered action potentials. The sustained rhythmic activity may continue for a variable number of impulses and terminates when repolarization of the initiating action potential returns membrane potential to a high level (Fig. 35-12C). As repolarization occurs, the rate of the triggered rhythm slows because the rate is dependent on the level of membrane potential in the same way as is abnormal automaticity. Sometimes repolarization to the high level of membrane potential may not occur, and membrane potential may remain at the plateau level or at a level intermediate between the plateau level and the resting potential[61] (Fig. 35-12*D*). The sustained rhythmic activity may then continue at the reduced level of membrane potential.[126]

The level of membrane potential at which the triggered action potentials occur determines both the rate of triggered activity and whether or not the triggered action potentials can propagate and excite adjacent normal regions.[192] At the more positive membrane potentials of the plateau, the rate of triggered activity is more rapid than later during phase 3. Triggered action potentials occurring at the plateau level have slow upstrokes, and therefore, conduction of these action potentials may sometimes block,[193,194] while the faster upstrokes of triggered action potentials occurring later during phase 3 enable them to propagate more easily. The ionic current responsible for the upstrokes of the action potentials during triggered activity caused by EADs is determined by the level of membrane potential at which the action potentials occur. Triggered action potentials occurring during the plateau phase and early during phase 3, at a time when most fast Na^+ channels are still inactivated, most likely have upstrokes caused by the inward L-type Ca^{2+} current.[4,195] At higher membrane potentials during late phase 3 of repolarization, where there is partial reactivation of the fast Na^+ channels, the upstrokes are caused by the fast inward Na^+ current. Current flowing through both L-type Ca^{2+} channels and partially reactivated fast Na^+ channels may be involved over intermediate ranges of membrane potential.

Causes of Early Afterdepolarizations and Triggered Activity Early afterdepolarizations and triggered activity have been produced in experimental studies under a variety of conditions, some of which would never be expected to be associated with naturally occurring arrhythmias in the in situ heart. Most of these conditions somehow delay repolarization of the action potential by increasing inward current or by decreasing outward current during the repolarization phases. Most often, EADs occur more readily in Purkinje fibers than in ventricular or atrial muscle.

Early afterdepolarizations may occur when the rate of stimulation is markedly slowed, reducing the outward current generated by the Na^+-K^+ pump, especially when K^+ in the extracellular environment is lower than normal, also reducing outward current.[127] At a "physiological range" of cycle lengths (a range that encompasses the normal sinus rhythm of the adult human heart, 1000 to 700 ms), EADs have rarely occurred in the studies on isolated preparations of cardiac fibers. As cycle length is increased and repolarization prolongs, EADs are more likely to occur.[196] The result is a bradycardia-induced tachycardia during which there may be very slow conduction. Another important characteristic is that the longer the basic drive cycle length, the greater the number of impulses that are triggered by EADs.[196]

Once EADs have achieved a steady-state magnitude at a constant drive cycle length, any event which shortens drive cycle length tends to reduce their amplitude.[196] Hence, initiation of a single premature depolarization, which is associated with an acceleration of repolarization, will reduce the magnitude of the EADs that accompany the premature action potential, and as a result, triggered activity is not expected to follow premature stimulation.

Polymorphic ventricular tachycardias that sometimes resemble torsades de pointes have been induced in dogs by infusing cesium, which blocks i_{K1} to cause EADs.[197] Occurrence of tachycardia is preceded by Q-T interval prolongation, a consequence of delayed repolarization, as is characteristically seen in patients with torsades de pointes.[198] The initial beat of the tachycardia caused by cesium often occurs during repolarization, i.e., during the T wave. Early afterdepolarizations and triggered activity have been seen in monophasic action potentials recorded from the ventricles in dogs with cesium-induced ventricular tachycardia.[199,200] Because the experimental arrhythmias caused by agents such as cesium, which are known to induce EADs, do resemble torsades de pointes, it has been proposed that clinically occurring torsades de pointes may sometimes be caused by EADs.

Other agents which can cause EADs and triggered activity are used therapeutically, and therefore, arrhythmias associated with their use may result from triggered activity. Antiarrhythmic drugs that prolong the duration of the action potential of Purkinje fibers (e.g., sotalol,[201,202] *N*-acetylprocainamide,[203] and quinidine[204,205] can cause EADs and triggered activity when administered to isolated preparations of Purkinje fibers, particularly when the rate of stimulation is low and the extracellular K^+ concentration is less than normal, e.g., <4 m*M*. The mechanisms by which these effects are exerted have been studied in detail for only some of these drugs. Both the d (no beta receptor blockade) and the l (beta blocking) forms of sotalol prolong the action potential duration by inhibiting the repolarizing K current, i_{K1}.[202] Similarly, the prolongation of the action potential by quinidine, which may lead to EADs, is related to quinidine's blocking effect on the outward membrane repolarizing K^+ current and not to quinidine's well-known blocking effect on the Na^+ channel.[206] It is known that quinidine may cause ventricular tachyarrhythmias in patients undergoing antiarrhythmic therapy with the drug. Interestingly, the arrhythmias may occur at low plasma quinidine concentrations that do not cause widening of the QRS complex in the ECG,[207] consistent with observations in superfused Purkinje fibers that afterdepolarizations due to quinidine occur without depression of the action potential upstroke. Hypokalemia and bradycardia both predispose to the occurrence of quinidine-induced torsades de pointes,[198,208] and both have been shown to potentiate induction of EADs in vitro by quinidine.[204,205] Torsades de pointes has also been associated with the administration to patients of *N*-acetylprocainamide[209] and sotalol.[210] Magnesium has been shown to abolish EAD-dependent triggered activity in experimental studies.[205,211] Magnesium also has been shown to provide effective therapy when used to treat some clinical cases of drug-induced torsades de pointes,[212,213] further evidence that this clinical arrhythmia may be a manifestation of triggered activity. (See also Chap. 36.)

Arrhythmias Caused by Reentry

Introduction

As discussed previously, the excitation wave front originating in the sinus node normally activates the cardiac tissues in an orderly sequence and then dies out. Thus, during normal sinus rhythm, each heart beat is generated by a new pacemaker impulse in the sinus node. There are, however, arrhythmias in which, in the presence of a requisite set of circumstances, an excitation wave front can continuously propagate and thereby continue to excite the heart because it always encounters excitable tissue. Such an arrhythmia is called reentrant.

Requisites for Reentrant Excitation

Perhaps the easiest way to illustrate this is to discuss again, but in more detail, the earliest description of reentrant excitation by Mayer[3] in 1906 in the excitable subumbrella ring of tissue of the scyphomedusae (the jellyfish) à la Fig. 35-4. This example well illustrates the requisites for reentrant excitation. First, a substrate must be present that would support reentrant excitation, in this case the subumbrella ring of excitable tissue of the jellyfish. Second, the excitation wave front must encounter unidirectional block (Fig. 35-4*B*). Unidirectional block must be present, or else the excitation wave fronts traveling around the ring will collide and extinguish each other (Fig. 35-4*A*). If the site of unidirectional block instead manifests bidirectional block, reentrant excitation also will not occur because the circulating excitation wave front will be unable to propagate through the area of block to reexcite the tissue initially excited.

Third, there must be a central area of block around which the reentrant excitation wave front can circulate. In this example, it was the hole in the center of the ring that clearly was inexcitable. Without a central area of block, the excitation wave front will not necessarily be limited to the outer ring of excitable tissue, but rather could take a short cut. This would permit the circulating excitation wave front to arrive quite early at the site where it originated, perhaps sufficiently early that the latter tissue will still be refractory. Reentrant excitation would not be possible. But even with the presence of a central area of block and without the presence of a short cut, the circulating wave front will only manifest reentrant excitation if the tissue it initially activated has had sufficient time to recover its excitability, i.e., to repolarize. Thus, conduction of the circulating excitation wave front must take long enough for this to happen, and there must always be a gap of excitable tissue (either fully or partially excitable) ahead of the circulating wave front (the so-called excitable gap). In the case of the subumbrella ring of excitable tissue of the jellyfish, conduction velocity was constant and the length of the ring long enough so that conduction time around the ring was longer than the effective refractory period of the excitable tissue comprising the ring, permitting reentry. Had the length of the ring been critically shorter or had conduction velocity been critically faster, the circulating excitation wave front would have arrived at the site of initial excitation before sufficient recovery of excitability had occurred, preventing reexcitation.

From these sorts of observations grew the concept of the wavelength of the circulating impulse.[214–216] The wavelength is the product of the conduction velocity of the circulating excitation wave front and the effective refractory period of the tissue in which the excitation wave front is propagating. Thus, the wavelength of the reentrant excitation wave front must be shorter than the length of the pathway of the potential reentrant circuit for reentrant excitation to occur. In the example of Mayer and the jellyfish ring experiment,[3] this was the case. For virtually all clinically important reentrant arrhythmias due to ordered reentry, however, in the presence of uniform conduction velocity along the reentrant pathway, the wavelength would be too long to permit reentrant excitation. Thus, virtually all these arrhythmias must have and, in fact, do have one or more areas of slow conduction as a part of the reentrant circuit. This permits the average wavelength of reentrant activation to be shorter than the path length. The fact that the reentrant circuit of virtually all clinically important reentrant arrhythmias has one or more areas of slow conduction serves to emphasize that the electrophysiological properties of the cardiac tissue comprising the reentrant circuit are not often uniform. In fact, there may be, and usually are, variations of conduction velocity and refractoriness along the course of the reentrant circuit.

An additional requisite for random reentry is the necessity of a critical mass of tissue in order to sustain the several simultaneously circulating reentrant excitation wavefronts.[217] Thus, it is essentially not possible to achieve sustained fibrillation of ventricles of very small normal mammalian hearts and equally difficult to achieve sustained fibrillation of the normal atria of humans or smaller mammals.

Finally, a usual requisite for reentrant excitation to occur is the presence of an initiating trigger. The trigger, usually the occurrence of one or more premature beats, frequently is required because it elicits or brings to a critical state one or more of the conditions necessary to achieve reentrant excitation. Thus, a premature impulse will arrive at one site in the potential reentrant circuit sufficiently early that it encounters unidirectional block because that tissue has had insufficient time following excitation by the prior beat to repolarize (Fig. 35-4). Furthermore, in the other limb of the potential reentrant circuit, the premature arrival of the excitation wave front at a site of slow conduction results in further slowing of conduction of the excitation wave front through the area of slow conduction. The resulting increase in conduction time around this limb of the potential reentrant circuit serves to allow the region of unidirectional block in the tissue in the other limb activated initially by the premature beat to recover excitability, i.e., to repolarize. Thus, when the circulating excitation wave front of the premature beat arrives at these tissue sites, the excitation wave front can reexcite the tissue, thereby manifesting reentrant excitation (Fig. 35-4). It should be noted that the mechanism of the premature beat may be different than the mechanism of the tachycardia. Thus, the premature beat may be an automatic or triggered beat or may be due to any mechanism. For instance, during cardiac catheterization, the premature beat may be due to the catheter forcefully hitting the heart wall, i.e., a mechanical cause.

The trigger to initiate reentrant excitation need not be a premature beat. The trigger to initiate reentrant excitation may be the normal sinus beat. One example is the rhythm known as permanent nonparoxysmal AV junctional reentrant tachycardia.[218,219] In this example, the potential reentrant circuit contains an area of permanent unidirectional block in an antegrade direction. Moreover, the potential reentrant circuit also has an area of very slow conduction, such that the wavelength of the propagating excitation wave front is shorter than the length of the potential reentrant circuit. In this circumstance, the normal sinus beat propagates around the reentrant circuit with sufficient delay that when it arrives in a retrograde direction at the area of permanent antegrade unidirectional block, the tissue at that site has recovered excitability. Furthermore, the conduction time around the reentrant circuit is such that the excitation wave front continually encounters excitable tissue in the direction in which it is propagating, resulting in continuous reentrant excitation and an incessant tachycardia. Another example is thought to be reentrant premature ventricular beats, e.g., as in ventricular bigeminy. (See also Chap. 36.)

Components of the Reentrant Circuit

The Substrate The cardiac tissue in which reentrant excitation can occur can be located almost anywhere in the heart. Furthermore, the reentrant circuit may consist of any number of shapes, sizes, and types of cardiac tissues. The reentrant circuit may be an anatomic structure, such as a loop of fibers in the Purkinje system.[220] The reentrant circuit may be a functionally rather than an anatomically defined pathway, with its existence, size, and shape determined by the electrophysiological properties of cardiac tissues in which the reentrant wave front circulates, such as has been shown in some models of atrial flutter.[221,222] Or it may be an anatomic-functional combination, as has been suggested for some intraatrial reentrant rhythms such as atrial flutter or ventricular tachycardia.

The Area(s) of Slow Conduction A condition necessary for reentry is that the impulse be delayed sufficiently in the alternate pathway(s) to allow elements proximal to the site of unidirectional block to recover from refractoriness. If reentry is to succeed, the impulse traveling around the reentrant circuit in one direction due to the unidirectional block must not return to this site of block before it and regions around it recover excitability. In the presence of normal conduction, sufficient time to accomplish repolarization might occur if the alternate pathway is long enough so that enough time can pass to allow recovery of excitability. Reentry is facilitated when conduction in all or a part of the alternate pathway is slow, since long pathways are then not necessary.

The area(s) of slow conduction may be an anatomic structure normally expected to manifest slow conduction, such as the AV node. Thus, the AV node is the area of slow conduction in AV reentrant tachycardia (a reentrant tachycardia in which the circuit involves the atria, the AV node, the His-Purkinje system, the ventricles, and an accessory AV connection). The area of slow conduction may be in cardiac tissue that normally does not manifest slow conduction. Such an area is not present during sinus rhythm (in contrast to the AV node) but is functionally present during the tachycardia. An example of a functionally determined area of slow conduction is found in the free wall of the right atrium of the canine sterile pericarditis model of atrial flutter.[222] Yet another example may be found in tissue that has been permanently damaged, as following a myocardial infarct. Such tissue normally would not manifest slow conduction but, following the injury, may remain an area of slow conduction even during sinus rhythm.[223] Slow conduction can be a consequence of active membrane properties determining the characteristics of inward currents depolarizing the membrane during the action potential, or it can be a consequence of passive properties governing the flow of current between cardiac cells.

Depression of Resting Membrane Potential An important feature of the transmembrane action potentials of atrial, ventricular, and Purkinje fibers that governs the speed of propagation is the magnitude of the inward Na^+ current flowing through the fast Na^+ channels in the sarcolemma during the upstroke. The magnitude of this current flow is reflected in the rate at which the cell depolarizes (V_{max} of phase 0).[224] The depolarization phase or upstroke of the action potential results from the opening of specific membrane channels (fast Na^+ channels) through which

Na^+ ions rapidly pass from the extracellular fluid into the cell.

During conduction of the impulse, the inward transmembrane Na^+ current flowing during the depolarization phase (phase 0) of the action potential results in the flow of axial current along the cardiac fiber through the cytoplasm and the gap junction of the intercalated disks connecting the cardiac cells. The current flows out of the cells through the membrane ahead as resistive and capacitive current. The conduction velocity depends both on how much capacitive current flows out of the cell at unexcited sites ahead of the propagating wave front and the distance at which the capacitive current can bring membrane potential to threshold. One important factor that influences the amount of current flowing through the sarcoplasm of a muscle fiber (axial current), and therefore capacitive current, is the amount of fast inward current causing the propagating action potential. A reduction in this inward current, leading to a reduction in the rate or amplitude of depolarization during phase 0, may decrease axial current flow, slow conduction, and lead to conduction block. Such a reduction may result from inactivation of Na^+ channels. The intensity of the inward Na^+ current depends on the fraction of Na^+ channels that open when the cell is excited and the size of the Na^+ electrochemical potential gradient (relative concentration of Na^+ in the extracellular space compared to Na^+ concentration inside the cell[225]). The fraction of Na^+ channels available for opening is determined largely by the level of membrane potential at which an action potential is initiated.[225] The Na^+ channels are inactivated either after the upstroke of an action potential or if the steady-state resting membrane potential is reduced. Immediately after the upstroke, cardiac fibers are inexcitable because of Na^+ channel inactivation at the positive level of membrane potential. During repolarization, progressive removal of inactivation allows increasingly large Na^+ currents to flow through the still partially inactivated Na^+ channels when the cells are excited. The inward Na^+ current, amplitude, and rate of rise of premature action potentials initiated during this relative refractory period is reduced because the Na^+ channels are only partly reactivated.[225] In Fig. 35-14*B*, premature action potentials a, b, and c have low amplitudes and slow rates of depolarization because they were initiated prior to full repolarization of the action potential. Hence, the conduction velocity of these premature action potentials is low. Premature activation of the heart may, therefore, induce reentry because premature impulses conduct slowly in regions of the heart where the cardiac fibers are not completely repolarized (where Na^+ channels are to some extent still inactivated).

Conduction slow enough to facilitate reentry might also occur in cardiac cells with persistently low levels of resting potential (which may be between −60 and −70 mV) caused by disease. At these resting potentials, about 50 percent of the Na^+ channels are inactivated,[225] and, therefore, are unavailable for activation by a depolarizing stimulus. Also, at these resting membrane potentials, recovery from inactivation is markedly prolonged and extends beyond complete repolarization.[226] The magnitude of the inward current during phase 0 of the action potential is reduced, and consequently, both the speed

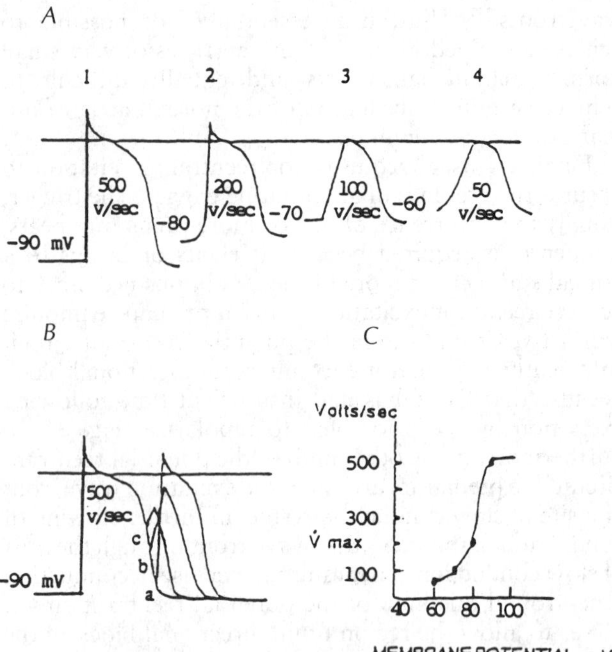

FIGURE 35-14 Diagrammatic representation of the relationship between the level of membrane potential at the onset of phase 0 and the maximum rate of depolarization during phase 0 (dv/dt_{max} or $\dot{V}_{max}$). *A.* Fiber has been depolarized by progressively increasing the extracellular potassium concentration. As resting membrane potential decreases, the rate of depolarization of the action potential upstroke decreases. *B.* Fiber is activated by premature stimuli that occur at different times during phase 3 (*a, b,* and *c*). The premature action potentials have reduced rates of depolarization because they arise at reduced membrane potentials. *C.* For both types of experiments the general relationship between $\dot{V}_{max}$ and membrane potential is shown.

and amplitude of the upstroke is diminished (Fig. 35-14*A*, action potentials 2, 3, and 4), decreasing axial current flow and slowing conduction significantly. Such action potentials with upstrokes dependent on inward current flowing via partially inactivated Na^+ channels are sometimes referred to as *depressed fast responses.* Further depolarization and inactivation of the Na^+ channel may decrease the excitability of cardiac fibers to such an extent that they may become a site of unidirectional conduction block.[227] Thus, in a diseased region with partially depolarized fibers, there may be some areas of slow conduction and some areas of conduction block, depending on the level of resting potential. This combination may cause reentry. The chance for reentry in such fibers is even greater during premature activation or during regular rhythms at a rapid rate because slow conduction or the possibility of block is increased even further, owing to the prolonged time for the channels to recover from inactivation.

After the upstroke of the normal action potential, membrane potential begins to return to the resting level because the Na^+ channels are inactivated and the fast (depolarizing) Na^+ current ceases to flow. This return, however, is slowed by a second inward current that is smaller and slower than the fast Na^+ current and probably is carried by both Na^+ and Ca^{2+} ions.[228] This secondary inward current flows through L-type Ca^{2+} channels that are distinct from the fast Na^+ channels.[19] The threshold for activation of the L-type Ca^{2+} current is in the range of −30 to −40 mV compared with about −70 mV for the fast Na^+ current. This current inactivates much more slowly than the fast Na^+ current and gradually diminishes as the cell repolarizes. Under special conditions, this Ca^{2+} current may also underlie the occurrence of the slow conduction that causes reentrant arrhythmias.[4] Although the fast Na^+ channel may be largely inactivated at membrane potentials near −50 mV, the L-type Ca^{2+} channel is not inactivated and is still available for activation.[4,228] Under certain conditions, in cells with resting potentials less than −60 mV (such as when membrane conductance is very low or when catecholamines are present), this normally weak inward Ca^{2+} current may give rise to regenerative action potentials that propagate very slowly and are prone to block. The propagated action potential, dependent on inward Ca^{2+} current, is referred to as the "slow response."[4] Slow response action potentials can occur in diseased cardiac fibers with low resting potentials, but they also occur in some normal tissue of the heart, such as cells of the sinus and AV nodes, where the maximum diastolic potential is normally less than about −70 mV.[4,229] In fact, slow conduction is a normal property of both the sinus and AV nodes. Thus, it should be of no surprise that either of these nodes may be a critical area of slow conduction in some reentrant circuits, e.g., the AV node in AV reentrant tachycardia involving an accessory AV connection.

Anisotropy The slow conduction that facilitates the occurrence of reentry can also be caused by factors other than a decrease in inward current during the transmembrane action potential. An increased resistance to axial current flow, which can be expressed as *effective axial resistance* (defined as resistance to current flow in the direction of propagation[230,231]) decreases the magnitude and spread of axial current along the myocardial fiber and may decrease conduction velocity. During conduction of the impulse, axial current flows from one myocardial cell to the adjacent cell through the gap junctions of the intercalated disks which form a major source of intracellular resistance to current flow along a fiber bundle.[224] Therefore, the structure of the myocardium which governs the extent and distribution of these gap junctions has a profound influence on axial resistance and conduction. This influence can be seen in normal atrial or ventricular myocardium. The atria and ventricles are composed of bundles of myocardial cells that have been called unit bundles by Sommer and Dolber.[232] Such bundles are comprised of 2 to 30 cells surrounded by a connective tissue sheath. Within a unit bundle, cells are tightly connected or coupled to each other through intercalated disks that contain the gap junctions. All the cells of a unit bundle are connected to each other within the space of 30 to 50 μm down the length of a strand.[232] An individual cardiac myocyte may be connected to as many as nine other myocytes through one or more intercalated disks.[233] These connections are mainly at the ends of the myocytes rather than along their sides, but the overlapping nature of the junctions effectively connects myocytes within a bundle in the transverse as well as the longitudinal direction. Therefore, as a consequence of the many intercellular connections, the myocytes in a unit bundle are activated uniformly and synchronously as an impulse propagates along the bundle. The unit bundles are also connected to each other. Unit bundles lying parallel to each other in normal atrial and ventricular muscle are connected in a lateral direction at intervals in the range of 100 to 150 μm.[232] As a consequence of this structure, the myocardium is better coupled in the direction of the long axis of its cells and bundles (because of the high frequency of the gap junctions within a unit bundle) than the direction transverse to the long axis (because of the low frequency of interconnections between the unit bundles). This is reflected in a lower axial resistivity in the longitudinal direction than in the transverse direction in cardiac tissues that are composed of many bundles.[234,235] As stated above, the effective axial resistivity is an important determinant of the conduction velocity, and therefore, conduction through atrial and ventricular myocardium is much more rapid in the longitudinal direction owing to the lower resistivity than in the transverse direction. Thus, cardiac muscle is anisotropic; its conduction properties vary depending on the direction in which they are measured. (See also Chap. 34.)

Spach et al.[230,231,236] have classified anisotropy into two major subdivisions: uniform and nonuniform. Uniform anisotropy is characterized by an advancing wave front that is smooth in all directions (longitudinal and transverse to fiber orientation), indicating relatively tight coupling between groups of fibers in all directions (although coupling is "tighter" in the longitudinal than in the transverse direction because of the myocardial structure discussed previously.[237] Uniform anisotropy is exemplified by the conduction properties of normal septal ventricular muscle shown in Fig. 35-15*A*. The muscle was stimulated in the center (pulse symbol), and activation spread away from this site in all directions, as indicated by the arrows. In the direction of the longitudinal axis of the fibers (along the length of the unit bundle) (from top to bottom) the activation isochrones are widely spaced, indicating rapid conduction, in this case 0.51 m/s. There is a relatively broad area of fast conduction with an elliptic shape of the isochrones that is characteristic of uniform anisotropy.[236] In the direction transverse to the long axis (between unit bundles) (to the right and to the left), the isochrones are spaced close together, indicating slower conduction, 0.17 m/s in this example. As the direction of propagation changes between these two axes, the apparent conduction velocity changes monotonically from fast to slow, another characteristic of uniform anisotropy.[230] The slow conduction in the direction transverse to the longitudinal fiber axis occurs despite action potentials with normal resting potentials and upstroke velocities. Associated with the differences in conduction velocity based on direction of propagation, however, are unexpected changes in the action potentials. Thus, when going from fast longitudinal conduction to slow transverse conduction, the rate of depolarization during the upstroke of the action potential (V_{max}) increases and the time constant of the foot of the upstroke decreases without any change in the resting potential, as shown in Fig. 35-15*C;* the upstroke that is dashed was recorded from a cell during longitudinal propagation, while the upstroke indicated by the solid line was recorded from the same

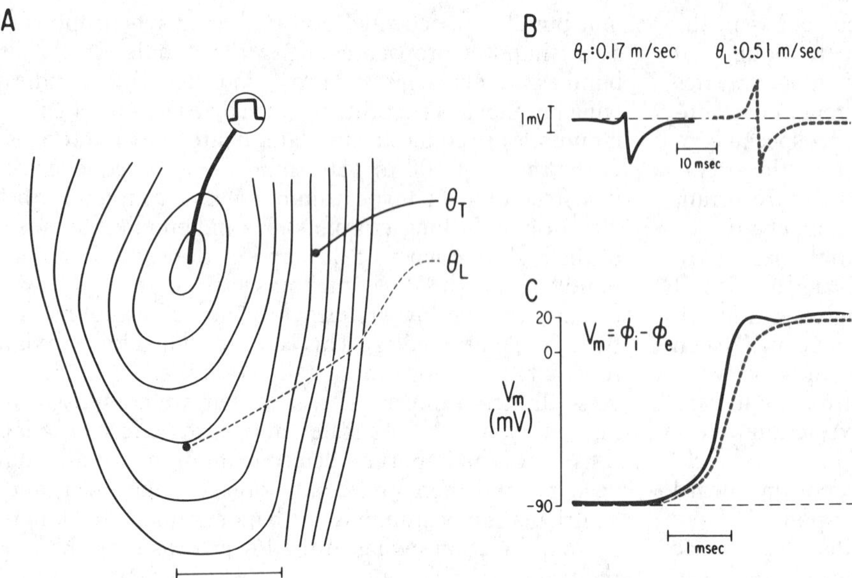

FIGURE 35-15 Relationship between the spread of excitation in uniform anisotropic ventricular muscle (*A*) and the extracellular (*B*) and the transmembrane potential waveforms (*C*). The excitation sequence in *A* was constructed from the extracellular waveforms measured at 100 positions on the endocardial surface of the right ventricular septum. The extracellular waveforms in *B* were measured at the sites indicated by the solid dots superimposed on the isochrones of *A*. The direction of propagation at the single transmembrane recording site was altered by initiating propagation at different locations, one to produce propagation along the longitudinal axis of the impaled fiber and the other to produce propagation along the transverse axis. Panel *C* shows the effects of the different directions of propagation on the upstroke of the action potential. [*From Spach MS, Dolber PC: In Zipes DP, Jalife J (eds): Cardiac Electrophysiology and Arrhythmias. New York, Grune & Stratton, 1985: 241–252. Reproduced with permission from the publisher and author.*]

cell during transverse propagation.[230] These characteristics are opposite to the changes in the action potentials associated with slowing of conduction when the membrane currents are altered (such as by membrane depolarization).[238,239] Despite the increase in V_{max}, when conduction is slowed in the transverse direction, the slowing of conduction is associated with a decrease in the amplitude of the extracellular electrogram, showing that there is a decrease in the extracellular current flow as a result of the increased axial resistivity. In uniformly anisotropic tissue, the extracellular unipolar waveform has a large-amplitude, smooth biphasic, positive-negative morphology during propagation in the fast longitudinal direction (Fig. 35-15*B*, dashed line) and a low-amplitude, smooth triphasic (negative-positive-negative) morphology in the transverse direction (Fig. 35-15*B*, solid line). The initial negativity of the electrogram in the transverse direction is a reflection of distant activity rapidly propagating along the longitudinal axis.[240]

Nonuniform anisotropy has been defined[231] as tight electrical coupling between cells in the longitudinal direction, but recurrent areas in the transverse direction in which side-to-side electrical coupling of adjacent groups (unit bundles) of parallel fibers is absent. Therefore, propagation of normal action potentials transverse to the long axis is interrupted such that adjacent bundles are excited in a markedly irregular sequence, or *zigzag conduction*.[231,236] In nonuniformly anisotropic muscle, there is also an abrupt transition in conduction velocity from the fast longitudinal direction to the slow transverse direction, unlike uniform anisotropic muscle, in which intermediate velocities occur between the two directions. This pattern of excitation in nonuniform anisotropic atrial pectinate bundles from older patients is diagrammed in Fig. 35-16*A*. The white arrow on the outline of the preparation indicates the narrow region of fast conduction down the long axis of the fibers when the bundle was excited at the asterisk. The zigzag arrow indicates the irregular course of excitation across the fibers, which occurred all along the length of the zone of fast conduction. Conduction in the transverse direction in these nonuniformly anisotropic bundles was nearly as slow as the slowest conduction associated with membrane depolarization and slow response action potentials.[4] In pectinate muscles from older patients, mean fast velocity was 0.69 m/s and slow velocity was 0.07 m/s, a ratio of almost 10,[236] despite the normal resting potential and the fast action potential upstroke of the atrial cells. As in uniform anisotropy, the upstroke velocity of the action potential is more rapid in the slow direction transverse to the long axis of the fibers than in the fast direction parallel to the long axis.

The morphologic basis for the nonuniform anisotropic properties in human atrial muscle is that the fascicles of muscle bundles are separated in the transverse direction by fibrous tissue that proliferates with aging to form longitudinally oriented insulting boundaries. Intercellular connections cannot occur where the cardiac fibers are separated by connective tissue septae and there is uncoupling between parallel oriented groups of fibers.[231,236] Part of the reduction of the conduction velocity in this transverse direction may be a result of the tortuous path length necessary for the wave front to propagate transversely from one bundle to another because of these septae, accounting for the zigzag activation pattern. Similar connective tissue septae cause nonuniform anisotropy in other normal cardiac tissues such as crista terminalis and the interatrial band in adult atria or ventricular papillary muscle as well as pathological situations in which fibrosis in the myocardium occurs (chronic ischemia). The irregular activation transversely is evident in the extracellular electrogram, which is characterized by a sequence of multiple deflections, each representing activation of a separate bundle of fibers, with the largest, most rapid intrinsic deflection produced by local excitation and less rapid and lower amplitude deflections produced by excitation of adjacent fascicles.[231] In Fig. 35-16*B*, the multiple deflections can be seen in electrograms recorded from sites 2 and 3 in the atrial pectinate muscle and are even more prominent in the derivatives

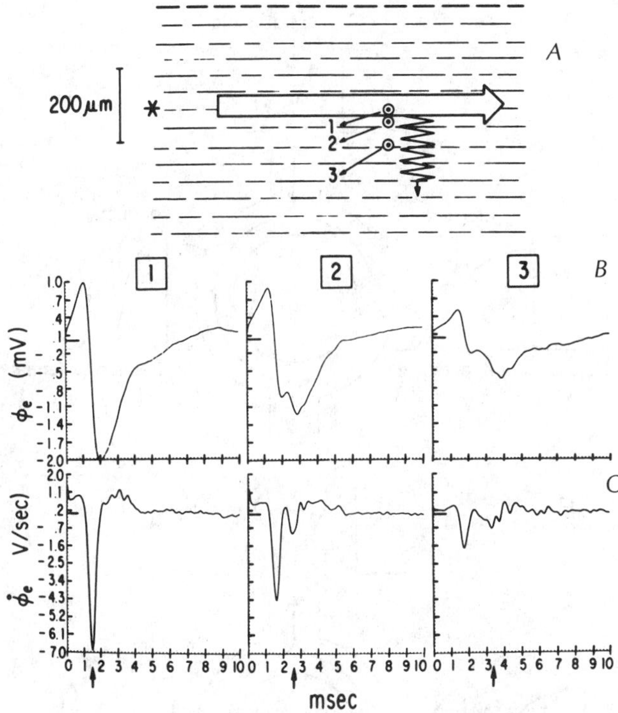

FIGURE 35-16 *A.* Diagram of a nonuniform anisotropic atrial muscle bundle with the long axis of the myocardial fibers indicated by the dashed lines. The bundle was stimulated at the asterisk. Propagation of the longitudinal wave front is shown by the large white arrow. Transverse propagation occurred as diagrammed by the "zigzag" arrow. *B.* Electrograms recorded from sites 1, 2, and 3 on the diagram. *C.* The first derivative of these electrograms is shown. (*From Spach MS, Dolber PC: Relating extracellular potentials and their derivatives to anisotropic propagation at a microscopic level in human cardiac muscle. Evidence for uncoupling of side-to-side fiber connections with increasing age. Circ Res 58:356, 1986. Reproduced with permission from the publisher and author.*)

of these electrograms (Fig. 35-16C). During longitudinal propagation, large biphasic electrograms are still evident (electrogram at site 1).

Anisotropy on a macroscopic scale can also influence conduction at sites where a bundle of cardiac fibers branches or where separate bundles coalesce. Marked slowing can occur when there is a sudden change in the fiber direction, causing an abrupt increase in the effective axial resistivity.[231] Figure 35-17 illustrates this point. The drawings show a small branch of an atrial pectinate muscle from the crista terminalis. The general direction of the fiber orientation is indicated by the thin broken lines and the pattern of propagation is illustrated by the thick solid lines with arrows. In *A*(1) at the left, wave fronts initiated by stimulation at the top propagate throughout the crista and its branch along the longitudinal axis of the fibers throughout so that there is no conduction delay entering the branch. At the right in *A*(2), wave fronts initiated by stimulation at the bottom propagate up the crista and into the branch, but they encounter a marked change in direction of the fibers from longitudinal to transverse while entering the branch, resulting in a slowing of conduction because of the sudden increase in axial resistance. Conduction block, which sometimes may be unidirectional, may occur at such junction sites, particularly when the inward current is decreased.

In addition to the structural features of the cellular interconnections influencing axial current flow and conduction as expressed in the anisotropic properties of cardiac muscle, the intercellular resistance may also increase because of an increase in gap junctional resistance that results from a decrease in the conductance of the junctions, i.e., a decrease of the ease with which the ions that carry axial current move through the junctions. In

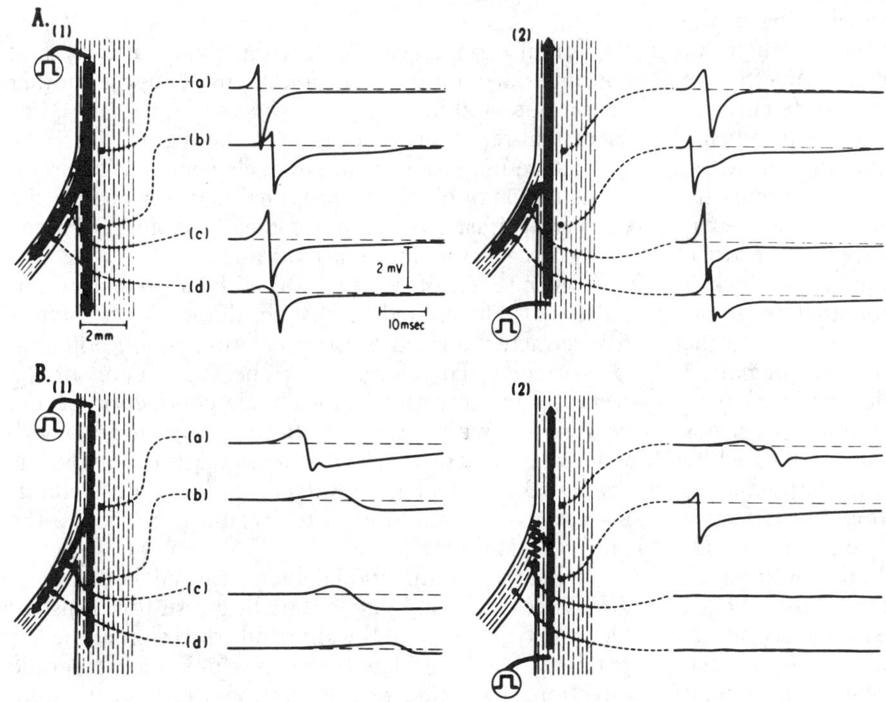

FIGURE 35-17 Conduction characteristics and unidirectional block at branch sites. The drawings represent a small branch formed by the origin of a pectinate muscle from the larger crista terminalis. The general direction of the fiber orientation is indicated by the broken lines. The patterns of propagation are shown by the solid arrows. Extracellular waveforms recorded at sites indicated by the dashed lines are also shown. (*From Spach MS et al: The functional role of structural complexities in the propagation of depolarization in the atrium of the dog: Cardiac conduction disturbances due to discontinuities of effective axial resistivity. Circ Res 50:175, 1982. Reproduced with permission from the publisher and authors.*)

a computer model, conduction velocity could be reduced by a factor of 20 by increasing disk resistance, and decremental conduction and block result.[241,242] Perhaps the most important influence on gap junctional resistance in pathological situations is the level of intracellular Ca^{2+}. A significant rise increases resistance to current flow through the junctions and eventually leads to physiological uncoupling of the cells.[243,244] Intracellular Ca^{2+} increases during ischemia and may be a factor causing slow conduction and reentry.

Thus, there are several causes for slow conduction that may lead to reentry: (1) slow responses that are a normal property of some regions of the heart such as the sinus and AV node; (2) depressed fast responses or slow responses caused by pathology-induced partial depolarization of the membrane potential; (3) anisotropy; and (4) changes in gap junctional resistance.

Unidirectional Block Unidirectional block occurs when an impulse cannot conduct in one direction along a bundle of cardiac fibers but can conduct in the opposite direction. This condition is necessary for the occurrence of classical reentrant rhythms. Thus, unidirectional block in part of the circuit leaves a return pathway through which the impulse conducts to reenter previously excited areas. There are a number of mechanisms that might cause unidirectional block. They involve both active and passive electrical properties of cardiac cells.

Regional Differences in Recovery of Excitability One cause of unidirectional block that enables the initiation of reentry is regional differences in recovery of excitability. When differences in the duration of the effective refractory period occur in adjacent areas, conduction of an appropriately timed premature impulse may be blocked in the region with the longest refractory period, which then becomes a site of unidirectional block, while conduction continues through regions with a shorter refractory period. Figure 35-18 is a schematic representation of the initiation and continuation of circus movement in an anatomically defined circuit, with differences in effective refractory period duration resulting from differences in the time course of action potential repolarization being the cause for unidirectional block in one of the pathways. The action potentials in various parts of the circuit are shown. In the upper panel (*A*), conduction of a premature impulse (which can be either induced by electrical stimulation or may occur "spontaneously") is blocked in the pathway with the long action potential durations and, therefore, long effective refractory periods (to the left), referred to as the blocked pathway. The premature impulse, however, conducts in the other pathway with shorter action potential durations and refractory periods (to the right). This pattern of activation is indicated by the arrows. In order for block to occur, the premature impulse must also arise in a region with a short effective refractory period so that it occurs before the action potentials in the left pathway repolarize. In the lower panel, which shows a continuation of these events, the blocked pathway is retrogradely invaded by the impulse conducting from the right to cause the second action potential (arrow at the left). The proximal region where the premature impulse originated is then reexcited (reentry), as

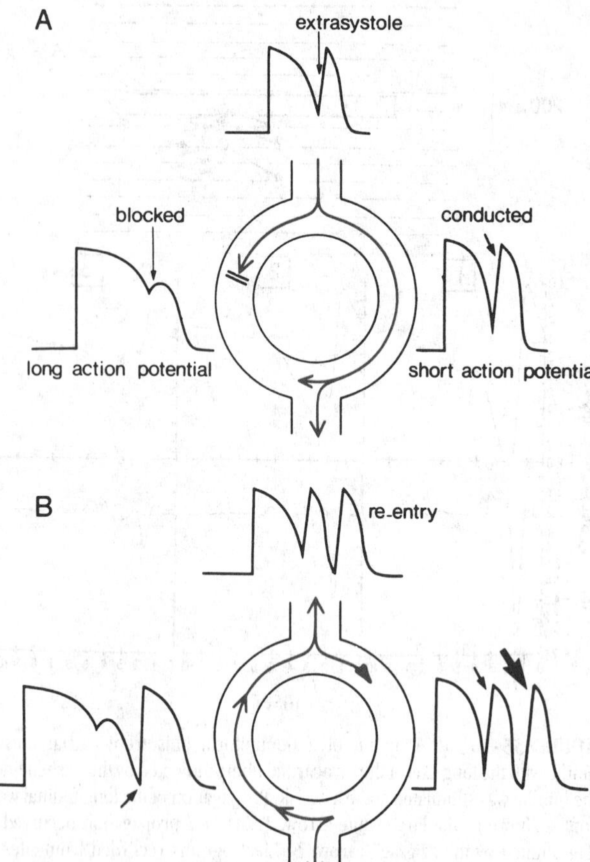

FIGURE 35-18 Diagram of reentry caused by dispersion in refractory periods. A ring of cardiac tissue is shown and the pattern of conduction is indicated by the arrows. Action potentials with different durations located in different regions of the ring are diagrammed. (*From Wit AL, Janse MJ: The Ventricular Arrhythmia of Ischemia and Infarction. The Electrophysiological Mechanisms. Mt Kisco, NY, Futura Publishing 1992. Reproduced with permission from the publisher and authors.*)

the impulse once again enters the right pathway and continues around the reentrant circuit, causing another action potential in the right pathway (large arrow). For successful reexcitation to occur in the region where the premature impulse was initiated, elements in the circuit at the region of block and proximal to it (toward the site of origin) must have regained their excitability by the time the cardiac impulse arrives there.

Continuation of reentry induced by a premature impulse is also facilitated because the duration of the effective refractory period of the premature action potential is shortened. Therefore, on the next excursion of the reentrant impulse around the circuit, conduction occurs in a circuit with a shorter effective refractory period. Finally, conduction velocity of premature impulses is decreased, shortening the wavelength[245,246] and facilitating successful excitation of the region proximal to the unidirectional block.

Therefore, unidirectional block caused by regional differences in excitability is actually a result of transient block. Block occurs in the antegrade direction in the left pathway while conduction is successful in the retrograde direction. This kind of unidirectional block can cause initiation of reentry not only in anatomic circuits, as shown in Fig. 35-18, but also in functional circuits. For reentrant arrhythmias to arise because of regional differences in effective refractory periods, a premature impulse that initiates reentry is as necessary a requirement as the conditions allowing perpetuation of reentrant activation. Thus, both a "trigger" (the premature impulse) and a "substrate" (the reentrant circuit) are needed. The mechanism causing the premature impulse may be quite different from the arrhythmia it initiates. It might arise spontaneously by automaticity or it might be a result of triggered activity. The premature impulse might also be induced by an electrical stimulus during a programmed stimulation protocol.

The degree of nonuniformity in effective refractory period duration necessary for a properly timed premature stimulus to cause reentry may be quite small. This degree of nonuniformity is often referred to as the dispersion in refractory periods or dispersion in recovery of excitability, meaning the difference between the shortest and longest refractory period. When stimuli were delivered at the border of two areas with different refractory periods in atrial tissue in the experiments of Allessie et al.,[247] the minimal difference in effective refractory period needed to cause block of an appropriately timed stimulated premature impulse was between 11 and 16 ms, well within the normal physiological range of variation of effective refractory period durations. A properly timed single premature stimulus can initiate reentry in the atria because the differences in refractory period may cause unidirectional block.[247] In the ventricles, where refractory periods are much longer than in the atria, the physiological differences between longest and shortest refractory period duration is on the order of 40 ms.[248,249] Unlike in the atria, dispersion of refractory periods in normal ventricles is not sufficiently large to allow initiation of reentry by premature impulses. When dispersion of refractory periods is increased by local cooling of the ventricles and a critical difference between shortest and longest effective refractory period ranging from 95 to 145 ms is reached, premature stimuli delivered at the site with the shortest effective refractory period can induce repetitive activity in the canine left ventricle, presumably because block of the premature impulses in the regions with a long effective refractory period creates unidirectional block and permits reentry.[250,251] Similarly, critical increases in the dispersion of refractory periods that are caused by acute or prolonged ischemia result in reentrant arrhythmias.

The difference between longest and shortest refractory period is not the only factor determining whether premature stimuli will induce reentry.[247] If the regions of long and short refractory periods are separated by a large distance, an early premature impulse arising in a region of short refractoriness may not be able to arrive in the region of long refractoriness sufficiently early to cause block because conduction between the regions may be slow. Regions of long and short refractory periods must, therefore, be relatively close to one another for block to occur. In addition, if block does occur, the size of the area of unidirectional block is of crucial importance. Even in the presence of large differences in effective refractory period duration, reentry may not occur when the area with long effective refractory periods is small, because the impulse traveling around the area of unidirectional block along alternate pathways will not be delayed sufficiently to reexcite the point of origin at the end of its effective refractory period. Thus, *dispersion in recovery of excitability* is in itself not a complete index for describing the propensity for induction of reentrant arrhythmias.

The regional differences in recovery of excitability that lead to unidirectional conduction block might also occur in the absence of regional differences in action potential duration. Computer models have shown that the activation sequence of a propagating impulse can lead to asynchronous repolarization and refractoriness even when membrane properties are homogeneous.[88,242] A stimulated premature impulse can block in a region that has been depolarized most recently by a prior wave of excitation and is therefore still refractory but may conduct into another region that was excited much earlier by the prior wave of excitation if it has had time to recover excitability. The conducting premature excitation wave then can later return to excite the area of block after it recovers, resulting in reentry.

Asymmetrical Depression of Excitability Unidirectional conduction block in a reentrant circuit can also be persistent and independent of premature activation. Persistent unidirectional block is often associated with depression of the transmembrane potentials and excitability of cardiac fibers.[252]

There are several possible mechanisms for the persistent unidirectional block in a region where action potentials are depressed. One mechanism is asymmetrical depression of excitability. Such asymmetrical depression might occur because of asymmetrical distribution of a pathological event. As a simple example, the action potential upstrokes in a bundle of fibers may be diminished as a result of a reduction of perfusion after coronary occlusion, but the depression of the upstroke may be more severe toward one end of the bundle than the other. This situation is diagrammed in Fig. 35-19. A propagating impulse consisting of an action potential with a normal upstrock velocity (site 1) enters the poorly perfused region (stippled in the diagram) and propagates through

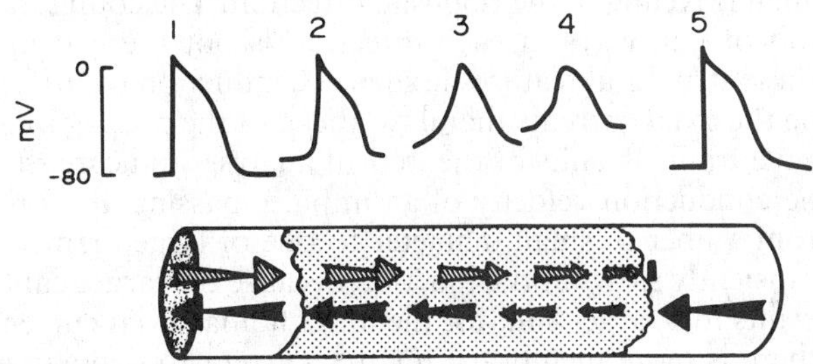

FIGURE 35-19 Asymmetrical depression of excitability as a mechanism for unidirectional conduction block in a bundle of cardiac muscle fibers. Action potentials shown above were recorded from sites on the fiber bundle. The stippled part of the bundle is depressed. Conduction from left to right along the bundle is indicated by the striped arrows, conduction from right to left by the black arrows. (*Modified after Wit AL, Rosen MR: In MacFarlane PW, Veitch Lawrie TD (eds): Comprehensive Electrocardiology, Theory and Practice in Health and Disease, vol 2. New York, Pergamon, 1989: 801–841. Reproduced with permission from the publisher and authors.*)

this region with decrement (from left to right or from site 1 to 4), i.e., as it conducts from the less depressed end (1) to the more severely depressed end (4), the action potential upstroke velocity and amplitude progressively decrease, as does the axial current flowing toward cells to be excited by the upstroke (as indicated by the decreasing size of the striped arrows). When the impulse arrives at the opposite end of the depressed segment of the bundle where there is suddenly a normally perfused bundle with normal action potentials (between action potential 4 and 5), the action potential amplitude is markedly reduced and the weak axial current from site 4 is not sufficient to depolarize the normal membrane to threshold at site 5. Conduction, therefore, blocks even though the normally perfused region is excitable. Conduction in the opposite direction (from right to left), however, might still succeed. The large axial current generated by the normal action potential at site 5 can flow for a considerable distance through the depressed region and may depolarize to threshold fibers at some distance from the most severely depressed region (perhaps as far as site 3). These cells, in turn, may be able to excite adjacent fibers in the direction of propagation (from right to left), and as a result, the impulse successfully propagates from site 3 to site 1, as indicated by the black arrows.

Geometrical Factors Causing Unidirectional Block Geometrical factors related to tissue architecture may also influence impulse conduction and under certain conditions lead to unidirectional block. An impulse can conduct rapidly in either direction along the length of a bundle of atrial, ventricular, or Purkinje fibers with normal electrophysiological properties. There is usually some asymmetry in the conduction velocity, however, meaning that conduction in one direction may take slightly longer than in the other direction.[4,224,227] This is usually of no physiological significance. The asymmetry of conduction can be the result of several factors. Bundles of cardiac muscle are composed of interconnecting myocardial fibers with different diameters packed in a connective tissue matrix. These bundles branch frequently (although the individual myocardial fibers do not branch). An impulse conducting in one direction encounters a different sequence of changes in fiber diameter, branching, and frequency and distribution of gap junctions than it does when traveling in the opposite direction. The configuration of pathways in each direction is not the same.[227] These structural features influence conduction by affecting the axial currents that flow ahead of the propagating wave front. Results of theoretical analyses indicate that the conduction velocity of an impulse passing abruptly from a fiber of small diameter to one of large diameter transiently slows at the junction because the larger cable results in a larger sink for the longitudinal axial current (there is more membrane for this current to depolarize to threshold if conduction of the impulse is to continue).[224,227,242,253,254] A similar slowing occurs when an impulse conducts into a region where there is an abrupt increase in branching of the myocardial syncytium; conduction transiently slows because of the larger current sink provided by the increased membrane area that must be depolarized. In the opposite direction, it can be predicted that conduction will speed transiently as the impulse moves from a larger to a smaller cable because the small sink for axial current results in more rapid depolarization of the membrane to threshold.[224,253,254] Theoretically, if there is a large enough difference in the diameter of the two cables, an impulse conducting from the small cable to the large cable should block at the junction, while conduction in the opposite direction (from large cable to small cable) is maintained.

A probable example of unidirectional block based on this geometrical factor in the normal heart is at the junctions between Purkinje and muscle cells. At certain sites, propagation from muscle to Purkinje fibers is possible while propagation from Purkinje fibers to muscle is not.[255] This asymmetry of conduction results from the difference in mass of the Purkinje and muscle layers. The smaller mass Purkinje fiber bundle is the small-diameter cable while the larger mass muscle is the larger diameter cable. It is unlikely that in normal circumstances these localized sites of unidirectional block predispose to reentry since the myocardium is quickly excited via the many other Purkinje-to-muscle junctions where the geometrical differences are not sufficient to cause block. It is possible, however, when conduction in ischemic myocardium is slow and coupling resistance at the junctions increases, that such sites of unidirectional block may become important in initiating reentry.[255–258]

It is doubtful that abrupt changes in geometrical properties such as fiber diameter of the magnitude required to cause block of the *normal* action potential often exist (except at some Purkinje fiber–muscle junctions as described above) because the safety factor for conduction is large, i.e., there is a large excess of activating current over the amount required for propagation.[224] Dodge and Cranefield[227] have pointed out that "only if an action potential is a relatively weak stimulus and the unexcited area is not easily excited will plausible changes in membrane resistance, cell diameter, or intercellular coupling produce block." There is a necessity for interaction of abnormal action potentials and decreased excitability with the preexisting anatomic impediments, such as will occur in acute ischemia. When the resting potential of fibers in a muscle or Purkinje bundle is decreased, the reduced action potential upstroke results in a decreased axial current, and therefore, the action potential is a weak stimulus. The normal directional differences in conduction are then exaggerated. At a critical degree of depression of the action potential upstroke, conduction may fail in one direction while being maintained in the other (although it may be markedly slowed). At this critical degree of depression, the reduced axial current might not be sufficient to depolarize the membrane to threshold where the current sink is increased because of the structural changes described above (increased fiber diameter), but the axial current is still more than adequate during conduction in the opposite direction.

The anisotropic properties of cardiac muscle also represent a geometrical factor that may sometimes contribute to the occurrence of unidirectional block. Spach et al.[230] have indicated that in anisotropic muscle, the safety factor for conduction is lower in the longitudinal direction of rapid conduction than in the transverse direction of slow conduction (opposite to that predicted on the basis of continuous cable theory). The low safety factor longitudinally is a result of a large current load on the membrane associated with the low axial resistivity and large membrane capacitance in the longitudinal direction. The low safety factor may result in preferential conduction block of premature impulses in the longitudinal direction under certain conditions. In uniformly anisotropic muscle, a decrease in inward current during the depolarization phase of an action potential, such as might result from premature activation, results in slowing of conduction in the longitudinal direction more than in the transverse direction, but propagation still continues as a spatially smooth process. Conduction block of early premature impulses occurs in both longitudinal and transverse directions nearly simultaneously in uniformly anisotropic muscle.[237] In nonuniformly anisotropic atrial muscle, however, premature activation can result in conduction block in the longitudinal direction even when the impulse is conducting from a region with a long refractory period into a region of shorter refractory period, while conduction in the transverse direction continues.[237] The site of block in the longitudinal direction can become a site of unidirectional block that leads to reentry, much like the block of premature impulses caused by a sudden increase in action potential duration and effective refractory period. It can be excited by an impulse propagating in the opposite direction, i.e., by the wave front initially launched successfully in the transverse direction and that later propagates to the distal side of the region of the block.

In contrast to the propensity of premature impulses to block in the longitudinal direction in nonuniformly anisotropic myocardium because of the decreased depolarizing current and low safety factor, when coupling resistance between cells is increased, conduction of all impulses will block first in the transverse direction. Preferential block in this direction occurs because there are fewer gap junctions connecting muscle bundles transversely than longitudinally. An increase in coupling resistance will reduce the number of functional transverse connections below the critical level needed to maintain conduction before the number of functional longitudinal connections is reduced to this critical level.[259,260] Unlike longitudinal block of a premature impulse which is transient block and which may lead to reentry, block in the transverse direction caused by increased coupling resistance is bidirectional and should not cause reentry.

Anisotropy can also result in unidirectional block at sites of muscle bundle branching or at the junction of muscle bundles.[231] It was shown in Fig. 35-17*A*(2) that when a wave front propagating in a bundle of parallel fibers enters a branch that is formed at an acute angle, the direction of propagation is quickly altered from longitudinal to transverse, causing an abrupt increase in the effective axial resistance in the direction of propagation and a slowing of conduction velocity. If the inward current is also reduced by partial depolarization such as after premature stimulation or elevation of extracellular K^+, conduction block may occur.[231] This is shown in Fig. 35-17*B*(2), where extracellular K^+ concentration was increased from 4.6 to 9.0 meq/liter. Failure of the stimulated impulse to enter the branch is shown by the absence of electrical activity at sites *c* and *d*. On the other hand, as shown in Fig. 35-17*B*(1), propagation from the other direction into the branch does not involve a change in the direction of the wave front relative to the fiber orientation since it continues in a parallel direction, and therefore, there is no block in this direction.[231] These sites can become areas of unidirectional block that are instrumental in the occurrence of reentry.

Alterations in Refractory Period Alterations of the effective refractory period may contribute to the occurrence of reentry. As indicated previously, a decrease in the effective refractory period decreases the wavelength of the reentrant impulse and, therefore, the necessary size of the reentrant circuit. If the refractory period is decreased, the degree of slow conduction needed for successful reentry is diminished. The effective refractory period of cardiac fibers in a reentrant circuit may be decreased during rapid tachycardias because of rate-dependent shortening of the action potential duration.[242,261] The computer model of Quan and Rudy[242] predict that in circuits with a small or no excitable gap, electrotonic interaction between the head and the tail of the reentrant wave front can also shorten action potential duration. If the effective refractory period is decreased sufficiently, more than one reentrant circuit can exist at a time in some regions.[262,263] The effective refractory period of atrial muscle, for example, is decreased by the acetylcholine released during vagal stimulation. As a result, reentry in atrial muscle causing atrial fibrillation is more easily induced during vagal stimulation.[264] Several reentrant circuits exist simultaneously during this arrhythmia.[263,265] Action potential duration and effective refractory period are decreased in the ventricle during reperfusion after brief periods of ischemia or in some of the ventricular muscle cells in chronically ischemic areas, probably contributing to the occurrence of reentry.

The Central Area of Block The central area of block may be anatomic, functional, or a combination of the two. Anatomic block is the result of a nonconductive medium in the center of the circuit. An example of an anatomically determined central area of block is in the tricuspid ring reentrant circuit found in a canine model of atrial flutter[261] and perhaps present in a clinical counterpart, atrial flutter found commonly in patients who have previously had a Mustard procedure to repair transposition of the great vessels.[266] The animal model depends critically on large incisions made in the right atrial free wall, which, in fact, are similar to those made by the surgeon during the Mustard procedure.

Functional block at the center of a circuit occurs when there is block of impulses in otherwise excitable cardiac muscle. An example of a functional center of block was first described by Allessie[267] in a model of reentrant excitation in the rabbit left atrium called the leading circle mechanism of reentry. Functional block has subsequently been described in several other models of atrial flutter.[221,222,268,269] The central area of functional block develops during the initiation of the reentrant circuit by the formation of a line of block most likely due to refractoriness. When the reentrant circuit forms, the line of block is then sustained by centripetal activation from the circulating reentrant wave front which, by repeatedly bombarding the central area of block, maintains the state of refractoriness of this region.

A combination of an anatomic and functional central area of block in the reentrant circuit has been described in some models of atrial flutter (e.g., the orifice of one of the cavae and an area of functional block continuous with or adjacent to the caval orifice).[270]

The Excitable Gap As indicated earlier, the excitable gap is the extent of excitable tissue along the reentrant pathway immediately ahead of the excitation wave front. The gap may be fully excitable, i.e., the tissue comprising the gap has fully repolarized following its previous period of excitation and is again normally excitable. The gap also may be partially excitable, i.e., the tissue comprising the gap of excitability is in its relative refractory period because it is incompletely repolarized from its previous period of excitation. Anatomically determined reentrant circuits may be characterized by a fully excitable gap or a partially excitable gap.[271] Functionally determined reentry of the leading circle type has a partially excitable gap,[267] but it is uncertain whether anisotropic reentry has only a partially excitable gap or may also have a fully excitable gap (see next section).

Types of Reentry

We have previously indicated that there are two types of reentry: ordered and random.[1] The reentrant circuits can be anatomically determined, functionally determined, or both anatomically and functionally determined. In anatomically determined circuits, the pathway is fixed and the characteristics of the reentrant circuit are determined by the characteristics of the anatomic components of the circuit. Anatomic circuits are, therefore, associated with ordered reentry. Perhaps the best example is that of AV reentrant tachycardia in which the reentrant circuit is composed of atrium, the AV node, the His-Purkinje system, ventricle, and an accessory AV connection. In functionally determined circuits, the pathway is formed because of the electrophysiological properties of the cardiac cells and not by a predetermined anatomic pathway. Functional circuits can be associated with ordered or random reentry.

Two types of functionally determined reentrant circuits are the leading circle type of reentry[267] and anisotropic reentry.[272] Allessie and co-workers[247,267,273] were able to induce stable reentrant tachycardia in small pieces of isolated rabbit left atrium by precisely timed premature impulses in regions that were activated normally at regular rates of stimulation. Initiation of reentry was made possible by the different refractory periods of atrial fibers in close proximity to one another. The premature impulse that initiated reentry blocked in fibers with long refractory periods and conducted in fibers with shorter refractory periods, eventually returning to the initial region of block after excitability recovered there. The impulse then continued to circulate around a central area which was kept refractory because it was constantly bombarded by impulses propagating toward it from all sides of the circuit. This central area provides a functional obstacle that prevents excitation from propagating across the fulcrum of the circuit. No anatomic obstacles or anatomically defined conducting pathways are present in the leading circle, and the reentrant circuit is completely defined by the electrophysiological properties of the tissue involved. The circumferences of the leading circle around a functional obstacle may be as little as 6 to 8 mm and represent a pathway in which the efficacy of stimulation of the circulating wave front is just sufficient to excite the tissue ahead, which is still in its relative refractory phase. Conduction through the functional reentrant circuit is slowed, therefore, because impulses are propagating in partially refractory tissue (a partially excitable gap). Reentrant excitation that has been mapped in the atria of canine models of atrial flutter may be caused by the leading circle mechanism.[221,268] The reentrant circuit remains in the same place during the flutter and is therefore ordered reentry. Functional reentrant circuits of the leading circle type may also change their size and location and, if they do, would fall under the general category of random reentry. This may occur when leading circle reentry causes fibrillation.

Anisotropy can cause conduction slow enough to result in reentry in small anatomic circuits. Reentrant circuits caused by anisotropy can also occur without well-defined anatomic pathways and might be classified as functional. Unlike the functional characteristic that leads to the leading circle type of reentry (local differences in membrane properties causing a difference in effective refractory periods in adjacent areas), in functional reentry caused by anisotropy the functional characteristic is the difference in effective axial resistance to impulse propagation dependent on fiber direction. This mechanism has been classified as anisotropic reentry.[272] In its pure form, both the unidirectional conduction block and slow conduction in the reentrant circuit are a result of anisotropic, discontinuous propagation, and there is no need for variations in membrane properties such as regional differences in effective refractory periods or depression of the resting and action potential.[237] On the basis of the longitudinal and transverse conduction velocities of premature impulses in nonuniform anisotropic muscle and of measurements of refractory periods in these experiments, Spach et al.[237] calculated that circuits in nonuniform anisotropic bundles can be as small as 2 to 4 mm^2 (transverse velocity of 0.5 m/s, dissociated longitudinal velocity of 0.2 m/s) in the absence of nonuniformities in repolarization. Furthermore, anisotropic circuits are elliptical or rectangular because of the directional differences in conduction velocities with the long axis of the ellipse in the fast, longitudinal direction. Circuits with this shape can have a smaller dimension than circular circuits such as the leading circle.[237]

Anisotropic reentrant circuits usually remain in a fixed position to cause ordered reentry.[274] The degree of anisotropy (ratio of longitudinal to transverse conduction velocity) varies in different regions of the heart, and the circuit can only reside in a region where the conduction transverse to the longitudinal axis is sufficiently slow to allow reentry. Stability of anisotropic reentrant circuits is also assisted by the presence of an excitable gap that does not occur in the leading circle functional circuit. The excitable gap is caused by the sudden slowing of conduction velocity and decrease in the wavelength of excitation as the reentrant impulse turns the corner from the fast longitudinal direction to the slow transverse direction and from the slow transverse direction to the fast longitudinal direction.[275,276]

Methods to Identify Mechanisms of Arrhythmias

Introduction

Since the early and classic experiments of Mayer[3,277] on reentry in the Medusa ring and later studies by Mines[214,278] on reentry in ring preparations cut from dog fish auricles or from canine right ventricles, it has been thought that mapping of the sequence of activation of the heart during a tachycardia should provide the best evidence for the presence of a reentrant circuit. Even so, the admonition of Mines[278] that "the chief error to be guarded against is that of mistaking a series of automatic beats originating in one point of a ring [substitute apparent reentrant circuit] and traveling around it in one direction only owing to a complete block close to the point of origin of the rhythm on one side of this point" for reentrant beats must be kept in mind. The point, of course, is that even sequence of activation mapping may not provide definitive proof of the presence of reentry even though it provides evidence consistent with reentry. Mines suggested that severing the ring (again, substitute the critical portion of the apparent reentrant circuit) and then demonstrating that no further reentrant excitation could occur was required for proof that reentrant excitation had been present. This, of course, has been accomplished in the example of AV reentrant tachycardia, with cure of the arrhythmia following catheter or surgical ablation of the accessory AV connection. Nevertheless, while "severing the ring" is both diagnostic and therapeutic when it can be accomplished to treat a tachyarrhythmia, it is virtually always clinically impractical as a diagnostic tool. Furthermore, until recently, precise sequence of activation cardiac mapping to identify reentry has been quite difficult to perform, particularly in patients. Although it is now possible to obtain remarkably precise sequence of cardiac activation maps in vivo using simultaneous multisite mapping techniques, it is only possible with use of sophisticated recording techniques that require the chest to be open and the heart exposed.

In fact, for the study of arrhythmias in the in situ heart, it is not routinely possible to obtain the direct electrical recordings (microelectrode studies, simultaneous multisite mapping, etc.) from the arrhythmogenic source that enable one to determine the electrophysiological mechanism causing the arrhythmias. Therefore, indirect approaches have evolved that can provide information that suggests the mechanism of an arrhythmia. These approaches include (1) the characterization of the arrhythmia from the ECG; (2) analyzing the effects of cardiac pacing on the arrhythmia; and (3) analyzing the effects of selected pharmacologic agents on the arrhythmia. Since cardiac pacing has long been an important tool in the study of mechanisms of both clinical and experimental arrhythmias and since it is also usually rather easy to apply, we present here a discussion of the use of this technique to identify the mechanism of an arrhythmia.

Cardiac Pacing to Determine Arrhythmogenic Mechanisms

The mechanism of an arrhythmia in the in situ heart can sometimes be deduced from the response of the arrhythmia to cardiac pacing. The ability to do this is based largely on studies in which the effects of electrical stimulation were determined on transmembrane action potentials recorded with microelectrodes in isolated and superfused cardiac tissues. Critical to the ability to use the response to electrical stimulation to study arrhythmia mechanisms is that the stimulated impulse(s) must reach the site of origin of the arrhythmia in order for this approach to be valid. There are many reasons why this might not happen. The stimulated impulse(s) might not reach the site at which the arrhythmia arises because of the electrophysiological properties of the intervening tissue between the stimulus site and the site of arrhythmia origin. An intervening region of prolonged refractoriness or depressed conduction might cause stimulated impulses to block before they reached the site of origin. If conduction time from the stimulation site to the site of arrhythmia origin is prolonged for any reason, impulses generated in the arrhythmogenic focus also may be able to leave that focus and depolarize large regions of myocardium around it, preventing the stimulated impulse from reaching the site of arrhythmia origin. Even when the stimulation site is close to the site of arrhythmia origin, areas of depressed conduction may prevent the stimulated impulses from reaching the arrhythmogenic cells.

Two basic patterns of stimulation are generally used to study the mechanisms of arrhythmias: (1) overdrive pacing (pacing at a rate or rates faster than the spontaneous rate of the tachycardia) and (2) introduction of a premature beat or beats using programmed stimulation. With either technique, the effects of the pacing on the spontaneous rhythm are observed following completion of the stimulation. Overdrive pacing is generally used during the arrhythmia to determine if the overdrive can terminate it or, if it does not, to determine the effect of the overdrive on characteristics of the arrhythmia. Overdrive pacing is sometimes used during sinus rhythm to determine whether or not the period of stimulation can induce an arrhythmia that has previously occurred spontaneously.

Introduction of a premature beat or beats at selected intervals during electrical diastole during programmed stimulation of the heart can be performed either during the spontaneous arrhythmia to test the effects of the premature beats or during sinus rhythm to see if the arrhythmia can be induced. For the latter, the premature beats usually are introduced following a basic drive train of 8 to 15 beats, although the premature beats may be introduced during sinus rhythm as well.

Effects of Electrical Stimulation on Arrhythmias Caused by Automaticity

The discussion of automaticity as an arrhythmogenic mechanism included a consideration of how the sinus node pacemaker and electrical stimulation (pacing) influence subsidiary pacemakers with different automatic mechanisms. Overdrive either by the sinus node or by electrical stimuli exerts an inhibitory effect on the normal automatic mechanism of subsidiary or latent pacemakers (overdrive suppression) that is primarily the result of enhanced Na^+-K^+ pump activity, but has less inhibitory effects on the abnormal automatic mechanism of subsidiary pacemakers. These known effects of overdrive on pacemaker mechanisms are sometimes useful in distinguishing automatic arrhythmias from arrhythmias caused by reentry or triggered activity in the in situ heart. The effects of overdrive pacing can also be of use in distinguishing arrhythmias caused by normal automaticity from those caused by abnormal automaticity.[85]

Based on the results of experimental studies, it can be assumed that arrhythmias caused by normal automaticity in the in situ heart cannot be initiated by overdrive pacing. Arrhythmias caused by normal automaticity can be suppressed transiently, but cannot be terminated by overdrive pacing. Based on microelectrode studies on isolated superfused pacemaker tissues, when overdrive pacing is applied during an ongoing arrhythmia caused by normal automaticity, the arrhythmia is expected to be transiently suppressed immediately after the overdrive pacing is stopped. This is manifest by a transient pause after overdrive and should be followed by a gradual speeding up of the rhythm (so-called warmup) until the original rate of the automatic rhythm is resumed. The duration of the transient pause and the time required for resumption of the original rate is expected to be directly related to the rate and duration of the overdrive. This behavior is mainly the result of the increased activity of the Na^+-K^+ pump, which is dependent both on the rate and duration of stimulation. This characteristic behavior of normally automatic pacemakers has been demonstrated in some clinical and experimental electrophysiological studies of both atrial and ventricular tachycardias.[180,279,280]

Like normal automaticity, arrhythmias caused by abnormal automaticity can neither be initiated nor terminated by overdrive pacing. On the other hand, arrhythmias caused by abnormal automaticity should not be suppressed by overdrive pacing unless the overdrive period is long and the rate of overdrive is fast.[85] The difficulty in suppressing such arrhythmias stems from the lesser amount of Na^+ entering the cells during the upstroke of the action potential and, therefore, less intense Na^+ pump stimulation by overdrive. Short periods of overdrive can even result in a transient speeding of the rate of impulse generation (overdrive acceleration).[85] Accelerated idioventricular tachycardia in myocardial infarction is not easily overdrive suppressed and, therefore, may be caused by abnormal automaticity.

The response of automatic arrhythmias to premature stimulation is also sometimes useful in distinguishing automaticity from other arrhythmogenic mechanisms. Of major importance, automatic rhythms caused by either normal or abnormal automaticity can neither be initiated nor terminated by premature stimuli, in contrast to reentry and triggered activity. Other than that, premature impulses induced at different times during diastole may transiently perturb an automatic rhythm for a few cycles. The characteristics of the perturbation may sometimes distinguish automaticity from other arrhythmogenic mechanisms. The response of normal and abnormal automaticity to premature stimulation may be somewhat similar. The characteristic response of an automatic pacemaker to premature stimulation is best exemplified by the response of the sinus node to atrial premature stimulation.[281] In Fig. 35-20 is plotted the normalized return cycle (cycle following the premature impulse) on the y axis versus the normalized premature cycle (test cycle) on the x axis for a study in which premature stimuli were applied to the atria of the human heart during sinus rhythm. The solid line (A) represents the line of identity; points falling on this line are compensatory (the sum of the premature cycle and the return cycle is equal to the sum of two spontaneous cycles). Premature impulses delivered late in the cycle length are followed by a compensatory pause and fall on this line (as the test cycle shortens, the return cycle lengthens in a reciprocal manner) because the premature impulses collide with the impulse emanating from the sinus node pacemaker without reaching and resetting the pacemaker. Therefore, the pacemaker discharge following the premature impulse occurs exactly on time. As the premature coupling interval is decreased, a point is reached in the basic cycle where the premature impulse reaches the pacemaker before it has spontaneously depolarized to threshold and depolarizes it early. The pacemaker is reset. When this occurs, the post-extrasystolic cycle (which is a result of the stimulated or reset pacemaker cells spontaneously depolarizing to threshold) is less than compensatory and the points fall below the line of identity. For the most part, the post-extrasystolic cycle

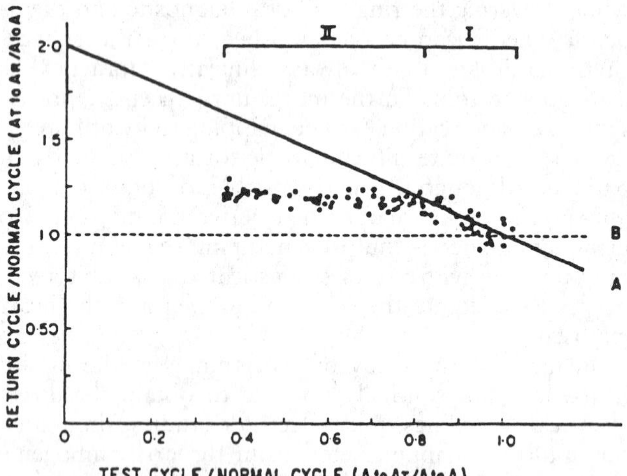

FIGURE 35-20 Return cycles as a function of premature stimulated cycles during premature atrial stimulation in a patient in sinus rhythm. The graph depicts the relationship of the normalized return cycle to the degree of prematurity of the test cycle, which is also normalized. Points falling on the line A represent nonreset of the sinus pacemaker (fully compensatory pause) and are in zone I. Premature stimulated atrial beats introduced earlier in atrial diastole fall in zone II. Line B, projected from the y axis, is a reference line indicating the spontaneous sinus cycle length. The distance the zone II points (reset points) are above line B is interpreted to indicate conduction time into and out of the sinus node, assuming the sinus node pacemaker cycle length immediately following the stimulated premature atrial beat is identical to the preceding sinus node pacemaker cycle length. (*From Strauss et al: Circulation 47:86, 1973. Reproduced with permission from the publisher and author.*)

length is expected to be equal to the unperturbed spontaneous cycle length. The dashed line (*B*) on the graph in Fig. 35-20 indicates the cycle length of the basic rhythm so that the return cycle length relative to the basic cycle length can be seen to be somewhat longer in this study. The prolonged return cycle has been proposed to result from slowed conduction of the premature impulse into the pacemaker site and the pacemaker impulse out of this site.[281] It might also result, at least partly, from depression of the rate of spontaneous diastolic depolarization. Further shortening of the premature coupling interval to midcycle results in points parallel to the dashed line and possibly slightly above it, which indicates no change in the post-extrasystolic cycle length over a wide range of coupling intervals. Finally, conduction of very early premature impulses might block prior to reaching the pacemaker, and the next pacemaker discharge would, again, occur on time and be compensatory. Of course, this relationship might be upset by changes in conduction of impulses into and out of the pacemaker site.

This same relationship between premature and return cycle length found in studies on sinus rhythm has also been shown in studies on some ectopic tachycardias and, when found, indicates that the tachycardias are likely to be caused by automaticity.[279,280,282] Ectopic pacemakers might also exist in an extensive region of slow conduction, much as the pacemaker in the sinus node, and conduction delays into and out of the pacemaker site may influence to some extent the relationship between return cycle and premature cycle. Conduction delays might cause some prolongation of the return cycle. When the above relationship is seen, however, it is probably indicative of automaticity (either normal or abnormal), since triggered activity and reentry are expected to show a different behavior.

In addition to the atrial arrhythmias discussed, some ventricular arrhythmias are likely to be caused by automaticity. Idioventricular rhythms in patients with complete heart block respond in the manner shown in microelectrode studies on slowly beating Purkinje fibers; the post-extrasystolic cycle following late premature impulses is longer than the cycle length of the basic rhythm but less than compensatory, while it is shorter than the basic cycle length following early premature impulses (and obviously less than compensatory).[283] Some exercise-provoked ventricular tachycardia might also be caused by normal automaticity.[284,285] On the other hand, there is some evidence that accelerated idioventricular rhythms in the clinical setting of myocardial infarction might be caused by abnormal automaticity.

Effects of Electrical Stimulation of Reentrant Excitation

A hallmark feature of reentry is that it can be induced and terminated by electrical stimuli (both overdrive pacing or introduction of premature stimuli), unlike automaticity. Initially it was thought sufficient to show that an arrhythmia could be initiated or terminated by overdrive pacing or programmed stimulation to demonstrate a reentrant mechanism.[286] That is because until the 1970s, the only other mechanism that was widely considered a cause of arrhythmias was automaticity, and automatic rhythms can neither be initiated nor terminated by pacing. After the 1970s, when the concept of afterdepolarization-induced arrhythmias was revived and expanded, these criteria alone were no longer sufficient, because triggered activity caused by DADs can also be initiated and terminated by pacing.

The induction of arrhythmias by overdrive pacing or introduction of a premature beat or beats can be used as an indicator of a reentrant mechanism if other characteristics are also present that eliminate the probability of triggered activity dependent on DADs. The ability to demonstrate directly that induction of an arrhythmia is related to a critical amount of slow conduction in the region where the arrhythmia originates adds credence to the interpretation that the arrhythmia is caused by reentry. The sudden large increase in the A-H interval associated with pacing induction of AV nodal reentrant tachycardia is one such example. The induction of triggered activity caused by DADs is not dependent on slowed conduction and should not show this relationship. Also, when a tachycardia is initiated by introduction of a premature beat over a wide range of coupling intervals, there may be an inverse relationship between the coupling interval of the premature impulse and the interval from the premature impulse to the first impulse of tachycardia.[287–289] This, too, is not found with the induction of triggered activity due to DADs.

Another feature of reentrant arrhythmias is that they can be terminated by overdrive pacing or premature stimulation. This is not specific for reentry, since triggered activity caused by DADs can also be terminated. As with initiation, termination by overdrive pacing requires a critical rate and duration of the stimulation train, while termination with stimulated premature impulses requires a critical coupling interval between the premature impulse and the previous impulse of the tachyarrhythmia. Failure to terminate an arrhythmia by stimulated impulses does not, per se, eliminate reentry as a mechanism for the arrhythmia. Termination of reentry requires that the stimulated impulse enter the reentrant circuit to cause the block of the reentrant wave front, and this requires that the circuit have an excitable gap. Some reentrant circuits, particularly if caused by the leading circle mechanism of reentry, may not have a gap of excitability large enough to allow a premature impulse to penetrate readily into the circuit. If a tachycardia is very rapid, the excitable gap also may be very small, again preventing ready entry into the circuit by stimulated impulses.

Entrainment In this context, the demonstration of transient entrainment of a tachycardia with or without its subsequent interruption is a relatively easy and reliable way to identify reentry as the mechanism of a tachyarrhythmia. Transient entrainment of a tachycardia was first described in 1977 during rapid pacing to interrupt classical (type I) atrial flutter.[290] At that time, although transient entrainment was not well understood, it was recognized as representing an increase in the rate of the tachycardia to the faster pacing rate, with resumption of the intrinsic rate of the tachycardia upon either abrupt cessation of pacing or slowing of the pacing rate below the intrinsic rate of the tachycardia.[290] On the basis of a series of clinical studies during rapid pacing of atrial flutter,[290–293] ventricular tachycardia,[294–296] AV reentry tachycardia involving an accessory AV connection,[297,298] AV nodal reentry tachycardia,[299] and intraatrial reentry tachycardia,[300] it was proposed that transient entrainment represents capture of a reentrant circuit by wave fronts generated by the pacing impulse without causing interruption of the tachycardia. This was confirmed during studies of transient entrainment in animal models of ventricular tachycardia[301–303] and atrial flutter[304,305] which utilized multiplexing techniques to record simultaneously from large numbers of electrodes in direct contact with cardiac tissue.

During transient entrainment of a reentrant tachycardia, the wave front from each pacing impulse enters into the excitable gap of the reentrant circuit. Once there, it travels in two directions: (1) antidromically, i.e., in the opposite direction of the circulating reentrant wave front of the spontaneous tachycardia, where it collides with the orthodromic wave front of the preceding beat, and (2) orthodromically, i.e., in the same direction as the circulating reentrant wave front of the spontaneous tachycardia, thereby both continuing the tachycardia and resetting it to the pacing rate. This explanation is universal for transient entrainment of any tachycardia due to reentry with an excitable gap and is diagrammatically illustrated in Fig. 35-21. The left panel is a diagrammatic representation of the reentrant circuit during a spontaneous ventricular tachycardia (VT) at an assumed rate of 145 beats per minute. The *X* represent the orthodromic wave fronts of the reentrant rhythm. The arrows indicate the direction of spread of the impulse, the box represents an area of slow conduction in the reentrant circuit, the serpentine line indicates slow conduction of the impulse in the area of slow conduction, and the dots represent recording sites along the course of the double arc of reentry from which ventricular electrograms (VEGs) are recorded. The middle panel is a diagrammatic representation of the introduction of the first pacing impulse ($X + 1$) during ventricular pacing at a rate of 150 beats per minute during the spontaneous ventricular tachycardia. The antidromic (anti) wave fronts ($X + 1$) collide with the orthodromic wave fronts from the previous spontaneous beat (X), resulting in fusion of ventricular activation. The orthodromic wave front (ortho) from the pacing impulse ($X + 1$) continues the ventricular tachycardia, resetting it to the pacing rate. The right panel shows a diagrammatic representation of the introduction of the second pacing impulse ($X + 2$) during ventricular pacing at a rate of 150 beats per minute during the spontaneous ventricular tachycardia. The antidromic wave fronts ($X + 2$) collide with the orthodromic wave fronts from the previous paced beat ($X + 1$), again resulting in ventricular fusion. Once again, the orthodromic wave front ($X + 2$) from the pacing impulse continues the ventricular tachycardia, resetting it to the pacing rate.

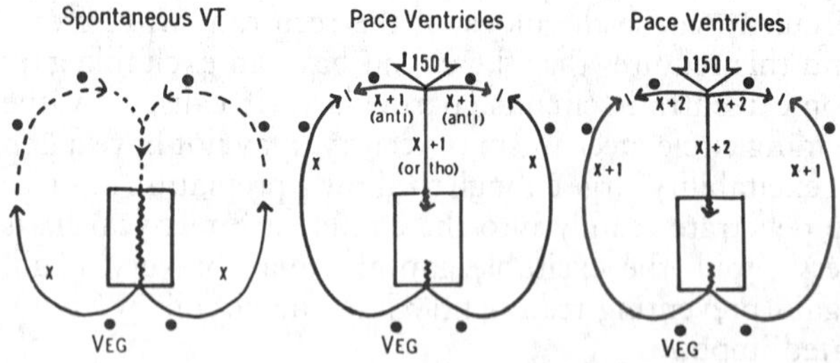

FIGURE 35-21 Diagrammatic representation of the reentrant circuit during spontaneous ventricular tachycardia (VT) and the first two beats of entrainment of the ventricular tachycardia at a rate of 150 beats per minute (middle and right panels, respectively). Each *X* represents the orthodromic wave fronts of the reentrant rhythm. In this and subsequent diagrams, the arrows indicate the direction of spread of the impulse, the box represents an area of slow conduction, the serpentine line indicates slow conduction of the impulse in the area of slow conduction, the dots represent recording sites along the course of the double arc of reentry from which ventricular electrograms (VEGs) are recorded, and the large arrow indicates the wave front from the pacing impulse entering into the ventricular tachycardia reentry circuit, where it is conducted orthodromically (ortho) and antidromically (anti). (*From Waldo AL, Henthorn RW: PACE 12:231, 1981. Reproduced with permission from the publisher and authors.*)

TABLE 35-2

Criteria to Establish the Presence of Transient Entrainment

1. The demonstration of constant fusion beats in the ECG during the period of rapid pacing at a constant rate except for the last captured beat, which is entrained but not fused (i.e., the last entrained beat demonstrates the ECG morphology of the spontaneous tachycardia)
2. The demonstration of constant fusion beats in the ECG during rapid pacing at any constant rate but different degrees of constant fusion at different rapid rates, i.e., progressive fusion
3. Interruption of the tachycardia associated with localized conduction block to a site(s) for one beat, followed by subsequent activation of that site(s) from a different direction, manifest by a change in morphology of the electrogram at the blocked site(s) and with a shorter conduction time
4. A change in conduction time to and electrogram morphology at one recording site when pacing from another site at two different constant pacing rates, each of which is faster than the spontaneous rate of the tachycardia but fails to interrupt it

Criteria to Establish Transient Entrainment There are four criteria established (Table 35-2), any one of which, if demonstrated, establishes the presence of transient entrainment and thereby the presence of a reentrant rhythm with an excitable gap. Figures 35-22 to 35-24 demonstrate the four criteria in diagrammatic fashion for the same ventricular tachycardia illustrated in Fig. 35-21. In Fig. 35-22, which illustrates the first criterion (Table 35-2), the left panel is a diagrammatic representation of the termination of ventricular pacing illustrated in Fig. 35-21. In the left panel, the large arrow indicates the wave front from the last pacing impulse delivered at a rate of 150 beats per minute entering into the reentrant circuit of the ventricular tachycardia, where it is conducted orthodromically and antidromically. The antidromic wave fronts (X_n[a]) collide with the orthodromic

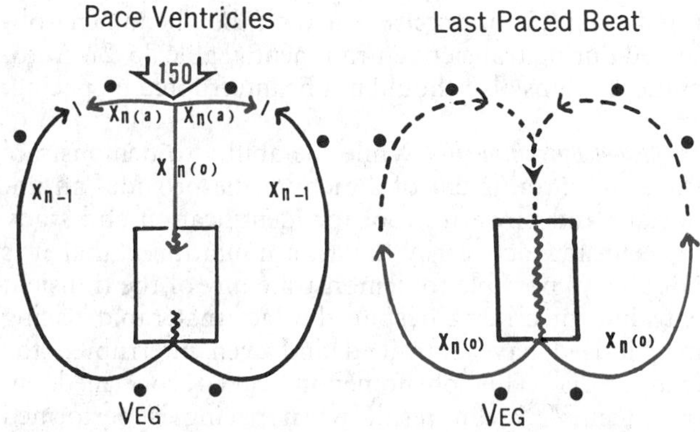

FIGURE 35-22 Diagrammatic representation of the first entrainment criterion during termination of ventricular pacing illustrated in Fig. 35-21. (*From Waldo AL, Henthorn RW: PACE 12:231, 1989. Reproduced with permission from the publisher and authors.*)

wave fronts (X_n[o]) of the previous beat (X_{n-1}), resulting in the fusion of ventricular activation, but the orthodromic wave front from the last pacing impulse continues and resets the tachycardia. The right panel shows that the orthodromic wave fronts from the last pacing impulse are now unopposed by any antidromic wave fronts because there is no subsequent pacing impulse. Thus, no fusion of ventricular activation occurs despite the presence of transient entrainment. This last entrained beat travels around the reentrant circuit, continuing the spontaneous tachycardia.

Figure 35-23 is a diagrammatic representation of entrainment in the same spontaneous ventricular tachycardia during pacing from the same site proximal to the area of slow conduction of the reentrant circuit at a rate of 150 (left panel), 155 (middle panel), and 160 beats per minute (right panel), demonstrating both the second and fourth entrainment criteria. When pacing at a rate of 155 beats per minute, the pacing cycle length is shorter than at 150 beats per minute, so that the antidromic wave front from each pacing impulse will penetrate the excitable gap of the reentrant circuit to a further degree in an antidromic direction compared to 150 beats per minute, resulting in a different degree of fusion of the QRS complex in the ECG than at a rate of 150 beats per minute. As a result, the QRS complex morphology in the ECG during pacing at 155 beats per minute will be different than at 150 beats per minute. This, then, is the demonstration of progressive fusion (Table 35-2). When pacing at 160 beats per minute, once again the antidromic wave front from each pacing impulse will collide with the orthodromic wave front, but at yet a different site. This occurs because the pacing cycle length is shorter than pacing at the previous rates, permitting greater penetration of the excitable gap by the antidromic wave front of the pacing impulse, illustrating yet more progressive fusion. These diagrams also illustrate the fourth criterion (Table 35-2): A site or sites activated by the orthodromic wave front of each pacing impulse during entrainment at one pacing rate will be activated by the antidromic wave front of each pacing impulse during entrainment at a faster pacing rate. This will be manifest both by a change in the morphology of the electrogram recorded at the site in question (it will have the same morphology during the spontaneous tachycardia as during pacing at the rate which results in activation of the site by the orthodromic wave front, but a different morphology when activated by the antidromic wave front of the pacing impulse at a faster pacing rate) and a change in conduction time to the recording site from the pacing site (the stimulus-to-recording site interval will be longer when activated by the orthodromic wave front of each pacing impulse than when activated by the antidromic wave front of each pacing impulse). Thus, note that the two middle recording sites denoted by black dots on each side of the reentrant circuit become activated in turn from a different direction and with a shorter conduction time when the pacing rate is increased from 150 to 155 beats per minute and then to 160 beats per minute.

Figure 35-24 is a diagrammatic representation of the third criterion and shows the events during interruption of the ventricular tachycardia by ventricular pacing at a rate of 165 beats per minute. In the left panel, the large arrow indicates the wave front from the pacing impulse delivered at a rate of 165 beats per minute entering into the reentrant circuit of the ventricular tachycardia, where it is conducted orthodromically ($X + 1$[o]) and antidromically ($X + 1$[a]). The antidromic wave fronts collide with the orthodromic wave fronts from the previous beats (X_n) resulting in fusion of ventricular activation. Note that this fusion of ventricular activation is at still a different site than during pacing at the previous pacing rates (Fig. 35-23). Thus, initially there is still more progressive fusion of the QRS complex morphology in the ECG. This time, however, the orthodromic wave front does not reset the tachycardia to the pacing rate. Rather, it too is blocked, presumably in the area of slow conduction, during the same beat. Note that each recording site

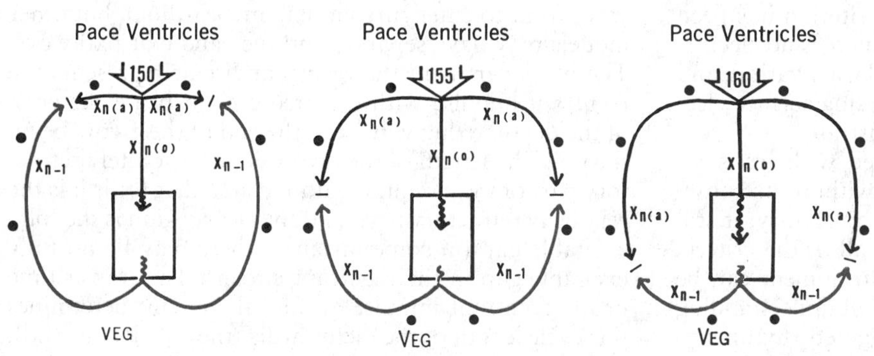

FIGURE 35-23 Diagrammatic representation of the second and fourth entrainment criteria during entrainment of the same spontaneous ventricular tachycardia shown in Fig. 35-21 by ventricular pacing at a rate of 150 (*left panel*), 155 (*middle panel*), and 160 (*right panel*) beats per minute. (*From Waldo AL, Henthorn RW: PACE 12:231, 1989. Reproduced with permission from the publisher and authors.*)

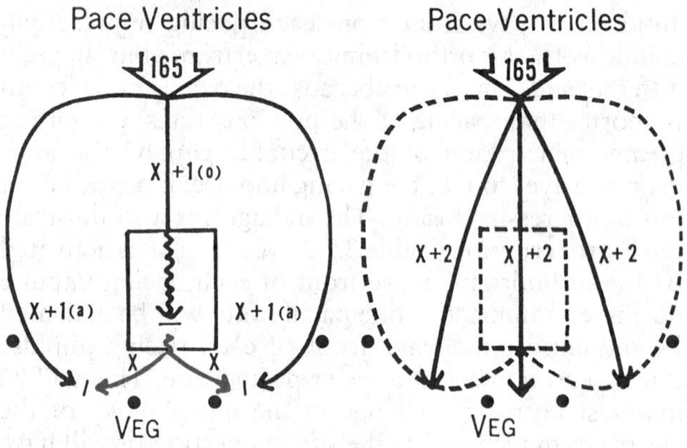

FIGURE 35-24 Diagrammatic representation of the third entrainment criterion during interruption of the ventricular tachycardia by ventricular pacing at a rate of 165 beats per minute. (*From Waldo AL, Henthorn RW: PACE 12:231, 1989. Reproduced with permission from the publisher and authors.*)

on each of the two arcs of reentry immediately distal to the area of slow conduction is activated by the orthodromic wave front of the previous beat (*X*) but is not activated by X + 1 because the orthodromic wave front (*X* + 1[o]) never reaches either site (there is localized conduction block for one beat). In the right panel, the large arrows indicate the next pacing impulse (*X* + 2) delivered at the same pacing rate (165 beats per minute) from the same pacing site as in the left diagram. The dashed lines indicate the reentrant circuit present during the previous periods of spontaneous ventricular tachycardia and transient entrainment of the ventricular tachycardia. Because the ventricular tachycardia has been interrupted by the previous pacing impulse (*X* + 1), the sequence of ventricular activation of the next pacing impulse (*X* + 2) is as one would expect during overdrive pacing of sinus rhythm from that same ventricular pacing site. Therefore, the two electrogram recording sites immediately distal to the previously but no longer present area of slow conduction are now activated from a different direction than during transient entrainment. In addition, because the presumed area of slow conduction is no longer functionally present, the stimulus-to-right-ventricular conduction time is shorter. Thus, the requirements for the third criterion of entrainment are fulfilled (Table 35-2).

Although these illustrative diagrams show the example of transient entrainment and interruption of ventricular tachycardia, the principles are the same for all the putative reentrant rhythms. For AV nodal reentrant tachycardia, however, only the third criterion has been demonstrated,[299] presumably because there is no electrocardiographic manifestation of AV nodal activation, and recording directly from the AV node using surface electrograms has not been reliably demonstrated.

Although the phenomena associated with transient entrainment of a tachycardia with or without its subsequent interruption are best explained by reentry, it still must be asked whether or not any or all of the criteria for the demonstration of transient entrainment can be explained by another mechanism. Present understanding of the response of automatic and triggered rhythms to rapid pacing is not consistent with the phenomena observed during transient entrainment (Table 35-2). Automatic rhythms also should not be interrupted by pacing.

Concealed Entrainment While the ability to demonstrate transient entrainment of a tachycardia provides an important and powerful tool for identification and study of reentrant tachyarrhythmias, a limitation is that it is not always possible to demonstrate any of the transient entrainment criteria despite the fact that rapid pacing may indeed have entrained and even interrupted the tachycardia. This phenomenon, called concealed entrainment,[296,298] can result when pacing is performed from a site which is orthodromically distal to the area of slow conduction in the reentry circuit, when pacing from a site which is rather distant from the reentrant circuit, or when pacing from an area of slow conduction in the reentrant circuit.[296,298,306–308] In order to label a response of a tachycardia to rapid pacing as concealed entrainment, except in the example of pacing from an area of slow conduction in the reentry circuit, one must also show that transient entrainment can be demonstrated when pacing from another site. Thus, it is clear that unless one is able to pace from an appropriate site, a reentrant circuit with an excitable gap may be present, but entrainment, though present, will not be demonstrable.

Resetting The response of an arrhythmia to a prematurely stimulated impulse that does not terminate the arrhythmia may still provide information useful for determining the mechanism of the arrhythmia. Information on the effects of stimulated premature impulses on reentry comes from studies on experimental preparations of isolated tissues or hearts in which reentrant excitation has been mapped. Other predictions concerning the effects of premature impulses on reentry are based mainly on theoretical considerations using a model of a reentrant circuit with a fixed pathway in which the circuit cannot change its dimensions and in which there is an excitable gap. Such circuits may have a single entrance and exit pathway leading into and out of the circuit, as illustrated in Fig. 35-25, or the entrance and exit pathways may be separate. These characteristics will influence the characteristics of the resetting response as seen on the ECG.

The theoretically possible responses of a tachycardia caused by reentrant excitation to premature stimulation are explained in the diagram in Fig. 35-25. An anatomic circuit with fixed dimensions and a single entrance pathway is diagrammed. In this diagram the entrance pathway also serves as an exit pathway for the reentrant wave front to enter surrounding myocardium, but other models may have separate entrance and exit pathways. The black arrow in the reentrant circuit represents the reentrant impulse with the arrow point being the crest of the depolarizing wave and the end of the arrow being the tail. The length of the arrow is the absolutely refractory part of the circuit, the dotted area that trails it is the relatively refractory part, and the clear region is the fully excitable gap (in some instances there may be no fully excitable gap in the reentrant circuit). The transit time of the reentrant impulse around the circuit determines one cycle length of the tachycardia (the $R_1 \rightarrow R_1$ interval).

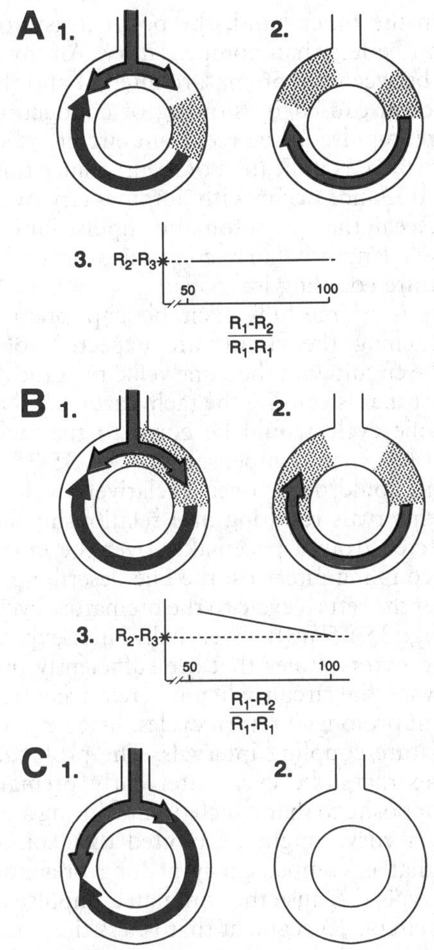

FIGURE 35-25 Effects of premature impulses on reentrant circuit with an excitable gap. In each panel, diagrams are shown of an anatomic circuit with a single entrance route from above. In *A1, B1,* and *C1*, black arrows in the circuit represent the reentrant impulse causing tachycardia. The length of the arrow is the wavelength of the impulse and shows the part of the circuit that is completely refractory. The part of the circuit that is stippled is relatively refractory and the part of the circuit that is clear is completely excitable (the fully excitable gap). Black arrows entering the circuit from above represent a prematurely stimulated impulse initiated outside the circuit. *A2* and *B2* show conduction of the premature impulse in the circuit. Graphs show the expected relationship between the return (premature impulse) cycle length ($R_2 - R_3$) and premature coupling interval ($R_1 - R_2/R_1 - R_1$) for premature impulses conducting in the fully excitable gap (*A3*) and in the relatively refractory tissue of a partially excitable gap (*B3*). (*Modified after Wit AL, Janse MJ: The Ventricular Arrhythmias of Ischemia and Infarction. The Electrophysiological Mechanisms. Mt. Kisco, NY, Futura Publishing, 1992. Reproduced with permission from the publisher and authors.*)

In panel *A*(1) a stimulated premature impulse (R_2) (black arrow from above) is shown to reach the circuit and enter it in the region of the fully excitable gap. The stimulated premature wave front may then propagate both in the orthodromic (to the right) and antidromic (to the left) direction in the reentrant pathway. In the antidromic direction, it collides with the oncoming reentrant wave front, extinguishing both stimulated and reentrant impulses at the point of collision. In the orthodromic direction, the stimulated impulse becomes the reentrant impulse and propagates through the circuit in completely excitable tissue of the gap (which also moves around the circuit), shown in panel *A*(2). This stimulated reentrant wave front would leave the circuit through the normal exit route and become the next tachycardia impulse. Since the stimulated impulse traveled through the circuit in completely excitable tissue at normal conduction velocity, the interval between the stimulated impulse (R_2) and the next impulse of tachycardia (R_3) is equal to the normal transit time around the circuit or the normal tachycardia cycle length ($R_1 \rightarrow R_1$). The rhythm, however, is reset, i.e., the sum of the curtailed (premature) cycle length and the return cycle length ($R1 \rightarrow R_2 + R_2 \rightarrow R_3$) (first poststimulus cycle) is less than two cycle lengths of the tachycardia [$2(R_1 \rightarrow R_1)$]. This holds throughout the range of premature coupling intervals at which the stimulated premature impulse is able to conduct around the circuit at a normal velocity in completely excitable tissue. Thus, a plot showing the relationship between the premature coupling intervals and the return (poststimulus) cycles over this range appears as a flat line. This plot is shown in Fig. 35-25*A*(3). The poststimulus cycle length is the $R_2 - R_3$ interval on the *y* axis. The normalized premature coupling interval is represented by $R_1 - R_1/R_1 - R_1$ on the horizontal axis where $R_1 - R_1$ is the basic cycle length of the tachycardia. In this graph, $R_2 - R_3$ remains constant (and equal to $R_1 - R_1$) over the entire range of premature coupling intervals, indicating conduction of the premature impulse in completely excitable tissue. Premature impulses entering the circuit in the relatively refractory part of the excitable gap (stippled region in the circuit) shown by the black arrow from above in Fig. 35-25*B*(1) also collide with the reentrant impulse in the antidromic direction, extinguishing it while conducting in the orthodromic direction. But conduction around the circuit is slower than normal because the impulse is activating relatively refractory tissue, indicated by the stippled area in Fig. 35-25*B*(2). Therefore, the return (poststimulus) cycle, which is dependent on the conduction time of the stimulated impulse in the circuit, is longer than the tachycardia cycle. As the coupling interval of the stimulated premature impulse is decreased and this impulse enters the circuit earlier and earlier in the relatively refractory period of the excitable gap, conduction time around the circuit and the return cycle progressively increase. Thus, a plot showing the relationship between the premature coupling interval and the return cycle length appears as shown in Fig. 35-25*B*(3). The line representing the $R_2 - R_3$ interval increases as the normalized premature coupling interval ($R_1 - R_2/R_1 - R_1$) decreases. It is also apparent on the graph that conduction time of the premature impulse around the circuit as measured by the $R_2 - R_3$ interval is greater than conduction time of the normal tachycardia impulse around the circuit, which is indicated by the dashed line. The sum of the premature and return cycle may either be less than compensatory or greater than compensatory depending on how slow conduction of the premature impulse is around the circuit. Extremely slow conduction may prolong the return cycle to such an extent that the sum of the premature and return cycles is greater than the sum of two spontaneous cycles. However, more often, despite slowing of conduction of the premature impulse in the circuit, the prolonged return cycle does not compensate for the shortened premature cycle.[309-312] Panel C shows what happens when an earlier premature impulse, indicated by the black arrow from above, reaches the circuit when it is even less excitable. It conducts antidromically into the circuit and collides with the wave front of the reentrant impulse but cannot excite the orthodromic path because it blocks in refractory tissue (black tail of the reentrant impulse). Thus, reentry is terminated (C2). The range of coupling intervals over which there is evidence that the premature impulse entered the reentrant circuit to reset the tachycardia prior to termination of reentry is a rough measurement of the duration of the excitable gap if the premature stimuli are applied close to the circuit.[312] Therefore, fixed reentrant circuits with excitable gaps have patterns of responses to premature stimulation that are characteristic for this mechanism.

In sum, the stable tachycardia cycle length ($R_1 - R_1$) is determined by the time it takes the reentrant wave front to travel one complete revolution around the circuit and reach an exit pathway to the ventricles. When such a circuit is the cause of a tachycardia, premature depolarizations delivered late in the cycle length are often followed by a post-extrasystolic pause that is compensatory for the same reason as described for automatic tachycardias, i.e., the stimulated impulse may not be able to reach the reentrant circuit, possibly due to collision between the stimulated impulse and the impulse coming from the circuit. The next tachycardia impulse then comes precisely on time. In this case, the tachycardia is not reset since the sum of the premature cycle length and the return cycle length is equal to two successive premature cycle lengths. Over the range of premature coupling intervals that do not reset the tachycardia, the relationship between the premature coupling interval and the following (return) cycle falls along the line of identity (see Fig. 35-20). Premature impulses delivered earlier in the tachycardia cycle might have several different effects that are dependent on some of the characteristics of the reentrant circuit. If there is virtually no excitable gap, as might be expected of some functional circuits, no resetting of the tachycardia will occur since the stimulated impulse cannot enter the circuit, and the return cycle will remain compensatory. If the excitable gap is partially excitable, e.g., composed of relatively refractory tissue, premature impulses that succeed in entering the circuit and traveling around it will do so at reduced conduction velocities, as diagrammed in Fig. 35-25*B*.[313] When they emerge from the circuit, they cause the first post-extrasystolic (tachycardia) impulse. As a result of the slowing of conduction of the premature impulse around the circuit, the post-extrasystolic cycle is longer than the basic cycle [represented by the dashed line in Fig. 35-25*B*(3)]. Conduction time of the premature impulse around the circuit should continue to increase as the premature impulse is delivered earlier and earlier in the cycle, since the premature impulse conducts in more refractory tissue, causing an inverse relationship between the premature coupling interval and the post-extrasystolic cycle [Fig. 35-25*B*(3)]. In the study of Bigger and Goldreyer[288] on AV nodal reentrant tachycardia, the prolongation of the post-extrasystolic cycle over the entire range of premature coupling intervals was sufficient to result in a greater than compensatory pause following the premature impulse. On the other hand, the post-extrasystolic cycle length can be less than compensatory. An inverse relationship between the premature interval and the return cycle interval caused by slowing of conduction of the premature impulse in the reentrant circuit, as shown in Fig. 35-25*B*(3), is indicative of reentry since this type of response does not occur with automaticity or triggered activity. Recall that for automatic impulse initiation, the return cycle length is fairly constant over a wide range of premature coupling intervals.

If there is a large fully excitable gap, premature impulses reaching the circuit are expected to conduct around the circuit with the same velocity as the reentrant wave front that is causing the tachycardia, and the post-extrasystolic cycle would be equal to the tachycardia cycle and less than compensatory [Fig. 35-25*A*(1) and *A*(2)]. This could occur over a relatively wide range of coupling intervals resulting in a relationship similar to that expected from a pacemaker over the intermediate range of coupling intervals; the line describing the relationship of the return cycle to the premature cycle would be flat [Fig. 35-25*A*(3)]. Eventually, it is expected that stimulated extrasystoles that are sufficiently premature would invade the circuit when it is relatively refractory, resulting in prolonged return cycles, inversely related to the premature coupling intervals. The prolongation of the post-extrasystolic cycle after early premature impulses is opposite to that which occurs during automaticity. Thus a curve might be plotted that consists of a segment that is compensatory at long premature coupling intervals (because the stimulated impulse does not reach the circuit), a segment that is less than compensatory and flat at intermediate premature coupling intervals (when the stimulated impulse is conducting in completely excitable tissue in the circuit), and a segment that is ascending at short premature coupling intervals (when the stimulated impulse is conducting in relatively refractory tissue in the circuit). Still earlier premature impulses might block prior to reaching a circuit, resulting in interpolation, as described for an automatic focus. A sufficiently early premature impulse could also terminate the tachycardia by blocking in the circuit and causing block of the reentrant wave front. This is not expected of automatic impulse initiation.

As mentioned above, the entrance route that a stimulated impulse takes into a reentrant circuit and the exit route from the circuit may be separate. When this occurs, the return cycle following a premature impulse may be less than the tachycardia cycle because the premature impulse, after entering the circuit, need not conduct around the entire circuit before exiting. The return cycle may still show any of the relationships to the premature cycle that is described in Fig. 35-25; i.e., it may be flat or show an inverse relationship to the premature coupling interval depending on whether it is conducting in partially or fully excitable tissue. This expected effect of premature impulses on the cycle length of reentry might also be altered in a functional circuit if the premature impulse can somehow cause a change in the size or shape of the circuit. It is not possible to predict easily what the effects would be.

In summary, the relationship between the post-extrasystolic cycle and the curtailed cycle when premature impulses are introduced during a tachycardia caused by reentry may be different than during automaticity. Therefore, premature stimulation during the study of a tachycardia may provide useful information that helps to determine whether or not reentry is the mechanism. There are, however, a number of confounding influences that, if present, can upset the theoretically predicted relationships. They include the absence of an excitable gap and properties of intervening tissue between the stimulus site and the site of the circuit that can slow or block conduction of premature impulses into and out of the circuit. Therefore, failure to find the relationships expected for a reentrant mechanism does not necessarily mean that the arrhythmia is caused by a mechanism other than reentry.

Effects of Electrical Stimulation on Arrhythmias Caused by Triggered Activity

Arrhythmias Caused by Delayed Afterdepolarizations The amplitude of DADs increases with a decrease in the cycle length at which the action potentials occur until the afterdepolarizations reach threshold to cause triggered activity. Therefore, triggered arrhythmias caused by DADs in the in situ heart should be initiated by either overdrive pacing or programmed premature stimulation. Since automatic arrhythmias are not initiated by pacing, they should be readily distinguished from triggered arrhythmias caused by DADs. Reentrant arrhythmias can also be induced by the same stimulation protocols, however, so whether or not there are any other characteristics during arrhythmia induction by pacing that might distinguish between triggered activity and reentry is important. An attempt to distinguish between the two mechanisms is further complicated by the fact that triggered activity caused by DADs may be due to different causes, e.g., digitalis and catecholamines, each with somewhat different characteristics. The following guidelines have been proposed to assist in distinguishing DAD-induced triggered activity from other causes of arrhythmias.[314,315] The guidelines are based on the characteristics of triggered activity determined from in vitro studies with microelectrodes.

Triggered activity caused by DADs has been more easily induced by rapid pacing or by several successive premature stimuli than by a single premature stimulus in studies on isolated tissue preparations. This characteristic, which should be expected to occur in the in situ human heart, is probably explained by the fact that rapid pacing or introduction of a number of premature stimuli are more effective than a single premature stimulus in increasing intracellular Ca^{2+} levels. The latter control the afterdepolarization amplitude. Also, arrhythmias caused by triggered activity should be more easily induced by premature stimuli superimposed on a rapid drive rate than on a slow one because during rapid pacing, the afterdepolarization amplitude is larger and membrane potential at the peak of the afterpolarization is closer to threshold. In contrast, ordered reentrant rhythms in humans (with the exception of atrial flutter) seem more easily and reproducibly induced by premature impulses than by rapid pacing, although several premature impulses in succession are sometimes necessary. One reason may be that premature impulses block more effectively in areas with long refractory periods than do impulses during rapid pacing, because rapid pacing can shorten refractory period duration. This, of course, is important because block is a prerequisite for initiation of reentry.

Both extrasystoles and the first beat of a tachycardia, when caused by DAD-dependent triggered activity initiated by pacing, are predicted to occur late in the cardiac cycle.[314] This proposal is based on experimental data from studies on isolated tissue that show that DADs rarely reach their peak amplitude at less than 50 percent of the cardiac cycle when the drive cycle length is shorter than 1000 ms. In contrast, reentrant beats often occur early in the cycle.

One would expect a direct relationship between the pacing cycle length that induces triggered activity due to DADs and the coupling interval from the last stimulated impulse to the first beat of the induced tachycardia. As the pacing cycle length decreases, the coupling interval from the last stimulated impulse to the first impulse of tachycardia should decrease because at short cycle lengths, the coupling interval of the afterdepolarizations to the proceeding action potential decreases. A direct relationship between pacing cycle length and coupling interval of the first impulse of the tachycardia has been shown to occur in arrhythmias caused by digitalis toxicity.[316] This relationship might sometimes be complicated by the presence of two afterdepolarizations and the possibility of a triggered impulse arising from either one.[317] No comparable data are available from pacing studies on digitalis toxic human hearts. The direct relationship has also been shown in some cases of idiopathic ventricular tachycardia believed to be caused by triggered activity.[165] Such a direct relationship is not expected during initiation of reentrant arrhythmias. Failure to show the direct relationship, however, cannot be taken as proof that the arrhythmia is not caused by triggered activity since slow conduction into or out of the triggerable focus can distort it. In microelectrode studies, during initiation of triggered activity with premature stimuli, no significant effects of the premature stimulus coupling interval were observed on the relationship (coupling interval) of the first triggered impulse to the premature stimulus.[187] On the basis of these data, it is expected that during initiation of arrhythmias caused by triggered activity in situ with programmed premature stimulation, the coupling interval of the first beat of tachycardia should remain relatively constant over a range of coupling intervals of introduced premature impulses. The response to premature stimulation is also contrary to that expected during initiation of reentrant arrhythmias, where an inverse relationship is expected between the premature stimulus coupling interval and the coupling interval between the premature impulse and the first impulse of tachycardia.

Triggered arrhythmias, unlike automatic arrhythmias but like reentrant arrhythmias, are predicted to be terminated by cardiac pacing. Single premature impulses may terminate triggered arrhythmias, but based on the results of microelectrode studies, termination should be infrequent and not usually reproducible at the same critical premature cycle length. In contrast, single premature impulses often terminate reentrant arrhythmias in a reproducible manner and over a consistent range of premature cycle lengths in any one individual as long as the reentrant circuit has an excitable gap.[318,319] Therefore, an arrhythmia that is readily terminated by a single prematurely stimulated impulse is more likely to be caused by reentry than by triggered activity. The effects of premature impulses that do not terminate sustained triggered activity have also been determined.[190] The response is almost identical to that of automaticity. The return cycle length remains fairly constant over a wide range of premature coupling intervals and nearly the same as the cycle length of the basic triggered rhythm (less than compensatory).

On the other hand, overdrive pacing should terminate triggered arrhythmias due to afterdepolarizations. Such termination requires a critical rate and duration of overdrive,[185–187] just as it does with reentry.[289,290,294] Overdrive stimulation may cause acceleration of triggered arrhythmias followed by gradual slowing and termination or rapid overdrive may cause abrupt termination. Although reentrant rhythms might be accelerated by overdrive pacing, a gradual slowing of the rate prior to termination is not expected. Overdrive pacing that does not terminate triggered activity, such as when the cycle length of the overdrive is too long or when the trains of stimuli are too short, does not entrain the arrhythmia either.[320] In fact, none of the characteristics of entrainment are expected during overdrive pacing of triggered activity caused by DADs.

It is therefore apparent that although the response of triggered arrhythmias caused by DADs to stimulation can be predicted from the experimental studies, there is no single feature that would positively enable a triggered rhythm to be distinguished from reentry except entrainment. Since the characteristics of initiation and termination of triggered rhythms by stimulation are very different from the characteristics of automatic rhythms, it should be easier to distinguish between these mechanisms by pacing techniques. This differentiation may be made more difficult when an arrhythmia is persistent and the initiation cannot be studied. Also, entrance block of stimulated impulses into arrhythmogenic foci, whether automatic, triggered, or reentrant, may negate the use of pacing techniques to distinguish between these mechanisms.

The characteristics of some clinical arrhythmias occasionally conform to those expected of DAD-dependent triggered activity.[127,321] In addition to digitalis toxicity, an example is some cases of exercise-induced ventricular tachycardia in patients with no structural heart disease.[165,285] This tachycardia, which occurs spontaneously during exertion, can sometimes be initiated by overdrive pacing or programmed premature stimulation. An isoproterenol infusion during stimulation may be required for successful initiation. Lerman et al.[165] have proposed that the tachycardias are caused by a catecholamine-induced increase in cyclic AMP, which is known to cause DADs. Evidence supporting this hypothesis is the termination of tachycardias by intravenous injection of adenosine, which antagonizes the electrophysiological effects of catecholamines mediated through the adenylate cyclase–cyclic AMP system. Jackman et al.[322] have proposed that some forms of ventricular tachycardia associated with the congenital long QT syndrome and dependent on adrenergic stimulation are a result of triggered activity caused by DADs. Cranefield and Aronson[127] have provided a detailed review of the clinical arrhythmias that may be caused by triggered activity. (See also Chaps. 34 and 36.)

Arrhythmias Caused by Early Afterdepolarizations Arrhythmias caused by EADs should not be inducible by overdrive pacing, similar to automatic arrhythmias and unlike arrhythmias caused by DADs or reentry. Likewise, triggered activity dependent on EADs is not expected immediately to follow the short cycle length of one or several prematurely stimulated impulses. As shown in the experimental studies, the appearance of EAD-induced triggered activity is facilitated by long cycle lengths. Therefore, this kind of triggered activity should be initiated by slowing the basic heart rate. Of course, if an increase in heart rate caused by pacing resulted in entrance block into a focus where EADs occur, the block could cause a prolongation of the cycle length in that focus that might result in triggered activity.[127] Prematurely stimulated impulses might also initiate triggered activity if there is a long compensatory pause following the stimulated impulse. The long cycle might trigger an arrhythmia that would follow it.[127] In the absence of such entrance block, bursts of tachycardia caused by EADs should occur more frequently when the heart rate is slowed, and pacing the heart at rates faster than the basic underlying rhythm is predicted to cause disappearance of the period of tachycardia. Increasing the basic heart rate shortens action potential duration and thereby suppresses EADs. When the pacing is stopped, arrhythmias should reappear, as the action potential returns to its original duration. The reappearance of the arrhythmias may not be immediate, however, since it requires some time for the action potential duration to lengthen owing to the enhanced pump current that follows a period of rapid stimulation.

Many of these characteristics have been shown to apply to the experimental triggered arrhythmias caused by cesium in the in situ canine heart[197] and have been demonstrated in some cases of torsades de pointes in patients. Acquired forms of the syndrome (e.g., prolonged QT and torsades de pointes caused by quinidine) exhibit all the features expected of triggered activity caused by EADs, whereas other forms (e.g., congenital) may not be due to this mechanism.[323] Torsades de pointes invariably occurs after a preceding long R – R interval,[198] is unlikely to be initiated by programmed stimulation,[324] and can be prevented from occurring by pacing the heart at a rapid rate.[198,324] In contrast, triggered arrhythmias caused by DADs may become more frequent as heart rate increases,[314] and the effect of increasing the heart rate on extrasystoles caused by reentry is variable; i.e., reentry might be exacerbated or it might stop.[220] There may be some difficulty in distinguishing EAD-dependent triggered arrhythmias from automatic arrhythmias only on the basis of their response to electrical stimulation, however, since the occurrence of automatic arrhythmias is facilitated by slow heart rates and increasing the basic heart rate by overdrive pacing may cause disappearance of automatic arrhythmias during the periods of pacing.

The electrocardiographic characteristics of arrhythmias caused by triggered activity due to EADs and by automaticity might be of additional help. The triggered rhythms are more likely to occur in bursts or salvos of different lengths with the first few cycle lengths of a burst decreasing progressively and the last few cycle lengths increasing progressively.

Triggered arrhythmias caused by EADs might not only occur in bursts, but might also be sustained. When sustained, their response to single premature stimuli or overdrive pacing can be predicted on the basis of the results of in vitro studies. Some arrhythmias might be terminated by premature stimuli, but this should be a relatively rare occurrence. The effects of premature stimulated impulses that do not terminate the arrhythmia are expected to be the same as their effects on automatic impulse initiation. Some arrhythmias also might be terminated by overdrive pacing, but termination should not be the usual effect. When termination occurs, it is expected to follow the overdrive immediately, whereas termination of triggered activity caused by DADs may sometimes be preceded by up to 10 triggered "afterbeats."[185,186] When termination does not occur, overdrive is not expected to cause any significant effect on the rhythm; the response should be more like that of an arrhythmia caused by abnormal automaticity[190] than normal automaticity, which is readily overdrive suppressed.[72] Because of this variability of response, stimulation during a sustained tachycardia caused by EADs is not much help in determining the mechanism.

Therefore, like the triggered arrhythmias caused by DADs, there is no single feature in the response to cardiac pacing that would positively enable EAD-induced triggered rhythms to be distinguished from other arrhythmogenic mechanisms. Early afterdepolarization–induced nonsustained arrhythmias can usually be differentiated from rhythms induced by DADs or automaticity at high membrane potentials and sometimes from reentry by pacing, but the response of sustained triggered activity to pacing is often indistinguishable from abnormal automaticity at low membrane potentials.

Summary of Effects of Electrical Stimulation

Despite the fact that there are exceptions and inconsistencies to virtually all the rules that can be proposed to distinguish among the different arrhythmogenic mechanisms using pacing techniques, determining the effects of electrical stimulation is really quite useful. The following is a summary of the most important points:

1. Initiation of a tachycardia by stimulation indicates that the arrhythmia is caused either by reentry or delayed afterdepolarization–induced triggered activity. Other characteristics of initiation are then useful in distinguishing between the two. Other mechanisms of arrhythmias such as automaticity and triggered activity caused by early afterdepolarizations are eliminated when a tachycardia is induced by cardiac pacing.
2. Termination of a tachycardia by overdrive pacing or premature stimulation is expected of reentry or triggered activity caused by delayed afterdepolarizations, but not of automaticity and early afterdepolarization–dependent triggered activity. Overdrive suppression is expected of arrhythmias caused by normal automaticity, and overdrive acceleration may occur with arrhythmias caused by abnormal automaticity.
3. Demonstration of entrainment of a tachycardia during overdrive pacing is indicative of a reentrant mechanism and is not expected of other mechanisms.
4. The response to premature stimulation is different during arrhythmias caused by automaticity and those caused by reentry. During automatic arrhythmias, the return cycle length should not increase as the premature coupling interval decreases. The return cycle should be less than compensatory. During reentrant arrhythmias, the return cycle length should increase as the premature impulse occurs earlier in the dominant cycle. The increase may sometimes begin to occur with late coupled premature impulses or it may not occur until premature impulses are early coupled. The return cycle length is often less than compensatory.

REFERENCES

1. Hoffman BF, Rosen MR: Cellular mechanisms for cardiac arrhythmias. *Circ Res* 1981; 49:1–15.
2. Waldo AL, Kaiser GA, Bowman FO Jr, Malm JR: Etiology of prolongation of the P-R interval in patients with an endocardial cushion defect: Further observations on internodal conduction and the polarity of the retrograde P wave. *Circulation* 1973; 48:19–27.
3. Mayer AG: Rhythmical pulsation in Scyphomedusae. Washington, Carnegie Institution of Washington, Publication no 47, 1906; 1–62.
4. Cranefield PF: *The Conduction of the Cardiac Impulse. The Slow Response and Cardiac Arrhythmia.* Mount Kisco, NY, Futura Publishing, 1975.
5. Schmitt FO, Erlanger J: Directional differences in the conduction of the impulse through the heart muscle and their possible relation to extrasystolic and fibrillary contractions. *Am J Physiol* 1928–1929; 87:326–347.
6. Wit AL, Hoffman BF, Cranefield PF: Slow conduction and reentry in the ventricular conduction system. I. Return extrasystole in canine Purkinje fibers. *Circ Res* 1972; 30:1–10.
7. Cranefield PF, Wit AL, Hoffman BF: Genesis of cardiac arrhythmias. *Circulation* 1973; 47:190–204.
8. Singer DH, Lazzara R, Hoffman BF: Interrelationships between automaticity and conduction in Purkinje fibers. *Circ Res* 1967; 21:537–558.
9. Di Francesco D: The hyperpolarization-activated current, i_f, and cardiac pacemaking. In: *Cardiac Electrophysiology; a Textbook.* Rosen MR, Janse MJ, Wit AL (eds): Mount Kisco, Futura Publishing, 1990: 117–132.
10. Yanagihara K, Irisawa H: Potassium current during the pacemaker depolarization in rabbit sinoatrial node cell. *Pflügers Arch* 1980; 388:255–260.
11. Di Francesco D: Characterization of single pacemaker channels in cardiac sinoatrial node cells. *Nature* 1986; 324:470–473.
12. Di Francesco D, Ferroni A, Massanti M, Tromba C: Properties of the hyperpolarizing-activated current (i_f) in cells isolated from the rabbit sino-atrial node. *J Physiol* 1986; 37:61–88.
13. Brown HF: Electrophysiology of the sinoatrial node. *Physiol Rev* 1982; 52:505–530.
14. Brown HF, Kmiura K, Noble SJ: The relative contributions of various time-dependent membrane currents to pacemaker activity in the sino atrial node. In: Bouman LN, Jongsma HJ (eds): *Cardiac Rate and Rhythm: Physiological, Morphological and Developmental Aspects.* Boston, Martinus-Nijhoff, 1982: 53–68.
15. Nakayama T, Kurachi Y, Noma A: Action potential and mem-

brane currents of single pacemaker cells of the rabbit heart. *Pflügers Arch* 1984; 402:248–257.
16. Shibasaki T: Conductance and kinetics of delayed rectifier potassium channels in nodal cells of the rabbit heart. *J Physiol* 1987; 387:227–250.
17. Irisawa H, Giles WR: Sinus and atrioventricular node cells: Cellular electrophysiology. In: Zipes DP, Jalife J (eds): *Cardiac Electrophysiology: From Cell to Bedside*. Philadelphia, Saunders, 1990: 95–102.
18. Reuter H: Ion channels in cardiac cell membranes. *Ann Rev Physiol* 1984; 46:473–484.
19. Bean BP: Two kinds of calcium channels in canine atrial cells. *J Gen Physiol* 1985; 85:1–30.
20. Hagiwara N, Irisawa H, Kameyama M: Contribution of two types of calcium currents to the pacemaker potentials of rabbit sino-atrial node cells. *J Physiol* 1988; 409:121–141.
21. Doerr T, Denger R, Trautwein W: Calcium currents in single SA nodal cells of the rabbit heart studied with action potential clamp. *Pflügers Arch* 1989; 413:599–603.
22. Hoffman BF, Cranefield PF: *Electrophysiology of the Heart*. New York, McGraw-Hill, 1960.
23. Trautwein W: Effects of acetylcholine on the SA node of the heart. In: Carpenter O (ed): *Cellular Pacemakers: Mechanisms of Pacemaker Generation*. New York, Wiley, 1981: 127–160.
24. Soejma M, Noma A: Mode of regulation of the ACh-sensitive K channel by the muscarinic receptor in rabbit atrial cells. *Pflügers Arch* 1984; 400:424–431.
25. Di Francesco D, Tromba C: Inhibition of the hyperpolarizing-activated current, i_f, induced by acetylcholine in rabbit sino-atrial node myocytes. *J Physiol* 1988; 405:477–491.
26. Noma A, Kotake H, Irisawa H: Slow inward current and its role mediating the chronotropic effect of epinephrine in the rabbit sinoatrial node. *Pflügers Arch* 1980; 388:1–9.
27. Di Francesco D: The cardiac-hyperpolarizing activated current, i_f. Origins and developments. *Prog Biophys Mol Biol* 1985; 46:163–183.
28. Hogan PM, David LD: Evidence for specialized fibers in the canine atrium. *Circ Res* 1968; 23:387–396.
29. Jones SB, Euler DE, Hardie E, Randall WC, Brynjolfsson G: Comparison of SA nodal and subsidiary pacemaker function and location in the dog. *Am J Physiol* 1978; 234:H471–H476.
30. Rozanski GJ, Lipsius SL: Electrophysiology of functional subsidiary pacemakers in canine right atrium. *Am J Physiol* 1985; 249:H594–H603.
31. Rozanski GJ, Lipsius SL, Randall WD: Functional characteristics of sinoatrial and subsidiary pacemaker activity in the canine right atrium. *Circulation* 1983; 67:1378–1387.
32. Wit AL, Cranefield PF: Triggered and automatic activity in the canine coronary sinus. *Circ Res* 1977; 41:435–445.
33. Wit AL, Fenoglio JJ Jr, Wagner BM, Bassett AL: Electrophysiological properties of cardiac muscle in the anterior mitral valve leaflet and the adjacent atrium in the dog. Possible implications for the genesis of atrial dysrhythmias. *Circ Res* 1973; 32:731–745.
34. Bassett AL, Fenoglio JJ, Wit AL, Myerburg RJ, Gelband H: Electrophysiologic and ultrastructural characteristics of the canine tricuspid valve. *Am J Physiol* 1976; 230:1366–1377.
35. Rozanski GJ: Electrophysiological properties of automatic fibers in rabbit atrioventricular valves. *Am J Physiol Heart Circ Physiol* 1987; 22:H720–H727.
36. Kokobun S, Nishimura M, Noma A, Irisawa H: The spontaneous action potential of rabbit atrioventricular node cells. *Jpn J Physiol* 1980; 30:529–540.
37. James TN, Isobe JH, Urthaler JH: Correlative electrophysiological and anatomical studies concerning the site of origin of escape rhythm during complete atrioventricular block in the dog. *Circ Res* 1979; 45:108–119.
38. Jones SB, Euler DE, Randall WC, Brynjolfsson G, Hardie EL: Atrial ectopic foci in the canine heart: Hierarchy of pacemaker automaticity. *Am J Physiol Heart Circ Physiol* 1980; 238:H788–H793.
39. Randall WC, Talano J, Kaye MP, Euler DE, Jones SB, Brynjolfsson G: Cardiac pacemakers in the absence of the SA node: Responses to exercise and autonomic blockade. *Am J Physiol* 1978; 234:H465–H470.
40. Wallick DW, Levy MN, Felder DS, Zieske H: Effects of repetitive bursts of vagal activity on atrioventricular junctional rate in dogs. *Am J Physiol* 1979; 237:H275–H281.
41. Spear JF, Moore EN: Influence of brief vagal and stellate nerve stimulation on pacemaker activity and conduction within the atrioventricular conduction system of the dog. *Circ Res* 1973; 32:27–40.
42. Rozanski GJ, Jalife J: Automaticity in atrioventricular valve leaflets of rabbit heart. *Am J Physiol Heart Circ Physiol* 1986; 19:H397–H406.
43. Weidmann S: *Elektrophysiologie Der Herzmuskelfaser*. Medizinischer Verlag Hans Huber Bern und Stuttgart, 1956.
44. Hope RR, Scherlag BJ, El-Sherif N, Lazzara R: Hierarchy of ventricular pacemakers. *Circ Res* 1976; 39:883–888.
45. Vassalle M, Levine MJ, Stuckey JH: On the sympathetic control of ventricular automaticity. The effects of stellate ganglia stimulation. *Circ Res* 1968; 23:249–258.
46. Levy MN: Sympathetic-parasympathetic interactions in the heart. *Circ Res* 1971; 29:437–445.
47. Levy MN, Blattberg B: Effect of vagal stimulation on the overflow of norepinephrine into the coronary sinus during cardiac sympathetic nerve stimulation in the dog. *Circ Res* 1976; 38:81–85.
48. Di Francesco D: A new interpretation of the pace-maker current in calf Purkinje fibers. *J Physiol* 1981; 314:359–376.
49. Di Francesco D: A study of the ionic nature of the pace-maker current in calf Purkinje fibers. *J Physiol* 1981; 314:377–393.
50. Noble D: The surprising heart: A review of recent progress in cardiac electrophysiology. *J Physiol* 1984; 353:1–50.
51. Di Francesco D, Noble D: A model of cardiac electrical activity incorporating ionic pumps and concentration changes. *Phil Trans R Soc Lond B* 1985; 307:353–398.
52. Gintant GA, Coehn IS: Advances in cardiac cellular electrophysiology: Implications for automaticity and therapeutics. *Ann Rev Pharmacol Toxicol* 1988; 28:61–81.
53. Hauswirth O, Noble D, Tsien RW. The mechanism of oscillatory activity at low membrane potentials in cardiac Purkinje fibers. *J Physiol* 1969; 200:255–265.
54. Imanishi S: Calcium-sensitive discharge in canine Purkinje fibers. *Jpn J Physiol* 1971; 21:443–463.
55. Noble D, Tsien RW: The kinetics and rectifier properties of the slow potassium current in cardiac Purkinje fibers. *J Physiol* 1968; 195:185–214.
56. Katzung BG, Morgenstern JA: Effects of extracellular potassium on ventricular automaticity and evidence for a pacemaker current in mammalian ventricular myocardium. *Circ Res* 1977; 40:105–111.
57. Escande D, Coraboeuf E, Planche C: Abnormal pacemaking is modulated by sarcoplasmic reticulum in partially depolarized myocardium from dilated right atria in humans. *J Mol Cell Cardiol* 1987; 19:231–241.
58. Kimura T, Imanishi S, Arita M, Hadama T, Shirabe J: Two differential mechanisms of automaticity in diseased human atrial fibers. *Jpn J Physiol* 1988; 38:851–867.
59. January CT, Fozzard HA: The effects of membrane potential, extracellular potassium and tetrodotoxin on the intracellular sodium ion activity in sheep cardiac muscle. *Circ Res* 1984; 54:652–665.
60. Carmeliet EE: *Chloride and Potassium in Cardiac Purkinje Fibers*. Thesis, Editions ARSCI, S.A. Bruxelles, Presses Academiques Europeennes, 1961.
61. Gadsby DC, Cranefield PF: Two levels of resting potential in cardiac Purkinje fibers. *J Gen Physiol* 1977; 70:725–746.
62. Hill JL, Gettes LS: Effects of acute coronary artery occlusion on local myocardial extracellular K+ activity in swine. *Circulation* 1980; 61:768–778.
63. Hirche HJ, Franz C, Bos L, Bissig R, Lang R, Schramm M: Myocardial extracellular K^+ and H^+ increase and noradrenaline release as possible cause of early arrhythmias following acute coronary artery occlusion in pigs. *J Mol Cell Cardiol* 1980; 12:579–593.
64. Kléber AG: Resting membrane potential, extracellular potassium activity and intracellular sodium activity during acute global ischemia in isolated perfused guinea-pig hearts. *Circ Res* 1983; 52:442–450.
65. Dresdner KP, Kline R, Wit AL: Intracellular K+ activity, intracellular Na activity and maximum diastolic potential of canine subendocardial Purkinje cells from one-day-old infarcts. *Circ Res* 1987; 60:122–132.
66. Dresdner KP, Kline RP, Wit AL: Cytoplasmic K^+ and Na^+ activity in subendocardial canine Purkinje fibers from one day old

infarcts using double-barrel ion sensitive electrodes. *Biophys J* 1985; 47:463a.

67. Friedman PL, Stewart JR, Wit AL: Spontaneous and induced cardiac arrhythmias in subendocardial Purkinje fibers surviving extensive myocardial infarction in dogs. *Circ Res* 1973; 33:612–626.
68. Lazzara R, El-Sherif N, Scherlag BJ: Electrophysiological properties of canine Purkinje cells in one day old myocardial infarction. *Circ Res* 1973; 33:722–734.
69. Hordof AJ, Edie R, Malm JR, Hoffman BF, Rosen MR: Electrophysiological properties and response to pharmacological agents of fibers from diseased human atria. *Circulation* 1976; 54:774–779.
70. TenEick RE, Singer DH: Electrophysiological properties from diseases human atria. I. Low diastolic potential and altered cellular response to potassium. *Circ Res* 1979; 44:545–557.
71. Singer DH, Baumgarten CM, TenEick RE: Cellular electrophysiology of ventricular and other dysrhythmias: Studies on diseased and ischemic hearts. *Progr Cardiovasc Dis* 1981; 24:97–156.
72. Vassalle M: Electrogenic suppression of automaticity in sheep and dog Purkinje fibers. *Circ Res* 1970; 27:361–377.
73. Vassalle M: The relationship among cardiac pacemakers. Overdrive suppression. *Circ Res* 1977; 41:269–277.
74. Vassalle M: Cardiac pacemaker potentials at different extra- and intracellular K concentrations. *Am J Physiol* 1965; 208:770–775.
75. Vassalle M, Caress DL, Slovin AJ, Stuckey JH: On the cause of ventricular asystole during vagal stimulation. *Circ Res* 1967; 20:228–241.
76. Randall WC, Rinkema LE, Jones SB, Moran JF, Brynjolfsson G: Overdrive suppression of atrial pacemaker tissues in the alert, awake dog before and chronically after excision of the sinoatrial node. *Am J Cardiol* 1982; 49:1166–1175.
77. Glitsch HG: Characteristics of active Na transport in intact cardiac cells. *Am J Physiol* 1979; 236:H189–H199.
78. Gadsby DC, Cranefield PF: Electrogenic sodium extrusion in cardiac Purkinje fibers. *J Gen Physiol* 1979; 73:819–837.
79. Jordan JL, Yamaguchi I, Mandel WJ, McCullen AE: Comparative effects of overdrive on sinus and subsidiary pacemaker function. *Am Heart J* 1977; 93:367–374.
80. Kodama I, Goto J, Ando A, Toyama I, Yamada K: Effects of rapid stimulation on the transmembrane action potentials of rabbit sinus node pacemaker cells. *Circ Res* 1980; 46:90–99.
81. Greenberg YJ, Vassalle M: On the mechanism of overdrive suppression in the guinea pig sino-atrial node. *J Electrocardiol* 1990; 37:53–67.
82. Gang ES, Reiffel JA, Livelli FD Jr, Bigger JT Jr: Sinus node recovery times following the spontaneous termination of supraventricular tachycardia and following atrial overdrive pacing. A comparison. *Am Heart J* 1983; 105:210–215.
83. Breithardt G, Seipel L, Loogen F: Sinus node recovery time and calculated sinoatrial conduction time in normal subjects and patients with sinus node dysfunction. *Circulation* 1977; 56:43–50.
84. Carmeliet E: The slow inward current: Non-voltage-clamp studies. In: Zipes DP, Bailey JC, Elharrar V (eds): *The Slow Inward Current and Cardiac Arrhythmias*. The Hague, Martinus Nijhoff Publishers, 1980: 97–110.
85. Hoffman BF, Dangman KH: Are arrhythmias caused by automatic impulse generation? In: Paes de Carvalho A, Hoffman BF, Lieberman M (eds): *Normal and Abnormal Conduction in the Heart*. Mount Kisco, NY, Futura Publishing, 1982: 429–448.
86. Dangman KH, Hoffman BF: Studies on overdrive stimulation of canine cardiac Purkinje fibers: Maximum diastolic potential as a determinant of the response. *J Am Coll Cardiol* 1983; 2:1183–1191.
87. Falk RT, Cohen IS: Membrane current following activity in canine cardiac Purkinje fibers. *J Gen Physiol* 1984; 83:771–799.
88. Van Capelle FJL, Durrer D: Computer simulation of arrhythmias in a network of coupled excitable elements. *Circ Res* 1980; 47:454–466.
89. Wit AL, Cranefield PF: Mechanism of impulse initiation in the atrioventricular junction and the effect of acetylstrophantidin (abstr.) *Am J Cardiol* 1982; 49:921.
90. Kirchhof CJ, Bonke FIM, Allessie MA: Evidence for the presence of electrotonic depression of pacemakers in the rabbit atrioventricular node. The effects of uncoupling from the surrounding myocardium. *Basic Res Cardiol* 1988; 83:190–201.
91. Opthof T, van Ginneken ACG, Bouman LN, Jongsma HJ: The intrinsic cycle length in small pieces isolated from the rabbit sinoatrial node. *J Mol Cell Cardiol* 1987; 19:923–934.
92. Janse MJ, Van Capelle FJL: Electrotonic interactions across an inexcitable region as a cause of ectopic activity in acute regional myocardial ischemia. A study in intact porcine and canine hearts and computer models. *Circ Res* 1982; 50:527–537.
93. Boineau JP, Schuessler RB, Mooney CR, Wylds AC, Miller CB, Hudson RD, et al: Multicentric origin of the atrial depolarization waves: The pacemaker complex. Relation to dynamics of atrial conduction, P wave changes and heart rate control. *Circulation* 1978; 58:1036–1048.
94. Toda N, West TC: Changes in sino-atrial node transmembrane potentials on vagal stimulation of the isolated rabbit atrium. *Nature* 1965; 205:808–809.
95. Ferrer II: The sick sinus syndrome. Mount Kisco, NY, Futura Publishing, 1974.
96. Katz LN, Pick A: *Clinical Electrocardiography. The Arrhythmias*. Philadelphia, Lea & Febiger, 1956.
97. Jalife J, Moe GK: Effect of electrotonic potentials on pacemaker activity of canine Purkinje fibers in relation to parasystole. *Circ Res* 1976; 39:801–808.
98. Jalife J, Moe GK: A biologic model of parasystole. *Am J Cardiol* 1979; 43:761–772.
99. Moe GK, Jalife J, Mueller WJ, Moe B: A mathematical model of parasystole and its application to clinical arrhythmias. *Circulation* 1977; 56:968–979.
100. Euler DE, Jones SB, Gunnar WP, Loeb JM, Murdock DK, Randall WC: Cardiac arrhythmias in the conscious dog after excision of the sinus node and crista terminalis. *Circulation* 1979; 59:468–475.
101. Loeb JM, Euler DE, Randall WC, Moran JF, Brynjolfsson G: Cardiac arrhythmias after chronic embolization of the sinus node artery: Alterations in parasympathetic pacemaker control. *Circulation* 1980; 61:192–198.
102. Randall WC, Rinkema LE, Jones SB, Moran JF, Brynjolfsson G: Functional characteristics of atrial pacemaker activity. *Am J Physiol* 1982; 242:H98–H106.
103. Gillette PC, Kugler JD, Garson A Jr, Gutgesell HP, Duff DF, McNamara DG: Mechanisms of cardiac arrhythmias after the Mustard operation for transposition of the great arteries. *Am J Cardiol* 1980; 45:1225–1230.
104. Klein HO, Lebson R, Cranefield PF, Hoffman BF: Effect of extrasystoles on idioventricular rhythm. Clinical and electrophysiologic correlation. *Circulation* 1973; 47:758–764.
105. Webb SW, Adgey AAJ, Pantridge JF: Autonomic disturbance of onset of acute myocardial infarction. *Br Med J* 1972; 3: 89–92.
106. Lie KI, Wellens HJJ, Schuilenburg RM: Mechanism and significance of widened QRS complexes during complete atrioventricular block in acute inferior myocardial infarction. *Am J Cardiol* 1974; 33:833–839.
107. Dahl G, Isenberg G: Decoupling of heart muscle cells: Correlation with increased cytoplasmic calcium activity and with changes of nexus ultrastructure. *J Membr Biol* 1980; 53:63–75.
108. Weingart R: The actions of ouabain on intercellular coupling and conduction velocity in mammalian ventricular muscle. *J Physiol* 1977; 264:341–365.
109. Ellis D: The effects of external cations and ouabain on the intracellular sodium activity of sheep heart Purkinje fibers. *J Physiol* 1977; 273:211–240.
110. Davis LD: Effects of autonomic neurohumors on transmembrane potentials of atrial plateau fibers. *Am J Physiol* 1975; 229:1351–1364.
111. Tsien RW: Effects of epinephrine on the pacemaker potassium current of cardiac Purkinje fibers. *J Gen Physiol* 1974; 64:293–319.
112. Pliam MB, Krellenstein DJ, Vassalle M, Brooks C McC: The influence of norepinephrine, reserpine and propranolol on overdrive suppression. *J Electrocardiol* 1975; 8:17–24.
113. Armour JA, Hageman GR, Randall WC: Arrhythmias induced by local cardiac nerve stimulation. *Am J Physiol* 1972; 223:1068–1075.
114. Katzung BG, Hondeghem LM, Grant AO: Cardiac ventricular automaticity induced by current of injury. *Pflügers Arch* 1975; 360:193–197.
115. Rosen MR, Gelband H, Hoffman BF: Correlation between the effects of ouabain on the canine electrocardiogram and trans-

membrane potentials of isolated Purkinje fibers. *Circulation* 1973; 47:65–72.
116. Rosen MR, Gelband H, Merker C, Hoffman BF: Mechanisms of digitalis toxicity: Effects of ouabain on phase four of canine Purkinje fiber transmembrane potentials. *Circulation* 1973; 47:681–689.
117. Deck KA: Aenderungen des Ruhepotentials und der Kabeleigenschaften von Purkinje-Fäden bei der Dehnung. *Pflügers Arch* 1964; 280:131–140.
118. Dudel J, Trautwein W: Das Aktionspotential und Mechanogramm des Herzmuskels unter dem Einflusz der Dehnung. *Cardiologia* 1954; 25:344–362.
119. Kaufmann R, Theophile U: Automatie fördernde Dehnungseffekte am Purkinje Faden, Papillarmuskeln und Vorhoftrabekeln von Rhesusaffen. *Pflügers Arch* 1967; 291:174–189.
120. Hansen DE, Craig CS, Hondeghem LM: Stretch-induced arrhythmias in the isolated canine ventricle. Evidence for the importance of mechanoelectrical feedback. *Circulation* 1990; 81:1094–1105.
121. Ferrier GR, Rosenthal JE: Automaticity and entrance block induced by focal depolarization of mammalian ventricular tissues. *Circ Res* 1980; 47:238–248.
122. Imanishi S, Surawicz B: Automatic activity in depolarized guinea-pig ventricular myocardium. *Circ Res* 1976; 39:751–759.
123. Brown HF, Noble SJ: Membrane currents underlying delayed rectification and pace-maker activity in frog atrial muscle. *J Physiol* 1969; 204:717–736.
124. Hume J, Katzung BG: Physiological role of endogenous amines in the modulation of ventricular automaticity in the guinea-pig. *J Physiol* 1980; 309:275–286.
125. Cranefield PF, Aronson RS: Initiation of sustained rhythmic activity by single propagated action potentials in canine cardiac Purkinje fibers exposed to sodium-free solution or to ouabain. *Circ Res* 1974; 34:477–481.
126. Cranefield PF: Action potentials, afterpotentials and arrhythmias. *Circ Res* 1977; 41:415–425.
127. Cranefield PF, Aronson RS: Cardiac arrhythmias: The role of triggered activity and other mechanisms. Mount Kisco, NY, Futura Publishing, 1988.
128. Cramer M, Siegal M, Bigger JT Jr, Hoffman BF: Characteristics of extracellular potentials recorded from the sinoatrial pacemaker of the rabbit. *Circ Res* 1977; 41:292–300.
129. Wit AL, Boyden PA, Gadsby CD, Cranefield PF: Triggered activity as a cause of atrial arrhythmias. In: Narula OS (ed): *Cardiac Arrhythmias: Electrophysiology, Diagnosis and Management.* Baltimore, Williams & Wilkins, 1979: 14–31.
130. Olsson SB, Blomström-Lundqvist C, Wohlfart B: Endocardial monophasic action potentials: Correlations with intracellular electrical activity. *Ann NY Acad Sci* 1990; 601:119–127.
131. Harriman RJ, Holzman R, Gough WB, Mehra R, Gomes JAC, El-Sherif N: In vivo demonstration of delayed afterdepolarization as a cause of ventricular rhythms in one day old infarction. *J Am Coll Cardiol* 1984; 3:478.
132. Priori SG, Mantica M, Schwartz PJ: Delayed afterdepolarizations elicited in vivo by left stellate ganglion stimulation. *Circulation* 1988; 78:178–185.
133. Fabiato A, Fabiato F: Contraction induced by a calcium-triggered release of calcium from the sarcoplasmic reticulum of single skinned cardiac cells. *J Physiol* 1975; 249:469–495.
134. Aronson RS, Gelles JM, Hoffman BF: Effect of ouabain on the current underlying spontaneous diastolic depolarization in cardiac Purkinje fibers. *Nature New Biol* 1973, 245:118–120.
135. Lederer WJ, Tsien RW: Transient inward current underlying arrhythmogenic effect of cardiotonic steroids in Purkinje fibers. *J Physiol* 1976; 263:73–100.
136. Kass RS, Lederer WJ, Tsien RW, Weingart R: Role of calcium ions in transient inward currents and after contractions induced by strophantidin in cardiac Purkinje fibers. *J Physiol* 1978; 281:187–208.
137. Kass RS, Tsien RW, Weingart R: Ionic basis of transient inward current induced by strophantidin in cardiac Purkinje fibers. *J Physiol* 1978; 281:209–226.
138. Karagueuzian HS, Katzung BG: Voltage clamp studies of transient inward current and mechanical oscillations induced by ouabain in ferret papillary muscle. *J Physiol* 1982; 327:255–271.
139. Vassalle M, Mugelli A: An oscillatory current in sheep cardiac Purkinje fibers. *Circ Res* 1981; 48:618–631.
140. Lipsius SL, Gobbins WR: Membrane currents, contractions and aftercontractions in cardiac Purkinje fibers. *Am J Physiol* 1982; 243:H77–H86.
141. Eisner DA, Lederer WJ: Inotropic and arrhythmogenic effects of potassium-depleted solutions on mammalian cardiac muscle. *J Physiol* 1979; 294:255–277.
142. Baker PF, Blaustein MP, Hodgkin AL, Steinhardt RA: The influence of calcium on sodium efflux in squid axons. *J Physiol* 1969; 200:431–458.
143. Mullins LJ: The generation of electrical currents in cardiac fibers by Na/Ca exchange. *Am J Physiol* 1979; 236:C103–C110.
144. Eisner DA, Lederer WJ: Na-Ca exchange: Stoichiometry and electrogenicity. *Am J Physiol* 1985; 248:C189–C202.
145. David LD: Effect of changes in cycle length on diastolic depolarization produced by ouabain in canine Purkinje fibers. *Circ Res* 1973; 32:206–214.
146. Ferrier GR, Saunders JH, Mendez C: A cellular mechanism for the generation of ventricular arrhythmias by acetylstrophantidin. *Circ Res* 1973; 32:600–609.
147. Ferrier GR, Moe GK: Effect of calcium on acetylstrophantidin-induced transient depolarizations in canine Purkinje tissue. *Circ Res* 1973; 33:508–515.
148. Hashimoto K, and Moe GK: Transient depolarizations induced by acetylstrophantidin in specialized tissue of dog atrium and ventricle. *Circ Res* 1973; 32:618–624.
149. Hogan PM, Wittenberg SM, Kocke FJ: Relationship of stimulation frequency to automaticity in the canine Purkinje fiber during ouabain administration. *Circ Res* 1973; 32:377–384.
150. Aronson RS, Cranefield PF: The effect of resting potential on the electrical activity of canine cardiac Purkinje fibers exposed to Na-free solution or to ouabain. *Pflügers Arch* 1974; 347:101–116.
151. Zipes DP, Arbel E, Knope RF, Moe GK: Accelerated cardiac escape rhythms caused by ouabain intoxication. *Am J Cardiol* 1974; 33:248–253.
152. Lown B, Cannon RL, Rossi MA: Electrical stimulation and digitalis drugs: Repetitive response in diastole. *Proc Soc Exptl Biol Med* 1967; 126:697–701.
153. Lown B: Electrical stimulation to estimate the degree of digitalization. II. Experimental studies. *Am J Cardiol* 1968; 22:251–259.
154. Castellanos A, Lemberg L, Centurion MJ, Berkovits BV: Concealed digitalis-induced arrhythmias unmasked by electrical stimulation of the heart. *Am Heart J* 1967; 73:484–490.
155. Deitmer JW, Ellis D: The intracellular sodium activity of cardiac Purkinje fibers during inhibition and re-activation of the Na-K pump. *J Physiol* 1978; 284:241–259.
156. Lee CO, Dagostino M: Effect of strophantidin on intracellular Na ion activity and twitch tension of constantly driven cardiac Purkinje fibers. *Biophys J* 1982; 40:185–198.
157. Lee CO, Kang DH, Sokol JH, Lee KS: Relation between intracellular Na ion activity and tension of sheep cardiac Purkinje fibers exposed to dihydro-ouabain. *Biophys J* 1980; 29:315–330.
158. Reuter H, Seitz N: The dependence of calcium efflux from cardiac muscle on temperature and external ion composition. *J Physiol* 1968; 195:451–470.
159. Mullins JL: *Ion Transport in Heart.* New York, Raven, 1981.
160. Wit A, Cranefield PF: Triggered activity in cardiac muscle fibers of the simian mitral valve. *Circ Res* 1976; 38:85–98.
161. Boyden PA, Tilley LP, Albala A, Liu SK, Fenoglio JJ Jr, Wit AL: Mechanisms for atrial arrhythmias associated with cardiomyopathy: A study of feline hearts with primary myocardial disease. *Circ Res* 1984; 69:1036–1047.
162. Malfatto G, Rosen TS, Rosen MR: The response to overdrive pacing of triggered atrial and ventricular arrhythmias in the canine heart. *Circulation* 1988; 77:1139–1148.
163. Belardinelli L, Isenberg G: Actions of adenosine and isoproterenol on isolated mammalian ventricular myocyte. *Circ Res* 1983; 53:287–297.
164. Lazzara R, Marchi S: Electrophysiological mechanisms for the generation of arrhythmias with adrenergic stimulation. In: Brachman J, Schomig A (eds): *Adrenergic System and Ventricular Arrhythmias in Myocardial Infarction.* Heidelberg, Springer Verlag, 1989: 231–238.
165. Lerman BB, Belardinelli L, West A, Berne RM, DiMarco JP: Adenosine-sensitive ventricular tachycardia: Evidence suggesting cyclic AMP–mediated triggered activity. *Circulation* 1986; 74:270–280.

166. El-Sherif N, Zeiler R, Gough WB: Effects of catecholamine, verapamil, and tetrodotoxin on triggered automaticity in canine ischemic Purkinje fibers (abstr). *Circulation* 1980; 62:III-281.
167. El-Sherif N, Gough WB, Zeiler RH, Mehra R: Triggered ventricular arrhythmias in one day old myocardial infarction in the dog. *Circ Res* 1983; 52:566–579.
168. Reuter H: Localization of beta adrenergic receptors and effects of noradrenaline and cyclic nucleotides on action potentials, ionic currents and tension in mammalian cardiac muscle. *J Physiol* 1974; 242:429–451.
169. Horn EM, Johnson NJ, Bilezikian JP, Rosen MR: Developmental changes in the electrophysiological properties and the beta-adrenergic receptor-effector complex in atrial fibers of the canine coronary sinus. *Circ Res* 1989; 65:325–333.
170. Morad M, Rolett E: Relaxing effect of catecholamine on mammalian heart. *J Physiol* 1972; 224:537–558.
171. Fabiato A: Calcium-induced release of calcium from the cardiac sarcoplasmic reticulum. *Am J Physiol* 1983; 245:C1–C14.
172. Saito T, Otoguro M, Matsubara T: Electrophysiological studies on the mechanism of electrically induced sustained rhythmic activity in the rabbit right atrium. *Circ Res* 1978; 42:199–206.
173. Mary-Rabine L, Hordof AJ, Danilo P, Malm JR, Rosen MR: Mechanisms for impulse initiation in isolated human atrial fibers. *Circ Res* 1980; 47:267–277.
174. Aronson RS: Afterpotentials and triggered activity in hypertrophied myocardium from rats with renal hypertension. *Circ Res* 1981; 48:720–727.
175. Nordin C, Gilat E, Aronson RS: Delayed afterdepolarizations and triggered activity in ventricular muscle from rats with streptozotocin-induced diabetes. *Circ Res* 1985; 57:28–34.
176. Arlock P, Katzung BG: Effects of sodium substitutes on transient inward current and tension in guinea-pig and ferret papillary muscle. *J Physiol* 1985; 360:105–120.
177. Ferrier G: Effects of transmembrane potential on oscillatory afterpotentials induced by acetylstrophantidin in canine ventricular tissues. *J Pharm Exp Ther* 1981; 215:332–341.
178. Wasserstrom JA, Ferrier GR: Voltage dependence of digitalis afterpotentials, aftercontractions, and inotropy. *Am J Physiol* 1981; 241:H646–H653.
179. Henning B, Wit AL: Action potential characteristics control afterdepolarization amplitude and triggered activity in canine coronary sinus. *Circulation* 1981; 64:IV-50.
180. LeMarec H, Dangman KH, Danilo P, Rosen MR: An evaluation of automaticity and triggered activity in the canine heart one to four days after myocardial infarction. *Circulation* 1985; 71:1224–1236.
181. Gough WB, El-Sherif N: Dependence of delayed afterdepolarizations on diastolic potentials in ischemic Purkinje fibers. *Am J Physiol* 1989; 257:H770–H777.
182. Wit AL, Tseng G-N, Henning B, Hanna MS: Arrhythmogenic effects of quinidine on catecholamine-induced delayed afterdepolarizations in canine atrial fibers. *J Cardiovasc Electrophysiol* 1990; 1:15–30.
183. Sheu SS, Lederer WJ: Lidocaine's negative inotropic and antiarrhythmic actions: Dependence on shortening of action potential duration and reduction of intracellular sodium activity. *Circ Res* 1985; 57:578–590.
184. Aronson RS: Characteristics of action potentials of hypertrophied myocardium from rats with renal hypertension. *Circ Res* 1980; 47:443–454.
185. Moak JP, Rosen MF: Induction and termination of triggered activity by pacing in isolated canine Purkinje fibers. *Circulation* 1984; 69:149–162.
186. Wit AL, Gadsby DC, Cranefield PF: Electrogenic sodium extrusion can stop triggered activity in the canine coronary sinus. *Circ Res* 1981; 49:1029–1042.
187. Johnson N, Danilo P, Wit A, Rosen MR: Response to pacing of triggered activity occurring in catecholamine-treated canine coronary sinus. *Circulation* 1986; 74:1168–1179.
188. Gadsby DC, Cranefield PF: Direct measurement of changes in sodium pump current in canine cardiac Purkinje fibers. *Proc Natl Acad Sci USA* 1979; 76:1783–1787.
189. Johnson N, Rosen MR: The distinction between triggered activity and other cardiac arrhythmias. In: Brugada P, Wellens HJJ (eds): *Cardiac Arrhythmias: Where to Go from Here.* Mount Kisco, NY, Futura Publishing, 1987: 129–145.
190. Dangman KH, Hoffman BF: The effects of single premature stimuli on automatic and triggered rhythms in isolated canine Purkinje fibers. *Circulation* 1985; 71:813–822.
191. Trautwein W: Mechanisms of tachyarrhythmias and extrasystoles. In: Sandoe E, Flenstad-Jenson E, Olesen K (eds): *Symposium on Cardiac Arrhythmias.* Sodertalje, Sweden, AB Astra, 1970: 53–66.
192. January CT, Shorofsky S: Early afterdepolarizations: Newer insights into cellular mechanisms. *J Cardiovasc Electrophysiol* 1990; 1:161–169.
193. Mendez C, Delmar M: Triggered activity: Its possible role in cardiac arrhythmias. In: Zipes DP, Jalife J (eds): *Cardiac Electrophysiology and Arrhythmias.* Orlando, FL, Grune & Stratton, 1985: 311–313.
194. Kupersmith J, Hoff P: Occurrence and transmission of localized repolarization abnormalities in vitro. *J Am Coll Cardiol* 1985; 6:152–160.
195. Wit AL, Wiggins JR, Cranefield PF: Some effects of electrical stimulation on impulse initiation in cardiac fibers: Its relevance for the determination of the mechanisms of clinical cardiac arrhythmias. In: Wellens JHH, Lie KI, Janse MJ (eds): *The Conduction System of the Heart.* Philadelphia, Lea & Febiger, 1976: 163–181.
196. Damiano BP, Rosen MR: Effects of pacing on triggered activity induced by early afterdepolarizations. *Circulation* 1984; 69:1013–1025.
197. Brachmann J, Scherlag BJ, Rosenshtraukh LV, Lazzara R: Bradycardia dependent triggered activity: Relevance to drug-induced multiform ventricular tachycardia. *Circulation* 1983; 68:846–856.
198. Kay GN, Plumb VJ, Arciniegas JG, Henthorn RW, Waldo AL: Torsade de pointes: The long-short initiating sequence and other clinical features: Observations in 32 patients. *J Am Coll Cardiol* 1983; 2:806–817.
199. Ben David J, Zipes DP: Differential response to right and left ansae subclaviae stimulation of early afterdepolarizations and ventricular tachycardia induced by cesium in dogs. *Circulation* 1988; 78:1241–1250.
200. Levine JH, Spear JF, Guarnieri T, Weisfeldt M, de Langen CDJ, Becker LC, Moore EN: Cesium chloride-induced long QT syndrome: Demonstration of afterdepolarizations and triggered activity in vivo. *Circulation* 1985; 72:1092–1104.
201. Strauss, HC, Bigger JT Jr, Hoffman BF. Electrophysiological and beta-blocking effects of MJ 1999 on dog and rabbit cardiac tissue. *Circ Res* 1970; 26:661–678.
202. Carmeliet E: Electrophysiologic and voltage clamp analyses of the effects of sotalol on isolated cardiac muscle and Purkinje fibers. *J Pharmacol Exptl Ther* 1985; 232:817–825.
203. Dangman KH, Hoffman BF: In vivo and in vitro antiarrhythmic and arrhythmogenic effects of *N*-acetylprocainamide. *J Pharmacol Exp Ther* 1981; 217:851–862.
204. Roden DM, Hoffman BF: Action potential prolongation and induction of abnormal automaticity by low quinidine concentrations in canine Purkinje fibers. Relationship to potassium and cycle length. *Circ Res* 1985; 56:857–867.
205. Davidenko JM, Cohen L, Goodrow R, Antzelevitch C. Quinidine-induced action potential prolongation, early afterdepolarizations, and triggered activity in canine Purkinje fibers: Effects of stimulation rate, potassium, and magnesium. *Circulation* 1989; 79:674–686.
206. Colatsky T: Mechanisms of action of lidocaine and quinidine on action potential duration in rabbit cardiac Purkinje fibers: An effect on steady-state sodium currents. *Circ Res* 1982; 50: 17–27.
207. Selzer A, Wray HW: Quinidine syncope. Paroxysmal ventricular fibrillation occurring during treatment of chronic atrial arrhythmias. *Circulation* 1964; 30:17–26.
208. Smith WM, Gallagher JJ: "Les torsades de pointes." An unusual ventricular arrhythmia. *Ann Intern Med* 1980; 93:578–584.
209. Olshansky B, Martins J, Hunt S: *N*-acetyl procainamide causing torsades de pointes. *Am J Cardiol* 1982; 50:1439–1441.
210. Kuck KH, Kunze DP, Roewer N, Bleifield W: Sotalol-induced torsade de pointes. *Am Heart J* 1984; 107:179–180.
211. Bailie DS, Inoue H, Kaseda S, Ben-David J, Zipes DP: Magnesium suppression of early afterdepolarizations and ventricular tachyarrhythmias induced by cesium in dogs. *Circulation* 1988; 77:1395–1402.
212. Tzivoni D, Keren A, Cohen AM, Loebel H, Zahavi I, Chenzbraun

A, et al: Magnesium therapy for torsade de pointes. *Am J Cardiol* 1984; 53:528–530.
213. Perticone F, Adinolfi L, Bonaduce D: Efficacy of magnesium sulfate in the treatment of torsade de pointes. *Am Heart J* 1986; 112:847–849.
214. Mines GR: On dynamic equilibrium in the heart. *J Physiol (Lond)* 1913; 46:349–383.
215. Lewis T: *The Mechanism and Graphic Registration of the Heart Beat,* 3d ed. London, Shaw & Sons, 1925.
216. Smeets JLRM, Allessie MA, Lammers WJEP, Bonke FIM, Hollen J: The wavelength of cardiac impulse and reentrant arrhythmias in isolated rabbit atrium: The role of heart rate, autonomic transmitters, temperature, and potassium. *Circ Res* 1986; 58:96–108.
217. Garrey W: The nature of fibrillary contraction of the heart. Its relation to tissue mass and form. *Am J Physiol* 1914; 33:397–414.
218. Coumel P, Cabrol C, Fabiato A, Gourgon R, Slama R: Tachycardie permanente par rhythme reciproque. *Arch Mal Coeur* 1967; 60:1830–1864.
219. Critelli G, Gallagher JJ, Monda V, Coltorti F, Scherillo M, Rossi L: Anatomic and electrohysiologic substrate of the permanent form of junctional reciprocating tachycardia. *J Am Coll Cardiol* 1984; 4:601–610.
220. Wit AL, Cranefield PF, Hoffman BF: Slow conduction and reentry in the ventricular conducting system. II. Single and sustained circus movement in networks of canine and bovine Purkinje fibers. *Circ Res* 1972; 30:11–22.
221. Boyden PA: Activation sequence during atrial flutter in dogs with surgically induced right atrial enlargement. I. Observations during sustained rhythms. *Circ Res* 1988; 62:596–608.
222. Shimizu A, Nozaki A, Rudy Y, Waldo AL: Onset of induced atrial flutter in the canine pericarditis model. *J Am Coll Cardiol* 1991; 17:1223–1234.
223. Klein H, Karp RB, Kouchoukus NT, Zorn GL Jr, James TN, Waldo AL: Intraoperative electrophysiological mapping of the ventricles during sinus rhythm in patients with a previous myocardial infarction. Identification of the electrophysiological substrate for the generation of ventricular arrhythmias. *Circulation* 1982; 66:847–853.
224. Fozzard HA: Conduction of the action potential. In: Berne RM (ed): *The Cardiovascular System.* The American Physiological Society, Bethesda, MD, 1979: 335–356.
225. Weidmann S: The effect of the cardiac membrane potential on the rapid availability of the sodium carrying system. *J Physiol* 1955; 127:213–224.
226. Gettes LS, Reuter H: Slow recovery from inactivation of inward currents in mammalian myocardial fibers. *J Physiol* 1974; 240:703–724.
227. Dodge FA, Cranefield PF: Nonuniform conduction in cardiac Purkinje fibers. In: Paes de Carvalho A, Hoffman BF, Lieberman M (eds): *Normal and Abnormal Conduction in the Heart.* Mount Kisco, NY, Futura Publishing, 1982: 379–395.
228. Tsien RW: Calcium channels in excitable cell membranes. *Ann Rev Physiol* 1983; 45:341–358.
229. Zipes DP, Mendez C: Action of manganese ions and tetrodotoxin on atrioventricular nodal transmembrane potentials in isolated rabbit hearts. *Circ Res* 1973; 32:447–454.
230. Spach MS, Miller WT, Geselowitz DB, Barr RC, Kootsey JM, Johnson EA: The discontinuous nature of propagation in normal canine cardiac muscle: Evidence for recurrent discontinuities of intracellular resistance that effect membrane currents. *Circ Res* 1981; 48:39–54.
231. Spach MS, Miller WT, Dolber PC, Kootsey JM, Sommer JR, Mosher EC: The functional role of structural complexities in the propagation of depolarization in the atrium of the dog: Cardiac conduction disturbances due to discontinuities of effective axial resistivity. *Circ Res* 1982; 50:175–191.
232. Sommer JR, Dolber PC: Cardiac muscle: The ultrastructure of its cells and bundles. In: Hoffman BF, Lieberman M, Paes de Carvallo A (eds): *Normal and Abnormal Conduction of the Heart Beat.* Mount Kisco, NY, Futura Publishing, 1982: 1–27.
233. Hoyt RH, Cohen ML, Saffitz JE: Distribution and three-dimensional structure of intercellular junctions in canine myocardium. *Circ Res* 1989; 64:563–574.
234. Roberts DE, Hersh LT, Scher AM: Influence of cardiac fiber orientation on wavefront voltage, conduction velocity and tissue resistivity in the dog. *Circ Res* 1979; 44:701–712.
235. Clerc L: Directional differences of impulse spread in trabecular muscle from mammalian heart. *J Physiol* 1976; 255:335–346.
236. Spach MS, Dolber PC: Relating extracellular potentials and their derivatives to anisotropic propagation at a microscopic level in human cardiac muscle. Evidence for uncoupling of side-to-side fiber connections with increasing age. *Circ Res* 1986; 58:356–371.
237. Spach MS, Dolber PC, Heidlage JF: Influence of the passive anisotropic properties on directional differences in propagation following modification of the sodium conductance in human atrial muscle: A model of reentry based on anisotropic discontinuous propagation. *Circ Res* 1988; 62:811–832.
238. Hunter Pj, McNaughten PA, Noble D: Analytical models of propagation in excitable cells. *Prog Biophys Mol Biol* 1975; 30:99–144.
239. Dominguez G, Fozzard HA: Influence of extracellular K^+ concentration on cable properties and excitability of sheep cardiac Purkinje fibers. *Circ Res* 1970; 26:565–574.
240. Spach MS, Miller WT, Miller-Jones E, Warren RB, Barr RC: Extracellular potentials related to intracellular action potentials during impulse conduction in anisotropic canine cardiac muscle. *Circ Res* 1979; 45:188–204.
241. Rudy Y, Quan W: A model study of the effects of the discrete cellular structure on electrical propagation in cardiac tissue. *Circ Res* 1987; 61:815–823.
242. Quan W, Rudy Y: Unidirectional block and reentry of cardiac excitation: A model study. *Circ Res* 1990; 60:367–382.
243. DeMello WC: Effect of intracellular injection of calcium and strontium in cell communication in heart. *J Physiol* 1975; 250:231–245.
244. Hess SP, Weingart R: Intracellular free calcium modified by pH_i in sheep cardiac Purkinje fibres. *J Physiol* 1980; 307:60P–61P.
245. Van Dam RTh: Experimenteel onderzoek naar het prikkelbaarheidsverloop van de hartspier. Thesis, University of Amsterdam, Klein Offsetdrukkerij Poortpers, Amsterdam, 1960.
246. Rensma PL, Allessie MA, Lammers WJEP, Bonke FIM, Schalij MJ: Length of excitation wave and susceptibility to reentrant atrial arrhythmias in normal conscious dogs. *Circ Res* 1988; 62:395–410.
247. Allessie MA, Bonke FIM, Schopman FJG: Circus movement in rabbit atrial muscle as a mechanism of tachycardia. 2. The role of nonuniform recovery of excitability in the occurrence of unidirectional block as studied with multiple microelectrodes. *Circ Res* 1976; 39:168–177.
248. Han J, Moe GK: Nonuniform recovery of excitability of ventricular muscle. *Circ Res* 1964; 14:44–60.
249. Janse MJ: The effects of changes in heart rate on the refractory period of the heart. Thesis, University of Amsterdam, Mondeel-Offsetdrukkerij, 1971.
250. Wallace AG, Mignone RS: Physiologic evidence concerning the reentry hypothesis for ectopic beats. *Am Heart J* 1966; 72:60–70.
251. Kuo C-S, Munakata K, Reddy CP, Surawicz B: Characteristics and possible mechanisms of ventricular arrhythmia dependent on the dispersion of action potential durations. *Circulation* 1983; 67:1356–1367.
252. Cranefield PF, Klein HO, Hoffman BF: Conduction of the cardiac impulse: 1. Delay, block and one-way block in the pressed Purkinje fibers. *Circ Res* 1971; 28:199–219.
253. Joyner RW, Overholt ED, Ramza B, Veenstra RD: Propagation through electrically coupled cells: Two inhomogeneously coupled cardiac tissue layers. *Am J Physiol* 1984; 247:H596–H609.
254. Goldstein SS, Rall W: Changes in action potential shape and velocity for changing core conductor geometry. *Biophys J* 1974; 14:731–757.
255. Overholt ED, Joyner RW, Veenstra RD, Rawling D, Wiedmann R: Unidirectional block between Purkinje and ventricular layers of papillary muscles. *Am J Physiol* 1984; 247:H584–H595.
256. Janse MJ, Wilms-Schopman F, Wilensky RJ, Tranum-Jensen J: Role of the subendocardium in arrhythmogenesis during acute ischemia. In: Zipes DP, Jalife J (eds): *Cardiac Electrophysiology and Arrhythmias,* Orlando, FL, Grune & Stratton, 1985: 353–362.
257. Gilmour RF, Evans JJ, Zipes DP: Purkinje-muscle coupling and endocardial response to hyperkalemia, hypoxia, and acidosis. *Am J Physiol* 1984; 247:H303–H311.
258. Gilmour RF, Evans JJ, Zipes DP: Preferential interruption of

impulse transmission across Purkinje-muscle junctions by interventions that depress conduction. In: Zipes DP, Jalife J (eds): *Cardiac Electrophysiology and Arrhythmias,* Orlando, FL, Grune & Stratton, 1985; 287–300.
259. Delmar M, Michaels DC, Johnson T, Jalife J: Effects of increasing intercellular resistance on transverse and longitudinal propagation in sheep epicardial muscle. *Circ Res* 1987; 60:780–785.
260. Delgado C, Steinhaus B, Delmar M, Chialvo DR, Jalife J: Directional differences in excitability and margin of safety for propagation in sheep ventricular epicardial muscle. *Circ Res* 1990; 67:97–110.
261. Frame LH, Page RL, Boyden PA, Fenoglio JJ Jr, Hoffman BF: Circus movement in the canine atrium around the tricuspid ring during experimental atrial flutter and during reentry in vitro. *Circulation* 1987; 76:1155–1175.
262. Moe GK: On the multiple wavelet hypothesis of atrial fibrillation. *Arch Int Pharmacodyn* 1962; 140:180–188.
263. Moe GK, Rheinboldt WC, Abildskov JA: A computer model of atrial fibrillation. *Am Heart J* 1964; 67:200–220.
264. Coumel P: Role of the autonomic nervous system in paroxysmal atrial fibrillation. In: Touboul P, Waldo AL (eds): *Atrial Arrhythmias.* Mosby-YearBook, St. Louis, 1990: 248–261.
265. Allessie MA, Lammers WJEP, Bonke FIM, Hollen J: Experimental evaluation of Moe's multiple wavelet hypothesis of atrial fibrillation. In: Zipes DP, Jalife J (eds): *Cardiac Electrophysiology and Arrhythmias.* New York, Grune & Stratton, 1985: 265–275.
266. Waldo AL: Mechanisms of atrial fibrillation, atrial flutter, and ectopic atrial tachycardia—A brief review. *Circulation* 1987; 75-III:37–40.
267. Allessie MA, Bonke FIM, Schopman FJG: Circus movement in rabbit atrial muscle as a mechanism of tachycardia. 3. The "leading circle" concept: A new model of circus movement in cardiac tissue without the involvement of an anatomical obstacle. *Circ Res* 1977; 41:9–18.
268. Allessie MA, Lammers WJEP, Bonke FIM, Hollen J: Intra-atrial reentry as a mechanism for atrial flutter by acetylcholine and rapid pacing in the dog. *Circulation* 1984; 70:123–135.
269. Okumura K, Plumb VJ, Pagé PL, Waldo AL: Atrial activation sequence during atrial flutter in the canine pericarditis model and its effects on the polarity of the flutter wave in the electrocardiogram. *J Am Coll Cardiol* 1991; 17:509–518.
270. Cosío FG: Endocardial mapping of atrial flutter. In: Touboul P, Waldo AL (eds): *Atrial Arrhythmias—Current Concepts and Management.* St. Louis, Mosby-YearBook, 1990: 229–240.
271. Spinelli W, Hoffman BF: Mechanisms of termination of reentrant atrial arrhythmias by Class I and Class III antiarrhythmic agents. *Circ Res* 1989; 65:1565–1579.
272. Wit AL, Dillon SM: Anisotropic reentry. In: Zipes DP, Jalife J (eds): *Cardiac Electrophysiology—From Cell to Bedside.* Philadelphia, Saunders, 1990: 353–364.
273. Allessie MA, Bonke FIM, Schopman FJG: Circus movement in rabbit atrial muscle as a mechanism of tachycardia. *Circ Res* 1973; 32:54–62.
274. Dillon S, Allessie MA, Ursell PC, Wit AL: Influence of anisotropic tissue structure on reentrant circuits and the sub-epicardial border zone of subacute canine infarcts. *Circ Res* 1988; 63:182–206.
275. Schalij MJ: Anisotropic conduction and ventricular tachycardia. Ph.D. Thesis, University of Limburg, Maastricht, The Netherlands, 1988.
276. Lammers WJEP, Wit AL, Allessie MA: Effects of anisotropy on functional reentrant circuits: Preliminary results of computer simulation studies. In: Sideman S, Beyar R (eds): *Activation, Metabolism, and Perfusion of the Heart.* Dordrecht, Martinus Nijhoff, 1987: 133–150.
277. Mayer AG: Rhythmical pulsation in Scyphomedusae: II. *Pap Tortugas Lab Carnegie Inst Wash.* 1908; 1: 113–131.
278. Mines GR: On circulating excitation in heart muscles and their possible relations to tachycardia and fibrillation. *Trans R Soc Can* 1914; 8(ser III, sec IV):43–52.
279. Goldreyer BN, Gallagher JJ, Damato AN: The electrophysiologic demonstration of atrial ectopic tachycardia in man. *Am Heart J* 1973; 85:205–215.
280. Scheinman MM, Basu D, Holenberg M: Electrophysiologic studies in patients with persistent atrial tachycardia. *Circulation* 1974; 50:266–273.
281. Strauss HC, Saroff AL, Bigger JT Jr, Giardina GV: Premature atrial stimulation as a key to the understanding of sinoatrial conduction in man. Presentation of data and critical review of the literature. *Circulation* 1973; 47:86–93.
282. Gillette PC, Garson A Jr: Electrophysiologic and pharmacologic characteristics of automatic ectopic atrial tachycardia. *Circulation* 1977; 56:571–575.
283. Klein HO, Cranefield PF, Hoffman BF: Effect of extrasystoles on idioventricular rhythm. *Circ Res* 1972; 30:651–665.
284. Palileo EV, Ashley WW, Swiryn S, Bauernfeind RA, Strasberg B, Petropoulis AT, et al: Exercise provokable right ventricular outflow tract tachycardia. *Am Heart J* 1982; 104:185–193.
285. Sung RJ, Shen EN, Morady F, Scheinman MM, Hess D, Botvinick CH: Electrophysiologic mechanism of exercise-induced sustained ventricular tachycardia. *Am J Cardiol* 1983; 51:525–530.
286. Wellens HJJ: Value and limitations of programmed electrical stimulation of the heart in the study and treatment of tachycardias. *Circulation* 1978; 57:845–853.
287. Goldreyer BN, Bigger JT Jr: Site of reentry in paroxysmal supraventricular tachycardia in man. *Circulation* 1971; 43:15–26.
288. Bigger JT Jr, Goldreyer BN: The mechanism of supraventricular tachycardia. *Circulation* 1970; 42:673–688.
289. Waldo AL: Cardiac pacing: Role in diagnosis and treatment of disorders of cardiac rhythm and conduction. In: Rosen MRR, Hoffman BF (eds): *Cardiac Therapy.* Boston, Martinus Nijhoff, 1983: 299–336.
290. Waldo AL, MacLean WAH, Karp RB, Kouchoukos NT, James TN: Entrainment and interruption of atrial flutter with atrial pacing. Studies in man following open heart surgery. *Circulation* 1977; 56:737–744.
291. Waldo AL, Plumb VJ, Henthorn RW: Observations on the mechanism of atrial flutter. In: Surawicz B, Reddy CP, Prystowsky EN (eds): *Tachycardias.* The Hague, Martinus Nijhoff, 1984: 213–229.
292. Olshansky B, Okumura K, Henthorn RW, Waldo AL: Characterization of double potentials in human atrial flutter: Studies during transient entrainment. *J Am Coll Cardiol* 1990, 15:833–841.
293. Olshansky B, Okumura K, Hess PG, Waldo AL: Demonstration of an area of slow conduction in human atrial flutter. *J Am Coll Cardiol* 1990; 16:1639–1648.
294. MacLean WAH, Plumb VJ, Waldo AL: Transient entrainment and interruption of ventricular tachycardia. *PACE* 1981; 4:358–366.
295. Waldo AL, Henthorn RW, Plumb VJ, MacLean WAH: Demonstration of the mechanism of transient entrainment and interruption of ventricular tachycardia with rapid atrial pacing. *J Am Coll Cardiol* 1984; 3:422–430.
296. Okumura K, Olshansky B, Henthron RW, Epstein AE, Plumb VJ, Waldo AL: Demonstration of the presence of slow conduction during sustained ventricular tachycardia in man. *Circulation* 1987; 75:369–378.
297. Waldo AL, Plumb VJ, Arciniegas JG, MacLean WAH, Cooper TB, Priest MF, et al: Transient entrainment and interruption of AV bypass pathway type paroxysmal atrial tachycardia. A model for understanding and identifying reentrant arrhythmias in man. *Circulation* 1982; 67:73–83.
298. Okumura K, Henthorn RW, Epstein AE, Plumb VJO, Waldo AL: Further observations on transient entrainment: Importance of pacing site and properties of the components of the reentry circuit. *Circulation* 1985; 72:1293–1307.
299. Brugada P, Waldo AL, Wellens HJJ: Transient entrainment and interruption of atrioventricular tachycardia. *J Am Coll Cardiol* 1987; 9:769–775.
300. Henthron RW, Okumura K, Olshansky B, Waldo AL: A fourth criterion for transient entrainment: The electrogram equivalent of progressive fusion. *Circulation* 1988; 77:1003–1012.
301. Chen P-S, Lowe JE, German LD, Vidaillet HJ Jr, Greer GS, Smith WM, et al: Mapping ventricular fusion beats during entrainment. *Circulation* 1986; 74-II:484.
302. El-Sherif N, Gough WB, Restivo M: Reentrant ventricular arrhythmias in the late myocardial infarction period: 14. Mechanisms of resetting, entrrainment, acceleration, or termination of reentrant tachycardia by programmed electrical stimulation. *PACE* 1987; 10:341–371.
303. Waldecker B, Coromilas J, Saltman AE, Dillon SM, Wit AL: Overdrive stimulation of functional reentrant circuits causing ventricular tachycardia in the infarcted canine heart—Resetting and entrainment. *Circulation,* 1993; 87:1286–1305.

304. Boyden PA, Frame LH, Hoffman BF: Activation mapping of reentry around an anatomic barrier in the canine atrium. *Circulation* 1989; 79:406–416.
305. Shimizu A, Nozaki A, Rudy Y, Waldo AL: Multiplexing studies of effects of rapid atrial pacing on the area of slow conduction during atrial flutter in canine pericarditis model. *Circulation* 1991; 83:983–994.
306. Frank R, Tonet JL, Kounde S, Farenq G, Fontaine G: Localization of the area of slow conduction during ventricular tachycardia. In: Brugada P, Wellen HJJ (eds): *Cardiac Arrhythmias: Where to Go From Here?* Mount Kisco, NY, Futura Publishing, 1987: 191–208.
307. Morady F, Frank R, Kou WH Tonet JL, Nelson SD, Kounde S, et al: Identification and catheter ablation of a zone of slow conduction in the reentrant circuit of ventricular tachycardia in humans. *J Am Coll Cardiol* 1988; 11:775–782.
308. Stevenson WG, Weiss JN, Wiener I, Nademanee K, Wohlgelernter D, Yeatman L, et al: Resetting of ventricular tachycardia: Implications for localizing the area of slow conduction. *J Am Coll Cardiol* 1988; 11:522–529.
309. Almendral JM, Rosenthal ME, Stamato NJ, Marchlinski FE, Buxton AE, Frame LH, et al: Analysis of the resetting phenomenon in sustained uniform ventricular tachycardia: Incidence and relation to termination. *J Am Coll Cardiol* 1986; 8:294–300.
310. Almendral JM, Stamato NJ, Rosenthal ME, Marchlinski FE, Miller JM, Josephson ME: Resetting response patterns during sustained ventricular tachycardia: Relationship to the excitable gap. *Circulation* 1986; 74:722–730.
311. Stamato NJ, Rosenthal ME, Almendral JM, Josephson ME: The resetting response of ventricular tachycardia to single and double extrastimuli: Implications for an excitable gap. *Am J Cardiol* 1987; 60:596–601.
312. Bernstein RC, Frame LH: Ventricular reentry around a fixed barrier: Resetting with advancement in an in vitro model. *Circulation* 1990; 81:267–280.
313. Frame LH, Page RL, Hoffman BF: Atrial reentry around an anatomic barrier with a partially refractory excitable gap. *Circ Res* 1986; 58:495–511.
314. Rosen MR, Fisch C, Hoffman BF, Danilo P, Lovace DE, Knoebel SB: Can accelerated atrioventricular junctional escape rhythms be explained by delayed afterdepolarizations? *Am J Cardiol* 1980; 45:1272–1284.
315. Rosen MR, Reder RF: Does triggered activity have a role in the genesis of cardiac arrhythmias? *Ann Intern Med* 1981; 94:794–801.
316. Gorgels APM, Beekman HDM, Brugada P, Dassen WRM, Richards DAB, Wellens HJJ: Extrastimulus-related shortening of the first post pacing interval in digitalis-induced ventricular tachycardia: Observations during programmed electrical stimulation in the conscious dog. *J Am Coll Cardiol* 1983; 1:840–857.
317. Wit AL, Rosen MR: Afterdepolarizations and triggered activity. In: Fozzard HA, Jennings RB, Haber E, et al (eds): *The Heart and Cardiovascular System. Scientific Foundations.* New York, Raven, 1986: 1449–1490.
318. Akhtar M: Supraventricular tachycardias. Electrophysiologic mechanisms, diagnosis, and pharmacologic therapy. In: Josephson ME, Wellens HJJ (eds): *Tachycardias: Mechanisms, Diagnosis, Treatment.* Philadelphia, Lea & Febiger, 1984: 137–169.
319. Josephson ME, Marchlinski FE, Buxton AE, Waxman HL, Doherty JU, Kienzle MG, et al: Electrophysiologic basis for sustained ventricular tachycardia—role of reentry. In: Josephson ME, Wellens HJJ (eds): *Tachycardias: Mechanisms, Diagnosis, Treatment.* Philadelphia, Lea & Febiger, 1984: 305–323.
320. Vos MA, Gorgels APM, Leunisse JDM, Brugada P, Wellens HJJ: The effect of an entrainment protocol on ouabain-induced ventricular tachycardia. *PACE* 1989; 12:1485–1493.
321. Brugada P, Wellens HJJ: Programmed electrical stimulation of the human heart. General principles. In: Josephson ME, Wellens HJJ (eds): *Tachycardias: Mechanisms, Diagnosis, Treatment.* Philadelphia, Lea & Febiger, 1984: 61–89.
322. Jackman WM, Clark M, Friday KJ, Aliot EM, Anderson J, Lazzara R: Ventricular tacharrhythmias in the long QT syndromes. *Med Clin N Am* 1984; 68: 1079–1109.
323. Schecter E, Freeman CC, Lazzara R: Afterdepolarizations as a mechanism for the long QT syndrome. Electrophysiologic studies of a case. *J Am Coll Cardiol* 1984; 3:1556–1561.
324. Coumel P, LeClercq J, Dessertenne F: Torsades de pointes. In: Josephson ME, Wellens HJJ (eds): *Tachycardia: Mechanisms, Diagnosis, Treatment.* Philadelphia, Lea & Febiger, 1984: 325–351.

Chapter 36

Recognition, Clinical Assessment, and Management of Arrhythmias and Conduction Disturbances

Robert J. Myerburg, M.D. ■ Kenneth M. Kessler, M.D.
Agustin Castellanos, M.D.

The principles used for the diagnosis and management of cardiac arrhythmias and conduction disturbances are structured around three interacting considerations: (1) electrocardiographic analysis of the rhythm disturbance, (2) assessment of the clinical setting, and (3) identification of an appropriate endpoint of therapy.[1]

- Electrocardiographic recognition of arrhythmias requires an organized system of analysis of atrial and ventricular muscle activation and deduction of atrioventricular (AV) conduction patterns. Forms of arrhythmias are separated into those that are considered *triggering arrhythmias*,[2] such as premature atrial or ventricular impulses, and those that are considered *sustained arrhythmias*, such as supraventricular or ventricular tachycardias, ventricular fibrillation, or bradycardias (Table 36-1).
- Clinical settings are broadly divided into those that cause *acute* or *transient* electrophysiological abnormalities, such as acute ischemia, the acute phase of myocardial infarction, electrolyte disturbances, or proarrhythmic effects of antiarrhythmic drugs, and those that are *chronic* and cause *persistent* or *recurrent* arrhythmias. Commonly, the latter include chronic ischemic heart disease, cardiomyopathies, and the anatomic and physiological substrate for the various paroxysmal supraventricular tachyarrhythmias.[3] Analogous to the "triggering" and "sustained" arrhythmia concept, transient ischemia or hemodynamic disturbances may be viewed as "triggering events" and chronic ischemic heart disease, or the hypertrophied or myopathic heart, as the "sustaining" substrate.
- The goals or endpoints of therapy of cardiac arrhythmias are dependent on the forms, clinical settings, and mechanisms of arrhythmia. Broadly, goals of treatment may be *antiarrhythmic* (targeted to the suppression of triggering arrhythmias or events) or *antitachycardiac*, *antifibrillatory*, or *heart rate supporting* (in which the goal is prevention or reversion of sustained arrhythmias, whether well-tolerated, symptomatic, or life threatening).

PRINCIPLES OF RHYTHM ANALYSIS

The Standard Electrocardiogram

Both historically and in current clinical practice, the standard 12-lead electrocardiogram (ECG) and rhythm strips provide a direct and easily accessible method for diagnosing disturbances of cardiac rhythm. The simultaneous 3-lead rhythm strip accompanying the 12-lead ECG on modern ECG machines, plus the option of recording a

TABLE 36-1
Assessment of Cardiac Arrhythmias

Forms of cardiac arrhythmias
Triggering arrhythmias (e.g., premature atrial or ventricular impulses)
Sustained or potentially lethal arrhythmias (e.g., supraventricular or ventricular tachycardias, ventricular fibrillation, sustained bradyarrhythmias)
Clinical settings in which arrhythmias occur
Acute, transient (e.g., acute ischemic events, metabolic disturbances)
Chronic, persistent, recurrent (e.g., chronic ischemic heart disease, cardiomyopathy, anatomic/physiological substrate for paroxysmal supraventricular tachycardia, chronic conducting system disease)
End-points of management
Antidysrhythmic (suppress triggering arrhythmias)
Antitachycardia/antifibrillatory (prevent or revert tachycardias or fibrillation)
Heart rate support (prevent symptomatic bradycardias)

SOURCE: Modified from R Myerburg et al.[1] With permission of the *American Heart Journal.*

longer 1-lead rhythm strip, will yield sufficient information for a prompt and accurate diagnosis of most cardiac rhythms.

For many arrhythmias, analysis requires only the recognition of P-wave and QRS morphology and their relative timing. Simple inspection of the tracing may be sufficient, but the analysis of more complex arrhythmias is facilitated by the use of *ladder diagrams*. First used extensively by Sir Thomas Lewis, they are also referred to as *Lewis lines*. The ladders are usually constructed with three tiers—A, AV, and V (Fig. 36-1*A*)—but additional tiers may be helpful in depicting events related to sinoatrial conduction (Fig. 36-1*B*) or ventricular ectopic rhythms (Fig. 36-1*C*).

The A and V tiers depict activation of atrial (A) and ventricular (V) muscle. The middle tier (AV) is used to infer conduction characteristics in the AV junction. Since atrial and ventricular activation are the only direct registrations of electrical activity on the ECG, they are diagrammed first. The "A" line is drawn from the beginning of the P wave, and the "V" line from the beginning of the QRS. Time is indicated by the slope of the line, and the site within a tier in which impulse propagation begins (upper, middle, or lower) shows the direction the impulse is traveling. The site of origin may be represented by a black dot. A blocked impulse is indicated by a short bar at a right angle to the main line, and aberrant intraventricular conduction is shown as a pair of slightly divergent lines. A variety of such examples are shown in Fig. 36-1.

In using the diagram, particularly for complex arrhythmias, the first caution is to draw only what can be seen or inferred with certainty. Subsequently, the AV tier can be filled with proposed mechanisms of conduction (Fig. 36-2).

Special Leads

When the standard ECG does not provide sufficient information to establish a diagnosis, usually due to inability to identify P waves, special lead systems may be used. A bipolar esophageal lead can record left atrial activity, and an intraatrial electrode catheter can record activity in the right atrium. For both techniques, it is necessary to have a standard surface ECG lead recorded simultaneously with the special lead.

Continuous Monitor Recordings

Constant monitoring of cardiac rhythm may be performed in hospital in special care units or in the outpatient using various types of ambulatory recording devices. Both types of systems now provide the capability for simultaneous two-lead recordings that considerably improve diagnostic yield. The addition of long-term stor-

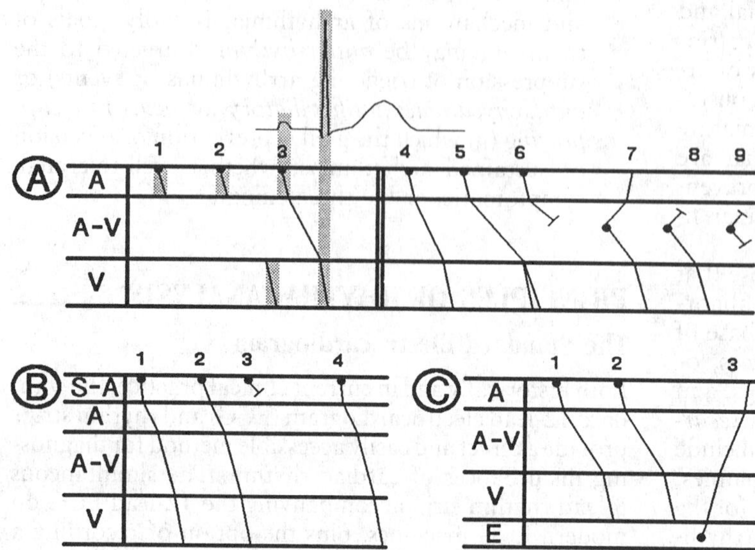

FIGURE 36-1 Ladder diagrams for analysis of cardiac arrhythmias. *A*. Charting of P-wave and QRS complexes and deduction of conduction relationships for a normal sinus impulse are demonstrated in A1 to A3. The diversion of lines shown in the V level in A5 is used to indicate aberrant intraventricular conduction, and the incomplete cross-hatched line in the AV level in A6 represents an impulse blocked in the AV junction. The AV junctional impulses with retrograde and antegrade conduction (A7), retrograde block and antegrade conduction (A8), and block in both directions resulting in a concealed extrasystole (A9) are shown next. *B*. Diagram used to analyze sinoatrial conduction is demonstrated. A sinus impulse that fails to conduct to the atrium is indicated as in B3. *C*. Ventricular ectopic activity (E) is depicted as shown in C3, which represents a premature ventricular contraction with retrograde conduction to the atrium.

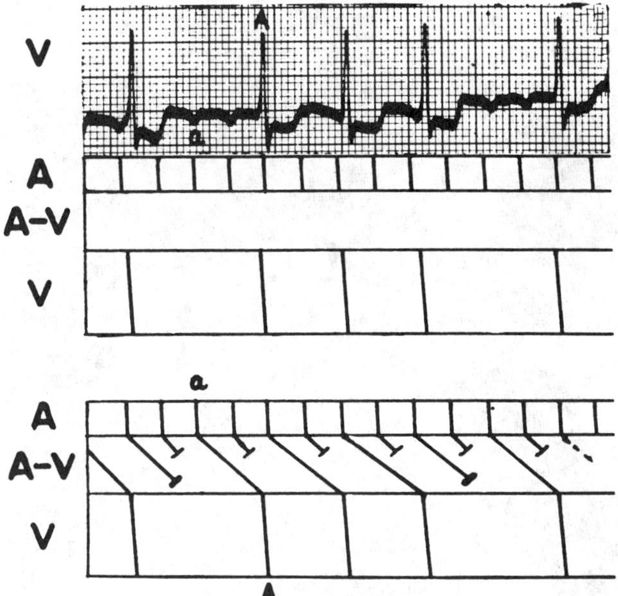

FIGURE 36-2 Construction of ladder diagrams for analyzing specific arrhythmias. *Stage 1*: Draw lines to represent atrial activity (seen and inferred by measurement) and ventricular complexes. *Stage 2*: Since in flutter the F-R interval usually ranges between 0.26 and 0.45 s, start by connecting the F wave *a* to the QRS *A* in this example. As successive impulses are diagrammed, it becomes apparent that there is a basic 2 : 1 AV conduction with a Wenckebach period of the alternate cycles. (*From HJL Marriott: Armchair arrhythmias. Tampa Tracings, 1966. Reproduced with permission.*)

age capabilities for inpatient monitoring systems permits off-line analysis of complex rhythm disturbances if the physician is not available at the time the arrhythmia occurs. The two most popular leads for use in bedside monitoring systems are lead II and MCL-I, the latter providing a pattern similar to V_1. For infrequently occurring arrhythmias, a number of "event recorders" are now available. They allow the patient to activate the device when an event occurs, providing internal storage that can be reviewed by the physician later. Transtelephonic transmitters can be used for more persistent events.

Exercise Testing for Cardiac Arrhythmias

Treadmill stress testing may be used to initiate an evanescent arrhythmia, document an exercise relationship to its onset, and evaluate efficacy of therapy and adverse responses in some circumstances. The standard treadmill is used, and thallium imaging is not necessary unless an ischemic basis correlating with the onset of arrhythmia is suspected. The procedure is especially useful for eliciting and evaluating therapy of exercise-induced ventricular arrhythmias [either premature ventricular contractions (PVCs) or ventricular tachycardia], to distinguish between autonomic and structural disease mechanisms for sinus node or AV node dysfunction, and to evaluate for adverse effects of drug therapy, such as possible rate-dependent proarrhythmic effects (see below). It can also be used to evaluate roughly the refractory periods of anomalous pathways in the Wolff-Parkinson-White (WPW) syndrome.

Intracardiac Electrocardiography and Electrophysiological Studies

These procedures, which are described in detail in Chap. 46, can be used to diagnose many rhythm and conduction disturbances for which surface electrocardiography is insufficient. Intracardiac electrophysiological studies are also used to define appropriate therapy and to test the results of therapy for various forms of supraventricular and ventricular arrhythmias. The use of multicatheter electrode systems, providing simultaneous recordings from many intracardiac sites (Fig. 36-3), allows mapping of the sequence of excitation in the atria, AV junction, and ventricle. Such intracardiac mapping procedures permit the identification of sites of anomalous pathways, mechanisms of ventricular tachyarrhythmias, and the site of origin of supraventricular tachyarrhythmias. In

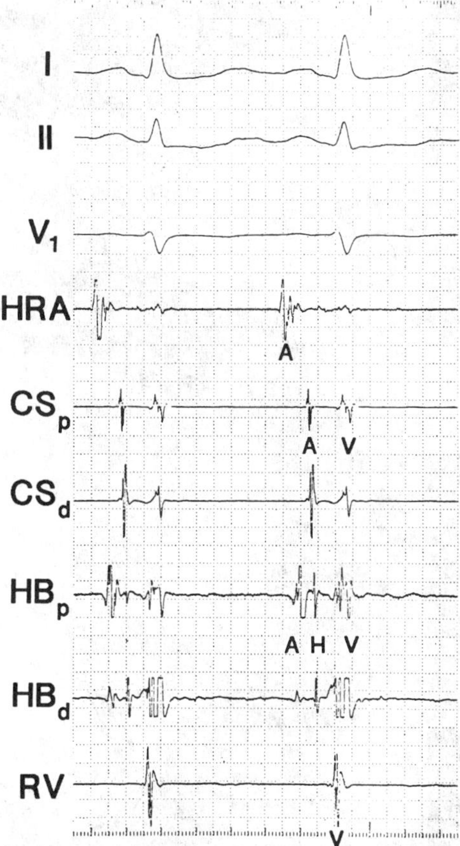

FIGURE 36-3 Intracardiac recordings during electrophysiological testing. Recordings during sinus rhythm in a multicatheter study are illustrated. The comprehensive intracardiac study includes the recording of atrial activity (A) from the high right atrium (HRA), a proximal (HB_p) and distal (HB_d) site in the His bundle region, proximal (CS_p) and distal (CS_d) sites recorded from within the coronary sinus, which record atrial and ventricular activity from the posterior/posteroseptal and posterolateral/lateral areas, respectively, and activity in the right ventricle (RV), either the apex or outflow tract, depending upon the study. For more detailed mapping procedures, more sites in the coronary sinus or sites around the tricuspid ring can be recorded or the left ventricle can be mapped by a retrograde recording catheter from the femoral artery. Less extensive studies using fewer catheters and recording sites can be used for different clinical settings. The configuration shown is standard for patients with supraventricular tachycardias. For ventricular tachycardia studies, three catheters can be used (HRA, HB, RV) for the diagnostic study. (A = atrial; H = His bundle deflection; V = ventricle).

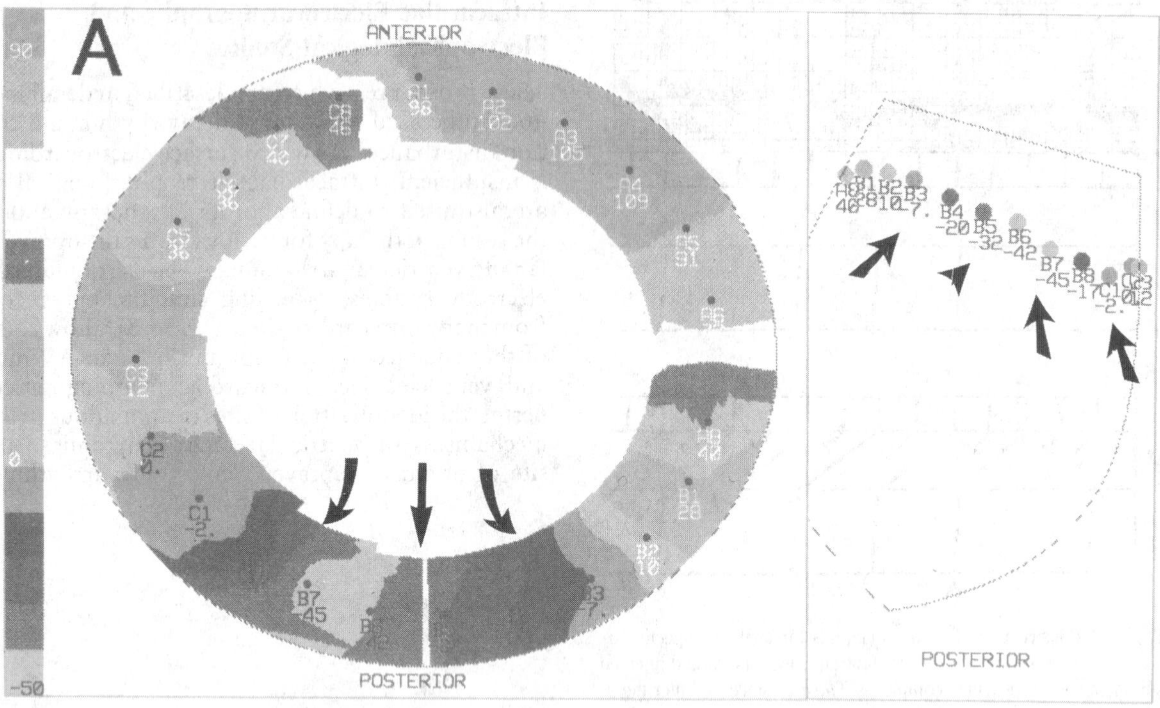

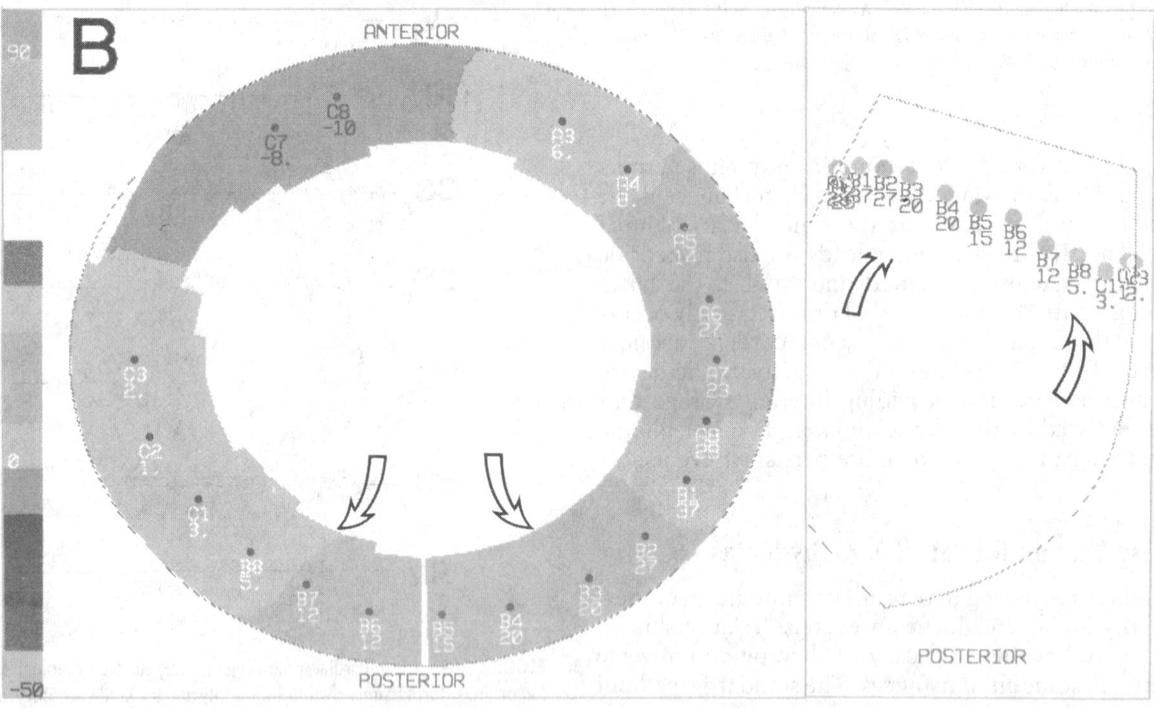

FIGURE 36-4 Computerized mapping of ventricular activation sequences during surgery for the WPW syndrome. Panel *A* demonstrates early activation in the posteroseptal region prior to surgical ablation of the bypass tract, and panel *B* demonstrates the map generated immediately after dividing the accessory pathway. The negative values in panel *A* represent early activation, with preexcitation indicated by the solid arrows; the same area in panel *B* demonstrates normal activation (open arrows) after the tract was divided.

addition, the distinction between AV block above and below the level of the bundle of His, and between true AV block and pseudo-AV block caused by concealed extrasystoles, is also possible. Specific clinical applications are provided in the appropriate sections below and in Chap. 46.

Intraoperative Mapping

Mapping of pathways and sites of origin for both ventricular and supraventricular tachyarrhythmias, including the WPW syndrome, has greatly improved surgical results. The use of hand-held probes for point-to-point recordings and the more recent multiple electrode arrays, which allow simultaneous recordings from many points during the same cardiac cycle, can be used to generate maps of activation quickly during the surgical procedure and allow the clinical electrophysiologist and surgeons to identify target areas for surgical ablation. Figure 36-4 is an example of a map from a multielectrode array demonstrating the sequence of activation in a patient with WPW syndrome undergoing surgical ablation of a bypass tract. (See also Chaps. 43 and 44.) Although quite successful in recent years, intraoperative mapping for WPW syndrome has been largely displaced by catheter mapping and ablation techniques, except for a few clinical circumstances (see below).

OVERVIEW OF MANAGEMENT STRATEGIES

Management strategies for cardiac arrhythmias have become far more complex in recent years, compared to the simple pharmacologic approaches of the past. There is better understanding of the underlying systemic and cardiac factors that can be modified to influence predisposition to arrhythmias, the range of indications for pharmacologic therapy has contracted, and nonpharmacologic interventions have been expanded (Table 36-2). Many patients now are managed with multiple interventions, with one therapeutic mode complementary to another.

A complete management plan for any arrhythmia must consider and distinguish between (1) an underlying structural etiology (e.g., coronary heart disease, cardiomyopathy, WPW syndrome, etc.) and (2) transient functional factors that interact with the underlying structural abnormality (e.g., hemodynamic, electrolyte, metabolic, and respiratory abnormalities) (see Table 36-3).[3,4] The identification of contributing factors, which interact with underlying etiology to initiate the proximate electrophysiological cause of an arrhythmia, is inherent to any treatment plan. Contributing factors may be systemic or cardiac. The major systemic abnormalities include hemodynamic dysfunction, hypoxia, acidosis, electrolyte disturbances, toxic or proarrhythmic drug effects, and endocrine abnormalities. Central nervous system factors, including fluctuations in autonomic tone, may cause or aggravate specific arrhythmias. Prompt reversal of serious arrhythmias may follow control of these disturbances.

Primary and secondary arrhythmias must be distinguished for both management and prognosis. An arrhythmia that results from an electrophysiological disturbance caused by a disease process, independent of a significant change in hemodynamic function, is defined as a *primary arrhythmia*; an arrhythmia that results from an electrical disturbance initiated by hemodynamic deterioration or metabolic abnormalities is a *secondary arrhythmia* (Fig. 36-5). In the former, antiarrhythmic drugs may be used prior to the development of a clinically manifest electrophysiological disturbance (e.g., the prophylactic use of lidocaine in acute myocardial infarction) or after an electrophysiological abnormality has developed in order to prevent or revert a sustained primary arrhythmia. In secondary arrhythmias, the use of hemodynamically active drugs to support the failing circulation may prevent electrical disturbances; but once electrical disturbances develop, antiarrhythmic and hemodynamically active drugs have complementary roles.

Direct cardiac interventions for control of arrhythmias include pharmacologic approaches, ablation of specific foci involved in arrhythmogenesis, antiarrhythmic surgical approaches, and implantable devices designed to respond to tachyarrhythmic events or to prevent symptomatic bradyarrhythmias (Table 36-2). The antiarrhythmic drugs may be classified into groups using the modified Vaughn Williams system, which categorizes

TABLE 36-2

Summary of Approaches to Arrhythmia Management

- General systemic interventions
  - Respiratory support
  - Hemodynamic support
  - Metabolic and electrolyte control
  - Neurophysiological control
- Electropharmacologic therapy
  - Control triggering events
    - Suppress triggering arrhythmias
    - Prevent/reverse arrhythmogenic factors (e.g., anti-ischemic therapy, electrolyte replacement)
  - Control sustained arrhythmias
    - Acute interventions
    - Chronic prevention
  - Control ventricular rate
- Catheter ablation procedures
  - Paroxysmal supraventricular tachycardia
    - AV nodal reentry
    - WPW syndrome
    - AV node modification in atrial fibrillation
    - Atrial flutter
  - Ventricular tachycardia*
- Surgical intervention
  - Antiarrhythmic surgery
    - Anomalous pathways, AV node ablation
    - Aneurysmectomy, endocardial resection
    - Cryoablation
    - Laser ablation†
  - Anti-ischemic surgery
  - Structural heart disease surgery
- Electronic devices
  - Acute applications
    - Cardioversion
    - Defibrillation
    - Temporary pacemakers
  - Chronic applications
    - Permanent pacemakers
    - Antitachycardia devices*
    - Implantable cardioverter defibrillators (with and without antitachycardiac pacing)

* Limited clinical application at the time of this writing)
† Early experimental/developmental clinical applications at the time of this writing)

TABLE 36-3
Causes of Cardiac Arrhythmias: Structure and Function

Structural Abnormalities	Functional Factors
Coronary heart disease	Transient ischemia/ reperfusion
Acute myocardial infarction	Substrate deprivation
Chronic ischemic heart disease	Injurious substances
Ventricular hypertrophy	Disturbed ionic homeostasis
Secondary left ventricular hypertrophy	Systemic abnormalities
Hypertrophic cardiomyopathy	Hemodynamic abnormalities
Obstructive	Electrolyte imbalance
Nonobstructive	Acidosis, hypoxia
Myopathic ventricles	Neurophysiological alterations
Dilated cardiomyopathy	Central nervous system influences
Pericarditis, myocarditis	Receptor function
Noninfectious inflammatory diseases	Neurotransmitters
Infiltrative diseases	Toxic substances
Structural electrophysiology abnormalities	Proarrhythmic drugs
Sinus node, AV node, and His-Purkinje disease	Idiosyncratic
Accessory pathways	Toxic
	Cardiotoxins

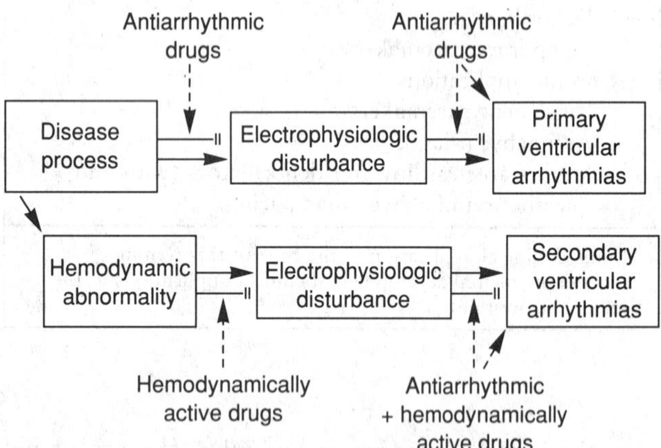

FIGURE 36-5 Primary and secondary arrhythmias. When a disease process directly initiates an electrophysiological disturbance, the resulting arrhythmia is referred to as *primary*. In contrast, when the disease process produces a hemodynamic abnormality that in turn initiates the electrophysiological disturbance, a resulting arrhythmia is referred to as *secondary*. Antiarrhythmic drugs may be used to prevent the electrophysiological disturbance, prevent the electrophysiologically unstable heart from developing a manifest arrhythmia, or reverse a primary arrhythmia. In secondary arrhythmias, hemodynamically active drugs may prevent the secondary electrophysiological disturbance or reverse secondary electrophysiological abnormalities, alone or in conjunction with antiarrhythmic drugs. (*Modified from RJ Myerburg, KM Kessler, et al: Pharmacologic approaches to management of arrhythmias in patients with cardiomyopathy and heart failure. Am Heart J 114:1273–1279, 1987. Reproduced with permission from the publisher.*)

them on the basis of electropharmacologic and electrophysiological properties (see Table 36-4). This classification is inherently useful and practical for the clinician but has increasingly evident shortcomings.[5] These include difficulty categorizing new drugs, exclusion of some drugs with obvious antiarrhythmic properties (e.g., adenosine), and inability to correlate drug class with specific effects as antiarrhythmic agents. The usual dosages and routes of administration for the antiarrhythmic agents approved by the U.S. Food and Drug Administration at the time of this writing are listed in Table 36-5. A number of other drugs are presently at various stages of study for ventricular and supraventricular arrhythmia indications. These include bethanidine, cibenzoline, imipramine, lorcainide, meobentine, nortriptyline, pirmenol, recainam, sematilide, and sotalol. (See also Chap. 38.)

SUPRAVENTRICULAR ARRHYTHMIAS

Sinus Rhythms and Sinus Tachycardia

The range of normal sinus rates is defined as 60 to 100 impulses per minute and the rhythm is regular. When the variation between the longest and shortest cycle on a resting tracing is above 0.12 s, *sinus arrhythmia* is present (Fig. 36-6*A*). This normal variant is most common in children and decreases with advancing age. It is defined as *phasic sinus arrhythmia* if the cycle lengths shorten with inspiration and lengthen with expiration. If unrelated to the respiratory cycle, it is referred to as *nonphasic*.

A sinus rhythm at a rate below 60 impulses per minute is defined as sinus bradycardia (Fig. 36-6*C*); its significance depends on the clinical circumstance (see section on bradycardias below). It may be normal, even at rates in the 30's, in highly trained young athletes, while it may be abnormal in the elderly. A sinus rate above 100 impulses per minute is sinus tachycardia. Occasional normal individuals will have resting sinus rates in excess of 100 per minute. In addition, sinus rates in excess of 100 per minute are normal in infants and children under 2 years of age. These examples fall into the category of *physiological* sinus tachycardias, which also include the normal sinus rate responses to exercise, excitement, anxiety, and other emotional stresses. *Pharmacologic* sinus tachycardias result from medications such as epinephrine, ephedrine, amyl nitrate, isoproterenol, and atropine and may occur upon exposure to alcohol, nicotine, or caffeine. The heart rate responses are a result of the pharmacologic properties of these drugs. *Pathological* sinus tachycardia may be secondary or noncardiac in origin or due to specific cardiac abnormalities. Among the secondary causes are fever, hypoxemia, hemorrhage, hypotension, thyrotoxicosis, and anemia. Cardiac causes include congestive heart failure, myocardial infarction, and pulmonary embolism.

Electrocardiographic Features

The ECG in sinus tachycardia reveals a rate in excess of 100 per minute accompanied by a normal P-R relationship and a normal P-wave vector (Fig. 36-6*B*). The upper

TABLE 36-4

Modified Vaughn Williams Classification of Drugs Approved for Antiarrhythmic Uses

Examples	Depolarization	Repolarization
Class I: Membrane-active drugs		
IA Quinidine (Quinaglute, Quinidex, Cardioquin) Procainamide (Pronestyl, Procan-SR) Disopyramide (Norpace) Moricizine (Ethmozine)	Moderate depression; intermediate kinetics	Prolonged
IB Lidocaine (Xylocaine) Tocainide (Tonocard) Mexiletine (Mexitil) Phenytoin (Dilantin)	Limited depression; rapid kinetics	No effect or shortened
IC Flecainide (Tambocor) Encainide (Enkaid) Propafenone (Rhythmol)	Marked depression; slow kinetics	Minimal effect
Class II: β-Adrenoceptor blocking drugs Propranolol (Inderal) Esmolol (Brevibloc) Acebutolol (Sectral)		
Class III: Drugs that prolong repolarization Amiodarone (Cordarone) Bretylium Tosylate (Bretylol) Sotalol (Betapacs)		
Class IV: Ca^{2+} entry blocking drugs Verapamil (Isoptin, Calan) Diltiazem (Cardizem)		
Unclassified in this system Digoxin (Lanoxin) Adenosine (Adenocard)		

Drugs identified by name are limited to those approved for antiarrhythmic use by the U.S. Food and Drug Administration at the time of this writing.

limit of sinus tachycardia varies according to the patient's clinical status and factors responsible for the tachycardia. For instance, in the physiological tachycardia group, the upper limit in the normal adult during exercise testing may range from 160 to 190 per minute, whereas the highly trained athlete may attain a rate of at least 200 per minute under maximal effort. In contrast, the pharmacologic tachycardias do not commonly induce a rate exceeding 130 per minute, whereas the rate that is secondary to pathological causes may range from 120 to 140 per minute (e.g., hypotension, hypoxemia, hemorrhage, fever) to 160 per minute (hyperthyroidism, severe heart failure). In a persistent sinus tachycardia, the rate characteristically varies during the course of the day, in contrast to the fixed rate that occurs in ectopic tachycardias or AV nodal reentrant tachycardia. Carotid sinus massage characteristically slows the sinus rate transiently with a return to the baseline rate after cessation of the procedure.

Management of Sinus Tachycardia

This modification in heart rate, except when it is an appropriate response to acute physical or emotional stress, is usually categorized as *persistent* and is easily recognized. Its management almost always depends on control of exogenous or endogenous systemic factors or of an underlying cardiac disease. Its differentiation from other supraventricular tachycardias (SVTs) at rates of 150 or more a minute may be achieved with carotid sinus massage, which produces a typical gradual slowing, followed by a gradual return to the baseline rate. Specific therapy is rarely required; when it is, beta-adrenergic blockade will often achieve at least partial control of the sinus rate. In uncomplicated acute myocardial infarction, the sinus rate may be controlled with small doses of propranolol (10 to 20 mg every 6 h). Persistent sinus tachycardia occurs in thyrotoxicosis, and higher doses of propranolol may be required for control. Persistent sinus tachycardia during heart failure or hypovolemic states will respond promptly to an improving hemodynamic status as the primary problem is corrected. A *chronic* form of nonparoxysmal sinus tachycardia has been reported[7] and is thought to be due to autonomic dysfunction.

Premature Atrial Impulses

Atrial extrasystoles or premature atrial contractions (PACs) are extremely common and may occur in normal individuals or in the presence of systemic or cardiac abnormalities. They occur at any age, including infancy, and were observed in 0.4 percent of 122,000 asymptomatic healthy males, 16 to 50 years of age, in the U.S. Air

TABLE 36-5
Antiarrhythmic Drugs: Dosage and Kinetics

Drug	Usual Dosing Range*	Half-Life (h)	Therapeutic Range (μg/mL)	Plasma Protein Binding (%)	Major Route of Excretion
Class IA					
Quinidine	Oral sulfate: 200–600 q 6 h Oral long acting: 330–660 mg, q 8 h or q 6 h	5–7	2.3–5	80	H
Procainamide	Oral: 250–750 mg, q 4 h or q 6 h Oral long acting: 500–1500, q 8 h or q 6 h IV: 10–15 mg/kg at 25 mg/min, then 1–6 mg/min	3–5	4–10	15	R†
Disopyramide	Oral: 100–200 mg q 8 h or q 6 h	8–9	2–5	35–95	H/R
Moricizine‡	Oral: 150–300 mg q 12 h to q 8 h	6–13	—	95	H
Class IB					
Lidocaine	IV: 1–3 mg/kg at 20–50 mg/min, then 1–4 mg/min	1–2	1–5	60	H
Tocainide	Oral: 400–600 q 8–12 h	15	4–10	10	H
Mexiletine	Oral: 200–400 mg q 8 h	10–12	0.5–2.0	55	H
Class IC					
Flecainide	Oral: 100–200 mg q 12 h	20	0.4–1.0	40	H
Encainide	Oral: 25–50 mg q 8 h	3–4+	0.5–1.0§	80	H
Propafenone	Oral: 150–300 mg q 8 h	2–10	0.5–1.5§	95	H
Class II					
Propanolol	Oral: 10–100 mg q 6 h IV: 0.1 mg/kg in divided 1-mg doses	4–6	0.04–0.10	95	H
Esmolol	IV: 500 mg/kg per min × 1 min followed by 50 mg/kg per min × 4 min, repeat with 50-mg increments to maintenance dose to 200 mg/kg per min	9 min	—	55	H
Acebutolol	Oral: 200–600 mg bid	3–4	—	26	H/R
Class III					
Amiodarone	Oral: 80–1600 mg/day × 1–3 weeks, then 600–800/day × 2–4 weeks, then 200–400 mg/day	50 days	1–2.5	96	H
Bretylium	IV: 5–10 mg/kg at 1–2 mg/kg, then 0.5–2.0 mg/min	8–14	0.5–1.5	—	R
Sotalol¶	Oral: 80–320 mg q 12 h	10–15	—	0	R
Class IV					
Verapamil	Oral: 80–120 mg q 6–8 h IV: 5–10 mg in 1–2 min	3–8	0.1–0.15	90	H
Diltiazem	IV: 0.25 mg/kg body wt over 2 min; if response inadequate, wait 15 min, then 0.35 mg/kg over 2 min; maintenance 10–15 mg/h	3.5–5.0	0.1–3.0	70–80	H
Other					
Digoxin	Oral: 1.25–1.5 mg in divided doses over 24 h followed by 0.125–0.375 mg/day IV: Approximately 70% of oral dose	36	0.8–1.4 ng/mL	30	R
Adenosine	IV: 6 mg rapidly; if unsuccessful within 1–2 min, 12 mg rapidly	10 s	—	—	—

H = hepatic; R = renal.
*All dosing should follow FDA-approved guidelines as outlined in package insert or *Physicians' Desk Reference*. See also Chap. 38.
†Parent compound metabolized to active metabolite (NAPA) in liver; both active metabolite and unmetabolized parent compound excreted by kidneys.
‡Shares classes IB, IC activities; §Active metabolite limits significance of these measurements; ¶Shares class II activity.

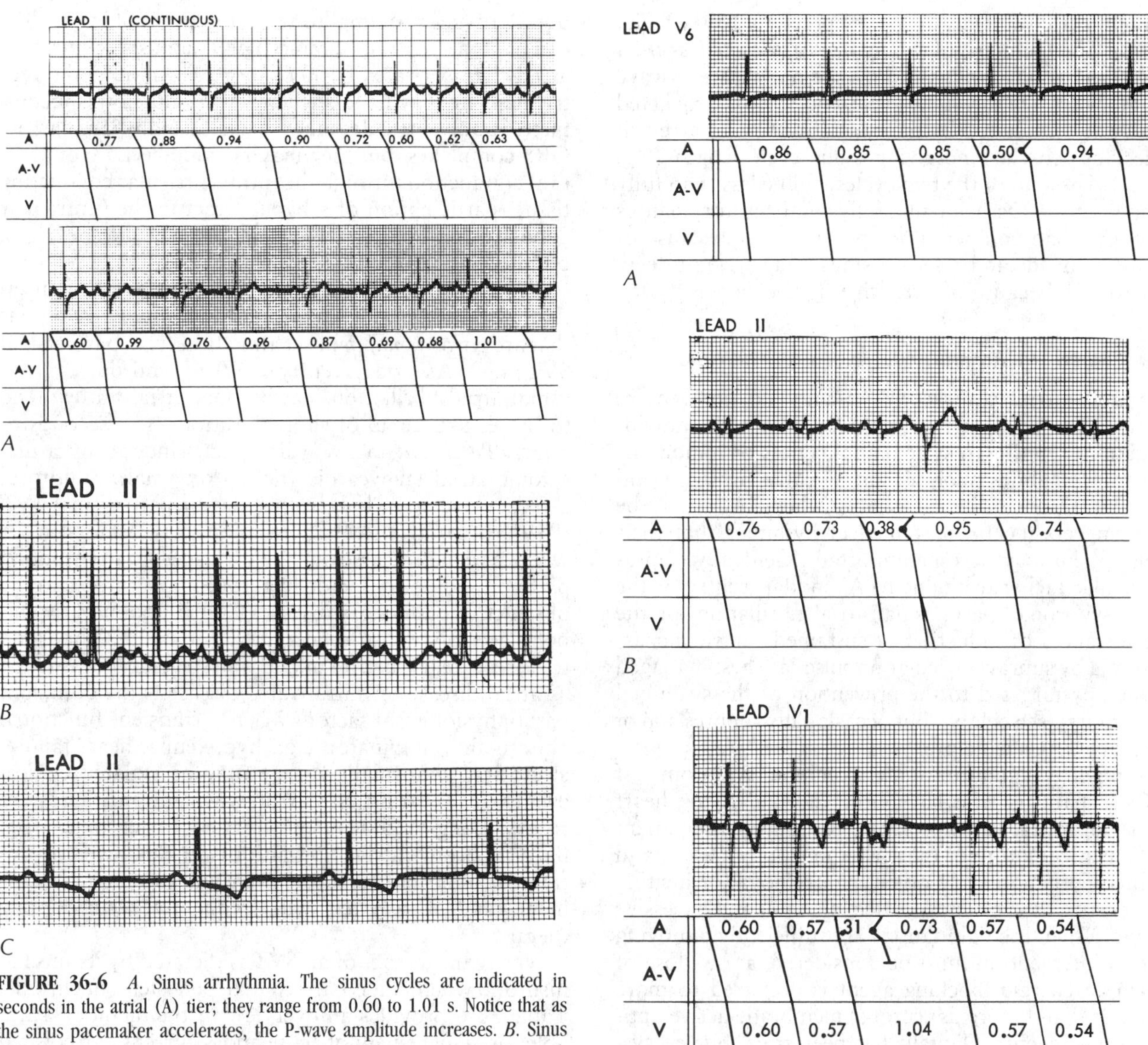

FIGURE 36-6 *A.* Sinus arrhythmia. The sinus cycles are indicated in seconds in the atrial (A) tier; they range from 0.60 to 1.01 s. Notice that as the sinus pacemaker accelerates, the P-wave amplitude increases. *B.* Sinus tachycardia. Note normally shaped and directed P waves, normal P-R interval, and a rate of almost 150 per minute. *C.* Sinus bradycardia. Note normally directed (but abnormally wide) P waves, normal P-R interval, and a rate of slightly more than 50 per minute.

FIGURE 36-7 *A.* The fifth impulse is an atrial premature beat; there is a premature P′ wave followed by a normal QRS-T complex, and the postextrasystolic pause is longer than the sinus cycle but less than compensatory. *B.* The fourth impulse is an atrial premature beat with aberrant intraventricular conduction; there is a premature P′ wave followed by an anomalous QRS-T complex; the postextrasystolic pause is less than compensatory. *C.* Nonconducted atrial premature beat. Following the third ventricular complex, a P′ wave negatively deforms the ST segment and is not followed by a ventricular response.

Force.[6] Because of the cross-sectional nature of this data base and the limited electrocardiographic sample size per individual, the actual prevalence is likely to be considerably higher. Both endogenous (febrile illnesses, thyrotoxicosis, emotional stress, etc.) and exogenous (alcohol, tobacco, or caffeine consumption) systemic factors may initiate or worsen atrial extrasystolic activity. Among cardiac causes, myopericarditis, ischemia, heart failure, and digitalis intoxication are all precipitating or contributing factors.

Electrocardiographic Features

The PAC is characterized by (1) a P wave that occurs before the next expected sinus impulse and (2) a change in the vector of the early P wave. The P-R interval of the conducted PAC is usually normal or minimally prolonged (see Fig. 36-7). Much more marked prolongation of the P-R interval occurs occasionally. More subtle electrocardiographic patterns include (1) superimposition of the premature P wave on the T wave of the preceding sinus impulse and (2) an unexpected pause due to failure of conduction of a PAC to the ventricles. In both instances, careful inspection of the T wave of the sinus impulse before the PAC will reveal a distortion of the T wave, sometimes minimal, indicating the presence of the PAC. When the coupling interval of the PAC to the previous sinus P wave is short, aberrant intraventricular conduction makes the diagnosis dependent upon recognition of the P wave distorting the previous T wave (Fig. 36-7*B*). The hallmark of timing of PACs is the *less than fully compensatory pause*. Since the premature P wave commonly resets the sinus cycle, the PAC is bracketed by a cycle terminated by the early P wave and a return cycle close to the underlying sinus cycle length (Fig. 36-7*A*). The sum of the two cycles will be less than fully compensatory. Occasionally, fully compensatory pauses or longer than compensatory pauses occur because of failure to invade and reset the sinus node cycle or delay of its return because of overdrive suppression.

Management of Premature Atrial Contractions

Premature atrial contractions usually do not require treatment, especially when they occur in normal individuals and when due to systemic influences or minor cardiac abnormalities such as mitral valve prolapse and acute viral pericarditis. It is only when PACs may be triggering events[2] for sustained arrhythmias that their management may become important. Generally, supraventricular tachycardia due to AV nodal reentry or the WPW syndrome, paroxysmal atrial fibrillation, or the rare instances of induction of sustained ventricular arrhythmia by supraventricular impulses are best managed by therapy targeted to the prevention of the sustained arrhythmias (see below). But occasionally suppression of triggering PACs is helpful.

Annoying palpitations are common symptoms of PACs in patients who have either no underlying heart disease or mitral valve prolapse. Reassuring the patient of the benign nature of the arrhythmia may suffice, and no therapy is necessary other than removal of inciting factors such as cigarettes, coffee, alcohol, and excessive fatigue. When the palpitations are sufficiently annoying that an intervention must be considered, a low dose of a beta-adrenergic blocking agent is preferred to more aggressive (and more dangerous) membrane-active antiarrhythmic agents. Digitalis has been tried, but no systematic studies of its efficacy has been reported.

When it is necessary to treat PACs to prevent initiation of sustained arrhythmias or because of intolerable palpitations, conventional antiarrhythmic agents may be effective. Depending upon tolerance and side effects, any of the membrane-active drugs or beta-adrenoceptor blocking agents may be considered. There are little data available on the efficacy of tocainide, mexiletine, flecainide, encainide, propafenone, or beta blockers for PACs, but clinical experience suggests that each may be effective for individual patients. At present, they have not been approved for this indication in the United States. Class IC drugs should be avoided for this indication in patients with even the remote possibility of coronary artery disease because of the adverse outcome in the Cardiac Arrhythmia Suppression Trial (CAST).[8,9] Atrial distension in heart failure may induce PACs; they usually disappear as hemodynamics improve, and antiarrhythmic drugs are avoided.

Supraventricular Tachyarrhythmias

This category includes all tachyarrhythmias that originate above the bifurcation of the bundle of His or incorporate tissues proximal to the bifurcation of the bundle of His in a reentrant circuit. The diagnosis requires an atrial chamber rate of 100 or more per minute; the ventricular rate may be less when AV conduction is incomplete. Supraventricular tachycardias usually have narrow QRS complexes, but they may be wide because of aberrant conduction through the intraventricular conducting tissue, participation of a bypass tract in the ventricular depolarization pattern, or in the presence of coexisting bundle branch block.

We categorize SVTs into three groups based on duration: *paroxysmal*, *persistent*, and *chronic*. Arrhythmias that are *paroxysmal* in onset and offset (e.g., paroxysmal SVT due to AV nodal reentry or WPW syndrome, paroxysmal atrial fibrillation, paroxysmal atrial flutter) tend to be recurrent and of short duration—i.e., seconds to hours. *Persistent* tachycardias [e.g., sinus tachycardia, ectopic atrial tachycardia (nonparoxysmal), multifocal atrial tachycardia, longer episodes of paroxysmal SVT (PSVT) or atrial flutter of fibrillation] may last for days or weeks and may be associated with a specific contributing pathophysiological factor [e.g., decompensated chronic obstructive pulmonary disease (COPD), pulmonary emboli, electrolyte disturbances, drug toxicity]. They tend to be recurrent when an underlying structural cause such as atrial disease or mitral valve disease is the dominant pathophysiological factor. When a transient functional abnormality dominates (e.g., hypoxemia, heart failure, electrolyte abnormality), they may be isolated clinical events, reappearing only if or when the inciting event recurs. Longstanding or *chronic* SVTs (chronic atrial flutter, chronic atrial fibrillation) do not revert if untreated, often fail to revert even with attempted treatment, and if reverted will frequently recur despite therapy.

The management of an SVT is dictated by its mechanism and whether it is paroxysmal, persistent, or chronic. Table 36-6 provides an overview of the methods available for management of acute and recurrent paroxysmal SVTs.

The Reentrant Paroxysmal Supraventricular Tachycardias

Paroxysmal supraventricular tachycardia may be due to AV nodal reentry, to WPW syndrome, or to intraatrial or sinus node reentry. Most of the interventions for SVT listed in Table 36-6 are applicable to these arrhythmias.

PSVT Due to AV Nodal Reentry Paroxysmal supraventricular tachycardia due to AV nodal reentry is the most common form of PSVT. The underlying pathophysiological disturbance in AV nodal reentry is the presence of dual AV nodal pathways. The AV node in patients with dual-pathway physiology behaves as though there are two types of conduction pathways in the AV node, one capable of faster conduction, which usually has a longer refractory period, and the other more slowly conducting and having a shorter refractory period. As illustrated in Fig. 36-8, a premature atrial impulse with a sufficiently short coupling interval may block in the fast pathway, allowing conduction to proceed through the slow pathway, with the impulse reentering the fast pathway in the

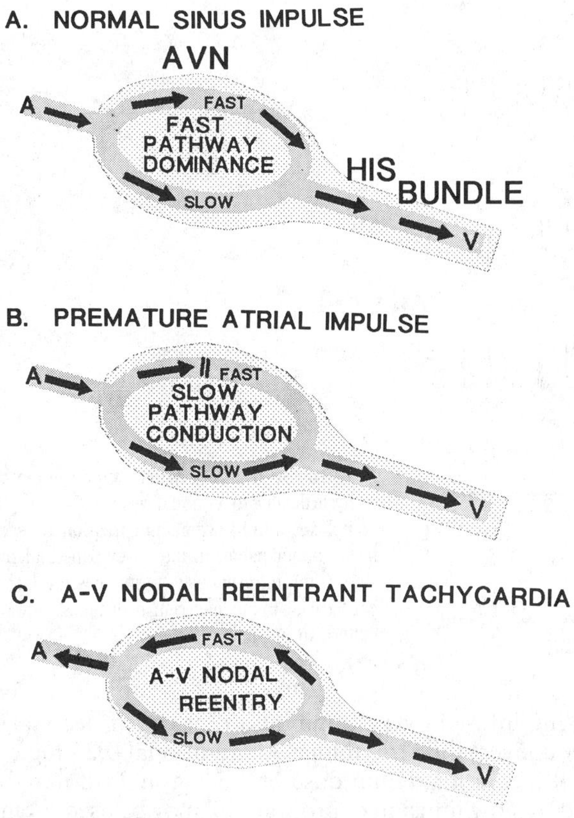

FIGURE 36-8 Mechanism of paroxysmal supraventricular tachycardia due to AV nodal reentry. PSVT due to AV nodal reentry is due to the presence of dual AV nodal pathways with different conduction properties and refractory periods. Although the slow AV nodal pathway is now thought not to be part of the anatomic AV node, the dual pathway physiology concept still appears to be valid. *A*. During sinus rhythm in the presence of dual AV nodal pathway, the fast pathway (which generally has a longer refractory period) is primarily responsible for AV transmission because of slower propagation in the other pathway. *B*. A premature atrial impulse blocks in the fast pathway because of its longer refractory period and propagates down the slow pathway prolonging the P-R interval and allowing retrograde invasion of the fast pathway because of its fully polarized tissue. *C*. Echo beats or AV nodal reentrant tachycardia will occur when the time relationships between slow pathway conduction and recovery of excitability at the site of block in the fast pathway allow the impulse to reenter the slow pathway after retrograde fast pathway transmission. The atria are also activated retrogradely. In a far less common form of AV nodal reentry, a shorter refractory period in the fast pathway reverses the loop, with antegrade conduction down the fast pathway and retrograde conduction up the slow pathway (see Fig. 36-10 for examples).

retrograde direction and arriving at the proximal end after it has recovered excitability. When this occurs, a circuit is completed and the impulse may then reenter the slow pathway if it too has regained excitability. Once established, this reentrant pattern will continue until the relationship between conduction velocities and refractory periods in the two pathways is disturbed so as to interrupt the cycle. The circulating impulse progresses through the His-Purkinje system to ventricular muscle each time it passes the distal end of the reentrant loop and provides retrograde atrial activation each time it passes the proximal end. Because antegrade conduction is slow and retrograde conduction rapid, atrial activity begins soon after ventricular activation, creating an inability to identify P waves on the standard ECG during AV nodal reentrant tachycardia (Fig. 36-9). The characteristic alignment of electrograms recorded during AV nodal reentrant tachycardia is shown in Fig. 36-10. In a much less common form of AV nodal reentry, the circulating wavefront proceeds antegradely down the fast pathway and retrogradely up the slow pathway, creating a sequence of excitation of atria that is delayed relative to ventricular activation because of slow retrograde conduction. This form of AV nodal reentrant tachycardia is characterized by a long R-P interval and a short P-R interval, with an inverted P wave in II, III, and aVF. (See also Chap. 35.)

Electrocardiographic Features Paroxysmal supraventricular tachycardia due to AV nodal reentry is characterized by an abrupt onset and offset and usually has a narrow QRS complex without clearly discernable P waves. The rate is usually in the range of 160 to 190 per minute but may be as slow as 120 to 130 per minute and occasionally as rapid as 200 per minute. When preexisting bundle branch block is present, the tachycardia will reflect the preexisting wide QRS complex, and functional bundle branch block due to tachycardia may also occur, making a distinction from ventricular tachyarrhythmias difficult (Fig. 36-11). Functional bundle branch block may have either a left or a right bundle pattern. Figures 36-10*A* and 36-10*B* contrast the electrophysiological findings in the common and uncommon form of AV nodal reentry.

Management of PSVT Due to AV Nodal Reentry Paroxysmal supraventricular tachycardia due to AV nodal reentry is a benign disturbance, requiring intervention primarily for the patient's comfort and sense of well-being, except when it coexists with other disease processes in which the tachyarrhythmia is poorly tolerated, such as ischemic heart disease or mitral stenosis. Occasionally, the rate is rapid enough to cause near syncope in otherwise normal individuals, although such rates are more common in PSVT due to WPW (see below).

Rest, sedation, and vagotonic maneuvers are simple means for reverting acute episodes, and patients can be taught self-administered vagotonic maneuvers for recurrences. Patients should be advised to avoid inciting factors such as smoking, alcohol, extreme fatigue, and stress. Many of the effective pharmacologic interventions for acute episodes used in the past have given way to new drug therapy. Infusions of sympathomimetic (phenylephrine, methoxamine) and parasympathomimetic drugs (edrophonium, neostigmine) have largely been supplanted by intravenous adenosine, Ca^{2+}-entry blockers, digoxin, or beta-adrenergic blockers for managing the acute episodes. Adenosine, 6 mg intravenous (see Fig. 36-9), followed by one or two 12-mg boluses if necessary, is effective and safe[12] for acute treatment. Because of its very short duration of action and lack of negative inotropic effects, it is now preferred to other acute pharmacologic therapies, especially when considering a differential diagnosis between SVT and ventricular tachycardia. A 5-mg bolus of verapamil, followed by one or two additional 5-mg boluses 10 min apart if the initial dose does not convert the arrhythmia, has been an effective regimen in up to 90 percent of patients with

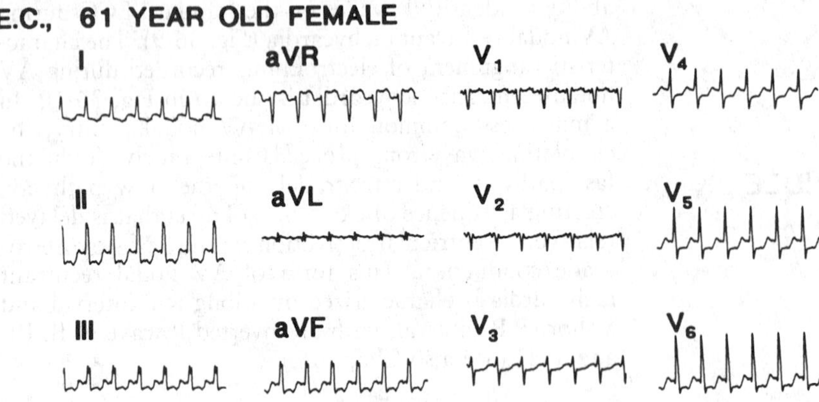

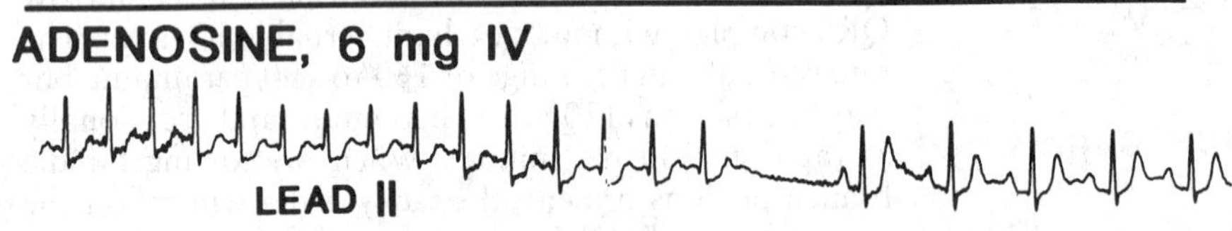

FIGURE 36-9 Paroxysmal supraventricular tachycardia due to AV nodal reentry. Narrow QRS complexes with ST segment depression are seen in the upper panel. In the lower panel, adenosine, 6 mg intravenously, terminates the tachycardia with immediate return of the ST-T wave pattern to normal.

PSVT due to AV node reentry.[10,11] However, it must not be used for an unknown wide QRS tachycardia because of risk of adverse effects when used in patients who have ventricular tachycardia.[13] Intravenous diltiazem is also effective.[14,15] Beginning treatment consists of a bolus of 0.25 mg/kg actual body weight over 2 min. If the response is inadequate, wait 15 min and then give a repeat bolus of 0.35 mg/kg over 2 min. Intravenous digoxin, 0.5 mg infused over 10 min and repeated if necessary, may convert the arrhythmia. An additional 0.25 mg every 4 h to a maximum dose of 1.5 mg in 24 h may be used. A slow infusion of propranolol may be used.[16] One milligram per minute is given to a total dose of 5 to 10 mg or a significant fall in blood pressure. The class IA antiarrhythmic agents, which appear to depress conduction in the fast pathway, may be tried if other drugs fail.[17]

A-V NODAL REENTRANT TACHYCARDIA

A COMMON TYPE B UNCOMMON TYPE

FIGURE 36-10 Common and uncommon forms of AV nodal reentrant tachycardia recorded during electrophysiological studies. *A*. The common type of AV nodal reentrant tachycardia, antegrade in the slow pathway and retrograde in the fast pathway, results in atrial (A) and ventricular (V) activation that are close in time to one another. Characteristically, intracardiac recordings demonstrate a "lining up" of atrial and ventricular electrograms. *B*. In the uncommon type of AV nodal reentrant tachycardia, antegrade fast pathway and retrograde slow pathway conduction change the relative timing pattern so that atrial activation is delayed relative to ventricular activation, and the electrograms are not in line. In this form of PSVT, the R-P interval is longer than the P-R interval on the ECG, which may result in the retrograde P wave appearing beyond the ST-T wave of the related ventricular impulse. The uncommon type of AV nodal reentrant tachycardia may be difficult to distinguish from other arrhythmias such as ectopic atrial tachyarrhythmias or concealed WPW syndrome (see text).

Several special points must be remembered. When the QRS complex is wide and ventricular tachycardia is mistakenly diagnosed as SVT with aberrant conduction, intravenous verapamil frequently causes a clinically significant fall in blood pressure and potentially lethal events.[13] Unless it is absolutely clear that a wide QRS tachycardia is due to aberrant intraventricular conduction or preexisting bundle branch block, verapamil should not be used. Similarly, in patients with coexisting hemodynamically significant underlying heart disease, intravenous propranolol must be used with caution, if at all. For those few patients in whom the clinical setting demands an immediate return to a normal sinus mechanism, DC cardioversion can be employed. A low-energy shock (10 to 50 W · s) may be sufficient; larger energies are used if necessary. If DC cardioversion should be avoided (e.g., because of possible adverse response after digitalis administration), pacing the right atrium or ventricle via a temporary pacing catheter is usually successful.[18] (See Chap. 39.)

Long-term control of recurrent PSVT due to AV nodal reentry may be achieved with pharmacologic therapy, catheter ablation or surgical techniques, or electronic devices. Patients who have infrequent, well-tolerated attacks that are short-lived and/or respond to self-administered physiological maneuvers (Table 36-6) may require no chronic interventions. In the majority of others, pharmacologic therapy is sufficient. Many patients will have reduced numbers and severity of attacks with simple medications such as digoxin in standard maintenance doses, propranolol, or verapamil. These drugs act by

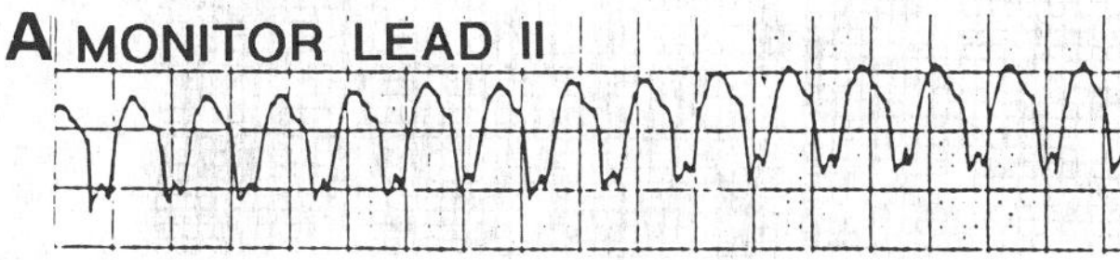

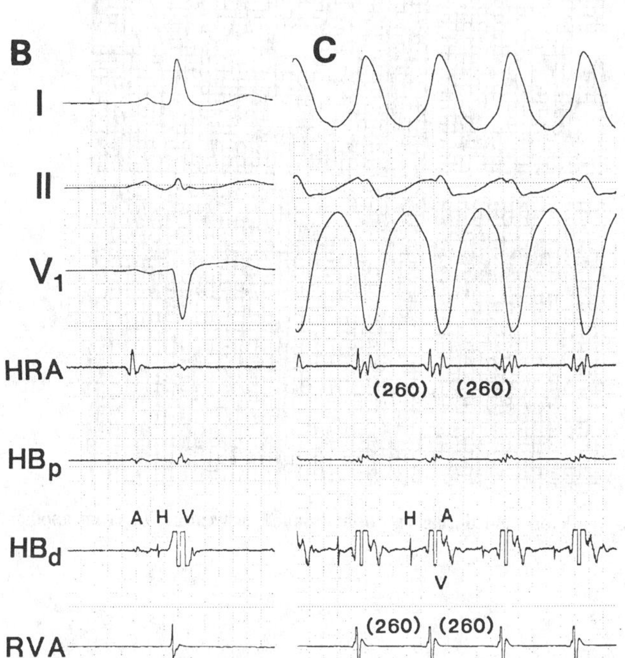

FIGURE 36-11 Paroxysmal supraventricular tachycardia due to AV nodal reentry. *A.* The initial presenting rhythm was a wide QRS tachycardia with a vertical axis and a left bundle branch block pattern. *B.* A sinus impulse with intracardiac recordings demonstrating normal sequences of AV conduction. *C.* Recording of a wide QRS tachycardia with a left bundle branch block pattern. The nearly simultaneous activation patterns in the retrograde and antegrade directions suggest the common form of AV nodal reentry, rather than ventricular tachycardia.

altering conduction in AV nodal pathways to prevent initiation or maintenance of sustained arrhythmias. Membrane-active antiarrhythmic drugs may prevent recurrences, both by suppressing triggering premature impulses and by depressing conduction in the retrograde (fast) pathway of the AV nodal reentrant circuit.[17] However, their efficacy, combined with the risk of potentially serious proarrhythmic side effects of membrane-active drugs, limits use of the latter to more difficult cases. Invasive electrophysiological studies to guide therapy[19] are also appropriate for difficult cases. Catheter ablation[20] or curative surgical techniques that may preserve AV node conduction[21] are available, as are antitachycardia pacing devices.[22] Recent experience with radiofrequency (RF) catheter ablation techniques has demonstrated that the procedure is safe and effective for PSVT due to AV nodal reentrant tachycardia.[23,24] It is emerging as the treatment of choice for patients with frequent arrhythmic episodes and/or poor tolerance of drugs. (See also Chap. 43.)

PSVT Due to WPW Syndrome Wolff-Parkinson-White syndrome appears to be the second most common cause of PSVT. Since it also occurs in a *concealed* form, in which the standard ECG is normal during sinus rhythm because of inability of the accessory pathway to conduct in the antegrade direction, the total number of PSVTs that are due to accessory pathways may approach or even exceed those due to AV nodal reentry. As in AV nodal reentry, the pathophysiology of reentrant tachyarrhythmias in WPW syndrome relates to the presence of two pathways between the atria and the ventricles that have different conduction properties and characteristics of refractoriness. In the majority of cases, the effective refractory period of the accessory pathway exceeds that of the normal AV nodal–His-Purkinje pathway. Therefore, a premature atrial impulse may block at the accessory pathway and conduct antegradely down the normal pathway, ultimately entering the accessory pathway in the retrograde direction and reentering the atrium to

TABLE 36-6
Management of Paroxysmal Supraventricular Tachycardias

	Acute	Long-term
Physiological interventions	Rest, sedation Valsalva maneuver Carotid sinus massage	Self-administered Valsalva maneuver, carotid sinus massage Avoid inciting factors
Pharmacologic therapy	Vagomimetic or sympathomimetic drugs* Direct effect on AV nodal or accessory pathway Slow ventricular rate	Suppress triggering arrhythmias Change properties of accessory pathways Control ventricular rate
Catheter ablation and surgical techniques	—	Ablation or sectioning of reentrant pathway Modification of AV node
Electronic devices	Temporary pacing Cardioversion	Permanent pacemaker Antitachycardia pacing*

*Limited use in current practice.

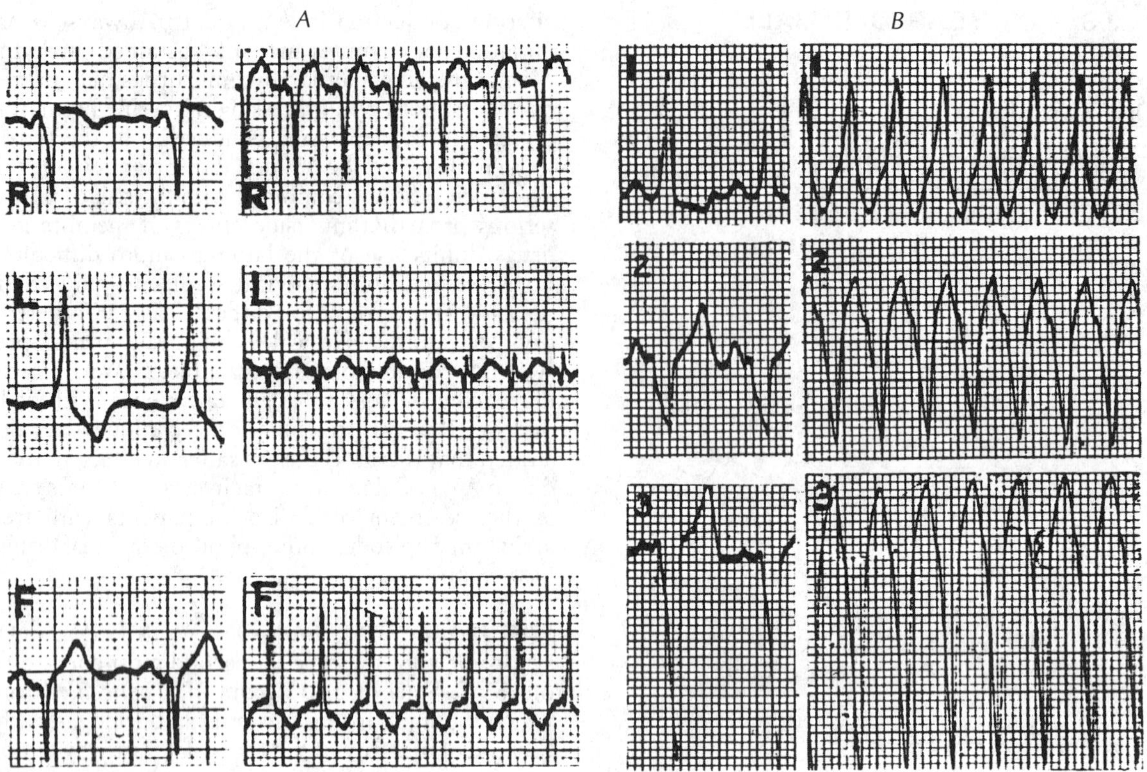

FIGURE 36-12 Wolff-Parkinson-White syndrome with reciprocating tachycardia. *A.* Before and during an "orthodromic" tachycardia. *B.* From another patient, before and during an "antidromic" tachycardia.

establish a circus movement tachycardia referred to as *orthodromic* (see Fig. 36-12*A*). Because the normal pathway is used for ventricular activation, the delta wave is lost, causing the QRS complex to normalize during orthodromic tachycardias. In addition, since the accessory pathway provides retrograde conduction to the atria, P waves, if seen, are usually inverted in the inferior and lateral leads. The stability of the reentrant circuit depends upon the conduction properties and refractory periods of the two pathways. In a less common form of PSVT, a shorter refractory period in the anomalous pathway results in block of an initiating premature atrial impulse in the normal pathway, with antegrade conduction down the anomalous pathway and then retrograde invasion of the normal AV nodal pathway to establish an *antidromic tachycardia.* The QRS complex is wide, having the characteristics of a ventricular complex originating near the insertion site of the anomalous pathway (Fig. 36-12*B*). These wide QRS tachycardias may be difficult to distinguish from ventricular tachyarrhythmias if the existence of WPW syndrome was not known prior to presentation with a tachyarrhythmia. In concealed WPW syndrome,[25] only orthodromic tachycardias can occur because of inability of the bypass tract to conduct in the antegrade direction. Distinction between concealed WPW syndrome and AV nodal reentrant tachycardia may be difficult, although a faster rate (>200 per minute) and a retrograde P wave after, rather than within, the QRS complex favor concealed WPW syndrome. When atrial flutter or fibrillation occurs in patients with WPW syndrome, the risk of potentially lethal arrhythmias due to very rapid conduction across accessory pathways must be considered. The risk is particularly treacherous in patients with short-refractory-period anomalous pathways since atrial fibrillation may induce ventricular fibrillation.

Paroxysmal supraventricular tachycardia in WPW syndrome may begin in childhood or not appear until middle age. In asymptomatic patients, the probability of losing the capacity for antegrade conduction across the accessory pathway increases with advancing age.[26] Symptomatic arrhythmias may be due to PSVT, atrial fibrillation or flutter, or both in individual patients. In a series of 212 patients with tachyarrhythmias and WPW, PSVT alone occurred in 64 percent, atrial fibrillation alone in 20 percent, and both in 16 percent.[27] Since the reentrant tachyarrhythmias tend to be more rapid than those in patients with AV nodal reentry, they may be more symptomatic. Light headedness, near syncope, and syncope appear to occur more commonly in WPW with PSVT or atrial fibrillation than in AV nodal reentry.

A risk of sudden death in patients with WPW has been emphasized, but the magnitude of the risk is unknown, even in those with short refractory periods. Other factors that appear to influence risk are multiple tracts and family history of premature sudden death.[28]

Electrocardiographic Features The most common patterns recorded during PSVT due to WPW syndrome are narrow QRS tachycardias at rates ranging from 160 to 240 per minute. Rates may occasionally be faster or somewhat slower. When the tachycardia is antidromic, the

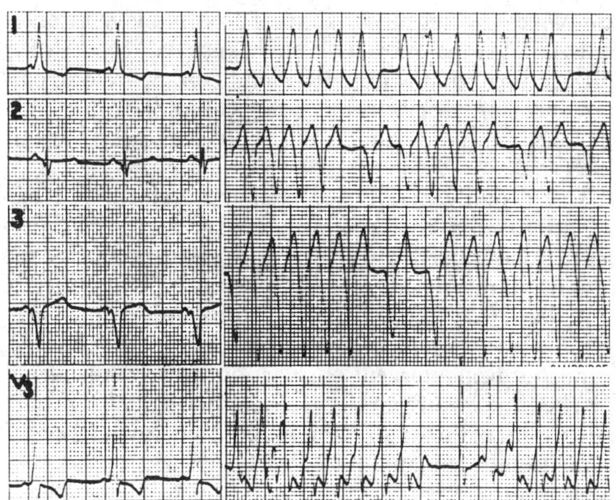

FIGURE 36-13 Atrial fibrillation in WPW syndrome with accessory pathway conduction. *Left*: Sinus rhythm with a typical preexcitation pattern. *Right*: Accessory pathway conduction during atrial fibrillation. The QRS axis has shifted to the left, and the ventricular rhythm is now irregular at a rate in excess of 200 per minute. (*From HJL Marriott, HM Rogers: Mimics of ventricular tachycardia associated with the W-P-W syndrome. J Electrocardiol 2: 77, 1969. Reproduced with permission from the publisher and author.*)

QRS complexes are wide and have characteristics similar to fully preexcited impulses during sinus rhythm or premature atrial contractions (see Fig. 36-12). In atrial fibrillation with WPW syndrome, if the accessory pathway has a refractory period longer than the normal pathway, the delta wave will disappear and typical atrial fibrillation with narrow QRS complexes will be recorded. In contrast, when the refractory period of the accessory pathway is shorter, wide QRS complexes dominate the tracing (Fig. 36-13). The grossly irregular rhythm, wide QRS complexes, and a mean ventricular rate in excess of 200 per minute are clues supporting WPW with atrial fibrillation in the differential diagnosis of a wide QRS complex tachycardia. Another form of wide QRS tachycardia in WPW is orthodromic tachycardia with functional bundle branch block. When a patient with left lateral bypass tract abruptly develops a left bundle branch block pattern during orthodromic tachycardia, the diagnosis of aberrancy is strongly suspected when the cycle length of the tachycardia lengthens when the QRS widens because of delayed return of the retrograde impulse to the accessory pathway. (See also Chap. 35.)

Management of PSVT Due to WPW Syndrome This form of reentrant SVT is amenable to a broad range of interventions. Careful attention to the details of therapy is required because a subgroup is at risk for potentially lethal arrhythmias due to very rapid conduction across the anomalous pathways during atrial flutter or fibrillation. This concern influences the pharmacologic approaches to PSVT in the WPW syndrome, since drugs have different effects on accessory pathways and the AV node and because reciprocating PSVT may convert to atrial flutter or fibrillation.[29]

The general physiological interventions and vagomimetic drugs can be used safely during acute episodes of reciprocating tachycardia. In addition, adenosine, verapamil, diltiazem, propranolol, and membrane-active antiarrhythmic agents such as procainamide, quinidine, or disopyramide may be used to convert acute reentrant tachycardias. Verapamil[30,31] and lidocaine[32] may accelerate the ventricular rate during atrial flutter or fibrillation in the WPW syndrome, however, and should be avoided if atrial fibrillation is present or if the patient has previously demonstrated alternation between atrial fibrillation and reciprocating tachycardia. Digoxin *must be avoided* in patients with WPW because it may shorten the refractory period of the accessory pathway[33] as well as atrial muscle. Should this occur in the presence of unrecognized atrial flutter or fibrillation or with the conversion of a reciprocating tachycardia to atrial fibrillation, the patient could develop a life-threatening tachyarrhythmia due to rapid accessory pathway conduction.[34] Whenever there is doubt, therapy should be limited to those drugs that will depress conduction in the accessory pathway or prolong its refractory period, such as the membrane-active antiarrhythmic agents, or to agents such as adenosine that have no effect on an accessory pathway. Electrical cardioversion should be used if other means have failed or as initial therapy if the patient has extremely rapid rates or is hemodynamically intolerant of the tachycardia.

The approach to long-term management of patients with WPW syndrome is determined by the physiological characteristics of the bypass tract and the frequency, duration, and symptoms of arrhythmias. Three choices of therapy are available: drugs, surgery, and catheter ablation. The latter, using an RF energy source, is rapidly evolving as the preferred method for treatment of patients with symptomatic or life-threatening arrhythmias in WPW (Fig. 36-14).[23,24,35] (See Chap. 43.) Intracardiac electrophysiological studies provide information on efficacy and pharmacologic effects on the bypass tract,[36] but this invasive procedure is not required for all patients.[37] Patients who demonstrate a good clinical response to therapy, measured in terms of reduced frequency or rate of tachyarrhythmic episodes, can be managed noninvasively; patients with intermittent delta wave and no clinical arrhythmia need no therapy. On the other hand, patients who have frequent or poorly tolerated tachyarrhythmias, those who are prone to episodes of atrial flutter or fibrillation[38] (particularly if they develop wide QRS complexes during their tachyarrhythmias, suggesting bypass tract conduction), or those who have a family history of WPW and sudden death[28,39] should be evaluated by electrophysiological testing. In such patients, catheter ablation using RF energy has rapidly emerged as the intervention of choice when available in an experienced laboratory and accepted by the patient.[24,35,40] When this is not available, or in the event of failure of the technique to ablate *the tract(s),* surgical interventions should be considered.[41,42] Among those with symptomatic or life-threatening arrhythmias for whom such interventions are not available or feasible, a clear-cut response to antiarrhythmic therapy is mandated. Among the antiarrhythmic agents, the class IA, IC, and III drugs (see Table 36-4) may be useful. At the time of this writing, not all of these drugs were approved for this indication in the United States, but efficacy stud-

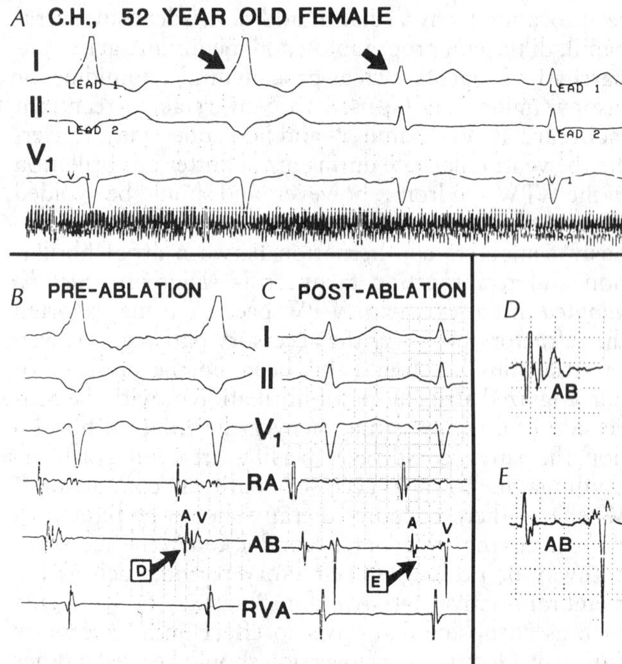

FIGURE 36-14 Radiofrequency ablation in WPW syndrome. The patient had frequent recurrent supraventricular tachycardias due to WPW syndrome. *A*. Standard leads I, II, and V_1 demonstrate disappearance of the delta wave from one impulse to the next, 5 s after beginning the application of radiofrequency energy (compare successive QRS complexes indicated by arrows). *B*. Prior to ablation, the interval between atrial (A) and ventricular (V) activation at the site of the ablation catheter is below 50 ms, and the sharp spike between A and V likely represents activity in the bypass tract. *C*. Immediately after ablation, the A-V interval at the site of the ablation catheter (AB) is lengthened to 150 ms, and the accessory pathway spike has disappeared. *D and E*. Enlargements of *D* and *E* from panels *B* and *C*, respectively. (RA = right atrium, AB = ablation catheter, RVA = right ventricular apex.)

ies are impressive.[43–47] Because of its side-effect profile, the threshold for use of amiodarone should be high, despite good efficacy.[45] (See also Chap. 38.)

Paroxysmal supraventricular tachycardia also occurs in patients with *concealed* WPW syndrome,[25,48] in which the bypass tract is incapable of conducting in the antegrade direction. Thus, there is no delta wave during sinus rhythm, but intact retrograde conduction permits reciprocating tachycardias. The diagnosis is suggested by longer RP intervals on the ECG during tachycardia than occur in AV nodal reentry[25] and can be established by electrophysiological testing. Management is similar to other WPW syndrome patients, except for the lack of concern about risk of atrial fibrillation degenerating to ventricular fibrillation.

Other Reentrant SVTs The other reentrant SVTs are far less common than PSVT due to AV node reentry or WPW syndrome. The *PSVT due to sinus node reentry*[49,50] may be difficult to distinguish clinically and by ECG from sinus tachycardia, except for its paroxysmal onset and offset. P-wave morphology is similar to that in sinus tachycardia. Intraatrial reentry[50,51] is difficult to distinguish from certain forms of automatic ectopic atrial tachycardia. Intraatrial or sinus node reentry are distinguished from PSVT due to AV node reentry or WPW on a standard ECG because P waves *precede* narrow QRS complexes during these tachycardias. Nodoventricular pathways (Mahaim tracts)[52] may cause PSVT with wide QRS complexes having a left bundle branch block pattern. Intracardiac electrophysiological studies are usually very helpful in distinguishing between these various PSVTs.

There is no generally accepted and predictably effective approach to therapy. Intraatrial reentrant tachycardia may be treated with conventional membrane-active antiarrhythmic agents, beta-adrenergic blocking agents, or perhaps Ca^{2+}-entry blockers. Sinus node reentry may respond to digoxin, propranolol, diltiazem, or verapamil. Surgical interventions[53] are only rarely considered for these arrhythmias because of their usually benign nature, but catheter ablation with RF energy may prove to be useful for many. (See also Chap. 43.)

Ectopic Atrial Tachycardias

These arrhythmias are usually persistent, are commonly referred to as "nonparoxysmal," and may be associated with specific inciting factors. There are experimental and clinical reasons to suspect that ectopic atrial tachycardia could be due to mechanisms of reentry[54] or automaticity (enhanced spontaneous phase 4 depolarization)[55] or a clinical expression of triggered activity.[56] An underlying toxic or metabolic cause is commonly identified as the factor responsible for ectopic atrial tachycardia. When an ectopic atrial rate is in the range of 160 to over 200 per minute and associated with 2 : 1 conduction or variable block in a patient receiving digitalis, a digitalis-toxic rhythm must be suspected strongly. Decompensated chronic lung disease, metabolic abnormalities (including acute alcohol abuse), electrolyte disturbances, and hypoxemia should be considered when digitalis toxicity has been excluded. Various forms of cardiac disease, including acute myocardial infarction, also may cause ectopic atrial tachycardia. Treatment is dictated by identification and reversal of inciting factors and by control of the heart rate when necessary.

Electrocardiographic Features P waves are usually normal to quite small in amplitude and may be difficult to identify when the ventricular rate is rapid (Fig. 36-15). Atrial activity does not slow during carotid sinus massage, but AV conduction is usually impeded, making P waves more evident. When due to digitalis intoxication, P waves may be "diminutive" and the ventricular rate slow (Fig. 36-16*A*) because of high grade block.

Management Temporary pacing is required infrequently. More commonly, the problem is one of a rapid ventricular rate. Attempts to control the atrial arrhythmia pharmacologically have not been uniformly successful with membrane-active drugs, beta-adrenergic blocking agents, or calcium-entry blocking agents, although all have been tried. Electrical cardioversion is not indicated because it is usually unsuccessful. The mainstay of therapy remains the removal or reversal of inciting factors. In the absence of identifying a reversible inciting factor, antiarrhythmic drugs may be tried. Surgical excision of the site of origin of a chronic ectopic atrial tachycardia can be achieved with intraoperative mapping.[57] It

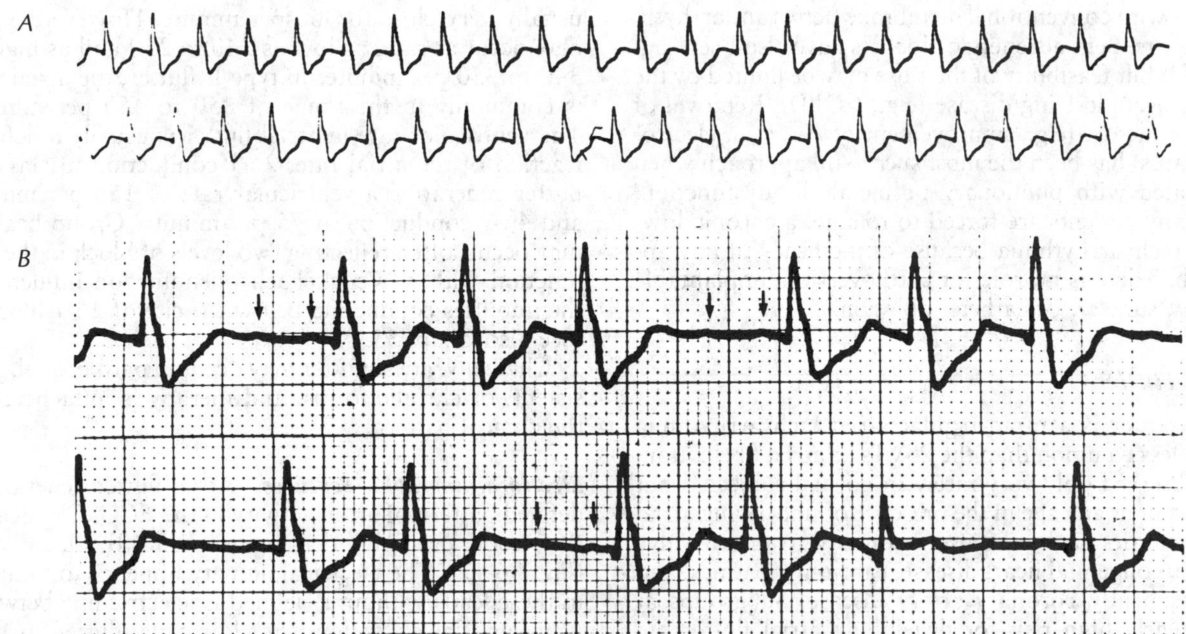

FIGURE 36-15 Ectopic atrial tachycardia. *A.* A 20-s continuous recording demonstrates a regular tachycardia at a ventricular rate of approximately 140 per minute. *B.* During carotid sinus massage, ventricular conduction becomes irregular and diminutive P waves at twice the basic ventricular rate are evident. Impaired AV conduction with little or no effect on atrial activity is characteristic of the response of an ectopic atrial tachycardia to carotid sinus massage.

should be used only under extraordinary circumstances, however, since atrial disease is commonly multicentric.

Multifocal Atrial Tachycardia; Chaotic Atrial Rhythm

The diagnosis requires the identification of P waves having three or more different morphologies that occur at different cycle lengths (Fig. 36-16*B*). The rhythm, as the name indicates, is usually chaotic, but the rate is not usually excessive (less than 140 per minute).[58] It is most commonly associated with underlying lung disease, metabolic abnormalities, electrolyte disturbances, and in rare instances toxic causes such as digitalis intoxication. Calcium-entry blockers have been tried with some success[59] when given acutely, but there is little or no

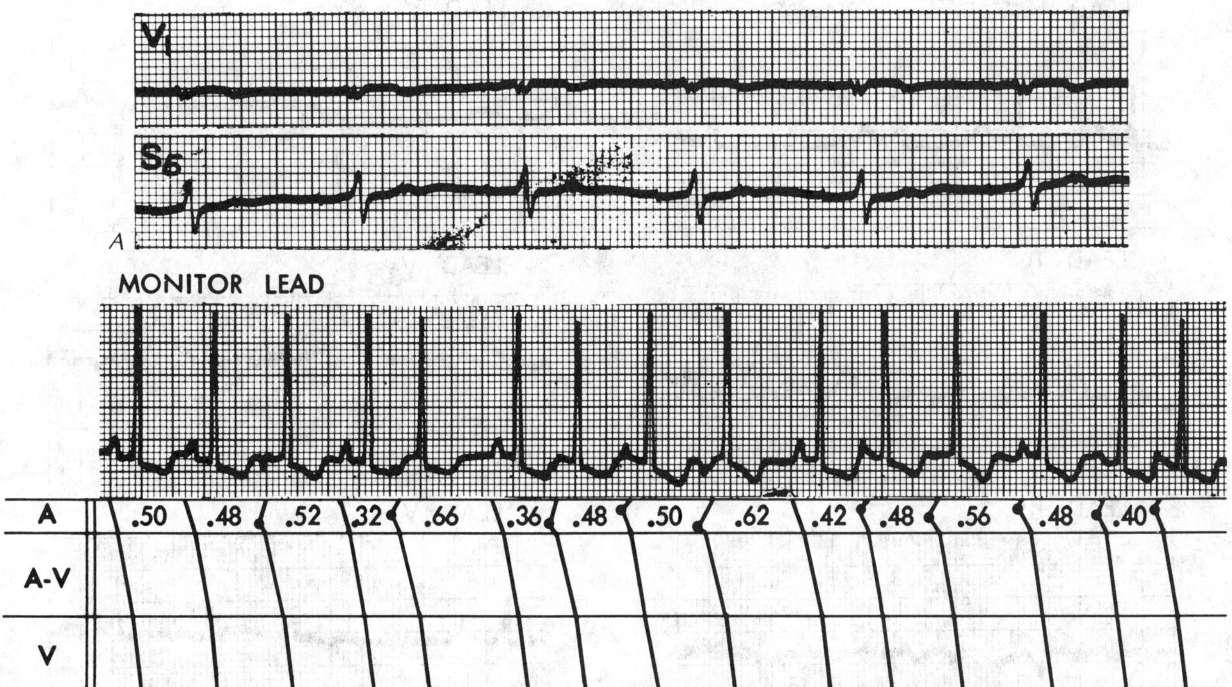

FIGURE 36-16 *A.* Atrial tachycardia with 2 : 1 AV block due to digitalis intoxication. Note the diminutive P waves, barely visible even in V_1. *B.* Multifocal (chaotic) atrial tachycardia. Note the constantly changing form of the ectopic P waves and the irregular rhythm at a mean rate of 122 per minute.

success with conventional membrane-active antiarrhythmic agents. Beta-adrenergic blockers have also been suggested,[60] but feasibility of their use may be limited by the nature of underlying disease (e.g., COPD). Removal of inciting factors (e.g., improvement of P_{O_2}, P_{CO_2}, electrolyte status) has been the most successful approach when associated with pulmonary or metabolic dysfunction, but many patients are forced to tolerate a chronic low-grade tachyarrhythmia because of inefficacy of any approach. There is no role for cardioversion, implantable devices, surgery, or catheter ablation.

Atrial Flutter

Atrial flutter is a rapid regular atrial tachyarrhythmia that is less common than the PSVTs or atrial fibrillation. It is observed only very rarely in normal subjects[61] but may occur at any age in the presence of underlying atrial abnormalities such as those secondary to mitral valve disease, congenital heart disease, cardiomyopathies, and less frequently coronary artery disease. Subgroups at particularly high risk for developing atrial flutter are children, adolescents, and young adults who have undergone corrective surgery for complex congenital heart diseases, most commonly transposition of the great vessels, tetralogy of Fallot, or atrial septal defects.[62]

Atrial flutter has been separated into two types, classical or type I and type II.[63] The distinction is not based upon differences in electrocardiographic morphology of atrial activity but rather upon (1) the ability to entrain and interrupt classical (type I) flutter with atrial pacing techniques and (2) a faster atrial rate in type II flutter compared to type I. Untreated classical type I flutter commonly has rates between 280 and 320 per minute, usually very close to 300 per minute. However, type I may occur at rates as low as 240 to 250 and as high as 340 to 350 per minute. In type II flutter, the atrial rate is commonly in the range of 350 to 450 per minute. The ventricular rate in atrial flutter is usually a defined fraction of the atrial rate, 2 : 1 conduction in classical flutter generating a ventricular rate of 150 per minute and 4 : 1 conduction at 75 per minute. Group beating may occur, often reflecting two levels of block in the AV junction with a Wenckebach phenomenon influencing the impulses conducting below the site of 2 : 1 block.[64] (See also Chap. 35.)

Clinically, atrial flutter may occur in paroxysmal, persistent, or chronic forms, and therapy is influenced by the clinical pattern.

Electrocardiographic Features Atrial flutter generates a defined pattern of atrial activity in the ECG. Classically, a sawtooth pattern is identifiable in leads II, III, and aVF (Fig. 36-17). The electrical activity appears continuous in these leads without a defined isoelectric line between wavelets. The exception is in slow atrial flutter, as may occur in the presence of antiarrhythmic drugs, in which a definite isoelectric line may appear in these leads. In contrast, other leads, most notably lead V_1, generally record discrete waves with an isoelectric line between them (Fig. 36-17). The pattern in leads II, III, and aVF may reflect the continuous electrical activity in the reentrant pathway in the low right atrium, while the pattern in lead V_1 reflects discrete signals approaching an area remote from the reentrant loop. Leads I and V_6 may generate intermediate patterns. In type II flutter, the electrocardiographic patterns are similar, except for the faster rate.

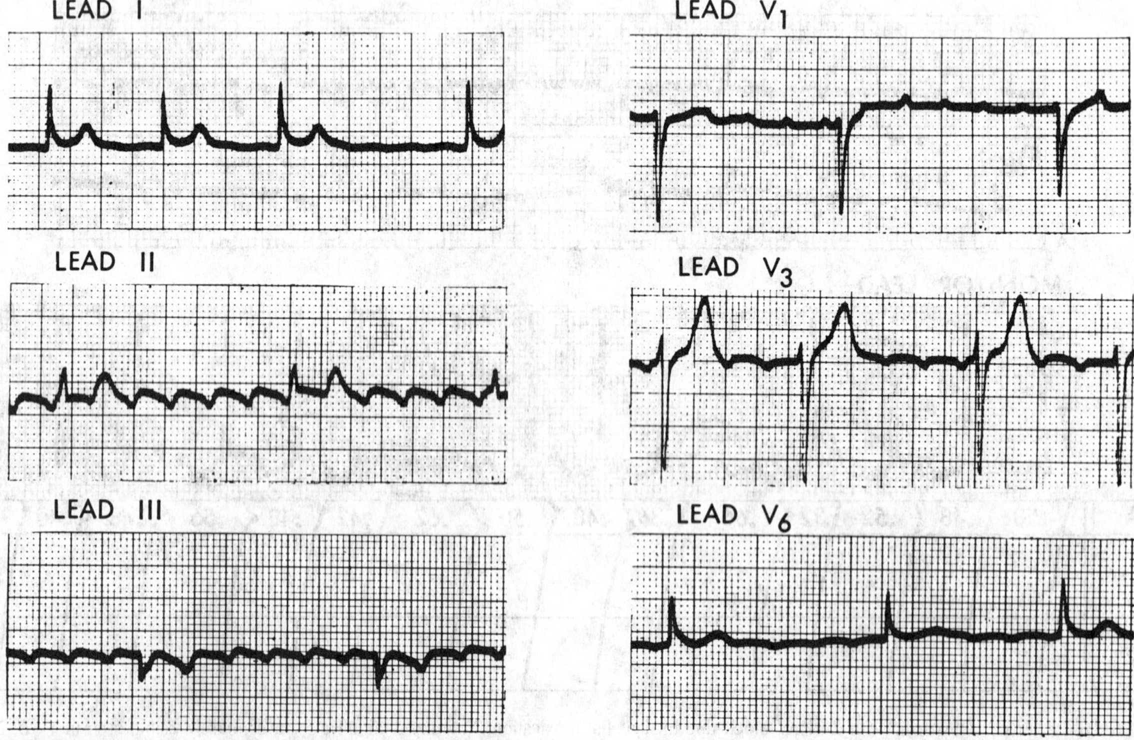

FIGURE 36-17 Atrial flutter. Note the "sawtooth" pattern in leads II and III, discrete atrial waves in V_1, and poorly registered atrial activity in leads I and V_6.

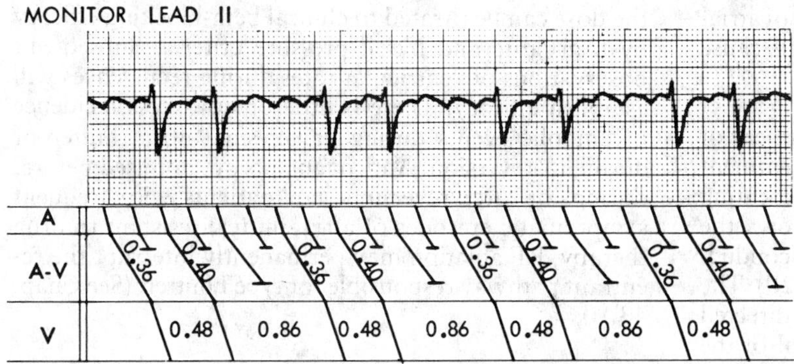

FIGURE 36-18 Atrial flutter with alternating 4 : 1 and 2 : 1 conduction. This common cause of bigeminal rhythm is almost always due to 2 : 1 AV conduction high in the AV junction and 3 : 2 Wenckebach periods at a lower level, as diagrammed.

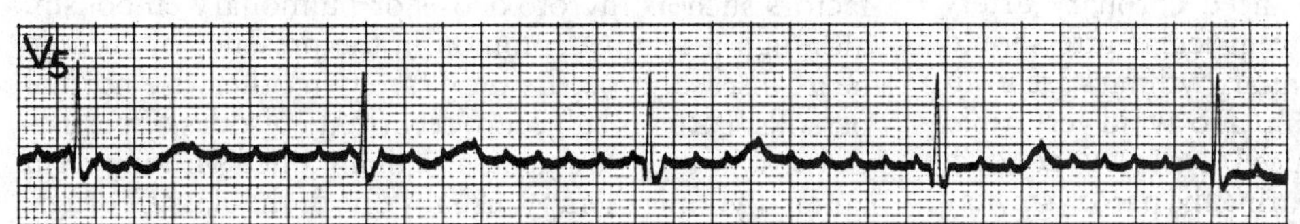

FIGURE 36-19 Atrial flutter (Type II) with complete AV block. The atrial rate is 366 per minute and the ventricular rate is 40 per minute. The ventricular rhythm remains regular while the relationship between atrial and ventricular complexes varies.

The most common AV conduction ratios in atrial flutter are 2 : 1 and 4 : 1, generating a ventricular rate of approximately 150 and 75 per minute. A 1 : 1 ratio may occur in young children and rarely in adults. Continuous 3 : 1 and 5 : 1 ratios are very rare, but alternating 2 : 1 and 4 : 1 ratios are common, generating a bigeminal pattern (Fig. 36-18). Occasionally, the second impulse of the bigeminal pattern is aberrantly conducted in the ventricles, requiring a distinction between the Ashman phenomenon and a ventricular ectopic beat. Atrial flutter associated with high-grade or complete AV block will produce a ventricular rate below 60 per minute with dissociation between flutter waves and QRS complexes (Fig. 36-19).

A narrow QRS complex tachycardia at a rate of 150 per minute should always lead to the consideration of atrial flutter. Carotid sinus massage may be helpful in distinguishing flutter from other mechanisms because of the characteristic response to the parasympathetic stimulus (see Fig. 36-20). Carotid sinus massage will not interrupt atrial flutter, but it will impair AV nodal conduction and cause an abrupt change from a rate of 150 per minute to one of 75 per minute or less. The unmasking of occult flutter waves at the slower ventricular rate will make the diagnosis obvious. In addition, the atrial rate in atrial flutter during carotid sinus massage tends to accelerate (Fig. 36-20). The combination of abrupt slowing of the ventricular rate and an increased rate of atrial

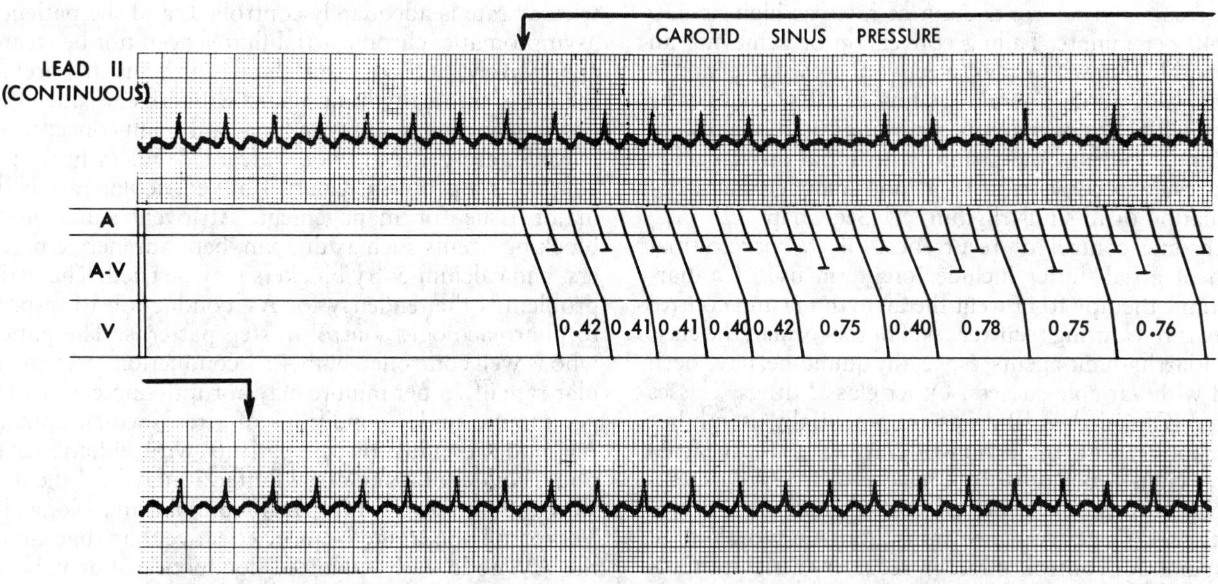

FIGURE 36-20 Atrial flutter and carotid sinus massage. At the beginning of the strip, AV conduction is occurring at the common 2 : 1 ratio, and flutter waves can be suspected but not proved; however, during carotid sinus massage, the conduction ratio increases to 4 : 1 and the flutter waves are clearly exposed. Note the tendency of the flutter rate to increase slightly during the parasympathetic stimulus.

electrical activity strongly supports the diagnosis of atrial flutter. Occasionally, carotid sinus massage will cause atrial flutter to convert to atrial fibrillation.

Management of Paroxysmal Atrial Flutter Treatment of acute paroxysmal atrial flutter differs from the treatment of PSVT due to AV nodal reentry or AV reciprocating mechanisms. Carotid sinus massage usually slows the ventricular rate by partially blocking AV nodal conduction but tends to increase the atrial rate (Fig. 36-20). The pharmacologic treatment of atrial flutter may be directed to reversion to a sinus mechanism or to control of the ventricular rate. The usual ventricular rate of 150 $\pm$ 10 per minute may be well tolerated in the absence of myocardial dysfunction, advanced coronary artery disease, or mitral stenosis. The ventricular rate should be slowed with digitalis before antiarrhythmics are instituted to convert the atrial arrhythmia to avoid very rapid rates associated with drug-induced 1 : 1 AV conduction.[65] Control of the heart rate during the paroxysm may also be achieved with calcium-entry blocking agents.[11] Verapamil has been studied in detail, and intravenous diltiazem is also successful. Nifedipine has little clinical effect on AV nodal conduction and therefore is not useful.

When the ventricular rate is poorly tolerated due to effects on hemodynamics or coronary blood flow, electrical cardioversion is used as initial treatment. An attempt at 10 to 20 W · s may be successful; higher energies may be used if necessary.

Conventional antiarrhythmic agents are used to convert flutter to sinus rhythm, but efficacy is unpredictable. Quinidine historically has been the initial drug of choice, but the other class IA antiarrhythmic agents may be equally effective. Conventional dosing schedules are now used, in contrast to the highly toxic aggressive quinidine protocols of the past. The class IC drugs (flecainide, encainide) may also be effective for pharmacologic reversion of atrial flutter,[43] although they slow intraatrial conduction without lengthening refractory periods, which may result in 1 : 1 conduction at rates as high as 220 to 240 per minute. Failing conversion or achieving an acceptable rate with drugs, elective DC cardioversion is usually successful. Energies as low as 10 W · s may be effective. If cardioversion is contraindicated or fails, an attempt to entrain the atrium with rapid atrial pacing may result in conversion to a more manageable atrial fibrillation or to sinus rhythm.[66,67] (See Chap. 39.)

Chronic control of recurrences of the paroxysmal form of atrial flutter include long-term use of antiarrhythmic therapy to prevent the arrhythmia and control of heart rate during recurrences. For the former, the class IA antiarrhythmic agents, especially quinidine, have been used with variable success. Other class I drugs (classes IB and IC) and class III drugs are potentially useful, but the concern with the action of class IC drugs in atrial flutter cited above must be considered. Control of ventricular rate is best achieved with digitalis because of safety and efficacy considerations. Long-term oral use of verapamil for control of rate in recurrent atrial flutter is less predictably effective than intravenous use to slow the rate during a paroxysm.[10] Beta-adrenergic blocking agents have been used, and if the drugs are well tolerated, the dose can be titrated to clinical beta-blocking efficacy by heart rate and blood pressure criteria. Subsequent observations of ventricular rates during recurrences will establish efficacy. There is little or no excess incidence of embolic events during paroxysmal atrial flutter or during its reversion. Anticoagulants are not used before, during, or after reversion. For patients with frequent symptomatic episodes of atrial flutter, resistant to drug therapy, RF ablation may permanently interrupt the reentrant pathway responsible for type I flutter. (See Chap. 43.)

Management of Persistent Atrial Flutter Atrial flutter may occur in a persistent form secondary to noncardiac factors such as thyrotoxicosis or pulmonary embolism, although it is most common in the presence of chronic heart disease. It occurs only rarely in otherwise normal persons. Patients subject to recurrent episodes of persistent atrial flutter are generally maintained on long-term antiarrhythmic therapy, usually one of the class IA drugs. Class IC and class III drugs may also be effective in some. If the arrhythmia continues to recur despite chronic drug treatment, therapeutic approaches during recurrences may include additional antiarrhythmic agents for reverting atrial flutter and agents that will control the ventricular rate. Electrical reversion, however, is commonly required. The same general approaches outlined for paroxysmal atrial flutter are applied. Surgical approaches are feasible and are being evaluated for patients with frequent symptomatic recurrences,[53] and catheter ablation has been successful.[68]

Management of Chronic Atrial Flutter Some patients will remain in atrial flutter despite aggressive therapy, and flutter will recur predictably shortly after DC cardioversion. This usually occurs in the setting of advanced heart disease and commonly is the forerunner of chronic atrial fibrillation. It may occur rarely in otherwise normal persons[61] and more commonly in association with other SVTs, such as WPW and AV nodal reentry.[69] If the ventricular rate is adequately controlled, and the patient is asymptomatic, chronic atrial flutter need not be treated aggressively. In these cases, there is little justification for the use of antiarrhythmic agents with adverse side-effect profiles; and surgical procedures, although conceptually feasible, are generally not warranted unless heart rate control is a problem. Control of ventricular rate is the major issue for management. Atrioventricular nodal blocking agents such as digoxin, beta-adrenergic blockers, and calcium-entry blockers may be tried. The major problem is the tendency for AV conduction to respond to pharmacologic control in step patterns. The patient who is well controlled with 4 : 1 conduction at a ventricular rate of 75 per minute may abruptly increase to 150 per minute under conditions of stress, which enhance AV nodal conduction. In patients with enhanced AV nodal conduction and atrial flutter, it may be difficult to slow the rate below 150 per minute pharmacologically. Verapamil appears to be more effective than digoxin for the AV node with enhanced conduction, but it is not uniformly effective. In some patients, catheter ablation for AV node modification is necessary for rate control, and direct surgical interruption is possible in some patients,[53] as is catheter ablation of the type I flutter pathway.[68] Long-term anticoagulation is not generally used for chronic atrial flutter.

Atrial Fibrillation

The prevalence, presentation, clinical significance, and long-term implications of atrial fibrillation depend heavily upon the clinical circumstance in which it occurs. Among the cross-sectional studies of prevalence, there is a large gradient across age categories, ranging from less than 0.5 percent in young adults to the range of 1 to 5 percent through the decades from 40 to 70 years and reaching rates in excess of 10 percent in some beyond age 70.[70] At each age, however, prevalence is powerfully influenced by the presence of disease, especially rheumatic mitral valve disease but also nonrheumatic abnormalities. The clinical presentation ranges from a minimally symptomatic or asymptomatic incidental finding to acute pulmonary edema in patients with advanced mitral or aortic stenosis. Between these extremes, atrial fibrillation may herald the presence of noncardiac disorders (e.g., thyrotoxicosis), alert to the significance of another cardiac disorder (e.g., WPW syndrome), constitute a transient complicating factor of another cardiac disorder (e.g., acute myocardial infarction or systemic arterial hypertension), or occur as an isolated event having no inherent significance (e.g., lone paroxysmal atrial fibrillation in healthy young adults). The hemodynamic consequences of atrial fibrillation are due to two factors: (1) the loss of atrial systole may impair ventricular function in the noncompliant ventricle [e.g., aortic stenosis, left ventricular hypertrophy (LVH)] or the dilated ventricle with systolic dysfunction and (2) a rapid ventricular rate encroaches upon diastolic filling of the left ventricle and the coronary arteries. The risk of embolism and stroke is a long-term concern of special importance (see below). Atrial fibrillation may occur in paroxysmal, persistent, and chronic patterns.

Electrocardiographic Features Atrial fibrillation is characterized electrocardiographically by grossly disorganized atrial electrical activity that is irregular in respect to both rate and rhythm. There is no visually discernible timing pattern to the atrial electrical activity on the surface ECG or to electrogram sequences recorded by catheter electrodes. Specific patterns of AV conduction sequences (ventricular responses) have been proposed as a result of sophisticated analytic techniques[71]; this appears to provide some physiological insight but does not yet have practical clinical value. Atrial fibrillatory waves are best seen in standard lead V_1 and are usually clearly evident in II, III, and aVF as well. They may be quite large and coarse or almost imperceptible (compare panels *A* and *B* in Fig. 36-21). In the absence of discernible atrial electrical activity, a grossly irregular ventricular rhythm still suggests the presence of atrial fibrillation. Coarse atrial fibrillation is occasionally difficult to distinguish from atrial flutter waves, but the irregular ventricular response is again helpful in making the distinction. In contrast, obvious coarse flutter waves with a regular ventricular response, especially when slow, suggests the

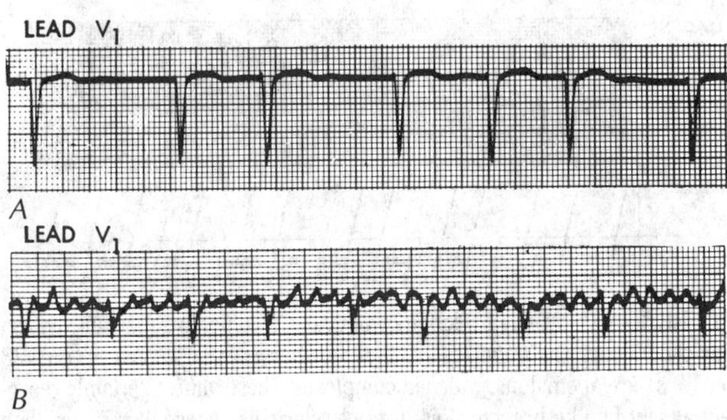

FIGURE 36-21 *A*. Fine atrial fibrillation, leaving virtually no imprint on the baseline ("straight-line" fibrillation). *B*. Coarse atrial fibrillation; the fibrillatory waves are the size of respectable flutter waves but are irregular.

coexistence of high-grade AV block with atrial fibrillation.

One of the more challenging exercises in clinical electrocardiography is the distinction between aberrant intraventricular conduction and ventricular ectopy in the presence of atrial fibrillation. Aberrant conduction tends to occur when a long ventricular cycle is followed by a short cycle. This long-short cycle sequence, with the short cycle terminated by an aberrantly conducted beat, is referred to as the *Ashman phenomenon*.[72] It is important to recognize that "long" and "short" cycles are relative terms and carry no implications of absolute value (see Figs. 36-22 and 36-23). A series of short cycles, if short enough, may generate runs of consecutively aberrant beats imitating ventricular tachycardia (Fig. 36-23). Thus, additional criteria for distinction between aberrancy and ectopy are required. In general, an initial QRS vector similar or identical to that of narrow QRS complexes and a typical right bundle branch block pattern, in association with a long-short cycle sequence, strongly favor aberrancy over ectopy.[73] Left bundle branch block aberrancy also occurs, but it is far less common. It is more likely when aberrant conduction is persistent (i.e., functional bundle branch block during a sustained supraventricular tachycardia) (Fig. 36-11), while it is unusual

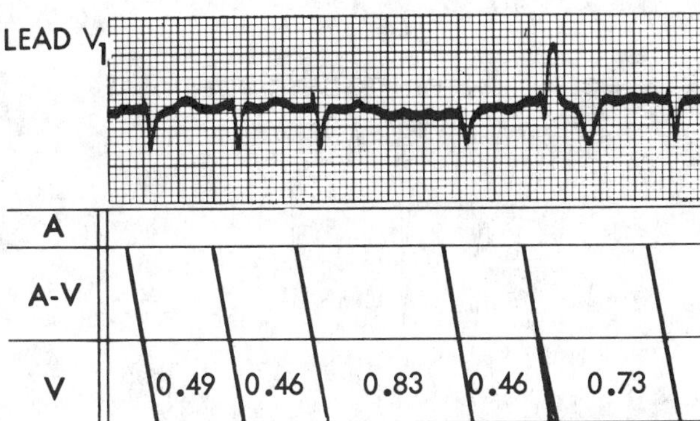

FIGURE 36-22 Ashman's phenomenon. During atrial fibrillation, the impulse ending a short cycle preceded by a relatively long cycle manifests aberrant intraventricular conduction. In this example, the aberrant beat shows typical right bundle branch block type aberration in lead V_1, with an rsR′ pattern and the initial deflection identical with that of the preceding and following normally conducted beats.

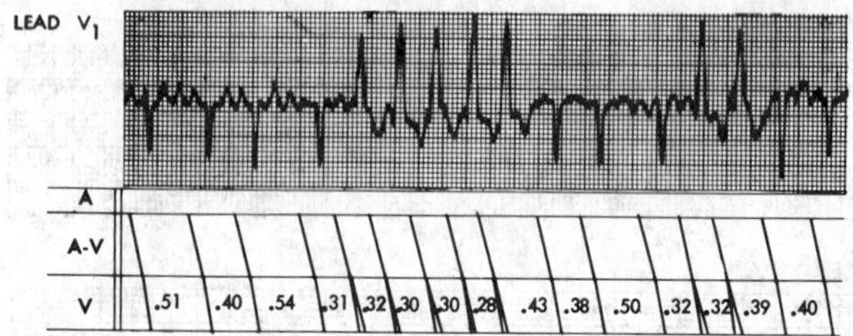

FIGURE 36-23 Atrial fibrillation complicated by repetitive aberrant ventricular conduction. The impulses that end the shortest ventricular cycles (0.28 to 0.32 s) are anomalous, widened complexes. These almost certainly represent a right bundle branch block type of ventricular aberration rather than ventricular ectopy. Note that the cycle preceding the onset of the salvos of anomalous beats is relatively long (0.54 and 0.50 s), in accordance with Ashman's phenomenon.

in single-cycle aberrancy (Fig. 36-22). Atrial fibrillation alters intraventricular conduction only through the mechanisms of (1) functional bundle branch block or aberrancy (Fig. 36-24), (2) loss of delta waves in WPW syndrome with normal pathway conduction during atrial fibrillation, or (3) totally preexcited QRS complexes during atrial fibrillation in WPW syndrome (Fig. 36-13). The QRS complex during atrial fibrillation will be similar to that recorded during sinus rhythm under all other circumstances. In patients with preexisting bundle branch block who develop atrial fibrillation with rapid ventricular responses, the distinction from ventricular tachycardia may be difficult.

Evaluation of the First Episode of Atrial Fibrillation

The first episode of atrial fibrillation requires special attention, in the form of a thorough investigation of the clinical status to determine whether the patient has a primary electrical cause, an event secondary to hemodynamic abnormalities, or a systemic abnormality that predisposes to atrial fibrillation. It is necessary to exclude previously unrecognized mitral or aortic stenosis or regurgitation, hypertension, coronary heart disease, cardiomyopathy, atrial septal defect, pericarditis, or atrial abnormalities secondary to left or right ventricular overload. Pulmonary emboli and metabolic abnormalities, such as thyrotoxicosis, also must be considered. The

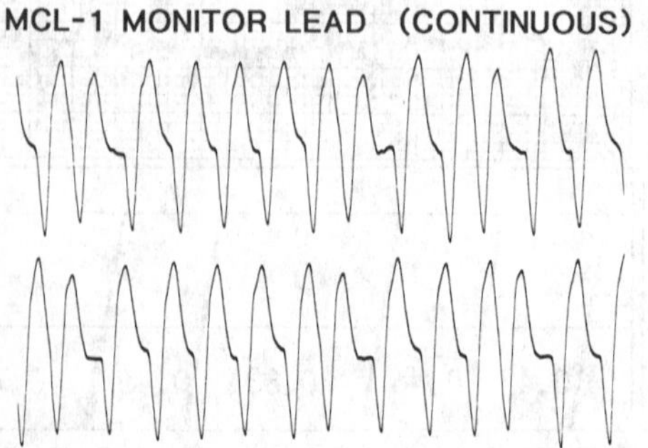

FIGURE 36-24 Irregular wide QRS tachycardia. A rapid irregular rhythm with wide QRS complexes having a left bundle branch block pattern is recorded. The rhythm is atrial fibrillation with abnormal intraventricular conduction. A similar pattern may occur in WPW syndrome with atrial fibrillation and conduction down the accessory pathway or in rare cases of irregular ventricular tachycardia.

identification of associated factors at the time of the first episode of atrial fibrillation will dictate future management. In the absence of an identifiable cause, so-called lone atrial fibrillation carries a good prognosis,[74] especially if it is a single event or intermittently recurrent. Chronic lone atrial fibrillation may indicate a higher risk,[75] although conflicting data[74] question the validity of this conclusion. In a young, healthy individual in whom there is no evidence of structural heart disease, paroxysmal episodes of lone atrial fibrillation may occur under conditions of exogenous precipitating factors, such as excessive cigarette, alcohol, and/or coffee consumption, stress or fatigue, and rarely upon cessation of extreme exercise.

In the absence of organic heart disease or coexistent WPW syndrome, long-term management after the first episode need include no more than avoidance or removal of precipitating factors and continuous observation of the patient to estimate the frequency of recurrences. In the presence of treatable cardiac or noncardiac causes, management must include attention to precipitating factors. For instance, in atrial fibrillation occurring during the acute phase of myocardial infarction, which has been observed in up to 18 percent of monitored patients, spontaneous reversion is very common and rate control is the only therapy needed. In the setting of thyrotoxicosis, there is little justification for trying to convert atrial fibrillation until the thyrotoxic state is controlled; the ventricular rate may be slowed with propranolol in the interim. When atrial fibrillation calls attention to previously undiagnosed mitral stenosis, the patient should be evaluated for surgery. If the patient is a candidate at that time, conversion of atrial fibrillation can await the postoperative period if the ventricular rate is controlled. In atrial septal defect, atrial fibrillation generally is a sign of advanced hemodynamic deterioration, and such patients must be considered for surgery promptly. In patients with advanced heart disease of any etiology, and dilated atria, the first episode may herald a chronic fibrillatory state. Some clinicians will make a first attempt at reversion, either pharmacologically or electrically, the latter usually with a concomitant pharmacologic agent, but the recurrence rate is high.[76,77] The recent onset of chronic atrial fibrillation has special implication for anticoagulation therapy (see below).

If it is felt that the patient will benefit from the hemodynamic advantage provided by an atrial contraction, one attempt at reversion during the first episode of atrial fibrillation is warranted. In hemodynamically significant mitral stenosis or aortic stenosis, acute pulmonary edema may follow the onset of the first episode of atrial fibrillation, making immediate electrical cardioversion mandatory. In mitral stenosis, recurrences can be expected; but even a short time in sinus rhythm can provide hemodynamic benefit and allow institution of therapy that will control the ventricular rate with the next episode. A longer diastolic filling period may prevent the recurrence of pulmonary edema. In aortic stenosis, dependence upon the atrial kick for optimal hemodynamic function of the noncompliant hypertrophied left ventricle, rather than encroachment on the diastolic filling period, is the major concern. In some patients, multiple cardioversions may be necessary while preparing for surgery.

Management of Paroxysmal Atrial Fibrillation Short paroxysms of atrial fibrillation in the absence of underlying heart disease are usually managed conservatively. Rest, mild sedation with 5 to 10 mg of diazepam, and digitalis for control of the ventricular rate is the usual approach. After the first episode, patients having lone atrial fibrillation can be reassured in respect to the absence of underlying organic heart disease and guided to avoid precipitating factors. In the presence of heart disease, particularly when the hemodynamic circumstances require either the mechanical benefit of atrial systole or a slow ventricular rate, immediate reversion to sinus rhythm or slowing of the ventricular rate may be mandatory. The presence of clinical signs of heart failure require immediate cardioversion to achieve either or both of these goals. If the patient is clinically stable, pharmacologic approaches to control the rate (digitalis or intravenous verapamil or diltiazem) may be attempted, as may antiarrhythmic agents.

Chronic pharmacologic therapy in the absence of underlying heart disease, or only trivial abnormalities, is based on the need to control ventricular rate during recurrences. Digitalis, beta blockers, or Ca^{2+}-entry blockers are used as described for atrial flutter. Prevention of episodes of atrial fibrillation may be achieved with class IA, IC, or III antiarrhythmic drugs. If episodes are clinically benign and infrequent, the threshold for such treatment should be high. Efficacy is uneven and proarrhythmic or toxic side effects are of concern. During short paroxysms of atrial fibrillation, anticoagulation is not required prior to reversion; and long-term anticoagulation is not necessary for patients subject to short paroxysmal attacks.[78]

Management of Persistent Atrial Fibrillation The decision to intervene in atrial fibrillation that has lasted for days is based on the balance between hemodynamic tolerance and the likelihood of being able to control future episodes. Many patients with organic heart disease have intermittent episodes of persistent atrial fibrillation prior to establishing chronic atrial fibrillation.[79] These are the most difficult patients for management since antiarrhythmic efficacy for control of recurrences is unpredictable. Prediction of the ability to control ventricular rate by AV nodal blocking agents is better but still imperfect. After the first episode of persistent atrial fibrillation, most clinicians avoid electrical cardioversion of recurrences of a persistent pattern if they are well tolerated hemodynamically. In view of the fact that they will revert and recur intermittently until the patient evolves into chronic atrial fibrillation, the best therapeutic approach is control of ventricular rate during recurrences. Membrane-active antiarrhythmic agents are often used in an attempt to limit the number of recurrences, but efficacy is unpredictable and risk of side effects is high. The flecainide data seem promising,[47,80] especially for patients with good left ventricular function and those free of underlying coronary artery disease.[8,9]

Management of Chronic Atrial Fibrillation The ventricular rate in chronic atrial fibrillation is more easily controlled than in recurrent episodes of paroxysmal or persistent atrial fibrillation. The only indication for attempting pharmacologic or electrical cardioversion in patients with advanced heart disease and atrial enlargement is the possibility of a hemodynamic benefit. This is a matter for individual clinical judgment, but most agree that no more than one attempt at electrical cardioversion is warranted in the presence of adequate levels of a membrane-active antiarrhythmic agent. Among patients with diverse diseases who have been electrically cardioverted, approximately one-third will revert back to atrial fibrillation within 1 week and two-thirds within 12 months.[76] If the patient reverts to chronic atrial fibrillation shortly after cardioversion, the probability of long-term maintenance of sinus rhythm is nearly nil. The ventricular rate is controlled as outlined above.

Anticoagulation of Patients with Atrial Fibrillation This is an important component in the management of patients with persistent or chronic atrial fibrillation. It is generally accepted that patients with atrial fibrillation have a greater than fivefold increase in risk of stroke, compared to control populations without atrial fibrillation.[81–84] In addition, there are specific high-risk subgroups. Among patients with rheumatic heart disease, the risk exceeds by up to 17 times that of a control group.[82,83] Other subgroups at high risk include patients with dilated cardiomyopathy, dilated left atrium of any cause, atrial fibrillation of recent onset, and a history of prior embolism. Atrial fibrillation in thyrotoxic patients is also accompanied by an increased incidence of embolic events.[85] The chronic form of "lone" atrial fibrillation has been reported to be associated with a relative increase in risk of embolic stroke,[86] although other studies have not identified an increased risk. As a group, the nonrheumatic disease states associated with atrial fibrillation tend to have excess risks in the range of five to six times among various studies.[70] However, absolute risks differ little between the various rheumatic and nonrheumatic etiologies, with event rates in the range of 4 to 6 percent for each, except for lone atrial fibrillation, which has a considerably lower rate.[70,74,86] The risk of embolic events tends to cluster around changes in rhythm—the highest incidence occurring within the first year after onset of chronic atrial fibrillation[82] and a concentrated 1- to 2-percent risk occurring in the first days after conversion to sinus rhythm.[87–89]

The issue of anticoagulation in atrial fibrillation hinges on a balance between efficacy of preventing embolic events and risk of bleeding. Until recently, most of the data on efficacy of anticoagulation for reducing incidence of embolic events in atrial fibrillation were from poorly controlled or uncontrolled studies, and there was no concensus based on the available data.[81] The available combination of risk and retrospective or uncontrolled efficacy data[77,78,81] tended to result in the practice of using long-term anticoagulation for patients with a rheumatic etiology, as well as those with advanced structural diseases, associated with atrial fibrillation. This included patients with coronary artery disease and a prior embolism, idiopathic dilated cardiomyopathy, and of course prosthetic cardiac valves. Several recent placebo-controlled studies have now provided considerable clarification of the role and methods for anticoagulation in patients with nonrheumatic atrial fibrillation.

In one multicenter randomized trial, the Stroke Prevention in Atrial Fibrillation (SPAF) Study, aspirin, 325 mg/day, and warfarin with prolongation of prothrombin times to 1.3 to 1.8 times control were each compared to placebo among a population of 1330 patients.[90] During a mean follow-up of 1.3 years, ischemic stroke or systemic embolization occurred at a rate of 6.3 percent per year in the placebo group, compared to 3.6 percent per year in the aspirin-treated group, a 42-percent reduction in the treated group ($p = .02$). Among the warfarin eligible patients, the event rate in the untreated group was 7.4 percent compared to 2.3 percent in the treated group, a 67-percent reduction ($p < .01$). Primary embolic events and deaths combined were reduced by 58 percent in the warfarin group and 32 percent in the aspirin group. Thus, both warfarin and aspirin were effective, but the design of the study prevented comparison of the two treatments. Although both chronic atrial fibrillation and intermittent atrial fibrillation were included in the study, the data reported do not permit a determination of any difference in risk or benefit for the two patterns. In another study, the Canadian Atrial Fibrillation Anticoagulation (CAFA) Study, the placebo group experienced a 5.2 percent embolism/stroke rate compared to 3.5 percent in a warfarin-treated group, a relative reduction of 37 percent with treatment.[91] The differences did not reach statistical significance since the study was prematurely terminated because of outcome data from other large studies suggesting benefit. Among two other studies, the Copenhagen AFASK Study[92] and the Boston Area Anticoagulation Trial in Atrial Fibrillation,[93] warfarin again demonstrated significant reductions in risk (82 and 87 percent, respectively), while aspirin demonstrated only a 14-percent reduction in the Copenhagen study (nonsignificant),[92] even though it was associated with a 42-percent reduction in the SPAF study.[90] In summary, these studies all show the same outcome—a significant benefit for reduction of embolism and stroke in nonrheumatic atrial fibrillation patients with the use of warfarin and likely with aspirin as an alternative. (See Chap. 122.)

Indications for anticoagulation prior to elective cardioversion have not undergone the same scrutiny for efficacy as has now been provided for chronic (and possibly intermittent) atrial fibrillation. Nonetheless, there is enough information available to warrant the routine use of anticogulation prior to elective cardioversion of recent onset, persistent atrial fibrillation, or chronic atrial fibrillation, particularly when associated with an enlarged left atrium, regardless of etiology. Anticoagulation with warfarin is started 3 to 4 weeks before elective cardioversion and is maintained for 3 to 4 weeks subsequently. Anticoagulation may be used less uniformly prior to elective cardioversion of atrial fibrillation of short duration (less than 2 to 3 days), particularly if it is lone atrial fibrillation or associated with minimal structure disease and normal atrial dimensions. The risk-benefit data are less clear under these conditions.

The potential efficacy of anticoagulation must be weighed against its risk. Patients receiving anticoagulants retain a risk of embolization in the range of 1 to greater than 3 percent,[70,77,89–93] depending upon disease states. Furthermore, there is a significant incidence of major bleeding events (requiring transfusion) or life-threatening events among patients on long-term anticoagulation. However, in one report,[94] the incidence was 4.3 percent per treatment year. However, in the SPAF study,[90] bleeding risk hovered around 1.5 percent and did not differ among aspirin-treated, warfarin-treated, and placebo groups. The less aggressive warfarin dosing than used previously (prothrombin times 1.3 to 1.8 times control) may be one reason for the absence of excess risk with warfarin. Since the risk is accentuated with prothrombin times greater than 2.5 times control, the inability to control the prothrombin time, including inability of the patient to comply with the prescribed dosages, must be considered relative contraindications. Intracranial bleeds are considered among the major complications and may have an incidence of 1 to 2 percent per treatment year.[95] Table 36-7 lists indications and relative contraindications for anticoagulation in patients with atrial fibrillation. The physician must balance accepted indications and risks in judging whether or not to use anticoagulation in individual patients. For instance, in intermittent lone atrial fibrillation, the risk of embolic events is so low that warfarin should be avoided. When anticoagulation is used, warfarin is given in sufficient doses to prolong the prothrombin time 1.3 to 1.8 times control [international normalized ratio (INR) of 2.0 to 3.0]. (See also Chap. 68.)

TABLE 36-7

Anticoagulation of Patients with Atrial Fibrillation

Indications
Rheumatic mitral valve disease with recurrent or chronic atrial fibrillation
Dilated cardiomyopathy with recurrent persistent or chronic atrial fibrillation
Prosthetic valves
Elective cardioversion of persistent or chronic atrial fibrillation, especially with mitral valve disease, prosthetic valves, dilated left atrium, or prior embolic events
Coronary heart disease or hypertensive heart disease with recurrent or chronic atrial fibrillation
Chronic or persistent lone atrial fibrillation
Controversial; or limited data
Coronary or hypertensive heart disease with normal left atrial size, after first episode of persistent atrial fibrillation
Atrial fibrillation in thyrotoxicosis (while awaiting long-term control; elective cardioversion)
Elective cardioversion of atrial fibrillation of short duration (2–3 days) with normal left atrial size with structural heart disease
Not indicated
Paroxysmal lone atrial fibrillation
Most clinical settings associated with short paroxysms in otherwise normal hearts
Relative contraindications
Difficulty controlling prothrombin times
Dementia
Malignancies
Prior bleeding events
Uncontrolled hypertension

ATRIOVENTRICULAR JUNCTIONAL AND ACCELERATED VENTRICULAR RHYTHMS

Rhythm disturbances that originate in the AV junction include premature AV junctional impulses, accelerated junctional rhythms, and AV junctional tachycardias that may be automatic or reentrant. Those arrhythmias that incorporate the AV junction as part of a larger reentrant pathway (i.e., various accessory pathway syndromes) and PSVT due to AV nodal reentry are discussed elsewhere. Junctional escape rhythms at rates of 40 to 60 per minute during sinus bradycardia or AV block are normal physiological phenomena; failure of normal junctional escape mechanisms resulting in significant bradycardia will be discussed later.

The normal inherent rate of AV junctional automatic activity is 40 to 60 per minute, and those of subordinate pacemakers at the fascicular or ventricular level are 20 to 40 per minute. Faster rates from either of these levels are considered "accelerated" rhythms up to 100 impulses per minute, at which point they take on the general definition of a tachycardia. Accelerated junctional and accelerated ventricular rhythms and most nonparoxysmal AV junctional tachycardias are thought to be due to enhanced automatic activity.[96,97] Clinical and experimental observations suggest that the mechanism of acceleration is enhanced phase 4 depolarization, although other forms of abnormal automaticity, including triggered activity initiated by afterdepolarizations, may also originate in the AV junction.[98,99] (See also Chap. 35.)

AV Junctional Premature Beats

These occur much less frequently than premature atrial or ventricular complexes. The timing of P waves and QRS complexes is variable, however. The P waves may precede QRS complexes by 0.12 s or less, may be concealed within the QRS complexes, or may appear in the ST segment following the QRS complex (Fig. 36-25). The P waves are usually inverted in leads II, III, and aVF, isoelectric to slightly inverted in leads I and V_6, and upright in the right precordial leads. The QRS complexes are narrow except when aberrant intraventricular conduction is present. When the P waves precede the QRS complex, distinction from premature atrial complexes may be difficult, and when aberrant intraventricular conduction is present and the P wave is within or after the QRS complex, the distinction from premature ventricular complexes may be impossible without intracardiac recordings. There are no special aspects to the management of AV junctional premature beats. They generally require no treatment; but when treated, they are approached using the same principles applied to the treatment of premature ventricular complexes (see below).

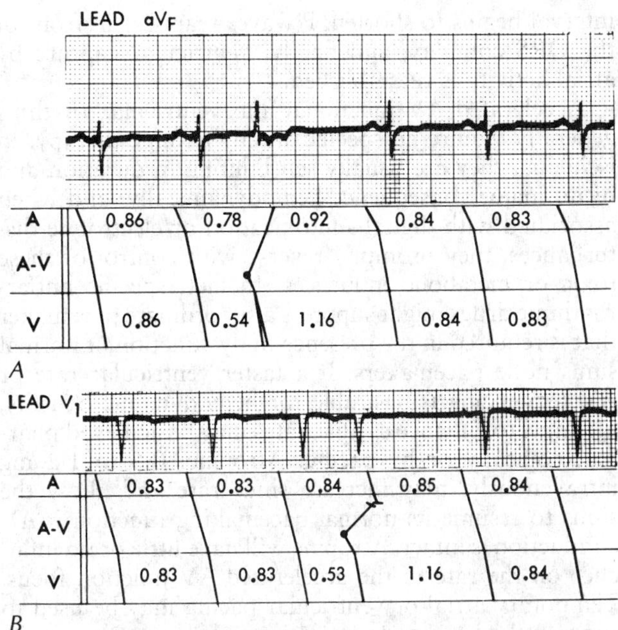

FIGURE 36-25 *A.* AV junctional extrasystole: The retrograde P wave follows the premature QRS complex, which shows some degree of ventricular aberration. *B.* The fourth complex is an AV premature impulse without retroconduction to the atria, leaving the sinus rhythm undisturbed.

Accelerated Junctional and Accelerated Ventricular Rhythms

Accelerated rhythms derive from subordinate pacemakers and emerge when the sinus rate is less than the normally suppressed focus. Sinus bradycardia combined with enhanced automaticity of the subordinate site is the common pathophysiology. Ischemia (especially inferior wall myocardial ischemia or infarction), digitalis intoxication, electrolyte disturbances (especially hypokalemia), and hypoxemia may enhance phase 4 depolarization in the AV junction or intraventricular specialized conducting system, accelerating the rate of impulse formation of the subordinate pacemakers located at these sites. Digitalis intoxication, various degrees of AV block, and sinus node depression may accompany AV junctional acceleration producing complex ECG patterns. In inferior wall ischemia, subordinate pacemaker acceleration is commonly associated with sinus node depression.

The typical electrocardiographic pattern is apparent shortening of the P-R interval as the P-P intervals prolong, leading to emergence of the subordinate QRS complexes as they assume the pacemaker function (Fig. 36-26). After a usually brief period of time, the P-P

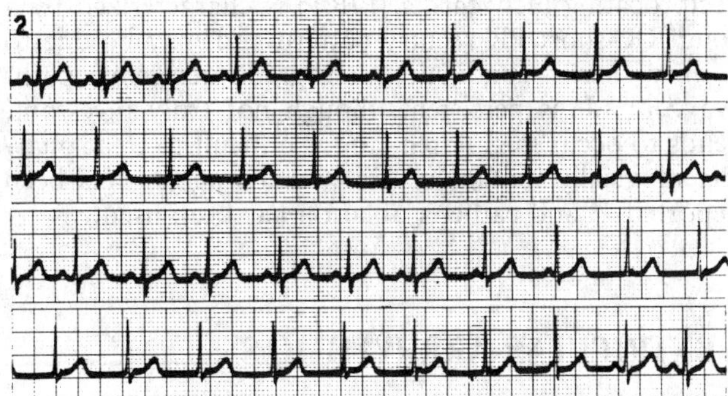

FIGURE 36-26 Accelerated idionodal rhythm with isorhythmic AV dissociation. After four sinus beats, the sinus rate slows slightly, enabling an accelerated junctional pacemaker to escape at a rate of 94 per minute. After several seconds the sinus pacemaker accelerates and recaptures the ventricles. The same sequence is then repeated (the strips are continuous). *(From HJL Marriott: Workshop in electrocardiography. Tampa Tracings, 1972. Reproduced with permission from the publisher and author.)*

interval begins to shorten, P waves reappear in front of the QRS complex, and finally, ventricular capture by atrial activity is reestablished.

Accelerated AV junctional and ventricular rhythms generally require no specific antiarrhythmic therapy. In ischemia, they are usually self-limiting in duration and of no major consequence hemodynamically; and when associated with digitalis intoxication or electrolyte disturbances, they promptly reverse with control of these toxic or metabolic influences. In fact, specific antiarrhythmic drugs might suppress a subordinate pacemaker that is required in the presence of dysfunction of normal sinus node pacemakers. If a faster ventricular rate or AV sequencing is desirable for hemodynamic benefits, attempts to enhance cardiac rates may be achieved pharmacologically or by pacing. Atropine, 0.6 to 1.2 mg intravenously, may increase sinus rate and allow the sinus to resume its normal pacemaking function if AV conduction is intact. Atropine will have little or no influence on the rate of the accelerated AV junction focus. Temporary atrial or ventricular pacing may be used to support the heart rate, but it is rarely necessary.

AV Junctional Tachycardia

Enhanced AV junctional rhythm may occasionally double its rate abruptly to a true tachycardic range.[100] This likely represents an automatic focus firing at the faster rate with 2 : 1 exit block, which abruptly changes to 1 : 1 conduction. In acute ischemic events, it may be desirable to reduce the rate with antiarrhythmic agents. However, these incidents are commonly self-limited and will usually cease spontaneously or revert back to 2 : 1 exit block.

Ectopic, or persistent nonparoxysmal, AV junctional tachycardia may occur intermittently in patients with chronic heart disease and appears to be more frequent and more important in children, particularly after surgical correction of congenital defects.[101,102] The response to treatment is unpredictable, and the rhythm may be resistant to conventional antiarrhythmic drugs. However, catheter ablation has been suggested for some patients.[102]

An arrhythmia referred to as permanent junctional reciprocating tachycardia (PJRT) is characterized by a long RR–short PR reentry pattern and may be due to a very slowly conducting retrograde accessory pathway.[103–105] It is persistent, though not truly incessant, tends to occur in children, and is difficult to treat pharmacologically. Some success with IC agents has been reported,[106] and catheter ablation has been used.

VENTRICULAR ARRHYTHMIAS

Attitudes and approaches to the evaluation and management of ventricular arrhythmias have undergone dramatic changes in recent years. New insight into the risk implied by ventricular arrhythmias in various clinical settings, some clarification of the risk-benefit ratio of antiarrhythmic drug treatment, and the refinement of nonpharmacologic methods of treatment all have developed in parallel in recent years. The equilibrium between the risk implied by an arrhythmia and the proarrhythmic risk of a drug[107–110] has been dramatically emphasized by the results of the CAST.[8,9] The implications of that study have resulted in major changes in indications and methods for treatment of some ventricular arrhythmias. The *urge* to treat, based upon limited scientific support in the past, has yielded to indications based upon the *need* to treat, with indications for treatment now modulated by a better definition of the risk of treatment. Clinical approaches to the patient with ventricular arrhythmias require a clear analysis of the interrelationships between electrocardiographic forms of arrhythmias, the specific clinical setting in which it occurs, and realistic goals of therapy (Tables 36-1 and 36-2).

Definitions, Classification of Risk, and Endpoints of Therapy

When the algorithm of electrocardiographic forms, clinical settings, and endpoints of treatment (Table 36-1) is applied to ventricular arrhythmias,[1] "forms" may be separated into the various patterns of triggering premature ventricular contractions (PVCs) and of potentially lethal sustained ventricular tachycardia or fibrillation (VT or VF) (Fig. 36-27). This distinction, however, is an oversimplification because of the lack of a uniformly accepted classification system to estimate risk and of the complexity of the interaction between chronic PVCs, the extent of underlying disease, and the severity of left ventricular dysfunction.

The conventional definition of VT—three or more consecutive ventricular ectopic impulses at a rate of 120 or greater—is too broad to apply to current evaluation and management procedures. A distinction between

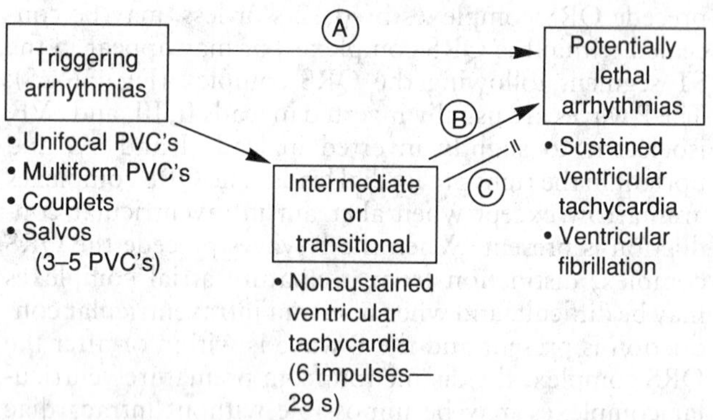

FIGURE 36-27 Forms of ventricular arrhythmias; triggering versus potentially lethal arrhythmias. A background of chronic, subacute, or acute forms of PVCs are viewed as triggering events, which may initiate potentially lethal arrhythmias at a time when the ventricular myocardium is susceptible to sustained VT or VF (arrows A and B). Unifocal and multiform PVCs, couplets, salvos (3 to 5 PVCs), and nonsustained ventricular tachycardia are included among the triggering forms, while sustained VT or VF are the potentially lethal sustained arrhythmias. Nonsustained VT may be considered an intermediate or transitional form, functioning as an intense trigger to initiate potentially lethal arrhythmias (B) or as an "incomplete" form of VT (C). Approaches to therapy may be targeted to suppression of triggering events or prevention of initiation of lethal arrhythmias by stabilizing the myocardial mass. (*Modified from RJ Myerburg et al: Pharmacologic approaches to management of arrhythmias in patients with cardiomyopathy and heart failure. Am Heart J 114: 1273–1279, 1987. Reproduced with permission from the publisher.*)

TABLE 36-8
Specific Forms of Ventricular Tachycardia

Duration	ECG Pattern
Salvo (3–5 impulses)	Uniform morphology VT
Nonsustained VT (6 impulses, 29 s)	Polymorphic VT Torsades de pointes
Sustained VT ($\geq$30 s)	Right ventricular outflow pattern Bidirectional tachycardia

VT, ventricular tachycardia

HIERARCHY OF FREQUENCIES

CLASS 0 – NIL

CLASS I – RARE
< 1 ectopic impulse/hour

CLASS II – INFREQUENT
1 to 9 ectopic impulses/hour

CLASS III – INTERMEDIATE
10 to 29 ectopic impulses/hour

CLASS IV – FREQUENT
$\geq$ 30 ectopic impulses/hour

HIERARCHY OF FORMS

CLASS A – UNIFORM MORPHOLOGY, UNIFOCAL

CLASS B – MULTIFORM, MULTIFOCAL

CLASS C – REPETITIVE FORMS
• COUPLETS
• SALVOS, REPETITIVE RESPONSES
(3–5 consecutive impulses)

CLASS D – NON-SUSTAINED VENTRICULAR TACHYCARDIA
(from 6 consecutive ectopic impulses to runs lasting up to 30 seconds)

CLASS E – SUSTAINED VENTRICULAR TACHYCARDIA
(runs of ectopic activity $\geq$ 30 seconds)

FIGURE 36-28 Classification of ventricular arrhythmias based on hierarchies of frequency and forms. Hierarchical schemes for estimating risk of ventricular arrhythmias have been developed based on frequency and forms of ventricular arrhythmias. In some clinical settings, frequencies in the range of 1 to 9 ectopic impulses per hour become significant, and in most settings of clinically significant heart disease, risk based on frequency plateaus in the range of 10 to 30 ectopic impulse per hour. Among forms of ventricular arrhythmias, the repetitive forms, particularly salvos or nonsustained VT, indicate high risk in most clinical settings. (*Modified from RJ Myerburg et al: Classification of ventricular arrhythmias based on parallel hierarchies of frequency and form. Am J Cardiol 54:1355, 1984. Reproduced with permission from the publisher.*)

short runs or *salvos* of three to five consecutive impulses, bursts of *nonsustained VT* lasting for up to 30 s, and *sustained VT* lasting 30 s or more (Table 36-8) is necessary to properly evaluate bedside clinical information, ambulatory monitoring data, the results of invasive electrophysiological testing, and responses to therapy. In addition to defining VT by its duration, useful information is contained in the definition of VT based on its ECG pattern.

Most studies of risk of chronic PVCs have used hierarchical schemes based on either frequency or forms of PVCs. In order to analyze and apply such data to the management of patients, parallel hierarchies of frequency and forms are useful.[111] Data on the risk of PVCs after convalescence from myocardial infarction have been analyzed on the basis of both frequency and forms.[112–116] Using the frequency hierarchy in Fig. 36-28, most studies demonstrate increased risk with frequencies of 10 or more ectopic impulses per hour, and one major study demonstrated a rapid increase in risk in the 1 to 9 impulses per hour range.[116] Similarly, in the hierarchy of forms, couplets indicate a small increase in risk over uniform or multiform single PVCs,[116] and salvos indicate a significantly higher risk.[115,116] There are insufficient data to determine whether or not longer runs (i.e., nonsustained VTs) constitute even higher risk. Within the hierarchy of forms, unifocal, multiform, couplets, and salvos are considered among the triggering PVCs, and sustained VT and VF are the potentially lethal forms. There may be justification for considering nonsustained VT as an intermediate or transitional form[1] (Fig. 36-27); pathophysiologically, it may be an "incomplete" form of sustained VT or an "intense trigger." Patterns such as bigeminy and trigeminy are simply an expression of frequency and contain no inherent form information.

When one evaluates or manages any form of ventricular arrhythmia, it is necessary to develop an approach based upon clinical information beyond the pattern of the arrhythmia itself. Very high frequencies and/or advanced forms connote little or no increased risk in the absence of organic heart disease. Risk begins to increase with the presence of organic heart disease and becomes prominent with falling ejection fractions.[87,88] A simplified but useful clinically based classification incorporates both form/frequency and clinical disease information. Bigger[117] suggested classifying ventricular arrhythmias as "benign," "potentially malignant," and "malignant" based on these considerations. As an extension of this concept, we have integrated frequency, forms, severity of cardiac disease, and left ventricular function (ejection fraction) into a *clinical* classification of *benign* (no independent increase in risk), *significant* (independent increase in risk), and *potentially lethal* (untreated, can lead to proximate fatality). While these clinically based approaches have not been quantitated, they do provide a conceptual framework for classifying arrhythmias.

Management of PVCs must be further analyzed in regard to specific etiology (e.g., low-risk mitral valve prolapse versus high-risk idiopathic dilated cardiomyopathy), and PVCs in acute or subacute clinical settings must be distinguished from those occurring in chronic settings. Finally, endpoints of therapy that are based upon suppression of underlying ectopy (i.e., background PVCs) are separated from endpoints based upon prevention of potentially lethal arrhythmias (i.e., sustained VT or VF) (see Table 36-1).

Premature Ventricular Contractions

Electrocardiographic Recognition of PVCs

Ventricular arrhythmias originate in the specialized conducting tissue distal to the bifurcation of the bundle of His or in true ventricular myocardium. Accordingly, they are characterized by prolonged ventricular depolarization time (i.e., wide QRS complex) and/or an alteration in the sequence of ventricular activation (i.e., a change in the QRS vector) and/or alterations in the timing sequence of consecutive QRS complexes (prematurity, escape rhythms). The caution implied by the "and/or" modifiers is intentional, because no one criterion or set of criteria are totally sensitive and specific for arrhythmias of ventricular origin. On occasion, PVCs demonstrate narrow QRS complexes, have vectors not different from the normal QRS vector, or have timing little changed from the normal sinus sequence. The majority of impulses originating in the ventricles have QRS complexes of at least 0.12 s and a shift in the QRS vector, and most single PVCs or initiating beats for runs of ventricular ectopic activity are premature. They may fail to conduct to the atria or may demonstrate retrograde atrial activation. In either case, the sinus cycle is usually not interrupted, resulting in a fully compensatory pause (Fig. 36-29). The pause is characterized by an interval between the P wave of the sinus impulse immediately before the PVC and the first sinus P wave after the PVC equal to twice the sinus cycle length (Fig. 36-29*A*). If the sinus rate is relatively slow, PVCs may be interpolated between two sinus beats with no alteration of the sinus cycle length (Fig. 36-29*B*). Exceptions to the compensatory pause rule do occur (Fig. 36-30) and occasionally complicate diagnostic criteria. Premature ventricular contractions that presumably originate in the fascicles of the specialized conducting system may have more narrow QRS complexes with only slight alterations in the QRS vector.

The common form of PVCs are coupled to the preceding sinus beat by a fixed coupling interval. This generalization has exceptions in that PVCs having different QRS morphologies may have different coupling intervals,[118] and PVCs having the same morphology in a given patient may have different coupling intervals under different pathophysiological conditions. The pattern of fixed coupling has led to a concept of a physiological relationship between the sinus beat and the PVC and is used as an argument in favor of a reentrant or triggered mechanism for common PVCs. In contrast, *parasystolic rhythms* refer to an independent ectopic rhythm, with the focus of origin being protected in the sense that descending impulses cannot enter and reset the parasystolic focus but can create a field of refractoriness around it limiting the rate and timing of existing impulses. Thus, the parasystolic focus, automatic in nature, can deliver impulses to the myocardium but cannot be reset by impulses originating elsewhere. Accordingly, the ECG reflects the presence of parallel competing pacemakers, the sinus node and a protected automatic ectopic ventricular focus, creating the classical triad of (1) variable coupling between sinus beats and ectopic QRS complexes, (2) fusion beats, and (3) a fixed common denominator of interectopic intervals between manifest parasystolic extrasystoles (Fig. 36-31). In recent years, however, classic concepts of parasystole have been altered by the discovery that parasystole may be modulated by relationships between the parasystolic focus and impulses originating in the sinus node. Sinus impulses occurring early in the parasystolic cycle tend to shorten the cycle length of the parasystolic focus, whereas those arriving in the latter half of the cycle tend to lengthen the cycle length of the parasystolic focus.[119] Parasystolic patterns may also occur with atrial extrasystolic activity.

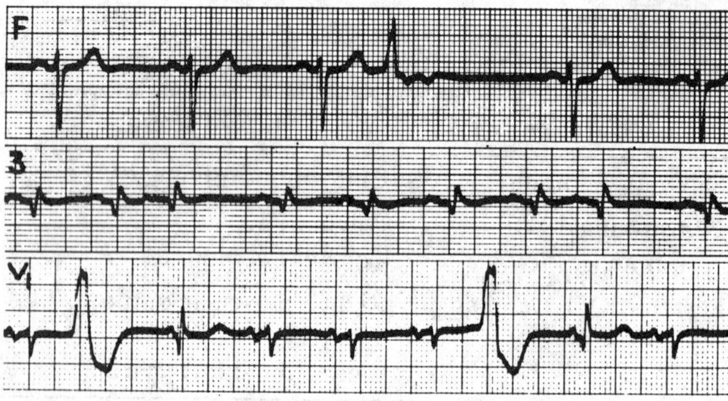

FIGURE 36-30 Exceptions to the rules for compensatory pauses. *Top*: Ventricular extrasystole with less than compensatory pause. Retrograde conduction to the atria (retrograde P wave deforms first part of ST segment) discharges the sinus pacemaker early and thus shortens the postextrasystolic cycle. *Middle*: Atrial premature contraction followed by fully compensatory pause. The third and eighth beats are atrial extrasystoles; but presumably because they suppress the sinus pacemaker, they are followed by compensatory pauses. *Bottom*: Ventricular extrasystoles with less than compensatory pauses. Each postextrasystolic cycle ends in an escape beat and so is slightly less than compensatory.

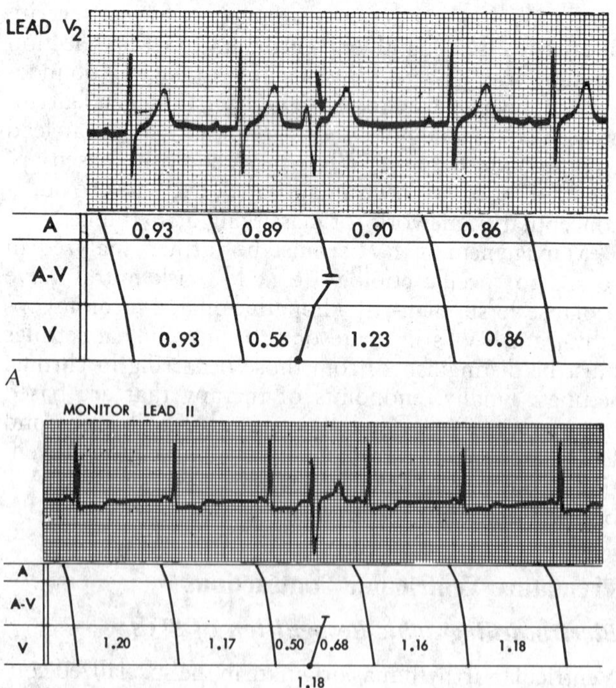

FIGURE 36-29 Ventricular premature contractions. *A*. The third impulse is wide and bizarre, and since the sinus rhythm is undisturbed (next sinus P wave indicated by arrow), the postextrasystolic pause is compensatory. *B*. The fourth impulse is an interpolated ventricular premature contraction; it is sandwiched between two consecutive sinus beats.

Management of PVCs

PVCs in the Absence of Significant Structural Heart Disease

Premature ventricular contractions occur in many healthy individuals. In the absence of heart disease, there is little or no increased risk,[120] and the risk-benefit ratio of antiarrhythmic therapy does not support routine treat-

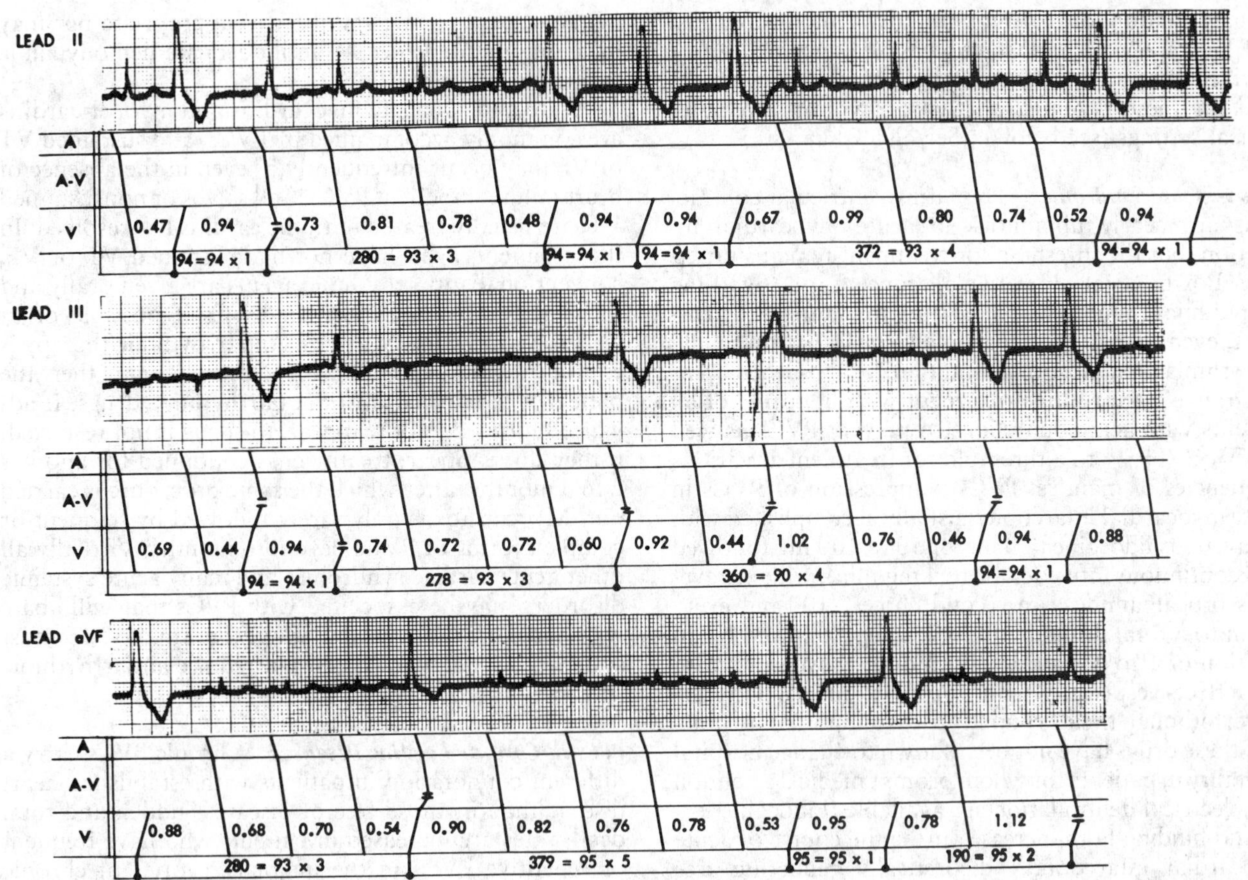

FIGURE 36-31 Ventricular parasystole. The strips are continuous. Note that (1) the interval between an ectopic beat and the preceding sinus beat varies; (2) the interectopic intervals all have a common denominator of 0.90 to 0.95 s; and (3) there are occasional fusion beats (third beat in top strip; fourth beat in second strip; last beat in bottom strip). (*From JW Hurst, R Myerburg: Introduction to Electrocardiography. New York, McGraw-Hill Book Company, 1973. Reproduced with permission from the publisher and authors.*)

ment. For the patient who complains of disturbing palpitations due to PVCs, however, the clinician may have to attempt to relieve the symptom. Reassurance and avoidance of potentially aggravating factors (e.g., tobacco, coffee, caffeine-containing soft drinks, environmental stress, stimulants) should be tried before specific pharmacologic therapy. For the latter, mild anxiolytic drugs or beta-adrenergic blockers (which may sedate, reduce PVC frequency, and decrease the strength of postextrasystolic impulses causing the perception of palpitations) are preferred. When used for this purpose, low doses of beta-adrenergic blockers are often sufficient—e.g., 5 to 20 mg of propranolol qid or an equivalent dose of other preparations. The endpoint, relief of symptoms, may not necessarily be accompanied by significantly reduced PVC frequency. The frequency of PVCs may be modulated by underlying heart rate,[121] and thus manipulations of sympathetic and parasympathetic balance may be useful. Because of their side-effect profiles, class I antiarrhythmic agents are rarely indicated in this clinical setting, and the class III agent, amiodarone, is unnecessarily potent. Premature ventricular contractions are often more prominent with pregnancy and premenstrually and increase in frequency with age.[122]

There may be an urge to be more aggressive in the management of patients who have advanced forms of PVCs (i.e., salvos, nonsustained VT) or a high frequency of PVCs (30 or more PVCs per hour) in the absence of structural disease. On the other hand, Kennedy et al.[120] reported no increased risk of death in a cohort of such persons followed for a mean of over 6 years.

The occurrence of PVCs in patients with *mitral valve prolapse* (MVP) has gained special attention for three reasons: (1) the high prevalence of MVP, (2) the prevalence of PVCs in patients with MVP, and (3) the very small risk of sustained VT or VF. Annoying palpitations are a common complaint, but the arrhythmia does not require treatment in the vast majority. There are limited data suggesting that the patients at highest risk for serious ventricular arrhythmias can be subgrouped by the presence of nonspecific ST-T wave changes in leads II, III, and aVF[123,124] in conjunction with advanced grades of ventricular arrhythmias and redundancy of the mitral valve echocardiographically.[125] The approach to treatment of patients with benign forms of PVCs in MVP should be no different than that outlined for individuals with no structural abnormalities. Beta-adrenergic blocking agents are often sufficient to control the symptoms, and membrane-active antiarrhythmic drugs should be avoided. Patients at risk for more serious arrhythmias, as outlined above, may require more aggressive treatment; membrane-active drugs are considered for use in this special situation for patients with salvos or nonsustained VT. The rare MVP patient who has had sustained VT or survived after VF is managed by the approaches generally used for these potentially lethal arrhythmias in other clinical settings (see below). (See also Chap. 80.)

PVCs in Acute Syndromes Premature ventricular contractions are nearly ubiquitous in acute myocardial infarction, but the threshold for treatment remains unsettled. Lown et al.'s[126] original concept of "warning arrhythmias" remains an indication for aggressive treatment, even though the predictive value of such warning arrhythmias remains unsubstantiated.[127,128] Other opinions range from routine treatment with lidocaine of all patients with acute infarctions to prevent PVCs as well as VT or VF[129,130] to a threshold for treatment at various frequencies of manifest PVCs. Suppression of PVCs in acute myocardial infarction is usually accomplished with intravenous lidocaine (a bolus of 50 to 100 mg followed by a continuous infusion of 2 to 4 mg/min), with intravenous procainamide as a second choice (100 mg every 5 min to a total dose of 500 to 750 mg, followed by an infusion of 1 to 4 mg/min). Both drugs have significant side effects, especially with improper dosing. Furthermore, although their "routine" use is supported by practice, these drugs have not been shown to change hospital mortality in patients for whom prompt medical attention and electrical defibrillation are available. Lidocaine levels and binding both increase during the course of acute myocardial infarction,[131] theoretically rendering free drug levels stable. The practice of tapering the lidocaine infusion to avoid toxicity[132] is not appropriate if free drug concentration represents active drug and does not rise. Caution is warranted until these points are confirmed. (See also Chap. 60.)

A number of other acute cardiac syndromes are associated with the emergence of PVCs. Transient acute ischemic syndromes have a high incidence of PVCs that are accompanied by a risk for sustained VT or VF.[133,134] The primary intervention for controlling PVCs in these settings is the control of transient ischemia.[133] On first contact, however, the use of intravenous lidocaine or procainamide to suppress ischemic arrhythmias is justified. Clinical settings characterized by myocardial reperfusion—e.g., Prinzmetal's angina, thrombolysis in acute myocardial infarction, balloon deflation during percutaneous transluminal coronary angioplasty (PTCA)—may be accompanied by risk of reperfusion arrhythmias. These arrhythmias are usually transient and self-limiting but may evolve into sustained VT or VF.[134] Although there are theoretic and experimental reasons to suspect that Ca^{2+}-mediated electrophysiological disturbances occur during reperfusion,[135,136] intravenous lidocaine is currently used to treat reperfusion arrhythmias. It is used in the same dose and infusion techniques as in acute myocardial infarction and may be used prophylactically during thrombolysis or PTCA.

Severe heart failure and acute pulmonary edema are commonly accompanied by frequent and advanced forms of PVCs,[137,138] and as in acute myocardial infarction with low-output states, the PVCs are considered secondary to the hemodynamic abnormality (Fig. 36-1). The use of antiarrhythmic agents while the hemodynamic status is being stabilized is appropriate but may have only limited success until adequate hemodynamic control is achieved.

Acute and subacute myocarditis and myopericarditis are commonly accompanied by PVCs, and sustained VT or VF may occur infrequently,[139] even in the absence of heart failure. Frequent PVCs, and salvos or nonsustained VT, are usually treated until the carditis has resolved. In those patients who have not had sustained VT or VF, conventional antiarrhythmic agents are given orally and titrated to suppression of the PVCs if possible or at least to suppression of salvos. Antiarrhythmic therapy is continued for a minimum of 2 months, and then the patient is monitored off of antiarrhythmic drugs. If advanced forms do not reappear, the drug is not restarted; if they do reappear, treatment is continued for another 2 to 3 months, after which the same procedure is carried out. Myocarditis is only rarely followed by frequent or complex forms of PVCs beyond 6 months. Virtually all other acute cardiac syndromes and many acute systemic disorders may be associated with PVCs that will abate with resolution of the initiating abnormality. In most systemic disorders, PVCs do not require antiarrhythmic therapy.

PVCs in Chronic Cardiac Diseases Chronic PVCs carry a different connotation in patients with established heart disease than in those free of disease. Sudden and total death rates are increased in patients who have frequent or repetitive PVCs in the major categories of chronic cardiac disease in the United States—chronic ischemic heart disease,[112–116] hypertensive heart disease, and the cardiomyopathies.[1,137,138,140,141] When frequent PVCs and/or salvos or runs of nonsustained VT are accompanied by a reduced ejection fraction (EF), the risk of sudden death is distinctly elevated.[115,116] Bigger et al.[116] observed a 42-percent 2-year mortality for postinfarction patients with salvos or nonsustained VT and an EF of less than 30 percent, compared to a 12-percent 2-year mortality for patients with salvos or nonsustained VT and an EF of 50 percent or more. The 2-year rate fell to 7 percent for patients with only single PVCs and an EF of 50 percent or more.

Attitudes and approaches to the management of frequent and repetitive forms of chronic PVCs after myocardial infarction have changed dramatically since the results of CAST were published.[8] Previous studies,[142,143] as well as CAST,[8] had demonstrated that PVC suppression was feasible in these patients, but CAST clearly demonstrated a significant excess risk of sudden and total cardiovascular mortality among the treatment groups receiving the 2 class IC agents (flecainide and encainide) evaluated in the study, and CAST II demonstrated a trend toward increased mortality risk for moricizine.[144] Metaanalyses of data derived from previous smaller randomized studies testing the effect of antiarrhythmic drugs on mortality after myocardial infarction also suggested an adverse effect of most antiarrhythmic drugs when used in the post–myocardial infarction patient.[145] Accordingly, the drugs used in CAST are now contraindicated in post–myocardial infarction patients with asymptomatic or mildly symptomatic PVCs, and there is a trend away from the use of any membrane-active antiarrhythmic agent in such patients. Beta-adrenoceptor blocking agents, however, have a beneficial effect on long-term outcome in the post–myocardial infarction patient.[146,147] In addition, they are effective in suppressing repetitive forms of PVCs in many patients[148] and significantly reduce total PVC frequency in some.[149] Beta blockers, therefore, have evolved as the drug category of choice for post–myocardial infarction patients with asymptomatic or mildly symptomatic PVCs. While no properly randomized study directed to a sudden and total death outcome as a result of PVC suppression using beta-adrenoceptor blocking agents has been reported, the existing randomized mortality data from the post–myocardial infarction population at large demonstrates beneficial effects.[146,147] The management problem becomes more difficult for postinfarction patients with symptomatic repetitive forms of PVCs, especially when accompanied by a low EF. Such patients have a higher risk of sudden death, and it is not known whether or not the CAST data should be extrapolated to this population as well. Because of CAST, the class IC agents are generally avoided in these patients, but clinicians may use other antiarrhythmic drugs if they are well tolerated and no adverse effects are observed soon after initiation of therapy. Regardless of EFs, beta-adrenergic blocking agents can be tried initially; if they are effective and well tolerated, they are the preferred treatment, even in this category. Another approach is the use of antiarrhythmic therapy guided by the results of programmed electrical stimulation in patients who have coronary heart disease, low EFs, nonsustained VT clinically, and induced VT during invasive electrophysiological testing.[150] The reported results appear beneficial, but the interpretation is limited, as in most electrophysiologically guided data for such patients, by the absence of concurrent placebo-controlled observations. The identification of patients at increased risk of developing VT or VF may be enhanced by the identification of late potentials by signal-averaged electrocardiography. (See Chap. 47.)

Chronic PVCs are very common in patients with advanced idiopathic dilated cardiomyopathy and in patients with hypertrophic cardiomyopathy, and both groups have a high risk of arrhythmic sudden death. In some reports, more than 90 percent of patients with dilated cardiomyopathy have frequent PVCs and over 50 percent have salvos or nonsustained VT.[137,138] Efficacy of antiarrhythmic therapy for both suppression of chronic PVCs and prevention of VT and VF is unclear and perhaps is quite limited in these patient categories. Nonetheless, treatment remains customary even though it is not known whether or not the CAST data can be extrapolated to this group. When treatment is prescribed, the patient should be hospitalized for initiation of antiarrhythmic therapy because of proarrhythmic risk in cardiomyopathy.[151] Secondary ventricular arrhythmias in patients who have chronic heart failure (Fig. 36-1) may respond to control of heart failure. In one carefully designed study, treatment with an angiotensin converting enzyme inhibitor had a very favorable effect on both parameters of heart failure and ventricular ectopy.[152]

When antiarrhythmic drugs are to be used, the selection of a drug or drug combination for high-risk patients with chronic PVCs is complex. The class IA drugs are moderately effective but have a high incidence of allergic reactions (e.g., procainamide), intolerable side effects (e.g., quinidine), or significant myocardial depression in patients with a reduced EF (e.g., disopyramide). Moricizine appears to be better tolerated, but all have significant risks of proarrhythmic effects, although the majority of these events are not life threatening.[106] Among the class IB agents (e.g., tocainide, mexiletine), efficacy might be quite good in some patients, but there is a high incidence of uncomfortable side effects; the proarrhythmic incidence is lower. The currently approved IC agents (flecainide, encainide, propafenone) are very effective in reducing ectopy and are well tolerated in patients with normal or only minimally depressed left ventricular dysfunction. Their use is limited for patients with recent myocardial infarction by the adverse outcome observed in CAST[8] and more generally by the fact that the incidence of proarrhythmic effects and myocardial depression is highest in the subgroup at greatest need for the intervention—i.e., those with repetitive forms and impaired left ventricular function. The long-term benefits of the class I agents in respect to reducing death rates, in patient groups other than the type enrolled in CAST and CAST II, are unknown at present. In regard to proarrhythmic risk, there are differences among the various groups. Class IA drugs are predominantly associated with classical proarrhythmia (torsades de pointes), which usually appears shortly after initiation of therapy.[153] Class III drugs have the same pattern of proarrhythmia. The common denominator between class IA and class III drugs, which likely contributes to this concordant proarrhythmic pattern, is moderate to marked prolongation of repolarization. In contrast, the class IC drugs, which have minimal effect on repolarization, have a low rate of classical proarrhythmia. They may, however, worsen clinical arrhythmias or generate a new rapid sinusoidal sustained VT[154] (Fig. 36-32). In addition, the excess death rate in CAST, attributed to proarrhythmia, extended over the entire period of drug exposure rather than close in time to the start of treatment. A possible explanation for this pattern is a tendency for the class IC drugs to interact with sporadic intercurrent events, such as transient ischemia or left ventricular dysfunction.[9] Such an explanation is consistent with disturbed conduction patterns (depolarization) contributing to proarrhythmia rather than repolarization abnormalities.[5] (See also Chap. 38.)

Combining drug classes has been found to be effective by some, although carefully controlled studies are limited;[155] combinations such as a class IA and a class IB drug may be tried. The class II drugs, beta-adrenergic blocking agents, have been mentioned earlier and many consider them the first choice of therapy even if the EF is not normal. They may be used in combination with class I drugs in some patients. Class III drugs have only been approved for use in life-threatening arrhythmias, although amiodarone may be appropriate for selected patients with longer runs of nonsustained VT and advanced left ventricular dysfunction. The available data on amiodarone is promising for patients with life-threatening arrhythmias,[156] but the specific benefit for patients with clinical nonsustained VT is unclear. The class IV

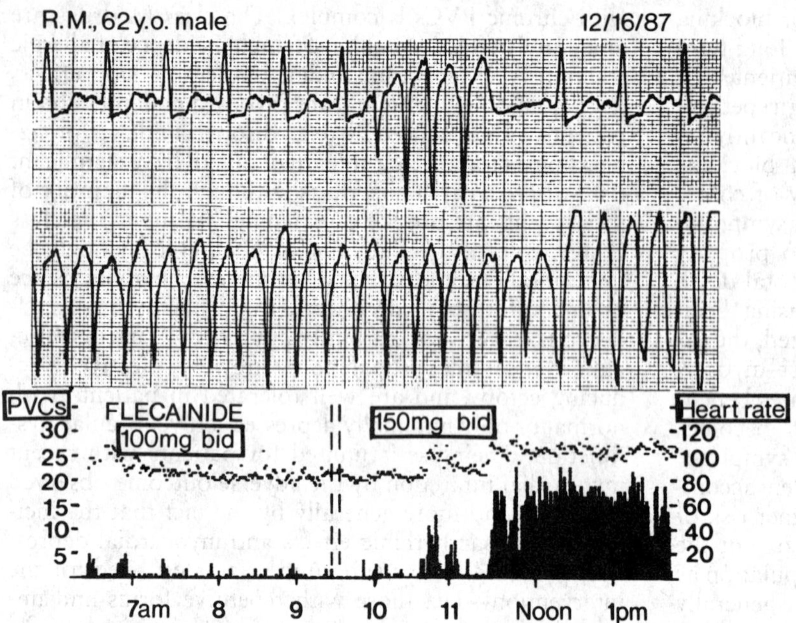

FIGURE 36-32 Proarrhythmic response to flecainide acetate. The trend recording demonstrates heart rate variations (dots) and PVC frequency (bars). While receiving flecainide acetate, 100 mg every 12 h, ventricular ectopic activity was of low frequency (mean 1.2 PVCs per minute) and the mean heart rate was 98 per minute. After increasing the dose to 150 mg every 12 h, there was a marked increase in total PVC frequency, including the generation of salvos (top tracing) and the emergence of runs of spontaneous sustained VT (lower tracing) that had not previously been present. The sustained VT was tolerated hemodynamically most of the time, but when cardioversion was necessary, multiple shocks had to be delivered. (*From Myerburg et al.,*[154] *with permission of the publisher.*)

drugs, calcium-entry blockers, have no role in the treatment of chronic PVCs.

With any of these drugs or drug combinations, attention to underlying heart disease and systemic factors is necessary. Treatment for limiting episodes of transient ischemia, maximizing left ventricular function, maintaining electrolyte balance, and controlling blood pressure, all may act in concert with antiarrhythmic agents to limit the risk of cardiac morbidity and mortality in patients with chronic PVCs.

The endpoint of treatment (see Table 36-1) of high-risk chronic PVCs is not fully understood. The pharmacodynamics of PVC suppression differ from those of VT prevention,[157] and quantitative PVC suppression is difficult to achieve. Suppression of advanced forms of PVCs (couplets, salvos, nonsustained VT) appears to be an acceptable and achievable endpoint for high-risk patients with these forms on baseline ambulatory monitoring,[158] even if quantitative PVC suppression cannot be achieved. General guidelines include suppression of 70 to 80 percent of total PVCs on a 24-h ambulatory monitor[159] and complete suppression of salvos or nonsustained VT.[160]

Unsustained Ventricular Tachycardia

Unsustained runs of VT (*salvos* of three to five consecutive impulses or nonsustained VT of six impulses to 30 s) (Fig. 36-33) are considered indicators of high risk for potentially lethal arrhythmias (sustained VT or VF) in most clinical settings. There are exceptions, however. Patients who have no organic disease or limited cardiac abnormalities do not appear to have increased risk, although some patients who have very rapid polymorphic VT may be at increased risk. At the other extreme, cardiomyopathy patients and those with advanced coronary artery disease with a poor EF are among the highest risk groups. Conceptually, nonsustained VT may be viewed as self-terminating VT or as an intense triggering event in a susceptible myocardium (Fig. 36-27).[1] Treatment is generally similar to that outlined for other patterns of PVCs, although it is suggested that patients with prior myocardial infarction who have nonsustained VT and are inducible into VT in the clinical electrophysiology laboratory are at higher risk.[150] However, it is suggested, but not certain, that they benefit from therapy guided by electrophysiological testing.

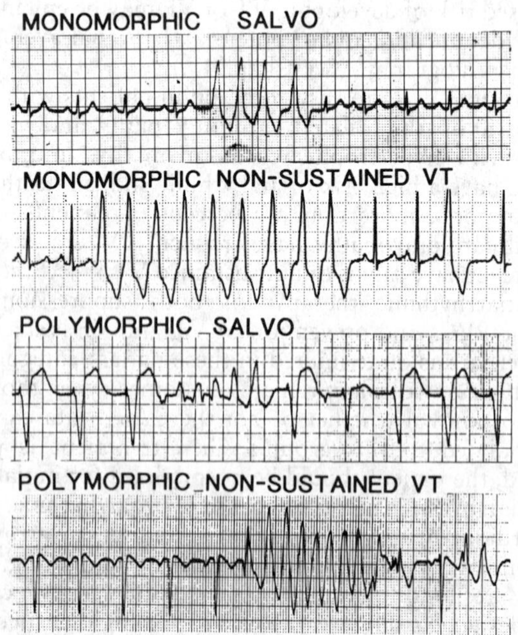

FIGURE 36-33 Unsustained forms of VT. Ventricular tachycardia below 30 s in duration is subgrouped into *salvos* of three to five consecutive impulses and *nonsustained VT* of six or more impulses up to 30 s in duration. Both forms may be further defined according to morphology as monomorphic or polymorphic.

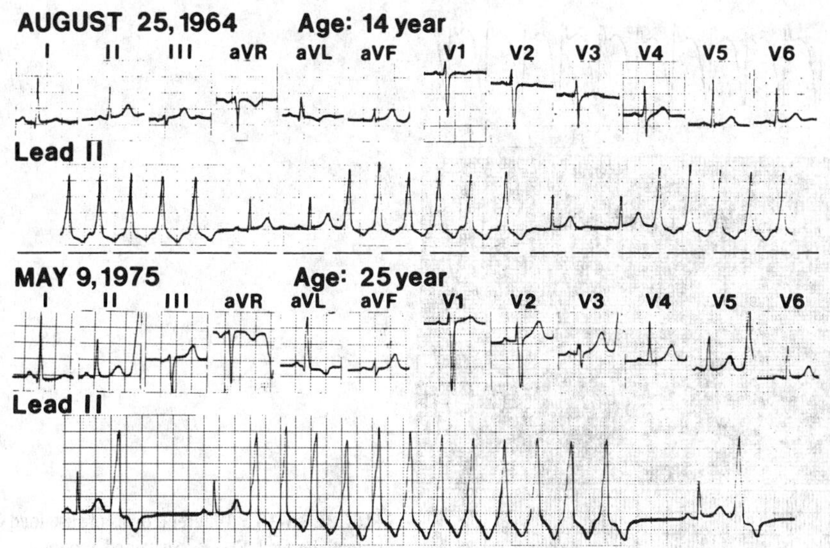

FIGURE 36-34 Repetitive monomorphic VT. This syndrome is characterized by runs of nonsustained VT, commonly separated by only a few sinus beats. It is occasionally sustained and usually suppresses with exercise. It is a benign arrhythmia, more common in women, and has a QRS morphology suggesting a right ventricular outflow origin. In this example, an 11-year follow-up shows persistence of the arrhythmia and no other significant ECG abnormalities and reflects the expected benign course.

Repetitive Monomorphic VT

This is an unusual form of repetitive salvos or nonsustained VT, often separated from one another by only a few sinus impulses (Fig. 36-34).[161] Occasionally, it is continuous and fulfills the definition for sustained VT. The tachycardia rate is usually 150 or less per minute but may be greater than 200 per minute in some. The syndrome is more common in women and is usually benign.[161-163] The QRS patterns of the tachycardia on 12-lead ECGs suggest a right ventricular outflow tract (RVOT) origin, and the mechanism is probably a form of enhanced automaticity.[164] Treatment is considered only when structural heart disease is also present or when the palpitations are intolerable. Membrane-active antiarrhythmic drugs should be avoided and beta-adrenoceptor and Ca^{2+}-entry blocking agents are effective in some. An attempt at catheter ablation may be considered for the more sustained patterns.

Sustained Ventricular Tachycardia

Overview

Sustained VT originates in the specialized conducting system distal to the bundle of His, in ventricular myocardium, or by an interaction between the two. By definition, it occurs at a heart rate of 100 per minute or more and lasts for 30 s or more. An abnormally rapid ventricular rhythm not meeting the strict definition of "tachycardia" (above 40 to 50 per minute but below 100 per minute) is referred to as an *accelerated* ventricular rhythm. Runs of VT below 30 s that are hemodynamically significant enough to cause symptoms of reduced peripheral blood flow are considered the functional equivalent of a sustained ventricular tachyarrhythmia. Although generally considered to be included among the life-threatening cardiac arrhythmias, benign forms of sustained VT do exist. They occur in persons without structural heart disease, and a functional basis can be identified in many instances (see below).

The etiology of VT will determine its mechanism and clinical presentation. For example, in the patient with prior myocardial infarction and a defined ventricular aneurysm, sustained monomorphic VT occurs at rates ranging from 140 to 200 per minute, most commonly in the range of 150 to 180 per minute (Fig. 36-35*A*). This arrhythmia is reentrant, the mechanism involving the interface between the area of the aneurysm and normal tissue. In contrast, patients with transient myocardial ischemia often have more rapid ventricular tachyarrhythmias (in excess of 250 per minute) that may be polymorphic or sinusoidal (Fig. 36-35*B*). The mechanism is not as clearly defined but likely may be either reentrant or automatic, including the possibility of triggered activity. They tend to be unstable, with a high risk of degenerating to VF and are accompanied by hemodynamic instability. They tend not to persist for long periods of time, in contrast to the sustained monomorphic VTs (which may persist for hours in some patients) but either degenerate to VF, convert to monomorphic VT, or spontaneously revert to sinus rhythm. (See also Chap. 35.)

Some patients will tolerate sustained monomorphic VT remarkably well, while most have accompanying hemodynamic disturbances causing light-headedness, dizziness, syncope, or clinical cardiac arrest. The risk that sustained VT will degenerate into VF must always be kept in mind. When the hemodynamic status is stable and there is no evidence of myocardial ischemia or infarction, or poor central nervous system (CNS) perfusion, electrical cardioversion can await a trial of intravenous drug therapy. With acute myocardial infarction, falling blood pressure, or evidence of ischemia, immediate cardioversion is indicated. In patients who are already receiving antiarrhythmic agents because of prior sustained VT or for treatment of other ventricular arrhythmias, recurrent sustained VT presents a challenging therapeutic problem. If it is known that the patient has not complied with antiarrhythmic regimens, standard intravenous regimens may be tried, but more commonly this is not the case. Plasma concentrations of the prescribed antiarrhythmics should be ordered at the time of presentation, even though the information usually will not be available for *initial* management. The distinction

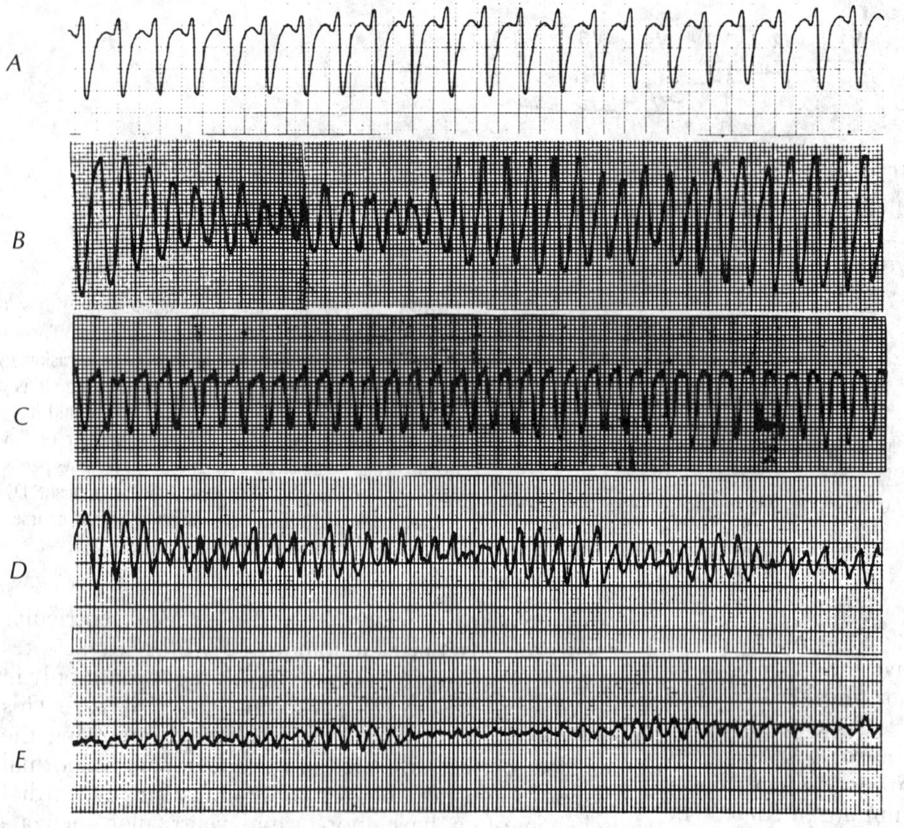

FIGURE 36-35 Different forms of sustained potentially fatal VTs. *A.* Sustained monomorphic VT recorded from a patient with a left ventricular aneurysm. *B.* Sustained polymorphic VT in a patient with myocardial ischemia. *C.* Ventricular flutter often has a sine wave configuration with a cycle length of 200 to 220 ms. *D.* Coarse VF. *E.* Fine VF. A careful distinction between the different morphologies and rates of tachyarrhythmia contains important information for prognosis and management.

between recurrence of the previous VT or proarrhythmic effects caused by antiarrhythmic agents is a major dilemma. Proarrhythmia should be suspected if the VT morphology is different from the previously identified clinical VT morphology, if antiarrhythmic agents have been recently prescribed or changed, if there is marked prolongation of the QT interval, or if the VT has a polymorphic or torsades de pointes configuration. If there are repeated recurrences after cardioversion, the possibility of proarrhythmia should be seriously entertained, and temporary pacing may be useful.

Electrocardiographic Recognition of Sustained VT

Having met the rate and duration criteria for a sustained tachyarrhythmia, the distinction between sustained ventricular tachyarrhythmias and supraventricular tachyarrhythmias with abnormal intraventricular conduction patterns is based upon a complex set of electrocardiographic criteria. The evaluation of the patient's general clinical status is only of limited value, since very rapid SVTs may cause hypotension or syncope; conversely, sustained monomorphic VT may be hemodynamically stable. Nonetheless, the distinction between SVTs and VTs at the bedside is important because of its clinical and therapeutic implications.

Electrocardiographic criteria derive from atrial/ventricular relationships and from QRS durations, configurations, and axes. The presence of ventricular/atrial dissociation, with clearly discernible P waves, independent of a regular QRS rhythm, is strongly suggestive of VT (Fig. 36-36*A*), as is the presence of P waves associated with alternate QRS complexes (see Fig. 36-37). The latter, best identified in lead V_1, is due to 2 : 1 retrograde block because of the rate of the tachycardia. The presence of a 1 : 1 relationship between P waves and QRS complexes, with a short R-P interval (as in Fig. 36-36*B*), is also considered supportive evidence for VT. A variety of SVTs with aberrant intraventricular conduction may mimic this pattern, however, and therefore it is not conclusive. Finally, in the presence of ventricular/atrial dissociation, a fortuitously timed sinus impulse may fuse with the wide QRS complex due to VT and produce a single cycle of an altered (usually narrowed) QRS complex (Fig. 36-36*C*). Such *fusion beats* are helpful when present but are not common.

A *QRS duration* above 0.14 s favors VT as the cause of a wide QRS complex tachyarrhythmia. It is nonspecific, however, and is commonly seen in patients with SVT in the presence of a preexisting bundle branch block. Supraventricular tachycardia with QRS complexes above 0.14 s occurs only rarely as a consequence of aberrant intraventricular conduction when QRS complexes are normal during sinus rhythm. In addition, antidromic tachycardias in WPW syndrome usually have QRS complexes in excess of 0.24 s and, therefore, may closely mimic VT. The *mean QRS axis* is also of limited help in distinguishing between SVT with aberration and VT. Abnormal axis deviation (−30° or beyond) favors VT but does not exclude SVT with preexisting bundle branch block or various supraventricular arrhythmias associated with accessory pathways. Some unusual VTs are associated with a left bundle branch block pattern and right-axis deviation.

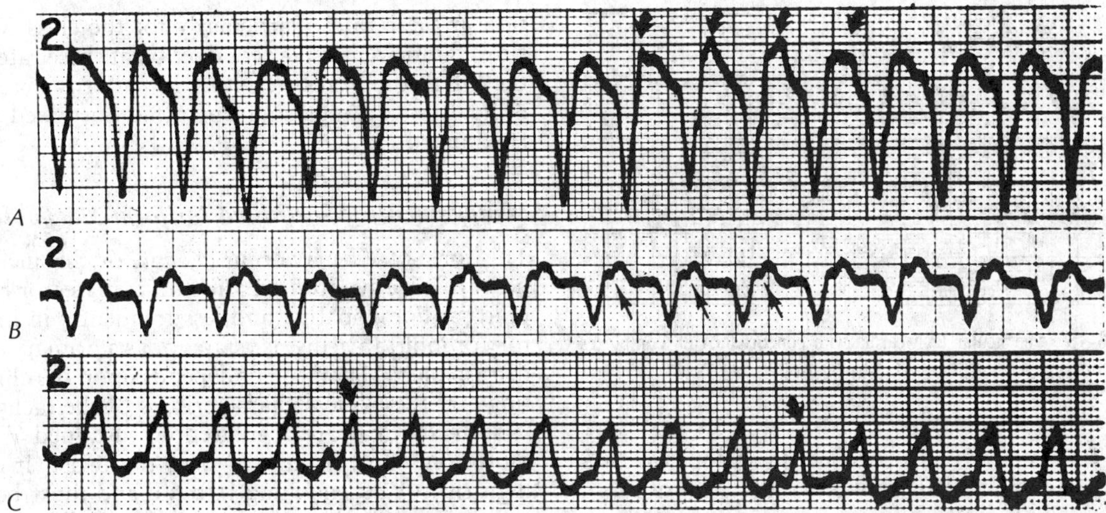

FIGURE 36-36 *A.* Ventricular tachycardia with regular independent P waves (arrows). *B.* Ventricular tachycardia with retroconduction to atria (retrograde P waves indicated by arrows). *C.* Ventricular tachycardia with fusion (Dressler's) beats (arrows). Note the sinus P wave preceding each fusion beat.

QRS configurations have been carefully studied in both VT and SVT with aberrant intraventricular conduction and are of considerable help in distinguishing between the two. Generally, concordantly positive or negative QRS complexes across the precordium from V_1 to V_6 strongly favor VT over aberrant intraventricular conduction (Fig. 36-38). In addition, patterns in specific leads may be helpful. In V_1, a right bundle branch block configuration that is monophasic (R) or biphasic (qR) suggests VT, while a triphasic pattern (rSR′) strongly favors aberrant intraventricular conduction. R-wave amplitude in V_1 during the tachycardia that exceeds that during sinus rhythm favors VT, and an initial R wave during the tachycardia of 30 ms duration or longer also

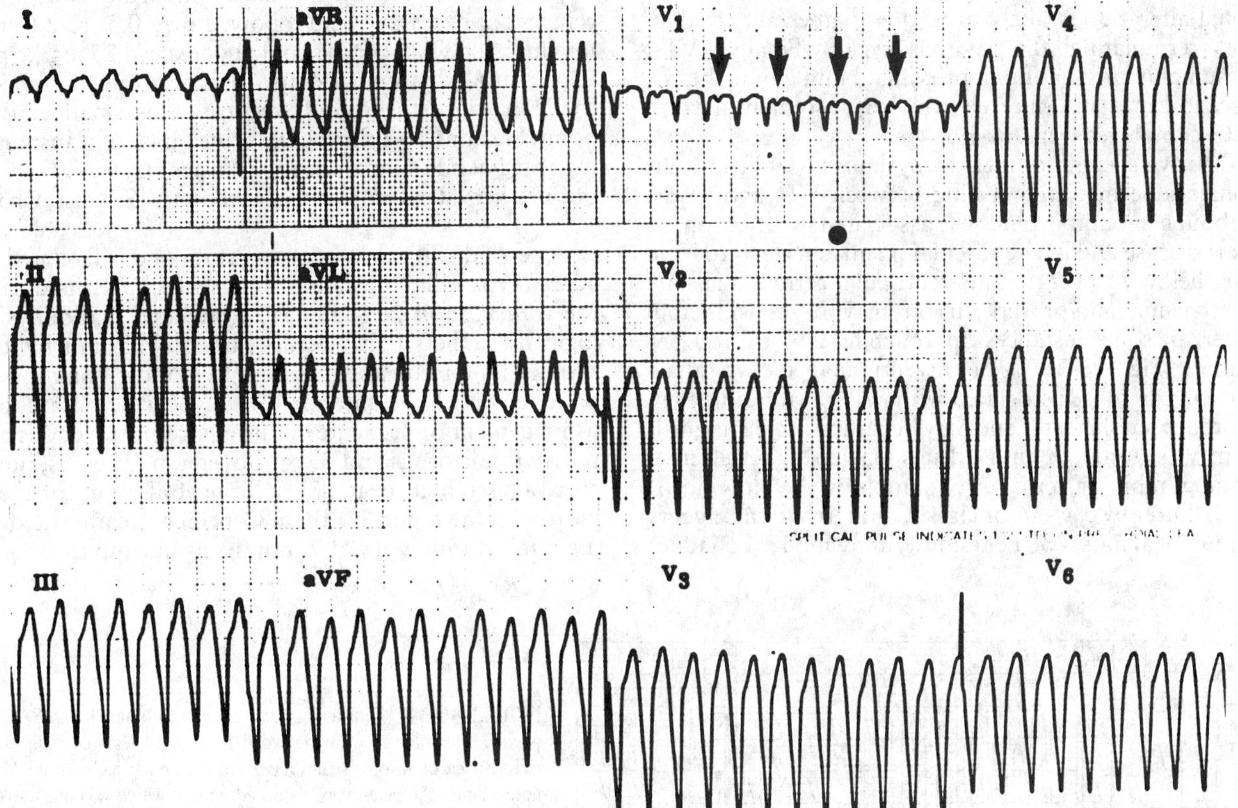

FIGURE 36-37 A rapid wide QRS tachycardia in a 22-year-old female with a history of prior chest wall trauma and a left ventricular aneurysm. Ventricular tachycardia is suggested by the history and QRS pattern (see text), but useful confirmatory information is present in the form of 2 : 1 retrograde conduction, resulting in P waves following alternate QRS complexes, most clearly seen in lead V_1. In difficult cases, the presence of a 2 : 1 V-A conduction pattern is strongly supportive of ventricular tachycardia.

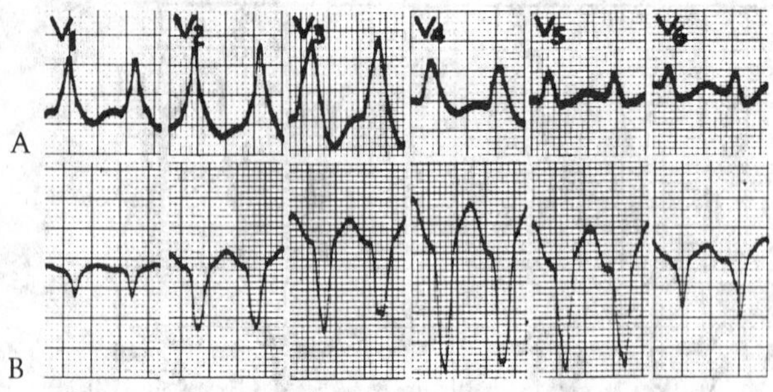

FIGURE 36-38 Ventricular tachycardia with concordant QRS complexes across precordium. *A*. All upright. *B*. All negative.

favors VT. In V_1 and V_2, a notched downslope on an S wave suggests VT, as does an interval of 70 ms or more from onset of the QRS to the negative peak of the S wave. In lead V_6, a deep S wave with an R : S ratio below 1 and a qR or QS pattern both favor VT.[165,166] Each of these criteria may be altered or modified by the presence of preexisting intraventricular conduction abnormalities in individual cases.

Several additional features of tachyarrhythmias may be helpful. Polymorphic tachyarrhythmias are almost exclusively ventricular in origin, as is a wide QRS tachycardia with a left bundle branch configuration in the precordial leads and right-axis deviation in the frontal plane leads. A regular rhythm with alternating QRS axes (a bidirectional pattern) alteration is likely to be ventricular in origin, while paired group beating with bidirectional alteration is likely to be due to aberrant conduction terminating the shorter cycles. Finally, VTs, presumably originating in proximal bundle branches or fascicles, may inscribe relatively or absolutely narrow QRS complexes (Fig. 36-39).

The cycle length of tachyarrhythmias is of little additional value in distinguishing between VTs and SVTs. Although monomorphic VT associated with coronary heart disease and left ventricular aneurysms tend to have rates below 220 per minute, ventricular arrhythmias due to ischemia and/or reperfusion may be considerably faster, in some instances approaching 250 to 280 per minute (Fig. 36-35*B*). Supraventricular tachycardias, particularly those associated with WPW syndrome, may approach similar rates and may be difficult to distinguish from VTs. Antiarrhythmic drugs may also alter electrocardiographic patterns. An example is the slowing of atrial flutter by class IA or class IC antiarrhythmic agents to rates of at most 230 per minute, allowing 1 : 1 conduction at these rates. Particularly for the class IC agents, slowed intraventricular conduction at these rates widens the QRS complexes, resulting in patterns that are very difficult to distinguish from rapid sustained tachyarrhythmias.

Management of Sustained Uniform Morphology VT

This form of VT may occur in acute or chronic ischemic heart disease syndromes, idiopathic dilated or hypertrophic cardiomyopathy, and less frequently in inflammatory or infiltrative disease states or as a primary electrical disturbance. Management depends upon the clinical setting and the clinical characteristics of the tachycardia.

In *acute* myocardial infarction, sustained VT occurs most commonly within 24 h of the onset. It carries a high risk of degenerating into VF and must be treated aggressively. If the patient is stable, a 75- to 100-mg bolus of intravenous lidocaine followed by a continuous infusion of 1 to 4 mg/min may be tried. The infusion dose depends upon the patient's age, size, and general clinical status.[167] If the VT does not revert immediately or if the patient is hypotensive, immediate DC cardioversion is required. Following cardioversion, intravenous lidocaine is continued to prevent recurrences. If VT recurs with lidocaine, 100-mg boluses of procainamide are infused at 5-min intervals to a total loading dose of 500 to 1000 mg, followed by a constant infusion of 2 to 4 mg/min.[168] If breakthroughs occur on both drugs, the next drug of choice is bretylium tosylate,[169] using a loading dose of 5 mg/kg intravenously infused over 15 min, repeated if necessary, and followed by a 0.5- to 2.0-mg/min infusion. Total dose should not exceed 25 mg/kg per 24 h. Antiarrhythmic therapy may be stopped after 48 to 72 h, since the risk of recurrence is small at that point. Sustained VT during the acute phase of transmural myocardial infarction is due to transient factors and does not predict later recurrent arrhythmias. (See also Chap. 60.)

A second clinical category of sustained VT related to acute myocardial infarction is that which occurs during the *convalescent* period.[170] It is unrelated pathophysiologically to the VT that occurs early and has much more serious long-term implications. It is most common in patients with large anterior wall myocardial infarction. Management of the acute event requires intravenous antiarrhythmic drugs and/or cardioversion. There is, however, a very high death rate during follow-up of these patients. One report cited an 83-percent death rate during a mean follow-up of 7 months using empiric antiar-

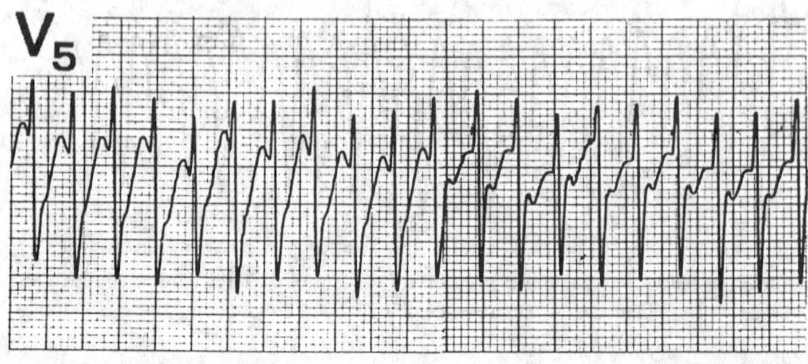

FIGURE 36-39 Ventricular tachycardia with narrow QRS complexes. The tracings were recorded from a 39-year-old male with ischemic cardiomyopathy and recurrent ventricular tachycardia. Multiple VT morphologies were recorded, one of which was this narrow QRS morphology. These may be recognized by their onset if the latter is available but often may be very difficult to distinguish from supraventricular tachycardia with altered repolarization patterns. The tachycardia shown was confirmed by invasive electrophysiological studies.

rhythmic therapy.[171] Others have reported a somewhat better outcome when such patients undergo electrophysiological testing for evaluation of drug therapy and/or surgical interventions,[172] although mortality is still high—approximately 25 percent total mortality during a mean follow-up of 16 months. Sustained VT in patients beyond the convalescent phase of myocardial infarction (6 to 8 weeks) has a somewhat less ominous prognosis than convalescent phase VT but is still considered life threatening and requires special interventions (see below).[171]

Sustained VT may complicate other acute or transient cardiac syndromes, including ischemia/reperfusion sequences associated with coronary spasm or thrombolysis early after the onset of myocardial infarction, heart failure,[173] acute myocarditis,[139] and almost any toxic or metabolic disturbance of sufficient severity. Therapeutic approaches include both conventional arrhythmia treatment, as described above for sustained VT in acute myocardial infarction, and careful attention to the underlying predisposing factors. Long-term survival is determined more by successful management of the underlying factors than by specific antiarrhythmic approaches.

Long-Term Management The long-term management of recurrent VT in patients with chronic ischemic heart disease has evolved into a complex clinical exercise. Antiarrhythmic therapy guided by invasive electrophysiological testing or by ambulatory monitoring or exercise testing, surgical procedures designed to excise or cryoablate reentrant pathways or automatic foci, and use of the implantable cardioverter defibrillator (ICD) all are applicable to individual patients. Invasive electrophysiological testing to guide therapy has become a standard part of treatment for patients with recurrent monomorphic sustained VT in ischemic heart disease. An initial study free of drugs to demonstrate baseline inducibility of VT and characteristics of the induced arrhythmia is required, with a few exceptions, before evaluating medical or surgical interventions. Baseline studies may be avoided in patients with left main coronary artery disease or unstable angina pectoris.

Although there is controversy about the validity of different protocols for programmed electrical stimulation in patients who had clinical VT,[174] up to 95 percent of inducible sustained monomorphic VTs can be induced by right ventricular stimulation alone, using up to two drive cycle lengths between 600 and 400 ms from two right ventricular locations (apex and outflow tract), with up to three extrastimuli. (See also Chap. 46.) At least 80 percent of patients with chronic ischemic heart disease and recurrent monomorphic sustained VT can be induced into their clinical tachyarrhythmias at baseline study off of antiarrhythmic agents. The subsequent identification of a drug, or combination of drugs, that will prevent reinduction into the same sustained monomorphic VT is associated with a reduction of risk of recurrent VT at 1 year of follow-up from 30 to 40 percent if VT remains inducible on therapy to 10 to 15 percent if therapy results in a noninducible status.[175] The left ventricular EF strongly influences outcome. Among cardiac arrest survivors, whether or not therapy is successful in the electrophysiology laboratory, an EF of 30 percent or less predicts a mortality rate approximately twice as high as patients in the same category with EFs above 30 percent.[176] A similar relationship likely exists for patients who present clinically with sustained VT. Unfortunately, all statements about the potential benefit of therapy guided by programmed electrical stimulation are based upon comparisons of groups who did or did not respond to therapy by converting to a noninducible status. Lacking is a randomized, placebo-controlled study of patients who convert to a noninducible status on therapy, with a similar strategy for patients with VT that remains inducible. Such a study would determine whether it is the therapy or simply the ability to change inducibility status that is determining outcome. Among VT and VF patients who met criteria for both the invasive electrophysiological approach (i.e., inducibility at baseline) and the ambulatory monitoring approach (30 or more PVCs per hour), a randomized comparison revealed a significantly lower VT recurrence rate with therapy guided by the invasive testing technique[177]—20 percent recurrence rate of symptomatic VT at 24 months with invasive procedures versus 50 percent with noninvasive procedures. The study, however, did not detect a difference in *death rate*, possibly because of the small number of patients randomized. In another study, a drug or drug combination that *did not prevent* inducibility during invasive electrophysiological study but did prolong the cycle length of induced VT by more than 100 ms with stable hemodynamics maintained, predicted a favorable mortality outcome, even though the incidence of recurrent VT was not different from those who failed to show any measure of a successful response.[178] Patients who have a partial response to a drug regimen (i.e., induced runs of six or more but not less than 15 impulses) also appear to have a lower risk of recurrent VT.[179] Most electrophysiologists currently will accept induced runs of up to nine impulses on therapy as a satisfactory endpoint, and all will accept less than six. Any change in therapy established by invasive electrophysiological testing because of drug intolerance or clinical failure should be evaluated by repeat testing.[175,180]

Noninvasive management strategies for VT require identification of frequent (i.e., 10 or more to 30 or more PVCs per hour) and/or complex PVC forms (i.e., salvos, nonsustained VT) at baseline monitoring, or VT induced during exercise testing. Reduction of PVC frequency (80 percent or more suppression) and abolition of complex forms is the usual endpoint for successful response. This approach has been reported to be successful in some studies,[158,181] even in patients who have failed to achieve a successful endpoint by invasive electrophysiological testing.[181] Unfortunately, it is not yet clear which patients who fail invasive electrophysiological testing require surgical or implantable device management, even when noninvasive methods are successful,[182] and many clinicians now use surgical treatment or implantable devices for such patients. (See Chap. 42.) Failure by *both* invasive and noninvasive criteria connotes a poor prognosis and requires other considerations for therapy—i.e., surgery or implantable devices.

Patients who have discrete ventricular aneurysms and bypassable coronary artery lesions are often considered for surgical interventions for recurrent sustained VT.

Surgery is recommended, absent contraindications, for such patients who fail electrophysiological testing with antiarrhythmic drugs.[175,183,184] It may also be recommended in lieu of successful drug therapy by electrophysiological criteria if the patient has exceptionally good surgical anatomy and/or requires revascularization. Patients without discrete aneurysms who have large dyskinetic areas may have sites of origin of VT mapped in the cardiac electrophysiology laboratory and operating room if they are inducible into stable tachycardias. Mapping allows the identification of areas that may be attacked by endocardial resection or surgical cryoablation.[185] Map-guided surgical procedures employing resection, cryoablation, and revascularization have markedly improved the clinical outcome of surgically treated patients[186] (Fig. 36-40). Overall surgical results have also benefited from the preferred use of ICDs in poor surgical candidates. (See Chaps. 42 and 44.)

Coronary bypass surgery may be helpful in a small group of patients when recurrent VT is initiated by transient ischemic episodes.[187] Catheter ablation techniques,[188] using electrical, radiofrequency, or possibly laser energy sources, appear to be of only limited value as primary therapy[189] but may be useful as an adjunct to ICD therapy (see Fig. 36-41).

Patients who have hemodynamically unstable VT before surgery may receive ICD electrode patches at the time of surgery. If they are reinducible into VT after surgery, an ICD should be implanted. The routine use of an ICD after antiarrhythmia surgery, even if successful by postsurgical programmed stimulation study, has been advocated[190] but has gained only limited acceptance. Implantable cardioverter defibrillators are indicated for patients with recurrent or unstable VT who have not been controlled surgically and do not respond to subsequent medical therapy[191,192] and perhaps for patients with EF below 30 percent even if they do respond to drug therapy. The development of ICDs with antitachycardia pacing (ATP) capabilities and programmable tiered therapy is expanding the scope of device therapy for recurrent sustained VT. The availability of ATP obviates the need for antiarrhythmic surgery in at least some (perhaps many) patients who have been considered surgical candidates on the basis of anatomy and physiology in the recent past (Fig. 36-42). (See also Chap. 42.)

Sustained VT in patients with idiopathic dilated car-

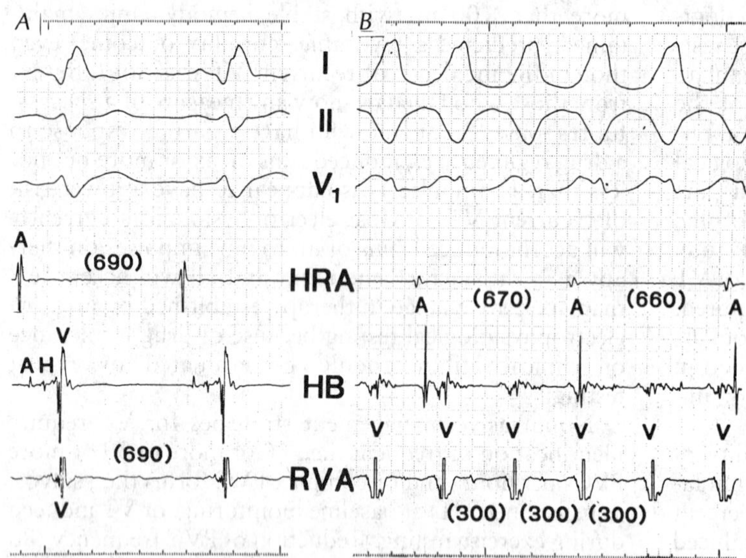

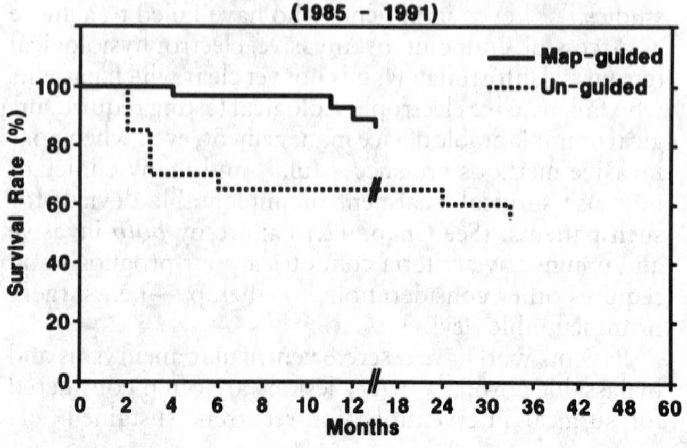

FIGURE 36-40 Benefit of mapped-guided antiarrhythmic surgery on outcome. *A* and *B* . Normal sinus rhythm and induced, hemodynamically stable VT in a patient with the same VT clinically. The ability to induce and sustain the clinical VT by programmed stimulation makes the patient a favorable surgical candidate if the appropriate surgical anatomy is present (see text). *C.* The actuarial curves show outcome at one institution of patients operated on for recurrent sustained VT, comparing outcome after mapped-guided surgery with intraoperative ablation procedures to the subgroup of patients who could not be mapped at the time of surgery. Primary surgical success rate and survival are markedly improved by intraoperative mapping.

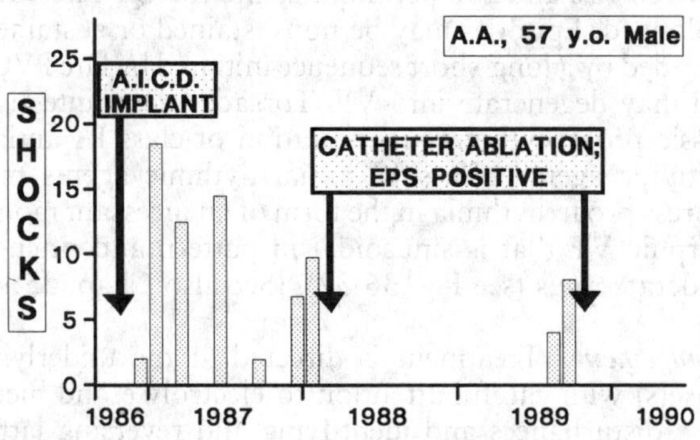

FIGURE 36-41 Catheter ablation for VT as an adjunct to an implantable cardioverter defibrillator. A patient with recurrent life-threatening episodes of sustained VT who received an implantable cardioverter defibrillator (ICD) had multiple shocks for recurrent arrhythmias that were resistant to all antiarrhythmic agents attempted. Ventricular mapping and catheter ablation of a VT focus provided freedom from recurrent ICD discharges for approximately 19 months, after which the multiple ICD discharges recurred. A second ablation procedure again provided relief from the recurrent discharges. While of limited value as primary therapy for life-threatening ventricular arrhythmias in patients with coronary heart disease or cardiomyopathy because of risk of recurrence, this procedure can provide some benefit as an adjunct to other primary forms of therapy by preventing frequent discharges and improving quality of life.

diomyopathy, dilated cardiomyopathies due to specific etiologies, or hypertrophic cardiomyopathies has a poor prognosis. Invasive electrophysiologically guided therapy is applicable to patients with dilated cardiomyopathy who have clinical sustained VT,[193,194] although it is not clear that the long-term outcome is altered by drug therapy. In a subgroup of these patients sustained VT is due to bundle branch reentry,[195] which may be cured by catheter ablation of the right bundle branch. Electrophysiologically guided management does not appear useful in idiopathic dilated cardiomyopathy patients who have had clinical *VF* or *nonsustained VT*.[196] There is almost no role for surgical therapy in these patients at present; but the ICD is an appropriate means of management. The device appears effective for reverting potentially fatal arrhythmias in cardiomyopathy, and most patients have appropriate use of the device,[197] but the long-term outcome may be dominated by left ventricular function. Ventricular tachycardia is also a late consequence and poor prognostic sign in patients with hypertrophic cardiomyopathy.[198–200] In this setting, the use of electrophysiological testing has been limited because of unvalidated concerns about the ability to cardiovert the severely hypertrophied and obstructed ventricle,[200,201] and there is no uniform opinion regarding the best approach to management of these patients, other than the accepted need for antiarrhythmic therapy. Preoperative electrophysiological testing is also avoided in patients with severe aortic stenosis who have survived sustained VT or VF.

Less Common Clinical Causes of Sustained VT

There are a limited number of patients in whom sustained VT appears to be mediated by catecholamines or other neurophysiological influences.[202,203] Sustained VT in these patients is commonly induced by physical or emotional stress. Isoproterenol infusions may be used to initiate the VT, which may then be suppressed and subsequently prevented by beta-adrenergic blocking agents (Fig. 36-43). Another small group of patients have sustained VT that may respond to Ca^{2+}-entry blockers.[203–205] This is a heterogeneous group that includes adenosine-sensitive VT[204] and an unusual VT with RBBB/left-axis deviation originating in the low interventricular septum.[206] Catecholamine-mediated VT may occur in the presence or absence of structural heart disease; those responsive to Ca^{2+}-entry blockers generally occur in the absence of structural heart disease.

Arrhythmogenic right ventricular dysplasia (ARVD) is commonly associated with nonsustained or sustained VT. It reportedly has a low mortality rate.[207] Pharmacologic and surgical approaches have been used for its management.[207,208] Amiodarone and class IC drugs have been suggested to be effective for ARVD patients with symptomatic arrhythmias. Sustained VT is also associated with isolated right ventricular cardiomyopathy,[209,210] which may be an extreme form of ARVD but has a significantly higher risk of lethal arrhythmias.

Sustained VT or VF may appear years after repair of complex congenital heart defects,[211] especially tetralogy of Fallot and transposition of the great vessels. The arrhythmias are potentially lethal and must be treated pharmacologically[212] or surgically.[213]

Bidirectional VT (Fig. 36-44) is usually a manifestation of digitalis intoxication and responds to standard measures.

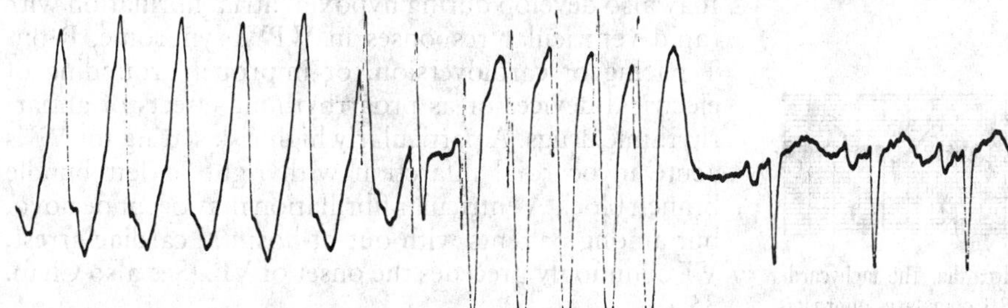

FIGURE 36-42 Implantable cardioverter defibrillator with antitachycardia pacing. The figure demonstrates the end of a run of induced sustained ventricular tachycardia (left) followed by antitachycardia pacing that converts the rhythm back to normal sinus (right). The device will revert to a defibrillator mode if programmed pacing sequences fail to convert the rhythm.

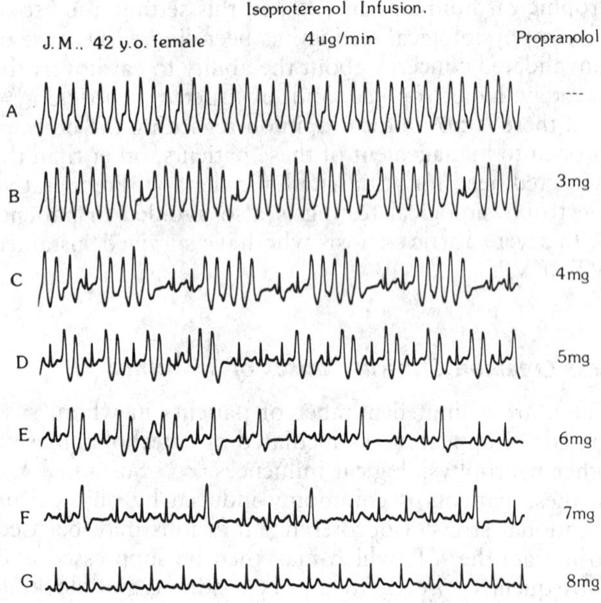

FIGURE 36-43 Catecholamine-mediated VT in an otherwise healthy female. Psychologic stress or isoproterenol infusion could initiate the arrhythmia in this patient. During this sequence, a 4-μg/min isoproterenol infusion initiated the VT (*A*), and the patient was treated with intravenous propranolol. After the first 3 mg of propranolol (*B*), occasional sinus beats interrupted the tachycardia. On a milligram-by-milligram basis up to a total dose of 8 mg of propranolol, there was further suppression of VT to the point of salvos (*C, D, E*), frequent PVCs (*E*), and complete abolition of ectopic activity (*G*).

Torsades de Pointes

This specific variant of polymorphic VT is characterized by QRS peaks that seem to "twist" around the baseline (Fig. 36-45). Torsades de pointes is usually considered as part of a syndrome that includes a prolonged QT interval plus a predisposing factor.[214] The same ECG pattern, however, may occur in the absence of QT prolongation. The most common predisposing factors are antiarrhythmic agents (classically quinidine, but also the other class IA agents, with QT prolongation frequently preceding the arrhythmia),[215] hypokalemia, severe bradycardias, and acquired or congenital prolonged QT syndromes.[216–220] Other associations include phenothiazines, hypomagnesemia, acute ischemia and reperfusion, acute central nervous system injury, class III and IV antiarrhythmic agents, liquid protein diets, and pacing stimuli interrupting T waves.

Electrocardiographic Features Torsades de pointes is characterized by axis variations over several beats causing the QRS complexes to appear to twist about the baseline (Fig. 36-45). Characteristically the rate varies between 150 and 250 per minute, and the QT interval is prolonged. Episodes may be nonsustained or sustained, preceded by a long-short sequence initiated by late PVCs, and may degenerate into VF. Torsades de pointes is a classic proarrhythmic manifestation of class IA antiarrhythmic agents. Class IC antiarrhythmic agents may express proarrhythmia in the form of an incessant monomorphic VT that is sinusoidal in pattern and often at moderate rates (see Fig. 36-32). (See also Chap. 35.)

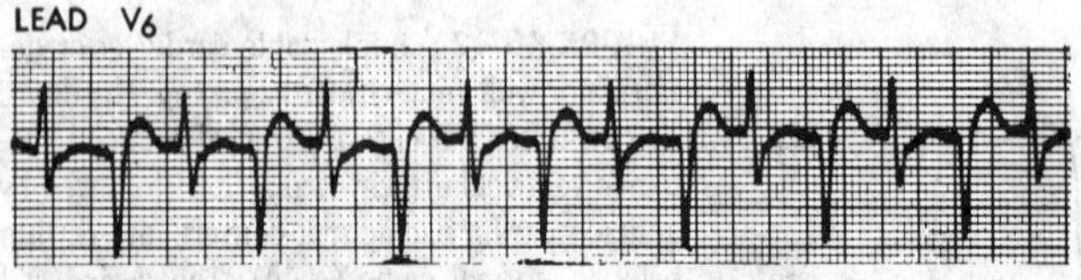

FIGURE 36-44 Bidirectional or alternating tachycardia. The tachycardia is regular at a rate of 160, but the form of the QRS-T complexes alternates.

Management Treatment is directed at the underlying cause(s) with careful attention to electrolyte and metabolic disturbances and identifying and reversing iatrogenic factors. Although cardioversion-defibrillation may interrupt torsades de pointes, it frequently recurs. Lidocaine may be beneficial, as may other class IB drugs, which tend to stabilize cell membranes while shortening the QT interval. Intravenous magnesium sulfate is often beneficial when the torsade is due to quinidine. It may be given in a dose of 2 g over 2 min followed by an infusion of 2 to 20 mg/min. Nevertheless, overdrive atrial or ventricular pacing is often required. Acceleration of the underlying heart rate with isoproterenol infusion to shorten the acquired QT interval prolongation may be effective but should be avoided in patients with symptomatic ischemic heart disease. Class IA and class III antiarrhythmic agents should be avoided. Careful long-term management of patients with congenital QT prolongation and symptomatic ventricular arrhythmias is important; therapy includes beta-adrenergic blockade and/or left cardiac sympathetic denervation.[219,221] Placement of an ICD should be considered for patients with resistant arrhythmias. There are two rare congenital syndromes that are both characterized by a prolonged QT interval and a tendency to sudden cardiac death. The *Ward-Romano syndrome* is not associated with deafness and is inherited as an autosomal dominant, whereas the *Jervell and Lange-Nielsen syndrome* is characterized by congenital deafness and an autosomal recessive pattern of inheritance.

Ventricular Fibrillation and Flutter

Ventricular fibrillation is a terminal arrhythmia, uniformly requiring rapid initiation of emergency measures. Ventricular flutter with loss of consciousness and rapid unstable VT may be clinically equivalent to VF and is treated identically when accompanied by the clinical picture of cardiac arrest. Ventricular fibrillation occurs commonly in the setting of acute ischemic events or unpredictably in advanced chronic ischemic heart disease. Moreover, it is the mode of death in 25 to 50 percent of fatalities among patients with cardiomyopathies.[222,223] It may also develop during hypoxia, atrial fibrillation with rapid ventricular responses in WPW syndrome, R-on-T pacing or cardioversion, or improper grounding of electrical devices or as proarrhythmic effects of antiarrhythmic drugs. A particularly high risk setting for VF is acute myocardial infarction with right or left bundle branch block. Ventricular fibrillation may occur de novo, but among patients with out-of-hospital cardiac arrest, VT commonly precedes the onset of VF. (See also Chap. 35.)

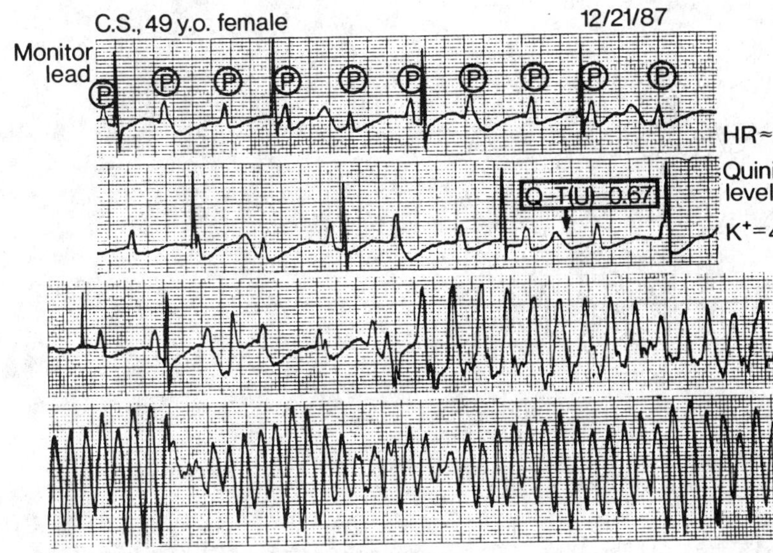

FIGURE 36-45 Torsades de pointes. The patient has complete heart block and was receiving quinidine sulfate for a ventricular arrhythmia. The rhythm shown in the bottom two strips occurred shortly after institution of therapy. Note the prolonged QT(U) interval (0.67 s) and the onset of classical torsades de pointes.

Electrocardiographic Features

The electrocardiographic pattern of VF is that of gross disorganization without identifiable repetitive waveforms or intervals (Fig. 36-35*D* and *E*). At the onset, VF may be "coarse" in pattern, but over time, it loses its amplitude and becomes "fine" ($<$0.2 mV). Successful defibrillation and survival rates are decreased in patients with the fine pattern of VF. In ventricular flutter (Fig. 36-35C), a sine wave configuration is present, having a cycle length in the range of 200 to 240 ms. Rapid polymorphic VTs may be difficult to distinguish from ventricular fibrillation or flutter. Hemodynamic findings may be marginally stable in ventricular flutter, but hypotension, loss of consciousness, and degeneration to VF are common.

Management

There are two major goals of therapy: (1) immediate resuscitation and (2) long-term prevention of recurrences. Basic life support with standard cardiopulmonary resuscitation (Chap. 52) is used only until emergency defibrillation at 200 or more joules can be carried out. (See Chap. 41.) Early defibrillation is essential to survival.[224] Resistance to defibrillation may occur due to patient size, improper paddle placement, improper use of conducting media, acidosis, hypoxemia, or electrolyte disturbances.[225] Some antiarrhythmic drugs may raise the defibrillation threshold. Defibrillation thresholds may be decreased by administration of bretylium, lidocaine, or epinephrine (the latter especially when the fibrillatory baseline is fine). Immediate steps to improve metabolic and electrolyte disturbances are required, paramount of which is to establish an airway, followed by techniques to support ventillation.[226] In rare instances, "spontaneous" reversion of VF[227] or "medical" defibrillation with bretylium[169] has been reported. A physiological or pharmacologic increase in catecholamines has been postulated as the underlying mechanism.

After successful defibrillation, careful attention to the total clinical status of the patient and prophylactic antiarrhythmic drugs are required. Lidocaine, procainamide, and in resistant cases, bretylium are useful. In addition to oxygenation and improving the metabolic milieu, the aggressive treatment or prevention of recurrent ischemia or heart failure is necessary, since they may act as pathophysiological triggers for recurrences.

In the in-hospital setting, early recognition and aggressive treatment of VT may prevent VF. In the patient with acute myocardial infarction, early VF, like VT, is associated with an increase in hospital mortality but does not independently influence posthospital mortality and does not justify long-term antiarrhythmic therapy.[228–230] When VF occurs as a convalescent-phase complication of acute myocardial infarction, aggressive long-term antiarrhythmic management is indicated (see above).[231,232] The vast majority of patients who have VT or VF in the convalescent phase of myocardial infarction (3 days to 8 weeks) will be inducible at baseline electrophysiological study.[172]

In survivors of out-of-hospital VF not caused by acute myocardial infarction, control of ischemia and heart failure is essential. The clinical context[233,234] is evaluated in terms of the interaction of structural (coronary heart disease, myopathy, hypertrophy, anatomic electrical abnormalities) and functional (ischemia/reperfusion, systemic factors including congestive heart failure, metabolic and electrolyte disturbances, neurophysiological interactions, and toxic effects) abnormalities. Long-term arrhythmia management guided by results of invasive electrophysiological testing is preferred.[235] However, only about 33 to 40 percent will be inducible into sustained monomorphic VT at baseline.[235,236] A similar fraction will be inducible into nonsustained VT or VF (Fig. 36-46), and 20 to 30 percent are noninducible. There are some data suggesting that the subgroup whose unexpected VF is related to transient ischemia, in contrast to an underlying structural basis, is less likely to be inducible at baseline.[237] Patients who do not have inducible arrhythmia at baseline invasive testing and who have high-risk forms on ambulatory monitoring or exercise testing may have drug therapy guided by suppression of these spontaneous arrhythmias by noninvasive tech-

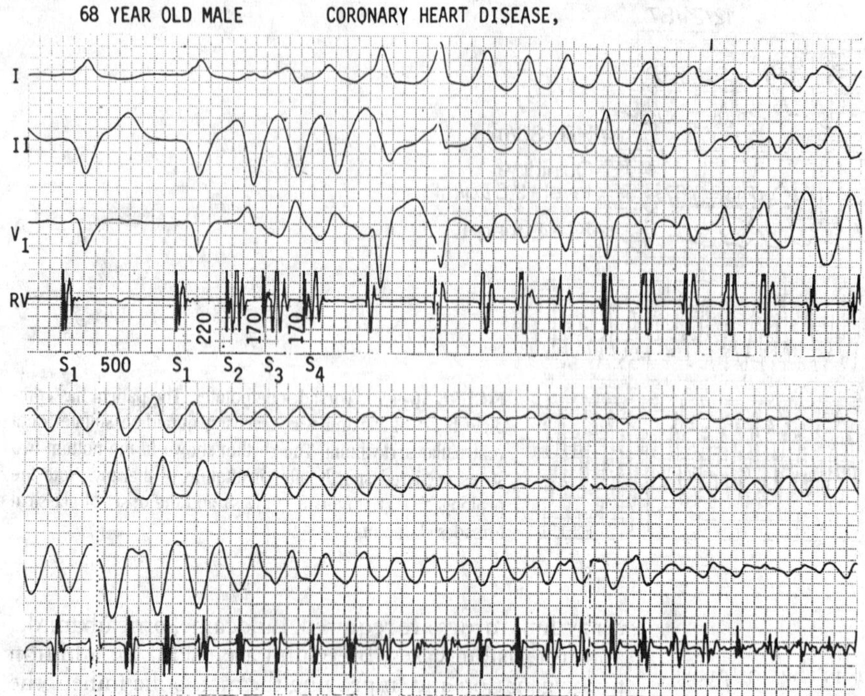

FIGURE 36-46 Programmed electrical stimulation study in a survivor of out-of-hospital cardiac arrest. The patient had ischemic heart disease and polymorphic VT degenerating to VF was reproducibily induced prior to bypass surgery. After surgery, the tachycardia was no longer inducible.

niques[158,181,182] if the EF is greater than 40 percent. For this circumstance with lower EFs, the use of ICDs is emerging as the preferred treatment. Patients who have recurrences despite drug therapy predicted to be effective during testing,[236] those in whom a reliable endpoint of therapy cannot be established, or those in whom the risk of recurrence remains high because underlying precipitating factors cannot be adequately controlled should generally be considered for ICD placement.[236] The development of programmable devices and transvenous lead systems is expanding the set of circumstances in which ICD is preferred therapy. (See Chap. 42.) Concomitant antiarrhythmic therapy may be required if surgery fails to achieve noninducibility or to prevent excessive shocks in those with ICDs. Defibrillation thresholds should be checked at steady-state drug levels, since antiarrhythmic drugs may increase threshold.

BRADYARRHYTHMIAS

Bradyarrhythmias may be due to depression or failure of impulse formation or to failure of AV conduction. They are often asymptomatic, but when symptoms of hypoperfusion occur (e.g., symptoms of inadequate cerebral or coronary blood flow, worsening of congestive heart failure) at rest or during exercise, treatment is required. Symptoms are almost always due to inadequate rate, although under some circumstances (e.g., aortic stenosis), loss of synchronized atrial contraction may contribute to symptoms. Bradyarrhythmias may be due solely to cardiac factors but are often caused or aggravated by noncardiac factors such as drugs, autonomic imbalance, hypothyroidism, hypothermia, or hyperkalemia.[238] Furthermore, the hypoperfusion associated with bradycardia may be multifactorial, such as in acute inferior wall infarction, in which manifest bradycardia and left ventricular dysfunction may be additive. In all cases, careful evaluation of both cardiac and noncardiac factors is necessary. If the patient is symptomatic, the first step in management is to increase the heart rate, which is readily accomplished by parasympatholytic drugs (e.g., atropine) or sympathomimetic drugs (e.g., isoproterenol). Underdosing with atropine (e.g., $\leq$0.3 mg) may cause a centrally mediated bradycardia and should be avoided. In addition, sympathomimetics must be used cautiously in all patients and avoided in the patient with ischemic symptoms. Temporary external pacing offers a logical alternative.[239,240] Stable, reliable increases in heart rate are afforded by temporary ventricular demand pacing. Temporary dual-chamber pacing is required for those cases in which synchronized atrial contraction is deemed beneficial, e.g., in bradycardia associated with inferior wall and right ventricular infarction.[241] General circulatory support and elimination of drugs that aggravate bradycardia is the second step in management. Rarely, permanent pacing may be obviated by substitution of a vasodilator drug that tends to increase heart rate (e.g., hydralazine)[242,243] for negative chronotropic antihypertensive agents. The administration of ephedrine has been used in the past for symptomatic bradycardia but is rarely superior to permanent pacing.

Failure of Impulse Formation

Sinus Bradycardia

Sinus bradycardia ranges from a benign asymptomatic physiological adjustment in heart rate to a symptomatic expression of sinus node dysfunction. The asymptomatic forms are most often benign and related to physiological (e.g., exercise training effect) or pathological (e.g., inferior wall infarction) excesses in vagal tone.[244–248] Although most commonly due to impaired impulse formation, it may also be caused by sinoatrial block.

Electrocardiographic Features of Sinus Bradycardia and Sinoatrial Block

Sinus bradycardia is defined as a rate less than 60 impulses per minute, with the pacemaker impulse originating in the sinus node, resulting in P waves of normal amplitude and vector. It is rarely considered outside of the physiological range until rates are under 50 per minute. In well-trained athletes (Fig. 36-6C) and during sleep, rates of 40 per minute or less may occur. Sinus bradycardia is commonly accompanied by some degree of sinus arrhythmia.

Sinoatrial (SA) block, referring to abnormal conduction of a sinus impulse from the SA node to the atrial muscle, is categorized as first-degree (delayed conduction), second-degree (intermittent), or third-degree (complete) block. Vagal stimulation, digitalis, and ischemia are the most common predisposing factors in these otherwise rare conduction disorders. Sinoatrial block may be recognized by the absence of expected P waves and the subsequent QRS complex. First- and third-degree SA blocks cannot be recognized on the standard clinical ECG, but second-degree SA block may be identified because of its intermittent pattern. Characteristically, in SA Wenckebach, the P-P and R-R intervals will progressively shorten together before a dropped P-QRS complex results in a pause; a recurrent pattern may be identified (Fig. 36-47*B*). Sinoatrial Wenckebach periods are frequently overlooked and mislabeled as sinus arrhythmia. Intermittent 2 : 1 block may also be deduced from standard rhythm strips (Fig. 36-48), but persistent 2 : 1 SA block may be indistinguishable from sinus bradycardia.

Management of Sinus Bradyarrhythmias

Treatment of asymptomatic bradycardic patients is often unnecessary and may even be detrimental, such as in those in whom an increase in rate may aggravate myocardial ischemia or failure. In the symptomatic patient, elimination of reversible aggravating factors is essential. When this is ineffective or negative chronotropic agents are essential to overall patient management, permanent pacing may be needed. (See Chap. 40.) A similar approach is taken for patients with sinus pauses, sinus arrest, or SA exit block, which may be associated with myocardial infarction, myocarditis, sinus node fibrosis, digitalis excess or excess vagal tone.[249,250] In the patient with symptomatic hypersensitive carotid sinus syndrome,[251,252] medical treatment is usually inadequate. Permanent ventricular or dual-chamber[253] pacing is indicated but may not relieve symptoms due to the coexisting

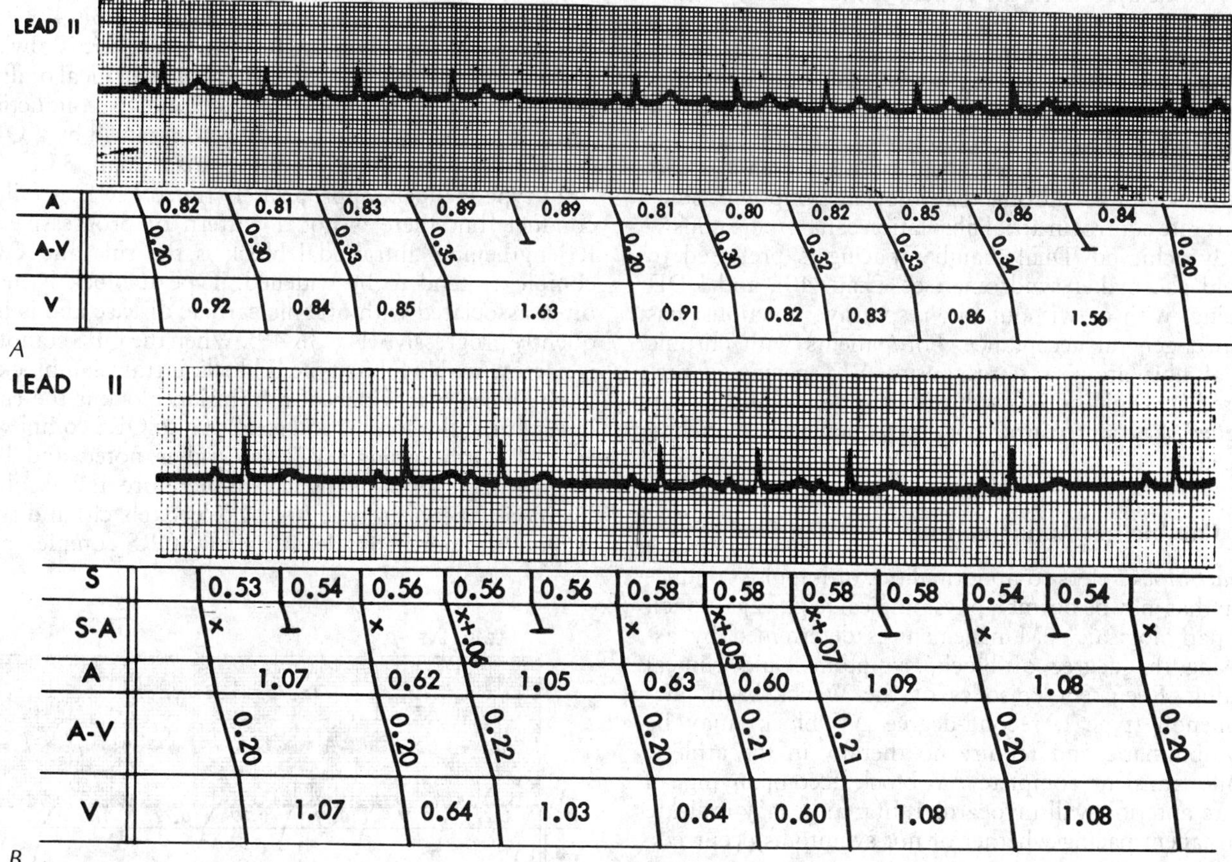

FIGURE 36-47 Wenckebach phenomenon. *A*. A 5 : 4 and 6 : 5 AV Wenckebach period. Note that the PR interval progressively lengthens but by a decreasing increment; therefore the ventricular cycle tends to shorten (at least for the first two cycles following the dropped beat). *B*. A 3 : 2 and 4 : 3 sinoatrial Wenckebach period with 2 : 1 sinoatrial block at beginning and end of strip. (*From JW Hurst, R Myerburg: Introduction to Electrocardiography. New York, McGraw-Hill,* 1973. *Reproduced with permission from the publisher and authors.*)

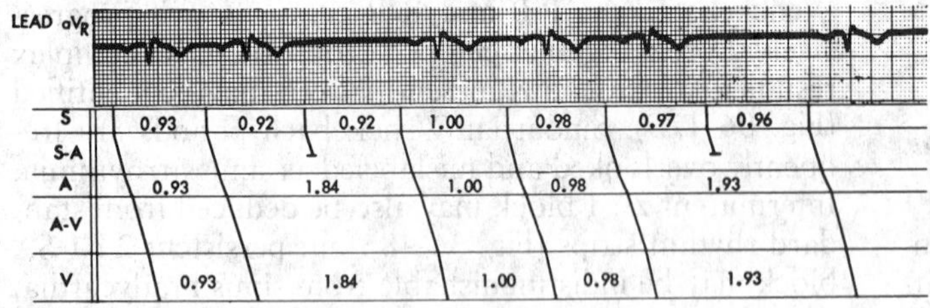

FIGURE 36-48 Sinoatrial (SA) block. In each pause the entire P-QRS-T sequence is missing, and the long cycle is approximately equal to two of the sinus cycles.

vasodepressor reflexes.[254] A distinct complex, referred to as neurally mediated vasodepressor syncope, has combined manifestations of sinus bradycardia and vasodepressor responses. It is revealed by the response to head-up tilt testing and is due to an abnormal reflex originating in the left ventricular wall.[255] (See Chap. 50.)

Sick-Sinus Syndrome

"*Sick-sinus*" *syndrome*[256–258] is a generalized abnormality of cardiac impulse formation and intraatrial and AV conduction abnormalities[244,259,260] that may be manifested by a wide range of combinations of brady- or tachyarrhythmias.[261] Treatment, therefore, must be individualized to each patient's manifested arrhythmias.[262] Often the patient is asymptomatic or the symptoms are mild and nonspecific. Negative chronotropic agents are avoided or discontinued,[258,263] and permanent pacing may be delayed until the patient is more clearly symptomatic.[264,265] In all patients, symptoms must be carefully correlated to arrhythmia manifestations. In the clearly symptomatic patient, treatment may include a combination of antiarrhythmic agents and permanent pacing (for intrinsic and drug-induced bradycardias). Ironically, the eventual development of atrial fibrillation in patients with sick-sinus syndrome may alleviate symptoms, since heart rate control in atrial fibrillation can be more consistently achieved. Dual-chamber pacing is preferred to avoid pacemaker syndrome (see Chap. 40), and DDD pacing, with or without rate-responsive functions, has gained general acceptance. For patients with chronic atrial fibrillation, rate-responsive VVI pacing is preferred.[266] Digitalis is used with caution[263] and, when needed, is easier to titrate once the patient is permanently paced.

AV Conduction Abnormalities

Heart block refers to abnormalities of impulse conduction that may be normal, physiological (e.g., vagal tone), or pathological.[267] Management is determined by assessing the degree of block, symptoms, and clinical setting. Recurrent episodes of the Wenckebach phenomenon (type I, second-degree AV block) may be asymptomatic and require no therapy in the athlete, while transient complete AV block accompanying an acute anterior wall myocardial infarction may indicate permanent pacing whether or not symptoms occurred.

Electrocardiographic Findings

In first-degree AV block, the P-R interval is prolonged (>200 ms at normal rates), indicating prolonged AV conduction, but there are no nonconducted sinus impulses. Second-degree block is characterized by intermittent failure of conduction from atria to ventricles and is further subdivided into type I (Wenckebach phenomenon) and Möbitz type II second-degree block. Type I block is characterized electrocardiographically by progressive lengthening of the P-R interval, eventually leading to a nonconducted P wave (Fig. 36-47*A*). This often recurs with regularity, and patterns of "group beating" are recognized. The degree of block can be quantified by the conduction ratio—the ratio of the number of P waves to the number of QRS complexes in each episode or period terminated by the pause. Because the magnitude of P-R lengthening typically is less with subsequent R-R intervals, the R-R intervals themselves characteristically shorten before the pause caused by the dropped QRS complex. The greatest decrement occurs in the second cycle of a Wenckebach period, and atypical patterns may actually demonstrate lengthening of R-R intervals in later cycles of a Wenckebach period (see Fig. 36-47). The shortening of the second R-R cycle, however, is always present. Wenckebach block is often physiological or digitalis induced. It is almost always due to conduction across the AV node and usually accompanied by a QRS complex of normal duration. (See also Chap. 35.)

In type II block, appropriately timed P waves fail to conduct, but there is not a pattern of progressive P-R lengthening. Infranodal block is the rule and QRS complexes tend to be widened. Type II block is most often associated with organic cardiac disease and is frequently progressive (Fig. 36-49). When the QRS complex is narrow with Möbitz type II block, intrahisian block is likely; when it is widened, infrahisian block is the rule.

At times, the conduction ratio of P to QRS complexes is 2 : 1. Only a single P-R interval is noted and P-R lengthening cannot be discerned; therefore, the absolute distinction between type I (2 : 1 Wenckebach) and type II block cannot be made. A narrow QRS complex and

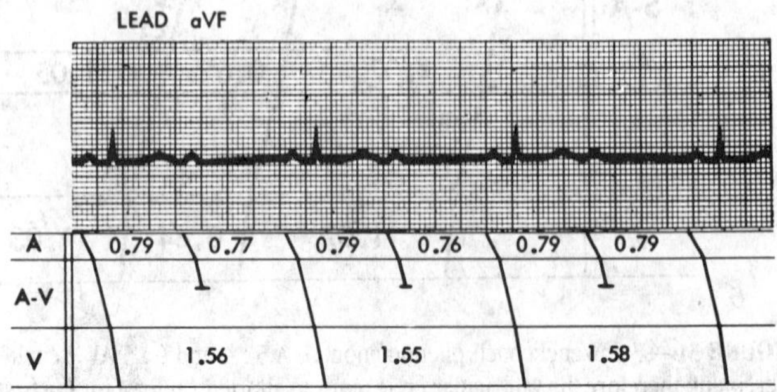

FIGURE 36-49 A form of second-degree AV block. There are two P waves to each QRS 2 : 1 AV block (alternate sinus impulses are blocked).

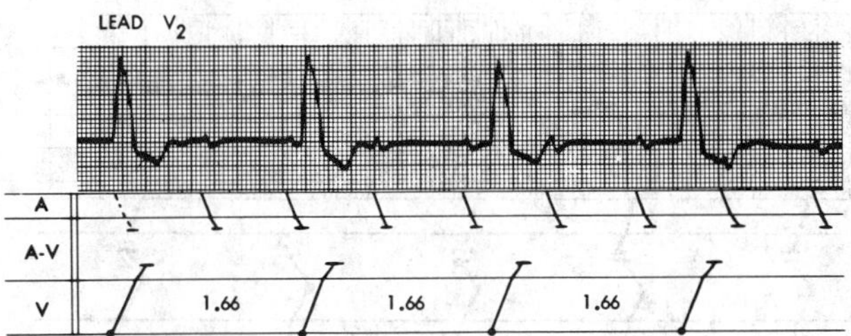

FIGURE 36-50 Complete (third-degree) AV block. There is a regular idioventricular rhythm at rate 36, and the P waves indicate their independence by changing their relation to the QRS complexes.

type I block at other times on the tracing suggest that 2 : 1 block is a manifestation of type I (Wenckebach–AV nodal) physiology. Wide QRS complexes favor type II block. High conduction ratios such as 3 : 1 and greater may be diagnosed simply as paroxysmal or high-grade AV block.

In complete, or third-degree, AV block, the atrial and ventricular rates are regular but dissociated (Fig. 36–50). At times, the P waves and QRS rates are so similar (isorhythmic dissociation) as to make this judgment difficult. QRS complexes represent the escape of junctional (narrow QRS) or ventricular (wide QRS) pacemakers. Complete AV block may be preceded by years of varying and/or progressive lower grades of block as well as bundle branch and fascicular blocks.

Management of AV Block

First-Degree Heart Block Isolated first-degree AV block is never symptomatic and is not an indication for temporary or permanent pacing.[268]

Second-Degree Heart Block Möbitz type I AV block, or the Wenckebach phenomenon is usually associated with an adequate ventricular rate and is rarely symptomatic.[269] It is seen in some athletes[270] and is a normal response to rapid atrial pacing. In most patients who have the Wenckebach phenomenon secondary to AV nodal disease, routine prophylactic pacing is not advised, as it tends not to progress.[271] Rarely, the effective ventricular rate is slow and patients are symptomatic, requiring pacing if vagolytic maneuvers are ineffective. The prognosis in patients who have underlying organic heart disease is dominated by the extent of the underlying disease, not the Möbitz type I block.[271] It is common in the acute phase of inferior wall myocardial infarction and rarely requires temporary pacing in this setting. Reversion is usually prompt (hours to days).

Möbitz type II block is less common but implies more significant conduction system disease. The site of block is almost always below the AV node and usually below the bundle of His; therefore, slower escape rhythms and risk of progression to complete heart block are of concern. It is almost always associated with a defined disease process. Permanent pacing is indicated,[268] except where Möbitz type II block is induced by rapid artificial pacing.[272,273] The purpose of pacing is primarily to protect against symptomatic events—e.g., syncope—and thus to protect the patient from injury to himself or herself or others. There are few data to suggest that pacemakers will prolong the life of patients with Möbitz type II block. The selection among specific designs of pacing devices is discussed in Chap. 40.

A special circumstance involves 2 : 1 AV block, in which the underlying mechanism of block remains obscure. The decision to treat is inferred from the clinical setting. Wide QRS complexes, sudden onset of periods of block, and inadequate escape rates favor type II block, whereas narrow complexes and coincident episodes of typical type I block favor Wenckebach block. His bundle electrograms may be diagnostic, but such invasive studies are indicated only when needed for a therapeutic decision.[274–276]

Paroxysmal AV Block Runs of consecutive atrial impulses that fail to conduct to the ventricles may last for up to 10 to 20 s and may be associated with syncope. Unless a clearly defined reversible cause is identified, permanent pacing is required.

Complete AV Block Complete heart block may be acute in onset and produce significant symptoms or may be chronic and discovered incidentally. When acute and symptomatic, evaluation and rate support are urgently needed. Pharmacologic intervention with atropine or isoproterenol is usually most readily available. The latter should be avoided in the ischemic setting and external pacing instituted if needed.[239,240] Reliable rate control is achieved by ventricular or dual-chamber temporary cardiac pacing. Permanent pacing is indicated unless those factors responsible for the heart block are reversible or when transient complete block complicates an acute inferior wall infarction.[268] The selection between ventricular and dual-chamber pacing and considerations for rate-responsive pacing are discussed in Chap. 40.

AV Dissociation

This diagnosis is not synonymous with AV block but occurs in conjunction with block as well as in its absence. It implies an abnormality of intrinsic pacemaker activity that may be slowing of normal pacemaker activity (default), acceleration of a normally subordinate or latent pacemaker (usurpation), AV block, or a combination of these.

Electrocardiographic Findings Atrioventricular dissociation implies that the atria and ventricles each have independent pacemakers. In the setting of AV block, a junctional or ventricular pacemaker emerges as an escape rhythm; if it fails or if the escape is too slow, AV block will become a symptomatic or terminal rhythm. The atria and ventricles may beat independently if a lower junctional or ventricular pacemaker discharges faster than the sinus or atrial pacemaker. Since AV block is not necessarily present, ventricular capture by impulses of sinus origin may occur as a result of fortuitous timing relationships between sinus node activity and ventricular refractoriness. At times, capture beats and junctional or ventricular beats coincide and generate fusion beats (Fig. 36-51).

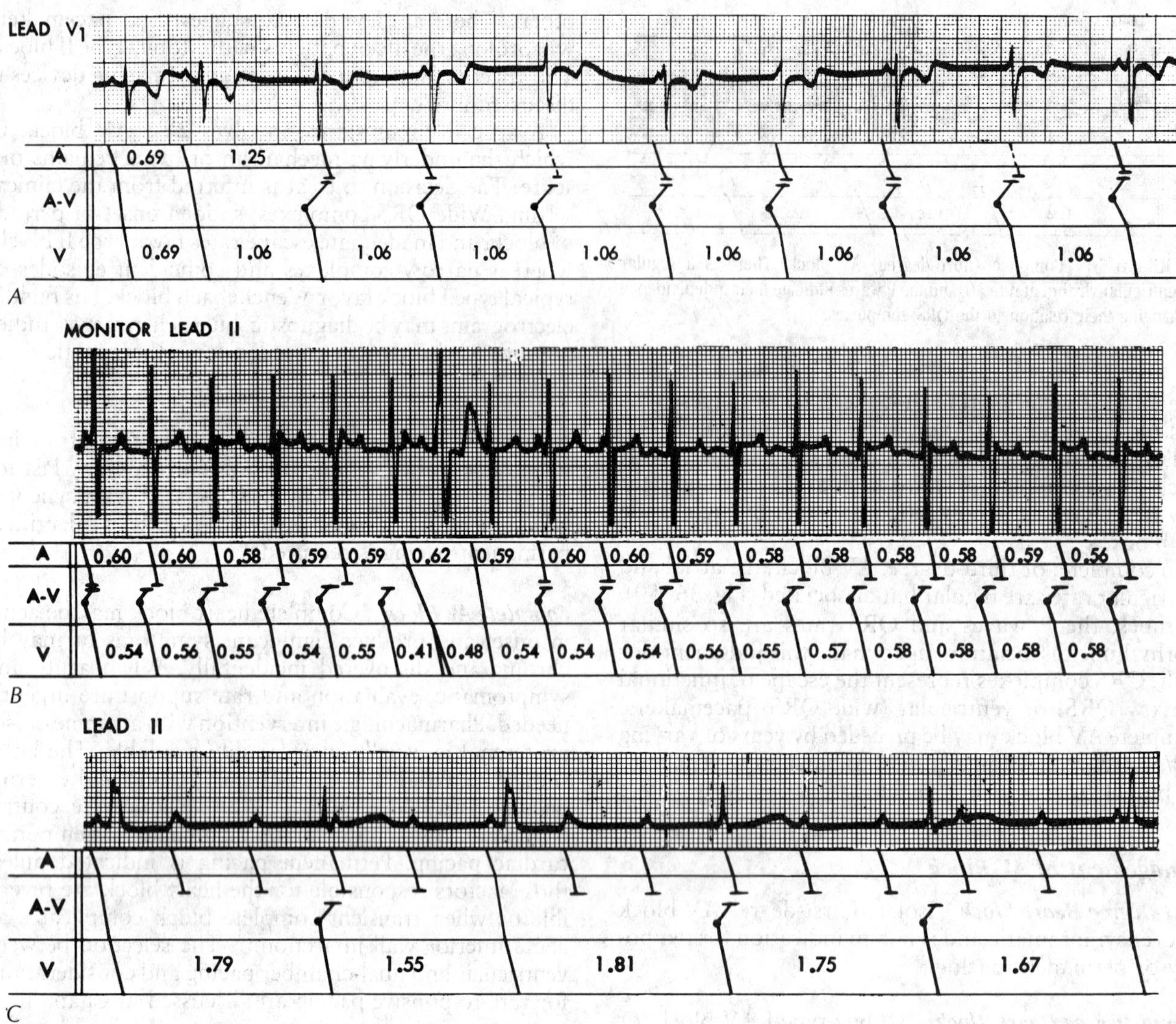

FIGURE 36-51 Atrioventricular dissociation. *A*. Sinus arrhythmia: The bradycardic phase enables the AV node to escape, with resulting dissociation. *B*. Atrioventricular tachycardia: The tachycardia enables the AV pacemaker to usurp control of the ventricles, with resulting dissociation; the seventh and eighth beats are ventricular captures, the seventh, ending the shorter cycle, showing ventricular aberration. *C*. High-grade AV block permits the AV node to escape (second, fourth, and fifth beats) with resulting dissociation.

Management Treatment, when needed, is directed to the underlying cause. It is important to evaluate whether symptoms are present and whether they are due to a rapid or slow rate. Suppression of tachyarrhythmias (e.g., AV dissociation in VT) is the primary goal when symptoms are related primarily to the tachyarrhythmia and an intact intrinsic or artificial pacemaker is present. Intermittent ventricular ectopy may be an escape phenomenon in an otherwise asymptomatic patient who has an underlying persistent bradycardia. In such a case, rate support (e.g., pacing) is indicated and will often relieve the symptoms and ventricular ectopy. If initial therapy is mistakenly targeted to tachycardia, the underlying bradycardia may worsen due to drug suppression of lower intrinsic pacemaker sites.[277]

Indication for Pacing

Pacing is indicated for symptomatic bradyarrhythmias that have no identifiable reversible cardiac or noncardiac cause.[278,279] Prophylactic pacing to prevent mortality or the onset of life-threatening symptoms is controversial, since increased risk of death is more likely related to underlying organic heart disease. The benefits of pacing, though theoretically sound, often lack rigorous proof of effectiveness. Less controversial is the use of permanent pacing to reduce symptomatic bradyarrhythmic events.[278,279] (See also Chap. 40.)

Temporary pacing is indicated for AV block associated with acute anterior wall infarction if the heart rate is excessively slow and/or associated with rate-dependent hypotension and is advanced in some newly acquired left or right bundle branch block accompanied by hemiblock.[280] The availability of external pacing techniques[239,240] has tended to relax the sense of urgency for prophylactic pacing catheters in these settings. New left bundle branch block or preexisting right or left bundle branch block does not require pacing. Permanent pacing is often recommended for those with acute anterior wall infarction who have had transient complete heart block.[281] However, the change in long-term survival is not well documented.[282] Temporary pacing can often be avoided in AV block associated with inferior infarction since block is often related to ischemia or parasympathetic reflexes, is often asymptomatic, and reverses with time.[283] If hypotension occurs in inferior infarction (not due to hypovolemia or right ventricular infarct), temporary pacing for severe sinus bradycardia or higher grades of AV block is often used. Permanent pacing after AV block in inferior infarction is required only very rarely. (See also Chap. 39.)

Permanent prophylactic pacing in bifascicular block is not routinely recommended.[284,285] In patients at high risk for complete heart block (e.g., Kearns-Sayre syndrome) or recurrent neurologic symptoms associated with advanced H-V prolongation (e.g., H-V longer than 70 ms), however, prophylactic pacing may be of benefit.[286] Guidelines for permanent cardiac pacemaker implantation have been published[268] and are further discussed in Chap. 40.

Pacemaker-Associated Arrhythmias

As pacemakers have become more sophisticated, there has been an increasing difficulty in being able to identify normal and abnormal pacemaker rhythms. The baseline pacing pattern is dependent on the pacemaker electronics and the interaction with the patient's intrinsic rhythm. These aspects, as well as pacemaker testing, are reviewed in detail in Chap. 40. Apparent pacemaker malfunctions are frequently due to observer inexperience and lack of knowledge of pacemaker electronics. Unusually rapid or slow rates may connote pacemaker malfunction, but programming changes, magnet activation, and over- and undersensing must be excluded. Fusion beats, pseudofusion, and ventricular triggered pacing may cause confusion. Fusion beats occur when there is overlap in the timing of paced and normal beats and the morphology of the fused complex is midway between the normal and paced QRS complexes. Ventricular triggered pacing becomes confusing when a PVC occurs and is thought to be triggered by the pacemaker because of the width of the complex and the presence of a pacemaker artifact. The pacing artifact occurs slightly after the initiation of the PVC, giving a clue to the fact that the ventricular ectopy is real. Inappropriate bradycardias may be induced by oversensing of the pacemaker or normal sensing of extracardiac stimuli such as myopotentials (skeletal muscle activity) or extracorporeal inhibition by electromagnetic or radiofrequency waves. "Cross talk" can result in arrhythmias, for instance, when the ventricular lead senses atrial activity.

Dual-chamber pacing may lead to a variety of arrhythmias that are actually an undesirable byproduct of normal pacemaker function. Arrhythmias may be initiated by asynchronous ventricular or atrial stimulation (DVI pacemakers), interruption of ventricular sensing during ventricular blanking (all dual-chamber pacemakers), or asynchronous atrial or ventricular stimulation in the magnet mode (all dual-chamber pacemakers). Furthermore, dual-chamber units create an artificial bypass tract that may become operative in the presence of ventriculoatrial conduction. A ventricular event, either paced or spontaneous, may trigger retrograde atrial activation, which is the retrograde limb of the circuit. This is sensed by the atrial electrode that initiates an AV delay. The ventricular stimulus (the antegrade limb of the circuit) follows, and the process continues to repeat itself. This artificial arrhythmia has been called an "endless loop" tachycardia[287] (Fig. 36-52). Spontaneous termination of the reentry tachycardia may occur by fatigue or block in the retrograde limb. Treatment includes reprogramming of pacemaker parameters, including extension of the atrial refractory period of the pacemaker or avoidance of the DDD or VDD mode (at the extreme, the VVI mode is used). In order to guard against rapid ventricular pacing and response to sudden increases in atrial rate, physiological pacemakers tend to have an upper rate limit control. Earlier models suddenly drop to 2 : 1 pacing rates, which could create confusion. Recent models often induce a gradual Wenckebach-type response. The pacemaker electronically creates a Wenckebach phenomenon with a gradually increasing number of dropped QRS complexes. (See also Chap. 40.)

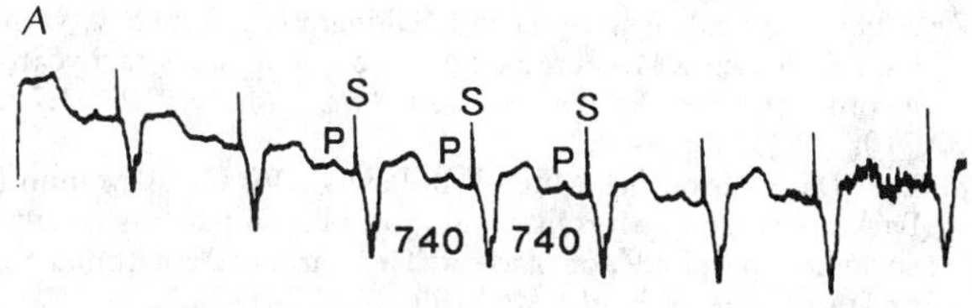

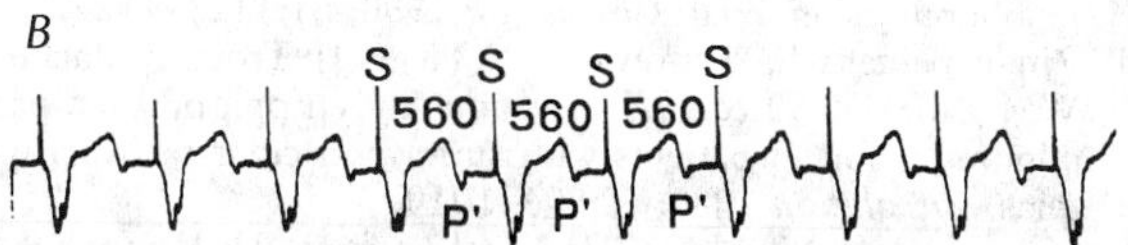

FIGURE 36-52 Pacemaker-mediated (endless-loop) tachycardia. The patient had a DDD pacemaker and presented with episodes of sustained rapid heart action. The tracing (lead II) demonstrates (*A*) atrial tracking with ventricular pacing at a cycle length of 740 ms and (*B*) ventricular pacing with retrograde atrial activation. The retrograde P waves (P′) following each paced QRS are sensed by the atrial sensing lead and trigger a ventricular pacing spike (S) followed by the paced QRS with repeated retrograde atrial activation.

REFERENCES

1. Myerburg RJ, Kessler KM, Zaman L, Fernandez P, DeMarchena E, Castellanos A: Pharmacologic approaches to management of arrhythmias in patients with cardiomyopathy and heart failure. *Am Heart J* 1987; 114:1273–1279.
2. Castellanos A, Aranda J, Befeler B, Myerburg RJ: Intraventricular reentrant tachycardias. In: Schlant RC, Hurst JW (eds): *Advances in Electrocardiography*. New York, Grune & Stratton, 1976: 131–142.
3. Myerburg RJ, Kessler KM, Bassett AL, Castellanos A: A biological approach to sudden cardiac death: Structure, function and cause. *Am J Cardiol* 1989; 63:1512–1516.
4. Myerburg RJ, Kessler KM, Castellanos A: Pathophysiology of sudden cardiac death. *PACE* 1991; 23:127–135.
5. Task Force of the Working Group on Arrhythmias of the European Society of Cardiology: The Sicilian gambit: A new approach to the classification of antiarrhythmic drugs based on their actions on antiarrhythmogenic mechanisms. *Circulation* 1991; 84:1831–1851.
6. Hiss RG, Lamb LE: Electrocardiographic findings in 122,043 individuals. *Circulation* 1962; 25:947–961.

7. Bauernfeind RA, Amat-y-Leon F, Dhingra RC, Kehoe R, Wyndham C, Rosen KM: Chronic nonparoxysmal sinus tachycardia in otherwise healthy persons. *Ann Intern Med* 1979; 91:702–710.
8. Echt DS, Liebson PR, Mitchell B, Peters RW, Obias-Manno D, Barker AH, et al: Mortality and morbidity in patients receiving encainide, flecainide, or placebo. The Cardiac Arrhythmia Suppression Trial. *N Engl J Med* 1991; 324:781–788.
9. Akhtar M, Breithardt G, Camm AJ, Coumel P, Janse MJ, Lazzara R, et al: CAST and beyond: Implications of the Cardiac Arrhythmia Suppression Trial. *Circulation* 1990; 81:1123–1127.
10. Rinkenberger RL, Prystowsky EN, Heger JJ, Troup PJ, Jackman WM, Zipes DP: Effects of intravenous and chronic oral verapamil administration in patients with supraventricular tachyarrhythmias. *Circulation* 1980; 62:996–1010.
11. Waxman HL, Myerburg RJ, Appel R, Sung RJ: Verapamil for control of ventricular rate in paroxysmal supraventricular tachycardia and atrial fibrillation or flutter: A double-blind randomized cross-over study. *Ann Intern Med* 1981; 94:1–6.
12. DiMarco JP, Sellers TD, Lerman BB, Greenberg ML, Berne RM, Belardinelli L: Diagnostic and therapeutic use of adenosine in patients with supraventricular tachyarrhythmias. *J Am Coll Cardiol* 1985; 6:417–425.
13. Stewart RB, Bardy GH, Greene LH: Wide complex tachycardia: Misdiagnosis and outcome after emergent therapy. *Ann Intern Med* 1986; 104:766–771.
14. Rozanski JJ, Zaman L, Castellanos A: Electrophysiologic effects of diltiazem hydrochloride in supraventricular tachycardia. *Am J Cardiol* 1982; 49:621–628.
15. Betriu A, Chaitman BR, Bourassa MG, Brevers G, Scholl J, Bruneau P, et al: Beneficial effect of intravenous diltiazem in the acute management of paroxysmal supraventricular tachyarrhythmias. *Circulation* 1983; 67:88–94.
16. Wu D, Denes P, Dhingra R, Khan A, Rosen KM: The effects of propranolol on induction of A-V nodal reentrant paroxysmal tachycardia. *Circulation* 1974; 50:665–677.
17. Wu D, Hung JS, Kuo CT, Hsu KS, Shieh WB: Effects of quinidine on atrioventricular nodal reentrant paroxysmal tachycardia. *Circulation* 1981; 64:823–831.
18. Batchelder J, Zipes DP: Treatment of tachyarrhythmias by pacing. *Arch Intern Med* 1975; 135:1115–1124.
19. Bauernfeind RA, Wyndham CR, Dhingra RC, Swiryn SP, Palileo E, Strasberg B, et al: Serial electrophysiologic testing of multiple drugs in patients with atrioventricular nodal reentrant paroxysmal tachycardia. *Circulation* 1980; 62:1341–1349.
20. Gallagher J, Svenson R, Kasell J, German L, Bardy G, Broughton A, et al: Catheter technique for closed-chest ablation of the atrioventricular conduction system: A therapeutic alternative for treatment of refractory supraventricular tachycardia. *N Engl J Med* 1982; 306:194–200.
21. Ross DL, Johnson DC, Denniss AR, Cooper MJ, Richards DA, Uther JB: Curative surgery for atrioventricular junctional ("AV nodal") reentrant tachycardia. *J Am Coll Cardiol* 1985; 6:1383–1392.
22. den Dulk K, Bertholet M, Brugada P, Bar FW, Richards D, Dennoulin JC, et al: Clinical experience with implantable devices for control of tachyarrhythmias. *PACE* 1984; 7:548–556.
23. Lee MA, Morady F, Kadish A, Schamp DJ, Chin MC, Sheinman MM, et al: Catheter modification of the atrioventricular junction with radiofrequency energy for control of atrioventricular nodal reentry tachycardia. *Circulation* 1991; 83:827–835.
24. Calkins H, Sousa J, El-Atassi R, Rosenheck S, deBuitleir M, Kou WH, et al: Diagnosis and cure of the Wolff-Parkinson-White syndrome or paroxysmal supraventricular tachycardias during a single electrophysiologic test. *N Engl J Med* 1991; 324:1612–1618.
25. Sung RJ, Castellanos A, Gelband H, Myerburg RJ: Mechanisms of reciprocating tachycardia initiated during sinus rhythm in concealed Wolff-Parkinson-White syndrome. *Circulation* 1976; 54:338–344.
26. Klein GT, Yee R, Sharma AD: Longitudinal electrophysiologic assessment of asymptomatic patients with the Wolff-Parkinson-White electrocardiographic pattern. *N Engl J Med* 1989; 320:1229–1233.
27. Wellens HJJ: Wolff-Parkinson-White syndrome: I. Diagnosis, arrhythmias and identification of the high risk patient. *Mod Concepts Cardiovasc Dis* 1983; 52:53–56.
28. Vidaillet HJ Jr, Pressley JC, Henke E, Harrell FE Jr, German LD: Familial occurrence of accessory A-V pathways (preexcitation syndrome). *N Engl J Med* 1987; 317:65–69.
29. Sung RJ, Castellanos A, Mallon SM, Bloom MG, Gelband H, Myerburg RJ: Mechanisms of spontaneous alternation between reciprocating tachycardia and atrial flutter-fibrillation in the Wolff-Parkinson-White syndrome. *Circulation* 1977; 56:409–415.
30. Gulamhusein S, Ko P, Carruthers SG, Klein GJ: Acceleration of the ventricular response during atrial fibrillation in the Wolff-Parkinson-White syndrome after verapamil. *Circulation* 1982; 65:348–354.
31. McGovern B, Garan H, Ruskin JN: Precipitation of cardiac arrest by verapamil in patients with Wolff-Parkinson-White syndrome. *Ann Intern Med* 1986; 104:791–794.
32. Akhtar M, Gilbert CJ, Shenasa M: Effect of lidocaine on atrioventricular response via the accessory pathway in patients with Wolff-Parkinson-White syndrome. *Circulation* 1981; 63:435–441.
33. Wellens HJJ, Durrer D: Effect of digitalis on atrioventricular conduction and circus movement tachycardias in patients with Wolff-Parkinson-White syndrome. *Circulation* 1973; 47:1229–1233.
34. Sellers TD, Bashore TM, Gallagher JJ: Digitalis in the preexcitation syndrome: Analysis during atrial fibrillation. *Circulation* 1977; 56:260–267.
35. Jackman WM, Wang X, Friday KJ, Roman CA, Moulton KR, Beckman KJ, et al: Catheter ablation of accessory atrioventricular pathways (Wolff-Parkinson-White syndrome) by radiofrequency current. *N Engl J Med* 1991; 324:1605–1611.
36. Wellens HJJ, Brugada P: Value of programmed stimulation of the heart in patients with the Wolff-Parkinson-White syndrome. In: Josephson ME, Wellens HJJ (eds): *Tachycardias: Mechanisms, Diagnosis, Treatment.* Philadelphia, Lea & Febiger, 1984: 199–221.
37. Prystowsky EN: Indications for intracardiac electrophysiologic studies in patients with supraventricular tachycardia. *Circulation* 1987; 75(suppl III):III-119–III-122.
38. Klein GJ, Bashore TM, Sellers TD, Pritchett ELC, Smith WM, Gallagher JJ: Ventricular fibrillation in the Wolff-Parkinson-White syndrome. *N Engl J Med* 1979; 301:1080–1075.
39. Castellanos A, Myerburg RJ: Changing perspectives in the preexcitation syndromes. *N Engl J Med* 1987; 317:109–111.
40. Scheinman MM: Catheter ablation for patients with ventricular preexcitation syndromes. In: Benditt DG, Benson DW (eds): *Cardiac Preexcitation Syndromes.* Boston, Martinus Nijhoff, 1986: 493–506.
41. Cox JL, Cain ME: Surgery for preexcitation syndromes. In: Benditt DG, Benson DW (eds): *Cardiac Preexcitation Syndromes.* Boston, Martinus Nijhoff, 1986: 527–534.
42. Guiraudon GM, Klein GJ, Sharma AD, Jones DL, McLellan DG: Surgery for Wolff-Parkinson-White syndrome: Further experience with an epicardial approach. *Circulation* 1986; 74:525–529.
43. Camm J, Hellestrand KJ, Nathan AW, Bexton RS: Clinical usefulness of flecainide acetate in the treatment of paroxysmal supraventricular arrhythmias. *Drugs* 1985; 29:7–13.
44. Prystowsky EN, Klein G, Rinkenberger RL, Heger JJ, Nacarelli GV, Zipes DP: Clinical efficacy and electrophysiologic effects of encainide in patients with Wolff-Parkinson-White syndrome. *Circulation* 1984; 69:278–287.
45. Fogoros RN, Anderson KP, Winkle RA, Swerdlow CD, Mason JW: Amiodarone: Clinical efficacy and toxicity in 96 patients with recurrent drug refractory arrhythmias. *Circulation* 1983; 68:88–94.
46. Breithardt G, Borggrefe M, Wiebringhaus E, Seipel L: Effect of propafenone in the Wolff-Parkinson-White syndrome: Electrophysiologic findings and long term followup. *Am J Cardiol* 1984; 54:29D–39D.
47. Pritchett EL, DaTorre SD, Platt ML, McCarville SE, Hougham AJ: Flecainide acetate treatment of paroxysmal supraventricular tachycardia and paroxysmal atrial fibrillation: Dose-response studies. *J Am Coll Cardiol* 1991; 17:297–303.
48. Neuss H, Schlepper M, Thormann J: Analysis of reentry mechanisms in the three patients with concealed Wolff-Parkinson-White syndrome. *Circulation* 1975; 51:75–81.
49. Wu D, Amat-y-Leon F, Denes P, Dhingra RC, Pietras RJ, Rosen

KM: Demonstration of sustained sinus and atrial reentry as a mechanism of paroxysmal supraventricular tachycardia. *Circulation* 1975; 51:234–243.

50. Wu D, Denes P, Amat-y-Leon, Dhingra RC, Wyndham CRC, Bauernfeind R, Latif P, Rosen KM: Clinical electrocardiographic and electrophysiologic observations in patients with paroxysmal supraventricular tachycardia. *Am J Cardiol* 1978; 41:1045–1051.
51. Coumel P, Flammang D, Attuel P, Leclercq JF: Sustained intra-atrial reentrant tachycardia: Electrophysiologic study of 20 cases. *Clin Cardiol* 1979; 2:167–178.
52. Gallagher JJ, Smith WM, Kassell JH, Benson DW, Sterba R, Grant RO: Role of Mahaim fibers in cardiac arrhythmias in man. *Circulation* 1981; 64:176–189.
53. Cox JL: The status of surgery for cardiac arrhythmias. *Circulation* 1985; 71:413–417.
54. Allessie MA, Bonke FIM, Schopman FJG: Circus movement in rabbit atrial muscle as a mechanism of tachycardia. III. The "leading circle" concept: A new model of circus movement in cardiac tissue without the involvement of an anatomical obstacle. *Circ Res* 1977; 41:9–18.
55. Gelband H, Bush HL, Rosen MR, Myerburg RJ, Hoffman BF: Electrophysiologic properties of isolated preparations of human atrial myocardium. *Circ Res* 1972; 30:290–300.
56. Mary-Rabine L, Hordof AJ, Danilo P Jr, Malm JR, Rosen MR: Mechanisms for impulse initiation in isolated human atrial fibers. *Circ Res* 1980; 47:267–277.
57. Josephson ME, Spear JF, Harken AH, Horowitz LN, Dorio RJ: Surgical excision of automatic atrial tachycardia: Anatomic and electrophysiologic correlates. *Am Heart J* 1982; 104:1076–1085.
58. Shine KI, Kastor JA, Yurchak PM: Multifocal atrial tachycardia. Clinical and electrocardiographic features in 32 patients *N Engl J Med* 1968; 279:344–349.
59. Salerno DM, Anderson B, Sharkey PJ, Iber C: Intravenous verapamil for treatment of multifocal atrial tachycardia with and without calcium pretreatment. *Ann Intern Med* 1987; 107:623–628.
60. Wang K, Goldfarb JL, Gobel F, Richman HG: Multifocal atrial tachycardia. *Arch Intern Med* 1977; 137:161–164.
61. Fosmoe RJ, Averill KH, Lamb LE: Electrocardiographic findings in 67,375 asymptomatic subjects. II: Supraventricular arrhythmias. *Am J Cardiol* 1960; 6:84–95.
62. Garson A, Bink-Boelkens M, Hesslein PS, Hordof AJ, Keane JF, Neches WH, et al: Atrial flutter in the young: A collaborative study of 380 cases. *J Am Coll Cardiol* 1985; 6:871–878.
63. Waldo AL, Henthorn RW, Plumb VJ: Atrial flutter: Recent observations in man. In: Josephson ME, Wellens HJJ (eds): *Tachycardias: Mechanisms, Diagnosis, Treatment.* Philadelphia, Lea & Febiger, 1982: 113–135.
64. Slama R, Leclercq JF, Rosengarten M, Coumel PH, Bouvrain Y: Multilevel block in the atrioventricular node during atrial tachycardia and flutter alternating with Wenckebach phenomenon. *Br Heart J* 1979; 42:463–470.
65. Robertson CE, Miller HC: Extreme tachycardia complicating the use of disopyramide in atrial flutter. *Br Heart J* 1980; 44:602–603.
66. Waldo AL, MacLean WH, Karp RP, Kouchoukos NT, James TN: Entrainment and interruption of atrial flutter with atrial pacing. Studies in man following open heart surgery. *Circulation* 1977; 56:737–745.
67. Camm J, Ward D, Spurrell R: Response of atrial flutter to overdrive atrial pacing and intravenous disopyramide phosphate, singly and in combination. *Br Heart J* 1980; 44:240–247.
68. Touboul P, Saoudi N, Georges A, Kirkorian G: Electrophysiological basis of catheter ablation in atrial flutter. *Am J Cardiol* 1989; 64:79J–82J.
69. Benditt DG, Pritchett EL, Gallagher JJ: Spectrum of regular tachycardias with wide QRS complexes in patients with accessory atrioventricular pathways. *Am J Cardiol* 1978; 42:828–838.
70. Cairns JA, Connolly ST: Nonrheumatic atrial fibrillation: Risk of stroke and role of antithrombotic therapy. *Circulation* 1991; 84:469–481.
71. Shrier A, Dubarsky H, Rosengarten M, Guevara MR, Nattal S, Glass L: Prediction of complex atrioventricular conduction rhythms in humans with use of the atrioventricular nodal recovery curve. *Circulation* 1987; 76:1196–1205.
72. Gouaux JL, Ashman R: Auricular fibrillation with aberration simulating ventricular paroxysmal tachycardia. *Am Heart J* 1947; 34:366–373.
73. Marriott HJL, Sandler LA: Criteria, old and new, for differentiating between ectopic ventricular beats and aberrant ventricular conduction in the presence of atrial fibrillation. *Prog Cardiovasc Dis* 1966; 9:18–28.
74. Kopecky SL, Gersh BJ, McGoon MD, Whisnant JP, Holmes DR, Ilstrup DM, et al: The natural history of lone atrial fibrillation: A population-based study over three decades. *N Engl J Med* 1987; 317:669–674.
75. Gajewski J, Singer RB: Mortality in an insured population with atrial fibrillation. *JAMA* 1981; 245:1540–1544.
76. Morris JM, Peter RH, Mcintosh HD: Electrical conversion of atrial fibrillation: Immediate and long-term results and selection of patients. *Ann Intern Med* 1966; 65:216–231.
77. Mancini GBJ, Goldberger AL: Cardioversion of atrial fibrillation: Consideration of embolization, anticoagulation, prophylactic pacemaker and long-term success. *Am Heart J* 1982; 104:617–621.
78. Dunn M, Alexandre J, DeSilva R, Hildner F: Antithrombotic therapy in atrial fibrillation. *Chest* 1986; 89:68s–73s.
79. Takahashi N, Seki A, Imataka K, Fuji J: Clinical features of paroxysmal atrial fibrillation: An observation of 94 patients *Jpn Heart J* 1981; 22:143–149.
80. Berns E, Rinkenberger RL, Jeang MK, Dougherty AH, Jenkins M, Naccarelli GV: Efficacy and safety of flecainide acetate for atrial tachycardia or fibrillation. *Am J Cardiol* 1987; 59:1337–1341.
81. Olshansky B, Waldo AL: Atrial fibrillation: Update on mechanism, diagnosis, and management. *Mod Conc Cardiovasc Dis* 1987; 56:23–27.
82. Wolf PA, Dawber TR, Thomas HE: Epidemiologic assessment of chronic atrial fibrillation and risk of stroke: The Framingham study. *Neurology* 1978; 28:973–977.
83. Wolf PA, Kannel WB, McGee DL, Meeks SL, Bharucha NE, McNamara PM: Duration of atrial fibrillation and imminence of stroke: The Framingham study. *Stroke* 1983; 14:664–667.
84. Kannel WB, Abbott RD, Savage DD, McNamara PM: Epidemiologic features of chronic atrial fibrillation. *N Engl J Med* 1982; 306:1018–1022.
85. Staffurth JS, Gibberd MC: Arterial embolism in thyrotoxicosis with atrial fibrillation. *Br Med J* 1977; 2:688–690.
86. Brand FN, Abbott RD, Kannel WB, Wolf PA: Characteristics and prognosis of lone atrial fibrillation. *JAMA* 1985; 254:3449–3453.
87. Lown B: Electrical reversion of cardiac arrhythmias. *Br Heart J* 1967; 29:469–489.
88. Resenkov L, McDonald L: Complications in 220 patients with cardiac dysrhythmias treated by phased direct current shock and indications for electrocardioversion. *Br Heart J* 1967; 29:926–936.
89. Bjerkelund CJ, Orning OM: The efficacy of anticoagulant therapy in preventing embolism related to DC electrical conversion of atrial fibrillation. *Am J Cardiol* 1969; 23:208–216.
90. Stroke Prevention in Atrial Fibrillation Investigators: Stroke prevention in atrial fibrillation study: Final results. *Circulation* 1991; 84:527–539.
91. Connolly SJ, Laupacis A, Gent M, Roberts RS, Cairns JA, Joyner C, for the CAFA Study Coinvestigators: Canadian atrial fibrillation anticoagulation (CAFA) study. *J Am Coll Cardiol* 1991; 18:349–355.
92. Peterson P, Boysen G, Godtfredsen J, Andersen ED, Andersen B: Placebo-controlled, randomized trial of warfarin and aspirin for prevention of thromboembolic complications in chronic atrial fibrillation: The Copenhagen AFASAK study. *Lancet* 1989; 1:175–179.
93. Boston Area Anticoagulation Trial in Atrial Fibrillation Investigators: The effect of low-dose warfarin on the risk of stroke in patients with non-rheumatic atrial fibrillation. *N Engl J Med* 1990; 323:1505–1511.
94. Forfar JC: A 7-year analysis of haemorrhage in patients on long-term anticoagulant treatment. *Br Heart J* 1979; 42:128–132.
95. Whisnant JP, Cartlidge NEF, Elveback LR: Carotid and vertibral-basilar transient ischemic attacks: Effect of anticoagulants, hypertension, and cardiac disorders on survival and stroke occurrence—a population study. *Ann Neurol* 1978; 3:107–115.

96. Hoffman BF, Rosen MR; Cellular mechanisms for cardiac arrhythmias. *Circ Res* 1981; 43:1–15.
97. Friedman PL, Stewart JR, Wit AL: Spontaneous and induced cardiac arrhythmias in subendocardial Purkinje fibers surviving extensive myocardial infarction in dogs. *Circ Res* 1973; 33:612–626.
98. Rosen MR, Fisch C, Hoffman BF, Danilo P Jr, Lovelace DE, Knoebel SB: Can accelerated atrioventricular junctional escape rhythms be explained by delayed afterdepolarizations? *Am J Cardiol* 1980; 45:1272–1284.
99. Sclarowsky S, Strasberg B, Fuchs J, Lewin RF, Arditi A, Klainman E, et al: Multiform accelerated idioventricular rhythm in acute myocardial infarction: Electrocardiographic characteristics and response to verapamil. *Am J Cardiol* 1983; 52:43–47.
100. deSoyza N, Bissett JK, Kane JJ, Murphy ML, Doherthy JE: Association of accelerated idioventricular rhythm and paroxysmal ventricular tachycardia in acute myocardial infarction. *Am J Cardiol* 1974; 34:667–670.
101. Garson A, Gillette PC: Junctional ectopic tachycardia in children: Electrocardiography, electrophysiology and pharmacologic response. *Am J Cardiol* 1979; 44:298–302.
102. Gillette PC, Garson A, Porter J, Ott D, McVey P, Zinner A, et al: Junctional automatic ectopic tachycardia: New proposed treatment of transcatheter His bundle ablation. *Am Heart J* 1983; 106:619–623.
103. Green M, Heddle B, Dassen W, Wehr M, V Abdollah H, Brugada P, et al: Value of QRS alternation in determining the site of origin of narrow QRS supraventricular tachycardia. *Circulation* 1983; 68:368–373.
104. Brugada P, Bar FWHM, Vanagt Ej, Friedman PR, Wellens HJJ: Observations in patients showing A-V junctional echoes with a shorter P-R than R-P interval: Distinction between intranodal reentry and reentry using an accessory pathway with a long conduction time. *Am J Cardiol* 1981; 48:611–622.
105. Brudaga P, Farre H, Green M, Heddle B, Roy D, Wellens HJJ: Observations in patients with supraventricular tachycardia having a P-R interval shorter than the R-P interval: Differentiation between atrial tachycardia and reciprocating atrioventricular tachycardia using an accessory pathway with long conduction times. *Am Heart J* 1984; 107:556–570.
106. Perry JC, McQuinn RL, Smith RT, Gothing C, Fredell P, Garson A: Flecainide acetate for resistant arrhythmias in the young: Efficacy and pharmacokinetics. *J Am Coll Cardiol* 1989; 14:185–191.
107. Velebit V, Podrid P, Lown B, Cohen BH, Graboys TB: Aggravation and provocation of ventricular arrhythmia by antiarrhythmic drugs. *Circulation* 1982; 65:886–894.
108. Ruskin JN, McGovern B, Garan H, DeMarco JP, Kelly E: Antiarrhythmic drugs: A possible cause of out-of-hospital cardiac arrest. *N Engl J Med* 1983; 309:1302–1306.
109. Myerburg RJ, Kessler KM, Prineas RJ: The cardiac arrhythmia suppression trial (letter). *N Engl J Med* 1989; 321:1754.
110. Starmer CF, Lastra AA, Nesterenko VV, Grant AO: Proarrhythmic response to sodium channel blockade: Theoretical model and numerical experiments. *Circulation* 1991; 84:1364–1377.
111. Myerburg RJ, Kessler KM, Luceri RFM, Zaman L, Trohman RG, Estes D, et al: Classification of ventricular arrhythmias based on parallel hierarchies of frequency and form. *Am J Cardiol* 1984; 54:1355–1358.
112. Moss AJ, Schnitzler R, Green R, DeCamilla J: Ventricular arrhythmias 3 weeks after acute myocardial infarction. *Ann Intern Med* 1971; 75:837–841.
113. Vismara LA, Amsterdam BA, Mason DT: Relation of ventricular arrhythmias in the late-hospital phase of acute myocardial infarction to sudden death after hospital discharge. *Am J Med* 1975; 59:6–12.
114. Rubermman W, Weinblatt, Goldberg JD, Frank CW, Chaudhary BS, Shapiro S: Ventricular premature complexes and sudden death after myocardial infarction. *Circulation* 1981; 64:297–305.
115. Schulze RA, Strauss HW, Pitt B: Sudden death in the year following myocardial infarction: Relationship of ventricular premature contractions in the late hospital phase and left ventricular ejection fraction. *Am J Med* 1977; 62:192–199.
116. Bigger JT, Fleiss JL, Kleiger R, Miller JP, Rolnitzky LM, and the Multicenter Post-infarction Research Group: The relationships among ventricular arrhythmias, left ventricular dysfunction, and mortality in the 2 years after myocardial infarction. *Circulation* 1984; 69:250–258.
117. Bigger JT Jr: Current approaches to drug treatment of ventricular arrhythmias. *Am J Cardiol* 1987; 60:10F–20F.
118. Kessler KM, McAuliff D, Chakko S, Castellanos A, Myerburg RJ: Multiform ventricular complexes: A transitional arrhythmia form? *Am Heart J* 1989; 118:441–444.
119. Castellanos A, Luceri RM, Moleiro F, Kayden DA, Trohman RG, Zaman L, et al: Annihilation, entrainment and modulation of ventricular parasystolic rhythms. *Am J Cardiol* 1984; 54:317–322.
120. Kennedy HL, Whitlock JA, Sprague MK, Kennedy LJ, Buckingham TA, Goldberg RJ: Long-term follow-up of asymptomatic healthy subjects with frequent and complex ventricular ectopy. *N Engl J Med* 1985; 313:193–197.
121. Winkle RA: The relationship between ventricular ectopic beat frequency and heart rate. *Circulation* 1982; 66:439–446.
122. Kostis JB, McCrone K, Moreyra AE, Gotzoyannis S, Aglitz NM, Natarajan N, et al: Premature ventricular complexes in the absence of identifiable heart disease. *Circulation* 1981; 63:1351–1356.
123. Campbell RWF, Godman MG, Fiddler GI, Marquis RM, Julian DG: Ventricular arrhythmias in the syndrome of balloon deformity of mitral valve: Definition of possible high risk group. *Br Heart J* 1976; 38:1053–1057.
124. Pocock WA, Bosman CK, Chesler E, Barlow JE, Edwards JE: Sudden death in primary mitral valve prolapse. *Am Heart J* 1984; 107:378–382.
125. Nishimura RA, McGoon MD, Shub C, Miller FA, Ilstrup DM, Tajik AJ: Echocardiographically documented mitral valve prolapse: Long-term follow-up of 237 patients. *N Engl J Med* 1985; 313:1305–1309.
126. Lown B, Fakhro AM, Hood WB, Thorn GW: The coronary care unit: New perspectives and directions. *JAMA* 1967; 199:156–166.
127. El-Sherif N, Myerburg RJ, Scherlag BJ, Befeler B, Aranda JM, Castellanos A, et al: Electrocardiographic antecedents of primary ventricular fibrillation. Value of the R-on-T phenomenon in myocardial infarction. *Br Heart J* 1976; 38:415–422.
128. DeSozya N, Meacham D, Murphy ML, Kane JJ, Doherty JE, Bissett JK: Evaluation of warning arrhythmias before paroxysmal ventricular tachycardia during acute myocardial infarction in man. *Circulation* 1979; 60:814–818.
129. Wyman MG, Hammersmith L: Comprehensive treatment plan for the prevention of primary ventricular fibrillation in acute myocardial infarction. *Am J Cardiol* 1974; 33:661–667.
130. Lie KI, Wellens HJJ, Van Capelli FJ: Lidocaine in the prevention of primary ventricular fibrillation. A double blind randomized study of 212 consecutive patients. *N Engl J Med* 1974; 291:1324–1326.
131. Routledge PA, Stargel WW, Wagner GS, Shand DG: Increased alpha-1-acid glycoprotein and lidocaine distribution in myocardial infarction. *Ann Intern Med* 1980; 293:701–704.
132. LeLorier J, Genon D, Latour Y: Pharmacokinetics of lidocaine after prolonged intravenous infusions in uncomplicated myocardial infarction. *Ann Intern Med* 1977; 87:700–702.
133. Maseri A, Severi S, Marzulio P: Role of coronary arterial spasm in sudden coronary ischemic death. *Ann NY Acad Sci* 1982; 382:204–217.
134. Tzivoni D, Keren A, Granot H, Gottlieb S, Benhorin J, Stern S: Ventricular fibrillation caused by myocardial reperfusion in Prinzmetal's angina. *Am Heart J* 1983; 105:323–325.
135. Kimura S, Bassett AL, Saoudi NC, Cameron JS, Kozlovskis PL, Myerburg RJ: Cellular electrophysiologic changes and "arrhythmias" during experimental ischemia and reperfusion in isolated cat ventricular myocardium. *J Am Coll Cardiol* 1986; 7:833–841.
136. Kimura S, Bassett AL, Kohya T, Kozlovskis PL, Myerburg RJ: Simultaneous recording of action potentials from endocardium and epicardium during ischemia in the isolated cat ventricle: Relation of temporal electrophysiologic heterogeneities to arrhythmias. *Circulation* 1986; 74:401–409.
137. Maskin CS, Siskin SJ, LeJemtal TH: High prevalence of nonsustained ventricular tachycardia in severe congestive heart failure. *Am Heart J* 1983; 207:896–901.

138. Chakko CS, Gheorghiade M: Ventricular arrhythmias in severe heart failure: Incidence, significance, and effectiveness of antiarrhythmic therapy. *Am Heart J* 1985; 109:497–504.
139. Vignola PA, Aonuma K, Swaye PS, Rozanski JJ, Blankstein RL, Benson J, et al: Lymphocytic myocarditis presenting as unexplained ventricular arrhythmias: Diagnosis with endomyocardial biopsy and response to immunosuppression. *J Am Coll Cardiol* 1984; 4:812–819.
140. Meinertz T, Hofmann T, Kasper W, Treese N, Bechtold H, Stienen U, et al: Significance of ventricular arrhythmias in idiopathic dilated cardiomyopathy. *Am J Cardiol* 1984; 53:902–907.
141. Holmes J, Kubo SH, Cody RJ, Kligfield P: Arrhythmias in ischemic and nonischemic dilated cardiomyopathy: Prediction of mortality by ambulatory electrocardiography. *Am J Cardiol* 1985; 55:146–151.
142. Bigger JT: Methodology for clinical trials with antiarrhythmic drugs to prevent cardiac deaths: U.S. experience. *Cardiology* 1987; 74(suppl 2):40–56.
143. The Cardiac Arrhythmia Pilot Study (CAPS) Investigators: Effects of encainide, flecainide, imipramine, and muricizime on ventricular arrhythmias during the year after acute myocardial infarction: The CAPS study. *Am J Cardiol* 1988; 61:501–509.
144. The Cardiac Arrhythmia Suppression Trial II Investigators: Effect of the antiarrhythmic agent moricizine in survival after myocardial infarction. *N Eng J Med* 1992; 327:227–233.
145. Hine LK, Laird NM, Hewitt P, Chalmers TC: Meta-analysis of empirical long-term antiarrhythmic therapy after myocardial infarction. *JAMA* 1989; 262:3037–3040.
146. Beta-Blocker Heart Attack Research Group: A randomized trial of propranolol in patients with acute myocardial infarction. 1. Mortality results. *JAMA* 1982; 247:1707–1714.
147. Pederson TR and the Norwegian Multicenter Study Group: Six-year follow-up of the Norwegian multicenter study on timolol after acute myocardial infarction. *N Engl J Med* 1985; 313:1055–1058.
148. Woosley RL, Kornhauser D, Smith R, Reele S, Higgins SB, Nies RS, et al: Suppression of chronic ventricular arrhythmias with propranolol. *Circulation* 1979; 60:819–827.
149. Lichstein E, Morganroth J, Harrist R, Hubble E, for the BHAT Study Study Group: Effect of propranolol on ventricular arrhythmia: The beta-blocker heart attack trial experience. *Circulation* 1983; 67(suppl I):I-5–I-10.
150. Gomes JA, Harriman RI, Kaing P, El-Sherif N, Chowdhry I, Lyons J: Programmed electrical stimulation in patients with high-grade ventricular ectopy: Electrophysiologic findings and prognosis for survival. *Circulation* 1984; 70:43–51.
151. Morganroth J, Anderson JL, Gentzkow CD: Classification by type of arrhythmia predicts frequency of adverse cardiac events from flecainide. *J Am Coll Cardiol* 1986; 8:607–615.
152. Webster MWI, Fitzpatrick MA, Nicholis MG, Ikram H, Wells JE: Effect of enalapril on ventricular arrhythmias in congestive heart failure. *Am J Cardiol* 1985; 56:566–569.
153. Minardo JD, Heger JJ, Miles WM, Zipes DP, Prystowsky EN: Clinical characteristics of patients with ventricular fibrillation during antiarrhythmic drug therapy. *N Engl J Med* 1988; 319:257–262.
154. Myerburg RJ, Kessler KM, Cox MM, Huikuri H, Terracall E, Interian A, et al: Reversal of proarrhythmic effects of flecainide acetate and encainide hydrochloride by propranolol. *Circulation* 1989; 80:1571–1579.
155. Anderson JL: Rationale of combination antiarrhythmic drug therapy. *Cardiovasc Clin* 1985; 16:307–327.
156. Herre JM, Sauve MJ, Malone P, Griffin JC, Helmy I, Laneberg JJ, et al: Long-term results of amiodarone therapy in patients with recurrent sustained ventricular tachycardia or ventricular fibrillation. *J Am Coll Cardiol* 1989; 13:442–449.
157. Myerburg RJ, Kessler KM, Kiem I, Pefkaros KC, Conde CA, Cooper D, et al: The relationship between plasma levels of procainamide, suppression of premature ventricular contractions, and prevention of recurrent ventricular tachycardia. *Circulation* 1981; 64:280–290.
158. Graboys TB, Lown B, Podrid PJ, DeSilva R: Long-term survival of patients with malignant ventricular arrhythmias treated with antiarrhythmic drugs. *Am J Cardiol* 1982; 50:437–443.
159. Morganroth J, Michelson EL, Horowitz LN, Josephson ME, Pearlman AS, Dankman WB: Limitations of routine long-term electrocardiographic monitoring to assess ventricular ectopic frequency. *Circulation* 1978; 58:408–414.
160. Vlay SC, Kallman CH, Reid RP: Prognostic assessment of survivors of ventricular tachycardia and ventricular fibrillation with ambulatory monitoring. *Am J Cardiol* 1984; 54:87–90.
161. Gallavardin L, Veil P: Deux nouveaux cas d'extrasystolic-ventriculaire avec salves tachycardiques. *Arch Mal Coeur* 1929; 22:738–741.
162. Buxton AE, Marchlinski FE, Doherty JU, Cassidy DM, Vassalo JA, Flores BT, et al: Repetitive monomorphic ventricular tachycardia: Clinical and electrophysiologic characteristics in patients with and without organic heart disease. *Am J Cardiol* 1984; 54:997–1002.
163. Coumel P, Leclercq JF, Attuel P, Rosengarten M, Milosevic D, Slama P, et al: Tachycardies ventriculaires en salves: Etude electrophysiologique et therapeutique. *Arch Mal Coeur* 1980; 73:155–164.
164. Rahilly GT, Prystowsky EN, Zipes DP, Naccerelli GV, Jackson WM, Heger JJ: Clinical and electrophysiologic findings in patients with otherwise normal electrocardiograms. *Am J Cardiol* 1982; 50:459–468.
165. Wellens HJJ, Bar FRWM, Lie KI: The value of the electrocardiogram in the differential diagnosis of a tachycardia with a widened QRS complex. *Am J Med* 1978; 64:27–33.
166. Wellens HJJ, Bar FRHM, Vanagt EJDM, Brugada P: Medical treatment of ventricular tachycardia: Considerations in the selection of patients for surgical treatment. *Am J Cardiol* 1982; 49:187–193.
167. Thompson PD, Melmon KL, Richardson JA, Cohn K, Cudihee R, Steinbrunn W, et al: Lidocaine pharmacokinetics in advanced heart failure, liver disease and renal failure in humans. *Ann Intern Med* 1973; 78:499–508.
168. Giardina EG, Heissenbuttel RH, Bigger JT: Intermittent intravenous procainamide to treat ventricular arrhythmias. Correlation of plasma concentration with effect on arrhythmia, electrocardiogram, and blood pressure. *Ann Intern Med* 1973; 78:183–193.
169. Holder DA, Sniderman AD, Fraser G, Fallen EL: Experience with bretylium tosylate by a hospital cardiac arrest team. *Circulation* 1977; 55:541–544.
170. Myerburg RJ, Zaman L, Luceri R, Kessler KM, Kayden D, Castellanos A: Antiarrhythmic drug therapy after myocardial infarction. In: Kulbertus HE, Wellens HJJ (eds): *The First Year after a Myocardial Infarction.* Mt. Kisco, NY, Futura, 1983: 321–339.
171. Wellens HJJ, Bar FWH, Vanagt EJDM, Brugada P: Medical treatment for ventricular tachycardia: Considerations in the selection of patients for surgical therapy. *Am J Cardiol* 1982; 49:186–193.
172. DiMarco JP, Lerman BB, Kron IL, Sellers TD: Sustained ventricular tachyarrhythmias within 2 months of acute myocardial infarction: Results of medical and surgical therapy in patients resuscitated from the initial episode. *J Am Coll Cardiol* 1985; 6:759–768.
173. Packer M: Sudden unexpected death in patients with congestive heart failure. A second frontier. *Circulation* 1985; 72:681–685.
174. Wellens HJJ, Brugada P, Stevenson WG: Programmed electrical stimulation of the heart in patients with life-threatening ventricular arrhythmias: What is the significance of induced arrhythmias and what is the correct stimulation protocol? *Circulation* 1985; 72:1–7.
175. Swerdlow CD, Winkle RA, Mason JW: Determinant of survival in patients with ventricular tachycardias. *N Engl J Med* 1983; 308:1436–1442.
176. Wilbur DJ, Garan H, Finkelstein D, Kelly E, Newell J, McGovern B, et al: Out-of-hospital cardiac arrest: Use of electrophysiologic testing in the prediction of long-term outcome. *N Engl J Med* 1988; 318:19–24.
177. Mitchell LB, Duff HJ, Manyari DE, Wyse DG: A randomized clinical trial of the noninvasive and invasive approaches to drug therapy of ventricular tachycardia. *N Engl J Med* 1987; 317:1681–1687.
178. Waller TJ, Kay HR, Spielman SR, Kutalek SP, Greenspan AM, Horowitz LN: Reduction in sudden death and total mortality by antiarrhythmic therapy evaluated by electrophysiologic drug testing: Criteria of efficacy in patients with sustained ventricular tachycardia. *J Am Coll Cardiol* 1987; 10:83–89.

179. Rae AP, Greenspan AM, Spielman SR, Sokoloff NM, Webb CR, Kay HR, et al: Antiarrhythmic drug efficacy for ventricular tachyarrhythmias associated with coronary artery disease as assessed by electrophysiologic studies. *Am J Cardiol* 1985; 55:1494–1499.
180. Myerburg RJ, Kessler KM, Estes D, Conde CA, Luceri RM, Zaman L, et al: Long-term survival after prehospital cardiac arrest: Analysis of outcome during an 8-year study. *Circulation* 1984; 70:538–546.
181. Kim SG, Seiden SW, Felder SD, Waspe LE, Fisher JD: Is programmed stimulation of value in predicting the long-term success of antiarrhythmic therapy for ventricular tachycardias? *N Engl J Med* 1986; 315:356–362.
182. Kim SG: The management of patients with life-threatening ventricular tachyarrhythmias: Programmed stimulation or Holter monitoring (either or both)? *Circulation* 1987; 76:1–5.
183. Weiner I, Mindich B, Pitchon R: Determinant of ventricular tachycardia in patients with ventricular aneurysms: Results of intraoperative epicardial and endocardial mapping. *Circulation* 1982; 65:856–861.
184. Josephson ME, Harken AH, Horowitz LN: Endocardial excision. A new surgical technique for the treatment of recurrent ventricular tachycardia. *Circulation* 1979; 60:1430–1439.
185. Gallagher JJ, Anderson RW, Kasell JH, Rice JR, Pritchett ELC, Gault JH, et al: cryoablation of drug resistant ventricular tachycardia in a patient with a variant of scleroderma. *Circulation* 1978; 57:190–197.
186. Cox JL: Ventricular tachycardia surgery: A review of the first decade and a suggested contemporary approach. *Semin Thorac Cardiovasc Surg* 1989; 1:97–103.
187. Condini MA, Sommerfeldt I, Eybel CE, DeLaria GA, Messer JV: Efficacy of coronary bypass grafting in exercise-induced ventricular tachycardia. *J Thorac Cardiovasc Surg* 1981; 81:502–506.
188. Fontaine G, Lechat PH, Cansell A, Guiraudon G, Linares-Cruz E, Kouliball M, et al: Advances in the treatment of cardiac arrhythmias in the last decade: Definition and role of ablative techniques. In: Fontaine G, Scheinman MM (eds): *Ablation in Cardiac Arrhythmias*. Mt. Kisco, NY, Futura, 1987: 5–20.
189. Garan H, Kuchar D, Freeman C, Finkelstein D, Ruskin JN: Early assessment of the effect of map-guided transcatheter intracardiac electric shock on sustained ventricular tachycardia secondary to coronary artery disease. *Am J Cardiol* 1988; 61:1018–1023.
190. Platia EV, Griffith LSC, Watkins L, Mower MM, Guarnieri T, Mirowski M, et al: Treatment of malignant ventricular arrhythmias with endocardial resection and implantation of the automatic cardioverter-defibrillator. *N Engl J Med* 1986; 314:213–216.
191. Mirowski M, Reid PR, Winkle RA, Mower MM, Watkins L, Stinson GB, et al: Mortality in patients with implanted automatic defibrillators. *Ann Intern Med* 1983; 98:585–588.
192. Echt DS, Armstrong K, Schmidt P, Oyer PE, Stinson EB, Winkle RA: Clinical experience, complications, and survival in 70 patients with the automatic implantable cardioverter/defibrillator. *Circulation* 1985; 7:289–296.
193. Poll DS, Marchinski FE, Buxton AE, Josephson ME: Usefulness of programmed stimulation in idiopathic dilated cardiomyopathy. *Am J Cardiol* 1986; 58:992–997.
194. Rae AP, Spielman SC, Kutalek SP, Kay HR, Horowitz LN: Electrophysiologic assessment of antiarrhythmic drug efficacy for ventricular tachyarrhythmias associated with dilated cardiomyopathy. *Am J Cardiol* 1987; 59:291–295.
195. Caceres J, Jazayeri M, McKinnie J, Avitall B, Denker ST, Tchou P, et al: Sustained bundle branch reentry mechanism of clinical tachycardia. *Circulation* 1989; 79:256–270.
196. Das SK, Morady F, DiCarlo L, Baerman J, Krol R, DeBultleir M, et al: Prognostic usefulness of programmed ventricular stimulation in idiopathic dilated cardiomyopathy without symptomatic ventricular arrhythmias. *Am J Cardiol* 1986; 58:998–1000.
197. Myerburg RJ, Luceri RM, Thurer R, Cooper DK, Zaman L, Interian A, et al: Time to first shock and clinical outcome in patients receiving automatic implantable cardioverter defibrillators. *J Am Coll Cardiol* 1989; 14:508–514.
198. Anderson KP: Sudden death, hypertension, and hypertrophy. *J Cardiovasc Pharm* 1984; 6:(suppl III):S498–S503.
199. Goodwin JF, Krikler DM: Arrhythmia as a cause of sudden death in hypertrophic cardiomyopathy. *Lancet* 1976; 2:937–940.
200. Kowey PR, Eisenberg R, Engel TR: Sustained arrhythmias in hypertrophic obstructive cardiomyopathy. *N Engl J Med* 1984; 310:1566–1569.
201. Anderson KP, Stinson EB, Derby GC, Oyer PE, Mason JW: Vulnerability of patients with obstructive hypertrophic cardiomyopathy to ventricular arrhythmia induction in the operating room. *Am J Cardiol* 1983; 51:811–816.
202. Coumel P, Rosengarten MD, Leciereq JF, Attuel P: Role of sympathetic nervous system in non-ischemic ventricular arrhythmias. *Br Heart J* 1982; 47:137–147.
203. Sung RJ, Shapiro WA, Shen EN, Morady F, Davis J: Effects of verapamil on ventricular tachycardias possibly caused by reentry, automaticity, and triggered activity. *J Clin Invest* 1983; 72:350–360.
204. Lerman BB, Belardinelli L, West A, Berne RM, DiMarco JP: Adenosine-sensitive ventricular tachycardia: Evidence suggesting cyclic AMP-mediated triggered activity. *Circulation* 1986; 74:270–280.
205. Ward DE, Nathan AW, Camm AJ: Fascicular tachycardia sensitive to calcium antagonists. *Eur Heart J* 1984; 5:896–905.
206. Ohe T, Shimomura S, Aihara N, Kamakura S, Matsuhisa M, Sato I, et al: Idiopathic sustained left ventricular tachycardia: Clinical and electrophysiologic characteristics. *Circulation* 1988; 77:560–568.
207. Marcus FI, Fontaine GH, Guiraudon G, Frank R, Laurenceau JL, Malergue C, et al: Right ventricular dysplasia: A report of 24 adult cases. *Circulation* 1982; 65:384–398.
208. Guiraudon GM, Klein GJ, Guiamhusein SS, Painvin GA, DelCampo C, Gonzales JC, et al: Total disconnection of the right ventricular free wall: Surgical treatment of right ventricular tachycardia associated with right ventricular dysplasia. *Circulation* 1983; 67:463–470.
209. Fitchett DH, Sugrue DD, MacArthur CG, Oakley CM: Right ventricular dilated cardiomyopathy. *Br Heart J* 1984; 51:25–29.
210. Thiene G, Nava A, Corrado D, Rossi L, Pinnelli N: Right ventricular cardiomyopathy and sudden death in young people. *N Engl J Med* 1988; 318:129–133.
211. Dunnigan A, Pritzker MR, Benditt DG, Benson DW: Life-threatening ventricular tachycardias in late survivors of surgically corrected tetralogy of Fallot. *Br Heart J* 1984; 52:198–206.
212. Garson A, Randall DC, Gillette PC, Smith RT, Moak JP, McVey P, et al: Prevention of sudden death after repair of tetralogy of Fallot: Treatment of ventricular arrhythmias. *J Am Coll Cardiol* 1985; 6:221–227.
213. Harken AH, Horowitz LN, Josephson ME: Surgical correction of recurrent sustained ventricular tachycardia on complete repair of tetralogy of Fallot. *J Thorac Cardiovasc Surg* 1980; 80:779–781.
214. Fontaine G, Frank R, Grosgogeat Y: Torsades de pointes: Definition and management. *Mod Conc Cardiovasc Dis* 1982; 51:103–108.
215. Denes P, Gabster A, Huang SK: Clinical, electrocardiographic and follow-up observations in patients having ventricular fibrillation during Holter monitoring. *Am J Cardiol* 1981; 48:9–27.
216. Krikler DM, Curry PVL: Torsades de pointes, an atypical ventricular tachycardia. *Br Heart J* 1976; 38:117–120.
217. Smith WM, Gallagher JJ: "Les torsades de pointes": An unusual ventricular arrhythmia. *Ann Intern Med* 1980; 93:578–584.
218. Keren A, Tzivoni D, Gavish D, Levi J, Gottlieb S, Benhorin J, et al: Etiology warning signs and therapy of torsades de pointes—a study of ten patients. *Circulation* 1981; 64:1167–1174.
219. Bhandari AK, Scheinman M: The long Q-T syndrome. *Mod Conc Cardiovasc Dis* 1985; 54:45–50.
220. Stratmann HG, Kennedy HL: Torsades de pointes associated with drugs and toxins: Recognition and management. *Am Heart J* 1987; 113:1470–1482.
221. Schwart PH, Locati EH, Moss AJ, Crampton RS, Trazzi R, Ruberti U: Left cardiac sympathetic denervation in the therapy of congenital long QT syndrome: A worldwide report. *Circulation* 1991; 84:503–511.
222. Packer M: Sudden unexpected death in patients with congestive heart failure. A second frontier. *Circulation* 1985; 72:681–685.
223. Luu M, Stevenson WG, Stevenson LW, Baron K, Walden J: Diverse mechanisms of unexpected cardiac arrest in advanced heart failure. *Circulation* 1991; 80:1675–1680.
224. Cummins RO, Ornato JP, Thies WH, Pepe PE: Improving survival from sudden cardiac arrest: The "chain of survival" concept. *Circulation* 1991; 83:1832–1847.

225. Creed JD, Packard JM, Lambrew CT, Lewis AJ: Defibrillation and synchronized cardioversion. In: McIntyre KM, Lewis AJ (eds): *Textbook of Advanced Cardiac Life Support*. Dallas, American Heart Association, 1983: 89–96.
226. Standard and guidelines for cardiopulmonary resuscitation (CPR) and emergency cardiac care (ECC). *JAMA* 1986; 255:2915–2954.
227. Interian A, Trohman RG, Castellanos A, Cox M, Zaman L, Myerburg RJ: Spontaneous conversion of ventricular fibrillation in cardiogenic shock for acute myocardial infarction. *Am J Cardiol* 1987; 50:1200–1201.
228. Behar S, Goldbourt U, Reicher-Reiss H, Kaplinsky E, The Principal Investigators of the SPRINT Study: Prognosis of acute myocardial infarction complicated by primary ventricular fibrillation. *Am J Cardiol* 1990; 66:1208–1211.
229. Volpi A, Cavalli A, Franzosi MG, Maggioni A, Mauri F, Santoro G, et al: One-year prognosis of primary ventricular fibrillation complicating acute myocardial infarction. *Am J Cardiol* 1989; 63:1174–1178.
230. Nicod P, Gilpin E, Nicod P, Gilpin C, Dittrich H, Wright M, et al: Late clinical outcome in patients with early ventricular fibrillation after myocardial infarction. *J Am Coll Cardiol* 1988; 11:464–470.
231. Lie KI, Leim KL, Schullenberg RM, David GK, Durrer D: Early identification of patients developing late in-hospital ventricular fibrillation after discharge from the coronary care unit. *Am J Cardiol* 1978; 41:674–677.
232. Hauer RNW, Lie KI, Liem KL, Durrer D: Long-term prognosis in patients with bundle branch block complicating acute anteroseptal infarction. *Am J Cardiol* 1982; 49:1581–1585.
233. Luceri RM, Castellanos A, Zaman L, Myerburg RJ: The arrhythmias of dual-chamber cardiac pacemaker and their management. *Ann Intern Med* 1983; 99:354–359.
234. Myerburg RJ, Kessler KM, Castellanos A: Sudden cardiac death: Structure, function and time-dependence of risk. *Circulation* 1992; 85(Suppl I): I-2–I-10.
235. Wilber DJ, Garan H, Finkelstein D, Kelly E, Newell J, McGovern B, et al: Out-of-hospital cardiac arrest: Use of electrophysiologic testing in the prediction of long-term outcome. *N Engl J Med* 1988; 318:19–24.
236. Myerburg RJ, Kessler KM: Management of patients who survive cardiac arrest. *Mod Conc Cardiovasc Dis* 1986; 55:61–66.
237. Morady F, DiCarlo L, Winston S, Davis JC, Scheinman MM: Clinical features and prognosis of patients with out-of-hospital cardiac arrest and a normal electrophysiologic study. *J Am Coll Cardiol* 1984; 4:39–44.
238. Kunis RL, Garfein OB, Pepe AJ, Dwyer EM: Deglutition syncope and atrioventricular block selectively induced by hot food and liquid. *Am J Cardiol* 1985; 55:613.
239. Falk RH, Zoll PM, Zoll RH: Safety and efficiency of noninvasive cardiac pacing. A preliminary report. *N Engl J Med* 1983; 309:1166–1168.
240. Zoll PM, Zoll RH, Falk RH, Clinton JE, Eitel DR: External noninvasive temporary cardiac pacing: Clinical trials. *Circulation* 1985; 71:937–944.
241. Love JC, Haffajee MD, Gore MD, Alpert JS: Reversibility of hypotension and shock by atrial or atrioventricular sequential pacing in patients with right ventricular infarction. *Am Heart J* 1984; 108:5–13.
242. Weiss AT, Rod JL, Gotsman MD, Lewis BS: Hydralazine in the management of symptomatic sinus bradycardia. *Eur J Cardiol* 1981; 12:261–170.
243. Lewis BS, Rozenman Y, Mardler A, Rodeanu ME, Shefer A, Halon DA: Chronotropic effect of hydralazine and its mechanism in symptomatic sinus bradycardia. *Am J Cardiol* 1987; 59:93–96.
244. Kang PS, Gomes JA, Kelen G, El-Sherif N: Role of autonomic regulatory mechanism in sinoatrial conduction and sinus nodal automaticity in sick sinus syndrome. *Circulation* 1981; 64:832–838.
245. Yabek SM, Swensson RE, Jarmakani JM: Electrocardiographic recognition of sinus node dysfunction in children and young adults. *Circulation* 1977; 56:235–239.
246. Mackintosh AF: Sinoatrial disease in young people. *Br Heart J* 1981; 45:62–66.
247. Rasmussen V, Haunso S, Skagen K: Cerebral attacks due to excessive vagal tone in heavily trained persons. A clinical and electrophysiologic study. *Acta Med Scand* 1978; 204:401–405.
248. Bharati S, Nordenberg A, Bauernfeind R, Varghese JP, Carvalho AG, Rosen KM, et al: The anatomic substrate for the sick sinus syndrome in adolescents. *Am J Cardiol* 1980; 46:156–172.
249. DeMoulin JC, Kulbertus HE: Histopathological correlates of sinoatrial disease. *Br Heart J* 1978; 40:1384–1389.
250. Thery C, Gosselin B, Lekieffre J, Warrenbourg H: Pathology of the sinoatrial node. Correlation with electrocardiographic findings in 111 patients. *Am Heart J* 1977; 93:735–740.
251. Walter PF, Crawley IS, Dorney ER: Carotid sinus hypersensitivity and syncope. *Am J Cardiol* 1978; 42:396–403.
252. Davies AB, Stephens MR, Davies AG: Carotid sinus hypersensitivity in patients presenting with syncope. *Br Heart J* 1979; 42:583–586.
253. Madigan NP, Fiaker GC, Curtis JJ, Reid J, Mueller KJ, Murphy BS: Carotid sinus hypersensitivity: Beneficial effects of dual-chamber pacing. *Am J Cardiol* 1984; 53:1034–1040.
254. Wenger TL, Dohrmann ML, Strauss HC, Conley MJ, Wechsler AD, Wagner GS: Hypersensitive carotid sinus syndrome manifested as cough syncope. *PACE* 1980; 3:332–339.
255. Sra JS, Anderson AJ, Sheikh SH, Avitall B, Tchou PJ, Troup PJ, et al: Unexplained syncope evaluated by electrophysiologic studies and head-up tilt testing. *Ann Intern Med* 1991; 114:1013–1019.
256. Bigger JT Jr, Reiffel JA: Sick sinus syndrome. *Annu Rev Med* 1979; 30:91–118.
257. Chung EK: Sick sinus syndrome: Current views. *Mod Conc Cardiovasc Dis* 1980; 49:61–66.
258. Crossen KJ, Cain ME: Assessment and management of sinus node dysfunction. *Mod Conc Cardiovasc Dis* 1986; 55:43–48.
259. Narula OS: Atrioventricular conduction disturbances in patients with sinus bradycardia. *Circulation* 1971; 44:1096–1110.
260. Jordan JA, Yamaguchi L, Mandel WJ: Studies on the mechanisms of sinus node dysfunction in a sick sinus syndrome. *Circulation* 1978; 57:217–223.
261. Rosenqvist M, Vallin H, Edhag O: Clinical electrophysiologic course of sinus node diseases: Five-year follow-up study. *Am Heart J* 1985; 109:513–522.
262. Benditt DG, Benson DW, Kreitt J, Dunnigan A, Pritzker MR, Crouse L, et al: Electrophysiologic effects of theophylline in young patients with symptomatic bradyarrhythmias. *Am J Cardiol* 1983; 52:1223–1229.
263. Gomes JA, Kang PS, El-Sherif N: Effects of digitalis on the human sick sinus node after pharmacologic autonomic blockade. *Am J Cardiol* 1981; 48:783–788.
264. Dhingra RC, Amat-y-Leon F, Wyndham C, Deedwania PC, Wu D, Denes P, et al: Clinical significance of prolonged sinoatrial conduction time. *Circulation* 1977; 55:8–15.
265. Gann D, Tolentino A, Samet P: Electrophysiologic evaluation of elderly patients with sinus bradycardia: A long-term follow-up study. *Ann Intern Med* 1979; 90:24–29.
266. Rosenqvist M, Brandt J, Schuller H: Atrial versus ventricular pacing in sinus node disease: A treatment comparison study. *Am Heart J* 1986; 111:292–297.
267. Denes P: Atrioventricular and intraventricular block. *Circulation* 1987; 75(suppl III):III-19–III-25.
268. Dreifus LS, Fisch C, Griffin JC, Gillette P, Mason JW, Parsonnet V: Guidelines for implantation of cardiac pacemakers and antiarrhythmic devices. *J Am Coll Cardiol* 1991; 18:1–13.
269. Zipes DP: Current topics. Second degree atrioventricular block. *Circulation* 1979; 60:465–472.
270. Zeppilli P, Feniel R, Sassara M, Pisrami MM, Casell G: Wenckebach second degree A-V block in top-ranking athletes: An old problem revisited. *Am Heart J* 1980; 100:281–294.
271. Strasberg B, Amat-y-Leon F, Dhingra RC, Palileo E, Swiryn S, Eayernfeind R, et al: Natural history of chronic second degree atrioventricular nodal block. *Circulation* 1981; 63:1043–1049.
272. Damato AN, Varghese PJH, Caracta AR, Akhtar M, Lau SH: Functional 2 : 1 A-V block within the His Purkinje system. Simulation of Type II A-V block. *Circulation* 1973; 47:534–542.
273. Woelfel A, Simpson RJ Jr, Foster JR: Functional "Type I-Like" distal atrioventricular block induced by atrial pacing. *Am J Cardiol* 1984; 54:1363–1364.
274. Rahimtoola SH, Zipes DP, Akhtar M, Burchell M, Mason J, Myerburg RJ, et al: Consensus statement of the Conference on the State of the Art of Electrophysiologic Testing in the Diagnosis

and Treatment of Patients with Cardiac Arrhythmias. *Circulation* 1987; 75(suppl III):3–11.

275. Gallastregui J, Hariman RJ: Indications for intracardiac electrophysiologic studies in patients with atrioventricular and intraventricular blocks not associated with acute myocardial infarction. *Circulation* 1987; 75(suppl III):III-103–III-106.
276. Bhandari AK, Rahimtoola SH: Intracardiac electrophysiologic studies in patients with atrioventricular and intraventricular blocks not associated with acute myocardial infarction. Discussion. *Circulation* 1987; 75(suppl III):III-107–III-109.
277. Tenczer J, Littmann L, Rohia N, Fenyvesi T: The effects of overdrive pacing and lidocaine on atrioventricular junctional rhythm in man: The role of abnormal automaticity. *Circulation* 1985; 72:480–486.
278. Mond HG: The bradyarrhythmias: Current indications for permanent pacing (Part I). *PACE* 1981; 4:432–442.
279. Mond GH: The bradyarrhythmias: Current indications for permanent pacing (Part II). *PACE* 1981; 4:538–547.
280. Gunnar RM, bourdillon, PVD, Dixon DW, Fuster V, Karp RB, Kennedy JW, Klocke FJ, et al: ACC/AHA guidelines for the early management of patients with acute myocardial infarction. *Circulation* 1990; 82:664–707.
281. Hindman MC, Wagner GS, Jaro M: The clinical significance of bundle branch block complicating acute myocardial infarction: 2. Indications for temporary and permanent pacemaker insertion. *Circulation* 1978; 58:689–699.
282. Watson RDS, Glober DR, Page AJF, Littier WA, Davies P, DeGiovanni J, et al: The Birmingham trial of permanent pacing in patients with intraventricular conduction disorders after acute myocardial infarction. *Am Heart J* 1984; 108:496–501.
283. Kastor JA: Atrioventricular block. *N Engl J Med* 1975; 292:462–465.
284. Dhingra RC, Palileo E, Strasberg B, Swiryn S, Bauerfeind RA, Wyndham C, et al: Significance of the HV interval in 517 patients with chronic bifascicular block. *Circulation* 1982; 64:1265–1271.
285. McAnulty JH, Rahimtoola DH, Murphy ES, Kauffman S, Ritzmann LW, Kanarek P, et al: A prospective study of sudden death in high risk bundle branch block. *N Engl J Med* 1978; 299:209–215.
286. Scheinman MM, Peters RW, Modin G, Brennan M, Mies C, O'Young J: Prognostic value of infranodal conduction time in patients with chronic bundle branch block. *Circulation* 1977; 56:240–244.
287. Furman S, Fischer JD: Endless loop tachycardia in the A-V universal (DDD) pacemaker. *PACE* 1982; 5:486–489.

Chapter 37

Electrolytes and the Heart

David P. Rardon, M.D. ■ Charles Fisch, M.D.

The normal contraction of the heart is accompanied by temporary changes in the transmembrane potential of cardiac cells. Microelectrode techniques have allowed the study of the sequential changes in the transmembrane voltage resulting in the transmembrane action potential (TAP). Sodium (Na), potassium (K), and calcium (Ca) are the major ions responsible for the normal electrical activity of the heart. In addition, Ca is the messenger that initiates excitation-contraction coupling and, along with magnesium (Mg) and phosphorus (P), is involved in steps leading to myocardial contraction. The normal ionic currents that give rise to the TAP may be altered by abnormally high or low K or Ca in the extracellular space or by abnormal intracellular concentrations of Mg or P. Clinically recognizable disturbances in cardiac electrical and mechanical function may occur secondary to abnormal concentrations of these ions.

In order to understand the effects of changing electrolyte concentrations on the mechanical and electrical behavior of the heart, one should understand (1) the sequence of transmembrane voltage changes resulting in the TAP and (2) the electrolyte fluxes generally responsible for such changes.

THE CARDIAC TRANSMEMBRANE ACTION POTENTIAL

The Resting Potential (Phase 4)

The transmembrane potential during electrical quiescence is referred to as the *resting potential* or *phase 4* of the cardiac action potential. In excitable cells, including cardiac cells, the intracellular and extracellular concentrations of Na,[1] Ca, K,[2] and chloride differ (Fig. 37-1*A*). However, the resting membrane potential is largely determined by the concentration gradient for K ions across the cell membrane. The cell membrane is permeable to K ions but is relatively impermeable to Na, Ca, and chloride (Cl). Outward diffusion of K ions causes the intracellular space to be negatively charged with respect to the extracellular space. Electroneutrality cannot be maintained by the outward movement of anions since these are largely associated with cellular proteins.[3] The resultant negative charge opposes the further diffusion of K out of the cell. The intracellular potential at which the net passive flux of K ions is zero is called the equilibrium potential for K ions (E_K), and its value is given by the Nernst equation,[4]

$$E_K = (RT/F)\ln[K]_o/[K]_i$$

where R is the gas constant, T is the absolute temperature, F is the Faraday constant, and $[K]_o$ and $[K]_i$ are the extracellular and intracellular concentrations of K ions, respectively. (See also Chap. 34.)

The resting membrane potential varies with the external K concentration. Elevation of extracellular K reduces the resting membrane potential. In the physiological range of extracellular K, particularly when extracellular K is decreased below 2.0, the inward movement of Na influences the resting membrane potential to a greater amount.[5,6] The depolarizing influence of Na is described by the Goldman[7] and Hodgkin and Katz[8] *constant field equation* for the resting potential V_r of a cell permeable to both K and Na,

$$V_r = \frac{RT}{F}\ln\frac{[K^+]_o + P_{Na}/P_K\,[Na^+]_o}{[K^+]_i + P_{Na}/P_K\,[Na^+]_i}$$

A

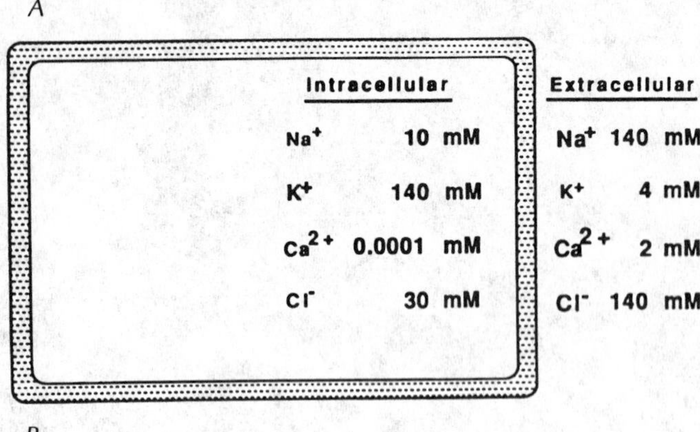

B

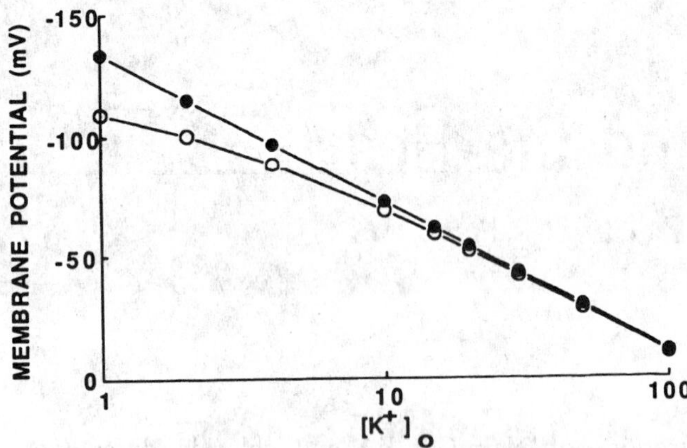

FIGURE 37-1 *A.* Approximate concentrations of Na^+, K^+, Ca^{2+}, and Cl^- in the extra- and intracellular fluid compartments. *B.* Effects of $[K^+]_o$ on resting membrane potential. (●) was determined from the Nernst equation in which resting membrane potential only depends on $[K^+]_o/[K^+]_i$. (○) was calculated from the Goldman equation in which resting membrane potential varies with the gradients of both K^+ and Na^+. (*Reprinted with permission from Ref. 34.*)

where P_{Na}/P_K is the ratio of the Na and K permeability coefficients of the cell membrane. Figure 37-1*B* illustrates V_r when calculated for a membrane permeable only to K compared to a membrane permeable to both Na and K.

The resting potential is an important determinant of the rate of rise of the TAP and thus an important determinant of the conduction velocity of the propagated cardiac action potential. Clinically, reduction of the resting potential may play an important role in the genesis of arrhythmias and conduction disturbances. (See also Chaps. 34 and 35.)

Rapid Depolarization (Phase 0)

When cardiac muscle is activated by a greater than threshold stimulus, there is a rapid influx of Na into the cell. Sodium moves inward through ion-specific channels, and V_m quickly changes to a positive value.[9] Inactivation of the Na current and a complex series of ionic events responsible for repolarization ensue, producing a TAP (Fig. 37-2*A*). The amount of Na that moves into the cell per unit time is an important determinant of normal and abnormal activation and conduction in heart muscle. The rate of influx of Na into the cell is dependent on the size of the Na electrochemical potential gradient and the available (or noninactivated) Na channels.[10] The rate of rise of phase 0, referred to as dV/dt_{max} or V_{max}, is directly related to the rate of Na influx into the cell. Here V_{max} is a significant determinant of the speed of conduction of the cardiac impulse. The greater (more negative) the V_m at the onset of phase 0, the greater the rate of rise of phase 0 and the greater the speed of conduction of the cardiac impulse.[11,12] The relationship of the rate of change of phase 0 to V_m expresses membrane responsiveness. Since an increase in extracellular K lowers V_m, the rate of rise of phase 0 and the amplitude of the TAP are reduced and conduction of the cardiac impulse is depressed.[13]

Reduction of V_m brings V_m closer to the threshold potential (approximately −60 mV), and the strength of the stimulus needed to bring V_m to threshold (excitability) is also decreased. Consequently, conduction depression due to reduction of V_m may, within narrow ranges of hyperkalemia, be preceded by an increase in excitability and conduction velocity.[13] As a result, conduction alterations due to changing K concentration may reflect altered rate of rise of phase 0 as well as changing excitability.

The Plateau (Phase 2)

When the V_m is reduced to about −40 mV, a second, slow inward current carried primarily by Ca through specific "slow channels" is activated.[14,15] The sarcolemmal Ca current is distinct from the Na current, which is responsible for the phase 0 of the TAP. Different types of voltage-sensitive Ca channels (classified as L, T, and N) are known to exist. In cardiac muscle, both L- and T-type but not N-type channels have been observed.[16–18] The L-type channel is activated at membrane potentials more positive than −10 mV and conducts a long-lasting current of large conductance.[19,20]

Whereas the Na current is inhibited by tetrodotoxin[21] and antiarrhythmic drugs such as quinidine, the L-type Ca current is selectively affected by a group of compounds referred to as Ca effectors. These drugs belong to three distinct chemical classes: (1) the 1,4-dihydropyridine derivatives like nitrendipine, nimodipine, and Bay K 8644; (2) the phenylalkylamines such as verapamil, D-600, and D-888; and (3) the benzothiazepines, typified by diltiazem. Clinically used drugs all inhibit the Ca channel, but activating compounds (e.g., Bay K 8644) also have been identified.

Under experimental conditions, cardiac action potentials primarily dependent of the influx of Ca rather than Na can be produced (Fig. 37-2*B*).[22] The Ca-dependent action potential is characterized by a low V_m, low amplitude of the action potential, slow rate of depolarization as compared with the rapid Na-dependent action potential, very slow propagation velocity, graded response to stimuli, refractoriness exceeding the duration of the TAP, and low safety factor for conduction. Sinus and atrioventricular (AV) nodal cells lack or have no significant inward Na or inward rectifying K channels. Therefore, the upstroke of these action potentials is generated entirely

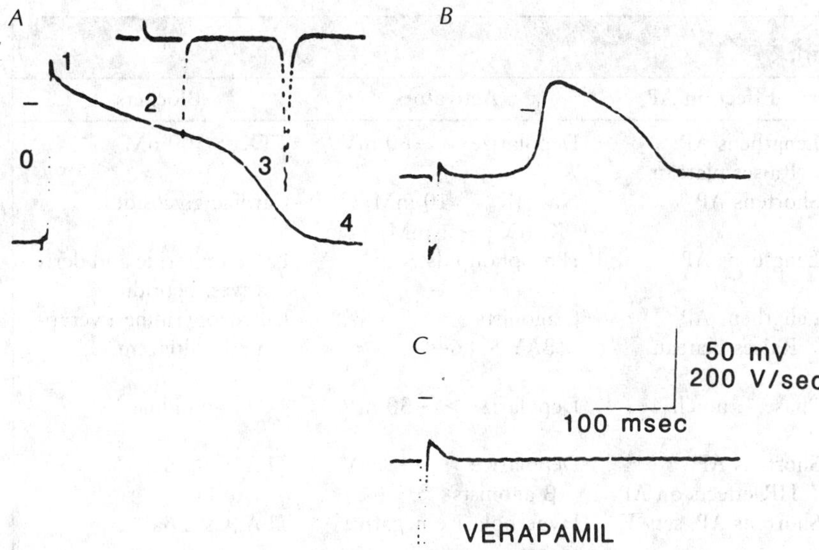

FIGURE 37-2 *A.* Normal cardiac Purkinje fiber transmembrane action potential. Phases of the action potential: 0, rapid depolarization; 1, early repolarization; 2, plateau; 3, rapid repolarization; 4, diastole. After superfusion with a high-K solution the transmembrane potential is reduced. *B.* Stimulation produces a TAP generated primarily by the influx of Ca. Characteristics of the Ca-dependent TAP are described in the text. *C.* Administration of verapamil, a Ca blocker, eliminates the Ca-dependent TAP.

by an inward Ca current, which exhibits the properties noted above.

The magnitude of the inward Ca current is influenced by both the sympathetic and parasympathetic limbs of the autonomic nervous system.[23] β-Adrenergic receptor agonists such as isoproterenol increase the inward Ca current, which in turn heightens the plateau and shortens the action potential duration of cardiac Purkinje fibers.[24,25] The effects of β agonists are secondary to cyclic adenosine monophosphate (AMP)–mediated phosphorylation of the L-type Ca channel proteins. Phosphorylation increases the probability that the L-type channel is in the open state.[24,25] Microinjection of the purified catalytic subunit of cyclic AMP–dependent protein kinase into isolated myocytes[26,27] mimics the effects of elevation of intracellular cyclic AMP and can be inhibited by phosphoprotein phosphatase 1 or 2A. Parasympathetic stimulation inhibits sympathetic-mediated increases in the magnitude of the inward Ca current.[23]

Other currents contribute to the prolonged plateau phase of the cardiac action potential. In cardiac tissue slowly inactivating Na current continues to enter the cell at plateau potentials and contributes to the plateau's long duration.[28,29] Action potential duration is also lengthened by Na entry via the Na/Ca exchanger.[30]

Repolarization (Phases 1 and 3)

Action potentials recorded in Purkinje fibers and in some ventricular muscle fibers show a brief, early phase of repolarization (phase 1) immediately following the action potential upstroke (Fig. 37-2*A*). This early repolarization is secondary to a transient outward K current.[31]

The rate of repolarization during the plateau of the TAP is slow. Incomplete inactivation of the fast Na ("late Na current" or "window current"), inward Ca currents, and Na entry via the Na/Ca exchanger contribute to the prolonged duration of the plateau. The influx of Ca via the L-type Ca channel is crucial for excitation-contraction coupling, providing an influx of Ca that triggers the release of Ca from the junctional sarcoplasmic reticulum.[32] The rise in cytosolic Ca affects the repolarization of the action potential. This Ca also activates a specific K channel whose opening is part of phase 3 repolarization of the TAP. Repolarization of the TAP is a complicated process due primarily to an outwardly directed K current. Potassium efflux through at least seven or eight different cardiac ventricular muscle and Purkinje cell K channels constitutes this repolarizing current.[33] Table 37-1 lists five of the K currents that seem to be major contributors to the repolarization of the action potential and outlines specific agents that regulate the kinetics of these channels.[34] (See also Chap. 34.)

POTASSIUM

Hyperkalemia

Electrophysiological Effects

An increased extracellular K concentration ($[K]_o$) produces two major changes in the TAP. Elevated $[K]_o$ increases membrane permeability to K,[35] thus increasing the rate of repolarization (more rapid slope of phase 3 of the TAP) and shortening the duration of the TAP. These changes in TAP characteristics are responsible for the electrocardiographic manifestations of hyperkalemia. As $[K]_o$ is increased, the resting membrane potential becomes less negative and alters the threshold potential. Hyperkalemia usually shifts the resting membrane potential more than the threshold potential; therefore, at modestly increased $[K]_o$ the difference between the resting and threshold potentials may decrease and myocardial excitability may actually be enhanced.[13] An increase in $[K]_o$ does not always decrease conduction velocity, but a modest improvement in conduction velocity may occur early during the rise of the K concentration.[13]

Electrocardiographic Manifestations

The earliest electrocardiographic manifestations of hyperkalemia are peaked or tented T waves.[36–40] Hyperkalemic T-wave changes may be manifest when plasma K

TABLE 37-1

Plateau and Repolarizing Currents in the Ventricle

Current Type	Direction	Effect on AP	Activators	Blockers
Late Na^+ current (window current)	Inward Na^+	Lengthens AP Raises plateau	Depolarize > −60 mV	TTX ≈ 100 nM
Na/K ATPase (pump current)	Net outward Na^+	Shortens AP	Na_i^+ (K_m ~ 10 mM) K_o^+ (K_m ~ 1 mM)	Cardiac glycosides
i_{NaCa} (Na/Ca exchange)	Net inward Na^+	Lengthens AP	?Phospholipids ?Ca_i^{2+}	La^{3+}; amiloride and derivatives; bepridil
L-type i_{Ca} (slow inward current)	Inward Ca^{2+}	Lengthens AP Raises plateau	β agonists BAY K 8644	Dihydropyridines; verapamil; diltiazem
i_A or i_{to} (transient outward)	Outward K^+	Phase 1; notch	Depolarize > −30 mV	4-AP, quinidine
i_K or i_X (delayed rectifier)	Outward K^+	Shortens AP; HR effects on AP	Depolarize > −45 mV β agonists	TEA, Cs^+, Ba^{2+}
i_{K1} (inward rectifier)	Small outward K^+	Shortens AP; sets V_r	Hyperpolarize negative to E_K	TEA, Cs^+, Ba^{2+}
$i_{K(Ca)}$ (Ca activated)	Outward K^+	Shortens AP	Ca_i^{2+} (K_m ~ 1 μM) Depolarize > −50 mV	TEA, charybdotoxin, Ba^{2+}
$i_{K(ATP)}$ (ATP activated)	Outward K^+	Shortens AP in ischemia	Diazoxide Nicorandil Pinacidil	ATP_i ≈ 500 μM Glibenclamide Tolbutamide

AP, action potential; TTX, tetrodotoxin; Na_i^+, intracellular [Na^+]; K_o^+, extracellular [K^+]; Ca_i^{2+}, intracellular [Ca^{2+}]; K_m, half-maximal activation; 4-AP, 4-aminopyridine; HR, heart rate; TEA, tetraethylammonium; V_r, resting potential; E_K, equilibrium potential for K^+. Only selected activators and blockers are shown.
SOURCE: DP Rardon and ML Pressler.[34]

levels exceed 5.5 to 6.0 meq/liter. Hyperkalemia usually produces T waves of increased amplitude; however, the T-wave amplitude may be normal and differ in appearance only in that they are narrow based and symmetrical.[41] Tented T waves are seen in approximately 20 percent of patients with hyperkalemia.[41,42] Because of the proximity effect, the T-wave changes of hyperkalemia are best noted in leads V_2 to V_4.

As extracellular K increases, the transmembrane diastolic K gradient is reduced and results in a decrease in the resting membrane potential. The decrease in membrane potential is responsible for decreasing the upstroke velocity of the action potential, which in turn slows the intraventricular conduction and increases the duration of the QRS complex. At a plasma K of 7 meq/liter the P wave is altered, becoming broad and of low amplitude as a result of depression of intraatrial conduction. The PR interval prolongs and not infrequently progresses to second-degree AV block. The P wave becomes unrecognizable at plasma levels over 8.5 meq/liter.

The QRS widens uniformly at a K level of 9 to 11 meq/liter. The intraventricular conduction defects can be differentiated from the classic bundle branch blocks because hyperkalemia induces uniform depression of conduction, resulting in aberration of both the initial and terminal portions of the QRS complex. Less commonly, hyperkalemia-induced depression of conduction may produce right bundle branch block, left bundle branch block,[43] anterior or posterior fascicular block, or a combination of the above. As the QRS complex widens, the T wave and QRS complex blend together to produce a record simulating a sine wave. Electrocardiographic changes induced by various levels of hyperkalemia are illustrated in Fig. 37-3. In the presence of advanced hyperpotassemia with a wide QRS complex, the T wave may lack its characteristic peaked and narrow configuration, probably because the T-wave abnormality secondary to the intraventricular conduction disturbance obscures the primary T-wave changes.

Administration of K to patients with physiologically inverted T waves often normalizes the T-wave vector. On the other hand, K has no effect on inverted T waves secondary to organic disease, which may result from ischemic heart disease or administration of drugs.[44–46]

The correlation between electrocardiogram (ECG) changes and plasma K concentration differs, depending on whether hyperkalemia is induced experimentally or results from clinical disorders such as renal failure. The electrocardiographic changes parallel the plasma K level when K is infused in animals or in the course of clinical studies in humans.[47] In clinical circumstances, however, the ECG changes of hyperkalemia often occur at much lower levels of K. The correlation of plasma K values with the ECG is based on a pure plasma K change, which rarely occurs clinically. Most patients with hyperkalemia have some degree of acidosis and may have hyponatremia as well. Both acidosis and hyponatremia augment the electrocardiographic changes of hyperkalemia. A plasma K of 6.0 meq/liter may be life threatening in association with hyponatremia and acidosis, and plasma K concentrations of 8.0 to 8.5 meq/liter have been reported with no electrocardiographic changes when pH and Na levels are normal.[48] Hypocalcemia may also potentiate the cardiotoxic effects of hyperkalemia.[48] A de-

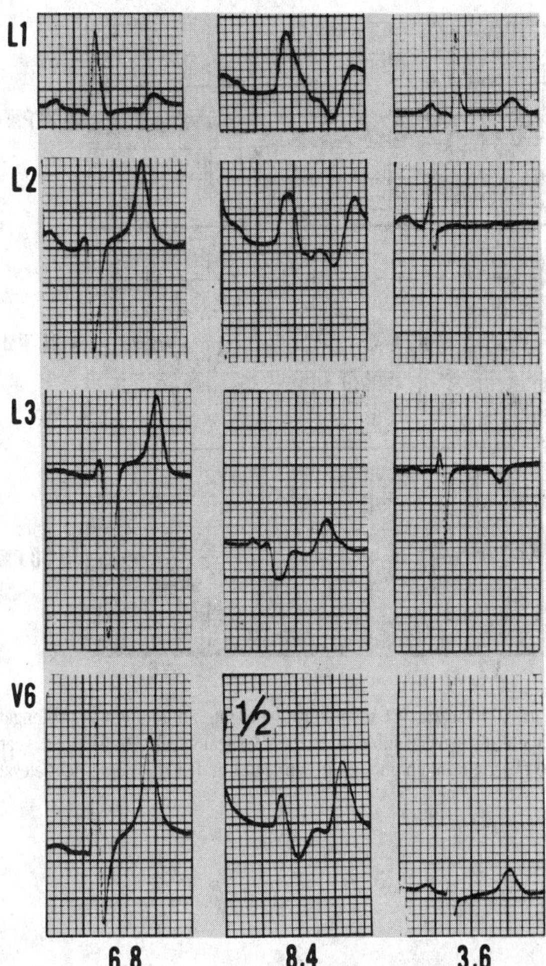

FIGURE 37-3 Potassium and the electrocardiogram (ECG). After treatment and at a level of 3.6 meq/liter, the PR, QRS, and T waves are normal. At 6.8 meq/liter, the PR and QRS are prolonged, with a shift of the QRS axis to the left, and the T waves are symmetrical, narrow based, and tall—the so-called tented T waves. At a K level of 8.4 meq/liter there is further prolongation of PR, the P wave becomes difficult to identify, the QRS axis shifts to the right, and the QRS prolongs to 0.20 s. The characteristic prolongation of both the initial and terminal portions of the QRS is best illustrated in V_6.

crease in plasma Ca in patients with hyperkalemia augments the development of intraventricular and AV block and facilitates the development of ventricular fibrillation.

The sequential changes of hyperkalemia are usually characteristic but on occasion may simulate other cardiac processes and may be overlooked. The usual effect of advanced hyperkalemia is depression of the R-ST segment. Occasionally ST-segment elevation may occur and the injury current may simulate either pericarditis or acute myocardial injury[49] (Fig. 37-4). Intraventricular conduction is usually uniformly suppressed, but in some cases the conduction defect may be selective and the possibility of hyperkalemia overlooked. Hyperkalemia has been reported to produce right and left axis deviation[50,51] as well as complete right and left bundle branch block.[43]

Other pathological states may produce tall peaked T waves simulating hyperkalemia. T-wave changes similar to hyperkalemic T-wave changes may be seen in patients with cerebral vascular accidents,[52,53] tachycardia,[54] and subendocardial ischemia. Two electrocardiographic criteria may be helpful in differentiating hyperkalemic T waves from those secondary to the aforementioned conditions. Hyperkalemic T waves are most often narrow based, and the QT_c interval in hyperkalemia is usually normal or slightly decreased. Cerebral vascular accidents and subendocardial ischemia often produce broad-based T waves, and the QT_c interval is frequently prolonged.

Ordinarily, the ventricular myocardium is less sensitive to changes in K than atrial myocardium, and the specialized fibers of the sinoatrial (SA) node and bundle of His are least sensitive.[55] Other electrolytes, pH, O_2 saturation, and the etiology and severity of the underlying heart disease may modify the sensitivity of the cardiac tissues to K and other electrolytes. Additionally, the rate of change of K and not the absolute level may determine the effect of K on impulse formation and conduction within the heart.

Hyperkalemia and Arrhythmias

The effect of hyperkalemia on cardiac rhythm is complex, and virtually any arrhythmia may be seen (Fig. 37-5). Various bradyarrhythmias, including impaired AV conduction and complete AV block, may occur.[56] Hyperkalemia may produce sinus bradycardia, sinus arrest, slow idioventricular rhythm, and asystole. In other circumstances, tachycardias may result, including sinus tachycardia, frequent ventricular extrasystole, ventricular tachycardia, and ventricular fibrillation.[57] The rate of K elevation appears to influence the type of arrhythmia produced. A slow elevation of K produces widespread block and depressed automaticity, and rapid infusions produce ventricular ectopic rhythms and terminally ventricular fibrillation. The fact that the ectopy following rapid elevation of plasma K is accompanied by K-induced depression of conduction suggests that the predominant mechanism of the arrhythmia may be reentry rather than automaticity. Ectopic rhythms other than junctional are relatively rare in clinical hyperkalemia, except as a terminal event.

Mathison[58] observed that infusion of K produced AV block in the cat heart. Since the specialized conduction tissue is more resistant to K than the myocardium, AV block due to hyperkalemia was considered rare. More recent studies have demonstrated a dual effect of K on AV conduction.[56,59] At plasma levels of 6.0 to 6.5 meq/liter, AV conduction is accelerated, but at levels of 7.5 meq/liter or higher, conduction is depressed. One can postulate an electrophysiological basis for this dual effect. As K is increased, the membrane potential becomes less negative and less current is required to depolarize the membrane to the threshold for generation of a cellular action potential. As K concentration rises further, the membrane potential becomes less negative and the conduction velocity of the cardiac impulse is diminished. At higher K levels this latter effect must predominate, resulting in depressed conduction of the cardiac impulse (Fig. 37-6). Additionally, in the intact animal, the antivagal effect of K contributes to enhancement of AV conduction.[60,61] At times, complete AV block is induced when

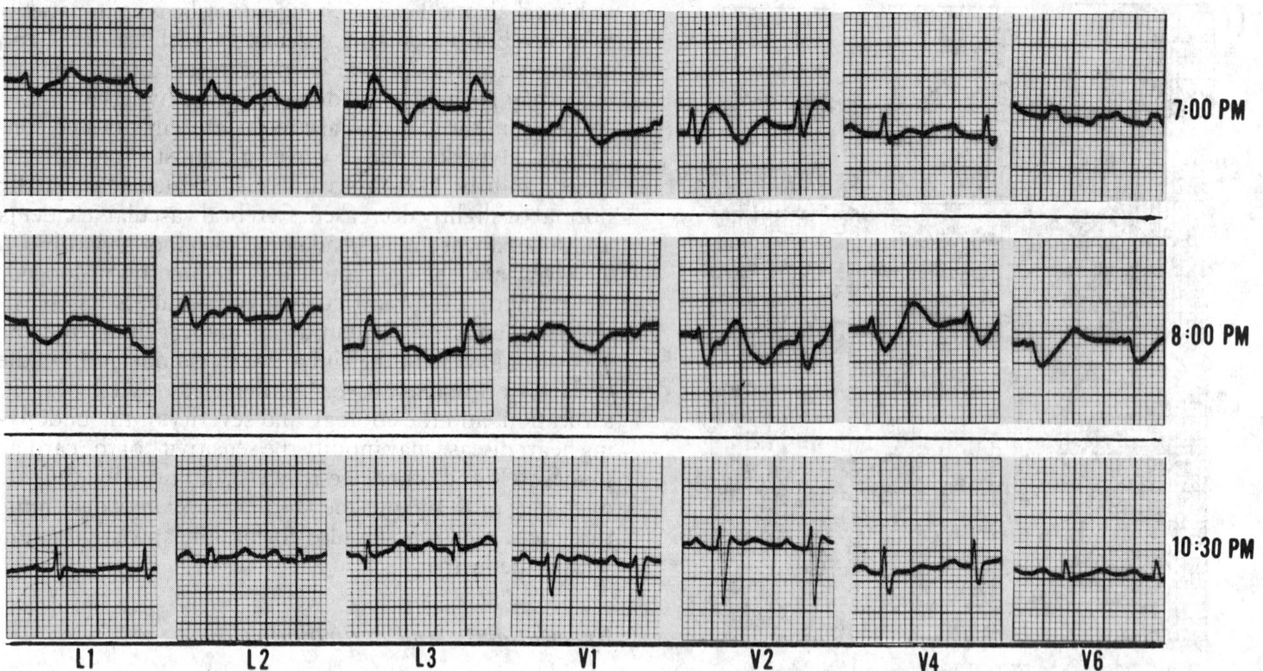

FIGURE 37-4 The current of injury occasionally seen in hyperkalemia. The plasma K at 7:00 P.M. was 9.1 meq/liter, illustrating, in addition to prolongation of the PR and diffuse intraventricular conduction delay, a current of injury simulating acute myocardial infarction. The ST-segment elevation is best seen in leads III, V_1, and V_2. After treatment of the hyperkalemia (10:30 P.M.), the tracing, with the exception of an abnormal T in lead I and slight ST-segment elevation in lead III, is normal.

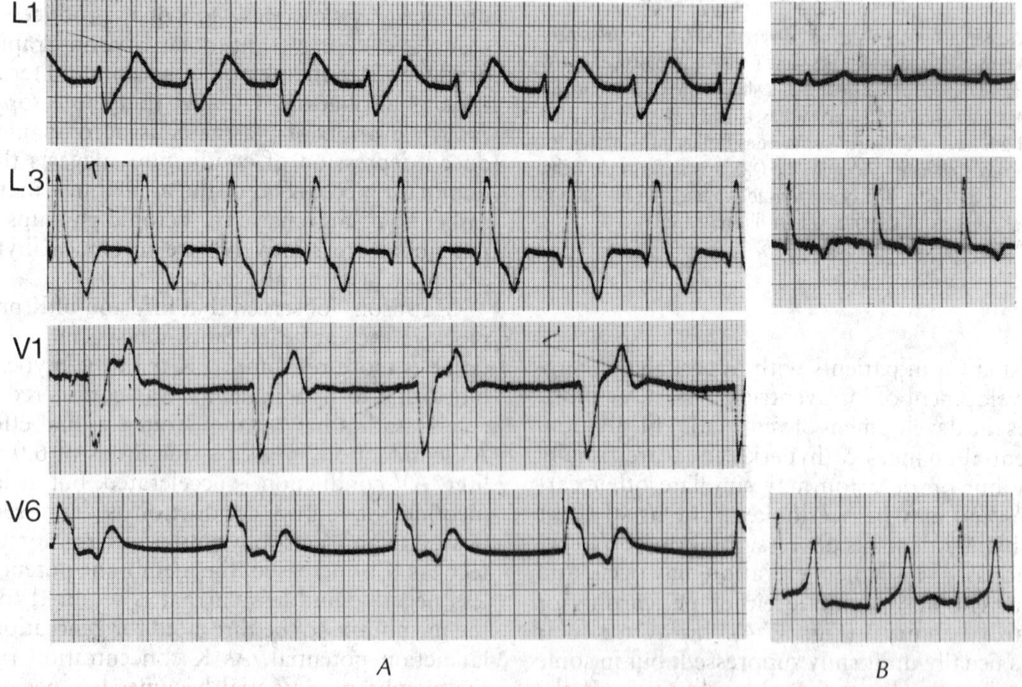

FIGURE 37-5 Difficulties encountered in analysis of the rhythm in presence of hyperkalemia. *A.* An ECG recorded at a plasma K level of 9.1 meq/liter with a blood urea nitrogen of 270 mg/dL and CO_2 of 10 meq/liter. The P waves are absent, making a definitive diagnosis of the rhythm difficult, if not impossible. The possible atrial rhythms include (1) SA rhythm without identifiable P waves with a 2 : 1 SA block in leads V_1 and V_6; (2) SA rhythm with 1 : 1 AV conduction in leads I and III with 2 : 1 conduction in V_1 and V_6; (3) sinus slowing in V_1 and V_6; (4) SA arrest or atrial fibrillation with a junctional tachycardia with 1 : 1 exit in leads I and III and 2 : 1 exit in leads V_1 and V_6. The QRS is prolonged to 0.20 s with prolongation of both the initial and terminal portions, best seen in leads III and V_6, respectively. *B.* Recorded after treatment of the hyperkalemia. *(From Fisch C: Relation of electrolyte disturbances of cardiac arrhythmias. Circulation 47:408, 1973. Reproduced by permission of the American Heart Association and the author.)*

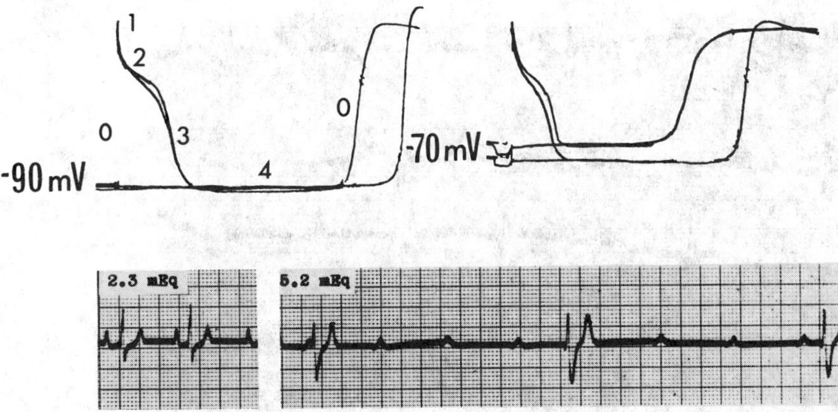

FIGURE 37-6 Electrophysiological basis for AV block due to K. *A.* Two TAPs are recorded about 1 mm apart, with a rapid sweep seen to the right. The latter shows the rapid upstroke of phase 0 and the delay of conduction between the two microelectrodes. *B.* Transmembrane resting potential is reduced to −70 mV by administration of K. This resulted in a slowing of the upstroke of phase 0 and a prolongation of conduction time between the two microelectrodes. *C.* Potassium-induced AV block in a digitalized animal. *(From Fisch C: Relation of electrolyte disturbances to cardiac arrhythmias. Circulation 47:408, 1973. Reproduced by permission of the American Heart Association and the author.)*

both P and QRS are still present, indicating that under certain circumstances the AV conduction system is less resistant to the depressing effects of K than either atrial or ventricular tissue[62,63] (Fig. 37-7). His bundle studies localize the initial AV delay or block above the bundle of His followed by block below the bundle of His. With rapid infusion, however, K preferentially depresses conduction below the bundle of His.[64]

As noted above, hyperkalemia may induce a number of arrhythmias and cardiac conduction disturbances. Moderate hyperkalemia, on the other hand, has been reported to suppress supraventricular and ventricular ectopic beats in about 80 percent of patients[65] (Figs. 37-8 and 37-9). Several potential effects of elevated K could suppress arrhythmias. Potassium depresses automaticity of ectopic pacemakers by decreasing diastolic depolarization and may terminate reentrant arrhythmias by either improving or impairing conduction.[60,61] Occasionally, the normal response to pacemaker stimulation can be restored by administration of K.[66] This may be secondary to a K-induced reduction in the excitability threshold. Though K may exert beneficial effects on arrhythmogenesis under certain circumstances, the therapeutic effect is usually transient and the therapeutic window is narrow.

Hypokalemia

Electrophysiological Effects

Hypokalemia decreases the rate of repolarization of the cardiac cell, thus prolonging recovery time.[67,68] Typically, hypokalemia produces a steeper slope of phase 2 and a less steep slope of phase 3, which produces a prolonged "tail" of the TAP. When the slope of phase 3 of the TAP is less steep, there is a longer interval during which the difference between the transmembrane potential and the threshold potential is small. This means that the period of increased excitability is prolonged and the appearance of ectopic complexes is facilitated.[67,69] A decrease in the extracellular K concentration increases the difference in K concentrations across the cell membrane and tends to

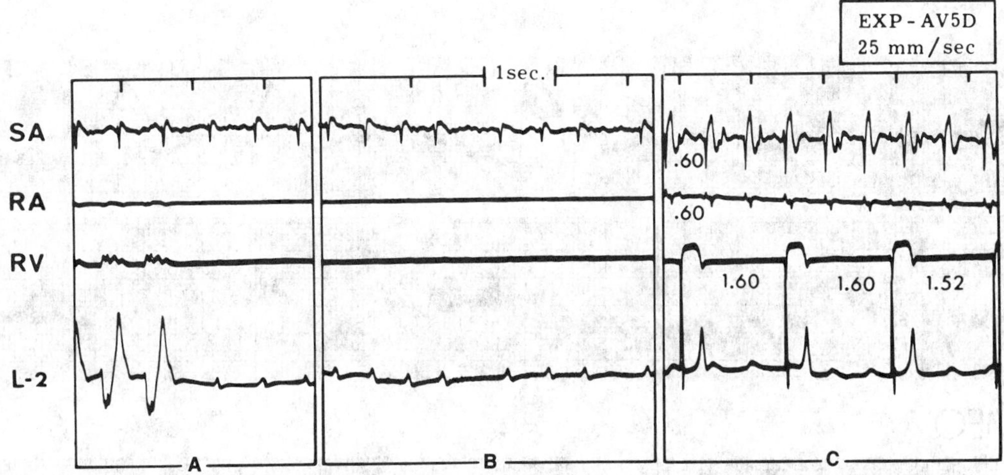

FIGURE 37-7 Potassium-induced AV block and differential sensitivity of various cardiac tissues to K. Records were obtained from the region of the SA node (SA), right atrium (RA), right ventricle (RV), lead II (L-2). *A,B.* The RA and RV leads fail to record electrical activity at a time when P waves are still present in L-2, indicating that the SA node and some parts of the atrium are less sensitive to K than the ventricular myocardium. *C.* Complete AV dissociation, recorded after the K infusion was discontinued, indicates that the junction is less resistant to K than either the SA node or the atrial and ventricular myocardium. Normal duration of the QRS in the presence of a prolonged P wave indicates that the ventricular myocardium is more resistant to K than the atrial myocardium. *(From Fisch C, Greenspan K, Edmands RR: Complete atrioventricular block due to potassium. Circ Res 19:373, 1966. Reproduced by permission of the American Heart Association and the author.)*

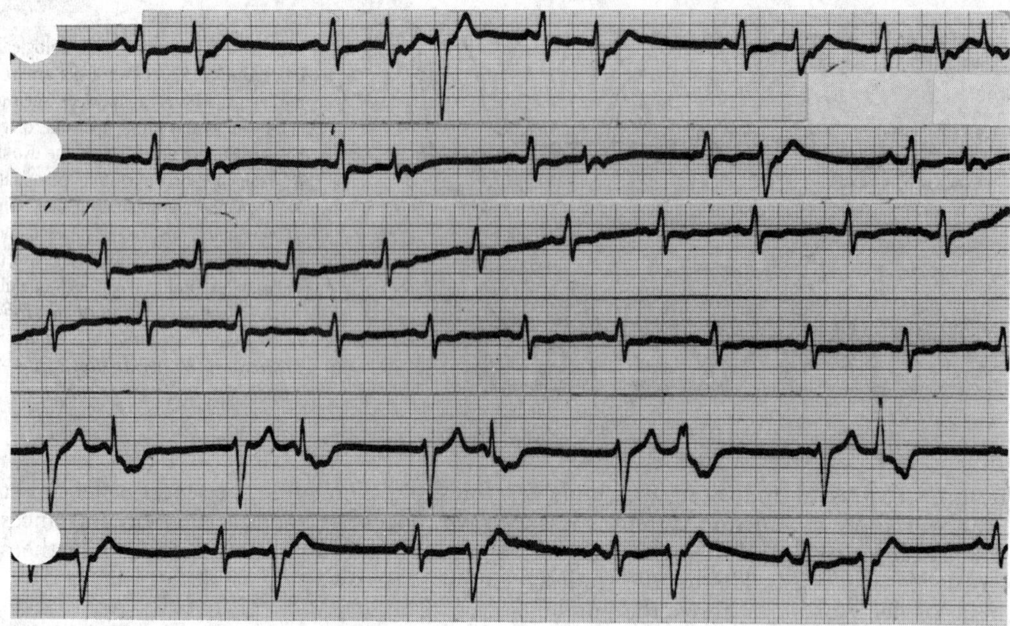

FIGURE 37-8 Effects in human beings of rapidly administered K. *A.* Control illustrates sinus rhythm with premature ventricular contraction (PVC), some followed by retrograde atrial activation. *B.* With rapid infusion of K, PVCs are promptly eliminated. Further infusion depresses the SA node and is followed by an idioventricular escape rhythm with ventricular bigeminy. It is possible that suppression is that of the atrial myocardium with SA block rather than depression of sinus node activity. *C.* After K infusion is discontinued, the rhythm returns to control. *(From Fisch C, Steinmetz EF, Chevalier RB: Transient effect of intravenous potassium on A-V conduction and ventricular ectopic beats: Clinical study. Am Heart J 60:220, 1960. Reproduced with permission from the publisher and author.)*

hyperpolarize the cell during diastole. At very low K concentrations the membrane potential depolarizes (deviation from values predicted by the Nernst equation) (Fig. 37-1*B*). Therefore, hypokalemia may slow conduction secondary to a reduction in the transmembrane resting potential or, alternatively, hypokalemia may slow conduction because depolarization may begin in completely repolarized tissue. Hypokalemia also increases diastolic depolarization in the Purkinje fibers[70,71] and therefore promotes automatic activity in normally quiescent Purkinje fibers.

Electrocardiographic Manifestations

The electrocardiographic recognition of hypokalemia is based on the presence of an exaggerated U wave without any significant change in the QT duration.[72] The U wave may be a normal finding, and its presence is not specific

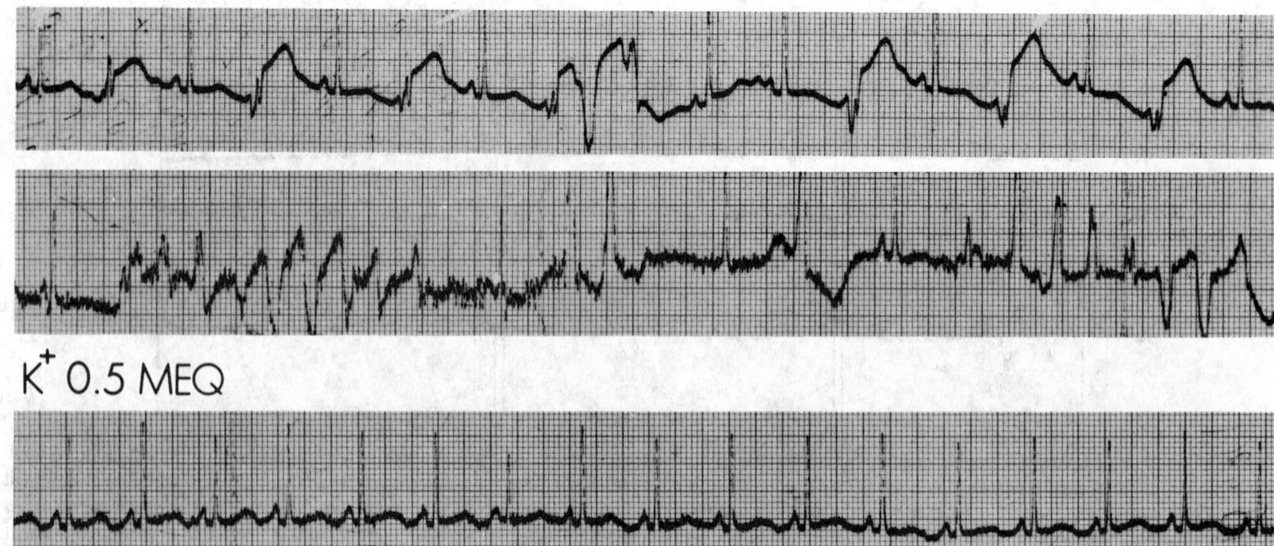

FIGURE 37-9 Antiarrhythmic properties of K in a digitalis-intoxicated patient. The plasma K is 4.0 meq/liter. The upper two strips represent the chaotic ventricular arrhythmia, which responded promptly to a 0.5-meq bolus of K. It is not advisable to administer K rapidly.

for hypokalemia. When the amplitude of the U wave exceeds the amplitude of the adjacent T wave, however, hypokalemia should be suspected. This change is usually most evident in lead II or III or the midprecordial leads. As hypokalemia becomes more severe, the T-wave amplitude decreases and may become inverted and the ST segment becomes depressed. Decreased amplitude of the T wave, an increase in U-wave amplitude, and ST-segment depression produce a rather characteristic undulating appearance to the baseline very suggestive of hypokalemia (Fig. 37-10). When hypokalemia is severe, the QRS complex may widen slightly in a diffuse manner. The P-wave amplitude may be increased and the PR interval is often slightly prolonged.[73]

The changes in the ECG correlate reasonably well with the plasma K level. Electrocardiographic changes of hypokalemia were found in 78 percent of patients with plasma K below 2.7 meq/liter, in 35 percent of patients with plasma K between 2.7 and 3.0 meq/liter, and in 10 percent of patients with plasma K between 3.0 and 3.5 meq/liter.[74] The electrocardiographic pattern of hypokalemia is not specific and may follow administration of digitalis, antiarrhythmic agents, or phenothiazines and in the presence of ventricular hypertrophy or bradycardia.[48,75]

Hypokalemia and Arrhythmias

Conduction disturbances with hypokalemia are rare. In experimental animals, hypokalemia may cause delay of AV conduction and block,[56,58] with delay of intraventricular conduction less common. The exact mechanism of conduction delay is not clear, though several hypotheses have been proposed to explain this experimental observation. Hyperpolarization of the myocardial cell increases the current requirement to bring the transmembrane potential to threshold. Excitation of the cell during the prolonged repolarization phase may reduce the takeoff potential and depress conduction. At very low extracellular K concentrations the membrane potential may depolarize and reduce conduction velocity. These explanations may, alone or in combination, account for hypokalemia-induced AV conduction delay or block.

Hypokalemia promotes the appearance of supraventricular and ventricular ectopic rhythms.[69,76] In hospitalized patients with plasma K levels less than 3.2 meq/liter who are not on digitalis, ectopic complexes occurred three times and AV conduction abnormalities two times more frequently than in the control hospital population.[77] These arrhythmias may be enhanced by hypokalemia-induced increased automaticity and/or facilitation of reentry. Perfusion of isolated hearts with potassium-deficient solutions produces ventricular fibrillation.[71,78]

Potassium and Digitalis

The effects of digitalis on the myocardium are modified by the extracellular K concentration. Digitalis glycosides bind to and inhibit the Na-K-ATPase, increasing intracellular Na and reducing intracellular K. This interrelation-

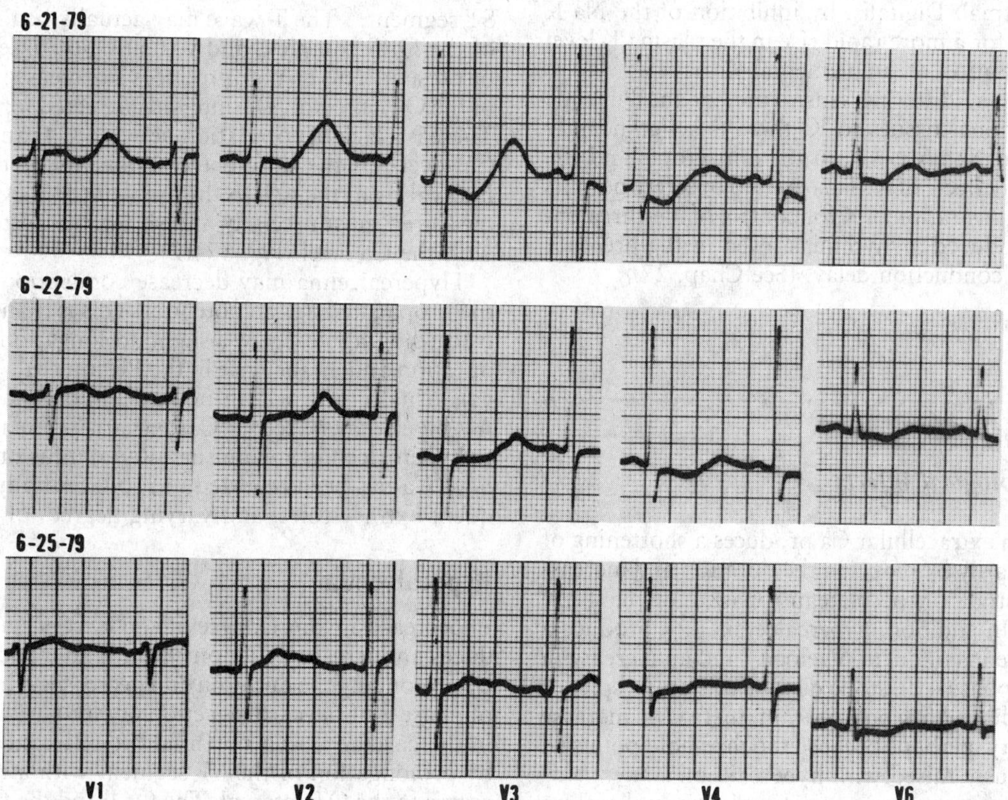

FIGURE 37-10 Electrocardiogram changes of hypokalemia. A striking U wave with a marked prolongation of a QU interval is recorded on June 21, 1979. The K level at that time was 1.3 meq/liter. With replacement of K, there was a gradual improvement with a normal QT and U wave recorded on June 25, 1979, at a plasma K of 3.9 meq/liter.

ship between digitalis and K is manifest by (1) depression of digitalis-induced ectopy by K, (2) emergence of digitalis-induced ectopy during hypokalemia,[79,80] and (3) enhancement of digitalis-induced depression of conduction by K.[81] Since diuretic therapy, insulin administration or carbohydrate loading, renal disease, and acid-base disturbances all potentially may induce significant alterations in K homeostasis, digitalis must be used with knowledge that the plasma K may be affected by these clinical circumstances.

The major manifestation of digitalis toxicity is increased automaticity with extrasystoles or tachycardias, both of which are potentiated by low serum K. The most characteristic arrhythmias in hypokalemic patients treated with digitalis are nonparoxysmal junctional tachycardia and atrial tachycardia with block. These arrhythmias are caused by a combination of enhanced automaticity and depressed AV conduction. The administration of K is safe and quite effective in suppressing these arrhythmias. Potassium suppression of digitalis-induced ectopic rhythm is most likely multifactorial. Potassium slows the rate of binding of cardiac glycosides to the myocardial Na-K-ATPase,[82–84] depresses digitalis-induced phase 4 depolarization, and likely interrupts reentrant pathways by altering conduction.

In patients whose major manifestations of digitalis toxicity is high-grade AV block, the rapid administration of K may enhance the depression of conduction further.[79,81] Rapid administration of K to humans or animals intoxicated with digitalis results in depression of SA, intraatrial, AV, and intraventricular conduction.[79,81,85] If the plasma K is low, there is little danger of raising the K level to normal. Digitalis, by inhibition of the Na-K pump, allows for a more rapid rise in the plasma K level with administration of supplemental K.

Because of the differing sensitivities of the Purkinje and AV junctional tissues to K, there is a significantly wide margin of safety between the antiectopic and the AV depressant effects of K. This margin of safety permits judicious administration of K for control of life-threatening digitalis-induced arrhythmias, even in the presence of simple AV conduction delay. (See Chap. 27.)

CALCIUM

Hypercalcemia

Electrophysiological Effects

An increase in extracellular Ca produces a shortening of the TAP primarily by reducing the duration and increasing the amplitude of the plateau (phase 2 of the TAP) (Fig. 37-11). In addition, hypercalcemia may produce a slight decrease in conduction velocity and an increase in spontaneous phase 4 diastolic depolarization. In spite of the effect on diastolic depolarization, there is no increase in automaticity, perhaps because the threshold potential is simultaneously raised with hypercalcemia.[86]

Calcium is important in normal and abnormal cardiac function. Influx of Ca via sarcolemmal Ca channels regulates the force of myocardial contraction. (See Chap. 5.) Calcium-dependent TAP and calcium-dependent triggered ventricular activity may be important in certain clinical arrhythmias. The role of Ca in these events is discussed in the sections that follow.

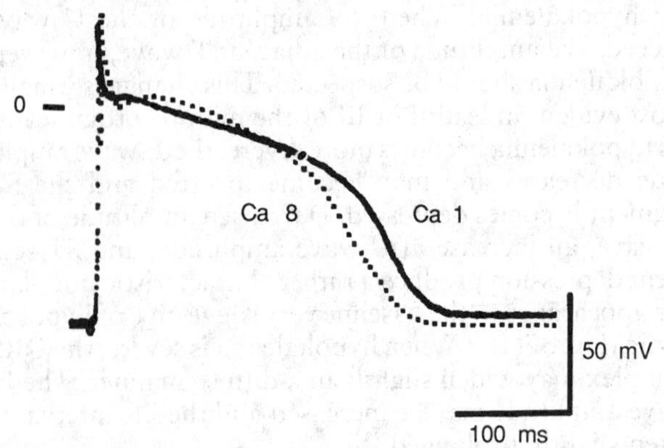

FIGURE 37-11 Effects of Ca^{2+} on the TAP of a dog Purkinje fiber. Solid lines represent TAP in $[Ca^{2+}]_o$ of 1 mM; dotted lines represent record in $[Ca^{2+}]_o$ of 8 m*M*. Increasing $[Ca^{2+}]_o$ raised the plateau potential, shortened TAP duration, and slightly hyperpolarized the maximum diastolic potential. Changes in $[Ca^{2+}]_o$ have been shown to elevate $[Ca^{2+}]_i$, and opening the Ca^{2+}-activated K^+ channels may explain the decrease in TAP duration. *(Reprinted with permission from Ref. 34.)*

Electrocardiographic Manifestations

The changes in the TAP produced by hypercalcemia are reflected in the ECG by altered duration of the ST segment and QT interval. The primary manifestation of hypercalcemia is a marked decrease in duration of the ST segment.[87] The T wave may actually begin at the end of the QRS complex, and virtually no ST segment may be present. This change produces a decrease in the length of the QT_c interval (QT interval corrected for heart rate). There is a lack of correlation between QT_c and the serum Ca level. Of the different components of the QT, the interval from the QT to the apex of the T (QaT) can be measured most precisely and shows the best correlation with the Ca level (Fig. 37-12).[88]

Hypercalcemia may decrease conduction velocity of the propagated action potential. This is manifested electrocardiographically by a slight prolongation of the QRS duration and an increase in the PR interval. These intervals usually stay within normal limits, but first-degree AV block may be seen.[89] Cardiac arrhythmias secondary to hypercalcemia are unusual. Rapid infusion of intravenous Ca has been reported to produce bradycardia, frequent extrasystoles, and varying degrees of AV block.

Hypocalcemia

A decrease in the extracellular Ca concentration produces an increase in action potential duration primarily by prolonging the duration and decreasing the amplitude of phase 2 of the cardiac action potential. These changes in the cardiac action potential are reflected in the ECG by prolongation of the ST segment with a resultant increase in the QT interval. The QaT and the QT intervals are prolonged. The QT_c, however, rarely exceeds 140 percent of the normal. If the QT exceeds that number, the U wave is likely to be included in the measurement.

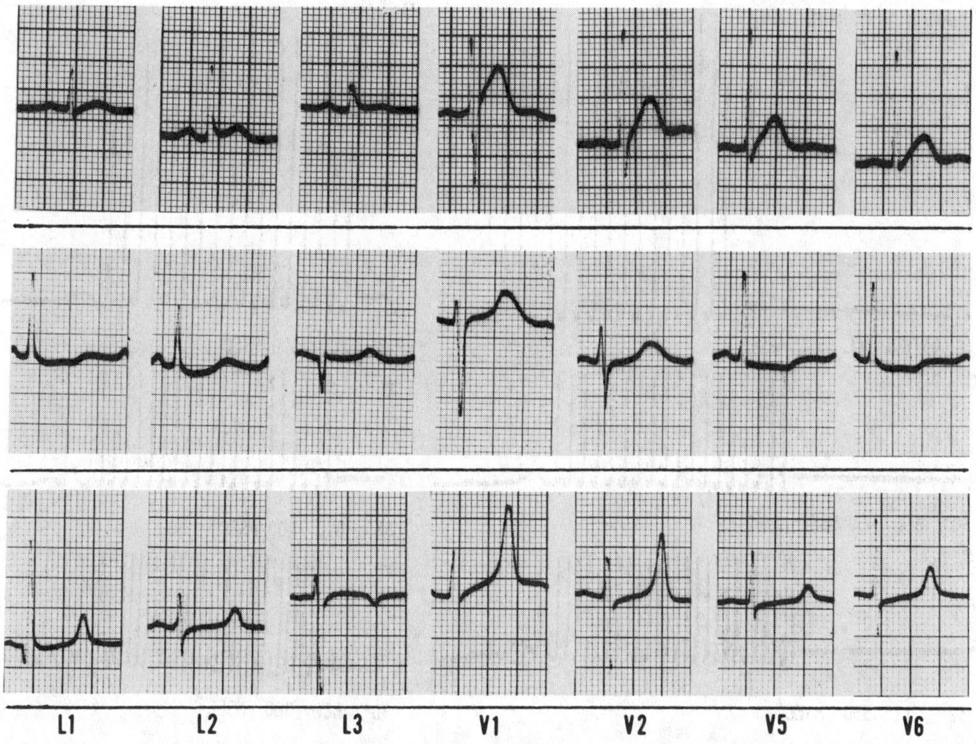

FIGURE 37-12 *A.* Recorded at a Ca level of 17.0 mg/dL. Illustrates the short ST segment characteristic of hypercalcemia. *B.* Recorded at a Ca level of 5.9 mg/dL. Shows prolongation of the ST segment of hypocalcemia. *C.* Recorded at a K level of 6.2 meq/liter, Ca of 5.3 mg/dL, and P of 12.2 mg/dL. The prolongation of QT due to hypocalcemia, terminated by the tented T of hyperkalemia, is characteristic of both hypocalcemia and hyperkalemia seen in chronic renal disease.

The T wave of the ECG is not altered by hypocalcemia (Fig. 37-12*B*). Hypocalcemia combines with hyperkalemia to produce an easily recognizable pattern and is most often seen in patients with chronic renal disease. This pattern is characterized by prolongation of the ST segment and appearance of a tented T wave (Fig. 37-12*C*). Similarly, hypocalcemia in association with hypokalemia may exhibit a prolonged ST segment with a prominent terminal wave consisting of both the T and the U waves. While the ST segment is prolonged, the total QU interval remains normal.

Calcium and Contractility

The need of Ca for proper mechanical function of cardiac tissue was demonstrated by Ringer.[90] The key event in initiation of contraction is a rise in intracellular Ca. Calcium, which enters the cell during the plateau phase of the cardiac action potential through the sarcolemmal Ca channels, in turn stimulates the junctional sarcoplasmic reticulum to release Ca via a ryanodine-sensitive Ca-release channel.[91] The Ca released from the sarcoplasmic reticulum significantly increases the free intracellular Ca (10^{-7} to $10^{-5}M$). This Ca diffuses into the myofibrils; combines with troponin, which in its Ca-free state inhibits the myosin actin interaction; and releases this inhibition. Actin combines with myosin, and adenosine triphosphate (ATP) is split by the Ca-dependent ATPase. The released energy is transformed into mechanical work, with the actin filament sliding over the myosin filaments, and shortening of the myofibrils results. (See also Chap. 5.)

Various interventions, including alterations in extracellular Ca concentrations, affect myocardial contractility. Increasing extracellular Ca increases the magnitude of contraction without altering the rate of myocardial relaxation. Sympathetic amines increase cyclic AMP, which increases the sarcolemmal Ca current and myocardial contractility. Sympathetic amines also increase the rate of myocardial relaxation, secondary to phosphorylation-dependent increases in Ca reuptake into sarcoplasmic reticulum.[92] (See also Chap. 28.)

Though Ca is fundamentally important in the process of contraction, chronic hypocalcemia has not been shown to result in heart failure. Occasionally, acutely induced hypocalcemia may be associated with depression of ventricular function.[93] Calcium channel antagonists decrease myocardial contractility, though in the absence of significant left ventricular dysfunction, it is unusual for the decrease to be clinically important. (See also Chap. 67.)

Calcium and Arrhythmias

Under normal circumstances atrial and ventricular fibers do not exhibit spontaneous phase 4 diastolic depolarization. Under abnormal conditions nonpacemaker atrial or ventricular fibers can acquire phase 4 depolarization and become transformed into spontaneously firing pacemaker fibers.[94] In general, these spontaneous action potentials arise from a less negative membrane potential, have a slower upstroke velocity, and are conducted at a slower rate than normal action potentials. Some data suggest that these automatic rhythms may be generated

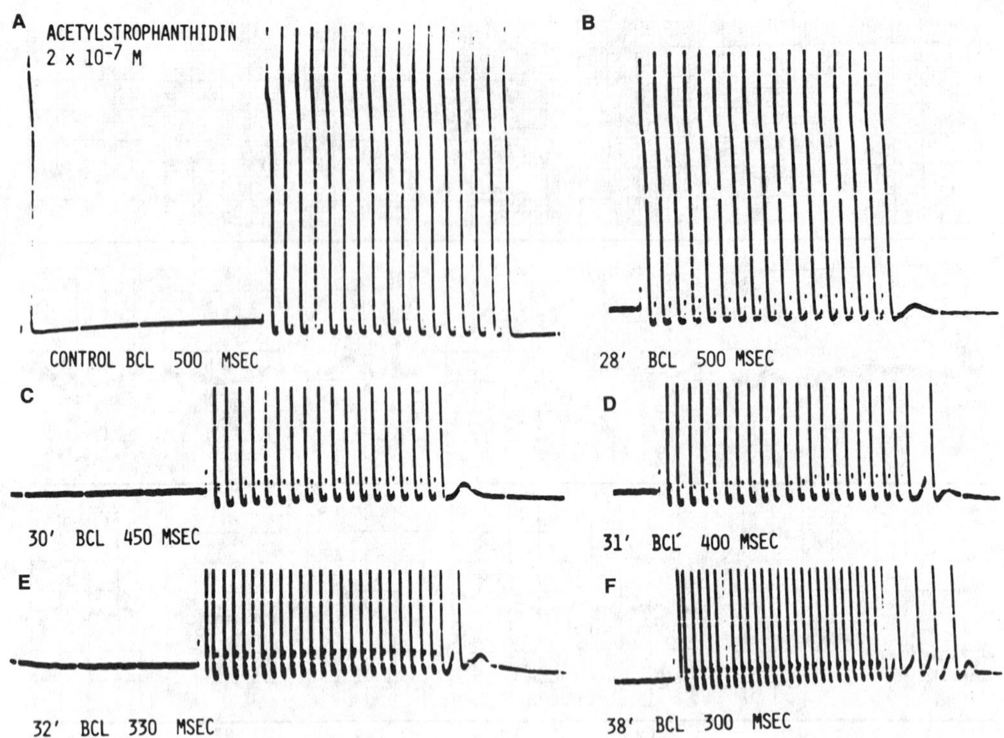

FIGURE 37-13 Diastolic afterpotentials (triggered automatically) very likely related to intracellular Ca shift. Purkinje fiber is superfused with 2×10^{-7} *M* acetylstrophanthidin. The basic driving cycle length is gradually shortened from 500 to 300 ms (*A*, 500 ms; *F*, 300 ms). At a cycle length of 500 ms, 28 min after onset of superfusion, cessation of pacing is followed by a nonpropagated diastolic afterpotential. *C–F.* Similar nonpropagated potential is noted. *F.* The afterpotential results in a full action potential with repetitive responses noted, paralleling the duration of superfusion with acetylstrophanthidin and the rate of stimulation.

by Ca-dependent action potentials,[95] though Na channel activity may also contribute to action potential generation. Depressed action potentials sensitive to verapamil have been observed in subendocardial fibers of infarcts taken from human hearts with ventricular aneurysms,[96] though the role of such slow-response-action potentials in the genesis of arrhythmias during life is still uncertain.

In vitro electrophysiological studies have demonstrated that cellular Ca overload may produce delayed afterdepolarizations and triggered cardiac activity. Transient depolarizations are postulated secondary to cellular Ca overload, which triggers release of Ca from the junctional sarcoplasmic reticulum via the ryanodine-sensitive Ca-release channel protein.[91] This Ca in turn activates a sarcolemmal channel[97] or Na-Ca exchange mechanism[98] that depolarizes the cell membrane transiently. When cells are stimulated rapidly, the delayed afterdepolarization amplitude can reach threshold and spontaneous triggered automatic activity can occur (Fig. 37-13).[99] Though no definite proof of clinical triggered automatic rhythms exists, clinical data suggest that this may play a role in the initiation of certain clinical arrhythmias.[100] (See also Chaps. 34 and 35.)

MAGNESIUM

Electrophysiological Effects

Magnesium is an important metallocoenzyme for many enzyme reactions. It activates ATPase, which is essential for normal cell membrane function and is the energy source for the Na-K pump. Intracellular Mg deficiency may be associated with an increase in intracellular Na and Ca and a loss of K. Similarly, an increase of Mg theoretically can result in an intracellular decrease of Na and Ca and an increase in K.[101,102]

Clinically encountered Mg concentrations have no effect on TAP characteristic when K and Ca concentrations are normal. Electrophysiological effects of low Ca are corrected by high Mg, suggesting some limited competition between Ca and Mg at the cell membrane.[103,104]

Electrocardiographic Manifestations

Because alterations in Mg levels affect Na, K, and Ca concentrations, it is rare to see isolated Mg derangements in clinical settings. The interdependence of the electrophysiological effects of Mg, Ca, Na, and K makes the ECG recognition of Mg alterations difficult, if not impossible. During the early course of Mg deficiency, the QRS complex narrows and the T wave becomes tall and peaked. The T wave is not narrow based but is of normal width, and the QT interval is normal. The change in T-wave morphology is attributed to impairment in the Na-K-ATPase, which results in a loss of intracellular K. When Mg deficiency is more severe, hypokalemia occurs. The ECG resembles that of hypokalemia with a wider QRS complex, ST-segment depression, and low-amplitude T waves.[105]

Elevation of extracellular Mg to a level of 6 to 10 meq/liter depresses AV and intraventricular conduction.[106–108]

This may be due to slowing of the upstroke velocity of phase 0, a mechanism similar or identical to that induced by hyperkalemia. Sinoatrial and AV block occur at 15 meq/liter, and cardiac arrest may be expected at levels of 15 to 22 meq/liter.[107] Neuromuscular and respiratory paralysis usually precedes cardiac arrest.

Magnesium and Arrhythmias

Hypomagnesemia may predispose to digitalis toxicity. Lowering the Mg level by dialyzing with an Mg-free solution reduces the amount of acetylstrophanthidin necessary to induce arrhythmias. The arrhythmia is promptly abolished in most, but not all, of the animals by administration of magnesium sulfate. Magnesium depletion may become clinically important with the chronic administration of diuretic agents and with gastrointestinal disease or diabetes mellitus. In patients with congestive heart failure, prolonged secondary aldosteronism may deplete total body Mg stores. Currently, the role of hypomagnesemia in potentiating digitalis toxicity is unresolved.[109] In one study approximately 20 percent of patients on digitalis were found to have hypomagnesemia, yet Mg levels did not differ between patients with and without digitalis toxicity.[110] Though this issue is unresolved, hypomagnesemia appears to potentiate digitalis-induced arrhythmias; and in patients with low Mg, administration of Mg may suppress digitalis-induced arrhythmias.

Administration of intravenous magnesium sulfate to patients with prolonged QT intervals and torsades de pointes, whether the initial Mg level is normal or low, may suppress the ventricular arrhythmia.[111] Recent evidence suggests that torsades de pointes is secondary to early afterdepolarizations.[112] Early afterdepolarizations are abnormal secondary repolarizations that occur prior to the full completion of repolarization in myocardial cells.[113] Early afterdepolarization amplitude and ventricular tachycardia induction can be facilitated by slow rates, low extracellular K and/or Ca concentrations, and increased catecholoamines and are depressed by Mg.[114] Though the exact mechanism of the Mg inhibition of early afterdepolarization amplitude and torsades de pointes is currently unknown, magnesium sulfate injection is a safe form of initial therapy for this arrhythmia. (See also Chaps. 36 and 60.)

PHOSPHORUS

Severe hypophosphatemia with serum levels below 1.0 mg/dL has been reported to alter myocardial performance.[115,116] Phosphorus is essential for production and utilization of high-energy phosphate compounds such as ATP and creatine phosphate. It is also important for the activity of ATP-dependent cation pump activity, such as that of Ca-ATPase. Presumably, decreased cellular levels of P-containing metabolites and membrane phospholipids result in altered myocardial performance as well as the other widespread consequences of hypophosphatemia. Animals with dietary-induced P depletion may exhibit evidence of depression of myocardial function, which is reversed with P repletion. The impairment of myocardial function associated with P depletion is independent of the left ventricular volume, resistance of ventricular ejection, or ventricular rate.[116]

Severe hypophosphatemia occurs in a variety of clinical settings, including hyperalimentation, nutritional recovery after starvation, treatment of diabetic ketoacidosis, alcoholic withdrawal, combination of phosphorus-binding antacids with dialysis, and prolonged respiratory alkalosis. In a group of severely ill patients with serum P levels less than 2.0 mg/dL, infusion of potassium phosphate has been demonstrated to increase stroke work.[117]

These observations suggest that myocardial contractility may be depressed by a depletion of body phosphate. The depressed cardiac function may be secondary to depletion of available ATP, and the depression of myocardial function may be reversed in some hypophosphatemic patients by phosphate.

LITHIUM

Although not a naturally occurring electrolyte, lithium (Li) has assumed an importance in cardiac electrophysiology because of its wide use in the management of depressive disorders.

Although reversible T-wave changes are the most common ECG abnormality due to Li,[118,119] dysfunction of the SA node has emerged as the characteristic and clinically significant complication of Li therapy. Disordered sinus node function may be manifested by sinus bradycardia, SA arrest, or exit block, either type I (Wenckebach) or type II (Mobitz II). These side effects occur most often with Li levels within the therapeutic range. The effect of Li on the SA node appears to be selective, as suggested by a normal PR, a normal QRS, and in the His electrogram,[120,121] a normal AH with only a slightly prolonged HV interval.

REFERENCES

1. Ellis D: The effects of external cations and ouabain on the intracellular sodium activity of sheep heart Purkinje fibers. *J Physiol (Lond)* 1977; 273:211–240.
2. Miura DS, Hoffman BF, Rosen MR: The effect of extracellular potassium on the intracellular potassium ion activity and transmembrane potentials of beating canine Purkinje fibers. *J Gen Physiol* 1977; 69:463–474.
3. Adrian RH: Potassium chloride movement and the membrane potential of frog muscle. *J Physiol (Lond)* 1960; 151:154–185.
4. Hodgkin AL: Ionic movements and electrical activity in giant nerve fibers. *Proc R Soc Lond (Biol)* 1958; 148:1–37.
5. Weidmann S: *Elektrophysiolgie der Herzmuskelfaser*. Bern and Stuttgart, Medizinisher Verlag Hans Huber, 1956.
6. Gadsby DC, Cranefield PF: Two levels of resting potential in cardiac Purkinje fibers. *J Gen Physiol* 1977; 70:725–746.
7. Goldman DE: Potential, impedance and rectification in membranes. *J Gen Physiol* 1943; 27:37–60.
8. Hodgkin AL, Katz B: The effect of sodium ions on the electrical activity of the giant axon of the squid. *J Physiol (Lond)* 1949; 108:37–77.
9. Draper MH, Weidmann S: Cardiac resting and action potentials recorded with an intracellular electrode. *J Physiol* 1951; 115:74–94.
10. Fozzard HA: Cardiac muscle: Excitability and passive electrical properties. *Prog Cardiovasc Dis* 1977; 19:343–359.

11. Weidmann S: The effect of the cardiac membrane potential on the rapid availability of the sodium carrying system. *J Physiol (Lond)* 1955; 127:213–224.
12. Walton MK, Fozzard HA: The conducted action potential. Models and comparison to experiments. *Biophys J* 1983; 44:9–26.
13. Dominguez G, Fozzard HA: Influence of extracellular K^+ concentration on cable properties and excitability of sheep cardiac Purkinje fibers. *Circ Res* 1970; 26:565–574.
14. Van Dam RT, Moore EN, Hoffman BF: Initiation and conduction of impulses in partially depolarized cardiac fibers. *Am J Physiol* 1963; 204:1133–1144.
15. Reuter H: The dependence of slow inward current in Purkinje fibers on the extracellular calcium concentration. *J Physiol (Lond)* 1967; 192:479–492.
16. Bean BP: Two kinds of calcium channels in canine atrial cells. Difference in kinetics, selectivity and pharmacology. *J Gen Physiol* 1985; 86:1–30.
17. Nilius B, Hess P, Lansman JB, Nilius B, Hess P, Lansman JB, Tsien RW: A novel type of cardiac calcium channel in ventricular cells. *Nature* 1985; 316:443–446.
18. Mitra R, Morad M: Two types of calcium channels in guinea pig ventricular myocytes. *Proc Natl Acad Sci USA* 1986; 83:5340–5344.
19. Nowycky MC, Fox AP, Tsien RW: Three types of neuronal calcium channels with different calcium agonist sensitivity. *Nature* 1985; 316:440–443.
20. Fox AP, Nowycky MC, Tsien RW: Single channel recordings of three types of calcium channels in chick sensory neurones. *J Physiol (Lond)* 1987; 394:173–200.
21. Kao CY: Tetrodotoxin, saxitoxin and their significance in the study of excitation phenomenon. *Pharmacol Rev* 1966; 18:997–1049.
22. Pappano AJ: Calcium dependent action potentials produced by catecholamines in guinea pig atrial muscle fibers depolarized by potassium. *Circ Res* 1970; 27:379–390.
23. Bailey JC, Watanabe AM, Besch HR Jr, Lathrop DA: Acetylcholine antagonism of the electrophysiological effects of isoproterenol on canine cardiac Purkinje fibers. *Circ Res* 1979; 44:378–393.
24. Reuter H: Calcium channel modulation by neurotransmitters, enzymes and drugs. *Nature* 1983; 301:569–574.
25. Tsien RW, Bean BP, Hess P, Lansman JB, Nilius B, Nowycky MC: Mechanisms of calcium channel modulation by beta-adrenergic agents and dihydropyridine calcium agonists. *J. Mol Cell Cardiol* 1986; 18:691–710.
26. Osterrieder W, Brum G, Hescheler J, Trautwein W, Flockerzi V, Hofmann F: Injection of subunits of cyclic AMP-dependent protein kinase into cardiac myocytes modulates Ca^{2+}-current. *Nature* 1982; 298:576–578.
27. Brum G, Osterrieder W, Trautwein W: β-Adrenergic increase in the calcium conductance of cardiac myocytes studied with the patch clamp. *Pflügers Arch* 1984; 401:111–118.
28. Coraboeuf E, Deroabaix E, Coulombe A: Effect of tetrodotoxin on action potentials of the conduction system in the dog heart. *Am J Physiol* 1979; 236:H561–H567.
29. Attwell D, Cohen I, Eisner D, Ohba M, Ojeda C: The steady state TTX-sensitive ("window") sodium current in cardiac Purkinje fibres. *Pflügers Arch* 1979; 379:137–142.
30. Egan TM, Noble SJ, Noble D, Powell T, Spindler AJ, Twist VW: Sodium-channel exchange during the action potential in guinea-pig ventricular cells. *J Physiol (Lond)* 1989; 411:639–661.
31. Kenyon JL, Gibbons WR: Effects of low chloride solutions on action potentials of sheep cardiac Purkinje fibers. *J Gen Physiol* 1977; 70:635–660.
32. Hess P: Elementary properties of cardiac calcium channels: A brief review. *Can J Physiol Pharmacol* 1988; 66:1218–1223.
33. Carmeliet EE: K^+ channels in cardiac cells: Mechanisms of activation, inactivation, rectification and K^+ sensitivity. *Pflügers Arch* 1989; 414(suppl 1):588–592.
34. Rardon DP, Pressler ML: Cardiac resting and action potentials: Current concepts. In: Fisch C, Surawicz B (eds): *Cardiac Electrophysiology and Arrhythmias: Current Topics in Cardiology.* New York, Elsevier Science, 1991: 3–12.
35. Carmeliet E: L'influence de la concentration extracellulaire du K sur la perméabilité de la membrane des fibres de Purkije de mouton pour les ions ^{42}K. *Helv Physiol Acta* 1960; 18:C15–C16.
36. Surawicz B: The interrelationship of electrolyte abnormalities and arrhythmias. In: Mandel WS (ed): *Cardiac Arrhythmias: Their Mechanisms, Diagnosis and Management.* Philadelphia, Lippincott, 1980: 83–106.
37. Thompson WAR: Potassium and the T wave of the electrocardiogram. *Lancet* 1939; 1:808–811.
38. Keith NM, Burchell HB, Baggenstoss AH: Electrocardiographic changes in uremia associated with a high concentration of serum potassium. A report of three cases. *Am Heart J* 1944; 27:817–844.
39. Nadier CS, Bellet S, Lanning M: Influence of the serum potassium and other electrolytes on the electrocardiogram in diabetic acidosis. *Am J Med* 1948; 5:838–848.
40. Braun HA, Surawicz B, Bellet S: T waves in hyperpotassemia. *Am J Med Sci* 1955; 230:147–156.
41. Levine HD, Jehangir P, Vazifdar JP, Lown B, Merrill JP: "Tent-shaped" T waves of normal amplitude in potassium intoxication. *Am Heart J* 1952; 43:437–450.
42. Merrill JP, Levine HD, Somerville W, Smith S: Clinical recognition and treatment of acute potassium intoxication. *Ann Intern Med* 1950; 33:797–830.
43. Levine HD, Merrill JP, Somerville W: Advanced disturbances of cardiac mechanism in potassium intoxication in man. *Circulation* 1951; 3:889–905.
44. Goldberger E, Pokress MJ, Stein R: Effect of potassium on downward T waves of precordial leads of normal children. *Am Heart J* 1949; 37:418–424.
45. Sharpey-Schafer EP: Potassium effects on T wave inversion in myocardial infarction and preponderance of a ventricle. *Br Heart J* 1943; 5:80–84.
46. Wasserberger RH, Corliss RJ: Value of oral potassium salts in differentiation of functional and organic T-wave changes. *Am J Cardiol* 1962; 10:673–687.
47. Winkler AW, Hoff HE, Smith PK: Electrocardiographic changes and concentration of potassium in serum following intravenous injection of potassium chloride. *Am J Physiol* 1938; 124:478–483.
48. Surawicz B: Relationship between electrocardiogram and electrolytes. *Am Heart J* 1967; 73:814–834.
49. Levine HD, Wanzer SH, Merrill JP: Dialyzable currents of injury in potassium intoxication resembling acute myocardial infarction or pericarditis. *Circulation* 1956; 13:29–36.
50. Pryor R, Blount SG: The clinical significance of true left axis deviation: Left intraventricular blocks. *Am Heart J* 1966; 72:391–413.
51. Awy GA, Karliner J, Bedynck JL: Electrocardiographic QRS axis shift as a manifestation of hyperkalemia. *JAMA* 1971; 215:429–432.
52. Burch GE, Meyers R, Abildskov JA: A new electrocardiographic pattern observed in cerebrovascular accidents. *Circulation* 1954; 9:719–723.
53. Runge PJ, Bousvaros G: Giant peaked upright T waves in cerebrovascular accident. *Br Heart J* 1970; 32:717–719.
54. Hoffman BF, Sucking EE: Effect of heart rate on cardiac membrane potentials and the unipolar electrogram. *Am J Physiol* 1954; 179:123–130.
55. Hoffman BF, Cranefield PF: *Electrophysiology of the Heart.* New York, McGraw-Hill, 1960.
56. Fisch C: Effect of potassium on AV conduction (editorial). *Circulation* 1970; 41:575–578.
57. Nahum LH, Hoff HE: Observations on potassium fibrillation. *J Pharmacol Exp Ther* 1939; 65:322–331.
58. Mathison GC: The effect of potassium salts upon the circulation and their action on plain muscle. *J Physiol (Lond)* 1911; 42:471–494.
59. Fisch C, Knoebel SB, Feigenbaum H, Greenspan K: Potassium and the monophasic action potential electrocardiogram, conduction and arrhythmias. *Prog Cardiovasc Dis* 1966; 8:387–418.
60. Feigenbaum H, Wunsch CM, Fisch C: Interrelationship of potassium and vagal action on the sinoatrial pacemaker and on atrioventricular conduction. *J Clin Invest* 1965; 44: 399–405.
61. Fisch C, Feigenbaum H, Bowers JA: The inhibition of acetylcholine-induced atrioventricular block by potassium. *J Clin Invest* 1963; 42:563–569.
62. Fisch C, Greenspan K, Edwards RE: Complete atrioventricular block due to potassium. *Circ Res* 1966; 19:373–377.

63. Fisch C, Feigenbaum H, Bowers JA: The effect of potassium on atrioventricular conduction of normal dogs. *Am J Cardiol* 1963; 11:487–492.
64. Cohen HC, Gozo EG, Pick A: The nature and type of arrhythmias in acute experimental hyperkalemia in the intact dog. *Am Heart J* 1971; 82:777–785.
65. Bettinger JC, Surawicz B, Bryfogle JW, Anderson BN, Bellet S: The effect of intravenous administration of potassium chloride on ectopic rhythms, ectopic beats and disturbances in A-V conduction. *Am J Med* 1956; 21:521–533.
66. Walker WJ, Elkins JT, Wood LW: Effect of potassium in restoring myocardial response to a subthreshold cardiac pacemaker. *N Engl J Med* 1964; 271:597–602.
67. Surawicz B, Lepeschkin E, Herrlich HC, Hoffman BF: Effect of potassium and calcium deficiency on the monophasic action potential, electrocardiogram and contractility of isolated rabbit hearts. *Am J Physiol* 1959; 196:1302–1307.
68. Hecht H, Heath JM, Maier ES, Lange RL, Nelson CV: The cellular basis for the electrocardiographic changes associated with alterations in serum potassium. *J Clin Invest* 1957; 36:897–898.
69. Gettes LS, Surawicz B, Schiue JC: Effect of high K, low K, and quinidine on QRS duration and ventricular action potential. *Am J Physiol* 1962; 203:1135–1140.
70. Gettes L, Surawicz B: Effects of low and high concentrations of potassium on the simultaneously recorded Purkinje and ventricular action potentials of the perfused pig moderator band. *Circ Res* 1968; 23:717–729.
71. Grumbach L, Howard JW, Merrill VI: Factors related to the initiation of ventricular fibrillation in the isolated heart: Effect of calcium and potassium. *Circ Res* 1954; 2:452–459.
72. Surawicz B, Lepeschkin E: Electrocardiographic pattern of hypopotassemia with and without hypocalcemia. *Circulation* 1953; 8:801–828.
73. Weaver WF, Burchell HB: Serum potassium and electrocardiogram in hypokalemia. *Circulation* 1960; 21:505–521.
74. Surawicz B, Braun HA, Crum WB, Kemp RL, Wagner S, Bellet S: Quantitative analysis of the electrocardiographic pattern of hypopotassemia. *Circulation* 1957; 16:750–763.
75. Van Buchem FSP: The electrocardiogram and potassium metabolism: Electrocardiographic abnormalities in primary aldosteronism and familial periodic paralysis. *Am J Med* 1957; 23:376–384.
76. Schwartz W, Levine HD, Relman AS: The electrocardiogram in potassium depletion: Its relation to the total potassium deficit and the serum concentration. *Am J Med* 1954; 16:395–403.
77. Davidson S, Surawicz B: Ectopic beats and atrioventricular conduction disturbances in patients with hypopotassemia. *Arch Intern Med* 1967; 120:280–285.
78. Surawicz B, Gettes LS: Two mechanisms of cardiac arrest produced by potassium. *Circ Res* 1963; 12:415–421.
79. Fisch C, Greenspan K, Knoebel SB, Feigenbaum H: Effect of digitalis on conduction of the heart. *Prog Cardiovasc Dis* 1964; 6:343–365.
80. Lown B, Weller JM, Wyatt N, et al: Effects of alterations of body potassium on digitalis toxicity (abstr). *J Clin Invest* 1952; 31:648.
81. Fisch C, Martz BL, Priebe FH: Enhancement of potassium-induced atrioventricular block by toxic doses of digitalis drugs. *J Clin Invest* 1960; 39:1885–1893.
82. Schwartz A, Matsui H, Laughter AH: Tritiated digoxin binding to (Na^+ + K^+)-activation adenosine triphosphatase. Possible allosteric site. *Science* 1968; 160:323–327.
83. Prindle KH Jr, Skelton CL, Epstein SE, Marcus FI: Influence of extracellular potassium concentration on myocardial uptake and inotropic effect of treated digoxin. *Circ Res* 1971; 28:337–345.
84. Goldman RH, Coltart DJ, Friedman JP, Nola GT, Berke DK, Schweizer E, et al: The inotropic effects of digoxin in hyperkalemia: Relation to (Na^+, K^+)-ATPase inhibition in the intact animal. *Circulation* 1973; 48:830–838.
85. Sampson JJ, Alberton EC, Kondo B: The effects on man of potassium administration in relation to digitalis glycosides, with special reference to blood serum potassium, the electrocardiogram, and ectopic beats. *Am Heart J* 1943; 26:164–179.
86. Pressler ML, Elharrar V, Bailey JC: Effects of extracellular calcium ions, verapamil, and lanthanum on active and passive properties of canine cardiac Purkinje fibers. *Circ Res* 1982; 51:637–651.
87. Surawicz B, MacDonald MG, Kaliot V, Bettinger JC: Treatment of cardiac arrhythmias with salts of ethylenediamine tetraacetic acid (EDTA). *Am Heart J* 1959; 58:493–503.
88. Nierenberg DW, Ransil BJ: QaT_c interval as a clinical indicator of hypercalcemia. *Am J Cardiol* 1979; 44:243–248.
89. Fisch C: Relation of electrolyte disturbances to cardiac arrhythmias. *Circulation* 1973; 47:408–419.
90. Ringer S: A further contribution regarding the influence of the different constituents of blood on the contraction of the heart. *J Physiol* 1883; 4:29–42.
91. Rardon DP, Cefali DC, Mitchell RD, Seiler SM, Jones LR: High molecular weight proteins purified from cardiac junctional sarcoplasmic reticulum vesicles are ryanodine-sensitive calcium channels. *Circ Res* 1989; 64:779–789.
92. Hicks MJ, Shigekauka M, Katz AM: Mechanism by which cyclic adenosine 3′,5′ monophosphate dependent protein kinase stimulates calcium transport in cardiac sarcoplasmic reticulum. *Circ Res* 1979; 44:384–391.
93. Layzer RB, Rowland LP: Cramps. *N Engl J Med* 1971; 285:31–40.
94. Surawicz B: Depolarization-induced automaticity in atrial and ventricular myocardial fibers. In: Zipes DP, Bailey JC, Elharrar V (eds): *The Slow Inward Current and Cardiac Arrhythmias.* The Hague, Martinus Nijhoff, 1980: 375–396.
95. Katzung BG: Effects of extracellular calcium and sodium on depolarization-induced automaticity in guinea pig papillary muscles. *Circ Res* 1975; 37:118–127.
96. Spear JF, Horowitz LN, Hodess AB, MacVaugh H, Moore EN: Cellular electrophysiology of human myocardial infarction I. Abnormalities of cellular activation. *Circulation* 1979; 59:247–256.
97. Kass RS, Lederer WJ, Tsien RW, Weingart R: Role of calcium ions in transient inward currents and after contractions induced by strophanthidin in cardiac Purkinje fibers. *J Physiol (Lond)* 1978; 281:187–208.
98. Arlock P, Katzurg BG: Effects of sodium substitutes on transient inward current and tension in guinea-pig and ferret papillary muscle. *J Physiol (Lond)* 1985; 360:105–120.
99. Ferrier GR, Saunders JH, Mendez C: A cellular mechanism for the generation of ventricular arrhythmias by acetylstrophanthidin. *Circ Res* 1973; 32:600–609.
100. Rosen MR, Fisch C, Hoffman BF, Danilo P, Lovelace E, Knoebel SB: Can accelerated AV junctional escape rhythms be explained by delayed afterdepolarizations? *Am J Cardiol* 1980; 45:1272–1283.
101. Kleeman C, Singh BN: Serum electrolytes and the heart. In: Maxwell MH, Kleeman CR (eds): *Clinical Disorders of Fluid and Electrolyte Metabolism.* New York, McGraw-Hill, 1979: 166.
102. Davis WH, Ziady F: The effect of oral magnesium chloride therapy on the QT_c and QU_c intervals of the electrocardiogram. *S Afr Med J* 1978; 53:591–593.
103. Hoffman BF, Suckling EE: Effect of several cations on transmembrane potentials of cardiac muscle. *Am J Physiol* 1956; 186:317–324.
104. Ternte JV, Davis LD: Effect of calcium concentration on the transmembrane potentials of Purkinje fibers. *Circ Res* 1967; 20:32–44.
105. Seeling MS: Electrocardiographic patterns of magnesium depletion in alcoholic heart disease. *Ann NY Acad Sci* 1969; 162:906–917.
106. Surawicz B, Chlebus H, Massellemi A: Hemodynamic and electrocardiographic effects of hyperpotassemia: Differences in response to slow and rapid increases in concentration of plasma K. *Am Heart J* 1967; 73:647–664.
107. Seta K, Kleiger R, Hellerstein EF, Lown B, Vitale JJ: Effect of potassium and magnesium deficiency on the electrocardiogram and plasma electrolytes of pure bred beagles. *Am J Cardiol* 1966; 17:516–519.
108. Smith PK, Winkler AW, Hoff HE: Electrocardiographic changes and concentration of magnesium in serum following intravenous injection of magnesium salts. *Am J Physiol* 1939; 126:720–730.
109. Hoh DW, Goulding R: Magnesium depletion and digoxin toxicity. *Br Med J* 1975; 1:627–628.
110. Beller GA, Hood WB Jr, Smith TW, Abelmann WH, Wacker WES: Correlation of serum magnesium levels and cardiac digitalis intoxication. *Am J Cardiol* 1975; 33:225–229.

111. Iseri LT: Magnesium in coronary artery disease. *Drugs* 1984; 28(suppl 1):151–160.
112. Jackman WM, Szabo B, Friday K, Margolis PD, Moulton K, Wang X, et al: Ventricular tachyarrhythmias related to early after depolarizations and triggered firing: Relation to QT interval prolongation and potential therapeutic role for calcium channel blocking agents. *J Cardiovasc Electrophysiol* 1990; 1:170–195.
113. Cranefield PF: Action potentials, after potentials, and arrhythmias. *Circ Res* 1977; 41:415–423.
114. Bailie DS, Inure H, Kaseda S, Ben-David J, Zipes DP: Magnesium suppression of early after depolarizations and ventricular tachyarrhythmias induced by cesium in dogs. *Circulation* 1988; 77:1395–1402.
115. Swaminathan R, Morgan DB, Ionescu M, Hill GL: Hypophosphatemia and its consequences in patients following open heart surgery. *Anaesthesia* 1978; 33:601–605.
116. Fuller TJ, Nichols WW, Brenner BJ, Peterson JC: Reversible depression in myocardial performance in dogs with experimental phosphorus deficiency. *J Clin Invest* 1978; 62:1194–1200.
117. O'Connor LR, Wheeler WS, Bethune JE: Effect of hypophosphatemia of myocardial performance in man. *N Engl J Med* 1977; 297:901–903.
118. Rector WG, Jarzobski JA, Levin HS: Sinus node dysfunction associated with lithium therapy: Report of a case and a review of the literature. *Nebr Med J* 1979; 64:193–196.
119. Tilkian AG, Schroeder JS, Kao J, Hultgren H: Effect of lithium on cardiovascular performance: Report on extended ambulatory monitoring and exercise testing before and during lithium therapy. *Am J Cardiol* 1976; 38:701–708.
120. Wellens HJ, Cats VM, Duren DR: Symptomatic sinus node abnormalities following lithium carbonate therapy. *Am J Med* 1974; 59:285–287.
121. Carmeliet EE: Influence of lithium ions on the transmembrane potential and cation content of cardiac cells. *J Gen Physiol* 1964; 47:501–530.

Chapter 38

Antiarrhythmic Drugs

Raymond L. Woosley, M.D., Ph.D.

Modern antiarrhythmic agents have the potential to extend and improve life for many patients with cardiovascular disease. However, for many their usefulness has been limited by ineffectiveness and/or toxicity. Care must be taken, therefore, in deciding the mode of treatment, or in fact whether or not to treat at all. Many antiarrhythmic agents are available today, and still more are under development; however, this abundance shows that no single agent is effective for all patients and that every agent has the potential for inducing serious adverse effects.

Since all of the currently available drugs have generally similar efficacy in a given patient population, drug selection is often empiric. The side-effect profiles of the available drugs are very different, however, and are often the determining factor in drug selection. Side effects may completely eliminate the use of certain classes of drugs for a specific patient. Because of the narrow margin between effective and potentially toxic dosages, it is essential that physicians be thoroughly familiar with the pharmacology, dosage, and adverse effect profile of any of these agents that they choose to prescribe.

The use of antiarrhythmic drugs has been dramatically altered by the findings of the Cardiac Arrhythmia Suppression Trial (CAST).[1] This study was designed to test the hypothesis that suppression of asymptomatic ventricular arrhythmias in patients with recent myocardial infarction will reduce mortality from cardiac arrest and/or arrhythmic sudden death. Prior to the CAST, it had become common practice to prescribe antiarrhythmic drugs for these patients in the hope that suppression of the risk factor, the arrhythmia, would lead to improved mortality. Based on the results of the Cardiac Arrhythmia Pilot Study (CAPS), a feasibility and planning trial, the CAST evaluated encainide, flecainide, and moricizine because they were all tolerated and had reasonable ability to suppress asymptomatic ventricular arrhythmias. In April 1989, the CAST was interrupted by the Data Safety and Monitoring Committee, and encainide and flecainide were removed because they were found to increase mortality two to threefold in patients whose arrhythmias had been effectively suppressed. The CAST II continued to evaluate the remaining drug, moricizine. The CAST II was finally terminated prematurely in August 1991 when it became apparent that moricizine was producing a similar trend toward harm and there was no reasonable chance that a beneficial effect on mortality could be detected. These results shocked the medical community but have influenced thinking in this and many other areas of medicine. Hine et al.[2] reported a metaanalysis of the CAST and similar studies with sodium channel-blocking drugs and found overall support for the conclusion of the CAST. The CAST has also led to recommendations by the Food and Drug Administration for more restrictive labeling for all antiarrhythmic drugs. In 1991, these drugs were given class labeling with indications for the treatment of documented ventricular arrhythmias that, in the judgment of the physician, are life threatening. The only exceptions are quinidine and flecainide, both of which have an indication for supraventricular arrhythmias.

CLASSIFICATION OF ANTIARRHYTHMIC DRUGS

Antiarrhythmic drugs are often classified according to their electrophysiological effects.[3] The most often described scheme, that of Vaughan Williams, was originally proposed as a classification of drug *actions* that should be antiarrhythmic, not a classification of drugs. This is a subtle but important distinction that is made for the following reasons:

- Most antiarrhythmic drugs have multiple actions, hence their pharmacology is more complex than indicated by a simple drug classification scheme.
- The actions of a given drug may differ in different tissues.
- Many antiarrhythmic agents have pharmacologically active metabolites whose activity may be quite different and in a class other than that of the parent compound.
- Production of these metabolites is genetically determined in some cases and often varies extensively within the population.

Drugs having *class I action* possess "local anesthetic" or "membrane-stabilizing" activity. Their predominant action is to block the fast inward sodium channel. This produces a decrease in the maximum depolarization rate ($\dot{V}_{max}$) of the action potential (phase 0) and slows intracardiac conduction. These agents can be further subclassified as belonging to class IA, IB, or IC on the basis of their effects on specific aspects of intracardiac conduction and refractoriness. Drugs having class IA action include quinidine, procainamide, and disopyramide. These agents also produce measurable increases in ventricular refractoriness and QT interval. Lidocaine, mexiletine, and tocainide have actions belonging to class IB. Their potency for blocking sodium channels is only moderate, and in isolated tissues, they shorten the action potential duration (APD) and refractoriness. They generally exert little effect on PR, QRS, or QT intervals. Drugs with class IC actions are the newer, more potent agents: flecainide, encainide, propafenone, and indecainide. Because these are potent sodium channel inhibitors, slowing conduction velocity while having little effect on repolarization, they increase the PR and QRS intervals but cause little change in QT.

Class II action refers to beta-adrenergic antagonism, possessed by agents such as propranolol, timolol, and metoprolol. While these drugs are effective for treatment of supraventricular arrhythmias and tachyarrhythmias secondary to excessive sympathetic activity, they are not very effective in the treatment of severe arrhythmias, such as recurrent ventricular tachycardia. Although the mechanism is unknown, they are the only drugs found effective in preventing sudden cardiac death in patients with prior myocardial infarction.

Drugs whose predominant effect is to prolong the duration of the cardiac action potential and refractoriness have *class III action.* Amiodarone, sotalol, bretylium, and *N*-acetylprocainamide (NAPA), a metabolite of procainamide, have class III action.

Class IV action is calcium channel antagonism. Drugs with this action include verapamil, diltiazem, nicardipine, and nifedipine.

Because of the many limitations of the Vaughan Williams classification of antiarrhythmic drugs, a new approach has been proposed.[4] The new classification system is based on the differential effects of antiarrhythmic drugs on (1) channels, (2) receptors, and (3) transmembrane pumps. The grouping is based first primarily on the drug's *predominant action* and second on the other actions that may be clinically relevant. As shown in Fig. 38-1, the primary actions are aligned diagonally. For example, in this system quinidine is a *sodium channel antagonist (moderate time constant for recovery) with potassium channel- and alpha-blocking activity.* This provides a more complete and accurate description of the pharmacologic actions of the drugs. When combined with an understanding of the electrophysiological role of these actions, one can predict the effects likely to occur in vivo. In this case one would expect conduction slowing, increased APD (and refractoriness), and vasodilation to result from these three actions of quinidine.

The new system creates a framework in which newly discovered actions of drugs can be readily added. It also emphasizes the multiple actions of drugs and the subtle differences and similarities that exist. It is more complex than the simple grouping of drugs in the Vaughan Williams classification. At present, our understanding of the pharmacology of these drugs has progressed to the point that the Vaughan Williams "short hand" is an oversimplification that can be misleading. The increased complexity of the new system reflects the current state of our knowledge at a level necessary for optimal use of these drugs. Unfortunately, we can no longer afford the convenience of the Vaughan Williams system as we attempt to understand and apply these drugs clinically.

Due to the low efficacy of any one agent, the treatment of acute or chronic ventricular arrhythmias frequently necessitates the use of multiple drugs, singly or in combination. One may produce increased sodium channel blockade and, hopefully, increase drug efficacy by using combinations of drugs with different kinetics of interaction with the sodium channel. Basic to these considerations is an understanding of the regulation of sodium channel function. Hodgkin and Huxley[5] proposed that sodium channels exist in three distinct states: open, closed, and inactivated. According to the modulated receptor theory (MRT) of cardiac sodium channel regulation proposed by Hille and Hondeghem and Katzung, sodium channels in each of these states have differing affinities for a given local anesthetic drug (Fig. 38-2).[6] Using these concepts, Hondeghem and Katzung[6] suggested that combining a drug such as lidocaine (which interacts predominantly with the inactivated sodium channel) with a drug such as quinidine or procainamide (which interact with the activated sodium channel) should provide synergistic blockade of sodium channels.[7] This has become the basis for many effective combinations in patients with arrhythmias.

Frequency dependence (use dependence) of antiarrhythmic drug action describes the increase in conduction block observed at increasing rate of stimulation in response to sodium channel-blocking antiarrhythmic agents. The MRT provides a potential explanation for this phenomenon. Since an increase in the rate of stimulation increases the number of sodium channels in the open and inactivated states, antiarrhythmic agents having greater affinity for activated (open) or inactivated channels (as opposed to rested channels) would have a greater opportunity to bind to the receptor and slow conduction. Therefore, greater block will occur during tachycardia,

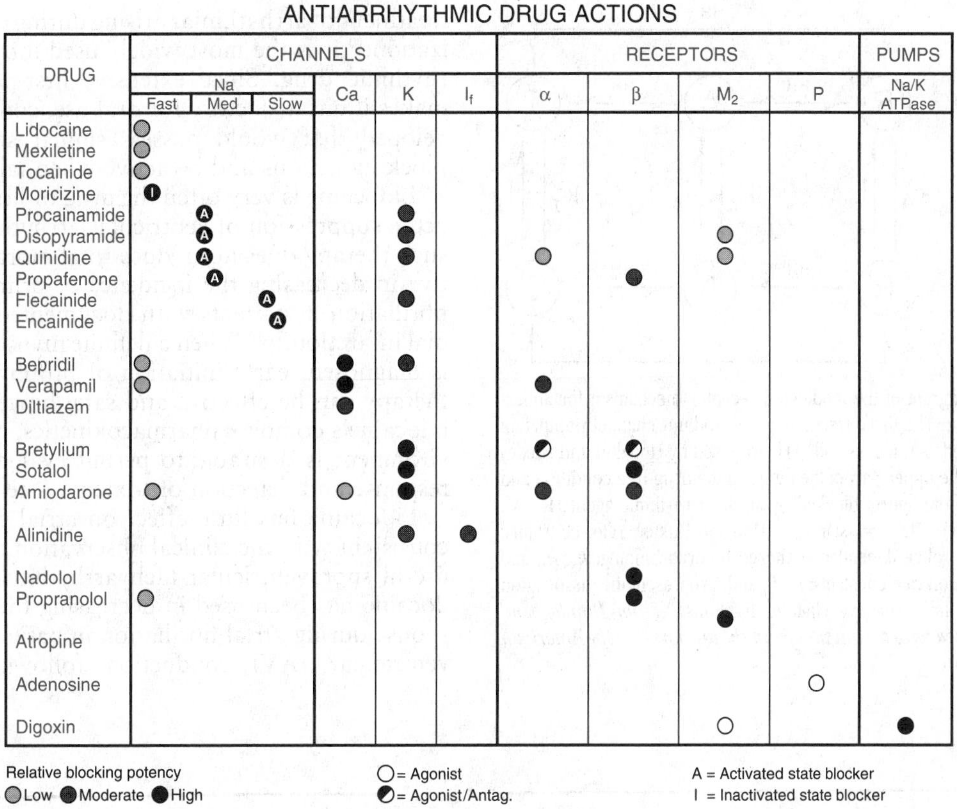

ANTIARRHYTHMIC DRUG ACTIONS

DRUG	CHANNELS						RECEPTORS				PUMPS
	Na			Ca	K	I_f	α	β	M_2	P	Na/K ATPase
	Fast	Med	Slow								
Lidocaine	Low										
Mexiletine	Low										
Tocainide	Low										
Moricizine	High (I)										
Procainamide		High (A)			Moderate						
Disopyramide		High (A)			Moderate				Low		
Quinidine		High (A)			Moderate		Low		Low		
Propafenone		High (A)						Moderate			
Flecainide			High (A)		Moderate						
Encainide			High (A)								
Bepridil	Low			High	Moderate						
Verapamil	Low			High			Moderate				
Diltiazem				Moderate							
Bretylium					High		Agonist/Antag.	Agonist/Antag.			
Sotalol					High			High			
Amiodarone	Low			Low	High		Moderate	Moderate			
Alinidine					Moderate	Moderate					
Nadolol								High			
Propranolol	Low							High			
Atropine									High		
Adenosine										Agonist	
Digoxin									Agonist		High

Relative blocking potency: Low, Moderate, High

○ = Agonist
◐ = Agonist/Antag.

A = Activated state blocker
I = Inactivated state blocker

FIGURE 38-1 Summary of the potentially most important actions of drugs on membrane channels, receptors, and ionic pumps in the heart. Included are examples of drugs used to modify cardiac rhythm. Most are already marketed as antiarrhythmic agents, but some are not yet approved for this purpose. The drugs (rows) are ordered in a fashion similar to the columns so that generally the entries for their predominant action(s) form a diagonal. Drugs with multiple actions (e.g., amiodarone) depart strikely from the diagonal trend. The actions of drugs on the sodium, calcium, potassium (I_K), and I_f channels are indicated. Sodium channel blockade is subdivided into three groups of actions characterized by fast (<300 ms), medium (Med)(200–1500 ms), and slow (>1500 ms) time constants for recovery from block. This parameter is a measure of use dependence and predicts the likelihood that a drug will decrease conduction velocity of normal sodium-dependent tissues in the heart and perhaps the propensity of a drug for causing bundle branch block or proarrhythmia. The rate constant for onset of block might be even more clinically relevant. Blockade in the inactivated (I) or activated (A) state is indicated. Information on the state dependency of the block caused by moricizine, propafenone, encainide, and flecainide is especially limited and may be altered with additional research. Drug interaction with receptors (α and β adrenergic, muscarinic subtype [M_2], and A_1 purinergic [P]) and drug effects on the sodium/potassium pump (Na/K, ATPase) are indicated. Filled circles indicate antagonist or inhibitory actions; unfilled circles indicate direct or indirect acting agonists or stimulators. The darkness of the symbol increases with the intensity of the action. Half-filled circles for bretylium indicate its biphasic action to initially stimulate α and β receptors by release of norepinephrine followed by subsequent block of norepinephrine release and indirect antagonism of these receptors. (*From Task Force of the Working Group on Arrhythmias of the European Society of Cardiology: The Sicilian gambit: A new approach to the classification of antiarrhythmic drugs based on their actions on arrhythmogenic mechanisms. Circulation 84:1831, 1991. Reproduced with permission of the American Heart Association.*)

leaving less drug action at normal heart rates. Also, antiarrhythmic drugs have different affinities for the sodium channel, and this is manifested as different rates for onset or recovery from block. Drugs that slowly associate with the receptor will cause block to accumulate over the first few stimulated beats, such as shown for procainamide in Fig. 38-3. Drugs that associate more rapidly, such as lidocaine, produce little additional block after the first beat in a train of stimuli. This is compared to procainamide in Fig. 38-3. Likewise, drugs dissociate from the sodium channel at different rates, leading to differences in rates of recovery from block. The rate of onset of block of sodium channels has been proposed as a means to subclassify antiarrhythmic drugs.[8] This is the correlate of the subclassification of sodium channel blockers proposed by Harrison and based on differences in clinical effects of the drugs.[9]

This chapter provides a review of the clinical pharmacology and applications of the currently available antiarrhythmic drugs, excluding digoxin, beta receptor antagonists, and calcium channel blockers that are addressed in other chapters. The drugs appear in the same order as listed in Fig. 38-1, the new classification system. The pharmacokinetics, usual dosages, and plasma concentration ranges for the major drugs are listed in Tables 38-1 and 38-2.

LIDOCAINE (Xylocaine)

Clinical Applications

Lidocaine was introduced as a local anesthetic and was first used as an antiarrhythmic agent in the 1950s for the

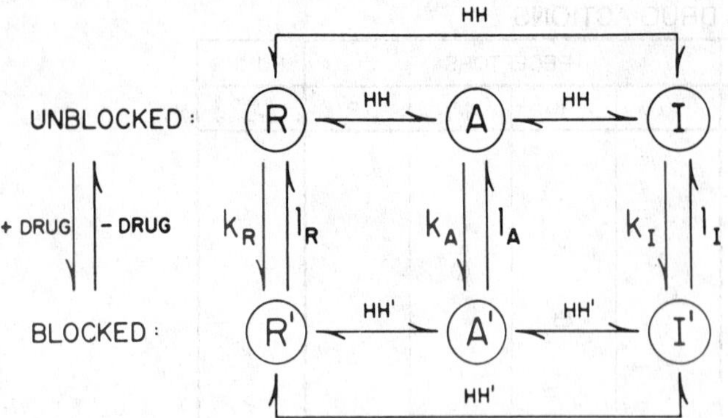

FIGURE 38-2 Diagram of the modulated receptor mechanism for antiarrhythmic drug action. The three fractions of the sodium channel population [rested (R), activated (A), inactivated (I)] proposed by Hodgkin and Huxley are represented in the upper part of the figure in the drug-free condition and in the lower part of the figure, blocked by an antiarrhythmic agent (R′, A′, and I′, respectively). HH = standard Hodgkin-Huxley rate constants; HH′ = same, with voltge dependence altered by drug binding; k_R, k_A, and k_I represent association rate constants; l_R, l_A, and l_I represent the dissociation rate constants for the respective channel fractions. (*From Hondeghem, Katzung.*[6] *Reproduced with permission from the authors and the American Heart Association.*)

treatment of arrhythmias arising during cardiac catheterization.[10] It is the most widely used intravenous antiarrhythmic drug. Since extensive first-pass metabolism makes it unsatisfactory for oral use, congeners were developed that would possess similar sodium channel-blocking actions and be active when taken orally.

Lidocaine is very often the drug of first choice for the acute suppression of ventricular arrhythmias. Although such therapy does not reduce total mortality, it is effective in decreasing the incidence of primary ventricular fibrillation in patients with documented acute myocardial infarction.[11,12] When a definite myocardial infarction is diagnosed, early initiation of prophylactic lidocaine therapy can be effective and safe; however, because of lidocaine's complex pharmacokinetics, a monitored environment is desirable to permit evaluation of patient response and detection of toxicity. (See Chap. 60.)

Lidocaine has little effect on atrial tissue in vitro,[13] consistent with the clinical observation that it is of little use in supraventricular tachyarrhythmias. Although lidocaine has been used in decreasing the ventricular response during atrial fibrillation in patients whose atrioventricular (AV) conduction follows an accessory

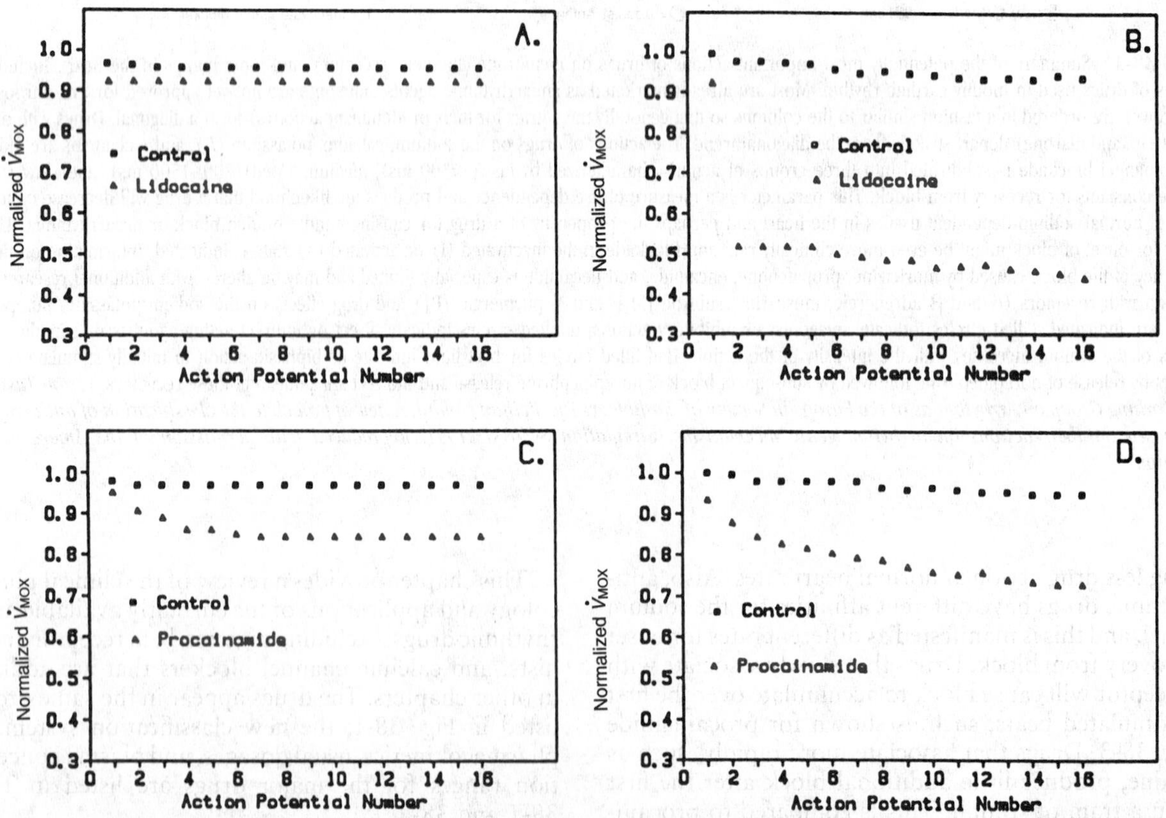

FIGURE 38-3 Rate- (interval-) dependent depression of $\dot{V}_{max}$ by lidocaine and procainamide. Following a 20-s rest period, a train of 16 action potentials were elicited using interstimulus intervals (ISIs) of 1 s or 200 ms, in the presence (triangles) or absence (squares) of lidocaine or procainamide. For the duration of the train $\dot{V}_{max}$ was relatively constant when measured at either ISI in the absence of drug. In the presence of lidocaine (22 μ*M*), stimulation at an ISI of 1 s (*A*) produced no use-dependent block. However, stimulation at 200 ms (*B*) produced a 50 percent reduction in $\dot{V}_{max}$ from baseline, which was first observed for the second action potentials and was constant thereafter. A different pattern is seen in the presence of 276 μ*M* procainamide, which produced a significant depression of $\dot{V}_{max}$ at an ISI of 1 s (*C*). This depression was more pronounced when the ISI was shortened to 200 ms (*D*). Unlike the case for lidocaine, the use-dependent depression of $\dot{V}_{max}$ due to procainamide required multiple action potentials to approach steady-state values. (*From GR Ehring, JW Moyer, LM Hondeghem: Quantitative structure activity studies of antiarrhythmic properties in a series of lidocaine and procainamide derivatives. J Pharmacol Exp Ther 244:479–492, 1989. Reproduced with permission from the authors and publisher.*)

TABLE 38-1

Pharmacokinetics of Antiarrhythmic Drugs

Agent	Inactivation or Elimination* (%)	Protein Binding (%)	V_D (liters/kg)	Elimination Half-life (h)	Bioavailability (%)	Apparent Oral Clearance (mL/min)
Quinidine	Hepatic (50–90) Renal (10–30)	80–90	2.5	3–19	70	200–400
Procainamide	Hepatic (40–70)† Renal (30–60)	15	2	2–4	100	400–700
Disopyramide	Hepatic (20–30) Renal (40–50)	20–50	0.6	6–8	80–90	90
Lidocaine	Hepatic (90)	40–70	1.1	1.5–4	35‡	700–1000‡
Tocainide	Hepatic (30–40) Renal (40)	10	1.5–3	8–20	90	150–200
Mexiletine	Hepatic (85–90)† Renal (10–15)	70	5.5–9.5	8–20	90	400–700
Flecainide	Hepatic (70)† Renal (30)	40	7–10	7–26	90–95	200–800
Propafenone	Hepatic (99)†	90	3–4	2–24†	10–50†	800–5000†
Amiodarone	Hepatic (99)	95	20–200	13–103 days	20–80	6500–11,000
Bretylium	Renal (90)	Low	3–4	4–16	25‡	1300

*Renal—elimination of unchanged drug.
†Dependent on metabolic phenotype (see text).
‡Not recommended for oral administration.

TABLE 38-2

Dosage and Plasma Concentration Ranges for Antiarrhythmic Agents*

Agent	Usual Initial Dosage†	Modification of Dosage in Disease‡	Dosage Range	Maximum Single Dose	Therapeutic Range§ (μg/mL)
Quinidine (sulfate)	200 mg q 6 h	None	800–2400 mg/day	600	0.7–5
Procainamide (sustained release)	500 mg q 6 h	↓ CHF ↓ RI	2000–6000 mg/day	1500	4–8
Disopyramide	100 mg q 6 h	↓ CHF ↓ HI ↓ RI	300–1200 mg/day	300	2–5
Lidocaine	See text	↓ CHF ↓ HI	1–4 mg/min IV	—	1.5–5
Tocainide	400 mg q 8 h	↓ HI ↓ RI	1200–2400 mg/day	800	4–10
Mexiletine	200 mg q 8 h	↓ CHF ↓ HI?	600–1200 mg/day	400	0.7–2
Flecainide	100 mg q 12 h	↓ CHF ↓ RI ↓ HI?	200–400 mg/day	200	0.2–1
Encainide	25 mg q 8 h	↓ RI	75–200 mg/day	75	—
Propafenone	150 mg q 8 h	See text	300–900 mg/day	300	0.5–3?
Amiodarone	600–1400 mg/day (load)	None	200–600 mg/day	600	1–2
Bretylium	See text	↓ RI	1–4 mg/min IV	—	—

*These are general guidelines only. Dosage should be determined for each patient based on clinical presentation, disease states, clinical response, and tolerance to the drug.
†Dosage usually recommended in absence of significant cardiac, renal, or hepatic failure.
‡CHF, congestive heart failure; HI, hepatic insufficiency; RI, renal insufficiency. See text for details.
§The range of therapeutic plasma concentrations is a statistical range that should be considered only a guideline to therapy.

pathway,[14,15] some workers have reported accelerated conduction,[16] and other drugs such as procainamide are probably preferred in this situation.

Mechanism of Action

In concentrations similar to those attained during clinical use, lidocaine reduces $\dot{V}_{max}$ and produces shortening or no change in APD and effective refractory period (ERP) of normal Purkinje fibers. This contrasts with quinidine and procainamide, which additionally block potassium channels and produce *lengthening* of APD.[17,18] Lidocaine has little effect on the electrophysiology of the normal conduction system. Studies on the effect of lidocaine in patients with conduction system abnormalities have produced variable results. Some studies have failed to detect significant changes in conduction,[19,20] while others have found slowing of ventricular rate or potentiation of infranodal block in patients with conduction system defects.[21,22] Variability in dosage and pharmacokinetics may explain some of these discrepancies.

Clinical Pharmacology

Orally administered lidocaine is well absorbed, but it has poor oral bioavailability because it undergoes extensive first-pass hepatic metabolism. Lidocaine clearance is well approximated by measurement of liver blood flow.[23,24] The deethylated metabolites, which are excreted by the kidneys, have less antiarrhythmic potency than the parent drug and may contribute to the production of central nervous system (CNS) side effects occurring with lidocaine.[25,26]

Following intravenous administration, lidocaine disposition is well represented by a two-compartment pharmacokinetic model.[27] Since antiarrhythmic activity is correlated with lidocaine's concentration in the central compartment and the half-life of distribution out of this compartment is rapid (8 min), regimens employing a series of multiple loading and maintenance infusions should be used to achieve quickly and then maintain a therapeutic plasma and myocardial lidocaine concentration.

Regardless of the loading regimen employed, the lidocaine concentration eventually reached at steady state will be dependent on only drug infusion rate and clearance. The time required to reach steady-state conditions is approximately 8 to 10 h in normal individuals and up to 20 to 24 h in some patients with heart failure and/or liver disease. This is longer than often anticipated because of the failure to recognize the relatively long *elimination* half-life of 1.5 to 2 h in normal subjects and even longer in patients with heart failure or hepatic disease.

Dosage and Administration

Lidocaine's primary use as an antiarrhythmic agent is for the acute suppression of rhythm disturbances. Obviously, under these circumstances a prompt effect is desirable. Single intravenous boluses will achieve only transient therapeutic effects because the drug is rapidly distributed out of the plasma and myocardium; therefore, multiple loading doses should be used in order to rapidly achieve more sustained therapeutic plasma levels of lidocaine. Based on pharmacokinetic analyses and clinical studies, several regimens have been designed to maintain a relatively constant therapeutic level. For a stable patient, a total loading dose of lidocaine is approximately 3 to 4 mg per kilogram of body weight administered over 20 to 30 min. After an initial dose of 1 mg/kg over 2 min, a series of three loading "boluses" should be administered slowly (50 mg each over 2 min) 8 min apart, while the patient is continuously observed for the development of side effects. Loading should be stopped should these occur.

One effective and well-tolerated loading regimen was outlined by Wyman et al.[28] For a 75-kg person, an initial bolus of 75 mg was given followed by 50 mg every 5 min to a total dose of 225 mg. This regimen usually achieves and maintains plasma concentrations within usual therapeutic guidelines (1.5 to 5 μg/mL). A priming dose of 75 mg followed by a loading infusion of 150 mg over 18 min has also been successfully used.[29] At the time of initiation of the loading regimen, a maintenance infusion, designed to replace ongoing losses due to drug elimination, should be started. This may be calculated as the product of the desired plasma concentration (about 3 μg/mL) times the expected clearance (usually yielding a dosage in the range of 20 to 60 μg per kilogram of body weight per minute).

Even among normal individuals there is tremendous variability in the calculated size of the central compartment for lidocaine and, consequently, in the peak plasma concentration. Therefore, during loading, the patient's electrocardiogram (ECG), blood pressure, and mental status should be monitored; the process should be stopped at the first sign of lidocaine excess. When symptomatic arrhythmias persist in the presence of documented adequate dosage (side effects present or plasma concentration in excess of 7μg/mL), another agent should be used.

If the maintenance infusion has reached steady state but is too low, so that arrhythmia reappears (side effects being absent), the appropriate action is (1) obtain a plasma sample for measurement of lidocaine concentration for future reference (if the patient's clinical condition permits), (2) administer a small bolus of lidocaine (25 to 50 mg), and (3) increase the maintenance infusion rate proportionally. The plasma concentration can be used to estimate clearance for calculation of the final maintenance infusion (i.e., clearance equals infusion rate divided by plasma concentration at steady state).

Little therapeutic effect is evident at lidocaine plasma concentrations below 1.5 μg/mL while the risk of toxicity increases at concentrations above 5 μg/mL. In some patients, however, concentrations in the range of 5 to 9 μg/mL may be required for arrhythmia suppression and can safely be achieved with cautious drug administration.[30]

Lidocaine infusions are often terminated by a practice of "tapering," based on the misconception that lidocaine is eliminated very rapidly. The rapid dissipation of lidocaine's effects following an intravenous bolus is due to distribution, however, not elimination. Simply terminating a lidocaine infusion once steady-state conditions have been achieved will result in a gradual decline in plasma levels over the next 8 to 10 h as elimination occurs. Not only is there no reason to taper lidocaine infusions, but it may be dangerous if oral antiarrhythmic therapy is initiated. Tapering in this case prolongs the period during which unpredictable additive effects may occur between lidocaine and newly started oral therapy. Likewise, tapering makes it difficult, if not impossible, to estimate when lidocaine levels have fallen below the range expected to be effective, a useful and practical application of pharmacokinetic principles.

If a patient has reached steady state-equilibrium, it is possible to estimate when the plasma lidocaine concentration will fall below usually therapeutic levels. The plasma lidocaine concentration should be determined at the time the infusion is terminated, and the number of half-lives needed for that level to reach approximately 1.5 μg/mL are estimated from the following equation:

$$t_{1/2} = \frac{\text{plasma concentration} \times V_D \times 0.693}{\text{infusion rate}}$$

Plasma concentration and infusion are known components of the equation. The volume of distribution (V_D) is usually 1.1 liters/kg but may be reduced by half in heart failure.

Prophylactic intramuscular injections of large doses of lidocaine by paramedical personnel for patients who have suspected myocardial infarction has been, and still is, the subject of controversy. This approach has been used in prehospital care, but the resultant plasma concentrations are generally variable and at the low end of the usual therapeutic range. One study demonstrated an apparent beneficial effect of lidocaine (400 mg) on the incidence of fibrillation when administered by paramedical personnel upon reaching possible myocardial infarction victims out of hospital.[31] Plasma levels from 369 patients were measured 11 to 20 min after injection and were found to average 3 μg/mL (304 patients had levels above 2 μg/mL). On the other hand, a pooled analysis of all trials of lidocaine in acute myocardial infarction indicated that lidocaine administration did not improve the overall mortality.[12]

Modification of Dosage in Disease States

Initial loading regimens require no adjustment in patients with renal or liver disease[27]; however, maintenance infusions must be decreased in liver disease and heart failure to compensate for decreased clearance. Since clearance alone is altered in liver disease with little change in the volume of distribution, the half-life of elimination is prolonged greatly (to almost 5 h) and steady-state conditions will not be achieved until 20 to 25 h following the institution of an intravenous infusion. Despite the fact that lidocaine metabolites are excreted by the kidneys, renal disease has not been reported to exert any significant effect on lidocaine dosing regimens.

In patients undergoing mechanical ventilation, there is a decrease in cardiac output and hepatic blood flow. Since lidocaine is extensively metabolized by the liver and clearance is influenced by liver blood flow, a decrease in its elimination is seen under these conditions; however, the clinical relevance of such a decrease is difficult to predict.[32]

Patients with congestive heart failure achieve lidocaine levels that are almost double those in normal individuals given the same dose. Not only is their volume of distribution for lidocaine significantly reduced, but a fall in cardiac output results in reduction in liver blood flow and lidocaine clearance.[27] Since the central volume of distribution is generally halved, loading doses should be reduced by 50 percent; since clearance is approximately halved, maintenance doses should be reduced proportionately from an infusion rate of 30 μg per kilogram of body weight per minute used for normal patients to about half that figure. The time required to achieve steady-state conditions following the institution of a maintenance infusion is still 8 to 10 h in many patients because of concomitant changes in V_D and a clearance leaving half-life similar to that seen in patients without heart failure.

These are general recommendations for initial lidocaine dosage selection; they should be adjusted for each patient based on clinical presentation, clinical response, and the results of plasma level monitoring. Even patients without complicating disease states will still have highly variable pharmacokinetics and response to lidocaine. Some patients with congestive heart failure may experience toxicity when given an infusion of 0.5 mg/mL. Therefore, blood level monitoring is essential for proper dosage adjustment.

In post–myocardial infarction patients receiving lidocaine infusions for more than 24 h, plasma lidocaine levels can increase and the elimination phase half-life can increase up to 50 percent.[33] This increase is due, in part, to changes occurring in protein binding of lidocaine during the first few days of therapy. Patients should be monitored and evaluated carefully. Assays for plasma lidocaine measure the sum of both protein-bound and free lidocaine as total lidocaine and thus do not give a true picture of the amount of free drug available. An increase in plasma lidocaine occurring at this time often reflects an elevation in plasma levels of alpha-1-acid glycoprotein (AAG) to which it binds[34] and does not always indicate an increase in free, active drug. In this case, the lidocaine dosage should not be reduced to compensate for the higher total plasma concentration as long as the patient displays no adverse effects. Subsequent decreases in AAG concentrations will result in an apparent decrease in plasma lidocaine, which may reflect a drop in only that fraction bound to AAG.

Adverse Reactions

Central nervous system symptoms are the most frequent side effects during lidocaine administration. If a bolus of lidocaine is administered very rapidly, seizures are likely to occur. With more gradual attainment of excessive plasma levels, symptoms are usually limited to drowsiness, dysarthria, and dysesthesia.

Excessive lidocaine can also cause coma and should enter into the differential diagnosis of postcardiac arrest encephalopathy. Excessive dosages of lidocaine can also depress cardiac function, which leads to decreased lidocaine clearance and an even greater increase in lidocaine concentrations—a vicious cycle.

The potential for advanced degrees of sinus node dysfunction has been reported in isolated instances.[35,36] Little data are available on the effects of lidocaine administration to patients with conduction system disturbances acquired during acute myocardial infarction. In this group, particularly in those with conduction abnormalities below the AV node, lidocaine should be administered cautiously, if at all, unless a temporary pacemaker is inserted.

Drug Interactions

An additive or synergistic depression of myocardial function or conduction may occur during combined therapy using lidocaine with other antiarrhythmic agents.[37] The possiblity of such an interaction should be considered during a patient's conversion from lidocaine to another antiarrhythmic agent.

A pharmacokinetic drug interaction between propranolol and lidocaine has been described experimentally in which beta-adrenergic blockade caused a decrease in cardiac output and liver blood flow. As a result, lidocaine clearance was reduced and lidocaine plasma concentrations were subsequently increased.[38] This phenomenon has been verified in humans.[39]

Cimetidine has been reported to decrease lidocaine's volume of distribution, decrease splanchnic (and hence liver) blood flow, and inhibit the enzymes responsible for lidocaine metabolism. All three effects serve to raise lidocaine plasma concentrations, and both loading and maintenance dosages may require downward adjustment in patients receiving cimetidine.[40] A recent study found less marked increases in total lidocaine over 24 h than had been previously reported and suggested that empiric dosage reductions of lidocaine in patients receiving cimetidine may not be appropriate.[41] Another study examining the effect of cimetidine on lidocaine pharmacokinetics found that lidocaine clearance under steady-state conditions was 34 percent lower than under single-dose conditions, but the effects of cimetidine on lidocaine disposition were similar under both circumstances.[42] A study of rifampicin-lidocaine interaction in animals has reported an increase in the total plasma concentration of lidocaine, reflecting a rifampicin-induced increase in AAG, accompanied by a fall in the percentage of free lidocaine from 50 to 30 percent. The net result, however, was little change in either free plasma concentration or pharmacologic effect.[43] (See also Chap. 109.)

Therapeutic interactions using lidocaine in synergistic combination with other antiarrhythmic agents such as quinidine or encainide have only been investigated in vitro or in small clinical studies.[6,7,44] The treatment of acute and chronic ventricular arrhythmias frequently necessitates combination therapy due to the low efficacy of single agents. Combination therapy using drugs with differing kinetics of sodium channel interaction should produce increased sodium channel blockade and, possibly, increased drug efficacy.

MEXILETINE (Mexitil)

Clinical Applications

Mexiletine is used in the treatment of ventricular arrhythmias, and has, on occasion, been effective in treating arrhythmias that were refractory to several other agents. Such studies have provided conflicting results, however, with success rates between 6 and 60 percent; and more than half of the studies suggest limited efficacy (less than 20 percent).[45] Mexiletine does not prolong the QT interval; therefore, it is useful in patients having a history of torsades de pointes or long QT syndrome, for whom quinidine, procainamide, or disopyramide are contraindicated. While the rate of response to mexiletine when used alone is low, it has been combined successfully with quinidine,[45] propranolol,[46] or procainamide.[47] This mode of therapy takes advantage of the additive, and perhaps synergistic, antiarrhythmic response produced by the combination of these agents. Lower than usual dosages of both agents can be used so that dosage-related adverse effects are reduced concomitantly.

Description

Mexiletine is an orally active lidocaine congener with class IB sodium channel-blocking activity and structural similarity to tocainide. It was originally developed as an anorexiant and anticonvulsant agent whose antiarrhythmic properties were only later recognized. Mexiletine exerts minimal effects on both hemodynamics and myocardial contractility, even in patients with severe congestive heart failure.[48]

Mechanism of Action

While mexiletine is twice as potent as tocainide, the drugs are very similar overall, with similar clinical efficacy. Both are classified as antiarrhythmic agents with type IB action. They block fast sodium channels, decreasing the maximal rate of depolarization ($\dot{V}_{max}$) and shortening the repolarization phase of ventricular myocardium.[49,50] Like lidocaine, the effects of mexiletine appear to be rate dependent and more noticeable in hypoxic tissue, although mexiletine has greater effect at slower pacing rates than does lidocaine.[51] In patients with preexisting impairment of impulse generation and conduction, mexiletine consistently lengthens conduction time between the His bundle and ventricular muscle and therefore may have the potential to produce AV block in such patients.[52] Mexiletine has little effect on the surface ECG. It does not prolong the QT interval and may, in some cases, shorten it. It, like tocainide, produces no clinically apparent effects on calcium-dependent channels or anticholinergic actions.

Clinical Pharmacology

Mexiletine's systemic bioavailability approximates 90 percent.[53] Mexiletine has a large volume of distribution (5.5 to 9.5 liters/kg), which reflects extensive tissue uptake of the drug. About 1 percent of total body content of mexiletine is in the plasma compartment, with approximately 70 percent of this bound to serum proteins. Mexiletine has little first-pass metabolism but is eliminated primarily by hepatic metabolism with only 10 to 15 percent being excreted unchanged in the urine.[54,55] Its half-life of elimination is similar to tocainide's, varying between 8 and 20 h (9 and 12 h for healthy subjects), with the time needed to reach steady state ranging between 1 and 3 days.[56] The most important difference between tocainide and mexiletine is that tocainide is eliminated to a large extent by the kidneys while mexiletine undergoes extensive hepatic metabolism.[54,57] Consequently, mexiletine clearance will be more variable. Like tocainide, mexiletine exists in two enantiomeric forms having different rates of elimination. Differences in antiarrhythmic potencies for *R*- and *S*-mexiletine probably contribute to the wide variability in "effective" mexiletine plasma concentrations. The major metabolites of mexiletine, *para*-hydroxymexiletine (PHM) and hydroxymethylmexiletine (HMM), and their corresponding alcohols appear to have no pharmacologic activity.[56,58] The conversion to PHM and HMM is genetically determined by the activity of $P450_{2D6}$.[59] Therefore, 7 percent of the Caucasian population who lack this enzyme have lower mexiletine clearance and higher plasma mexiletine concentrations.

Dosage and Administration

Mexiletine therapy should be initiated with a low dosage, which is increased at 2- to 3-day intervals until efficacy or intolerable side effects (usually tremor or other CNS symptoms) develop. For the average patient with normal renal function, the recommended initial oral mexiletine dosage is 200 mg every 8 h.

Several factors influence the dosage. First, as with most drugs having extensive liver metabolism, clearance will be widely variable within the population. This is especially true for mexiletine because $P450_{2D6}$, responsible for its metabolism, is missing in 7 percent of the Caucasian population. Second, consideration of dosage adjustment to compensate for the action of agents (discussed below) that induce or inhibit hepatic mexiletine metabolism is required.

Modification of Dosage in Disease States

In general, mexiletine's kinetics is not markedly different in most patients with renal failure,[60] although patients with renal failure who also inherit a deficiency of hepatic $P450_{2D6}$ are likely to have extremely slow elimination for mexiletine. For this reason, patients with renal failure should be given low initial doses. Elimination half-life and clearance may be prolonged by overt congestive heart failure,[61] and dosage reduction is necessary in this instance. Dosage reduction is required for patients with hepatic failure to compensate for reduced mexiletine clearance and impaired elimination.[62]

Adverse Reactions

Most of the adverse reactions to mexiletine are dose-related neurologic symptoms: tremor, visual blurring, dizziness, dysphoria, and nausea. These can sometimes be reduced by administering mexiletine with food to slow absorption. Limited comparative data are available, but mexiletine seems to be less allergenic than tocainide, causing rash less frequently. Thrombocytopenia has been reported to occur infrequently with mexiletine therapy,[63,64] and a positive antinuclear antibody test occurs rarely. Severe bradycardia and abnormal prolongation of sinus node recovery time have been reported in patients with the "sick-sinus" syndrome.[52] At high concentrations, mexiletine has been reported to cause worsening of heart block.[65]

No effect of oral mexiletine was observed on ventricular function even in patients having ejection fractions less than 50 percent,[66] and long-term oral therapy with mexiletine has not been associated with the development of congestive heart failure.[67] Depression of cardiac function after intravenous mexiletine (not available in the United States), however, has been noted in some patients with a history of either pulmonary edema or congestive heart failure.[68]

Drug Interactions

Mexiletine's hepatic metabolism can be induced. Agents such as phenobarbital, phenytoin (Dilantin), or rifampicin will increase clearance and reduce the half-life of mexiletine, possibly reducing an effective does to an ineffective one.[56,58,69] Conversely, if treatment with an inducing agent is stopped, an effective dose may become toxic.

There appears to be no pharmacokinetic interaction between mexiletine and digoxin,[70] and except for a slowing of mexiletine absorption, there is no significant interaction between mexiletine and cimetidine.[71,72] This delay of absorption probably explains the early mistaken impression that cimetidine increased the mexiletine plasma concentration. Concomitant administration of atropine-like drugs, which slow gastric emptying, or antacids has been reported to delay absorption of mexiletine, although bioavailability is not altered.[53] Mexiletine decreased the clearance and increased the plasma concentrations of theophylline in eight normal subjects.[73] Inhibition of *N*-demethylation of theophylline was the proposed mechanism. Quinidine inhibits the $P450_{2D6}$ enzyme partially responsible for mexiletine clearance, and plasma concentration of mexiletine may increase in those individuals who have the enzyme (93 percent of Caucasians). (See also Chap. 109.)

Mexiletine and quinidine have been used in low doses in combination therapy to produce a synergistic or additive antiarrhythmic effect. While both agents block sodium channels, they exert opposite effects on repolarization time.[3,74] Preliminary reports suggest similar results for mexiletine and disopyramide combined therapy.[75]

MORICIZINE (Ethmozine)

Clinical Applications

Moricizine has the structural characteristics of the phenothiazine class of antipsychotic drugs but has modest efficacy as an antiarrhythmic agent. It was first discovered and developed in the former Soviet Union and has been extensively tested in patients with stable or refractory ventricular arrhythmias using ambulatory monitoring and/or exercise testing to determine response to therapy.[76] It has been found to have a relatively high degree of efficacy in these studies and was very well tolerated.[76,77] It was compared to placebo, encainide, flecainide, and imipramine in the Cardiac Arrhythmia Pilot Study[78,79] sponsored by the National Institutes of Health (NIH).

Moricizine was found to be moderately effective (less than encainide and flecainide) in suppressing ventricular ectopy but equally well tolerated. For these reasons it was selected as one of three drugs to be used in the CAST. As discussed earlier, the second phase of the study was terminated prematurely because moricizine was producing a similar trend and had no chance of ever producing a beneficial effect on mortality. Moricizine has had only limited evaluation in the treatment of life-threatening ventricular arrhythmias such as sustained ventricular tachycardia but does not appear to be more effective than other agents with class I activity.[80–82] In preliminary studies it seems to lack any efficacy for supraventricular arrhythmias.

Mechanism of Action

Moricizine has electrophysiological actions similar to several drugs and produces block of sodium channels by predominately binding to the sodium channel while it is in the open and inactivated state.[83,84] Lee and Rosen[84] have compared the electrophysiological effects of moricizine, encainide, and flecainide in canine Purkinje fibers and found moricizine's actions to be a hybrid of characteristics seen with several other drugs with time constants for onset and recovery of block clearly intermediate to those for encainide and lidocaine. It would not be classified as a IC agent in the modified Vaughan Williams system.

Clinical Pharmacology

Moricizine's use is complicated by the formation of active metabolites that require several days for the attainment of steady-state equilibrium. The concept of active metabolites is supported by the observation that while cimetidine blocks elimination of moricizine, there is no increase in pharmacologic effects with the higher moricizine plasma concentrations.[85] The half-life of moricizine in normal volunteers is 3.4 ± 0.5 h and ranges from 0.8 to 4.2 h in patients with cardiac disease. Several days are required for accumulation of maximum drug effects. Specific recommendations for dosage adjustments in patients with cardiac, hepatic, or renal disease are not well established.

Dosage and Administration

The usual range of dosages of moricizine, which has been found effective for suppression of ventricular arrhythmias, is 5 to 15 mg/kg per day. As with other antiarrhythmic agents, its dosage should be titrated carefully with time allowed for attainment of steady-state conditions before any dose increment.

Adverse Reactions

The side-effect profile for moricizine is similar to other antiarrhythmic agents, but the frequency of their occurrence seems to be lower. The CAPS, which comprised patients with relatively well-preserved myocardial function and no other serious disease, provides the only currently available controlled comparison to newer agents.[86,87]

Drug Interactions

Preclinical studies in animals have found that moricizine induces hepatic metabolism of several drugs.[88] For example, moricizine treatment of normal volunteers led to enhanced elimination and a reduction in plasma concentrations of theophylline.[89] Although carefully conducted studies are not available, clinical experience has not detected interactions between moricizine and propranolol or warfarin.[88] Also, there does not appear to be a pharmacokinetic interaction between digoxin and moricizine.[90,91] Yet, coadministration of moricizine and digoxin leads to significant increases in PR intervals, and isolated cases of first-degree AV block and bundle branch block have been reported in patients with cardiac disease.[92] Cimetidine pretreatment caused a 51 percent reduction in moricizine clearance in normal volunteers. There was, however, no evidence of a pharmacodynamic interaction because prolongation of electrocardiographic intervals (PR and QRS) was not altered.[85] This implies that the metabolites of moricizine may be active. Therefore, the potential clinical relevance of a pharmacokinetic interaction must be considered before alterations in dosing recommendations are made. (See also Chap. 109.)

PROCAINAMIDE (Pronestyl-SR, Procan-SR)

Clinical Applications

Procainamide, like quinidine, is effective against both supraventricular and ventricular arrhythmias.[93,94] Although the two drugs have similar electrophysiological effects, they are clinically different, and one agent may be effective for a patient when the other is not. Procainamide is useful in acute management of patients with reentrant supraventricular tachycardia and atrial fibrillation and flutter associated with Wolff-Parkinson-White syndrome.[95–98]

Although lidocaine is more often used, procainamide is also used intravenously to suppress ventricular arrhythmias occurring immediately following myocardial infarction or to convert sustained ventricular tachycardia. Under these conditions, it takes approximately 20 min to safely administer a loading dose of procainamide, so its use is limited to those situations in which adequate time is likely to be available. The advantage to its use in this setting instead of lidocaine is the potential for conversion to oral therapy using the same agent. In most such patients, however, lidocaine is usually used because the initial loading dose can be given within a 2- to 5-min period.

The active metabolite of procainamide, *N*-acetylprocainamide (acecainide, NAPA), is currently an investigational drug. It has been shown to be effective in the treatment of ventricular arrhythmias, but its use is limited by a narrow therapeutic index.[97–99]

Description

The development of procainamide as an antiarrhythmic agent resulted from a systematic search for a useful congener of procaine, whose use was precluded by adverse reactions.[100] Nearly 40 years later, procainamide is still used extensively. *N*-acetylprocainamide, the major metabolite of procainamide, produces antiarrhythmic activity in some patients, although not always those who respond to procainamide. This is most likely due to the drug's very different electrophysiological actions. Since procainamide is an effective agent but is not without adverse effects, it has served as a prototype for development of several of the newer antiarrhythmic agents.

Mechanism of Action

Like other agents processing class I activity, procainamide slows conduction and decreases automaticity and excitability of atrial and ventricular myocardium and Purkinje fibers.[93,94,101–103] Because of its effect on potassium channels, it also prolongs APD and refractoriness. Compared to quinidine procainamide has very little vagolytic activity and does not prolong the QT interval to as great an extent.[93] Its major metabolite, NAPA, has predominantly class III antiarrhythmic activity; it prolongs APD and refractoriness in both atrial and ventricular myocardium and prolongs the QT interval.[95,96,99,104–106] It has little or no effect on $\dot{V}_{max}$, in either Purkinje fibers or ventricular cells, and does not alter His-Purkinje conduction velocity because of its very low potency as a sodium channel antagonist.

Clinical Pharmacology

Procainamide is rapidly absorbed and 100 percent bioavailable when taken orally. About 15 percent of procainamide is bound to serum proteins. Procainamide's short half-life of elimination (2 to 4 h) in patients with normal renal function necessitates dosing every 3 to 6 h. Dosing every 6 to 8 h is possible with sustained-release preparations.

Slightly more than half of the general population are phenotypic rapid acetylators of procainamide and quickly convert it to NAPA, a metabolite with very pure class III antiarrhythmic action.[97] As expected, however, the response to one agent does not predict response to the other. When each is given as the sole agent, the usually effective plasma concentration is 4 to 8 μg/mL for procainamide and 7 to 15 μg/mL for NAPA.[97] During oral procainamide therapy, both agents are present in variable amounts, and there is no way to determine the contribution of NAPA to arrhythmia suppression under these conditions. Consequently, the utility of measuring plasma levels of procainamide during chronic therapy is limited because of this variable hepatic conversion to NAPA. Monitoring plasma concentrations for determination of compliance or prevention of toxicity is feasible and recommended (see below).

Dosage and Administration

Procainamide is available for either intravenous or oral use. In patients with normal renal and cardiac function, initial oral maintenance dosage of 50 mg per kilogram of body weight per day has been recommended. Frequent administration is required for oral procainamide, which is inconvenient and makes compliance difficult for the patient. A sustained-release form of procainamide is available, which permits dosing every 6 to 8 h. During chronic therapy, levels of NAPA may accumulate to effective or toxic levels in some individuals, resulting in achievement of maximum pharmacologic effect long after the time procainamide itself reaches steady state.[97,107] Therefore, the elimination half-life for procainamide may be misleading as a predictor of time to the occurrence of stable pharmacologic action. For these reasons, dosage should be initiated at conservative levels, and the patient should be monitored carefully until both procainamide and its metabolite reach steady state. The range of plasma concentrations of procainamide usually associated with an antiarrhythmic effect is from 4 to 8 μg/mL.[97] Patients with ventricular tachycardia may need higher levels for prevention of induction by programmed stimulation,[108] although such dosage frequently leads to adverse effects. Patients receiving higher doses should be carefully monitored. Since the electrophysiological effects of procainamide and NAPA are quite different, monitoring of patients receiving procainamide should at some point include measurement of plasma concentrations of both agents to determine their relative concentrations. Patients who are rapid acetylators or who have impaired renal function have plasma concentrations of NAPA higher than procainamide. These individuals should be monitored for excessive accumulation of NAPA during dose titration to maintain plasma levels below 20 μg/mL. The practice of using the sum of the plasma concentration of procainamide and NAPA is not recommended (see above discussions).

When administered intravenously, procainamide can be given as a constant 25-min loading infusion of 275 μg/min per kilogram of body weight or by a series of doses (≤100 mg delivered over 3 min) given every 5 min, up to a total dose of 1 g.[109,110] If the loading infusion is well tolerated (no hypotension and less than 25 percent QRS or QT widening), a maintenance intravenous infusion of 20 to 60 μg per kilogram of body weight per minute can then be given. Larger and more rapid loading infusions of 1 g over 15 to 20 min have been given in the electrophysiology laboratory to prevent induction of ventricular tachycardia by programmed ventricular stimulation. A second loading infusion of 0.5 to 1 g has been given in some instances where an initial loading infusion was well tolerated but ineffective. These large dosages are accompanied by a higher incidence of hypotension and conduction disturbance and often result in attainment of unacceptably high plasma concentration.

Modification of Dosage in Disease States

Both procainamide and NAPA accumulate to high and potentially toxic concentrations when patients with renal dysfunction are given usual dosages. Dosage should be lowered in patients with renal failure or low cardiac output.[111]

Increased plasma levels for procainamide and/or NAPA may also be seen in patients with congestive heart failure due to decreased urinary excretion and hydrolysis of procainamide.[112] On the other hand, one study of procainamide pharmacokinetics following a single intravenous bolus revealed no difference in volume of distribution, clearance, elimination half-life, unbound drug fraction, and peak procainamide concentrations between patients with congestive heart failure and normal individuals.[113]

Although intravenous procainamide does depress myocardial contractility and lower blood pressure, worsening of heart failure is uncommon during oral therapy when usual dosages and plasma concentrations are maintained.

Adverse Reactions

The incidence of side effects associated with long-term procainamide therapy limits its usefulness. A high percentage (up to 40 percent) of patients discontinue therapy in the first 6 months due to adverse reactions. The potential exists for arrhythmia aggravation, including the development of torsades de pointes due to procainamide or, more often, NAPA.[114,115] Therefore, just as with all agents possessing class IA activity, procainamide should not be used in patients with a long QT syndrome, a history of torsades de pointes, or hypokalemia.[116] In order to reduce the occurrence of proarrhythmia, potassium levels should be maintained at not less than 4 meq/liter in patients taking procainamide.

Fifteen to 20 percent of patients receiving procainamide develop a lupuslike syndrome, which often is difficult to recognize but regresses with discontinuation of treatment. The syndrome begins insidiously as mild arthralgia but progresses to frank arthritis, fever, malar erythematous rash, pleural and/or pericardial effusions, and antibodies against nucleoprotein (histone) in serum appearing as antinuclear antibodies with a "smooth" or "diffuse" pattern. These symptoms abate if procainamide is discontinued and generally resolve at a rate proportional to their duration. (See also Chap. 109.)

Almost all patients treated chronically develop detectable antinuclear antibodies, but only 15 to 20 percent develop symptoms of the lupus syndrome. Therefore, it is unnecessary to discontinue therapy solely due to the positive antinuclear antibody titer. The patient should be fully informed of the symptoms, which should be reported, so therapy can be discontinued at the earliest symptoms or signs of the lupus syndrome. Continuing procainamide after the development of the early symptoms of the lupus syndrome is dangerous because of the above-noted possibility of pleural effusion and potentially lethal pericardial tamponade.[117]

More recently, procainamide therapy has been associated with the development of agranulocytosis. It has been suggested, but not proven, that the sustained-release form of the drug may be especially capable of inducing this toxicity.[118] The manufacturer recommends that a white blood count be obtained every 2 weeks for the first 3 months. Heart block and sinus node dysfunction can occur in patients with preexisting conduction system abnormalities.[119]

Drug Interactions

Unlike quinidine, procainamide does not cause an increase in digoxin levels. There are few reports of interactions between procainamide and other drugs. Its clearance is reduced between 30 and 50 percent by cimetidine, which blocks the renal tubular secretion of procainamide.[120,121] A similar competition has been found between procainamide and its predominate metabolite, NAPA.[107] Ranitidine affects procainamide pharmacokinetics by reducing both its renal clearance and its absorption, the former by 14 to 23 percent and the latter by 10 to 24 percent, depending on the dose.[122]

DISOPYRAMIDE (Norpace)

Clinical Applications

Disopyramide is effective against a broad range of supraventricular and ventricular arrhythmias, its antiarrhythmic profile being similar to that of quinidine and procainamide.

Description

Disopyramide has class IA action and, in contrast to quinidine and procainamide, is better suited for long-term therapy, having relatively little associated chronic toxicity. While newer than quinidine or procainamide, disopyramide is still one of the older antiarrhythmic agents, having been in use in the United States since 1977. Its negative inotropic and anticholinergic actions occur frequently and limit its usefulness.

Mechanisms of Action

Disopyramide's antiarrhythmic effects are predominately those associated with sodium and potassium channel blockade. Its effects are similar to those of quinidine and procainamide on automaticity, conduction, and refractoriness in atrial and ventricular tissue.[123,125] Disopyramide prolongs the APD of normal and ischemic cells and reduces dispersion of repolarization between ischemic and normal tissues.[126,127] Its direct action on the sinus node tends to slow the heart rate,[128] but this is counteracted by disopyramide's potent anticholinergic actions[124,125,128,129] so that there is either a tendency for a small net increase or no change in heart rate. The enantiomers and metabolites of disopyramide differ in their pharmacodynamic effects. Those predominately responsible for the anticholinergic effects associated with disopyramide therapy are *l*-disopyramide and *l*-nor-disopyramide.[130] Prolongation of action potential duration is caused mainly by *d*-disopyramide,[131,132] whereas *d*- and *l*-disopyramide have similar potency for blocking the fast sodium channel.

Clinical Pharmacology

Disopyramide's oral bioavailability is 80 to 90 percent.[133] Its half-life of elimination, usually 6 to 8 h, is lengthened to as much as 15 h in cardiac patients.[134] About half of the compound is eliminated by the kidneys unchanged and the remainder as an active metabolite (resulting from hepatic *N*-dealkylation).[135-137] Protein binding of disopyramide is complex with between 20 and 50 percent of disopyramide being bound to plasma proteins. This variability is due in part to interindividual differences in affinity and capacity of alpha-1-acid glycoprotein (AAG) to bind the drug and to the nonlinear saturable (concentration-dependent) binding profile seen at plasma concentrations achieved during standard therapy.[138–142] For most drugs, the percentage bound to plasma protein is a constant over the usual range of therapeutic concentrations. The saturation of disopyramide-binding sites on plasma proteins means that there are disproportionate increases in levels of free drug in plasma compared to the magnitude of dosage increment[135,138] and that values obtained for free drug levels may better correlate with drug action than do values for total drug levels.

Dosage and Administration

Careful monitoring of patients, cautious dose titration, and the avoidance of loading doses are essential to safe and effective disopyramide therapy. For reasons discussed above, use of loading doses or rapid dose escalation is likely to lead to unexpectedly high free drug concentrations and unwanted actions.

The usually effective dosage for disopyramide is 100 to 400 mg three to four times daily, and the usual maximal dose is 800 mg/day. Therapy should be very carefully titrated beginning with low doses, allowing ample time for achievement of steady-state equilibrium.

While rapid fluctuations in plasma concentration are undesirable, they are difficult to avoid because of disopyramide's saturable protein binding. The controlled-release form of disopyramide may be useful in reducing adverse effects by decreasing fluctuations in the concentration of free disopyramide in plasma.[143] Because of saturable protein binding,[13] the generally accepted therapeutic range for (total) disopyramide plasma concentration (2 to 5 μg/mL) should not be strictly relied on. While monitoring the plasma concentrations of free disopyramide has been recommended,[144] the range of concentrations associated with arrhythmia suppression has not been clearly delineated and overlaps with that causing adverse effects.

Modification of Dosage in Disease States

Patient response to disopyramide should be monitored especially closely following acute myocardial infarction because both the absorption and elimination of disopyramide are decreased at this time.[145,146] In fact, in view of disopyramide's negative inotropic actions and changes in plasma AAG concentrations following a myocardial infarction, other antiarrhythmic agents should be considered first. While it is possible that the changes in absorption and elimination might balance each other, the potential exists for drug accumulation to toxic levels or a return of the patient's arrhythmia due to subtherapeutic plasma levels.

Disopyramide is contraindicated in patients with uncompensated heart failure because it can worsen the failure.[147] The initial dosage of disopyramide should be reduced (to 50 to 100 mg every 12 h) in patients with renal insufficiency[134] or decreased hepatic function.[148]

Adverse Reactions

When disopyramide was first marketed in the United States, the incidence of side effects was high. This probably resulted from three factors:

1. Loading doses, now known to significantly decrease myocardial contractility, were used.
2. Dosage recommendations were based upon pharmacokinetic studies in normal subjects, whereas we now know that the handling of the drug in cardiac patients is significantly different.
3. Binding of disopyramide to plasma proteins is nonlinear.

Understanding these factors has led to more conservative dosage regimens as well as heightened appreciation of the need for patient monitoring.

Disopyramide's side effects predominately include new or worsened congestive heart failure and symptoms resulting from the drug's dose-related anticholinergic actions (urinary retention, constipation, dry mouth, and esophageal reflux).[149] Because of this anticholinergic action, patients with obstructive uropathy or glaucoma should not receive this agent.[149] For some patients, the anticholinergic side effects can be prevented or alleviated by concomitant use of cholinesterase inhibitors such as physostigmine and neostigmine without reduction in antiarrhythmic efficacy.[150] As with all agents that prolong repolarization, disopyramide should not be used in patients with long QT syndrome, hypokalemia, or a history of torsades de pointes[151] because of the potential for arrhythmia aggravation. It is also possible that the direct actions of disopyramide on the sinus node can lead to excessive bradycardia in patients with sinus nodal dysfunction,[152] not only a problem in itself but possibly a contributing factor to development of torsades de pointes in patients with hypokalemia.[153]

Drug Interactions

Disopyramide does not increase digoxin levels,[154] and the effects of warfarin are not potentiated by disopyramide.[155] Phenytoin, rifampicin, and phenobarbital induce hepatic metabolism of disopyramide, thus increasing its elimination and leading to loss of antiarrhythmic effect.[156–158] Significant depression of myocardial contractility may result from the combined administration of disopyramide with beta-adrenergic or calcium channel antagonists and should be avoided in patients with any impairment of ventricular function.[159] (See also Chap. 109.)

QUINIDINE

Clinical Applications

Quinidine has been used successfully for a variety of supraventricular and ventricular arrhythmias, including conversion of atrial fibrillation or flutter,[160,161] supraventricular tachycardia,[93,162] ventricular extrasystoles,[163–165] and ventricular tachycardia and fibrillation.[166,167] On the other hand, a grouped analysis of six small placebo-controlled trials in patients with atrial fibrillation showed a statistically significant increase in mortality for the patients treated with quinidine.[168] Because of the similarity to the results in the CAST and CAST II, one must assume that the results of this metaanalysis are valid until a definitive prospective study is available.

Quinidine has been found effective, in combination with other antiarrhythmic agents, especially agents with class IB action, for treatment of life-threatening arrhythmias refractory to single-agent therapy.[7,169]

Description

Quinidine, one of the three optical isomers of quinine, historically was noticed to suppress atrial fibrillation in some patients receiving it for malaria.[170] This led to its use in the treatment of arrhythmias. Perhaps because of its long history and familiarity, it is considered by many clinicians in the United States to be the drug of choice for initial oral therapy of many arrhythmias. It is one of the most widely used antiarrhythmic agents, being effective in the treatment of a variety of supraventricular and ventricular arrhythmias. As with all antiarrhythmic drugs, however, both a narrow therapeutic window and the potential for lethal side effects make it imperative that its dosage and the patient's response be monitored closely. A great deal of controversy exists over its use and whether or not it should ever be initially prescribed to outpatients. Many physicians who feel comfortable with quinidine regularly prescribe it to outpatients, whereas many other physicians contend that the incidence of torsades de pointes (see below) justifies hospitalization of the patient before initiating therapy.[171] This concern is reflected in the current revised labeling for quinidine and all other antiarrhythmic drugs in which initiation of therapy in the hospital is recommended.

Mechanism of Action

Quinidine has multiple actions, but the action thought to be primarily responsible for its efficacy is block of the rapid inward sodium channel. This results in a decrease in $\dot{V}_{max}$ of action potential upstroke and slowed conduction, more marked in the His-Purkinje system than in the atria. Quinidine's effects on sodium channels are greatest at increased heart rate and less negative membrane potential, i.e., they are pH, rate, and voltage dependent. The ERP and, to a lesser degree, the APD are also increased, resulting in an increase in the ratio of ERP to APD. These effects on ERP and APD are most likely due to quinidine's ability to block potassium channels responsible for the delayed rectifier current. Dose-related changes in the ECG are increases in PR, QRS, and QT_c intervals, which reflect quinidine's multiple actions.

Antiarrhythmic therapies using low doses of quinidine in combination with other agents are currently being investigated. The rationale for combining quinidine with lidocaine-like drugs was first proposed by Hondeghem and Katzung[6] and was based on their ability to block the different states of the sodium channel. Another factor that may have a similar mechanistic basis is their different rates for interacting with the sodium channel. Quinidine is among those agents for which the recovery of $\dot{V}_{max}$ (the index of sodium conductance) is prolonged,[6] and its use in combination with agents for which recovery of $\dot{V}_{max}$ occurs quickly (for example, lidocaine or mexiletine) holds promise.

Clinical Pharmacology

Quinidine's effective dosage varies among individuals because of several factors. Although quinidine sulfate is usually administered every 6 h, there is wide variation in its elimination half-life (3 to 19 h).[172] Plasma protein binding also varies widely, ranging from 50 to 95 percent.[172] Oral bioavailability is approximately 70 percent and oral clearance ranges from 200 to 400 mL/min. Quinidine is inactivated or eliminated by both hepatic metabolism (50 to 90 percent) and renal elimination (10 to 30 percent). Several potentially active metabolites are formed in amounts that vary among individuals,[173] but for most, their clinical role has not been determined. One of quinidine's metabolites, 3-hydroxyquinidine, has been shown to possess antiarrhythmic activity in humans.[173] Experimental data indicate some contribution by metabolites of quinidine to its antiarrhythmic action.[174–176]

Dosage and Administration

Quinidine therapy (as the sulfate) is usually initiated with an oral dosage of 200 mg every 6 h, and the dosage is carefully titrated every 3 or more days. Elderly patients often require lower dosages of quinidine because of both reduced clearance and volume of distribution. Quinidine is available commercially in at least three different forms: quinidine sulfate, gluconate, and polygalacturonate. Since the quinidine content varies among these at 83, 62, and 60 percent, respectively, the need for dosage adjustment should be considered if one form is substituted for another. The usually effective dosage of quinidine sulfate ranges from 800 to 2400 mg/day, with the maximum recommended single dose being 600 mg. Because the half-life varies from 3 to 19 h, one should wait 2 to 4 days between dosage increases to prevent unexpected drug accumulation. The range of therapeutic plasma concentrations (measured using assays that differentiate quinidine from its metabolites) is 0.7 to 5.5 μg/mL.[172,177,178] Rapid escalation in quinidine dosage has been used to convert atrial fibrillation, but this therapy is no longer recommended because of unnecessary toxicity.

Intravenous therapy with quinidine is usually avoided if alternatives are feasible. Vasodilation and hypotension result from quinidine-induced alpha-adrenergic blockade. If quinidine is given intravenously (as quinidine gluconate), the patient should be carefully monitored and the infustion rate should be no greater than 16 mg/min. This should be discontinued if hypotension is observed or the QRS is prolonged by more than 25 percent.

Modification of Dosage in Disease States

No adjustment in initial dosage is usually needed for patients with renal or hepatic disease,[179,180] although due to decreased protein binding in patients with hepatic failure, lower than usual total plasma concentration can produce toxicity.[181] Slower dose titration is advisable to permit attainment of steady state and accumulation of active metabolites; however, because the usual range of effective dosages is wide, dosage for these patients is not markedly different. Patients with rapid elimination, often due to induction of hepatic metabolism by other drugs, may require higher dosages (up to 600 mg every 6 h).

Patients with congenital long QT syndrome, hypokalemia, or a history of torsades de pointes[182] should not be given quinidine because of their increased risk for this form of proarrhythmic event. For patients with congestive heart failure, problems associated with use of quinidine are proarrhythmia and digitalis (either digitoxin or digoxin) toxicity. Prudent use of quinidine in these individuals requires that titration begin at a reduced dosage; that dosage of any cardiac glycoside being administered concomitantly be reduced (see Chap. 109); and that plasma electrolyte levels, especially potassium, be maintained in the normal range and above 4 meq/liter.

Plasma levels of quinidine in patients with congestive heart failure are usually higher than in control subjects, even though absorption may be reduced.[183] This suggests a reduced volume of distribution. There are conflicting data concerning the elimination half-life in these patients. In some studies the elimination half-life has been reported as unchanged, implying that perhaps clearance and volume of distribution are both reduced. Other studies have found great variation in both half-life and quinidine blood levels among patients with congestive heart failure, although blood levels are generally higher than in normal subjects given comparable dosages.[184] Although quinidine does possess some direct negative inotropic effects, this is usually counteracted by its vasodilatory effect; therefore oral quinidine appears to be well tolerated hemodynamically when given at dosages producing usual plasma concentrations, even in patients with reduced ventricular function.[48,185,186] In a study of over 650 patients, 35 percent of whom had congestive heart failure, quinidine therapy resulted in no induction or worsening of congestive heart failure.[185] On the other hand, a significant problem for patients with congestive heart failure receiving quinidine therapy is proarrhythmia, with quinidine-induced torsades de pointes being potentiated in the setting of bradycardia and low serum magnesium or potassium.[153,187]

Adverse Reactions

Marked prolongation of the QT interval is seen in some patients receiving low or usual dosages of quinidine, and the risk of torsades de pointes is markedly increased in these patients. This arrhythmia may be responsible for *quinidine syncope*, which occurs in as many as 5 to 10 percent of patients within the first days of quinidine treatment, and quinidine-induced sudden death.[188] Torsades de pointes usually occurs in patients with low serum concentrations of quinidine, hypokalemia, and bradycardia.[188] Using an in vitro model, Roden and Hoffman[153] demonstrated that low concentrations of quinidine, when coupled with low extracellular potassium and slow stimulation rate, produced early afterdepolarizations in isolated Purkinje fibers. For patients who develop torsades de pointes, treatment with pacing, sodium bicarbonate, and/or isoproterenol is very effective. Magnesium sulfate injection has also been used, although controlled trials are not available. Of course these measures should also include discontinuation of quinidine and correction of hypokalemia. Clinically, it is essential to distinguish torsades de pointes from polymorphic ventricular tachycardia occurring in the setting of a normal QT interval because the latter should be treated with local anesthetic antiarrhythmic drugs and may be worsened by the above treatment for torsades de pointes. (See Chap. 36.)

Since quinidine acts via alpha-adrenergic blockade to produce vasodilatation,[189] hypotension may occur, especially in patients concomitantly receiving nitrates or other vasodilators. Other adverse effects include a high incidence of diarrhea and vomiting, tinnitus at high plasma levels, rare thrombocytopenia,[190] and in unusual cases, conduction block in patients with existing conduction system disease.[185] In patients treated with quinidine for atrial flutter (without prior AV nodal blockade by digitalis*), there have been reports of sudden increases in AV conduction and the rate of ventricular response.[189] This results from a slight reduction of the flutter rate and enhanced AV nodal conduction due to quinidine's anticholinergic effects. This permits 1 : 1 conduction through the AV node, often at 200 to 250 beats per minute. This may be of particular concern for patients receiving other drugs that increase conduction through the AV node, such as beta-adrenergic agonists.

Drug Interactions

Quinidine metabolism is inhibited by cimetidine[191] and induced by phenytoin, phenobarbital,[192] and rifampicin,[190] with the latter agents leading to reduced, subtherapeutic quinidine concentrations.

Clinical digoxin toxicity has been described in 20 to 40 percent of patients receiving quinidine and digoxin concurrently.[191] This interaction is dependent on quinidine dosage, and in some patients it may not appear until the dosage is increased to higher levels. The addition of quinidine can produce an approximate doubling of plasma digoxin levels paralleled by an increase in the cardiac effects of digoxin,[193] although the latter is controversial. The mechanism involved in this drug interaction includes displacement of digoxin from noncardiac tissue stores, resulting in a 30 to 40 percent reduction in the apparent volume of distribution for digoxin, increased gastrointestinal absorption, decreased biliary excretion, and a 30 to 50 percent decrease in renal tubular secretion of the digoxin.[194] The rise in digoxin levels appears with the first dose of quinidine; therefore, it is suggested that digoxin dosage be halved when quinidine therapy is initiated. A similar interaction has been reported for quinidine and digitoxin. While this interaction is less well studied than that of digoxin and quinidine, it is probable that the mechanisms involved differ from those of the quinidine-digoxin interaction. (See also Chap. 109.)

*Digitalis is used in the treatment of atrial fibrillation, atrial flutter, and other arrhythmias. It is discussed in Chaps. 27 and 36.

Quinidine is a potent inhibitor of the hepatic cytochrome P450 specific for debrisoquin metabolism ($P450_{2D6}$),[195-197] although it is not metabolized by this enzyme.[198,199] Thus, it may interfere with the biotransformation and actions of pharmacologic agents dependent on this cytochrome for their metabolism (e.g., including encainide, propafenone, mexiletine, flecainide, metoprolol, timolol, sparteine, and bufuralol.[200] Quinidine worsens neuromuscular blockade in patients with myasthenia gravis[201] and may prolong the effects of succinylcholine.[202]

PROPAFENONE (Rythmol)

Clinical Applications

Propafenone is a very interesting agent developed in Germany and marketed there since 1977 and is similar to other antiarrhythmic agents in overall efficacy and patient tolerance. Since it has been found effective in patients refractory to other agents, it is likely to have a role in the treatment of many types of arrhythmias, including supraventricular arrhythmias.[203-206]

Clinical Pharmacology

It has been described as having class IC antiarrhythmic activity because of its potent ability to slow conduction velocity with little change in APD.[207,208] The time constants for onset and recovery of sodium channel block are intermediate between quinidine and flecainide. Therefore, compared to flecainide, slightly less prolongation of the QRS is seen at effective dosages. While it has a marked structural similarity to propranolol, in vitro and single-dose studies in normal volunteers initially concluded that it had only one-fortieth of the beta receptor blocking potency of propranolol and that there was little likelihood that it would produce clinically significant beta-adrenergic receptor blocking activity.[209,210] Subsequent studies, however, have shown that propafenone can accumulate during continued administration to levels capable of producing clinically significant beta-adrenergic inhibition.[207,211]

Propafenone, like encainide, is eliminated by a metabolic pathway that has a polymorphic pattern of inheritance. Seven percent of the population, those deficient in activity of the cytochrome $P450_{2D6}$ responsible for the metabolism of debrisoquin, encainide, metoprolol, flecainide, mexiletine, sparteine, and many other drugs, have very slow elimination of propafenone and fail to form measurable quantities of the potentially active metabolite, 5-hydroxypropafenone.[212] The accumulation of high concentrations of propafenone leads to significant beta receptor antagonism at both low and high dosages in poor metabolizers but only at high dosages in extensive metabolizers of propafenone.[212] Although metabolic phenotype does not seem to dramatically influence the antiarrhythmic response to propafenone,[212] it clearly influences the degree of beta blockade occurring during therapy.

Dosage and Administration

Effective dosages range from 300 to 900 mg/day in two to four divided dosages. In order to prevent unexpected accumulation of pharmacologic action, propafenone dosage should not be changed more frequently than every 3 days; there is slow elimination of the parent drug in poor metabolizers and slow accumulation of the metabolite(s) in extensive metabolizers.

Patients receiving propafenone should be carefully monitored for deterioration in ventricular function, which may result from beta-adrenergic receptor antagonism and/or the direct negative inotropic effect and be manifest in patients with reduced ventricular function.[213]

Modification of Dosage in Disease States

Dosage recommendations for patients with cardiac, renal, or hepatic dysfunction are not yet available.

Drug Interactions

It is very likely that there will be drug interactions between propafenone and other agents that utilize or inhibit cytochrome $P450_{2D6}$ for their metabolism. Such an interaction has been documented already between propafenone and metoprolol[214] and should be expected with timolol, encainide, tricyclic antidepressants, and perhaps other agents. Quinidine, which inhibits this cytochrome, inhibits the formation of 5-hydroxypropafenone in extensive metabolizers[215]; however, the clinical consequence of such inhibition is unknown and difficult to predict. One would expect greater beta blockade to occur after combining quinidine with propafenone therapy because of the higher propafenone concentrations.

FLECAINIDE (Tambocor)

Clinical Applications

Flecainide is very effective in suppressing a variety of ventricular and supraventricular tachycardias.[216,217] The finding of increased mortality when given to patients with ischemic heart disease has led to restricted usage (see above); however, there has been no evidence to indicate that this increase in mortality is seen when flecainide is given to patients with supraventricular arrhythmias in the absence of coronary artery disease.[218] Overall, the antiarrhythmic response to flecainide in patients with symptomatic life-threatening ventricular arrhythmias is not markedly better than with agents that have predominant class IA or IB activity.[216,219] Its negative inotropic actions restrict its use to patients having moderately well-preserved ventricular function. Likewise, its potential to increase mortality in patients with ischemic heart disease limits its usefulness.

Description

Flecainide has sodium channel blocking activity and is considered to have class IC actions. It has also been found to block the delayed rectifier potassium channel in feline ventricular myocytes, and this action may be clinically relevant.[220] It also has weak calcium antagonist properties that are probably not manifest clinically. Like encainide, it is highly effective at suppressing asymptomatic premature ventricular contractions (PVCs) and is well tolerated. Although it had a high degree of potency in the classical arrhythmia models it appeared to increase the incidence of ventricular fibrillation in animal models of acute ischemia.[221] In retrospect, this is entirely consistent with the effects observed in the CAST.

Flecainide is a sodium channel antagonist whose predominant activity belongs to class IC. It markedly depresses $\dot{V}_{max}$ in Purkinje fibers and ventricular muscle.[222] As with other sodium channel blockers, this effect is frequency dependent, with more inhibition occurring at rapid stimulation rates. Flecainide, however, dissociates more slowly from the sodium channel than do other agents with class IA or IB activity. This results in the rate dependence of sodium channel blockade appearing at heart rates within the normal range and, therefore, more conduction slowing with flecainide than with other agents. This characteristic most likely explains flecainide-induced lengthening of the QRS interval on the surface ECG observed at normal heart rates.[216]

Flecainide slows intraventricular conduction velocity more than it prolongs effective refractory periods.[223] It prolongs AH and HV intervals and measurably increases PR and QRS intervals on the surface ECG at therapeutic doses. The QT_c interval is slightly increased, primarily due to prolongation of the QRS.

Clinical Pharmacology

Flecainide is reliably absorbed after oral administration, and its systemic bioavailability is 90 to 95 percent.[224] Most of flecainide is metabolized in the liver to compounds that are not pharmacologically active at the concentrations usually found in plasma.[216] Thus, measurement of the parent compound correlates reasonably well with QRS prolongation and antiarrhythmic effect.[225] Flecainide, like many other antiarrhythmic agents, is metabolized by the debrisoquin $P450_{2D6}$ enzyme.[226] Because flecainide is also eliminated by the kidneys to a considerable extent, the enzyme deficiency seen in 7 percent of Caucasians has little effect on the pharmacokinetics of flecainide. If, however, those patients without the enzyme develop renal insufficiency or if renal patients are given a drug that blocks the metabolism, extremely high plasma concentrations are likely to occur. Twenty-seven percent of flecainide is excreted unchanged in the urine. Alkalinization of urine reduces renal elimination of flecainide, probably by increasing the amount of the drug present as the nonionized form and hence increasing tubular reabsorption.[227] A potential advantage of flecainide is its very slow elimination, with half-life ranging from 7 to 23 h in normal subjects and tending to be even longer (14 to 26 h) in patients with cardiac disease (even in the absence of heart failure).[224,228] Plasma protein binding is moderate (40 percent) and is only minimally affected by elevations in AAG. Flecainide has a very large volume of distribution, indicative of its high degree of tissue uptake.[224]

Dosage and Administration

The usual dosage of flecainide is 100 to 150 mg every 12 h in patients without cardiac or renal failure. A total daily dosage of more than 400 mg may sometimes be used but should be administered only under close medical monitoring (see below). The range of therapeutic plasma concentrations of flecainide is reported to be between 200 and 1000 ng/mL, although adverse effects may occur in some patients at concentrations within this range,[229,230] and many patients tolerate concentrations well above this range. To reduce the incidence of adverse effects, flecainide therapy should start with a low dosage that is maintained until steady state has been reached (at least 4 days). As with other antiarrhythmic agents, monitoring of the patient's clinical condition remains the cornerstone of evaluation.

Modification of Dosage in Disease States

The usual initial dosage for flecainide for patients with cardiac failure is 50 to 100 mg every 12 h. Since 7 percent of Caucasian patients with renal failure will not have the $P450_{2D6}$ enzyme and because flecainide is usually eliminated by both metabolism and renal excretion, all patients with renal failure should be given very low dosages and titrated very carefully. Plasma concentration monitoring will be essential in patients with renal disease or cardiac or hepatic dysfunction. Any significant reduction in ejection fraction should be expected to lengthen elimination half-life and hence the time needed to attain steady-state equilibrium. Reductions in clearance occur in renal or hepatic dysfunction and lead to higher plasma concentrations at steady state. Flecainide should probably not be used in patients with congestive heart failure.

Adverse Reactions

Although aggravation of arrhythmias seen in the early days of flecainide's evaluation was often due to excessive initial doses and frequent dose increments, flecainide has a potential to induce proarrhythmic events even when prescribed as currently recommended. This is especially true in patients with severe heart disease and if flecainide is given in higher dosages.[234]

Flecainide, because of its negative inotropic effects at dosages necessary to suppress arrhythmias, produces a measurable decrease in left ventricular function in most patients.[232,233] In the premarketing experience, it was found that new or worsened congestive heart failure occurred in 5 percent of those receiving flecainide, and therapy was discontinued in 1.4 percent because of these effects.[234]

The classification of patients according to their type of ventricular arrhythmia has been found useful in predicting the frequency of adverse cardiac effects from flecainide.[234] Sustained ventricular tachycardia and structural heart disease were both associated with an increased incidence of lethal or serious proarrhythmic events. The increased mortality seen in the CAST seems to be confined to patients with structural heart disease (see above).[218] A retrospective study of five multiple-dose efficacy trials showed that of patients with a history of congestive heart failure, oral flecainide precipitated heart failure in 15 percent.[235] A dose-related depression of myocardial performance was found after rapid (1 to 2 mg per kilogram of body weight) intravenous injections.[236]

Other side effects of flecainide include those one would expect from its effect on intracardiac conduction. Flecainide can depress sinus node activity in patients with preexisting sinus node dysfunction.[237] Prolongation of QRS and PR intervals on the surface ECG is common and, if below 25 percent, does not necessarily indicate excessive dosage.

Flecainide increases pacing thresholds by as much as 200 percent and should therefore be used with caution in patients dependent upon pacemakers.[238,239] It also increases the threshold for electrical defibrillation so patients with implanted devices should be evaluated carefully.[240]

Drug Interactions

Cimetidine reduces flecainide clearance and prolongs flecainide elimination half-life.[241] Studies in normal volunteers have demonstrated an increase in the plasma concentrations of digoxin and propranolol when flecainide is coadministered.[242,243] Not unexpectedly, propranolol and flecainide have been found to have additive negative inotropic effects. An interaction with amiodarone, resulting in elevation of plasma flecainide concentration and necessitating reduction of flecainide dosage, has been described.[244]

ENCAINIDE (Enkaid)

Clinical Applications

Encainide is a highly effective, well-tolerated agent used for the treatment of ventricular and supraventricular arrhythmias, including those associated with the Wolff-Parkinson-White syndrome.[245] Encainide and flecainide are quite similar in terms of efficacy.[246] Encainide was one of the drugs evaluated in the CAST, and it proved to increase mortality in patients with ventricular arrhythmias after myocardial infarction. Because of the restrictions in its use, it was removed from the market by its manufacturer in September 1991 and will only be clinically available for patients who cannot be treated with other available agents.

CALCIUM CHANNEL BLOCKERS

Some calcium channel blockers are also used as antiarrhythmic agents.[247,248] (See Chap. 67.) Verapamil and diltiazem are useful in the management of supraventricular tachycardia, where they are administered to slow the ventricular rate in patients with atrial fibrillation or flutter and to treat and prevent AV nodal reentrant tachycardia. Intravenous diltiazem is useful for the temporary control of rapid ventricular rate during atrial fibrillation and flutter. In controlled clinical trials, conversion to sinus rhythm occurred with diltiazem and placebo with equal frequency.

Although the intravenous administration of verapamil is extremely dangerous in the acute treatment of ventricular tachycardia in patients with chronic or acute ischemic heart disease, verapamil has been shown to suppress a rare form of ventricular tachycardia with right bundle branch block pattern and left axis deviation,[249] often seen in patients with structurally normal hearts.

Both verapamil and diltiazem have been shown to decrease antipyrine clearance, often considered a rough index of oxidative metabolism in the liver[250]; but only verapamil increases liver blood flow.[250] Verapamil thus may increase the systemic elimination of drugs with high hepatic extraction ratio. Both agents can raise the plasma concentration of digoxin. (See Chaps. 67 and 109.)

BRETYLIUM (Bretylol)

Clinical Applications

Bretylium is effective for acute therapy of ventricular tachycardia and/or ventricular fibrillation. Because it produces complex indirect effects via the autonomic nervous system, it should be reserved for patients who have failed to respond to lidocaine.

Description

Because of its sympatholytic activity, bretylium tosylate was first evaluated in the 1950s for the treatment of hypertension; however, a very high incidence of orthostatic hypotension and unreliable oral absorption led to its disfavor for chronic therapy. After its antiarrhythmic activity was discovered in animals,[251] it was eventually marketed in the United States as intravenous therapy for life-threatening ventricular arrhythmias. Bretylium is usually employed only after patients have not responded to lidocaine.

Mechanism of Action

In addition to the indirect electrophysiological changes caused by the drug's action on postganglionic autonomic neurons, bretylium has a direct class III action that causes an increase in APD and refractoriness in ventricular muscle and Purkinje fibers.[252] When clinically relevant concentrations of bretylium are studied in normal tissues, no changes are seen in $\dot{V}_{max}$, maximum diastolic potential, or conduction velocity. Studies have found that bretylium acts predominantly on normal tissue to reduce the degree of dispersion of repolarization across the boundary between normal and ischemic tissue.[253] Transient increases in membrane potential and conduction velocity are seen early after bretylium administration and are presumed to be due to the local release of catecholamines. Bretylium has been found to elevate the threshold for electrically induced difibrillation in a variety of animal models.

When initially administered, bretylium causes the release of norepinephrine from postganglionic adrenergic neurons.[254] Bretylium is transported into the neuron by the norepinephrine pump, and extensive accumulation in the neuron is then associated with a blockade of further release or uptake of norepinephrine by the neuron. The blockade of uptake of circulating or infused catecholamines leads to supersensitivity that is functionally similar to a denervated state.

In assessing the effects of bretylium, one should distinguish between its direct effects and its indirect effects via the autonomic nervous system. This may be difficult because, in clinical research, patients are often studied under conditions very different from the usual clinical situation. In clinical use patients experiencing ventricular tachycardia or recurrent ventricular fibrillation have striking adrenergic stimulation, and the potential effects of bretylium on the autonomic nervous system may be overwhelmed. In serial evaluations of the electrophysiological actions of bretylium in patients given a loading dose of 5 mg per kilogram of body weight and again 5 mg/kg after a 1-h infusion at 1.5 mg/min, changes were found that were compatible with catecholamine release during both periods, i.e., shortening of the refractory periods of the AV node, right atrium, and right ventricle.[255]

Clinical Pharmacology

Bretylium is poorly absorbed after oral administration with bioavailability of approximately 25 percent and is therefore available only for parenteral administration. It is eliminated almost entirely unchanged in the urine, and clearance correlates well with creatinine clearance.[256] It is probably actively secreted by the base transport system in the distal tubules of the kidney.

Dosage and Administration

The usual intravenous dosage for bretylium is 5 mg per kilogram of body weight given at a rate dependent upon the clinical setting.[257] During cardiac emergencies, it should be given by rapid injection into a central intravenous line. In less acute situations, giving a loading infusion of the same dose but over 10 to 20 min will reduce the incidence of nausea and vomiting. The loading dose should be repeated after 20 min if the arrhythmia is still present. A total loading dose of 20 mg per kilogram of body weight may be required and dosages up to 9 g in 24 h have been given without serious adverse effects. Maintenance infusions of 1 to 4 mg/min should be given depending upon body size and renal function. Heart rhythm and blood pressure should be monitored carefully, especially during the first few hours of bretylium therapy.

Studies in animals have found that early after the first dose, the electrophysiological effects of bretylium correlate better with myocardial concentrations than with plasma concentrations. Plasma concentrations of 1 to 2 μg/mL have been reported in a few patients with antiarrhythmic response to bretylium.[255] Unfortunately, the wide therapeutic index and myocardial accumulation make plasma level monitoring of limited clinical utility.

Modification of Dosage in Disease States

In patients with renal insufficiency, bretylium clearance is reduced and half-life prolonged; therefore, the maintenance infusion for bretylium should be reduced to the lowest effective dosage. There are no data to guide dosage adjustment in cardiac or hepatic impairment, but it is unlikely that the dosage should be altered in these patients.

Adverse Reactions

When bretylium is given by rapid intravenous injection, many patients experience nausea and vomiting. The release of norepinephrine by bretylium has the potential to cause increased blood pressure, but severe hypertension has not been described. Increased frequency of ventricular arrhythmias is often seen at this time and can lead to the need for more frequent cardioversion. The reduction in peripheral vascular resistance can cause symptomatic hypotension in volume-depleted patients, but this can be readily corrected if recognized. Hypotension could prove dangerous in patients with fixed valvular obstruction. Bradycardia has been reported in some patients with abnormalities of the conduction system when given large intravenous dosages of bretylium.

Studies in stable patients found that either low or high dosages of bretylium cause a transient increase in heart rate, blood pressure, contractility, peripheral vascular resistance, and arrhythmia frequency. This was followed by a fall in standing blood pressure and peripheral vascular resistance.[258] Orthostatic hypotension is almost uniformly seen in patients receiving bretylium and sometimes lasts for days after discontinuation of therapy. Dosages that are well below those required for antiarrhythmic efficacy are capable of causing orthostatic hypotension. When hypotension develops during bretylium therapy, it should be corrected with intravenous volume expansion, and adequate doses of bretylium should be given to suppress arrhythmias. After the initial phase of catecholamine release, bretylium has little effect on myocardial contractility at clinically achieved levels.

Drug Interactions

Other than those with tricyclic antidepressants, no drug interactions have been reported. One would expect, however, that there might be competition for renal tubular secretion with procainamide, NAPA, cimetidine, and other organic bases.

SOTALOL (Betapace)

Clinical Applications

Sotalol has been used for up to 20 years in many countries for angina and hypertension, and it was in this setting that its value as an antiarrhythmic agent was first observed. Sotalol is unlike other beta-adrenergic antagonists in that it prolongs the action potential, producing a parallel increase in refractoriness of cardiac tissues.[259] This unique combination of properties makes sotalol effective in a variety of supraventricular and ventricular arrhythmias. It has been found to be effective in patients with sustained ventricular tachycardia evaluated by programmed ventricular stimulation. In a controlled comparison to procainamide, sotalol was effective in 30 percent of patients with inducible sustained ventricular tachycardia whereas only 20 percent responded to procainamide ($P < .2$).[260] This is consistent with the response rate for sotalol (31 percent) in the NIH-sponsored ESVEM trial, which compared therapy guided by programmed electrical stimulation to therapy guided by ambulatory monitoring.[261] In this study, a mean of only 12 percent of patients responded to the other antiarrhythmic drugs evaluated.

Mechanism of Action

Sotalol has two main actions each of which can contribute to its antiarrhythmic efficacy.[262] The drug was originally synthesized for its actions as a beta-adrenergic receptor antagonist. Unlike other beta receptor antagonists, it markedly prolongs refractoriness in atrial and ventricular tissues, a class III antiarrhythmic action that is thought to be due to block of the delayed rectifier potassium current, the major current responsible for repolarization of cardiac tissue. In patients these actions slow heart rate, decrease AV nodal conduction, and increase refractoriness of atrial, ventricular, AV nodal, and AV accessory pathways in both the anterograde and retrograde directions.[263] When given in dosages between 160 and 640 mg per day there are increases of 40 to 100 ms in the QT interval and 10 to 40 ms in QT_c.

Clinical Pharmacology

Sotalol has a desirable pharmacokinetic profile. Oral bioavailability is greater than 90 percent, and peak concentrations are seen 2.5 to 4 h after a dose. It is not bound to plasma proteins and is eliminated by the kidneys unchanged, with an elimination half-life of approximately 12 h. Because of the relatively long half-life and bid dosing regimen, it is recommended that testing for efficacy be conducted near the end of the dosing interval at steady state. Age, per se, does not influence the pharmacokinetics of sotalol other than that due to the natural decline in renal function that occurs with age. Dosage adjustment must be made for alterations in renal function (see below).

Dosages and Administration

Sotalol is only available in the oral form in the United States, although the intravenous form is available in Canada and many other countries. The recommended initial dose of sotalol is 80 mg every 12 h. In patients with relatively normal renal function steady state will occur in 2 to 3 days. If evaluation on this dosage indicates lack of response without evidence of excessive effects on repolarization (QT below 550 ms), the dosage may be increased to 160 mg bid and if necessary to 240 mg bid. Some patients with life-threatening arrhythmias have required dosages of 640 mg/day.

Modification of Dosage in Disease States

Because sotalol is mainly eliminated unchanged in the urine, the dosage must be adjusted for altered renal function. For patients with a creatinine clearance greater than 60 mL/min, the usual dosing interval is every 12 h. If the creatinine clearance (CL_{CR}) is between 30 and 60 mL/min, however, the recommended interval between doses is 24 h. For patients with CL_{CR} between 10 and 30 mL/min, the interval should be every 36 to 48 h or the usual dose halved and given every 24 h. The dosage for patients with CL_{CR} below 10 mL/min should be individualized. There is no theoretical reason to use lower doses in patients with liver disease, and pharmacokinetic studies in patients with liver disease have not found differences from normal populations. Because of the increased risk of proarrhythmia and congestive heart failure, patients with reduced cardiac output should be given lower doses and monitored carefully.

Adverse Reactions

A major concern with sotalol treatment has been the occurrence of torsades de pointes (TdP). Reports of this syndrome have predominantly been cases of suicidal overdoses or in patients who were receiving concomitant diuretics and inadequate potassium replacement. Clearly, hypokalemia and bradycardia are predisposing factors for the development of this arrhythmia during sotalol therapy, as they are with quinidine, disopyramide, and procainamide. The manufacturer observed an overall incidence of TdP of 2 percent (in patients with sustained ventricular tachycardia 4 percent and in those with supraventricular arrhythmia 1.5 percent). It is more common in patients with congestive heart failure and a history of sustained ventricular tachycardia (7 percent). The incidence of TdP can be held to a minimum by careful screening for predisposing factors (bradycardia, baseline prolongation of the QT interval, and electrolyte disturbances, especially hypokalemia), careful dose escalation beginning at 160 mg/day and limiting the maximum QT interval prolongation to less than 550 ms.

Serious proarrhythmic events tend to occur within 7 days of initiating therapy or increasing the dosage. They occur at low dosage but are progressively more common at increasing dosages, reaching a high of 4.5 percent at doses above 640 mg/day. The incidence of new or worsened congestive heart failure is only about 3 percent. This is somewhat lower than expected for a drug with potent beta-blocking actions but may be attenuated because of the increased inotropy produced by its action to prolong repolarization. Other side effects typical of beta blockers are to be expected (bronchospasm in asthmatic patients, masking the signs and symptoms of hypoglycemia in diabetics, and catecholamine hypersensitivity withdrawal syndrome).

Discontinuation of therapy due to adverse effects is relatively uncommon and was lower for sotalol than for any other antiarrhythmic agent in the ESVEM trial. During development of sotalol, the manufacturer observed an overall discontinuation rate of 13 percent due to adverse effects and the following as the most common causes of discontinuation: dyspnea, 3 percent; fatigue, 3 percent; proarrhythmia, 3 percent; asthenia, 2 percent; bradycardia, 2 percent; congestive heart failure, 1 percent.[261]

Drug Interactions

Concomitant use with agents that prolong repolarization have the potential to increase the likelihood of torsades des pointes. No pharmacokinetic interactions have been seen with sotalol and/or warfarin, digoxin, cholestyramine, or hydrochlorothiazide. Because of the beta-blocking actions of sotalol, it is likely that there would be increased pharmacologic effect if the drug is combined with calcium channel blockers, antihypertensive agents, or antiarrhythmic agents.

AMIODARONE (Cordarone)

Clinical Applications

Although amiodarone has been reported to have efficacy in a wide range of arrhythmias, the Food and Drug Administration in the United States has recommended it only as oral therapy for life-threatening ventricular arrhythmias refractory to all other available forms of therapy. Nevertheless, there are numerous reports in the literature describing the efficacy of amiodarone in the conversion and slowing of atrial fibrillation, AV nodal reentrant tachycardia, and tachycardias associated with the Wolff-Parkinson-White syndrome.[264,265] The reasons for amiodarone's limited labeling are (1) the lack of requisite controlled trials to support its use for other indications, (2) the documented potentially lethal complications of chronic amiodarone therapy, (3) the difficulties associated with its variable time for onset of action, and (4) multiple dangerous drug interactions. The effects of amiodarone on mortality are currently being investigated in several multicenter studies of patients at increased risk for sudden cardiac death. A pilot study of amiodarone in patients with prior myocardial infarction and ventricular ectopy has been reported.[266] Although only a small number of patients in the study received amiodarone ($n = 48$) and rather severe side effects were seen, the authors concluded that a full-scale trial was in order and feasible.

Description

Amiodarone is an iodinated benzofuran that has structural similarity to thyroxine and procainamide and was originally developed as an antianginal agent. It was incidentally noted to effectively suppress a wide variety of ventricular and supraventricular arrhythmias. This efficacy has been assumed to be due to its prolongation of refractoriness and APD in myocardial tissue (Vaughan Williams class III antiarrhythmic activity), although amiodarone has been found to have many diverse pharmacologic actions (see Table 38-1); the one(s) responsible for its high degree of antiarrhythmic efficacy remain unidentified.

Mechanism of Action

Intracellular recordings in cardiac tissues from rabbits chronically treated with amidarone demonstrated prolongation of APD and increased refractoriness of both atrial and ventricular myocardium, Purkinje fibers, and sinus and AV nodal tissues. Amiodarone decreases phase 0 depolarization of myocardial cells and blocks sodium channels that are in the inactivated state.[267,268] It also slows phase 4 depolarization of the sinus node as well as conduction through the AV node. The electrophysiological actions of the major metabolite of amiodarone, desethylamiodarone (DEA), differ from those of amiodarone, with the metabolite having greater effects on conduction due to effects on sodium channels and, hence, upon conduction.[269]

The electrophysiological changes seen in humans must be considered with respect to the route of drug administration and the duration of therapy. Following acute intravenous amiodarone administration, prolongation of the AH interval and an increase in the refractory periods of the AV node and bypass tracts are seen, but some of these changes may be due to the presence of the solubilizing agent, polysorbate 80 (Tween 80), in the intravenous formulation. No changes are seen in either sinus rate or atrial or ventricular refractoriness, whereas these are prolonged during chronic oral therapy. Chronic amiodarone therapy also prolongs the AH and HV intervals and the PR and QT intervals of the surface ECG. There are conflicting data on the time course of the development of these changes and how they might relate to the antiarrhythmic efficacy of amiodarone. Changes in APD and refractoriness are seen in hypothyroidism, similar to changes resulting from oral amiodarone therapy.[270] Since these changes can be prevented in animals by coadministration of thyroid hormone with amiodarone,[271] some have concluded that amiodarone's antiarrhythmic efficacy is due to production of "cardiac hypothyroidism." This is supported by the observation that amiodarone's major metabolite causes noncompetitive inhibition of thyroid hormone binding to nuclear receptors.[272] On the other hand, amiodarone also causes noncompetitive blockade of alpha and beta receptors,[273] muscarinic receptors,[274] and both calcium and sodium channel blockade, any combination of which may contribute to its antiarrhythmic efficacy.

Clinical Pharmacology

Amiodarone is a highly lipid-soluble compound having extremely variable and complex pharmacokinetics. It is slowly absorbed from the gastrointestinal tract, and bioavailability varies over a fourfold range.[275] Amiodarone is extensively metabolized to DEA, and little if any is excreted unchanged in the urine. Concentrations of DEA in plasma vary from 0.4 to 2.0 times that of amiodarone during chronic therapy.[276] This metabolite has antiarrhythmic potency equal or greater to amiodarone when compared in in vitro and animal models.[277] Amiodarone is rapidly concentrated in some tissues (including myocardium) but accumulates more slowly in others (adipose tissue). It redistributes out of myocardial tissue while still accumulating in adipose and other tissues.[276,278] Until all tissues are saturated, rapid redistribution out of the myocardium may be responsible for early recurrence of arrhythmias after discontinuation of therapy or rapid reduction of dosage. Because of drug accumulation in tissues, the volume of distribution for amiodarone is very large, 20 to 200 liters/kg.[278] After intravenous administration, the measured half-life in plasma is from 4.8 to 68.2 h,[279] with tissue uptake being the primary factor responsible for the decline in plasma concentration. As tissues become saturated, however, the decline in plasma levels is slow, reflecting mainly elimination and slow redistribution of drug out of adipose and muscle tissues. This leads to slow and extremely variable elimination from plasma, with half-lives ranging from 13 to 103 days at steady state.[278] It is also possible that amiodarone inhibits its own elimination after chronic therapy, contributing to the differences between half-life early in therapy to that after prolonged therapy.

Dosage and Administration

Without a loading dose, amiodarone requires several weeks to months before producing its antiarrhythmic action. Large intravenous dosages or oral loading dosages can hasten the onset of therapeutic effects; however, only small prospective studies are available evaluating the optimal method for administering loading dosages. Loading dosages reported in the literature have varied from 600 to 1400 mg/day for 2 to 21 days.[280] Because of relatively rapid redistribution out of myocardial tissue, the dosage should be tapered over a period of several weeks. The usual maintenance dose varies from 200 to 600 mg/day, and because of the severe nature of adverse reactions, the lowest effective dosage should be prescribed. It is thought that patients with supraventricular arrhythmias will respond to lower dosages than those with ventricular arrhythmias, but there are many exceptions, and no comparative trials are available. Because of the variable pharmacokinetics and oral bioavailability, it is unlikely that generalizations such as this will be reliable. Some patients with extensive absorption (80 percent bioavailabilty) of low doses may have the same drug exposure as a person with limited bioavailability given a high dose.

Plasma concentrations of amiodarone are usually between 1 and 2 μg/mL during effective therapy.[281,282] Similar concentrations of the desethyl metabolite accumulate during therapy and, although unproven, are likely to contribute to the antiarrhythmic efficacy. Because of extensive overlap between the range of concentrations required for arrhythmia suppression and those associated with toxicity, monitoring of plasma concentrations is of limited value. Clearly, levels of amiodarone above 3 to 4 μg/mL for prolonged periods of time are associated with a higher incidence of adverse effects.[283]

Modification of Dosage in Disease States

Long-term oral therapy with amiodarone appears to be well tolerated hemodynamically in patients with congestive heart failure. An uncontrolled retrospective study has suggested that amiodarone therapy has prolonged life for congestive heart failure patients with arrhythmias.[284] These data only support the need for an adequate study to evaluate amiodarone's effects in congestive heart failure patients who have refractory symptomatic arrhythmias. Such studies are being performed at this time.

Adverse Reactions

Intravenous administration of amiodarone at dosages greater than 5 mg/kg decreases contractility and peripheral vascular resistance, producing severe hypotension in some instances. It is possible that some of this effect, like the electrophysiological effects described earlier, may be due to the effects of polysorbate 80 or benzyl alcohol present in the formulation. After oral administration, at usual dosages, no change in myocardial contractility has been observed.

The medical literature for amiodarone is replete with conflicting opinions regarding its safety. The early reports found it to be very well tolerated, one report even describing it as the "ideal antiarrhythmic drug." Some studies continue to find that it is safe and effective, even in the treatment of arrhythmias in children.[285] The reason for these differences is not apparent, but clearly the experience with amiodarone in the United States, with a very high incidence of intolerable and sometimes lethal reactions, is different from that in Europe. The discrepancy may be due to differences in dosage, the patient population, drug interactions, or some unknown genetic or geographic factors. It is very difficult to determine the incidence of these adverse reactions because most studies in the literature report the incidence in populations having highly variable durations of treatment. An actuarial analysis of the rate of occurrence would be much more helpful, and data from such an analysis indicate that the toxicity may be more frequent than previously appreciated.[267,286]

The most serious reaction is potentially lethal interstitial pneumonitis,[267,287] which may be more common in patients with preexisting lung disease. It is important that physicians monitor their patients carefully because the pneumonitis is reversible if detected early. Serial pulmonary function tests are of little value for follow-up of patients because of the nonspecific nature of the changes that are seen and their cost. Most physicians familiar with the drug monitor their patients by having them obtain a chest x-ray every 3 months. Hyper- or hypothyroidism is seen in about 4 percent of patients.[270] Accumulation of corneal microdeposits is almost uniform during long-term therapy and in many cases can progress to the point of interfering with vision.[288] Some Caucasian patients notice a slate-gray or bluish discoloration of sun-exposed areas of the skin.[289] Many also complain of photosensitivity, which can sometimes be prevented or alleviated with sunscreens and garments. Thirty percent or more of patients have abnormally elevated hepatic enzyme levels in their serum, and progression to jaundice and cirrhosis has been reported.[290,291] Serial laboratory tests to screen for amiodarone toxicity can be costly and generally are of little value; however, it is wise to obtain a reliable assessment of baseline tests (complete blood count, blood chemistry, tests of thyroid and pulmonary function, a slit lamp examination, and measurement of blood levels of other drugs whenever possible). Careful instructions to patients and their family members are important in screening for toxicity.

Drug Interactions

Amiodarone has been found to interfere with the clearance of many drugs. A partial explanation for these interactions may involve the formation of a metabolically inactive cytochrome P450(II)–metabolite complex that has been described in animals treated with amiodarone.[292] This may explain the unexpected accumulation of warfarin,[293] quinidine, procainamide, disopyramide, mexiletine, and propafenone[294] and the resulting bleeding, heart block, or torsades de pointes. However, it does not explain the interaction between amiodarone and drugs eliminated predominantly by the kidneys such as digoxin.[295] It is likely that the elimination of many other drugs can be impaired by amiodarone, and the physician should titrate any concomitant therapy to the lowest effective dosage. (See also Chapter 109.)

BETA RECEPTOR ANTAGONISTS

The beta receptor antagonists are the only agents that have been shown to reduce mortality in the early period and during the 1 to 2 years following acute myocardial infarction.[296] (See Chap. 66.) Even this benefit is confined to those beta receptor antagonists that lack intrinsic sympathomimetic activity. Studies have shown that chronic ventricular arrhythmias can be suppressed by propranolol,[297] metoprolol,[298] timolol,[299] acebutolol,[300] pindolol,[301] nadolol,[302] and atenolol.[303] These agents have proven to be very useful as an adjunct to therapy with agents with class I antiarrhythmic actions.[304,305]

Beta receptor antagonists can also be very useful for control of ventricular rate in atrial fibrillation or flutter, paroxysmal supraventricular tachycardia, symptomatic sinus tachycardia, and the management of catecholamine-related ventricular arrhythmias and ischemia-related arrhythmias.

It has been suggested that this aspect of these agents' action is an antiarrhythmic effect of adrenergic blockade.[296] It has been consistently noted that beta receptor antagonists suppress repetitive ventricular arrhythmias more effectively than they suppress isolated ectopic beats. The finding that the non-beta-blocking dextroisomer of propranolol has antiarrhythmic activity suggests that some of the antiarrhythmic effects of propranolol may be due to other mechanisms.[306]

ADENOSINE (Adenocard)

Clinical Applications

Adenosine is very effective for the acute conversion of paroxysmal supraventricular tachycardia (PSVT) due to reentry involving the AV node. Sixty percent of patients respond at a dose of 6 mg, and an additional 32 percent respond when given a higher dose of 12 mg. Some patients with PSVT associated with the Wolff-Parkinson-White syndrome have also been found to respond to adenosine. Because of the fleeting and relatively selective action of adenosine on the AV node, many cardiologists suggest that it be used as a diagnostic tool in patients with narrow and wide complex tachycardia.[307] On the other hand, it would seem much more reasonable and safer to use the appropriate diagnostic procedures to make the correct diagnosis and not entail the risk of adverse drug reactions, even if transient.

Description

Adenosine is a nucleoside formed in the body by serial dephosphorylation of adenosine triphosphate (ATP) for cyclic adenosine monophosphate or from hydrolysis of *S*-adenosylhomocysteine. It is formed both intra- and extracellularly, and its actions are rapidly terminated by transport into cells followed by metabolism by adenosine deaminase to inosine or phosphorylated to adenosine monophosphate. The actions of adenosine are highly dependent on the rate and route of administration. A rapid intravenous injection into a central venous line is thought to activate carotid body chemoreceptors and usually produces an initial increase in blood pressure of 10 to 15 mmHg followed by a small and transient decrease in pressure. These reflexes are attenuated during surgery, and in this setting, adenosine decreases peripheral vascular resistance, increases cardiac output, and moderately increases heart rate. Bolus injections also produce biphasic effects on heart rate. Approximately 20 s after injection, sinus bradycardia occurs for 10 to 15 s followed by sinus tachycardia (thought to be due to chemoreceptor activation). Activation of the carotid chemoreceptors stimulates respiration and causes secondary activation of pulmonary stretch receptors. Adenosine has a direct effect of slowing AV nodal conduction, which can result in transient AV block. Although adenosine has no direct effect on the His-Purkinje system, it does attenuate the effects of catecholamine stimulation and, in patients with heart block, can block acceleration of the ventricular escape rate by isoproterenol. Adenosine usually has no effect on anterograde or retrograde accessory pathway conduction. Pathways that demonstrate decremental conduction often respond to adenosine, probably because they are partially depolarized and can be hyperpolarized by adenosine. Slow injections into a peripheral line often produce no clinical benefit or changes in blood pressure or heart rate.

Mechanism of Action

The development of synthetic agonists and antagonists of adenosine receptors has made possible the subclassification of A_1 and A_2 receptor subtypes. The A_1 receptors are present in myocardial cells and mediate the negative inotropic, dromotropic, and chronotropic actions of adenosine. The A_2 receptors are present in the endothelium and vascular smooth muscle cells and cause coronary vasodilatation, when activated.

The efficacy of adenosine in PSVT is most likely due to the following actions in atrial myocardium and the AV node: (1) hyperpolarization of sinoatrial nodal cells and slowing of rate of firing, (2) shortening of the action potential of atrial cells, and (3) depression of conduction velocity in the AV node. These actions are due to activation of A_1 adenosine receptor subtypes, which leads to activation of cyclic adenosine monophosphate– (cAMP-)

independent, acetylcholine/adenosine-regulated potassium current, $I_{ACh, Ado}$. Although it may be unrelated to the mechanism of action, adenosine also causes a small inhibition of basal calcium currents in atrial tissue. The A_2 receptors mediate the coronary vasodilator actions of adenosine. Many other actions of adenosine vary with the origin of the tissue and the conditions of the experiment.[307]

Clinical Pharmacology

After intravenous injection adenosine is rapidly transported into red blood cells and endothelial cells. It is difficult to determine accurately a half-life of elimination, but it has been estimated to be from 1.5 to 10 s. The drug is rapidly metabolized in the plasma and in cells to form inosine and adenosine monophosphate. Maximal pharmacologic effects are seen within 30 s after injection into a peripheral intravenous line but occur within 10 to 20 s when given into a central line.

Dosage and Administration

Adenosine should be injected intravenously into a proximal tubing site and flushed quickly with saline. For adults the recommended initial dose is 6 mg injected over 1 to 2 s. If the arrhythmia persists, a 12-mg dose can be injected 1 to 2 min later. This can be repeated, but doses larger than 12 mg are not recommended by the manufacturer. A dosage regimen based on body weight has been proposed, with an initial dose of 50 μg/kg incremented by 50 μg/kg until the PSVT is terminated or side effects become intolerable.[307] Higher doses may be required for patients who have received caffeine or theophylline because of their antagonistic effects at A_1 receptors. Lower doses are recommended if the patients are receiving dipyridamole or carbamazepine.

Modification of Dosage in Disease States

Although the pharmacokinetics of adenosine are unlikely to be altered in patients with renal or hepatic disease, these patients often have electrolyte imbalances that could alter the clinical response. Experience in these patient populations is limited, but preliminary results have not detected any substantial differences in response. Although patients with congestive heart failure have not been reported to respond abnormally, cardiac transplant patients appear to require one-third to one-fifth of the usual dose because of denervation hypersensitivity.[308]

Adverse Reactions

Adenosine is contraindicated in patients with sick-sinus syndrome or second- or third-degree heart block unless the patient has a functioning artificial pacemaker. Because of the rapid clearance of adenosine, side effects last less than 60 s. The most common side effects of adenosine are facial flushing, dyspnea, or chest pressure. Although intrapulmonary administration of adenosine has precipitated bronchospasm in asthmatic patients, this has not been reported with intravenous administration. The manufacturer recommends caution when treating patients with asthma. Other less frequent side effects include the following: nausea, lightheadedness, headache, sweating, palpitations, hypotension, and blurred vision. Intravenous theophylline, which has been recommended to reverse the effects of adenosine, should be prepared and ready for injection.

Drug Interactions

There are several proven interactions that can increase or decrease the activity of adenosine. There are also several other theoretical interactions that could occur but have not been identified. It is clear that dipyridamole pretreatment increases the potency of adenosine, probably because it blocks cellular uptake of adenosine.[309] On the other hand, caffeine and theophylline antagonize the actions of adenosine.[310] The manufacturer cautions that carbamazepine may potentiate the actions of adenosine but that it has been used without obvious problems in patients who have been treated with beta receptor antagonists, calcium entry blockers, digitalis glycosides, quinidine, and angiotensin converting enzyme inhibitors. (See also Chap. 109.)

INVESTIGATIONAL

There are many new agents under development in the United States at this time. Several of these, such as sematilide or E-4031, are analogs of sotalol and/or NAPA, which have been selected for testing because they have class III activity but lack the other actions such as beta-adrenergic receptor inhibition or sodium channel-blocking activity.[311,312] Some impetus for the development of these sotalol-like agents lies in the hope that they will have amiodarone's efficacy without its toxicity. Amiodarone is a very effective antiarrhythmic, and an agent possessing a similar degree of efficacy but lacking in toxicity would be extremely valuable. Unfortunately, it seems unlikely that these new drugs will have markedly improved efficacy because of their electrophysiological similarity to modest agents such as NAPA, clofilium and *d*-sotalol.[99,311,313]

REFERENCES

1. CAST investigators: Preliminary report: Effect of encainide and flecainide on mortality in a randomized trial of arrhythmia suppression after myocardial infarction. *N Engl J Med* 1989; 32:406–412.
2. Hine LK, Laird NM, Hewitt P, Chalmers TC: Meta-analysis of empirical long-term antiarrhythmic therapy after myocardial infarction. *JAMA* 1989; 262(21):3037–3040.
3. Vaughan Williams EM: A classification of antiarrhythmic actions reassessed after a decade of new drugs. *J Clin Pharmacol* 1984; 24:129–147.
4. Task Force of the Working Group on Arrhythmias of the European Society of Cardiology: The Sicilian gambit: A new approach to the classification of antiarrhythmic drugs based on their actions on arrhythmogenic mechanisms. *Circulation* 1991; 84:1831–1851.
5. Hodgkin AL, Huxley AF: A quantitative description of mem-

brane current and its application to conduction and excitation in nerve. *J Physiol* 1952; 117:500–544.
6. Hondeghem LM, Katzung BG: Test of a model of antiarrhythmic drug action: Effects of quinidine and lidocaine on myocardial conduction. *Circulation* 1980; 61:1217–1224.
7. Duff HJ, Roden DM, Primm RK, Carey EL, Oates JA, Woosley RL: Mexiletine for resistant ventricular tachycardia: Comparison with lidocaine and enhancement of efficacy by combination with quinidine (abstr). *Am J Cardiol* 1981; 47:438.
8. Campbell TJ: Kinetics of onset of rate-dependent effects of class I antiarrhythmic drugs are important in determining their effects on refractoriness in guinea-pig ventricle, and provide a theoretical basis for their subclassification. *Cardiovasc Res* 1983; 17:344–352.
9. Harrison DC: Antiarrhythmic drug classification: New science and practical applications. *Am J Cardiol* 1985; 56:185–187.
10. Southworth JL, McKusick VA, Pierce EC II, Rawson FL Jr: Ventricular fibrillation precipitated by cardiac catheterization. *JAMA* 1950; 143:717–720.
11. Lie KI, Wellens JH, van Capelle FJ, Durrer D: Lidocaine in the prevention of primary ventricular fibrillation. A double-blind, randomized study of 212 consecutive patients. *N Engl J Med* 1974; 291:1324–1326.
12. MacMahon S, Collins R, Peto R, Koster RW, Yusuf S: Effects of prophylactic lidocaine in suspected acute myocardial infarction. *JAMA* 1988; 260:1910–1916.
13. Pedersen LE, Bonde J, Graudal NA, Backer NV, Hansen J-ES, Kampmann JP: Quantitative and qualitative binding characteristics of disopyramide in serum from patients with decreased renal and hepatic function. *Br J Clin Pharmacol* 1987; 23:41–46.
14. Rosen KM, Barwolf C, Ehsani A, Rahimtoola SH: Effects of lidocaine and propranolol on the normal and anomalous pathways in patients with preexcitation. *Am J Cardiol* 1972; 30:801–809.
15. Josephson ME, Kastor JA, Kitchen JG III: Lidocaine in Wolff-Parkinson-White syndrome with atrial fibrillation. *Ann Intern Med* 1976; 84:44–45.
16. Akhtar M, Gilbert CJ, Shenasa M: Effect of lidocaine on atrioventricular response via the accessory pathway in patients with Wolff-Parkinson-White syndrome. *Circulation* 1981; 63:435–441.
17. Davis LD, Temte JV: Electrophysiological actions of lidocaine on canine ventricular muscle and Purkinje fibers. *Circ Res* 1969; 24:639–655.
18. Bigger JT Jr, Mandel WJ: Effect of lidocaine on the electrophysiological properties of ventricular muscle and Purkinje fibers. *J Clin Invest* 1970; 49:63–77.
19. Kunkel F, Rowland M, Scheinman MM: The electrophysiologic effects of lidocaine in patients with intraventricular conduction defects. *Circulation* 1974; 49:894–899.
20. Bekheit S, Murtagh JG, Morton P, Fletcher E: Effect of lignocaine on conducting system of human heart. *Br Heart J* 1973; 35:305–311.
21. Gupta PK, Lichstein E, Chadda KD: Lidocaine-induced heart block in patients with bundle branch block. *Am J Cardiol* 1974; 33:487–492.
22. Aravindakshan V, Kuo C-S, Gettes LS: Effect of lidocaine on escape rate in patients with complete atrioventricular block. A. Distal His block. *Am J Cardiol* 1977; 40:177–183.
23. Stenson RE, Constantino RT, Harrison DC: Interrelationships of hepatic blood flow, cardiac output, and blood levels of lidocaine in man. *Circulation* 1971; 43:205–211.
24. Zito RA, Reid PR: Lidocaine kinetics predicted by indocyanine green clearance. *N Engl J Med* 1978; 298:1160–1163.
25. Blumer J, Strong JM, Atkinson AJ Jr: The convulsant potency of lidocaine and its N-dealkylated metabolites. *J Pharmacol Exp Ther* 1973; 186:31–36.
26. Narang PK, Crouthamel WG, Carliner NH, Fisher ML: Lidocaine and its active metabolites. *Clin Pharmacol Ther* 24:654–662.
27. Thomson PD, Melmon KL, Richardson JA, Cohn K, Steinbrunn W, Cudihee R, et al: Lidocaine pharmacokinetics in advanced heart failure, liver disease and renal failure in humans. *Ann Intern Med* 1973; 78:499–508.
28. Wyman MG, Slaughter RL, Farolino DA, Gore S, Cannom DS, Goldreyer BN, et al: Multiple bolus technique for lidocaine administration in acute ischemic heart disease. II. Treatment of refractory ventricular arrhythmias and the pharmacokinetic significance of severe left ventricular failure. *J Am Coll Cardiol* 1983; 2:764–769.
29. Stargel WW, Shand DG, Routledge PA, Barchowsky A, Wagner GS: Clinical comparison of rapid infusion and multiple injection methods for lidocaine loading. *Am Heart J* 1981; 102:872–876.
30. Alderman EL, Kerber RE, Harrison DC: Evaluation of lidocaine resistance in man using intermittent large-dose infusion techniques. *Am J Cardiol* 1974; 34:342–349.
31. Koster RW, Dunning AJ: Intramuscular lidocaine for prevention of lethal arrhythmias in the prehospitalization phase of acute myocardial infarction. *N Engl J Med* 1985; 313:1105–1110.
32. Richard C, Berdeaux A, Delion F, Riou B, Rimailho A, Giudicelli JF, et al: Effect of mechanical ventilation on hepatic drug pharmacokinetics. *Chest* 1986; 90:837–841.
33. LeLorier J, Grenon D, Latour Y, Caille G, Dumont G, Brosseau A, et al: Pharmacokinetics of lidocaine after prolonged intravenous infusions in uncomplicated myocardial infarction. *Ann Intern Med* 1977; 87:700–702.
34. Routledge PA, Shand DG, Barchowsky A, Wagner G, Stargel WW: Relationship between alpha 1-acid glycoprotein and lidocaine disposition in myocardial infarction. *Clin Pharmacol Ther* 1981; 30:154–157.
35. Cheng TO, Wadhwa K: Sinus standstill following intravenous lidocaine administration. *JAMA* 1973; 223:790–792.
36. Marriott HJL, Phillips K: Profound hypotension and bradycardia after a single bolus of lidocaine. *J Electrocardiol* 1974; 7:79–82.
37. Cote P, Harrison DC, Basile J, Schroeder JS: Hemodynamic interaction of procainamide and lidocaine after experimental myocardial infarction. *Am J Cardiol* 1973; 32:937–942.
38. Branch RA, Shand DG, Wilkinson GR, Nies AS: The reduction of lidocaine clearance by dl-propranolol: An example of hemodynamic drug interaction. *J Pharmacol Exp Ther* 1973; 184:515–519.
39. Ochs HR, Carstens G, Greenblatt DJ: Reduction in lidocaine clearance during continuous infusion and by coadministration of propranolol. *N Engl J Med* 1980; 303:373–377.
40. Feeley J, Wilkinson GR, McAllister CB, Wood AJJ: Increased toxicity and reduced clearance of lidocaine by cimetidine. *Ann Intern Med* 1982; 96:592–593.
41. Berk SI, Gal P, Bauman JL, Douglas JB, McCue JD, Powell JR: The effect of oral cimetidine on total and unbound serum lidocaine concentration in patients with suspected myocardial infarction. *Int J Cardiol* 1987; 14:91–94.
42. Powell JR, Foster JR, Patterson JH, Cross R, Wargin W: Effect of duration of lidocaine infusion and route of cimetidine administration on lidocaine pharmacokinetics. *Clin Pharm* 1986; 5:993–998.
43. De Rick AF, Belpaire FM, Dello C, Bogaert MG: Influence of enhanced alpha-1-acid glycoprotein concentration on protein binding, pharmacokinetics and antiarrhythmic effect of lidocaine in the dog. *J Pharmacol Exp Ther* 1987; 241:289–293.
44. Lineberry MD, Davies RF, Chaffin PL, et al: Safety and efficacy of combining encainide and lidocaine. *Circulation* 1987; 76(suppl IV):IV-511.
45. Duff HJ, Roden D, Primm RK, Oates JA, Woosley RL: Mexiletine in the treatment of resistant ventricular arrhythmias: Enhancement of efficacy and reduction of dose-related side effects by combination with quinidine. *Circulation* 1983; 67: 1124–1128.
46. Leahey EB Jr, Heissenbuttel RH, Giardina E-GV, Bigger JT Jr: Combined mexiletine and propranolol treatment of refractory ventricular arrhythmia. *Br Med J* 1980; 281:357–358.
47. Ruskin JN, DiMarco JP, Garan H: Out-of-hospital cardiac arrest: Electrophysiologic observations and selection of long-term antiarrhythmic therapy. *N Engl J Med* 1980; 303:607–613.
48. Stein J, Podrid P, Lown B: Effects of oral mexiletine on left and right ventricular function. *Am J Cardiol* 1984; 54:575–578.
49. Yamaguchi I, Singh BN, Mandel WJ: Electrophysiological effects of mexiletine on isolated rabbit atria and canine ventricular muscle Purkinje fiber. *Cardiovasc Res* 1979; 13:288–296.
50. Weld FM, Bigger JT Jr, Swistel D, Bordiuk J, Lau YH: Electrophysiological effects of mexiletine (KO1173) on ovine cardiac Purkinje fibers. *J Pharmacol Exp Ther* 1979; 210:222–228.
51. Frame L, Gintant G, Hoffman BF: Mexiletine and tocainide differ from lidocaine in their use-dependent kinetics (abstr). *Circulation* 1982; 66(suppl):II-292.

52. Roos JC, Paalman ACA, Dunning AJ: Electrophysiological effects of mexiletine in man. *Br Heart J* 1976; 38:1262–1271.
53. Prescott LF, Clements JA, Pottage A: Absorption, distribution, and elimination of mexiletine. *Postgrad Med J* 1977; 53(suppl 1):50–55.
54. Beckett AH, Chidomere EC: The distribution, metabolism and excretion of mexiletine in man. *Postgrad Med J* 1977; 53(suppl 1):60–66.
55. Campbell NPS, Kelley JG, Adgey AAJ, Shanks RG: The clinical pharmacology of mexiletine. *Br J Clin Pharmacol* 1978; 6:103–108.
56. Woosley RL, Wang T, Stone W, Siddoway L, Thompson K, Duff HJ, et al: Pharmacology, electrophysiology, and pharmacokinetics of mexiletine. *Am Heart J* 1984; 107:1058–1065.
57. Brown JE, Shand DG: Therapeutic drug monitoring of antiarrhythmic agents. *Clin Pharmacokinet* 1982; 7:125–148.
58. Campbell RWF: Mexiletine. *N Engl J Med* 1987; 316:29–34.
59. Broly F, Vandamme N, Caron J, Libersa C, Lhermitte M: Single-dose quinidine treatment inhibitis mexiletine oxidation in extensive metabolizers of debrisoquine. *Life Sci* 1991; 48:PL-123–PL-128.
60. el Allaf D, Henrard L, Crochelet L, Delapierre D, Carlier J, Dresse A: Pharmacokinetics of mexiletine in renal insufficiency. *Br J Clin Pharmacol* 1982; 14:431–435.
61. Leahey EB Jr, Giardina E-GV, Bigger JT Jr: Effect of ventricular failure on steady state kinetics of mexiletine (abstr). *Clin Res* 1980; 26:239A.
62. Pentikainen PJ, Hietakorpi S, Halinen MO, Lampinen LM: Cirrhosis of the liver markedly impairs the elimination of mexiletine. *Eur J Clin Pharmacol* 1986; 30:83–88.
63. Fasola GP, D'Osualdo F, de Pangher V, Barducci E: Thrombocytopenia and mexiletine (letter). *Ann Intern Med* 1984; 100:162.
64. Girmann G, Pees H, Scheurlen PG: Pseudothrombocytopenia and mexiletine (letter). *Ann Intern Med* 1984; 100:767.
65. Campbell RWF, Dolder MA, Prescott LF, Talbot RG, Murray A, Julian DG: Comparison of procainamide and mexiletine in prevention of ventricular arrhythmias after acute myocardial infarction. *Lancet* 1975; 1:1257–1259.
66. Klein MD, Levin PA, Ryan TJ: Antiarrhythmic efficacy, pharmacokinetics and clinical safety of tocainide in convalescent myocardial infarction patients. *Chest* 1980; 77:726–730.
67. Stein J, Podrid PJ, Lampert S, Hirsowitz G, Lown B: Long-term mexiletine for ventricular arrhythmia. *Am Heart J* 1984; 107:1091–1098.
68. Saunamaki KI: Hemodynamic effects of a new anti-arrhythmic agent mexiletine (Ko 1173) in ischaemic heart disease. *Cardiovasc Res* 1975; 9:788–792.
69. Pentikainen PJ, Koivula IH, Hiltunen HA: Effect of rifampicin treatment on the kinetics of mexiletine. *Eur J Clin Pharmacol* 1982; 23:261–266.
70. Bigger JT Jr: The interaction of mexiletine with other cardiovascular drugs. *Am Heart J* 1984; 107:1079–1085.
71. Klein AL, Sami MH: Usefulness and safety of cimetidine in patients receiving mexiletine for ventricular arrhythmia. *Am Heart J* 1985; 109: 1281–1286.
72. Klein AL, Sami M, Selinger K: Mexiletine kinetics in healthy subjects taking cimetidine. *Clin Pharmacol Ther* 1985; 37:669–673.
73. Hurwitz A, Vacek JL, Botteron GW, Sztern MI, Hughes EM, Jayaraj A: Mexiletine effects on theophylline disposition. *Clin Pharmacol* 1991; 50:299–307.
74. Kaplan HR, Mertz TE, Steffe TJ: New class I antiarrhythmic agents. In: Lucchesi BR, Dingle JV, Schwartz RP Jr (eds): *Clinical Pharmacology of Antiarrhythmic Therapy.* New York, Raven, 1984:77–94.
75. Kim SG, Mercando AD, Fisher JD: Combination of tocainide and quinidine for better tolerance and additive effects in patients with coronary artery disease. *J Am Coll Cardiol* 1987; 9:1369–1374.
76. Singh SN, DiBianco R, Gottdiener JS, Ginsberg R, Fletcher RD: Effect of moricizine-hydrochloride in reducing chronic high-frequency ventricular arrhythmia: Results of a prospective, controlled trial. *Am J Cardiol* 1984; 53:745–750.
77. Shand DG, McLeod AA: Human beta-adrenoceptor antagonism by the Class I antiarrhythmic drug propafenone; Clinical study. *II World Conf Clin Pharmacol Ther 1983*; 54.
78. CAPS Investigators: The Cardiac Arrhythmia Pilot Study. *Am J Cardiol* 1986; 57:91–95.
79. Cardiac Arrhythmia Pilot Study (CAPS) Investigators: The Effect of encainide, flecainide, imipramine and moricizine on ventricular arrhythmias during the year after myocardial infarction. The CAPS. *Am J Cardiol* 1988; 61:501–509.
80. Miura DS, Wynn J, Torres V, Laux B, Keefe DL, Somberg JC: Antiarrhythmic efficacy of Ethmozine in patients with ventricular tachycardia as determined by programmed electrical stimulation. *Am Heart J* 1986; 111:661–666.
81. Wyndham CRC, Pratt CM, Mann DE, Winkle RA, Somberg J, DeMaria AN, et al: Electrophysiology of Ethmozine (moricizine HCl) for ventricular tachycardia. *Am J Cardiol* 1987; 60(suppl F):67F–72F.
82. Dorian P, Echt DS, Mead RH, Lee JT, Lebsack CS, Winkle RA: Ethmozine: Electrophysiology, hemodynamics, and antiarrhythmic efficacy in patients with life-threatening ventricular arrhythmias. *Am Heart J* 1986; 112:327–332.
83. Schubert B, Hering S, Bodewei R, Rosenshtraukh LV, Wollenberg A: Use- and voltage-dependent depression by Ethmozine (moricizine) of the rapid inward sodium current in single rat ventricular muscle cells. *J Cardiovasc Pharmacol* 1986; 8:358–366.
84. Lee JH, Rosen MR: Use-dependent actions and effects on transmembrane action potentials of flecainide, encainide, and ethmozine in canine Purkinje fibers. *J Cardiovasc Pharmacol* 1991; 18(2)285–292.
85. Biollaz J, Shaheen O, Wood AJ: Cimetidine inhibition of Ethmozine metabolism. *Clin Pharmacol Ther* 1985; 37:665–668.
86. Doherty JE: Clinical use of digitalis glycosides. An update. *Cardiology* 1985; 72:225–254.
87. Piepho RW: Individualization of calcium entry-blocker dosage for systemic hypertension. *Am J Cardiol* 1985; 56(suppl):105H–111H.
88. Siddoway LA, Schwartz SL, Barbey JT, Woosley RL: Clinical pharmacokinetics of moricizine. *Am J Cardiol* 1990; 65(suppl D):21D-25D.
89. Benedek IH, Pieniaszek HJ, Davidson AF: Effect of moricizine on the pharmacokinetics of theophylline in healthy volunteers. *Pharm Res* 1989; 6:s243.
90. Antman EM, Arnold JMO, Friedman PL, White H, Bosak M, et al: Drug interactions with cardiac glycosides: Evaluation of a possible digoxin-Ethmozine pharmacokinetic interaction. *J Cardiovasc Pharmacol* 1987; 9:622–627.
91. MacFarland RT, Moeller VR, Pieniaszek HJ, Whitney CC Jr, Marcus FI: Assessment of the potential pharmacokinetic interaction between digoxin and Ethmozine. *J Clin Pharmacol* 1985; 25:138–143.
92. Woosley RL, Morganroth J, Fogoros RN, McMahon FG, Humphries JO, Mason DT, et al: Pharmacokinetics of moricizine HCl. *Am J Cardiol* 1987; 60(suppl F):35F–39F.
93. Hoffman BF, Rosen MR, Wit AL: Electrophysiology and pharmacology of cardiac arrhythmias. VII. Cardiac effects of quinidine and procaine amide. *Am Heart J* 1975; 90:117–122.
94. Wellens HJJ, Durrer D: Effect of procaine amide, quinidine and ajmaline in the Wolff-Parkinson-White syndrome. *Circulation* 1974; 50:114–120.
95. Elson J, Strong JM, Lee W-K, Atkinson AJ Jr: Antiarrhythmic potency of *N*-acetylprocainamide. *Clin Pharmacol Ther* 1975; 17:134–140.
96. Dangman KH, Hoffman BF: In vivo and in vitro antiarrhythmic and arrhythmogenic effects of *N*-acetyl procainamide. *J Pharmacol Exp Ther* 1981; 217:851–862.
97. Roden DM, Reele SB, Higgins SB, Wilkinson GR, Smith RF, Oates JA, et al: Antiarrhythmic efficacy, pharmacokinetics and safety of *N*-acetylprocainamide in human subjects: Comparison with procainamide. *Am J Cardiol* 1980; 46:463–468.
98. Kluger J, Drayer DE, Reidenberg M, Ellis G, Lloyd V, Tyberg T, et al: The clinical pharmacology and antiarrhythmic efficacy of acetylprocainamide in patients with arrhythmias. *Am J Cardiol* 1980; 45:1250–1257.
99. Jaillon P, Rubenson D, Peters F, Mason JW, Winkle RA: Electrophysiologic effects of *N*-acetylprocainamide in human beings. *Am J Cardiol* 1981; 47:1134–1140.
100. Mark LC, Kayden HJ, Steele JM, Cooper JR, Berlin I, Rovenstine EA, et al: The physiologic disposition and cardiac effects of procaine amide. *J Pharmacol Exp Ther* 1951; 102:5–15.
101. Rosen MR, Gelband H, Hoffman BF: Canine electrocardiographic and cardiac electrophysiologic changes induced by procainamide. *Circulation* 1972; 46:528–536.

102. Rosen MR, Merker C, Gelband H, Hoffman BF: Effects of procaine amide on the electrophysiologic properties of the canine ventricular conduction system. *J Pharmacol Exp Ther* 1973; 185:438–446.
103. Arnsdorf MF, Bigger JT Jr: The effect of procaine amide on components of excitability in long mammalian cardiac Purkinje fibers. *Circ Res* 1976; 38:115–122.
104. Jaillon P, Winkle RA: Electrophysiologic comparative study of procainamide and *N*-acetylprocainamide in anesthetized dogs: Concentration-response relationships. *Circulation* 1979; 60:1385–1394.
105. Lee W-K, Strong JM, Kehoe RF, Dutcher JS, Atkinson AJ Jr: Antiarrhythmic efficacy of *N*-acetylprocainamide in patients with premature ventricular contractions. *Clin Pharmacol Ther* 1976; 19:508–514.
106. Winkle RA, Jaillon P, Kates RE, Peters F: Clinical pharmacology and antiarrhythmic efficacy of *N*-acetylprocainamide. *Am J Cardiol* 1981; 47:123–130.
107. Funck-Brentano C, Jared LL, Roden DM, Woosley RL: Interaction of procainamide and *N*-acetylprocainamide in man. *Circulation* 1987; 76(suppl):IV-520.
108. Myerburg RJ, Kessler KM, Kiem I, Pefkanos KC, Conde CA, Cooper D, et al: Relationship between plasma levels of procainamide, suppression of premature ventricular complexes and prevention of recurrent ventricular tachycardia. *Circulation* 1981; 64:280–290.
109. Giardina E-GV, Heissenbuttel RH, Bigger JT Jr: Intermittent intravenous procainamide to treat ventricular arrhythmias. Correlation of plasma concentration with effect on arrhythmia, electrocardiogram and blood pressure. *Ann Intern Med* 1973; 78:183–193.
110. Lima JJ, Goldfarb AL, Conti DR, Golden LH, Bascomb BL, Benedetti GM, et al: Safety and efficacy of procainamide infusions. *Am J Cardiol* 1979; 43:98–105.
111. Karlsson E: Clinical pharmacokinetics of procainamide. *Clin Pharmacokinet* 1978; 3:97–107.
112. du Souich P, Erill S: Metabolism of procainamide in patients with chronic heart failure, chronic respiratory failure and chronic renal failure. *Eur J Clin Pharmacol* 1978; 14:21–27.
113. Kessler KM, Kayden DS, Estes DM, Koslovskis PL, Sequeira R, Trohman RG, et al: Procainamide pharmacokinetics in patients with acute myocardial infarction or congestive heart failure. *J Am Coll Cardiol* 1986; 7:1131–1139.
114. Jackman WM, Clark M, Friday KJ, Aliot EM, Anderson JL, Lazzara R: Ventricular tachyarrhythmias in the long QT syndrome. *Med Clin North Am* 1984; 68:1079–1109.
115. Olshansky B, Martins J, Hunt S: *N*-acetyl procainamide causing torsades de pointes. *Am J Cardiol* 1982; 50:1439–1441.
116. Brachmann J, Scherlag BJ, Rosenshtraukh LV, Lazzara R: Bradycardia-dependent triggered activity: Relevance to drug-induced multiform ventricular tachycardia. *Circulation* 1983; 68:846–856.
117. Kosowsky BD, Taylor J, Lown B, Ritchie RF: Long-term use of procaine amide following acute myocardial infarction. *Circulation* 1973; 47:1204–1210.
118. Ellrodt AG, Murata GH, Riedinger MS, Stewart ME, Mochizuki C, Gray R: Severe neutropenia associated with sustained-release procainamide. *Ann Intern Med* 1984; 100:197–201.
119. Wyse DG, McAnulty JH, Rahimtoola SH: Influence of plasma drug level and the presence of conduction disease on the electrophysiologic effects of procainamide. *Am J Cardiol* 1979; 43:619–626.
120. Somogyi A, McLean A, Heinzow B: Cimetidine-procainamide pharmacokinetic interaction in man: evidence of competition for tubular secretion of basic drugs. *Eur J Clin Pharmacol* 1983; 25:339–345.
121. Christian CD Jr, Meredith CG, Speeg KV Jr: Cimetidine inhibits renal procainamide clearance. *Clin Pharmacol Ther* 1984; 36:221–227.
122. Somogyi A, Bochner F: Dose and concentration dependent effect of ranitidine on procainamide disposition and renal clearance in man. *Br J Clin Pharmacol* 1984; 18:175–181.
123. Danilo P Jr, Hordof AJ, Rosen MR: Effects of disopyramide on electrophysiologic properties of canine cardiac Purkinje fibers. *J Pharmacol Exp Ther* 1977; 201:701–710.
124. Mirro MJ, Watanabe AM, Bailey JC: Electrophysiological effects of disopyramide and quinidine on guinea pig atria and canine Purkinje fibers. *Circ Res* 1980; 46:660–668.
125. Befeler B, Castellanos A, Wells DE, Vagueiro MC, Yeh BK: Electrophysiologic effects of the antiarrhythmic agent disopyramide phosphate. *Am J Cardiol* 1975; 35:282–287.
126. Kus T, Sasyniuk BI: Electrophysiological actions of disopyramide phosphate on canine ventricular muscle and Purkinje fibers. *Circ Res* 1975; 37:844–854.
127. Levites R, Anderson GJ: Electrophysiological effects of disopyramide phosphate during experimental myocardial ischemia. *Am Heart J* 1979; 98:339–344.
128. Birkhead JS, Vaughan Williams EM: Dual effects of disopyramide on atrial and atrioventricular conduction and refractory periods. *Br Heart J* 1977; 39:657–660.
129. Josephson ME, Caracta AR, Lau SH, Gallagher JJ, Damato AN: Electrophysiological evaluation of disopyramide in man. *Am Heart J* 1973; 86:771–780.
130. Giacomini KM, Cox BM, Blaschke TF: Comparative anticholingergic potencies of *R*- and *S*-disopyramide in longitudinal muscle strips from guinea pig ileum. *Life Sci* 1980; 27:1191–1197.
131. Kidwell GA, Schaal SF, Muir WW III: Stereospecific effects of disopyramide enantiomers following pretreatment of canine cardiac Purkinje fibers with verapamil and nisoldipine. *J Cardiovasc Pharmacol* 1987; 9:276–284.
132. Dubray C, Boucher M, Paire M, Pinatel H, Duchene-Marullaz P: Comparative effects of disopyramide and its mono-*N*-dealkylated metabolite in conscious dogs with chronic atrioventricular block: Plasma concentration-response relationships. *J Cardiovasc Pharmacol* 1986; 8:1229–1234.
133. Dubetz DK, Brown NN, Hooper WD, Eadie MJ, Tyrer JH: Disopyramide pharmacokinetics and bioavailability (letter). *Br J Clin Pharmacol* 1978; 6:279–281.
134. Johnston A, Henry JA, Warrington SJ, Hamer NAJ: Pharmacokinetics of oral disopyramide phosphate in patients with renal impairment. *Br J Clin Pharmacol* 1980; 10:245–248.
135. Rangno RE, Warnica W, Ogilvie RI, Kreeft JH, Bridger E: Correlation of disopyramide pharmacokinetics with efficacy in ventricular tachyarrhythmia. *J Int Med Res* 1976; 4(suppl1):54–58.
136. Hinderling PH, Garrett ER: Pharmacokinetics of the antiarrhythmic disopyramide in healthy humans. *J Pharmacokinet Biopharm* 1976; 4:199–230.
137. Hinderling PH, Garrett ER: Pharmacodynamics of the antiarrhythmic disopyramide in healthy humans. Correlation of the kinetics of the drug and its effect. *J Pharmacokinet Biopharm* 1976; 4:231–242.
138. Meffin PJ, Robert EW, Winkle RA, Harapart S, Peters FA, Harrison DC: The role of concentration-dependent plasma protein binding in disopyramide disposition. *J Pharmacokinet Biopharm* 1979; 7:29–46.
139. Lima JJ, Boudoulas H, Blanford M: Concentration-dependence of disopyramide binding to serum protein and its influence on kinetics and dynamics. *J Pharmacol Exp Ther* 1981; 219:741–747.
140. Haughey DB, Lima JJ: Influence of concentration dependent protein binding on serum concentrations and urinary excretion of disopyramide and its metabolite following oral administration. *Biopharm Drug Dispos* 1983; 4:103–112.
141. Bredeson JE, Kierulf P: Relationship between alpha 1-acid glycoprotein and distribution of disopyramide and mono-*N*-dealkyldisopyramide in whole blood. *Br J Clin Pharmacol* 1986; 22:281–286.
142. Upton RA, Williams RL: The impact of neglecting nonlinear plasma-protein binding on disopyramide bioavailability studies. *J Pharmacokinet Biopharm* 1986; 14:365–379.
143. Davies RF, Siddoway LA, Shaw L, Barbey JT, Lineberry MD, Roden DM, et al: An assessment of the pharmacokinetic and pharmacodynamic consequences of concentration dependent plasma binding of disopyramide: A comparison of regular with sustained (abstr). *Clin Res* 1986; 34:396A.
144. Edvardsson N, Olsson SB: Clinical value of plasma concentrations of antiarrhythmic drugs. *Eur Heart J* 1987; 8(suppl A):83–89.
145. Kumana CR, Rambihar VS, Tanser PH, Cairns JA, Gupta RN, Wildeman RA, et al: A placebo-controlled study to determine the efficacy of oral disopyramide phosphate for the prophylaxis of ventricular dysrhythmias after acute myocardial infarction. *Br J Clin Pharmacol* 1982; 14:519–527.
146. Ilett KF, Madsen BW, Woods JD: Disopyramide kinetics in patients with acute myocardial infarction. *Clin Pharmacol Ther* 1979; 26:1–7.

147. Podrid PJ, Schoenberger A, Lown B: Congestive heart failure caused by oral disopyramide. *N Engl J Med* 1980; 302:614–617.
148. Bonde J, Gradual NA, Pedersen LE, Balslov S, Angelo HR, Svendsen TL, et al: Kinetics of disopyramide in decreased hepatic function. *Eur J Clin Pharmacol* 1986; 31:73–77.
149. Mokler CM, Hillman RA: Nature of the anticholinergic action of some antiarrhythmic drugs. *Pharmacol Res Commun* 1972; 4:171–178.
150. Teichman SL, Ferrick A, Kim SG, Matos JA, Waspe LE, Fisher JD: Disopyramide-pyridostigmine interaction: Selective reversal of anticholinergic symptoms with preservation of antiarrhythmic effect. *J Am Coll Cardiol* 1987; 10:633–641.
151. Schweitzer P, Mark H: Torsades de pointes caused by disopyramide and hypokalemia. *Mt Sinai J Med* 1982; 49:110–114.
152. LaBarre A, Strauss HC, Scheinman MM, Evans GT, Bashore T, Tiedman JS, et al: Electrophysiologic effects of disopyramide phosphate on sinus node function in patients with sinus node dysfunction. *Circulation* 1979; 59:226–235.
153. Roden DM, Hoffman BF: Action potential prolongation and induction of abnormal automaticity by low quinidine concentrations in canine Purkinje fibers. Relationship to potassium and cycle length. *Circ Res* 1985; 56:857–867.
154. Risler T, Burk M, Peters U, Grabensee B, Seipel L: On the interaction between digoxin and disopyramide. *Clin Pharmacol Ther* 1983; 34:176–180.
155. Sylven C, Anderson P: Evidence that disopyramide does not interact with warfarin. *Br Med J* 1983; 286:1181.
156. Kessler JM, Keys PW, Stattford RW: Disopyramide and phenytoin interaction. *Clin Pharm* 1982; 1:263–264.
157. Aitio M-L, Mansury L, Tala E, Haataja M, Aitio A: The effect of enzyme-induction on the metabolism of disopyramide in man. *Br J Clin Pharmacol* 1981; 11:279–285.
158. Aitio M-L, Vuorenmaa T: Enhanced metabolism and diminished efficacy of disopyramide by enzyme induction. *Br J Clin Pharmacol* 1980; 9:149–152.
159. Cumming AD, Robertson C: Interaction between disopyramide and practolol. *Br Med J* 1979; 2:1264.
160. Sodermark T, Edhag O, Sjogren A, Jonsson B, Olsson A, Oro L, et al: Effect of quinidine on maintaining sinus rhythm after conversion of atrial fibrillation or flutter: A multicenter study from Stockholm. *Br Heart J* 1975; 37:486–492.
161. Levi GF, Proto C: Combined treatment of atrial fibrillation with quinidine and beta-blockers. *Br Heart J* 1972; 34:911–914.
162. Wu D, Kou H-C, Hung J-S: Exercise-triggered paroxysmal ventricular tachycardia. *Ann Intern Med* 1981; 95:410–414.
163. Bloomfield SS, Romhilt DW, Chou T-C, Fowler NO: Natural history of cardiac arrhythmias and their prevention with quinidine in patients with acute coronary insufficiency. *Circulation* 1973; 47:967–973.
164. Yount E H, Rosenblum M, McMillan RL: Use of quinidine in treatment of chronic auricular fibrillation. *Arch Intern Med* 1952; 89:63–69.
165. Weisman SA: Do's and don'ts in the treatment of auricular fibrillation with quinidine. *Am J Cardiol* 1959; 3:333–335.
166. Carliner NH, Crouthamel WG, Fisher ML, Mugmon MA, Vassar DL, Narang PK, et al: Quinidine therapy in hospitalized patients with ventricular arrhythmias. *Am Heart J* 1979; 98:708–715.
167. Winkle RA, Gradman AH, Fitzgerald JW: Antiarrhythmic drug effect assessed from ventricular arrhythmia reduction in the ambulatory electrocardiogram and treadmill test: Comparison of propranolol, procainamide and quinidine. *Am J Cardiol* 1978; 42:473–480.
168. Coplen SE, Antman EM, Berlin JA, Hewitt P, Chalmers TC: Efficacy and safety of quinidine therapy for maintenance of sinus rhythms after cardioversion. A meta-analysis of randomized control trials. *Circulation* 1990; 82:1106–1114.
169. Fasola AF, Noble RJ, Zipes DP: Treatment of recurrent ventricular tachycardia and fibrillation with aprindine. *Am J Cardiol* 1977; 39:903–909.
170. Wenckebach KF: *Die unregelmassige Herztatigkeit und ihre klinische Bedeutung*. Leipzig, W. Engelmann, 1914.
171. Denes P, Gabster A, Huang SK: Clinical, electrocardiographic and follow-up observations in patients having ventricular fibrillation during Holter monitoring. Role of quinidine therapy. *Am J Cardiol* 1981; 48:9–16.
172. Sokolow M, Edgar AL: Blood quinidine concentrations as a guide in the treatment of cardiac arrhythmias. *Circulation* 1950; 1:576–592.
173. Vozeh S, Uematsu T, Follath F: Antiarrhythmic activity of two quinidine metabolites in experimental reperfusion arrhythmia: Relative potency and pharmacodynamic interaction with the parent drug. *J Pharmacol Exp Ther* 1987; 243:297–301.
174. Vozeh S, Bindschedler M, Huy-Riem HA, Kaufmann G, Guentert TW, Follath F: Pharmacodynamics of 3-hydroxyquinidine alone and in combination with quinidine in healthy persons. *Am J Cardiol* 1987; 59:681–684.
175. Kavanagh KM, Wyse DG, Mitchell LB, Gilhooly T, Gillis AM, Duff HJ: Contribution of quinidine metabolites to electrophysiologic responses in human subjects. *Clin Pharmacol Ther* 1989; 46:352–358.
176. Thompson KA, Blair IA, Woosley RL, Roden DM: Comparative in vitro electrophysiology of quinidine, its major metabolites and dihydroquinidine. *J Pharmacol Exp Ther* 1987; 241:84–90.
177. Cramer G, Isaksson B: Quantitative determination of quinidine in plasma. *Scand J Clin Lab Invest* 1963; 15:553–556.
178. Drayer DE, Lorenzo B, Reidenberg MM: Liquid chromatography and fluorescence spectroscopy compared with a homogeneous enzyme immunoassay technique for determining quinidine in serum. *Clin Chem* 1981; 27:308–310.
179. Drayer DE, Lowenthal DT, Restivo KM, Schwartz A, Cook CE, Reidenberg MM: Steady-state serum levels of quinidine and active metabolites in cardiac patients with varying degrees of renal function. *Clin Pharmacol Ther* 1978; 24:31–39.
180. Kessler KM, Humphries WC, Black M, Spann JF: Quinidine pharmacokinetics in patients with cirrhosis or receiving propranolol. *Am Heart J* 1978; 96:627–635.
181. Ochs HR, Greenblatt DJ, Woo E: Clinical pharmacokinetics of quinidine. *Clin Pharmacokinet* 1980; 5:150–168.
182. Kay GN, Plumb VJ, Arciniegas JG, Henthorn RW, Waldo AL: Torsades de pointes: The long-short initiating sequence and other clinical features: Observations in 32 patients. *J Am Coll Cardiol* 1983; 2:806–817.
183. Crouthamel WG: The effect of congestive heart failure on quinidine pharmacokinetics. *Am Heart J* 1975; 90:335–339.
184. Conrad KA, Molk BL, Chidsey CA: Pharmacokinetic studies of quinidine in patients with arrhythmias. *Circulation* 1977; 55:1–7.
185. Cohen IS, Jick H, Cohen SI: Adverse reactions to quinidine in hospitalized patients: Findings based on data from the Boston Collaborative Drug Surveillance Programs. *Prog Cardiovasc Dis* 1977; 20:151–163.
186. Sami MH: Acute intravenous and long-term oral hemodynamic effects of encainide. *Am J Cardiol* 1986; 58(suppl):25C–30C.
187. Dargie HJ, Cleland JGF, Leckie BJ, Inglis CG, East BW, Ford I: Relation of arrhythmias and electrolyte abnormalities to survival in patients with severe chronic heart failure. *Circulation* 1987; 75(suppl):IV-98–IV-107.
188. Roden DM, Woosley RL, Bostick D, Bernard Y, Primm RK: Quinidine-induced long QT syndrome: Incidence and presenting features (abstr). *Circulation* 1983; 68(suppl):III-276.
189. Schmid PG, Nelson LD, Mark AL, Heistad DD, Abboud FM: Inhibition of adrenergic vasoconstriction by quinidine. *J Pharmacol Exp Ther* 1974; 188:124–134.
190. Nair MR, Duvernoy WF, Leichtman DA: Severe leukopenia and thrombocytopenia secondary to quinidine. *Clin Cardiol* 1981; 4:247–257.
191. Polish LB, Branch RA, Fitzgerald GA: Digitoxin-quinidine interaction: Potentiation during administration of cimetidine. *South Med J* 1981; 74:633–634.
192. Data JL, Wilkinson GR, Nies AS: Interaction of quinidine with anticonvulsant drugs. *N Engl J Med* 1976; 294:699–702.
193. Leahey EB Jr, Reiffel JA, Drusin RE, Heissenbuttel RH, Lovejoy WP, Bigger JT Jr: Interactions between quinidine and digoxin. *JAMA* 1978; 240:533–534.
194. Bussey HI: The influence of quinidine and other agents on digitalis glycosides. *Am Heart J* 1982; 104:289–302.
195. Brinn R, Brosen K, Gram LF, Haghfelt T, Otton SV: Spartine oxidation is practically abolished in quinidine-treated patients. *Br J Clin Pharmacol* 1986; 22:194–197.
196. Inaba T, Tyndale RE, Mahon WA: Quinidine: Potent inhibition of sparteine and debrisoquine oxidation in vivo (letter). *Br J Clin Pharmacol* 1986; 22:199–200.
197. Spiers CJ, Murray S, Boobis AR, Seddon CE, Davies DS: Quinidine and the identification of drugs whose elimination is impaired in subjects classified as poor metabolizers of debrisoquine. *Br J Clin Pharmacol* 1986; 22:739–743.

198. Guengerich FP, Muller-Enoch D, Blair IA: Oxidation of quinidine by human liver cytochrome P-450. *Mol Pharmacol* 1986; 30:287–295.
199. Mikus G, Ha HR, Vozeh S, Zekorn C, Follath F, Eichelbaum M: Pharmacokinetics and metabolism of quinidine in extensive and poor metabolizers of sparteine. *Eur J Clin Pharmacol* 1986; 31:69–72.
200. Brosen K, Gram LF, Haghfelt T, Bertilsson L: Extensive metabolizers of debrisoquin become poor metabolizers during quinidine treatment. *Pharmacol Toxicol* 1987; 60:312–314.
201. Kornfeld P, Horowitz SH, Genkins G, Papatestas AE: Myasthenia gravis unmasked by antiarrhythmic agents. *Mt Sinai J Med* 1976; 43:10–14.
202. Grogono AW: Anesthesia for atrial fibrillation. Effect of quinidine on muscle relaxation. *Lancet* 1963; 2:1039–1040.
203. Dinh H, Murphy ML, Baker BJ, deSoyza N, Franciosa JA: Efficacy of propafenone compared with quinidine in chronic ventricular arrhythmias. *Am J Cardiol* 1985; 55:1520–1524.
204. Chilson DA, Heger JJ, Zipes DP, Browne KF, Prystowsky EN: Electrophysiologic effects and clinical efficacy of oral propafenone therapy in patients with ventricular tachycardia. *J Am Coll Cardiol* 1985; 5:1407–1413.
205. Connolly SJ, Mulji AS, Hoffert DL, Davis CA, Schragge BW: Randomized placebo-controlled trial of propafenone for treatment of atrial tachyarrhythmias after cardiac surgery. *J Am Coll Cardiol* 1987; 10:1145–1148.
206. Breithardt G, Borggrefe M, Wiebringhaus E, Seipel L: Effect of propafenone in the Wolff-Parkinson-White syndrome: Electrophysiologic findings and long-term follow-up. *Am J Cardiol* 1984; 54(suppl D):29D–39D.
207. von Philipsborn G, Gries J, Hofmann HP, Kreiskott H, Kretzschmar R, Muller CD, et al: Pharmacological studies on propafenone and its main metabolite 5-hydroxypropafenone. *Arzneimittelforschung* 1984; 34:1489–1497.
208. Valenzuela C, Delgado C, Tamargo J: Electrophysiological effects of 5-hydroxypropafenone on guinea pig ventricular muscle fibers. *J Cardiovasc Pharmacol* 1987; 10:523–529.
209. McLeod AA, Stiles GL, Shand DG: Demonstration of beta adrenoceptor blockade by propafenone hydrochloride: Clinical pharmacologic, radioligand binding, and adenylate cyclase activation studies. *J Pharmacol Exp Ther* 1984; 228:461–466.
210. Muller-Peltzer H, Greger G, Neugebauer G, Hollman M: Beta-blocking and electrophysiological effects of propafenone in volunteers. *Eur J Clin Pharmacol* 1983; 25:831–833.
211. Lee JT, Funck-Brentano C, Lineberry MD, Chaffin PL, Roden DM, Woosley RL: Beta receptor antagonism by propafenone in man: Influence of polymorphic metabolism (abstr). *Clin Res* 1988; 36:294A.
212. Siddoway LA, Thompson KA, McAllister CB, Wang T, Wilkinson GR, Roden DM, et al: Polymorphism of propafenone metabolism and disposition in man: Clinical and pharmacokinetic consequences. *Circulation* 1987; 75: 785–791.
213. Baker BJ, Dinh H. Kroskey D, deSoyza NDB, Murphy ML, Franciosa JA: Effect of propafenone on left ventricular ejection fraction. *Am J Cardiol* 1984; 54:(suppl D):20D–22D.
214. Wagner F, Kalusche D, Trenk D, Jahnchen E, Roskamm H: Drug interaction between propafenone and metoprolol. *Br J Clin Pharmacol* 1987; 24:213–220.
215. Funck-Brentano C, Kroemer HK, Pavlou H, Wright GM, Woosley RL, Roden DM: Inhibition of propafenone metabolism by low doses of quinidine in man (abstr). *Clin Res* 1988; 36:363A.
216. Roden DM, Woosley RL: Flecainide. *N Engl J Med* 1986; 315:36–41.
217. Hellestrand KJ, Nathan AW, Bexton RS, Spurrell RAJ, Camm AJ: Cardiac electrophysiologic effects of flecainide acetate for paroxysmal reentrant junctional tachycardias. *Am J Cardiol* 1983; 51:770–776.
218. Pritchett EL, Wilkinson WE: Mortality in patients treated with flecainide and encainide for supraventricular arrhythmias. *Am J Cardiol* 1991; 67:976–980.
219. The Flecainide-Quinidine Research Group: Flecainide versus quinidine for treatment of chronic ventricular arrhythmias. A multicenter clinical trial. *Circulation* 1983; 67:1117–1123.
220. Follmer CH, Colatsky TJ: Block of delayed rectifier potassium current, IK, by flecainide and E-4031 in cat ventricular myocytes. *Circulation* 1990; 82:289–293.
221. Kou H, Nelson SD, Lynch JJ, Montgomery DG, DiCarlo L, Lucchesi BR: Effect of flecainide acetate on prevention of electrical induction of ventricular tachycardia and occurrence of ischemic ventricular fibrillation during the early postmyocardial infarction period: Evaluation in a conscious canine model of sudden death. *J Am Coll Cardiol* 1987; 9:359–365.
222. Ikeda N, Singh BN, Davis LD, Hauswirth O: Effects of flecainide on the electrophysiologic properties of isolated canine and rabbit myocardial fibers. *J Am Coll Cardiol* 1985; 5:303–310.
223. Estes NAM III, Garan H, Ruskin JN: Electrophysiological properties of flecainide acetate. *Am J Cardiol* 1984; 53(suppl B):26B–29B.
224. Conrad GJ, Ober RE: Metabolism of flecainide. *Am J Cardiol* 1984; 53(suppl B):41B–51B.
225. Guehler J, Gornick CC, Tobler HG, Almquist A, Schmid JR, Benson DW Jr, et al: Electrophysiologic effects of flecainide acetate and its major metabolites in the canine heart. *Am J Cardiol* 1985; 55:807–812.
226. Haefeli WE, Bragetzi MJ, Follath F, Meyer UA: Potent inhibition of cytochrome P450IID6 (debrisoquin 4-hydroxylase) by flecainide in vitro and in vivo. *J Cardiovasc Pharmacol* 1990; 15:776–779.
227. Johnston A, Warrington S, Turner P: Flecainide pharmacokinetics in healthy volunteers: The influence of urinary pH. *Br J Clin Pharmacol* 1985; 20:333–338.
228. Franciosa JA, Wilen M, Weeks CE, Tannenbaum R, Kvam DC, Miller AM: Pharmacokinetics and hemodynamic effects of flecainide in patients with chronic low output heart failure (abstr). *J Am Coll Cardiol* 1983; 1:699.
229. Winkelman BR, Leinberger H: Life-threatening flecainide toxicity. A pharmacodynamic approach. *Ann Intern Med* 1987; 106:807–814.
230. Salerno DM, Granrud GA, Sharkey P, Krejci J, Larson T, Erlien D, et al: Pharmacodynamics and side effects of flecainide acetate. *Clin Pharmacol Ther* 1986; 40:101–107.
231. Morganroth J, Horowitz LN: Flecainide: Its proarrhythmic effect and expected changes on the surface electrocardiogram. *Am J Cardiol* 1984; 53(suppl B):89B–94B.
232. Josephson MA, Kaul S, Hopkins J, Kvam DC, Singh BN: Hemodynamic effects of intravenous flecainide relative to the level of ventricular function in patients with coronary artery disease. *Am Heart J* 1985; 109:41–45.
233. Muhiddin KA, Turner P, Blackett A: Effect of flecainide on cardiac output. *Clin Pharmacol Ther* 1985; 37:260–263.
234. Morganroth J, Anderson JL, Gentzkow GD: Classification by type of ventricular arrhythmia predicts frequency of adverse cardiac events from flecainide. *J Am Coll Cardiol* 1986; 8:607–615.
235. Rotmensch HH, Belhassen B, Ferguson RK: Amiodarone—benefits and risks in perspective. *Am Heart J* 1982; 104:1117–1119.
236. Josephson MA, Ikeda N, Singh BN: Effects of flecainide on ventricular function: Clinical and experimental correlations. *Am J Cardiol* 1984; 53:95B–100B.
237. Vik-Mo H, Ohm O-J, Lund-Johansen P: Electrophysiological effects of flecainide acetate in patients with sinus nodal dysfunction. *Am J Cardiol* 1982; 50:1090–1094.
238. Hellestrand KJ, Nathan AW, Bexton RS, Camm AJ: Electrophysicologic effects of flecainide acetate on sinus node function, anomalous atrioventricular connections and pacemaker thresholds. *Am J Cardiol* 1984; 53(suppl B):30B–38B.
239. Hellestrand KJ, Burnett PJ, Milne JR, Bexton RS, Nathan AW, Camm AJ: The effect of the antiarrhythmic agent flecainide on acute and chronic pacing thresholds. *PACE* 1983; 6:892–899.
240. Hernandez R, Mann DE, Breckinridge S, Williams GR, Reiter MJ: Effects of flecainide on defibrillation thresholds in the anesthetized dog. *J Am Coll Cardiol* 1989; 14:777–781.
241. Tjandra-Maga TB, van Hecken A, van Melle P, Verbesselt R, deSchepper PJ: Altered pharmacokinetics of oral flecainide by cimetidine. *Br J Clin Pharmacol* 1986; 22:108–110.
242. Weeks CE, Conrad GJ, Kvam DC, Fox JM, Chang SF, Paone RP, et al: The effect of flecainide acetate, a new antiarrhythmic, on plasma digoxin levels. *J Clin Pharmacol* 1986; 26:27–31.
243. Lewis GP, Holtzman JL: Interaction of flecainide with digoxin and propranolol. *Am J Cardol* 1984; 53(suppl B):52B–57B.
244. Shea P, Lal R, Kim SS, Schechtman K, Ruffy R: Flecainide and amiodarone interaction. *J Am Coll Cardiol* 1986; 7:1127–1130.
245. Somberg JC, Zanger D, Levine E, Tepper D: Encainide: A new and potent antiarrhythmic. *Am Heart J* 1987; 114:826–835.
246. Morganroth J: Encainide for ventricular arrhythmias: Placebo-controlled and standard comparison trials. *Am J Cardiol* 1986; 58(suppl):74C–82C.

247. Rowland E: Antiarrhythmic drugs—class IV. *Eur Heart J* 1987; 8(suppl A):61–63.
248. Singh BN, Nademanee K, Baky SH: Calcium Antagonists. Clinical use in the treatment of arrhythmias. *Drugs* 1983; 25:125–153.
249. Ward DE, Nathan AW, Camm AJ: Fascicular tachycardia sensitive to calcium antagonists. *Eur Heart J* 1984; 5:896–905.
250. Bauer LA, Stenwall M, Horn JR, Davis R, Opheim K, Greene L: Changes in antipyrine and indocyanine green kinetics during nifedipine, verapamil, and diltiazem therapy. *Clin Pharmacol Ther* 1986; 40:239–242.
251. Bacaner MB: Treatment of ventricular fibrillation and other acute arrhythmias with bretylium tosylate. *Am J Cardiol* 1986: 21:530–543.
252. Bigger JT Jr, Jaffe CC: The effect of bretylium tosylate on the electrophysiologic properties on ventricular muscle and Purkinje fibers. *Am J Cardiol* 1971; 27:82–92.
253. Cardinale R, Sasyniuk BI: Electrophysiological effects of bretylium tosylate on subendocardial Purkinje fibers from infarcted canine hearts. *J Pharmacol Exp Ther* 1978; 204:159–174.
254. Nishimura M, Watanabe Y: Membrane action and catecholamine release action of bretylium tosylate in normoxic and hypoxic canine Purkinje fibers. *J Am Coll Cardiol* 1983; 2:287–295.
255. Anderson JL, Brodine WN, Patterson E, Marshall HW, Allison SD, Lucchesi BR: Serial electrophysiologic effects of bretylium in man and their correlation with plasma concentrations. *J Cardiovasc Pharmacol* 1982; 4:871–882.
256. Narang PK, Adir J, Josselson J, Yacobi A: Pharmacokinetics of bretylium in man after intravenous administration. *J Pharmacokinet Biopharm* 1980; 8:363–372.
257. Chow MSS, Kluger J, DiPersio DM, Lawrence R, Fieldman A: Antifibrillatory effects of lidocaine and bretylium immediately postcardiopulmonary resuscitation. *Am Heart J* 1985; 110: 938–943.
258. Duff HJ, Roden DM, Yacobi A, Robertson D, Wang T, Maffucci RJ, et al: Bretylium: Relations between plasma concentrations and pharmacologic actions in high-frequency ventricular arrhythmias. *Am J Cardiol* 1985; 5:395–401.
259. Singh BN, Nademanee K: Sotalol: A beta-blocker with unique antiarrhythmic properties. *Am Heart J* 1987; 114:121–139.
260. Quart B: Sotalol-procainamide comparison in sustained ventricular tachycardia. Personal communication, 1991.
261. The ESVEM Investigators: Determinants of predicted efficacy of antiarrhythmic drugs in the electrophysiologic study versus electrocardiographic monitoring trial. *Circulation* 1993; 87:323–329.
262. Wang T, Bergstrand RH, Thompson KA, Siddoway LA, Duff HJ, Woosley RL, et al: Concentration-dependent pharmacologic properties of sotalol. *Am J Cardiol* 1986; 57:1160–1165.
263. Kopelman HA, Woosley RL, Lee JT, Roden DM, Echt DS: Electrophysiologic effects of intravenous and oral sotalol for sustained ventricular tachycardia secondary to coronary artery disease. *Am J Cardiol* 1988; 61:1006–1011.
264. Graboys TB, Podrid PJ, Lown B: Efficacy of amiodarone for refractory supraventricular tachyarrhythmias. *Am Heart J* 1983; 106:870–876.
265. Horowitz LN, Spielman SR, Greenspan AM, Mintz GS, Morganroth J, Brown R, et al: Use of amiodarone in the treatment of persistent and paroxysmal atrial fibrillation resistant to quinidine therapy. *J Am Coll Cardiol* 1985; 6:1402–1407.
266. Cairns JA, Connolly SJ, Gent M, Roberts R: Post-myocardial infarction mortality in patients with ventricular premature depolarizations. *Circulation* 1991; 84:550–557.
267. Mason JW: Amiodarone. *N Engl J Med* 1987; 316:455–466.
268. Mason JW, Hondeghem LM, Katzung BG: Amiodarone blocks inactivated cardiac sodium channels. *Pflugers Arch* 1983; 396:79–81.
269. Talajic M, DeRoode MR, Nattel S: Comparative electrophysiologic effects of intravenous amiodarone and desmethylamiodarone in dogs: Evidence for clinically relevant activity of the metabolite. *Circulation* 1987; 75:265–271.
270. Albert SG, Alves LE, Rose EP: Thyroid dysfunction during chronic amiodarone therapy. *J Am Coll Cardiol* 1987; 9:175–183.
271. Singh BN, Nademanee K: Amiodarone and thyroid function: Clinical implications during antiarrhythmic therapy. *Am Heart J* 1983; 106:857–869.
272. Latham KR, Sellitti DF, Goldstein RE: Interaction of amiodarone and desethylamiodarone with solubilized nuclear thyroid hormone receptors. *J Am Coll Cardiol* 1987; 9:872–876.
273. Charlier R, Deltour G, Baudine A, Chaillet F: Pharmacology of amiodarone, an anti-anginal drug with a new biological profile. *Arzneimittelforschung* 1986; 18:1408–1417.
274. Cohen-Armon M, Schreiber G, Sokolovsky M: Interaction of the antiarrhythmic drug amiodarone with the muscarinic receptor in rat heart and brain. *J Cardiovasc Pharmacol* 1984; 6:1148–1155.
275. Pourbaix S, Berger Y, Desager J-P, Pacco M, Harvengt M: Absolute bioavailability of amiodarone in normal subjects. *Clin Pharmacol Ther* 1985; 37:118–123.
276. Adams PC, Holt DW, Storey GC, Morley AR, Callaghan J, Path MRC, et al: Amiodarone and its desethyl metabolite: Tissue distribution and morphologic changes during long-term therapy. *Circulation* 1985; 72:1064–1075.
277. Nattel S, Davies M, Quantz M: The antiarrhythmic efficacy of amiodarone and desethylamiodarone, alone and in combination, in dogs with acute myocardial infarction. *Circulation* 1988; 77:200–208.
278. Holt DW, Tucker GT, Jackson PR, McKenna WJ: Amiodarone pharmacokinetics. *Br J Clin Pract* 1986; 44(symp suppl):109–114.
279. Plomp TA, van Rossum JM, Robles de Medina EO, van Lier T, Maes RA: Pharmacokinetics and body distribution of amiodarone in man. *Arzneimittelforschung* 1984; 34:513–520.
280. Siddoway LA, McAllister CB, Wilkinson GR, Roden DM, Woosley RL: Amiodarone dosing: A proposal based on its pharmacokinetics. *Am Heart J* 1983; 106:951–956.
281. Escoubet B, Coumel P, Poirier J-M, Maison-Blanche P, Jaillon P, LeClercq J-F, et al: Suppression of arrhythmias within hours after a single oral dose of amiodarone and relation to plasma and myocardial concentration. *Am J Cardiol* 1985; 55:696–702.
282. Mostow ND, Vrobel TR, Noon D, Rakita L: Rapid suppression of complex ventricular arrhythmias with high-dose oral amiodarone. *Circulation* 1986; 73:1231–1238.
283. Greenberg ML, Lerman BB, Shipe JR, Kaiser DL, DiMarco JP: Relation between amiodarone and desethylamiodarone plasma concentrations and electrophysiological effects, efficacy and toxicity. *J Am Coll Cardiol* 1987; 9:1148–1155.
284. Neri R, Mestroni L, Salvi A, Pandullo C, Camerini F: Ventricular arrhythmias in dilated cardiomyopathy: Efficacy of amiodarone. *Am Heart J* 1987: 113:707–715.
285. Coumel P, Fidelle J: Amiodarone in the treatment of cardiac arrhythmias in children: One hundred thirty-five cases. *Am Heart J* 1980; 100:1063–1069.
286. Mason JW, the Amiodarone Toxicity Study Group: Toxicity of amiodarone (abstr). *Circulation* 1985; 72(suppl):III-272.
287. Veltri EP, Reid PR: Amiodarone pulmonary toxicity: Early changes in pulmonary function tests during amiodarone rechallenge. *J Am Coll Cardiol* 1985; 6:802–805.
288. Orlando RG, Dangel ME, Schaal SF: Clinical experience and grading of amiodarone keratopathy. *Ophthalmology* 1984; 91:1184–1187.
289. Zachary CB, Slater DN, Holt DW, Storey GCA, MacDonald DM: The pathogenesis of amiodarone-induced pigmentation and photosensitivity. *Br J Dermatol* 1984; 110:451–456.
290. Simon JB, Manley PN, Brien JF, Armstrong PW: Amiodarone hepatotoxicity simulating alcoholic liver disease. *N Engl J Med* 1984; 311:167–172.
291. Rigas B, Rosenfeld LE, Barwick KW, Enriquez R, Helzberg J, Batsford WP, et al: Amiodarone hepatotoxicity: A clinicopathologic study of five patients. *Ann Intern Med* 1986; 104: 348–351.
292. Larrey D, Tinel M, Letteron P, Geneve J, Descatoire V, Pessayer D: Formation of an inactive cytochrome P-450 Fe(II)–metabolite complex after administration of amiodarone in rats, mice and hamsters. *Biochem Pharmacol* 1986; 35:2213–2220.
293. Almog S, Shafran N, Halkin H, Weiss P, Farfel Z, Martinowitz U, et al: Mechanism of warfarin potentiation by amiodarone: Dose- and concentration-dependent inhibition of warfarin elimination. *Eur J Clin Pharmacol* 1985; 28:257–261.
294. Marcus FI: Drug interactions with amiodarone. *Am Heart J* 1983; 106:924–930.
295. Fenster PE, White NW Jr, Hanson CD: Pharmacokinetic evaluation of the digoxin-amiodarone interaction. *J Am Coll Cardiol* 1985; 5:108–112.

296. Yusuf S, Peto R, Lewis J, Collins R, Sleight P: Beta blockade during and after myocardial infarction: An overview of the randomized trials. *Prog Cardiovasc Dis* 1985; 27:335–371.
297. Duff HJ, Mitchell LB, Wyse DG: Antiarrhythmic efficacy of proparanolol: Comparison of low and high serum concentrations. *J Am Coll Cardiol* 1986; 8:959–965.
298. Pratt CM, Yepson SC, Bloom MGK, Taylor AA, Young JB, Quinones MA: Evaluation of metoprolol in suppressing complex ventricular arrhythmias. *Am J Cardiol* 1983; 52:73–78.
299. Von Der Lippe G, Lund-Johansen P, Kjekshus J: Effect of timolol on late ventricular arrhythmias after acute myocardial infarction. *Acta Med Scand* 1981; 651(suppl):253–263.
300. deSoyza N, Shapiro W, Chandraratna PAN, Aronow WS, Laddu AR, Thompson CH: Acebutolol therapy for ventricular arrhythmia. A randomized, placebo-controlled, double-blind multicenter study. *Circulation* 1982; 65:1129–1133.
301. Podrid PJ, Lown B: Pindolol for ventricular arrhythmia. *Am Heart J* 1982; 104:491–496.
302. Nademanee K, Schleman NM, Singh BN, Morganroth J, Reid PR, Stritar JA: Beta-adrenergic blockage by nadolol in control of ventricular tachyarrhythmias. *Am Heart J* 1984; 108:1109–1115.
303. Fenster PE, Reynolds D, Horwitz LD, Morrison D, Goldman S, Thadani U, et al: Atenolol for ventricular ectopy: A dose-response study. *Clin Pharmacol Ther* 1987; 41:118–123.
304. Graboys TB, Lown B, Podrid PJ, DeSilva R: Long-term survival of patients with malignant ventricular arrhythmias treated with antiarrhythmic drugs. *Am J Cardiol* 1982; 50:437–443.
305. Tonet JL, Cazaux P, Chevalier B: Efficacy of low dose of beta-blocker agents combined with amiodarone in refractory ventricular tachycardia. *Circulation* 1987; 76(suppl):IV–367.
306. Thompson KA, Roden DM, Wood AJJ, Siddoway LA, Barbey JT, Woosley RL: Suppression of ventricular arrhythmias by dextropropranolol in man independent of beta-adrenergic receptor blockade, *J Clin Invest* 1990; 85:836–842.
307. Lerman BB, Belardinelli L: Cardiac electrophysiology of adenosine; basic and clinical concepts. *Circulation* 1991; 83:1499–1509.
308. Ellenbogen KA, Thames MD, DiMarco JP, Sheehan H, Lerman BB: Electrophysiologic effects of adenosine in the transplanted human heart: Evidence for supersensitivity. *Circulation* 1990; 81:821–828.
309. Lerman BB, Wesley RC, Belardinelli L: Electrophysiologic effects of dipyridamole on atrioventricular nodal conduction and supraventricular tachycardia: Role of endogenous adenosine. *Circulation* 1989; 80:1536–1543.
310. DiMarco JP, Sellers TD, Lerman BB, Greenberg ML, Berne RM, Belardinelli L: Diagnostic and therapeutic use of adenosine in patients with supraventricular tachyarrhythmias. *J Am Coll Cardiol* 1985; 6:417–425.
311. Baskin EP, Serik CM, Wallace AA, Brookes LM, Selnick HG, Claremon DA, et al: Effects of new and potent methanesulfonanilide class III antiarrhythmic agents on myocardial refractoriness and contractility in isolated cardiac muscle. *J Cardiovasc Pharmacol* 1991; 18:406–414.
312. Wettwer E, Scholtysik G, Schaad A, Himmel H, Ravens U: Effects of the new class III antiarrhythmic drug E-4031 on myocardial contractility and electrophysiological parameters. *J Cardiovasc Pharmacol* 1991; 17:480–487.
313. Steinberg MI, Sullivan ME, Wiest SA, Rockhold FW, Molloy BB: Cellular electrophysiology of clofilium, a new antifibrillatory agent, in normal and ischemic canine purkinje fibers. *J Cardiovasc Pharm* 1981; 3:881–895.

Chapter 39

Temporary Cardiac Pacing

Ross D. Fletcher, M.D., ■ *Marc Wish, M.D.,*
E. Pendleton Alexander, M.D.

Temporary pacing, first described by Zoll in 1952,[1] was noninvasive and used transthoracic energy. While lifesaving in many instances, this form of external pacing was poorly tolerated. Transvenous temporary pacing was introduced by Furman in 1959.[2] For several years thereafter some patients were paced transvenously with external generators on a long-term basis. Implantable permanent pacemakers were developed in 1960.[3]

INDICATIONS

Long after the development of permanent implantable pacemaker generators and leads, temporary pacemakers are still required for many indications (Table 39-1). Temporary pacing systems are often a bridge to permanent pacing, especially for patients who are unable to undergo immediate permanent implantation or for patients whose bradycardia is severe and hemodynamically unstable. Temporary pacing is required most frequently in patients with severe infranodal block and less frequently with AV nodal block and sick sinus syndrome.

Temporary pacing is also indicated when symptomatic or hemodynamically significant bradycardia is due to drugs such as an excess of digitalis. Pacing may be required as the drug is discontinued and agents such as Digibind are used to counter the drug-induced bradyarrhythmia (see also Chap. 27).

Anticipated or actual bradyarrhythmia during acute myocardial infarction also may require temporary pacing. (See Chap. 60.) The most serious bradyarrhythmias occur with anterior myocardial infarction. The left anterior descending artery supplies both the right bundle branch and the anterior, superior division of the left bundle branch (Chap. 4). The onset of right bundle branch block and especially left axis deviation often precedes infranodal heart block.[4] An abrupt transition can occur from 1:1 conduction, to Mobitz II second degree block, or complete asystole. The lack of escape rhythm makes this particularly dangerous and warrants temporary pacing even with only the onset of right bundle

TABLE 39-1
Indications for Temporary Cardiac Pacing

1. Permanent symptomatic bradycardia as a bridge to permanent pacing
   a. Complete heart block
      (1) Infranodal
      (2) AV nodal
   b. Sick sinus syndrome
2. Temporary bradycardia due to drugs
   a. Digoxin
   b. Antiarrhythmic agents
3. Acute myocardial infarction (MI)
   a. Antero-septal MI: Infranodal RBBB with left axis deviation
   b. Inferior MI: Hemodynamically unstable complete AV nodal block
4. Post operative—cardiac surgery
5. Tachyarrhythmia control with overdrive
   a. Long QT
   b. Blocked atrial premature complexes (APCs)
   c. Incessant ventricular tachycardia (VT)
   d. When late-coupled premature ventricular contractions (PVCs) induce VT

branch block in the presence of an anterior myocardial infarction. The presence of a prolonged HV time increases the likelihood of developing infranodal heart block.[4] Only 4 percent of patients with a normal HV time went on to heart block while 75 percent of those with a long HV time progressed to heart block. No patient with a long HV had a PR interval less than 0.15. Thus, a patient with new right bundle and a PR interval less than 0.15 is unlikely to progress to distal heart block.

Less serious bradyarrhythmias occur with inferior myocardial infarction. The AV nodal artery arises from the crux just before the posterior descending artery. Heart block involving the AV node is usually tolerated and develops more gradually with good ventricular escape. In some patients, however, the onset of junctional rhythm produces marked hypotension. If atropine does not restore a sinus mechanism and blood pressure, temporary ventricular or dual chamber pacing may be necessary.

Temporary pacing of either atrium or ventricle frequently is useful after cardiac surgery.[5-7] Transient bradyarrhythmias are common. Even more common are episodes of atrial flutter which can be diagnosed and treated with temporary removable pacing wires attached to the atrium.[8,9] Atrial pacing at rates of 90 to 100 are routinely employed by some surgeons to maximize cardiac output and to suppress arrhythmia. Pacing of both atrium and ventricle is preferred in the presence of AV block.[10]

While temporary pacing is used primarily for bradyarrhythmia, increasingly tachyarrhythmias are controlled with temporary pacemakers.[11] Pacing is specifically recommended for recurrent tachyarrhythmia due to a long QT. Even bradycardia temporarily caused by blocked atrial premature complexes (APCs) can cause long QT and *torsade de pointe.* Preventing long pauses helps to prevent ventricular tachyarrhythmia. Incessant ventricular tachycardia can be treated by recurrent reversion with pacing but also can be prevented by pacing faster than the sinus rate. This is particularly true when the ventricular tachycardia starts with a long coupling interval.

METHODS OF TEMPORARY PACING

Leads (Table 39-2)

As in permanent pacing (Chap. 40) each system requires leads and a pacing generator. Standard transvenous pacing leads (often 4F) are inserted percutaneously into femoral, internal jugular, or subclavian veins. The groin is preferred if the subclavian areas are to be used for permanent implantation. The ports of the side arm introducer are capped and no infusions are made to avoid the possibility of contamination. The sites of a temporary pacing catheter are well shaven and prepared with sterile solutions. The site should be changed after 3 to 4 days. Unless the temporary pacing catheter is placed in a truly emergency situation, fluoroscopy assures adequate positioning in the right ventricular apex. Balloon-tipped, flow-directed catheters are often difficult to position in the right ventricular apex and often require repositioning. A Swan Ganz catheter with two electrodes incorporated in the body of the catheter spaced to lie within the right ventricle allows simultaneous hemodynamic monitoring and pacing. Thresholds with this form of pacing, however, are high and often unreliable. The "Pace-Port" Swan Ganz catheter developed by BARD (Billerica, MA) has an extra lumen through which a #2.5 French bipolar pacing wire is advanced. The extra lumen ends in the right ventricle and the wire is directed at the right ventricular wall. The Swan Ganz is more stable when inserted from the jugular or subclavian veins than from the femoral vein.

TABLE 39-2
Methods: Leads

1. Transvenous
   a. Standard pacing leads—4F fluoroscopy
   b. Flow directed with balloon tip
   c. Pacing Swan-Ganz
   d. Pace port Swan-Ganz—single and dual
   e. Littleford J lead—atrium
2. Temporary suture leads
3. Esophageal
   a. Pill electrode
   b. Catheter with deflectable tip
4. Transthoracic
   a. High impedance patch electrodes
   b. Combined defibrillation and pacing patch electrodes

Single temporary leads can be placed in the atrium. Temporary atrial pacing catheters placed from the groin run a higher risk of dislodgement and loss of capture than ventricular leads. To provide increased stability to atrial leads, the atrial appendage has been used. Littleford[12] developed a "J" lead which is placed from the subclavian or jugular vein. The tip is placed into the right atrial appendage. Proper placement can be accomplished without fluoroscopy but is more reliable with fluoroscopy.

Esophogeal pacing has been used particularly for atrial pacing.[13,14] This can be used for either temporary bradycardia support or overdrive pacing of regular atrial tachyarrhythmias such as atrial flutter. A standard bipolar pill electrode[15] and more recently tip deflecting catheters have been used to improve atrial and ventricular capture.

In 1985, Zoll[16] reported the use of a newer form of noninvasive external transthoracic pacing. This form of external pacing uses large antero-posterior electrode skin patches (5 to 10 cm in diameter) connected to the pulse generator. High impedance electrodes were initially used to improve patient comfort.[17] These leads should not be used for defibrillation. A newer lead allows combined defibrillation and pacing through the same patches. The placement posteriorly and anteriorly to the left of the sternum is preferable to placement apically and under the right clavicle. The negative or cathodal patch should be closest to the heart (anterior or apical).

GENERATORS

Single Chamber Generators

Single chamber VVI generators are most common with individual controls for output, rate in beats per minute (bpm) and sensitivity to 2 millivolts (mv). Output should be 3 times threshold but pacing is usually performed at a minimum of 3 milliamps (ma) since minor dislodgement can cause major changes in threshold. When the lead is in the atrium, AAI and AOO pacing is possible. AOO generators are utilized for rapid pacing required to revert flutter to sinus rhythm. Usually the reversion rate is 140 percent faster than the flutter rate. Care should be taken to insure capture. Careful gradual increases in rate not exceeding 360 bpm have the highest yield of direct reversion to sinus rhythm rather than reversion from flutter to atrial fibrillation.

Dual Chamber Temporary Pacing Generators

While dual chamber pacing is as beneficial in temporary pacing as it is in permanent pacing, it has been used infrequently.[18] The most common generator available is DVI. Lack of atrial sensing eliminates P wave tracking and may lead to pacing on the atrial vulnerable period. This may precipitate atrial fibrillation. True DDD temporary pacemakers have recently become available and are software controlled, allowing all of the options available to permanent DDD pacemakers. This includes the post V atrial refractory period (PVARP). As in permanent pacing the PVARP device should be programmed longer than retrograde conduction of V to atrium in order to eliminate pacemaker mediated tachycardia. The AV interval, RR interval, and upper rate limits are also independently programmable.

Esophageal and Transthoracic Generators

Generators for esophageal pacing allow long pulse widths and can pace at rapid rates. Transthoracic generators also require long pulse widths (20–40) msec at outputs up to 200 ma. Comfortable pacing is achieved if the output is less than 75 ma. Special filters are required for clear electrocardiograms; however, documentation of capture may require observation of repolarization (T waves) (Fig. 39-1). A common error is 2 : 1 capture which is detected by palpating the pulse as well as examining the ECG. Increasing output often allows 1 : 1 capture. The captured QRS can be dissimilar from beat to beat especially when pacing close to threshold, which occurs commonly when one attempts to minimize patient discomfort. Prophylactic transvenous pacing can be largely avoided if a transthoracic pacing system can be proven to capture. A short period of pacing can often be tolerated during acute bradycardia while a standard transvenous lead is inserted. Some transthoracic generators allow rapid rates or can be triggered from standard laboratory pacemakers. On occasion a brief transthoracic burst can revert ventricular tachycardia[19] (Fig. 39-2).

COMPLICATIONS AND MALFUNCTION

Care of temporary pacing systems includes inspection for infection, daily pacing thresholds, sensing thresholds, and tightening of all connections. A change in the pacing axis on a 12-lead ECG can reveal migration of the pacing lead and impending dislodgement (Fig. 39-3). Unipolar recordings from the lead are made with an alligator clip connector between the lead and the V_1 lead of the ECG. The ECG should be checked to have low leakage current less than 10 micro amps. The unipolar recordings normally show more pronounced ST elevation on the tip than on the proximal electrode (Fig. 39-4*B*). ST inversion on the tip electrode is associated with perforation (Fig. 39-4*A*).[20,21] Bipolar recordings using the proximal electrode attached to the right arm (RA) lead of an ECG and the distal electrode attached to the left arm (LA) record in lead I the voltage seen by the pacing system (Fig. 39-5*A*). When this bipolar voltage is less than 2mv, inadequate sensing will occur in standard temporary systems (Fig. 39-5*B*). Temporary pacing frequently occurs in situations with low fibrillation thresholds such as digitalis toxicity, acute myocardial infarction,[22] and acutely post cardiac surgery. Consequently, the maintenance of adequate sensing is as important as in a permanent pacing system. The standard bipolar pacing lead includes anodal pacing which is more likely to cause ventricular fibrillation[23] (Fig. 39-6).

Monitoring should be set to demonstrate the pacemaker spike. Pacing failure with a visible spike is likely

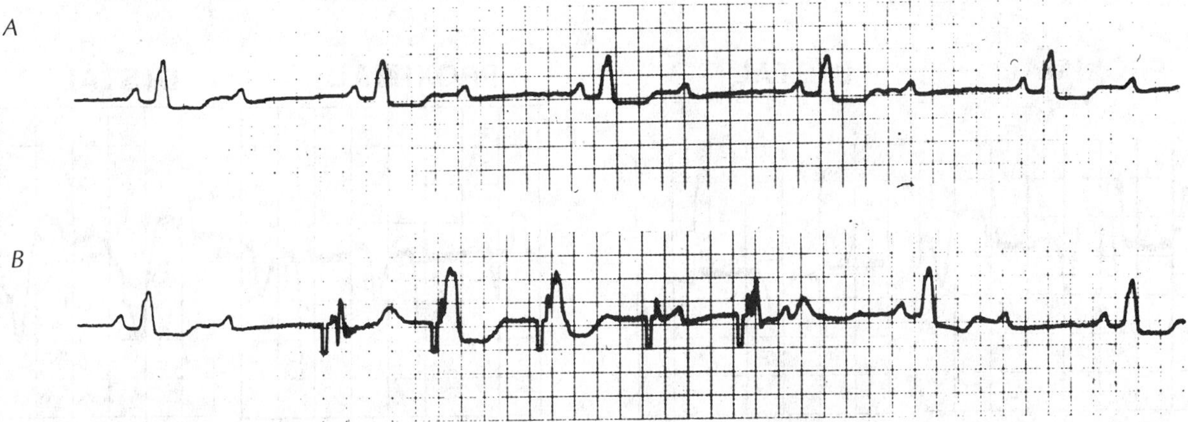

FIGURE 39-1 Trial of external transthoracic pacing in a patient with 2 : 1 AV block *(A)*. In *B* the first three paced beats are captured as noted by QRS and T wave. The fourth paced beat failed to produce either a QRS or a T wave while number 5 captured again. Paced QRS morphology changes when pacing nears threshold.

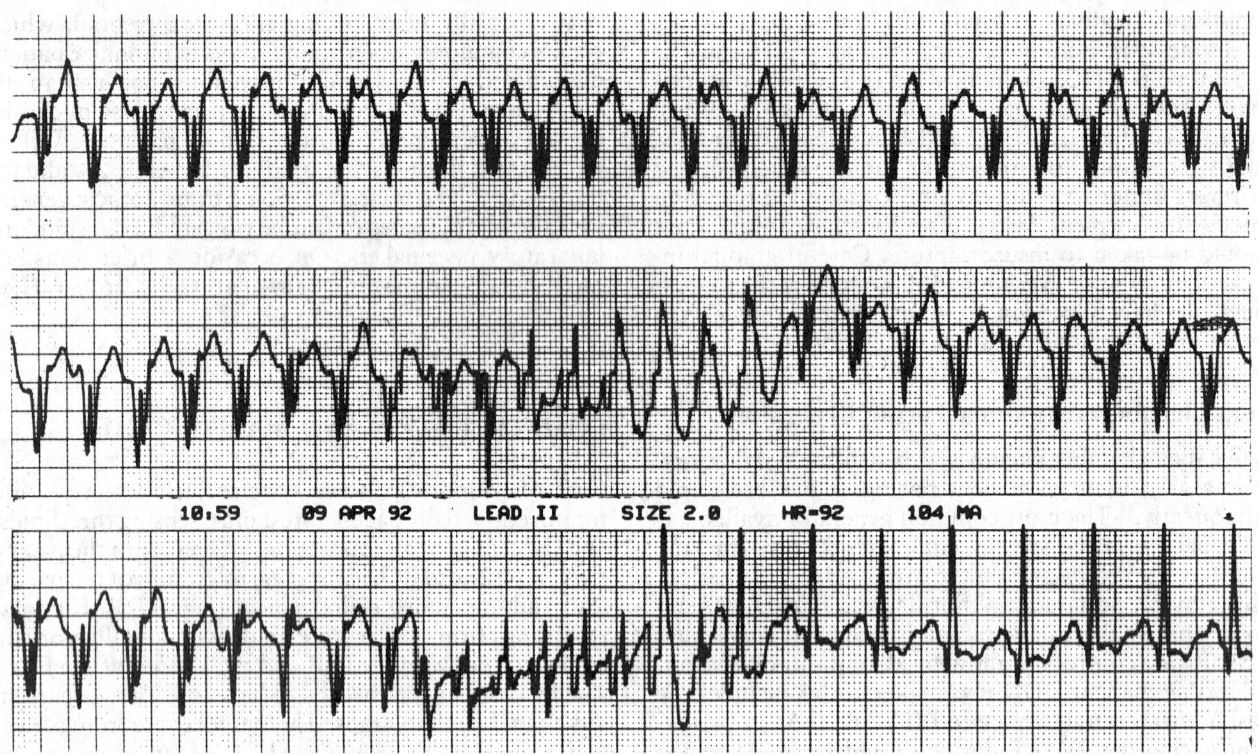

FIGURE 39-2 The ventricular tachycardia on the first strip had pacing reversion attempted with transthoracic pacing on the middle strip. Pacing at a faster rate in the lower strip at 105 ma captured the ventricle and restored sinus rhythm.

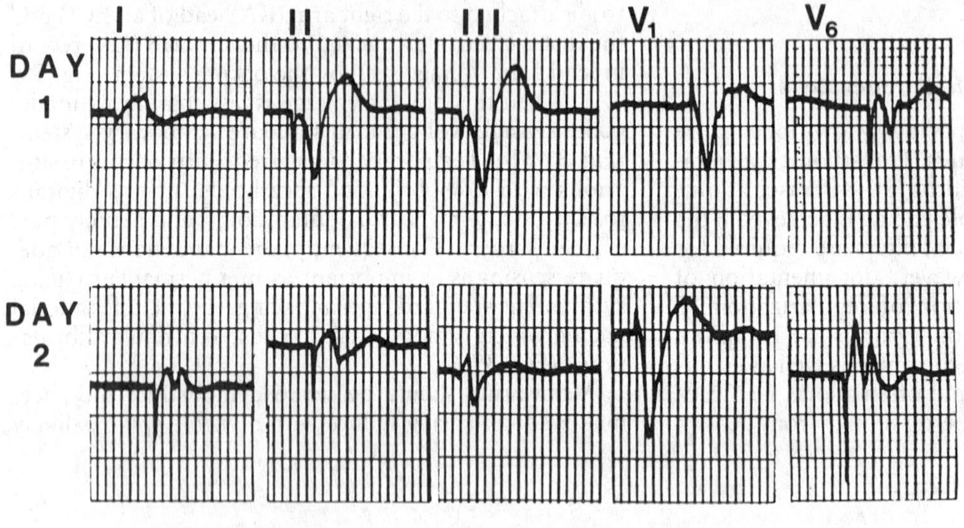

FIGURE 39-3 The axis shifted from superior to lateral. This axis shift seen in the frontal plane was likely due to migration of the catheter from RV apex to RV midseptum. Dislodgement of temporary wires is a prelude to loss of capture, sensing or electrode-induced PVCs.

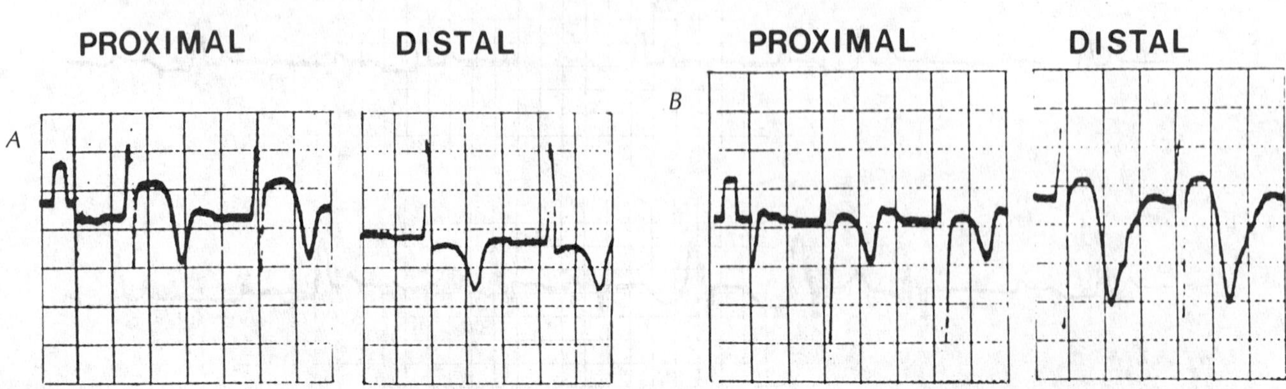

FIGURE 39-4 Unipolar pacing lead electrogram (UPLE) were obtained by attaching the tip and the proximal ring to V leads in the ECG. ST depression from the tip and elevation on the proximal lead indicate perforation *(A)*. After withdrawal the normal ST elevation at the tip greater than at the proximal lead is restored *(B)*.

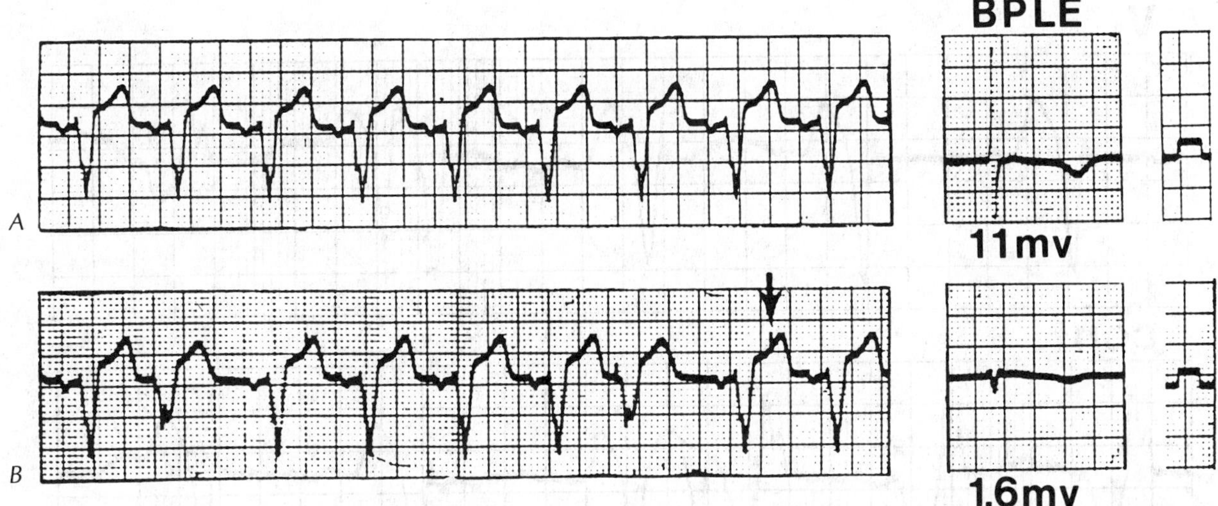

FIGURE 39-5 Sensing suppressed the pacing spike in *A* predicted by the bipolar pacing lead electrogram (BPLE of 11 ms). The tip connected to the LA and the proximal ring electrode connected to the RA produced a BPLE on channel I. In *B* undersensing was predicted by a BPLE of less than 11 mv.

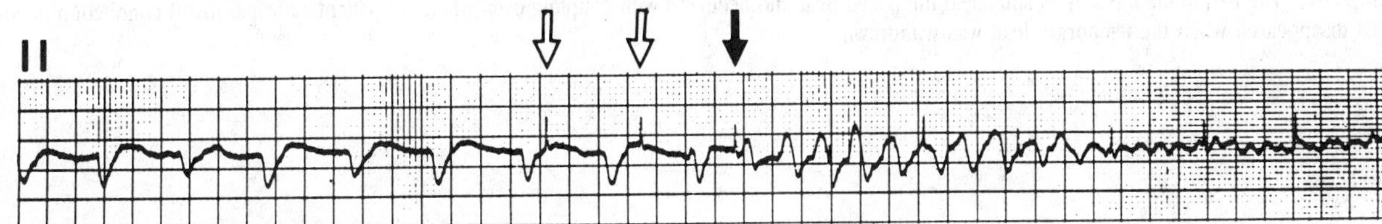

FIGURE 39-6 Sensing failure produced pacing on the T wave without capture (open arrows) until capture (closed arrow) in the vulnerable period caused ventricular fibrillation. The patient was more susceptible to ventricular fibrillation because of digitalis toxicity.

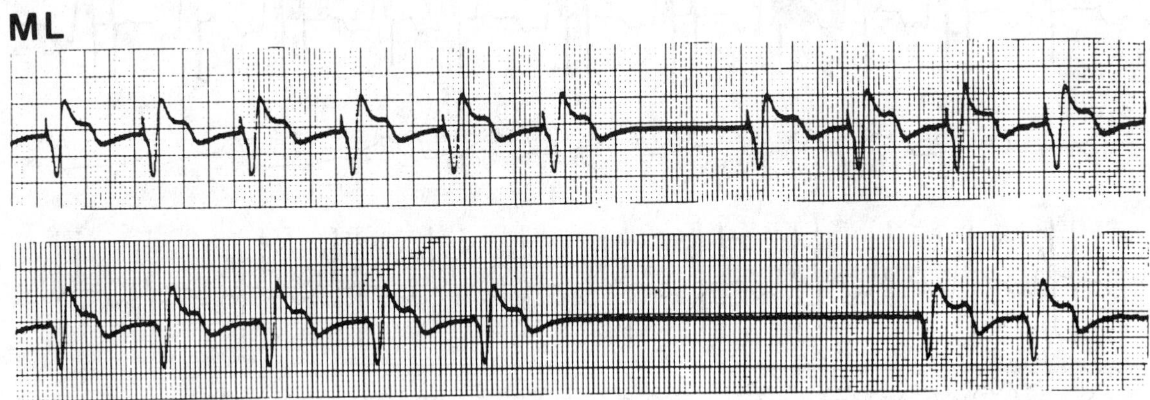

FIGURE 39-7 Failure to pace with no pacing spike did not recur after the connections between generator and pacing leads was tightened.

to be due to dislodgement. Failure to pace with pacing spike absent is due to inhibition (oversensing) or a disconnected lead (Fig. 39-7). Inhibition can be caused by static charge, T waves, P waves, and make break potentials from a fractured lead. Other problems can occur when premature ventricular complexes (PVCs) are induced by the pacemaker lead and appear similar to paced beats (Fig. 39-8). Serious lead induced ectopy should be treated by repositioning the lead.

Temporary and permanent pacemakers can complicate the use of other systems requiring adequate sensing of the cardiac rhythm. Intraortic balloon pumps can be timed with one of three triggers: the arterial pressure, the V paced ECG or the AV paced ECG. When the pacemaker changes from pacing both A and V (DVI) to sensing A and triggering V (VDD), the standard intraortic balloon loses its timing (Fig. 39-9*A*). The rate of the pacemaker should be set either above the intrinsic atrial rate in constant DVI with AV trigger or below the atrial rate for V trigger or be set in VVI mode. Newer balloon pumps have algorithms that permit changing the trigger for the balloon automatically when the DDD pacemaker changes from DVI to VDD mode. Arterial pressure will also trigger the units accurately even if the patient changes from DVI to VDD (Fig. 39-9*B*).

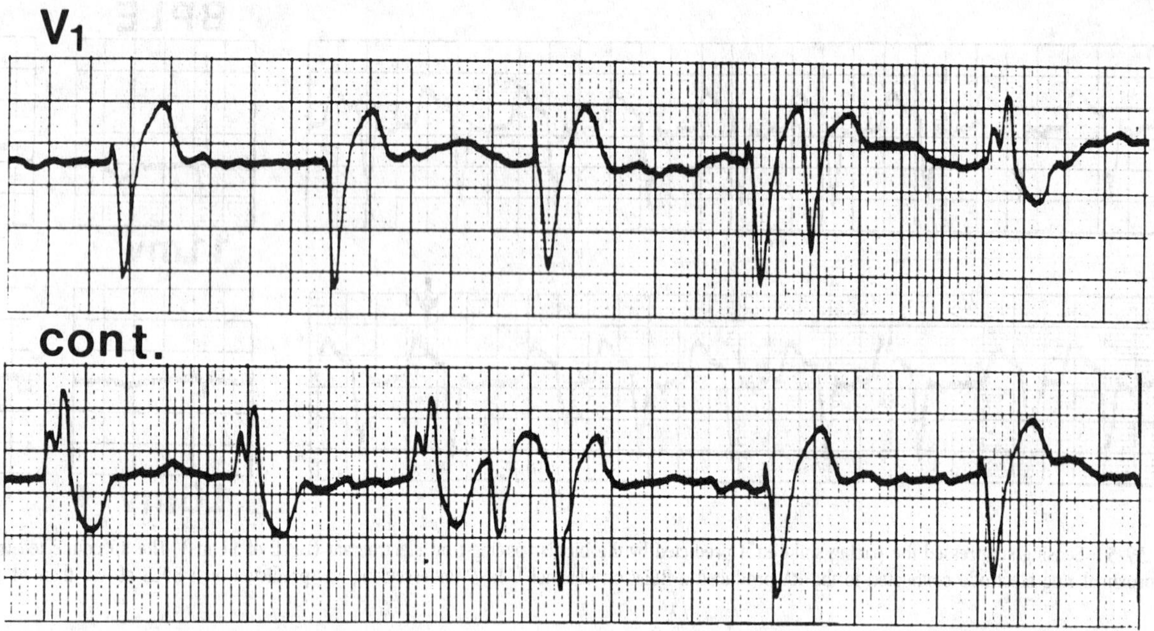

FIGURE 39-8 The PVC in the top strip is similar to the paced beat and occurred with coupling even when the patient's normal RBBB conduction occurred. The PVCs disappeared when the temporary lead was withdrawn.

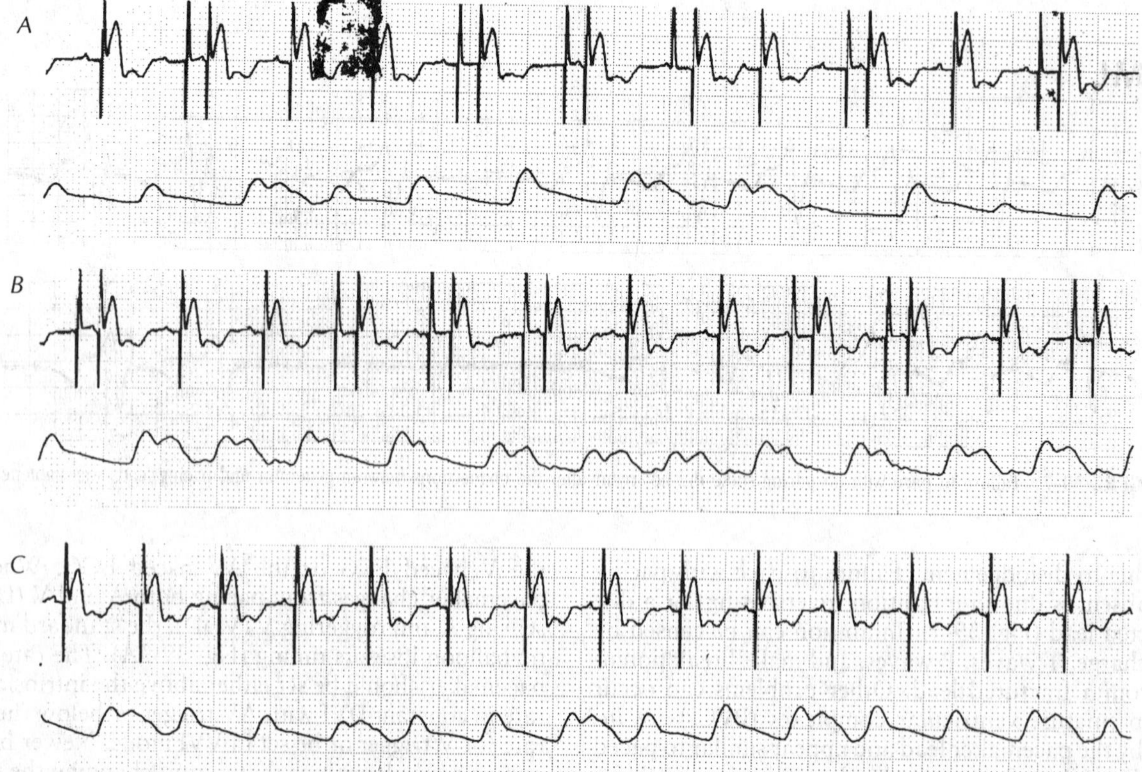

FIGURE 39-9 Temporary dual chamber pacing after cardiac surgery with an aortic balloon pump. In *A* the balloon was triggered by AV pacing (DVI) and failed to augment arterial pressure when the atrium triggered ventricular pacing VDD. Failure to sense the P wave was the reason for AV pacing. In *B* when arterial pressure triggered the balloon, augmentation occurred with each paced QRS regardless of VDD or DVI mode. In *C* after atrial sensing was improved, balloon augmentation was required every third QRS and was consistently triggered by V pacing alone.

REFERENCES

1. Zoll P: Resuscitation of the heart in ventricular standstill by external electric stimulation. *N Engl J Med* 1952;247:768–771.
2. Furman S, Schwedel J: An intracardiac pacemaker for Stokes-Adams seizures. *N Engl J Med* 1959;261:943–948.
3. Chardack W, Gage A, Greatbatch W: A transistorized selfcontained implantable pacemaker for the long-term correction of complete heart block. *Surgery* 1960;48:643–654.
4. Lie K, Wellens J, Shiulenberg R: Bundle branch block in acute myocardial infarction, In: Wellens, Lie, and Janse (eds): *The Conduction System of the Heart.* Philadelphia, Lea & Febiger, 1976:662–672.
5. Curtis JJ, Maloney JD, Barnhorst DA, Pluth JR, Hartzler GO, Wallace RB: A critical look at temporary ventricular pacing following cardiac surgery. *Surgery* 1977;82:888–893.
6. Waldo AL, MacLean WH, Cooper TB, Kouchoukos NT, Karp RB: Use of temporarily placed epicardial atrial wire electrodes for the diagnosis and treatment of cardiac arrhythmias following open heart surgery. *J Thorac Cardiovasc Surg* 1978;76:500–505.
7. Edgeton JR, Kanuf DG, Alexander JA: Temporary pacemaker wire insertion: A simple, safe, and effective technique. *Ann Thorac Surg* 1981;32:615–617.
8. Cooper TB, MacLean WAH, Waldo AL: Overdrive pacing for supraventricular tachycardia: A review of theoretical implications and therapeutic techniques. *PACE* 1978;1:196–221.
9. Waldo AL, MacLean WAH: *Diagnosis and Treatment of Cardiac Arrhythmia Following Open Heart Surgery: Emphasis on the Use of Atrial and Ventricular Epicardial Wire Electrodes.* Mount Kisco, NY, Futura, 1980.
10. Fields J, Berkovitz BV, Matloff JM: Surgical experience with temporary and permanent AV sequential demand pacing. *J Thorac Cardiovas Surg* 1973;66:865–877.
11. Barold S: Therapeutic use of cardiac pacing in tachyarrhythmias. In: Narula OS (ed): *His Bundle Electrocardiography and Clinical Electrophysiology.* Philadelphia, F.A. Davis, 1975.
12. Littleford PO, Pepine CJ: A new temporary atrial pacing catheter inserted percutaneously into the subclavian vein without fluoroscopy. *PACE* 1981;4:458–464.
13. Montoyo JV, Angel J, Valle V, Causi C: Cardioversion of tachycardias by transesophageal atrial pacing. *Am J Cardiol* 1973;32: 85–90.
14. Galagher JJ, Smith W, Kerr C, Kasell J, Cook L, Reiter M, et al: Esophageal pacing: A diagnostic and therapeutic tool. *Circulation* 1982;65:336–341.
15. Arzbaecher R, Collins S, Brown D: Transesophageal recording and pacing with a new pill electrode. (abstr). *Circulation* 1978;58:ii.
16. Zoll PM, Zoll RH, Falk RH, Clinton JE, Eitel DR, Antman EM: External noninvasive temporary cardiac pacing: Clinical trials. *Circulation* 1985;71:937–944.
17. Falk RH, Zoll PM, Zoll RH: Safety and efficacy of noninvasive cardiac pacing. A preliminary report. *N Engl J Med* 1983; 309:1166–1168.
18. Littleford PO, Pepine CJ: A new temporary (external) DDD pacing unit. *Am J Cardiol* 1984;53:1041–1043.
19. Luck JC, Davis D: Termination of sustained tachycardia by external noninvasive pacing. *PACE* 1987;10:125–129.
20. Nathan D, Center S, Pina R, Medow A, Keller W: Perforation during indwelling catheter pacing. *Circulation* 1966;33:128–130.
21. Barold S, Center S: Electrocardiographic diagnosis of perforation of the heart by pacing catheter electrode. *Am J Cardiol* 1969;24:274–278.
22. Wiggers CJ, Wegria R, Pinera B: The effects of myocardial ischemia on the fibrillation threshold. The mechanism of ventricular fibrillation following coronary occlusion. *Am J Physiol* 1940;131:309–316.
23. Preston TA: A new temporary pacing catheter with improved sensing and safety characteristics. *Am Heart J* 1974;88:289–293.

Chapter 40

Permanent Cardiac Pacemakers: Techniques of Implantation, Testing, and Surveillance

Harry G. Mond, M.D.

The marked advances in pacemaker technology in recent years has resulted in new lead designs, microprocessor-based electronic circuitry, long-life power sources, multi-programmability, telemetry, and highly sophisticated dual-chamber and rate-responsive pacing systems. These advances coupled with a manufacturing reliability and quality control unparalleled in any other industry have allowed many more patients to benefit from cardiac pacing, particularly in the pediatric age group. Today, an estimated two million people throughout the world have received a permanent cardiac pacemaker.

HISTORICAL ASPECTS OF CARDIAC PACING

In 1932 Hyman was credited with the design and use of the first pacemaker,[1] but he acknowledged an earlier device developed in Australia by Lidwill during the mid-1920s,[2] and used successfully to resuscitate a stillborn infant.[3] For the next 20 years, almost no work was done in this field because of the unavailability of electronic equipment and appropriate surgical techniques. In 1952, Zoll demonstrated his high-voltage external pacemaker with plate electrodes strapped to the chest wall.[4] Using epicardial leads, in 1957 Lillehei and others paced patients who developed heart block at cardiac surgery.[4] The following year, Furman and Schwedel developed a transvenous endocardial electrode for long-term use.[4] By the late 1950s, the first transistors had become available, allowing for development of implantable, battery-operated pulse generators. The first design, using a rechargeable power source, was implanted in Sweden by Senning and Elmquist in 1958.[4] In 1959, in the United States, Greatbatch developed the first self-contained implantable pulse generator using zinc-mercury batteries.[4] By 1968, QRS sensing circuits had been designed for "demand" pacemaker systems. Some remarkable pacing developments since the 1970s are discussed in this chapter.

INDICATIONS FOR PERMANENT CARDIAC PACING

During the early 1960s, the only indication for permanent cardiac pacing was incapacitating Stokes-Adams attacks, usually resulting from complete heart block.[5] (See also Chap. 36.) In patients who remained nonpaced, there was a high incidence of sudden death and a profound morbidity usually because of severe heart failure and frightening and debilitating syncopal episodes. Such patients were shown to have an improved survival with permanent pacing.[6] Before long, it was recognized that a number of other, less serious bradyarrhythmias could also cause debilitating symptoms and could be eradicated by appropriate cardiac pacing. With the advent of programmability and dual-chamber and rate-responsive systems, the range of pacing options and modalities has increased substantially, creating a new pacing art form: selecting the most appropriate pacemaker for the individual patient.

Despite well-defined indications for permanent pacing, there still exist a number of grey zones and in particular the use and value of permanent pacing in apparently asymptomatic patients or markedly symptomatic patients with a normal resting electrocardiogram (ECG). In a discussion on guidelines for cardiac pacing, Roberts[7] has emphasized that, even with clinical bradycardia, the indications for cardiac pacing are not always clearcut and physicians often have an honest difference of opinion. It therefore behooves each cardiologist to fully record the diagnosis and detailed indications for cardiac pacing prior to pacemaker implantation.

In most patients, the decision for permanent pacing is made on assessment of the resting ECG, symptoms, predicted patient prognosis, and physical state. In more complex cases, the final decision depends on the results of ECG monitoring, electrophysiological studies, the continuing need for cardiac drugs, the state of the underlying myocardium, the desire to operate a motor vehicle, and even knowledge of the long-term follow-up with similar patients.[6] Relative contraindications to permanent pacing include debilitating general disease, very poor left ventricular function, dementia, and advanced cancer. Patients with such contraindications, however, should not necessarily be deprived of a pacemaker if the indications are significant and the management of these other problems can be simplified. In some countries, the cost of the pacing hardware is quoted as a relative contraindication to permanent pacing. In this situation refurbishing of pulse generators where practiced has been found to be safe and economical.[8] It should not be forgotten that the cost of prolonged intensive nursing of patients with Stokes-Adams attacks, intractable cardiac failure, arrhythmias, or severe weakness is far greater than the cost of implanting a permanent pacemaker and transferring the patient to a less intensive nursing environment.

The two major indications for permanent cardiac pacing today are failure of impulse formation and failure of cardiac conduction. These usually result from degenerative, fibrotic, or atherosclerotic processes that damage pacemaker cells, the surrounding tissue, and the conductive elements. Other less common etiologies include infective, rheumatic, vascular, infiltrative, or neoplastic processes.[9] At the time of clinical presentation, although ECG features are usually straightforward, the exact etiology is usually obscure. Electrocardiographic disorder of the sinus node is called the "sick sinus syndrome," whereas disorders of the atrioventricular (AV) node and distal conducting system are referred to as heart block. The term *high-degree AV block* will be used as a major heading for a variety of electrocardiographic patterns, including complete heart block, second-degree AV block, bundle branch blocks, or combinations of these. The sick sinus syndrome and high-degree AV block are frequently associated, this being referred to as a pan-conduction defect. Both tend to occur in advanced age groups with similar pathological processes. Despite this, diseases of the components of the pacemaker and conducting system continue to be differentiated into separate clinical, pathological, and electrocardiographic entities. (See Chap. 36.)

Symptomatic Acquired High-Degree AV Block

Complete Heart Block

Patients with fixed, chronic, complete heart block with a slow ventricular response (below 40 beats per minute) should be paced irrespective of symptoms. Although asymptomatic patients exist, careful history taking suggests that this is unusual. Often, asymptomatic patients attribute their slowing down to advancing age or factors other than the bradycardia, and the results of permanent pacing in these patients can be very impressive.

Second-Degree AV Block

Second-degree AV block can be divided into Mobitz types 1 and 2. Mobitz type 1, or Wenckebach, block most frequently results from a conduction disturbance in the AV node. A normal width QRS complex is usually present, and progression to complete heart block with a marked symptomatic bradycardia is unusual and therefore permanent pacing is usually unnecessary. With Mobitz type 2 block, the conduction disturbance is distal and the QRS is widened unless the block is at the level of the common His bundle. In general, Mobitz type 2 block is progressive, is unpredictable, and may result in Stokes-Adams attacks, thus necessitating permanent pacing.

Bundle Branch Blocks

Although the various types of bundle branch blocks are frequently and easily recognized on the ECG, the natural history and the progression of the lesions are not well understood. Electrophysiological investigations of patients with a bundle branch block on the ECG, although helpful, cannot by themselves be used as accurate predictors of complete heart block. Therapeutic decisions require clinical data. Symptomatic patients with bifascicular block or intermittent complete heart block and a wide QRS will have a prolonged infranodal conduction time, and pacing is indicated without electrophysiological studies.

A more difficult clinical situation is chronic bifascicular block without demonstrable ECG evidence of disease in the third fascicle. Here, knowledge of the infranodal conduction time is of value. Narula[10] showed that patients with bifascicular block and a prolonged HV interval who are not permanently paced have a 23 percent mortality per year compared to those with a normal HV interval, whether symptomatic (8 percent) or asymptomatic (6 percent). The actual measured HV interval also appears important. Scheinman et al.[11] demonstrated that in patients with bifascicular block, the incidence of progression to higher degrees of heart block was much higher if the HV interval was equal to or greater than 70 ms. Patients who show alternating right and left bundle branch block have significant bilateral bundle branch block disease, and permanent pacing is usually indicated.

Congenital High-Degree AV Block

This uncommon entity is present at birth. Complete heart block detected in the young, however, may result from myocarditis, rheumatic heart disease, trauma, or vascular, neoplastic, or infiltrative disorders. If surgically uncorrected congenital cardiac malformations are also present, the term *congenital heart block* can be applied even if not detected at birth. Congenital complete heart block as an isolated anomaly is usually well tolerated in childhood. The ventricular rate is usually stable and may range from 40 to 90 beats per minute, often increasing modestly with exercise. Most infants and children with isolated congenital complete heart block grow and develop normally and can lead active lives. Permanent cardiac pacing is indicated in all symptomatic cases of congenital heart block irrespective of age. The asymptomatic child with complete heart block, whether congenital or acquired, may also require permanent pacing. In these cases, the prognosis must be considered. The site and particularly the stability of the ventricular pacemaker can be assessed by ambulatory monitoring and, if necessary, electrophysiological studies.[12] A single pacemaker focus usually lies in the AV junctional tissue or His bundle. An additional ectopic ventricular focus may predispose to instability and consequently life-threatening ventricular tachyarrhythmias and Stokes-Adams attacks. With the development of sophisticated physiological pacing systems, it has become popular to recommend permanent pacing in all children with complete heart block if ambulatory monitoring reveals additional unstable ventricular ectopic foci.

High-Degree AV Block Following Acute Myocardial Infarction

A major controversy in pacemaker therapy is the role of prophylactic, temporary, or permanent cardiac pacing following an acute myocardial infarction. The physician is dealing with a difficult clinical situation involving both a myocardial conduction defect and a prognosis limiting myocardial contraction abnormality with a propensity for further acute infarction. Any attempt to evaluate the effects of pacing will be hampered by the myocardial dysfunction, manifested by pump failure, angina, arrhythmias, and sudden death.

In the early 1970s it became popular to pace, on a temporary basis, all patients who developed complete heart block following an acute inferior myocardial infarction. However, because of the transient nature of this block and its usually benign hemodynamic consequences, temporary pacing is now performed only when significant hemodynamic indications prevail. High-degree AV block complicating an acute anterior myocardial infarction is only one-third as common but three times as lethal as the acute inferior type.[13] Unlike inferior myocardial infarction, it is advisable to predict which patients with anterior myocardial infarction will develop complete heart block and to institute prophylactic temporary pacing. Patients most likely to require temporary pacing are those who develop a combination of a new right bundle branch block and a left hemiblock or a pattern of alternating left and right bundle branch blocks.[14] Patients who survive Mobitz type 2 block or complete heart block during the course of an acute anterior myocardial infarction should be monitored for 7 to 10 days prior to making a decision regarding permanent pacing. Patients should be considered for permanent pacing even if the block complicating the anterior infarction was transient.[14] (See also Chap. 39.)

Sick Sinus Syndrome

The sick sinus syndrome entails episodic or persistent sinus bradycardia together with periods of sinus arrest or sinoatrial block with or without an escape AV junctional rhythm and with varying degrees of AV block.[15] Paroxysmal supraventricular and even ventricular tachyarrhythmias may alternate with the bradycardia. Termination of the tachyarrhythmias may reveal failure or slow recovery of sinus node function, and the resultant profound bradycardia may result in Stokes-Adams attacks.

With regard to clinical presentation and prognosis, the sick sinus syndrome can be divided into three groups. Patients with the most benign course are those with sinus bradycardia. A second patient group exhibits sinus arrest or sinoatrial block with or without the sinus bradycardia. The most severe group is a combination of both bradyarrhythmias and paroxysmal tachyarrhythmias and is called the tachycardia-bradycardia syndrome. Pathologically, chronic sinoatrial bradyarrhythmias are associated with extensive degenerative lesions within and around the sinus node. The tachycardia-bradycardia syndrome, however, is also associated with lesions in atrial tissue.[16] Patients with the sick sinus syndrome are usually elderly and form a group similar to those who present with complete heart block. Sinus node dysfunction may be familial,[17] has been reported in children and young adults,[18] and in particular may follow corrective congenital heart surgery.[19]

Symptomatic patients with sick sinus syndrome may present with syncope or dizziness resulting from a bradycardia or even a tachycardia with a reduced cardiac output. Other symptoms include palpitations, tiredness, lethargy, heart failure, and angina. The asymptomatic patient with electrocardiographic features of sick sinus syndrome usually does not require permanent pacing unless beta-adrenergic blockade or antiarryhthmic drugs are required for other reasons. Pacemaker therapy is highly successful in patients with sick sinus syndrome and syncopal episodes.[16,20] In the majority of cases, the syncopal episodes are abolished, accompanied by marked physical and psychologic improvement. Because of atrial arrhythmias and frequent association of distal conduction tissue disturbances, ventricular pacing usually with a rate-responsive sensor is recommended rather than pure atrial pacing. In elderly patients with impaired left ventricular function, the atrial boost provided with atrial pacing may be valuable for congestive cardiac failure. In these cases, as well as young patients and those with retrograde conduction, rate-responsive dual-chamber pacing may be recommended, provided frequent or established atrial fibrillation is not present.

The long-term prognosis of patients with sick sinus syndrome, whether paced or not, depends on the patient's age, the presence or absence of cardiac failure, and the nature of the underlying pathology.[21] Because of diffuse atrial disease, patients with tachycardia-bradycardia syndrome have the worst prognosis. Despite an overall high mortality in patients with the sick sinus syndrome, symptomatic patients, irrespective of the underlying myocardial pathology, should not be denied the benefits of permanent pacing.

Slow Junctional Rhythm

Slow junctional rhythm is usually a manifestation of the sick sinus syndrome but can also occur in normal patients such as athletes. Symptomatic patients with either a failure of sinus node activity or an insignificant rise in pulse rate with exercise may require permanent pacing.

Slow Atrial Fibrillation or Flutter

Without the influence of drugs such as digitalis or beta-adrenergic blockade, this condition usually reflects extensive AV nodal block. When the ventricular response is regular and slow, complete heart block is usually present. On occasion, patients with atrial fibrillation demonstrate symptomatic prolonged asystolic pauses even when the atrial fibrillation rate is otherwise rapid. These patients require permanent ventricular pacing to correct the pauses and allow the atrial fibrillation rate to be controlled pharmacologically.

Atrial Inexcitability

Atrial inexcitability, a condition in which the atria cannot be stimulated by pacing, is rare and results from a diffuse abnormality of atrial muscle. Usually the etiology is obscure, although it has been reported with cardiomyopathies, amyloid heart, atherosclerotic heart disease, and muscular dystrophies.[22] On the ECG, there is no P wave, and electrophysiological studies show a complete lack of electrical and mechanical activity in the atrium. Rate-responsive ventricular pacing is indicated in symptomatic patients.

Recurrent Ventricular Standstill

When not due to drug toxicity, recurrent ventricular standstill reflects extensive pacemaker and conduction tissue degeneration and belongs to the pan-conduction disease group. Although pacing can successfully abolish symptoms, the prognosis depends on the underlying pathology.

Ablation of His Bundle and/or Adjoining Tissue

Successful His bundle ablation has been performed for a variety of intractable atrial arrhythmias and in particular atrial fibrillation. All patients who undergo His bundle ablation should receive an implanted cardiac pacemaker even if their spontaneous heart rhythm appears satisfactory.

Hereditary Prolongation of QT Interval

These patients are prone to syncope and sudden death. Permanent atrial or ventricular pacing has been used together with beta-adrenergic blockade in an attempt to override the drug-induced bradycardia that may encourage ventricular ectopics.

Carotid Sinus Hypersensitivity and Vasovagal Syncope

Carotid sinus hypersensitivity is a common problem in elderly patients with coronary atherosclerosis and hypertensive heart disease. Syncope is usually due to a combination of a bradycardia and vasodilatation and may be induced by shaving, micturition, sneezing, head turning, looking up, exercise, and tight neck collars.[23] Asymptomatic or mildly symptomatic patients with carotid sinus hypersensitivity do not require therapy apart from avoidance of the precipitating factors. Dual-chamber pacing is usually successful in preventing syncope due to bradycardia. Pure atrial pacing is contraindicated because of a high incidence of associated AV nodal block.

Profound vasovagal syncope is a very distressing and potentially dangerous syndrome often found in young females and frequently responds to high-rate dual-chamber pacing. Many of the symptoms are common to carotid sinus syncope, although the factors that precipitate syncope usually remain obscure.

Tachyarrhythmias

Cardiac pacing for the treatment of both supraventricular and ventricular tachyarrhythmias has been used for many years with limited success. Most earlier techniques were temporary, although occasionally permanent pacemakers were implanted for overdrive suppression. Recent developments in the field of clinical electrophysiology have resulted in marked progress in the understanding of tachyarrhythmias, especially with regard to the initiation and termination of re-entry pathways. As a result, many pacing systems have been described, but only overdrive suppression, radiofrequency-induced rapid atrial pacing, and specialized complex automatic systems have been successful.[15] The use of these systems has been limited to those patients who are resistant to, refuse, or cannot tolerate drug therapy. Today, with successful surgery or ablative techniques for atrial tachyarrhythmias, permanent pacing techniques are rarely required. For ventricular tachycardia, pacing techniques have now been incorporated into cardioverter-defibrillators in an attempt to revert the tachyarrhythmia with complicated pacing algorithms or for bradycardia support following reversion or defibrillation. (See also Chap. 42.)

IMPLANTABLE PACEMAKER SYSTEM

Pacemaker Pulse Generator

Modern pulse generators are sophisticated power packs that are small, compact, reliable, long-lived, and multiprogrammable. Within the pulse generator lies the power source and electronics, hermetically sealed in a titanium or stainless steel casing to protect the contents from a hostile environment of body tissues.

Pulse Generator Power Source

The original power source that sustained the pacemaker industry for 15 years was the zinc-mercury battery. This chemical battery had an unpredictable failure mode and an average life of only 2 to 4 years. By the mid-1970s a number of other power sources were being considered. The rechargeable nickel-cadmium battery was reliable, but patients resented having to frequently recharge their power source. Nuclear power cells first used in 1970 were also reliable and had projected implant lives up to 20 years. Unfortunately, because of expense, limited implant indications, nuclear radiation fear, strict nuclear regulatory controls, and failure of the manufacturers to keep abreast of other technologies, nuclear-powered pulse generators are rarely used today.

The lithium anode battery has completely revolutionized the pacemaker industry because of its reliability and longevity. The main battery used for implantable pulse generators has been the lithium-iodine cell. Although there is a gradual fall in voltage output as the lithium and iodine are consumed in the chemical reaction, nevertheless a satisfactory voltage output is retained for 90 percent of the battery's life, and this is used by manufacturers to monitor pulse generator progress and impending power source depletion.

Pulse Generator Circuitry

There are three essential electronic circuits in a pulse generator. The timing circuit controls the pacing rate, the output circuit controls the charging and discharging of the impulse, and the sensing circuit is responsible for the recognition of spontaneous intracardiac electrical signals. There are time constraints on the functioning of the timing and sensing circuits. During depolarization and for a set period after atrial and ventricular myocardial depolarization, whether it be paced or spontaneous, there are protective periods of nonsensing in both the atrium and ventricle called refractory periods.

Pacing circuits are further complicated by a variety of other electronic accessories including filtering devices, voltage multipliers, reed switches, and complex circuitry required for programmability, telemetry, memory, and dual-chamber and rate-responsive sensor control. In order to confirm cardiac pacing when the pulse generator output is inhibited, a reed switch is used to convert the pulse generator to the asynchronous mode. This switch is actuated by positioning a test magnet over the implanted pulse generator. The removal of the magnetic field allows the reed switch to assume its base status, and the pulse generator sensing circuit will respond in a synchronous manner.

Pacemaker Lead

The pacemaker lead delivers the pulse generator charge to the myocardium and conducts intracardiac potentials back to the sensing circuit. Originally epicardial or epimyocardial leads were used, but because of the necessity for a thoracotomy, transvenous leads gradually became popular. Today, epimyocardial leads are rarely used except in the pediatric population.

Bipolar and Unipolar Electrode Systems

There are two major types of lead systems. A unipolar lead has only one electrode on the lead itself: the cathode, or active pole. Current flows from the cathode, stimulates the heart, and returns to the anode on the casing of the pulse generator to complete the circuit. A bipolar lead has two poles on the lead a short distance from each other at the distal end, and both electrodes lie within the heart. The original bipolar lead was bulky and had two connectors. By arranging the two conductors in a coaxial fashion and creating a single low-profile in-line connector, the size of bipolar leads has been significantly reduced. With modern pacing systems, there is little difference between unipolar and bipolar lead systems. Both are reliable and suitable for long-term pacing in both the atrium and ventricle. Because of their size, unipolar leads became popular. Coaxial bipolar leads with low-profile in-line connectors, however, are now being used more frequently, and with single-coil multiconductor technology, future bipolar leads will be the same size as unipolar.[24]

The major disadvantage of unipolar pacing is oversensing. Although unipolar sensing is theoretically superior because of the large interelectrode distance, this is not a problem with modern programmable pacemakers. The enhanced sensing capability of unipolar leads, however, makes such systems more sensitive to extracardiac electrical potentials, in particular skeletal myopotentials, crosstalk, and far-field sensing.[24] Another disadvantage of unipolar pacing is the proximity of skeletal muscle to the anode plate. Frequently local skeletal muscle contractions occur when current is returning to the anode after myocardial stimulation. Although this can be prevented by having the pulse generator anode facing subcutaneous tissues, this nevertheless prevents unipolar pacemakers from being buried deep in skeletal muscle.

Probably the only significant advantage of unipolar pacing is the size of the stimulus artifact during pacemaker testing. This can be overcome by programming a bipolar pacing system to the unipolar mode if polarity programming is available.[24]

Cardiac Electrode

The stimulating tip electrode or cathode is responsible for delivery of charge to the myocardium. The original designs had large surface areas approximating 100 mm^2. With such electrodes, the pacing impedance was low, the current drain was high, and the current dispersion over the large electrode resulted in a high-voltage stimulation threshold.[25] By reducing the cathode surface area, high-impedance, low-stimulation-threshold, more energy efficient electrodes were created.[26] Today, most pacing electrode designs have cathodes with surface areas of 5 to 8 mm^2 with even smaller electrodes entering clinical trials.

Although the reduction in cathode size results in a significant reduction in stimulation threshold, this does not necessarily produce a low-energy lead. Such small electrodes may result in increased energy losses from polarization. Electrical current within metal conductors is due to the flow of electrons, but in body tissues it is due to the movement of charged molecules or ions. At the electrode-tissue interface, there is a transfer of electron energy to ionic energy, and hence, an intense chemical reaction occurs. Polarization is due to the alignment of oppositely charged particles at this interface and is a capacitance effect. During discharge it rises only to fall away at the time of the afterpotential due to dissipation of ions. The polarization effect increases as the electrode size is reduced and is also dependent on other factors.[27,28] Porous electrodes have been found to have low polarization properties.[26] With porous leads, the actual electrode-tissue interface is small; yet the electrode area includes the internal space between the pores, thereby creating a relatively large, low-polarization, electrolytic surface area. A popular microporous platinized platinum electrode has a very fine platinum powder electroplated to a solid metal base. The electrode appears black because the surface particles are smaller than the wavelength of visible light and are therefore absorbed.

The shape of the stimulating electrode helps define the electrode-tissue interface or area of stimulation contact with the endomyocardium. A variety of electrode shapes have been designed to create zones of high current density, where highly concentrated electron energy can depolarize adjacent myocardium. One popular design is shaped like a target with shallow grooves separated by peaks that are the zones of high current density (Fig. 40-1). However, once the electrode becomes very small, the whole surface area is high current density, and therefore specific and complicated shapes become irrelevant.

The composition of the electrode material is critical to the long-term function of a lead. Some metals, such as stainless steel and zinc, cause excessive corrosion resulting in an intense foreign body reaction and a thick fibrous capsule around the electrode. Platinum and its alloys are commonly used as cathode materials because they are relatively unreactive and act as a catalyst for the breakdown or re-formation of water. Lightly alloying platinum with up to 10 percent iridium increases its strength without altering its electromechanical performance. In Europe, vitreous carbon has been extensively used as a cathode for low-stimulation-threshold, low-polarization electrodes.[29] Titanium, titanium oxide, and titanium alloys have been found to be suitable for use as electrode materials, as both anode and cathode.[30,31] A platinum-coated titanium electrode has been in use since 1983. The low chronic thresholds obtained with this lead result from steroid elution and not the electrode materials.[32]

In the search for the low-stimulation-threshold, low-polarization electrode, the electrode-tissue interface has represented the greatest challenge. The inflammatory response and the subsequent development of a fibrous capsule between electrode and endomyocardium is an obvious impediment to current flow and is responsible for the unpredictable rise in stimulation threshold postimplantation. The answer to this problem lay in the use of pharmacologic agents. Many anti-inflammatory, anticoagulant, and antiextracellular matrix formation agents have been investigated, and only the glucocorticosteroid dexamethasone sodium phosphate resulted in a significant reduction in stimulation threshold levels.[33,34] As a result of this work, a number of steroid-eluting electrode systems have been developed. The original design was composed of a platinum-coated titanium electrode, hemispherical in shape, with a geometric surface of about 8 mm^2 (Fig. 40-2). The electrode surface is porous, and immediately behind it lies a plug of silicone rubber impregnated with less than 1 mg of dexamethasone sodium phosphate.[35]

Following implantation, tissue fluids traverse the electrode via the porous matrix and dissolve the steroid in the silicone rubber plug, which gradually elutes into the surrounding electrode-tissue interface. Initial experience with this electrode in the experimental animal and human beings has demonstrated very low acute and chronic stimulation thresholds in both the atrium and ventricle with virtual elimination of the early postoperative peak in stimulation threshold.[32,35-40] In particular, excellent results have been obtained in children[41] and in patients with a previous history of high threshold exit block.[33,42] Double-blind clinical trials comparing electrodes with and without steroid have confirmed that it is the steroid and not the electrode that has the threshold-lowering effect.[32,43] This effect has now been shown to persist for at least 6 years of follow-up.[26]

Second- and third-generation platinized microporous platinum, steroid-eluting electrodes, some with surface

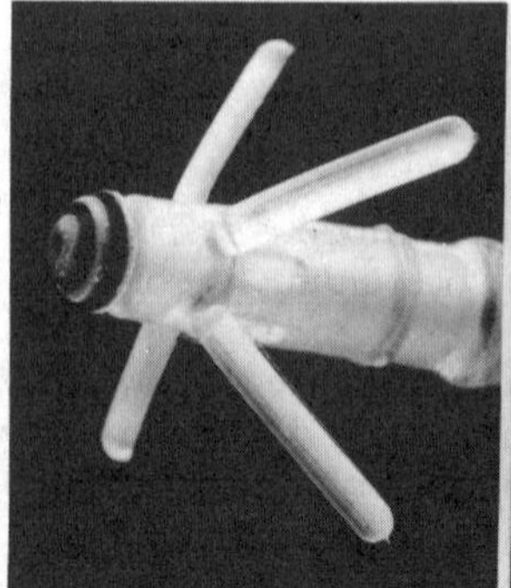
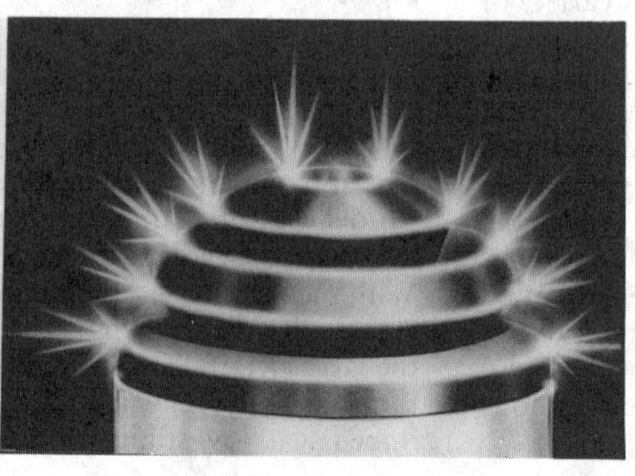

FIGURE 40-1 Microporous, platinized platinum electrode (Medtronic Target Tip). The target appearance is due to shallow grooves separated by peaks. (*Courtesy Medtronic, Inc.**)

*Medtronic Inc., Minneapolis, MN.

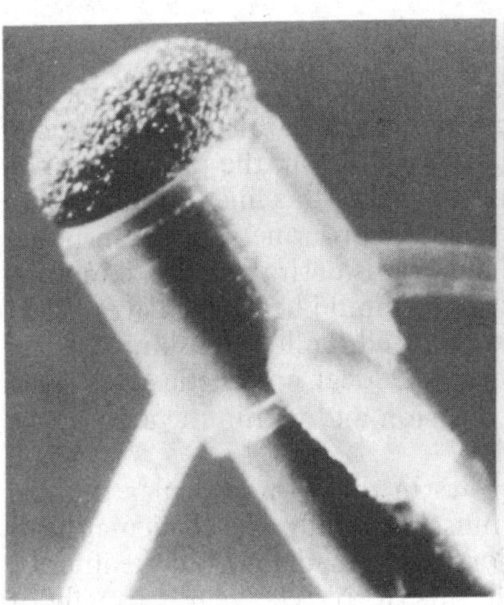

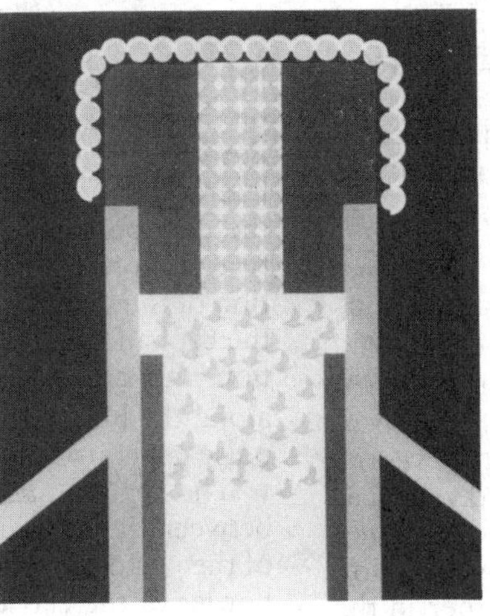

FIGURE 40-2 *Left:* Steroid eluting, porous, platinum-coated titanium electrode (Medtronic Capsure). *Right:* Cross-sectional diagram of the same electrode. Behind the electrode is the silicone rubber plug compounded with dexamethasone sodium phosphate. (*Courtesy Medtronic, Inc.**)

areas as small as 1.5 mm^2, are now being implanted. Another steroid-eluting electrode design uses a silicone rubber ring or collar positioned immediately behind the electrode. Human implant data have shown a significant reduction in stimulation threshold values for those electrodes containing steroid, with both unipolar[44,45] and bipolar[46] leads. Steroid-eluting collars have also been incorporated into active fixation screw-in leads (Fig. 40-3).

Lead Conductor

The lead conductor delivers current to the electrode-tissue interface. In the past, conductor fractures were responsible for a significant proportion of late lead complications.[47] Today pacing leads have conductors with immense strength and flexibility as well as high fracture and corrosion resistance. These lead conductors are composed of one or more strands of wire, tightly coiled around a hollow core to allow removable stylets to pass all the way to the distal electrode. Materials used included stainless steel and complex alloys. Bipolar leads require two conductors, usually in a coaxial design. A new design involves a single coil with multiple strands allowing it to be a multiconductor system.[24] Epimyocardial leads do not require a stylet, and there is consequently more flexibility with lead conductor design.

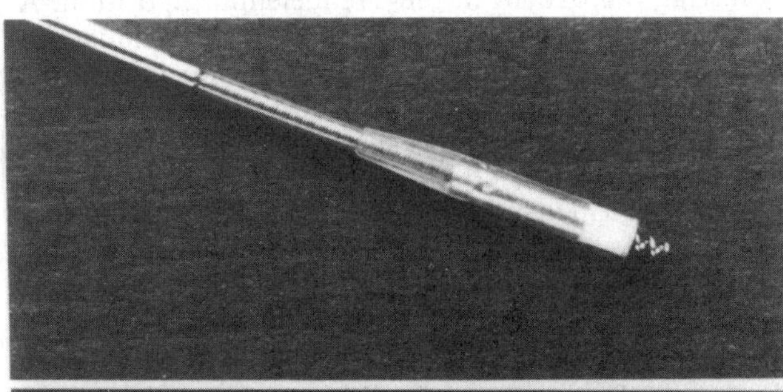

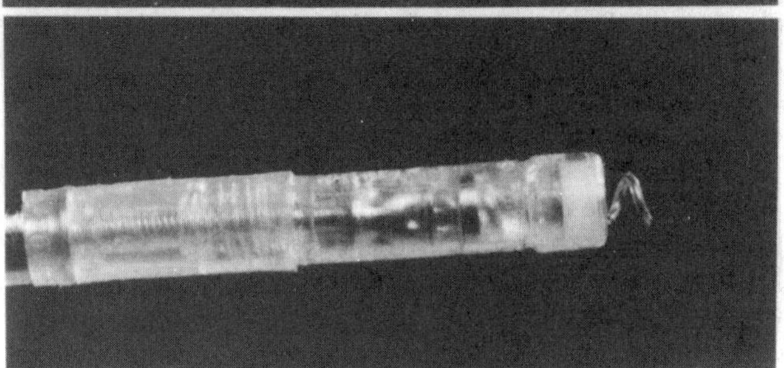

FIGURE 40-3 *Top:* Active fixation lead with a porous electrode and an electrically inert screw. Surrounding the electrode is a silicone rubber collar impregnated with dexamethasone sodium phosphate. (*Courtesy Telectronics Pacing Systems.**) *Bottom:* Active fixation lead with an electrically active screw. There is a steroid eluting collar surrounding the screw. (*Courtesy Medtronic, Inc.*)

*Telectronics Pacing Systems, Denver, CO.

Lead Insulator

The earliest insulating material was polyethylene, which had poor long-term insulation properties. Silicone rubber was substituted, but because of its tendency to tear and cut, the insulation layer was made thicker. Several polyurethanes have also been found to be suitable for pacemaker lead insulation. These polyurethanes are tougher and stiffer than silicone rubber, and the insulation thickness can be reduced.

Lead Connector

The connector joins the lead to the pulse generator. The ideal connector is small, compact, reliable, and universally compatible, allowing any lead to be attached to the pulse generator of any manufacturer. In an attempt at some conformity within the industry, most pacemaker companies used 5- or 6-mm unipolar connectors with bipolar leads having a bifurcated arrangement. A major improvement has been the development of low-profile in-line connectors. An in-line connector places both poles on a single lead pin with an insulating barrier separating them. An international standard, called IS-1 for unipolar and bipolar low-profile connectors, has recently been ratified.

Lead Fixation

Lead fixation may be passive or active. Passive-fixation leads promote fixation to the endocardium by indirect means, whereas active-fixation leads penetrate the endomyocardium. Passive-fixation leads include wedge,[47] tines,[47] balloons,[48] and helifix designs.[25] By far the most common means of lead fixation in the ventricle are tines (Figs. 40-1 and 40-2). The most frequently used active-fixation lead has been the screw-in design (Fig. 40-3).[49]

Transvenous Atrial Leads

The right atrial appendage is trabeculated and suitable for atrial pacing and sensing. A number of endocardial atrial J leads have been developed for use in this area. Although clinically successful, the incidence of complications remains higher than with similar leads in the ventricle. A number of authors prefer to use standard ventricular tined leads positioned in the atrial appendage using a J-shaped stylet.[50,51] In recent years, active-fixation screw-in leads have been successfully used either in the appendage or any other appropriate position in the right atrium.[52] Although rarely used today, leads can be placed in the coronary sinus for atrial pacing.[53]

A single-pass lead incorporates both the atrial and ventricular leads within a single body. For atrial pacing, the atrial electrode must make contact with the atrial wall, and for this reason single-pass leads have not been widely used. Most designs are simple with the bipolar atrial electrodes lying within the cavity of the atrium and used for atrial sensing only.[54,55]

Epimyocardial Leads

Direct suturing of the pacemaker lead to the epicardial surface was the original method of permanent lead implantation. As transvenous leads improved, they gradually began to dominate pacemaker implants, despite the initial success of the sutureless epimyocardial screw-in electrode introduced in 1971.[56] Today, epimyocardial lead implantation should be relegated to those situations where the transvenous approach is technically impossible or has failed.

PACEMAKER IMPLANTATION

Transvenous Ventricular Lead Implantation

Unlike the implantation of an epimyocardial lead, the evolution of the endocardial lead implantation technique from a highly complicated, time-consuming procedure to a rapid, relatively uncomplicated transvenous routine has been dramatic. Major reasons for this improvement include small pulse generators and sophisticated transvenous leads that utilize a stiffening and directing stylet. Consequently, transvenous lead implantation has become the routine practiced in most pacemaker centers. The following is an outline of the techniques generally used, although a more detailed description is available.[25]

On the day of surgery, the surgical site is prepared and an appropriate premedication ordered. Preoperative antibiotics, although not universally recommended, may be prescribed as a single dose or a short, broad-spectrum course. The operating room should have fluoroscopy, ECG monitoring, a pacing system analyzer, and resuscitative equipment. The room should have a unipotential ground and be regularly inspected for electrical hazards.

Lead Introduction

Prior to skin sterilization, a 4-cm incision line is marked on the chest wall 2 cm below and parallel to the clavicle. For cephalic vein lead introduction, the junction of the lateral third and middle third of this line should lie over the deltopectoral groove. For routine subclavian puncture, a more medial incision is desirable. The skin position of the subclavian vein should be marked even when the cephalic vein is to be used. Following skin sterilization and drape placement, local anesthetic is injected along the line of the incision and within the area of the pulse generator pocket.

The *cephalic vein* lies in the infraclavicular triangle between the deltoid muscle laterally, the clavicular head of the pectoralis major muscle medially, and the inferior border of the clavicle superiorly. The vein is usually of sufficient size to accept one or more pacing leads. Once isolated, the distal end of the cephalic vein is ligated and the proximal end secured. A small venous incision is made with fine scissors, and using an introducer, the pacing lead is placed within the vein and passed via the subclavian vein to the right atrium.

Subclavian vein puncture was originally applied in cases of failed cephalic vein insertion, but now many operators use this as their primary method of lead insertion. Because the technique is potentially more dangerous than cephalic vein insertion, experience and understanding of the local anatomy are key factors to success.[57,58] Because of potential complications, it is recommended that all cardiac pacemaker implanters learn the cephalic vein technique as their primary method of transvenous lead insertion.[59]

The subclavian vein arches over the first rib deep to the medial third of the clavicle and should be distended by having the patient in the Trendelenburg position. A rolled towel should be placed between the scapulae to force the shoulders back and elevate the subclavian vein from the apex of the lung. Instead of the standard skin incision, some operators prefer to make a very small cut and extend this after the vein has been punctured. To puncture the subclavian vein, the needle and syringe are placed below the inferior border of the clavicle at the junction of its medial and middle thirds. The needle is advanced under the clavicle with the tip aimed at the sternal notch, keeping the syringe parallel to the anterior chest wall. The operator should gently aspirate the syringe until venous blood is freely obtained. Firmly securing the needle, a J guide wire is passed into the vein. Over the guide wire, a vein dilator and sheath are passed. With finger pressure to control bleeding, the guide wire and dilator are removed, the pacemaker lead introduced into the right atrium, and the introducer peeled away. Prior to this, a second guide wire may be placed in order to pass a second dilator and sheath for two-lead, dual-chamber pacing.[60] Reported and potential complications of subclavian puncture include pneumothorax,[58] wound hematoma,[61] subclavian arterial puncture,[58,61] hemopneumomediastinum, air embolism, arteriovenous fistula, thoracic duct injury, subcutaneous emphysema, infection, and nerve injury. Difficulties may occur in patients with a previous fractured clavicle or chronic airway disease.

Other venous entry sites are rarely used due to the success of the cephalic and subclavian routes. The external jugular vein has many disadvantages, including difficult venous cannulation and lead manipulation, two incisions, and the formation of a loop of lead in the neck that may be uncomfortable and result in conductor fracture or lead erosion. The internal jugular vein, anterior pectoral veins, and femoral vein have all been used for transvenous lead insertion.

Lead Positioning

Once in the right atrium, the tip of the lead must be directed across the tricuspid valve and positioned at the apex of the right ventricle. To prevent coronary sinus placement, the lead with a curved stylet can be directed across the tricuspid valve and positioned in the right ventricular outflow tract or pulmonary artery. With a straight stylet inserted just beyond the tricuspid valve position, the lead is gradually retracted until the electrode is directed toward the right ventricular apex. The lead, again with stylet slightly retracted, is advanced and the electrode positioned at the apex. A tined lead should be gently retracted to demonstrate lead entrapment beneath ventricular trabeculae. Other endocardial lead fixation devices should now be activated.

Coronary venous pacing should be excluded. In the posteroanterior view, a lead in the coronary sinus is directed superiorly toward the left shoulder.[62] Electrodes in the middle or posterior cardiac veins, however, mimic the right ventricular apical position in the posteroanterior view. In the lateral view, right ventricular leads are directed anteriorly (Fig. 40-4), whereas those in the coronary venous system lie posteriorly.[62] Depending on its position, a lead in the coronary sinus will usually give atrial pacing, whereas an electrode in a cardiac vein will pace the ventricle with a right bundle branch block appearance, sometimes with an elevated pacing threshold and a characteristic endocardial electrogram.[25]

Lead Testing

Electrical testing of the lead at the time of pacemaker implantation allows for selection of the optimal electrode stimulation and sensing site. The threshold voltage and current, R-wave sensitivity, system impedance, and integrity of the pulse generator can all be determined using a pacing system analyzer. The endocardial R-wave size should have a value greater than 4 mV for adequate sensing by the pulse generator sensing circuit. The slew rate, which is the maximum rate of voltage change (*dv/dt*), in the ventricular electrogram can be measured by the cardiac pacing system analyzer or directly from the intracardiac electrogram. An adequate R-wave slew rate required to inhibit a pulse generator is 0.5 V/s. An intracardiac electrogram should also be recorded. The most common appearance of the ventricular electrogram is a biphasic wave with a dominant S wave. Once contact is made with the endocardium, ST elevation and T-wave inversion occur. In comparison, the epicardial ventricular pattern (coronary sinus tributary or lead perforation of the right ventricle) almost always has a dominant R wave without ST elevation and T-wave inversion.

To measure "stimulation threshold," the voltage output is slowly reduced until loss of capture occurs (consistent pacing not present).[63] Both voltage and resultant current are noted. By increasing the voltage output until consistent pacing is reestablished, the "pacing threshold" is obtained.[63] There is often a difference in the two threshold levels, the pacing threshold being higher by about 0.1 to 0.3 V. The usual acceptance range for acute stimulation threshold recordings at 0.5 ms pulse duration is from 0.3 to 1.0 V with a resultant current of 0.3 to 2.0 mA.

The impedance (resistance) of the implanted system is measured by pacing the heart at 5 V to offset the effects of polarization potentials at the electrode-tissue interface.[64] If a direct measurement is not available on the pacing system analyzer, the current is recorded and the impedance calculated using Ohm's law. The usual range for impedance is from 250 to 1000 Ω. Low imped-

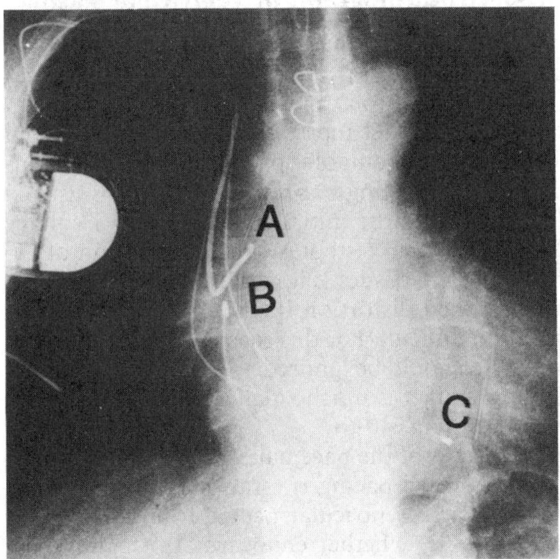

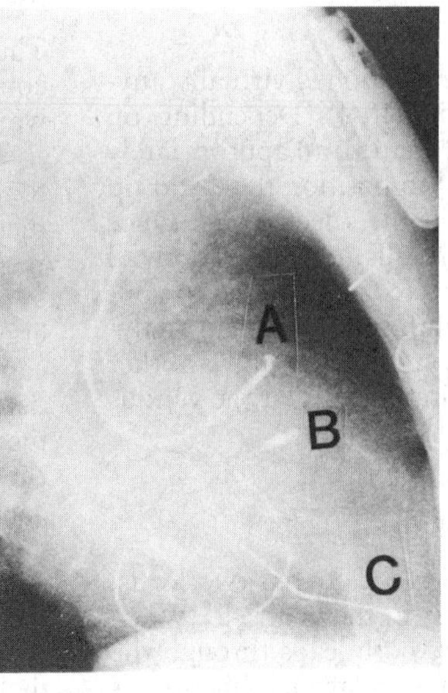

FIGURE 40-4 Posteroanterior (*left*) and lateral (*right*) chest radiographs illustrating three pacing leads: two in the atrium and one in the ventricle. The atrial appendage lead (*A*) lies above the atrial screw-in lead (*B*) secured to the anterior right atrial wall. The ventricular lead (*C*) lies at the apex of the right ventricle. In the lateral view (right) all electrodes lie anterior.

ance levels are found with large electrodes with a surface area of 25 to 100 mm^2. High impedance levels up to 1000 Ω occur with electrode surface areas as low as 4 mm^2. A diaphragmatic pacing threshold can be obtained by pacing the ventricle at 10 V and observing diaphragmatic contractions by fluoroscopy. If diaphragmatic stimulations occur, the pacing voltage should be reduced and the threshold determined. A low diaphragmatic pacing threshold of 5 to 6 V usually necessitates repositioning of the lead. After fluoroscopic examination to determine if sufficient loop or slack is left in the atrium and across the tricuspid valve, the lead is secured with nonabsorbable sutures around the supplied collar.

Transvenous Atrial Lead Implantation

Tined Atrial J Lead

Using a straight stylet, the operator directs the lead to the right atrium. By partially withdrawing the stylet, the operator reforms the J and the electrode positioned adjacent to the tricuspid valve lying anterior and to the left. When the lead is gradually retracted the electrode moves superiorly into the right atrial appendage (Fig. 40-4). Once in the appendage, retracting the lead straightens the J, confirming correct positioning. The lead also demonstrates a characteristic rocking lateral-medial motion with each atrial and ventricular contraction. The lead should be gently jerked upward to anchor the tines well into the appendage. Lead stability can be assessed by vigorous coughing. A number of other active- and passive-fixation leads, in particular, the standard tined ventricular lead or screw-in leads, can be placed in the right atrial appendage. With straight leads, a J stylet should be used for atrial appendage positioning.

The lead is tested for atrial sensing and pacing. Atrial signals are small, but most multiprogrammable pulse generators cater to the specific sensing needs of the atrium. The atrial signals are usually biphasic, and values greater than 2 mV should be recorded. The atrial threshold at 0.5 ms pulse duration usually ranges from 0.3 to 1.5 V and the resultant current is from 0.5 to 2.0 mA.

Atrial Screw-in Lead

The atrial screw-in lead can be positioned virtually anywhere in the right atrium (Fig. 40-4). Depending on whether the lead is straight or J shaped, an appropriately curved or straight stylet is used to position the distal tip of the lead on the atrial wall at the selected site. Once the position is chosen, the screw is activated for wall fixation. The lead is gently retracted and rotated to confirm attachment. If the results of the pacing system analysis are unsuitable, the lead is unscrewed and another position sought. Prior to securing the lead at the venous insertion site, a loop is left in the atrium.

Dual-Chamber Cardiac Pacing

A dual-chamber pacing system generally has two leads, one in the atrium and the other in the ventricle. When possible, it is desirable to insert both leads through the cephalic vein. Alternatively, a subclavian puncture is used. The order of insertion and positioning depends on the preference of the operator.

Pulse Generator Implantation

With the introduction of small lithium pulse generators, the subclavicular area has become an ideal pulse generator implantation site. The pulse generator rarely erodes and is comfortable and accessible for magnet testing and reprogramming. For the pulse generator pocket, a plane is found deep in adipose tissue and superficial to pectoralis major fascia and is best prepared using blunt-finger dissection. For bipolar pacing systems, the pocket can be made deep to the pectoralis muscle. After the pulse generator is tested, the lead or leads are connected to the pulse generator, which is buried in the prepared pocket. For unipolar systems, the indifferent plate should lie against the subcutaneous tissue to prevent muscle stimulation. Pacing should be confirmed and the lead position checked by fluoroscopy. The wound is closed in layers, cleaned, and covered.

Postoperative Care

Postoperatively the patient should be observed for bleeding or tense hematoma, which can be minimized by nursing the patient sitting up in order to lower the venous pressure. Electrocardiographic monitoring is desirable for 24 h. Most patients can be mobilized as soon as the effects of the premedication have disappeared. Prior to discharge, the pacemaker system should be tested, a full 12-lead ECG taken, and a chest radiograph performed. If a subclavian puncture was used, a pneumothorax should be excluded. In general, patients are ready for hospital discharge the next day. The patient should be given information regarding the identification of the pacing system, the results of the initial testing, and the programmable parameters chosen.

PACEMAKER ELECTROCARDIOGRAPHY

Normal Electrocardiograph of Ventricular Pacing

The ventricular paced ECG is composed of three major components: stimulus artifact, depolarization (QRS) wave, and repolarization (T) wave (Fig. 40-5).

The stimulus artifact represents the energy delivered to the heart, and with unipolar pacing a biphasic perpendicular voltage deflecting of about 2 to 3 mV is usually recorded. Following the initial spike, there is a voltage exponential decay curve representing dissipation of energy through body tissues (Fig. 40-5). This decay curve can cause marked distortion of the QRS, making axis determination difficult. For this reason, the first 40 to 60 ms of the QRS should be ignored.[25] With bipolar pacing, the stimulus artifact is much smaller and in some leads cannot be seen (Fig. 40-6).

Vector analysis of the pacemaker QRS reveals typical characteristics when pacing is established from various parts of the heart. Ventricular pacing from the apex of the right ventricle, whether endocardial or epimyocardial, should give a left bundle branch block configura-

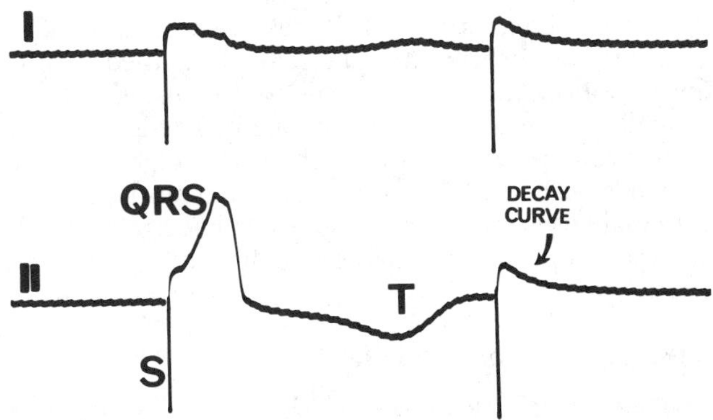

FIGURE 40-5 Electrocardiogram leads I and II (simultaneous). Unipolar endocardial lead in the right ventricle. The pacemaker ECG consists of a stimulus artifact (S), depolarization (QRS), and repolarization (T). In lead I, the first complex, the stimulus artifact is followed by a small QRS and T wave. The second complex is composed of a stimulus artifact and no QRS or T wave, i.e., failure to pace. The stimulus artifact is composed of the spike followed by an exponential decay curve, and this decay curve deforms the subsequent QRS. In lead I the decay curve could be confused with a small, almost isoelectric QRS. In lead II, however, the QRS and T waves are prominent, and despite the decay curve, there is no doubt about failed pacing.

tion, and the frontal plane vector is to the extreme left (Fig. 40-6). If endocardial pacing is established from the right ventricular outflow tract, then the QRS appearance still has a left bundle branch block configuration but the axis is to the right.[25] With epimyocardial left ventricular pacing or positioning the pacing lead in a cardiac vein via the coronary sinus, there is a right bundle branch block configuration and the axis is dependent on the position of the lead on the left ventricular surface.

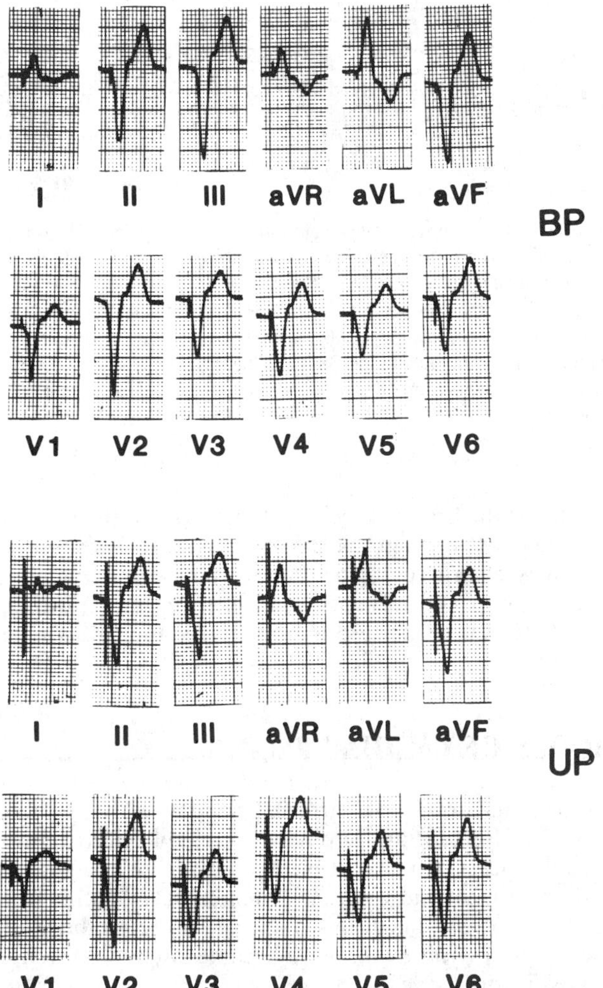

FIGURE 40-6 Twelve-lead ECGs demonstrating the differences between bipolar (BP) and unipolar (UP) pacing. The illustrations are from the same patient with endocardial pacing from the apex of the right ventricle. In BP pacing (*top*), small stimulus artifacts are seen except over the anterolateral leads (V_3 to V_6), which physically lie closest to the lead poles. In UP pacing (*bottom*), stimulus artifacts are prominent in all leads. In both ECGs, there is a left bundle branch block appearance with no R wave in the lateral chest leads. The frontal plane axis is to the extreme left.

Fusion and Pseudofusion Beats

A true pacing fusion beat results from the simultaneous activation of the atrium or ventricle by a spontaneous impulse and a paced one. Both foci contribute in varying amounts to the total chamber depolarization. It is important to recognize that this is not a malfunction of the pacemaker system but that the spontaneous impulse occurs at a similar time as the paced one, leaving insufficient time for the spontaneous impulse to be sensed and for the pulse generator to respond (Fig. 40-7).

Pseudofusion beats are more complicated and can masquerade as pacemaker malfunction, which may lead to pulse generator replacement.[65] A ventricular pseudofusion beat results when there is electrocardiographic superimposition of the stimulus artifact on a QRS complex which is generated from a single nonpaced focus. The stimulus artifact does not contribute to ventricular depolarization. Pseudofusion beats do not necessarily indicate failure of the sensing mechanism but may constitute a normal manifestation of demand pacing.[25]

Diagnosis of Acute Myocardial Infarction in Pacemaker Patients

In pacemaker patients with suspected acute myocardial infarction, the diagnosis depends on the history, clinical findings, serial serum enzymes, and occasionally other investigations such as myocardial imaging. This is because of the left bundle branch block configuration seen on the ECG with most pacing rhythms. With atrial pacing the QRS is not altered, and acute myocardial infarction changes may be seen. With the sick sinus syndrome, the pacing rhythm may be slowed or inhibited by suitable programming and the underlying rhythm inspected. This is usually of no value if complete heart block is present. Irrespective of the pattern of the underlying rhythm, long-term ventricular pacing generally results in marked T-wave changes in this underlying rhythm that can be very confusing.[66]

Marked ST changes may occasionally be seen on the ECG of a pacing rhythm during the evolution of an acute myocardial infarction, and provided the changes are acute and transient, the diagnosis of an acute myocardial infarction can be made. In nonpaced patients with extensive anteroseptal transmural myocardial infarction and

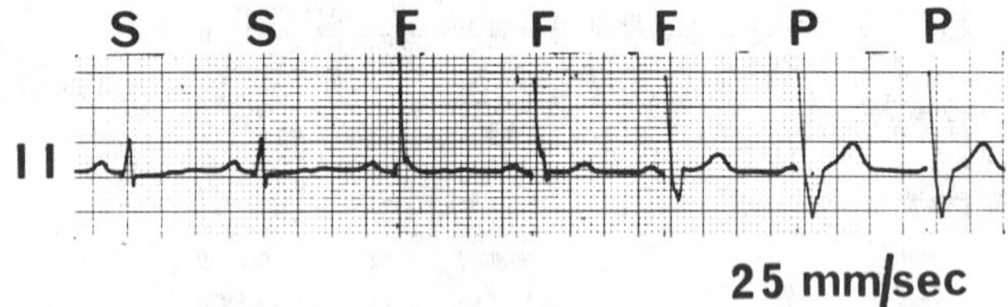

FIGURE 40-7 Electrocardiogram lead II demonstrating normal ventricular inhibited (VVI) pacing. The first two complexes are sensed (S) and there is pulse generator output inhibition. The last two complexes show ventricular pacing (P). Complexes 3 to 5 are fusion beats (F), although complex 3 may more correctly be called a pseudofusion beat as the stimulus artifact is late and does not contribute to the QRS. This can be clearly seen by observing the T-wave changes from the sinus complexes through the fusion beats to the paced beats.

a left bundle branch block configuration on the ECG, Q waves may occur in leads I, aV_L, V_5, and V_6.[67] Similar changes can therefore be seen in right ventricular pacing.[68] For paced patients with inferior infarction, the presence of a qR pattern in leads II, III, and aV_F appears specific.[69]

MODES OF CARDIAC PACING

The original mode of cardiac pacing was ventricular without QRS sensing. Today, with reliable electrogram sensing and sophisticated endocardial leads, pacing of both the atrium and ventricle can be achieved with a low incidence of complications. Because of the plethora of pacing modes now available, it became essential to create a classification code to describe simply a mode of pacing. The original and still most frequently used nomenclature involves a three-letter identification code.[70] The first position refers to the chamber paced and three letters are used: V (ventricle), A (atrium), and D (dual chamber). The second letter refers to the chamber sensed, and the same three letters are used. Where there is no sensing capability (asynchronous), the letter O is used. In the third position, the mode of response to sensing is documented using four letters: I (inhibited), T (triggered), O (asynchronous), and D (more than one response). The code has been extended to five positions to define programmable functions, rate-responsive pacing, and antitachycardia pacing systems (Table 40-1).[71]

Ventricular Pacing Systems

Ventricular Asynchronous (VOO)

There is ventricular pacing but no sensing (Fig. 40-8). Although virtually obsolete, VOO pacing can be programmed for troublesome pulse generator inhibition due to skeletal myopotential oversensing.

Ventricular Inhibited (VVI)

This is the most common pacing system used today. Spontaneous QRS potentials are sensed by the pacemaker and the subsequent pacing stimulus inhibited. The output circuit of the pulse generator is recycled, and a pacing stimulus will then occur at a set rate unless further spontaneous QRS potentials fall within that period (Fig. 40-8). This mode is frequently used with rate-responsive pacing.

Ventricular Triggered (VVT)

This system was popular during the late 1960s when QRS sensing was unreliable but is rarely used today. The sensing mechanism is similar to the VVI system, but the response is the reverse. Instead of inhibition, the full output of the pulse generator is delivered into the spontaneous QRS during the absolute refractory period (Fig. 40-8). Ventricular triggered pacing can be used for symptomatic skeletal myopotential oversensing.

TABLE 40-1
The North American Society of Pacing and Electrophysiology/British Pacing and Electrophysiology Group Generic Pacemaker Code*

Position I† (Chamber Paced)	Position II† (Chamber Sensed)	Position III (Responding to Sensing)	Position IV (Programmable Functions; Rale Modulation)	Position V (Antitachyarrhythmia Functions)
V—ventricle A—atrium D—double O—none	V—ventricle A—atrium D—double O—none	T—triggers pacing I—inhibits pacing D—triggers and inhibits pacing O—none	P—programmable rate and/or output M—multiprogrammability of rate, output sensitivity, etc. C—communicating functions (telemetry) R—rate modulation O—none	P—antitachyarrhythmia S—shock D—dual (P + S) O—none

*Positions I–III are used exclusively for antibradarrhythmia pacing.
†Manufacturers often use S for single-chamber (A or V).
SOURCE Bernstein et al.[71]

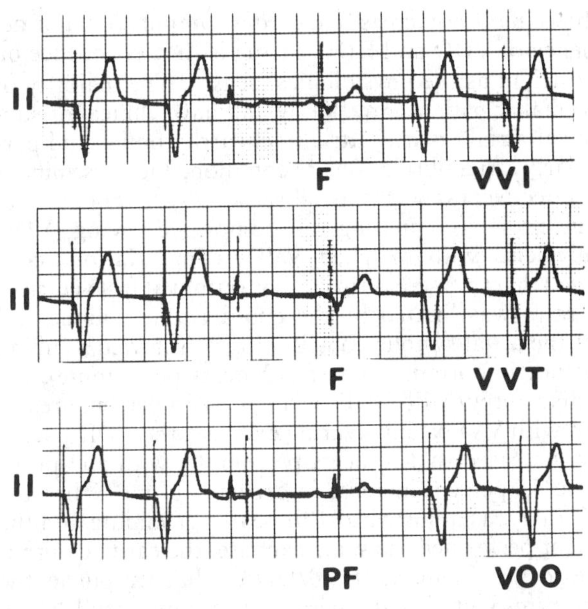

FIGURE 40-8 Electrocardiogram lead II demonstrating three modes of ventricular pacing. In each example the first two and the last two beats are paced. The third and fourth beats are sinus beats. *Top:* VVI pacing. The third beat is sensed with inhibition of ventricular output. The fourth beat is a fusion beat (F). *Middle:* VVT pacing. The third beat is sensed and the pulse generator discharges into the latter part of the QRS but, unlike a fusion beat, does not contribute to the wave of depolarization. Depending on the timing of QRS detection, VVT pacing may deform the QRS complex. The fourth beat is a true fusion beat. *Bottom:* VOO pacing. There is no QRS sensing and the stimulus artifact falls after the QRS in the refractory period. With the fourth beat the stimulus artifact is close to the QRS and is therefore a form of pseudofusion (PF).

Atrial Pacing Systems

Atrial Asynchronous (AOO) and Triggered (ATT)

Like their ventricular counterparts these modes are virtually obsolete.

Atrial Inhibited (AAI)

This is the most common form of atrial pacing with or without the addition of rate-responsive pacing (Fig. 40-9). Atrial inhibited pacing has not been widely utilized because of the unknown long-term results with atrial leads, the high incidence of AV conduction abnormalities, and atrial arrhythmias in patients with sick sinus syndrome. The advantage of AAI pacing is the maintenance of the atrial contribution of ventricular filling.

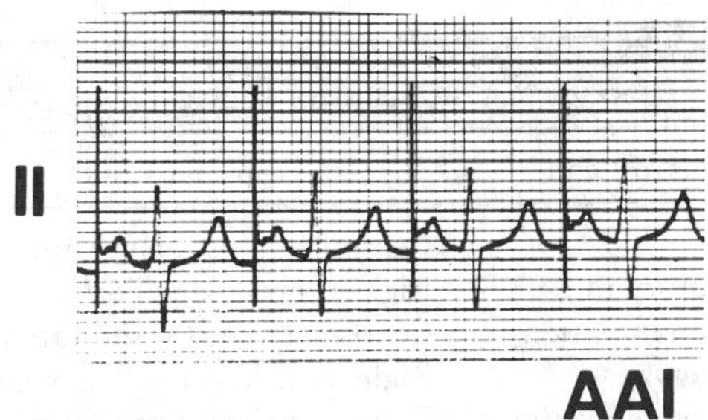

FIGURE 40-9 Electrocardiogram lead II demonstrating atrial pacing. Following the stimulus artifact there are P waves with normal AV conduction. In this example, there are no sinus P waves and thus no pacemaker inhibition.

Dual-Chamber Pacing Systems

Although many pacing modes can be used with dual-chamber pacing systems, all of these can be incorporated into a single multiprogrammable pulse generator with or without an added rate-responsive function. Chronologically, atrial and ventricular pacing was developed first with sensing functions added later.

AV Asynchronous Sequential (DOO)

This was the earliest form of sequential pacing and is now of academic interest only. The atrium is paced and after a set period, called the AV delay, the ventricle is stimulated. There is no sensing in either chamber (Fig. 40-10).

AV Sequential (DVI)

In this mode, both chambers are paced but only the ventricle is capable of sensing, responding in both a ventricular inhibited and atrial inhibited fashion. The atrial and ventricular pulse rates are identical and separated by a fixed AV delay (Fig. 40-10). Atrioventricular sequential pacing is used in the pacemaker syndrome,

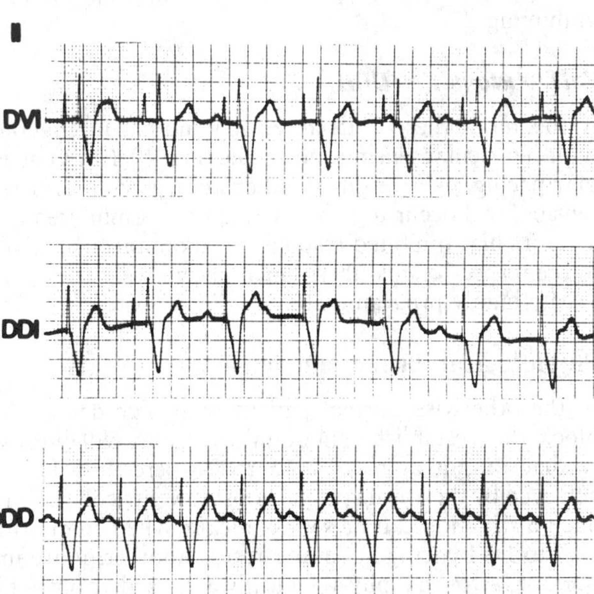

FIGURE 40-10 Electrocardiogram lead II demonstrating dual-chamber pacing. *Top:* DVI pacing. There is no atrial sensing and atrial pacing is committed. In this illustration, there are no spontaneous QRS complexes and ventricular inhibition is not demonstrated. This example could also be called DOO pacing. *Middle:* DDI pacing. Although there is atrial sensing, the pacing system can only inhibit the next atrial paced beat. Ventricular pacing will occur after a set period provided ventricular sensing does not occur. Like DVI, the pacing rate is fixed. *Bottom:* DDD pacing. There is normal atrial sensing followed by ventricular pacing. In this illustration, there is no atrial pacing because the sinus rate exceeds the atrial pacing escape rate. This example could also be called VDD pacing.

where atrial pacing, prior to ventricular pacing, prevents retrograde conduction. A variation of this system is DDI pacing. As the nomenclature suggests, there is atrial sensing, which results in inhibition of atrial pacing, but there is no AV synchrony (with atrial sensing) and no change in the ventricular pacing rate (Fig. 40-10). Although rarely used, DDI pacing is useful in patients with chronotrophic incompetence, requiring dual-chamber pacing but suffering from intermittent atrial arrhythmias.

Atrial Synchronous Ventricular Inhibited (VDD)

P-wave sensing results in ventricular pacing after an appropriate AV delay. Ventricular pacing inhibition will occur in the presence of spontaneous ventricular activity (Fig. 40-10). In the presence of normal sinus node function, VDD pacing is an excellent pacing mode for the management of complete heart block. There are two important programmable functions with VDD pacemakers. The first is the atrial upper rate limit to which the ventricle will respond. This protects the ventricle from rapid triggering that might occur with atrial arrhythmias and is usually set between 120 and 175 beats per minute. The second is the atrial lower rate limit that the ventricle will respond to before escape ventricle pacing (VVI) occurs and is usually set at a rate of 50 to 70 beats per minute. This is important in the event of atrial sensing failure or atrial bradyarrhythmias. A disadvantage of VDD pacing is the absence of atrial backup pacing in the event of sinus bradycardia. In the presence of retrograde conduction, VDD pacing may result in the troublesome pacemaker-mediated reentry tachyarrhythmia that can usually be rectified with appropriate programming.[72]

Fully Automatic (DDD)

In this mode there is atrial sensing and pacing together with ventricular sensing and pacing (Fig. 40-10). Ventricular pacing, as a result of either atrial pacing or atrial sensing, will occur together with an atrial inhibited and a ventricular inhibited response to spontaneous activity in the respective chambers. Such pacemakers are by necessity highly programmable.

Physiological Pacing and Sensors

In the otherwise normal patient with high-degree AV block, the reestablishment of AV synchrony will improve cardiac output at rest by 15 to 20 percent.[73] This is achieved by the atrial systolic boost to ventricular filling. Such a situation can be seen clinically when comparing VVI to DVI pacing at similar rates. Another, more important factor that physiologically aids cardiac output is rate responsiveness. The atrium via sinus node modulation will alter its rate according to hemodynamic requirements, and because of AV synchrony, the ventricular pacing rate alters accordingly. Pacing modes that are rate responsive include VDD and DDD and are dependent on the sinus node as the physiological sensor. The major advantage of such pacing is the ability in appropriate patients under extreme stress to increase cardiac output by 200 to 300 percent. Under similar stress with pacemaker-dependent patients, VVI and DVI pacing can only achieve modest increases in cardiac output. A major deficiency of VDD and DDD pacing is the dependence on the atrium as the physiological sensor. The majority of pacemaker patients are elderly and have clinical or subclinical atrial disease. Atrial tachyarrhythmias and particularly atrial fibrillation are common, and these hinder the effectiveness of the atrial sensor.

In a study comparing rate-responsive pacing (VDD equivalent) with matched VVI pacing, Karlof[74] concluded that the increase in cardiac output at fast ventricular rates was limited by the end-diastolic volume and that the atrial systolic contribution to ventricular filling was not important. At rest (72 beats per minute), the cardiac output with VDD pacing was 15 percent greater than with VVI pacing. During exercise, the VDD pacing rate increased to 120 beats per minute with an appropriate 75 percent increase in cardiac output. When the VVI rate was adjusted to 120 beats per minute and the patient performed the same exercise, the cardiac output rose to almost match the VDD cardiac output at the same rate. Santini et al.[75] performed a similar study using VVI pacing. During exercise, at 70 beats per minute, the cardiac output rose to 10 liters/min. When the VVI pacing rate was increased to 115 beats per minute, the cardiac output rose to 17 liters/min and there was 100 percent improvement in exercise capacity. From these studies, it can be concluded that the normal sinus node sensor as seen with atrial synchrony is not essential for physiological pacing. Increasing the atrial and ventricular rate alone by the use of other sensors will also result in an adequate hemodynamic response to stress.

Nonatrial Mediated Rate-Responsive Pacing (VVIR, AAIR, DDDR, etc.)

The search for stable, reliable, implantable sensors other than the sinus node for automatic rate-responsive cardiac pacing has resulted in the creation of at least 10 sensor-based systems (Table 40-2). These sensors can be divided into those using a standard pacing lead and those requiring the sensor to be incorporated into a special pacing lead. To date only those systems using a standard pacing lead have survived the initial clinical evaluation.

By far the most frequently used rate-responsive pacing system uses an activity sensor such as a piezoelectric crystal or an accelerometer bonded to the inner surface of the pulse generator can or electronic circuitry.[76] Following detection of movement, there is an increase in pacing rate. This sensor is nonmetabolic and nonphysio-

TABLE 40-2
Sensors Used for Rate-Responsive Pacing

Standard Lead	Special Lead
Activity	Central venous temperature
Respiratory rate	Right ventricular *dP/dt*
Minute ventilation	Central venous O_2 saturation
QT interval	Right ventricular stroke volume
Paced depolarization integral	Right ventricular preejection period
	Right ventricular pH period

logical, but because of its inherent simplicity, it has been widely accepted by pacemaker physicians and represents by far the main sensor-based pacemaker produced by major pacing companies. The activity sensor has a very rapid response time, and the rate acceleration appears appropriate for most patients. The system is limited by its failure to regularly achieve pacing rates above 120 pulses per minute and is also subject to inappropriate pacing tachycardia from external vibrational forces such as vehicular motion. The activity sensor works equally well for atrial (AAIR) and ventricular (VVIR) pacing and is particularly successful with dual-chamber (DDDR, DDIR) pacing.

The use of respiratory rate as a sensor for rate-responsive pacing involves the implantation of a specific sensor in the subcutaneous tissues across the anterior chest wall.[77] This sensor acts as a strain gauge that alters its impedance with respiration when a small current is passed through it. The pacing rate increases in response to a rise in respiratory rate above a programmable preset tidal volume threshold. A standard unipolar pacing lead is used. Respiratory rate is not a good physiological variable, and the system is only rarely used today. The rate-responsive pacing system using minute ventilation, the product of respiratory rate and tidal volume, is physiologically preferable to respiratory rate alone,[78] and the sensor technology is far superior and much simpler. A standard bipolar lead is used, a low-energy current is generated from the indifferent ring electrode, and measurement of transthoracic impedance is made between the tip electrode and the pulse generator casing.[79] The changes in measured transthoracic impedance have been shown to correlate very closely with tidal volume,[80] while at the same time the system can measure respiratory rate. Pacing can reach the programmed upper rate, but the response time and rate acceleration are slower than activity-based systems. This will hopefully be overcome in newer models. With this sensor, AAIR, VVIR, and DDDR pacing can be successfully performed.

The QT-interval rate-responsive pacing system measures the endocardial evoked response of paced beats using a standard unipolar lead.[81] The endocardial electrogram measurements are made from the ventricular pacing stimulus to the peak of the T wave. This interval, which is under the influence of catecholamines and sympathetic drive, alters with exertion and emotion and can be used to vary the pacing rate. The system depends on ventricular pacing and has a slow response time, and only VVIR pacing is available. This sensor has been incorporated into a dual-sensor system with activity being used to increase the pacing rate at the commencement of exercise. The paced depolarization integral rate-responsive system also uses the pacemaker-evoked response but measures the integral of the QRS complex. This measurement, which is the area under the paced endocardial electrogram, falls with exertion and increases again with rest. A closed-loop system can be developed to maintain a constant integral by altering the ventricular pacing rate. The system is extremely simple, highly physiological, but dependent on and limited to ventricular pacing. Whether this system can stand alone or requires a second sensor for support in a dual-sensor system is still unknown.

Rate-responsive pacing systems requiring special leads are highly physiological but inappropriately sensitive to the pathological processes common to the elderly, in particular congestive cardiac failure. The result is that these systems with unique noninterchangeable leads have highly complex algorithms, generally slow response times, and occasionally attenuated or erratic pacing rate changes with exertion. Only central venous temperature using a small thermistor embedded in the pacemaker lead behind the electrode achieved any level of clinical usage, but this is rarely prescribed today.[82] Right ventricular *dP/dt* uses a pressure sensor[83] and central venous oxygen saturation an oxygen sensor[84] in similar positions behind the cathode. Right ventricular stroke volume and preejection period use a tripolar lead to measure intravascular impedance.[85] Although their usage will be limited with cardiac pacing, these systems may find application with other implantable devices such as the cardioverter-defibrillator.

Pacing Systems for Treatment of Tachyarrhythmias

The use of complex, automatic, antitachycardia pacemakers has diminished in recent years because of the success of cardiac surgical and catheter ablative techniques to treat tachyarrhythmias. In general, the use of these pacemakers has been limited to those patients with hemodynamically disabling tachycardias resistant to or intolerant of drug therapy and physiological proof of repeated tachycardia interruption by the pacing method. A number of highly sophisticated automatic antitachycardia pacing systems were found to be clinically successful in selected patients.[86]

PACEMAKER PROGRAMMABILITY

Pacemaker programmability is a noninvasive, stable, reversible change in the operating parameter of an implanted pulse generator.[87] The vast majority of pulse generators manufactured today have one or more functions that are programmable. When three or more functions can be altered, the system is called multiprogrammable. To program an implanted pulse generator, a hand-held programmer is necessary. These programmers range from powerful magnets to highly sophisticated benchtop computers. For telemetry, printers are necessary, adding further bulk and expense to the equipment. For programming, the programmer must transmit a preselected coded message, with radio-frequency signals being the easiest, most efficient, and most commonly used. Major advantages of programmability include selection of the most appropriate pacing parameters or mode, noninvasive diagnosis and correction of pacing malfunction, and extension of pulse generator longevity by the reduction of energy output.

Rate Programming

Alteration of the pacing rate is the most widely available and used programmable function. Fast pacing rates are suggested for pediatric use, following general or open heart surgery, in serious infections, and for overdrive suppression particularly of ectopic beats or tachyarrhythmias. Increasing the pacing rate may be useful for the analysis of pacing rhythm problems and in particular fusion beats. Slowing the pacing rate is useful to encourage sinus rhythm in patients with sick sinus syndrome and to extend pulse generator life. A slow pacing rate will also allow observation of the underlying rhythm and will test sensing function.

Output Programming

The pulse generator output is dependent on the voltage and the time for the energy to be delivered, called the pulse duration. In multiprogrammable pulse generators, either or both of these may be programmable. The normal pacemaker voltage output is 5 V. A number of programmable pulse generators provide a 2.5-V output setting for patients with low chronic stimulation threshold leads and a high output setting of 7.5 or 10 V for high stimulation thresholds. It is not unusual for manufacturers today to provide a broad range of programmable voltage outputs starting at 0.8 V. Pulse duration is also a common programmable function. There is a wide range of values available, the most frequently used being 0.5 ms. Major indications for output programming include prolonging the power source life, treating high stimulation threshold exit block, correcting diaphragmatic pacing, and reducing the output to below stimulation threshold, such as at open heart surgery.

Sensitivity Programming

Multiprogrammable pulse generators generally have a broad range of sensitivity values useful for correcting sensing problems and allowing the pulse generator to be used for both atrial and ventricular pacing.

Hysteresis Programming

In cardiac pacing, hysteresis refers to an escape interval that differs from the set pacing rate. The escape interval is the period from the sensed beat to the next paced beat. With hysteresis this escape interval is longer than the pacing rate. For example, 60 to 70 hysteresis indicates that pacing at a rate of 70 beats per minute will occur when the sinus rate falls below 60 beats per minute. Sinus beats will reemerge when the rate exceeds 70 beats per minute. Hysteresis is particularly useful for patients with sick sinus syndrome with a sinus rate marginally slower than the pacing rate. In this situation it is preferable to keep the patient in sinus rhythm, but when cardiac pacing is required because of bradyarrhythmias, the pacing rate should be adequate to maintain a satisfactory cardiac output. Hysteresis is not desirable in patients with atrial fibrillation because of the resultant long pulses. Recently atrial hysteresis has been incorporated into dual-chamber pacemakers particularly for patients with vasovagal syncope.

Dual-Chamber, Rate-Responsive, and Antitachycardia Pacemaker Programming

The newer, more complex, dual-chamber, rate-responsive, and automatic antitachycardia pulse generators must be highly multiprogrammable. With dual-chamber systems, specific programmable features include the upper and lower atrial sensed rate, AV delay, sensitivity, and pacing mode. Rate-responsive systems have programmable features linked to the sensor algorithm in order to tailor the rate response to the patient's needs. Automatic antitachycardia systems have programmable functions specific to the methods of reversion.

Telemetry

Telemetry is a noninvasive function linked to programmability, where pacemaker status can be telemetered (transmitted) to the programmer on interrogation of the pulse generator. Telemetry includes programmed information, pulse generator identification, battery status, lead impedance, threshold measurement, rate-responsive features, intracardiac electrogram, event marking, percentage pacing, and arrhythmia documentation. Also included are special data such as details about the individual patient or implantation, which can be programmed into the pulse generator memory for later retrieval. The standard information available by telemetry is the programmed settings. A more recent function is real-time telemetry, which provides measured performance data including the battery and lead measurements, output energy, and pulse amplitude. This capability may eventually supersede electronic testing and will accurately determine pulse generator end-of-life. Lead impedance data obtained by telemetry have been helpful in evaluating new electrodes. An unexpected rise in lead impedance suggests a partial lead fracture and a fall may indicate insulation rupture. Telemetry of the pacemaker identification and serial number makes it simple to interface directly with a software-based follow-up system.[88]

Telemetered main timing events and endocardial electrograms have proved to be extremely valuable tools, particularly in the interpretation of complex dual-chamber pacing rhythms and sensing problems (Fig. 40-11).[89,90] The incorporation of random-access memory into pulse generator circuitry allows the storage of large amounts of data and, in particular, accumulated totals of sensed and paced events. With this information a record of intervals between such events can also be compiled and rate histograms generated. Pacemaker function, the effectiveness of rate-responsive pacing, and intrinsic P and QRS sensing can be evaluated and arrhythmias monitored.[91,92]

CARDIAC PACEMAKER TESTING AND SURVEILLANCE

Until the early 1970s, the safety of a pacemaker implant was dependent on the rapid detection and correction of malfunctions as they arose. The ECG confirmed an intact pacing system, and the oscilloscope was used to visualize

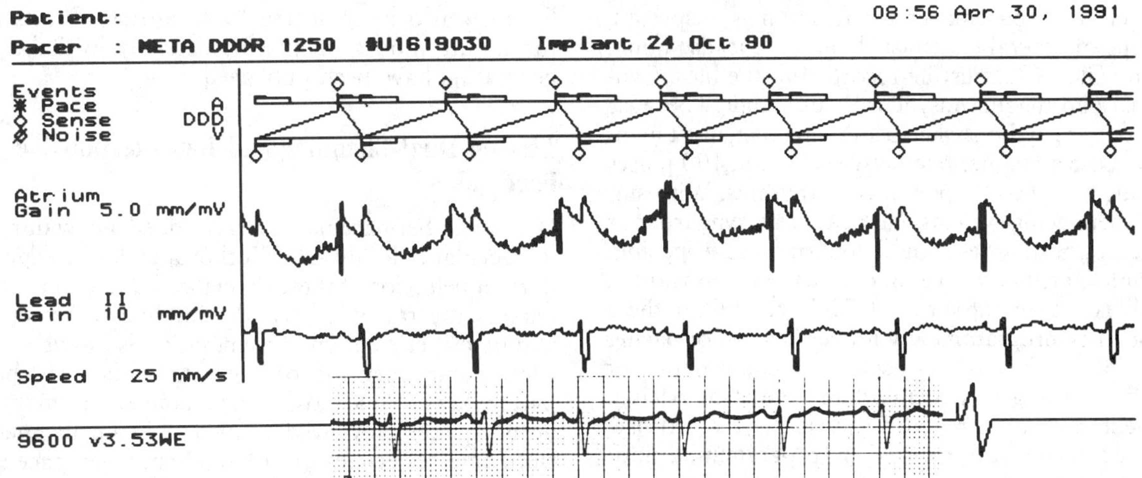

FIGURE 40-11 Telemetered main timing events and calibrated atrial endocardial electrogram documented with a simultaneous ECG lead II from a patient with a dual-chamber rate-responsive pacing system (META DDDR, Telectronics Pacing Systems). A separate ECG lead II is also shown. There is sensing in both atrium and ventricle and the ECGs show sinus rhythm with normal conduction. The main timing events demonstrate on the ladder diagram sensing in both channels, the AV delay, and the refractory periods. The atrial electrogram is over 2 mV and a far-field ventricular electrogram can be seen in the refractory period.

the stimulus artifact and help establish end-of-life characteristics.[93] In practice, these testing methods were unpredictable, and many pacing centers explanted pulse generators on an elective basis after a fixed implant time. Modern routine pacemaker testing is remarkably simple, quick, and highly accurate. Some older testing methods, such as vector analysis, have been abandoned, whereas other tests such as fluoroscopy, oscilloscopic examination, and chest wall stimulation, although not routine, nevertheless remain valuable investigative tools for suspected malfunction.

Pacemaker Clinic

A well-organized pacemaker follow-up clinic is essential for the long-term management of pacemaker patients,[25,94,95] particularly for complex dual-chamber systems.[96] A number of different clinic structures have been described, but the most important common feature is a central reviewing clinic. Such a clinic is conducted by a physician and nursing or technical staff who are experienced in pacemaker testing. Although the major function of the clinic is a mechanical one, the physician must be prepared to educate and reassure as well as deal with associated medical and psychological problems.

Pacemaker patients should be examined within 2 weeks postimplantation to inspect the operation site, remove external sutures, and test the pacing system. Subsequent clinic visits should be at 3- to 6-month intervals. Toward the end of the pacemaker battery life, more frequent visits may become necessary. In general, the lithium power source is very reliable and has a very predictable failure mode.[25,97]

Many patients live far from a central pacemaker clinic and have difficulty attending regularly. For these patients, the most common means of follow-up is transtelephonic monitoring.[98,99] The advantage of this system is that it provides for home testing, and makes emergency services available. The disadvantages are that physical examination cannot be carried out, the pacemaker cannot be programmed, and telemetry data usually cannot be determined.[94] In addition, some elderly patients or relatives have difficulty using the equipment. Transtelephonic monitoring, however, can be used in conjunction with occasional clinic visits. The cost of a transtelephone monitoring service run by a hospital with only a small cardiac pacemaker clinic can be exorbitant. However, large, central, commercial telephone monitoring services have been both successful and economical.[98] On occasion, the transmitting equipment may reside at a regional pacemaker clinic such as the office of a local primary physician or small hospital. Local pacemaker patients can attend at regular intervals and the information can be sent to the central clinic. A traveling pacemaker clinic is another means of monitoring patients who live far from a central clinic.[100] Here members of the central clinic visit regional centers for testing.

Recordkeeping is an integral function of the pacemaker follow-up clinic. Patient, pacemaker, and programmed details together with the results of all testing must be recorded. Simple, user-friendly computer programs for pacemaker data storage and follow-up have become essential components of the large central clinics.[101]

Patient self-testing is a controversial issue. Patients may be instructed to take their pulse and notify the clinic of any change. Frequently, confusion between sensed and paced beats causes anxiety. Because of the reliability of modern pacing systems and the use of rate-responsive and dual-chamber pacemakers, patients are now usually advised not to regularly take their peripheral pulse rate.

Routine Cardiac Pacemaker Electrocardiography

An electrocardiographic rhythm strip is essential to document pacemaker function and in most cases can be performed with the patient sitting. Although lead II is usually adequate, in cases where the stimulus artifacts are not clear or pacemaker malfunction is suspected, long strips of several electrocardiographic leads should be taken. The ECG must be recorded in the base (synchronous) and magnet (asynchronous) modes. Because of competitive rhythms when using a magnet, most manufacturers use a magnet rate between 90 and 100 pulses per minute to override spontaneous rhythms. With single-chamber pacing systems, the ECG in the synchronous or asynchronous modes should confirm normal pacing. The stimulus artifact of the bipolar lead system is often impossible to see on the surface ECG (Fig. 40-6). In these cases, polarity programming with verification of pacing in the unipolar mode is very useful. For confirmation of pacemaker sensing in patients with consistent pacing, the patient can be exercised to accelerate the intrinsic rate or the pacing rate reduced by programming until the intrinsic rate emerges.

Cardiac Pacemaker Electronic Testing

The pacing rate and pulse duration can be measured with a simple electronic tester. For dual-chamber pacemakers, the equipment should measure both atrial and ventricular pulses and the AV delay. Measurements must be obtained in the magnet mode, but also in the base mode in pacemaker-dependent patients. Bipolar measurements and in particular pulse duration may be difficult to measure, and new equipment is now available to overcome these problems (Fig. 40-12). The results of electronic testing and electrocardiographic recordings should be documented in the patient's record and/or on the computer data base. Comparison with previous data is essential. Pacemaker manufacturers have incorporated changes in pacemaker pacing rate and pulse duration as indicators of impending power source depletion. In general, this is a slowing of the pacing rate, usually in the magnet mode, together with widening of the pulse duration in order to maintain a constant energy output as the power source voltage falls. Power source end-of-life may also be indicated by telemetry. Charts listing the failure modes of all commercially available pulse generators have been published.[97]

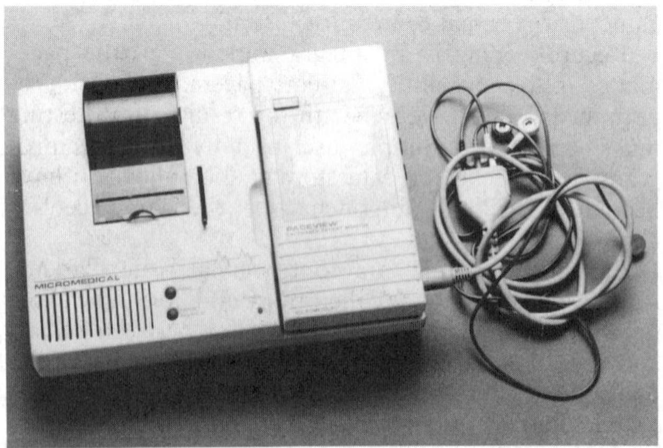

FIGURE 40-12 Pacemaker patient monitor, Paceview. On the back of the monitor are four electrodes that must make contact with the patient's skin. The monitor is particularly effective for measuring the bipolar stimulus artifact. An ECG rhythm strip and the oscilloscopic appearance of the stimulus artifact can also be visualized. The electrode cable is optional, and the recorded information can be stored in the monitor and printed on the accompanying printer, which uses ECG paper. (*Courtesy Micromedical, Sydney, Australia.*)

Testing Dual-Chamber and Rate-Responsive Pacemakers

Dual-chamber pacemakers have added a new dimension to pacemaker follow-up.[96] A thorough knowledge of the normal behavior of these specialized and complex pacemakers, together with an understanding of the individual manufacturer's design idiosyncrasies, is essential for the routine management of patients with dual-chamber pacemakers. While most single-chamber pacemakers can be adequately reviewed using the ECG, magnet, and electronic tester, testing of dual-chamber pacemakers also requires the use of the pacemaker programmer.

Routine testing of dual-chamber pacemakers requires confirmation of atrial and ventricular pacing and, where possible, atrial and ventricular sensing. In the DDD mode, if there is atrial pacing, atrial sensing may be documented by programming the escape atrial pacing rate to a lower setting. The sensing threshold can be determined by gradually reducing atrial sensitivity until atrial sensing is lost or a telemetered atrial electrogram is performed (Fig. 40-11). The sensitivity value then chosen should allow for a broad range of P-wave voltages to be sensed. Atrial capture is often difficult to confirm because of the small size of the P wave. Programming the atrial pacing rate to a value considerably faster than the sinus rate and prolonging the AV delay may make atrial pacing easier to confirm. In the presence of intact AV conduction, atrial pacing can usually be determined using AAI pacing and observing absent AV conduction.

Ventricular pacing should be clear from the ECG in either the base or magnet mode. Determination of ventricular sensing is dependent on whether or not the patient has an underlying rhythm. As with atrial sensing, the sensing threshold can be determined by increasing the programmed settings until sensing failure occurs or a telemetered electrogram is performed. The AV delay is an important programmable function, particularly in patients with intact AV conduction. With normal AV conduction, the set pacemaker AV delay should be longer than the patient's PR interval so that ventricular sensing is the normal operation. This will optimize ventricular depolarization as well as preserve pacemaker battery life.

Testing rate-responsive pacing systems involves confirmation of an adequate pacing rate response with appropriate stimuli, in particular exertion. Simple measures include tapping an activity pulse generator or asking the patient with a minute ventilation pacemaker to hyperventilate. These confirm that the sensor-based system is functioning. Exercise testing, ambulatory electrocardiographic monitoring, and when available, telemetered histograms are valuable to determine if the rate response is adequate with exertion and normal daily activities.

Noninvasive Threshold Measurement

Measurement of stimulation threshold obtained by noninvasive techniques allows multiprogrammable pulse generators to be programmed to low-energy output levels to extend battery life. Routine threshold measurements can also be used to monitor high stimulation thresholds and adjust energy outputs appropriately. A simple magnet-actuated threshold-measuring method is the Vario system in Siemens and Telectronics pulse generators.[25,88] In the magnet mode after 16 beats at 99 pulses per minute, the pacing rate increases to 120 pulses per minute for another 16 beats with the amplitude of each pulse falling by one-sixteenth of the programmed output. For a pulse generator with 5 V output, each stimulus is decremented by approximately 0.3 V. On the recorded ECG, loss of capture is seen when the pulse amplitude is below threshold. A more sophisticated, highly accurate, programmer-based atrial and ventricular threshold measuring system is now available with new model Telectronics pacemakers (Fig. 40-13).

The Medtronic threshold margin test is another magnet approach to threshold testing; the third beat in the magnet mode is delivered with only 75 percent of the programmed pulse duration. Failure to capture suggests that a higher energy output be programmed. A third method of threshold testing is the autothreshold feature available on Medtronic pulse generators. Using the ECG and appropriate programmer key, the displayed pulse duration is decremented automatically every few seconds. When capture is lost, the key is released and the pulse duration returns to its set value.[88]

Ambulatory Monitoring

Ambulatory electrocardiographic or Holter monitoring has been found to be very useful in the investigation of pacemaker patients with syncope, dizziness, and palpitations.[102,103] Before considering ambulatory monitoring, the patient must undergo a thorough history, examinations, and pacemaker testing. Because of the low-pass filter cutoff with ambulatory monitoring, there may be difficulty identifying the stimulus artifact on pacemaker electrocardiographic recordings, particularly with bipolar pacing. A solution is to separately process and record the pacing spike.[104,105] The stimulus artifact is sensed by the recorder, and a pulse is placed on a separate channel to the ECG.

Ambulatory monitoring is most helpful when symptoms occur during the monitored period. Documented abnormalities may include failure to pace or sense during symptoms. In dual-chamber pacemakers, episodes of pacemaker-mediated tachycardia or skeletal myopotential-triggered tachycardia may be recorded. The cause of the symptoms may also be due to supraventricular or ventricular tachyarrythmias.[103] The documentation of a normal ambulatory electrocardiographic tracing during symptoms may exclude a cardiac cause.[103] Interpretation of ambulatory electrocardiographic abnormalities in the absence of symptoms must be done cautiously. It is not uncommon to have abnormal ambulatory monitoring without correlation to symptoms.[106,107] This suggests that minor abnormalities in pacemaker function are not uncommon, and provided the patients remain asymptomatic, there may be no cause for alarm. Another indication for ambulatory monitoring is the assessment of dual-chamber and rate-responsive pacing systems to ensure the best possible programming for that system and the patient's needs.

Chest Radiography and Fluoroscopy

This is an essential part of any investigation of suspected or proven pacemaker malfunction. Visualization of the lead and pulse generator by radiographic means will help confirm an intact pacemaker system. Poor lead positioning, lead fracture, and failure of contact between the lead pin and pulse generator connector block can be readily diagnosed.

Oscilloscopic Examination

The use of a high-speed storage oscilloscope to visualize the stimulus artifact originally played a major role in the pacemaker follow-up clinic.[93] Today, it is only occasionally performed on a routine basis, and the examination remains useful primarily in the evaluation of pulse gener-

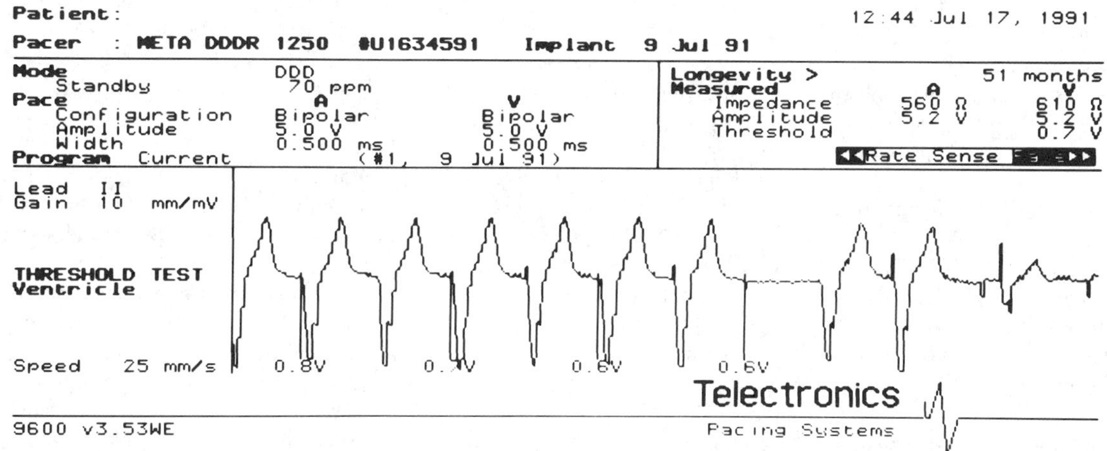

FIGURE 40-13 Ventricular threshold testing (Telectronics Pacing Systems). At the commencement of testing, the pacing rhythm becomes VVI at 100 beats per minute or a chosen value. The voltage of alternate paced beats is reduced until there is failure of pacing, and the voltage of each beat is shown by the programmer. Upon recognition of failed pacing, the appropriate key is pressed and normal pacing resumes. The value is documented. For atrial threshold testing (not shown), the pacing rhythm is either DOO or AOO and the voltage falls with consecutive beats.

ator electronic malfunction, lead conductor fracture, and lead insulation breakdown.

Chest Wall Stimulation

Stimulations to the chest wall using an external pulse generator can be used to assess the sensing function of an implanted pulse generator as well as to inspect the underlying intrinsic cardiac rhythm.[88] The external stimulations are sensed by the implanted VVI pulse generator whose output is then inhibited, confirming normal sensing. The technique can only be used with unipolar pacing systems and is today rarely used because of simpler methods using programmers.

Carotid Sinus Pressure

Carotid sinus pressure will slow a sinus rhythm in order to inspect a pacing rhythm. The procedure must be performed gently, never on both sides simultaneously, and resuscitation equipment should be available because severe bradycardia may occur in the event of pacemaker malfunction.

Invasive Investigations

Surgical Exploration

After appropriate noninvasive investigations, surgical intervention may become necessary on occasion to identify or correct a pacemaker malfunction. Prior to the surgery the full pacemaker records and previous operation notes should be reviewed. At operation, the pulse generator and lead system are mobilized and inspected; both are tested using the pacing system analyzer and an intracardiac electrogram may be performed. The lead system is carefully observed under fluoroscopy, and where necessary, traction is applied to demonstrate a lead fracture. Any site where nonabsorbable suture material is tied around the lead should be carefully inspected. Any area where there is an acute bend, such as in the neck with an external jugular venous entry approach, is a likely site of lead fracture. Blood inside the lead insulation suggests an insulation break and a possible site for current leakage. All suspected malfunctioning pulse generators should be tested to document the fault. This can be performed at surgery using the pacing system analyzer and faults confirmed by a biomedical engineering department or the pulse generator manufacturer.

Pacing System Analysis

Table 40-3 summarizes the pacing system analysis of a number of more common cardiac pacemaker malfunctions. Such malfunctions are related to the pulse generator, the lead, the myocardium, or a combination of these. The inoperative pacemaker can be easily differentiated into a lead or pulse generator fault. The finding of a high-voltage stimulation threshold, low current, and a very

TABLE 40-3
Pacing System Analysis of Common Pacemaker Malfunctions

	Variable Voltage, 0.5 ms Pulse Duration		Impedance (Ω)	Recorded P- or R-Wave Value	Pulse Generator Testing
	Voltage Threshold	Resultant Current			
Normal range (chronic lead)	Less than 3.5 V	Less than 6 mA	250–1000	Greater than 4 mV (ventricle) and 2mV (atrium)	5 V output, 2 mV sensing
Lead fracture (no conduction)	Pacing not possible	Pacing not possible	Infinity	0	Normal
Lead fracture (intermittent conduction)	High	Low	Very high	Normal (if retained)	Normal
Lead displacement	Very high (if pacing possible)	Very high (if pacing possible)	Normal	Variable	Normal
Exit block	High	High	Normal	Variable	Output may be low
Lead insulation break	Normal or low	High	Low	Usually low	Output may be low (high current drain)
Undersensing (synchronous)	Normal	Normal	Normal	Low (myocardial cause)	Sensing fault (pulse generator cause)
Oversensing (synchronous)	Normal	Normal	Normal	Normal (may sense large P or T waves)	Normal (unless programmed very sensitive)
Pulse generator inoperative	Normal	Normal	Normal	Normal	No output
Reduced pulse repetition rate (asynchronous)	Normal	Normal	Normal	Normal	Low output (power source depletion)

high impedance suggests a lead fracture with current conduction due to contact of the fractured ends or a fluid bridge. A high-voltage stimulation threshold also occurs with lead displacement or exit block, and in both of these situations the impedance remains normal. Lead displacement and exit block can be differentiated with fluoroscopy. A lead insulation break results in a low impedance due to current leak and thus high-current requirements. A thorough review of these pacing complications is available.[25]

PACEMAKER FUNCTION AND MALFUNCTION

In devising a practical classification of pacemaker malfunction, the electrocardiographic appearances of pacing in the synchronous (demand) and asynchronous (magnet or test) modes are used. Three principles must be fulfilled to establish normal pacing:

- A normal stimulus artifact is produced regularly at the preset rate in the asynchronous mode.
- The stimulus artifact is followed by ventricular depolarization (QRS) and repolarization (T).
- The pacemaker senses normally.

Using these principles, a flow diagram has been constructed (Fig. 40-14). The first step investigates the stimulus artifact, and the magnet must be applied. The second step investigates the QRS and T wave, and magnet application is not essential. The third step investigates demand function, and the magnet must be removed. Within each section of the flow diagram there are a number of endpoints. One is "normal," indicating that the pacemaker malfunction under investigation is not within this section, since the basic principle being examined had been fulfilled. The other endpoints represent pacemaker mal-

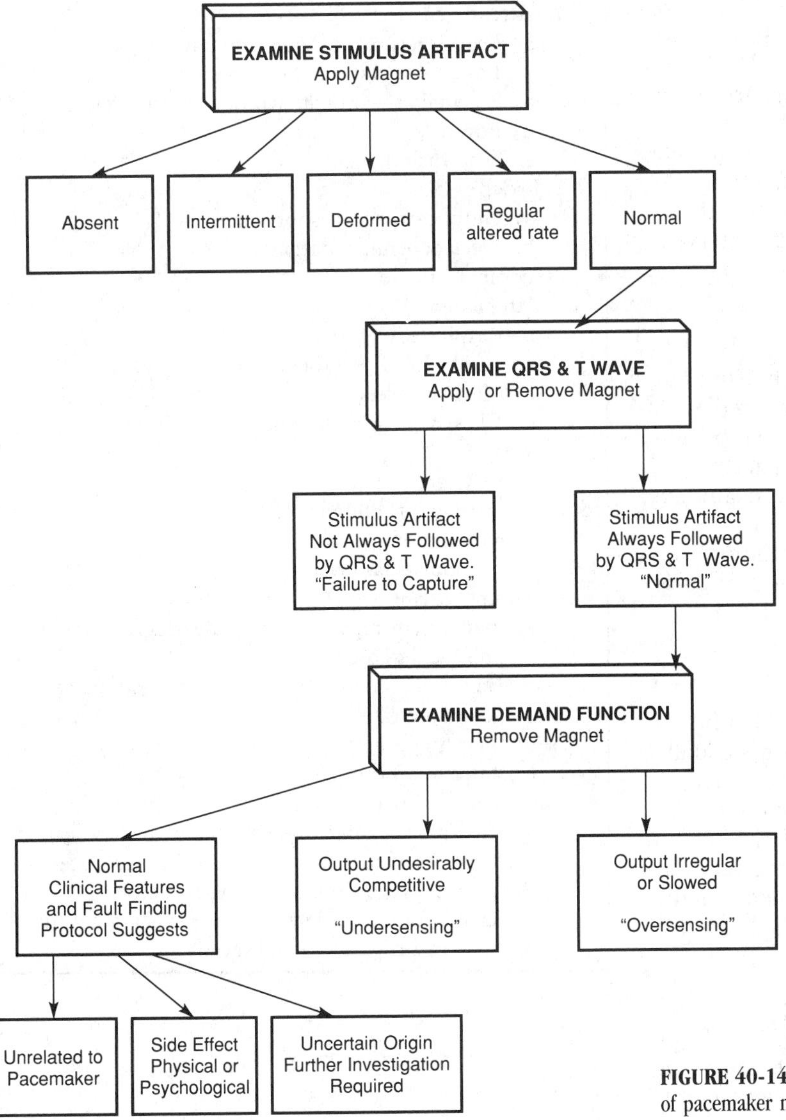

FIGURE 40-14 Flow diagram demonstrating the protocol for investigation of pacemaker malfunction using the ECG and electronic testing.

function groups as identified by an ECG or electronic testing abnormality, and specific causes of each malfunction are tabulated (Tables 40-4 to 40-6). The tables are subdivided into true malfunctions and pseudomalfunctions. Pseudomalfunctions usually result from misinterpretation or faulty documentation of test data or from a poor understanding of the pacemaker system. If the ECG and electronic testing are normal, clinical features may suggest that the problem is not strictly a pacemaker malfunction but rather physical or psychological side effects of pacing (Table 40-7). The symptoms may also suggest that the problem is not related to the pacemaker system or is of an uncertain origin and that further investigation is warranted.

Stimulus Artifacts

Four abnormalities of the stimulus artifact are recognized: absent, intermittent, deformed, and present but at an altered rate (Table 40-4).

Stimulus Artifact Absent (Inoperative Pacemaker System)

There is no detectable stimulus artifact and no pulse generator output in the asynchronous mode. There are three major true malfunctions listed in Table 40-4. Diagnosis of the actual malfunction may be difficult by routine noninvasive testing because the stimulus artifact is absent. Chest radiography and fluoroscopy are usually diagnostic for lead conductor fractures with complete discontinuity. Treatment of all true malfunctions requires surgical intervention. Identifying pseudomalfunctions is extremely important because surgical intervention is not indicated.

Stimulus Artifact Intermittent

Intermittently in the asynchronous mode, the stimulus artifact is not recorded on the ECG or detected with electronic testing equipment (Table 40-4). The most important cause is an intermittent break in the pacemaker-patient electrical circuit, such as a fractured lead conductor in which the fractured ends intermittently make contact. Provocative maneuvers and ambulatory monitoring may be helpful in making the diagnosis. Of particular value is the telemetered measured lead impedance.

Stimulus Artifact Deformed

A deformed stimulus artifact may be attenuated or broad (Table 40-4). The attenuated stimulus artifact is usually subthreshold and represents reduced current reaching the heart. A common cause is a fractured lead conductor in which the ends make contact but result in a high lead impedance as determined by telemetry or directly at surgery. A broad stimulus artifact is rare and usually represents direct current (DC) leakage into the heart due to a short circuit in the output circuit.

Stimulus Artifact Present but Altered Rate

True malfunctions are peculiar to the pulse generator (Table 40-4). A marked fall in pacing rate suggests im-

TABLE 40-4
Malfunctions Related to Stimulus Artifact

- Stimulus artifact absent (inoperative pacemaker system)
  - True malfunction
    1. Power source failure
    2. Output circuit failure
    3. Pacemaker—patient electrical circuit incomplete, e.g., lead conductor fracture
  - Pseudomalfunction
    1. Misinterpretation, ECG (e.g., pulse artifact overlooked)
    2. Testing equipment problem (e.g., equipment failure)
- Stimulus artifact intermittent
  - True malfunction
    1. Pacemaker—patient electrical circuit incomplete, intermittent
    2. Timing or output circuit, intermittent component failure
    3. Pacemaker—patient electrical short circuit, intermittent
  - Pseudomalfunction
    1. Same as for stimulus artifact absent
- Stimulus artifact deformed
  - True malfunction
    1. Attenuated
       - a. Lead fracture with some contact
       - b. Loss of insulation
       - c. Pacemaker—patient electrical short circuit
       - d. Power source failure
       - e. Lead dislodgment
    2. Broad
       - a. Output capacitor short circuit
       - b. Electrochemical potentials
  - Pseudomal function
    1. Attenuated
       - a. Respiratory effect
       - b. Faulty ECG recorder
       - c. Marker spikes
       - d. Chest wall stimulation
    2. Broad
       - a. ECG artifacts
- Stimulus artifact at altered rate
  - True malfunction
    1. Power source failure (rate slow)
    2. Timing circuit
       - a. Inadvertent reprogramming of programmable pulse generator
       - b. Random component failure—runaway pulse generator rate slow
  - Pseudomal function
    1. Misinterpretation
       - a. Lack of understanding of rate changes with temperature change, power source depletion, and activation of reed switch (magnet or test rate)
    2. Faulty ECG recording or testing equipment
       - a. Asynchronous and synchronous testing confused
       - b. ECG recorder—variable speed

pending power source depletion. The runaway pulse generator is a rare problem and refers to an increase in pacing rate beyond 150 pulses per minute with sufficient output to capture the heart.[108]

P, QRS, and T Waves

Pacemaker malfunction can be recognized when the stimulus artifact in the asynchronous or synchronous mode demonstrates intermittent or absent capture. An example of intermittent capture is shown in Fig. 40-15 and the causes are listed in Table 40-5. Because this malfunction is unrelated to demand function, sensing may be retained.[25] The problem of a lead incorrectly placed at implant should be overcome by proper surgical technique. With the use of tines, ventricular lead dislodgment is now unusual, although atrial lead dislodgment still remains a problem.

TABLE 40-5

Malfunctions Related to QRS and T Waves
Capture intermittent or absent
1. True malfunction
a. Improper electrode-lead position: incorrectly placed at implant, e.g., coronary sinus displacement; dislodgment or perforation
b. Pulse generator voltage output to heart below pacing threshold
Power source failing
Current leakage, loss of insulation
Output circuit random component failure
c. Increased pacing threshold
Exit block—fibrosis?
Myocardial infarction
Severe metabolic imbalance
Drug overdose, e.g., antiarrhythmics, antidepressants
d. High impedance in electrode-lead system (e.g., lead conductor partial fracture)
2. Pseudomalfunction
a. Misinterpretation of ECG (e.g., threshold testing)

Demand Function

The two major abnormalities of sensing function are undersensing (output undesirably competitive) or oversensing (synchronous output slowed or irregular).

Undersensing

Failure to sense P or QRS waves may result from a fault in the pulse generator or electrode lead system or from the size and type of potentials produced by the myocardium (Table 40-6). Rate programming or chest wall stimulation can be used to differentiate a pulse generator defect from a myocardial cause.

Oversensing

Slowing of the pulse generator output only in the synchronous mode implies oversensing. Intermittent oversensing produces an irregular output whereas persistent oversensing may appear as a decreased rate or total inhibition of the synchronous output. As seen in Table 40-6, oversensing may occur from four sources: cardiac, pacemaker, skeletal, and extracorporeal. Myopotentials produced by contracting skeletal muscle represent a common cause of oversensing, but despite an apparently high incidence of this problem, significant clinical symptoms are unusual. A form of oversensing peculiar to dual-chamber pacing is crosstalk, which is an alteration in pacemaker timing induced as a result of inappropriate sensing of the atrial stimulus artifact by the ventricular channel. This results in inhibition of ventricular output, either intermittent or persistent, and can be life threatening in the pacemaker-dependent patient.[109] Because of the large stimulus artifact, crosstalk is usually restricted to unipolar dual-chamber pacing systems. Apart from polarity, other factors important in creating crosstalk include the AV delay, the atrial stimulus artifact voltage, pulse duration, waveform and afterpotentials, and the ventricular blanking period and sensitivity. In most cases, more than one factor is necessary to develop inappropriate ventricular sensing of the atrial stimulus artifact, although unipolar ventricular sensing appears to be particularly important.

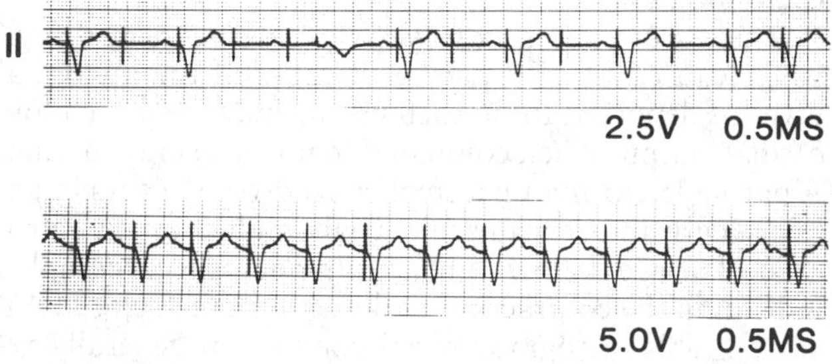

FIGURE 40-15 Electrocardiogram lead II demonstrating intermittent failure of ventricular capture at 2.5 V (*top*). The pacing mode is DDD, the sinus rate is almost 100 beats per minute, and the underlying rhythm is complete heart block. After two failed paced beats, there is a spontaneous QRS. Following programming to 5 V output, normal ventricular pacing returns (*bottom*).

Extracorporeal pulse generator interference resulting in oversensing is rarely a significant clinical problem today. Protection devices include electronic barriers, metal encapsulation of the pulse generator, and reversion to the asynchronous mode in the presence of recognized interference. A number of common potential problems appear unfounded. Microwave oven irradiation represents high-frequency interference that is easily rejected by modern pacemaker systems.[25] Airport security devices do not affect implanted pulse generators.[110] However, potential and documented interference may still occur with surgical diathermy, arc welding, radar installations, telephone transformers, and high-tension electric fields.[25,111]

Pacemaker System Produces Side Effects

Pacemaker side effects can be physical or psychological (Table 40-7).

TABLE 40-6

Malfunctions Related to Sensing

Malfunctions Related to Sensing
Output undesirably competitive (undersensing)
True malfunction
1. Pulse generator
a. Power source failure
b. Reed switch stuck in asynchronous mode
c. Sensing circuit random component failure
d. Reprogramming sensitivity
2. Electrode-lead system
a. Loss of insulation
b. Improper electrode-lead position
3. Myocardium (size of QRS)
a. Broad QRS (poor slew rate)
b. Reduced size of QRS
Pseudomalfunction
1. Misinterpretation ECG
a. Fusion beats
b. Ventricular triggered pacing
2. Faulty recording
a. Magnet applied during test or synchronous mode
b. Asynchronous testing labeled as synchronous mode
Synchronous output slowed or irregular (oversensing)
True malfunction
1. Cardiac source: P wave, T wave, or concealed ventricular ectopics
2. Pacemaker source: afterpotentials, partial lead fracture, current leakage from pulse generator, loose connections, insulation break
3. Skeletal source: muscle beneath implanted pulse generator
4. Extracorporeal source: electromagnetic or radio-frequency
Pseudomalfunction
1. Misinterpretation of ECG
a. Pulse generator inhibition owing to test magnet placement or removal
b. Hysteresis interpreted as oversensing
c. VVT interpreted as VVI
2. Faulty recording
a. Monitoring equipment faulty
b. ECG recorder speed variable

TABLE 40-7

Pacemaker Side Effects (Normal Pacemaker Function)

Pacemaker Side Effects (Normal Pacemaker Function)
Physical side effects
Placement of pacemaker system, causing:
1. Erosion or preerosion
2. Infection
a. Local
b. Septicemia or endocarditis
3. Failure to heal
4. Pain
a. Local
b. Remote, anginal, or pericardial
5. Venous thrombosis or stenosis
6. Pulmonary emboli or lead migration into pulmonary artery
7. Pacemaker twiddler's syndrome (lead dislodgment may occur)
8. Allergy to components
9. Pericardial tamponade owing to lead perforation
10. Carcinoma of breast
Pacing causing undesirable stimulation
1. Skeletal muscle stimulation
2. Diaphragmatic, direct, or via phrenic nerve
3. Ventricular fibrillation with asynchronous pacing
Defibrillation of electrosurgery, causing:
1. Pacemaker malfunction
2. Cardiac burning or infarction at electrode site
Physiotherapy short-wave treatment with local heat production
Pacemaker syndrome
Psychological side effects
Frequent self-detection of ectopic beats, distressing patient
Enforced reliance on pacing system by patient, causing psychological disturbance
Attempted suicide using pacemaker system

Physical Side Effects

The problems of pulse generator erosion and infection have diminished significantly in recent years. Pre-erosion can be diagnosed when an area of reddening develops, usually on a corner of an implanted pulse generator site where the skin has become firmly attached to the pulse generator. Although bacterial endocarditis on an endocardial lead is rare, sustained bacteremia or septicemia can occur in 1 to 3 percent of patients; the usual organism is *Staphylococcus*.[112] Clinical evidence of recurrent pulmonary emboli secondary to thrombosis around a permanent lead is surprisingly rare, even if the thrombotic material is infected. Symptomatic local venous thrombosis induced by pacemaker leads is also very uncommon. The pacemaker-twiddler's syndrome is due to repeated turning of the implanted pulse generator under the skin, which results in lead retraction from the endocardium.[25] Myocardial burning may occur with DC electrocardioversion or surgical diathermy and is due to the electric discharge being transmitted along the lead. Physiotherapy short-wave treatment may result in local heat production, thus damaging the pulse generator or surrounding tissues.

The *pacemaker syndrome* is a physiological disturbance caused by VVI pacing. Because of the abnormal wave of depolarization, such pacing may result in a low cardiac output when compared to normal sinus rhythm. A particular form of pacemaker syndrome occurs in patients with intact ventriculoatrial conduction. A retrograde P wave follows each ventricular paced complex indicating the contraction of the atria against closed AV valves. This retrograde atrial conduction generally results in a reduced cardiac output and blood pressure. The result is vertigo, light-headedness, and occasionally syncope.[113] This problem can be rectified by pacing the atrium prior to the ventricle using DVI or appropriately programmed DDD pacing. The problem can be exacerbated with VVIR pacing.

Psychological Side Effects

Psychological side effects following pacemaker system implantation can be minimized through careful explanation of the procedure to the patient and relatives beforehand. In the elderly age group, depression is common. The patient may fear that the inevitable battery failure will produce a further crisis in his or her life and that he or she is being run by an artificial device. There have been suicide attempts by patients endeavoring to damage the pacemaker system.

REFERENCES

1. Schecter DC: Background of clinical cardiac electrostimulation. V. Direct electrostimulation of heart without thoracotomy. *NY State J Med* 1972; 72:605–619.
2. Hyman AS: Resuscitation of the stopped heart by intracardial therapy. II. Experimental use of an artificial pacemaker. *Arch Intern Med* 1932; 50:283–305.
3. Mond HG, Sloman JG, Edwards RH: The first pacemaker. *PACE* 1982; 5:278–282.
4. Schecter DC: Background of clinical cardiac electrostimulation. VII. Modern era of artificial cardiac pacemakers. *NY State J Med* 1972; 72:1166–1191.
5. Pomerantz B, O'Rourke RA: The Stokes-Adams syndrome. *Am J Med* 1969; 46:941–960.
6. Dreifus LS, Fisch C, Griffin JC, Gillette PC, Mason JW, Parsonnet V: Guidelines for implantation of cardiac pacemakers and antiarrhythmic devices. *J Am Coll Cardiol* 1991; 18:1–13.
7. Roberts WC: Guidelines for cardiac pacing. *J Electrophysiol* 1987; 1:35–46.
8. Mond H, Tartaglia S, Cole A, Sloman G: The refurbished pulse generator. *PACE* 1980; 3:311–317.
9. Lev M, Bharati S: Atrioventricular and intraventricular conduction disease. *Arch Intern Med* 1975; 135:405–410.
10. Narula OS: Prognostic value of H-V interval and new interpretations of bundle branch block patterns. In: Kelly D (ed): *Advances in the Management of Arrhythmias.* Sydney, Australia, Telectronics Pty, 1978: 374–387.
11. Scheinman MM, Peters RW, Modin G, Brennan M, Mies C, 'O'Young J: Prognostic value of infranodal conduction time in patients with chronic bundle branch block. *Circulation* 1977; 56:240–244.
12. Levy AM, Camm AJ, Keane JF: Multiple arrhythmias detected during nocturnal monitoring in patients with congenital complete heart block. *Circulation* 1977; 55:247–253.
13. Brown RW, Hunt D, Sloman JG: The natural history of atrioventricular conduction defects in acute myocardial infarction. *Am Heart J* 1969; 78:460–466.
14. Hindman MC, Wagner GS, JaRo M, Atkins JM, Scheinman MM, DeSanchis RW, et al: The clinical significance of bundle branch block complication in acute myocardial infarction: 2. Indications for temporary and permanent pacemaker insertion. *Circulation* 1978; 58:689–699.
15. Mond HG: Indications for cardiac pacing. In: Hurst JW (ed): *Update V: The Heart.* New York, McGraw-Hill, 1981: 131–157.
16. Kaplan BM, Langendorf F, Lev M, Pick A: Tachycardia bradycardia syndrome (so-called "sick sinus syndrome"): Pathology, mechanisms and treatment. *Am J Cardiol* 1973; 31:497–508.
17. Caralis DG, Vanghese PJ: Familial sinoatrial node dysfunction, increased vagal tone and possible aetiology. *Br Heart J* 1976; 38:951–956.
18. Ferrer MI: The sick sinus syndrome. *Circulation* 1973; 47:635–641.
19. Greenwood RD, Rosenthal A, Sloss LJ, LaCorte M, Nadas A: Sick sinus syndrome after surgery for congenital heart disease. *Circulation* 1975; 52:208–213.
20. Chokshi DS, Mascarehnas E, Samet P, Center S: Treatment of sinoatrial rhythm disturbances with permanent cardiac pacing. *Am J Cardiol* 1973; 32:215–220.
21. Wohl AJ, Laborde NJ, Atkins JM, Blomquist CG, Mullins CB: Prognosis of patients permanently paced for sick sinus syndrome. *Arch Intern Med* 1976; 136:406–408.
22. Amram SS, Vagueiro MC, Pimenta A, Machado HB: Persistent atrial standstill with atrial inexcitability. *PACE* 1978; 1:80–89.
23. Walter PF, Crawley IS, Dorney ER: Carotid sinus hypersensitivity and syncope. *Am J Cardiol* 1978; 42:396–403.
24. Mond HG: Unipolar versus bipolar pacing—poles apart. *PACE* 1991; 1411–1424.
25. Mond H: *The Cardiac Pacemaker. Function and Malfunction.* New York, Grune & Stratton, 1983.
26. Mond H: Development of low-stimulation-threshold, low-polarization electrodes. In: Barold S, Mugica J (eds): *New Perspectives in Cardiac Pacing,* vol 2. New York, Futura, 1991: 133–162.
27. Barold SS, Ong LS, Heinle RA: Stimulation and sensing thresholds for cardiac pacing: Electrophysiologic and technical aspects. *Prog Cardiovasc Dis* 1981; 24:1–24.
28. Tyres GFO, Torman HA, Hughes HC Jr: Comparative studies of "state of art" and presently used clinical cardiac pacemaker electrodes. *J Thorac Cardiovasc Surg* 1974; 67:849–856.
29. Elmqvist H, Schueller H, Richter G: The carbon tip electrode. *PACE* 1983; 6:436–439.
30. Timmis GC, Helland J, Westveer DC: The evolution of low threshold leads. *Clin Prog Pacing Electrophysiol* 1983; 1:313–333.
31. Hirshorn MS, Holley LK, Hales JRS, Money DK, Young FA, Spector M, et al: Screening of solid and porous materials for pacemaker electrodes. *PACE* 1981; 4:380–390.
32. Mond H, Stokes K, Helland J, Grigg L, Kerles P, Pate B, et al: The porous titanium steroid eluting electrode: A double blind study assessing the stimulation threshold effects of steroid. *PACE* 1988; 11:214–219.
33. Stokes K, Bornzin G: The electrode-biointerface: Stimulation. In: Barold SS (ed): *Modern Cardiac Pacing.* New York, Futura, 1985: 33–77.
34. Brewer G, McAuslan BR, Skalsky M, Mathiuanar R: Initial screening of bio-active agents with potential to reduce stimulation threshold. *PACE* 1988; 11:509.
35. Stokes KB, Bornzin GA, Wiebusch WA: A steroid-eluting, low-threshold, low-polarising electrode. In: Steinbach K, Glogar D, Laszkovics A, et al (eds): *Cardiac Pacing. Proceedings of the VIIth World Symposium on Cardiac Pacing.* Vienna, Steinkopff Verlag, 1983: 369–376.
36. Kruse I, Terpstra B: Clinical experience with a steroid-eluting electrode for atrial and ventricular pacing. In: Aubert AE, Ector H (eds): *Pacemaker Leads.* Amsterdam, Elsevier BV, 1985: 255–260.
37. Hoff PI, Breivik K, Tronstad A, Andersen KS, Ohm O-J: A new steroid-eluting lead for low-threshold pacing. *PACE* 1985; 8:A-4.
38. Kruse IM: Long-term performance of endocardial leads with steroid-eluting electrodes. *PACE* 1986; 9:1217–1219.
39. Church T, Martinson M, Rueter J, Watson W, Lathrop T: A multi-center clinical trial of unipolar steroid-eluting electrodes. *PACE* 1987; 10:659.
40. Pirzada FA, Moschitto LJ, Diorio D: Clinical experience with steroid-eluting unipolar electrodes. *PACE* 1988; 11:1739–1744.
41. Till JA, Jones S, Shinebourne EA, Rowland E, Ward DE: Clinical experience with a steroid eluting lead in children. *Circulation* 1989; 80:II-389.
42. Stokes K, Church T: The elimination of exit block as a pacing complication using a transvenous steroid eluting lead. *PACE* 1987; 10:748.
43. Tronstad A, Hoff PI, Ohm O-J: Myocardial excitability thresholds of a new steroid lead compared to two non-steroid leads: A double blind study. *PACE* 1987; 10:754.
44. Brewer G, Mathivanar R, Skalsky M, Anderson N: Composite electrode tips containing externally paced drug releasing collars. *PACE* 1988; 11:1760–1769.
45. Wilson A, Kay N, Padeletti L, Michelucci A, Ferri F, Baird D, et al: A multicentre study of steroid eluting collar leads. *PACE* 1991; 14:629.
46. Skalsky M, Mathivanar R, Anderson N, et al: Threshold performance of bipolar leads with a drug eluting collar (DEC). Cardiostim 90. *RBM* 1990; 12:108.
47. Kertes P, Mond H, Sloman JG, Vohra J, Hunt D: Comparison of lead complications with polyurethane tined, silicone rubber

tined and wedge tip leads: Clinical experience with 882 ventricular endocardial leads. *PACE* 1983; 6:957–962.
48. Sloman JG, Mond HG, Bailey B, Cole A, Duffield A: The use of balloon tipped electrodes for permanent cardiac pacing. *PACE* 1979; 2:579–585.
49. Bisping HJ, Kreuger J, Krikenheier H: Three years' clinical experience with a new endocardial screw-in lead with introduction protection for use in the atrium and ventricle. *PACE* 1980; 3:424–435.
50. Kruse I, Ryden L, Ydse B: A new lead for transvenous atrial pacing and sensing. *PACE* 1980; 3:395–405.
51. Curzio G, Alliengro A, Santini M, Caprioli V: A new passive fixation transvenous atrial lead: Clinical experience. *PACE* 1981; 4:A-39.
52. Mond H, Kertes P, Strathmore N, Chong KC, Vohra J, Hunt D: Endocardial screw in lead. Clinical experience in the atrial position. *PACE* 1987; 10:719.
53. Daubert C, Mabo P, De Place C, Lelong B, Paillard F, Kermarrec A: Permanent left atrial pacing via the coronary sinus: Use of "J" shaped leads. Cardiostim 90. *RBM* 1990; 12:60.
54. Percoco GF, Lansani L, Barbieri D, Guardigli G, Toselli T, Audoglio R, et al: Twinal 30: A new single lead VDD pacing system. Cardiostim 90. *RBM* 1990; 12:64.
55. Eng TS: The multicenter experience with the single lead VDD Phymos system experimented on 244 patients. Cardiostim 90. *RBM* 1990; 12:65.
56. Mansour KA, Fleming W, Hatcher CR: Initial experience with a sutureless screw-in electrode for cardiac pacing. *Ann Thorac Surg* 1973; 16:127–135.
57. Linos DA, Mucha P, VanHeerdon JA: A golden route. *Mayo Clin Proc* 1980; 55:315–321.
58. Miller FA, Holmes DR, Gersh BJ, Maloney, JD: Permanent transvenous pacemaker implantation via the subclavian vein. *Mayo Clin Proc* 1980; 55:309–314.
59. Furman S: Subclavian puncture for pacemaker lead placement (editorial). *PACE* 1986; 9:467.
60. Bellot PH: A variation on the introducer technique for unlimited access to the subclavian vein. *PACE* 1981; 4:43–48.
61. Janchuck SJ, Gill BS, Petty AH: Pacing through the subclavian vein. *Br J Surg* 1974; 61:373–376.
62. Kaul TK, Bain WH: Radiographic appearances of implanted transvenous endocardial pacing electrodes. *Chest* 1977; 72:323–326.
63. Smyth NPD: Techniques on implantation: Atrial and ventricular thoracotomy and transvenous. *Prog Cardiovasc Dis* 1981; 23:435–450.
64. Byrd C: Permanent pacemaker implantation techniques. In: Samet P, El-Sherif N (eds): *Cardiac Pacing*, 2d ed. New York, Grune & Stratton, 1980: 229–253.
65. Martin CM, Kleid JJ: Pseudofusion beats masquerading as a pacemaker failure. *J Electrocardiol* 1974; 7:179–181.
66. Chatterjee K, Harris AM, Davies JG, Leatham A: T wave changes after artificial pacing. *Lancet* 1969; 1:759–760.
67. Barold SS, Ong LS, Heinle RA: Electrocardiographic diagnosis of myocardial infarction in patients with transvenous pacemakers. *J Electrocardiol* 1976; 9:99–102.
68. Castellanos A, Zoble R, Procacci PM, Myerburg RJ, Berkovits BV: ST-QR pattern: New sign of diagnosis of anterior myocardial infarction during right ventricular pacing. *Br Heart J* 1973; 35:1161–1165.
69. Barold SS, Ong LS, Banner RL: Diagnosis of inferior wall myocardial infarction during right ventricular apical pacing. *Chest* 1976; 69:232–235.
70. Parsonnet V, Furman S, Smyth NPD: Implantable cardiac pacemakers: Status report and resource guideline. *Circulation* 1974; 50:A21–A35.
71. Bernstein AD, Camm AJ, Fletcher RD, Gold RD, Rickards AF, Smyth NPD, et al: The NASPE/BPEG generic pacemaker code for antibradyarrhythmias and adaptive-rate pacing and antitachyarrhythmias devices. *PACE* 1987; 10:794–799.
72. Tolentino AO, Javier RP, Byrd C, Samet P: Pacer-induced tachycardia associated with an atrial synchronous ventricular inhibited (ASVIP) pulse generator. *PACE* 1982; 5:251–259.
73. Goldreyer BN: Physiologic pacing: The role of AV synchrony. *PACE* 1982; 5:613–615.
74. Karlof I: Haemodynamic effect of atrial triggered versus fixed rate pacing at rest and during exercise in complete heart block. *Acta Med Scan* 1973; 197:195–206.
75. Santini M, MacCarter D, Knudson M, Alliegrto A, Camillo S: Automatic atrial rate responsive VVI pacing: A simple physiologic approach. *PACE* 1981; 4:a-72.
76. Humen DP, Anderson K, Brumwell D, Huntley S, Klein GJ: A pacemaker which automatically increases its rate with physical activity. In: Steinbach K, Glogan D, Lasykovics A, et al (eds): *Proceedings of the VIIth World Symposium on Cardiac Pacing*. Darmstadt, Steinkopff Verlag, 1983: 259–264.
77. Rossi P, Plicchi G, Canducci G, Ragnoni G, Aina F: Respiratory rate as a determinant of optimal pacing rate. *PACE* 1983; 6:502–507.
78. Alt E, Volker R, Wirtzfeld A: Directly and indirectly measured respiratory parameters compared with oxygen uptake and heart rate. *PACE* 1985; 8:A-21.
79. Mond H, Strathmore N, Kertes P, Hunt D, Baker G: Rate responsive pacing using a minute ventilation sensor. *PACE* 1988; 11:1866–1874.
80. Nappholz T, Lubin M, Maloney J, Simmons T: Measuring minute ventilation with a pacing catheter. *PACE* 1985; 8:785.
81. Rickards AF, Donaldson M, Thalen HJ Th: The use of QT interval to determine pacing rate: Early clinical experience. *PACE* 1983; 6:346–354.
82. Griffin JC, Jutzy KR, Claude JP, Knutti JW: Central body temperature as a guide to optimal heart rate. *PACE* 1983; 6:498–501.
83. Sutton R, Sharma A, Ingram A, Camm J, Lindemans F, Bennett T: First derivative of right ventricular pressure as a sensor for an implantable rate responsive VVI pacemaker. *PACE* 1987; 10:1230.
84. Stangl K, Wirtzfeld A, Heinze, R, Laule M: First clinical experience with an oxygen saturation controlled pacemaker in man. *PACE* 1988; 11:1882–1887.
85. Olson WH, Bennett TD, Beck RC, Erickson MK, Biallas RM: Stroke volume controlled rate responsive pacing in exercising heart-blocked canines. *Circulation* 1985; 72(suppl III):432.
86. Fisher JD, Furman S, Kim SG, Ferrick KJ, Roth JA, Gross J, et al: Tachycardia management by devices. In: Barold SS, Mugica J (eds): *New Perspectives in Cardiac Pacing*, vol 2. New York, Futura, 1991: 359–404.
87. Furman S: Pacemaker programmability. *PACE* 1978; 1:161–162.
88. Strathmore NF, Mond HG: Non-invasive monitoring and testing of pacemaker function. *PACE* 1987; 10:1359–1370.
89. Kruse I, Markowitz T, Ryden L: Timing markers showing pacemaker behaviour to aid in the follow up of a physiological pacemaker. *PACE* 1983; 6:801–805.
90. Levine PA, Sholder J, Duncan JL: Clinical benefits of telemetered electrograms in assessment of DDD function. *PACE* 1984; 7:1170–1177.
91. Sanders R, Martin R, Frumin H, Goldberg M: Data storage and retrieval by implantable pacemakers for diagnostic purposes. *PACE* 1984; 7:1228–1233.
92. Adler S, Whistler S, Martin R: Advances in single-chamber pacemaker diagnostic data. *PACE* 1986; 9:1141–1146.
93. Mond H, Twentyman R, Smith G, Sloman G: The pacemaker clinic. *Cardiology* 1972; 57:262–276.
94. Levine PA, Belott PH, Bilitch M, Boal B, Escher D, Furman S, et al: Recommendations of the NASPE policy conference on pacemaker programmability and follow up. *PACE* 1983; 6:1222–1223.
95. Byrd CL, Schwartz SJ, Gonzales M, Byrd CB, Sivina M, Yahr WZ, et al: Pacemaker clinical evaluations: Key to early identification of surgical problems. *PACE* 1986; 9:1259–1264.
96. Luceri RM, Hayes DL: Follow-up of DDD pacemakers. *PACE* 1984; 7:1187–1194.
97. Levine PA: Magnet rates and recommended replacement time indicators of lithium pacemakers 1986. *Clin Prog Electrophysiol Pacing* 1986; 4:608–618.
98. Dreifus LS, Zinberg A, Hurzeler P, Puziak AD, Pennock R, Feldman M, et al: Transtelephonic monitoring of 25,919 implanted pacemakers. *PACE* 1986; 9:371–378.
99. Zinberg A: Transtelephonic follow up. *Clin Prog Pacing Electrophysiol* 1984; 2:177–179.
100. Mond H, Gerloff J, Flower D, Kerles P, Hunt D: The travelling pacemaker clinic. A ten year appraisal. *PACE* 1983; 6:A-30.

101. Strathmore N, Mond H, Hunt D, Graham D, Cowling R, Hale G, et al: "Pacecare"—A computerized database for pacemaker follow-up. *PACE* 1990; 13:1787–1791.
102. Famularo MA, Kennedy HL: Ambulatory electrocardiography in the assessment of pacemaker function. *Am Heart J* 1982; 104:1086–1094.
103. Hoffman A, Jost M, Pfisterer M, Bukart F, Burckhardt D: Persistent symptoms despite permanent pacing. *Chest* 1984; 85: 207–210.
104. Kelen GJ, Bloomfield DA, Hardage M, Gomes JA, Kahn R, Gopalaswamy C, et al: A clinical evaluation of an improved Holter monitoring technique for artificial pacemaker function. *PACE* 1980; 3:192–197.
105. Tranesjö J, Faåhracus T, Nygaårds ME, Wigertz O: Automatic detection of pacemaker pulses in ambulatory ECG recording. *PACE* 1982; 5:120–123.
106. Breivik K, Ohm OJ: Myopotential inhibition of unipolar QRS-inhibited (VVI) pacemakers, assessed by ambulatory Holter monitoring of the electrocardiogram. *PACE* 1980; 3:470–478.
107. Secemsky SI, Hauser RG, Denes P, Edwards, LM: Unipolar sensing abnormalities: Incidence and clinical significance of skeletal muscle interference and undersensing in 228 patients. *PACE* 1982; 5:10–19.
108. *Runaway Protection of CPI Implantable Pacemakers*. CPI Tech. Issues, No. 11. St. Paul, MN, Cardiac Pacemakers.
109. Levine PA, Venditti FJ, Podrid PJ, Klein MD: Therapeutic and diagnostic benefits of intentional crosstalk mediated ventricular output inhibition. *PACE* 1988; 11:1194–1201.
110. Smyth NPD, Keshishian JM, Hood OC, Hoffman AA, Baker NR, Podolak E: Effect of an active magnetometer on permanently implanted pacemakers. *JAMA* 1972; 221:162–166.
111. Butrous GS, Male JC, Webber RS, Barton DG, Meldrum SJ, Bonnell JA, et al: The effect of power frequency high intensity electric fields on implanted cardiac pacemakers. *PACE* 1983; 6:1282–1292.
112. Morgan G, Ginks W, Siddons H, Learham A: Septicemia in patients with an endocardial pacemaker. *AM J Cardiol* 1979; 44:221–224.
113. Miller M, Fox S, Jenkins R, Schwartz, J Toonder FG: Pacemaker syndrome: A noninvasive means to its diagnosis and treatment. *PACE* 1981; 4:503–506.

Chapter 41

Cardioversion and Defibrillation

Bernard Lown, M.D. ■ *Regis A. de Silva, M.D.*

The use of direct electrical current for elective and emergency reversion of cardiac arrhythmias has become standard therapy clinically during the past 25 years.[1-3] This chapter will deal with external cardioversion and defibrillation and will not discuss reversion of arrhythmias with pacing methods or implanted devices.

The discharge of electrical energy synchronized on the R wave of the electrocardiogram (ECG) is known as *cardioversion,* while unsynchronized discharge is referred to as *defibrillation.* Energy level is measured in watt-seconds (W·s) or joules (J), which are numerically interchangeable. The objective of both cardioversion and defibrillation is to provide an electrical pulse transthoracically so as to completely depolarize the heart during passage of the current through the chest. Electrode placement is therefore a critical determinant of the amount of energy used as well as of the success rate for electrical reversion. The physiological basis for cardioversion is probably the closure of the excitable gap in a reentrant pathway by the electrical discharge. This explanation accounts for the fact that a small discharge such as 1 J may be sufficient to terminate an arrhythmia such as atrial flutter or ventricular tachycardia, since these arrhythmias are due to reentrant mechanisms. Removal of the circuit for the arrhythmia permits the reemergence of sinus rhythm. Defibrillation, which often requires 100 J or more, is probably due to the necessity of depolarizing a multiplicity of out-of-phase circuits before the normal pacemaker can assert its dominance. Low-energy defibrillation may succeed because a substantial part of the myocardium may be disengaged from the fibrillatory process, thereby depriving the arrhythmia of a critical mass to sustain reentry.

PROCEDURE

Elective cardioversion should be done in the morning after overnight fasting. In urgent cases, meals should be withheld for as long as possible. Serum levels for electrolytes, digoxin, blood urea nitrogen, and creatinine should be obtained whenever possible; hypokalemia should be corrected to prevent arrhythmic complications. Digitalis glycosides need be withheld only on the day of cardioversion. If digitalis toxicity is suspected, elective cardioversion is deferred until the problem is corrected. An intravenous line is started, and equipment for cardiopulmonary resuscitation should be available. Blood pressure and heart rate are monitored frequently before and after the procedure, and the patient should be observed on a monitor for 24 h after the procedure to avoid late arrhythmic complications, especially when digitalis, quinidine, or other antiarrhythmic drug toxicity is suspected. Sedation is administered by an anesthesiologist. Otherwise, sedation with diazepam (Valium) or miazolam (Versed) intravenously may be given in incremental doses until the patient is slightly drousy in order to provide sedation with amnesia.

Synchronization of the discharge with the tallest R wave of the ECG prevents accidental triggering of ventricular fibrillation. Improper synchronization may occur when there are artifactual spikes from a malfunctioning pacemaker, bundle branch block with the R′ wave being taller than the R wave, and when the T wave is tall and peaked. Synchronization should be checked before each successive discharge.

Electrodes may be placed either in an anterior/posterior or in an anterior/lateral position. The anterior electrode is placed over the second and third right intercostal spaces, and the posterior electrode is placed at the tip of the scapula. In the anterior/lateral configuration, the second electrode is placed at the cardiac apex. In either configuration, the path of current flow is along the long axis of the heart, encompassing the bulk of the cardiac mass and minimizing travel through high-impedance bony tissue such as the sternum and the vertebral column. Placement of electrodes side by side is not effective as such positioning may result in short-circuiting due to bridging between electrodes by conductive paste.

Energy titration minimizes energy use and reduces complications. Experimental evidence shows that repeated low-energy shocks cause less damage than a higher energy shock of similar total aggregate energy.[4] The initial setting may be as low as 10 J (for atrial flutter and stable ventricular tachycardia), and the level is increased successively to 25, 50, 100, 200, 300, and 360 J. Lead II of the ECG is monitored to determine if sinus rhythm has been established. If ventricular arrhythmia occurs after a discharge, a lidocaine bolus is administered before the next discharge. When it is possible to measure transthoracic impedance prior to discharge using a suitably modified cardioverter-defibrillator, unnecessary shocks may be avoided and success rates improved.[5]

ANTICOAGULATION

Atrial fibrillation (AF) is the arrhythmia most likely to be associated with embolism during cardioversion. Anticoagulation reduces the incidence of emboli and is recommended in the absence of contraindications.[6] Anticoagulation with warfarin (Coumadin) should be started 3 weeks before cardioversion to maintain a prothrombin time of approximately 1.3 to 1.5 times the control level or an international normalized ratio (INR) of 2.0 to 3.0 using rabbit brain thromboplastin.[7] Treatment is continued for 4 weeks after cardioversion because of the possibility of delayed embolism. Following cardioversion, atrial mechanical activity may not resume for several days despite sinus rhythm on the ECG. Because of electromechanical dissociation in the atrium, thrombus may be released in the days or weeks following cardioversion. Doppler echocardiography for documenting the presence of the atrial A wave is useful in assessing the absence or presence of atrial contraction if electromechanical dissociation is suspected postcardioversion.[8] Anticoagulation beyond 4 weeks may be indicated in the presence of prosthetic valves, cardiomyopathy, atrial or ventricular clot, or a history of previous embolization.

For emergency cardioversion, heparin therapy alone should be used with the simultaneous initiation of warfarin to enable long-term anticoagulation. Transthoracic and transesophageal echocardiography are helpful in decision making, but the absence of thrombus does not exclude the possibility that embolism may still occur. For AF of short duration, no reliable data exist. Anticoagulation for 3 weeks is considered unnecessary if AF has been present for less than 3 days, but heparin should be started in anticipation of cardioversion to avoid formation of thrombus.[7] Warfarin therapy is initiated if the circumstances suggest that AF may recur or if long-term anticoagulation is necessary for other reasons. If warfarin is contraindicated for long-term anticoagulation, there is some evidence that aspirin may help prevent thromboembolic complications. There is, however, no evidence that aspirin, dipyridamole, or a combination is helpful acutely in preventing embolism in patients undergoing cardioversion when warfarin and heparin anticoagulation are contraindicated. Unless other indications exist, anticoagulation for pure atrial flutter and supraventricular tachycardia is unnecessary[7]. (See also Chaps. 36, 68 and 122.)

TREATMENT OF SPECIFIC ARRHYTHMIAS

Atrial Fibrillation

The risk for stroke in atrial fibrillation increases from 6.7 percent in the sixth decade to 36.2 percent in the ninth decade of life.[9] Atrial fibrillation, therefore, when newly diagnosed, deserves at least one attempt at reversion if no specific contraindications exist, since such treatment may avoid the need for a lifetime of anticoagulation. Moreover, maximal exercise capacity and improvement in cerebral blood flow from 13 to 30 percent also result after cardioversion from atrial fibrillation.[10,11] Decreases in atrial natriuretic peptide after cardioversion, regardless of the presence of heart failure, suggest desirable improvements in cardiac hemodynamics, even when heart failure is absent.[12]

Pretreatment of the patient with quinidine, disopyramide, or another suitable agent for 48 h before cardioversion is useful, as an adequate blood level of the antiarrhythmic agent prevents early recurrence. Though quinidine is effective in maintaining sinus rhythm, a metaanalysis of six randomized trials with the drug suggested that mortality was increased in the quinidine-treated group compared to a control group.[13]

Success rate of cardioversion for atrial fibrillation is variable and is considered to be dependent on factors such as duration of arrhythmia, size of left atrium, presence of underlying conduction system disease, presence of valvular disease, and patient's age. In one study, however, multifactorial linear regression analysis showed that the only factor significantly associated with prediction of success of cardioversion was duration of atrial fibrillation.[14] Overall success rates may be as high as 94 percent of cases, with 40 percent reverting to sinus rhythm with the use of 50 J or less and 95 percent reverting with 200 J or less.[2] When atrial fibrillation has been present for 3 months or less, the success rate is 98 percent and the mean energy level required is 87 J. Left atrial size of 45 mm or greater and a less than 10 percent increase in the A wave on Doppler echocardiography postcardioversion have a positive predictive value for recurrence of the arrhythmia.[8]

In patients with congestive heart failure, higher energy levels may not succeed or relapse may occur. Rapid digitalization may reduce pulmonary congestion and heart failure and allow successful cardioversion. Acute myocardial infarction is not a contraindication to cardioversion. Indeed, prompt reversion terminates sustained tachycardia and prevents infarct extension.

In patients with conduction system disease, arrhythmias such as atrial ectopic activity, severe sinus bradycardia, sinus arrest, junctional rhythm, or multifocal atrial tachycardia may follow cardioversion, and sinus rhythm may be only gradually restored. In such cases, atropine or isoproterenol is administered and cardioversion terminated. Prophylactic pacing before cardioversion is generally unnecessary. Careful energy titration anticipates complications and prevents asystole. If, however, major conduction system disease is suspected, accepting AF as the rhythm of choice is preferable to cardioversion. Other patients who may not benefit from cardioversion include those with mitral valve disease and a "giant" left atrium or following mitral valve replacement, those with recurrent paroxysmal atrial tachyarrhythmias (Parkinson-Papp syndrome), and those with an intolerance to antiarrhythmic drugs.

Atrial Flutter

If drug reversion is unsuccessful, cardioversion is the procedure of choice. Though often benign and asymptomatic, this arrhythmia may have serious life-threatening consequences if 1:1 conduction at rates of 300 or more occurs, especially in the presence of myocardial impairment. Low-energy shocks easily produce reversion to sinus rhythm with success rates approaching 100 percent.[15] The mean energy level required is 25 J, and usually one shock suffices. With shocks of 50 J or less, 95 percent of cases revert to sinus rhythm.

Supraventricular Tachycardia

Because of its response to vagal maneuvers and the availability of numerous drugs such as verapamil, beta-adrenergic blockers, and adenosine to treat this arrhythmia, supraventricular tachycardia does not often require cardioversion. When digitalis toxicity is the cause of the arrhythmia, cardioversion is contraindicated as ventricular fibrillation may be precipitated. If it is not possible to ascertain whether or not digitalis toxicity is the inciting cause, energy titration is cautiously performed and lidocaine pretreatment given to suppress ventricular arrhythmias. If low-energy discharges result in high-grade atrioventricular block or in serious ventricular arrhythmias, digitalis toxicity is suspected and cardioversion discontinued.

Ventricular Tachycardia

When ventricular tachycardia is unresponsive to intravenous administration of lidocaine, bretylium, tosylate, or procainamide or the patient is becoming hemodynamically unstable, cardioversion is performed promptly if a chest thump fails to terminate the arrhythmia. If the patient is clinically stable, prior sedation should be administered. Energy titration is performed and levels as low as 1 to 5 J may terminate ventricular tachycardia; in over 90 percent of the cases, 10 J or less is successful; only rarely is more than 100 J necessary. When ventricular tachycardia is rapid and the QRS complex very broad or indistinguishable from the T wave, synchronization has an equal chance of being triggered on the T wave. In such cases, or if the patient is clinically unstable, unsynchronized discharge with 100 J reduces the risk of ventricular fibrillation. If the shock fails to terminate the arrhythmia or if ventricular fibrillation is provoked, the shock strength should be increased and immediate defibrillation performed at 200, 300, and 360 J until sinus rhythm is restored. Polymorphic ventricular tachycardia, hemodynamically unstable rapid ventricular tachycardia, and torsades de pointes that is not self-terminating should be treated similarly. Torsades de pointes may be refractory to electric shock and might be amenable to overdrive pacing or to treatment with magnesium sulfate. (See Chap. 36.)

Ventricular Fibrillation

Unsynchronized discharge is used only for ventricular fibrillation or for pulseless ventricular tachycardia. This setting is also used for "blind defibrillation" in an unmonitored patient who has had cardiac arrest. The electrode positions used are as for cardioversion. The American Heart Association algorithm for defibrillation suggests an initial shock of 200 J following institution of cardiopulmonary resuscitation. A second shock of 200 to 300 J followed by 360 J is given if ventricular fibrillation persists.[16] If there is failure to defibrillate after three shocks, epinephrine, 0.5 to 1.0 mg intravenously, is given and defibrillation attempted with 360 J. (See also Chap. 52.)

The appropriate energy dose for successful defibrillation remains to be established. In children, as little as 10 to 100 J is sufficient. As a guideline, 1 J/lb or 2 J/kg is recommended. Prospective clinical studies have shown that 200 J or less is often sufficient for defibrillation of adults of normal weight and have not borne out assumptions that heavier individuals require high-energy discharges beyond 400 J.[17] When ventricular fibrillation of prolonged duration is refractory to defibrillation, correction of hypoxia and acid-base imbalance with administration of a beta-adrenergic agonist such as isoproterenol may convert fine-grain fibrillation to a coarse form that is more susceptible to defibrillation. If this approach is unsuccessful, rapid serial delivery of two or three 360-J shocks may occasionally succeed. Rarely, fine ventricular fibrillation may appear as asystole on a monitor, and defibrillation should be attempted.

COMPLICATIONS

Both morphologic and functional cardiac damage may follow the use of high-energy shocks.[3] After electric discharge, catecholamines, acetylcholine, creatine kinase, and other enzymes are released. Creatine kinase elevation following cardioversion is transient, derives from skeletal muscle, and usually does not obscure the diagnosis of myocardial infarction. Electric shock also releases myocardial potassium, and such release is accentuated in the digitalized heart. Electrocardiographic signs of hyperkalemia are occasionally detected after high-energy shocks; in these cases much of the released potassium derives from electrical trauma to intercostal muscle.

Benign arrhythmias such as atrial, ventricular, and junctional premature beats may occur transiently. Asystole with cardiac arrest occurs rarely in severe conduction system disease. Occurrence of serious ventricular arrhythmias is related to level of the electrical discharge, overdigitalization, severity of heart disease, and electrolyte imbalance. When ventricular fibrillation occurs, it is often due to improper synchronization, with delivery of the discharge in the vulnerable period, and the arrhythmia follows instantly after the shock. When ventricular fibrillation and sudden death occur hours after cardioversion, it is often presumed to be toxicity from digitalis, quinidine, or both drugs. Experimental studies suggest that ventricular arrhythmias following cardioversion may be due to myocardial potassium release from the electric shock upon an excessively digitalized myocardium. On the other hand, mild hypokalemia following cardioversion for ventricular tachycardia has also been described. If high-energy levels are used for cardioversion and defibrillation, prolonged periods of asystole may result, which in the ischemic or infarcted heart may provoke serious ventricular arrhythmias.

Pulmonary edema following cardioversion has been noted most often in the presence of mitral or aortic valvular disease or left ventricular dysfunction. It is likely that these factors in conjunction with alterations in ventricular function, delayed return of atrial function, fluid overload prior to cardioversion, and pulmonary embolism contribute to precipitation of pulmonary edema. Systemic embolization is a serious complication and has been discussed earlier. Unexplained hypotension may occur after cardioversion; if the condition does not resolve spontaneously, treatment with fluids may be necessary. Pacemakers may show loss of function or exhibit transient or chronic increases in stimulation threshold. This effect is probably due to current flow through the casing to the electrode lead causing a myocardial burn. Because the increase in threshold may be gradual, serial measurements of the stimulation threshold for 2 months is recommended.[18] Implantable cardioverter-defibrillator devices contain diode circuits, which generally protect against damage from external electrical shock; on rare occasions, malfunction may occur. Electrodes should therefore be placed at least 12 cm from implanted devices before discharge.

Cardioversion has been safely performed during pregnancy, and fetal death has not been reported as a direct consequence of treatment. Nonetheless, in the interest of safety, fetal heart rate monitoring should be performed when possible. Despite adverse effects, the use of electrical energy for the reversion of arrhythmias, when properly utilized, can be safely accomplished with a low incidence of complications.

REFERENCES

1. Lown B, Amarasingham R, Neuman J: New method for termination of cardiac arrhythmias. *JAMA* 1962; 182:548–555.
2. Lown B: Electrical reversion of cardiac arrhythmias. *Br Heart J* 1967; 29:469–489.
3. DeSilva RA, Graboys TB, Podrid PJ, Lown B: Cardioversion and defibrillation. *Am Heart J* 1980; 100:881–895.
4. Patton JN, Allen D, Pantridge JF: The effects of shock energy, propranolol and verapamil on cardiac damage caused by transthoracic countershock. *Circulation* 1984; 69:357–368.
5. Kerber RE, Martins JB, Kienzle MG, Constantin L, Olshansky B, Hopson R, et al: Energy, current, and success in defibrillation and cardioversion: Clinical studies using an automated impedance-based method of energy adjustment. *Circulation* 1988; 77:1038–1046.
6. Bjerkelund CJ, Orning OM: The efficacy of anticoagulant therapy in preventing embolism related to DC electrical cardioversion of atrial fibrillation. *Am J Cardiol* 1969; 23:208–216.
7. Dunn M, Alexander J, DeSilva RA, Hildner F: Antithrombotic therapy in atrial fibrillation. *Chest* 1989; 95(suppl):118S–127S.
8. Dethy M, Chassat C, Roy D, Mercier LA: Doppler echocardiographic predictors of recurrence of atrial fibrillation. *Am J Cardiol* 1988; 62:723–726.
9. Wolf PA, Abbott RD, Kannel WB: Atrial fibrillation: A major contribution to stroke in the elderly. The Framingham Study. *Arch Intern Med* 1987; 147:1561–1564.
10. Atwood JE, Myers J, Sullivan M, Forbes S, Sandhu S, Callahan P, et al: Effect of cardioversion on maximal exercise capacity after cardioversion of atrial fibrillation to sinus rhythm. *Am Heart J* 1989; 118:913–918.
11. Petersen P, Kastrup J, Videback R, Boysen G: Cerebral blood flow before and after cardioversion of atrial fibrillation. *J Cereb Blood Flow Metab* 1989; 9:422–425.
12. Petersen P, Kastrup J, Vilhelmsen R, Schoutten HJ: Atrial natriuretic peptide in atrial fibrillation after electrical cardioversion therapy. *Eur Heart J* 1988; 9:639–641.
13. Coplen SE, Antman EM, Berlin JA, Hewitt P, Chalmers TC: Efficacy and safety of quinidine therapy for maintenance of sinus rhythm after cardioversion. *Circulation* 1990; 82:1107–1115.
14. Dalzell GW, Anderson J, Adgey AAJ: Factors determining success and energy requirements for cardioversion of atrial fibrillation. *Q J Med* 1990; 76:903–913.
15. Guiney TE, Lown B: Electrical conversion of atrial flutter to atrial fibrillation. Flutter mechanism in man. *Br Heart J* 1972; 34:1215–1224.
16. *Textbook of Advanced Cardiac Life Support,* 2d ed. Dallas, TX, American Heart Association, 1987: 238.
17. Gascho JA, Crampton RS, Cherwek ML, Sipes JN, Hunter FP, O'Brien WM: Determinants of ventricular defibrillation in adults. *Circulation* 1979; 60:231–240.
18. Levine PA, Barold S, Fletcher RD, Talbot P: Adverse acute and chronic effects of electrical defibrillation and cardioversion on implanted unipolar cardiac pacing systems. *J Am Coll Cardiol* 1983; 1:1413–1422.

Chapter 42

The Implantable Cardioverter-Defibrillator

Ross Brooks, M.D. ■ *Jeremy N. Ruskin, M.D.*

Sudden cardiac death claims between 350,000 and 400,000 lives annually in the United States and represents a major contemporary public health problem.[1] The principal cause of sudden cardiac death remained unclear until in-field electrocardiogram (ECG) monitoring demonstrated a high prevalence of ventricular fibrillation in victims of out-of-hospital cardiac arrest.[2] (See also Chap. 51.) In the vast majority of cases (greater than 80 percent), sudden death is caused by the abrupt onset of ventricular tachycardia that either persists or more commonly progresses to ventricular fibrillation.[3] Since self-termination of ventricular fibrillation is exceedingly rare, it is recognized that the single most important factor determining survival in individuals with ventricular fibrillation is the time interval between the onset of collapse and the first defibrillation attempt.[4] Overall mortality associated with out-of-hospital cardiac arrest remains high (above 75 percent), mainly because of delay in providing effective therapy to afflicted individuals.[5] As originally conceived by Mirowski,[6] the implantable defibrillator was designed to circumvent the delay in providing definitive therapy to ambulatory individuals with malignant ventricular arrhythmias. The internal defibrillator responds by delivering an initial electrical countershock within 10 to 20 s of arrhythmia onset, a time frame in which the potential for arrhythmia reversal approaches 100 percent. Because these remarkable devices are capable of responding immediately to spontaneous ventricular fibrillation, they represent the most effective method for aborting sudden death in individuals with life-threatening ventricular arrhythmias. In the first decade of clinical usage, the implantable cardioverter-defibrillator (ICD) has proved to be a reliable and effective means of preventing subsequent sudden death in survivors of out-of-hospital cardiac arrest.[7] Implantable cardioverter-defibrillator technology is evolving rapidly, and newer devices with expanded diagnostic and therapeutic capabilities continue to emerge. Therefore, the indications for these devices will continue to broaden. In the 1990s, the extent to which this technology will impact the global problem of sudden cardiac death should become clearer, as increasing numbers of patients with potential or manifest life-threatening arrhythmias are treated with implantable arrhythmia control devices. (See also Chap. 36.)

HISTORICAL PERSPECTIVE

Interest in the use of intrathoracic electrical countershock to defibrillate the heart dates back to the work of Hobbs and Bigelow[8] in the 1950s. The feasibility of this approach was demonstrated in the subsequent decade by separate groups led by Mirowski[9] and Schuder,[10] who achieved successful internal defibrillation with electric shocks delivered between two intravascular electrodes positioned in the superior vena cava and at the apex of the right ventricle. The initial work by Mirowski and coworkers[11] was carried out at Sinai Hospital in Baltimore, where the first experimental model of the implantable defibrillator was built and successfully tested in 1969 in a dog. After 10 years of research and development, Mirowski and coworkers[12] performed the first automatic defibrillator implantation in a human at the Johns Hopkins University Medical Center on February 4, 1980. For the first year, defibrillator implantation was performed only at the Johns Hopkins Hospital, with expansion to Stanford University Medical Center in 1981. Investigational implantation of the automatic implantable cardioverter-defibrillator (AICD) was limited to 35 institutions until the device was approved by the U.S. Food and Drug Administration (FDA) in October 1985.[13] By the end of the last decade, more than 400 centers worldwide had implanted in excess of 10,000 units. According to an industry analyst's projections, the number of new implants may reach 100,000 by 1995.

SYSTEM COMPONENTS AND FUNCTION

The ICD system is comprised of two basic components: a pulse generator and lead electrodes for arrhythmia detection and for delivery of the cardioverting/defibrillating pulse. The original system (AID) was designed to serve only as a defibrillator and did not contain any cardioverting functions. Synchronized cardioverting capabilities are a feature present in all devices manufactured since 1982. The pulse generator contains the energy source consisting of two lithium–silver vanadium pentoxide cells connected in series, the energy-storing electrolytic capacitors, and various electronic components. The outer covering of the pulse generator is made of titanium with a header made of epoxy. The header has three or four electrode receptacles to receive the defibrillation and sensing lead electrodes. Depending on the particular manufacturer and the specific model under consideration, the pulse generator weighs between 190 and 260 g with a volume of 113 to 165 mL. All ICD systems utilize endocardial or epicardially placed rate-sensing leads for arrhythmia detection. Newer systems may also use these leads for antitachycardia and VVI pacing functions (Table 42-1). A variety of electrode configurations may be used for delivering electric shock energy to the myocardium. The particular configuration chosen is defined at the time of implantation when defibrillation threshold (DFT) testing is performed (see next section). Currently available systems utilize heart rate criteria as the primary arrhythmia sensing parameter. When heart rate exceeds a preset value and the arrhythmia detection algorithm is satisfied, an internal charge cycle is initiated that culminates in the delivery of a shock across the defibrillating electrodes. If the first shock is

TABLE 42-1
Features of ICD Devices Currently in Use and of Those Undergoing Clinical Evaluation

Manufacturer	Model	High-*E* CV/DF	Detention Morph	Detention Rate	Low-*E* CV	Holter Monitor	Second Look	VVI Pacing	A-T Pacing	Shock Charac-teristics	Status (US)
First generation											
MEDRAD/ INTEC	AID	−/+	+	−	−	−	−	−	−	m	N/A
Second generation											
INTEC/CPI	B1400	+/+	+	+	−	−	−	−	−	m	N/A
INTEC/CPI	B1410	+/+	+	+	−	−	−	−	−	m	N/A
INTEC/CPI	BR1420	−/+	−	+	−	−	−	−	−	m	N/A
CPI	Ventak 1550	+/+	+	+	−	−	−	−	−	m	N/A
CPI	Ventak 1510*	+/+	+	+	−	−	−	−	−	m	N/A
CPI	Ventak 1520	+/+	−	+	−	−	−	−	−	m	N/A
Third generation											
CPI	Ventak 1550	+/+	+	+	+	−	−	−	−	m	A
CPI	Ventak P 1600	+/+	+	+	+	−	−	−	−	m	A
Telectronics	Guardian 1402	+/+	−	+	+	−	+	+	−	m	CT-89
Fourth generation											
Ventritex	Cadence V-100	+/+	−	+	+	+	+	+	+	m/b	A
CPI	PRX/PRX-II	+/+	+	+	+	+	+	+	+	m/b	CT-90
CPI	P-2	+/+	+	+	+	+	+	+	−	b	CT-92
Medtronic	PCD 7217B	+/+	−	+	+	−	+/−	+	+	m/s	A
Telectronics	Guardian ATP 4210	+/+	−	+	+	+	+	+	+	m/b	CT-90
Intermedics	Res-Q 102-02	+/+	−	+	+	+	−	+	+	m/b	CT-91

A = available; A-T = antitachycardia; b = biphasic pulses; CPI = Cardiac Pacemakers Incorporated; CT = clinical trials; CV = cardioversion; DF = defibrillation; *E* = energy; ICD = implantable cardioverter/defibrillator; m = monophasic pulses; morphology N/A = not available; prog = programmable; pac = morphology pacing; s = sequential; + = present; − = absent
* high-energy device (first shock = 30 j).

unsuccessful, the ICD will recycle and deliver additional countershocks. The latest series of devices have antitachycardia pacing capabilities in addition to cardioverting/defibrillating functions. These units are capable of different initial responses to one or more tachycardias (classified by rate) as well as a programmable sequence of responses ("tiered" or "graded" therapy) to a particular arrhythmia (e.g., adaptive or autodecremental pacing sequences to low-energy cardioversion to high-energy defibrillation). The characteristics of the shock waveform (e.g., monophasic vs. biphasic) and the current pathway (single, bidirectional, sequential) used in the ICD vary depending on the specific model and lead configuration chosen (Table 42-1). Recent experimental data have shown that biphasic shock waveforms are generally superior to monophasic shocks and result in lower DFTs.[14] The amount of energy delivered to the myocardium at the time of shock delivery is a programmable feature of all current devices. For ventricular fibrillation, an initial shock energy level between 25 and 35 J is generally used, while a lower initial energy may be selected for monomorphic ventricular tachycardia.

TABLE 42-2
Guidelines for ICD Implantation

Currently Accepted Indications for ICD Implantation

1. Following one or more episodes of spontaneously occurring and inducible VF or syncopal or hypotensive VT that is (i) not associated with acute myocardial infarction, (ii) not due to a remediable cause (e.g., drug toxicity, electrolyte derangement, ischemia), and (iii) neither controlled by acceptable drug therapy after serial testing nor amenable to definitive therapy (e.g., surgical ablation).
2. Following spontaneously occurring but noninducible documented syncopal or hypotensive VT that was not due to (i) to (iii) above.
3. Following VT/VF cardiac arrest that was not due to (i) to (iii) above and not associated with an inducible ventricular arrhythmia.
4. Following surgery for VT or VF if the ventricular arrhythmia remains inducible.

Situations in which an ICD May Be Indicated (Patient Characteristics Determine Appropriateness)

1. Following one or more episodes of spontaneously occurring and inducible VF or syncopal or hypotensive VT that is (i) associated with an acute myocardial infarction (within 1 month but more than 2 days after the infarct), (ii) not due to a remediable cause, and (iii) neither controlled by acceptable drug therapy after multiple trials nor amenable to definitive treatment.
2. Following unexplained syncope, which by history and clinical circumstances was probably due to a ventricular tachyarrhythmia, and in the presence of reproducible inducible syncopal or hypotensive VT or VF that is not due to (i) to (iii) above.
3. Following VF or syncopal or hypotensive VT that is apparently controlled by drug, surgical, or ablative therapy but in which the results of treatment are too unpredictable to justify withholding ICD therapy.

ICD Not Indicated

1. Other disease processes that clearly and severely limit life expectancy.
2. Asymptomatic VT or symptomatic VT/VF that is (i) associated with acute myocardial infarction within 2 days, (ii) due to a remediable cause, (iii) controlled by acceptable drug therapy, or (iv) amenable to definitive treatment (i.e., ablative procedures, surgery).

PATIENT SELECTION

The first patients who received implantable defibrillators were required to have drug-refractory recurrent ventricular tachycardia or fibrillation and to have survived at least two episodes of cardiac arrest. This strict criterion was then liberalized to permit inclusion of patients surviving only one episode of cardiac arrest or hemodynamically compromising sustained ventricular tachycardia in whom the arrhythmia was unresponsive to drug therapy and not amenable to surgical therapy. Indications for the ICD continue to broaden, particularly with the availability of fourth-generation devices with antitachycardia pacing capabilities (Table 42-1). Current guidelines for cardioverter-defibrillator implantation are listed in Table 42-2. Candidates for ICD therapy generally fall into one of three patient subsets: (1) survivors of cardiac arrest with documented ventricular tachycardia/fibrillation; (2) patients with drug refractory, clinical and induced sustained ventricular tachycardia; and (3) patients without documented sustained clinical ventricular arrhythmias who are deemed at high risk for future life-threatening arrhythmic events because of inducible arrhythmias at electrophysiological study.

Cardiac Arrest Survivors

Survivors of out-of-hospital cardiac arrest owing to ventricular fibrillation are recognized as being at high risk for recurrent arrhythmic events and sudden cardiac death.[15] Data from Seattle in the 1970s showed a 30 to 40 percent 1-year mortality rate in untreated patients following an episode of out-of-hospital ventricular fibrillation unassociated with a new transmural myocardial infarction, emphasizing the need to define appropriate therapy for these individuals during the initial hospitalization postcardiac arrest.[16] (See also Chap. 51.) The ICD is now considered the treatment of choice for survivors of out-of-hospital ventricular fibrillation with drug-refractory arrhythmias not associated with a reversible predisposing cause (e.g., acute myocardial ischemia). Indeed, analysis of published ICD series in the 1980s showed that a prior history of cardiac arrest was present in the vast majority (80 percent) of patients who received these devices.[17-22] A majority of patients undergoing electrophysiological testing following out-of-hospital cardiac arrest will manifest inducible rapid sustained ventricular arrhythmias in response to programmed electrical stimulation, while in 15 to 30 percent of cases, no sustained arrhythmia will be induced.[23] Earlier studies in this patient population showed that patients whose arrhythmias were suppressed by electrophysiologically guided drug therapy had a much improved long-term prognosis relative to those patients in whom no suppressive antiarrhythmic therapy could be found.[23-29] (See also Chap. 36.) The ICD is now considered the next step in the management of patients with arrhythmias unresponsive to drug therapy.[30] Implantable cardioverter-defibrillators should also be considered for a majority of patients with cardiac arrest due to documented ventricular fibrillation in whom no inducible sustained arrhythmia is found during electrophysiological testing, since these individuals also remain at risk for recurrent arrhythmic events and sudden death. This consideration also applies to patients in whom the role of electropharmacologic testing is currently less certain (e.g., idiopathic dilated cardiomyopathy, hypertrophic cardiomyopathy, long QT syndrome). Finally, since data show that patients with drug-suppressed arrhythmias and very poor left ventricular function have higher rates of recurrent arrhythmias and sudden death than corresponding patients with well-preserved left ventricular function, the ICD should also be considered for any patient in whom the long-term effectiveness of pharmacologic therapy remains in doubt.[23]

Patients with Symptomatic Sustained Ventricular Tachycardia

Another subset of patients in whom the ICD is being used with increasing frequency is those with spontaneous and induced sustained monomorphic ventricular tachycardia. In this subset of patients potential therapeutic options are more numerous and may include (1) antiarrhythmic drug therapy, (2) surgical map-guided aneurysmectomy/endocardial resection, (3) transcatheter ablation, and (4) ICD systems with antitachycardia pacing capabilities. Most patients with recurrent sustained monomorphic ventricular tachycardia receive antiarrhythmic drugs as initial therapy. (See Chap. 36.) Patients with ventricular tachycardia resistant to conventional antiarrhythmic agents are eventually selected for amiodarone therapy, at which time nonpharmacologic options should be considered. Although amiodarone may be effective, up to 50 percent of patients are eventually withdrawn from this agent within 5 years because of toxic side effects, indicating that this therapy may not represent a long-term solution for many patients.[31] (See Chap. 38.) Appropriately selected patients with recurrent monomorphic ventricular tachycardia may be candidates for surgical or radiofrequency catheter ablative procedures that offer the potential for arrhythmia cure. Patients with drug-resistant tachycardias that are reliably terminated by overdrive ventricular pacing are also candidates for an ICD with antitachycardia pacing (ATP) functions. Antitachycardia pacing is highly effective in a majority of patients with recurrent monomorphic ventricular tachycardia and is usually imperceptible to the patient, a feature that enhances patient acceptance of these devices. The superiority of the ICD over other forms of therapy in this patient subset has not been as clearly demonstrated as in the groups previously discussed, and requires further study.

High-Risk Patients without a History of Sustained Arrhythmias

A majority of patients at high risk for sudden cardiac death have not previously experienced a sustained ventricular arrhythmia. Since current mortality rates associated with out-of-hospital cardiac arrest are in the range of 70 to 85 percent, it is evident that primary prevention strategies will have the greatest impact on reducing mortality from sudden cardiac death.[32] Primary prevention of sudden cardiac death will therefore require the detection of individuals at high risk for life-threatening arrhythmias before cardiac arrest occurs. A majority of patients at risk for life-threatening arrhythmias have underlying structural heart disease, but up to 20 percent may have no previous history. (See also Chap. 51.) Potential target populations for "prophylactic" cardioverter-defibrillator implantation include high-risk postinfarction and postsurgical patients and patients with advanced ischemic and nonischemic cardiomyopathy. The Cardiac Arrhythmia Suppression Trial (CAST) has emphasized the potential dangers of using class IC antiarrhythmic drug therapy in this patient population, suggesting that alternative, pharmacologic and nonpharmacologic approaches to the prevention of sudden cardiac death must be considered.[33] Prospective controlled studies will be required to define the role of electrophysiological testing and prophylactic ICD use in patients at high risk for sudden cardiac death who have not yet experienced a life-threatening arrhythmia. Toward this end, a number of trials [e.g., Coronary Artery Bypass Grafting (CABG) Patch, Multicenter Automatic Defibrillator Implantation (MADIT), Multicenter Unsustained Tachycardia Trial (MUSTT), and Dilated Cardiomyopathy Trials] are currently in progress or under consideration to test the hypothesis that the ICD will decrease sudden death mortality in these high-risk patient subsets.[34] In the future, nonthoracotomy lead systems, which simplify the implantation procedure and reduce hospital length of stay and cost, will facilitate these and other studies designed to test the efficacy of ICD therapy in high-risk patients.

DEVICE SELECTION

As ICD devices with an increasing array of sophisticated diagnostic and therapeutic features become available from a variety of manufacturers, device selection will become a more relevant consideration. Currently, three ICDs are approved by the FDA for clinical use (CPI Ventak 1550, 1555, and 1600), although at least five additional devices are currently in various phases of clinical investigation (Table 42-1). When fourth-generation devices become clinically available, a number of considerations will govern the choice of a particular system. These include (1) the approach used for lead implantation (nonthoracotomy vs. thoracotomy); (2) whether or not ATP and VVI pacing functions are desirable; and (3) cost considerations. All current ICDs have programmable rate detection parameters and first shock energy levels that permit an appropriate detection rate cutoff and initial shock energy to be selected for a variety of tachyarrhythmias. The needs of patients with spontaneous or inducible ventricular fibrillation can be satisfactorily met with standard defibrillator devices that may not have advanced functions. Patients with sustained monomorphic ventricular tachycardia may benefit additionally from devices capable of antitachycardia pacing in addition to cardioverter-defibrillator functions. Patients with a history of chronic sinus bradycardia, A-V conduction system disease, or severe postshock bradyarrhythmias may benefit from devices with VVI pacing capabilities. (See also Chap. 40.) Devices with integrated defibrillator/pacemaker capabilities will also eliminate potentially dangerous interactions between separately implanted units.[35] Since none of the currently approved or investigational devices have dual-chamber pacing capabilities, those patients who require DDD pacing will still require separate defibrillator and pacemaker devices. Patients with higher than usual defibrillation energy requirements (20 to 25 J) may benefit from an ICD capable of delivering biphasic shock waveforms and/or a high-energy output pulse generator available from some manufacturers.

IMPLANTATION AND TESTING PROCEDURES

Approximately 80 percent of patients have the ICD implanted as the sole procedure, while in the other 20 percent an additional surgical intervention is performed, most frequently coronary artery revascularization.[17–19] Patients undergoing combined revascularization and ICD insertion usually receive extrapericardial ventricular patch electrodes and screw-in epimyocardial bipolar rate-sensing leads at the initial operation after the revascularization procedure is completed. The ICD pulse generator is often implanted subsequently as a separate procedure. In many patients, pulse generator implantation is deferred until the antiarrhythmic effects of bypass graft surgery or other procedures (e.g., endocardial resection) alone can be assessed by postoperative electrophysiological testing. The placement of extrapericardial patches is not associated with significant alterations in regional or global ventricular function, although late development of constrictive pericarditis or infection are recognized as potential, although rare, complications.[36] Therefore, in potential ICD recipients, it is usually prudent to place one or more patch-lead electrodes at the time of the initial surgical procedure (*leads-only implant*) rather than run the risk that the patient will require a thoracotomy at a later date.

Thoracotomy System

In patients undergoing ICD implantation alone, a number of surgical approaches have been used for patch-lead placement. For intrathoracic placement of the patch electrodes, a left thoracotomy, left subcostal, or subxiphoid approach may be employed.[37] A left anterior thoracotomy is the preferred surgical approach at many institutions since it generally permits the best exposure for patch-lead placement.[17–19] During the early years of ICD implantation, the standard lead configuration consisted of a transvenous superior vena cava coil electrode in conjunction with placement of one epicardial patch (coil-patch configuration).[12,18] Subsequently, two patches were used that generally resulted in lower DFTs in most patients.[38] Two extrapericardial patches (patch-patch configuration) have now become the standard configuration at most centers. In the two-patch lead configuration, one small or large patch is placed anteriorly over the right ventricle while the other is placed over the posterolateral left ventricle. The usual electrode polarity is anterior or right ventricular patch as anode (+) and the posterior or left ventricular patch as cathode (−). In recent years there has been a trend toward extrapericardial rather than epicardial placement of patch electrodes. This is preferable in patients who may later require coronary artery bypass grafting or other cardiac surgery. Rate-sensing leads used in conventional thoracotomy systems may be implanted in either an epicardial or transvenous endocardial position. At our institution the latter is preferred because of greater long-term signal stability. The pulse generator is usually inserted into a left paraumbilical subcutaneous pocket and the leads are tunneled subcutaneously from the chest to the abdominal pocket. For cosmetic reasons, implantation behind the abdominal rectus muscle may be performed in selected patients. Output signals from the rate-sensing lead are measured during sinus rhythm and ventricular tachycardia/fibrillation to ensure adequate slew rate and amplitude for reliable arrthythmia detection. Intraoperative testing to determine the DFT is carried out with an external cardioverter-defibrillator. Although DFT testing practices vary widely among institutions, three consecutive defibrillations with 20 J or less is considered by many investigators to be a minimum requirement for pulse generator implantation in most patients. In our institutions, a goal of 15 J or less is felt to be desirable. This former requirement generally ensures a minimum 10-J "safety margin" between the DFT and the maximal stored energy of currently approved devices (30 J) and predicts greater than 95 percent probability of defibrillation at the maximal energy level. Newer devices have higher energy ratings (35 to 40 J) and may permit implantation of ICD units in patients with higher than usual DFTs (20 to 25 J). The ICD pulse generator is then connected to the implanted leads and tested for appropriate arrhythmia detection and conversion immediately before implantation. In most large series the operative mortality associated with primary ICD implantation is less than 2 percent.[17–23] Complications associated with ICD implantation occur in 15 to 20 percent of patients and are mainly related to the surgical procedure involved (e.g., thoracotomy).

Nonthoracotomy Lead Systems

Clinical experience with nonthoracotomy lead systems dates back to 1988 when CPI first introduced the Endotak system. The Endotak program was suspended in 1989 due to malfunction of some devices caused by lead fractures. Modified sensing and subcutaneous patch electrodes are now available from the manufacturer, and a larger clinical trial of this system is nearing completion.

To date, more than 800 patients have been enrolled into this program. The Endotak system incorporates a modified rectangular patch-lead that is implanted subcutaneously on the lateral chest wall outside the thorax (Fig. 42-1).[39] This patch electrode is used in conjunction with a transvenous endocardial electrode, the tripolar Endotak C-lead. The tip of the Endotak lead consists of a bipolar sensing electrode used for arrhythmia detection. Proximal and distal coil electrodes for cardioversion/defibrillation are located in the superior vena cava and at the right ventricular apex (Fig. 42-1). In some patients, satisfactory DFTs may be achieved using the proximal and distal coil electrodes alone. In most patients, however, the subcutaneous patch must be incorporated into the final electrode configuration. A specially designed "Y" adaptor allows for the creation of a variety of electrical vectors and bidirectional current delivery using this three-electrode system. The most successful configuration has incorporated the subcutaneous patch and proximal coil electrodes as common anodes (+) and the distal coil electrode as the cathode (−).[40] Preliminary data in a selected patient population indicate that more than 70 percent of all nonthoracotomy systems attempted are successful, indicating that this approach is possible for most patients.[41] In the future, far higher success rates may be possible with careful testing and multiple patch-electrode positions and the use of biphasic shocks. If satisfactory DFTs cannot be achieved with this system, open thoracotomy becomes necessary. In most patients requiring thoracotomy, a "hybrid" system consisting of a single epicardial patch in conjunction with two coil electrodes can be successfully implanted. No long-term data on the durability of these leads are available, nor is the long-term efficacy of this system known. Nonthoracotomy systems developed by Medtronic, Intermedics, and Telectronics are also under clinical investigation.

At most centers, a postimplant electrophysiological study is performed before the patient is discharged home. Ventricular tachycardia and/or fibrillation is induced, and the efficacy of the implanted device in detecting the arrhythmia and in delivering pacing and/or cardioversion/defibrillation therapy is evaluated. The antitachycardia pacing functions of newer devices may be more extensively tested and reprogrammed during the predischarge electrophysiological study than at the time of implantation.

PERFORMANCE OF THE ICD

Currently reported series of patients with ICDs show sudden death–free survival rates between 90 and 98 percent over follow-up periods of 1 to 5 years.[17–22] The manufacturer of the currently approved ICD (CPI) has reported 5-year sudden death–free, total cardiac, and overall survival rates of 98, 92, and 84 percent, respectively, among more than 25,000 patients worldwide through March 1993.[41] It should be noted that these results are pooled from all patients receiving ICDs. Since the vast majority of patients in these series (over 75 percent) had a history of prior cardiac arrest, however, the results are skewed in the direction of this patient population. Survival data in these series are also reported from the time of implant rather than from the time of the first appropriate discharge of the device. To derive benefit from the ICD, there must be not only an appropriate discharge but also prolonged survival after this

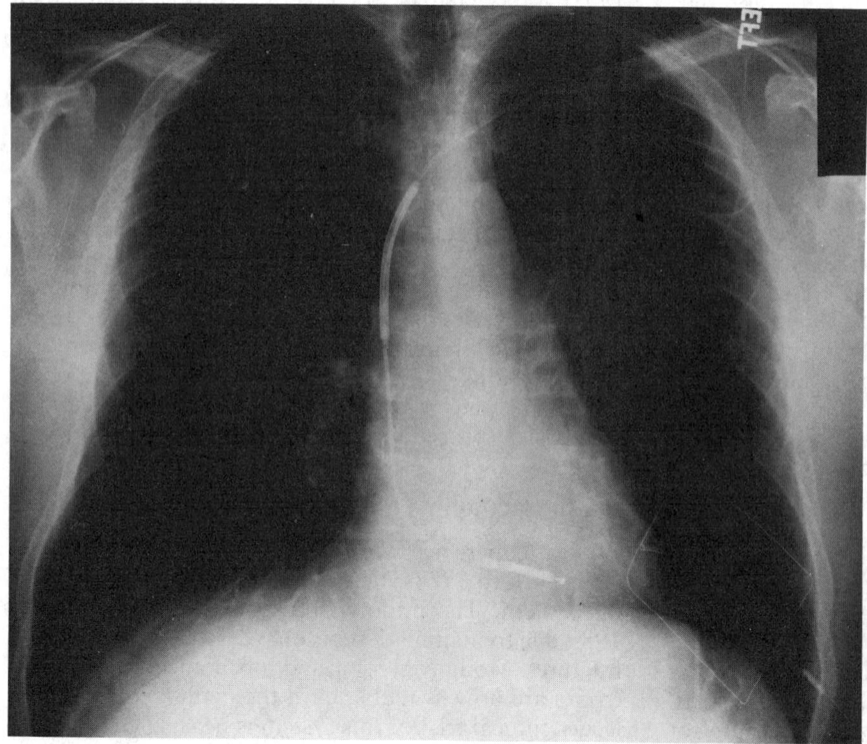

FIGURE 42-1 Posteroanterior chest x-ray film of a patient implanted with an Endotak AICD lead system. A tripolar transvenous lead is shown with the tip implanted at the apex of the right ventricle. The proximal coil electrode is positioned in the superior vena cava. The distal coil electrode is located in the right ventricle. A subcutaneous patch electrode is implanted on the left posterolateral chest wall outside the thorax. In this particular patient the right ventricular coil electrode served as the cathode [−], with the superior vena cava coil and subcutaneous patch electrodes serving as a combined anode [+].

discharge. A more recent study[43] demonstrated a mean survival of 23.8 months after the first ICD discharge, which occurred a mean of 9.1 months after implantation. In survivors of cardiac arrest, these survival figures generally surpass those achieved with other treatment modalities and confirm the efficacy of these devices in preventing sudden death in this high-risk patient population. (See also Chap. 51.) The follow-up of patients with devices produced by other manufacturers is shorter but to date has shown similar results. Ventritex has cited a 99 percent sudden death–free actuarial survival after 20 months for 337 patients receiving the Cadence V-100 ICD.[44] It should be noted that only 30 percent of the patients receiving this investigational Cadence device had a history of prior cardiac arrest. Future studies will be aimed at determining more precisely the relative benefits of these devices in patients with sustained ventricular tachycardia without a history of cardiac arrest. Low left ventricular ejection fraction and advanced congestive heart failure functional class are associated with early ICD discharges and shortened survival,[22,43] while coronary artery bypass grafting and the use of beta receptor blocking agents are associated with later discharges.[43] Surgical revascularization is also associated with longer survival in patients with coronary artery disease receiving ICDs.[43] The cause of most deaths in patients with ICDs is congestive heart failure resulting from advanced pump dysfunction.

Although the ICD provides a highly effective therapy for reducing mortality from sudden cardiac death in high-risk patients, a small incidence of sudden death remains in patients with these devices.[45] Device failures are extremely rare (below 1 percent) and may be attributed to factors such as lead fracture or migration, premature battery depletion, and generator malfunction.[46] Deaths in the setting of documented refractory ventricular fibrillation and normal device function are also described.[45] The factors accounting for the resistance to defibrillation in these cases are incompletely understood and may, in some cases, result from severe ischemia and/or end-stage pump failure. High DFTs at the time of implantation or a rise in the DFT postimplant as well as asystole and electromechanical dissociation may account for other instances of sudden death. The occurrence of clinically significant bradyarrhythmias after device discharge is rare, and combination devices with backup bradyarrhythmia pacing capability to treat this problem are in clinical trials. A better understanding of the pathogenesis of sudden death in patients with normally functioning devices will allow for measures that may further improve survival.

OUTPATIENT EVALUATION AND ICD REPLACEMENT PRACTICES

Because electrolytic capacitors require periodic reformation and because of the need to assess battery reserve by measuring the time required to charge the capacitors, patients must return every 2 to 3 months after ICD implantation for a noninvasive outpatient test of device battery status. The estimated battery life of current ICD devices ranges between 3 and 6 years. All current devices are interrogated and programmed by means of an external programmer. All units are also temporarily modified by placing a magnet over the pulse generator (Table 42-3). Tachycardia detection and therapy are temporarily suspended by magnet placement in all currently approved and investigational devices.

As of this writing, almost all patients with an ICD should be considered for pulse generator replacement when there is evidence of battery depletion. About 50 percent of patients undergoing replacement of approved pulse generators will have received appropriate shock or pacing therapy in the intervening period, indicating an ongoing need for the system. The decision to replace the device in patients without previous shocks must be individualized and depends on factors such as the presenting arrhythmia, the circumstances of its occurrence, the nature and severity of underlying heart disease, the results of electrophysiological testing, and the presence of other co-morbid factors. The vast majority of patients who have not received therapy in the intervening period should also be considered for reimplantation, since late shocks occurring many years after primary implantation appear to define a continuing need for this therapy in many patients.[47] Patients requiring generator replacement are electively admitted and have the same generator or an upgraded model implanted. All current investigational devices can be adapted to most existing lead configurations. Our practice is to perform generator replacements under general anesthesia to facilitate patient comfort and DFT testing. Lead electrodes are not routinely changed at the time of generator replacement unless a problem is identified. Confirmation of previously established rate-sensing lead electrogram amplitude in addition to DFTs are performed, followed by testing of the new pulse generator. Several studies have confirmed the stability over time of lead systems implanted at thoracotomy as well as DFTs in most patients.[48,49] In occasional patients, however, DFTs may be unexpectedly elevated at the time of generator replacement, supporting the practice of routine DFT testing.[50]

TABLE 42-3
Responses of ICD Devices to Magnet Application

Device	Suspends Tachycardia Detection and Therapy	Suspends Bradycardia Therapy
CPI 1550/1600	Yes*	—
CPI PRX-I/II	Yes*	No
CPI P2	Yes*	No
Ventritex-Cadence V-100	Yes†	No
Telectronics 4202/4203	Yes†	Yes
Telectronics 4210	Yes†	No
Medtronic PCD 7216/7217b	Yes†	No
Intermedics RES Q	Yes†	No

* Magnet will inactivate device after 30 seconds. To reactivate AICD, magnet must be reapplied for 30 seconds.
† Tachyarrhythmia therapy will be temporarily inhibited for as long as magnet is applied.

Many potential factors including the type and severity of underlying heart disease, mass of the myocardium, ventricular function, intracellular electrolyte concentration, configuration of the lead system, characteristics of the shock waveform and current pathway, and the presence of drugs may account for individual variability in DFTs. Following implantation, most variables remain fixed although drug therapy may change and underlying disease processes may worsen. Drugs may have variable effects on DFTs, and effects may be different in experimental models and human patients. The most significant DFT interaction noted to date has occurred in patients receiving the drug amiodarone.[19] Chronic amiodarone therapy has been shown to be associated independently with significantly higher DFTs in patients undergoing ICD implantation as compared with patients not receiving this drug.[51] Defibrillation thresholds may also increase in patients receiving class IC agents[52] and mexiletine.[53] Repeat testing of the ICD is recommended in these individuals to confirm adequate function, especially in those with minimal safety margins established at the time of intraoperative DFT testing.

INTERPRETATION OF ICD DISCHARGES AND TROUBLE SHOOTING

The first three generations of ICD devices did not contain any arrhythmia memory (Holter monitor) functions, and electrograms were not recorded or stored at the time of shock delivery (Table 42-1). All current devices, however, contain an event counter that records the cumulative number of shocks delivered to the patient. Whether or not a shock was actually delivered can be confirmed easily by interrogating the unit. Clinical findings may be helpful in the interpretation of ICD discharges when electrocardiographic correlation is not available. A history of palpitations in conjunction with lightheadedness, near syncope, or syncope immediately before device discharge is consistent with a ventricular tachyarrhythmia. It has also become apparent that many so-called asymptomatic ICD discharges are in fact appropriate discharges in response to ventricular tachycardia.[54] Appropriate, undesirable discharges may sometimes be difficult to distinguish from appropriate, desirable shocks. For example, atrial fibrillation with a rapid ventricular rate exceeding the programmed rate cutoff may trigger an appropriate (although undesirable) discharge and may account for repetitive discharges experienced in close succession. Nonsustained ventricular tachycardia may sometimes result in undesirable shocks in patients with earlier "committed" devices that do not contain "second-look" features. Devices with second-look features that require arrhythmia reconfirmation immediately prior to shock delivery have largely eliminated the problem of undesirable discharges due to nonsustained ventricular tachycardia (Table 42-2). Sensing lead malfunction (oversensing) resulting from lead fractures may be the cause of inappropriate discharges triggered by sensing artifact. Lead disruption may be diagnosed on the basis of overpenetrated x-ray findings, by analyzing audible tones emitted in synchrony with sensed events ("beepograms"), or by examining the telemetered records of stored or real-time intracardiac electrograms. Discharge of the ICD during sinus rhythm is strong evidence for sensing malfunction. Analysis of electrograms or rate intervals recorded by the newer devices during sinus rhythm and at the time of therapy delivery has allowed for better correlation between arrhythmic events and device responses and has greatly facilitated the diagnosis of lead or pulse generator malfunction.

PSYCHOSOCIAL ISSUES

The ICD is generally well accepted in the vast majority of patients for whom this therapy is recommended. Before implantation, the implications of having an ICD must be thoroughly discussed with the patient and his or her family. It is important for patients to understand that the ICD represents potentially lifelong therapy. The issue causing the greatest ambivalence among patients with these devices is the potential restriction of life-style related to automobile driving. Because of the potential risk of an arrhythmia recurrence and the delivery of high-energy shocks, most physicians who implant ICDs agree that some restriction on driving should be considered. Since the risk of a recurrent arrhythmic event may persist indefinitely and because the timing of recurrent events cannot be predicted accurately, some physicians argue that patients with ICDs should not be allowed to drive again. Other physicians permit driving in patients who do not lose consciousness with their arrhythmias or who have not experienced a discharge after an arbitrary length of follow-up (e.g., 6 to 12 months). This approach is also problematic, however, since recurrent arrhythmic events may still occur despite a long initial shock-free interval.[47] Patients receiving implantable defibrillators comprise a heterogeneous population, and one set of guidelines may not serve all cases. At one end of the spectrum is the patient with impaired ventricular function, documented recurrent sustained ventricular arrhythmias causing syncope or cardiac arrest, and persistently inducible ventricular tachycardia at the time of electrophysiological testing. Patients with these characteristics are more likely to be "high-frequency" device users, because of the increased probability of recurrent spontaneous arrhythmic events. At the other end of the spectrum is the patient lacking any history of prior sustained arrhythmic events but with an inducible arrhythmia defined by electrophysiological testing. The probability of a future arrhythmic episode in the latter patient is undefined but is considered lower. A more restrictive approach to the issue of automobile driving seems appropriate for the former group of patients but is perhaps inappropriate for the latter and may make patients unwilling to accept the ICD as "prophylactic" therapy. At present only a few states in the United States have specific laws for patients with life-threatening arrhythmias, and no state makes any distinction between patients managed with an ICD versus those managed medically.[55] Therefore there is no legal consensus to guide physicians in advising patients with ICDs. Until more data become available about the pattern and frequency of device usage in various patient subsets, a conservative approach seems prudent, particularly for patients with a history of previous sustained arrhythmias who are deemed at high risk for recurrent arrhythmic events.

Many implanting centers have ICD support groups that meet several times a year to discuss issues relating to these devices. These groups provide a forum for patients with ICDs to discuss issues with one another and with implanting physicians and nurses. Support groups of this nature provide an invaluable service to patients with these devices.

ECONOMIC CONSIDERATIONS

Inevitably, therapeutic efficacy associated with such highly sophisticated technology necessarily comes at a substantial price. The cost of the ICD with leads ranges between $16,000 and $20,000. Hospital costs associated with the evaluation of patients with life-threatening arrhythmias and subsequent ICD implantation may exceed these figures. There is no indication from the manufacturers that the cost of these devices will be lower in the future, and hospital costs associated with the care of these patients will likely continue to escalate. Because of the propensity for such devices to consume a large percentage of health care dollars, their utilization will continue to undergo close scrutiny by third-party payers. Novel ways of reducing the costs associated with these devices will be necessary in order for the full impact of this therapy to be realized. Earlier decision making resulting in shorter hospital stays as well as the use of nonthoracotomy lead systems (when available) will reduce substantially the costs associated with initial implantation of these devices.[39] A recent analysis shows that the cost effectiveness of the implantable defibrillator is well within the range of currently accepted life-saving technology.[56] Moreover, as this technology evolves, it is likely to become more cost effective. For instance, newer devices with noninvasive programmed stimulation capabilities ("NIPS") will permit outpatient evaluation and re-programming. Devices capable of delivering antitachycardia pacing therapy may reduce the frequency of re-hospitalization in patients with recurrent ventricular tachycardia. Units with ambulatory electrocardiographic (Holter) monitoring functions will facilitate the interpretation of device responses, facilitate trouble shooting, and should potentially reduce the need for ambulatory or in-hospital ECG monitoring in many patients. Devices with "second look" features may eliminate the need for concomitant antiarrhythmic drugs to suppress nonsustained ventricular tachycardia. Devices with combined VVI pacemaker and ICD functions may obviate the need for separate pacemaker and ICD implantation in patients requiring both therapies. Nonthoracotomy systems, because of their ease of implantation, should decrease the postoperative length of stay and reduce overall hospital costs. Improvements in capacitor and battery technology forthcoming in current investigational and future devices will increase battery longevity, lengthen the interval between generator changes, and result in substantial savings.

Future Directions of ICD Therapy

The last decade began with a single ICD manufacturer and a simple defibrillator, and ended with 5 separate manufacturers involved in the development and testing of highly sophisticated, versatile arrhythmia control devices. Fourth generation implantable cardioverter-defibrillator systems with advanced diagnostic and therapeutic features are currently under investigation by a number of manufacturers, and some are likely to become approved for marketing within one to two years. Several manufacturers are also active in the development and testing of non-thoracotomy lead systems. Advances in shock waveform technology (e.g., biphasic, quadraphasic shocks) and current delivery systems (e.g., bidirectional, sequential current pathways), may reduce energy requirements, improve the efficiency of defibrillation, and permit the use of smaller batteries and capacitors. Devices of smaller size will simplify further the implantation procedure and ultimately permit pectoral placement of the pulse generator. Recent studies in animals have shown that thorascopically implanted patch electrodes may be feasible in the future, thereby simplifying the implantation of extrapericardial leads. Newer devices will contain advanced arrhythmia detection algorithms capable of reliably distinguishing between supraventricular and ventricular arrhythmias. Subsequent generations of devices will also incorporate an atrial electrode resulting in "DDD-ICDs". An atrial electrode will enable reliable differentiation between ventricular and supraventricular tachycardias, and permit antitachycardia atrial pacing in response to supraventricular arrhythmias. In addition, these units will provide dual chamber pacing functions that are necessary in about 10 to 15% of patients currently receiving ICDs.[18] Although somewhat more speculative, some future devices may also contain closed-loop drug infusion systems, permitting adjunctive drug therapy to be delivered in response to spontaneous arrhythmias. This system potentially might minimize or eliminate altogether the need for chronic oral antiarrhythmic drug therapy in some patients, and may improve further the ability of these devices to provide effective pacing and defibrillation therapy. The ultimate challenge for the future will lie in the detection of premonitory biological signals that will trigger electrical and/or pharmacologic interventions directed at the prevention of ventricular tachycardia and fibrillation.[57]

REFERENCES

1. WHO Scientific Group: Sudden cardiac death. *WHO Tech Rep Ser* 1985; 726:5.
2. Kerber RE, Jensen SR, Gascho JA, Grayzel J, Hoyt R, Kennedy J: Determinants of defibrillation: A prospective analysis of 183 patients. *Am J Cardiol* 1983; 52:739–745.
3. DeLuna AB, Coumel P, Leclercq JF: Ambulatory sudden cardiac death: Mechanisms of production of fatal arrhythmias on the basis of 157 cases. *Am Heart J* 1989; 117:151–159.
4. Pionkowski RS, Thompson BM, Gruchow HW, Aprahamian CV, Darin JC: Resuscitation time in ventricular fibrillation—a prognosis indicator. *Ann Emerg Med* 1983; 12:733–738.
5. Weaver WD, Cobb LA, Hallstrom AP, Fahrenbruch C, Copass MK, Ray R: Factors influencing survival after out-of-hospital cardiac arrest. *J Am Coll Cardiol* 1986; 7:752–757.

6. Mirowski M: The automatic implantable cardioverter/defibrillator: An overview. *J Am Cardiol* 1985; 6:461–466.
7. Brooks R, McGovern BA, Garan H, Ruskin JN. Current treatment of patients surviving out-of-hospital cardiac arrest. *JAMA* 1991; 265:762–768.
8. Hobbs JA, Bigelow WG: Electrical treatment of cardiac arrest: A cardiac stimulator-defibrillator. *Surgery* 1954; 36:833–849.
9. Mirowski M, Mower MM, Staewen WS, Denniston RH, Mendelhoff AI: The development of the transvenous automatic defibrillator. *Arch Intern Med* 1972; 129:773–779.
10. Schuder JC, Stoeckle H, Gold JH, West JA, Keskar PY: Experimental ventricular defibrillation with an automatic and completely implanted system. *Trans Am Soc Artif Intern Org* 1970; 16:207–214.
11. Mirowski M, Mower MM, Langer A, Hellman MS, Schreibman J: A chronically implanted system for automatic defibrillation in active conscious dogs. Experimental model for treatment of sudden death from ventricular fibrillation. *Circulation* 1978; 58:90–93.
12. Mirowski M, Reid PR, Mower MM, Watkins L, Gott VL, Schauble JF, et al: Termination of malignant ventricular arrhythmias with an implanted automatic defibrillator in human beings. *N Engl J Med* 1980; 303:322–324.
13. Federal Register, November 15, 1985.
14. Winkle RA, Mead RH, Ruder MA, Gaudiani V, Buch WS, Pless B, et al: Improved low energy defibrillation efficacy in man with the use of biphasic truncated exponential waveform. *Am Heart J* 1989; 117:122–127.
15. Schaffer WA, Cobb LA: Recurrent ventricular fibrillation and modes of death in survivors of out-of-hospital ventricular fibrillation. 1975; *N Engl J Med* 293:259–262.
16. Cobb LA, Baum RS, Alvarez H, Schaffer WA: Resuscitation from an out-of-hospital ventricular fibrillation: Four years follow-up. *Circulation* 1975; 52:III-223.
17. Winkle RA, Mead RH, Ruder MA, Gaudiani VA, Smith NA, Buch WA, et al: Long-term outcome with the automatic implantable cardioverter/defibrillator. *J Am Coll Cardiol* 1989; 13:1353–1361.
18. Reid PR, Griffith LSC, Platia EV, Borggrefe M, Zipes DP: The automatic implantable cardioverter/defibrillator: five-year clinical experience. In: Breithardt G, Borggrefe M, Zipes DP (eds): *Nonpharmacological Therapy of Tachyarrhythmias*. London, England: Futura Publishing, 1987:477–485.
19. Kelly PA, Cannom DS, Garan H, Mirabal GS, Harthorne WJ, Hurtivz RJ, et al: The automatic implantable cardioverter-defibrillator: Efficacy, complications, and survival in patients with malignant ventricular arrhythmias. *J Am Coll Cardiol* 1988; 11:1278–1286.
20. Manolis AS, Tan-DeGuzman W, Lee MA, Rastegar H, Haffajee CI, Huang JKS, et al: Clinical experience in seventy-seven patients with the automatic implantable cardioverter/defibrillator. *Am Heart J* 1989; 118:445–449.
21. Tchou PJ, Kadri N, Anderson J, Caceres JA: Jazayeri M, Akhtar M: Automatic implantable cardioverter/defibrillators and survival of patients with left ventricular dysfunction and malignant ventricular arrhythmias. *Ann Intern Med* 1988; 109:529–534.
22. Myerburg RJ, Luceri RM, Thurer R, Couper DK, Zaman L, Interian A, et al: Time to first shock and clinical outcome in patients receiving an automatic implantable cardioverter/defibrillator. *J Am Coll Cardiol* 1989; 14:508–514.
23. Wilber DJ, Garan H, Finkelstein D, Kelly E, Newell J, McGovern BA, et al: Out-of-hospital cardiac arrest: Use of electrophysiologic testing in the prediction of long-term outcome. *N Engl J Med* 1988; 318:19–24.
24. Myerberg RJ, Conde CA, Sung RJ, Mayorga-Cortes A, Mallon SM, Sheps DS, et al: Clinical, electrophysiologic, and hemodynamic profile of patients resuscitated from pre-hospital cardiac arrest. *Am J Med* 1980; 68:568–576.
25. Morady F, Scheinman MM, Hess DS, Sung RJ, Shen E, Shapiro W: Electrophysiologic testing in the management of survivors of out-of-hospital cardiac arrest. *Am J Cardiol* 1983; 51:85–89.
26. Roy D, Waxman HL, Kienzle MG, Buxton AE, Marchlinski FE, Josephson ME: Clinical characteristics and long-term follow-up in 119 survivors of cardiac arrest: Relation to inducibility at electrophysiologic testing. *Am J Cardiol* 1983; 52:969–974.
27. Benditt DG, Benson DW, Klein GJ, Pritzker MR, Kreitt JM, Anderson RW: Prevention of recurrent sudden cardiac death: Role of provocative electropharmacologic testing. *J Am Coll Cardiol* 1983; 2:418–425.
28. Skale BT, Miles WM, Heger JJ, Zipes DP, Prystowsky EN: Survivors of cardiac arrest: Prevention of recurrence by drug therapy as predicted by electrophysiologic testing or electrocardiographic monitoring. *Am J Cardiol* 1986; 57:113–119.
29. Eldar M, Sauve MJ, Scheinman MM: Electrophysiologic testing and follow-up of patients with aborted sudden death. *J Am Coll Cardiol* 1987; 10:291–298.
30. Lehmann MH, Steinman RT, Shuger CD, Jackson K: The automatic implantable cardioverter/defibrillator as antiarrhythmic treatment modality of choice for survivors of cardiac arrest unrelated to acute myocardial infarction. *Am J Cardiol* 1988; 62:803–805.
31. Herre JM, Sauve MJ, Malone P, Griffin JS, Helmy I, Langberg JJ, et al: Long-term results of amiodarone therapy in patients with recurrent sustained ventricular tachycardia or fibrillation. *J Am Coll Cardiol* 1989; 13:442–449.
32. Eisenberg MS, Hallstrom A, Bergner L: Long-term survival after out-of-hospital cardiac arrest. *N Engl J Med* 1982; 306:1340–1343.
33. Cardiac Arrhythmia Suppression Trial (CAST) Investigators: Preliminary report: Effect of encainide and flecainide on mortality in a randomized trial of arrhythmia suppression after myocardial infarction. *N Engl J Med* 1989; 321:406–412.
34. Nisam S, Thomas A, Mower M, Hauser R: Identifying patients for prophylactic automatic implantable cardioverter defibrillator therapy: Status of prospective studies. *Am Heart J* 1991; 122:607–612.
35. Kim SG, Furman S, Waspe L, Brodman R, Fisher JD: Unipolar pacer/artifacts induced failure of an automatic implantable cardioverter/defibrillator to detect ventricular fibrillation. *Am J Cardiol* 1986; 57:880–881.
36. Almassi GH, Chapman PD, Troup PJ, Whetherbee JN, Olinger GN: Constrictive pericarditis associated with patch electrodes of the automatic implantable cardioverter-defibrillator. *Chest* 1987; 92:369–371.
37. Thurer RJ, Luceri RM, Bolooki H: Automatic implantable cardioverter/defibrillator: Techniques of implantation and results. *Ann Thorac Surg* 1986; 42:143–147.
38. Troup PJ, Chapman PD, Olinger GN, Kleinman LH: The implantable defibrillator: Relation of defibrillating lead configurations and clinical variables to defibrillation thresholds. *J Am Coll Cardiol* 1985; 6:1315–1321.
39. McGowan R, Maloney J, Wilkoff B, Simmons T, Khoury D, McAlister H, et al: Automatic implantable cardioverter-defibrillator without thoracotomy using an endocardial and submuscular patch system. *J Am Coll Cardiol* 1991; 17:415–421.
40. Winkle RA, Bach SM, Mead H, Guadiani VA, Stinson EB, Fain ES, et al: Comparison of defibrillation efficacy in humans using a new catheter and superior vena cava spring—left ventricular patch electrode. *J Am Coll Cardiol* 1988; 11:365–370.
41. Data on File, Cardiac Pacemakers Incorporated, Minneapolis, MN.
42. Saksena S, Mehta D, Krol RB, Tullo NG, Saxena A, Kaushik R, et al: Experience with a third generation implantable cardioverter-defibrillator. *Am J Cardiol* 1991; 67:1375–1384.
43. Levine JH, Mellits D, Baumgardner RA, Veltri EP, Mower M, Grunwald BA, et al: Predictors of first discharge and subsequent survival in patients with automatic implantable cardioverter-defibrillators. *Circulation* 1991; 84:558–566.
44. Data on file, Ventritex Corporation, Sunydale, CA.
45. Steinman RT, Thomas AC, Schuger C, Lehmann MH: Clinical findings in monitored cases of sudden cardiac death in patients with an automatic implantable defibrillator (abstr). *PACE* 1989; 12:646.
46. Vlay S, Olson LC, Burger L. Internal cardioverter defibrillator component failure. *PACE* 1990; 13:1086–1087.
47. Fogros RN, Ebson JJ, Bonnett CA: Actuarial incidence and pattern of occurrence of shocks following implantation of the automatic implantable cardioverter defibrillator. *PACE* 1989; 12:1465
48. Wetherbee JN, Chapman PDm, Troup PJ, Veneth-Rogers, Thakur RK, Hossein TG, et al: Long-term internal cardiac defibrillation threshold stability. *PACE* 1989; 12:443
49. Joachim-Trappe H. Klein H. Frank G, Wenzlaff P: Do the defibrillation thresholds of an automatic defibrillator remain acceptable with time? (abstr). *PACE* 1989; 12:664.
50. Vlay SC: Defibrillation testing. Necessary but evil. *Am Heart J* 1989; 117:499–504.
51. Guarnieri T, Levine JH, Veltri E, Griffith LSC, Watkins L, Juan-

teguy J, et al: Success of chronic defibrillation and the role of antiarrhythmic drugs with automatic implantable cardioverter/defibrillator. *Am J Cardiol* 1987 60:1061–1064.

52. Echt DS, Black JN, Barbey JT, Coxe DR, Cato E: Evaluation of antiarrhythmic drugs on defibrillation energy requirements in dogs. *Circulation* 1989; 79:1106–1117.
53. Marinchak RA, Friehling TD, Kline RA, Stohler J, Kowey PR: Effect of antiarrhythmic drugs on defibrillation threshold: Case report of an adverse effect of Mexiletine and review of the literature. *PACE* 1988; 11:7–12.
54. Masterson M, Maloney J, Wilkoff B, Simmons T, Morant V, Golding LAR, et al: Clinical performance of the automatic implantable cardioverter-defibrillator: Electrocardiographic documentation of 82 spontaneous discharges. *J Am Coll Cardiol* 1988; 11:18A.
55. Strickberger SA, Cantillon CO, Friedman PL: When should patients with lethal ventricular arrhythmias resume driving. An analysis of state regulations and physician practices. *Ann Intern Med* 1991; 115:560–563.
56. Kuppermann M, Luce BR, McGovern B, Podrid PJ, Bigger JT, Ruskin JN: An analysis of the cost effectiveness of the implantable defibrillator. *Circulation* 1990: 81:91–100.
57. Prystowsky EN, Miles WM, Windle JR, Gilmour RF, Skale BT, Kammerling J, et al: Electrical inhibition of the myocardium: A mode to prevent the occurrence of tachyarrhythmias? In: Breithardt G, Borggrefe M, Zipes DP (eds): *Nonpharmacologic Therapy of Arrhythmias*. Mt. Kisco, NY, Futura Publishing, 1987; 359–367.

Chapter 43

Treatment of Cardiac Arrhythmias with Catheter Ablative Techniques

Melvin M. Scheinman, M.D.

Over the past several years various techniques have been introduced using catheter ablative procedures for patients with cardiac arrhythmias. Particularly impressive are some of the newer techniques utilizing radiofrequency energy sources for patients with supraventricular arrhythmias. In this chapter we will review the techniques, results, and clinical indications for these procedures.

TECHNIQUES

Ablation of the Atrioventricular Junction

Our laboratory introduced the technique of catheter ablation of the atrioventricular (AV) junction in canines.[1] This technique was subsequently utilized for the control of drug-refractory atrial arrhythmias in patients.[2,3] Multipolar electrode catheters are inserted by vein and positioned just across the tricuspid valve and against the apex of the right ventricle. A short intraarterial cannula is used for continuous monitoring of the arterial pressure. The catheter across the tricuspid valve is manipulated to allow the recording of the largest unipolar His bundle potential (Fig. 43-1).[2,3] Radiofrequency energy 350 to 500 kHz is applied between the distal electrode and a large back patch. After persistent AV block is observed, a permanent cardiac pacemaker is inserted.

Ablation of Accessory Pathways

Patients with accessory extranodal pathways often experience reentrant arrhythmias with tachycardia circuit involving antegrade conduction over the normal AV nodal conduction system and retrograde conduction over the accessory pathway.[4] Surgical techniques have proved very effective and safe in the interruption of these pathways.[5] More recently, a variety of catheter techniques have been introduced for attempted catheter ablation of these pathways. Fisher et al.[6] were the first to use this technique for attempted ablation of left free wall accessory pathways via the coronary sinus. Accessory AV pathways occur anywhere along the cardiac annulus or in the septum. The majority of pathways are found traversing the left AV groove. These pathways are currently approached by inserting a steerable multipolar electrode catheter into the femoral artery and retrograde catheterization of the left ventricle. The catheter is then placed under the mitral annulus in the putative site of the accessory pathway. One or more applications of radiofrequency energy are applied in order to ablate the pathways. In contrast, most septal and all right free wall pathways are approached from right-sided catheterization.

Modification of the Atrioventricular Node in Atrioventricular Nodal Reentrant Tachycardia

Patients with AV nodal reentrant tachycardia are thought to have two pathways within or in close proximity to the AV node. These pathways show fast and slow conducting properties and have different refractory periods. Techniques have been introduced that allow for selective ablation of either pathway. The fast pathway is

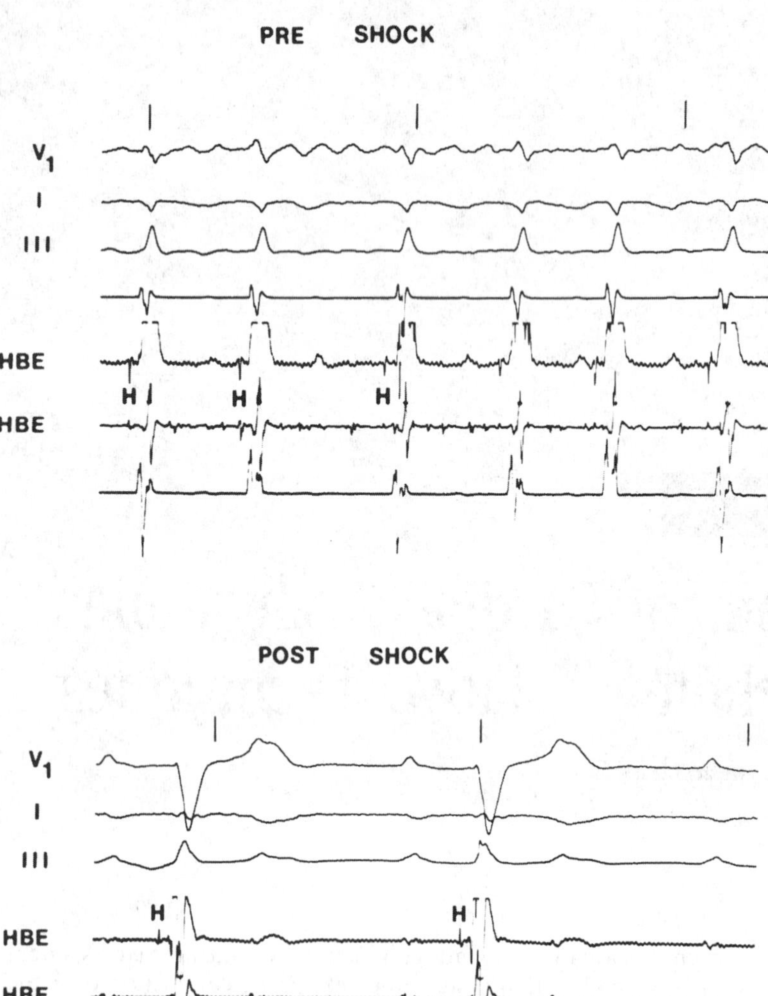

FIGURE 43-1 *Top panel:* Atrial fibrillation with rapid ventricular response with a His bundle deflection recorded prior to each ventricular depolarization. *Bottom panel:* After delivery of 300 J to the AV junction, complete AV block is present and atrial fibrillation has reverted to sinus rhythm. Note the P wave located in the T wave.

approached by withdrawing the catheter recording the His bundle potential to a more proximal location that is associated with a large-amplitude atrial electrogram and a very small (<100 mV) or absent His deflection.[7] Application of radiofrequency energy to this area results in abrupt prolongation of the PR or AH since ablation of the fast pathway forces conduction over the slow pathway. An alternative technique for ablation of the slow pathway was introduced by Roman and associates.[8] In this procedure, the radiofrequency energy is applied posteriorly between the os of the coronary sinus and the septal leaflet of the tricuspid valve. Successful application of the latter technique does not result in a change in the PR or AH.

Ablation of Ventricular Tachycardia Foci

The most demanding of the catheter ablative techniques is attempted ablation of ventricular tachycardia foci. For this procedure, multipolar electrode catheters are inserted into the right ventricle, coronary sinus, and left ventricle. Ventricular tachycardia is induced by using standard stimulation protocols, and the catheters are manipulated within the ventricles in order to determine the earliest ventricular endocardial electrogram (during ventricular tachycardia) in relation to at least three reference orthogonal surface leads.[9] Ventricular overdrive pacing is used in an attempt to entrain the tachycardia and to prove that the earliest endocardial potentials precede (rather than follow) the tachycardia complex. In addition, the putative ventricular tachycardia focus is paced in an effort to determine whether the paced complexes are identical or similar to the induced tachycardia.[10] The latter procedure is known as pace mapping. Once the earliest site is found, one or more direct current shocks or radiofrequency applications are delivered from the distal electrode near this endocardial site to a chest wall patch placed closest to the distal electrode. A subset of patients with ventricular tachycardia particularly amenable to catheter ablation are those with bundle branch reentrant arrhythmias. In these patients the tachycardia mechanism involves bundle-to-bundle conduction.[11] Catheter cure may be achieved by ablation of the right bundle branch. The right bundle is usually draped superficially over the right septal surface of the ventricular septum and the right bundle potential is usually easily located. The right bundle may be ablated either by direct current or preferably by radiofrequency discharges.[12]

RESULTS OF CATHETER ABLATIVE PROCEDURES

Atrioventricular Junctional Ablation

To date, the largest experience relating to the various ablative procedures has been accumulated from a worldwide voluntary ablation registry.[13] At present, over 500 attempted catheter ablations of the AV junction using direct-current shocks have been reported to the registry. Analysis of the first consecutive 367 patients[12] has shown the following results: Complete permanent AV block was achieved in 231 (63 percent) patients. In 37 (10 percent), AV conduction resumed after the procedure but conduction was sufficiently modified so that no further antiarrhythmic drug therapy was required. In 44 (12 percent), AV conduction resumed but arrhythmia control was achieved by drug therapy, while the procedure proved unsuccessful in 55 (15 percent). Overall, an excellent or good response in terms of arrhythmia control was achieved in 85 percent of patients. Similar results have been reported using radiofrequency discharges.[14] The advantages of the latter technique include obviation of barotraumatic injury as well as the need for general anesthesia.

Ablation of Accessory Pathways

Results from a number of centers have documented the remarkable efficacy of catheter ablative techniques. Warin and others[15] reported a consecutive series of 248 patients who underwent direct current ablation of accessory pathways with a success rate of 96 percent. Significant complications of direct-current shock include rare episodes of cardiac tamponade, coronary artery spasm, and two episodes of late sudden death. Similar success rates have been reported by others using radiofrequency ablative techniques without any reports of sudden cardiac death.[16,17]

Modification of the Atrioventricular Junction for Atrioventricular Nodal Reentrant Tachycardia

Several groups have reported success rates of from 85 to 100 percent for attenuation of AV nodal function resulting in tachycardia cure. Although initial reports used high-energy direct-current discharges,[18,19] more recent results suggest that radiofrequency techniques are equally effective and have less side effects.[7,8] The chief adverse effect of this technique is the potential for producing complete AV block, which has been reported to be as high as 8 percent for attempted fast pathway ablation.[7] A lower incidence of AV block has been reported for attempted slow pathway conduction.[20]

Ablation of the Ventricular Tachycardia Foci

Attempts at catheter ablation of ventricular tachycardia foci have been reported by a number of groups with varying success.[20,21] The largest aggregate experience to date is reported from the worldwide registry.[13] In the 150 reported ablative attempts, 33 percent of patients had arrhythmia control without the need for antiarrhythmic drugs, an additional 20 percent had arrhythmia control with continued drug therapy, and the remainder failed ablative therapy. The series reported by Morady et al.[20] showed similar results; however, significantly better results were reported by Fontaine et al.[22] Reported serious complications include induction of severe low-output states, malignant ventricular arrhythmias, electromechanical dissociation, and cerebrovascular accidents. The catheter technique has proven to be most successful for patients with bundle branch reentry tachycardia. Selective destruction of the right bundle branch is easy to perform and curative. More recent reports have documented successful ablation in patients with right ventricular outflow tract tachycardias.

ADVANTAGES AND DISADVANTAGES OF CATHETER ABLATIVE TECHNIQUES

Advantages

The use of catheter ablative techniques has greatly impacted on our approach to the management of patients with supraventricular tachycardia. Catheter ablation of the AV junction has replaced the need for surgical ablation of the His bundle for patients with atrial arrhythmias refractory to drug therapy. Catheter procedures may cure patients with reentrant supraventricular arrhythmias. The initial reports suggest a cure rate of 90 to 100 percent with minimal serious adverse effects.[16,17] For selected patients with ventricular tachycardia, catheter ablative procedures may obviate the need for surgical intervention. This is particularly true for patients with bundle branch reentry or with right ventricular outflow tract tachycardias.

Disadvantages

The chief disadvantage of AV junctional ablation is the need for chronic cardiac pacing after successful ablation. Another serious adverse effect is the reported 2 to 4 percent incidence of polymorphous ventricular tachycardia occurring in the postablative period.[23] This arrhythmia is more common in patients with severe myocardial disease, bradycardia, and electrolyte abnormalities and may be enhanced by use of class IA antiarrhythmic agents. The chief complication reported for patients undergoing AV modification procedures is the risk for complete AV block. Attempted ablation of the slow AV nodal pathway as well as more meticulous attention to the proper technique for fast pathway ablation promises to diminish or obviate this risk.

The chief risk of catheter ablation of accessory pathways appears to be induction of coronary spasm when energy is applied in close proximity to the coronary arteries. In addition, the prolonged exposure to irradiation, which is at times required for pathway ablation, is of concern.

Major complications have been reported in the use of catheter-delivered direct-current shocks for treatment of ventricular tachycardia. Such complications include shock-induced ventricular arrhythmias, depression of ventricular function, cardiac tamponade, cerebral embolism, and electromechanical dissociation.

CONCLUSION

Catheter ablative techniques have revolutionized our approach to the management of patients with supraventricular tachycardia. These techniques have evolved to the point where curative ablative procedures are recommended as the treatment of choice for all symptomatic patients with accessory pathway-mediated tachycardias and for most patients with symptomatic AV nodal reentrant tachycardia. Complete AV junctional ablation is the procedure of choice for patients with drug refractory atrial arrhythmias. While selected patients with ventricular arrhythmias may benefit from catheter ablative techniques, the majority of these patients are best managed by drug, device, or surgical therapy.

REFERENCES

1. Gonzalez R, Scheinman M, Margaretten W, Rubinstein M: Closed-chest electrode-catheter technique for His bundle ablation in dogs. *Am J Physiol* 1981; 241:H283–H287.
2. Scheinman MM, Morady F, Hess DS, Gonzalez R: Catheter-induced ablation of the atrioventricular junction to control refractory supraventricular arrhythmias. *JAMA* 1982; 248:851–855.
3. Gallagher JJ, Svenson RH, Kasell JH, et al: Catheter technique for closed-chest ablation of the atrioventricular conduction system: A therapeutic alternative for the treatment of refractory supraventricular tachycardia. *N Engl J Med* 1982; 306:194–200.
4. Gallagher JJ, Gilbert M, Swenson RH, Sealy WC, Kasell J, Wallace AG: Wolff-Parkinson-White syndrome: The problem, evaluation, and surgical correction. *Circulation* 1975; 51:767–785.
5. Gallagher JJ, Sealy WC, Cox JL, Kasell JH: Results of surgery for preexcitation in 200 consecutive cases. In: Levy S, Scheinman MM (eds): *Cardiac Arrhythmias: From Diagnosis to Therapy.* Mt. Kisco, NY, Futura Publishing, 1984: 323–340.
6. Fisher JD, Brodman R, Kim SG, Matos JA, Brodman E, Wallerson D: Attempted nonsurgical electrical ablation of accessory pathways via the coronary sinus in the Wolff-Parkinson-White syndrome. *J Am Coll Cardiol* 1984; 4:685–694.
7. Lee MA, Morady F, Kadish A, Schamp DJ, Chin MC, Scheinman MM: Catheter modification of the atrioventricular junction with radiofrequency energy for control of atrioventricular nodal reentry tachycardia. *Circulation* 1991; 83:827–835.
8. Roman CA, Wang X, Friday KJ, Moulton KP, Margolis PD, Klonis D: Catheter technique for selective ablation of slow pathway in AV nodal reentrant tachycardia. *PACE* 1990; 13:498 (abstr).
9. Marchlinski FE, Almendrah JM, Cassidy DM, et al: Localization of endocardial site for catheter ablation of ventricular tachycardia. In: Fontaine G, Scheinman MM (eds): *Ablation in Cardiac Arrhythmias.* Mt. Kisco, New York, Futura Publishing, 1987: 289–302.
10. Josephson ME, Waxman HL, Cain ME, Gardner MJ, Buxton AE: Ventricular activation during ventricular endocardial pacing: II. Role of pacemapping to localize origin of ventricular tachycardia. *Am J Cardiol* 1982; 50:11–22.
11. Tchou P, Jazayeri M, Denker S, Dongas J, Caceres J, Akhtar M: Transcatheter electrical ablation of right bundle branch: A method of treating macroreentrant ventricular tachycardia attributed to bundle branch reentry. *Circulation* 1988; 78:246–257.
12. Langberg JJ, Desai J, Dullet N, Scheinman MM: Treatment of macroreentrant ventricular tachycardia with radiofrequency ablation of the right bundle branch. *Am J Cardiol* 1989; 63:1010–1013.
13. Scheinman MM, Evans-Bell T, The Executive Committee of the Percutaneous Mapping and Ablation Registry: Catheter ablation of the atrioventricular junction: A report of the Percutaneous Mapping and Ablation Registry. *Circulation* 1984; 70:1024–1029.
14. Langberg JJ, Chin MC, Rosenqvist M, Cockrell J, Dullet N, Van Hare G: Catheter ablation of the atrioventricular junction with radiofrequency energy. *Circulation* 1989; 80:1527–1535.
15. Warin J-F, Haissaguerre M, D'Ivernois C, LeMetayer P, Montserrat P: Catheter ablation of accessory pathways: Technique and results in 248 patients. *PACE* 1990; 13:1609–1614.
16. Calkins H, Sousa J, El-Atassi R, Rosenheck S, deBuitleir M, Kou WH: Diagnosis and cure of the Wolff-Parkinson-White syndrome or paroxysmal supraventricular tachycardias during a single electrophysiologic test. *N Engl J Med* 1991; 324:1612–1618.
17. Jackman WM, Wang XH, Friday KJ, Roman CA, Moulton KP, Beckman KJ: Catheter ablation of accessory atrioventricular pathways (Wolff-Parkinson-White syndrome) by radiofrequency current. *N Engl J Med* 1991; 324:1605–1611.
18. Haissaguerre M, Warin JF, Lematayer P, Saoudi N, Guillem JP, Blanchot P: Closed-chest ablation of retrograde conduction in patients with atrioventricular nodal reentrant tachycardia. *N Engl J Med* 1989; 320:426–433.
19. Epstein LM, Scheinman MM, Langberg JJ, Chilson D, Goldberg HR, Griffin JC: Percutaneous catheter modification of the atrioventricular node: A potential cure for atrioventricular nodal reentrant tachycardia. *Circulation* 1989; 80:757–768.
20. Morady F, Scheinman MM, DiCarlo LA Jr, Davis JC, Herre JM, Griffin JC: Catheter ablation of ventricular tachycardia with intracardiac shocks: Results in 33 patients. *Circulation* 1987; 75:1037–1049.
21. Belhassen B, Miller HI, Geller E, Laniado S: Transcatheter electrical shock ablation of ventricular tachycardia. *J Am Coll Cardiol* 1986; 7:1347–1355.
22. Fontaine G, Tonet JL, Frank R, Gallais Y, Farenq G, Grosgogeat Y: La fulguration endocavitaire: Une nouvelle methode de traitement des troubles du rhythme? *Ann Cardiol Angeiol (Paris)* 1984; 33:543–561.
23. Scheinman MM: Catheter ablation: present role and projected impact on health care for patients with cardiac arrhythmias. *Circulation* 1991; 83:1489–1498.

Chapter 44

Surgical Treatment of Cardiac Arrhythmias

James L. Cox, M.D.

During the past two decades, the evolution of cardiac arrhythmia surgery has paralleled the progressive elucidation of the anatomic and electrophysiologic abnormalities responsible for supraventricular tachyarrhythmias. The development of sophisticated electrophysiologic mapping systems and anatomically precise surgical techniques combined to provide the ability to cure the Wolff-Parkinson-White (WPW) syndrome, atrioventricular (AV) node reentry tachycardia, automatic atrial tachycardias, and ischemic and nonischemic ventricular tachyarrhythmias. Knowledge gained from the electrophysiologically guided surgical approaches to the WPW syndrome and AV node reentry tachycardia contributed in part to the more recent development of endocardial catheter techniques capable of curing these arrhythmias without the need for surgical intervention (see Chap. 43).[1,2] In addition, the increasing sophistication and availability of antitachycardia pacemakers and implantable cardioverter-defibrillator devices[3] have narrowed the indications for surgical intervention for refractory ventricular tachyarrhythmias.

Despite these technological advances, surgery remains an important therapeutic modality for the treatment of cardiac arrhythmias. Indeed, the recent development of a surgical technique for the treatment of atrial fibrillation[4-8] represents perhaps the only means by which this most common of all cardiac arrhythmias can be cured. Moreover, the present results of surgery for ventricular tachycardia, in properly selected patients, are comparable to those once attainable only in patients with supraventricular arrhythmias. Thus, the contemporary therapy for cardiac arrhythmias includes a variety of therapeutic options that, when used in a complementary fashion, are capable of curing virtually all supraventricular and ventricular tachyarrhythmias.

SURGERY FOR SUPRAVENTRICULAR ARRHYTHMIAS

The introduction of endocardial catheter techniques utilizing radiofrequency energy has had its most dramatic impact on the treatment of supraventricular arrhythmias, particularly those associated with the WPW syndrome and AV node reentry.[2] Despite the rather dramatic decrease in the number of patients who now require surgery for these arrhythmias, a thorough knowledge of the anatomy, electrophysiology, and surgical techniques remains of paramount importance not only to the surgeon but also the interventional electrophysiologist.

WPW Syndrome

The WPW syndrome is caused by accessory connections ("accessory pathways") that span the AV groove and connect the atrium to the ventricle electrically. Traditionally, the location of accessory pathways in the WPW syndrome has been based on the site of insertion of the ventricular end of the pathway. This arbitrary classification of accessory pathway locations into left free-wall, posterior septal, right free-wall, and anterior septal spaces (in decreasing order of frequency) has proven to be advantageous, not only because of the dissimilarities of the electrophysiological manifestations of pathways located in each of these four areas but also because the surgical approach to each of these four spaces is unique. The four anatomical spaces in which a given accessory pathway may reside are identified by viewing the AV groove in the horizontal plane (Fig. 44-1).[9] Both the preoperative catheter electrophysiology study and the intraoperative mapping procedure are directed toward localizing an accessory pathway to one of these four anatomic spaces.

Surgical therapy for the WPW syndrome is directed at locating and dividing the accessory AV connections, thus leaving the patient with normal AV conduction via the AV node–His bundle complex. The first successful surgical procedure for the WPW syndrome was performed by Sealy in 1968,[10] an event that ushered in the modern era of cardiac arrhythmia surgery. Two surgical approaches have evolved into current use.[11] Most commonly, surgery to interrupt these pathways by the standard endocardial approach originally described by Sealy and coworkers[12] and modified by the author in 1981.[9] The alternative surgical approach is an epicardial one, described by Giuraudon and associates in 1984 (Fig. 44-2).[13] The endocardial technique is designed to divide the ventricular end of the accessory pathway, and the epicardial technique divides the atrial end of the pathway. Although the epicardial technique has been described as a "closed-heart cryosurgical technique," it is neither closed-heart nor cryosurgery-dependent in the majority of patients. Detailed descriptions of both of these techniques can be found elsewhere.[14,15]

Certain types of congenital heart abnormalities are frequently associated with the WPW syndrome, the most common being Ebstein's anomaly, in which the septal leaflet, and occasionally the posterior leaflet, of the tricuspid valve is displaced downward into the right ventricle (see also Chap. 97).[16] The position of the AV node and conduction bundles in patients with Ebstein's anomaly is normal, although the right bundle branch may be compressed by thickened endocardium. In our experience, a distinct association between patients with Ebstein's anomaly and the specific location of the accessory pathways exists. Most commonly, patients with this anomaly have posterior septal accessory pathways. However, in our series a majority of patients with Ebstein's anomaly have also had a combination of right free-wall and posterior septal accessory pathways.[9] This correlation is so high that if a patient is found to have this combination of pathways on the preoperative electrophysiologic study, an echocardiogram is indicated to determine the presence or absence of Ebstein's anomaly.

Standard endocardial techniques are used to interrupt these accessory pathways. If valve replacement or placement of an annuloplasty ring is necessary to correct severe Ebstein's anomaly, the valve or annuloplasty ring should be placed below the coronary sinus by sutures placed through the true tricuspid annulus. Plication of the atrialized ventricle may or may not be necessary.

The incidence of successful surgical correction of the WPW syndrome now approaches 100 percent, with an operative mortality that ranges from 0 to 0.5 percent. Both early and late recurrences following surgery utilizing either the endocardial or the epicardial technique are extremely unusual.[14,15] Problems such as the inadvertent creation of heart block are now of historical interest only. While similar results have not yet been achieved with radiofrequency catheter ablation techniques, the avoidance of a thoracotomy and major surgery in the

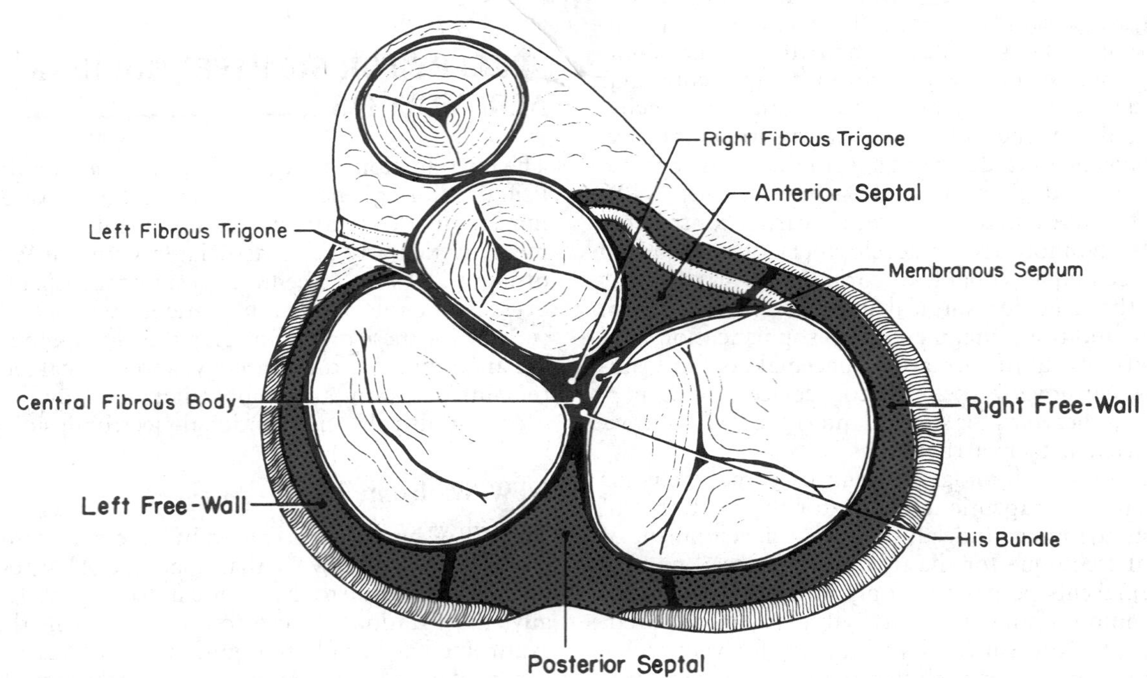

FIGURE 44-1 Diagram of the superior view of the heart with the atria cut away, demonstrating the boundaries of each of the four anatomic areas where accessory pathways can occur in the WPW syndrome. (Reproduced with permission from Cox et al.[9])

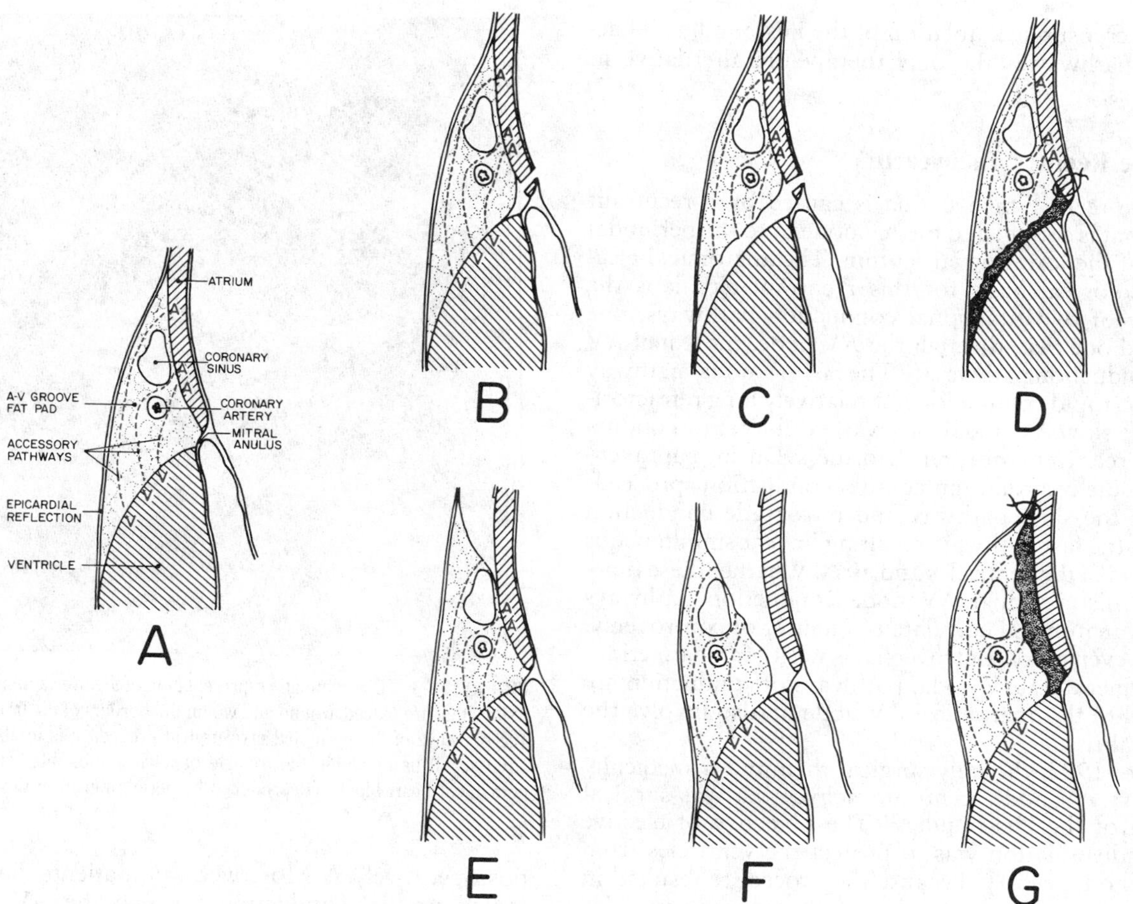

FIGURE 44-2 Diagrammatic representation of a cross section of the posterior left heart showing the various depths at which left free-wall pathways can be located in relation to the mitral annulus and the epicardial reflection. *B–D.* The endocardial surgical technique. *E–G.* The epicardial technique. (Reproduced by permission from Cox et al.[11])

majority of patients has revolutionized the nonpharmacologic treatment of this syndrome. Surgery is currently indicated primarily when catheter ablation (Chap. 43) has failed or when concomitant surgery for other cardiac conditions is required.

Mahaim Fibers

Nodofascicular and fasciculoventricular connections, as described by Mahaim, occur between the nodal and fascicular components of the AV node–His bundle complex and the ventricular septum. Classically, these fibers have been depicted as originating from the AV node or its penetrating (His) bundle and then perforating the central fibrous body to insert into the ventricular myocardium. More recently, the appropriateness of depicting these accessory pathways as nodoventricular has been questioned. Tchou and colleagues[17] have suggested that such pathways represent atriofascicular connections with decremental conduction properties without direct anatomic connection to the AV nodal tissue, and Klein and coworkers[18] have suggested that "typical" nodoventricular connections may be atypical accessory pathways with decremental conduction properties and a distal right ventricular insertion site. Whatever the substrate, from a surgical point of view, Mahaim fibers may connect the His bundle to the ventricular septum by traversing the posterior septal space or the anterior septal space, in which case the Mahaim fiber is anterior to the His bundle. In addition, right free-wall accessory pathways with typical "Mahaim-like" characteristics have been reported,[18] and left-sided nodoventricular connections have recently been described as well.[19]

Depending on the spatial separation of the Mahaim fiber and the His bundle, these accessory connections can be interrupted using standard endocardial surgical dissection techniques in combination with cryosurgery. The surgical approach depends on the location of the accessory pathway as determined by preoperative and intraoperative electrophysiological mapping. When the posterior septal space is involved, a combination of discrete cryosurgery[20] and a posterior septal space dissection is required in some patients, while in others cryosurgery alone is sufficient to interrupt the pathway. In still other patients, a combination of cryosurgery with both anterior and posterior septal dissections is necessary. Finally, a subset of patients have what should be classified as "para-Hisian" connections, since despite all maneuvers the accessory connection is so closely juxtaposed to the His bundle that it cannot be separated surgically. Simultaneous cryosurgical ablation of the His bundle and accessory pathway is the only therapeutic alternative in such cases.

AV Node Reentry Tachycardia

AV node reentry tachycardia is caused by a reentrant circuit that is confined to the AV node or to the perinodal tissues of the lower atrial septum. The anatomical-electrophysiological basis for this reentrant circuit is the presence of two functional conduction pathways, one slow and one fast, through the AV node, the "dual AV node conduction pathways." The fast AV nodal pathway manifests rapid conduction but relatively long refractoriness. The slow AV nodal pathway exhibits slow conduction but relatively short refractoriness. During supraventricular tachycardia, antegrade conduction proceeds through the slow pathway and retrograde conduction through the fast pathway, resulting in near simultaneous activation of the ventricles and atria. Whether these functionally distinct dual AV node conduction pathways have an anatomical correlate is a matter of controversy. Perhaps even more controversial is whether the functionally distinct dual AV nodal pathways of conduction are confined to the anatomical AV node or also involve the perinodal tissues.

Before 1982, the only surgical therapy for medically refractory AV node reentrant tachycardia was surgical division of the His bundle.[21] The objective of elective His-bundle ablation was to protect the ventricles from the AV node reentry. Because the procedure resulted in complete heart block, however, a permanent ventricular pacemaker was required postoperatively in all patients, In 1982, Scheinman described a technique for ablating the His bundle by introducing an electrical shock through a catheter placed adjacent to the His bundle.[22] This closed-chest procedure immediately replaced the open heart surgical method of interrupting the His bundle. However, since the catheter fulguration technique also created complete heart block, all of those patients also required implantation of permanent pacemaker systems.

Although both the surgical technique and the catheter ablative technique for His bundle interruption ameliorated the unpleasant and detrimental effects of AV node reentry tachycardia, both procedures replaced one type of arrhythmia (tachycardia) with another (heart block). In 1982, we attained the first clinical cure of AV node reentry tachycardia utilizing a discrete cryosurgical technique (Fig. 44-3).[23] Ross and colleagues subsequently reported the cure of AV node reentry tachycardia utilizing surgical dissection of the perinodal tissues.[24] Guiraudon and colleagues have reported success with a similar surgical dissection technique.[25]

Although the surgical techniques designed to cure AV node reentry tachycardia have been employed for only a short period of time, the results have been excellent. There have been no operative deaths in any of the three major series reported. After a perinodal cyrosurgical procedure, smooth AV node conduction curves through the remaining single conduction pathway have been demonstrated in all 38 patients in our series, and none of the patients has had inducible AV node reentry tachycardia postoperatively.[26] Moreover, all patients have maintained normal conduction through the AV node–His bundle complex with no recurrent AV node reentry tachycardia. The surgical dissection techniques have been associated with a low incidence of permanent complete heart block and a low incidence of recurrent AV node reentry tachycardia.[24,25]

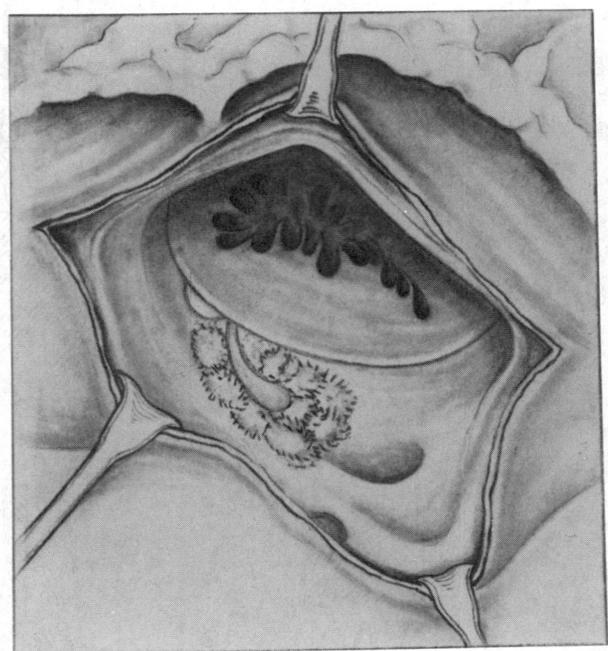

FIGURE 44-3 Diagrammatic representation of the overlapping 3-mm cryolesions that are placed around and within the borders of the triangle of Koch. The objective of the perinodal cryosurgical procedure is to ablate as much atrial septal tissue within the triangle of Koch as possible without causing permanent heart block. (Reproduced by permission from Cox et al.[26])

Currently, radiofrequency catheter techniques (Chap. 43) have replaced surgery as the procedure of choice for AV node reentry tachycardia. However, the incidence of heart block that accompanies the radiofrequency catheter procedures justifies continued consideration of the safer and more effective surgical approaches.

Automatic (Ectopic) Atrial Tachycardia

Clinical data suggest that derangements in automaticity, and not reentry, underlie the genesis of automatic, or ectopic, atrial tachycardias (Chap. 36). These tachycardias appear to have a focal origin and usually originate from the body of the right atrium or left atrium, although they may occasionally arise from the interatrial septum. Accurate preoperative localization is particularly important for patients with automatic atrial tachycardias if surgical ablation of the ectopic focus is contemplated. These tachycardias are frequently suppressed with general anesthesia, and, as a result, intraoperative mapping to localize their site of origin may not be possible. In addition, automatic tachycardias are not inducible by standard programmed stimulation techniques. Without accurate intraoperative localization, elective His bundle ablation was once the only surgical alternative; however, alternative surgical techniques that leave the normal AV conduction intact while isolating the arrhythmogenic atrial myocardium from the remainder of the heart have not been developed. If the site of origin of an automatic atrial tachycardia can be localized precisely by intraoperative mapping, the arrhythmogenic focus may be either excised or cryoablated.[27] Automatic foci located in the free wall of the left atrium or in either of the atrial appendages are ideal for excision or cryoablation. Automatic atrial tachycardias arising near the orifices of the pulmonary veins are best treated either by pulmonary vein isolation or by left atrial isolation.[28]

Theoretically, if intraoperative mapping properly localizes automatic foci in the free wall of the body of the right atrium, those foci can be either excised or cryoablated. However, automatic right atrial tachycardias are frequently multifocal in origin, and the ablation or excision of one automatic focus may be followed by the appearance of another at a later date. Thus, the recurrence rate following local excision or cryoablation of automatic right atrial tachycardias is unacceptably high. As a result, we prefer to perform a right atrial isolation procedure, even though the site of origin of the tachycardia may be well defined by intraoperative computerized mapping.[29,30]

Atrial Flutter and Fibrillation

At least 0.4 percent of the United States population, 1 million people, suffer from atrial fibrillation.[31] There are three detrimental side effects when one converts from normal sinus rhythm to atrial fibrillation: (1) a rapid, irregular heartbeat; (2) impaired cardiac hemodynamics due to a loss of AV synchrony; and (3) an increased vulnerability to thromboembolism.

Elective His bundle ablation, either by open heart surgical techniques or by endocardial catheter fulguration, has been the only nonpharmacologic method of treating refractory atrial fibrillation until recently. Unfortunately, His bundle ablation does not protect the patient from all three of the detrimental effects of atrial fibrillation. The patients remain at significant risk for thrombus formation in the fibrillating atrial cavity with the subsequent risk of thromboembolism, and the loss of atrial transport function in certain patients, particularly those with impaired ventricular function, may result in significant symptoms of congestive heart failure that are difficult to control medically.

During the past decade, three more specific surgical procedures have been developed and applied clinically for the treatment of atrial fibrillation. However, neither the left atrial isolation procedure nor the corridor procedure satisfies all of the requirements for the cure of atrial fibrillation, namely, (1) restoration of normal sinus rhythm mechanism, (2) restoration of atrial transport function, and (3) reduction in the risk of thromboembolism.

The left atrial isolation procedure, which was first introduced experimentally in 1980[28] and clinically in 1982,[23] is capable of confining atrial fibrillation to the left atrium, but, because the left atrium continues to fibrillate postoperatively, it has not been applied routinely to control the detrimental effects of atrial fibrillation clinically. In 1985, Guiraudon introduced the corridor procedure,[32] in which a strip of atrial septum between the sinoatrial node and the AV node was isolated from the remainder of the atrial myocardium in patients with atrial fibrillation. Although this procedure has now been performed in several patients, it alleviates only the rapid, irregular ventricular response to atrial fibrillation. Since both atria may continue to fibrillate, however, it does not restore AV synchrony, nor does it reduce the vulnerability of patients to thromboembolic problems. For these reasons, this operation offers little advantage over catheter His bundle ablation and insertion of a rate-responsive pacemaker system.

The limitations of the above-mentioned surgical procedures and the documentation that human atrial fibrillation, once established, is perhaps too complex to be amenable to map-guided surgery, led to our development of the maze procedure (Fig 44-4).[4-7] Between September 25, 1987, and September 1, 1991, 25 patients underwent this procedure for atrial fibrillation.[8] The presenting preoperative arrhythmia was paroxsymal atrial fibrillation in 12 patients (48 percent), chronic atrial fibrillation in 11 patients (44 percent), and paroxysmal atrial flutter in 2 patients (8 percent). Of the 11 patients who underwent surgery for chronic atrial fibrillation, 1 of the patients had experienced continuous atrial fibrillation for 10 years and another for 16 years preoperatively. Treatment of patients with an average of five antiarrhythmic medications each prior to surgical therapy had failed. There were no operative deaths, and all patients have been documented to have preserved atrial transport function postoperatively. In addition, high-frequency endocardial

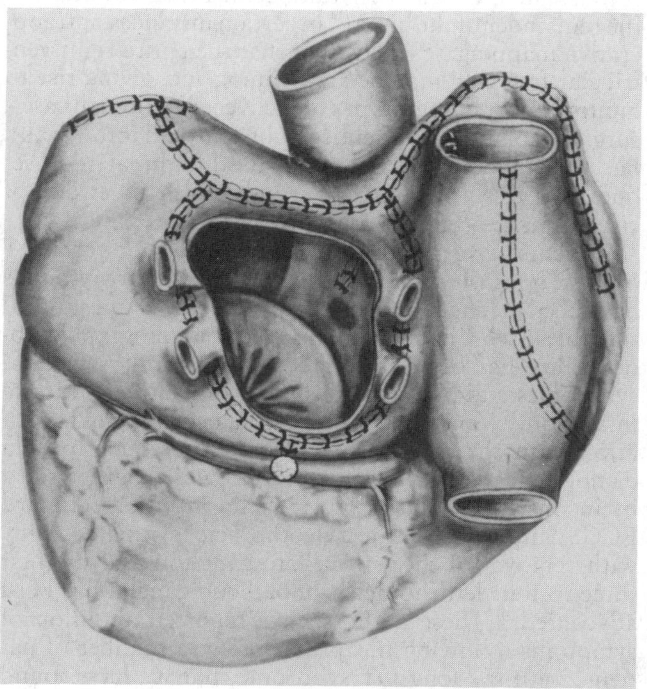

FIGURE 44-4 Three-dimensional depiction of the incisions used for performing the maze procedure. Note the presence of the transmural cryolesion (white dot) of the coronary sinus at the site of the posteroinferior left atriotomy. Both atrial appendages have been excised. The only completely isolated portions of the atrium are the orifices of the pulmonary veins. (Reproduced by permission from Cox et al.[8])

catheter stimulation of multiple sites of the atrium has been unsuccessful in inducing atrial fibrillation in any of the patients postoperatively. Moreover, no patient beyond the 3-month postoperative period has experienced a recurrence of atrial fibrillation. Since AV synchrony with preserved atrial transport function is retored following the maze procedure, it alleviates all three of the detrimental sequelae of this most common of cardiac arrhythmias.

SURGERY FOR VENTRICULAR TACHYARRHYTHMIAS

Nonischemic Ventricular Tachycardia

Nonischemic forms of ventricular tachyarrhythmias usually arise in the right ventricle and in general are extremely resistant to medical therapy. Fontaine and associates described a previously unrecognized form of cardiomyopathy localized to the right ventricle, termed *arrhythmogenic right ventricular dysplasia,* that is frequently responsible for nonischemic ventricular tachycardia.[33] This congenital myopathy is remarkable pathologically for transmural infiltration of adipose tissue resulting in weakness and aneurysmal bulging of three pathologic areas of the right ventricle: the infundibulum, the apex, and the posterior basilar region. Because the origin of the tachycardia is the right ventricle, the standard ECG shows a pattern consistent with a left bundle branch block pattern during the tachycardia.

The objective of surgical intervention in these patients is to isolate the local arrhythmogenic myocardium from the remainder of the heart.[34] In certain instances, intraoperative mapping has suggested that the entire right ventricular free wall may be arrhythmogenic, giving rise to multiple morphologic types of tachycardia. In such cases, surgical isolation of the entire right ventricular free wall[23] has been undertaken to relieve the life-threatening sequelae of this arrhythmia, but only in the most dire of circumstances (Fig. 44-5).

Patients with familial or idiopathic *prolonged QT interval syndrome* and recurrent ventricular arrhythmias have been managed with a variety of medical and surgical therapies (see Chap. 36). This electrocardiographic abnormality has been associated with several congenital syndromes and noted as a sequelae of acute myocardial infarction.[35] Ventricular tachycardia occurring in association with the lone QT syndrome is frequently of a distinct type called *torsades de pointes,* characterized by inconsistent polarity of the tachycardia on standard ECG. Surgically, left cervicothoracic sympathectomy with removal of the left stellate ganglion and the first three to four left thoracic sympathetic ganglia has been advocated.[36] These authors have reported abolition of symptoms following this procedure in a number of patients with the long QT syndrome, but we have found the results to be characterized by early success and late failure.[37] Because of these equivocal surgical results, implantation of a cardioverter-defibrillator device (Chap. 42) has been advocated as an adjunct to sympathectomy to serve as backup therapy for these life-threatening arrhythmias.[38]

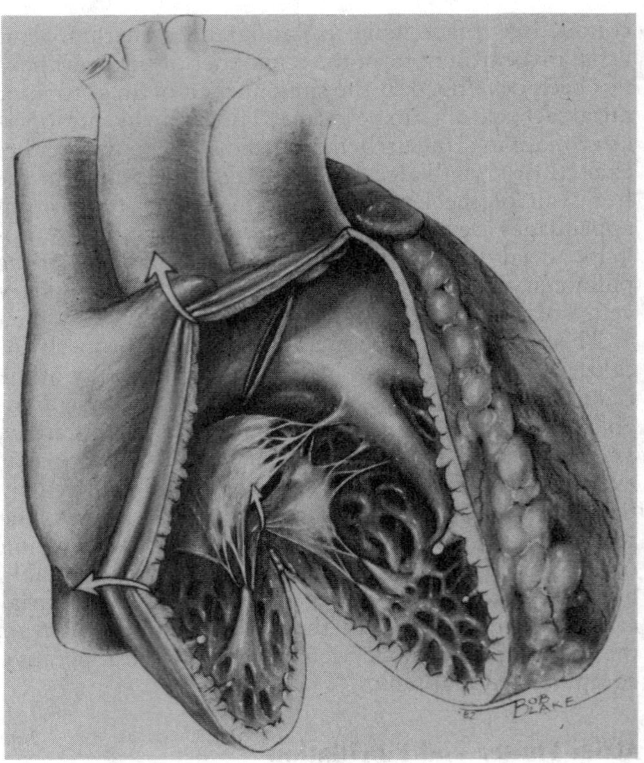

FIGURE 44-5 Surgical technique for right ventricular isolation. Both ventriculotomies extend from the pulmonary valve to the tricuspid valve annulus. The arrows represent the direction of retraction required to visualize the dissection. (Reproduced by permission from Cox et al.[23])

Ischemic Ventricular Tachycardia

The most common ventricular tachyarrhythmias are those that occur in association with ischemic heart disease. Serious ventricular arrhythmias of this type are harbingers of sudden cardiac death within the first year after an acute myocardial infarction and are frequently unresponsive to medical management.[39] Surgical treatment of ventricular tachycardias in the setting of ischemic heart disease dates to 1959, when Couch and associates[40] performed a simple aneurysmectomy in an attempt to ablate the tachycardia. Since then, much progress has been made through the development of a number of surgical procedures designed to cure the patient of the tachycardia (Fig. 44-6). In 1978, Guiraudon and associates[41] introduced the encircling endocardial ventriculotomy (EEV) as the first direct surgical technique for ablation of malignant ventricular tachyarrhythmias. Subsequent experience showed that the EEV was associated with an unacceptable incidence of postoperative left ventricular dysfunction,[42] and it has not been abandoned. In 1979, Josephson and Harken described the subendocardial resection (SER) procedure.[43] This operation, based on intraoperative mapping findings and thus an electrophysiologically guided procedure, continues to be one of the most important procedures used for control of ischemic ventricular tachyarrhythmias. In 1982, Moran and coworkers[44] reported a modification of the original subendocardial resection procedure in which all of the endocardial fibrosis associated with an aneurysm or in-

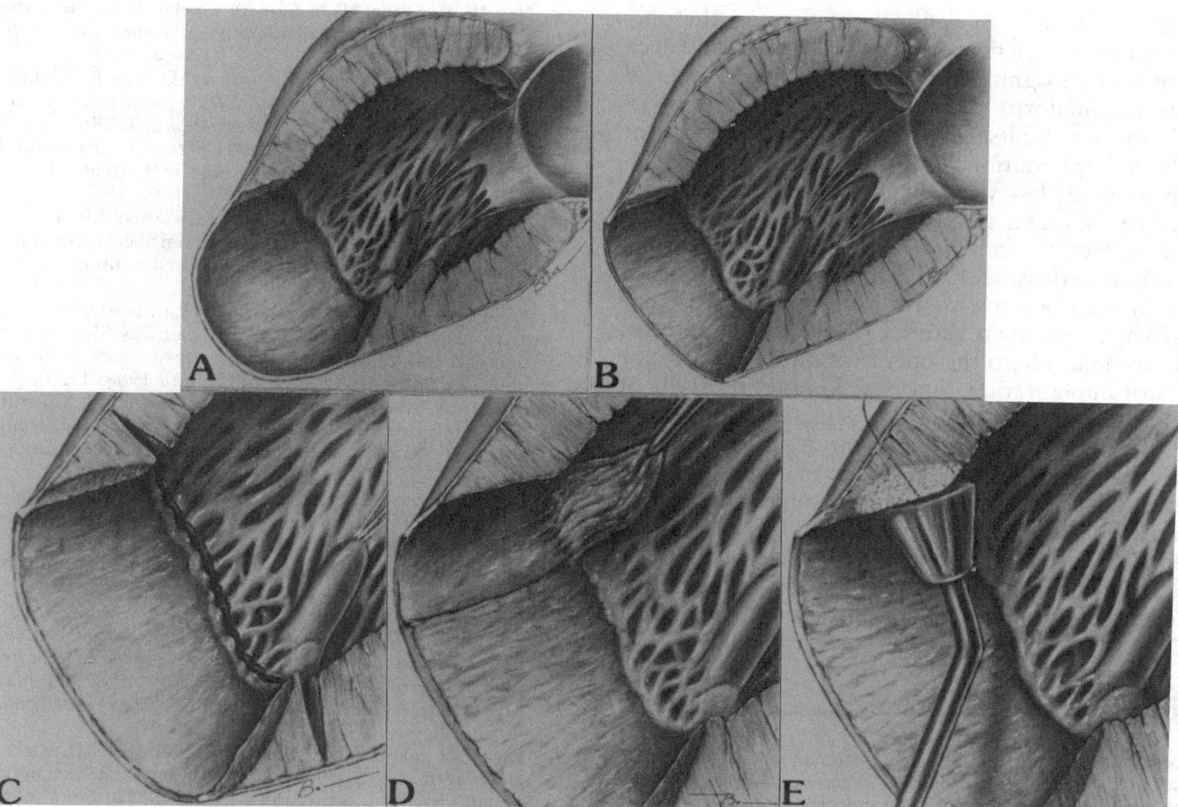

FIGURE 44-6 *A.* Diagrammatic cross section of an anterior left ventricular aneurysm showing more proximal extension of associated fibrosis at the endocardial level than at the epicardial level. *B.* Because reentrant circuits responsible for ischemic ventricular tachycardia occur most commonly at the junction of this endocardial fibrosis and normal myocardium, standard left ventricular aneurysm resection does not ablate or remove them. *C.* Encircling endocardial ventriculotomy; *D,* localized endocardial (or "subendocardial") resection; and *E,* endocardial cryoablation were all introduced specifically to ablate ventricular tachycardia associated with left ventricular aneurysms or infarcts. (Reproduced by permission from Cox et al.[49])

farct was resected, the so-called extended endocardial resection procedure (EERP). Other modifications of the original SER operation have included the addition of endocardial cryoablation as an adjunctive procedure. In 1984, Ostermeyer and colleagues[45] introduced the partial EEV with excellent surgical results. Our approach has been to perform extensive intraoperative mapping followed by an EERP followed by extensive cryosurgical ablation. This technique has been used since 1979 with excellent results.[46]

A review of the cumulative experience with these direct surgical procedures for the treatment of ventricular tachyarrhythmias during the first decade of their application (1979–1898) reveals two problems that made ventricular tachycardia surgery less attractive as a therapeutic option than surgery for supraventricular tachycardia.[46] The operative mortality rate averaged 12.4 percent, and 23.8 percent of patients still had inducible ventricular tachycardia postoperatively. Despite the reinducibility of ventricular tachycardia postoperatively in one out of four survivors, the long-term follow-up revealed an extremely low incidence of sudden death in these patients. The five reported series with over 50 patients and greater than a 5-year follow-up period showed that 96 percent of the survivors were either cured by surgery alone or were able to have their arrhythmia controlled postoperatively by medical therapy, a remarkable success rate in these patients with a life-threatening problem.

Because the operative mortality rate associated with these direct surgical procedures for the treatment of refractory ischemic ventricular tachyarrhythmias was higher than that for routine coronary artery bypass surgery, some authors in the late 1980s began to advocate routine implantation of an automatic defibrillator and performance of coronary artery bypass surgery as the primary therapy for patients with ischemic ventricular tachyarrhythmias.[47] However, the sudden death rate following defibrillator implantation (Chap. 42) is 1.5 to 2.0 percent per year, or 7.5 to 10.0 percent over a 5-year period.[48] The sudden death rate in the survivors of ventricular tachyarrhythmia surgery is less than 1 percent per year and less than 5 percent for 5 years. Thus, while the sudden death rate following defibrillator implantation is excellent, it remains approximately twice the sudden death rate following successful VT surgery.[46]

Paradoxically, the clinical availability of implantable defibrillator devices is perhaps the most important single development that has made ventricular tachyarrhythmia surgery safer today than it was in the 1980s. These devices represent a previously missing therapeutic option that can now be applied to patients with intractable, medically refractory ventricular tachycardia who are inoperable because of severe left ventricular dysfunction.

Before the availability of defibrillator devices, the only recourse for such patients was surgical intervention even though it was recognized to entail inordinate surgical risk. The vast majority of the operative mortalities occurred in those patients.[46] By selecting such patients for defibrillator implantation, only those patients with acceptable levels of left ventricular dysfunction are now subjected to the direct surgical procedures for the treatment of refractory ischemic ventricular tachycardia. Such a selective therapeutic approach has resulted in a decrease in the operative mortality rate for ventricular tachycardia in our own series to less than 3 percent, which is comparable to the operative mortality rate for defibrillator implantation. Since the long-term results of ventricular tachycardia surgery are superior to the long-term results of defibrillator implantation in terms of the prevention of sudden death, such surgery should be applied to any patient considered a reasonable operative candidate. Thus, the two therapeutic modalities, surgery and defibrillator implantation, should be viewed as complementary, not competing, procedures for the treatment of medically refractory ischemic ventricular tachycardia.

REFERENCES

1. Jackman WM, Wang XZ, Friday KJ, Roman CA, Moulton KP, Beckman KJ, et al: Catheter ablation of accessory atrioventricular pathways (Wolff-Parkinson-White syndrome) by radiofrequency current. *N Engl J Med* 1991; 324:1605–1611.
2. Lee MA, Morady F, Kadish A, Schamp DJ, Chin MC, Scheinman MM, et al: Catheter modification of the atrioventricular junction with radiofrequency energy for control of atrioventricular nodal reentry tachycardia. *Circulation* 1991; 83:827–835.
3. Mirowski M: The automatic implantable cardioverter-defibrillator: An overview. *J Am Coll Cardiol* 1985; 6:461–466.
4. Cox JL, Schuessler RB, Boineau JP: The surgical treatment of atrial fibrillation: 1. Summary of the current concepts of the mechanisms of atrial flutter and atrial fibrillation. *J Thorac Cardiovasc Surg* 1991; 101:402–405.
5. Cox JL, Canavan TE, Schuessler RB, Cain ME, Lindsay BD, Stone C, et al: The surgical treatment of atrial fibrillation: 2. Intraoperative electrophysiologic mapping and description of the electrophysiologic basis of atrial flutter and atrial fibrillation. *J Thorac Cardiovasc Surg* 1991; 101:406–426.
6. Cox JL, Schuessler RB, D'Agostino HJ Jr, Stone CM, Chang BC, Cain ME: The surgical treatment of atrial fibrillation: 3. Development of a definite surgical procedure. *J Thorac Cardiovasc Surg* 1991; 101:569–583.
7. Cox JL: The surgical treatment of atrial fibrillation: 4. Surgical technique. *J Thorac Cardiovasc Surg* 1991; 101:584–592.
8. Cox JL, Boineau JP, Scheussler RB, Ferguson TB Jr, Cain ME, Lindsay BD, et al: Successful surgical treatment of atrial fibrillation. *JAMA* 1991; 266:1976–1980.
9. Cox JL, Gallagher JJ, Cain ME: Experience with 118 consecutive patients undergoing surgery for the Wolff-Parkinson-White syndrome. *J Thorac Cardiovasc Surg* 1985; 90:490–501.
10. Cobb FR, Blumenschein SD, Sealy WB, Boineau JP, Wagner GS, Wallace AG: Successful surgical interruption of the bundle of Kent in a patient with Wolff-Parkinson-White syndrome. *Circulation* 1968; 38:1018–1029.
11. Cox JL: The surgical management of cardiac arrhythmias. In: Sabiston DC Jr, Spencer FC (eds): *Gibbon's Surgery of the Chest*, 5th ed. Philadelphia, Saunders, 1990:1861–1900.
12. Sealy WC, Hattler BG, Blumenschein SD, Cobb FR: Surgical treatment of Wolff-Parkinson-White syndrome. *Ann Thorac Surg* 1969; 8:1–11.
13. Guiraudon GM, Klein GJ, Gulamhusein S, Jones DL, Yee R, Perkins DG, et al: Surgical repair of Wolff-Parkinson-White syndrome: A new closed-heart technique. *Ann Thorac Surg* 1984; 37:67–71.
14. Cox JL, Ferguson TB Jr: Surgery for the Wolff-Parkinson-White syndrome: The endocardial approach. *Semin Thorac Cardiovasc Surg* 1989; 1:34–46.
15. Guiraudon GM, Klein GJ, Sharma AD, Yee R, McLellan DG: Surgery for the Wolff-Parkinson-White syndrome: The epicardial approach. *Semin Thorac Cardiovasc Surg* 1989; 1:21–33.
16. Lev M, Liberthson RR, Joseph RH, Setan CE, Eekner FA, Kunske RD, et al: The pathologic anatomy of Ebstein's disease. *Arch Pathol* 1970; 90:334–343.
17. Tchou P, Lehmann MJ, Jazayeri M, Akhtar M: Atriofascicular connection or a nodoventricular Mahaim fiber? Electrophysiologic elucidation of the pathway and associated reentrant circuit. *Circulation* 1988; 44:837–848.
18. Klein GJ, Guiraudon GM, Kerr CR, Sharma AD, Yee R, Szabo T, et al: "Nodoventricular" accessory pathway: Evidence for a distinct accessory atrioventricular pathway with atrioventricular node-like properties. *J Am Coll Cardiol* 1988: 11:1035–1040.
19. Abbott JA, Scheinman MM, Morady F, Shen EN, Miller R, Ruder MA, et al: Coexistent Mahaim and Kent accessory connections: Diagnostic and therapeutic implications. *J Am Coll Cardiol* 1987; 10:364–372.
20. Cox JL, Ferguson TB Jr: Surgery for atrioventricular node reentry tachycardia: The discrete cryosurgical technique. *Semin Thorac Cardiovasc Surg* 1989; 1:47–52.
21. Sealy WC, Gallagher JJ, Kasell JH: His bundle interruption for control of inappropriate ventricular responses to atrial arrhythmias. *Ann Thorac Surg* 1981; 32:429–438.
22. Scheinman MM, Morady F, Hess DS, Gonzalez R: Catheter-induced ablation of the atrioventricular junction to control refractory supraventricular arrhythmias. *JAMA* 1982; 248:851–855.
23. Cox JL: Surgery for cardiac arrhythmias. *Curr Probl Cardiol* 1983; 8(4):1–60.
24. Ross DL, Johnson DC, Denniss AR, Cooper MJ, Richards DA, Uther JB: Curative surgery for atrioventricular junctional ("A-V nodal") reentrant tachycardia. *J Am Coll Cardiol* 1985; 6:1383–1392.
25. Fujimara O, Guiraudon GM, Yee R, Sharma AD, Klein GK: Operative therapy of atrioventricular node reentry and results of an anatomically guided procedure. *Am J Cardiol* 1989; 64:1327–1332.
26. Cox JL, Ferguson TB Jr, Lindsay BD, Cain ME: Perinodal cryosurgery for AV node reentry tachycardia in 23 patients. *J Thorac Cardiovasc Surg* 1990; 99:440–449.
27. Gallagher JJ, Cox JL, German LD, Kasell JH: Non-pharmacologic treatment of supraventricular tachycardia. In: Josephson ME, Wellens HJJ (eds.): *Tachycardias: Mechanisms, Diagnosis, and Treatment.* Philadelphia, Lea & Febiger, 1984:271–285.
28. Williams JM, Ungerleider RM, Lofland GK, Cox JL: Left atrial isolation: New technique for the treatment of supraventricular arrhythmias. *J Thorac Cardiovasc Surg* 1980; 80:373–380.
29. Harada A, D'Agostino HJ Jr, Boineau JP, Cox JL: Right atrial isolation: A new surgical treatment for supraventricular tachycardia: 1. Surgical technique and electrophysiologic effects. *J Thorac Cardiovasc Surg* 1988; 95:643–650.
30. Harada A, D'Agostino HJ Jr., Boineau JP, Cox JL: Right atrial isolation: A new surgical treatment for supraventricular tachycardia: 2. Hemodynamic effects: *J Thorac Cardiovasc Surg* 1988; 95:651–657.
31. Savage DD, Garrison RJ, Castelli WP, McNamara PM, Anderson SJ, Kannel WB, et al: Prevalence of submitral (annular) calcium and its correlates in a general population-based sample (the Framingham Study). *Am J Cardiol* 1983; 51:1375–1378.
32. Guiraudon GM, Campbell CS, Jones DL, McLellan JL, MacDonald JL: Combined sinoatrial node atrioventricular node isolation: A surgical alternative to His bundle ablation in patients with atrial fibrillation (abstract). *Circulation* 1985; 72 (suppl 3):220.
33. Fontaine G, Guiraudon G, Frank R, et al: Epicardial mapping and surgical treatment in six cases of resistant ventricular tachycardia not related to coronary artery disease. In Wellens HJJ, Lie KI, Janse MJ (eds): *The Conduction System of the Heart.* Philadelphia, Lea & Febiger, 1976: 545–563.
34. Cox JL, Bardy GH, Damiano RJ, German LD, Fedor JM, Kisslo JA, et al: Right ventricular isolation procedures for nonischemic ventricular tachycardia. *J Thorac Cardiovasc Surg* 1985; 90:212–224.
35. Schwartz PJ, Periti M, Malliani A: The long Q-T syndrome. *Am Heart J* 1975; 89:378–390.

36. Moss AJ, Schwartz PJ, Crampton RS, Locati E, Carleen E: The long QT syndrome: A prospective international study. *Circulation* 1985; 71:17–21.
37. Benson DW Jr, Cox JL: Surgical treatment of cardiac arrhythmias. In: Roberts NK, Gelband H (eds): *Cardiac Arrhythmias in the Neonate, Infant and Child,* 2d ed. New York, Appleton-Century-Crofts, 1982: 341–366.
38. Platia EV, Griffith LSC, Watkins L, Mirowski M, Mower MM, Reid PR: Management of the prolonged QT syndrome and recurrent ventricular fibrillation with an implantable automatic cardioverter-defibrillator. *Clin Cardiol* 1985; 8:490–493.
39. Breithardt G, Broggrefe M, Podczeck A, et al: Prognostic significance of programmed ventricular stimulation for identification of patients at risk of ventricular tachyarrhythmias. In: Iwa T, Fontaine G (eds): *Cardiac Arrhythmias: Recent Progress in Investigation and Management.* Amsterdam, Elsevier, 1988: chap 13.
40. Couch OA Jr: Cardiac aneurysm with ventricular tachycardia and subsequent excision of aneurysm. *Circulation* 1959; 20:251–253.
41. Guiraudon G, Fontaine G, Frank R, Escande G, Elievent P, Cabrol C: Encircling endocardial ventriculotomy: A new surgical treatment of life-threatening ventricular tachycardias resistant to medical treatment following myocardial infarction. *Ann Thorac Surg* 1978; 26:438–444.
42. Cox JL, Gallagher JJ, Ungerleider RM: Encircling endocardial ventriculotomy (EEV) for refractory ischemic ventricular tachycardia: 4. Clinical indications, surgical technique, mechanism of action, and results. *J Thorac Cardiovasc Surg* 1982; 83:865–872.
43. Josephson ME, Harken AH, Horowitz LN: Endocardial excision: A new surgical technique for the treatment of recurrent ventricular tachycardia. *Circulation* 1979; 60:1430–1439.
44. Moran JM, Kehoe RF, Loeb JM, Lichenthal PR, Sanders JH Jr, Michaelis LL: Extended endocardial resection for the treatment of ventricular tachycardia and ventricular fibrillation. *Ann Thorac Surg* 1982; 34:538–552.
45. Ostermeyer J, Breithardt G, Borggrefe M, Godehardt E, Seipel L, Bricks W: Surgical treatment of ventricular tachycardias: Complete versus partial encircling ventriculotomy. *J Thorac Cardiovasc Surg* 1984; 87:517–525.
46. Cox JL: Patient selection criteria and results of surgery for refractory ischemic ventricular tachycardia. *Circulation* 1989; 79(suppl 1):163–177.
47. Fonger JD, Guarnieri T, Griffith LSC, Veltri E, Levine J, Mower M, et al: Impending sudden cardiac death: Treatment with myocardial revascularization and automatic implantable cardioverter defibrillator. *Ann Thorac Surg* 1988; 46:13–19.
48. Echt DS, Armstrong K, Schmidt P, Oyer PE, Stinson EB, Winkle RA: Clinical experience, complications, and survival in 70 patients wtih the automatic implantable cardioverter/defibrillator. *Circulation* 1985; 71:289–296.
49. Cox JL: Anatomic-electrophysiologic basis for the surgical treatment of refractory ischemic ventricular tachycardia. *Ann Surg* 1983; 198:119–129.

SECTION B
Special Diagnostic Procedures

Chapter 45

Long-Term Continuous Electrocardiographic Recording

R. Joe Noble, M.D. ■ *Douglas P. Zipes, M.D.*

Long-term electrocardiographic recording (Holter monitoring) is a method of recording the electrocardiogram (ECG) for extended periods of time; the recording is subsequently analyzed for rhythm and ST-segment and T-wave alterations.[1-3] Technological advances in the past few years have provided a diversity of recording and analysis systems.

The indications for long-term electrocardiographic recording as well as the information provided by extended electrocardiographic recording and the sensitivity and specificity of the technique are discussed in Chap. 36. The reader is also referred to *Guidelines for Ambulatory Electrocardiography*, published jointly by the American College of Cardiology and American Heart Association, for a consideration of clinical indications for ambulatory ECG recordings.[4] This chapter will deal with the technical aspects of long-term electrocardiographic recording: the recording systems, analyzer systems, comparison of different techniques, optimal duration of recording, and artifacts and errors in long-term electrocardiographic recording and analysis.

RECORDING TECHNIQUES

Two general methods of acquiring data are currently available: continuous recorders and intermittent, or "event," recorders.

Continuous Recorders

The ECG can be recorded continuously on tape (either reel to reel or cassette) or digitally in solid-state memory in more recently developed models. The tape recorder is a battery-powered miniaturized device with very slow tape speed and is small enough to be suspended by a strap over the shoulder or around the waist. All-digital recording systems amplify, digitize, and store the ECG in solid-state memory. Most current systems provide channels sufficient to record at least two ECG leads, which are essential to differentiate between ventricular arrhythmias and supraventricular arrhythmias with aberrancy, and also to assess ST-T segments. The frequency response of older models was limited in the lower ranges, so that accurate ST-T configuration could not be recorded[5,6]; current tape systems should conform to accepted ECG standards,[7,8] and digital records should eliminate distortion of low-frequency signals. Most current recorders are equipped with an event marker, consisting of a button the patient pushes to note the time of a symptom. Activation of the event recorder marks the tape so that the symptom and recording can be correlated during analysis. The patient carries a diary in which are entered any symptoms experienced during the recording period, the patient's activities, and the time at which the symptoms occurred.

When incorporated into an ambulatory recording system, microcomputers and microelectronic circuits sample the cardiac rhythm at real time as it is being recorded, convert the analog signal into a digital signal, and analyze the data in terms of maximal or minimal rates, RR intervals, and changes in RR intervals. Selected, brief segments of the patient's ECG, e.g., 6- to 10-s intervals, can also be stored. Within minutes of disconnection from the patient, the information can be retrieved in the form of a histogram covering the entire recording period, and a write-out in real time of selected segments can be obtained. Thus, this instrument records the analysis of the entire recording period, which in this sense is similar to continuous tape recording. It is dissimilar in that the actual ECG has not been recorded on tape. Microcomputers that can analyze electronic data over prolonged periods—even several days—have been developed.

The lead systems on recorders vary from one manufacturer to another. As mentioned, at least two leads should be simultaneously recorded, either V_1 and V_5, or a bipolar limb and unipolar chest lead. Meticulous attention must be paid to placing the electrodes on the patient's chest, since poor electrode contact will produce technically inadequate recordings (Fig. 45-1).

Event Recorders

An alternative method records only *abnormalities* in rhythm or conduction or records when the patient senses symptoms. Of the numerous event recorders available, there are two basic types, with several variations within each type. In the first, the rhythm is monitored continuously. Operators select those parameters they wish the recorder to recognize as abnormal and, hence, print out, such as a maximum or minimum rate, a premature complex or a pause exceeding the predetermined limit. Patients can also activate the unit when they experience symptoms. Thus, an abnormal rhythm or an ECG synchronous with a symptom can be recorded either automatically or in response to patient activation. More recently developed instruments incorporate a "memory" in the form of a loop recorder, which is capable of recording information several seconds or minutes before or after a recognized event; the number of events that can be recorded and the allotment of recording time prior to and after the abnòrmality is "sensed" are programmable.

In the second variety, the unit does not automatically recognize abnormalities and does not continuously monitor the ECG. The patient can wear the recorder continuously, activating it when symptomatic. Alternately, the patient can carry a miniature, solid-state recorder (sufficiently small to fit into his or her pocket or purse) with which the rhythm can be recorded, whenever the patient is symptomatic, by simply placing the unit on the precordium. The recorded data are stored in memory until the patient submits the information either directly or transtelephonically to an electrocardiographic receiver, where it is recorded. When a tape is employed, the tape is then erased, and subsequent data may be recorded and transmitted to facilitate the recording of rhythm or pattern during several symptomatic episodes; when digital acquisition devices are used, a prolonged, continuous event can be recorded and stored or up to three separate events may be acquired. As another variation, the device that acquires data can transmit the ECG information directly and transtelephonically, in real time, and without recording the data in the unit.

SCANNING AND ANALYSIS TECHNIQUES

The recording can be analyzed by scanning the tape at high speed, by writing it out directly, or as in the case of microcomputers, by processing during the recording and writing out the analysis at the termination of the sampling.

Scanning techniques include technician-dependent analysis, in which a technician interprets the cardiac

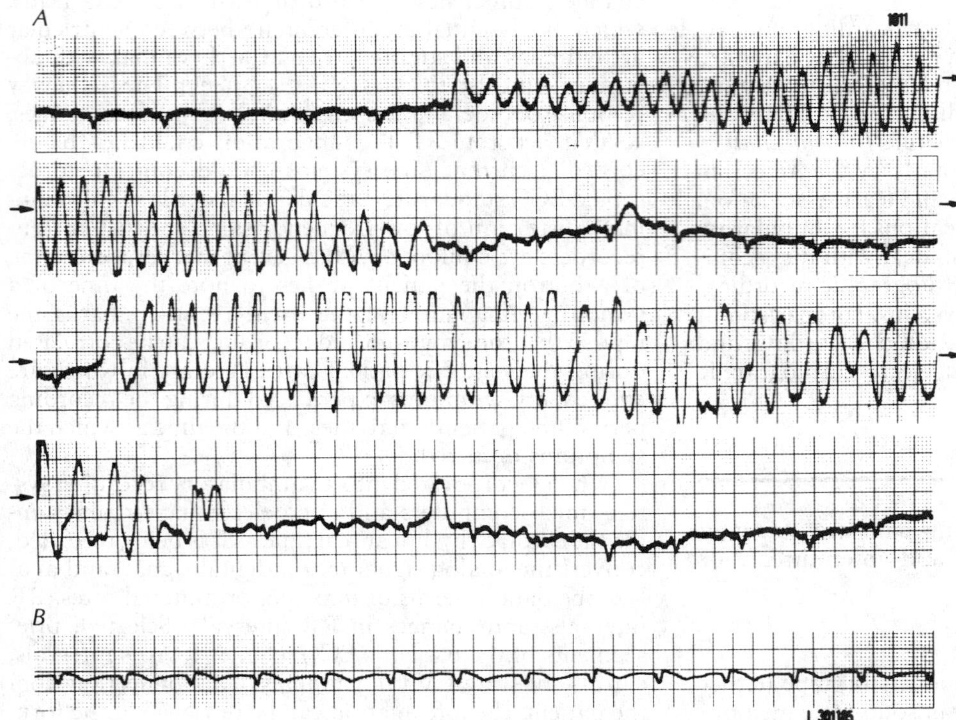

FIGURE 45-1 Artifact recorded on Holter monitor. *A.* A loose electrode was responsible for the artifactual tracing mimicking ventricular flutter-fibrillation recorded by the monitor. *B.* A simultaneous electrocardiogram confirmed continuous sinus rhythm, and the patient remained asymptomatic.

rhythm as it is played back at high speed on an oscilloscope at 30 to 120 times real time. One commonly used method of scanning superimposes each QRS complex on the immediately preceding complex, so that identical QRS contours present as a stationary image. Variations in QRS contour then become readily apparent. Simultaneously displayed on the oscilloscope for each cardiac cycle is a vertical bar graph, the height of which is directly proportional to each RR interval and QRS morphology. Thus, the occurrence of a premature ventricular extrasystole would alter the stationary image by producing a variation in the QRS contour, would alter the pitch and sound of the audio signal, and would shorten the vertical bar reflecting cycle lengths. When such an abnormal event is noted, the tape can be played in real time for analysis on a standard electrocardiographic machine.

To minimize the human factor and provide accurate quantitative data, the tape can be analyzed by a semiautomated electronic analyzer, which quantitates the number of abnormalities it recognizes. The accuracy of the system depends on the system's ability to distinguish abnormal from normal.

A computer can be interfaced with the scanner to quantitate the data even more accurately. The playback analysis can be as rapid as 240 times real time. Electronic analyzers and computers, as well as the scanner, can be "taught" to recognize the patient's own QRS complex and then to recognize any deviation from the normal. The computer program can provide summaries of heart rates, frequency of premature atrial or ventricular extrasystoles, coupling intervals, runs of tachycardia or other arrhythmias, and variations in QRS, ST, or T patterns during any time period; hard copies can be written out for verification. When arrhythmias or pattern changes are detected, automatic electrocardiograph write-out can be triggered by the event marker or by the computer.

Scanning services are available and can generally provide reasonably accurate analysis at less cost than can small institutions or offices with smaller volumes of long-term electrocardiographic recordings. Recorders can be purchased, leased, or rented.

An alternative method to scanning is the *direct write-out* of the entire record. The electrocardiogram is compressed to reduce the amount of paper that the physician must examine. By directly writing out the entire ECG, the need for a trained technician and scanners may be obviated.

Since *microcomputers* assess the electrocardiogram in real time, as it is recorded, there is no need for a scanner or expert technician when the results are written out. The physician evaluates the trend chart or any recorded rhythm strip.

Comparison of Techniques for Prolonged Electrocardiographic Recording

Operator-dependent, high-speed audiovisual analysis of the tape, without direct write-out or electronic analysis, probably recognizes serious rhythm disturbances. On the other hand, the operator can miss as many as one-third to two-thirds of ventricular and supraventricular arrhythmias.[7] Operator-dependent systems are affected by the capabilities of this person. If quantitation is unimportant, this system of analysis is quite adequate.

Electronic analysis systems improve upon the sensitivity and specificity of interpretation of long-term electrocardiographic recordings. Computer analysis systems are said to be 90 to 95 percent accurate in quantitating ectopic complexes.[9-11] Current computer-based systems that permit operator editing are even more sensitive and accurate, but both electronic and computer analysis systems increase cost. One reason for the stated accuracy of computer interpretations is that ventricular ectopy is responsible for most broad complex beats. Supraventricular ectopy with aberrancy or intermittent preexcitation is not accurately diagnosed by computer, but the relatively low frequency of these complexes does not statistically alter sensitivity calculations. Both electronic and computer analysis systems increase cost.

"Full disclosure"—i.e., hard-copy write-out of the entire record—provides a visual analysis of the record to identify immediately complex disturbances such as ventricular tachycardia or prolonged asystolic intervals. In addition, it is often useful to have hard-copy ECG data available (as opposed to that derived from analysis of the ECG data) with which to compare subsequent records. The direct write-out does not quantitate the actual number of events. Assuming care in interpretation, the direct write-out may be more sensitive than high-speed, operator-dependent, and semiautomated systems and as accurate as computer-based systems with operator editing in identifying pairs or triplets of consecutive ectopic complexes.[9]

An event recorder does not require a scanner or an experienced technician; however, the continuously recording event recorder itself is more expensive than a continuously recording tape recorder. The recorder that the patient applies only when symptomatic and does not have continuous tape recording capability is less expensive. Both types of event recorders provide an electrocardiographic record more quickly than a system that requires scanning,[12] but neither creates a long-term record of the ECG during asymptomatic intervals. The automatic event recorder is limited by the accuracy and sensitivity of the algorithm used to detect abnormalities. Either event recorder clearly allows correlation between the patient's symptoms and the rhythm. The only technique currently available to record rhythm events leading up to and following infrequently occurring symptoms is the memory loop event recorder.

When a more rapid identification of a rhythm abnormality is essential, such as in the patient with a potentially dangerous rhythm disturbance, a new development permits frequent and automatic transtelephonic transmission of the ambulatory record to a hospital telemetry receiver. The monitor technician can then quickly identify a serious rhythm abnormality and arrange for the patient's proper management.

Those microcomputers that analyze the rhythm in real time, simultaneous with the recording, should prove at least as accurate as other high-speed playback analysis systems. More importantly, longer periods can be monitored than are practical for other systems. The cost of the analysis is independent of the duration of recording, so that patient cost should be less for prolonged periods of monitoring. Finally, the analysis of the entire recording and the actual write-out of the specific ECG segment are available within minutes of the recording. On the other hand, only limited segments of actual ECG records are generally available, and the accuracy of abnormal rhythm or pattern recognition remains dependent upon the computer algorithm; this recognition is far from perfect, since many problems of computer analysis of complex rhythm disturbances remain unsolved.

Whichever system is employed, the ultimate accuracy of ECG interpretation depends on the technician and overreading physician; scanners and computers cannot differentiate complex patterns (supraventricular arrhythmias with aberrancy as opposed to ventricular arrhythmias or preexcitation) or even artifact. The clinical application of the data is solely the function of the responsible physician. No data acquisition system or scanner, no computer, and no technician can substitute for the well-trained physician in determining the significance of any recorded data and their clinical utility.

Selection of Device

The ultimate selection of a long-term ECG recording system depends on individual patient needs. If a precise count of ectopy is required, then a continuous recorder with computer-based analysis is essential. On the other hand, if the purpose of the recording is to detect ventricular tachycardia or asystole, then an event recorder, a microcomputer, or direct write-out of the entire record would be an excellent choice. Either a microcomputer or an event recorder provides an opportunity to monitor over prolonged periods of time, and it is beneficial to the patient whose rhythm disturbance occurs infrequently. When the goal is to correlate the patient's rhythm or ECG pattern with symptoms that are very infrequent (at weekly intervals or less), the patient-applied and patient-activated recorder is the optimal choice. However, if the patient's symptoms are of such brief duration (seconds) or severity (frank syncope) to preclude capture by such a unit, then a loop event recorder is preferred. This and the direct write-out are less expensive for an individual physician's or small clinic's use.

Except with large scanning services, it is impractical for an individual physician to have available all the monitoring techniques for each individual patient's needs. Hence, the physician's selection of a system is based upon his or her own patient population, the frequency of using this test, the availability of dependable scanning services, and his or her own cost analysis. The physician would do well to realize that any or all of the above systems are available alone or in combination. The more detailed and precisely quantitated the final report, generally the more expensive the equipment and personnel required. All systems recognize ventricular tachycardia or marked bradycardia and, qualitatively at least, detect ectopy. For clinical purposes, this amount of information is usually sufficient. The practicing physician does not really require precise quantitation since the therapeutic and prognostic significance of such quantitation is not yet known. In short, technology exceeds clinical assimilation of the results at the present time.

DURATION OF RECORDING

A standard resting ECG, which records less than 1 min of cardiac rhythm, detects ventricular premature systoles in about 8 percent of patients with known coronary artery disease; this frequency doubles if the recording period is extended to 12 h.[13] A 48-h electrocardiographic recording period detects additional and more complex ventricular arrhythmias and supraventricular tachyarrhythmias and also displays the character and frequency of rhythm disturbances during sleep as well as during awake periods.

Arrhythmias are often evanescent, occurring only rarely. In such patients, 24-h electrocardiographic recordings are unlikely to detect the abnormal rhythm. Even when arrhythmias are frequent, marked variation in the frequency and complexity of the rhythm disturbance is expected, with variations occurring during and between days. Spontaneous reduction in the frequency of ventricular ectopy of 50 to 90 percent is common.[14,15] For screening purposes, 24-h electrocardiographic tape recording seems an optimal compromise between the practical limits of recording and the point of diminishing return.[13,16,17]

If a reduction in total number of premature ventricular complexes is the goal of antiarrhythmic therapy, then more than one control 24-h electrocardiographic recording and several recordings while the patient is receiving therapy are required to prove efficacy. The total number of premature ventricular complexes must be reduced by about 80 percent.[14,15,18] On the other hand, since it has not yet been demonstrated that reducing the total number of premature ventricular complexes necessarily implies an elimination of more dire ventricular rhythm disturbances or sudden death, this is often not the goal of the physician. Instead, simply preventing sustained, symptomatic ventricular tachycardia may be the therapeutic goal,[19] in which case multiple 24-h recordings are less essential.

The ideal duration of recording varies from patient to patient, depending on the physician's goals. If the objective is to correlate the cardiac rhythm or pattern with a symptom such as syncope, palpitations, or chest pain, then the recording period must be extended sufficiently to incorporate a symptomatic period, whether these intervals occur with a frequency of hours or days.

RECORDINGS OF ST SEGMENTS AND T WAVES

For several reasons, both technical and physiological, long-term ECG recording devices do not provide the same degree of reliability in the interpretation of the pattern of the ST segment and T wave as in the detection of rhythm disturbances. Technical limitations have included unsatisfactory low-frequency responses, which have precluded accurate display of the very low frequency ST segment and T waves.[4–6] Another limitation has been the use of a one-lead system. Just as a single lead on a standard ECG might not record "ischemic" ST-segment and T-wave changes during myocardial isch-

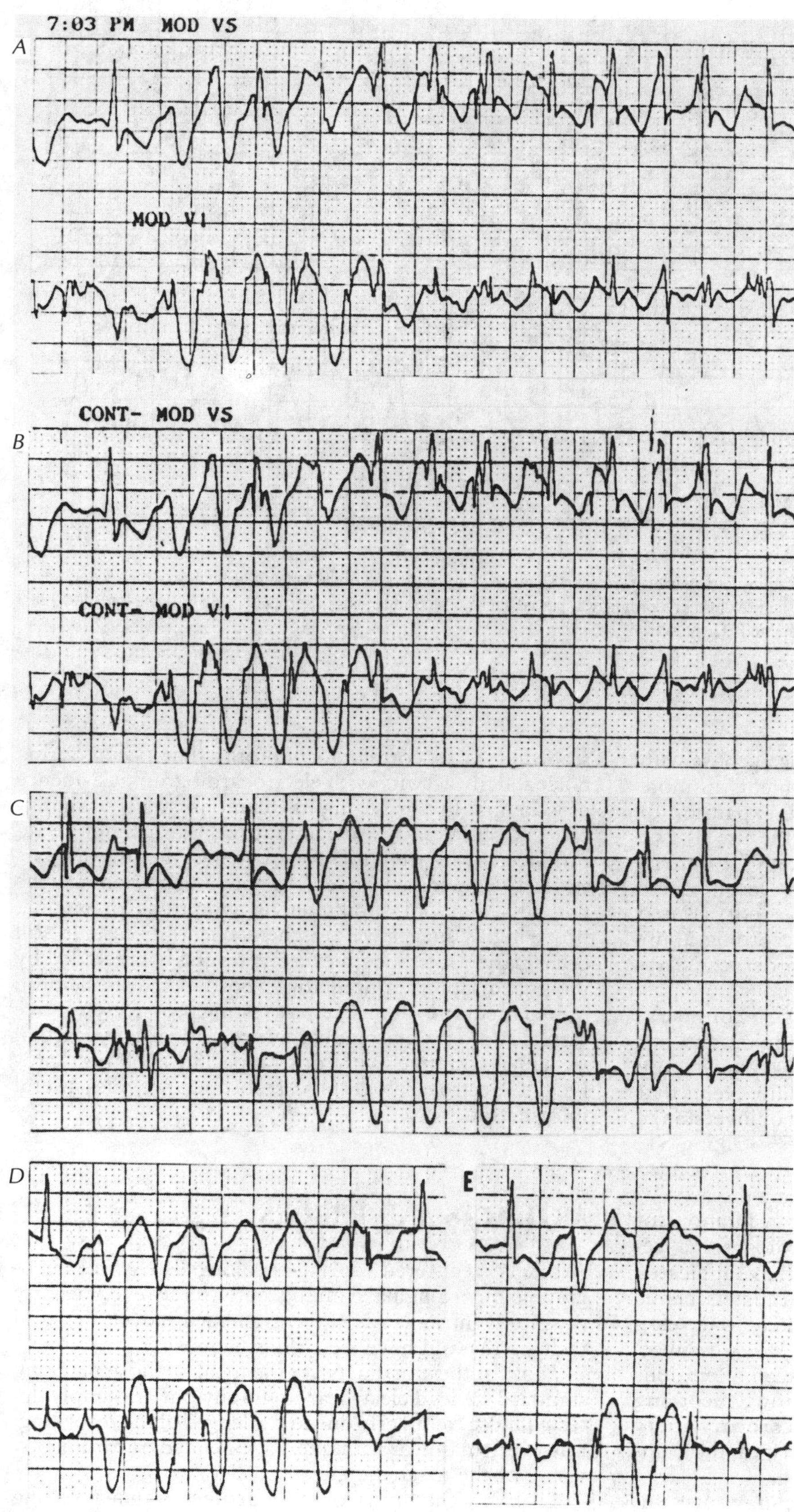

FIGURE 45-2 Mechanical stimulation of electrodes mimicking ventricular tachycardia. Regular, rapid (160 per minute) broad QRS complexes were repeatedly recorded in both leads V_1 and V_5 and interpreted as ventricular tachycardia (A through D) or pairs of premature ventricular complexes (PVCs) (E). Antiarrhythmic therapy was administered. However, the clue to the artifactual recording is the normal QRS "marching through" the "ventricular tachycardia" and the fact that the coupling interval between the last normal complex preceding the "tachycardia" and the first complex following it are often so short as to be unphysiological. Intense pruritus from the electrodes elicited scratching, which explained the artifacts.

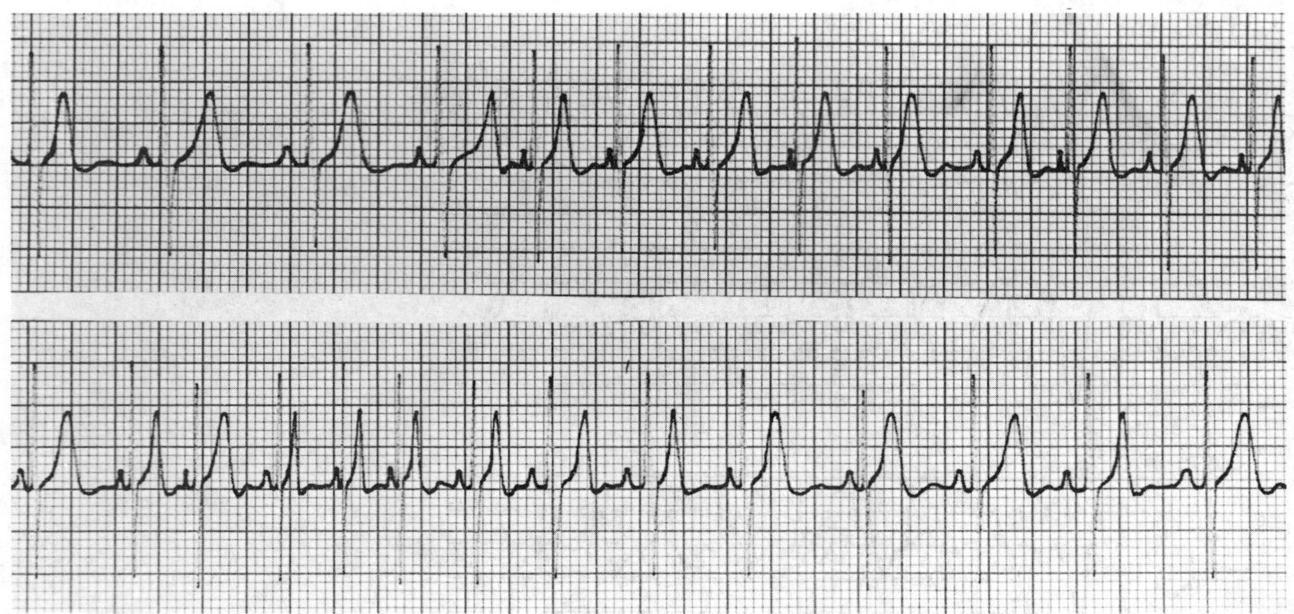

FIGURE 45-3 Deceleration of tape during recording. Supraventricular tachycardia is simulated toward the end of the top and beginning of the second trace, as the tape, which transiently slowed as a result of battery failure during recording, was played back on recording paper at proper speed. Note the foreshortening of the duration of the P wave, PR interval, QRS complex, and QT interval.

emia, so a single lead is inadequate for this purpose with prolonged recording. Technical improvements in more recently developed models, including the expansion of the lower limit frequency response and the use of two leads, have enhanced the reliability of QRS-ST-T pattern interpretation with long-term recording. Despite these improvements, most manufacturers have not assured that the appropriate specifications for recording apply not only to the amplifier, but to the recorder, the playback system, and the printout device.[20]

Even more important than these technical considerations, however, are certain physiological limitations. For instance, standing, hyperventilation, eating, anxiety, use of drugs, and change in heart rate are all daily events that may result in depression of the ST segment or inversion of the T wave to simulate ischemic changes. Striking ST-segment elevation has been recorded during prolonged recording in patients without organic heart disease.[21]

Despite these limitations, preliminary evaluations of the technique of prolonged electrocardiographic recording to detect ischemic heart disease have indicated in some instances (1) that patients who display ischemic ST segment–T wave changes are more likely to develop overt manifestations of ischemic heart disease subsequently than those who do not display such alterations and (2) that a similar ECG pattern during recording correlates with angiographic evidence of coronary artery disease.[22–24] The sensitivity and specificity of the technique, however, remain to be determined.

Long-term electrocardiographic recording proves superior to exercise testing in detecting angina at rest accompanied by ST-segment elevation, which cannot be reproduced with exercise (Prinzmetal's variant angina). Another potential use of prolonged electrocardiographic recording is to correlate symptoms that occur during normal daily activity with electrocardiographic evidence of ischemia. In this setting, the demonstration of significant ST segment–T wave alterations that cannot be reproduced by hyperventilation or change in position, particularly when reinforced by documentation in the patient's diary of simultaneous symptoms of angina, prove highly suggestive of ischemic heart disease. In still other patients, in whom exercise testing is precluded by physical disability, ambulatory recording may be helpful; or in patients in whom exercise testing produces negative results and yet symptoms highly suggestive of myocardial ischemia continue with other specific activities, prolonged electrocardiographic recording provides useful information.

ARTIFACTS AND ERRORS

Artifacts registered during prolonged electrocardiographic recording have mimicked virtually every variety of supraventricular and ventricular bradycardia and tachycardia and have led to misdiagnosis.[25,26]

Most of these artifacts are identical to those plaguing standard 12-lead electrocardiography but are simply detected more frequently due to the length of the recording; however, many are unique to extended recording by virtue of the magnetic tape recorder.

Probably the most common artifact is that resulting from a loose electrode (Fig. 45-1) or mechanical "stimulation" of the electrode. In Fig. 45-2, ventricular tachycardia is simulated by the patient "scratching" the electrodes. Failure of either the battery or the motor of the

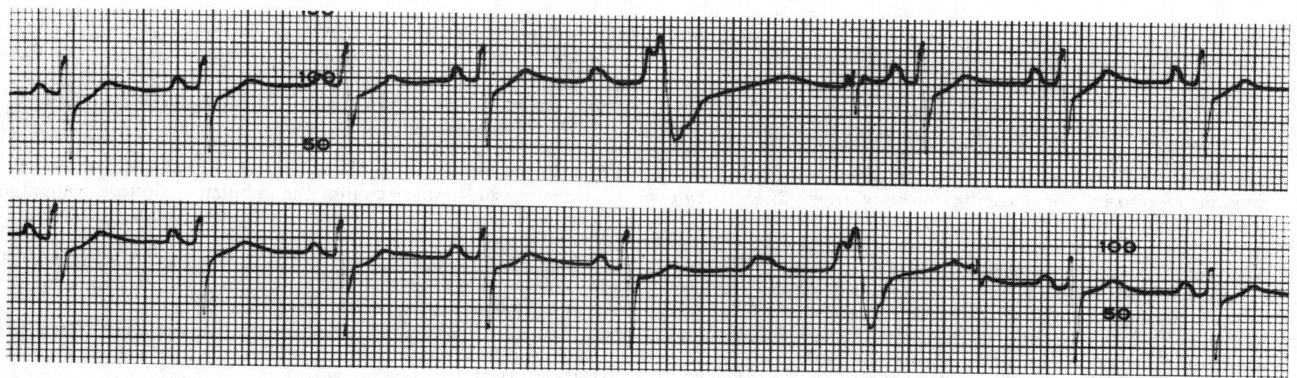

FIGURE 45-4 Deceleration of tape during playback. Slowing or sticking of the tape during playback spreads out the P wave, PR interval, and QRS complex to resemble sinus deceleration, or transient atrioventricular or intraventricular conduction delay. (Fifth complex in top trace; sixth complex in bottom trace.)

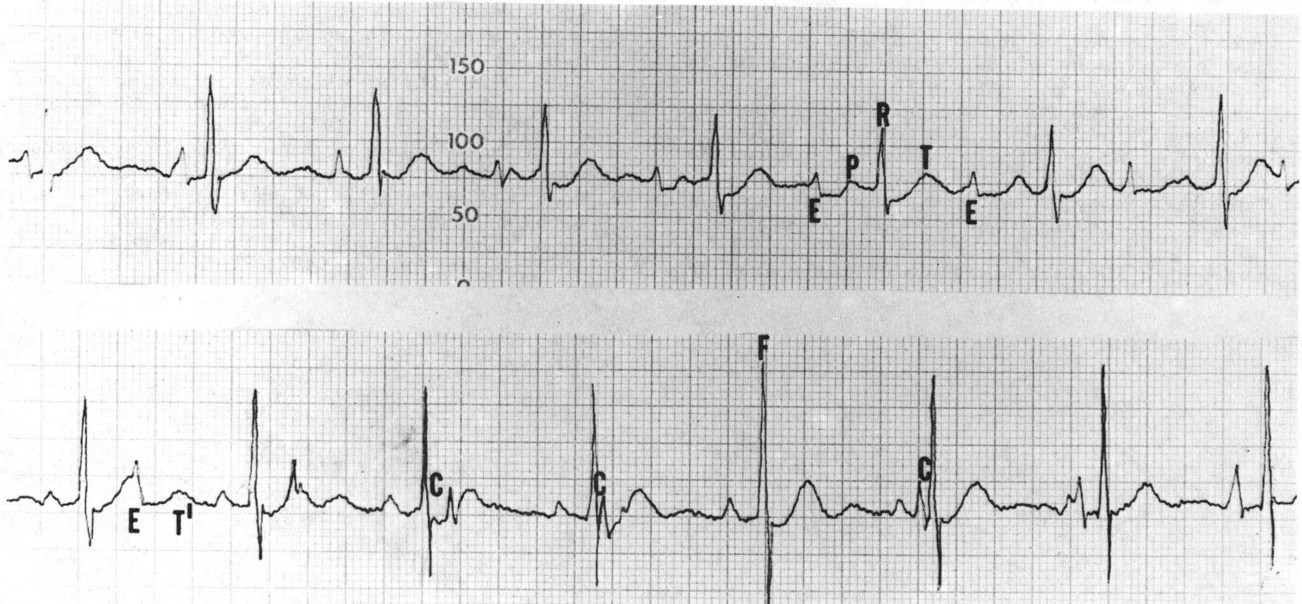

FIGURE 45-5 Incomplete erasure of tape. Two independent ventricular rhythms are identified: a larger QRS, labeled R, whose P wave and T wave are also labeled, and a smaller QRS, considered "ectopic," and labeled E; its T wave is labeled T′. The sequence could be recorded with a piggyback heart transplant, or in Siamese twins. Alternately, ectopic complex E might be misinterpreted to represent a parasystolic rhythm even fusing with complex R at F. The very short coupling intervals (C) preclude this possibility and indicate that the ECG record of one patient is superimposed on that of another.

recorder generally results in a slowing of the tape speed as the ECG is recorded. When played back, the heart rate will appear fast; i.e., it will mimic a tachycardia (Fig. 45-3). The interpreter may be alerted to the artifact by the concomitant shortening of all electrocardiographic intervals (PR, QRS, QT, and RR) and decrease in QRS voltage. Conversely, transient slowing or sticking of the tape during playback will suggest bradycardia or atrioventricular (AV) or intraventricular conduction disturbances (Fig. 45-4). Recording an ECG on a previously used tape that is incompletely erased results in the simultaneous registration of two ECGs and potentially the misinterpretation of a "parasystolic" ectopic rhythm (Fig. 45-5). Digital recording in solid-state memory eliminates these various mechanical failures of tape recordings.

The technician and/or physician who interprets prolonged ECG recordings must have a working knowledge of these and other potential artifacts in order to interpret the records properly.

REFERENCES

1. Holter NJ: New method for heart studies: Continuous electrocardiography of active subjects over long periods is now practical. *Science* 1961; 134:1214–1220.
2. Gilson JS, Holter NJ, Glassock WR: Clinical observations using this electrocardiocorder—AVSEP continuous electrocardiographic system. *Am J Cardiol* 1964; 14:204–217.
3. Winkle RA: Curriculum in cardiology, current status of ambulatory electrocardiography. *Am Heart J* 1981; 102:757–768.
4. Guidelines for Ambulatory Electrocardiography: A report of the American College of Cardiology/American Heart Association

Task Force on Assessment of Diagnostic and Therapeutic Cardiovascular Procedures (Subcommittee on Ambulatory Electrocardiography), *J Am Coll Cardiol* 1989; 13:249–258.
5. Hinkle LE Jr, Meyer J, Stevens M, Carver ST: Recordings of the ECG of active men. *Circulation* 1967; 36:752–765.
6. Crawford MH, Mendoza CA, O'Rourke RA, White DH, Boucher CA, Gorwit J: Limitations of continuous ambulatory electrocardiogram monitoring for detecting coronary artery disease. *Ann Intern Med* 1978; 89:1–5.
7. Report of Committee on Electrocardiography, American Heart Association: Recommendations for standardization of leads and of specifications for instruments in electrocardiography and vectorcardiography. *Circulation* 1967; 35:583–602.
8. Sheffield LT, Berson A, Bragg-Remschel D, Gillette PC, Hermes RE, Hinkle L, et al: Recommendations for standards of instrumentation and practice in the use of ambulatory electrocardiography. *Circulation* 1985; 71:626A–636A.
9. Stein IM, Plunkett J, Troy M: Comparison of techniques for examining long-term ECG recordings. *Med Instrum* 1980; 14:69–72.
10. Fitzgerald JW, Spitz AL, Winkle RA, Harrison DC: Quantitation of ambulatory electrocardiograms. *Circulation* 1977; 56(suppl 3):178 (abstract).
11. Knoebel SB, Lovelace DE, Rasmussen S, Wash SE: Computer detection of premature ventricular complexes: A modified approach. *Am J Cardiol* 1976; 38:440–447.
12. Dreifus LS, Pennock R: Newer techniques in cardiac monitoring. *Heart Lung* 1975; 4:568–572.
13. Lown B, Wolf M: Approaches to sudden death from coronary heart disease. *Circulation* 1971; 14:130–142.
14. Winkle RA: Antiarrhythmic drug effect mimicked by spontaneous variability of ventricular ectopy. *Circulation* 1978; 57:1116–1121.
15. Morganroth J, Michelson EL, Horowitz LN, Josephson ME, Pearlman, AS, Dunkman, WB: Limitations of routine long-term ambulatory electrocardiographic monitoring to assess ventricular ectopic frequency. *Circulation* 1978; 58:408–414.
16. Lopes MG, Runge P, Harrison DC, Schroeder JS: Comparison of 24 versus 12 hours of ambulatory ECG monitoring. *Chest* 1975; 67:269–273.
17. Kennedy HL, Chandra V, Sayther KL, Caralis DG: Effectiveness of increasing hours of continuous ambulatory electrocardiography in detecting maximal ventricular ectopy. *Am J Cardiol* 1978; 42:925–930.
18. Sami M, Kraemer H, Harrison DC, Houston, N, Shimasaki C, DeBusk RF: A new method for evaluating antiarrhythmic drug efficacy. *Circulation* 1980; 62:1172–1179.
19. Winkle RA, Alderman EL, Fitzgerald JW, Harrison DC: Treatment of recurrent symptomatic ventricular tachycardia. *Ann Intern Med* 1976; 85:1–7.
20. Berman DA, Rozanski AL, Knoebel SB: The detection of silent ischemia: Cautions and precautions. *Circulation* 1987; 75:101–105.
21. Golding B, Wolf E, Tzivoni D, Stern S: Transient S-T elevation detected by 24-hour ECG monitoring during normal daily activity. *Am Heart J* 1973; 86:501–507.
22. Stern S, Tzivoni D: Early detection of silent ischaemic heart disease by 24-hour electrocardiographic monitoring of active subjects. *Br Heart J* 1974; 36:481–486.
23. Wolf E, Tzivoni D, Stern S: Comparison of exercise tests and 24-hour ambulatory electrocardiographic monitoring in detection of ST-T changes. *Br Heart J* 1974; 36:90–95.
24. Stern S, Tzivoni D: Dynamic changes in the ST-T segment during sleep in ischemic heart disease. *Am J Cardiol* 1973; 32:17–20.
25. Krasnow AZ, Bloomfield DK: Artifacts in portable electrocardiographic monitoring. *Am Heart J* 1976; 91:349–357.
26. Malek J, Glushien A: To the editor: Artifacts in portable ECG monitoring. *Ann Intern Med* 1972; 77:1004.

Chapter 46

Technique of Electrophysiological Testing

Masood Akhtar, M.D.

Recording intracavitary electrocardiographic signals along with various forms of pacing programs has experienced enormous growth during the last 25 years. Clinical recording of intracardiac signals from the region of the His bundle was initially done by Scherlag et al.[1] Its clinical value was immediately established in various situations including atrioventricular (AV) blocks and supraventricular and ventricular tachyarrhythmias.[1-10] Recording methods were complemented by pacing to unmask sinus node dysfunction and AV conduction abnormalities and to initiate supraventricular tachycardias.[3-8] These techniques of intracardiac electrophysiological studies (EPSs) now find utility in a variety of cardiac arrhythmias including sinus node dysfunction, intraventricular and AV conduction disturbances, supraventricular tachycardias (SVTs), ventricular tachycardias (VTs), preexcitation syndromes, and ventricular fibrillation (VF). In addition to the diagnostic value, these studies are now also employed for correction of arrhythmic substrates. This chapter addresses recording and pacing techniques along with their clinical utility.

TECHNIQUES OF INTRACARDIAC ELECTROPHYSIOLOGICAL STUDIES[11]

The exact type of electric signal recordings, specific equipment used, and pacing protocol depend upon the nature of the clinical problem, the type of electrophysiological assessment, and the anticipated course of action. Routine cardiac electrophysiological studies are performed in a nonsedated postabsorptive state. Although some degree of sedation is advisable in apprehensive patients, drugs that may alter the properties of the cardiac conduction system should be avoided. Antiarrhythmic drugs are usually eliminated. In selected cases antiarrhythmic drugs may be continued if a clinical event occurred while the patient was on a specific agent. Customarily, other cardiac active drugs that are necessary for nonarrhythmic cardiovascular problems such as hypertension, angina, and heart failure are continued.

The typical electrode catheters used for both recording and cardiac stimulation are multipolar (sizes varying from 4 to 8 F). Catheters can be inserted via peripheral veins such as the antecubital, femoral, and at times subclavian and internal jugular. When a catheter is intended to be left in place for several days, subclavian and internal jugular veins are preferable. Using local anesthesia, a guide wire is inserted percutaneously through a needle and a dilator and sheath are advanced over the guide wire. Through the sheath a catheter is fluoroscopically guided to position in the appropriate cardiac chamber. For most electrophysiological testing the catheter locations are in the high right atrium, His bundle, or right bundle branch region across the tricuspid valve and right ventricle apex or outflow. In patients suspected of accessory pathways or AV junctional tachycardias, a catheter in the region of the coronary sinus is desirable. Heparinization is recommended by continuous infusion of approximately 1000 units per hour. For electrophysiological studies, good contact between the electrodes and the walls of the various chambers is critical. For His bundle and right bundle branch recording, the catheter is introduced via the femoral vein, advanced across the tricuspid valve, and gradually withdrawn until an appropriate recording from the right bundle and/or the His bundle is obtained (Fig. 46-1). Placement of a coronary sinus catheter can be accomplished via an arm, internal jugular, or subclavian vein. If necessary, coronary sinus catheterization can also be accomplished via a femoral approach. For a routine study left-sided heart catheterization is seldom necessary. However, in patients with ventricular tachycardia and/or left-sided accessory pathways this is performed for diagnostic or therapeutic purposes. Continuous heparinization is desirable for left-sided heart catheterization to avoid thromboembolic complications.

Electrophysiological Recordings

Once the electrode catheters are placed appropriately, the connections are made via a junction box and isolation units to prevent excess current in the event of random electrical surges. All of the electrograms are displayed simultaneously on a multichannel oscilloscopic recorder. In addition to the intracardiac signals, several unfiltered surface electrocardiographic leads, i.e., X, Y, Z or leads 1, 2, or AVF and V_1, are recorded. To reduce the noise generated with the low-frequency signals, the usual filtering frequency for intracardiac signals is between 30 and 40 Hz for the high-pass and 500 Hz for the low-pass filters. Although appropriately placed electrode catheters will record appropriate signals at any filtering frequency, filter settings between 30/40 and 500 Hz are best suited

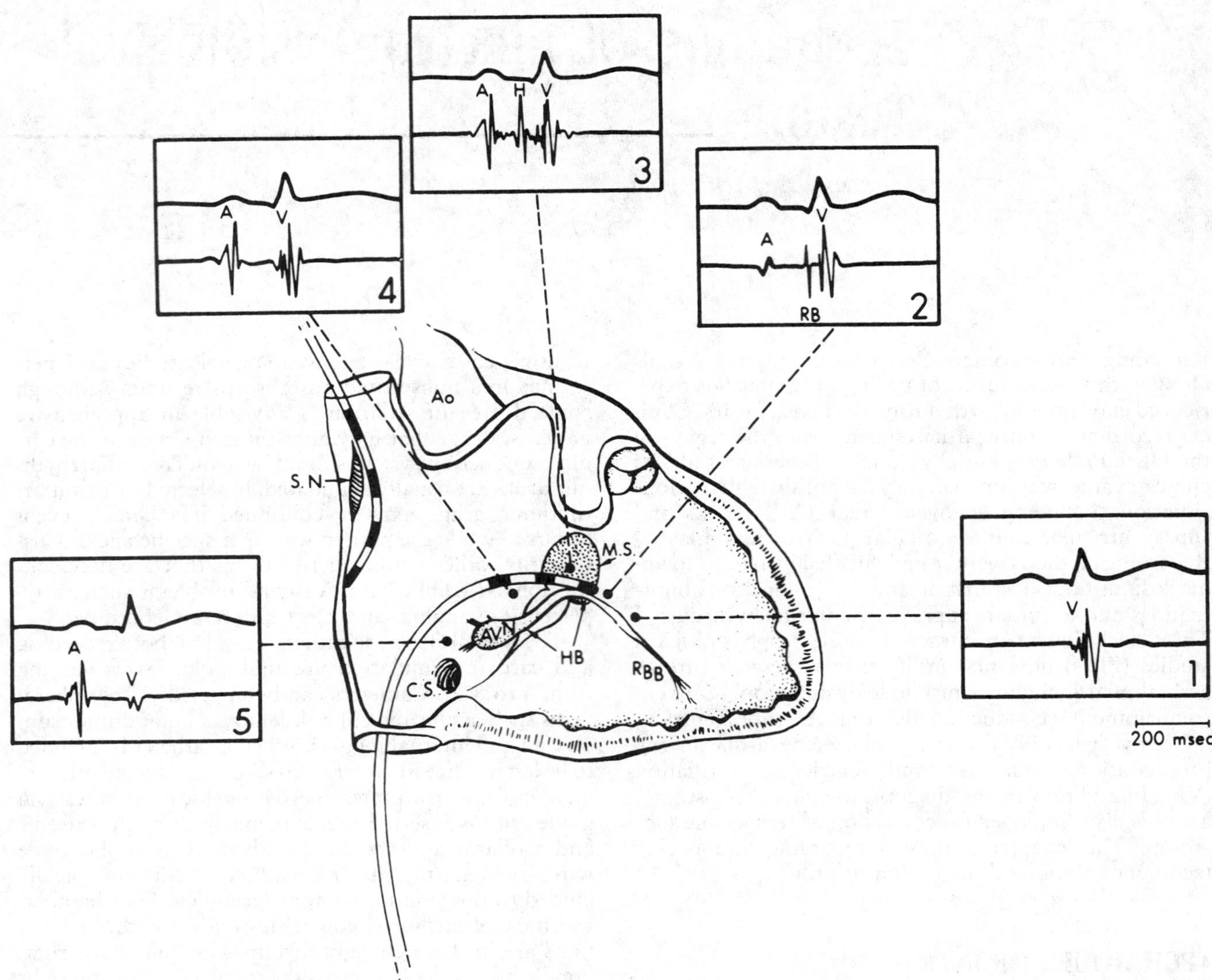

FIGURE 46-1 Intracardiac recordings from the specialized conduction system in the AV junction. The recording of various electrograms along the right side of the interventricular septum with gradual withdrawal of the catheter across the tricuspid valve is shown. The intracardiac recordings are labeled. Numbers 1 through 5 refer to intracardiac location of catheters along with corresponding electrogram. (CS, coronary sinus; SN, sinus node; Ao, aorta; MS, membranous septum; AVN, atrioventricular node; HB, His bundle; RBB, right bundle branch, A, atrial deflection; H and RB, His and right bundle potentials; V, ventricular deflection.) [*From JJ Gallagher, AN Damato: Technique of recording His bundle activity in man. In: W Grossman (ed): Cardiac Catheterization and Angiography. Philadelphia, Lea & Febiger, 1980: 283–301. Reproduced with permission from the publisher and authors*].

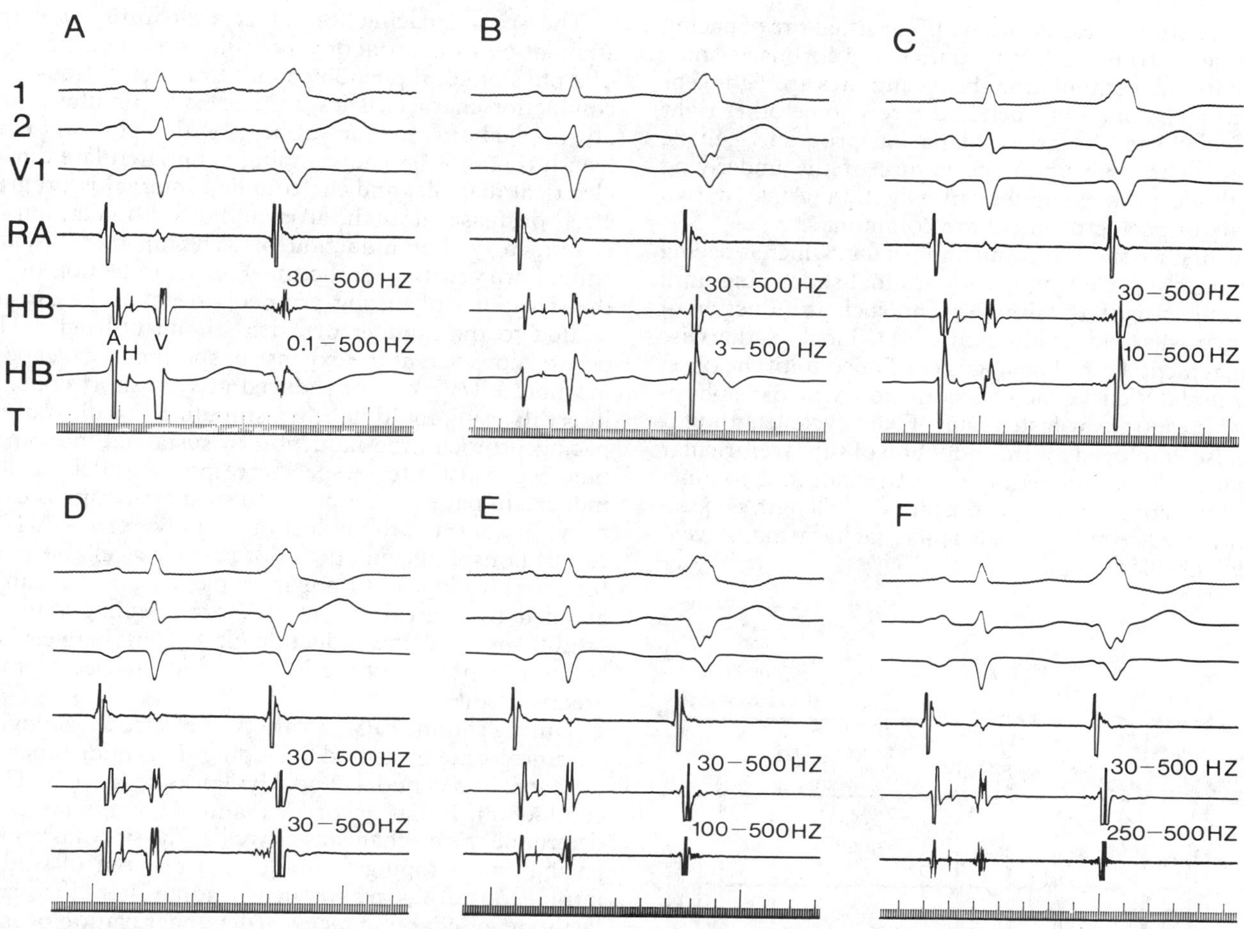

FIGURE 46-2 Effects of various filtering frequencies on the morphologic appearance of intracardiac electrograms *A* through *F*. The tracings from top to bottom are ECG leads I, II, V_1, right atrial (RA), two His bundle (HB) electrograms, and time (T) line. Similar abbreviations are used in subsequent figures and tracings. In each panel the first beat is of sinus origin and is followed by a spontaneous ventricular premature beat. The top HB, RA, and RV are filtered at 30 to 500 Hz (i.e., the usual filtering frequencies). The bottom HB tracing shows the effect of various filtering frequencies on the appearance. The low-frequency signals are mostly eliminated at high-bandpass filter frequency settings above 10 Hz (*C*). The low-bandpass filter settings above 500 Hz generally do not have a significant effect on the intracardiac electrogram appearance. It should be pointed out that the high-bandpass setting reduces the overall magnitude of the electrogram, necessitating an increase in amplification. It should also be noted that at all frequencies depicted, the HB deflection can be clearly identified. [*From M Akhtar: Invasive cardiac electrophysiologic studies: An introduction. In: WW Parmley, K Chatterjee, (eds): Cardiology, vol 1: Physiology, Pharmacology, Diagnosis. Philadelphia, JB Lippincott, 1991: Chap. 64: 1–17. Reproduced with permission from the publisher and authors*].

for sharp intracardiac signals such as those from the His bundle and accessory pathways (Fig. 46-2). Undesirable low-frequency signals can be reduced by a high-pass filter setting of more than 50 to 100 Hz. On the other hand, 60-cycle interference can be eliminated with a low-pass filter setting at 50 Hz. Alteration in the high-bandpass filter for surface electrocardiography can markedly alter the scalar electrocardiographic morphology. Amplification is frequently necessary to identify desirable signals from the specialized conduction system. This can lead to superimposition of the larger myocardial signals on various electrocardiographic tracings. In most recording equipment, however, there are limiting filters that allow the adjustment of amplitude limits.

The main value of intracardiac/electrocardiographic tracings is timing of electric events. To acquire true local electrical activity, a bipolar electrogram with an inter-electrode distance of less than 1 cm is desirable. When unipolar electrograms are obtained, a rapid intrinsic deflection will identify a local activation point. For routine intracardiac electrocardiographic studies, unipolar electrograms provide relatively limited advantage over bipolar signals, and therefore, the latter are more often utilized. In other clinical situations different types of diagnostic methods are utilized. For example, during intraoperative mapping, direct placement of electrodes over the epicardium or endocardium is necessary to get appropriate signals to identify the origin and route of impulse propagation during the tachycardia. These electrodes can be in the form of either hand-held probes or plaques that can be placed or sutured over the myocardium. All electrical signals can be recorded on either a disk or frequency-modulated tape for permanent storage.

Programmed Electrical Stimulation

After satisfactory placement of the electrode catheters, patches, or other forms of recording equipment, programmed stimulation is initiated. The usual site of pacing is the right atrium or left atrium via the coronary sinus. For ventricular stimulation the pacing sites are right ventricular apex, outflow tract, and rarely some other right ventricular site. A variety of pacing programs can be utilized depending upon the nature of the underlying arrhythmic problem under investigation. At least two formats of pacing protocol are common.

The first format is incremental pacing, which is pacing at a constant cycle length with gradual shortening until the occurrence of a desirable event, such as induction of a tachycardia and production of AV block. Otherwise the incremental atrial pacing is continued until the onset of AV nodal Wenckebach phenomenon, which is a physiological response at faster rates. Fixed cycle length pacing is also employed for the induction of supraventricular tachyarrhythmias and study of ventriculoatrial conduction. Bursts of pacing at a constant cycle length is occasionally used to induce ventricular tachycardia or ventricular fibrillation.

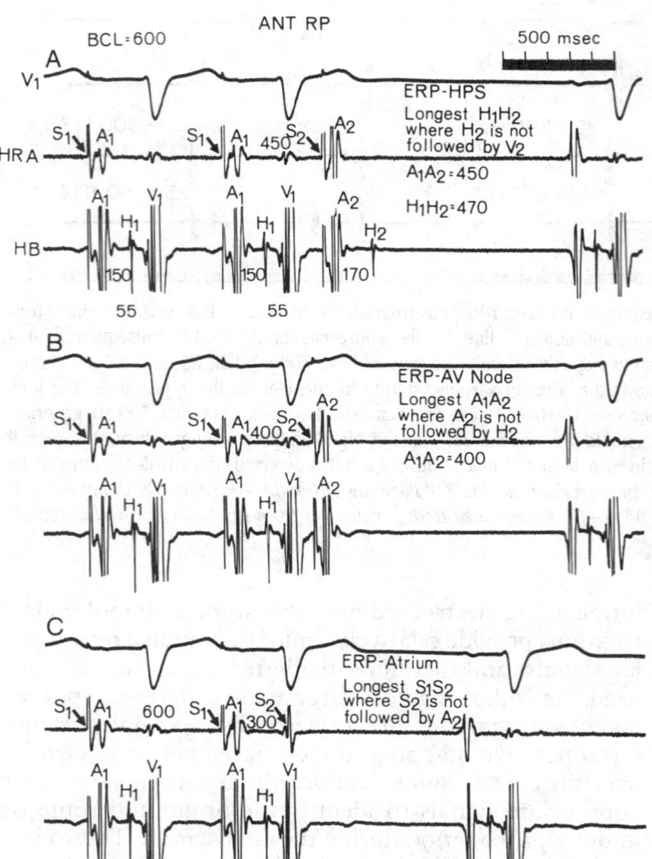

FIGURE 46-3 Determination of cardiac refractory periods during atrial pacing (*A* through *C*). During a basic cycle length pacing at 600 ms (S_1S_1 or A_1A_1), atrial premature stimulation (S_2 or A_2) at progressively shorter coupling intervals (S_1S_2 or A_1A_2) is depicted. The definition of the effective refractory period (ERP) of the His-Purkinje system (HPS), AV node, and atrium are labeled. (ANT RP, antegrade refractory period.) [*From M Akhtar: Invasive cardiac electrophysiologic studies: An introduction. In: WW Parmley, K Chatterjee (eds): Cardiology, vol 1: Physiology, Pharmacology, Diagnosis. Philadelphia, JB Lippincott, 1991: Chap. 64, 1–17. Reproduced with permission from the publisher and authors*].

The second pacing format is premature (or extra) stimulation from atrial or ventricular sites. For the study of a physiological phenomenon, refractory periods, and conduction characteristics, a single extra stimulus is usually applied after a series of beats with a constant cycle length (Fig. 46-3). The scanning is initiated late during electrical diastole, and the coupling interval is progressively decreased until the atrial and/or ventricular muscle is refractory. For induction of SVTs up to two extra stimuli are generally sufficient. For the induction of VT the sensitivity of pacing protocols seems to be directly related to the number of extra stimuli utilized.[12] This occurs, however, at the expense of specificity when polymorphic VT/VF can be induced at very short coupling intervals using multiple extra stimuli. Regardless of the pacing protocol, the induction of sustained monomorphic VT constitutes a specific response and is seldom induced in patients not prone to such arrhythmias clinically. In contrast, the induction of polymorphic VT/VF can be nonspecific and does not provide a reliable guide for serial testing. Both polymorphic VT and VF can be avoided to a great extent if short coupling intervals (<200 ms) and the induction of latency between the stimulus artifact and the local ventricular electrograms are avoided.[13]

During routine EPSs, a variety of electrophysiological parameters are measured, including sinus node function, intraatrial, AV nodal, and His-Purkinje system (HPS) conduction. Initiation of SVT and VT is attempted to determine the mechanisms as well as the site of origin by pacing and mapping techniques. After control studies, intravenous drugs are frequently administered either to facilitate induction of tachycardias, aggravation of sinus node function, and production of AV block (Fig. 46-4) or to determine drug efficacy.[14] At the completion of testing, the catheters are withdrawn and gentle pressure is applied at the area of catheter insertion. Unless arterial catheterization is performed, the patients are usually allowed to ambulate after 4 to 6 h.

There has been a significant evolution in the role of EPSs in patient management over the last decades. The technique has evolved from a purely diagnostic method to a frequently applied therapeutic tool. A brief outline of the value of clinical EPSs in various arrhythmia settings is outlined separately under diagnostic and therapeutic categories.

INVASIVE ELECTROPHYSIOLOGICAL STUDIES FOR DIAGNOSIS

Sinus Node Dysfunction[3,4]

Electrophysiological studies are generally performed to detect sinus node dysfunction, i.e., in patients with dizziness, presyncope, syncope, etc., in whom the diagnosis cannot be made noninvasively. The demonstration of sinus node dysfunction at EPS is often used to facilitate decision making regarding therapy. Electrophysiological studies are not indicated in asymptomatic patients with sinus node dysfunction or those who have obvious sinus node dysfunction demonstrable from the surface electrocardiogram (ECG). Invasive EPS is also done to test the sinus node automaticity, or sinoatrial conduction time.

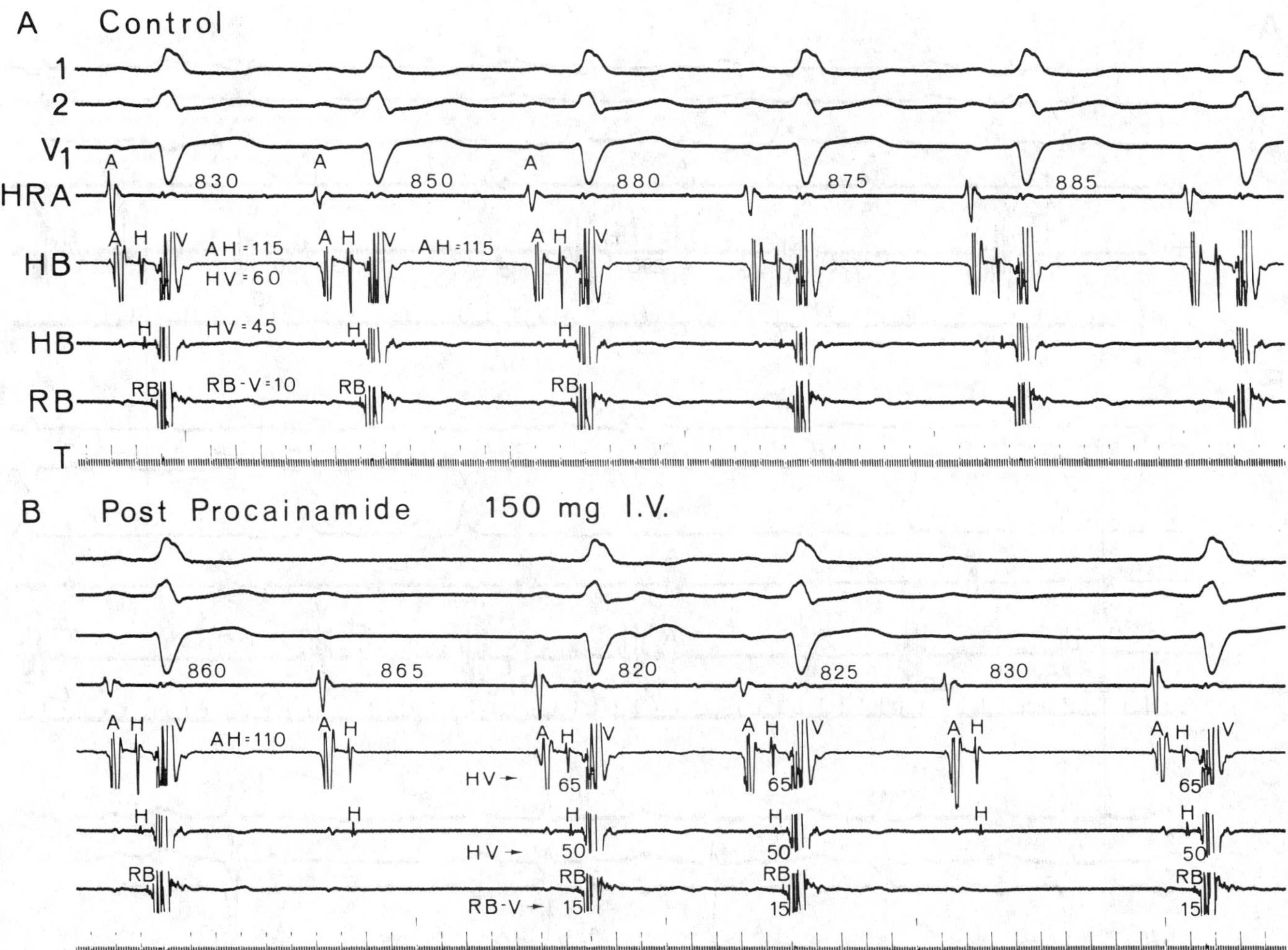

FIGURE 46-4 Atrioventricular block in the HPS. (*A*) 1 : 1 AV conduction is depicted in A in a patient with unexplained syncope. Following 150 mg of intravenous procainamide (*B*) a second-degree AV block in the HPS is noted (i.e., His bundle potential is not followed by a QRS complex), an abnormal response to a small dose of procainamide suggesting AV block in the HPS as a potential cause of syncope.

The most frequently performed test is that of sinus node suppression utilizing overdrive atrial pacing. After pacing at several basic cycle lengths for a period of approximately 30 s or longer, the pacing is interrupted. The resultant escape interval, which is called sinus node recovery time, is measured. By deducting the predominant sinus cycle length from this interval, one can obtain the so-called corrected sinus node recovery time. A sinus node recovery time in patients with sinus node disease was reported by Mandel et al. to average 3087 ms.[3] Normal patients in the same study averaged 1073 ms. In the series by Narula et al.[6] the value for corrected sinus node recovery time was less than 525 ms in normal individuals and exceeded those values in patients with overt sinus node dysfunction. More recently, direct sinus node recordings have been obtained by amplification of recording from catheters placed in a closed proximity to the sinus node.[15,16]

By the use of such direct recordings, both the sinus node automaticity and sinoatrial conduction can be precisely determined. In the vast majority of patients with true sinus node disease, sinoatrial conduction abnormalities are the predominant reason for sinus node dysfunction. The sinoatrial conduction time in normal individuals without obvious sinus node disease is less than 100 ms. The sensitivity of sinus node recovery time for the detection of sinus node dysfunction is 54 percent while that of sinoatrial conduction time is 51 percent with a combined sensitivity of the two tests of around 64 percent. The specificity of the two tests combined is approximately 88 percent. In patients with sinus node dysfunction it is important to test the AV conduction since the latter is also frequently abnormal. In patients with brady-cardia/tachycardia syndrome, tachycardias particularly arising in the atrium are frequent, and testing may also be necessary for the proper diagnosis and therapy of the concomitant tachyarrhythmia.

Atrioventricular Block

In asymptomatic patients with first-degree AV block (prolonged PR interval), electrophysiological assessment is unnecessary regardless of the QRS morphology of the

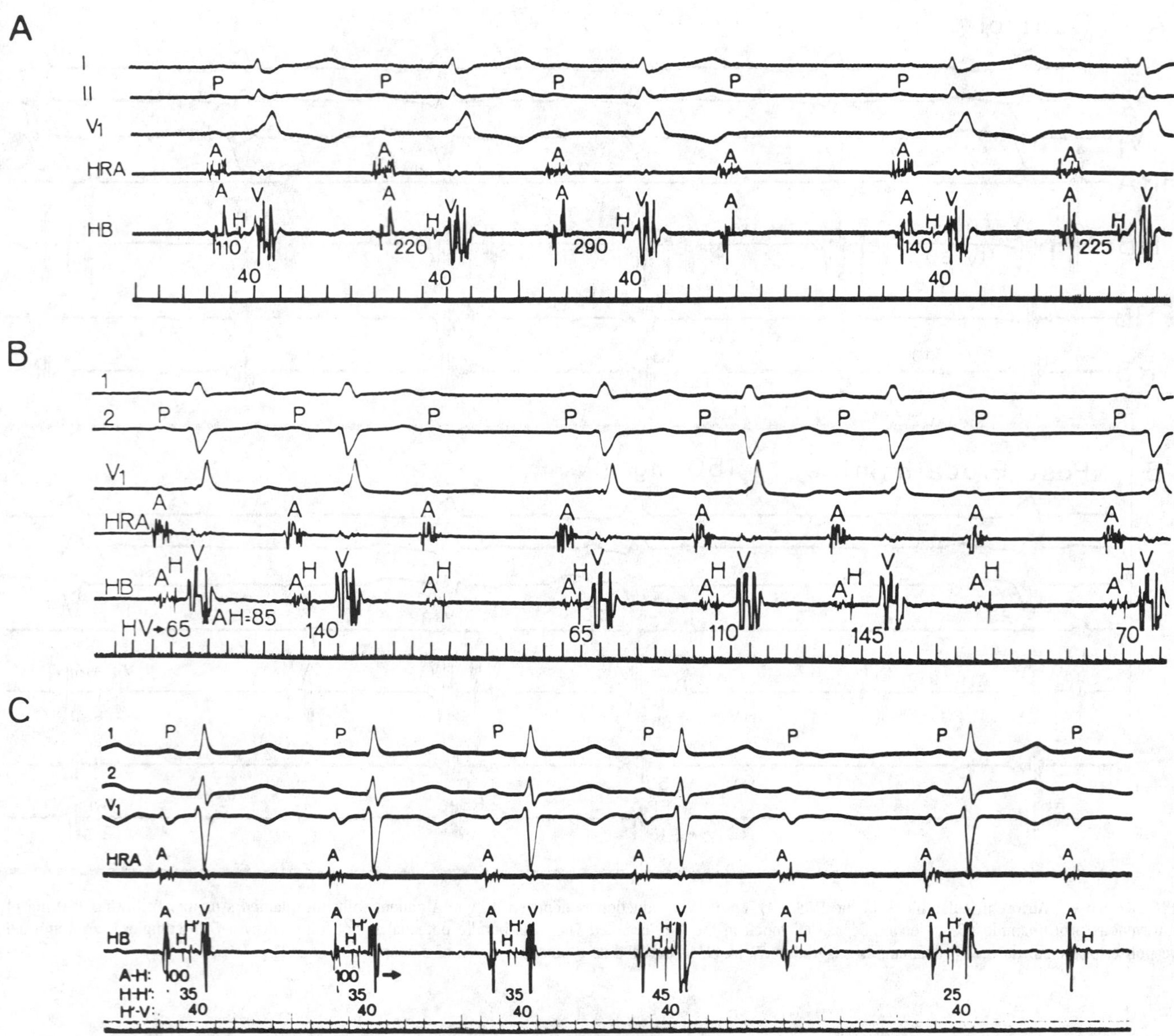

FIGURE 46-5 HB electrograms in AV block. The tracings are from three different patients with second-degree AV block. In *A* and *B* the conducted QRS complexes are wide and associated with bundle branch block (BBB). In *A* the block is within the AV node (i.e., the A wave on HB is not followed by an HB deflection). In *B* it can be appreciated that the block is distal to the HB even though the surface ECG demonstrates a Wenckebach phenomenon. The latter can obviously occur in the HPS as well, as depicted in this figure. *C.* Site of block is within the HB. This is suggested by split HB potentials (labeled H and H′), and the block is distal to the H but proximal to the H′. Intra-His block is difficult to diagnose from the surface ECG but can be suspected when a Mobitz type II occurs in association with a normal PR interval and a narrow QRS complex. [*From M Akhtar: Clinical application of electrophysiologic studies in the management of patients requiring pacemaker therapy. In: SS Barold (ed): Modern Cardiac Pacing. Mount Kisco, NY, Futura, 1985: 3–17. Reproduced with permission from the publisher and author*].

conducted beats. With second-degree AV block, the main role of electrophysiological assessment is finding the site of block (Figs. 46-4 and 46-5). Patients with intra-Hisian or infra-Hisian block tend to have a more unpredictable course, and permanent pacing is usually desirable.[17] On the other hand, asymptomatic patients with AV nodal block generally do not require permanent pacing. Even though the intranodal block usually presents as Wenckebach phenomenon or Mobitz type I, it is not uncommon to see Wenckebach phenomena within the HPS or within the His bundle. There is no difference in prognosis regardless of how the infra- or intra-Hisian second-degree block manifests itself i.e., type I versus type II. On occasion, intranodal blocks are preceded by no discernible change in PR interval and from a surface ECG may appear as forms of Mobitz type II. The absolute length of the PR interval is usually quite diagnostic in that it is prolonged (≥250 ms) and there is a shortening exceeding 100 ms of the PR interval following the block beat. In symptomatic patients with second-degree AV block the role of EPS is limited because permanent pacing is the appropriate intervention. On the other hand, if the patient's symptom cannot be explained on the basis of AV block and may be related to another arrhythmia, such

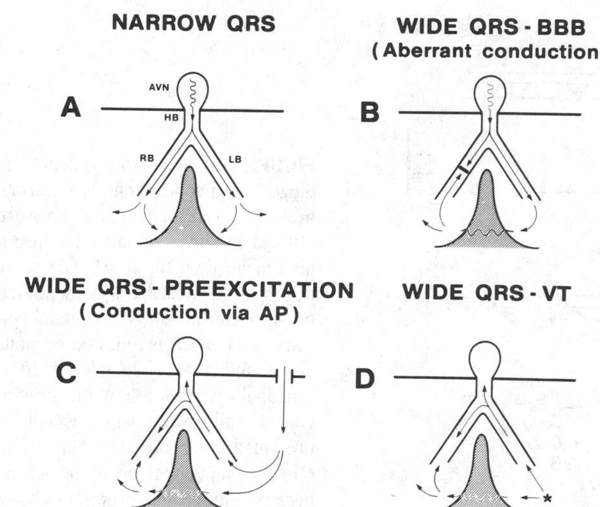

FIGURE 46-6 Wide QRS tachycardia. Routes of impulse propagation during a wide QRS tachycardia in various settings are depicted. It should be noted that only in *A* and *B* is His bundle activation expected to precede ventricular activation. This helps the delineation from other causes of wide QRS tachycardia shown in *C* and *D*.

as ventricular tachycardia, EPS should be considered. In patients with third-degree or complete AV block EPSs are seldom required and permanent pacing is the obvious option in symptomatic patients.

For EPS to determine the site of AV block it is critical to have the catheter across the AV junction that records the His bundle. A discernible His bundle recording allows one to determine the exact site of AV conduction abnormality, i.e., proximal to, within, or distal to the His bundle region. This, in combination with surface electrocardiographic morphology of conducted beats, allows one to identify precisely the location of conduction abnormality. The normal atrial to His bundle activation time (A-H) is approximately 50 to 140 ms, while the His to ventricular myocardial depolarization interval (H-V) measures 35 to 55 ms.

Wide QRS Tachycardia

Wide QRS tachycardia occurs from a variety of electrophysiological mechanisms both of supraventricular and ventricular origin in the presence, as well as the absence, of accessory pathways (Fig. 46-6).[18] (See also Chap. 36.) The underlying nature of the wide QRS tachycardia is critical for both prognosis and therapy. Electrophysiological studies have proven invaluable in distinguishing the various etiologies (Fig. 46-7). With few exceptions, when the nature of the arrhythmic problem is not well known and the direction of therapy is not clear, patients with wide QRS tachycardia should undergo EPS. This is particularly true in situations where nonpharmacologic therapy is the desired goal.

Unexplained Syncope

Unexplained syncope is commonly due to cardiovascular mechanisms. The two most common reasons for cardiovascular syncope are cardiac arrhythmias and neurocardiogenic dysfunction, referred to as vasodepressor syncope.[19–22] Electrophysiological study constitutes an integral part of the workup and evaluation of patients with unexplained syncope. During such studies, all arrhythmic potential possibilities such as sinus node dysfunction, AV conduction abnormalities, SVT, and VT should be excluded. Neurocardiogenic mechanisms constitute the most common causes of syncope in patients without structural heart disease, and incomplete assessment in these patients may lead to inappropriate therapy (Fig. 46-8).[19] The possibility of neurocardiogenic dysfunction can be unmasked on a tilt table. The triage of patients toward one or the other, i.e., electrophysiological testing versus head-up tilt, is fairly simple and predicted by clinical history and the presence or absence of structural heart disease.[19] Patients with underlying structural heart disease such as old myocardial infarction or primary myocardial disease generally have underlying VT to explain the symptoms of syncope (Fig. 46-9). When arrhythmias occur in patients without overt struc-

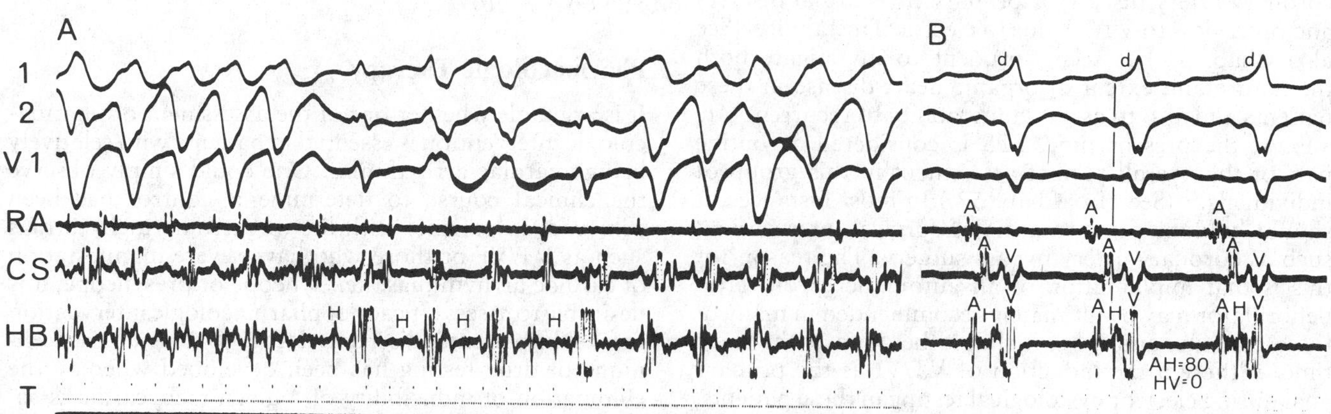

FIGURE 46-7 Wide QRS tachycardia. *A*. Wide QRS complexes of at least two varieties. Those showing a left bundle branch block pattern are due to conduction over an accessory pathway, while those with a right bundle branch pattern are aberrant in nature. Note the His bundle activation prior to the QRS in narrow and aberrant complexes but not before preexcited complexes. A right posteroseptal preexcitation can be appreciated in *B* with a short PR, a delta wave (*d*), an HV of zero and negative delta wave in lead V_1.

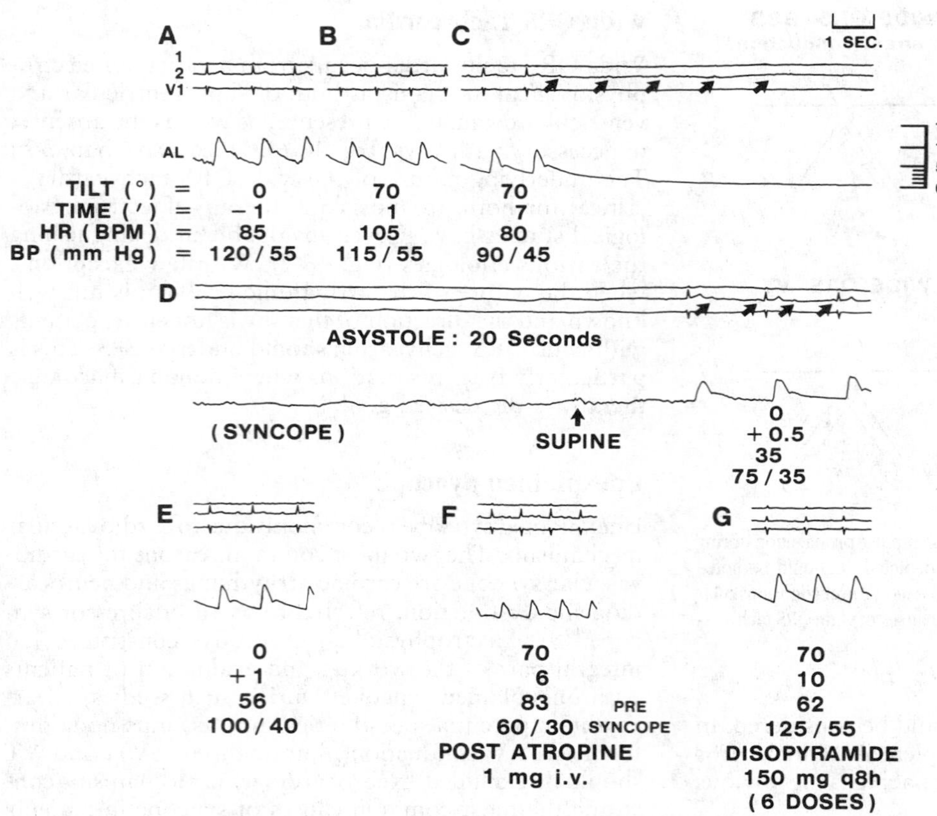

FIGURE 46-8 Asystole in neurocardiogenic syncope. Note the normal heart rate (HR) and blood pressure (BP) at supine position. At the beginning of head-up tilt at 70° (*B*) some degree of tachycardia is noted. Seven minutes after the tilt (*C*) an initial episode of AV block is followed by sinus arrest and a total asystole of 20 s. Syncopal episodes follow but presyncope is still present when asystole is prevented by atropine (*F*). Findings in *C* might tempt one to prescribe permanent pacing, an inappropriate choice of therapy. In this patient with neurocardiogenic syncope, disopyramide (*G*) prevented hypotension and syncope without the need for a permanent pacemaker. (*From J Sra, AJ Anderson, SH Sheikh, B Avitall, PJ Tchou, P Troup, et al: Unexplained syncope evaluated by electrophysiologic studies and head-up tilt testing. Ann Intern Med 114:1013–1019, 1991. Reproduced with permission from the publisher and authors.*)

tural heart disease sinus node dysfunction, AV conduction, particularly intra-Hisian block or SVTs are likely. On rare occasion, VT can occur in the absence of an overt structural heart disease. (See also Chap. 50.)

Survivors of Sudden Cardiac Death

In most patients with documented episodes of cardiac arrest, VF can be documented at the time of collapse. When the rescue squad has available monitor strips, VF is commonly demonstrated. Patients dying suddenly generally have underlying structural heart disease (usually coronary artery disease or primary myocardial disease) and proneness to VT/VF due to electrical instability. (See also Chap. 51.) It seems prudent to investigate both the nature and extent of organic heart disease in these patients and also to assess vulnerability to recurrent VT/VF. At the present time, EPS is considered a routine part of the overall patient assessment in this group of individuals.[23] (See also Chap. 52.) In most instances, it should be done prior to a major surgical intervention, such as coronary artery bypass surgery. The reason for this is that implantation of an automatic cardioverter defibrillator may be ultimately recommended in many of these patients, and if so, it should be done at the same time. Although the induction of VT/VF is the primary goal during electrophysiological testing in these patients, other arrhythmic possibilities such as sinus node dysfunction and AV block should also be evaluated. In some cases another rhythm abnormality may trigger cardiac arrest and lead to VT/VF due to prolonged pauses and, on rare occasions, from SVT. (See also Chap. 35.)

INVASIVE CARDIAC ELECTROPHYSIOLOGICAL STUDIES FOR THERAPEUTIC INTERVENTION

Because of the episodic nature of most cardiac arrhythmias, it is difficult to assess the efficacy of any therapeutic intervention unless the arrhythmia in question can be replicated. Diagnostic EPS provides that opportunity, and it seems logical to use the same tool to assess therapeutic interventions.[24–26] This method to assess efficacy can be applied for both pharmacologic and nonpharmacologic therapy.

Pharmacologic Therapy

It is arguable whether or not the assessment of pharmacologic intervention is essential in patients with relatively benign cardiac arrhythmias. One could simply observe the clinical course to determine if control has been achieved. In patients with life-threatening tachycardias such as VT/VF or those who have severe manifestation of cardiac arrhythmias, i.e., syncope or presyncope, it is desirable to assess efficacy of pharmacologic intervention before the patient is discharged (Fig. 46-10.)[25,26] The technique of drug testing has been developed whereby the elimination of inducibility of a given tachycardia is assessed following a drug administration. This can be done following intravenous drugs as well as oral agents. Both the drug efficacy and the lack thereof can be evaluated using this method. When drug therapy does eliminate induction of a previously inducible tachycardia, the addi-

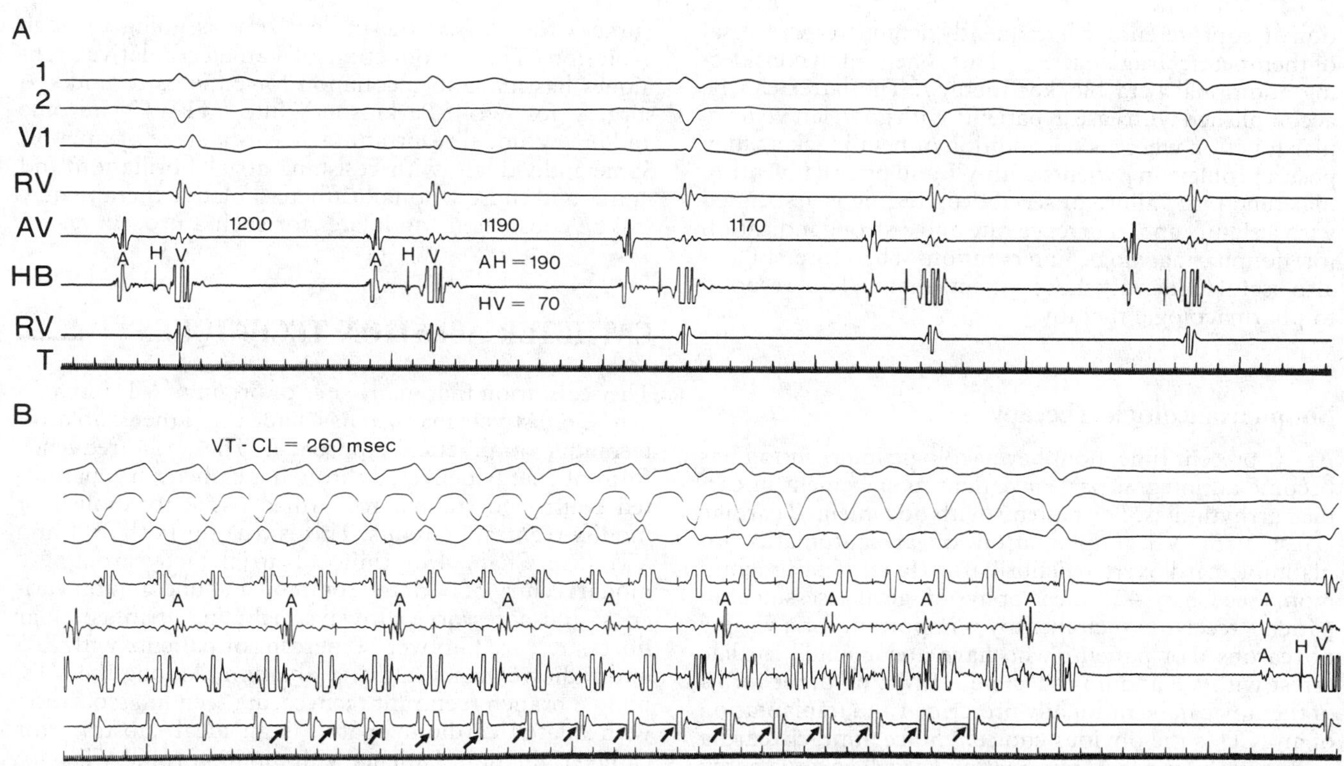

FIGURE 46-9 Arrhythmic causes of syncope. *A*. Sinus rhythm in a patient with unexplained syncope. Sinus bradycardia, bifascicular block, and a long PR interval from surface ECG suggest possible AV block as the cause. In this patient, however, ventricular tachycardia (*B*) was the actual cause. Control of ventricular tachycardia (VT) without a pacemaker was sufficient to prevent syncope in this patient. Termination of tachycardia and restoration of sinus rhythm is shown in *B*.

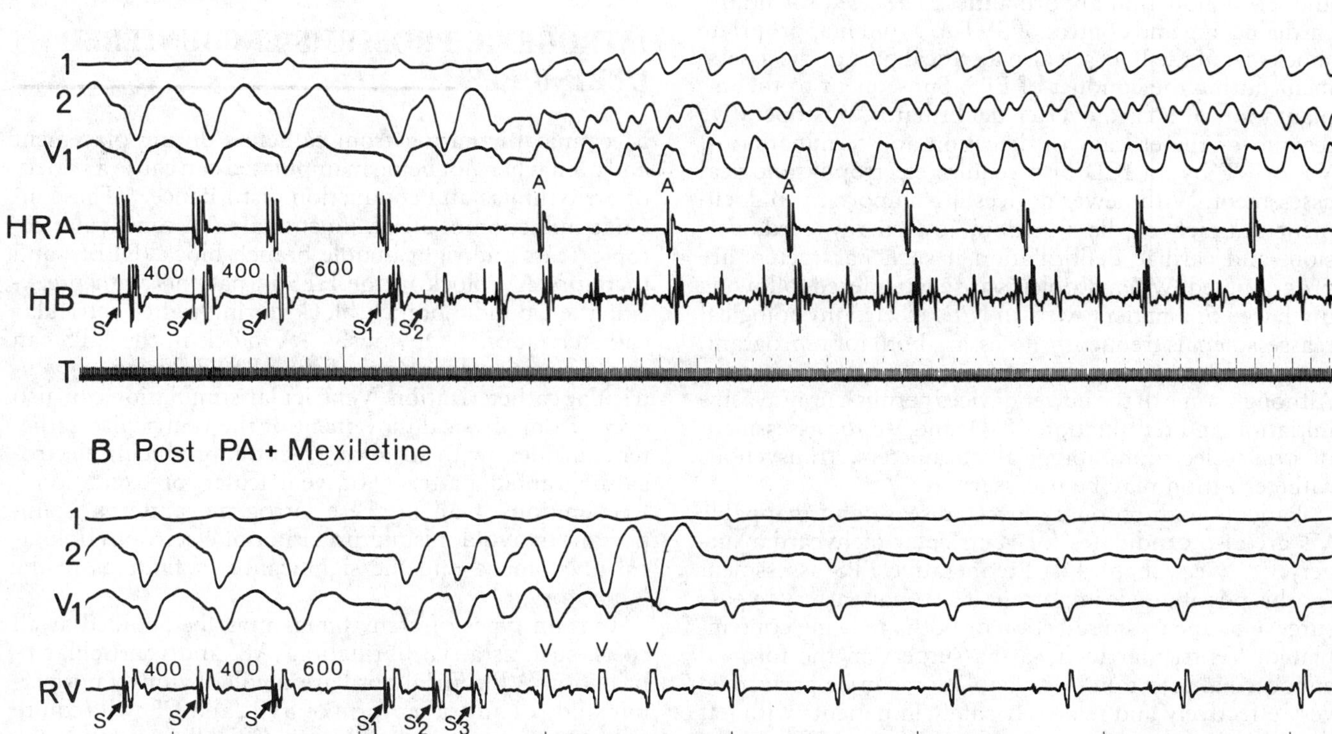

FIGURE 46-10 Initiation of sustained monomorphic VT is shown in *A*. After oral procainamide and mexiletine the sustained VT could not be induced despite using more aggressive pacing protocol.

tion of isoproterenol will frequently demonstrate reversal of therapeutic drug effect.[27,28] This is helpful in considering additional beta blocker therapy. The latter can be accomplished with ease in patients with good left ventricular function whereas the addition of beta blockers may pose a problem in patients with VT and poor left ventricular function. Failure of serial drug testing is associated with a significant recurrence rate and a strong indication for nonpharmacologic intervention. Therefore, EPS is also useful to identify those patients that will not respond to pharmacologic therapy.

Nonpharmacologic Therapy

At the present time, nonpharmacologic intervention has become an integral part of patient management in cardiac arrhythmias. For patients with documented cardiac arrest with VF, implantation of an automatic implantable cardioverter defibrillator (ICD) is fairly common. (See Chap. 42.) Electrophysiological assessment in patients receiving such therapy is important for a variety of reasons. For patients who have documented cardiac arrest with VF and no inducible VT/VF, no other forms of therapy can be rationally prescribed and implantation of an ICD is the obvious choice.[29] Since antitachycardia pacing with overdrive termination as well as low-energy cardioversion have become available in ICD devices, testing for the hemodynamic stability of VT, cycle length, and the ability to terminate are key pieces of information and should be obtained prior to implant. In addition to VT, these patients also have a variety of other abnormalities including proneness to SVT, sinus node dysfunction, and AV conduction abnormalities. The need for bradycardia pacing and control of SVT to avoid inappropriate shocks from the ICD are also a critical part of the assessment during the conduct of EPS. Subsequent to the implantation of a cardioverter defibrillator, postoperative testing for the efficacy of detection and termination of VT or VF by an ICD also require electrophysiological assessment. With newer devices it is important to document antitachycardia function, low-energy cardioversion, and cardiac defibrillation if such parameters are programmed. When problems are encountered following discharge of a patient with an ICD, electrophysiological reassessment is frequently necessary both for reprogramming and for the detection of any unexplained events. Although some of the newer devices permit a noninvasive initiation and termination of VT and VF for assessment of other electrophysiological parameters, transvenous catheterization may be necessary.

Patients with coronary artery disease and mappable VT are also candidates for ventricular tachycardia surgery.[30–32] (See Chap. 44.) Preoperative EPS assessment for this possibility is important if coronary artery bypass surgery or aneurysm resection or both are being contemplated. Ventricular tachycardia surgery in the form of endocardial resection or cryoablation can be performed very effectively and relatively safely in patients with left ventricular ejection fraction of greater than 20 percent. This curative procedure will provide effective control in approximately 75 percent of the patients who have monomorphic VT that can be appropriately mapped. Surgery for SVT at the present time is going through evolution. The introduction of catheter ablative techniques has made it uncommon for patients to undergo surgery for Wolff-Parkinson-White (WPW) syndrome and/or AV nodal reentrant tachycardia. (See Chap. 43.) Some individuals with resistant atrial fibrillation and flutter and those who fail catheter ablative therapy may still be considered candidates for such a procedure.

CATHETER ABLATION TECHNIQUES[33–35]

The realization that many sites of origin of VT and SVT can be effectively mapped has made the catheter ablative technique a practical approach. The radiofrequency form of energy delivered through a catheter has permitted controlled trauma to cardiac tissue to abolish or modify reentrant circuits. This is true for both SVT and VT. (See Chap. 43.) Unifocal atrial tachycardia, AV modal reentry of both the common and uncommon varieties, and accessory pathways including atriofascicular fibers are cured in over 90 percent of patients with EPS and radiofrequency catheter ablation. Among the VTs, bundle branch reentrant tachycardia seen in association with dilated cardiomyopathy is an ideal substrate for catheter ablation. Patients with monomorphic VT associated with myocardial scarring or other substrates can also be considered candidates, particularly when they are not suitable for VT surgery and have failed drug therapy. In all of these patient subsets, initial EPS evaluation is crucial.

IATROGENIC PROBLEMS ENCOUNTERED DURING EPS

Mechanical irritation from catheters during placement and even when not being manipulated can cause a variety of arrhythmias and conduction disturbance.[36] These include induction of atrial, junctional, and ventricular ectopic beats and right bundle branch block (RBBB) and therefore AV block in the HPS in patients with preexisting left bundle branch block during right ventricular catheterization.[36] Obviously, AV block in the HPS can occur in patients with preexisting RBBB during left ventricular catheterization. Ventricular stimulation can also occur from physical movement of the ventricular catheter coincident with atrial contraction, producing electrocardiographic patterns of ventricular preexcitation.[36] Recognition of all of these iatrogenic patterns is important to avoid misinterpretation of electrophysiological phenomena and the significance of findings in the laboratory.

Certain types of arrhythmias must be avoided at all costs, such as atrial fibrillation (AF) and ventricular fibrillation (VF). Atrial fibrillation will obviously not permit study of any other form of SVT, and VF will require prompt cardioversion, making it difficult to continue the EPS. If AF must be initiated for diagnostic purposes (i.e., to assess ventricular response over the accessory pathway in WPW syndrome), it should be done at the end of the study. Patients with a prior history of AF are more prone to the occurrence of sustained AF in the laboratory. Frequently, this will occur during initial placement of catheters, and excessive manipulation of catheters in the atria should therefore be avoided.

Risks

When only right-sided heart catheterization is done for EPS, the complication rate is relatively low, with almost negligible mortality.[37,38] In our own experience with more than 8000 EPS procedures, no mortality has been encountered. Other complications include deep venous thrombosis, pulmonary embolism, infection at catheter sites, systemic infection, pneumothorax, and perforation of a cardiac chamber or coronary sinus.

The occurrence of potentially lethal arrhythmias such as rapid VT or VF is common in the laboratory. These are not necessarily countered as complications, however, but are often expected and anticipated events. Nonetheless, the common occurrence of these events makes the electrophysiology laboratory a place for only highly trained personnel equipped to handle such problems.

REFERENCES

1. Scherlag BJ, Lau SH, Helfant RH, Berkowitz WD, Stein E, Damato AN: Catheter technique for recording His bundle activity in man. *Circulation* 1969; 39:13–18.
2. Goldreyer BN, Bigger JT: Spontaneous and induced reentrant tachycardia. *Ann Intern Med* 1969; 70:87–98.
3. Mandel WJ, Hayakawa H, Danzig R, Marcus HS: Evaluation of sinoatrial node function in man by overdrive suppression. *Circulation* 1971; 44:59–66.
4. Narula OS, Samet P, Javier RP: Significance of the sinus node recovery time. *Circulation* 1972; 45:140–158.
5. Damato AN, Lau SH, Helfant RH, Stein E, Patton RD, Scherlag BJ, et al: A study of heart block in man using His bundle recordings. *Circulation* 1969; 39:297–305.
6. Narula OS, Scherlag BJ, Samet P, Javier RP: Atrioventricular block: Localization and classification by His bundle recordings. *Am J Med* 1971; 50:146–165.
7. Goldreyer BN, Damato AN: The essential role of atrioventricular conduction delay in the initiation of paroxysmal supraventricular tachycardia. *Circulation* 1971; 43:679–687.
8. Wellens HJJ, Schuilenberg RM, Durrer D: Electrical stimulation of the heart in patients with the Wolff-Parkinson-White syndrome type A. *Circulation* 1971; 43:99–114.
9. Mason JW, Winkel RA: Electrode catheter arrhythmia induction in the selection and assessment of antiarrhythmic drug therapy for recurrent ventricular tachycardia. *Circulation* 1978; 58:971–985.
10. Ruskin JN, DiMarco JP, Garan H: Out of hospital cardiac arrest: Electrophysiologic observations in selection of long-term antiarrhythmic therapy. *N Engl J Med* 1980; 303:607–613.
11. Akhtar M: Invasive cardiac electrophysiologic studies: An introduction. In: Parmley WW, Chatterjee K (eds): *Cardiology*, vol 1: *Physiology, Pharmacology, Diagnosis*. Philadelphia, Lippincott, 1991: 64, 1–17.
12. Brugada P, Green M, Abdollah H, Wellens HJ: Significance of ventricular arrhythmias initiated by programmed ventricular stimulation: The importance of the type of ventricular arrhythmia induced and the number of premature stimuli required. *Circulation* 1984; 69:87–92.
13. Avitall B, McKinnie J, Jazayeri M, Akhtar M, Tchou P: Induction of ventricular fibrillation versus monomorphic ventricular tachycardia during programmed stimulation: Role of premature beat conduction delay. *Circulation* 1992; 85:1271–1278.
14. Akhtar M: Clinical application of electrophysiologic studies in the management of patients requiring pacemaker therapy. In: Barold S (ed): *Modern Cardiac Pacing*. Mount Kisco, NY, Futura, 1985: 3–17.
15. Hariman RJ, Krongrad E, Boxer RA, Weiss MB, Steeg CN, Hoffman BF: Method for recording electrical activity of the sinoatrial node and automatic atrial foci during cardiac catheterization in human subjects. *Am J Cardiol* 1980; 45:775–781.
16. Gomes JA: The sick sinus syndrome and evaluation of the patient with sinus node disorders. In: Parmley WW, Chatterjee K (eds): *Cardiology*, vol 1: *Physiology, Pharmacology, Diagnosis*. Philadelphia, Lippincott, 1991: 67, 1–15.
17. Dhingra RC, Wyndham CRC, Bauernfiend R, Swiryn S, Deedwania PC, Smith T, et al: Significance of block distal to the His bundle induced by atrial pacing in patients with chronic bifascicular block. *Circulation* 1979; 60:1455–1464.
18. Akhtar M, Jazayeri M, Avitall B, McKinnie J, Tchou P: Electrophysiologic spectrum of wide QRS complex tachycardia. In: Zipes DP, Jalife J (eds): *Cardiac Electrophysiology: From Cell to Bedside*. Orlando, FL, WB Saunders, 1990: 635–646.
19. Sra J, Anderson A, Sheikh S, Avitall B, Tchou P, Troup P, et al: Unexplained syncope evaluated by electrophysiologic studies and head-up tilt testing. *Ann Intern Med* 1991; 114:1013–1019.
20. DiMarco JP, Garan H, Ruskin JN: Cardiac electrophysiologic techniques in recurrent syncope of unknown cause. *Ann Intern Med* 1981; 95:542–548.
21. Akhtar M, Shenasa M, Denker S, Gilbert CJ, Rizwi N: Role of cardiac electrophysiologic studies in patients with unexplained recurrent syncope. *PACE* 1983; 6:192–201.
22. Morady F, Scheinman MM: The role and limitations of electrophysiologic testing in patients with unexplained syncope. *Int J Cardiol* 1983; 4:229–234.
23. Akhtar M, Garan H, Lehmann MH, Troup PJ: Sudden cardiac death: Management of high-risk patients. *Ann Intern Med* 1991; 114:499–512.
24. Wu D, Wyndham CR, Denes P, Amat-y-Leon F, Miller RH, Dhingra RC, et al: Chronic electrophysiological study in patients with recurrent paroxysmal tachycardia: A new method for developing successful oral antiarrhythmic therapy. In: Kulbertus HE (ed): *Reentrant Arrhythmias*. Baltimore, University Park Press, 1976: 294.
25. Horowitz LN, Josephson ME, Farshidi A, Spielman SR, Michelson EL, Greenspan AM: Recurrent sustained ventricular tachycardia: Role of the electrophysiologic study in selection of antiarrhythmic regimens. *Circulation* 1978; 58:986–997.
26. Mason JW, Winkle RA: Accuracy of ventricular tachycardia induction study for predicting long term efficacy and inefficacy of antiarrhythmic drugs. *N Engl J Med* 1980; 303:1073–1077.
27. Niazi I, Naccarelli G, Dougherty A, Rinkenberger R, Tchou P, Akhtar M: Treatment of atrioventricular node reentrant tachycardia with encainide: Reversal of drug effect with isoproterenol. *J Am Coll Cardiol* 1989; 13:904–910.
28. Jazayeri M, Van Wyhe G, Avitall B, McKinnie J, Tchou P, Akhtar M: Isoproterenol reversal of antiarrhythmic effects in patients with inducible sustained ventricular tachyarrhythmias. *J Am Coll Cardiol* 1989; 14:705–711.
29. Akhtar M, Avitall B, Jazayeri M, Tchou P, Troup P, Sra J, et al: Role of implantable cardioverter defibrillator therapy in the management of high risk patients. *Circulation* 1992; 85(suppl I): I-131–I-139.
30. Josephson ME, Harken AH, Horowitz LN: Long-term results of endocardial resection from sustained ventricular tachycardia in coronary disease patients. *Am Heart J* 1982; 104:51–57.
31. Caceres J, Werner P, Jazayeri M, Akhtar M, Tchou P: Efficacy of cryosurgery alone for refractory monomorphic sustained ventricular tachycardia due to inferior wall infarct. *J Am Coll Cardiol* 1988; 11:1254–1259.
32. Caceres J, Akhtar M, Werner P, Jazayeri M, McKinnie J, Avitall B, et al: Cryoablation of refractory sustained ventricular tachycardia due to coronary artery disease. *Am J Cardiol* 1989; 63:296–300.
33. Jackman WM, Wang X, Friday KJ, Roman CA, Moulton KP, Beckman KJ, et al: Catheter ablation of accessory atrioventricular pathways (Wolff-Parkinson-White syndrome) by radiofrequency current. *N Engl J Med* 1991; 324:1605–1611.
34. Calkins H, Sousa J, El-Atassi R, Rosenheck S, de Buitleir M, Kou WH, et al: Diagnosis and cure of the Wolff-Parkinson-White

syndrome or paroxysmal supraventricular tachycardias during a single electrophysiologic test. *N Engl J Med* 1991; 324:1612–1618.

35. Jazayeri M, Hempe SL, Sra JS, Dhala AA, Blanck Z, Deshpande SS, et al: Selective transcatheter ablation of the fast and slow pathways using radiofrequency energy in patients with atrioventricular nodal reentrant tachycardia. *Circulation* 1992; 85:1318–1328.
36. Akhtar M, Damato AN, Gilbert-Leeds CJ, Batsford WP, Reddy CP, Gomes JA, et al: Induction of iatrogenic electrocardiographic patterns during electrophysiologic studies. *Circulation* 1977; 56:60–65.
37. Di Marco JP, Garan H, Ruskin JN: Complications in patients undergoing cardiac electrophysiologic procedures. *Ann Intern Med* 1982; 97:490–493.
38. Horowitz L: Risks and complications of clinical cardiac electrophysiologic studies. A prospective analysis of 1000 consecutive patients. *J Am Coll Cardiol* 1987; 9:1261–1268.

Chapter 47

Technique of Signal-Averaged Electrocardiography

Paul F. Walter, M.D.

During the past decade, many investigators have discovered low-amplitude, high-frequency waveforms in the terminal QRS complex, both in laboratory models of myocardial infarction and in patients vulnerable to sustained ventricular tachycardia (VT).[1] These microvolt-level signals are called ventricular late potentials. They are continuous with the QRS complex and persist for tens of milliseconds into the ST segment. Late potentials are detectable from leads of the surface electrocardiogram (ECG) with a signal-averaging technique described under 'Technique."

PATHOPHYSIOLOGICAL BASIS OF LATE POTENTIALS

Ventricular late potentials on the body surface appear to arise from small areas of abnormal myocardium in which ventricular activation is delayed and asynchronous.[2] Structural myocardial abnormality is an important determinant of delayed activation.[3] When surviving myocardial bundles are separated by connective tissue, heterogeneous activation patterns may occur. The result is a low-amplitude, fragmented local electrogram.

Late potentials in patients correlate temporally with delayed, fragmented electrogram activity recorded directly from the heart. Fragmented electrogram activity can be recorded in most patients with remote myocardial infarction but is detected at fewer recording sites and is of shorter duration in infarction patients without clinical VT. Late potentials imply that the substrate for reentry is present, and VT may then be precipitated by such triggers as premature ventricular beats, myocardial ischemia, electrolyte imbalance, or autonomic nervous system instability. (See also Chap. 35.)

Healthy volunteers rarely have abnormal signal-averaged electrocardiograms (SAECGs). Patients with sustained, inducible monomorphic VT after myocardial infarction have abnormal SAECGs in 79 to 92 percent of cases.[1] Late potentials occur more frequently and are of greater duration in patients with monomorphic sustained VT than in patients with ventricular fibrillation, a rhythm less associated with conduction delay.

TECHNIQUE

A major problem in recording small bioelectric cardiac signals is interference from extraneous noise. The purpose of signal averaging is to decrease the amount of noise that contaminates the surface ECG. Skeletal muscle activity is the primary source of noise. The problem of noise contamination is partially solved when signal averaging is used. This technique averages together multiple samples of a repeating waveform, and so randomly occurring noise is diminished. Ectopic ventricular beats and excessively noisy beats must be rejected by the computer before averaging. Noise reduction is primarily dependent on the number of cycles to be summed. The signal-to-noise ratio improves in proportion to the square root of the number of averaged signals. Noise is measured in the averaged signal over an interval of at least 40 ms in the ST or TP segment with a four-pole Butterworth filter. The residual high-frequency noise content should be less than 1.0 μV with a 25-Hz high-pass cutoff or less than 0.7 μV with a 40-Hz high-pass cutoff as measured by the root-mean-square method from a vector magnitude of the X, Y, and Z orthogonal leads. After signal averaging, the ECG is high-pass filtered to reduce the low-frequency signals contained in the QRS complex and ST segment. High-pass filtering is necessary because the plateau, or repolarization phases, of the action potential produces slowly changing and lower frequency signals that would interfere with the measurement of microvolt signals corresponding to the delayed depolarization of small areas of myocardium.[4] A bidirectional digital filter free of ringing or overshoot artifact has been used in most studies.

High-pass filtering is called time domain analysis since the filter output corresponds in time with the input signal. Any time domain signal is the sum of many independent sinusoidal components of different amplitudes and frequencies. Timing information, such as the duration of the filtered QRS complex, can be obtained after filtering (Fig. 47-1).

Frequency domain analysis, usually performed by the Fourier transform, is another means to extract diagnostic high-frequency content from the SAECG. The fast Fourier transform is a mathematical algorithm that separates the signal into its individual sinusoids and provides information regarding the amplitudes and frequency of these individual components. The analysis of multiple segments (spectrotemporal mapping) is frequently used and may allow better separation between noise and late potentials (Fig. 47-2)[5].

Orthogonal X, Y, and Z leads are recorded in most studies of late potentials. After filtering, signals from the three leads are combined into a vector magnitude, $\sqrt{X^2+Y^2+Z^2}$, a summation of high-frequency information contained in all leads. The vector magnitude is called the filtered QRS complex.

VENTRICULAR LATE POTENTIALS

Ventricular late potentials are high-frequency waveforms that extend from the terminal QRS complex into the ST segment. The definition of a late potential and the scoring of the SAECG as normal or abnormal are not standardized. Common criteria defining late potentials

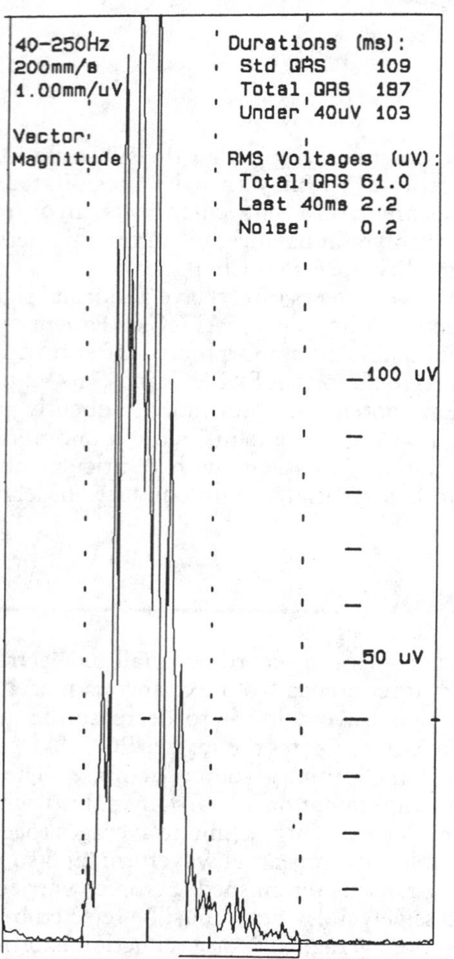

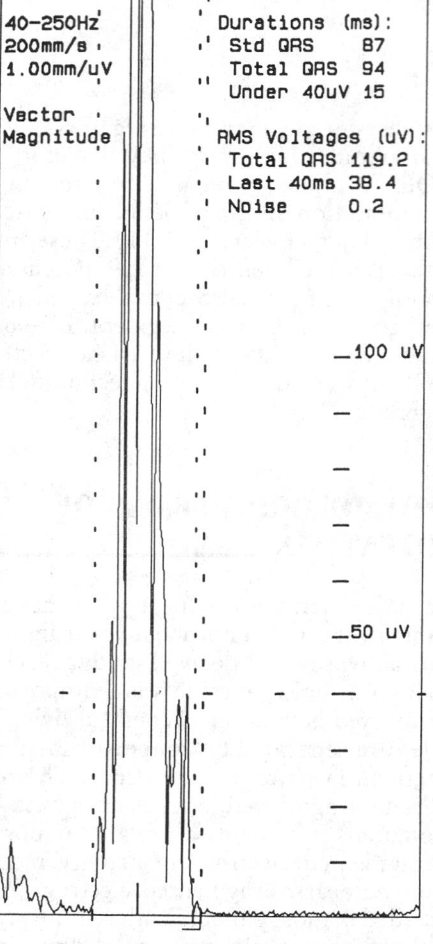

FIGURE 47-1 *A.* Normal signal-averaged vector complex. *B.* Abnormal signal-averaged vector complex. All three signal-averaged measurements are abnormal. The signal averaged QRS duration is 187 ms, low-amplitude signals are 103 ms in duration, and the root-mean—square voltage is 2.2 μV.

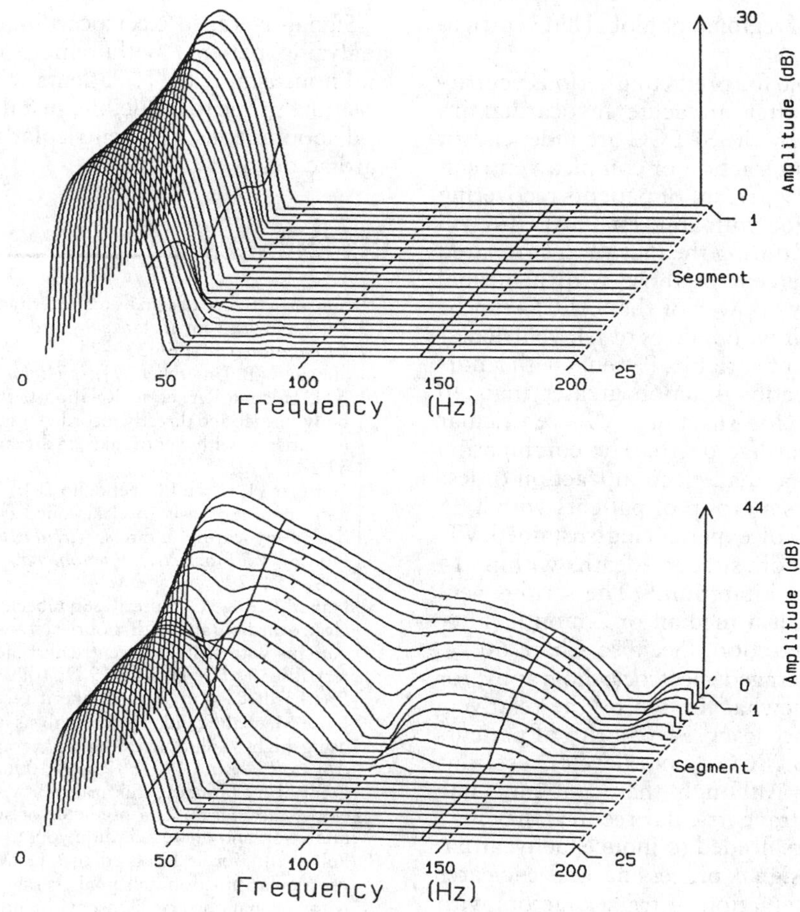

FIGURE 47-2 *A.* Normal spectral temporal map of the signal-averaged electrocardiogram. *B.* Abnormal spectral temporal map. An increase in the spectral amplitudes between 40 and 200 Hz in the earlier segments of the spectral temporal map is indicative of late potentials.

include the following: (1) the filtered QRS complex is longer than 114 ms, (2) the terminal filtered QRS complex remains below 40 μV for more than 38 ms, and (3) there is less than 20 μV of signal in the last 40 ms of the filtered QRS complex.[6] Some investigators require that two of the three criteria be abnormal. The duration of the filtered QRS complex is the most diagnostic parameter in patients without bundle branch block. When the terminal QRS and ST segment are analyzed by the Fourier transform, an increase in the 20- to 50-Hz components is seen in patients with VT. Other investigators have found an increase in the spectral amplitudes between 40 and 160 Hz as indicative of late potentials.[5] In the presence of bundle branch block, the diagnostic utility of time domain analysis is limited and it appears that frequency domain analysis is preferred.

Late potentials are not present universally in patients with recurrent VT. In some instances the fragmented activity may be too brief or the late potential may be masked by bundle branch block. The signal amplitude may be too low to be differentiated from noise. Delayed, fragmented electrical activity is probably related to reentrant ventricular arrhythmias. Other potential electrophysiological mechanisms of VT, such as increased automaticity or triggered activity, may not be associated with late potentials. Patients with VT in the absence of demonstrable structural heart disease rarely have late potentials.

The SAECG may have some utility in identifying patients with nonischemic cardiomyopathy and sustained VT. A prospective study of patients with dilated cardiomyopathy showed that the SAECG was useful for predicting sudden death, but not death from congestive heart failure.[7] On the other hand, the clinical value of the SAECG for detecting patients with nonischemic cardiomyopathy at risk for ventricular arrhythmias is not established.

PROGNOSTIC VALUE OF LATE POTENTIALS AFTER ACUTE MYOCARDIAL INFARCTION

Several prospective studies in postmyocardial infarction patients have shown an increased likelihood of spontaneous sustained VT or sudden cardiac death in patients who have an abnormal SAECG. Abnormal SAECGs are found in 26 to 40 percent of postmyocardial infarction patients when the recording is made prior to hospital discharge. Successful thrombolytic therapy with patency of the infarct artery seems to be associated with a lower incidence of late potentials. The presence of an abnormal

SAECG is independent of regional or global left ventricular function.[8]

The SAECG is valuable for predicting serious ventricular tachyarrhythmias after an acute myocardial infarction. Data provided by the SAECG are independent of left ventricular ejection fraction or complex ventricular ectopy. Fourteen to 29 percent of patients recovering from myocardial infarction with abnormal SAECGs will experience sustained VT during the first year, compared with only 0.8 to 4.5 percent of those with a normal recording.[9] The predictive power of the SAECG can be increased by combining it with indices of left ventricular function as an independent variable. Patients with a normal SAECG and an ejection fraction greater than 40 percent are at low risk for sustained VT, ventricular fibrillation, or sudden cardiac death. The combination of an abnormal SAECG and an ejection fraction of less than 40 percent identifies a group of patients with a 35 to 36 percent likelihood of experiencing sustained VT, ventricular fibrillation, or sudden death within 14 months after myocardial infarction.[10] The serious ventricular arrhythmias occur a median of 2 months after the acute myocardial infarction. (See also Chap. 60.)

The use of signal-averaged electrocardiography for risk stratification is somewhat limited by the relatively low positive predictive accuracy. A majority of patients who have an abnormal SAECG do not develop a serious ventricular arrhythmia. Although these patients may have the substrate for intraventricular reentry, they may lack the triggering factors needed to induce tachycardia. Further refinements of signal processing and a clearer understanding of the interaction of trigger factors with regional, delayed activation should increase the predictive accuracy of this technique.

Although the positive predictive accuracy of the SAECG is not high, the negative predictive accuracy exceeds 95 percent. A negative SAECG coupled with normal left ventricular function suggests less need for concern about arrhythmias and less need for ambulatory monitoring and drug therapy of ventricular ectopy. In general, there is a need for more data regarding the sensitivity/specificity of SAECG.

Signal-averaged electrocardiography is also useful in analyzing patients with remote myocardial infarction and nonsustained VT. Patients with abnormal SAECGs are more prone to inducible, sustained monomorphic VT and spontaneous VT, ventricular fibrillation, or sudden cardiac death.[11]

REFERENCES

1. Simson MB: Use of signals in the terminal QRS complex to identify patients with ventricular tachycardia after myocardial infarction. *Circulation* 1981; 64:235–242.
2. Simson MB, Untereker WJ, Spielman SR, Horowitz LN, Marcus NH, Falcone RA, et al: Relation between late potentials on the body surface and directly recorded fragmented electrocardiograms in patients with ventricular tachycardia. *Am J Cardiol* 1983; 51:105–112.
3. Gardner PI, Ursell PL, Fenoglio JJ Jr, Wit AL: Electrophysiologic and anatomic basis for fractioned electrograms recorded from healed myocardial infarcts. *Circulation* 1985; 72:596–611.
4. Plonsey R: *Bioelectric Phenomena.* New York, McGraw-Hill, 1969:281–299.
5. Haberl R, Jilge G, Pulter R, Steinbeck G: Spectral mapping of the electrocardiogram with Fourier transform for identification of patients with sustained ventricular tachycardia and coronary artery disease. *Eur Heart J* 1989; 10:316–322.
6. Breithardt G, Cain ME, El-Sherif N, Flowers NC, Hombach V, Janse M, et al: Standards for analysis of ventricular late potentials using high-resolution or signal-averaged electrocardiography. *J Am Coll Cardiol* 1991; 17:999–1006.
7. Ohnishi Y, Inoue T, Fukuzaki H: Value of the signal-averaged electrocardiogram as a predictor of sudden death in myocardial infarction and dilated cardiomyopathy. *Jpn Circ J* 1990; 54:127.
8. Pollak SJ, Kertes PJ, Bredlau CE, Walter PF: Influence of left ventricular function on signal averaged late potentials in patients with coronary artery disease with and without ventricular tachycardia. *Am Heart J* 1985; 110:747–752.
9. Breithardt G, Borggrefe M: Recent advances in the identification of patients at risk of ventricular tachyarrhythmias: Role of ventricular late potentials. *Circulation* 1987; 75:1091–1096.
10. Kuchar DL, Thorburn CW, Sammel NL: Prediction of serious arrhythmic events after myocardial infarction: Signal-averaged electrocardiogram, Holter monitoring and radionuclide ventriculography. *J Am Coll Cardiol* 1987; 9:531–538.
11. Turitto G, Fontaine JM, Ursell SW, Caref EB, Henkin R, El-Sherif N: Value of the signal-averaged electrocardiogram as a predictor of the results of programmed stimulation in nonsustained ventricular tachycardia. *Am J Cardiol* 1988; 61:1272–1278.

Chapter 48

Technique of Esophageal Electrocardiography

Ross D. Fletcher, M.D. ■ *Robert C. Saunders, M.D.*

P-wave timing and occasionally vector are needed to analyze disturbances of cardiac rhythm. Accordingly, many approaches have been developed to detect atrial activity (Table 48-1).[1–20] Standard electrocardiogram (ECG) and bipolar chest leads often do not disclose P waves, and invasive intracardiac atrial recording may not be practical or available. Recording atrial electrical activity from the esophagus, however, is simple, noninvasive, and effective.

DESCRIPTION

Recent developments facilitate clinical application of esophageal leads. Three-channel ECG recorders now in general use permit simultaneous surface and esophageal recording. Filtered preamplifiers and bipolar recording eliminate baseline drift. Recording electrodes are small, easily positioned, and tolerated by the patient.

While other systems are useful, the esophageal pill electrode developed by Arzbaecher is also easily swallowed and well-tolerated.[21] This insulated lead system consists of long, filamentous wires connected to a cylinder 3 mm in diameter and 1.9 cm long with a 6-mm electrode on each end (Fig. 48-1, lower panel). A gelatin capsule encloses the electrode and dissolves in the stomach. The pill may be swallowed with liquid or embedded in ice cream, although many patients swallow it without capsule or liquid. The wires are usually comfortable but

TABLE 48-1

Methods of Detecting Atrial Activity

1. Jugular venous pulse tracings
2. Standard electrocardiographic leads (II, V_1, aV_R)
3. Bipolar chest leads
   a. Lewis lead
   b. Right parasternal bipolar leads
4. Intracavitary atrial electrocardiogram
   a. Pacing electrode catheter
   b. Saline solution-filled polyethylene tubing
   c. Temporary atrial pacing electrode
   d. Quadripolar catheter for pacing and recording
   e. Zucker catheter with lumen
   f. Balloon-tipped, flow-directed catheter with electrodes 25–30 cm from the catheter tip
5. Esophageal electrode
   a. Solid nasogastric tube with multiple electrodes: Nyboer tube
   b. Standard nasogastric tube with conductive paste and cotton wick
   c. Silastic bipolar pacemaker lead
   d. Esophageal "pill" electrode
6. Echocardiography: detection and timing of right and left AV valves with dual echocardiogram

SOURCE: Fletcher R, Saunders R: Esophageal electrocardiography: 1981. In: Hurst JW (ed): *Update V: The Heart*. New York, McGraw-Hill, 1981. Reproduced with permission from the publisher and author.

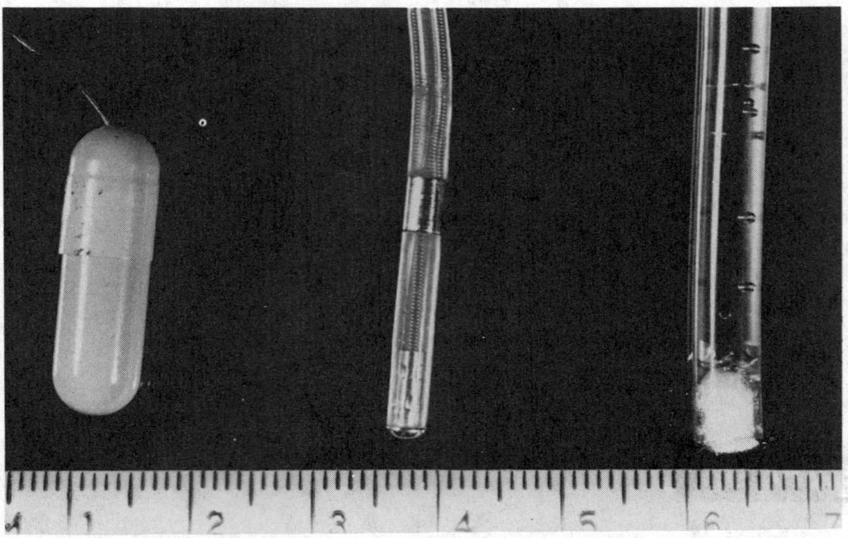

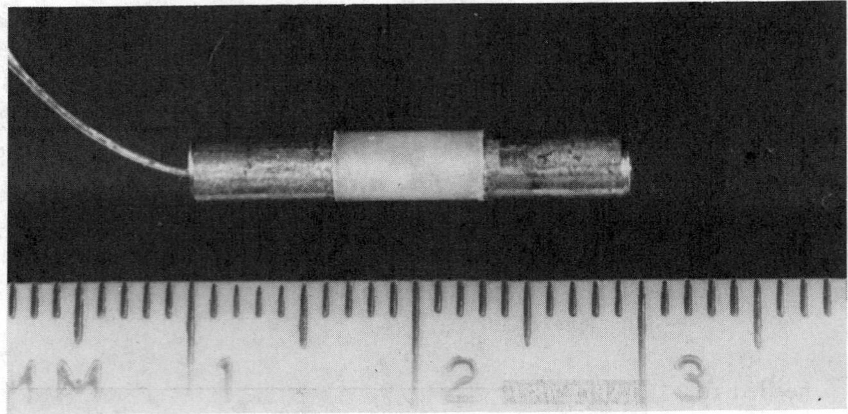

FIGURE 48-1 The upper panel compares the encapsulated pill electrode, an implantable pacemaker lead, and a conductive-gel-filled nasogastric tube with cotton plug. The pill is swallowed. The others are inserted by the nasal route. The lower panel enlarges the pill electrode without its gelatin capsule. *(From R Fletcher, R Saunders: Esophageal electrocardiography: 1981. In JW Hurst (ed): Update V: The Heart. New York, McGraw-Hill, 1981. Reproduced with permission from the publisher and author.)*

may produce a scratchy sensation that can be relieved with anesthetic gargle. The pill is swallowed to 45 cm, noted by a marker on the wire. The leads are connected to a single or three-channel ECG recorder. Permanent pacemaker leads are also effective and not subject to lead fracture. Simultaneous unipolar and bipolar esophageal recording is achieved with an implantable lead designed for bipolar pacing and endocardial shock.

While all recording systems described in Table 48-2 are effective, a three-channel recorder in the lead I-II-III position with the Arzco preamplifier consistently provides a useful record. The preamplifier sends a moderately filtered bipolar esophageal signal to channel I, a normal lead II to channel II, and a compound signal (an inverted bipolar esophageal lead superimposed on lead II) to channel III (Fig. 48-2). Alternatively, the distal and proximal esophageal leads may be attached directly to the right and left arm leads of an ECG patient cable, producing a bipolar esophageal trace in channel I (no low-frequency filtering) and a compound left leg to esophageal trace on channels II and III. Best results are obtained with the right and left arm leads disconnected from the arms. Proximal and distal unipolar tracings are obtained simultaneously with V_2 attached to the proximal esophageal electrode and V_3 attached to the distal esophageal electrode. Then, V_1, V_2, and V_3 are simultaneously visualized on a three-channel recorder.

TABLE 48-2

Esophageal Recording Systems

1. Single-channel recorder
   a. Unipolar: attach to V lead
   b. Bipolar: attach distal to left arm and proximal to right arm; record lead I
2. Standard three-channel ECG recorder
   a. Unipolar
      (1) V_1: normal position
      (2) V_2: distal esophageal electrode
      (3) V_3: proximal esophageal electrode
   b. Bipolar
      (1) Lead I: bipolar esophageal (attach as single-channel bipolar)
      (2) Lead II: compound leg and proximal electrode
      (3) Lead III: compound leg and distal electrode
3. Standard three-channel ECG recorder with preamplifier
   a. Lead I: bipolar esophageal
   b. Lead II: standard lead II
   c. Lead III: compound esophageal and lead II

SOURCE: Fletcher R, Saunders R: Esophageal electrocardiography: 1981. In: Hurst JW (ed): *Update V: The Heart*. New York, McGraw-Hill, 1981. Reproduced with permission from the publisher and author.

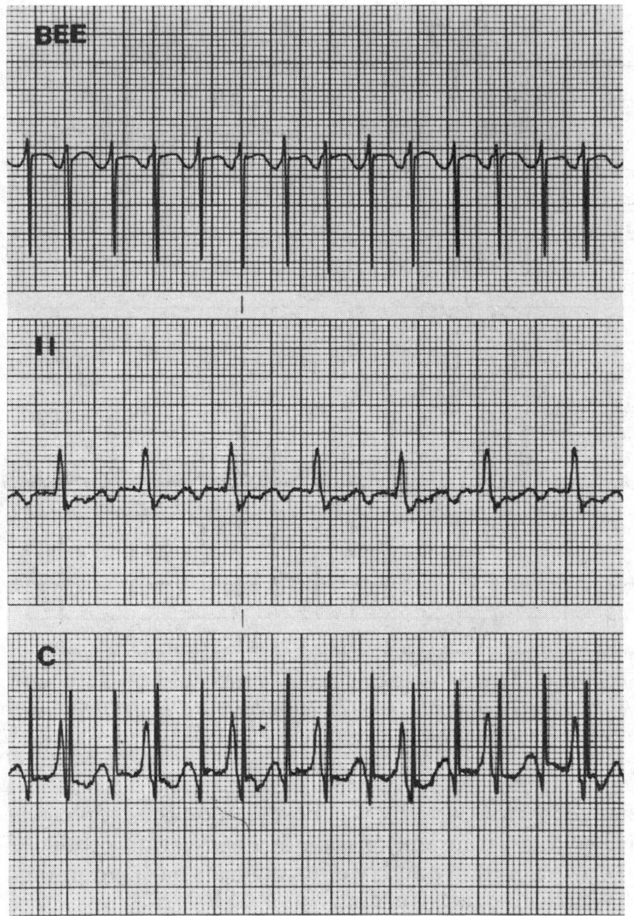

FIGURE 48-2 Simultaneous bipolar esophageal electrogram (BEE), standard lead II, and compound lead. Atrial tachycardia of 200 beats per minute is clearly seen on the bipolar esophageal trace. *(From R Fletcher, R Saunders: Esophageal electrocardiography: 1981. In: JW Hurst (ed): Update V: The Heart. New York, McGraw-Hill, 1981. Reproduced with permission from the publisher and author.)*

Careful withdrawal of the pill from the stomach will yield deflections first from the left ventricle and then the low interatrial septum. As the electrode is positioned 35 to 42 cm from incisor teeth, maximal atrial deflection with minimal ventricular contamination is seen on the bipolar trace (Fig. 48-3). In this position, remote ventricular activity is recorded on both unipolar leads. During bipolar esophageal electrode (BEE) recording, the similar ventricular deflections cancel when proximal and distal electrodes are assigned negative and positive polarity and added algebraically by the differential ECG amplifier.[17,22,23] Figure 48-3 presents a bipolar esophageal trace with lead II, recorded as the pill was placed at different distances from the incisors. Low in the esophagus the ventricular deflection is larger than the atrial deflection. As the pill passes the atrioventricular (AV) groove to the atrium (37 cm), the atrial deflection is enlarged. The best position for bipolar atrial monitoring in this patient is at 36 cm, where the bipolar electrogram writes a minimal QRS. Similar QRS morphologies from the remote ventricle are canceled, and the local atrial deflection is accentuated. While atrial activity recorded from the lowest possible lead position may be the goal in some studies, usually the largest atrial deflection is desired. In one report, the most distal lead position recorded the earliest retrograde atrial electrogram (46 ± 6 cm), but the largest P waves were recorded between 37 ± 6 cm and 41 ± 4 cm from the incisors.[20]

Tracing artifacts can be minimized in several ways.[24] The baseline is often erratic when recordings are made from the stomach. Contact with the esophageal wall is necessary for good-quality recordings. Peristalsis, left ventricular pulsations, or aortic pulsations may cause artifacts that can be minimized with mild filtering. Low-frequency filters, commonplace with intracavitary recording,[25,26] were adapted for esophageal recording by Barold[18] and later by Arzbaecher,[21] who incorporated mild (5-Hz) low-frequency filters into a preamplifier.

APPLICATIONS

Esophageal recordings have many applications (Table 48-3), particularly when P-wave activity cannot be delineated on an external tracing. The presence of atrial tachycardia can be revealed on a bipolar esophageal electrogram while external leads show no rapid atrial activity.

The nature of pauses seen on a surface recording may be determined using the esophageal lead. Blocked premature atrial beats obscured by the preceding T wave or second-degree AV block with 2:1 conduction may be seen on an esophageal trace but missed with a standard surface lead. The presence or absence of atrial activity associated with an anomalous QRS helps differentiate beats initiated in the ventricles from beats of supraventricular origin with aberrant conduction to the ventricles.[27] Antecedent P waves, with prolonged AV conduction times, confirm the supraventricular origin of anomalous QRSs occurring as single beats or bursts. Atrial activity dissociated from an anomalous QRS tachycardia confirms the diagnosis of ventricular tachycardia. Atrial activity associated 1:1 with sustained anomalous QRS tachyarrhythmia is seen with supraventricular rhythms but can also be present during ventricular tachycardia with 1:1 retrograde conduction to the atrium. Vagal maneuvers, intravenous propranolol, or intravenous verapamil may increase retrograde block or dissociate the atrium from the ventricle, making more firm the diagnosis of ventricular tachycardia.

Difficulty discerning these rhythms is illustrated by a patient we studied. A tentative diagnosis of supraventricular tachycardia was established because a triphasic rSR′ was seen on lead MCL_1 and the esophageal lead showed P waves associated with every QRS (Fig. 48-4*A*). Carotid sinus pressure, however, eliminated all atrial activity for a short period, after which P waves reappeared with 3:1 retrograde conduction and finally 1:1 with the QRS (Fig. 48-4*B*). Atrial activity was altered without any change in the anomalous QRS tachyarrhythmia, confirming a ventricular rhythm independent of the atrium. The 1:1 relationship of P wave to QRS was due to retrograde conduction. Although uncommon, this rhythm could be junctional with aberrant conduction. In this patient, ventricular tachycardia was confirmed by intracavitary re-

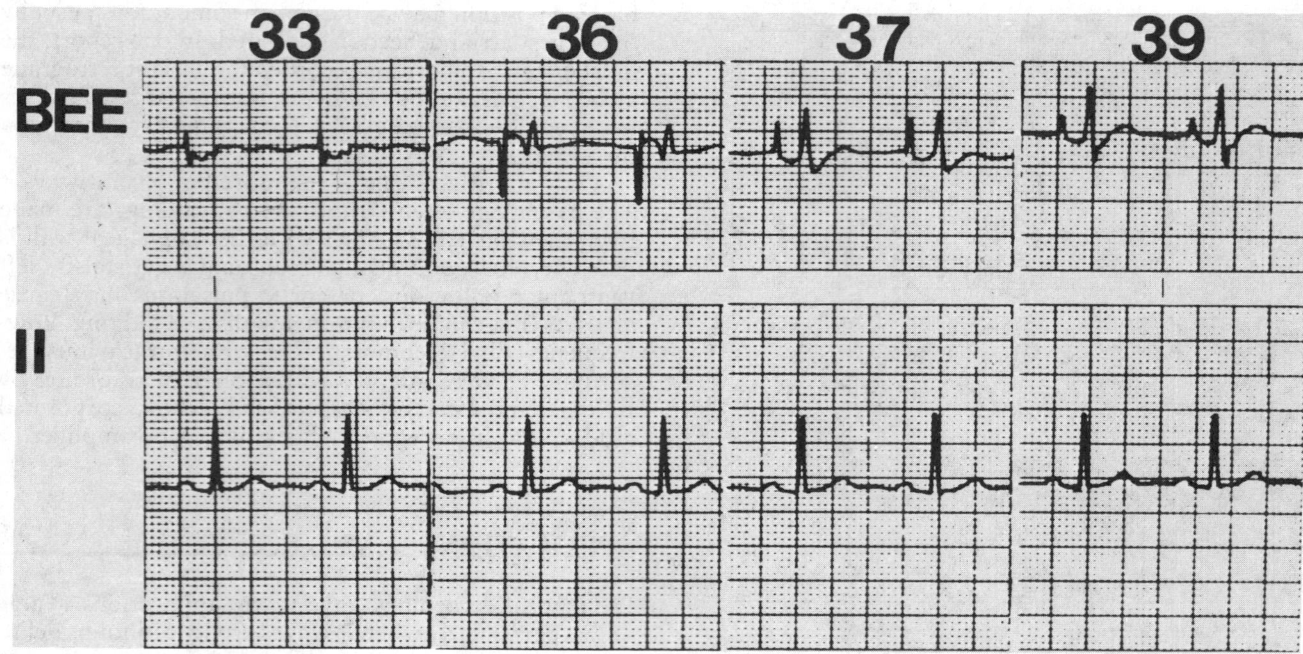

FIGURE 48-3 Recording at intervals of 39 to 33 cm from the teeth during withdrawal of the bipolar esophageal electrode (BEE) shows pure left atrial activity (with smallest QRS) to occur at 36 cm in this patient. *(From R Fletcher, R Saunders: Esophageal electrocardiography: 1981. In: JW Hurst (ed): Update V: The Heart. New York, McGraw-Hill, 1981. Reproduced with permission from the publisher and author.)*

cording in which no antecedent His bundle deflection was seen before the anomalous QRS.

In another patient with wide QRS tachycardia and association between atrium and ventricle (Fig. 48-5*A*), carotid pressure slowed only the atrial rate. While the change in atrial activity was best seen on the esophageal electrogram, transient retrograde dissociation produced an obvious capture and two fusion beats pathognomonic of ventricular tachycardia (Fig. 48-5*B*).

Sustained atrial pacing should be accomplished by the

TABLE 48-3

Application of Esophageal Leads

I. Detect or confirm inapparent atrial activity
  A. Atrial tachycardias
    1. Flutter
    2. Fibrillation
    3. Reentrant atrial AV nodal tachycardia
  B. Pauses: Detect P wave in the pause
    1. Blocked premature atrial beat
    2. Inapparent AV block with 2:1 conduction
  C. Anomalous QRS beats
    1. Atrial activity controlling aberrant ventricular depolarization
    2. Ventricular depolarization dissociated from atrial activity
    3. Ventricular tachycardia with 1:1 retrograde conduction to atrium: dissociated or blocked with carotid sinus pressure or propranolol
  D. Pauses during atrial pacing
    1. Confirms atrial capture but with AV block
    2. Confirms lack of atrial capture by pacemaker
      a. Normal atrial refractory period
      b. Hidden reentrant or premature P making the atrium refractory
  E. Detect atrial activity during noninvasive programmed stimulation of atrium or ventricle using permanent pacemakers

II. Temporary pacing
  A. Atrium: 70 percent successful at 20–30 mA
    1. Temporary support of atrial bradycardias
    2. Revert atrial tachycardias
  B. Ventricle: rarely necessary: 50 mA

III. Record specific posterior cardiac structures (low atrial septum on left atrium)
  A. Dissimilar atrial rhythms
    1. Right and left atrial tachycardia mimicking atrial flutter
    2. Right sick sinus with left atrial flutter
  B. Measure intraatrial and left atrium to left ventricle conduction times
  C. Timing of retrograde P wave obscured by QRS
    1. Junctional ventricular beats
    2. Wolff-Parkinson-White syndrome

SOURCE: Fletcher R, Saunders R: Esophageal electrocardiography: 1981. In: Hurst JW (ed): *Update V: The Heart.* New York, McGraw-Hill, 1981. Reproduced with permission from the publisher and author.

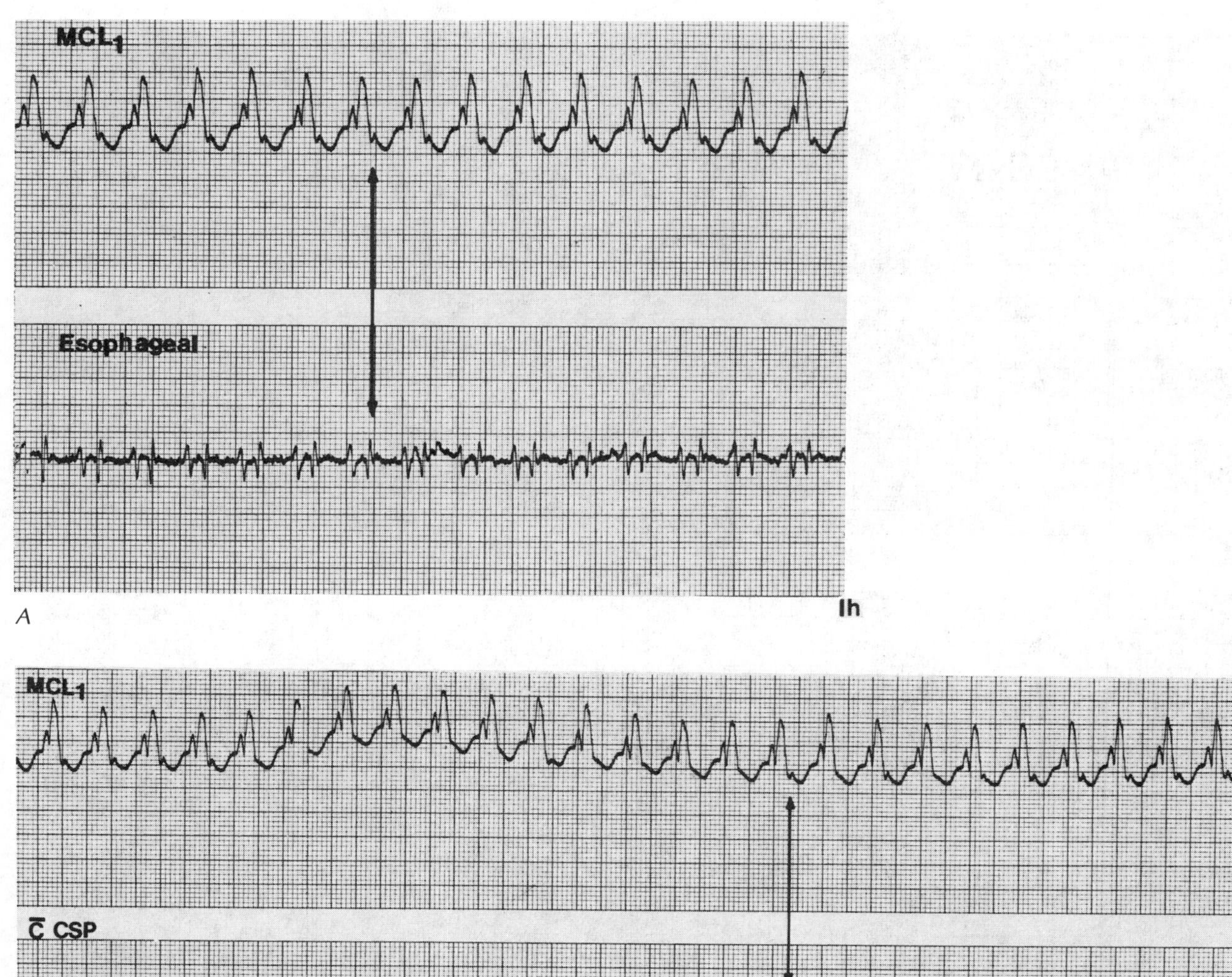

FIGURE 48-4 *A.* Lead MCL_1 shows tachycardia with a wide rsR′ QRS pattern. A simultaneous bipolar esophageal trace recorded from the transitional zone shows P waves associated 1:1 with each QRS. Supraventricular tachycardia with aberrant conduction to the ventricles is suggested. *B.* Carotid sinus pressure (CSP) did not change the rate of ventricular complexes *(open arrows)* but produced a striking decrease in atrial activity *(black arrows),* confirming complete retrograde (VA) block and dissociation followed by 2:1 and finally 1:1 retrograde conduction. P waves are seen on the MCI_1 lead *(double arrows).*

intracardiac route, but the esophageal lead may provide temporary atrial pacing or pace-out of atrial tachycardias.[28–33] The lowest pacing threshold (12 mA) was achieved using a 2-cm spaced bipolar electrode and a 7-ms pulse width, while 19 mA are required for a pulse width of 1 ms.[30] At lower pulse widths, pacing was only 70 percent reliable.[34,35] The esophageal route for ventricular pacing has been used by Lubell and by Burack and Furman at even higher current levels (50 mA).[36,37] This is accomplished in lower lead positions where large ventricular deflections are recorded using the bipolar configuration. Pacing from the esophagus is usually limited to short-term supportive pacing for bradycardias and conversion of atrial arrhythmia. Atrial flutter has been terminated in 43 percent of patients using the pill electrode.[38] The efficacy of pacing from esophageal leads for ventricle and atrium has been improved using an electrode with a deflectable tip. In usual invasive electrophysiology laboratory procedures, a quadripolar catheter records the presence of atrial capture from two proximal electrodes after bipolar pacing from two distal electrodes. In patients in whom implanted single- and dual-chamber pacemakers are used for temporary electrophysiology studies, the esophageal leads are equiva-

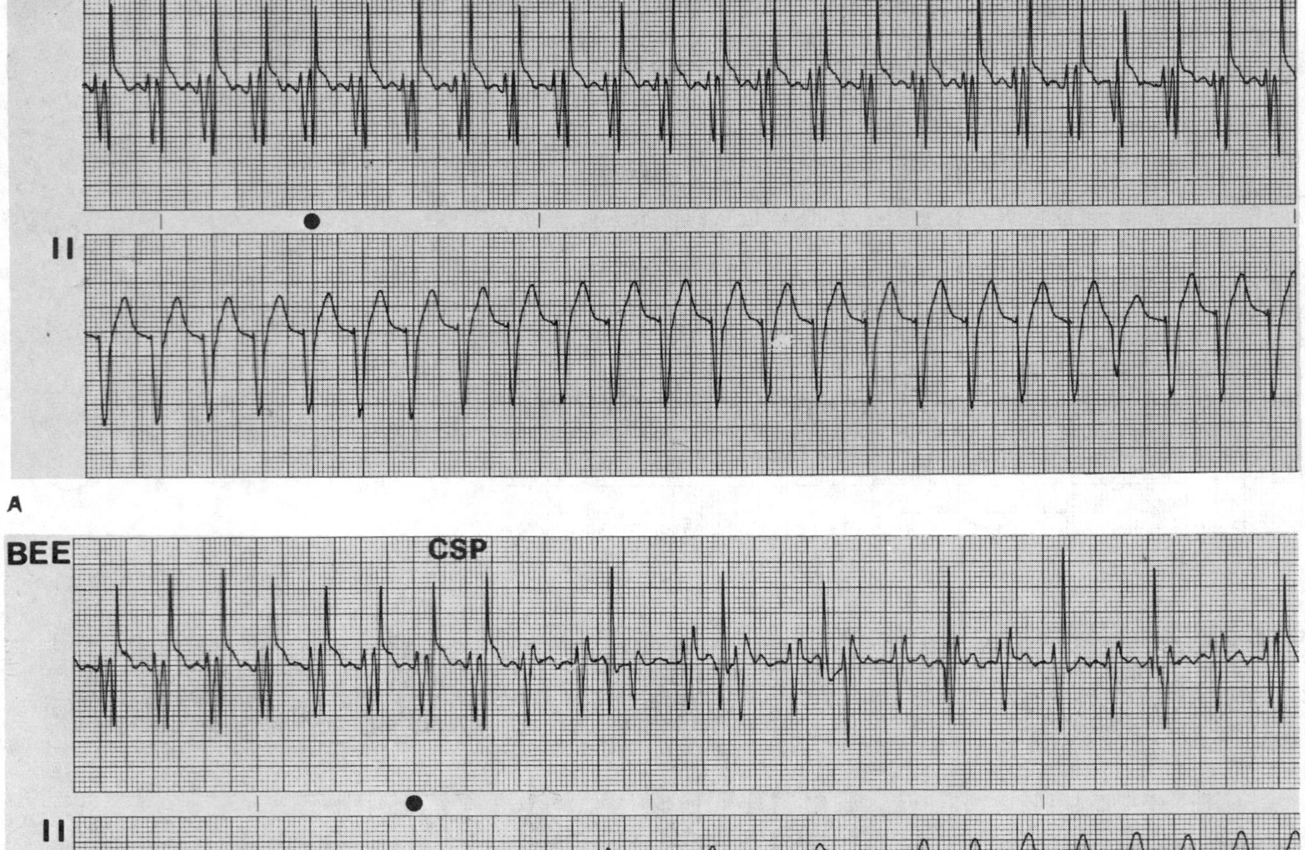

FIGURE 48-5 *A.* The esophageal lead reveals one P wave for each QRS, representing 1:1 antegrade conduction with first-degree block of 1:1 retrograde conduction in a patient with ventricular or junctional tachycardia. *B.* Carotid sinus pressure (CSP) produced ventriculoatrial dissociation, which allowed one pure capture (C) and two fusion beats (F) to reveal the diagnosis of ventricular tachycardia.

lent to the atrial recording electrodes, thus providing information similar to that obtained by an invasive study.

Commercially available, programmable, permanent atrial and AV synchronous pacemakers allow complete testing for inducible tachycardia and for pace-out with test-made pacing rates above 300 beats per minute.[39] This testing requires simultaneous recording of atrial activity for evidence of retrograde conduction, dissociation, atrial tachycardia, and atrial capture during rapid atrial stimulation. Lack of capture during the unsuccessful attempt to pace-out these tachycardias can frequently be improved by increasing stimulation strength. The addition of antiarrhythmic drugs such as procainamide or quinidine may decrease the atrial rate and allow atrial capture.

Trouble-shooting permanent dual-chamber pacemakers is enhanced with esophageal leads clearly showing the presence or absence of atrial capture (Fig. 48-6). Loss of atrial capture leads not only to loss of atrial kick but can also allow the P wave to appear after the post V atrial refractory period (PVARP). In this position the sensed P wave can trigger pacing of the ventricle, and, if retrograde conduction is intact, pacemaker-mediated tachycardia can be started at or just below the upper rate limit of the pacemaker.

The hemodynamic effect of dual-chamber pacing is influenced by the programmed AV delay but may be enhanced by controlling the relationship of left atrial to left ventricular events,[40] a relationship not always predictable from knowledge of the right atrium-to-left ventricle (RA-LV) time (i.e., AV delay). Intraatrial and left

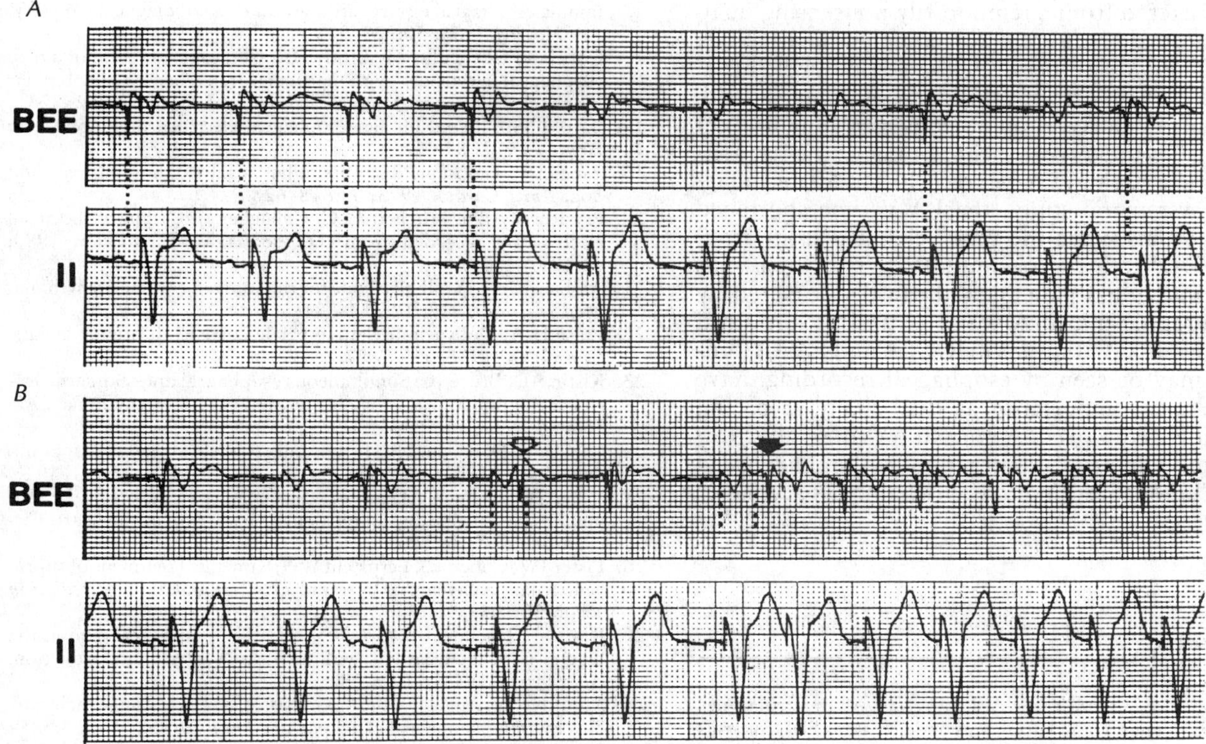

FIGURE 48-6 *A.* In lead II, the sinus P wave triggers fourth ventricular pacing (VDD) and then defaults to AV sequential (DVI) pacing on the fourth beat. Loss of atrial capture, which is difficult to see in lead II, is clear in the simultaneous bipolar esophageal electrogram (BEE) with no atrial activity recorded for beats 5, 6, 7, and 9. *B.* The loss of atrial capture places the slow sinus P wave after the QRS *(open arrow),* where it is not sensed by the pacemaker because it falls within the post V atrial refractory period (PVARP, *dotted bars*). The next P wave to fall after the QRS *(closed arrow)* is now outside the PVARP. After being sensed, the pacemaker triggers a paced ventricular beat that conducts retrograde to the atrium. Subsequent triggered ventricular pacing and retrograde conduction to the atrium produces sustained pacemaker-mediated tachycardia.

atrium-to-left ventricle (LA-LV) timing may be determined by using the BEE to record left atrial events. Right atrial timing is marked by the beginning of programmed AV delay, seen in the DVI mode as an atrial pacing output or, in the VDD mode, as a sensed local right atrial depolarization, which may be revealed by a telemetered right electrogram (A-EGM) available from some permanent single- or dual-chamber pacemakers. In Fig. 48-7 simultaneous recording of left atrial activity from the esophagus and a right atrial appendage electrogram (A-

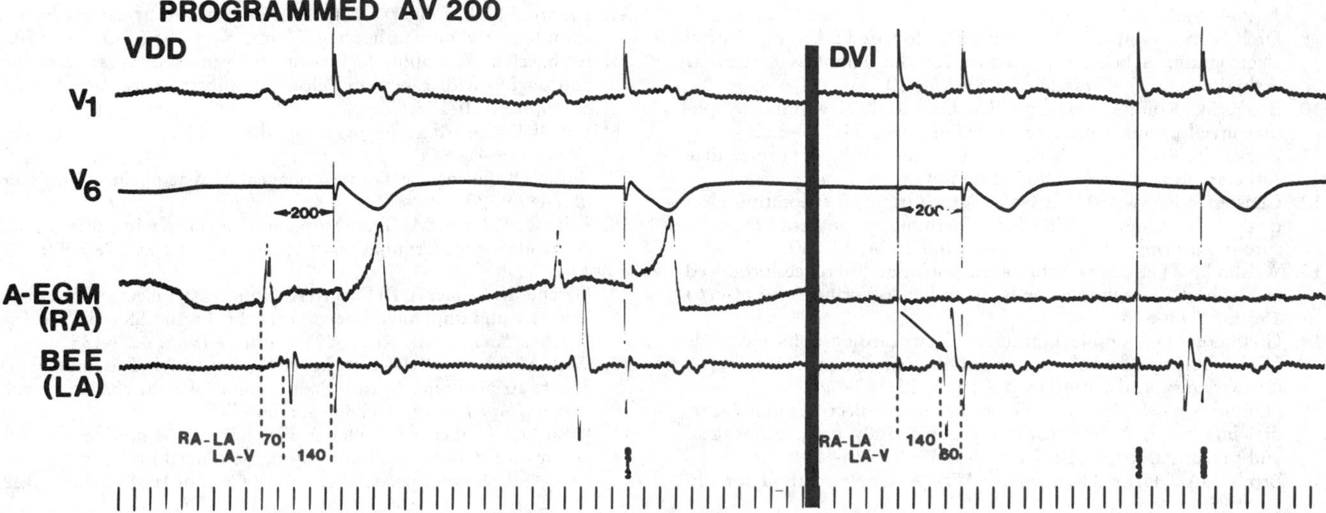

FIGURE 48-7 The DDD pacemaker is operating with a programmed AV delay of 200 ms in VDD mode on the left panel and DVI mode on the right panel. The sensed right atrial electrogram (A-EGM) occurs 70 ms before the left atrial bipolar esophageal lead electrogram (BEE; LA). The left atrium-to-ventricle (LA-V) pace decreases from 140 ms in VDD to 60 ms in DVI mode.

EGM) telemetered from a temporarily nonsensing dual-chamber pacemaker inserted for complete heart block reveals a 70 ms delay between the sensed right atrial electrogram and the left atrial bipolar esophageal lead. At a constant AV delay, simultaneous recording of right and left atrial events revealed shortening of the left atrium-to-ventricle pacing (LA-V) from 140 to 60 ms in Fig. 48-7. In a systematic study, the LA-V time shortened an average 80 ms when the mode changed from atrial tracking (VDD) to atrial pacing (DVI). This interval is variable in individual patients and can be measured by echocardiographic mitral A wave as well as left atrial esophageal leads.[41] Variations in RA-LA and LA-LV timing, which may be seen by esophageal recording, have increased clinical importance as dual-chamber pacing becomes widely employed. A normal AV interval of 150 ms can place left atrial contraction within the paced QRS in DVI mode, leading to dual-chamber pacemaker syndrome.

REFERENCES

1. Cremer M: Ueber die direkte Ableitung der Akionsstrome des menslichen Herzens vom Oesophagus und ueber das Elektrokardiogramm des Fotus. *Munch Wochensch* 1906; 53:811–813.
2. Brown WH: A study of the esophageal lead in clinical electrocardiography. *Am Heart J* 1906; 12:307–308.
3. Smith C: An endo-oesophageal stethoscope. *Anesthesiology* 1954; 15:566.
4. Matsumoto M, Oka Y, Lin YT, Strom J, Sonnenblick EH, Frater RW: Transesophageal echocardiography for assessing ventricular performance. *N Y State J Med* 1979; 79:19–21.
5. Wenckebach EF: Ueber Verkehrasstorungen in Herzen. *Wien Med Wochenschr* 1927; 77:1307–1311.
6. Lewis T, Meakings J, White PD: The excitatory process in the dog's heart: I. The auricle. *Philos Trans R Soc Lond [Biol]* 1914; 205:375–420.
7. Wilson FN, McLeod AG, Baker PS: The order of ventricular excitation in human bundle branch block. *Am Heart J* 1931; 7:305–330.
8. Vogel JHK, Tabari K, Averile KH, Blount SG Jr: A simple technique for identifying P waves in complex arrhythmias. *Am Heart J* 1964; 67:158–161.
9. Dreifus LS, Najmi M, Pomerantz D, Novack P: The right atrial electrogram: A bedside procedure for the diagnosis of cardiac arrhythmias. *Dis Chest* 1965; 48:617–620.
10. Berens SC, Kolin A, MacAlpin RN, Lenz MW: New stable temporary atrial pacing loop. *Am J Cardiol* 1974; 34:325–332.
11. Zucker R, Rothfeld E, Bernstein A: A new multipurpose cardiac catheter. *Am J Cardiol* 1965; 15:45–47.
12. Chatterjee K, Swan HJC, Ganz W: Multipurpose flotation electrode catheter-new catheter for arrhythmia and intracardiac pressure monitoring (abstr.). *Am J Cardiol* 1974; 33:130.
13. Wilson FN: The distribution of the potential differences produced by the heart beat within the body and at its surface. *Am Heart J* 1930; 5:599–616.
14. Goldberger E: A simple, indifferent electrocardiographic electrode of zero potential and a technique of obtaining, augmented, unipolar extremity leads. *Am Heart J* 1942; 23:483–492.
15. Hamilton JGM, Nyboer J: The ventricular deflections in myocardial infarction: An electrocardiographic study using esophageal and precardial leads. *Am Heart J* 1938; 15:414–424.
16. Brody DA, Harris TR, Romans WE: A simple method for obtaining esophageal electrocardiograms of good diagnostic quality. *Am Heart J* 1955; 50:923–926.
17. Copeland GD, Tullis EF, Brody DA: Clinical evaluation of a new esophageal electrode, with particular reference to the bipolar esophageal electrocardiogram. *Am Heart J* 1959; 57:862–873.
18. Barold SS: Filtered bipolar esophageal electrocardiography. *Am Heart J* 1972; 83:431.
19. Zipes DP, DeJoseph RL: Dissimilar atrial rhythms in man and dog. *Am J Cardiol* 1973; 32:618–628.
20. Prystowsky EN, Pritchett ELC, Gallagher JJ: Origin of the atrial electrogram recorded from the esophagus. *Circulation* 1980; 61:1017–1023.
21. Arzbaecher R: A pill-electrode for the study of cardiac arrhythmia. *Med Instrum* 1978; 12:277–281.
22. Luisada A: Derivazioni elettive per le correnti di origine atriale. *Cuore Circ* 1935; 19:77–87.
23. Kistin AD, Bruce JC: Simultaneous esophageal and standard electrocardiographic leads for the study of cardiac arrhythmias. *Am Heart J* 1957; 53:65–73.
24. Oblath R, Darpman H: The normal esophageal lead electrogram. *Am Heart J* 1951; 369–381.
25. Lister JW, Delman AJ, Stein E: Dominant pacemaker of the Human heart: Antegrade and retrograde activation of the heart. *Circulation* 1967; 35:22–31.
26. Lister JW, Cohen LS, Bernstein WH, Samet P: Treatment of supraventricular tachycardia by rapid atrial stimulation. *Circulation* 1968; 38:1044–1059.
27. Rubin L, Jagendorf B, Goldberg AL: The esophageal lead in the diagnosis of tachycardias with aberrant ventricular conduction. *Am Heart J* 1956; 57:19–28.
28. Montoyo JV, Angel J, Valle V, Gausi C: Cardioversion of tachycardias by transesophageal atrial pacing. *Am J Cardiol* 1973; 32:85–90.
29. Hartzler GO, Maloney JD: Transesophageal atrial pacing in the Wolff-Parkinson-White syndrome. *Mayo Clin Proc* 1977; 52:576–581.
30. Gallagher JJ, Smith WM, Kerr CR, Kasell J, Cook L, Reiter M, et al: Esophageal pacing: A diagnostic and therapeutic tool. *Circulation* 1982; 65:336–341.
31. Critelli G, Grassi G, Perticone F, Coltoriti F, Monda V, Condurelli M: Transesophageal pacing for prognostic evaluation of preexcitation syndrome and assessment of protective therapy. *Am J Cardiol* 1983; 51:513–518.
32. Benson DW, Dunnigan A, Sterba R, Benditt DG: Atrial pacing from the esophagus in the diagnosis and management of tachycardia and palpitations. *J Pediatr* 1983; 102:40–46.
33. Kerr CR, Gallagher JJ, Smith WM, Sterba R, German LD, Cook L, et al: The induction of atrial flutter and fibrillation and the termination of atrial flutter by esophageal pacing. *PACE* 1983; 6:60–72.
34. Shafiroff BGP, Linder J: Effects of external electrical pacemaker stimuli on the human heart. *J Thorac Surg* 1957; 33:544–550.
35. Arzbaecher R, Collins S, Brown D: Transesophageal recording and pacing with a new pill electrode (abstr.) *Circulation* 1978; 58(suppl. II):II-173.
36. Lubell DL: Cardiac pacing from the esophagus. *Am J Cardiol* 1971; 27:641–644.
37. Burack B, Furman S: Transesophageal cardiac pacing. *Am J Cardiol* 1969; 23:469–472.
38. Falk R, Werner M: Transesophageal atrial pacing using a pill electrode for the termination of atrial flutter. *Chest* 1987; 92:110–114.
39. Fletcher R, Cohen A, DelNegro A: Noninvasive electrophysiologic studies using implanted pacemakers. In: Barold SS (ed): *Modern Cardiac Pacing.* Mt. Kisco, NY, Futura, 1985: 421–438.
40. Wish M, Fletcher RD, Gottdiener JS, Cohen AI: The importance of left atrial timing in the programming of dual chamber pacemakers. *Am J Cardiol* 1987; 60:566–571.
41. Wish M, Gottdiener J, Cohen A, Fletcher RD: M-mode echocardiograms for determination of optimal left atrial timing in patients with dual chamber pacemakers. *Am J Cardiol* 1988; 61:317–322.

PART VI

Shock, Syncope, Sudden Death, and Cardio-Pulmonary Resuscitation

Chapter 49

Pathophysiology, Diagnosis, and Management of Cardiogenic Shock

Joseph S. Alpert, M.D. ■ *Richard C. Becker, M.D.*

Shock is one of the most feared medical conditions. If left untreated, almost all patients who develop shock will eventually die. Although the clinical syndrome has been recognized since antiquity, the first description of shock in the medical literature was in the middle of the eighteenth century.[1]

DEFINITION

Shock is currently defined as a syndrome, i.e., a recognizable collection of symptoms, signs, and laboratory abnormalities, that results from systemic hypoperfusion associated with widespread cellular and organ dysfunction. Patients are usually hypotensive, and cardiac output is frequently depressed. In some shock states, however, cardiac output is normal despite hypotension and/or evidence for organ dysfunction.

With some notable exceptions, e.g., skeletal muscle, most cells are dependent on a continuous supply of blood-borne oxygen and nutrients in order to generate the high-energy phosphate compounds essential for normal function. In most shock states, organs, tissues, and cells receive inadequate blood perfusion and hence an inadequate supply of oxygen and nutrients. Cellular, tissue, and organ dysfunction develop. This dysfunction is initially reversible. Persistent hypoperfusion, however, leads to irreversible, permanent cellular injury and necrosis. Widespread cellular necrosis with consequent organ dysfunction leads to death.

Cardiogenic shock is any shock state in which abnormal cardiac function plays a major role in the genesis of the shock syndrome.

ETIOLOGY OF SHOCK SYNDROME

A number of pathophysiological states can result in shock (Table 49-1). The most important entity is abnormal myocardial function. The causes of myocardial dysfunction that may result in shock are listed in Table 49-2. Patients with septic and hemorrhagic shock in which the heart is not primarily involved have also been shown to have abnormal myocardial function.[2–4]

Other initiating processes leading to cardiovascular shock (Table 49-1) include hypovolemia, e.g., hemorrhage or severe dehydration; maldistribution of blood volume, e.g., adverse reactions to anesthetic agents or vasodilators; increased resistance to blood flow in the systemic or pulmonary circulations, e.g., myxoma, coarctation of the aorta, pulmonary embolism; abnormal capillary function, e.g., anaphylaxis, adult respiratory distress syndrome (ARDS); and arteriovenous shunting of blood, e.g., sepsis, pneumonia, peritonitis.

Once a primary process has initiated the shock syndrome, tissue hypoperfusion leads to abnormal organ

TABLE 49-1

Primary or Initiating Pathophysiological Mechanisms in Shock Syndrome

1. Depressed myocardial performance—heart failure
2. Reduced or maldistributed intravascular volume
3. Increased resistance to blood flow in the systemic or pulmonary circulation
4. Abnormal capillary function
5. Arteriovenous shunting of blood

function which reinforces and exacerbates the shock state. Increased levels of circulating catecholamines lead to systemic arteriolar vasoconstriction that further impairs tissue perfusion. Abnormalities of carbohydrate and lipid metabolism develop, i.e., hyperglycemia followed by hypoglycemia when glycogen stores are exhausted and hypertriglyceridemia.[5–7] A variety of vasoactive substances are released during shock states, including histamine, various kinins, serotonin, prostaglandins, endorphins, proteases, free oxygen radicals, activated complement components, and tumor necrosis factor.[4, 8–12] Recent work suggests that excessive nitric oxide [also known as endothelium-derived relaxing factor (EDRF)] production by endothelial cells and macrophages mediates the hypotensive effect of tumor necrosis factor.[13] On the other hand, nitric oxide may also have a beneficial action in shock since it helps to maintain vascular integrity in the intestinal mucosa following endotoxin challenge.[14] Of interest in this regard is the finding that glucocorticoids inhibit nitric oxide synthetase, an essential enzyme in the production of nitric oxide. Inhibition of this enzyme may explain, at least in part, some of the therapeutic and adverse effects of steroids in shock patients.[15] Once the shock state is present, major, secondary dysfunction can develop in the myocardium, kidneys, liver, lungs, stomach and intestine, pancreas, and brain.[4, 16–26] The summated abnormalities sustain and deepen the shock state, eventually leading to irreversible damage.

TABLE 49-2

Etiologies of Cardiovascular Shock

I. Acute myocardial infarction
   A. Markedly reduced left ventricular function
   B. Ventricular septal rupture, acute
   C. Mitral regurgitation, acute
   D. Right ventricular infarction
   E. Ventricular free-wall rupture
II. Other cardiac entities associated with inadequate ventricular function
   A. Dilated cardiomyopathy/severe myocarditis
   B. End-stage valvular heart disease—aortic stenosis, mitral stenosis, aortic regurgitation, mitral regurgitation
   C. Myocardial dysfunction in septic shock
   D. Tachyarrhythmia or bradyarrhythmia
   E. Following cardiopulmonary bypass
III. Cardiac obstruction or compression
   A. Pericardial tamponade or constriction
   B. Pulmonary embolism
   C. Severe pulmonary hypertension, e.g., primary pulmonary hypertension
   D. Coarctation of the aorta
   E. Myxoma
   F. Severe hypertrophic cardiomyopathy
   G. Tension pneumothorax
IV. Hypovolemia related to cardiovascular pathology
   A. Ruptured abdominal aortic aneurysm, dissecting aneurysm
   B. Hemorrhagic shock

COMPENSATORY MECHANISMS

The hypotensive state with accompanying tissue hypoperfusion leads to activation of a number of defense mechanisms that attempt to restore circulatory homeostasis and/or preserve perfusion to heart and brain (Table 49-3). In the early phases of the shock syndrome, these compensatory mechanisms are more or less successful in preserving cardiac output and a marginally adequate systemic blood pressure. If the shock state persists, however, gradual erosion of the efficacy of compensatory mechanisms develops. Finally, the shock state worsens, compensatory mechanisms become ineffective, and irreversible shock supervenes. Mortality from shock increases progressively in direct relationship to the severity and duration of the syndrome. The major homeostatic defense mechanism in shock is activation of the sympathetic nervous system. The signal for activation of increased adrenergic nervous activity is decreased cardiac output and systemic arterial blood pressure.[27] A decline ... systemic arterial blood pressure and/or blood volume activates stretch baroreceptors in the aortic arch, carotid sinus, and splanchnic arterial bed.[28,29] Volume-sensitive baroreceptors within the heart can also be activated.[28] Increased signals from these baroreceptors to the central nervous system lead to increased sympathetic nerve efferent responses and decreased parasympathetic activity. A number of different peripheral events are produced by increased sympathetic nerve traffic: (1) arteriolar vasoconstriction with resultant decreased perfusion to skin, skeletal muscle, kidney, and splanchnic organs[28,30]; (2) increased heart rate and myocardial contractility[28]; (3) venoconstriction with a resultant increase in venous return and central blood volume[28,31]; (4) increased release of adrenal hormones[32]; and (5) activation of the renin-angiotensin-aldosterone axis.[33] Activation of the latter mechanism in response to shock produces immediate arteriolar vasoconstriction and in the long term seeks to restore normal circulatory blood volume and cardiac output through sodium and water retention.[33,34] Simultaneous release of arginine vasopressin from the posterior pituitary also occurs during the shock syndrome. Vasopressin binds to specific receptors in splanchnic, renal, and other vascular territories, further increasing vascular resistance in order to maintain systemic blood pressure and decreasing renal water clearance in order to augment blood volume.[35]

Another compensatory mechanism that is observed in response to decreased cardiac output is transcapillary

TABLE 49-3

Compensatory Responses in Shock Syndrome
1. Preservation of coronary and cerebral perfusion at the expense of skin, skeletal muscle, kidney, and splanchnic perfusion
2. Preservation of cardiac output through increased sympathetic nervous system activity: increased heart rate and myocardial contractility
3. Preservation of intravascular volume: venoconstriction and transcapillary refill, activation of the renin-angiotensin-aldosterone axis

refill. This factor involves the decrease in capillary hydrostatic pressure that results from adrenergic vasoconstriction of the precapillary sphincters. Decreased luminal capillary hydrostatic pressure favors movement of fluid and solutes from the interstitial space into the capillary, thereby increasing circulating blood volume.[36]

Mechanisms Working Against Compensation in Shock Syndrome

A number of factors augment and intensify the harmful effects of the shock state, ultimately leading to the irreversible, fatal nature of the syndrome. The first of these decompensating factors is loss of adrenergic vasoconstriction.[37] Mechanisms responsible for this loss of peripheral vascular tone are listed in Table 49-4.[38–44] Other microcirculatory phenomena that accentuate and/or amplify the shock syndrome include increased capillary permeability, obstruction of the microvasculature by platelet and white cell aggregates, decreased red blood cell deformability, and swelling of endothelial cells.[45–48]

Animal and clinical studies support the concept of progressive myocardial depression during shock. A number of factors apparently contribute to this derangement in cardiac performance:

1. A decrease in coronary perfusion secondary to systemic arterial hypotension and circulating coronary arterial vasoconstrictors, e.g., leukotrienes.
2. Presence in the blood of circulating myocardial depressant substances, e.g., tumor necrosis factor.[4,49–52] Occasional patients develop marked bradycardia during shock.[53] This phenomenon has also been observed in experimental animal models of shock.[54] This inappropriate bradycardia is apparently the result of activation of inhibitory cardiac vagal afferent nerve fibers perhaps secondary to vigorous myocardial contraction around nearly empty cardiac chambers.[55]
3. Acidosis may also interfere with responsiveness of beta receptors.

TABLE 49-4

Factors Leading to Loss of Peripheral Vascular Vasoconstriction during Shock
1. Release of vasodilating prostaglandins
2. Enhanced release of nitric oxide
3. Catecholamine depletion from vascular smooth-muscle adrenergic nerve endings
4. Decreased sympathetic nervous system activity secondary to cerebral ischemia
5. Antiadrenergic action of increasing peripheral and central nervous system levels of endorphins
6. Acidosis

Dysfunction in other organs can also contribute to persistence and/or worsening of the shock state. Increased capillary permeability and respiratory muscle fatigue lead to hypoxemia and respiratory failure (ARDS).[56] Acute renal failure secondary to acute tubular necrosis is a common event in shock patients. Metabolic acidosis and hyperkalemia often accompany acute renal failure.[57,58] Splanchnic vasoconstriction with resultant visceral ischemia can lead to erosive gastritis, pancreatitis, acalculous cholecystitis, and loss of the barrier function of the gastrointestinal tract with secondary release of bacteria into the circulation.[59]

Hepatic hypoperfusion can result in centrilobular liver necrosis (so-called shock liver) characterized by modest elevations in serum bilirubin and alkaline phosphatase and marked increases in serum transaminase values.[60] Cerebral hypoperfusion can lead to restlessness, agitation, mental obtundation, and even coma. Cerebral infarction in a "watershed" distribution may also occur.

Some patients with shock develop disseminated intravascular coagulation (DIC) with resultant consumption of clotting factors. However, DIC is usually seen in septic or endotoxic shock and only occasionally in cardiogenic shock. Functional derangement of the reticuloendothelial system (RES) often accompanies shock. Phagocytic activity by cells of the RES is transiently depressed in patients who recover; irreversible shock is associated with persistently depressed RES function that lasts until the patient's death.[61–63] Immune function is also depressed in shock patients, leading to delayed recovery even if hypotension and hypoperfusion are reversed.[64] A wide variety of derangements of immune function have been described in patients with the shock syndrome.[64–67]

Clinical Presentation of Shock Syndrome

The two cardinal manifestations of the shock syndrome that enable the clinician to establish the diagnosis are (1) hypotension and (2) hypoperfusion. Hypotension is usually defined as a blood pressure less than 90 mmHg, although patients may manifest the shock syndrome with systemic blood pressures above 90 mmHg if previous basal values were *above* the usual normal range, i.e., 100 to 140/60 to 90 mmHg. Moreover, some patients may tolerate pressures of 80 mmHg systolic without evidence of hypoperfusion. Some authorities have advocated a definition of hypotension that includes any individual whose mean blood pressure is 30 mmHg below previous basal values.[68]

The presence of hypoperfusion is usually diagnosed from one or more readily obtained clinical observations: (1) altered mental status—restlessness, agitation, obtundation; (2) cool, clammy skin, and (3) reduced urine output (below 20 mL/h.) Most patients with cardiogenic shock have sinus tachycardia; peripheral pulses are often weak and thready. Many patients also demonstrate tachypnea (respiratory rate above 20 per minute) and hypo- or hyperthermia. Confirmatory laboratory findings are listed in Table 49-5.

EPIDEMIOLOGY OF CARDIOGENIC SHOCK

Epidemiologic analysis of most forms of shock are unavailable. Cardiogenic shock following myocardial infarction, however, has been studied.[69-75] Cardiogenic shock complicates 5 to 15 percent of all acute myocardial infarctions without major changes in incidence over the years.[69] Despite recent technological advances in the diagnosis and treatment of patients with acute myocardial infarction, in-hospital and long-term mortality remains very high.[69] In-hospital case fatality rates in various series range from 70 to nearly 100 percent. For the few survivors, the 5-year survival rate following discharge from the hospital is approximately 40 percent. These grim statistics are undoubtedly a reflection of the major myocardial insult that leads to cardiogenic shock.

PATHOPHYSIOLOGY OF SPECIFIC ENTITIES THAT RESULT IN CARDIOGENIC SHOCK

A number of pathological conditions can lead to cardiogenic shock (Table 49-2). Many are associated with injured and/or markedly depressed left and/or right ventricular function. Less common are conditions that relate to cardiac compression with inadequate ventricular filling or severe ventricular inflow or outflow obstruction, e.g., left atrial myxoma and coarctation of the aorta. Yet another cardiovascular cause for the shock syndrome is intravascular hypovolemia secondary to blood loss, e.g., a ruptured aortic aneurysm.

Acute Myocardial Infarction

A variety of events and/or complications can occur in the setting of acute myocardial infarction that result in cardiogenic shock (Table 49-6). The commonest cause of infarct-related cardiogenic shock is permanent (necrosis) or transient (ischemically stunned) myocardial injury that prevents 40 percent or more of the left ventricular myocardium from contracting.[76,77] Once extensive left ventricular dysfunction develops, associated arterial hypoxemia and decreased cardiac output combine to depress further left ventricular systolic function. A vicious downward spiral is generated: left ventricular dysfunction leads to worsening cardiac output and progressive hypotension and arterial hypoxemia, which in turn decrease myocardial blood flow and oxygenation, thereby further depressing left ventricular function. Myocardial necrosis, recent and old, and myocardial ischemia all have the same additive effect: decreased left ventricular systolic and diastolic function. Depressed diastolic function elevates left atrial and consequently pulmonary capillary wedge pressure with resultant pulmonary interstitial edema and progressive arterial hypoxemia.

TABLE 49-5
Laboratory Findings in Cardiogenic Shock

1. Arterial blood gases: metabolic acidosis, hypoxemia, hypocarbia (compensatory respiratory alkalosis)
2. Elevated blood lactate levels
3. Leukocytosis; thrombocytopenia when DIC is present
4. Electrocardiogram may reveal infarction, LBBB, sinus tachycardia, or dysrhythmia (e.g., ventricular tachycardia)
5. Chest x-ray may reveal pulmonary edema or ARDS
6. Hemodynamic monitoring usually demonstrates reduced cardiac output, arterial hypotension, and elevated pulmonary capillary wedge and pulmonary arterial pressures

DIC = disseminated intravascular coagulation, LBBB = left bundle branch block, ARDS = adult respiratory distress syndrome.

Some patients have a single, large, and catastrophic infarct leading to cardiogenic shock while others have a stuttering course with progressive or repetitive elevations in serum levels of myocardial enzymes.[78] The majority of patients who develop this type of cardiogenic shock have multivessel coronary artery disease usually involving the left anterior descending coronary artery.[79] Left ventricular ejection fraction is almost always less than 0.20 to 0.30. Cardiac output is less than 2.2 liters/min per m^2 and pulmonary capillary wedge pressure exceeds 18 mmHg. Right-sided pressures (right ventricular, right atrial) are usually normal or only slightly elevated initially.

Mechanical defects can also lead to cardiogenic shock. Table 49-6 lists the various defects that are commonly associated with cardiogenic shock. Papillary muscle rup-

TABLE 49-6
Pathogenesis of Cardiogenic Shock after Acute Myocardial Infarction

1. Extensive left ventricular dysfunction
   a. Myocardial infarction (MI) with extension or associated ischemic dysfunction
   b. Massive MI
   c. Small MI on top of extensive earlier myocardial damage
   d. Small/moderate size MI with metabolic derangements or dysrhythmia
2. Mechanical defects
   a. Rupture of interventricular septum resulting in large left-to-right shunt
   b. Rupture of part or all of papillary muscle resulting in severe mitral regurgitation
   c. Ischemic dysfunction of papillary muscle resulting in severe mitral regurgitation
   d. Rupture of free ventricular wall resulting in cardiac tamponade
3. Extensive right ventricular infarction

ture accounts for 5 percent of all cardiac ruptures while ventricular septal and free wall ruptures account for 10 and 85 percent, respectively.

The posteromedial papillary muscle is 5 to 10 times more prone to ischemia, infarction, and/or rupture compared with the anterolateral papillary muscle, possibly because it receives blood from only one coronary artery. Thus, clinically important mitral regurgitation usually occurs in patients with inferoposterior myocardial infarction. Papillary muscle ischemia or infarction by itself is rarely sufficient to produce severe mitral regurgitation. Concomitant left ventricular myocardial dysfunction at the base of the papillary muscle must be present in order for there to be significant mitral regurgitation.[80]

Rupture of the interventricular septum occurs with both anterior and inferoposterior myocardial infarction. Multivessel coronary artery disease is common, but single-vessel disease can also lead to this complication. Rupture of the septum can occur 1 to 14 days after infarction; however, this complication usually develops 3 to 7 days after infarction. A large left-to-right shunt is almost always present; left ventricular ejection fraction may be surprisingly normal since the left ventricle "unloads" into the low-pressure right ventricle. Adequacy of right ventricular function is a major determinant of survival in patients with ventricular septal rupture.[81] (See also Chap. 60.)

Right Ventricular Infarction

Although right ventricular infarction may complicate up to one-third of inferoposterior left ventricular infarcts, the volume of injured right ventricular myocardium is usually moderate.[82] An occasional patient with inferoposterior infarction develops extensive necrosis/ischemia of the right ventricle with resultant cardiogenic shock. These patients present with the clinical picture of isolated right-sided heart failure: jugular venous distension, clear lungs, right ventricular S_3 and S_4, and hepatic congestion. Kussmaul's sign (inspiratory increase in jugular venous pressure) may be seen. Cardiac output is markedly depressed (usually less than 2.0 liters/min per m^2); pulmonary capillary wedge pressure is normal or slightly elevated. Right atrial pressure is significantly elevated and exceeds pulmonary capillary wedge pressure while pulmonary arterial pressure is surprisingly normal. Pulmonary arterial pulse pressure is diminished (usually less than 15 to 20 mmHg). The hemodynamic findings often resemble those seen with tamponade or constriction. Radionuclide right ventricular ejection is usually less than 0.39 while left ventricular ejection fraction exceeds 0.45. Tricuspid regurgitation is often present.

Low systemic arterial blood pressure is the result of decreased left ventricular filling secondary to diminished right ventricular cardiac output and increased intrapericardial pressure from the dilated right ventricle, which produces in effect a tamponade of the left ventricle.[83–85] The reverse Bernheim phenomenon (septal bulging into the left ventricle) may also play a role in diminished left ventricular volumes and stroke output. Bradyarrhythmias with loss of an appropriately timed atrial "kick" also contribute to the decrease in right ventricular function.[86] (See also Chap. 60.)

Dilated Cardiomyopathy/Myocarditis

Patients with end-stage idiopathic dilated cardiomyopathy and markedly depressed left (and often right) ventricular function may develop terminal cardiogenic shock. Left ventricular ejection fraction is usually less than 0.20 and substantial left ventricular dilatation is usually present. Chest roentgenography demonstrates marked cardiomegaly and pulmonary interstitial edema. Fulminant acute viral myocarditis can also lead to cardiogenic shock, although this scenario is unusual.

Valvular Heart Disease

End-stage chronic valvular heart disease involving one or more valves, stenotic and/or regurgitant, or acute, massive regurgitant lesions can terminate with cardiogenic shock. Patients with chronic volume overload, i.e., mitral and aortic regurgitation, resemble dilated, congestive cardiomyopathy terminally. Massive left ventricular dilatation and biventricular failure are often present. At this stage, the regurgitant volume of blood may be modest, thereby confusing the clinician as to the etiology of the congestive cardiomyopathy.

Acute aortic and/or mitral regurgitation may also cause cardiogenic shock. These lesions are usually the result of infectious endocarditis, dissection of the aorta, or spontaneous rupture of a myxomatous valve or chordae tendineae. The left ventricle is not dilated since the regurgitant lesion is acute.[87] Severe pulmonary edema is invariably present.

Patients with end-stage stenotic valvular lesions may also develop cardiogenic shock. Individuals with severe aortic stenosis and shock have a small gradient across the aortic valve (usually less than 20 to 30 mmHg) and markedly depressed cardiac output and left ventricular ejection fraction. End-stage mitral stenosis leading to cardiogenic shock is associated with marked right ventricular dilatation and failure producing severe tricuspid regurgitation. Cardiac output is severely depressed (often less than 1.0 liter/min per m^2), resulting in marked prerenal azotemia.

Myocardial Dysfunction in Septic Shock

Normal or even elevated cardiac output is usually present in patients with septic shock. The peripheral vascular bed, however, is markedly vasodilated, resulting in arterial hypotension and hypoperfusion despite the apparently adequate ventricular output. In fact, cardiac output is inadequate for the degree of peripheral vasodilatation; myocardial depression is indeed present.[3,4,88–90] Biventricular depression of ejection fraction that resolves over 10 to 14 days has been documented in septic patients without prior cardiac disease who recover. The mechanism of myocardial depression in septic shock is not well understood but may involve a circulating substance that decreases myocardial contractility, e.g., tumor necrosis factor.[4,91,92]

Tachyarrhythmias or Bradyarrhythmias

Arrhythmias may produce cardiogenic shock by markedly depressing cardiac output. This may occur because of (1) inadequate ventricular diastolic filling (atrial and ventricular tachyarrhythmias), (2) abnormal ventricular contraction patterns resulting from abnormal electrical activation patterns in the ventricle (ventricular tachyarrhythmias), and (3) inadequate heart rate in the face of adequate ventricular function (bradyarrhythmias). Abnormal ventricular function prior to the development of an arrhythmia predisposes to more severe hemodynamic derangement once an arrhythmia develops.

Myocardial Depression Following Cardiopulmonary Bypass

Shock following cardiopulmonary bypass is usually multifactorial with both cardiogenic and hypovolemic components. The cardiogenic factors contributing to shock in this setting include arrhythmias, tamponade, myocardial ischemic dysfunction or stunning, and/or myocardial infarction. In general, left ventricular dysfunction predominates in this setting, but right ventricular dysfunction in the face of postoperative pulmonary hypertension may also contribute to the shock syndrome following cardiopulmonary bypass.[93,94]

Pericardial Tamponade or Constriction

Myocardial function is often normal in patients with pericardial tamponade or constriction. Depressed cardiac output is the result of markedly impaired ventricular diastolic filling secondary to the pericardial abnormality. Severe tamponade and shock can develop within seconds to minutes, e.g., myocardial rupture, or it may occur following days or even weeks of subacute, more moderate, restriction of ventricular filling. (See also Chap. 90.)

Pulmonary Embolism

Massive pulmonary embolism obstructing more than 60 percent of the pulmonary vascular bed can produce syncope, hypotension, or the shock syndrome. Occasionally, pulmonary embolism presents as cardiogenic shock. The right ventricle fails acutely secondary to the sudden increase in afterload: cardiac output falls and right ventricular filling pressures rise. The increase in right ventricular afterload is the result of mechanical obstruction of the pulmonary arterial bed. Release of vasoactive substances following an episode of pulmonary embolism probably plays little or no role in the pathophysiology of shock secondary to massive pulmonary embolism. Pulmonary arterial and right ventricular systolic pressure does not exceed 50 to 60 mmHg in individuals with previously normal pulmonary arterial pressure. Left-sided heart pressures are normal or subnormal because of inadequate left ventricular filling. Arterial hypoxemia is invariably present. There may be a small to moderate right-to-left shunt of deoxygenated blood through a patent foramen ovale. (See also Chap. 100.)

Primary Pulmonary Hypertension/Severe Pulmonary Hypertension

Cardiogenic shock may result from severe pulmonary hypertension, primary or other etiology, with marked, chronic right ventricular failure. The right ventricle is markedly dilated with high filling pressures. Pulmonary arterial and right ventricular systolic pressure often exceeds 100 mmHg. Left ventricular filling pressures are low or normal secondary to left ventricular hypovolemia. Right-to-left shunting of blood through a patent foramen ovale may be present. (See also Chap. 99.)

Coarctation of the Aorta

Coarctation of the aorta may cause cardiogenic shock early in life as the ductus arteriosus closes and the left ventricle is unable to adapt to the markedly increased aortic resistance/afterload. In this setting, the left ventricle may fail acutely. Adults with coarctation of the aorta do not develop cardiogenic shock because they have developed left ventricular hypertrophy that is adequate to maintain peripheral perfusion despite the marked increase in aortic resistance. (See Chap. 97.)

Myxoma

Atrial myxomas may suddenly prolapse into the mitral (usual) or tricuspid (rare) valve orifice, thereby totally or nearly totally obstructing blood flow into the affected ventricle. Cardiac output fills precipitously as does systemic arterial blood pressure. (See also Chap. 111.)

Hypertrophic Cardiomyopathy

A rare individual with hypertrophic obstructive cardiomyopathy may develop cardiogenic shock if or when very severe, sudden-onset left ventricular outflow obstruction occurs. Since left ventricular outflow obstruction is dynamic in these individuals, severe obstruction with resultant shock may be transient or it may lead to potentially lethal dysrhythmias. (See also Chap. 90.)

Tension Pneumothorax

In patients with tension pneumothorax, the great veins within the thorax are subjected to very high levels of intrapleural pressure. These high pressures cause the veins to collapse, thereby markedly decreasing venous return to the heart. Cardiac output declines precipitously and cardiogenic shock develops.

Cardiovascular Causes of Hypovolemic Shock

Hypovolemic shock secondary to a cardiovascular etiology may be the result of ruptured aortic aneurysm or traumatic disruption of the aorta or other major artery or vein.

EVALUATION OF THE CARDIOGENIC SHOCK PATIENT

Before evaluation of the patient with cardiogenic shock, stabilization and some degree of reversal of shock must be effected (Table 49-7). It too often happens that diagnostic zeal prompts the physician to obtain various non-

TABLE 49-7
Stabilization of Patient with Cardiogenic Shock

1. Establish effective ventilation and oxygenation: arterial P_{O_2} above 70 mmHg
2. Restore adequate central blood pressure (mean arterial blood pressure above 70 mmHg) with pressors, e.g., dopamine, norepinephrine
3. If hypovolemia is present, infuse volume replacement
4. Treat pain, arrhythmias, acid-base abnormalities

invasive and invasive tests before some level of circulatory homeostasis has been reestablished. The result is that an exact diagnosis is ascertained but the patient succumbs to irreversible shock.

RECOGNITION OF SPECIFIC ENTITIES PRODUCING CARDIOGENIC SHOCK

The various clinical entities listed in Table 49-2 can usually be distinguished from each other by history, physical examination, and various laboratory tests.

Acute Myocardial Infarction

Patients with acute myocardial infarction and cardiogenic shock usually present with a history of recent and/or past episodes of chest discomfort. The heart rate is usually 100 beats per minute or more with sinus tachycardia as the underlying rhythm. The physical examination usually reveals extensive pulmonary rales, S_3/S_4 gallops, as well as the findings associated with the shock syndrome (peripheral cyanosis; cool, clammy skin; decreased mental status). In patients with extensive left ventricular dysfunction and no mechanical defect, the electrocardiogram (ECG) usually reveals anterior infarction with extensive loss of R waves in leads I, AV_L, or V_{1-6} or both anterior and inferoposterior infarction. Left or right bundle branch block may also be observed. Noninvasive (echocardiography, radionuclide ventriculography) or invasive (catheterization/angiography) tests of left ventricular wall motion disclose marked reduction in systolic contractile function. Cardiac output is usually less than 2.0 liter/min per m^2; left ventricular filling pressure exceeds 20 mmHg.

Patients with cardiogenic shock and a mechanical defect (mitral regurgitation or ventricular septal rupture) usually demonstrate all of the findings just described as well as a loud systolic murmur. Patients with ventricular septal rupture almost invariably have a palpable precordial thrill. The ECG reveals either anterior or inferoposterior infarction in patients with ventricular septal rupture; 80 percent of patients with severe mitral regurgitation will have inferoposterior infarction. Noninvasive and invasive cardiac tests demonstrate the mechanical lesion and quantitate shunt or regurgitant blood flow. Left ventricular systolic function may be mildly or markedly reduced. Forward cardiac output is low, usually less than 2.0 liters/min per m^2; left ventricular filling pressures are elevated, usually more than 20 mmHg; right ventricular filling pressures may be normal or abnormal. (See also Chaps. 60 and 74.)

Individuals with *right ventricular infarction* with marked dysfunction but without a mechanical defect usually have distended neck veins, clear lungs, and bradyarrhythmias. The ECG in these patients invariably reveals an inferoposterior infarction. Noninvasive and invasive tests of cardiac function demonstrate a dilated right ventricle with markedly reduced systolic function. Left ventricular function is usually adequate. Cardiac output is markedly reduced, usually less than 2.0 liters/min per m^2; left ventricular filling pressures are often normal or only slightly elevated; right ventricular filling pressures are often markedly elevated (>10 mmHg). (See also Chap. 60.)

Dilated Cardiomyopathy/Myocarditis

Patients with idiopathic dilated cardiomyopathy often have a history consistent with chronic heart failure. The physical examination discloses sinus tachycardia, a narrow pulse pressure, jugular venous distension, pulmonary rales, S_3 and S_4 gallops, murmurs of mitral and/or tricuspid regurgitation, and peripheral edema. Electrocardiographic findings are usually nonspecific, i.e., low-voltage, left bundle branch block, diffuse ST-T wave changes. The chest roentgenogram reveals marked cardiomegaly; cardiac tests (invasive and noninvasive) demonstrate very poor left and often right ventricular systolic function. Cardiac output is very low (often below 1.0 liter/min per m^2); left and often right ventricular filling pressures are abnormally high (left ventricular exceeding 25 mmHg; right ventricular above 8 to 10 mmHg). (See also Chap. 89.)

Individuals with myocarditis report the rather sudden onset of heart failure symptoms with or without a prior history of a viral syndrome. Physical findings include sinus tachycardia, narrow pulse pressure, pulmonary rales, S_3 and S_4 gallops, and at times, murmurs of mitral and/or tricuspid regurgitation. Electrocardiographic findings are nonspecific. Left ventricular systolic function is poor. Myocardial biopsy discloses inflammatory infiltrates in the myocardium. (See also Chap. 88.)

End-stage Valvular Heart Disease

Patients with terminal mitral and/or aortic regurgitation usually have a history compatible with chronic heart failure. Results of the physical examination and laboratory tests are similar to those described for dilated cardiomyopathy. Atrial fibrillation is often present. The murmurs of mitral and/or aortic regurgitation may not be prominent. Patients with aortic stenosis may report angina pectoris and/or syncope. Physical findings include sinus tachycardia or atrial fibrillation, a narrow pulse pressure, pulmonary rales, a soft or absent murmur of aortic stenosis, and S_3/S_4 gallops. The ECG usually demonstrates left ventricular hypertrophy (LVH) with ST-T changes or left bundle branch block. Noninvasive and invasive cardiac testing often discloses marked left ventricular hypertrophy and systolic dysfunction as well as severe aortic stenosis.

Patients with end-stage mitral stenosis also have a history of chronic heart failure. They may report prior episodes of arterial embolism and/or hemoptysis. Physical findings usually suggest that severe pulmonary hypertension and right ventricular dysfunction are present: cachexia, irregularly irregular pulse, cyanosis, jugular venous distension, right ventricular heave, an increased P_2, right ventricular S_3 and S_4, hepatomegaly with or without ascites, and peripheral edema. The murmur of mitral stenosis is often soft or inaudible. Noninvasive and invasive cardiac tests document the presence of severe mitral stenosis. (See also Chap. 80.)

Septic Shock

Patients with septic shock will usually have an associated or antecedent illness leading to sepsis such as cholecystitis, pyelonephritis, etc. These patients usually manifest fever, tachypnea, and sinus tachycardia. Their skin is warm and moist and their pulse is bounding. Other physical findings usually pertain to the underlying illness that is causing sepsis. The ECG demonstrates nonspecific findings, e.g., sinus tachycardia and ST-T wave changes. Ventricular contractile function is initially hyperdynamic by noninvasive and invasive cardiac testing in patients without heart disease. Cardiac output is usually normal or elevated; left and right ventricular filling pressures are normal or low.

Tachyarrhythmias or Bradyarrhythmias

The diagnosis is rarely in doubt when bradyarrhythmias or tachyarrhythmias lead to the shock syndrome. Accurate, rapid electrocardiographic diagnosis is essential followed by prompt therapy.

Cardiopulmonary Bypass

The unique setting of postbypass cardiogenic shock presents special challenges and opportunities for diagnosis. Left and right ventricular function can be assessed visually and hemodynamically. Transesophageal echocardiography is useful in determining the adequacy of ventricular and valvular function.

Pericardial Tamponade/Constriction

The history of individuals with pericardial tamponade is usually dominated by symptoms related to the underlying illness involving the pericardium, e.g., malignant neoplasm and dissection of the aorta. Physical findings related to pericardial tamponade include sinus tachycardia, narrow pulse pressure, pulsus paradoxus, jugular venous distension, and a small quiet heart. The ECG reveals low-voltage and nonspecific ST-T changes. Chest roentgenography demonstrates cardiomegaly. Echocardiography is the diagnostic test of choice since it demonstrates the pericardial effusion and its effects on atrial and ventricular filling. Cardiac output is reduced; left and right ventricular filling pressures are moderately elevated and approximately equal.

Patients with constrictive pericarditis usually have a history and physical examination consistent with chronic, severe right ventricular failure. Patients may be cachectic with moderate to large ascitic fluid collections. Jugular and peripheral veins are usually distended; the lungs are clear. Echocardiography, computerized tomography (CT) scanning or magnetic resonance imaging (MRI), and invasive hemodynamic measurements may help distinguish constrictive pericarditis from restrictive cardiomyopathy. (See Chaps. 91 and 92.)

Pulmonary Embolism

Patients with massive pulmonary embolism present with sudden-onset syncope and/or shock. The history usually points to some predisposition to deep venous thrombosis, e.g., an orthopedic surgical procedure with subsequent bed rest. Physical findings include sinus tachycardia, jugular venous distension, clear lungs, and a right ventricular summation gallop. The ECG demonstrates acute cor pulmonale, e.g., S_1-Q_3-T_3. Echocardiography reveals a dilated right ventricle and normal left ventricular function in the absence of preexisting heart disease. There is arterial hypoxemia and respiratory alkalosis. Cardiac output is markedly reduced; left ventricular filling pressures are low; right ventricular filling pressures are often markedly elevated. A ventilation-perfusion (V/Q) lung scan demonstrates large, mismatched, ventilation/perfusion defects. (See also Chap. 100.)

Severe Pulmonary Hypertension

Patients with end-stage pulmonary hypertensive disease and shock have a history compatible with chronic cor pulmonale, i.e., dyspnea on exertion, fatigue, and peripheral edema. Physical examination often discloses sinus tachycardia, cyanosis, jugular venous distension, clear lungs, right ventricular S_3 and S_4 gallops, ascites, and peripheral edema. Clubbing may be noted if chronic arterial hypoxemia has been present. Noninvasive and invasive cardiac testing demonstrates right ventricular hypertrophy, dilatation, and systolic dysfunction. Cardiac output is markedly reduced; left ventricular filling pressures are normal or low; right ventricular filling pressures are elevated. (See also Chap. 99.)

Coarctation of the Aorta

Infants with severe coarctation, left ventricular failure, and shock present with respiratory distress and cyanosis. Echocardiography usually discloses the coarctation.

Myxoma

Myxomatous tumors can produce acute-onset symptoms including respiratory distress and peripheral cyanosis. Patients may have a chronic history of dyspnea on exertion or a lupuslike syndrome. Physical examination may reveal only findings associated with the shock syndrome; however, a diastolic murmur of mitral or tricuspid stenosis may be heard. Echocardiographic examination reveals tumor. (See also Chap. 111.)

Hypertrophic Cardiomyopathy

Severe dynamic obstruction of the left ventricular outflow tract may produce a sudden-onset shock syndrome

suscitation. Patients with massive pulmonary embolism complicated by systemic hypotension and acute cor pulmonale also require an increased preload to maintain an effective cardiac output. (See also Chap. 60.)

Caution regarding the use of intravenous diuretics is recommended in patients with systemic hypotension and mildly increased filling pressures; a decrease in preload may cause progressive declines in systemic blood pressure and coronary arterial perfusion pressure. Small intravenous doses of furosemide (10 to 20 mg) or bumetanide (0.5 mg) can be administered if the pulmonary capillary wedge pressure is above 20 mmHg and pulmonary edema is present. Larger doses can be used subsequently as the systemic blood pressure allows. Patients with cardiogenic shock solely on the basis of diastolic dysfunction, e.g., hypertrophic obstructive cardiomyopathy, are particularly sensitive to changes in preload.

Increases in afterload depress myocardial fiber shortening, stroke volume, and cardiac output. When left ventricular systolic function is impaired, afterload becomes a primary determinant of overall cardiac performance. Therefore, pharmacologic reduction of afterload may improve cardiac index and decrease pulmonary wedge pressure by as much as 30 and 40 percent, respectively. The observed hemodynamic improvements may be accompanied by a reduction in heart rate and a decrease in myocardial oxygen demand without compromising coronary arterial perfusion (Fig. 49-2). Hemodynamic monitoring is recommended.

In patients with fixed, increased afterload, e.g., critical aortic stenosis, pharmacologic agents are minimally effective. Therefore, emergent intervention with either balloon valvuloplasty or surgical aortic valve replacement is required. (See also Chap. 79.)

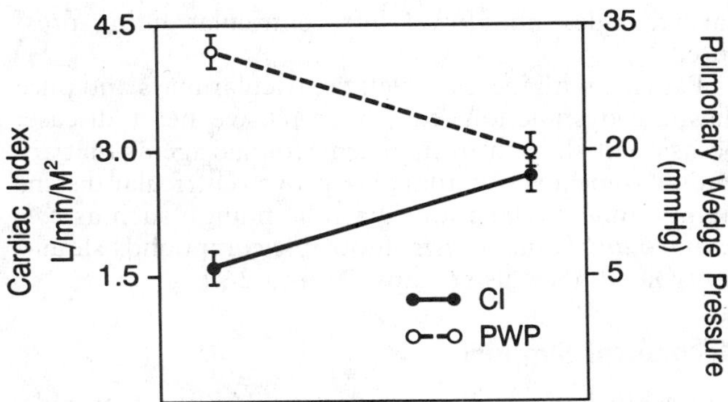

FIGURE 49-2 Hemodynamic effects of afterload reduction with intravenous nitroprusside in patients with pulmonary congestion and peripheral hypoperfusion. A progressive decrease in pulmonary wedge pressure (PWP) concomitant with a steady increase in cardiac index (CI) is observed (*From JS Forrester et al: N Engl J Med 295:1404, 1976. Reproduced with permission.*)

Pharmacologic Therapy

Persistent systemic hypotension, particularly when accompanied by signs of poor peripheral perfusion and an elevated pulmonary capillary wedge pressure, is an indication for pharmacologic therapy. As discussed previously, agents with peripheral vasodilating capacity such as nitroprusside or nitroglycerin should be considered in patients with poor systolic function and myocardial ischemia or infarction, respectively. If the systemic blood pressure or cardiac output cannot be maintained, however, inotropic support with catecholamines or other sympathomimetic amines should be added. The maintenance of systemic blood pressure (mean blood pressure exceeding 70 mmHg) is of particular importance in patients with obstructive coronary artery disease.

Dopamine (3,4-dihydroxyphenylethylamine) is an immediate precursor of norepinephrine. Its major cardiovascular effects are the result of both α- and β-adrenergic receptor stimulation as well as dopaminergic receptor stimulation within the mesenteric and renal vascular beds. At doses required to increase mean arterial blood pressure and cardiac output (5 to 8 μg/kg per min), heart rate and myocardial oxgen demand may be increased substantially.[98] In the presence of acidosis, larger doses may be required. In contrast, *dobutamine*, a synthesized derivative of isoproterenol primarily with β-adrenergic receptor activity, is frequently able to increase cardiac index (initial dose 2.5 to 5.0 μg/kg per min) with small increases in heart rate and myocardial oxygen demand.[99–101] It has been shown to increase cardiac output in patients with acute myocardial infarction complicated by cardiogenic shock without increasing infarct size or the occurrence of malignant ventricular arrhythmias.[100,101] Therefore, in this setting it is considered the inotropic agent of choice. Caution is recommended, however, in patients with profound systemic hypotension (systolic blood pressure at most 80 mmHg) in whom the peripheral β_2-stimulating effects of dobutamine may cause further reductions in blood pressure and coronary arterial perfusion pressure. *Amrinone*, which blocks the breakdown of cyclic adenosine monophosphate (AMP) induced by dobutamine (β_1 stimulation), amplifies the effects of dobutamine and produces a decrease in both preload and afterload. (See also Chaps. 28 and 30.)

Levarterenol (norepinephrine), a chemical mediator liberated by postganglionic adrenergic nerves, acts primarily on peripheral α receptors, increasing peripheral vascular resistance. It does, however, exhibit some myocardial β_1-receptor activity as well. Norepinephrine is not a first-line agent in the treatment of cardiogenic shock. Its use is reserved more commonly for patients with systemic hypotension refractory to inotropic agents and other supportive measures. (See also Chap. 30.)

Isoproterenol, a pure β-adrenergic receptor agonist, does not have a primary role in the management of patients with cardiogenic shock.[102]

Digitalis glycosides are ineffective in cardiogenic shock. In addition, the incidence of toxicity is increased in this setting. Uncontrolled or recurrent supraventricular tachyarrhythmias are the principal indications for the use of intravenous digitalis glycosides.

The efficacy of dobutamine and dopamine may decline with continued use, a reflection, at least theoretically, of decreased myocardial adrenergic receptor responsiveness. Phosphodiesterase inhibitors also increase myocyte cyclic AMP concentrations but do not rely on surface receptors. *Amrinone* and *milrinone* have been used successfully in the treatment of cardiogenic shock.[103] Enoximone, administered either alone or in combination with an adrenergic agent, has been shown to increase cardiac index and lower left ventricular filling pressure.[104,105]

Patients with increased left ventricular mass and pure diastolic dysfunction, e.g., hypertensive heart disease, occasionally benefit from pharmacologic agents that are said by some investigators to improve ventricular distensibility and/or relaxation (diastolic filling), such as *calcium channel antagonists*. Inotropic compounds should be avoided. (See also Chaps. 25 and 26.)

Mechanical Support

Intraaortic balloon counterpulsation (IABP) can provide rapid stabilization of patients with cardiogenic shock, particularly those with global myocardial ischemia or infarction complicated by mechanical defects such as papillary muscle rupture causing acute, severe mitral regurgitation or a moderate to large ventricular septal defect. In most instances it can be inserted percutaneously either with or without fluoroscopic guidance, although the latter is preferred. The augmented coronary perfusion pressure during diastole facilitates coronary arterial blood flow. Since the balloon deflates rapidly at the onset of ventricular systole, left ventricular impedance is reduced (decreased afterload). Hemodynamic changes typically include a 10 to 20 percent increase in cardiac output, a reduction in systolic and increase in diastolic blood pressures, a diminution in heart rate, and an increase in urine output. In some patients, continued inotropic support is required to maintain an acceptable blood pressure (>90 mmHg systolic) and cardiac index (>2.2 liters/min per m^2) even after IABP insertion. (See also Chap. 31.)

Intraaortic balloon counterpulsation was first used in the treatment of cardiogenic shock by Kantrowitz and colleagues in 1968.[106] Clinical improvement occurs in a large percentage (approximately 75 percent) of patients; however, in-hospital mortality remains high and many patients cannot be removed successfully from mechanical support.[107] Although recently more powerful circulatory-assist devices providing flow rates of 8 to 10 liters/min have been developed, similar limitations have been recognized with the Hemopump[108,109] and percutaneous cardiopulmonary support system.[110–112] Some patients who do not stabilize with IABP will improve following insertion of the Hemopump. Mechanical assistance with these devices, therefore, should be considered in patients with cardiogenic shock who need temporary support while preparation for definitive, corrective intervention is being made.

Surgical Intervention

Surgical intervention in the treatment of cardiogenic shock is most successful when mechanical defects such as acute mitral regurgitation are present. Patients can be stabilized initially with an IABP (or another circulatory-assist device) and inotropic support; however, surgery should not be delayed. There is substantial evidence that patients with either an isolated mechanical defect or severe coronary artery disease derive the greatest benefit when surgical intervention is undertaken promptly.[113–115] Prompt surgery also may reduce the risks and complications of prolonged end-organ hypoperfusion such as infections, ARDS, and renal insufficiency. The importance of early cardiovascular support with IABP prior to and following surgery has also been recognized.[116] (See also Chap. 74.)

Patients with acute aortic regurgitation and severe hemodynamic compromise, regardless of the etiology, are not candidates for IABP.

Cardiac transplantation is a surgical option for a small select group of individuals with cardiogenic shock. Currently, there are two basic approaches to mechanical circulatory support as a bridge to cardiac transplantation: (1) the total artificial heart and (2) ventricular-assist devices. Biventricular circulatory support may be particularly beneficial in potential heart transplant candidates with life-threatening, refractory ventricular arrhythmias.[117,118] In select cases, ventricular-assist devices can effectively replace left-sided heart function for prolonged periods of time (weeks to months) until a donor heart can be found. (See also Chap. 32.)

Reperfusion Strategies

Cardiogenic shock following acute myocardial infarction results from extensive myocardial necrosis. Unfortunately, patients receiving standard supportive therapy have an in-hospital mortality approaching 80 percent.

There is mounting evidence that infarct-related coronary arterial patency is a primary determinant of clinical outcome in acute myocardial infarction[119,120] (Table 49-8). Although the efficacy of thrombolytic therapy in patients with overt cardiogenic shock has not been critically evaluated, available data are encouraging.[121] Analysis of data from the Society for Cardiac Angiography[122] and the ISIS-2 trial[123] suggests a survival benefit for patients with cardiogenic shock in whom successful thrombolysis and coronary arterial reperfusion are achieved. A number of large clinical trials, including GISSI-1[124] and GISSI-2,[125] have identified high mortality rates, typically exceeding 70 percent, for patients with cardiogenic shock despite thrombolytic therapy. (See also Chap. 60.)

Improved survival appears to be contingent on early and sustained reperfusion of the infarct-related coronary artery. Experience suggests that early reperfusion, achieved in 50 to 80 percent of patients depending on the thrombolytic agent and the dosing regimen chosen, limits the incidence of cardiogenic shock. However, these agents may be more effective in preventing rather than treating cardiogenic shock.

Early coronary angiography can identify patients not responding to thrombolytic therapy and may, therefore,

TABLE 49-8

Benefits of Patent Infarct-Related Coronary Artery in Patients with Acute Myocardial Infarction

Limit infarct size
Preserve left ventricular function
Prevent infarct expansion, aneurysm formation, and progressive ventricular dilation
Enhance electrical stability
Maintain collateral circulation

be an important step in early management. This approach should be considered in patients with persistent systemic hypotension, evidence of ongoing myocardial ischemia, and/or clinical instability. In such cases, rescue coronary angioplasty may improve survival.[126,127] Although randomized studies have not yet been undertaken, retrospective analyses of patients with acute myocardial infarction complicated by cardiogenic shock suggest that successful coronary balloon angioplasty of the infarct-related artery is associated with a significant reduction in mortality.[128,129] (See also Chap. 70.)

Patients undergoing emergent coronary angioplasty may benefit from initial stabilization with IABP.[130–132] Additional modalities used for circulatory support or as a bridge to emergent bypass surgery include coronary arterial autoperfusion[133–135] or hemoperfusion[136–138] catheters, synchronized coronary sinus retroperfusion,[139,140] percutaneous cardiopulmonary bypass,[141] and partial left-sided heart bypass.[142] (See Chap. 31.)

A generalized approach to treatment among patients with cardiogenic shock is outlined in Table 49-9. The subsets refer to those in Fig. 49-1.

TABLE 49-9

Approach to Treatment Among Patients with Cardiogenic Shock

Patient Classification†	Historical Features and Physical Findings	Diagnostic Screening Tools	Definitive Diagnostic Studies	Treatment Considerations
Subset 1				
Volume depletion (subacute) chronic	Dry mucous membranes Tending of skin Lethargy Obtundation (elderly) Tachycardia (moderate)	Hemoglobin, hematocrit Serum electrolytes, blood urea nitrogen Hemoccult stool	Upper/lower GI series Blood, urine, sputum, stool Iron studies	Volume replacement (0.9% NaCl, D_5W, Blood products
Acute	Anxious Skin cool/clammy Tachycardia (moderate) Localized pain	Hemoglobin, hematocrit Chest x-ray Abdominal x-ray (KUB) Arterial blood gas Hemoccult stool	Nasogastric tube Upper GI endoscopy CT Exploratory surgery (trauma)	Rapid volume replacement (0.9% NaCl, dextran, blood products) Surgical intervention (trauma, ruptured viscus, mesenteric ischemia/infarction, uncontrollable GI bleed)
Ruptured abdominal aneurysm	Anxious Skin cool/clammy Tachycardia (moderate) Abdominal, flank, or lower quadrant pain Flank ecchymosis	Hemoglobin, hematocrit Electrocardiogram Chest x-ray Abdominal x-ray (KUB) Arterial blood gas	CT, abdomen Aortography Surgery (exploratory)	Blood pressure support (dopamine, norepinephrine) Volume replacement Emergent surgical intervention Volume replacement (0.9% NaCl, dextran, blood products)
Pericardial tamponade	Anxious Skin moist Tachycardia (variable) Distant heart sounds (acute tamponade) Jugular venous distension Pulsus paradoxus (>10 mmHg)	Chest x-ray Electrocardiogram Arterial blood gas PT, PTT, platelet count	Echocardiogram Transthoracic or transesophageal if aortic dissection CT chest x-ray Pericardial window (trauma)	Intravenous fluids Pericardiocentesis Pericardiostomy (purulent pericarditis) Pericardial window (trauma) Dopamine
Tension pneumothorax	Anxious Shortness of breath (variable) Chest/back pain Absent breath sounds (unilateral) Hypoxemia (variable)	Arterial blood gas Electrocardiogram	Chest x-ray CT chest (trauma)	Chest tube placement Supplemental oxygen Volume replacement Blood pressure support Pleural tap

TABLE 49-9

Approach to Treatment Among Patients with Cardiogenic Shock *(continued)*

Patient Classification†	Historical Features and Physical Findings	Diagnostic Screening Tools	Definitive Diagnostic Studies	Treatment Considerations
Massive pulmonary embolism	Chest pain (pleuritic) Shortness of breath Tachycardia (variable) Jugular venous distension "Kussmaul's sign" (variable) Hypoxemia	Electrocardiogram Arterial blood gas Chest x-ray	Pulmonary angiogram Ventilation/perfusion scan	Intravenous fluids Supplemental oxygen Thrombolytic therapy Anticoagulation Embolectomy Extraction thrombectomy
Right ventricular infarction	Chest pain Skin cool, moist Variable heart rate (bradycardia/tachycardia) AV block Jugular venous distension "Right sided" S_3, S_4 gallop	Electrocardiogram (with right-sided leads) Arterial blood gas Chest x-ray	Right-sided heart catheterization Echocardiogram Radionuclide ventriculogram	Intravenous fluids Inotropic support (Dobutamine) Intraaortic balloon pump Thrombolytic therapy Coronary angioplasty
Ventricular septal defect (acute)	Chest pain (variable) Tachycardia (moderate) Localized "new" murmur	Electrocardiogram Chest x-ray Arterial blood gas	Right-sided heart catheterization (with saturations) Electrocardiogram with Doppler flow Contrast ventriculogram	Intravenous fluids Intraaortic balloon pump Blood pressure support Surgical intervention Intrapulmonary balloon pump
Subset II Left-sided heart failure (systolic)	Shortness of breath	Electrocardiogram	Pulmonary artery catheterization	Inotropic support (Dopamine, Dobutamine, Amrinone)
Mitral regurgitation MI, ventricular septal defect	Anxious Skin moist; livedo reticularis Cyanosis Pulmonary rales S_3 gallop Heart murmur (MR, VsD) Tachycardia Hypoxemia/acidemia (variable)	Arterial blood gas Chest x-ray Echocardiogram (with Doppler flow)	Left-sided heart catheterization Coronary Angiography	Supplemental oxygen Intraaortic balloon pump Diuretics Morphine sulfate† Nitrate preparations† Coronary reperfusion Surgical intervention
Aortic regurgitation (acute)	Shortness of breath Chest pain/back pain (with aortic dissection) Skin moist Stigmata of endocarditits Diastolic murmur Pulse pressure narrow S_3 gallop (variable) Pulmonary rales Tachycardia Hypoxemia	Arterial blood gas Electrocardiogram Chest x-ray Blood cultures	Echocardiogram (transthoracic/transesophageal) Aortic root flush Cine MRI CT chest (trauma)	Inotropic support Blood pressure support Supplemental oxygen Surgical intervention

TABLE 49-9

Approach to Treatment Among Patients with Cardiogenic Shock *(continued)*

Patient Classification†	Historical Features and Physical Findings	Diagnostic Screening Tools	Definitive Diagnostic Studies	Treatment Considerations
Critical aortic stenosis	Shortness of breath Pulmonary rales Jugular venous distension Tachycardia (variable) Late-peaking systolic murmur Diminished carotid upstroke Hypoxemia	Electrocardiogram Chest x-ray Arterial blood gas	Echocardiogram (with Doppler flow) Pulmonary artery catheterization	Inotropic support Supplemental oxygen Control Surgical intervention Balloon valvuloplasty
Critical mitral stenosis	Shortness of breath Tachycardia (variable) Jugular venous distension Diastolic murmur (variable) Opening snap (variable) Previous thromboembolic events Pulmonary rales Hypoxemia	Electrocardiogram Chest x-ray Arterial blood gas	Echocardiogram Left-sided heart catheterization Pulmonary artery catheterization	Supplemental oxygen Control arrhythmias Diuretics Morphine sulfate Balloon valvuloplasty Surgical intervention
Volume overload	Shortness of breath Tachycardia (variable) S_3 gallop Pulmonary rales Jugular venous distension Hypoxemia (variable)	Chest x-ray Arterial blood gas Electrocardiogram Echocardiogram Hematocrit Serum electrolytes	Pulmonary artery catheterization	Supplemental oxygen Inotropic support Diuretics Morphine sulfate Nitrate preparations
Left-sided heart failure (diastolic)	Shortness of breath Pulmonary rales S_4 gallop Jugular venous distension Hypoxemia (variable)	Chest x-ray Arterial blood gas Electrocardiogram	Pulmonary artery catheterization Echocardiogram (with Doppler flow)	Supplemental oxygen Control arrhythmias Nitrate preparations Beta-blockers Calcium channel blockers
Noncardiogenic shock (septic, neurogenic)	Mental status (variable) Anxious → obtunded Focal neurologic exam (in neurogenic shock) Hypoxemia (variable) Acidemia (variable)	Arterial blood gas Chest x-ray Blood sugar CBC with differential Toxic screen (blood/ urine) Blood, urine, sputum cultures (others as indicated) electrocardiogram DIC screen	Pulmonary arterial catherization CT, head MRI, head Lumbar puncture	Blood pressure support (Dopamine, norepinephrine, Neosynephrine) Supplemental oxygen Intravenous fluids (septic shock) Antibiotics (septic shock) Surgical intervention (as indicated)

* From Fig. 49-1.
GI, gastrointestinal; KUB, kidney-ureter-bladder (film); CT, computerized tomography; PT, prothrombin time; PTT, partial thromboplastin time; MRI, magnetic resonance imaging; DIC, disseminated intravascular coagulation.
† Diuretics, morphine sulfate, and nitrate preparations must be used cautiously in the setting of left-sided heart failure when the systolic blood pressure is at most 100 mmHg.

REFERENCES

1. Fink MP: Shock: An overview. In: Rippe JM, Irwin RS, Alpert JS, Fink MP (eds): *Intensive Care Medicine*. Boston, Little Brown, 1991: 1417–1435.
2. Crowell JW, Guyton AC: Further evidence favoring a cardiac mechanism in irreversible hemorrhagic shock. *Am J Physiol* 1962; 203:248–252.
3. Vincent J-L, Weil MH, Puri V, Carlson RW: Circulatory shock associated with purulent peritonitis. *Am J Surg* 1981; 142:262–270.
4. Snell RJ, Parrillo JE: Cardiovascular dysfunction in septic shock. Chest 1991; 99:1000–1009.

5. Naylor JM, Kronfeld DS: In vivo studies of hypoglycemia and lactic acidosis in endotoxic shock. *Am J Physiol* 1985; 248:E309–E316.
6. Togari H, Sugiyama S, Ogino T, Suzuki S, Ito T, Echiki T, et al: Interactions of endotoxin with cortisol and acute phase proteins in septic shock neonates. *Acta Paeditr Scand* 1986; 75:69–74.
7. Bagby GJ, Spitzer JA: Decreased myocardial extracellular and muscle lipoprotein lipase activities in endotoxin-treated rats. *Proc Soc Exper Biol Med* 1981; 168:395–398.
8. Miller RL, Reichgott MJ, Melmon KL: Biochemical mechanisms of generation of bradykinin by endotoxin. *J Infect Dis* 1973; 128:S144–S156.
9. Carmona RH, Tsao TC, Trunkey DD: The role of prostacyclin and thromboxane in sepsis and septic shock. *Arch Surg* 1984; 119:189–192.
10. Berton EW, Long JB, Holaday JW: Opioids and neuropeptides: Mechanisms in circulatory shock. *Fed Proc* 1985; 44:290–299.
11. Krausz MM, Utsunomiya T, Feuerstein G, Wolfe JHN, Shepro N, Hechtman HB: Prostacyclin reversal of lethal endotoxemia in dogs. *J Clin Invest* 1981; 67:1118–1125.
12. Siegal T, Seligsohn U, Aghai E, Modan M: Clinical and laboratory aspects of disseminated intravascular coagulation (DIC): A study of 118 cases. *Thromb Haemost* 1978, 39: 122–134.
13. Kilbourn RG, Gross SS, Jubran A, Adams J, Griffith OW, Levi R, et al: N^G-methyl-L-arginine inhibits tumor necrosis factor–induced hypotension: Implications for the involvement of nitric oxide. *Proc Natl Acad Sci USA* 1990; 87:3629–3632.
14. Hutcheson IR, Whittle BJR, Boughton-Smith NK: Role of nitric oxide in maintaining vascular integrity in endotoxin-induced acute intestinal damage in the rat. *Br J Pharmacol* 1990; 101:815–820.
15. Radomski MW, Palmer RMJ, Moncada S: Glucocorticoids inhibit the expression of an inducible, but not the constitutive, nitric oxide synthase in vascular endothelial cells. *Proc Natl Acad Sci USA* 1990; 87:10043–10047.
16. Donohoe JF, Venkatachalam MA, Bernard DB, Levinsky NG: Tubular leakage and obstruction after renal ischemia: Structural-functional correlations. *Kidney Int* 1978; 13:208–222.
17. Brezis M, Rosen S, Silva P, Epstein FH: Selected vulnerability of the medullary thick ascending limb to anoxia in the isolated perfused rat kidney. *J Clin Invest* 1984; 73:182–190.
18. Brezis M, Rosen S, Spokes K, Silva P, Epstein FH: Renal ischemia: A new perspective. *Kidney Int* 1984; 26:375–383.
19. Lucas CE, Harrigan C, Denis R, Ledgerwood AM: Impaired renal concentrating ability during resuscitation from shock. *Arch Surg* 1983; 118:642–645.
20. Bor NM, Alvur M, Ercan MT, Bekdik CF: Liver blood flow rate and glucose metabolism in hemorrhagic hypotension and shock. *J Trauma* 1982; 22:753–758.
21. Rinaldo JE, Rogers RM: Adult respiratory-distress syndrome. Changing concepts of lung injury and repair. *N Engl J Med* 1982; 306:900–909.
22. Bhagwat AG, Hawk WA: Terminal hemorrhagic necrotizing enteropathy (THNE). *Am J Gastroenterol* 1966; 45:163–188.
23. Cuevas P, Fine J: Demonstration of a lethal endotoxemia in experimental occlusion of the superior mesenteric artery. *Surg Gynecol Obstet* 1971; 133:88–83.
24. Spath JA Jr, Gorczynski RJ, Lefer AM: Pancreatic perfusion in the pathophysiology of hemorrhagic shock. *Am J Physiol* 1974; 226:443–451.
25. Herlihy BL, Lefer AM: Alterations in pancreatic acinar cell organelles during circulatory shock. *Circ Shock* 1975; 2:143–153.
26. Tindall GT, Greenfield JC Jr, Dillon ML, Odom GL: Effect of hemorrhage on blood flow in the carotid arteries. Studies in ten rhesus monkeys. *J Neurosurg* 1964; 21:763–768.
27. Green HD: Circulatory systems: Physical principals. In: Glasser O (ed): *Medical Physics*, vol 2. Chicago, Yearbook Publishers, 1950:228–241.
28. Chien S: Role of the sympathetic nervous system in hemorrhage. *Physiol Rev* 1967; 47:214–288.
29. Bond RF, Green HD: Cardiac output redistribution during bilateral common carotid occlusion. *Am J Physiol* 1969; 216:393–403.
30. Forsyth RP, Hoffbrand BI, Melmon KL: Redistribution of cardiac output during hemorrhage in the unanesthetized monkey. *Circ Res* 1970; 27:311–320.
31. Rothe CF: Reflex control of veins and vascular capacitance. *Physiol Rev* 1983; 63:1281–1342.
32. Bereiter DA, Zaid AM, Gann DS: Effect of rate of hemorrhage on sympathoadrenal catecholamine release in cats. *Am J Physiol* 1986; 250:E69–E75.
33. Davis JO, Freeman RH: Mechanisms regulating renin release. *Physiol Rev* 1976; 56:1–56.
34. Abboud FM, Thames MD: Interaction of cardiovascular reflexes in circulatory control. In: *Handbook of Physiology: The Cardiovascular System. Peripheral Circulation and Organ Blood Flow*, vol III. Bethesda, MD, American Physiological Society, 1984: section 2, pt 2, chap 19, pp 675–753.
35. Liard JF: Vasopressin in cardiovascular control: Role of circulating vasopressin. *Clin Sci* 1984; 67:473–481.
36. Gann DS, Carlson DE, Byrnes GJ, Pickle JC Jr, Allen-Rowlands CF: Role of solute in the early restitution of blood volume after hemorrhage. *Surgery* 1983; 94:439–446.
37. Bond RF, Johnson G III: Vascular adrenergic interactions during hemorrhagic shock. *Fed Proc* 1985; 44:281–289.
38. Bond RF, Bond CH, Peissner LC, Manning ES: Prostaglandin modulation of adrenergic vascular control during hemorrhagic shock. *Am J Physiol* 1981; 241:H85–H90.
39. Hift H, Campos HA: Changes in the subcellular distribution of cardiac catecholamines in dogs dying in irreversible hemorrhagic shock. *Nature* 1962; 196:678–679.
40. Coleman B, Glaviano VV: Tissue levels of norepinephrine in hemorrhagic shock. *Science* 1962; 139:54.
41. Koyama S, Aibiki M, Kanai K, Fujita T, Miyakawa K: Role of central nervous system in renal nerve activity during prolonged hemorrhagic shock in dogs. *Am J Physiol* 1988; 254:R761–R769.
42. Holaday JW, Faden AI: Naloxone reversal of endotoxin hypotension suggests role of endorphins in shock. *Nature* 1978; 275:450–451.
43. Reynods DG, Gurll NJ, Vargish T, Lechner RB, Faden AI, Holaday JW: Blockade of opiate receptors with naloxone improves survival and cardiac performance in canine endotoxic shock. *Circ Shock* 1980; 7:39–48.
44. Schadt JC, Gaddis RR: Endogenous opiate peptides may limit norepinephrine release during hemorrhage. *J Pharmacol Exp Ther* 1985; 232:656–660.
45. Carden DL, Smith JK, Zimmerman BJ, Korthuis RJ, Granger DN: Reperfusion injury following circulatory collapse: The role of reactive oxygen metabolites. *J Crit Care* 1989; 4:294–307.
46. Barroso-Aranda J, Schmid-Schonbein GW, Zweifach BW, Ensler RL: Granulocytes and no-reflow phenomenon in irreversible hemorrhagic shock. *Circ Res* 1988; 63:437–447.
47. Barroso-Aranda J, Schmid-Schonbein GW: Transformation of neutrophils as indicator of irreversibility in hemorrhagic shock. *Am J Physiol* 1989; 257:H846–H852.
48. Hurd TC, Dasmahapatra KS, Rush BF Jr, Machiedo GW: Red blood cell deformability in human and experimental sepsis. *Arch Surg* 1988, 123:217–220.
49. Sarnoff SJ, Case RB, Waitag PE, Issacs J: Insufficient coronary flow and myocardial failure as a complicating factor in late hemorrhagic shock. *Am J Physiol* 1954; 176:439–444.
50. Horton J, Landreneau, R, Tuggle D: Cardiac response to fluid resuscitation from hemorrhagic shock. *Surg Gynecol Obstet* 1985; 160:444–452.
51. Lefer AM: Interaction between myocardial depressant factor and vasoactive mediators with ischemia and shock. *Am J Physiol* 1987; 252:R193–R205.
52. Parrillo JE, Burch C, Shelhamer JH, Parker MM, Natanson C, Schuette W: A circulating myocardial depressant substance in humans with septic shock: Septic shock patients with a reduced ejection fraction have a circulating factor that depresses in vitro myocardial cell performance. *J Clin Invest* 1985; 76:1539–1553.
53. Sander-Jensen K, Secher NH, Bie P, Warbers J, Schwartz TN: Vagal slowing of the heart during hemorrhage: Observations from twenty consecutive hypotensive patients. *Br Med J* 1986; 295:364–366.
54. Skoog P, Mansson J, Thoren P: Changes in sympathetic outflow during hypotensive haemorrhage in rats. *Acta Physiol Scand* 1985; 125:655–660.
55. Morgan DA, Thoren P, Wilczynski EA, Victor RG, Mark AL:

Serotonergic mechanisms mediate renal sympathoinhibition during severe hemorrhage in rats. *Am J Physiol* 1988; 255:H496–H502.
56. Roussos C, Macklem PT: The respiratory muscles. *N Engl J Med* 1982; 307:786–797.
57. Rasmussen HH, Ibels LS: Acute renal failure. Multivariate analysis of causes and risk factors. *Am J Med* 1982; 73:211–218.
58. Menashe PI, Ross SA, Gottlieb JE: Acquired renal insufficiency in critically ill patients. *Crit Care Med* 1988; 16:1106–1109.
59. Montgomery A, Hartmann M, Jonsson K, Haglund U: Intramucosal pH measurement with tonometers for detecting gastrointestinal ischemia in porcine hemorrhagic shock. *Circ Shock* 1989; 29:319–327.
60. Bulkley GB, Oshima A, Bailey RW: Pathophysiology of hepatic ischemia in cardiogenic shock. *AM J Surg* 1986; 151:87–97.
61. Saba TM: Fibronectin: Relevance to phagocytic post-response to injury. *Circ Shock* 1989; 29:257–278.
62. Altura BM, Hershey SG: Reticuloendothelial function in experimental injury and tolerance to shock. *Adv Exp Med Biol* 1973; 33:545–569.
63. Kaplan JE, Saba TM: Humoral deficiency and reticuloendothelial depression after traumatic shock. *Am J Physiol* 1976; 230:7–14.
64. Abraham E: Host defense abnormalities after hemorrhage, trauma, and burns. *Crit Care Med* 1989; 17:934–939.
65. Abraham E, Freitas AA: Hemorrhage produces abnormalities in lymphocyte function and lymphokine generation. *J Immunol* 1989; 142:899–906.
66. Abraham E, Chang Y-H: Cellular and humoral bases of hemorrhage-induced depression of lymphocyte function. *Crit Care Med* 1986; 14:81–86.
67. Baker CC, Miller CL, Trunkey DD: Correlation of traumatic shock with immunocompetence and sepsis. *Surg Forum* 1979; 30:20–21.
68. McCall D, O'Rourke RA: Hypotension and cardiogenic shock. In: Stein JH (ed): *Internal Medicine*. Boston, Little, Brown, 1990:97–108.
69. Goldberg RJ, Gore JM, Alpert JS, Osganian V, deGroot J, Bade J, et al: Cardiogenic shock resulting from acute myocardial infarction: A fourteen year community-wide perspective. *N Engl J Med* 1991; 325:1117–1122.
70. Agress CM, Binder MJ: Cardiogenic shock. *Am Heart J* 1957; 54:458–77.
71. Kuhn LA: The treatment of cardiogenic shock. Part 1. The nature of cardiogenic shock. *Am Heart J* 1967; 74:578–581.
72. Kobayashi M, Niitani H, Hasegawa M, Goto H, Kuwahara K: Effect of medical treatment of acute myocardial infarction in coronary care unit: Study on its effect mainly on the cases with complication. *Jpn Circ J* 1984; 48:650–58.
73. Jugdutt BI, Warnica JW: Intravenous nitroglycerin therapy to limit myocardial infarct size, expansion, and complications. Effect of timing, dosage and infarct location. *Circulation* 1988; 78:906–919.
74. Meinertz T, Kasper W, Schumacher M, Just H, for the APSAC Multicenter Trial Group: The German multicenter trial of anisoylated plasminogen streptokinase activator complex versus heparin for acute myocardial infarction. *Am J Cardiol* 1988; 62:347–351.
75. Takano T, Endo T, Saito H, Ida T, Tanaka K, Osaka S, et al: Clinical usefulness of intraaortic balloon pumping in acute myocardial infarction complicated with cardiogenic shock, ventricular septal perforation and mitral regurgitation. *Jpn Circ J* 1984; 48:678–689.
76. Page DL, Caulfield JB, Kastor JA, DeSanctis RW, Sanders CA: Myocardial changes associated with cardiogenic shock. *N Engl J Med* 1971; 285:133–137.
77. Alonso DR, Scheidt S, Post M, Killip T: Pathophysiology of cardiogenic shock: Quantification of myocardial necrosis: Clinical, pathologic and electrocardiographic correlation. *Circulation* 1973; 48:588–596.
78. Gutovitz AL, Sobel BE, Roberts R: Progressive nature of myocardial injury in selected patients with cardiogenic shock. *Am J Cardiol* 1978; 41:469–475.
79. Wackers FJ, Lie KI, Becker AE: Coronary artery disease in patients dying from cardiogenic shock or congestive heart failure in the setting of acute myocardial infarction. *Br Heart J* 1976; 38:906–910.
80. Shelburne JC, Rubinstein D, Gorlin R: A reappraisal of papillary muscle dysfunction: Correlative clinical and angiographic study. *Am J Med* 1969; 46:862–871.
81. Held AC, Cole PL, Lipton B, Gore JM, Antman EM, Hochman JS, et al: Rupture of the interventricular septum complicating acute MI: A multicenter analysis of clinical findings and outcome. *AM Heart J* 1988; 116:1330–1336.
82. Barnard D, Alpert JS: Right ventricular infarction. In: *Intensive Care Medicine*, 2d ed. Boston, Little, Brown, 1991: 381–391.
83. Shah PK, Maddahi J, Berman DS, Pichler M, Swan HJ: Scintigraphically detected predominant right ventricular dysfunction in acute myocardial infarction: Clinical, hemodynamic correlates and implications for therapy and prognosis. *J Am Coll Cardiol* 1985; 6:1264–1272.
84. Lorrell B, Leinbach RC, Pohost GM, Gold HK, Dinsmore RE, Hutter AM Jr, et al: Right ventricular infarction: Clinical diagnosis and differentiation from cardiac tamponade and pericardial constriction. *Am J Cardiol* 1979; 43:465–471.
85. Goldstein JA, Vlahakes GJ, Verrier ED, Schiller NB, Tybers JV, Ports TA, et al: The role of right ventricular systolic dysfunction and elevated intrapericardial pressure in the genesis of low cardiac output in experimental right ventricular infarction. *Circulation* 1982; 65:513–522.
86. Love JC, Haffajee CI, Gore JM, Alpert JS: Reversibility of hypotension and shock by atrial or atrioventricular sequential pacing in patients with right ventricular infarction. *Am Heart J* 1984; 108:5–13.
87. Benotti JR: Acute aortic insufficiency. In: Dalen JE, Alpert JS (eds): *Valvular Heart Disease*, 2d ed. Boston, Little, Brown, 1987: 319–351.
88. Ellrodt AG, Riedinger MS, Kimchi A, Berman DS, Maddahi J, Swan HJ, et al: Left ventricular performance in septic shock: Reversible segmental and global abnormalities. *Am Heart J* 1985; 110:402–409.
89. Kimchi A, Ellrodt GA, Berman DS, Riedinser MS, Swan HJ, Murata GH: Right ventricular performance in septic shock: A combined radionuclide and hemodynamic study. *J Am Coll Cardiol* 1984; 4:945–951.
90. Parker MM, McCarthy KE, Ognibene FP, Parrillo JE: Right ventricular dysfunction and dilatation, similar to left ventricular changes, characterize the cardiac depression of septic shock in humans. *Chest* 1990; 97:126–131.
91. Reilly JM, Cunnion RE, Burch-Whitman C, Parker MM, Shelhamer JH, Parrillo JE: A circulating myocardial depressant substance is associated with cardiac dysfunction and peripheral hypoperfusion (lactic acidemia) in patients with septic shock. *Chest* 1989; 95:1072–1080.
92. Natanson C, Eichenholz PW, Danner RL, Eichacker PQ, Hoffman WD, Kuo GC, et al: Endotoxin and tumor necrosis factor challenges in dogs simulate the cardiovascular profile of human septic shock. *J Exp Med* 1989; 169:823–832.
93. D'Ambra MN, LaRaia PJ, Philbin DM, Watkins WD, Hilsenberg AD, Buckley MJ: Prostaglandin E_1: A new therapy for refractory right heart failure and pulmonary hypertension after mitral valve replacement. *J Thorac Cardiovasc Surg* 1985; 89:567–572.
94. Morel DR, Lowenstein E, Nguyenduy T, Robinson DR, Repino JE, Chenoweth DE, et al: Acute pulmonary vasoconstriction and thromboxane release during protamine reversal of heparin anticoagulation in awake sheep. Evidence for the role of reactive oxygen metabolites following nonimmunological complement activation. *Circ Res* 1988; 62:905–915.
95. Topol EJ, Goldschlager N, Ports TA, Dicarlo LA Jr, Schiller NB, Botvinick EH, et al: Hemodynamic benefit of atrial pacing in right ventricular myocardial infarction. *Ann Intern Med* 1982; 96:594–597.
96. Forrester JS, Diamond G, Chatterjee K, Swan HJ: Medical therapy of acute myocardial infarction by application of hemodynamic subsets (First of Two Parts). *N Engl J Med* 1976; 295:1356–1362.
97. Forrester JS, Diamond G, Chatterjee K, Swan HJC: Medical therapy of acute myocardial infarction by application of hemodynamic subsets (Second of Two Parts). *N Engl J Med* 1976; 295:1404–1413.
98. Mueller HS, Evans R, Ayres SM: Effect of dopamine on hemodynamics and myocardial metabolism in shock following acute myocardial infarction in man. *Circulation* 1978; 57:361–365.

99. Maekawa K, Liang C, Hood WB: Comparison of dobutamine and dopamine in acute myocardial infarction. Effects of systemic hemodynamics, plasma catecholamines, blood flows and infarct size. *Circulation* 1983; 30:371–377.
100. Gillespie TA, Ambos HD, Sobel BE, Roberts R: Effects of dobutamine in patients with acute myocardial infarction. *Am J Cardiol* 1977; 39:588–594.
101. Francis GS, Sharma B, Hodges M: Comparative hemodynamic effects of dopamine and dobutamine in patients with acute cardiogenic circulatory collapse. *Am Heart J* 1982; 103:995–1000.
102. Gunnar RM, Loeb HS, Petras RJ, Tobin JR: Ineffectiveness of isoproterenol in shock due to acute myocardial infarction. *JAMA* 1967; 202:1124–1128.
103. Klocke RK, Mager G, Kux A, Hopp HW, Hilser HH: Effects of a 24-hour milrinone infusion in patients with severe heart failure and cardiogenic shock as a function of the hemodynamic initial condition. *Am Heart J* 1991; 121:1965–1973.
104. Vincent JL, Carlier E, Berre J, Armistead CW, Kahn RJ, Coussaert E, et al: Administration of enoximone in cardiogenic shock. *Am J Cardiol* 1988; 62:419–423.
105. Vincent JL, Leon M, Berre J: The role of enoximone in the treatment of cardiogenic shock. *Cardiology* 1990; 77 (suppl 3): 21–26.
106. Kantrowitz A, Tjonneland S, Krakauer JS, Phillips SJ, Freed PS, Butner AN: Mechanical intraaortic cardiac assistance in cardiogenic shock. Hemodynamic effects. *Arch Surg* 1968; 97:1000–1004.
107. Scheidt S, Wilner G, Mueller H, Summers D, Lesch M, Wolff G, et al: Intra-aortic balloon counterpulsation in cardiogenic shock. *N Engl J Med* 1973; 288:979–984.
108. Merhige ME, Smalling RW, Cassidy D, Barrett R, Wise G, Short J, et al: Effect of the hemopump left ventricular assist device on regional myocardial perfusion and function: Reduction of ischemia during coronary occlusion. *Circulation* 1989; 80(suppl III):III-158–II-166.
109. Frazier OH, Nakatan T, Duncan JM, Parnis SM, Fuqua SM: Clinical experience with the hemopump. *ASAIO Trans* 1989; 35:604–606.
110. Phillips SJ, Ballentine B, Slonine D, Hall J, Vandehaar J, Kongtahworn C, Zeff RH, et al: Percutaneous initiation of cardiopulmonary bypass. *Ann Thorac Surg* 1983; 36:223–225.
111. O'Neill P, Menendez T, Hust R, Howell J, Espada R, Pacifico A: Prolonged ventricular fibrillation-salvage using a new percutaneous cardiopulmonary support system. *Am J Cardiol* 1989; 64:545.
112. Phillips SJ, Zeff RH, Kongtahworn C, Skinner J, Toon R, Grignon A, et al: Percutaneous cardiopulmonary bypass: Application and indication for use. *Ann Thorac Surg* 1989; 47:121–123.
113. Bert RJ, Selinger SL, Leonard JL, Grunwald RP, O'Grady WP: Immediate coronary artery bypass for acute evolving myocardial infarction. *J Thorac Cardiovasc Surg* 1981; 81:493–497.
114. Phillips SJ, Konstahworn C, Skinner JR, Zeff MT: Emergency coronary artery reperfusion: A choice therapy for evolving myocardial infarction. Results in 339 patients. *J Thorac Cardiovasc Surg* 1983; 86:679–688.
115. DeWood MA, Notske RN, Hensley GR, Shields JP, O'Grady WP, Spores J, et al: Intra-aortic balloon counterpulsation with or without reperfusion for myocardial shock. *Circulation* 1980; 61:1105–1112.
116. Alcan KE, Stertzer SH, Wallsh E, Bruno MS, DePasquale NP: Current status of intraaortic balloon counterpulsation in critical care cardiology. *Crit Care Med* 1984; 12:489–495.
117. Joyce LD, Johnson KE, Pierce WS, Semb BK, Copeland JG, Griffith BP, et al: Summary of the world experience with clinical use of total artificial hearts as heart support devices. *J Heart Transplant* 1986; 5:229–235.
118. Farrar DJ, Hill JD, Gray LA, Gailbraith TA, Chow E, Hershon JJ: Successful biventricular circulatory support as a bridge to cardiac transplantation during prolonged ventricular fibrillation and asystole. *Circulation* 1989; 80(suppl III):III-147–III-151.
119. Fortin DF, Califf RM: Long-term survival from acute myocardial infarction: Salutary effect of an open coronary vessel. *Am J Med* 1990; 88:1-9N–1-15N.
120. Ohman EM, Califf RM, Topol EJ, Candela R, Abbottsmith C, Ellis S, et al: Consequences of reocclusion after successful reperfusion therapy in acute myocardial infarction. *Circulation* 1990; 82:781–791.
121. Lew AS, Weiss AT, Shah PK, Fishbein MC, Berman DS, Maddahi J: Extensive myocardial salvage and reversal of cardiogenic shock after reperfusion of the left main coronary artery by intravenous streptokinase. *Am J Cardiol* 1984; 54:450–452.
122. Kennedy JE, Gensini CG, Timmis GC, Maynard C: Acute myocardial infarction treated with intracoronary streptokinase: A report from the Society for Cardiac Angiography. *Am J Cardiol* 1985; 55:871–877.
123. ISIS-2 Collaborative Group: Randomized trial of intravenous streptokinase, oral aspirin, both or neither among 17,187 cases of suspected acute myocardial infarction. ISIS-2. *Lancet* 1988; 2:349–360.
124. Gruppo Italiano per lo Studio della Streptochinas, nell'Infarcto Miocardico (GISSI): Effectiveness of intravenous thrombolytic treatment in acute myocardial infarction. *Lancet* 1986; 1:397–401.
125. Gruppo Italiano per lo Studio della Sofravivenza nell' Infarto Miocardico (GISSI-2): A factorial randomized trial of alteplase versus streptokinase and heparin versus no heparin among 12490 patients with acute myocardial infarction. *Lancet* 1990; 336:65–71.
126. Abbottsmith CW, Topol EJ, George BS, Stack RS, Kereiakes DJ, Candela RJ, et al: Fate of patients with acute myocardial infarction with patency of the infarct-related vessel achieved with successful thrombolysis versus rescue angiography. *J Am Coll Cardiol* 1990; 16:770–778.
127. Stack RS, Califf RM, Hinohara R, Phillips HR, Pryor DB, Simonton CA, et al: Survival and cardiac event rates in the first year after emergency coronary angioplasty for acute myocardial infarction. *J Am Coll Cardiol* 1988; 11:1141–1149.
128. Lee L, Bates ER, Pitt B, Walton JA, Laufer N, O'Neill WW: Percutaneous transluminal coronary angioplasty improves survival in acute myocardial infarction complicated by cardiogenic shock. *Circulation* 1988; 78:1345–1351.
129. Lee L, Erbel R, Brown TM, Laufer N, Meyer J, O'Neill WW: Multicenter registry of angioplasty therapy of cardiogenic shock: Initial and long-term survival. *J Am Coll Cardiol* 1991; 17:599–603.
130. Szatmary LJ, Marco J, Fajadet J, Caster L: The combined use of diastolic counterpulsation and coronary dilation in unstable angina due to multivessel disease under unstable hemodynamic conditions. *Int J Cardiol* 1988; 19:59–66.
131. Voudris V, Marco J, Morice MC, Fajadet J, Royer T: "High-risk" percutaneous transluminal coronary angioplasty with preventive intraaortic balloon counterpulsation. *Cathet Cardiovasc Diagn* 1990; 19:160–164.
132. Kahn JK, Rutherford BD, McConahay Dr, Johnson WL, Giorsi LV, Hartzler GO: Supported "high risk" coronary angioplasty using intraaortic ballon pump counterpulsation. *J Am Coll Cardiol* 1990; 15:1151–1155.
133. Hinohara T, Simpson JB, Phillips HR, Behar VS, Peter RH, Kons Y, et al: Transluminal catheter reperfusion: A new technique to reestablish blood flow after coronary occlusion during percutaneous transluminal coronary angioplasty. *Am J Cardiol* 1986; 57:684–686.
134. Christensen CW, Lassar TA, Daley LC, Reider MA, Schmidt DH: Regional myocardial blood flow with a reperfusion catheter and an autoperfusion balloon catheter during total coronary occlusion. *Am Heart J* 1990; 119:242–248.
135. Sundram P, Harvey JR, Johnson RG, Schwartz MJ, Baim DS: Benefit of the perfusion catheter for emergency coronary artery grafting after failed percutaneous transluminal coronary angioplasty. *Am J Cardiol* 1989; 63:282–285.
136. Banka VS, Trivedi A, Patel R, Ghossan M, Voci G: Prevention of myocardial ischemia during coronary angioplasty: A simple new method for distal antegrade arterial blood perfusion. *Am Heart J* 1989; 118:830–836.
137. Heibig J, Angelini P, Leachman R, Beall MM, Beall AC Jr: Use of mechanical devices for distal hemoperfusion during balloon catheter coronary angioplasty. *Cathet Cardiovasc Diagn* 1988; 15:143–149.
138. Lehmann KG, Atwood JE, Snyder EL, Ellison RL: Autologous blood perfusion for myocardial protection during coronary angioplasty: A feasibility study. *Circulation* 1987; 76:312–323.
139. Drury JK, Yamazaki S, Fishbein MC, Meebaum S, Corday E: Synchronized diastolic coronary venous retroperfusion: Results

of a preclinical safety and efficacy study. *J Am Coll Cardiol* 1985; 6:328–335.

140. Hajduczki I, Kar S, Areeda J, Ryden L, Corday S, Haendchen R: Reversal of chronic regional myocardial dysfunction (hibernating myocardium) by synchronized diastolic coronary venous retroperfusion during coronary angioplasty. *J AM Coll Cardiol* 1990; 15:238–242.

141. Shawl FA, Domanski MJ, Punja S, Hernandez TJ: Percutaneous cardiopulmonary bypass support in high-risk patients undergoing percutaneous transluminal coronary angioplasty. *Am J Cardiol* 1988; 62:811:813.

142. Glassman E, Chinitz L, Levite H, Slater J, Winer H: Partial left heart bypass support during high-risk angioplasty (abstr). *Circulation* 1989; 80(suppl II):II-272.

Chapter 50

Diagnosis and Management of Syncope

Richard P. Lewis, M.D. ■ *Harisios Budoulas, M.D.*
Stephen F. Schaal, M.D. ■ *Arnold M. Weissler, M.D.*

Syncope is a sudden and transient loss or depression in the state of consciousness. The occurrence of syncope in the general population, as reflected in the 26-year surveillance of the Framingham Study, is 3.0 percent in men and 3.5 percent in women.[1] The initial episode of syncope occurs most commonly in adult life (mean age 52 in men and 50 in women), and the prevalence of syncope in the general population increases with age.

As a presenting complaint, syncope connotes a diversity of disorders ranging from a benign episode to catastrophic sudden death. Studies in recent years have documented the multiple causes and the widely divergent mortality risks associated with an episode of syncope. On the basis of these studies, patients with a transient episode of altered consciousness (presyncope) and those with complete loss of consciousness (syncope) can be classified into three broad categories (Table 50-1): syncope unassociated with heart disease, syncope associated with heart disease, and syncope of undetermined cause.[2–8] The relative incidence of these categories varies with the clinical site from which the patients are selected (Table 50-2). In the emergency room, syncope unassociated with cardiac disease is most common. For patients admitted to the hospital, cardiac syncope is the most common diagnosis. Among all patients in whom syncope or presyncope is the presenting symptom, a diagnosis cannot be readily established in one-third.

The 1-year mortality for patients with syncope associated with cardiac disease varies from 19 to 33 percent, while in patients with syncope unassociated with cardiac disease, it varies from 0 to 12 percent. In patients with syncope of undetermined cause, 1-year mortality clusters about 6 percent (Table 50-3). Clearly, the highest mortality occurs among those with syncope-associated cardiac disease. Elderly patients (aged 60 years and older) with syncope, irrespective of its cause, have a distinctly high morbidity and mortality.[9] Among all patients with syncope associated with cardiac disease, sudden death is inordinately frequent.

TABLE 50-1

Classification of Syncope
Syncope unassociated with cardiac disease
Syncope associated with cardiac disease
Syncope of undetermined cause

SYNCOPE UNASSOCIATED WITH CARDIAC DISEASE

Sudden transient loss or impairment of consciousness in the absence of associated cardiac disease occurs under a wide variety of circumstances (Table 50-4). The pathophysiologic mechanisms, diagnostic features, and therapy for these disorders will be discussed below.

TABLE 50-2
Distribution of Patients by Cause of Syncope: Summary of Recent Studies

Cause	All Patients (N = 1153), %	Emergency Room Patients (N = 544), %
Syncope Unassociated with Cardiac Disease		
Vasodepressor	20.0	33.8
Seizures	7.5	13.8
Orthostatic	6.4	4.6
Situational	4.0	1.7
Drugs/ethanol	2.5	2.9
Cerebrovascular	1.5	0.9
Psychogenic	1.1	1.8
Carotid sinus	0.7	0.0
Hyperventilation	0.7	1.3
Hypoglycemia	0.6	1.3
Gastrointestinal hemorrhage	0.5	1.1
Migraine	0.3	0.6
Neuralgia	0.1	0.0
Subgroup total	46	64
Syncope Associated with Cardiac Disease: Obstructive		
Aortic stenosis	1.6	0.9
Pulmonary embolism	0.6	0.4
Pulmonary hypertension	0.2	0.0
Mitral stenosis	0.1	0.2
Subgroup total	2.5	1.5
Syncope Associated with Cardiac Disease: Arrhythmic		
Ventricular tachycardia	6.8	2.4
Bradycardia/sick sinus	2.9	1.0
Sinoventricular tachycardia/atrial fibrillation	2.0	0.8
AV block	1.6	0.9
Myocardial infarction	1.3	0.6
Pacemaker-induced	0.6	0.0
Multiple premature ventricular complexes	0.3	0.0
Mitral stenosis	0.1	0.2
Mitral prolapse	0.1	0.0
Subgroup total	16	6
Syncope of Undetermined Cause		
Subgroup total	36	29

SOURCE: Eagle et al.[2]; Martin et al.[3]; Day et al.[4]; Silverstein et al.[5]; Kapoor et al.[6]; and Ben-Chetrit et al.[7]

Vasodepressor Syncope

Diagnosis

Transient unconsciousness unassociated with cardiac disease is most commonly caused by vasodepressor syncope (the common faint).[1–3,9] While vasodepressor syncope frequently occurs early in life, it is not uncommon in older patients. It is often a familial trait and in a given individual may be a lifelong symptom. Vasodepressor syncope is generally benign, particularly when it occurs in the absence of associated cardiac disease, and its prompt recognition can avoid unnecessary psychological stress and expensive laboratory studies. A thorough knowledge of the clinical picture of the common faint is critical in establishing the correct diagnosis.

Vasodepressor syncope often occurs as a response to sudden physiologic stress or in a setting of real, threatened, or fantasied injury.[10] The reaction is frequently brought on by venipuncture or the sight of blood, or after a sudden, painful experience or following severe tissue injury. It commonly occurs in an uncomfortable environment such as a hot, crowded room and is often preceded by excessive fatigue, hunger, dehydration, malaise, fever, or recent blood loss. The common faint usually occurs when the patient is upright or sitting but rarely may occur while the patient is recumbent. Clinically it is characterized by a fall in arterial pressure associated with impairment or loss of consciousness. Transient convulsive movements and, rarely, incontinence may accompany the episode.

Rather than sudden collapse, premonitory symptoms of vasodepressor syncope may appear for several minutes before loss of consciousness. The patient is often aware that syncope is imminent. Pallor accompanied by cold perspiration is noted first, followed by epigastric discomfort, frequently likened to nausea. Pupillary dilatation and perhaps visual blurring occur just prior to loss of consciousness. While bradycardia is characteristically present at the time of impaired consciousness, the premonitory phase of fainting is most often associated with a relatively rapid heart rate. When the individual suffering vasodepressor syncope is allowed to rest in the head-down position, consciousness is rapidly regained; however, the relative bradycardia persists. Of additional importance in identifying vasodepressor syncope are the postsyncopal findings of persistent pallor, perspiration, nausea, weakness, and a tendency toward recurrence of syncope if the individual prematurely returns to an upright posture.

Although it was first thought that vasodepressor syncope might be caused by a severe depression of cardiac output, laboratory-induced syncope shows only a slight decline in cardiac output beyond that which occurs with the assumption of the head-up posture.[11] Rather, a marked fall in total peripheral vascular resistance is the major hemodynamic perturbation in vasodepressor syncope,[12] and the consequent fall in perfusion of the brain results in the loss of consciousness. It is important to note that the fall in arterial resistance is not compensated for by a rise in cardiac output. Why the usual regulatory mechanisms fail to induce an immediate cardiac output response is not entirely clear. Vagal-induced bradycardia is a contributing, but not a causal, factor, since vasodepressor syncope occurs even when bradycardia is prevented by atropine.

In subjects prone to vasodepressor syncope, sudden withdrawal of sympathetic vasoconstrictor activity occurs at the onset of syncope.[13–15] In addition, a diminution in the normal rise in plasma renin activity during an

TABLE 50-3

One-Year Mortality in Patients Presenting with Syncope: Percent Mortality by Diagnostic Category

Reference	Noncardiac	Cardiac	Undetermined
Eagle et al.[2]	0	21	6
Silverstein et at.[5]	6	19	6
Kapoor et al.[6]	12	30	6

upright tilt has been suggested as a predisposing cause.[16] Recently it has been suggested that the peripheral arterial dilatation and bradycardia in vasodepressor syncope are caused by activation of unmyelinated left ventricular vagal fibers, the C fibers, which are stimulated by catecholamines, nicotine, and hypercontractility of the ventricles.[17–19] Such C-fiber activation reduces efferent sympathetic tone and increases efferent vagal tone.

Vasodepressor syncope related to stress was first described by Charles Darwin and in later years elaborated by Engel and Romano.[10] The neural pathways linking the psychological arousal and the inhibition of sympathetic vasoconstrictor activity in this setting have not been elucidated.

The onset of unconsciousness in syncope is associated with the sudden appearance in the electroencephalogram of large-amplitude slow-wave activity. This dramatic change occurs with a profound diminution in mean arterial pressure (average mean arterial pressure of 25 mmHg at heart level) accompanied by a 50 to 70 percent fall in cerebral blood flow. Recently, inappropriate cerebral vasoconstriction has been documented with vasodepressor syncope.[20]

The common faint is associated with a moderate-to-severe degree of hyperventilation, most probably the result of the associated anxiety and the cerebral hypoxia. Arterial carbon dioxide content falls with hyperventilation which independently reduces cerebral blood flow.

TABLE 50-4

Syncope Unassociated with Cardiac Disease

- Vasodepressor syncope
- Orthostatic syncope
- Syncope in cerebrovascular disease
- Carotid sinus syncope
- Reflex syncope
- Other causes of noncardiac syncope
  - Cough syncope
  - Valsalva syncope
  - Micturition syncope
  - Defecation syncope
  - Diver's syncope
  - Hypoxia
  - Hypoglycemic
  - Hyperventilation
  - Convulsive disorders
  - Vertigo
  - Hysterical syncope
  - Syncopal migraine

Predisposition to vasodepressor syncope occurs under a wide variety of clinical circumstances. Indeed, the vasodepressor reaction per se may be the ultimate cause of most types of syncope (see below). Vasodepressor syncope is often noted in individuals receiving sympathetic blocking agents and vasodilator drugs for hypertension, in elderly individuals receiving tranquilizers, in patients with acute or chronic anemia, and with transient reductions in blood volume, such as those that occur following a brisk diuresis or blood donation. Vasodepressor syncope of an unusual type may occur in pregnancy, being precipitated when the patient is supine and reversed when the patient assumes a lateral decubitus or upright posture (see also Chap. 113). Vasodepressor syncope has also been noted to follow strenuous exercise. The common faint complicates acute febrile infections and occurs with prolonged recumbency in chronic illness. Normal individuals at prolonged bed rest have a propensity for fainting, particularly when they arise abruptly from a sitting or recumbent position. Vasodepressor syncope occurs during rapid acceleration in air flight, particularly when centrifugal force is applied in the head-to-foot position. It is probably the most frequent cause of cardiovascular collapse during dental manipulations (dental syncope).

Passive head-up tilt testing is extremely useful for the identification of patients with vasodepressor syncope and for the evaluation of therapy.[21–28] Passive upright tilt to 60 or 80° is maintained for a period of 20 to 60 min. Combining tilt with isoproterenol infusion may yield as high as 80 percent positive responses in patients with a likelihood of vasodepressor syncope. The specificity of the isoproterenol challenge, however, requires more study. The reproducibility of the response to upright tilt in approximately 75 percent and false-positive results have ranged from 0 to 11 percent, the latter reported with the use of tilt plus isoproterenol.

Therapy

Immediate therapy for the common faint consists of placing the patient in a recumbent position with the head down. With profound and persistent bradycardia, intravenously administered atropine may be required. Vasopressor therapy is rarely needed to reverse hypotension. The management of recurrent vasodepressor syncope is challenging and sometimes unsatisfactory. Several pharmacologic and nonpharmacologic options are available. The choice of therapy should be based on an understanding of the cardiovascular-autonomic cascade that eventually culminates in vasodepressor syncope. Head-up tilt testing can be used to predict the clinical response to pharmacologic interventions. In addition, certain subsets of patients, for instance, those with prolonged periods of asystole that accompany peripheral vasodilation, may require combination therapy designed not only to prevent vasodilation (vasodepressor component) but also to prevent the bradycardia (cardioinhibitory component), which can contribute to hypotension.

One of the most important aspects in the management of vasodepressor syncope is education of the patient. In the vast majority of patients, vasodepressor syncope is not life-threatening (unfortunately, if the onset of unconsciousness is sudden, it occasionally results in trauma). A thorough history is of crucial importance to identify a trigger, or provocative situation. Avoidance of the trigger is one mainstay of therapy. When premonitory symptoms occur, the patient should be instructed to lie down immediately, with elevation of the feet, and to cough in order to maintain cerebral blood flow.

Because the severity and frequency of vasodepressor syncope is highly variable, many patients do not require pharmacologic therapy. Indeed, younger adults may have a flurry of spells that resolve spontaneously and never recur. Therefore, the pharmacologic management of vasodepressor syncope must be highly individualized and not necessarily lifelong.

Therapeutic options include volume expansion, beta-adrenergic receptor blockade, anticholinergic agents, methylxanthines, and artificial cardiac pacing. The initial dose of medication should be low and can be gradually increased until the frequency and severity of spells is diminished. Several centers use head-up tilt table testing to predict the clinical outcome of therapy. If one class of drugs is ineffective, a combination of drugs, each acting on different limbs of the vasodepressor syncope reflex, may be beneficial.

Because a significant portion of patients with vasodepressor syncope have evidence of mild reduction in central plasma volume, plasma volume expansion can prevent vasodepressor syncope. Simple measures, such as liberalizing salt intake and avoidance of dieting and fluid restriction, may suffice. Custom-fitted support garments that extend from the ankle to the waist may be of benefit in the highly motivated individual. In some instances, fludrocortisone acetate may be required for augmenting salt retention and volume expansion.

Because increased adrenergic tone is believed to be an important early step in the pathophysiologic cascade that culminates in vasodepressor syncope, beta-adrenergic blocking agents have been used. Beta blockers, which diminish increased cardiac contractility induced by increased sympathetic tone, prevent activation of ventricular mechanoreceptors and decrease recurrent symptoms.[29]

The antiarrhythmic drug disopyramide, whose anticholinergic and negative inotropic properties also prevent the activation of cardiopulmonary mechanoreceptors, can also reduce the frequency of vasodepressor syncope[30]; however, disopyramide must be used with caution because of its potential for proarrhythmia.

Theophylline also reduces the frequency of vasodepressor syncope, although the mechanism is unclear.[31,32] Even low-dose theophylline (6 to 12 mg/kg per day) is of benefit in those patients who cannot tolerate higher doses.

During vasodepressor syncope, certain subsets of patients experience profound bradycardia.[33] The profound bradyarrhythmias are primarily observed in the younger and healthier age group. In such patients, anticholinergic agents such as propantheline bromide may be efficacious.[34] In difficult patients, a pacemaker may be required (see below).

Orthostatic Syncope (Orthostatic Hypotension)

Diagnosis

Orthostatic hypotension is a disorder in which assumption of the upright posture is associated with a fall in arterial pressure associated with lightheadedness, blurring of vision, and a sense of weakness and unsteadiness.[35–38] Hypotension is progressive over a period of seconds to minutes, depending upon the degree of loss in reflex adaptation. If the fall in perfusion pressure to the brain is profound, syncope occurs. If the individual assumes the recumbent posture, arterial pressure rapidly normalizes and consciousness is restored.

From the diagnostic viewpoint, orthostatic hypotension is conveniently classified under three major causes: venous pooling and/or blood volume depletion, drugs, and neurogenic causes. Excessive venous pooling accounts for the postural hypotension accompanying sustained bed rest, prolonged standing, pregnancy, and marked venous varicosities. Tall, asthenic individuals with poorly developed musculature are particularly prone to this form of postural hypotension. In patients with diabetes mellitus, multiple factors, including insulin administration, can result in postural hypotension.[39–42]

Blood volume depletion accounts for the orthostatic hypotension associated with dehydration, excessive diuresis, anemia, hemorrhage, excessive gastrointestinal fluid loss, third-space sequestration, prolonged fever, renal dialysis, excessive perspiration, weightlessness, adrenal insufficiency, pheochromocytoma, and diabetes insipidus.

Pharmacologically induced postural hypotension is a complicating side effect in the administration of several classes of drugs, including antihypertensives, sympathetic blocking agents, diuretics, nitrates, calcium channel blockers, converting enzyme inhibitors, antidepressants, phenothiazines, tranquilizers, antipsychotic drugs, antiparkinsonian drugs, and central nervous system depressants.

Neurogenic postural hypotension has been observed in a wide variety of diseases affecting the autonomic nervous system. Specific entities include diabetes mellitus, alcoholic neuropathy, hydrocephalus, Guillain-Barré syndrome, syringomyelia, multiple sclerosis, Holmes-Adie syndrome, tabes dorsalis, and familial dysautonomia (Riley-Day syndrome). Deconditioning of normal autonomic reflex vasoconstriction may contribute to the orthostatic hypotension associated with prolonged bed rest and following extended periods of weightlessness in astronauts. Administration of adrenergic blocking drugs and vasodilators may accentuate the predisposition to orthostatic hypotension in patients with primary neurogenic postural hypotension.

Two syndromes in which orthostatic hypotension is a dominant manifestation have been widely investigated in recent years. An idiopathic form of chronic autonomic failure in which postural hypotension is accompanied by relatively fixed heart rate, heat intolerance, anhidrosis, nocturnal polyuria, urinary and anal sphincter dysfunction, and impotency was reported in 1925 by Bradbury and Eggleston.[43] In 1960, Shy and Drager[44] reported a syndrome of orthostatic hypotension accompanied by multiple central nervous system manifestations. In recent years the former syndrome has been termed *idiopathic orthostatic hypotension* (IOH), while the latter is referred to as *multiple system atrophy* (MSA). These syndromes usually begin in middle age and occur more commonly in men than in women. Symptoms appear gradually over a period of years. The central nervous system manifestations in MSA may be indistinguishable from those of idiopathic Parkinson's disease and may precede or follow the onset of orthostatic hypotension. The prognosis appears to be worse in patients with MSA than in those with IOH, death often resulting from general debilitation and its complications, pulmonary embolism, malnutrition, and pneumonia. Severe supine hypertension may complicate the presence of orthostatic hypotension. In IOH, the pathologic process is predominantly in the efferent sympathetic pathway, while in MSA degenerative pathologic changes are found centrally in the basal ganglia, substantia nigra, cerebellum, dorsal nucleus of the vagus, pigmented brain stem nuclei, intermediate and lateral columns of the spinal cord, and sympathetic ganglia. Present evidence is consistent with the hypothesis that, in patients with IOH, the orthostatic hypotension is caused by a primary defect in the efferent limb of the sympathetic nervous system, resulting in a loss of neurotransmitter (norepinephrine) from the nerve endings, while the autonomic defect in patients with MSA appears to reside predominantly in the afferent pathways controlling autonomic reflex adjustment to changes in posture.[45–48] Some overlap of the sites of the neurologic disorder prompts caution in invoking a simple differentiation of all patients with IOH and MSA. The fact that some patients may present with isolated peripheral autonomic deficiency only to develop manifestations of central nervous system disease years later further complicates a simple clinical differentiation of these syndromes. Several studies have implicated the presence of profound defects in the parasympathetic system in patients with orthostatic hypotension, providing evidence of a global deficiency in autonomic function in patients with these disorders.[49,50]

When total or central blood volume is depleted in the presence of an intact autonomic nervous system, pallor, coldness of the extremities, tachycardia, and sweating are evident. Relative bradycardia may occur at the time of syncope, and the clinical presentation may be identical to that of vasodepressor syncope. When orthostatic hypotension is due to loss or severe impairment of autonomic reflexes, the syncope is associated with little or no change in heart rate, and there is an absence of the pallor, sweating, and other manifestations observed in patients with intact autonomic reflexes.

Therapy

Effective therapy in postural hypotension is closely linked to an accurate diagnosis. Primary emphasis must be based on treatable causes, in particular pharmacologically induced postural hypotension, blood volume loss, venous pooling, and reversible disease entities. A summary of treatment modalities currently applied among patients with chronic orthostatic hypotension is presented in Table 50-5. The wide variety of recommended approaches reflects the frequently disappointing therapeutic response to each of these modalities. Commonly, multiple maneuvers are necessary to achieve optimum control of postural hypotension. Of singular importance is the need to have the patient avoid experiences, such as dehydration, that accentuate postural hypotension and to restrict the use of pharmacologic agents that induce blood volume depletion, vasodilation, and sympathetic blockade. The patients should be instructed about simple adaptive maneuvers, including slow rising from a recumbent or sitting position, flexing of the calf muscles during assumption of the upright posture, and avoidance of prolonged immobility during standing. The use of atrial tachypacing has been used to maintain effective sympathetic and hemodynamic improvement in orthostatic hypotension.

Syncope in Cerebrovascular Disease

In patients with extensive occlusive disease of the origins of the brachiocephalic vessels, such as pulseless disease (e.g., aortic arch syndrome and Takayasu's arteritis), syncope occurs with a high degree of frequency. With

TABLE 50-5

Treatment of Chronic Orthostatic Hypotension

I. Evaluation for reversible and accentuating disease entities
II. Specific modalities for irreversible orthostatic hypotension
   A. Mechanical measures
      1. Head-up position of bed
      2. Lower body compression garment
      3. Slow motion and calf muscle flexing on arising
   B. Volume expansion
      1. High-salt diet
      2. Fludrocortisone acetate
   C. Pharmacologic agents
      1. Sympathomimetics
      2. Vasoconstrictors
      3. Beta-receptor blockers
      4. Alpha$_2$-receptor agonists
      5. Prostaglandin synthesis inhibitors
      6. Antiserotonergics
      7. Monoamine oxidase inhibitors and tyramine
      8. Vasopressin
   D. Atrial pacing

lesser degrees of cerebral occlusive disease, as in cerebrovascular atherosclerotic narrowing, transient lowering of arterial pressure such as that immediately following assumption of the upright posture may be followed by vague symptoms suggesting impaired cerebral blood flow. In patients with cerebrovascular occlusive disease, a transient decrease in cardiac output and arterial pressure may provoke syncope at levels of arterial pressure that would otherwise be tolerated.

Impairment or loss of consciousness in relation to changing positions of the head, particularly hyperextension and lateral rotation, has been attributed to mechanical narrowing of the vertebral arteries by skeletal deformities of the cervical spine. Such symptoms have been observed in patients with Klippel-Feil deformity, cervical spondylosis, and severe cervical osteoarthritis. Altered consciousness is often preceded by vestibular symptoms. When vertigo is a predominant symptom, the syndrome of benign postural vertigo must be ruled out.

Among patients with major occlusive disease of the carotid-vertebrobasilar arterial system, manual compression of the carotid artery as a test for carotid sinus hypersensitivity may induce syncope, at times associated with focal neurologic signs. The occurrence of syncope under such circumstances may be misdiagnosed as *carotid sinus syndrome*. The occurrence of a cerebrovascular accident following manual compression of the carotid sinus has been reported in patients with carotid disease, and carotid sinus massage should be avoided in patients with symptomatic or suspected occlusive carotid vascular disease.

Syncope in the *subclavian steal syndrome* is caused by major occlusive disease of the subclavian artery proximal to the origin of the vertebral artery. During upper extremity exercise, blood flow is shunted retrograde, by the circle of Willis, to the distal subclavian artery. The consequent decrease in cerebral circulation induces cerebral ischemia. This syndrome is suggested by the findings of diminished brachial arterial pressure on the affected side, a bruit that is maximal over the supraclavicular area adjacent to the origin of the vertebral artery, and the induction of symptoms by exercise of the involved extremity.

While focal neurologic symptoms and signs are the usual neurologic manifestations of cerebral emboli, transient loss of consciousness can be a primary presenting symptom. In study of 557 episodes of ischemic stroke and transient ischemic attack, transient loss of consciousness occurred in 6.5 percent.[51]

Syncopal episodes are more likely to occur when atherosclerotic occlusive disease involves the vertebrobasilar system with compromised perfusion to the medullary arousal center. In vertebrobasilar vascular insufficiency, syncope or presyncope is often preceded by symptoms of vertigo, diplopia, dysarthria, and ataxia. The episodes are generally attributed to microemboli arising from an atherosclerotic plaque, although vasospasm or postural hypotension may contribute.

Therapy

The treatment of recurrent syncope in cerebrovascular disease is predicated on an accurate diagnosis. In this regard, it is essential to segregate the potential contribution of cardiac and vascular factors and their interplay. Anticoagulants and/or platelet antiaggregant agents are recommended for the prevention of embolic disease from the heart or central vessels (see Chap. 68). Surgical endarterectomy should be considered in carotid arterial occlusive disease for transient ischemic attacks unresponsive to antiplatelet or anticoagulant therapy.

Carotid Sinus Syncope

Diagnosis

Compression of the carotid sinus in normal persons is often associated with transient slowing of the heart and mild hypotension. In some patients, such stimulation is followed by a profound slowing of heart rate and/or a marked diminution of arterial pressure. This disorder is referred to as carotid sinus hypersensitivity. Carotid sinus syncope is the term applied when a hypersensitive carotid sinus reflex is demonstrated to be the cause of syncope.[52–54] Recent studies suggest it is more common than previously thought.[55]

There are three forms of carotid sinus syncope, as originally described by Weiss and Baker: cardioinhibitory, vasodepressor, and mixed type.[52] The cardioinhibitory type of carotid sinus syncope is the most common. It is associated with slowing of the heart rate secondary to marked sinus bradycardia, sinoatrial block, and/or high-degree atrioventricular (AV) block. Here, syncope is related to the prolonged asystole rather than to a fall in peripheral vascular resistance. The vasodepressor type of carotid sinus syncope is that form of the syndrome in which fainting occurs as a result of a primary decrease in arterial pressure in the absence of profound bradycardia. Presyncopal signs, such as nausea, sweating and pallor, are usually not observed, and the fall in arterial pressure may be precipitous. In the mixed form of carotid sinus syncope with bradycardia and hypotension, the vasodepressor component may not be evident until after atropine blockade or during cardiac pacing. Under such circumstances, carotid sinus massage uncovers the hypotension in the absence of bradycardia.

Carotid sinus syncope and presyncope are commonly found in elderly patients in whom symptoms of lightheadedness and impaired consciousness may be initiated by relatively minor stimulation of the carotid sinus. Classically, an episode is precipitated by head motion, shaving, and wearing a tight collar. In patients with a history of syncope and the presence of a hypersensitive carotid sinus reflex, a direct cause-and-effect relationship between the hypersensitivity and the syncope must be documented before a firm diagnosis of carotid sinus syncope can be established.

The frequency of a hypersensitive response to manual carotid sinus compression in elderly persons enjoins caution whenever this maneuver is attempted. Digital carotid massage should first be attempted with a very gentle and brief (2 to 4 s) compression, always when the patient is supine and ideally with monitoring of the heart rate and blood pressure.

Carotid sinus syncope has been observed in patients with neoplasms, inflammatory masses, and lymph nodes in the neck adjacent to the carotid sinus.[56–58] Carotid sinus syncope is well established as a complication of carotid body and parotid tumors.

Therapy

Thorough patient education concerning avoidance of carotid sinus pressure may be effective in preventing syncopal episodes. Anticholinergic and sympathomimetic agents may be tried, but inadequacy of drug therapy and the occurrence of side effects may necessitate pacemaker therapy. Implantation of a permanent transvenous ventricular demand (VVI) pacemaker was the earliest form of pacemaker therapy for intractable carotid sinus syncope.[59] This therapy has been effective for the cardioinhibitory type of carotid sinus syncope. In patients with the mixed form of carotid sinus syncope, ventricular demand pacing may pose serious therapeutic problems.[60] Not only does the vasodepressor response to carotid stimulation persist, but it may be induced by ventricular pacing per se (pacemaker syndrome). AV sequential pacing appears to minimize the hypotensive effect of cardiac pacing and hence is the preferred form of pacemaker therapy in the mixed form of carotid sinus syncope.[61] It is essential that pacemaker effectiveness be verified objectively through observation of the effect of carotid sinus stimulation on cardiac rhythm and arterial pressure following pacemaker insertion.

Reflex Syncope

Diagnosis

Syncope or presyncope may occur in individuals without evidence of heart disease as a result of profound reflex-induced bradycardia. The term *vagovagal syncope* is applied to such episodes because the entire reflex arc is located within the vagal system. Syncopal episodes associated with painful stimulation of the endobronchial, pharyngeal, laryngeal, or esophageal mucosa are most probably based on this mechanism. Vagally induced sinus bradycardia, sinus arrest, nodal bradycardia, second-degree AV block, and asystole are the mechanisms responsible for the profound bradycardia and syncope. Similar mechanisms have been implicated in syncope following distension of the viscera, fainting associated with irritation of the pleura or peritoneum, and cardiac asystole associated with esophagoscopy or bronchoscopy.

Swallowing or deglutition syncope has been reported in association with tumor, diverticulum, achalasia, stricture, and spasm of the esophagus. In some patients no abnormality can be identified radiologically or endoscopically. In the latter group, symptoms of dysphagia or pain on swallowing food or beverages in common, and dilatation of the esophageal wall activates the afferent limb of the reflex arc. Cardiac arrhythmias responsible for swallow syncope include sinus or nodal bradycardia, sinoatrial and AV block, ventricular tachycardia, and asystole.[62,63]

Glossopharyngeal neuralgia is an extremely painful syndrome that may occur as an isolated entity or with neoplasms of the oropharynx and base of the skull.[64,65] It is associated with recurrent episodes of syncope caused by sinus bradycardia, sinus arrest, or high-degree AV block frequently accompanied by arterial hypotension. The triggering mechanism is most commonly swallowing, and attacks may be provoked by tactile stimulation in the region of the tonsil. Severe lancinating pain in the neck, tonsillar area, ear, and jaw upon swallowing distinguish this form of syncope from deglutition syncope.

Therapy

Treatment of recurrent reflex syncope necessitates interventions directed at the initiating mechanisms, namely, esophageal tumor or stricture. Episodes of syncope may be prevented by anticholinergic drugs such as atropine (commonly used prior to procedures). In glossopharyngeal neuralgia, anticonvulsants (e.g., carbamazepine and diphenylhydantoin) have been effective in relieving episodes of neuralgia and syncope. In some patients, however, thermocoagulation of the ganglion of the glossopharyngeal nerve or resection of the ninth nerve and rostral fibers of the vagus may be the only effective means of controlling the neuralgia and syncope. Pacemaker therapy has been used in patients with uncontrolled syncopal episodes related to glossopharyngeal neuralgia.[65]

Other Causes of Noncardiac Syncope

The term *situational syncope* has been applied to a group of syndromes that are defined by the circumstances that precipitate the event. In the past, the syncope in these disorders has been attributed mainly to mechanical factors. Recent observations suggest that, at least in part, vagovagal or vasodepressor reactions contribute to the syncope.

Cough Syncope

In cough syncope (also termed *laryngeal vertigo, tussive syncope,* and *posttussive syncope*), loss of consciousness occurs following a paroxysm of vigorous coughing. It is often seen in robust men and children but rarely in women. This syndrome is particularly frequent among individuals with chronic bronchitis and a persistent "hacking cough." Cerebral blood flow is impaired by the marked increase in cerebrospinal fluid pressure during coughing, which increases cerebrovascular resistance. There is also a "concussive effect" transmitted via the cerebrospinal fluid. Reflex-induced sinus bradycardia, sinus arrest, and AV block have been observed in patients with cough syncope.[66,67] Episodes of syncope following sneezing (sneeze syncope) probably have a similar mechanism. Basilar invagination of the brain has been implicated as a causal mechanism of sneeze syncope in patients with Arnold-Chiari malformation or syringomyelia.[68,69]

In the treatment of cough syncope, the patient should be informed of the deleterious effects of vigorous coughing. Cessation of smoking and initiation of bronchodilator and anti-inflammatory therapy for associated bronchitis is mandatory for the prevention of cough-induced syncope.

Valsalva Syncope

Syncope related to prolonged increases in intrathoracic pressure may be observed during a sustained Valsalva maneuver. With prolonged exhalation against a closed glottis, there is a progressive fall in venous return, arterial pressure, and cardiac output. These hemodynamic changes may be sufficient to impair cerebral circulation. Associated post-Valsalva sinus bradycardia adds to the impairment in cerebral blood flow. An episode of Valsalva syncope may be the first indication of the presence of a disorder predisposing to syncope (e.g., cerebrovascular occlusive disease and sick sinus syndrome). Instruction to the patient regarding avoidance of sustained Valsalva maneuvers is essential in preventing recurring episodes.

Micturition Syncope

Micturition syncope is often seen in adult men with nocturia. During or immediately following voiding there is a loss of consciousness, often without premonitory symptoms.[70] The ingestion of large quantities of alcoholic beverages before retiring is common. A similar type of syncope may be observed following drainage of the distended bladder or after removal of large quantities of ascitic fluid. The loss of consciousness in these circumstances may be related to bradycardia and a sudden reflex decrease in peripheral arterial resistance induced by the precipitous fall in intraabdominal volume. The loss of consciousness to typical vasodepressor syncope is associated by such factors as the Valsalva maneuver in the upright posture and the peripheral vasodilation associated with a warm bed and recent alcohol consumption.

Defecation Syncope

Syncope during defecation occurs most commonly in the elderly, usually after arising from bed at night or during manual disimpaction of the rectum. It has been attributed to sudden decompression of the rectum.[71] Valsalva-related syncope could also explain defecation syncope. Many patients with defecation syncope have underlying gastrointestinal or cardiovascular disease. Syncope during defecation should suggest pulmonary embolism as a possible underlying cause (see also Chap. 100).

Diver's Syncope

Unusual and poorly understood forms of loss of consciousness and even sudden death may occur in underwater diving. Some may be forms of vasodepressor syncope. Hypoxia and bradycardia of the diving reflex may be contributing factors.

Hypoxia and Syncope

Fainting due to hypoxia may be related directly to a lack of oxygen or to an episode of vasodepressor syncope initiated during a period of oxygen lack. In the presence of cardiovascular disease, pulmonary insufficiency, and anemia, symptoms of hypoxia occur at lesser levels of oxygen deprivation. The impairment of consciousness due to hypoxia is accompanied by sinus tachycardia, while arterial pressure is usually normal. The environmental setting in which impaired consciousness due to hypoxia occurs usually leaves little difficulty in its differentiation from other forms of syncope.

Hypoglycemia and Syncope

Severe hypoglycemia is associated with weakness, sweating, a sensation of hunger, confusion, and altered consciousness. The symptoms are unrelated to posture and usually respond promptly to food ingestion or intravenous glucose administration. Impaired consciousness is usually associated with sinus tachycardia and is rarely accompanied by hypotension. In contrast to syncope of circulatory origin, it is gradual in onset.

Hyperventilation, Panic Attacks, and Syncope

In normal persons, anxiety is accompanied by varying degrees of hyperventilation. In the hyperventilation syndrome or in a panic episode, anxiety is associated with an inordinate degree of hyperventilation. Symptoms of hypocapnia may dominate the clinical picture. During the episode, the patient complains of a tightness in the chest and a feeling of suffocation. This is followed by confusion, a sense of unreality, bewilderment, lightheadedness, and a feeling of panic. Symptoms of palpitation, precordial oppression, and dyspnea may suggest an acute cardiac or pulmonary catastrophe. Associated with the abovementioned symptoms are sensations of numbness or coldness of the extremities and circumoral areas. The symptoms may be protracted and persist while the subject is sitting or in recumbency (see also Chap. 118). During hyperventilation, there is slight hypotension but no profound fall in arterial pressure, while the heart rate is rapid. The episode usually terminates when the patient's anxiety is allayed and the hyperventilation ceases. One may assist in the resolution of symptoms of hypocapnia by having the patient rebreathe in a paper or plastic bag. Although mentation is impaired, complete loss of consciousness rarely occurs. Typical vasodepressor syncope may be superimposed, making identification of the syndrome more difficult. The induction of a typical episode by voluntary hyperventilation is helpful in distinguishing this syndrome and aids in educating the patient regarding the prevention and control of attacks.

Convulsive Disorders and Syncope

Differentiation of the various forms of syncope from the loss of consciousness during a generalized convulsive seizure is often made on the basis of history alone. Grand mal epilepsy as a cause of sudden loss of consciousness is suggested by the dramatic nature of the onset of the attack, which is often preceded by an aura. Other observations that aid in distinguishing epilepsy are the absence of hypotension and cardiac arrhythmia (other than sinus tachycardia); the presence of sustained tonic-clonic convulsive movements with upturning of the eyes; prolonged unconsciousness; urinary incontinence; and postictal drowsiness, headache, and confusion. While any of the abovementioned findings occasionally occur in episodes of syncope, the frequent association of these several events generally allows differentiation of epilepsy as its cause.[72] Akinetic seizures and absence (petite mal) seizures may be difficult to differentiate from syncope. The occurrence in childhood, a past history of recurrent episodes, and the absence of pallor in witnessed episodes are helpful diagnostic findings. Temporal lobe seizures are the most likely form of epilepsy to masquerade as syncope.[73]

An abnormal electroencephalogram (EEG) between episodes of altered consciousness can aid in distinguishing a seizure disorder when clinical observations are not definitive, and in some instances continuous EEG and electrocardiogram (ECG) monitoring is required.[74] On the other hand, routine use of the EEG in patients presenting with syncope is costly and rarely yields a definitive diagnosis when employed indiscriminately in all patients.[75] In fact, it is probably more common for patients with true syncope to be incorrectly diagnosed as having a seizure disorder (see also Chap. 122).

Vertigo and Syncope

Although recurrent episodes of vertigo may first be described by the patient as a loss or impairment of consciousness, careful attention to the history will usually reveal the true nature of this symptom. In true vertigo there is a keen sense of movement, either of the environment or of the patient. Falling may be abrupt; it is due, not to weakness of postural tone, but to a loss of balance. Nausea, pallor, and cold perspiration suggest vasodepressor syncope, but the lack of true loss or impairment of consciousness, the increased distress with head movement, the associated nystagmus, and the findings of normal arterial pressure and pulse during an attack help differentiate vertigo from syncope.

Hysterical Syncope

Hysterical syncope may mimic altered consciousness of circulatory origin. Hysterical episodes occur most frequently in young adults, often with severe emotional illness, and generally in the presence of an audience. The individual slumps gently, even gracefully, to the floor or in a convenient chair or sofa, typically without injury or awkwardness. The patient may be motionless or may exhibit symbolic resistive movements.

Episodes are of varying duration and may last an hour or more. Although the patient is unresponsive to verbal stimulation, there is evidence that consciousness is well preserved, and no abnormalities in pulse, arterial pressure, or skin color are evident. There is no sharp recovery with recumbency. A distinctive characteristic is the calm emotional detachment with which the patient describes the symptoms.

Migraine and Syncope

Symptoms suggesting syncope are unusual in ordinary types of migraine. In rare instances in which the basilar arterial system is involved (as opposed to the more usually affected carotid system), the premonitory aura of migraine terminates in a period of unconsciousness of several minutes' duration. The unconsciousness is slow in onset and may be preceded by a dreamlike state. When the patient awakens, there is severe headache, typically in the occipital area. This form of migraine usually afflicts young women and has a strong menstrual association. In the original description of the syndrome, the period of unconsciousness was apparently unassociated with circulatory alterations.[76] The symptoms in syncopal migraine may suggest hyperventilation and/or hysterical syncope. Recently, hyperresponsiveness to dopamine receptors (tested by the administration of bromocriptine, a dopamine receptor agonist), with inhibition of the vasomotor center, has been proposed as an alternative explanation for syncope in patients with migraine.[77]

SYNCOPE ASSOCIATED WITH CARDIAC DISEASE

Either severe obstruction of cardiac output or disturbances of cardiac rhythm can produce syncope of cardiac origin. Obstructive lesions and arrhythmias frequently coexist; indeed, one abnormality may accentuate the other. Common disorders associated with cardiac syncope are listed in Table 50-6.

TABLE 50-6

Common Disorders Associated with Cardiac Syncope
Obstruction of cardiac output
Left-sided heart
Aortic stenosis
Hypertrophic cardiomyopathy
Prosthetic valve malfunction
Mitral stenosis
Left atrial myxoma
Right-sided heart
Eisenmenger syndrome
Tetralogy of Fallot
Pulmonary embolism
Pulmonary stenosis
Primary pulmonary hypertension
Cardiac tamponade
Cardiac arrhythmia
Conduction system disease (primary or secondary)
Sick sinus syndrome
AV block
AV node disease
His-Purkinje disease
Paroxysmal supraventricular tachycardias
WPW syndrome
Paroxysmal ventricular tachycardia/fibrillation
Long QT syndromes
Congenital
Acquired
Pharmacologic and metabolic disorders
Pacemaker-induced syncope
Malfunction
Pacemaker-induced arrhythmias
Pacemaker syndrome

Syncope Related to Obstruction of Cardiac Output

Obstruction to cardiac output sufficient to cause syncope may occur on the left or right side of the heart. Syncope, particularly that occurring with effort, is a major symptom of aortic stenosis and often is the initial presentation. The mechanisms are unclear, but studies suggest a reflex fall in peripheral vascular resistance as the usual cause.[78] Failure of cardiac output to increase adequately during exercise, while peripheral resistance decreases, may play a role. Transient arrhythmias can also induce syncope in aortic stenosis (see also Chap. 79).[79] Syncope associated with effort (often occurring immediately after effort) is observed in patients with hypertrophic cardiomyopathy as well.[80] Nonexertional syncope related to acute decreases in preload or afterload, to inotropic stimulation, or to transient arrhythmias may also occur in hypertrophic cardiomyopathy (see also Chap. 90). Left-sided heart prosthetic valve malfunction can produce transient and at times profound obstruction to blood flow with syncope (see also Chap. 83). A left atrial myxoma may obstruct left ventricular filling, leading to low cardiac output and syncope. The obstruction of left ventricular inflow in atrial myxoma may be posturally induced (see also Chap. 111). Mitral stenosis can produce cardiac syncope but usually does so only when tachycardia or other arrhythmias supervene (see also Chap. 80).

Primary pulmonary hypertension and pulmonary hypertension secondary to congenital heart disease may both be complicated by syncope, particularly effort-related syncope.[81] In these conditions limitation of right ventricular outflow markedly inhibits the cardiac output response during increased peripheral demand. The fall in peripheral resistance in the presence of a limited cardiac output response may result in profound hypotension. A reflex fall in peripheral resistance similar to that which occurs with aortic stenosis may play a role (see also Chap. 99). In pulmonary stenosis and pulmonary embolism, similar mechanisms may account for syncope. In a young patient without a cardiac murmur who presents with syncope during or shortly after exertion, primary pulmonary hypertension should be considered. In tetralogy of Fallot, the magnitude of flow through the right-to-left shunt increases when systemic resistance falls with effort, since the right ventricular outflow obstruction is usually fixed. This results in marked arterial hypoxia, which may precipitate a syncopal episode (see also Chap. 97).

Cardiac tamponade, which affects both the right and the left side of the heart, can produce syncope, but this is extremely rare. The likelihood of syncope is increased by concomitant arrhythmias.

Syncope Related to Cardiac Arrhythmia

Arrhythmias are a common cause of syncope and must be considered in all patients, particularly when cardiac disease is present.[8,82,83] Either extreme of ventricular rate—bradycardia or tachycardia—can depress cardiac output to the point of critical hypotension and syncope. As noted earlier for other forms of syncope, a vasodepressor reaction may be precipitated by the hemodynamic effects of arrhythmias (see also Chaps. 35 and 36).

The most common arrhythmias producing syncope or presyncope are profound sinus bradycardia, high-grade AV block, supraventricular tachycardia, ventricular tachycardia, and the pacemaker syndrome. Although arrhythmias occur in the absence of demonstrable underlying cardiac disease, they are usually secondary to such disorders as ischemic heart disease, cardiomyopathy, valvular heart disease, and primary conduction system disease.

Primary degenerative lesions in the sinus node and the specialized conduction tissue are the most frequent causes of the sick sinus syndrome.[84] The sick sinus syndrome may be manifested by persistent or episodic sinus bradycardia, sinoatrial exit block, impaired junctional escape rhythm, and reentrant supraventricular tachycardias. The appearance of alternating sinus bradycardia with paroxysmal supraventricular tachycardia is quite common and is referred to as the bradycardia-tachycardia syndrome.[85] Syncope often occurs after abrupt termination of a tachycardia, when there is overdrive suppression of the sinoatrial or junctional pacemakers or of AV conduction. Transient increases in vagal tone may be responsible for episodes of more severe bradycardia. A high incidence of associated AV block and intraventricular conduction defects occur in the sick sinus syndrome. Thus, AV block, impaired junctional escape rhythm, or ventricular arrhythmias may actually be responsible for syncope in the sick sinus syndrome.

High-grade AV block may be due either to disease of the AV node or of the His-Purkinje system. Disease of the AV node is associated with an intact junctional pacemaker and a normal QRS complex, while AV block due to disease of the His-Purkinje system is usually associated with a wide, complex idioventricular rhythm, which may be quite slow. Syncope due to high-grade AV block (Adams-Stokes syndrome) most likely occurs when AV block is due to His-Purkinje disease. Progression to high-grade AV block in patients with bifascicular block and a normal PR interval is uncommon, but if bifascicular block is associated with a prolonged PR interval, the risk of developing high-grade AV block is substantially higher.[86–88] As noted above, ventricular tachycardia may be the cause of syncope with AV block.[89]

Sinus bradycardia, AV block, or cardiac asystole may be mediated by reflex vagal mechanisms and have been observed in a variety of disease states or during diagnostic procedures (see above). Paroxysmal vagal bradycardia or AV block can also occur in apparently healthy young individuals, although these patients often have mitral valve prolapse.[90–95]

Paroxysmal supraventricular tachycardias usually do not produce syncope in young individuals. Syncope, however, may occur in younger individuals who have accessory AV pathways due to the Wolff-Parkinson-White (WPW) syndrome, wherein supraventricular tachycardia is associated with a very rapid ventricular response. In older individuals less rapid heart rates may produce hypotension and lead to syncope.

Paroxysmal ventricular tachycardia may produce syncope at any age and can occur as a manifestation of most types of cardiac disease in which there is ventricular hypertrophy, ischemia, or fibrosis, and adrenergic hyperactivity. Ventricular tachycardia is the commonest arrhythmic cause of syncope in most series. In many patients ventricular and supraventricular tachycardias coexist.[96]

The long QT interval syndrome may be congenital or acquired.[97] The recognition of long QT syndromes depends on demonstration of QT prolongation and recurrent syncope, which is almost always due to ventricular arrhythmia.[98] The ventricular arrhythmia is usually torsade de pointes ventricular tachycardia.[99] The congenital long QT syndromes include the autosomal recessive Jervell and Lange-Nielson syndrome with deafness and the autosomal dominant Romano-Ward syndrome without deafness.

It is particularly important to recognize the acquired long QT syndrome because it is a common and life-threatening side effect of many antiarrhythmic drugs and metabolic abnormalities. The most frequent causes of acquired long QT syndromes are class I antiarrhythmic drugs and electrolyte disorders (hypokalemia and hypomagnesemia). Additional causes are antidepressant drugs, phenothiazines, liquid protein diet, acute ischemia, and myocarditis. Chronic myocardial disease, especially when left ventricular hypertrophy is present, may result in prolongation of the QT interval (see also Chap. 36).

Digitalis may be responsible for ventricular or supraventricular tachycardias, AV dissociation, and AV block, especially in patients with antecedent AV node disease. Beta-blocking agents and calcium channel blocking agents may cause profound bradycardia and AV block, particularly in patients with conduction system disease. Theophylline and beta agonists, used for therapy of chronic obstructive pulmonary disease, may precipitate ventricular or supraventricular arrhythmias. Therapy with diuretics often causes hypokalemia and hypomagnesemia, which predispose to supraventricular and ventricular arrhythmias. Both caffeine and alcohol may precipitate either atrial or ventricular tachycardia.

In patients with an artificial pacemaker, syncope may be secondary to pacemaker malfunction or to the pacemaker syndrome.[100,101] Dual-chamber pacemakers can produce pacemaker-mediated tachycardias when there is retrograde conduction of the ventricular impulse to the atria. Improvements in technology have reduced the incidence of this complication.

Several mechanisms are responsible for the so-called pacemaker syndrome. Cardiac output in patients with ventricular pacemakers may decrease owing to loss of normal AV synchrony. Loss of the atrial contribution to ventricular filling is only part of the problem. When there is intact ventriculoatrial conduction of the pacemaker impulse and an atrial contraction occurs during ventricular systole, mitral and tricuspid regurgitation may result. Finally, atrial contraction against closed AV valves may decrease the peripheral arterial resistance by a reflex mechanism, particularly in patients with carotid sinus hypersensitivity (see also Chap. 40).

Diagnostic Evaluation of Syncope Associated with Cardiac Disease

While the history and physical examination often establish the diagnosis of obstructive cardiac syncope, laboratory studies are usually required for the determination of the severity of the disorder (see also Chap. 90). Cardiac catheterization is required when corrective cardiac surgery is contemplated.

By far the most challenging diagnostic evaluation occurs when arrhythmic cardiac syncope is suspected. Such patients often have evidence of underlying cardiovascular disease, which when present carries a distinctly poorer prognosis. Thus, diagnostic studies directed to the nature and severity of the underlying cardiac disease must be pursued in addition to the arrhythmia evaluation.

The various diagnostic tests used for the evaluation of arrhythmic syncope are listed in Table 50-7. Because of the transient nature of most arrhythmias, the routine ECG is generally of limited value. It is, however, very useful in identifying patients with abnormalities that may predispose to syncope, such as prior infarction, WPW pattern, and AV or bundle branch block.

The technique of signal averaging the ECG for detecting late potentials can be used as a noninvasive screening test for detecting a high-risk subset of patients prone to lethal ventricular arrhythmias.[102–105] The accu-

TABLE 50-7
Diagnostic Tests for Evaluation of Arrhythmic Causes of Syncope

Test	Use
ECG	Documents conduction disease, WPW syndrome, ischemic heart disease, ventricular hypertrophy, atrial and ventricular ectopy; occasionally defines arrhythmia
Signal-averaged ECG	Screen for ventricular tachycardia
Exercise testing	May document exertional arrhythmias
Ambulatory monitoring	Records rhythm disturbances during one or more 24-h cycles; relates arrhythmia to symptoms; aids in defining response to therapy
Patient-activated monitors	May document paroxysmal arrhythmias in low-risk subsets
Upright tilt	Elicits vasodepressor/vasovagal reaction
Invasive electrophysiologic	Defines conduction system study disease when noninvasive studies are inconclusive in high-risk patients; elicits supraventricular and ventricular tachycardias; measures hemodynamic effects of arrhythmias and responses to pharmacologic and pacing interventions

racy of the signal-averaged ECG in predicting the induction of sustained monomorphic ventricular tachycardia in high-risk patients who undergo electrophysiologic studies is approximately 90 percent. The predictive power of the signal-averaged ECG has been shown to be independent of other risk variables, including the status of left ventricular function, the presence of left ventricular aneurysm, myocardial infarction, and clinical risk indicators. Thus, it has become a useful screening test in detecting patients who require invasive electrophysiologic evaluation (see also Chap. 47).

Exercise testing can directly provoke arrhythmias in patients with a history suggesting exercise-induced tachycardia, but it is of limited use for bradyarrhythmias.[106] It should be performed when exertional arrhythmias are suspected but not documented by ambulatory monitoring or when ischemia is suspected (see also Chap. 16).

Continuous ECG monitoring is the most widely used screening test for suspected arrhythmic syncope.[107–111] While such observation can be made in a hospital monitoring unit, ambulatory monitoring is more efficacious when the patient is allowed to perform ordinary daily activities. It is important to recognize that one 24-h monitoring period may not be sufficient for detecting transient rhythm disturbances. However, the diagnostic yield increases only slightly with more prolonged monitoring. Continuous ECG monitoring has limited sensitivity (15 to 20 percent) in *unselected* patients with a history of syncope. In patients suspected of having arrhythmic syncope, however, the sensitivity is in the range of 50 percent. A major advantage of this technique is that it relates the presence of arrhythmia to symptoms (see also Chap. 45).

When ambulatory monitoring does not document an arrhythmia, a patient-activated electrocardiographic device may prove efficacious.[112–114] A device with recording capabilities is preferred. This type of monitoring is effective in documenting infrequent arrhythmia and may establish the diagnosis of arrhythmic syncope in up to one-third of those studied. It should not be used in patients with suspected life-threatening arrhythmias.

As noted earlier, head-up tilt has proved extremely useful for identification of primary vasodepressor syncope or for documenting the presence of a vasodepressor reaction accompanying other forms of syncope. Thus, this test is indicated in most patients with syncope and is often performed in conjunction with an electrophysiologic study.

When noninvasive testing is inconclusive for the diagnosis of arrhythmic syncope, an electrophysiologic study should be performed on high-risk patients (i.e., those with underlying heart disease, suspicious arrhythmia by ECG monitoring, or bodily injury associated with syncope). The identification of a probable cause for syncope by electrophysiologic study has ranged from 30 to 75 percent.[107,113,115–126] This variance in percentage of positive responses depends primarily on the definition of a positive finding and the patient population studied. The patient without identifiable heart disease is less likely to have the cause of syncope identified by electrophysiologic study (see also Chap. 46).

Electrophysiologic studies involve the placement of electrode catheters for the recording in intracardiac electrograms as well as atrial and ventricular pacing. Evaluation of sinus node function involves pacing near the high right atrium with measurement of sinus node recovery time. Sinoatrial function is evaluated by the application of atrial premature depolarizations in sinus rhythm for the measurement of sinoatrial conduction time. AV conduction is separated between AV node conduction (low atrium to His bundle depolarization) and His-Purkinje conduction (His-ventricular activation) by means of His bundle recording. The effect of atrial pacing on these intervals and the pacing rate required to provoke AV block provide additional assessment of AV conduction.

Tachyarrhythmias are usually induced with atrial or ventricular premature stimulation. The type of supraventricular tachycardia is readily identified by the ventricular-atrial timing relationships in tachycardia and the influence of premature ventricular or atrial stimulation during tachycardia. Ventricular tachycardia (unimorphic or polymorphic) is usually provoked by ventricular premature stimulation during sinus rhythm or after a train of paced beats, although burst pacing may at times provoke tachycardia. As many as three premature stimuli are routinely tested. Tachycardia duration of six beats to 30 s is termed nonsustained tachycardia; sustained tachycardia lasts more than 30 s or requires termination because of symptoms or hemodynamic instability. The provocation of ventricular fibrillation is often an indeterminate endpoint, particularly in the patient with syncope and no prior ECG evidence of ventricular tachyarrhythmia. Isoproterenol infusion or upright tilt is often required to provoke a tachyarrhythmia or to assess the potential for acceleration of heart rate during tachycardia or the attendant hemodynamic sequelae.

The cause of syncope most commonly identified by electrophysiologic study is ventricular tachycardia, which is present in approximately 50 percent of positive studies. Bradycardiac rhythms (sinoatrial and AV abnormalities) account for approximately 30 percent of identifiable causes for syncope, while supraventricular tachycardia at a rate to cause symptoms during the supine or the upright state or with isoproterenol challenge is identified as a cause of syncope in approximately 20 percent (see also Chap. 46).

The recurrence of syncope in patients with syncope who had positive electrophysiologic findings and treatment based on those findings ranges from 15 to 25 percent. Patients who continue to have arrhythmic syncope despite negative electrophysiologic study results usually have recurrence due to bradycardiac rhythms. It is noteworthy that such patients often have several mild abnormalities of sinoatrial or AV conduction, the consequence of which is to make bradycardiac syncope likely to occur (Fig. 50-1).[127]

Electrophysiologic studies are useful in stratifying risk among symptomatic patients with bundle branch block. Patients with normal electrophysiologic study results have a favorable prognosis even without treatment. Patients undergoing permanent pacing on the basis of electrophysiologic testing also have a favorable prognosis with a low rate of symptom recurrence.

The prognosis in patients with syncope due to supraventricular tachycardia is usually good, since a variety

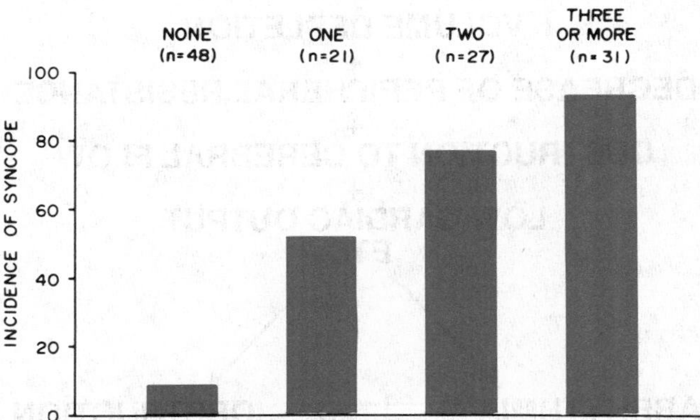

FIGURE 50-1 Relationship between the number of abnormalities on electrophysiologic testing and incidence of syncope in patients with syncope on the basis of transient sinoatrial dysfunction or AV conduction defect. Electrophysiologic data include sinoatrial conduction time, atrial-to-His interval, His-to-ventricular depolarization interval, or AV block at slow rates during atrial pacing. *(From Boudoulas et al.*[127] *Reproduced with permission from the publisher and author.)*

of therapeutic approaches are available (i.e., drugs, pacemaker, and radiofrequency ablation). The prognosis in patients with inducible ventricular tachycardia is less favorable but is improved when specific therapy can be demonstrated to inhibit the inducibility of ventricular tachycardia.[128] Long-term follow-up of patients undergoing electrophysiologic study shows a higher mortality in those with positive findings (13 to 48 percent) than in those with negative results (2 to 9 percent).[118,126,129] The 5-year cumulative survival of patients with syncope is as follows: ventricular tachycardia, 37 percent ± 28 percent; supraventricular tachycardia, 90 percent ± 9 percent; bradyarrhythmias, 71 percent ± 10 percent; and normal study, 96 percent ± 4 percent.[20]

Treatment of Cardiac Syncope

A detailed discussion of therapy for cardiac arrhythmias is presented in Chap. 36. Some general principles of arrhythmia management as they apply to patients with syncope will be summarized here. For the patient with syncope caused by obstructive heart disease, cardiac surgery is often the treatment of choice. Patients with hypertrophic cardiomyopathy and syncope may respond well to pharmacologic therapy; however, if the obstruction is severe and the patient remains symptomatic, surgery must be considered (see Chap. 90). Among all patients with obstructive heart disease and recurrent syncope, the diagnosis of fixed pulmonary hypertension is most difficult to treat because effective therapeutic options are limited (see Chap. 99).

Therapy for syncope caused by arrhythmia should first be addressed to the therapy for underlying cardiovascular disease and to the mitigation of precipitating or initiating events (especially ischemia). The ingestion of caffeine or other arrhythmia-inducing agents (i.e., alcohol) should be interdicted when an association with the arrhythmia is uncovered or suspected. During therapy with antiarrhythmic drugs, efficacy should be documented objectively (through ambulatory monitoring, exercise testing, or electrophysiologic studies). In patients with the tachycardia-bradycardia syndrome, antiarrhythmic drugs that suppress the tachyarrhythmia may aggravate the bradyarrhythmia. Thus, a permanent transvenous pacemaker may be necessary to make it possible to administer appropriate antiarrhythmic agents.

One of the most controversial areas of therapy is in the use of pacemakers for patients with syncope associated with bradycardiac syndromes.[130,131] Such controversy is especially evident in the treatment of older patients with sinus bradycardia, patients with sick sinus syndrome, and patients with syncope who exhibit bifascicular or trifascicular block on ECG. In general, since these disorders have low short-term mortality, pacemaker placement must be justified largely on the basis of a reduction of symptoms. Although the decision to insert a pacemaker in such patients is often contested, it would appear that severe syncopal episodes can be averted. Experience with pacemakers capable of recording bradyarrhythmic events indicates that the initial judgment for artificial cardiac pacing in such patients was usually appropriate.[132] Care must be taken to avoid pacemaker syndromes, especially in those patients with carotid sinus hypersensitivity or postural hypotension (see also Chap. 40).

In patients with the congenital long QT syndromes and syncope, beta-adrenergic blocking drugs usually control the symptoms.[133] If syncope persists despite therapy, left sympathetic stellectomy with or without beta-blockade therapy may be effective. In some patients, implantation of a permanent pacemaker may be effective.[134] In syncope due to the acquired long QT syndrome, discontinuation of the offending drugs and restoration of metabolic balance usually prevents recurring episodes.

In patients with recurrent tachyarrhythmias that are refractory to antiarrhythmic drugs, nonpharmacologic interventions have proved useful. These interventions include revascularization in patients with ischemic disease and viable myocardium, automatic defibrillator implantation for ventricular tachycardia (see Chap. 42), and radiofrequency ablation of accessory pathways or the AV node in patients with supraventricular tachycardia (see Chap. 43).[135–141]

SPECIAL PROBLEMS IN SYNCOPE

Syncope in the Elderly

Elderly persons are particularly prone to develop syncope or presyncope.[142–146] The aging process can result in diminished cerebral oxygen delivery by a variety of physiologic mechanisms, including decreased cerebral blood flow from low cardiac output, cerebral vascular disease, decreased hemoglobin, and lower arterial P_{O_2}. In addition, cerebral arteriolar sclerosis may be present and may necessitate a higher arterial perfusion pressure. Thus, many older patients have only marginal cerebral oxygen delivery at rest.

Physiologic defenses against a fall in blood pressure may also be impaired. These defenses include diminished baroreceptor responsiveness, sinus bradycardia from sinus node dysfunction, impaired adrenergic responsiveness, impaired renal sodium conservation, and impaired renin-angiotensin-aldosterone responsiveness. In addition, autonomic neuropathy may be present (see also Chap. 115).

The aged may also suffer from multiple sensory deficits (e.g., in vision, vestibular function, peripheral sensory nerve function, etc.), variable degrees of dementia, bradykinesis, arthritis, and muscle weakness, all of which enhance the likelihood of a fall when cerebral perfusion is marginal. "Drop" attacks, in which muscle tone in the lower extremities is lost, are frequent in the elderly and must be distinguished from syncope. Carotid sinus sensitivity also is more common in the elderly. Postprandial syncope (most likely due to reflex sympathetic withdrawal after large meals) is common in the elderly.[147] The elderly frequently have multisystem disease and are likely to be taking several medications, often in excessive amounts, that may aggravate the tendency to syncope (e.g., antihypertensive drugs, diuretics, vasodilators, antiarrhythmic drugs, or psychoactive drugs).

Arrhythmias are common in elderly subjects, especially in those presenting with syncope. This makes assigning a diagnosis of arrhythmic syncope on the basis of ECG monitoring extremely difficult. The proarrhythmic effect of antiarrhythmic drugs is an especially notable problem for the elderly.

In the elderly, syncope may be the presenting complaint for common disorders such as pneumonia, viral illness, acute myocardial infarction, occult hemorrhage, or urinary tract infection. Thus, the management of syncope in the aged often requires initial management of underlying diseases with subsequent close follow-up to determine if such therapy controls syncope.

Multiple Causes of Syncope

In many instances, syncope requires that a constellation of events occur, either simultaneously or in sequence. Without the full complex, the patient may note only lightheadedness or perhaps no definable symptoms. A careful history is required to elucidate such complex presentations.

Transient abnormalities such as fever, fatigue, hypoglycemia, or pharmacologic agents may increase the likelihood of syncope. Coexisting diseases may decrease the patient's physiologic defenses for maintaining adequate cerebral perfusion to sustain consciousness. A cardiac arrhythmia that ordinarily would not produce syncope may become a contributory factor when other predisposing factors are present (Fig. 50-2). With respect to combined causes of syncope, it is notable that in the original description of Adams-Stokes syncope, the patients exhibited a permanently slow pulse accompanied by aortic stenosis.[148,149]

The development of either a vasodepressor or a vagovagal reaction (or both) may determine whether a given stimulus initiates syncope. This relationship has been shown in such diverse causes of syncope as aortic stenosis, vasodilator drug therapy, volume loss, pulmonary embolism, tachyarrhythmias, pacemaker syndrome, postprandial state in the elderly, and postexercise. A common pathophysiologic mechanism that may trigger the vasodepressor reaction is diminished venous return to the right side of the heart.

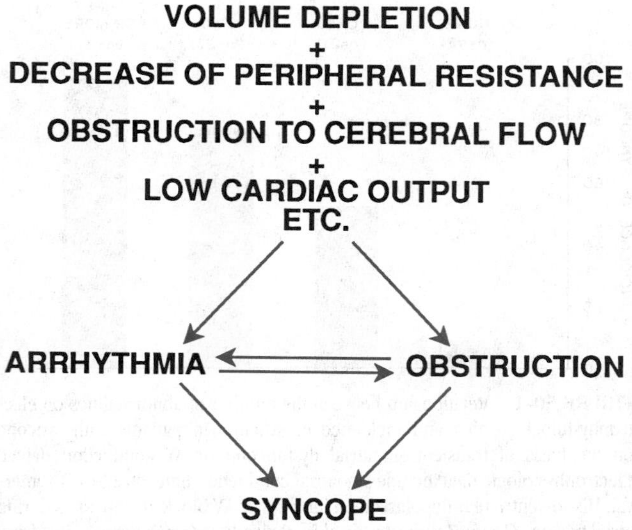

FIGURE 50-2 Frequently, multiple factors must be present simultaneously or in sequence for syncope to occur as a result of an arrhythmia or obstruction to cardiac output. *(From Boudoulas et al.[151] Reproduced with permission from the publisher and author.)*

Syncope and Sudden Death

As noted previously, sudden death is more common in those with known cardiac syncope (both obstructive and arrhythmic), but it can also occur in noncardiac syncope and syncope of unknown cause. It would appear, therefore, that in some patients, syncope is a harbinger of sudden death. It is not always clear to what extent the occurrence of syncope per se is a risk factor for sudden death or whether the risk is more related to the underlying disease (see also Chap. 51).

Recurrent Syncope

In up to one-third of all patients with syncope, it is a recurring event.[150] Of interest for most patients is the fact that the persistence of syncope increases morbidity from trauma but does not increase mortality. Such recurrences most often reflect a lack of effective therapy and/or a failure to establish the correct diagnosis. Recurrent syncope is particularly common in patients with mitral valve prolapse in whom dysautonomia, arrhythmia, and hypovolemia all play a role (see also Chap. 80). For patients with recurrent syncope, advice regarding the avoidance of certain activities, such as working with dangerous equipment, is needed, and, in some cases in which public safety is involved, a change in jobs is required (e.g., pilots or bus drivers).

DIAGNOSTIC EVALUATION OF SYNCOPE: AN OVERVIEW

In the initial approach to the diagnosis of syncope, it is essential to distinguish the underlying cause in terms of

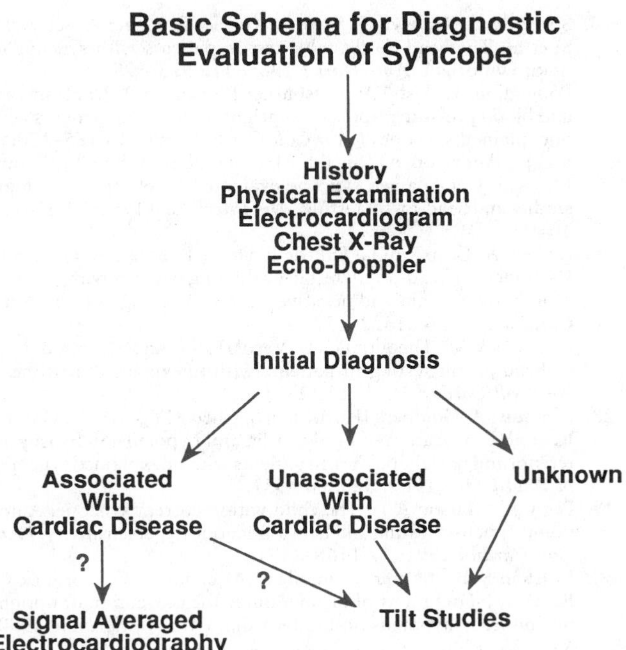

FIGURE 50-3 Differentiation of the three major diagnostic categories of syncope is accomplished in the majority of patients with the history, physical examination, ECG, chest X-ray, and routine laboratory studies. The echo Doppler study is often decisive for either diagnosis or assessment of the severity of underlying cardiac disease. The signal-averaged ECG should be considered in patients with underlying heart disease. Head-up tilt studies should be considered in most patients in whom the mechanism of syncope is not clearly defined.

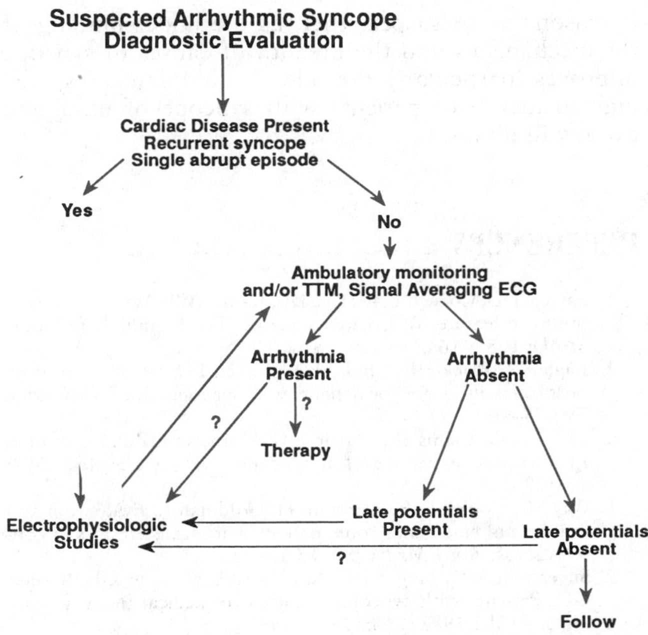

FIGURE 50-4 Approach to the patients with suspected arrhythmic syncope. Many patients with underlying cardiac disease, recurrent syncope, or abrupt syncope should be considered for an electrophysiologic study as an initial step. In less severe patients, noninvasive evaluation should be performed initially. *(From Boudoulas.[152] Reproduced with permission from the publisher and author.)*

the three basic categories outlined in Table 50-1. This differentiation is accomplished in a majority of patients by a history and physical examination supplemented by routine laboratory studies, including echocardiography (Fig. 50-3).

The data in Table 50-2 provide a useful framework for initiating a diagnostic evaluation of syncope and underscore the importance of a thorough knowledge of the diverse causes of syncope. The extent of evaluation should initially be predicated on the estimation of mortality and morbidity risk (high in cardiac syncope and low in noncardiovascular syncope and syncope of unknown cause). While dose effectiveness in diagnosis must be practiced, the need for an assiduous search should not be dismissed when lethal disease is suspected.

Hospitalization for more complete evaluation of syncope is generally required for the elderly, for patients with suspected cardiac causes, and for those who incur severe bodily injury regardless of suspected etiology (Fig. 50-4). Recurrent syncope in the absence of a diagnosis may also be an indication for admission. When patients in such a selected group undergo a thorough evaluation, including an electrophysiologic study, an arrhythmic basis for syncope can be found in the majority of patients (Fig. 50-5). Negative results are often as important as actual identification of an arrhythmia, since they usually denote a favorable long-term prognosis. Long-term follow-up suggests that a reduction in both morbidity and mortality can be achieved by therapy guided by electrophysiologic study results. Unfortunately, no controlled studies exist (or are likely to be done) to conclusively establish these benefits.

The diagnostic evaluation of the patient with syncope of unknown cause presents a perplexing problem, particularly when syncope occurs repeatedly. The varying mortality (0 to 12 percent) in the patient with syncope so categorized undoubtedly reflects the varying incidence of undetected cardiac syncope despite careful evaluation. It

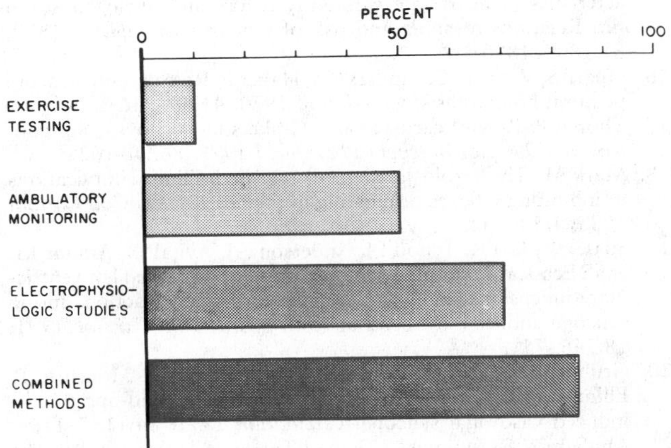

FIGURE 50-5 The sensitivity of exercise testing, ambulatory monitoring (including use of transtelephonic devices), and electrophysiologic testing singly and in combination in detecting arrhythmia as a cause of syncope in patients suspected of having arrhythmic syncope. *(From Boudoulas et al.[82] Reproduced with permission from the publisher and author.)*

is reasonable to suspect that, as the understanding of the mechanisms and the breadth of causes of syncope improves (particularly the role of multiple causes), the high incidence of patients with syncope of unknown cause will diminish.

REFERENCES

1. Savage DD, Corwin L, McGee DL, Kannel WB, Wolf PA: Epidemiologic features of isolated syncope: The Framingham Study. *Stroke* 1985; 16:626–629.
2. Eagle KA, Black HR, Cook EF, Goldman L: Evaluation of prognostic classifications for patients with syncope. *Am J Med* 1985; 79:455–460.
3. Martin GJ, Adams SL, Martin HG, Mathews J, Zull D, Scanlon PJ: Prospective evaluation of syncope. *Ann Emerg Med* 1984; 13:499–504.
4. Day SC, Cook EF, Funkenstein H, Goldman L: Evaluation and outcome of emergency room patients with transient loss of consciousness. *Am J Med* 1982; 73:15–23.
5. Silverstein MD, Singer DE, Mulley AG, Thibault GE, Barnett GO: Patients with syncope admitted to medical intensive care units. *JAMA* 1982; 248:1185–1189.
6. Kapoor WN, Karpf M, Wieland S, Peterson JR, Levey GS: A prospective evaluation and follow-up of patients with syncope. *N Engl J Med* 1983; 309:197–204.
7. Ben-Chetrit E, Flugelman M, Eliakim M: Syncope: A retrospective study of 101 hospitalized patients. *Isr J Med Sci* 1985; 21:950–952.
8. Manolis AS, Linzer M, Deeb S, Estes NA III: Syncope: Current diagnostic evaluation and management. *Ann Intern Med* 1990; 112:850–864.
9. Kapoor W, Snustad D, Peterson J, Weiland HS, Cha R, Karpf M: Syncope in the elderly. *Am J Med* 1986; 80:419–428.
10. Engel GL, Romano J: Studies of syncope: 4. Biologic interpretations of vasodepressor syncope. *Psychosom Med* 1947; 9:288–294.
11. Weissler AM, Warren JV, Estes EH, McIntosh HD, Leonard JJ: Vasodepressor syncope: Factors influencing cardiac output. *Circulation* 1957; 15:875–882.
12. Weissler AM, Warren JV: Vasodepressor syncope. *Am Heart J* 1959; 57:786–791.
13. Wallin BG, Sundloff G: Sympathetic outflow to muscles during the vasovagal syncope. *J Auton Nerv Syst* 1982; 6:287–291.
14. Goldstein DS, Spanarkel M, Pitterman A, Toltzis R, Gratz E, Epstein S, et al: Circulatory control mechanisms in vasodepressor syncope. *Am Heart J* 1982; 104:1071–1075.
15. Lipsitz LA, Mietus J, Moody GB, Goldberger AL: Spectral characteristics of heart rate variability before and during postural tilt: Relations to aging and risk of syncope. *Circulation* 1990; 81:1803–1810.
16. Oparil S, Vassaux C, Sanders CA, Haber E: Role of renin in acute postural homeostasis. *Circulation* 1970; 41:89–94.
17. Thoren P: Role of cardiac vagal C-fibers in cardiovascular control. *Rev Physiol Biochem Pharmacol* 1979; 86:90–102.
18. Mark AL: The Bezold-Jarish reflex revisited: Clinical implications of inhibiting reflexes originating in the heart. *J Am Coll Cardiol* 1983; 1:50–102.
19. Shalev Y, Gal R, Tchou PJ, Anderson AJ, Avitall B, Ahktar M, et al: Echocardiographic demonstration of decreased left ventricular dimensions and vigorous myocardial contraction during syncope induced by head-up tilt. *J Am Coll Cardiol* 1991; 18:746–751.
20. Grubb BP, Gerard G, Roush K, Tenesy-Armos P, Montford P, Elliott L, et al: Cerebral vasoconstriction during head-upright tilt-induced vasovagal syncope. *Circulation* 1991; 84:1157–1164.
21. Abi-Samra F, Maloney J, Fouad-Tarazi FM, Castle LW: The usefulness of head-up tilt testing and hemodynamic investigations in the workup of syncope of unknown origin. *PACE* 1988; 11:1202–1214.
22. Kenny RA, Bayliss J, Ingram A, Sutton R: Head-up tilt: A useful test for investigating unexplained syncope. *Lancet* 1986; 1:1352–1355.
23. Strasberg B, Rechavia E, Sagie A, Kusniec F, Mager A, Sclarvsky S, et al: The head-up tilt table test in patients with syncope of unknown origin. *Am Heart J* 1989; 118:923–927.
24. Pongiglione G, Fish FA, Strasburger JF, Benson W Jr: Heart rate and blood pressure response to upright tilt in young patients with unexplained syncope. *J Am Coll Cardiol* 1990; 16:165–170.
25. Sra JS, Anderson AJ, Sheikh SH, Avitall B, Tchou PJ, Troup PJ, et al: Unexplained syncope evaluated by electrophysiologic studies and head-up tilt testing. *Ann Intern Med* 1991; 114:1013–1019.
26. Raviele A, Gasparini G, DiPede F, Delise P, Bonso A, Piccolo E: Usefulness of head-up tilt test in evaluating patients with syncope of unknown origin and negative electrophysiologic study. *Am J Cardiol* 1990; 65:1322–1327.
27. Fitzpatrick AP, Theodorakis G, Vardis P, Sutton R: Methodology of head-up tilt testing in patients with unexplained syncope. *J Am Coll Cardiol* 1991; 17:125–130.
28. Almquist A, Goldberg IF, Milstein S, Chen MY, Chen X, Hansen R, et al: Provocation of bradycardia and hypotension by isoproterenol and upright posture in patients with unexplained syncope. *N Engl J Med* 1989; 320:346–351.
29. Perry JC, Garson A Jr: The child with recurrent syncope: Autonomic function testing and beta adrenergic hypersensitivity. *J Am Coll Cardiol* 1991; 17:1168–1171.
30. Milstein S, Buetikofer J, Dunnigan A, Benditt DG, Gormick C, Reyes WJ: Usefulness of disopyramide for prevention of upright tilt-induced hypotension-bradycardia. *Am J Cardiol* 1990; 65:1339–1344.
31. Benditt DG, Benson W, Dreitt J, Dunnigan A, Pritzker MR, Crouse L, et al: Electrophysiologic effects of theophylline in young patients with recurrent symptomatic bradyarrhythmias. *Am J Cardiol* 1983; 52:1223–1229.
32. Nelson SD, Stanley MR, Love CJ, Coyne KS, Schaal SF: The autonomic and hemodynamic effects of oral theophylline in patients with vasodepressor syncope. *Arch Intern Med* 1991; 151:2425–2429.
33. Milstein S, Buetikofer J, Lesser J, Goldenberg IF, Benditt DG, Gornick CC, et al: Cardiac asystole: A manifestation of neurally-mediated hypotension-bradycardia. *J Am Coll Cardiol* 1989; 14:1626–1632.
34. McLaran CJ, Gersch BJ, Osborn MJ: Increased vagal tone as an isolated finding in patients undergoing electrophysiologic testing for recurrent syncope: Response to long-term anticholinergic agents. *Br Heart J* 1986; 55:53–57.
35. Schatz IJ: Orthostatic hypotension. *Arch Intern Med* 1984; 144:773,1037–1043.
36. Thomas JE, Schirger A, Fealey RD, Sheps SG: Orthostatic hypotension. *Mayo Clin Proc* 1981; 156:117–125.
37. Johnson RH: Orthostatic hypotension in neurological disease. *Cardiology* 1976; 61(suppl 1):150–152.
38. Ziegler MG: Postural hypotension. *Ann Rev Med* 1980; 31:239–245.
39. Hilsted J, Parving HH, Christensen NJ, Galbo H: Hemodynamics in diabetic orthostatic hypotension. *J Clin Invest* 1981; 68:1427–1434.
40. Page MM, Watkins PJ: Provocation of postural hypotension by insulin in diabetic autonomic neuropathy. *Diabetes* 1976; 25:90–95.
41. Polinsky RJ, Taylor IL, Chew P, Weise V, Kopin IJ: Pancreatic polypeptide responses to hypoglycemia in chronic autonomic failure. *J Clin Endocrinol Metab* 1982; 54:48–52.
42. Cryer PE, Silverberg AB, Santiago JV, Shah SD: Plasma catecholamines in diabetes: The syndromes of hypoadrenergic and hyperadrenergic postural hypotension. *Am J Med* 1978; 64:407–416.
43. Bradbury S, Eggleston C: Postural hypotension: A report of three cases. *Am Heart J* 1925; 1:73–86.
44. Shy GM, Drager GA: A neurologic syndrome associated with orthostatic hypotension. *Arch Neurol* 1960; 2:511–527.
45. Kontos HA, Richardson DW, Norvell JE: Norepinephrine depletion in idiopathic orthostatic hypotension. *Ann Intern Med* 1975; 82:336–341.
46. Ziegler MG, Lake CR, Kopin IJ: The sympathetic-nervous-system defect in primary orthostatic hypotension. *N Engl J Med* 1977; 296:293–297.
47. Bannister R, Crowe R, Eames R, Burnstock G: Adrenergic innervation in autonomic failure. *Neurology* 1981; 31:1501–1506.
48. Kopin IJ, Polinsky RJ, Oliver JA, Oddershede IR, Eberj MH:

Urinary catecholamine metabolites distinguish different types of sympathetic neuronal dysfunction in patients with orthostatic hypotension. *J Clin Endocrinol Metab* 1983; 57:632–637.

49. Khurana RK, Nelson E, Azzarelli B, Garcia JH: Shy-Drager syndrome: Diagnosis and treatment of cholinergic dysfunction. *Neurology* 1980; 30:805–809.
50. McGrath BP, Stern AI, Esler M, Hansky J: Impaired pancreatic polypeptide release to insulin hypoglycaemia in chronic autonomic failure with postural hypotension: Evidence for parasympathetic dysfunction. *Clin Sci* 1982; 63:321–323.
51. Bousser MG, Dubois B, Castaigne P: Transient loss of consciousness in ischemic cerebral events: A study of 557 ischemic strokes and transient ischemic attacks. *Ann Med Intern* 1980; 132:300–307.
52. Weiss S, Baker JP: The carotid sinus reflex in health and disease: Its role in the causation of fainting and convulsions. *Medicine* 1933; 12:297–354.
53. Davies AB, Stephens MR, Davies AG: Carotid sinus hypersensitivity in patients presenting with syncope. *Br Heart J* 1979; 42:583–586.
54. Walter PF, Crawley IS, Dorney ER: Carotid sinus hypersensitivity and syncope. *Am J Cardiol* 1978; 42:396–403.
55. Huang SK, Erzi MD, Hauser RG, Davis P: Carotid sinus hypersensitivity in patients with unexplained syncope: Clinical, electrophysiologic, and long-term follow-up observations. *Am Heart J* 1988; 116:989–996.
56. Patel AK, Yap VU, Fields J, Thomsen JH: Carotid sinus syncope induced by malignant tumors in the neck: Emergence of vasodepressor manifestations following pacemaker therapy. *Arch Intern Med* 1979; 139:1281–1288.
57. Matthew TK, Huang MT, Mathew PK: Carotid sinus syncope as a manifestation of parotid tumors. *Am Heart J* 1982; 104:316–319.
58. Muntz HR, Smith PG: Carotid sinus hypersensitivity: A cause of syncope in patients with tumors of the head and neck. *Laryngoscope* 1983; 93:1290–1293.
59. Peretz DI, Abdulla A: Management of cardioinhibitory hypersensitive carotid sinus syncope with permanent cardiac pacing: A seventeen year prospective study. *Can J Cardiol* 1985; 1:86–93.
60. Morley CA, Perrins EJ, Grant P, Chan SL, McBrien DJ, Sutton R: Carotid sinus syncope treated by pacing analysis of persistent symptoms and role of atrioventricular sequential pacing. *Br Heart J* 1982; 47:411–418.
61. Brignole M, Menozzi C, Lolli G, Sartore B, Barra M: Natural and unnatural history of patients with severe carotid sinus hypersensitivity: A preliminary study. *PACE* 1988; 11:1628–1635.
62. Levin B, Posner JB: Swallow syncope. *Neurology* 1972; 22:1086–1093.
63. Bortolotti M, Cirignotta F, Labo G: Atrioventricular block induced by swallowing in a patient with diffuse esophageal spasm. *JAMA* 1982; 248:2297–2299.
64. Dykman TR, Montgomery IB, Gerstenberger PD, Zeiger HE, Clutter WE, Cryer PE: Glossopharyngeal neuralgia with syncope secondary to tumor. *Am J Med* 1981; 71:165–170.
65. St John JN: Glossopharyngeal neuralgia associated with syncope and seizures. *Neurosurgery* 1982; 10:380–383.
66. Hart G, Oldershaw PJ, Cull RE, Humphrey P, Ward D: Syncope caused by cough-induced complete atrioventricular block. *PACE* 1982; 5:564–566.
67. Saito D, Matsuno S, Matsushita K, Takeda H, Hyodo T, Haraoka S, et al: Cough syncope due to atrioventricular conduction block. *Jpn Heart J* 1982; 23:1015–1020.
68. Hampton B, Williams B, Loizou L: Syncope as a presenting feature of hindbrain herniation with syringomyelia. *J Neurol Neurosurg Psychiatry* 1982; 45:919–922.
69. Corbett JJ, Butler AB, Kaufman B: "Sneeze syncope," basilar invagination and Arnold-Chiari type I malformation. *J Neurol Neurosurg Psychiatry* 1976; 39:381–384.
70. Godec CJ, Cass AS: Micturition syncope. *J Urol* 1981; 126:551–556.
71. Kapoor WN, Peterson J, Karpf M: Defecation syncope: A symptom with multiple etiologies. *Arch Intern Med* 1986; 146:2377–2382.
72. Aminoff MJ, Scheimman MM, Griffin JC, Herre JM: Electrocerebral accompaniments of syncope associated with malignant ventricular arrhythmias. *Ann Intern Med* 1988; 108:791–796.
73. Constantin L, Martins JB, Fincham RW, Dagli RD: Bradycardia and syncope as manifestations of partial epilepsy. *J Am Coll Cardiol* 1990; 15:900–905.
74. Lai C-W, Ziegler DK: Syncope problem solved by continuous ambulatory simultaneous EEG/ECG recording. *Neurology* 1981; 31:1152–1154.
75. Davis TL, Jreeman FR: Electroencephalography should not be routine in the evaluation of syncope in adults. *Arch Intern Med* 1990; 150:2027–2029.
76. Bickerstaff ER: Impairment of consciousness in migraine. *Lancet* 1961; 2:1057–1059.
77. Sicuteri E, Boccuni M, Fanciullacci M, D'Egidio P, Bonciani M: A new nonvascular interpretation of syncopal migraine. *Adv Neurol* 1982; 33:199–208.
78. Grech ED, Ramsdale DR: Exertional syncope in aortic stenosis: Evidence to support inappropriate left ventricular baroreceptor response. *Am Heart J* 1991; 121:603–606.
79. Schwartz LS, Goldfisher J, Sprague GJ, Schwartz SP: Syncope and sudden death in aortic stenosis. *Am J Cardiol* 1969; 23:647–658.
80. Nienaber CA, Hiller S, Speilmann RP, Geiger M, Kuck KH: Syncope in hypertrophic cardiomyopathy: Multivariate analysis of prognostic determinants. *J Am Coll Cardiol* 1990; 15:948–955.
81. Dressler W: Effort syncope as an early manifestation of primary pulmonary hypertension. *Am J Med Sci* 1952; 223:131–143.
82. Boudoulas H, Weissler AM, Lewis RP, Warren JV: The clinical diagnosis of syncope. *Curr Probl Cardiol* 1982; 7(7):6–40.
83. Medine RP, Dreifus LS: Syncope. *Curr Probl Cardiol* 1983; 8(6):1–50.
84. Scarpa WJ: The sick sinus syndrome. *Am Heart J* 1983; 92:648–651.
85. Moss AJ, Davis RJ: Brady-tachy syndrome. *Prog Cardiovasc Dis* 1974; 16:439–454.
86. McAnulty JH, Kauffman S, Murphy E, Kassebaum DG, Rahimtoola SH: Survival in patients with intraventricular conduction defects. *Arch Intern Med* 1978; 138:30–35.
87. Scheinman MM, Peters RW, Sauve MJ, Gonzalez R: Value of the H-Q interval in patients with bundle branch block and the role of prophylactic permanent pacing. *Am J Cardiol* 1982; 50:1316–1322.
88. Kaul U, Dev V, Narula J, Malhotra AK, Talwar KK, Bahatia ML: Evaluation of patients with bundle branch block and "unexplained" syncope: A study based on comprehensive electrophysiologic testing and ajmaline stress. *PACE* 1988; 11:289–297.
89. Steinbrecher UP, Fitchett DH: Torsade de pointes: A cause of syncope with atrioventricular block. *Arch Intern Med* 1980; 140:1223–1226.
90. Kadish AH, Wechsler L, Marchlinski FE: Swallowing syncope: Observations in the absence of conduction system or esophageal disease. *Am J Med* 1986; 81:1098–1103.
91. Kofflard M, DeBoer H, Van Mechelen R: Reflex cardiac asystole. *PACE* 1986; 9:908–911.
92. Talwar KK, Edvardsson N, Varnauskas E: Paroxysmal vagally mediated AV block with recurrent syncope. *Clin Cardiol* 1985; 8:337–340.
93. Albin G, Hayes DL, Holmes DR Jr: Sinus node dysfunction in pediatric and young adult patients: Treatment by implantation of a permanent pacemaker in 39 cases. *Mayo Clin Proc* 1985; 60:667–672.
94. Beder SD, Cohen MH, Riemenschneider TA: Occult arrhythmias as the etiology of unexplained syncope in children with structurally normal hearts. *Am Heart J* 1985; 109:309–313.
95. Boudoulas H, Wooley CF: *Mitral Valve Prolapse and the Mitral Valve Prolapse Syndrome.* Mt Kisco, NY, Futura Publishing, 1988.
96. Ezri MD, Jacobs LG, Denes P: Unexpected coexistence of supraventricular and ventricular tachycardia in patients with syncope. *PACE* 1985; 8:329–340.
97. Moss AJ, Schwartz PJ, Crampton RS, Tzivoni D, Locati EH, MacCluer J, et al: The long QT syndrome: Prospective longitudinal study of 328 families. *Circulation* 1991; 84:1136–1144.
98. Soffer J, Dreifus LS, Michelson EL: Polymorphous ventricular tachycardia associated with normal and long QT intervals. *Am J Cardiol* 1982; 138:30–35.
99. Krikler DM, Curry PV: Torsade de pointes: An atypical ventricular tachycardia. *Br Heart J* 1976; 38:117–120.
100. Alicandri C, Fouad FM, Tarazi RC, Castle L, Morant V: Three

cases of hypotension and syncope with ventricular pacing: Possible role of atrial reflexes. *Am J Cardiol* 1978; 42:137–142.
101. Ausubel K, Boal BH, Furmen S: Pacemaker syndrome: Definition and evaluation. *Cardiol Clin* 1985; 3:587–589.
102. Kuchar DL, Thorburn CW, Sammel NL: Signal averaged electrocardiogram for evaluation of recurrent syncope. *Am J Cardiol* 1986; 58:949–953.
103. Gang ES, Peter T, Rosenthal ME, Oseran D, Mandel WJ, Deng ZW, et al: Detection of late potentials on the surface electrocardiogram in unexplained syncope. *Am J Cardiol* 1986; 58:1014–1020.
104. Winters SL, Stewart D, Gomes JA: Signal averaging of the surface QRS complex predicts inducibility of ventricular tachycardia in patients with syncope of unknown origin: A prospective study. *J Am Coll Cardiol* 1987; 10:775–781.
105. Nalos PC, Gang ES, Mandel WJ, Laddenheim ML, Lass Y, Peter T: The signal averaged electrocardiogram as a screening test for inducibility of sustained ventricular tachycardia in high risk patients: A prospective study. *J Am Coll Cardiol* 1987; 9:539–548.
106. Boudoulas H, Schaal SF, Lewis RP, Robinson JL: Superiority of 24-hour outpatient monitoring over multi-stage exercise testing for the evaluation of syncope. *J Electrocardiol* 1979; 12:103–108.
107. Boudoulas H, Geleris P, Schaal SF, Leier CV, Lewis RP: Comparison between electrophysiologic studies and ambulatory monitoring in patients with syncope. *J Electrocardiol* 1983; 16:91–96.
108. Dewey RC, Capeless MA, Levy AM: Use of ambulatory electrocardiographic monitoring to identify high risk patients with congenital complete heart block. *N Engl J Med* 1987; 316:835–839.
109. Kapoor WN, Cha R, Peterson JR, Wieand HS, Karpf M: Prolonged electrocardiographic monitoring in patients with syncope: Importance of frequent or repetitive ventricular ectopy. *Am J Med* 1987; 82:20–28.
110. Hysing J, Grendahl H: Ambulatory 24 hour ECG in patients with a history of syncope: A retrospective follow-up study over 2 years. *Eur Heart J* 1985; 6:120–122.
111. Gibson TC, Heitzman MR: Diagnostic efficacy of 24 hour electrocardiographic monitoring for syncope. *Am J Cardiol* 1984; 53:1013–1017.
112. Linzer M, Prystowsky EN, Brunetti LL, Varia IM, German LD: Recurrent syncope of unknown origin diagnosed by ambulatory continuous loop ECG recording. *Am Heart J* 1988; 116:1632–1634.
113. Lewis RP, Boudoulas H, Voto S, Schaal SF, Stang JM: Arrhythmic syncope: What to do when ambulatory monitoring is non-diagnostic. *Trans Am Clin Climatol Assoc* 1985; 96:131–140.
114. Shen WK, Holmes DR Jr, Hammill SC: Transtelephonic monitoring: Documentation of transient cardiac rhythm disturbances. *Mayo Clin Proc* 1987; 63:109–112.
115. DiMarco JP, Garan H, Harthorne JW, Ruskin JN: Intracardiac electrophysiologic techniques in recurrent syncope of unknown cause. *Ann Intern Med* 1981; 95:542–548.
116. Bhandari AK, Shapiro, WA, Shen EN, Morady F, Mason J, Scheinman MM: Electrophysiologic testing in patients with the long QT syndrome. *Circulation* 1985; 71:63–71.
117. Reiffel JA, Wang P, Bower R, Bigger JT, Livelli F Jr, Ferrick K, et al: Electrophysiologic testing in patients with recurrent syncope: Are results predicted by prior ambulatory monitoring? *Am Heart J* 1985; 110:1146–1153.
118. Teichman SL, Felder SD, Matos JA, Kim SG, Waspe LE, Fisher JD: The value of electrophysiologic studies in syncope of undetermined origin: Report of 150 cases. *Am Heart J* 1985; 110:469–479.
119. Denes P, Ezri MD: The role of electrophysiologic studies in management of patients with unexplained syncope. *PACE* 1985; 8:424–435.
120. Olshansky B, Mazuz M, Martins JB: Significance of inducible tachycardia in patients with syncope of unknown origin: A long-term follow-up. *J Am Coll Cardiol* 1985; 5:216–223.
121. Kaul U, Karla GS, Talwar KK, Bhatia ML: The value of intracardiac electrophysiologic techniques in recurrent syncope of "unknown cause." *Int J Cardiol* 1986; 10:23–31.
122. Click RL, Gersh BJ, Sugrue DD, Holmes DR Jr, Wood KL, Osburn MJ, et al: Role of invasive electrophysiologic testing in patients with symptomatic bundle branch block. *Am J Cardiol* 1987; 59:817–823.
123. Krol RB, Morady F, Flaker G, DiCarlo LA Jr, Baerman JM, Hewett J, et al: Electrophysiologic testing in patients with unexplained syncope: Clinical and noninvasive predictors of outcome. *J Am Coll Cardiol* 1987; 10:358–363.
124. Doherty JU, Pembrook-Rogers D, Grogan EW, Falcone R, Buxton AE, Marchlinski FE, et al: Electrophysiologic evaluation and follow-up characteristics of patients with recurrent unexplained syncope and presyncope. *Am J Cardiol* 1985; 55:703–708.
125. Kushner JA, Kou WH, Kadish AM, Moran F: Natural history of patients with unexplained syncope and a nondiagnostic electrophysiologic study. *J Am Coll Cardiol* 1989; 74:391–396.
126. Bass EB, Elson JJ, Fogoros RN, Peterson J, Arena VC, Kapoor WN: Long-term prognosis of patients undergoing electrophysiologic studies for syncope of unknown origin. *Am J Cardiol* 1988; 62:1922–1928.
127. Boudoulas H, Schaal SF, Lewis RP: Electrophysiologic risk factors in syncope. *J Electrocardiol* 1978; 11:339–342.
128. Mitchell LB, Duff HJ, Manyari DE, Wyse DG: A randomized clinical trial of the noninvasive and invasive approaches to drug therapy of ventricular tachycardia. *N Engl J Med* 1987; 317:1681–1687.
129. Morady F, Shen E, Schwartz A: Long-term follow-up of patients with recurrent unexplained syncope evaluated by electrophysiologic testing. *J Am Coll Cardiol* 1983; 2:1053–1059.
130. Baedeker W, Stein H, Theiss W, Geodel-Meimer L, Schmidt G, Blomer H: Syncopes of unclear etiology: Diagnosis, follow-up observations and pacemaker therapy. *Dtsch Med Wochenschr* 1987; 112:128–134.
131. Bellinder G, Nordlander R, Pehrsson SK, Astrom H: Atrial pacing in the management of sick sinus syndrome: Long-term observation for conduction disturbances and supraventricular tachyarrhythmias. *Eur Heart J* 1986; 7:105–109.
132. Langenfeld H, Grimm W, Marsch B, Dochsiek K: Course of symptoms and spontaneous ECG in pacemaker patients: A 5-year follow-up study. *PACE* 1988; 11:2198–2206.
133. Bhandari AK, Scheinman M: The long QT syndrome. *Mod Concepts Cardiovasc Dis* 1985; 54:45–51.
134. Moss AJ, Liu JE, Gottlieb S, Locati EH, Schwartz PJ, Robinson JL: Efficacy of permanent pacing in the management of high-risk patients with long QT syndrome. *Circulation* 1991; 84:1524–1529.
135. Weiner DA, Levine SR, Klein MD: Ventricular arrhythmias during exercise testing: Mechanism, response to coronary bypass surgery and prognostic significance. *Am J Cardiol* 1984; 53:1553–1559.
136. Echt DS, Armstrong K, Schmidt P, Dyer PE, Stinson EB, Winkle RA: Clinical experience, complications, and survival in 70 patients with the automatic implantable cardiovertor/defibrillator. *Circulation* 1985; 71:289–296.
137. Scheinman MM: Nonpharmacologic treatment of life-threatening cardiac arrhythmias. *Am Heart J* 1987; 114:1291–1298.
138. Manolis AS, Rastegar H, Estes NA: Automatic implantable cardiovertor defibrillator: Current status. *JAMA* 1989; 262:1362–1368.
139. Mirowski M, Reid PR, Mower MM, Watkins L, Gott VL, Schauble JF, et al: Termination of malignant ventricular arrhythmias with an implanted automatic defibrillator in human beings. *N Engl J Med* 1980; 330:322–324.
140. Jackman WM, Xunzhang W, Friday K, Roman C, Moulton KP, Beckman KJ, et al: Catheter ablation of accessory atrioventricular pathways (Wolff-Parkinson-White syndrome) by radiofrequency current. *N Engl J Med* 1991; 324:1605–1611.
141. Calkins H, Sousa J, El-Atassi R, Rosensheck S, de Buitleir H, Kou WH, et al: Diagnosis and cure of the Wolff-White-Parkinson syndrome or paroxysmal supraventricular tachycardia during a single electrophysiologic test. *N Engl J Med* 1991; 324:1612–1618.
142. Lipsitz LA: Syncope in the elderly. *Ann Intern Med* 1983; 99:92–105.
143. Lipsitz LA: The drop attack: A common geriatric symptom. *J Am Geriatr Soc* 1983; 31:617–620.
144. Rubenstein LZ, Robbins AS, Josephson KR, Schulman BL, Osterweil D: The value of assessing falls in an elderly population: A randomized clinical trial. *Ann Intern Med* 1990; 113:308–316.
145. Lipsitz LA, Marks ER, Koestner J, Jonsson PV, Wei JY: Reduced susceptibility to syncope during postural tilt in old age: Is beta-blockade protective? *Arch Intern Med* 1989; 149:2709–2712.

146. Jonsson PV, Lipsitz LA, Kelley M, Koestner J: Hypotensive responses to common daily activities in institutionalized elderly. *Arch Intern Med* 1990; 150:1518–1524.
147. Lipsitz LA, Nyquist RP Jr, Wei JY, Rowe JW: Postprandial reduction in blood pressure in the elderly. *N Engl J Med* 1983; 309:81–83.
148. Adams R: Cases of diseases of the heart, accompanied with pathological observations. *Dublin Hospital Reports* 1827; 4:353–453.
149. Stokes W: Observations on some permanently slow pulse. *Dublin Quarterly J C Med Sci* 1846; 2:73–85.
150. Kapoor WN, Peterson J, Wieand HS, Karpf M: Diagnostic and prognostic implications of recurrences in patients with syncope. *Am J Med* 1987; 83:700–708.
151. Boudoulas H, Lewis RP: Cardiac syncope: Diagnosis, mechanism, and management. In: Hurst JW (ed): *The Heart,* 6th ed. New York, McGraw-Hill, 1986: 321–529.
152. Boudoulas H: Should patients with cardiovascular disease and unexplained syncope undergo invasive electrophysiologic study? In: Gitnick G (ed): *Debates in Medicine,* vol 4. St. Louis, Mosby Year Book, 1991: 4–14.

Chapter 51

The Mechanisms, Predictors, and Prevention of Sudden Cardiac Death

Leonard A. Cobb, M.D.

DEFINITION OF SUDDEN CARDIAC DEATH

Sudden cardiac death results from diverse mechanisms and conditions; accordingly, none of several proposed definitions is entirely satisfactory. For epidemiologic purposes and for practical considerations, however, this disorder may be defined as unexpected cardiac death, occurring outside of hospital and preceded by no apparent symptoms or by symptoms less than 1 h in duration.[1–4] Most episodes are considered to be the result of cardiac arrhythmias.

COMMUNITY IMPACT OF SUDDEN CARDIAC DEATH

Of all deaths from coronary atherosclerotic heart disease, one-half to two-thirds can be classified as sudden cardiac deaths. In the United States the incidence of sudden cardiac death approximates 400,000 per year, an estimated 80 percent due to atherosclerotic coronary heart disease. It is important to note that there appears to have been a decline in the incidence of out-of-hospital cardiac arrest in the past decade,[5,6] probably reflecting the substantial reduction in age-adjusted mortality attributable to atherosclerotic coronary heart disease in the United States as well as in other Western nations. Most victims have had prior signs or symptoms of cardiovascular disease; however, in 20 to 25 percent of cases, cardiac arrest is the first such manifestation. There is a distinct predominance of males, whose average age approximates 65 years.[1,5] Although sudden cardiac death typically occurs during the routine activities of daily life,[7,8] there appears to be an additional risk for sudden cardiac arrest during physical exertion.[9–11] The net effect of that additional hazard is probably not great, considering the limited exposure to vigorous exercise in most persons. It is important to note that approximately one-half the victims of sudden cardiac death are under age 65 and that a large proportion do not have major functional impairment. Accordingly, a concept of "premature" death requires emphasis.

MECHANISMS UNDERLYING SUDDEN CARDIAC DEATH

Importance of Ventricular Fibrillation

The majority of sudden cardiac deaths are thought to be precipitated by ventricular fibrillation.[7,11] Although the electrical events immediately prior to collapse have been recorded and reported in only a small number of patients, ventricular fibrillation has often been confirmed.[12,13] Asystole or profound bradycardia has occasionally been recorded shortly after the onset of unexpected cardiac arrest, but those conditions are most likely to be encountered in situations in which there has been substantial delay in initiating emergency care or where an abrupt collapse has terminated an illness with an anticipated fatal outcome.[7,14,15] In the setting of acute myocardial ischemia the sudden onset of electromechanical dissociation is usually fatal but, on occasion, may be impressively reversible.[16]

Ventricular Fibrillation versus Ventricular Tachycardia

Although much attention has been focused on the management of patients referred to tertiary care centers because of recurrent, symptomatic ventricular tachycardia, those patients represent only a very small proportion of persons who develop unexpected cardiac arrest, probably less than 5 percent.[5,17] It is noteworthy that electrocardiograms recorded at the onset of cardiac arrest often demonstrate that ventricular fibrillation was preceded by a few beats of ventricular tachycardia.[12,13]

Myocardial Ischemia

A relationship between ventricular fibrillation and acute myocardial ischemia has been convincingly shown in animal experiments in which a major coronary artery is acutely occluded. In such models, ischemia quickly leads to intracellular and extracellular acidosis, loss of cellular membrane integrity, and lowering of the resting transmembrane potential.[18] As depolarization and conduction are slowed, conditions are created for fragmented electrical activity and local reentrant pathways, thereby facilitating the emergence of ventricular fibrillation. Such experimentally produced arrhythmias appear relevant to acute myocardial infarction secondary to occlusion of a coronary artery and also to transient myocardial ischemia due either to fixed or dynamic coronary arterial narrowing. (See also Chaps. 34 and 35.)

From a clinical point of view, however, the importance of transient myocardial ischemia in precipitating cardiac arrest is unclear. It is certainly reasonable to consider ischemia, or subsequent reperfusion, as potentially causal for the development of ventricular fibrillation in patients with atherosclerotic coronary heart disease; but at the same time, it is difficult to estimate the magnitude of that relationship in victims of sudden cardiac death.[19,20]

Neural and Neurohumoral Influences

For decades, clinicians have considered arousal of the autonomic nervous system to be a potential factor in the genesis of ventricular (as well as supraventricular) arrhythmias,[21] and the abundance of experimental evidence for that interaction is striking. In models of myocardial ischemia catecholamines, sympathetic stimulation, or perturbation of parasympathetic tone may all influence the development of ventricular arrhythmias.[22,23] Interestingly, the propensity for sudden death to occur in the morning hours has been tentatively linked to increases in plasma catecholamines and enhancement of platelet aggregation.[24] (See also Chaps. 58 to 60.)

Microscopic Correlates of Sudden Cardiac Death

Scattered areas of selective myocardial cell necrosis (myocytolysis) are present in most sudden death victims[25] (Fig. 51-1). There is also evidence for a relationship between microscopic areas of cellular necrosis and platelet emboli, particularly in deaths related to unstable angina.[20] Although direct evidence is lacking, it is possible that such lesions represent the consequences of neurohumoral stimulation, akin to the experimentally induced lesions that may follow several interventions, including catecholamine infusion.[26] Similar lesions have been described in patients with subarachnoid hemorrhage or pheochromocytoma and have also been observed in about one of four randomly selected patients undergoing autopsy. Hence, this microscopic lesion, possibly with

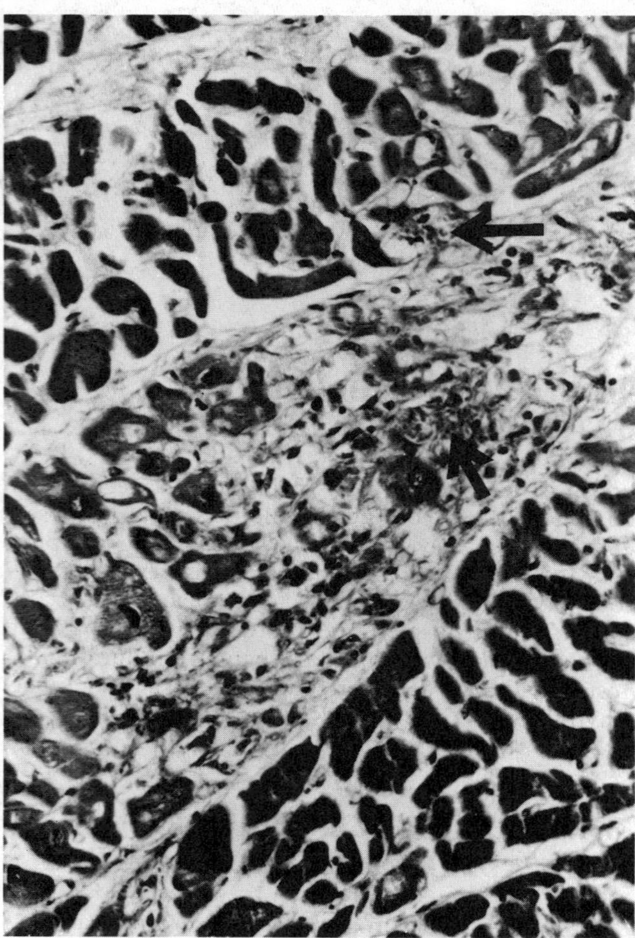

FIGURE 51-1 Left ventricular myocardium from a 53-year-old victim of sudden cardiac arrest due to coronary atherosclerosis. Relatively normal myocardial cells are present at the top and bottom. The central diagonal area shows changes indicative of cellular injury ranging from approximately 2 (arrows) to 7 days. Such patchy areas of selective myocardial cellular necrosis were present in 88 percent of consecutive victims.[25] Gomori Trichrome stain, approximately 150×. (*Photomicrograph kindly provided by D. D. Reichenbach, M.D.*)

important pathophysiological significance, is not specific for sudden cardiac death. Reichenbach and Moss[25] emphasized, however, that in sudden cardiac death, selective myocardial cell necrosis appears to antedate cardiac arrest.

Unstable Coronary Arterial Lesions

In patients with atherosclerotic coronary heart disease platelet turnover is typically accelerated, probably reflecting consumption and aggregation related to the atherosclerotic plaque. Although complete thrombotic occlusion of a coronary artery is likely responsible for only about one-quarter of sudden cardiac deaths,[27] one autopsy-based study has shown a considerably greater incidence of partially occlusive coronary arterial thrombi related to "unstable" atherosclerotic plaques.[28] At this time it is conjectural whether or not such thrombi represent a basis for ischemia-related arrhythmias. The relationship of these lesions to platelet aggregation and embolization also warrants further clarification.[29,30]

Predisposing Myocardial Substrate

Normal hearts rarely develop spontaneous ventricular fibrillation; and the most frequent clinical correlate of the sudden cardiac death syndrome is chronic myocardial dysfunction secondary to atherosclerotic coronary vascular disease, cardiomyopathic disorders, or valvular lesions. Myocardial hypertrophy is a special situation in which sudden death commonly occurs.[2,31] Although the linkage of these correlations to specific mechanisms is tentative, there is reason to implicate several pathological findings as being important in the establishment of reentrant pathways. For example, myocardial fibrosis, edema, or infiltrative processes might each lead to fractionated and nonhomogeneous conduction, thereby facilitating reentry and ventricular fibrillation. (See also Chap. 35.)

PERSONS AT RISK FOR SUDDEN CARDIAC DEATH

More than three-fourths of sudden cardiac deaths in the United States can be attributed to atherosclerotic coronary heart disease, typically with major obstruction of two or three coronary arteries.[1,27] On the other hand, a host of other cardiac lesions may also lead to unexpected cardiac arrest.[32] In the absence of structural heart disease or evident conduction abnormalities, sudden death is unusual, particularly when the event occurs nearly instantaneously.

Sudden Cardiac Death in Patients with Cardiac Disease Other Than Atherosclerotic Coronary Heart Disease

Approximately 20 percent of victims have cardiac diagnoses other than atherosclerotic coronary heart disease. Uncommon causes of sudden death include congenital anomalies of the coronary arteries (Chap. 97) and Marfan's syndrome (Chap. 123). For the purposes of this section, three major, noncoronary classifications are briefly considered: (1) cardiomyopathic syndromes, (2) valvular lesions, and (3) primary arrhythmic disturbances.

Cardiomyopathic Syndromes

Virtually any form of cardiomyopathy may culminate in unexpected cardiac arrest. Sudden cardiac death, however, assumes a particularly prominent role in the natural history of hypertrophic cardiomyopathy. Indeed, sudden death, probably due to ventricular fibrillation, is the most common mode of death in those patients, with or without subvalvular systolic pressure gradients. It is not clear if treatment, particularly with beta blockade or calcium channel blocking agents, affects either the prevalence of arrhythmias or the development of sudden death in these disorders.[31] The use of amiodarone in hypertrophic cardiomyopathy has been proposed as being useful in preventing cardiac arrest in patients with ventricular arrhythmias, but the available data are inconclusive.[33] (See also Chap. 90.)

Valvular Lesions

Sudden collapse is a relatively frequent mode of death in patients with aortic stenosis or aortic regurgitation. (See also Chap. 79.) Additionally, mitral valve prolapse syndromes have also been indicted as a cause of sudden death. In view of the large number of persons with mitral valve prolapse, however, sudden death is a rare complication in that disorder. (See also Chap. 80.)

Primary Arrhythmic Disturbances

Of the primary arrhythmic syndromes responsible for sudden death, atrioventricular block, ventricular preexcitation, and prolonged QT syndromes are most commonly described. While the latter are frequently associated with other cardiac or metabolic abnormalities, the congenitally prolonged QT syndromes are often isolated abnormalities. Drug therapy in the form of beta-blocking agents and/or excision of the left thoracic sympathetic chain may be effective in preventing cardiac arrest and recurrent syncope in patients with idiopathic QT prolongation.[34] (See also Chaps. 35 and 36.)

A perplexing form of nocturnal sudden cardiac death, without evident cardiomyopathy, was noted in the United States among Southeast Asian immigrants following the war in Vietnam.[35,36] That disorder has largely become extinct in the United States, presumably because of the declining rate of immigration. The syndrome probably continues to occur among the susceptible indigenous populations in Southeast Asia.

Significance of Coronary Risk Factors

In view of the very high proportion of sudden deaths due to atherosclerotic coronary heart disease, it is to be expected that established coronary risk factors would be prevalent in patients likely to develop sudden cardiac death. Indeed, hypertension, hypercholesterolemia, and/

or a history of cigarette smoking are commonly present in such persons.[2,37] An important observation in the Framingham experience was an association with cigarette smoking: Each of the men who died before age 65 of atherosclerotic coronary heart disease but without prior cardiovascular signs or symptoms was a cigarette smoker.[2]

Systemic Arterial Hypertension

Arterial hypertension warrants special comment because it may be the sole manifestation of cardiovascular disease prior to sudden cardiac death. Thus, in the Framingham cohort, high blood pressure was the only recognized cardiovascular abnormality in nearly one-fourth of sudden deaths due to atherosclerotic coronary heart disease in men aged 65 and younger. Furthermore, left ventricular hypertrophy on the electrocardiogram was present in an additional 19 percent, also without symptomatic heart disease.[2]

Cardiovascular Manifestations Prior to Sudden Death

Patients successfully resuscitated from out-of-hospital ventricular fibrillation usually have had one or more manifestations of cardiovascular disease prior to cardiac arrest. Histories of remote heart attack, angina, congestive heart failure, or hypertension were present in over 80 percent of Seattle patients who survived an aborted episode of sudden death; in the remaining patients, out-of-hospital cardiac arrest was the first indication of cardiovascular disease.[5] Comparable data were reported in the Framingham study; of 59 men who died suddenly, sudden cardiac arrest was the first manifestation of cardiovascular disease in 20 percent of men younger than 65 years.[2]

Recognition of High-Risk Patients

In groups of patients with atherosclerotic coronary heart disease and/or hypertension, four major characteristics have been shown to be associated with enhanced risk for sudden cardiac death: (1) ventricular electrical instability, (2) extensive coronary arterial narrowings, (3) abnormal left ventricular function, and (4) electrocardiographic conduction and repolarization abnormalities. Although these predictors have statistical significance in identifying groups of patients at risk for sudden cardiac death, they are less than satisfactory in both sensitivity and specificity, reflecting the seemingly erratic manner in which that disorder occurs.

Ventricular Electrical Instability Since ventricular fibrillation appears to underlie most episodes of sudden cardiac death, manifestations of myocardial electrical instability have been considered as potential harbingers; indeed, ventricular ectopy is commonly present in patients with atherosclerotic coronary heart disease who are likely to develop sudden cardiac death.[38–41] In particular, so-called complex forms of ventricular ectopy, i.e., multiform beats, repetitive forms, or early (R on T) ventricular depolarizations, have been recognized as statistical predictors of patients at high risk.

Although complex forms of ventricular ectopy are predictors of sudden cardiac death in patients with known atherosclerotic coronary heart disease, ventricular ectopic activity in persons without demonstrable heart disease appears to have little, if any, prognostic import.[38,42] At one time it was hoped that ventricular ectopic activity, detected by ambulatory electrocardiographic monitoring or during exercise, might prove to be a sensitive and specific marker of patients at risk for sudden cardiac death. Arrhythmias in patients with recognized coronary atherosclerotic heart disease are ubiquitous, however, and even high grades of ventricular ectopy fail to be useful predictors of patients at high risk. For example, in a carefully performed study by Ruberman et al.,[39] the detection of complex forms of ventricular ectopy was a statistically significant predictor of sudden cardiac death in ambulatory patients after myocardial infarction. On the other hand, 51 percent of the sudden deaths occurred in patients who *did not* have complex ventricular ectopy during the hour of monitoring. Furthermore, only 15 percent of those with complex ectopy developed sudden cardiac death during 4 years of observation.

Coronary Arterial Narrowing Patients who develop sudden cardiac death on the basis of atherosclerotic coronary heart disease typically have major obstruction (70 percent or greater diameter narrowing) in two or three coronary arteries.[1,27,43] Although some reports have described victims of sudden death as having most involvement in the left anterior descending coronary artery,[44] others have indicated that all three of the major coronary arterial systems appear to be equally affected.[27,43] Severe obstruction of the left main coronary artery is infrequently encountered in either survivors or nonsurvivors of out-of-hospital cardiac arrest.[27,43]

The extent of coronary artery narrowing, independent of other clinical findings, is not a specific predictor of sudden cardiac death.[45] There may, however, be a gradient for risk within specific subgroups.[43,46] For example, in ambulatory patients who had been resuscitated from an episode of out-of-hospital ventricular fibrillation, recurrent cardiac arrest was reported in nearly 50 percent of patients with triple-vessel narrowing, compared to only 10 percent of patients with single-vessel narrowing.[43]

Abnormal Ventricular Function In patients who had been resuscitated from ventricular fibrillation, Ritchie et al.[47] reported a high prevalence of left ventricular wall motion abnormalities, particularly in patients who later developed recurrent cardiac arrest. Also in that study there was a striking correlation between worsening left ventricular ejection fraction and recurrent cardiac arrest (Fig. 51-2). Another example of the association between impaired ventricular function and sudden cardiac death is found in the post–hospital phase of acute myocardial infarction where there is a relatively high mortality, commonly sudden death, during the first year after infarction.[48]

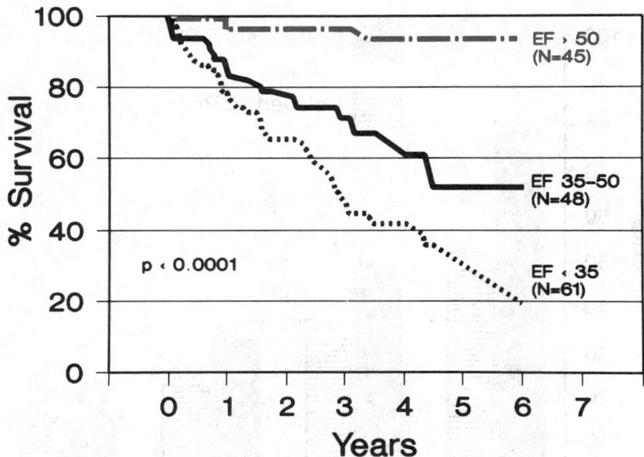

FIGURE 51-2 Survival in 154 patients with coronary atherosclerosis resuscitated from out-of-hospital cardiac arrest. The patients are grouped according to the radionuclide left ventricular ejection fraction performed an average of 4 months after resuscitation. During follow-up there were a total of 54 fatal events: 42 recurrences of sudden cardiac arrest, 6 other cardiac causes, and 6 noncardiac causes. (*From Ritchie et al: Out-of-hospital sudden coronary death: Rest and exercise radionuclide left ventricular function in survivors. Am J Cardiol 55:645, 1985. Reproduced with permission from the publisher and authors.*)

Because of the association between ventricular ectopic activity and abnormal ventricular function, it is debatable whether complex forms of ventricular ectopy are *independent* predictors of sudden death or whether the arrhythmias are merely reflective of a predisposing and vulnerable myocardial substrate. Ruberman and colleagues[39] reported that the predictive value of complex ventricular ectopy in identifying patients who later developed sudden death was independent of clinical manifestations of heart failure. When ventricular function is quantified by measurement of left ventricular ejection fraction, however, ventricular ectopy emerges as a much less powerful (but nonetheless independent) predictor in postinfarct patients[48] as well as survivors of out-of-hospital cardiac arrest.[47] Although there is clearly an interaction between ventricular ectopy and ventricular dysfunction, their ability to predict sudden cardiac death appears additive, the latter being of much greater significance.

Electrocardiographic Abnormalities of Conduction and Repolarization Resting electrocardiographic markers of patients with atherosclerotic coronary heart disease who are at greater than average risk for sudden death include abnormalities of conduction, prolongation of QT intervals, and ST-T changes.[37,41] On the other hand, it has yet to be shown that these are independent markers able to provide additional prognostic information beyond that obtained by other assessments. Interestingly, an abnormal electrocardiogram (ECG) was a significant predictor of recurrent cardiac arrest in patients with normal or near normal ventricular function and without significant coronary artery disease.[49] Whereas signal-averaged late potentials are commonly observed in patients with recurrent ventricular tachycardia, these abnormalities are less frequently evident in patients who have been resuscitated from ventricular fibrillation. Hence, signal-averaged late potentials appear to be, at best, an insensitive marker for patients at risk for sudden cardiac death.[50]

LESSONS LEARNED FROM SURVIVORS OF THE SUDDEN CARDIAC DEATH SYNDROME

When patients with ventricular fibrillation are treated with early initiation of cardiopulmonary resuscitation (CPR) and promptly defibrillated, a substantial proportion can be resuscitated and ultimately discharged home after hospitalization.[5,11,51–53]

Treatment of Out-of-Hospital Ventricular Fibrillation

When one treats out-of-hospital ventricular fibrillation, it is imperative that resuscitation be initiated as rapidly as possible. This is demonstrated in Fig. 51-3, which shows a clear relationship between survival and the rapidity of response in a medium-sized U.S. city. Such emergency care systems operate effectively with a tiered response, quickly providing both basic and advanced life support. The major goal of paramedic staffed units is to deliver emergency care comparable to that which a well-trained physician would provide on the scene. Paramedics are trained in a number of skills including tracheal intubation, use of common emergency drugs, arrhythmia recognition, and defibrillation. (See also Chap. 52).

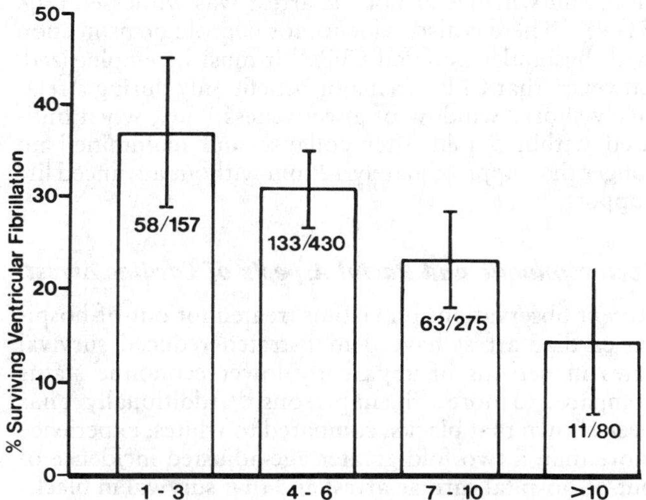

FIGURE 51-3 Nine hundred forty-two patients with out-of-hospital cardiac arrest whose first recorded rhythm was ventricular fibrillation. The patients are grouped according to the response time of the first arriving fire department unit able to provide defibrillation. The proportions of patients who were ultimately discharged home fell proportionately to the delay in providing defibrillation. (*From Weaver et al: Factors influencing survival after out-of-hospital cardiac arrest. J Am Coll Cardiol 7:752, 1986. Reproduced with permission from the publisher and authors.*)

In Seattle, the community represented in Fig. 51-3, the response time from dispatch until arrival of the first fire department unit averages 3 to 4 min, and the advanced life support units arrive on the scene approximately 4 min later. Except for cardiac arrest and hypovolemic shock, all therapy is carried out in conjunction with a physician who is in communication by radio or telephone with the paramedics.[51,53] Each year the fire department paramedics treat 200 to 300 patients who are in cardiac arrest with ventricular fibrillation when first examined (4 to 6 cases per 10,000 population per year). (An additional 40 to 50 patients typically develop ventricular fibrillation after arrival of the mobile units.) In the initial years of the Seattle experience, 10 to 12 percent of patients found in ventricular fibrillation were ultimately discharged home; subsequently, this figure has ranged from 24 to 33 percent.[5] Unfortunately, the outcome is dismal for patients whose first recorded rhythm is asystole or electromechanical dissociation.[5,14,15]

Bystander-Initiated Cardiopulmonary Resuscitation

The involvement of the general public in the initiation of CPR is a useful adjunct to an emergency care system.[52,54] In the Seattle area, for example, over 500,000 persons of high school age and older have received CPR training during the past 20 years. More than 40 percent of resuscitations in this city are initiated by bystanders prior to arrival of the fire department, and survival in patients with ventricular fibrillation is approximately 40 percent greater in those patients who received early initiation of CPR. Improved survival rates have now been reported in several communities, and the benefit of early CPR has been shown to be independent of associated factors such as age of the victim, time to defibrillation, and whether or not the arrest was witnessed (Fig. 51–4).[52] There is also evidence for neurologic protection with bystander-initiated CPR.[54] It must be emphasized, however, that CPR has major benefit only during a relatively short "window of effectiveness," i.e., when initiated within 5 min after collapse and maintained no longer than approximately 12 min without advanced life support.[52]

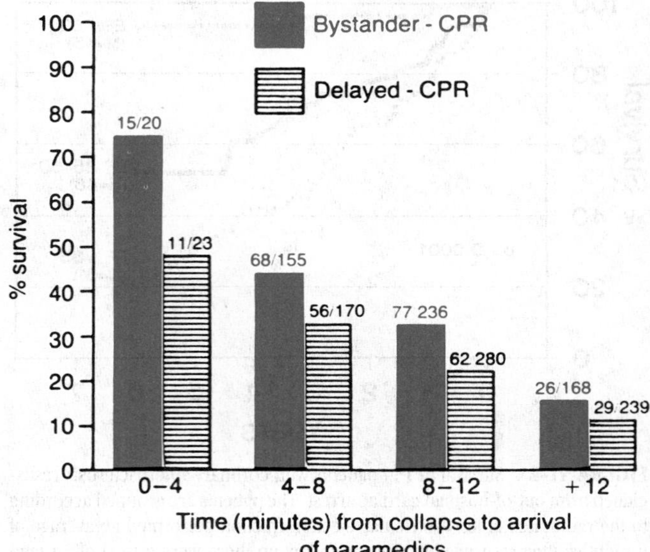

FIGURE 51-4 Comparison of survival in patients treated for out-of-hospital cardiac arrest. Patients who received bystander-initiated CPR had significantly improved survival to hospital discharge. Represented here are witnessed arrests attributed to cardiac etiology without restriction of initial cardiac rhythm. (*From Cummins et al: Automatic external defibrillators: Clinical, training, psychological, and public health issues. Ann Emerg Med 14:755, 1985. Reproduced with permission from the publisher and authors.*)

Socioeconomic and Racial Aspects of Cardiac Arrest

Recent observations on victims treated for out-of-hospital cardiac arrest have demonstrated reduced survival rates in persons of apparently lower economic status compared to more affluent persons.[54a] Additionally it has been shown that blacks, compared to whites, experience more than a two-fold greater age-adjusted incidence of out-of-hospital cardiac arrest and that survival in blacks is markedly reduced.[54b] The explanations for these findings are not evident. Service factors such as response time were unrelated to these differences in outcome.

Distinction between Acute Myocardial Infarction and Sudden Cardiac Death

Although atherosclerotic coronary heart disease is responsible for most episodes of out-of-hospital ventricular fibrillation, only a minority of resuscitated patients appear to have developed ventricular fibrillation as a consequence of *acute* myocardial infarction. In the days following resuscitation, new Q waves developed in only 19 percent of patients and lactate dehydrogenase isoenzyme patterns of myocardial necrosis were found in 38 percent of patients. The majority of patients had ST and/or T wave changes or no appreciable electrocardiographic changes during the postresuscitation hospitalization.[4,51] The disparity between the incidence of acute Q-wave infarction and the occurrence of isoenzyme evidence for necrosis may be explained by either non-Q-wave infarction or, perhaps more likely, enzymatic elevation secondary to cardiac arrest and resuscitation. In either case, it is apparent that the majority of patients developed ventricular fibrillation without acute myocardial infarction as a precipitating event.[44,51,55] This is in accord with the observation that most victims of sudden cardiac death do not have antecedent chest pain[3] and also is consistent with the findings from autopsy series.[1,27]

Recurrence of Sudden Cardiac Death Syndrome

During the 1970s resuscitated patients experienced approximately a 25 percent 1-year mortality rate; the majority of these deaths were due to recurrent cardiac arrest, usually with ventricular fibrillation as the first recorded rhythm.[5,7,17] Subsequent reports from Seattle and Miami have noted that recurrences of cardiac arrest had declined in recent years to levels of 10 to 15 percent by 1 year.[5,56] It is possible that the better outcome is due to improved therapy, but that conclusion remains conjectural.

Predictors of Recurrent Cardiac Arrest

Using easily obtained information from survivors of out-of-hospital ventricular fibrillation, risk profiles have been developed and validated.[57,58] As shown in Table 51-1, the sudden cardiac death syndrome recurred predominantly in patients whose initial episode of ventricular fibrillation was *not* associated with acute Q-wave infarction. Historical factors associated with recurrences included remote myocardial infarction and congestive heart failure prior to the episode of ventricular fibrillation. Other predictors of recurrence were abnormal left ventricular function, extensive coronary artery narrowing, complex ventricular ectopy, and continued smoking of cigarettes.[43,47,54,55,58] In a multivariate analysis, resting left ventricular ejection fraction emerged as an extremely powerful independent predictor, which in large part overshadowed electrocardiographic and clinical markers[47] (Fig. 51-2).

Vulnerability to Recurrent Ventricular Fibrillation

The contrasting rates of recurrent cardiac arrest in patients stratified according to the presence of acute Q-wave myocardial infarction (Table 51-1) are striking and warrant comment. First, this simple stratification provides useful prognostic information, in part presumably reflecting the likelihood that cardiac arrest victims with acute infarction of large size are not often effectively resuscitated. Additionally, however, the comparison emphasizes a concept of sustained propensity to develop ventricular fibrillation. Thus, in patients with acute myocardial infarction, there is a transiently enhanced likelihood of developing ventricular fibrillation during the initial hours or days. On the other hand, when ventricular fibrillation is precipitated by mechanisms other than acute infarction, there appears to be a residual state of electrical instability that predisposes to recurrences of cardiac arrest. Whether that propensity is related to scars from previous infarction, to chronic ischemia, or to intermittent acute ischemia is often difficult to determine. Other factors that may modulate myocardial vulnerability include physical and psychological "stress," arousal of the autonomic nervous system, metabolic derangements such as potassium or magnesium depletion, and the effects of many pharmacologic agents.

TABLE 51-1

One-Year Risk of Recurrent SCD Syndrome in 425 VF Survivors with Coronary Atherosclerotic Heart Disease

Type of Survivor	Recurrence
AQMI	2% (2 of 85 patients)
No AQMI	22% (75 of 340 patients)
History of remote MI	30%
No history of remote MI	14%
With CHF	30%
Without CHF	11%

NOTES: VF = ventricular fibrillation; AQMI = acute Q-wave myocardial infarction associated with VF; MI = myocardial infarction; CHF = history of congestive heart failure.
SOURCE: Modified slightly from Cobb et al.,[51] Reproduced with permission from the American Heart Association, Inc., and authors.

PREVENTION OF SUDDEN CARDIAC DEATH

The containment of sudden cardiac death largely lies with the prevention, slowing, or reversal of the atherosclerotic process. Until that can be attained, however, other approaches must be pursued. Because ventricular fibrillation is usually the immediate cause of sudden death, it follows that efforts to prevent the latter disorder should be directed to the treatment and prevention of ventricular fibrillation.

Resuscitation

Sudden cardiac death, in its simplest expression, can be viewed as a primary arrhythmic event that is potentially responsive to electrical defibrillation. Unfortunately, the difficulties in aborting an episode of sudden death are compounded by the inherent nature of the disorder, first by the location of the incident, which is typically removed from a conventional site of medical care, and second by the lack of warning symptoms in 70 percent or more of cases.[3] Nonetheless, as discussed previously in this chapter, the development of systems to provide advanced level prehospital emergency care has resulted in the resuscitation of many persons who otherwise would certainly have died.

The effectiveness of emergency medical systems in managing cardiac arrest depends largely on the rapidity of response. Since logistic considerations may often preclude a quick response, other means of providing defibrillation have been proposed. Simple, portable defibrillators placed, under medical supervision, in the homes of "high-risk" patients or in public places has been considered, and pilot programs have been initiated.[59–61] Additionally, Mirowski and colleagues[62] developed an implantable defibrillator that provides electronic sensing of ventricular fibrillation (or ventricular tachycardia) and delivery of a defibrillatory current through surgically implanted electrodes. While these latter devices can effect reversion of an arrhythmia moments after onset, their application is limited, at least for the time being, to patients at high risk for developing recurrent cardiac arrest or to selected patients with recurrent ventricular tachycardia. Hence, the current devices have not had a major impact on the incidence of out-of-hospital cardiac arrest. The use of implantable defibrillators will likely be extended now that the availability of catheter systems for implantation of devices can obviate the need for thoracotomy. (See Chap. 47.)

Prevention of Ventricular Fibrillation

Ventricular fibrillation can be prevented in the setting of experimentally induced myocardial ischemia or infarction, and laboratory studies have shown that the propensity to develop ventricular fibrillation can be modified by such diverse measures as psychological adaptations, beta-adrenergic blocking agents, and antiarrhythmic drugs. Furthermore, clinical studies in patients with acute myocardial infarction have shown that the prophylactic use of lidocaine, in some circumstances, may prevent the development of ventricular fibrillation. (See Chap. 60.)

The paradox of an acute lethal event arising in the setting, of long-standing ventricular dysfunction and chronic ventricular ectopy has stimulated a search for precipitating factors. Current knowledge suggests that the events leading to ventricular fibrillation may be electrical or mechanical, both of which are likely mediated at the cellular level and modulated by neural traffic.

Measures to Prevent Sudden Cardiac Death

Clinical trials aimed at the reduction of sudden death have been carried out predominantly in ambulatory patients who had recovered from an acute myocardial infarction. Although such studies have an important bearing on the problem of sudden death, the characteristics of patients in the postinfarction period may not be representative of the large number of patients with chronic coronary atherosclerotic heart disease who are at risk for sudden death. Also, it is noteworthy that, in patients resuscitated from out-of-hospital ventricular fibrillation in Seattle, only 15 percent had sustained a recognized acute myocardial infarction in the year preceding the episode of ventricular fibrillation, and 60 percent had no history of *ever* having an acute infarction. Hence, at this time it would be prudent to be somewhat cautious in extrapolating interventions in postinfarction patients to the broad spectrum of patients with atherosclerotic coronary heart disease.

Beta-Adrenergic Blocking Agents Studies carried out in Europe in the 1970s indicated that two beta-blocking drugs, alprenolol and practolol, appeared to reduce mortality during the first year or two following myocardial infarction. Subsequently, these observations were confirmed in several large, well-controlled trials employing other beta blockers.[63] Thus, the chronic administration of most beta blockers can be expected to extend the survival of perhaps 2 to 4 percent of patients 1 year after myocardial infarction. A major proportion of that benefit is due to a reduction of sudden death. Although the mechanisms underlying this protection are not known, it seems relevant to note that the incidence of recurrent, nonfatal myocardial infarction is also lowered by the use of beta blockers. (See also Chaps. 60 and 63.)

Antiarrhythmic Drug Therapy It is of interest that ventricular ectopic activity was not used as a major endpoint in the trials of beta-blocking drugs cited above. This contrasts to the approaches of others who have vigorously investigated and treated patients considered to be at increased risk for sudden death because of advanced grades of ventricular ectopy.[64] It is important to note that the use of antiarrhythmics in postinfarction patients did not improve survival in trials using mexiletine, aprindine, flecainide, encainide, or moricizine.[65–68] In fact, there was significant *excess* mortality in patients treated with 1-cc antiarrhythmic agents or moricizine compared to those who received placebo.[67,68]

Several investigators have advocated the use of arrhythmia-provoking, cardiac pacing techniques as a means of recognizing myocardial electrical instability. That approach (programmed ventricular stimulation) is thought to facilitate the recognition of a state of electrical instability and the susceptibility for developing ventricular fibrillation. Such techniques also have therapeutic implications since the provoked ventricular arrhythmias may be modified by pharmacologic interventions. Studies in survivors of cardiac arrest point to a relatively low rate of recurrent arrest among those patients in whom ventricular tachycardia could no longer be induced after receiving an antiarrhythmic regimen[69] (Fig. 51-5). Although this observation offers potentially useful prognostic information, it is not clear whether the antiarrhythmic agents are responsible for the improved outcome or whether the modified electrophysiological responses simply represent a risk stratification process. (See also Chap. 46.)

Unfortunately, the use of antiarrhythmic agents to reduce the incidence of sudden death is hampered, not only by unacceptable and sometimes dangerous side effects, but also by substantial uncertainty in therapeutic guidelines. At this time there is no convincing evidence that antiarrhythmic agents prevent sudden cardiac death, with the possible exception of that relatively small group who have received antiarrhythmics according to the results of programmed electrical stimulation. Although there is evidence of efficacy when the latter procedure is used to guide therapy for recurrent, symptomatic ventricular tachycardia (see Chap. 36), that arrhythmia is not often recognized prior to out-of-hospital cardiac arrest.[5]

Heart Surgery Since most victims of sudden cardiac death have atherosclerotic coronary artery obstruction, it might follow that improvement in coronary blood flow would enhance the survival of these patients, particularly by preventing or forestalling sudden death. Since coronary bypass surgery is performed on more than 300,000 patients each year in the United States, it is proper to ask if this operation will prevent sudden cardiac death. Randomized, prospective trials of coronary artery bypass grafting have been carried out in patients with stable angina pectoris. In spite of appreciable symptomatic relief from angina, the effects on long-term mortality have not consistently favored the surgically treated groups except for patients with left main coronary artery obstruction. In the European Coronary Surgery Study Group trial, there was a reduction in mortality, including sudden deaths, in a major subgroup of surgically treated patients who had triple-vessel disease.[70,71] In the Coronary Artery Surgery Study (CASS) carried out in the United States, survival following coronary artery bypass grafting was not significantly different in the patients treated surgically or medically.[45] (See also Chap. 73.) It is important to point out, however, that the medically treated patients in the CASS had excellent survival rates and that the life-extending effect of any intervention, regardless of its value, would have been difficult to recognize in those selected patients. In a retrospective study of patients resuscitated from out-of-hospital cardiac arrest,

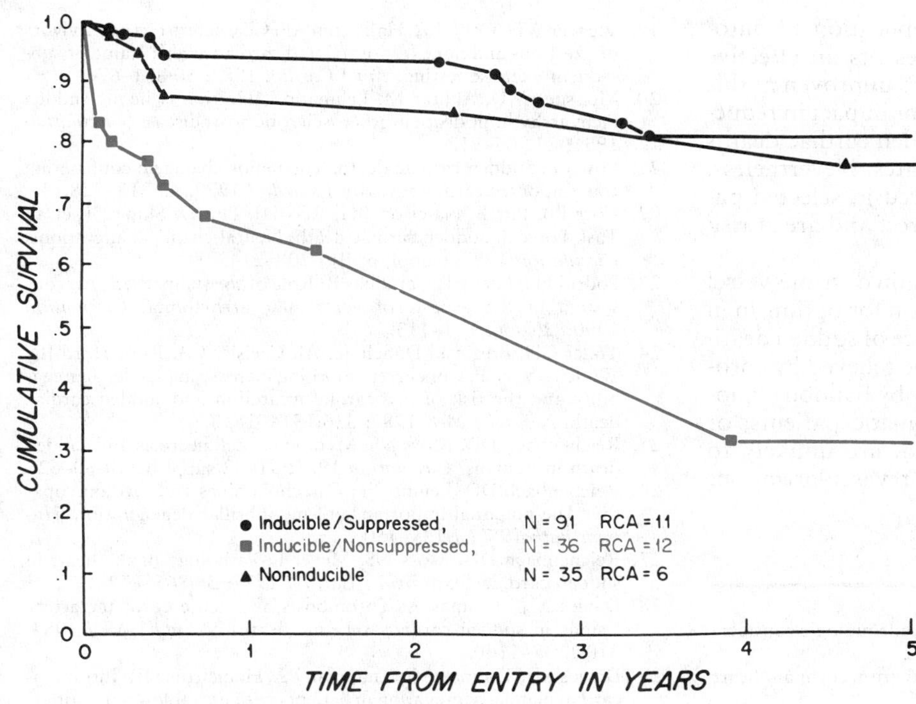

FIGURE 51-5 Survival without cardiac arrest in 162 patients resuscitated from out-of-hospital cardiac arrest. The patients are grouped according to the responses elicited by programmed electrical stimulation and subsequent antiarrhythmic drug testing. The persistence of inducible ventricular arrhythmias increased the risk of recurrent cardiac arrest (RCA) independently of left ventricular ejection fraction. (*From Wilber et al: Out-of-hospital cardiac arrest: Use of electrophysiologic testing in the prediction of long-term outcome. N Engl J Med 318:19, 1988. Reproduced with permission from the publisher and author.*)

survival was improved in comparable patients who received coronary bypass surgery compared to those treated medically.[72] Although uncertainties remain, evidence to date indicates that sudden death may be forestalled or prevented in subgroups of symptomatic patients treated surgically for left main and triple-vessel coronary artery obstruction. On the other hand, the role of balloon angioplasty in preventing sudden death has not yet been established. Although there are encouraging reports concerning the efficacy of myocardial surgery for patients with recurrent, drug-resistant ventricular tachycardia (see Chap. 44), the strategy for managing patients with ventricular tachycardia is usually not relevant to the much larger numbers of patients who typically develop sudden cardiac death without previously recognized cardiac arrhythmias.

Automatic Implantable Cardioverter/Defibrillators To date there have been no published results of randomized, controlled trials using implantable cardioverter/defibrillators. Case series of patients at high risk for death, mostly due to recurrent ventricular arrhythmias, however, have strongly suggested a life-extending benefit.[73,74] Controlled clinical trials are now in progress and should prove useful in defining the role of these devices. Additionally, a trial of implantable devices in high-risk postinfarction patients is now underway. Improving technology to permit nonsurgical implantation and reduced cost may extend this promising approach. (See also Chap. 42.)

Other Therapies Several additional interventions have been proposed to reduce the likelihood of sudden death following myocardial infarction e.g., anticoagulants, hygienic measures, lipid-lowering drugs, and antiplatelet agents. To date none of these measures has shown a clear-cut effect on mortality, although salutary effects on morbidity have been demonstrated.[75,76] Importantly, a number of observational studies have shown a reduction in both morbidity and mortality when patients stop cigarette smoking.[58]

SUMMARY

A large proportion of deaths from atherosclerotic coronary heart disease are sudden, unexpected events that occur outside the hospital and are thought to be precipitated by ventricular fibrillation. In approximately 80 percent of instances, the patients have had prior manifestations of heart disease or systemic arterial hypertension or both. In patients with recognized cardiovascular disease, complex ventricular ectopy has a statistical relationship to sudden cardiac death. That marker, however, is only a weak predictor when adjusted for the severity of myocardial dysfunction, which is the most useful predictor of sudden cardiac death.

Following acute myocardial infarction, beta-blocking drugs have been shown to prevent or forestall sudden death in the initial 2 years. On the other hand, there is little evidence for a life-extending benefit accompanying the use of antiarrhythmic drugs; in fact, the bulk of evidence suggests a detrimental effect. In patients at risk for sudden death, cessation of cigarette smoking and treatment of high blood pressure are prudent, preventive measures.

The application of emergency medical services represents a major advance in averting sudden cardiac death. Further strategies to facilitate prompt initiation of CPR and rapid defibrillation will likely be accompanied by improved rates of resuscitation and survival.

Whereas the development and application of automatic implantable defibrillators represents an effective application of modern technology, it is unproven at this time that these devices will have a major impact in reducing the hundreds of thousands of sudden cardiac deaths that occur each year in the United States. Nevertheless, their use should be strongly considered in selected patients who have survived a cardiac arrest and are at risk for recurrences.

In symptomatic patients with left main or triple-vessel coronary atherosclerosis, there is reason for optimism in anticipating a reduction in the incidence of sudden death if transient myocardial ischemia can be relieved by coronary artery bypass grafting or possibly by balloon angioplasty. On the other hand, asymptomatic patients, or those with mild symptoms of angina, are unlikely to derive a life-extending effect by such revascularization.

REFERENCES

1. Kuller LH: Sudden death—definition and epidemiologic considerations. *Prog Cardiovasc Dis* 1980; 23:1–12.
2. Gordon T, Kannell WB: Premature mortality from coronary heart disease. *JAMA* 1971; 215:1617–1625.
3. Gillum RF, Feinleid M, Margolis JR, Fabsitz RR, Brasch RC: Delay in the prehospital phase of acute myocardial infarction. *Arch Intern Med* 1976; 136:649–654.
4. Baum RS, Alvarez H, Cobb LA: Survival after resuscitation from out-of-hospital ventricular fibrillation. *Circulation* 1974; 50:1231–1235.
5. Cobb LA, Weaver DW, Fahrenbruch CE, Hallstrom AP, Copass MK: Community based interventions for sudden cardiac death: Impact, limitations and changes. *Circulation* 1992; 85(suppl I):I-98–I-102.
6. Gillum RF: Sudden coronary death in the United States 1980–1985. *Circulation* 1989; 79:756–765.
7. Schaffer WA, Cobb LA: Recurrent ventricular fibrillation and modes of death in survivors of out-of-hospital ventricular fibrillation. *N Engl J Med* 1975; 293:260–262.
8. Wikland B: Medically unattended fatal cases of ischemic heart disease in a defined population. *Acta Med Scand* 1971; 524(suppl):23–30.
9. Cobb LA, Weaver WD: Exercise: A risk for sudden death in patients with coronary heart disease. *J Am Coll Cardiol* 1986; 7:215–219.
10. Siscovick DS, Weiss NS, Fletcher RH, Lasky T: The incidence of primary cardiac arrest during vigorous exercise. *N Engl J Med* 1984; 311:874–877.
11. Hossack KF, Hartwig R: Cardiac arrest associated with supervised cardiac rehabilitation. *J Cardiac Rehab* 1982; 2:402–408.
12. Nikolic G, Bishop RL, Singh JB: Sudden death recorded during Holter monitoring. *Circulation* 1982; 66:218–225.
13. Pratt CM, Francis MJ, Luck JC, Wyndham CR, Miller RR, Quinones MA: Analysis of ambulatory electrocardiograms in 15 patients during spontaneous ventricular fibrillation with special reference to preceding arrhythmic events. *J Am Coll Cardiol* 1983; 2:789–797.
14. Iseri LT, Humphrey SB, Sinner EJ: Prehospital bradyasystolic cardiac arrest. *Ann Intern Med* 1978; 88:741–744.
15. Myerburg RJ, Estes D, Zaman L, Luceri RM, Kessler KM, Trohman RG, et al: Outcome of resuscitation from bradyarrhythmic or asystolic cardiac arrest. *J Am Coll Cardiol* 1984; 4:1118–1122.
16. Dexter L: Cardiac arrest. In: Mandell H, Spiro H (eds): *When Doctors Get Sick*. New York, Plenum, 1987: 39–43.
17. Weaver WD, Hill D, Fahrenbruch CE, Copass MK, Martin JS, Cobb LA, Hallstrom AP: Use of automatic external defibrillator in the management of out-of-hospital cardiac arrest. *N Engl J Med* 1988; 319:661–666.
18. Lazzara R, El-Sherif N, Hope RR: Ventricular arrhythmias and electrophysiological consequences of myocardial ischemia and infarction. *Circ Res* 1978; 42:740–756.
19. Weaver WD, Cobb LA, Hallstrom AP: Characteristics of survivors of exertion- and nonexertion-related cardiac arrest: Value of subsequent exercise testing. *Am J Cardiol* 1982; 50:671–676.
20. Meissner MD, Akhtar M, Lehmann MH: Non-ischemic sudden tachyarrhythmic death in atherosclerotic heart disease. *Circulation* 1991; 84:905–912.
21. Lown B: Sudden cardiac death: The major challenge confronting contemporary cardiology. *Am J Cardiol* 1979; 43:313–328.
22. Corr PB, Pitt B, Natelson BH, Reis DJ, Phil D, Shine KI, et al: Task Force 3: Sudden cardiac death: Neural-chemical alterations. *Circulation* 1987; (suppl, pt II):I-208–214.
23. Podrid PH, Fuchs T, Candinas R: Role of the sympathetic nervous system in the genesis of ventricular arrhythmia. *Circulation* 1990:82(suppl 1):1–113.
24. Tofler GH, Brezinski D, Schafer AI, Czeisler CA, Rutherford JD, Willich SN, et al: Concurrent morning increase in platelet aggregability and the risk of myocardial infarction and sudden cardiac death. *N Engl J Med* 1987; 316:1514–1518.
25. Reichenbach DD, Moss NS: Myocardial cell necrosis and sudden death in humans. *Circulation* 1975; 51–52(suppl III):III-60–62.
26. Reichenbach DD, Benditt EP: Catecholamines and cardiomyopathy: The potential importance of myofibrillar degeneration. *Human Path* 1970; 1:125–150.
27. Reichenbach DD, Moss NS, Meyer E: Pathology of the heart in sudden cardiac death. *Am J Cardiol* 1977; 39:865–872.
28. Davies MJ, Thomas A: Thrombosis and acute coronary artery lesions in sudden cardiac ischemic death. *N Engl J Med* 1984; 310:1137–1140.
29. Davies MJ, Thomas AC, Knapman PA, Hangartner JR: Intramyocardial platelet aggregation in patients with unstable angina suffering sudden ischemic cardiac death. *Circulation* 1986; 73:418–427.
30. Hammon JW, Oates JA: Interaction of platelets with the vessel wall in the pathophysiology of sudden cardiac death. *Circulation* 1986; 73:224–226.
31. Maron BJ, Roberts WC, Epstein SE: Sudden death in hypertrophic cardiomyopathy: A profile of 78 patients. *Circulation* 1982; 65:1388–1394.
32. Goldstein S: *Sudden Death Coronary Heart Disease*. Mt. Kisco, NY, Futura Publishing, 1974: 22–36.
33. McKenna WJ, Harris L, Rowland E, Kleinebenne A, Krikler DM, Oakley M, et al: Amiodarone for long term management of patients with cardiomyopathy. *Am J Cardiol* 1984; 54:802–810.
34. Moss AM, Schwartz PJ, Crampton RS, Tzivoni D, Locati EH, MacCluer J, et al: The long QT syndrome prospective longitudinal study of 328 families. *Circulation* 1991; 84:1136–1144.
35. Otto CM, Tauxe RV, Cobb LA, Greene HL, Gross BW, Werner JA, et al: Ventricular fibrillation causes sudden death in Southeast Asian immigrants. *Ann Intern Med* 1984; 101:45–47.
36. Kirschner RH, Eckner FA, Baron RC: The cardiac pathology of sudden, unexplained nocturnal death in Southeast Asian refugees. *JAMA* 1986; 256:2700–2705.
37. Friedman GD, Klatsky AL, Siegelaub AB: Predictors of sudden cardiac death. *Circulation* 1975; 51–52(suppl 3):164–170.
38. Moss AJ: Clinical significance of ventricular arrhythmias in patients with and without coronary artery disease. *Prog Cardiovasc Dis* 1980; 23:33–40.
39. Ruberman W, Weinblatt E, Goldberg JD, Frank CW, Chaudhary BS, Shapiro S: Ventricular premature complexes and sudden death after myocardial infarction. *Circulation* 1981; 64:297–305.
40. Weaver WD, Cobb LA, Hallstrom AP: Ambulatory arrhythmias in resuscitated victims of cardiac arrest. *Circulation* 1982; 66:212–218.
41. Haynes RE, Hallstrom AP, Cobb LA: Repolarization abnormalities in survivors of out-of-hospital ventricular fibrillation. *Circulation* 1978; 57:652–658.
42. Kennedy HL, Whitlock JA, Sprague MK: Long-term follow-up of asymptomatic healthy subjects with frequent and complex ventricular ectopy. *N Engl J Med* 1985; 312:193–199.
43. Weaver WD, Lorch GS, Alvarez HA, Cobb LA: Angiographic findings and prognostic indicators in patients resuscitated from sudden cardiac death. *Circulation* 1976; 54:895–900.
44. Liberthson RR, Nagel EL, Hirschman JC, Nussenfeld SR, Blackbourne BD, Davis JH: Pathophysiologic observations in prehospital ventricular fibrillation and sudden cardiac death. *Circulation* 1974; 49:790–798.
45. Fisher LD, Kronmal RA, Davis KB, Gillespie MJ, Kennedy JW, Rogers WJ, et al: Coronary Artery Surgery Study (CASS): A Ran-

domized Trial of Coronary Artery Bypass Surgery Survival Data. *Circulation* 1983; 68:939–950.

46. Oberman A, Ray M, Turner ME, Barnes G, Grooms C: Sudden death in patients evaluated for ischemic heart disease. *Circulation* 1975; 52(suppl III):170–175.
47. Ritchie JL, Hallstrom AP, Trobaugh GB, Caldwell JH, Cobb LA: Out-of-hospital sudden coronary death: Rest and exercise radionuclide left ventricular function in survivors. *Am J Cardiol* 1985; 55:645–651.
48. The Multicenter Postinfarction Research Group: Risk stratification and survival after myocardial infarction. *N Engl J Med* 1983; 309:331–336.
49. Kudenchuk PJ, Cobb LA, Greene HL, Fahrenbruch CE, Sheehan FH: Late outcome of survivors of out-of-hospital cardiac arrest with left ventricular ejection fractions 50% or greater and without significant coronary arterial narrowing. *Am J Cardiol* 1991; 67:704–708.
50. Dolack GL, Callahan DB, Bardy GH, Greene HL: Signal-averaged electrocardiographic late potentials in resuscitated survivors of out-of-hospital ventricular fibrillation. *Am J Cardiol* 1990; 65:1102–1104.
51. Cobb LA, Werner JA, Trobaugh GB: Sudden cardiac death, I. A decade's experience with out-of-hospital resuscitation. *Mod Concepts Cardiovasc Dis* 1980; 19:31–36.
52. Cummins RO, Eisenberg MS, Hallstrom AP, Litwin P: Survival of out-of-hospital cardiac arrest with early initiation of cardiopulmonary resuscitation. *Am J Emerg Med* 1985; 3:114–119.
53. Weaver WD, Cobb LA, Hallstrom AP, Fahrenbruch CE, Copass MK, Ray R: Factors influencing survival after out-of-hospital cardiac arrest. *J Am Coll Cardiol* 1986; 7:752–757.
54. Cobb LA, Hallstrom AP: Community-based cardiopulmonary resuscitation: What have we learned? *Ann NY Acad Sci* 1982; 382:330–342.

54a. Hallstrom A, Boutin P, Cobb L, Johnson E: Socioeconomic status and prediction of ventricular fibrillation survival. *Am J Public Health* 1993; 83:245–248.

54b. Cowie M, Fahrenbruch C, Cobb L, Hallstrom A: Out-of-hospital cardiac arrest: Racial differences in outcome in Seattle. *Am J Public Health* 1993; 83:955–959.

55. Goldstein S, Landis R, Leighton R, Ritter C, Vasu CM, Wolfe RA, et al: Predictive survival models for resuscitated victims of out-of-hospital cardiac arrest with coronary heart disease. *Circulation* 1985; 71:873–880.
56. Myerburg RJ, Kessler KM, Estes D, Conde CA, Luceri RM, Zaman L, et al: Long-term survival after prehospital cardiac arrest: Analysis of outcome during an 8 year study. *Circulation* 1984; 70:538–546.
57. Cobb LA, Werner JA, Trobaugh GB: Sudden cardiac death: II. Outcome of resuscitation: Management, and future directions. *Mod Concepts Cardiovasc Dis* 1980; 49:37–42.
58. Hallstrom AP, Cobb LA, Ray R: Smoking as a risk factor for recurrence of cardiac arrest. *N Engl J Med* 1986; 314:271–275.
59. Eisenberg MS, Moore J, Cummins RO, Andersen E, Litwin PE, Hallstrom AP, et al: Use of the automated external defibrillator in homes of survivors of out-of-hospital ventricular fibrillation. *Am J Cardiol* 1989; 63:443–446.
60. Cummins RO, Eisenberg MS, Moore JE, Hearne TR, Andersen E, Wendt R, et al: Automatic external defibrillators: Clinical, training, psychological, and public health issues. *Ann Emerg Med* 1985; 14:755–560.
61. Chadda KD, Kammerer R: Early experiences with the portable automatic external defibrillator in the home and public places. *Am J Cardiol* 1987; 60:732–733.
62. Mirowski M: The automatic implantable cardioverter—Defibrillator: An overview. *J Am Coll Cardiol* 1985; 6:461–466.
63. Frishman WH, Furberg CD, Friedewald WT: Beta-adrenergic blockade for survivors of acute myocardial infarction. *N Engl J Med* 1984; 310:830–841.
64. Graboys TB, Lown B, Podrid PJ, Desilva R: Long-term survival of patients with malignant ventricular arrhythmia treated with antiarrhythmic drugs. *Am J Cardiol* 1982; 50:437–443.
65. Impact Research Group: International mexiletine and placebo antiarrhythmic coronary trial: I. Report on arrhythmia and other findings. *J Am Coll Cardiol* 1984; 4:1148–1163.
66. Gottlieb SH, Achuff SC, Mellits ED, Gerstenblith G, Baughman KL, Becker L, et al: Prophylactic antiarrhythmic therapy of high risk survivors of myocardial infarction: Lower mortality at 1 month but not at 1 year. *Circulation* 1987; 75:792–799.
67. The Cardiac Arrhythmia Suppression Trial (CAST) Investigators: Preliminary Report: Effect of encainide and flecainide on mortality in a randomized trial of arrhythmia suppression after myocardial infarction. *N Engl J Med* 1989; 321:406–412.
68. Cardiac Arrhythmia Suppression Trial II Investigators: Effect of the antiarrhythmic agent moricizine on survival after myocardial infarction. *N Engl J Med* 1992; 327:227–233.
69. Wilber DJ, Garan H, Finkelstein D, Kelly E, Newell J, McGovern B, et al: Out-of-hospital cardiac arrest: Use of electrophysiologic testing in the prediction of long-term outcome. *N Engl J Med* 1988; 318:19–24.
70. European Coronary Surgery Study Group: Long-term results of prospective randomized study of coronary artery bypass surgery in stable angina pectoris. *Lancet* 1982; 2:1173–1179.
71. Varnauskas E, the European Coronary Surgery Study Group: Twelve-year follow-up of survival in the randomized European coronary surgery study. *N Engl J Med* 1988; 6:332–337.
72. Every NE, Fahrenbruch CE, Hallstrom AP, Weaver WD, Cobb LA: Influence of coronary bypass surgery on subsequent outcome of patients resuscitated from out of hospital cardiac arrest. *J Am Coll Cardiol* 1992; 19:1435–1439.
73. Myerburg RJ, Luceri RM, Thurer R, Cooper DK, Zaman L, Interian A, et al: Time to first shock and clinical outcome in patients receiving an automatic implantable cardioverter-defibrillator. *J Am Coll Cardiol* 1989; 14:508–514.
74. Kupperman M, Luce BR, McGovern B, Podrid PJ, Bigger T, Ruskin JN: An analysis of the cost effectiveness of the implantable defibrillator. *Circulation* 1990; 81:91–100.
75. May GS, Eberlein KA, Furburg CD, Passamini ER, DeMets DL: Secondary prevention after myocardial infarction: A review of long-term trials. *Prog Cardiovasc Dis* 1982; 24:331–352.
76. Oliver MF: Lack of impact of prevention on sudden cardiac death. *J Am Coll Cardiol* 1985; 5:150B–154B.

Chapter 52

Cardiopulmonary Resuscitation and the Subsequent Management of the Patient

Nisha Chibber Chandra, M.D. ■ *Myron L. Weisfeldt, M.D.*

Since biblical times, humans have attempted to restore life to the dead or nearly dead individual. In the eighteenth century, it was a common practice in Europe to throw unconscious persons over the back of trotting horses or roll them over barrels in an attempt to move air in and out of their chests. Bellows were also used to inflate the lungs. One technique that gained broad use in this century was the Schafer prone pressure method of artificial respiration, in which the lower back was pressed cyclically, thus forcing air from the lungs.[1] At the time, all these methods were viewed as a means for primarily providing lung ventilation. In 1954, Elam and colleagues[2] showed that mouth-to-mouth or mouth-to-nose resuscitation was superior to the Schafer method in terms of efficacy of ventilation. The importance of circulation of blood was also recognized, and direct or internal cardiac massage became an accepted technique as early as 1916. Despite proven efficacy, internal massage remains fraught with complications and should only be employed by trained personnel.[3,4]

In the 1930s, Wiggers pioneered the study of ventricular fibrillation and elucidated its mechanisms and treatment.[5] It was not until 1960 that Kouwenhoven, Jude, and Knickerbocker developed the present technique of external chest compression in the supine position and coupled this with artificial respiration.[6] These investigators proposed that during chest compression in the arrested state, the heart was squeezed or massaged between the sternum and vertebral column resulting in the forward flow of blood. This technique of cardiopulmonary resuscitation (CPR) gained rapid popularity and was shown to be effective.[7]

MECHANISMS OF MOVEMENT OF BLOOD DURING CPR

The original hypothesis, as mentioned above, suggested that blood flow to the periphery during external chest compression resulted from direct compression of the heart between the sternum and the vertebral column.[6] According to this concept, chest compression ("systole"), similar to internal cardiac massage, resulted in blood being squeezed from both ventricles into the great arteries as the pulmonary and aortic valves opened. Retrograde flow of blood was prevented by closure of the mitral and tricuspid valves. During the release phase of chest compression ("diastole"), the ventricles recoiled to their original shape and filled by a suction effect while elevated arterial pressure was thought to close both the pulmonic and aortic valves.

This widely held concept is not, however, consistent with a number of observations in animal models[8] and humans[9] that suggest a correlation between the rise in intrathoracic pressure during chest compression and the apparent magnitude of carotid flow and pressure. The importance of fluctuations in intrathoracic pressure, as a means for generating blood flow, is further supported by the observations of Criley et al. that, by the continuous and early initiation of coughing, patients in ventricular fibrillation can maintain consciousness as long as cough is continued.[10] The critical ingredient of the cough is clearly a rise in intrathoracic pressure with likely no cardiac compression. Criley's observations strongly suggest that following cardiac arrest a rise in intrathoracic pressure is a potent mechanism for the movement of blood to the brain in humans.

EXPERIMENTAL OBSERVATIONS

For brain blood flow to occur during CPR, a carotid arterial-to-jugular pressure gradient must be present during chest compression. In large animals, chest compression during CPR results in an essentially equal rise in central venous, right atrial, pulmonary artery, aortic, esophageal, and lateral pleural space pressures with no transcardiac gradient being developed (Fig. 52-1).[11]

In such animals, aortic pressure is transmitted efficiently to the carotid arteries but retrograde transmission of intrathoracic venous pressure into the jugular veins is prevented by valves at the thoracic inlet and also venous collapse. Thus, during chest compression ("systole"), a peripheral arterial venous pressure gradient appears, and blood flow occurs consequent to this gradient. In such a system, there is no pressure gradient across the heart; therefore, the heart cannot be the pump responsible for generating blood flow during CPR. In fact, the heart functions merely as a passive conduit. When chest compression is released ("diastole"), intrathoracic pressures fall toward zero, and venous flow into the right side of the heart and lungs occurs. During diastole, a modest gradient also develops between the intrathoracic aorta and the right atrium and determines myocardial flow. Retrograde flow into the aorta from extrathoracic arteries also occurs but is limited by the relative low capacitance of the intrathoracic arterial bed and closure of the aortic valve. The rise in intrathoracic pressure during chest compression is likely a consequence of airway collapse that occurs at the small bronchiolar level and results in air trapping. With the release of chest compression, this airway collapse is relieved.[12]

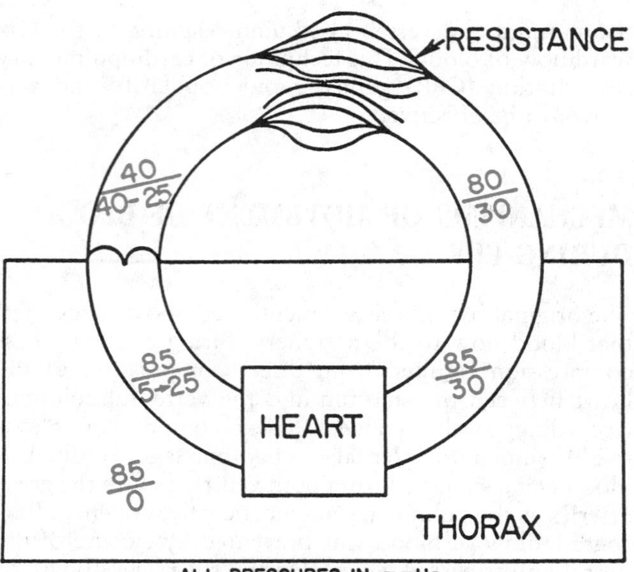

FIGURE 52-1 Representative pressures recorded during conventional cardiopulmonary resuscitation with forward carotid flow. Pressures are those recorded during compression. Intrathoracic pressures were indexed from esophageal pressures. There is no significant pressure gradient across the heart. The extrathoracic arterial pressure is similar to the intrathoracic aortic pressure. The extrathoracic venous pressure is markedly lower than the intrathoracic venous (right atrial) pressure. There is an extrathoracic arterio-venous pressure gradient that results in forward flow.

Unlike the hemodynamic pattern described above, intrathoracic vascular pressures during vigorous chest compression are much higher than pleural pressure in small animals and, rarely, in large dogs.[13] In such animals the rise in vascular pressures probably results from compression of the heart during chest compression and is not principally due to a rise in intrathoracic pressure. The classic mechanism of direct cardiac compression is likely operating in these animals. Even during cardiac compression, however, venous valves at the thoracic inlet remain essential for establishing a peripheral arterio-venous pressure gradient which facilitates peripheral flow.

Cineangiographic studies during CPR in animals demonstrate that the mitral and aortic valves are open during chest compression, when the mechanism for blood flow is manipulation of intrathoracic pressure. Based on these and other observations, the position of the mitral valve during chest compression came to be regarded as a "marker" for the mechanism of blood flow during CPR, with mitral valve closure suggesting direct cardiac compression.[14] Some investigators have demonstrated mitral valve closure during CPR in humans using transesophageal echocardiography.[15] Others have reported that the mitral valve remains open during chest compression.[16] Recent animal studies have shown that changes in intrathoracic pressure can cause the mitral valve to open or close, depending on how the rise in pressure is generated.[17] Thus, mitral valve closure or position cannot be used to identify the primary mechanism for blood flow during CPR.

Studies of vital organ perfusion indicate that during CPR (irrespective of the primary mechanism for blood flow), cerebral flow is dependent on the gradient between the carotid artery and the intracranial pressure during "systole," with myocardial flow being dependent on the gradient between the aorta and right atrium during "diastole."[18]

Building on these concepts, experimental maneuvers and techniques have been developed to increase arterial pressure during chest compression. One such technique, peri-thoracic high pressure vest inflation without airway manipulation (vest CPR), allows safe cyclical increments in intrathoracic pressure to 100 to 150 mmHg during external chest compression by the vest and has been shown to significantly increase cerebral and myocardial flow during CPR.[19] Initial human data, using a specially designed pneumatic vest, confirms higher vascular pressures during vest CPR as compared to conventional resuscitation.[20] "High impulse CPR" has also been shown to improve vascular pressures.[13] Clinical experience with this technique is limited. Interposed abdominal compression (IAC) CPR in animals increases carotid flow and improves survival in humans as compared to conventional CPR.[21] The mechanism of benefit with IAC-CPR in humans is unclear, but may relate to improved venous return and decreased arterial run off. Active compression-decompression CPR incorporates a negative pressure "pull" on the thorax during the release phase of chest compression and improves vascular pressures during CPR.[22] The mechanism of benefit from this technique of resuscitation may relate to improved venous return and/or increased intrathoracic pressure during chest compression as a consequence of changes in the bony thorax.

Epinephrine is a potent pharmacological means for increasing arterial pressure and cerebral and myocardial flow during CPR. Its hemodynamic effects are additive to those of other maneuvers.[23] With vest CPR and epinephrine infusion, 100 percent of prearrest cerebral flow and 40 percent of prearrest myocardial flow can be achieved (vs. 15 and 5 percent during conventional CPR and epinephrine infusion) (see Fig. 52-2).[19] Epinephrine is discussed in detail below.

Studies have shown that there are several aspects of external chest compression alone that can be manipulated and are critical in determining vital organ perfusion pressures.[24] First, greater sternal force augments myocardial and cerebral perfusion but can also result in greater tissue injury. Secondly, adequate compression duration during each chest compression-release cycle is critical for maintaining maximal myocardial and cerebral flow during resuscitation. Myocardial and brain flow are optimal at chest compression durations of approximately 50 percent of cycle length. Short-duration, low-force chest compression cycles are undesirable, as they result in a considerable reduction in both cerebral and myocardial flow. It is important to note that in dogs, at optimal chest compression force and duration, vital organ perfusion is not greatly influenced by compression rate.[24] If there is direct cardiac compression, however, higher compression rates augment vital organ flow. At higher chest compression rates, an optimal chest compression duration of 50 percent of cycle time is more easily achieved. Based on these data, changes in the AHA recommendations regarding chest compression rate evolved.[25] The 1986 standards recommended an increase in the rate of chest compression from the historical 60 beats per minute to 80 to 100 beats per minute. This higher rate more easily ensures a prolonged compression duration and, thus, facilitates vital organ flow if blood moves due to changes in intrathoracic pressure. It also serves to facilitate vital organ blood flow, if direct vascular compression occurs during CPR.

Observations in Humans

Unfortunately, at this point, in humans we can draw no final conclusion as to the frequency or importance of the two mechanisms (cardiac compression or generalized increase in intrathoracic pressure) during conventional

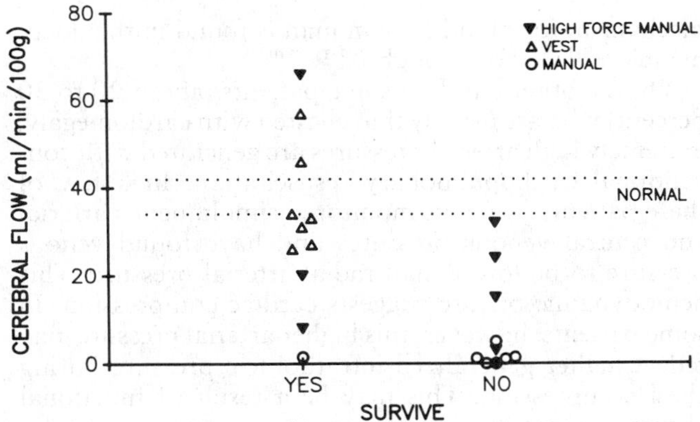

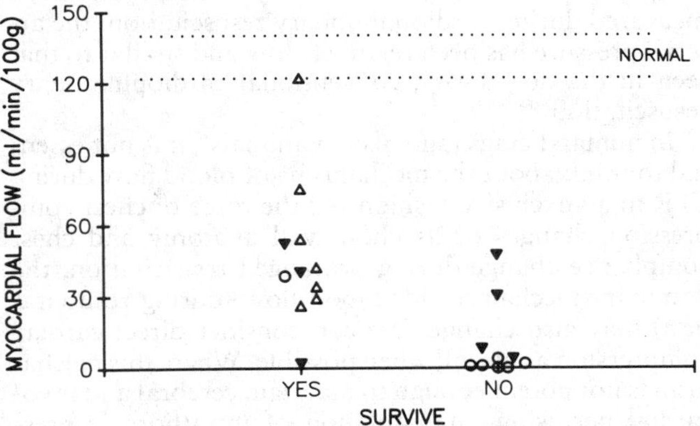

FIGURE 52-2 Myocardial and cerebral blood flow during two forms of manual CPR at normal compression and high compression force and during vest cardiopulmonary resuscitation. Dogs were anesthetized and ventricular fibrillation was induced. Defibrillation was attempted after 25 min and survival was assessed at 24 h. All of the vest CPR dogs survived whereas only about one-third of those dogs receiving usual force or high force manual CPR survived. Improved survival is related to greater cerebral and myocardial blood flow in the vest CPR animals. Those animals having high flows but not surviving manual CPR had severe trauma. None of the vest dogs suffered trauma and all survived.

cardiopulmonary resuscitation. Published studies, however, suggest that manipulation of intrathoracic pressure is likely the dominant mechanism.[26–28]

In a number of patients, comparable arterial and right atrial pressures have been observed as well as the presence of a pressure gradient at the thoracic inlet upon withdrawing intravascular catheters from the superior vena cava to the extrathoracic internal jugular vein.[11,27,28] This hemodynamic pattern favors the concept of forward flow of blood through manipulation of intrathoracic pressure. This concept is further strengthened by the observation that maneuvers designed to increase intrathoracic pressure during chest compression such as prolonged compression duration, abdominal binding, simultaneous compression ventilation CPR, or vest CPR are rewarded by a significant increase in peripheral arterial pressure.[29,30] Prehospital trials of simultaneous compression ventilation CPR, however, failed to show improved survival, though trials with IAC-CPR appear more promising.[31,21] Perhaps the strongest evidence supporting the theory of manipulation of intrathoracic pressure as a mechanism for blood flow in man is found in the documented efficacy of "cough CPR."[10]

On the other hand, in some patients (about 20 to 30 percent) who are usually thin chested with cardiomegaly, extremely high arterial pressures are generated with conventional cardiopulmonary resuscitation. In a few of these patients, we have monitored simultaneous arterial and central venous pressures and have found venous pressure to be lower than radial arterial pressure. This hemodynamic picture suggests cardiac compression. In some patients, however, this higher arterial pressure may reflect higher generalized intrathoracic pressure during chest compression. This may be a result of functional airway obstruction due to airway collapse, pulmonary congestion, and/or bronchospasm.[12] In the majority of the patients in whom radial artery pressure has been measured during cardiopulmonary resuscitation, the arterial pressure has been relatively low and similar to that seen in the dog during conventional cardiopulmonary resuscitation.[26–28]

In human beings (and also in animals), it is not essential to think about the mechanisms of blood flow during CPR in an exclusive fashion. As the force of chest compression changes or as chest wall anatomy and chest compliance change during prolonged resuscitation, the dominant mechanism for blood flow (during resuscitation) may also change. We can consider direct cardiac compression as useful, when possible. Where this mechanism is not potent enough to maintain cerebral and myocardial perfusion, manipulation of intrathoracic pressures may have a favorable additive effect on vital organ and peripheral blood flow.

DIAGNOSIS AND IDENTIFICATION OF CARDIAC ARREST

Cardiac arrest is defined as the sudden cessation of effective cardiac pumping function as a result of either ventricular asystole (electrical or mechanical) or ventricular fibrillation. Rapid diagnosis and treatment are essential because (1) more than a few minutes of total cardiac arrest results in permanent cerebral anoxic damage, and (2) the success of resuscitative measures is related to the rapidity with which they are instituted following arrest. Based on these and other observations, the concept of early activation of Emergency Medical Systems (EMS) has evolved for victims of out-of-hospital cardiac arrest[32] (see also Chap. 51).

Cardiac arrest should be considered in the differential diagnosis of sudden collapse in any patient. It can be clinically confirmed by pulseless major vessels and absent heart sounds. Although respirations (agonal respirations) may continue for a minute or two, the patient with cardiac arrest becomes rapidly cyanotic and unconscious.

If available, an electrocardiogram can confirm the diagnosis and identify asystole, ventricular fibrillation, or electromechanical dissociation as the mechanism of arrest. Cardiopulmonary resuscitation (CPR), however, should be initiated immediately once the clinical diagnosis is made without delaying to obtain this information. If a defibrillator but not an ECG is immediately available, a 200-J countershock should be administered without delay. Prehospital CPR studies confirm in several patients that the mechanism of cardiac arrest is usually ventricular fibrillation, and survival is critically dependent on the time to defibrillation.[33] Based on these observations, automatic external defibrillators (AED) were developed for use by first (minimally trained) responders, and were shown to dramatically improve survival from prehospital arrest.[34] AEDs have a >90 percent sensitivity and specificity for successfully recognizing ventricular fibrillation. They are designed for use by first responders or persons with little medical training (e.g., firemen, Emergency Medical Technicians). These devices have varying degrees of automation, and can deliver several successive defibrillatory shocks by two selfadhesive electrodes that are placed by the user on the left anterior chest. It is highly recommended that all first responder units be equipped with AEDs.

RESPIRATORY ARREST

Respiratory arrest is the cessation of effective respiratory effort. It can result from airway obstruction (due to a foreign-body or other causes), drowning, smoke inhalation, drug overdose, head trauma, cerebrovascular accident, or suffocation. When respiratory arrest occurs suddenly (as with foreign-body obstruction), the patient rapidly becomes cyanotic, though a palpable pulse with blood pressure, consciousness, and ineffective respiratory efforts may be maintained for several minutes. Opening the airway and/or rescue breathing may be all that is necessary to resuscitate such a patient.

The Heimlich maneuver is recommended for relieving foreign body airway obstruction. It is implemented by standing behind the victim[35] and delivering a series of sharp thrusts to the upper abdomen with a closed fist. Abdominal thrusts can also be used directly in the unconscious supine patient to help dislodge a foreign body mechanically. The Heimlich maneuver can also be self administered by placing the fist between the navel and xiphoid process, and delivering a series of quick upward thrusts. If incorrectly administered, this maneuver can lead to visceral damage.[36] When properly used, however, the technique is both safe and effective. Manual removal of a foreign body should only be used in the unconscious victim. This can be achieved by opening the victim's mouth and manually attempting to dislodge any obvious foreign body with a finger. As a single method, back blows may not be as effective as the Heimlich maneuver in adults. For this reason, the Heimlich maneuver is considered the technique of choice.

VENTILATION DURING CARDIOPULMONARY RESUSCITATION

Clearing the airway is of the utmost importance. Foreign bodies, loose dentures or any other oral obstruction should be removed. Next, the *head tilt-chin lift technique,* which causes the tongue to move anteriorly, is used to open the airway. The chin is lifted forward with the fingers of one hand supporting the jaw, and the head tilted back by the other hand on the forehead of the patient.[37] The *head tilt-neck lift method* of opening the airway is also commonly employed and is an acceptable technique for use by the skilled rescuer. Here, the head is tilted back with one hand on the forehead; the other hand is placed behind the neck, lifting it upward to open the airway. If no spontaneous respirations are present, mouth-to-mouth (or mouth-to-nose) ventilation is immediately initiated, with adequacy being judged by the rise and fall of the patient's chest with each breath. To minimize gastric distension, it is necessary to deliver slow ($1\frac{1}{2}$ to 2 s) ventilatory breaths.

Equipped rescuers will use a barrier device or a bag-mask technique of ventilation together with a small plastic oral "airway," which moves the tongue anteriorly. Adequate ventilation is difficult with the bag-mask technique, since a single rescuer often has difficulty maintaining an adequate seal on the face, and rapid bag deflation commonly results in gastric distension and aspiration. Slow ($1\frac{1}{2}$ to 2 s) ventilation must be employed if a bag-mask is used. Several invasive airway adjuncts have also been developed for use by nonphysician health care providers in prehospital situations. The esophageal obturator airway (EOA), esophageal gastric tube airway (EGTA), and the pharyngotracheal lumen airway are among those that have been used in the prehospital setting. The EOA or EGTA with balloon obstruction of the esophagus and ventilation through proximal ports in the mouth avoids aspiration and appears to provide some but not optimal ventilation.[38] Both have been used extensively in the field. Considerable training and skill is needed in placing and using these devices properly. Serious life-threatening complications occur often and, after successful resuscitation, balloon deflation frequently results in the regurgitation of gastric contents.

Endotracheal intubation remains the ideal technique for ensuring adequate ventilation during CPR. It can be rapidly implemented, but much valuable time can be wasted by repeated unskilled attempts at intubation. If this technique is used, cardiopulmonary resuscitation should be discontinued for no more than 20 s while the tube is being passed into the airway. If more than 20 s elapse without successful intubation, the laryngoscope should be withdrawn and cardiopulmonary resuscitation reinstituted. Whenever possible, a nasogastric tube should be inserted to drain the stomach and thus decrease the chances of aspiration.

The optimal requirements for ventilation during CPR in human beings remain unknown. No study has clearly identified the optimal timing, sequence in relation to chest compression, or tidal volume needed during CPR. American Heart Association (AHA) recommendations advise 10 to 12 slow ventilatory breaths per minute with a tidal volume of 800 to 1200 mL per breath.[32]

CHEST COMPRESSION DURING CARDIOPULMONARY RESUSCITATION

In 1974, 1980, 1986, and 1992 (revised), the American Heart Association published "Standards for Cardiopulmonary Resuscitation and Emergency Cardiac Care."[32] In reference to external chest compression, they advised: (1) 80 to 100 sternal compressions per minute, (2) 50 percent of each compression-relaxation cycle to be compression, and (3) one slow ($1\frac{1}{2}$ to 2 s) ventilation for every five compressions if two trained rescuers are performing CPR, and two slow ($1\frac{1}{2}$ to 2 s) ventilatory breaths every 15 chest compressions if lay rescuers or one trained person is performing CPR. As mentioned earlier, at such faster chest compression rates, a prolongation of chest compression duration is more easily achieved by most individuals. In addition to these recommendations, it is critical when performing chest compression to use sufficient force to depress the sternum by 2 to $2\frac{1}{2}$ in (5 to 6 cm). As this is usually difficult to gauge, sufficient chest compression force should be used to generate a palpable femoral or carotid arterial pulse.

*A*irway-*B*reathing-*C*hest compression, "ABC," is the specific sequence used to initiate CPR in the U.S. and many other countries. However, in the Netherlands, "CAB" is the common technique for CPR implementation with resuscitation outcomes similar to those reported for "ABC" in the United States. No human studies have compared the "ABC" technique of resuscitation with "CAB." Both techniques are effective. "ABC" CPR remains the dominant technique for CPR implementation in the United States with survival rates as high as 40 percent in cities with advanced EMS systems[33,34] (see Chap. 51).

The 1990s, however, have brought a new challenge to the implementation of CPR in the field. Despite its proven efficacy, the perceived risk of infectious disease transmission during CPR has reduced the willingness of both lay and medical personnel to initiate mouth-to-mouth ventilation and CPR in unknown victims of cardiac arrest. In an effort to respond to these concerns and encourage layman CPR, some cities have mandated the public availability and use of barrier devices during mouth-to-mouth ventilation. The effectiveness of such barrier devices is, however, unknown. To overcome this limitation, potential rescuers who are reticent to initiate CPR because of the perceived risk of infection should be encouraged to activate the EMS system immediately, open the victim's airway, and then initiate and continue chest compressions only until paramedics arrive. The paramedics can then initiate ventilation with the necessary protective equipment.

DEFINITIVE THERAPY

The 1992 AHA Standards Guidelines for Emergency Cardiac Care have adopted a new classification for therapeutic recommendations.[32] This classification allows a relative therapeutic value to be assigned to a given strategy of treatment:

Class I:	Definitely helpful
Class IIA:	Acceptable, probably helpful
Class IIB:	Acceptable, possibly helpful, probably not harmful
Class III:	Not indicated, may be harmful

In the text that follows, when appropriate, these specific therapeutic classifications will be mentioned.

During cardiac arrest, the ECG will usually show rapid ventricular tachycardia or fibrillation, asystole, or heart block, or it may be near normal.

Ventricular Tachycardia or Fibrillation

With ventricular fibrillation, an attempt at electrical defibrillation should be made as quickly as possible. Successful defibrillation is accomplished by the passage of adequate electrical current (amperes) through the heart (see also Chap. 41). Current flow is dependent on the energy chosen (joules) and the transthoracic impedance (ohms), or resistance to current flow. Factors that affect transthoracic impedance include the energy selected, electrode size, skin-paddle coupling material, the number and time interval of previous shocks, the distance between the electrodes (size of the chest), phase of ventilation, and paddle electrode pressure.[39] Human transthoracic impedance ranges from 15 to 150 Ω with the average adult impedance being 70 to 80 Ω. If transthoracic impedance is high, low energy shocks are ineffective in generating enough current to achieve successful defibrillation. Transthoracic impedance can be reduced by firm pressure on hand-held electrode paddles and a gel/cream, or saline-soaked gauze pads, between the electrode and the skin.[39] In addition, proper electrode/paddle placement is essential; one electrode should be placed right of the upper sternum below the clavicle and the other left of the nipple with the center of the electrode in the midaxillary line. An acceptable alternative is one electrode anteriorly over the left precordium and the other posteriorly behind the heart in the right infrascapular location.[39] The latter positioning is best achieved by using preadhesive rather than hand-held electrodes. Direct current is employed during defibrillation. The paddles, coated with low-resistance gel, are applied firmly to the chest and then discharged with 200 J which is repeated at 200 to 300 J if the first shock is unsuccessful. The current AHA standards suggest that a third 360 J shock be delivered if ventricular fibrillation persists.[32] These three shocks should be delivered in rapid succession. Prospective studies by Adgey and others[40,41] have shown 85 to 90 percent successful defibrillation using only 200 J in patients weighing up to 90 kg. Some advocate higher-energy defibrillation,[42] but few currently use more than 400 J. High-energy defibrillation may cause more cardiac injury, and there is no clear evidence that it increases the frequency of successful resuscitation.[43] The importance of transthoracic impedance as a determinant of successful defibrillation has led to the concept of "current-based" defibrillation. Here, the operator selects electric current (amperes) instead of energy (joules). Such an approach avoids the problem of an inappropriately low energy selection in patients with high impedance (with consequent low current flow and failure to defibrillate), or high energy selection in patients with low impedance, which could result in excessive current flow, myocardial injury, and failure to defibrillate. Recent advances in defibrillator design have made such an approach feasible by displaying an instantaneous measurement of transthoracic impedance. Clinical studies with this technique support its effectiveness.[44]

When ECG shows "fine" fibrillation waves, defibrillation efforts are often unsuccessful. The administration of epinephrine (5 to 10 mL of 1:10,000) intravenously (IV) results in a more vigorous and coarse fibrillation that is more responsive to defibrillation. This effect is likely due to improved coronary flow following epinephrine administration (see below). If defibrillation fails, it is likely that marked acidosis or hypoxemia is present. Emphasis should be on hyperventilation with supplemental oxygen to correct both hypoxemia and metabolic acidosis.[45] Sodium bicarbonate might then be administered (1 meq/kg) to aid in the management of acidosis, and defibrillation should be repeated with 320 to 400 J.

For recurrent ventricular fibrillation, the administration of 75 to 100 mg of lidocaine IV followed by repeat defibrillation may increase the likelihood of returning to a stable rhythm. Lidocaine is the antiarrhythmic agent of choice for recurrent ventricular fibrillation. Bretylium tosylate is a second-line drug for recurrent ventricular fibrillation in patients failing treatment with lidocaine alone. It can be used either in addition to or in place of lidocaine. Haynes et al. have shown comparable survival from ventricular fibrillation in patients receiving either lidocaine or bretylium.[46] Initially, 5 mg/kg of bretylium is given IV followed by electrical defibrillation. The dose can be increased to 10 mg/kg and repeated at 15- to 30-min intervals until a maximum dose of 30 mg/kg has been given. Procainamide can be used in patients failing lidocaine and bretylium therapy. For recurrent ventricular fibrillation, propranolol is another effective drug. It seems particularly helpful in the setting of primary ventricular fibrillation complicating acute myocardial infarction. Although available only on an investigational basis, amiodarone IV may also be very useful.

Hyperkalemia is a readily treated condition that can cause AV block, impaired intraatrial and intraventricular conduction, and occasionally leads to ventricular fibrillation or, less commonly, asystole. It can be recognized by the development of tall, peaked T waves with a normal QT interval and sine wavelike ventricular tachycardia. Life-threatening hyperkalemia responds most readily to calcium infusion; 10 to 30 mL of 10% calcium gluconate is infused intravenously over 1 to 5 min under constant electrocardiographic monitoring. Calcium counteracts the adverse effects of potassium on the neuromuscular membranes, but does not alter plasma potassium. Its effect, though immediate, is transient. Hyperkalemia should subsequently be treated by glucose-insulin infusion, or ion-exchange resins. (See also Chaps. 36 and 37.) Sodium bicarbonate also is used as an agent to lower potassium.

With ventricular tachycardia, cough[47] may revert the arrhythmia without defibrillation, and repeated cough will maintain the conscious state as a result of the rise in intrathoracic pressure.[10] The efficacy of the precordial thump (precordial chest blows) has been variably reported in patients with ventricular tachycardia. A thump is generally ineffective for terminating prehospital ventricular fibrillation and may be deleterious for ventricular tachycardia, converting it to ventricular fibrillation or asystole. Hence, it should never be used in the patient with ventricular tachycardia and a pulse unless defibrillator is available immediately.

ASYSTOLE OR HEART BLOCK

For patients with prehospital cardiac arrest, asystole has been shown to be an ominous rhythm with a very low likelihood of successful resuscitation.[33] On the other hand, asystole due to vagal stimulation is the commonest cause of cardiac arrest associated with anesthesia induction and surgical procedures. Asystole also occurs as a result of heart block or sinus node disease (see Chaps. 35 and 36). Atropine (0.5 mg) given IV and repeated in 5 min can be used acutely to prevent or reverse severe bradycardia in many of these settings.

If asystole is witnessed or of short duration, vigorous blows to the precordium may sometimes restart the heart. Rhythmic chest blows may maintain limited perfusion and can be continued if needed while palpating the femoral or carotid pulse until other treatment is available. If the chest blow fails, cardiopulmonary resuscitation should be initiated and intravenous epinephrine (5 to 10 mL of 1:10,000) administered. Possible treatable causes of asystole such as acidosis, hypoxemia, hyper- or hypokalemia, and hypothermia should be considered and appropriately treated if suspected. If calcium channel blocker overdose is suspected, calcium chloride, 1 gm IV bolus, may be very effective (Class IIA recommendation). Resuscitation measures may result in a slow ventricular rhythm returning, which can subsequently be supported with atropine (1 to 2 mg IV) until a temporary pacemaker is placed.

Temporary pacing is the optimal treatment for true asystole or profound bradycardia. Obviously, considerable skill and training are required for temporary transvenous pacemaker placement (see Chap. 39). Transcutaneous pacing has been developed as a noninvasive and simple pacing technique that can be rapidly implemented. The technique uses external surface electrodes with a high voltage pacing source. Higher voltages are required to overcome transthoracic resistance, but they are painful and are therefore used mainly on unconscious patients. The energy delivered to the heart by this technique is variable, as is its efficacy. Recently, pacing sources with longer pacing stimulus duration have been developed and may offer less painful and more effective pacing. It may be of some benefit for patients in asystole (Class IIB intervention). Clinical evidence does not support its routine use in all patients with asystole. Transesophageal pacing is an infrequently used alternative technique for noninvasive pacing, but its clinical applicability has been limited.

In rare instances, very fine ventricular fibrillation may result in a near straight line on a single lead ECG and, thus, be mistaken for "asystole." In such cases where the diagnosis of asystole in question, it is suggested that a perpendicular ECG lead be viewed. Rotation of "quick look" ECG paddles by 90 degrees easily achieves this. If ventricular fibrillation is present, the perpendicular ECG lead will demonstrate a typical fibrillation pattern, whereas in true asystole, a straight line will be seen in all ECG leads. If ventricular fibrillation is diagnosed, the initial treatment should be according to the outline above; i.e., three successive countershocks. There is little value of defibrillating true asystole.

ELECTROMECHANICAL DISSOCIATION

In electromechanical dissociation (EMD), there is evidence of organized electrical activity on the ECG at a reasonable rate but failure of effective perfusion (no pulse or blood pressure). The most treatable causes of this condition are hypovolemia due to severe hemorrhage, pericardial tamponade, tension pneumothorax, hypoxia, hypothermia, acidosis, hyperkalemia, and massive pulmonary embolism. Signs of these problems should be sought and definitive therapy undertaken with fluids and/or blood replacement, pericardiocentesis, placement of a pleural needle or tube, endotracheal intubation, and other maneuvers as deemed necessary. These conditions should also be strongly considered if cardiopulmonary resuscitation results in no palpable pulse or evidence of perfusion. Unfortunately, many patients with electromechanical dissociation have primary myocardial failure. Following diagnosis, ventilation should be optimized and epinephrine administered. Calcium chloride was used for EMD, but in prospective studies has not been shown to improve survival.[48] In acute myocardial infarction, sudden electromechanical dissociation is a sign of myocardial rupture. In such cases, pericardiocentesis and surgical repair can rarely result in survival.

ESTABLISHMENT OF AN INTRAVENOUS ROUTE

While external chest compression and artificial ventilation are continued, a plastic catheter should be inserted into a large peripheral vein. Drug administration during CPR should only be accomplished from a source above the diaphragm, since there is little cephalad flow from veins below the diaphragm. If a peripheral vein cannot be cannulated, a cutdown should be attempted or a central venous line placed by a percutaneous route. If cardiopulmonary resuscitation is properly performed, drugs administered through a peripheral line will often reach the arterial circulation within 15 to 30 s.[45] Recent data suggest that a 20-mL fluid bolus significantly improves peripheral drug delivery to the central compartment. Intracardiac injections are unnecessary except when there is no intravenous access. If an intravenous route is unavailable, epinephrine (1 to 2 mg in 10 mL of sterile distilled water) and lidocaine (50 to 100 mg in 10 mL of sterile distilled water) can be administered by way of the endotracheal tube into the bronchial tree. The drug should be injected through a long catheter passed beyond the tip of the endotracheal tube. Cardiac compression should be withheld, and several insufflations with an Ambu bag should immediately follow drug administration to aid drug absorption through aerosolization.

MAJOR DRUGS USED DURING CARDIOPULMONARY RESUSCITATION

Drugs that are used for the treatment of various arrhythmias are mentioned above.

Catecholamines are used in cardiac arrest to (1) increase arterial and coronary perfusion during and following cardiopulmonary resuscitation, (2) stimulate spontaneous contraction during asystole, (3) make fine ventricular fibrillation more responsive to defibrillation, and (4) act as an inotropic agent.

Epinephrine is effective in achieving all these goals. Recent studies have extensively evaluated the hemodynamic effects of epinephrine during resuscitation and have clearly shown it to be the singularly most important drug for common use during CPR.[23] Animal studies show that during conventional CPR, cerebral and myocardial perfusion pressures are low. Epinephrine increases brain and heart flow by two mechanisms:

(1) It prevents carotid artery collapse and raises arterial pressure during both chest compression and the release phase of chest compression (i.e., "systole" and "diastole," respectively). This results in higher carotid arterial "systolic" and aortic "diastolic" pressures, which, in turn, is reflected in higher cerebral perfusion and myocardial perfusion pressures and flow.[23]

(2) It preferentially reduces blood flow to the external carotid, renal, and splanchnic beds, thereby redirecting flow towards the brain and heart.[23]

Arterial collapse at the thoracic inlet has been shown to be the critical limiting factor for cerebral perfusion pressure and flow during prolonged CPR. Arterial collapse results from high extravascular intrathoracic pressures, low intravascular volumes, and loss of arterial tone. Collapse results in a precipitous fall in carotid arterial and, hence, cerebral perfusion pressure. Epinephrine during CPR can not only reverse arterial collapse but also prevent it from developing.[23] With the administration of epinephrine during conventional manual CPR in the dog, cerebral blood flow can be maintained at ≃15 percent and myocardial flow at ≃5 percent of prearrest values for 20 min (Fig. 52-2). If the experimental technique of vest CPR is used along with the frequent administration of epinephrine in dogs, cerebral flow can be maintained at normal levels and myocardial flow >40 percent of prearrest values at 20 min (Fig. 52-2).[19]

These data strongly support the early and frequent use of epinephrine during CPR in an effort to optimize vital organ perfusion. Hence, once the diagnosis of cardiac arrest is established and CPR initiated, epinephrine should be administered as soon as possible. The recommended dose is 0.5 to 1 mg IV, and this dose should be repeated at approximately 3- to 5-min intervals unless effective cardiac activity is restored. If an intravenous route is not available, epinephrine can be administered down the endotracheal tube; 10 mL of a 1:10,000 solution should be used, and this can also be repeated every 3 to 5 min.

The benefits of epinephrine are principally due to the alpha vasoconstriction induced by this agent. The inotropic effects of the drug may not be helpful, since these effects increase myocardial oxygen demand, even during ventricular fibrillation when supply or blood flow is limited. Consequently, there is some interest in using a pure vasoconstrictor during CPR rather than epinephrine. Animal studies of vital organ perfusion comparing epinephrine and phenylepinephrine (a pure alpha vasoconstrictor) have yielded similar results. With asystole, the chronotropic effects of epinephrine may be useful.

The recommended dose of epinephrine—1 mg IV every 3 to 5 min—is comparable to a 0.007 to 0.014 mg/kg dose in a 70-kg person. This dose has been questioned since animal studies using higher doses of epinephrine have shown improved vital organ flow and survival.[49] Other studies of higher doses of epinephrine, however, have shown increased myocardial oxygen demand despite this improved blood flow.[50] Higher than recommended doses of epinephrine have been reported to increase arterial pressure and coronary perfusion pressure in a small number of human studies.[51] These studies spawned an intense interest in the use of higher doses of epinephrine during CPR. Preliminary results from four prospective randomized clinical trials of more than 2400 adult cardiac arrest victims, however, have shown no statistically significant improvement in survival to hospital admission or discharge when higher doses of epinephrine (0.1 to 0.2 mg/kg) were compared to standard doses.[52,53] On the other hand, these trials did not demonstrate any obvious deleterious effect of the higher doses of epinephrine. Hence, higher dose epinephrine should be considered a Class IIB recommendation. Its use in patients failing the initial standard doses of epinephrine during cardiac arrest is discretionary.

Norepinephrine is a potent vasoconstrictor and generally produces a rise in blood pressure; it is also an inotropic agent. Its disadvantage is renal and mesenteric vasoconstriction, and it should not be used in the initial phase of resuscitation. This agent is most useful where severe hypotension is present but where the chronotropic effects of epinephrine are not desirable (such as in acute myocardial infarction or severe ischemia). This agent should be cautiously administered since severe tissue injury results from extravasation around an intravenous site.

Similarly, dopamine (a chemical precursor of norepinephrine) and dobutamine (a synthetic catecholamine) are preferred for use as inotropic agents because of their lesser chronotropic effect. Both these drugs, however, have little use in the initial phases of resuscitation when peripheral vasoconstriction is of primary importance. Isoproterenol (a synthetic catecholamine) is a pure β-adrenergic agonist and effective vasodilator. Therefore, its use during CPR is contraindicated since it can significantly decrease vital organ perfusion pressures. In patients with a palpable pulse, however, it is useful for treatment of bradycardia due to heart block or asystole until a temporary pacemaker is placed (see also Chap. 39).

SODIUM BICARBONATE

The recent AHA recommendations have de-emphasized the role of sodium bicarbonate and suggest that much less sodium bicarbonate should be used than previously advocated for acid-base control during cardiac arrest. As with other types of metabolic acidosis, if adequate alveolar ventilation is achieved, the metabolic acidosis of arrest is partially corrected through P_{CO_2} excretion.[45] No study has clearly demonstrated improved outcome from cardiac arrest with buffer therapy. Rather, several deleterious effects of bicarbonate administration including metabolic acidosis, hypernatremia, hyperosmolality have been reported. Ideally, sodium bicarbonate should be given according to the results of measurement of arterial blood pH, P_{CO_2} determination, and calculation of the base deficit. Bicarbonate should be used, if at all, only after more established interventions such as defibrillation, ventilation with endotracheal intubation, and pharmacological therapies (epinephrine and antiarrhythmic drugs) have been tried.[32] If needed, 1 meq/kg of sodium bicarbonate should be administered; then no more than half this dose repeated every 15 min. Excessive use of sodium bicarbonate can result in metabolic alkalosis, hypernatremia, and hyperosmolality. On the other hand, bicarbonate may be most useful during the immediate post resuscitation period when a profound metabolic acidosis occurs. In most instances during CPR, its use should be considered as a Class IIB recommendation.[32]

Calcium chloride (5 to 7 mg/kg) enhances the contractile state of the heart and is indicated in treating severe hypotension due to calcium channel blocker overdose or hyperkalemia. It is no longer recommended for use in asystole or electromechanical dissociation.[32,48]

TERMINATION OF CARDIOPULMONARY RESUSCITATION

Despite resuscitative efforts, the patient in cardiac arrest may not regain spontaneous circulation. The decision to end cardiopulmonary resuscitation should be based on a physician's assessment of the cerebral, cardiovascular, and general status of the patient.[54,55] Failure is likely if there is absence of organized ventricular electrocardiography activity and/or peripheral perfusion after 10 to 15 min of adequate cardiopulmonary resuscitation and appropriate therapy. Persistent deep unconsciousness and absence of respiration, reflex response, or pupillary reaction suggest cerebral death, and resuscitative efforts are usually unproductive. These guidelines, however, should be altered in patients with hypothermia, barbiturate overdose, and, perhaps, following electrocution, where recovery has been seen even after hours of resuscitation.[56]

POSTARREST CARE

Patients who have been successfully resuscitated usually require monitoring in an intensive care setting. These patients are prone to cardiac arrhythmias, hemodynamic and ventilatory instability, and ischemic encephalopathy. Ventilatory support with a respirator may well be necssary initially. Serial arterial blood gas determinations should be made to identify hypoxemia and assess the rapidly changing acid-base status.

Several therapeutic strategies have been employed in animal models to help reduce postcardiac-arrest hypoxic encephalopathy. None (including emergency cardiopulmonary bypass that is currently undergoing clinical testing) have clearly been shown to be beneficial in man. The treatment of post-cardiac-arrest encephalopathy involves the prevention of further hypoxia and hypotension. For cerebral edema after cardiac arrest, methylprednisolone (60 to 100 mg) or dexamethasone sodium phosphate (12 to 20 mg IV every 6 h) has been recommended, but there is no conclusive evidence that these agents are beneficial. High-dose barbiturates or lidoflazine have also been shown to reduce postarrest brain injury in animal studies[57]; the value of this therapy in human beings is negligible.[58] The prognosis of the patient with anoxic encephalopathy is related to the depth and continued duration of cerebral dysfunction (see also Chap. 122).

Animal data suggest that reperfusion injury may contribute significantly to postarrest encephalopathy. Treatment with free radical scavengers to reduce reperfusion injury has been shown to significantly improve brain function post arrest in animals. The usefulness of such therapy in humans, however, remains to be evaluated.

Other potential life-threatening problems in the postarrest period include acute renal failure, bowel infarction, infection, and sepsis. Patients regaining consciousness may have postarrest amnesia or may develop psychotic behavior.

OUTCOME OF RESUSCITATION

In their initial study, Kouwenhoven, Jude, and Knickerbocker reported a 24 percent successful resuscitation and discharge rate from the hospital. Recent studies have shown that with a paramedical response system, a near 40 percent successful out-of-hospital resuscitation rate can be achieved.[33,34] More than 50 percent of these patients die in hospital, however, with the dominant cause of death being anoxic encephalopathy.[59] The critical factors for successful out-of-hospital resuscitation include <7 min total duration of CPR, <4 min from collapse to the initiation of CPR, and <10 min to successful delivery of first countershock. It is important to point out, however, that the quality of life for patients surviving to hospital discharge is often quite good, with most discharged patients being able to return to gainful employment.[60]

REFERENCES

1. Comroe JH: Retrospectroscope, ". . . In Comes the Good Air." *Am Rev Respir Dis* 1979; 119:803–809.
2. Elam JO, Brown ES, Elder JD: Artificial respiration by mouth-to-mask method. *N Engl J Med* 1954; 250:749–754.

3. Sanders AB, Kern KB, Ewy GA: Open chest massage for resuscitation from cardiac arrest. *Resuscitation* 1988; 16:153–154.
4. Eldor J, Frankel DZN, Davidson JT: Open chest cardiac massage: A review. *Resuscitation* 1988; 16:155–162.
5. Wiggers CJ: The physiologic basis for cardiac resuscitation from ventricular fibrillation—method of serial defibrillation. *Am Heart J* 1940; 20:413–422.
6. Kouwenhoven WB, Jude JR, Knickerbocker GG: Closed chest cardiac massage. *JAMA* 1960; 173:1064–1067.
7. Jude JR, Kouwenhoven WB, Knickerbocker GG: Cardiac Arrest: Report of application of external cardiac massage on 118 patients. *JAMA* 1961; 178:1063–1071.
8. Weale FE, Rothwell-Jackson RL: The efficiency of cardiac massage. *Lancet* 1962; 1:990–992.
9. MacKenzie GJ, Taylor SH, McDonald AH, Donald KW: Hemodynamic effects of external cardiac compression. *Lancet* 1964; 1:1342–1345.
10. Criley JM, Blaufuss AN, Kissel GL: Cough-induced cardiac compression. *JAMA* 1976; 236:1246–1250.
11. Rudikoff MT, Maughan WL, Effron M, Freund P, Weisfeldt ML: Mechanisms of flow during cardiopulmonary resuscitation. *Circulation* 1980; 61:345–351.
12. Halperin H, Brower R, Weisfeldt ML, Tsitlik J, Chandra N, Cristiano L, et al: Air trapping in the lungs during cardiopulmonary resuscitation in dogs: A mechanism for generating changes in intrathoracic pressure. *Circulation Res* 1989; 65:946–954.
13. Maier GW, Tyson GS, Olsen CO, Kerstein KH, Davis JW, Conn EH, et al: The physiology of external cardiac massage: High impulse cardiopulmonary resuscitation. *Circulation* 1984; 70:86–101.
14. Feneley MP, Maier GW, Gaynor JW, Gall SA, Kisslo JA, Davis JW, et al: Sequence of mitral valve motion and transmitral blood flow during manual cardiopulmonary resuscitation in dogs. *Circulation* 1987; 76:363–375.
15. Deshmukh HG, Weil MH, Gudipati CV, Trevino RP, Bisera J, Rackow EC: Mechanism of blood flow generated by precordial compression during CPR. I. Studies on closed chest precordial compression. *Chest* 1989; 95:1092–1099.
16. Werner JA, Greene HL, Janko CL, Cobb LA: Visualization of cardiac valve motion in man during external chest compression using two-dimensional echocardiography. Implications regarding the mechanism of blood flow. *Circulation* 1981; 63:1417–1421.
17. Halperin HR, Weiss JL, Guerci AD, Chandra N, Tsitlik JE, Brower R, et al: Cyclic elevation of intrathoracic pressure can close the mitral valve during cardiac arrest in dogs. *Circulation* 1988; 78:754–760.
18. Koehler RC, Chandra N, Guerci AD, Tsitlik J, Traytsman RJ, Rogers MC, et al: Augmentation of cerebral perfusion by simultaneous chest compression and lung inflation with abdominal binding following cardiac arrest in dogs. *Circulation* 1983; 67:266–275.
19. Halperin HR, Guerci AD, Chandra N, Herskowitz A, Tsitlik JE, Niskanen RA, et al: Vest inflation without simultaneous ventilation during cardiac arrest in dogs: Improved survival from prolonged cardiopulmonary resuscitation. *Circulation* 1986; 74:1407–1415.
20. Guerci A, Chandra N, Gelfand M, Gruben K, Scott C, Weisfeldt M, et al: Vest CPR increases aortic pressure in humans (Abstract). *Circulation* 1989; 80:II–496.
21. Sack J, Kesselbrenner M, Bergman D: Survival from in-hospital arrest with interposed abdominal counterpulsation during cardiopulmonary resuscitation. *JAMA* 1992; 276:379–385.
22. Cohen TJ, Tucker KJ, Lurie KG, Redberg RF, Dutton JP, Dwyer KA, et al: Active compression-decompression resuscitation: A new method of cardiopulmonary resuscitation. JAMA 1992; 267:2916–2923.
23. Michael JR, Guerci AD, Koehler RC, Shi AY, Tsitlik J, Chandra N, et al: Mechanisms by which epinephrine augments cerebral and myocardial perfusion during cardiopulmonary resuscitation in dogs. *Circulation* 1984; 69:822–835.
24. Halperin HR, Tsitlik JE, Guerci AD, Levin HR, Shi AY, Chandra N, et al: Determinants of blood flow to vital organs during cardiopulmonary resuscitation in dogs. *Circulation* 1986; 73:539–551.
25. Standards and Guidelines for cardiopulmonary resuscitation (CPR) and emergency cardiac care (ECC). *JAMA* 1986; 255:2905–2989.
26. Swenson RD, Weaver WD, Nisaken RA, Martin J, Dahlberg S: Hemodynamics in humans during conventional and experimental methods of cardiopulmonary resuscitation. *Circulation* 1988; 78:630–639.
27. Chandra NC, Tsitlik JE, Halperin HR, Guerci AD, Weisfeldt ML: Observations of hemodynamics during cardiopulmonary resuscitation. *Crit Care Med* 1990; 18:929–934.
28. Paradis N, Martin G, Goetting M, Rosenberg J, Rivers E, Appleton T, et al: Simultaneous aortic, jugular bulb, and right atrial pressures during cardiopulmonary resuscitation in humans: Insights into mechanisms. *Circulation* 1989; 80:361–368.
29. Chandra N, Snyder LD, Weisfeldt ML: Abdominal binding during CPR in man. *JAMA* 1981; 246:351–353.
30. Chandra N, Rudikoff M, Weisfeldt ML: Simultaneous chest compression and ventilation at high airway pressure during cardiopulmonary resuscitation. *Lancet* 1980; 1:175–178.
31. Krischer JP, Fine EG, Weisfeldt ML, Guerci AD, Nagel E, Chandra N: Comparison of prehospital conventional and simultaneous compression-ventilation cardiopulmonary resuscitation. *Crit Care Med* 1989; 17:1263–1269.
32. Emergency Cardiac Care Committee and Subcommittees, American Heart Association: Guidelines for cardiopulmonary resuscitation and emergency cardiac care. *JAMA* 1992; 268:2171–2302.
33. Cobb LA, Werner JA, Trobaugh GB: Sudden cardiac death: parts 1 and 2. *Mod Concepts Cardiovasc Dis* 1980; 49:31–36, 37–42.
34. Eisenberg MS, Copass MK, Hallstrom AP, Blake B, Bergner L, Short FA, et al: Treatment of out-of-hospital cardiac arrest with rapid defibrillation by emergency medical technicians. *N Engl J Med* 1980; 302:1379–1383.
35. Heimlich HJ: A life saving maneuver to prevent from choking. *JAMA* 1975; 234:398–401.
36. Visintine RE, Baick CH: Ruptured stomach after Heimlich maneuver. *JAMA* 1975; 234:415.
37. Greene DG, Elam JO, Dobkin AB, Studley CL: Cine-fluorographic study of hypertension of the neck and upper airway patency. *JAMA* 1961; 176:570–573.
38. Bass RR, Allison EJ, Hunt RC: The esophageal obturator airway: A reassessment of use by paramedics. *Ann Emerg Med* 1983; 11:358–360.
39. Sirna SJ, Fergusson DW, Charbonnier F, Kerber RE: Electrical cardioversion in humans: Factors affecting transthoracic impedance. *Am J Cardiol* 1988; 62:1048–1052.
40. Adgey AAJ, Patton JN, Campbell NPS, Webb SW: Ventricular defibrillation: Appropriate energy levels. *Circulation* 1979; 60:219–223.
41. Gascho JA, Crampton RS, Cherwek ML, Sipes JM, Hunter FP, O'Brien WM: Determinants of ventricular defibrillation in adults. *Circulation* 1979; 60:231–240.
42. Tacker WA, Ewy GA: Emergency defibrillation dose, recommendation and rationale. *Circulation* 1979; 60:223–225.
43. Weaver WD, Cobb LA, Copass MK, Hallstrom AP: Ventricular defibrillation—a comparative trial using 175-J and 320-J shocks. *N Engl J Med* 1982; 307:1101–1106.
44. Lerman BB, DiMarco JP, Haines D: Current-based versus energy-based ventricular defibrillation: A prospective study. *J Am Coll Cardiol* 1988; 12:1259–1264.
45. Bishop RL, Weisfeldt ML: Sodium bicarbonate administration during cardiac arrest. Effect of arterial pH, P_{CO_2} and osmolality. *JAMA* 1976; 235:506–509.
46. Haynes RE, Copass MK, Chinn TL, Cobb LA: Comparison of bretylium tosylate and lidocaine in management of out-of-hospital ventricular fibrillation. A randomized clinical trial. *Am J Coll* 1981; 48:353–356.
47. Wei JY, Greene HL, Weisfeldt ML: Cough-facilitated conversion of ventricular tachycardia. *Am J Cardiol* 1980; 45:174–176.
48. Stueven HA, Thompson BM, Aprahamian C, Tonsfeldt DJ: Calcium chloride, reassessment of use in asystole. *Ann Emerg Med* 1984; 13:820–822.
49. Brown CG, Wermn HA, Davis EA, Hobson J, Hamlin RL: The effects of graded doses of epinephrine on regional myocardial blood flow during cardiopulmonary resuscitation in swine. *Circulation* 1987; 75:491–497.
50. Ditchey RV, Lindenfeld J: Failure of epinephrine to improve the balance between myocardial oxygen supply and demand during closed chest resuscitation in dogs. *Circulation* 1988; 78:382–389.
51. Paradis NA, Martin GB, Rivers EP, Goetting MG, Appleton TH,

Feingold M, et al: Coronary perfusion pressure and the return of spontaneous circulation in human cardiopulmonary resuscitation. *JAMA* 1990; 263:1106–1113.

52. Stiell IG, Hebert PC, Weitzman BN, Wells GA; Raman S, Stark RM, et al: High-dose epinephrine in adult cardiac arrest. *N Engl J Med* 1992; 327:1045–1050.
53. Brown CG, Martin DR, Pepe PE, Steuven H, Cummins RO, Gonzalez E, et al: A comparison of standard-dose and high-dose epinephrine in cardiac arrest outside the hospital. *N Engl J Med* 1992; 327:1051–1055.
54. Luce JM, Raffin TA: Withholding and withdrawal of life support from critically ill patients. *Chest* 1988; 94:621–626.
55. Niemann JT: Cardiopulmonary resuscitation. *N Engl J Med* 1992; 327:1075–1080.
56. Ravitch MM, Lane R, Safar P, Steichen FM, Knowles P: Lightning stroke. Report of a case with recovery after cardiac massage and prolonged artificial respiration. *N Engl J Med* 1961; 264:36–38.
57. Safar P, Bleyart A, Nemoto EM, Moossy J, Snyder JV: Resuscitation after global brain ischemia-anoxia. *Crit Care Med* 1978; 6:215–227.
58. Safar P: Resuscitation from clinical death: pathophysiologic limits and therapeutic potentials. *Crit Care Med* 1988; 16:923–941.
59. Chandra NC, Fine EG, Guerci AD, Nagel EL, Krischer JP: Hospital mortality in survivors of out-of-hospital resuscitation (abstract). *Circulation* 1987; 76:IV-220.
60. Eisenberg MS, Hallstrom A, Bergner L: Long-term survival after out-of-hospital cardiac arrest. *N Engl J Med* 1982; 306:1340–1343.

PART VII

Coronary Heart Disease

SECTION A

Basic Considerations

Chapter 53

The Biochemistry of Blood Lipid Regulation and the Assessment of Lipid Abnormalities

Peter H. Jones, M.D. ■ *Josef Patsch, M.D.* ■ *Antonio M. Gotto, Jr., M.D., D. Phil.*

Atherosclerotic coronary heart disease (CHD) is a major health problem in the United States and other industrialized countries. Most epidemiologic data in single and cross-cultural populations have strongly linked untreated hypertension, cigarette smoking, and elevated total and low-density lipoprotein (LDL) cholesterol levels to the subsequent development of CHD. Evidence supporting the relation between blood cholesterol level and CHD risk has been strengthened by numerous animal studies showing progression and regression of atherosclerotic lesions as cholesterol levels rise and fall and by natural-history studies of genetic hypercholesterolemias (such as familial hypercholesterolemia), in which marked cholesterol elevations caused premature atherosclerosis even in the absence of other risk factors.

In asymptomatic patients deemed at high risk for CHD, drugs have been shown to reduce total and LDL cholesterol levels and subsequently to decrease CHD risk. The Lipid Research Clinics Coronary Primary Prevention Trial (LRC-CPPT) used the bile acid sequestrant cholestyramine in a randomized, double-blind, placebo-controlled study conducted over a 7- to 10-year period in 3806 men aged 35 to 59 years with total cholesterol values above 265 mg/dL (6.8 mmol/liter). The treated group had a significant (19 percent) reduction in fatal and nonfatal CHD events compared with the placebo group.[1,2] The Helsinki Heart Study, conducted among 4081 men aged 40 to 55 years, was similar in design but used the drug gemfibrozil, a fibric acid derivative. The treated men had 34 percent fewer fatal and nonfatal CHD events, associated with the combination of lowering LDL cholesterol levels and raising high-density lipoprotein (HDL) cholesterol levels.[3] Although these two studies did not show a reduction in total mortality by the use of hypocholesterolemic medications, a 15-year follow-up of the patients in the Coronary Drug Project, a secondary prevention trial, who took nicotinic acid only for the initial 5 years showed a significant reduction in overall mortality.[4] Several studies, including the Cholesterol-Lowering Atherosclerosis Study (CLAS),[5,6] the Familial Atherosclerosis Treatment Study (FATS),[7] and the U.S. National Heart, Lung, and Blood Institute (NHLBI) Type II Coronary Intervention Study,[8] have provided strong evidence that the progression of angiographically documented coronary atherosclerotic lesions in native and bypass grafts is slowed, and in some cases halted or even reversed, by drug-induced reductions of total cholesterol.

There is no longer a question as to whether one should attempt to detect and treat hypercholesterolemia.[9,10] The Adult Treatment Panel II of the National Cholesterol Education Program (NCEP) has provided specific guidelines for the assessment and treatment of hyperlipidemia in adults age 20 or older. The guidelines include specific recommendations on how and when to use dietary and drug interventions.[11] This chapter reviews the biochemistry and metabolic regulation of lipoproteins as well as the clinical assessment of lipoprotein abnormalities. A review of the lipid-modulating medications and recommended first-line treatments is in Chap. 65.

BIOCHEMISTRY OF BLOOD LIPID REGULATION

The five major classes of lipids in blood plasma are cholesterol, cholesteryl ester, phospholipid, triglyceride, and unesterified fatty acids. Unesterified fatty acids are transported with plasma albumin. All of the other major plasma lipids are packaged in micelle-like structures called lipoproteins.

Plasma lipoproteins were first recognized by Macheboeuf in the 1920s.[12] He found that treating serum with ammonium sulfate under specific conditions led to the precipitation of a fraction of relatively constant composition containing lipid and protein. Further advances in the study of lipoproteins came in the 1940s, when Oncley[13] applied the technique of Cohn fractionation to separate lipoproteins and Gofman and coworkers[14] separated lipoproteins on the basis of density and sedimentation velocity in the analytical ultracentrifuge. Because their lipid content gives them a low density, plasma lipoproteins can float in a salt gradient; the other, lipid-free proteins settle. Havel et al.[15] introduced the procedure of preparative ultracentrifugation to isolate lipoproteins. Ultracentrifugation is needed to separate all the lipoproteins except chylomicrons, which can be isolated by overnight refrigeration of plasma. The density of normal protein-free plasma or serum is approximately 1.006 g/mL. At this density, the very low density lipoproteins (VLDLs) float to the top of the ultracentrifuge. At a density of 1.063 g/mL, two lipoprotein classes float in the ultracentrifuge: intermediate-density lipoprotein (IDL) (density 1.006 to 1.019 g/mL) and LDL (density 1.019 to 1.063 g/mL). Finally, at a density of 1.21 g/mL, the HDLs float to the top. The HDLs are subdivided as HDL_2 (density 1.063 to 1.125 g/mL) and HDL_3 (density 1.125 to 1.210 g/mL).

Ultracentrifugation is one of two classic methods used to separate and identify lipoproteins; the other is electrophoresis. Lees and Hatch[16] improved the technique of paper electrophoretic separation of plasma lipoproteins through the use of an albuminated buffer. Fredrickson et al.[17] then used paper electrophoresis in conjunction with heparin/manganese precipitation and preparative ultracentrifugation to establish a system for classifying plasma lipoprotein disorders based on which family or families of lipoproteins were elevated. In this technique, called beta quantification, chylomicrons remain at the origin, while VLDLs migrate in front of the beta-globulins. The VLDL mobility is called pre-beta. The LDLs comigrate with the beta-globulins and thus are sometimes referred to as beta-lipoproteins. IDLs, too, have beta mobility. HDLs migrate with the alpha-globulins (hence, "alpha-lipoproteins").

All lipoproteins that contain apolipoprotein B species (apo B-48 and/or apo B-100) can be precipitated under specified conditions, leaving HDL in solution. This method makes it possible to determine the HDL cholesterol content in plasma after the removal of all the other lipoproteins. The method usually employs either heparin and manganese or phosphotungstate.[18]

Lipoproteins are high-molecular-weight particles that transport water-insoluble nonpolar lipids (primarily triglycerides and cholesteryl esters) through the plasma. The general structure of a lipoprotein particle is shown in Fig. 53-1. Each lipoprotein particle has a nonpolar core containing various amounts of triglyceride and cholesteryl ester molecules that form an oily droplet. The core is surrounded by a monolayer of phospholipids. The polar head groups of phospholipids are oriented toward the aqueous phase of the plasma, which stabilizes the lipoprotein particle so that it can remain in solution in plasma. Unesterified cholesterol and proteins are also present in the surface monolayer. The proteins, termed apolipoproteins, are amphipathic in character, in part embedded in the lipid domain of the lipoprotein and in

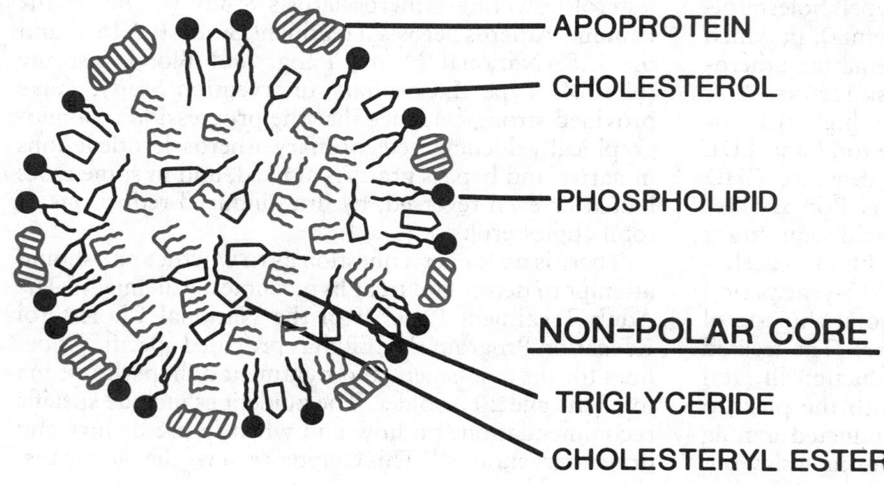

FIGURE 53-1 General structure of a lipoprotein particle.

TABLE 53-1
Classification and Properties of Plasma Lipoproteins

Lipoprotein Class	Major Lipids	Apolipoproteins	Density (g/mL)	Diameter (Å)	Electrophoretic Mobility
Chylomicrons	Dietary triglycerides, cholesteryl esters	A-I, A-II, A-IV, B-48, C-I, C-II, C-III, E	<0.95	800–5000	Origin
Remnants	Dietary cholesteryl esters	B-48, E	<1.006	>300	Origin
VLDL	Endogenous triglycerides	B-100, C-I, C-II, C-III, E	<1.006	300–800	Pre-β
IDL	Cholesteryl esters, triglycerides	B-100, E	1.006–1.019	250–350	Pre-β/β
LDL	Cholesteryl esters	B-100	1.019–1.063	180–280	β
HDL_2	Cholesteryl esters	A-I, A-II	1.063–1.125	90–120	α
HDL_3	Cholesteryl esters	A-I, A-II	1.125–1.210	50–90	α

HDL, high-density lipoprotein; IDL, intermediate-density lipoprotein; LDL, low-density lipoprotein; VLDL, very low density lipoprotein.

part protruding from the surface of the lipoprotein into the aqueous phase of the plasma. The latter nature allows the lipoprotein particle to be soluble and to interact with enzymes and cell membrane receptors.[19] Thus, the apolipoproteins hold a key function for the metabolic fate of the lipoprotein.

The properties of the various human plasma lipoproteins are summarized in Table 53-1. Triglycerides dominate in the cores of chylomicrons and VLDL, and cholesteryl esters are the major core constituent of LDL and HDL. Since the thickness of the monomolecular surface coat is the same in all lipoproteins, the variability in lipoprotein particle size is a variability in core size. With the exception of the subset of HDL particles that is extremely small, the hydrophobic core accounts for most of the mass of a lipoprotein particle.

Transport of Exogenous Lipids

In the intestine, dietary cholesteryl esters are mixed with a similar amount of endogenous cholesterol from saliva, gastric secretions, bile, and sloughed intestinal epithelial cells.[20] Cholesterol can also be synthesized de novo by enterocytes.[21] Within the enterocyte, dietary triglycerides and cholesterol are packaged into a core and wrapped into a surface film of phospholipids, cholesterol, and apo B-48 to form a chylomicron (apo B-48 is the principal apolipoprotein of chylomicrons). The nascent chylomicron particles are secreted from the Golgi vacuoles into the intercellular spaces, where they reach the intestinal lymph, pass through the thoracic duct, and enter the general circulation through the subclavian vein. The appearance of chylomicrons in plasma begins within 1 h after fat ingestion and is called postprandial lipemia. Chylomicrons transport about 100 g triglyceride as dietary fat and 0.5 to 1.0 g cholesterol per day.

The catabolism of chylomicrons is basically a two-step process (Fig. 53-2). First, the enzyme lipoprotein lipase located in extrahepatic tissues hydrolyzes the triglycerides from the chylomicron particles to form the triglyceride-depleted chylomicron remnants. The $t_{1/2}$ of chylomicron triglycerides in the circulation is about 5 min. Second, chylomicron remnants are taken up by remnant receptors in the liver. After entering the circulation, a nascent chylomicron undergoes rapid modification, with some components released from the particle and others joining it. Apo B-48 remains an integral component, but the soluble apolipoproteins A-I, A-II, and A-IV quickly leave the chylomicron to associate with HDL. Newly secreted chylomicrons gain apolipoproteins C-I, C-II, C-III, and E from VLDL and HDL.

In the capillaries, the chylomicrons adhere to binding sites on the vessel walls, where they are exposed to lipoprotein lipase.[22] For lipoprotein lipase to act on the chylomicron particle, apo C-II is required. The lipoprotein lipase causes lipolysis of triglycerides, resulting in the formation of free fatty acids and monoglycerides, which are quickly removed from the blood. The fatty acids pass through the endothelial cell layer and enter the underlying cells such as adipocytes or muscle cells. The major sites of lipoprotein lipase activity are adipose tissue, skeletal muscle, the myocardium, and the mammary gland. These tissues are known to take up triglycerides for storage (adipose tissue), oxidation (muscle work), or secretion (milk).

The chylomicron remnant is the end result of the first step of chylomicron catabolism (i.e., lipolysis) and contains cholesteryl esters as the predominant core component. As lipolysis proceeds, additional modifications occur.[20] As the size of the chylomicron is reduced, surface phospholipids become redundant and are transferred to HDL. The activator protein of lipoprotein lipase, apo C-II, is also shuttled back to HDL. The same is true for apo C-III, which functions to prevent premature removal of the chylomicron by the liver. Thus, most chylomicron constituents not cleared with the remnant are transferred to HDL. With most of the triglyceride hydrolyzed and many of the surface components dissociated, the chylomicron particle will have lost about 95 percent of its mass. The remaining chylomicron remnant, enriched in cholesteryl esters and containing apos B-48 and E, dissociates from the capillary endothelium to reenter the circulation.

The remnant particle is removed from the circulation by the liver. This uptake appears to be mediated by apo E. The remnant's other major apolipoprotein, B-48, is necessary for secretion of the chylomicron by the enterocyte but is not required for chylomicron removal. Al-

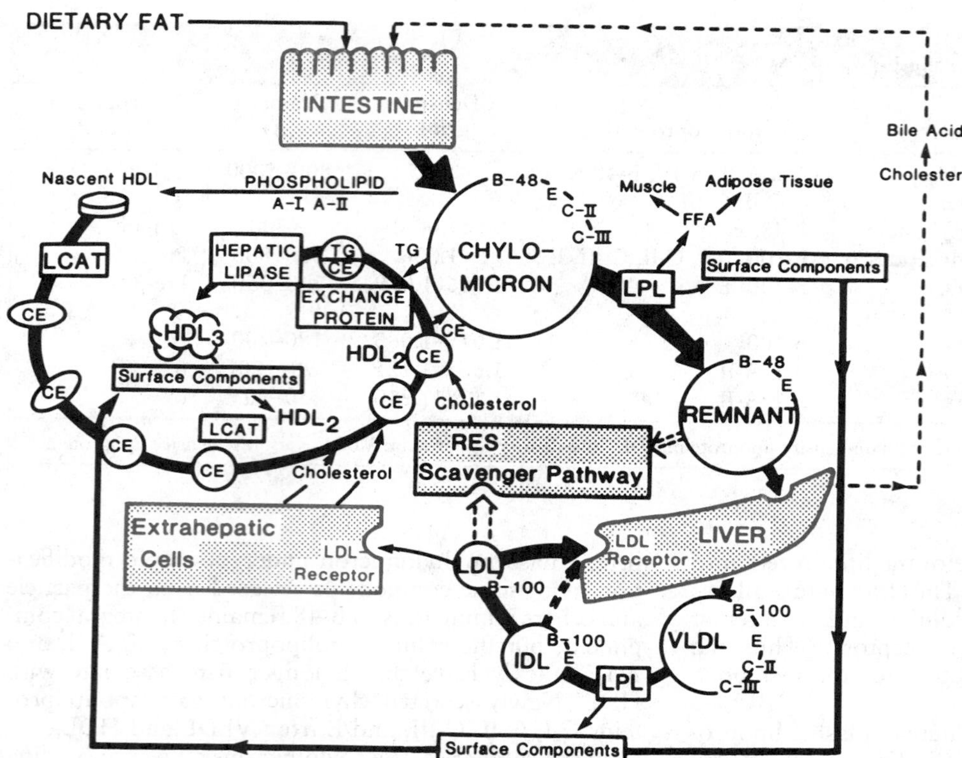

FIGURE 53-2 Lipid transport by plasma lipoproteins. CE = cholesteryl ester; FFA = free fatty acids; HDL = high-density lipoprotein; LCAT = lecithin:cholesterol acyltransferase; LDL = low-density lipoprotein; LPL = lipoprotein lipase; RES = reticuloendothelial system; TG = triglyceride; VLDL = very low density lipoprotein. Surface components include phospholipids, unesterified cholesterol, and apolipoproteins C liberated from the surface of triglyceride-rich lipoproteins during lipolysis.

though B-48 is a product of the same gene as B-100, which binds to the LDL receptor (a protein molecule), it lacks the COOH terminal receptor-binding domain of B-100.[23] Chylomicron remnants are internalized into the hepatocytes by receptor-mediated endocytosis and subsequently degraded within lysosomes. The cholesterol directed through chylomicron remnants to the liver is converted to bile acids or excreted into the bile without conversion to bile acids. An additional fraction of the chylomicron cholesterol can be incorporated into VLDL particles and secreted by the liver into the bloodstream.

The body synthesizes 60 to 80 percent of its cholesterol, primarily in the liver and intestine, and derives the remainder from the diet. The uptake of cholesterol by the liver from chylomicron remnants reduces both the hepatic synthesis of cholesterol and LDL receptor activity.[24] Chylomicron remnants are more effective than LDL or HDL in suppressing cholesterol biosynthesis by the liver.[25] Provision of excess dietary cholesterol to the liver not only suppresses the liver's endogenous synthesis of cholesterol but also decreases the activity of the LDL receptors, which bind apo B-100 and apo E. Chronic suppression of hepatic LDL receptor activity by dietary cholesterol or saturated fat may lead to elevated levels of LDL in the blood and thus predispose to atherosclerosis. The relationship between dietary intake of cholesterol and/or saturated fat and atherosclerosis is well established; linking that relationship with suppression of the LDL receptor provides one plausible hypothesis for dietary effects on lipids and atherogenesis.

Chylomicron remnants can also interact with receptors other than those on hepatocytes. The uptake of these remnants—by macrophages in particular—can lead to the overloading of cells with both triglyceride and cholesterol,[26] raising the possibility that these lipoproteins contribute to atherosclerosis.[27]

Transport of Endogenous Lipids

Triglycerides synthesized in the liver are incorporated into the cores of VLDLs and secreted into the bloodstream. This synthesis is enhanced in the postprandial state or when the diet contains excess carbohydrates. In these situations, excess fatty acids are generated and incorporated by the liver into triglycerides. Cholesteryl esters are packed into the VLDL core and constitute about one-tenth of the triglyceride in VLDL.

The principal apolipoprotein of VLDL is B-100. With 4536 amino acid residues, B-100 is a very large protein molecule.[28–30] It contains many lipid-binding domains and also a domain on its COOH terminal end that binds to the LDL receptor.[28] When the VLDL particles reach the capillaries, they are hydrolyzed by the same lipoprotein lipase enzyme that catabolizes chylomicrons. Analogous to chylomicron metabolism, the VLDL particle during lipolysis loses most of its apolipoprotein components other than B-100 (Fig. 53-2). Redundant surface phospholipids, generated during the reduction of VLDL size through lipolysis of triglyceride, are transferred to HDL. The same is true for apo C-II and apo C-III. Removal of much of the triglyceride from the VLDL particle core results in the formation of the VLDL remnant particle called IDL. The IDL particle is similar to the chylomicron remnant but has a different metabolic fate. Only some of the IDL particles are catabolized by the liver; the route is interaction with LDL receptors on hepatocyte membranes. These receptors bind either to apo B-100 or apo E, more likely to the latter in the case of IDL. In the

IDL particles that remain in the plasma, triglyceride is removed until LDL particles are formed, with a major core constituency of cholesteryl ester and with B-100 as the only protein component.

One function of LDL is to supply cholesterol to cells for the synthesis of cell membranes and steroid hormones. Many cell surfaces contain LDL receptors, the number of which is thought to be a major determinant of the concentration of LDL in the blood. The number and activity of receptors are high early in life and tend to diminish with age. As discussed above, a diet rich throughout life in saturated fat and cholesterol may lead to chronic suppression of LDL receptor activity. Factors that diminish intrahepatic cellular concentration of cholesterol will lead to an increase in receptor activity, whereas an increase in intrahepatic cellular cholesterol will down-regulate the receptors. Hepatocytes contain LDL receptors and use much of the LDL cholesterol for the synthesis of bile acids. The LDLs bind to LDL receptors and are internalized into the cells by receptor-mediated endocytosis[31] (Fig. 53-3). Subsequently, LDL receptors are recycled to the cell surface. In the lysosomes, the cholesteryl esters of LDL are hydrolyzed by a lysosomal cholesteryl esterase (acid lipase) into unesterified cholesterol, thus converting cholesterol from its transport form to its metabolically active form.

Cholesterol and Atherosclerosis

As noted above, it is well established that hypercholesterolemia due to elevated blood levels of LDL is a major cause of CHD and that lowering elevated levels of cholesterol will reduce the risk of coronary disease.[1,3,9,10] In healthy humans, more than 70 percent of the LDL particles circulating in plasma are removed through LDL receptors. The remainder are removed by alternative pathways, some receptor mediated and others nonspecific. This alternative removal of LDL from the circulation, chiefly by cells of the reticuloendothelial system, has been termed collectively the scavenger-cell pathway[31]; it is thought to function as a removal mechanism for excess LDL and apparently is not needed to satisfy the physiological requirements of cells for cholesterol.

The "scavenger receptor" of the receptor-mediated alternative route is also called the "acetyl LDL receptor"[32] because it recognizes chemically modified LDL. Exposure of LDL to endothelial cells results in its peroxidation.[33] The peroxidation process includes a number of structural changes of LDL, including peroxidation of polyunsaturated fatty acids of its lipid moieties, a conversion of much of its lecithin to lysolecithin, oxidation of cholesterol, and fragmentation of apo B-100, with a decrease in the content of histidine, lysine, and proline. Fragmentation of fatty acids can lead to formation of shorter chain aldehydes.

Some of these lipid peroxidation products can attach covalently to B-100,[34] thus masking lysine ε-amino groups of the apolipoprotein or of its fragments.[35,36] These structural changes mean an increased negative charge and density of the peroxidized LDL particles and hence major changes in biologic activity, including chemotactic activity for circulating blood monocytes, the ability to become substrates for the scavenger receptor, and cytotoxicity.[33] Oxidation of LDL—or other modifications of LDL, including glycation of B-100[37]—could thus lead to accumulation of cholesteryl esters in macrophages and smooth-muscle cells and the development of atherosclerotic plaque. An alternative mechanism for foam cell genesis could be the formation of immune complexes between oxidized LDL and autoantibodies against oxidized LDL[38,39] and the uptake of the complexes by macrophages through the Fc receptor.[40] It appears that normal, unmodified LDL particles do not go through the scavenger pathway or lead to the formation of foam cells.[31]

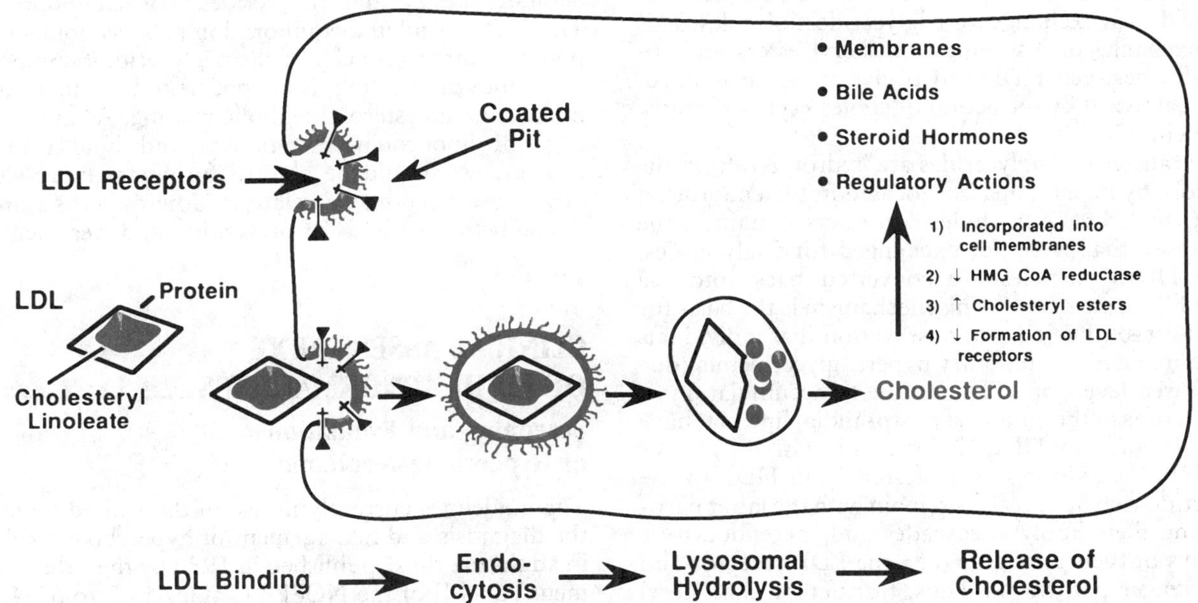

FIGURE 53-3 The low-density lipoprotein (LDL) receptor pathway. HMG-CoA = 3-hydroxy-3-methylglutaryl coenzyme A. *(Adapted from Goldstein JL, Brown MS: The LDL receptor defect in familial hypercholesterolemia. Med Clin North Am 1987; 66:335. Reproduced with permission from the publisher and the authors.)*

HDL Cholesterol and Reverse Cholesterol Transport

A strong negative correlation has been demonstrated between plasma level of HDL cholesterol and CHD.[41] Most of the variability in HDL cholesterol level reflects HDL_2 level; plasma levels of the other major HDL subclass, HDL_3, are fairly constant both intra- and interindividually.[42]

HDL particles are not secreted into the circulation as mature, spherical lipoproteins but as discoidal, precursor particles devoid of cholesteryl esters.[43] These nascent HDL particles—secreted by intestine, liver, and cholesteryl ester–enriched macrophages—are complexes of apolipoproteins and phospholipids and acquire unesterified cholesterol originating in cell membranes during cell renewal or death. Their major phospholipid is phosphatidylcholine, or lecithin.

Both lecithin and unesterified cholesterol serve as substrates for the cholesterol-esterifying enzyme lecithin: cholesterol acyltransferase (LCAT),[44] which circulates with HDL in the plasma. LCAT acts on the nascent HDL particles to generate a core of cholesteryl esters and to effect the structural transition to mature, spherical HDL particles. LCAT also acts on mature HDL_3 particles, i.e., after they have acquired cholesterol and lecithin not only from cell membranes but also from chylomicrons and VLDLs during those particles' lipolysis.[45] Generation of cholesteryl esters by the LCAT reaction leads to enlargement of the small HDL_3 particles such that they are converted into the larger HDL_2 particles. Formation of HDL_2 increases the cholesterol-carrying capacity of HDL, and HDL cholesterol levels rise; this drives the process termed reverse cholesterol transport, in which HDL returns cholesterol from peripheral tissues to the liver for excretion into the bile.

The cholesteryl esters of HDL, particularly of HDL_2 formed de novo by the LCAT action,[44] need not remain within the HDL core. They can be transferred from HDL to the triglyceride-rich lipoproteins—i.e., chylomicrons and VLDL—in exchange for triglyceride molecules. This heteroexchange of insoluble cholesteryl esters and triglycerides between HDL and triglyceride-rich lipoproteins is catalyzed by the action of cholesteryl ester transfer protein (CETP).[46–48]

The transferred triglycerides are hydrolyzed from the HDL core by hepatic lipase,[22] located in the endothelial cells of the liver. Only cholesteryl esters remain in the core—those that were not exchanged for triglycerides. Hence, HDL_2 particles are converted back into the smaller HDL_3 particles.[49] This mechanism is the basis for the well-established clinical observation that individuals with permanent or temporary hypertriglyceridemia (due to increased levels of VLDL or due to accumulation of chylomicrons in the course of postprandial lipemia) have low HDL_2 and low HDL cholesterol levels.

The cholesteryl esters transferred from HDL to the triglyceride-rich lipoproteins remain with the latter particles along their lipolytic cascades and the endocytotic pathways of their remnants (i.e., the LDL receptor and the scavenger pathways). Thus, transfer of cholesteryl esters from HDL to triglyceride-rich lipoproteins may contribute to the atherogenic potential of chylomicrons and VLDL, in that "good" cholesterol is turned into "bad" cholesterol.[50]

A splicing defect of the CETP gene that leads to CETP deficiency appears to be a frequent cause of increased HDL levels in Japan.[51,52] The heritable deficiency seems to disenable triglyceride-rich lipoproteins from directing triglycerides into HDL_2 (thus preventing their catabolism) and from robbing HDL of its cholesteryl esters—i.e., from switching antiatherogenic into potentially atherogenic cholesterol. Indeed, the CETP-deficient Japanese patients exhibit high HDL cholesterol levels and an overwhelming preponderance of HDL_2 and even larger HDL particles and present no evidence of premature atherosclerosis.

Mechanisms in Overview

The above brief review of the structure of the plasma lipoproteins and the transport of exogenous and endogenous lipids makes clear that each lipoprotein family has a specific lipid transport function. The plasma levels of lipoproteins are under complex regulation by the dietary intake of cholesterol, monounsaturated and polyunsaturated fats, and the pathways of lipoprotein clearance involving specific hepatic receptors, tissue receptors, and low-affinity pathways of macrophages and the reticuloendothelial system. A knowledge of the biochemistry of lipid regulation is necessary for a rational understanding of the mechanisms of hyperlipoproteinemia and hyperlipidemia. An excess of circulating chylomicron remnants, IDL, or LDL predisposes to atherosclerosis whether the mechanism is an oversynthesis of the lipoprotein, a decrease in catabolism, or a combination of the two defects.

Regarding the relation between atherosclerosis and blood lipids, important progress has recently been made in two areas: the recognition of the potential atherogenicity of oxidized or otherwise modified LDL and the recognition of CETP as the means of equilibration of cholesteryl esters and triglycerides between lipoproteins. The CETP-regulated equilibration process points to the potential atherogenicity of the triglyceride-rich lipoproteins since their metabolism appears to be a major determinant of cholesterol metabolic routing. As our knowledge of lipoprotein metabolism and lipid transport evolves, we should be able to formulate more clearly how these phenomena relate to atherosclerosis and to devise better methods of prevention and treatment.

CLINICAL ASSESSMENT OF LIPID ABNORMALITIES

Screening and Evaluation of Hypercholesterolemia

The guidelines currently in use in the United States for the diagnosis and management of hypercholesterolemia in adults are those published in 1993 by the Adult Treatment Panel II of the NCEP[11] (Tables 53-2 to 53-4) and revolve around elevations of LDL cholesterol. They are part of a four-panel effort to educate the general U.S.

TABLE 53-2

Initial Classifications and Recommended Follow-up for Patients without Definite Coronary Heart Disease. National Cholesterol Education Program Adult Treatment Panel II 1993 Guidelines.

Total Cholesterol (mg/dL)	Risk Classification	Low HDL Cholesterol* (<35 mg/dL)	Recommended Follow-up
<200	Desirable	No	Provide risk reduction materials and repeat total cholesterol and HDL cholesterol within 5 years.
		Yes	Provide information on risk factor reduction; reevaluate in 1 to 2 years.
200–239	Borderline-high	No	If fewer than two other risk factors present, provide risk reduction materials and reevaluate in 1 to 2 years. If two or more risk factors present, do lipoprotein analysis.
		Yes	Do lipoprotein analysis.
≥240	High	No	Do lipoprotein analysis.
		Yes	Do lipoprotein analysis.

Conversions: 200 mg/dL cholesterol corresponds to 5.2 mmol/liter; 240 mg/dL cholesterol corresponds to 6.2 mmol/liter.
*Nonfasting measurements acceptable.
SOURCE: Adapted from the Expert Panel.[11]

population about hypercholesterolemia and to develop an overall approach to the detection and management of hypercholesterolemia for the health care profession. The other panels have addressed population-based screening strategies, the evaluation of hypercholesterolemia in children, and the standardization of cholesterol measurements in the laboratory.

The Adult Treatment Panel II recommends that total and HDL cholesterol levels be measured in all adults age 20 and over at least once every 5 years. The measurement in this screening format may be nonfasting and part of an automated panel of blood chemistry determinations or a fingerstick determination. The total cholesterol value found is classified as desirable, borderline-high, or high in relation to CHD risk (Table 53-2), categories that do not take into account age or sex (although both age and sex affect risk—see below).

When the total cholesterol value exceeds 200 mg/dL, the measurement should be repeated within several weeks. The average of the values should be used unless the two are very different (>30 mg/dL, or 0.8 mmol/liter), in which case a third cholesterol measurement should be made and the three averaged. This procedure should compensate enough for the inherent variability in cholesterol values that the baseline achieved can be used with confidence. (See Chap. 65.)

When total cholesterol is found to be at a desirable level i.e., <200 mg/dL (5.2 mmol/liter), the HDL cholesterol level determines follow-up. Patients with HDL cholesterol greater than or equal to 35 mg/dL (0.9 mmol/liter) should be given general dietary and risk reduction information and have another serum cholesterol test within 5 years. If HDL levels are less than 35 mg/dL, lipoprotein analysis should be performed.

TABLE 53-3

Subsequent Classification Based on LDL Cholesterol Level for Patients without Definite Coronary Heart Disease. National Cholesterol Education Program Adult Treatment Panel II 1993 Guidelines.

Lipoprotein Analysis after Fasting for 9 to 12 h		
LDL Cholesterol (mg/dL)	**Risk Classification**	**Recommended Follow-up**
<130	Desirable	Provide risk reduction materials and repeat total cholesterol and HDL cholesterol within 5 years.
130–159	Borderline-high	If fewer than two other risk factors present, provide information on the Step One Diet and exercise. Reevaluate annually, repeating lipoprotein analysis. If two or more other risk factors present, do clinical evaluation and initiate dietary therapy.
≥160	High	Do clinical evaluation and initiate dietary therapy.

LDL = low-density lipoprotein. Conversions: 130 mg/dL cholesterol corresponds to 3.4 mmol/liter; 160 mg/dL cholesterol corresponds to 4.1 mmol/liter; 190 mg/dL cholesterol corresponds to 4.9 mmol/liter.
SOURCE: Adapted from the Expert Panel.[11]

TABLE 53-4

Other Risk Factors* for Consideration in Application of the National Cholesterol Education Program 1993 Adult Treatment Guidelines

Positive	Age
	Men ≥45
	Women ≥55 or those in premature menopause without estrogen replacement therapy
	Family history of CHD
	Smoking
	Hypertension
	HDL cholesterol <35 mg/dL (0.9 mmol/liter)
	Diabetes
Negative	HDL cholesterol ≥60 mg/dL (1.6 mmol/liter)

*Besides total and low-density lipoprotein cholesterol elevations and definite coronary heart disease (characteristic clinical picture and objective laboratory findings of myocardial ischemia or prior myocardial infarction).
SOURCE: Adapted from the Expert Panel.[11]

For individuals with total cholesterol levels between 200 and 239 mg/dL (5.2 to 6.2 mmol/liter), follow-up is determined by HDL cholesterol levels and by other CHD risk factors (Table 53-4). Those with HDL cholesterol of or exceeding 35 mg/dL and with fewer than two risk factors are instructed in dietary modification, physical activity, and other risk reduction activities and are advised to repeat screening in 1 to 2 years. Those with HDL cholesterol levels below 35 mg/dL or with two (or more) other risk factors require a complete lipid profile and should be further stratified by LDL cholesterol level (Table 53-3). This analysis is also necessary for all patients with total cholesterol value exceeding 240 mg/dL (6.2 mmol/liter). (See also Chap. 62.)

The complete lipid profile measures serum total cholesterol, HDL cholesterol, and triglycerides. LDL cholesterol level is calculated from these values by the Friedewald formula:

$$\text{LDL cholesterol (mg/dL)} = \text{total cholesterol} - \text{HDL cholesterol} - (\text{triglycerides}/5)$$

(The triglycerides divisor is 2.2 if values are in SI units.) The formula does not apply if the triglyceride level exceeds 400 mg/dL (4.5 mmol/liter) or the patient has type III hyperlipoproteinemia (phenotype definitions are given below). The profile should be performed after a 12-h fast. The patient should not be acutely ill and should be at a stable weight. A confirming profile should be performed within several weeks to establish baselines.

The management of patients whose LDL level is in the NCEP desirable range (<130 mg/dL, or 3.4 mmol/liter) is the same as that for patients with a desirable level of total cholesterol: education on diet, physical activity, and risk reduction and retesting within 5 years. Patients with a borderline-high LDL level (130 to 159 mg/dL, or 3.4 to 4.1 mmol/liter) without definite CHD or two risk factors should be informed about and advised to follow a fat-modified diet (Step One Diet; see Table 53-5) and reassessed annually (or more often, depending on the complete clinical picture).

Patients at higher risk—those with borderline-high LDL cholesterol and CHD or two other risk factors and those with high LDL cholesterol (≥160 mg/dL)—are assigned to treatment designed to affect LDL cholesterol specifically.

In patients thus stratified to LDL-lowering therapy, a full clinical evaluation, including history, physical examination, and basic laboratory tests, is necessary for two reasons. First, it is important to determine whether the LDL cholesterol elevation is secondary to a disease state, drug treatment, or diet. Consideration of, and appropriate testing for, the following more common disease states is warranted: hypothyroidism, nephrotic syndrome, chronic obstructive liver disease (e.g., primary biliary cirrhosis), and diabetes mellitus. Appropriate treatment and/or control of these conditions can greatly improve LDL cholesterol levels. Thiazide diuretics, progestins, anabolic steroids, and 13-*cis*-retinoic acid are commonly prescribed drugs that can raise LDL cholesterol levels. When possible, the offending drug should be discontinued and LDL cholesterol reevaluated. A diet history that includes high fat intake, particularly of saturated fat, and large amounts of cholesterol can be a cause of sporadic hypercholesterolemia. Second, it is necessary to consider the possibility of a genetic cause of hypercholesterolemia (see below), and a complete family history is helpful.

Managing Hypercholesterolemia

Treatment goals recommended by the NCEP for adults with elevated LDL cholesterol levels are included in Table 53-3. Clinical trial evidence shows that aggressive cholesterol reduction slows the progression or even enhances the regression of atherosclerosis in patients with definite CHD; thus LDL cholesterol levels below 100 mg/dL (2.6 mmol/liter) are recommended.[5–8,11] For those without CHD but with two risk factors, LDL cholesterol

TABLE 53-5

Nutrient Intake Guidelines of the Step One and Step Two Diets for Management of Hypercholesterolemia

Nutrient	Recommended Intake* (% of total calories except as specified)
Saturated fatty acids	<8–10% Step One <7% Step Two
Polyunsaturated fatty acids	≤10%
Monounsaturated fatty acids	15%
Total fat	≤30%
Carbohydrates	55% or more
Protein	Approximately 15%
Cholesterol	<300 mg/day Step One <200 mg/day Step Two

SOURCE: Adapted from the Expert Panel.[11]
* Identical for Step One and Step Two except as indicated.

levels below 130 mg/dL (3.4 mmol/liter) are sought to alleviate the synergy between LDL cholesterol elevation and other risk factors in atherosclerosis development.[53]

Initial management strategy is hygienic, and all subjects should be advised about diet and risk factor modification. Patients with high risk and those with borderline-high risk and two risk factors should begin the Step One Diet (Table 53-5) to reduce total fat, saturated fat, and cholesterol intake and to achieve a reasonable body weight. Serum total cholesterol level should be measured and adherence to the diet assessed at 4 to 6 weeks and at 3 months (monitoring may be by total cholesterol level). If a satisfactory reduction in cholesterol is not achieved within 3 months, the patient should be referred to a dietician. With the dietician's supervision, the patient should again try the Step One Diet or undertake the more rigorous Step Two Diet (Table 53-5). Patients with established CHD or other atherosclerotic disease should immediately begin the Step Two Diet. (See Fig. 62-3, 62-4, and 62-5.)

Sufficient time to make dietary changes should be given, particularly if a large weight loss is anticipated. A 6-month minimum of intensive dietary therapy and counseling generally should be carried out in primary prevention before initiating drug therapy; shorter periods can be considered in patients with LDL cholesterol levels greater than 220 mg/dL (5.7 mmol/liter). Also, if the physician is certain that a high-risk patient with severe hypercholesterolemia has a genetic dyslipidemia and dietary changes are not expected to normalize the LDL cholesterol level, drug treatment may be initiated sooner.

After a sufficient attempt at dietary modification, drug therapy should be considered in addition to diet if LDL cholesterol levels remain above the NCEP cutpoints for drug therapy [≥ 130 mg/dL (3.4 mmol/liter) if CHD is present; ≥ 160 mg/dL (4.1 mmol/liter) if two other risk factors are present; and ≥ 190 mg/dL (4.9 mmol/liter) if fewer than two other risk factors are present; see Table 53-3]. Several factors enter into the clinical decision to initiate drug therapy. Foremost is the consideration that drug treatment commits the patient to long-term and possibly lifelong therapy that can be costly. In patients taking medications for other medical conditions, the addition of hypolipidemic drugs can complicate compliance and increase drug interactions. Age is another consideration. Drug therapy can often be delayed in adult men under age 35, and in premenopausal women with LDL cholesterol levels below 220 mg/dL (5.7 mmol/liter) and no other risk factors. Furthermore, asymptomatic high-risk patients over age 65 who do not have other CHD risk factors may not need therapy beyond good diet habits, weight maintenance, and exercise. For high-risk patients in this age group who do have CHD or other risk factors, however, lipid-lowering medications should be considered when diet has not been sufficient, given that the patient has the life expectancy to encompass the approximately 2 years[54] required for CHD benefit from lipid-lowering drug therapy. (See also Chap. 62.)

Some patients will not reach their minimal LDL cholesterol goal with nonpharmacological measures, yet they will not have an LDL cholesterol level as high as the NCEP cutpoint for drug treatment. For such patients—i.e., those without CHD or two other risk factors whose LDL level is in the 160 to 189 mg/dL (4.14 to 4.89 mmol/liter) range [190 to 219 mg/dL (4.9 to 5.7 mmol/liter) for young adults] and those with two risk factors with LDL levels of 130 to 159 mg/dL (3.36 to 4.11 mmol/liter)—use of medication may be considered according to the physician's judgment and the patient's desire. That use must be in conjunction with the nonpharmacological treatments. The Adult Treatment Panel II guidelines suggest low-dose bile acid sequestrants if drug treatment is to be considered in such patients, especially in men.

Heritable Hypercholesterolemia

Several of the recognized genetic types of hypercholesterolemia deserve special mention here. Beyond consideration of the genetic component in the index patient, it is also highly desirable to measure cholesterol in all first-degree relatives to identify those who would benefit from cholesterol-lowering maneuvers. Severe or complicated hyperlipidemia may require referral to a lipid specialist.

Familial Hypercholesterolemia

Familial hypercholesterolemia is an autosomal dominant disorder involving a mutation of the gene that encodes for the specific cell surface receptor responsible for LDL uptake.

The heterozygous form is the more common, affecting about 1 in 500 people. That the normal number of LDL receptors is halved in these people means total cholesterol levels are twice acceptable levels and LDL cholesterol levels are elevated two to three times or more. Physical examination may show tendon xanthomas, corneal arcus, and xanthelasma. Male heterozygotes develop CHD in their thirties and forties, whereas female heterozygotes develop CHD about a decade later.

Homozygous familial hypercholesterolemia is rare, with an occurrence of about 1 in 1 million. LDL cholesterol may be elevated sixfold, since there is a total or almost-total deficiency of functioning LDL receptors. Homozygotes develop severe aortic stenosis and proximal coronary artery atherosclerosis before age 20 if untreated.

Polygenic Hypercholesterolemia

Autosomal dominant inheritance is probably operative in polygenic hypercholesterolemia, or primary moderate hypercholesterolemia. Unlike in familial hypercholesterolemia, single-gene abnormalities have not been described. Most likely an interaction of several genes with environmental factors such as diet and obesity leads to a suppression of normal LDL receptor activity.

Total cholesterol values range from 240 to 325 mg/dL (6.2 to 8.4 mmol/liter) despite good dietary habits, and CHD before age 60 is usual in this disorder. Penetrance of the suspected multiple gene defects is quite variable; hence, fewer than 50 percent of first-degree relatives are found to have hypercholesterolemia.

Familial Combined Hyperlipidemia

Familial combined hyperlipidemia is found in 10 to 15 percent of patients diagnosed with CHD before age 60 and may be present in 1 to 2 percent of the general population.[55] It is characterized by multiple lipoprotein phenotypes (types IIa, IIb, IV) in a single family. Thus, some family members may have elevated cholesterol alone, elevated triglycerides alone, or elevated cholesterol and triglycerides together. Also, the lipoprotein phenotype in any given patient may change over time. The genetic defect is poorly understood but probably involves increased production of apo B–containing lipoproteins, possibly in conjunction with a defect in VLDL catabolism.[56]

Some lipid experts believe that a subset of familial combined hyperlipidemia patients have overproduction of apo B as their only lipid abnormality.[57] These patients present with desirable total cholesterol and triglyceride levels, yet have a significant elevation of apo B. This disorder has been termed hyperapobetalipoproteinemia (or hyper–apo B syndrome) and appears to be associated with an increased risk of premature CHD.

Last, elevation of LDL cholesterol has been noted in a few patients who have a single amino acid substitution (glutamine for arginine) at residue 3500 of the apo B molecule.[58] This defect occurs in the apo B–binding domain that attaches to the LDL receptor, resulting in reduced receptor-mediated removal of LDL particles and has been called familial defective apo B. Its frequency in the general population is unknown, but it appears to be present in less than 4 percent of patients with hypercholesterolemia.

Evaluation of Other Lipid Disorders

The primary thrust of the assessment of lipid abnormalities has been to identify and correct hypercholesterolemia due to LDL cholesterol elevation. However, there are other lipoprotein disorders that can be identified during the screening process, categorized by Fredrickson phenotype (Table 53-6).

In most instances, the standard lipid profile—comprising measured total cholesterol, HDL cholesterol, and triglyceride levels and calculated LDL cholesterol level—will be sufficient to determine the lipoprotein phenotype. However, elevations of both total cholesterol and triglycerides (the latter exceeding 300 mg/dL, or 3.4 mmol/liter) can make the assessment more complicated. Marked hypertriglyceridemia in association with elevated total cholesterol (in an approximately 10:1 triglyceride-to-cholesterol ratio) may be due to VLDL and chylomicron accumulations (type V), which can be detected by one of two methods. Serum stored overnight at 4°C will have a white floating layer (chylomicrons) over a cloudy supernatant (VLDL). Serum lipoprotein electrophoresis, as described at the beginning of this chapter, will also detect these two lipoproteins. Elevations in cholesterol and triglycerides in fairly equal proportion can be due to increased LDL and VLDL (type IIb) or to the presence of IDL (type III). Again, serum lipoprotein electrophoresis is very helpful in separating these disorders, the "broad-beta" band representing IDL. Certain specialized laboratories may also use ultracentrifugation for lipoprotein analysis, particularly for the accurate measurement of LDL cholesterol.

TABLE 53-6

Fredrickson Classification of the Hyperlipidemias

Phenotype	Lipoprotein Abnormality	Result
Type I	Chylomicrons elevated	Very high TG
Type IIa	LDL elevated	High cholesterol
Type IIb	LDL and VLDL elevated	High cholesterol and TG
Type III	IDL elevated	High cholesterol and TG
Type IV	VLDL elevated	High TG; normal to slightly high cholesterol
Type V	Chylomicrons present and VLDL elevated	Very high TG and cholesterol

IDL, intermediate-density lipoprotein; LDL, low-density lipoprotein; TG, triglyceride; VLDL, very low density lipoprotein.
SOURCE: Adapted from Herbert PN, Assmann G, Gotto AM Jr, Fredrickson DS: Familial lipoprotein deficiency: Abetalipoproteinemia, hypobetalipoproteinemia, and Tangier disease. In: Stanbury JB, Wyngaarden JB, Fredrickson DS, Goldstein JL, Brown MS (eds): *The Metabolic Basis of Inherited Disease*, 5th ed. New York, McGraw-Hill, 1983: 594.

Hypertriglyceridemia

There is considerable debate about the association of hypertriglyceridemia and CHD. In most population studies, triglyceride level is positively associated with increased CHD risk on univariate analysis[59,60]; however, the independent predictive power is often lost when other factors such as total cholesterol, HDL cholesterol, cigarette smoking, hypertension, and obesity are considered.[61] Some studies suggest that triglyceride level is an independent risk factor for myocardial infarction in men and for CHD in women.[62–64]

Many experts believe that triglyceride elevation may not be a direct cause of atherosclerosis but rather a marker of certain conditions that predispose to atherogenesis, such as diabetes mellitus, chronic renal failure, obesity, and low HDL cholesterol levels.[60] Recent clinical work suggests that fasting hypertriglyceridemia may indicate underlying metabolic abnormalities that increase the potential for atherogenesis, such as prolonged postprandial lipemia, presence of small, dense LDL particles, and peripheral insulin resistance with hyperinsulinemia.[65–69]

The 1992 National Institutes of Health (NIH) Consensus Conference on hypertriglyceridemia classified triglyceride levels below 250 mg/dL (2.8 mmol/liter) as acceptable, 250 to 500 mg/dL (2.8 to 5.6 mmol/liter) as borderline-high, and above 500 mg/dL (5.6 mmol/liter) as definite hypertriglyceridemia.[73] Other bodies, such as the European Atherosclerosis Society[71] and the International Committee for the Evaluation of Hypertriglyceridemia as a Vascular Risk Factor,[72] have set a lower limit—200 mg/dL (2.3 mmol/liter)—for triglyceride elevation. Because of its intraindividual variability, triglyceride should be determined on fasting measurement, with persistent hypertriglyceridemia defined by at least two fasting measurements on separate occasions.

In most patients, the triglyceride elevation will not exceed 750 mg/dL (8.5 mmol/liter), secondary to VLDL elevation (type IV hyperlipoproteinemia). At higher triglyceride levels, chylomicrons are frequently increased in addition to VLDL (type V). Very rarely, extreme chylomicron elevations alone can occur (type I).

A specific indication to treat triglyceride elevations above 500 mg/dL, especially those due to chylomicron elevation, is to decrease the potential for acute pancreatitis. This disease can cause considerable morbidity and occasional mortality. In most patients with borderline hypertriglyceridemia, the triglyceride elevation is secondary to a condition such as obesity, excessive alcohol intake, poorly controlled diabetes mellitus, chronic renal failure, nephrotic syndrome, or use of certain drugs such as beta-blocking agents, estrogens, and corticosteroids. Modification of the underlying conditions should be attempted before any medical therapy is contemplated. A complete dietary change, particularly for weight control, is essential.

If diet, exercise, and control of an underlying condition do not lower the triglyceride level significantly, the physician should entertain the possibility that a familial form of hypertriglyceridemia exists. One such form is familial combined hyperlipidemia,[55] as described above. Family screening is most helpful in detecting this condition. Since there is increased risk of premature CHD is this disorder, even in patients with isolated triglyceride elevations, medical therapy is justified. Another hereditary disorder, familial hypertriglyceridemia, can cause borderline or definite hypertriglyceridemia. These patients appear to be at less risk for CHD than those with familial combined hyperlipidemia. Total cholesterol and LDL cholesterol levels are usually within the normal range in the patient and in family members.

Type III hyperlipoproteinemia, or dysbetalipoproteinemia, is uncommon. The metabolic defect appears to be a combination of VLDL oversynthesis and homozygosity for a specific apo E isoform, ϵ_2, that results in decreased binding of the apo E–containing lipoproteins to hepatic LDL receptors. Type III hyperlipoproteinemia confers increased risk of premature CHD and peripheral vascular disease. That type III hyperlipoproteinemia is rare even though apo E_2 homozygosity occurs in about 1 percent of the general population indicates environmental or other genetic factors are required for expression of the disease. There may be a role for conditions associated with VLDL overproduction (e.g., obesity, diabetes, and hypothyroidism) in its etiology. Intensive management of type III hyperlipoproteinemia with diet and nicotinic acid or a fibric acid derivative such as gemfibrozil is recommended.

Recent recommendations regarding the management of hypertriglyceridemia and low HDL cholesterol have come from the 1992 NIH Consensus Development Conference on Triglyceride, High Density Lipoprotein, and Coronary Heart Disease,[73] with the intent of extending but not replacing the 1988 NCEP adult guidelines. The panel recommended that HDL cholesterol measurement be incorporated into routine screening for CHD if accuracy of measurement, appropriate counseling, and follow-up can be assured. Further, it delineated additional clinical circumstances under which HDL cholesterol and triglyceride should be measured—among them, in known CHD, in the setting of a desirable total cholesterol level (as defined by the NCEP) when two or more CHD risk factors are present, and in such disorders as diabetes mellitus and hypertension (Table 53-7).

The panel used as its definitions of borderline and distinct hypertriglyceridemia those given by the 1983 NIH consensus conference and as its definition of low HDL that of the 1988 NCEP adult guidelines. It recommended hygienic intervention (in chief diet and weight control, exercise, and stopping smoking) whenever serum triglyceride is elevated or HDL is low. For borderline hypertriglyceridemia occurring with low HDL and a desirable LDL cholesterol level (as defined by the NCEP), the panel noted that the mainstay of hygienic therapy may need to be extended by pharmacologic therapy if the hygienic measures fail and CHD or a strong risk profile is present. Drug therapy may be required as initial therapy together with hygienic measures if distinct hypertriglyceridemia is accompanied by a history of pancreatitis (Table 53-8).

Low HDL Cholesterol Levels

That HDL cholesterol has a strong, independent inverse association with CHD risk may derive from a role in the posited reverse cholesterol transport system, described in the first half of this chapter. The NCEP Adult Treatment Panel II defines a low HDL cholesterol level as below 35 mg/dL (0.9 mmol/liter) and considers it a major risk factor for CHD, whereas a value of 60 mg/dL (1.6 mmol/liter) or greater is considered a negative risk factor.[11] Although there is no clinical trial directly demonstrating the benefit of increasing HDL cholesterol alone, Helsinki Heart Study results suggest that increasing HDL adds benefit to lowering LDL in CHD risk reduction.[3] Similarly, data from the Prospective Cardiovascular Muenster (PROCAM) Study have shown that the combination of LDL elevation, hypertriglyceridemia, and low HDL confers greater risk of CHD than elevated LDL alone.[54,74]

There are several causes for low serum HDL cholesterol levels. Heavy cigarette smoking is a documented cause. Obesity is an apparent association, as is a sedentary lifestyle. As noted above, hypertriglyceridemia is frequently associated with very low HDL levels. Certain drugs can also have an appreciable depressing effect on HDL. Finally, there is evidence that isolated low HDL cholesterol, termed hypoalphalipoproteinemia, may be genetically transmitted in an autosomal dominant fashion. Patients with this disorder have a normal lipid profile other than the low HDL but an apparently increased risk for atherosclerosis.

The recommended methods for improving HDL cholesterol values are nonpharmacologic: smoking cessation, weight reduction, regular and vigorous exercise, and alteration of offending drugs, if possible. As yet, there is no direct evidence that drug-induced increases of low HDL cholesterol in the setting of normal LDL cholesterol and triglyceride levels are beneficial in CHD

TABLE 53-7

Additional Lipid Measurements Recommended by the 1992 NIH Consensus Development Conference on Triglyceride, High Density Lipoprotein, and Coronary Heart Disease*

Measure HDL-C (nonfasting sample acceptable)	
Healthy individuals	In addition to TC to assess CAD risk *if accuracy of HDL-C measurement, appropriate counseling, and follow-up can be assured*
Measure HDL-C and TG (fasting sample)[†]	
Known CAD	To assess risks for progression of CAD and development of additional cardiovascular complications
Increased TC	To identify patients with high HDL-C and desirable LDL-C, as at low to average lipid risk for CAD[‡]
Desirable TC + ≥ 2 risk factors[§]	To identify patients with low HDL-C and/or high TG, as at possible additional risk for CAD
Other disorders that may be associated with increased TG and known to be associated with increased CAD risk, including diabetes, peripheral vascular disease, hypertension, central obesity, chronic renal disease	To refine CAD risk assessment
Lactescent serum, lipemia retinalis, xanthomas, pancreatitis	To identify familial hyperlipidemic disorders and/or likelihood of recurrence of pancreatitis; to follow response to treatment
On hygienic or drug therapy for high TG and/or low HDL-C	To follow results of therapy

**Data from* National Institutes of Health.[73]
[†]It is generally recommended that at least two (ideally three) samples be taken at least 1 week apart before a treatment decision is finalized.
[‡]Under NCEP adult guidelines,[11] lipoprotein analysis is performed if there is high TC, or borderline-high TC and ≥ 2 other risk factors, to identify patients with increased LDL-C (Table 53-2).
[§]The 1992 NIH panel notes that accumulating evidence suggests that postmenopausal status be considered an additional risk factor for CAD. CAD = coronary artery disease; HDL-C = high-density lipoprotein cholesterol; LDL-C = low-density lipoprotein cholesterol; NCEP = National Cholesterol Education Program; NIH = U.S. National Institutes of Health; TC = total cholesterol; TG = triglyceride.
SOURCE: Adapted from Gotto AM Jr: Primary and secondary prevention of coronary artery disease. *Current Opinion in Cardiology* 1992; 7:553–562. Used with permission.

risk reduction. HDL cholesterol levels can be increased with gemfibrozil (the agent used in the Helsinki study) or nicotinic acid. The 1992 NIH consensus conference's screening and treatment recommendations for low HDL and hypertriglyceridemia are reviewed above and in Tables 53-7 and 53-8.

Abnormal Levels of Apolipoproteins and Lipoprotein[a]

Several clinical studies have recently focused on the strong correlation of certain apolipoprotein levels with the incidence and severity of CHD.[75,76] Apo B, the only protein component of the LDL particle, is the apolipoprotein with the strongest positive correlation with severity of coronary atherosclerosis. In the aforementioned FATS trial, apo B level correlated independently on multivariate analysis with regression of coronary lesions, as did systolic blood pressure and increased HDL cholesterol level.[7] Apo A-I, the major protein of HDL particles, has just as strong a negative association with CHD severity. Levels of these apolipoproteins can be determined on commercially available analyzers; however, there is no standardization of normal ranges and no consensus on predictive or treatment value. Further study is needed to determine the usefulness of such apolipoprotein measurement as an adjunct to risk evaluation by routine lipid measurements.

Lipoprotein[a] (Lp[a]) has also been identified as an independent risk factor for the development of CHD.[77–79] This unusual plasma lipoprotein consists of an LDL particle that carries an additional protein, apo[a]. Apo[a] is linked by a disulfide bond to the apo B-100 of LDL and has considerable structural homology to plasminogen. It may compete with plasminogen in the fibrinolytic pathway and thus perhaps enhance thrombosis. Lp[a] may confer a direct atherogenic effect because of its LDL core.

Epidemiologic evidence suggests that Lp[a] levels in the top quartile increase CHD risk anywhere from two- to fivefold.[80] At present, however, Lp[a] measurement is considered to be a research tool, and studies of methods to reduce Lp[a] levels are limited. Further studies on Lp[a]'s origins, metabolism, and physiological functions and on modulation of its plasma levels are necessary before routine use of this risk factor can be recommended. Lp[a] measurement has not been standardized.

TABLE 53-8

Treatment Recommendations of the 1992 NIH Consensus Development Conference on Triglyceride, High Density Lipoprotein, and Coronary Heart Disease*

Lipid value(s)†	Treatment‡§
Borderline HTG (250–500 mg/dL) + Low HDL-C (< 35 mg/dL) + Desirable LDL-C (< 130 mg/dL)	Hygienic measures. No consensus for the use of drug therapy, but may be considered in unusual cases when hygienic measures fail and CAD or strong risk profile is present
Distinct HTG (> 500 mg/dL)	Hygienic measures are initial therapy. If hygienic measures fail, drug therapy is warranted to reduce the risk of pancreatitis. Drugs should be considered as initial therapy with hygienic measures if history of pancreatitis is present.
Special Cases	
Very low or absent HDL-C + Desirable LDL-C (< 130 mg/dL) Distinct HTG (> 500 mg/dL)	Probably represents rare genetic disorders, which require expert evaluation; no specific therapy
Primary hypoalphalipoproteinemia: Low HDL-C (< 35 mg/dL); TG and LDL-C usually in desirable range	Hygienic measures and control of coexisting risk factors for CAD. Drugs that ordinarily raise HDL-C may be ineffectual.

**Data from* National Institutes of Health.[73]
†The values defining borderline and distinct HTG are the same as set forth by the 1983 NIH Consensus Development Conference on HTG.[70] The cut-point for low HDL-C is not changed from the 1988 NCEP adult guidelines[81]; the 1992 NIH panel notes that this cut-point may be too low for women and other subpopulations. The definition of desirable LDL-C is from the 1988 NCEP adult guidelines.
‡TG and HDL-C cannot be interpreted in the absence of LDL-C.
§Beyond the clinical situations listed here, there is no consensus for treating isolated mild, sporadic HTG and/or low HDL-C with drugs in the general population. Hygienic measures should always be employed when TG is elevated or HDL-C is low, regardless of TC level.
CAD = coronary artery disease; HDL-C = high-density lipoprotein cholesterol; HTG = hypertriglyceridemia; LDL-C = low-density lipoprotein cholesterol; NCEP = National Cholesterol Education Program; NIH = U.S. National Institutes of Health; TC = total cholesterol; TG = triglyceride.
SOURCE: Adapted from Gotto AM Jr: Primary and secondary prevention of coronary artery disease. *Current Opinion in Cardiology* 1992; 7:553–562. Used with permission.

SUMMARY

All of the major lipids in the blood except unesterified fatty acids are carried in complexes called lipoproteins. Hyperlipidemia is defined as an elevation of cholesterol and/or triglyceride. Translating hyperlipidemia into hyperlipoproteinemia depends on which class or classes of lipoproteins are elevated.

Lipid transport may be divided into an exogenous pathway, which involves chylomicrons and chylomicron remnants, and an endogenous pathway, which involves VLDL, IDL (VLDL remnants), LDL, and HDL. Transport of triglyceride provides the body with energy and also represents a response to excessive caloric intake. The free fatty acids that are not metabolized are converted into triglyceride and stored in adipose tissue. The cells and tissues of the body obtain their cholesterol either by endogenous synthesis from acetate to cholesterol or from the LDL receptor on the surface of the cell.

The relationship of lipids and lipoproteins to CHD is very complex. Current evidence suggests that LDL particles are atherogenic. Oxidation or other chemical modification of LDL may increase its atherogenicity by enhancing its interaction with tissue macrophages and monocytes. A great deal of evidence also suggests that remnant lipoproteins from chylomicrons or VLDL are atherogenic. On the other hand, HDL is inversely correlated with CHD risk. The mechanism by which HDL confers such a protective effect is not known. Reverse cholesterol transport is one postulated mechanism; another is that a high level of HDL represents effective metabolism of the triglyceride-rich lipoproteins.

Hyperlipoproteinemia can be categorized by phenotype. Also, several genetic disorders of lipid transport have been well characterized. The approach to hypercholesterolemia recommended by the Adult Treatment Panel of the NCEP focuses on the patient with type IIa hyperlipoproteinemia. Treatment by the NCEP algorithm depends primarily on concentrations of total cholesterol, HDL cholesterol, and LDL cholesterol, but a patient may be reassigned from the medium-risk to the high-risk category according to the presence of at least two additional risk factors for CHD.

Treatment may have its basis in whether the dyslipidemia is primary or secondary. Heritable forms of elevated cholesterol include familial hypercholesterolemia, familial combined hyperlipidemia, familial defective apo B, and polygenic hypercholesterolemia. In familial dysbetalipoproteinemia, both serum cholesterol and triglyceride are elevated as a result of an increase in remnant lipoproteins. Other genetic disorders involving triglycerides include familial combined hyperlipidemia, familial hypertriglyceridemia, familial hyperchylomicronemia due to a deficiency of either lipoprotein lipase or apo C-II, and familial type V hyperlipidemia, in which both chylomicrons and VLDL are elevated. Low levels of HDL may also predispose to CHD, particularly if accompanied by an increase in LDL or the triglyceride-rich lipoproteins.

The cornerstone of treatment of hyperlipidemia is diet. A number of medications are effective as adjunctive treatment if diet alone is insufficient. (See Chap. 65.) Extensive data now exist that show that aggressive lowering of lipid and lipoprotein levels can reduce the risk of myocardial infarction in patients with and without coronary disease and can decrease the progression of coronary blockage in patients with established coronary disease. (See also Chap. 62.)

REFERENCES

1. Lipid Research Clinics Program: The Lipid Research Clinics Coronary Primary Prevention Trial results. I. Reduction in incidence of coronary heart disease. *JAMA* 1984; 251:351–364.
2. Lipid Research Clinics Program: The Lipid Research Clinics Coronary Primary Prevention Trial results. II. The relationship of reduction in incidence of coronary heart disease to cholesterol lowering. *JAMA* 1984; 251:365–374.
3. Frick MH, Elo O, Haapa K, Heinonen OP, Heinsalmi P, Helo P, et al: Helsinki Heart Study: Primary-prevention trial with gemfibrozil in middle-aged men with dyslipidemia. Safety of treatment, changes in risk factors, and incidence of coronary heart disease. *N Engl J Med* 1987; 317:1237–1245.
4. Canner PL, Berge KG, Wenger NK, Stamler J, Friedman L, Prineas RJ, et al: Fifteen year mortality in Coronary Drug Project patients: Long-term benefit with niacin. *J Am Coll Cardiol* 1986; 8:1245–1255.
5. Blankenhorn DH, Nessim SA, Johnson RL, Sanmarco ME, Azen SP, Cashin-Hemphill L: Beneficial effects of combined colestipol-niacin therapy on coronary atherosclerosis and coronary venous bypass grafts. *JAMA* 1987; 257:3233–3240.
6. Cashin-Hemphill L, Mack WJ, Pogoda JM, Sanmarco ME, Azen SP, Blankenhorn DH: Beneficial effects of colestipol-niacin on coronary atherosclerosis. A 4-year follow-up. *JAMA* 1990; 264:3013–3017.
7. Brown G, Albers JJ, Fisher LD, Schaefer SM, Lin JT, Kaplan C, et al: Regression of coronary artery disease as a result of intensive lipid-lowering therapy in men with high levels of apolipoprotein B. *N Engl J Med* 1990; 323:1289–1298.
8. Brensike JF, Levy RI, Kelsey SF, Passamani ER, Richardson JM, Loh IK, et al: Effects of therapy with cholestyramine on progression of coronary arteriosclerosis: Results of the NHLBI Type II Coronary Intervention Study. *Circulation* 1984; 69:313–324.
9. LaRosa JC, Hunninghake D, Bush D, Criqui MH, Getz GS, Gotto AM Jr, et al: The cholesterol facts. A summary of the evidence relating dietary fats, serum cholesterol, and coronary heart disease. A joint statement by the American Heart Association and the National Heart, Lung, and Blood Institute. The Task Force on Cholesterol Issues, American Heart Association. *Circulation* 1990; 81:1721–1733.
10. Consensus Conference. Lowering blood cholesterol to prevent heart disease. *JAMA* 1985; 253:2080–2086.
11. The Expert Panel: Summary of the second Report of the National Cholesterol Education Program (NCEP) Expert Panel on detection, evaluation, and treatment of high blood cholesterol in adults (Adult Treatment Panel II). *JAMA* 1993; 269:3015–3023.
12. Macheboeuf MA: Recherches sur les phosphoaminolipides et les sterides du serum et du plasma sanguins: Entrainement des phospholipides, des sterols et des sterides par les diverses fractions au cours du fractionnement des proteides du serum. *Bull Soc Chim Biol* 1929; 11:268.
13. Oncley JL: *Brain Lipids and Lipoproteins and Leukodystrophies.* Amsterdam, Elsevier, 1963.
14. Gofman JW, Lindgren FT, Elliott H: Ultracentrifugal studies of lipoproteins. *J Biol Chem* 1949; 179:973.
15. Havel RJ, Eder HA, Bragdon JH: Distribution and chemical composition of ultracentrifugally separated lipoproteins in human serum. *J Clin Invest* 1955; 34:1345.
16. Lees RS, Hatch FT: Sharper separation of lipoprotein species by paper electrophoresis in albumin-containing buffer. *J Lab Clin Med* 1963; 61:518.
17. Fredrickson DS, Levy RI, Lees RS: Fat transport in lipoproteins—An integrated approach to mechanisms and disorders. *N Engl J Med* 1967; 276:148–156.
18. Burstein M, Scholnick HR, Morfin R: Rapid method for the isolation of lipoproteins from human serum by precipitation with polyanions. *J Lipid Res* 1970; 11:583–595.
19. Bradley WA, Gotto AM Jr: Structure of intact human plasma lipoproteins. In: Dietschy JM, Gotto AM Jr, Ontka TA (eds): *Disturbances in Lipid and Lipoprotein Metabolism.* New York, American Physiological Society, 1978: 111.
20. Patsch JR: Postprandial lipaemia. *Baillieres Clin Endocrinol Metab* 1987; 1:551–580.
21. Sviridov DD, Safonova IG, Talalaev AG, Repin VS, Smirnov VN: Regulation of cholesterol synthesis in isolated epithelial cells of human small intestine. *Lipids* 1986; 21:759–763.
22. Jackson RL: Lipoprotein lipase and hepatic lipase. In: Boyer PD (ed): *Lipid Enzymology. The Enzymes,* vol 16. New York, Academic, 1983: 141.
23. Chen SH, Habib G, Yang CY, Gu ZW, Lee BR, Weng SA, et al: Apolipoprotein B-48 is the product of a messenger RNA with an organ-specific in-frame stop codon. *Science* 1987; 238:363–366.
24. Angelin B, Raviola CA, Innerarity TL, Mahley RW: Regulation of hepatic lipoprotein receptors in the dog. Rapid regulation of apolipoprotein B,E receptors, but not of apolipoprotein E receptors, by intestinal lipoproteins and bile acids. *J Clin Invest* 1983; 71:816–831.
25. Andersen JM, Turley SD, Dietschy JM: Low and high density lipoproteins and chylomicrons as regulators of rate of cholesterol synthesis in rat liver in vivo. *Proc Natl Acad Sci USA* 1979; 76:165–169.
26. Bates SR, Murphy PL, Feng ZC, Kanazawa T, Getz GS: Very low density lipoproteins promote triglyceride accumulation in macrophages. *Arteriosclerosis* 1984; 4:103–114.
27. Zilversmit DB: Atherogenesis: A postprandial phenomenon. *Circulation* 1979; 60:473–485.
28. Yang CY, Chen SH, Gianturco SH, Bradley WA, Sparrow JT, Tanimura M, et al: Sequence, structure, receptor-binding domains and internal repeats of human apolipoprotein B-100. *Nature* 1986; 323:738–742.
29. Knott TJ, Pease RJ, Powell LM, Wallis SC, Rall SC Jr, Innerarity TL, et al: Complete protein sequence and identification of structural domains of human apolipoprotein B. *Nature* 1986; 323:734–738.
30. Higuchi K, Monge JC, Lee N, Law SW, Brewer HB Jr, Sakaguchi AY, et al: The human apoB-100 gene: ApoB-100 is encoded by a single copy gene in the human genome. *Biochem Biophys Res Commun* 1987; 144:1332–1339.
31. Brown MS, Goldstein JL: A receptor-mediated pathway for cholesterol homeostasis. *Science* 1986; 232:34–47.
32. Kodama T, Freeman M, Rohrer L, Zabrecky J, Matsudaira P, Krieger M: Type I macrophage scavenger receptor contains alpha-helical and collagen-like coiled coils. *Nature* 1990; 343:531–535.
33. Steinberg D, Parthasarathy S, Carew TE, Khoo JC, Witztum JL: Beyond cholesterol. Modifications of low-density lipoprotein that increase its atherogenicity. *N Engl J Med* 1989; 320:915–924.
34. Fong LG, Parthasarathy S, Witztum JL, Steinberg D: Nonenzymatic oxidative cleavage of peptide bonds in apoprotein B-100. *J Lipid Res* 1987; 28:1466–1477.
35. Steinbrecher UP, Witztum JL, Parthasarathy S, Steinberg D: Decrease in reactive amino groups during oxidation or endothelial cell modification of LDL. Correlation with changes in receptor-mediated catabolism. *Arteriosclerosis* 1987; 7:135–143.
36. Steinbrecher UP: Oxidation of human low density lipoprotein results in derivatization of lysine residues of apolipoprotein B by lipid peroxide decomposition products. *J Biol Chem* 1987; 262:3603–3608.
37. Steinbrecher UP, Witztum JL: Glucosylation of low-density lipoproteins to an extent comparable to that seen in diabetes slows their catabolism. *Diabetes* 1984; 33:130–134.

38. Palinski W, Rosenfeld ME, Yla Herttuala S, Gurtner GC, Socher SS, Butler SW, et al: Low density lipoprotein undergoes oxidative modification in vivo. *Proc Natl Acad Sci USA* 1989; 86:1372–1376.
39. Mitchinson MJ, Ball RY, Carpenter KLH, Parums DV: Macrophages and ceroid in atherosclerosis. In: Suckling KE, Groot PHE (eds): *Hyperlipidaemia and Atherosclerosis.* London, Academic, 1988: 117.
40. Parums D, Mitchinson MJ: Demonstration of immunoglobulin in the neighbourhood of advanced atherosclerotic plaques. *Atherosclerosis* 1981; 38:211–216.
41. Gordon T, Castelli WP, Hjortland MC, Kannel WB, Dawber TR: High density lipoprotein as a protective factor against coronary heart disease. The Framingham Study. *Am J Med* 1977; 62:707–714.
42. Patsch JR, Gotto AM Jr: Metabolism of high density lipoproteins. In: Gotto AM Jr (ed): *Plasma Lipoproteins. New Comprehensive Biochemistry,* vol 14. Amsterdam, Elsevier, 1987: 221–259.
43. Eisenberg S: High density lipoprotein metabolism. *J Lipid Res* 1984; 25:1017–1058.
44. Glomset JA: The plasma lecithins: Cholesterol acyltransferase reaction. *J Lipid Res* 1968; 9:155–167.
45. Patsch JR, Gotto AM Jr, Olivercrona T, Eisenberg S: Formation of high density lipoprotein$_2$-like particles during lipolysis of very low density lipoproteins in vitro. *Proc Natl Acad Sci USA* 1978; 75:4519–4523.
46. Morton RE, Zilversmit DB: Inter-relationship of lipids transferred by the lipid-transfer protein isolated from human lipoprotein–deficient plasma. *J Biol Chem* 1983; 258:11751–11757.
47. Albers JJ, Tollefson JH, Chen CH, Steinmetz A: Isolation and characterization of human plasma lipid transfer proteins. *Arteriosclerosis* 1984; 4:49–58.
48. Tall AR: Plasma lipid transfer proteins. *J Lipid Res* 1986; 27:361–367.
49. Patsch JR, Prasad S, Gotto AM Jr, Patsch W: High density lipoprotein$_2$. Relationship of the plasma levels of this lipoprotein species to its composition, to the magnitude of postprandial lipemia, and to the activities of lipoprotein lipase and hepatic lipase. *J Clin Invest* 1987; 80:341–347.
50. Miesenboeck G, Patsch JR: Coronary artery disease: Synergy of triglyceride-rich lipoproteins and HDL. *Cardiovasc Risk Factors* 1991; 1:293.
51. Brown ML, Inazu A, Hesler CB, Agellon LB, Mann C, Whitlock ME, et al: Molecular basis of lipid transfer protein deficiency in a family with increased high-density lipoproteins. *Nature* 1989; 342:448–451.
52. Inazu A, Brown ML, Hesler CB, Agellon LB, Koizumi J, Takata K, et al: Increased high-density lipoprotein levels caused by a common cholesteryl-ester transfer protein gene mutation. *N Engl J Med* 1990; 323:1234–1238.
53. Kannel WB, Stokes J III: The epidemiology of coronary artery disease. In: Cohn PF (ed): *Diagnosis and Therapy of Coronary Artery Disease.* London, Martinus Nijhoff, 1985: 63–88.
54. Assmann G, Schulte H: Triglycerides and atherosclerosis: Results from the Prospective Cardiovascular Münster Study. *Atheroscler Rev* 1991; 22:51–63.
55. Goldstein JL, Schrott HG, Hazzard WR, Bierman EL, Motulsky AG: Hyperlipidemia in coronary heart disease. II. Genetic analysis of lipid levels in 176 families and delineation of a new inherited disorder, combined hyperlipidemia. *J Clin Invest* 1973; 52:1544–1568.
56. Sniderman AD, Wolfson C, Teng B, Franklin FA, Bachorik PS, Kwiterovich PO Jr: Association of hyperapobetalipoproteinemia with endogenous hypertriglyceridemia and atherosclerosis. *Ann Intern Med* 1982; 97:833–839.
57. Sniderman A, Shapiro S, Marpole D, Skinner B, Teng B, Kwiterovich PO Jr: Association of coronary atherosclerosis with hyperapobetalipoproteinemia. *Proc Natl Acad Sci USA* 1980; 77:604–608.
58. Soria LF, Ludwig EH, Clarke HR, Vega GL, Grundy SM, McCarthy BJ: Association between a specific apolipoprotein B mutation and familial defective apolipoprotein B-100. *Proc Natl Acad Sci USA* 1989; 86:587–591.
59. Austin MA: Plasma triglyceride and coronary heart disease. *Arterioscler Thromb* 1991; 11:2–14.
60. Austin MA: Plasma triglyceride as a risk factor for coronary heart disease. The epidemiologic evidence and beyond. *Am J Epidemiol* 1989; 129:249–259.
61. Hulley SB, Rosenman RH, Bawol RD, Brand RJ: Epidemiology as a guide to clinical decisions. The association between triglyceride and coronary heart disease. *N Engl J Med* 1980; 302:1383–1389.
62. Carlson LA, Bottiger LE: Risk factors for ischaemic heart disease in men and women. Results of the 19-year follow-up of the Stockholm Prospective Study. *Acta Med Scand* 1985; 218:207–211.
63. Aberg H, Lithell H, Selinus I, Hedstrand H: Serum triglycerides are a risk factor for myocardial infarction but not for angina pectoris. Results from a 10-year follow-up of Uppsala primary preventive study. *Atherosclerosis* 1985; 54:89–97.
64. Cambien F, Jacqueson A, Richard JL, Warnet JM, Ducimetiere P, Claude JR: Is the level of serum triglyceride a significant predictor of coronary death in "normocholesterolemic" subjects? The Paris Prospective Study. *Am J Epidemiol* 1986; 124:624–632.
65. Zilversmit DB: Postprandial hyperlipidemia and its relationship to atherosclerosis. In: deGennes JL (ed): *Latent Dyslipoproteinemias and Atherosclerosis.* New York, Raven, 1984: 1–8.
66. Austin MA, King MC, Vranizan KM, Krauss RM: Atherogenic lipoprotein phenotype. A proposed genetic marker for coronary heart disease risk. *Circulation* 1990; 82:495–506.
67. Austin MA, Breslow JL, Hennekens CH, Buring JE, Willett WC, Krauss RM: Low-density lipoprotein subclass patterns and risk of myocardial infarction. *JAMA* 1988; 260:1917–1921.
68. Kaplan NM: The deadly quartet. Upper-body obesity, glucose intolerance, hypertriglyceridemia, and hypertension. *Arch Intern Med* 1989; 149:1514–1520.
69. Modan M, Halkin H, Almog S, Lusky A, Eshkol A, Shefi M, et al: Hyperinsulinemia. A link between hypertension, obesity and glucose intolerance. *J Clin Invest* 1985; 75:809–817.
70. Consensus Conference: Treatment of hypertriglyceridemia. *JAMA* 1984; 251:1196–1200.
71. European Atherosclerosis Study Group: The recognition and management of hyperlipidaemia in adults: A policy statement of the European Atherosclerosis Society. *Eur Heart J* 1988; 9:571–600.
72. Assmann G, Betteridge DJ, Gotto AM Jr, Steiner G: Management of hypertriglyceridemic patients. A. Treatment classifications and goals. *Am J Cardiol* 1991; 68:30A–34A.
73. National Institutes of Health: *Conference Statement: Triglyercide, High Density Lipoprotein, and Coronary Heart Disease. JAMA* 1993; 269:505–510.
74. Assmann G, Schulte H: The importance of triglycerides: Results from the Prospective Cardiovascular Muenster (PROCAM) Study. *Eur J Epidemiol,* in press.
75. Avogaro P, Bon GB, Cazzolato G, Rorai E: Relationship between apolipoproteins and chemical components of lipoproteins in survivors of myocardial infarction. *Atherosclerosis* 1980; 37:69–76.
76. Maciejko JJ, Holmes DR, Kottke BA, Zinsmeister AR, Dinh DM, Mao SJ: Apolipoprotein A-I as a marker of angiographically assessed coronary-artery disease. *N Engl J Med* 1983; 309:385–389.
77. Morrisett JD, Guyton JR, Gaubatz JW, Gotto AM Jr: Lipoprotein(a): Structure, metabolism and epidemiology. In: Gotto AM Jr (ed): *Plasma Lipoproteins. New Comprehensive Biochemistry,* vol 14. Amsterdam, Elsevier, 1987: 129–152.
78. Utermann G: The mysteries of lipoprotein(a). *Science* 1989; 246:904–910.
79. Scanu AM, Fless GM: Lipoprotein (a). Heterogeneity and biological relevance. *J Clin Invest* 1990; 85:1709–1715.
80. Scanu AM, Lawn RM, Berg K: Lipoprotein(a) and atherosclerosis. *Ann Intern Med* 1991; 115:209–218.
81. The Expert Panel: Report of the National Cholesterol Education Program Expert Panel on detection, evaluation, and treatment of high blood cholesterol in adults. (*Arch Intern Med* 1988; 148:36–69.

Chapter 54

Factors Influencing Atherogenesis

Russell Ross, Ph.D.

THE LESIONS OF ATHEROSCLEROSIS

Atherosclerosis is not a single disease entity. The lesions of atherosclerosis take different forms, depending on their anatomic site; the age, genetic, and physiological status of the affected individual; and, presumably, the so-called risk factors to which each individual may have been exposed. Examination of atherosclerotic lesions with modern techniques of cell and molecular biology has revealed that each lesion contains significant elements of three cellular phenomena. These are smooth-muscle proliferation; formation by the proliferated cells of large amounts of connective tissue matrix including collagen, elastic fibers, and proteoglycans; and accumulation of intracellular and extracellular lipid.[1] In each instance, the relative degree to which each of the cells responds to different atherogenic stimuli determines the unique combination that defines the type and extent of the resulting lesion.

The lesions of atherosclerosis occur principally within the innermost layer of the artery wall, the intima. They include the fatty streak, the fibrous plaque, and the so-called complicated lesions[2] (see Chap. 55). Secondary changes have been noted in the media of the artery underlying the lesion, principally in association with the more advanced lesions of atherosclerosis (Fig. 54-1).

The Fatty Streak

The process of atherosclerosis begins in childhood with the development of flat, lipid-rich lesions called *fatty streaks* (see Chap. 55). Studies using monoclonal antibodies specific for macrophages and for smooth-muscle cells have shown that early fatty streaks appear to consist of macrophages together with variable numbers of T lymphocytes. As the lesions expand, they appear to contain smooth-muscle cells that have migrated into the intima as well. As a consequence, these lesions become mixed macrophage–T lymphocyte–smooth-muscle lesions in which both macrophages and smooth muscle are lipid laden. Each of these cell types contains deposits of cholesterol and cholesterol oleate. Fatty streaks can be found in the aorta shortly after birth and appear in increasing numbers between the ages of 8 and 18 years. Fatty streaks appear in the coronary arteries at about age 15 and continue to increase in amount in these vessels through the third decade of life.[3]

The lesions are yellowish and sessile in appearance and cause little or no obstruction of the affected artery and no clinical sequelae. The fatty streak is ubiquitous in young people and even in those populations that do not appear to develop severe atherosclerosis. This observation suggests that lipid deposition does not inevitably lead to the advanced lesions of atherosclerosis but that a number of other factors are associated with the progression of the lesions and with the development of the more complex form of atherosclerosis, the fibrous plaque.

The Fibrous Plaque

More advanced lesions begin to develop around the age of 25 in those populations in which there is a high incidence of atherosclerosis and its clinical sequelae. The fibrous plaque is grossly white in appearance and becomes elevated so that it may protrude into the lumen of the artery (see Chap. 55). If this lesion progresses sufficiently, it can occlude the lumen and compromise

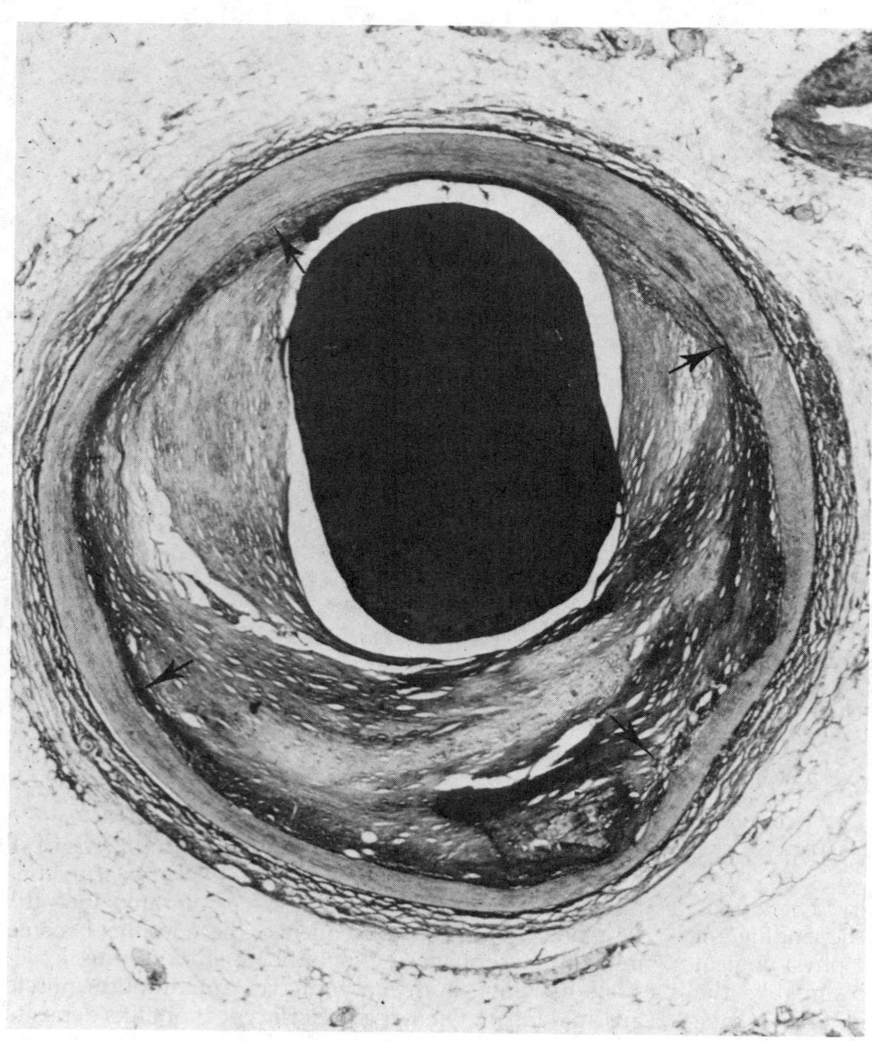

FIGURE 54-1 Classical light micrograph of a cross section of a coronary artery that contains a large atherosclerotic lesion. The lumen of the artery is relatively small. The original lumen is indicated by the arrows. In this preparation, it is virtually impossible to see cellular detail and, in particular, to determine the type of cells involved in the formation of the lesion.

the vascular supply of the involved tissue. The principal change that occurs within the arterial intima during the development of the fibrous plaque consists of migration and proliferation of smooth-muscle cells. These cells usually form a fibrous cap owing to the deposition by the cells of new connective tissue matrix and to the accumulation of intracellular and extracellular lipids. This fibrous cap covers a deeper deposit of varying amounts of extracellular lipid and cell debris[4] (Fig. 54-2).

It has been suggested that fibrous plaques are derived from fatty streaks that continue the process of cell proliferation, lipid accumulation, and connective tissue formation and that the deep core of lipid and cell debris results from inadequate blood supply and cell necrosis. Such a relation has not been proved but has been questioned because, although fatty streaks in young individuals are often found in the same anatomic location in the coronary and extracranial cerebral arteries as fibrous plaques in older individuals, fatty streaks can also occur in anatomic sites that are different from those in which fibrous plaques appear. The reasons for these differences are not understood. It has been suggested that in those instances where their location is different, the fatty streaks may have simply regressed and disappeared, whereas in the instances where the anatomic location is the same, lesion progression has occurred. This remains a matter of controversy. There is a lesion that is generally accepted as a forerunner of the fibrous plaque. This is known as the *fibromusculoelastic lesion* of the intima, which consists of proliferated smooth-muscle cells surrounded by connective tissue and contains little to no lipid.[5]

Immunohistochemical examination of fibrous plaques with cell-specific monoclonal antibodies has shown that the fibrous cap of the lesion consists of numerous smooth-muscle cells surrounded by a dense connective tissue matrix and intermixed with numerous macrophages. This cap covers a deeper layer of macrophages (many of which are filled with lipid in hypercholesterolemic individuals) that are often intermixed with variable numbers of T lymphocytes. Deeper in the lesion there may be necrotic debris and extracellular lipid, and deeper still, there may be numerous proliferated smooth-muscle cells. The presence of T lymphocytes in the lesions raises the possibility that the immune response may be important in lesion genesis or progression and that some lesions may represent an autoimmune response.

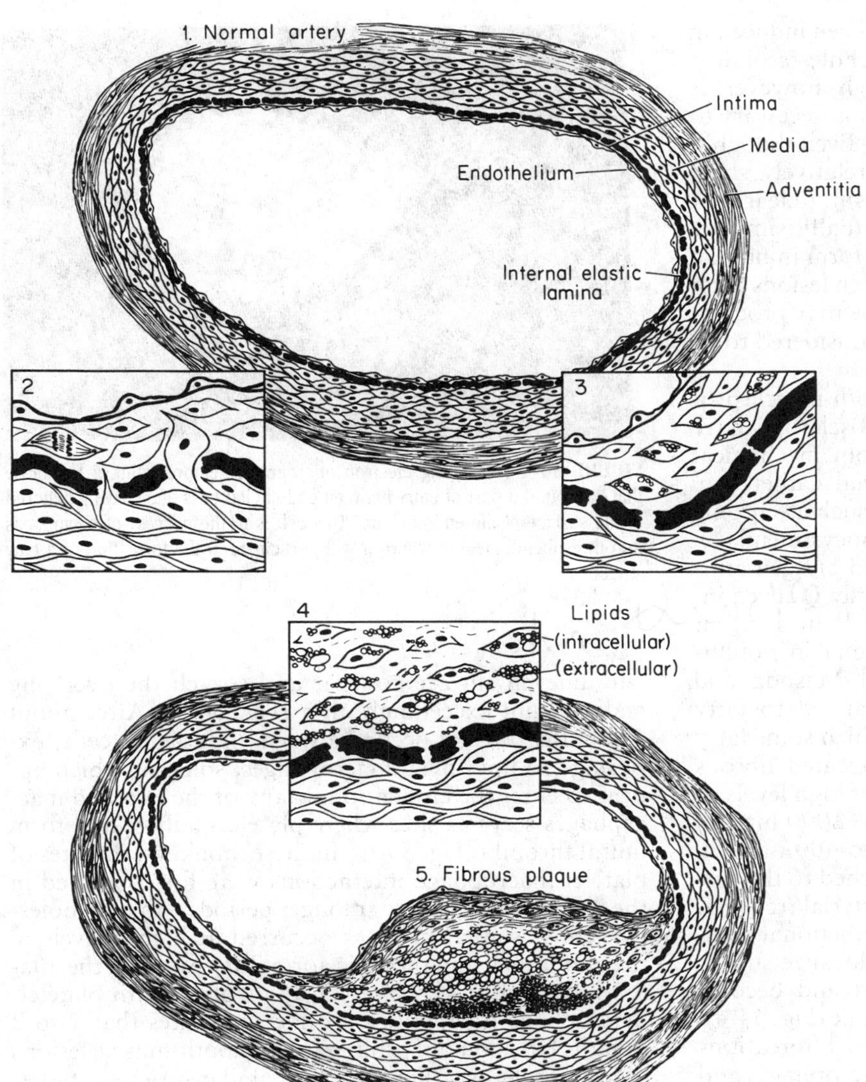

FIGURE 54-2 A series of possible stages in the development of the various lesions of atherosclerosis. (1) The appearance of a normal muscular artery and its component layers; the intima bounded by endothelium and internal elastic lamina, the media, and adventitia. In children and young adults the intima is thin and contains only an occasional smooth-muscle cell; with age it slowly and uniformly increases in thickness and cell content. It is important to note that there are no fibroblasts present in either the intima or the media of mammalian arteries. Fibroblasts are found only in the adventitia. (2) The first phase of a developing lesion in atherosclerosis; a focal thickening of the intima consists of an increase in smooth-muscle cells and extracellular matrix. Smooth-muscle cells are shown proliferating within the intima; two are in the process of migrating through fenestrae of the internal elastic lamina. Subsequent to or possibly concomitant with intimal smooth-muscle proliferation, accumulation of intercellular lipid deposits (3) or extracellular lipid (4) or both occurs resulting in a fatty streak. A fibrous plaque (5) may result from a continued accumulation of a connective tissue cap covering increased numbers of smooth-muscle cells laden with lipids, extracellular lipid, and cell debris overlying a deeper extracellular pool of lipid. A complicated lesion may form as a result of continuing cell degeneration, ingress of blood constituents, and calcification superimposed upon the elements present in the fibrous plaque. Observations made at necropsy and experiments such as those described in the text suggest that this may represent the sequence of events that occurs in humans. (*From JA Glomset, R Ross: Atherosclerosis and the arterial smooth muscle cell, Science 180:1332, 1973. Copyright 1973 by the American Association for the Advancement of Science. Reproduced with permission from the publisher and authors.*)

The Advanced (Complicated) Lesion

The complicated lesions of atherosclerosis (see Chap. 55) occur in increasing frequency with increasing age. The fibrous plaque can become vascularized both from the luminal as well as its medial aspects. In the complicated lesion, the necrotic "lipid-rich core" increases in size and often becomes calcified. The lesions may become increasingly complex as a result of hemorrhage and calcification, and the intimal surface may develop fissures or cracks, may disintegrate and ulcerate, and may become involved with thrombotic episodes that can lead to occlusive disease. Such thrombi may then organize and further increase the thickness of the plaque while progressively reducing the size of the arterial lumen. It is not uncommon that as the intimal lesions progress, the number of smooth-muscle cells in the underlying media decreases and the media undergoes atrophy, which can sometimes result in aneurysmal changes rather than lead to thrombotic occlusion of the artery.

There is quite a range of variability in the degree of severity of the lesions of atherosclerosis in different arteries. Recognition that the components of smooth-muscle proliferation, connective tissue formation, and lipid accumulation represent the key elements of the developing lesions of atherosclerosis has led to the utilization of a number of models of experimentally induced atherosclerosis to study this process in different animal species.

EXPERIMENTALLY INDUCED ATHEROSCLEROSIS

Four species have been widely used in studying atherogenesis: rabbits, chickens, swine, and nonhuman primates. Most early work was performed in rabbits; however, swine and nonhuman primates are generally considered to develop lesions that correspond more closely with those that occur in human beings. A great deal of new information has been gained from studies of swine and primates, although rabbits continue to provide important data in terms of understanding a number of cellular phenomena. Atherosclerosis has been induced in most animal models by a high-fat, high-cholesterol diet. A principal shortcoming of this approach, however, is that to produce more advanced lesions, it is necessary to maintain animals on such diets for years. Even though it is possible to induce the lesions in a relatively short period (1 to 3 years in the monkey), it is not clear that the lesions produced in this manner actually simulate those that may require 20 to 30 years to form in human beings. On the other hand, the rate at which lesions form in humans is not entirely clear, since some may progress more rapidly than had heretofore been considered to be possible.[6]

Other approaches to studying the smooth-muscle proliferative changes associated with atherosclerosis have included endothelial injury resulting from mechanical injury from varying types of intraarterial catheters,[7,8] chemically induced injury (from sources such as chronic hypercholesterolemia[9] or chronic homocystinemia[10]), immune-type injuries[11] (from exposure to antigen-antibody complexes), and more recently, virally induced injury in entities such as Marek's disease.[12] In a recent study of diet-induced hypercholesterolemia in nonhuman primates, Faggiotto et al.[13,14] and Masuda and Ross[15,16] have described the changes that led to fatty streak development and the manner in which some fatty streaks progress to become more complicated fibrous plaques. Within 12 days after induction of high levels of plasma cholesterol (approximately 700 to 1000 mg/dL) or within 1 month at lower levels (200 to 400 mg/dL), numerous monocytes were observed attached to the surface of the endothelium throughout the arterial tree (Fig. 54-3). These monocytes probe between junctional complexes of the endothelium, migrate, and localize subendothelially, where they accumulate lipid and become foam cells to establish the initial fatty streak (Fig. 54-4). These fatty streaks form at branches and bifurcations and accumulate increasing numbers of macrophages and smooth-muscle cells; in the process they create a markedly uneven surface contour and stretch the overlying endothelium exceedingly thin (Fig. 54-5). After about 5 months, breaks occur between endothelial cells, exposing the lipid-filled macrophages, some of which appear to enter the circulation. Many of the exposed macrophages serve as sites where platelets adhere and form mural thrombi (Fig. 54-6). In these monkeys, the sites of platelet-macrophage interactions were first observed in the iliac arteries, and after longer periods of hypercholesterolemia, similar changes occurred at higher levels in the abdominal and thoracic aorta. Interestingly, the anatomic sites that were previously involved with platelet-macrophage interactions are the same sites that 1 to 2 months later contain proliferative smooth-muscle lesions of atherosclerosis (Fig. 54-7). A similar series of studies of chronic hypercholesterolemia in nonhuman primates has recently been published by Masuda and Ross.[15,16] These studies examined monkeys that were fed a high-fat, high-cholesterol diet that led to cholesterol levels ranging between 200 and 400 mg/dL. The same cellular interactions and process of lesion progression from fatty streak to intermediate lesion to fibrous plaque were observed in these monkeys as those observed at the much higher levels of cholesterol by Faggiotto et al.[13,14] They also showed the same increase in lesion progression in a cephalad direction that was observed in the earlier studies, suggesting a relationship between the early fatty streak and the ultimate advanced lesion, or fibrous plaque.

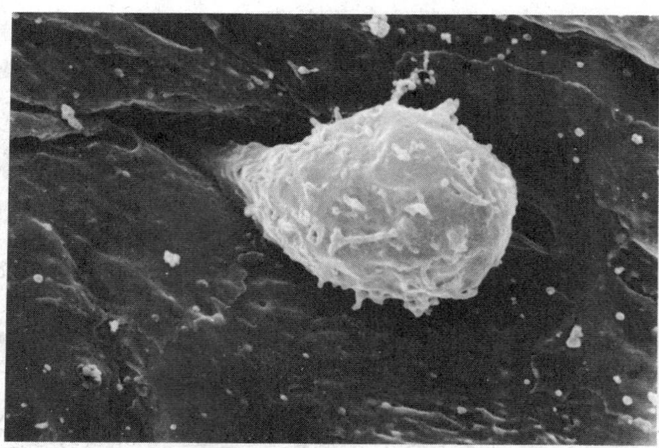

FIGURE 54-4 Scanning electron micrograph demonstrating a leukocyte that has found a port of entry between endothelial cells after having adhered to the surface of the endothelium. This cell is in the process of chemotaxis into the subendothelium where it will participate in the formation of a fatty streak.

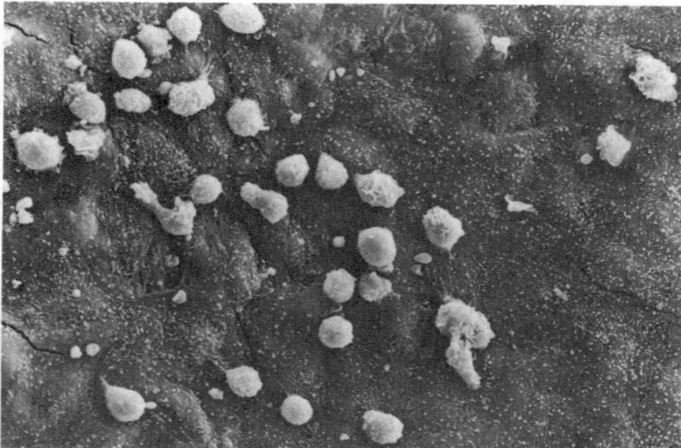

FIGURE 54-3 Scanning electron micrograph demonstrating the adherence of leukocytes (monocytes and T lymphocytes) to the endothelium in a segment of the aorta from a nonhuman primate that had been hypercholesterolemic (250 mg/dL) for 1 month. Most of the cells are rounded; however, a few of them have begun to spread on the surface over which they migrate prior to entry into the artery wall between the endothelial cells.

These studies further support observations that endothelial injury and platelet and macrophage interactions may be important in atherogenesis. This causal relation is exceedingly difficult to establish, however. It is probable that the derivation of most fibrous plaques from fatty streaks is the result of direct progression of the fatty streak. A biologic basis for this possibility has been demonstrated by the fact that both activated endothelial cells and activated macrophages can produce growth factors that can have a profound effect by inducing smooth-muscle cell migration, proliferation, and connective tis-

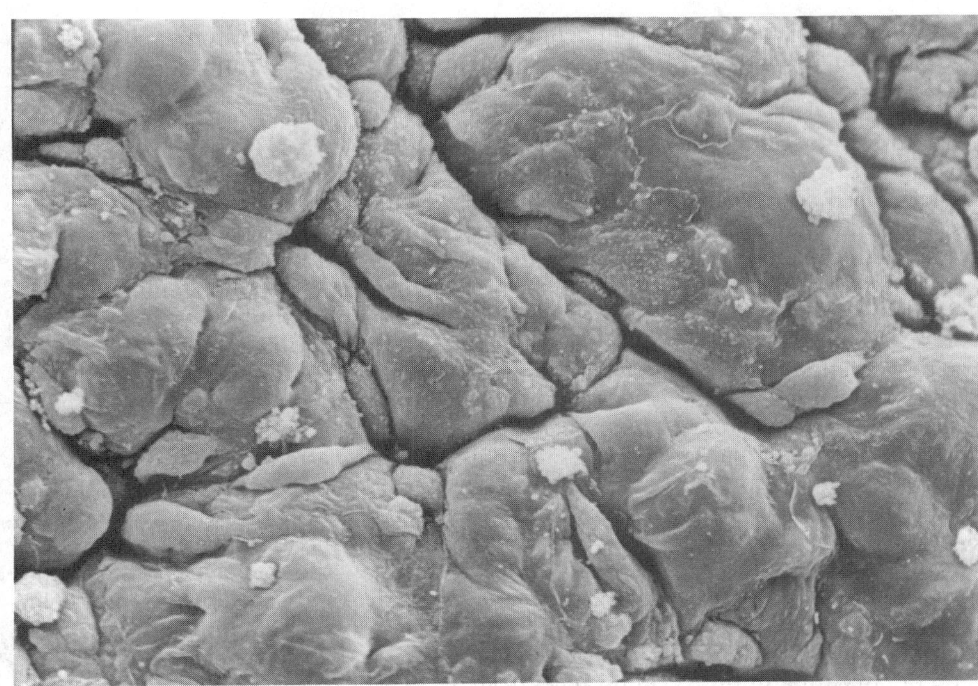

FIGURE 54-5 Scanning electron micrograph demonstrating the uneven appearance of the surface of a fatty streak in a hypercholesterolemic nonhuman primate. The domelike configurations and deep folds between these elevated regions represent accumulations of lipid-filled macrophages (foam cells) and T lymphocytes beneath the endothelial cells. Additional adherent leukocytes can be seen on the surface of the fatty streak that may potentially participate in the expansion of the lesion. Thus, the endothelium covering the surface of the fatty streak is altered and induces additional leukocyte adhesion, chemotaxis, and foam cell formation so that the fatty streak can expand.

sue formation. Virtually identical observations concerning the cellular interactions that lead to lesions of atherosclerosis have also been made in the Watanabe Heritable Hyperlipidemic (WHHL) rabbit (an animal model of homozygous familial hypercholesterolemia), in fat-fed rabbits,[17,18] and in hypercholesterolemic swine.

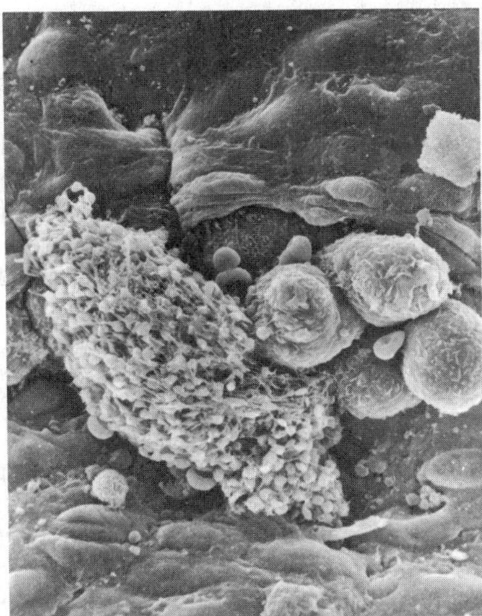

FIGURE 54-6 Scanning electron micrograph of a portion of a fatty streak that has become exposed due to separation between endothelial cells at their junctional attachment sites. The expanding lesion appears to somehow induce this separation, leading to exposure of the underlying lipid-filled macrophages, several of which have become a site for thrombus formation. The mural platelet thrombus that has formed on the left side of the micrograph demonstrates that many of these macrophages can become thrombogenic sites and potentially represent sites where the platelets may release their products including several growth regulatory molecules.

Each animal model has its shortcomings; however, important new information has been obtained from these approaches, particularly when they can be studied in correlation with in vitro models using cell culture techniques. The latter have permitted in-depth studies of endothelium, smooth muscle, macrophages, and platelets. The interrelationships among these cells and among observations resulting from in vivo studies of atherogenesis and cell culture are discussed later in this chapter.

The cellular responses described in hypercholesterolemic nonhuman primates and rabbits have now been

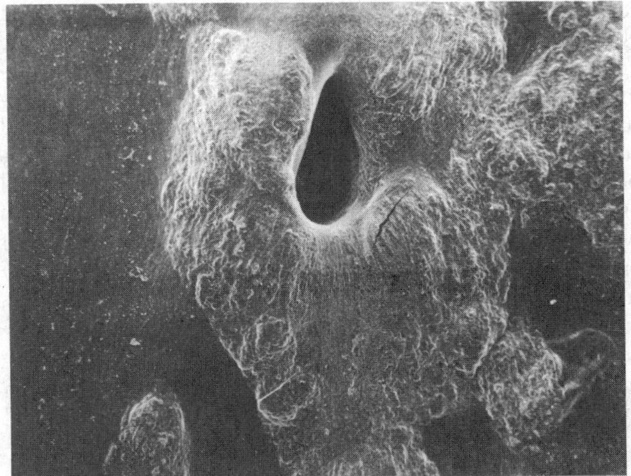

FIGURE 54-7 Low-power scanning electron micrograph of an intermediate or fibrofatty lesion that has formed at the inflow track of one of the intercostal arteries in the thoracic aorta of a chronically hypercholesterolemic nonhuman primate. The elevation due to the fibroproliferative response and continuing accumulation of macrophages in this lesion can be seen at this site. This may potentially go on to become a fibrous plaque.

verified in humans. Davies et al.[19] examined a series of hearts that contained advanced coronary atherosclerosis that were removed for transplant purposes. The hearts were perfuse fixed as rapidly as possible after their removal and examined by light microscopy and scanning and transmission electron microscopy. Virtually, the same cellular responses, including increased adherence of monocytes and T lymphocytes, transendothelial migration by these adherent leukocytes, and localization in the intima to form the early fatty streaks, were observed. Further, sites of endothelial separation over expanding fatty streaks were observed to be covered by platelet mural thrombi, similar to the mural thrombi that formed on the exposed migrating macrophages in the nonhuman primates and rabbits. Ultimately, the cellular makeup of the advanced lesions of atherosclerosis in the human lesions are essentially identical to those observed in the experimental animals. In essence, these observations represent the hallmarks of a marked, chronic inflammatory process associated with a subsequent fibroproliferative process. Due to the excessive nature of both the inflammation and the fibroproliferative processes, the incursion of the lesion into the lumen of the artery, and secondary changes that lead to thrombosis and organization of the thrombi, these lesions continue to expand. When there is no compensatory arterial dilation, they will encroach upon the lumen and lead to clinical sequelae. Thus, atherosclerosis represents an excessive, chronic inflammatory-fibroproliferative response that begins as a protective response but in its excess becomes the disease process.

HYPOTHESES OF ATHEROGENESIS

Historical View of Atherogenesis

Atherosclerosis has been recognized in humans for thousands of years. Lesions of atherosclerosis were identified in Egyptian mummies dating from as early as the fifteenth century B.C. Long[20] has discussed the development of clinical-pathological correlations that evolved during the era when autopsy examination permitted the development of an understanding between the degree of atherosclerosis and the incidence of myocardial infarction and stroke. In the mid-nineteenth century, Virchow[21] proposed the idea that some form of injury to the artery wall associated with an inflammatory response resulted in what was then considered to be a degenerative lesion of atherosclerosis. This idea was subsequently modified by Anitschkow[22] and further included the role of platelets and thrombogenesis in atherosclerosis, as expanded by Duguid[23] in 1948.

Many of the modern views of atherogenesis stem from the work of John French,[24] who noted that the structural integrity of the endothelial lining of the artery represented a key element in the maintenance of normal arterial function and that alterations in endothelial integrity might precede a sequence of events that would lead to the various forms of the lesions of atherosclerosis. Thus, over the years a number of theories concerning the etiology and pathogenesis of atherosclerosis have been developed. At least three of these deserve elaboration and comment. These are the response-to-injury hypothesis, the monoclonal hypothesis, and the lipogenic hypothesis.

The Response-to-Injury Hypothesis

One basis for the *response-to-injury hypothesis* of atherosclerosis[1,9,25,26] lies in the marked similarity observed by many investigators between the ubiquitous fibromusculoelastic lesions noted at autopsy and a similar lesion that can be induced in a number of animal species, including nonhuman primates, rabbits, and swine, after different forms of arterial endothelial injury.

The hypothesis (Fig. 54-8) states that some form of "injury" to the endothelium results in structural and/or functional alterations in the endothelial cells. Factors such as chronic hypercholesterolemia[9]; altered shear stress from the flow of blood over the endothelial cells, as may occur at branch points or bifurcations in arteries in hypertension[27]; and dysfunction induced by toxins or other injurious agents may lead to changes in the nature of the permeability barrier established by the endothelial cells. In the normal artery, the endothelial cells form a continuous monolayer that regulates the passage of substances from the plasma to the underlying artery wall. Injury to the endothelial cells may alter their permeability characteristics and change endothelial cell–cell or endothelial cell–connective tissue relations, permitting hemodynamic forces to induce focal endothelial cell detachment and thus permit interactions to occur between elements from the blood and the wall of the artery. (See also Chap. 2.)

Not only do the endothelial cells play an important role as a permeability barrier but they also form a thromboresistant surface that promotes the continuous flow of blood throughout the vascular tree. The thromboresistant character of the endothelium appears to be due principally to two factors produced by the cells. Both of these have been identified, but their physiological roles are relatively poorly understood. They are the cell surface glycoproteins and proteoglycans that form the surface coat of the endothelial cells and a prostaglandin derivative, prostacyclin (PGI_2).[28] Prostacyclin is one of the most potent vasodilatory agents thus far isolated and is a potent inhibitor of platelet aggregation. Both endothelial cells and smooth-muscle cells are capable of synthesizing prostacyclin: this is discussed in greater detail below. The endothelium also produces endothelium-derived relaxing factor (EDRF), which produces vascular vasodilatation and also inhibits platelet function.

Injury to the endothelium that results in alterations in permeability would permit plasma constituents such as lipoproteins to have more ready access to the artery wall. Such injury, and others that affect endothelial function, may not result in any changes in the morphology of the endothelial monolayer that lines the artery. Endothelial dysfunction could also alter the thromboresistant character of the lumen of the artery so that platelets could interact directly at sites of endothelial injury. If the injury were sufficiently severe, the endothelial cells might desquamate and be lost into the bloodstream, leading to exposure of the underlying connective tissue to platelets and to other elements in the circulation. The response-to-injury hypothesis suggests that the interaction between

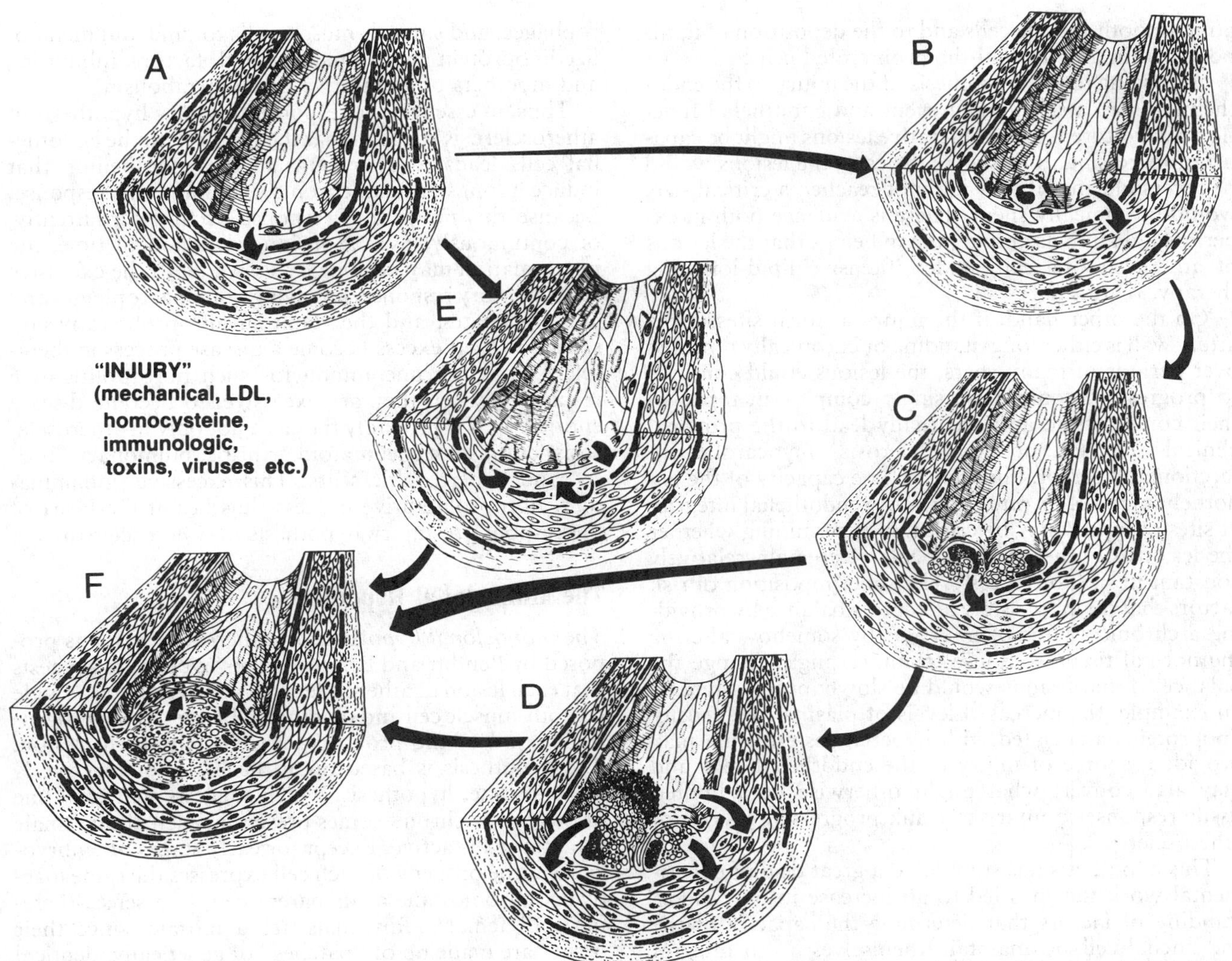

FIGURE 54-8 Revised response-to-injury hypothesis. Advanced intimal proliferative lesions of atherosclerosis may occur by at least two pathways. The pathway demonstrated by the clockwise (long) arrows to the right has been observed in experimentally induced hypercholesterolemia. Injury to the endothelium (*A*) may induce growth factor secretion (short arrow). Monocytes attach to endothelium (*B*), which may continue to secrete growth factors (short arrow). Subendothelial migration of monocytes (*C*) may lead to fatty-streak formation and release of growth factors such as PDGF (short arrow). Fatty streaks may become directly converted to fibrous plaques (long arrow from *C* to *F*) through release of growth factors from macrophages or endothelial cells or both. Macrophages may also stimulate or injure the overlying endothelium. In some cases, macrophages may lose their endothelial cover and platelet attachment may occur (*D*), providing three possible sources of growth factors—platelets, macrophages, and endothelium (short arrows). Some of the smooth-muscle cells in the proliferative lesion itself (*F*) may form and secrete growth factors such as PDGFs (short arrows).

An alternative pathway for development of advanced lesions of atherosclerosis is shown by the arrows from *A* to *E* to *F*. In this case, the endothelium may be injured but remain intact. Increased endothelial turnover may result in growth factor formation by endothelial cells (*A*). This may stimulate migration of smooth-muscle cells from the media into the intima, accompanied by endogenous production of PDGF by smooth muscle as well as growth factor secretion from the "injured" endothelial cells (*E*). These interactions could then lead to fibrous plaque formation and further lesion progression (*F*). (*From R Ross: The pathogenesis of atherosclerosis: An update.* N Engl J Med 314:488, 1986. *Reproduced with permission from the publisher and author.*)

constituents in the plasma, platelets and monocyte/macrophages, and the endothelium or the connective tissue, principally collagen, could result in platelet adherence, aggregation, and release of contents normally stored within the granules of the platelets or released from activated intimal macrophages, or foam cells. In most cases, the advanced lesions probably form due to macrophage–smooth muscle interactions. The early fatty streak contains principally macrophages. Furthermore, platelet interactions may be relatively rare unless thrombosis occurs, and direct progression of fatty streaks to fibrous plaques probably represents the most common course of atherogenesis in hypercholesterolemia. The exposure of the artery wall at sites of injury to factors derived from the platelets and/or macrophages, together with components from the plasma such as lipoproteins and hormones, would then lead to focal proliferation of arterial smooth-muscle cells. According to the hypothesis, this smooth-muscle proliferation would be derived from two sources: preexisting intimal smooth-muscle cells and medial smooth-muscle cells that are attracted to and migrate and proliferate within the intima at sites of "injury." Such a local stimulus could also lead to the formation of new connective tissue matrix constituents by the proliferating smooth-muscle cells and to the deposition of lipids both within and around the proliferated cells.

According to this hypothesis, if the injury to the endothelium were a self-limited event and endothelial function was restored, the proliferative lesions might be capable of regressing. If this were the case, the lesions would be reversible and, if they had not reached a critical size, would be clinically silent. There is evidence both in experimental animals and in human beings that the lesions of atherosclerosis can, under intensive lipid-lowering therapy, regress.[29,30]

On the other hand, if the injury at focal sites in the artery wall is either long-standing or chronically repeated over periods of many years, the lesions could continue to progress, become increasingly complex in terms of their composition, and eventually lead to the principal clinical sequelae of atherosclerosis, myocardial infarction and cerebral infarction. The capacity of the endothelium to regenerate and restore endothelial integrity at sites of injury may be critical in determining whether the lesions of atherosclerosis enlarge, remain relatively constant in size, or regress. The superimposition of risk factors that might possibly affect this balance by providing a chronic source of injury or by somehow altering the normal tissue response to injury might change the balance so that lesions would be slowly progressive. As an example, the increased levels of plasma low-density lipoproteins associated with hypercholesterolemia may provide a source of injury to the endothelial cells and may also convert what might otherwise be a limited tissue response to injury to frank progressive lesions of atherosclerosis.

This hypothesis has stimulated a great deal of experimental work that has led to an increase in our understanding of factors that determine the capacity of the endothelial cells to maintain themselves as an integral continuous cell layer and to studies of those factors that control the growth of endothelium. Of equal importance, many studies have elucidated the factors that modify the capacity of arterial smooth-muscle cells to form connective tissue proteins, to synthesize and metabolize lipids and lipoproteins, and to proliferate in response to different mitogenic factors.

One of the more important observations that has resulted from examination of this hypothesis is the discovery that platelets, macrophages, and some smooth-muscle cells can release a potent mitogen, the platelet-derived growth factor (PDGF).[31] It has been suggested that this factor may play an important role in inducing the intimal smooth-muscle proliferative response seen in experimentally induced atherosclerosis and in atherosclerosis in human beings. This is discussed in greater detail below.

A number of important questions have arisen concerning the factors that promote proliferation of smooth-muscle and endothelial cells and the mechanisms whereby lesions of atherosclerosis may regress. More is becoming known concerning the factors responsible for the turnover of connective tissue matrix within the artery wall and concerning the mechanisms responsible for removing either this matrix or cholesterol from lesions. The response-to-injury hypothesis has provided explanations for some of these phenomena. Much has been learned regarding the capacity of endothelial cells, macrophages, and smooth-muscle cells to bind and metabolize lipoprotein and to make growth factors, inhibitors, and modifiers of connective tissue metabolism.

Thus, in essence, the response-to-injury hypothesis of atherosclerosis suggests that the "injury" to the endothelial cells leads to alterations in the endothelium that induce a longstanding, chronic, inflammatory response. Because this injury and response occur intermittently, or continuously, over a prolonged period of time, the inflammation may become excessive. Both the excessive inflammatory response, involving both macrophages and T lymphocytes, and the resulting fibroproliferative response in their excess become a disease process in themselves. It is not uncommon for such fibroproliferative responses, when they are excessive, to become disease entities. This is probably the case, not only in atherosclerosis, but also in rheumatoid arthritis, pulmonary fibrosis, and hypertrophic scars. This excessive, inflammatory, fibroproliferative process thus lies at the heart of the response-to-injury hypothesis of atherosclerosis.

The Monoclonal Hypothesis

The *monoclonal hypothesis* of atherosclerosis was proposed by Benditt and Benditt.[32] This hypothesis suggests that each lesion of atherosclerosis is derived from a single smooth-muscle cell and that this cell serves as the progenitor for all of the proliferating cells within the lesion. The hypothesis is based upon the Lyon, or inactive X chromosome, hypothesis, which suggests that only one of the two X chromosomes present in each adult female somatic cell is active. Except for early stages of embryogenesis, the progeny of each cell expresses the same inactive X chromosome as its parent cell. In a sense, therefore, all female individuals are a mosaic, since their tissues are made up of "patches" of genetically identical cells that have either an active maternal or an active paternal X chromosome. This observation makes little to no metabolic difference, since both X chromosomes code for similar enzymes. The Bendits, however, took advantage of the fact that a special case exists for the enzyme glucose-6-phosphate dehydrogenase (G6PD). The genes for this enzyme are located in the X chromosome and in humans can occur in two forms of isoenzyme that can be separated by paper electrophoresis. Some black females have been found to be heterozygous for these two isoenzymes so that they represent a mosaic of the two isoenzymes in various somatic cell populations. Consequently, it is possible to distinguish different cell patches within this mosaic by identification of the appropriate isoenzyme. This was originally taken advantage of by Linder and Gartler,[33] who examined multiple samples of uterine leiomyomas and found that they were composed of cells that contained the same active X chromosome, whereas comparable samples of normal myometrium contained a mixture of cells derived from both types of progenitor cells. Studies of some other tumors have demonstrated similar phenomena, and in some cases there are data supporting the notion that all the cells of a given tumor originate from a single cell and are therefore monoclonal.[34]

More recently, Benditt and others have referred to this character of lesions as *monotypic*. Additional research has produced data that both support and negate this hypothesis. Pearson et al.[35] observed that the majority of atherosclerotic lesions examined from a series of autopsied black females contained either one or the other of the two isoenzymes of G6PD but that fatty streaks from these individuals and the noninvolved, or normal, arterial tissue contained both isoenzymes and therefore did not appear to be monotypic. Thomas et al.[36] examined the lesion and nonlesion areas of arteries from black females at autopsy in a slightly different manner and obtained data that are at variance with the data supporting the hypothesis and that have been interpreted differently. Thomas et al. examined multiple samples of lesions versus nonlesion areas and found a much higher percentage of both isoenzymes within lesions than had been reported in the earlier studies.

Benditt[37] has interpreted his data to signify that since each lesion of atherosclerosis is monotypic and is presumably derived from a single smooth-muscle cell, each lesion is a benign neoplasm that may have occurred as a result of cell transformation by agents such as viruses or chemicals.

Fialkow[34] has pointed out that the observation of a single enzyme phenotype in a lesion does not necessarily imply a clonal origin for such a lesion. He stresses that each lesion could arise from a population of genetically identical cells that contained the same isoenzyme rather than from a single cell. These two possibilities could not be distinguished from one another using the single technique of paper electrophoresis. In the artery wall, the possibility of a monoclonal origin would presumably depend on the mosaic composition of the artery wall and therefore the distribution of cells with one or the other isoenzyme within the normal intima or media. Unfortunately, relatively little is known concerning the distribution of isoenzymes within the artery, and the possibility that sparsely distributed, single progenitor cells in the normal intima could give rise to smooth-muscle cell patches that are appreciably larger than those in the media deserves to be explored. If lesion development were characterized by repeated cycles of cell death and growth, according to Fialkow, "repetitive sampling could lead to a single enzyme phenotype, despite multicellular origin."[34] It is therefore possible that under those circumstances clonal selection with evolution toward a single enzyme phenotype within the lesion could conceivably occur in some kinds of hyperplastic responses. Therefore it is likely that the lesions of atherosclerosis are derived not from a single cell, but rather from a population of cells of identical phenotype or some combination of these events. It is probable that the bulk of the lesions of atherosclerosis are hyperplastic rather than neoplastic, which provides further reason for developing means of intervention and treatment leading to lesion regression.

The Lipogenic Hypothesis

Both lesion initiation and lesion progression in atherosclerosis appear somehow to be associated in many individuals with markedly increased elevations of plasma low-density lipoproteins (LDLs). The accumulation of lipid within proliferated smooth-muscle cells, within macrophages in the lesions, and within the extracellular connective tissue matrix is a common finding, particularly in the lesions of atherosclerosis.[38] The presence of elevated levels of LDL suggest that cholesterol internalization and esterification by cells may be accelerated to such a degree that proliferated smooth-muscle cells within lesions become filled with cholesterol oleate. Many of the cells may go on to become necrotic and may release their lipid into the extracellular spaces. In the presence of excess plasma LDL, which is relatively rich in cholesterol linoleate, the debris may be a mixture of both types of cholesteryl esters.

Some studies have suggested that modified or oxidized LDL in hyperlipemic animals may promote endothelial injury and indirectly proliferation of smooth-muscle cells and the production of new connective tissue components by these cells.[39,40] Thus, a sequence of events involving injury to the endothelium by chronic elevated levels of modified LDL and continuing progression of lesions of atherosclerosis by exposure to elevated levels of LDL and, presumably, by decreased levels of high-density lipoproteins (HDLs) could provide a sequence of events leading to the development of advanced lesions of atherosclerosis. This hypothesis might explain how some fatty streaks could progress to become fibrous plaques, but it fails to take into account many of the other components of the lesions of atherosclerosis. In particular, it fails to explain, in addition to the proliferative response of smooth-muscle cells, the basis for other phenomena such as the stimulation of new connective tissue formation.

It is possible that the different lesions of atherosclerosis may occur by any of the mechanisms suggested in these different hypotheses or by different combinations of them. It is also clear that as many aspects of our understanding of the biology of smooth-muscle cells and endothelium continue to be expanded, new factors that have not been anticipated may be revealed that may play a role in the pathogenesis of atherosclerosis.

The Role of Risk Factors

A number of risk factors of atherosclerosis have become reasonably well established on the basis of their relation in epidemiologic studies to the incidence of clinically manifest disease. Unfortunately, there is no basis for comparison between risk factors and the severity or extent of the lesions of atherosclerosis. Among many factors that are considered to be important are hyperlipidemia, hypertension, cigarette smoking, male sex, and diabetes mellitus. These have in general been associated with an increased incidence of fibrous plaques and their sequelae. The associations are relatively strong when they are made on a group comparison basis, although all of the studies have demonstrated a high degree of variability among individuals within even the most homogeneous of groups.[41] (See Chap. 62.)

Hyperlipidemia

Dietary lipids are considered to be one of the most important environmental agents responsible for severe atherosclerosis and for the high frequency of atherosclerotic disease in industrially developed parts of the world. Saturated fats became associated with increased incidence of atherosclerosis when it was found that they elevated the concentration of plasma cholesterol; however, the specific contributions of cholesterol, saturated fats, polyunsaturated fats, and total fats in atherosclerosis are still unclear. It has become possible to demonstrate an unequivocal association between ingestion of dietary cholesterol and plasma cholesterol levels and the incidence and prevalence of coronary disease within population groups. The results of the Lipid Research Clinics Trial[42,43] demonstrated for the first time a direct association between the plasma lipoprotein profile, cholesterol levels, and morbidity and mortality from coronary atherosclerosis. By means of the combination of diet and cholestyramine, a decrease in plasma cholesterol of 8 percent was obtained, which led to a decrease in the incidence of myocardial infarction and in the need for coronary bypass surgery. Thus, for the first time, there are unequivocal data demonstrating that lowering of plasma cholesterol in humans will have beneficial effects in reducing the incidence of atherosclerosis and its sequelae. (See also Chaps. 53 and 65.)

Even more recently, Brown et al.[44] have demonstrated that some semiocclusive lesions of atherosclerosis, followed in individuals by angiography, can be induced to regress and decrease in size during a sufficient period of reduced plasma cholesterol levels. Those studies provided an unequivocal demonstration that some lesions of atherosclerosis can regress under appropriate conditions. New guidelines have been issued by the National Institutes of Health related to plasma cholesterol and lipoproteins. All individuals should have these measured as a routine part of their physical examination. Cholesterol levels below 200 mg/dL are considered normal, 200 to 240 mg/dL are considered borderline and should be treated by diet modification, and levels greater than 240 mg/dL should be treated with drug therapy. Similarly, LDL levels less than or equal to 130 mg/dL are considered normal, 130 to 159 borderline, and greater than 160 mg/dL require therapy. (See Chap. 62.[45])

Unfortunately, there is a great deal of variation from individual to individual in terms of dietary intake of fats and plasma cholesterol levels on a daily basis. There is also intrinsic variation in plasma cholesterol levels among individuals who consume the same diet but respond differently to it.

There is little question that dietary cholesterol directly affects the levels of plasma cholesterol.[46] Dietary cholesterol may also affect the incidence of atherosclerosis by altering the profile of plasma lipoproteins and possibly by changing the structural or functional properties of these lipoproteins.[47] Increased dietary cholesterol generally results in an increase in LDL cholesterol with a lesser increase in HDL cholesterol. Low-density lipoprotein leads to increased uptake of lipid in cells, whereas HDL plays a role in removing lipid from cells and is thus protective. (See Chap. 53.)

The Role of Oxidized LDL

Studies with WHHL rabbits showed that use of the antioxidant probucol had a statistically significant effect in reducing both lesion size and incidence in these genetically, endogenously hypercholesterolemic rabbits.[40,48] Subsequent to this observation, a great many animal studies have demonstrated that oxidized LDL (oxLDL) may play an important role in this disease in animals as well as humans. Oxidized LDL has been observed immunohistochemically in macrophages in both human and experimental atherosclerosis. Oxidized LDL is injurious to endothelium and smooth-muscle cells, and LDL oxidation can take place during the transport of LDL through endothelial cells and after its uptake by macrophages. The ability of antioxidants, such as probucol, to diminish lesion size suggests that by protecting the lipoproteins from oxidation, both at the level of the endothelium and within the lesions by the macrophages and potentially the smooth-muscle cells themselves, it may be possible both to prevent lesion formation and potentially induce lesion regression. Intensive studies are underway in numerous laboratories to determine the specific roles played by oxLDL in atherogenesis and the potential usefulness of various approaches to prevent oxidation and free-radical formation in reducing lesion size and incidence.[49]

Hypertension

Hypertension has been established unequivocally as an associated risk factor in that individuals with elevated blood pressure show accelerated atherogenesis, an increased incidence of coronary heart disease, and in particular, increased incidence of cerebrovascular disease. The effects of hypertension appear to be independent of other risk factors in an epidemiologic sense; however, it does not appear to be a primary cause of advanced atherosclerosis in those populations in which the incidence of clinically manifest atherosclerosis is less than average.

The means by which hypertension induces atherogenesis are not clear, although there are many humoral mediators of blood pressure that may participate in this process. For example, renin, angiotensin, β-adrenergic substances, and other hypertensive agents may induce cellular changes that lead to atherogenesis. Fry[27] and his colleagues, as well as others, have suggested that altered flow characteristics, including the eddy currents and backflow of blood, particularly in hypertensive individuals, at selected anatomic sites within the arterial tree may result in focally altered endothelium and in the development of atherosclerotic lesions very much as suggested in the response-to-injury hypothesis discussed earlier.

Cigarette Smoking

Cigarette smoking provides perhaps the strongest and most consistent correlation with the increased incidence of atherosclerotic disease and appears to be a major contributor to increased risk of disease, generally in combination with other risk factors. Unfortunately, there is relatively little information concerning the means by which cigarette smoking exerts an impact at the cellular level. Early studies suggested that carbon monoxide might be a causative agent; however, these have not been confirmed. Becker et al.[50] identified agents derived from cigarette smoke that may be injurious to the artery wall. It has also been suggested that inhalation of cigarette smoke may result in the exposure of arterial cells to mutagens that transform the smooth-muscle cells and result in the stimulation of their proliferation. Apparently, cessation of cigarette smoking decreases the risk for development of the clinical sequelae of atherosclerosis and possibly may augment regression of lesions. Further research is clearly required to identify the factors in cigarette smoke that are responsible for its cardiovascular effects and to determine the mechanisms by which these factors alter cellular metabolism. (See also Chap. 62.)

Male Sex

Perhaps one of the best-documented and most consistent risk factors for coronary atherosclerosis is male sex. This differential is accentuated in nonwhite populations, and it has been suggested that females have a decreased incidence because of a protective function exerted by estrogens. Paradoxically, unfortunately, large doses of estrogenic hormones appear to increase cardiovascular mortality in men who have had one myocardial infarct and among men under treatment for prostatic cancer. Consequently, the reason for the sex difference is not understood and remains to be elucidated.

Diabetes

Another risk factor known to be associated with increased incidence of atherosclerosis and myocardial infarction is diabetes mellitus. The mechanisms involved are poorly understood. There is, unfortunately, no consistency in the evidence related to whether elevated concentrations of plasma cholesterol and lipoproteins occur in diabetics whose concentrations of blood and urine glucose are carefully regulated. There does appear to be some evidence suggesting a decreased concentration of HDL cholesterol in diabetics and a high prevalence of hypertension associated with hyperglycemia. The basic mechanisms associated with the proliferation of smooth-muscle-type cells in the mesangium of the kidney in renal complications of diabetes and in increased thickness of capillary basement membrane in diabetics with microvascular disease may bear some similarity to smooth-muscle proliferation in atherogenesis. In general, the alterations in the arterial tree in diabetics that precede the lesions of atherogenesis are not well documented and are poorly understood. (See also Chap. 62.)

Although a great deal of new information, to be discussed below, has evolved concerning our understanding of endothelial cells, smooth-muscle cells, macrophages, and platelets and the interactions among these cells, the specific role of each of the risk factors that are associated with increased incidence of atherosclerosis on an epidemiologic basis remains, for the most part, to be investigated and elucidated. This information will be critical if we are to proceed with the development of improved means of diagnosis, prevention, and intervention in this disease process. (See also Chap. 56.)

CELLULAR MODULATIONS IN ATHEROSCLEROSIS

Endothelium

The Barrier Role

Endothelial cells provide a selective permeability barrier, a blood-compatible interface, and a thromboresistant lining to the artery wall and are metabolically active. A number of studies of endothelial permeability using various tracer molecules have demonstrated the presence of pinocytotic vesicles, transendothelial channels, and intracellular clefts in different kinds of endothelium. The junctional complexes between endothelial cells and the artery wall appear to be functionally dynamic structures that can respond to stimuli such as changes in blood pressure and pharmacologic agents. The surface components, at the molecular level, of the endothelial cells appear to influence the selective permeability of the endothelium.[51,52] Endothelial cells have been shown by the Steins[53] to be capable of transporting plasma lipoproteins of given sizes into the artery wall via vesicles. Thus, molecules like HDL would be transported, but larger lipoproteins the size of very low density lipoproteins (VLDLs) or chylomicrons would have difficulty in crossing the endothelial barrier without some kind of alteration of these lipid-rich particles. (See also Chap. 2.)

The disruption of this barrier has been shown, in a number of experimental animals, to result in opportunities that permit interactions between platelets and the artery wall at sites of endothelial injury resulting in the formation of an intimal smooth-muscle proliferative response. Stemerman and Ross[7] observed that if endothelial cells were removed by abrasion with an intraarterial catheter, sites of exposure of the subendothelial connective tissue were quickly coated with a "carpet" of degranulated platelets (Fig. 54-9). The interaction of products released from the platelets and plasma constituents at such sites of endothelial injury precedes a sequence of events that begins with focal smooth-muscle migration and proliferation and that eventually leads to the development of a fibromusculoelastic lesion. If this mechanical injury is modified by the addition of a high-fat, high-cholesterol diet to the experiment, the hyperlipemic animals whose endothelium has been mechanically injured develop intimal proliferative lesions essentially identical to fibrous plaques. In the normocholesterolemic animals, such endothelial injury leads to a fibromusculoelastic proliferative lesion that, over a period of 6 months, may undergo regression, whereas in hypercholesterolemic animals, the lesions become slowly progressive and show no signs of regression (Figs. 54-10 and 54-11).

Ross and Harker[9] observed that monkeys that received no mechanical injury but that were only fed a high-fat, high-cholesterol diet for a year or longer showed signs of endothelial injury as determined morphologically and by measurements of endothelial cell turnover at selected sites in the arterial tree.

Faggiotto et al.[13,14] and Masuda and Ross[15,16] have observed a sequence of events in chronic hypercholesterolemic monkeys that culminates in dysjunction of endo-

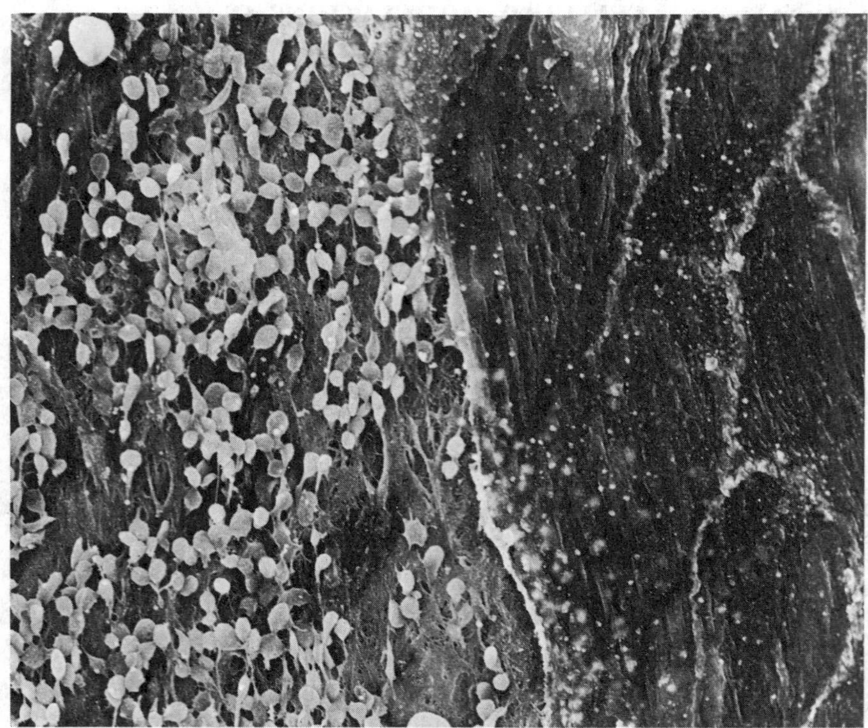

FIGURE 54-9 Scanning electron micrograph presenting a surface view of an artery in which the endothelial cells shown on the right have been removed with a catheter in the left portion of the micrograph. Demonstrates platelets, seen as the small ovoid bodies that have attached to the subendothelial connective tissue that was exposed upon injury to the endothelium. These platelets tend to adhere to the exposed connective tissue and to one another and, in the process of doing so, release their intracellular contents.

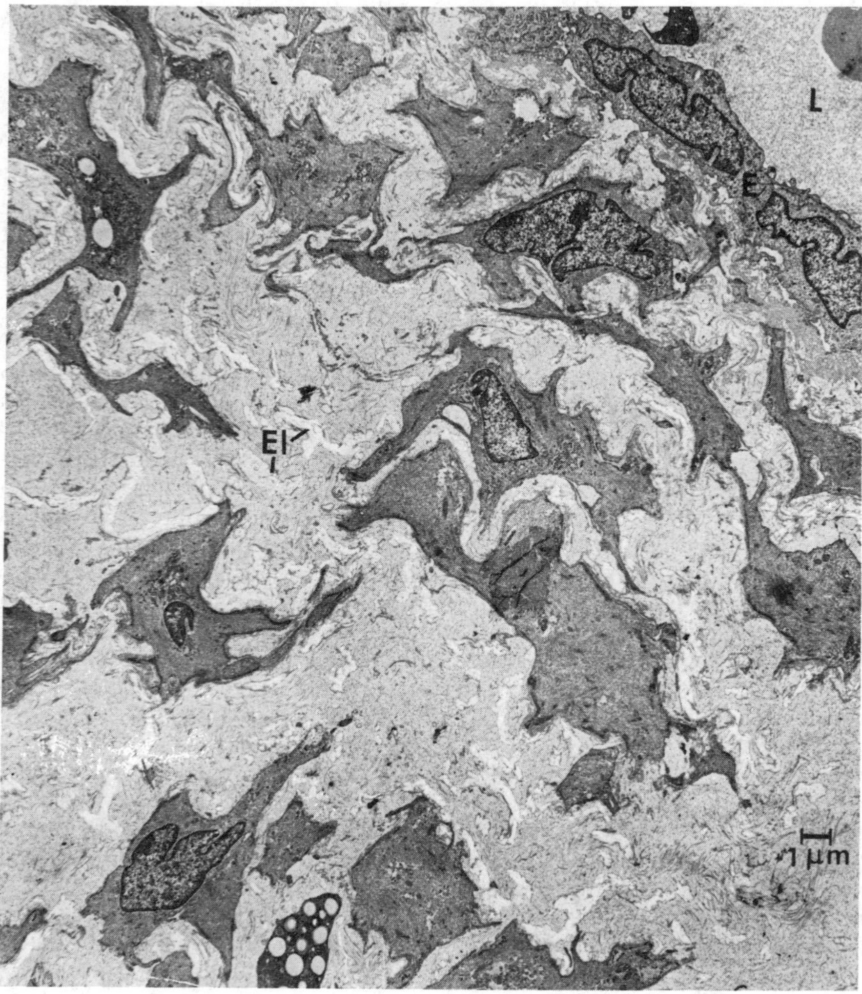

FIGURE 54-10 Electron micrograph of part of the intima from the right iliac artery of a macaque 3 months after the endothelium was removed with an intravascular balloon catheter. The lumen (L) is to the upper right. Endothelial cells cover the markedly thickened intima, which contains large numbers of smooth-muscle cells surrounded by a matrix of small elastic fibers (El), collagen, and proteoglycan.

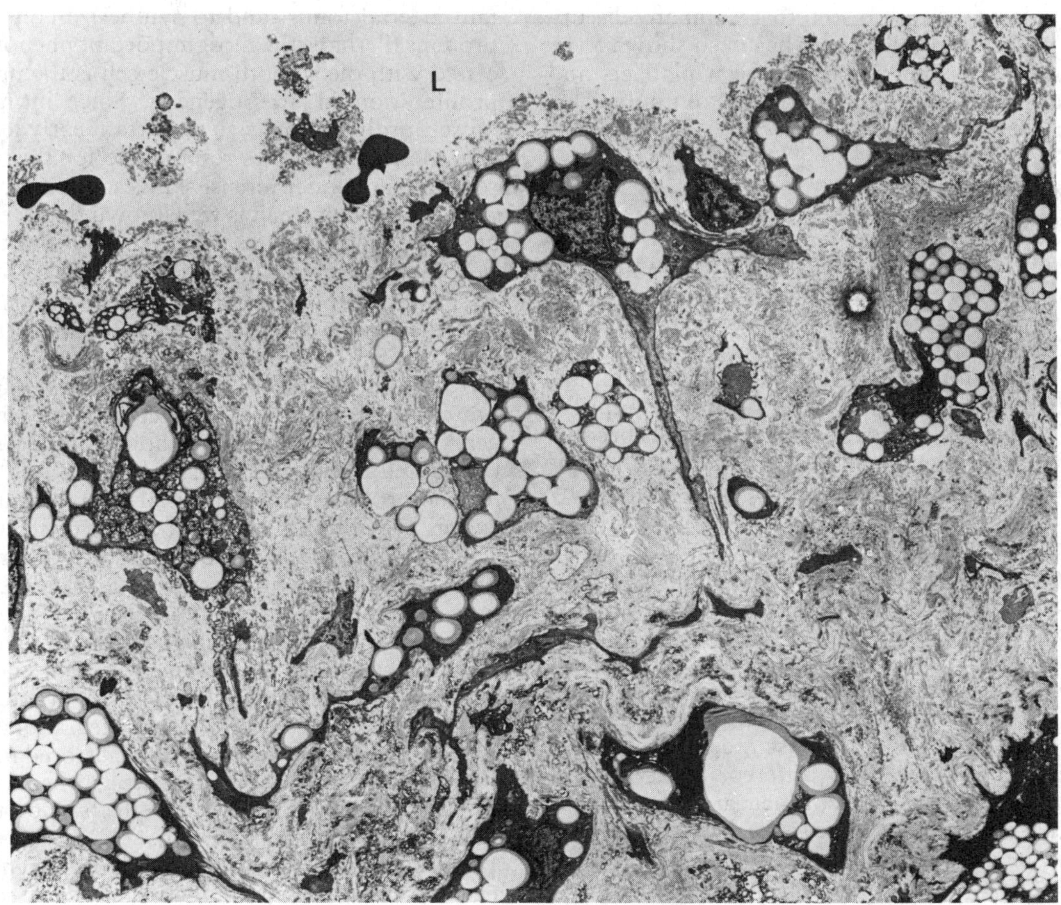

FIGURE 54-11 Electron micrograph of a portion of an intimal lesion in the iliac artery of a monkey on a hyperlipidemic diet 6 months after balloon injury. Most of the smooth-muscle cells in the lesion contain large lipid deposits. The cells are surrounded by small globular membranous deposits in the connective tissue. An endothelial cover is lacking at the luminal surface (L) at the crest of the lesion.

thelium overlying foam cells in fatty streaks that are derived from blood monocytes. Exposure of the foam cells leads to platelet interactions with both the macrophages and the exposed connective tissues. These interactions occur at the same anatomic sites that 1 to 2 months later are occupied by extensive smooth-muscle proliferative lesions of atherosclerosis. Virtually identical observations also have been made in hypercholesterolemic rabbits[17,18] and in human coronary arteries with lesions of atherosclerosis.

It is now recognized that one of the principal changes that occurs in the endothelium after hyperlipidemia or in hypertensive individuals is increased adherence of leukocytes, specifically monocytes and T lymphocytes, to the endothelial cells at particular sites in the artery wall. These adherent leukocytes occur in clusters and appear to do so due to the formation of increased amounts of specific cell surface glycoproteins that are responsible for the leukocyte adhesion (Fig. 54-3). Several of the cell surface glycoproteins that form on both the leukocytes and the endothelial cells have been identified, isolated, and purified. One form, called VCAM (vascular cell adhesion molecule), or alternately athero-ELAM (atherosclerosis-endothelial leukocyte adhesion molecule), has been shown to be present lining the surface of endothelium over lesions of atherosclerosis in rabbits. These molecules on the leukocytes and on the endothelium interact in a ligand-receptor-type manner and may be critical in the initial phases of the specialized, chronic, inflammatory response that is part of the atherogenic process. Thus, the earliest phase of the chronic, inflammatory response that has become recognized to be the hallmark of atherogenesis is represented by leukocyte adhesion due to the formation of these adherence molecules on the surfaces of the endothelium and the leukocytes. (See also Chap. 56.)

A second factor is transmigration of these adherent leukocytes between endothelial cells to localize in the subendothelial matrix where they establish the first lesion of atherosclerosis, the fatty streak (Fig. 54-4). This transmigration of leukocytes is mediated by chemotactic factors that can be generated both by the endothelial cells and by the underlying smooth-muscle cells. Oxidized LDL, referred to above, can act as one of these chemotactic reagents and can also induce the endothelial cells and the underlying smooth-muscle cells to form a second, very potent, chemotactic factor, monocyte chemotactic protein-1 (MCP-1), which may also actively participate in this inflammatory process.

Thus, in addition to leukocyte adhesion, the intimal

smooth-muscle proliferation seen to accompany disruption of the endothelial cell barrier has been shown to be associated with the interactions between platelets and the exposed subendothelium at such sites of injury. This will be discussed below.

Endothelial Cell Culture

Arterial endothelial cells have been successfully cultured from a number of species, including the cow, rabbit, swine, nonhuman primate, and human being.[54,55] Endothelial cells from each of these species demonstrate a number of common characteristics. They grow, as they do in vivo, in a unique, continuous monolayer and, unlike cells such as smooth muscle or fibroblasts, appear to be truly "contact inhibited." That is, the cells become quiescent when they remain in contact and become confluent. If the monolayer is disrupted, for example, by wounding, the cells are stimulated to synthesize new deoxyribonucleic acid (DNA) and to proliferate and restore the continuity of the monolayer. Only those cells in the culture next to the margins of the wound appear to undergo DNA synthesis and proliferation, whereas those in the monolayer at a distance from the wound appear to remain relatively quiescent. This peculiar characteristic of the growth of endothelium is so strikingly different from that of smooth-muscle cells that it has been suggested that these two different cell types are under different sets of controls of their growth and that somehow cell–cell contact appears to be important in determining the state of quiescence of endothelial cells. Endothelial cells grown in culture have been shown to be capable of forming a number of connective tissue matrix macromolecules including particular types of collagen[56]; of transporting lipids; of synthesizing prostacyclin,[28] factor VIII,[57] and angiotensin converting enzyme[58]; and in maintaining many aspects of their differentiated phenotype through several passages. (See also Chap. 2.)

Endothelial-Derived Growth Factors

Recently, endothelial cells have been shown to be capable of forming growth factors in culture. One of these substances is a form of *PDGF*, which is capable of stimulating cells such as fibroblasts and smooth muscle to proliferate.[59] Endothelial cells in culture release PDGF into the medium after they have been exposed to plasma or to serum-free medium.[60] It is not as yet known whether it is formed by endothelial cells in vivo, although in situ hybridization techniques have demonstrated the presence of messenger ribonucleic acid (mRNA) for both chains of PDGF in arterial endothelium.[61] This observation could have potential importance in atherogenesis because PDGF formation could induce lesion progression.

Smooth Muscle

Smooth-Muscle Proliferation

Smooth-muscle cells have long been recognized to possess a number of features important to normal arterial function, including their capacity to contract, to maintain arterial tonus, and to synthesize connective tissue proteins. Perhaps the most important phenomenon associated with the smooth-muscle cell is the process of cell proliferation in atherogenesis. Since intimal smooth-muscle proliferation is an important early feature in atherogenesis, the factors responsible for this proliferative response are under intensive investigation in vivo and in vitro. In cell culture, it is well known that serum provides all of the factors necessary for smooth-muscle proliferation. Arterial smooth-muscle cells from a large number of species can be grown in culture and are able to maintain their differentiated phenotype under these conditions.[62,63]

Ross and coworkers,[31] together with several other laboratories,[64,65] have demonstrated that the principal mitogenic component present in whole blood serum and missing in cell-free plasma-derived serum and responsible for the proliferation of arterial smooth-muscle cells in culture is a mitogen derived from the platelet, the PDGF. The observation that smooth-muscle proliferation in culture is stimulated principally by this mitogen led to a series of studies to examine the role of platelets in smooth-muscle proliferation induced in vivo.

As described above, several forms of endothelial injury result in adherence of platelets at sites of injury. Platelet adherence is followed by degranulation and release into the artery wall of material stored in the platelet granules. Together with plasma constituents, these platelet products have far-reaching effects upon the smooth-muscle cells of the artery wall.

Harker et al.[10] demonstrated that in homocystinuria, a genetic disease of childhood commonly associated with markedly increased incidence of arteriosclerosis, platelets appear to interact at sites where the endothelium has somehow been injured by increased levels of plasma homocysteine. Harker et al.[10] demonstrated this association by measuring the survival of autologous ^{51}Cr-labeled platelets in homocystinuric children and observed that the greater the levels of plasma homocysteine, the greater the decrease in platelet survival. As a result of these observations, they developed an animal model of homocystinuria by chronically infusing homocysteine in baboons. In this model they showed a similar correlation between elevated levels of plasma homocysteine and decreased levels of platelet survival (or increased platelet utilization). When they maintained the baboons on a homocystinemic regimen for 3 months, they observed an increased incidence of missing endothelial cells by morphometric examination of whole-mount preparations of the aorta. Their studies established a correlation between the amounts of injured endothelium, the decrease in platelet survival, and the formation of proliferative smooth-muscle atherosclerotic lesions at the sites of endothelial injury. Harker and his colleagues[10] went on to demonstrate that if they administered to the homocystinemic baboons one of two pharmacologic agents that could inhibit platelet interactions with the injured artery wall, they could prevent the intimal smooth-muscle proliferative lesions that otherwise developed. One of these agents, dipyridamole, returned platelet survival to normal levels and is known because of its capacity to inhibit platelet phosphodiesterase activity and to inhibit platelet adherence. The other agent, sulfinpyrazone, appeared to somehow protect the endothelial cells, since the sulfinpyrazone-treated homocystinemic baboons demonstrated fewer areas of endothelial injury. In both approaches, platelet survival levels were normalized, and the proliferative lesions of atherosclerosis were prevented. These were the first data to correlate a requirement for platelet function with experimentally induced atherosclerosis. (See also Chap. 7.)

Other approaches to examining these same phenomena were taken by Moore and his colleagues[66] and by Friedman et al.[67] In both of their studies, atherosclerosis was induced in rabbits by injuring the endothelium with an intraarterial catheter. In each case, the investigators induced a thrombocytopenia by administration of a specific antiplatelet antiserum. The animals made thrombocytopenic in this manner had no proliferative atherosclerotic lesions, whereas the control animals had extensive lesions.

Using a different approach, Fuster and his colleagues[68] examined the incidence of atherosclerosis in the aortas of swine fed a high-fat, high-cholesterol diet. They were able to study the role of platelets in these swine by trying to induce atherosclerosis with a high-cholesterol diet in a group of swine that were homozygous for von Willebrand's disease, as compared with a group of normal swine. The swine with severe von Willebrand's disease had essentially no factor VIII—von Willebrand's factor—in their plasma. Normally this factor is required for platelet adherence and release. The control animals on the high-lipid diet developed extensive proliferative lesions of atherosclerosis, whereas the von Willebrand's swine developed intimal infiltrates of lipid but no smooth-muscle proliferative lesions. In the absence of von Willebrand's factor, platelet interactions may be somewhat inhibited in the hypercholesterolemic von Willebrand's diseased swine.

All of these studies point to the importance of platelet interactions at sites of endothelial alterations that precede the formation of experimentally induced proliferative lesions of atherosclerosis. (See Chap. 56.)

Lipid Metabolism

Since lipids are essential components of all cells, it is not surprising that they are involved in a number of cell functions and metabolic processes, as they represent the principal constituent of all cell membranes. Both the plasma membrane and the internal membranous compartments of all cells, including smooth muscle, are composed of phospholipids, proteins, and cholesterol, principally unesterified cholesterol. Esterified cholesterol is found in smooth muscle only under abnormal conditions. Accumulations of cholesteryl ester in smooth-muscle cells and macrophages lead to the development of foam cells found in the lesions of atherosclerosis. Some experiments have shown that smooth-muscle cells can acquire cholesterol both by de novo synthesis[69] and from an exogenous source of cholesterol-carrying lipoproteins.[70] Such a dual mechanism may help the cell to protect itself against possible deficits in cholesterol.

Smooth-muscle cells and many other cells can also protect themselves against excess cholesterol. The mechanism that has evolved for this purpose is the surface-located, high-affinity LDL receptor.[71,72] These receptors bind LDL, and the cell then internalizes the bound LDL by the process of endocytosis and transports it to lysosomes where the LDL is degraded and free cholesterol is liberated for use by the cell. If the cell is exposed to excess LDL, there is a feedback inhibitory pathway in the cell that inhibits the synthesis of LDL receptors. In addition, the presence within the cell of excess cholesterol provides a signal that inhibits cholesterol synthesis by the rate-limiting intracellular enzyme, hydroxymethylglutaryl-coenzyme A reductase (HMG-CoA reductase). (See also Chap. 53.)

Under normal circumstances, sterol balance in the cell maintains a given receptor level for LDL at the cell surface. In this way the requirements for extracellular cholesterol are met by concentrations of plasma LDL that are not atherogenic. Increased concentrations of plasma LDL may alter the endothelial barrier and bring large amounts of LDL in direct contact with the smooth-muscle cell, which may ingest much of the LDL by bulk-phase endocytosis, bypassing the high-affinity receptor mechanism and leading to increased esterification and storage of cholesterol esters and the development of foam cells. (See also Chap. 56.)

As discussed above, two laboratories[39,48] have observed that antioxidant drugs may protect hyperlipidemic rabbits by decreasing lesion formation due to decrease in oxidized LDL. The oxidized LDL may act primarily as an injurious agent in hypercholesterolemia to endothelium and is taken up by macrophages via their scavenger receptors. The elucidation of the effects of oxidized LDL may be important in understanding the basis of the atherogenic effect of hyperlipidemia.

Evidence is accumulating in favor of the notion that HDL, in contrast to LDL, is a negative factor in the development of atherosclerosis. Two mechanisms have been proposed to explain how HDL might be a deterrent against atherosclerosis. The first suggests that HDL augments the removal of cholesterol from cells such as smooth muscle. The second mechanism involves the apparent ability of HDL to influence the binding and absorption of LDL by cells such as smooth muscle. Neither of these mechanisms, however, has been shown to be responsible for control of cellular cholesterol.

In addition to metabolizing and responding to growth regulatory molecules, it has now been shown that smooth-muscle cells themselves can form PDGF A chain. Smooth-muscle cells can be induced to form PDGF-AA by other growth regulatory molecules, such as transforming growth factor β, or by the cytokines, interleukin-1 (IL-1), and tumor necrosis factor (TNF). In each case, the cells proliferate in culture due to autocrine stimulation by the PDGF-AA that the smooth-muscle cells themselves form. Thus, under appropriate stimulation, it is entirely possible that smooth-muscle cells may continue to proliferate in the artery wall if they are exposed to agents that appropriately induce them to stimulate themselves in an autocrine fashion.

The Macrophage

Macrophages are commonly found in early lesions of atherosclerosis as well as in advanced lesions like the fibrous plaque. They are probably the principal cell responsible for advanced lesion formation. In their studies of hypercholesterolemia in nonhuman primates, Faggiotto et al.[13,14] and Masuda and Ross[15,16] found that monocyte-derived macrophages were a major component of the fatty streaks in these animals and were found in abundance in fibrous plaques as well. A new observation made in those studies was the separation of endothelium over advancing lesions leading to exposure of subendothelial lipid-laden macrophages (foam cells) that sometimes became the foci for platelet adherence and formation of mural thrombi. Such cellular interactions were often found at anatomic sites (branches and bifurcations) that 1 to 2 months later were sites of advanced proliferative smooth-muscle lesions. The expansion of the macrophage-rich fatty streaks appeared to possibly predispose to rupture of endothelial junctions of overlying, thinly stretched endothelium. This established the conditions for macrophage exposure and for macrophage-platelet interactions. Macrophages could conceivably play several roles in lesion progression and possibly in regression as well. In tissue culture, macrophages have been shown to release mitogens as potent as those derived from platelets into the culture medium.[73] It has recently been shown that the mitogens formed by appropriately activated macrophages include both forms of PDGF (that is, dimers of both the A and B chains of the molecule),[74] transforming growth factor alpha,[75] transforming growth factor beta,[76] IL-1, and possibly fibroblast growth factor. Since the macrophage is the principal cell of the fatty streak and is located throughout the fibrous plaque, it would appear that it may, in fact, be the principal source of growth factors responsible for the progression of fatty streaks to fibrous plaques.

This concept is further supported by the recent observations that macrophages in all stages of atherogenesis contain reasonably large amounts of PDGF B-chain protein.[77] This discovery was made using a monoclonal antibody specific for PDGF B chain, which when used for immunohistochemistry demonstrates the presence of this protein in a Golgi, rough endoplasmic reticulum–type distribution within the cells. Furthermore, using complementary DNA probes for PDGF B chain and in situ hybridization, mRNA for PDGF-B (presumably PDGF-BB) can be shown to be present in these cells as well. Thus, the fact that both the message and the protein are present in these cells and that they have the capacity to secrete PDGF-BB in culture supports the notion that the macrophages are a principal source of this mitogen in the lesions of atherosclerosis as well. Although platelets are also a potent source of mitogens, platelet interactions may only occur under certain circumstances, whereas macrophages are always present. Thus the majority of lesions may progress due to macrophage activation. This could occur through direct secretion of growth factors by the macrophages themselves or by macrophage secretion of cytokines such as tumor necrosis factor alpha (TNFα) and IL-1. Tumor necrosis factor alpha has been shown to affect profoundly endothelial cells and to induce them to make PDGF.[78] Interleukin-1 induces smooth-muscle cells also to make PDGF. Thus macrophage activation and endothelial or smooth-muscle interactions such as those that could occur in the fatty streak may lead to oxidation of lipid (which in turn could injure endothelium) and to formation and release of cytokines that result, directly or indirectly, in smooth-muscle proliferation.

Macrophages have long been known to be largely responsible for tissue debridement. There is increasing evidence in experimental studies and in human beings[29] that some lesions of atherosclerosis are capable of regression. The potential role of the macrophage in this phenomenon remains to be elucidated.

T Lymphocytes

T lymphocytes have also been observed in all lesions during all phases of atherogenesis. Their presence suggests that some form of an immune response may play a role in the pathogenesis of the lesions. This is clearly the case in the specialized lesion of atherosclerosis that forms during cardiac transplant rejection, in which the lesion is a concentric, neointimal proliferative, macrophage- and T-cell-rich lesion. In common atherosclerosis, however, where the lesion tends to be eccentric, there are still numerous T lymphocytes present. It is not yet clear whether specific antigens induce this response and thus participate in the process of atherogenesis or the T cells are present for other reasons. Nevertheless, their presence suggests that T cell–macrophage interactions and the formation of substances that are readily synthesized by T cells, such as interferon γ, could play roles in either lesion progression or regression. Interferon γ can be a potent inhibitor of cell proliferation but can also be a potent activator of macrophages, resulting in further lesion progression. The role of T cells in the pathogenesis of atherosclerosis, particularly as they may be related to the different causative agents, remains an important, as yet unsolved area of investigation in this disease process.

Platelets

Aggregates of platelets, or mural thrombi, are commonly observed in every phase of lesion formation during atherogenesis in nonhuman primates, and similar aggregates have been observed in human lesions, as described above. Since platelets can provide a number of growth regulatory molecules and cytokines to the tissues upon their activation and release, the presence of these platelets may be important in lesion progression. This is particularly the case in a special type of neointimal smooth-muscle proliferative response that forms after balloon catheter angioplasty and also may be critical in lesion progression of advanced lesions of atherosclerosis, which characteristically develop fissures, cracks, or ulcerations, which serve as sites for mural thrombosis. If the mural thrombus is not occlusive, it could serve as a rapid means of increase in lesion size due to the organization of the thrombus by smooth-muscle cells that migrate from the lesion adjacent to the thrombus into the thrombus due to the presence of numerous growth regulatory molecules and, in particular, PDGF. (See also Chaps. 7 and 55.)

GROWTH REGULATORY MOLECULES, CYTOKINES, AND OTHER LOW MOLECULAR WEIGHT SUBSTANCES

A number of cytokines and other growth regulatory molecules have been shown to be capable of either directly or indirectly influencing smooth-muscle cell replication and connective tissue formation. For example, TGFβ is a potent inhibitor of cell replication. It also will induce secondary gene expression of PDGF A chain in smooth-muscle cells, PDGF-AA secretion, and smooth-muscle proliferation at low doses. At high doses it inhibits smooth-muscle replication. At the same time, TGFβ is probably the most potent molecule known to induce the synthesis of connective tissue molecules, such as collagen, proteoglycans, and elastic fiber proteins.

Similar to TGFβ, the cytokines, IL-1 and TNFα, also induce secondary gene expression for PDGF in smooth-muscle cells and endothelium, respectively, as noted previously. These two molecules also can have other profound effects on cells. Since they represent principal products of activated macrophages, they could play critical roles in lesion progression or regression. Finally, fibroblast growth factor (FGF) appears to be present in many cells, which can be released during cell injury. This is true for endothelium, smooth muscle, and macrophages. Thus, injury sufficient to induce increased cell permeability or, if severe enough, cell lysis and release of FGF could also be important in furthering proliferation of both the smooth-muscle cells and potentially even endothelial cells, should this occur within the tissues. Additionally, other molecules have been discovered whose functions in atherosclerosis are not clear but that may be important. An example is heparin-binding EGF-like growth factor. This molecule is as potent a mitogen for smooth muscle as is PDGF, binds to the EGF receptor, and can be formed by smooth-muscle cells or activated macrophages. Northern analysis of human atherosclerotic lesions has demonstrated the presence of this molecule. Thus, its potential role in atherogenesis is under active investigation.

Platelet-Derived Growth Factor

The PDGF is a mitogen that is stored in the alpha granule of the platelets and that has been purified to homogeneity. It consists of two highly homologous chains (A and B) of 16,000 and 14,000 molecular weight, has a molecular weight of approximately 32,000, and is a highly cationic (pI 9.8), stable, disulfide-bonded protein. This growth factor is extremely potent, as it will cause proliferation of all susceptible cells in culture at a level of 5 ng/mL of culture medium (equivalent to addition of 5 percent whole blood serum). As discussed earlier in this chapter, PDGF is the principal mitogen in whole blood serum to which cells characteristically respond by cell proliferation. Exposure of smooth muscle to this factor results in a sequence of events that includes binding of the molecule to the surface of the cells. This then causes the cell to traverse the cell cycle leading to DNA synthesis and cell multiplication.

The PDGF stimulates a number of phenomena upon exposure to smooth-muscle cells in addition to DNA synthesis. It causes increases in pinocytosis, protein synthesis, RNA synthesis, and lipid metabolism. Chait et al.[70] have observed that exposure of arterial smooth-muscle cells to this growth factor results in increased binding of LDL to the cells due to the formation of an increased number of high-affinity receptors for LDL at the cell surface. This increased binding of LDL permits the cells to utilize exogenous sources of cholesterol for cell multiplication more effectively. Habenicht et al.[69] have demonstrated that this mitogen also stimulates increased cholesterol synthesis by cells if an exogenous source of cholesterol is not available to them. Davies and Ross[79] observed that smooth-muscle cells exposed to the PDGF undergo a marked increase in the rate of endocytosis of tracer molecules. In other words, exposure to this mitogen results in an increase in a number of cellular activities, many of which are associated with cell proliferation and with new protein synthesis and therefore with connective tissue formation.[80] Thus, exposure to this factor could potentially provide the trigger that results in the initiation of all of the components of a proliferative lesion. The PDGF is clearly operative in cell culture and has recently been shown to be formed by endothelium, macrophages, and even appropriately activated smooth-muscle cells. Thus most of the cells involved in lesion development are probably involved in PDGF generation during the process of atherogenesis.[81] Formation of this growth factor, together with others elaborated by the cells, is probably dependent upon particular cellular interactions. The role of functional platelets and macrophages in inducing experimental atherosclerosis in vivo is unquestioned. The role of the PDGF in stimulating mitogenesis in cell culture is clear and is rapidly becoming clarified in vivo, particularly in view of its presence in macrophages in the lesions, as noted above. (See also Chaps. 2 and 7.)

Prostaglandins

A great deal has been learned during the past 20 years about a new category of substances, the prostaglandins, that may play critical roles in the metabolism of platelets, endothelium, and smooth muscle. All three cell types are capable of converting the fatty acid, arachidonic acid, into prostaglandin endoperoxides. Studies of these endoperoxides identified a number of unstable intermediates in the metabolic pathway of arachidonic acid that lead to the formation of two important end products: thromboxane A_2 (formed by platelets) and prostacyclin (formed by endothelium and smooth muscle). Understanding these two end products has greatly expanded our view of the role potentially played by platelets in thrombosis and by endothelium and smooth muscle in prevention of thrombosis and potentially atherosclerosis.

Arachidonic acid is derived either from linoleic acid, an essential fatty acid in the membranes of cells, or from arachidonic acid in the diet. Thromboxane A_2 is a powerful vasoconstrictor and, therefore, is capable of stimulating smooth-muscle contraction and platelet aggregation.

It has a short half-life (30 s) and breaks down spontaneously into a stable substance, thromboxane B_2. A number of inhibitors of thromboxane synthesis markedly reduce platelet aggregation. These include aspirin and indomethacin.[82,83]

Prostacyclin is the principal product of cyclooxygenase activity in the walls of arteries and veins. Endothelium and smooth muscle synthesize PGI_2 from arachidonic acid and may also be able to synthesize this prostaglandin derivative from endoperoxides released from platelets. Prostacyclin is also unstable and is an extremely potent vasodilator as well as an inhibitor of platelet aggregation.

It is possible that an imbalance in the relative amounts of thromboxane A_2 versus PGI_2 may provide part of the explanation of the involvement of platelets in cardiovascular diseases. Since platelets contain thromboxane synthetase, the enzyme responsible for synthesis of thromboxane A_2, and since inhibition of the activity of this enzyme does not interfere with cyclooxygenase activity, it has been speculated that platelets could potentially donate endoperoxides to endothelial cells that then use them as substrates for PGI_2 production. Therefore, specific inhibitors of thromboxane synthesis are being developed that would not affect PGI_2 production by cells of the blood vessel wall.

Prostaglandin biosynthesis may be important not only in thrombosis (in terms of platelet adherence and aggregation) but also in prevention of atherogenesis (by formation of PGI_2). This has led to speculation that alterations in the contents of fatty acids in the diet might offer some protection against the development of atherosclerosis. Populations that consume diets principally composed of marine animals often replace arachidonic acid, the normal substrate for prostaglandin synthesis, with eicosapentaenoic acid. This fatty acid is not completely metabolized by platelets and, instead, produces a relatively inert form of thromboxane, thromboxane A_3. Eicosapentaenoic acid appears to inhibit the capacity of platelets to metabolize arachidonic acid. When eicosapentaenoic acid is exposed to cells of the blood vessel, they will form an analogue of prostacyclin, PGI_3, which appears to be as effective as PGI_2 in preventing platelet aggregation and in inducing vasodilatation. Thus, further studies of the role of this fatty acid derived from marine animals could have implications for individuals who consume a marine diet in terms of being protected against atherogenesis. Clearly, there is much to be learned in prostaglandin metabolism before the agents that have thus far been discovered, and those that are yet undiscovered, can be understood, both in atherogenesis and in protection against this disease process. (See also Chaps. 53 and 62.)

REFERENCES

1. Ross R, Glomset JA: The pathogenesis of atherosclerosis. *N Engl J Med* 1976; 295:420–425.
2. McGill HC Jr: Atherosclerosis: Problems in pathogenesis. *Atherosclerosis Rev* 1977; 2:27–65.
3. Bierman EL, Ross R: Aging and atherosclerosis. *Atherosclerosis Rev* 1977; 2:79–111.
4. Geer JC, Haust MD: Smooth muscle cells in atherosclerosis. *Monogr Atherosclerosis* 1972; 2:1–88.
5. *Arteriosclerosis: A Report by the National Heart and Lung Institute Task Force on Arteriosclerosis*, vol. 2 DHEW pub. (NIH) 72–219, 1971: 1–365.
6. Debakey ME: Patterns of atherosclerosis and rates of progression. *Atherosclerosis Rev* 1976; 3:1–56.
7. Stemerman MB, Ross R: Experimental arteriosclerosis. I. Fibrous plaque formation in primates, an electron microscope study. *J Exp Med* 1972; 136:769–789.
8. Bjorkerud S, Bondjers G: Arterial repair and atherosclerosis after mechanical injury: I. Permeability and light microscopic characteristics of endothelium in non-atherosclerotic and atherosclerotic lesions. *Atherosclerosis* 1971; 13:355–363.
9. Ross R, Harker LA: Hyperlipidemia and atherosclerosis. *Science* 1976; 193:1094–1100.
10. Harker LA, Ross R, Slichter SJ, Scott CR: Homocystine-induced arteriosclerosis: The role of endothelial cell injury and platelet response in its genesis. *J Clin Invest* 1976; 58:731–741.
11. Minick CR, Murphy GE: Experimental induction of atheroarteriosclerosis by the synergy of allergic injury to arteries and lipid-rich diet. II. Effect of repeated injections of horse serum in rabbits fed a lipid-rich, cholesterol-poor diet. *Am J Pathol* 1973; 73:265–300.
12. Fabricant CG, Fabricant J, Litrenta MM, Minick CR: Virus-induced atherosclerosis. *J Exp Med* 1978; 48:335–340.
13. Faggiotto A, Ross R, Harker L: Studies of hypercholesterolemia in the nonhuman primate. I. Changes that lead to fatty streak formation. *Arteriosclerosis* 1984; 4:323–340.
14. Faggiotto A, Ross R: Studies of hypercholesterolemia in the nonhuman primate. II. Fatty streak conversion to fibrous plaque. *Arteriosclerosis* 1984; 4:341–356.
15. Masuda J, Ross R: Atherogenesis during low-level hypercholesterolemia in the nonhuman primate. I. Fatty streak formation. *Arteriosclerosis* 1990; 10:164–177.
16. Masuda J, Ross R: Atherogenesis during low-level hypercholesterolemia in the nonhuman primate. II. Fatty streak conversion to fibrous plaque. *Arteriosclerosis* 1990; 10:178–187.
17. Rosenfeld ME, Tsukada T, Gown AM, Ross R: Fatty streak initiation in Watanabe heritable hyperlipemic and comparably hypercholesterolemic fat-fed rabbits. *Arteriosclerosis* 1987; 7:9–23.
18. Rosenfeld ME, Tsukada T, Chait A, Bierman EL, Gown AM, Ross R: Fatty streak expansion and maturation in Watanabe heritable hyperlipemic and comparably hypercholesterolemic fat-fed rabbits. *Arteriosclerosis* 1987; 7:24–34.
19. Davies MJ, Woolf N, Rowles PM, Pepper J: Morphology of the endothelium over atherosclerotic plaques in human coronary arteries. *Br Heart J* 1988; 60:459–464.
20. Long ER: The development of our knowledge of arteriosclerosis. In: EV Cowdry (ed): *Arteriosclerosis. A Survey of the Problem.* New York, Macmillan, 1933: 19–52.
21. Virchow R: *Gesammelte Adhandlungen zur Wissenschaftlichen Medicin.* Frankfurt-am-Main, Meidinger Sohn and Company, 1856:458–636.
22. Anitschkow NN: A history of experimentation on arterial atherosclerosis in animals. In: HT Blumenthal (ed): *Cowdry's Arteriosclerosis*, 2d ed. Springfield, CC Thomas, 1967: 21–44.
23. Duguid JB: Thrombosis as a factor in the pathogenesis of coronary atherosclerosis. *J Pathol Bacteriol* 1946: 58:207–212.
24. French JE: Atherosclerosis in relation to the structure and function of the arterial intima, with special reference to the endothelium. *Int Rev Exp Pathol* 1966; 5:253–353.
25. Ross R, Glomset JA: Atherosclerosis and the arterial smooth muscle cell. *Science* 1973; 180:1332–1339.
26. Ross R: The pathogenesis of atherosclerosis—an update. *N Engl J Med* 1986; 314:488–500.
27. Fry DL: Hemodynamic forces in atherogenesis. In: P Scheinberg (ed): *Cerebrovascular Diseases, Tenth Princeton Conference.* New York, Raven, 1976: 77–95.
28. Moncada S, Higgs EA, Vane JR: Human arterial and venous tissue generate prostacyclin (prostaglandin x), a potent inhibitor of platelet aggregation. *Lancet* 1977; 2:18–20.
29. Wissler RW, Vesselinovitch D: Studies of regression of advanced atherosclerosis in experimental animals and man. *Ann NY Acad Sci* 1976; 275:363–378.
30. Blankenhorn DH, Nessim SA, Johnson RL, Sanmarco ME, Azen SP, Cashin-Hemphill L: Beneficial effects of combined colestipol-

niacin therapy on coronary atherosclerosis and coronary venous bypass grafts. *JAMA* 1987; 257:3233–3240.

31. Ross R, Glomset JA, Kariya B, Harker L: A platelet-dependent serum factor that stimulates the proliferation of arterial smooth muscle cells in vitro. *Proc Natl Acad Sci USA* 1974; 71:1207–1210.
32. Benditt EP, Benditt JM: Evidence for a monoclonal origin of human atherosclerotic plaques. *Proc Natl Acad Sci USA* 1973; 70:1753–1756.
33. Linder D, Gartler SM: Glucose-6-phosphate dehydrogenase mosaicism: Utilization as a cell marker in the study of leiomyomas. *Science* 1965; 150:67–69.
34. Fialkow PJ: The origin and development of human tumors studied with cell markers. *N Engl J Med* 1974; 291:26–35.
35. Pearson TA, Wang A, Solez K, Heptinstall RH: Clonal characteristics of fibrous plaques and fatty streaks from human aortas. *Am J Pathol* 1975; 81:379–387.
36. Thomas WA, Reiner JM, Janakidevi K, Florentin RA, Lee KT: Population dynamics of arterial cells during atherogenesis: X. Study of monotypism in atherosclerotic lesions of black women heterozygous for glucose-6-phosphate dehydrogenase. *Exp Mol Pathol* 1979; 31:367–386.
37. Benditt EP: The monoclonal theory of atherogenesis. *Atherosclerosis Rev* 1978; 3:77–85.
38. Geer JC, McGill HC Jr, Strong JP: The fine structure of human atherosclerotic lesions. *Am J Pathol* 1961; 38:263–287.
39. Wissler RW: Interaction of low-density lipoproteins from hypercholesterolemic serum with arterial wall cells and their extracellular products in atherogenesis and regression. *Biochem Atherosclerosis* 1979; 7:345–368.
40. Carew TE, Schwenke DC, Steinberg D: Antiatherogenic effect of probucol unrelated to its hypocholesterolemic effect: Evidence that antioxidants in vivo can selectively inhibit low density lipoprotein degradation in macrophage-rich fatty streaks and slow the progression of atherosclerosis in the Watanabe heritable hyperlipidemic rabbit. *Proc Natl Acad Sci USA* 1987; 84:7725–7729.
41. McGill HC Jr: Risk factors for atherosclerosis. *Adv Exp Med Biol* 1978; 104:273–280.
42. Lipid Research Clinics Program, Lipid Metabolism-Atherogenesis Branch, National Heart, Lung, and Blood Institute: The lipid research clinics coronary primary prevention trial results. I. Reduction in incidence of coronary heart disease. *JAMA* 1984; 251:351–364.
43. Lipid Research Clinics Program, Lipid Metabolism-Atherogenesis Branch, National Heart, Lung, and Blood Institute: The lipid research clinics coronary primary prevention trial results. II. The relationship of reduction in incidence of coronary heart disease to cholesterol lowering. *JAMA* 1984; 251:365–374.
44. Brown BG, Albers JJ, Fisher LD, Schaefer FM, Lin J-T, Kaplan C: Regression of coronary artery disease as a result of intensive lipid-lowering therapy in men with high levels of apolipoprotein B. *N Engl J Med* 1990; 323:1289–1298.
45. National Cholesterol Education Program: Report of the National Cholesterol Education Program Expert Panel on detection, evaluation and treatment of high blood cholesterol in adults. *Arch Intern Med* 1988; 148:36–69.
46. Grundy SM: Dietary fats and sterols. In: R Levy, B Rifkind, B Dennis, N Ernst (eds): *Nutrition, Lipids, and Coronary Heart Disease.* New York, Raven, 1979: 89–118.
47. McGill HC Jr: The relationship of dietary cholesterol to serum cholesterol concentration and to atherosclerosis in man. *Am J Clin Nutr* 1979; 32(suppl):2664–2702.
48. Kita T, Nagano Y, Yokode M, Ishii K, Kume H, Ooshima A: Probucol prevents the progression of atherosclerosis in Watanabe heritable hyperlipidemic rabbit, an animal model for familial hypercholesterolemia. *Proc Natl Acad Sci USA* 1987; 84:5928–5931.
49. Steinberg D: Antioxidants and atherosclerosis: A current assessment. *Circ* 1991; 84:1420–1425.
50. Becker CG, Dubin T, Wiedemann HP: Hypersensitivity to tobacco antigen. *Proc Natl Acad Sci USA* 1976; 73:1712–1716.
51. Simionescu N, Simionescu M, Palade GE: Permeability of muscle capillaries to small heme-peptides: Evidence for the existence of patent transendothelial channels. *J Cell Biol* 1975; 64:586–607.
52. Renkin EM: Multiple pathways of capillary permeability. *Circ Res* 1977; 41:735–743.
53. Stein Y, Stein O: Interaction between serum lipoproteins and cellular components of the arterial wall. *Biochem Atherosclerosis* 1979; 7:313–344.
54. Gimbrone MA Jr: Culture of vascular endothelium. *Prog Hemost Thromb* 1976; 3:1–28.
55. Jaffe EA, Nachman RL, Becker CG, Minick CR: Culture of human endothelial cells derived from umbilical veins: Identification by morphologic and immunologic criteria. *J Clin Invest* 1973; 52:2745–2756.
56. Jaffe EA, Adelman B, Minick CR: Synthesis of basement membrane by cultured human endothelial cells. *Circulation* 1975; 51(suppl 1):11.
57. Jaffe EA, Hoyer LW, Nachman RL: Synthesis of antihemophilic factor by antigen cultured human endothelial cells. *J Clin Invest* 1973; 52:2757–2764.
58. Gimbrone MA Jr, Alexander RW: Angiotensin II stimulation of prostaglandin production in cultured human vascular endothelium. *Science* 1975; 189:219.
59. Gajdusek C, DiCorleto P, Ross R, Schwartz SM: An endothelial cell derived growth factor. *J Cell Biol* 1980; 85:467–472.
60. DiCorleto PE, Bowen-Pope DF: Cultured endothelial cells produce a platelet-derived growth factor–like protein. *Proc Natl Acad Sci USA* 1983; 80:1919–1923.
61. Wilcox JN, Smith KM, Williams LT, Schwartz SM, Gordon D: Platelet-derived growth factor mRNA detection in human atherosclerotic plaques by in situ hybridization. *J Clin Invest* 1988; 82:1134–1143.
62. Ross R, Kariya B: Morphogenesis of vascular smooth muscle in atherosclerosis and cell culture. In: DF Bohr, AP Somlyo, HV Sparks (eds): *Handbook of Physiology—The Cardiovascular System II: Circulation, Vascular Smooth Muscle.* Bethesda, American Physiological Society, 1980: 69–91.
63. Chamley-Campbell J, Campbell GR, Ross R: The smooth muscle cell in culture. *Physiol Rev* 1979; 59:1–61.
64. Kohler N, Lipton A: Platelets as a source of fibroblast growth-promoting activity. *Exp Cell Res* 1974; 87:297–301.
65. Heldin C-H, Wasteson Å, Westermark B: Partial purification and characterization of platelet factors stimulating the multiplication of normal human glial cells. *Exp Cell Res* 1977; 109:429–437.
66. Moore S, Friedman RJ, Singal DP, Gauldie MA, Blajchman MA, Roberts RS: Inhibition of injury induced thromboatherosclerotic lesions by anti-platelet serum in rabbits. *Thromb Haemostasis* 1976; 35:70–81.
67. Friedman RJ, Stemerman MB, Wenz B, Moore S, Gauldie J, Gent M: The effect of thrombocytopenia on experimental atherosclerotic lesion formation in rabbits. Smooth muscle cell proliferation and re-endothelialization. *J Clin Invest* 1977; 60:1191–1201.
68. Fuster V, Bowie EJW, Lewis JC, Fass DN, Owen CA Jr, Brown AL: Resistance to arteriosclerosis in pigs with von Willebrand's disease. Spontaneous and high cholesterol diet-induced arteriosclerosis. *J Clin Invest* 1978; 61:722–730.
69. Habenicht AJR, Glomset JA, Ross R: Relation of cholesterol and mevalonic acid to the cell cycle in smooth muscle and Swiss 3T3 cells stimulated to divide by platelet-derived growth factor. *J Biol Chem* 1980; 255:5134–5140.
70. Chait A, Ross R, Albers JJ, Bierman EL: Platelet-derived growth factor stimulates activity of low density lipoprotein receptors. *Proc Natl Acad Sci USA* 1980; 77:4084–4088.
71. Brown MS, Faust JR, Goldstein JL: Role of the low density lipoprotein receptor in regulating the content of free and esterified cholesterol in human fibroblasts. *J Clin Invest* 1975; 55:783–793.
72. Goldstein JL, Brown MS: The low-density lipoprotein pathway and its relation to atherosclerosis. *Annu Rev Biochem* 1977; 46:897–930.
73. Leibovich SJ, Ross R: A macrophage-dependent factor that stimulates the proliferation of fibroblasts in vitro. *Am J Pathol* 1976; 84:501–513.
74. Shimokado K, Raines EW, Madtes DK, Barrett TB, Benditt EP, Ross R: A significant part of macrophage-derived growth factor consists of at least two forms of PDGF. *Cell* 1985; 43:277–286.
75. Madtes DK, Raines EW, Sakariassen KS, Assoian RK, Sporn MB, Bell GI, Ross R: Induction of transforming growth factor-alpha in activated human alveolar macrophages. *Cell* 1988; 53:285–293.
76. Assoian RK, Fleurdelys BE, Stevenson HC, Miller PJ, Madtes DK, Raines EW: Expression and secretion of type β transforming growth factor by activated human macrophages. *Proc Natl Acad Sci USA* 1987; 84:6020–6024.

77. Ross R, Masuda J, Raines EW, Gown AM, Katsuda S, Sasahara M: Localization of PDGF-B protein in macrophages in all phases of atherogenesis. *Science* 1990; 248:1009–1012.
78. Hajjar KA, Hajjar DP, Silverstein RL, Nachman RL: Tumor necrosis factor–mediated release of platelet-derived growth factor from cultured endothelial cells. *J Exp Med* 1987; 166:235–245.
79. Davies PF, Ross R: Mediation of pinocytosis in cultured arterial smooth muscle and endothelial cells by platelet-derived growth factor. *J Cell Biol* 1978; 79:663–671.
80. Burke JM, Ross R: Synthesis of connective tissue macromolecules by smooth muscle. *Int Rev Connect Tissue Res* 1979; 8:119–157.
81. Ross R: Platelet-derived growth factor. *Annu Rev Med* 1987; 38:71–79.
82. Moncada S, Vane JR: Arachidonic acid metabolites and the interactions between platelets and blood-vessel walls. *N Engl J Med* 1979; 300:1142–1147.
83. Moncada S, Vane JR: Mode of action of aspirin-like drugs. *Adv Intern Med* 1979; 24:1–22.

Chapter 55

The Pathology of Coronary Atherosclerosis

Michael J. Davies, M.D.

Consideration of the mechanisms by which atherosclerosis produces clinical symptoms must begin with a basic definition of the disease.

Atherosclerosis is a disease of medium and large arteries; the aorta and cerebral and epicardial coronary arteries are prime targets while small arteries, such as those within the myocardium, are spared. Atherosclerosis is a focal *intimal* disease. The focal nature of the disease is highlighted by the term *plaque*, used first by pathologists who observed elevated oval lesions up to 1 cm in length dotted over the intimal surface of an aorta opened longitudinally and viewed "enface" in the autopsy room. In medium-sized arteries such as the coronary vessels the focal nature of plaque is also expressed by only part of the circumference of the vessel wall being involved, thus retaining an arc of normal vessel wall.

Plaque is in part made up of collagen with other connective tissue components such as elastin and glycosoaminoglycans, all being produced by smooth-muscle cells acting in their synthetic phenotype. Another major component of plaque by volume is lipid, either contained within foam cells, predominantly of monocyte/macrophage origin, or lying free within the intima as crystalline cholesterol esters.

An additional process complicates atherosclerosis but is not part of the basic disease. The *media* behind plaques shows a striking atrophy with loss of smooth-muscle cells, and thus the artery dilates. Even before this final phase, remodeling of the media occurs, tending to enlarge the vessel to accommodate the plaque and thus to preserve the dimensions of the lumen.[1] The ultimate production of segmental stenosis occurs only when smooth-muscle proliferation within the intimal plaque itself exceeds the remodeling capacity of smooth-muscle cells in the media.

Plaques must not be regarded as static. Plaques are the site of a complex interreaction between smooth-muscle cells, T lymphocytes, macrophages, and monocytes involving inflammatory mediators, cytokines, and growth factors analogous in many ways to the synovial membranes in rheumatoid arthritis.[2] Like rheumatoid joints plaques may have active or more quiescent phases and can finally become a relatively inert mass of collagen.

A paradox is presented by the fact that plaques contain a large amount of plasma-derived lipid and a florid inflammatory response involving predominantly the monocyte/macrophage while native plasma low-density lipoproteins (LDLs) move freely in and out of the intima and are inert with regard to the monocyte. Once oxidized within the intima, however, LDL becomes a monocyte chemoattractant factor and is avidly taken up via the scavenger receptor of macrophages. This receptor is not down regulated, and the massive accumulation of intracellular lipid that ensues leads to foam cell formation. Oxidized lipids are activators of monocytes as well as being cytotoxic and are now believed to be a major factor in plaque progression.[3] The development of atherosclerosis is therefore seen not only as a consequence of plasma lipids entering the vessel wall in large amounts but also as a consequence of oxidation and retention of lipid within the intima by macrophages.

Epidemiologic studies of necropsy material[4,5] show

that in any particular geographic or ethnic population the mean number of plaques present in the coronary arteries is a predictor of the risk of expressed coronary heart disease in that population. Moreover subjects with hypertension or diabetes, who smoke, or who have high plasma lipid levels have more plaques than individuals without these factors.[6,7] Thus the overall total number of atherosclerotic plaques in populations or in an individual is a measure of the risk of clinical symptoms developing. This does not, however, preclude the unlucky individual who develops a thrombus over a lone plaque in a key position, such as the main left coronary artery, and dies.

CORONARY ATHEROSCLEROSIS IN RELATION TO CLINICAL SYMPTOMS

The clinical features of coronary atherosclerosis cover a wide spectrum. On one hand there are patients with chronic exertional angina, while on the other hand patients experience the sudden onset of unstable angina or acute infarction. The distinction is however less clear-cut than perceived a decade ago. Patients with chronic exertional angina or a healed myocardial infarct may develop episodic silent attacks of transient acute ischemia unrelated to an increase in myocardial oxygen demand. Some patients with atherosclerosis have ischemia related to demonstrable epicardial coronary artery spasm. All these phenomena relate to one or more of three pathophysiological subsets (Fig. 55-1). First, the stable plaque, by virtue of its volume, encroaches sufficiently on the lumen of epicardial coronary arteries to be flow limiting when myocardial oxygen demand rises. Second, there is a plaque that is suddenly complicated by a thrombus that protrudes into the lumen, and finally atherosclerotic vessels have abnormalities of tone leading to inappropriate vasoconstriction.

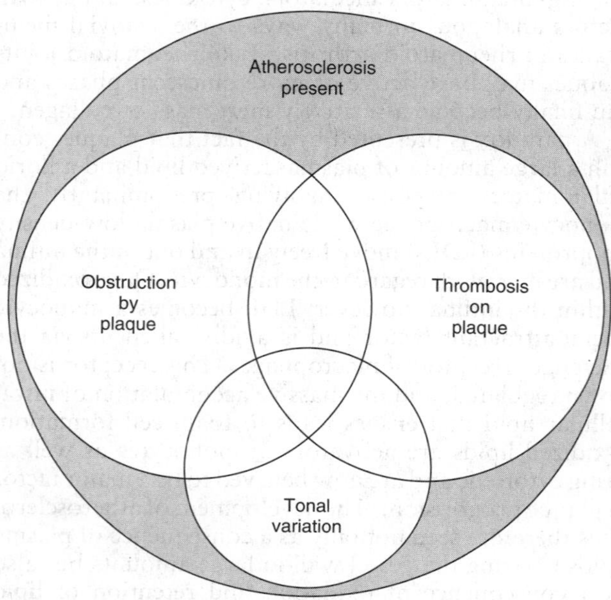

FIGURE 55-1 Interrelation of the three vascular mechanisms causing acute myocardial ischemia.

It is conceptually helpful to consider stable angina, coronary thrombosis, and vasomotor tonal abnormalities separately, bearing in mind that they overlap in terms of their clinical symptoms.

STABLE ANGINA

Clinical and necropsy studies[8,9] both show that the majority of patients with stable exertional angina have one or more coronary artery segments with stenosis in excess of 50 percent by diameter. The majority of these patients have a range of angiographic lesions varying in severity from a slight irregularity of the lumen through increasing degrees of narrowing up to chronic total occlusion.

Clinical angiographic studies in living individuals report less stenoses in terms of the relative proportions of single-, double-, and triple-vessel disease than necropsy studies. In part this reflects the inevitable selection of necropsy series toward end-stage disease. In part, however, it reflects the relative insensitivity of clinical angiography in demonstrating atherosclerosis.

Morphologic Characteristics of Stable Coronary Stenoses

Cross sections of the arterial wall and lumen in coronary arteries that have been distended at physiological pressures show that stenoses of between 20 and 70 percent by diameter have combinations of two sets of variables. The plaque may be eccentric with regard to the lumen occupying only a segment of the circumference of the vessel wall or be circumferential. Eccentric stenoses (Figs. 55-2 and 55-3), which have retained an arc of normal vessel wall opposite the plaque, have the potential for tonal variations in medial muscle to alter both the shape and cross-sectional area of the lumen. Concentric stenoses are more likely to be fixed owing to the splinting

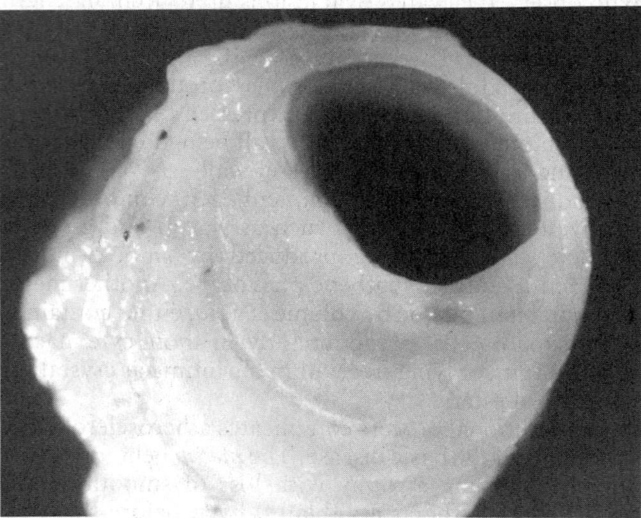

FIGURE 55-2 Eccentric human coronary artery plaque with displacement of the lumen from the midline of the vessel and retention of an arc of normal vessel wall.

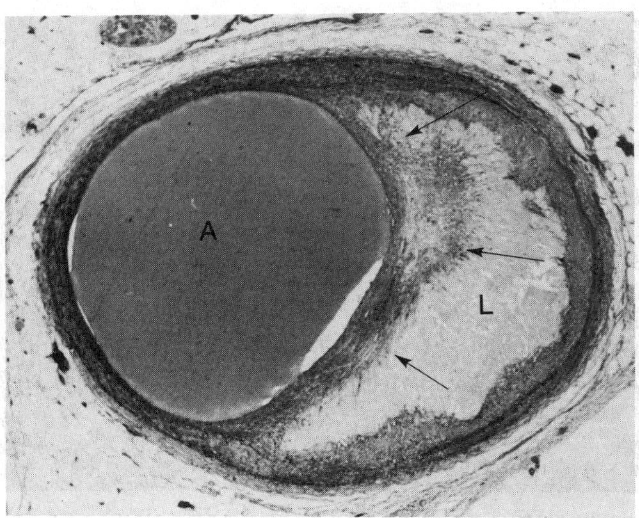

FIGURE 55-3 Histological cross section of human coronary artery plaque. The lumen contains residual barium from postmortem angiography (A). Stenosis is caused by a large atherosclerotic plaque with a core of lipid (L) separated from the lumen by a cap of fibrous tissue (arrows). Opposite the plaque there is a normal thin-walled segment of artery wall.

effect of the diffuse intimal thickening. The arc of retained normal vessel wall in eccentric lesions can occupy up to 70 percent of the vessel circumference; this arc tends to be smaller with higher grades of stenosis. Theoretical calculations suggested that with a fixed element of stenosis of more than 75 percent by cross-sectional area due to the plaque volume itself, combined with an arc of normal media of more than 60°, tonal variations in the physiological range will alter flow significantly.[10] Hypercontraction of the medial segment, i.e., spasm, would have more striking effects on flow. There is conflicting evidence in the literature of the frequency of eccentric stenoses that have the potential for variation of lumen cross-sectional area. One necropsy study of 54 patients who had stable angina[9] put the figure at 24 percent of all high-grade lesions (>50 percent diameter) and found that 56 percent of the patients had at least one high-grade stenosis that was potentially variable. Other series that included surgical and acute infarction deaths record a far higher proportion of up to 70 percent of stenoses to be eccentric.[11-13] The variation reflects both different patient selection and different morphologic definitions of what is a variable stenosis; but from the clinical context the important facts are that patients with stable angina differ in the type of lesions present, but many patients with stable angina will have at least one variable stenosis in series with a fixed stenosis. Clinical studies confirm that the diameter of the lumen over eccentric stenoses can be varied by pharmacologic means.[14] In this context it must be appreciated that the lumen at points of high-grade stenosis may be displaced from the center point of the original lumen and appear eccentric on angiography without there being a retained arc of normal media; thus not all lesions that are eccentric on angiography would be expected to vary.

The second major element of coronary plaques causing stenosis that differs between lesions is the relative proportion of lipid and connective tissue. At one extreme there are "soft" plaques with between 40 and 70 percent of their volume made up of extracellular cholesterol. At the other extreme are "hard" plaques with less than 10 percent by volume of extracellular cholesterol. Plaques that have a significant proportion of extracellular lipid have the highest risk of subsequent thrombosis.

Lipid-rich plaques have a very characteristic microanatomy (Figs. 55-3 and 55-4) in arteries that have been distended at physiological pressures. The lumen is rounded in shape although reduced in dimensions as compared to adjacent normal segments. The plaque is convex with regard to the adventitia, i.e., it bulges outward rather than inward. Extracellular lipid (much of it in a crystalline form) makes up the core of the plaque. In this lipid core collagen is often sparse; thus in many plaques the lipid occupies a potential space within the intima. At necropsy or at operation the lipid of the central core can be felt to be soft, like toothpaste, and is easily deformed. The physiochemical properties of the lipid core suggest it is in fact semifluid at body tempera-

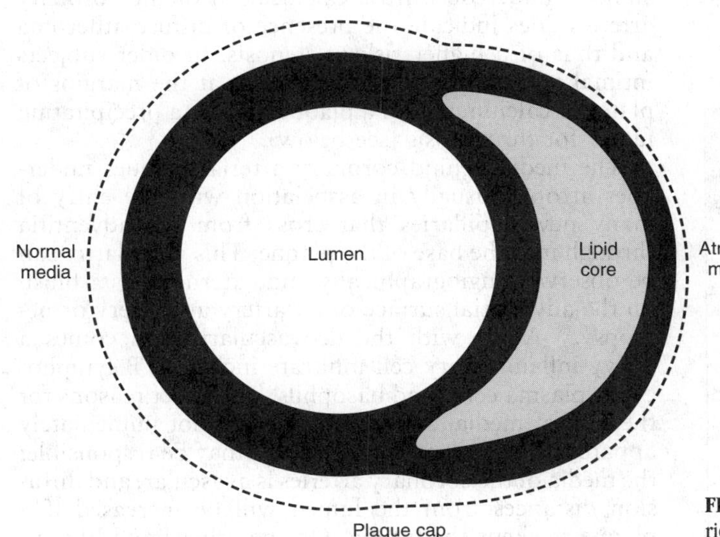

FIGURE 55-4 Diagrammatic representation of the microanatomy of a lipid-rich coronary plaque.

ture.[15] The plaque core is highly thrombogenic because it contains lamellar lipid, fragments of collagen, and Tissue Factor.[16] Fortunately this thrombogenic core is separated from the lumen of the artery by the fibromuscular cap of the plaque, itself covered in turn by a monolayer of endothelial cells. The mechanical strength of the fibrous cap is dependent on the presence of high concentration of collagen and elastin produced by smooth-muscle cells. The macrophage/foam cells within the plaque are concentrated around the margins of the lipid pool while the smooth-muscle cells predominantly occupy the base, shoulder areas, and cap of the plaque.

The relative proportions of extracellular lipid, smooth-muscle cells, macrophages, and collagen vary widely from plaque to plaque even within one individual coronary artery. This variation, illustrated in Table 55-1, is the rule rather than the exception. The plaques of some individuals, however, contain virtually no extracellular lipid and vice versa.[9]

On the basis of the two variables of eccentric versus concentric and lipid-rich versus fibrous, it is possible to make a classification of plaque as concentric fibrous, concentric lipid rich, eccentric fibrous, and eccentric lipid rich. Such a scheme has two limitations. First it applies to lesions over the middle range of stenoses; very high grade lesions have additional characteristics. Second the variables themselves cover a wide range. The arbitrary cutoff point of, for example, what is called lipid rich could be made at any percentage by volume between 30 and 50 percent.

Higher Grade Stenoses: Morphology of Coronary Lesions

Stenoses in excess of 70 percent by diameter are more complex in structure than those of lesser degree. The proportion of collagen is far higher, and that of lipid is a less striking feature. The plaques are often complex with several layers of fibrous tissue superimposed on each other; the lumen is often represented by two more channels. All these appearances and in particular a multichannel lumen (Fig. 55-5) are suggestive that recanalization of previous episodes of thrombosis has occurred. The presence of such recanalized segments in necropsy studies is by no means confined to arteries supplying scars of previous infarction. In one study of necropsy material 62.5 percent of subjects with stable angina in life without infarct scars had recanalized segments of coronary artery.[9]

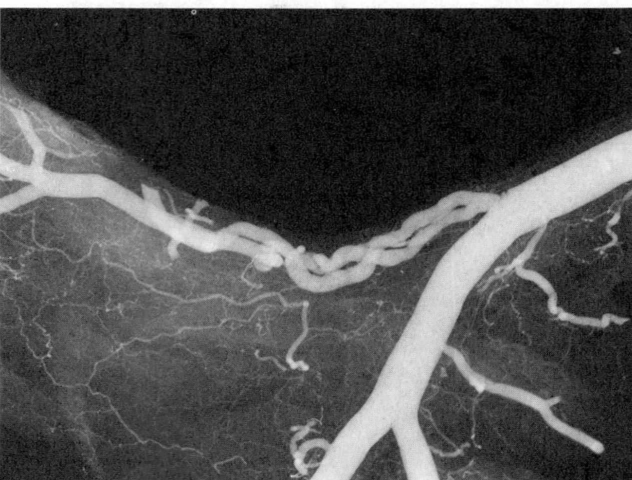

FIGURE 55-5 Angiographic appearance of a multichanneled lumen characteristic of recanalization by new vessels within the original lumen after an episode of occlusive thrombus.

TABLE 55-1

Volume Composition of Eight Human Coronary Artery Plaques Causing Stenosis between 20 and 50% by Diameter in One Individual

Plaque No.	Percentage of Lipid	Percentage of Collagen
A	2.6	72.5
B	5.6	76.1
C	6.9	71.2
D	10.5	60.6
E	20.8	52.2
F	32.6	48.6
G	44.5	41.0
H	54.3	33.5

Secondary Complications of Atherosclerosis

A number of processes complicate the process of atherosclerosis in advanced plaques without directly contributing to clinical symptoms. Calcification develops as a dystrophic process at two sites. It may occur either as nodular masses within the lipid pool or as irregular plates within the dense collagen of advanced plaques. Calcification has no direct relation to stenosis and does not contribute to an increase in plaque volume because it is laid down within preexisting tissue components. In clinical terms calcification is age related and is thus widely prevalent in the coronary arteries of subjects over 70 years of age irrespective of the degree of stenosis.[17] In subjects under 60 diffuse calcification of the coronary arteries does indicate the presence of diffuse atheroma and thus of a higher risk of stenosis. In older subjects intimal tearing due to shear stresses at the margins of plates of calcium within a plaque may be a precipitating factor for thrombosis (see below).

The media behind coronary arterial plaques undergoes atrophy usually in association with the entry of many new capillaries that cross from the adventitia through into the base of the plaque. This vascularity can be observed angiographically and externally as a blush on the adventitial surface of an artery at surgery or necropsy.[18] Along with the neovascularization comes a heavy inflammatory cell infiltrate including B lymphocytes, plasma cells, and basophils. The exact reasons for the loss of medial smooth muscle are not immediately apparent. On the one hand hypoxia may be responsible; the media of the coronary arteries is avascular, and diffusion distances from the lumen will be increased if a plaque thickens the intima. On the other hand, the inflammatory process in the adventitia may be cytotoxic for the smooth-muscle cells. Media smooth-muscle loss is the mechanism by which coronary arteries become ectatic, particularly in old age.

Angiographic Assessment of Coronary Atherosclerosis in Stable Angina

Current clinical practice uses angiography primarily to demonstrate segmental stenoses and to estimate indirectly the physiological significance of such stenoses, but a secondary purpose is to assess the overall amount of wall disease present and to follow progression or regression. Comparison of successive angiograms for the appearances of "new" lesions has become a tool in following the natural history and response to antiatherogenic drugs. The serious limitations of the angiogram, which is no more than an outline of lumen, with regard to these objectives should be realized.

The localized medial atrophy that develops behind eccentric plaques allows the plaque to bulge outward rather than inward. In extreme cases the internal elastic lamina is ruptured and the plaque virtually extruded from the vessel. Thus an angiographically normal artery can harbor large plaques. Apart from this localized medial response, a general remodeling of the whole artery occurs in atherosclerosis. This response is such that the intimal mass can be increased by up to 40 percent of the original volume before any encroachment on the lumen develops.[19] This process leads to an increase in the external dimensions of the artery with an increase in wall thickness that cannot be appreciated from the angiogram. In this context estimation of plaque volume from an angiogram is as relevant as measuring the mass of an iceberg from what is above the surface. "New" angiographic lesions, i.e., 10 to 20 percent stenoses appearing in the interval between two successive examinations, are not new in terms of plaque inception but indicate accelerated growth in an already established plaque.

Errors Introduced by Reference Segment Comparison

The conventional method of measuring stenosis compares the diameter of the test segment with an adjacent external reference segment adjudged to be normal. The method is dependent on the reference segment being normal; it may in fact be diffusely narrowed or more commonly dilated, introducing errors.[20,21] Computer construction of a predicated taper to the vessel over several centimeters improves the measurement unless there is very diffuse disease present.

Pathologists who measure stenosis in histological sections adopt an internal reference using the area of the vessel wall within the internal elastic lamina. Because of the overall dilatation, this is an exaggerated dimension leading to an overcall on the degree of stenosis. Despite all these caveats, once stenoses are over 50 percent by diameter (75 percent by cross-sectional area), correlation of angiographic studies in life, flow measurements, and necropsy studies improves and becomes largely concordant.

Errors Induced by Lumen Shape

Normal vessels have a round lumen that is independent of filling pressure; in abnormal vessels this is not so. The crescentic and slit-shaped lumens illustrated in pathology texts are largely artifacts of examining empty vessels, but the lumen in atherosclerotic arteries does deviate from being circular.[22] In vitro studies show that atherosclerotic arteries perfused at pressure around 100 mgHg have D-shaped or oval lumens in relation to some plaques.[20] Elevation of the filling pressure to 200 mgHg does not significantly alter these findings. The deviation from a circular shape occurs particularly over eccentric hard plaques that retain a straight edge, while the normal segment of vessel wall adopts a circular profile. Two plaques on opposing sides of the vessel give an oval lumen. These noncircular lumens are likely to occur in life and may be altered in shape by tone in the normal segments, thus deviating further from a circular profile. Such stenoses require examination in exactly the same plane and degree of medial tone if they are to be compared in sequential angiograms.

Endothelial Status over Stable Human Coronary Plaques

In animal models of atherosclerosis, whether in the rabbit, pig, or primate, the clear message emerges that the integrity of the endothelial surface is maintained during plaque initiation, but once raised plaques are formed, a secondary phenomenon of endothelial denudation occurs, exposing the underlying intima.[23,24] The implication is that platelet interaction with the collagen beneath the endothelium cannot be an initiating factor for a plaque but may enhance the growth of already established plaques. This does not imply that the endothelium in early atherosclerotic lesions is functionally normal and indeed ample evidence exists for the abnormal endothelial expression of adhesion molecules for monocytes over very early plaques[25] but that the endothelial "barrier" function of keeping the platelet away from collagen and tissue factor is still preserved. Studies of the endothelial surface of human atherosclerotic arteries by scanning electron microscopy indicate that the same is true in humans.[26] The endothelial cells over all forms of plaques in human coronary arteries are irreguarly arranged, vary in shape and size, as well as show evidence of monocyte adhesion and migration. Simple fatty streaks, regarded as the earliest lesions of atherosclerosis, have an intact endothelial surface, but more advanced plaques show endothelial denudation injury. This injury ranges from loss of single endothelial cells (Fig. 55-6) to larger areas of denudation that expose the underlying connective tissue over which a monolayer of platelets forms. Denudation injury is more directly associated with heavy concentrations of monocytes in the intima rather than the size of the plaque or degree of stenosis.

In patients with stable angina due to atherosclerosis there will therefore be ultramicroscopic deposition of platelets occurring on the endothelial surface of the coronary arteries. The potential pathophysiological importance of this process is considerable. Endothelial injury implies enhanced endothelial regeneration; recently re-

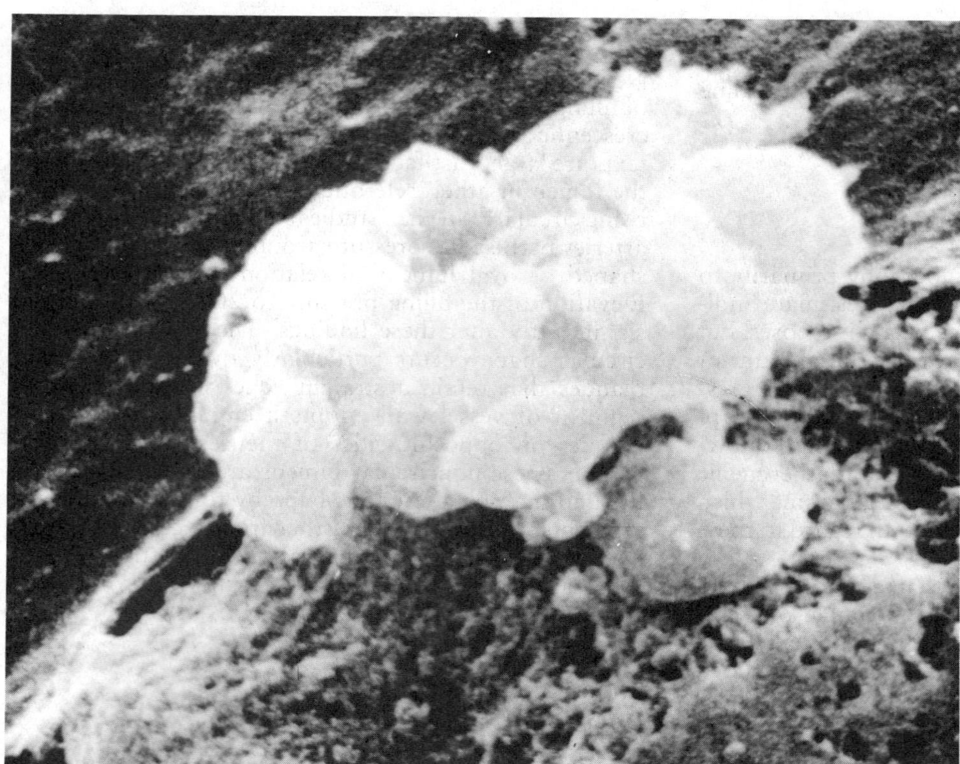

FIGURE 55-6 Scanning electron micrograph of human coronary artery. A single endothelial cell has undergone denudation. Over the exposed subendothelial tissue a small clump of platelets has formed. No platelets adhere to adjacent intact endothelial cells.

generated endothelium is deficient in endothelium-derived relaxing factor (EDRF) production. Platelets are a source of growth factors stimulating smooth-muscle proliferation, and finally small thrombi may grow into large thrombi that influence blood flow.

ACUTE ISCHEMIC SYNDROMES

There is now overwhelming evidence that the major factor initiating acute ischemia in unstable angina, acute myocardial infarction, and a proportion of sudden ischemic deaths is a thrombus of a sufficient size to protrude into the arterial lumen and thus influence blood flow. This does not imply thrombosis is the only factor, but necropsy studies including angiography,[27-31] angiography in life,[32-34] angioscopy,[35] and the success of fibrinolytic therapy in restoring patency all indicate a predominant role for thrombosis. Given these facts, understanding why a major thrombus capable of being demonstrated by angiography should form is of considerable importance.

Factors Inducing Plaque Thrombosis

Reconstruction of human coronary thrombi causing death shows that two processes within the vessel wall are responsible.[36]

In superficial plaque injury there is a thrombus superimposed on the surface of an otherwise intact plaque. The process is a continuation and extreme expression of the endothelial denudation that occurs over many plaques in subjects with coronary atherosclerosis. Factors associated with this form of coronary thrombosis include significant preexisting stenosis, heavy monocyte infiltration of the intima of the type often seen in diabetes, and high plasma lipid levels. Smaller epicardial arteries such as the posterior descending and left marginal branches are often involved. This process is responsible for approximately 30 percent of major thrombi.

The more common factor precipitating major coronary thrombi is intimal tearing with deep injury to the plaque.[37-39] The process of tearing has been called cracking, splitting, fissuring, or plaque rupture, indicating that the tears range in size from a few hundred micrometers to loss of the whole cap of a plaque 2 cm long in the carotid artery. The intimal tear allows blood from the lumen to dissect into the plaque itself and thus come into contact with the intensely thrombogenic lipid core. Thrombosis initially occurs within the substance of the plaque, expanding and changing its configuration. Subsequently the plaque may either reseal and then heal by smooth-muscle proliferation or progress to the formation of additional thrombosis within the lumen itself (Fig. 55-7). The intraluminal thrombosis will initially protrude into the lumen while still allowing some antegrade blood flow. At this stage distal embolization of platelet aggregates from the surface of the thrombus may occur.[39,40] Intraluminal thrombus may finally grow to completely occlude the lumen. The dynamic nature of the thrombotic process following the stimulus of the plaque tearing cannot be overemphasized. Thrombus may build up within the lumen to occlude the vessel; the thrombus then breaks up, and flow is restored followed by a further phase of thrombus formation. There is good

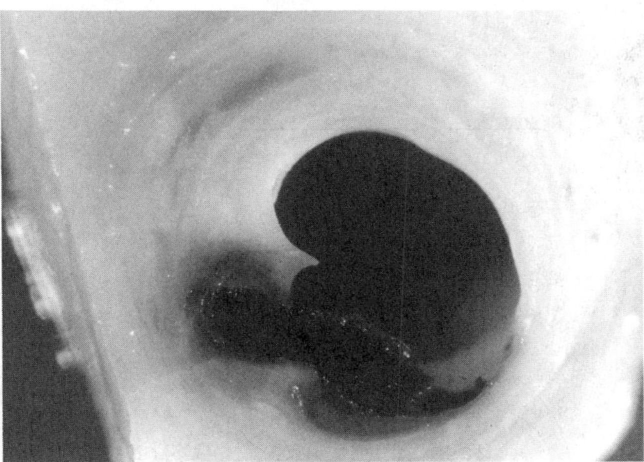

FIGURE 55-7 Human coronary artery supplying an area of regional infarction 5 days previously. There is a plaque that has undergone fissuring, and the torn end of the plaque cap is visible (arrow). A mass of thrombus within the original lipid core protrudes out into the lumen. Much of the lipid from the core has washed out to leave an "aneurysmal" cavity.

experimental evidence of these changes following wall injury[41] and good clinical evidence of intermittent thrombotic occlusion in humans.[42] The formation of intraluminal thrombus, as distinct from intraplaque thrombus after plaque tearing, is by no means inevitable, and the process can be aborted and healed by smooth-muscle proliferation at any stage. The end results of an episode of plaque thrombosis covers a wide spectrum from minor plaque growth to chronic total occlusion (Fig. 55-8). Plaques that reseal will have shown an abrupt increase in volume that may later diminish as internal thrombus is organized by smooth-muscle ingrowth. Subclinical plaque fissuring and intraplaque thrombosis is an important factor in disease progression (see below).

Mechanism of Intimal Tears

Reconstruction of human atherosclerotic plaque that has undergone tearing shows that the majority has a large pool of extracellular cholesterol occupying over 40 percent of the plaque by volume.[43,44] The common site of tearing in eccentric lesions is at the insertion of the plaque cap into the more normal vessel wall.

Mechanical tearing of tissue usually results from a combination of excess stress on an abnormally weak structure; plaque caps are no exception. On one hand, computer reconstruction of the circumferential wall stress during systole over plaque that has a soft and thus non-load-bearing core shows that stress is elevated and concentrated on the tissue of the plaque cap. On the other hand, the cap of plaque that has undergone fissuring can be shown to be mechanically weak when tested in vitro and to have a reduced collagen content, an increased macrophage density,[45] and a reduced smooth-muscle density. These changes in the cap tissue probably indicate a change in the balance of smooth-muscle proliferation and collagen production with collagenolysis by proteolytic enzymes following inflammatory activity within the plaque. The ability of the plaque to retain its integrity by smooth-muscle proliferation has been overcome.

Bleeding from transmedial vessels into the plaque has been postulated to be a factor in initiating expansion of plaque. Two facts militate against this view. First, the transmedial vessels are capillary with filling pressure below that of the circumferential hemodynamic force exerted across the arterial wall from the lumen. Second, studies in which the whole plaque is reconstructed inevitably show a break in the plaque cap joining the interior of the plaque to the lumen in cases where there is a large thrombus within a plaque.

A small minority of coronary thrombi are caused by tears that develop at the margins of plates of calcium within fibrous plaque that does not contain large amounts of lipid. This form of mechanical injury probably represents the action of shear stress between two tissues with very different mechanical properties. It may be a more important cause of thrombosis in the ectatic calcified coronary arteries of subjects over 75 years of age than in those in middle life with conventional stenosing disease.

UNSTABLE ANGINA

Intermittent resting ischemia, which is the hallmark of unstable angina, is related to "dynamic" stenosis, i.e., the obstruction to flow varies rather than being fixed. Two main mechanisms are proposed: intermittent thrombosis at the site of a culprit plaque and varying vasomotor tone either within the main epicardial arteries or within the distal vascular bed. Neither process is exclusive and both may operate contiguously.

Angiographic studies in unstable angina of the crescendo (type B) form[46] in which there is a known risk of subsequent acute infarction emphasize the presence of eccentric stenoses with ragged outlines, designated as type II (Fig. 55-9), and intraluminal filling defects.[47–49] Angioscopy and necropsy studies confirm that these angiographic appearances are due to nonocclusive thrombi developing over a fissured plaque.[31,50] A major cause of unstable angina is therefore a culprit plaque over which thrombus is arrested at an intermediate stage in which it is neither occlusive nor resolved sufficiently to allow the plaque to reseal. Pathological studies show that platelet emboli into the distal myocardium lead to small foci of acute myocardial necrosis in subjects dying suddenly after unstable angina.[39,40] Clinical studies[51] suggest that episodes of pain coincide with episodes of platelet activation, as shown by the presence of metabolites of thromboxane in the urine. Ultimately the thrombotic lesion either progresses to become occlusive or regresses to allow healing. The concept has thus emerged that unstable angina is predominantly due to an unstable plaque undergoing thrombosis that is in turn predominantly due to plaque fissuring. The presence of thrombus and intimal tearing may well be associated with enhanced local vasomotor hyperactivity at the site, further reducing blood flow and initiating myocardial infarction. Platelet adhesion to the vessel wall in experimental models is known to be associated with a marked increase in local vasomotor tone.[52]

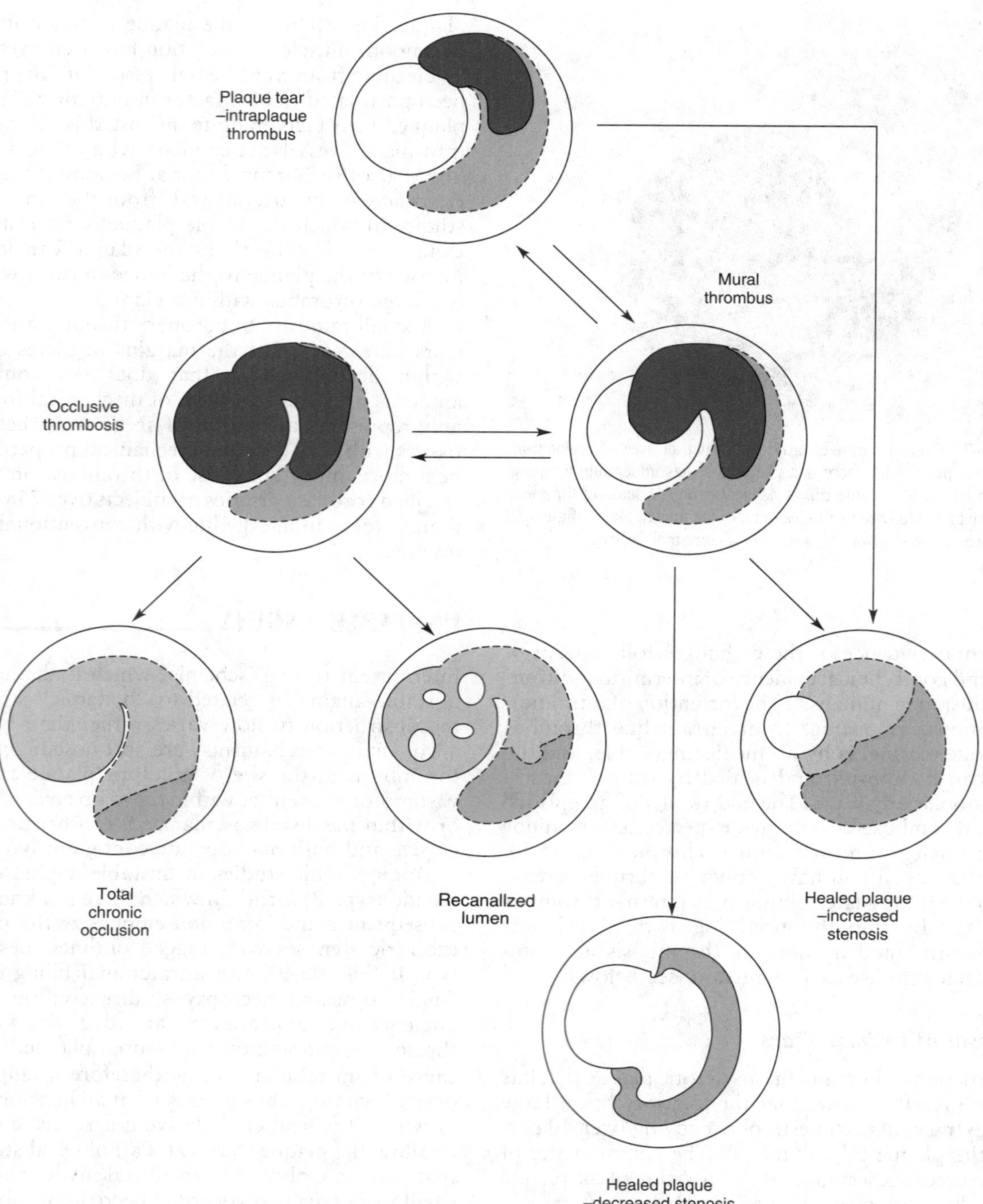

FIGURE 55-8 Diagrammatic representation of the possible outcomes of an episode of plaque fissuring.

ACUTE MYOCARDIAL INFARCTION

The blood supply of the mammalian myocardium is regional; each major branch of the coronary arteries supplies its own specific segment of myocardium. There is considerable interspecies variation in the degree of innate crossflow between epicardial arteries; humans and the pig share the property of having little natural collateral development. The only way to produce regional infarction in experimental models is to occlude a regional coronary artery.

Clinical studies of regional myocardial infarction in humans confirm the importance of occlusion of the subtending artery. Angiography during the early hours of regional infarction show the subtending artery to be occluded.[32,33,53] The frequency of occlusion falls with time, and as antegrade flow returns, filling defects are seen within the lumen over a type II stenosis.[34,54] Fibrinolytic therapy increases the number and speed with which the subtending artery reopens.[55] These data suggest a dynamic thrombotic process is occurring within the subtending artery.[42,56] Necropsy studies that have been spe-

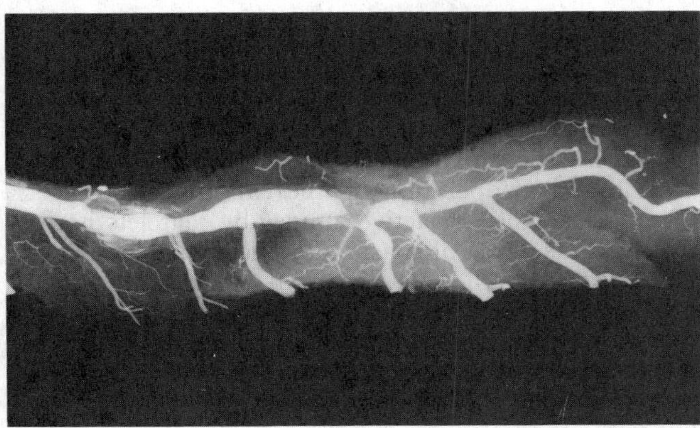

FIGURE 55-9 Postmortem angiogram showing a type II lesion in a subject dying suddenly after intermittent resting chest pain.

cifically directed to regional acute infarction confirm this view.[57,58] It is interesting, however, that necropsy studies show a higher frequency of residual total thrombotic occlusion than equivalent angiographic studies of survivors of acute infarction. This suggests that persistent occlusion has an adverse influence on survival, probably by being linked to larger infarct size and thus cardiogenic shock.

The only questions that remain are whether thrombosis could conceivably be a secondary phenomenon following reduced flow occurring *after* infarction had occurred.

Reconstruction of the microanatomy of occlusive coronary thrombi from serial histological sections shows the majority to be due to plaque ruptures in which there is both an intraplaque component and an intraluminal component.[29,30] The thrombus varies in age, suggesting that it is formed by an intermittent process taking place over some days. The intraplaque component of the thrombus is predominantly platelets; the thrombus within the fissure site is formed of densely packed fibrin, while within the lumen there is a more loosely packed fibrin network interlaced with red cells. These morphologic appearances suggest both a difference in time and the mechanisms by which the thrombus forms. Much of the intraluminal thrombus, particularly that distal to the fissured plaque, is "venous" in type, suggesting it has formed in a static column of blood. At least part of the intraluminal thrombus may thus be a late phenomenon. In vivo radiolabeling studies in subjects who subsequently died of acute infarction show that both fibrinogen and platelets given after the onset of the infarction can be incorporated into the coronary thrombus.[59,60] More detailed studies, however, showed that the thrombus within the fissured plaque is not labeled, i.e., predates infarction while a proportion of thrombus in the lumen is labeled, i.e., postdates infarction.[57]

Pathological evidence therefore shows that coronary thrombi that cause infarction evolve with time. Clinical studies show that prior to infarction occlusion is often intermittent. The initiating nidus of thrombus over the plaque is an early initiating event, while propagating thrombus in the lumen is a later secondary event.

Reconstruction of plaque that has fissured and underlies coronary thrombi shows considerable heterogeneity. At one extreme there are plaques with a minor intraplaque component of thrombus, a small fissure, and a large intraluminal thrombotic component. Such thrombi would be very susceptible to lysis with a good chance of restoring flow. In the middle range are plaques in which both thrombotic components are equal in size, while at the other extreme are plaques in which the major factor in occlusion is expansion of the plaque by thrombus from within, extrusion of its lipid content into the lumen, and elevation of flaps of intima. This latter group may be those lesions that are very resistant to lytic therapy.[61]

Interrelation of Infarct Morphology and Arterial Thrombi

The simplicity of dog models in which regional infarction is produced by sudden ligation of a normal coronary artery has given pathophysiological insight into the mechanisms of myocyte injury but perhaps has led to an oversimplified view of the pathogenesis of human infarcts.

Human regional infarcts may indeed be formed of myocardial necrosis of uniform age extending through the full-wall thickness. Such infarcts are closely analogous to the dog lesions and represent thrombus occurring suddenly and progressing to occlusion over a very short time in a vessel in which there was no preexisting stenosis. The variables found within the human coronary artery are, in many cases, more complex. There may be preexisting high-grade stenosis that has invoked collateral formation; in such arteries thrombosis may occur without causing any infarction. Thrombosis may be mural and associated with distal embolization of platelet masses or intermittently occlusive prior to the final occlusive episode. Antegrade flow may or may not be restored spontaneously within a period of hours. These more complex developmental patterns of thrombosis are associated with regional infarcts that are built up by the coalescence of small, often microscopic, areas of necrosis of different ages. Retention of areas of viable myocardium mixed with necrotic areas is common. Infarcts that are regional but confined to the subendocardial zone (nontransmural) are almost always of this type. In humans nontransmural infarction when compared with transmural infarction has a higher frequency of previously established collateral flow and/or restoration of antegrade flow over the culprit plaque.[62,63] The sinister complications of infarct expansion, infarct rupture, and cardiogenic shock are virtually confined to transmural infarcts and are associated with persistent total occlusion of long segments of coronary artery.

SUDDEN ISCHEMIC DEATH

A proportion of sudden deaths due to coronary atherosclerosis is the result of ventricular fibrillation induced by new sudden acute myocardial ischemia whose pathogenesis is not different from that found in unstable angina or developing infarction. A proportion of sudden ischemic deaths, however, have no cause of acute ischemia, and death results from ventricular fibrillation supervening on reentrant tachycardias in a scarred and/or hypertrophied left ventricle. The exact proportions of each group are contentious, and there is no agreement on this matter between either individual necropsy studies or studies of the resuscitated survivors of out-of-hospital cardiac arrest subsequently shown to have coronary atherosclerosis by angiography. The disagreements between series almost certainly reflect large selection biases operating in favor of one or other mechanism. Two large necropsy series[38,64,65] found the frequency of a new thrombotic arterial lesion potentially causing acute ischemia to be 93 and 20 percent. The latter, however, excluded patients with any chest pain immediately prior to the cardiac arrest; the former did not. Another necropsy series of sudden ischemic death found an overall rate of new acute ischemia to be 73.3 percent and showed that major factors predicting that acute thrombi will be found are prodromal chest pain and a subject not known to have previous ischemic heart disease.[66] Conversely, subjects without warning pain who are known to have had a previous healed infarct have a lower incidence of coronary thrombi. Clinical series are equally lacking in agreement; the frequency of electrocardiographic (ECG) and enzyme evidence of new myocardial damage in resuscitated victims of out-of-hosptial arrest varies from 20 to 78 percent.[66,67] Such resuscitated individuals have been found to have an increase of angiographic lesions with a morphology similar to those seen in unstable angina, and this frequency is higher in those in whom reentry tachycardias cannot be initiated during a subsequent electrophysiological investigation.[68,69] (See Chaps. 51 and 52.)

VASOMOTOR TONAL ABNORMALITIES IN ATHEROSCLEROSIS

There is now abundant evidence both in humans and in animals that atherosclerotic arteries have abnormal and inappropriate vasoconstrictor responses. These responses, which have been induced both by exercise and intracoronary infusion of acetylcholine, are characterized as failure of the normal vasodilatory response due to EDRF release. (See Chaps. 2 and 56.) Pathological studies can have a minor role only in elucidating the role of abnormal tone in producing symptoms in ischemic heart disease. On morphological grounds it is possible to say that good reasons exist for a failure of EDRF production in atherosclerotic arteries. The endothelium is regenerating at an enhanced rate, and such cells may take some weeks to acquire normal EDRF production. In a normal artery endothelial cells may actually be in contact with medial smooth muscle via gaps in the internal elastic lamina; in atherosclerosis the endothelial surface is physically separated from the muscle cells in the media by the bulk of the plaque. Free-radical production or hemoglobin within plaques may neutralize the EDRF produced. The uptake of oxidized LDL by coronary artery endothelial cells in vitro may inhibit nitric oxide formation.[70,71]

Cases of unstable angina are clearly described in which localized vasoconstriction at a site of eccentric stenosis in a major coronary artery was responsible.[72] It is less clear why one such lesion should acquire such vasomotor excitability. In one case small amounts of thrombus, too small to be detected angiographically, were found at operation on the endothelial surface.[72] Local release of vasoactive amines by platelets is thus one possible cause of spasm. Another postulated cause is related to the heavy adventitial inflammation; mast cells may release pharmacologically active substances that directly act on adventitial nerve tissue.[73,74] The Prinzmetal variant form of angina frequently occurs in arteries that have some angiographic evidence of atherosclerosis but without an element of high-grade fixed stenosis.[75,76]

The final unresolved issue concerning the mechanisms by which atherosclerosis induces clinical symptoms lies in the status of the peripheral vascular bed within the myocardium itself. In acute thrombotic situations the peripheral vascular bed suffers morphologic damage, which is associated with a steep rise in resistance and a decline in coronary flow reserve. Platelet emboli and white cell plugging of small vessels are both observed phenomena in subjects dying of unstable angina and myocardial infarction. In stable states very little is known about the function of the peripheral vascular bed in the myocardium; abnormal tonal responses redistributing blood flow within the myocardium itself may be a mechanism capable of inducing transient ischemia in subjects with atherosclerosis.

MECHANISMS OF ATHEROSCLEROTIC PROGRESSION AND REGRESSION

Clinical angiographic studies are one way of studying disease progression and show that it is phasic and unpredictable in any particular arterial segment.[77-82] High-grade lesions do not necessarily appear at sites where previous lower grade lesions were present. Many new lesions causing over 50 percent diameter stenosis appear between two angiographic examinations in normal segments of artery. The sites of future acute occlusions cannot be predicted. The progression of separate lesions in an individual is unrelated, and the progression of normal segments is often greater than in areas recognized to have an irregular outline.[81] Thus individual plaques can enter an accelerated growth phase that is unrelated to the degree of stenosis they are causing. One explanation for this erratic and stepwise progression is that subclinical episodes of thrombosis are responsible for plaque growth.[82] It is clearly recognized clinically that large intraluminal thrombi causing infarction do result in plaque growth and considerable residual stenosis, which may remodel and modify over some months. The evidence that smaller subclinical thrombi cause similar plaque growth is largely derived from pathology studies. Demonstration of buried thrombi incorporated into large plaques has been reported very widely since the pioneer studies of Duguid in 1948.[83] A study of the coronary arteries of subjects with coronary atherosclerosis but who died of noncardiac causes and in whom no symptoms of acute ischemia were noted showed an episode of recent intraplaque thrombus in 16 percent of those with hypertension and diabetes and in 8 percent of those without these factors.[66] These data suggest that subclinical plaque thrombosis occurs in all subjects with extensive coronary plaque formation and will thus inevitably cause plaque growth. The only alternative view for intermittent plaque growth is that the plaque enters a sudden phase of smooth-muscle proliferation associated with a greatly accelerated lipid accumulation unrelated to thrombus deposition. If such sudden acceleration in these two processes can occur, the mechanism is unknown. The dynamics of lipid exchange in vivo in human lesions is virtually unknown.

Primate and porcine models of atherosclerosis induced by high-fat diets lead to the creation of lipid-rich plaques. The fate of these plaques can be followed after lowering plasma lipid levels, as a result of which plaque extracellular lipids are mobilized[84] with some reduction in plaque volume. At the same time smooth-muscle proliferation and collagen synthesis within the plaque increases.[85] This leads to a more solid plaque that decreases in size very slowly. If the same evolutionary process occurs in humans, lowering plasma lipid levels would lead to a decrease in plaque volume and an increase in lumen size only in the minority of high-grade lesions that have a high lipid component. Plaque stabilization would, however, occur with a more striking effect on both the slowing of angiographic progression and reducing the frequency of major thrombotic/ischemic events.

REFERENCES

1. Zarins C, Weisenberg E, Kolettis G, Strankunavicius R, Glagov S: Differential enlargement of artery segments in response to enlarging atherosclerotic plaques. *J Vasc Surg* 1988; 7:386–394.
2. Libby P, Hansson G: Involvement of the immune system in human atherogenesis: Current knowledge and unanswered questions. *Lab Invest* 1991; 64:5–15.
3. Steinberg D, Parthasarathy S, Carew TE, Khoo JC, Witztum JL: Beyond cholesterol. Modifications of low-density lipoprotein that increase its atherogenicity. *New Engl J Med* 1989; 320:915–924.
4. Strong J, Solberg L, Restrepo C: Atherosclerosis in persons with coronary heart disease. *Lab Invest* 1968; 18:527–537.
5. Deupree R, Fields R, McMahon C, Strong J: Atherosclerotic lesions and coronary heart disease. Key relationships in necropsied cases. *Lab Invest* 1973; 28:252–262.
6. Robertson W, Strong J: Atherosclerosis in persons with hypertension and diabetes mellitus. *Lab Invest* 1968; 18:538–551.
7. PDAY Research G: Relationship of atherosclerosis in young men to serum lipoprotein cholesterol concentrations and smoking. A preliminary report from the pathological determinant of atherosclerosis in youth study. *JAMA* 1990; 264:3018–3024.
8. Roberts W: The coronary arteries and left ventricle in clinically isolated angina pectoris. *Circulation* 1976; 54:388–390.
9. Hangartner J, Charleston A, Davies M, Thomas A: Morphological characteristics of clinically significant coronary artery stenosis in stable angina. *Br Heart J* 1986; 56:501–508.
10. Brown B, Bolson E, Dodge H: Dynamic mechanisms in human coronary stenosis. *Circulation* 1984; 70:917–922.
11. Saner H, Gobel F, Salomonowitz E, Erlien D, Edwards J: The disease free wall in coronary atherosclerosis: Its relation to degree of obstruction. *J Am Coll Cardiol* 1985; 6:1096–1099.
12. Waller BF: The eccentric coronary atherosclerotic plaque: Morphologic observations and clinical relevance. *Clin Cardiol* 1989; 12:14–20.
13. Freudenberg H, Lichtlen P: The normal wall segment in coronary stenosis: A post mortem study. *Z Kardiol* 1981; 70:836–839.
14. Kaski JC, Tousoulis D, Haider AW, Gavrielides S, Crea F, Maseri A: Reactivity of eccentric and concentric coronary stenoses in patients with chronic stable angina. *J Am Coll Cardiol* 1991; 17:627–633.
15. Lundberg B: Chemical composition and physical state of lipid deposits in atherosclerosis. *Atherosclerosis* 1985; 56:93–110.
16. Wilcox J, Smith K, Schwartz S, Gordon D: Localisation of tissue factor in the normal vessel wall and in the atherosclerotic plaque. *Proc Natl Acad Sci USA* 1989; 86:2839–2843.
17. Agatston AS, Janowitz WR, Hildner FJ, Zusmer NR, Viamonte M, Detrano R: Quantification of coronary artery calcium using ultrafast computed tomography. *J Am Coll Cardiol* 1990; 15:827–832.
18. Barger A, Beeuwkes RI, Lainey L, Silverman K: Hypothesis: Vasa vasorum and neovascularization of human coronary arteries. A possible role in the pathophysiology of atherosclerosis. *N Engl J Med* 1983; 310:175–177.
19. Glagov S, Weisenberd E, Zarins C, Stankunavicius R, Kolettis G: Compensatory enlargement of human atherosclerotic coronary arteries. *N Engl J Med* 1987; 16:1371–1375.
20. Stiel G, Ludmilla S, Schofer J, Konath K, Mathey D: Impact of compensatory enlargement of atherosclerotic coronary arteries on angiographic assessment of coronary artery disease. *Circulation* 1989; 80:1603–1609.
21. de Feyter P, Serruys P, Davies M, Richardson P, Lubsen J, Oliver M: Quantitative coronary angiography to measure progression and regression of coronary atherosclerosis. Value, limitations, and implications for clinical trials. *Circulation* 1991; 84:412–423.
22. Thomas A, Davies M, Dilly S, Dilly N, Franc F: Potential errors in the estimation of coronary arterial stenosis from clinical arteriography with reference to the shape of the coronary arterial lumen. *Br Heart J* 1986; 55:129–139.
23. Faggiotto A, Ross R, Harker L: Studies of hypercholesterolaemia in the non-human primate. I. Changes that lead to fatty streak formation. *Arteriosclerosis* 1984; 4:323–340.
24. Faggiotto A, Ross R: Studies of hypercholesterolaemia in non-human primates. II. Fatty streak conversion to fibrous plaque. *Arteriosclerosis* 1984; 4:341–356.
25. Cybulsky M, Gimbrone M: Endothelial expression of a mononuclear leucocyte adhesion molecule during atherogenesis. *Science* 1991; 251:788–791.
26. Davies M, Woolf N, Rowles P, Pepper J: Morphology of the endothelium over atherosclerotic plaques in human coronary arteries. *Br Heart J* 1988; 60:459–464.
27. Davies M, Woolf N, Robertson W: Pathology of acute myocardial infarction with particular reference to occlusive coronary thrombi. *Br Heart J* 1976; 38:659–664.
28. Horie T, Sekiguchi M, Hirosawa K: Coronary thrombosis in pathogenesis of acute myocardial infarction. Histopathological study of coronary arteries in 108 necropsied cases using serial section. *Br Heart J* 1978; 40:153–161.
29. Falk E: Plaque rupture with severe pre-existing stenosis precipitating coronary thrombosis. Characteristics of coronary atherosclerotic plaque underlying fatal occlusive thrombi. *Br Heart J* 1983; 50:127–131.
30. Davies M, Thomas A: Plaque fissuring—the cause of acute myocardial infarction, sudden ischaemic death and crescendo angina. *Br Heart J* 1985; 53:363–373.
31. Levin D, Fallon J: Significance of the angiographic morphology of localized coronary stenosis: Histopathologic correlations. *Circulation* 1982; 66:316–320.
32. DeWood M, Spores J, Notske R, Mouser LT, Burroughs R, Golden MS, et al: Prevalence of total coronary occlusion during the early hours of transmural myocardial infarction. *N Engl J Med* 1980; 303:897–902.
33. Stadius M, Maynard C, Fritz J: Coronary anatomy and left ventricular function in the first 12 hours of acute myocardial infarction: The Western Washington randomized intracoronary streptokinase trial. *Circulation* 1985; 72:292:301.
34. Ambrose J, Hjemdahl-Monsen C, Borrico S, Gorlin R, Fuster V: Angiographic demonstration of a common link between unstable angina pectoris and non Q-wave acute myocardial infarction. *J Am Coll Cardiol* 1988; 12:244–247.
35. Forrester J, Litvak F, Grundfest W, Hickey A: A perspective of coronary disease seen through the arteries of a living man. *Circulation* 1987; 75:505–513.
36. Davies MJ: A macroscopic and microscopic view of coronary thrombi. *Circulation* 1990; 82:1138–1146.

37. Constantinides P: Plaque fissures in human coronary thrombosis. *J Atheroscler Res* 1966; 6:1–17.
38. Davies MJ, Thomas A: Thrombosis and acute coronary artery lesions in sudden cardiac ischemic death. *N Engl J Med* 1984; 310:1137–1140.
39. Falk E: Unstable angina with fatal outcome: Dynamic coronary thrombosis leading to infarction and/or sudden death. *Circulation* 1985; 71:699–708.
40. Davies MJ, Thomas A, Knapman P, Hangartner R: Intramyocardial platelet aggregation in patients with unstable angina suffering sudden ischemic cardiac death. *Circulation* 1986; 73:418–427.
41. Folts J: An in vivo model of experimental arterial stenosis intimal damage and periodic thrombosis. *Circulation* 1991; 83:IV.3–IV.14.
42. Maseri A, Chierchia S, Davies G: Pathophysiology of coronary occlusion in acute infarction. *Circulation* 1986; 73:233–239.
43. Richardson P, Davies M, Born G: Influence of plaque configuration and stress distribution on fissuring of coronary atherosclerotic plaques. *Lancet* 1989; ii:941–944.
44. Tracy R, Devaney K, Kissling G: Characteristics of the plaque under a coronary thrombus. *Virch Arch Pathol Anat* 1985; 405:411–427.
45. Lendon C, Davies M, Born G, Richardson P: Atherosclerotic plaque caps are locally weakened when macrophage density is increased. *Atherosclerosis* 1991; 65:302–310.
46. Brumwald E: Unstable angina, a classification. *Circulation* 1989; 80:410–414.
47. Ambrose J, Winters S, Stern A: Angiographic morphology and the pathogenesis of unstable angina. *J Am Coll Cardiol* 1985; 5:609–616.
48. Williams A, Freeman M, Chisholm R, Patt N, Armstrong P: Angiographic morphology in unstable angina pectoris. *Am J Cardiol* 1988; 62:1024–1027.
49. Rehr R, Discuascio G, Vetrovec G, Cowley M: Angiographic morphology of coronary artery stenoses in prolonged rest angina: Evidence of intracoronary thrombosis. *J Am Coll Cardiol* 1989; 14:1429–1437.
50. Sherman C, Litvack F, Grundfest W: Coronary angioscopy in patients with unstable pectoris. *N Engl J Med* 1986; 315:913–919.
51. Fitzgerald D, Roy L, Catella F, Fitzgerald A: A platelet activation in unstable coronary disease. *N Engl J Med* 1986; 315:983–989.
52. Lam J, Chesebro J, Steele P, Dadimon L, Fuster V: Is vasospasm related to platelet deposition. Relationship in a porcine preparation of arterial injury in vivo. *Circulation* 1987; 75:243–248.
53. Bertrand M, Lefebvre J, Laisne C, Rousseau M, Carre A, Lekieffre J: Coronary arteriography in acute transmural myocardial infarction. *Am Heart J* 1979; 97:61–69.
54. Wilson R, Holida M, White C: Quantitative angiographic morphology of coronary stenoses leading to myocardial infarction or unstable angina. *Circulation* 1986; 73:286–293.
55. Brown BG, Gallery CA, Badger RS, Kennedy JW, Mathey D, Bolson EL, et al: Incomplete lysis of thrombus in the moderate underlying atherosclerotic lesions during intracoronary infarction: Quantitative angiographic observations. *Circulation* 1986; 73:653–661.
56. Hackett D, Davies G, Chierchia S, Maseri A: Intermittent coronary occlusion in acute myocardial infarction. Value of combined thrombolytic and vasodilator therapy. *N Engl J Med* 1987; 317:1055–1059.
57. Davies M, Fulton W, Robertson W: The relationship of coronary thrombosis to ischaemic myocardial necrosis. *J Pathol* 1979; 127:99–110.
58. Ridolfi R, Bulkley B, Hutchins G: The relationship between coronary lesions and myocardial infarct, ulceration of atherosclerotic plaques precipitating coronary thrombosis. *Am Heart J* 1977; 93:1977–1986.
59. Erhardt L, Unge G, Bowman G: Formation of coronary arterial thrombi in relation to onset of necrosis in acute myocardial infarction in man. *Am Heart J* 1976; 91:592–598.
60. Henriksson P, Edhag O, Jansson B: A role for platelets in the process of infarct extension. *N Engl J Med* 1985; 313:1660.
61. Davies MJ: Successful and unsuccessful coronary thrombolysis. *Br Heart J* 1989; 61:381–384.
62. Piek J, Becker A: Collateral blood supply to the myocardium at risk in human myocardial infarction: A quantitative postmortem assessment. *J Am Coll Cardiol* 1988; 11:1290–1296.
63. Levine H: Subendocardial infarction in retrospect: Pathologic, cardiographic and axillary features. *Circulation* 1985; 72:790–800.
64. Warnes C, Roberts W: Sudden coronary death: Relation of amount and distribution of coronary narrowing at necropsy to previous symptoms of myocardial ischemia, left ventricular scarring and heart weight. *Am J Cardiol* 1984; 54:65–73.
65. Warnes C, Roberts W: Sudden coronary death: Comparison of patients with to those without coronary thrombus at necropsy. *Am J Cardiol* 1984; 54:1206–1211.
66. Davies M, Bland J, Hangartner J, Angelini A, Thomas A: Factors influencing the presence or absence of acute coronary artery thrombi in sudden ischaemic death. *Eur Heart J* 1989; 10:203–208.
67. Goldstein S, Landis J, Leighton R, et al: Characteristics of the resuscitated out-of-hospital cardiac arrest victim with coronary heart disease. *Circulation* 1981; 64:977–984.
68. Lo Y-SA, Cutler J, Blake K, Wright A, Kron J, Swerdlow C: Angiographic coronary morphology in survivors of cardiac arrest. *Am Heart J* 1988; 115:781–785.
69. Stevenson W, Wiener I, Yeatman L, Wohlgelernter D, Weiss J: Complicated atherosclerotic lesions: A potential cause of ischaemic ventricular arrhythmias in cardiac arrest survivors who do not have inducible ventricular tachycardia? *Am Heart J* 1988; 116:1–6.
70. Tanner F, Noll G, Boulanger C, Luscher T: Oxidized low density lipoproteins inhibit relaxations of porcine coronary arteries. Role of scavenger receptor and endothelium-derived nitric oxide. *Circulation* 1991; 83:2012–2020.
71. Rosenfeld M: Oxidized LDL affects multiple atherogenic cellular responses. *Circulation* 1991; 83:2137–2140.
72. Brown B: Observations linking the clinical spectrum of ischaemic heart disease to the dynamic pathology of coronary atherosclerosis. *Arch Intern Med* 1981; 141:716–722.
73. Kohchi K, Takebayashi S, Hiroki T, Nobuyoshi M: Significance of adventitial inflammation of the coronary artery in patients with unstable angina: Results at autopsy. *Circulation* 1985; 71:709–716.
74. Forman M, Oates J, Robertson D: Increased adventitial mast cells in a patient with coronary spasm. *N Engl J Med* 1985; 313:1138–1141.
75. Maseri A, Severi S, Nes MD, Labbate A, Chierchia S, Marzilli M, et al: "Variant" angina: One aspect of a continuous spectrum of vasospastic myocardial ischaemia. *Am J Cardiol* 1978; 42:1019–1035.
76. Roberts W, Curry R, Isner J: Sudden death in Prinzmetal's angina with coronary spasm documented by arteriography: Analysis of three necropsy cases. *Am J Cardiol* 1982; 50:203–210.
77. Bruschke A, Wijers T, Kolsters W, Landmann J: The anatomic evaluation of coronary artery disease demonstrated by coronary angiography in 256 non-operated patients. *Circulation* 1981; 63:527–540.
78. Bruschke A, Kramer J, Bal E, Haque I, Detranto R, Goormastic M: The dynamics of progression of coronary atherosclerosis studied in 168 medically treated patients who underwent coronary arteriography three times. *Am Heart J* 1989; 117:296–305.
79. Rafflenbeul W, Nellessen U, Galvao P, Kreft M, Peters S, Lichtlen P: Progression and regression of coronary artery disease as assessed with sequential coronary angiography. *Z Kardiol* 1984; 73:33–40.
80. Little W, Constantinescu M, Applegate R: Can coronary arteriography predict the site of subsequent myocardial infarction in a patient with mild to moderate coronary artery disease? *Circulation* 1988; 78:1157–1166.
81. Gibson M, Stonbe P, Pasternak R, Sandor T, Rosner B, Sacks F: The natural history of coronary atherosclerosis using quantitative angiography: Implications for regression trials. *J Am Coll Cardiol* 1991; 17:231A.
82. Singh R: Progression of coronary atherosclerosis. Clues to pathogenesis from serial coronary arteriography. *Br Heart J* 1984; 52:451–461.
83. Duguid J: Thrombosis as a factor in the pathogenesis of aortic atherosclerosis. *J Pathol Bact* 1984; 60:57–61.
84. Small D: George Lyman Duff Memorial Lecture. Progression and regression of atherosclerotic lesions: Insights from lipid physical biochemistry. *Arteriosclerosis* 1988; 8:103–129.
85. Blankenhorn D, Kramsch D: Reversal of atherosis and sclerosis. The two components of atherosclerosis. *Circulation* 1989; 79:1–7.

Chapter 56

The Coronary Ischemic Syndromes: Relationship to the Biology of Atherosclerosis

R. Wayne Alexander, M.D., Ph.D.

INTRODUCTION

The coronary ischemic syndromes, which include stable angina, unstable angina, and myocardial infarction, have been extensively studied and characterized. Their pathophysiological basis may be related to increased oxygen demand in the setting of a flow-limiting lesion or, especially in unstable angina or myocardial infarction, there may be primary decreases in blood flow caused by vasospasm and thrombosis. Although the clinical syndromes are almost exclusively associated with atherosclerosis of the epicardial coronaries, efforts have been made only in recent years to relate the syndromes of coronary ischemia to the biology of atherosclerosis. There has been increasing interest in explaining the clinical syndromes in terms of the biology of the underlying disease for two major reasons. First, the clinical cardiologist has a need to understand the episodic nature of, in particular, the unstable ischemic syndromes, while at the same time appreciating that there is a dynamism to even the so-called "stable anginal syndromes." Second, the extraordinary progress in understanding the basic pathobiology of atherosclerosis has now made the attempts to reconcile the clinical cardiologist's observations with those of the experimental and clinical pathologist worthwhile.

The pathologist and cardiologist traditionally have had very different views of atherosclerosis. The pathologist views the disease as chronic, and frequently considers that there is a linear growth in lesion size and lumenal encroachment. The cardiologist, on the other hand, sees the disease in its late stages as an episodic event presenting frequently with acute myocardial infarction or the subacute development of unstable angina pectoris. Although both of these clinical entities may be superimposed upon stable angina, their cyclic and episodic nature is still one of the most prominent manifestations of chronic coronary atherosclerosis. One of the most intriguing conundrums in cardiovascular medicine involves the problem of understanding the cellular mechanisms by which a chronic stable atherosclerotic lesion is transformed to a state in which it fissures or ruptures and supports clot formation—the substrate for the development of unstable angina or myocardial infarction. The process in the lesion leading to unstable angina or infarction has been referred to generically as "activation," and the lesion has been called "active."

This chapter will provide a mechanistic framework that will permit conceptualization of the process in cell biological terms. It will also provide an explanation for the spectrum of the ischemic coronary syndromes in the context of the rapidly expanding body of knowledge concerning the cell biology of atherosclerosis.

BIOLOGY OF ATHEROSCLEROSIS

The fundamental features of atherosclerosis are discussed in detail in Chaps. 54 and 55. The atherosclerotic lesion occurs almost exclusively in the large conduit and conduction vessels of the arterial system. The distribution is nonrandom. It occurs predominantly at flow dividers in areas of low shear stress. The lesion is characterized by the proliferation of medial smooth muscle cells that have been changed into a growth phenotype referred to as the "modulated state."[1] Smooth muscle cells migrate into the intima and contribute to intimal thickening. Another major feature of an atherosclerotic lesion is the presence of blood monocytes that have adhered to the endothelium and migrated into the intima. These monocytes are transformed into tissue macrophage-like cells. These cells are the major source of the typical lipid-laden foam cells of the atherosclerotic lesion. The foam cells are caused primarily by the uptake of modified or oxidized LDL. Macrophages express the so-called scavenger receptor, which is a receptor that recognizes modified, but not native, LDL. More recently, it has been appreciated that atherosclerotic lesions have T cells as important constituents.[2] Furthermore, these are frequently memory T cells that express late activation antigens suggesting that they have been immunologically activated.[3] An additional significant characteristic of an atherosclerotic lesion is neovascularization that is developed from new capillary vessel growth from the adventitial surface.[4] Thus, the atherosclerotic lesion has many features typical of inflammation.

The evolving concept that atherosclerosis is an inflammatory response to injury has led to considerable progress in the understanding of the basic pathogenesis of the disease.[5] As will be developed, this concept is also particularly relevant to the understanding of the episodic nature of clinical coronary disease. The artery exhibits a rather limited repertoire of responses to multiple injuries, all manifesting as an atherosclerotic lesion. The major injuries constitute the well-recognized risk factors. There is the metabolic injury of hyperlipidemia and the injury of physical forces induced by hypertension. As alluded to, physical forces—both shear and pressure—are thought to play a major role in the nonrandom distribution in the arterial system. The vessel may also respond to injury from smoking or to immune injury as in transplant atherosclerosis. In addition, it may respond to the direct physical insult of balloon angioplasty.

As noted, viewing the lesion as an inflammatory response provides an important basis for considering the episodic nature of clinical coronary disease. An atherosclerotic lesion may be viewed as a chronic inflammatory nidus that may be quiescent or subject to periodic activation.

One of the most important of the new discoveries about the fundamental nature of atherosclerosis has come from work initiated by Steinberg and his colleagues.[6] Initially they observed that native low density lipoprotein (LDL) was not taken up readily by monocytes/macrophages in vitro, but that LDL modified by endothelial cells was readily taken up and foam cells were formed.[7] It was found subsequently that one of the mechanisms involved in modification of LDL that would alter its handling by monocytes was oxidation of the particle with a marked increase in the content of lysophosphatidylcholine (LPC).[8] Modified LDL and LPC elicit a number of responses that are important in the pathogenesis of atherosclerosis including stimulation of endothelial monocyte and lymphocyte adhesion molecules[9] and monocyte chemotactic protein expression.[10] These compounds will also stimulate growth factor production by the endothelium.[11] The central importance of enhanced oxidation mechanisms in atherosclerosis is emphasized by animal studies in which antioxidants, such as probucol, inhibit atherosclerotic lesion formation.[12]

ENDOTHELIUM

The endothelium plays the central role in controlling the biology of the vessel wall. It has been one of the main tenets in the study of atherosclerosis that a healthy endothelium is crucial to the prevention of disease development. This view evolved from early studies that demonstrated that mechanical removal of the endothelium facilitated lesion development in hypercholesterolemic monkeys. For a period of time, it was assumed that lesion development, in most instances, was associated with endothelial cell detachment exposing the subendothelial surface and permitting platelet adherence and clot formation with the release of growth factors.[13]

The concept of "dysfunction" of the endothelium developed when it became apparent that the endothelium, over many lesions, was intact morphologically.[14] Endothelial dysfunction implies that the normal functions of the endothelium may be modified or modulated to a maladaptive phenotypic state. This concept is central to the major, current views of the pathogenesis of the disease. The normal functions of the endothelium and the consequences of the development of dysfunction are summarized in Table 56-1.

Endothelial-Dependent Vasodilation

The endothelium has a number of critical functions. One of the most important of these is endothelial-dependent vasodilation. (See Chap. 2.) In 1982, Furchgott and Zawadzki demonstrated the existence of an endothelial-derived humoral factor, which they termed endothelial-derived relaxing factor (EDRF), that caused the dilatation of blood vessels by diffusing to the underlying smooth muscle cells and increasing cGMP.[15] Agents such as the muscarinic cholinergic agonist, acetylcholine, caused dilatation with an intact endothelium and contraction when the endothelium was removed (Fig. 56-1). Many, if not most, vasodilators including serotonin, thrombin, flow, substance P, and adenine nucleotides act through this mechanism.

Early work characterizing EDRF suggested similarities to nitric oxide (NO).[16] Nitric oxide has proven to be the most important of the endothelial-derived vasodilator substances. One of the characteristics of EDRF that was known to be shared with NO was its ease of degradation by oxygen-free radicals.[17] This susceptibility of this important endogenous vasodilator to degradation by an oxidative environment is central to the understanding of disordered control of vasomotor tone clinically.

TABLE 56-1
Normal and Dysfunctional Arterial Endothelium

Normal Function	Dysfunction in Atherosclerosis	Cause(s) of Dysfunction
Antithrombotic	Potentially prothrombotic	Inflammatory cytokines Oxygen free radical production
Vasodilator	Decreased vasodilation ? constrictor	Oxygen free radicals—degradation of NO causing decreased vasodilator activity
Growth inhibition	Growth promotion Loss of inhibition	Increased growth factor release; ? decreased inhibitor release
Antiinflammatory	Proinflammatory—supports monocyte and T-cell localization into lesion	Increased leukocyte adhesion molecule and chemotactic protein expression

Inflammation

The endothelium also has a central role in controlling the development of inflammation by controlling the localization of circulating leukocytes. For example, localization of monocytes and lymphocytes to atherosclerotic lesion-prone areas is controlled by the expression by the endothelium of leukocyte adhesion molecules, such as vascular cell adhesion molecule 1 (VCAM-1). (See Chap. 2.)[18] In response to metabolic stress such as hyperlipidemia, the endothelium may also express chemotactic proteins such as monocyte chemotactic protein-1.[19] Inflammatory cytokines, such as tumor necrosis factor, interleukin-1, and γ-interferon, may be produced in the injured vessel and target the endothelium, potentially stimulating expression of adhesion molecules and chemotactic proteins.[20] Thus, the inflammatory response in, for example, an atherosclerotic lesion, may be self-perpetuating during active phases of the disease and result in recruitment of additional inflammatory cells by cells resident in the lesion.

Thrombosis

As discussed in Chaps. 2 and 7, endothelium is the prototypic nonthrombogenic surface. It produces agents that inhibit platelet aggregation and clot formation and also produces thrombolytic agents such as tissue-plasminogen activator. Under the influence of inflammatory mediators, the endothelium may become either frankly prothrombogenic or less antithrombogenic.[21,22] This regulated property may be important in clot formation in the unstable anginal syndromes.

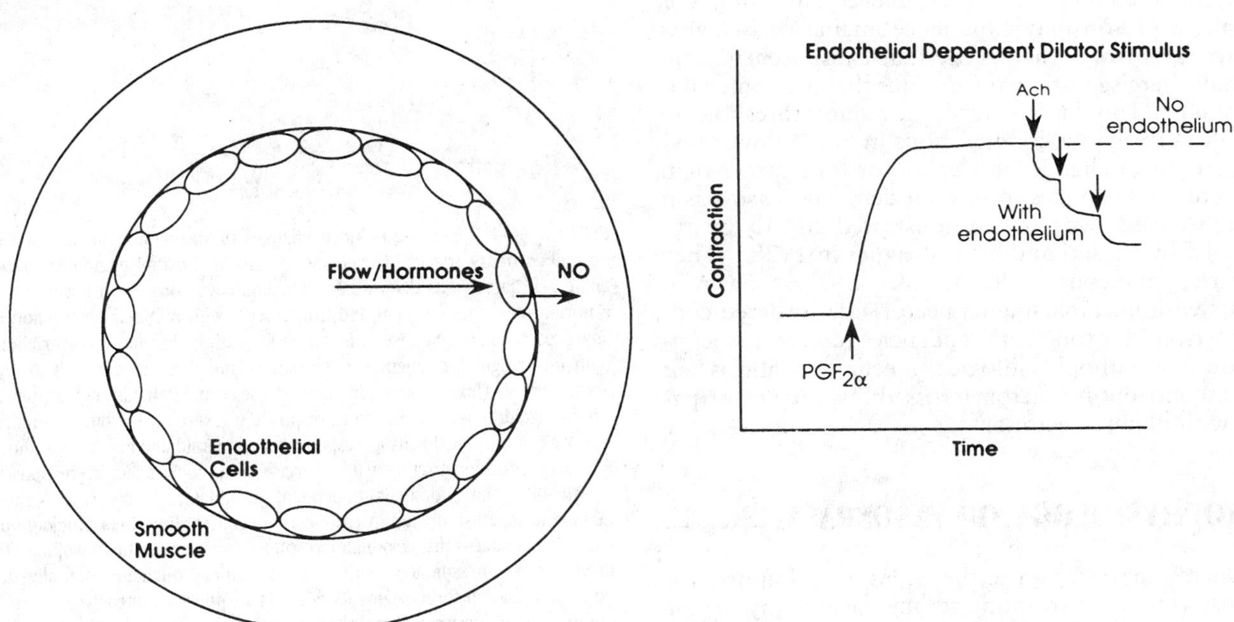

FIGURE 56-1 Endothelial-dependent dilatation. The left panel shows an artery with stimuli acting upon the endothelium to cause the release of EDRF or nitric oxide. This diffuses to the underlying smooth muscle to increase cyclic GMP and cause relaxation. The right panel depicts the effects of the endothelial-dependent vasodilator acetylcholine (Ach) on an artery precontracted with $PGF_2\alpha$. In the presence of an intact endothelium, acetylcholine results in a dose-dependent relaxation. When endothelium is removed, acetylcholine no longer induces relaxation.

Growth Control

The normal endothelium is primarily growth-inhibitory. Blood vessels with a normal functional endothelium respond minimally to direct growth factor stimulation.[23] An important property of dysfunctional endothelium in disease is the shift from an antigrowth mode to a mode that promotes growth, in particular, of vascular smooth muscle in the vessel wall. The growth-inhibitory properties are not understood well. It is likely that the growth-promoting properties of the endothelium reflect stimulated production of growth factors such as PDGF-B, insulin-like growth factor-1, and fibroblast growth factor.

STABLE ANGINA PECTORIS

Stable angina is characterized by a consistent pain pattern that does not change over 6 to 8 weeks in either threshold, duration, or the setting in which it occurs. Pain characteristically occurs with exertion, emotional upset, or other stimuli that increase myocardial oxygen consumption. The threshold for pain is characteristically, not absolutely, fixed, but is somewhat variable; that is, a stimulus that causes angina on one occasion may not on another, although a consistent pattern can usually be determined. Furthermore, when assessed by ambulatory monitoring, ischemia may be noted to occur at different heart rates.[24]

Hemodynamically significant obstructive disease of the coronary artery contributes to angina in situations where myocardial oxygen consumption is increased. Such obstructions account for the relatively reproducible time to onset of ischemia on treadmill exercise testing. A variability in angina threshold and setting in which pain occurs is common, however, in everyday living. For example, a person may experience angina or ischemia at heart rates lower than those that cause ischemia on treadmill exercise testing and at rates that are somewhat inconstant.[24] This inconsistency in angina threshold in daily life is likely due to alterations in blood flow delivery—a result of changes in vasomotor tone rather than to unperceived changes in oxygen demand. Vasospasm causing ischemia was first demonstrated directly by angiography by Maseri and his colleagues in 1978.[25] They showed spontaneous occlusive coronary vasospasm in patients with unstable angina pectoris. Disordered control of vasomotor tone with tendencies toward vasoconstriction is a pathophysiological mechanism and is felt to be a contributing factor across the spectrum of patients with angina pectoris.[26]

PATHOPHYSIOLOGY OF VASOSPASM

The general appreciation of the widespread importance of vasospasm in contributing to angina in many, if not most, patients coincided with the discovery by Furchgott and Zawadzki[15] of the new endothelial-dependent vasodilator system. Since endothelial dysfunction was generally assumed by experimentalists to contribute to the pathogenesis of atherosclerosis, it was thought that this dysfunction might extend broadly and encompass the endothelial dependent vasodilator functions.[27] In other words, atherosclerosis might compromise this dilator system and provide the substrate for abnormal control of vasomotor tone. Thus, vasospasm might result from loss of endothelial-dependent dilator function.

This hypothesis has been tested and found to be true in a variety of clinical studies. Initially, acetylcholine, an endothelial-dependent vasodilator, was shown angiographically to dilate normal coronary arteries and to constrict both minimal and advanced stenoses.[27] The pathophysiological importance of these observations was emphasized by the findings that exercise[28] and cold pressor testing[29] dilated normal coronary arteries but constricted both minimally and advanced stenotic lesions (Figs. 56-2 and 56-3). Endothelial abnormalities were inferred in the exercise studies since acetylcholine and exercise had qualitatively identical effects on segments

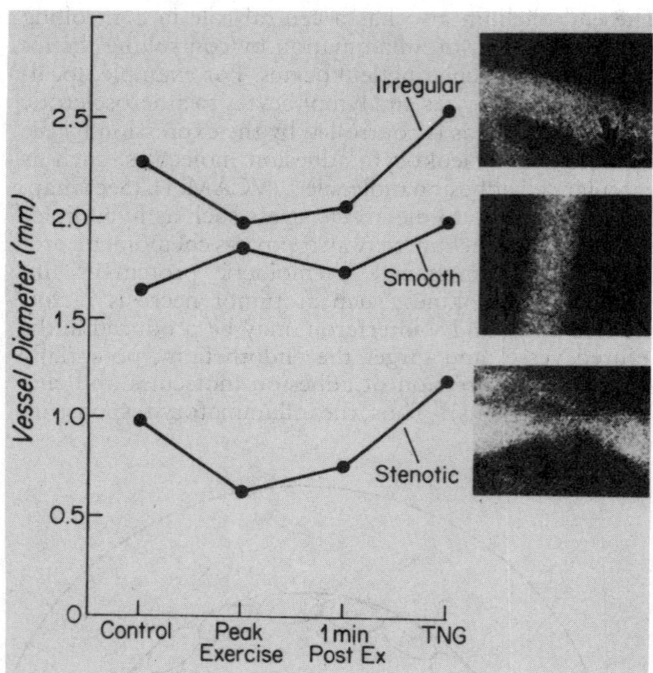

FIGURE 56-2 Exercise-induced changes in vasomotion in diseased and normal coronary arteries. The effects are shown of exercise and nitroglycerin on vessel diameter as determined by quantitative coronary arteriography in a normal coronary segment and in segments with minimal obstruction and advanced stenosis. Exercise induced on the cath table caused constriction of both the irregular segment (upper panel) and the segment with the high grade stenosis (lower panel). In contrast, the segment that is angiographically smooth (middle panel) dilated in response to exercise. Endothelial dysfunction was implicated in these responses since simultaneous studies showed that segments constricting with exercise also constricted in response to acetylcholine, an endothelial-dependent vasodilator. In contrast, segments dilating to exercise dilated in response to acetylcholine. Beta blockade only partially attenuated the vasodilator response to exercise, thus invoking other mechanisms—presumably endothelial-dependent dilatation stimulated by flow. Note that all three segments dilate in response to nitroglycerin, an NO donor, which bypasses the defective endothelial control mechanism and dilates directly the smooth muscle. (From Gordon JB, Ganz P, Nabel EG, Fish RD, Zebede J, Mudge GH, et al: Atherosclerosis influences the vasomotor response of epicardial coronary arteries to exercise. *J Clin Invest* 1989; 83:1946–1952. Reproduced with permission of the publisher and the authors.)

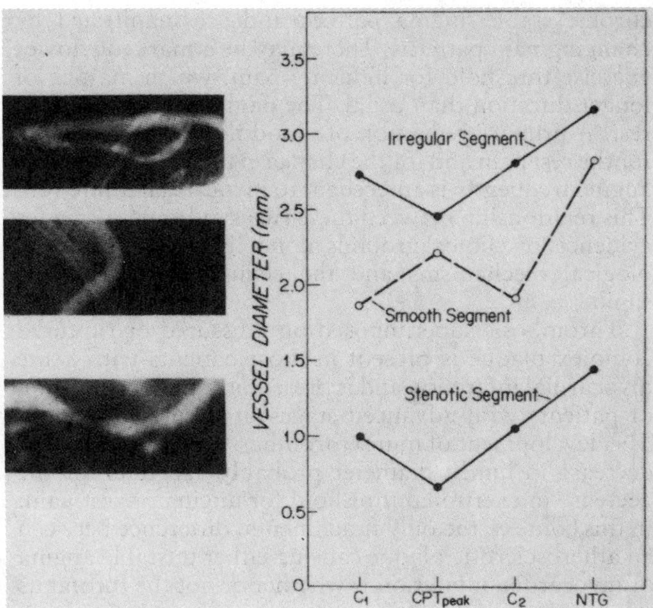

FIGURE 56-3 Effects of stimulation of the sympathetic nervous system by cold presser testing of coronary artery diameter. At catheterization, the sympathetic nervous system was stimulated by the emersion of a hand in an ice slurry for 90 s. The middle panel shows a normal adaptative response to increase diameter at a time when myocardial oxygen consumption is increased, thus contributing to increased flow. This response in a perfectly smooth segment is contrasted with the response in a minimally diseased segment (upper panel) and a segment with advanced stenosis (lower panel). In both of these instances, there was constriction of the artery. In the case of the stenotic segment, this extent of constriction contributed importantly to a decrease in blood flow and might precipitate ischemia. The mechanisms mediating the dilator response undoubtedly include endothelial-dependent stimulation to dilatation caused by an increase in blood flow. The constrictor responses reflect, at least in part, the loss of endothelial-dependent dilatation. As in the case of exercise depicted in Fig. 56–2, nitroglycerin dilates both diseased and normal vessels by delivering nitric oxide directly to the smooth muscle. (*From Nabel EG, Ganz P, Gordon JB, Alexander RW, Selwyn AP: Dilatation of normal and constriction of atherosclerotic coronary arteries caused by the cold pressor test. Circulation 1988; 77:43–52. Reproduced with permission of the publisher and the authors.*)

that dilated or constricted. Furthermore, endothelial-dependent relaxation of coronary arteries becomes defective with the presence of increasing numbers of risk factors, such as smoking and a family history for coronary artery disease, even before disease is angiographically apparent.[30] Recent preliminary studies using B mode scanning of brachial arteries of young people with hypercholesterolemia indicated that flow-mediated dilatation, which is endothelial dependent, is impaired, even at an early age.[31] This endothelial dysfunction is likely the substrate upon which more advanced coronary disease develops. Thus, endothelial-dependent dilation, probably the single most important intrinsic vasodilator system, is defective in atherosclerosis and undoubtedly contributes to the increased vasoconstriction and disordered vasomotor control in the disease.

Enhanced vasoconstrictor tone due to either increased local concentration of vasoconstrictor agonist or increased sensitivity of coronary vascular smooth muscle to vasoconstrictors might also contribute to vasospasm.[32] These possibilities have been somewhat more difficult to prove. The enhanced sensitivity to nonspecific vasoconstrictors, such as ergonovine, and the therapeutic efficacy in angina pectoris of vasodilators, such as calcium-entry blockers, are consistent with the possibility that contraction-mediating mechanisms are augmented in atherosclerosis.

Cellular Mechanisms of Vasospasm

Both the clinical data already cited and data from hypercholesterolemic animals indicate that there is decreased activity of EDRF (NO) released by the endothelium. There are two possible explanations for this: (1) there is a decrease in production of NO; or, (2) alternatively, there is normal or increased production of NO by the endothelial cell with increased degradation to inactive metabolites before it can produce its effect on smooth muscle. There are data in experimental animals showing reversal of the endothelial-dependent vasodilator defect with administration of the NO precursor, the amino acid arginine.[33,34] Other evidence, however, favors the proposition that there is normal, or even increased, production of NO with enhanced degradation leading to decreased vasodilator activity.[35] In hypercholesterolemic rabbits, increased levels of NO metabolites were measured in a setting of decreased EDRF dilator activity. Hypercholesterolemic rabbits have been shown to exhibit dramatic increase in oxygen-free radical production after only 1 month of cholesterol feeding.[36] The idea that free radical degradation of NO contributes to the contractile abnormality in atherosclerosis receives support from experiments on cholesterol-fed rabbits in whichthe defect in endothelial-dependent relaxation was largely reversed by superoxide dismutase, which scavenges the free radicals.[37] In the context of the previously reviewed data indicating that an abnormal redox state with enhanced oxidation in the atherosclerotic artery is central to the molecular mechanisms involved in the pathogenesis of atherosclerosis, the data on contraction are consistent with the presence of enhanced production of oxygen free radicals. Recent in situ hybridization and immunohistochemistry studies of human atherosclerotic lesions indicate increased, not decreased, expression of NO synthase in diseased arteries relative to normal arteries.[35] These clinical and experimental data confirm the existence of a fundamental defect in endothelial-dependent vasodilatation is atherosclerosis. A likely mechanism for this defect is increased degradation of NO by oxygen free radical production that is probably a fundamental characteristic of the disease.

The possibility of increased sensitivity of vascular smooth muscle constrictors as a contributor to vasospasm has been noted. The efficacy of calcium-entry blockers in decreasing vasospasm suggests that there may be abnormal expression of voltage-dependent calcium channels that could enhance contractility. Mechanisms potentially contributing to vasospasm are summarized in Fig. 56-4.

Clinical Implications of Vasospasm

Abnormal control of vasomotor tone with a predominance of vasoconstrictor activity is present in virtually all

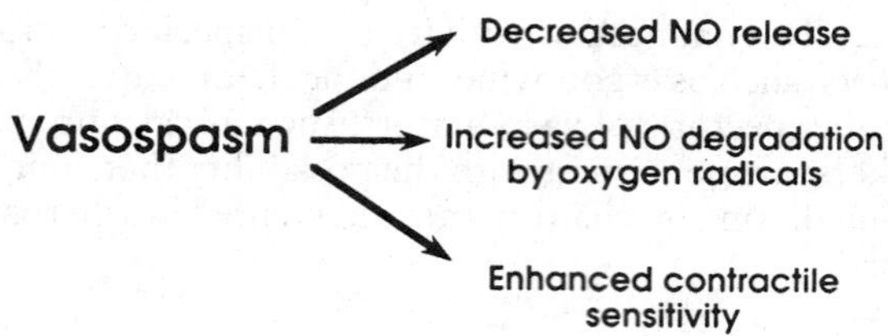

FIGURE 56-4 Mechanisms accounting for vasospasm. Decreased endothelial-dependent vasodilator function is a major contributor to the vasomotor abnormality in most patients with coronary artery disease. This may be associated with decreased nitric oxide release. A considerable amount of data suggests that the endothelium may produce normal, or even increased, amounts of nitric oxide. The vasodilator activity, however, is lost by enhanced degradation by the abnormal redox environment of the diseased artery with increased production of oxygen radicals. There may be also enhanced direct contractile sensitivity of vascular smooth muscle cells in diseased arteries. Increased local concentration of vasoconstrictor agents is possible.

patients with coronary artery disease, and this enhanced vasoconstrictor tone probably accounts for the efficacy of vasodilators, such as nitrates and calcium-entry blockers, in treating angina. The mechanisms defined in animal models involving excessive production of oxygen radicals with degradation of NO are in agreement with the developing concept that one of the fundamental metabolic defects in the atherosclerotic artery is an enhanced oxidative state. Increased understanding of the biology of vasospasm should lead rapidly to therapeutic strategies to treat the primary abnormality of the underlying atherosclerosis. Experience in monkeys demonstrates that the defect in endothelial-dependent relaxation induced by hypercholesterolemia can be reversed by stopping cholesterol feeding which forces serum cholesterol levels to return to their normal values.[39] Thus, lipid lowering may be shown to be an effective therapy to correct the vasomotor control abnormalities in coronary artery disease. In the future, antioxidants may also prove to be effective. Importantly, correction of disordered endothelial-dependent vasomotor abnormalities may provide eventually a therapeutic end-point for evaluating the effectiveness of treatment of atherosclerosis.

UNSTABLE ANGINA AND MYOCARDIAL INFARCTION

These syndromes are considered together because, from a biological point of view, it is likely that the underlying cellular mechanisms in the atherosclerotic plaque are similar, if not identical. The presence of mural thrombus is the common pathological feature uniting the two syndromes.[40] It may be partially or transiently occlusive in unstable angina and totally occlusive for an extended period in myocardial infarction. The syndromes also share the underlying cellular mechanisms associated with conversion of the lesion from the stable state to one that has a propensity to fracture or rupture. (See also Chap. 55.)

Unstable angina and myocardial infarction are episodic events that frequently are superimposed upon a chronic stable angina pattern and are manifested by changing pain patterns. There may be a markedly lower exercise threshold for inducing pain, which may be of longer duration than usual. The pain may also occur at rest. A primary reduction of blood flow likely accounts for the rest pain and for the change in threshold. Unstable angina frequently is antecedent to myocardial infarction. This relationship between these two syndromes provides evidence, on clinical grounds alone, that the pathophysiological mechanisms and the cellular basis must be similar.

Thrombosis superimposed on a fissured or ruptured complex plaque is present in most patients with acute myocardial infarction and is present in a high proportion of patients with advanced stages of unstable angina.[40] The development of mural thrombus with the associated decrease in lumen diameter probably accounts for the decrease in exertional threshold for angina or rest pain. In this context, the only fundamental difference between an atherosclerotic plaque causing either unstable angina or myocardial infarction is whether or not the thrombus is occlusive for a sufficient time to cause tissue death downstream. The thrombus most commonly occurs with disruption of the plaque or desquamation of endothelial cells[41] to expose thrombogenic surfaces and tissue thromboplastins. Clot could theoretically occur with intact endothelium since inflammatory mediators, such as interleukin-1 (IL-1) and tumor necrosis factor, which are expressed in active, inflammatory lesions, can stimulate expression of the procoagulant tissue factor in human endothelial cells in culture.[21] Such a mechanism has not been demonstrated definitively in diseased arteries. Other products of inflammatory cells may contribute to the breakdown of the connective tissue skeleton of the plaque, compromising its structural integrity and predisposing it to fracture and fissuring.

Vasospasm also plays an important role in unstable angina, as already discussed.[25] The constrictor predominance present in stable angina may be enhanced further in the unstable state by increased sensitivity to vasoconstrictors. Furthermore, the presence of clot with thrombin and platelet products such as 5-HT and thromboxane A_2 also may provide increased vasoconstrictor stimuli.[42]

Cellular Mechanisms of Unstable Angina and Myocardial Infarction

One of the more intriguing issues in cardiovascular medicine is why a chronic atherosclerotic lesion is converted to an active state, leading to enhanced vasoconstriction and thrombus formation with the resultant unstable angina and/or myocardial infarction. There is a compelling body of evidence that is consistent with enhanced inflammatory activity in these unstable states. In 1958, Pomerance showed increased inflammatory cell number in the adventitia of the infarct-related artery of patients who had died suddenly, thus minimizing the possibility that inflammatory response was secondary to the infarct.[43] The implication was that the inflammatory cells might, in fact, be a contributing factor. Increased subendothelial infiltration of the coronary arteries with monocytes and macrophages and also increased adventitial inflammatory cell numbers have been observed at autopsy in patients who had unstable angina.[44,45] A recent study showed that pultaceous plaques were frequent at sites of thrombosis and ulceration, and T-cells and macrophages were prominent in other areas.[46] TNF-alpha and IL-2 were expressed in these plaques.

Altered Plaque Structural Integrity

The increased numbers of inflammatory cells and their activation may be related directly to plaque instability, fracture or fissuring, and thrombus formation. Macrophages, for example, may have protean effects on the vessel wall, the understanding of which may provide mechanistic insights into the relationship between the activation of the inflammatory response and development of the unstable coronary syndromes. Interactions between macrophages and lymphocytes are likely to be particularly important. As noted, there are resident macrophages and T-cells in most atherosclerotic lesions.[2] Activation of the inflammatory response by whatever stimulus may precipitate expression of factors that recruit the additional leukocytes into the lesion in unstable angina.[44,45] For example, release of IL-1 or TNF by lymphocytes or macrophages (or endothelium) could increase expression of endothelial adhesion molecules to cause attachment to the overlying endothelium, resulting in movement of additional mononuclear cells into the intima. Similarly, production of chemotactic factors, such as monocyte chemotactic protein-1, which may be stimulated by cytokines, may also contribute to monocyte recruitment.[19] Activation of lymphocytes and macrophages results in release of a number of additional substances that could be directly related to the pathogenesis of the unstable coronary syndromes. The release of oxygen free radicals and formation of H_2O_2, together with the secretion of degradative enzymes such as collagenase and haluronidase, can degrade connective tissue and compromise the structural integrity of the plaque, which, in the stable state with a dense connective tissue skeleton, may be quite resistant to rupture or fissuring. Davies and colleagues have described the fissuring of plaque at sites in the cap where there were increased concentration of macrophages/foam cells.[47] They suggested the macrophages may be degrading the collagen consequently compromising the structural integrity of the plaque at that location. When the plaque does fracture because of compromise of its connective tissue skeletal framework or for other reasons, the clotting factors derived from macrophages and from the lipid core in the vessel wall contribute to lumenal clot formation. As detailed previously, thrombus theoretically might also occur on a morphologically intact endothelium because of the capacity of cytokines to induce tissue factor production by endothelial cells in vitro.[21] Finally the neovascularization of the plaque with thin-walled vessels penetrating from the adventitial surface can lead to rupture, resulting in intramural hemorrhage and thrombus formation with disruption of plaque structure. The cellular events postulated to occur in an "active" atherosclerotic lesion are summarized in Fig. 56-5.

Episodic Thrombosis

Studies by Falk[48] have provided compelling evidence that clot formation in unstable angina is episodic, hence providing a potential explanation for the cyclic nature of the clinical manifestations of the disease. Autopsies of patients with a history of one or more episodes of unstable angina before dying of their ischemic heart disease showed a layering of thrombi of different ages in the epicardial infarct-related artery. Furthermore, downstream from the epicardial lesion, pathological changes were observed ranging from fibrotic areas of healed microinfarctions to recent platelet-rich isoemboli in the microvasculature. These pathological data viewed in the context of the evidence of episodic disease activation clinically suggest that the cyclic nature of the clinical presentation reflects recurrent changes in the biologic state of the atherosclerotic lesion leading to recurrent thrombosis.

According to the above synthesis, plaque rupture, and thus the propensity for infarction, would be a function of the biologic (inflammatory) state of the lesion rather than being closely related to the extent of stenosis. This concept has very important clinical implications as discussed below.

Clinical Implications

The suggestion of an inflammatory cause of the unstable coronary syndromes is based upon the premise that conversion of a stable coronary atherosclerotic lesion to an unstable one may be caused by an activation of the resident and newly recruited monocytes/macrophages and T-cells to cause an enhanced inflammatory response. Thus, it may be that the recurrent nature of the unstable coronary syndromes may be related to the cyclic activation of a chronic inflammatory focus in a manner that might be analogous to the episodic activation of other chronic inflammatory diseases such as rheumatoid arthritis. While the initiating factors for this episodic activation are unknown, and details need to be confirmed, the proposed scenario is consistent with the available evidence about the pathogenesis of atherosclerosis and provides a synthesis and reconciliation with clinical observations.

PRECIPITATING EVENTS FOR LESION ACTIVATION

The mechanisms underlying lesion activation remain obscure. Clearly, the view of the process as having an inflammatory basis provides a conceptual framework for a better understanding. There are several possibilities. First, local mechanisms that are currently not known could initiate inflammatory cell activation and recruitment. Another consideration is the possibility that there is an antigen generated within the lesion that is presented by macrophages to T-cells leading to activation of the inflammatory response (Fig. 56-5). Although there is no firm basis for speculating about any specific antigen, it is interesting to note that oxidized LDL is a potent

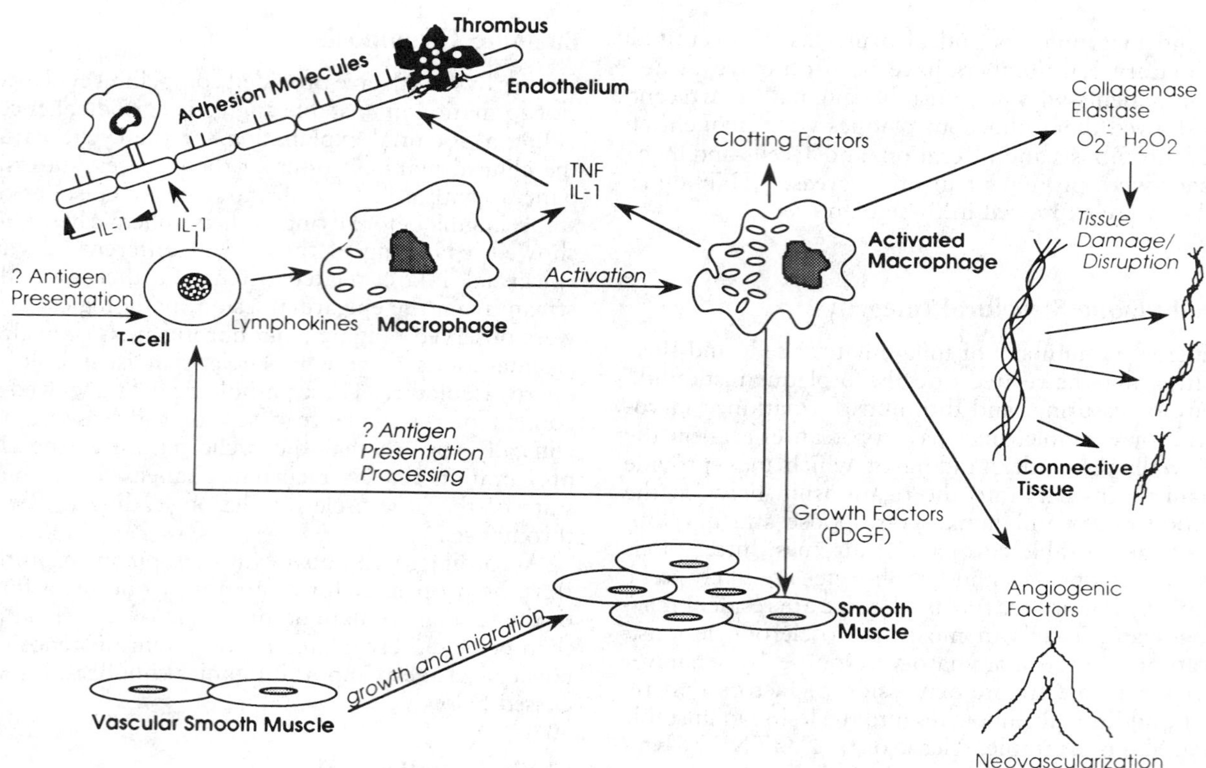

FIGURE 56-5 Postulated cellular mechanism in an "active" atherosclerotic lesion leading to mononuclear cell recruitment, lesion disruption, and clot formation. Activation of the lesion is thought to be associated with enhanced production of growth factors contributing to lesion growth through smooth muscle cell migration and proliferation. It is very likely that there is interaction between resident T cells and macrophages, and this may perhaps involve antigen presentation and/or processing that contributes to activation of the cells. Cytokine production will result in increased adhesion molecule expression and further recruitment of mononuclear cells and lymphocytes. The activated macrophage will produce procoagulant factors and growth factors. Importantly, the activated macrophage is likely to produce proteolytic agents, such as collagenase, elastase, and free radicals, that will lead to tissue damage and disruption. Fracture of the connective tissue can interfere with structural integrity of the plaque, leading to plaque fissuring and mural thrombus formation. The macrophages may also contribute angiogenic factors that increase the neovascularization of the plaque. This may be a source of intramural hemorrhage that can also compromise the structural integrity of the plaque. Decreasing inflammatory response in the plaque will, in the future, be a therapeutic objective, and possibly is a major contributor to the decrease in cardiac event rates that have been reported in lipid-lowering trials.

immunogen[49] and that some patients with atherosclerosis have circulating antibodies against the molecule.[50] At present, oxidized or modified LDL must be considered only a potential candidate antigen for stimulating local inflammation. It is also possible that modified lipids may generate an immune response within an atherosclerotic lesion. Cytokines produced during this activation could markedly affect growth and differentiation of vascular cells and mediate the response to injury.

There are data that raise intriguing questions concerning the possibility of systemic triggers of lesion activation. Spodick has called attention to the frequency with which patients who have had a myocardial infarction have a history of an antecedent febrile illness.[51] More recently, there have been reports that patients suffering acute cardiac events have a statistically significant increase in antibody titers to *Chlamydia pneumoniae* relative to controls.[52] Moreover, other analyses have suggested that chronic infection with *Chlamydia pneumoniae* may be a risk factor for coronary artery disease.[53] It is difficult for one to conceive, at present, of a mechanistic relationship between infection with this particular organism and lesion activation. Precipitation by infectious illness of acute episodes of other inflammatory diseases, such as rheumatoid arthritis, is a well-known phenomenon. In some cases of the unstable coronary syndromes, activation of the resident inflammatory cells in a previously quiescent coronary lesion by an infection triggering systemic inflammatory responses may occur.[54] There is some direct evidence of systemic activation of inflammatory responses during unstable angina. The acute phase reactant, C-reactive protein, has been reported to be elevated in this circumstance.[55] Furthermore, incubation of lymphocytes and mononuclear cells from patients with unstable angina is associated with production of tissue factor-like activity.[56] Tissue factor production was not observed six weeks later when the instability had resolved. Whether or not this evidence of systemic inflammatory response bears a cause and effect relationship to unstable angina remains to be determined. Nonetheless, these data also support the concept that the active coronary syndromes have an inflammatory component.

OVERVIEW

Two major propositions emerge from the synthesis of the clinical and experimental data reviewed here. First,

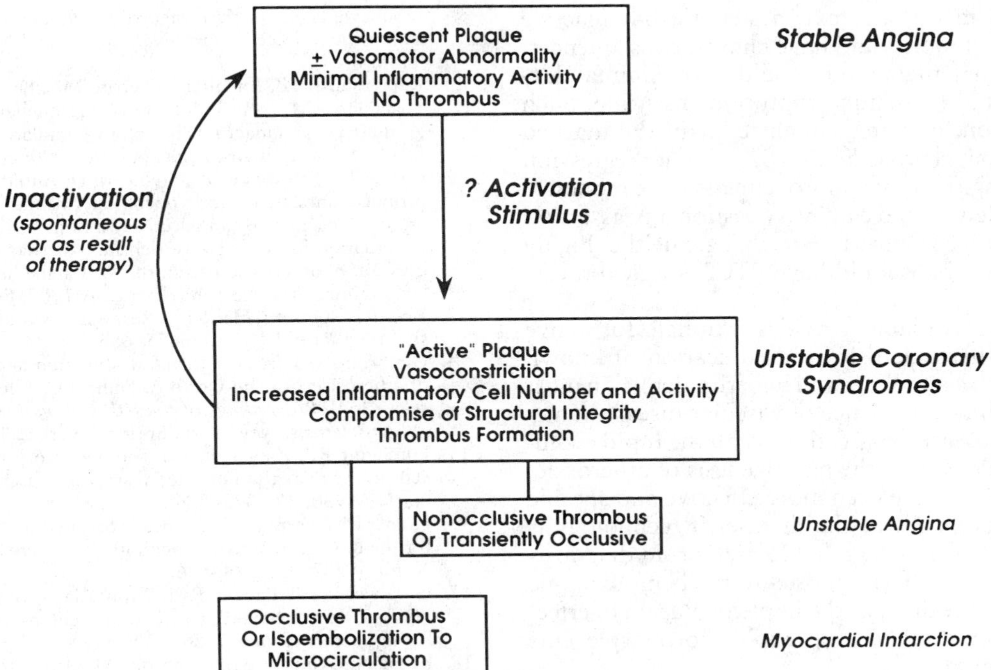

FIGURE 56-6 Cyclic nature of the coronary ischemic syndromes. Stable angina is associated with a plaque that has intact structural integrity and probably minimal inflammatory activity. Resident inflammatory cells are not in an active state. Effort angina is a result of the hemodynamic consequences of lumenal narrowing as well as the loss of endothelial-dependent vasodilator mechanisms that may be chronic. An activation stimulus, the nature of which is not yet understood, likely causes increased inflammatory activity. There is increased recruitment of inflammatory cells, and there is activation of these cells. As a result of the activation, the tendencies for enhanced vasoconstriction become even more prominent. Because of the inflammatory response, there may be compromise of the structural integrity of the plaque that may be associated with fissuring or fracture with thrombus formation. A mural nonocclusive thrombus (or one that is only transiently occlusive) would be associated with unstable angina, whereas prolonged occlusion, or isoembolization, and microvascular occlusion would manifest as myocardial infarction. Inactivation of the plaque inflammatory activity would result in termination of the unstable state. The mechanisms for termination of lesion activity are also unknown but may be analogous to spontaneous inactivation, or quiescence, of inflammatory responses elsewhere. Plaque inactivation may account for the dramatic lowering of cardiac event rates in lipid-lowering regression trials.

the manifestly episodic nature of the ischemic coronary syndromes and, in particular, the unstable syndromes reflects cyclic changes in the cell biology of the atherosclerotic plaque (Fig. 56-6). Second, this cell biology is fundamentally an inflammatory response to metabolic and/or physical injury to, initially, the endothelium. It follows then that the state of inflammatory activity of the lesion is critically important in determining the clinical course, and that the extent of stenosis of a lesion may be of secondary importance as to whether or not a lesion is life threatening. This view is consistent with the observations that the residual infarct-related lesion after thrombolysis sometimes is minimally stenotic,[57,58] and that assessment of location and severity of stenosis angiographically does not permit reliable prediction of the location of subsequent myocardial infarction.[59] This formulation is also consistent with the observations in angiographic coronary regression trials with aggressive lipid lowering regimens. For example, in the Familial Atherosclerosis Treatment Trial, rather modest improvement (2 to 3 percent) in lumenal diameter and/or lack of progression was associated with very substantial (~75 percent) reduction in cardiac event rates for death, myocardial infarction, or requirement for percutaneous transluminal coronary angioplasty (PTCA) or coronary artery bypass grafting.[60] Similarly, in the St. Thomas Atherosclerosis Regression Study (STARS), lowering cholesterol with diet, or diet plus cholestyramine, was associated with about a 75 percent reduction in cardiovascular events over 3 years while showing only modest improvement in lesion diameter or lack of progression.[61] Thus, lipid lowering may favorably affect the biology of coronary lesions making them less prone to activation and more resistant to structural breakdown and thrombus formation. This interpretation is consistent with the view that *the biologic state, or activity, of an atherosclerotic lesion is a more important determinant of clinical course than is the extent of stenosis.*

These observations have considerable clinical significance. If, in fact, the life history of an atherosclerotic plaque is not one of continuous linear growth and lumenal narrowing but, as the evidence suggests, consists of cyclic periods of growth associated with inflammatory activation and enhanced potential for catastrophic clinical events, then therapeutic objectives in the future may focus not so exclusively on the hemodynamic consequences of a lesion but rather on the prevention of lesion activation and on inactivation of an unstable lesion. An inactive lesion would be one with a minimal number of inflammatory cells in a quiescent state with an intact connective tissue framework and a relatively healthy overlying endothelium. This description applies to the coronary artery lesions of monkeys approximately 1 year after cessation of a high cholesterol diet that, during the hypercholesterolemic stage, had been highly cellular with marked impairment of endothelial vasodilator function.[62] Viewed in this context, a stenotic but inactive coronary artery lesion could have clinical consequences, such as exertional angina, but would have minimal devastating potential for plaque rupture or fissuring. Such an interpretation, as noted, might explain the marked reduction of clinical events in FATS, and other regression trials, where angiographic improvements were modest.[60] This point of view would call into question any assertion that patients with coronary lesions that are neither highly stenotic nor unstable should have PTCA surgical revascularization.

The evidence available provides rationale for active treatment of atherosclerosis by modification of known risk factors, such as smoking and hyperlipidemia, in most patients with clinical evidence of vascular disease at any stage of life or disease progression. With the rapid evolution of knowledge about the pathogenesis of atherosclerosis, one can anticipate even more effective and specific therapeutic approaches to the disease. If technology is developed that permits the reliable premorbid diagnosis of atherosclerosis itself as opposed to the hemodynamic consequences of the disease, the implementation of effective therapy should make catastrophic coronary events much less common.

ACKNOWLEDGMENT

I thank Barbara Merchant for her excellent editorial assistance.

REFERENCES

1. Ross R, Masuda J, Raines EW: Cellular interactions, growth factors, and smooth muscle proliferation in atherogenesis. *Ann NY Acad Sci* 1990; 598:102–112.
2. Hansson GK, Jonasson L, Seifert PS, Stemme S: Immune mechanisms in atherosclerosis. *Arteriosclerosis* 1989; 9:567–578.
3. Stemme S, Holm J, Hansson GK: T lymphocytes in human atherosclerotic plaques are memory cells expressing CD45RO and the integrin VLA-1. *Arterioscler Thromb* 1992; 12:206–211.
4. Kamat BR, Galli SJ, Barger AC, Lainey LL, Silverman KJ: Neovascularization and coronary atherosclerotic plaque: Cinematographic localization and quantitative histologic analysis. *Human Pathol* 1987; 18:1036–1042.
5. Munro JM, Cotran RS: The pathogenesis of atherosclerosis: Atherogenesis and inflammation. *Lab Invest* 1988; 58:249–261.
6. Steinberg D, Parthasarathy S, Carew TE, Khoo JC, Witztum JL: Beyond cholesterol. Modifications of low-density lipoprotein that increase its atherogenicity. *N Engl J Med* 1989; 320:915–924.
7. Henriksen T, Mahoney EM, Steinberg D: Enhanced macrophage degradation of low density lipoprotein previously incubated with cultured endothelial cells: Recognition by receptor for acetylated low density lipoprotein. *Proc Natl Acad Sci USA* 1981; 78:6499–6503.
8. Steinbrecher UP, Parthasarathy S, Leake DS, Witztum JL, Steinberg D: Modification of low density lipoprotein by endothelial cells involves lipid peroxidation and degradation of low density lipoprotein phospholipids. *Proc Natl Acad Sci USA* 1984; 81:3883–3887.
9. Fostegard J, Haegerstrand A, Gidlund M, Nilsson J: Biologically modified LDL increases the adhesive properties of endothelial cells. *Atherosclerosis* 1991; 90:112–126.
10. Cushing SD, Berliner JA, Valente AJ, Territo MC, Naval M, Parhami F, et al: Minimally modified low density lipoprotein induces monocyte chemotactic protein-1 in human endothelial cells and smooth muscle cells. *Proc Natl Acad Sci USA* 1990; 85:5134–5138.
11. Rajavashirth TB, Andalibi A, Territo MC, Berliner JA, Navab M, Fogelman AM, et al: Induction of endothelial cell expression of granulocyte and macrophage colony stimulating factors by modified low-density lipoproteins. *Nature* 1990; 344:254–257.
12. Carew TE, Schwenke DC, Steinberg D: Antiatherogenic effect of probucol unrelated to its hypocholesterolemic effect; evidence that antioxidants in vivo can selectively inhibit low density lipoprotein degradation in macrophage-rich fatty streaks and slow the progression of atherosclerosis in the Watanabe heritable hyperlipidemic rabbit. *Proc Natl Acad Sci USA* 1987; 84:7725–7729.
13. Ross R, Glomset J, Harker L: Response to injury and atherogenesis. *Am J Pathol* 1977; 86:675–684.
14. Gimbrone MA Jr: Endothelial dysfunction and the pathogenesis of atherosclerosis. In: Gotto A, Smith LC, Allen B (eds): *Atherosclerosis-V. Proceedings of the Vth International Symposium on Atherosclerosis*. New York, Springer-Verlag, 1980; 415–425.
15. Furchgott RF, Zawadzki JV: The obligatory role of endothelial cells in the relaxation of arterial smooth muscle by acetylcholine. *Nature* 1980; 288:373–376.
16. Palmer RM, Ferrige AG, Moncada S: Nitric oxide release accounts for the biological activity of endothelium-derived relaxing factor. *Nature* 1987; 327:524–526.
17. Gryglewski RJ, Palmer RM, Moncada S: Superoxide anion is involved in the breakdown of endothelium-derived vascular relaxing factor. *Nature* 1986; 320:454–456.
18. Kume N, Cybulsky MI, Gimbrone MA Jr.: Lysophosphatidylcholine, a component of atherogenic lipoproteins, induces mononuclear leukocyte adhesion molecules in cultured human and rabbit arterial endothelial cells. *J Clin Invest* 1992; 90:1138–1144.
19. Cushing SD, Berliner JA, Valente AJ, Territo MC, Navab M, Parhami F, et al: Minimally modified low density lipoprotein induces monocyte chemotactic protein-1 in human endothelial cells and smooth muscle cells. *Proc Natl Acad Sci USA* 1990; 87:5134–5138.
20. Libby P, Hansson GK: Involvement of the immune system in human atherogenesis: current knowledge and unanswered questions. *Lab Invest* 1991; 64:5–15.
21. Bevilacqua MP, Gimbrone MA Jr: Inducible endothelial functions in inflammation and coagulation. *Semin Thromb Hemost* 1987; 13:425–433.
22. Bevilacqua MP, Schleff RR, Gimbrone MA Jr., Loskutoff DJ: Regulation of the fibrinolytic system of cultured human vascular endothelium by interleukin 1. *J Clin Invest* 1986; 78:587–591.
23. Edelman ER, Nugent MA, Smith LT, Karnovsky MJ: Basic fibroblast growth factor enhances the coupling of intimal hyperplasia and proliferation of vaso vasorum in injured rat arteries. *J Clin Invest* 1992; 89:465–473.
24. Deanfield JE, Maseri A, Selwyn AP, Ribeiro P, Chierchia S, Krikler S, et al: Myocardial ischaemia during daily life in patients with stable angina: Its relation to symptoms and heart rate changes. *Lancet* 1983; 2:753–758.
25. Maseri A, Labbate A, Baroldi G, Chierchia S, Marzilli M, Ballestra AM, et al: Coronary vasospasm as a possible cause of myocardial infarction. A conclusion derived from the study of "preinfarction" angina. *N Engl J Med* 1978; 299:1271–1277.
26. Antman E, Muller J, Goldberg S, MacAlpin R, Rubenfire M, Tabatznik B, et al: Nifedipine therapy for coronary artery spasm. *N Engl J Med* 1980; 302:1269–1273.
27. Ludmer PL, Selwyn AP, Shook TL, Wayne RR, Mudge GH, Alexander RW, et al: Paradoxical vasoconstriction induced by acetylcholine in atherosclerotic coronary arteries. *N Engl J Med* 1986; 315:1046–1051.
28. Gordon JB, Ganz P, Nabel EG, Fish RD, Zebede J, Mudge GH, et al: Atherosclerosis influences the vasomotor response of epicardial coronary arteries to exercise. *J Clin Invest* 1989; 83:1946–1952.
29. Nabel EG, Ganz P, Gordon JB, Alexander RW, Selwyn AP: Dilation of normal and constriction of atherosclerotic coronary arteries caused by the cold pressor test. *Circulation* 1988; 77:43–52.
30. Vita JA, Treasure CB, Nabel EG, McLenachan JM, Fish RD, Yeung AC, et al: Coronary vasomotor response to acetylcholine relates to risk factors for coronary artery disease. *Circulation* 1990; 81:491–497.
31. Celermajer DS, Sorensen KE, Gooch VM, Spiegelhalter DJ, Miller OI, Sullivan ID, et al: Non-invasive detection of endothelial dys-

function in children and adults at risk of atherosclerosis. *Lancet* 1992; 340:1111–1115.

32. Ganz P, Alexander RW: New insights into the cellular mechanisms of vasospasm. *Am J Cardiol* 1985; 56:11E–15E.
33. Cooke JP, Singer AH, Tsao P, Zera P, Rowan RA, Billingham ME: Antiatherogenic effects of L-arginine in the hypercholesterolemic rabbit. *J Clin Invest* 1992; 90:1168–1172.
34. Rossitch E Jr., Alexander E 3d., Black PM, Cooke JP: L-arginine normalizes endothelial function in cerebral vessels from hypercholesterolemic rabbits. *J Clin Invest* 1991; 87:1295–1299.
35. Minor RL Jr., Myers P, Guerra R Jr., Bates JN, Harrison DG: Diet-induced atherosclerosis increases the release of nitrogen oxides from rabbit aorta. *J Clin Invest* 1990; 86:2109–2116.
36. Ohara Y, Peterson TE, Harrison DG: Hypercholesterolemia increases endothelial superoxide anion production. *J Clin Invest,* 1993; 91:2546–2551.
37. Mugge A, Elwell JH, Peterson TE, Hofmeyer TG, Heistad DD, Harrison DG: Chronic treatment with polyethylene-glycolated superoxide dismutase partially restores endothelium-dependent vascular relaxations in cholesterol-fed rabbits. *Circulation Research* 1991; 69:1293–1300.
38. Sundell CL, Marsden PA, Subramanian RR, Pollock JS, Harrison DG, Wilcox JN: Nitric oxide synthase is expressed by endothelial cells overlying human atherosclerotic plaques. *Circulation* 1992; 86:I–473.
39. Freiman PC, Mitchell GG, Heistad DD, Armstrong ML, Harrison DG: Atherosclerosis impairs endothelium-dependent vascular relaxation to acetylcholine and thrombin in primates. *Circulation Research* 1986; 58:783–789.
40. Mizuno K, Stomura K, Miyamoto A, Arakawa K, Shibuya T, Arai T, et al: Angioscopic evaluation of coronary-artery thrombi in acute coronary syndromes. *N Engl J Med* 1992; 326:287–291.
41. Sherman CT, Litvack F, Grundfest W, Lee M, Hickey A, Chaux A, et al: Coronary angioscopy in patients with unstable angina pectoris. *N Engl J Med* 1986; 315:913–919.
42. Willerson JT, Yao SK, McNatt J, Benedict CR, Anderson HV, Golino P, et al: Frequency and severity of cyclic flow alternations and platelet aggregation predict the severity of neointimal proliferation following experimental coronary stenosis and endothelial injury. *Proc Natl Acad Sci (USA)* 1991; 88:10624–10628.
43. Pomerance A: Periarterial mast cells in coronary atheroma and thrombosis. *J Pathol Bacteriol* 1958; 76:55–70.
44. Sato T, Takebayashi S, Kohchi K: Increased subendothelial infiltration of the coronary arteries with monocytes/macrophages in patients with unstable angina. *Atherosclerosis* 1987; 68:191–197.
45. Kohchi K, Takebayashi S, Hiroki T, Nobuyoshi M: Significance of adventitial inflammation of the coronary artery in patients with unstable angina: Results at autopsy. *Circulation* 1985; 71:709–716.
46. Arbustini E, Grasso M, Diegoli M, Pucci A, Bramerio M, Ardissino D, et al: Coronary atherosclerotic plaques with and without thrombus in ischemic heart syndromes: A morphologic, immunohistochemical, and biochemical study. *Am J Cardiol* 1991; 68:36B–50B.
47. Richardson PD, Davies MJ, Born GV: Influence of plaque configuration and stress distribution of fissuring of coronary atherosclerotic plaques. *Lancet* 1989; 2:941–944.
48. Falk E: Unstable angina with fatal outcome: Dynamic coronary thrombosis leading to infarction and/or sudden death. Autopsy evidence of recurrent mural thrombosis with peripheral embolization culminating in total vascular occlusion. *Circulation* 1985; 71:699–708.
49. Palinski W, Yla-Herttuala S, Rosenfeld ME, Butler SW, Socher SA, Parthasarathy S, et al: Antisera and monoclonal antibodies specific for epitopes generated during oxidative modification of low density lipoprotein. *Arteriosclerosis* 1990; 10:325–335.
50. Salonen JT, Yla-Herttuala S, Yamamoto R, Butler S, Korpela H, Salonen R, et al: Autoantibody against oxidised LDL and progression of carotid atherosclerosis. *Lancet* 1992; 339:883–887.
51. Spodick DH: Infection and infarction. Acute viral (and other) infection in the onset, pathogenesis and mimicry of acute myocardial infarction. *Am J Med* 1986; 81:661–668.
52. Saikku P, Leinonen M, Tenkanen L, Linnanmaki E, Ekman MR, Manninen V, et al: Chronic *Chlamydia pneumoniae* infections as a risk factor for coronary heart disease in the Helsinki Heart Study. *Ann Intern Med* 1992; 116:273–278.
53. Thom DH, Wang SP, Grayston JT, Siscovick DS, Stewart DK, Kronmal RA, et al: Chlamydia pneumoniae strain TWAR antibody and angiographically demonstrated coronary heart disease. *Arterioscler Thromb* 1991; 11:547–551.
54. Valtonen VV: Infection as a risk factor for infarction and atherosclerosis. *Ann Med* 1991; 23:539–543.
55. Berk BC, Weintraub WS, Alexander RW: Elevation of C-reactive protein in "active" coronary artery disease. *Am J Cardiol* 1990; 65:168–172.
56. Serveri GG, Abbate R, Gori AM, Attanasio M, Martini F, Giusti B, et al: Transient intermittent lymphocyte activation is responsible for the instability of angina. *Circulation* 1992; 86:790–797.
57. Ganz W, Buchbinder N, Marcus H, Mondkar A, Maddahi J, Charuzi Y, et al: Intracoronary thrombolysis in evolving myocardial infarction. *Am Heart J* 1981; 101:4–13.
58. Hackett D, Davies G, Maseri A: Pre-existing coronary stenoses in patients with first myocardial infarction are not necessarily severe. *Eur Heart J* 1988; 9:1317–1323.
59. Little WC, Constantinescu M, Applegate RJ, Kutcher MA, Burrows MT, Kahl FR, et al: Can coronary angiography predict the site of a subsequent myocardial infarction in patients with mild to moderate coronary artery disease? *Circulation* 1988; 78:1157–1166.
60. Brown G, Albers JJ, Fisher LD, Schaefer SM, Lin JT, Kaplan C, et al: Regression of coronary artery disease as a result of intensive lipid-lowering therapy in men with high levels of apolipoprotein B. *N Engl J Med* 1990; 323:1289–1298.
61. Watts GF, Lewis B, Brunt JNH, Lewis ES, Coltart DJ, Smith LDR, et al: Effect on coronary artery disease of lipid-lowering diet, or diet plus cholestyramine, in the St. Thomas Atherosclerosis Regression Study (STARS). *Lancet* 1992; 339:563–569.
62. Harrison DG, Armstrong ML, Freiman PC, Heistad DD: Restoration of endothelium-dependent relaxation by dietary treatment of atherosclerosis. *J Clin Invest* 1987; 80:1808–1811.

Chapter 57

Pathophysiology of Myocardial Ischemia

Stephen M. Factor, M.D. ■ *Robert J. Bache, M.D.*

PATHOPHYSIOLOGY OF MYOCARDIAL ISCHEMIA

The heart functions almost exclusively as an aerobic organ with little capacity for anaerobic metabolism. Even during resting conditions 70 to 80 percent of the oxygen in the blood perfusing the coronary arteries is extracted by the myocardium.[1] Because there is little capacity to increase oxygen availability by increasing oxygen extraction, increases of myocardial demands during exercise or other stress must be met by equivalent increases of coronary blood flow. Myocardial ischemia results when the arterial blood supply fails to meet the needs of the heart muscle for oxygen and metabolic substrate. Since direct measurements of myocardial blood flow are not generally available in the clinical setting, myocardial ischemia is recognized by the consequences that it produces. Even limited ischemia is likely to be evident from anginal pain, electrocardiographic and metabolic changes, and a decrease in cardiac diastolic and contractile function, while severe sustained ischemia is likely to result in myocardial infarction. Persistent systolic dysfunction resulting from cumulative and recurrent ischemia may result in left ventricular failure. (See also Chap. 58.)

Primary Causes of Myocardial Ischemia

Under normal circumstances coronary blood flow closely parallels myocardial metabolic demands despite wide fluctuations in oxygen consumption of the heart.[1] Cardiac metabolism appears unable to outstrip its blood supply in normal individuals, even at extreme limits of activity, so that excessive demand is never a primary cause of ischemia.[2,3] The most frequently recognized cause of myocardial ischemia is occlusive coronary atherosclerosis, which either causes direct arterial narrowing or produces coronary obstruction by inducing thrombus formation. Coronary narrowing may also occur secondary to stenosis of the coronary ostia produced by primary disease of the aorta, coronary embolism, inflammatory disease of the coronary arteries, and congenital syndromes such as anomalous origin of a coronary artery from the pulmonary artery. Vasoconstriction of an epicardial artery at the site of an atherosclerotic plaque may significantly aggravate obstruction to blood flow.[4] Coronary artery spasm, either in an angiographically normal coronary artery or at the site of an atherosclerotic plaque, may transiently interrupt blood flow and produce severe transmural myocardial ischemia.[5] In occasional individuals small coronary vessel constriction may limit myocardial blood flow and lead to ischemia during exercise or other stress.[6] Regardless of the precise cause, a limited arterial blood supply is common to both mild or incipient ischemia and to severe ischemia, so that factors that determine blood flow will be central foci in the consideration of myocardial ischemia. Consequently, it is appropriate to review the mechanisms responsible for normal regulation of coronary blood flow. (See also Chap. 5.)

Coronary Autoregulation

A fundamental property of the coronary circulation is the almost complete independence of blood flow from changes in perfusion pressure. If cardiac function and the composition of arterial blood remain constant, steady-state values of coronary blood flow are remarkably constant.[7] Coronary perfusion pressure is normally identical to aortic pressure and is maintained, within narrow limits by arterial baroreceptor activity. When an atheroma causes coronary artery narrowing, pressure distal to the obstruction is reduced by the resistance of the obstruction, but ischemia is avoided by a compensatory decrease in resistance in the distal arteriolar bed.[8] This autoregulatory response is a fundamental mechanism for maintaining myocardial perfusion in the presence of occlusive coronary artery disease.

The mechanism that allows coronary flow to be independent of perfusion pressure is probably identical to the mechanism that adjusts the tone of the coronary vessels relative to the metabolic needs of the myocardium. The precise relationship between coronary blood flow and myocardial metabolism suggests that coronary autoregulation involves a metabolite. Attention has been directed toward chemicals that induce relaxation of coronary vascular smooth muscle. When flow is insufficient, a metabolite may accumulate in the myocardium, reduce vascular tone, and thus restore normal flow. The most carefully documented paradigm for this type of negative-feedback control of the coronary circulation is the adenosine hypothesis (Fig. 57-1). This hypothesis proposes that adenosine, a powerful coronary vasodilator, is continuously released into the interstitial fluid by the myocardial cells and that its release is enhanced in response to either an increase in myocardial metabolism or a reduction in arterial blood supply.[9] An increase in the interstitial fluid adenosine decreases the resistance of the coronary vessels, augments flow, and thus restores the balance between supply and demand. (See also Chap. 2.)

These considerations, although appealing in their simplicity, probably obscure a series of complex, integrated feedback loops involved in vascular control. There may be significantly different control mechanisms for vessels that are normal vs. diseased. There are numerous mediators of vascular tone: These include those derived from or dependent on endothelium, adrenergic receptors, prostaglandins, serotonin, platelets, and possibly even cholesterol.[10–13] (See also Chap. 56.)

Effect of Myocardial Contraction on Coronary Blood Flow

Unlike other organs in which blood flow varies directly with arterial driving pressure so that greatest flow occurs in systole when arterial pressure is highest, in the heart systolic contraction throttles blood flow, so that coronary flow normally occurs predominantly during diastole.[14] Impedance to coronary blood flow produced by the contracting myocardium is not uniform across the left ventricular wall. Thus, when coronary inflow is limited to systole, a steep transmural gradient of perfusion occurs, with selective reduction of flow to the subendocardium.[15,16] Impedance to blood flow produced by the contracting myocardium could result from shearing forces within the left ventricular wall that could pinch off intramural vessels or from the compressing effects of the myocardium acting on vessels within the left ventricular wall. Shearing forces have been found to account for only a small fraction of the total systolic impedance to coronary flow.[17] Furthermore, the effects of shearing forces on coronary flow are uniform transmurally, and so could not explain the progressively increasing impedance to flow from epicardium to endocardium produced by cardiac contraction.[17] (See also Chap. 5.)

During systole the left ventricular subendocardium is exposed to cavitary pressure, while the subepicardium is exposed to intrathoracic pressure. It is not surprising that myocardial perfusion during systole would reflect this pressure difference across the left ventricular wall. Although the magnitude and pattern of intramyocardial pressure within the wall is uncertain, it is clear that effective intramyocardial pressure is highest in the subendocardial myocardium and falls progressively in the more superficial myocardial layers.[18] The blood vessels within the left ventricular wall act as collapsible tubes, and flow in collapsible tubes is inhibited in direct proportion to the magnitude of the external forces compressing the vessels. This phenomenon is termed the *vascular waterfall* and explains the increasing impedance to blood flow during systole in proportion to the depth of the muscle layer.[19] Impedance to blood flow produced by the

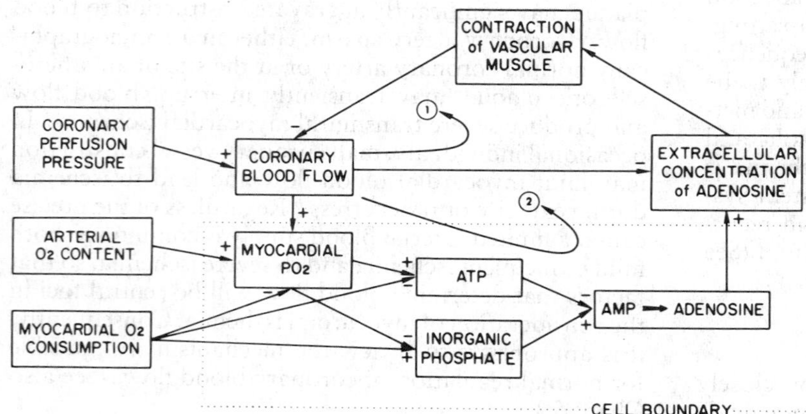

FIGURE 57-1 Diagram of feedback mechanism of regulation of coronary blood flow by adenosine.[1] Each variable is characterized as to its effect, that is, whether it increases (+) or decreases (−) the variable it acts on. In this type of diagram, negative feedback is characterized by having an odd number of negative signs in the feedback loop. Two negative-feedback loops involving coronary blood flow are indicated: involving (1) only extracellular variables and (2) intracellular variables. In this diagram the balance between supply and demand is represented in terms of delivery and utilization of oxygen.[1]

vascular waterfall is additive to vasomotor tone in the coronary resistance vessels, but even during maximal coronary vasodilation the extravascular component of coronary resistance in the beating heart remains 25 to 35 percent of total coronary resistance.[19] With maximal coronary vasodilation, the extravascular compressive forces become the principal determinant of the transmural distribution of blood flow and may significantly influence the balance of supply and demand in the subendocardium.[20] Systole does not normally inhibit the blood supply to the right ventricle, since right ventricular intracavitary pressure (and thus tissue pressure) remains well below coronary perfusion pressure throughout the cardiac cycle.[21] In pulmonary hypertension, however, the increased right ventricular systolic pressure may impede blood flow in a manner similar to that in the left ventricle.[22] During acute severe elevation of right ventricular systolic pressure secondary to acute pulmonary artery obstruction, systolic impairment of right ventricular myocardial blood flow may contribute to the development of right ventricular failure by limiting right ventricular blood flow and contributing to the development of ischemia.[22,23] (See also Chap. 99.)

Subendocardial Ischemia

In the normal heart, blood flow to the subendocardium is maintained equal to or greater than subepicardial flow, reflecting slightly greater systolic stress development and oxygen consumption in the subendocardium.[24] Maintenance of uniform transmural myocardial blood flow despite systolic underperfusion in the subendocardium indicates that a perfusion gradient favoring the subendocardium must exist during diastole. This diastolic gradient of blood flow favoring the subendocardium requires that the resistance vessels maintain a greater state of vasodilation in the subendocardium than in the subepicardium. Because of the need for greater vasodilation of the subendocardial resistance vessels during basal conditions, the vasodilator reserve available to increase flow during periods of stress is least in this region.[25] As noted below, this loss of coronary vasodilator reserve is even more marked in the presence of left ventricular hypertrophy. (See also Chap. 58.)

In response to a proximal arterial stenosis, the distal coronary vessels undergo vasodilation to compensate for the resistance offered by the stenosis in an attempt to maintain adequate myocardial blood flow.[8] This compensatory vasodilation of the resistance vessels compromises the capacity for additional vasodilation during subsequent increases of myocardial oxygen demands. The degree of coronary artery stenosis that elicits maximal vasodilation of the resistance vessels is termed a *critical stenosis*, since any further reduction of luminal area will cause a decrease in coronary blood flow. In the presence of a critical stenosis, an increase of myocardial oxygen demands cannot be met by an increase in coronary blood flow, since the distal vasculature has fully utilized its vasodilator capability. (See also Chaps. 2 and 56.)

When blood flow is limited by a proximal stenosis rather than by the coronary resistance vessels, myocardial hypoperfusion and ischemia occur preferentially in the subendocardium. Redistribution of blood flow away from the subendocardium is the result of several interrelated pathophysiological mechanisms that occur when arterial inflow is insufficient to meet myocardial demands. First, since vasodilator reserve is least in the subendocardium, maximal vasodilation occurs first in this region, so that further reductions of perfusion pressure distal to the stenosis cannot be met by further vasodilation.[25] In contrast, residual vasodilator reserve may still exist in the subepicardium, allowing further vasodilation in this region to maintain blood flow. Second, the presence of a flow-limiting coronary stenosis alters the phasic pattern of coronary blood flow. Since the stenosis limits maximum blood flow rates through the proximal artery, and since maximal coronary flow rates occur in diastole, the influence of the stenosis is to preferentially decrease flow in diastole while allowing a greater fraction of flow to occur in systole.[26] Because cardiac contraction selectively impedes blood flow to the subendocardium, the increased systolic component of flow is delivered preferentially to the subepicardium. Finally, at the very low levels of perfusion pressure that exist distal to a flow-limiting coronary stenosis, extravascular forces may influence the transmural distribution of blood flow during diastole.[27] Since diastolic extravascular pressure is highest in the subendocardium, interaction between this compressive force and the low intravascular distending pressure that exists distal to a flow-limiting coronary stenosis preferentially impedes perfusion of the subendocardium. This effect is augmented with the onset of ischemia, because of the ischemia-induced increase in diastolic intracavitary pressure secondary to decreased myocardial compliance. The subendocardium is especially susceptible to ischemia because not only is this region most vulnerable to hypoperfusion, but oxygen requirements are greatest in the subendocardium owing to the greater systolic tension development in this region.[24]

Myocardial Oxygen Supply

Myocardial oxygen supply can be approximated by the product of myocardial blood flow and arterial oxygen content. Precise evaluation of myocardial oxygen supply, however, must be made at the level of the capillary bed. As oxygen diffuses from the capillaries to the mitochondria within the myocardial cells, ischemia occurs when the partial pressure of oxygen (P_{O_2}) falls below a critical level at the mitochondria. In broad terms, this level is equal to that required to rephosphorylate the adenosine triphosphate (ATP) load being utilized by myocardial work.[28] In vitro experiments have shown that the critical level of P_{O_2} in the mitochondria is much less than the lowest levels of P_{O_2} observed in coronary venous blood. The discrepancy between critical levels of intracellular P_{O_2} and coronary venous P_{O_2} suggests that the diffusion of oxygen from the capillary bed has a decisive role in myocardial oxygen supply.[29]

Anatomic evidence of closed metarterioles and precapillary sphincters in the beating heart indicates that myocardial capillaries are not all functional at all times.[30] These findings are supported by physiological evidence of variability of blood flow to different regions of the heart (spatial heterogeneity) and, in any given region, variability of blood flow with time (temporal heterogeneity).[31,32] Analysis of these findings in terms of a diffusion model for oxygen suggests that changes in the number of open capillaries may be as important in maintaining myocardial P_{O_2} as changes in coronary vascular resistance.[29] With myocardial ischemia all of the available capillaries are likely to be recruited so that the diffusion of oxygen is limited by the anatomic capillary density. Myocardial capillaries parallel myocytes with a ratio of approximately one capillary for each myocardial cell, which places each cell in contact with three to four capillaries.[33] This ratio of one capillary per myocyte remains constant in adults and is unchanged with cardiac hypertrophy.[33,34] The decreased capillary density may contribute to increased vulnerability to ischemia in the hypertrophied heart.[35] Other factors that limit exchange between myocardium and blood, such as myocardial edema, fibrosis, capillary obstruction by microemboli, or precapillary vasoconstriction, could also contribute to development of myocardial ischemia. Decreases in arterial oxygen content (which can result from a variety of causes including anemia, hypoxia, and carbon monoxide poisoning) reduce myocardial oxygen supply and would also precipitate ischemia if not compensated for by an increase in flow.

Coronary Vasoconstriction

In the normal heart the proximal coronary arteries contribute only a small fraction of total vascular resistance so that normal vasomotor activity can occur without significantly affecting blood flow. In the presence of atheromatous disease, however, a significant portion of the total resistance to blood flow may reside at the proximal coronary artery. Approximately 70 percent of coronary atheromata are eccentric in location, leaving the remaining circumference of the artery able to undergo vasomotor changes.[36] In this situation even modest degrees of coronary vasomotion may markedly influence the resistance offered by the proximal stenosis. Thus, coronary vasoconstriction produced by alpha-adrenergic activity or circulating vasoactive peptides that would be benign in a normal coronary artery could significantly impair blood flow when the lumen is nearly obstructed by disease.[37] In addition to this modest vasoconstrictor activity, in occasional susceptible individuals coronary artery spasm may occur in either an angiographically normal or atheromatous coronary artery to produce the severe primary reduction of coronary blood characteristic of Prinzmetal's variant angina.[5]

The vascular endothelium contributes importantly to modulation of vasomotor tone in the coronary arterial system. Furchgott and Zawadski[38] demonstrated that acetylcholine caused relaxation of isolated coronary artery rings when the endothelium was intact but contraction if the endothelium was removed. Subsequent studies have demonstrated that a number of agents including acetylcholine, bradykinin, and histamine cause coronary vasodilation indirectly by engaging specific receptors on the endothelium that then cause release of an endogenous vasodilator termed endothelium-derived relaxing factor (EDRF).[39] Endothelium-derived relaxing factor appears to be nitric oxide, or a closely related compound with a very short half-life, which is produced by the endothelial cells and diffuses to the underlying smooth muscle to cause vasodilation.[40] The shearing force of the flowing blood also modulates EDRF production, forming a mechanism by which the proximal coronary arteries undergo vasodilation in response to the increased blood flow during exercise or other stress.[41] Normal EDRF production is impaired or lost in atherosclerotic coronary arteries.[42] This has been demonstrated by the finding that the vasodilator response to intraarterial acetylcholine, which is observed in patients with angiographically normal coronary arteries, is converted to vasoconstriction in patients with atherosclerotic coronary artery disease.[43] In addition to vasodilator factors, the endothelium produces vasoconstrictor peptides called endothelins.[44] Although circulating endothelin levels are increased in myocardial infarction and shock, the role of these agents in control of the coronary circulation is at present unclear. Nevertheless, it is likely that endothelial dysfunction, especially with failure of normal EDRF production, contributes to abnormal vasoconstrictor activity in some patients with coronary atherosclerosis. (See also Chaps. 2 and 56.)

It has generally been assumed that during ischemia local metabolic influences would cause maximal vasodilation of the coronary resistance vessels. Recent studies in experimental animals, however, have demonstrated residual vasomotor tone even in the presence of a coronary artery stenosis sufficiently severe to cause myocardial hypoperfusion, lactate production, and depression of contractile function.[45] Small-vessel vasoconstriction in ischemic myocardium is mediated, at least in part, by alpha-adrenergic activity.[46] Coronary resistance vessels in regions of ischemic myocardium also retain ability to respond to other vasoconstrictors including thromboxane A_2.[47] It is thus possible that sympathetic influences or vasoconstrictors released in the proximal coronary artery by activated platelets could worsen myocardial hypoperfusion by causing vasoconstriction of the distal coronary resistance vessels. (See also Chap. 55.)

Coronary Collateral Blood Flow

With total occlusion of a major coronary artery, severe ischemia and infarction of the dependent myocardium will occur unless alternative arterial pathways exist. Although the normal human heart has preexisting connections between distal coronary artery branches, these native collateral vessels are usually insufficient to prevent infarction. In response to gradual obstruction of a coronary artery, however, collateral vessels may undergo sufficient growth to maintain or restore an adequate blood supply to the dependent myocardium. Transformation of the native rudimentary intercoronary anastomotic channels into mature collateral vessels involves a complex sequence of vessel injury, inflammation, and cellular proliferation.[48] Within the first 2 to 3 days after coronary occlusion, the small preexisting collateral vessels show extensive damage with rupture of the internal elastic lamina and appear as thin-walled, overstretched arterioles. This period of early transformation is marked by extensive perivascular inflammation with infiltration of monocytes and macrophages. Mitotic activity is seen in endothelial and smooth-muscle cells, with prominent intimal proliferation and subintimal hyperplasia. As growth continues and inflammation subsides, the collateral channels take on an organized smooth-muscle coat, so that within 6 to 12 months after coronary occlusion they are similar in appearance to small arteries of comparable size.[48] As would be inferred from their appearance, these mature collateral channels do not function as passive conduits but have considerable vasomotor capability. Thus, developed collateral channels have been shown to undergo vasoconstriction in response to the vasoactive peptides angiotensin II and vasopressin and vasodilation in response to nitroglycerin and atrial natriuretic peptide.[49] In addition, collateral vessels undergo vasoconstriction in response to serotonin and thromboxane A_2, suggesting that these platelet products may be capable of impairing perfusion of collateral-dependent myocardium.[50]

There is considerable evidence that a functioning coronary collateral system can provide protection against myocardial ischemia in humans. Pathologic studies have shown that approximately 20 percent of all chronic total coronary artery occlusions found at autopsy are not associated with infarction of the dependent myocardium.[51] Presumably, in these patients coronary occlusion proceeded gradually, allowing sufficient time for an effective collateral circulation to develop before total occlusion occurred. Both in experimental animals and in patients, even acute coronary occlusion frequently does not result in infarction of all of the dependent myocardium. Preservation of myocardium in the ischemic region is quantitatively related to the degree of coronary collateral inflow.[52] In patients undergoing angioplasty, the presence of well-developed collateral vessels minimized or prevented the development of a regional left ventricular wall motion abnormality during occlusion of the coronary artery with the angioplasty balloon.[53] Similarly, in patients undergoing thrombolytic therapy to interrupt the course of acute myocardial infarction, an effective coronary collateral system has been shown to delay the progression of ischemic injury, thereby extending the period during which reperfusion can result in salvage of ischemic myocardium.[54]

The usual stimulus for development of an effective coronary collateral circulation is the presence of high-grade occlusive coronary artery disease. Cohen et al.[55] demonstrated that angiographically well-developed collateral vessels are found regularly only in patients with greater than 80 percent stenosis of a major coronary artery. Although the rate of development of collateral vessels in response to high-grade coronary artery stenosis is unknown, approximately three-quarters of patients suffering acute myocardial infarction develop angiographically well-functioning collaterals within 2 to 5 weeks after acute coronary occlusion.[56] The rate of collateral vessel development in response to stenotic lesions may proceed at a slower rate. McHenry et al.[57] have provided evidence that antecedent exercise-induced myocardial ischemia can modify the syndrome that occurs in response to total coronary occlusion. Thus, when apparently healthy individuals with a previously positive exercise stress test experienced a coronary event, they were likely to suffer the onset of new or unstable angina, whereas similar individuals with a previously normal stress test were more likely to suffer myocardial infarction or sudden death. This finding suggests that the presence of a coronary stenosis sufficient to result in an ischemic response during exercise was also sufficient to cause development of coronary collateral vessels, which then exerted a protective influence when the coronary stenosis went to total occlusion. These observations indicate that development of a functioning collateral circulation is an effective long-term adaptation to occlusive coronary artery disease.

Although well-developed coronary collateral vessels can provide an alternative arterial blood supply to maintain perfusion of the dependent myocardium during resting conditions, patients with viable but collateral dependent myocardium will commonly have evidence of stress-induced myocardial ischemia. Collateral perfusion may be further compromised by disease in the coronary artery supplying the collateral vessels. When collateral channels are unable to increase blood flow adequately to the dependent myocardium during exercise, the distribution of blood flow will be similar to that observed when perfusion is limited by an arterial stenosis, with ischemia occurring preferentially in the subendocardium.[58] The maximum capacity for blood flow through collateral channels is not fixed but may be increased in response to collateral vasodilators such as nitroglycerin, while exercise capacity may be decreased following administration of collateral vasoconstrictors such as vasopressin.[59]

Coronary Steal

Under certain conditions an increase in blood flow in one region of the myocardium can decrease flow in another region as the result of *coronary steal*. The conditions necessary for coronary steal include (1) a common coronary artery having some resistance to flow that supplies two myocardial regions in parallel and (2) vasodilatation in only one of the two parallel regions.[60] The key to interpreting coronary steal is the coronary pressure at the point where the common vessel branches into the parallel circulations. A decrease in pressure at this point will decrease flow in the already vasodilated passive circulation. This occurs when flow increases through the common vessel as a result of vasodilatation in the active circulation.

The resistance of the common supply vessel is a critical determinant of the potential for coronary steal.[60] If the proximal artery has minimal resistance, large increases in flow will cause only minor decreases in pressure at the branch point. Conversely, if resistance in the proximal artery is markedly increased by occlusive atherosclerotic disease, autoregulation will recruit increasing portions of the vasodilator reserve in both distal branches and diminish the potential for steal.[8] Thus, there appears to be an optimal degree of common coronary resistance corresponding to some degree of partial coronary obstruction. Although vasodilatation in one of two parallel regions is often used as evidence of coronary steal, small concomitant decreases in resistance in the common vessel or in the other parallel vascular bed could completely offset the tendency for a flow reduction. This possibility may be difficult to exclude whenever a coronary steal mechanism is considered to result from a coronary vasodilator drug. Drugs such as nitroglycerin elicit a selective long-acting vasodilation in larger coronary vessels and therefore tend to prevent coronary steal. The drugs with the greatest potential for eliciting coronary steal are those that override the normal autoregulatory mechanisms, such as dipyridamole.

The conditions governing collateral blood flow are frequently conducive to the development of coronary steal. Collateral blood flow always occurs in parallel with flow to an adjacent normally perfused region, and often the adjacent region has a large vasodilator reserve.[61] In fact, steal of collateral blood can be ruled out following a stimulus for small-vessel vasodilation only if both regions are ischemic or if the collateral vessels are so well developed that no ischemia occurs. On the other hand, when a critical level of collateral blood flow results in a region's being balanced on the verge of ischemia, changes in demand or effective coronary perfusion pressure could be more significant determinants of myocardial ischemia than changes in supply caused by a steal mechanism.

Left Ventricular Hypertrophy

Left ventricular hypertrophy confers an increased risk for the development of myocardial ischemia. In hypertensive patients left ventricular hypertrophy detected echocardiographically is associated with a substantially increased incidence of angina pectoris, myocardial infarction, and sudden death.[62] In dogs with left ventricular hypertrophy secondary to renovascular hypertension acute coronary artery occlusion results in larger infarcts and a greater incidence of sudden death than in normal animals.[63] A coronary stenosis that results in similar reductions of distal pressure produces more severe subendocardial ischemia during exercise in animals with left ventricular hypertrophy than in normal animals.[64]

Increased vulnerability to ischemia results from both structural and functional abnormalities in the hypertrophied heart. Although both epicardial arteries and intramural vessels increase in size during hypertrophy, this vascular growth appears to be less than would be expected from the increase in myocardial mass.[63] In agreement with this, studies in both human subjects and experimental animals with chronic pressure overload have demonstrated impaired coronary vasodilator reserve in the hypertrophied left ventricle.[65] The capillary-to-myocyte ratio remains near unity during hypertrophy, so that intercapillary diffusion distances for oxygen are increased in proportion to the increased myocyte diameter.[34] In addition to these structural alterations, functional abnormalities may result in subendocardial ischemia during exercise.[66] Methods that measure only total coronary inflow may fail to detect this abnormality, since normal or supranormal subepicardial flow may exist in parallel with an underperfused subendocardium, resulting in a normal mean blood flow. This transmural redistribution of blood flow away from the subendocardium during exercise or other stress appears to be the result of abnormally increased extravascular forces resulting from decreased compliance and increased cavitary pressure in the hypertrophied left ventricle.[66] These structural and functional abnormalities in the pressure-overloaded hypertrophied left ventricle cause increased sensitivity to the effects of occlusive coronary artery disease and, if sufficiently severe (as in critical aortic stenosis), may be sufficient to result in exercise-induced myocardial ischemia even in the absence of coronary disease. (See also Chap. 58.)

Determinants of Myocardial Oxygen Consumption

Although the primary cause of myocardial ischemia is a defect in arterial blood supply, ischemia does not occur until the tissue demand for oxygen to support energy generation outstrips its supply of oxygen. Thus the determinants of myocardial oxygen consumption play a decisive role in setting the threshold for ischemia. The normal heart is dependent on aerobic metabolism for contractile function; therefore oxygen consumption closely parallels energy production. Energy production within the myocytes can be predicted from certain easily measurable hemodynamic variables. Although the exact relationship between myocardial mitochondrial respiration and measurements of cardiac pump function is not known, good correlations exist between myocardial oxygen consumption and indexes based on pressure and volume measurements.[67,68] At the risk of oversimplifying a complex and often empirical body of knowledge, three factors can be indentified as having important, and possibly independent, effects on myocardial oxygen consumption. A discussion of each follows. (See also Chap. 5.)

Heart Rate

Heart rate bears a strong direct relationship to the rate of myocardial energy utilization. The effect of heart rate can be factored out by expressing myocardial oxygen consumption per cardiac stroke, but it is generally easier to relate the balance of demand and supply in per minute units.

Systolic Wall Tension

Systolic wall tension is proportional to ventricular systolic pressure and, according to the Laplace relationship, is also proportional to the ventricular radius. Since systolic wall tension cannot be directly measured, approximations derived from ventricular systolic pressure are used. Usually the important effect of ventricular radius is neglected, with the result that the relationship is imprecise. Wall tension is inversely proportional to wall thickness and consequently decreases with increased wall thickness. With compensated hypertrophy secondary to pressure overload, wall thickness is increased in proportion to the increase in systolic pressure, so that systolic wall stress (force per unit area) is generally normal during resting conditions.

Myocardial Contractility

Myocardial contractility is a concept with general utility but for which there is no easily obtained measure. There is no unique index that can be derived from pressure and/or volume measurements that quantitates changes in myocardial contractility. Indexes that rely on the velocity of the contractile process, such as the rate of rise of pressure during isovolumic contraction, *dP/dt*, have been widely used and are helpful in estimating changes in myocardial oxygen consumption produced by alterations of contractility.

The combination of heart rate, systolic wall tension, and contractility can be used to estimate directional changes in myocardial oxygen consumption, but it is impractical to balance quantitatively the factors determining myocardial blood flow against the factors determining demand.[68] Exact relationships are not known, and the measurements available are seldom equal to the task. Under favorable conditions, changes in the determinants of oxygen demand and myocardial blood flow may not oppose each other, and the change in the balance of supply and demand can be clearly interpreted. With severe ischemia aerobic metabolism of the myocardium rapidly decreases and anaerobic glycolysis becomes the predominant form of energy production. (See Chap. 6A.) In the absence of adequate oxygen, contractile failure ensues and electrical inexcitability may ultimately follow. Under these conditions the determinants of myocardial need are likely to be unrelated to mechanical function in the normal myocardium.

Supply-and-Demand Considerations in the Therapy of Coronary Artery Disease

The preceding analysis of the physiological and pathological mechanisms that apply at the onset of myocardial ischemia are summarized diagrammatically in Fig. 57-2. This diagram is a model that can be used to assess the effect of an intervention on the balance of myocardial supply and demand. Based on the preceding analysis, the three underlying conditions of the model are that (1) the critical regions to analyze are the subendocardial layers in segments of the heart supplied by obstructed arteries, (2) the availability of oxygen to the myocardium determines the adequacy of supply, and (3) the resistance vessels in the ischemic myocardium are vasodilated as the result of autoregulation. In the model the effect of each of the factors on the balance of oxygen supply and demand in the ischemic subendocardium is shown by arrows. An increase in each variable is characterized as to whether it causes an increase (+) or a decrease (−) in the variable(s) it acts upon, which (depending on the side of the equation affected) either raises or lowers the balance in favor of oxygen supply. Several factors, such as aortic pressure and coronary artery obstruction, act only on one side of the balance and therefore have predictable effects on myocardial ischemia. Other variables affect both supply and demand and tend to shift the balance in an additive manner, i.e., ventricular size and heart rate. Contractility has by far the most complex interaction with the factors determining supply and demand. Although contractility has a direct effect on myocardial oxygen consumption, the end result of a positive inotropic intervention on oxygen demand could be offset, particularly in the failing dilated ventricle, by a reduction of ventricular size and, consequently, wall tension. In addition, increased contractility tends to increase the blood supply by (1) reducing both systolic and diastolic compression of the subendocardial layers, (2) shortening systole with a resultant increase in the diastolic perfusion interval, and (3) decreasing ventricular volume. To further complicate the analysis, many interventions have effects on more than one variable. The model is helpful to understand the complexity of the balance between oxygen supply and demand and to caution against oversimplified interpretations of the effect of an intervention.

PATHOLOGY OF MYOCARDIAL ISCHEMIA AND INFARCTION

Introduction

Coronary ischemia that develops rapidly and then persists for a sufficient period leads to the evolution of cardiac tissue necrosis known as *myocardial infarction*. A myocardial infarction is both a spatial and a temporal event, the size and histopathology of which are dependent on the availability of coronary collateral blood sup-

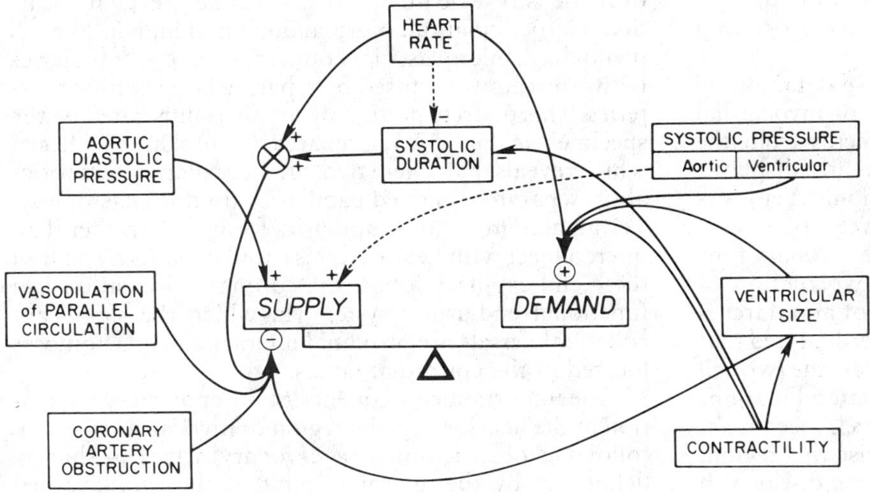

FIGURE 57-2 Diagram summarizing the factors in the balance of oxygen supply and demand in ischemic subendocardium. An increase in each variable is characterized as to its effect in increasing (+) or decreasing (−) the variables it acts on. The product (×) of heart rate and systolic duration decreases the relative diastolic time and thereby decreases supply. Interactions of secondary importance are shown by dotted lines. Some interactions have direct effects on the balance of oxygen supply and demand (e.g., effect of aortic diastolic pressure on supply), while other interactions have a secondary effect on supply or demand (e.g., contractility effect on ventricular size).

ply and the metabolic demands of the tissue. As discussed above, the primary determinant of myocardial necrosis is blood flow; a diminution of coronary supply below a critical but often not predictable threshold leads to cell death. It is clear from studies on brief transient coronary artery occlusion[69] as well as from observations in animals and patients subjected to complete cessation of coronary flow during open heart surgery, however, that myocardial necrosis is not inevitable if blood flow is restored within a finite period of time. The complex pathophysiological interrelationships among the underlying coronary anatomy, the development of transient or permanent coronary occlusion leading to myocellular necrosis, and the identification and evolution of the infarction process will be explored in the succeeding section. (See also Chap. 55.)

Coronary Artery Anatomy and Pathology

Sudden obstruction of any coronary artery or a smaller branch vessel theoretically would not cause myocardial ischemia or necrosis if the coronary circulation were *diffusely* interconnected at all levels and if flow were homogeneous across the collateralized vascular bed. Even if myocardial infarction did develop because of *inadequate* collateralization of inhomogeneous flow, the pattern of tissue necrosis would likely be irregular and patchy, with indistinct borders possibly representing ischemic but surviving myocardium. Although larger collateral vessels can be demonstrated in the epicardial and subepicardial layers, the critical determinant of adequate blood supply to the myocardium is at the microcirculatory level where capillaries provide oxygen to myocytes. If capillaries were diffusely interconnected and were derived from both occluded and patent stem vessels, myocardial cells might be maintained in an ischemic but viable state despite coronary artery occlusion. Two hypothetical capillary patterns are illustrated in Fig. 57-3, either of which could account for ischemic and surviving myocells at the lateral border of an infarct, e.g., *a lateral border zone*. A gradual but progressive diminution of blood flow could then extend from the periphery of the perfusion field of an obstructed coronary artery toward the center until the ischemic threshold was reached and the myocardial cells were irreversibly injured. Thus, multiple layers of ischemia would exist in a continuum from the lateral to the central zone, thereby giving rise to a "bullseye" patten of infarction.

Is such a view consistent with objective data? Blood flow, which is the primary determinant of myocardial survival, when measured with microspheres from the normal to the ischemic zone, does apparently display a gradual falloff toward the central infarction.[70] Yet gross myocardial sampling at the border between two coronary artery territories in order to measure coronary flow fails to take account of an alternative explanation of intermediate levels: Tissue at the border of an infarct is discretely necrotic or normal and is so interdigitated that bulk analysis cannot be employed to separate the two cell populations. Thus, gross sampling at the lateral margins invariably gives intermediate marker levels because it averages the two tissue types that comprise this region.

A number of sensitive techniques that can distinguish

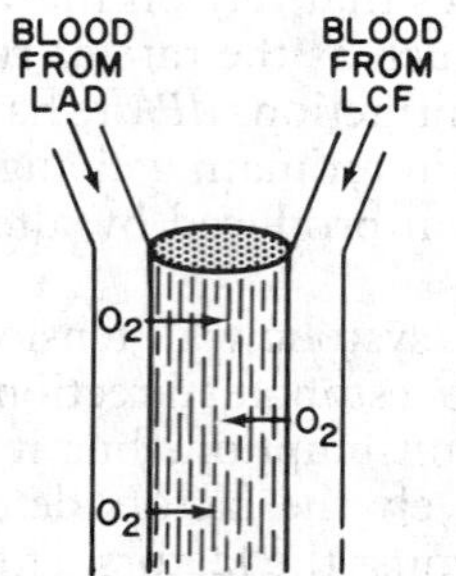

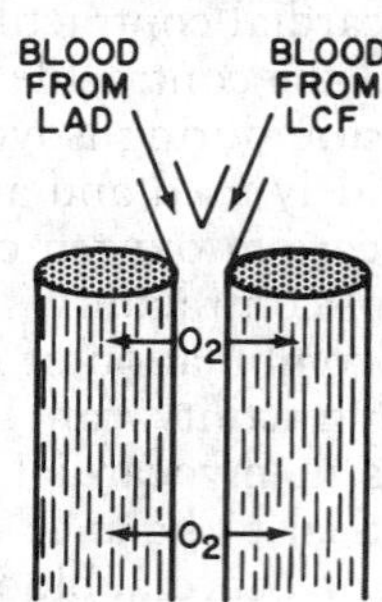

FIGURE 57-3 Two hypothetical capillary anatomic patterns that could explain the existence of surviving but ischemic myocardium at the lateral border of an acute myocardial infarction. On the left, each myocardial cell is intimately associated with interdigitating or overlapping capillaries derived from separate large coronary arteries. Occlusion of one main vessel would allow the cell to be supplied by oxygenated blood from the patent artery in diminished amounts as compared with normal. On the right, capillaries derived from two major vessels are interconnected, so that occlusion of one coronary artery would allow cells to be partially supplied by the patent vessel. With both patterns, enough substrate might be provided from the nonoccluded vascular bed to keep the myocardial cells viable, though ischemic. LAD = left anterior descending coronary artery; LCF = left circumflex artery. (*From SM Factor, EM Okun, T Minase, ES Kirk: The microcirculation of the human heart; end-capillary loops with discrete perfusion fields. Circulation 66:1241–1248, 1982. Reproduced with permission from the American Heart Association, Inc., and the authors.*)

ischemic tissue have shown that there is a sharp transition between normal and ischemic myocardium.[71–76] Serial section analysis of completed infarcts with three-dimensional reconstruction has revealed that infarcts are remarkably complex along their lateral borders, with numerous interdigitating *peninsulas* of histologically normal or necrotic myocardium.[77] Routine two-dimensional histologic sections tend to give a false impression of the spatial characteristics of an infarct; e.g., small regions of normal or necrotic myocardium appear as "islands" separated from homologous tissue. Reconstruction, however, demonstrates that this impression is due to an artifact of examining a three-dimensional structure in two dimensions and the border between normal and necrotic tissue is very sharp (Fig. 57-4).

An anatomic explanation for this discrete separation of tissue is revealed by perfusion studies of the myocardial microcirculation. Normal dog[78] and human[79] hearts do not have microvascular connections at the boundaries between regions perfused by separate large coronary arteries. This discrete pattern of supply is illustrated by the specimen in Fig. 57-5, prepared from a human heart, which reveals that where two microcirculatory territories abut, separately derived capillaries do not anastomose. Terminal homologous capillaries form loops rather than interconnect with heterologous capillaries. As a result of these end-capillary loops, the coronary circulation is a functional end-artery system, in which the significant collateral vessels are proximal interarterial anastomoses located in the epicardial layers.

One important consequence of the end-artery circulation in the heart is that the region of myocardium at risk following obstruction of a coronary artery is sharply delineated by the anatomic limit of the capillary bed

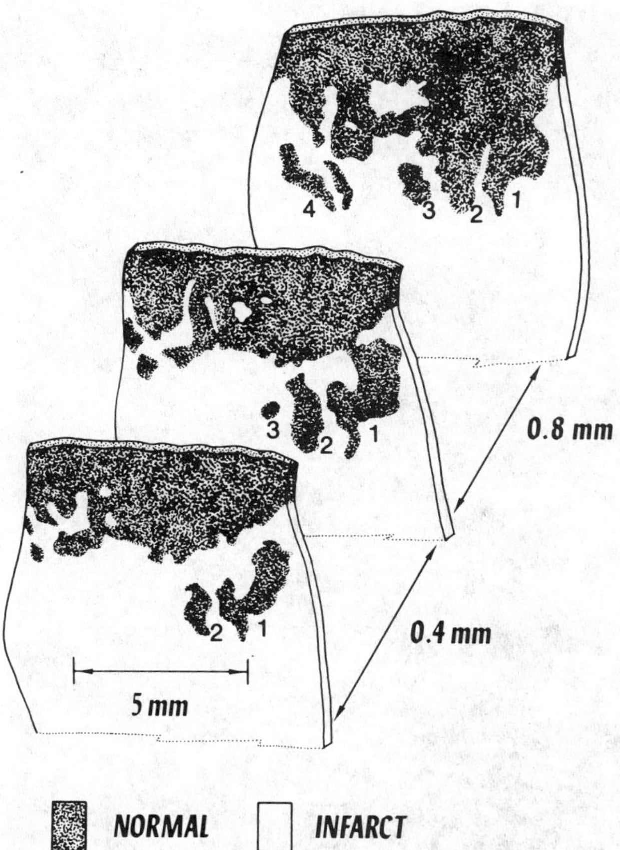

FIGURE 57-4 Composite illustration, based on original drawings of three myocardial sections. Intervening sections have been omitted for clarity. Preserved subepicardial normal myocardium (shaded area) can be seen at the top of each section. In the foreground, two islands of normal tissue (1 and 2) are completely separated from the subepicardial normal zone. Two sections deeper within the block, island 2 is still isolated. At the same level, a new island (3) becomes apparent. The last drawing, four sections away, shows complete continuity between islands 1 and 2 and the overlying subepicardial myocardium. Island 3 is larger at this level and becomes attached in subsequent sections. Several islands on the left (4) progressively enlarge and eventually become peninsulas. Additionally, the islands of necrotic tissue (unshaded) within the subepicardial zone demonstrate continuity with the infarct region at various levels and therefore are also peninsulas. The reconstruction illustrates that the border region consists of numerous interdigitated peninsulas that may appear as islands of normal or necrotic tissue when any one section is viewed. (*From SM Factor, EH Sonnenblick, ES Kirk: The histologic border zone of acute myocardial infarction: Islands or peninsulas? Am J Pathol 92:111–124, 1978. Reproduced with permission from the publisher and authors.*)

supplied by the artery. Tissue outside the artery bed is not made ischemic and is therefore not directly jeopardized. The concept of a region at risk determined by the arterial anatomy is emphasized by finding a close correlation between the size of an infarct and the size of the occluded artery bed.[80] Its relevance to humans is demonstrated by a recent autopsy study showing that Q-wave infarcts involve essentially the entire region of the occluded artery bed, with minimal surviving tissue at lateral margins of the area at risk.[81] When the cellular histology of infarcted or normal myocardium is correlated with the microvascular supply, there is an extremely close relationship between the microcirculation derived from the occluded artery and the necrotic tissue.[82] Analysis demonstrated that the highly complex, interdigitated histologic border results from an equally complex, interdigitated microvascular supply.

One can conclude from these observations that the preexisting coronary anatomy organized into an end-vessel system determines the area at risk of infarction if the supply vessel becomes occluded. Although preformed collaterals may mitigate the consequences of coronary occlusion, they are predominantly epicardial vessels, which as previously discussed, are affected by intraventricular and intramural pressures that limit their perfusion of the subendocardium. In addition, since they are located proximal to the terminal capillary loops, their distal effects may be attenuated where they are most required to keep tissue viable. The result of this anatomic arrangement of the coronary circulation is the presence of numerous areas at risk progressing from the subendocardium to the subepicardium and potentially involving the tissue supplied by a single arteriolar-capillary unit up to the largest stem coronary vessel.

Coronary Artery Occlusion

Previous sections have emphasized that the primary determinant of myocardial tissue viability is blood flow. Abrupt coronary occlusion in an experimental animal such as a dog leads to a transmural gradient of ischemia within the myocardium with lowest blood flows in the subendocardial zone and relatively higher flows in the subepicardial region. In the sheep, without significant preformed collateral vessels, occlusion of a coronary artery leads to dense ischemia throughout the transmural risk region. In humans, the situation is more complex: collateral vessels may or may not be present, several coronary arteries may have multiple areas of partial or complete occlusion, and the arteries supplying the collaterals may themselves be diseased. Thus, the risk region may be more difficult to ascertain, and the beneficial effect of the collateral supply may not be predictable.

In experimental animals myocardial infarcts generally are produced by *sudden* occlusion of an anatomically normal coronary artery. In humans, the time course of subtotal or complete coronary obstruction associated with an acute infarction is less easy to ascertain, but it appears to occur over a relatively brief interval (minutes or hours). Observations of human coronary arteries at postmortem generally reveal complete luminal occlusion with thrombosis in association with transmural myocardial infarction. Subtotal thrombotic occlusions also may be observed (Fig. 57-6), however, suggesting that human infarcts may occur in a progressive, "stuttering" pattern. Infarcted tissue that has different stages of myocardial necrosis provides further evidence that animal models of sudden occlusion leading to myocardial infarction are not entirely characteristic of clinical infarcts. (See also Chap. 55.)

As a rule, the coronary vessel supplying the area at risk in most patients with transmural infarction reveals characteristic atherosclerosis with luminal narrowing.[83] Yet atherosclerosis is a chronic process that takes months or years to evolve. If slowly progressing atherosclerosis causes ischemia, collateral development also may be

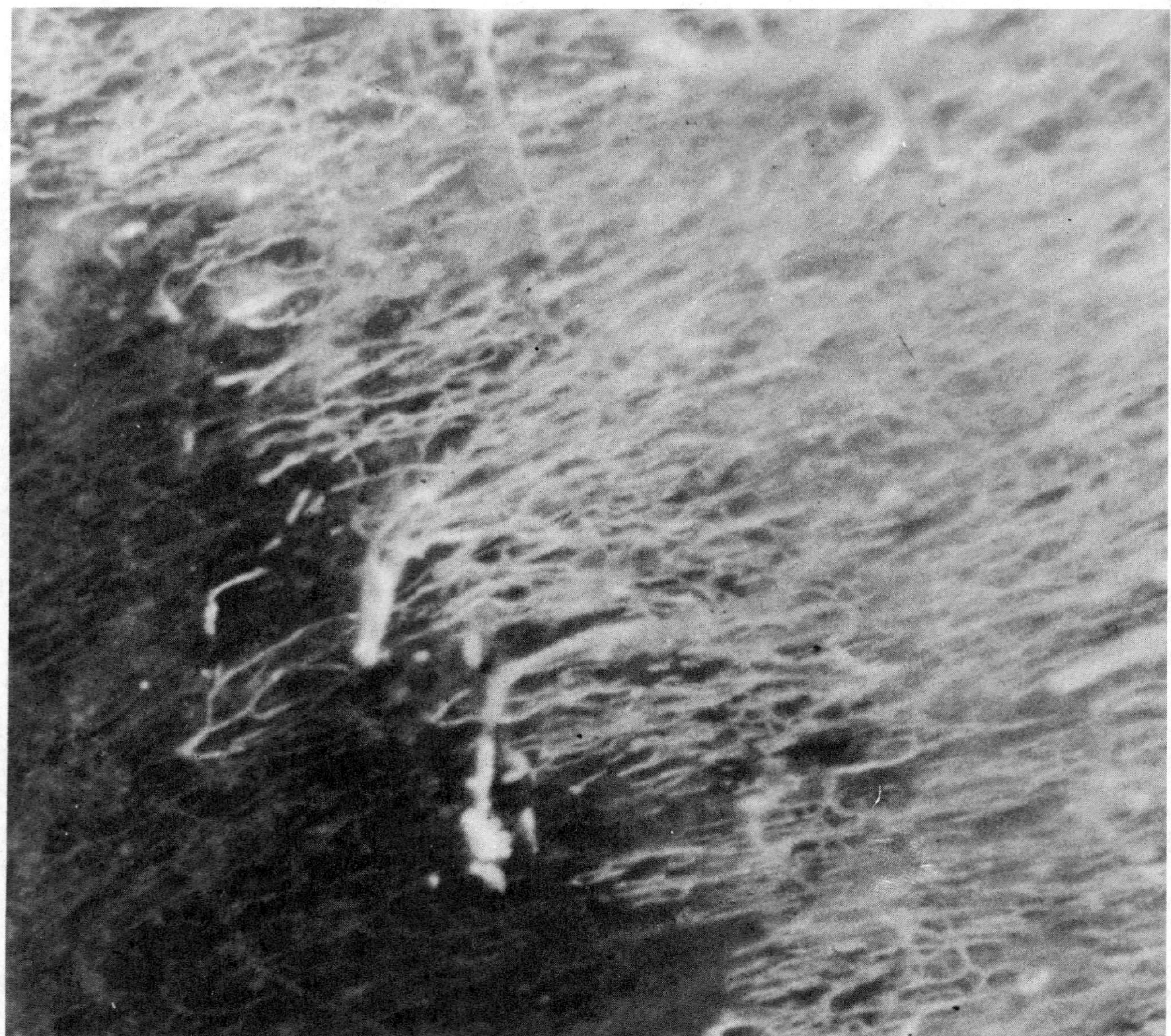

FIGURE 57-5 Multiple capillaries filled with white silicone rubber (Microfil) via injection of one coronary artery approach a zone perfused by an adjacent artery that is filled with red silicone rubber (reproduced here as gray). Where the white- and red-filled capillaries abut, they loop back on themselves, forming sharp hairpin turns. Some loops appear incomplete because they extend out of the section or out of the plane of focus. No anastomosis with capillaries perfused with different colors are noted, nor is there a complex alternation of red- and white-filled capillaries in this border region.

stimulated to provide alternative blood flow to the region, thus preventing tissue necrosis. Since atherosclerosis and infarction occur over different time frames, their frequent association is not reasonable proof of causation. Accordingly, in most instances the atherosclerotic coronary artery must have an acute, superimposed occlusive lesion to account for the development of a myocardial infarction. Recent observations support this conclusion. (See Chap. 55.)

Coronary Thrombosis

There has been considerable controversy and cyclical interest in the role played by coronary thrombosis in the causation of acute myocardial infarction.[84] Although a number of autopsy studies during the last two decades[85-87] suggested that coronary thrombi were secondary to infarction, there is now general agreement that in fatal acute transmural myocardial infarction more than 90 percent have associated coronary thrombosis.[88] Significantly fewer thrombi (less than 33 percent) are found in cases of either subendocardial infarction or sudden death,[88] thus suggesting different pathophysiological mechanisms for these latter two events.

Rapid patient triage, because of the potential for interventions that may salvage acutely infarcting myocardium, have led a number of groups to perform coronary angiography during the early period after infarct onset. These studies have generally reported frequencies of occlusive coronary thrombosis to be greater than 70 to 80 percent in patients studied during the first 6 h after onset of symptoms. DeWood et al.[89] evaluated patients in the

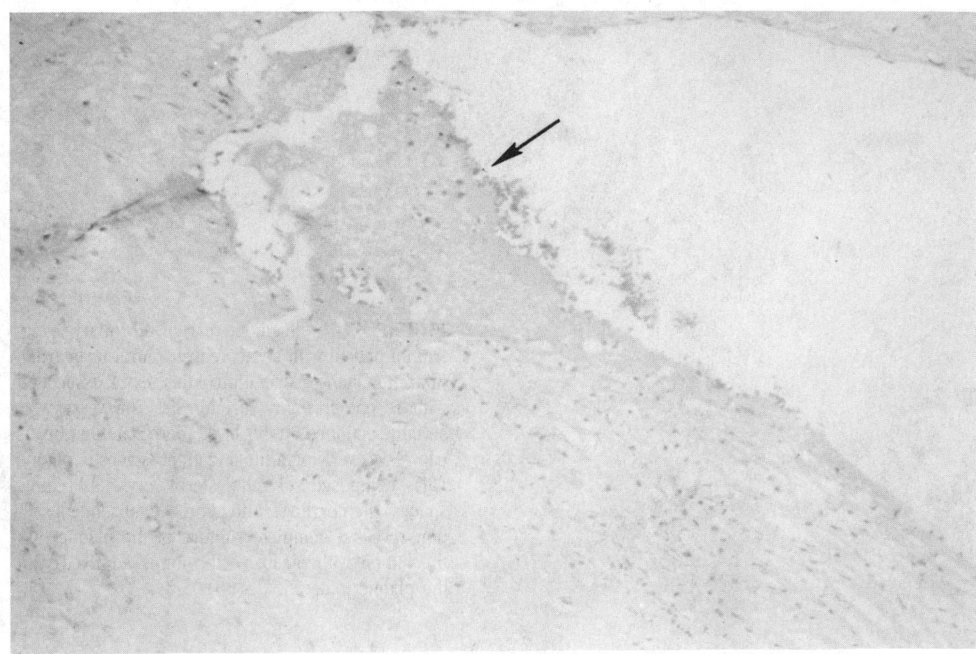

FIGURE 57-6 Platelet and fibrin nonocclusive thrombus present in the lumen of a moderately atherosclerotic coronary artery (arrow). Such nonocclusive thrombi may be found in coronary arteries of patients with subendocardial myocardial infarctions with areas of multifocal necrosis or with transmural infarctions of different histologic ages. This type of coronary artery thrombus may indicate an "unstable" vessel with spasm leading to endothelial damage and platelet adherence. (×150)

first 4 h and found 87 percent thrombotic occlusion, whereas this percentage decreased to 65 percent when patients were studied 12 to 24 h after onset. These observations suggest that thrombi may undergo spontaneous thrombolysis, fragmentation, and distal embolization with infarct evolution to account for their diminished frequency in older infarcts.

These data provide the rationale and basis for rapid intervention with thrombolytic agents in the early hours of myocardial infarction; furthermore, the efficacy of such agents as intravenous streptokinase or tissue plasminogen activator, in a circular fashion, provides evidence that coronary thrombosis is involved in infarct development.[90] The ability to reestablish coronary flow with these agents or with the technique of percutaneous transluminal angioplasty (PCTA) is predicated on the concept that the coronary occlusion is due to an intraluminal thrombus or an acutely unstable atherosclerotic plaque (see below). The rationale for such therapy is to preserve myocardium by preventing necrosis of jeopardized tissue. Improvement of left ventricular function and in-hospital mortality[91] support the efficacy of these procedures and suggest that reperfusion occurred by clot lysis. (See also Chap. 60.)

Even if it is accepted that coronary thrombosis is a primary cause of sudden coronary obstruction, it is clear that thrombus occurs often in a diseased vessel with subtotal atherosclerotic luminal compromise.[83] Although alterations of blood flow including diminished velocity and turbulence, and direct atherosclerotic injury to the vessel intima may induce platelet adherence to subendothelial collagen with subsequent initiation of the coagulation process, other dynamic mechanisms may be involved. It is beyond the scope of this chapter to review the complex interrelationships between cellular, humoral, cytokine, and coagulability parameters that may be associated with coronary thrombosis. Equally complex, but somewhat easier to study, plaque rupture and coronary artery spasm are two possibly related pathophysiological events that also have attained recent prominence because of their potential role in thrombus development. (See Chap. 55.)

Atherosclerotic Plaque Rupture

The human coronary atherosclerotic plaque is a complex structure composed of connective tissue, calcium, lipid, and inflammatory cells in differing proportions from patient to patient. Thin-walled vessels may enter the plaque and be potential sources of mural hemorrhage. Plaques may be eccentric (localized primarily along one segment of the wall) or concentric (localized circumferentially); regardless of their orientation, some intact smooth muscle usually is present in the residual medial layer, which may be a source of vessel vasomotion or vascular spasm under the appropriate stimulus. The consistency of plaques depends on the proportion of their component elements: A heavily calcified and fibrotic plaque is hard, while the plaque composed predominantly of cholesterol ester and lipid-containing macrophages is soft. Not infrequently, this soft lipid core of a plaque may be covered by a relatively thin cap of fibrous connective tissue separating the plaque material from the luminal blood flow (Fig. 57-7). (See also Chap. 55.)

A number of studies have associated acute coronary thrombosis with rupture or cracks of the thin fibrous cap and release of the plaque material into the vascular lumen. Carefully performed studies have found between 78 and 93 percent[92–94] of acute coronary thrombi at postmortem can be identified as secondary to plaque rupture. This work essentially confirms the findings of Friedman and Van den Bovenkamp, [95] early proponents of this concept, who found 98 percent concordance between thrombi and plaque rupture. Plaque rupture may induce thrombosis by any one or a combination of several mech-

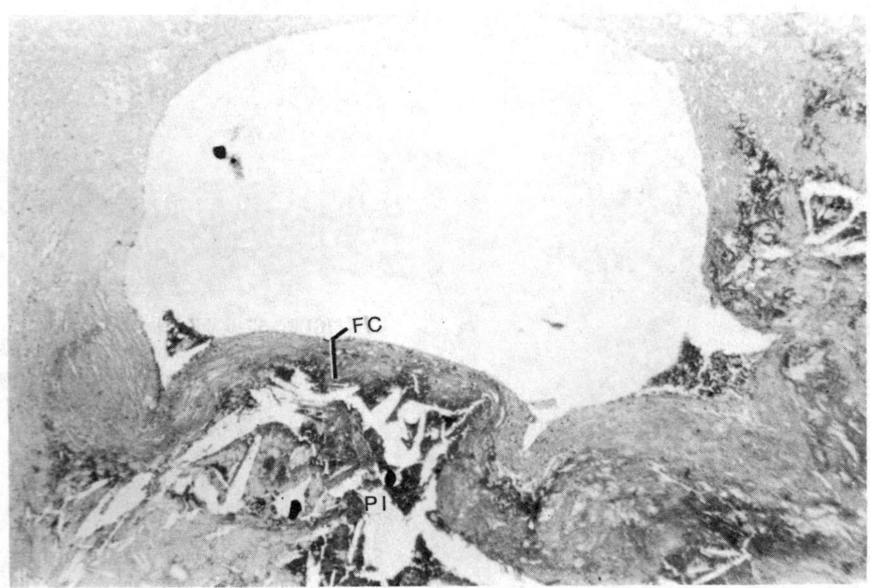

FIGURE 57-7 Segment of right coronary artery from a patient with an acute transmural myocardial infarction in the distribution of this vessel, associated with recent coronary thrombosis. The vessel was serially sectioned. At this level, there is a thin fibrous cap (FC) overlying a bulging atherosclerotic plaque (Pl) composed of cholesterol crystals (empty spaces), hemorrhage, and debris. A subsequent section revealed complete rupture of the plaque into the lumen with occlusive thrombus admixed with the plaque material. (×60)

anisms: (1) contact of platelets with exposed collagen leading to thrombocyte adherence and the buildup of a platelet plug; (2) release of tissue thromboplastin from the plaque material inducing the initiation of the clotting cascade; and (3) mechanical obstruction of the vessel lumen by the plaque components. Although what causes the thin-walled fibrous cap to crack or rupture leading to release of the plaque debris is still unknown, recent postmortem evidence suggests that coronary spasm may play a role.[96] Coronary artery atherosclerotic plaques are often eccentric with adequate smooth muscle remaining in the unaffected or less affected segment of the wall. Contraction of this muscle could lead to distortion and rupture of the thin plaque cap, thereby causing admixture of blood and plaque contents. Conversely, abnormal spasm could cause rupture of thin-walled vessels in the plaque, leading to an elevation of intraplaque pressure with eventual surface disruption.

Coronary Artery Spasm

The knowledge that coronary thrombosis is linked to the pathogenesis of acute myocardial infarction has developed in parallel with evidence that ischemic syndromes can be produced by coronary artery spasm, an old idea originally proposed by Latham[97] over a century ago and subsequently elaborated on by Sir William Osler[98] in 1910. There are now firm data that coronary artery spasm plays a major role in classical and variant angina pectoris as well as in acute myocardial infarction.[99–101] Angiographic studies performed in patients with clinical symptomatology or during provoked attacks have provided direct evidence that vasospasm can cause partial or complete coronary obstruction. Led by the pioneering efforts of Maseri et al.[102] in Europe and Oliva and Breckenridge[103] in the United States, there is now general acceptance for this view. What induces the vasospasm in most instances remains unknown[101]; however, preventive therapy with calcium channel blocking agents and nitrates has now entered the standard armamentarium for the treatment and prevention of the ischemic syndromes. Whether or not spasm due to a pathological contraction of medial smooth muscle in one or several segments of a vessel and lasting for a brief or indeterminate period is *solely* responsible for dynamic coronary obstruction is also not known.

Recent observations have altered the emphasis on medial smooth muscle in the pathogenesis of coronary artery spasm and have focused attention on the critical role of endothelial cells in the maintenance of vascular homeostasis. Endothelial cells not only play a role in the adhesion of platelets and inflammatory cells to the luminal surface but also serve to elaborate a number of mediators that can relax (prostacyclin and EDRF) or constrict (endothelins) vessels.[104] These mediators provide exquisite control of vascular tone in normal blood vessels, but with derangements of endothelial integrity induced by trauma, toxins, or atherosclerosis among others, the balance may be upset, leading to loss of vasodilatory capacity.[105,106] Since endothelial integrity is also critical for the prevention of atherosclerosis and its alteration may initiate atherosclerosis through elaboration of multiple inflammatory cytokines and cell surface adhesion molecules[107] it can be seen that two of the major pathologic processes affecting coronary artery patency (e.g., atherosclerosis and spasm) are interrelated, with the common pathway being the endothelial cell. (See also Chaps. 2 and 56.)

Though coronary artery spasm may occlude a vessel without any other associated vascular pathology, most often the spasm occurs in the setting of coronary atherosclerosis. If the occlusion is of sufficient duration (see below), tissue injury or necrosis may supervene before vascular relaxation restores blood flow. There is also evidence that coronary vasospasm is often the initiating event in the development of an acute thrombus.[108] Support for this concept comes from experimental studies demonstrating that arterial constriction induced with norepinephrine[109] or nonocclusive ligation[110] can lead to vessel wall damage including endothelial injury and subsequent thrombosis. As suggested above, coronary vasospasm also may be implicated in the frequent plaque ruptures associated with thrombi. Thus, endothelial integrity, vasospasm, atherosclerosis, and coronary thrombosis are all related phenomena that can act together to enhance the occurrence of any single event leading to coronary artery occlusion.

With the latter hypothesis, we have come full circle. Myocardial ischemia and infarction require a diminution of blood flow below a critical level before they occur. This process develops relatively suddenly, but in most instances, in the setting of chronic atherosclerosis. A significant body of evidence suggests that temporally abrupt coronary occlusion is related to thrombosis, plaque rupture, and vasospasm. It appears increasingly apparent that these pathophysiological processes are not mutually exclusive but may be intimately related. Thus, plaque rupture can induce thrombosis, which can be caused by vasospasm, and platelet adherence to an atherosclerotic vessel wall can lead to the release of vasoactive substances causing vasospasm and plaque rupture. Both vasospasm and nonocclusive thrombosis may even be implicated in the development or enlargement of an atherosclerotic plaque. It is the interplay of complex static and dynamic events in the coronary vessel that produces obstructive vascular changes intimately associated with the pathogenesis and pathophysiology of myocardial ischemia.

Patterns of Acute Myocardial Infarction

The onset of abrupt coronary obstruction, induced by the mechanisms discussed in the previous sections, leads to the development of transmural ischemia within the area at risk determined by the coronry anatomy. At least partially because collateral flow increases from the deepest subendocardial layers to the subepicardium, the jeopardized myocardium within the risk region dies in a transmural pattern beginning in the subendocardium. This progression of necrosis has been termed a "wavefront" by Jennings and coworkers.[111–112] They showed that in the open chest, anesthetized dog a 40-min occlusion of the left circumflex coronary artery followed by 2 to 4 days of reperfusion resulted in subendocardial necrosis involving 38 percent of the transmural dimension.[111] Subsequent occlusions of 3 or 4 h duration followed by reperfusions produced transmural infarcts of 57 and 71 percent, respectively; 6 h reperfused infarcts did not differ from a 24-h infarct produced by permanent occlusions.[111] These observations have been confirmed by several laboratories,[113,114] strongly indicating that this temporal and spatial progression of necrosis across the ventricular wall represents a fundamental pathophysiological phenomenon. This phenomenon also appears to be applicable to human infarcts. A comparative study of human subendocardial infarct extension following permanent coronary artery occlusion revealed an identical pattern to that seen in dogs with 40-min subendocardial infarcts and subsequent transmural extension.[114]

There are several important implications that can be drawn from this work. Most significant is the conclusion that jeopardized myocardium undergoes necrosis in a sequential fashion beginning in the subendocardium and extending toward the epicardium. The salvage of tissue in the epicardial layers is dependent either on the restoration of blood flow to this zone through the transiently occluded coronary artery or the presence of sufficient collateral supply to this area to prevent necrosis. By inference, then, *subendocardial infarctions in humans are likely to be secondary to intermittent coronary artery occlusions*. This may occur due to coronary artery spasm with spontaneous or drug-induced relaxation or to luminal thrombosis with clot lysis; in either case, the restoration of blood flow most likely must occur within a narrow time frame of several hours. Of interest, despite the evidence favoring blood flow–mediated transmural extension of myocardial necrosis, a recent study showed that the subendocardium was more vulnerable to damage than the subepicardium even in the absence of all blood flow in the tissue.[115] This suggests that subendocardial vulnerability may be due to metabolic or other unknown factors.

Because of the complexity of atherosclerotic coronary disease in humans and the unpredictability of collateral supply, it is difficult to know whether or not the relatively short time course available for reperfusion and salvage of subepicardial myocardium demonstrated experimentally also applies to clinical subjects. If transmural necrosis is essentially completed within 3 to 6 h, there is little time available for institution of measures that will restore blood flow to the area at risk. Early reperfusion in animals has been shown to salvage myocardial function[116] and to have positive effects on survival even when infarct size did not significantly differ from that produced by permanent coronary occlusion.[117] In contrast, early reperfusion may lead to preservation of increased numbers of myocytes in the immediate subendocardial zone[114]; it has been suggested that these cells may be responsible for ventricular arrhythmias that may have adverse consequences in the postinfarction period.[118,119] Thus, although it seems logical to believe that reperfusion is invariably beneficial, the preservation of jeopardized tissue otherwise destined to die may have unanticipated adverse results. (See also Chap. 60.)

Morphologic Effects of Reperfusion

Myocardial infarction secondary to *complete* obstruction of a coronary artery is not entirely devoid of blood flow if collateral vessels are present, but the flows are below the threshold required to maintain viability. Despite this insufficient circulation, an infarct in which minimal reperfusion occurs evolves into a relatively pale yellow-white zone of necrotic muscle over several days, with demarcation from the normal muscle by a rim of hyperemia. Mottling and hemorrhage may be present focally, but they are only due to residual flow and stasis. In contrast, a reperfused infarct is hemorrhagic (Fig. 57-8) with the hemorrhage localized within the necrotic tissue in the subendocardium; the hemorrhage is due to microvascular injury. There has been considerable debate over whether reperfusion and the elicited intramyocardial hemorrhage have immediate or more chronic adverse consequences. The weight of evidence now strongly supports the view that reperfusion does not affect the ultimate evolution and healing of the infarct. This point

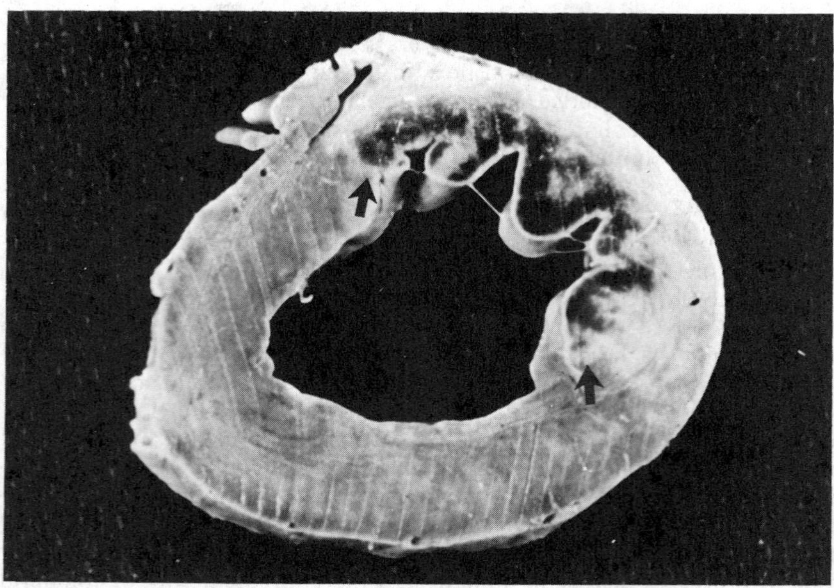

FIGURE 57-8 Left ventricle of a dog following a 40-min occlusion of the left anterior descending coronary artery (LAD) with 24 h of reperfusion. The region of risk has been delineated by perfusing the LAD with white silicone rubber. Note the dark subendocardial hemorrhage, which was histologically verified to be within the necrotic zone. Laterally, the hemorrhage and necrosis closely approach the lateral extent of the risk region (arrows).

is of considerable practical importance because of the clinical application of techniques to reestablish blood flow to infarcting myocardium during the active phase of necrosis.

Reperfusion has a number of other consequences that may be related primarily to cell membrane damage.[120] The pathogenesis of the membrane damage remains in dispute, although the involvement of free oxygen radicals following reoxygenation of ischemic tissue has been promoted actively over the last decade. Whether or not oxygen and/or hydroxyl free radicals are generated during ischemia-reperfusion and whether or not they are deleterious to cells that would otherwise be viable are still areas of considerable debate and practical importance. Several recent commentaries have reviewed the salient issues on both sides.[121,122] Regardless of the cause, reperfusion leads to development of myocardial cell swelling,[123] accumulation of calcium in mitochrondria,[124] accelerated washout of cellular enzymes,[125] and the presence of characteristic contraction bands.[126,127] These contraction bands are the morphologic marker of reperfusion injury, indicating that myocardial cells were ischemically damaged and then subsequently supplied with oxygenated blood. For example, they are seen in acute subendocardial infarction throughout the necrotic zone, and they have been described following coronary bypass grafting of patients with acute myocardial ischemia, where they are secondary to surgical reperfusion.[122] They may also be observed along the periphery of transmural infarctions, often associated with focal mitochondrial calcification (Fig. 57-9). In this location, they are probably related to diffusion of oxygenated substrate from the normally perfused tissue.

Morphology of Nonreperfused Infarcts

There are several characteristic features of predominantly nonreperfused infarctions that permit histologic identification and approximate dating. These features were outlined by Mallory et al.[128] in a classic paper in 1939, and they were verified more recently by Fishbein and colleagues.[129] The major limitation of histology is the insensitivity of light microscopy in early infarctions; morphologic alterations are not clearly defined in the first 6 to 12 h of infarct development. A variety of histochemical and ultrastructural methods have been employed to circumvent these problems, but light microscopy with hematoxylin-eosin staining still remains the "gold standard" for infarcts older than 12 to 24 h. The primary advantage of histology, particularly when compared with ultrastructure, is the ability to examine large regions of myocardium and to correlate the changes with vascular markers that can identify the area at risk. For early infarcts of less than 6 h duration, however, other methods are required.

The most significant histologic marker of infarction is the presence of increased sarcoplasmic eosinophilia, or hypereosinophilia, characteristic of coagulation necrosis, which can be appreciated within the first 24 h (Fig. 57-9). Myocytes at this stage also may be attenuated and aligned in parallel bundles of wavy fibers,[130] but this is not a constant finding. The waviness is related to stretching of the necrotic tissue by the surrounding viable myocardium, with subsequent relaxation postmortem. Because of stretching, cross-striations are less prominent, but they are still present with increased sarcomeric spacing. Nonreperfused infarcts may have congested vessels and interstitial edema, but prominent intercellular hemorrhage is usually absent. Even without reperfusion, however, some blood flow is usually present in the infarct zone unless collaterals are absent; because of this, some viable myocytes may be seen surrounding vessels deep within the necrotic tissue. Focal contraction bands and myocytolytic changes typical of reperfusion are usually seen along the periphery of the infarction. Whether this is related to reperfusion through collaterals or diffusion from the noninfarcted zone or is due to the effects of catecholamines is not known. As previously noted, this is also the region where focal cellular calcification can be identified.

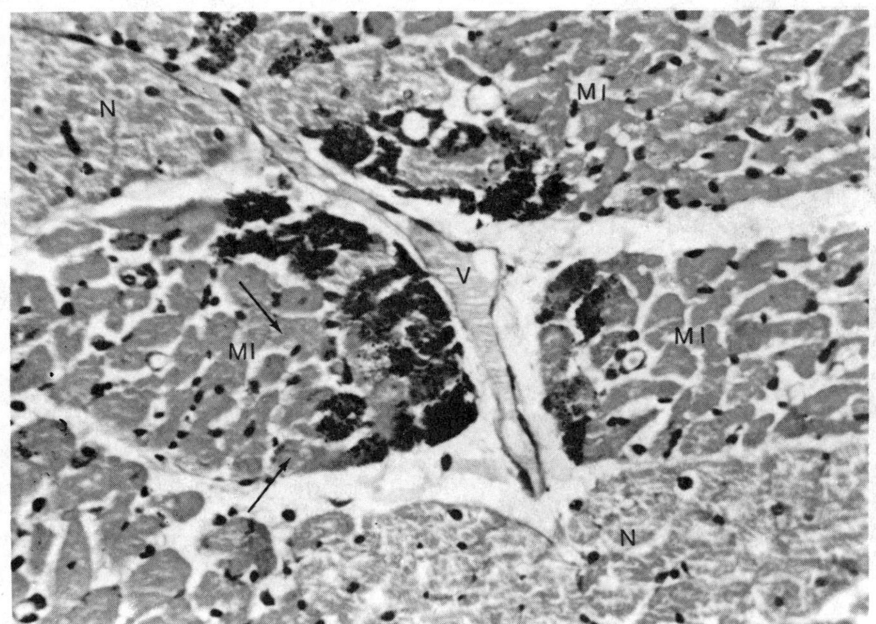

FIGURE 57-9 Histologic border of the 24-h canine transmural infarction. The darker, hypereosinophilic necrotic myocardial cells (MI) are sharply delimited from peninsulas of normal myocardium (N). In the region surrounding a thin-walled patent vessel (V), the necrotic cells contain finely granular calcium precipitate (black in this photomicrograph), which extends two to three cells away from the vessel. A few contraction bands are observed in the same area (arrows). The spatial orientation of the calcification and contraction bands suggests that they were secondary to diffusion of substrate from the noninfarcted zone or the patent vessel. (×150)

Within the first 12 h polymorphonuclear leukocytes (PMNs) marginate in vessels and begin to migrate into the interstitial spaces; this PMN response is most likely mediated by cytokine release from the ischemically injured tissues, and it plays a role in further damage to the myocardium.[131] By 24 to 48 h, all infarcts have infiltrates of PMNs at variable depths within the necrotic tissue moving from the periphery toward the center. The variability probably reflects the extent of local blood flow, which may not be sufficient to keep the myocardium viable but may be capable of bringing inflammatory cells into the area. Lymphatic and venous drainage from the infarct zone carries away cellular proteins and enzymes that leak through damaged membranes and that may be measured systemically as markers of necrosis [e.g., creatine kinase (CK)]. Serial sectioning of acute infarcts demonstrates that the PMN collections are not homogeneous but discontinuous.[77] Absent blood flow related to microcirculatory damage (no-reflow phenomenon[132]), vascular thrombi within the infarct region, or inadequate collaterals may account for this discontinuity.

By 2 to 4 days of age the degree of PMN inflammation has increased and inflammatory cells begin to undergo necrosis and fragmentation. Centripetal degeneration of necrotic myocytes is observed, and the peripheral infarct begins to demonstrate admixtures of mononuclear inflammatory cells including lymphocytes, mast cells, and macrophages. The latter often contain lipofuscin pigment from the breakdown of myocytes. Eosinophils are an inconstant feature, but they may be observed in this early period.

Within the first 4 to 7 days, although PMNs are still present, chronic inflammatory infiltration increases. At the periphery of the infarct, progressing toward the central zone, fibroblasts and new capillaries can be identified. By 1 week, this granulation tissue is well defined, and loose collagen is being deposited in the interstitium. This process of scar formation progresses for weeks until a densely collagenized healed infarct is present. In very large infarctions, presumably where there is complete absence of blood flow in the center of the risk region, mummified necrotic myocytes surrounded by scar may be seen months or years after healing is complete. For most infarctions, scarring is generally completed within 6 to 8 weeks.

Alterations in Postinfarct Period

Although we have stressed that myocyte necrosis secondary to ischemia is a temporal event that takes a minimum of several hours for completion across the ventricular wall, it is equally true that once the infarct has developed fully, there may be associated remodeling changes with time in the immediate and distant regions of the ventricle that have adverse consequences for the heart. There has been recent popularization of this concept in descriptions of infarct expansion and extension.[133] *Expansion* refers to the dilatation and thinning of the infarct without superimposed new myocyte necrosis. In one study,[134] infarct expansion was identified in 59 percent of 76 consecutive acute transmural myocardial infarcts, with severe expansion occurring in infarcts greater than 5 days old. We have observed marked infarct thinning within the first 3 days (Fig 57-10) and even as early as 1 day after onset, particularly if the infarct results in ventricular rupture. The pathogenesis of this pronounced thinning is unknown. Although it may be related to attenuation and disruption of myocardial fibers, recent observations suggest that it may be secondary to disruption or destruction of the interstitial connective tissue matrix of the heart. Myocardial cells are surrounded by a complex connective tissue skeleton that serves to attach myocytes to each other and to other structures in the heart.[135] This skeleton is not observable with the commonly used staining procedures for connective tissue, and therefore it has not been evaluated routinely in myocardial infarction. It appears, however, that even in very early infarction, there is loss or damage to this skeleton,

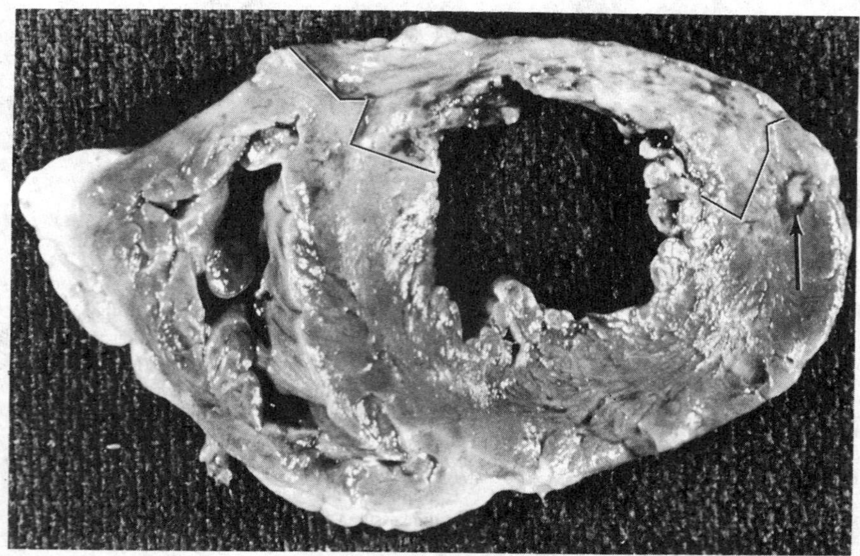

FIGURE 57-10 There is marked thinning of the posterior free wall secondary to a transmural acute myocardial infarction (approximately 72 h old). There was ventricular rupture present at another level. The infarct is demarcated at its gross lateral borders; a region of acute necrosis (arrow) is present peripheral to the main infarct.

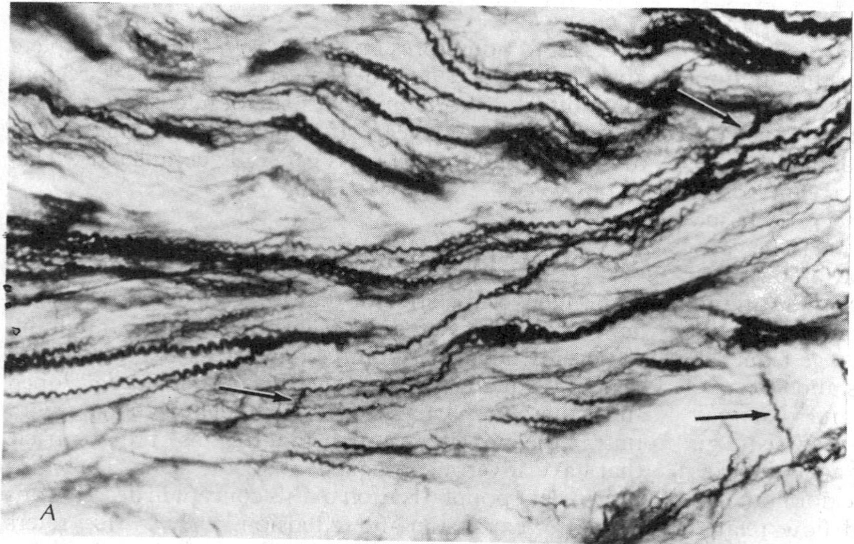

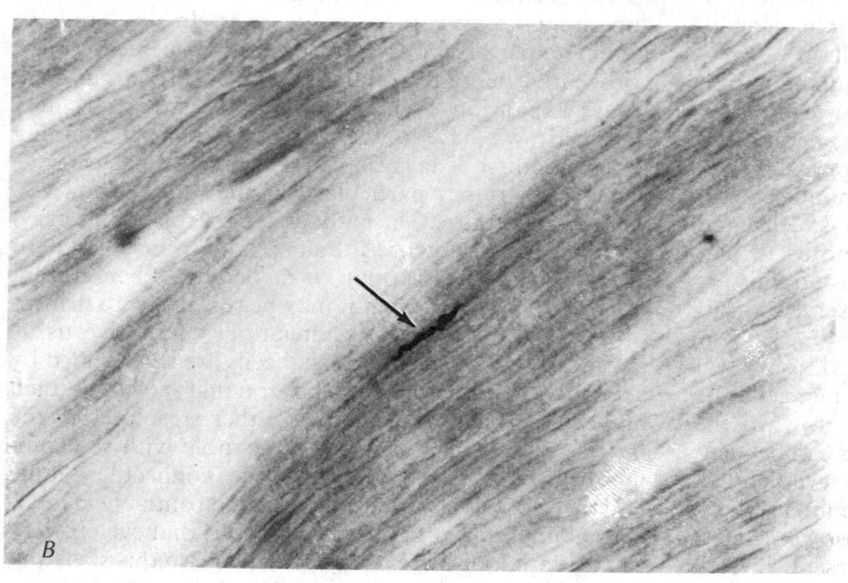

FIGURE 57-11 *A*. Section of normal myocardium from a patient with a 27-h-old ruptured infarct has been reacted with the del Rio Hortega silver stain to demonstrate the extent of the extracellular skeletal framework in this specimen.[136] Note the dark silver-positive collagen fibers in the extracellular space, some of which (arrows) act as struts between myocardial cells. (×150) *B*. Section from the same heart taken from the myocardial rupture site. With the exception of a single silver-positive fiber (arrow), none of the skeletal framework is apparent in this area. (×150)

suggesting profound alterations in its composition and integrity (Fig. 57-11). Disruption of the matrix holding myocardial cells to each other may account for their slippage during infarction, leading to expansion and wall thinning, ventricular aneurysm formation, or myocardial rupture.[136]

In contrast to infarct thinning without new necrosis, *extension* refers to the development of additional myocardial necrosis adjacent to the initial infarct.[133] In the study reported by Hutchins and Bulkley, they described relatively small zones of contraction band necrosis in 17 percent of 76 acute infarctions and ascribed its occurrence to transient hypoperfusion.[134] Because of the small volume of myocardium involved, they believed that this process was probably hemodynamically insignificant. A clinical study by Fraker et al.,[137] however, identified acute extension in 13 percent of 458 patients with acute infarction and observed a fourfold increase in in-hospital mortality and decreased 1-year survival. Although the mechanism for extension is unknown, experimental infarcts in which the risk region is precisely defined reveal that extension can occur in the normal nonrisk zone.[138] The contraction band morphology of the necrosis and its localization suggest that catecholamines and/or microvascular spasm may be implicated.

Identification of the vascular area at risk with histologic infarct extension into the normal region links this phenomenon to the development of new necrosis at a distance from the initial infarct. This necrosis may represent a second myocardial infarction due to transient or complete obstruction of a main coronary artery with features of a non-Q-wave or Q-wave infarction. Not infrequently, however, new necrosis is identified with contraction band or myocytolytic morphology in the epicardium or mid–ventricular wall and this is not in the vascular distribution expected with main coronary artery occlusion. The pathogenesis of this necrosis is unknown, but it may be similar to that proposed for acute extension. (See also Chap. 60.)

Ischemic Myocardial Dysfunction without Necrosis (Stunned Myocardium)

There has been increasing recent interest in the phenomenon of stunned myocardium, or the development of persistent mechanical dysfunction of the ventricle with ischemic insults insufficient to produce necrosis.[139] The dysfunctional stunned myocardium has contractile abnormalities with systolic bulging and wall thinning. Although originally described in experimental animals, stunning may have important clinical implications. Patients may develop transient or persistent dysfunction secondary to intermittent coronary occlusions with angina pectoris or incipient infarction interrupted by coronary thrombolysis or PCTA. Global ventricular dysfunction following cardiac surgery with cardiopulmonary bypass also may be a form of stunning. Regardless of the underlying precipitating event, the pathogenesis of stunned myocardium is unknown. A metabolic cause has been suggested due to depression of adenosine triphosphate levels.[140] Other postulated mechanisms include damage due to oxygen free radicals or abnormal sarcoplasmic reticulum calcium transport.[141] Against a primary metabolic defect, however, is the fact that inotropic stimulation with dopamine or epinephrine can lead to marked functional improvement,[142,143] suggesting that the contractile machinery is intact.

An alternative explanation for this paradox has been proposed by Zhao et al.,[144] who demonstrated striking alterations of intercellular connective tissue in stunned canine myocardium. Focal connective tissue fibers were destroyed or absent without evidence of myocardial cell damage (Fig 57-12). This observation suggests that the contractile dysfunction may result from an *untethering* of connections between viable myocytes, leading to cell and mural layer slippage. The implication of these observations is that active collagenolysis is provoked by ischemia even without necrosis or inflammation. Because of the significant clinical implications, more investigations

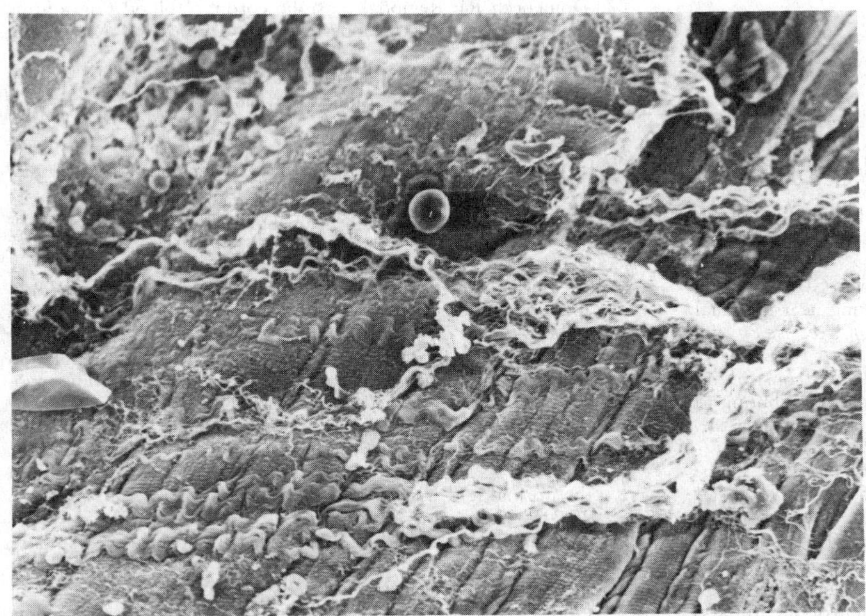

FIGURE 57-12 Scanning electron micrograph from the stunned region of canine myocardium following 12 episodes of transient 5 min ischemia with 10 min of reperfusion after each occlusion. The myocardium is viable; however, there is severe degeneration and unraveling of the surface connective tissue fibers. This degradation of collagen may account for the marked increase of compliance in the stunned region. [*From M Zhao, Z Hong, TF Robinson, et al: Profound structural alterations of the extracellular collagen matrix in postischemic dysfunctional ("stunned") but viable myocardium. J Am Coll Cardiol 10:1322–1334, 1987. Reproduced with permission from the publisher and authors.*]

are needed to elucidate the pathogenesis and possible prevention of myocardial stunning.

ISCHEMIC PRECONDITIONING

In addition to causing myocardial stunning, a transient coronary occlusion insufficient to produce infarction has been found to convey a protective effect against subsequent ischemic injury.[145] Thus, coronary occlusions as brief as 5 min in duration followed by a short period of reperfusion cause a marked reduction in infarct size during a subsequent more prolonged coronary occlusion.[146] This protective effect, termed *ischemic preconditioning*, is relatively short-lived, lasting no more than 1 to 2 h after the initial brief period of ischemia.[146] The preconditioning effect is distinct from stunning, since stunning can persist long after preconditioning has disappeared.[146] Furthermore, interventions which prevent or attenuate stunning do not necessarily interfere with the preconditioning effect. The mechanism for preconditioning is not completely elucidated, but may be dependent on a reduction of myocardial metabolic demands; this is supported by a decreased rate of ATP utilization and slowed anerobic glycolysis during ischemia in the preconditioned heart.[147] This protective effect appears to be mediated through adenosine, since preconditioning can be blocked with adenosine receptor inhibitors, while specific adenosine A_2 receptor agonists are capable of mimicking the preconditioning effect.[148] Adenosine production is dependent on the ectoenzyme 5′-nucleotidase associated with the myocardial cell membrane; recent evidence indicates that this enzyme is activated during the initial ischemic episode, resulting in increased adenosine production and preconditioning.[149] Although the clinical importance of the preconditioning phenomenon is as yet unclear, it is possible that transient ischemia that may precede total coronary occlusion can modify the subsequent course of myocardial infarction.

REFERENCES

1. Berne RM, Rubio R: Coronary circulation. In: Berne RM, Sperelakis S, Geiger SR (eds): *Handbook of Physiology*, sec 2: *The Cardiovascular System*, vol 1: *The Heart*. Bethesda, *MD, American Physiological Society*, 1979: 873–952.
2. Sanders M, White FC, Bloor CM: Myocardial blood flow distribution in miniature pigs during exercise. *Basic Res Cardiol* 1977; 72:326–331.
3. Barnard RN, Duncan WH, Livesay JJ, Buckbert GD: Coronary vasodilator reserve and flow distribution during near-maximal exercise in dogs. *J Appl Physiol: Respir Environ Exercise Physiol* 1977; 43:988–992.
4. Brown BG, Lee AB, Bolson EL, Dodge HT: Reflex constriction of significant coronary stenosis as a mechanism contributing to ischemic left ventricular dysfunction during isometric exercise. *Circulation* 1984; 70:18–24.
5. Maseri A, Mimmo R, Chierchia S, Marchesi C, Pesola A, L'Abbate A: Coronary artery spasm as a cause of acute myocardial ischemia in man. *Chest* 1975; 68:625–633.
6. Cannon RO, Leon MB, Watson RM, Rosing DR, Epstein SE: Chest pain in patients with "normal" coronary arteries—the role of small coronary arteries. *Am J Cardiol* 1985; 55:50B–60B.
7. Mosher P, Ross J Jr, McFate PA, Shaw RF: Control of coronary blood flow by an autoregulatory mechanism. *Circ Res* 1964; 14:250–259.
8. Gould KL, Lipscomb K, Calvert C: Compensatory changes of the distal coronary vascular bed during progressive constriction. *Circulation* 1975; 51:1085–1094.
9. Berne RM: The role of adenosine in the regulation of coronary blood flow. *Cir Res* 1980; 47:807–813.
10. Feigl EO: Coronary physiology. *Physiol Rev* 1983; 63:54–96.
11. Furchgott RF: Role of endothelium in responses of vascular smooth muscle. *Circ Res* 1983; 53:557–573.
12. Moncada S, Vane JR: Pharmacology and endogenous roles of prostaglandin endoperoxides, thromboxane A_2 and prostacyclin. *Pharmacol Rev* 1978; 30:293–331.
13. Heistad DD, Armstrong ML, Marcus ML, Piegors DJ, Mark AL: Augmented responses to vasoconstrictor stimuli in hypercholesterolemic and atherosclerotic monkeys. *Circ Res* 1984; 54:711–718.
14. Sabiston DC, Gregg DE: Effects of cardiac contraction on coronary blood flow. *Circulation* 1957; 15:14–20.
15. Downey JM, Kirk ES: Inhibition of coronary blood flow by a vascular waterfall mechanism. *Circ Res* 1975; 36:753–760.
16. Hess DS, Bache RJ: Transmural distribution of myocardial blood flow during systole in the awake dog. *Circ Res* 1976; 38:5–15.
17. Downey JM, Downey HF, Kirk ES: Effect of myocardial strains on coronary blood flow. *Circ Res* 1974; 34:286–292.
18. Brandi G, MacGregor M: Intramural pressure in the left ventricle of the dog. *Cardiovasc Res* 1969; 3:472–475.
19. Permutt S, Riley RL: Hemodynamics of collapsible vessels with tone: The vascular waterfall. *J Appl Physiol* 1963; 18:924–932.
20. Bache RJ, Cobb FR: Effect of maximal coronary vasodilation on transmural myocardial perfusion during tachycardia in the awake dog. *Circ Res* 1977; 41:648–653.
21. Hess DS, Bache RJ: Transmural right ventricular myocardial blood flow during systole in the awake dog. *Circ Res* 1979; 45:88–94.
22. Gold FL, Bache RJ: Transmural right ventricular blood flow during acute pulmonary artery hypertension in the sedated dog: Evidence for subendocardial ischemia despite residual vasodilator reserve. *Circ Res* 1982; 51:196–204.
23. Brooks H, Kirk ES, Vokanas PS, Urschel CW, Sonnenblick EH: Performance of the right ventricle under stress: Relation to right coronary flow. *J Clin Invest* 1971; 50:2176–2183.
24. Weiss HH, Neubauer JD, Lipp JD, Sinha AK: Quantitative determination of regional oxygen consumption in the dog heart. *Circ Res* 1978; 42:394–401.
25. Hoffman JIE: Determinants and prediction of transmural myocardial perfusion. *Circulation* 1978; 58:381–391.
26. Bache RJ, McHale PA, Greenfield JC Jr: Transmural myocardial perfusion during restricted coronary inflow in the awake dog. *Am J Physiol* 1977; 232:H645–H651.
27. Domenech RJ: Regional diastolic coronary blood flow during diastolic ventricular hypertension. *Cardiovasc Res* 1978; 12:639–645.
28. Chance B: Pyridine nucleotide as an indicator of the oxygen requirements for energy-linked functions of mitochondria. *Circ Res* 1976, 38(suppl 1):31–38.
29. Myers WW, Honig CR: Number and distribution of capillaries as determinants of myocardial oxygen tension. *Am J Physiol* 1964; 207:653–660.
30. Provenza DV, Scherlis S: Coronary circulation in dog's heart: Demonstration of muscle sphincters in capillaries. *Circ Res* 1959; 7:318–324.
31. Austin RE, Aldea GS, Coggins DL, Flynn AE, Hoffman JI: Profound spatial heterogeneity of coronary reserve. *Circ Res* 1990; 67:319–331.
32. Sestier FJ, Mildenberger RR, Klassen GA: Role of autoregulation in spatial and temporal perfusion heterogeneity of canine myocardium. *Am J Physiol* 1978; 235:H64–H71.
33. Shipley RA, Shipley LJ, Wearn JT: The capillary supply in normal and hypertrophied hearts of rabbits. *J Exp Med* 1937; 65:29–42.
34. Rakusan K, Moravec J, Hatt PY: Regional capillary supply in the normal and hypertrophied rat heart. *Microvasc Res* 1980; 20:319–326.
35. Turek Z, Rakusan K: Log normal distribution of intercapillary distance in normal and hypertrophic rat heart as estimated by the method of concentric circles. Its effect on tissue oxygenation. *Pflugers Arch* 1981; 391:17–21.

36. Freudenberg H, Lichtlen PR: The normal wall segment in coronary stenosis—a postmortem study. *Z Kardiol* 1981; 70:863–870.
37. Hossack KF, Brown BG, Stewart DK, Dodge HT: Diltiazem-induced blockade of sympathetically mediated constriction of normal and diseased coronary arteries: Lack of epicardial coronary dilatory effect in humans. *Circulation* 1984; 70:465–471.
38. Furchgott RF, Zawadski JV: The obligatory role of endothelial cells in the relaxation of arterial smooth muscle by acetylcholine. *Nature* 1980; 288:373–376.
39. Furchgott RF, Vanhoutte PM: Endothelium-derived relaxing and contracting factors. *FASEB J* 1989; 3:2007–2018.
40. Ignarro LJ, Byrns RE, Buga GM, Wood KS: Endothelium-derived relaxing factor from pulmonary artery and vein possesses pharmacologic and chemical properties identical to those of nitric oxide radical. *Circ Res* 1987; 61:866–879.
41. Bassenge E: Flow-dependent regulation of coronary vasomotor tone. *Eur Heart J* 1989; 10(suppl F): 22–27.
42. Friedman PC, Mitchell GC, Heistad DD, Armstrong ML, Harrison DO: Atherosclerosis impairs endothelium-dependent vascular relaxation to acetylcholine and thrombin in primates. *Circ Res* 1988; 58:783–789.
43. Ludmer PL, Selwyn AP, Shook TL, Wayne RR, Mudge GH, Alexander RW, et al: Paradoxical vasoconstriction induced by acetylcholine in atherosclerotic coronary arteries. *N Engl J Med* 1986; 315:1046–1051.
44. Yanagisawa M, Masaki T: Endothelin, a novel endothelium-derived peptide. Pharmacological activities, regulation and possible roles in cardiovascular control. *Biochem Pharmacol* 1989; 38:1877–1883.
45. Aversano T, Becker LC: Persistence of coronary vasodilator reserve despite functionally significant flow reduction. *Am J Physiol* 1985; 248:H403–H411.
46. Laxson DD, Dai X, Homans DC, Bache RJ: The role of alpha$_1$- and alpha$_2$-adrenergic receptors in mediating coronary vasoconstriction in hypoperfused ischemic myocardium during exercise. *Circ Res* 1989; 65:1688–1697.
47. Bache RJ, Dai X: The thromboxane A_2 mimetic, U46619, worsens myocardial hypoperfusion during exercise in the presence of a coronary stenosis. *Cardiovasc Res* 1992; 26:351–356.
48. Schaper W: The collateral circulation of the heart. Amsterdam, Elsevier North-Holland, 1971.
49. Hautamaa PV, Dai X, Homans DC, Bache RJ: Vasomotor activity of the moderately well-developed canine coronary collateral circulation. *Am J Physiol* 1989; 256(*Heart Circ Physiol* 25):H890–H897.
50. Wright L, Homans DC, Laxson DD, Dai X, Bache RJ: Effect of serotonin and thromboxane A_2 on blood flow through moderately well developed coronary collateral vessels. *J Am Coll Cardiol* 1992; 19:687–693.
51. Baroldi G, Scomazzoni G: Coronary circulation in the normal and the pathologic heart. Washington, DC, Department of the Army, 1967: 217–228.
52. Rivas F, Cobb FR, Bache RJ, Greenfield JC Jr: Relationship between blood flow to ischemic regions and extent of myocardial infarction. *Circ Res* 1976; 38:439–447.
53. Cohen M, Rentrop KP: Limitation of myocardial ischemia by collateral circulation during sudden controlled coronary artery occlusion in human subjects: A prospective study. *Circulation* 1986; 74:469–476.
54. Rentrop KP, Feit F, Sherman W, Stecy P, Hosat S, Cohen M, et al: Late thrombolytic therapy preserves left ventricular function in patients with collateralized total coronary occlusion: Primary endpoint findings of the second Mount Sinai—New York University reperfusion trial. *J Am Coll Cardiol* 1989; 14:58–64.
55. Cohen M, Sherman W, Rentrop KP, Gorlin R: Determinants of collateral filling observed during sudden controlled coronary artery occlusion in human subjects. *J Am Coll Cardiol* 1989; 13:297–303.
56. Schwartz H, Leiboff RH, Bren GB, Wasserman AG, Katz RJ, Varghese PJ, et al: Temporal evolution of the human coronary collateral circulation after myocardial infarction. *J Am Coll Cardiol* 1984; 4:1088–1093.
57. McHenry PL, O'Donnell J, Morris SN, Jordan JJ: The abnormal exercise electrocardiogram in apparently healthy men: A predictor of angina pectoris as an initial coronary event during long-term follow-up. *Circulation* 1984; 70:547–551.
58. Bache RJ, Schwartz JS: Myocardial blood flow during exercise after gradual coronary occlusion in the dog. *Am J Physiol* 1983; 245(*Heart Circ Physiol* 14):131–138.
59. Foreman BW, Dai X, Bache RJ: Vasoconstriction of canine coronary collateral vessels with vasopressin limits blood flow to collateral dependent myocardium during exercise. *Circ Res* 1991; 69:657–664.
60. Becker LC: Conditions for vasodilator-induced coronary steal in experimental myocardial ischemia. *Circulation* 1978:57:1103–1110.
61. Schaper W: Influence of chronic coronary occlusion on maximal blood flow to normal areas. In: Schaper W (ed): *The Pathophysiology of Myocardial Perfusion.* Amsterdam, New York, Oxford, Elsevier North-Holland Biomedical, 1979:444.
62. Koren MJ, Devereux RB, Casale PN, Savage DD, Laragh JH: Relation of left ventricular mass and geometry to morbidity and mortality in uncomplicated essential hypertension. *Ann Intern Med* 1991; 114:345–352.
63. Mueller TM, Tomanek RJ, Kerber RE, Marcus ML: Myocardial infarction in dogs with chronic hypertension and left ventricular hypertrophy. *Am J Physiol* 1980; 239:H731–H735.
64. Bache RJ, Wright L, Laxson DL, Dai X: Effect of a coronary stenosis on myocardial blood flow during exercise in the chronically pressure overloaded hypertrophied left ventricle. *Circulation* 1990; 81:1967–1973.
65. Bache RJ: Effects of hypertrophy on the coronary circulation. *Prog Cardiovasc Dis* 1988; 31:403–440.
66. Bache RJ, Vrobel TR, Ring WS, Emery RW, Andersen RW: Regional myocardial blood flow during exercise in dogs with chronic left ventricular hypertrophy. *Circ Res* 1981; 48:76–87.
67. Sarnoff SJ, Braunwald E, Welch GH Jr, Case RB, Stainsby WN, Marcruz R: Hemodynamic determinates of oxygen consumption of the heart with special reference to the tension time index. *Am J Physiol* 1958; 192:148–156.
68. Rook GA, Feigl EO: Work as a correlate of canine left ventricular oxygen consumption, and the problem of catecholamine wasting. *Circ Res* 1982; 50:273–286.
69. Jennings RB, Sommers HM, Smyth GA, Flack HA, Linn H: Myocardial necrosis induced by temporary occlusion of a coronary artery in the dog. *Arch Pathol* 1960; 70:68–78.
70. Hirzel HO, Sonneblick EH, Kirk ES: Absence of a lateral border zone of intermediate creatine phosphokinase depletion surrounding a central infarct 24 hours after acute coronary occlusion in the dog. *Circ Res* 1977; 673–683.
71. Marcus ML, Kerber RE, Ehrhardt J, Abboud FM: Three dimensional geometry of acutely ischemic myocardium. *Circulation* 1975; 52:254–263.
72. Barlow CH, Chance B: Ischemic areas in perfused rat hearts: Measurement by NADH fluorescence photography. *Science* 1976; 193:909–910.
73. Harken AH, Barlow CH, Harden WR 3d, Chance B: Two- and three-dimensional display of myocardial ischemic "border zone" in dog. *Am J Cardiol* 1978; 42:954–959.
74. Janse MJ, Cinca J, Morena H, Fiolet JWT, Kleber AG, DeVries GP, et al: The "border zone" in myocardial ischemia. An electrophysiological, metabolic, and histochemical correlation in the pig heart. *Circ Res* 1979; 44:576–588.
75. Harken AH, Simson MB, Haselgrove J, Wetstein L, Harden WR III, Barlow CH: Early ischemia after complete coronary litigation in the rabbit, dog, pig, and monkey. *Am J Physiol* 1981; 241:H202–H210.
76. Yellon DM, Hearse DJ, Crome R, Grannel J, Wyse RKH: Characterization of the lateral interface between normal and ischemic tissue in the canine heart during evolving myocardial infarction. *Am J Cardiol* 1981; 47:1233–1239.
77. Factor SM, Sonnenblick EH, Kirk ES: The histologic border zone of acute myocardial infarction: Islands or peninsulas? *Am J Pathol* 1978; 92:111–124.
78. Okun EM, Factor SM, Kirk ES: End-capillary loops in the heart: An explanation for discrete myocardial infarctions without border zones. *Science* 1979; 206:565–567.
79. Factor SM, Okun EM, Minase T, Kirk ES: The microcirculation of the human heart: End-capillary loops with discrete perfusion fields. *Circulation* 1982; 66:1241–1248.
80. Lowe JE, Reimer KA, Jennings RB: Experimental infarct size as a function of the amount of myocardium at risk. *Am J Pathol* 1978; 90:363–378.

81. Lee JT, Ideker RE, Reimer KA: Myocardial infarct size and location in relation to the coronary vascular bed at risk in man. *Circulation* 1981; 64:526–534.
82. Factor SM, Okun EM, Kirk ES: The histologic border of acute canine myocardial infarction: A function of microcirculation. *Circ Res* 1981; 48:640–649.
83. Brosius FC III, Roberts WC: Significance of coronary arterial thrombus in transmural acute myocardial infarction. A study of 54 necropsy patients. *Circulation* 1981; 63:810–816.
84. Muller JE: Coronary artery thrombosis: Historical aspects. *J Am Coll Cardiol* 1983; 1:893–896.
85. Erhlich JC, Shinohara Y: Low incidence of coronary thrombosis in myocardial infarction. A restudy by serial block technique. *Arch Pathol* 1964; 78:432–445.
86. Roberts EC, Buja M: The frequency and significance of coronary arterial thrombi and other observations in fatal acute myocardial infarction: A study of 107 necropsy patients. *Am J Med* 1972; 52:425–443.
87. Silver MD, Baroldi G, Mariani F: The relationship between acute occlusive coronary thrombi and myocardial infarction studies in 100 consecutive patients. *Circulation* 1980; 61:219–227.
88. Buja LM, Willerson JT: The role of coronary artery lesions in ischemic heart disease. *Hum Pathol* 1987; 451–461.
89. DeWood MA, Spores J, Notske R, Mouser LT, Burroughs R, Golden MS, et al: Prevalence of total coronary occlusion during the early hours of transmural myocardial infarction. *N Engl J Med* 1980; 303:897–902.
90. Rapaport E: Thrombolytic agents in acute myocardial infarction. *N Engl J Med* 1989; 320:861–864.
91. White HD, Norris RM, Brown MA, Takayama M, Maslowski A, Bass NM, et al: Effect of intravenous streptokinase on left ventricular function and early survival after acute myocardial infarction. *N Engl J Med* 1987; 317:850–855.
92. Ridolfi RL, Hutchins GM: The relationship between coronary artery lesions and myocardial infarcts: Ulceration of atherosclerotic plaques precipitating coronary thrombosis. *Am Heart J* 1977; 93:468–486.
93. Horie T, Sekiguchi M, Hirosawa K: Coronary thrombosis in pathogenesis of acute myocardial infarction. *Br Heart J* 1978; 40:153–161.
94. Falk E: Plaque rupture with severe pre-existing stenosis precipitating coronary thrombosis. Characteristics of coronary atherosclerosis plaques underlying fatal occlusive thrombi. *Br Heart J* 1983; 50:127–134.
95. Friedman M, Van den Bovenkamp GJ: The pathogenesis of coronary thrombus. *Am J Pathol* 1966; 48:19–45.
96. Factor SM, Cho S: Smooth muscle contraction bands in the media of coronary arteries: A post-mortem marker of ante-mortem spasm? *J Am Coll Cardiol* 1985; 6:1329–1337.
97. Latham PM: Lecture 37. In: *Collected Works*. London, New Sydenham Society, 1886; 1:445.
98. Osler W: Lumleian lectures on angina pectoris. *Lancet* 1910; 1:839.
99. Buja LM, Hillis LD, Petty CS, Willerson JT: The role of coronary arterial spasm in ischemic heart disease. *Arch Pathol Lab Med* 1981; 105:221–226.
100. Gorlin R: Role of coronary vasospasm in the pathogenesis of myocardial ischemia and angina pectoris. *Am Heart J* 1982; 103:598–603.
101. Yasue H, Omote S, Takizawa A, Nagao M: Coronary arterial spasm in ischemic heart disease and its pathogenesis. A review. *Circ Res* 1983; 52(suppl 1):147–152.
102. Maseri A, L'Abbate A, Baroldi G, Chierchia S, Marzilli M, Ballestra AM, et al: Coronary vasospasm as a possible cause of myocardial infarction. A conclusion derived from the study of "preinfarction" angina. *N Engl J Med* 1978; 299:1271–1277.
103. Oliva JPB, Breckenridge JC: Arteriographic evidence of coronary arterial spasm in acute myocardial infarction. *Circulation* 1977; 56:366–374.
104. Rubanyi GM, Botelho LHP: Endothelins. *FASEB J* 1991; 5:2713–2720.
105. Forstermann U, Mugge A, Alheid U, Haverich A, Frolich JC: Selective attenuation of endothelium-mediated vasodilation in atherosclerotic human coronary arteries. *Circ Res* 1988; 62:185–190.
106. Harrison DG: From isolated vessels to the catheterization laboratory. Studies of endothelial function in the coronary circulation of humans. *Circulation* 1989; 80:703–706.
107. Berman JW, Calderon TM: The role of endothelial adhesion molecules in the development of atherosclerosis. *Cardiovasc Pathol* 1992; 1:17–28.
108. Dalen JE, Ockene IS, Alpert JS: Coronary spasm, coronary thrombosis, and myocardial infarction: A hypothesis concerning the pathophysiology of acute myocardial infarction. *Am Heart J* 1982; 104:1119–1124.
109. Joris I, Majno G: Endothelial changes induced by arterial spasm. *Am J Pathol* 1981; 102:346–358.
110. Gertz SD, Uretsky G, Wajnberg RS, Navot N, Gotsman MS: Endothelial cell damage and thrombus formation after partial arterial constriction: Relevance to the role of coronary artery spasm in the pathogenesis of myocardial infarction. *Circulation* 1981; 63:476–486.
111. Reimer KA, Lowe JE, Rasmussen MM, Jennings RB: The wavefront phenomenon of ischemic cell death: I. Myocardial infarct size vs. duration of coronary occlusion in dogs. *Circulation* 1977, 56:786–794.
112. Reimer KA, Jennings RB: The "Wavefront Phenomenon" of myocardial ischemic cell death: II. Transmural progression of necrosis within the framework of ischemic bed size (myocardium at risk) and collateral flow. *Lab Invest* 1979; 40:633–664.
113. Schaper W, Frenzel H, Hort W, Winkler B: Experimental coronary artery occlusion: II. Spatial and temporal evolution of infarcts in the dog heart. *Basic Res Cardiol* 1979; 74:233–239.
114. Forman R, Cho S, Factor SM, Kirk ES: Acute myocardial infarct extension into a previously preserved subendocardial region at risk in dogs and patients. *Circulation* 1983; 67:117–183.
115. Eng C, Cho S, Factor SM, Kirk S: A non-flow basis for the vulnerability of the subendocardium. *J Am Coll Cardiol* 1987; 9:374–379.
116. Lavellee M, Cox D, Patrick TA, Vatner SF: Salvage of myocardial function by coronary artery reperfusion 1, 2, and 4 hours after occlusion in conscious dogs. *Circ Res* 1983; 53:235–247.
117. Baughman KL, Maroko PR, Vatner SF: Effects of coronary artery reperfusion on myocardial infarct size and survival in conscious dogs. *Circulation* 1981; 63:317–322.
118. Fenoglio JJ, Karagueuzian HS, Friedman PL, Albala A, Wit AL: Time course of infarct growth toward the endocardial surface during the first 24 hours after coronary occlusion. *Am J Physiol* 1979; 236:H356–H370.
119. Karagueuzian HS, Fenoglio JJ, Weiss MB, Wit AL: Coronary occlusion and reperfusion: Effects on subendocardial cardiac fibers. *Am J Physiol* 1980; 236:H581–H593.
120. Frame LK, Lopez JA, Khaw BA, Fallon JT, Haber E, Powell WJ Jr: Early membrane damage during coronary reperfusion in dogs. Detection by radiolabeled anticardiac myosin. *J Clin Invest* 1983; 72:535–544.
121. Kloner RA, Przyklenk K, Whittaker P: Deleterious effects of oxygen radicals in ischemia/reperfusion. Resolved and unresolved issues. *Circulation* 1989; 80:1115–1127.
122. Kehrer JP: Concepts related to the study of reactive oxygen and cardiac reperfusion injury. *Free Radic Res Commun* 1989; 5:305–314.
123. Whalen DA, Hamilton DG, Ganote CE, Jennings RB: Effect of a transient period of ischemia on myocardial cells. Effects on cell volume regulation. *Am J Pathol* 1974; 74:381–398.
124. Shen AC, Jennings RB: Myocardial calcium and magnesium in acute ischemic injury. *Am J Pathol* 1972; 67:414–440.
125. Hearse DJ: Reperfusion of the ischemic myocardium. *J Mol Cell Cardiol* 1977; 9:605–616.
126. Sommers HM, Jennings RB: Experimental acute myocardial infarction, histologic and histochemical studies of early myocardial infarcts induced by temporary or permanent occlusion of a coronary artery. *Lab Invest* 1964; 13:1491–1503.
127. Bulkley BH, Hutchins GM: Myocardial consequences of coronary artery bypass graft surgery: The paradox of necrosis in areas of revascularization. *Circulation* 1977; 56:906–913.
128. Mallory GK, White PD, Salcedo-Salgar J: The speed of healing of myocardial infarction: A study of the pathologic anatomy in 72 cases. *Am Heart J* 1939; 18:647–671.
129. Fishbein MC, MacLean D, Maroko PR: The histopathologic evolution of myocardial infarction. *Chest* 1978; 73:843–849.
130. Bouchardy B, Majno C: Histopathology of early myocardial infarcts: A new approach. *Am J Pathol* 1974; 74:301–330.
131. Weiss SJ: Tissue destruction by neutrophils. *N Engl J Med* 1989; 320:365–376.
132. Kloner RA, Ganote CE, Jenning RB: The "no-reflow" phenome-

non after temporary coronary occlusion in the dog. *J Clin Invest* 1974; 54:1496–1508.

133. Weisman HF, Healy B: Myocardial infarct expansion, infarct extension, and re-infarction: Pathophysiologic concepts. *Prog Cardiovasc Dis* 1987; 30:73–110.
134. Hutchins GM, Bulkley BH: Infarct expansion versus extension: Two different complications of acute myocardial infarction. *Am J Cardiol* 1978; 41:1127–1132.
135. Robinson TF, Cohen-Gould, Factor SM: Skeletal framework of mammalian heart muscle. Arrangement of inter- and pericellular connective tissue structures. *Lab Invest* 1983; 49:482–498.
136. Factor SM, Robinson TF, Dominitz R, Cho S: Alterations of the myocardial skeletal framework in acute myocardial infarction with and without ventricular rupture. *Am J Cardiovasc Pathol* 1987; 1:91–98.
137. Fraker TD Jr, Wagner GS, Rosati RA: Extension of myocardial infarction: Incidence and prognosis. *Circulation* 1979; 60:1127–1129.
138. Factor SM, Okun EM, Kirk ES: Microextension of acute myocardial necrosis into the normal zone of 7 day canine infarcts. *Circulation* 1979; 60(suppl 2):114.
139. Braunwald E, Kloner RA: The stunned myocardium: Prolonged, post-ischemic ventricular dysfunction. *Circulation* 1982; 66:1146–1149.
140. DeBoer LWV, Ingwall JS, Kloner RA, Braunwald E: Prolonged derangements of canine myocardial purine metabolism after a brief coronary artery occlusion not associated with anatomic evidence of necrosis. *Proc Natl Acad Sci USA* 1980; 77:5471–5475.
141. Przyklenk K, Kloner RA: Superoxide dismutase plus catalase improve contractile function in the canine model of the "stunned myocardium." *Circ Res* 1986; 58:148–156.
142. Ellis SG, Wynne J, Braunwald E, Henschke CI, Sandor T, Kloner RA: Response of reperfusion salvaged, stunned myocardium to inotropic stimulation. *Am Heart J* 1984; 107:13–19.
143. Becker LC, Levine JH, DiPaula AF, Guarnieri T, Aversano T: Reversal of dysfunction in postischemic stunned myocardium by epinephrine and postextrasystolic potentiation. *J Am Coll Cardiol* 1986; 7:580–589.
144. Zhao M, Hong Z, Robinson TF, Factor SM, Sonnenblick EH, Eng C: Profound structural alterations of the extracellular collagen matrix in postischemic dysfunctional ("stunned") but viable myocardium. *J Am Coll Cardiol* 1987; 10:1322–1334.
145. Murry CE, Jennings RB, Reimer KA: Preconditioning with ischemia: A delay of lethal cell injury in ischemic myocardium. *Circulation* 1986; 74:1124–1136.
146. Murry CE, Richard VJ, Jennings RB, Reimer KA: Myocardial protection is lost before contractile function recovers from ischemic preconditioning. *Am J Physiol (Heart Circ Physiol)* 1991; 260:H796–H804.
147. Murry CE, Richard VJ, Reimer KA, Jennings RB: Ischemic preconditioning slows energy metabolism and delays ultrastructural damage during a sustained ischemic episode. *Circ Res* 1990; 66:913–931.
148. Lui GS, Thornton J, Van Winkle DM, Stanley AWH, Olsson RA, Downey JM: Protection against infarction afforded by preconditioning is mediated by A1 adenosine receptors in rabbit heart. *Circulation* 1991; 84:350–356.
149. Kitakaze M, Hori M, Takashima S, Sato H, Inoue M, Kamada T: Ischemic preconditioning increases adenosine release and 5′-nucleotidase activity during myocardial ischemia and reperfusion in dogs. *Circulation* 1993;87:208–215.

SECTION B

Clinical Considerations

Chapter 58

Diagnosis and Management of Chronic Ischemic Heart Disease

Robert C. Schlant, M.D. ■ *R. Wayne Alexander, M.D.*

DEFINITION

Angina pectoris (literally "strangling" in the chest) is a recurrent symptom complex of discomfort in the chest or related areas associated with myocardial ischemia and dysfunction but without myocardial necrosis. Characteristically, the discomfort is produced by exertion and is promptly relieved by rest or nitroglycerin.

HISTORICAL PERSPECTIVE

There were references to what would be recognized today as angina pectoris, myocardial infarction, and sudden death in ancient Egyptian, Greek, Biblical, and Talmudic sources. In 1768 William Heberden presented his classic description of angina pectoris in a lecture before the Royal College of Physicians and it was published in 1772.[1] This classic description was again published with additions and minor changes in a chapter entitled "Pectoris Dolor" in his *Commentaries on the History and Cure of Diseases*, which was translated from the Latin and published by his son, also called William Heberden, in 1802, a year after Heberden's death.[2] The following quotation is from his original lecture:

> **There is a disorder of the breast, marked with strong and peculiar symptoms, considerable for the kind of danger belonging to it, and extremely rare, of which I do not recollect any mention among medical authors. The seat of it, and sense of strangling and anxiety with which it is attended, may make it not improperly be called angina pectoris.**
>
> **Those who are afflicted with it, are seized, while they are walking, and more particularly when they walk soon after eating, with a painful and most disagreeable sensation in the breast, which seems as if it would take their life away, if it were to increase or to continue: the moment they stand still all this uneasiness vanishes. In all other respects the patients are at the beginning of this disorder perfectly well, and in particular have no shortness of breath, from which it is totally different.**
>
> **After it has continued some months, it will not cease so instantaneously upon standing still; and it will come on, not only when the persons are walking, but when they are lying down, and oblige them to rise up from their beds every night for many months together; and in one or two very inveterate cases it has been brought on by the motion of a horse or a carriage, and even by swallowing, coughing, going to stool or speaking, or by any disturbance of mind. I have heard once, and only one person, say that he had known it to attack him when he was up and standing still or sitting. But most, whom I have seen, have been perfectly unaffected with riding in any manner, with speaking, swallowing, laughing, sneezing, or vomiting. One has told me that his complaint was greatest in winter; another, that it was aggravated by warm weather; in the rest the seasons were not suspected of making any difference.**
>
> **I have observed something like this affection of the breast in one woman who was paralytic, and have heard one or two young men complain of it in a slight degree; but all the rest, whom I have seen, who are at least twenty,**

were men, and almost all above 50 years old, and most of them with a short neck, and inclining to be fat.

When a fit of this sort comes on by walking, its duration is very short, as it goes off almost immediately upon stopping. If it comes on in the night, it will last an hour or two; and I have met with one, in whom it once continued for several days, during all which time the patient seemed to be in imminent danger of death.

When I first took notice of this distemper, and could find no satisfaction from books, I consulted an able physician of long experience, who told me that he had known several ill of it, and that all of them had died suddenly. This observation I have reason to think is generally true of such patients; having known six of those, for whom I have been consulted, die in this manner; and more perhaps may have experienced the same death, which I had no opportunity of knowing. But the natural tendency of this illness be to kill the patients suddenly, yet unless it have a power of preserving a person from all other ails, it will easily be believed that some of those, who are afflicted with it, may die in a different manner, since this disorder will last, as I have known it more than once, near twenty years, and most usually attacks only those who are above fifty years of age. I have accordingly observed one, who sunk under a lingering illness of a different nature.

The os sterni is usually pointed to as the seat of this malady, but it seems sometimes as if it was under the lower part of it, and at other times under the middle or upper part, but always inclining more to the left side, and sometimes there is with it a pain about the middle of the left arm. What the particular mischief is, which is referred to these different parts of the sternum, it is not easy to guess, and I have had no opportunity of knowing with certainty. It may be a strong cramp, or an ulcer, or possibly both.

For the interested reader, Leibowitz has published an excellent history of coronary heart disease.[3]

The syndrome of angina pectoris was described as rare in textbooks of medicine in 1866 (Austin Flint) and 1892 (William Osler). P.D. White wrote that "(angina pectoris) was still uncommon in my early professional years. But when the automobile came in the 1920s and the population at large became more prosperous and overnourished, the current epidemic of coronary heart disease, as shown prevailingly by the symptom angina pectoris, began and incidentally involved younger and younger men."[4] In the United States the peak mortality rate from coronary heart disease (CHD) occurred about 1962 to 1965, since when it has been steadily decreasing.[5]

ETIOLOGY

Angina pectoris is caused by coronary atherosclerosis in the vast majority of patients. (See Chaps. 53 to 57, 62.) Many nonatherosclerotic causes of coronary artery disease (CAD) (Tables 64-1 and 64-2) can also produce angina pectoris or myocardial infarction; these are discussed in Chap. 64. Other conditions particularly associated with angina pectoris include congenital coronary artery abnormalities (Chaps. 64 and 97), aortic stenosis (Chap. 79), mitral stenosis that produces severe right ventricular hypertension (Chap. 80), hypertrophic cardiomyopathy (Chap. 90), and systemic arterial hypertension (Chaps. 75 and 76). Conditions in which angina occurs less often include aortic regurgitation (Chap. 79), idiopathic dilated cardiomyopathy and specific forms of heart muscle disease (Chaps. 88 and 89), and syphilitic heart disease (Chap. 106). Mitral valve prolapse (Chap. 80) is rarely a cause of true angina pectoris. Many conditions may alter the myocardial oxygen supply-demand relationship and worsen angina pectoris, including severe anemia, tachycardia, fever, hyperthyroidism, hypothyroidism, and Paget's disease of bone. Many of these are associated with a high cardiac output. (See also Chap. 24.)

CLASSIFICATION

The Canadian Cardiovascular Society Grading Scale (Table 19-2) is currently widely used to classify the severity of angina pectoris.[6]

DIAGNOSIS OF ANGINA PECTORIS

Symptoms

Angina pectoris is classified as *stable* when its characteristics (frequency, severity, duration, time of appearance, and precipitating factors) have not changed for the previous 60 days. Angina pectoris ("angina") may be described by the patient using a variety of descriptors, (Table 58-1). The discomfort is often not painful. The wide variety of terms used to describe the discomfort at times reflects the patient's cultural background and life experience. Certain descriptors of discomfort suggest that the discomfort is not angina pectoris (Table 58-2).[7] Other important characteristics of angina pectoris include its precipitating factors, location, mode of onset and duration, and disappearance. (See Chap. 19.)

Classically, the discomfort of chronic stable angina pectoris is precipitated by physical activity, emotions, eating, or cold weather. Some patients are able to describe fairly precisely the amount of exercise (length of walking or number of stairs) at which they reproducibly experience their discomfort. In some patients the amount of exertion that produces angina is much less in the morning soon after arising. Upper extremity exertion may induce angina, at times more readily than walking.

TABLE 58-1
Common Terms Used to Describe Angina Pectoris

Pressure	Uncomfortable	Ache
Tightness	Swelling	Weight
Heaviness	Burning	Heartburn
Constricting	Dull	Soreness
Compressing	Searing	Bursting
Fullness	Hard	Like a toothache
Choking	Strangling	
Discomfort	Indigestion	Like a vise

TABLE 58-2

Descriptors of Discomfort Not Likely to Be Angina Pectoris

Needlelike	Shooting	Pricking
Sticking	Jabbing	Cutting
Stabbing	Twitching	Like an ice pick
Knifelike	Itching	
Stinging	Tingling	

Angina may be precipitated by cold temperatures or cold wind, which may also be associated with a decrease in the duration of exercise before the onset of discomfort. Angina may also occur after meals (prandial or postprandial angina) due to the increase in cardiac output.[8,9] Many patients with angina will have symptoms if they walk up a hill after a large meal with a cold wind blowing in their face. Emotions, particularly anger, excitation, and frustration, may also precipitate angina in patients with significant coronary atherosclerosis. Cigarette smoking can also precipitate or lower the exertion threshold for angina pectoris in some patients.[10,11] In most patients a combination of factors is present, and the amount of exertion associated with discomfort frequently varies. Very often, an episode occurs after performing a certain amount of a particular activity at a certain time of the day, but not while performing even more strenuous activity at another time of day. (See below.)

In most instances, stable angina pectoris develops and increases to a plateau over 10 to 30 s and usually disappears after several minutes if the exertion is discontinued. Occasionally, the angina will disappear despite physical activity, so-called walk-through angina. Most patients have discomfort that lasts a few minutes or up to 10 to 15 min and, rarely, up to 30 min. When discomfort is documented to last more than 15 min, one should have a strong suspicion that there may have been necrosis of at least a few myocytes, which may be too few to be diagnosed as myocardial infarction (see Chaps. 59 and 60). Discomfort that is sharp and stabbing, like an ice pick, and that has a sudden onset and lasts a few seconds is usually not due to myocardial ischemia (Table 58-2).

The discomfort of angina is most often located substernally or just to the left of the sternum. Some patients clench their fist over their sternum (Levine's sign) as they describe their discomfort. This sign has a high diagnostic accuracy. Less often, angina is located over the precordium. It is unusual for the discomfort to be located only at the apex of the heart. It can be located anywhere from the epigastrium to the neck and rarely it may be located only in the neck, throat, arm, or back. Some patients state that they have a "funny" or "different" feeling that they cannot describe further. It is very rare that angina pectoris is located only below the costal margin. The discomfort of angina pectoris often radiates down the arms or to the neck, jaw, teeth, shoulders, or back. Radiation to the left side is more common than to the right, but both sides can be involved. The radiation is characteristically down the ulnar aspect of the arm; frequently, the radiation is described as a numbness.

Increased heat or humidity may also lower the exertional threshold at which angina occurs. Amphetamines and across-the-counter cold remedies, which may increase the arterial blood pressure and heart rate, may precipitate angina, as can cocaine, which can also increase heart rate and blood pressure and produce coronary artery vasoconstriction or thrombosis. (See Chap. 110.)

Nocturnal angina is the occurrence of angina at night. In some patients it may be related to an increase in blood volume and in cardiac output as the result of assuming the recumbent position. Other possible causes include dreaming, unrecognized tachycardia, or a marked decrease in systemic arterial blood pressure. Some patients who have nocturnal angina as a consequence of the increase in blood volume respond to therapy with digoxin and diuretics. In general, both nocturnal and rest angina are strongly suggestive of unstable angina pectoris, which usually requires a prompt and thorough evaluation. (See Chap 59.)

Conditions that increase myocardial oxygen requirements may exacerbate the occurrence of angina pectoris and, occasionally, may be associated with angina in the absence of significant coronary artery disease on routine coronary arteriography.

Angina Equivalents

As noted below, patients with stable angina have many episodes of myocardial ischemia that are asymptomatic or silent. In addition, patients may have episodes of myocardial ischemia that result in symptoms from either systolic or diastolic left ventricular dysfunction but that are not associated with chest discomfort or symptoms characteristic of angina pectoris. Like other types of angina, "angina equivalent" symptoms usually are associated with exertion and are relieved by rest and nitroglycerin. The most common symptoms are (1) exertional dyspnea, which is probably related to alterations in diastolic relaxation and compliance due to myocardial ischemia; and (2) exertional fatigue or exhaustion, which is probably related to an acute decrease in cardiac output related to decreased systolic left ventricular function and/or associated mitral regurgitation from transient papillary muscle dysfunction. Myocardial ischemia results in a slowing of the isovolumic relaxation rate and an upward shift of the left ventricular diastolic pressure-volume relation, together with a variable degree of depression of systolic function and changes in end-systolic volume.[12–18]

In general, when myocardial ischemia is produced, diastolic dysfunction occurs before systolic dysfunction, which in turn often occurs prior to electrocardiographic (ECG) changes and before the symptom of angina pectoris (Fig. 58-1).

Patients with angina pectoris due to atherosclerosis have an increased frequency of the usual risk factors for atherosclerosis including hypercholesterolemia, cigarette smoking, systemic arterial hypertension, diabetes mellitus, physical inactivity, and a family history of CAD in a parent or close relative before the age of 55. In women, the use of oral birth control pills and the postmenopausal state without estrogen replacement may contribute to the development and progression of atherosclerosis. These factors are discussed in Chaps. 53 and 62.

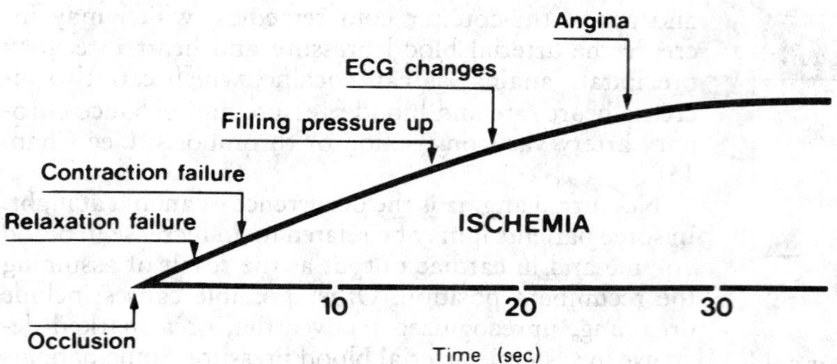

FIGURE 58-1 Appearance of events during transient coronary occlusion. (*From Sigwart et al.*[112] *Reproduced with permission from the publisher and authors.*)

Physical Examination

During an attack of angina pectoris, many patients appear somewhat pale and quiet. They are frequently sweating. The heart rate and blood pressure are both often slightly elevated, and occasionally there are atrial or ventricular premature contractions. Abnormal systolic bulges may be present at the apex or at ectopic precordial areas. A new gallop, usually an S_4 and occasionally an S_3, may be transiently present as well as an apical systolic murmur of mitral regurgitation from papillary muscle dysfunction.[19] Rarely, the second heart sound may demonstrate reversed splitting.[20,21]

A useful test to confirm the diagnosis in a patient experiencing discomfort is to perform carotid sinus massage for a few seconds while listening to the heart. If the patient experiences significant cardiac slowing, the physician should discontinue the massage and ask the patient whether the massage made the discomfort worse. If the patient replies "no" and adds that the massage made the discomfort go away, the diagnosis of angina pectoris is virtually established. On the other hand, if no slowing of the heart rate occurs, the test is indeterminate. Carotid sinus massage should not be performed until one has examined both carotid arteries for evidence of disease. In some patients, angina pectoris is relieved by performing a Valsalva maneuver, presumably by a decrease in myocardial oxygen requirements due to the decrease in left ventricular volume and wall stress produced by the decreased venous return. Patients with angina pectoris may have physical signs associated with hyperlipidemia, including arcus senilis, xanthelasma, eruptive xanthomata, tendon xanthomata, and tuberous xanthomata. (See Chap. 10.)

Special Tests

Introduction

Most special tests in patients with suspected stable angina pectoris are performed either to establish the diagnosis or to obtain prognostic information.[22] In general, men with a history of classic angina pectoris have a higher probability of having significant CAD on coronary arteriography than do women.[23,24] The gender difference is even greater for patients with atypical angina pectoris. Table 58-3 and Fig. 58-2 provide the likelihood for each gender by age and characteristics of the chest discomfort. They also illustrate one reason why women have more false-positive responses to ECG exercise testing than do men. (See also Chap. 16.) Table 58-4 provides a glossary of terms useful in the evaluation and selection of diagnostic tests. Bayes' theorem states that the pretest disease prevalence influences the posttest like-

TABLE 58-3

Pretest Likelihood of Coronary Disease According to Age, Sex, and Symptoms*†

Age, Years	Asymptomatic		Nonanginal Chest Pain		Atypical Angina		Typical Angina	
	Men	Women	Men	Women	Men	Women	Men	Women
35–45	0.037 ±0.024	0.007 ±0.006	0.105 ±0.063	0.027 ±0.024	0.428 ±0.144	0.155 ±0.111	0.809 ±0.104	0.454 ±0.186
45–55	0.077 ±0.040	0.021 ±0.018	0.206 ±0.090	0.069 ±0.051	0.601 ±0.129	0.317 ±0.160	0.907 ±0.049	0.677 ±0.167
55–65	0.111 ±0.049	0.054 ±0.042	0.282 ±0.100	0.127 ±0.080	0.690 ±0.106	0.465 ±0.174	0.939 ±0.029	0.839 ±0.108
65–75	0.113 ±0.050	0.115 ±0.078	0.282 ±0.100	0.171 ±0.097	0.700 ±0.103	0.541 ±0.169	0.943 ±0.026	0.947 ±0.057

SOURCE: Adapted from Diamond GA: A clinically relevant classification of chest discomfort. *J Am Coll Cardiol* 1983; 1:574. Reproduced with permission from the author and the American College of Cardiology.
* Each value represents the percentage ± standard error of the percentage.
† Assessment of anginal symptoms: (1) Is chest pain substernal? (2) Is it precipitated by exertion? (3) Is it relieved within 10 min by rest or nitroglycerin? Answers to three of three questions "yes" = typical angina. Answers to two of three questions "yes" = atypical angina. Answers to one of three questions "yes" = nonanginal chest pain. No complaints of chest discomfort above the diaphragm = asymptomatic.

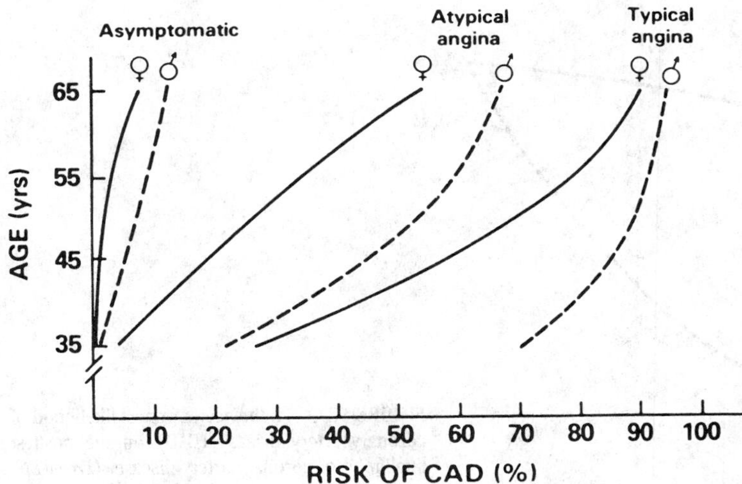

FIGURE 58-2 Influence of age, sex, and symptoms of coronary artery disease (CAD) derived from data of Diamond and Forrester.[23] *(From Epstein SE: Implications of probability analysis on the strategy used for noninvasive detection of coronary artery disease. Am J Cardiol 1980; 46:491–499. Reproduced with permission from the publisher and author.)*

lihood of significant CAD. This is illustrated in Fig. 58-3. In this figure, the posttest likelihood of CAD is plotted as a function of the pretest likelihood of disease, assuming that the test has a sensitivity of 75 percent or a specificity of 85 percent, which are reasonable figures for ECG exercise testing. The positive test curve illustrates that the posttest likelihood of CAD must be very high in patients with a high pretest likelihood of disease. Figure 58-4 illustrates the varying probabilities obtained with ECG exercise testing using different criteria for a positive test. Note that a "positive" test result consisting of a 1-mm ST-segment depression in an asymptomatic 50-year-old man has a very low probability of being associated with coronary artery disease and therefore is of questionable diagnostic importance, whereas an ST-segment depression of 2 mm or more in the same patient has a very high probability of indicating coronary artery disease. Note that when the pretest likelihood of disease is 40 to 80 percent, an ECG exercise test resulting in an ST-segment depression greater than 1 mm but less than 2 mm is still associated with considerable uncertainty, as is a negative test (Fig. 58-4). It should be noted that the values assumed for the sensitivities and specificities are assumed values and that these may vary in individual laboratories. In addition, this discussion has pertained only to the diagnosis of CAD. In many patients with known CAD, exercise testing is performed not for diagnostic but rather for prognostic purposes.

Figure 58-5 illustrates the impact of Bayes' theorem when evaluating several diagnostic tests for coronary artery disease. If one were to perform an exercise ECG test on a 55-year-old woman with a typical chest pain, with a pretest likelihood for coronary disease of 0.46, a positive test response would indicate her posttest likelihood to be 0.86. If she were then to have a thallium scan, her pretest likelihood would be 0.86. If she had a positive thallium scan, her likelihood of disease would increase to 0.98, whereas if her thallium scan were negative, her likelihood of disease would decrease to 0.63. As long as additional tests meet the criterion of conditional independence and are based on different aspects of the pathophysiological process, this principle can be applied with additional tests to establish a diagnosis more firmly. On the other hand, diagnostic tests should only be performed to answer a specific clinical question.

From the above discussion, it should be apparent that a diagnostic test may be of limited additional diagnostic value in patients with either a very high or very low pretest risk for coronary artery disease. On the other hand, an exercise test may give valuable prognostic information, and nuclear scintigraphy may provide valuable information about the functional aspects of the coronary circulation.

TABLE 58-4

Glossary of Terms

True positive (TP): Positive result in patient with disease

True negative (TN): Negative result in patient without disease

False positive (FP): Positive result in patient without disease

False negative (FN): Negative result in patient with disease

Sensitivity: $\dfrac{TP}{TP + FN}$

Specificity: $\dfrac{TN}{TN + FP}$

Predictive value of a positive test: $\dfrac{TP}{TP + FP}$

Predictive value of a negative test: $\dfrac{TN}{TN + FN}$

Bayes' theorem:

Probability of disease presence with a positive test =

$$\frac{\text{sensitivity} \times \text{prevalence}}{(\text{sensitivity} \times \text{prevalence}) + [(1 - \text{specificity}) \times (1 - \text{prevalence})]}$$

Probability of disease presence with a negative test =

$$\frac{(1 - \text{sensitivity}) \times \text{prevalence}}{(1 - \text{sensitivity} \times \text{prevalence}) + [\text{specificity} \times (1 - \text{prevalence})]}$$

Exercise-Stress Electrocardiography

Exercise-stress electrocardiography is the most widely applied test used to obtain objective evidence of myocardial ischemia and significant CAD. It is also employed to obtain prognostic data regarding ventricular performance in patients with known CAD.[25] See Chap. 16 for

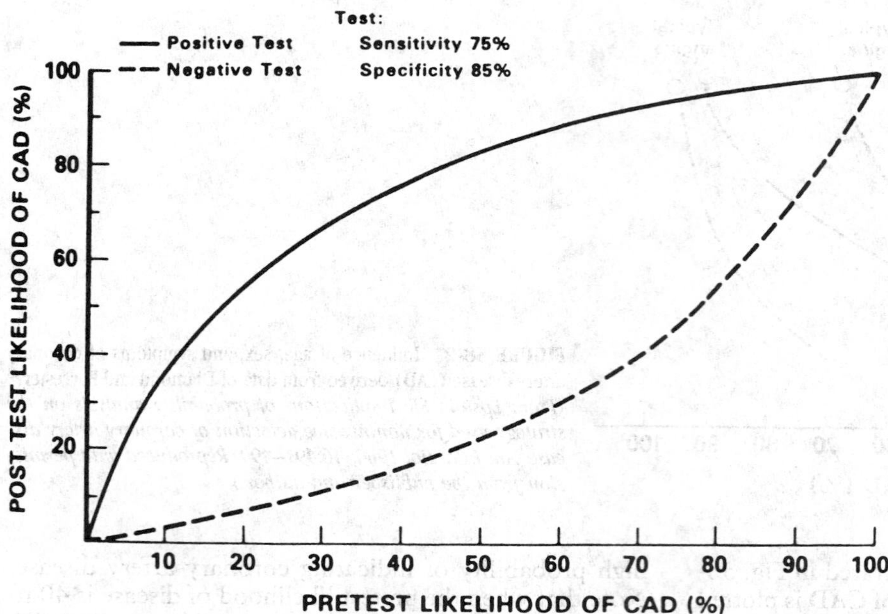

FIGURE 58-3 Influence of pretest likelihood of coronary artery disease (CAD) on the posttest likelihood of coronary artery disease. *(From Epstein SE: Implications of probability analysis on the strategy used for noninvasive detection of coronary artery disease. Am J Cardiol 1980; 46:491–499. Reproduced with permission from the publisher and author.)*

a more thorough discussion of exercise treadmill testing (ETT). Figure 58-4 illustrates the data for the conclusion that a greater ST-segment depression is associated with a significantly greater posttest likelihood of CAD.

The sensitivity and specificity of exercise ECG testing have been stated to be 55 to 70 percent and 85 to 90 percent.[26] On the other hand, an extensive meta-analysis of 147 consecutive reports comparing exercise-induced

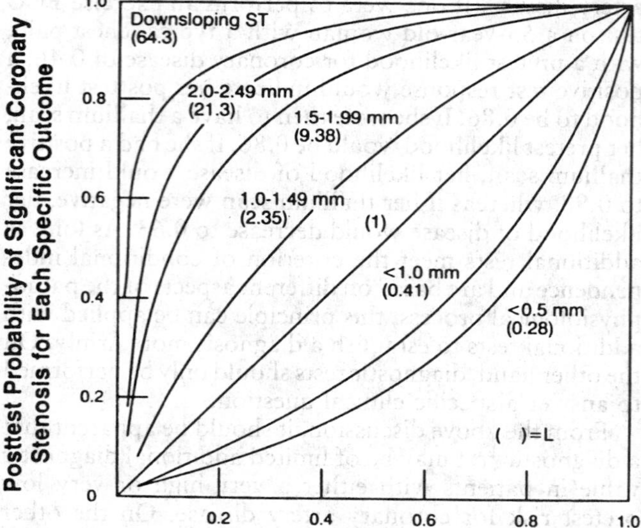

FIGURE 58-4 Curves showing the posttest risk of disease (P) as a function of pretest risk for the test outcomes indicated. The curves are based on the empirical values of the likelihood ratios (L) associated with these test outcomes according to published data. It is noted that greater degrees of ST-segment depression within the range 1.0 to 2.49 mm are associated with larger values of likelihood ratio and, correspondingly, increased probability of disease as compared to pretest risk. Conversely, ST-segment depression of <1.0 mm or <0.5 mm is associated with a likelihood ratio of less than unity and a modest reduction in probability of disease as compared to pretest risk. *(From Rifkin RD, Hood WB Jr.[24] Reproduced with permission from the publisher and authors.)*

ST depression with coronary arteriography in 24,074 patients found a wide variability in both sensitivity and specificity. The mean sensitivity was 68 percent [range, 23 to 100 percent; standard deviation (SD), 16 percent], and the mean specificity was 77 percent (range 17 to 100 percent; SD, 17 percent).[27,28]

Efforts to improve the clinical usefulness of exercise ECG testing in the diagnosis of CAD include development of a treadmill score[29,30] and a prognostic score and predicted 5-year survival determined from the amount of ST-segment depression, the degree of angina during exercise, and the duration of exercise (or equivalent).[31] Other techniques include the ST/HR slope (ST = ST-segment depression; HR = heart rate) calculated from linear regression of ST-segment depression against heart rate during peak exercise[32] and the simple ST/HR index in which additional ST-segment depression is divided by the overall change in HR throughout the exercise period.[33–35] To date none of these promising techniques has been clearly shown to be cost effective in daily practice.

Exercise ECG testing is of greatest diagnostic value in the evaluation of middle-aged men with atypical angina and a pretest probability of significant disease of 30 to 70 percent. Exercise ECG testing for diagnosis is somewhat more controversial when performed in women with typical or atypical angina; in men with atypical chest pain and complete right bundle branch block; in apparently healthy men more than 40 years old in special occupations (e.g., pilot, police officer, fire fighter, traffic controller); and in asymptomatic men with two or more major risk factors for coronary disease. Exercise ECG testing is not indicated for diagnostic purposes in asymptomatic men and women who are apparently healthy or who have marginal chest pain.[36] The overall clinical usefulness of exercise ECG testing for diagnostic purposes has been well reviewed.[23–25,27,28,37–40] It is relatively safe when performed using established guidelines and precautions.[41] (See also Chap. 16.)

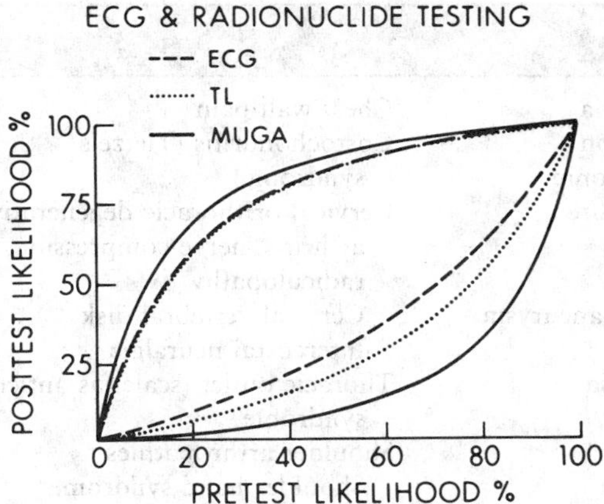

FIGURE 58-5 The use of Bayes' theorem in the diagnosis of coronary artery disease. The impact of exercise ECG, thallium (Tl), and ventriculographic (MUGA) test results as a function of pretest disease likelihood is shown. The curves above the line of identity represent positive test results. See text for additional discussion. (*Adapted from Epstein SE: Implications of probability analysis on the strategy used for noninvasive detection of coronary artery disease. Am J Cardiol 46:491, 1980. Reproduced with permission from the publisher and author.*)

Radionuclide Scintigraphy

Radionuclide techniques are discussed in detail in Chap. 134. Although it is more expensive, stress myocardial perfusion imaging provides higher sensitivity and specificity for the diagnosis of CAD than exercise ECG testing.[42–45] It may also be less dependent upon the level of exercise achieved.[46,47] Some of the findings that indicate a poor prognosis include an increased lung thallium 201 uptake, extensive perfusion defects, and postexercise transient left ventricular dilatation.[48–50] In general, a normal thallium 201 perfusion scan indicates that the likelihood of the patient experiencing a cardiac event is similar to the likelihood of the general population, even if the patient has known CAD.[47,51,52]

Pharmacologic stress testing, usually using dipyridamole, dobutamine, or adenosine, and thallium 201 can be employed in patients unable to exercise because of peripheral vascular disease, poor exercise tolerance, arthritis, neurologic disorders, or other contraindications. Stress scintigraphy is useful in the study of selected patients with chronic stable angina, patients with suspected CAD prior to noncardiac surgery (Chap. 139), or patients following myocardial infarction.[53–58] The use of technetium 99m sestamibi and other new agents may significantly improve imaging capabilities, particularly if they are used in combination with thallium 201.[59] (See Chap. 134.)

Positron Emission Tomography

Positron emission tomography (PET) promises to be even more accurate than standard thallium 201 single-photon emission computed tomography (SPECT) for the detection of CAD. It may also provide an estimate of coronary blood flow and coronary flow reserve as well as myocardial viability.[60–62] (See Chap. 137.)

Patients with stable angina may have persistent defects on 3-h redistribution imaging with thallium 201. About 30 to 40 percent of such patients may show improved perfusion and function after revascularization.[63] Viability can also be assessed using technetium 99m methoxyisobutyl isonitrile (^{99m}Tc sestamibi) or PET with fluorine-18, 2-deoxyglucose.[64]

Radionuclide Angiography

Radionuclide angiography, with the determination of peak exercise ejection fraction, is also useful for the diagnosis of CAD, although the presence of irregular heart rhythms, left bundle branch block, or marked left ventricular dysfunction limits its diagnostic value.[65] (See also Chap. 134.)

Echocardiography

Echocardiography (Chap. 14), Doppler echocardiography (Chap. 130), transesophageal echocardiography (Chap. 131), stress echocardiography (Chap. 132), and intravascular echocardiography (Chap. 133) are all useful in the assessment of one or more subsets of patients with CAD. Routine echocardiography provides a good estimate of ventricular size and of regional and generalized left ventricular wall motion. This can be performed at rest, during exercise, or immediately afterwards.[66] Either routine echocardiography or Doppler echocardiography can also be performed during or following pharmacologic stress with doubutamine, dipyridamole, or adenosine.[67–72] If adequate images can be obtained, exercise echocardiography has been reported to be comparable to radionuclide testing for the evaluation of CAD.[62] (See Chap. 132.)

Coronary Arteriography

It is controversial whether or not all patients with stable angina pectoris should undergo coronary arteriography. Some physicians routinely have cardiac catheterization and coronary arteriography performed to obtain an estimate of left ventricular regional and generalized wall motion and an evaluation of the extent and location of coronary artery disease. Other physicians are more selective and obtain coronary arteriography only if the diagnosis is in doubt or if revascularization by coronary artery bypass surgery or coronary angioplasty is contemplated. In general, patients whose symptoms are well controlled by medications and who have a good exercise tolerance are less likely to benefit significantly from revascularization. We would tend toward earlier cardiac catheterization in many patients since exercise ECG testing, radionuclide testing, and echocardiographic testing may not always properly identify patients who are good candidates for revascularization.

DIFFERENTIAL DIAGNOSIS

Table 58-5 lists the differential diagnosis of angina pectoris. In most instances, the distinction is clear if one is able to obtain an accurate history and perform a complete physical examination.

TABLE 58-5

Differential Diagnosis of Angina Pectoris

- Cardiovascular
  - Myocardial ischemia
    - Coronary atherosclerosis
    - Coronary vasospasm
    - Congenital coronary artery disease
      - Anomalous origin
      - Aberrant coronary artery
      - Coronary arteriovenous fistula
    - Kawasaki's disease
    - Small vessel disease
    - Microvascular angina (syndrome X)
    - Systemic arterial hypertension
    - Hypertrophic cardiomyopathy
    - Idiopathic dilated cardiomyopathy
    - Aortic valve disease
    - Coronary artery dissection (Marfan's syndrome)
    - Pulmonary hypertension
    - Right ventricular hypertension
    - Chronic obstructive pulmonary disease
    - Syphilitic aortitis, coronary ostial disease
    - Collagen-vascular disease
      - Periarteritis nodosa
      - Systemic lupus erythematosus
      - Rheumatoid arthritis
    - Cardiac amyloid
    - Cardiac tumors
    - Hereditary connective tissue disorders
      - Pseudoxanthoma elasticum
      - Cystic medial necrosis
      - Homocystinuria
      - Gargoylism
    - Severe anemia, hypoxia
    - High-dose x-irradiation
    - Withdrawal from chronic nitroglycerin exposure
  - Nonmyocardial ischemia
    - Aortic dissection
    - Discrete thoracic aortic aneurysm
    - Mitral valve prolapse
    - Tachycardia, bradycardia
    - Palpitations
    - Pericarditis
- Thoracic-respiratory
  - Pulmonary embolism, infarction
  - Pneumothorax
  - Pneumomediastinum (mediastinal emphysema)
  - Pleuritis
  - Epidemic pleurodynia (Bornholm's disease)
  - Mediastinitis
  - Intrathoracic malignancy
  - Café Coronary
- Gastrointestinal
  - Gastroesophageal reflux, esophagitis
  - Esophageal spasm
  - Esophageal rupture (Mallory-Weiss syndrome; Boerhaave's syndrome)
  - Esophageal impaction
  - Hiatal hernia
  - Cholecystitis, gallstones
  - Gastritis
  - Peptic ulcer disease
  - Pancreatitis
  - Splenic infarction
  - Splenic flexure syndrome
- Neuromuscular/skeletal
  - Chest wall pain
  - Costochondritis (Tietze's syndrome)
  - Cervical or thoracic degenerative arthritis, nerve compression, radiculopathy
    - Cervical vertebral disk
    - Intercostal neuralgia
  - Thoracic outlet (scalenus anticus) syndrome
  - Shoulder arthropathies
    - Shoulder hand syndrome
  - Fibromyalgia (myofascial pain syndrome; fibromyositis)
    - Pectoral, intercostal, serratus anterior
    - Precordial catch syndrome
  - Cardiac causalgia
  - Bursitis
  - Superficial thrombophlebitis of thoracic veins (Mondor's syndrome)
  - Xiphoidalgia
  - Diaphragmatic flutter
- Neurocutaneous
  - Herpes zoster
- Breast
  - Pendulous breast syndrome
  - Brassiere syndrome
- Psychologic
  - Anxiety
  - Hyperventilation
  - Panic attacks
  - Depression
  - Self-gain
  - Munchhausen syndrome

Patients with hypertensive or valvular heart disease may have chest pain that is located at the apex rather than substernally and that is often associated with hyperesthesia of the left breast or precordium. Some patients with functional heart disease have apical pain that often occurs at rest. Chest wall pain, cervical arthritis, and subdeltoid bursitis can occur with exertion and be relieved by rest. It should be emphasized that not infrequently patients will have more than one type of chest discomfort. See Chap. 19 for a discussion of the differential diagnosis of chest pain.

PATHOPHYSIOLOGY

In patients with stable angina pectoris due to atherosclerotic CAD, there is little correlation between the severity and extent of the atherosclerosis and the severity of the angina symptoms. There is also no apparent correlation between the location of the angina discomfort and the location of the myocardial ischemia. Women have angina as the initial manifestation of coronary heart disease more often than men, who commonly have acute myocardial infarction. The pathology of coronary atherosclerosis is discussed in detail in Chap. 55. The nonatherosclerotic causes of coronary heart disease are discussed in Chap. 64.

The fundamental feature of ischemic heart disease is the imbalance between the supply of coronary blood flow and the metabolic demands of the myocardium. This imbalance may be manifested episodically as angina pectoris or arrhythmias or chronically as congestive heart failure. The clinical evidence of ischemia is exhibited when myocardial demand exceeds the capacity of the coronary arteries to deliver an adequate supply of oxygen. In normal hearts there is excess capacity on the supply side so that ischemia does not occur even with very vigorous exercise.[73] The presence of disease in either the epicardial coronary arteries or, as has become apparent recently, in the coronary microvasculature may result in imbalance between supply and demand at even modest levels of exercise. Understanding the determinants of coronary blood supply and myocardial metabolic demand is important in the management of chronic ischemic heart disease.

Myocardial Oxygen Demand

The major, clinically relevant determinants of oxygen demand are heart rate, contractility, and systolic wall tension (Table 5-2 and Fig. 58-6). A detailed discussion of the major and minor determinants of demand is presented in Chap. 5. Heart rate is one of the most important determinants of myocardial oxygen consumption (MV_{O_2})[74] and is the one that is most easily manipulated pharmacologically in most patients. Myocardial contractility, which is reflected in the rate of change of pressure (dP/dt), is a major determinant of oxygen consumption that is ordinarily not an important direct target for therapeutic manipulation. On the other hand, systolic wall tension is frequently an important factor in therapeutic considerations.

Systolic wall tension is directly related to the left ventricular systolic pressure and radius and inversely related to wall thickness. It follows that oxygen consumption can be decreased by decreasing systolic pressure and afterload. Reduction of preload, through venodilation, and thus of left ventricular distension and oxygen consumption is one of the important mechanisms for the therapeutic efficacy of nitrates in angina pectoris (see below). Positive inotropic agents may actually decrease oxygen consumption in patients with enlarged ventricles because the effects of decreasing radius may outweigh those of increasing contractility.

Myocardial Oxygen Supply

Oxygen supply to the myocardium is dependent upon the oxygen-carrying capacity of the blood and on blood flow. Decreased oxygen-carrying capacity may contribute to the development or exacerbation of myocardial ischemia in severe anemia. Most commonly, however, ischemia related to oxygen supply results from compromised coronary blood flow. Normally the arteriolar resistance vessels are the primary regulators of myocardial blood flow since the epicardial arteries are low resistance conduits. Narrowing of the large coronary arteries transiently by vasospasm or permanently by structural changes, as in atherosclerosis, may cause the development of resistance that is high enough to restrict blood flow. Until relatively recently, consideration of the factors limiting blood supply in ischemic heart disease has focused on the epicardial coronaries. There has been increasing appreciation in ischemic disease of a pathophysiological role of the microvasculature,[75] either concomitantly with atherosclerotic narrowing of the large conduit arteries or predominantly, in anginal syndromes with normal epicardial arteries (syndrome X—discussed subsequently).[76,77]

The determinants of myocardial blood flow are relatively complex[78] and include: (1) metabolic control, (2) autoregulation, (3) extravascular compressive forces, (4) duration of diastole, (5) humoral agents composed of both circulating hormones and autocrine and paracrine factors produced within the arterial wall and in particu-

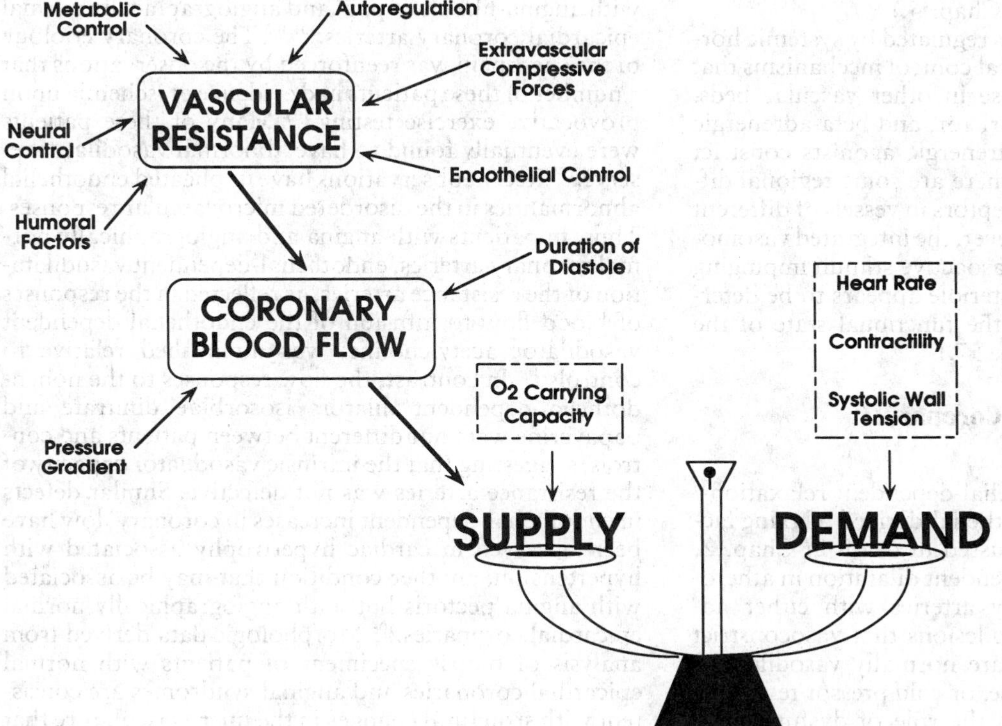

FIGURE 58-6 Factors controlling myocardial oxygen supply and demand. (*From Ardehali A, Ports TA.*[78] *Modified with permission from the author and publisher.*)

lar by the endothelium, (6) neural control, and (7) the pressure difference between aortic diastolic pressure and right atrial pressure. The factors controlling myocardial blood flow are depicted in Fig. 58-6. For a more complete discussion see Chaps. 5 and 57.

Myocardial blood flow is matched closely with myocardial work and metabolism.[74] The molecular mechanism(s) involved has not been completely defined but likely includes adenosine, a degradation product of ATP that is released into the interstitium and is a potent dilator of microvessels.[79,80] (See also Chaps. 5 and 57.)

Myocardial blood flow is relatively constant (autoregulated) over a range of perfusion pressures between 60 and 160 mmHg.[81] Below a perfusion pressure of about 60 mmHg, vasodilator reserve is consumed and blood flow is directly related to perfusion pressure. Experimentally, loss of vasodilator reserve occurs distal to lesions with an 85 percent decrease in diameter.[82] A decrease in coronary blood flow, presumably due to vasoconstriction and loss of vasodilator reserve, has been observed in spite of an increase in blood pressure in response to cold pressor stimulation in patients with significant coronary artery disease.[83]

Extravascular compressive forces, including intrapericardial, intramyocardial, and intraventricular pressures, are important in the control of coronary blood flow and account for 30 to 50 percent of vascular resistance.[84] Since the intramyocardial and intraventricular pressures are maximal during systole and are exerted maximally on the subendocardium, the effects on blood flow are greatest on subendocardial vessels. Subendocardial blood flow ceases during systole.[85] Thus, the subendocardial blood flow is most vulnerable in any circumstance in which total blood flow is decreased or in which metabolic demands are increased and blood flow is limited. Because of the systolic compressive forces, the subendocardium is also critically dependent on the duration of diastole for its blood flow. (See also Chap. 5.)

The coronary circulation is regulated by systemic hormonal influences and by neural control mechanisms that are not dissimilar from those in other vascular beds. Angiotensin II is a vasoconstrictor, and beta-adrenergic agonists dilate and alpha-adrenergic agonists constrict coronary arteries, although there are some regional differences in distribution of receptors in vessels of different sizes. Very importantly, however, the integrated vasomotor response to the various vasoactive stimuli impinging upon a coronary artery or arteriole appears to be determined to a great extent by the functional state of the endothelium. (See also Chap. 57.)

Endothelial Function and Coronary Vasomotor Control

The phenomenon of endothelial-dependent relaxation[86] and the identification of endothelial-derived relaxing factor as nitric oxide[87] are discussed in detail in Chap. 2. The defect in endothelial-dependent dilatation in atherosclerotic epicardial coronary arteries with either advanced or minimally stenotic lesions that vasoconstrict in response to stimuli that are normally vasodilatory, such as acetylcholine, exercise, or cold pressor testing, is discussed in Chap. 56, as is the role of dysfunctional endothelium in both the stable and unstable coronary syndromes. The prevailing view is that in nondiseased epicardial coronary arteries endothelial-dependent vasodilator mechanisms are predominant. Thus, interventions such as exercise,[88–92] mental stress,[93–95] cold pressor testing,[96,97] or even pacing-induced tachycardia[98] that normally induce increases in MV_{O_2} and in flow are normally associated with epicardial dilatation that is, at least in part, endothelial-dependent. The presence of even nonocclusive, early atherosclerosis as well as of more advanced stenoses appears to attenuate this vasodilator mechanism and to result in the predominance of constrictor forces. In illustration of this point, local infusion of the alpha-adrenergic agonist phenylephrine does not constrict normal coronary arteries of patients with intact endothelial-dependent dilatation.[99] In patients with even minimally diseased coronary arteries, however, constriction occurs at low concentrations of phenylephrine. Thus, in coronary artery disease there appears to be not only loss of endothelial-dependent dilatation but also enhanced vasoconstrictor sensitivity to catecholamines. This disordered vasomotor control is almost certainly an important contributor to the variability in anginal threshold that is seen commonly in many patients; it has been called *mixed angina* because it is felt to involve both high-grade stenoses and variable vasoconstrictor activity.[100] (It is discussed in more detail subsequently.) Moderate vasoconstriction of a minimal stenosis may have little hemodynamic importance, whereas the same degree of vasoconstriction on a higher grade stenosis may markedly decrease blood flow and induce ischemia.

The Microvasculature and Coronary Ischemia

The realization of the potential importance of the coronary microvascular resistance vessels in the pathogenesis of angina pectoris developed from studies of patients with angina-like chest pain and angiographically normal epicardial coronary arteries.[101,102] The coronary etiology of the chest pain was reenforced by the observations that a number of these patients had evidence of ischemia upon provocative exercise testing.[103] Many of these patients were eventually found to have abnormal vasodilator reserve.[104] Recent observations have implicated endothelial abnormalities in the disordered microvascular responses. Thus, in patients with angina and angiographically normal coronary arteries, endothelial-dependent vasodilatation of the resistance arteries, as reflected in the responses of blood flow to infusion of the endothelial-dependent vasodilator acetylcholine, was diminished relative to controls.[105] In contrast, the flow responses to the nonendothelial-dependent dilators isosorbide dinitrate and papaverine were not different between patients and controls, suggesting that the intrinsic vasodilator capacity of the resistance arteries was not defective. Similar defects in endothelial-dependent increases in coronary flow have been observed in cardiac hypertrophy associated with hypertension, another condition that may be associated with angina pectoris but with angiographically normal epicardial coronaries.[106] Morphologic data derived from analysis of biopsy specimens of patients with normal epicardial coronaries and anginal syndromes are consistent with structural changes in the microvasculature that may reflect the observed functional abnormalities. In these patients there was capillary narrowing with swollen endothelium encroaching on the lumen as well as decreased capillary density.[107] Taken together, these data are consistent with the notion that the coronary microvasculature can develop dysfunction of vasomotor control mechanisms and, in particular, of endothelial-dependent vasodilatation that may become clinically significant in the setting of increased demand or MV_{O_2}. In this case loss of vasodilator reserve and/or the actual constriction of resistance arterioles might induce ischemia and chest pain.

Spectrum of Pathophysiological Mechanisms Associated with the Stable Coronary Ischemic Syndromes

Symptomatic coronary ischemia associated with predominantly microvascular abnormalities in control of tone likely represents, pathophysiologically, one end of the spectrum of the anginal syndromes. Angina pectoris or anginal equivalents, with a rather constant threshold for inducing symptoms that likely results from a fixed stenosis of an epicardial coronary, can be viewed as the other end of the spectrum. In between lie most patients who have a threshold for inducing angina that is somewhat variable from day to day or even at different times of the day as discussed subsequently. For example, the same activity that produces angina in the early morning may not do so in the afternoon or evening. These same patients may have a reproducible exercise level for inducing ischemia on formal exercise testing because of the increased myocardial oxygen consumption resulting from increases in heart rate, contractility, and blood pressure, which is associated with an increase in wall tension. This apparent paradox is explained by the presence of flow-limiting epicardial stenosis or stenoses and the concomitant association of episodic vasoconstriction. This clinical scenario has been termed *mixed angina* by Maseri.[100] These patients have ischemia induced by both increase in demand and by a decrease in flow. The site(s) of vasoconstriction may be at an epicardial stenosis, in the microvasculature, or at both locations.[108] The concept of a variable flow reserve that interacts with differing metabolic demands to produce intermittent ischemia is depicted in Fig. 58-7. Variability of the flow reserve is undoubtedly a major contributor to such phenomena as the precipitation of angina by an activity that, even when repeated soon thereafter, subsequently does not cause angina. A classic example is of the golfer who develops angina on the first or second hole and later, after resolution of the episode, can complete the round free of pain. Although loss or attenuation of endothelial-dependent vasodilator mechanisms is undoubtedly an important substrate permitting expression of vasoconstrictor stimuli, the predominant vasoconstrictors have not been identified. In the stable anginal syndromes these are likely neural and hormonal, whereas in the unstable syndromes platelet and coagulation products and inflammatory mediators are thought to be additional contributors. Patients with predominantly vasoconstrictor pathophysiology in an epicardial vessel have been classified as having *vasospastic angina*. Many of these patients may have unstable angina or Prinzmetal's variant angina (see Chap. 59).

Cellular Bases for the Clinical Manifestations of Ischemia

The cellular effects of myocardial ischemia are discussed in detail in Chaps. 57 and 60. The rapid decreases in systolic function and in diastolic compliance that are associated with creatine phosphate depletion and ionic shifts will increase end-diastolic pressure. This pressure increase will be reflected in the pulmonary vascular pressures and may ultimately stimulate mechanoreceptors mediating dyspneic responses (see Chap. 20). Dyspnea may be an associated symptom with angina or may be present as an anginal equivalent in patients who do not develop pain.

The metabolic abnormalities induced by ischemia lead to cellular depolarization and the flow of electrical currents between normal and ischemic areas that are reflected on the ECG. ST-segment depression reflecting subendocardial hypoperfusion is the most common ECG manifestation of ischemia in chronic, stable angina during ambulatory monitoring or exercise testing.[109] Somewhat surprisingly, the electrical inhomogeneity inferred

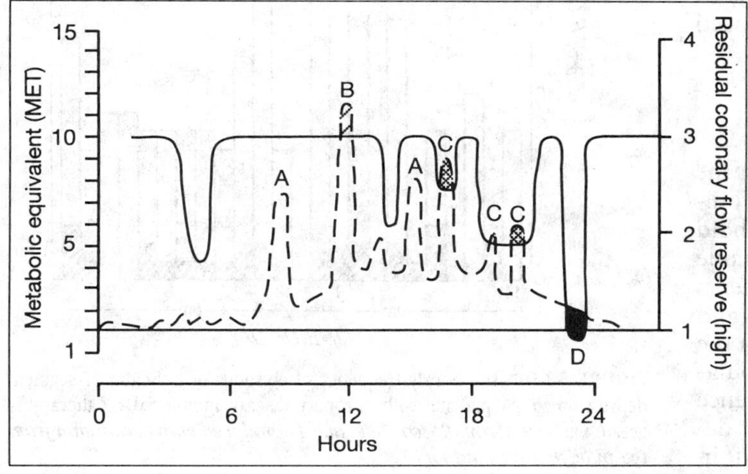

FIGURE 58-7 Concept of variable coronary flow reserve in presence of variable atherosclerotic obstruction. A: Episodes not associated with ischemia; B: ischemic episode occurring at levels of exercise exceeding threshold of residual coronary flow reserve; C: ischemic episodes occurring at lower levels of exercise when residual coronary flow is reduced; D: ischemic episodes occurring at rest in presence of maximal reduction in residual coronary flow reserve; (——) residual coronary flow reserve; (– – –) variable atherosclerotic obstruction, as measured by MET. (*From Cohn PF: Mechanisms of myocardial ischemia. Am J Cardiol 1992; 70:14G–18G. Adapted from Maseri A: Role of coronary artery spasm in symptomatic and silent myocardial ischemia. J Am Coll Cardiol 1987; 9:249–262. Reproduced with permission from the authors and publishers.*)

by ST-segment depression observed during exercise testing or ambulatory monitoring is not commonly associated with ventricular arrhythmias, especially of the complex or life-threatening type.[110] Exercise-induced ventricular ectopic activity is not a reliable predictor of cardiac events in asymptomatic persons.[111]

Sequence of Events during Coronary Ischemia

Studies in which hemodynamic and ECG monitoring have been performed during spontaneous episodes of ischemia, usually in unstable patients or during balloon inflation at angioplasty, have provided insights into the sequential responses evoked at the onset of ischemia. After balloon inflation, as implied above, relaxation failure or a decrease in compliance is the earliest event, occurring within seconds, and is followed by contractile dysfunction with a decrease in ejection fraction of up to one-third within 10 s.[112] ECG changes occur at about 20 s, and angina, if it occurs, does so beyond 25 s. These sequential events are depicted in Fig. 58-1. It is implicit from considering this sequence that there are likely to be ischemic episodes that do not progress to angina. Since there are many patients who do not perceive coronary ischemic pain or have high pain thresholds, it follows that there is likely to be a substantial frequency of silent ischemia in the population with CAD. This, in fact, is the case as will be discussed subsequently.

The various studies of patients with spontaneous or exercise-induced ischemia that have included hemodynamic and ECG monitoring have provided insights into and confirmed assumptions about the physiological basis for a number of classic clinical observations about angina. For example, as noted above, an anginal attack may be associated with new physical findings, including the development of an atrial gallop, systolic bulging of the precordium, mitral regurgitation due to papillary muscle dysfunction, and paradoxical splitting of the second sound. The atrial gallop reflects diastolic dysfunction and decreased compliance while the remaining features reflect systolic dysfunction, including prolonged left ventricular ejection time accounting for the paradoxical splitting. In addition, the crescendo-decrescendo nature of anginal pain that is one of its most important differentiating characteristics is reflected in the crescendo-decrescendo pattern of the development and resolution of ischemic ST-segment changes and elevations of left ventricular filling pressure during exercise-induced angina (Fig. 58-8).

Circadian Rhythm of Coronary Ischemia

The incidence of myocardial infarction is highest in the morning in the first few hours after awakening.[113] Similarly, as many clinicians have observed, the threshold for precipitating anginal attacks in patients with stable angina appears to be lowest in the morning. Patients are more likely to develop ST-segment depression and angina at lower thresholds during exercise testing in the morning than in the afternoon.[114] Studies with ambulatory ECG monitoring have confirmed that the incidence of both painful and painless episodes of ST-segment depression is highest in the morning[115] (Fig. 58-9) and, in

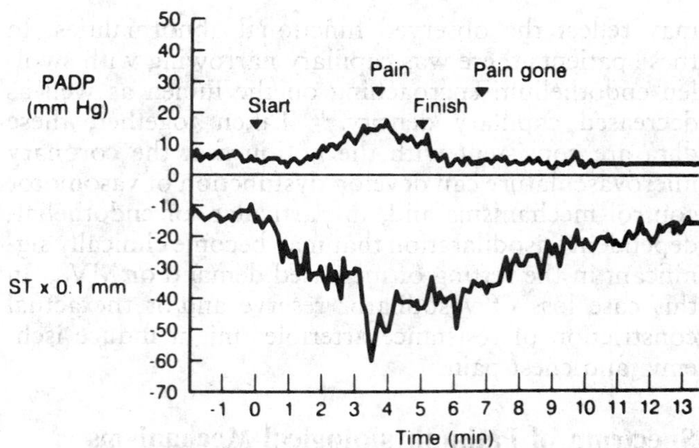

FIGURE 58-8 Changes in pulmonary artery diastolic pressure (PADP) and the ST segment in a patient with coronary artery disease who performed treadmill exercise (modified Bruce protocol) for 5 mins. Note again the crescendo-decrescendo pattern of the temporal sequence of change in the parameters recorded during an episode of myocardial ischemia. *(From Levy RD, Shapiro LM, Wright C, et al.: Hemodynamic response to myocardial ischemia during unrestricted activity, exercise testing and atrial pacing assessed by ambulatory pulmonary artery pressure monitoring. Br Heart J 1986; 56:1218. Reproduced with permission from the publisher and authors.)*

particular, in the first few hours after awakening (Fig. 58-10).

The diurnal variation in ischemic threshold is likely related to endogenous rhythms of catecholamine secretion, which are highest in the morning, and to sensitivity to coronary vasoconstrictors, which appears to be highest in the morning since the dilating response to nitroglycerin is highest in patients at this time of day.[116] The

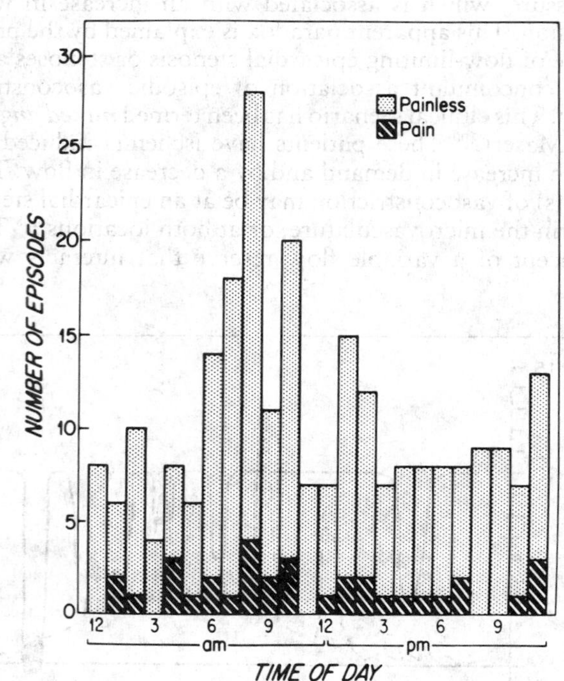

FIGURE 58-9 The hourly frequency of episodes of ischemic ST-segment depression in 24 patients with coronary disease monitored off therapy is greatest at 8 A.M. *(From Rocco MB et al.[115] Reproduced with permission from the publisher and authors.)*

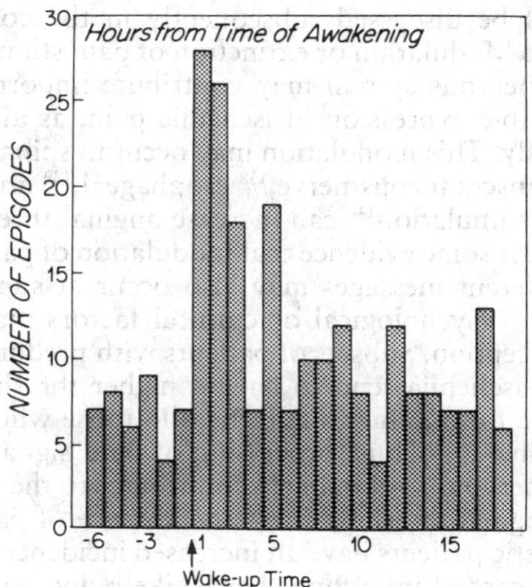

FIGURE 58-10 When the frequency of episodes is displayed hourly from the time of awakening, the peak activity occurs in the first and second hour after rising. (*From Rocco et al.*[115] *Reproduced with permission from the publisher and authors.*)

increase in sympathetic nervous system activity is associated with increases in heart rate, blood pressure, and contractility. Taken together with the myocardial demands associated with activities of daily living, these various factors may converge to cause the morning increase in ischemic episodes. Factors potentially contributing to the lowered morning ischemic threshold are depicted in Fig. 58-11.[117,118]

The lowered morning anginal threshold has important therapeutic implications. A decrease in the frequency of ischemia can be achieved by blunting of the morning surge of beta-adrenergic stimulation with beta blockers chosen and administered in a manner to provide adequate pharmacologic effects in the morning. Furthermore, in patients with rather predictable morning angina, the use of nitroglycerin soon after awakening may be useful in preventing angina in many instances.

Mechanisms of Anginal Pain

Anginal pain may be a very useful warning system, although it is frequently insufficiently sensitive. Pain stimuli arise within the myocardium and most likely stimulate free nerve endings in the vicinity of small coronary vessels.[115] Impulses travel in afferent unmyelinated or small myelinated cardiac sympathetic nerves through the upper five thoracic sympathetic ganglia to dorsal horn cells and through the spinothalamic tract to the thalamus and then to the cortex.[119] There is thought to be integration and modulation of these impulses at several levels including the cerebral cortex. This modulation may also contribute importantly to the variability in anginal threshold alluded to previously. At the cortical level psychosocial and cultural factors may modulate the perception of pain. The radiation patterns of angina are determined by the levels of the thoracic spinal cord that share the sensory inputs from the heart and from somatic structures. It was proposed that radiation of angina to the neck and jaw might be via vagal afferents since this radiation pattern became more prominent after thoracic sympathectomy when this procedure was used to treat refractory angina.[120] This supposition has been challenged.[104]

The nature of the stimuli causing angina has been difficult to delineate. The causes are almost certainly chemical, and a number of candidate molecules including kinins, serotonin, hydrogen ions, and inflammatory mediators have been proposed. The usual lack of an association of, for example, inflammatory myocarditis either with pain in general or with anginal type pain specifically has directed attention away from inflammatory mediators. Substance P has been implicated as a potential cause of angina but does not provoke chest pain when infused into humans.[121] On the other hand adenosine, which is increased during ischemia, as discussed previously, has been shown to cause anginal type pain during intravenous infusion in normal volunteers.[122] The definitive nature of the stimuli causing anginal pain remains to be determined.

SILENT ISCHEMIA IN STABLE CORONARY ARTERY DISEASE

The presence of clinically silent ischemic heart disease has intrigued physicians for decades, and the presence of unrecognized myocardial infarction was commented upon by Herrick in 1912.[123] The presence of extensive coronary disease and myocardial infarction at autopsy of apparently asymptomatic persons was emphasized subsequently.[124] Direct evidence of silent or asymptomatic ischemia during exercise testing[125,126] or during ambulatory monitoring[127] heightened interest in the subject.[128]

Prevalence

Silent ischemic episodes may be present in patients across the spectrum of the ischemic coronary syndromes from stable to unstable angina or after myocardial infarction and may be observed in patients who are totally asymptomatic or are symptomatic with some episodes of ischemia but not with others.[129] Recent evidence suggests

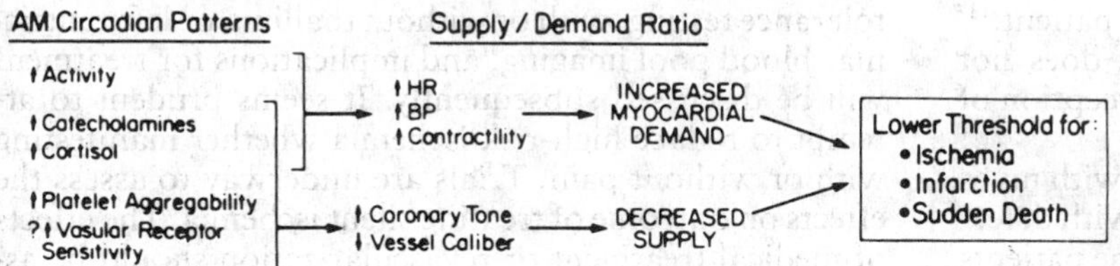

FIGURE 58-11 Hypothetical mechanisms causing morning increases in symptomatic and asymptomatic ischemic coronary events. (*From Rocco MB, Selwyn AP.*[117] *Reproduced with permission from the publisher and authors.*)

that silent ischemic episodes are present in virtually all patients with active unstable angina and in 36 to 38 percent of patients with stable, effort angina or in those with a remote (greater than 4 weeks previously) history of instability.[130] Cohn has estimated the prevalence in an adult population of asymptomatic coronary artery disease of an extent capable of inducing ischemia at approximately 5 percent.[131] ST-segment depression on ambulatory monitoring is rare in patients with proven absence of coronary artery disease[132] but has been reported to be more common in a general population, raising questions about the use of ambulatory monitoring as a screening mechanism.[133] A more recent prospective study of 68-year-old men with a 9.9 percent and a 6.6 percent prevalence of a history of angina pectoris or myocardial infarction, respectively, reported that 25 percent exhibited ST-segment depression on ambulatory electrocardiographic monitoring.[134] Ninety two percent of the "ischemic" episodes were asymptomatic. ST-segment depression was associated with increased cardiovascular risk, as discussed subsequently. The true prevalence of silent ischemia is difficult to discern in the population and will obviously depend on age and the presence and activity of coronary artery disease. In the presence of coronary disease, however, it is apparent that episodes of asymptomatic ischemia are more common than are painful ones.[135]

Pathophysiology

Imbalance between coronary blood supply and myocardial oxygen demand in silent ischemia likely has the same fundamental causes as in stable angina in general, as discussed previously. There are unique aspects that must be considered. Why are some episodes of ischemia appreciated as pain (approximately 25 percent)[136] whereas others are asymptomatic? Why do some patients not experience pain with ischemia at all? Are the causes and functional consequences of silent ischemia the same as for painful ischemia, or is there something unique about this portion of the spectrum of ischemic manifestations?

An obvious possible explanation for painful as opposed to asymptomatic ischemia is that the ischemia, and thus the noxious stimulus, is more severe in the former than in the latter. There is, however, no strong correlation between the duration and severity of an ischemic episode and the development of anginal pain in chronic stable angina.[136] Symptomatic episodes lasted slightly longer and had a slightly higher frequency of severe ST-segment depression than did painless ones, but there was considerable overlap. Chierchia et al. have assessed painful and asymptomatic ischemic episodes as follows: (1) Ischemic episodes of less than 3 min duration that are associated with less than a 7-mmHg rise in end-diastolic pressure are usually painless; (2) episodes that are more severe and perhaps much more severe and/or longer may be painless or painful in the same patient.[137] Thus, the intensity of the ischemic stimulus does not appear to account for the variability of the perception of pain in angina.[104]

An alternative explanation for lack of pain with myocardial ischemia is neurologic.[104] Neuropathy with defective sensory efferent nerves likely occurs in some patients and will be discussed subsequently in the context of diabetes. Modulation or extinction of pain stimuli in the central nervous system may contribute importantly to the variable expression of ischemic pain, as alluded to previously. This modulation may occur in spinal centers since transcutaneous nerve,[138] esophageal,[139] and dorsal column stimulation[140] can increase anginal threshold.

There is some evidence that modulation of pain-mediating efferent messages may also occur at supraspinal centers.[104] Psychological or cultural factors may affect pain perception. Subsets of patients with predominantly painless ischemia tend to have a higher threshold and tolerance for painful stimuli than do those who experience pain.[141–143] Thus, processing of pain signals in the central nervous system likely contributes to the variability of anginal threshold or to the absence of pain.

Diabetic patients have an increased incidence of painless myocardial infarction that is likely due, in part, to cardiac autonomic neuropathy.[144,145] They have an increased prevalence, relative to nondiabetic patients, of silent ischemia on exercise testing and ambulatory ECG monitoring.[146,147]

Causes and Functional Consequences of Silent Ischemia

Ischemia caused by the increased demand associated with exercise testing may be silent.[148] Ambulatory ECG monitoring has provided insights into potential mechanisms of many episodes of ischemia—painless or painful—during daily living. The heart rate at the onset of ischemia is generally lower with ambulatory than with exercise testing.[136,148] These observations suggest that increased vascular tone likely contributes to many episodes of ischemia.

The consequences for myocardial perfusion appear to be similar whether or not the ischemia is associated with chest pain and whether it is provoked or spontaneous. Thus perfusion measured by rubidium 82 PET was decreased to a similar extent by exercise, cold pressor testing, and mental arithmetic or during spontaneous ischemia.[136,149]

Clinical Implications

The available data indicate that silent ischemia is a common, almost ubiquitous, component of the whole spectrum of the coronary syndromes. It thus appears to have no special implications but, in terms of predicting adverse events, has approximately the same significance as symptomatic ischemia.[150,151] The fundamental issues appear to be the extent and severity of ischemia, regardless of how it is detected or manifested, and whether the disease is in a stable or unstable phase. Unstable angina is discussed in Chap. 59.

Evidence of high-risk ischemia detected by exercise tolerance testing, with or without thallium or left ventricular blood pool imaging, and implications for treatment will be discussed subsequently. It seems prudent to attempt to reduce high-risk ischemia whether manifesting with or without pain. Trials are underway to assess the effects on outcome of treating silent ischemia. The effects of medical treatment or revascularization should be assessed with follow-up evaluation for ischemia. Persistent severe ischemia in spite of medical therapy should lead to consideration of revascularization.

The role of ambulatory ECG monitoring for ischemia in routine patient care remains to be defined. At present there appears to be no obligatory, noninvestigational indication for its use.

Treatment of Silent Ischemia

Most medical or interventional strategies that reduce symptomatic ischemia will also reduce silent ischemia and are discussed subsequently. The available data from clinical trials of treatment of silent ischemia in stable coronary disease have been summarized by Bertolet et al.[151] and are depicted in Fig. 58-12. Nitroglycerin is highly effective. Somewhat surprisingly, beta blockers appear to be somewhat more effective than calcium-entry blockers. Calcium antagonists may be most effective in preventing ischemia that occurs at lower heart rates when vasoconstriction may be a predominant factor, as discussed previously.

There has been a considerable evolution conceptually in the approaches to stable ischemic coronary disease with the appreciation that the total ischemic burden, and not just symptoms, may be the appropriate therapeutic target. While this concept is still being tested, other current developments are likely to revolutionize the approach to ischemic coronary disease. The fundamental interrelationship between the biology of the atherosclerotic lesion and the coronary ischemic syndromes has been alluded to previously in the context of the contribution of endothelial dysfunction to disordered control of vasomotor tone and, in detail, in the broader scope in Chap. 56. Aggressive lipid lowering in coronary regression trials has shown dramatic lowering of subsequent cardiac event rates, even in the context of modest angiographic improvements.[152] The observations suggest that the biology of atherosclerotic lesions is being favorably influenced. Preliminary evidence suggests that ischemia can be diminished by marked life-style changes.[153] As discussed below, the treatment of atherosclerosis through risk factor modification should become a fundamental component of the treatment regimen for stable coronary disease with or without painful manifestations. (See Chap. 62.)

MEDICAL THERAPY

General

All patients with stable angina pectoris should have an evaluation of risk factors for coronary heart disease (see Chap. 62). Whenever possible, risk factors should be corrected. Of particular importance is the cessation of tobacco smoking or exposure to tobacco products in any other form, such as snuff, chewing tobacco, or passive smoking. Achievement of ideal body weight and optimal control of diabetes mellitus and of systemic arterial hypertension are very important. In a randomized clinical trial of 333 male physicians with angina pectoris, low-dose aspirin (325 mg every other day) decreased the incidence of a first myocardial infarction by 87 percent.[154] In the Swedish Angina Pectoris Aspirin Trial (SAPAT), a double-blind trial involving 2035 men and women, optimal symptom control was first obtained in all patients with sotalol (median dose, 160 mg/day), following which the patients were randomized to aspirin (75 mg/day) or placebo. The median duration of follow-up was 50 months. Compared to the placebo plus sotalol group, the aspirin plus sotalol group had a 34 percent reduction

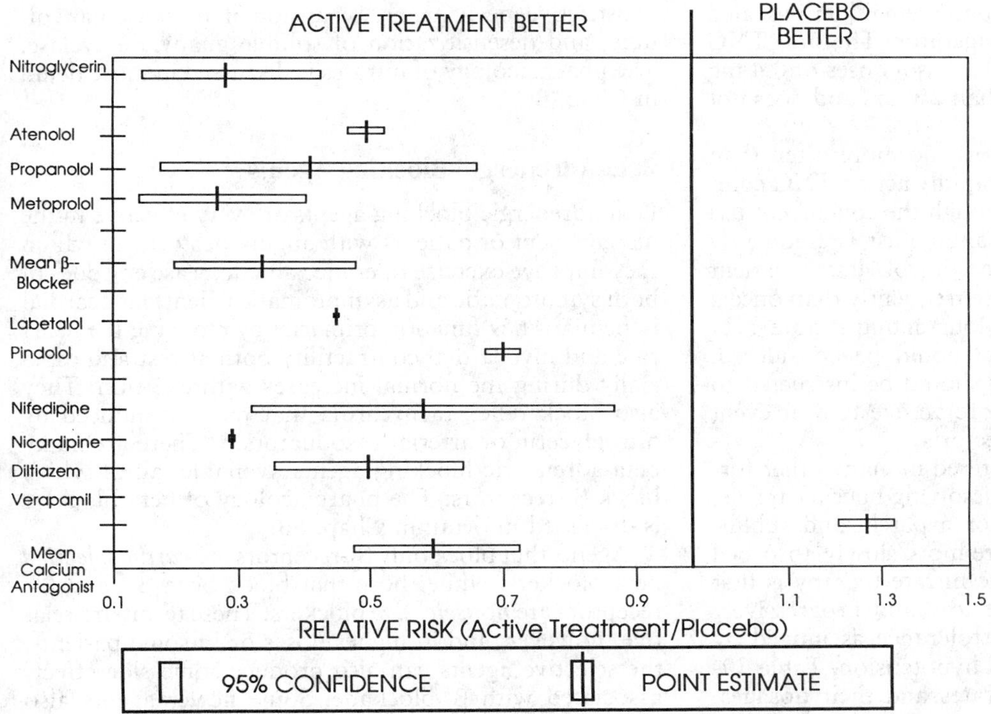

FIGURE 58-12 Pooled data analysis of the relative risk of silent ischemia during various drug regimens as compared with placebo in stable coronary artery disease syndromes. Beta blockers appear more effective than calcium antagonists. (*From Bertolet et al.*[151] *Reproduced with permission from the publisher and authors.*)

in primary outcome events (myocardial infarction and sudden death).[155] Accordingly, patients with stable angina pectoris should be given aspirin in the absence of contraindications. The daily dose of aspirin should be individualized. A reasonable dose is 160 to 325mg/day.[156,157] (See also Chap. 68.)

The Second Adult Treatment Panel[158] has recommended that dietary and, if necessary, drug therapy be employed to lower the low-density lipoprotein (LDL) cholesterol to or below 100 mg/dL (2.6 mmol/liter) in patients with documented CHD. (See Chaps. 53 and 62.) For many patients, drug therapy (Chap. 65) will be required to reach this goal. In a randomized clinical trial of 113 male patients with stable angina pectoris, 56 men assigned to a program of low-fat diet and intensive physical exercise had significantly slower progression of their coronary artery disease than 57 patients in the control group on usual care.[159]

An active exercise program, either individually directed or as part of a formal rehabilitation program (Chap. 63), is very helpful in achieving ideal body weight, decreasing coronary risk factors, and possibly even decreasing the risk of recurrent myocardial infarction.[160] Exercise training also increases the functional capacity of patients with stable angina pectoris.[159,161–167]

Nitrates

The standard first-line therapy of patients with stable angina pectoris is nitroglycerin (TNG), which usually relieves the symptoms in about 1 to 5 min.[168–173] TNG may be self-administered in the form of a sublingual tablet (0.3 to 0.6 mg) or as an oral spray, each puff of which delivers approximately 0.4 mg. Sublingual TNG tablets lose their potency over time and may require prescription refills every 2 to 3 months. Although new formulations may have a longer shelf life, it is appropriate to advise the patient to keep only a small supply of tablets with them and to keep the remainder in sealed small brown bottles in the refrigerator. The oral TNG spray, which provides over 200 aerosol doses of 0.4 mg TNG, has a shelf life of more than 2 years and does not require refrigeration.

If patients have angina pectoris no more often than once a week, the use of only a rapidly acting TNG compound may be satisfactory, although the concurrent use of a beta blocker or calcium antagonist is frequently appropriate for blood pressure control. If the patient experiences angina pectoris more frequently than once a week, the additional use of a long-acting nitrate beta blocker or calcium antagonist should be considered. Whenever possible, the patient should be instructed to take TNG prophylactically before an exertion or event known to precipitate angina pectoris.

Nitrates can also be administered in many other formulations, including a slowly dissolving buccal capsule, transdermally as an ointment or a patch, and sublingually or orally in forms that are more slowly absorbed and metabolized. When chronic nitrate therapy is first initiated, the dosage should be low and progressively increased to near the point of tolerance as judged by headache, dizziness, or postural hypotension. Table 30-1 lists the commonly used nitrates and their dosages. The use of a long-acting nitrate compound decreases the frequency of angina attacks and increases the amount of effort before angina (or angina equivalent) occurs.

The development of tolerance is a major disadvantage to chronic nitrate therapy.[168,174] In general, decreased effectiveness of TNG is encountered whenever a nitrate compound is regularly given without a 10- to 12-h nitrate-free period. The rate of development of nitrate tolerance increases with higher and more continuous dosages of nitrate compounds. For most patients, a satisfactory nitrate-free period is from about 9 P.M. to about 7 A.M. If the patients are taking an oral nitrate in a form that is slowly metabolized, it may be necessary to administer the last dosage in the early evening. For example, isosorbide dinitrate (ISDN) (10 to 60 mg) may be taken in doses of 30 mg twice a day at 8 A.M. and 5 P.M. or three times a day (8 A.M., 1 P.M., and 5 P.M.).[175] Nitroglycerin ointment or patches should usually be removed about 8 P.M. to 9 P.M. The administration of 20 mg isosorbide-5-mononitrate, which is the most important metabolite of ISDN, at 7 A.M. and 2 P.M. appears to prevent the development of tolerance in most patients. It is important to be sure that the patient is on other antianginal therapy, such as a beta blocker or calcium antagonist, during the 10- to 12-h nitrate-free period. In patients who experience more episodes of angina between 9 P.M. and 7 A.M. than at other times, the nitrate-free period should be scheduled during other hours, often from about noon to 10 P.M. The physician should determine the ideal nitrate-free period in each individual patient. The interval is 8 to 12 h in most patients.

Nitrate tolerance is thought to be related to oxidation or depletion of sulfhydryl groups. The results of clinical trials to prevent tolerance by administering sulfhydryl donors such as acetylcysteine or methionine are variable, with some reports suggesting benefit[176–179] and others finding none.[180–182] Other postulated mechanisms of nitrate tolerance include activation of neurohumoral vasoconstrictive mechanisms, expansion of intravascular volume, and desensitization of soluble guanylate cyclase. The pharmacology of nitrates is discussed in more detail in Chap. 30.

Beta-Adrenergic Blocking Agents

Beta-adrenergic blocking agents are very effective in the management of patients with angina pectoris, in whom they improve exercise tolerance and decrease episodes of both symptomatic and asymptomatic (silent) myocardial ischemia. They function primarily by reducing the heart rate and myocardial contractility both at rest and especially during the normal increases with exertion. They also block reflex tachycardia that may be induced by nitroglycerin or arterial vasodilators.[183] There are many beta-adrenergic blocking agents available, all of which block β_1-receptors. The pharmacology of beta blockers is discussed in detail in Chap. 66.

Agents that block only β_1-receptors are *cardioselective* beta blockers, while those that block both β_1- and β_2-receptors are *nonselective* blockers. These terms are relative, however, and in higher doses or in some patients, the selective agents can also produce some side effects associated with β_2-blockade. Some newer agents also block α_1-receptors or dilate blood vessels directly and are "vasodilator" beta blockers. Beta blockers also differ in whether or not they have some intrinsic sympathomimetic activity (ISA); agents with ISA tend to produce less slowing of the resting heart rate. Beta blockers vary in their lipid and water solubility, a quality that can affect their duration of action and perhaps side effects. The membrane-stabilizing (or local anesthetic or quinidine-like) effect, which is unrelated to beta blockade, does not appear to be of clinical significance. (See also Chap. 66.)

Adverse effects of beta blockers related to beta blockade include excess bradycardia, hypotension, ventricular dysfunction, bronchospasm, inhibition of metabolic and circulatory response to hypoglycemia, and cold extremities. Adverse effects that are apparently unrelated to beta blockade include impotence, lethargy, depression, confusion, hallucination, and constipation.

In general, all beta blockers are effective in the management of patients with stable angina pectoris. It is generally appropriate to select agents that have been shown to be effective in clinical trials and that have properties least likely to produce adverse effects in an individual patient. Thus, cardioselective agents are preferred in patients who have a history of bronchospastic disease, diabetes mellitus, or peripheral vascular disease. Even cardioselective beta blockers, however, can worsen bronchial constriction. Similarly, all beta blockers can worsen heart block and left ventricular function and worsen heart failure in patients with severe left ventricular dysfunction.

Beta blockers are usually administered in a dosage to lower the resting heart rate to 50 to 60 per minute; in some patients, even lower resting heart rates can be tolerated without symptoms. When beta-blocker therapy is discontinued, the dosage should be tapered over 4 to 10 days to avoid a rebound worsening of angina pectoris and possible myocardial infarction. The characteristics and dosages of individual beta blockers are shown in Tables 66-1, 66-2, 66-3, 66-7, and 66-10. Additional discussion of the selection of different beta blockers is provided below.

Calcium Antagonists

Calcium antagonists (or calcium channel entry blockers) are diverse compounds that impede the entry of calcium into myocytes and smooth muscle cells. In general, they decrease myocardial oxygen requirements by producing arterial dilatation and reducing arterial blood pressure and afterload and by reducing myocardial contractility. Some, such as diltiazem and verapamil, also tend to reduce heart rate. Many calcium antagonists also produce coronary vasodilatation and prevent coronary artery spasm. Different calcium antagonists appear to interact with different receptors; they also vary significantly in their relative effects upon different vascular beds and the myocardium. They may be classified into papaverine derivatives (verapamil), dihydropyridines (nifedipine, nicardipine), benzodiazepine derivatives (diltiazem), mixed calcium and sodium channel blockers (bepridil), and some antihistamines (flunarizine). The pharmacology and recommended dosages of the calcium antagonists are discussed in detail in Chap. 67 and summarized in Tables 67-1 to 67-4.

Adverse effects include ankle edema, headache, palpitations, flushing, hypotension, and aggravation of angina due to coronary steal, especially with dihydropyridine derivatives (nifedipine, nicardipine, etc.). Atrioventricular nodal delay may occur with verapamil and diltiazem; rarely, higher degrees of heart block occur, particularly when these agents are used concurrently with a beta blocker. All currently available calcium antagonists can have a negative inotropic effect, particularly verapamil. Other side effects include constipation, particularly with the use of verapamil.

All classes of calcium antagonists are effective in the management of patients with stable angina pectoris. In general, they are as effective as beta blockers, with which they are frequently used concurrently. Calcium antagonists are of special value in patients who have conditions that may be made worse by beta blockers, such as asthma, chronic obstructive pulmonary disease, or peripheral vascular disease. Elderly patients often tolerate calcium antagonists better than beta blockers. Verapamil, which has a stronger negative inotropic effect, is useful in the management of patients with angina pectoris due to hypertrophic obstructive cardiomyopathy (see Chap. 90).

Combination Drug Therapy for Stable Angina Pectoris

Patients with infrequent episodes of angina can be managed effectively with short-acting nitrates. In patients with more frequent episodes of angina who may require a combination of a short-acting and a long-acting nitrate, the use of a long-acting beta blocker or a calcium antagonist is advisable during a nitrate-free period initiated to prevent the development of nitrate tolerance. The use of a beta blocker or either diltiazem or verapamil tends to block the reflex tachycardia that is produced by nitrates in some patients. In general, the combination of nitrates and nifedipine is more likely to be associated with reflex tachycardia or even supraventricular tachycardias than the combination of nitrates with other calcium antagonists. Table 67-6 presents the rationale for combining nitrates and calcium antagonists in the therapy of patients with angina pectoris.

The combination of beta blocker and calcium antagonist therapy is widely employed in the management of patients with stable angina pectoris. Table 67-5 presents the hemodynamic effects of beta blockers, calcium antagonists, and combination treatment. The combination of a beta blocker with verapamil is particularly likely to worsen heart failure and should be used with special caution in patients with left ventricular dysfunction. Similarly, the combination of a beta blocker and verapamil can produce heart block in some patients, particularly the elderly. The combination of a beta blocker and diltiazem is usually well tolerated, although it too can produce heart failure and heart block.

Triple therapy of patients with severe stable angina pectoris is relatively frequent, although often it is no more effective than double therapy. The physician should be especially cautious whenever employing triple therapy because of the increased likelihood of adverse side effects. The selection of the particular beta blocker and calcium antagonist should be individualized, and the determination of the optimal combination often requires a series of therapeutic trials with various combinations.

Digitalis

Although digitalis is an inotrope and therefore would be expected to increase myocardial contractility and myocardial oxygen requirements, it may actually decrease myocardial oxygen requirements if it results in a decrease in left ventricular endiastolic volume. This occurs because of the Laplace relationship (Chap. 5) wherein systolic wall tension is directly related to mean ventricular diameter. In addition, the perfusion of the subendocardium of the left ventricle may be improved if the digoxin decreases the left ventricular diastolic pressure.

Revascularization

Patients with stable angina pectoris may be appropriate candidates for revascularization either by coronary artery bypass surgery (CABS) or percutaneous transluminal coronary angioplasty (PTCA) (coronary angioplasty). In general, this is an individual decision to be made by the patient with knowledge of the advantages and disadvantages either of medical therapy alone or of revascularization with either CABS or coronary angioplasty. While there are guidelines for indications for performing each of these procedures,[184,185] the guidelines are necessarily broad and do not include the many important variables for an individual patient. The indications for surgical revascularization are classified as shown in Table 58-6.

There are two general indications for a revascularization procedure: (1) the presence of symptoms that are not acceptable to the patient either because of restriction of physical activity and life-style or because of restrictions or side effects from medications, or (2) the presence of findings that indicate clearly that the patient would have a better prognosis with revascularization than with medical therapy. For some patients the occurrence of angina may be so incapacitating despite optimal double or triple drug therapy that revascularization is desired. In other patients, the side effects from the medications necessary to control symptoms may be such that the patient prefers surgery.

Anatomic considerations for revascularization are based upon an assessment of the grade or class of angina experienced by the patient, the presence and severity of evidence of myocardial ischemia on noninvasive stress testing, the degree of left ventricular function, and the distribution and severity of coronary artery disease. The indications for surgical revascularization and the results of such surgery are discussed in detail in Chap. 73.

Tables 58-7 and 58-8 show the guidelines for CABS in patients with stable angina pectoris recommended by the joint American College of Cardiology/American Heart Association Task Force in 1991.[185]

A review of randomized trials and registry studies revealed a trend for CABS to prolong survival in patients at high risk on the basis of clinical, functional, and anatomic characteristics in a comparison with medical therapy alone.[186–191] The 18-year follow-up of the Veterans Affairs Cooperative Study of Coronary Artery Bypass Surgery for Stable Angina found increased survival for patients with left main coronary artery disease and that other patients had relief of angina and better exercise performance for 5 years but that there was no difference at 10 years, presumably due to graft closure. Low-risk patients derived no survival benefit with surgical therapy at any time during the 18 years of follow-up.[192]

Coronary angioplasty (see Chaps. 70 and 71) has produced excellent results in patients with stable angina pectoris. Initially, it was used primarily in patients with single-vessel disease and it is still the preferred technique of revascularization in most patients with single-vessel disease other than left main. Subsequently, coronary angioplasty has been widely employed in patients with multivessel disease.[184] At present, there are a number of ongoing randomized studies comparing the long-term results of coronary angioplasty and CABS in patients with lesions that are favorable to both procedures.[193] Until the long-term follow-up results of these studies are available in patients with stable angina pectoris and multivessel disease, it is not possible to select one procedure over the other with a great deal of confidence. Certainly, coronary angioplasty is extremely valuable in many patients with moderate-to-severe angina and suitable coronary anatomy.[184] A 6-month follow-up report of a randomized comparison of coronary angioplasty with medical therapy in patients with single-vessel disease indicated that angioplasty provided earlier and more complete relief of angina and was associated with better performance on the exercise test but that it was more expensive and associated with more complications.[194] Table 58-9 lists clinical features and the results of testing that have been found to indicate an increased risk and mortality over the next several years in patients with coronary heart disease.[36,151,184,185,195–197] These fea-

TABLE 58-6

Classification of Indications for the Coronary Artery Bypass Graft Operation

Treatment Class	Description
I	Conditions for which the operation is indicated on the basis of a demonstrated advantage over medical treatment in terms of longevity or relief of symptoms, or both.
II	Conditions for which the operation is acceptable treatment but for which its advantages over medical treatment have not yet been fully defined.
III	Conditions for which the operation is not generally considered to be indicated, because of lack of demonstrated advantage over medical treatment.

SOURCE: American College of Cardiology/American Heart Association Task Force on Assessment of Diagnostic and Therapeutic Cardiovascular Procedures.[185] Reproduced with permission from the publisher.

TABLE 58-7

Treatment Class of the Coronary Artery Bypass Operation in Patients with Chronic Stable Class I or II Angina

	Indication Class Left Ventricular Dysfunction			
CAD	None	Mild	Moderate	Severe (but EF >0.20)
No or Mild Myocardial Ischemia with Noninvasive Stress Testing				
Left main	I	I	I	I
3 vessel	II*	II*	I	I
2 vessel	II*	II*	II*	II*
1 vessel	III†	III†	II*	II*
Moderate or Severe Myocardial Ischemia with Noninvasive Stress Testing				
Left main	I	I	I	I
3 vessel	I	I	I	I
2 vessel	II*	II*	II*	II*
1 vessel	III†	III†	II*	II*

SOURCE: American College of Cardiology/American Heart Association Task Force on Assessment of Diagnostic and Therapeutic Cardiovascular Procedures.[185] Reproduced with permission from the publisher.
* Class I if there is severe proximal stenosis in a large left anterior descending coronary artery.
† Class II if there is severe proximal stenosis in a large left anterior descending coronary artery.
NOTES: Angina classified by Canadian Cardiovascular Society grades (Campeau[6]). Noninvasive stress testing includes exercise ECG testing, radionuclide scintigraphy, and radionuclide ventriculography. CAD = coronary artery disease; EF = ejection fraction.

tures are useful in evaluating patients for coronary arteriography and possible coronary revascularization.

External Counterpulsation

External counterpulsation has been used in China for the treatment of patients with angina pectoris with some success. A recent report described a clinical trial of 18 patients using a device employing air counterpulsation of balloons around the calves, thighs, and buttocks for 1 h daily for a total of 36 h. In 14 patients, thallium scintigraphy showed a decrease in myocardial ischemia and an increase in exercise duration on maximal stress testing.[198] This innovative technique needs much more study before it can be recommended.

MANAGEMENT OF SPECIAL CATEGORIES OF PATIENTS WITH STABLE ANGINA PECTORIS

Systemic Arterial Hypertension

Patients with systemic arterial hypertension (SAH) often have angina pectoris. In most such patients, significant coronary atherosclerosis of the epicardial blood vessels is present, but some patients with SAH may have angina pectoris or even fatal myocardial infarction without significant obstruction of the large epicardial vessels. In some patients this may be due to the marked increase in myocardial oxygen requirements which exceed the coronary blood flow reserve, whereas others may have microvascular angina ("syndrome X") and abnormalities of the small coronary blood vessels (see below). In many patients treatment of the SAH with a beta blocker, calcium antagonist, or angiotensin-converting enzyme (ACE) inhibitor will also decrease myocardial oxygen requirements and prevent the development of angina pectoris. In general, efforts should be made to control the blood pressure both at rest and during exertion. (See also Chap. 77.)

Chronic Obstructive Pulmonary Disease (COPD); Asthma

In general, beta blockers should be avoided in this subset of patients, and preference should be given to the use of nitrates and calcium antagonists. Since many of these patients receive medications for their pulmonary disease that may increase their heart rate or even produce supraventricular tachycardia, such as sinus tachycardia or multifocal atrial tachycardia, it is preferable to use diltiazem or verapamil rather than nifedipine. The tachycardia can markedly increase myocardial consumption and precipitate myocardial ischemia. Some patients with a history of only asthma or only mild COPD may be able to tolerate small dosages of cardioselective beta blockers. When beta blockers are used in such patients, however, special caution and careful patient monitoring are appropriate. At times, very small dosages can prevent much of the tachycardia induced by the medications given for asthma or COPD.

Elderly Patients

In general, elderly patients tolerate calcium antagonists better than beta blockers. The presence of sinus tachycardia or atrial fibrillation is a relative contraindication to the selection of nifedipine; in such patients, diltiazem or verapamil or even a beta blocker would be preferable. On the other hand, beta blockers, verapamil, and diltiazem can exacerbate heart block, and verapamil can produce troublesome constipation in some elderly patients.

TABLE 58-8
Treatment Class of the Coronary Artery Bypass Operation in Patients with Chronic Stable Class III or IV Angina

CAD	Indication Class Left Ventricular Dysfunction: None	Mild	Moderate	Severe (but EF >0.20)
No or Mild Myocardial Ischemia with Noninvasive Stress Testing				
Left main	I	I	I	I
3 vessel	I	I	I	I
2 vessel	II*	II*	II*	II*
1 vessel	II*	II*	II*	II*
Moderate or Severe Myocardial Ischemia with Noninvasive Stress Testing				
Left main	I	I	I	I
3 vessel	I	I	I	I
2 vessel	II*	II*	II*	II*
1 vessel	II*	II*	II*	II*

SOURCE: American College of Cardiology/American Heart Association Task Force on Assessment of Diagnostic and Therapeutic Cardiovascular Procedures.[185] Reproduced with permission from the publisher.
* Class I if there is severe proximal stenosis in a large left anterior descending coronary artery.
NOTES: Angina classified by Canadian Cardiovascular Society grades (Campeau). Noninvasive stress testing includes exercise ECG testing, radionuclide scintigraphy, and radionuclide ventriculography. CAD = coronary artery disease; EF = ejection fraction.

Some elderly patients are very sensitive to postural hypotension from short-acting nitrates.

Peripheral Vascular Disease

Although satisfactory clinical trials are lacking, many physicians have noted that patients with peripheral vascular disease may have a worsening of their symptoms when treated with a nonselective beta blocker, which might allow unopposed alpha-induced vasoconstriction. Alternatively, the worsening symptoms may be due to the decrease in arterial perfusion pressure. In general, it is preferable to treat patients with chronic stable angina who have peripheral vascular disease with nitrates and a calcium antagonist.

Diabetes Mellitus

Patients with chronic stable angina pectoris who have diabetes mellitus should preferably be treated with nitrates. A calcium antagonist may be used as a second drug. If it is necessary to use a beta blocker, one should use a cardioselective agent, which would be less likely to impair recognition of and recovery from insulin-induced hypoglycemia.

Chronic Renal Disease

While beta blockers and calcium antagonists can normally be used effectively in patients with chronic angina and chronic renal insufficiency, careful monitoring may be necessary since many beta blockers (Chap. 66) and calcium antagonists (Chap. 67) are excreted primarily by the kidneys. In addition, the decrease in arterial blood pressure can sometimes lower renal blood flow and worsen renal function. (See also Chap. 108.)

OTHER MANIFESTATIONS OF CHRONIC ISCHEMIC HEART DISEASE

Heart Failure

Patients with severe coronary artery disease that produces a loss of left ventricular myocardium, usually at least more than approximately 20 percent, or that results in a ventricular septal defect or significant mitral regurgitation may have significant left ventricular failure. While there may be significant hypertrophy of the remaining myocytes and interstitium (Chap. 5), the ventricle is unable to compensate fully, and there is often a syndrome of heart failure with decreased stroke volume and elevated diastolic filling pressures in the left ventricle. This can produce a syndrome of heart failure (see Chaps. 25 and 26) that is clinically predominant and often more incapacitating than the symptom of angina pectoris. Extremely rarely, patients may present with a syndrome of heart failure that can even resemble constrictive pericarditis and have no history of angina or myocardial infarction. Such patients were some of the first to be referred to by the term *ischemic cardiomyopathy*. In the past three decades, however, this term has been overused and now is sometimes used in reference to virtually any systolic or diastolic left ventricular dysfunction in patients with CAD. Ideally, it would be preferable to restrict the term *cardiomyopathy* to refer to primary conditions of heart muscle disease and not to use it to refer to the end results of coronary, hypertensive, or valvular disease. (See Chap. 87.)

Patients who have severe left ventricular dysfunction due to CAD have a poor prognosis. (See Chap. 61.) In most instances, it reflects permanent, irreversible loss of myocytes. In a small percentage of patients, severe chronic CAD is associated with significant depression of

TABLE 58-9

Major Prognostic Variables in Patients with Chronic Stable Angina

Clinical	ST-segment elevation
Congestive heart failure	Inability to attain target heart rate (off medication)
NYHA Functional class	Exercise-induced ventricular couplets or tachycardia at a low work load
Prior myocardial infarction	ST/HR Slope ≥ 6 V per beat per min
Diuretic use	Angina
Digitalis use	Thallium 201 scintigraphy
Cardiomegaly	Multiple severe initial thallium defects
S_3 gallop	Multiple areas showing thallium redistribution
Ventricular arrhythmias	Increased lung/heart thallium ratio
ST-segment depression on resting ECG	Transient left ventricular dilatation
Angina frequency	Radionuclide left ventricular imaging
Angina duration	Ejection fraction ≤ 35 percent
Exercise ECG testing	Multiple regional wall motion abnormalities
Inability to exercise	Exercise-induced reduction in ejection fraction ≥ 10 percent
Poor exercise capacity (<5 METS) or maximal work (<100 W)	Failure to increase ejection fraction ≥ 5 percent during exercise if ≤ 70 years age
≥ 2 mm of ischemic ST-segment depression at a low work load (≤ stage 2 or ≤ 130 beats per min)	Exercise-induced left ventricular cavity dilatation
Failure to increase blood pressure (>130 mmHg) or a fall in blood pressure during exercise	Ambulatory ECG Monitoring
Early onset (stage1) or prolonged duration (>5 min) of ST-segment depression	Prolonged ST-segment depression (≥ 60 min per 24 h)
Multiple leads (≥ 5) with ST-segment depression	Marked ST-segment depression (≥ 2 mm)
	Frequent transient ischemic episodes (> 6 per 24 h)

NOTES: NYHA = New York Heart Association; METS = metabolic equivalents; HR = heart rate.

left ventricular function, referred to by Rahimtoola as "hibernating myocardium."[199] This concept is important because there can be a significant improvement following good left ventricular revascularization. While this does not occur often, it is important to take it into account before concluding that the left ventricular function of an individual patient is too low to consider revascularization surgery or that the etiology of the heart failure is not CHD. At times, the latent function of the left ventricle can be detected following a premature ventricular contraction. Radionuclide techniques (Chap. 134) and especially PET (Chap. 137) may also be useful in detecting myocardial viability.

The therapy of patients with heart failure due to ischemic heart disease is the same as for most patients with combined systolic and diastolic left ventricular failure, i.e., triple therapy with one or more diuretics, an ACE inhibitor, and digoxin (see Chap. 26). Because these patients frequently have overt or latent renal insufficiency, it may be necessary to use a combination of a long-acting nitrate (such as isosorbide dinitrate) and oral hydralazine in place of the ACE inhibitor. In addition, since the remaining left ventricular myocardium usually has significant areas that are chronically or intermittently ischemic, these patients tend to be more sensitive to electrolyte disturbances, particularly hypokalemia and hypomagnesemia. The ischemic myocardium may also be more susceptible than the normal myocardium to arrhythmias and conduction disturbances from digitalis. Nevertheless, it is useful and should be given with appropriate monitoring. Recent studies have reconfirmed the worsening of many patients with systolic heart failure and normal sinus rhythm when digoxin was discontinued.[200]

Therapy with a beta blocker, particularly metoprolol, should also be considered. Such therapy, which is currently experimental and not an approved use of these medications, has been found to be efficacious in recent studies. The beta blocker must be started in extremely low dosage and the dosage very slowly increased over several months. At present, such therapy should be administered with very great care because of the danger of precipitating severe, acute heart failure. (See Chap. 89.)

A new agent, vesnarinone, has been found to improve 6-month survival in a randomized double-blind clinical trial involving patients with moderate to severe heart failure and on triple therapy.[201] A small percentage of the patients developed reversible neutropenia on larger doses. Many of the patients studied had CAD as the etiology of their heart failure.

Cardiac transplantation is also frequently performed for severe heart failure due to CAD. The indications for, exclusions from, and results of cardiac transplantation are discussed in Chap. 32.

A patient with heart failure who has a large ventricular aneurysm may benefit from aneurysmectomy if there is sufficient remaining functioning left ventricular tissue. (See Chap. 74.) Similarly, heart failure due to severe mitral regurgitation can sometimes be significantly improved by corrective mitral valve surgery, which is often combined with coronary revascularization. The operative mortality for this procedure can be high. (See Chap. 74.)

Cardiac Arrhythmias, Conduction Disturbances

Chronic ischemic heart disease is a cause of many cardiac arrhythmias, including atrial and ventricular premature contractions, atrial fibrillation, sustained and nonsustained ventricular tachycardia, and ventricular fibrillation. The basic management is discussed in Chap. 36. In general, beta blockers should be employed whenever there is no strong contraindication, and type IC agents (Chap. 38) should be avoided unless the patient is symptomatic (see Chap. 36). In patients with atrial fibrillation, the ventricular response rate should be controlled with digoxin. Patients with chronic atrial fibrillation should also be maintained on warfarin (INR = 2 to 3) unless there is a contraindiction, in which case aspirin (81 to 325 mg/day) should be used. Patients in heart failure who have atrial fibrillation may benefit from electrical cardioversion (Chap. 41), although a very high percentage revert in the next few months. Nevertheless, cardioversion can sometimes significantly improve overall cardiac function, even though for a short time.

Patients with recurrent symptomatic ventricular tachycardia or ventricular fibrillation can be treated with an automatic implantable cardioverter defibrillator. The use of these devices is discussed in Chap. 42.

Conduction abnormalities are generally managed as described in Chap. 36 and 40.

Embolic Disease

Patients with ischemic heart disease are likely to have systemic emboli, particularly patients with a history of systemic embolus, chronic atrial fibrillation, ventricular aneurysm, a large dyskinetic or hypokinetic area of myocardium, or a severely depressed left ventricular ejection fraction. Such patients should be considered for chronic, long-term, low-dose warfarin therapy (INR = 2 to 3). (See Chap. 68.)

CHEST PAIN WITH NORMAL CORONARY ARTERIES

The combination of chest pain with many of the features of angina pectoris, although frequently atypical, and normal epicardial coronary arteries at cardiac catheterization has attracted a great deal attention since the entity was first noted in the 1960s.[101,102] These early studies identified many of the characteristics of what was subsequently characterized as a syndrome: female predominance; the frequent presence of ischemic ST-segment changes on the exercise electrocardiogram; inconsistent relationship between ECG changes and metabolic or hemodynamic evidence of ischemia; and pain that could be very severe, prolonged, atypical in location and precipitating events, and unresponsive commonly to usual anti-ischemic therapy.

The term *syndrome* X was applied to this diagnostic conundrum in 1973[202]; it is usually used to describe patients with the common features of angina-like pain and normal epicardial coronaries, as noted, but is also used to categorize groups that undoubtedly are pathophysiologically heterogeneous.[77] The continued use of the term is thus unfortunate and has been discouraged,[203] especially since there is another syndrome X, characterized by insulin resistance, hyperinsulinemia, and diabetes, that is associated with dyslipidemia, hypertension, and abdominal obesity.[204] There may be some overlap between the two syndromes because a group of patients has been reported that has hyperinsulinemia, dyslipidemia, angina with normal coronary arteriograms, and presumed microvasculopathy.[205] A more specific terminology such as *angina with normal coronary arteriography* is preferable.[203]

Clinical Presentation and Characteristics

The essential features of the clinical presentation of patients with chest pain and normal coronary arteriograms were described previously. Patients, about 70 percent of whom are women with an average age of approximately 50 years, complain of pain that is frequently consistent with, but not typical of, angina pectoris that is associated with epicardial coronary artery disease. It may be precipitated by exertion, although the threshold for precipitating pain is highly variable.[75] As noted, its duration may be uncharacteristically long and it may be unusually severe and is not commonly associated with symptoms such as diaphoresis. Nitroglycerin frequently does not give the characteristic rapid relief seen in usual angina pectoris. Approximately one-third of patients have hypertension or a history of hypertension without evidence of left ventricular hypertrophy.[77] The presence of left ventricular hypertrophy would result in the classification of patients as having hypertensive heart disease, which can result in similar chest pain syndromes and which probably overlaps mechanistically with the syndrome of chest pain with normal coronary arteriograms.[206]

Evidence for Ischemia

Ischemic ST-segment depression on exercise testing in the absence of epicardial coronary disease has been one of the hallmarks of syndrome X and has frequently been one of the criteria for its diagnosis.[77] More than 50 percent of patients evaluated at the National Institutes of Health for chest pain and normal coronaries had an ischemic ST-segment response.[207] Ischemic ST-segment depression and chest pain have been observed in two-thirds of patients but in no controls during the infusion of the vasodilator papaverine.[105] Thallium perfusion abnormalities have been observed commonly in patients with chest pain and normal arteriograms, but no consistent correlation could be made among the extent of the defect, the positivity of the exercise test, and exercise tolerance.[208] In such patients there is a relatively high frequency of abnormal ventricular responses (decreased ejection fraction or regional wall motion abnormality) to exercise.[207] Thus in many of these patients there is compelling evidence of perfusion abnormalities and ischemia that inferentially are related to abnormalities in the microvasculature.

Metabolic studies have been performed in patients with chest pain and normal coronaries to evaluate evidence of ischemia developing during stress. Results assessing lactate production have been inconsistent. Rapid atrial pacing has been reported not to increase lactate production in this setting[209] or to increase it in about one-third of patients, while intracoronary papaverine infusion consistently increased cardiac lactate production.[105] The available metabolic data do not permit definitive conclusions about the presence of ischemia. The methodologies used, however, may be insufficiently sensitive to detect the metabolic manifestations of ischemia if they are limited to relatively small areas of myocardium.

Abnormalities in the Coronary Flow Reserve in Chest Pain with Normal Coronary Arteriograms

Decreased coronary flow reserve has been the pathophysiological abnormality that has been observed most consistently, but not universally, in the chest pain–normal coronary arteriogram syndrome. Relative to normal individuals, flow increases less in response to vasodilators or to rapid pacing.[104,210] Enhanced vasoconstrictor responsiveness to ergonovine in the resistance vessels after vasodilator stimulation by rapid pacing that precipitated pain has been observed.[104] Such observations led to the proposal that these patients be classified as having *microvascular angina*.[211,212] Differences in flow reserve between controls and patients have also been observed using PET.[61]

The mechanisms of the microvascular dysfunction have not been completely defined. The increased contractile responsiveness to ergonovine was alluded to previously.[104] Recent evidence has been presented that implicates defective endothelial-dependent vasodilator mechanisms in the microvasculature. In a somewhat heterogeneous patient population with respect to concomitant diseases such as hypertension and diabetes, Motz et al. demonstrated defective endothelial-dependent microvascular dilation in a subset of patients with chest pain and normal epicardial coronaries.[213] In a more homogeneous population in which associated diseases were rigorously excluded, abnormalities in endothelial-dependent microvascular dilation were observed consistently.[105]

In summary, there is compelling evidence for abnormalities in coronary microvascular vasomotor control mechanisms in the syndrome of chest pain with normal coronary arteriograms. Dysfunction of endothelial-dependent vasodilator mechanisms is likely important pathogenetically. Nevertheless, the syndrome is probably not homogeneous with respect to etiology.

Myocardial Dysfunction

There is a growing body of data that is consistent with the notion that the myocardium is not normal in many patients with the chest pain–normal coronary artery syndrome, and a cardiomyopathic component of the syndrome has been implicated.[214] Endocardial biopsy has been reported to show mitochondrial swelling in myocardial cells[210] or hypertrophy and patchy fibrosis.[77,215] Although patients with the syndrome have been said to have consistently normal left ventricular response to exercise,[216] development of wall motion abnormalities or a decrease in ejection fraction in sizeable subsets of patients with angina and normal epicardial coronaries has been reported.[207,217] Those patients with abnormalities of flow reserve were most likely to have abnormal ventricular responses and, among these, two-thirds of those with left bundle branch block exhibited exercise-induced ventricular dysfunction. The presence of resting or exercise-induced left bundle branch block has been shown by others to identify a subgroup within the syndrome to be at particularly high risk for the chronic deterioration in left ventricular ejection fraction.[214,218] Romeo et al. also noted the relatively high frequency with which hypertension developed in these patients,[214] an association noted by others and alluded to previously. In analyzing their population they confirmed the heterogeneity of the syndrome and considered that it encompasses three groups: patients with ischemia who remain relatively stable, with or without worsening of the chest pain; those with borderline hypertension; and those with early cardiomyopathy. This formulation also implies that the long-term prognosis is not as favorable as generally thought in all subsets of the syndrome.

Disordered Pain Perception with Chest Pain and Normal Coronary Arteries

The intensity of the chest pain in the syndrome associated with normal coronary arteries, especially relative to stimuli that may appear mild or are not apparent, has led to speculation that there may be enhanced pain perception in many of these patients.[108] Patients with the syndrome have a low threshold for pain induction by stimuli such as forearm ischemia, cold pressor testing, or skin electrical stimulation.[219] They also may exhibit abnormal sensitivity to catheter manipulation, injection of normal saline into the atrium, pacing at the right ventricular apex, or injection of contrast into the left coronary artery.[220,221]

It has been proposed that release of high concentrations of adenosine in ischemic areas may account for the pain in many cases.[108] Thus, it may be that with respect to the cause of chest pain, patients with angina and normal coronary arteries can be divided into two groups—those with microvascular dysfunction and ischemia and those with neither.[77] The release of adenosine and stimulation of pain receptors may be related to pain in the former case, whereas nocioceptive hypersensitivity with triggers such as ectopic beats, changes in loading conditions, or changes in heart rhythm, rate, or contractility may be involved in the latter.

Approach to the Patient with Chest Pain and Normal Coronary Arteriograms

The ideal approach to these patients would be to assess abnormalities of flow reserve using Doppler catheters and endothelial-dependent and endothelial-independent dilators. This approach is not practical, however, in most clinical environments. Evidence of ischemia should be sought using exercise echocardiogram, nuclear angiography, or exercise perfusion thallium imaging. Those with evidence of ischemia should be given a trial of anti-ischemic therapy preferably including nitrates and calcium-entry blockers. Such trials are arguably indicated in most of these patients because of the relative insensitivity in detecting what may be small areas of ischemia. Borderline hypertensive patients or patients who become hypertensive should be treated effectively to keep blood pressure well within the normal range. For those without evidence of ischemia and/or who do not respond to anti-ischemic therapy, general supportive therapy and reassurance should be provided. Narcotics and repeat hospitalization should be avoided. Noncardiac causes of chest pain obviously should be rigorously sought early in the course.

REFERENCES

1. Heberden W: Some account of disorder of the breast. *Med Traus R Col Physicians (London)* 1772; 2:59–67.
2. Heberden W: *Commentaries on the History and Care of Disease.* London, T. Payne, 1802.
3. Leibowitz JO: *The History of Coronary Heart Disease.* Berkeley, Univ Calif Press, 1970: 1–227.
4. White PD: Angina pectoris: Historical background. In: Paul O (ed): *Angina Pectoris.* New York, Medcom Press, 1974: 1–11.
5. *1993 Heart and Stroke Facts Statistics.* Dallas, American Heart Association, 1992.
6. Campeau L: Grading of angina pectoris (letter). *Circulation* 1976; 54:522–523.
7. Willis PW III: Diagnosing angina pectoris. In: Paul O (ed): *Angina Pectoris.* New York, Medcom Press, 1974: 19–32.
8. Cowley AJ, Fullwood LJ, Stainer K, Harrison E, Muller AF, Hampton JR: Postprandial worsening of angina: All due to changes in cardiac output? *Br Heart J* 1991; 66:147–150.
9. Colles P, Juneau M, Gregoire J, Lariver L, Desideri A, Waters D: Effect of a standardized meal on the threshold of exercise-induced myocardial ischemia in patients with stable angina. *J Am Coll Cardiol* 1993; 21:1052–1057.
10. Winniford MD, Wheelan KR, Kremers MS, Ugolini V, van den Berg E, Niggemann EH, et al: Smoking-induced coronary vasoconstriction in patients with atherosclerotic coronary artery disease: Evidence for adrenergically mediated alterations in coronary artery tone. *Circulation* 1986; 73:662–667.
11. Winniford MD, Jansen DE, Reynolds GA, Apprill P, Black WH, Hillis LD: Cigarette smoking–induced coronary vasoconstriction in atherosclerotic coronary artery disease and prevention by calcium antagonists and nitroglycerin. *Am J Cardiol* 1987; 59:203–207.
12. Parker JO, Ledwich JR, West RO, Case RB: Reversible cardiac failure during angina pectoris: Hemodynamic effects of atrial pacing in coronary artery disease. *Circulation* 1969; 39:745–757.
13. McLaurin LP, Rolett EL, Grossman W: Impaired left ventricular relaxation during pacing-induced ischemia. *Am J Cardiol* 1973; 32:751–757.
14. Barry WH, Books JZ, Alderman EL, Harrison DC: Changes in diastolic stiffness and tone of the left ventricle during angina pectoris. *Circulation* 1974; 49:255–263.
15. Mann T, Brodie BR, Grossman W, McLaurin LP: Effect of angina on the left ventricular diastolic pressure-volume relationship. *Circulation* 1977; 55:761–766.
16. Bourdillon PD, Lorell BH, Mirsky I, Paulus WJ, Wynne J, Grossman W: Increased regional myocardial stiffness of the left ventricle during pacing-induced angina in man. *Circulation* 1983; 67:316–323.
17. Carroll JD, Hess OM, Hirzel HO, Krayenbuehl HP: Exercise-induced ischemia: The influence of altered relaxation on early diastolic pressures. *Circulation* 1983; 67:521–528.
18. Lorrell B: Significance of diastolic dysfunction of the heart. *Annu Rev Med* 1991; 42:411–436.
19. Kono T, Sabbah HN, Rosman H, Alam M, Jafri S, Stein PD, et al: Mechanism of functional mitral regurgitation during acute myocardial ischemia. *J Am Coll Cardiol* 1992; 19:1101–1105.
20. Fowler NO: Clinical diagnosis. *Circulation* 1972; 42:1079–1097.
21. Martin CE, Shaver JA, Leonard JJ: Physical signs, apex cardiography, phonocardiography, and systolic time intervals in angina pectoris. *Circulation* 1972; 46:1098–1114.
22. Shub C: Stable angina pectoris: 2. Cardiac evaluation and diagnostic testing. *Mayo Clin Proc* 1990; 65:243–255.
23. Diamond GA, Forrester JS: Analysis of probability as an aid in the clinical diagnosis of coronary-artery disease. *N Engl J Med* 1979; 300:1350–1358.
24. Rifkin RD, Hood WB Jr: Bayesian analysis of electrocardiographic exercise stress testing. *N Engl J Med* 1977; 297:681–686.
25. Reeves TJ: Use of stress electrocardiography in practice. *Heart Dis Stroke* 1992:13–18.
26. Levinson JR, Guiney TE, Boucher CA: Functional tests for myocardial ischemia. *Annu Rev Med* 1991; 42:119–126.
27. Gianrossi R, Detrano R, Mulvihil D, Lehmann K, Dubach P, Colombo A, et al: Exercise-induced ST depression in the diagnosis of coronary artery disease: A meta-analysis. *Circulation* 1989; 80:87–98.
28. Detrano R, Gianrossi R, Froelicher V: The diagnostic accuracy of the exercise electrocardiogram: A meta-analysis of 22 years of research. *Prog Cardiovasc Dis* 1989; 32:173–206.
29. Hollenberg M, Budge WR, Wisneski JA, Gertz EW: Treadmill score quantifies electrocardiographic responses to exercise and improves test accuracy and reproductibility. *Circulation* 1980; 61:276–285.
30. Veragari J, Hakki AH, Heo J, Iskandrian AS: Merits and limitations of quantitative treadmill exercise score. *Am Heart J* 1987; 114:819–826.
31. Mark DB, Shaw L, Harrell FE, Hlatky MA, Lee KL, Bengtson JR, et al: Prognostic value of a treadmill exercise score in outpatients with suspected coronary artery disease. *N Engl J Med* 1991; 325:849–853.
32. Kligfield P, Ameisen O, Okin PM: Heart rate adjustment of ST segment depression for improved detection of coronary artery disease. *Circulation* 1989; 79:245–255.
33. Lachterman B, Lehmann KG, Detrano R, Neutel J, Froelicher VF: Comparison of the ST/heart rate index to standard ST criteria for analysis of the exercise electrocardiogram. *Circulation* 1990; 82:44–50.
34. Bobbio M, Detrano R, Schmid J-J, Janosi A, Righetti A, Pfisterer M, et al: Exercise-induced ST depression and ST/heart rate index to predict triple-vessel or left main coronary disease: A multicenter analysis. *J Am Coll Cardiol* 1992; 19:11–18.
35. Kligfield P, Okin PM, Goldberg HL: Value and limitations of heart rate–adjusted ST segment depression criteria for the identification of anatomically severe coronary obstruction: Test performance in relation to method of rate correction, definition of extent of disease, and β-blockade. *Am Heart J* 1993; 125:1262–1268.
36. American College of Cardiology/American Heart Association Task Force on Assessment of Cardiovascular Procedures: Guidelines for exercise testing. *J Am Coll Cardiol* 1986; 8:725–738.
37. Bartel AG, Behar VS, Peter RH, Orgain ES, Kong Y: Graded exercise stress tests in angiographically documented coronary artery disease. *Circulation* 1974; 49:348–356.
38. Goldschlager N, Selzer A, Cohn K: Treadmill stress tests as indicators of presence and severity of coronary artery disease. *Ann Intern Med* 1976; 85:277–286.
39. McNeer JF, Margolis JR, Lee KL, Kisslo JA, Peter RH, Kong Y, et al: The role of the exercise test in the evaluation of patients for ischemic heart disease. *Circulation* 1978; 57:64–70.
40. Froelicher VF: *Exercise and the Heart: Clinical Concepts.* Chicago, Yearbook Medical Publishers, 1987.
41. Gibbons L, Blair SN, Kohl HW, Cooper K: The safety of maximal exercise testing. *Circulation* 1989; 80:846–852.
42. Ladenheim ML, Pollack BH, Royanski A, Berman DS, Staniloff HM, Forrester JS, et al: Extent and severity of myocardial reperfusion as predictors of prognosis in patients with suspected coronary artery disease. *J Am Coll Cardiol* 1986; 7:464–471.
43. Kaul S: A look at 15 years of planar thallium-201. *Am Heart J* 1989; 118:581–601.
44. Lotler TS, Diamond GA: Exercise thallium-201 scintigraphy in the diagnosis and prognosis of coronary artery disease. *Ann Intern Med* 1990; 113:684–702.

45. Beller GA: Pharmacologic stress imaging. *JAMA* 1991; 265:633–638.
46. Esquivel L, Pollock SG, Beller GA, Gibson RS, Watson DD, Kaul S: Effect of the degree of effort on the sensitivity of the exercise thallium-201 stress test in symptomatic coronary artery disease. *Am J Cardiol* 1989; 63:160–165.
47. Iskandrian AS, Hakki AH, Kane-Marsh S: Exercise thallium-201 scintigraphy in men with non-diagnostic exercise electrocardiograms: Prognostic implications. *Arch Intern Med* 1986; 146:2189–2193.
48. Boucher CA, Zin LM, Beller GA, Okada RD, McKusick KA, Strauss HW, et al: Increased lung uptake of thallium-201 during exercise myocardial imaging: Clinical, hemodynamic and angiographic implications in patients with coronary artery disease. *Am J Cardiol* 1980; 46:189–196.
49. Kaul S, Finkelstein DM, Homma S, Leavitt M, Okada RD, Bousher CA: Superiority of quantitative exercise thallium-201 variables in determining long-term prognosis in ambulatory patients with chest pain: A comparison with cardiac catheterization. *J Am Coll Cardiol* 1988; 12:25–34.
50. Brown K: Prognostic value of thallium-201 myocardial perfusion imaging: A diagnostic tool comes of age. *Circulation* 1991; 83:363–381.
51. Pamelia FX, Gibson RS, Watson DD, Craddock GB, Sirowatka J, Beller GA: Prognosis with chest pain and normal thallium-201 exercise scintigrams. *Am J Cardiol* 1985; 55:920–926.
52. Staniloff HM, Forrester JS, Berman DS, Swan HJC: Prediction of death, myocardial infarction, and worsening chest pain using thallium scintigraphy and exercise electrocardiography. *J Nucl Med* 1986; 27:1842–1848.
53. Gibson RS, Watson DD, Craddock GB, Crampton RS, Kaiser DL, Denny MJ, et al: Prediction of cardiac events after uncomplicated myocardial infarction: A prospective study comparing predischarge exercise thallium-201 scintigraphy and coronary angiography. *Circulation* 1983; 68:321–336.
54. Boucher CA, Brewster DC, Darling RC, Okada RC, Strauss HW, Pohost GM: Determination of cardiac risk by dipyridamole-thallium imaging before peripheral vascular surgery. *N Engl J Med* 1985; 312:389–394.
55. Leppo J, Plaja J, Goinet M, Tumolo J, Paraskos JA, Cutler BS: Noninvasive evaluation of cardiac risk before elective surgery. *J Am Coll Cardiol* 1987; 9:269–276.
56. Hays JT, Mahmarian JJ, Cochran AJ, Verani MS: Dobutamine thallium-201 tomography for evaluating patients with suspected coronary artery disease unable to undergo exercise or vasodilator pharmacologic stress testing. *J Am Coll Cardiol* 1993; 21:1583–1590.
57. Forster T, McNeil AJ, Salustri A, Reijs AEM, el-Said EM, Roelandt JRTC, et al: Simultaneous dobutamine stress echocardiography and technetium-99m isonitrile single-photon emission computed tomography in patients with suspected coronary artery disease. *J Am Coll Cardiol* 1993; 21:1591–1596.
58. O'Keefe JH Jr, Bateman TM, Barnhard CS: Adenosine thallium-201 is superior to exercise thallium-201 for detecting coronary artery disease in patients with left bundle branch block. *J Am Coll Cardiol* 1993; 21:1332–1338.
59. Friedman J, VanTrain K, Kiat H, Wang FP, Nyun M, Silagan G, et al: Simultaneous dual isotope rest/stress myocardial perfusion scintigraphy: A feasibility study abstract. *J Am Coll Cardiol* 1991; 17(suppl A):390A.
60. Hutchins GD, Schwaiger M, Rosenspire KC, Krivokapich J, Schelbert HR, Kuhl DE: Non-invasive quantification of regional blood flow in the human heart using N-13 ammonia and dynamic position emission tomographic imaging. *J Am Coll Cardiol* 1990; 15:1031–1042.
61. Geltman EM, Hennes GC, Senneff MJ, Sobel BE, Bergmann SR: Increased myocardial perfusion at rest and diminished perfusion reserve in patients with angina and angiographically normal coronary arteries. *J Am Coll Cardiol* 1990; 16:586–595.
62. Quinones MA, Verani MS, Haichin RM, Mahmarian JJ, Suarez J, Zoghbi W: Exercise echocardiography versus ^{201}Tl single-photon emission computed tomography in evaluation of coronary artery disease: Analysis of 292 patients. *Circulation* 1992; 85:1026–1031.
63. Beller GA: Evaluation of myocardial viability using thallium-201 imaging. *Cardiol Rev* 1993; 1:78–86.
64. Bonow RO, Dilsizian V, Cuocolo A, Bacharach SL: Identification of viable myocardium in patients with chronic coronary artery disease and left ventricular dysfunction: Comparison of thallium scintigraphy with reinjection and PET imaging with ^{18}F-fluorodioxide glucose. *Circulation* 1991; 83:26–37.
65. Gibbons RJ: Rest and exercise radionuclide angiography for diagnosis in chronic ischemic heart disease. *Circulation* 1991; 84(suppl l):l-93–l-99.
66. Marwick TH, Nemec JJ, Pashkow FJ, Stewart WJ, Salcedo EE: Accuracy and limitations of exercise echocardiography in a routine clinical setting. *J Am Coll Cardiol* 1992; 19:74–81.
67. Berthe C, Pierard LA, Hiernaux M, Trotteur G, Lempereur P, Carlier J, et al: Predicting the extent and location of coronary artery disease in acute myocardial infarction by echocardiography during dobutamine infusion. *Am J Cardiol* 1986; 58:1167–1172.
68. Harrison MR, Smith MD, Friedman BJ, DeMaria AN: Uses and limitations of exercise Doppler echocardiography in the diagnosis of ischemic heart disease. *J Am Coll Cardiol* 1987; 10:809–817.
69. Cohen JL, Greene TO, Ottenweller J, Binenvaum SZ, Wilchfort SD, Kim CS: Dobutamine digital echocardiography for detecting coronary artery disease. *Am J Cardiol* 1991; 67:1311–1318.
70. Mazeika P, Nihoyannopoulos P, Nadazdin A, Oakley CM: Pharmacological stress echocardiography in the evaluation of coronary artery disease. *Postgrad Med J* 1991; 67(suppl 1):S21–S35.
71. Mazeika PK, Nadazdin A, Oakley CM: Stress Doppler echocardiography using dobutamine in coronary patients with and without ischaemia induction. *Eur Heart J* 1992; 13:1020–1027.
72. Martin TW, Seaworth JF, Johns SP, Pupa LE, Condos WR: Comparison of adenosine, dipyridamole, and dobutamine in stress echocardiography. *Ann Intern Med* 1992; 116:190–196.
73. Barnard RJ, Duncan HW, Livesay JJ, Buckberg GD: Coronary vasodilator reserve and flow distribution during near-maximal exercise in dogs. *J Appl Physiol: Resp Environ Exercise Physiol* 1977; 43:988–992.
74. Boerth RC, Covell JW, Pool PE, Ross J Jr: Increased myocardial oxygen consumption and contractile state associated with increases in heart rate in dogs. *Circ Res* 1969; 24:725–734.
75. Pupita G, Maseri A, Kaski JC, Galassi AR, Gavrielides S, Davies G, et al: Myocardial ischemia caused by distal coronary artery constriction in stable angina pectoris. *N Engl J Med* 1990; 323:514–520.
76. Egashira K, Inou T, Hirooka Y, Yamada A, Urabe Y, Takeshita A: Evidence of impaired endothelium-dependent coronary vasodilatation in patients with angina pectoris and normal coronary angiograms. *N Engl J Med* 1993; 328:1659–1664.
77. Cannon RO III, Camici PG, Epstein SE: Pathophysiological dilemma of syndrome X. *Circulation* 1992; 85:883–892.
78. Ardehali A, Ports TA: Myocardial oxygen supply and demand. *Chest* 1990; 98:699–705.
79. Rubio R, Berne RM: Release of adenosine by normal myocardium and its relationship to the regulation of coronary resistance. *Circ Res* 1969; 25:407–415.
80. Berne RM: The role of adenosine in the regulation of coronary blood flow. *Circ Res* 1980; 47:807–813.
81. Mosher P, Ross J Jr, McFate PA, Shaw RF: Control of coronary blood flow by an autoregulatory mechanism. *Circ Res* 1964; 14:250–259.
82. Gould KL, Lipscomb K, Calvert C: Compensatory changes of the distal coronary vascular bed during progressive coronary constriction. *Circulation* 1975; 51:1085–1094.
83. Mudge GH Jr, Grossman W, Mills RM Jr, Lesch M, Braunwald E: Reflex increase in coronary vascular resistance in patients with ischemic heart disease. *N Engl J Med* 1976; 295:1333–1337.
84. Sabiston DC, Gregg DE: Effects of cardiac contraction on coronary blood flow. *Circulation* 1957; 15:14–20.
85. Lewis FB, Coffmann JD, Gregg DE: Effect of heart rate and intracoronary isoproterenol, levarterenol, and epinephrine on coronary flow and resistance. *Circ Res* 1961; 9:89–95.
86. Furchgott RF, Zawadzski JV: The obligatory role of endothelial cells in the relaxation of arterial smooth muscle by acetylcholine. *Nature* 1980; 288:373–376.
87. Palmer RMJ, Ferrige AG, Moncada S: Nitric oxide release accounts for the biological activity of endothelium-derived relaxing factor. *Nature* 1987; 327:524–526.
88. Brown BG, Bolson EL, Dodge HT: Dynamic mechanisms in human coronary stenosis. *Circulation* 1984; 42:917–922.

89. Gage JE, Hess OM, Murakami T, Ritter M, Grimm J, Krayenbuehl HP: Vasoconstriction of stenotic coronary arteries during dynamic exercise in patients with classic angina pectoris: Reversibility by nitroglycerin. *Circulation* 1986; 73:865–876.
90. Gordon JB, Ganz P, Nabel EG, Fish RD, Zebede J, Mudge GH, et al: Atherosclerosis influences the vasomotor response of epicardial coronary arteries to exercise. *J Clin Invest* 1989; 83:1946–1952.
91. Bortone AS, Hess OM, Eberli FR: Abnormal coronary vasomotion during exercise in patients with normal coronary arteries and reduced coronary flow reserve. *Circulation* 1991; 83:26–37.
92. Hess OM, Büchi M, Kirkeeide R, Niederer P, Anliker M, Gould KL, et al: Potential role of coronary vasoconstriction in ischemic heart disease: Effect of exercise. *Eur Heart J* 1900; 11(suppl B):58–64.
93. Bassen M, Marcus H, Ganz W: The effect of mild to moderate mental stress on coronary hemodynamics in patients with coronary artery disease. *Circulation* 1980; 62:933–935.
94. Deanfield JE, Kensett M, Wilson RA, Shea M, Horlock P, deLandsheere CM et al: Silent myocardial ischaemia due to mental stress. *Lancet* 1984; 2:1001–1005.
95. Yeung AC, Vekshtein VI, Krantz DS, Vita JA, Ryan TJ, Ganz P, et al: The effect of atherosclerosis on the vasomotor response of coronary arteries to mental stress. *N Engl J Med* 1991; 325:1551–1556.
96. Zeiher AM, Drexler H, Wollschlaeger H, Saubier B, Just H: Coronary vasomotion in response to sympathetic stimulation in humans: Importance of the functional integrity of the endothelium. *J Am Coll Cardiol* 1989; 14:1181–1190.
97. Nabel EG, Ganz P, Gordon JB, Alexander RW, Selwyn AP: Dilation of normal and constriction of atherosclerotic coronary arteries caused by the cold pressor testing. *Circulation* 1988; 77:43–52.
98. Nabel EG, Selwyn AP, Ganz P: Paradoxical narrowing of atherosclerotic coronary arteries induced by increases in heart rate. *Circulation* 1990; 81:850–859.
99. Vita JA, Treasure CB, Yeung AC, Vekshtein VI, Fantasia GM, Fish RD, et al: Patients with evidence of coronary endothelial dysfunction as assessed by acetylcholine infusion demonstrate marked increase in sensitivity to constrictor effects of catecholamines. *Circulation* 1992; 85:1390–1397.
100. Maseri A, Chierchia S, Kaski JC: Mixed angina pectoris. *Am J Cardiol* 1985; 56:30E–33E.
101. Likoff W, Segal BL, Kasparian H: Paradox of normal selective coronary arteriograms in patients considered to have unmistakable coronary heart disease. *N Engl J Med* 1967; 276:1063–1066.
102. Kemp HG, Elliott WC, Gorlin R: The anginal syndrome with normal coronary arteriography. *Trans Assoc Am Physicians* 1967; 80:59–70.
103. Legrand V, Hodgson JM, Bates ER, Aueron FM, Mancini GBJ, Smith JS, et al: Abnormal coronary flow reserve and abnormal radionuclide exercise test results in patients with normal coronary angiograms. *J Am Coll Cardiol* 1985; 6:1245–1253.
104. Cannon RO III, Watson RM, Rosing DR, Epstein SE: Angina caused by reduced vasodilator reserve of the small coronary arteries. *J Am Coll Cardiol* 1983; 1:1359–1373.
105. Egashira K, Inou T, Hirooka Y, Yamada A, Urabe Y, Takeshita A: Evidence of impaired endothelium-dependent coronary vasodilatation in patients with angina pectoris and normal coronary angiograms. *N Engl J Med* 1993; 328:1659–1664.
106. Treasure CB, Klein JL, Vita JA, Manoukian SV, Renwick GH, Selwyn AP, et al: Hypertension and left ventricular hypertrophy are associated with impaired endothelium-mediated relaxation in human coronary resistance vessels. *Circulation* 1993; 87:86–93.
107. Mosseri M, Schaper J, Admon D, Hasin Y, Gotsman MS, Sapoznikov D, et al: Coronary capillaries in patients with congestive cardiomyopathy or angina pectoris with patent main coronary arteries. Ultrastructural morphometry of endomyocardial biopsy samples. *Circulation* 1991; 48:203–210.
108. Maseri A, Crea F, Kaski JC, Davies G: Mechanisms and significance of cardiac ischemic pain. *Prog Cardiovasc Dis* 1992; 35:1–18.
109. Deanfield JE: Characteristics of silent and symptomatic ischemia in chronic stable angina: Comparison with unstable and vasospastic angina. In: Singh BM (ed): *Silent Myocardial Ischemia and Angina. Prevalence, Prognostic, and Therapeutic Significance*. New York, Pergamon, 1988:104–111.
110. Stern S, Tzivoni D: Ventricular arrhythmias, sudden death, and silent myocardial ischemia. *Prog Cardiovasc Dis* 1992; 35:19–26.
111. Nair CK, Aronow MH, Sketch R, Pagano JD, Lynch AN, Moose D, et al: Diagnostic and prognostic significance of exercise-induced premature ventricular complexes in men and women: A four year follow-up *J Am Coll Cardiol* 1983; 1:1201–1206.
112. Sigwart U, Grbic M, Payot J, Goy A, Essinger A, Fischer A. Ischemic events during coronary artery balloon occlusion. In: Rutishauser W, Roskamm H (eds): *Silent Myocardial Ischemia*. Berlin, Springer-Verlag, 1984:29–36.
113. Muller JE, Stone PH, Turi ZG, Rutherford JD, Czeisler CA, Parker C, et al: Circadian variation in the frequency of onset of acute myocardial infarction. *N Engl J Med* 1985; 313:1315–1322.
114. Kenkels U, Blumchen G, Ebner F: Zur Probleme von Belastungsprofungen in abhängigkeit von der Tageszeit bei Patienten mit Koronarinsuffizienz. *Herz Kreisal* 1977; 9:343–346.
115. Rocco MB, Barry J, Campbell S, Nabel E, Cook EF, Goldman L, Selwyn AP: Circadian variation of transient myocardial ischemia in patients with coronary artery disease. *Circulation* 1987; 75:395–400.
116. Yasue H, Omote S, Takizawa A, Nagao M, Miwa K, Tanaka S: Circadian variation of exercise capacity in patients with Prinzmetal's variant angina: Role of exercise-induced coronary arterial spasm. *Circulation* 1979; 59:938–948.
117. Rocco MB, Selwyn AP: Circadian rhythms and ischemic heart disease with particular reference to transient myocardial ischemia. In: Singh B (ed): *Silent Myocardial Ischemia and Angina*. New York, Pergamon, 1988:70–81.
118. Deanfield JE: Characteristic of silent and symptomatic ischemia in chronic stable angina: Comparison with unstable and vasospastic angina. In: Singh BM (ed): *Silent Myocardial Ischemia and Angina*. New York, Pergamon, 1988:104–111.
119. White JC: Cardiac pain: Anatomic pathways and physiologic mechanisms. *Circulation* 1957; 16:644.
120. Lindgren I, Olivecrona H: Surgical treatment of angina pectoris. *J Neurosurg* 1947; 4:19–39.
121. Crossman DC, Larkin SW, Fuller RW: Substance P dilates epicardial coronary arteries and increases coronary blood flow in humans. *Circulation* 1989; 80:475–484.
122. Sylven C, Beerman B, Jonzon B: Angina pectoris-like pain provoked by intravenous adenosine in healthy volunteers. *Br Med J* 1986; 293:227–230.
123. Herrick JB: Clinical features of sudden obstruction of the coronary arteries. *JAMA* 1912; 59:2015–2020.
124. Roseman MD: Painless myocardial infarction: A review of the literature and analysis of 220 cases. *Ann Intern Med* 1954; 41:1–8.
125. Master AM, Geller AM: The extent of completely asymptomatic coronary artery disease. *Am J Cardiol* 1969; 23:173–179.
126. Froelicher VF, Yanowitz FG, Thompson AJ: The correlation of coronary angiography and the electrocardiographic response to maximal treadmill testing in 76 asymptomatic men. *Circulation* 1973; 48:597–604.
127. Stern S, Tzivoni D: Early detection of silent ischaemic heart disease by 24-hour electrocardiographic monitoring of active subjects. *Br Heart J* 1974; 36:481–486.
128. Gettes LS: Painless myocardial ischemia. *Chest* 1974; 66:612–613.
129. Cohn PF: Asymptomatic coronary artery disease: Pathophysiology, diagnosis, management. *Mod Conc Cardiovasc Dis* 1981; 50:55–60.
130. Serneri GGN, Doddi M, Arata L, Rostagno C, Dabizzi P, Coppo M, et al: Silent ischemia in unstable angina is related to an altered cardiac norepinephrine handling. *Circulation* 1993; 87:1928–1937.
131. Cohn PF: Prevalence of silent myocardial ischemia. In: Cohn PF (ed): *Silent Myocardial Ischemia and Infarction*. New York, Marcel Dekker, 1986:71–80.
132. Deanfield JE, Ribiero P, Oakley K, Krikler S, Selwyn AP: Analysis of ST-segment changes in normal subjects: Implications for ambulatory monitoring in angina pectoris. *Am J Cardiol* 1984; 54:1321–1325.

133. Armstrong WF, Jordan JW, Morris SN, McHenry PL: Prevalence and magnitude of ST segment and T wave abnormalities in normal men during continuous ambulatory electrocardiography. *Am J Cardiol* 1982; 49:1639–1642.
134. Hedblad B, Juul-Möller S, Svensson K, Hanson BS, Isacsson SO, Janzon L: Increased mortality in men with ST segment depression during 24 h ambulatory long-term ECG recording: Results from prospective population study 'Men born in 1914,' from Malmo, Sweden. *Eur Heart J* 1989; 10:149–158.
135. Pepine CJ, Coy K, Lambert C: Silent myocardial ischemia during daily activities in asymptomatic patients with positive treadmill tests. In: Singh B (ed): *Silent Myocardial Ischemia and Angina.* New York, Pergamon, 1988:93–103.
136. Deanfield JE, Maseri A, Selwyn AP, Ribeiro P, Chierchia S, Krikler S, et al: Myocardial ischemia during daily life in patients with stable angina: Its relation to symptoms and heart rate changes. *Lancet* 1983; 2:753–758.
137. Chierchia S, Lazzari M, Freedman B, Brunelli C, Maseri A: Impairment of myocardial perfusion and function during painless myocardial ischemia. *J Am Coll Cardiol* 1983; 1:924–930.
138. Mannheimer C, Carlsson CA, Vedin A, Wilhelmsson C: Transcutaneous electrical nerve stimulation (TENS) in angina pectoris. *Pain* 1986; 26:291–300.
139. Davies HA, Page Z, Rush EM, Brown AL, Lewis MJ: Esophageal stimulation lowers exertional angina threshold. *Lancet* 1985; 1:1011–1014.
140. Murphy DF, Giles KE: Dorsal column stimulation for pain relief from intractable angina pectoris. *Pain* 1987; 28:365–368.
141. Droste C, Roskamm H: Experimental pain measurements in patients with asymptomatic myocardial ischemia. *J Am Coll Cardiol* 1983; 1:940–945.
142. Glazier JJ, Chierchia S, Brown MJ, Maseri A: Importance of generalized defective perception of painful stimuli as a cause of silent myocardial ischemia in chronic stable angina pectoris. *Am J Cardiol* 1986; 58:667–672.
143. Falcone C, Sconocchia R, Guasti L, Codega S, Montemartini C, Specchia G: Dental pain threshold and angina pectoris in patients with coronary artery disease. *J Am Col Cardiol* 1988; 12:348–352.
144. Bradley RF, Partamian JO: Coronary heart disease in the diabetic patient. *Med Clin North Am* 1993; 78:1093–1104.
145. Fearman I, Faccio E, Melei J: Autonomic neuropathy and painless myocardial infarction in diabetic patients: Histologic evidence of their relationships. *Diabetes* 1977; 26:1147–1158.
146. Nesto RW, Phillips RT, Kett KG: Angina and exertional myocardial ischemia in diabetic and nondiabetic patients: Assessment by exercise thallium scintigraphy. *Ann Intern Med* 1988; 108:170–175.
147. Chiariello M, Indolfi C, Cotecchia MR: Asymptomatic transient ST changes during ambulatory ECG monitoring in diabetic patients. *Am Heart J* 1985; 110:529–534.
148. Coy KM, Imperi GA, Lambert CR, Pepine CJ: Silent myocardial ischemia during daily activities in asymptomatic men with possitive exercise test responses. *Am J Cardiol* 1987; 59:45–49.
149. Deanfield JE, Kensett M, Wilson RA, Shea M, Horlock P, deLandsheere CM, et al: Silent myocardial ischaemia due to mental stress. *Lancet* 1984; 2:1001.
150. Pepine CJ: Is silent ischemia a treatable risk factor in patients with angina pectoris? *Circulation* 1990; 82(suppl ll):ll-135–ll-142.
151. Bertolet BD, Hill JA, Pepine CJ: Treatment strategies for daily life silent myocardial ischemia: A correlation with potential pathogenic mechanisms. *Prog Cardiovasc Dis* 1992; 35:97–118.
152. Brown BG, Zhao XQ, Sacco DE, Albers JJ: Lipid lowering and plaque regression: New insights into prevention of plaque disruption and clinical events in coronary disease. *Circulation* 1993; 87:1781–1791.
153. Ornish D, Brown SE, Scherwitz LW, Billings JH, Armstrong WT, Ports TA, et al: Can lifestyle changes reverse coronary heart disease? *Lancet* 1990; 336:129–133.
154. Ridker PM, Manson JE, Gaziano JM, Buring JE, Hennekens CH: Low-dose aspirin therapy for chronic stable angina: A randomized, placebo-controlled clinical trial. *Ann Intern Med* 1991; 114:835–839.
155. Juul-Möller S, Edvardsson N, Jahnmatz B, Rosén A, Sørensen S, Ömblus R: Double-blind trial of aspirin in primary prevention of myocardial infarction in patients with stable chronic angina pectoris. *Lancet* 1992; 340:1421–1425.
156. Stein B, Fuster V: Anticoagulants and platelet inhibitors. *Curr Opin Cardiol* 1990; 5:461–474.
157. Willard JE, Lange RA, Hillis LD: The use of aspirin in ischemic heart disease. *N Engl J Med* 1992; 327:175–181.
158. Summary of the Second Report of National Cholesterol Education Program (NCEP) Expert Panel on Detection, Evaluation, and Treatment of High Blood Cholesterol in Adults (Adult Treatment Panel II). *JAMA* 1993; 269:3015–3023.
159. Schuler G, Hambrecht R, Schlierf G, Niebauer J, Hauer K, Neumann J, et al: Regular physical exercise and low-fat diet. Effects on progression of coronary artery disease. *Circulation* 1992; 86:1–11.
160. Fletcher GF, Blair SN, Blumenthal J, Caspersen C, Chaitman B, Epstein S, et al: Statement on exercise benefits and recommendations for physical activity programs for all Americans. A statement for health care professionals by the Committee on Exercise and Cardiac Rehabilitation of the Council on Clinical Cardiology. American Heart Association. *Circulation* 1992; 86:340–344.
161. Redwood DR, Rosing DR, Epstein SE: Circulatory and symptomatic effects of physical training in patients with coronary artery disease and angina pectoris. *N Engl J Med* 1972; 286:959–965.
162. Amsterdam EA, Hughes JL III, DeMaria AN: Indirect assessment of myocardial oxygen consumption in the evaluation of mechanisms and therapy of angina pectoris. *Am J Cardiol* 1974; 33:737–743.
163. Sim DN, Neill WA: Investigation of the physiological basis for increased exercise threshold for angina pectoris after physical conditioning. *J Clin Res* 1974; 54:763–770.
164. Clausen JP: Circulatory adjustments to dynamic exercise and the effect of physical training in normal subjects and in patients with coronary artery disease. *Prog Cardiovasc Dis* 1976; 18:459–495.
165. Kennedy CC, Spiekerman RE, Lindsay MI, Mankin HT, Frye RL, McCallister BD: One-year graduated exercise program for men with angina pectoris. *Mayo Clin Proc* 1976; 51:231–236.
166. Ehsani AA, Health GW, Hagberg JM, Sobel BE, Holoszy JO: Effects of 12 months intense exercise training on ischemic ST segment depression in patients with coronary artery disease. *Circulation* 1981; 64:1116–1124.
167. Froelicher V, Jensen D, Genter F, Sullivan M, McKirnan MD, Witztum K, et al: A randomized trial of exercise training in patients with coronary artery disease. *JAMA* 1984; 252:1291–1297.
168. Parker JO: Nitrate therapy in stable angina pectoris. *N Engl J Med* 1987; 316:1635–1642.
169. Abrams J: A reappraisal of nitrate therapy. *JAMA* 1988; 259(3):396–401.
170. Abrams J: Transdermal nitroglycerin in angina pectoris. *Eur Heart J* 1989; 10(suppl A):11–19.
171. Abrams J: Use of nitrates in ischemic heart disease. *Curr Probl Cardiol* 1992; 17:487–542.
172. Abrams J(ed): A symposium:Third North American conference on nitroglycerin therapy. *Am J Cardiol* 1992; 70(suppl B):1B-103B.
173. Frishman W(ed): Optimizing anti-anginal therapy: A consensus conference. *Am J Cardiol* 1992; 70(suppl G); 1G-76G.
174. Leier CV: Nitrate tolerance. *Am Heart J* 1985; 110:224–232.
175. Parker JO, Farrell B, Lahey K, Moe G: Effect of intervals between doses on the development of tolerance to isosobide dinitrate. *N Engl J Med* 1987; 316:1440–1444.
176. Horowitz JD, Antman EM, Lorell BH, Barry WH, Smith TN: Potentiation of the cardiovascular effects of nitroglycerin by *n*-acetylcysteine. *Circulation* 1983; 68:1247–1253.
177. Torresi J, Horowitz JD, Dusting GJ: Prevention and reversal of tolerance to nitroglycerin with *n*-acetylcysteine. *J Cardiovasc Pharmacol* 1985; 7:777–783.
178. Packer M, Lee WH, Kessler PD, Gottlieb SS, Medina N, Yushak M: Prevention and reversal of nitrate tolerance in patients with congestive heart failure. *N Engl J Med* 1987; 17:799–804.
179. Levy WS, Katz RJ, Ruffalo RL, et al: Potentiation of the hemodynamic effects of acutely administered nitroglycerin by methionine. *Circulation* 1988; 78:640–645.
180. Parker JO, Farrell B, Labey KA, Rose BF: Nitrate tolerance: The lack of effect of *n*-acetylcysteine. *Circulation* 1987; 76:572–576.

181. Munzel T, Holtz J, Mulsch A, Stewart DJ, Bassenge E: Nitrate tolerance in epicardial arteries or in the venous system is not reversed by *n*-acetylcysteine in vivo, but tolerance-independent interactions exist. *Circulation* 1989; 79:188–197.
182. Dupris J, Lalonde G, Lemieux R, Rouleau JL: Tolerance to intravenous nitroglycerin in patients with congestive heart failure. Role of increased volume, neurohumoral activation and lack of prevention with *n*-acetylcysteine. *J Am Cardiol* 1990; 16:932–934.
183. Thadani U, Davidson C, Singleton W, Taylor SH: Comparison of the immediate effects of five beta-adrenoreceptor–blocking drugs with different ancillary properties in angina pectoris. *N Engl J Med* 1979; 300:750–755.
184. Ryan TJ, Faxon DP, Gunnar RM, Kennedy JW, King SB, Loop FD, et al: Guidelines for percutaneous transluminal coronary angioplasty: A report of the American College of Cardiology/American Heart Association Task Force on Assessment of Diagnostic and Therapeutic Cardiovascular Procedures (Subcommittee on Percutaneous Transluminal Angioplasty). *Circulation* 1988; 78:486–502.
185. American College of Cardiology/American Heart Association Task Force on Assessment of Diagnostic and Therapeutic Cardiovascular Procedures: Guidelines and indications for coronary artery bypass graft surgery. *J Am Coll Cardiol* 1991; 17:543–584.
186. Varnauskas E and the European Coronary Surgery Study Group: Twelve-year follow-up of survival in the randomized European Coronary Surgery Study. *N Engl J Med* 1988; 319:332–337.
187. Alderman EL, Bourassa MG, Cohen LS, Davis KB, Kaiser GG, Killip T, et al: Ten-year follow-up of survival and myocardial infarction in the randomized coronary artery surgery study. *Circulation* 1990; 82:1629–1646.
188. Rogers WJ, Coggin CJ, Gersh BJ, Fisher LD, Myers WO, Oberman A, et al: Ten-year follow-up of quality of life in patients randomized to receive medical therapy or coronary artery bypass graft surgery: The coronary artery surgery study. *Circulation* 1990; 82:1647–1658.
189. Gersh BJ, Califf RM, Loop FD, Akins CW, Pryor DB, Takaro TC: Coronary bypass surgery in chronic stable angina. *Circulation* 1989; 79(suppl l):l-46–l-59.
190. Hammermeister KE, Morrison DA: Coronary bypass surgery for stable and unstable angina pectoris. *Cardiol Clin* 1991; 9:135–155.
191. Nwasokwa ON, Koss JH, Friedman GH, Grunwald AM, Bodenheimer MM: Bypass surgery for chronic stable angina: Predictors of survival benefit and strategy for patient selection. *Ann Intern Med* 1991; 114:1035–1049.
192. Veterans Affairs Coronary Artery Bypass Surgery Cooperative Study Group: Eighteen-year Follow-up in the Veterans Affairs Cooperative Study of Coronary Artery Bypass Surgery for Stable Angina. *Circulation* 1992; 86:121–130.
193. BARI, CABRI, EAST, GABI, and RITA: Coronary angioplasty on trial (editorial). *Lancet* 1990; 335:1315–1316.
194. Parisi AF, Folland ED, Hartigan P: A comparison of angioplasty with medical therapy in the treatment of single-vessel coronary artery disease. *N Engl J Med* 1992; 326:10–16.
195. Guidelines for coronary angiography. A report of the ACC/AHA Task Force on Assessment of Diagnostic and Therapeutic Cardiovascular Procedures. *J Am Coll Cardiol* 1987; 10:935–950.
196. Pryor DB, Bruce RA, Chaitman BR, Fisher L, Gajewski J, Hammermeister KE, et al: Task Force I: Determination of prognosis in patients with ischemic heart disease. *J Am Coll Cardiol* 1989; 14:1016–1025.
197. Weiner DA: Risk stratification in angina pectoris. *Cardiol Clin* 1991; 9:39–47.
198. Lawson WE, Hui JCK, Soroff HS, Zheng ZS, Kayden DS, Sasvary D, et al: Efficacy of enhanced external counterpulsation in the treatment of angina pectoris. *Am J Cardiol* 1992; 70:859–862.
199. Rahimtoola SH: The hibernating myocardium. *Am Heart J* 1989; 117:211–221.
200. Packer M, Gheorghiade M, Young JB, Costantini PJ, Adams KF, Cody RJ, et al: Withdrawal of digoxin from patients with chronic heart failure treated with angiotensin-coverting-enzyme inhibitors. *N Engl J Med* 1993; 329:1–7.
201. Feldman AM, Bistow MR, Parmley WW, Carson PE, Gilbert EM, Strobeck JE, et al: Effects of vesnarinone on morbidity and mortality in patients with heart failure. *N Engl J Med* 1993; 329:149–155.
202. Kemp GH: Left ventricular function in patients with the anginal syndrome and normal coronary arteriograms. *Am J Cardiol* 1973; 32:375–376.
203. Kaplan MN: Syndromes X: Two too many. *J Am Coll Cardiol* 1992; 69:1643–1644.
204. Reaven GM: Role of insulin resistance in human disease. *Diabetes* 1988; 37:1595–1607.
205. Dean JD, Jones CJH, Hutchison SJ, Peters JR, Henderson AH: Hyperinsulinaemia and microvascular angina ("syndrome X"). *Lancet* 1991; 337:456–457.
206. Brush JE, Cannon RO, Schenke WH, Bonow RO, Leon MB, Maron BJ, et al: Angina due to coronary microvascular disease in hypertensive patients without left ventricular hypertrophy. *N Engl J Med* 1988; 319:1302–1307.
207. Cannon RO: Microvascular angina: Cardiovascular investigation regarding pathophysiology and management. In: Richter JE, Cannon RO, Reitman B (eds): *Unexplained Chest Pain*. Philadelphia, Saunders, 1991: 1097–1118.
208. Tweddel AC, Martin W, Hutton 1: Thallium scans in syndrome X. *Br Heart J* 1992; 68:48–50.
209. Camici PG, Marraccini P, Lorenzoni R, Buzzligoli G, Pecori N, Perissinotto A, et al: Coronary hemodynamics and myocardial metabolism in patients with syndrome X. Response to pacing stress. *J Am Coll Cardiol* 1991; 17:1461–1470.
210. Opherk D, Zebe H, Weihe E, Mall G, Durr C, Gravert B, et al: Reduced coronary dilatory capacity and ultrastructural changes of the myocardium in patients with angina pectoris but normal coronary arteriograms. *Circulation* 1981; 63:817–825.
211. Cannon RO, Epstein SE: "Microvascular angina" as a cause of chest pain with angiographically normal coronary arteries. *Am J Cardiol* 1988; 61:1338–1343.
212. Epstein SE, Cannon RO: Site of increased resistance to coronary flow in patients with angina pectoris and normal epicardial coronary arteries. *J Am Coll Cardiol* 1986; 8:459–461.
213. Motz W, Vogt M, Rabenay O, Scheler S, Luckhoff A, Straver BE: Evidence of endothelial dysfunction in coronary resistance vessels in patients with angina pectoris and normal coronary angiograms. *Am J Cardiol* 1991; 68:996–1003.
214. Romeo F, Rosano G, Martuscelli E, Lombardo L, Valente A: Long-term follow-up of patients initially diagnosed with syndrome X. *Am J Cardiol* 1993; 71:669–673.
215. Cannon RO, Dilsizian V, Correa R, Epstein SE, Bonow RO: Chronic deterioration in left ventricular function in patients with microvascular angina (abstr). *J Am Coll Cardiol* 1991; 17:28A.
216. Nihoyannopoulos P, Kaski JC, Crake T, Maseri A: Absence of myocardial dysfunction during stress in patients with syndrome X. *J Am Coll Cardiol* 1991; 18:1463–1470.
217. Opherk D, Zebe H, Schuler G, Weihe E, Mall G, Kubler W: Reduced coronary reserve and abnormal exercise left ventricular reserve in patients with syndrome X. *Arch Mal Cocur* 1983; 76:231–235.
218. Opherk D, Schuler G, Wetterauer K, Manthey J, Schwarz F, Kubler W: Four-year follow-up in patients with angina pectoris and normal coronary arteriograms ("syndrome X"). *Circulation* 1989; 80:1610–1616.
219. Turiel M, Galassi AR, Glazier JJ, Kaski JC, Maseri A: Pain threshold and tolerance in women with Syndrome X and women with stable angina pectoris. *Am J Cardiol* 1987; 60:503–508.
220. Shapiro LM, Crake T, Poole-Wilson PA: Is altered cardiac sensation responsible for chest pain in patients with normal coronary arteries? Clinical observation during catheterization. *Br Med J* 1988; 296:170–171.
221. Cannon RO, Quyyumi AA, Schenke WH, Fananapazir L, Tucker EE, Gaughan AM, et al: Abnormal cardiac sensitivity in patients with chest pain and normal coronary arteries. *J Am Coll Cardiol* 1990; 16:1359–1366.
222. Maseri A, Crea F, Kaski JC, Davies G: Mechanisms of angina pectoris in syndrome X. *J Am Coll Cardiol* 1991; 17:499–506.

Chapter 59

Diagnosis and Management of Patients with Unstable Angina

Pierre Théroux, M.D. ■ David Waters, M.D.

Unstable angina is diagnosed clinically as angina pectoris in an accelerating pattern. Because of its uncertain etiology, the understanding and treatment of unstable angina have lagged behind other aspects of coronary disease. New insights, however, suggest that unstable angina represents the change of coronary artery disease from a chronic to an acute stage. Recognizing unstable angina before the occurrence of myocardial necrosis permits therapeutic intervention that may profoundly modify the natural course of coronary disease.

HISTORICAL PERSPECTIVE

Understanding of the syndrome of unstable angina originated from early clinical observations of a high frequency of prodromal symptoms preceding myocardial infarction. Thus, Osler,[1] in the Lumleian lectures on angina pectoris in 1910, described the progression of symptoms sometimes followed by acute myocardial infarction. Parkinson and Bedford[2] in 1928 suggested that the prodromal pain heralds the beginning of coronary artery thrombosis based on clinicopathological observations. In 1937 Sampson and Eliaser[3] reported prolonged chest pain or progressively more severe symptoms preceding acute myocardial infarction, and Feil[4] reported the occurrence of angina unrelated to effort and emotion, clearly delineating the syndrome of unstable angina. A frequency of 44 to 70 percent of prodromal symptoms preceding the infarction was subsequently described.[5,6] These observations led to prospective studies of patients presenting with a changing pattern of chest pain. Levy[7] in 1956 reported a 38 percent incidence of myocardial infarction and a 32 percent mortality rate within 3 months of diagnosis. Subsequent advances in our understanding of unstable angina can be divided into three overlapping decades of clinical research.

From 1960 to 1970 unstable angina became a well-established clinical syndrome as more studies were performed on the natural history and authors groped for a proper definition. Vakil[8] confirmed the unfavorable prognosis in 251 patients. Beamish and Storrie[9] reported an 80 percent infarction and a 60 percent mortality rate at 15 months. The terminology used to define the syndrome was either descriptive with such terms as *crescendo angina, status anginosus,* and *accelerated angina* or referred to pathophysiological mechanisms (*coronary failure, acute coronary insufficiency*) or to prognostic implications (*impending myocardial infarction, preinfarction angina*). The term of *unstable angina,* proposed by Fowler,[10] was eventually retained. Oral anticoagulants were proposed as effective therapy during this era.[11]

From 1970 to 1980, the disease was further defined, classified, and stratified for risk.[12-14] New treatments developed for chronic stable angina were cautiously applied, including beta blockers and coronary bypass surgery.[15] The latter part of the decade saw an attempt at defining the pathophysiological mechanisms involved, with emphasis on the role of a primary decrease in myocardial oxygen supply possibly due to coronary vasoconstriction.[16]

From 1980 to 1990 pathological studies,[17,18] the aggressive use of coronary angiography,[19] balloon angioplasty, coronary angioscopy,[20] and laboratory measurement of platelet function and of coagulation greatly increased our understanding of the cause of unstable angina. It became demarcated from stable angina by the loss of endothelial integrity and activation of the cellular components of the plaque. Increasingly sophisticated clinical trials have more accurately defined useful treatments as detailed in this chapter.

DEFINITION AND INCIDENCE

Inherent to the definition of unstable angina is the evolving pattern of chest pain with multiple manifestations that depart from the usual pattern of angina. Many patients with symptoms will not seek medical advice; others will be treated out of hospital or in a regular hospital ward. Patients with clearly manifested unstable angina will be hospitalized in a coronary care unit; such patients now account for approximately half of the admissions to these units, and the relative proportion compared to myocardial infarction is steadily increasing, suggesting greater awareness. In the United States, unstable angina is responsible for about 750,000 hospitalizations per year and non Q-wave myocardial infarction for an additional 250,000 hospitalizations.[21] Unstable angina can also recur many times in the natural history of coronary artery disease in the same patient, an important point when considering the natural history and pathobiology of coronary artery disease as described in Chaps. 54, 55, 56, 57, and 61.

CLASSIFICATION

All proposed classifications of unstable angina distinguish between primary and secondary forms. The former reflects primary pathological changes at a plaque level, whereas the latter involves factors affecting myocardial oxygen demand and delivery, with no change in plaque activity.

Primary Unstable Angina

Various classifications have been proposed for primary unstable angina. One was based on clinical presentation.[14] Three subgroups were defined: (1) initial onset of progressive, crescendo angina and pain at rest in a patient previously free of symptoms; (2) the same as 1 but occurring in a patient with known stable angina; and (3) episodes of chest pain at rest more than 15 min duration not related to any obvious precipitating factor. Another classification proposed considering the circumstances of occurrence of angina and its severity.[22] The clinical situations are an extracardiac condition intensifying myocardial ischemia, no contributing extracardiac condition, and unstable angina within 2 weeks after myocardial infarction. The severity gradings are new onset of severe angina without rest pain, angina at rest within the past month but not within 48 h, and angina at rest within 48 h. Subclassifications referred to the intensity of previous treatment from none to standard and to intensive treatment with further subdivision depending on ST-T wave changes during pain.

The clinical classification proposed by Gazes et al.[14] is updated in Table 59-1 to include more recently recognized *clinical presentations* and *clinical background* on which unstable angina develops. This is further extended in Table 59-2 to include descriptors of unstable angina for a comprehensive approach to the patient, including angina equivalents, medication used, severity, provocative factors, extent of coronary atherosclerosis, and dynamics of the coronary artery obstructions. Objective documentation of ischemia during chest pain is usually obtained by the 12-lead electrocardiogram (ECG). Continuous ECG monitoring[23] and myocardial imaging can also be used.[24] Assessment of the early clinical evolution should be part of any classification. It is usually evaluated

TABLE 59-1
Clinical Classification of Unstable Angina*

1. Primary unstable angina pectoris
   Clinical presentation
   A. Onset of angina within 60 days
   B. Crescendo angina pectoris
   C. Angina pectoris at rest
   Clinical background
   A. Post–myocardial infarction angina pectoris
   B. Post–coronary angioplasty angina pectoris
   C. Post–bypass surgery angina pectoris
   D. Variant (Prinzmetal's) angina pectoris
2. Secondary unstable angina pectoris

* Patients with primary angina pectoris may have characteristics of more than one class.

TABLE 59-2
Subclassification/Descriptors of Primary Unstable Angina Pectoris

1. Presence or absence of a history of stable angina pectoris, myocardial infarction, or revascularization procedure
2. Duration of episodes of pain, or of angina equivalents
3. Occurrence of symptoms or evidence of asymptomatic myocardial ischemia on or off pharmacologic therapy for angina pectoris and the characteristics of such therapy
4. Presence or absence of electrocardiographic changes at rest and/or during episodes of pain or angina equivalents
5. Objective evidence of asymptomatic, silent myocardial ischemia
6. Electrocardiographic and functional (echocardiographic, nuclear) response to exercise or to pharmacologic stress testing
7. Detailed characteristics of coronary artery atheromata and obstructions
8. Extent of coronary artery narrowing, coronary artery flow reserve, and response to vasoactive drugs such as nitroglycerin, acetylcholine, and ergonovine

TABLE 59-3

Evaluation of the Early Clinical Evolution

Class 0:	No recurrent angina, no angina equivalents
Class 1:	Occasional pain, not requiring modification of treatment
Class 2:	Recurrent pain and/or ischemia controlled by intensification of medical treatment
Class 3:	Recurrent angina, or ischemia, persisting despite intensive medical treatment
Class 4:	Recurrent, severe ischemia, requiring urgent intervention

by recurrence of ischemia in-hospital and by its severity. A grading system in four classes is suggested in Table 59-3.

The initial classification of unstable angina does not use provocative testing, which is more useful for subsequent risk stratification in stabilized patients. The functional classification of the Canadian Cardiovascular Society, useful to document the clinical status of a patient before an episode of unstable angina, is of little help and may be misleading during the acute phase of the disease where episodes of ischemia can occur unpredictably at rest with, at times, paradoxically no symptoms during physical activities. (See Chaps. 19 and 58.)

Secondary Unstable Angina

Extracoronary Causes

This form of unstable angina is partly a misnomer because it is provoked by fundamentally different pathophysiological mechanisms than those involved in primary unstable angina. Any factor causing excessive increase in myocardial oxygen demand can lead to worsening of angina, usually in the presence of coronary artery disease but also in its absence. The major determinants of myocardial oxygen consumption are heart rate, the inotropic state of the myocardial fiber, and the loading conditions of the left ventricle. Typical conditions associated with a rapid heart rate are anemia, thyrotoxicosis, tachyarrhythmias, and fever. The inotropic state is increased by catecholamine stimulation, afterload by left ventricular outflow tract obstruction and severe hypertension, and preload by congestive heart failure and left ventricular dilatation. Other conditions influencing oxygen delivery such as low arterial P_{O2}, anemia, polycythemia, and high blood viscosity may also be contributive. A more exhaustive listing of aggravating conditions is provided in Table 59-4.

Intracoronary Causes

The coronary circulation, particularly in diseased coronary artery segments, can be influenced by extracardiac conditions. Coronary disease is accompanied by endothelial dysfunction with impaired production of the endothelium-derived relaxing factor.[25] Thus, vasoconstriction induced by alpha-adrenergic stimulation can be exaggerated in these segments, with a potential for intense vasoconstriction. The production of endothelin, a potent endothelium-derived vasoconstrictor peptide, may also be increased.[26] Exercise,[27] cigarette smoking,[28] and exposure to cold[29] induce more vasoconstriction at sites of coronary stenoses. Severe vasoconstriction per se can cause endothelial damage, setting the stage for plaque fissure, platelet aggregation, and thrombus formation. Systemic conditions can further enhance local platelet aggregability. (See Chaps. 54 to 57.)

TABLE 59-4

Precipitating Factors for Unstable Angina

Extracoronary factors
- Increase in myocardial oxygen demand
  - Increase in heart rate
    - Anemia
    - Fever
    - Tachyarrhythmias
    - Thyrotoxicosis
  - Higher inotropic state
    - High adrenergic state
    - Use of sympathicomimetic drugs
  - Higher afterload
    - Aortic stenosis
    - Hypertrophic cardiomyopathy
    - Severe hypertension
  - High preload
    - Severe congestive heart failure
    - High output states
- Interference with oxygen delivery
  - Anemia
  - Hypoxemia
  - Polycythemia
  - High blood viscosity

Intracoronary factors (external factors interfering with coronary artery tone or reactivity, endothelial function, and/or intravascular coagulation)
- Adrenergic stimulation
- Cocaine intoxication
- Hypercoagulability state

These physiopathological mechanisms provide multiple triggers for unstable angina. For example, cocaine can cause unstable angina, myocardial infarction, and death in otherwise healthy persons.[30] Coronary angiography in cocaine users have shown arterial spasm or acute thrombosis with minimal coronary atherosclerosis.[31] Cocaine affects both central and peripheral control of adrenergic stimulation; the presynaptic reuptake of catecholamines is blocked, leaving excessive adrenergic stimulation at the postsynaptic receptors. Enhanced vasoconstriction at sites of significant coronary artery stenoses has been demonstrated in humans[32] as has enhanced platelet responsiveness to aggregating stimuli in experimental models.[33] (See Chap. 110.)

DIAGNOSIS

The diagnosis is primarily clinical, based on symptoms and supported by diagnostic procedures. Clinical signs are those of coronary artery disease, which may be neither highly sensitive nor specific.

Clinical Manifestations

The term *unstable angina* refers to a distinctive increase in the number, severity, or duration of anginal episodes; angina occurs at a decreasing level of exercise, sometimes at minimal exercise. In its more typical form, it occurs *at rest.* Angina may also occur at night. The episodes of chest pain may also be more severe, more prolonged, and less responsive to nitroglycerin, often with attacks recurring shortly after initial relief. They can also be unresponsive with episodes of prolonged chest pain. An episode of chest pain that lasts a few hours can often be differentiated clinically from myocardial infarction by its fluctuating character. The angina is said to be of *new onset* or *de novo* when it developed in the previous 2 months and to be *crescendo angina* when occurring in the setting of a prior history of angina. Angina equivalents are important to recognize. The distinction between a *prolonged chest pain* (30 min or more in duration) and non-Q-wave myocardial infarction is often made a posteriori when the results of the cardiac enzymes become available. Progress in the enzymatic diagnosis of myocardial infarction has increased the sensitivity of our diagnosis and has narrowed the margins between the two clinical syndromes. It is likely that the pathophysiological basis of the two conditions is similar and that the differentiating feature of enzyme elevation merely reflects the extent and duration of compromise of coronary blood flow. (See also Chap. 60.)

Prinzmetal's variant angina is a clinical syndrome with a peculiar pattern of chest pain occurring mainly in the early morning and marked by transient ST segment elevation during pain. Because of its very distinctive features compared to other forms of unstable angina, variant angina is discussed in the last section of this chapter.

Three specific clinical backgrounds should also be recognized in the classification of unstable angina. *Early postinfarction ischemia* refers to patients with recurrent chest pain developing between 24 h and 1 month after an acute myocardial infarction.[34] It occurs in 20 percent of infarct patients, and the incidence is probably slightly reduced with fibrinolytic therapy.[35] Ischemia at a distance is defined by transient ST-T changes occurring in ECG leads away from the original infarct; it is more frequent in inferior infarcts and in patients with two or three-vessel disease.[36] Ischemia in the infarct zone occurs in the same electrocardiographic leads as the original infarct; it is more often associated with viable myocardium at jeopardy by a critical stenosis of the infarct-related artery and is more frequent in anterior myocardial infarction.[36]

Unstable angina in patients with previous coronary bypass surgery now accounts for up to 20 percent of all patients admitted for unstable angina in active cardiology centers.[37] Although the early in-hospital course is similar in these patients, the long-term prognosis is worse, with twice as many events. The reasons are probably related to more rapid progression of disease in venous grafts and reduced possibility for a new revascularization procedure.[38]

Recurrent angina after coronary angioplasty is encountered in approximately 20 to 30 percent of patients within the first 6 months after the procedure and is associated with angiographic restenosis.[39] Although the clinical presentation may resemble unstable angina, the pathophysiological and prognostic implications are different. Myocardial infarctions are unusual in these patients because the stenosis reflects vascular smooth muscle proliferation rather than thrombus formation on an unstable lesion. Complications associated with a repeat coronary angioplasty are also infrequent. When unstable angina occurs 6 months or more after the procedure, a new active lesion is likely present.[40] (See also Chap. 70.)

DIAGNOSTIC AIDS

The diagnosis of the unstable state can be difficult and somewhat imprecise if based mainly on symptoms, as is frequently the case. Indeed, features such as variable threshold, duration, and settings such as chest pain at rest are atypical in otherwise stable angina; yet these symptoms may assume diagnostic importance if they truly indicate unstable angina. Thus, false-positive diagnoses will occur commonly, and normal coronary angiograms will be found in 10 to 20 percent of patients with the clinical diagnosis.[41] The 12-lead ECG can provide extremely useful diagnostic information if ST-segment depression or elevation is present.[14] Myocardial scintigraphy has also been used to confirm the presence of ischemia.[24] Detection of elevated blood levels of specific cardiac enzymes such as MB-creatine kinase or troponin T can confirm the presence of coronary disease and myocardial necrosis.[42] Other blood markers of myocardial ischemia or of an ongoing thrombotic process have been described, but their diagnostic yield in a clinical setting remains to be investigated.[43,44]

Twelve-Lead Electrocardiography

In the 12-lead ECG, ST-segment depression is the most frequent finding, occurring in 30 percent of patients; T-wave inversion has been reported in 20 percent and ST-segment elevation in 4 percent.[14] The ST-segment elevation reflects transient total occlusion of a major epicardial coronary artery segment without significant collateral flow, implying transmural myocardial ischemia. When reversible, it is the hallmark of variant angina, but it can also be found with transient thrombotic occlusion. Tall upright T waves and pseudonormalization of previously negative T waves can also indicate transmural ischemia and are frequently encountered in variant angina and as the initial changes in acute myocardial infarction.

On the other hand, ST-segment depression and T-wave inversion indicate subendocardial ischemia. These changes tend to be more transient in unstable angina; they are more sustained in non-Q-wave myocardial infarction and may last for few days or more.

Some ECG patterns are useful for the diagnosis of specific coronary artery lesions (Fig. 59-1). Deeply negative T waves in the precordial leads with the ST-segment

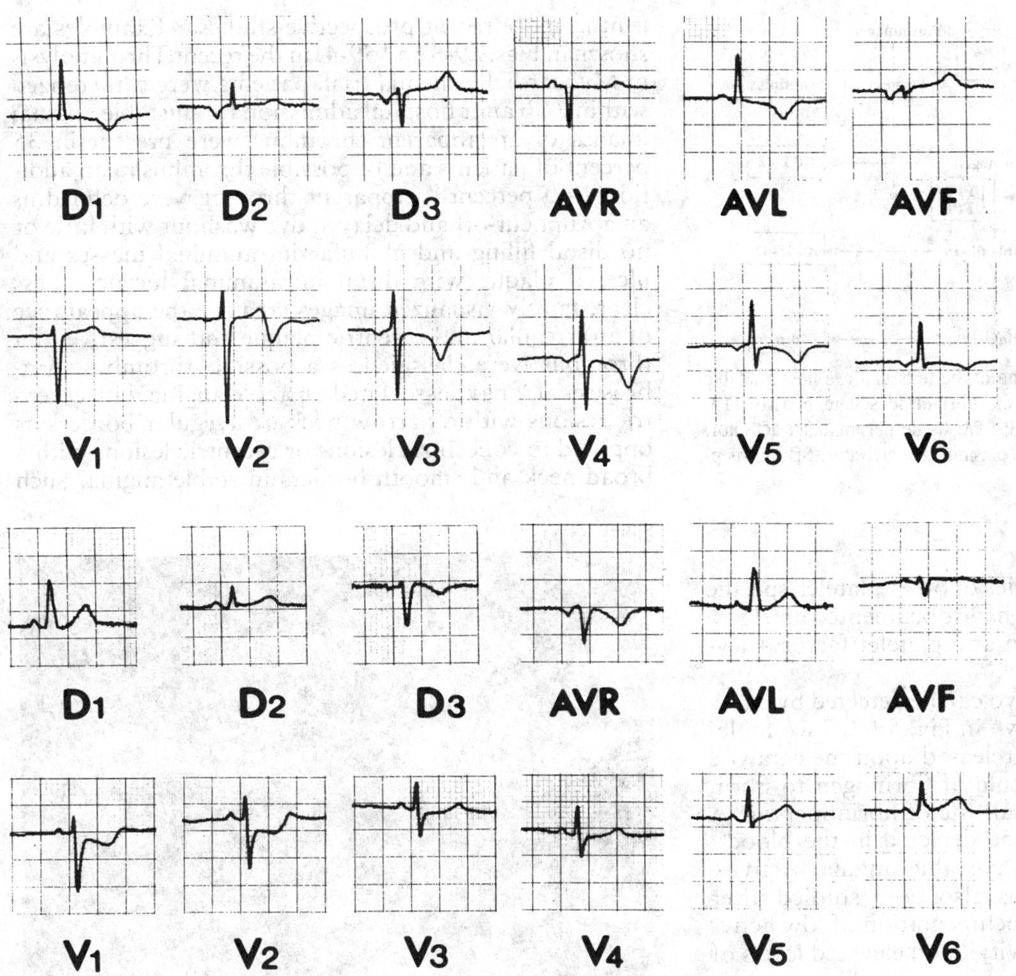

FIGURE 59-1 Specific ECG patterns in unstable angina. *Top:* The ECG shows deep T-wave inversion in the anterior lead extending to leads D_1 and AVL. It is strongly suggestive of a significant involvement of the proximal left anterior descending coronary artery and a large area of myocardium at risk. *Bottom:* The ST segment is depressed in leads V_1 and V_2. Closer inspection also revealed some ST elevation in the inferior leads. This ECG pattern in a patient with a prolonged chest pain indicates a true posterior wall infarct with an indication for fibrinolytic therapy.

isoelectric or slightly elevated in leads V_2 and V_3 or depressed in leads V_4 or V_5 indicates critical reduction of flow in the left anterior descending coronary artery, with proximal involvement when the changes include all anterior and anterolateral leads.[45] These patients are at high risk of a more severe event. The ST-segment depression in the right precordial leads when accompanied with prolonged chest pain most often represents the reciprocal change of a posterior wall infarction. These patients most often have thrombotic occlusion of the left circumflex coronary artery and should be considered for fibrinolytic therapy.

Myocardial Scintigraphy

Both thallium-201 and technetium-99m sestamibi have been studied in patients with unstable angina. In selected patients with variant angina, thallium-201 injected during an episode of chest pain documented a perfusion defect with a sensitivity of 95 percent.[46] Injections during pain-free intervals documented defects in 40 to 60 percent of patients.[47,48] Washout abnormalities of thallium-201 have also been described.[49]

The early redistribution with thallium-201 necessitates immediate imaging, which may interfere with patient management. Redistribution is minimal with 99m sestamibi. The agent can thus be administered at the time of chest pain and scintigraphies obtained up to 6 h later, perhaps in a more stable condition. (See Chap. 134.) Single-photon-emission computed tomography with this agent in patients hospitalized for spontaneous chest pain suggestive of unstable angina has shown high sensitivity and specificity for the detection of significant coronary artery disease, significantly enhancing the predictive value of the 12-lead ECG.[24] (See Chap. 137.)

Surrogate Markers of Blood Activation

There is evidence of platelet activation, thrombin generation, and fibrin formation in patients with unstable angina. Thromboxane A_2 is a potent stimulus to platelet aggregation and also induces vasoconstriction. It is released by activated platelets through the action of cyclooxygenase and thromboxane synthetase on arachidonic acid and endoperoxide intermediates. The blood levels of thromboxane B_2, the main metabolite of thromboxane A_2, and the urine content of 2,3-dinor thromboxane B_2 are elevated in unstable angina, indicating platelet activation.[43] This elevation in thromboxane levels is frequently associated with angiographic evidence of thrombus formation[50] and can coincide with episodes of myo-

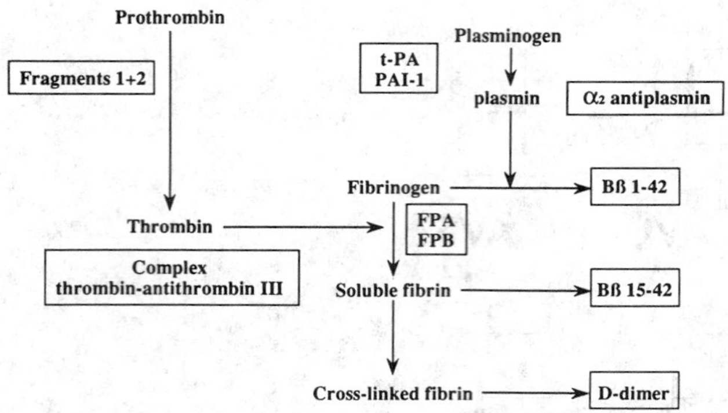

FIGURE 59-2 Diagram showing some of the tests that are now available to evaluate thrombin generation and the fibrinolytic system in vivo. FPA: fibrinopeptide A; FPB: fibrinopeptide B; t-PA: tissue plasminogen activator; PAI-I: fast-acting inhibitor of tissue-type plasminogen activator; Bβ: polypeptide chain of fibrinogen.

cardial ischemia.[43] Some studies of other platelet-specific proteins released into plasma have documented an elevation of beta-thromboglobulin and platelet factor 4 levels[51]; others have not.[44]

Thrombin generation in vivo can be detected by many tests, some of which are shown in Fig. 59-2. Two molecules of fibrinopeptide A are released upon the catalytic transformation of one molecule of fibrinogen to fibrin by thrombin. Although the half-life of fibrinopeptide A is short, elevated levels can be detected in the blood[44] and urine[51] of patients with unstable angina. Activity of the fibrinolytic system has also been studied after myocardial infarction with documentation of low activity of tissue plasminogen activity[52] and elevated levels of its fast inhibitor.[53]

These surrogate markers have the potential of improving the diagnosis and the evaluation of the response to treatment. These tests, which are easily affected by the technique of blood sampling and unknown variables, remain a research tool. They are consistent, however, with the thrombogenic etiology of unstable angina. (See also Chaps. 7 and 68.)

Coronary Angiography

The traditional analysis of coronary angiograms in terms of severity and extent of coronary artery disease does not provide useful information for the diagnosis of unstable angina. Indeed, the extent and severity of coronary lesions do not distinguish among patients with unstable angina, stable angina, or myocardial infarction.[41] Plaque morphology and quantitative angiographic analysis, however, are useful to define the culprit coronary lesion responsible for the ischemic state. These observations imply that the biologic and rheologic characteristics of the plaque and not the severity of stenosis are critical determinants for the development of unstable angina. (See Chap. 55.)

The concept of the culprit lesion forms the basis for the new approach to the diagnosis and treatment of acute coronary artery syndromes. The reported incidence of intracoronary thrombus in unstable angina has increased from 1 percent in early retrospective studies[54] to 52 percent in more recent prospective studies.[55] Examples are shown in Figs. 59-3 and 59-4. In the recent Thrombolysis in Myocardial Ischemia trial, patients were catheterized within 24 h after hospital admission for unstable angina; images of an apparent thrombus were present in 35 percent of patients and of possible thrombus in an additional 40 percent.[56] Apparent thrombi were defined as an abrupt cut-off and delayed dye washout with little or no distal filling and globular intraluminal masses and ulcered plaque with distal intraluminal lucency. Less clear, faintly visualized images creating the appearance of an irregular and eccentric plaque and suggestive of a thrombus were classified as a possible thrombus. Ambrose et al.[57] have associated unstable angina with eccentric lesions with a narrow neck or irregular borders as opposed to concentric lesions or eccentric lesions with a broad neck and smooth borders in stable angina. Such

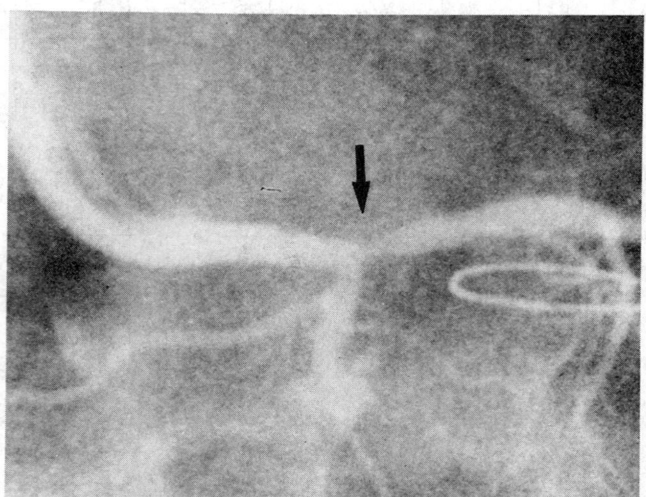

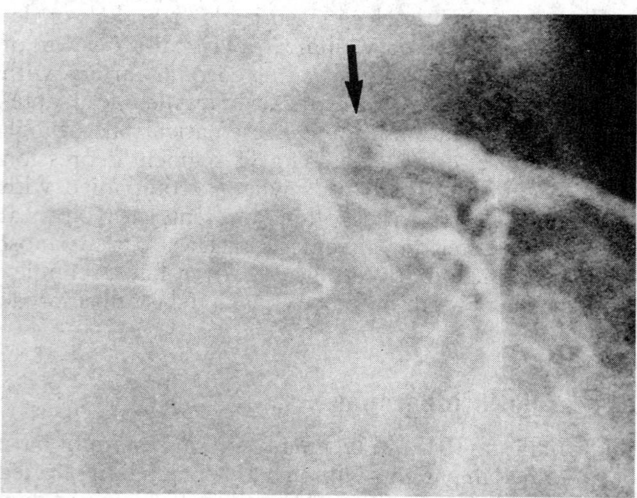

FIGURE 59-3 Left coronary dye injections obtained in a patient with stable angina who subsequently developed unstable angina. The injection during the stable state shows a 60 percent stenosis of the proximal left anterior descending coronary artery (*left*). One week later, the patient experienced a 30-min episode of chest pain at rest with transient ST-T changes in the anterior leads but no enzyme elevation. The angiogram obtained 2 h later displays an intraluminal globular radiotranslucent mass just distal to the previously described narrowing (*right*). This image represents a thrombus partially occluding the lumen.

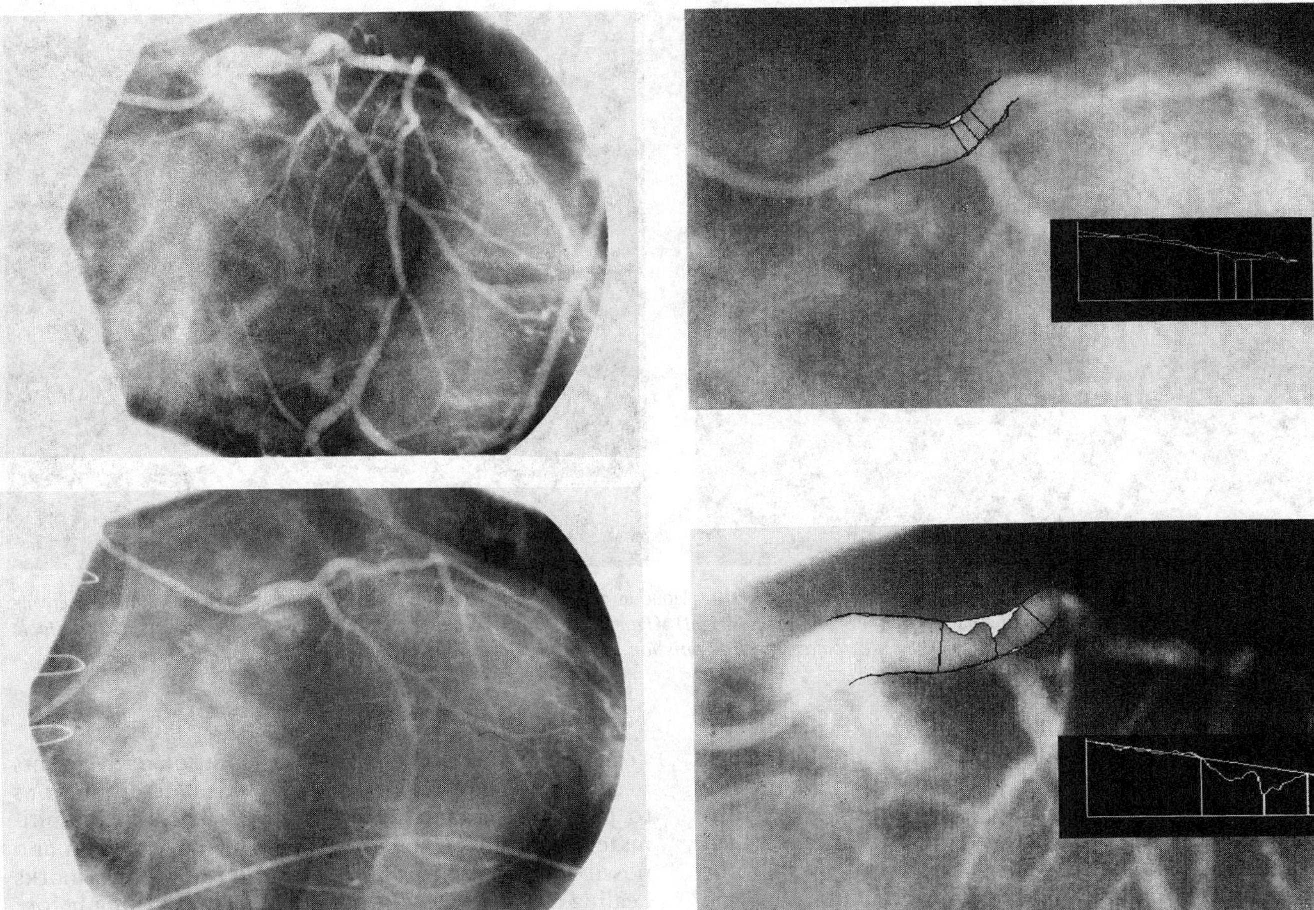

FIGURE 59-4 Computer-assisted analysis of two left coronary angiograms obtained at 1-year interval in the same patient. The angiogram at the top shows a minimal plaque on the distal left main vessel, well delineated by the computer analysis (*top right*). The second angiogram at the bottom was obtained after stabilization of crescendo angina. The plaque has progressed to cause a 60 percent obstruction showing further the aspect of a complex, asymmetric, and ulcerated crater, representing a nidus for platelet aggregation and thrombus formation.

angiographic features likely represent changes in the structural integrity of the plaque.

The coronary anatomy preceding the unstable angina episode is important to define the high-risk plaque. Plaque features favoring higher shear stress and flow separation, such as the severity of stenosis, the acuteness of the stenosis angles, and the presence of a division branch originating within the stenosis, are associated with a higher risk of thrombosis.[58] Interestingly, lesions that occlude to produce acute syndromes are only moderately severe, typically 45 to 50 percent lumen diameter reduction,[58] and patients with clinical events have a higher number of diseased coronary artery segments.[59]

Angiographic studies performed after the acute phase have also documented that unstable angina is associated with a higher risk of subsequent progression of coronary artery disease compared to matched patients with stable angina.[60,61] Possibly also relevant to the underlying pathophysiology is the observation that progression can occur at many coronary artery sites and in normal and nonsignificantly diseased segments.[60]

The present main use of coronary angiography is risk evaluation and the selection of optimal long-term treatment.

Other Methods to Visualize Coronary Lesions

Coronary angioscopy has been successfully used intraoperatively for the study of the culprit lesion, as illustrated in Fig. 59-5.[20] Partial thrombi and complex plaques have been described as opposed to smooth plaques with no red discoloration, no endothelial hemorrhage, and no adherent thrombus in stable angina. Percutaneous fiberoptic angioscopes are now available providing the means to characterize the culprit lesion in the catheterization laboratory. Grayish white thrombi have been associated with unstable angina and reddish thrombi with myocardial infarction.[62] Intravascular ultrasound is also valuable for the study of the vessel wall with the additional potential of identifying the inner core of the higher risk plaque.[63] (See Chap. 133.)

PATHOPHYSIOLOGICAL MECHANISMS

Unstable angina, like myocardial infarction, is an acute manifestation of coronary artery disease, clearly related to a regional decrease in blood flow caused by acute focal coronary obstruction. The mechanisms for thrombotic

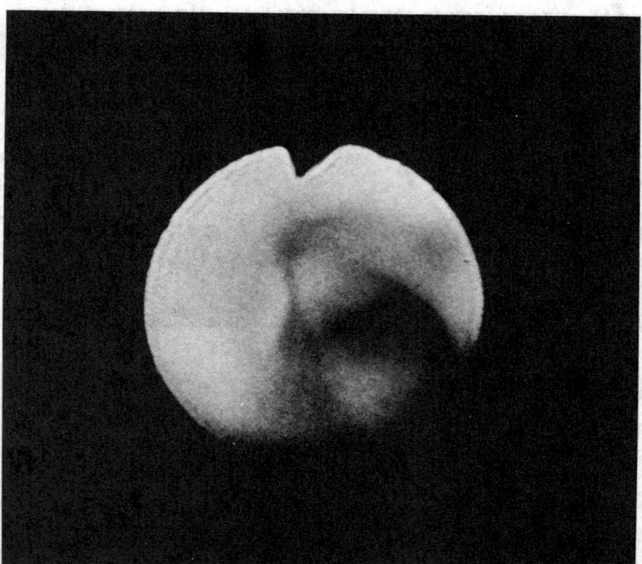

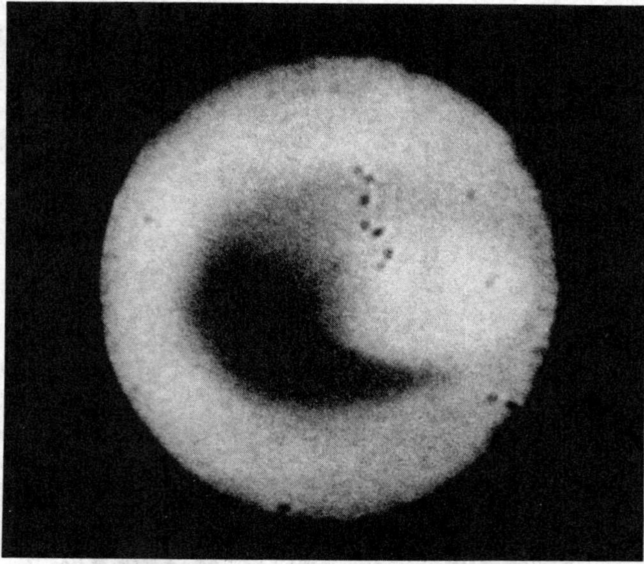

FIGURE 59-5 Angioscopic images of a noncomplicated atherosclerotic plaque in a patient with stable angina (*left*) and of a plaque with an overlying thrombus creating lumen obstruction in a patient with unstable angina (*right*). (*From CT Sherman, et al: Coronary angioscopy in patients with unstable angina pectoris. N Engl J Med 315:913–919, 1986. Reproduced with permission of the author and the publisher.*)

occlusion are complex and require further elucidation of the close interdependence between the plaque, the endothelium, platelets, coagulation factors, and the fibrinolytic system. This interrelation is further influenced by hemodynamic and rheologic factors, the vasomotor response of the vessel, and systemic circulating factors, including epinephrine levels and lipoprotein characteristics.

In patients dying suddenly there is a high incidence of complicated atherosclerotic plaques with fissure and rupture and intraluminal thrombus (Fig. 59-6)[17,18] and with thrombi of various age indicating the cyclic nature of thrombosis in unstable angina.[64] Plaques that undergo rupture are relatively small, are softer, and contain a deformable cavity filled with crystalline cholesterol and its ester within the intima.[65] Exposed collagen after rupturing triggers platelet deposition, the rate of which increases with higher shear rate,[66] leading to thrombin generation, further platelet aggregation, deposition of fibrin, and an occlusive blood clot. Partial growth or regression of these intracoronary thrombi could explain some of the clinical features of unstable angina including the intermittent clinical manifestations, the often unpredictable course, and the response to therapy. Once initiated, the thrombotic process can perpetuate itself. Indeed, the thrombus per se is a strongly thrombogenic surface acting as a reservoir for the progressive exposure of the thrombin bound to fibrin leading to further thrombogenesis.[67,68] Other mechanisms can also act in unstable angina. Such mechanisms can be intraplaque hemorrhage by rupture of a vasa vasorum, distal coronary embolization of platelet aggregates, functional loss of the antithrombotic properties of the endothelium, and focal vasoconstriction induced by the release of local vasoactive agents.[69] The degree to which vasoconstriction contributes to the pathogenesis of unstable angina is likely variable.

Figure 59-7 is a schematic representation of the events in unstable angina to correlate the clinical manifestations to pathophysiological mechanisms.[68] The process ultimately would lead to complete coronary occlusion and possibly to myocardial infarction. Its resolution marks healing and a return to the clinical status existing before the unstable state. The acute process by the release of platelet-derived growth factor and other mitogenic factors and the healing process with the fibrotic organization of intracoronary thrombi[70] can be associated with more severe stenosis, leading to rapid progression of coronary artery stenosis.[60,61] Inherent to this perspective is the view that coronary artery disease is an episodic phenomenon associated with periodic plaque activation and growth that may be subclinical. (See also Chaps. 53 to 57.)

NATURAL HISTORY AND PROGNOSIS

Unstable angina carries a high risk of myocardial infarction and death. Early studies have reported an infarction rate between 6 weeks and 3 months of 20 to 40 percent and a mortality rate of 1 to 60 percent.[7–11] Subsequent natural history studies have documented a 3-month incidence of myocardial infarction of 10 to 20 percent and a mortality rate of 4 to 10 percent.[71–73] Similar figures are found in the placebo groups of more recent studies evaluating the efficacy of newer forms of therapy (Table 59-5).[74–78] The risk of nonfatal or fatal myocardial infarction can now be estimated to be 10 percent in the first week and 15 percent at 3 to 6 months. Additional events in these patients are a 20 to 25 percent incidence of recurrent severe refractory angina in the hospital and a 30 to 50 percent incidence of residual ischemia with a positive treadmill test. (See also Chap. 61.)

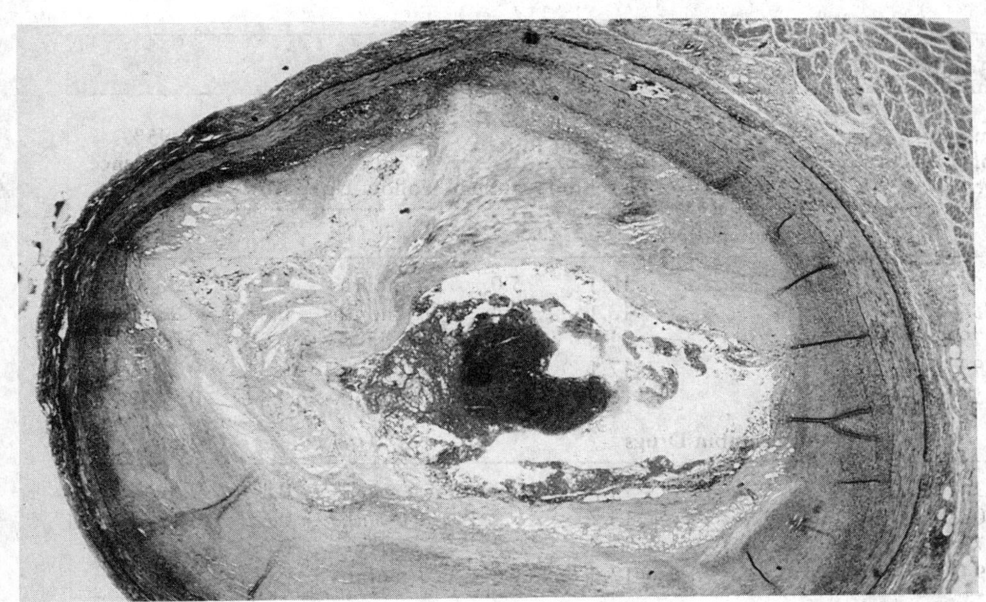

FIGURE 59-6 Histopathology of coronary arterial stenoses causing unstable coronary artery clinical states. An atherosclerotic plaque filled with lipid and cholesterol showed a superficial fissure (arrow), which is the site of a mural thrombosis protruding into the lumen. (*Courtesy of Dr. B. C. Solymoss.*)

RISK EVALUATION

Risk evaluation in unstable angina is approached in two steps. Early prognosis includes evaluation of the severity of the underlying disease process, of its control by treatment, and of the area of myocardial mass at jeopardy by the active lesion. After the acute phase, the determinants of prognosis are more those of chronic coronary artery disease or those of postmyocardial infarction. Such patients are stratified before hospital discharge with exercise or other provocative tests.

Early Prognosis

Clinical Features

In general, the more severe the clinical presentation, the more severe is the prognosis. Thus increasingly worse prognosis has been reported from new-onset angina to crescendo angina to angina at rest and to prolonged chest pain as the presenting symptoms.[12–14,71] The early in-hospital evolution also reflects disease activity. Chest pain present for more than 48 h in hospital was associated with a 1-month mortality of 20 percent, in contrast to 2 percent without early in-hospital angina.[14] In another study, persisting pain after 12 h identified 86 percent of the patients with subsequent in-hospital myocardial infarction.[12] In a multivariate analysis of clinical electrocardiographic, and angiographic characteristics, recurrence of chest pain was the single most powerful predictor of prognosis in the acute phase[79]; and in a 12-month natural history study, early angina that did not resolve early in the hospital course was the only predictive feature of subsequent cardiac events, occurring during the early posthospital phase in 35 percent of patients with angina as compared to 13 percent without.[72]

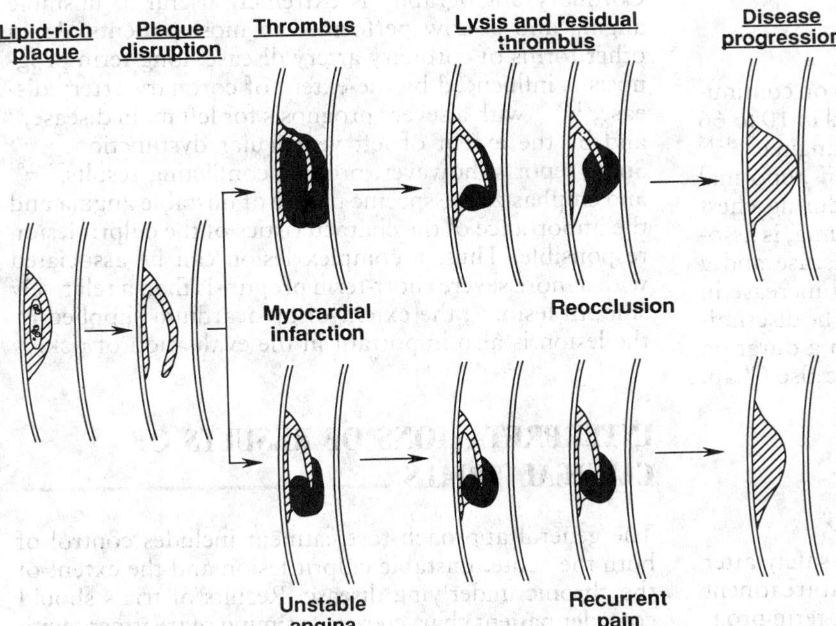

FIGURE 59-7 Schematic representation of plaque events leading to acute coronary syndromes. Plaque rupture is favored by its lipid content and by external forces applied. A deep fissure is a powerful stimulus for thrombus formation. A more superficial fissure leads to mural thrombus. The evolution is influenced by systemic factors and the balance between thrombogenic stimulation and plasma antithrombin and fibrinolytic activity. The healing process is associated with progression of atherosclerosis. (*Adapted from V Fuster et al: The pathogenesis of coronary artery disease and the acute coronary syndromes. N Engl J Med 326:242–250, 1992. Reproduced with permission of the author and the publisher.*)

TABLE 59-5
Clinical Trials on Prevention of Fatal and Nonfatal Myocardial Infarction

Authors	Year Published	Number of Patients	Time of Entry			Percentage of Event Rate		Duration of Follow-Up	Relative Risk	95% Confidence Limits
			<24 h	24–72 h	>72 h	Placebo	Treatment			
Antiplatelet Drugs										
Lewis et al[74]	1983	1266		X		10.1	5.0	3 months	0.45	0.28–0.73
Cairns et al[75]*	1985	555			X	13.1	6.4	18 months	0.48	0.28–0.82
Théroux et al[76]	1988	479	X			11.8	3.3	5 days	0.29	0.08–0.8
RISC Study Group[77]	1990	794		X		17.1	6.5	90 days	0.36	0.23–0.57
Balsano et al[78]†	1990	657		X		10.9	5.1	6 months	0.44	0.24–0.79
Antithrombin Drugs										
Telford and Wilson[96]	1981	214	X			14.9	3	1 week	0.12	0.02–0.61
Williams[98]	1986	102	X			13.7	5.9	6 months	0.67	0.12–3.8
Théroux et al[76]	1988	479	X			11.8	0.8	5 days	0.06	0.14–0.61
RISC Study Group[77]	1990	794		X		12.6	11.0	3 months	—	—

* Results analyzed by drug efficacy.
† Ticlopidine used as the antiplatelet agent.

Electrocardiographic Changes

The presence of ischemic ST-T changes on the basal electrocardiogram has prognostic value. When transient changes develop during chest pain, further information is added.[14] The combination of these changes with ongoing ischemia predicted a death rate of 42 percent at 1 year as compared to 5 percent at 2 years when absent.[80] In early postinfarction angina the prognosis is also better when no ECG changes are present, rivaling the prognosis without early postinfarction angina.[81] The prognostic implications of ST-T changes are likely related to a greater likelihood of more significant coronary artery disease, to a more extensive ischemic zone, and possibly also to inadequate collaterals or to collaterals jeopardized by multivessel disease.

Silent Ischemia

Transient episodes of ST-segment depression on continuous ambulatory ECG recordings are reported in 10 to 66 percent of patients hospitalized for unstable angina.[23,82,83] The incidence is highest in patients with an abnormal baseline ECG or with an abnormal ECG during chest pain.[84] Silent ischemia, as symptomatic ischemia, is associated with more severe coronary artery disease and a worse prognosis with, in general, a twofold increase in the risk of myocardial infarction and death. The discriminative power may be higher in patients with a duration of silent ischemia of 60 min or more.[23,83,84] (See also Chap. 58.)

Late Prognosis: Risk Stratification

Exercise Test and Myocardial Scintigraphy

Treadmill exercise testing can be performed safely after stabilization of unstable angina with medical treatment and has shown usefulness for predicting long-term prognosis. Cardiac events during a 1-year follow-up occurred in 87 percent of patients with angina or ST-segment depression during the test compared to 29 percent of patients with a negative test.[83] Exercise thallium-201 myocardial perfusion studies may provide additional prognostic information, and dipyridamole perfusion scintigraphy is a useful alternative to treadmill exercise testing.[85] The prognostic value of different testing modalities to detect myocardial ischemia is likely related to their ability to determine the severity of underlying coronary disease.[86,87] (See also Chaps. 16 and 134.)

Coronary Angiography and Left Ventricular Function

Coronary angiography is extremely useful in unstable angina and is now performed in most patients. As in other forms of coronary artery disease, long-term prognosis is influenced by the extent of coronary artery disease,[71,88–90] with a severe prognosis for left main disease,[89] and by the extent of left ventricular dysfunction.[72,90,91] Some reports, however, provide conflicting results[79,92,93] and emphasize the specific nature of unstable angina and the importance of the characteristics of the culprit lesion responsible. Thus, a complex lesion can be associated with a more severe short-term prognosis than a relatively smooth lesion[94]; the extent of myocardium supplied by the lesion is also important in the evaluation of risk.[88]

INTERPRETATIONS OF RESULTS OF CLINICAL TRIALS

The general approach to treatment includes control of both the acute, unstable culprit lesion and the extent of the chronic underlying disease. Results of trials should consider patient characteristics, timing of treatment with

TABLE 59-6

Protocol Considerations for the Interpretation of Clinical Trials in Unstable Angina

Population characteristics
- Clinical classification (Table 59-1)

Timing of study
- Acute (early entry trials)
- Subacute
- Chronic (late entry trials)

Endpoints
- Related to unstable angina
  - Death
  - Myocardial infarction
  - Severe recurrent ischemia (classes 3 and 4, Table 59-3)
  - Silent ischemia (≥60 min in duration)
  - Need for intraaortic balloon pump, coronary angioplasty, or bypass surgery for recurrent symptoms
- Related to either unstable angina or underlying disease
  - Recurrent ischemia (classes 1 and 2, Table 59-3)
  - Silent ischemia (<60 min in duration)
  - Positive provocative testing
  - Coronary angioplasty or bypass surgery for severity of disease

TABLE 59-7

Specific Therapy in Unstable Angina

Intervention	Mechanisms
Control of Symptoms	
Nitroglycerin	Preload and afterload reduction Coronary vasodilatation Spasm relief Favorable redistribution of blood flow *Antiplatelet effect*
Beta blockers	Slowing in heart rate Afterload reduction Negative inotropic effect Myocardial cell protection
Calcium antagonists	Coronary vasodilatation Spasm relief Afterload reduction Slowing in heart rate (diltiazem)
Heparin	*Prevention of thrombus growth*
Coronary angioplasty	Relief of obstruction Plaque remodeling
Coronary bypass surgery	Bypass of culprit lesion
Intraaortic balloon	Enhanced diastolic flow Afterload reduction *Prevention of intermittent occlusion*
Control of Disease Process	
Heparin	*Antithrombin effects* *Antiplatelet effects* *Endothelial stabilization* (?)
Aspirin	*Antiplatelet effects*

regard to a more acute or more chronic phase of disease, and endpoints analyzed (Table 59-6). For example, the results of a treadmill test may be meaningless when performed acutely but significant when performed once the acute disease process has been controlled.

THERAPEUTIC OPTIONS

Treatment of unstable angina can be divided into three categories: (1) pharmacologic agents to control the pathogenic thrombotic process, (2) antianginal drugs to control chest pain, and (3) interventional procedures to address the underlying extent and severity of coronary artery disease. Specific treatments and their mechanisms of action are listed in Table 59-7.

CAUSE-SPECIFIC TREATMENT

Aspirin

Aspirin has unequivocally been demonstrated to be useful for the early and late management of unstable angina. Four major trials have shown consistent benefits despite differences in populations studied, doses of aspirin used, time of initiation of treatment, and duration of follow-up.[74–77] These trials are summarized in Table 59-5. The Veterans Administration Cooperative Study was a double-blind, randomized study of aspirin, 324 mg daily, versus placebo that enrolled 1266 men within 48 h after admission to hospital for unstable angina.[74] Aspirin reduced the incidence of fatal and nonfatal myocardial infarction from 10.1 to 5 percent. Although the study drugs were discontinued after the 12 weeks, the mortality rate remained 43 percent lower after 1 year follow-up in the aspirin group.

The second trial involved 555 patients of either sex, randomized to aspirin (325 mg four times daily), sulfinpyrazone (200 mg four times daily), both drugs, or neither.[75] The study was initiated within 8 days after hospitalization and lasted 18 months. Gastrointestinal side effects were frequent with these high doses of aspirin, occurring in 44 percent of patients. There was no evidence of a benefit from sulfinpyrazone or of a favorable interaction of this drug with aspirin. With aspirin, the incidence of cardiac death and nonfatal myocardial infarction was reduced from 17 to 8.6 percent by drug efficacy analysis and from 14.7 to 10.5 percent by intention-to-treat analysis.

In a study of 479 patients during the hospital phase, aspirin, 325 mg twice a day, compared to no aspirin reduced the risk of fatal and nonfatal myocardial infarction from 6.4 to 2.5 percent.[76]

The most recent trial tested a low dose of aspirin of 75 mg daily in 945 men with unstable angina or non-Q-wave myocardial infarction and confirmed a reduction in the rate of fatal and nonfatal myocardial infarction at 5 days from 5.7 to 2.5 percent and at 90 days from 17 to 6.5 percent.[77] The beneficial effects were limited during the first 2 days of therapy, possibly because of the absence of a loading dose of aspirin.

Aspirin likely exerts its beneficial effect by irreversibly inhibiting the cyclooxygenase pathway in platelets and inhibiting thromboxane-induced aggregation. Experimental models of partly obstructed coronary arteries support this conclusion since aspirin inhibited the cyclic reductions observed in coronary blood flow that are likely caused by platelet aggregates.[95] (See Chap. 68.)

Ticlopidine, 250 mg bid, was also documented to be useful with a reduction in the rate of fatal and nonfatal myocardial infarction at 6 month follow-up from 13.6 to 7.3 percent in a population of 652 unstable angina patients of either sex.[78] This drug, unlike aspirin, does not block cyclooxygenase but appears to interfere with the platelet activation mechanism mediated by adenosine diphosphate (ADP) and with the fibrinogen receptors. (See also Chaps. 7 and 68.)

Heparin

Trials testing heparin in unstable angina have been more limited but have also shown benefit (Table 59-5). In a first report of 214 patients, heparin (5000 units intravenously every 6 h) compared to a beta blocker reduced the in-hospital incidence of fatal and nonfatal myocardial infarction from 15 to 3 percent.[96] These results were criticized because 46 percent of randomized patients were excluded from analysis. A more recent study of 479 patients has confirmed a reduction in the incidence of fatal and nonfatal myocardial infarction from 12 to 0.8 percent with heparin infused at therapeutic doses.[76] The incidence of severe refractory angina was also reduced with heparin.

Dissimilar results were observed in a more recent study that showed a reduction of fatal and nonfatal myocardial infarction in the first 5 days only when aspirin was used conjointly with heparin.[77] Treatment was initiated relatively late in this trial and addressed less unstable patients since a treadmill exercise test was often used for the diagnosis. Further, heparin was administered as intermittent bolus injections of 3750 to 5000 units every 6 h. A continuous ECG monitoring study has documented the efficacy of an intravenous infusion of heparin to control episodes of ST-segment shifts but no effect of intermittent heparin, recombinant tissue plasminogen activator, or aspirin.[97] (See Chap. 68.)

Oral Anticoagulants

No trials have adequately tested the value of oral anticoagulants for the longer term management of unstable angina, although early and more recent noncontrolled trials have suggested benefit.[8,10,11,98] Trials testing the efficacy of long-term anticoagulants as well as the safety and usefulness of a combined use with antiplatelet drugs are warranted and some are currently underway.

Fibrinolytic Therapy

Early small clinical and angiographic studies have suggested some usefulness of fibrinolysis.[99–101] The benefits were not confirmed in subsequent studies that showed little improvement in lumen diameter of the culprit lesion compared to heparin alone.[101,102] The angiographic part of the Thrombolysis in Myocardial Ischemia (TIMI 3A) trial has suggested that patients with an apparent thrombus and patients with a non-Q-wave myocardial infarction may benefit from the fibrinolytic therapy.[56] Angiographic improvement, however, may not correspond to clinical improvement.[103] A clinical benefit, when detected, is usually limited to the first 24 h after treatment.[97,100,101] The role of thrombolytic therapy in unstable angina remains uncertain, with the need for further investigation to define subsets of patients who may benefit. Patients with recurrent angina in hospital, class 3 and 4 (Table 59-3), and possibly also patients with previous bypass surgery with the culprit lesion involving a venous graft may be candidates for investigation. At present, thrombolytic therapy for unstable angina cannot be generally recommended. It would appear that patients with unstable angina need an agent to prevent the thrombus from progressing. Antiplatelet and antithrombin therapy is most appropriate; in contrast, the partial lysis induced by thrombolytic therapy may stimulate thrombin generation. (See also Chap. 68.)

ANTIANGINAL THERAPY

Nitroglycerin

The benefits of nitroglycerin for controlling chest pain were documented in many studies although of small sample sizes.[104–106] A decrease in angina episodes has been reported in between 15 and 94 percent of patients with refractory angina treated with intravenous nitroglycerin for periods varying between 24 h and 3 weeks. Nitroglycerin is the cornerstone of therapy for the management of angina pectoris. It reduces preload and afterload of the heart, produces coronary vasodilatation, relieves vasospasm, and favors preferential flow to the ischemic zones. It is the exogenous equivalent of the endothelium-derived relaxing factor and acts by increasing intracellular levels of cyclic guanosine monophosphate (GMP).[107] The precise mechanisms of benefit of nitroglycerin remain unclear in unstable angina. Continuous infusions over several days are useful in spite of the almost certain development of some tolerance. Indeed, paradoxically, chest pain frequently recurs following discontinuation of nitroglycerin, even after prolonged use. The beneficial effect could be related, at least in part, to an inhibition of platelet aggregation. This inhibitory effect has been well documented in vitro[108] and in the Folts' model of stenosed canine coronary arteries with intimal damage in which nitroglycerin abolished acute platelet thrombus formation and cyclical flow reductions.[109] Recent studies in humans suggest that a similar effect based on inhibition of platelet aggregation by nitroglycerin could be present in patients with unstable angina administered therapeutic doses (Fig. 59-8).[110] (See Chap. 30.)

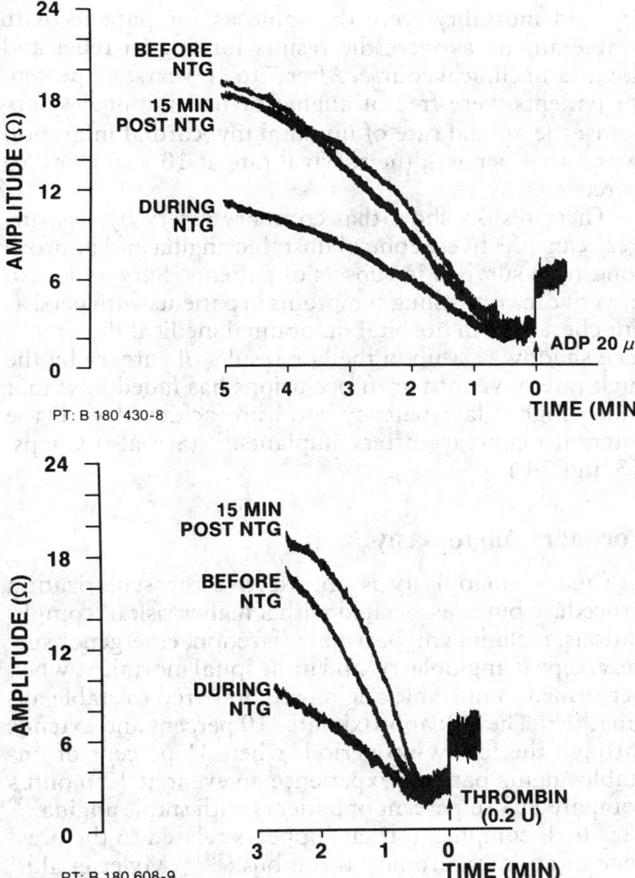

FIGURE 59-8 Platelet aggregation measured on whole blood at bedside with the impedance aggregometer before, during a 30-min intravenous infusion of nitroglycerin, and 15 min after its discontinuation. Platelet aggregation to ADP (*top*) and to thrombin (*bottom*) is reduced by 50 percent with nitroglycerin. (*From J Diodati et al: Effects of nitroglycerin at therapeutic doses on platelet aggregation in unstable angina pectoris and acute myocardial infarction. Am J Cardiol 66:683–687, 1990. Reproduced with permission of the author and the publisher.*)

Beta-Adrenergic Blockers

Although no major trial has tested specifically their benefit in reducing major cardiac events in unstable angina, beta blockers have become part of standard therapy. They are used to prevent and control recurrent chest pain, based on the results of small studies that have shown their usefulness.[111,112] They are most useful in a patient with a high sympathetic tone manifested by sinus tachycardia and elevated blood pressure. They reduce myocardial oxygen demand and may also possess a myocardial protective effect. In a specific subset of patients with chest pain suggestive of myocardial infarction, the risk of developing myocardial infarction was reduced by 13 percent.[111,112] Beta blockers may be associated with an unopposed alpha-adrenergic vasoconstriction and, very rarely, may exacerbate coronary artery spasm.[113] (See also Chap. 66.)

Calcium Antagonists

Calcium antagonists have been studied extensively in unstable angina.[114–118] Many trials have shown that verapamil, nifedipine, and diltiazem can efficiently control chest pain in unstable angina with striking results in Prinzmetal's variant angina. These trials, however, have generally failed to document a reduction in the rate of myocardial infarction, death, and severe refractory angina. In some studies using nifedipine as a single therapy an unfavorable trend was found.[114,117] The combination of propranolol with nifedipine, however, may be superior to either drug alone for the prevention of angina.[114,117] In general, diltiazem and propranolol are equally effective in controlling recurrent ischemia and preventing cardiac events.[118]

The antianginal effects of nitroglycerin, beta blockers, and calcium antagonists are additive, and triple therapy is often recommended during acute unstable angina, reaping benefit from the effects of each drug. This approach is largely empirical but is widely used and felt to be effective. (See also Chap. 67.)

Intraaortic Balloon Pump

Intraaortic balloon counterpulsation can now be easily performed at bedside using the transcutaneous approach. The augmented diastolic pressure favors diastolic flow through severe stenoses and may prevent complete occlusion, while cardiac work is decreased by systolic unloading. The efficacy of intraaortic balloon pump has not been evaluated in randomized studies, but clinical experience shows that it can be extremely efficacious in controlling recurrent ischemia. Unfortunately, the technique is associated with a complication rate of 10 percent and is only useful as a bridge to more definitive procedures.[119] The local complications are usually controlled by removing the catheter. The intraaortic balloon is used in 1 to 5 percent of patients to control severe recurrent ischemia and to stabilize hemodynamically unstable patients, reducing also the complication rates associated with coronary angiography, coronary angioplasty, and coronary bypass surgery. (See also Chap. 31.)

REVASCULARIZATION PROCEDURES

Coronary artery bypass surgery has been applied to the management of unstable angina since the early 1970s, a few years after its introduction in clinical practice. Coronary angioplasty was applied in the early 1980s, immediately after documentation of its feasibility in stable angina. These revascularization procedures are now widely used in the management of unstable angina and are extremely useful.

Coronary Artery Bypass Surgery

Early reports have shown that bypass vein graft surgery could be performed with a low operative mortality with substantial relief of symptoms; the results were, however, offset by a high perioperative infarction rate of 15 to 20 percent.[15,120–122] Subsequent studies have compared the results of surgical and medical treatment. In one series, the 23-month mortality was 21 percent in medically treated patients and 5.8 percent in surgical patients.[121]

Five randomized studies, however, failed to demonstrate a benefit of surgery on survival. In the National Cooperative Study, mortality was the same in surgically and medically treated patients.[92] In the larger Veterans Administration Cooperative Study of 468 men, the rates of nonfatal myocardial infarction at 2 years were 11.7 percent in patients treated surgically and 12.2 percent (NS) in patients treated medically.[123] Patients with left main disease and patients with a low ejection fraction were excluded from this study. Further, subset analyses showed a favorable trend for surgery in patients with three-vessel disease and a significant benefit in patients with abnormal left ventricular function. The 5-year survivals in patients with three-vessel disease were 89 percent with surgical and 75 percent with medical treatment. Prognosis was determined by the ejection fraction in medically treated patients, but not in surgical patients (Fig. 59-9). Comparative mortalities were 27 and 14 percent in patients with ejection fractions between 30 and 49 percent ($p = .03$).[123]

All randomized studies have shown a better long-term control of angina with surgical treatment with a high crossover rate of medical patients to surgery: 36 percent in the National Cooperative Study and 43 percent at 5 years in the Veterans Administration Cooperative Study. The latter study also reported a better quality of life in surgical patients.[124]

Kaiser et al.[125] recently reviewed 14 reports published from 1978 to 1988 involving 6136 patients with unstable angina treated by coronary artery bypass grafting. Patients with recent myocardial infarction and patients operated electively after stabilization with medical therapy were excluded. Mean operative mortality was 4.1 percent. Mean incidence of perioperative infarction was 9.9 percent, and mean incidence of postoperative low cardiac output was 16 percent. The risk factors for morbidity and mortality were the same as for patients with stable angina as were the results for angina relief and long-term clinical course. After 7 to 10 years, 80 percent of patients were free of angina or had minimal symptoms; the annual rate of nonfatal myocardial infarction was 3 to 4 percent; the survival rate at 10 years was 80 percent.

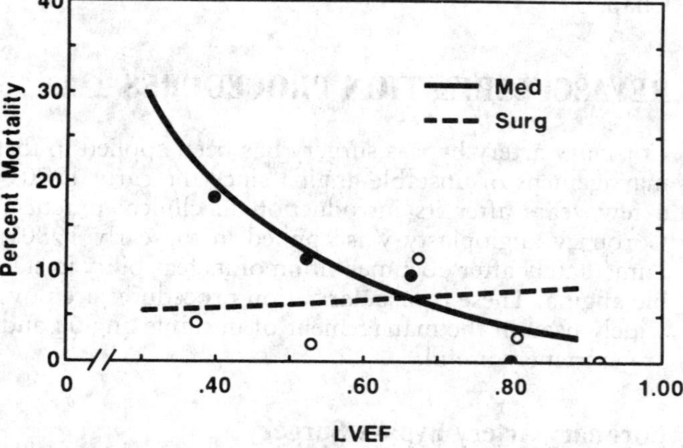

FIGURE 59-9 Results of the Veterans Administrative study on the 2-year survival of patients with unstable angina randomized to medical or surgical treatment. No difference in survival rate existed between the two study groups. However, the ejection fraction influenced the results. The survival rate was poor in medically treated patients with a low ejection fraction. In surgically treated patients, survival was good and independent of a lower ejection fraction. (*From RJ Luchi et al: Comparison of medical and surgical treatment for unstable angina pectoris. N Engl J Med 316:977–984, 1987. Reproduced with permission of the author and the publisher.*)

These results show that coronary artery bypass surgery can effectively control unstable angina and improve long-term survival in subsets of patients. Surgery is also effective in controlling symptoms in patients with persistent chest pain in hospital on optimal medical therapy.[126] The shadow cast upon the late results of surgery by the high rate of venous graft occlusions has faded now that much higher late patency rates are achieved with the internal mammary artery implants.[127] (See also Chaps. 73 and 74.)

Coronary Angioplasty

Coronary angioplasty is an effective revascularization procedure but is associated with a higher risk of complications, including myocardial infarction, emergency surgery, repeat angioplasty, and in-hospital mortality, when performed in unstable angina as compared to stable angina.[128,129] The risk approximates 10 percent and extends through the follow-up period, when 31 percent of unstable angina patients experience an event at 12 months compared to 16 percent of patients with stable angina.[130] This high complication rate appears related to the presence of an intracoronary thrombus.[131–133] Myler et al.[131] reported an incidence of Q-wave myocardial infarction of 6.5 percent, of emergency surgery of 9.4 percent, and a follow-up mortality of 5.8 percent with the procedure performed with 1 week after the onset of unstable angina as opposed to respectively 1.6, 4.8, and 1.7 percent when delayed for 2 to 4 weeks. Coronary artery bypass may be a better choice in patients with multivessel disease because it is less risky, but dilatation limited to the culprit coronary lesion has been recommended as an initial approach to stabilize the unstable clinical status.[129–134] This strategy is successful in many patients, although it is associated with more frequent recurrence of angina requiring later elective bypass surgery or angioplasty of other diseased coronary sites. Other interventional procedures in unstable angina such as laser angioplasty, atherectomy, and stent implantations remain investigational. (See Chap. 71.)

Coronary angioplasty is thus an option to consider in the management of patients with unstable angina when the coronary anatomy is suitable, preferably as a semielective procedure after initial medical stabilization or more acutely in patients refractory to pharmacologic treatment. Nonrandomized studies have suggested that 3 to 6 days of heparin pretreatment may reduce the incidence of abrupt vessel closure from 8 to 10 percent to 1 to 2 percent.[135] Intracoronary fibrinolytic agents are often useful when angioplasty is complicated by an early acute thrombotic occlusion.[136] Prophylactic use of these agents is currently under investigation. In the future, new clot-active antithrombin agents or more potent antiplatelet drugs could be useful to prevent procedure-related thrombotic occlusion. (See also Chap. 70.)

MANAGEMENT

General Measures

Unstable angina in the active phase requires hospitalization, preferably in the coronary care unit, with bed rest and general measures to assure well being, including relief of pain, control of anxiety, and attention to other medical problems such as constipation. Potential secondary causes of exacerbation of angina should be excluded. Bleeding tendency or contraindications to the use of antiplatelet drugs, anticoagulants, or fibrinolytic agents should be assessed.

Treatment in the Acute Phase

Specific treatment to prevent growth of the thrombotic process should be initiated early. Aspirin and heparin are useful in this regard. In the more acute phase and in the more unstable patient, heparin at therapeutic intravenous doses is favored, based on its superiority to aspirin in preventing myocardial infarction and recurrent severe angina. A bolus of 5000 units is first administered followed by an infusion at a rate of 1000 units per hour subsequently adjusted to maintain the activated partial thromboplastin time (APTT) at 1.5 to 2.5 times the control values. Aspirin is also useful during the acute phase and is the treatment of choice thereafter and in the long term. It can be used safely in combination with heparin for a few days.

Antianginal therapy is also indicated. Nitrates, beta blockers, and calcium antagonists as a single therapy or in combination can be used. We favor first the routine use of intravenous nitroglycerin, which is highly efficacious and possesses coronary vasodilator properties and possibly antiplatelet effects. Beta blockers are also indicated for angina control and, when prolonged pain is present, for their protective effect on the ischemic myocardium. The dose is adjusted to maintain heart rate in the low range of normal. Diltiazem is a good second choice if beta blockers are contraindicated. Triple therapy should be used in the patient with recurrent angina; nifedipine in combination with beta blockers has been shown useful in this setting.

The duration of this acute phase is empirical. Clinical experience suggests that it may extend to 48 to 96 h past the last episode of pain, which probably reflects the time required for a plaque rupture to heal. Recurrent ischemia (of types 3 and 4 of the classification of Table 59-3) is an indicator of ongoing active disease, and these patients should have coronary arteriography.

Subacute Phase

Past the acute phase, management is progressively adjusted to the long term. Intravenous nitroglycerin is weaned and may be replaced by oral or transdermal treatment. Heparin is continued until definitive treatment is selected. Most patients undergo coronary arteriography, although the cost effectiveness of this routine has not been documented. If patients do not have coronary arteriography, risk stratification with exercise testing or with pharmacologic provocation such as dipyridamole thallium scintigraphy (Chap. 134) or stress echocardiography (Chap. 132) should be performed. The goal at this stage is to detect patients with severe underlying coronary artery disease or with residual latent ischemia who could benefit from more aggressive therapy. A high percentage of patients have severe underlying disease even though the unstable angina is controlled.

If medical therapy is selected, aspirin should be initiated before the discontinuation of heparin to prevent reactivation of the disease following heparin discontinuation.[137] Aspirin should be given in combination with heparin if coronary angioplasty is performed. If coronary artery bypass surgery is contemplated, heparin alone should be continued up to the procedure to prevent the increase in blood loss associated with aspirin use. (See also Chap. 68.)

Prompt fibrinolytic therapy is indicated if an acute myocardial infarction complicates the clinical course. Recurrent ischemia at rest with optimal therapy is an indication for urgent coronary angiography with a view to coronary angioplasty and/or coronary bypass surgery. These maneuvers may be performed under the protection of intraaortic balloon counterpulsation for the most unstable patients.

Chronic Therapy

Aspirin should be administered long term following an episode of unstable angina. If aspirin is contraindicated, ticlopidine administration should be considered. The indication for antiplatelet treatment is prevention of recurrence of unstable angina and of myocardial infarction and also as general secondary prevention for coronary artery disease. Antianginal drugs are also prescribed and subsequently may be adjusted to the clinical evolution. The clinical condition of these patients should be reassessed after a few weeks to adjust therapy. Indeed, the unstable angina episode may have led to progression of the underlying coronary disease and be a manifestation of accelerated atherosclerosis.[60] In addition, the acute disease process that has provoked the unstable state may show recurrence. An aggressive program of control of risk factors should be instituted, including discontinuation of cigarette smoking, control of plasma lipoproteins, which can prevent progression of disease and favor plaque regression, and stress management. This program can not only halt progression of coronary artery disease but possibly also stabilize an atherosclerotic plaque preventing rupture. (See Chaps. 62 and 65.)

Despite our successes in the management of unstable angina with specific treatment now available, the high failure rate justifies continued efforts for primary and secondary prevention and the search for more specific and more potent antithrombin and antiplatelet drugs. The ultimate goal of secondary prevention is to prevent reactivation of the disease. Altering plaque composition and its lipid content may be an effective approach for the secondary prevention of acute coronary syndromes.

VARIANT ANGINA

In 1959 Prinzmetal et al.[138] described a syndrome characterized by angina at rest associated with transient ST-segment elevation. In most cases exercise tolerance was well preserved and the attacks were cyclical in nature, often occurring in the early morning hours. The attacks did not last longer than ordinary anginal episodes and the ST-segment elevation rapidly normalized as the chest pain receded. Ventricular arrhythmias and atrioventricular block sometimes occurred at the height of an attack, and both myocardial infarction and sudden death were common complications.

With the advent of coronary arteriography it soon became apparent that the syndrome was caused by transient coronary artery spasm, usually focal, and often at the site of coronary stenosis.[139] The underlying coronary disease can vary from a subtotal occlusion to a very mild stenosis, however, and in some cases the coronary arteries are angiographically normal. Coronary artery spasm has been demonstrated to be the cause of myocardial ischemia in some patients who have only ST depression or pseudonormalization of abnormal T waves during episodes of angina.[140]

Pathophysiology

A central neural mechanism is unlikely involved since coronary spasm can occur in the denervated transplanted heart.[141] The frequency of attacks of variant angina is not reduced by alpha-adrenergic blockade,[142] blockade of serotonin receptors,[143] inhibition of thromboxane A_2 production,[144] or administration of prostacyclin.[145]

Coronary spasm is usually localized to the site of an atherosclerotic lesion. Even variant angina patients with normal appearing arteries at angiography may have underlying atherosclerosis at autopsy.[146] The response of other coronary segments to vasoconstrictive stimuli is normal, indicating that a generalized abnormality of coronary reactivity is not present.[147]

Normal endothelium modulates coronary tone by releasing endothelium-derived relaxing factors (EDRFs); this function is lost at sites of early atherosclerosis and is impaired by hypercholesterolemia.[26] The EDRFs inhibit platelet aggregation; aggregating platelets release vasoconstricting substances that can act unopposed in the absence of EDRFs. Acetylcholine dilates arterial segments with normal endothelium by stimulating EDRF release but constricts segments with dysfunctional endothelium.[25] It is likely that loss of endothelial vasodilator function contributes to constriction in variant angina. Increased smooth-muscle contractility also probably plays an important role. (See also Chaps. 2 and 54 to 57.)

The pathophysiological consequences of coronary spasm are well understood. Severe spasm rapidly induces transmural ischemia, resulting in regional dyskinesia and ST elevation. If the ischemic zone is large, cardiac output and systemic arterial pressure will decrease. The risk of serious ventricular arrhythmias increases with the severity and extent of ischemia. Intraarterial stasis due to spasm can generate local thrombotic activity that can be detected as increased circulating fibrinopeptide A levels.[148]

Clinical Features

Variant angina is uncommon, and the presenting symptoms are usually not remarkable enough to be distinguished immediately from unstable angina. Angina at rest occurs with a cyclical pattern and often with attacks occurring in the early morning hours. Exertional angina coexists in slightly more than half of the patients, but the ischemic threshold is extremely variable.[149] Variant angina can occur during the recovery phase of myocardial infarction[150] or in patients who have had coronary bypass surgery[151] or recent angioplasty.[152]

Most patients with variant angina are heavy cigarette smokers, but their age, gender, and risk factor profiles are otherwise similar to other coronary patients.[153] Those with angiographically normal coronary arteries tend to be younger and more often women and often do not have more risk factors than noncoronary controls.[154] One-quarter of variant angina patients have a history of migraine headaches and one-quarter have symptoms of Raynaud's phenomenon.[155] Thus, variant angina in some cases may be part of a more generalized vasospastic diathesis. Syncope during rest angina is a useful diagnostic clue.

Physical examination of variant angina patients between attacks reveals no abnormalities. Routine laboratory tests, including cardiac enzymes, are likewise normal.

Variant angina can be most easily diagnosed by recording an ECG during an episode of rest angina. The ST-segment elevation that occurs during an attack will disappear promptly with the administration of nitroglycerin. As illustrated in Fig. 59-10, coronary spasm can induce ST elevation, ST depression, or pseudonormalization of abnormally negative T waves. Atrioventricular block may develop when the site of ST elevation is the

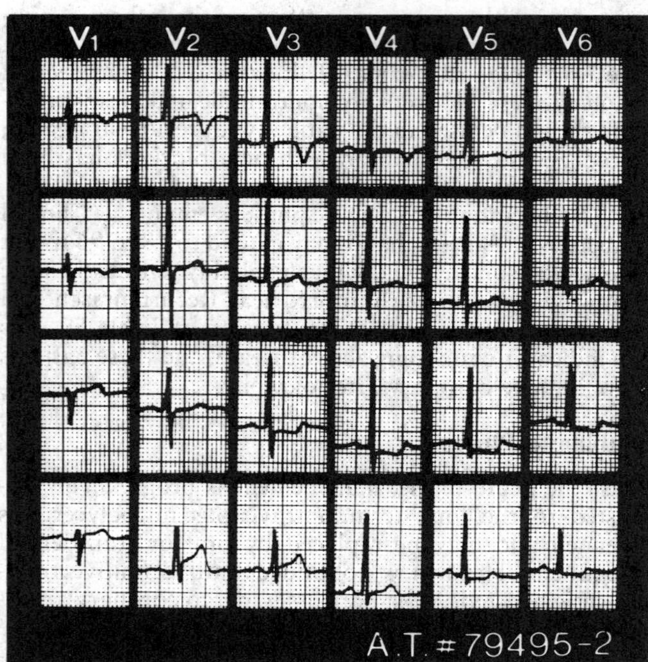

FIGURE 59-10 Electrocardiograms (leads V_1 to V_6) from a patient with active variant angina. Negative T waves are present in the control tracing (*top*). The other three tracings were recorded during separate episodes of rest angina and show (respectively) pseudonormalization of T waves, ST depression, and ST elevation.

inferior leads; ventricular arrhythmias, including ventricular fibrillation, can occur with ST elevation in any territory. The risk of these arrhythmias and conduction disturbances increases with the degree of ST elevation.[155]

Diagnostic Procedures

The most important diagnostic procedure to obtain during an episode of pain at rest is a 12-lead ECG. When variant angina is suspected, ambulatory electrocardiographic monitoring can be useful to confirm the diagnosis. Exercise testing will provoke angina with ST elevation in approximately one-third of variant angina patients during an active phase of their disease.[149–156] The cold pressor test induces a variant angina attack in only 10 percent of patients.[156]

Several different pharmacologic agents have been used to induce episodes of variant angina. Histamine[157] and dopamine[158] provoke attacks in only one-quarter to one-half of variant angina patients. Intracoronary acetylcholine has a much higher sensitivity, 90 percent in one large series,[159] but cannot be used without a temporary pacemaker because of the high incidence of bradyarrhythmias and conduction disturbances after right coronary artery injection.

Ergonovine, an ergot alkaloid that constricts vascular smooth muscle by stimulating both alpha-adrenergic and serotonergic receptors, is the agent most commonly used. When administered intravenously to patients with active variant angina at the time of coronary arteriography, more than 90 percent of patients will develop severe, focal coronary spasm.[160] Spontaneous and ergonovine-induced episodes of variant angina are very much similar. Examples of spontaneous and ergonovine-induced coronary spasm are illustrated in Fig. 59-11. Ergonovine causes physiological coronary vasoconstriction and in-

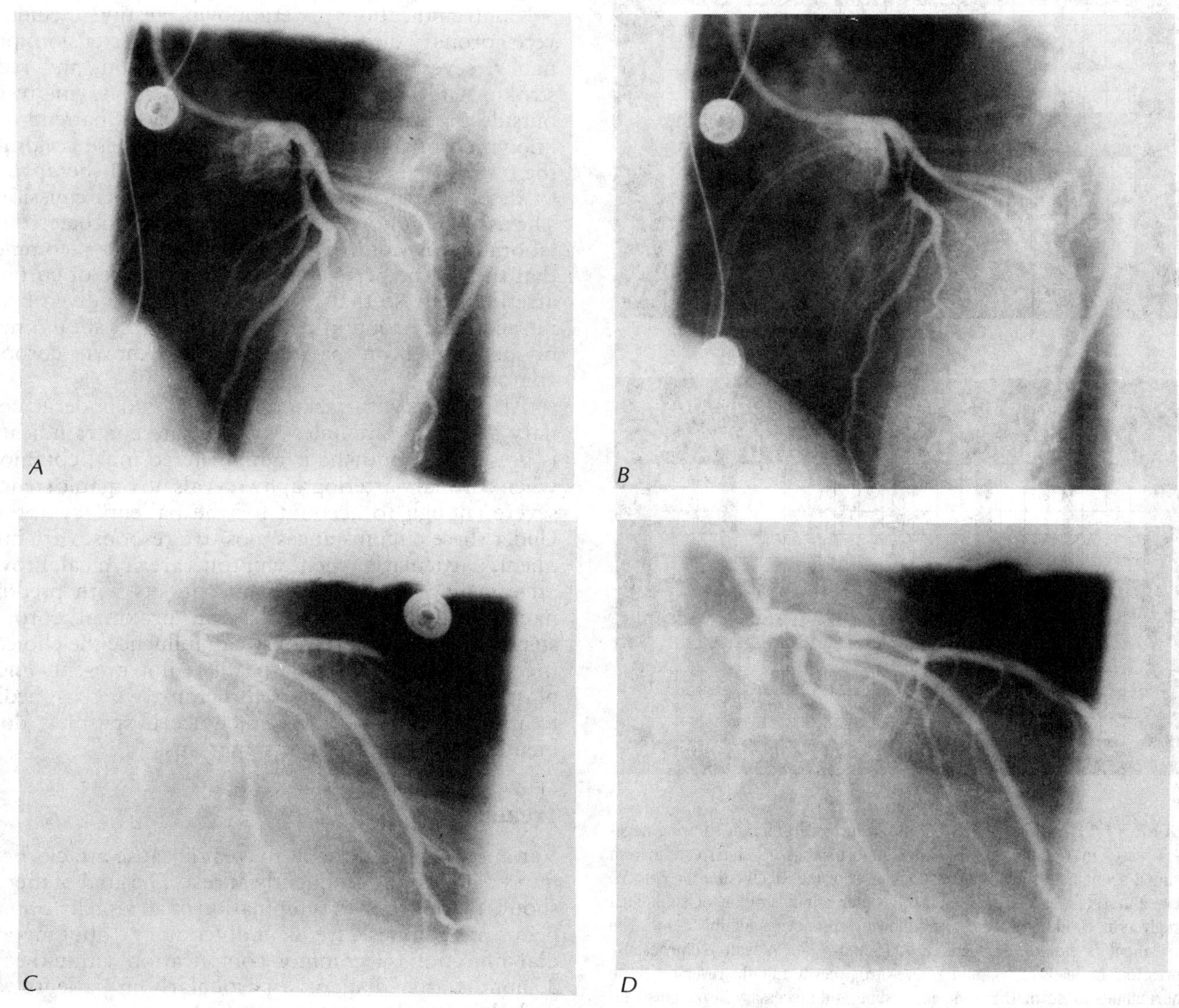

FIGURE 59-11 *A.* Left coronary arteriogram (45° LAD view with 25° craniocaudal angulation) of a 47-year-old man with active variant angina. A 40 percent proximal LAD stenosis is present. The coronary arteries are otherwise normal angiographically. *B.* The control angina and ST elevation developed spontaneously during coronary arteriography. Repeat injections reveal severe focal spasm at the site of the lesion. The coronary spasm resolved immediately after nitroglycerin administration. *C.* Left coronary arteriogram in the RAO view after ergonovine administration. Severe coronary spasm is present both at the site of the LAD stenosis and distal to it. *D.* Resolution of ergonovine-induced spasm following nitroglycerin administration.

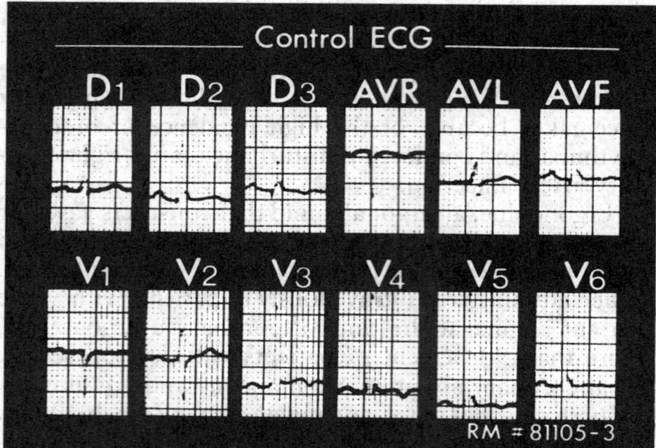

E

F

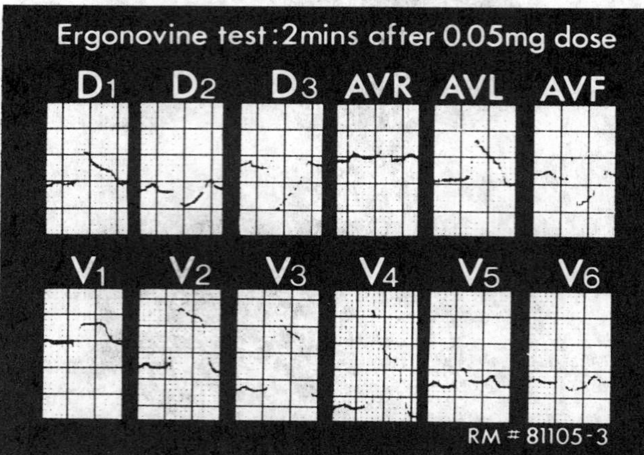

G

FIGURE 59-11 *(continued)* *E.* Control electrocardiogram showing negative T waves in V_3 to V_6 with no other abnormalities. *F.* Electrocardiogram during a spontaneous attack of rest angina showing ST elevation in V_2 to V_5. These abnormalities disappeared 2 min after administration of sublingual nitroglycerin. *G.* Electrocardiogram following ergonovine administration. The ST segment is elevated in leads 1, AVL, and V_1 to V_5 with reciprocal ST depression in leads 2, 3, and AVF. Nitroglycerin rapidly reversed these abnormalities to normal. Ergonovine testing is unnecessary in patients with documented spontaneous attacks. [*From DD Waters, P Théroux: The role of coronary artery spasm in Prinzmetal's angina. In: RA Chahine (ed): Coronary Artery Spasm, vol 6. Mount Kisco, Futura, 1983: 119–140. Reproduced with permission of the author and the publisher.*]

creases peripheral vascular resistance; these changes can induce myocardial ischemia with ST-segment depression if the underlying coronary stenoses are severe.[161] In a study in which ergonovine was administered to more than 1000 patients with various types of cardiac disease, coronary spasm was provoked in 38 percent of those with angina at rest, 14 percent of those with rest and effort angina, 4 percent of those with effort angina only, 20 percent of recent infarct patients, 1 percent of those with atypical chest pain, and almost no patients without coronary disease.[162] A negative ergonovine test in the absence of coronary vasodilators in a patient with recent chest pain provides compelling evidence against coronary spasm as the cause.

Ergonovine testing has occasionally caused refractory coronary spasm resulting in death[163] and can induce multivessel coronary spasm.[159] Selective intracoronary administration eliminates this risk and the systemic effects of the agents. The cumulative intracoronary dose of ergonovine is 50 μg compared to the cumulative intraarterial or intravenous dose of 0.3 to 1 mg.[139]

Contraindications to ergonovine testing include severe coronary disease, uncontrolled hypertension, pregnancy, severe left ventricular dysfunction, and recent stroke. A few investigators perform ergonovine testing outside the catheterization laboratory in patients with known coronary anatomy.[164,165] Under these conditions the test can be used to assess the effect of therapy[166] or to detect the occurrence of spontaneous remission.[167] The use of ergonovine testing outside the catheterization laboratory is controversial; most experts recommend that the test be performed only at the time of coronary arteriography so that nitroglycerin can be given by the intracoronary route if necessary. The test should never be performed on patients with unknown coronary anatomy.

All patients with variant angina should undergo coronary arteriography unless an absolute contraindication is present. Ergonovine is administered most commonly when coronary arteriography reveals no organic stenoses severe enough to account for the patient's symptoms. Under these circumstances, positive responses are infrequent, particularly when symptoms are atypical. Provocative testing is often useful in patients with predominantly rest angina and a focal, proximal coronary stenosis because the response can influence the choice of therapy. For example, if spasm is not present, angioplasty might be the preferred therapy, whereas medical treatment might be a better choice if spasm is documented to be the cause of symptoms.

Treatment

Variant angina is difficult to treat because attacks occur unpredictably and frequently at rest. The goal of therapy should therefore be the elimination of all attacks. Spontaneous remission is a frequent outcome,[168,169] but myocardial infarction is a common complication within the first 3 months after diagnosis, particularly in patients with underlying multivessel disease.[170]

Nitroglycerin relieves variant angina attacks within minutes and should be used promptly. Long-acting nitrates are effective in preventing variant angina attacks, but the development of nitrate tolerance limits their usefulness. Beta-adrenergic blocking drugs are often of little value in patients with predominantly vasospastic angina and may be dangerous by increasing the duration of attacks.[117,171]

The calcium channel blockers nifedipine,[172] diltiazem,[173] and verapamil[174] are very effective in preventing attacks of variant angina. More than half of the patients treated with one of these drugs become completely asymptomatic. The response is better at high doses; for example, nifedipine, 80 mg per day, diltiazem, 360 mg per day, or verapamil, 480 mg per day. Patients with an incomplete response to one drug often become angina free on a combination of nifedipine with either diltiazem or verapamil. The efficacy of these three drugs in preventing variant angina is roughly equal.[166] Evidence from uncontrolled studies[175] suggests that treatment with calcium channel blockers reduces the risk of myocardial infarction. (See also Chap. 67.)

Approximately 20 percent of variant angina patients will not respond to treatment with two calcium channel blockers plus long-acting nitrates. Although not approved in the United States for this indication, amiodarone,[176] guanethidine, and clonidine[177] have been reported to be effective in some such refractory patients. Therapy for ventricular arrhythmias and conduction disturbances that complicate attacks in some cases should be directed toward the elimination of all episodes of spasm. Patients with variant angina should be treated with low-dose aspirin, as are other patients with coronary disease, to reduce the risk of myocardial infarction, even though very high doses of aspirin may aggravate coronary spasm.[178]

Coronary bypass surgery should be considered in most patients with variant angina and significant multivessel atherosclerotic disease. Operative mortality and the perioperative infarction rate are, however, higher than for comparable patients without variant angina.[179,180] For example, in the Duke series 3 deaths and 3 nonfatal infarctions occurred perioperatively in 48 surgically treated patients.[179] Surgery almost invariably eliminates variant angina, and long-term outcome is excellent. Only one myocardial infarction and no deaths were observed over 5 years of follow-up.

Bypass surgery will be successful when the anastomosis can be situated distal to the site of focal spasm but not when diffuse spasm involves the entire artery. Cardiac denervation by plexectomy in association with bypass surgery has yielded excellent results,[181] but this procedure has not been evaluated in a controlled study. The occurrence of spasm after cardiac transplantation or autotransplantation[182] argues against a beneficial effect from denervation. Bypass surgery is not indicated for variant angina in the absence of significant organic stenoses.

Many patients with variant angina have coronary lesions that are ideal for angioplasty. When such patients are pretreated with calcium channel blockers and given intravenous or intracoronary nitroglycerin during the procedure, the primary success rate is high.[152,183,184] Coronary spasm may persist or recur after successful angioplasty, however, and calcium channel blockers should therefore be continued. The restenosis rate is significantly higher than usual in patients with variant angina.[152,185] As with bypass surgery, coronary angioplasty is not indicated for patients with coronary spasm who have normal or nearly normal arteries on coronary arteriography.

Prognosis

The long-term prognosis of variant angina has been reported for several large series of patients from different countries.[170,179,186–188] The extent and severity of the underlying coronary disease appear to be the most important factors influencing outcome. As illustrated in Fig. 59-12, survival without myocardial infarction at 1 year in 217 consecutive patients was 93 percent for those without stenoses of 70 percent or more, 86 percent for patients with one-vessel disease, and 65 percent for those with multivessel disease.[170] At 5 years the corresponding figures were 83, 74, and 44 percent, respectively. Other

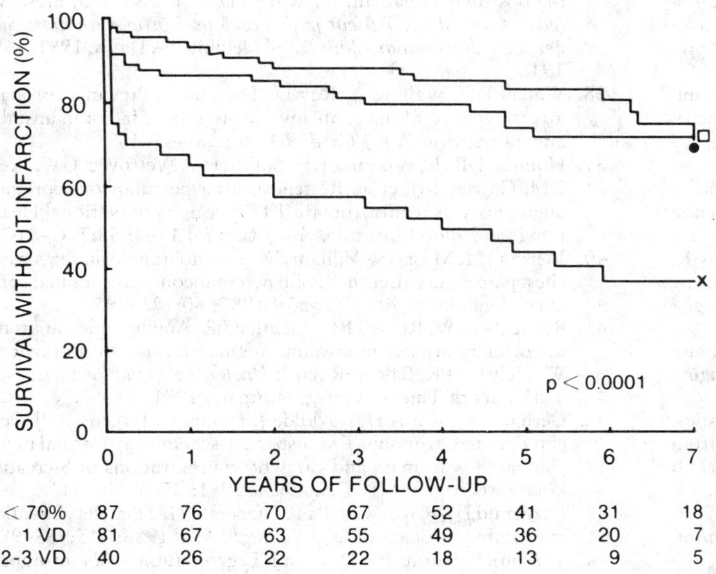

FIGURE 59-12 Survival without myocardial infarction in variant angina patients with no stenoses of 70 percent or more (●), those with one vessel disease (□), and those with multivessel disease (×). The outcome in the latter group of patients is much worse than in the other two groups. Events are clustered early in the follow-up period. (*From A. Walling, DD Waters, DD Miller, D Roy, GB Pelletier, P Théroux: Long-term prognosis of patients with variant angina. Circulation 76:990–997, 1987. Reproduced with permission of the author and the American Heart Association.*)

variables that correlate with a poor outcome include the presence of abnormal left ventricular function, ventricular arrhythmias during attacks, multivessel spasm and the absence of treatment with calcium channel blockers. Patients who become angina free may later experience recurrence of variant angina or may develop other manifestations of coronary artery disease. (See also Chap. 61.)

REFERENCES

1. Osler W: The Lumleian lectures on angina pectoris. *Lancet* 1910; 1:697–701.
2. Parkinson J, Bedford DE: Cardiac infarction and coronary thrombosis. *Lancet* 1928; 1:4–11.
3. Sampson JJ, Eliaser M Jr: The diagnosis of impending acute coronary artery occlusion. *Am Heart J* 1937; 13:675–686.
4. Feil H: Preliminary pain in coronary thrombosis. *Am J Med Sci* 1937; 193:42–48.
5. Master AM, Dack S, Jaffe HL: Premonitory symptoms of acute coronary occlusion; a study of 260 cases. *Ann Intern Med* 1941; 14:1115–1165.
6. Solomon HA, Edwards AL, Killip T: Prodromata in acute myocardial infarction. *Circulation* 1969; 40:463–471.
7. Levy H: The natural history of changing pattern of angina pectoris. *Ann Intern Med* 1956; 44:1123–1135.
8. Vakil RJ: Intermediate coronary syndrome. *Circulation* 1961; 24:557–571.
9. Beamish RE, Storrie VM: Impending myocardial infarction. Recognition and management. *Circulation* 1960; 21:1107–1115.
10. Fowler NO: "Preinfarctional" angina: A need for an objective definition and for a controlled clinical trial of its management. *Circulation* 1971; 44:755–758.
11. Wood P: Acute and subacute coronary insufficiency. *Br Med J* 1961; 1:1779–1782.
12. Krauss KR, Hutter AM, De Sanctis RW: Acute coronary insufficiency course and follow-up. *Circulation* 1972; 45(suppl I):I-66–I-71.
13. Fulton M, Lutz W, Donald KM, Kirby BJ, Duncan B, Morrison SL, et al: Natural history of unstable angina. *Lancet* 1972; 1:800–865.
14. Gazes PC, Mobly FM, Faris HM, Duncan RC, Humphries GB: Pre-infarctional (unstable angina)—a prospective study—10 year follow-up. Prognostic significance of electrocardiographic changes. *Circulation* 1973; 48:331–337.
15. Scanlon PJ, Nemickas R, Moran JF, Talano JV, Amirparviz F, Pifarre R: Accelerated angina pectoris: Clinical, hemodynamic, arteriographic and therapeutic experience in 85 patients. *Circulation* 1973; 47:19–26.
16. Maseri A, L'Abbate A, Baroldi G, Chierchia S, Marzilli M, Ballestra AM, et al: Coronary vasospasm as a possible cause of myocardial infarction: Conclusion derived from the study of "preinfarction angina." *N Engl J Med* 1978; 299:1271–1277.
17. Falk E: Plaque rupture with severe pre-existing stenosis precipitating coronary thrombosis: Characteristics of coronary atherosclerotic plaques underlying fatal occlusive thrombi. *Br Heart J* 1983; 50:127–134.
18. Davies MJ, Thomas AC: Plaque fissuring—the cause of acute myocardial infarction, sudden ischemic death, and crescendo angina. *Br Heart J* 1985; 53:363–373.
19. De Wood MA, Spores J, Notske R, Mouser LT, Burroughs R, Golden MS, et al: Prevalence of total coronary occlusion during the early hours of transmural myocardial infarction. *N Engl J Med* 1980; 303:897–902.
20. Sherman CT, Litvack F, Grundfest W, Lee M, Hickey A, Chaux A, et al: Coronary angioscopy in patients with unstable angina pectoris. *N Engl J Med* 1986; 315:913–919.
21. National Center for Health Statistics: Vital and health statistics: Detailed diagnosis and procedures for patients discharged from short stay hospitals. Hyattsville, MD, U.S. Department of Health and Human Services, Public Health Service, Series 13, No. 90, 1987.
22. Braunwald E: Unstable angina. A classification. *Circulation* 1989; 80:410–414.
23. Gottlieb SO, Weisfeldt, ML, Ouyang P, Mellitis ED, Gerstenblith G: Silent ischemia as a marker for early unfavorable outcomes in patients with unstable angina. *N Engl J Med* 1986; 314:1214–1219.
24. Bilodeau L, Théroux P, Grégoire J, Gagnon D, Arsenault A: Technetium-99m Sestamibi tomography in patients with spontaneous chest pain: Correlations with clinical, electrocardiographic and angiographic findings. *J Am Coll Cardiol* 1991; 18:1684–1691.
25. Vanhoutte PM, Shimokawa H: Endothelium-derived relaxing factor and coronary vasospasm. *Circulation* 1989; 80:1–9.
26. Lerman A, Edward BS, Hallett JW, Heublein DM, Sandberg SM, Burnett CJ Jr: Circulating and tissue endothelin immunoreactivity in advanced atherosclerosis. *N Engl J Med* 1991; 325:997–1001.
27. Brown BG, Lee AB, Bolson EL, Dodge HT: Reflex vasoconstriction of significant coronary artery stenosis as a mechanism contributing to ischemic left ventricular dysfunction during isometric exercise. *Circulation* 1984; 70:18–24.
28. Winniford MD, Wheelan KR, Kremers MS, Ugolini V, van den Berg E, Niggemann EH, et al: Smoking-induced coronary vasoconstriction in patients with atherosclerotic coronary artery disease: Evidence for adrenergically mediated alterations in coronary artery tone. *Circulation* 1986; 73:662–667.
29. Mudge GH, Grossman W, Mills RM, Braunwald E: Reflex increase in coronary vascular resistance in patients with ischemic heart disease. *N Engl J Med* 1976; 295:1333–1337.
30. Isner JM, Estes NAM III, Thompson PD, Costanzo-Nordin MR, Subramanian R, Miller G, et al: Acute cardiac events temporally related to cocaine abuse. *N Engl J Med* 1986; 315:1438–1443.
31. Hadjimihiades S, Covalesky V, Manno OV, Haaz WS, Mintz GS: Coronary arteriographic findings in cocaine abuse–induced myocardial infarction. *Cathet Cardiovasc Diag* 1988; 14:33–36.
32. Flores ED, Lange RA, Cigarroa RG, Hillis LD: Effect of cocaine on coronary artery dimensions in atherosclerotic coronary artery disease: Enhanced vasoconstriction at sites of significant stenoses. *J Am Coll Cardiol* 1990; 16:74–79.
33. Togna G, Tempesta E, Togna AR, Dolci N, Cebo B, Caprino L: Platelet responsiveness and biosynthesis of thromboxane and prostacyclin in response to in vitro cocaine treatment. *Haemostasis* 1985; 15:100–107.
34. Schuster EH, Bulkley B: Early post-infarction angina: Ischemia at a distance and ischemia in the infarct zone. *N Engl J Med* 1981; 305:1101–1105.
35. Théroux P, Morissette D, Juneau M, de Guise P, Pelletier G, Waters DD: Influence of fibrinolysis and percutaneous transluminal coronary angioplasty on the frequency of ventricular premature complexes. *Am J Cardiol* 1989; 63:797–801.
36. Bosch X, Théroux P, Waters D, Pelletier GB, Roy D: Early postinfarction ischemia: Clinical, angiographic, and prognostic significance. *Circulation* 1987; 75:988–995.
37. Théroux P, Waters D: Unstable angina: Special considerations in the post-bypass patient. In: Waters D, Bourassa MG, Brest AN (eds): *Care of the Patient with Previous Coronary Bypass Surgery. Cardiovascular Clinics.* Philadelphia, FA Davis, 1991: 169–191.
38. Waters DD, Walling A, Roy D, Théroux P: Previous coronary artery bypass grafting as an adverse prognostic factor in unstable angina pectoris. *Am J Cardiol* 1986; 58:465–469.
39. Holmes DR Jr, Vliestra RE, Smith HV, Vetrovec GW, Kent KM, Cowley MJ, et al: Restenosis after percutaneous coronary angioplasty: A report from the PTCA registry of National Heart, Lung, and Blood Institute. *Am J Cardiol* 1984; 53:77C–81C.
40. Joelson JM, Most AS, Williams DO: Angiographic findings when chest pain recurs after successful percutaneous transluminal coronary angioplasty. *Am J Cardiol* 1987; 60:792–795.
41. Rafflenbeul W, Russell RO, Lichtlen PR: Angiographic anatomy of coronary arteries in unstable angina pectoris. In: Rafflenbeul W, Lichtlen PR, Balcon R (eds): *Unstable Angina Pectoris.* New York, Georg Thieme Verlag, Stuttgart, 1981: 51–57.
42. Gerhardt W, Katus H, Ravkilde J, Hamm C, Jorgensen PJ, Peheim E, et al: S-troponin T in suspected ischemic myocardial injury compared with mass and catalytic concentrations of S-creatine kinase isoenzyme MB. *Clin Chem* 1991; 37:1405–1411.
43. Fitzgerald DJ, Roy L, Catella F, Fitzgerald GA: Platelet activation in unstable coronary disease. *N Engl J Med* 1986; 315:983–989.
44. Théroux P, Latour JG, De Lara J, Léger-Gauthier C: Fibrinopep-

tide A and platelet factor levels in unstable angina pectoris. *Circulation* 1987; 75:156–162.

45. de Zwaan C, Bär FW, Janssen JHA, Cherier EC, Dassen WRM, Brugada P, et al: Angiographic and clinical characteristics of patients with unstable angina showing an ECG pattern indicating critical narrowing of the proximal LAD coronary artery. *Am Heart J* 1989; 117:657–664.
46. Maseri A, Parodi O, Severi S, Pesola A: Transient transmural reduction of myocardial blood demonstrated by thallium-201 scintigraphy, as a cause of variant angina. *Circulation* 1976; 54:280–288.
47. Wackers FJT, Lie KI, Liem KL, Sokole EB, Samson G, Van de Shoot JB, et al: Thallium-201 scintigraphy in unstable angina pectoris. *Circulation* 1978; 57:738–741.
48. Brown KA, Okada RD, Boucher CA, Phillips HR, Strauss HW, Pohost GM: Serial thallium-201 imaging at rest in patients with unstable and stable angina pectoris: Relationship of myocardial perfusion at rest to presenting clinical syndrome. *Am Heart J* 1983; 106:70–77.
49. Freeman MR, Williams AE, Chisholm RJ, Patt NL, Greyson MD, Armstrong PW: Role of resting thallium-201 perfusion in predicting coronary anatomy, left ventricular wall motion, and hospital outcome in unstable angina pectoris. *Am Heart J* 1989; 117:306–314.
50. Hamm CW, Lorenz RL, Bleifeld W, Kupper W, Wober E, Weber PC: Biochemical evidence of platelet activation in patients with persistent unstable angina. *J Am Coll Cardiol* 1987; 10:998–1006.
51. Gallino A, Haeberli A, Baur HR, Straub PW: Fibrin formation and platelet aggregation in patients with severe coronary artery disease: Relation with the degree of myocardial ischemia. *Circulation* 1985; 72:27–30.
52. Gram, J, Jespersen J: A selective depression of tissue plasminogen activator (t-PA) activity in euglobulins characterizes a risk group among survivors of acute myocardial infarction. *Thromb Haemost* 1987; 57:137–139.
53. Hamsten A, Wiman B, de Faire U, Blomback M: Increased plasma levels of a rapid inhibitor of tissue plasminogen activator in young survivors of myocardial infarction. *N Engl J Med* 1985; 313:1557–1563.
54. Holmes DR Jr, Hartzler GO, Smith HG, Fuster V: Coronary artery thrombosis in patients with unstable angina. *Br Heart J* 1981; 45:411–416.
55. Capone G, Wolf NM, Mayer B, Meister SG: Incidence of intracoronary filling defects by angiography in angina pectoris at rest. *Am J Cardiol* 1985; 56:403–406.
56. The TIMI Investigator Group: Thrombolysis in Myocardial Ischemia. TIMI 3A trial. Angiographic findings. *N Engl J Med* (in press).
57. Ambrose JA, Winters SL, Stern A, Eng A, Teichholtz LE, Gorlin R, et al: Angiographic morphology and the pathogenesis of unstable angina pectoris. *J Am Coll Cardiol* 1985; 5:609–616.
58. Taeymans Y, Théroux P, Lespérance J, Waters DD: Quantitative angiographic morphology of the coronary artery lesions at risk of thrombotic occlusion. *Circulation* 1992; 85:78–85.
59. Moise A, Lespérance J, Théroux P, Taeymans Y, Goulet C, Bourassa MG: Clinical and angiographic predictors of new total coronary occlusion in coronary artery disease: Analysis of 313 non-operated patients. *Am J Cardiol* 1984; 54:1176–1181.
60. Moise A, Théroux P, Taeymans Y, Descoings B, Lespérance J, Waters DD, et al: Unstable angina and progression of coronary atherosclerosis. *N Engl J Med* 1983; 309:685–689.
61. Ambrose JA, Winters SL, Arora RR, Eng A, Riccio A, Gorlin R, et al: Angiographic evolution of coronary artery morphology in unstable angina. *J Am Coll Cardiol* 1986; 7:472–478.
62. Mizuno K, Satomura K, Miyamoto A, Arakawa K, Shibuya T, Arai T, et al: Angioscopic evaluation of coronary-artery thrombi in acute coronary syndromes. *N Engl J Med* 1992; 326:287–291.
63. Pandian NG, Kreis A, Brockway B: Detection of intraarterial thrombus by intravascular high frequency two-dimensional ultrasound imaging in vitro and in vivo studies. *Am J Cardiol* 1990; 65:1280–1283.
64. Falk E: Unstable angina with fatal outcome: Dynamic coronary thrombosis leading to infarction and/or sudden death. Autopsy evidence of recurrent mural thrombosis with peripheral embolization culminating in total vascular occlusion. *Circulation* 1985; 50:127–134.
65. Davies MJ, Woolf N, Rowles PM, Peper J: Morphology of the endothelium over atherosclerotic plaques in human coronary arteries. *Br Heart J* 1988; 60:459–464.
66. Badimon L, Badimon JJ, Turrito VT, Vallabhajosula S, Fuster V: Platelet thrombus formation on collagen type I: A model of deep vessel injury: Influence of blood rheology, von Willebrand factor and blood coagulation. *Circulation* 1988; 78:1431–1442.
67. Francis CW, Markham RE Jr, Barlow GH, Florack TM, Dobrzynski DM, Marder VJ: Thrombin activity of fibrin thrombi and soluble plasmic derivatives. *J Lab Clin Med* 1983; 102:220–230.
68. Fuster V, Badimon L, Badimon JJ, Chesebro JH: Mechanisms of disease: The pathogenesis of coronary artery disease and the acute coronary syndromes. *N Engl J Med* 1992; 326:310–318.
69. Lam JYT, Chesebro JH, Steele PM, Badimon L, Fuster V: Is vasospasm related to platelet deposition? Relationship in a porcine preparation of arterial injury in vivo. *Circulation* 1987; 75:243–248.
70. Fuster V, Badimon L, Badimon JJ, Chesebro JH: The pathogenesis of coronary artery disease and the acute coronary syndromes. *N Engl J Med* 1992; 326:242–250.
71. Bertolasi CA, Tronge JE, Riccitelli MA, Villamayor RM, Zuffardi E: Natural history of unstable angina with medical or surgical treatment. *Chest* 1976; 70:596–605.
72. Plotnic GD, Conti DR: Unstable angina: Angiography, short and long term morbidity, mortality, and symptomatic status of medically treated patients. *Am J Med* 1977; 63:870–873.
73. Mulcahy R, Daly L, Graham L, Hickey N, O'Donoghue S, Owens A, et al: Unstable angina: Natural history and determinants of prognosis. *Am J Cardiol* 1981; 48:525–528.
74. Lewis HD, Davis JW, Archibald DG, Steinke WE, Smitherman TC, Doherty JE, et al: Protective effects of aspirin against myocardial infarction and death in men with unstable angina. *N Engl J Med* 1983; 309:396–403.
75. Cairns JA, Gent M, Singer J, Finnie KJ, Frogatt GM, Holder DA, et al: Aspirin, sulfinpyrazone, or both in unstable angina. *N Engl J Med* 1985; 313:1369–1375.
76. Théroux P, Ouimet H, McCans J, Latour JG, Joly P, Lévy G, et al: Aspirin, heparin, or both to treat acute unstable angina. *N Engl J Med* 1988; 319:1105–1111.
77. The RISC Group: Risk of myocardial infarction and death during treatment with low dose aspirin and intravenous heparin in men with unstable coronary disease. *Lancet* 1990; 336:827–830.
78. Balsano F, Rizzon P, Violi F, Scrutinio D, Cimminiello C, Aguglia F, et al: Antiplatelet treatment with ticlopidine in unstable angina. A controlled multicenter clinical trial. *Circulation* 1990; 82:17–26.
79. Théroux P, Ouimet H, Latour JG, McCans J, Pelletier GB, Juneau M, et al: Prediction and prevention of myocardial infarction during the acute phase of unstable angina (abstr). *J Am Coll Cardiol* 1989; 13:192A.
80. Olson HG, Lyons KP, Aronow WS, Stinson PJ, Kuperus J, Waters HJ: The high risk angina patient. Identification by clinical features, hospital course, electrocardiography and technetium-99m stannous pyrophosphate scintigraphy. *Circulation* 1981; 64:674–684.
81. Bosch X, Théroux P, Pelletier GB, Waters D: Clinical and angiographic features and prognostic significance of early postinfarction angina with and without electrocardiographic signs of transient ischemia. *Am J Med* 1991; 91:493–501.
82. Nademanee K, Intarachot V, Josephson MA, Rieders D, Vaghaiwalla F, Singh BN: Prognostic significance of silent ischemia in patients with unstable angina. *J Am Coll Cardiol* 1987; 10:1–9.
83. Langer A, Freeman MR, Armstrong PW: ST segment shift in unstable angina: Pathophysiology and association with coronary anatomy and hospital outcome. *J Am Coll Cardiol* 1989; 13:1495–1502.
84. Wilcox I, Freedman SB, Kelly DT, Harris PJ: Clinical significance of silent ischemia in unstable angina pectoris. *Am J Cardiol* 1990; 65:1313–1316.
85. Zhu YY, Chung WS, Botvinick EH, Dae MW, Lim AD, Ports TA, et al: Dipyridamole perfusion scintigraphy: The experience with the application in one hundred seventy patients with known or suspected unstable angina. *Am Heart J* 1991; 121:33–43.
86. Butman SM, Olson HG, Gardin JM, Piters KM, Hullett M, Butman LK: Submaximal exercise testing after stabilization of unstable angina pectoris. *J Am Coll Cardiol* 1984; 4:667–673.

87. Brown KA: Prognostic value of thallium-201 myocardial perfusion imaging in patients with unstable angina who respond to medical treatment. *J Am Coll Cardiol* 1991; 17:1053–1057.
88. Ouyang P, Brinker JA, Mellits ED, Weisfeldt ML, Gerstenblith G: Variables predictive of successful medical therapy in patients with unstable angina: Selection by multivariate analysis from clinical, electrocardiographic and angiographic evaluations. *Circulation* 1984; 70:367–376.
89. Alison HW, Russell RO, Mantle JA, Kouchoukos NT, Morashi RE, Rackley CE: Coronary anatomy and arteriography in patients with unstable angina pectoris. *Am J Cardiol* 1978; 41:204–209.
90. De Servi S, Berzuini C, Poma E, Fenario M, Ghio S, Scire A, et al: Long-term survival and risk stratification in patients with angina at rest undergoing medical treatment. *Int J Cardiol* 1989; 22:43–50.
91. Scott SM, Luchi RJ, Deupree RH, Veterans Administration Unstable Angina Cooperative Study Group: Veterans Administration Cooperative Study Group for treatment of patients with unstable angina. Results in patients with abnormal left ventricular function. *Circulation* 1988; 78(suppl I):I-113–I-121.
92. Russell RO, Moraski RE, Kouchoukos N, Karp R, Mantle JA, Rogers WJ, et al: Unstable angina pectoris: National Cooperative Study Group to compare surgical and medical therapy. II. In-hospital experience and initial follow-up results in patients with one, two and three vessel disease. *Am J Cardiol* 1978; 42:839–848.
93. Castaner A, Roig E, Serra A, De Flores T, Magrina J, Azqueta M, et al: Risk stratification and prognosis of patients with recent onset angina. *Eur Heart J* 1990; 11:868–875.
94. Bugiardini R, Pozzati A, Borghi A, Morgagni GL, Ottani F, Muzi A, Puddu P: Angiographic morphology in unstable angina and its relation to transient myocardial ischemia and hospital outcome. *Am J Cardiol* 1991; 67:460–464.
95. Folts JD, Crowell EB Jr, Rowe GG: Platelet aggregation in partially obstructed vessels and its elimination with aspirin. *Circulation* 1976; 54:365–370.
96. Telford AM, Wilson C: Trial of heparin versus atenolol in prevention of myocardial infarction in intermediate coronary syndrome. *Lancet* 1981; 1:1225–1228.
97. Neri-Serneri GG, Gensini GR, Poggesi L, Trotta F, Modesti PA, Boddi M, et al: Effect of heparin, aspirin or alteplase in reduction of myocardial ischemia in refractory unstable angina. *Lancet* 1990, 335:615–618.
98. Williams DO, Kirby MG, McPherson K, Phear DM: Anticoagulant treatment in unstable angina. *Br J Clin Pract* 1986; 40:114–116.
99. Lawrence JB, Sheperd JT, Bone I, Rogen AS, Fulton WFM: Fibrinolytic therapy in unstable angina pectoris—a controlled clinical trial. *Throm Res* 1990; 17:767–777.
100. Gold HK, Johns JA, Leinbach RC, Yasuda T, Grossbard E, Zusman R, et al: A randomized, placebo-controlled trial of recombinant human tissue–type plasminogen activator in patients with unstable angina pectoris. *Circulation* 1987; 75:1192–1199.
101. Nicklas JM, Topol EJ, Kander N, O'Neil WW, Walton JA, Ellis SG, et al: Randomized double-blind placebo-controlled trial of tissue plasminogen activator in unstable angina. *J Am Coll Cardiol* 1989; 13:434–441.
102. Ambrose JA, Hjemdahl-Monsen C, Borrico S, Sherman W, Cohen M, Gorlin R, et al: Quantitative and qualitative effects of intracoronary streptokinase in unstable angina and non-Q wave infarction. *J Am Coll Cardiol* 1987; 9:1156–1165.
103. Freeman MR, Langer A, Wilson RF, Morgan CD, Armstrong PW: Thrombolysis in unstable angina. Randomized double-blind trial of t-PA and placebo. *Circulation* 1992; 85:150–157.
104. Dauwe F, Affaki G, Waters DD, Théroux P, Mizgala HF: Intravenous nitroglycerin in refractory unstable angina (abstr). *Am J Cardiol* 1979; 43:416.
105. Kaplan K, Davison R, Parker M, Przybylek J, Teagarden JR, Lesch M: Intravenous nitroglycerin for the treatment of angina at rest unresponsive to standard nitrate therapy. *Am J Cardiol* 1983; 51:694–698.
106. Curfman GD, Heinsimer JA, Lozner EC, Fung HL: Intravenous nitroglycerin in the treatment of spontaneous angina pectoris: A prospective randomized trial. *Circulation* 1983; 67:276–282.
107. Palmer RMJ, Ferrige AG, Moncada S: Nitric oxide release accounts for the biologic activity of endothelium-derived relaxing factor. *Nature* 1987; 327:524–526.
108. Schafer AI, Alexander RW, Handin RI: Inhibition of platelet function by organic nitrate vasodilators. *Blood* 1980; 55:649–654.
109. Folts JD, Stamler J, Loscalzo J: Intravenous nitroglycerin infusion inhibits cyclic blood flow responses caused by periodic platelet thrombus formation in stenosed coronary canine arteries. *Circulation* 1991; 83:2122–2127.
110. Diodati J, Théroux P, Latour JG, Lacoste L, Lam JYT, Waters D: Effects of nitroglycerin at therapeutic doses on platelet aggregation in unstable angina pectoris and acute myocardial infarction. *Am J Cardiol* 1990; 66:683–687.
111. Yusuf S, Wittes J, Friedman L: Overview of results of randomized trials in heart disease. II. Unstable angina, heart failure, primary prevention with aspirin, and risk factor modification. *JAMA* 1988; 260:2259–2263.
112. Yusuf S, Ramsdale D, Peto R, Furse L, Bennett D, Bray C, et al: Early intravenous atenolol treatment in suspected acute myocardial infarction. *Lancet* 1980; 2:273–276.
113. Robertson RM, Wood AJJ, Vaughn WK, Robertson D: Exacerbation of vasotonic angina pectoris by propranolol. *Circulation* 1982; 65:281–285.
114. Muller JE, Turi ZG, Pearle DL, Schneider JF, Sekfas DH, Morison J: Nifedipine and conventional therapy for unstable angina pectoris: A randomized, double-blind comparison. *Circulation* 1984; 69:728–739.
115. Gerstenblith G, Ouyang P, Achuff SC, Bulkley BH, Becker LC, Mellits ED, et al: Nifedipine in unstable angina: A double-blind randomized trial. *N Engl J Med* 1982; 306:885–889.
116. Gottlieb SO, Weisfeldt ML, Ouyang P, Achuff SC, Baughman KL, Traill TA, et al: Effect of the addition of propranolol to therapy with nifedipine for unstable angina pectoris: A randomized, double-blind, placebo-controlled trial. *Circulation* 1986; 73:331–337.
117. Report of the Holland Interuniversity Nifedipine/Metoprolol Trial. Holland Interuniversity Nifedipine/Metoprolol Trial (HINT) Research Group: Early treatment of unstable angina in the coronary care unit: A randomized, double blind, placebo controlled comparison of recurrent ischemia in patients treated with nifedipine or metoprolol or both: Report of the Holland Interuniversity Nifedipine/Metoprolol Trial (HINT) Research Group. *Br Heart J* 1986; 56:400–413.
118. Théroux P, Taeymans Y, Morissette D, Bosch X, Pelletier GB, Waters DD: A randomized study comparing propranolol and diltiazem in the treatment of unstable angina. *J Am Coll Cardiol* 1985; 5:717–722.
119. Weintraub RM, Arvesty JM, Paulin S, Levine FH, Markis JE, LaRala PJ, et al: Medically refractory unstable angina. 1. Long-term follow-up of patients undergoing intra-aortic balloon counterpulsation and operation. *Am J Cardiol* 1979; 43:877–882.
120. Bonchek LI, Rahimtoola S, Anderson RP, McAnulty JA, Rosch J, Bristow JD, et al: Late results following emergency saphenous vein bypass grafting for unstable angina. *Circulation* 1974; 50:972–977.
121. Hultgren HN, Pfeifer JF, Angel WW, Lipton MJ, Bilisoly J: Unstable angina: Comparison of medical and surgical patients. *Am J Cardiol* 1977; 39:734–740.
122. Selden R, Neill WA, Rizmann LW, Okies JE, Anderson RP: Medical versus surgical therapy for acute coronary insufficiency: A randomized study. *N Engl J Med* 1975; 293:1329–1333.
123. Luchi RJ, Scott SM, Deupree RH, Principal Investigators and their Associates of Veterans Administration Cooperative Study No. 28: Comparison of medical and surgical treatment for unstable angina pectoris. *N Engl J Med* 1987; 316:977–984.
124. Booth DC, Deupree RH, Hultgren HM, De Maria AN, Scott SM, Luchi RJ, et al: Quality of life after bypass surgery for unstable angina. 5-year follow-up results of a Veterans Affairs Cooperative Study. *Circulation* 1991; 83:87–95.
125. Kaiser GC, Schaff HV, Killip T: Myocardial revascularization for unstable angina pectoris. *Circulation* 1989; 79(suppl I):I-60–I-67.
126. Rankin JS, Newton JR, Califf RM, Jones RH, Wechsler AS, Oldham N, et al: Clinical characteristics and current management of medically refractory unstable angina. *Ann Surg* 1984; 200:457–464.

127. Loop FD, Lytle BW, Cosgrove DM, Stewart RW, Goormastic M, Williams GW, et al: Influence of the internal-mammary-artery graft on 10-year survival and other cardiac events. *N Engl J Med* 1986; 314:1–6.
128. Dorros G, Cowley MJ, Simpson J, Bentivoglio LG, Block PC, Bourassa M, et al: Percutaneous transluminal coronary angioplasty: Report of complications from the National Heart, Lung, and Blood Institute PTCA Registry. *Circulation* 1983; 67:723–730.
129. de Feyter PJ, Suryapranata H, Serruys PW, Beatt K, van Domburg R, van den Brand M, et al: Coronary angioplasty for unstable angina: Immediate and late results in 200 consecutive patients with identification of risk factors for unfavorable early and late outcome. *J Am Coll Cardiol* 1988; 12:324–333.
130. Rupprecht HJ, Brennecke R, Koitmeyer M, Bernhard G, Erbel R, Pop T, et al: Short- and long-term outcome after PTCA in patients with stable and unstable angina. *Eur Heart J* 1990; 11:964–973.
131. Myler RK, Shaw RE, Stertzer SH, Bashover TT, Ryan C, Hecht HS, et al: Unstable angina and coronary angioplasty. *Circulation* 1990; 82(suppl II):II-88–II-95.
132. de Guise P, Théroux P, Bonan R, Lévy G, Côté G, Crépeau J: Rethrombosis after successful thrombolysis and angioplasty in acute myocardial infarction (abstr). *J Am Coll Cardiol* 1988; 11:192A.
133. Mabin TA, Holmes DR, Smith HC: Intracoronary thrombus: Role in coronary occlusion complicating percutaneous transluminal coronary angioplasty. *J Am Coll Cardiol* 1985; 5:198–202.
134. de Feyter PJ, Serruys PW, van den Brand M, Balakumaran K, Mochtar B, Soward AL, et al: Emergency coronary angioplasty in refractory unstable angina. *N Engl J Med* 1985; 313:342–346.
135. Lukas MA, Deutsch E, Hirshfeld JW Jr, Kussmaul WG, Barnathan E, Laskey WK: Influence of heparin therapy on percutaneous transluminal coronary angioplasty outcome in patients with coronary arterial thrombus. *Am J Cardiol* 1990; 65:179–182.
136. Suryapranata H, de Feyter PJ, Serruys PW: Coronary angioplasty in patients with unstable angina: Is there a role for thrombolysis. *J Am Coll Cardiol* 1988; 12:69A–77A.
137. Théroux P, Waters D, Lam J, Juneau M, McCans J: Reactivation of unstable angina following discontinuation of heparin. *N Engl J Med* 1992; 327:141–145.
138. Prinzmetal M, Kennamer R, Merliss R, Wada T, Bor N: Angina pectoris: I. A variant form of angina pectoris. *Am J Med* 1959; 27:375–388.
139. MacAlpin RN, Kattus AA, Alvaro AB: Angina pectoris at rest with preservation of exercise capacity. Prinzmetal's variant angina. *Circulation* 1973; 47:946–958.
140. Maseri A, Severi S, De Nes M, L'Abbate A, Chierchia S, Marzilli M, et al: "Variant" angina: One aspect of a continuous spectrum of vasospastic myocardial ischemia. *Am J Cardiol* 1978; 42:1019–1035.
141. Kushwaha S, Mitchell AG, Yacoub MH: Coronary artery spasm after cardiac transplantation. *Am J Cardiol* 1990; 65:1515–1518.
142. Chierchia S, Davies G, Berkenboom G, Crea F, Crean P, Maseri A: α-Adrenergic receptors and coronary spasm: An elusive link. *Circulation* 1984; 69:8–14.
143. Freedman SB, Chierchia S, Rodriguez-Plaza L, Bugiardini R, Smith G, Maseri A: Ergonovine-induced myocardial ischemia: No role for serotonergic receptors? *Circulation* 1984; 70:178–183.
144. Robertson RM, Robertson D, Roberts LJ, Maas RL, FitzGerald GA, Friesinger GC, et al: Thromboxane A_2 in vasotonic angina pectoris. Evidence from direct measurements and inhibitor trials. *N Engl J Med* 1981; 304:998–1003.
145. Chierchia S, Patrono C, Crea F, Ciabattoni G, De Caterina R, Cinotti GA, et al: Effects of intravenous prostacyclin in variant angina. *Circulation* 1982; 65:470–477.
146. Roberts WC, Curry RC Jr, Isner JM, Waller BF, McManus BM, Mariani-Constantini R, et al: Sudden death in Prinzmetal's angina with coronary spasm documented by angiography. Analysis of three necropsy patients. *Am J Cardiol* 1982; 50:203–210.
147. Kaski JC, Tousoulis D, Gavrielides S, McFadden E, Galassi AR, Crea F, et al: Comparison of epicardial coronary artery tone and reactivity in Prinzmetal's variant angina and chronic stable angina pectoris. *J Am Coll Cardiol* 1991; 17:1058–1062.
148. Irie T, Imaizumi T, Matuguchi T, Koyanagi S, Kanaide H, Takeshita A, et al: Increased fibrinopeptide A during anginal attacks in patients with variant angina. *J Am Coll Cardiol* 1989; 14:589–594.
149. Waters DD, Szlachcic J, Bourassa MG, Scholl JM, Théroux P: Exercise testing in patients with variant angina: Results, correlation with clinical and angiographic features and prognostic significance. *Circulation* 1982; 65:265–274.
150. Koiwaya Y, Torii S, Takeshita A, Nakagaki O, Nakamura M: Postinfarction angina caused by coronary arterial spasm. *Circulation* 1982; 65:275–280.
151. Waters DD, Théroux P, Crittin J, Dauwe F, Mizgala HF: Previously undiagnosed variant angina as a cause of chest pain after coronary artery bypass surgery. *Circulation* 1980; 61:1159–1164.
152. David PR, Waters DD, Scholl JM, Crépeau J, Szlachcic J, Lespérance J, et al: Percutaneous transluminal coronary angioplasty in patients with variant angina. *Circulation* 1982; 66:695–702.
153. Scholl JM, Benacerraf A, Ducimetiere P, Chabas D, Brau J, Chapelle J, et al: Comparison of risk factors in vasospastic angina without significant fixed coronary narrowing to significant fixed coronary narrowing and no vasospastic angina. *Am J Cardiol* 1986; 57:199–202.
154. Miller D, Waters DD, Warnica W, Szlachcic J, Kreeft J, Théroux P: Is variant angina the coronary manifestation of a generalized vasospastic disorder? *N Engl J Med* 1981; 304:763–766.
155. Miller DD, Waters DD, Szlachcic J, Théroux P: Clinical characteristics associated with sudden death in patients with variant angina. *Circulation* 1982; 66:588–592.
156. Waters DD, Szlachcic J, Bonan R, Miller DD, Dauwe F, Théroux P: Comparative sensitivity of exercise, cold pressor and ergonovine testing in provoking attacks of variant angina in patients with active disease. *Circulation* 1983; 67:310–315.
157. Okumura K, Yasue H, Matsuyama K, Matsuyama K, Morikami Y, et al: Effect of H1 receptor stimulation on coronary artery diameter in patients with variant angina: Comparison with effect of acetylcholine. *J Am Coll Cardiol* 1991; 17:338–345.
158. Crea F, Chierchia S, Kaski JC, Davies GJ, Margonato A, Miran DO, et al: Provocation of coronary spasm by dopamine in patients with active variant angina pectoris. *Circulation* 1986; 74:262–269.
159. Okumura K, Yasue H, Matsuyama K, Goto K, Miyagi H, Ogawa H, et al: Sensitivity and specificity of intracoronary injection of acetylcholine for the induction of coronary artery spasm. *J Am Coll Cardiol* 1988; 12:883–888.
160. Heupler FA Jr, Proudfit WL, Razavi M, Shirey EK, Greenstreet R, Sheldon WC: Ergonovine maleate provocative test for coronary arterial spasm. *Am J Cardiol* 1978; 41:631–640.
161. Crea F, Davies G, Romeo F, Chierchia S, Bugiardini R, Kaski JC, et al: Myocardial ischemia during ergonovine testing: Different susceptibility to coronary vasoconstriction in patients with exertional and variant angina. *Circulation* 1984; 69:690–695.
162. Bertrand ME, LaBlanche JM, Tilmant PY, Thieuleux FA, Delforge MR, Carre AG, et al: Frequency of provoked coronary arterial spasm in 1089 consecutive patients undergoing coronary arteriography. *Circulation* 1982; 65:1299–1306.
163. Buxton A, Goldberg S, Hirshfeld JW, Wilson J, Mann T, Williams DO, et al: Refractory ergonovine-induced coronary vasospasm: Importance of intracoronary nitroglycerin. *Am J Cardiol* 1980; 46:329–334.
164. Waters DD, Théroux P, Szlachcic J, Dauwe F, Crittin J, Bonan R, et al: Ergonovine testing in a coronary care unit. *Am J Cardiol* 1980; 46:922–930.
165. Ginsburg R, Lamb IH, Bristow MR, Schneder JS, Harrison DC: Application and safety of outpatient ergonovine testing in accurately detecting coronary spasm in patients with possible variant angina. *Am Heart J* 1981; 102:698–702.
166. Waters DD, Théroux P, Szlachcic J, Dauwe F: Provocative testing with ergonovine to assess the efficacy of treatment with nifedipine, diltiazem and verapamil in variant angina. *Am J Cardiol* 1981; 48:123–130.
167. Waters DD, Szlachcic J, Théroux P, Dauwe F, Mizgala HF: Ergonovine testing to detect spontaneous remissions of variant angina during long-term treatment with calcium antagonist drugs. *Am J Cardiol* 1981; 47:179–184.
168. Waters DD, Bouchard A, Théroux P: Spontaneous remission is

a frequent outcome of variant angina. *J Am Coll Cardiol* 1983; 2:195–199.
169. Previtali M, Panciroli C, Ardissino D, Chimienti M, Angoli L, Salerno JA: Spontaneous remission of variant angina documented by Holter monitoring and ergonovine testing in patients treated with calcium antagonists. *Am J Cardiol* 1987; 59:235–240.
170. Walling A, Waters DD, Miller DD, Roy D, Pelletier GB, Théroux P: Long-term prognosis of patients with variant angina. *Circulation* 1987; 76:990–997.
171. Tilmant PY, Lablanche JM, Thieuleux FA, Dupuis BA, Bertrand ME: Detrimental effect of propranolol in patients with coronary arterial spasm countered by combination with diltiazem. *Am J Cardiol* 1983; 52:230–233.
172. Morikami Y, Yasue H: Efficacy of slow-release nifedipine on myocardial ischemic episodes in variant angina pectoris. *Am J Cardiol* 1991; 68:580–584.
173. Pepine CJ, Feldman RL, Whittle J, Curry C, Conti CR: Effect of diltiazem in patients with variant angina: A randomized double-blind trial. *Am Heart J* 1981; 101:719–725.
174. Johnson SM, Mauritson DR, Willerson JT, Hillis LD: A controlled clinical trial of verapamil for Prinzmetal's variant angina. *N Engl J Med* 1981; 304:862–866.
175. Yasue H, Takizawa A, Nagao M, Nishida S, Horie M, Kubota J, et al: Long-term prognosis for patients with variant angina and influential factors. *Circulation* 1988; 78:1–9.
176. Rutitzky B, Girotti AL, Rosenbaum MB: Efficacy of chronic amiodarone therapy in patients with variant angina pectoris and inhibition of ergonovine coronary constriction. *Am Heart J* 1982; 103:38–43.
177. Frenneaux M, Kaski JC, Brown M, Maseri A: Refractory variant angina relieved by guanethidine and clonidine. *Am J Cardiol* 1988; 62:832–833.
178. Miwa K, Kambara H, Kawai C: Exercise-induced angina provoked by aspirin administration in patients with variant angina. *Am J Cardiol* 1981; 47:1210–1214.
179. Mark DB, Califf RM, Morris KG, Harrell FE Jr, Pryor DB, Hlatky MA, et al: Clinical characteristics and long-term survival of patients with variant angina. *Circulation* 1984; 69:880–888.
180. Shubrooks SJ Jr, Bete JM, Hutter AM Jr, Block PC, Buckley MJ, Daggett WM, et al: Variant angina pectoris: Clinical and anatomic spectrum and results of coronary bypass surgery. *Am J Cardiol* 1975; 36:142–147.
181. Bertrand ME, Lablanche JM, Tilmant PY: Treatment of Prinzmetal's variant angina. Role of medical treatment with nifedipine and surgical coronary revascularization combined with plexectomy. *Am J Cardiol* 1981; 47:174–178.
182. Bertrand ME, Lablanche JM, Tilmant PY, Ducloux G, Warembourg H Jr, Soots G: Complete denervation of the heart (autotransplantation) for treatment of severe, refractory coronary spasm. *Am J Cardiol* 1981; 47:1375–1378.
183. Leisch F, Schützenberger W, Kerschner K, Herbinger W: Influence of a variant angina on the results of percutaneous transluminal coronary angioplasty. *Br Heart J* 1986; 56:341–345.
184. Bertrand ME, Lablanche JM, Thieuleux FA, Fourrier JL, Traisnel G, Asseman P: Comparative results of percutaneous transluminal coronary angioplasty in patients with dynamic versus fixed coronary stenosis. *J Am Coll Cardiol* 1986; 8:504–508.
185. Bertrand ME, Lablanche JM, Fourrier JL, Gommeaux A, Ruel M: Relation to restenosis after percutaneous transluminal coronary angioplasty to vasomotion of the dilated coronary arterial segment. *Am J Cardiol* 1989; 63:277–281.
186. Severi S, Davies G, Maseri A, Marzullo P, L'Abbate A: Long-term prognosis of "variant" angina with medical treatment. *Am J Cardiol* 1980; 46:226–232.
187. Nakamura M, Takeshita A, Nose Y: Clinical characteristics associated with myocardial infarction, arrhythmias, and sudden death in patients with vasospastic angina. *Circulation* 1987; 75:1110–1116.
188. Waters DD, Szlachcic J, Miller D, Théroux P: Clinical characteristics of patients with variant angina complicated by myocardial infarction or death within 1 month. *Am J Cardiol* 1982; 49:658–664.

Chapter 60

Pathophysiology, Recognition, and Treatment of Acute Myocardial Infarction and its Complications

Robert Roberts, M.D. ■ *Doug Morris, M.D.*
Craig M. Pratt, M.D. ■ *R. Wayne Alexander, M.D., Ph.D.*

This section provides overview of important issues concerning myocardial infarction. The pathophysiological processes contributing to the pathogenesis of myocardial infarction have been described elsewhere: hyperlipidemia (Chapter 53), atherosclerosis (Chapter 55), endothelial dysfunction (Chapter 54 and 56), thrombosis (Chapter 7), and decreasing coronary flow (Chapter 57).

The following are important general facts about myocardial infarction:

1. The major cause of myocardial infarction is atherosclerotic coronary artery disease, which contributes to hemodynamically significant narrowing of the artery lumen, disordered control of vasomotor tone, and a propensity for plaque disruption and thrombus formation.
2. Myocardial ischemia or infarction is a segmental disease with a focal occlusion of only one of the three large coronary vessels or branches during any particular event. The resulting impaired contractility occurs within seconds and is initially restricted to the affected segment.
3. Myocardial ischemia and/or subsequent infarction usually begins in the endocardium and spreads toward the epicardium.
4. Irreversible cardiac injury occurs if occlusion is complete for at least 15 to 20 min. Irreversible injury occurs maximally in the area at risk and when occlusion is sustained for 4 to 6 h, but most of the damage occurs in the first 2 to 3 h. Thus, restoration of flow within the first 4 to 6 h is associated with salvage of myocardium, but the salvage is exponentially greater if restoration occurs in 1 to 2 h.
5. The percentage of the tissue at risk that undergoes necrosis (infarct size) depends on existing collateral flow, which is highly variable and difficult to predict.
6. A major determinant of mortality and morbidity is the extent of myocardial damage (infarct size). The temporal evolution of myocardial necrosis and the resulting extent of damage are influenced by factors that alter myocardial oxygen supply and demand. An increase in myocardial oxygen demand during evolution appears to increase infarct size, while a decrease in myocardial oxygen demand tends to decrease infarct size. Decreased oxygen demand, however, is much less effective in salvaging myocardium already at risk than is increased oxygen supply by coronary reperfusion.
7. The onset of acute Q-wave myocardial infarction occurs commonly in the morning hours soon after arising, a period of increasing adrenergic activity, increased plasma fibrinogen levels, and increased platelet adhesiveness. Non-Q-wave infarction does not exhibit this circadian rhythm.
8. Until a decade ago, myocardial infarction was con-

sidered primarily a disease of the left ventricle. Today it is recognized that right ventricular infarction is frequently associated with inferior infarction.

9. With their initial myocardial infarction, more than half of all patients have significant obstructive atherosclerosis in only one vessel. This fact emphasizes the potential for secondary prevention.
10. Coronary thrombosis undergoes spontaneous lysis, even if untreated, in about 50 percent of cases within 10 days. Patients who exhibit minimal myocardial damage may have experienced early spontaneous lysis, which may account for many cases of non-Q-wave infarction.
11. Q-wave and non-Q-wave infarctions have distinctly different short-term prognoses. When untreated, Q-wave infarction is associated with a high in-hospital mortality rate and a highly vulnerable period of 6 to 12 weeks. In contrast, non-Q-wave infarction is associated with a lower acute mortality and complication rate but a longer period of vulnerability to death and reinfarction. As a result, 1- to 2-year survival rates are similar to those for Q-wave infarction. Thus, there is significant potential for prevention of death and morbidity after non-Q-wave infarction. The prognosis of Q-wave infarction following thrombolysis, however, appears to be different than in the era prior to thrombolytic therapy. The vulnerable period appears to be shorter if the artery is opened by thrombolysis with or without angioplasty, particularly in patients with subsequent ischemia who undergo angioplasty. (See also Chap. 57.)

In addition to thrombosis superimposed on atherosclerosis, several other causes may induce coronary obstruction (see also Chap. 64.) Thrombus formation in an otherwise normal coronary artery has been associated with use of the birth control pill. Spontaneous coronary dissection, aortic dissection, emboli, congenital coronary anomalies, metabolic abnormalities, blunt chest or penetrating trauma, vasculitides, and, increasingly, drug abuse, particularly cocaine abuse, are nonatherosclerotic causes of myocardial infarction (see Chap. 64). Cocaine probably induces coronary occlusion by vasoconstriction and thrombus formation (see Chap. 110). The cocaine-induced increase in myocardial oxygen demand due to tachycardia and increased blood pressure enhances the potential for cell death. Coronary spasm in the absence of demonstrable atherosclerosis as a cause of myocardial infarction is more common in Japan than in North America.

PATHOGENESIS OF CORONARY OCCLUSION

Occlusive thrombosis on a coronary artery atheromatous plaque is the usual reason for myocardial infarction. The reasons for thrombus formation are incompletely understood (see Chaps. 55 and 56). In many patients, postmortem analysis shows a thrombus overlying a ruptured plaque.[1,2] In addition to the propensity for plaque rupture, the atheroma induces other conditions that favor thrombosis. Vasospasm due, at least in part, to loss of endothelium-dependent dilator mechanisms in atherosclerosis may predispose to thrombus formation.[3–6] Thrombosis and acute myocardial infarction have been observed in the setting of vasospasm, defined by persistently abnormal ergonovine test results with nearly normal coronary arteries, as determined by angiographic studies.[7] Synthesis of endothelial factors that act as anticoagulants, such as tissue plasminogen activator[8] and prostacyclin,[9] is also significantly decreased by atherosclerosis. Thus, the vasoconstriction and increased thrombogenicity of the lesion surface predispose the patient to decreased coronary flow and to thrombus formation.[10] Acute vasoconstriction may also induce plaque rupture. Once thrombus formation is initiated, activation of platelets releases substances, such as thromboxane A_2 and serotonin, that induce vasoconstriction and further platelet aggregation.[11] Recent studies have also suggested a potential causal link between lipoproteins and thrombosis.[12,13] Elevated plasma levels of lipoprotein (a) [Lp(a)], a complex of apoB-100 protein bound to apo(a) by a disulfide bridge, is a coronary risk factor. There is a 96 percent homology between the amino acid sequence of Lp(a) and plasminogen in the protease-serine domain. Lp(a) has been shown to bind to plasminogen and fibrinogen. Fatty streaks and atheroma removed from the vessels of humans contain fibrin and plasminogen. Lp(a), by binding to plasminogen, inhibits activation by the naturally secreted tPA and as such inhibits or attenuates clot lysis. The clinical relevance of this hypothesis is under investigation.

PATHOPHYSIOLOGY OF MYOCARDIAL ISCHEMIA AND INFARCTION

Experimental and Clinical Syndromes Following Coronary Occlusion

The consequences of coronary occlusion are determined by the degree and duration of occlusion (Fig. 60-1). The clinically relevant consequences include transient ischemia, myocardial stunning, myocardial hibernation, necrosis, and reperfusion necrosis. There is an almost linear relationship between the percentage decrease in regional myocardial perfusion and in regional function as reflected by a decrease in ventricular wall thickening. A decrease in myocardial perfusion of 80 percent is associated with complete cessation of function with no wall thickening or shortening. If perfusion is reduced further (90 percent), dyskinesis or systolic bulging occurs. Sudden, complete occlusion of the coronary artery for 15 to 20 min or less, as may occur with unstable angina, is associated with impaired regional myocardial function due to *myocardial ischemia.* Restoration of coronary flow within this interval is associated with no irreversible injury, but there is reversible impairment of ventricular function, which may require hours or days to recover and is referred to as *myocardial stunning* or *postischemic dysfunction.* Complete coronary occlusion lasting beyond 20 min is generally associated with *necrosis* (myocardial infarction) despite restoration of flow; however, the surrounding ischemic but viable myocardium may

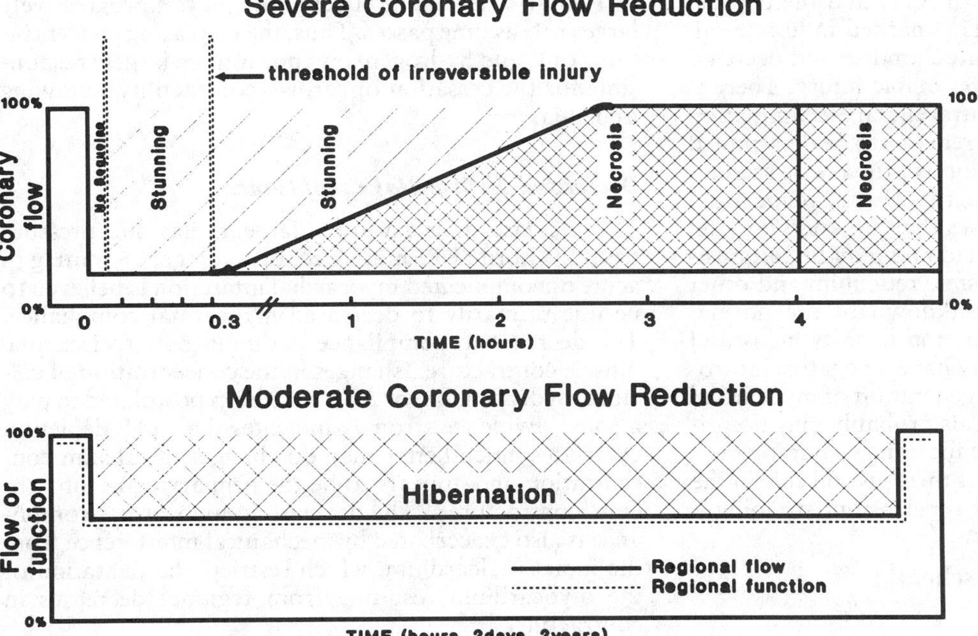

FIGURE 60-1 Illustrated here is the spectrum of consequences for the myocardium resulting from alteration in coronary flow. In the *top panel*, a severe reduction in flow for 2 to 3 min is associated with no alteration in function. A severe reduction in flow for up to 20 min is associated with no irreversible injury but is associated with reversible impaired ventricular function (stunning) that requires hours to days for full recovery. Severe reduction of flow after 20 min is associated with some degree of irreversible injury and the surrounding surviving myocardium exhibits varying degrees of stunning. Sustained moderate reduction of coronary flow is associated with downregulation of function but no irreversible injury either during the reduction or following restoration of flow (hibernation) (*lower panel*).

exhibit stunning. Restoration of flow within 6 h of the onset of occlusion is associated with *significant salvage of myocardium*. Restoration of flow after 6 h is usually too late to salvage myocardium in experimental models, and whether or not late opening of the vessel provides some long-term protective effect remains to be determined.

Reduction in coronary flow to 30 to 40 percent below normal induces the myocardial region to decrease or cease contractions so that the energy stores are adequate to maintain survival of the myocardium. When coronary blood flow is chronically limited, myocardial contractility may be diminished; the resultant state is referred to as *myocardial hibernation. Reperfusion necrosis* is postulated to occur as a result of reperfusion. Thus, while early restoration of flow is associated with significant salvage of ischemic myocardium, the actual extent of salvage may be somewhat less than maximal because of necrosis induced by the reperfusion per se. The issue of whether or not reperfusion necrosis is important remains controversial, both experimentally and clinically. Extensive experimental studies together with the results of thrombolytic therapy in humans indicate that reperfusion necrosis, if it does occur, is probably minimal and of questionable consequence.

Metabolic Consequences of Myocardial Ischemia

The heart is an aerobic organ and gets most of its energy from oxidative phosphorylation of fatty acids (see Chap. 6A).[14] Glucose is also utilized for energy, especially under anaerobic conditions such as ischemia. The heart can also use other carbohydrates, such as glycogen, lactic acids, pyruvate, and, under severe conditions, amino acids. Following coronary occlusion, myocardial oxygen tension drops to zero within seconds, and there is a rapid shift to anaerobic metabolism. The labile form of high-energy phosphate, adenosine triphosphate (ATP), and the energy storage form of phosphate, creatine phosphate (CP), are depleted in minutes.[14a] Lactic acid accumulates, and the resulting decreased pH stimulates glycolysis by its effect on the rate-limiting enzyme phosphofructokinase; however, marked increases in hydrogen ion concentration inhibit this enzyme and glycolysis (see also Chap. 6A).

Following coronary artery occlusion, ventricular function in the ischemic area is impaired within a few seconds and is completely reversible if flow is promptly restored.[15,16] This initial sudden dysfunction occurs before the depletion of the high-energy phosphates and appears to be mediated via ionic change, such as alteration of calcium homeostasis, although the mechanism is not precisely known. A mechanical decrease in sarcomere length with a reduction in coronary perfusion pressure (the "garden hose effect") may also contribute to the dysfunction.[14b] In the early minutes of ischemia, creatine phosphate is depleted at a more rapid rate than is ATP, which indicates that ATP is replenished from creatine phosphate stores. If ischemia is reversed in the first 10 to 15 min, all alterations in the biochemical processes and myocardial function are fully reversible, although it may take several hours for contractility to return fully to normal. If ischemia is prolonged, however, irreversible damage occurs despite subsequent restoration of coronary perfusion. Irreversible injury is characterized by structural alterations, including marked glycogen depletion, diffuse mitochondrial swelling, accumulation of amorphous densities in the mitochondria, peripheral aggregation of nuclear chromatin, and loss of cellular integrity, manifested by small breaks in the cytoplasmic membrane and in membranes of intracellular organelles (see Chap. 55).

The factors that make injury irreversible are unknown. Potential causes include the accumulation of lactic acid, the marked depletion of ATP, and the net loss of total adenine nucleotides! The marked influx of calcium ions may overload the mitochondria and decrease ATP production, leading to irreversible injury. There is extensive evidence showing intracellular accumulation of calcium with necrosis, but it remains to be determined whether or not this accumulation is primary or secondary to loss of cell membrane integrity. During myocardial ischemia, various phospholipases that are known to degrade phospholipids are activated and may be responsible for disrupting the sarcoplasmic reticulum and other membranes, resulting in a breakdown of the normal barriers. There is also accumulation of fatty acids and phosphatidylcholine, which may have a negative inotropic effect and play a role in the generation of myocardial arrhythmias. Oxygen free radicals probably play no primary role in irreversible ischemic injury, but there is considerable evidence to support their pivotal role in the reversible injury observed after reperfusion (stunning).

Hemodynamic Sequelae of Ischemia and Its Molecular Basis

The functional effects of ischemia on the performance of the heart are that (1) the contractile force decreases within seconds and practically ceases within 10 min; (2) the diastolic intracavitary pressure increases gradually, due primarily to impaired relaxation, decreased myocardial compliance, or ischemic contracture; and (3) electrophysiological abnormalities develop that impair conduction and induce arrhythmias.

Decreased Systolic Contraction

As noted, impairment of calcium homeostasis has been implicated for many years in the sudden decrease in contractility induced by ischemia.[17] With the onset of myocardial ischemia, there is an increase in the calcium influx during systole, and the overall calcium transient reaches a maximum in 15 to 30 min. Following this, there is a progressive shortening of the action potential with a decline in the intracellular concentration of calcium during systole and eventual cessation of the calcium transient. In contrast, there is a slow, gradual rise in intracellular calcium levels during diastole which continues beyond the evolution of the increase in systolic calcium. The initial increase in the concentration of calcium during systole may be accentuated by the increasing acidosis.[18,19] Thus, the early decrease in the force of contraction induced by ischemia is not due to a reduction in the calcium transient, nor is it due to inadequate levels of ATP, since concentrations appear to be adequate.[20,21] Moreover, acidosis could only account for a small fraction of the early decrease in force.[22] The most likely explanation for the immediate decrease in contractility is the significant increase in intracellular inorganic phosphate (P_i), which occurs due to phosphocreatine breakdown[23,24] together with the small contribution from the intracellular increase in hydrogen ions.[25] In vitro studies have shown that P_i, normally present at about a 2 m*M* concentration, can increase during ischemia to 15 to 16 m*M* in association with a 50 to 80 percent reduction in contractile force.[23] The effect of P_i is greater in the initial 5 to 10 min, whereas the effect of pH plays a progressively larger role as time passes. Thus, the increasing concentrations of P_i and hydrogen ion appear to be largely responsible for the cessation of cardiac contractility following ischemia.[23,24,26]

Decreased Myocardial Compliance

The increase in left ventricular end-diastolic pressure from the normal 12 mmHg to, on average, 16 mmHg in acute uncomplicated myocardial infarction is believed to be due primarily to decreased myocardial compliance. The decrease in compliance is due in part to ischemic muscle contracture. Changes in the concentration of calcium, hydrogen ion, or ATP have been postulated to play a role.[17] Evidence strongly indicates that ATP depletion correlates much better than do changes in calcium concentration and appears to be the primary cause of ischemic contracture.[21] The decrease in myocardial compliance is also exacerbated by mechanical interference from the intact pericardium, which restricts the dilatation of the myocardium resulting from regional decreases in contractility.[27,28]

Development of Arrhythmias

Ischemia is a major cause of ventricular arrhythmias that can lead to ventricular fibrillation and death. The electrophysiological changes associated with ischemia are (1) shortening of the action potential, (2) depolarization of the resting potential, (3) slowing of the rate of initial depolarization, and (4) impaired conduction.[29] The molecular and/or cellular mechanisms involve potassium and calcium ions.[30] The onset of myocardial ischemia is associated with a large increase in extracellular potassium levels due to an efflux of potassium, partly because of the loss of inhibition of the ATP-sensitive potassium channel.[31,32] Arrhythmias develop from either automaticity from a single focus or reentry. Elevated extracellular potassium levels induce resting depolarization, which, in turn, inactivates the Na^+ channel and contributes to the reduced rate of rise of the action potential, slowing conduction and facilitating reentry arrhythmias.[33] The current between the normal and the potassium-depolarized region can lead to automaticity in the normal region.[34] Both of these mechanisms can be induced by decreased intracellular potassium levels. The temporal increase in calcium transient may in part be responsible for the onset of early ventricular arrhythmias.[35] Recently, reperfusion has been shown to be associated with the onset of arrhythmias, which is also correlated with an increased influx of calcium into the ischemic cell.[36] The evidence for calcium as a precipitant of arrhythmias is further supported by the observation that pretreatment with calcium channel blockers attenuates the arrhythmia response to reperfusion. Depletion of myocardial magnesium, which is known to occur with ischemia, and elevated levels of circulating catecholamines and free fatty acids may also be involved in the genesis of arrhythmias (see also Chap. 35).

Subsequent to myocardial injury from ischemia, there is loss of membrane integrity and breakdown of phospholipids with release of lysophospholipids such as lysophosphatidylcholine (LPC). LPC generates ventricular arrhythmias in vitro and in vivo and is postulated to play a pivotal role in the genesis of ischemic arrhythmias.[37–39]

Irreversible Myocardial Injury

Irreversible necrosis may occur after 20 to 30 min of ischemia, spreading from the endocardium to the epicardium (see Chap. 57). If complete coronary occlusion is sustained for 6 to 8 h in experimental models, a variable amount of up to 70 to 80 percent of the area at risk will undergo necrosis, depending on the coronary collateral flow.[40] The mortality, morbidity, and overall quality of life and residual impairment of the patient with myocardial infarction are heavily determined by the extent of myocardial damage.[41,42] Infarction of more than 40 to 45 percent of the left ventricle is likely to be associated with death, whereas 5 to 10 percent damage is associated with very little functional impairment following the healing phase.[43–45] Patients with 25 percent or more involvement of the ventricle who survive are likely to have residual impairment of cardiac performance and will develop cardiac failure.

Myocardial Stunning

Reduction of coronary flow induces myocardial dysfunction, the nature and severity of which is related to the extent and duration of the reduction. Occlusion of a coronary artery for at least 2 min and up to a maximum of 15 to 20 min followed by restoration of flow results in impaired ventricular function that may require up to 24 to 48 h of reperfusion to recover.[46–49] The duration of the return of function is related to the duration of ischemia and the severity of the perfusion deficit, which is related to collateral flow.[50]

While myocardial stunning is not associated with irreversible morphologic changes, biochemically it is associated with a reduction in ATP and CP. Restoration of flow is associated with an immediate increase in CP to levels slightly above normal, while the return of ATP to normal requires several days.[51–53] The total adenine nucleotide pool is significantly depressed and requires several days to return to normal,[54,55] but depressed levels of high-energy phosphate are not the mechanism responsible for stunning.[49,56,57] Other suggested mechanisms have been alterations in sarcoplasmic calcium ATPase[58] or calcium metabolism.[59,60] In addition to the changes in nucleotide levels, there is an up-regulation of several genes, including that for heat shock protein following transient ischemia and reperfusion.[61–63] It is possible that recovery of contractile function is delayed because of the slow resynthesis of proteins damaged during acute ischemia and/or reperfusion. A likely mechanism is related to the generation of oxygen free radicals. Reaction of a radical with, for example, fatty acids in a lipid membrane may produce another free radical, which may result in a chain reaction. The major oxygen radicals consist of superoxide ($O_2\cdot$) and the hydroxyl ($OH\cdot$) radicals. Normally, oxygen undergoes reduction to water via the cytochrome c chain in the mitochondria, with less than 5 percent resulting in oxygen free radical formation. This leakage of 5 percent is eliminated by the body's scavengers, primarily superoxide dismutase, catalase, and glutathione peroxidase.[64] It is postulated that, upon reperfusion, there is saturation of the normal scavenger mechanisms, with the result that the excess oxygen generates a massive burst of oxygen free radicals, as observed in experimental studies.[65–67] Oxygen free radicals are minimally present during the ischemic phase but undergo an abrupt, marked increase upon reperfusion.[68,69] Experimentally, recovery is enhanced by free radical scavenging agents such as superoxide dismutase and catalase,[59,70,71] *N*-2-mercaptopropionylglycine,[65,72] and dimethylthiourea[73] or by agents preventing free radical generation, such as allopurinol,[74] oxypurinol,[75] and desferrioxamine.[76] Such a protective effect has also been shown in conscious animals.[77–79] The actual mechanism whereby oxygen free radicals induce ventricular dysfunction remains unknown, but possibly peroxidation of unsaturated fatty acids of the sarcolemma membrane or that of intracellular organelles is involved and requires hours to days to be repaired.[80,81] Other proposed mechanisms of myocardial stunning include excess accumulation of calcium, decreased sensitivity of the myofibrils to calcium, and impaired release of calcium by the sarcoplasmic reticulum.[82] There is also some evidence of impairment in substrate utilization and availability.[83,84] It appears from available data that free radicals play a prominent role in this impairment, but the cause is probably multifactorial.

Several studies have shown delay in return of regional myocardial function to normal levels following prolonged periods of ischemia in humans[85–87] after cardiac surgery, cardiac transplantation, and myocardial infarction.[88,89] Exercise-induced ischemia in humans may also be associated with stunning.[90,91] The recognition of the existence of stunning of viable myocardium in association with infarction dictates caution in making a final assessment of ventricular function until there is complete recovery. The role of free radical scavengers in attenuating stunning in humans has yet to be properly evaluated.

Myocardial Hibernation

Hibernating myocardium manifests as a persistent contractile dysfunction, due to reduced coronary flow, that can be completely reversed by restoring perfusion.[92,93] The presumption is that coronary flow is decreased to the point where the myocardium down-regulates contraction to match its blood supply in order to survive. There is an almost linear relationship between the decrease in coronary flow and the corresponding decrease in ventricular function. Reduction of coronary flow to about 20 percent of normal base-line values is associated with complete cessation of contractile function with absence of wall thickening or shortening.[94–97] Moreover, if flow is reduced to about 5 percent of normal, dyskinesis and wall thinning occur.[98] Only about 15 to 20 percent of the normal perfusion is necessary to prevent myocardial necrosis.[87] The term "hibernating myocardium" implies that mechanical function will return to normal when adequate perfusion is restored. "Hibernation" was first used by Rahimtoola to indicate impaired ventricular function without overt clinical evidence of ischemia that was reversed by coronary bypass surgery.[93,99] There are several reports of hibernating myocardium occurring in patients[100–107] in whom depressed regional myocardium had persisted for what was estimated to be several months or even years. Whether depressed ventricular function results from decreased flow (hibernation) or from necrosis is clinically significant, since revascularization may restore contraction to hibernating myocardium. Distinguishing hibernating from stunned myocardium may be difficult. Positive emission tomography (PET) scanning (Chap. 137) and nuclear scintigraphy (Chap. 134) may be useful in this regard.

Reperfusion Injury

Initial animal studies established that reperfusion following prolonged periods of coronary occlusion was associated with significant salvage of ischemic myocardium.[108–110] These findings have been confirmed in animals and humans with thrombolytic therapy and have been extensively reviewed.[111,112] Further investigations, however, have raised questions about possible deleterious effects of reperfusion, such as myocardial hemorrhaging,[113–115] the "no-reflow" phenomenon,[116] and myocardial stunning, as discussed. Myocardial hemorrhage after reperfusion refers to exudation of red blood cells and contracture necrosis. Most of the reperfusion hemorrhage, however, occurs in the area undergoing necrosis and thus may not contribute to further irreversible injury.[117,118] The "no-reflow" phenomenon is a lack of perfusion despite restoration of flow in the conductance artery. Platelet thrombi, vasoconstriction, and leukocyte aggregates that temporarily block the arterioles are implicated.[119] Several experimental studies have suggested that reperfusion did not salvage the anticipated amount of myocardium because of some small component of necrosis induced by reperfusion itself.[120–124] Initial studies with oxygen free radical scavenger and reperfusion[125–127] showed enhanced salvage of myocardium. Subsequent studies in the conscious dog from several laboratories consistently showed no effect of the radical scavengers on infarct size after reperfusions.[75,128–130] Thus, it would appear that reperfusion injury is probably minimal (10 to 15 percent) and less than originally thought. Any such effect would not be detectable clinically. Whether or not reperfusion necrosis occurs and to what extent remains to be determined (see also Chap. 57).

Preconditioning is another response of the myocardium to interruption of the blood supply. In animals, repeated brief interruption of coronary blood flow prior to prolonged occlusion is associated with less myocardial damage than when occlusion is not preceeded by the brief conditioning occlusions. This phenomenon is discussed in more detail in Chap. 58.

Hyperfunctioning Myocardium and Compensatory Growth

Following myocardial infarction, the surrounding intact myocardium almost always exhibits increased contractility.[131–134] The compensatory hyperfunction in surrounding tissue is usually observed transiently within seconds to minutes of the onset of ischemia and then recedes toward the control level over days to weeks. The mechanism initiating hyperfunction is not known but may be related to unloading, since it is no longer restricted by the adjacent area of myocardium that is noncontracting. It may also be a response to increased levels of catecholamines or other factors. The compensatory hyperfunctioning of surrounding viable myocardium may in part explain why the left ventricular ejection fraction, a measure of global ventricular function, does not correlate well with infarct size in the acute phase of myocardial infarction.

The most important and sustained adaptive myocardial mechanism following infarction is compensatory growth or hypertrophy. Compensatory hypertrophy is the universal response of the heart to all forms of injury, including hypertension, valvular heart disease, and heart muscle disease. While the normal surviving myocyte may not be able to replicate (see Chap. 25), increased protein and DNA synthesis occurs, resulting in a much enlarged cell with altered gene expression in which a variety of proteins expressed during fetal life are now reexpressed. These proteins include atrial natriuretic factor, skeletal and smooth muscle actin, and a host of oncogenes. The mechanism of the hypertrophic stimulus is unknown; however, in pressure-induced hypertrophy, intrinsic paracrine and autocrine factors are involved (see Chap. 6B). It remains to be determined why hypertrophy following myocardial infarction appears to be an essential compensatory mechanism yet subsequently plays a major role in cardiac failure. Compensatory hypertrophy has been documented in experimental studies[135,136] and to a lesser extent in humans.[137–140] The hypertrophy is usually most significant in the areas immediately adjacent to the region of infarction.[136,141,142]

CLINICAL RECOGNITION OF MYOCARDIAL INFARCTION

Electrocardiographic Classification of Myocardial Infarction: Q-Wave versus Non-Q-Wave

Myocardial infarctions have traditionally been classified as transmural or subendocardial based on the presence or absence of pathological Q waves on the electrocardiogram (ECG). This concept is misleading, since autopsy studies have demonstrated convincingly that pathological Q waves may be associated with nontransmural infarction and may be absent with transmural infarction.[143–145] These misnomers have been replaced by the terms *Q-wave infarction* and *non-Q-wave infarction* for *transmural* and *nontransmural infarction*, respectively.[146] Differentiating these two types of infarction has become entrenched, since there are major differences in pathogenesis, clinical manifestations, treatment, and prognosis (Table 60-1). The initiating events in the pathogenesis of Q-wave and non-Q-wave infarction are thought to be identical, namely, coronary occlusion induced by a thrombus superimposed on a plaque together with vasoconstriction (see Chap. 55). There is considerable evidence, however, to indicate that in non-Q-wave infarction, early spontaneous reperfusion occurs, the mechanism of which remains uncertain. In contrast, in Q-wave infarction, the coronary occlusion is sustained at least for a time sufficient to cause extensive necrosis.

TABLE 60-1
Differences between Patients with Q-Wave and Non-Q-Wave Myocardial Infarction

Characteristic	Q-Wave	Non-Q-Wave
Prevalence	47%	53%
Incidence of coronary occlusion	80–90%	15–25%
ST-T segment elevation	80%	25%
ST-T segment depression	20%	75%
Postinfarction angina	15–25%	30–40%
Incidence of early reinfarction	5–8%	15–25%
1-Month mortality	10–15%	3–5%
2-Year mortality	30%	30%
Infarct size	Moderate to large	Usually small
Residual ischemia	10–20%	40–50%
Acute complication	Common	Uncommon
Therapy		
Thrombolysis	Indicated	Not indicated
Beta-adrenergic blockers	Indicated	Retrospective analysis shows ineffective
Calcium channel blockers		
Nifedepine	Possibly detrimental	Not determined
Diltiazam	Not indicated	Recommended
Verapamil	Beneficial	Possibly beneficial but not established

One explanation for early spontaneous reperfusion is lack of sustained vasoconstriction, which may contribute to occlusion.[147] The evidence supporting the existence of early spontaneous reperfusion in non-Q-wave infarction is as follows: (1) coronary angiographic studies performed in the early hours after onset show that only about 20 to 30 percent of patients have complete coronary occlusion of infarct-related vessel, whereas, for Q-wave infarction, it is about 80 to 90 percent; (2) infarct size is routinely much less than that observed with Q-wave infarction, which is consistent with salvage by early reperfusion; (3) peak plasma creatine kinase (CK) levels are reached on an average of 12 to 13 h after onset of symptoms, indicating early washout of the enzyme, as opposed to about 27 h after Q-wave infarction; (4) reperfusion-induced contraction necrosis is extremely common, as it is in patients who undergo early reperfusion induced by thrombolytic therapy;[153] (5) acute mortality rates are around 2 to 3 percent, compared to 10 percent for Q-wave infarction; (6) the complications are minimal compared to those after a Q-wave infarction; and (7) the long-term prognosis is characterized by recurrent episodes of reinfarction so that, after about 2 years, survival is the same as that after Q-wave infarction.[148–152]

The difference in the long-term prognosis has significant implications for treatment in terms of preventing reinfarction. It is also of interest that treatment of patients after non-Q-wave infarctions with calcium blockers reduces the incidence of reinfarction and death, while beta-blockers are ineffective.[149]

Precipitating Factors

The risk factors for the development of atherosclerotic coronary heart disease (i.e., hypercholesterolemia, family history, male gender, cigarette smoking, diabetes mellitus, and hypertension) are well defined (see Chap. 62). The precipitating factors triggering acute myocardial infarction are much less well understood. The likely biologic bases are discussed in Chap. 56. Most myocardial infarctions occur at rest (51 percent), and nearly as many occur during sleep as during heavy physical activity (8 and 13 percent, respectively).[154] Distressing or changing life events reportedly occur with increased frequency in the months preceding a myocardial infarction.[155–157]

Besides the customary thrombotic occlusion of a coronary artery, coronary spasm,[158] coronary embolism,[159] primary dissection of a coronary artery,[160] traumatic occlusion of a coronary artery, and drugs such as cocaine,[161] as indicated earlier, are also primary causes of myocardial infarction (see also Chap. 64).

Life-Styles

The typical life-style of the "coronary-prone" individual seems to be one characterized by sedentary habits, overwork with a lack of relaxing pastimes, overeating, smoking, and inadequate coping mechanisms. From observational studies, it does appear that the habitually active person has a lower risk of coronary death.[162] Work overload has been implicated as a coronary risk factor, but a lack of sufficient relaxation and inadequate coping mechanisms may be decisive elements. Perhaps even the energetic and competitive (type A) person, with adequate relaxation to counter the effects of daily stresses, can avoid ischemic events.[163] In fact, the evidence linking the type A personality to coronary disease has been somewhat discredited in recent years.[164] The association between personality and heart disease is probably more complex than originally proposed (see Chap. 62).

Circadian Rhythm

Results of the Multicenter Investigation of Limitation of Infarct Size (MILIS) showed a marked circadian periodicity in the occurrence of myocardial infarction, with a peak prevalence between 6:00 A.M. and noon. The circadian rhythm was present whether the onset of the infarction was marked subjectively by the appearance of pain or objectively by plasma MB-CK levels. There was a threefold increase in the frequency of infarction at peak (9:00 A.M.) as compared with trough (11:00 P.M.) periods.[165] This circadian variation in the occurrence of myocardial infarction was first evident in a 1960 report on coronary occlusion by Master.[166] Three years later, Pell and D'Alonza recognized and discussed this phenomenon.[167] As a corollary, sudden death attributed to ischemic heart disease has a similar circadian periodicity. Available data suggest that the rhythms for both the occurrence of myocardial infarction and deaths from ischemic events are actually bimodal. The rhythms are characterized not only by the morning peak but also by a secondary, less pronounced, late afternoon or early evening peak (6:00 to 8:00 P.M.).[168]

The explanation for this temporal distribution of ischemic events remains obscure but probably is related to an early tendency toward thrombosis. There is both an increase in the tendency toward platelet aggregability[169] and a trough in intrinsic fibrinolytic activity during the morning hours.[170] A similar circadian variation is observed for cerebral infarction,[171] which further implicates an increased propensity for thrombosis in the morning hours.

Other endogenous daily rhythms may be causally related. A study of ambulatory ST-segment changes in patients with coronary artery disease demonstrated a close correlation between basal heart rate and the frequency of ischemic ST changes.[172] Another study found a circadian variation in arterial pressure that parallels the observed rhythms in ischemic events.[173] These observations reflect the diurnal variation in levels of plasma catecholamines.[174] The morning increase in sympathetic activity not only increases the metabolic demand but may cause coronary vasoconstriction. A blunting of the morning peak in myocardial infarction by beta-adrenergic blocking agents implies a role for increased sympathetic activity in the circadian rhythm. While there are also exogenous daily rhythms that might play a role in this periodicity, none have yet been incriminated. The MILIS data indicate that the circadian pattern is not related to smoking tobacco or drinking alcohol.

Symptoms

The classic history of an acute myocardial infarction (AMI) is retrosternal or precordial discomfort that is described as aching, burning, crushing, squeezing, heavy, or swelling up.[175,176] The discomfort often radiates over the anterior of the chest and frequently into the left or both arms (particularly the medial aspect) and/or into the neck or jaw. In unusual instances, the pain may be in the back, particularly between the scapulae. A common feature of pain occurring in the chest due to cardiac ischemia is the pressure of a retrosternal component. Pain restricted to the inframammary region is frequently not cardiac in origin. Patients may describe their pain with a clenched fist and point toward their chest (Levine's sign). There may be skip areas with retrosternal pain associated with jaw, antecubital fossa, or wrist pain and no pain in between the two sites. Moreover, the pain may appear only in the referral area. A recent report concluded that the occluded artery could be predicted by the site of pain, but a nonoffending artery could not be eliminated.[177] The duration of the pain of infarction is prolonged, lasting by definition longer than 15 min. While the intensity of the pain is usually steady following an initial crescendo, there is occasionally some waxing and waning in intensity. Accompanying symptoms may include dyspnea, diaphoresis, nausea, vomiting, belching, and an urge to defecate. Occasionally, presenting symptom include syncope, acute confusion, agitation, stroke, or palpitations.

Approximately 23 percent of myocardial infarctions go unrecognized because of the absence of symptoms or the absence of classic chest pain.[178] The common symptoms in the latter group are atypical pain, dyspnea, nausea, vomiting, and/or epigastric pain. A myocardial infarction may also masquerade as the development or worsening of congestive heart failure, the appearance of an arrhythmia, an overwhelming sense of apprehension, profound weakness, acute indigestion, pericarditis, stroke, or peripheral embolus.[179] The majority of patients experiencing an acute myocardial infarction have prodromal symptoms, the most frequent being new or worsening angina. Other symptoms commonly noted to precede an infarction are new or worsening exertional fatigue, weakness, or dyspnea.[180] Elderly patients are particularly likely to present with atypical symptoms.

Physical Findings

General Examination

Features of the physical examination during AMI have been the subject of several reviews.[181–183] The patient is frequently sitting up because of a sense of suffocation or a feeling of shortness of breath. Most patients with cardiac pain or myocardial infarction have some sense of impending doom that is reflected in their facial expression. They may have a grayish appearance or one of panic or exhaustion. Diaphoresis is frequent. In severe cases, patients may be quite anxious, with an ashen or pale face beaded with perspiration.

The patient should be examined in both the supine and left lateral decubitus position. The major findings pertaining to the heart are found on palpation of the precordium in the left lateral position. It is important to ascertain rapidly the vital signs and the nature, character, and rhythm of the arterial pulse and to observe the jugular venous pulse, check the peripheral pulses, palpate the precordium, and auscultate the chest and precordium. Examination of the extremities should include subjective assessment of the temperature and color of the feet. Very cool feet, especially with acrocyanosis in the setting of tachycardia, suggest low cardiac output.

The heart rate and rhythm are very important indicators of cardiac function in the initial hours of myocardial infarction. A normal rate usually indicates that the patient is not under significant hemodynamic compromise. In patients with inferior myocardial infarction, heart rates in the fifties and sixties are very common in the initial hours. Up to 60 percent of these patients initially have bradycardia, which increases gradually over the next few hours. The bradycardia, which may be associated with secondary hypotension, results from stimulation of myocardial receptors with vagal afferents. Persistent sinus tachycardia beyond the initial 12 to 24 h is predictive of a very high mortality rate. The pulse may be low in volume, reflecting decreased stroke volume. The blood pressure is usually normal but may be increased secondary to anxiety or decreased from cardiac failure. Blood pressure frequently normalizes temporarily with acute infarction in patients with hypertension. All peripheral pulses should be examined to observe their presence, and their status should be noted both to exclude current occlusion and to provide a baseline in case of future embolic events. The carotid pulse is most useful in assessing systolic upstroke time and stroke volume, which is decreased in the patient with a low output state.

The rhythm of the pulse is very important because of the frequency of ectopic atrial and, in particular, ventricular beats in AMI. Observation of the jugular venous pulse is useful in determining whether ectopic beats are atrial or ventricular. A large A wave, indicating that the right atrium is contracting against a closed atrioventricular valve, suggests that the ectopic beat is ventricular.

The respiratory rate is usually within the normal range. However, patients who are extremely anxious often exhibit hyperventilation, and those with pulmonary edema and cardiac failure have an increased respiratory rate associated with shallow inspirations. Abnormal breathing patterns, such as Cheyne-Stokes respirations, are rare unless the patient is in cardiogenic shock.

Examination of the jugular venous pulse is important with AMI, especially in patients with an inferior infarction, because insights can be gained into possible involvement of the right ventricle. The right ventricle is commonly involved with inferior infarction, but right-sided failure is seen only with major right ventricular involvement. It may be manifested by an elevated jugular venous pressure. In addition, in many patients with right ventricular infarction there is also a prominent A wave because of the decreased compliance of the right ventricle.[184] Kussmaul's sign, or an increase in the venous pressure on inspiration, may also be seen in right ventricular infarction because of decreased right ventricular compliance. Generally, right ventricular failure commonly reflects left ventricular failure with secondary elevation in pulmonary and right ventricular pressures. This circumstance occurs usually with large anterior or anterolateral infarction.

Examination of the Lungs

Basilar rales are frequently detected in AMI. Cardiac failure diagnosed on the basis of mild signs of pulmonary congestion occurs in 30 to 40 percent of patients with otherwise uncomplicated myocardial infarction. A clinical classification proposed by Killip provides some uniformity in terms of describing cardiac failure and pulmonary congestion. Class I patients do not have any pulmonary rales or a third heart sound. Class II patients have rales of a mild-to-moderate degree, involving less than 50 percent of the lung fields, and may or may not have an S3 gallop. Class III patients have rales more than halfway up the lung fields and an S3 gallop. Class IV patients are those in cardiogenic shock.

Cardiac Examination

Palpation of the precordium may reveal evidence of regional wall motion abnormalities. Palpation should be performed with the patient initially lying in the supine position; this often is adequate to ascertain whether there is a localized normal apical impulse and also permits assessing for dyskinetic impulses (see Chap. 10). Frequently, one may not feel any precordial impulse with the patient in the supine position because of the decreased intensity of contraction and/or body habitus. With the patient in the left lateral decubitus position, one may palpate a diffuse rather than a localized apical impulse; akinesis or paradoxical bulging during late systole; and, in some patients, a palpable atrial contraction corresponding to an audible S4 gallop due to the decreased compliance of the left ventricle. One or more of these features of decreased contractility or lusitrophy and dyssynergy are frequently present in the early hours of acute myocardial infarction, particularly with extensive damage.

The first and second heart sounds are often very soft because of decreased contractility. The first heart sound may also be diminished because of a prolonged PR interval. If there is a tachycardia, a shortened PR interval may result in a somewhat accentuated first heart sound. The second heart sound is usually normal; however, with extensive damage there may be a single second sound. Rarely, paradoxical splitting may reflect severe left ventricular dysfunction. A fourth heart sound is often audible in patients with AMI. A third heart sound is heard in probably only about 15 to 20 percent of patients with acute infarction. A pericardial friction rub is usually not heard until 48 to 72 h after onset of myocardial infarction and occurs in only about 10 percent of patients. The murmur of papillary muscle dysfunction is relatively common early in the course of infarction. This crescendo-decrescendo, midsystolic murmur often reflects ischemia of the papillary muscles or the myocardial attachment rather than irreversible injury to these structures. This murmur usually disappears after the first 12 to 24 h if it is soft; however, if the murmur is moderate to loud in intensity, it may persist much longer, possibly throughout the patient's life. Mitral regurgitation is most commonly due to ischemia of the posteromedial papillary muscle (see also Chap. 11). Other findings on physical examination, such as the murmur of papillary muscle rupture or ruptured ventricular septum, are described in appropriate sections under "Complications."

Right Ventricular Infarction

Until about a decade ago, right ventricular infarction was recognized infrequently and usually thought not to be of great consequence. Subsequently, it was shown that the majority of patients with acute inferior infarction had abnormal regional function of the right ventricle.[185–187] The incidence of right ventricular infarction in patients with obstruction of the right coronary artery and inferior infarction is in the 70 to 80 percent range.[184] Occasionally, patients may have predominantly right ventricular involvement and exhibit right ventricular failure with signs of systemic congestion without pulmonary congestion.[188] The infarction usually involves the posterior septum and posterior wall rather than the right ventricular free wall. The blood supplies of the right and left ventricles differ.[189–191] In addition to supply from the right coronary artery, the anterior free wall of the right ventricle receives perfusion from the conus artery, which frequently originates independently from the aorta, as well as from the septal branches of the left anterior descending coronary artery. Perfusion of the free wall is also enhanced because the right ventricle is thin and often gets significant blood flow from the thebesian vessels and the passive diffusion from the ventricular cavity blood. These characteristics, together with the relatively low work load of the right ventricle, minimize myocardial injury and provide relative protection of the anterior free wall (see also Chap. 4).

Knowledge of the pathogenesis of right ventricular infarction with inferior myocardial infarction is important in making management decisions. For example, vasodilator therapy is unlikely to be beneficial but may significantly reduce venous return. In contrast, these patients frequently require additional fluid to maintain adequate cardiac output. Thus, the volume status in patients with inferior infarction with right ventricular involvement should be carefully assessed before initiating therapy with diuretics or vasodilators.

Clinical features of right ventricular infarction that occur in conjunction with inferior infarction or a true posterior infarction are few unless there is severe involvement and right ventricular failure. There is often a prominent A wave in the jugular venous pressure pulse, and a positive Kussmaul's sign may be noted. Additional signs in patients with severe right ventricular dysfunction, or right-sided failure, include elevated jugular venous pressure, a steep *y* descent, hypotension, the absence of pulmonary edema, and, rarely, a paradoxical pulse.[192,193] Severe right ventricular dysfunction, however, is uncommon and probably occurs in less than 10 percent of the cases. The presence of right-sided S3 or S4 sounds may aid in assessing severity. Occasionally, there is a right-sided papillary muscle dysfunction, which gives rise to a systolic murmur that may increase with inspiration, as with tricuspid regurgitation of other etiologies (see Chap. 11).

The diagnosis of right ventricular infarction is very difficult to establish on the basis of clinical findings alone. Electrocardiographic findings as well as hemodynamic manifestations are frequently very helpful. The diagnosis may be confirmed with radionuclide or echocardiographic assessment. An ECG using right-sided chest leads in the midclavicular line of the fifth intercostal space may detect ST-T segment elevation (see Chap. 13). A postmortem study has shown that a 25 percent or greater involvement of the right ventricle was necessary to produce ST-T segment elevation.[194] It is important, however, to rule out constrictive pericarditis, cardiac tamponade, pulmonary emboli, and restrictive cardiomyopathy as causes of marked elevation of right-sided pressure. Echocardiographic studies may show a dilated or enlarged right ventricle, regional right ventricular dysfunction, or abnormal motion of the atrial septum (see Chap. 15).[195-197] The management of right ventricular infarction is discussed in more detail later in this chapter.

Diagnosis of Acute Myocardial Infarction

Differential Diagnosis

Myocardial infarction has typically been diagnosed on the basis of the triad of chest pain, ECG changes, and elevated plasma enzyme activity. Although AMI occurs without chest pain (20 to 25 percent of cases), chest pain remains the most common symptom and is usually responsible for the patient's seeking medical help. The differential diagnosis of prolonged chest pain is presented in Table 60-2. Chest pain, however, is not specific for cardiac disease, and it is often impossible on the basis of history alone to distinguish ischemia or infarction from other causes of chest pain. The differential diagnosis of chest pain is discussed in Chap. 19. Of patients presenting to the emergency room with chest pain, only about 14 percent are subsequently documented to have AMI.[198-201] Most patients at risk for myocardial infarction will be admitted to evaluate their chest pain unless definite noncardiac causes of chest pain—such as chest wall pain, hyperventilation, pleurisy, gastrointestinal pain, and so on—that are not imminently dangerous can be identified. In the coronary care unit, only about 20 percent of patients admitted with chest pain have AMI.

TABLE 60-2

Differential Diagnosis of Prolonged Chest Pain

AMI
Aortic dissection
Pericarditis
Atypical anginal pain associated with hypertrophic cardiomyopathy
Esophageal, other upper gastrointestinal, or biliary tract disease
Pulmonary disease
- Pleurisy: infectious, malignant, or immune disease-related
- Embolus with or without infarction
- Pneumothorax

Hyperventilation syndrome
Chest wall
- Skeletal
- Neuropathic

Psychogenic

Electrocardiographic Diagnosis

The ECG is very sensitive for detecting myocardial ischemia and infarction but frequently is not powerful in differentiating ischemia from necrosis (see Chap. 13).[199,200,202] An ECG obtained during cardiac ischemic pain frequently, but not always, exhibits changes in repolarization. The absence of ECG changes during pain provides evidence, but not proof, that the pain is not ischemic in nature. The early ECG changes of T-wave inversion or ST-T segment depression may reflect ischemia or infarction. ST-T segment elevation is more specific for AMI and reflects the epicardial injury–associated total occlusion of an epicardial coronary artery. The hallmark of AMI is development of abnormal Q waves,[203,206] which appear, on the average, 8 to 12 h from onset of symptoms but may not develop for 24 to 48 h. Abnormal Q waves usually reflect tissue death and the development of an electrical dead zone. Since abnormal Q waves do not develop immediately, they are not very helpful for initial diagnostic management and therapeutic triage except to signify the presence or absence of prior myocardial infarction. The diagnostic serial ECG changes consist of ST-segment elevation with the development of T-wave inversion and with the evolution of abnormal Q waves (Fig. 60-2). The appearance of abnormal Q waves is very specific for AMI; however, they are present in less than 50 percent of patients with documented AMI.[207] Most of the other patients who have AMI will have ECG changes restricted to T-wave inversion or ST-segment depression or no change at all.[202] These patients represent the group with non-Q-wave infarction.[152] A small percentage of patients will have left bundle branch block that masks the development of abnormal Q waves. It is important to obtain frequent ECGs, since any change may have significant diagnostic and management implications. In view of the lack of sensitivity and specificity of chest pain or the ECG, confirmation of the diagnosis of AMI is based on elevated plasma enzyme activity, particularly of cardiac-specific isoenzymes.

The resting ECG is insensitive for detecting the presence of atherosclerotic coronary heart disease; it is normal in 50 percent of patients with angiographically significant coronary obstruction.[208] Nevertheless, an abnormally wide Q wave on a resting ECG has been the standard criterion for the diagnosis of a myocardial infarction for over 60 years.[209]

The ECG criteria for the diagnosis of AMI as outlined in the MILIS study are the presence, in the setting of chest pain, of any one of the following: (1) new, or presumably new, Q waves (at least 30 ms wide and 0.20 V deep) in at least two leads from any of the following: (a) leads II, III, or aV_F; (b) leads V_1 through V_6; or (c) leads I and aV_L; (2) new, or presumably new, ST-T segment elevation or depression ($\geq$0.10 mV measured 0.02 s after the J point in two contiguous leads of the abovementioned lead combinations); or (3) complete left bundle branch block in the appropriate clinical setting. An evaluation of these criteria in 1809 enzyme-confirmed infarctions found that 21 percent of the patients with an infarction had none of these changes.[210] Conversely, over 90 percent of patients who had ST-segment elevation of 0.1 mV, as described previously, were confirmed to have an AMI. If the patients also had ST depression in the so-called reciprocal leads, the infarction rate was 3 percent higher. Patients with left branch bundle block or ST segment depression without other abnormalities had a lower rate of infarction (46 and 52 to 56 percent, respectively). Furthermore, the presence of abnormal Q waves on the resting ECG accurately predicts the presence and location of left ventricular contraction abnormalities. In a study of 64 patients with abnormal Q waves on the ECG, all patients with abnormal Q waves in the anterior leads and 30 of 33 with abnormal Q waves in the inferior leads demonstrated contraction abnormalities in the corresponding left ventricular segments.[211] The evolution of a Q-wave myocardial infarction can be separated electrocardiographically into four phases: (1) hyperacute, (2) acute, (3) subacute, and (4) chronic stabilized (Fig. 60-2; see Chap. 13).

In the hyperacute phase (Fig. 60-2), usually the earliest ECG manifestation of an acute infarction is straightening of the normal upward concavity of the ST-T segment.[212] With further evolution, the straightened ST-T segment becomes elevated. The ST-T segment usually slopes upward, since the portion of the ST-T segment nearest the T wave is more elevated than the proximal portion. The amplitude of the T wave is usually also increased. Occasionally, the ST-T segment may be markedly elevated and yet retain its upward concavity. ST-T depressions in leads oriented toward the presumably noninfarcted myocardium were traditionally termed "reciprocal changes." Recent studies have indicated that such ST-T depressions usually reflect more extensive infarction. In the subacute phase, the abnormal Q wave representing myocardial necrosis begins to appear, but the T-wave sector still points toward the infarct zone (Fig. 60-2). In the fully evolved phase, the ST-T segment begins to diminish in amplitude and becomes coved or convex upward. It blends into the now symmetrically inverted T waves (see Fig. 60-2). The abnormal Q waves (>0.03 s in duration and more than 30 percent of the R-wave amplitude) appear during this stage. During the chronic phase (Fig. 60-2), there is generally resolution of the ST- and T-wave changes, with the only residual change being an abnormal Q wave. Although the ST-T segments again become isoelectric, they are frequently horizontal with a sharp-angled ST-T junction, rather than exhibiting the normal concavity. Occasionally, in small inferior infarctions, even the abnormal Q waves resolve.

Posterior myocardial infarction occurs in the posterior left ventricular wall. An isolated true posterior infarction is quite uncommon, since such an infarction is usually associated with an inferior or lateral infarction. Since there are no ECG leads oriented toward the posterior left ventricular wall, the ECG changes of a true posterior infarction are seen as mirror-image representations in leads V_1 to V_3. Perloff described the criteria for a true posterior infarction as follows: R waves of 0.04 s in lead V_1 and in contiguous right precordial leads with upright T waves and, in the acute phase, ST-segment depression and a R/S ratio equal to or greater than 1 in leads V_1 and V_2.[212] Usually there are associated changes of an inferior or lateral infarction. As the infarction evolves, the ST-segment depression decreases and the upright T-wave amplitude increases. It is helpful to turn the ECG upside down and look at it from the back while holding it to a strong light. The changes in leads V_1 and V_2, which might be overlooked on a direct glance, are seen as abnormal Q waves, ST elevation, and T-wave inversion when viewed from this perspective.

The evolution of a non-Q-wave infarction is characterized by a lack of development of an abnormal Q wave and the appearance of reversible ST-T wave changes that usually return to normal over a few days but occasionally are permanent.

Enzymatic Diagnosis

Myocardial necrosis is associated with release of a variety of macromolecules, including enzymes, myoglobin, and contractile proteins that have been evaluated as potential diagnostic markers for AMI. Most have been of limited diagnostic value because their presence in noncardiac tissue results in elevated plasma levels from injury other than that of the myocardium.[213] Three enzymes have been routinely used for the diagnosis of AMI: aspartate transaminase (AST), lactate dehydrogenase (LDH), and creatine kinase (CK). AST, formerly referred to as

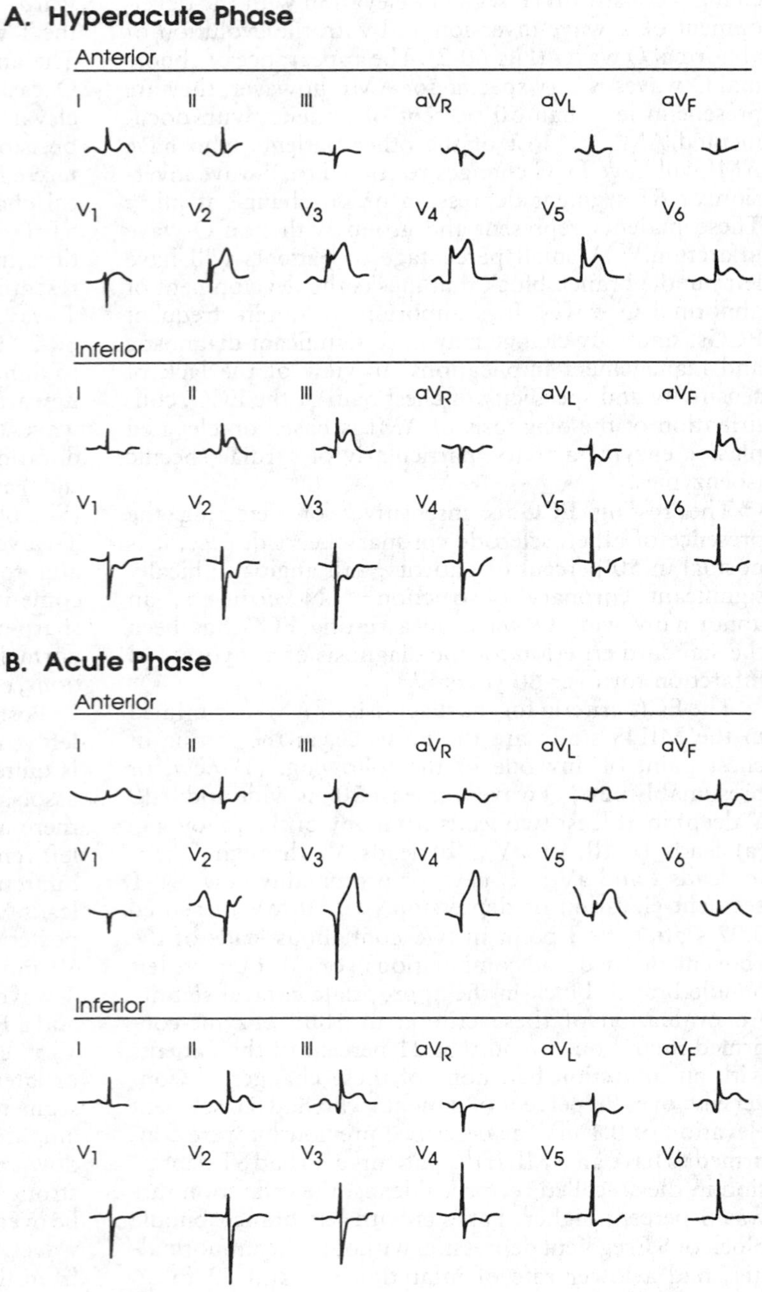

FIGURE 60-2 Electrocardiographic Evolution of Acute Anterior and Inferior Myocardial Infarction. *A*). Hyperacute phase: There is marked ST segment elevation in V_2 to V_5 in the anterior infarction and in II, III, and aVf in the inferior infarction. In the inferior infarction, there are reciprocal changes or posterior involvement as reflected in the ST depression in the precordial leads. There are no QRS changes in either case; *B*). Acute phase: Q waves indicating myocardial necrosis develop during this phase. There is some persistent ST elevation and the T wave vector generally points toward the infarct zone; *C*). Subacute phase: QRS changes are well developed and ST elevation is still present. The T vector, or more precisely the terminal portion of the T vector, begins to point away from the infarct zone; *D*). Chronic phase: Minimal or no ST elevation is present and the T wave is directed away from the infarct zone. (*Modified with permission from Wagner NB, White RD, Wagner GS: The 12-lead ECG and the extent of myocardium at risk of acute infarction: Cardiac anatomy and lead locations, and the phases of serial changes during acute occlusion. In: Califf RM, Mark DB, Wagner GS (eds): Acute Coronary Care in the Thrombolytic Era. Chicago, Year Book Medical Publishers, 1988:31–45.*)

SGOT, has been shown to be too insensitive and, because of its ubiquitous distribution, too nonspecific; therefore, it is no longer recommended for the diagnosis of myocardial infarction. Lactate dehydrogenase (LDH) and its isoenzymes are used primarily in patients who are admitted to the hospital late (48 to 72 h after onset of symptoms). In contrast, the use of CK and MB-CK has become routine and is regarded as the most sensitive, specific, and cost-effective means of diagnosing myocardial infarction.[214–216] The use of total CK alone without MB-CK yields a similar sensitivity, but specificity is markedly lower, in the range of 70 percent.[217]

Creatine kinase is an enzyme that catalyzes the reversible transfer of high-energy phosphate from ATP to creatine and is highly concentrated in organs, such as muscle, where there is high utilization of energy. Creatine kinase consists of two monomers, each having a molecular weight of 43,000.[218] The isoenzymes of CK are formed by the association of two M monomers (MM-CK), that predominate in muscle (hence the name) or of two B monomers (BB-CK), that predominate in the brain and internal visceral organs, and a hybrid form (MB-CK) composed of one M subunit and one B subunit. There are also two other CKs, that are located in the mitochondria[219,220] and are encoded by separate genes.[221,222] One mitochondrial CK isoenzyme has a ubiquitous distribution in the body, while the other predominates in mitochondria of muscle tissue. The mitochondrial CKs have recently been studied as markers for the diagnosis of myocardial infarction and also for the diagnosis of cere-

C. Subacute Phase

Anterior

I II III aV$_R$ aV$_L$ aV$_F$

V$_1$ V$_2$ V$_3$ V$_4$ V$_5$ V$_6$

Inferior

I II III aV$_R$ aV$_L$ aV$_F$

V$_1$ V$_2$ V$_3$ V$_4$ V$_5$ V$_6$

D. Chronic Phase

Anterior

I II III aV$_R$ aV$_L$ aV$_F$

V$_1$ V$_2$ V$_3$ V$_4$ V$_5$ V$_6$

Inferior

I II III aV$_R$ aV$_L$ aV$_F$

V$_1$ V$_2$ V$_3$ V$_4$ V$_5$ V$_6$

bral infarction. The mitochondrial form offers significant potential as an independent marker of cell necrosis.[223,224]

Fifteen percent of the CK in the myocardium is in the form of MB-CK, which provides for its sensitivity and specificity as a diagnostic marker of AMI. Several investigators have found small amounts of MB-CK in normal adult skeletal muscle,[225,226] whereas others have failed to detect any cytosolic CK other than MM-CK.[227,228] On the other hand, there are data indicating that 5 to 7 percent of the CK in skeletal muscle can become MB-CK following various forms of skeletal muscle injury, such as after chronic exercise,[229,230] inflammation,[231] trauma,[232] and electrical injury.[233] It is known that in certain hereditary muscle diseases, such as Duchenne's muscular dystrophy (DMD), there is an increased amount of MB-CK, in the range of 4 to 5 percent. During the first 6 weeks of life in utero, only BB-CK is synthesized, while at about the eighth week, M-CK synthesis is induced and rapidly supplants the B-CK in skeletal and cardiac muscle such that by about the twelfth week MM-CK predominates.[234,235] In DMD, it is believed that these muscles do not develop normally and retain increased expression of the B-CK gene. In the case of a reaction to muscle injury, it is postulated that undifferentiated skeletal muscle cells differentiate to form mature skeletal myocytes and thus repeat the developmental program of fetal skeletal muscle but the expression of B-CK is probably transient.[236]

The tradition of assaying three enzymes—LDH, CK, and AST (SGOT)—daily or twice daily has been abandoned. Plasma total CK and MB-CK activity should be analyzed immediately upon admission and followed by serial analysis.[237] Total plasma CK activity, although a highly sensitive index of infarction, is less specific, as noted, and may be elevated after a variety of conditions, such as intramuscular injections, trauma, cardiac catheterization, surgery, cerebrovascular accidents, rhabdomyolysis, or thyroiditis.[238] Electrocardioversion also causes significant elevation of total CK activity, but it does not elevate plasma MB-CK activity significantly unless the procedure is repeated several times. It is also important that MB-CK be analyzed even if total CK activities are within the normal range. In patients with low base-line levels of total CK, the plasma MB-CK activity may increase two- to threefold while total CK activity remains in the normal range. In patients with very low levels of plasma MB-CK, it is preferable that the CK isoforms be analyzed, as discussed below.

Plasma MB-CK activity, as assessed by conventional techniques, is significantly elevated within 6 to 10 h of onset of symptoms of infarction, and maximal levels are reached between 14 and 36 h, with return to normal levels after 48 to 72 h (Fig. 60-3).[237] In patients with non-Q-wave infarction, plasma MB-CK activity peaks on average at about 15 h. In contrast, after Q-wave infarction, MB-CK levels peak at an average of 28 h. It is recommended that samples be analyzed immediately on admission and approximately every 6 to 8 h for the initial 24 h. The diagnosis is usually evident within 16 h. If plasma MB-CK activity is not elevated by 24 h, further sampling is unnecessary. If plasma total CK and MB-CK activity remains within the normal range, the reliability of excluding myocardial infarction is 95 percent or greater.

An elevated plasma MB-CK level as a diagnostic marker for myocardial infarction is associated with a very low incidence of false-negative results if samples are collected frequently and appropriately. False-positive results may occur, since MB-CK can be released from tissues other than the heart. As outlined previously, skeletal muscle injury may induce the synthesis of MB-CK, and elevated levels have been documented after crush injury,[232] electrical injury,[233] dermatomyositis, polymyositis,[231] and DMD,[239] as well as in professional athletes and marathon runners.[229,230] The following characteristics suggest that the source of the elevated plasma MB-CK activity is skeletal, rather than cardiac, muscle: (1) the appropriate clinical setting, namely, skeletal muscle disease or trauma; (2) an atypical time course for the increase and decrease in plasma MB-CK activity, particularly if prolonged, as might be seen in inflammatory disorders; (3) MB-CK activity of less than 10 to 15 percent of the total CK activity; and (4) a marked elevation of total CK activity of 20- to 30-fold. An elevated plasma MB-CK level may also be due to artifact. Assays using anion exchange columns may give spurious increases in MB-CK due to spilling of MM into the MB-CK fraction.[240] Electrophoresis with fluorescence detection may show an artifact in the region of the MB-CK band in patients undergoing renal dialysis[241] and in those taking chlordiazepoxide, tricyclic antidepressants, or aspirin in high doses. Those assays that do not differentiate the B from the M subunit may show elevations in MB-CK levels because of detection of B-CK in the circulation resulting from injury to the prostate, uterus, gastrointestinal tract, or brain,[242–245] which are known to be rich in MM-CK. Similar artifactual elevations of plasma MB-CK levels may be seen in women following vaginal or cesarean delivery of a baby.[246] Release of BB-CK from the brain is seldom observed following cerebrovascular accidents,[247] but it may occur after trauma and infection or diffuse brain injury.[248] Finally, certain tumors, including those of the lung, brain, and breast, abnormally synthesize BB-CK, which is released into the circulation.[249] Hypothyroidism is associated with elevated levels of both plasma total CR and MB-CK due to diminished clearance.[250] Occasionally one sees what is referred to as a *macro CK-1*, a complex of CK and macroglobulins, which migrates to the position of MB-CK on electrophoresis,[251,252] which results in a false-positive diagnosis of AMI. Macro CK-1 is more common in elderly women and in patients who are chronically ill and is said to have an incidence of 1.6 percent in hospitalized patients.[251]

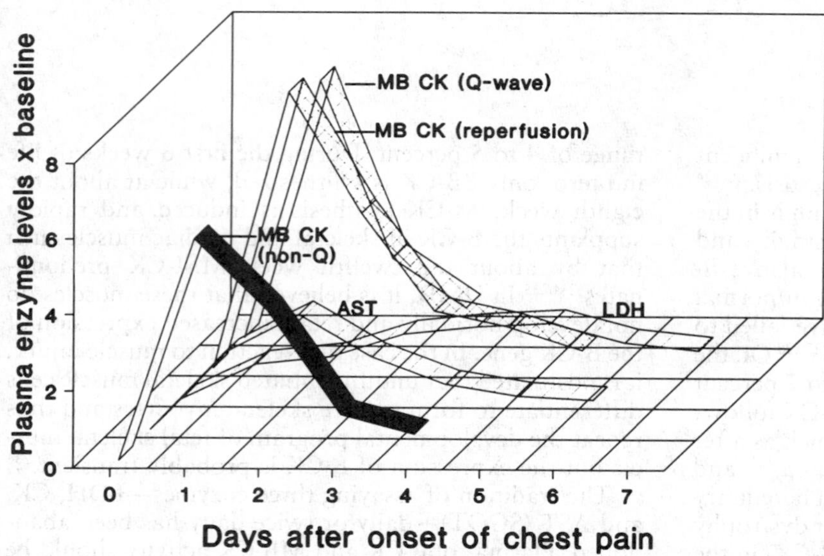

FIGURE 60-3 Typical plasma profiles for the MB isoenzyme of creatine kinase (MB CK), aspartate amino transferase (AST), and lactate dehydrogenase (LDH) activities following onset of acute myocardial infarction.

Usually the correct diagnosis can be made by electrophoretic demonstration that the band is intermediate between MM and MB-CK.

The upper limit of normal for plasma total CK activity is around 120 IU/L and for plasma MB-CK activity, 10 to 13 IU/L, but these values vary from laboratory to laboratory. Elevated plasma MB-CK activity indicative of myocardial infarction should exceed 5 percent of total CK activity. At the time of peak plasma CK after myocardial infarction, MB-CK levels usually make up 10 to 15 percent of the total CK activity.

The following are the enzymatic criteria for the diagnosis of myocardial infarction (Table 60-3):

1. There is a serial elevation in plasma MB-CK levels followed by a decrease to baseline with a change of 25 percent or more between two values.
2. Plasma MB-CK activity increases 50 percent or more between two samples separated by at least 4 h and not more than 12 h.
3. Preferably, the diagnosis is made based on no fewer than two samples in a 24-h period separated by at least 4 h.
4. If only a single sample is present, the diagnosis must be made on the basis of an elevation of MB-CK levels above normal by at least twofold.
5. In patients admitted beyond 72 h from the onset of infarction, LDH isoenzyme analysis is preferred, since MB-CK levels may have returned to normal.

Diagnosis of Myocardial Infarction after 48 to 72 h

By 72 h after myocardial infarction, particularly when associated with minimal myocardial damage, plasma MB-CK may have returned to normal levels. In this situation, LDH-1 activity, which peaks between 48 and 72 h and remains elevated for 10 to 14 days, should be assessed serially.[253] Sampling for LDH activity due to its long half-life can be much less frequent than for CK; sampling every 12 to 24 h is adequate. A value of LDH-1 greater than that of LDH-2 is considered significant.

Diagnosis of Early Reinfarction

The diagnosis of early reinfarction is difficult, since it may be associated with an elevation in enzyme activity superimposed on elevated plasma enzyme activity.[254,255] It may be difficult to interpret a secondary elevation of MB-CK levels if it occurs within the initial 24-h period. However, if MB-CK levels have returned to normal, the diagnosis is relatively easy, since a secondary increase is seen. Diagnosis of reinfarction is based on an increase of 50 percent or more of the plasma MB-CK activity above the preceding baseline (the mean of the two preceding samples) in at least two samples separated by a minimum of 4 h within a 24-h interval with an absolute value of ±14 IU/L in at least one sample.[237] If the MB-CK activity is on the downslope from the antecedent infarction, a 25 percent increase is considered diagnostic; however, this criterion is always less reliable than is a secondary elevation after the return of MB-CK activity to baseline. These criteria were found to be reliable in three large clinical trials.[152,252,256]

TABLE 60-3

Enzymatic Criteria for Diagnosis of Myocardial Infarction

Serial increase, then decrease of plasma MB-CK, with a change > 25% between any two values
MB-CK > 10–13 units/liter or > 5% total CK activity
Increase in MB-CK activity > 50% between any two samples, separated by at least 4 h
If only a single sample available, MB-CK elevation > twofold
Beyond 72 h, an elevation of LDH-1 > LDH-2

Diagnosis of Myocardial Infarction after Surgery

Myocardial infarction after noncardiac surgery is reliably determined from serial analysis of plasma MB-CK levels every 6 to 8 h.[217,257] There is marked elevation of enzymes, including total CK level, due to tissue trauma, but MB-CK is highly specific for myocardium. In the setting of cardiac surgery, however, MB-CK levels, like those of other cardiac enzymes, are frequently elevated and are not a reliable diagnostic index.[258,259] Myocardial infarction after cardiac surgery that is not associated with the development of abnormal Q waves is best diagnosed by radionuclide techniques. Pyrophosphate imaging provides a reasonably reliable diagnosis (see also Chap. 134). Nevertheless, the elevation of plasma MB-CK levels several-fold, even in the absence of abnormal Q waves, is highly suggestive of perioperative infarction, although as a sole criterion it lacks specificity.

Diagnosis of Remote Infarction

Determining whether or not a patient has had remote myocardial infarction can be difficult in the absence of abnormal Q waves.[260,261] The diagnosis of remote infarction by thallium 201 perfusion scanning or gated blood pool scanning with technetium 99-labeled red blood cells has been shown to be extremely reliable, sensitive, and specific based on a prospective study in patients whose infarct size was estimated enzymatically at the time of the acute episode.[262] Perfusion defects were detected (at an average time of 11 months after infarction) in 94 percent of patients with infarction, and corresponding wall motion abnormalities were noted in 78 percent. In patients with a small infarct, wall motion abnormalities were found in only 50 percent. The ECG showed abnormal Q waves in only 56 percent. In the patients with persistent abnormal Q waves (30 percent), infarct size was consistently rather large. Thallium 201 perfusion imaging is sensitive in detecting remote infarction (see Chap. 134).

MB-CK Subforms for Early Diagnosis of Infarction and Assessment of Reperfusion

MM and MB-CK, although present in tissue in single forms, are converted by plasma proteolytic activity to various electrophoretic forms.[263,264] MM-CK is converted into MM-3, MM-2, and MM-1; and MB CK is converted into MB-2 and MB-1.[265,266] The development of a new high-voltage electrophoresis technique permits separation of the MM and MB subforms within about 25 min.[267] Normally, in the plasma the various subforms are in equilibrium such that the ratio of MB-1 to MB-2 is 1. When infarction occurs, MB-2, the tissue form, is released into the circulation initially in minute amounts so that the absolute level of MB-CK may remain within the normal range but the ratio of MB-2 to MB-1 may change drastically. As noted above, the diagnosis of myocardial infarction based on conventional MB-CK analysis is not reliable until 8 to 10 h after onset of symptoms.[267] However, when the subform assay of the ratio of MB-2 to MB-1 exceeds 1.5 or greater, it is diagnostic of infarction. Initial studies indicate that a reliable diagnosis can be established within 6 h with a sensitivity and specificity of greater than 95 percent.[268] This assay may be an effective approach to triage and permit an earlier diagnosis than previously used techniques.[269,270]

Nondiagnostic General Responses to Myocardial Infarction

Myocardial infarction elicits nonspecific generalized responses to the injury. An elevated temperature of 38 to 38.5°C may develop at 12 to 24 h and last up to 8 to 10 days after infarction. The white blood cell count may be mildly elevated after several days, and levels of acute-phase reactants, such as C-reactive protein, are usually increased. Initially lipoprotein and cholesterol levels may be normal but may decrease very quickly after infarction, and levels determined during the early recovery period may not provide an adequate basis for assessing risk factors and planning secondary prevention strategies. The final assessment of base-line lipid status should be based on measurement either at admission or, preferably, 6 to 8 weeks after the event.[271,272] Acute myocardial infarction can either precipitate or worsen glucose intolerance.[273,274]

Estimates of Infarct Size

Enzymatic Estimates of Infarct Size

It has been established experimentally[275,276] and clinically[41,42] that the major determinant of both acute and long-term prognoses following myocardial infarction is the extent of myocardial damage. In the early 1970s there was a major effort to quantify infarct size through a variety of techniques, such as utilizing the degree of ST-segment elevation[277] on the ECG, myocardial radioisotope uptake,[278–280] and the kinetics of cardiac enzyme release into the circulation.[281] Enzymatic estimates of infarct size based on plasma estimates of the total MB-CK released into the circulation[282] emerged as a technique to estimate accurately the amount of myocardial damage that occurs during myocardial infarction and was shown to correlate closely with clinical manifestations, such as impairment of ventricular function,[283] the incidence of ventricular arrhythmias, the incidence of ventricular failure,[285] the acute mortality rate,[286] and the long-term mortality rate.[41,42] The precision of the enzymatic estimates was confirmed by postmortem studies in humans showing a close correlation between histological estimates of infarct size and those of enzymatic estimates using MB-CK.[287] The basis for enzymatic estimates of infarct size was validated in animals.[275,276] Enzymatic estimates of infarct size were used experimentally and clinically to assess a variety of interventions designed to salvage ischemic myocardium.[288–292] However, with the advent of thrombolytic therapy to induce reperfusion, it was observed that there was more rapid washout of CK, and the ratio of CK released into the circulation to that depleted from the myocardium was altered, and estimates of infarct size in this clinical setting may not be reliable.[293]

Electrocardiographic Estimates of Infarct Size

The ECG has long been used to obtain a semiquantitative assessment of the extent of myocardial infarction. Patients with anterior infarction who develop abnormal Q waves from leads V_1 to V_6 usually have extensive damage and an unfavorable prognosis. Earlier studies had demonstrated that the sum of ST-segment elevations measured from the precordial leads was useful in assessing the extent of myocardial injury in patients with anterior myocardial infarction.[294] This technique, however, was found to be very limited because it does not distinguish between reversible and irreversible ischemic changes and depends on the overall influence of the myocardial geometry.[295] In an attempt to provide a more quantitative method, a QRS scoring system with planer[296,297] or electrocardiographic[298] techniques to estimate infarct size was developed. These techniques are probably not accurate enough to provide quantitative estimates of infarct size in assessing interventions such as thrombolytic therapy.

For routine clinical purposes, there are useful indicators of the size of an infarction. In an acute anterior infarction, the extent of jeopardized myocardium correlates with the number of precordial leads showing ST and QRS changes and with the extent of those changes.[298a] The presence of right bundle branch block is associated with a large anterior infarct because it indicates that the occlusion of the left anterior descending artery may be proximal to the first septal perforator.[298b] In acute inferior infarction, elevation of the ST segment in lead V_{4R}, indicating the involvement of the right ventricle, is associated with proximal occlusion of the proximal right coronary artery and thus with a large infarct and a poor prognosis.[298c]

Radionuclide Estimates of Infarct Size

There is a continuing need for estimates of infarct size for prognostic purposes and to provide insights into the effects of thrombolytic therapy. In view of the unproven reliability of enzymatic estimates of infarct size during reperfusion in assessing thrombolytic therapy,[293,299] several attempts have been made based on imaging of various radionuclides, such as thallium[300] and pyrophosphate.[301] The more reliable approach has been that of positron emission transaxial (PET) tomography (see Chap. 137).[278] This technique, however, while accurate and quantitative, is not practical on a routine basis and is used primarily as a research tool. Technetium-99m sestamibi (Tc-99m hexakis 2-methoxy-2-isobutyl isonitrile) has undergone extensive testing recently and offers considerable promise as an agent for estimating both the area at risk and the actual ultimate necrosis. This agent is taken up by the myocardium in proportion to blood flow[302,303] and demonstrates minimal redistribution.[303,304] It has been validated in animal models with permanent occlusion[305] and reperfusion[303,306] and has been demonstrated to be reliable in estimating the area at risk and ultimate infarct size in patients during AMI.[307–309] This technique provides a routinely available method of estimating infarct size and could prove to be a reliable prognostic indicator (see Chap. 134).[310]

Noninvasive Imaging in Acute Myocardial Infarction

Chest Roentgenogram

The chest roentgenogram (x-ray) provides very important information in the evaluation of chest pain and in contributing to an integrative assessment of the clinical situation after a diagnosis of myocardial infarction has been made. A chest x-ray may assist in the initial evaluation of chest pain to exclude diagnoses such as pneumothorax, pulmonary infarction with effusions, aortic dissection, skeletal fractures, and so on. In the patient with acute infarction, the x-ray can be useful in establishing the presence of pulmonary edema and cardiac size to assist in assessing whether or not cardiomegaly is present and whether heart failure or myocardial or valvular disease is acute or chronic. It must be emphasized that severe left ventricular failure can be present without manifesting pulmonary edema on the chest x-ray and, conversely, that improvement in the chest x-ray can lag behind hemodynamic resolution of pulmonary congestion (see also Chap. 14).

Radioisotopic Studies

Many radioisotope techniques are useful cardiac assessment, and they are discussed in detail in Chap. 134. Evaluation of ejection fraction and regional wall motion abnormalities is essential in establishing a prognosis and planning therapy in post myocardial infarction patients prior to discharge. The role of echocardiography in this regard is discussed subsequently. The use of Tc-99m-labeled red blood cells for blood pool labeling is very helpful in assessing ejection fraction and regional wall motion abnormalities in both the left and right ventricles. This approach is still regarded as the most reliable means of diagnosing right ventricular infarction.[181,188,311] An alternative is to use thallium scintigraphy, which detects reperfusion defects in both the right and left ventricles and also outlines the septum. Perhaps the least sensitive imaging agent for assessing infarct size is technetium pyrophosphate uptake.[312] Two new radionuclides for myocardial imaging have become available. One is Tc-99m sestamibi. Technetium-99m sestamibi offers a means of estimating infarct size, as mentioned earlier, and is being explored as a means of estimating myocardial salvage with thrombolytic therapy.[310] Teboroxine is now being examined as a possible agent for imaging myocardial infarction and for assessing infarct size but may be less suitable than Tc-99m sestamibi due to its short half-life.

Echocardiography

M-mode, two-dimensional, and Doppler echocardiographic studies have become routine in overall cardiac evaluation and also in the assessment of myocardial infarction. Echocardiography offers the most reliable noninvasive and rapid means of assessing ventricular function, excluding other possible diagnoses, and assessing certain complications in myocardial infarction.[313] The uses and limitations of the technique are discussed in detail in Chap. 15. In the emergency room, the echocardiogram is being explored as a possible means of rapidly diagnosing infarction, particularly in the assessment for thrombolytic therapy.[314,315] This technique is particularly useful in detecting even small pericardial effusions in patients postinfarction or in patients in whom pericarditis, rather than myocardial infarction, is suspected as the primary abnormality. Echocardiography provides a means of quantitating regional and global function of the left and right ventricles[316–319] and of diagnosing and assessing right ventricular infarction.[320] The echocardiogram is particularly helpful in detecting intraventricular thrombi, in excluding such diagnoses as aortic dissection, cardiac tamponade, bacterial endocarditis, and ventricular aneurysm; and in assessing right ventricular failure secondary to pulmonary emboli. Doppler echocardiography (see Chap. 130) provides quantitation of valvular regurgitation and assessment of other hemodynamic parameters, such as cardiac output, left ventricular diastolic function, and pulmonary artery systolic pressure.[321–323] Transesophageal echocardiography (see Chap. 131) can be a powerful tool for assessing the hemodynamically unstable patient in whom transthoracic imaging may be suboptimal.[324] The ready availability of echocardiography makes it extremely valuable in AMI. It is extremely useful in detecting and qualifying such complications as ruptured chordae tendineae or ruptured ventricular septum. It provides much of the information necessary should surgery be contemplated.[325] The use of sonicated albumin in conjunction with echocardiography for assessing coronary flow is being intensely explored.[326]

Magnetic Resonance Imaging

In both the assessment of infarct size[327] and the estimation of coronary blood flow,[328] magnetic resonance imaging (MRI) is being employed extensively in the experimental assessment of myocardial infarction (see Chap. 136). It offers potential for differentiating noninfarcted viable ischemic myocardium from necrosis and ultimately for assessing myocardial perfusion.[329] It also offers improvement over present techniques for assessing wall thickness and making overall estimates of chamber size. The role, if any, of MRI in the routine assessment of AMI is under investigation.

MANAGEMENT OF MYOCARDIAL INFARCTION

Objectives of Early Treatment

The immediate management of the patient with AMI has at least five major goals: (1) provide cardiac resuscitation if necessary, (2) transfer the patient immediately to a hospital, (3) treat life-threatening arrhythmias, (4) alleviate pain and anxiety, and (5) preserve as much myocardium as possible.

Rationale for Cardioprotection

The premise that a myocardial infarction might be aborted prior to destruction of all ischemic tissue arose from studies in which infarct size was estimated by a variety of techniques.[40,43–45,280–284,330,331] These investigations gave rise to several tenets:

1. Myocardial damage as a result of coronary occlusion evolves from endocardium to epicardium and is time-dependent, requiring four to six h for completion of necrosis. This necrosis begins after 15 to 20 min near the subendocardium and progresses toward the epicardium in a "wave front" of cell death.
2. The immediate hemodynamic consequences of this cell death include both systolic and diastolic dysfunction. Over a period of 1 to 3 min, the regional disturbance of contraction progresses to dyskinesia. The diastolic impairment often precedes the systolic dysfunction, resulting ultimately in decreased distensibility of the involved segment.[331]
3. The extent of damage can be markedly limited by early restoration of coronary blood flow.[332,333] Restoration of flow within 15 to 20 min was associated with minimal necrosis, and salvage of myocardium decreased exponentially with time such that two-thirds of the myocardium was salvaged if reperfusion occurred after 40 min, with less than 20 percent salvaged after 4 h, and insignificant salvage was achieved after 6 h of coronary occlusion.[40]
4. The extent of infarct size could also be limited or at least delayed by decreasing myocardial oxygen demand.[334] Decreasing myocardial oxygen demand by use of a variety of drugs and techniques limited infarct size but was not as effective as increasing oxygen supply via early reperfusion.
5. Infarct size correlated with mortality. Prospective in vivo studies in humans showed that enzymatic estimates of infarct size correlated closely with mortality rates[280,281] and with clinical manifestations reflective of morbidity, such as the incidence of cardiac failure,[285] the frequency and severity of arrhythmias,[34,284] and the degree of impairment of ventricular function.[283] Postmortem studies showed that with destruction of 40 percent or more of the left ventricle death was inevitable (see Chap. 57).[43–45]

Cardioprotection by Decreased Myocardial Oxygen Consumption

While beta blockers clearly have been shown to reduce mortality following myocardial infarction and are of tremendous clinical benefit in disorders such as angina and hypertension, their role in the limitation of infarct size is probably slight. Initial animal studies showing that beta blockers limit infarct size were based on assessment by ST-segment elevation and CK release without accounting for the overall area at risk and collateral flow.[294] It was soon recognized that infarct size in the commonly used dog model was extremely variable and dependent on collateral flow.[335,336] Studies in which infarct size was estimated as a percentage of the total area at risk failed to show any significant reduction of infarct size.[337–339] The lack of effect of blocking sympathetic input on salvaging myocardium has been confirmed, since whole body sympathectomy failed to limit infarct size.[340] The consensus is that, in animal models, beta blockers do not limit infarct size.[338]

The results of clinical trials assessing the effect of beta blockers on infarct size have been inconsistent.[292,341] Furthermore, in the TIMI-2 thrombolytic trial, metoprolol given intravenously within 3 to 4 h of onset of infarction in conjunction with tissue plasminogen activator (t-PA) had no effect on infarct size or mortality.[342] There is a consensus, however, that acute beta-blocker administration to appropriate patients with Q-wave infarction is safe and reduces the incidence of reinfarction by about 18 percent and 1 week mortality by about 14 percent. The major mechanism for the reduction in mortality is a reduction in the incidence of ventricular fibrillation and sudden death.[342] The effect of reducing reinfarction is by reduction of myocardial ischemia.[342]

While decreasing myocardial oxygen consumption ($\dot{M}V_{O_2}$) does not appear to salvage myocardium significantly, agents that decrease coronary flow and/or increase MV_{O_2} by increasing heart rate, blood pressure, or contractility may increase myocardial necrosis as well as increase the incidence of ventricular arrhythmias and cardiac failure. Thus, every effort should be made to maintain adequate systemic and cardiac perfusion with minimal adverse effects on contractility, heart rate, blood pressure, arterial resistance, or impedance to coronary flow.

Cardioprotection by Increasing Coronary Flow: Thrombolysis

The advent of thrombolytic therapy ushered in a new therapeutic era, analogous to the introduction of the coronary care unit. Three facts provide the foundation for the success of thrombolytic therapy: (1) the evolution of myocardial necrosis (the animal model) following coronary occlusion is time-dependent over 4 to 6 h; (2) the restoration of coronary blood flow within this 4- to 6-hour interval salvages myocardium, but in a time-dependent fashion; and (3) the proximate cause of myocardial infarction in humans is generally an occlusive thrombus within the coronary artery.[110,299,343–346]

The results from clinical trials have confirmed that early reperfusion in humans induced by a thrombolytic agent—recombinant tissue plasminogen activator (rt-PA), streptokinase (SK), urokinase, or anisoylated plasminogen streptokinase activator complex (APSAC)—is associated with limitation of infarct size, preservation of ventricular function, and improved survival. In the

GISSI-1 trial, which enrolled patients with AMI, mortality was reduced 47 percent in those patients receiving SK within 1.5 h of onset of symptoms, compared to a reduction of 23 percent in those treated within the first 3 h and 13 percent in patients treated between 3 and 6 h; no significant benefit was noted in those treated after 6 h.[347] The parallel between the time-dependent presumed salvage of myocardium in humans with that observed in animals is illustrated in Fig. 60-4. In the top panel, the extent of necrosis in the animal is illustrated as a function of time from the onset of coronary occlusion until the restoration of flow. The bottom panel shows the reduction of mortality rates in humans versus the time from the onset of symptoms until the initiation of thrombolytic therapy. A similar but less striking association between the time until treatment and a reduction of mortality rates was found in the European Cooperative Study (ECSG),[348] the Second International Study of Infarct Survival (ISIS-2),[349] and the ISIS-3 trial.[350] In the ECSG, mortality at 3 months was reduced by 36 percent in the entire group receiving rt-PA, but among patients treated within 3 h, mortality was reduced by 59 percent. In ISIS-2, the overall mortality at 5 weeks was reduced by 23 percent in patients treated with SK, but in those treated within 3 h of onset of symptoms it was reduced by 34 percent.

Comparable data showing the limitation of infarct size by reperfusion therapy to be time-dependent is more difficult to obtain in humans, since quantitative estimation of infarct size, particularly during reperfusion, is imprecise. Nevertheless, in the Netherlands Interuniversity Cardiology Institute Trial, patients treated with SK within the first hour after the onset of symptoms had a 51 percent decrease in enzymatically determined infarct size compared with those treated with conventional therapy; those treated between the first and second hours

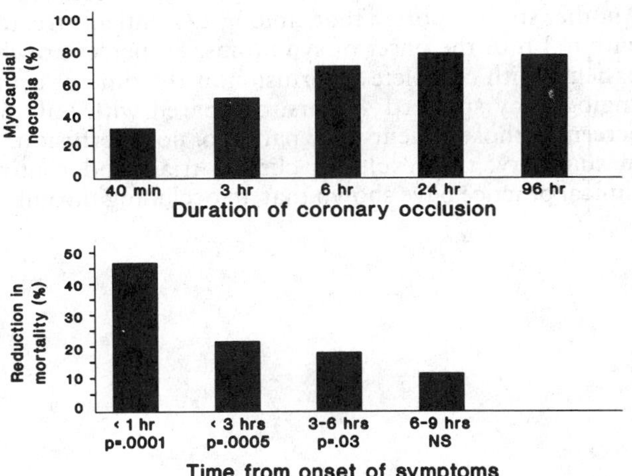

FIGURE 60-4 Shown in the *top panel* is the relationship between the extent of myocardial necrosis and the duration of coronary occlusion in the dog (Reimer et al[110].). The *bottom panel* presents the relationship between the reduction in mortality and the time of initiating thrombolytic therapy (streptokinase) from onset of symptoms (GISSI-1[347]). The parallelism between salvage of myocardium in the dog and salvage in man as reflected by infarct size is striking. This parallelism is evidence that evolution of infarction has a similar temporal profile in both humans and animals.

had a 31 percent reduction; and those treated later than 2 h had a 13 percent reduction.[351] In a small trial,[352] peak plasma CK activity was significantly lower in patients who underwent early reperfusion compared to those undergoing late reperfusion or those without reperfusion. Similar findings were observed in the Western Washington trial[353] and the results of the Intravenous Streptokinase in Acute Myocardial Infarction Study (ISAM)[354] are concordant. In the Tissue Plasminogen Activator Toronto placebo-controlled trial (TPAT),[355] patients treated within 4 h of onset of symptoms underwent coronary angiography on the first day. In patients in whom the patency of the infarct-related artery had been restored, a reduction of infarct size, measured by thallium scintigraphy, was associated with improvement in regional ventricular function.

Ventricular function, although a less sensitive indicator of myocardial salvage than infarct size, reflects myocardial salvage and is similarly dependent on early reperfusion. The initial studies showing improvement in global and regional function in patients treated with thrombolytic therapy were those of Khoran and coworkers,[356] who showed that SK given intravenously within 1.5 h of onset of symptoms was associated with a global ejection fraction of 56 ± 15 percent, compared with 47 ± 14 percent in the placebo group ($p < .05$). Similar findings were reported in patients treated with rt-PA.[357] The results of studies by Guerci and associates[358] and those of the National Heart Foundation of Australia study[359] were concordant and indicated that preservation of ventricular function is observed only when patency is restored within the first 2 to 4 h of the onset of symptoms.

The time window of 4 to 6 h during which reperfusion will limit infarct size has been confirmed in humans in the recent trial referred to as EMERAS (Estudio Multicenter Estreptoquinasa Republicas Americas Sud).[360] In this study, over 3600 patients were randomized to either SK or a placebo. All were patients who presented to the hospital between 6 and 24 h from the onset of symptoms. At the end of 1 month, the mortality rate was the same in the group treated with SK as in the conventionally (placebo-) treated group. Subgroup analysis also found no difference between patients treated between 7 and 12 h and those treated between 12 and 24 h. Thus, these data indicate that significant preservation of ventricular function and reduction of mortality from limitation of infarct size is possible only in patients in whom reperfusion is established within the first 4 to 6 h after the onset of symptoms. In the more recent Late Assessment of Thrombolytic Efficacy (LATE) trial,[361] patients received rt-PA or placebo between 6 and 24 h after the onset of symptoms. While no benefit in left ventricular function was observed with thrombolytic therapy after 12 h from onset, there was a significant reduction in mortality in patients receiving rt-PA between 6 and 12 h from onset. It must be emphasized, however, that the salvage of myocardium is more extensive in the initial 1 to 2 h than in the subsequent hours of this interval. Anecdotal studies report that very early thrombolysis (within 20 to 30 min of symptom onset) in patients with infarction can completely abort the attack, leaving no evidence of irreversible myocardial injury, as detected by ventriculography and serial analysis of plasma enzymes.

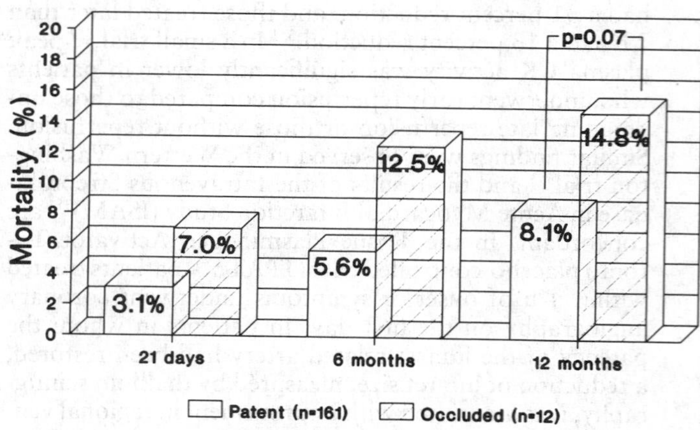

FIGURE 60-5 Comparison of mortality in TIMI-1 based on the patency status of the infarct-related artery. Striking reductions are seen in short- and long-term mortality only when thrombolysis was successful.[365]

That thrombus is the proximate cause of myocardial infarction was reconfirmed and emphasized by the results of the clinical trials. Coronary angiography performed within the first hours of onset of AMI in patients presenting with ST-T-segment elevation shows a thrombus occluding the infarct-related artery in 80 to 90 percent of patients.[362] The relationship between the restoration of flow in the occluded artery and the salvage of myocardium is demonstrated by the correlation between patency and improved mortality rates. In a study of 204 patients treated with intracoronarily administered SK,[363] the hospital mortality rate was 24 percent in patients with occlusion of the infarct-related artery in whom recanalization could not be achieved, compared to 5.4 percent in patients in whom patency was successfully restored within the first 3 to 6 h. In a similar study,[364] the hospital mortality rate was 7.3 percent in patients with a patent artery following administration of SK, compared with 25 percent in patients in whom reperfusion was not possible. Another study[86] showed that patients with an occluded infarct-related artery had a mortality rate of 17 percent, compared to 7 percent in patients with a patent vessel. In the TIMI-1 study,[365] in which patients underwent cardiac catheterization 90 min after initiation of thrombolytic therapy, the mortality rate at 21 days was 3.1 percent in patients with patent vessels, compared to 7 percent in patients in whom the vessel was occluded; and at 1 year the mortality rate was 14.8 percent in patients with an occluded artery, as opposed to only 8.5 percent in patients with an open vessel (Fig. 60-5). In the first Thrombolysis and Angioplasty in Myocardial Infarction (TAMI) trial,[366] a patent infarct-related vessel on the first angiogram was associated with a lower mortality rate (5.2 percent) than was an occluded artery (10.4 percent). In the accumulated data[367] from the first four TAMI trials of 810 patients presenting within 6 h of the onset of symptoms, cardiac catheterization performed at 90 min following initiation of thrombolytic therapy showed that patients with a patent artery had a hospital mortality rate of 4.5 percent, which was three times lower than that observed in the patients with persistent coronary occlusion. Furthermore, it was shown that patients who had undergone successful thrombolysis but in whom the vessel reoccluded had an overall mortality rate of 11 percent, compared to a mortality rate of 4.5 percent in patients whose vessels remained patent. These findings are illustrated in Fig. 60-6. In the t-PA and APSAC Patency Study (TAPS),[398] the importance of early versus late patency is again confirmed. Another study reported that, among 227 patients treated within 3 h of the onset of symptoms, 84 percent of the patients with complete reperfusion at the time of acute angiography survived 4 years, compared with only 63 percent of those patients with partial or no reperfusion.[369] In summary, the results of clinical trials and routine clinical practice have shown that an occluding thrombus

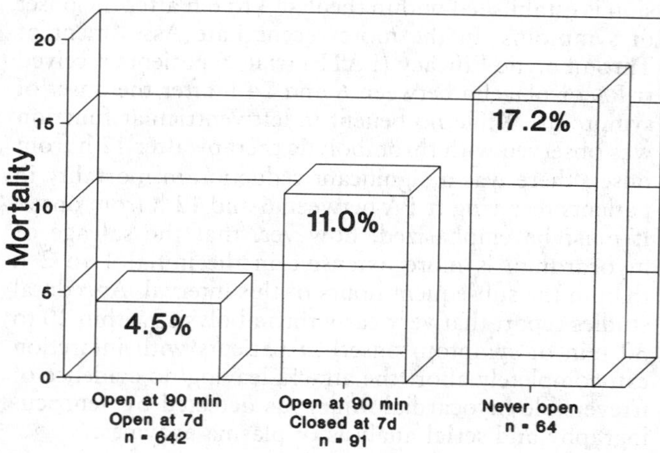

FIGURE 60-6 Composite analysis of data from the TAMI trials, phases one through four. Lowest hospital mortality is associated with early and sustained patency of the infarct artery. This benefit is markedly attenuated by subsequent reocclusion.

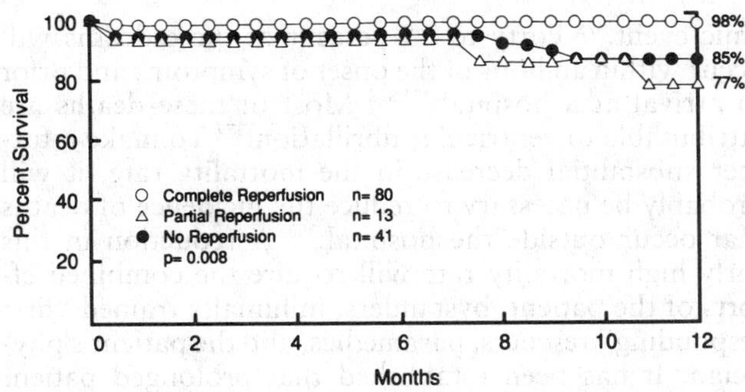

FIGURE 60-7 One year survival curves for streptokinase-treated patients in the Western Washington trial according to reperfusion status.[371]

is the proximate cause of myocardial infarction in patients who evolve Q-wave infarction and that early lysis of the thrombus leads to limitation of infarct size, improved ventricular function, and a marked reduction in acute and long-term mortality rates.

Sustained Patency and the Impact of Reocclusion

In the initial trials assessing thrombolytic therapy, the incidence of coronary reocclusion from rethrombosis was approximately 20 percent, and the incidence of reinfarction was approximately 10 percent.[370] Most of these occlusions occur within the first 24 h. In the initial TIMI trial, the ventricular global and regional ejection fractions increased significantly between the acute and the convalescent phases in patients with early and sustained reperfusion. In contrast, patients with reocclusion had no improvement. Patients having a patent artery at 90 min which remained patent had a mortality rate of 5.4 percent at 1 year, compared to 8.4 percent in patients in whom the vessel reoccluded. In a similar study,[367] the hospital mortality rate in patients with a patent artery at both 90 min and 7 days was 4.5 percent, compared with 11 percent in patients with a vessel that was patent at 90 min but was shown by angiographic studies to be occluded at follow-up on angiography. Similarly, recovery of the global and regional ejection fraction was impaired in patients with evidence of reocclusion at 1 week compared to those with sustained reperfusion. The beneficial effect on long-term survival of maintaining patency was shown in the Western Washington trial,[371] as illustrated by the data in Fig. 60-7.

Spontaneous Reperfusion

It is well established by coronary angiographic studies performed early in the course of an AMI that the infarct-related artery is patent in 20 percent of patients, presumably reflecting spontaneous reperfusion.[362,365] Moreover, there is a progressive increase in the percentage of arteries that are patent from 6 to 24 h to 4 weeks, reflecting an increase in spontaneous thrombolysis over time (Fig. 60-8).[372]

Late Reperfusion: The Open Artery Hypothesis

Early reperfusion is a prerequisite for limitation of infarct size, which accounts for the acute benefit of thrombolytic therapy.[343] Other mechanisms may also contribute to the beneficial effect of reperfusion. The benefit of late thrombolysis is suggested by mortality figures from clinical trials demonstrating reperfusion performed too late in the course of an evolving myocardial infarction to limit infarct size. Subgroup analysis from two trials, the APSAC Intervention Mortality Study (AIMS)[373] and the Anglo Scandinavian Study of Early Thrombolysis (ASSET),[374] noted a reduction in mortality in the 4-to-6 h window that was similar to that in the initial 4 h. In AIMS, mortality was reduced by 41 percent among patients treated within the first 4 h and 53 percent in those treated between 4 and 6 h. Similarly, in the ASSET trial, mortality was reduced approximately 25 percent whether patients were treated within the first or second 3 h from the onset of symptoms. The ISIS-2 study[349] extended the concept of beneficial late reperfusion with its analysis revealing a significant benefit at 6 to 12 h and even from 12 to 24 h. Yusuf and colleagues,[112] in a meta-analysis of several trials, concluded that a significant reduction in mortality of 22 percent was demonstrable in patients treated between 12 and 24 h with thrombolytic therapy. There is also a suggestion that late reperfusion may be beneficial in patients presenting with AMI who were treated with rt-PA or urokinase and/or angioplasty.[366] There are also retrospective data to suggest that patency restored late is better than persistent occlusion. In an analysis of patients managed in the prethrombo-

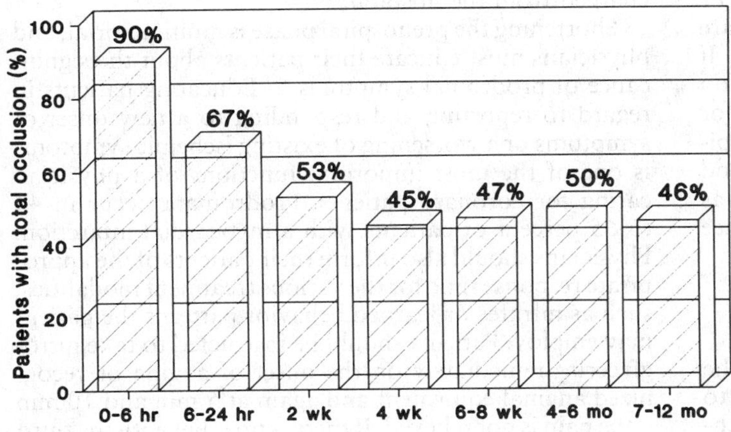

FIGURE 60-8 Percentage of patients with total coronary occlusion at different time intervals after the onset of symptoms of acute myocardial infarction. (*From deFeyter PJ, van den Brand M, Serruys PW, Wijns W: Am Heart J 1985; 109:194. Reproduced with permission from the publisher and authors.*)

lytic era, Cigarroa and coworkers[375] observed that an open artery following myocardial infarction was the most significant predictor of long-term survival in patients who had single-vessel disease.

It should be noted that the benefit of late reperfusion is debatable. It has been argued that in the ISIS-2 trial, since patients were enrolled on the basis of chest pain with or without ECG changes, some of the patients may have not yet developed myocardial infarction and the benefit resulted from the treatment of preinfarction syndromes. In this regard, it should be noted that in the ISIS-3 trial, however, no significant benefit was observed in those treated with SK, APSAC, or rt-PA in either the 6-to-12 or the 12-to-24 h interval. This finding is in keeping with the results of the prospective study, the EMERAS trial. This study was a multicenter trial conducted in South America consisting of 3600 patients with ST-T segment elevation who were enrolled between 6 and 24 h after onset of symptoms and randomized to conventional treatment or SK. The 1-month hospital mortality rate was 11.2 percent in the group receiving SK and 11.8 percent in the group receiving placebo. In subgroup analysis, patients treated with SK between 7 and 12 h had a mortality of 11.3, versus 12.8 percent in the conventionally treated group, which was not statistically significant. It is possible at this time only to speculate on the possible mechanisms mediating the benefit of late reperfusion. Such mechanisms could include the prevention of postinfarction remodeling by promoting better healing and stronger scar formation, providing a scaffolding effect for the necrotic region, or salvaging an intact rim of myocardium. It could also be a protective mechanism to reduce the frequency of ventricular fibrillation by some yet unexplained electrical stabilizing effect. It is also possible that the open infarct-related artery can provide collateral flow to other areas of the myocardium and offer protection in the event of an occlusion of the artery serving these areas.

Specific Therapies: Initial Assessments

Since the establishment of thrombolytic therapy as routine for myocardial infarction, triaging for appropriate candidates must be performed within minutes of the initial assessment. The patient's vital signs must be assessed rapidly, ECG electrodes applied to record a 12-lead ECG and for monitoring, and an intravenous access route established for subsequent therapy. Pain should be relieved immediately. If life-threatening arrhythmias are present, treatment is initiated usually with lidocaine. If the patient is at home, the patient is transferred as soon as possible to the nearest hospital having facilities for treatment of AMI. If there are no contraindications, aspirin and thrombolytic therapy, along with analgesic and antiarrhythmic therapy, if required, should be given as soon as possible after the diagnosis is established (see below).

Prehospital Care

An AMI will occur in 1.2 to 1.5 million people in the United States each year. Five hundred thousand to 600,000 of these people will die during this acute ischemic event.[376] Forty to 65 percent of these deaths will occur within an hour of the onset of symptoms and prior to arrival at a hospital.[377,378] Most of these deaths are attributable to ventricular fibrillation.[379] To make a further substantial decrease in the mortality rate, it will probably be necessary to reduce the incidence of deaths that occur outside the hospital.[380] A reduction in this early high mortality rate will require the combined efforts of the patient, bystanders, minimally trained "first responding" rescuers, paramedics, and the patient's physician. It has been established that prolonged patient delay time is the rate-limiting step in defining the prehospital phase of myocardial infarction. In a recent study the mean patient delay time was 2.7 h,[381] while an earlier study found that 4 h had elapsed before 70 percent of patients obtained medical consultations or were traveling to a hospital.[378] Recently, only 20 percent of patients were found to present within 2 h.[198] Most of this patient delay time is consumed in decision making.[382] The patient must perceive the symptoms, recognize their possible significance, and conclude that medical help is appropriate. In some patients, the decision time is prolonged by a lack of knowledge. It is interesting, however, that patient delay time is not dependent on education level, occupation, socioeconomic class, or past history of cardiac disease. In fact, patients with a past history of myocardial infarction or angina have an unexpectedly long decision time.[383] In other patients, the decision time is prolonged by denial or by "diagnostic trials" with household remedies, patent medications, or previously prescribed drugs. It has been noted that only 10 percent of patients arriving at the hospital within 1 h of the onset of pain utilized nonprescription medications, while 41 percent of those arriving after 12 h did so.[378] The remainder of the delay time is consumed by "human factors," including the time a patient takes to modify existing social obligations and the time a patient uses to prepare for going to the hospital. There is evidence, however, that public education can reduce the time required for decision making.[382]

The bystander can play an important role both in shortening patient delay time and responding to an arrest. It has been shown that a spouse's presence accelerated the hospital arrival time.[379] Furthermore, if basic life support is initiated by a bystander within 4 min of cardiac arrest and if defibrillation is accomplished within 8 min, 40 percent of the patients will survive to be discharged from the hospital.[384]

Shortening the prehospital phase is multifactorial, and physicians must educate their patients about the significance of prodromal symptoms.[380] Educating patients in regard to reporting and responding to a new onset of symptoms or a worsening of existing ischemic symptoms is one of the most important functions of a physician caring for coronary patients. Prodromata occur in 44 to 65 percent of patients with a myocardial infarction. Physicians should also inform their patients of the appropriate response time for the various treatment modalities, such as nitrates or learned behavior patterns the patient may employ. Patients should be instructed to take nitroglycerin immediately on the onset of angina or recognized anginal equivalent and again at 5 min and 10 min if the pain is not relieved. If there is no relief with the third dose of nitroglycerin, the patient should be transported immediately to the nearest emergency facility. The physician and patient must be aware that attempts at consultation with a physician during the patient decision time is likely to inordinately prolong hospital arrival time.[379]

Many communities in the United States are served by a two-tier ambulance service consisting of basic life support units and advanced life support units. Since there are usually more basic support units, the response times for these units are shorter than for advanced support units (3 min versus 6 min[385] or 6.8 min versus 8.4 min). A marked improvement in neurological recovery has been documented if these minimally trained "first-responding rescuers" are permitted to defibrillate ventricular fibrillation. The goal of any emergency medical system (EMS) should be to have individuals who are trained in advanced life support techniques, including the use of antiarrhythmics, intravenous fluid administration, and analgesics, and who can reach the patient as soon as possible in a vehicle equipped as a coronary care unit. These paramedics should have a physician-directed plan for evaluating the nature of the problem, initiating basic treatment, and transporting the patient. While the medical community often views the EMS as a "scoop and run" operation, the total time consumed from the reception of the 911 call until hospital arrival averaged 46.1 min in eight cities. The time was substantially longer than paramedics' perception of their field time (28 min).[386] Most of this field time was consumed by the medic on-scene time, which averaged 25.8 minutes. This total field time was not prolonged by acquisition in the field of a 12-lead ECG.[382] The National Registry of Myocardial Infarction found in a review of 48,128 patients with confirmed AMI that the average duration of the prehospital phase defined as onset of chest pain to hospital presentation was 5.1 h (National Registry of Myocardial Infarction; unpublished data). Upon arrival in the hospital emergency room, patients must be assessed rapidly and those suspected to have myocardial infarction identified immediately. Those suspected of having an infarction should have ECG monitoring from the time of entry, have their rhythm stabilized, and, when appropriate, have thrombolytic therapy initiated. Delays in evaluation and treatment related to hospital administrative procedures (e.g., establishing insurance coverage) or acquisition of nonmedical information should not delay initial arrhythmic or thrombolytic therapy. It is surprising to note that the National Registry of Myocardial Infarction found the time from hospital arrival to initiation of thrombolytic therapy to be 104 min in 13,718 patients (unpublished data), while in eight U.S. cities the time was found to be 83.8 min, with no difference in community hospitals and tertiary care facilities.[385]

Alleviation of Pain and Anxiety

The alleviation of pain and anxiety remains an essential element in the care of the patient with an acute myocardial infarction. The pain and the accompanying anxiety contribute to excessive activity of the autonomic nervous system and to restlessness. These factors, in turn, increase the metabolic demands of the myocardium. Physician assurance from the beginning is an essential part of treatment and should be provided with compassion, patience, and confidence. Optimal care of a patient with AMI requires a team of experienced individuals.

Hypoxemia is common in patients with AMI and in itself may be a cause for anxiety or chest pain. Thus, it has been routine to give oxygen through a nasal catheter for 24 to 48 h. Since oxygen may increase vascular resistance, there may not be a significant increase in oxygen delivery to the tissues, especially if the patient is not hypoxemic. There is increasing concern about the routine use of oxygen. One approach in the uncomplicated patient is to obtain blood gas values before initiating the use of oxygen. In patients who are anxious, have pain, or have any degree of obvious respiratory distress, administration of oxygen at 2 to 4 liters/min by mask or nasal prongs is mandatory. In patients with normal arterial gas values, the nasal prongs may be a source of irritation rather than benefit, and in such patients oxygen may not be necessary. In patients with severe respiratory distress or in pulmonary edema, endotracheal intubation is required, together with administration of 100 percent oxygen.

Narcotics remain the drugs of choice in the treatment of pain and anxiety with acute infarction. Among the available narcotics (meperidine, pentazocine, nalbuphine, and morphine), morphine seems to be particularly well tolerated. This drug offers significant analgesia with little cardiac depression.[387] Morphine does have respiratory depressant action and can cause hypotension by its peripheral vasodilator effects. Consequently, it is preferably administered in small repeated doses rather than a large single dose. Since intravenous morphine reaches its peak effect in 15 to 20 min, it should be titrated to the desired level of analgesia by administering 2 to 4 mg every 15 to 30 min.[382] In patients with an acute inferior myocardial infarction with bradycardia with or without hypotension, the vagolytic narcotic meperidine may be substituted for the parasympathomimetic morphine.

If the patient's anxiety is not controlled by the administration of narcotics, mild sedation with a benzodiazepine agent is appropriate. Diazepam in doses of 5 mg orally every 8 to 12 h or alprazolam in doses of 0.25 mg every 8 h are most often used. The other agent which has become important in managing the pain of the evolving myocardial infarction is intravenous nitroglycerin. While the predominantly antianginal effect of nitroglycerin is due to a reduction in myocardial oxygen demand, the drug appears to act on the coronary circulation primarily by dilating the large epicardial capacitance vessels and possibly the large collateral channels. Consequently, in patients with good collateral vessels, nitroglycerin is likely to increase flow into the ischemic regions.[389,390] Apart from relieving pain, intravenous nitroglycerin reduces the likelihood of developing cardiac failure, infarct extension, or cardiac death. Both clinical data,[391–393] and studies in animals suggest that the early administration of nitroglycerin limits the extent of myocardial damage and favorably affects survival.[391]

A reasonable approach is to initiate intravenous nitroglycerin therapy in any patient with discomfort thought to be due to myocardial ischemia that lasts longer than 15 to 30 min, particularly if the patient is hypertensive. The initial dose of 5 mg/min should be increased by 5 mg/min every 10 min until the pain is resolved or the desired reduction in arterial pressure is obtained. The adverse effect most frequently encountered is headache, which can usually be controlled with mild analgesics. Sinus tachycardia and hypotension may be avoided by careful titration of the dose. While the magnitude of potential benefit of intravenous nitroglycerin is open to question, the very low risk of its use when the dosage is carefully controlled results in a favorable risk-to-benefit ratio. The proper duration of its use in these circumstances remains unresolved, but it is usually given intravenously for 24 to 48 h, followed by transdermal or oral administration. The American Heart Association and the American College of Cardiology, in a joint statement on the management of AMI, recommended that nitroglycerin be used routinely.[394] The objective is not necessarily to limit infarct size but, rather, to relieve ischemia. Another approach is to add a beta blocker, preferably intravenously, particularly if the patient has tachycardia and ongoing chest pain.

Thrombolysis: Indications for Therapy

Reperfusion therapy should be given immediate consideration in all patients presenting with AMI. The primary indication for attempts at reperfusion given an appropriate history is the findings on the ECG. Patients with ST-segment elevation are candidates for thrombolytic therapy, whereas patients with ST-segment depression, T-wave inversion, or no ECG changes have not been shown to benefit from such therapy. A portion of this group with ST-T segment depression or T-wave inversion are subsequently confirmed to be non-Q-wave myocardial infarctions. Early spontaneous reperfusion is the likely scenario in these patients; consequently, the administration of a thrombolytic agent would be unlikely to hasten this process. Patients with ongoing symptoms suggestive of myocardial ischemia should be repeatedly evaluated by 12-lead ECGs as frequently as every 10 to 15 min in order to identify ST-segment elevation as soon as possible. Conversely, ST-segment elevation in the absence of suggestive symptoms should raise such possibilities as early repolarization, pericarditis, and previous infarction with aneurysm formation.

Patients presenting with the clinical features of AMI and left bundle branch block on their ECGs should also be considered candidates for thrombolytic therapy. In the ISIS-2 trial,[349] patients fitting this description had a mortality rate of 28 percent treated with placebo, versus 19.8 percent treated with SK and aspirin. A similar beneficial effect was noted in ISIS-3.[350] Echocardiographic studies in such patients may provide evidence compatible with acute myocardial ischemia.

Initially, elderly patients were excluded from thrombolytic therapy primarily because of a perceived increased risk of bleeding. More recent clinical trials have not excluded elderly patients, and the data derived from these studies indicate that thrombolytic therapy is even more beneficial in the elderly than in the young.[395] In patients over 75 years of age enrolled in the GISSI-2 trial, there were 4.2 fewer deaths per 100 patients in those treated with SK than in the controls,[396] while in ISIS-2 there were 3.3 fewer deaths per 100 patients in those patients over 70 years of age who were treated.[349] In the ISIS-2 trial, among patients 80 years of age or older who received SK and aspirin, as compared with placebo, the 1-month mortality rate was reduced from 37 to 20 percent. In contrast, in patients 60 years of age or younger, the mortality rate was reduced from 6 percent to only 4 percent. The ISIS-3 study confirmed this increased benefit of thrombolytic therapy in the elderly.[350] Advanced age should therefore no longer be considered a contraindication to thrombolysis, despite the increased risk of intracerebral bleeding.[397]

Large, placebo-controlled clinical trials have consistently demonstrated reduced mortality in patients receiving thrombolytic therapy within 6 h of the onset of an AMI.[347,373,374] These data are in concert with the data from animal models establishing the completion of transmural necrosis within 3 to 6 h of coronary occlusion. The question as to whether or not thrombolysis is beneficial when given more than 6 h after the onset of an infarction remains unresolved. The EMERAS trial[360] showed an insignificant (14 percent) reduction in survival using SK between 6 and 12 h after an infarction, while the LATE trial[361] observed a significant reduction (22 percent) in patients treated with rt-PA up to 12 h after infarction. When the data from the LATE, EMERAS, and ISIS trials are pooled, it presents the suggestion that there is improvement in survival with the use of thrombolytics up to 12 h postinfarction. Both the GISSI-1 and GUSTO trials establish that the benefit of thrombolysis is time-dependent. Thrombolytic therapy is most effective in the first 3 h, has significant benefit up to 6 h, and possibly has continued benefit up to 12 h. The benefit of thrombolysis given between 6 and 12 h postinfarction is likely to be confined to high-risk infarctions, such as large anterior infarctions or those associated with class III or IV heart failure. In weighing the risk of late thrombolytic therapy, such as at 7 or 8 h, the likely consequences of the myocardial infarction versus the possible complication of intracerebral bleeding must be considered. In patients who are known to be at high risk for complications and death, such as those with anterior infarction, left bundle branch block, or severe hypotension, thrombolytic therapy should be considered despite not knowing the precise time of onset of symptoms. Conversely, the young patient with inferior infarction having ST-T segment elevation in II, II, and aV_F leads only would not warrant receiving thrombolytic therapy after 6 h from the onset of symptoms.

Contraindications to Thrombolytic Therapy

The major contraindication to thrombolytic therapy is cerebrovascular accident (CVA) within the last 3 months. A hemorrhagic CVA in the past is an absolute contraindication, whereas a nonhemorrhagic CVA in the more distant past with complete or nearly complete recovery is only a relative contraindication.[398] Patients who have undergone recent (2 weeks) major surgery or delivery are not candidates for thrombolytic therapy, and neither are those with active internal bleeding or bleeding from a peptic ulcer. Puncture of a noncompressible vessel within the previous 10 days makes thrombolytic therapy inadvisable. Other absolute contraindica-

TABLE 60-4

Absolute and Relative Contraindications to Thrombolytic Therapy

Absolute Contraindications	Relative Contraindications
Active internal bleeding	History of nonhemorrhagic cerebrovascular accident in distant past with complete recovery
Intracranial neoplasm or recent head trauma	Recent trauma or surgery >2 weeks previously
Prolonged, traumatic CPR	Active peptic ulcer disease
Suspected aortic dissection	Hemorrhagic retinopathy
Pregnancy	History of severe hypertension with diastolic blood pressure >100
History of hemorrhagic cerebrovascular accident or recent nonhemorrhagic cerebrovascular accident	Bleeding diathesis or concurrent use of anticoagulants
Recorded blood pressure >200/120	Previous treatment with SK or APSAC if being considered (does not apply to rt-PA)
Trauma or surgery that is a potential bleeding source within previous 2 weeks	
Allergy to SK or APSAC if being considered	

tions to thrombolytic therapy include suspected aortic dissection, recent head trauma or known intracranial neoplasm, and pregnancy. Previous exposure to SK or APSAC requires the use of rt-PA in subsequent attempts at thrombolysis. Systemic arterial hypertension and cardiopulmonary resuscitation should no longer be regarded as absolute contraindications to thrombolytic therapy. The ISIS-2 trial found that, among patients with a systolic blood pressure greater than 175 mmHg, the mortality rate was lower in those receiving SK than in control subjects (5.7 percent versus 8.7 percent).[349] Some practitioners consider a recorded blood pressure greater than 200/120 an absolute contraindication. A history of chronic severe hypertension with diastolic blood pressure greater than 100 mmHg, with or without drug therapy, is a relative contraindication. Most clinicians proceed with thrombolytic therapy if elevated blood pressure normalizes promptly with the easing of pain and anxiety through the use of narcotics. Califf and associates noted that patients who had brief (<10 min), nontraumatic cardiopulmonary resuscitation (CPR) had no evidence of tamponade or hemothorax with thrombolytic therapy.[399] Prior administration of CPR should be considered a relative contraindication, since the risk of further bleeding in the chest may not outweigh the benefit. Other relative contraindications include hemorrhagic retinopathy, trauma or surgery more than 2 weeks previously, active peptic ulcer disease, and bleeding diathesis or current use of anticoagulants. The absolute and relative contraindications for thrombolytic therapy are summarized in Table 60-4.

Choice of Thrombolytic Agent

Three thrombolytic agents are currently approved for routine use: SK, rt-PA, and APSAC. Each has been shown to limit infarct size, preserve ventricular function, and improve survival rates. These drugs and their pharmacologic properties are discussed in detail in Chap. 69.

In angiographic studies,[343,400,401] rt-PA recanalized the coronary artery at 90 min in about 70 to 75 percent of patients, compared to 55 to 60 percent of those receiving SK or APSAC. Patency determined at 24 to 36 h is essentially the same for all three agents. The time course for this "catch-up" phenomenon in vessel patency, as defined by the GUSTO angiographic substudy, occurs within the first 3 h after administration of the lytic agent.[402] Since rapid lysis appears essential for limitation of infarct size, it was surprising that the initial large comparative trials of the three agents found the reduction in mortality to be identical for each of the three agents. In the GISSI-2 International rt-PA/SK Mortality trial, the mortality rate with SK therapy (8.5 percent) was the same as with rt-PA (8.9 percent).[396] Likewise, the ISIS-3 trial reported a 30-day mortality rate, which was the same for all three agents (10.5 percent for SK, 10.6 percent for APSAC, and 10.3 percent for rt-PA).[350] The mortality rates and adverse effects observed in the ISIS-3 trial are tabulated in Table 60-5. Conversely, the GUSTO trial found a 30-day mortality rate of 6.3 percent for the accelerated rt-PA regimen, which was significantly less than the 7.2 percent mortality with SK and subcutaneous heparin and the 7.4 percent mortality with SK and intra-

TABLE 60-5

Mortality Rates and Complications at 35 Days from the ISIS-3 Trial

Characteristic, %	Streptokinase	Anistreplase	Duteplase
Mortality			
All patients	10.5	10.6	10.3
Patients ≤6 h with ST elevation	9.9	10.1	9.6
Adverse reactions and reinfarction			
Allergic reaction causing persistent shock	0.3	0.6	0.1
Profound hypotension requiring drugs	6.8	7.2	4.3
Major bleeds requiring blood transfusions	0.9	1.0	0.9
Reinfarction	3.6	3.8	3.1
Any stroke	1.1	1.5	1.5
Probable cerebral hemorrhage	0.3	0.6	0.7
Other stroke	0.8	0.9	0.8

TABLE 60-6

30-Day Mortality Rates from the GUSTO Trial

Regimen	Mortality, %
SK and subcutaneous heparin	7.2
SK and intravenous heparin	7.4
Accelerated rt-PA and intravenous heparin	6.3*
Combination rt-PA and SK with intravenous heparin	7.0

* 4% reduction in mortality rate was achieved with the accelerated rt-PA regimen versus the SK strategies ($p = .001$).

venous heparin (Table 60-6).[403] The reasons for the discrepancies in these megatrials with regard to survival are probably related both to the more accelerated regimen of rt-PA administration in GUSTO and to the much more aggressive use of intravenous heparin in the rt-PA limb in GUSTO. While rt-PA induces patency in a greater percentage of patients than SK or APSAC, recent data indicate that the higher patency rate of rt-PA is maintained if the partial thromboplastin time (PTT) is maintained at at least 1.5 to 2.0 times normal. In the GISSI-2 International trial, heparin was not given until 12 h after thrombolytic therapy and was administered in doses of 12,500 units subcutaneously twice a day; in the ISIS-3 trial, it was also given subcutaneously but was initiated 4 h after thrombolytic therapy. It has been shown that heparin given subcutaneously does not reach adequate therapeutic levels for 24 to 36 h and that, at the dose used in these trials, adequate levels even after 24 h occur in only 50 percent of patients.[404] In the rt-PA limb of the GUSTO trial, a bolus of heparin was administered immediately and followed by intravenous heparin monitored closely by serial determinations of PTT.

The selection of a thrombolytic agent must be based on its adverse effects as well as its efficacy. The major risk with any thrombolytic agent is its propensity for causing bleeding, with the most devastating bleed being a hemorrhagic stroke. In the GUSTO trial, the frequency of hemorrhagic stroke was 0.49 percent for SK and subcutaneous heparin, 0.54 percent for SK and intravenous heparin, 0.72 percent for rt-PA, and 0.94 percent for combined SK and rt-PA. There was a small but significant excess of hemorrhagic strokes for rt-PA and for the combined rt-PA and SK strategy ($p < .001$) compared with SK arms. The combined end point of death or nonfatal hemorrhagic stroke was, however, significantly reduced in the rt-PA group compared with the SK groups (6.6 percent versus 7.5 percent; $p = .004$).[403]

Dose and Administration of Thrombolytic Agents

Streptokinase is given in a dose of 1.5 million units intravenously over 30 to 60 min. Since antibodies develop and may persist for several years, a subsequent need for thrombolytic therapy, such as for early or late reocclusion, would require the use of rt-PA. If the patient has had a streptococcal infection within 3 to 6 months, the use of rt-PA is preferable. APSAC is anisoylated streptokinase that is identical to SK as a thrombolytic agent but can be given as a rapid infusion of 30 units over 5 to 10 min. Its therapeutic half-life is similar to that of SK, which is about 90 min, in contrast that of rt-PA, which is about 5 min. The FDA-approved dose of rt-PA is a total of 100 mg given in initial bolus of 10 mg followed by 50 mg in the first hour and 20 mg per hour for the subsequent 2 h. The GUSTO trial, however, in establishing the superiority of rt-PA to SK in terms of a 30-day mortality rate reduction, used an accelerated dosing regimen for rt-PA.[403] This accelerated regimen, proposed by Neuhaus, consists of a bolus of 15 mg, an infusion of 50 mg or 0.75 mg per kilogram of body weight over the next 30 min, and an infusion of 35 mg or 0.50 mg per kilogram of body weight over the subsequent 60 min for a total of up to 100 mg given over 90 min. A recent study performed in 122 patients comparing various regimens of rt-PA showed that a bolus of 50 mg followed by a second bolus of 50 mg in 30 min was most effective, with a patency of 90 percent at 60 min.[405]

Thrombolytic therapy is rapidly evolving, and both the specific agent and various combinations as well as the specific doses and regimens of administration are changing rapidly. The overall trend at this time indicates that SK in a dose of 1.5 million units is more likely to be given over 30 to 45 min rather than 60 min. In the case of rt-PA, the total dose is likely to be given over 90 min, rather than the present 3 h, and the loading bolus is likely to be 15 to 20 mg, rather than the present 10 mg. Extensive ongoing research that involves molecular engineering of agents such as rt-PA may also have significant impact. In addition, urokinase has been used extensively in clinical trials and, although not approved for routine use, is frequently used as an intracoronary as well as an intravenous agent. Urokinase as an agent for thrombolytic therapy appears to be similar in efficacy and safety to SK but is more expensive. Another recombinant product is single-chain prourokinase, which has been studied as a single agent and in combination with either SK or rt-PA, but is not approved for routine use. Earlier data suggesting that the combination of SK with rt-PA provided greater benefit than either agent alone was not substantiated by the GUSTO trial.[403]

Conjunctive and Adjunctive Therapy

Lysis of a thrombus by any thrombolytic agent induces a surface which is perhaps the most thrombogenic known.[343,406] Furthermore, lysis with either rt-PA or SK has been shown to be associated with marked elevation of plasma levels of thrombin, which return to normal after 24 h.[407] Since aspirin has no effect on thrombin-induced platelet aggregation,[408] the use of heparin during the initial 24 to 48 h was assumed to be critical to prevent rethrombosis and reocclusion.

The necessity of heparin for maintaining coronary patency induced by rt-PA was established in the HART trial.[401] In this trial, 208 patients received rt-PA within 4 h of the onset of their infarction. Simultaneously, 50 percent of these patients received heparin administered as a bolus followed by an intravenous infusion, while

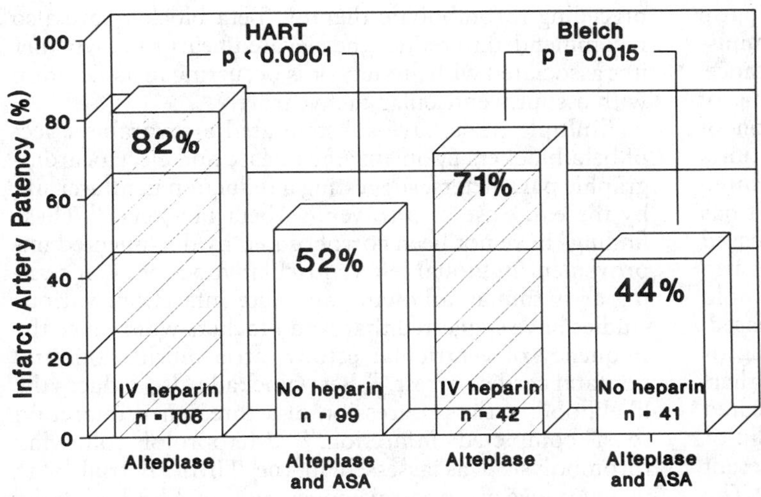

FIGURE 60-9 Influence of effective anticoagulation on early patency rates with t-PA. Patency assessed angiographically at an average of 18 to 81 h is significantly greater in patients treated with intravenous heparin.

the remainder received only oral aspirin in a dose of 81 mg/day. Coronary angiographic studies performed at 18 h showed a patency of 82 percent in the group receiving heparin and 52 percent in the group receiving aspirin (Fig. 60-9). Stratifying the group on the basis of PTT established an excellent correlation between patency and PTT (Fig. 60-10). In patients with a PTT of less than 45 s, the patency was only 45 percent; patency was 85 percent or greater in patients with a PTT over 45 s.[409] The findings of HART were confirmed by Bleich and associates,[410] who showed that rt-PA given with heparin had a patency of greater than 90 percent; without heparin, the patency rate was 44 percent (Fig. 60-9). In the National Heart Foundation of Australia Study,[359] all patients received TPA, followed by intravenous heparin for 24 h. They were then randomized to continue heparin for 72 h or switched to antiplatelet agents. The study found the patency rate at 72 h to be the same for both groups.

The TAMI-3 study showed that immediate intravenous heparin administration with rt-PA did not result in higher patency at 90 min than did the use of rt-PA alone,[411] indicating that heparin does not act by enhancing lysis. Heparin appears to act by preventing early reocclusion, at least after rt-PA.[412] The adjunctive heparin therapy in both GISSI-2 and ISIS-3 was administered by the subcutaneous route (12 h after thrombolytic therapy in GISSI-2 and 4 h afterward in ISIS-3). Such a heparin regimen seems to be suboptimal adjunctive therapy for rt-PA. A subcutaneous heparin dose of 12,500 units twice a day as used in the megatrials failed to provide therapeutic anticoagulation for at least 24 h in various cohort analytic studies.[404,413] Furthermore an analysis of the anticoagulant response to subcutaneous heparin in a subset of patients in ISIS-3 indicated a marked variation in response.[350] The administration of SK without adjunctive heparin has not been properly tested, but the ISIS data raise the possibility that it may not be necessary in the early hours, since the marked increase in plasma levels of fibrinogen breakdown products, known to inhibit platelet aggregation, may prevent rethrombosis and reocclusion. In contrast to the fibrin-selective agents rt-PA and prourokinase, SK and APSAC are nonspecific and attack circulating fibrinogen as well as clot-bound fibrinogen, which leads to high levels of breakdown products that inhibit platelet aggregation. The results of the SCATI trial argue for the existence of a beneficial effect of heparin even in patients treated with SK. In the SCATI trial, patients receiving SK with subcutaneous heparin had a mortality rate of 4.5 percent, while those receiving SK without heparin had a mortality rate of 8.8 percent.[414] The combined data from these studies suggest that heparin is not necessary to achieve reperfusion but is essential in the first 24 h to maintain

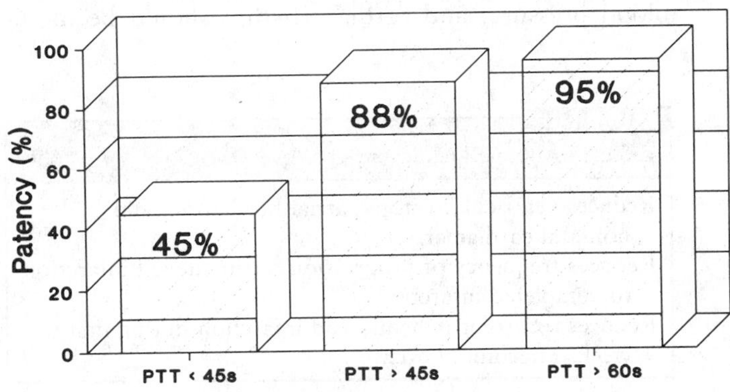

FIGURE 60-10 Retrospective analysis of the HART Trial showing the relationship between increased PTT and coronary artery patency (n = 94). This illustrates the importance of heparin.

patency rates of 80 percent with TPA. While heparin may be beneficial when using SK, subcutaneous administration of heparin appears adequate in this circumstance.

At present, heparin is recommended in a bolus of 5,000 units intravenously followed by an infusion of 1000 to 1200 units/h to keep the PTT at 1.5 to 2.0 times normal. It is recommended that the PTT not be measured until 6 h after initiating heparin therapy because it has not yet reached a steady state. If the PTT has increased more than twofold over normal, the same dose of heparin should be continued; if PTT exhibits less than a twofold increase, the infusion rate of heparin should be increased. Initiation of heparin is recommended either during or immediately following completion of thrombolytic therapy, and it should be maintained in the uncomplicated patient for 24 to 48 h. It is highly likely that hirudin or hirulog will replace heparin in the future, but at present both are undergoing validation in clinical trials.[406] The advantage of hirudin over heparin is due to its direct inhibition of thrombin and its activity against both fibrin-bound and free thrombin. Hirulog is similar to hirudin but has a half-life of 30 min, which makes it much easier to titrate than either heparin or hirudin (see Chap. 7).

Aspirin

After 24 to 48 h, aspirin is more effective than heparin, since the plasma thrombin levels have returned to normal by this time. Aspirin following thrombolytic therapy reduces the incidence of reocclusion and reinfarction.[349,415] In a summary of 33 trials, the incidence of reinfarction in the group receiving aspirin was 11 percent, as opposed to 25 percent in the group receiving conventional therapy without aspirin.[416] In the ISIS-2 pilot study, it was shown that aspirin 160 mg/day was effective. In the TIMI trials (I, II, and III), 80 mg/day was used and most recently has been shown to be beneficial.[417] A 40-mg dose of aspirin is estimated to acetylate adequately all of the platelet cyclooxygenase, the irreversible reaction responsible for the drug's platelet inhibitory effect.[408] It is perhaps prudent to use the lowest dose that is effective, since side effects of bleeding are probably dose-related. Furthermore, production of prostacyclin in the vessel wall is beneficial by virtue of its antiplatelet and vasodilator properties, and the higher doses of aspirin are more likely to inhibit prostacyclin production. A need for a loading dose of aspirin has been proposed, but it seems unnecessary in view of recent data showing that 80 mg of aspirin in normal volunteers induced complete inhibition of platelet aggregation in 15 to 30 min.[418] An upper limit of 80 to 160 mg of aspirin daily is recommended for life. Some physicians recommended 325 mg daily. In patients allergic to aspirin, ticlopidine (150 mg twice a day) can be considered (see also Chaps. 58 and 68).

Beta-Adrenergic Blockers

Beta blockers have been shown to be safe when administered in the setting of an evolving myocardial infarction and are effective in relieving pain, anxiety, and myocardial ischemia and in reducing the incidence of reinfarction following Q-wave infarction with or without preceding thrombolytic therapy. Beta blockers are also recommended to reduce the elevated heart rate, whether it is associated with anxiety or is occurring in association with a supraventricular tachycardia.

Multiple trials have substantiated a favorable effect of beta blockers upon enzyme release and electrocardiographic parameters, suggesting a reduction in infarct size by the early use of intravenous beta blockers.[341] These findings have not been corroborated by documented improvement in global left ventricular function. Concerning arrhythmias following an acute infarction, various studies have suggested that beta blockers will reduce the frequency of ventricular ectopy, atrial fibrillation, and nonfatal cardiac arrest.[419] Beta blockade also reduces the likelihood of the progression of a threatened infarction to a completed infarction.[341] Metoprolol following thrombolysis was assessed in the TIMI-2B trial,[342] in which it was given intravenously within 2 h of administering rt-PA in a total dose of 15 mg separated into three 5-mg doses given 5 to 10 min apart, followed by 50 mg twice the next day and subsequently 100 mg twice a day. In the other group of patients, metoprolol was initiated orally, 100 mg twice a day on the sixth day after thrombolytic therapy. Metoprolol given immediately did not improve ventricular function or survival but significantly decreased the incidence of myocardial ischemia and reinfarction over the initial 6-week period. It was the conclusion of the TIMI-2B trial that metoprolol did not necessarily need to be given routinely but, if used, should be given early in the course of a Q-wave myocardial infarction. The effects of beta blockers in AMI are summarized in Table 60-7. As discussed previously, beta blockers have not been shown to be effective in reducing the incidence of reinfarction in patients evolving non-Q-wave infarction, and thus this group of patients, most of whom will not get thrombolytic therapy, should be considered for a calcium channel blocker, preferably diltiazem or verapamil. While metoprolol and atenolol are the only FDA approved beta blockers for use in AMI, it is thought that all the beta blockers have a similar effect, except those that possess intrinsic sympathomimetic activity. The use of the beta blocker esmolol has also been shown to be safe in patients with AMI. In patients with borderline contraindications, such as borderline or questionable left ventricular function, esmolol can be used to assess patient tolerance of beta blockers. This agent has a rapid onset of action within 5 to 10 min and a half-life of about 30 min, affording a rapid resolution of its side effects should the hemodynamics be comprised. During the administration of any beta blocker, the heart rate, blood pressure, and cardiac rhythm should be moni-

TABLE 60-7

Effects of Beta Blockade in Q-Wave AMI
Reduces ventricular ectopy, atrial fibrillation, and nonfatal cardiac arrest
Reduces frequency of progression of threatened infarction to completed infarction
Reduces recurrent ischemia and infarction during first 6 weeks after initial event

tored. Beta-blocker therapy is contraindicated in the presence of (1) heart block of second degree or greater, (2) rales extending more than one-third of the way up the lung fields, (3) wheezes or development of bronchial asthma, (4) heart rate below 50 beats per minute, (5) systolic arterial pressure below 90 mmHg, (6) pulmonary artery wedge pressure greater than 24 mmHg, and (7) moderate-to-severe chronic obstructive lung disease.

It is preferable that the beta blocker be administered such that the heart rate is kept between 50 and 75 beats per minute and the systolic blood pressure does not go below 90 to 100 mmHg. In patients presenting with or developing severe pulmonary edema in the setting of AMI in whom beta blockade is considered to be aggravating or in any way precipitating the cardiac failure, it may be advantageous to administer intravenously a non-beta receptor-dependent agonist, such as milrinone, or increasing doses of dobutamine to overcome the beta blockade.

Magnesium

Magnesium ion has several cardiovascular effects, including coronary and systemic vasodilatation, antiarrhythmic action, and inhibition of platelet functions. It is also myocardium-protective and has been viewed as a calcium antagonist.[420] These pharmacologic actions in general and the antiarrhythmic effects in particular led to the clinical investigation of the efficacy of magnesium in AMI. Initial small clinical trials suggested a beneficial effect but were underpowered to prove the point. The second Leicester Intravenous Magnesium Intervention Trial (LIMIT-2) was a double-blind, randomized, placebo-controlled trial in over 2300 patients that was designed to address definitively the issue of whether intravenous magnesium was beneficial in the treatment of acute AMI.[421] The magnesium-treated group had a 24 percent reduction of all causes of mortality at 28 days, a 36 percent reduction in coronary care unit mortality rates, and a 25 percent reduction in the incidence of congestive heart failure in the coronary care unit. The effect was independent of thrombolytic therapy. There were no significant effects on arrhythmias, and the most likely explanation of efficacy was thought to be myocardial protection. A subsequent meta-analysis of previous trials concluded that intravenous magnesium gave a 54 percent reduction in mortality rates and approximately a 50 percent reduction in ventricular tachycardia and fibrillation and in cardiac arrest.[422] The effects of intravenous magnesium in AMI are summarized in Table 60-8. The most significant side effects of intravenous magnesium have been flushing with initial injection, bradycardia which occurs in a small number of cases, and a slight fall in blood pressure. Contraindications have not been established but have included high-degree atrioventricular block and systolic blood pressure of less than 80 to 90 mmHg in several trials. Regimens of administration have varied widely in published trials, but in LIMIT-2 the regimen was 8 mmol in 4 mL injected over 5 min with 65 mmol infused over the next 24 h. Given the very encouraging recent results, it seems reasonable to consider magnesium treatment of AMI less than 6 to 8 h from onset. More definitive or confirmatory data may be anticipated from ISIS-4.

TABLE 60-8

Beneficial Effects of Intravenous Magnesium in AMI
Reduces all causes of death and coronary care unit mortality rates
Reduces congestive heart failure in the coronary care unit
Probably acts to preserve myocardium
May reduce ventricular arrhythmias (data contradictory)

Angioplasty and Surgical Revascularization as Primary or Adjunctive Therapy to Thrombolysis

Detailed discussions of percutaneous transluminal coronary angioplasty (PTCA) and its indications appear in Chaps. 70 and 71. The role of coronary angioplasty in the treatment of the AMI is continuing to be evaluated. The circumstances in which angioplasty may be performed are (1) direct angioplasty, the use of angioplasty as the primary reperfusion technique; (2) immediate angioplasty, the use of angioplasty immediately following the administration of a thrombolytic agent; (3) rescue angioplasty, the use of angioplasty only in patients who do not reperfuse with a thrombolytic agent; (4) delayed angioplasty, the routine application of angioplasty in all patients 2 to 7 days after reperfusion; and (5) elective angioplasty, the use of angioplasty only in patients manifesting ischemia following reperfusion. Recognizing that the reperfusion rate with coronary angioplasty is probably superior to that with thrombolysis, some physicians have suggested that direct angioplasty be considered in certain circumstances, including the following: (1) presentation of a high-risk patient early (1 to 2 h) in the course of an AMI at a facility in which coronary angioplasty is immediately available; (2) a patient in whom coronary angiographic studies are necessary to make the diagnosis; and (3) a patient with a contraindication to thrombolytic therapy (see Chap. 70).

The issue of the role of direct angioplasty in the treatment of AMI has been reinvigorated by three papers describing the results of this approach. Direct angioplasty was compared[423–425] in randomized trials with thrombolytic therapy. Two[423,424] of the three trials reported better results with direct angioplasty than with thrombolytic therapy, whereas the third reported no difference.[425] The largest (395 patients) of these studies was the Primary Angioplasty in Myocardial Infarction study (PAMI).[423] There was a higher success rate for establishing reperfusion with angioplasty. The in-hospital mortality rate was 6.5 percent for the rt-PA group and 2.6 percent for the PTCA group. Higher-risk subgroups had a mortality rate of 10.4 percent with rt-PA versus a 2.6 percent rate with PTCA. Reinfarction or death in the hospital occurred in 12 percent and 5.1 percent of patients treated with rt-PA and PTCA, respectively. Treatment with PTCA was associated with a lower incidence of intracranial bleeding than was that with rt-PA. There was no difference in myocardial salvage, but there was a higher reinfarction and death rate at 6 months with rt-PA than with PTCA.

The results of the recent trials evaluating direct angioplasty in the treatment of AMI lead to the following conclusions: acute PTCA should be considered if the patient presents to a center with expertise in PTCA that is organized logistically to provide rapid intervention if the patient is high-risk (e.g., with a large anterior myocardial infarction or cardiogenic shock) or has a contraindication to thrombolytic therapy. Because of the limited availability of PTCA and because of the demonstrable efficacy of thrombolysis, thrombolytic therapy remains the standard of care.

Routine immediate or delayed angioplasty is not recommended as a standard mode of therapy following thrombolytic therapy. TIMI-2A and -2B trials,[426] the TAMI study,[411] the European Cooperative Study Group trial,[427] and the Should We Intervene Following Thrombolysis (SWIFT) trial[428] all showed no reduction in the incidence of coronary reocclusion or hospital mortality rates and no evidence of improved ventricular function with immediate or delayed angioplasty compared to elective angioplasty following thrombolytic therapy. Rescue angioplasty would seem to offer the benefit of improved early patency. However, the technique is not universally applicable and increases the risk of bleeding, and the means of detecting the necessity for its application are currently lacking.[429] With the exception of coronary angiography, there is no proven, accurate method of rapidly ascertaining whether or not a patient achieves perfusion (see Chap. 137). The TIMI-2 trial found that angioplasty either performed routinely at 18 to 48 h when anatomically appropriate or in response to induced or spontaneous ischemia did not improve survival or reduce the reinfarction rate at either 6 weeks or 1 year,[430] and neither did it reduce the need for surgery (Fig. 60-11). At present, the most widely accepted recommendation is to perform cardiac catheterization for possible angioplasty or bypass surgery in patients who develop angina or manifest evidence of myocardial ischemia during submaximal exercise testing.

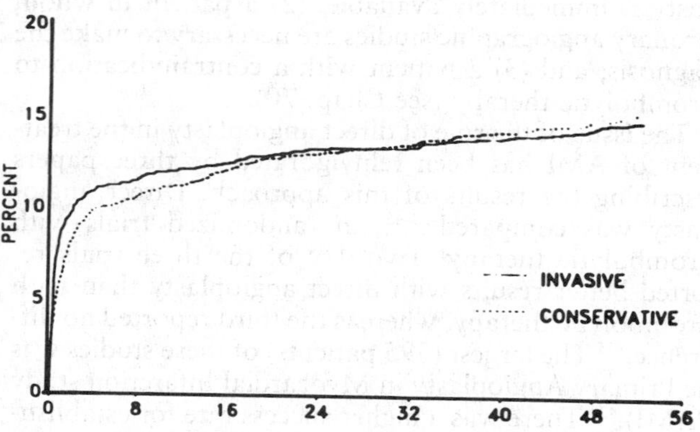

FIGURE 60-11 Kaplan Meier curves for death and infarction in patients assigned to the invasive or conservative strategies in TIMI-2. Routine cardiac catheterization after thrombolytic therapy and revascularization with PTCA or bypass grafting (when anatomically appropriate) was not a superior strategy to catheterization and revascularization when there is development of spontaneous ischemia or ischemia induced by exercise testing. *(From Williams DO, Braunwald E, Knatterud G, Babb J, Bresnahan J, Greenberg MA, et al.: One-year results of the thrombolysis in myocardial infarction investigation (TIMI) phase II trial. Circulation 1992:85:533–542. Reproduced with permission from the publisher and authors.)*

Overall Strategy for Reperfusion of Patients with Acute Myocardial Infarction

The criteria for initiating thrombolytic therapy are as follows (Table 60-9):

1. Patients presenting with chest pain suggestive of myocardial ischemia, having ST-T segment elevation greater than 1 mm in two continguous limb leads or greater than 2 mm in two contiguous precordial leads or new left bundle branch block and who are within 6 h of the onset of symptoms should receive thrombolytic therapy if there are no contraindications. In patients presenting between 6 and 12 h of the onset of symptoms, one must weigh more heavily the risk versus the benefit. Patients presenting after 12 h are no longer routinely considered for thrombolytic therapy.
2. Contraindications for thrombolytic therapy are absolute or relative, as discussed earlier (Table 60-4).
3. Whether the patient receives SK, APSAC, or rt-PA, it is recommended that heparin be given as a bolus infusion of 5000 units initially followed, by a continuous infusion of 1000 units/h, adjusted to keep the APTT at one-half to 2 times the normal control for 24 to 48 h. Aspirin (80 to 160 mg) should be administered as soon as possible and continued indefinitely. The use of beta blockers, nitrates, calcium, and intravenous magnesium may be given as indicated with or without thrombolytic therapy. Many patients with Q-wave infarction routinely receive nitroglycerin and a beta blocker orally.
4. Patients who received SK or APSAC and who again require thrombolytic therapy should receive rt-PA.
5. Patients presenting with ST-T segment depression and chest pain are not candidates for thrombolytic therapy. These patients need to be triaged as to whether their pain is of cardiac or noncardiac origin, and, if due to the latter, those with either unstable angina or non-Q-wave infarction should be treated as previously discussed and as illustrated in Fig. 60-12.[431] Heparin is given, together with diltiazem and aspirin, in conjunction with conventional therapy as needed.
6. PTCA generally is not a primary procedure, except in unusual cases and only then when there is a very

TABLE 60-9

Criteria for Initiating Thrombolytic Therapy
Chest pain consistent with angina
ECG changes
ST ↑ ≥ 1mm, ≥ 2 contiguous limb leads
ST ↑ ≥ 2mm, ≥ 2 contiguous precordial leads
New left bundle branch block
Absence of contraindications

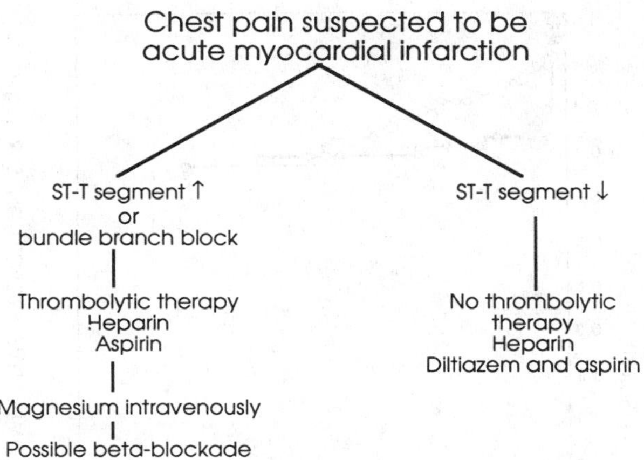

FIGURE 60-12 An algorithm for selection of patients for thrombolytic and other acute therapy.

skilled team readily available to perform the procedure. The role of this strategy is still being evaluated, as discussed above. PTCA is indicated in patients with a contraindication to thrombolytic therapy, such as an allergy to SK or APSAC, or in those with a severe bleeding diathesis. In centers where primary angioplasty is performed commonly, it perhaps should still be reserved for patients with more severe ischemia rather than for uncomplicated patients, such as those with inferior infarction.

7. Elective angioplasty should be reserved for patients who develop ischemia or reinfarction or in whom thrombolytic therapy appears ineffective. In patients in whom angioplasty cannot be performed and who develop recurrent ischemia with possible infarction, the possibility of readministering a thrombolytic agent should be considered; rt-PA may be given in a full dose if the patient has not received it for 24 to 48 h.

Management of Inferior Infarction Associated with Right Ventricular Infarction

Acute inferior myocardial infarction is generally felt to have a more benign course than acute anterior infarction. This purported difference in prognosis primarily reflects the fact that inferior infarctions are frequently smaller than anterior infarctions and are less commonly associated with congestive heart failure. If heart failure and low cardiac output do occur in acute inferior infarction, one or more of the following complications should be sought:[431a] (1) arrhythmia, such as atrial fibrillation, sustained ventricular arrhythmia, or high-degree atrioventricular block; (2) ongoing ischemia, such as ischemia at a distance if the occluded artery to the inferior wall was also supplying, through collaterals, the anterior wall; (3) previous infarction at another location; (4) a mechanical complication, such as papillary muscle dysfunction or, less commonly, a ventricular septal defect; or (5) right ventricular infarction. This differential diagnosis of causes of congestive heart failure in acute inferior myocardial infarction is summarized in Table 60-10.

TABLE 60-10

Differential Diagnosis of Congestive Heart Failure in Inferior AMI
Arrhythmia: high-degree AV block, atrial fibrillation, or sustained ventricular tachycardia
Ischemia at a distance, with the occluded artery to the inferior wall supplying the anterior wall via collaterals
Previous infarction at another location
Mechanical complication, such as papillary muscle dysfunction
Right ventricular infarction

As noted previously, right ventricular infarction commonly occurs in acute inferior infarction, presumably when the right coronary artery is occluded proximally. In a series of 200 patients with acute inferior infarction, 57 percent had evidence of right ventricular infarction, as manifested by ST-segment elevation in lead V_{4R}.[431b] The overall in-hospital mortality rate was 19 percent. ST-segment elevation in lead V_{4R} was the single most powerful independent indicator of a high-risk subgroup with an in-hospital mortality rate of 31 percent, versus 6 percent in those without V_{4R} ST-segment elevation. Those patients with V_{4R} ST-segment elevation had a higher incidence of major in-hospital complications (64 percent) than did those without (28 percent). The post-hospital course was similar in the two groups.

Wellens[431a] has made the following recommendations for the management of acute inferior myocardial infarction:

1. Lead V_{4R} should be assessed, in addition to the usual 12-lead ECG, to detect right ventricular involvement.
2. Thrombolytic therapy should be administered in the absence of contraindications if the right ventricle is involved.
3. If there is right ventricular involvement and there are contraindications to thrombolytic therapy, angioplasty should be attempted immediately in the setting, if possible, to open the proximal right coronary artery.
4. If there is no evidence of reperfusion after thrombolysis (reperfusion ventricular arrhythmia or resolution of pain and ST segment elevation), angioplasty should be considered.
5. In right ventricular infarction in which reperfusion has been unsuccessful and low cardiac output persists, fluid should be administered intravenously to increase right ventricular filling pressure and output. A pulmonary artery catheter should be inserted for hemodynamic monitoring. Vasodilation and especially venodilation, as with nitrates, should be avoided because of the potential for worsening hypotension by decreasing right ventricular filling pressure. If low cardiac output persists after increasing intravascular volume, dobutamine or dopamine should be administered. If high-degree atrioventricular block is associated with hemodynamic compromise, transvenous pacing should be started.

These recommendations are summarized in Table 60-11.

TABLE 60-11

Strategy for Management of Inferior AMI Complicated by Right Ventricular Infarction

Evaluate V_{4R} in addition to 12-lead ECG.
Administer thrombolytic therapy in the absence of contraindications, especially with right ventricular involvement.
Attempt PTCA if there is right ventricular involvement and if contraindications to thrombolysis are present.
Attempt PTCA when there is right ventricular involvement and if thrombolysis is unsuccessful.
Expand intravascular volume if reperfusion is unsuccessful and there is hemodynamic compromise; add positive inotropic agents if low cardiac output persists.
Avoid vasodilators, especially venodilators.
Institute transvenous pacing if high-degree AV block is associated with hemodynamic compromise.

Management of Non-Q-Wave Infarction

Patients with non-Q-wave infarction, with their high potential for recurrent infarction, present an opportunity for secondary prevention (Fig. 60-13). The incidence of non-Q-wave infarction is about 50 percent.[149] Most patients (75 percent) with non-Q-wave infarction present with ST-T segment depression[152] and are not candidates for thrombolytic therapy (Fig. 60-12), as demonstrated by the lack of benefit of lytic therapy in this setting in the TIMI-3 trial.[432] In contrast, the calcium entry blocker diltiazem has been shown to be effective in reducing reinfarction in the Diltiazem Reinfarction Study (DRS)[152] and in the MDPIT trial.[433] In the DRS (Fig. 60-14), diltiazem given in the initial 24 to 48 h after non-Q-wave infarction reduced the reinfarction rate during hospitalization (14 days) by 47 percent compared to conventional therapy.[152] In the MDPIT study, diltiazem reduced reinfarction and death by 40 percent at the end of 1 year and 34 percent at the end of 4.5 years in patients without evidence of pulmonary congestion.[434] The AHA/ACC Joint Task Force recommended that diltiazem be given routinely to patients with non-Q-wave infarction who do not have pulmonary congestion and cardiac failure and be continued for at least 1 year.[394] There has been no prospective trial assessing aspirin in non-Q-wave infarction, but retrospective analysis showed significant benefit.[435] It seems prudent to recommend aspirin (80 to 325 mg/day) along with diltiazem (120 to 240 mg/day) to patients with non-Q-wave infarction. It is also recommended that heparin be given intravenously for the initial 24 to 48 h, although there has been no prospective clinical trial to demonstrate effectiveness. Heparin should be given as a bolus of 5000 units, followed by 1000 to 1200 units/h titrated to increase the PTT to 1.5- to twofold over the normal range. Verapamil has been shown also to reduce long-term reinfarction and death by 23 percent compared to conventional therapy in the patients following both Q-wave and non-Q-wave infarction. In contrast, nifedipine is not indicated in patients with AMI either for cardioprotection or to reduce the reinfarction rate or to prolong survival.[436] There have been no pro-

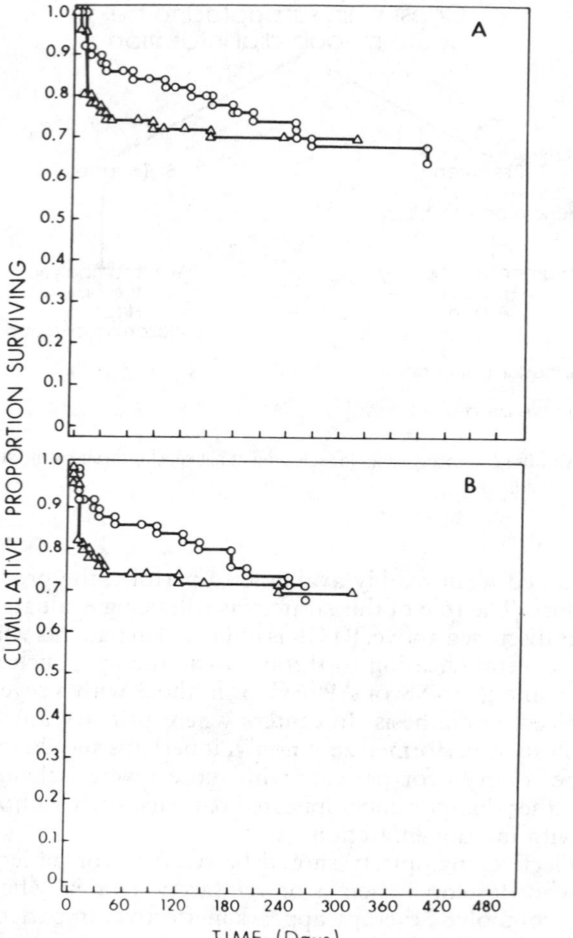

FIGURE 60-13 Comparison of the survival of patients with Q-wave infarction (triangles) to that of patients with non-Q-wave infarction with (circles) and without (squares) early recurrent infarction. Early mortality was higher after Q-wave infarction than after non-Q-wave infarction and no recurrence (*A*), but survival was identical for patients with Q-wave infarction and those with non-Q-wave infarction and an early recurrent infarction (*B*). Longer term mortality rates are similar in Q-wave infarction and non-Q-wave infarction with or without early recurrence.

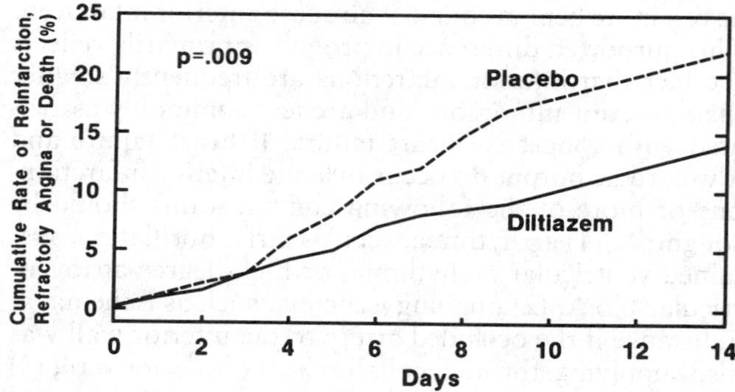

FIGURE 60-14 Life table cumulative rates of reinfarction, refractory angina, or death according to treatment group in patients receiving diltiazem (solid line) or placebo (dashed line). This shows a statistical reduction in favor of diltiazem that is maintained throughout the duration of therapy. (*From: J Cardiovasc Pharmacol 1989;13:S36. Reproduced with permission from the publisher and the authors.*)

spective studies of beta blockers performed solely in patients with non-Q-wave infarction, but retrospective analyses of trials performed prospectively involving both Q and non-Q-wave infarction consistently show no effect of beta blockers on the reinfarction rate in patients recovering from non-Q-wave infarction.[150] In the BHAT trial,[437] propranolol reduced the mortality and reinfarction rate in Q-wave infarction but had no effect on either endpoint in non-Q-wave infarction. Similarly, the MIAMI trial found no effect of metoprolol in non-Q-wave infarction.[466] In contrast, in the Norwegian Multicenter Study, timolol increased survival in both Q-wave and non-Q-wave infarction but decreased reinfarction only in patients with Q-wave infarction.[439] Beta blockers may be given to relieve pain or arrhythmia, as discussed previously for Q-wave infarction.

Nitroglycerin and Acute Infarction

Intravenous nitroglycerin has been used for more than a decade to prevent or reduce ischemia in patients with unstable angina and postinfarction. The effects of intravenous nitroglycerin on mortality and infarct size have been assessed in a number of trials.[391,440–448,468,469] Definitive conclusions regarding effect on infarct size could not be reached because of the small sample size. Nevertheless, in each of these studies infarct size assessed enzymatically or by ST-segment elevation was frequently less in patients treated with nitroglycerin than in those treated with placebo. In a recent study,[445] the use of nitroglycerin resulted in a significant reduction in the incidence of the end point: a combination of clinical events including mortality. Although definitive evidence of the efficacy of nitroglycerin in reducing infarct size or improving mortality is lacking, the AHA/ACC Task Force recommended that it be given routinely in AMI in the absence of contraindications, such as hypotension. Nitroglycerin relieves spasm, improves ischemia and pain, and decreases afterload and preload. Nitroglycerin is the drug of choice for vasodilation in the control of cardiac failure in the setting of AMI. While the preferred route of administration in the initial 24 to 48 h is intravenous, nitroglycerin may be given sublingually, orally, or percutaneously, provided that vital signs are monitored carefully. Oral and/or percutaneous routes of administration of nitroglycerin should be reserved for patients in whom the circulatory status is stable. Tolerance to nitroglycerin given intravenously develops as soon as 12 to 24 h, and the dose may have to be increased. The VA Cooperative trial evaluated intravenous nitroprusside in postinfarction patients whose left ventricular filling pressures exceeded 12 mmHg[440] and found no significant reduction in mortality rates. In a meta-analysis of all available clinical trials of nitroprusside and nitroglycerin, an overall reduction in mortality of 29 percent was demonstrated.[449,450]

Role of Calcium Channel Blockers

None of the calcium channel blockers is indicated in the initial hours of an evolving myocardial infarction. Dihydropyridines may have deleterious effects in this setting.[436] The role of diltiazem and verapamil in the long-term treatment of non-Q-wave infarction has been discussed. All of the calcium channel blockers are helpful and safe for use in the control of cardiac pain and ischemia after the acute phase in the absence of congestive heart failure, particularly when occurring in patients requiring control of hypertension.

COMPLICATIONS OF ACUTE MYOCARDIAL INFARCTION

Arrhythmias and Conduction Disturbances Complicating Myocardial Infarction

The basic mechanisms for conduction disturbances and arrhythmias in AMI were discussed earlier in this chapter; more extensive discussions of their recognition and management appear in Chaps. 34 through 38. Most patients with an AMI have some abnormality of cardiac conduction (about 25 percent) or rhythm (greater than 90 percent) during the first 24 h. These abnormalities of rhythm and conduction are the result of ischemia and necrosis as well as of altered autonomic tone, hypoxia, electrolyte, and acid-base disturbances, or are the result of concomitant therapies.

Ventricular Arrhythmias and Acute Myocardial Infarction

Lidocaine: Administration and Indications

Despite the fact that lidocaine has been used extensively for over two decades to treat or prevent ventricular arrhythmias, its role is being redefined. Lidocaine can reduce the incidence of primary ventricular fibrillation, yet patient benefit is unclear, since toxicities tend to offset the antifibrillatory effects.

A small, early study demonstrated that early administration of lidocaine in AMI was very effective in preventing ventricular fibrillation.[451] Subsequently, the Amsterdam Lidocaine Intervention trial was designated to assess in 6000 patients the effect of prophylactic lidocaine, given as an intramuscular bolus within the first hour of onset of pain, on the frequency of ventricular fibrillation.[452] The incidence of ventricular fibrillation was reduced by prophylactic lidocaine, but the mortality rate was unchanged, and patients on lidocaine had more asystole. The results of this, the largest prehospital trial conducted, are consistent with the disappointing results from two independent meta-analyses reported in over 9000 patients.[453,454] While an overview of all the clinical trials is consistent with some beneficial effect of lidocaine on a reduction of primary ventricular fibrillation, there is no mortality rate benefit. This appears to be a result of the toxic effects of lidocaine, resulting in conduction abnormalities and occasional asystole.[452–454] Thus, the controlled clinical trials provide no evidence that lidocaine is beneficial when given routinely or prophylactically early in the evolution of myocardial infarction.

Administration of lidocaine in AMI is recommended under the following circumstances: (1) frequent, multiform ventricular premature complexes (VPCs), especially with the R-on-T phenomenon or short runs of nonsustained ventricular tachycardia; or (2) after an episode of ventricular tachycardia or ventricular fibrillation requiring electrical defibrillation or cardiopulmonary resuscitation.[394]

It is usually recommended that multiple small bolus injections over the first 20 to 30 min be given in addition to a continuous intravenous infusion. While blood levels of 2 μg/mL may reduce VPCs and runs of nonsustained ventricular tachycardia, levels as high as 5 μg/mL may be necessary to prevent recurrent ventricular fibrillation in some patients.[455,456] An initial bolus injection of 1 mg per kilogram of body weight, not to exceed 100 mg, is usually recommended, followed 5 to 10 min by one additional bolus injection of 0.5 mg per kilogram of body weight, usually with the simultaneous initiation of a 2-mg/min infusion. Lidocaine may accumulate during prolonged infusion or when drip rates exceed 2 mg/min even in uncomplicated myocardial infarction.[447] Thus, the treatment indication after 12 to 24 h should be reevaluated, and therapy stopped if possible.

Lidocaine is metabolized in the liver. The elimination half-life for lidocaine is usually less than 2 h, but patients with progressive degrees of left ventricular dysfunction have increasingly prolonged plasma half-lives. The need for continued therapy should be reevaluated frequently because of the risk of toxicity. Early signs of elevated plasma lidocaine concentration include perioral numbness, gastrointestinal upset, drowsiness, confusion, and slurred speech. More severe neurological complications include respiratory failure, respiratory arrest, altered consciousness, or convulsions. Sinus pauses, sinus arrest, bradycardia, and asystole are cardiovascular complications of excessive lidocaine administration (see also Chap. 38).[458,459]

Ventricular Premature Complexes, Nonsustained Ventricular Tachycardia, Ventricular Fibrillation, and Idioventricular Rhythm

Lidocaine is the drug of choice for the management of ventricular ectopy and nonsustained ventricular tachycardia in the setting of AMI.[394,460] Before deciding to begin administration of lidocaine, it is important to consider ancillary factors that may increase the likelihood of ventricular arrhythmias, including inadequate oxygenation; electrolyte disturbances, such as hypokalemia and hypomagnesemia; cardiac failure; digitalis toxicity; and recurrent myocardial ischemia.[461–463]

Ventricular Fibrillation

Primary ventricular fibrillation occurring in the early hours of AMI should be treated, after defibrillation, with a bolus followed by a continuous intravenous infusion of lidocaine, as stated previously. The incidence of primary ventricular fibrillation is highest in the first hour after AMI and decreases dramatically thereafter. The majority of episodes of primary ventricular fibrillation occur in the first 4 to 6 h. While primary ventricular fibrillation can be initiated by either a premature ventricular beat occurring on the T-wave or a run of nonsustained ventricular tachycardia, it can also occur without previous ectopy.[464–466] Thus, it is difficult to identify those at high risk of developing ventricular fibrillation who might benefit from prophylactic administration of lidocaine.

Alternative drugs for sustained ventricular tachycardia or primary ventricular fibrillation unresponsive to maximal doses of lidocaine include procainamide and bretylium. Routine algorithms for the administration of these and all other medications used in a cardiac arrest have been reviewed in the standard guidelines for cardiopulmonary resuscitation by the American Heart Association (see also Chap. 52).[467]

The long-term prognosis of patients with an episode of primary ventricular fibrillation was reviewed recently by the GISSI investigators. In patients experiencing primary ventricular fibrillation within 48 h of the AMI, the prognosis at 6 and 12 months was the same as in patients without primary ventricular fibrillation.[468] In the SPRINT trial, although the long-term prognosis was unaffected by primary ventricular fibrillation, the in-hospital mortality rate was doubled.[469] In these two trials (>12,000 patients), the incidence of primary ventricular fibrillation was between 2.1 and 4.4 percent.[468,469] It is interesting that in a recent analysis of the GISSI-2 study, thrombolytic therapy with SK appeared to reduce the incidence of late in-hospital ventricular fibrillation.[468]

Accelerated Idioventricular Rhythm

Transient ventricular rhythms at rates between 60 and 110/min occur frequently in the setting of AMI, particularly with inferior infarction. These episodes are usually of short duration and terminate spontaneously. In general, they do not result in symptoms or significant hypotension. Treatment is not indicated, since there are no data to show that treatment improves prognosis. Commonly, patients have this arrhythmia in association with other types of bradycardia, as discussed previously. Runs of accelerated idioventricular rhythm can frequently be eliminated by increasing the heart rate[470,471] with atropine. Rarely, this rhythm may deteriorate into ventricular tachycardia, which does require treatment.

Supraventricular Tachyarrhythmias in Acute Myocardial Infarction

Sinus Tachycardia or Atrial Premature Beats

Sinus tachycardia following AMI is common and is frequently an unfavorable prognostic sign. The increased heart rate enhances myocardial oxygen demand, while the decreased diastolic time decreases diastolic coronary flow. Patients with a large area of infarcted myocardium may have sinus tachycardia on the basis of left ventricular dysfunction. Other obvious causes of sinus tachycardia, such as fever, anxiety, pain, pulmonary embolism, anemia, hypovolemia, or hypoxemia, must be evaluated and treated. Drugs such as dobutamine, dopamine, theophylline, and atropine may be responsible for sinus tachycardia.[472] Once these other potential causes are excluded, a persistent sinus tachycardia most likely reflects progressive left ventricular dysfunction. In patients with suspected left ventricular dysfunction as a cause of sinus tachycardia, a Swan-Ganz catheter frequently is inserted to assess the underlying hemodynamics.

Atrial ischemia or infarction and pericarditis are relatively common in AMI and may cause atrial premature complexes (APCs).[473–476] No specific therapy is indicated; rather, attention should be given to the underlying disease process.

Paroxysmal Supraventricular Tachycardia

Episodes of paroxysmal supraventricular tachycardia occur rather commonly and usually are transient.[473] Many of the factors associated with APCs may also precipitate brief episodes of supraventricular tachycardia. For reasons mentioned previously, persistent and rapid supraventricular tachycardia may precipitate further ischemia or worsen cardiac failure. Rate control is mandatory. Carotid sinus massage can be tried to break the rhythm. Other potential therapies include digoxin, beta blockers, adenosine, verapamil, or diltiazem. Adenosine and/or digitalis are preferable in the setting of left ventricular dysfunction, especially if hypotension exists. If recurrent ischemia precipitates episodes of supraventricular tachycardia, the therapeutic focus is directed to ischemia.

Atrial Flutter and Atrial Fibrillation

Atrial flutter is relatively uncommon in AMI, whereas atrial fibrillation has an incidence of 10 to 15 percent.[473,477] Atrial fibrillation is associated with an increased in-hospital mortality rate, probably because it is associated with large infarcts and is seen relatively more commonly in patients with cardiac failure.[477] The onset of atrial fibrillation in the first hours of AMI is probably a consequence of left atrial ischemia.[478] Both pericarditis or any condition leading to elevated left atrial pressure are frequent causes of atrial fibrillation in AMI.[479,480]

A rapid ventricular response will increase myocardial oxygen demand while decreasing diastolic coronary flow. The loss of atrial transport may further compromise cardiac output. Both of these consequences can have untoward effects early in the course of myocardial infarction. The most urgent considerations clinically depend upon whether the ventricular response is rapid and whether ischemia is being precipitated or worsened by the increased oxygen demand. An additional issue is whether cardiac output is being seriously compromised. If the patient is experiencing new or worsening ischemic pain or hypotension or both, electrical cardioversion is the most prudent course (see Chap. 41). Concurrent digitalization and initiation (preferably IV) of therapy with a class Ia antiarrhythmic, such as procainamide, is desirable to prevent recurrence and to slow the ventricular response should atrial fibrillation recur. Antiarrhythmic therapy in this setting can be short-term and can frequently be terminated prior to discharge. Atrial fibrillation with onset during the course of AMI is frequently not a long-term problem requiring chronic antiarrhythmic therapy, and the issues involving the use of class Ic agents to treat chronically ventricular ectopic activity after myocardial infarction, as in the Cardiac Arrhythmia Suppression Trial (CAST),[481,482] are not relevant in this setting. If left ventricular function has been documented to be preserved, intravenous diltiazem or a beta blocker can be used in patients with atrial fibrillation to slow ventricular rate effectively. The clinical issues with atrial flutter complicating AMI are the same as for atrial fibrillation, except that overdrive atrial pacing is available as an additional therapeutic option (see Chaps. 36 and 39).

Junctional Rhythm

An escape atrioventricular (AV) junctional rhythm at a rate of 40 to 60 beats per minute in patients with inferior myocardial infarction and a high degree of heart block is not uncommon.[473] Usually therapy is not required, since blood pressure and perfusion are maintained. A second type of junctional rhythm is an accelerated form, with rates of 70 to 130 beats per minute and with potential for increasing ischemia.[483] In general, treatment is aimed at the underlying conditions (see Chap. 36).[475,483]

An uncommon rhythm in AMI is paroxysmal junctional tachycardia. It is a potentially harmful arrhythmia, since the rate is frequently between 150 to 220 beats per minute. Therapy should be aimed at the underlying conditions, which include digitalis toxicity and myocardial ischemia.[484]

Sinus Bradycardia, Sinus Pauses, and Asystole

Sinus bradycardia, defined as any sinus rate less than 60 beats per minutes, is the most common arrhythmia in patients with AMI[485,486] and is especially associated with inferior infarction. In the initial 1 to 2 h after the onset of inferior infarction, bradycardia is present in about 40 percent of patients, but by 4 h the prevalence has decreased to about 20 percent.[379,485] The important clinical issue is whether or not the bradycardia itself is producing symptoms, which may include dizziness, near or frank syncope or confusion from cerebral hypoperfusion and low cardiac output, and congestive heart failure.[487] Sinus bradycardia, if profound, may increase the likelihood of repetitive ventricular arrhythmias.

In the absence of adverse signs or symptoms, therapy is not indicated. If therapy is indicated, atropine sulfate may be given as a bolus intravenously at a dose of 0.2 to 0.5 mg every 3 to 5 min for up to a total dose of 2 to 3 mg, depending on the rate of response. Every effort should be made to keep the heart rate in the range of 50 to 70 beats per minute and not to induce a tachycardia. Occasionally, a low dose of atropine may further aggravate sinus node slowing, whereas a high dose of 0.75 mg or more may produce sinus tachycardia, resulting in increased ischemia and/or ventricular arrhythmias.[488] In patients with hypotension associated with sinus bradycardia and inferior myocardial infarction, the inability to reverse the hypotension with atropine suggests volume depletion, right ventricular infarction, or both.

While sinus bradycardia in the first few hours of AMI is frequently attributable to increased vagal tone, transient sinus node dysfunction occurring later after AMI may be due to sinus node or atrial ischemia. Although this arrhythmia is usually transient and does not require therapy, if the patient develops "symptomatic hypotension," as defined above, the treatment would be similar with intravenous atropine. At times, the sinus node dysfunction may lead to a type I or type II second-degree sinoatrial block and sinus pauses, which may become symptomatic. Severe symptomatic episodes and even transient atrial asystole may require temporary pacemaker insertion (see Chap. 39).[489,490]

First-Degree AV Block

First-degree AV block or prolongation of the PR interval to greater than 0.20 s is common with AMI, especially inferior infarction. Frequently, this is attributable to acute ischemia, although often concomitant therapy with beta blockers or calcium entry blockers such as diltiazem or verapamil is at least partially responsible. In addition, digitalis can prolong the PR interval either as a result of its therapeutic effect or as a manifestation of intoxication. Although first-degree AV block is seen frequently (10 to 15 percent of cases), its clinical significance is usually minimal, and no specific therapy is indicated.

Second-Degree AV Block

Second-degree AV block manifests as intermittent failure of atrial impulses to conduct to the ventricles and exists in two forms (Chap. 36). The more benign type is Mobitz type I or Wenckebach AV block, which accounts for the majority of second-degree AV blocks. As many as 10 percent of patients with AMI develop Mobitz type I block.[491] There are several features distinguishing Mobitz type I from Mobitz type II block. Mobitz type I block (1) occurs as a result of ischemia of the AV node, (2) is relatively common in AMI, (3) is associated with a narrow QRS, (4) is most commonly caused by inferior infarction, and (5) usually has a varying PR interval, with the nonconducted beat usually following a progressive lengthening of the PR interval. Although progression to complete heart block may occur, it is usually transient, and greater than 90 percent return to normal within 5 days. Development of type I Mobitz block does not adversely affect prognosis.

Mobitz type II AV block is uncommon. As opposed to Mobitz type I, type II AV block (1) is associated with widening of the QRS, indicating that the lesion is in the conducting system below the bundle of His; (2) is usually associated with anterior infarction; (3) generally reflects trifascicular block; and (4) is characterized by a nonvarying PR interval before the nonconducted atrial beat. Heart block, if it develops, is sudden, without lengthening of the PR interval or increase in the ratio of conducted to nonconducted beats. The mortality rate associated with progression of Mobitz type II block to complete heart block is about 80 percent. In contrast to Mobitz type I block, Mobitz type II block is seldom reversible.

Third-Degree AV Block

Third-degree AV block, or complete heart block, occurs in about 5 percent of patients with AMI and is most commonly seen with inferior infarction. In patients with inferior myocardial infarction, this usually implies a block at or above the bundle of His. As indicated earlier, the prognosis of heart block depends on whether it is anterior or inferior infarction. Complete heart block with inferior infarction often results in only a modest asymptomatic bradycardia (with junctional or escape rhythm rates of 40 to 60 beats per minute) and is usually transient. The QRS complex is narrow, because of the site of block above the His bundle, in about 70 percent of the cases; the mortality rate is only about 15 percent but is higher if there is extensive right ventricular infarction. Complete heart block with inferior myocardial infarction may occur early or later in the hospitalization with the same prognosis. It is important to rule out volume depletion as a cause of hypotension in the setting of inferior infarct and high-degree heart block. This is especially true if concomitant right ventricular infarction is suspected. Therefore, a volume challenge is a reasonable clinical strategy prior to consideration of drug therapy or temporary pacing.[492–494] The combination of inferior myocardial infarction and complete heart block increases in-hospital mortality rates, but the presence of complete heart block is not an independent predictor of poor prognosis.[495] In contrast, patients with anterior infarction who develop third-degree AV block have a high mortality rate of 80 percent.[496] Implications for temporary and permanent pacing are discussed as follows and are also presented in Table 60-12 (see also Chaps. 39 and 40).

Intraventricular Conduction Disturbances

Conduction from the His bundle is relayed throughout the two ventricles via the three fascicles (the anterior and posterior divisions of the left bundle and the right bundle; see Chap. 34). It is estimated that disturbances occur in one or more of these fascicles in about 15 percent of patients with AMI. The right bundle branch and the left posterior division have a dual blood supply from the left anterior descending and the right coronary arteries. The septal perforators of the left anterior descending coronary artery supply the left anterior fascicle.

The development of bundle branch block during AMI usually signifies an extensive infarct. In one multicenter trial, the presence of bundle branch block was associated with a twofold increase in the in-hospital mortality rate (28 versus 14 percent) compared with the absence of bundle branch block.[497,498] Whether a bundle branch block is new or old is often unclear or difficult to document. Data from the detailed multicenter study by Hindman and coworkers[498] indicate that the presence of bundle branch block identifies patients who (1) are more likely to develop congestive heart failure, (2) are more likely to develop high-degree heart block, (3) are more likely to have an episode of ventricular fibrillation, and (4) have a higher mortality rate. In a retrospective and prospective study of 1897 patients with AMI, an increased incidence of ventricular fibrillation in the first 6 weeks was noted in patients presenting with anteroseptal myocardial infarction complicated by either right or left bundle branch block.[499]

Indications for Temporary Pacing

A summary of the general guidelines for temporary and permanent pacing in patients with AMI is contained in Table 60-12 (see also Chap. 39).[387,394] In addition to the general guidelines in Table 60-12, a number of consider-

TABLE 60-12

Conduction Disturbances Complicating AMI: Guidelines for Pacing

ECG Abnormality Observed	Indication for Temporary Pacing*	Indication for Permanent Pacing*
Disturbances of AV Conduction		
First-degree AV block	No	No
Second-degree AV block		
Mobitz I: no symptomatic bradycardia or hypotension	No	No
Mobitz II: symptomatic bradycardia and hypotension unresponsive to atropine	+ +	+ **
Third-degree (complete) AV block		
Inferior MI: narrow QRS, no symptomatic hypotension, and bradycardia	+	No
Inferior MI: narrow QRS, symptomatic hypotension, and bradycardia	+ +	+ **
Anterior MI: wide QRS	+ +	+ +
Disturbances of Intraventricular Conduction		
New fascicular block	No	No
New LBBB	+	No
New RBBB with LAFB or LPFB	+	No
Old/indeterminate LBBB or RBBB and either LAFB or LPFB	No	No
LBBB or RBBB with LAFB or LPFB and Mobitz II or complete heart block	+ +	+ +
Other Bradyarrhythmias		
Symptomatic bradycardia, sinus pauses (≥3.5 seconds), and transient asystole unresponsive to atropine	+ +	+ + **

ABBREVIATIONS: AV, atrioventricular; LAFB, left anterior fascicular block; LBBB, left bundle branch block; LPFB, left posterior fascicular block; MI, myocardial infarction; RBBB, right bundle branch block.
* No, pacing not indicated; +, pacing may be useful; + +, general agreement that pacing is indicated.
** Must be considered in light of persistent symptomatic bradycardia and/or conduction abnormalities.

ations may affect decisions in a specific patient. Overall, prognosis may be an important issue, and pacing may be withheld if the clinical situation is deemed hopeless because of the cardiac or other conditions. Pacing may sometimes be indicated because of aggravation or induction of severe bradycardia by antiischemic medications, such as beta blockers.[394,487]

The generally agreed on indications for temporary pacemaker insertion in AMI include: asystole, complete heart block in the setting of anterior myocardial infarction, new onset of right or left bundle branch block with persistent Mobitz II second-degree AV block in the setting of anterior myocardial infarction, or other symptomatic bradycardias unresponsive to atropine.[394] Any bradycardia unresponsive to atropine that is responsible for symptoms or is associated with hypotension may require temporary pacing (see also Chap. 39).

Bundle branch block in the setting of AMI identifies a population at risk for both electrical and mechanical complications. Such patients must be monitored for evidence of transient high-degree heart block. Prolonged intermediate care with telemetry monitoring and repeat assessments of heart failure status are important.

Indications for Permanent Pacing

There is general agreement that the following groups of patients should receive a permanent pacemaker[394,487] after AMI: (1) those with persistent high-degree block (Mobitz II or third-degree heart block) with a wide QRS complex and (2) those with transient advanced AV block associated with bundle branch block.[487,500–503] In addition, other persistent symptomatic bradycardias or conduction defects merit consideration for permanent pacing (Table 60-12), (see also Chap. 40).

Postinfarction Pain and Reinfarction

Early postinfarction angina requires immediate treatment, since it is an important predictor of the severity of coronary artery disease and has an overall incidence of about 18 percent.[504] Postinfarction angina is defined as chest pain that frequently is similar to the original discomfort, with or without transient ST-T changes and occurring 24 h or more after the onset of AMI. The pain is usualiy a result of ischemia in the territory of the myocardium supplied by the vessel that precipitated the initial myocardial infarction. At least three categories of patients are at high risk of postinfarction angina and reinfarction: (1) patients with non-Q-wave infarction, (2) patients who have received thrombolysis, and (3) patients with multiple risk factors.[149,152,255] The incidence of postinfarction angina is almost twice as high after non-Q-wave infarction (25 to 35 percent) than after Q-wave infarction (15 to 20 percent). Thrombolytic therapy for AMI created a new high-risk group for postinfarction angina (35 to 45 percent incidence) with a 12 to 15 percent incidence of reinfarction.[151] In the initial TIMI-1 trial,[400] the incidence of postinfarction angina was 43 percent, the cumulative incidence of postinfarction angina after the initial SK trials was 35 percent, and the incidence of reinfarction was 12 percent. Regardless of whether postinfarction angina occurs after Q-wave infarction, non-Q-wave infarction, or thrombolytic therapy, it is more likely to occur in patients with two- or three-vessel disease than in patients with single-vessel disease.[504] The importance of postinfarction angina is emphasized by the observation that it is associated with a twofold increase in the incidence of reinfarction. The 1-year mortality rate and acute risk of reinfarction is two- to fourfold greater in patients with postinfarction angina associated with ECG changes than in patients without chest pain or patients with chest pain but without associated ST-T segment changes.[505,506]

Postinfarction angina is an ominous clinical development and must be treated aggressively. Pain should be relieved by attempting to decrease oxygen demand by decreasing heart rate with beta blockers and by increasing coronary flow and decreasing preload with, initially, sublingual nitroglycerin and subsequently with reinstitution of intravenous nitroglycerin. Calcium channel blockers may be added, and the patient should be mildly sedated with, for example, benzodiazepines. Intravenous heparin should be started. Myocardial infarction should be ruled in or out with enzyme and serial ECGs, as described previously. In general, these patients should have cardiac catheterization and have high-grade stenoses treated with PTCA or coronary artery bypass grafting.

The incidence of reinfarction following non-Q-wave infarction has been reported to be as high as 40 percent in the first month following infarction,[148] but with proper treatment using heparin and diltiazem the incidence is less than 10 percent, as discussed previously. The incidence of reinfarction following thrombolytic therapy has been reduced from 12 to 15 percent to 5 to 7 percent with the use of adjunctive therapy including heparin, aspirin, nitroglycerin, and beta blockers, as previously discussed. Nevertheless, reinfarction, despite the use of heparin and aspirin, still accounts for a quarter of all of the deaths that occur following thrombolytic therapy and thus remains a major concern.[367] Patients presenting with Q-wave infarction who do not receive thrombolytic therapy are likely to have an incidence of postinfarction angina of only about 12 to 15 percent and a reinfarction rate of about 5 to 7 percent. Postinfarction ischemia is also a harbinger of ventricular arrhythmias and sudden death and thus may represent the first indication for the administration of antiarrhythmic therapy. Factors that may aggravate ischemia include anemia, electrolyte imbalance, hypoxia, and medications that may induce ischemia.

The place of reinfarction in risk stratification and management strategies with respect to cardiac catheterization and revascularization is discussed later. The use of beta blockers in patients with Q-wave infarction at risk of reinfarction must be emphasized, since all studies have shown that beta blockers without intrinsic sympathomimetic activity reduce the incidence of reinfarction. Similarly, aspirin has been shown to reduce markedly the incidence of reinfarction with or without thrombolytic therapy. In patients with persistent angina with ECG changes and/or threatened reinfarction, revascularization is recommended. If this is not possible, thrombolytic therapy should be given, and the choice of agent depends on the patient's history. If either SK or APSAC was previously used, neither should be used again, and rt-PA should be the choice. Treatment with rt-PA can be repeated. Another approach would be to proceed directly to cardiac catheterization and PTCA or surgery if these options are immediately available.

Recently it has been shown that the angiotensin-converting enzyme (ACE) inhibitors evaluated in several trials for their effect on chronic heart failure were shown to reduce the incidence of reinfarction by 25 percent in both the SAVE[507] and the SOLVD[508] trials. These observations may have little relevance for early reinfarction, but they do have implications for the prevention of late reinfarction, especially in patients with congestive heart failure.

Acute Cardiac Failure: Hemodynamics

The immediate hemodynamic consequences of myocardial infarction include both systolic and diastolic dysfunction. Systolic dysfunction is secondary to a loss of contractile function of the infarcted and ischemia myocardium.[139] Over a period of 1 to 3 min, the regional disturbance of contraction progresses from dyssynchrony (disturbed temporal sequence of contraction) through hypokinesis (diminished motion) and akinesis (total lack of motion) to dyskinesia (paradoxical systolic expansion).[509] This loss of contractile function results in a decreased systolic ejection, increased end-systolic volume, increased end-diastolic volume, and a secondary increase in diastolic filling pressure caused by the increase in ventricular volume. The diastolic impairment often precedes the systolic dysfunction. The diastolic dysfunction is characterized immediately by a transient increase in left ventricular diastolic distensibility,[510,511] followed by decreased distensibility due in part to ATP depletion and restraint by the pericardium, and perhaps ultimately contributed to by the infiltration of inflammatory fluid and cells. The hemodynamic consequence of the reduced distensibility is increased diastolic pressure. The adrenergic system, which is activated to maintain arterial blood pressure and cardiac output, increases the heart rate and afterload and increases preload. The systolic stress on the ischemic segment contributes to "cell stretch" and "cell slippage," results in expansion of the infarcted segment,[512] and provides the stimulus for volume overload hypertrophy characterized by sarcomere replication, fiber elongation, and chamber enlargement (see Chap. 6B). The growth response is prompt and, in addition to increased protein synthesis, is characterized by the reexpression of fetal proteins (see Chap. 1). The chamber enlargement accommodates the increased volume and allows the diastolic pressure to return toward normal.[509]

Cardiac failure develops when ventricular function is reduced to 30 percent or more of normal and usually occurs within minutes or hours of onset of a large infarction (see Chap. 25). Since even with sustained coronary occlusion only 60 to 70 percent of the ischemic region undergoes necrosis, compromise of cardiac function associated with AMI is transient (24 to 72 h) in perhaps more than two-thirds of the cases. Unlike the situation with chronic heart failure, the circulatory volume is normal or decreased in acute ventricular dysfunction associated with myocardial infarction. The usual clinical scenario is one of left ventricular dysfunction with pulmonary congestion without hypoperfusion. There is sometimes biventricular failure, and in about 5 to 10 percent of cases there is predominantly right ventricular failure. The severity of the failure, its duration, and whether or not it is reversible are predominantly dependent on infarct size.[41,42] If more than 40 percent of the myocardium is destroyed, decompensation occurs, resulting in shock.[43–45] In a few patients, failure develops later as a consequence of expansion of the infarcted segment, reinfarction, or ischemia.[510] Less commonly, failure is precipitated by papillary muscle dysfunction or ventricular septal rupture. The compromised heart will also be negatively affected by supraventricular or ventricular arrhythmias, conduction disturbances, drugs with negative inotropic effects, fever, and hypovolemia.

Left ventricular dysfunction with the clinical signs of failure is said to occur in 30 to 40 percent of patients and usually develops when the abnormally contracting segment exceeds 30 percent of the left ventricular circumference.[513] Another factor contributing to cardiac failure is residual scarring from previous episodes of infarction which limits the extent of compensation.

Decreased Myocardial Function and Heart Failure in Myocardial Infarction

After myocardial infarction, adjacent normal myocardium increases contractility because of increased stimulation by catecholamines and also utilizes the Starling mechanism in an attempt to maintain cardiac output. The pathophysiology of heart failure is discussed in Chap. 25. An important difference between acute heart failure after myocardial infarction and chronic heart failure is that intravascular volume is expanded in the latter situation but may be normal or decreased in the former. This fact is important in considering the therapeutic approach to low cardiac output and pulmonary congestion in acute infarction.

Diuretics and Cardiac Failure in Acute Myocardial Infarction

As alluded to, patients with failure due to AMI have normal total body water, and transudation of fluid into the lungs may induce hypovolemia. Since ventricular compliance is decreased, an increased left ventricular end-diastolic pressure is necessary to maintain cardiac output, since the heart operates on the steep portion of the ascending limb of Starling's curve.[514,515] The administration of a diuretic in this setting may be associated with a decrease in cardiac output.[516–518] Thus, diuretics should not be the drugs used initially in the treatment of pulmonary congestion in AMI. Their use early in the course should usually be guided by hemodynamic measurements from a Swan-Ganz catheter. Diuretic therapy may become appropriate later if salt and water retention develop.

Inotropic Agents in Congestive Heart Failure Associated with Acute Myocardial Infarction

Digoxin is not the inotropic agent of choice in acute heart failure in myocardial infarction. It is a relatively weak inotropic agent. In a direct comparison, dobutamine was shown to increase cardiac output by 40 percent and to decrease left ventricular filling pressure, whereas digoxin increased cardiac output by only 10 percent and did not decrease filling pressure.[519] Since endogenous catecholamine levels can be quite elevated, digoxin may contribute little. The primary use of digoxin in AMI is to control heart rate in atrial fibrillation.

Dobutamine has favorable pharmacologic properties for use in heart failure in myocardial infarction (see Chap. 28). It has a rapid onset of action and increases cardiac output because of its positive inotropic properties. It is a vasodilator and increases coronary flow. It decreases filling pressure, as noted. Dopamine has a tendency to increase heart rate more than dobutamine. With higher doses, it may increase peripheral resistance and increased filling pressures, offsetting some of the positive inotropic effects. The phosphodiesterase inhibitor amrinone increases contractility and is a vasodilator that has been used in patients with heart failure due to AMI. There is concern that positive inotropic agents may increase infarct size. Evaluation of dobutamine in AMI showed that, as long as heart rate was not increased more than 10 percent above baseline, there was no increase in infarct size or in incidence of reinfarction or arrhythmia.[520]

Management of Uncomplicated Cardiac Failure

The major determinant of left ventricular dysfunction is the extent of myocardial injury (Fig. 60-15).[41,42,521] The loss of contractile function in the initial minutes or hours (1 to 4) is potentially reversible and accounts in part for the transient nature of cardiac failure in the setting of uncomplicated AMI. The presence of cardiac failure and its severity depends not only on the extent of damage but also upon the extent of injury from previous episodes.

Since the introduction of the Swan-Ganz catheter, considerable data have accumulated correlating hemodynamics with clinical features. In 1967, prior to invasive monitoring, Killip and Kimball[522] devised a clinical classification based on physical findings on admission that provided a prognostic guide. That guide was followed by the classification of Forrester and colleagues,[523,524] based on extensive data obtained from invasive monitoring of patients with acute AMI (Table 60-13). The latter classification combined the presence or absence of pulmonary congestion with the presence or absence of systemic hypoperfusion. Forrester and colleagues added the underlying hemodynamics to this classification based on the pulmonary arterial occlusive pressure and the cardiac index. These classifications also provide important diagnostic and therapeutic guidelines, despite the observation that patients frequently cross over from one class to the other and are seldom restricted to one particular hemodynamic subset. Each classification illustrated that with increasing severity of ventricular dysfunction there is increased risk of mortality. Nevertheless, there is im-

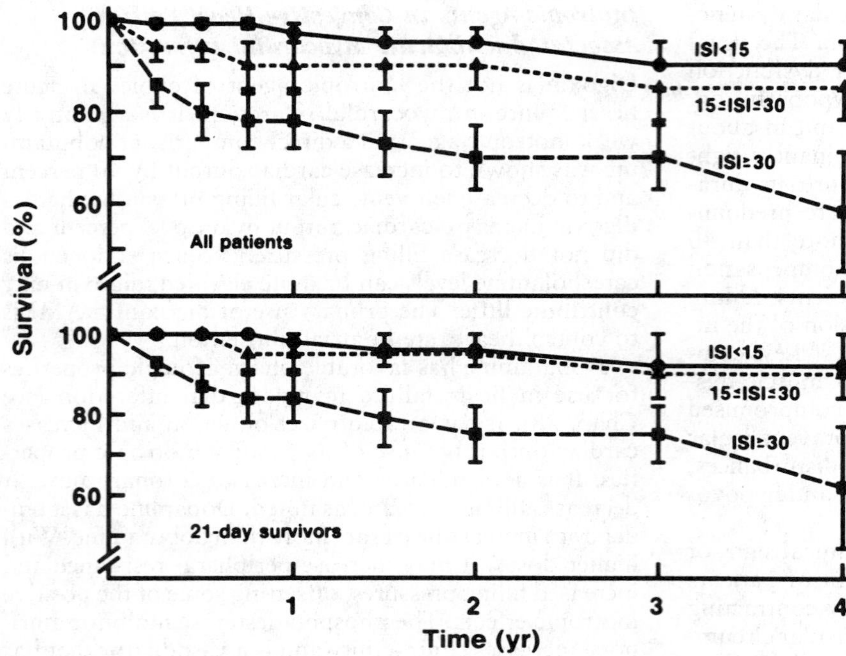

FIGURE 60-15 The effects of infarct size on survival. Distinct survival curves are evident based on infarct size as shown by patients whose infarct size corrected for body surface area (ISI) was less than 15 CK-g-Eq/m^2 (circles), modest (15≤ISI<30, triangles), and large (ISI≥30). Brackets indicate standard errors. Survival curves of all patients surviving 24 h are shown in the *top panel*, and those of patients surviving 21 days are shown in the *bottom panel*. Survival curves were similar for patients with small and modest-sized infarcts but significantly less for patients with large infarcts whether or not early deaths were excluded [*From Kelley WN (ed), Textbook of Internal Medicine, Lippincott, Philadelphia 1989. Reproduced with permission from publisher and authors.*]

precision in predicting mortality rates from hemodynamics. Rackley and coworkers[525] observed that patients with a ventricular filling pressure over 29 mmHg had a 100 percent mortality rate; those with a filling pressure over 15 mmHg and a cardiac index of less than 2 L/min per square meter of body surface had a mortality rate of 93 percent; while those with a ventricular filling pressure less than 15 and a cardiac index under 2 L/min per square meter of body surface had a mortality rate of 63 percent.

In patients with uncomplicated AMI, there is no need to perform invasive monitoring if careful clinical observations are made. There should be repeated assessment of the heart and lungs; examination of the skin and mucous membranes; monitoring of the systemic arterial

TABLE 60-13
Clinical and Hemodynamic Subsets in AMI

Subset	Clinical Features	Approximate % of Patients with AMI	Hospital Mortality, %
	Killip Class		
1	No signs of congestive heart failure	40–50	6
2	S_3 gallop and bibasilar rales	30–40	17
3	Acute pulmonary edema	10–15	38
4	Cardiogenic shock	5–10	81
	Cedars-Sinai Clinical Subsets		
1	No pulmonary congestion or tissue hypoperfusion	25	1
2	Pulmonary congestion only	25	11
3	Tissue hypoperfusion only	15	18
4	Pulmonary congestion and tissue hypoperfusion	35	60
	Cedars-Sinai Hemodynamic Subsets		
	Hemodynamic features		
1	PCW ≤ 18; CI > 2.2	25	3
2	PCW > 18; CI > 2.2	25	9
3	PCW ≤ 18; CI ≤ 2.2	15	23
4	PCW > 18; CI ≤ 2.2	35	51

ABBREVIATIONS: CI, cardiac index (L/min/m^2); PCW, pulmonary capilary wedge pressure (mmHg).

pressure, cardiac rhythm, and heart rate; and routine laboratory examinations including chest x-ray and determinations of urine output and arterial blood gas values. If there are clinical indications of pulmonary congestion and/or decreased peripheral perfusion, invasive monitoring may be indicated to obtain data upon which to base decisions for therapeutic intervention. Invasive monitoring includes the insertion of a Swan-Ganz catheter to monitor right ventricular hemodynamics and pulmonary artery occlusive pressure, which will reflect left ventricular end-diastolic pressure, and to obtain serial determinations of the cardiac output (see Chap. 18). The general guidelines for indications for invasive monitoring appear in Table 60-14. Occasionally it may be necessary to insert an arterial catheter to measure the arterial pressure; however, one can usually follow the arterial pressure adequately with the use of a sphygmomanometer or an automatic blood pressure monitoring device. Frequently, it is also essential to insert a Foley catheter to follow the urine output, particularly in patients with sustained hypotension or cardiogenic shock.

In most patients in whom cardiac failure is not complicated by mechanical factors, such as mitral valve rupture, ventricular septal rupture, pulmonary embolus, or tamponade, the failure is transient and of mild to moderate severity. If the cardiac output is normal, aggressive treatment is often not recommended.[237] In patients with rales at the base of the lungs with only minimal increase in heart rate and no other signs of hypoxemia (Killip class II), conventional therapy with morphine, nasal oxygen, intravenous, oral, or transdermal nitrates, and bed rest is adequate without any specific therapy for failure. In patients with extensive pulmonary edema exhibiting hypoxia and dyspnea who are normotensive (Forrester class II), the treatment of choice is nitroglycerin given intravenously at 0.1 μg per kilogram of body weight per minute and increased in increments of 5 to 10 mg/min, stopping at a dose that does not decrease the systolic blood pressure below 100 mmHg. On the average, nitroglycerin in a dose of 0.5 μg per kilogram of body weight per minute is required in patients with evolving acute infarction and failure. Another vasodilator that has been used extensively in the past in AMI is sodium nitroprusside, which is initiated at 0.5 μg per kilogram of body weight per minute and increased by 10- to 20-mg/min increments every 10 to 15 min until the desired therapeutic point or a maximum of 10 μg per kilogram of body weight per minute is reached. Nevertheless, nitroglycerin is the preferred agent, since it has been shown to offer some cardioprotection when given in the early phase of myocardial infarction and has been shown to be reliable and safe. In contrast, in experimental infarction in the dog it has been shown that nitroprusside is more likely to redirect coronary flow away from the ischemic area to normal areas and to induce coronary steal.[526] The effect of nitroprusside on cardioprotection has been inconsistent and in one large study was shown to be detrimental.[440] In view of the recent data showing ACE inhibitors to be very effective in cardiac failure, one can anticipate that an intravenous preparation such as is available for enalapril will soon be evaluated in this setting. It is preferable that hemodynamics be monitored invasively (Swan-Ganz catheter) when one gives a vasodilator to reduce the ventricular filling pressure to 15 to 17 mmHg while maintaining adequate cardiac output and coronary perfusion. Whether or not one monitors hemodynamics invasively will depend in part on the confidence that clinical features reflect the volume status. Mitral valve regurgitation due to papillary muscle dysfunction is commonly an aggravating factor even in mild to moderate cardiac failure and responds well to a vasodilator, as does systemic hypertension. Usually a vasodilator is not adequate, and an intravenous inotropic agent should be added. The inotropic agents are generally those of sympathomimetic drugs, including dobutamine, dopamine, and norepinephrine (see Chap. 28). Dobutamine, a synthetic direct acting agent, is the preferred agent and has actions that include vasodilatation, increased cardiac output, decreased ventricular filling pressure, and increased coronary flow.[527] The infusion should be initiated at 2 to 5 mg per kilogram of body weight per minute and should be increased such that adequate systemic pressure is maintained and the heart rate does not increase by more than 10 to 15 percent. Dobutamine is preferably titrated to cardiac output and ventricular filling pressure. The ventricular filling pressure should be decreased to a range of 14 to 18 mmHg while maintaining adequate CO and blood pressure. In general, the objective is to maintain an adequate cardiac output and blood pressure without inducing tachycardia and while maintaining a filling pressure that is normal or minimally increased.

TABLE 60-14

Indications for Invasive Monitoring in AMI

Persistent hypotension
Cardiac failure unresponsive to therapy
Persistent sinus tachycardia
Left ventricular failure in combination with severe lung disease
Right ventricular failure from suspected right ventricular infarction
To monitor the response to vasodilator therapy with systolic blood pressure of <100 mmHg
To monitor the response of the cardiac output and ventricular filling pressure to inotropic therapy
Acute rupture of mitral valve or ventricular septum
Cardiac failure with unexplained coma, restlessness, hypoxia, acidosis, or oliguria
AMI occurring during or after surgery

In patients with inferior infarction and low cardiac output, right ventricular infarction should be suspected. If it is present, a Swan-Ganz catheter should be inserted to determine the filling pressure. Therapy with a positive inotropic agent, such as dobutamine, should be used after assuring that there is appropriate intravascular volume to facilitate right ventricular filling.[528,529]

In patients with borderline blood pressure and evidence of peripheral hypoperfusion, therapy should be initiated with an inotropic agent and not a vasodilator. Similarly, in patients with left ventricular failure and frank hypotension (<95 mmHg), a vasodilator must be avoided, and initial therapy should be with a positive inotropic agent. Dopamine frequently would be the choice under these circumstances, since it exerts similar cardiovascular effects to those of dobutamine, but it also possesses an alpha-1-adrenergic activity and releases endogenous norepinephrine from sympathetic nerve endings. Low doses of dopamine (2 to 7 μg per kilogram of body weight per minute) are associated with an increase in stroke volume, increased cardiac output, increased renal blood flow, and moderate effects to increase peripheral resistance. Higher doses of dopamine induce significant vasoconstriction and may increase the left ventricular filling pressure due to increased afterload, which further exacerbates pulmonary congestion. Dopamine also has a more positive chronotropic effect than does dobutamine, which can be a disadvantage in AMI. Norepinephrine, which produces potent arteriolar and venous constriction, is used for hypotension in other settings but otherwise is relatively contraindicated in AMI. It is seldom used unless patients are hypotensive and do not respond to dopamine, amrinone or milrinone, or dobutamine. It is used in cardiogenic shock after dopamine has failed, since it is the major alternative to maintain adequate perfusion pressure.

As indicated earlier, diuretics should be used with more caution in acute heart failure associated with AMI than in chronic heart failure, since volume expansion is usually not the primary problem. If high filling pressure (>18 to 20 mmHg) persists after achieving adequate output with positive inotropic agents and/or vasodilators, diuretics may be added. However, this effect can be achieved by vasodilator therapy, which avoids hypovolemia and hypotension may occur secondary to the subsequent diuresis (1 to 2 h). The diuretics preferred are intravenous furosemide or ethacrynic acid.[530] These drugs also provide some acute venodilation (see Chap. 29).

Complicated Heart Failure after Myocardial Infarction

Some AMI patients present with acute, fulminating pulmonary edema (with severe respiratory distress; generalized inspiratory crackles and wheezing; expectoration of pink, frothy sputum; cool, clammy, diaphoretic skin; and cyanosis) and require much more aggressive therapy than do patients with uncomplicated AMI. The condition is usually associated with pulmonary artery wedge pressure exceeding 25 mmHg and an in-hospital mortality rate of at least 15 to 20 percent.[531] The systolic blood pressure usually is either low normal or borderline normal (95 to 105 mmHg). The maintenance of adequate oxygenation must be the primary concern. Administration of high concentrations (60 to 100 percent) of oxygen via a face mask is essential. If the patient appears moribund, endotracheal intubation should be performed. While an assessment of arterial blood gases is appropriate, the speed with which clinical events change in these emergent situations may demand that decisions be made without benefit of these values. After the institution of mechanical ventilation, positive end-expiratory pressure (PEEP) may be needed to maintain adequate oxygenation while keeping the inspired oxygen concentration within safe levels ($FI_{O_2} < 60$ percent). Positive end-expiratory pressure should be applied only with an awareness of its risks of pneumothorax and reduction in cardiac output secondary to decreased left ventricular preload.[531] Invasive hemodynamic monitoring is particularly useful in these patients. Therapeutic interventions, however, should not be delayed until the monitoring is established. The therapy for severe pulmonary edema should include intravenous morphine unless the patient is known to have chronic CO_2 retention. From 5 to 10 mg of morphine sulfate should be given slowly with careful observation for evidence of respiratory depression. If the systolic blood pressure is adequate (≥100 mmHg), nitroglycerin is administered intravenously. In the patient with severe pulmonary edema, the improvement in left ventricular pump performance afforded by prompt reduction in systemic vascular resistance by nitroprusside[532] may be essential for the rapid reversal of this life-threatening situation (particularly if systemic hypertension had been present). Either nitroglycerin or nitroprusside will provide a reduction in preload. If the systolic blood pressure is 100 mmHg or less, treatment probably should be initiated with a positive inotropic agent, with the subsequent addition of a vasodilator or an agent to improve cardiac output. The adjunctive use of intravenous diuretics is the same as outlined for milder degrees of heart failure.

Peripheral Hypoperfusion without Pulmonary Congestion

Patients with clinical hypoperfusion without pulmonary congestion (with cool, cyanotic extremities, somnolence or confusion, and decreased urine flow) usually have a cardiac index of less than 2.2 liters/min. The mortality rate in these patients is four times greater than in those patients without hypoperfusion.[531] Invasive hemodynamic monitoring of the pulmonary capillary pressure is essential. Volume augmentation is the initial therapeutic step in patients with a pulmonary capillary pressure of less than 15 mmHg. If possible, this pressure should be maintained below the level of pulmonary congestion (>20 mmHg). Vasodilators are usually not indicated at least until adequate filling pressures have been achieved and cardiac output is augmented with positive inotropic agents. This situation is commonly seen with severe biventricular infarction and thus should be suspected with inferior and right ventricular infarction. In this case, bradycardia should be treated with atropine if it is thought to be contributing to the systemic hypoperfusion. Excessive treatment with nitroglycerin and volume contraction from previous diuretic therapy can also contribute to systemic hypotension.

Hypotension and Cardiogenic Shock

Cardiogenic shock may occur when 40 percent or more of the left ventricle is destroyed.[43,44,533] It is the most common cause of in-hospital death with myocardial infarction. The incidence of cardiogenic shock was about 15 percent in the early 1970s, but it has now decreased to approximately 5 to 7 percent.[531] The mortality rate is frequently over 80 percent.[534] The most effective therapy in the treatment of cardiogenic shock is prevention, since its major determinant is infarct size.[41,535] Cardiogenic shock usually occurs within hours of onset of infarction due to massive ischemia and necrosis.[535] In other cases, a relatively small infarction that is superimposed on extensive previous damage may precipitate cardiogenic shock. Less commonly, cardiogenic shock may develop days after the initial event. This occurrence is almost always due to development of new necrosis (extension or early reinfarction) in the area of the preceding infarction. The decrease in the incidence of cardiogenic shock is believed to be in part due to better treatment of angina and ischemia, together with the widespread use of thrombolytic therapy and other cardioprotective agents. Cardiogenic shock by definition represents a more severe form of cardiac failure, resulting in decreased organ perfusion in addition to the conventional features of pulmonary congestion and left ventricular dysfunction. The distinction between cardiac failure with hypoperfusion and that regarded as cardiogenic shock may differ only in the severity of decreased perfusion. Clearly, every effort must be made to treat hypotension whether or not it satisfies the strict criteria of cardiogenic shock. Characteristics of cardiogenic shock are (Table 60-15) (1) evidence of organ hypoperfusion with cold, clammy skin, especially on the feet and hands, that may be associated with peripheral cyanosis of the nail beds; (2) oliguria and disordered mentation and systolic blood pressure of less than 80 to 90 mmHg; (3) left ventricular end-diastolic pressure or, more commonly, pulmonary capillary wedge pressure of greater than 18 mmHg; (4) evidence of a primary cardiac abnormality; and (5) a cardiac index not greater than 1.8 L/min per square meter of body surface. Hypotension or shock due to a primary abnormality of cardiac rhythm or conduction is not considered cardiogenic shock.

Since the prognosis is extremely poor for patients with cardiogenic shock due primarily to loss of muscle mass, reversible causes associated with a better prognosis must be excluded. Potentially reversible causes include mitral valve rupture, ventricular septal rupture, right ventricular infarction, pulmonary embolus, and cardiac tamponade. While the mortality associated with surgical correction of infarct-associated mitral rupture or ventricular septal defect is still high, it is far less than that associated with cardiogenic shock due solely to myocardial injury (see Chap. 74). The details of management of these mechanical causes for shock are discussed later. Hypotension may be due to inadequate fluid administration; to vasodilatation induced by such drugs as morphine and vasodilators; and, occasionally, to depressed contractility due to antiarrhythmic therapy. Inadequate filling pressure represents a very important cause for hypotension and should be corrected immediately. It is particularly common in patients with inferior infarction, as noted. A Swan-Ganz catheter (Chap. 18) should be inserted to determine the circulatory status and assess the response to therapy.

TABLE 60-15

Characteristics of Cardiogenic Shock

Evidence of hypoperfusion: cold clammy skin, especially of feet and hands; impaired mentation; and oliguria
Systolic blood pressure $< 80–90$ mmHg
LVED pressure (or PCW pressure) ≥ 18 mmHg
Evidence of primary cardiac abnormality
Cardiac index ≤ 1.8 L/m/m^2

Therapeutic objectives are to establish and maintain a systemic arterial pressure adequate to perfuse the vital organs and to reduce pulmonary congestion. The approaches to the pulmonary congestion include the judicious use of morphine and the maintenance of adequate oxygenation together with endotracheal intubation and mechanical ventilation if necessary. In addition to instituting hemodynamic monitoring, one should assess urinary output using an indwelling catheter. If the pulmonary artery wedge pressure is less than 15 mmHg, prompt volume expansion to raise the capillary pressure to 18 to 20 mmHg should be initiated. The cornerstones of therapy are inotropic and vasopressor agents. If the systemic arterial vasopressure is below 80 to 90 mmHg, a pressor agent such as dopamine should be infused.[536] At relatively low doses of 2 to 5 μg per kilogram of body weight per minute, increases in stroke volume and cardiac output are mediated by beta-adrenergic stimulation and increases in renal blood flow are mediated by the dopaminergic-specific receptors. The alpha-adrenergic vasoconstrictor effects are manifested progressively as doses above 5 μg per kilogram of body weight per minute. The use of intravenous dopamine requires careful titration, beginning with a low dose and gradually increasing until an adequate (90 to 100 mmHg) systemic pressure is achieved. If high doses of dopamine are necessary to maintain adequate perfusion, a change to norepinephrine infusion should be considered. This drug is a potent arteriolar and venous constrictor that is mediated through alpha-adrenergic stimulation. It demonstrates relatively modest beta-adrenergic stimulation. It is, therefore, a very potent pressor agent with less chronotropic or arrhythmogenic effects than dopamine.[40] The drug should be started at low doses of 1 to 4 μg/min. Extravasation should be avoided, since it will produce tissue sloughing (see also Chaps. 28 and 30).

When the systemic blood pressure is 90 mmHg or more, dobutamine is frequently the preferred agent. By increasing cardiac output, dobutamine may produce a rise in systemic blood pressure, but this increase would not be expected to be greater than 10 to 15 mmHg.[537,538] Dobutamine will not support arterial pressure except by its effect on cardiac output. As the cardiac output rises, the left ventricular filling pressure should decline. Dobutamine therapy should begin with a dose of 2 to 5 μg per kilogram of body weight per minute, with increases every 5 to 10 min. Inappropriate increases in heart rate are unlikely to occur with doses less than 15 to 20 μg per kilogram of body weight per minute.[520]

On occasion, the severity of cardiac pump dysfunction will require the use of two divergent therapeutic modalities in order to facilitate left ventricular emptying.[539] The most commonly utilized of these combined therapies is nitroprusside and dopamine. The principal advantage offered by nitroprusside in this combination is a reduction in left ventricular preload. The cardiac output is not appreciably increased by the addition of nitroprusside to dopamine therapy. The advantage offered by dopamine in this combination is an augmentation of cardiac output and the maintenance of systemic arterial pressure.[540] A less frequently used combination, dobutamine and nitroprusside, has been shown to result in higher cardiac output and lower pulmonary capillary pressures than either drug alone.[539]

Stabilization of the patient with cardiogenic shock may be achieved by mechanical circulatory assist devices, such as the intraaortic balloon (see Chap. 31). Aortic balloon counterpulsation reduces afterload while simultaneously improving coronary perfusion by increasing diastolic aortic pressure. It is the only intervention that will increase diastolic aortic pressure without increasing myocardial oxygen demand. Aortic counterpulsation is usually reserved for patients in cardiogenic shock due to a potentially reversible condition or in whom cardiac transplantation is being considered. Such conditions include an acute, but still evolving, myocardial infarction, or AMI with a severe mechanical complication (e.g., mitral regurgitation or ventricular septal defect). In such cases, aortic counterpulsation should be used to stabilize the patient's condition in preparation for salvage of the jeopardized but still viable myocardium or correction of the mechanical defect.[40] The use of aortic counterpulsation in patients without a reversible defect has been shown not to prolong life significantly or to provide long-term benefit and thus should not be instituted unless there is reasonable expectation of correcting the underlying problem or of transplantation.

Restoration of coronary blood will probably be the most effective therapy in salvaging patients with cardiogenic shock who are unresponsive to fluid and pharmacologic management in the early hours after a myocardial infarction. If angioplasty and/or coronary artery bypass grafting is not readily available, thrombolytic therapy should be tried if it has not already been utilized—although it has not been shown to improve survival in this setting.[541,542] These patients should be transferred quickly to a tertiary center. Blood pressure should be stabilized with an intraaortic balloon pump and cardiac catheterization performed as soon as possible. Assessment of correctable mechanical lesions, such as ruptured papillary muscles, can be made together with evaluation of coronary anatomy. Depending upon this anatomy, a judgment can be made as to whether to attempt PTCA or to proceed to coronary artery bypass surgery. Mechanical revascularization appears to improve survival in cardiogenic shock complicating AMI.[543]

Mechanical Dysfunction Contributing to Cardiac Failure

Papillary Muscle Rupture Rupture of the left ventricular papillary muscle occurs in approximately 1 percent of myocardial infarctions and accounts for 0.4 to 5.0 percent of infarct-related deaths.[544] It occurs slightly less frequently than ventricular septal rupture. The posteromedial papillary muscle is involved 6 to 12 times more frequently than the anterolateral muscle.[545] Thus, papillary muscle rupture with an acute anterior myocardial infarction is uncommon. The rupture may occur distally and involve one or several of the smaller heads of the muscle or, less commonly, may occur proximally and produce complete dehiscence of the papillary muscle.

Papillary muscle rupture is manifested by the sudden appearance of pulmonary edema, usually 2 to 7 days after the infarction. The abruptness of onset and severity of pulmonary edema are usually greater than seen with ventricular septal rupture. A mid- or holosystolic murmur with wide radiation is usually audible. Although the murmur is generally loud, a thrill is rarely present, and the murmur may seem inconsequential. The diagnosis can be established by Doppler echocardiographic studies (see Chap. 130). The two-dimensional echocardiogram will generally show a flail mitral leaflet and may reveal a portion of the papillary muscle visualized as a mass attached to the chordae. Even when the flail leaflet is not observed, documentation of relatively intact ventricular systolic function in the postinfarction patient with pulmonary edema should suggest the diagnosis. The Doppler study will establish the presence and severity of the mitral regurgitation. Bedside right heart catheterization can be used to exclude an oxygen stepup from the right atrium to right ventricle, indicative of ventricular septal rupture, and to confirm elevated pulmonary capillary wedge pressures with tall V (regurgitant) waves characteristic of acute mitral regurgitation.

Studies in the presurgical era demonstrated a poor prognosis for these patients, with a 50 percent mortality rate in the first 24 h and a 6 percent survival rate for longer than 2 months.[546] Thus, immediate recognition and treatment are essential. Intraaortic counterpulsation alone or with vasodilator and inotropic therapy are frequently required for temporary stabilization. During this period, the patient should undergo cardiac catheterization to define coronary anatomy and be transferred to surgery for mitral valve replacement or repair.

Papillary Muscle Dysfunction The sudden development of an apical systolic murmur after a myocardial infarction is much more often secondary to papillary muscle dysfunction than to rupture. Twenty percent of patients who die from infarction have histologic evidence of papillary muscle necrosis, usually without rupture.[547] Papillary muscle dysfunction is frequently compatible with long-term survival.

The posteromedial papillary muscle is involved with ischemia or infarction more commonly than the anterolateral muscle because the latter receives blood from two arteries (left anterior descending and circumflex), whereas the posteromedial muscle is supplied predominantly from the circumflex.[548] Dysfunction may be transient during ischemia. Papillary muscle ischemia is usually accompanied by ischemia of the contiguous ventricular wall.[549] Involvement of the contiguous ventricular wall is a key factor in the development of significant mitral regurgitation, since isolated papillary muscle ischemia or even infarction is usually not sufficient to cause important mitral regurgitation.[550]

Papillary muscle dysfunction typically presents with an apical systolic murmur. The murmur may be holosystolic, late systolic, or even early systolic. Echocardiographic coupled with Doppler flow studies will confirm the presence of mitral regurgitation, grade its severity, and permit assessment of left ventricular function. There is generally no hemodynamic deterioration associated with the appearance of the murmur. It is the unusual patient who develops pulmonary congestion or edema or hypotension due to papillary muscle dysfunction, and these patients usually have concomitant significant left ventricular dysfunction. The usual patient with papillary muscle dysfunction will require no specific therapy for the regurgitation, while the unusual patient with severe regurgitation should be treated like papillary muscle rupture. In intermediate cases with moderate to moderately severe regurgitation in whom cardiac surgery is not contemplated, afterload reduction with ACE inhibitors should be considered.

Ventricular Septal Rupture Rupture of the interventricular septum is estimated to occur in 1 to 3 percent of AMIs and accounts for approximately 5 percent of all infarct-related deaths.[551] Ventricular septal rupture occurs with an approximately equal frequency between anterior and inferior infarctions. There is a higher prevalence in first infarctions. The majority of ventricular septal ruptures occur within the first week, and 20 to 30 percent may develop as early as the first 24 h after the infarction.[552,553] Septal rupture rarely occurs after 2 weeks. Ventricular septal rupture is usually manifested by the appearance of a new harsh, holosystolic murmur along the left sternal border (often associated with a thrill) and sudden clinical deterioration with hypotension and pulmonary congestion. Right ventricular volume overload secondary to the shunt may produce signs of systemic venous congestion out of proportion to those of pulmonary venous congestion. Often the event is heralded by a recurrence of chest pain.

The diagnosis can be established by two-dimensional and Doppler echocardiographic studies that will demonstrate the site and approximate size of the rupture as well as the left-to-right shunt. Bedside right-sided heart catheterization is useful in confirming the diagnosis (an increase in O_2 saturation of >5 percent from right atrium to right ventricle) and is an aid in managing the patient. The primary diagnostic concern is to exclude rupture of the papillary muscle. The presence of a thrill or an anterior infarction would be unusual with papillary muscle rupture, and result of the Doppler echocardiographic studies and/or the oxygen stepup on right heart catheterization would confirm the presence of septal rupture.

When medical therapy alone is used, most patients with ventricular septal rupture deteriorate rapidly and virtually all patients die, many within 24 hours after rupture. Except for the rare case in which there is no clinical or hemodynamic deterioration, medical therapy can be expected to be ineffective. Intravenous sodium nitroprusside may improve forward cardiac output and reduce the shunt, but severe systemic hypotension frequently precludes its use. Inotropic and vasopressor agents may be required to sustain arterial blood pressure but can increase the left-to-right shunt. Prompt but temporary stabilization can be achieved with intraaortic balloon counterpulsation alone or in conjunction with vasodilator and inotropic drug therapy. Once the patient is stabilized, cardiac catheterization as a prelude to surgery should be performed in an expeditious manner. The cardiac catheterization should define cardiac anatomy, left ventricular function, and mitral valve competence. An aggressive approach of immediate operative repair of these patients results in a short-term survival rate of 42 to 75 percent.[554–556] The 5-year actuarial survival rate for the operative survivors has been reported to be as high as 88 percent.[557] Surgical results are worse when ventricular septal rupture complicates inferior infarction and when there is combined right ventricular and septal dysfunction.[556]

Cardiac Rupture Postinfarction Cardiorrhexis, or rupture of the heart, occurs in up to 24 percent of fatal AMIs. After cardiogenic shock and arrhythmias, it is the most common cause of death. The free wall of the ventricle is the most common site of rupture, and rupture there occurs 8 to 10 times more frequently than rupture of a papillary muscle or the ventricular septum.[558]

Rupture of the free wall generally occurs within the first 2 weeks of the infarction and may occur within the first 24 h.[559,560] Rupture occurring after this interval usually represents extension of the infarction or rupture through a false aneurysm.[561]

The rupture occurs primarily in the left ventricle, with a fairly even distribution between the anterior, inferior, and lateral walls. Given the relatively smaller number of lateral infarctions, the incidence of rupture with lateral wall infarctions would presumably be relatively greater than at other sites.[562] Free wall rupture is more likely to occur with the initial myocardial infarction, in women, in the sixth decade of life or later, and in patients with systemic arterial hypertension, particularly if there is no associated ventricular hypertrophy.[559] The prolonged use of corticosteroids might predispose a patient to rupture.

Cardiac rupture generally presents as sudden unanticipated death. Symptoms such as pain, agitation, sinus tachycardia, or vagally mediated bradycardia seldom precede death by more than minutes. Occasionally, intermittent chest pain and/or transient hypotension may precede and portend the final catastrophic event. Cardiac rupture is diagnosed terminally by development of electromechanical disassociation in the setting of recurrent chest pain. Few cases, and only those with immediate recognition, can be salvaged. Even these few cases require heroic measures, such as immediate pericardiocentesis, emergency thoracotomy, and surgical repair.

Other Complications

Pericarditis

Pericardial involvement associated with a myocardial infarction assumes one of two forms. The more common type is pericardial inflammation overlying the necrotic segment of a transmural myocardial infarction. This particular pericarditis is usually an incidental finding in the course of a more significant illness. The less frequent form of postinfarction pericarditis is generally a delayed complication that may represent an immunologic or autoimmune reaction. This pericarditis generally represents a major complication that often outlasts the basic illness.

Early Postinfarction Pericarditis The prevalence of early postinfarction pericarditis is 6 to 11 percent.[563,564]

The general consensus among cardiologists, however, is that this entity occurs far more frequently than it is clinically recognized. This suspicion is supported by postmortem studies finding evidence of postinfarction pericarditis when it was not recognized clinically.[565] The pericarditis usually becomes evident between the second and the fourth day following the infarction.

The most common manifestation of pericarditis is a scratchy two- or three-component friction rub along the left sternal border. The friction rub may have only a single component and be erroneously dismissed as a systolic murmur. The rub is evanescent, lasting 1 to 6 days. The pain of pericarditis is generally perceived by the patient to be different from that of the infarction. The location of the pain may be the same, but any radiation is usually to the neck, shoulder, or scapula rather than to the arms or jaw. Characteristically, the pain is aggravated by inspiration, swallowing, coughing, or recumbency. Fever, usually less than 39°C, generally accompanies the pericardial inflammation and typically lasts longer than 3 days, unlike the fever in an uncomplicated myocardial infarction.[566] The ECG is frequently not helpful in these patients, partially because it is usually distorted by the infarction and perhaps because of the localized nature of the inflammation. The cardiac rhythm is generally sinus tachycardia, but there is an increased prevalence of atrial fibrillation.[567] Since significant effusion is unusual with this form of pericarditis, the echocardiogram is of limited diagnostic value.

The pain of pericarditis usually responds promptly to aspirin or a nonsteroidal anti-inflammatory agent which should be administered for 5 to 7 days. In those infrequent cases in which severe symptoms do not resolve rapidly with nonsteroidal agents, a few doses of intravenous corticosteroids should be considered. Prolonged corticosteroid therapy should be avoided, since myocardial healing might be impaired. The use of anticoagulants is relatively contraindicated in AMI complicated by pericarditis. Situations ordinarily calling for anticoagulation, such as mural thrombosis seen on an echocardiogram, require excellent clinical judgment in assessing the risk-benefit ratio if pericarditis is also present.

Postmyocardial Infarction Syndrome (Dressler's Syndrome) The clinical features of this syndrome are fever, chest pain, evidence of polyserositis, and a tendency to recur.[568] The reported frequency is 1 to 3 percent of myocardial infarctions.[567,568] While there is usually a latency period of at least 1 week before its appearance, the pleuropericarditis may develop within the first week following the infarction.[569] The syndrome can occur in association with non-Q-wave infarctions. The absence of fever is rare. Generally the temperature is in the range of 38 to 39°C and occasionally rises to 40°C. The chest pain is the most sensitive index of this syndrome and often precedes the fever. Aggravation of the pain by deep inspiration and turning is its most distinctive feature. The pericarditis is manifested by a friction rub usually occurring between the second and eleventh week after the infarction and lasting from 3 days to 3 weeks. Pericardial effusion is common. While pericarditis is the dominant feature, as many as two-thirds of the patients have pleural effusions. These effusions are usually small and frequently bilateral but may be large and hemorrhagic. About one-quarter of the patients have linear or patchy infiltrates in the lung bases.

The clinical features, pathological findings, and prompt response to steroids all suggest an immunologic or autoimmune reaction. The presence of antimyocardial antibodies has been demonstrated in the majority of patients tested with this syndrome.

The treatment of Dressler's syndrome is similar to that of early postinfarction pericarditis but is more likely to require a course of oral corticosteroid therapy. If nonsteroidal anti-inflammatory agents fail to relieve symptoms, corticosteroids should be given and gradually tapered over 2 to 4 weeks. Recurrences are common for several months and require reinstitution of corticosteroids with a more gradual tapering. Anticoagulants generally should be discontinued in the presence of the postmyocardial infarction syndrome.[546]

Pulmonary Embolism

The prevalence of deep venous thrombosis (DVT) in AMI is reported to be between 12 and 38 percent. Patients with large infarctions in any location, anterior infarctions, evidence of congestive heart failure, and complicated infarctions have a greater frequency of DVT.[570,571] Reduced cardiac output and immobilization are additional predisposing factors for DVT (see Chap. 100).

The venous thrombosis is usually a minor and frequently an unrecognized complication of infarction but is potentially life-threatening. A prevalence of pulmonary embolism of 10 to 15 percent and a prevalence of fatal embolism in 3 to 6 percent has been reported in the past.[572] More recently, pulmonary embolism has been reported to account for less than 1 percent of deaths in myocardial infarction, probably because of earlier ambulation and better therapy of low output.[561]

Early mobilization combined with therapy directed toward improving cardiac output when appropriate is probably the most effective means of preventing pulmonary emboli. Prophylactic anticoagulant therapy is not routinely recommended for all patients after a myocardial infarction but is advisable for patients with increased risk factors for DVT and pulmonary embolism.

Systemic Emboli

Emboli to the cerebrovascular, renal, mesenteric, iliofemoral, or other arterial systems may complicate the AMI. The reported prevalence of clinically apparent systemic emboli in patients with myocardial infarction varies from 0.6 to 6.4 percent.[573,574]

These emboli result from dislodgment of left ventricular thrombi, that are found in 20 to 40 percent of anterior myocardial infarctions. A ventricular thrombus is unusual in patients with an inferior infarction.[574,575] The predilection of the apical wall for thrombus development appears to be related to a combination of stagnant blood flow and poor wall contractility. Severe depression of left ventricular function is not a prerequisite for thrombus formation. The development of a mural thrombus in a small infarction (CK <1000 units), however, is unusual.[576,577] Thrombus morphology and mobility do seem to correlate with systemic embolization.[573,578,579] Pedunculated and freely mobile thrombi have been thought to have a greater chance of embolization. At least two studies, however, could not correlate risk of embolization to any particular thrombus morphology.[574,577]

Left ventricular thrombosis usually occurs within the first 3 days after a myocardial infarction[577,580] but may occur at any time during the hospital course. Early mural thrombosis occurs in large infarctions that have an unfavorable prognosis.[577] Systemic embolization occurs an average of 14 days after AMI and is unlikely to occur after more than 4 to 6 weeks.[581]

Anticoagulation appears to reduce the incidence of mural thrombosis formation[582] and the prevalence of systemic embolization.[573,575,576] All patients with an anterior myocardial infarction should have two-dimensional echocardiography performed within 24 to 72 h following the infarction, with particular emphasis on the two-chamber and four-chamber apical views. Those with a severe apical wall contraction abnormality (akinesis or dyskinesis) should receive heparin for several days, followed by warfarin (INR 2 to 3) for 1 to 3 months. In patients with a left ventricular thrombus demonstrated by echocardiographic studies, chronic warfarin therapy (Chap. 68) is continued for 3 to 6 months. Warfarin administration should be maintained indefinitely for atrial fibrillation.

Two-dimensional echocardiography has a sensitivity of 83 to 95 percent and a specificity of 86 to 90 percent in diagnosing a mural thrombus.[574,576,578,583] Angiography has a sensitivity of 20 to 63 percent and a specificity of 67 to 75 percent.[573,584] Occasionally, a technically unsatisfactory echocardiogram may require the use of alternative noninvasive imaging modalities. Both computed tomography (CT) and magnetic resonance imaging (MRI) offer a similar sensitivity and perhaps superior specificity to echocardiography in this setting.[584]

Ventricular Aneurysm

The true prevalence of ventricular aneurysm after myocardial infarction is not well defined. Probably the best approximation comes from postmortem studies that estimate a 3 to 15 percent prevalence.[580,585] The CASS registry documented angiographically defined left ventricular aneurysms in 7.6 percent of patients with coronary artery disease. The location of the aneurysm is usually anterior, anteroapical, or apical. True posterior ventricular aneurysms located in the diaphragmatic wall between the septum and insertion of the posterior papillary muscle have been observed but are quite uncommon.[586]

Pathologically, the aneurysmal area is characterized by a thinned-out transmural scar that has lost completely its trabecular pattern. The scar, which may eventually calcify, is clearly delineated from surrounding ventricular muscle. Aneurysms characteristically have a wide base (the diameter of the mouth is equal to or larger than its greatest internal diameter), and one-half are lined by a laminated thrombus.[587]

As many as 80 percent of chronic ventricular aneurysms can be diagnosed clinically by the presence of an abnormal precordial impulse; a typical bulge on the left ventricular border on chest x-ray, frequently with calcification around the apex; and ECG evidence of a large anterior infarction with ST-segment elevation persisting beyond 2 weeks following the infarction. Two-dimensional echocardiographic studies can confirm the diagnosis.[588] Left ventricular aneurysms are associated with a reduced survival rate. The prognosis for these patients, however, is primarily related to the left ventricular dysfunction and not to the presence of the aneurysm. True ventricular aneurysms rarely rupture. In fact, the survival rate for patients with an aneurysm is no different than for patients without an aneurysm but a similar degree of left ventricular dysfunction. Moreover, the incidence of sudden death is no different. Whether or not clinical recognition of the presence of a ventricular aneurysm is important in the management of the patient after an AMI remains to be answered.[583]

Most patients with ventricular aneurysm should be treated the same as any other postinfarction patient with a similar degree of left ventricular dysfunction. Vasodilators, digoxin, anticoagulants, and antiarrhythmics should be used based, not on the presence of the aneurysm, but as dictated by presence of heart failure, mural thrombi, and life-threatening arrhythmias. Occasionally, surgical resection of the aneurysm is justified to correct refractory heart failure, recurrent life-threatening arrhythmias, or multiple systemic emboli (see Chap. 74). The aneurysm resection should usually be combined with coronary bypass grafting, and in cases of ventricular arrhythmias should be guided by electrophysiologic mapping.

Pseudoaneurysm

A pseudoaneurysm is a rare complication of myocardial infarction the prevalence of which is not known. The probable sequence of events in the development of a pseudoaneurysm is as follows: occurrence of a transmural infarction with localized pericarditis arising at the site of infarction; development of adhesions between the visceral and parietal pericardium; rupture of the infarcted myocardium, with the extravasated blood confined by the adherent pericardium; progressive enlargement of the aneurysmal sac; and development of thrombus within the sac.[589]

Unlike a true ventricular aneurysm, a pseudoaneurysm has a narrow base (site of rupture). The wall is composed only of thrombus and pericardium, and the risk of rupture is high.[590] While the neck is small (its diameter is less than 50 percent of the diameter of the fundus), the pseudoaneurysm may progressively enlarge to become larger than the left ventricle. The pseudoaneurysm may be clinically silent or may present as progressively worsening heart failure, an abnormal bulge on the cardiac border, persistent ST-segment elevation in the area overlying the infarction, or systolic murmurs.[591]

The diagnosis can be established by two-dimensional echocardiographic studies, ventriculographic radionuclide studies, MRI, or left ventriculographic contrast studies.[590]

Discharge from the Coronary Care Unit

The length of stay in the coronary care unit should be based on the risk of developing ventricular tachycardia and ventricular fibrillation. The risk of developing primary ventricular fibrillation after AMI decreases exponentially with the majority of arrhythmic deaths occurring within the first 24 h. After the third day, the episodes of life-threatening arrhythmias are fairly evenly distributed over the remainder of the hospitalization.[592] Thus, a patient with an uncomplicated infarction can be transferred from the coronary care unit on the third day. Since 31 to 34 percent of in-hospital deaths from AMI occur after discharge from the coronary care unit and since half of them are sudden and unexpected, certain patients need more prolonged cardiac monitoring.[593,594] Those patients who are prime candidates for late-hospital sudden deaths manifest, while in the coronary care unit, one or more of the following: (1) the arrhythmias of pump failure (sinus tachycardia, atrial flutter, or atrial fibrillation); (2) the arrhythmias of electrical instability (ventricular tachycardia or ventricular fibrillation); (3) acute interventricular conduction disturbances; (4) evidence of circulatory failure (congestive heart failure, pulmonary edema, or significant hypotension); or (5) large anterior infarction. The effectiveness of prolonged monitoring of this select group of patients in an intermediate care unit following coronary care unit discharge is evident in a doubling of the rate of successful resuscitations.[595,596] Patients who do not fit into these high-risk subgroups can be discharged from the coronary care unit to a medical unit without continuous monitoring. The wide availability of continuous monitoring in many hospitals in nonacute care units permits easy further monitoring on even lower risk patients.

The activity permitted the patient with uncomplicated infarction has changed immensely during the last two decades. In an uncomplicated myocardial infarction, the patient does not need to be confined to bed for longer than 24 h. In fact, the patient may use a bedside commode from the time of admission. The safety and benefits of chair rest were initially promoted by Samuel Levine and Bernard Lown in 1951.[597] Upon transfer from a coronary care unit, the patient should be started on a progressive ambulation program (Table 60-16). The speed with which the patient progresses from one stage to the next depends on the severity of the infarction, the presence or absence of complications, the age of the patient, and the presence of comorbid conditions. The length of hospitalization following an AMI should likewise depend on these same factors. If the patient has not manifested the arrhythmias of pump failure or electrical instability, evidence of circulatory failure, or advanced AV block during the first 4 days of hospitalization, he or she is very unlikely to do so at any later time.[598] This patient could probably be discharged after 7 days in the hospital.[599] The last 2 to 3 days of the hospitalization are generally necessary to resolve the questions pertaining to residual ventricular function, the presence or absence of ventricular ectopy, and the adequacy of the remainder of the coronary circulation. In addition, time is needed for instruction in risk-factor modification (see Chaps. 62 and 63).

RISK STRATIFICATION AND SECONDARY PREVENTION IN PATIENTS SURVIVING ACUTE MYOCARDIAL INFARCTION

Survivors of myocardial infarction have substantial risk of future cardiovascular events. The purpose of noninvasive risk assessment is to individualize the extent of further work-up and therapy. Risk stratification provides information useful in counseling the patient on prognosis and returning to work, developing an exercise program, and planning modifications of cardiovascular risk factors.

Three interrelated prognostic factors should be the focus of predischarge assessment: (1) measurement of left ventricular function,[600] (2) detection of residual myocardial ischemia (jeopardized myocardium),[601] and (3) assessment of risk of arrhythmic (sudden) death.[600,601] Most proposed algorithms of noninvasive test selection focus on these three important clinical areas.[602–605] The highest-risk patients are clinically identified by evidence of one or more of the following: congestive heart failure, angina associated with electrocardiographic changes, in-hospital cardiac arrest, or an episode of spontaneous sustained ventricular tachycardia. The mortality rate in this group exceeds 25 percent in 1 year, justifying an aggressive diagnostic and therapeutic approach.[606] In contrast to the high-risk group, most patients have a relatively benign hospital course. In these patients, noninvasive testing can accurately identify a very low-risk group, whose annual mortality is 1 to 3 percent.[601,607–610] The practical consequences of identifying this group are that emphasis is focused on risk-factor modification (Chaps. 52, 62, 63, and 65) and targeted prophylactic medical therapy rather than expensive, invasive diagnostic testing.

Noninvasive measurement of left ventricular ejection fraction (LVEF) should be obtained by radionuclide ventriculographic or two-dimensional echocardiographic studies.[318] Both techniques also provide a description of the segmental wall motion abnormalities. Myocardial ischemia has traditionally been assessed by the electrocardiographic response to a submaximal exercise test prior to hospital discharge,[611–616] but when it is available and practical to obtain, a myocardial perfusion scan with thallium is preferable for providing information on the extent of fixed (scar) and reversible (ischemic) perfusion defects (Chap. 134).[617] Several provocative pharmacologic techniques, including infusions of dipyridamole, adenosine, and dobutamine,[618–621] have extended the flexibility of thallium scintigraphy and permitted assessment of ischemia in patients who cannot exercise. A proliferation of new tests are available to identify patients at risk of sudden death. Ambulatory ECG recordings were initially used to measure asymptomatic spontaneous ventricular arrhythmia (see Chap. 45). Additional measurements from the ambulatory ECG recording include the detection of silent ischemic episodes[622] and assessment of heart rate variability.[623–625] The signal-averaged ECG (SAECG) is an additional useful tool for assessing sudden death risk, allowing more precise selection of patients for invasive electrophysiologic assessment (see Chap. 47).[626] The role of these

TABLE 60-16
Post Myocardial Infarction Ambulatory Activity Protocol

Steps	Activity	Observation	Education
I	Bedrest May use bedside commode May stand to void if necessary Complete bath Assistance with oral hygiene May wash hands, face, and personal areas May feed self Exercise 1: ankle flexion × 5 q 2 h Turning Passive range of motion	Chest discomfort Dysrhythmias Dyspnea on exertion Orthostatic hypotension	Orientation to CCU Instruction to inform staff of chest pain or shortness of breath
II	Dangle 5 min with BP check Upright in chair for 20 min t.i.d.; then recline in cardiac chair or bed Prefer patient did not eat a meal first time in chair May bathe face, arms, chest, and personal areas May use bedside commode Exercise 1: ankle flexion ×10 q 2 h Exercise 2: bilateral knee flexes × 5 q 2 h Passive range of motion if unable to do upper body movement	Orthostatic hypotension Chest discomfort/dyspnea on exertion Heart rate changes/ arrhythmias	Anatomy and physiology of the heart What is a heart attack?
III	Up in chair 45 min with or without meals t.i.d. May shave May bathe face, arms, and chest while sitting at bedside Bedside commode/bathroom with assistance Ankle flexion exercises ×10 q 2 h Continue knee flexes	Heart rate and arrhythmias during activity Chest discomfort Dyspnea on exertion	Reinforce step II topics The healing process Rationale for diagnostic procedures Risk factor identification
IV	Chair as tolerated Up to bathroom with assistance Assist with bath Begin exercises including feet/leg flexion, arm abduction, and leg extension each ×5 t.i.d.	Heart rate and arrhythmias during exercise Chest discomfort Dyspnea on exertion	Same as step IV
V	Ambulate from bed to door ×2 t.i.d. May stand at sink to shave Bathroom without assistance Continue exercises as above	Same as step IV	Risk factor reduction Current medications Educate as to results of diagnostic procedures Dietary instruction
VI	Ambulate in hall 50 ft. b.i.d. Up in room, as desired Bathe/shower self with assistance Continue exercises as above	Same as step IV	Same as step V
VII	Ambulate in hall 100 ft. t.i.d. Up in room, as desired Bathe/shower self Continue exercises as above Begin exercises including trunk rotation and neck flexion	Same as step IV	Symptoms to limit activity Activity progression at home Sexual activity progression
VIII	Ambulate length of hall b.i.d. Continue all exercises b.i.d. Stair climbing 3 steps	Same as step IV	Same as step VII

newer tests in risk-factor modification remains to be precisely defined.

It is important to understand the limitations of any proposed risk stratification algorithm. One significant issue is that many of the pivotal studies on risk stratification were in the prethrombolytic era. Extrapolation of such results to patients receiving thrombolytic therapy may have less validity. From an epidemiologic perspective, each noninvasive test identifies a *population* at increased risk for mortality or cardiovascular events following myocardial infarction but does not identify *specific patients* who will have a cardiac event within a certain time frame. Thus, the appropriate term is *relative risk*, and the lack of precision provides ample room for practicing the art of medicine. A comprehensive plan of diagnostic and therapeutic management of patients with AMI provides many useful guidelines and references.

Exercise Testing

Timing of Exercise Testing and Protocol Selection

During hospitalization, in patients recovering from AMI, a practical and safe approach to exercise testing has been to utilize a submaximal treadmill exercise protocol (modified Naughton or modified Bruce protocol) rather than the standard Bruce protocol. The target for completing the test is often symptom-limited exercise to a specific heart rate goal (e.g., 70 to 75 percent age-predicted) or to a specific oxygen consumption, such as 5 METs (see Chap. 16). In the typical postinfarction patient not on beta blockers, the target heart rate range is 110 to 125 beats per minute. In those patients taking beta blockers, exercise is frequently performed to a heart rate of at least 30 beats per minute over the resting heart rate. Depending on the exercise protocol used, exercise duration can also be to a specified work load or oxygen consumption. The exercise ECG is most accurately interpreted in the absence of baseline ST abnormalities or bundle branch block. Variables of clinical importance to evaluate include ST depression (magnitude, onset, and time to normalization during recovery), blood pressure response, exercise duration, the development of chest pain during exercise, and ventricular arrhythmias during exercise. Exercise testing is also useful in planning the exercise prescription for a cardiac rehabilitation program (see Chap. 63). Patients should be angina-free for 3 to 4 days and free of cardiac failure before exercise testing. Patients selected in this fashion under the supervision of a physician are at minimal risk of complications.[601,607–616,627]

Clinical Significance of Predischarge Submaximal Exercise Testing

The studies depicted in Table 60-17 have analyzed the predictive value of predischarge exercise testing during a 6- to 12-month follow-up after acute AMI. As seen, exercise variables that were found to be prognostically significant were exercise-induced ST-segment depression, ST-segment elevation, development of angina during exercise, inadequate blood pressure response to exercise, or exercise of short duration. From the practical standpoint, it is important to consider all of these exercise variables rather than to focus solely on the presence or absence of ST-segment depression during exercise. Exercise testing consistently identifies a high-risk group for recurrent cardiac events (myocardial infarction, unstable angina, etc.) or mortality over the next 12 months. However, the relative risk associated with a "positive exercise test" varies greatly (twofold to more than 15-fold). In one study, the presence of ST-segment shift or

TABLE 60-17

Submaximal Early Exercise Testing after Myocardial Infarction

Author	*n*	Actual Follow-up, Months	Predictive Exercise Variables	ID High Risk	ID Low Risk*	Predicts Total Mortality	Predicts Sudden Death
Theroux[601]	210	12	ST ↓, angina	+	2.1%	+	+
DeBusk[611]	200	3	ST ↓	+	–	–	–
Starling[612]	130	11	ST ↓, angina, inadequate BP response	+	–	+	–
Murray[613]	300	12	ST ↓, angina, hypotension, short duration	+	–	+	–
Krone[607]	207	12	Duration <9 min, ST ↓, angina	+	<2%**	+	–
Fuller[614]	40	7	ST ↓, angina	+	–	–	–
Schwartz[608]	48	14	Angina	+	≤3%	+	–
Weld[627]	250	12	Duration <6 min, VPCs	+	≤1%	+	–
Sami[615]	200	24	ST ↓	+	–	–	–
Smith[616]	62	21	ST↓, ST ↑	+	–	–	–
Fioretti[609]	405	12	Inability to raise systolic BP 30 mmHg	+	≤3%	+	–
Krone[610]	667	12	BP response, duration <9 min, VPCs	+	1%	+	–

ABBREVIATIONS: BP, blood pressure; ID, identifies; ST ↓, ST depression; ST ↑, ST elevation; VPC, ventricular premature complexes.
* 1-year mortality.
** Subgroup taking beta blockers.

angina during exercise also predicted sudden (arrhythmic) death.[601] Exercise testing also identifies a very low-risk group (<3 percent mortality rate for the first year).[601,607–610,627] Therefore, a negative test result is reassuring and should discourage the premature use of expensive and potentially dangerous testing and/or therapies. All uncomplicated patients with no contraindication to exercise should have submaximal exercise testing performed before discharge.

For patients with a normal exercise test before discharge, symptom-limited maximal exercise testing (preferably with thallium scintigraphy) should be repeated 4 to 6 weeks after AMI. The purpose of this test in some patients is to assess the adequacy of pharmacologic therapy for ischemia. If the issue is whether or not there is residual ischemic potential, antianginal medications may be discontinued for 24 h. A number of clinical trials have compared the value of maximal exercise testing 4 to 6 weeks after hospital discharge to predischarge exercise testing; most studies have concluded that the maximal exercise test identifies additional high-risk patients.[628–632] The magnitude of this additional ischemia detection, however, as compared to a submaximal exercise test prior to hospital discharge is modest. Since many cardiovascular events can occur in the first 4 to 6 weeks, predischarge exercise testing is preferred. The presence of ischemia on either the pre- or the postdischarge exercise test will in general lead to the decision to perform cardiac catheterization to define the coronary anatomy and to consider revascularization.

Exercise Thallium-201 Scintigraphy and Other Techniques in Predischarge Risk Stratification

There are several alternatives to standard exercise testing that have not yet become standard procedures in all centers. The best-studied technique generally is that of exercise thallium-201 scintigraphy (see Chap. 134). Exercise thallium-201 scintigraphy has a number of potential advantages over routine exercise testing: (1) it can be used when the 12-lead ECG is uninterpretable for ischemic ST-segment shifts because of baseline changes such as left bundle branch block; (2) it allows assessment of reversible and irreversible perfusion defects, both within and outside the vascular region involved in the AMI; and (3) the technique of SPECT thallium scintigraphy provides a semiquantitative evaluation of ischemia.[51,618,620,633]

Submaximal exercise scintigraphy appears to enhance the ability to identify high-risk, postmyocardial infarction in patients. High-risk patients were identified if (1) perfusion defects existed in more than one discrete vascular zone, (2) there was distinct evidence of redistribution, or (3) there was evidence of increased lung uptake.[617] Of patients with recurrent cardiac events, 94 percent were prospectively identified as having at least one of these factors. Low-risk patients as defined by a thallium scintigram showed involvement of a single vascular region without redistribution and no evidence of increased lung uptake. A thallium-201 scintigram indicating patients at high risk correlated with multivessel coronary disease. Thallium scintigraphy has been shown to be excellent at identifying high-grade stenoses of 90 percent or greater, especially high-grade lesions of the left anterior descending coronary artery.[618,620] Submaximal exercise thallium testing has not been generally used in predischarge risk stratification.

Exercise Echocardiography

Exercise two-dimensional echocardiography is an alternative technique for identifying ischemia.[634,635] A reversible segmental wall motion defect is felt to represent an area of significant ischemia. The limitation of this technique is the substantial subjectivity in interpreting echocardiographic wall motion abnormalities. Studies from specialized centers with expertise in echocardiography have shown that exercise or dobutamine echocardiographic studies have a high sensitivity and specificity in identifying patients with multivessel coronary disease (see Chap. 132).[635] Its role, if any, in early risk stratification remains to be determined.

Assessment of the Risk of Arrhythmic Death

Ambulatory Electrocardiogram Recordings: Ventricular Arrhythmias

Asymptomatic spontaneous ventricular arrhythmias detected on ambulatory ECG (AECG) recordings (Chap. 45) are predictive of an increased risk of arrhythmic (sudden) death in at least the first 2 years following AMI.[600,636,637] The mechanism responsible for the majority of arrhythmic deaths in post-AMI patients is sustained ventricular tachycardia or ventricular fibrillation.[638] The majority of patients who die of arrhythmic death or sudden cardiac death in the United States have a history of myocardial infarction. Vulnerability for arrhythmic death is highest in the first year after AMI, probably accounting for one-half the mortality. Thus, it is clinically relevant to attempt to assess potential arrhythmic death risk prior to hospital discharge. The use of AECG recording to identify a "high-risk" group, however, has poor positive predictive value, since the majority of patients with these "warning arrhythmias" will not incur arrhythmic death in the next few years.[639,640] As seen in Table 60-18, patients with no baseline ventricular arrhythmia on AECG recording are at very low risk for arrhythmic death.[641] The majority of uncomplicated patients following AMI have some ventricular premature complexes (VPCs). The presence of 3 to 10 VPCs per hour identifies at least a twofold increased risk for arrhythmic death, whereas the presence of nonsustained ventricular tachycardia is associated with a threefold increase in arrhythmic death risk. Even when patients with high risk are identified, the problem of defining rational prophylactic therapy has not been solved. As can be deduced from the data in Table 60-18 for every 100 patients identified with "warning arrhythmias," such as 10 or more VPCs per hour, only 4 to 7 of them will have an arrhythmic death in the following 1 to 2 years.[600,636,637,639–641] Thus, any prophylactic administration of an antiarrhythmic drug must be very safe, since the remaining 93 to 96 patients will be exposed to unnecessary, potentially dangerous therapy. This hazard is illustrated in the Cardiac Arrhythmia Suppression Trial (CAST), in which the treatment with encainide or flecai-

TABLE 60-18
Risk of Sudden Death Based on VPCs Detected on AECG in Patients Surviving AMI

Trial	Sample Size	Arrhythmic Death Mortality Rate, %*	Total Mortality Rate, %*	Actual Follow-up Months
CAST[639] (≥6 VPCs/h)				10
Encainide or flecainide	730	5.4**	9.2**	
Placebo	725	1.5	3.6	
CAPS[640] (≥10 VPCs/h)				12
All patients	502	4.6	9.0	
Placebo	100	—	7.0	
Bigger et al[600]				24
All patients	819	3.8	5.9	
0 VPC	112	1.5	3.0	
>3 VPCs/h	245	6.1	9.8	
>10 VPCs/h	162	6.3	9.4	
>30 VPCs/h	89	7.0	10.5	24
BHAT[714] (placebo group)				25
0 VPCs	260	1.2	2.5	
Any VPCs	1380	2.6	5.5	
≥10 VPCs/h	211	4.5	10.0	
≤10 VPCs/h	1429	2.0	4.3	
Moss et al[636]	759	6.8	11.0	6
Ruberman et al[637]				24
≤10 VPCs/h	1285	2.3	6.4	
≥10 VPCs/h	454	7.6	13.6	

* All corrected to an estimated 1-year mortality rate.
** End point of death or cardiac arrest.
ABBREVIATION: VPCS, ventricular premature complexes.

nide of postmyocardial infarction patients who had more than six asymptomatic VPCs per hour but did not have sustained or symptomatic ventricular tachycardia appeared actually to increase total mortality and sudden death.[639]

The prognostic significance of asymptomatic ventricular arrhythmias is more meaningfully interpreted with knowledge of the LVEF.[600] The presence of nonsustained ventricular tachycardia in patients with a LVEF of 30 percent or less increases the risk of arrhythmic death to 7 to 8 percent per year. A similar LVEF in the absence of nonsustained ventricular tachycardia or of frequent VPCs is associated with a 50 percent lower mortality rate. Data from CAST show that patients with frequent VPCs (six or more per hour) and relatively preserved left ventricular function (LVEF ≥ 40 percent) have a low risk of arrhythmic death.[639] Patients with LVEF of 40 percent or less after infarction should have AECG recordings taken to assess the presence of asymptomatic ventricular arrhythmias (see also Chap. 45).

Ambulatory Electrocardiogram Recordings: Silent Ischemia

One postmyocardial infarction trial provides evidence that the assessment of asymptomatic ST-segment depression (≥0.1 mV, ≤1 min) detected on AECG recordings can identify a population at increased risk for subsequent cardiovascular events.[642] Confirmation of this conclusion and further investigations describing any additive value of ischemia detected on AECG to that detected on exercise testing will clarify the value of analyzing the AECG for "silent ischemia." At present, the routine evaluation of silent ischemia on AECG is not recommended.

Ambulatory Electrocardiogram Recordings: Heart Rate Variability

Heart rate variability, measured by the standard deviation of the RR interval on monitored ECG leads, is an indirect assessment of proportional autonomic tone. Extensive variability in the heart rate connotes a preponderance of parasympathetic activity, whereas less variability in the heart rate is consistent with proportionately more sympathetic activity.[623–625] In animal models, enhanced sympathetic activity increases the vulnerability of ischemic myocardium to the development of ventricular fibrillation (see also Chap 35).[643,644]

Clinical trials have assessed the relationship of heart rate variability to mortality rate in patients surviving AMI. In the largest of these trials, heart rate variability was found to be an independent predictor of total mortality. A low heart rate variability observed in patients unable to perform low-level exercise was associated with a 54 percent mortality rate. In contrast, there was a 3 percent or lower mortality rate in patients with a high heart rate variability who could complete the low-level exercise test.[625] Decreased heart rate variability as an independent predictor of arrhythmic death has not been established, and defining its role, if any, awaits further investigation.

Signal-Averaged Electrocardiography

Time-domain analysis of the signal-averaged ECG (SAECG) can be used to detect low-amplitude, high-frequency potentials at the end of the QRS complex, termed *ventricular late potentials* (see Chap. 47). The presence of late potentials identifies patients likely to have inducible sustained monomorphic ventricular tachycardia during programmed electrical stimulation and who have an increased likelihood of subsequent arrhythmic events (Table 60-19).[623,626,645–652] The predictive value of late potentials is highest in patients with AMI and of less-established value in other patient populations. Time-domain analysis of the SAECG in the presence of left bundle branch block appears to be much less useful. Frequency-domain analysis of the SAECG may provide useful information in patients with left bundle branch block.

In some studies, an abnormal SAECG, the presence of frequent VPCs on the AECG recording, and the presence of left ventricular aneurysm were independent predictors of ventricular tachycardia.[652] The most practical

TABLE 60-19

Predictive Value of the Signal-Averaged Electrocardiogram after Acute Myocardial Infarction
Predictive of inducible ventricular tachycardia on EPS
Predictive of arrhythmic events
Not strongly predictive of total mortality rate or arrhythmic deaths

clinical advantage of SAECG is that it can identify a group at low risk of arrhythmic death. If results of the SAECG are negative, that is, there are no after-depolarizations, the negative predictive value in this population is excellent; and the likelihood of subsequent arrhythmic death is low.

Invasive Electrophysiologic Testing (Programmed Electrical Stimulation)

Invasive electrophysiological assessment has been evaluated in two distinct populations surviving AMI. The first and relatively small group had a cardiac arrest or an episode of sustained ventricular tachycardia following an AMI. In such patients, the risk of recurrent cardiac arrest or arrhythmic events is very high, and selection of therapy should be made utilizing electrophysiologic studies (EPS).[653] Patients presenting with sustained monomorphic ventricular tachycardia are very likely (approximately 90 percent) to have the ventricular tachycardia induced during programmed electrical stimulation. For patients whose presenting arrhythmia is cardiac arrest, the frequency of inducing sustained monomorphic VT decreases to a probability of 50 to 60 percent.[654] Indications for EPS after myocardial infarction are shown in Fig. 60-16 (see also Chap. 46).

A second patient population sometimes considered for EPS are those identified as having increased risk of an arrhythmic death based on the noninvasive tests discussed previously. Performing EPS on all asymptomatic "high-risk" patients is probably not justified at present. Reports on the utility of EPS have been inconsistent in predicting total mortality and are only slightly more consistent in identifying patients likely to have subsequent arrhythmic events.[648,655–664] These conclusions are summarized in Table 60-20.

TABLE 60-20

Electrophysiologic Study after Acute Myocardial Infarction
Predictive of total mortality
Not consistently predictive of arrhythmic deaths or events

Patients with preserved left ventricular function are at such a low risk of arrhythmic death that an AECG and a SAECG should not be routinely obtained. The high negative predictive valve of a normal SAECG result should discourage the routine use of EPS in patients with nonsustained ventricular tachycardia on AECG and an LVEF of 40 percent or less. Electrophysiologic studies should be considered for patients with an LVEF of 40 percent or less and a positive SAECG result. If sustained monomorphic ventricular tachycardia is not induced, antiarrhythmic therapy is not needed. As suggested in Fig. 60-16, asymptomatic patients with LVEF of 40 percent or less, positive SAECG results, and nonsustained ventricular tachycardia are at high risk (≥25 percent in first year) of an arrhythmic event; therefore, EPS is recommended. A negative EPS result (no inducible sustained ventricular tachycardia) should encourage a conservative therapeutic approach. There is no established beneficial therapeutic approach for patients who have inducible sustained ventricular tachycardia without an antecedent arrhythmic event. Antiarrhythmic drugs have been standard therapy although efficacy has not been established. The optimal treatment for asymptomatic patients with inducible sustained monomorphic ventricular tachycardia is not established, but continuing studies may provide some answer. Definitive recommendations to perform EPS in high risk post-AMI patients without a previous arrhythmic event are not possible (see Chap. 46). Although EPS may identify high-risk patients, its utility in guiding therapy has been questioned by the results of the ESVEM,[665] in which arrhythmia recurrence was unacceptably high regardless of whether ambulatory monitoring or electrophysiologic testing was used to guide therapy.

Q-Wave versus Non-Q-Wave Myocardial Infarction

A large number of studies support a difference in pathophysiology, clinical course, and management between

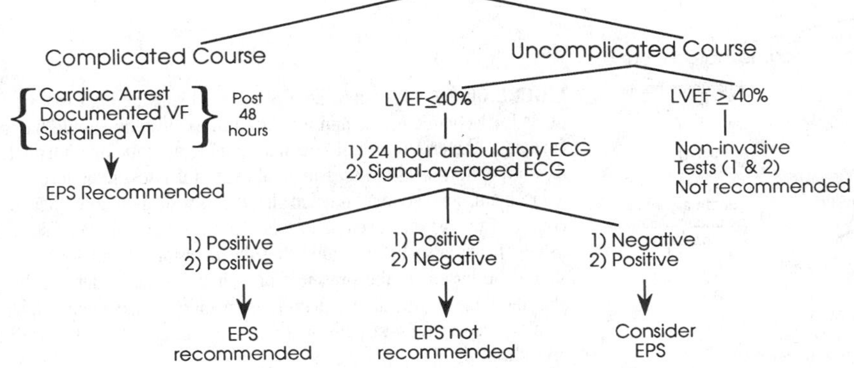

FIGURE 60-16 Assessing arrhythmic death risk: Noninvasive tests (24-h ambulatory ECG and signal-averaged ECG) and electrophysiologic study (EPS) should be targeted at appropriate high risk subsets. A positive ambulatory ECG (AECG) is defined as exhibiting nonsustained or sustained ventricular tachycardia. This proposed algorithm assumes LVEF (left ventricular ejection fraction) has been measured by some technique and appropriate tests for myocardial ischemia have been performed. The cost effectiveness of this algorithm has not been established. See text for explanation.

patients who incur a Q-wave infarction and those who incur a non-Q-wave myocardial infarction.[666] Coronary angiographic studies show that most patients (80 to 90 percent) with Q-wave myocardial infarction have an occluding thrombus of the infarct-related artery.[362] In contrast, in the early hours of a non-Q-wave myocardial infarction, only a partially occluding thrombus is present[667] in the majority of patients. Patients with Q-wave and non-Q-wave infarction have a similar extent of coronary atherosclerosis with a similar number of vessels involved. Both non-Q and Q-wave-infarction are precipitated by a thrombosis on an atheromatous plaque in conjunction with vasoconstriction, but indirect evidence indicates that early lysis of the thrombosis occurs with spontaneous restoration of coronary flow in patients with non-Q-wave infarction.

The differences in the acute and long-term mortality rates for Q-wave and non-Q-wave infarction have been studied extensively.[148,150,152,668–681] Patients with Q-wave infarction have more extensive initial myocardial damage and have a higher in-hospital mortality rate. The frequency of recurrent myocardial infarction, however, is greater in patients with non-Q-wave infarction such that the long-term mortality rates of Q-wave and non-Q-wave infarction are similar.

The fact that patients with non-Q-wave infarction have a greater amount of residual ischemic myocardium, as assessed by thallium scintigraphic studies, than Q-wave infarction patients accounts for the higher reinfarction rate.[678] Therefore, some clinicians recommend routine predischarge coronary angiographic studies in patients with a non-Q-wave infarction. The cost effectiveness of this strategy is not established but is being evaluated in an ongoing trial. An algorithm of patient selection for coronary angiography is presented in Fig. 60-17. Patients with a non-Q-wave infarction should have submaximal exercise testing (with thallium, if available), and those with evidence of ischemia should undergo coronary angiographic studies. Routine coronary angiographic studies for all non-Q-wave infarctions is still optional, although this strategy has not been shown to be cost effective.

Coronary Angiography

Selecting patients for cardiac catheterization and coronary angiographic studies prior to hospital discharge should be based on identifying patients at risk for ischemic events and whether or not the information provided by cardiac catheterization and coronary angiography will change patient management.

Studies analyzing the prognostic utility of cardiac catheterization prior to hospital discharge are from prethrombolytic era and demonstrated that the angiographic extent of coronary artery disease was related to survival.[617,629,682–686] Other trials have addressed the utility of routine coronary angiographic studies in patients who have received thrombolytic therapy.[687–692] The timing of cardiac catheterization during hospitalization has been addressed in several studies. In general, studies that have compared acute or early cardiac catheterization to a more conservative approach of performing cardiac catheterization and coronary angiographic studies only for patients with spontaneous recurrent angina or exercise-induced ischemia have demonstrated no benefit to the strategy of routine catheterization.[693]

Figure 60-17 presents a strategy for identifying symptomatic and asymptomatic high-risk patients who should have cardiac catheterization and coronary angiographic studies before discharge. Patients who have a complicated clinical course characterized by refractory cardiac failure, unstable angina, an episode of sustained ventricular tachycardia or cardiac arrest should be studied. An aggressive approach to these patients is justified because of the observed 1-year mortality rate, ranging from 10 to 25 percent.[694,695] In the case of patients with symptomatic cardiac failure, right heart catheterization should be included.

The recommended algorithm for selecting asymptomatic, uncomplicated post-AMI patients for cardiac catheterization is also presented in Fig. 60-17. Decision making focuses on the presence or absence of myocardial ischemia. Because of the high incidence of residual ischemia in patients with a non-Q-wave infarction, the task force for guidelines for coronary angiographic studies after myocardial infarction recommended such studies in all non-Q-wave infarctions.[696] The more conservative recommendation here emphasizes evidence of objective ischemia. In patients who have received thrombolytic therapy, it seems reasonable that patients who have evidence of residual ischemia are still at increased risk of future ischemic events and should undergo coronary angiography prior to discharge (Fig. 60-17). Consideration of PTCA following coronary angiographic studies should be based on established clinical and anatomic guidelines (see Chaps. 70 and 71).[697] Coronary artery

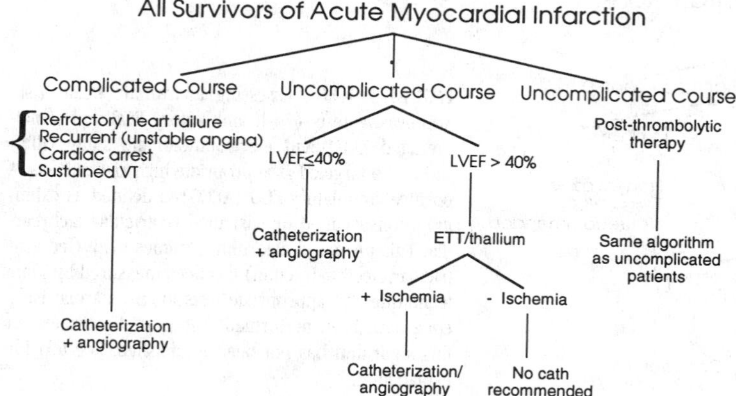

FIGURE 60-17 Proposed algorithm for identifying high risk patients for ischemic events and increased mortality who should have cardiac catheterization and coronary angiography before hospital discharge. Non-invasive assessment of LVEF and assessment of residual ischemia are recommended in all patients with an uncomplicated course. The cost effectiveness of this algorithm has not been established. It has also been argued that the decision for angiography should be based on the presence of ischemia independent of the alteration in the ejection fraction. Indication of ischemia might include recurrent chest pain or a positive exercise stress test with or without thallium.

bypass surgery should be considered in those groups in whom it has been shown to be of proven benefit: patients with triple-vessel disease, patients with ischemia, and patients with significant left ventricular dysfunction (see also Chap. 73).[683,698,699]

Combining Test Results for Assessing Risk

In clinical practice, multiple noninvasive tests to define risk more precisely are routinely performed. The studies in Table 60-21 have reported the cumulative value of a variety of multiple noninvasive tests for assessing risk. Some combination studies have focused either on myocardial ischemia or the risk of arrhythmic death, combined with assessment of the LVEF.[600,617,623–626,647,649,700,701] A number of the studies have compared the results of ventricular arrhythmias on AECG recordings with either SAECGs or heart rate variability.[600,623–626,647,649,700] The improved predictive value of these parameters was considered in creating the algorithm in Fig. 60-16 for selecting

TABLE 60-21
Studies Utilizing Multiple Non-Invasive Tests* for Risk Stratification

Author (ref)	(yr)	(*n*)	1	2	3	4	5	6	Follow-up (Months)	Predicts Ischemic Events	Predicts Arrhythmic Events	Predicts CV Mortality	Comments
Bigger[600]	(1984)	766	X	—	—	—	—	X	24		Yes	Yes	LVEF and VPCs are independent predictors of mortality. Predicts arrhythmic death mortality.
Gibson[617]	(1983)	140	—	—	—	X	X	—	15	Yes			Exercise thallium scintigraphy superior to EXT/angiography in predicting ischemic events
Kuchar[640]	(1987)	210	X	X	—	—	—	X	14		Yes		VPCS, SAECG, and LVEF are all independent predictors of arrhythmic events
Farrell[623]	(1991)	416	X	X	X	—	—	X	(1-37)		Yes		HRV and SAECG, when both are positive, have a risk ratio of 18.5 for arrhythmic events vs both negative
Gomes[700]	(1989)	102	X	X	—	—	—	X	12		Yes		NSVT, SAECG, and LVEF are all independent predictors of arrhythmic events
Kleiger[624]	(1987)	808	X	—	X	—	—	X	31		Yes		HRV <50 msec increases mortality risk 5.3-fold
Gomes[620]	(1989)	115	X	X	—	—	—	X	15		Yes		SAECG superior to NSVT and LVEF in predicting arrhythmic events
Starling[631]	(1986)	72	—	—	—	X	—	X	12	Yes		Yes	Mortality predicted by LVEF <40 and EXT ST depression (ischemia)
Kleiger[625]	(1990)	808	X	—	X	X	—	X	31			Yes	HRV is an independent risk, as is inability to perform low level EXT
Cripps[149]	(1988)	176	X	—	—	X	—	—	15	Yes	Yes		Ischemic events predicted by EXT, arrhythmic events by SAECG, anterior MI, complicated course Non-Q, and Killip class

* Non-invasive tests: 1. Holter; 2. signal-averaged ECG; 3. heart rate variability; 4. low level exercise test; 5. exercise/thallium; 6. left ventricular ejection fraction (various methods)
NOTE: Abbreviations: CV = cardiovascular; LVEF-left ventricular ejection fraction; VPC = ventricular premature complexes; EXT = exercise test; SAECG = signal-averaged ECG; HRV = heart rate variability; NSVT = nonsustained ventricular tachycardia; MI = myocardial infarction.

patients for EPS. Measurement of heart rate variability may provide additional discriminative information.

Other studies in Table 60-21 examine the combination of ischemia detection and the measurement of LVEF.[625,701] These two factors are essential to assess accurately cardiovascular risk; they are the pivotal tests used in creating the algorithm in Fig. 60-17. Patients recommended for coronary angiographic studies are those in whom noninvasive tests indicate an annual cardiac event rate of 10 percent or greater.

Secondary Prevention: Pharmacologic Therapy after Myocardial Infarction

Beta Blockers

The role of prophylactic beta blockade in patients surviving AMI is being clarified. Although a number of small randomized clinical trials suggest a modest benefit,[702–712] recommendations are based on large, randomized, multicenter clinical trials presented in Table 60-22.[438,439,713–720] The weight of the evidence suggests that beta-blocker therapy after AMI substantially reduces mortality rates. In the Norwegian timolol trial,[439] mortality was reduced by 36 percent over 17 months, with patients in high-risk subsets (complicated infarction and previous myocardial infarction) having the greatest benefit. In addition to total mortality, arrhythmic death was reduced. The Beta Blocker Heart Attack Trial (BHAT)[714] was similar in study design but used propranolol. The mortality rate in BHAT was reduced 30 percent. Nonfatal reinfarctions were also reduced in both trials (Norwegian, 26 percent; BHAT, 16 percent). Patients benefiting most from propranolol had previous infarctions or were patients with in-hospital electrical or mechanical complications, and a history of heart failure.[439,714]

The benefit of beta blockers applies only to patients similar to those in these trials. Many patients were excluded from these trials and thus are not necessarily candidates for prophylactic beta-blocker therapy. Contraindications to beta-blocker therapy include (1) symptomatic cardiac failure, (2) evidence of significant reactive airway disease, (3) insulin-dependent diabetes, and (4) significant bradycardia, heart block, or hypotension.

The Norwegian timolol and BHAT studies taken together represent a wide spectrum of risk. Both trials document a reduction in total mortality, arrhythmic death, and reinfarction. In both trials, the benefit to patients with non-Q-wave infarction seemed to be proportionally less than those with Q-wave infarction, although this may be related to a lower mortality rate and to problems of subset analysis. Meta-analysis of the beta-blocker experience shows a 34 percent reduction in sudden death ($p < .001$).[449,450] A review of many beta-blocker trials has led to other important observations that have implications for the mechanism of mortality reduction. There is a definite relationship between heart rate reduction and mortality reduction ($r = 0.60$; $p < .05$) and reduction in nonfatal myocardial infarction ($r = 0.59$; $p < .05$).[721] It is estimated that, in appropriately selected patients without contraindication who receive beta blockers, one can expect an overall 25 percent reduction in long-term mortality rates.

A practical clinical question is whether beta blockers should be administered acutely or later during the hospitalization. The potential benefits of early use of intravenous beta blockers have been investigated in the ISIS-1 (atenolol), Goteborg (metoprolol), and TIMI-2B (metoprolol) trials.[342,715,716,720] There appears to be a modest incremental benefit from acute administration of beta blockers; and in those patients deemed at high risk and appropriate for beta blockade, it is recommended that they be initiated within the first 24 h. Timolol, metoprolol, propranolol, and atenolol have been demonstrated to reduce mortality rates. Beneficial effects of beta blockade appear to be a class effect of the drugs. Beta blockers with intrinsic sympathomimetic activity should be avoided (see also Chap. 66).

Which patients should be selected for empiric prophylactic long-term beta-blocker therapy? In most of the large randomized clinical trials, patients at higher risk appeared to benefit the most from beta-blocker therapy. A long-term cost-effectiveness analysis estimated that the cost of beta-blocker therapy per year of a life saved

TABLE 60-22
Results of Beta Blocker (>1000 Patients) Treatment after Myocardial Infarction

	Placebo			Beta Blocker			
Trial (Ref)	N	Deaths	Mortality (%)	N	Deaths	Mortality (%)	p value
Multicenter International Study[713]	1520	78	5	1533	48	3	<.01
Norwegian Multicenter Study[439]	939	152	18	945	98	11	.0003
BHAT[714]	1921	188	10	1916	133	7	.005
Goteborg Metoprolol Trial*[716]	697	62	9	698	40	6	.03
Sotalol Trial[717]	582	52	9	874	64	7	.3
Metoprolol Intervention Trial[718]	1200	62	5	1195	65	5	NS
European Infarction Study[719]	883	45	5	858	57	7	.14
ISIS-1[720]	7990	367	5	8037	317	4	<.05
		951	12		866	11	.01
MIAMI[438]	2901	142	5	2877	123	4	.29

* Three month data.

would be $13,000 in low-risk, $3600 in moderate-risk, and $2400 in high-risk patients.[722] Beta blockers are definitely recommended in Q-wave infarction (if tolerated) if one of the following is present: LVEF of 40 percent or less, in-hospital electrical complications (ventricular tachycardia or cardiac arrest), a history of heart failure now compensated, asymptomatic nonsustained ventricular tachycardia, frequent ventricular premature beats, objective evidence of ischemia, or recurrent myocardial infarction. In patients with uncomplicated Q-wave infarction, the long-term benefit of beta blockers is less certain. Decisions to begin beta-blocker therapy can be individualized based on the results of noninvasive testing.

There are no prospective data on the use of beta blockers in patients surviving non-Q-wave infarction. Retrospective analyses have shown no benefit from beta blockers in non-Q-wave infarction.[437,714,723,724]

Unfortunately, many patients at high risk (e.g., patients with severe left ventricular dysfunction, patients with clinical congestive heart failure, insulin-dependent diabetics, and patients with known reactive airway disease) have contraindications to beta blockade. When indicated, beta blockers should be initiated before discharge and continued indefinitely. Because of the nature of clinical trials, it is very difficult to make firm recommendations beyond 2 years, although data from the Norwegian timolol trial show sustained benefit up to 6 years.[725]

Calcium Blockers

In contrast to the unequivocal benefit of prophylactic beta blockade on mortality rates, the data on calcium channel blockers in postinfarction patients is less compelling. The design of a number of trials using nifedipine often focused on acute administration (oral or sublingual),[252,726-729] but long-term clinical trials with nifedipine have also been completed[730-732] and have also not demonstrated a reduction in infarct size, frequency of recurrent myocardial infarction, or mortality rate reduction. The consistent lack of benefit in these trials indicates that dihydropyridine calcium blockers have no role in secondary prevention of recurrent infarction or death after myocardial infarction.

Two trials using verapamil have shown a trend toward a reduction in recurrent infarction (DAVIT I) and a marginal effect on mortality (DAVIT II).[733,734] Given such equivocal benefits, the prophylactic use of verapamil is not recommended.

There have also been two studies assessing the effect of diltiazem in patients after myocardial infarction. The Diltiazem Reinfarction Study (DRS), a prospective double-blind study limited to patients (n = 576) surviving non-Q-wave myocardial infarction demonstrated a statistically significant (50 percent) reduction in recurrent myocardial infarction over the 14-day interval of the study.[152] Analysis also showed a marked reduction ($p <$ .02) in the incidence of refractory angina and postinfarction angina independent of recurrent infarction. In the 1-year follow-up of these patients[505] it was found that the risk of death increased fourfold in patients experiencing recurrent infarction within the 2 weeks, in those with recurrent angina associated with ECG changes, and in those with persistent ST-T segment depression. Thus, patients with these manifestations are considered at high risk and should be considered for cardiac catheterization.

The MDPIT trial with diltiazem was a long-term study and included patients with both Q-wave (n = 1757) and non-Q-wave (n = 634) infarction who were followed for an average of 30 months. Overall, there was no significant reduction in mortality rate,[434] but analysis of several prospectively planned subgroup analysis showed that about 20 percent of the patients enrolled had cardiac failure and pulmonary congestion, and in this group diltiazem increased the mortality rate over that of the placebo. In the remaining 80 percent of patients, diltiazem was associated with a 27 percent reduction in nonfatal reinfarction and death. In the subgroup of patients with non-Q-wave infarction (n = 634) at the end of the first year, diltiazem was associated with a 43 percent reduction in reinfarction and death and a 34 percent reduction at the end of $4\frac{1}{2}$ years. The basis for the lack of effect of beta blockers after non-Q-wave infarction and the beneficial effect of diltiazem is a matter of speculation. The joint task force of the American Heart Association and American College of Cardiology recommended that patients with non-Q-wave infarction be given diltiazem in the first 24 h routinely and that therapy be continued for at least 1 year.[696] It is important to emphasize, however, that the data on which this recommendation is based are clearly weaker than the unequivocal benefit seen for beta blockade in selected groups of patients with Q-wave infarction. Two independent meta-analyses, which combined the results of the clinical trials of all calcium blockers, concluded that no overall benefit was demonstrated in patients postinfarction.[449,735]

Nitroglycerin

The clinical trials utilizing nitroglycerin and nitroprusside have been limited primarily to intravenous administration in the initial hours following the AMI. There are no large multicenter clinical trials evaluating the long-term effect of long-acting nitrates. Orally administered nitrates are routinely recommended for ischemia, left ventricular dysfunction, and cardiac failure (see Chaps. 26 and 30).

Angiotensin-Converting Enzyme Inhibitors

A number of clinical trials have evaluated the benefits of angiotensin-converting enzyme (ACE) inhibitors in patients with left ventricular dysfunction.[507,508,736-739] Two of these trials, the cooperative North Scandinavian Enalapril Survival Study (CONSENSUS II)[736] and the Survival and Ventricular Enlargement trial (SAVE),[507] limited enrollment to patients with myocardial infarction. SAVE enrolled 2231 patients with an LVEF of 40 percent or less an average of 11 days postinfarction who were randomized to captopril (50 mg three times a day) or placebo. The group receiving captopril had a significant reduction in mortality rate over 42 months as well as a significant decrease in recurrent myocardial infarction and hospitalization for heart failure. In contrast, CONSENSUS II, enrolled patients in the first 24 h (mean, 15

h) of infarction but had no LVEF limitation.[736] Treatment with enalapril (5 to 20 mg twice a day) for 6 months failed to result in a mortality rate benefit compared to placebo.

In Studies of Left Ventricular Dysfunction (SOLVD), enrollment was not limited exclusively to postinfarction patients, although the prevention limb of SOLVD, which compared enalapril (10 mg twice a day) to placebo, included primarily patients at least 4 weeks postinfarction, all of whom had a LVEF of 35 percent or less but no symptoms thought to be from heart failure.[508] There was a 12 percent reduction in mortality rate, which was not significant, but there was a significant reduction in the initial development of congestive heart failure. In an otherwise identical fashion, the SOLVD treatment limb enrolled symptomatic patients with a LVEF of 35 percent or less. A significant reduction in mortality rate was documented. In addition, the combined SOLVD studies show a significant reduction in recurrent myocardial infarction.[508] Other trials assessing ACE inhibitors or other vasodilators in congestive heart failure[736-738] have also shown a reduction in mortality rate with vasodilators. Patients surviving AMI with a LVEF of 40 percent or less with no contraindication to an ACE inhibitor should be given prophylactic enalapril or captopril, titrated to achieve doses of up to 20 mg twice a day or 50 mg three times a day, respectively. Therapy should be initiated during the hospitalization, once the patient is clinically stable, and continued indefinitely.

Antiarrhythmic Drugs

Many studies have attempted empiric, prophylactic use of antiarrhythmic drugs in patients surviving AMI. A meta-analysis of postinfarction clinical trials of antiarrhythmic therapy failed to reveal any mortality benefit with electrophysiologic class IA, IB, or IC antiarrhythmic drugs.[740] The majority of the clinical trials[741-750] had a number of major design disadvantages. Although many were placebo-controlled and double-blind, sample size was often very small, and the studies were underpowered for mortality end points. The vast majority of these trials did not limit randomization to patients at increased risk for sudden death but, rather, focused on all myocardial infarction survivors.

The Cardiac Arrhythmia Pilot Study (CAPS) was conducted from 1983 through 1985.[640] Based on information from this pilot study, the Cardiac Arrhythmia Suppression Trial (CAST) was implemented in 1987.[481] In this trial, patients with asymptomatic spontaneous ventricular arrhythmia, as detected by AECG monitoring, and who had survived AMI were randomized to one of four treatment strategies. The treatment strategies were selected (encainide, flecainide, moricizine, or placebo) based on efficacy of treating arrhythmias during an open-label experience. CAST had a number of unique features: (1) it was a large clinical trial designed for a mortality end point, (2) only patients at increased risk of arrhythmic death (ventricular arrhythmia on AECG recording) were randomized, (3) reduction of spontaneous ventricular ectopy was the end point of antiarrhythmic therapy, and (4) a parallel, placebo control group was included.

The results from CAST dramatically changed the perception of the risk-benefit ratio of empiric antiarrhythmic therapy. Both the encainide and flecainide limbs of CAST were prematurely discontinued (mean, 10 months of therapy) due to a 2.5-fold increase in mortality rate compared to placebo. In addition, a unique observation was that the excessive mortality persisted throughout the duration of the study (Fig. 60-18). The excess mortality was in deaths classified as arrhythmic deaths. Thus, a clinical trial had established that at least two antiarrhythmic drugs were responsible for late lethal proarrhythmia. These two antiarrhythmic drugs, both electrophysiologic IC antiarrhythmics, may have this lethal proarrhythmic effect due to (1) an interaction with transient ischemia, (2) effects on left ventricular function, (3) interaction with the autonomic nervous system, or (4) the electrophysiologic characteristics of use-dependence.[482] In the CAST II (moricizine-placebo comparison), the patient population was at higher risk (all had LVEF $\leq$ 40 percent), and recruitment was limited to the first 60 days postinfarction. The moricizine-placebo comparison in CAST II was also discontinued prematurely.[482] There was a small early increase in mortality rate in the moricizine group; however, there was no additional significant long-term mortality difference between placebo and moricizine. Thus, despite the fact that all three antiarrhythmic drugs had been shown to suppress VPCs better than the placebo did in the pilot study, all three were associated with a higher mortality than was the placebo. Although sudden or arrhythmic death is responsible for at least 40, and perhaps 50, percent of the long-term mortality rate in patients surviving AMI, there is *no proven benefit* of prophylactic antiarrhythmic drugs in this clinical setting, and *none are recommended*. Only the long-term use of beta blockers has been established to reduce the incidence of sudden death (estimated reduction, one-third).[449] At present, no treatment strategy has been shown further to reduce sudden death.[751] Promising preliminary results have been obtained with prophylactic oral amiodarone.[743,744] Long-term, large clinical trials are under way to clarify the risk-benefit ratio of this strategy. On the other hand, antiarrhythmic therapy is still appropriate in patients who have had an episode of spontane-

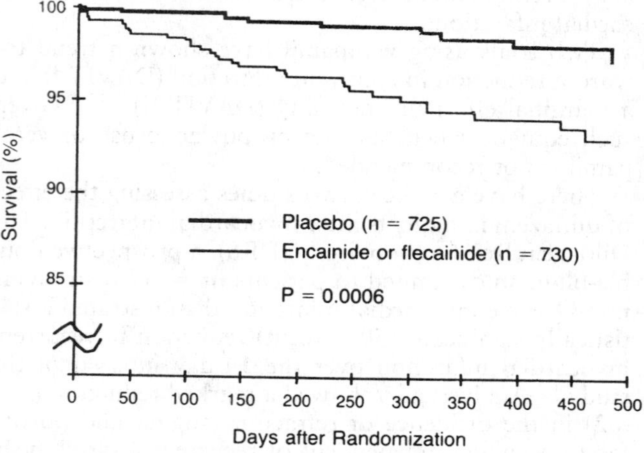

FIGURE 60-18 Survival comparison of enoainide/flecainide treatment patients to placebo (primary endpoint of CAST was arrhythmic or cardiac death).

ous sustained ventricular tachycardia and/or ventricular fibrillation or cardiac arrest after AMI. In such patients, the decision regarding antiarrhythmic therapy, mapping, and surgery or defibrillator implantation is best made on the results of electrophysiologic testing (see Fig. 60-16 and Chap. 46).

Aspirin

Aspirin plays a pivotal role as secondary prevention therapy in patients surviving AMI. Even early studies tended to show some improvement in long-term mortality. The doses of aspirin have varied greatly in different trials. The wide dose range (more than tenfold) may explain some of the inconsistencies.[415,752–756] It is also clear that trials have been of vastly different sample size and that many are underpowered.[435,757–759] The most definitive information can be obtained from the ISIS-2 trial. In this trial of more than 17,000 patients, aspirin or a placebo was given to patients immediately upon the diagnosis of AMI and continued for 5 weeks. The impressive 25 percent reduction in mortality rate on 160 mg aspirin compared to placebo is striking. The additive benefit of aspirin and SK was also demonstrated, reducing mortality by 42 percent compared to the placebo group. Thus, ISIS-2 provides a sound basis for strongly recommending aspirin in patients with AMI.[415] It is strongly recommended that all patients without an absolute contraindication be given aspirin (160 mg/day), starting immediately upon admission to the hospital. The ISIS-2 study documented a mortality rate benefit for a period of 5 weeks. It seems reasonable to continue aspirin indefinitely, at a dose of 80 to 160 mg daily.[449] See Chap. 68 for additional discussion of the use and dosage of aspirin.

Lipid-Lowering Agents after Myocardial Infarction

Secondary Prevention Trials Two secondary prevention trials of lipid lowering are notable (see also Chap. 62). The most aggressive postinfarction study was the Program on the Surgical Control of Hyperlipidemias (POSCH), which was a randomized trial to study the effects of partial ileal bypass operation on mortality and morbidity rates.[760] In this trial, 838 patients were randomized to either a control or a surgical group, with a mean follow-up of nearly 10 years. The long-term results of this trial included a 23 percent reduction in total plasma cholesterol levels and a reduction of low-density lipoprotein (LDL) cholesterol levels of nearly 38 percent. Although the mortality rate tended to be lower in the surgical group, the reduction did not reach statistical significance. When the combined end point was death due to coronary heart disease and nonfatal recurrent myocardial infarction was analyzed, a 35 percent reduction in mortality rate in the surgical group was noted. However, angiographic progression of coronary atherosclerosis was not different between the study groups. Although certainly not justifying an aggressive surgical approach, this study suggests that an aggressive reduction in blood lipid levels may result in a reduction in subsequent cardiovascular events.[760]

The Coronary Drug Project assessed the long-term efficacy of five plasma lipid-influencing therapies on 8341 men with a previous myocardial infarction. The most favorable treatment was niacin, which, when compared to a placebo, showed a modest reduction in the frequency of recurrent nonfatal myocardial infarction.[756,761–765] A 15-year follow-up of these patients indicates that mortality for all causes in the niacin group was 11 percent lower than in the placebo group. The mortality difference (52 versus 58.2 percent) was highly significant (p = .0004).[766] In a review of secondary prevention trials of cholesterol lowering, a meta-analysis of 7837 patients in eight trials revealed a significant reduction of both nonfatal ($p < .001$; odds ratio = 0.75) and fatal ($p < .01$; odds ratio = 0.84) infarctions. In those trials cardiovascular deaths were reduced (odds ratio = 0.77 to 0.99), although the total mortality rate did not reach statistical significance (odds ratio = 0.82 to 1.02).[767]

Primary Prevention Trials The more extensive experience from primary prevention trials is useful and consistent with the more modest experience in secondary prevention trials (see also Chap. 62). The Lipid Research Clinics Coronary Primary Prevention Trial (LRC-CPPT) was a multicenter, randomized double-blind study assessing the efficacy of lowering plasma lipids with cholestyramine versus a placebo group treated with diet alone.[768] A significant reduction in the combined end point of coronary heart disease death and/or definite nonfatal myocardial infarction was demonstrated over a treatment period of 7.4 years. There was an internal consistency of the data in that patients demonstrating the greatest cholesterol and LDL reductions had the greatest benefit.[768]

Gemfibrozil, a fibric acid derivative, was also shown to reduce cardiac end points in the Helsinki Heart Study, a primary prevention trial of middle-aged asymptomatic men with LDL cholesterol of 200 mg/dL or more.[769,770] Other trials of patients at high risk of developing symptomatic coronary atherosclerosis have shown that a number of drugs (colestipol, lovastatin, and niacin) that reduce LDL cholesterol may result in either lack of progression or regression of atherosclerotic lesions of the coronary arteries.[771–774]

The CLAS-1 trial of cholesterol lowering with the combination of colestipol and niacin included 162 men with previous coronary bypass surgery. A reduction of apolipoprotein B levels and an increase of high-density lipoprotein (HDL) levels were associated with favorable changes in both the native coronary arteries and the bypass grafts.[771]

The most significant additions to the pharmacologic armamentarium for lowering lipid levels are the 3-hydroxy-3-methylglutaryl-coenzyme A (HMG CoA) reductase inhibitors. The HMG CoA reductase inhibitors are powerful in reducing LDL cholesterol and offering compliance benefits.[775] The Familial Atherosclerosis Treatment Study (FATS) involved 146 men with angiographically proven coronary artery disease, high apolipoprotein B levels ($\geq$125 mg/mL), and a positive family history. FATS compared a combination of diet and placebo to the following lipid-lowering strategies: (1) lovastatin 20 mg twice a day and colestipol 10 g three times a day, (2) niacin 1 g four times a day and colestipol 10 g three times a day, and (3) placebo (and colestipol if LDL cholesterol was elevated). Compared to the diet-placebo combination over the $2\frac{1}{2}$-year study interval, the two active treatment strategies resulted in (1) LDL reduction and HDL increase; (2) more frequent regression of coronary atherosclerosis, as shown by angiographic study; and (3) reduction in cardiovascular events.[776]

Similarly, the St. Thomas Atherosclerosis Regression Study (STARS) showed in patients with coronary artery disease and high cholesterol levels that a low-fat diet with or without bile acid-sequestering resin was associated not only with regression or lack of progression of coronary lesions but with a significant reduction in clinical events and in angina frequency.[777] Thus, there is a rapidly accumulating body of data suggesting that the clinical course of coronary artery disease can be affected favorably by lipid-lowering therapy.

Lipid profiles should be obtained 2 to 3 months following the myocardial infarction (see also Chap. 53). All patients surviving AMI should have their fasting plasma lipids measured, including measurements of total cholesterol, HDL cholesterol, and triglycerides and estimation of LDL cholesterol. Every effort should be made to encourage maintenance of ideal body weight. Patients should be given instructions in following a low-fat, low-cholesterol diet. In general, not more than 20 percent of the caloric intake should be in the form of dietary fats. If, despite alterations of diet and weight, patients have a LDL cholesterol level above 140 mg/dL or a total cholesterol level of 210 mg/dL or more, they should be considered for pharmacologic lipid reduction (see Chap. 65). The goal of therapy should be to reduce the LDL level to less than 100 mg/dL.

Modification of Life-style and Cardiac Rehabilitation

After recovery from AMI, all cardiovascular risk factors should be evaluated. There are no adequate secondary prevention trials of all the risk factors to support specific recommendations. The recommendations regarding lipids are given above. There is strong evidence from both primary and secondary prevention trials that cessation of tobacco smoking will reduce the occurrence cardiac events.[772] Data from multiple controlled clinical trials of hypertension support the control of blood pressure to the normal range.[778]

A meta-analysis of randomized trials of exercise after myocardial infarction suggests that regular exercise may have a favorable effect on survival rates.[779] Another overview of 22 randomized trials of exercise after myocardial infarction included 4554 patients and showed a trend toward the reduction of cardiovascular death, sudden death as well as reinfarction.[780] Since many of these trials included many aspects of risk factor intervention other than exercise alone, the independent contribution of the exercise component to an improved outcome is not clear.[780] On the other hand, regular low-level exercise appears to be a positive aspect in developing an overall secondary prevention program for patients postinfarction. Other studies support the efficacy and safety of exercise rehabilitation programs.[781,782] A comprehensive review of recommendations for cardiac rehabilitation services has been published by the American College of Physicians.[783] While low-risk patients can benefit from home exercise, this review suggests that certain higher-risk postinfarction patients have medically supervised cardiac rehabilitation.[783]

Medically supervised cardiac rehabilitation after myocardial infarction should be limited specifically to high-risk patients who require telemetric monitoring or close medical observation. Cardiac rehabilitation classes should also be considered for individual patients who require additional incentive to modify risk factors. Although there is no definitive evidence that exercise prolongs survival, it has many benefits: (1) it facilitates the return to a desirable level of activity, (2) it reduces the patients' anxiety level, (3) it provides the physician with the opportunity to make detailed observations of the adequacy of pharmacologic therapy, and (4) it may increase levels of HDL and reduce blood pressure. An individualized exercise program should be planned and recommend to every ambulatory patient after myocardial infarction, and high-risk patients should be considered for medically supervised exercise with telemetric monitoring (see Chap. 63).

REFERENCES

1. Ross R: The pathogenesis of atherosclerosis: An update. *N Engl J Med* 1986; 314:488–500.
2. Davies MJ, Woolf N, Rowles P, Pepper J: Morphology of the endothelium over atherosclerotic plaques in human coronary arteries. *Br Heart J* 1988; 60:459–464.
3. Furchgott RF, Zawadzki JV: The obligatory role of endothelial cells in the relaxation of arterial smooth muscle by acetylcholine. *Nature* 1980; 288:373–376.
4. Furchgott RF: Role of endothelium in response of vascular smooth muscle. *Circ Res* 1983; 53:557–573.
5. Margolis B, Lucas C, Henry PD: Effects of Ca-antagonists on platelet aggregation and secretion. *Circulation* 1980; 62:191.
6. Freiman PC, Mitchell GG, Heistad DD, Armstrong ML, Harrison DG: Atherosclerosis impairs endothelium-dependent vascular relaxation to acetylcholine and thrombin in primates. *Circ Res* 1986; 58:783–789.
7. Benacerral A, Scholl JM, Achard P, Tenneiler M, Lavergne G: Coronary spasm and thrombosis associated with myocardial infarction in a patient with nearly normal coronary arteries. *Circulation* 1983; 67:1147–1150.
8. Verheugt FWA, Wouter ten Cat J, Sturk A, Imandt L, Verhorst PMJ, van Eenige MJV, et al: Tissue plasminogen activator activity and inhibition in acute myocardial infarction and angiographically normal coronary arteries. *Am J Cardiol* 1987; 59:1075–1079.
9. Coller BS: Platelets and thrombolytic therapy. *N Engl J Med* 1990; 322:33–42.
10. Fuster V, Badimon L, Cohen M, Ambrose JA, Badimon JJ, Chesebro J: Insights into the pathogenesis of acute ischemic syndromes. *Circulation* 1988; 77:1213–1220.
11. Golino P, Ashton JH, Glas-Greenwalt P, McNatt J, Buja LM, Willerson JR: Mediation of reocclusion by thromboxane A2 and serotonin after thrombolysis with tissue-type plasminogen activator in a canine preparation of coronary thrombosis. *Circulation* 1988; 77:678–684.
12. Simon DI, Fless GM, Scanu AM, Loscalzo J: Tissue-type plasminogen activator binds to and is inhibited by surface-bound lipoprotein(a) and low-density lipoprotein. *Biochemistry* 1991; 30:6671–6677.
13. Loscalzo J: Lipoprotein(a): A unique risk factor for atherothrombotic disease. *Arteriosclerosis* 1990; 10:672–679.
14. Neely JR, Grotyohann LW: Role of glycotic products in damage to ischemic myocardium: Dissociation of adenosine triphosphate

levels and recovery of function of reperfused ischemic hearts. *Circ Res* 1984; 55:816–824.

14a. Heyndrickx GR, Millard RW, McRitchie RJ, Maroko PR, Vatner SF: Regional myocardial function and electrophysiological alterations after brief coronary artery occlusion in conscious dogs. *J Clin Invest* 1975; 56:978–985.

14b. Katz AM: *Physiology of the Heart*, 2d ed. New York, Raven, 1992:1–434.

15. Reimer KA, Jennings RB: Myocardial ischemia, hypoxia and infarction. In: Fozzard HA, Haber E, Jennings RB, Katz AM, Morgan HE, (eds): *The Heart and Cardiovascular System: Scientific Foundations*. New York, Raven, 1992: 1133–1202.

16. Allen EG, Orchard CH: Myocardial cell function during ischemia and hypoxia. *Circ Res* 1987; 60:153–168.

17. Lee JA, Allen DG: Mechanisms of acute ischemic contractile failure of the heart: Role of intracellular calcium. *J Clin Invest* 1991; 88:361–367.

18. Allen DG, Lee JA, Smith GL: The consequences of simulated ischemia on intracellular Ca^{2+} and tension in isolated ferret ventricular muscle. *J Physiol (London)* 1989; 410:297–323.

19. Lee JA, Allen DG: The effects of repeated exposure to anoxia on intracellular Ca, glycogen and lactate in isolated ferret heart muscle. *Pfluegers Arch Eur J Physiol* 1988; 413:83–89.

20. Marban E, Kitakaze M, Koretsune Y, Yue DT, Chacko VP, Pike MM: Quantification of $[CA^{2+}]$ in perfused hearts: Critical evaluation of the 5F-BAPTA and nuclear magnetic resonance method as applied to the study of ischemia and reperfusion. *Circ Res* 1990; 66:1255–1267.

21. Koretsune Y, Marban E: Mechanisms of ischemic contracture in ferret hearts: Relative roles of $[CA^{2+}]_i$ elevation and ATP depletion. *Am J Physiol* 1990; 258:H9–H16.

22. Jacobus WE, Pores IH, Lucas SK, Kallman CH, Weisfeldt, Flaherty JT: The role of intracellular pH in the control of normal and ischemic myocardial contractility: A "P nuclear magnetic resonance and mass spectroscopy study. In: Nuccitelli R, Deamer DW (eds): *Intracellular pH: Its measurement, Regulation and Utilization in Cellular Function*. New York, Alan R. Liss, 1982:

23. Kentish JC: The effects of inorganic phosphate and creatine phosphate on force production in skinned muscles from rat ventricle. *J Physiol (London)* 1986; 370:585–604.

24. Godt RE, Nosek TM: Changes of intracellular milieu with fatigue or hypoxia depress contraction of skinned rabbit skeletal and cardiac muscle. *J Physiol (London)* 1989; 412:155–180.

25. Elliot AC (ed): *Phosphorus nuclear magnetic resonance studies of metabolite levels and intracellular pH in muscles*, University of London, 1987.

26. Kusuoka H, Weisfeldt ML, Szeier J, Jacobus WE, Marban E: Mechanism of early contractile failure during hypoxia in intact ferret heart: Evidence for modulation of maximal Ca^{2+}-activated force by inorganic phosphate. *Circ Res* 1986; 59:270–282.

27. Tybert JV, Smith ER: An evaluation of the pericardial hypothesis: The relevance of transmural right ventricular end-diastolic pressure. *Cor Artery Dis* 1991; 2:717–722.

28. Tyberg JV, Misbach GA, Glantz SA, Moores WY, Parmley WW: A mechanism for shifts in the diastolic left ventricular pressure-volume curve: The role of the pericardium. *Eur J Cardiol* 1987; 7:163–175.

29. Janse MJ, Wit AL: Electrophysiology mechanisms of ventricular arrhythmias resulting from myocardial ischemia and infarction. *Physiol Rev* 1989; 69:1049–1169.

30. Hill JL, Gettes LS: Effect of acute coronary artery occlusion on local myocardial extracellular K^+ activity in swine. *Circulation* 1980; 61:768–778.

31. Kantor PF, Coetzee WA, Carmeliet EE, Dennise SC, Opie LH: Reduction of ischemic K^+ loss and arrhythmias in rat hearts: Effect of glibenclamide, a sulphonylurea. *Circ Res* 1990; 66:478–485.

32. Wilde AAM, Escande M, Schumacher CA, Thuringer D, Mestre M, Fiolet JWT, et al: Potassium accumulation in the globally ischemic mammalian heart: A role for the ATP-sensitive potassium channel. *Circ Res* 1990; 67:835–843.

33. Kleber AG: Resting membrane potential, extracellular potassium activity and intracellular sodium activity during acute global ischemia in isolated perfused guinea-pig hearts. *Circ Res* 1983; 52:442–450.

34. Katzung BG, Hondeghem LM, Grant AO: Cardiac ventricular automaticity induced by current of injury. *Pfluegers Arch Eur J Physiol* 1975; 260:193–197.

35. Kaumann AJ, Aramendia P: Prevention of ventricular fibrillation induced by coronary ligation. *J Pharmacol Exp Ther* 1968; 164:326–332.

36. Thandroyen FT, McCarthy J, Burton KP, Opie LH: Ryanodine and caffeine prevent ventricular arrhythmias during acute myocardial ischemia and reperfusion in rat heart. *Circ Res* 1988; 62:306–314.

37. Sobel BE, Corr PB, Robinson AK, Goldstein RA, Witkowski RX, Klein MS: Accumulation of lysophosphyglycerides with arrhythmogenic properties in ischemic myocardium. *J Clin Invest* 1978; 62:546–553.

38. Corr PB, Cain MB, Witkowski FX, Price DA, Sobel BE: Potential arrhythmogenic electrophysiological derangements in canine Purkinje fibers induced by lysophosphyglycerides. *Circ Res* 1979; 44:822–832.

39. Elharrar V, Zipes DP: Cardiac electrophysiological alterations during myocardial ischemia. In: Levy MN, Vassalle M, (ed): *Excitation and Neural Control of the Heart*. Baltimore, Williams & Wilkins, 1982: 149–180.

40. Reimer KA, Lowe JE, Rasmussen MM, Jennings RB: The wavefront phenomenon of ischemic cell death. I. Myocardial infarct size vs duration of coronary occlusion in dogs. *Circulation* 1977; 56:786–794.

41. Sobel BE, Bresnahan GF, Shell WE, Yoder RD: Estimation of infarct size in man and its relation to prognosis. *Circulation* 1972; 46:640–648.

42. Roberts R, Henry PD, Sobel BE: An improved basis for enzymatic estimation of infarct size. *Circulation* 1975; 52:743–754.

43. Page DL, Caulfield JB, Kastor JA, DeSanctis RW, Sanders CA: Myocardial changes associated with cardiogenic shock. *N Engl J Med* 1971; 285:133–137.

44. Alonso DR, Scheidt S, Post M, Killip T: Pathophysiology of cardiogenic shock: Quantification of myocardial necrosis, clinical, pathologic and electrocardiographic correlations. *Circulation* 1973; 48:588–596.

45. Harnarayan C, Bennett MA, Pentecost BL, Brewer DB: Quantitative study of infarcted myocardium in cardiogenic shock. *Br Heart J* 1970; 32:728–732.

46. Braunwald E, Kloner RA: The stunned myocardium: Prolonged, post-ischemic ventricular dysfunction. *Circulation* 1982; 66:1146–1149.

47. Heyndrickx GR, Millard RW, McRitchie RJ, Maroko PR, Vatner SF: Regional myocardial functional and electrophysiological alterations after a brief coronary artery occlusion in conscious dogs. *J Clin Invest* 1975; 56:978–985.

48. Heyndrickx GR, Baig H, Nellers P, Leusen I, Fishbein MC, Vatner SF: Depression of regional myocardial blood flow and wall thickening after brief coronary occlusions. *Am J Physiol* 1978; 234:H653–H659.

49. Bolli R, Zhu WX, Myers HL, Hartley CJ, Roberts R: Beta-adrenergic stimulation reverses postischemic myocardial dysfunction without producing subsequent functional deterioration. *Am J Cardiol* 1985; 56:964–968.

50. Bolli R, Zhu WX, Thornby JI, O'Neill PG, Roberts R: Time course and determinants of recovery of function after reversible ischemia in conscious dogs. *Am J Physiol* 1988; 254:H102–H114.

51. Jennings RB, Murry CE, Steenbergen C Jr, Reimer KA: Development of cell injury in sustained acute ischemia. *Circulation* 1990; 82:II2–II12.

52. Jennings RB, Schaper J, Hill ML, Steenbergen C Jr, Reimer KA: Effect of reperfusion late in the phase of reversible ischemic injury: Changes in cell volume, electrolytes, metabolites, and ultrastructure. *Circ Res* 1985; 56:262–278.

53. Lange R, Ingwall JS, Hale SL, Alker KJ, Kloner RA: Effects of recurrent ischemia on myocardial high energy phosphate content in canine hearts. *Basic Res Cardiol* 1984; 79:469–478.

54. Reimer KA, Hill ML, Jennings RB: Prolonged depletion of ATP and of the adenine nucleotide pool due to delayed resynthesis of adenine nucleotides following reversible myocardial ischemic injury in dogs. *J Mol Cell Cardiol* 1981; 13:229–239.

55. Carmeliet E: Myocardial ischemia: Reversible and irreversible changes. *Circulation* 1984; 70:149–151.

56. Arnold JMO, Braunwald E, Sandor T, Kloner RA: Inotropic stimulation of reperfused myocardium with dopamine: Effects

on infarct size and myocardial function. *J Am Coll Cardiol* 1985; 6:1026–1043.

57. Ellis SG, Wysone J, Braunwald E, Henschke CJ, Sandor T, Kloner RA: Response of the reperfusion-salvaged, stunned myocardium to inotropic stimulation. *Am Heart J* 1984; 107:13–19.
58. Krause SM, Jacobus WE, Becker LC: Alterations in sarcoplasmic reticulum CA^{2+} transport in the postischemic "stunned" myocardium. *Circulation* 1986; 74:II-67.
59. Przyklenk K, Kloner RA: Superoxide dismutase plus catalase improves contractile function in the canine model of the "stunned myocardium." *Circ Res* 1986; 58:148–156.
60. Przyklenk K, Kloner RA: Effect of verapamil on postischemic "stunned" myocardium: Importance of the timing of treatment. *J Am Coll Cardiol* 1988; 11:614–623.
61. Knowlton AA, Brecher P, Ngou S, Apstein CS: Brief cardiac ischemia induces expression of heat shock protein. *Circulation* 1989; 80:II237.
62. Fleischmann KE, Brand T, Sharma HS, Duncker DJ, Sassen LMA, McFalls EO, et al: Gene expression in a preconditioning model. *Circulation* 1990; 82:III-464.
63. Yellon DM, Latchman DS: Stress proteins and myocardial protection. *J Mol Cell Cardiol* 1992; 24:113–124.
64. McCord JM: Oxygen-derived free radicals in postischemic tissue injury. *N Engl J Med* 1985; 312:159–163.
65. Bolli R, Patel BS, Jeroudi MO, Lai EK, McCay PB: Demonstration of free radical generation in "stunned" myocardium of intact dogs with the use of the spin trap A-phenyl *N*-Tert-Butyl nitrone. *J Clin Invest* 1988; 82:476–485.
66. Bolli R, Jeroudi MO, Patel BS, DuBose CM, Lai EK, Roberts R, et al: Direct evidence that oxygen-derived free radicals contribute to postischemic myocardial dysfunction in the intact dog. *Proc Natl Acad Sci USA* 1989; 86:4695–4699.
67. Zughayb M, Seikili S, Li XY, Traian JF, McCay PB, Bolli R: Detection of free radical generation in the "stunned" myocardium in the conscious dog using spin trapping techniques (abstr). *FASEB J* 1991; 5:A704.
68. Bolli R: Mechanism of myocardial "stunning." *Circulation* 1990; 82:723–738.
69. Hearse DJ: Reperfusion-induced injury: A possible role for oxidant stress and its manipulation. *Cardiovasc Drugs Ther* 1991; 5:225–236.
70. Myers ML, Bolli R, Lekich RF, Hartley CJ, Roberts R: Enhancement of recovery of myocardial function by oxygen free-radical scavengers after reversible regional ischemia. *Circulation* 1985; 72:915–921.
71. Gross GJ, Farber NE, Hardman HF, Warltier DC: Beneficial actions of superoxide dismutase and catalase in stunned myocardium of dogs. *Am J Physiol* 1986; 250:H372–H377.
72. Myers ML, Bolli R, Lekich RF, Hartley CJ, Roberts R: *N*-2-mercaptopropionylglycine improves recovery of myocardial function following reversible regional ischemia. *J Am Coll Cardiol* 1986; 8:1161–1168.
73. Bolli R, Zhu W, Hartley CJ, Michael LH, Repine JE, Hess ML, et al: Attenuation of dysfunction in the postischemic "stunned" myocardium by dimethylthiourea. *Circulation* 1987; 76:458–468.
74. Charlat ML, O'Neill PG, Egan JM, Abernethy DR, Michael LH, Myers ML, et al: Evidence for a pathogenetic role of xanthine oxidase in the "stunned" myocardium. *Am J Physiol* 1987; 252:H566–H577.
75. Puett DW, Forman BM, Cates CU, Wilson BH, Hande KR, Friesinger GC, et al: Oxypurinol limits myocardial stunning but does not reduce infarct size after reperfusion. *Circulation* 1987; 76:678–686.
76. Bolli R, Patel BS, Zhu W, O'Neill PG, Charlat ML, Roberts R: The iron chelator desferrioxamine attenuates postischemic ventricular dysfunction. *Am J Physiol* 1987; 253:H1372–H1380.
77. Triana JF, Li XY, Jamaluddin U, Thornby JI, Bolli R: Postischemic myocardial "stunning": Identification of major differences between the open-chest and the conscious dog and evaluation of the oxygen radical hypothesis in the conscious dog. *Circ Res* 1991; 69:731–747.
78. Bolli R, Jeroudi MO, Patel BS, Aruoma OI, Halliwell B, Lai EK, et al: Marked reduction of free radical generation and contractile dysfunction by antioxidant therapy began at the time of reperfusion: Evidence that myocardial "stunning" is a manifestation of reperfusion injury. *Circ Res* 1989; 65:607–622.
79. Bolli R, Patel BS, Jeroudi MO, Li XY, Triana JF, Lai EK, et al: Iron-mediated radical reactions upon reperfusion contribute to myocardial "stunning." *Am J Physiol* 1990; 259:H1901–H1911.
80. Romaschin AD, Rebeyka I, Wilson GJ, Mickle DAG: Conjugated dienes in ischemic and reperfused myocardium: An in vivo chemical signature of oxygen free radical mediated injury. *J Mol Cell Cardiol* 1987; 19:289–302.
81. Shlafer M, Kane PF, Wiggins VY, Kirsh MM: Possible role for cytotoxic oxygen metabolites in the pathogenesis of cardiac ischemic injury. *Circulation* 1982; 66:I-85–I-91.
82. Kusuoka H, Marban E: Cellular mechanisms of myocardial stunning. *Annu Rev Physiol* 1992; 54:243–256.
83. Lewandowski ED, Chari MV, Roberts R, Johnson LD: NMR studies of beta-oxidation and short-chain fatty acid metabolism during recovery of reperfused hearts. *Am J Physiol* 1991; 30:H354–H363.
84. Lewandowski ED, Johnston DL, Roberts R: Effects of inosine on glycolysis and contracture during myocardial ischemia. *Circ Res* 1991; 68:578–587.
85. Anderson JL, Marshall HW, Bray BE, Lutz JR, Frederick PR, Yanowitz FG, et al: A randomized trial of intracoronary streptokinase in the treatment of acute myocardial infarction. *N Engl J Med* 1983; 308:1313–1318.
86. Stack RS, Phillips H III, Grierson DS, Behar VS, Kong Y, Peter RH, et al: Functional improvement of jeopardized myocardium following intracoronary streptokinase infusion in acute myocardial infarction. *J Clin Invest* 1983; 72:84–95.
87. Bolli R: Myocardial "stunning" in man. *Circulation* 1992; 86:1671–1691.
88. Satler LF, Kent KM, Fox LM, Goldstein HA, Green CE, Rogers WJ, et al: The assessment of contractile reserve after thrombolytic therapy for acute myocardial infarction. *Am Heart J* 1986; 111:831–835.
89. Nixon JV, Brown CN, Smitherman TC: Identification of transient and persistent segmental wall abnormalities in patients with unstable angina by two-dimensional echocardiography. *Circulation* 1982; 65:1497–1503.
90. Robertson WS, Feigenbaum H, Armstrong WF, Dillon JC, O'Donnell J, McHenry PW: Exercise echocardiography: A clinically practical addition in the evaluation of coronary artery disease. *J Am Coll Cardiol* 1983; 2:1085–1089.
91. Kloner RA, Allen J, Cox TA, Zheng Y, Ruiz CE: Stunned left ventricular myocardium after exercise treadmill testing in coronary artery disease. *Am J Cardiol* 1991; 68:329–334.
92. Braunwald E, Rutherford JD: Reversible ischemic left ventricular dysfunction: Evidence for "hibernating myocardium." *J Am Coll Cardiol* 1986; 8:1467–1470.
93. Rahimtoola SH: The hibernating myocardium. *Am Heart J* 1989; 117:211–221.
94. Cox DA, Vatner SF: Myocardial function in areas of heterogeneous perfusion after coronary artery occlusion in conscious dogs. *Circulation* 1982; 66:1154–1158.
95. Kanaide H, Yashimura R, Makio N, Nakamura M: Regional myocardial function and metabolism during acute coronary artery occlusion. *Am J Physiol* 1982; 242:H980.
96. Kerber RE, Marcus ML, Erhardt J, Wilson R, Abboud FM: Correlation between echocardiographically demonstrated segmental dyskinesis and regional myocardial perfusion. *Circulation* 1975; 52:1097–1104.
97. Pagani M, Vatner SF, Baig H, Braunwald E: Initial myocardial adjustments to brief periods of ischemia and reperfusion in the conscious dog. *Circ Res* 1978; 43:83–92.
98. Vatner SF: Correlation between acute reductions in myocardial blood flow and function in conscious dogs. *Circ Res* 1980; 47:201–207.
99. Li X-Y, Jeroudi MO, Zughayb M, Sekili S, Sun J-Z, Bolli R: Stunned and hibernating myocardium: Pathophysiology, pathogenesis, and clinical implications. In: Buller N, Henderson AH, Krayenbul HP (eds): *Left Ventricular Dysfunction in Stunned and Hibernating Myocardium.* Amsterdam, Excerpta Medica, 1991: 6–18.
100. Rahimtoola SH: A perspective on the three large multicenter randomized clinical trials of coronary bypass surgery for chronic stable angina. *Circulation* 1985; 72:V123–V135.
101. Helfant RH, Pine R, Meister SG, Feldman MS, Trout RG, Banka VS: Nitroglycerin to unmask reversible asynergy: Correlation

with post-coronary bypass ventriculography. *Circulation* 1974; 50:108–113.

102. Brundage GH, Massie BM, Botvinick EH: Improved regional ventricular function after successful surgical revascularization. *J Am Coll Cardiol* 1984; 3:902–908.
103. Marshall RC, Tillisch JH, Phelps ME, Huang SC, Carson R, Henze E, et al: Identification and differentiation of resting myocardial ischemia and infarction in man with positron computed tomography ^{18}F-labeled flurodeoxyglucose and N-13 ammonia. Circulation 1983; 67:766–778.
104. Schelbert HR: Myocardial ischemia and clinical applications of positron emission tomography. *Am J Cardiol* 1989; 64:46E.
105. Tillisch JH, Brunken R, Marshall R, Schwaiger M, Mandelkern M, Phelps M, et al: Reversibility of cardiac wall-motion abnormalities predicted by positron tomography. *N Engl J Med* 1986; 314:884–888.
106. Bodenheimer MM, Banka VS, Fooshee C, Hermann GA, Helfant RH: Relationship between regional myocardial perfusion and the presence, severity and reversibility of asynergy in patients with coronary heart disease. *Circulation* 1978; 58:789–795.
107. Baker WB, Klein MS, Reardon MJ, Verani MS, Zoghbi WA: Reversible cardiac dysfunction (hibernation) from ischemia due to compression of the coronary arteries by a pseudoaneurysm. *N Engl J Med* 1991; 325:1858–1861.
108. Ginks WR, Sybers HD, Maroko PR, Covell JW, Sobel BE, Ross J Jr: Coronary artery reperfusion. II. Reduction of myocardial infarct size at 1 week after coronary occlusion. *J Clin Invest* 1972; 51:2717–2723.
109. Bergmann SR, Lerch RA, Fox KA, Ludbrook PA, Welch MJ, Ter-Pogossian MM, et al: Temporal dependence of beneficial effects of coronary thrombolysis characterized by positron tomography. *Am J Med* 1982; 73:573–581.
110. Reimer KA, Jennings RB: The "wavefront phenomenon" of myocardial ischemic cell death. II. Transmural progression of necrosis within the framework of ischemic bed size (myocardium at risk) and collateral flow. *Lab Invest* 1979; 40:633–644.
111. Mueller HS, Roberts R, Sobel BE (eds): *Thrombolytic Therapy in Acute Myocardial Infarction. CME Monograph, Albert Einstein College of Medicine/Montefiore Medical Center*. Greenwich, Connecticut, Mason Medical Communications, 1987.
112. Yusuf S, Collin R, Peto R, Furberg CD, Stampfer MJ, Goldhaber SZ, et al: VII. Intravenous and intracoronary fibrinolytic therapy in acute myocardial infarction: Overview of results on mortality, reinfarction and side effects from 33 randomized controlled trials. *Eur Heart J* 1985; 6:556–585.
113. Bresnahan GF, Roberts R, Shell WE, Ross J, Jr., Sobel BE: Deleterious effects due to hemorrhage after myocardial reperfusion. *Am J Cardiol* 1974; 33:82–86.
114. Roberts R, Sobel BE: Coronary revascularization during evolving myocardial infarction: The need for caution. *Circulation* 1974; 50:867–870.
115. West PN, Connors JP, Clark RE, Weldon CS, Ramsey DL, Roberts R, et al: Compromised microvascular integrity in ischemic myocardium. *Lab Invest* 1978; 38:677–684.
116. Fukuyama T, Sobel BE, Roberts R: Microvascular deterioration: Implications for reperfusion. *Cardiovasc Res* 1984; 18:310–320.
117. Laffel GL, Braunwald E: Thrombolytic therapy: A new strategy for treatment of acute myocardial infarction. *N Engl J Med* 1984; 311:770–776.
118. Gertz SD, Kalan JM, Kragel AH, Roberts WC, Braunwald E: Cardiac morphologic findings in patients with acute myocardial infarction treated with recombinant tissue plasminogen activator. *Am J Cardiol* 1990; 65:953–961.
119. Kloner RA, Ganote CE, Jennings RB: The "no-reflow" phenomenon after temporary coronary occlusion in the dog. *J Clin Invest* 1974; 54:1496–1508.
120. Hearse DJ: The protection of the ischaemic myocardium: Surgical success versus clinical failure. *Prog Cardiovasc Dis* 1988; 6:381–402.
121. Becker LC, Ambrosio G: Myocardial consequences of reperfusion. *Prog Cardiovasc Dis* 1987; 30:23–44.
122. Opie LH: Reperfusion injury and its pharmacological modification. *Circulation* 1989; 80:1049–1062.
123. Hearse DJ: Reperfusion of ischemic myocardium. *J Mol Cell Cardiol* 1977; 9:605–616.
124. Hearse DJ, Humphrey SM, Bullock GR: The oxygen paradox and the calcium paradox: Two facets of the same problem? *J Mol Cell Cardiol* 1978; 10:641–668.
125. Jolly SR, Kane WJ, Bailie MD, Abrams GD, Lucchesi BR: Canine myocardial reperfusion injury: Its reduction by the combined administration of superoxide dismutase and catalase. *Circ Res* 1984; 54:277–285.
126. Forman MB, Puett DW, Cates CU, McCroskey DE, Beckman JK, Greene HL, et al: Glutathione redox pathway and reperfusion injury: Effect of *N*-acetylcysteine on infarct size and ventricular function. *Circulation* 1988; 78:202–213.
127. Bolli R: Oxygen-derived free radicals and myocardial reperfusion injury: An overview. *Cardiovasc Drugs Ther* 1991; 5:249–268.
128. Nejima J, Knight DR, Fallon JT, Uemura N, Manders WT, Canfield DR, et al: Superoxide dismutase reduces reperfusion arrhythmias but fails to salvage regional myocardial function or myocardium at risk in conscious dogs. *Circulation* 1989; 79:143–153.
129. Patel BS, Jeroudi MO, O'Neil PG, Roberts R, Bolli R: Effect of human recombinant superoxide dismutase on canine myocardial infarction. *Am J Physiol* 1990; 258:H369–H380.
130. Downey JM: Free radicals and their involvement during long-term myocardial ischemia and reperfusion. *Annu Rev Physiol* 1990; 52:487–504.
131. Pandian NG, Koyanagi S, Skorton DJ, Collins SM, Eastham CL, Kieso RA, et al: Relations between two-dimensional echocardiographic wall thickening abnormalities, myocardial infarct size and coronary risk area in normal and hypertrophied myocardium. *Am J Cardiol* 1983; 52:1318–1325.
132. Cribier A, Berland J, Champoud O, Moore N, Behar P, Letac B: Intracoronary thrombolysis in evolving myocardial infarction: Sequential angiographic analysis of left ventricular performance. *Br Heart J* 1983; 50:401–410.
133. Hajduczok Z, Weiss RM, Stanford W, Marcus ML: Ventricular remodeling following infarction (abstr). *Circulation* 1988; 78:II-400.
134. Serruys PW, Simoons ML, Suryapranata H, Vermeer F, Wijns w, van den Brand M, et al: Preservation of global and regional left ventricular function after early thrombolysis in acute myocardial infarction. *J Am Coll Cardiol* 1986; 7:729–742.
135. Ginzton LE, Tigpen T, Garner D, Laks MM: Post-infarction hypertrophy of the non-infarcted myocardium: A compensatory response? (Abstr) *Circulation* 1985; 72:III-66.
136. Hood WB Jr: Experimental myocardial infarction. III. Recovery of left ventricular function in the healing phase: Contribution of increased fiber shortening in noninfarcted myocardium. *Am Heart J* 1970; 79:531–538.
137. Homans DC, Sublett E, Dai X-Z, Bache RJ: Persistence of regional left ventricular dysfunction after exercise-induced myocardial ischemia. *J Clin Invest* 1986; 77:66–73.
138. Henning H, O'Rourke RA, Crawford MH, Righetti A, Karliner JS: Inferior myocardial infarction as a cause of asymmetric septal hypertrophy. *Am J Cardiol* 1978; 41:817–822.
139. McKay RG, Pfeffer MA, Pasternak RC, Markis JE, Come PC, Nakao S, et al: Left ventricular remodeling after myocardial infarction: A corollary to infarct expansion. *Circulation* 1986; 74:693–702.
140. Stern A, Kessler KM, Hammer WF, Kruelen TH, Spann JF: Septal-free wall disproportion in inferior infarction: The echocardiographic differentiation from hypertrophic cardiomyopathy. *Circulation* 1978; 58:700–706.
141. Anversa P, Beghi C, Kikkawa Y, Olivetti G: Myocardial infarction in rats: Infarct size, myocyte hypertrophy and capillary growth. *Circ Res* 1986; 58:26–37.
142. Anversa P, Lond AV, Levicky V, Guiden G: Left ventricular failure induced by myocardial infarction. I. Myocyte hypertrophy. *Am J Physiol* 1986; 248:H876.
143. Pratt CM, Roberts R: Non-Q-wave myocardial infarction: Recognition, pathogenesis, prognosis and management. In: McIntosh HD (ed): *Baylor Cardiology Series*, 8th ed. Houston, Baylor College of Medicine, 1985: 5–19.
144. Bodenheimer MM, Banka VS, Trout RG, Hermann GA, Pasdar H, Helfant RH: Relationship between myocardial fibrosis and epicardial and surface electrocardiographic Q-waves in man. *J Electrocardiol* 1979; 12:205–210.
145. Wilson FN, Johnston FD, Hill IGW: The form of the electrocardiogram in experimental myocardial infarction. IV. Additional observations with later effects produced by ligation of the ante-

rior descending branch on the left coronary artery. *Am Heart J* 1935; 10:1025.
146. Spodick DH: Q-wave infarction versus S-T infarction: Nonspecificity of electrocardiographic criteria for differentiating transmural and nontransmural lesions. *Am J Cardiol* 1983; 51:913–915.
147. Roberts R: Nontransmural myocardial infarction. *Newsletter of the Council on Clinical Cardiology, American Heart Association* 1985; 11:1–17.
148. Marmor A, Sobel BE, Roberts R: Factors presaging early recurrent myocardial infarction ("extension"). *Am J Cardiol* 1981; 48:603–610.
149. Gibson RS: Non-Q-wave myocardial infarction diagnosis, prognosis and management. *Curr Probl Cardiol* 1988; 13:9–72.
150. Marmor A, Geltman EM, Schechtman K, Sobel BE, Roberts R: Recurrent myocardial infarction: Clinical predictors and prognostic implications. *Circulation* 1982; 66:415–421.
151. Schaer DH, Ross AM, Wasserman AG: Reinfarction, recurrent angina and reocclusion after thrombolytic therapy. *Circulation* 1987; 76:II-57.
152. Gibson RS, Boden WE, Theroux P, Strauss HD, Pratt CM, Gheorghiade M, et al: Diltiazem and reinfarction in patients with non-Q-wave myocardial infarction. Results of a double-blind, randomized, multicenter trial. *N Engl J Med* 1986; 315:423–429.
153. Eaton LW, Bulkley BH: Extension of acute myocardial infarction: Its relationship to infarct morphology in a canine model. *Circ Res* 1981; 49:80–88.
154. Phipps C: Contributory causes of coronary thrombosis. *JAMA* 1936; 106:761.
155. Rahe RH, Romo M, Siltanen P: Recent life changes, myocardial infarction, and abrupt coronary death. *Arch Intern Med* 1974; 133:221–228.
156. Lundberg U, Theorell T, Linda E: Life changes and myocardial infarction: Individual differences in life changes scaling. *J Psychosom Res* 1975; 37:27–32.
157. Jenkins CD: Recent evidence supporting psychologic and social risk factors for coronary disease. *N Engl J Med* 1976; 294:1033–1038.
158. Lambert CR, Jr., Pepine CJ: Coronary artery spasm and acute myocardial infarction. *Cardiovasc Clin* 1989; 20:131–140.
159. Herzog CA, Henry TD, Zimmer SD: Bacterial endocarditis presenting as acute myocardial infarction: A cautionary note for the era of reperfusion. *Am J Med* 1991; 90:392–397.
160. Bulkley BH, Roberts WC: Dissecting aneurysm (hematoma) limited to coronary artery: A clinicopathologic study of six patients. *Am J Cardiol* 1973; 55:747–756.
161. Foussas SG, Athanasopoulas GD, Cokkinos DV: Myocardial infarction caused by blunt chest injury: Possible mechanisms involved—case reports. *Angiology* 1989; 313–318.
162. Blackburn H, Jacobs R: Physical activity and the risk of coronary heart disease. *N Engl J Med* 1988; 319:1217–1219.
163. Wielgosz AT, Wielgosz M, Biro E, Nicholls E, MacWilliam L, Haney T: Risk factors for myocardial infarction: The importance of relaxation. *Br J Med Psychol* 1988; 61:209–217.
164. Dimsdale JE: A perspective on type A behavior and coronary disease. *N Engl J Med* 1988; 318:110–112.
165. Muller JE, Stone PH, Turi ZG, Rutherford JD, Czeisler C, Parker C, et al: Circadian variation in the frequency of onset of acute myocardial infarction. *N Engl J Med* 1985; 313:1315–1322.
166. Master AM: The role of effort and occupation (including physicians) in coronary occlusion. *JAMA* 1960; 174:942–948.
167. Pell S, D'Alonzo CA: Acute myocardial infarction in a large industrial population: Report of a 6 year study of 1,356 cases. *JAMA* 1963; 185:831–838.
168. Mitler MM, Kripke DF: Circadian variation in myocardial infarction. *N Engl J Med* 1986; 314:1187–1188.
169. Petralito A, Mangiafico RA, Giblino S, Cuffari MA, Miano MF, Piore CE: Daily modifications of plasma fibrinogen, platelet aggregation, Howell's time, PTT, PT, and antithrombin III in normal subjects and in patients with vascular disease. *Chronobiologia* 1982; 9:195–201.
170. Rosing DR, Brakma P, Redwood DR, Goldstein RE, Beiser GD, Astrup T, et al: Blood fibrinolytic activity in man: Diurnal variation and the response to varying intensities of exercise. *Circ Res* 1970; 27:171–184.
171. Marshall J: Diurnal variation in occurrence of strokes. *Stroke* 1977; 8:230–231.
172. Quyyumi AA, Mockus L, Wright, Fox KM: Morphology of ambulatory ST segment changes in patients with varying severity of coronary artery disease: Investigation of the frequency of nocturnal ischemia and coronary spasm. *Br Heart J* 1985; 53:186–193.
173. Millar-Craig MW, Bishop CN, Raftery EB: Circadian variation of blood pressure. *Lancet* 1978; 1:795–797.
174. Turton MB, Deegan T: Circadian variations of plasma catecholamine, cortisol, and immunoreactive insulin concentrations in supine subjects. *Clin Chim Acta* 1974; 55:389–397.
175. Maseri A, Crea F, Kaski JC, Davies G: Mechanisms and significance of cardiac ischemic pain. *Prog Cardiovasc Dis* 1992; 35:1–18.
176. Maseri A: The changing face of angina pectoris: Practical implications. *Lancet* 1983; 1:746–749.
177. Lichstein E, Breilbant S, Shani J, Hollander G, Greengart A: Relationship between location of chest pain and site of coronary artery occlusion. *Am Heart J* 1988; 115:564–568.
178. Margolis JR, Kannel WB, Feinleich M, Dawber TR, McNamara PM: Clinical features of unrecognized myocardial infarction—silent and symptomatic. *Am J Cardiol* 1973; 32:1–7.
179. Bean WB: Masquerades of myocardial infarction. *Lancet* 1977; 1:1044–1045.
180. Alonzo AA, Simon AB, Feinleib M: Prodromata of myocardial infarction and sudden death. *Circulation* 1975; 52:1056–1062.
181. Jaffe AS, Roberts R: Precordial inspection and palpation in patients with acute myocardial infarction. *Prac Cardiol* 1981; 7:46–50.
182. Fowler NO: Physical signs in acute myocardial infarction and its complications. *Prog Cardiovasc Dis* 1968; 10:287–297.
183. Harvey WP: Some pertinent physical findings in the clinical evaluation of acute myocardial infarction. *Circulation* 1969; 40:170.
184. Roberts R, Marmor AT: Right ventricular infarction. *Ann Rev Med* 1983; 34:377–390.
185. Marmor A, Geltman EM, Biello DR, Sobel BE, Siegel BA, Roberts R: Functional response of the right ventricle to myocardial infarction: Dependence on the site of left ventricular infarction. *Circulation* 1981; 64:1005–1011.
186. Wackers FJT, Lie KI, Sokole EB, Res J, Van der Schoot IB, Durrer D: Prevalence of right ventricular involvement in inferior wall infarction assessed with thallium 201 and technetium-99m pyrophosphate. *Am J Cardiol* 1978; 42:358–362.
187. Rigo P, Murray M, Taylor DR, Weisfeldt ML, Kelly DT, Strauss HW, et al: Right ventricular dysfunction detected by gated scintiphotography in patients with acute inferior myocardial infarction. *Circulation* 1975; 52:268–274.
188. Cohn JN, Guiha NH, Broder MI, Limas CJ: Right ventricular infarction. Clinical and hemodynamic features. *Am J Cardiol* 1974; 33:209–214.
189. Wade WG: The pathogenesis of infarction of the right ventricle. *Br Heart J* 1959; 21:545.
190. Farrer-Brown G: Vascular pattern of myocardium of right ventricle of human heart. *Br Heart J* 1968; 30:679–686.
191. Rotman M, Ratliff NB, Hawley J: Right ventricular infarction: A haemodynamic diagnosis. *Br Heart J* 1974; 36:941–944.
192. Raabe DS Jr, Chester AC: Right ventricular infarction. *Chest* 1978; 73:96–99.
193. Lorell B, Leinbach RC, Pohost GM, Gold HK, Dinsmore RE, Hutter AM Jr, et al: Right ventricular infarction: Clinical diagnosis and differentiation from cardiac tamponade and pericardial constriction. *Am J Cardiol* 1979; 43:465–471.
194. Erhardt LR, Sjogren A, Wahlberg I: Single right-sided precordial lead in the diagnosis of right ventricular involvement in inferior myocardial infarction. *Am Heart J* 1976; 91:571–576.
195. Dellitalia LJ, Lembo NJ, Starling MR, Crawford MH, Simmons RS, Lasher JC, et al: Hemodynamically important right ventricular infarction: Follow up evaluation of right ventricular systolic function at rest and during exercise with radionuclide ventriculography and respiratory gas exchange. *Circulation* 1987; 75:996–1003.
196. Andersen HR, Nielsen O, Lund O, Falk E: Prognostic significance of right ventricular infarction diagnosed by ST elevation in right chest lead V3R to V7R. *Int J Cardiol* 1989; 23:349–356.
197. Geft I, Shah PK, Rodriguez L, Hulse S, Maddahi J, Berman DS, et al: ST elevations in lead V1 to V5 may be caused by right coronary artery occlusion and acute right ventricular infarction. *Am J Cardiol* 1984; 53:991–996.

198. Lee TH, Weisberg MC, Brand DA, Rouan GW, Goldman L: Candidates for thrombolysis among emergency room patients with acute chest pain. *Ann Intern Med* 1989; 110:957–962.
199. Goldman L, Cook EF, Brand DA, Lee TH, Rouan GW, Weisberg MC, et al: A computer protocol to predict myocardial infarction in emergency department patients with chest pain. *N Engl J Med* 1988; 318:797–803.
200. Lee TH, Rouan GW, Weisberg MC, Brand DA, Cook EF, Acampora D, et al: Sensitivity of routine clinical criteria for diagnosing myocardial infarction within 24 hours of hospitalization. *Ann Intern Med* 1987; 106:181–186.
201. Lee TH, Juarez G, Cook EF, Weisberg MC, Rouan GW, Brand DA, et al: Ruling out acute myocardial infarction. *N Engl J Med* 1991; 324:1239–1246.
202. Roberts R: The two out of three criteria for the diagnosis of infarction—Is it passe? *Chest* 1984; 86:511–513.
203. Cook RW, Edwards JE, Pruitt RD: Electrocardiographic changes in acute subendocardial infarction. I. Large subendocardial and large transmural infarcts. *Circulation* 1958; 18:603.
204. Abildshov JA, Wilkinson RS Jr, Vincent WA, Cohen W: An experimental study of the electrocardiographic effects of localized myocardial lesions. *Am J Cardiol* 1961; 8:485.
205. Wagner GS, Ro CR, Limbird LE, Rosati RA, Wallace AG: The importance of identification of myocardial specific isoenzymes of creatine phosphokinase (MB form) in the diagnosis of acute myocardial infarction. *Circulation* 1973; 47:263–269.
206. Gunnar RM, Pietras RJ, Blackaller J, Dadmun SE, Szanto PB, Tobin JR Jr: Correlation of vectocardiographic criteria for myocardial infarction with autopsy findings. *Circulation* 1967; 35:158–171.
207. Ambos HD, Moore P, Roberts R: A database for analysis of patient diagnostic data. In: *Computers in Cardiology*. Long Beach, IEEE Computer Society, 1978.
208. Helfant RH, Banka VS (eds): *A Clinical and Angiographic Approach to Coronary Heart Disease*. Philadelphia, F.A. Davis, 1978.
209. Fenichel NM, Kugell VH: The large Q wave of the electrocardiogram. A correlation with pathologic observations. *Am Heart J* 1931; 7:235.
210. Rude RE, Poole WK, Muller JE, Turi Z, Rutherford J, Parker C, et al: Electrocardiographic and clinical criteria for recognition of acute myocardial infarction based on analysis of 3697 patients. *Am J Cardiol* 1983; 52:936–942.
211. Bodenheimer MM, Banka VS, Helfant RH: Q-waves and ventricular asynergy: Predictive value and hemodynamic significance of anatomic localization. *Am J Cardiol* 1975; 35:615–618.
212. Schamroth L: The 12-lead electrocardiogram. In: Book 1. Boston, Blackwell Scientific Publications, 1989:
213. Roberts R: Measurement of enzymes in cardiology. In: Linden RJ (ed): *Techniques in the Life Sciences*. Ireland, Elsevier Scientific Publishers, 1983: P312/1–P312/24.
214. Roberts R, Gowda KS, Ludbrook PA, Sobel BE: Specificity of elevated serum MB CPK activity in the diagnosis of acute myocardial infarction. *Am J Cardiol* 1975; 36:433–437.
215. Lee TH, Goldman L: Serum enzyme assays in the diagnosis of acute myocardial infarction. *Ann Intern Med* 1986; 105:221–233.
216. Grande P, Christiansen C, Pedersen A, Christensen MS: Optimal diagnosis in acute myocardial infarction. A cost effectiveness study. *Circulation* 1980; 61:723–728.
217. Klein MS, Shell WE, Sobel BE: Serum creatine phosphokinse (CPK) isoenzymes after intramuscular injections, surgery, and myocardial infarction. Experimental and clinical studies. *Cardiovasc Res* 1973; 7:412–418.
218. Dawwon DM, Epenberger HM, Kaplan NO: Creatine kinase: Evidence for the dimeric structure. *Biochem Biophys Res Commun* 1965; 21:346.
219. Roberts R, Grace AM: Purification of mitochondrial creatine kinase: Biochemical and immunological characterization. *J Biol Chem* 1980; 225:2870–2877.
220. Grace AM, Perryman MB, Roberts R: Purification and characterization of human mitochondrial creatine kinase. A single enzyme form. *J Biol Chem* 1983; 258:15346–15354.
221. Haas RC, Strauss AW: Separate nuclear genes encode sarcomere-specific and ubiquitous human mitochondrial creatine kinase isoenzymes. *J Biol Chem* 1990; 265:6921–6927.
222. Friedman DL, Perryman MB: Compartmentation of multiple forms of creatine kinase in the distal nephron of the rat kidney. *J Biol Chem* 1991; 266:22404–22410.
223. Grace A, Fukuyama T, Roberts R: Detection of elevated mitochondrial CK in plasma after infarction by a specific radioimmunoassay (abstr). *Am J Cardiol* 1980; 45:414.
224. Ishikawa Y, Grace A, Saffitz J, Roberts R: Elevated plasma mitochondrial creatine kinase: An in vivo marker of irreversible injury. *Am J Cardiol* 1982; 49:1038.
225. Tsung JS, Tsung SS: Creatine kinase isoenzymes in extracts of various human skeletal muscles. *Clin Chem* 1986; 32:1568–1570.
226. Wilhelm AH, Albers KM, Toss JK: Creatine phosphokinase isoenzyme distribution in human skeletal and heart muscles. *IRCS Med Sci* 1976; 4:418.
227. Yasmineh WG, Ibrahim GA, Abbasnezhad MA, Awad EA: Isoenzyme distribution of creatine kinase and lactate dehydrogenase in serum and skeletal muscle in Duchenne muscular dystrophy, collagen disease, and other muscular disorders. *Clin Chem* 1978; 24:1985–1989.
228. Roberts R, Henry PD, Witteveen SAGJ, Sobel BE: Quantification of serum creatine phosphokinase (CPK) isoenzyme activity. *Am J Cardiol* 1974; 33:650–654.
229. Apple FS, Robers MA, Sherman WM, Costill DL, Hagerman FC, Ivy JL: Profile of creatine kinase isoenzymes in skeletal muscles of marathon runners. *Clin Chem* 1984; 30:413–416.
230. Siegel AJ, Silverman LM, Evans WJ: Elevated skeletal muscle creatine kinase MB isoenzyme levels in marathon runners. *JAMA* 1983; 250:2835–2837.
231. Keshgegian AA, Feiberg NW: Serum creatine kinase MB isoenzyme in chronic muscle disease. *Clin Chem* 1984; 30:575–578.
232. Shahangian S, Ash KO, Wahlstrom NO, Jr., Warden GD, Saffle JR, Taylor AA, et al: Creatine kinase and lactate dehydrogenase isoenzymes in serum of patients suffering burns, blunt trauma, or myocardial infarction. *Clin Chem* 1984; 30:1332–1338.
233. McBride JW, Labrosse KR, Mccoy HG, Ahrenholz DH, Solem LD, Goldenberg IF: Is serum creatine kinase MB in electrically injured patients predictive of myocardial injury? *JAMA* 1986; 255:764–768.
234. Foxall CD, Emery AE: Changes in creatine kinase and its isoenzymes in human fetal muscle during development. *J Neurol Sci* 1975; 24:483–492.
235. Tzvetanova E: Creatine kinase isoenzymes in muscle tissue of patients with neuromuscular diseases and human fetuses. *Enzyme* 1971; 12:279.
236. Sadeh M, Stern LZ, Czyzewski K, Finley PR, Russell DH: Alterations of creatine kinase, ornithine decarboxylase, and transglutaminase during muscle regeneration. *Life Sci* 1984; 34:483–488.
237. Roberts R: Enzymatic diagnosis of acute myocardial infarction. *Chest* 1988; 93:3S–6S.
238. Puleo PR, Roberts R: Plasma enzymes in acute myocardial infarction. In: Francis GS, Alpert JS (eds): *Modern Coronary Care*. Boston, Little, Brown and Company, 1990: 95–121.
239. Somer H, Dubowitz V, Donner M: Creatine kinase isoenzymes in neuromuscular diseases. *J Neurol Sci* 1976; 29:129–136.
240. Henry PD, Roberts R, Sobel BE: Rapid separation of plasma creatine kinase isoenzymes by batch adsorption with glass beads. *Clin Chem* 1975; 21:844–849.
241. Jaffe AS, Ritter C, Meltzer V, Harter H, Roberts R: Unmasking artifactual increases in creatine kinase isoenzymes in patients with renal failure. *J Lab Clin Med* 1984; 104:193–202.
242. Karmen A, Wroblewski F, LaDu J: Transaminase activity in human blood. *J Clin Invest* 1954; 34:126.
243. Apple FS, Greenspan NS, Dietzler DN: Elevation of creatine kinase BB CK in hospitalized patients. *Ann Clin Lab Sci* 1982; 12:398–402.
244. Kimler SC, Sandhu RS: Circulating CK-MB and CK-BB isoenzymes after prostate resection. *Clin Chem* 1980; 26:55–59.
245. Tsung SH: Several conditions causing elevation of serum CK-MB and CK-BB. *Am J Clin Pathol* 1981; 75:711–715.
246. Laboda HM, Britton VJ: Creatine kinase isoenzyme activity in human placenta and in the serum of women in labor. *Clin Chem* 1977; 23:1329–1332.
247. Somer H, Kaste M, Troupp H, Konttinen A: Brain creatine kinase in blood after acute brain injury. *J Neurol Neurosurg Psychiatry* 1975; 38:572–576.

248. Kaste M, Some H, Konttine A: Brain-type creatine kinae isoenzyme. *Arch Neurol* 1977; 34:142–144.
249. Tsung SH: Creatine kinase activity and isoenzyme pattern in various normal tissues and neoplasms. *Clin Chem* 1983; 29:2040–2043.
250. Goldman J, Matz R, Mortimer R, Freeman R: High elevations of creatine phosphokinase in hypothyroidism: An isoenzyme analysis. *JAMA* 1977; 238:325–326.
251. Urdal P, Landaas S: Macro creatine kinase BB in serum, and some data on its prevalence. *Clin Chem* 1979; 25:461–465.
252. Muller JE, Morrison J, Stone PH, Rude RE, Rosner B, Roberts R, et al: Nifedipine therapy for patients with threatened and acute myocardial infarction: A randomized, double-blind, placebo-controlled comparison. *Circulation* 1984; 69:740–747.
253. Roberts R: Diagnostic assessment of myocardial infarction based on lactate dehydrogenase and creatine kinase isoenzymes. *Heart Lung* 1981; 10:486–506.
254. Turi ZG, Rutherford JD, Roberts R, Muller JE, Jaffe AS, Rude RE, et al: Electrocardiographic, enzymatic and scintigraphic criteria of acute myocardial infarction as determined from study of 726 patients (a MILIS Study). *Am J Cardiol* 1985; 55:1463–1469.
255. Roberts R: Recognition, diagnosis, and prognosis of early reinfarction: The role of calcium-channel blockers. *Circulation* 1987; 75:V-139–V-147.
256. MILIS Study Group: Multicenter Investigation of the Limitation of Infarct Size: Design, Methods and Endpoints. American Heart Association Monograph 1984;
257. Roberts R, Sobel BE: Elevated plasma MB creatine phosphokinase activity. A specific marker for myocardial infarction in perioperative patients. *Arch Intern Med* 1976; 136:421–424.
258. Klein MS, Coleman RE, Weldon CS, Sobel BE, Roberts R: Concordance of electrocardiographic and scintigraphic criteria of myocardial injury after cardiac surgery. *J Thorac Cardiovasc Surg* 1976; 71:934–937.
259. Righetti A, O'Rourke RA, Schelbert H, Henning H, Hardarson T, Daily PO, et al: Usefulness of preoperative and postoperative Tc-99m (Sn)-pyrophosphate scans in patients with ischemic and valvular heart disease. *Am J Cardiol* 1977; 39:43–49.
260. Sullivan W, Vlodaver Z, Tuna N, Long L, Edwards JE: Correlation of electrocardiographic and pathologic findings in healed myocardial infarction. *Am J Cardiol* 1978; 42:724–731.
261. Goldberger AL (ed): *Myocardial Infarction: Electrocardiographic Differential Diagnosis*. New York, CV Mosby, 1979.
262. Tiefenbrunn AJ, Biello DR, Geltman EM, Sobel BE, Siegel BA, Roberts R: Gated cardiac blood pool imaging and thallium-201 myocardial scintigraphy for detection of remote myocardial infarction. *Am J Cardiol* 1981; 47:1–6.
263. Wevers RA, Delsing M, Klein-Gebbink JA, Soons JB: Post-synthetic changes in creatine kinase isoenzymes. *Clin Chim Acta* 1978; 86:323–327.
264. Wevers RA, Olthuis HP, Van Niel JCC, Van Wilgenberg MG, Soons JB: A study on the dimeric structure of creatine kinase. *Clin Chim Acta* 1977; 75:377–385.
265. George S, Ishikawa Y, Perryman MB, Roberts R: Purification and characterization of naturally occurring and in vitro induced multiple forms of MM creatine kinase. *J Biol Chem* 1984; 259:2667–2674.
266. Perryman MB, Knell JD, Roberts R: Carboxypeptidase-catalyzed hydrolysis of C-terminal lysine: Mechanism for in vivo production of multiple forms of creatine kinase in plasma. *Clin Chem* 1984; 30:662–664.
267. Puleo PR, Guadagno PA, Roberts R, Perryman MB: A sensitive and rapid assay for the plasma subforms of MB creatine kinase. *Clin Chem* 1989; 35:1452–1455.
268. Puleo PR, Guadagno PA, Scheel MV, Roberts R, Perryman MB: Rapid and convenient assay of MB creatine kinase (CK) subforms in the initial hours of myocardial infarction. *Circulation* 1989; 80:II-354.
269. Roberts R: Reperfusion and the plasma isoforms of creatine kinase isoenzymes: A clinical perspective. *J Am Coll Cardiol* 1987; 9:464–466.
270. Puleo PR, Roberts R: Advances in the early diagnosis of acute myocardial infarction and reperfusion: The need for a new "mind set." *Circulation* 1992;
271. Gore JM, Goldberg RJ, Matsumoto AS, Castelli WP, McNamara PM, Dalen JG: Validity of serum total cholesterol level obtained within 24 hours of acute myocardial infarction. *Am J Cardiol* 1984; 54:722–725.
272. Ryder RE, Hayes TM, Mulligan IP, Kingswood JC, Williams S, Owens DR: How soon after myocardial infarction should plasma lipid values be assessed? *Br Med J* 1984; 289:1651–1653.
273. Ceremuzynski L: Hormonal and metabolic reactions evoked by acute myocardial infarction. *Circ Res* 1981; 48:767–776.
274. Goldberger E, Alesio J, Woll F: The significance of hyperglycemia in myocardial infarction. *NY State Med J* 1945; 45:391.
275. Kjekshus JK, Sobel BE: Depressed myocardial creatine phosphokinase activity following experimental myocardial infarction in rabbit. *Circ Res* 1970; 27:403–414.
276. Shell WE, Kjekshus JK, Sobel BE: Quantitative assessment of the extent of myocardial infarction in the conscious dog by means of analysis of serial changes in serum creatine phosphokinase (CPK) activity. *J Clin Invest* 1971; 50:2614–2625.
277. Maroko PR, Kjekshus JK, Sobel BE: Factors influencing infarct size following experimental coronary artery occlusion. *Circulation* 1972; 43:67–82.
278. Geltman EM, Roberts R, Sobel BE: Cardiac positron tomography: Current status and future directions. *Herz* 1980; 5:107–119.
279. Sobel BE, Kjekshus KJ, Roberts R: Enzymatic estimation of infarct size. In: Hearse DJ, De Leiris J (eds): *Enzymes in Cardiology: Diagnosis and Research*. Chichester, John Wiley and sons, 1979: 257–289.
280. Geltman EM, Ehsani AA, Campbell MK, Schechtman K, Roberts R, Sobel BE: The influence of location and extent of myocardial infarction on long-term ventricular dysrhythmia and mortality. *Circulation* 1979; 60:805–814.
281. Roberts R: Creatine kinase isozymes as diagnostic and prognostic indices of myocardial infarction. In: Rattazzi MC, Scandalios JG, Whitt GS (ed): *Isozymes: Current Topics in Biological and Medical Research*. New York, Alan R. Liss, 1979: 115–154.
282. Roberts R, Ambos HD, Sobel BE: Estimation of infarct size with MB rather than total CK. *Int J Cardiol* 1983; 2:479–489.
283. Rogers WJ, McDaniel HG, Smith LR, Mantle JA, Russell RO Jr, Rackley CE: Correlation of CPK-MB and angiographic estimates of infarct size in man. *Circulation* 1977; 56:199–205.
284. Roberts R, Husain R, Ambos HD, Oliver GC, Cox JR Jr, Sobel BE: Relation between infarct size and ventricular arrhythmia. *Br Heart J* 1975; 37:1169–1175.
285. Bleifeld W, Mathey D, Hanrath P, Buss H, Effert S: Infarct size estimated from serial serum creatine phosphokinase in relation to left ventricular hemodynamics. *Circulation* 1977; 55:303–311.
286. Gillespie IA, Sobel BE: A rationale for therapy of acute myocardial infarction: Limitation of infarct size. In: Stollerman GH (ed): *Advances in Internal Medicine*. Chicago, Year Book Medical Publishers, 1977:
287. Hackel DB, Reimer KA, Ideker RE, Mikat EM, Hartwell TD, Parker CB, et al: Comparison of enzymatic and anatomic estimates of myocardial infarct size in man. *Circulation* 1984; 70:824–835.
288. Fukuyama T, Schechtman KB, Roberts R: The effects of intravenous nitroglycerin on hemodynamics, coronary blood flow and morphologically and enzymatically estimated infarct size in conscious dogs. *Circulation* 1980; 62:1227–1238.
289. Mogelson S, Davidson J, Sobel BE, Roberts R: The effect of hyperbaric oxygen on infarct size in the conscious animal. *Eur J Cardiol* 1980; 12:135–146.
290. Clark RE, Christlieb IY, Ferguson TB, Weldon CS, Marbarger JP, Sobel BE, et al: Laboratory and initial clinical studies of nifedipine, a calcium antagonist for improved myocardial preservation. *Ann Surg* 1981; 193:719–732.
291. Jaffe AS, Geltman EM, Tiefenbrunn AJ, Ambos HD, Strauss HD, Sobel BE, et al: Reduction of infarct size in patients with inferior infarction with intravenous nitroglycerin. *Br Heart J* 1983; 49:452–460.
292. Roberts R, Croft C, Gold HK, Hartwell TD, Jaffe AS, Muller JE, et al: Effect of propranolol on myocardial infarct size in a randomized, blinded, multicenter trial. *N Engl J Med* 1985; 312:932–936.
293. Roberts R, Ishikawa Y: Enzymatic estimation of infarct size during reperfusion. *Circulation* 1919; 68:I-83–I-89.
294. Maroko PR, Libby P, Covell JW, Sobel BE, Ross J Jr, Braunwald E: Precordial ST-T segment elevation mapping: An atraumatic

method for assessing alterations in the extent of myocardial ischemic injury. *Am J Cardiol* 1972; 29:223–230.

295. Lekven J, Chatterje K, Tyberg JV, Parmley WW: Influence of left ventricular dimensions on endocardial and epicardial QRS amplitude and ST segment elevations during acute myocardial ischemia. *Circulation* 1980; 61:679–689.
296. Ideker RE, Wagner GS, Ruth WK, Alonso DR, Bishop SP, Bloor CM, et al: Evaluation of a QRS scoring system for estimating myocardial infarct size. II. Correlation with quantitative anatomic findings for anterior infarcts. *Am J Cardiol* 1982; 49:1604–1614.
297. Roark SF, Ideker RE, Wagner GS, Alonso DR, Bishop SP, Bloor CM, et al: Evaluation of a QRS scoring system for estimating myocardial infarct size. III. Correlation with quantitative anatomic findings for inferior infarcts. *Am J Cardiol* 1983; 51:382–389.
298. Cowan MJ, Bruce RA, Reichenback DD: Validation of computerized QRS criterion for estimating myocardial infarction size and correlation with quantitative morphologic measurements. *Am J Cardiol* 1986; 57:60–65.
298a. Bar FW, Vermeer F, de Zwaan C: Value of admission electrocardiogram in predicting outcome of thrombolytic therapy in acute myocardial infarction: A randomized trial conducted by The Netherlands Interuniversity Cardiology Institute. *Am J Cardiol* 1987; 59:6–13.
298b. Lie KI, Wellens HJJ, Schuilenburg RM, Becker AE, Durrer D: Factors influencing prognosis of bundle branch block complicating acute anteroseptal infarction: The value of the His bundle recordings. *Circulation* 1974; 50:935–941.
298c. Braat SH, Gorgels APM, Bar FW, Wellens HJJ: Value of the ST-T segment in lead V_4R in inferior wall acute myocardial infarction to predict the site of coronary arterial occlusion. *Am J Cardiol* 1988; 62:140–142.
299. Roberts R: Enzymatic estimation of infarct size. Thrombolysis induced its demise: Will it now rekindle its renaissance? *Circulation* 1990; 81:707–710.
300. Mahmarian JJ, Pratt CM, Borges-Neto S, Cashion WR, Roberts R, Verani MS: Quantification of infarct size by ^{201}Tl single-photon emission computed tomography during acute myocardial infarction in humans: Comparison with enzymatic estimates. *Circulation* 1988; 78:831–839.
301. Corbett JR, Lewis M, Willerson JT, Nicod PH, Huxley RL, Simon T, et al: ^{99m}Tc-pyrophosphate imaging in patients with acute myocardial infarction: Comparison of planar imaging with single-photon tomography with and without blood pool overlay. *Circulation* 1984; 69:1120–1128.
302. Li QS, Frank TL, Franceschi D, Wagner HN, Becker LC: Technetium-99m methyoxy isobutyl isonitril (RP30) for quantification of myocardial ischemia and reperfusion in dogs. *J Nucl Med* 1988; 29:1539–1548.
303. DeCoster PM, Wijns W, Cauwe F, Robert A, Beckers C, Melin J: Area-at-risk determination by technetium-99m-hexakis-2-methoxyisobutylisonitrile in experimental reperfused myocardial infarction. *Circulation* 1990; 82:2153–2162.
304. Okada RD, Glover D, Saffne T, Williams S: Myocardial kinetics of technetium-99m-hexakis-2-methyl-propyl-isonitrile. *Circulation* 1988; 77:491–498.
305. Verani MS, Jeroudi MO, Mahmarian JJ, Boyce TM, Borges-Neto S, Patel BS, et al: Quantitation of myocardial infarction during coronary occlusion and myocardial salvage after reperfusion using cardiac imaging with technetium-99m hexakis 2-methoxyisobutyl isonitrile. *J Am Coll Cardiol* 1988; 12:1573–1581.
306. Sinusas AJ, Trautman KA, Bergin JD, Watson DD, Ruiz M, Smith WH, et al: Quantification of "area at risk" during coronary occlusion and degree of myocardial salvage after reperfusion with technetium-99m-methoxy isobutyl isonitrile. *Circulation* 1990; 82:1424–1437.
307. Gibbons RJ, Verani MS, Behrenbeck T: Feasibility of tomographic 99Tc-hexakis-2-methoxy-2-methylpropyl-isonitrile imaging for the assessment of myocardial area at risk and the effect of treatment in acute myocardial infarction. *Circulation* 1989; 80:1277–1286.
308. Wackers FJ, Gibbons RJ, Kayden DS, Pellikka PA, Behrenbeck T, Mahmarian JJ, et al: Serial quantitative planar technetium-99m-isonitril imaging in acute myocardial infarction: Efficacy for noninvasive assessment of thrombolytic therapy. *J Am Coll Cardiol* 1989; 14:861–873.
309. Santoro GM, Bisi G, Sciagra R, Leoncini M, Fazzini PF, Meldolesi U: Single photon emission computed tomography with technetium-99m hexakis-2-methoxyisobutyl isonitril in acute myocardial infarction before and after thrombolytic treatment: Assessment of salvaged myocardium and pediction of late functional recovery. *J Am Coll Cardiol* 1990; 15:301–314.
310. Huber KC, Bresnahan JF, Bresnahan DR, Pellikka PA, Behrenbeck T, Gibbons RJ: Measurement of myocardium at risk by technetium-99m sestamibi: Correlation with coronary angiography. *J Am Coll Cardiol* 1992; 19:67–73.
311. Marmor A, Biello DR, Sampathkumaran KS, Geltman EM, Siegel BA, Roberts R: A new scintigraphic technique for assessment of right atrial function. *Radiology* 1981; 139:719–723.
312. Jaffe AS, Klein MS, Patel BR, Siegel BA, Roberts R: Abnormal technetium-99m pyrophosphate images in unstable angina: Ischemia versus infarction? *Am J Cardiol* 1979; 44:1035–1039.
313. Quiñones MA: Echocardiography in acute myocardial infarction. *Cardiol Clinics* 1984; 2:123–134.
314. Horowitz RS, Morganroth J, Parrotto C, Chen CC, Soffer J, Pareletto FJ: Immediate diagnosis of acute myocardial infarction by two-dimensional echocardiography. *Circulation* 1982; 65:323–329.
315. Oh JK, Miller PA, Shub C, Reeder GS, Tajik AJ: Evaluation of acute chest pain syndromes by two-dimensional echocardiography: Its potential application in the selection of patients for acute reperfusion therapy. *Mayo Clin Proc* 1987; 62:59–66.
316. Zoghbi WA, Charlat ML, Bolli R, Zhu W, Hartley CJ, Quiñones MA: Quantitative assessment of left ventricular wall motion by two-dimensional echocardiography: Validation during reversible ischemia in the conscious dog. *J Am Coll Cardiol* 1988; 11:851–860.
317. Van Reet RE, Quiñones MA, Poliner LR, Nelson JG, Waggoner AD, Kanon D, et al: Comparison of two-dimensional echocardiography with gated radionuclide ventriculography in the evaluation of global and regional left ventricular function in acute myocardial infarction. *J Am Coll Cardiol* 1984; 3:243–252.
318. Quiñones MA, Waggoner AD, Reduto LA, Nelson JG, Young JB, Winters WL Jr, et al: A new, simplified and accurate method for determining ejection fraction with two-dimensional echocardiography. *Circulation* 1981; 64:744–753.
319. Schiller NB, Shah PM, Crawford M, DeMaria A, Devereux R, Feigenbaum H, et al: Recommendations for quantitation of the left ventricle by two-dimensional echocardiography. *J Am Soc Echo* 1989; 5:358–367.
320. D'Arcy B, Nanda NC: Two-dimensional echocardiographic features of right ventricular ejection fraction in patients with coronary artery disease. *J Am Coll Cardiol* 1983; 2:911–918.
321. Rokey R, Sterling LL, Zoghbi WA, Sartori MP, Limacher MC, Kuo LC, et al: Determination of regurgitant fraction in isolated mitral or aortic regurgitation by pulsed-Doppler two-dimensional echocardiography. *J Am Coll Cardiol* 1986; 7:1273–1278.
322. Zoghbi WA, Quiñones MA: Determination of cardiac output by Doppler echocardiography: A critical appraisal. *Herz* 1986; 11:258–268.
323. Nishimura R, Abel MD, Hatle LK, Tajik AJ: Assessment of diastolic function of the heart: Background and current applications of Doppler echocardiography, Part II. Clinical studies. *Mayo Clin Proc* 1989; 64:181–204.
324. Oh KJ, Seward JB, Khandheria BK, Gersh BJ, McGregor GA, Freeman WK, et al: Transesophageal echocardiography in critically ill patients. *Am J Cardiol* 1990; 66:1492–1495.
325. Miyatake K, Okamota M, Kinoshita N, Park YD, Nagata S, Izumi S, et al: Doppler echocardiographic features of ventricular septal rupture in myocardial infarction. *J Am Coll Cardiol* 1985; 5:182–187.
326. Quiñones MA, Cheirif JB: New perspectives for perfusion imaging in echocardiography. *Circulation* 1991; 83:III-104–III-110.
327. Rokey R, Johnston DL, Wendt RE III, Quiñones MA, Roberts R: MRI of ischemic heart disease in man. Part 1. *Appl Radiol* 1987; 31–39.
328. Rokey R, Verani MS, Boli R, Kuo LC, Ford JJ, Wendt RE, et al: Quantification of myocardial infarct size by magnetic resonance imaging early after coronary artery occlusion in dogs. *Radiology* 1986; 158:771–774.
329. Johnston DL, Rice L, Vick GW, Hedrick TD, Rokey R: Assessment of tissue iron overload by nuclear magnetic resonance imaging. *Am J Med* 1989; 87:4–47.

330. Cox JL, McLaughlin VW, Flowers NC, Horan LG: The ischemic zone surrounding acute myocardial infarction: Its morphology as detected by dehydrogenase staining. *Am Heart J* 1968; 76:650–659.
331. Tennant R, Wiggers CJ: The effect of coronary occlusion on myocardial contractions. *Am J Physiol* 1935; 112:351.
332. Maroko PR, Libby P, Ginks WR, Bloor CM, Shell WE, Sobel BE, et al: Coronary artery reperfusion. I. Early effects on local myocardial function and the extent of myocardial necrosis. *J Clin Invest* 1972; 51:2710–2716.
333. Constantino C, Corday E, Lang TW, Meerbaum S, Brasch J, Kaplan L, et al: Revascularization after three hours of coronary arterial occlusion: Effects on regional cardiac metabolic function and infarct size. *Am J Cardiol* 1975; 36:368–384.
334. Maroko PR, Braunwald E: Modification of myocardial infarct size after coronary occlusion. *Ann Intern Med* 1973; 79:720–733.
335. Yellon DM, Miura T, Hearse DJ, Downey JM: Factors influencing infarct size: Is coronary collateral flow the key determinant? *J Cell Cardiol* 1986; 18:101.
336. Lowe JE, Reimer KA, Jennings RB: Experimental infarct size as a function of the amount of myocardium at risk. *Am J Pathol* 1978; 90:363–379.
337. Kudoh Y, Maxwell MP, Hearse DJ, Downey JM, Yellon DM: Failure of metoprolol to limit infarct size during 24 hours of coronary artery occlusion in a closed chest dog. *J Cardiovasc Pharmacol* 1984; 6:1201–1209.
338. Hearse DJ, Yellon DM, Downey JM: Can beta blockers limit myocardial infarct size? *Eur Heart J* 1986; 7:925–930.
339. Jennings RB, Reimer KA: Effects of beta adrenergic blockade on acute myocardial injury. In: Gross F (ed): *Modulation of Sympathetic Tone in the Treatment of Cardiovascular Diseases.* Berne, Hans Huber, 1979: 103–114.
340. Matsuki T, Cohen MV, Holt G, Ayling J, Hearse DJ, Downey JM: Chronic whole body sympathectomy fails to protect ischemic rabbit hearts. *Am J Physiol* 1989; 256:H1322–H1327.
341. ISIS-1 (First International Study of Infarct Survival) Collaborative Group: Randomized trial of intravenous atenolol among 16,027 cases of suspected acute myocardial infarction. ISIS-I. *Lancet* 1986; 2:57–66.
342. Roberts R, Rogers WJ, Mueller HS, Lambrew CT, Diver DJ, Smith HC, et al: Immediate versus deferred beta-blockade following thrombolytic therapy in patients with acute myocardial infarction: Results of the Thrombolysis In Myocardial Infarction (TIMI) II-B subgroup analyses. *Circulation* 1991; 83:422–437.
343. Roberts R, Kleiman N (eds): *The Open Artery: Perspectives on Coronary Reperfusion in Acute Myocardial Infarction.* Hamilton, Ontario, Canada, Decker Periodicals, 1992.
344. Braunwald E: Myocardial reperfusion, limitation of infarct size, reduction of left ventricular dysfunction, and improved survival: Should the paradigm be expanded? *Circulation* 1989; 79:441–444.
345. Tiefenbrunn AJ, Sobel BE: Thrombolysis and myocardial infarction. *Fibrinolysis* 1991; 5:1–15.
346. Verstraete M: Thrombolytic treatment in acute myocardial infarction. *Circulation* 1990; 82:96–109.
347. GISSI Group (Gruppo Italiano per lo studio della streptochinasi nell infarto miocardico): Effectiveness of intravenous thrombolytic treatment in acute myocardial infarction. *Lancet* 1986; 1:397–402.
348. Van de Werf F, Arnold AER: Intravenous tissue plasminogen activator and size of infarct, left ventricular function, and survival in acute myocardial infarction. *Br Med J* 1988; 297:1374–1379.
349. ISIS-2 (Second International Study of Infarct Survival): Collaborative Group: Randomized trial of intravenous streptokinase, oral aspirin, both or neither among 17,187 cases of suspected acute myocardial infarction ISIS-2. *Lancet* 1988; 2:349–360.
350. ISIS-3 Collaborative Group: ISIS-3: A randomized comparison of streptokinase vs tissue plasminogen activator vs anistreplase and of aspirin plus heparin vs aspirin alone among 41,299 cases of suspected acute myocardial infarction. *Lancet* 1992; 339:753–770.
351. Simoons ML, Serruys PW, van den Brand M, Res J, Verheugt FW, Krauss XH, et al: Early thrombolysis in acute myocardial infarction: Limitation of infarct size and improved survival. *J Am Coll Cardiol* 1986; 7:717–728.
352. Schwarz F, Faure A, Katus H, Von Olshausen K, Hoffmann M, Schuler G, et al: Intracoronary thrombolysis in acute myocardial infarction: An attempt to quantitate its effect by comparison of enzymatic estimate of myocardial necrosis with left ventricular ejection fraction. *Am J Cardiol* 1983; 51:1573–1578.
353. Ritchie JL, Cerquiera M, Maynard C, Davis K, Kennedy JW: Ventricular function and infarct size: The Western Washington intravenous streptokinase in myocardial infarction trial. *J Am Coll Cardiol* 1988; 11:689–697.
354. ISAM Study Group: A prospective trial of intravenous streptokinase in acute myocardial infarction: Mortality, morbidity and infarct size at 21 days. *N Engl J Med* 1986; 314:465–471.
355. Morgan CD, Roberts RS, Haq A, Baigrie RS, Daly PA, Gent M, et al: Coronary patency, infarct size and left ventricular function after thrombolytic therapy for acute myocardial infarction: Results from the tissue plasminogen activator: Toronto (TPAT) placebo-controlled trial, coronary perfusion and ventricular function. *J Am Coll Cardiol* 1991; 17:1451–1457.
356. Koren G, Weiss AT, Hasin Y, Appelbaum D, Welber S, Rosenman Y, et al: Prevention of myocardial damage in acute myocardial ischemia by early treatment with intravenous streptokinase. *N Engl J Med* 1985; 313:1384–1389.
357. O'Rourke M, Daron D, Koegh A, Kelly R, Nelson G, Barnes C, et al: Limitation of myocardial infarction by early infusion of recombinant tissue-type plasminogen activator. *Circulation* 1988; 77:1311–1315.
358. Guerci AD, Gerstenblith G, Brinker JA, Chandra NC, Gottlieb SO, Bahr RD, et al: A randomized trial of intravenous tissue plasminogen activator for acute myocardial infarction with subsequent randomization to elective coronary angioplasty. *N Engl J Med* 1987; 317:1613–1618.
359. National Heart Foundation of Australia: Coronary thrombolysis and myocardial salvage by tissue plasminogen activator given up to four hours after onset of myocardial infarction. *Lancet* 1988; 1:203–208.
360. Piegas LS, Canon SJF, AVezum AJ and EMERAS Investigators: Arterial patency and ejection fraction after late thrombolysis with streptokinase. Results from EMERAS (abstr.) *Eur Heart J* 1991; 12:97.
361. Wilcox RG: LATE assessment of thrombolytic efficacy: Randomized trial of altepase or placebo 6–24 hours after symptoms of acute myocardial infarction (abstr). *Eur Heart J* 1992; 13:423.
362. DeWood MA, Spores J, Notske R, Mouser LT, Burroughs R, Golden MS, et al: Prevalence of total coronary occlusion during the early hours of transmural myocardial infarction. *N Engl J Med* 1980; 303:897–902.
363. Merx W, Dorr R, Rentrop P, Blanke H, Karsch KR, Mathey DG, et al: Evaluation of the effectiveness of intracoronary streptokinase infusion in acute myocardial infarction: Postprocedure management and hospital course in 204 patients. *Am Heart J* 1981; 102:1181–1987.
364. Lew AS, Gelt I, Rodriguez L, Shah PK, Swan HJC, Ganz W: Short- and long-term mortality following intracoronary or intravenous streptokinase in acute myocardial infarction. *J Am Coll Cardiol* 1985; 5:496.
365. Chesebro JH, Knatterud G, Roberts R, Borer J, Cohen LS, Dalen J, et al: Thrombolysis in Myocardial Infarction (TIMI) Trial, Phase I: A comparison between intravenous tissue plasminogen activator and intravenous streptokinase. Clinical findings through hospital discharge. *Circulation* 1987; 76:142–154.
366. Ohman EM, Califf RM: Thrombolytic therapy: Overview of clinical trials. *Cor Artery Dis* 1990; 1:223–233.
367. Ohman EM, Califf RM, Topol EJ, Candela R, Abbottsmith C, Ellis S, Sigmon KN, Kereiakes D, George B, Stack R: Consequences of reocclusion after successful reperfusion therapy in acute myocardial infarction. *Circulation* 1990; 82:781–791.
368. Neuhaus KL, von Essen R, Tebbe U, Vogt A, Roth M, Riess M, et al: Improved thrombolysis in acute myocardial infarction with front-loaded administration of alteplase: Results of the rt-PA-APSAC Patency Study (TAPS). *J Am Coll Cardiol* 1991; 19:885–891.
369. Mathey DG, Schofer J, Sheehan FH, Krebber HJ, Justen M, Rodewald G, et al: Improved survival up to four years after early coronary thrombolysis. *Am J Cardiol* 1988; 61:524–529.
370. Roberts R: Thrombolysis and its sequelae: Calcium antagonists as potential adjunctive therapy. *Circulation* 1989; 80:IV-93–IV-101.

371. Kennedy JW, Ritchie JL, Davis KB, Fritz JK: Western Washington randomized trial of intracoronary streptokinase in acute myocardial infarction. *N Engl J Med* 1988; 309:1477–1482.
372. De Feyter PJ, Van Eenige MJ, van der Wall EE, Bezemer PD, van Engelen CL, Funke-Kupper AJ, et al: Effects of spontaneous and streptokinase-induced recanalization on left ventricular function after myocardial infarction. *Circulation* 1983; 67:1039–1044.
373. AIMS Trial Study Group: Effect of intravenous APSAC on mortality after acute myocardial infarction: Preliminary report of a placebo-controlled trial. *Lancet* 1988; 1:545–549.
374. Wilcox RG, von der Lippe G, Olsson CG, Jensen G, Skene AM, Hampton JR: Trial of tissue plasminogen activator for mortality reduction in acute myocardial infarction. *Lancet* 1988; 2:525–530.
375. Cigarroa RG, Lang RA, Hillis LD: Prognosis after acute myocardial infarction in patients with and without residual anterograde coronary blood flow. *Am J Cardiol* 1989; 64:155–160.
376. American Heart Association (ed): *Heart Facts 1983*. Dallas, American Heart Association, 1982.
377. Kuller L: Sudden death in arteriosclerotic heart disease; the case for preventive medicine. *Am J Cardiol* 1969; 24:617–628.
378. Fulton M, Julian DG, Oliver MF: Sudden death and myocardial infarction. *Circulation* 1969; 40:182–191.
379. Adgey AAJ, Allen JD, Geddes JS, James RG, Webb SW, Zaidi SA, et al: Acute phase of myocardial infarction. *Lancet* 1971; 2:501–504.
380. Simon AB, Feinleib M, Thompson HK Jr: Components of delay in the pre-hospital phase of acute myocardial infarction. *Am J Cardiol* 1972; 30:476–482.
381. Pressley JC, Severance HW Jr, Raney MP, McKinnis RA, Smith MW, Hindman MC, et al: A comparison of paramedic versus basic emergency medical care of patients at high and low risk during acute myocardial infarction. *J Am Coll Cardiol* 1988; 12:1555–1561.
382. Kareiakes DJ, Weaver WD, Anderson JL, Feldman T, Gibler B, Aufderheide T, et al: Time delays in the diagnosis and treatment of acute myocardial infarction: A tale of eight cities. Report from the Pre-hospital Study Group and the Cincinnati Heart Project. *Am Heart J* 1990; 120:773–780.
383. Goldstein S, Moss AJ, Greene W: Sudden death in acute myocardial infarction: Relationship to factors affecting delay in hospitalization. *Arch Intern Med* 1972; 129:720–724.
384. ACC/AHA: ACC/AHA Guidelines for the early management of patients with acute myocardial infarction. *Circulation* 1990; 82:664–707.
385. Lewis RP, Lanese RR, Stang JM, Chirikos TN, Keller MD, Warren JV: Reduction of mortality from prehospital myocardial infarction by prudent patient activation of mobile coronary care system. *Am Heart J* 1982; 103:123–130.
386. Weaver WD, Copass MK, Bufi D, Ray R, Hallstrom AP, Cobb LA: Improved neurologic recovery and survival after early defibrillation. *Circulation* 1984; 69:943–948.
387. Lowenstein E: Morphine "anesthesia"—a perspective. *Anesthesiology* 1971; 35:890.
388. Roberts R: Serum enzyme determinations in the diagnosis of acute myocardial infarction. In: Karliner JS, Gregoratos G (ed): *Coronary Care*. New York, Churchill Livingstone, 1980:213–237.
389. Mann T, Cohn PF, Holman L, Green LH, Markis JE, Phillips DA: Effect of nitroprusside on regional myocardial blood flow in coronary artery disease: Results in 25 patients and comparison with nitroglycerin. *Circulation* 1978; 57:732–738.
390. Chiariello M, Gold HK, Leinbach RC, Davis MA, Maroko PR: Comparison between the effects of nitroprusside and nitroglycerin on ischemic injury during acute myocardial infarction. *Circulation* 1976; 54:766–773.
391. Flaherty JT, Becker LC, Bulkley BH, Weiss JL, Gerstenblith G, Kallman CH, et al: A randomized prospective trial of intravenous nitroglycerin in patients with acute myocardial infarction. *Circulation* 1983; 68:576–588.
392. Bussmann WD, Passek D, Seidel W, Kaltenbach M: Reduction of CK and CK-MB indexes of infarct size by intravenous nitroglycerin. *Circulation* 1981; 63:615–622.
393. Jugdutt BI, Becker LC, Hutchins GM, Bulkley BH, Reid PR, Kallman CH: Effect of intravenous nitroglycerin on collateral blood flow and infarct size in the conscious dog. *Circulation* 1981; 63:17–28.
394. American College of Cardiology/American Heart Association Task Force: Guidelines for the early management of patients with acute myocardial infarction. *Circulation* 1990; 82:664–707.
395. Grimes CL, De Maria AN: Optimal utilization of thrombolytic therapy for acute myocardial infarction: Concepts and controversies. *J Am Coll Cardiol* 1990; 16:223–231.
396. Gruppo Italiano per lo Studio della Sopravvivenza nell'Infarto Miocardico. GISSI-2: A factorial randomised trial of alteplase versus streptokinase and heparin versus no heparin amount 12,490 patients with acute myocardial infarction. *Lancet* 1990; 336:65–71.
397. Krumholz HM, Pasternak RC, Weinstein MC, Friesinger GC, Ridker PM, Tosteson ANA, et al: Cost effectiveness of thrombolytic therapy with streptokinase in elderly patients with suspected acute myocardial infarction. *N Engl J Med* 1992; 327:7–13.
398. Grines CL, DeMaria AN: Optimal utilization of thrombolytic therapy for acute myocardial infarction: Concepts and controversies. *J Am Coll Cardiol* 1990; 16:223–231.
399. Califf RM, Topol EJ, Kereiakes DJ, Abbottsmith CW, George BS, Candela RJ, et al: Cardiac resuscitation should not be a contraindication to thrombolytic therapy for myocardial infarction. *Circulation* 1988; 78:II-127.
400. The TIMI Study Group: The Thrombolysis in Myocardial Infarction (TIMI) Trial: Phase I findings. *N Engl J Med* 1985; 312:932–936.
401. Hsia J, Hamilton WP, Kleiman NS, Roberts R, Chaitman B, Ross AM, et al: A comparison between heparin and low-dose aspirin as adjunctive therapy with tissue plasminogen activator for acute myocardial infarction. *N Engl J Med* 1990; 323:1433–1437.
402. The GUSTO Investigators: An international randomized trial comparing four thrombolytic strategies for acute myocardial infarction. *N Engl J Med* 329:673–682.
403. Granger CG, Califf RM, Hirsch J, Woodlief LH, Topol EJ, GUSTO Investigators: APTTs after thrombolysis and standard intravenous heparin are often low and correlate with body weight, age and sex: Experience from the GUSTO Trial. *Circulation* 1992; 86:I-258.
404. Hull RD, Raskob GE, Hirsh J, Jay RM, Leclerc JR, Geerts WH, et al: Continuous intravenous heparin compared with intermittent subcutaneous heparin in the initial treatment of proximal vein thrombosis. *N Engl J Med* 1986; 315:1109–1114.
405. Purvis JA, Trouton TG, Roberts MJ, McKeown P, Mulholland MG, Daizell GW, et al: Effectiveness of double bolus alteplase in the treatment of acute myocardial infarction. *Am J Cardiol* 1991; 68:1570–1574.
406. Roberts R: Heparin and aspirin in thrombolysis: Biological and clinical issues. *Clin Challenges* 1992; 1:1–7.
407. Francis CW, Markham RE, Jr., Barlow GH, Florack TM, Dobrzynski DM, Marder VJ: Thrombin activity of fibrin thrombi and soluble plasmic derivatives. *J Lab Clin Med* 1983; 102:220–230.
408. Funk CD, Funk LB, Kennedy ME, Pong AS, Fitzgerald GA: Human platelet/erythroleukemia cell prostaglandin G/H synthase: cDNA cloning, expression, and gene chromosomal assignment. *FASEB J* 1991; 5:2304–2312.
409. Hsia J, Kleiman NS, Aguirre FV, Chaitman BR, Roberts R, Ross AM, et al: Heparin-induced prolongation of partial thromboplastin time after thrombolysis: Relation to coronary artery patency. *J Am Coll Cardiol* 1992; 20:31–35.
410. Bleich SD, Nichols TC, Schumacher RR, Cooke DH, Tate DA, Teichman SL: Effect of heparin on coronary arterial patency after thrombolysis with tissue plasminogen activator in acute myocardial infarction. *Am J Cardiol* 1990; 66:1412–1417.
411. Topol EJ, George BS, Kereiakes DJ, Stump DC, Candela RJ, Abbottsmith CW, et al: A randomized controlled trial of intravenous tissue plasminogen activator and early intravenous heparin in acute myocardial infarction. *Circulation* 1989; 79:281–286.
412. Kander NH, Holland KJ, Pitt B, Topol EJ: A randomized pilot trial of brief versus prolonged heparin after successful reperfusion in acute myocardial infarction. *Am J Cardiol* 1990; 65:139–142.
413. Prins MH, Hirsh J: Heparin as an adjunctive treatment after thrombolytic therapy for acute myocardial infarction. *Am J Cardiol* 1991; 67:3A–11A.
414. The SCATI Group: Randomised controlled trial of subcutaneous calcium-heparin in acute myocardial infarction. *Lancet* 1989; 2:182–186.
415. ISIS-2 (Second International Study of Infarct Survival) Collabora-

tive Group: Randomized trial of intravenous streptokinase, oral aspirin, both, or neither among 17,187 cases of suspected acute myocardial infarction: ISIS-2. *J Am Coll Cardiol* 1988; 12:3A–13A.
416. Roux S, Christeller S, Ludin E: Effects of aspirin on coronary reocclusion and recurrent ischemia after thrombolysis: A meta-analysis. *J Am Coll Cardiol* 1992; 19:671–677.
417. TIMI IIIA Investigators: Early effects of tissue-type plasminogen activator added to conventional therapy on the culprit coronary lesion in patients presenting with ischemic cardiac pain at rest: Results of the Thrombolysis in Myocardial Ischemia (TIMI IIIA) Trial. *Circulation* 1993; 87:38–52.
418. Dabaghi SF, Kamat S, Hendricks O, Payne J, Kleiman NS: Low dose aspirin inhibits in vitro platelet aggregation within minutes after ingestion. *Circulation* 1992; 86:I-261.
419. Yusuf S, Peto R, Lewis J, Collins R, Sleight P: Beta blockade during and after myocardial infarction: an overview of the randomized trials. *Prog Cardiovasc Dis* 1985; 27:335–371.
420. Shechter M, Kaplinsky E, Rabinowitz B: The rationale of magnesium supplementation in acute myocardial infarction; a review of the literature. *Arch Intern Med* 1992; 152:2189–2196.
421. Woods KL, Fletcher S, Roffe C, Haider Y: Intravenous magnesium sulphate in suspected acute myocardial infarction; results of the second Leicester Intravenous Magnesium Intervention Trial (LIMIT-2). *Lancet* 1992; 339:1553–1558.
422. Horner SM. Efficacy of intravenous magnesium in acute myocardial infarction in reducing arrhythmia and mortality; meta analysis of magnesium in acute myocardial infarction. *Circulation* 1992; 86:774–779.
423. Grines CL, Browne KF, Marco J, Rothbaum D, Stone GW, O'Keefe J, et al: A comparison of immediate angioplasty with thrombolytic therapy for acute myocardial infarction. *N Engl J Med* 1993; 328:673–679.
424. Zijlstra F, deBoer MJ, Hoorntje JCA, Reiffers S, Rieber JHC, Suryapranata H: A comparison of immediate coronary angioplasty with intravenous streptokinase in acute myocardial infarction. *N Engl J Med* 1993; 328:680–684.
425. Gibbons RJ, Holmes DR, Reeder GS, Gailey KR, Hopfenspirger MR, Gersh BJ: Immediate angioplasty compared with the administration of a thrombolytic agent followed by conservative treatment for myocardial infarction. *N Engl J Med* 1993; 328:685–691.
426. Simoons MS, Arnold AER, Betriu A, de Bono DP, Col JJ, Dougherty FC, et al: Thrombolysis with tissue plasminogen activator in acute myocardial infarction. No additional benefit from immediate percutaneous coronary angioplasty. *Lancet* 1988; 1:197–203.
427. Verstraete M, Bory M, Collen D, Erbel R, Lennane RJ, Mathey D, et al: Randomized trial of intravenous recombinant tissue-type plasminogen activity versus intravenous streptokinase in acute myocardial infarction. Report from the European Cooperative Study Group for Recombinant Tissue-Type Plasminogen Activator. *Lancet* 1985; I:842–847.
428. SWIFT Trial Study Group: SWIFT trial of delayed elective intervention versus conservative treatment after thrombolysis with anistreplase in acute myocardial infarction. *Br Med J* 1991; 302:555–560.
429. TIMI Study Group: Comparison of invasive and conservative strategies after treatment with intravenous tissue plasminogen activator in acute myocardial infarction: Results of the thrombolysis in myocardial infarction (TIMI) phase II trial. *N Engl J Med* 1989; 320:618–626.
430. Williams DO, Braunwald E, Knatterud G, Babb J, Bresnahan JF, Greenberg MA, et al: One-year results of the Thrombolysis in Myocardial Infarction (TIMI) Phase II trial. *Circulation* 1992; 85:533–542.
431. Boden WE, Roberts R: Prognosis and management of patients with non-Q-wave myocardial infarction. In: Zipes DP, Rowlands DJ, (ed): *Progress in Cardiology*. Philadelphia, Lea & Febiger, 1991: 143–160.
431a. Wellens H: Right ventricular infarction. (editorial) *N Engl J Med* 1993; 328:1036–1038.
431b. Zehender M, Kasper W, Kauder E, Schonthaler M, Geibel A, Olschewski M, et al.: Right ventricular infarction as an independent predictor of prognosis after acute inferior myocardial infarction. *N Engl J Med* 1993; 328:981–988.
432. Diver DJ, Bier JD, Williams DO, McCabe CH, Braunwald E, TIMI-3A Study Group: Characterization of patients angiographically excluded from the TIMI-3A Trial. *Circulation* 1992; 86:I-454.
433. Boden WE, Krone RJ, Oakes D, Greenberg H, Dwyer EM Jr, Miller JP, et al: Electrocardiographic subset analysis of diltiazem administration on long-term outcome after acute myocardial infarction. *Am J Cardiol* 1991; 67:335–342.
434. The Multicenter Diltiazem Postinfarction Trial Research Group: The effect of diltiazem on mortality and reinfarction after myocardial infarction. *N Engl J Med* 1988; 319:385–392.
435. Klimt CR, Knatterud GL, Stamler J, Meier P: Persantine-aspirin reinfarction study. Part II. Secondary coronary prevention with persantine and aspirin. *J Am Coll Cardiol* 1986; 7:251–269.
436. Roberts R: Preventing recurrent myocardial infarction: Use of calcium-channel blockers. *Postgrad Med* 1988; 83:249–256.
437. Gheorghiade M, Schultz L, Tilley B, Kao W, Goldstein S: Natural history of the first non-Q-wave myocardial infarction in the placebo arm of the Beta-Blocker Heart Attack Trial. *Am Heart J* 1991; 122:1548–1553.
438. The MIAMI Trial Research Group: Metoprolol in acute myocardial infarction (MIAMI): A randomized placebo-controlled international trial. *Eur Heart J* 1985; 6:199–226.
439. The Norwegian Multicenter Study Group: Timolol-induced reduction in mortality and reinfarction in patients surviving acute myocardial infarction. *N Engl J Med* 1981; 304:801–807.
440. Cohn JN, Franciosa JA, Francis GS, Archibald D, Tristani F, Fletcher R, et al: Effect of short-term infusion of sodium nitroprusside on mortality rate in acute myocardial infarction complicated by left ventricular failure. *N Engl J Med* 1982; 306:1129–1135.
441. Durrer JD, Lie KI, van Capelle FJL, Durrer D: Effect of sodium nitroprusside on mortality in acute myocardial infarction. *N Engl J Med* 1982; 306:1121–1128.
442. Bussman W, Passek D, Seidel W, Kaltenbach M: Reduction of CK and CK-MB indexes of infarct size by intravenous nitroglycerin. *Circulation* 1981; 63:615–622.
443. Jaffe AS, Geltman EM, Tiefenbrunn AJ, Ambos HD, Strauss HD, Sobel BE, et al: Reduction of infarct size in patients with inferior infarction with intravenous glyceryl trinitrate. *Br Heart J* 1983; 49:452–460.
444. Chiche P, Derrida JP, Baligadoo S, Sal R: The treatment of recent myocardial infarction by prolonged infusion of trinitrin. *Novr Presse Med* 1977; 6:4119–4122.
445. Jugdutt BI, Warnica JW: Intravenous nitroglycerin therapy to limit myocardial infarct size, expansion, and complications. Effect of timing, dosage, and infarct location. *Circulation* 1988; 78:906–919.
446. Lis Y, Bennett D, Lambert G, Robson D: A preliminary double-blind study of intravenous nitroglycerin in acute myocardial infarction. *Intensive Care Med* 1984; 10:179–184.
447. Nelson GIC, Silke B, Ahuja RC, Hussain M, Taylor SH: Haemodynamic advantages of isosorbide dinitrate over furosemide in acute heart-failure following myocardial infarction. *Lancet* 1983; 730–733.
448. Hockings BEF, Cope GD, Clarke GM, Taylor DR: Randomized controlled trial of vasodilator therapy after myocardial infarction. *Am J Cardiol* 1981; 48:345–352.
449. Yusuf S, Wittes J, Friedman L: Overview of results of randomized clinical trials in heart disease: Treatments following myocardial infarction. *JAMA* 1988; 260:2088–2093.
450. Yusuf S, Peto R, Lewis J, Collin R, Sleight P: Beta-blockade during and after myocardial infarction: An overview of the randomized trials. *Prog Cardiovasc Dis* 1985; 27:335–371.
451. Lie KI, Wellens HJ, Van Capelle FJ, Durrer D: Lidocaine in the prevention of primary ventricular fibrillation: A double-blind, randomized study of 212 consecutive patients. *N Engl J Med* 1974; 291:1324–1326.
452. Koster RW, Dunning AJ: Intramuscular lidocaine for prevention of lethal arrhythmias in the prehospitalization phase of acute myocardial infarction. *N Engl J Med* 1985; 313:1105–1110.
453. MacMahon S, Collins R, Peto R, Koster RW, Yusuf S: Effects of prophylactic lidocaine in suspected acute myocardial infarction: An overview of results from the randomized, controlled trials. *JAMA* 1988; 260:1910–1916.
454. Hine LK, Laird N, Hewitt P, Chalmers TC: Meta-analytic evidence against prophylactic use of lidocaine in acute myocardial infarction. *Arch Intern Med* 1989; 149:2694–2698.

455. Wyman MG, Lalka D, Hammersmith L, Cannom DS, Goldreyer BN: Multiple bolus technique for lidocaine administration during the first hours of an acute myocardial infarction. *Am J Cardiol* 1978; 41:313–317.
456. Gianelly R, von der Groeben JO, Spivack AP, Harrison DC: Effect of lidocaine on ventricular arrhythmias in patients with coronary heart disease. *N Engl J Med* 1967; 277:1215–1219.
457. LeLorier J, Grenon D, Latour Y, Caille G, Dumont G, Brouseau A, et al: Pharmacokinetics of lidocaine after prolonged intravenous infusions in uncomplicated myocardial infarction. *Ann Intern Med* 1977; 87:700–706.
458. Zipes DP: Management of cardiac arrhythmias: Pharmacological, electrical and surgical techniques. In: Braunwald E (ed): *Heart Disease: A Textbook of Cardiovascular Medicine*, 3d ed. Philadelphia, Saunders, 1988: 625–627.
459. Prescott LF, Adjepon-Yamoah KK, Talbot RG: Impaired lignocaine metabolism in patients with acute myocardial infarction and cardiac failure. *Br Med J* 1976; 1:939–941.
460. Lown B, Vassaux C: Lidocaine in acute myocardial infarction. *Am Heart J* 1968; 76:586–587.
461. Nordrehaug JE, Johannessen KA, von der Lippe G: Serum potassium concentration as a risk factor of ventricular arrhythmias early in acute myocardial infarction. *Circulation* 1985; 71:645–649.
462. Lazzara R, El-Sherif N, Hope RR, Scherlag BJ: Ventricular arrhythmias and electrophysiological consequences of myocardial ischemia and infarction. *Circ Res* 1978; 42:740–749.
463. Gettes LS, Hill JL, Saito T, Kagiyama Y: Factors related to vulnerability to arrhythmias in acute myocardial infarction. *Am Heart J* 1982; 103:667–672.
464. Lie KI, Wellens HJJ, Downar E, Durrer D: Observations on patients with primary ventricular fibrillation complicating acute myocardial infarction. *Circulation* 1975; 52:755–759.
465. Campbell RWF, Murray A, Julian DG: Ventricular arrhythmias in first 12 hours of acute myocardial infarction. *Br Heart J* 1981; 46:351–357.
466. Campbell RWF, Murray A, Julian DG: Ventricular arrhythmias and ventricular fibrillation in acute myocardial infarction. *Am J Cardiol* 1979; 45:462.
467. Standards and guidelines for cardiopulmonary resuscitation (CPR) and emergency cardiac care (ECC). *JAMA* 1986; 255:2905–2989.
468. Volpi A, Cavalli A, Franzosi MG, Maggioni A, Mauri F, Santoro E, et al: One-year prognosis of primary ventricular fibrillation complicating acute myocardial infarction. *Am J Cardiol* 1989; 63:1174–1178.
469. Behar S, Goldbourt U, Reicher-Reiss H, Kaplinsky E, and the Principal Investigators of the SPRINT Study: Prognosis of acute myocardial infarction complicated by primary ventricular fibrillation. *Am J Cardiol* 1990; 66:1208–1211.
470. Bigger JT, Dresdale FJ, Heissenbuttel RH, Weld FM, Wit AL: Ventricular arrhythmias in ischemic heart disease: Mechanism, prevalence, significance, and management. *Prog Cardiovasc Dis* 1977; 19:255–300.
471. Sclarovsky S, Strasberg B, Martonovich G, Agmon J: Ventricular rhythms with intermediate rates in acute myocardial infarction. *Chest* 1978; 74:180–182.
472. Liberthson RR, Salisbury KW, Hutter AM, DeSanctis RW: Atrial tachyarrhythmias in acute myocardial infarction. *Am J Med* 1976; 60:956–960.
473. Zoni-Berisso M, Carratino L, Ferroni A, Mela GS, Mazzotta G, Vecchio C: Frequency, characteristics and significance of supraventricular tachyarrhythmias detected by 24-hour electrocardiographic recording in the late hospital phase of acute myocardial infarction. *Am J Cardiol* 1990; 65:1064–1070.
474. Gordon S, Finck DR, Perera RD, Levine J, Barnes SJ: Atrial infarction complicating an acute inferior myocardial infarction. *Arch Intern Med* 1984; 144:193.
475. Nielsen FE, Andersen HH, Gram-Hansen P, Sorensen JT, Klausen IC: The relationship between ECG signs of atrial infarction and the development of supraventricular arrhythmias in patients with acute myocardial infarction. *Am Heart J* 1992; 123:69–72.
476. James TN: Myocardial infarction and atrial arrhythmias. *Circulation* 1961; 24:761–776.
477. Goldberg RJ, Seeley D, Becker RC, Chen ZY, Osganian V, Gore JM, et al: Impact of atrial fibrillation on the in-hospital and long-term survival of patients with acute myocardial infarction: A community-wide perspective. *Am Heart J* 1990; 119:996–1001.
478. Hod H, Lew AS, Keltai M, Cercek B, Geft IL, Shah PK, et al: Early atrial fibrillation during evolving myocardial infarction: A consequence of impaired left atrial perfusion. *Circulation* 1987; 75:146–150.
479. Sugiura T, Iwasaka T, Takahashi N, Yuasa F, Takeuchi M, Hasegawa T, et al: Factors associated with atrial fibrillation in Q wave anterior myocardial infarction. *Am Heart J* 1991; 121:1409–1412.
480. Sugiura T, Iswasaka T, Takahashi N, Nakamura S, Taniguichi H, Nagaham Y, et al: Atrial fibrillation in inferior wall Q-wave acute myocardial infarction. *Am J Cardiol* 1991; 67:1135–1136.
481. Cardiac Arrhythmias Suppression Trial Investigators: Effect of encainide and flecainide on mortality in a randomized trial of arrhythmia suppression after myocardial infarction. *N Engl J Med* 1989; 321:406–412.
482. The Cardiac Arrhythmia Suppression Trial II Investigators: Effect of the antiarrhythmic agent moricizine on survival after myocardial infarction. *N Engl J Med* 1992; 327:227–233.
483. Konecke LL, Knoebel SB: Nonparoxysmal junctional tachycardia complicating acute myocardial infarction. *Circulation* 1972; 45:367–374.
484. DeSanctis RW, Block P, Hutter AM Jr: Tachyarrhythmias in myocardial infarction. *Circulation* 1972; 45:681–702.
485. Grauer LE, Gershen BJ, Orlando MM, Epstein SE: Bradycardia and its complications in the prehospital phase of acute myocardial infarction. *Am J Cardiol* 1973; 32:607–611.
486. Pantridge JF, Webb SW, Adgey AAJ: Arrhythmias in the first hours of acute myocardial infarction. *Prog Cardiovasc Dis* 1981; 23:265–278.
487. Dreifus LS, Fisch C, Griffin JC, Gillette PC, Mason JW, Parsonnet V: Guidelines for implantation of cardiac pacemakers and antiarrhythmic devices. A report of the American College of Cardiology/American Heart Association Task Force on assessment of diagnostic and therapeutic cardiovascular procedures. (Committee on Pacemaker Implantation). *Circulation* 1991; 84:455–467.
488. Chadda KD, Lichstein E, Gupta PK, Kourtesis P: Effects of atropine in patients with bradyarrhythmias complicating myocardial infarction. *Am J Med* 1977; 63:503–510.
489. Hatle L, Bathen J, Rokseth R: Sinoatrial disease in acute myocardial infarction: Long-term prognosis. *Br Heart J* 1976; 38:410–414.
490. Parameswaran R, Ohe T, Goldberg H: Sinus node dysfunction in acute myocardial infarction. *Br Heart J* 1976; 38:93–96.
491. Meltzer LE, Cohen HE: The incidence of arrhythmias associated with acute myocardial infarction. In: Meltzer LE, Dunning AJ (ed): *Textbook of Coronary Care*. Philadelphia, Charels Press, 1972:
492. Clemmensen P, Bates ER, Califf RM, Hlatky MA, Aronson L, George BS, et al: Complete atrioventricular block complicating inferior wall acute myocardial infarction treated with reperfusion therapy. *Am J Cardiol* 1991; 67:225–230.
493. Mavric Z, Zaputovic L, Matana A, Kucic J, Roje J, Marinovic D, et al: Prognostic significance of complete atrioventricular block in patients with acute inferior myocardial infarction with and without right ventricular involvement. *Am Heart J* 1990; 119:823–828.
494. Sugiura T, Iwasaka T, Takahashi N, Hata T, Hasegawa T, Matsutani M, et al: Factors associated with late onset of advanced atrioventricular block in acute Q wave inferior infarction. *Am Heart J* 1990; 119:1008–1013.
495. Nicod P, Gilpin E, Dittrich H, Polikar R, Henning H, Ross J Jr: Long-term outcome in patients with inferior myocardial infarction and complete atrioventricular block. *J Am Coll Cardiol* 1988; 12:589–594.
496. Kostuk WJ, Beanlands DS: Complete heart block associated with acute myocardial infarction. *Am J Cardiol* 1970; 26:380–384.
497. Hindman MC, Wagner GS, JaRo M, Atkins JM, Scheinman MM, DeSanctis RW, et al: The clinical significance of bundle branch block complicating acute myocardial infarction: Clinical characteristics, hospital mortality, and one-year follow-up. *Circulation* 1978; 58:679–688.
498. Hindman MC, Wagner GS, JaRo M, Atkins JM, Scheinman MM,

DeSanctis RW, et al: The clinical significance of bundle branch block complicating acute myocardial infarction: Indications for temporary and permanent pacemaker insertion. *Circulation* 1978; 58:689–699.
499. Lie KI, Liem KL, Schuilenburg RM, David GK, Durrer D: Early identification of patients developing late in-hospital ventricular fibrillation after discharge from the Coronary Care Unit: A $5\frac{1}{2}$ year retrospective and prospective study of 1,897 patients. *Am J Cardiol* 1978; 41:674–677.
500. Col JJ, Weinberg SL: The incidence and mortality of intraventricular conduction defects in acute myocardial infarction. *Am J Cardiol* 1972; 29:344–350.
501. Ritter WS, Atkins J, Blomqvist CG, Mullins CB: Permanent pacing in patients with transient trifascicular block during acute myocardial infarction. *Am J Cardiol* 1976; 38:205–208.
502. Domenighetti G, Perret C: Intraventricular conduction disturbances in acute myocardial infarction: Short- and long-term prognosis. *Eur J Cardiol* 1980; 11:51–59.
503. Lamas GA, Muller JE, Turi ZG, Stone PH, Rutherford JD, Jaffe AS, et al: A simplified method to predict occurrence of complete heart block during acute myocardial infarction. *Am J Cardiol* 1986; 57:1213–1219.
504. Bosch X, Theroux P, Waters DD, Pelletier GB, Roy D: Early postinfarction ischemia: Clinical, angiographic, and prognostic significance. *Circulation* 1987; 5:988–995.
505. Gibson RS, Young PM, Boden WE, Schechtman K, Roberts R, and the Diltiazem Reinfarction Study Group: Prognostic significance and beneficial effect of diltiazem on the incidence of early recurrent ischemia after non-Q-wave myocardial infarction: Results of the Diltiazem Reinfarction Study. *Am J Cardiol* 1987; 60:203–209.
506. Schechtman KB, Capone RJ, Kleiger RE, Gibson RS, Schwartz DJ, Roberts R, et al: Differential risk patterns associated with 3 month as compared with 3 to 12 month mortality and reinfarction after non-Q wave myocardial infarction. The Diltiazem Reinfarction Study Group. *J Am Coll Cardiol* 1990; 15:940–947.
507. St John Sutton M, Pfeffer MA, Plappert T, Arnold MO, Basta LL, Bittar N, et al: Survival and ventricular enlargement (SAVE) quantitative 2D echo substudy: Effects of ACE inhibition therapy on ventricular enlargement. *J Am Coll Cardiol* 1992; 19:767–772.
508. The SOLVD Investigators: Effect of enalapril on survival in patients with reduced left ventricular ejection fractions and congestive heart failure. *N Engl J Med* 1991; 325:293–302.
509. Forrester JS, Wyatt HL, da Luz PL, Tyberg JV, Diamond GA, Swan HJC: Functional significance of regional ischemic contraction abnormalities. *Circulation* 1976; 54:64–70.
510. Aroesty JM, McKay RG, Heller GV, Royal HD, Als AV, Grossman W: Simultaneous assessment of left ventricular systolic and diastolic dysfunction during pacing-induced ischemia. *Circulation* 1985; 71:889–900.
511. Tyberg JV, Forrester JS, Wyatt HL, Goldner SJ, Parmley WW, Swan HJC: An analysis of segmental ischemic dysfunction utilizing the pressure-length loop. *Circulation* 1974; 49:748–754.
512. Weisman HF, Healey B: Myocardial infarct expansion, infarct extension, and reinfarction: Pathophysiologic concepts. *Prog Cardiovasc Dis* 1987; 30:73–110.
513. Rigaud M, Rocha P, Boschat J, Farcot JC, Bardet J, Bourdarias JP: Regional left ventricular function assessed by contrast angiography in acute myocardial infarction. *Circulation* 1979; 60:130–139.
514. Parmley WW, Chuck L, Chatterjee K, Swan HJ, Klausner C, Glantz SA: Acute changes in the diastolic pressure-volume relationship of the left ventricle. *Eur J Cardiol* 1976; 4:105–120.
515. Smiseth OA, Rufsum H, Junemann J, Sievers RE, Lipton MJ, Carlsson E, et al: Ventricular diastolic pressure-volume shifts during acute ischemic left ventricular function in dogs. *J Am Coll Cardiol* 1984; 3:966.
516. Dikshit K, Vyden JK, Forrester JS, Chatterjee K, Prakash R, Swan HJC: Renal and extrarenal hemodynamic effects of furosemide in congestion heart failure after acute myocardial infarction. *N Engl J Med* 1973; 288:1087–1090.
517. Biddle TL, Yu PN: Effect of furosemide on hemodynamics and lung water in acute pulmonary edema secondary to myocardial infarction. *Am J Cardiol* 1979; 43:86.
518. Kiel J, Kelly DT, Taylor DR, Pitt B: The role of furosemide in the treatment of left ventricular dysfunction associated with acute myocardial infarction. *Circulation* 1973; 48:581.
519. Goldstein RA, Passamani ER, Roberts R: A comparison of digoxin and dobutamine in patients with acute infarction and failure. *N Engl J Med* 1980; 303:846–850.
520. Gillespie TA, Ambos HD, Sobel BE, Roberts R: Effects of dobutamine in patients with acute myocardial infarction. *Am J Cardiol* 1977; 39:588–594.
521. Kahn JC, Gueret P, Menier R, Giraudet P, Farhat MB, Bourdarias JP: Proganostic value of enzymatic (CPK) estimation of infarct size. *J Mol Med* 1977; 2:223–231.
522. Killip T, Kimbal JT: Treatment of myocardial infarction in a coronary care unit: A two year experience with 250 patients. *Am J Cardiol* 1967; 20:457.
523. Forrester JS, Diamond GA, Chatterjee K, Swan HJ: Medical therapy of acute myocardial infarction by application of hemodynamic subsets (first of two parts). *N Engl J Med* 1976; 295:1356–1362.
524. Forrester JS, Diamond GA, Chatterjee K, Swan HJ: Medical therapy of acute myocardial infarction by application of hemodynamic subsets (second of two parts). *N Engl J Med* 1976; 295:1404–1413.
525. Rackley CE, Satler LF, Pearle DL, Del Negro AA, Pallas RS, Kent KM: Use of hemodynamics measurements for management of acute myocadial infarction. *Cardiovasc Clin* 1986; 16:3–15.
526. Chiariella M, Gold HK, Leinbach RC, Davis MA, Maroko PR: Comparison between the effects of nitroprusside and nitroglycerine on ischemic injury during acute myocardial infarction. *Circulation* 1976; 54:766–773.
527. Roberts R, Ambos D: Evaluation of dobutamine in patients with cardiac failure and acute myocardial infarction. In: *International Dobutamine Symposium*. Munich, 1980: 208–216.
528. Clark G, Strauss HD, Roberts R: Dobutamine versus furosemide in the treatment of cardiac failure due to right ventricular function. *Chest* 1980; 77:220–223.
529. Roberts R: Inotropic therapy for cardiac failure associated with acute myocardial infarction. *Chest* 1988; 93:22S–24S.
530. Young JB, Roberts R: Heart failure. In: Dirks JH, Sutton RAL (eds): *Diuretics: Physiology, Pharmacology and Clinical Use*. Philadelphia, Saunders, 1986: 151–167.
531. Schreiber TL, Miller DH, Zola B: Management of myocardial infarction shock: Current status. *Am Heart J* 1989; 117:435–443.
532. Hill NS, Antman EM, Green LH, Alpert JS: Intravenous nitroglycerin: A review of pharmacology, indications, therapeutic effects and complications. *Chest* 1981; 79:69–76.
533. Wackers FJ, Lie KI, Becker AE, Durrer D, Wellens HJ: Coronary artery disease in patients dying from cardiogenic shock or congestive heart failure in the setting of acute myocardial infarction. *Br Heart J* 1976; 38:906–910.
534. Cercek B, Shah PK: Complicated acute myocardial infarction: Heart failure, shock, mechanical complications. *Cardiol Clinics* 1991; 9:569–593.
535. Gutovitz AL, Sobel BE, Roberts R: The progressive nature of myocardial injury in selected patients with cardiogenic shock. *Am J Cardiol* 1978; 41:469–475.
536. Goldberg LI: Cardiovascular and renal actions of dopamine: Potential clinical application. *Pharmacol Rev* 1972; 21:1–29.
537. Gunnar R, Mond Loeb HS: Shock in acute myocardial infarction: Evaluation of physiologic therapy. *J Am Coll Cardiol* 1983; 1:154–163.
538. Mikulic E, Cohn JN, Franciosa JA: Comparative hemodynamic effects of inotropic and vasodilator drugs in severe heart failure. *Circulation* 1977; 56:528–533.
539. Miller RR, Awan NA, Joyce JA, Maxwell KS, DeMaria AN, Amsterdam EA, et al: Combined dopamine and nitroprusside therapy in congestive heart failure. *Circulation* 1977; 55:881–884.
540. Richard C, Ricome JL, Rimailho A, Bottineau G, Auzepy P: Combined hemodynamic effects of dopamine and dobutamine in cardiogenic shock. *Circulation* 1983; 67:620–626.
541. Lee L, Erbel R, Brown TM, Laufer N, Meyer J, O'Neill WW: Multicenter registry of angioplasty therapy of cardiogenic shock: Initial and longerm survival. *J Am Coll Cardiol* 1991; 17:599–603.
542. Waller BF, Rothbaum DA, Pinkerton CA, Cowley MJ, Linnemeier TJ, Orr C, et al: States of the myocardium and infarct-related coronary artery is 19 necropsy patients with acute recanalization

using pharmacologic (Streptokinase, recombinant tissue plasminogen activator), mechanical (percutaneous transluminal coronary angioplasty) or combined types of reperfusion therapy. *J Am Coll Cardiol* 1987; 9:785–801.

543. Brodie BR, Weintraub RA, Stuckey TD, LeBauer EJ, Katz JD, Kelly TA, et al: Outcomes of direct coronary angioplasty for acute myocardial infarction in candidates and noncandidates for thrombolytic therapy. *Am J Cardiol* 1991; 67:7–12.
544. Wei JY, Hutchins GM, Buckley BH: Papillary muscle rupture in fatal acute myocardial infarction: A potentially treatable form of cardiogenic shock. *Ann Intern Med* 1979; 90:149–152.
545. Nishimura RA, Schoff HV, Shub C, Gersh BJ, Edwards WD, Tajik AJ: Papillary muscle rupture complicating acute myocardial infarction: Analysis of 17 patients. *Am J Cardiol* 1983; 51:373–377.
546. Kossowsky WA, Epstein PJ, Levine RS: Post myocardial infarction syndrome: An early complication of acute myocardial infarction. *Chest* 1973; 63:35–39.
547. Lie JT, Wright KE Jr, Titus JL: Sudden appearance of a systolic murmur after acute myocardial infarction. *Am Heart J* 1975; 90:507–512.
548. Shelburne JC, Rubinstein D, Gorlin R: A reappraisal of papillary muscle dysfunction: Correlative clinical and angiographic study. *Am J Med* 1969; 46:862–871.
549. DeBusk RF, Harrison DC: The clinical spectrum of papillary-muscle disease. *N Engl J Med* 1969; 281:1458–1467.
550. Burch GE, DePasquale NP, Phillips JH: The syndrome of papillary muscle dysfunction. *Am Heart J* 1968; 75:399–414.
551. Radford MJ, Johnson RA, Daggett WM, Fallon JT, Buckley MJ, Gold HK, et al: Ventricular septal rupture: A review of clinical and physiologic features and an analysis of survival. *Circulation* 1981; 64:545–553.
552. Rasmussen S, Leth A, Kjoller E, Pedersen A: Cardiac rupture in acute myocardial infarction: A review of 72 consecutive cases. *Acta Med Scand* 1979; 205:11–16.
553. Maker JF, Mallory GK, Laurenz GA: Rupture of the heart after myocardial infarction. *N Engl J Med* 1956; 255:1–10.
554. Held AC, Cole PL, Lipton B, Gore JM, Antman EM, Hochman JS, et al: Rupture of the interventricular septum complicating acute myocardial infarction: A multicenter analysis of clinical findings and outcome. *Am Heart J* 1988; 116:1330–1336.
555. Gaudiani VA, Miller DG, Stinson EB, Oyer PE, Reitz BA, Moreno-Cabral RJ, et al: Postinfarction ventricular septal defect: An argument for early operation. *Surgery* 1981; 89:48–54.
556. Gray RJ, Sethna D, Matloff JM: The role of cardiac surgery in acute myocardial infarction. I. With mechanical complications. *Am Heart J* 1983; 106:723–728.
557. Moore CA, Nygard TW, Kaiser DS, Cooper AA, Gibson RS: Postinfarction ventricular septal rupture: The importance of location of infarction and right ventricular function in determining survival. *Circulation* 1986; 74:45–55.
558. Bates RJ, Beutler S, Resnekor L, Anagnostopoulos CE: Cardiac rupture—challenge in diagnosis and management. *Am J Cardiol* 1970; 40:429–437.
559. Rasmussen S, Leth A, Kjoller E, Pedersen A: Cardiac rupture in acute myocardial infarction: A review of 72 consective cases. *Acta Med Scand* 1979; 205(102):11–16.
560. Maker JS, Mallory GK, Laurenz GA: Rupture of heart after myocardial infarction. *N Engl J Med* 1956; 255:1–10.
561. Roberts WG, Morrow AG: Pseudoaneurysm of the left ventricle: An unusual sequel of myocardial infarction and rupture of the heart. *Am J Med* 1967; 43:639–644.
562. Cabin HS, Roberts WC: Left ventricular aneurysm, intraaneurysmal thrombus and systemic embolus in coronary heart disease. *Chest* 1980; 77:586–589.
563. Krainin FM, Flessas AP, Spodick DH: Infarction-associated pericarditis: Rarity of diagnostic electrocardiogram. *N Engl J Med* 1984; 311:1211–1214.
564. Thadani U, Chopra MP, Aber CP, Portal RW: Pericarditis after acute myocardial infarction. *Br Med J* 1971; 2:135–137.
565. Erhardt LR: Clinical and pathological observations in different types of acute myocardial infarction: A study of 84 patients deceased after treatment in a coronary care unit. *Acta Med Scand* 1974; 560:1–78.
566. Barman PC, Krishnaswami V, Geraci AR: Pericarditis in acute myocardial infarction. *NYS J Med* 1973; 73:645–648.
567. Guillevin L, Valere PE: Pericarditis in acute myocardial infarction. *Lancet* 1976; 1:429.
568. Berman J, Haffajee CI, Alpert JS: Therapy of symptomatic pericarditis after myocardial infarction: Retrospective and prospective studies of aspirin, indomethacin, prednisone, and spontaneous resolution. *Am Heart J* 1981; 101:750–753.
569. Dressler W: The post-myocardial-infarction syndrome. *Arch Intern Med* 1959; 103:28–42.
570. Hayes MJ, Morris GK, Hampton JR: Lack of effect of bed rest and cigarette smoking on development of deep venous thrombus after myocardial infarction. *Br Heart J* 1976; 38:981–983.
571. Miller RR, Lies JE, Carretta RF, Wampold DB, DeNardo GL, Kraus JF, et al: Prevention of lower extremity venous thrombus by early mobilization. *Ann Intern Med* 1976; 84:700–703.
572. Emerson PA, Marks P: Preventing thromboembolism after myocardial infarction: Effect of low-dose heparin or smoking. *Br Med J* 1977; 1:18–20.
573. Weinreich DJ, Burke JF, Pauletto FJ: Left ventricular mural thrombi complicating acute myocardial infarction. *Ann Intern Med* 1984; 100:789–794.
574. Visser CA, Kan G, Meltzer RS, Dunning AJ, Roelandt J: Embolic potential of left ventricular thrombus after myocardial infarction: A two-dimensional echocardiographic study of 119 patients. *J Am Coll Cardiol* 1985; 5:1276–1280.
575. Kouvaras G, Chronopoulas G, Soufras G, Sofronas G, Solomos D, Bakirtzis A, et al: The effects of long term antithrombotic treatment on left ventricular thrombi in patients after an acute myocardial infarction. *Am Heart J* 1990; 119:73–78.
576. Keating EC, Gross SA, Schlamowitz RA, Glassman J, Mazur HJ, Pitt WA, et al: Mural thrombi in myocardial infarctions: Prospective evaluation by two dimensional echocardiography. *Am J Med* 1983; 74:989–995.
577. Spirito P, Bellotti P, Chiarella F: Prognostic significance and natural history of left ventricular thrombi in patients with acute anterior myocardial infarction: A two-dimensional echocardiographic study. *Circulation* 1985; 72:774–780.
578. Jugdutt BI, Sivaram CA: Prospective two-dimensional echocardiographic evaluation of left ventricular thrombus and embolism after acute myocardial infarction. *J Am Coll Cardiol* 1989; 13:554–564.
579. Johannssen KA, Nordrehoug JE, Vonder Lippe G, Vollset SE: Risk factors for embolization in patients with left ventricular thrombi and acute myocardial infarction. *Br Heart J* 1988; 60:104–110.
580. Davis MJE, Ireland MA: Effect of early anticoagulation on the frequency of left ventricular thrombi after anterior wall acute myocardial infarction. *Am J Cardiol* 1986; 57:1244–1247.
581. Lapeyre AC, III, Steele PM, Kazmier FJ, Chesebro JH, Vlietstra RE; Fuster V: Systemic embolism in chronic left ventricular aneurysm: Incidence and the role of anticoagulation. *J Am Coll Cardiol* 1985; 6:534–538.
582. Turpie ACG, Robinson JG, Doyle DJ, Mulji AS, Mishkel GJ, Sealey BJ, et al.: Comparison of high-dose with low-dose subcutaneous heparin to prevent left ventricular mural thrombosis in patients with acute transmural anterior myocardial infarction. *N Engl J Med* 1989; 320:352–357.
583. Takamoto T, Kim D, Urie PM, Guthaner DF, Gordon HJ, Keren A, et al: Comparative recognition of left ventricular thrombi by echocardiography and cineangiography. *Br Heart J* 1985; 53:36–42.
584. Sechtem U, Theissen P, Heindel W, Hungerberg K, Deutsch HJ, Welslau R, et al: Diagnosis of left ventricular thrombi by magnetic resonance imaging and comparison with angiocardiography, computed tomography and echocardiography. *Am J Cardiol* 1989; 64:1195–1199.
585. Faxon DP, Ryan TJ, Davis KB, McCabe CH, Myers W, Lesperance J, et al: Prognostic significance of angiographically documented left ventricular aneurysm from the coronary artery surgery study (CASS). *Am J Cardiol* 1982; 50:157–164.
586. Loop FD, Effler DB, Webster JS, Groves LK: Posterior ventricular aneurysms. Etiologic factors and surgical treatment. *N Engl J Med* 1973; 288:237–239.
587. Loop FD, Effler DB, Navia JA, Sheldon WC, Groves LK: Aneurysms of the left ventricle: Survival and results of a ten-year surgical experience. *Ann Surg* 1973; 178:399–405.
588. Visser CA, Kan G, David GK, Lie KI, Durrer D: Echocardiographic-cineangiographic correlation in detecting left ventricular

aneurysm: A prospective study of 422 patients. *Am J Cardiol* 1982; 50:337–341.

589. Roberts WC, Morrow AG: Pseudoaneurysm of the left ventricle: An unusual sequel of myocardial infarction and rupture of the heart. *Am J Med* 1967; 43:639–644.
590. Catherwood E, Mintz GS, Kotler MN, Parry WR, Segal BL: Two-dimensional echocardiographic recognition of left ventricular pseudo-aneurysm. *Circulation* 1980; 62:294–303.
591. Martin RH, Almond CH, Saab S, Watson LE: True and false aneurysms of the left ventricle following myocardial infarction. *Am J Med* 1977; 62:418–424.
592. Goble AJ, Sloman G, Robinson JS: Mortality reduction in a coronary care unit. *Br Med J* 1966; 1:1005–1009.
593. Graboys TB: In-hospital sudden death after coronary care unit discharge: A high risk profile. *Arch Intern Med* 1975; 135:512–514.
594. Grace WJ, Yarvote PM: Acute myocardial infarction: The course of the illness following discharge from the coronary care unit. A description of the intermediate coronary care unit. *Chest* 1971; 59:15–17.
595. Christensen D, Ford M, Reading J, Castle CH: Sudden death in the late hospital phase of acute myocardial infarction. *Arch Intern Med* 1977; 137:1675–1679.
596. Frieden J, Cooper JA: The role of the intermediate cardiac care unit. *JAMA* 1976; 235:816–819.
597. Levine A, Lown B: The "chair" treatment of coronary thrombosis. *Trans Assoc Am Phys* 1951; 64:316.
598. McNeer JF, Wagner GS, Ginsburg PB, Wallace AG, McCants CB, Conley MJ, et al: Hospital discharge one week after acute myocardial infarction. *N Engl J Med* 1978; 298:229–232.
599. Madsen EB, Hougaard P, Gilpin E, Pedersen A: The length of hospitalization after acute myocardial infarction determined by risk calculation. *Circulation* 1983; 68:9–16.
600. Bigger JT, Fleiss JL, Kleiger R, Miller JP, Rolnitzky LM, the Multicenter Post-Infarction Research Group: The relationships among ventricular arrhythmias, left ventricular dysfunction, and mortality in the 2 years after myocardial infarction. *Circulation* 1984; 69:250–258.
601. Theroux P, Waters DD, Halphen C, Debaisieux J, Mizgala HF: Prognostic value of exercise testing soon after myocardial infarction. *N Engl J Med* 1979; 301:341–345.
602. Epstein SE, Palmeri ST, Patterson RE: Evaluation of patients after acute myocardial infarction, Indications for cardiac catheterization and surgical intervention. *N Engl J Med* 1982; 307:1487–1492.
603. Henning H, Gilpin EA, Covell JW, Swan EA, O'Rourke RA, Ross J Jr: Prognosis after acute myocardial infarction: A multivariate analysis of mortality and survival. *Circulation* 1979; 59:1124–1134.
604. Iskandrian AS, Hakki AH, Kotler MN, Segal BL, Herling I: Evaluation of patients with acute myocardial infarction: Which test, for whom and why? *Am Heart J* 1985; 109:391–394.
605. Pratt CM, O'Rourke R: Application and interpretation of submaximal exercise testing and ambulatory ECG recordings in patients with acute myocardial infarction. *Chest* 1988; 93:29S–32S.
606. Madsen EB, Gilpin E: How much prognostic information do exercise test data add to clinical data after acute myocardial infarction? *Int J Cardiol* 1983; 4:15–27.
607. Krone RJ, Miller JP, Gillespie JA, Weld FM, Multicenter Post-Infarction Research Group: Usefulness of low-level exercise testing early after acute myocardial infarction in patients taking beta-blocking agents. *Am J Cardiol* 1987; 60:23–27.
608. Schwartz KM, Turner JD, Sheffield LT, Roitman DI, Kansal S, Papapietro SE, et al: Limited exercise testing soon after myocardial infarction. *Ann Intern Med* 1981; 94:727–734.
609. Fioretti P, Brower RW, Simoons ML, Bos RJ, Baardmen T, Beelen A, et al: Prediction of mortality during the first year after acute myocardial infarction from clinical variables and stress test at hospital discharge. *Am J Cardiol* 1985; 55:1313–1318.
610. Krone RJ, Gillespie JA, Weld FM, Miller JP, Moss AJ: Low-level exercise testing after myocardial infarction: Usefulness in enhancing clinical risk stratification. *Circulation* 1985; 71:80–89.
611. DeBusk RF, Haskell W: Symptom-limited vs. heart-rate-limited exercise testing soon after myocardial infarction. *Circulation* 1980; 61:738–743.
612. Starling MR, Crawford MH, Kennedy GT, O'Rourke RA: Exercise testing early after myocardial infarction: Predictive value for subsequent unstable angina and death. *Am J Cardiol* 1980; 46:909–914.
613. Murray DP, Salih M, Tan LB, Derry S, Murray RG, Littler WA: Which exercise test variables are of prognostic importance post-myocardial infarction? *Int J Cardiol* 1988; 20:353–363.
614. Fuller CM, Raizner AE, Verani MS, Nahormek PA, Chahine RA, McEntee CW, et al: Early post-myocardial infarction treadmill stress testing. *Ann Intern Med* 1981; 94:734–739.
615. Sami M, Kraemer H, DeBusk RF: The prognostic significance of serial exercise testing after myocardial infarction. *Circulation* 1979; 60:1238–1246.
616. Smith JW, Dennis CA, Gassmann A, Gaines JA, Staman M, Phibbs B, et al: Exercise testing 3 weeks after myocardial infarction. *Chest* 1979; 75:12–16.
617. Gibson RS, Watson DD, Craddock GB, Crampton RS, Kaiser DL, Denny MJ, et al: Prediction of cardiac events after uncomplicated myocardial infarction: A prospective study comparing predischarge exercise thallium-201 scintigraphy and coronary angiography. *Circulation* 1983; 68:321–336.
618. Jain A, Suarez J, Mahmarian JJ, Zoghbi WA, Quiñones MA, Verani MS: Functional significance of myocardial perfusion defects induced by dipyridamole using thallium-201 single-photon emission computer tomography and two-dimensional echocardiography. *Am J Cardiol* 1990; 66:802–806.
619. Cheirif J, Zoghbi WA, Bolli R, O'Neill PG, Hoyt BD, Quiñones MA: Assessment of regional myocardial perfusion by contrast echocardiography. II. Detection of changes in transmural and subendocardial perfusion during dipyridamole-induced hyperemia in a model of critical coronary stenosis. *J Am Coll Cardiol* 1989; 14:1555–1565.
620. Abreu A, Mahmarian JJ, Nishimura S, Boyce TM, Verani MS: Tolerance and safety of pharmacologic coronary vasodilation with adenosine in association with thallium-201 scintigraphy in patients with suspected coronary artery disease. *J Am Coll Cardiol* 1991; 18:730–735.
621. Fung AY, Gallagher KP, Buda AJ: The physiologic basis of dobutamine as compared with dipyridamole stress interventions in the assessment of critical coronary stenosis. *Circulation* 1987; 76:943–951.
622. Gottlieb SO, Weisfeldt ML, Ouyang P, Mellits ED, Gerstenblith G: Silent ischemia as a marker for early unfavorable outcomes in patients with unstable angina. *N Engl J Med* 1986; 314:1214–1219.
623. Farrell TG, Bashir Y, Cripps T, Malik M, Poloniecki J, Bennett ED, et al: Risk stratification for arrhythmic events in postinfarction patients based on heart rate variability, ambulatory electrocardiographic variables and the signal-averaged electrocardiogram. *J Am Coll Cardiol* 1991; 18:687–697.
624. Kleiger RE, Miller JP, Bigger JT, Moss AJ, the Multicenter Post-Infarction Research Group: Decreased heart rate variability and its association with increased mortality after acute myocardial infarction. *Am J Cardiol* 1987; 59:256–262.
625. Kleiger RE, Miller JP, Krone RJ, Bigger JT, the Multicenter Postinfarction Research Group: The independence of cycle length variability and exercise testing on predicting mortality of patients surviving acute myocardial infarction. *Am J Cardol* 1990; 65:408–411.
626. Gomes JA, Winters SL, Martinson M, Machac J, Stewart D, Targonski A: The prognostic significance of quantitative signal-averaged variables relative to clinical variables, site of myocardial infarction, ejection fraction and ventricular premature beats: A prospective study. *J Am Coll Cardiol* 1989; 13:377–384.
627. Weld FM, Chu KL, Bigger JT, Rolnitzky LM: Risk stratification with low-level exercise testing 2 weeks after acute myocardial infarction. *Circulation* 1981; 64:306–314.
628. Senaratne MPJ, Hsu L, Rossall RE, Kappagoda CT: Exercise testing after myocardial infarction: Relative values of the low level predischarge and the postdischarge exercise test. *J Am Coll Cardiol* 1988; 12:1416–1422.
629. De Feyter PJ, Van Eenige MJ, Dighton DH, Visser FC, de Jong J, Roos JP: Prognostic value of exercise testing, coronary angiography and left ventriculography 6–8 weeks after myocardial infarction. *Circulation* 1982; 66:527–536.
630. Stone PH, Turi ZG, Muller JE, Parker C, Hartwell T, Rutherford JD, et al: Prognostic significance of the treadmill exercise test

performance 6 months after myocardial infarction. *J Am Coll Cardiol* 1986; 8:1007–1017.

631. Starling MR, Crawford MH, Kennedy GT, O'Rourke RA: Treadmill exercise tests predischarge and six weeks post-myocardial infarction to detect abnormalities of known prognostic value. *Ann Intern Med* 1981; 94:721–727.
632. Davidson DM, DeBusk RF: Prognostic value of a single exercise test 3 weeks after uncomplicated myocardial infarction. *Circulation* 1980; 61:236–242.
633. Leppo J, Plaja J, Gionet M, Tumolo J, Paraskos JA, Cutler BS: Noninvasive evaluation of cardiac risk before elective vascular surgery. *J Am Coll Cardiol* 1987; 9:269–276.
634. Pines A, Fisman EZ, Ben-Ari E, Modan M, Kessler G, Drory Y, et al: Usefulness of immediate postexercise two-dimensional echocardiography in post-myocardial infarction patients without ischemic ECG changes in stress testing: Comparison with radionuclide angiography. *Angiology* 1989; 40:605–612.
635. Limacher MC, Quiñones MA, Poliner LR, Nelson JG, Winters WL, Waggoner AD: Detection of coronary artery disease with exercise two-dimensional echocardiography: Description of a clinicallly applicable method and comparison with radionuclide ventriculography. *Circulation* 1983; 67:1211–1218.
636. Moss AJ, DeCamilla J, Davis H: Cardiac death in the first 6 months after myocardial infarction: Potential for mortality reduction in the early posthospital period. *Am J Cardiol* 1977; 39:816–820.
637. Ruberman W, Weinblatt E, Goldberg JD, Frank CW, Shapiro S: Ventricular premature beats and mortality after myocardial infarction. *N Engl J Med* 1977; 297:750–757.
638. Pratt CM, Francis MJ, Luck JC, Wyndham CR, Miller RR, Quiñones MA: Analysis of ambulatory electrocardiograms in 15 patients during spontaneous ventricular fibrillation with special reference to preceding arrhythmic events. *J Am Coll Cardiol* 1983; 2:789–797.
639. The Cardiac Arrhythmia Suppression Trial (CAST) Investigators: Preliminary report: effect of encainide and flecainide on mortality in a randomized trial of arrhythmia suppression after myocardial infarction. *N Engl J Med* 1989; 321:406–412.
640. The Cardiac Arrhythmia Pilot Study (CAPS) Investigators: Effects of encainide, flecainide, imipramine, and moricizine on ventricular arrhythmias during the year after acute myocardial infarction: The CAPS. *Am J Cardiol* 1988; 61:501–509.
641. Friedman LM, Byington RP, Capone RJ, Furberg CD, Goldstein S, Lichstein E, et al: Effect of propranolol in patients with myocardial infarction and ventricular arrhythmia. *J Am Coll Cardiol* 1986; 7:1–8.
642. Gottlieb SO, Weisfeldt M, Achuff SC, Baumgardner R, Mellits ED, Weisfeldt M, et al: Silent ischemia on Holter monitoring predicts mortality in high-risk postinfarction patients. *JAMA* 1988; 259:1030–1035.
643. Schwartz PJ, Vanol E, Stramba-Badiale M, De Ferrari GM, Billman GE, Foreman RD: Autonomic mechanisms and sudden death: New insights from analysis of baroreceptor reflexes in conscious dogs with and without a myocardial infarction. *Circulation* 1988; 78:669–679.
644. Lown B, Verrier RL: Neural activity and ventricular fibrillation. *N Engl J Med* 1976; 294:1165–1170.
645. Turritto G, Fontaine JM, Ursell S, Caref EB, Bekheit S, El-Sherif N: Risk stratification and management of patients with organic heart disease and nonsustained VT: Role of programmed stimulation, LVEF, and the signal-averaged electrocardiogram. *Am J Med* 1990; 88:35N–41N.
646. El-Sherif N, Ursell SN, Bekheit S, Fontaine J, Turrit G, Henkin R, et al: Prognostic significance of the signal-averaged ECG depends on the time of recording in the postinfarction period. *Am Heart J* 1989; 118:256–264.
647. Kuchar DL, Thorburn CW, Sammel NL: Prediction of serious arrhythmic events after myocardial infarction: Signal-averaged electrocardiogram, Holter monitoring and radionuclide ventriculography. *J Am Coll Cardiol* 1987; 9:531–538.
648. Denniss AR, Richards DA, Cody DV, Russell PA, Young AA, Cooper MJ, et al: Prognostic significance of ventricular tachycardia and fibrillation induced at programmed stimulation and delayed potentials detected on the signal-averaged electrocardiograms of survivors of acute myocardial infarction. *Circulation* 1986; 74:731–745.
649. Cripps T, Bennett D, Camm J, Ward D: Prospective evaluation of clinical assessment, exercise testing and signal-averaged electrocardiogram in predicting outcome after acute myocardial infarction. *Am J Cardiol* 1988; 62:995–999.
650. Breithardt G, Schwarzmaier J, Borggrefe M, Haerten K, Seipel L: Prognostic significance of late ventricular potentials after acute myocardial infarction. *Eur Heart J* 1983; 4:487–495.
651. Simson MB: Use of signals in the terminal QRS complex to identify patients with ventricular tachycardia after myocardial infarction. *Circulation* 1981; 64:235–242.
652. Kanovsky MS, Falcone RA, Dresden CA, Josephson ME, Simson MB: Identification of patients with ventricular tachycardia after myocardial infarction: Signal-averaged electrocardiogram, Holter monitoring, and cardiac catheterization. *Circulation* 1984; 70:264–270.
653. Zipes DP, Akhtar M, Denes P, DeSanctis RW, Garson A, Gettes LS, et al: Guidelines for clinical intracardiac electrophysiologic studies: A report of the American College of Cardiology/American Heart Association Task Force on assessment of diagnostic and therapeutic cardiovascular procedures. *J Am Coll Cardiol* 1989; 14:1827–1842.
654. Pratt CM, Thornton BC, Magro SA, Wyndham CRC: Spontaneous arrhythmia detected on ambulatory electrocardiographic recording lacks precision in predicting inducibility of ventricular tachycardia during electrophysiologic study. *J Am Coll Cardiol* 1987; 10:97–104.
655. Bourke JP, Richards DAB, Ross DL, Wallace EM, McGuire MA, Uther JB: Routine programmed electrical stimulation in survivors of acute myocardial infarction for prediction of spontaneous ventricular tachyarrhythmias during follow-up: Results, optimal stimulation protocol and cost-effective screening. *J Am Coll Cardiol* 1991; 18:780–788.
656. Kowey PR, Waxman HL, Greenspon A, Greenberg R, Poll D, Kutalek S, et al: Value of electrophysiologic testing in patients with previous myocardial infarction and nonsustained ventricular tachycardia. *Am J Cardiol* 1990; 65:594–598.
657. Gonzalez R, Arriagada D, Corbalan R, Chamorro G, Fajuri A, Rodriguez JA: Role of programmed electrical stimulation of the heart in risk stratification post-myocardial infarction. *PACE* 1988; 11:283–288.
658. Roy D, Marchand E, Theroux P, Waters DD, Pelletier GB, Bourassa MG: Programmed ventricular stimulation in survivors of an acute myocardial infarction. *Circulation* 1985; 72:487–494.
659. Santarelli P, Bellocci F, Loperfido F, Mazzari M, Mongiardo R, Montenero AS, et al: Ventricular arrhythmia induced by programmed ventricular stimulation after acute myocardial infarction. *Am J Cardiol* 1985; 55:391–394.
660. Waspe LE, Seinfeld D, Ferrick A, Kim SG, Matos JA, Fisher JD: Prediction of sudden death and spontaneous ventricular tachycardia in survivors of complicated myocardial infarction: Value of the response to programmed stimulation using a maximum of three ventricular extra stimuli. *J Am Coll Cardiol* 1985; 5:1292–1301.
661. Bhandari AK, Rose JS, Kotlewski A, Rahimtoola SH, Wu D: Frequency and significance of induced sustained ventricular tachycardia or fibrillation two weeks after acute myocardial infarction. *Am J Cardol* 1985; 56:737–742.
662. Richards DA, Cody DV, Denniss AR, Russell PA, Young AA, Uther JB: Ventricular electrical instability: A predictor of death after myocardial infarction. *Am J Cardiol* 1983; 51:75–80.
663. Marchlinski FE, Buxton AE, Waxman HL, Josephson ME: Identifying patients at risk of sudden death after myocardial infarction: Value of the response to programmed stimulation, degree of ventricular ectopic activity and severity of left ventricular dysfunction. *Am J Cardiol* 1983; 52:1190–1196.
664. Hamer A, Vohra J, Hunt D, Sloman G: Prediction of sudden death by electrophysiologic studies in high risk patients surviving acute myocardial infarction. *Am J Cardiol* 1982; 50:223–229.
665. The ESVEM Investigators: Determinants of predicted efficacy of antiarrhythmic drugs in the electrophysiologic study versus electrocardiographic monitoring trial. *Circulation* 1993; 87:323–329.
666. Pratt CM, Roberts R: Non-Q-wave myocardial infarction: Recognition, pathogenesis, prognosis, and management. In: McIntosh HD, (ed): *Baylor Cardiology Series*, 8th ed. Houston, Baylor College of Medicine, 1985: 5–19.
667. DeWood MA, Stifter WF, Simpson CS, Spores J, Eugster GS, Judge TP, et al: Coronary arteriographic findings soon after non-

Q-wave myocardial infarction. *N Engl J Med* 1986; 315:417–423.

668. Nicod P, Gilpin E, Dittrich H, Polikar R, Hjalmarson A, Blacky AR, et al: Short- and long-term clinical outcome after Q wave and non-Q wave myocardial infarction in a large patient population. *Circulation* 1989; 79:528–536.
669. Maisel AS, Ahnve S, Gilpin E, Henning H, Goldberger AL, Collins D, et al: Prognosis after extension of myocardial infarct: The role of Q wave or non-Q wave infarction. *Circulation* 1985; 71:211–217.
670. Krone RJ, Friedman E, Thanavaro S, Miller JP, Kleiger RE, Oliver GC: Long-term prognosis after first Q-wave (transmural) or non-Q-wave (nontransmural) myocardial infarction: Analysis of 593 patient. *Am J Cardiol* 1983; 52:234–239.
671. Hutter AM, DeSanctis RW, Flynn T, Yeatman LA: Nontransmural myocardial infarction: A comparison of hospital and late clinical course of patients with that of matched patients with transmural anterior and transmural inferior myocardial infarction. *Am J Cardiol* 1981; 48:595–602.
672. Thanavaro S, Krone RJ, Kleiger RE, Province MA, Miller JP, deMello VR, et al: In-hospital prognosis of patients with first nontransmural infarctions. *Circulation* 1980; 61:29–33.
673. Fabricius-Bjerre N, Munkvad M, Knudsen JB: Subendocardial and transmural myocardial infarction. *Am J Med* 1979; 66:986–990.
674. Cannom DS, Levy W, Cohen LS: The short- and long-term prognosis of patients with transmural and nontransmural myocardial infarction. *Am J Med* 1976; 61:452–458.
675. Scheinman MM, Abbott JA: Clinical significance of transmural versus nontransmural electrocardiographic changes in patients with acute myocardial infarction. *Am J Med* 1973; 55:602–607.
676. Rigo P, Murray M, Taylor DR, Weisfeldt ML, Strauss HW, Pitt B: Hemodynamic and prognostic findings in patients with transmural and nontransmural infarction. *Circulation* 1975; 51:1064–1070.
677. Madias JE, Chahine RA, Gorlin R, Blacklow DJ: A comparison of transmural and nontransmural acute myocardial infarction. *Circulation* 1974; 49:498–507.
678. Gibson RS, Beller GA, Gheorghiade M, Nygaard TW, Watson DD, Huey BL, et al: The prevalence and significance of residual myocardial ischemia 2 weeks after uncomplicated non-Q wave infarction: A prospective natural history study. *Circulation* 1986; 73:1186–1198.
679. Eisenberg MJ, Barbash GI, Hod H, Roth A, Schachar A, Zolti L, et al: Prognostic importance of delayed Q-wave evolution 3 to 24 hours after initiation of thrombolytic therapy for acute myocardial infarction. *Am J Cardiol* 1991; 67:231–235.
680. Szklo M, Goldberg R, Kennedy HL, Tonascia JA: Survival of patients with nontransmural myocardial infarction: A population based study. *Am J Cardiol* 1978; 42:648–652.
681. Pohjola S, Siltanen P, Romo M: Five-year survival of 728 patients after myocardial infarction. *Br Heart J* 1980; 43:176–183.
682. Sanz G, Castaner A, Betriu A, Magrina J, Roig E, Coll S, et al: Determinants of prognosis in survivors of myocardial infarction. *N Engl J Med* 1982; 306:1065–1070.
683. Davis K, Kennedy JW, Kemp HG, Judkins MP, Gosselin AJ, Killip T: Complications of coronary arteriography from the collaborative study of coronary artery surgery (CASS). *Circulation* 1979; 59:1105–1112.
684. Abraham RD, Roubin GS, Harris PJ, Bernstein L, Kelly DT: Coronary and left ventricular angiographic anatomy and prognosis of survivors of first acute myocardial infarction. *Am J Cardiol* 1983; 52:257–260.
685. Taylor GJ, Humphries JO, Mellits ED, Pitt B, Schulze RA, Griffith LS, et al: Predictors of clinical course, coronary anatomy and left ventricular function after recovery from acute myocardial infarction. *Circulation* 1980; 62:960–970.
686. Turner JD, Rogers WJ, Mantle JA, Rackley CE, Russell RO Jr: Coronary angiography soon after myocardial infarction. *Chest* 1980; 77:58–64.
687. Grines CL, Topol EJ, Bates ER, Juni JE, Walton JA, O'Neill WW: Infarct vessel status after intravenous tissue plasminogen activator and acute coronary angioplasty: Prediction of clinical outcome. *Am Heart J* 1988; 115:1–7.
688. Topol EJ, Califf RM, George BS, Kereiakes DJ, Abbottsmith CW, Candela RJ, et al: A randomized trial of immediate versus delayed elective angioplasty after intravenous tissue plasminogen activator in acute myocardial infarction. *N Engl J Med* 1987; 317:581–588.
689. Muller DW, Topol EJ, Ellis SG, Sigmon KN, Lee K, Califf RM, et al: Multivessel coronary artery disease: A key predictor of short-term prognosis after reperfusion therapy for acute myocardial infarction. *Am Heart J* 1991; 121:1042–1049.
690. Aguirre FV, Kern MJ, Hsia J, Serota H, Janosik D, Greenwalt T, et al: Importance of myocardial infarction artery patency on the prevalence of ventricular arrhythmia and late potentials after thrombolysis in acute myocardial infarction. *Am J Cardiol* 1991; 68:1410–1416.
691. Stack RS, O'Connor CM, Mark DB, Hinohara T, Phillips HR, Lee MM, et al: Coronary perfusion during acute myocardial infarction with a combined therapy of coronary angioplasty and high-dose intravenous streptokinase. *Circulation* 1988; 77:151–161.
692. Stadius ML, Davis K, Maynard C, Ritchie JL, Kennedy JW: Risk stratification for 1 year survival based on characteristics identified in the early hours of acute myocardial infarction: The Western Washington Intracoronary Streptokinase Trial. *Circulation* 1986; 74:703–711.
693. The TIMI Study Group: Comparison of invasive and conservative strategies after treatment with intravenous tissue plasminogen activator in acute myocardial infarction: Results of the Thrombolysis in Myocardial Infarction (TIMI) Phase II Trial. *N Engl J Med* 1989; 310:618–627.
694. The Multicenter Postinfarction Research Group: Risk stratification and survival after myocardial infarction. *N Engl J Med* 1983; 303:331–336.
695. Davis HT, DeCamilla J, Bayer LW, Moss AJ: Survivorship patterns in the posthospital phase of myocardial infarction. *Circulation* 1979; 6:1252–1258.
696. Ross J Jr, Brandenburg RO, Dinsmore RE, Friesinger GC, Hultgren HH, Pepin CJ, et al: Guidelines for coronary angiography: A report of the American College of Cardiology/American Heart Association Task Force on assessment of diagnostic and therapeutic cardiovascular procedures. *J Am Coll Cardiol* 1987; 10:935–950.
697. Ryan TJ, Faxon DP, Gunnar RM, Kennedy JW, King SB, Loop FD, et al: Guidelines for percutaneous transluminal coronary angioplasty: A report of the American College of Cardiology/American Heart Association Task Force on the assessment of diagnostic and therapeutic cardiovascular procedures. *J Am Coll Cardiol* 1988; 12:529–545.
698. European Coronary Surgery Study Group: Coronary artery bypass surgery in stable angina pectoris: Survival at two years. *Lancet* 1979; 1:889–893.
699. European Coronary Surgery Study Group: Prospective randomized study of coronary artery bypass surgery in stable angina pectoris: a progress report on survival. *Circulation* 1982; 65:II-67–II-71.
700. Gomes JA, Winters SL, Stewart D, Horowitz S, Milner M, Barreca P: A new noninvasive index to predict sustained ventricular tachycardia and sudden death in the first year after myocardial infarction: based on signal-averaged electrocardiogram, radionuclide ejection fraction and Holter monitoring. *J Am Coll Cardiol* 1987; 10:349–357.
701. Starling MR, Crawford MH, Henry RL, Lembo NJ, Kennedy GT, O'Rourke RA: Prognostic value of electrocardiographic exercise testing and noninvasive assessment of left ventricular ejection fraction soon after acute myocardial infarction. *Am J Cardiol* 1986; 47:532–537.
702. Vedin A. Wilhelmsson C, Werko L: Chronic alprenolol treatment of patients with acute myocardial infarction after discharge from hospital. *Acta Med Scand* 1975; 575:3–56.
703. Andersen MP, Bechsgaard P, Frederiksen J, Hansen DA, Jurgensen HJ, Nielsen B, et al: Effect of alprenolol on mortality among patients with definitive or suspected acute myocardial infarction. *Lancet* 1979; 2:865–868.
704. Baber NS, Evans DW, Howitt G, Thomas M, Wilson C, Lewis JA, et al: Multicentre post-infarction trial of propranolol in 49 hospitals in the United Kingdom, Italy, and Yugoslavia. *Br Heart J* 1980; 44:96–100.
705. Barber JM, Boyle DM, Chaturvedi NC, Singh N, Walsh MJ: Practolol in acute myocardial infarction. *Acta Medica Scand* 1976; 587:213–219
706. Ahlmark G, Saetre H: Long-term treatment with Beta-Blockers

after myocardial infarction. *Eur J Clin Pharmacol* 1976; 10:77–83.

707. Olsson G, Rehnqvist N, Sjogren A, Erhardt L, Lundman T: Long-term treatment with metoprolol after myocardial infarction: effect on 3 year mortality and morbidity. *J Am Coll Cardiol* 1985; 5:1428–1437.
708. Wilcox RG, Roland JM, Banks DC, Hampton JR, Mitchell JR: Randomised trial comparing propranolol with atenolol in immediate treatment of suspected myocardial infarction. *Br Med J* 1980; 280:885–888.
709. Australian and Swedish Pindolol Study Group: The effect of pindolol on the two years mortality after complicated myocardial infarction. *Eur Heart J* 1983; 4:367–375.
710. Coronary Prevention Research Group: An early intervention secondary prevention study with oxprenolol following myocardial infarction. *Eur Heart J* 1981; 2:389–393.
711. Boissel JP, Leizorovicz A, Picolet H, Ducruet T, the APSI Investigators: Efficacy of acebutolol after acute myocardial infarction (the APSI trial). *Am J Cardiol* 1990; 66:24C–31C.
712. Hansteen V: Beta blockade after myocardial infarction: The Norwegian Propranolol Study in high-risk patients. *Circulation* 1983; 67:I57–I60.
713. Multicentre International Study: Reduction in mortality after myocardial infarction with long-term beta-adrenoreceptor blockade. *Br Med J* 1977; 2:419–421.
714. Beta-Blocker Heart Attack Trial Research Group: A randomized trial of propranolol in patients with acute myocardial infarction. Mortality Results. *JAMA* 1982; 247:1707–1714.
715. Herlitz J, Pennert K, Wedel H, Vedin A, Wilhelmsson C, Wilhelmsen L, et al: Goteborg metoprolol trial: tolerance. *Am J Cardiol* 1984; 53:46D–50D.
716. Hjalmarson A, Herlitz J, Holmberg S, Ryden L, Swedberg K, Vedin A, et al: The Goteborg metoprolol trial, effects on mortality and morbidity in acute myocardial infarction. *Circulation* 1983; 67:26I–31I.
717. Julian DG, Jackson FS, Szekely P, Prescott RJ: A controlled trial of sotalol for 1 year after myocardial infarction. *Circulation* 1983; 67:61I–67I.
718. Lopressor Intervention Trial Research Group: The lopressor intervention trial: Multicentre study of metoprolol in survivors of acute myocardial infarction. *Eur Heart J* 1987; 8:1056–1064.
719. Bethge KP, Andersen D, Boissel JP, von Leitner ER, Peyrieux JC, Schroder R, et al: Effect of oxprenolol on ventricular arrhythmias: the European infarction study experience. *J Am Coll Cardiol* 1985; 6:963–972.
720. First International Study of Infarct Survival Collaborative Group: Randomised trial of intravenous atenolol among 16027 cases of suspected acute myocardial infarction: ISIS-1. *Lancet* 1986; 57–66.
721. Kjekshus JK: Importance of heart rate in determining beta-blocker efficacy in acute and long-term acute myocardial infarction intervention trials. *Am J Cardiol* 1986; 57:43F–49F.
722. Goldman L, Sia STB, Cook F, Rutherford JD, Weinstein MC: Costs and effectiveness of routine therapy with long-term beta-adrenergic antagonists after acute myocardial infarction. *N Engl J Med* 1988; 319:152–157.
723. Overskeid K, Abrahamsen AM, Frisvold OJ, von der Lippe G, Lund-Johansen P, Petersen S: Timolol after myocardial infarction. *N Engl J Med* 1981; 305:406–408.
724. The MIAMI Trial Research Group: Development of myocardial infarction. *Am J Cardiol* 1985; 56:23G–26G.
725. Pedersen TR, and the Norwegian Multicenter Study Group: Six-year follow-up of the Norwegian multicenter study on timolol after acute myocardial infarction. *N Engl J Med* 1985; 313:1055–1058.
726. Gottlieb SO, Becker LC, Weiss JL, Shapiro EP, Chandra NC, Flaherty JT, et al: Nifedipine in acute myocardial infarction: an assessment of left ventricular function, infarct size, and infarct expansion. *Br Heart J* 1988; 59:411–418.
727. Walker LJE, MacKenzie G, Adgey AAJ: Effect of nifedipine on enzymatically estimated infarct size in the early phase of acute myocardial infarction. *Br Heart J* 1988; 59:403–410.
728. Erbel R, Pop T, Meinertz T, Olshausen KV, Treese N, Henrichs KJ, et al: Combination of calcium channel blocker and thrombolytic therapy in acute myocardial infarction. *Am Heart J* 1988; 115:529–538.
729. Branagan JP, Walsh K, Kelly P, Collins WC, McCafferty D, Walsh MJ: Effect of early treatment with nifedipine in suspected acute myocardial infarction. *Eur Heart J* 1986; 7:859–865.
730. Neufeld HN: Calcium antagonists in secondary prevention after acute myocardial infarction: The Secondary Prevention Reinfarction Nifedipine Trial. *Eur Heart J* 1986; 7:51–52.
731. Neufeld HN: Calcium antagonists in secondary prevention after acute myocardial infarction: The Secondary Prevention Reinfarction Nifedipine Trial (SPRINT). *Eur Heart J* 1986; 7B:51–52.
732. The Israeli Sprint Study Group: Secondary prevention reinfarction Israeli nifedipine trial (SPRINT). A randomized intervention trial of nifedipine in patients with acute myocardial infarction. *Eur Heart J* 1988; 9:354–364.
733. The Danish Study Group: Verapamil in acute myocardial infarction. *Eur Heart J* 1984; 5:516–528.
734. The Danish Study Group: Secondary prevention with verapamil after myocardial infarction. *Am J Cardiol* 1990; 66:33-I–40-I.
735. Held PH, Yusuf S, Furberg CD: Calcium channel blockers in acute myocardial infarction and unstable angina: An overview. *Br Med J* 1989; 299:1187–1192.
736. The CONSENSUS Trial Study Group: Effects of enalapril on mortality in severe congestive heart failure. Results of the Cooperative North Scandinavian Enalapril Survival study (CONSENSUS). *N Engl J Med* 1987; 316:1429–1435.
737. Cohn JN, Archibald DG, Ziesche S, Franciosa JA, Harston WE, Tristani FE, et al: Effect of vasodilator therapy on mortality in chronic congestive heart failure. Results of a Veterans Administration Cooperative Study. *N Engl J Med* 1986; 314:1547–1552.
738. Cohn JN, Johnson G, Ziesche S, Cobb F, Francis G, Tristani F, et al: A comparison of enalapril with hydralazine-isosorbide dinitrate in the treatment of chronic congestive heart failure. *N Engl J Med* 1991; 325:303–310.
739. Pfeffer MA, Lamas GA, Vaughan DE, Parisi AF, Braunwald E: Effect of captopril on progressive ventricular dilatation after anterior myocardial infarction. *N Engl J Med* 1988; 319:80–86.
740. Hine LK, Laird NM, Hewitt P, Chalmers TC: Meta-analysis of empirical long-term antiarrhythmic therapy after myocardial infarction. *JAMA* 1989; 226:3037–3040.
741. IMPACT Research Group: International Mexiletine and placebo antiarrhythmic coronary trial: I. Report on arrhythmia and other findings. *J Am Coll Cardiol* 1984; 4:1148–1163.
742. IMPACT Research Group: International Mexiletine and placebo antiarrhythmic coronary trial (IMPACT): II. Results from 24-hour electrocardiograms. *Eur Heart J* 1986; 7:749–759.
743. Burkart F, Pfisterer M, Kiowski W, Follath F, Burckhardt D, Jordi H: Effect of antiarrhythmic therapy on mortality in survivors of myocardial infarction with asymptomatic complex ventricular arrhythmias: Basel antiarrhythmic study of infarct survival (BASIS). *J Am Coll Cardiol* 1990; 16:1711–1718.
744. Ceremuzynski L, Kleczar E, Krzeminska-Pakula M, Kuch J, Nartowicz E, Smielak-Korombel J, et al: Low dose Amiodarone decreases mortality after myocardial infarction. *Circulation* 1991; 84:II-347.
745. Cosin J, Bayes de Luna A, Navarro F, Guindo J, Marrugat J, Spanish Trial on sudden death: Follow-up of 382 patients. *Circulation* 1991; 84:II-348.
746. Nicholls DP, Haybyrne T, Barnes PC: Intravenous and oral disopyramide after myocardial infarction. *Lancet* 1980; 2:936–938.
747. Wilcox RG, Rowley JM, Hampton JR, Mitchell JR, Roland JM, Banks DC: Randomised placebo-controlled trial comparing oxprenolol with disopyramide phosphate in immediate treatment of suspected myocardial infarction. *Lancet* 1980; 765–769.
748. Chamberlain DA, Jewitt DE, Julian DG, Campbell RWF, Boyle DMC, Shanks RG: Oral mexiletine in high-risk patients after myocardial infarction. *Lancet* 1980; 1324–1327.
749. Lubsen J: Clinical trials of antiarrhythmic therapy—an improper answer to a proper question? *Cardiology* 1987; 74:32–39.
750. Echt DS, Liebson PR, Mitchell LB, Peters RW, Obias-Manno D, Barker AH, et al: Mortality and morbidity in patients receiving encainide, flecainide, or placebo. The Cardiac Arrhythmia Suppression Trial. *N Engl J Med* 1991; 324:781–788.
751. Furberg CD: Effect of antiarrhythmic drugs on mortality after acute myocardial infarction. *Am J Cardiol* 1983; 52:32C–36C.
752. ISIS Pilot Study Investigators: Randomized factorial trial of high-dose intravenous streptokinase, or oral aspirin and of intravenous

heparin in acute myocardial infarction. *Eur Heart J* 1987; 8:634–642.

753. Aspirin Myocardial Infarction Study Research Group: A randomized, controlled trial of aspirin in persons recovered from myocardial infarction. *JAMA* 1980; 243:661–669.
754. Elwood PC, Sweetnam PM: Aspirin and secondary mortality after myocardial infarction. *Lancet* 1979; 1313–1315.
755. Elwood PC, Cochrane AL, Burr ML, Sweetnam PM, Williams G, Welsby E, et al: A randomized controlled trial of acetylsalicylic acid in the secondary prevention of mortality from myocardial infarction. *Br Med J* 1974; 1:436–440.
756. The Coronary Drug Project Research Group: Aspirin in coronary heart disease. *J Chron Dis* 1976; 29:625–642.
757. The Anturane Reinfarction Trial Research Group: Sulfinpyrazone in the prevention of cardiac death after myocardial infarction. *N Engl J Med* 1978; 298:298–295.
758. The Persantine Aspirin Reinfarction Study Research Group: Persantine and aspirin in coronary heart disease. *Circulation* 1980; 62:449–461.
759. Breddin K, Loew D, Lechner K, Oberla K, Walter E: The German-Austrian aspirin trial: A comparison of acetylsalicylic acid, placebo and phenprocoumon in secondary prevention of myocardial infarction. *Circulation* 1980; 62:V63–V72.
760. Buchwald H, Varco RL, Matts JP, Long JM, Fitch LL, Campbell GS, et al: Effect of partial ileal bypass surgery on mortality and morbidity from coronary heart disease in patients with hypercholesterolemia: Report of the Program on the Surgical Control of Hyperlipidemias (POSCH). *N Engl J Med* 1990; 323:946–955.
761. The Coronary Drug Project Research Group: The coronary drug project. Design, methods and baseline results. *Circulation* 1973; 47:1–50.
762. The Coronary Drug Project Research Group: The coronary drug project. Initial findings leading to modifications of its research protocol. *JAMA* 1970; 214:1303–1313.
763. The Coronary Drug Project Research Group: The coronary drug project. Findings leading to discontinuation of 2.5 mg/day estrogen group. *JAMA* 1973; 226:652–657.
764. The Coronary Drug Project Research Group: The coronary drug project. Clofibrate and niacin in coronary heart disease. *JAMA* 1975; 231:360–381.
765. The Coronary Drug Project Research Group: The coronary drug project. Findings leading to further modifications of its protocol with respect to dextrothyroxine. *JAMA* 1972; 220:996–1008.
766. Canner PL, Berge KG, Wenger NK, Stamler J, Friedman L, Prineas RJ, et al: Fifteen year mortality in coronary drug project patients: Long term benefit with niacin. *J Am Coll Cardiol* 1986; 8:1245–1255.
767. Rossouw JE, Lewis B, Rifkind BM: The value of lowering cholesterol after myocardial infarction. *N Engl J Med* 1990; 323:1112–1119.
768. Lipid Research Clinics Program: The Lipid Research Clinics Coronary Primary Prevention Trial Results: The relationship of reduction in incidence of coronary heart disease to cholesterol lowering. *JAMA* 1984; 251:365–374.
769. Brown WV: Clinical trials including an update on the Helsinki Heart Study. *Am J Cardiol* 1990; 66:11A–15A.
770. Manttari M, Romo M, Manninen V, Koskinen P, Huttunen JK, Heinonen OP, et al: Reduction in Q wave myocardial infarctions with gemfibrozil in the Helsinki Heart Study. *Am Heart J* 1990; 119:991–995.
771. Blankenhorn DH, Nessim SA, Johnson RL, Sanmarco ME, Azen SP, Cashin-Hemphill L: Beneficial effects of combined colestipol-niacin therapy on coronary atherosclerosis and coronary venous bypass grafts. *JAMA* 1987; 257:3233–3240.
772. Hjermann I, Velve-Byre K, Holme I, Leren P: Effect of diet and smoking intervention on the incidence of coronary heart disease: Report from the Oslo Study Group of a randomized trial in healthy men. *Lancet* 1981; 2:1303–1310.
773. Leren P: The Oslo Diet-Heart Study. Eleven-year report. *Circulation* 1970; 42:935–942.
774. Committee of Principal Investigators WHO Clofibrate Trial: W.H.O. Cooperative Trial on primary prevention of ischaemic heart disease using clofibrate to lower serum cholesterol: Mortality follow-up report. *Lancet* 1980; 2:379–385.
775. Grundy SM: HMG-CoA reductase inhibitors for treatment of hypercholesterolemia. *N Engl J Med* 1988; 319:24–33.
776. Brown G, Albers JJ, Fisher LD, Schaefer SM, Lin JT, Kaplan C, et al: Regression of coronary artery disease as a result of intensive lipid-lowering therapy in men with high levels of apolipoprotein B. *N Engl J Med* 1990; 323:1289–1298.
777. Watts GF, Lewis B, Brunt JN, Lewis ES, Coltart DJ, Smith LD, et al: Effects on coronary artery disease of lipid-lowering diet, or diet plus cholestyramine, in the St. Thomas Atherosclerosis Regression Study (S.T.A.R.S.). *Lancet* 1992; 339:563–569.
778. Hypertension Detection and Follow-up Program Cooperative Group: Five-year findings of the hypertension detection and follow-up program. Reduction in mortality of persons with high blood pressure, including mild hypertension. *JAMA* 1979; 242:2562–2571.
779. Yusuf S, Wittes J, Friedman L: Overview of results of randomized clinical trials in heart disease: Unstable angina, heart failure, primary prevention with aspirin, and risk factor modification. *JAMA* 1988; 260:2259–2263.
780. O'Connor GT, Buring JE, Yusuf S, Goldhaber SZ, Olmstead EM, Paffenbarger RS, et al: An overview of randomized trials of rehabilitation with exercise after myocardial infarction. *Circulation* 1989; 38:234–244.
781. Oldridge NB, Guyatt GH, Fischer ME, Rimm AA: Cardiac rehabilitation after myocardial infarction: A combined experience of randomized clinical trails. *JAMA* 1988; 260:945–950.
782. Van Camp SP, Peterson RA: Cardiovascular complications of outpatient cardiac rehabilitation programs. *JAMA* 1986; 256:1160–1163.
783. American College of Physicians: Health and Public Policy Committee: Cardiac rehabilitation services. *J Am Coll Phys* 1988; 671–673.

Chapter 61

The Natural History of Atherosclerotic Coronary Heart Disease

Gottlieb C. Friesinger, M.D.

BACKGROUND AND PRINCIPLES

Establishing prognosis with reasonable confidence is particularly difficult in patients with atherosclerotic coronary heart disease (CHD). The principal factors contributing to difficulties are the inherent complexity of the condition, its propensity to pursue a long and relapsing course, and the lack of fully satisfactory, easily available techniques to obtain objective data in many patients. A large number of patients will follow a course of many years (often greater than 10) with long periods of stability interrupted by apparently unpredictable (sometimes catastrophic) intercurrent events. These intercurrent and unpredictable events and the propensity for sudden death, which is present in all groups with atherosclerotic CHD, are a disconcerting element and add an emotional feature to prognosis not present in most diseases.

Our ability to judge prognosis has greatly improved during recent years as better objective data have become available on large numbers of patients and a clearer understanding of the most important determinants of prognosis has developed. Clinical therapeutic trials, often including hundreds or several thousands of patients, have provided invaluable information on prognosis. In addition, clinical data bases have been used as an alternative approach to develop prognostic information.[1] Multiple variables are fastidiously collected on each patient with subsequent critical follow-up and sophisticated data analyses. There are strong merits and significant limitations to each approach.

Randomized controlled trials (RCTs) provide the best approach to evaluate therapy, but entry selection criteria often exclude large numbers of patients and entire important clinical subsets. Registries can be much more inclusive, and therefore representative, of the entire population with the condition. Registries are best suited to assess risk factors for events and provide natural history data, but registries pose major problems in evaluating therapy, since treatment interventions are not standardized, and even the most sophisticated attempts at matching treated and nontreated patients cannot be as precise and certain as randomization.

The most useful approach in assessing prognosis is to divide patients into subsets using multiple factors, clinical descriptors, and laboratory data that have independent importance.[2,3] Objective and quantitative data are superior to subjective qualitative data. Since silent myocardial ischemia is common, and patients with significant left ventricular dysfunction and arrhythmias may not be symptomatic, the duration of treadmill exercise testing, degree of ST-segment depression on exercise, an estimate of left ventricular dysfunction, and characterization of ventricular arrhythmias on ambulatory monitoring are of greater value than merely eliciting the patient's complaint. Clinical and symptomatic evaluations of each patient are important, however, and patients with symptoms of breathlessness and ischemia tend to have a poorer prognosis than peer patients who have similar objective evidences of disease but who are symptomless. Hence, symptoms often have prognostic value in addition to the objective data obtained through testing.

Multiple methods for inducing ischemia and detecting arrhythmias in stable subsets are widely used. However, most of our best prognostic data on exercise-induced ischemia has been obtained by exercise electrocardiographic study. In the last decade, a wide variety of techniques, such as exercise or dipyridamole/adenosine-induced ischemia using thallium-201, radionuclide ventriculography, and stress echocardiography, have become popular. Many studies of ambulatory electrocardiographic monitoring for ventricular arrhythmias or evidence of a symptomatic ischemia have been reported. In general, these studies involve relatively small numbers of highly selected patients and short follow-up periods (often not more than 1 or 2 years). In patients with chronic CHD, such studies provide useful clinical information but very limited prognostic data, since the disease is so diverse in its clinical presentation and long-term course. In reference to prognosis, it is not possible to substitute directly one method for detecting ischemia for another, e.g., thallium-201 perfusion defect for exercise-induced ST-segment shift. The methods evaluate different pathophysiological manifestations of the same phenomena but are not directly comparable in reference to prognosis. Unfortunately, we do not have techniques to assess several other important factors in the natural history of patients with CHD, such as impaired reactivity of the coronary vasculature and increased tendency for intravascular arterial thrombosis.

Table 61-1 lists the principal prognostic determinants in patients whose symptoms are stable. Although the order of importance for the factors listed will differ from patient to patient, the *degree of left ventricular dysfunction* tends to be the most powerful predictive item in most patients in stable phases.

TABLE 61-1

Principal Prognostic Determinants of Stable Subsets

- Degree of left ventricular dysfunction
- Objective severity of ischemia
  - Duration of treadmill
  - Degree of ST shift
- Extent of coronary atherosclerosis
- Recent (6–9) month intercurrent ischemic events
  - Myocardial infarction
  - Unstable angina
  - Sudden cardiac death with resuscitation
- Additional factors
  - Hypertension
  - Cardiomegaly
  - Congestive heart failure
  - Diabetes mellitus
  - Electrocardiographic abnormalities
    - Ventricular arrhythmias
    - Conduction defects
    - Remote infarction
    - ST-segment depression
  - Cigarette smoking
  - Age
  - Gender
  - Blood lipids

The most important historical factor in prognosis is a *change in the patient's symptoms*. When a patient with stable angina pectoris has a change in symptoms or a patient with asymptomatic coronary arteriosclerosis develops complaints, the prognosis worsens for the next 3 to 6 months. This is the unstable phase. (See also Chap. 59.) Similarly, a patient who has experienced a myocardial infarction has a worse prognosis in the 6 to 9 months following that infarct compared to a more remote time. Such patients may be considered to be in a "transition zone," a situation depicted in Fig. 61-1.

The physician should assume that most patients with atherosclerotic CHD, even those who express no curiosity, have concern about their prognosis. Denial and/or fear may prevent patients from asking the physician about outcome. The physician's willingness to discuss prognosis in a realistic and sympathetic manner, with as much optimism as is warranted, at the appropriate time, and under proper circumstances, is important to the overall management of patients with atherosclerotic CHD.

The availability of coronary artery bypass (CAB) surgery and percutaneous transluminal angioplasty (PTCA) has increased the importance of estimating prognosis in each patient. The indications for these invasive and expensive procedures include relief of symptoms, prevention of complications, improvement of quality of life, and prolongation of life. The most objective and important is prolongation of life except in the very old. Because many patients pursue a long, relapsing course and because grafts fail and restenosis is common with PTCA, the timing of these procedures is the critical issue. The decision to intervene should be influenced heavily by the patient's prognosis.

the subsequent sections a brief summary of how these principles can be utilized in assessing prognosis in a variety of subsets of patients with atherosclerotic CHD is given. Although probabilities are cited, it should be emphasized that it is unwise to take a rigid statistical approach. At best, the probabilities cited are approximations obtained from groups of patients in which the selection process is frequently not clear.

This chapter relies heavily on data collected during the period 1960 to 1970, especially for chronic CHD syndromes. During that period objective methods for assessing CHD were developing rapidly, and the importance of careful data collection was appreciated. The enthusiasm and wide availability of interventions, such as CAB and PTCA, had not yet evolved. In addition, the development of new cardiovascular drugs, especially beta blockers, calcium channel blockers, and angiotensin converting enzyme (ACE) inhibitors, as well as the use of aspirin in ischemic syndromes, was just beginning. These phenomena made it possible to follow patients without interventions that modify prognosis for the periods of time needed to assess prognosis with some accuracy. Drug therapy, changes in lifestyle, and alteration in risk factors may significantly improve prognosis for patients with any given finding, such as an abnormal-

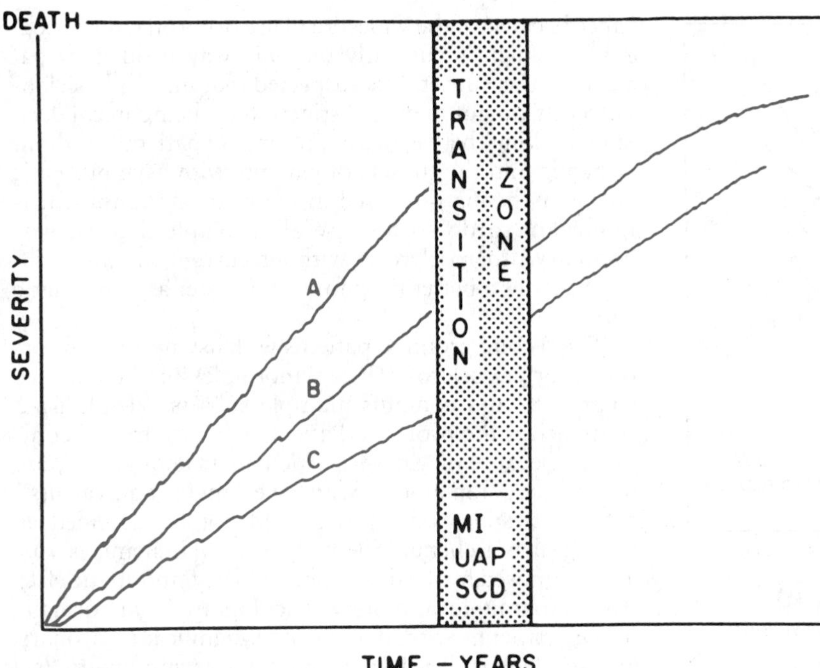

FIGURE 61-1 The hypothetical course of three patients (A,B,C) with atherosclerotic coronary heart disease. The slope of the lines is related to risk factors and other unknown items which determine the progression of coronary atherosclerosis. All three patients enter the transition zone, a time when they develop new manifestatons. Patient A died with acute myocardil infarction, or suffered sudden cardiac death. Patient B continued at a slope unchanged after having experienced a period of unstable angina pectoris but without myocardial necrosis. Patient C had a large myocardial infarction with considerable myocardial necrosis resulting in reduced ventricular function which made the slope of his line steeper and the severity of his disease worse. A patient is in the transition zone for a variable period, probably 3 or 4 stable angina pectoris and perhaps 6 to 12 months for the patient who has survived acute myocardial infarction. MI = myocardial infarction; UAP = unstable angina pectoris; SCD = sudden cardiac death. *(From Friesinger GC.*[2] *Reproduced with permission from the author.)*

ity on exercise testing or arteriography. Adequate data concerning these matters are not available and may never be.

Prognosis is of particular importance in patients with early manifestations of disease, often with minimal or no symptoms and only minor abnormalities on objective testing. In this stage of the disease, prognostic implications must be carefully weighed against the risks of the therapy as well as the cost. Clinical decision-making is too frequently predicated on a specific finding, e.g., premature ventricular complexes (PVCs) on ambulatory monitoring, a thallium regional perfusion defect, and a lesion on coronary arteriography, rather than on the composite overall view that determines the patient's prognosis.

Within the context of probabilities given, an individualized approach is possible. Finally, *prognosis in each patient needs to be reassessed continually because important changes may occur in the extent of the coronary atherosclerosis, exercise tolerance, frequency of arrhythmia, coronary vasomotor tone, tendency for arterial thrombosis, and status of left ventricular function—without change in symptoms or complaints.* In addition, a change in symptoms, even if very subtle, may herald the entry into the unstable phase and demand reassessing the prognosis.

PROGNOSTIC CONSIDERATIONS RELATED TO AGING

The frequency and severity of CHD increases with age. The number of individuals in the older segment of our society, arbitrarily defined as those greater than 65 years, is increasing at a more rapid rate than in any other segment. This is particularly true of people over the age of 75 years and the "oldest of the old," those greater than 85 years. The complications of CHD, as well as the complications related to invasive procedures, interventions, and drug therapy, are all higher in older persons.[4–8] The mortality from acute myocardial infarction (AMI) is extremely high. From Fig. 61-2 it is clear that the mortality under the age of 60 is relatively low but steadily increases with age, particularly after the age of 75. In most reports, especially those involving relatively small numbers with specific interventions, comorbidity is usually cited as a reason for the high mortality and complication rates. When the data are adequate, however, age per se is always shown to be an independent risk factor. There are a variety of changes in the cardiovascular system, as well as all other organs, that make it reasonable to assume that aging constitutes a major reason for the increasing morbidity and mortality in older persons. The heterogeneity of old age makes chronology an inadequate surrogate for aging. (See also Chap. 115.)

A number of important features differentiate old persons from younger patients in reference to prognosis. The presentation of their coronary heart syndrome is often different. More old patients present with silent myocardial infarction and with presentations (painless but not silent) that involve dyspnea, worsening heart failure, central nervous system symptoms, or other systemic manifestations than younger patients. In some reports, not more than 50 percent of older patients will present with the typical chest discomfort of myocardial infarction. Functional tests of ventricular function and induced ischemia have not been utilized in the systematic or comprehensive way in large numbers of older patients. Where data are available, it is suggested that the *ability to exercise* is a favorable prognostic feature, with much higher mortality in those not performing the exercise test, regardless of the reason why exercise is not possible. Noncardiac reasons for inability to perform an exercise test seem equally important to cardiac limitations. In addition, changes in the ST segment seem much less

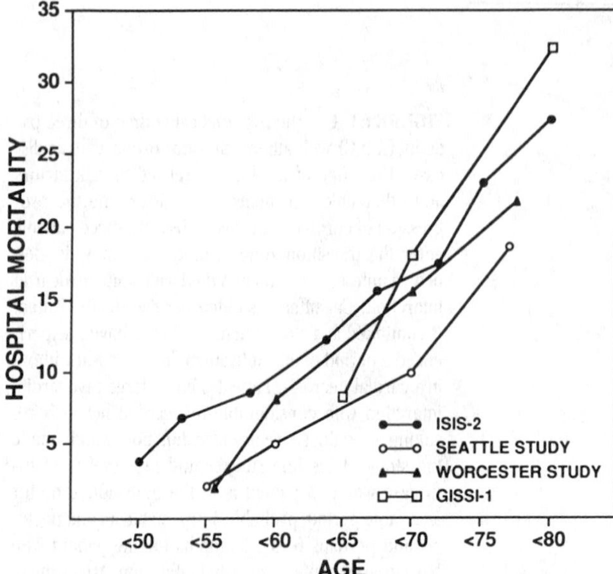

FIGURE 61-2 Hospital mortality for two community-wide registries and the placebo arm of two large randomized clinical trials. All study data are not directly comparable, but slopes of lines are similar and demonstrate the dramatic increase in mortality with age.

predictive for events than in younger persons.[9,10] Peak levels of enzymes released in myocardial infarction are lower in older persons compared to the young; yet the incidence of congestive heart failure and shock is very much higher, often two to four times as high in patients over the age of 75 compared to those under the age of 55.[11]

For the multiple reasons outlined above, older persons require special consideration and a highly individualized approach when considering prognosis. Although the principles involved in establishing prognoses in older persons do not differ from those applied to their younger cohorts, the issues are more complicated because of their presentation, the evaluation of functional tests, the response to the ischemic syndrome (particularly AMI), the higher incidence of complications related to interventions, and the much shorter life expectancy in patients over the age of 75 or 80.

ASYMPTOMATIC (SILENT) CORONARY ATHEROSCLEROSIS

The natural history of asymptomatic coronary atherosclerosis is unknown. The studies of Zoll, Blumgart, and Edwards and others[12–15] demonstrated that moderately severe or severe coronary atherosclerosis is common in our population, particularly with increasing age in males, but frequently is not associated with symptoms. This asymptomatic population contains two major subsets. One group of patients has never been symptomatic and has no evidence of ischemia (e.g., no ST-segment shift or ventricular functional abnormalities on exercise). This group has coronary atherosclerosis without ischemia. We have little prognostic information on this group. Prognosis in these patients has assumed greater importance because of the widespread use of coronary arteriography, which is currently the only way to identify patients in this subset. It is suspected that many physicians currently do not make a distinction in their clinical decision making between asymptomatic patients without ischemia and the subsets of patients with asymptomatic (silent) ischemia discussed in the next paragraphs. It is important to do so because all available data suggest coronary atherosclerosis without current or past ischemia carries a better prognosis than other asymptomatic subsets.

The second group of patients with asymptomatic coronary arteriosclerosis has symptomless ischemia (see Chap. 58) and contains multiple subsets.[19] Table 61-2 summarizes the problem. Patients who are free of complaints because they never participate in enough exercise to produce complaints or who have "angina equivalents" such as dyspnea on effort should not be classified as having silent ischemia. Silent myocardial ischemia is usually diagnosed by the development of asymptomatic electrocardiographic and/or ventriculographic abnormalities in patients with documented significant coronary arteriosclerosis. It is noteworthy that asymptomatic (silent) myocardial ischemia virtually always occurs in patients who also have symptomatic angina pectoris except for some patients who have silent angina pectoris and who may also have had silent myocardial infarction. Many of these patients have diabetes mellitus or are older. It is estimated that 2 to 4 percent of the adult male population older than 40 years may have asymptomatic (silent) myocardial ischemia. Their prognosis is a matter of controversy, but the limited data available suggest that the incidence of sudden death and myocardial infarction 8 to 10 years after discovery of the problem is very low. Two studies[16–18] suggest that the development of angina pectoris is more frequent than other symptomatic events.

An additional subset of patients includes those who have had previous symptoms of myocardial ischemia but who are currently totally free of symptoms and/or exercise-induced functional abnormalities when evaluated and who are on no medications. This latter group contains a substantial number of patients (perhaps as many as 50 percent of patients with remote myocardial infarction), in whom symptom-free periods may last for many months or several years. The prognosis in all these subsets is related to the extent of left ventricular dysfunction and coronary atherosclerosis in addition to the other factors in Table 61-1.

Although it has been impossible to match precisely patients with and without symptoms, the best data indicate that the presence of symptoms, whether related to ventricular arrhythmias, reduced ventricular performance, or to ischemia, predicts a higher mortality and a greater number of events when all other prognostic factors are the same. When objective manifestations of CHD are present, long term follow-up is no longer feasible. The presence of the abnormality leads to therapy and management decisions that almost certainly alter the course of the disease.

Finally, when using the term asymptomatic (silent) myocardial ischemia, it is important to remember that all patients with symptomatic myocardial ischemia may

TABLE 61-2
Subsets of Silent Myocardial Ischemia

Category	Estimated Frequency
I. Never symptomatic:	15–25% of all myocardial infarcts
Electrocardiographic evidence of ischemic heart disease, particularly of old myocardial infarction	
No clinical evidence of ischemic heart disease	2–4% of males over 40 years of age
II. Not currently symptomatic but previously symptomatic:	
Remote myocardial infarction	No good estimates are available; it is assumed the frequency is relatively low but highly variable
Remote unstable angina pectoris	
Remote stable angina pectoris	
III. Concomitant symptomatic episodes:	
Stable phase of ischemic heart disease with angina	Variable, up to 75–80%
Unstable phase of ischemic heart disease	
Unstable angina pectoris	Probably about 50%
Recent myocardial infarction	Probably up to 50%
Coronary artery spasm	Probably a majority of cases

SOURCE: Friesinger and Robertson.[19]

have concomitant silent episodes. In stable angina pectoris, this is estimated to be as high as 75 percent of patients. These matters are discussed in subsequent sections and in Chap. 58.

CORONARY ATHEROSCLEROSIS WITH REVERSIBLE ISCHEMIA

Stable Angina Pectoris

The key pathophysiological feature in this large group of patients, estimated to be as many as 5,000,000 in the United States, is the relationship between an increase in myocardial oxygen demand and the development of ischemia. Fixed coronary arteriosclerotic lesions, usually multiple and severe, are the principal anatomic abnormality accounting for the predictable appearance of ischemia when a certain myocardial oxygen demand is exceeded. Apparent variability in threshold for ischemia can often be related to the presence of several factors (e.g., anxiety on effort) combining to produce the increased myocardial oxygen demand. Variable threshold related to changes in coronary arterial tone is a feature of many patients with stable angina pectoris. It is estimated that up to 75 percent of patients also have *silent myocardial ischemia* as manifested by electrocardiographic ST-segment shifts and/or alteration in left ventricular function during exercise. Silent episodes are more likely to occur in the morning with a circadian variation and are apt to occur at lower MV_{O_2} threshold, suggesting that increased coronary tone is present.[19] (See also Chap. 58.)

When estimating prognosis, one must consider the "total ischemic burden," i.e., symptomatic plus silent episodes. Currently available data do not allow precise quantitative estimates of the importance of the total ischemic burden, but one study demonstrated a close inverse relationship between the time of occurrence of ST segment depression on the treadmill and the number of silent ischemic episodes and/or the total time of ischemia per 24 h determined by ambulatory monitoring.[20]

Some patients with reversible myocardial ischemia have *angina equivalents,* dyspnea, or fatigue with effort, which usually indicate the presence of severe disease with considerable left ventricular dysfunction and portends a poor prognosis despite the absence of the typical angina complaint.

Given a history of *stable angina pectoris,* the annual mortality rate in patients with angiographically proven coronary atherosclerosis but without left main coronary artery obstruction is 3 to 4 percent. The presence of hypertension and abnormalities on the resting electrocardiogram (ECG), such as nonspecific ST-T wave changes and/or Q waves, worsens the prognosis. If neither hypertension nor electrocardiographic abnormality is present, the mortality rate is as low as 2 percent per year. If both are present, the mortality is substantially higher, probably at least 5 percent annually.[21–24]

The severity and frequency of symptoms are of limited assistance in assessing prognosis in stable angina pectoris. Although profound symptoms and symptoms of long duration (more than 5 years) tend to worsen prognosis, there is a poor correlation between prognosis and the patient's symptoms. Many patients can effectively prevent or minimize symptoms by using nitroglycerin prophylactically and/or avoiding activities that provoke angina. Such patients appear to have mild infrequent complaints, yet objective data, such as exercising on the treadmill, may indicate marked diminution in exercise tolerance. The additional problem of silent ischemic episodes provides a confounding factor when assessing prognosis on the basis of symptoms.

Interesting and important observations have been reported by Califf et al.[25] Angina was classified on a scale of 0 to 3, class 0 being *truly stable angina,* class 3 being unstable or variant angina, and classes 1 and 2 being intermediate progressive symptoms. This was a complex and sophisticated retrospective analysis of 5886 patients in the Duke data bank. Forty-four percent of the symptomatic patients had class 0 angina, i.e., truly stable symptoms. In this group, the number of daily episodes of angina did not have independent prognostic implications. As in all studies, left ventricular (LV) function (in this instance judged by ejection fraction) was the most important prognostic factor. In angina groups 1 to 3, the number of daily episodes did provide prognostic information in addition to the other independent variables, such as LV function and the extent of coronary arteriosclerosis.

Ambient ventricular ectopy, as a separate prognostic factor, is controversial because it tends to be associated with ventricular dysfunction and other prognostic factors. On the other hand, it is probable that certain types of complex ventricular ectopy worsen prognosis.[26]

The widespread use of exercise testing and coronary angiography has provided extensive prognostic data in patients with stable angina pectoris. Unfortunately, comprehensive studies relating symptoms, arteriographic severity of atherosclerosis, left ventricular function, and exercise tolerance and ST-segment shift to prognosis have not been reported in any substantial number of patients. In the subsequent paragraphs these features will be discussed independently, with the full appreciation that a discriminant analysis is important and should be applied insofar as feasible in individual patients when these multiple variables are known.

Of the multiple examinations available, exercise testing provides the most overall information. The single most important prognostic determinant with exercise is exercise tolerance. There are many exercise protocols, and controversy exists as to whether exercise duration on a standard protocol or METS (Metabolic Equivalent System, 3.5 ml O_2/kg per min, the oxygen required at rest) should be used. Blood pressure response also can be factored into prognostic considerations (see Chap. 16). Multiple studies demonstrate the relationship between exercise tolerance and the 4- to 5-year outcome.[27-30] Patients with superb exercise tolerance, as judged by the heart rate achieved or exercise duration, in general have an excellent prognosis. A steadily worsening prognosis occurs as exercise tolerance lessens. Achieving a heart rate of 160 or reaching stage 4 in the Bruce protocol is associated with a short-term annual mortality rate of not more than 1 or 2 percent. Failure to achieve stage 2 on the Bruce protocol because of cardiac limitation is accompanied by an annual mortality rate as high as 6 to 10 percent, depending on other features, especially left ventricular function. These estimates are independent of the presence or degree of ST-segment depression, since the failure of ST-segment depression to occur does not necessarily denote a good prognosis. In reference to prognosis, a reduced exercise duration can be the result of poor ventricular function, induced ischemia, or a combination of the two. A study of 220 patients, all of whom had 2 mm ST-segment depression with exercise, demonstrated an excellent correlation between 5-year outcome and duration of exercise on the treadmill.[28] One large study provides an intercorrelation among duration of exercise on the treadmill, extent of ST-segment depression, coronary arteriographic abnormalities, and left ventricular function. A large group of patients (4083) from the CASS Registry,[30] had 30 clinical and exercise variables analyzed. Exercise duration was confirmed as the important exercise test variable, but ST-segment response also proved to have independent prognostic value. The overall mortality, with a minimum of 3 years follow-up, was low; 212 patients died (5 percent). On the basis of only the two exercise variables, a high-risk subset with an annual mortality of more than 5 percent consisted of 492 patients with 1 mm or greater of ST-segment depression at a low level of exercise (stage 1 or less). A low-risk subset with an annual mortality of less than 1 percent contained 1302 patients who had less than 1 mm ST-segment depression in the final exercise stage 3 or higher. Hence, in this very large sample, nearly 50 percent of the patients could be divided into high-and low-risk subsets on the basis of these two simply obtained exercise variables. From this study, a variety of other subsets can be evaluated. In 572 patients with three-vessel disease and good ventricular function, a wide spectrum of 4-year survival was seen. A small group of this subset achieved stage 5 on the Bruce protocol and had no mortality, while only 53 percent of the patients who were unable to achieve stage 1 survived 4 years. This is a very powerful approach to prognosis, and it is unfortunate that so few studies have multiple variables available for such sophisticated analyses.

It is important to remember that all studies have *excluded* some patients. When data are available in the reports, excluded patients *virtually always have a worse prognosis* than study patients, irrespective of the reason(s) for lack of participation, whether cardiac or noncardiac (age, comorbidity, etc.).

No systematically collected data are available concerning the importance of exercise-induced arrhythmias as an independent prognostic factor. The appearance of significant exercise-induced hypotension is a powerful adverse prognostic factor as it indicates that the ischemic process and/or scarring from past infarction is so severe that the stress exceeds the ability of the left ventricle to meet the demand. *Exercise testing is more valuable and more easily interpreted if used to estimate prognosis in patients with manifestly stable ischemic heart disease than it is in establishing the diagnosis of the condition.* The extensive data available can be summarized by stating that the functional capacity of patients with stable disease is a powerful prognostic factor and is additive to any other prognostic factor, including anatomic abnormalities.

Exercise radionuclide studies, utilizing tagged red blood cells to determine ejection fraction or thallium-201 injections to estimate regional myocardial perfusion, are widely used. (See also Chap. 134.) There are many reports concerning correlations among the radionuclide studies, angiographic finding, symptoms, and functional capacity. On the other hand, systematic studies involving large numbers of well-characterized patients who have not been selected in some biased way and who have been followed for more than 2 or 3 years are not available. Thallium scintigraphy has proved useful in identifying areas of ischemic myocardium, but the limitations, which involve technical problems in obtaining good imaging, interpretation problems related to data processing, and readings by nonexperts, as well as high cost, are special problems with the method. Radionuclide ventriculography with tagged red blood cells gives information about ejection fraction and its response during exercise, which is probably additive to the prognostic data from exercise duration, ST-segment shifts, and resting ventricular function. Systematic data in adequate numbers of patients are not available to assess this point. The use and limitations of these techniques are discussed elsewhere. (See Chap. 134.) A combination of clinical evaluation, determination of rest and exercise ejection fraction by radionuclide ventriculography, and exercise tolerance testing with study of ST-segment shift would provide the information needed to develop a sophisticated, and probably very reliable, noninvasive prognostic index in stable patients.

The use of angiographic information and the extent of coronary atherosclerosis and left ventricular contractile patterns in estimating prognosis in patients with reversible stable myocardial ischemia have been studied since 1970,[31–35] but the most extensive and valuable information reported has been accumulated through the National Heart, Lung, and Blood Institute CASS[35–37] (Fig. 61-3). Data on 25,000 patients have been collected and submitted to sophisticated statistical analyses. The criteria utilized to define a significant coronary arterial narrowing is important. The CASS utilized 70 percent or more reduction in internal diameter of the epicardial vessels, except for the left main coronary artery, where 50 percent or more reduction in internal diameter was judged significant. Other studies have utilized a 50 percent reduction in internal diameter (75 percent cross-sectional area reduction) as significant. It is interesting that findings related to outcome are similar despite these differences, since the measurements have a subjective element and other items such as the length of the narrowing, the presence of collateral vessels, and overall extent of disease in a given vessel are not usually considered. It can be assumed that prognosis worsens as narrowings become more severe by any criteria. Even allowing for the interobserver differences,[38,39] the simplified classification of patients with stable reversible myocardial ischemia into single-, double-, and triple-vessel disease is useful and widespread. However, data do exist to indicate that lesions of less than 50 percent narrowing also contribute to prognosis.[32]

So-called single-vessel disease carries a mortality rate of 1 to 3 percent per year over a 5-year period follow-up, provided left ventricular function is well preserved. In single-vessel disease, as in all subsets, prognosis is adversely affected by left ventricular dysfunction.

Two- and three-vessel disease can have an annual mortality as high as 6 to 9 percent (but often much lower), and mortality is significantly less when no left anterior descending (LAD) disease is present.[21] Moreover, as arteriographic findings become advanced, there is no direct relationship between the extent of arteriographic abnormality and prognosis because the multiple factors listed in Table 61-1 assume greater importance and need to be carefully assessed in reference to arteriographic abnormality. As discussed above, exercise tolerance is of major importance in determining prognosis in all subsets and regardless of the extent of arteriographic abnormality.

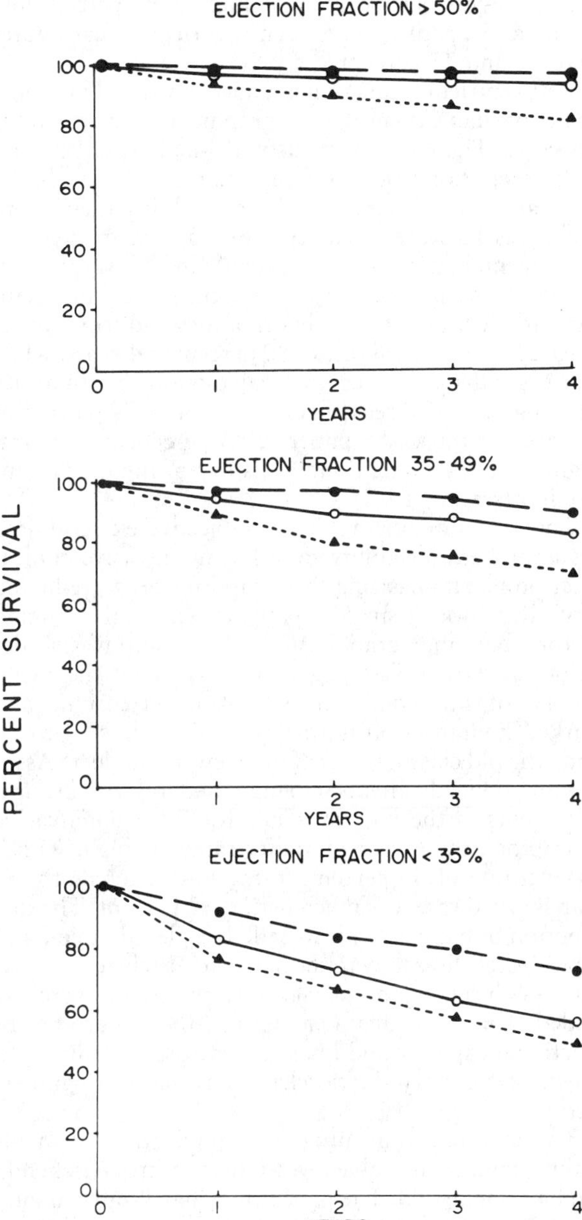

FIGURE 61-3 The 4-year survival in stable patients from the CASS registry: 6791 patients, 73 percent with typical angina pectoris, are included. The importance of left ventricular performance, judged on the basis of ejection fraction, is illustrated. Regional wall motion abnormalities showed a similar trend, i.e., worsening prognosis with increasing wall motion abnormalities for all grades of coronary arteriosclerosis. Single vessel disease = - • -; double vessel disease = - ○ -; triple vessel disease = - ▲ -. *(From Mock MB et al.*[36] *Redrawn and reproduced with permission from the American Heart Association, Inc., and the author.)*

Significant left main coronary arterial narrowing is a very powerful arteriographic prognostic factor. Ordinarily, left main disease is accompanied by extensive disease in other trunks. Regardless, in some reports this lesion carries the poorest prognosis, as high as 15 to 20 percent annual mortality rate. There is a spectrum of rates of survival even in patients with left main coronary artery disease, depending on its association with other factors such as ventricular function and exercise tolerance. One-year survivorship as high as 97 percent and as low as 59 percent have been reported; 3-year figures were 74 and 25 percent.[40]

Left ventricular function is a more powerful prognostic factor than extent of ateriographic narrowing. In the CASS (see Fig. 61-3), patients with single-vessel disease with an ejection fraction of less than 35 percent had a survival rate of 72 percent at 4 years, while patients with triple-vessel disease and an ejection fraction greater than 50 percent had a 4-year survival rate of 82 percent. Regional wall motion scores make the same point. Subsets with no wall motion abnormalities and triple-vessel disease had a survival rate of 80 percent at 4 years, while patients with marked regional wall motion abnormalities and single-vessel disease had a survival of 74 percent at 4 years. Of the CASS patients, 73 percent had typical angina and 48 percent had a history of myocardial infarction (see Fig. 61-3).

The use of angiographic and objective exercise data has improved our ability to utilize noninvasive clinical descriptors, emphasizing their importance in predicting survival.[41] More than 500 patients with stable angina pectoris had angiographic study. Four noninvasive descriptors, resting ST-segment depression on the ECG, history of infarction, history of hypertension, and marked limitation on normal activities (class III to IV using the old classification of the New York Heart Association), divided patients into high- and low-risk groups. In patients in the highest tercile for these noninvasive descriptors, the 6-year mortality rate was high, with a survival rate of 60 percent. In the lowest tercile the 6-year survival rate was much better, 92 percent. The distribution of patients with so-called single-, double-, and triple-vessel disease was the same for each tercile. Patients with left main coronary artery disease were excluded. This study again emphasizes the importance of functional capacity and historical factors in addition to extent of coronary arteriosclerosis as major prognostic factors.

The data concerning prognostic implications of angiographic findings in stable reversible myocardial ischemia can be summarized. The patient may have stable angina pectoris, no angina but objective evidence of ischemia, or angina equivalents (dyspnea or exhaustion with effort). The prognosis worsens as the extent of arteriographic abnormality increases, as LV dysfunction increases, and as exercise tolerance is reduced. The outlook for so-called single-vessel disease and good ventricular function is good, less than 1 to 2 percent mortality rate each year for the 5 years after presentation. Disease localized to the LAD artery carries a poorer prognosis than a similar degree of disease localized to the right coronary artery. Left main coronary artery lesions carry a very poor prognosis. So-called double- and triple-vessel diseases are intermediate. The prognosis of patients with angina equivalents may be poor because the complaints are sometimes due to severe disease with global myocardial ischemia. There are, however, inadequate reports on such patients.

Ventriculographic abnormalities are additive and even more powerful in predicting outcome than extent of atherosclerotic lesions. Exercise tolerance is an important independent prognostic factor.

Stable patients can be placed in low (1 to 2 percent annual mortality) and high (greater than 5 percent annual mortality) prognostic subsets by utilizing these principles and methods. The importance of reassessing prognosis on a timely basis in all stable patients cannot be overemphasized.

Unstable Angina Pectoris

Unstable angina pectoris and prolonged myocardial ischemia without objective evidence of infarction are clinical entities that carry similar connotations in reference to prognosis during the 3 to 6 months following their onset. (See also Chap. 59.) Retrospective studies, some done more than 50 years ago, emphasized that a change in symptoms occurs in 50 to 75 percent of patients preceding myocardial infarction.[42–44] Prospective data concerning the frequency of infarction and sudden death in patients who are experiencing the unstable anginal syndromes are fragmentary, but it is clear that such patients experience a significantly higher rate of complications than do patients with stable angina during the 3 to 6 months following the onset of the syndrome. When considering prognoses in unstable syndromes, it is important to remember that all the features listed in Table 61-1 must be considered. In that sense, the change in symptoms that heralds the onset of the unstable state represents an additive prognostic feature.

Gazes et al.[45] studied 140 patients judged to have unstable angina severe enough to require hospitalization during a period prior to evolution of our current concepts of pathophysiology and management. There was an 18 percent 1-year mortality in patients who had preexisting stable angina or pectoris and/or who persisted with frequent episodes of ischemia accompanied by ST-segment elevation after hospitalization. A prospective study by Duncan et al.[46] in Edinburgh examined 251 patients with new or worsening angina who were not hospitalized. In this mildly symptomatic group, the prognosis was better, but 4 percent died, and 12 percent developed myocardial infarction during a 6-month follow-up. Thirty-one percent were angina free at the end of the 6-month period. Other studies[47,48] have also determined a higher incidence of events, not surprisingly, because patient selection will influence the data gathered on outcome of unstable angina. In an interesting retrospective study by Roberts et al.,[49] 329 patients with new onset (less than 3 months) angina were compared with 1398 patients with chronic angina. At the end of 1 year, 16 percent of the new onset angina patients had suffered a cardiac event (nonfatal myocardial infarction or death), while 7 percent in the chronic angina group had such complications. Of particular interest is the finding that the new onset angina group had less severe anatomic disease. These studies emphasized the hazardous nature of the unstable phase and demonstrated substantially increased mortality and morbidity when compared with the stable phase.

Other prospectively designed studies have provided useful information, but patient selection, protocol design, and therapeutic interventions prevent direct comparison of studies and/or accurate estimate of prognosis for broad groups of patients. The National Cooperative Study[50] excluded patients with left main coronary arteriosclerosis and the protocol design prevented a true assessment of natural history because "crossover" to surgery from the medical treatment group was permitted when symptoms exacerbated. In this study patients assigned to medical therapy had a 10 percent mortality rate, a 19 percent incidence of myocardial infarction, and a 36 percent crossover to surgery for persistent angina during an average follow-up of 30 months after randomization. As would be anticipated, the incidence of these events was higher in the first few months following randomization and greater than expected for patients with stable angina.

The prospective study by Gerstenblith et al.[51] has a different experimental design and allowed inclusion of patients who had had myocardial infarction in the previous 3 months (35 percent of patients), patients over the age of 70, and those who were not candidates for bypass surgery on the basis of poor distal vessels. The principal reason for the study was an evaluation of drug therapy. Of 138 patients in the study, however, 19 percent had sudden death or myocardial infarction and an additional 30 percent (excluding those with left main coronary artery disease) required bypass surgery in a 4-month follow-up. Although the study suggested that therapy with a calcium channel blocker improved outcome when added to other medical therapy, it emphasized the hazardous nature of the unstable phase. Patients with ST-segment elevation during episodes of pain had a more serious prognosis than those who did not. The incidence of events, sudden cardiac death, myocardial infarction, and symptoms requiring bypass surgery, lessened with time; and by 3 to 4 months after the onset of the unstable phase, the number of events was at a very low frequency. These data suggest that the unstable period in such patients may last for 3 to 4 months, an important consideration in reference to therapy and prognosis.

An additional prospective study of unstable angina with a different experimental design yields similar information.[52] In a protocol designed to assess the efficacy of low-dose aspirin, 1266 men were selected from the 13,666 who were screened. Selection criteria excluded patients with recent myocardial infarction (6 weeks) and any clinical factor that might have resulted in an increase in myocardial oxygen consumption (such as paroxysmal tachycardia, anemia, hypoxia, or congestive heart failure). The patients were younger than in the Gerstenblith study. In a 12-week follow-up of this highly selected sample, 6.7 percent died or experienced acute myocardial infarction as compared to 10.1 percent in a control placebo group. The death rate in the control group of patients was 3.3 percent during the 3-month study period. These event rates, with or without drug treatment, are substantially higher than would be anticipated in patients with stable angina pectoris.

Silent myocardial ischemia occurs in all subsets of patients with manifest ischemic heart diesase. (See Chaps. 58 to 60.) One study found that 50 percent of patients with unstable angina had concomitant silent episodes as judged by ambulatory monitoring. As in the stable syndrome, the total ischemic burden, or the total of combined symptomatic plus silent episodes, was an important prognostic determinant.[53]

An intriguing area of current research concerns hypotheses that might explain why patients enter the unstable phase of disease and provide clues to how long the unstable phase persists. Where data are available, it appears the unstable phase usually persists for about 3 months. After that period, the occurrence of "events"—myocardial infarction, sudden cardiac death, ischemic episodes occurring at rest—diminishes to the level seen in the stable phase. Several angiographic and angioscopic studies[54,55] demonstrate lesions of a different morphology in the unstable phase when compared with lesions from patients in the stable phase. A variety of endothelial abnormalities, including plaque ulceration and rupture and filling defects suggestive of thrombus, are frequently seen in patients in the unstable phase but are only rarely present in those with stable complaints. These so-called acute, active, complex lesions could be responsible for episodic thrombus formation and spasm and account for the clinical manifestations of the unstable phase. It is reasonable to speculate that such lesions may heal over a period of several months or become even more active and provoke sinister events, such as infarction or sudden death.[56–58] In either instance, these lesions and their subsequent healing would account for the evanescent nature of the unstable phase. (See also Chaps. 55, 56, and 59.)

The information available regarding prognosis of patients with the unstable angina syndrome can be summarized. Clinical recognition and *prompt attention to evaluation and therapy are of critical importance in patients with new onset or change in symptoms because the incidence of sudden cardiac death and myocardial infarction in the 3 to 6 months following onset of an unstable anginal syndrome is higher than in stable patients.* Patients experiencing this presentation of atherosclerotic CHD represent a broad spectrum. Some will have had stable angina pectoris and/or previous myocardial infarction while others will be experiencing their first manifestation of disease. Patients who experience ST-segment elevation during episodes or who have episodes that persist despite excellent drug therapy or who have had previous symptomatic ischemic heart disease tend to have worse prognosis than those without such features. Left ventricular function is an important prognostic factor. Finally, the unstable state is a transient phase expected to persist 3 to 4 months in most patients, following which the patient develops stable angina and/or becomes asymptomatic. The prognosis then becomes the prognosis of the new clinical subset. (See Chap. 59.)

Variant (Prinzmetal's) Angina

Variant Prinzmetal's angina[59] (see Chap. 59) deserves comment for historical and pathophysiological reasons. These patients represent an unstable angina subset with ST-segment elevation during attacks that are not precipitated by an increase in myocardial oxygen demand. These episodes are due to coronary spasm. Coronary spasm is not unique to variant angina and may occur in a variety of other unstable angina states and also as a prelude to myocardial infarction. Coronary artery narrowing may also occur during exertion in patients with stable angina pectoris. Arteriographic study may reveal normal vessels in patients with variant angina. Most patients with variant angina in the United States have significant coronary atherosclerosis. Patients with variant angina and angiographically normal or near normal coronary arteries on arteriography may be more common in certain countries, i.e., Japan. Hence, as is true with any clinical descriptor, the subset of variant angina has multiple subsets. The first 3 months following the onset of variant angina is a hazardous time. During this period the incidence of sudden death or myocardial infarction is high and has been reported to be 18 percent in 132 patients studied by Waters et al.[60] The more severe the coronary atherosclerosis, the more disturbed the left ventricular dysfunction, and the less the response to appropriate therapy, the worse the prognosis.[60–63] The most intriguing aspect of variant angina is its cyclic nature. Regardless of the background anatomic features, the disease is often phasic, and when patients are in a period of remission, even ergonovine infusions may not provoke spasm and ST-T changes. Active phases usually persist 3 to 6 months. Many of the episodes while the patients are in the active phase of their disease are asymptomatic since monitoring often discloses episodes of ST-segment elevation unaccompanied by any symptoms.

Prolonged Ischemic Discomfort

An additional large, unstable subset of patients is comprised of those who have isolated, sometimes single, episodes of prolonged ischemic discomfort without objective evidence of myocardial infarction. These patients are frequently admitted to coronary care units to "rule out myocardial infarction." Although it is difficult to define definitively that these isolated episodes of prolonged chest discomfort are due to myocardial ischemia, the available data indicate that the mortality rate and incidence of myocardial infarction in this group at 1 to 2 years following the episodes are very similar to those of patients who are discharged following recovery from a documented myocardial infarction.[64,65] (See also Chap. 60.)

CORONARY ATHEROSCLEROSIS WITH MYOCARDIAL INFARCTION

The prognosis in patients with myocardial infarction may be considered in three phases: very early profound ischemia, evolving infarction, and completed infarction.

Very Early Profound Ischemia

Most patients who die in the first few minutes or several hours after the onset of an attack may not have myocardial necrosis or infarction demonstrable by routine study techniques. Most die of a catastrophic arrhythmia, primarily ventricular fibrillation, prior to the development of overt necrosis; some die with overwhelming pulmonary edema and shock. Lethal arrhythmias due to ischemia are as often a cause of death, as is AMI (necrosis). (See section below on sudden cardiac death and Chaps. 36 and 51.)

In a careful study in Edinburgh, nearly 50 percent of the total 30-day mortality occurred in the first 1 to 2 h after the onset of the episode and 70 to 80 percent during the first 24 h. Hence, of the 30 to 40 percent total mortality rate at 30 days, 15 to 20 of every hundred patients with an acute heart attack will die in the first 1 to 2 h, often before reaching a medical facility.[64,65] (See also Chap. 51.)

This statistic and the pattern of death suggest that mortalities reported by the coronary care unit have relatively little significance and will vary widely unless the time between the onset of the patient's complaint and arrival at the coronary care unit is known. If admission to the coronary care unit is delayed for some hours, the period of highest mortality is passed, and the mortality in such a coronary care unit will be lower than in a unit whose location and/or admitting arrangements allow arrival of patients very early following the onset of symptoms.

Evolving Myocardial Infarction

The concept of evolving infarction has assumed major importance, because thrombolytic therapy is most effective in the first several hours. While it is understood that the evolution of an infarction may take place over several days, it is clinically useful to consider the first 4 to 6 h as the critical time for myocardial salvage. (See also Chaps. 60 and 69.)

The principal determinants of mortality on patient arrival at the emergency room are shown in Table 61-3. Most relate to infarct size, which can be estimated only indirectly in the clinical setting. Older age is a very powerful prognostic factor. (See Fig. 61-1.)

The pain and/or discomfort of acute infarction are important in helping to establish the diagnosis, but the ischemic discomfort per se is of no major prognostic significance. *Many patients with extensive and even fatal infarction have little discomfort, sometimes none whatsoever (particularly the elderly).* It is estimated that 25 percent of infarcts are silent. Prognosis has been shown to be unrelated to the character or occurrence of pain. In addition, other problems during the course of infarction

TABLE 61-3

Prognostic Determinants: Evolving Myocardial Infarction
Age
Gender
Electrocardiographic changes (infarct location, conduction defects, number of leads with ST shifts, previous MI)
Blood pressure
Clinical manifestations (especially left ventricular failure)
Preexisting disease
Stable angina
Previous myocardial infarction
Cardiomegaly
Peak enzyme level (requires 24–36 h)
Associated diseases
Diabetes
Hypertension
Pulmonary disease

may produce chest discomfort; such complicating factors include pulmonary embolism, pericarditis, and upper gastrointestinal disease, especially peptic ulcer problems.

Cardiac arrhythmias are of enormous importance, but there is uncertainty concerning the prognostic implications of arrhythmias. The arrhythmias that occur with advanced left ventricular failure and are associated with other evidence of extensive infarction, including intraventricular conduction defects, do not have independent additional prognostic significance. Similarly, so-called primary ventricular fibrillation, which occurs early in the course of infarction without associated left ventricular dysfunction and responds promptly to defibrillation in the coronary care unit, does not measurably worsen the prognosis. In one study of 2088 myocardial infarctions,[66] 147 patients (7 percent) had ventricular fibrillation (VF) during the first 48 h. Although there was a hospital mortality of 25 percent in the fibrillation patients (compared to 13 percent in those without early fibrillation), 50 percent of the VF patients had accompanying left ventricular failure and/or cardiogenic shock, which was the immediate cause of death. Of all the patients discharged, the 1-year mortality and causes of death after hospital discharge were not different in patients with early VF compared to the total sample. The arguments concerning arrhythmia as an independent prognostic factor in its relationship to myocardial infarction size have been summarized by Cox et al.[67] Since most arrhythmias are reasonably easily controlled and those not readily controlled often have their genesis in a large infarction, usually associated with left ventricular dysfunction, it seems probable that arrhythmias per se are not important prognostic determinants in evolving myocardial infarction. There are occasional spectacular exceptions in patients who otherwise are judged to have a favorable prognosis but experience refractory ventricular arrhythmias and die as a consequence of them.

Serial electrocardiographic studies may provide additional insights into infarct size. Q-wave infarction denotes a larger area of necrosis than non-Q-wave infarction. Q-wave anterior infarction tends to result in larger infarcts than Q-wave inferior infarction, although there are *important exceptions.* Inferior infarction accompanied by right ventricular infarction, complete heart block, and/or striking reciprocal depression of anterior ST segments have a very unfavorable prognosis.[68] In addition, the relatively favorable prognosis of inferior myocardial infarction is lost in older patients. Intriguing data suggest that anterior infarction carries a more serious prognosis even if estimates of infarction size are similar.[69] The degree of ST-segment elevation and the number of leads with ST-segment elevation in initial tracings give a crude estimate of the infarct size and often presage the development of Q waves and eventual scarring. Past disease, the presence of pericarditis, occasional electrolyte disturbances, and the exact time at which the ECG is recorded all influence the information obtained. Even with complicated techniques and sophisticated analyses, involving extensive mapping using multiple precordial leads, no easily applicable reliable method for clinical use has evolved. (See also Chap. 60.)

Multiple studies have shown that the peak enzyme level is roughly correlated with infarct size.[70,71] As a clinically useful prognostic feature, a markedly elevated (five or six times normal) value indicates a large infarct and is associated with more frequent complications and higher mortality. On the other hand, a lower value does not necessarily guarantee a favorable prognosis, a conclusion apparent from the prognostic determinants in Table 61-3, which include past infarction and age. Older patients have more complications and higher mortality for the same degree (or less) of enzyme release.[11]

Other clinical findings, including a pericardial friction rub, leukocytosis greater than 20,000 per mm^3, and high fever (39° or greater without complicating cause) are features indicating poor prognosis. Since these features accompany evidence of a large infarction and/or congestive heart failure, they are prognostic indicators, but only when considered in light of the total picture.

Increasing age has an important adverse effect on prognosis. Patients over the age of 70 with Q-wave infarction have a high mortality rate, more than 25 percent in a number of series. A variety of disease states, particularly diabetes mellitus (primarily in patients requiring insulin), hypertension, and chronic pulmonary disease, tend to worsen prognosis by producing altered myocardial metabolism or hypoxia and/or by increasing myocardial oxygen requirements.

Major prognostic determinants have been combined to develop an index that can be easily obtained. One such index was devised by Norris and his colleagues.[72] The approach assesses simple major prognostic factors evaluated by discriminant analysis (Table 61-4). In this study six factors that can be obtained in the emergency room and that proved to have additive significance in establishing prognosis were selected from several hundred that were recorded in a large group of patients with myocardial infarction. Sophisticated analyses of the data give a numerical weighing (X) from 0 (absent) to 1. Each of the six items is further weighted according to the effect it has on morality (Y). The prognostic index is arrived at by adding the values of the products XY, i.e., $X_1Y_1 \pm \cdots = X_nY_n$ (prognostic index).

Noninvasive clinical indices such as the Norris index have provided the opportunity to study the prognosis of myocardial infarction over time and to do comparative studies among institutions. One important and interesting study has been done at the Royal Melbourne Hospital in Melbourne, Australia.[73] All 4253 infarction patients were studied prospectively from 1969 to 1983. Striking reduction in overall hospital mortality was seen in men, from 16.7 percent from 1969 to 1973 to 8.5 percent for the period 1979 to 1983. There were far fewer women (only 887 of the sample), but the mortality in women was constant at 19.2 percent during both periods. The higher mortality in women compared to that in men is a finding in many studies. Utilizing the Norris infarct severity indices, one could not account for the reduction in mortality on the basis of case mix, and the better outcomes must be related to management. This interesting and important study makes clear why historical controls cannot be used to assess prognosis in comparative studies, with or without therapeutic interventions. Some of the data from this study are summarized in Fig. 61-4.

Table 61-5 provides a combination of clinical descriptors and hemodynamic measurements that relate to

TABLE 61-4
Discriminant Analysis in a Prognostic Index

Factor	X	Y
Age (yr) (X_1, Y_1)		
<50	0.2	
50–59	0.4	
60–69	0.6	3.9
70–79	0.8	
80–89	1.0	
Position of infarct (X_2, Y_2)		
Anterior transmural	1.0	
Left bundle branch block	1.0	
Posterior transmural	0.7	2.8
Anterior subendocardial	0.3	
Posterior subendocardial	0.3	
Admission systolic blood pressure (mmHg) (X_3, Y_3):		
<55	1.0	
55–64	0.7	
65–74	0.6	
75–84	0.5	
85–94	0.4	10.0
95–104	0.3	
105–114	0.2	
115–125	0.1	
≥125	0	
Heart size (X_4, Y_4)		
Normal	0	
Doubtfully enlarged	0.5	1.5
Definitely enlarged	1.0	
Lung fields (X_5, Y_5)		
Normal	0	
Venous congestion	0.3	3.3
Interstitial edema	0.6	
Pulmonary edema	1.0	
Previous ischemia (X_6, Y_6)		
No ischemia	0	0.4
Previous angina or infarction	1	

NOTE: See explanation in text.
SOURCE: Norris RM, Brandt PWT, Caughey DE, et al.[72] Reproduced with permission from the publisher and author.

short-term (30-day) prognosis.[74] The Killip classification,[75] which utilizes only clinical descriptions (i.e., rales and peripheral perfusion), provides a reasonable separation for severe and mild cases; however, the lack of an age component reduces its usefulness.

Completed Myocardial Infarction

Since most of the myocardial damage occurs in the initial 6 h after the onset of chest discomfort, it is reasonable to consider the infarct as "complete" after that time. Additional evolutionary changes continue for some days and "stuttering" infarction occurs in some patients. In addition, myocardial stunning persists for as long as 10 days in some patients. These matters are of importance in timing the assessment of prognosis following completed myocardial infarction.

The 9 to 12 months following hospital discharge is a hazardous time. Following first myocardial infarction, a 6 to 10 percent mortality occurs, with most of the deaths in the first 6 months. In the second and third year following acute myocardial infarction, mortality rate is reduced to 3 to 4 percent per year. Extensive investigation of patients 2 to 4 weeks postinfarction has clarified the factors that allow a prediction of long-term prognosis.

Multiple studies have indicated that left ventricular function is a powerful determinant of postmyocardial infarction outcome. The study by a group of Spanish investigators[76] is particularly instructive. Ejection fraction, angiographically determined, was the most powerful predictor of 5-year outcome. Patients who had a resting ejection fraction of greater than 50 percent had an extremely low mortality rate while there was increasing mortality as resting ejection fraction reduced. Although the extent of coronary angiographic abnormality was additive, the ejection fraction was a much more powerful discriminator than angiographic abnormality. Figure 61-5 illustrates the point.

The occurrence of angina is generally a poor prognos-

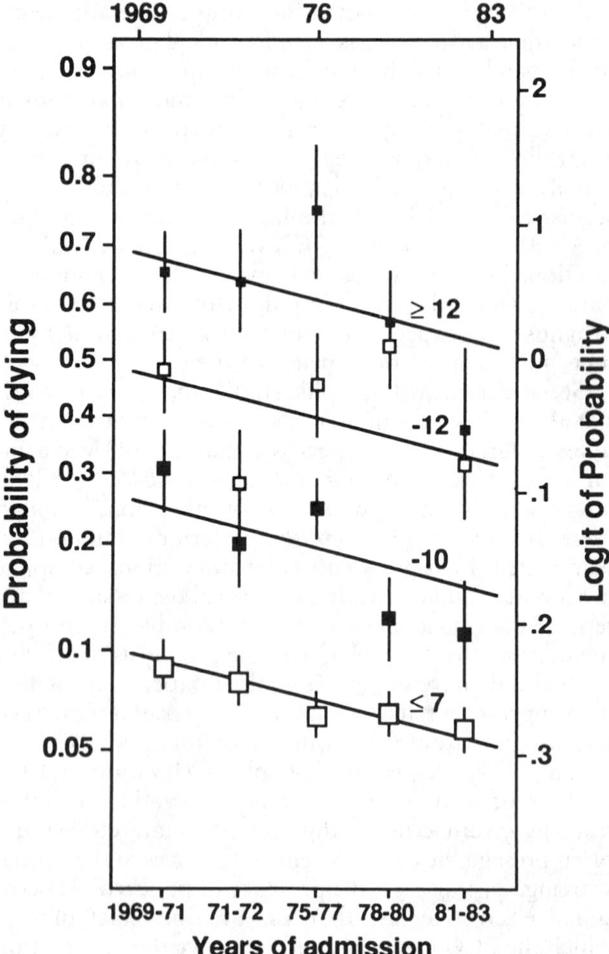

FIGURE 61-4 The graph demonstrates the in-hospital mortality for four prognostic subsets during the years 1969–1983. The same prognostic variables (age, site of MI or ECG, admitting BP, heart size and pulmonary congestion on chest x-ray, and history of previous ischemic disease) were used in the prognostic index. Applying the index at a single institution, there is a trend toward lower mortality in all prognostic subsets.

TABLE 61-5
Mortality Rates in Clinical and Hemodynamic Subsets

Subset	Pulmonary Congestion*	Peripheral Hypoperfusion†	% Mortality	
			Clinical	Hemodynamic
I	−	−	1	3
II	+	−	11	9
III	−	+	18	23
IV	+	+	60	51

* Pulmonary-capillary pressure > 18 mmHg.
† Cardiac index < 2.2 liters/min per m².
SOURCE: Forrester JS, Diamond G, Chatterjee K, et al.[74] Abstracted by permission of the *New England Journal of Medicine* and the author.

tic sign since it suggests the propensity for additional infarction. In some patients spasm may be the explanation rather than critical fixed narrowing.

Objective, rather than subjective, estimates of ischemia are preferred when assessing prognosis. Treadmill exercise testing in the early postinfarction period is popular and useful. Multiple studies indicate that ST-segment depression and angina during exercise and/or reduced exercise tolerance connote a poor prognosis. An early study of 210 patients[77] showed a favorable prognosis if no ST-segment depression was present (2.1 percent mortality rate in the year following infarction) but an extremely high (27 percent) mortality rate in the 64 patients with ST-segment depression. Although multiple studies have confirmed these observations, some have not. When reported, exercise capacity and appropriate blood pressure increase are always predictive variables.[78,79]

The predictive value of PVCs is highly variable in reference to prognosis. Many of the reports do not include enough variables to know the independent effect of PVCs. The PVCs are highly correlated with ventricular dysfunction as well as exercise-induced ischemia. In a multicenter trial involving 866 patients, careful postinfarction clinical assessment disclosed four descriptors, including PVCs at a rate of more than 10 per hour, to be important prognostic determinants.[80] The other variables were an ejection fraction of less than 40 percent, rales in the upper lung field *during the course of acute infarction,* and New York Heart Association functional classes II to IV *before admission.* An ejection fraction less than 40 percent was the single most powerful item in this study. One-third of the patients had none of the four factors present, and their mortality in the 2 years following the infarct was less than 3 percent.

Attempts to use electrophysiological testing with programmed ventricular stimulation to define further the implications of arrhythmias in the postinfarction period have resulted in conflicting evidence. Variables in interpreting such studies include the stimulation protocols utilized, patient selection, and treatment programs. Additional information and further refinement concerning the role of arrhythmias in the postinfarction patients can be expected, since this is an area of intense clinical investigation. Some reports are most enthusiastic.[81] There are currently underway large multicenter trials concerning this issue. Similarly, data related to the prognostic implications of late potentials detected by signal averaging are accumulating but incomplete. (See also Chaps. 47 and 60.)

Further refinement and extension of the risk stratification concept has been attempted utilizing radionuclide techniques.[82,83] Using ^{201}Tl scintigraphy, one can identify high-risk postinfarction patients by the development of more than one discrete defect (redistribution) or increased lung uptake. Exercise-induced reduction in ejection fraction and/or contractile state in studies using ^{99m}Tc-labeled red blood cells has been associated with an increased risk of events. On the other hand, the selection criteria for patients were variable, and the numbers of patients involved have been relatively small. The critical items are an objective estimate of ischemia and ventricular function during exercise rather than the specific technique or endpoint used. Since the best endpoints are those that are objectively quantitative, this makes radionuclide studies appealing, although there are interpretative problems especially with ^{201}Tl studies. (See also Chap. 134.) Whether or not data from such studies add independent prognostic information to more simple and less expensively obtained studies is unanswered. In one study of 351 hospital survivors of myocardial infarction who could perform exercise, it was concluded that prognostic stratification was not significantly improved by adding ambulatory electrocardiographic monitoring and radioventriculographic study to the more simply obtained clinical and exercise variables.[84]

It is important to differentiate non-Q-wave infarctions (formerly termed "subendocardial" or "nontransmural" infarction) from Q-wave infarctions. Non-Q-wave infarctions tend to involve a lesser amount of myocardium and to have a more favorable short-term outlook. Multiple studies have demonstrated, however, a higher incidence of late reinfarction and a higher mortality during the subsequent 2 to 3 years than for Q-wave infarctions.[85-88] It is, perhaps, most appropriate to consider non-Q-wave infarction as a relatively unstable phase of ischemic heart disease requiring risk stratification and a relatively more aggressive diagnostic approach, similar to that for a patient with unstable angina. Angiographic findings support this concept and approach, demonstrating "active, acute" lesions as in unstable angina.[88] (See Chaps. 59 and 60.)

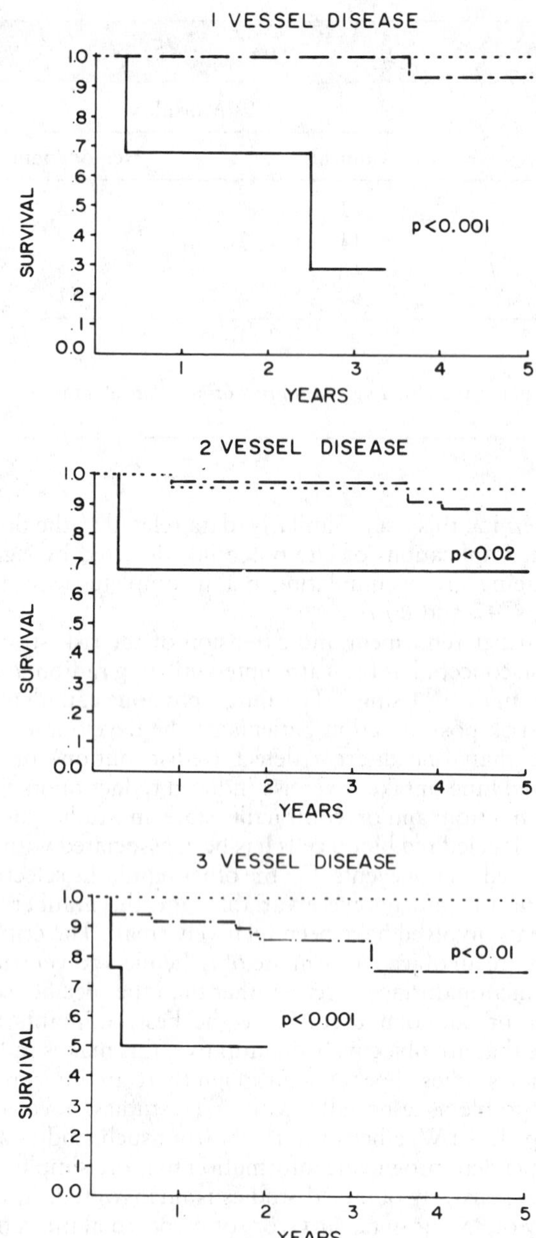

FIGURE 61-5 The relation among coronary atherosclerosis, resting ejection fraction, and 5-year survival in 241 patients evaluated following recovery from acute myocardial infarction. *P* values represent differences (long-rank test) between the group with an ejection fraction of 50 percent and the other two groups. Ejection fraction > 50 percent = ----; ejection fraction 21–49 percent = • - • -; ejection fraction < 21 percent = ———. *(From Sanz G et al.*[76] *Abstracted by permission of The New England Journal of Medicine and the author.)*

The information concerning prediction of outcome in the completed postinfarction period can be summarized as follows. Left ventricular function and objective evidence of ischemia as judged by exercise testing are the most important determinants. Ventricular ectopy appears to be an independent additive factor. Preexisting disease, particularly myocardial infarction, and the occurrence of heart failure during the acute infarction are additive factors. When all factors are taken into account, the extent of coronary atherosclerosis on arteriography appears to be a relatively weak contributing factor. Perhaps this is not surprising since a majority, usually 60 to 70 percent, of patients who have suffered myocardial infarction have two- or three-vessel disease, and one would not anticipate this to be a highly discriminatory factor. Refinements in the arteriographic classification of disease may enhance the prognostic value of this factor. Additional items such as age, diabetes, cardiomegaly, and hypertension aid in prognosis. Unfortunately, we do not currently have methods that can be readily utilized routinely to assess the tendency to produce arterial thrombosis or the vasomotor responsiveness of the coronary circulation.

A variety of approaches and methods are used to assess prognosis, but the four key determinants include left ventricular function, the presence of ischemia, the extent of coronary arteriosclerosis, and ventricular ectopy. Again, the variables listed in Table 61-1 should all be considered. How these factors are assessed in each patient is a matter of debate, experience, and physician choice. Regardless of the approach used, an evaluation resulting in risk stratification is important. Special attention should be given to patients who have non-Q-wave infarction since they represent a borderline situation between unstable angina and Q-wave infarction with the propensity for additional complications in the few months following diagnosis. (See also Chaps. 60 and 63.)

Complicated Myocardial Infarction

In many instances it is not simple to differentiate uncomplicated myocardial infarction from complicated infarction. A patient who is pursuing an uncomplicated course may suddenly experience an important new event or some subtle finding, not previously appreciated may become apparent, placing the patient in a high-risk group. (See also Chap. 60.)

Physicians have long appreciated that a significant proportion of patients with AMI suffer a "recurrent" infarction or "extension" within a few hours or several days. Careful serial enzyme and electrocardiographic methods in small numbers of patients indicate that extension may affect 30 to 50 percent of cases in the first week following infarcts.[89,90] This unexpectedly high incidence of infarct extension is likely related to case selection. The propensity for non-Q-wave infarction to extend is an important consideration in evaluating these kinds of data.[91] Diagnosing myocardial extension is not always simple, since ventricular remodeling and infarct expansion may occur and be a confounding factor. (See also Chap. 60.)

With the advent of thrombolytic therapy, "reinfarction" has become a better understood entity. In early thrombolytic trials, it occurred in as many as 15 to 20 percent of patients who had successful thrombolysis. The incidence is much lower with more effective use of adjunctive therapy, especially aspirin and intravenous heparin. It is suspected that infarction extension in Q and non-Q infarction is related to the same mechanism as reinfarction after successful thrombolysis, i.e., reocclusion of the infarct-related vessel. (See also Chap. 56.)

Many of the complications that occur in myocardial infarction can be related to the prognostic factors previously discussed. There are, however, many additional specific complications. The appearance, usually during the first week, of a new (sometimes, but not always) loud systolic murmur that is associated with the development of acute left ventricular failure in a patient with acute myocardial infarction arouses great interest. This is most likely to be a ventricular septal defect or a rupture of a papillary muscle or portion of the mitral valve apparatus. Probably less than 1 percent of patients have these complications. Both papillary muscle rupture and ventricular septal defect are potentially amenable to surgical therapy. Without surgery, both carry an extremely poor prognosis, with mortality rates in the range of 80 to 90 percent in the several weeks following the event unless recognized and treated surgically. The management of ruptured ventricular septum requires considerable judgment and individualization and is discussed later in this chapter and in Chap. 74.

SUDDEN DEATH

Sudden death is a major consideration when discussing the prognosis of atherosclerotic coronary heart disease since more than half of patients with known ischemic heart disease die suddenly. (See also Chaps. 51 and 60.) Of all the patients presenting with ischemic heart disease, sudden death is the initial and final event in nearly one-third. Many descriptions for sudden death have been proposed; unexpected cardiac death in a patient with or without preexisting disease within 1 h of having been free of symptoms is a reasonable definition. It is difficult, however, to get agreement on either a definition of sudden cardiac death or, among independent observers, on the cause of death in specific patients, even when definitions have been established.[92] Since patients who are victims of sudden cardiac death regularly have both serious diminution of ventricular function as well as ischemia, the precise cause of death is more difficult to ascertain than might be suspected. Estimates vary, but it is possible than at least 400,000 sudden cardiac deaths occur in the United States each year. The overwhelming majority are due to atherosclerotic CHD. This complex topic is considered in Chap. 51.

Most patients with ischemic heart disease who suffer sudden cardiac death have extensive coronary arteriosclerosis, frequently associated with ventricular scarring and reduced left ventricular function. In the Cardiac-Arrhythmia Suppression Trial (CAST) 23 baseline characteristics were prospectively assessed in the 743 patients randomized to the placebo arm.[93] All patients in the CAST had six or more PVCs per hour but no runs of ventricular tachycardia of 15 or more beats at a rate of at most 120 per minute, and all had a myocardial infarction in the last 2 years. All study patients had PVCs that could be suppressed by therapy. Patients in the placebo group proved to be in a low-risk group, with a 1-year mortality of 3.9 percent. Multivariate analysis demonstrated that the presence of a past Q-wave infarction, history of heart failure, use of digitalis, diabetes, and prolonged QRS duration were associated with substantial increased risk. On univariate analysis, other features indicative of ischemia or poor ventricular function, such as ejection fraction less than 30 percent or ST-segment depression of 1 mm greater on the resting ECG, were additional poor prognostic features.

Patients with sudden cardiac death infrequently experience prodromal symptoms, unlike patients who experience myocardial infarction, where a large majority have prodromal symptoms. Obviously, these data are difficult to obtain. This brief discussion will not include sudden cardiac death as related to diagnosable AMI. (See also Chap. 51.)

The majority of sudden cardiac deaths occur outside the hospital, and valuable information has been provided by an extensive community-wide program of resuscitation in Seattle, Washington. This program demonstrated that the majority of patients who suffer sudden cardiac death outside the hospital but are resuscitated do not have myocardial infarction and that there is a high propensity for suffering recurrent sudden cardiac death after the resuscitation if myocardial necrosis is not found during subsequent hospitalization. In survivors of out-of-hospital sudden cardiac death, the 1-year mortality rate is 4 percent if AMI occurred compared to 26 percent (nearly all of the deaths sudden) for the entire group.[94–97] This interesting statistic might be predicted on the basis of coronary care unit experience, where so-called primary ventricular fibrillation, occurring very early in the course of AMI and unaccompanied by other complications of ventricular dysfunction, does not carry an ominous long-term prognosis when treated promptly.[98–100] *The high incidence of recurrent ventricular fibrillation in the year following resuscitation is almost certainly associated with chronic advanced ventricular dysfunction and/or persistent propensity for ischemia.*

Attempts to improve our ability to predict which patients might suffer cardiac death, particularly as the first manifestation of their ischemic heart disease, have resulted in the hypothesis that the risk factors for sudden cardiac death are the same as those for other manifestations of atherosclerotic CHD. However, because only a minority, probably less than 20 percent, of patients with sudden cardiac death have a demonstrable AMI at postmortem examination, it seems likely that additional "risk factors" beyond those customarily considered are important in this subset of patients. The elegant postmortem studies of Davies[57] demonstrate a high incidence of platelet thrombi. (See also Chap. 55.)

The other major subset of patients suffering sudden cardiac death includes those who have previously manifested and/or currently experience symptomatic ischemic heart disease. The items listed in the Table 61-1 apply to this subset of patients. Multiple studies have demonstrated that left ventricular dysfunction and/or clinical symptoms accompanying left ventricular dysfunction are powerful predictors of sudden cardiac death. In groups of patients with manifest disease and poor ventricular function, the presence of PVCs particularly complex forms, is an independent additive feature in most studies. Although it has been difficult to establish PVCs as an independent risk factor, there is now general agreement that such is the case. To date, the important issues concerning the effectiveness of antiarrhythmic drugs in suppressing premature ventricular depolarizations and the influence of such suppression on the incidence of sudden cardiac death have not been resolved.

In the largest and most carefully done randomized trial, CAST, the suppression of asymptomatic PVCs by flecainide, encainide, or moricizine was not associated with a decrease in mortality during the subsequent follow-up period, but rather their use was associated with an increase in mortality.[101-103] (See also Chap. 50.)

ISCHEMIC CARDIOMYOPATHY

The imprecise term *ischemic cardiomyopathy* has been used by some in reference to a subset of patients in whom atherosclerotic coronary heart disease is manifested primarily, or exclusively, by myocardial dysfunction and congestive heart failure. It is caused by diffuse fibrosis and/or multiple infarctions. Unfortunately, the term is frequently used incorrectly in reference to any chronic decrease in left ventricular function in patients with coronary artery disease. (See also Chaps. 58, 60, and 87.)

There are subsets of patients with CHD and congestive heart failure who should not be considered as "ischemic cardiomyopathy." Some patients with an important degree of mitral regurgitation, those with discrete aneurysms, and patients who have some degree of myocardial scarring but who manifest an important element of dyspnea accompanying effort angina pectoris (indicating persistent viable myocardium at risk) must be identified. Such patients benefit from medical therapies and particularly surgical interventions that are not appropriate for patients who have ischemic cardiomyopathy.

Another interesting but poorly understood consideration in the area of chronic CHD or ischemic cardiomyopathy is persistent left ventricular dysfunction in the absence of extensive scarring resulting from long continued myocardial flow reduction. The term "hibernating myocardium" has been used to describe this situation. Its frequency is not yet known, and precise methods to determine its presence, which include coronary arteriography, estimates of left ventricular wall thickness, PET and nuclear medicine techniques, and ability of the "hibernating myocardium" to respond to inotropic stimuli, have not been well studied. (See Chap. 57.)

Some patients with coronary heart muscle disease or ischemic cardiomyopathy have congestive heart failure that is indistinguishable from that of an idiopathic primary cardiomyopathy or, rarely, even restrictive cardiomyopathy. This rare presentation is related to patchy fibrosis associated with diffuse severe coronary atherosclerosis in the absence of transmural myocardial infarction. In addition, some patients may have two conditions, diffuse coronary atherosclerosis and an independent cardiomyopathy or secondary heart muscle disease.

The more common manifestation of ischemic cardiomyopathy occurs following one, or more frequently multiple, myocardial infarctions with major areas of regional scars. It is possible that this condition is becoming more common in recent years. It is suspected that the use of coronary bypass surgery, which prolongs life in some subsets, may provide an opportunity for developing multiple small myocardial infarctions and areas of fibrosis that eventually result in coronary heart muscle disease or ischemic cardiomyopathy.

Although the term *ischemic cardiomyopathy* has been used to include multiple subsets, even after excluding complications not related primarily to left ventricular scarring, the prognosis in these subsets is generally very poor. Studies on relatively large numbers of patients in the mid-1970s indicated that very poor ventricular function, estimated from angiographic studies or left ventricular diastolic pressure, was associated with very high 5-year mortality rates.[32-35] In patients with so-called single-vessel disease, if there was associated marked global left ventricular dysfunction, the 5-year mortality rate was in excess of 50 percent. In one study, 84 percent of the patients were dead 5 years after presentation if clinical congestive heart failure was utilized as the descriptor.[32] In another study, a 31 percent 1-year mortality rate was reported.[104]

Patients with left ventricular resting ejection fraction less than 35 percent have been described from the CASS.[105] In this study 420 patients were followed with medical therapy, approximately one-half for a minimum of 3 years. Analyses of the data are complicated by the fact that slightly more than 50 percent had angina as a primary symptom, and only 20 percent reported congestive heart failure as the principal symptom. In slightly more than 25 percent, the angina was class III or class IV. At a 3-year follow-up 69 percent of patients who had chest discomfort and severe left ventricular dysfunction survived, while only 55 percent who had principally dyspnea or fatigue (ischemic cardiomyopathy) survived. Too few patients are reported to allow meaningful survival data beyond 3 years. Despite complexities in interpretation, the extremely poor prognosis is clear. In addition, symptoms are unremitting and progressive when clinical congestive failure is present.

Patients with CHD or ischemic cardiomyopathy may die as a consequence of unremitting refractory heart failure or recurrent myocardial infarction, but more suffer sudden cardiac death due to ventricular fibrillation. All patients with ischemic cardiomyopathy have PVCs, often complex forms, but carefully collected data on the independent importance of this feature have not been obtained.

The advent of better pharmacologic therapy for heart failure has resulted in randomized trials and provided additional and more precise prognostic data. Such studies emphasize the need to consider multiple risk factors in addition to the degree of left ventricular dysfunction. Randomized controlled trials with ACE inhibitors are particularly instructive. The Cooperative North Scandinavian Enalapril Survival Study (CONSENSUS)[106] included patients with far-advanced symptoms, New York Heart Association class IV within several weeks of entry into the study, and older persons (a mean age of 70 years) as well as many patients with atrial fibrillation (50 percent) and hypertension (20 percent). Sixty percent of the sample had coronary artery disease, and most of these had previous myocardial infarction. Although not a pure sample of ischemic cardiomyopathy, the mortality in the CONSENSUS placebo group of 126 patients was 52 percent at 1 year.

The Studies of Left Ventricular Dysfunction (SOLVD) selected a different set of patients. In one substudy, all patients had an ejection fraction less than 35 percent and had symptoms of heart failure and a mean age of 60 years.[107] Seventy-one percent of the sample had ischemic heart disease, and nearly 90 percent of the sample were in New York Heart Association class II or III. In the placebo group of 1284 patients the mortality was much lower than in the CONSENSUS group. About 12 to 14 percent per year died, giving a total mortality of 39.7 percent, during an average follow-up of 41.4 months. In another arm of the SOLVD study,[108] the placebo group also had an ejection fraction of less than 35 percent but were not receiving therapy for heart failure (New York Heart Association class I or II). The mean age of this group was 59 years, and 82 percent had ischemic heart disease. This large group of 2117 patients had a much lower mortality, 5 percent per year. In both of these placebo arms of the SOLVD substudies, in which all patients had ejection fractions less than 35 percent, a higher mortality occurred in patients with the lowest ejection fractions.

In the Survival and Ventricular Enlargement (SAVE) study, patients with left ventricular ejection fractions of 40 percent or less but without overt heart failure or symptoms of myocardial ischemia were identified 3 to 16 days after myocardial infarction. In the placebo group of 1116 patients, the all-cause mortality rate was 25 percent during an average follow-up of 42 months. In 1115 patients treated with captopril, there was an improvement in survival and a reduced morbidity and mortality due to major cardiovascular events.[109] (See also Chap. 60.)

The data available can be summarized. It is important to be specific if one uses the term ischemic cardiomyopathy and to exclude patients who have reversible myocardial ischemia, major mitral regurgitation, or discrete aneurysms. Even with such exclusions, some patients with coronary heart muscle disease or ischemic cardiomyopathy will have diffuse ventricular dysfunction with small scars and patchy fibrosis, while others will have large scarred areas with regions of well-functioning myocardium, usually with compensatory hypertrophy. It is possible that patients with the well-demarcated scars have a better outlook than those with diffuse dysfunction, but the rate of survival is very poor in both groups once symptoms of failure are present. With overt congestive heart failure, an annual mortality under 10 to as much as 50 percent may be found, depending on the degree of left ventricular dysfunction, the age of the patient, the occurrence of arrhythmia, the presence of hypertension, and the *degree of symptoms*. The presence of overt clinical congestive heart failure worsens the prognosis in groups of patients identified by objective measures of left ventricular dysfunction such as end-diastolic pressure, ejection fraction, or wall motion abnormalities.

REFERENCES

1. Califf RM, Pryor DB, Greenfield JC Jr: Beyond randomized clinical trials: Applying clinical experience in the treatment of patients with coronary artery disease. *Circulation* 1986; 74:1191–1194.
2. Friesinger GC: Prognosis in chronic ischemic heart disease. *Trans Am Clin Climatol Assoc* 1981; 91:98–107.
3. Friesinger GC: The reasonable workup before recommending medical or surgical therapy: An overall strategy. *Circulation* 1982; 65:21–26.
4. Feit F, Breed J, Anderson JL, Attubato MJ, Davison R, Sherrid MV: The TTOPP study. (abstr) *Circulation* 1990; 82 (suppl. III): III-666.
5. Gurwitz JH, Goldberg RJ, Gore JM: Coronary thrombolysis for the elderly? *JAMA* 1991; 265:720.
6. Solomon CG, Lee TH, Cook EF, Weisberg MC, Brad DA, Rouan GW, et al: Comparison of clinical presentation of acute myocardial infarction in patients older than 65 years of age to younger patients: The multicenter chest pain study experience. *Am J Cardiol* 1989; 63:772–776.
7. Tofler GH, Muller JE, Stone PH, Willich SN, Davis VG, Poole WK, et al: Factors leading to shorter survival after acute myocardial infarction in patients ages 65 to 75 years compared with younger patients. *Am J Cardiol* 1988; 62:860–867.
8. Weaver WD, Litwin PE, Martin JS, Kudenchuk PJ, Maynard C, Eisenberg MS, et al: Effect of age on use of thrombolytic therapy and mortality in acute myocardial infarction. *J Am Coll Cardiol* 1991; 18:657–662.
9. Saunamaki KI: Early post-myocardial infarction exercise testing in subjects 70 years or more of age. Functional and prognostic evaluation. *Eur Heart J* 1984; 5:93–96.
10. Podczeck A, Frohner K, Foderler G, Meisl K, Unger G, Steinbach K: Exercise test in patients over 65 years of age after the first myocardial infarction. *Eur Heart J* 1984; 5:89–92.
11. Goldberg RJ, Gore JM, Gurwitz JH, Alpert JS, Brady P, Strohsnitter W, et al: The impact of age on the incidence and prognosis of initial acute myocardial infarction: The Worcester Heart Attack Study. *Am Heart J* 1989; 117:543–549.
12. Ackerman RF, Dry TJ, Edwards JE: Relationship of various factors to the degree of coronary atherosclerosis in women. *Circulation* 1950; 1:1345–1354.
13. White NK, Edwards JE, Dry TJ: The relationship of the degree of coronary atherosclerosis with age, in men. *Circulation* 1950; 1:645–654.
14. Enos WF, Holmes RH, Byer J: Coronary disease among United States soldiers killed in action in Korea. *JAMA* 1953; 152:1090–1093.
15. Blumgart HL, Schlesinger MJ, Zoll PM: Angina pectoris, coronary failure and acute myocardial infarction. *JAMA* 1941; 116:91–97.
16. Erikssen J, Enge I, Forfang K, Storstein O: False positive diagnostic tests and coronary angiographic findings in 105 presumably healthy males. *Circulation* 1976; 54:371–376.
17. McHenry PL, O'Donnell J, Morris SN, Jordon JJ: The abnormal exercise electrocardiogram in apparently healthy men: A predictor of angina pectoris as an initial coronary event during long-term follow-up. *Circulation* 1984; 70:547–551.
18. Erikssen J, Thaulow E: Follow-up of patients with asymptomatic myocardial ischemia. In: Rutishaner W, Roskamon K (eds): *Silent Myocardial Ischemia.* Berlin, Springer-Verlag, 1984: 156–164.
19. Friesinger GC, Robertson RM: Silent myocardial ischemia. *Curr Opinion Cardiol* 1987; 2:961.
20. Rocco MB, Barry J, Campbell S, Nabel E, Cook EF, Goldman L, et al: Circadian variation of transient myocardial ischemia in patients with coronary artery disease. *Circulation* 1987; 75:395–400.
21. European Coronary Surgery Study Group: Prospective randomized study of coronary artery bypass surgery in stable angina pectoris: Second interim report. *Lancet* 1980; 2:491–495.
22. Murphy ML, Hultgren HN, Detre K, Thomsen J, Takaro T: Treatment of chronic stable angina: A preliminary report of survival data of the randomized Veterans Administration Cooperative Study. *N Engl J Med* 1977; 297:621–627.
23. Proudfit WJ, Bruschke AV, MacMillan JP, Williams GW, Sones FM Jr: Fifteen-year survival study of patients with obstructive coronary artery disease. *Circulation* 1983; 68:986–997.
24. Frank CW, Weinblatt E, Shapiro S: Angina pectoris in men: Prognostic significance of selected medical factors. *Circulation* 1973; 47:509–517.
25. Califf RM, Mark DB, Harrell FE Jr, Hlatky MA, Lee KL, Rosati RA, et al: Importance of clinical measures of ischemia in the prognosis of patients with documented coronary artery disease. *J Am Coll Cardiol* 1988; 11:20–26.
26. Ruberman W, Weinblatt E, Goldberg JD, Frank CW, Shapiro S, Chaudhary BS: Ventricular premature complexes in prognosis of angina. *Circulation* 1980; 61:1172–1178.
27. McNeer JF, Margolis JR, Lee KL, Kisslo JA, Peter RH, Kong Y,

et al: The role of the exercise test in the evaluation of patients for ischemic heart disease. *Circulation* 1978; 57:64–70.
28. Dagenais GR, Rouleau JR, Christen A, Fabia J: Survival of patients with a strongly positive exercise electrocardiogram. *Circulation* 1982; 65:452–456.
29. Gohlke H, Samek L, Betz P, Roskamm H: Exercise testing provides additional prognostic information in angiographically defined subgroups of patients with coronary artery disease. *Circulation* 1983; 68:979–985.
30. Weiner DA, Ryan TJ, McCabe CH, Chaitman BR, Sheffield T, Ferguson JC, et al: Prognostic importance of a clinical profile and exercise test in medically treated patients with coronary artery disease. *J Am Coll Cardiol* 1984; 3:772–779.
31. Friesinger GC, Page EE, Ross RS: Prognostic significance of coronary arteriography. *Trans Assoc Am Phys* 1974; 49:489–497.
32. Bruschke AV, Proudfit WL, Sones FM Jr: Progress study of 590 consecutive nonsurgical cases of coronary disease followed 5–9 years: I. Arteriographic correlations. *Circulation* 1973; 47:1147–1153.
33. Burggraf GW, Parker JO: Prognosis in coronary artery disease: Angiographic, hemodynamic and clinical factors. *Circulation* 1975; 51:146–156.
34. Oberman A, Jones WB, Riley CP, Reeves TJ, Sheffield T: Natural history of coronary artery disease. *Bull NY Acad Med* 1972; 48:1109–1125.
35. Killip T: National Heart, Lung, and Blood Institute Coronary Artery Surgery Study. *Circulation* 1981; 63(suppl 1):1.
36. Mock MB, Ringqvist I, Fisher LD, Davis KB, Chaitman BR, Kouchoukos NT, et al: Survival of medically treated patients in the Coronary Artery Surgery Study (CASS) registry. *Circulation* 1982; 66:562–568.
37. Coronary Artery Surgery Study (CASS): A randomized trial of coronary artery bypass surgery: Survival data. *Circulation* 1983; 68:939–950.
38. Zir LM, Miller SW, Dinsmore RE, Gilbert JP, Harthorne JW: Interobserver variability in coronary arteriography. *Circulation* 1976; 53:627–632.
39. Detre KM, Wright E, Murphy ML, Takaro T: Observer agreement in evaluating coronary angiograms. *Circulation* 1975; 52:979–986.
40. Conley MJ, Ely RL, Kisslo JA, Lee KL, McNeer JF, Rosati RA: The prognostic spectrum of left main stenosis. *Circulation* 1978; 57:947–952.
41. Detre K, Peduzzi P, Murphy M, Hultgren H, Thomsen J, Oberman A, et al: Effect of bypass surgery on survival in patients in low- and high-risk subgroups delineated by the use of simple clinical variables. *Circulation* 1981; 63:1329–1338.
42. Feil H: Preliminary pain in coronary thrombosis. *Am J Med Sci* 1937; 193:42–48.
43. Sampson JJ, Eliaser M Jr: The diagnosis of impending acute coronary artery occlusion. *Am Heart J* 1937; 13:675–686.
44. Solomon HA, Edwards AL, Killip T: Prodromata in acute myocardial infarction. *Circulation* 1969; 40:463–471.
45. Gazes PC, Mobley EM Jr, Faris MH Jr, Duncan RC, Humphries GB: Preinfarctional (unstable) angina: A prospective study: Ten-year follow-up. *Circulation* 1973; 48:331–337.
46. Duncan B, Fulton M, Morrison SL, Lutz W, Donald KW, Kerr F, et al: Prognosis of new and worsening angina pectoris. *Br Med J* 1976; 1:981–985.
47. Mulcahy R, Al-Awadhi AH, DeBuitleor M, Tobin G, Johnson H, Contoy R: Natural history and prognosis of unstable angina. *Am Heart J* 1985; 109:753–758.
48. Telfod AM, Wilson C: Trial of heparin versus atenolol in prevention of myocardial infarction in intermediate coronary syndrome. *Lancet* 1981; 1:1225–1228.
49. Roberts KB, Califf RM, Harrell FE Jr, Lee KL, Pryor DB, Rosati RA: The prognosis for patients with new-onset angina who have undergone cardiac catheterization. *Circulation* 1983; 68:970–978.
50. Unstable angina pectoris: National Cooperative Study Group to compare medical and surgical therapy: I. Report of protocol-patient population. *Am J Cardiol* 1976; 37:896–902.
51. Gerstenblith G, Ouyang P, Achuff SC, Bulkley BH, Becker LC, Mellits ED, et al: Nfedipine in unstable angina: A double-blind, randomized trial. *N Engl J Med* 1982; 306:885–889.
52. Lewis HD, Jr, Davis JW, Archibald DG, Steinke WE, Smitherman TC, Doherty JE III, et al: Protective effects of aspirin against acute myocardial infarction and death in men with unstable angina. Results of a Veterans Administration Cooperative Study. *N Engl J Med* 1983; 309:396–403.
53. Gottlieb SO, Weisfeldt ML, Ouyang P, Mellits ED, Gerstenblith G: Silent ischemia as a marker for early unfavorable outcomes in patients with unstable angina. *N Engl J Med* 1986; 314:1214–1219.
54. Ambrose JA, Winters SL, Arora RR, Eng A, Riccio A, Gorlin R, et al: Angiographic evolution of coronary artery morphology in unstable angina. *J Am Coll Cardiol* 1986; 7:472–478.
55. Cowley MJ, DiSchiascio G, Vetrovec GW: Coronary morphology in unstable angina: Angiographic findings and clinical relevance. *Circulation* 1985; 72:112.
56. Davies MJ, Thomas AC, Knapman PA, Hangartner JR: Intramyocardial platelet aggregation in patients with unstable angina suffering sudden ischemic cardiac death. *Circulation* 1986; 73:418–427.
57. Davies MJ, Thomas A: Thrombosis and acute coronary artery lesions in sudden cardiac ischemic death. *N Engl J Med* 1984; 310:1137–1140.
58. Davies MJ, Thomas AC: Plaque fissuring–the cause of acute myocardial infarction, sudden ischaemic death, and crescendo angina. *Br Heart J* 1985; 53:363–373.
59. Prinzmetal M, Kennamer R, Merliss R, Wada T, Bor N: Angina pectoris: I. A variant form of angina pectoris: Preliminary report. *Am J Med* 1959; 27:375–388.
60. Waters DD, Szlachcic J, Miller DD, Theroux P: Clinical characteristics of patients with variant angina complicated by myocardial infarction or death within one month. *Am J Cardiol* 1982; 49:658–664.
61. Waters DD, Miller DD, Szlachcic J, Bouchard A, Methe M, Kreeft J, et al: Factors influencing the long-term prognosis of treated patients with variant angina. *Circulation* 1983; 68:258–265.
62. Mark DB, Califf RM, Morris KG, Harrell FE Jr, Pryor DB, Hlatky MA, et al: Clinical characteristics and long-term survival of patients with variant angina. *Circulation* 1984; 69:880–888.
63. Miller DD, Waters DD, Szlachcic J, Theroux P: Clinical characteristics associated with sudden death in patients with variant angina. *Circulation* 1982; 66:588–592.
64. Armstrong A, Duncan B, Oliver MF, Julian DG, Donald KW, Fulton M, et al: Natural history of acute coronary heart attacks: A community study. *Br Heart J* 1972; 34:67–80.
65. Fulton M, Julian DG, Oliver MF: Sudden death and myocardial infarction in AHA Monograph no. 27, Research in Acute Myocardial Infarction. *Circulation* 1969; 40(suppl 4):182–193.
66. Nicod P, Gilpin E, Dittrich H: Late clinical outcome in patients with early ventricular fibrillation after myocardial infarction. *J Am Coll Cardiol* 1988; 1:464–470.
67. Cox JR Jr, Roberts R, Ambos HD, Oliver GC, Sobel BE: Relations between enzymatically estimated myocardial infarct size and early ventricular dysrhythmia. *Circulation* 1976; 53:I-150–155.
68. Berger PB, Ryan TJ: Inferior myocardial infarction. High risk groups. *Circulation* 1990; 81:401–411.
69. Stone PH, Raabe DS, Jaffe AS, Gustafson N, Muller JE, Turi ZG, et al: Prognostic significance of location and type of myocardial infarction: Independent adverse outcome associated with anterior location. *J Am Coll Cardiol* 1988; 11:453–463.
70. Chapman BL: Correlation of mortality rate and serum enzymes in myocardial infarction: Test of efficiency of coronary care. *Br Heart J* 1971; 33:643–646.
71. Rogers WJ, McDaniel HG, Smith LR, Mantle JA, Russell RO Jr, Rackley CE: Correlation of CPK-MB and angiographic estimates of infarct size in man. *Circulation* 1976; 54:II-28.
72. Norris RM, Brandt PWT, Caughey DE, Lee AJ, Scott PJ: A new coronary prognostic index. *Lancet* 1969; 1:274–281.
73. Hopper JL, Pathik B, Hunt P, Chan WW: Improved prognosis since 1969 of myocardial infarction treated in a coronary care unit: Lack of relation with changes in severity. *Br Med J* 1989; 299:892–896.
74. Forrester JS, Diamond G, Chatterjee K, Swan HJC: Medical therapy of acute myocardial infarction by application of hemodynamic subsets. *N Engl J Med* 1976; 295:1356–1362, 1404–1413.
75. Killip T, Kimball JT: Treatment of myocardial infarction in a coronary care unit; a two year experience with 250 patients. *Am J Cardiol* 1967; 20:457–464.

76. Sanz G, Castaner A, Betriu A, Magrina J, Roig E, Coll S, et al: Determinants of prognosis in survivors of myocardial infarction. *N Engl J Med* 1982; 306:1065–1070.
77. Theroux P, Waters DD, Halphen C, Debaisieux J, Mizgala HF: Prognostic value of exercise testing soon after myocardial infarction. *N Engl J Med* 1979; 301:341–345.
78. Froelicher VF, Perdue S, Pewen W, Risch M: Application of meta-analysis using an electronic spread sheet to exercise testing in patients after myocardial infarction. *Am J Med* 1987; 83:1045–1054.
79. Gianrossi R, Detrano R, Mulvihill D, Lehmann K, Dubach P, Colombo A, et al: Exercise-induced ST depression in the diagnosis of coronary artery disease. A meta-analysis. *Circulation* 1989; 80:87–98.
80. Multicenter Post Infarction Research Group: Risk stratification and survival after myocardial infarction. *N Engl J Med* 1983; 309:331–336.
81. Richards DAB, Byth K, Ross DL, Uther JB: What is the best predictor of spontaneous ventricular tachycardia and sudden death of the myocardial infarction. *Circulation* 1991; 83:756–763.
82. Gibson RS, Watson DD, Craddock GB, Crampton RS, Kaiser DL, Denny MJ, et al: Prediction of cardiac events after uncomplicated myocardial infarction: A prospective study comparing predischarge exercise thallium-201 scintigraphy and coronary angiography. *Circulation* 1983; 68:321–336.
83. Corbett JR, Dehmer GJ, Lewis SE, Woodward W, Henderson E, Parkey RW, et al: The prognostic value of submaximal exercise testing with radionuclide ventriculography before hospital discharge in patients with recent myocardial infarction. *Circulation* 1981; 64:535–544.
84. Fioretti P, Brower RW, Simoons ML, ten-Katen H, Beelen A, Baardman T, et al: Relative value of clinical variables, bicycle ergometry, rest radionuclide ventriculography and 24-hour ambulatory electrocardiographic monitoring at discharge to predict one-year survival after myocardial infarction. *J Am Coll Cardiol* 1986; 8:40–49.
85. Madigan NP, Rutherford BD, Frye RL: The clinical course, early prognosis and coronary anatomy of subendocardial infarction. *Am J Med* 1976; 60:634–641.
86. Madias JE, Chahine RA, Gorlin R, Blacklow DJ: A comparison of transmural and nontransmural acute myocardial infarction. *Circulation* 1974; 49:498–507.
87. Gibson RS, Boden WE, Theroux P, Strauss HD, Pratt CM, Gheorghiade M, et al: Diltiazem and reinfarction in patients with non-Q-wave myocardial infarction. Results of a double-blind, randomized, multicenter trial. *N Engl J Med* 1986; 315:423–429.
88. DeWood MA, Stifter WF, Simpson CS, Spores J, Eugster GS, Judge TP, et al: Coronary arteriographic findings soon after non-Q-wave myocardial infarction. *N Engl J Med* 1986; 315:417–423.
89. Reid PR, Taylor DR, Kelly DT, Weisfeldt ML, Humphries JO, Ross RS: Myocardial-infarct extension detected by precordial ST-segment mapping. *N Engl J Med* 1974; 290:123–128.
90. Buda AJ, Macdonald IL, Dubbin JD, Orr SA, Strauss HD: Myocardial infarct extension: Prevalence, clinical significance, and problems in diagnosis. *Am Heart J* 1983; 105:744–749.
91. Maisel AS, Ahnve S, Gilpin E, Henning H, Goldberger AL, Collins D, et al: Prognosis after extension of myocardial infarct: The role of Q wave or non-Q wave infarction. *Circulation* 1985; 71:211–217.
92. Greene HL, Richardson DW, Barker AH, Roden DM, Capone RJ, Echt DS, et al: Classification of deaths after myocardial infarction as arrhythmic or nonarrhythmic (The Cardiac Arrhythmia Pilot Study). *Am J Cardiol* 1989; 63:1–6.
93. Capone RJ, Pawitan Y, El-Sherif N, Geraci TS, Handshaw K, Morganroth J, et al: Events in the Cardiac Arrhythmia Suppression Trial: Baseline predictors of mortality in placebo-treated patients. *J Am Coll Cardiol* 1991; 18:1434–1438.
94. Cobb LA, Conn RD, Samson WE: Prehospital coronary care: The role of rapid response mobile intensive coronary care system. *Circulation* 1971; 43:11-139.
95. Cobb LA, Baum RS, Alvarez HA III, Schaffer WA: Resuscitation from out-of-hospital ventricular fibrillation: 4 years follow-up. *Circulation* 1985; 52:III-223–III-235.
96. Schaffer WA, Cobb LA: Recurrent ventricular fibrillation and modes of death in survivors of out-of-hospital ventricular fibrillation. *N Engl J Med* 1975; 293:259–262.
97. Weaver DW, Lorch GS, Alvarez HA III, Cobb LA: Angiographic findings and prognostic indicators. *Circulation* 1976; 54:895–900.
98. Nicod P, Gilpin E, Dittrich H, Wright M, Engler R, Rittlemeyer J, et al: Late clinical outcome in patients with early ventricular fibrillation after myocardial infarction. *J Am Coll Cardiol* 1988; 11:464–470.
99. Volpi A, Maggioni A, Franzosi MG, Pampallona S, Mauri F, Tognoni G: In-hospital prognosis of patients with acute myocardial infarction complicated by primary ventricular fibrillation. *N Engl J Med* 1987; 317:257–261.
100. Volpi A, Cavalli A, Franzosi MG, Maggioni A, Mauri F, Santoro E, et al: One-year prognosis of primary ventricular fibrillation complicating acute myocardial infarction. *Am J Cardiol* 1989; 63:1174–1178.
101. The Cardiac Arrhythmia Suppression Trial (CAST) Investigators: Preliminary report: Effect of encainide and flecainide on mortality in a randomized trial of arrhythmia suppression after myocardial infarction. *N Engl J Med* 1989; 321:406–412.
102. Echt DS, Liebson PR, Mitchell LB, Peters RW, Obias-Manno D, Barker AH, et al: Mortality and morbidity in patients receiving encainide, flecainide or placebo: The Cardiac Arrhythmia Suppression Trial. *N Engl J Med* 1991; 324:781–788.
103. The Cardiac Arrhythmia Suppression Trial II Investigators: Effect of the antiarrhythmic agent moricizine on survival after myocardial infarction. *N Engl J Med* 1992; 327:227–233.
104. Yatteau RF, Peter RH, Behar VS, Bartel AG, Rosati RA, Kong Y: Ischemic cardiomyopathy: The myopathy of coronary artery disease, natural history and results of medical versus surgical treatment. *Am J Cardiol* 1974; 34:520–525.
105. Alderman EL, Fisher LD, Litwin P, Kaiser GC, Myers WO, Maynard C, et al: Results of coronary artery surgery in patients with poor left ventricular function (CASS). *Circulation* 1983; 68:785–795.
106. CONSENSUS Trial Study Group: Effects of enalapril on mortality in severe congestive heart failure. *N Engl J Med* 1987; 316:1429–1435.
107. The SOLVD Investigators: Effect of enalapril on survival in patients with reduced left ventricular ejection fractions and congestive heart failure. *N Engl J Med* 1991; 325:293–302.
108. SOLVD Investigators: Effect of enalapril on mortality and the development of heart failure in asymptomatic patients with reduced left ventricular ejection fraction. *N Engl J Med* 1992; 327:685–691.
109. Pfeffer MA, Braunwald E, Moye LA, Basta L, Brown EJ Jr, Cuddy TE, et al: Effect of captopril on mortality and morbidity in patients with left ventricular dysfunction after myocardial infarction. *N Engl J Med* 1992; 327:669–677.

Chapter 62

Prevention of Coronary Artery Disease

Charles E. Rackley, M.D. ■ *Robert C. Schlant, M.D.*

INTRODUCTION

The major therapeutic advances in the treatment of coronary artery disease in the 20th century include coronary artery bypass surgery, percutaneous transluminal angioplasty, and thrombolytic treatment for acute myocardial infarction. Despite the impressive symptomatic benefits from these therapies, they do not influence the underlying disease mechanism nor alter atherosclerotic progression in the remaining coronary arteries. Risk characteristics for development of coronary artery disease include cigarette smoking, hypertension, family history, diabetes, obesity, and inactivity. Abnormal elevations of cholesterol have been consistently identified with these risks in the development of coronary artery disease as well as with a significant role in progression of the disease process. This chapter will examine the role of lipids in atherosclerosis, epidemiology studies on coronary heart disease, risk characteristics and modification, primary and secondary prevention trials, regression of coronary atherosclerosis, and, finally, future roles for lipid modification.

THE ROLE OF LIPIDS IN ATHEROSCLEROSIS

Theories on the cause of atherosclerosis include the incorporation of lipids, circulating blood elements, abnormal cells within the vascular wall, and the influence of mechanical forces and ischemic disease conditions.[1] The lipid theory includes the attraction, deposition, and modification of lipid substances within the arterial wall.[2,3] Lipids initially accumulate in monocytes that are subsequently converted to fat-laden macrophages or foam cells. A current theory proposed by Steinberg is that oxidation of LDL-cholesterol within the vascular wall serves as a stimulus for further recruitment of monocytes and further accumulation of modified LDL as well as cellular growth and proliferation.[4] (See also Chaps. 53 to 56.)

Extensive animal and clinical studies have provided evidence to support the lipid hypothesis. Feeding high-fat diets to primates and other model species produces atherosclerotic lesions.[5,6] In primates, atherosclerosis regresses when serum cholesterol is reduced by dietary changes and drug therapy.[7–10] In clinical studies, total cholesterol and LDL-cholesterol have been correlated directly with risk for coronary artery disease in various cross-cultural population studies. In people migrating from countries where cholesterol levels and coronary heart disease rates tend to be low, studies have shown that risk increases when these people adopt lifestyle patterns of the higher risk population. Finally, familial studies of inherited LDL-cholesterol metabolism abnormalities have identified families with a high incidence of severe premature atherosclerosis (Chap. 96).

In addition to their role in the genesis of atherosclerosis, cholesterol abnormalities have been shown to influence platelet function and vascular reactivity.[11] In the presence of high cholesterol levels platelet aggregation is increased. In experimental animals and human beings elevated cholesterol levels have been associated with abnormal vasoconstriction of coronary arteries when challenged by acetylcholine, a neurotransmitter that causes vasodilation in the normal vessel.[12,13] (See also Chap. 56.) Thus, experimental animal and clinical investigative studies continue to emphasize the primary role of lipid abnormalities in the development and progression of atherosclerosis in the coronary arteries.

EPIDEMIOLOGIC STUDIES

An important long-term study was initiated in 1958 under Keys that involved 16 cohorts spread over seven countries, with 12,095 subjects enrolled who were free of coronary heart disease.[14,14a] Selection was confined to men aged 40 to 59 years. Countries represented were the United States, the Netherlands, Finland, Greece, Japan, Italy, and Yugoslavia with a range of urban and rural lifestyles. Risk factors such as smoking, body weight, age, and physical activity varied from country to country. These broad characteristics assigned even greater significance to the finding that serum cholesterol was related to the rate of coronary heart disease death. The mortality was spread over cholesterol values beginning at less than 200 mg/dL (5.17 mmol/liter) and exceeding 250 mg/dL (6.47 mmol/liter). Hypertension and smoking were risk factors but had far less impact in people with low serum cholesterol, and thus emphasized the central significance of cholesterol in the development of coronary heart disease. The Japanese cohorts, who had very low serum cholesterol [median 160 mg/dL (4.14 mmol/liter)] but a high prevalence of hypertension and heavy smoking, had a mere 7 coronary deaths in 5 years among the 1005 men rated as free of coronary heart disease at the start of the trial. In contrast, the 1534 equivalent men in the two Finnish cohorts [median cholesterol 259 mg/dL (6.7 mmol/liter)] experienced 67 coronary heart disease deaths.

A large study in the United States examined the relationship of cholesterol to coronary heart disease and was designated the Multiple Risk Factor Intervention Trial (MRFIT).[15] In recruiting individuals for risk factor reduction, 361,662 men aged 35 to 57 were screened, and data used to examine the relationship of serum cholesterol to coronary heart disease (Fig. 62-1). The 6-year follow-up for this large study of middle-aged men demonstrated that baseline serum total cholesterol was a strong predictor of coronary heart disease mortality. Even at levels below 200 mg/dL (5.17 mmol/liter) there was a slight increase in the risk of coronary heart disease, and above this level the risk increased rapidly so that at 250 and 300 mg/dL (6.47 and 7.76 mmol/liter) the risk was respectively two- and fourfold greater than at 200 mg/dL (5.17 mmol/liter). Subjects with mean cholesterol levels of 167 mg/dL (4.32 mmol/liter) fared best in the analyses, but even at levels of 180 mg/dL (4.66 mmol/liter) blood cholesterol posed an increased coronary heart disease risk in middle-aged American men.

These and other epidemiologic surveys, including the Framingham Study and the U.S. Pooling Project, have all been concordant with the Seven Countries Study in identifying serum cholesterol as a major risk factor for coronary heart disease (Fig. 62-2).[16] In men total mortality and coronary heart disease mortality are both related to serum cholesterol.[17]

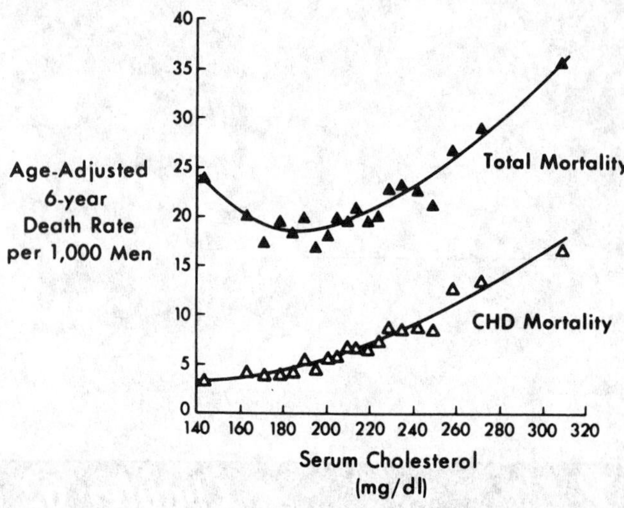

FIGURE 62-1 Age-adjusted 6-year CHD and total mortality rate per 1000 men screened for MRFIT according to serum cholesterol. The relationships of serum cholesterol to total mortality from all causes (upper curve) and from coronary heart disease (lower curve) were obtained in 361,662 men, 35 to 57 years of age, during an average follow-up of 6 years. Each point represents the median value for 5 percent of the population. Note that the risk of coronary heart disease increases steadily, particularly above levels of 200 mg/dL; and that the magnitude of the increased risk is large, fourfold in the top 10 percent as compared with the bottom 10 percent. The increased total mortality at the lowest cholesterol levels, which has been previously noted and is probably explained by a cholesterol-lowering effect of cancer, does not appear to persist beyond 5 years of follow-up in the MRFIT cohort. (*From Martin MJ, Browner WS, Hulley SB, et al: Serum cholesterol, blood pressure, and mortality: implications from a cohort of 361,662 men. Lancet 2:993, 1986. Reproduced with permission of the publisher and authors.*)

RISK CHARACTERISTICS FOR CORONARY ARTERY DISEASE

The most consistently recognized factors influencing coronary atherosclerosis are elevated lipids, smoking, and hypertension (Table 62-1). Additional risk factors include a family history of premature coronary disease, diabetes mellitus, low HDL-cholesterol, and age: male over 45 or female over 55 years. The National Cholesterol Education Program has identified these characteristics as potential risks for development of coronary artery disease.

Cigarette smoking can exert deleterious effects on the coronary artery, circulating elements, and viable myocardium.[18] Vascular endothelium can be damaged by cigarette smoking, which can cause thromboxane A_2 release, decrease prostacyclin production, induce alpha-adrenergic stimulation, enhance vasopressin generation, and finally provoke constriction of the vessel itself.[19] Platelet aggregation is increased and survival altered by cigarette smoking. Cigarettes elevate the circulating level

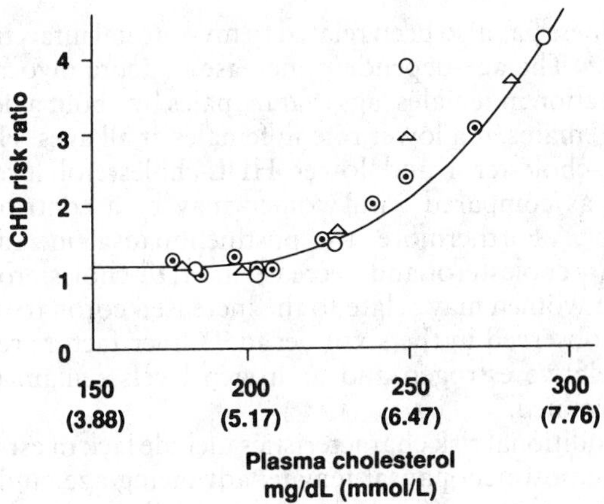

FIGURE 62-2 Relationship between plasma cholesterol level and relative risk of coronary heart disease in three prospective studies. (*From Stason WB: Costs and benefits of risk factor reduction for coronary heart disease: Insights from screening and treatment of serum cholesterol. Am Heart J 1990; 119:718–724. Reporduced with permission from the publisher and author.*)

TABLE 62-1

Risk Status Based on Presence of CHD Risk Factors Other Than Low-Density Lipoprotein Cholesterol*

Positive Risk Factors
Age (y) Male ≥45 Female ≥55 or premature menopause without estrogen replacement therapy Family history of premature CHD (definite myocardial infarction or sudden death before 55 y of age in father or other male first-degree relative, or before 65 y of age in mother or other female first-degree relative) Current cigarette smoking Hypertension (blood pressure ≥ 140/90 mm Hg,† or taking antihypertensive medication) Low HDL cholesterol (<35 mg/dL† [0.9 mmol/L]) Diabetes mellitus
Negative Risk Factor‡
High HDL cholesterol (≥60 mg/dL [1.6 mmol/L])

* High risk, defined as a net of two or more coronary heart disease (CHD) risk factors, leads to more vigorous intervention, shown in Figs. 62-3 and 62-4. Age (defined differently for men and women) is treated as a risk factor because rates of CHD are higher in the elderly than in the young, and in men than in women of the same age. Obesity is not listed as a risk factor because it operates through other risk factors that are included [hypertension, hyperlipidemia, decreased high-density lipoprotein (HDL) cholesterol, and diabetes mellitus], but it should be considered a target for intervention. Physical inactivity is similarly not listed as a risk factor, but it too should be considered a target for intervention, and physical activity is recommended as desirable for everyone. High risk due to coronary or peripheral atherosclerosis is addressed directly in Fig. 62-5.

† Confirmed by measurements on several occasions.

‡ If the HDL cholesterol level is ≥60 mg/dL (1.6 mmol/L), subtract one risk factor (because high HDL cholesterol levels decrease CHD risk).

SOURCE: From the Summary of the Second Report of the National Cholesterol Education Program (NCEP) Expert Panel on Detection, Evaluation, and Treatment of High Cholesterol in Adults (Adult Treatment Panel II). JAMA 1991;269:3015–3023. Reproduced with permission from the publisher and authors.

of catecholamines and free-fatty acids, which can further alter vascular tone. As a result heart rate, blood pressure, and myocardial contractility rise with a concomitant increase in vascular resistance, thereby leading to significant elevations in myocardial oxygen demand. Cigarette consumption is associated with reduced levels of HDL-cholesterol,[20,21] which may also correlate with abnormal vasoconstriction of both manifestly diseased and normal-appearing coronary artery segments.[13] Continuation of cigarette smoking after myocardial infarction is associated with the highest mortality of any of the other associated features, and an increased frequency of restenosis after angioplasty is reported in individuals who continue to smoke.[22,23]

Hypertension can predispose to atherosclerosis when coexistant risk characteristics are present, although the incidence of coronary artery disease is low in populations where hypertension is associated with cholesterol levels lower than 160 mg/dL (4.1 mmol/liter). Both fixed and labile hypertension increase the risk of coronary disease, as does elevated systolic blood pressure in older individuals. Hypertension is an additive risk factor when superimposed upon cigarette smoking, cholesterol elevation, glucose intolerance, and other risk characteristics.[24] Hypertension, in some instances, is associated with a reduction in HDL-cholesterol that can contribute to atherogenesis and abnormal vasoactivity.[25] Some antihypertensive drugs can worsen risk factors by causing hyperglycemia, elevating cholesterol and triglycerides, and lowering HDL levels.[26] (See Chap. 77.)

Total cholesterol levels above 160 mg/dL (4.1 mmol/liter) are associated with an increased risk for the development of coronary disease throughout the world.[27] The risk has been attributed primarily to total and LDL-cholesterol levels in epidemiologic studies. In addition, the Framingham Study earlier identified an abnormally low HDL-cholesteral as a risk for coronary atherosclerosis.[28] Recent studies have identified both male and female patients with total cholesterol levels under 200 mg/dL in whom an abnormally low HDL-cholesterol was the sole lipid abnormality correlating angiographically with coronary artery disease.[29] Low HDL-cholesterol values have been associated with cigarette smoking, hypertension, diabetes, and sedentary activity.

An unusual protein, LP_a, which is a combination of apo B 100 protein from LDL and apo_a and is structually analogous to plasminogen, is an additional risk factor for coronary artery disease.[30,31] Lp_a represents a potential linkage between lipoprotein metabolism and thrombosis as it may interfere with plasmin generation and thrombolysis.[32,32a]

Even though hypertriglyceridemia has not been consistently identified in the past as a significant coronary risk characteristic, recent studies suggest that this lipid may also contribute to coronary disease in both sexes.[33-36]

Values for HDL-cholesterol less than 35 mg/dL (0.9 mmol/liter) were identified by the National Cholesterol Education Program as a coronary risk factor, and in the 1993 recommendations an HDL-cholesterol value above 60 mg/dL (1.6 mmol/liter) was considered a nonrisk factor.[37,38] In addition to these epidemiologic associations, a high incidence of coronary disease has been found at cardiac catheterization in men and women with low HDL-cholesterol.[39] Low HDL-cholesterol was associated with abnormal endothelial-dependent vasoresponsiveness as assessed by acetylcholine challenge in both manifestly diseased and angiographically normal-appearing arteries.[13] Thus, the endothelial vasodilator dysfunction associated with low HDL-cholesterol may reflect the more generalized dysfunction, permitting the development of atherosclerosis.[39] A causal relationship, however, has not been proven. (See Chap. 56.)

A history of premature coronary disease in a family member before the age of 55 or 60 years is a risk characteristic and may or may not be associated with a manifest familial disorder of lipid metabolism, hypertension, or diabetes. Studies continue to link cholesterol elevation and lipid abnormalities with development of atherosclerosis in both young and elderly patients.[40-43] (See also Chaps. 96 and 102.) Cigarette smoking further enhances the atherogenic influence of diabetes, hypertension, hypercholesterolemia, or undefined hereditary traits.

Glucose intolerance furthers the risk of coronary artery disease, more so in women than in men. In addition to the risk factors of cigarette smoking, hypertension, or hypercholesterolemia, diabetes mellitus accelerates the development of atheromatous changes in coronary arteries in both sexes, but the threat is three to four times greater in women prior to age 50.[44] Diabetes mellitus influences the development of coronary artery disease through mechanisms such as lipid abnormalities, hypertension, obesity, and abnormally low HDL-cholesterol values.[45] It is important to note, however, that diabetes mellitus increases coronary artery disease risk even in patients without manifest abnormalities in plasma lipids.[46] In addition, insulin resistance in the nondiabetic individual with hypertension may also contribute to coronary atherosclerosis. (See also Chap. 102.)

Obesity has long been recognized for its relationship to coronary heart disease morbidity and mortality.[47,48] The contributions of obesity to the atherosclerotic process include the mechanisms of hypertension, impaired glucose tolerance, insulin resistance, hyperglycemia, and hyperlipidemia with elevated LDL-cholesterol and decreased HDL-cholesterol levels.[44] One-third of the adult population in the United States is estimated to be overweight. There is evidence that abdominal obesity (with an increased waist:hip ratio) is more strongly associated with coronary artery disease than obesity that is most marked in the hips.

A sedentary life-style increases the risk for coronary artery disease.[49] A low level of physical activity is associated with lower HDL-cholesterol levels, increased blood pressure, an increase in some clotting factors, and increased body weight.[50-52]

Male sex is a nonmodifiable coronary risk factor. Baldness has also been related to myocardial infarction in men.[53] The age-dependent increase in acute myocardial infarction in females lags that in males by about a decade but remains at a lower rate in females at all ages. Higher LDL-cholesterol and lower HDL-cholesterol levels in men as compared with women may be a contributing factor.[54] Furthermore, the postmenopausal increase in LDL=cholesterol and decrease in HDL-cholesterol levels in women may relate to the increased coronary event rate observed in the sixth decade. Other factors related to relative estrogen and androgen levels remain to be determined.

Additional risk characteristics include lack of estrogen in the postmenopausal female, advancing age, and psychological stress. Studies have reported that postmenopausal females on estrogen replacement have a significantly lower incidence of coronary artery disease than females not taking replace hormones.[55-58] Estrogen elevates HDL-cholesterol, which may confer protection as implied above.[59] Age is associated with coronary artery disease in all angiographic studies. Although controversial, the original characterization of type A and type B personalities may help identify coronary-prone individuals in some studies.[60] One trial of risk factor modification identified stress management as a significant modifiable risk in terms of slowing progression and inducing regression in anatomic coronary disease.[61] (See Chap. 117.)

MODIFICATION OF RISK CHARACTERISTICS

With the exceptions of genotype, sex, and age, risk factors can be modified by changes in life-style and diet and by the use of pharmacologic agents. Cessation of cigarette smoking decreases coronary risk almost 50 percent within the first year and to near that of nonsmokers within 2 to 10 years.[62] Many hospital and community programs are available to assist with smoking cessation. Although measures such as group support, hypnosis, and the use of nicotine gum or patches may sometimes be helpful, the emphasis placed by the physician on the importance of discontinuation of cigarette smoking is critically important. Cessation of smoking raises the HDL-cholesterol approximately 10 percent in 1 month and reduces platelet aggregability.

Although early trials of antihypertensive therapy demonstrated that control of moderate and severe hypertension resulted in decreased mortality from stroke and heart failure, no significant effect on myocardial infarction rates was observed.[63] More recently, however, treatment of mild diastolic hypertension (blood pressure of 95 mmHg) has been shown to reduce cardiovascular and all-cause mortality.[64] These observations have resulted in a reassessment of the previous negative results with respect to coronary events. In the opinion of many, the difficulty initially in demonstrating a reduction in cardiac events in hypertension treatment may have been due to the metabolic effects of the thiazide diuretics and beta blockers that were used commonly. Thiazides, for example, elevate triglycerides and cholesterol, while beta blockers increase triglycerides. Decreased use of thiazides and increased use of calcium entry blockers and angiotensin-converting enzyme (ACE) inhibitors that have fewer potentially adverse metabolic effects may decrease cardiac events more convincingly. (See also Chap. 77).

Weight reduction, caloric restriction, and decreased salt intake should be initial therapy in treatment of patients with mild hypertension.[65] Regular exercise decreases blood pressure, and studies employing biofeedback and stress relaxation suggest that they can contribute to the control of blood pressure in selected patients.[50–52,66]

The National Cholesterol Education Program recommends dietary management and regular exercise as initial steps to reduce abnormally elevated cholesterol values.[37] The American Heart Association Step-I Diet provides for a caloric intake consisting of less than 30 percent of total calories from fat, with 7 to 10 percent saturated fat, 50 to 60 percent of calories from carbohydrate, 10 to 20 percent of calories from protein, and with less than 300 mg of cholesterol per day. In the Step-II Diet total calories from fat remain at 30 percent, with less than 7 percent saturated fat, along with 50 to 60 percent carbohydrate, 10 to 20 percent protein, and less than 200mg of cholesterol per day. Regular exercise is recommended and can range from 15 to 20 minutes of walking per day to more vigorous levels for caloric expenditure.[67] In addition to its role in weight and blood pressure reduction, regular exercise will increase the HDL-cholesterol component.[68] Current guidelines recommend dietary changes and regular exercise for periods of 4 to 6 months for treatment of abnormally elevated lipids in patients with two or more risk characteristics. Pharmacologic agents can be instituted after this initial diet and exercise period or even earlier in the individual with documented coronary artery disease.

As alluded to previously, diabetes mellitus as well as subclinical insulin resistance increase risk of coronary artery disease. Although the ability to decrease the risk of coronary artery disease in patients with diabetes mellitus has not yet been demonstrated definitively, it is logical, in light of recent clinical trials of lipid lowering in nondiabetics, that improved metabolic control of both glucose and lipid metabolism would improve the outlook for control of coronary artery disease progression. (See Chap. 102.) Both diet modification and weight control can make important contributions to glucose control. Improved glucose tolerance can raise HDL-cholesterol. Current trials are evaluating the effects of lipid-lowering strategies on vascular disease risk in diabetic patients.

Weight reduction with a low-fat diet can reduce coronary events by influencing a number of coronary risk factors.[47,48] In addition, exercise and behavior modification techniques can facilitate weight reduction. Epidemiologic data suggest that occupational and recreational physical activity reduce the risk of coronary artery disease independently of other major characteristics.[69] A modest inverse relationship between leisure activity of high-risk middle-aged men and their overall coronary mortality was observed in the Multiple Risk Factor Intervention Trial.[70] Comparable protection in this study was offered by moderate and high levels of physical activity. Walking 15 to 20 min each day an average of 5 days each week can elevate HDL-cholesterol levels. Exercise can also modify physiological stress and promote a sense of well-being. In addition to enhanced caloric expenditure, exercise may further inhibit appetite.

Although emphasis was initially placed primarily on abnormal elevations of total cholesterol and LDL-cholesterol as major lipid abnormalities in coronary artery disease, an abnormally low HDL-cholesterol was found to be an important risk factor in the Framingham Study and the National Cholesterol Education Program (Table 62-2).[28,37,38] Efforts to raise HDL-cholesterol through regular exercise and smoking cessation and control of elevated blood pressure, glucose intolerance, and obesity are important interventions in selected patients.

The role of estrogen replacement in the postmenopausal female in decreasing the risk of coronary artery disease is being increasingly considered and examined.[56–58,71] Even though postmenopausal females on estrogen have been shown to have a lower incidence of angiographic coronary artery disease compared to individuals without estrogen replacement, concerns about breast and uterine cancer in patients on replacement hormones have hindered trials on estrogen replacement in coronary disease.[59] This question will have to be answered since the beneficial role of estrogen in the postmenopausal female may not only reduce the development of coronary artery disease but may also provide additional benefits such as prevention of osteoporosis. Some studies have found an increased incidence of breast cancer and uterine malignancy in subjects on long-term estrogen therapy. The potential benefits of hormone replacement therapy in reducing coronary artery disease versus the potential hazards of an increase in breast and endometrial cancer is currently being evaluated in ongoing studies. Additional issues being addressed are to define the role of combination therapy with progestin and to define the role of replacement therapy in high-risk women or in women with established vascular disease.

TABLE 62-2

Initial Classification Based on Total Cholesterol and HDL Cholesterol Levels*

Cholesterol Level	Initial Classification
Total Cholesterol	
<200 mg/dL (5.2 mmol/liter)	Desirable blood cholesterol
200–239 mg/dL (5.2–6.2 mmol/liter)	Borderline-high blood cholesterol
≥240 mg/dL (6.2 mmol/liter)	High blood cholesterol
HDL Cholesterol	
<35 mg/dL (0.9 mmol/liter)	Low HDL cholesterol

* HDL indicates high-density lipoprotein.

SOURCE: From the Summary of the Second Report of the National Cholesterol Education Program (NCEP) Expert Panel on Detection, Evaluation, and Treatment of High Cholesterol in Adults (Adult Treatment Panel II). JAMA 1991;269:3015–3023. Reproduced with permission from the publisher and authors.

PRIMARY PREVENTION

Primary prevention trials are those carried out on individuals who at the outset have no clinical manifestation of coronary heart disease. Significant primary prevention trials include the Los Angeles Veterans Administration Study,[72] the Oslo Primary Prevention Trial,[73] The World Health Organization (WHO) Cooperative Trial of Clofibrate,[74] the Multiple Risk Factor Intervention Trial (MRFIT),[15] the Lipid Research Clinics Coronary Primary Prevention Trial,[75] and the Helsinki Heart Study.[76] These trials involved two types of lipid-lowering therapy, one consisting of diet and the other drug therapy. Diet therapy was employed in the Los Angeles study,[72] the Oslo study,[73] and the MRFIT.[15] Lipid-lowering drugs were used in the WHO trial of clofibrate,[74] the Lipid Research Clinics trial,[75] and the Helsinki study.[76]

In the Los Angeles Veterans Administration Study the effects of a cholesterol-lowering, fat-modified diet on the incidence of atherosclerosis events and mortality were measured.[72] This randomized study started in 1959 and lasted 8½ years. Cohorts consisted of 840 male residents with a median age of 65½ years. Four hundred and twenty-four men were assigned to the intervention group and received a fat-modified diet in which the content of saturated fat and cholesterol was reduced and the amount of polyunsaturated fat was increased. The control group received their regular diet. The diet intervention group demonstrated a significant reduction in serum cholesterol, although in later years of the trial the difference between the serum cholesterol levels in the treatment and the control groups tended to narrow. In the intervention group there was a 31 percent reduction in the incidence of atherosclerosis-related cardiovascular events and a 31 percent reduction in mortality. There was also a significant increase in the mortality from cancer in the treatment group, which caused considerable concern at the time. Subsequent studies, however, showed no linkage between cholesterol reduction and cancer incidence. Indeed, a low serum cholesterol may reflect or result from the presence of cancer, rather than causing it.

The Oslo Primary Prevention Trial started in 1973 and was a 5-year, multifactorial, randomized controlled trial.[73] This study examined the impact on coronary heart disease of reduction in the intake of saturated fat and cholesterol, some increase in the intake of polyunsaturated fats, and of cessation of smoking. Subjects were 1232 normotensive men from 40 to 49 years old who were initially free of overt coronary heart disease but at high risk because of elevated cholesterol. Baseline serum cholesterol values for these men ranged from 290 to 380 mg/dL (7.5 to 9.8 mmol/liter) with a mean value of 329 mg/dL (8.5 mmol/liter), and 79 percent were cigarette smokers. Over the 5 years, there was a net reduction in serum cholesterol of 13 percent in the treatment group compared to controls. This group also showed a 20 to 25 percent reduction in serum triglyceride levels. Total coronary events, which included sudden coronary death, sudden unexplained death, and fatal and nonfatal myocardial infarction, numbered 19 in the intervention group and were significantly fewer than the 36 events in the control group. An inverse relationship was demonstrated between percent change in serum cholesterol and the incidence of coronary heart disease. Approximately 60 percent of the total benefit in the intervention group could be related to reduced serum cholesterol levels, whereas reduction in cigarette consumption accounted for another 25 percent lower incidence of coronary heart disease. Of interest were the 38 percent fewer deaths from cancer in the intervention group, in contrast with the results of the Los Angeles study.

In the Multiple Risk Factor Intervention Trial reduction of serum cholesterol, control of blood pressure, and cessation of smoking were essential elements.[15] In the randomized control trial 12,866 men aged 35 to 57 years were drawn from an initial population of 361,662 individuals. Men selected were at high risk for coronary artery disease and were in the upper 10 to 15 percent of risk distribution based on serum cholesterol level, blood pressure, and cigarette smoking. Subjects were assigned either to special intervention or to usual care groups and were followed for an average of 7 years. For usual care the men were referred to their family practitioners. Special intervention consisted of dietary restrictions to reduce saturated fat and cholesterol and increase polyunsaturated fat intake. Cholesterol levels in the intervention group declined by an average of 12 mg/dL at 6 years. Diastolic blood pressure also declined an average of 10.5 mmHg at 6 years, and 50 percent of individuals had discontinued smoking at 6 years.

There was unexpected improvement in the usual care group, with a decline in serum cholesterol level of 7.5 mg/dL, diastolic blood pressure by 7 mmHg, and smoking frequency by 29 percent. Thus, the final differences between the groups were smaller than had been expected, making difficult the demonstration of beneficial effect on risk factor modification on the incidence of coronary heart disease. Special intervention was projected to reduce coronary heart disease mortality by 22 percent relative to the usual care group, and the observed 7 percent difference was not statistically significant. Subset analysis, however, was consistent with there being a benefit in some groups. For example, there was an apparent reduction in coronary artery disease mortality in nonhypertensive men with initial serum cholesterol greater than 250 mg/dL (6.46 mmol/liter) or in those who smoked at the onset of the trial.

The World Health Organization Cooperative Trial of Clofibrate was designed to examine the effect on coronary heart disease rates of reducing serum cholesterol.[74] Hypercholesterolemia was defined as the upper third of the cholesterol distribution of the screened population in Edinburgh, Budapest, and Prague, and 10,627 men were enrolled. The trial was initiated in 1965 and concluded in 1976, with a mean duration of active treatment of 5.3 years. In the clofibrate treatment group the incidence of nonfatal myocardial infarction was reduced by 25 percent but there was no reduction in coronary heart disease mortality. A surprising observation in this study was the statistically significant increased mortality from all causes observed during the period of active treatment. No specific cause could be identified to explain this excess mortality, and there was no final proof of clofibrate toxicity. Nevertheless, the concern raised by increased mortality in the clofibrate treatment group diverted attention from the hypothesis that the trial was designed to test, i.e., that a reduction in cholesterol would reduce the incidence of coronary events, which the trial did confirm.

A major study performed in the United States was The Lipid Research Clinics Coronary Primary Prevention Trial, which was a multicenter, randomized, double-blind study designed to test the impact of reduction of serum cholesterol and, in particular, LDL-cholesterol on the risk of coronary heart disease.[75] The trial involved 3086 men ranging in ages from 39 to 59 years who had primary hypercholesterolemia but were asymptomatic for coronary heart disease. All patients were advised on dietary modification, and half the treatment group also received a bile acid sequestrant. The duration of treatment averaged slightly over 7 years. Dietary changes in the control group produced slight benefits with total serum cholesterol and LDL-cholesterol falling by 3.5 percent and 4.0 percent respectively. In the treatment group total cholesterol and LDL-cholesterol declined by 13 percent and 20 percent from their respective baseline values. In the group treated with diet modification and colestipol, definite coronary heart disease death and/or nonfatal myocardial infarction were 19 percent lower than in the control group. Other manifestations of heart disease such as angina, coronary artery bypass surgery, and positive exercise tests also showed treatment-related reductions from 20 to 25 percent relative to the control group. The general hypothesis, that reduction of total serum cholesterol and LDL-cholesterol is associated with reduced risk of major coronary heart disease events, was supported further by the observation that reduction of coronary heart disease incidence was greatest in patients showing greatest decrease in cholesterol. A 10 percent reduction in serum cholesterol resulted in a 20 percent reduction in the incidence of coronary heart disease. This study established the useful clinical guideline that a 1 percent reduction in serum cholesterol will produce a 2 percent reduction in coronary risk (Table 62-3).

The Helsinki Heart Study was a randomized, double-blind 5-year trial of 4081 asymptomatic men aged 40 to 55 years who were at high risk for coronary disease due to elevated blood lipids.[76] Gemfibrozil was given to 2051 men, while the remainder received a placebo. All subjects were advised to follow a lipid-lowering diet. In both groups initial serum cholesterol levels were over 285 mg/dL (7.4 mmol/liter); HDL-cholesterol levels were approximately 47 mg/dL (1.2 mmol/liter) and triglyceride levels were just over 175 mg/dL (2 mmol/liter). After 6 months, gemfibrozil had reduced total cholesterol, LDL-cholesterol, and triglycerides relative to control, while a 15 percent increase in HDL-cholesterol was noted. For the course of the trial, overall reductions in total cholesterol, LDL-cholesterol, and triglycerides were respectively 8 percent, 8 percent, and 35 percent, while the increase in HDL-cholesterol was about 10 percent. The greatest benefit was recorded for nonfatal myocardial infarctions, with 45 incidents in the treatment group and 71 in the control group. Overall, total cardiac events were reduced by 34 percent, fatal myocardial infarction by 26 percent, nonfatal infarction by 37 percent, and death due to coronary artery disease by 28 percent. Somewhat surprisingly, there was no reduction in overall mortality. Most of the benefit in the Helsinki study occurred in men who had an LDL-cholesterol/HDL-cholesterol ratio >5 and a serum triglyceride level >204 mg/dL (>2.3 mmol/liter).[76a] The trial provided convincing evidence that pharmacologic manipulation of lipoprotein cholesterol levels could produce a substantial reduction in coronary heart disease incidence. Furthermore, the study provided evidence, especially in retrospect, of the potential importance of HDL-cholesterol levels in treating coronary artery disease. The Helsinki Heart Study was important in that it substantiated the hypothesis that manipulating serum lipids could reduce coronary event rates. The precise contribution of each lipid fraction would require further study.

Although many of the earlier primary prevention trials on the effect of blood cholesterol lowering on the incidence of coronary heart disease had weaknesses in statistical design, later trials overcame these limitations to a large extent. Thus, conclusions from primary prevention studies have demonstrated that: (1) elevated blood cholesterol is a major risk factor for coronary heart disease, (2) primary preventive measures can greatly reduce coronary heart disease risk, and (3) a 1 percent reduction in blood cholesterol reduces coronary heart disease risk by 2 percent.

TABLE 62-3
Lipid Research Clinics Coronary Primary Prevention Trial*

Changes in Plasma Lipid Fractions	Reduction in Coronary Risk†
8 percent ↓ in cholesterol	19 percent
11 percent ↓ in LDL	19 percent

* Results at 7 to 10 years of follow-up in 1906 men treated with diet and cholestyramine.
† One percent Reduction in cholesterol = 2 percent Reduction in Coronary Risk.
SOURCE: From Lipid Research Clinics Program.[75]

SECONDARY PREVENTION

Secondary prevention is directed at forestalling a second or subsequent major cardiac event in patients who have already experienced at least one coronary episode. Thirteen secondary prevention studies have been conducted: seven involved fat-modified diets and six examined the use of drugs such as niacin, clofibrate and bile acid sequestrants. Secondary prevention trials utilizing dietary manipulation have involved rather small numbers of patients, usually several hundred, and dietary manipulation consisted of greatly reducing the proportion of fat in the diet or increasing the ratio between polyunsaturated and saturated fats. Such trials included studies by Morrison in 1955, Rose et al. in 1965, The Medical Research Council of the United Kingdom in 1965 and again in 1968, Leren in The Oslo Diet Heart Study in 1970, Bierenbaum and colleagues in 1973, and Woodhill and coworkers in 1978.[77–83] Serum cholesterol was generally reduced by 10 to 30 percent, but the small numbers of patients precluded establishing significant statistical conclusions as to any potential benefit. Some trials reported a reduction of coronary heart disease incidence while others did not. Two possible reasons were proposed for the lack of consistent findings. First, the time after myocardial infarction at which patients entered the trial was variable. As expected, studies of patients who had already survived a year after myocardial infarction described better survival than those in which patients enrolled earlier after the acute event. Second, the extent of myocardial damage incurred varied considerably and could have profoundly affected long-term survival.

The majority of the secondary prevention studies using drugs also involved relatively small numbers of patients. Such trials included those of Schoch for the Veterans Administration Drug Lipid Study in 1968, the Newcastle physicians' study in 1971, the Scottish physicians' study in 1971, studies by Door and colleagues in 1978 and Rosenhamer and coworkers in 1980, and The Coronary Drug Project.[84–89] Generally, these early prevention trials using drugs produced reductions in serum cholesterol between 10 and 15 percent but did not demonstrate evidence of reduction in coronary heart disease risk, although in some instances beneficial effects were confined to patients with preexisting angina rather than myocardial infarction. An exception to the pattern of small patient numbers was the Coronary Drug Project in which 8000 patients aged from 30 to 64 years, were enrolled between 1966 and 1969. The participants were randomized to receive conjugated estrogens, dextrothyroxine, niacin, or clofibrate for 5 years. Estrogens and dextrothyroxine were discontinued early due to serious excess mortality, and only the clofibrate and niacin treatments were completed. Clofibrate lowered the cholesterol by about 6 percent but produced only a small reduction in coronary heart disease morbidity and had no affect on total mortality. Niacin, on the other hand, reduced cholesterol levels by 10 percent and lowered the 5-year incidence of nonfatal myocardial infarction to 8.9 percent, which represented a significant improvement over the 12 percent incidence in the control group. Although niacin did not affect the 5-year mortality, an apparent benefit of niacin therapy in overall mortality was present at the end of a drug-free followup period of nearly 10 years.[89a] Thus, niacin, in addition to being the first agent to demonstrate cholesterol reduction in humans, also was shown to be the first agent that significantly reduced the recurrence of acute myocardial infarction.

REGRESSION STUDIES IN CORONARY ARTERY DISEASE

In recent years the demonstration of anatomic regression of atheromatous lesions in the coronary arteries has become an important objective for cholesterol-lowering trials in coronary heart disease.[90] Although the duration of some of these trials has been brief, the application of quantitative computerized techniques for analyzing the angiograms has enhanced their significance. Therapeutic interventions have involved diet alone, gastrointestinal surgery, and the use of lipid-lowering agents.

The earliest coronary angiographic study was initiated in 1975 in Finland and included 28 hyperlipidemic patients with symptomatic coronary artery disease.[91] Dietary therapy was used alone or in combination with either clofibrate or clofibrate plus niacin. Progression was evaluated over a 7-year period and compared to changes observed in 20 nonrandomized control patients with coronary artery disease. Average reductions of total cholesterol, triglyceride, and LDL-cholesterol were 18 percent, 38 percent, and 19 percent, respectively, and mean HDL-cholesterol rose 10 percent. Nine of twenty-eight treated patients evaluated at 7 years had no evidence of coronary artery disease progression, whereas lack of progression was seen in only 1 of 13 surviving controls evaluated at 5 years. The number of arterial segments showing progression was significantly reduced by treatment in 46 out of 278 (17 percent) compared to 50 out of 132 (38 percent) in control subjects. Low levels of total cholesterol and triglyceride, high levels of HDL-cholesterol, and a low LDL/HDL ratio were associated with reduced severity of progression. Levels of total cholesterol above 243 mg/dL (6.3 mmol/liter) were associated with a twofold increase in the number of coronary artery segments showing progression when compared to levels less than 243 mg/dL. Similarly, HDL-cholesterol levels less 42.5 mg/dL (1.1 mmol/liter) also showed a twofold increase in coronary segments exhibiting progression when compared to levels of HDL-cholesterol greater than 42.5 mg/dL. Finally, favorable effects were associated with reductions of combined levels of very low density lipoprotein cholesterol plus LDL-cholesterol.

The Leiden Intervention Trial involved 39 patients with angina pectoris and established coronary artery disease who were enrolled in a 2-year study consisting of a very strict vegetarian diet.[92] The ratio of polyunsaturated/saturated fats was about 2.5, and coronary angiography was employed to evaluate coronary patency before the trial and after 2 years of diet therapy. Reductions in serum total cholesterol were produced as expected, but the serum HDL-cholesterol did not change. Progression was shown in 21 patients, but no lesion growth was observed in the remaining 18. The 18 subjects in whom atherosclerosis did not progress revealed significantly lower levels of serum total cholesterol, lower serum total cholesterol/HDL-cholesterol ratio, and higher levels of HDL-cholesterol at the inception of the trial as well as after 2 years of dietary intervention. A significant association was observed between the average value of the serum total cholesterol/HDL-cholesterol ratio and lesion growth. Although these initial cholesterol treatment trials did not document regression of coronary artery disease, they introduced angiography as the basis for measuring the influence of cholesterol reduction on coronary atherosclerosis.

The National Heart Lung Blood Institute (NHLBI) Type II Coronary Intervention Study was a major effort to examine the effect of cholesterol-lowering (with cholestyramine) on the progression of coronary artery disease.[93] This study was a randomized, placebo-controlled, double-blind protocol over a period of 5 years that included 143 people with primary type II hypercholesterolemia. All patients were placed on a low-fat diet. Mean LDL-cholesterol levels were 253 mg/dL (6.5 mmol/liter) when patients were initially selected and remained at 237 mg/dL (6.1 mmol/liter) after 2 months of dietary therapy. Thus, subjects were in the upper 10 percent of LDL-cholesterol distribution. Treatment group baseline levels of total cholesterol, triglycerides, LDL-cholesterol, and HDL-cholesterol were 310, 156, 242, and 38 mg/dL, respectively. Baseline values in the control group were 293, 131, 229, and 39 mg/dL. Cholestyramine induced significant reduction in total cholesterol and LDL-cholesterol, although the extent of the reductions diminished over the duration of the trial. Decreases in LDL-cholesterol or total cholesterol and increases in HDL-cholesterol were independently associated with lower rates of coronary artery disease progression. Progression was observed in 35 percent of controls and 25 percent of the treatment group. Although this difference was not statistically significant, when incidences of definite plus probable regression were combined, the incidence rate of the treatment group was significantly lower than in the controls. Treatment benefits were more marked in those patients who initially had one lesion causing greater than 50 percent reduction in vessel lumen, and in this subgroup definite/probable progression occurred in 14 of 42 controls but in only 5 of 41 treated patients.

The Cholesterol-Lowering Atherosclerosis study (CLAS) tested the hypothesis that intervention to reduce LDL-cholesterol and increase HDL-cholesterol would arrest or reverse the development of atherosclerotic lesions.[94] This was a 2 year, randomized, placebo-controlled angiographic study in which participants were preselected to ensure compliance with the treatment. All participants had undergone previous coronary bypass surgery and had blood cholesterol levels between 185 and 300 mg/dL (4.8 and 7.8 mmol/liter). The 188 nonsmoking men were treated with a combination of dietary modification, colestipol, and niacin. Controls consisted of 162 men subject to dietary modifications only. Reductions of total cholesterol by 26 percent, triglycerides by 22 percent, and LDL-cholesterol by 43 percent were obtained in the treatment group. HDL-cholesterol rose by 37 percent. Coronary artery disease regression was documented in 16 percent of treated subjects compared to only 2 percent of controls. In native coronary vessels, treatment reduced both the average number of lesions that progressed per subject and the percentage of subjects with new lesions. In patients with grafted vessels, treatment also significantly reduced the percentage of patients showing adverse changes in these graft vessels as well as the percentage of subjects with new lesions in native vessels. Therapy not only produced benefits in those with exceptionally high cholesterol levels but also in patients with serum cholesterol from 185 to 240 mg/dL (4.8 to 6.2 mmol/liter). A subgroup of 103 men continued in the study for 4 years in CLAS-II.[94a] The results of CLAS-II confirm CLAS-I findings and indicate that regression can continue for 4 years. CLAS-I and CLAS-II reaffirmed the need for vigorous long-term lipid-lowering therapy in patients who undergo coronary bypass surgery. This clinical decision was strengthened by the observation that patients whose grafts showed no progression of atherosclerosis also had a lower rate of myocardial infarction.

The Program on the Surgical Control of the Hyperlipidemias (POSCH) was a prospective, randomized secondary atherosclerosis intervention trial by Buchwald and coworkers.[95] Between 1975 and 1983, 838 survivors of single myocardial infarction entered the study at four different centers. The 417 control group patients were randomly assigned to treatment by diet instruction only, and the 421 intervention group patients were randomized to partial ileal bypass in addition to diet therapy. The follow-up period ranged from 7 to almost 15 years, with a mean follow-up of 9 years. Compared to the control group at 5 years, the surgically treated group had a total cholesterol level 23 percent lower, an LDL-cholesterol level 38 percent lower, and an HDL-cholesterol level 4 percent higher. Overall mortality and mortality due to coronary heart disease, however, were not significantly reduced. The combined endpoint of death due to coronary disease and confirmed nonfatal myocardial infarction was 35 percent lower in the surgery group. Common side effects of partial ileal bypass were diarrhea, kidney stones, gall stones, and intestinal obstruction. When individual lesion analyses were used and patients with coronary bypass surgery or angioplasty excluded, for all coronary artery segments there was significantly less disease progression in the surgery group: 30 percent, 42 percent, 30 percent, and 32 percent less at 3, 5, 7, and 10 years, respectively.

Similarly a decrease in the percentage of patients with new coronary lesion formation in the surgery group was 44 percent, 50 percent, 28 percent, and 57 percent at 3, 5, 7, and 10 years, respectively. For coronary artery disease regression by global assessment, there were significant differences at 5 and 7 years of follow-up: 5 percent in the control group versus 13 percent in the surgery group at 5 years, and 6 percent control versus 14 percent surgery at 7 years. The investigators concluded that atherosclerosis progression could be slowed and that individual lesions could be stabilized and even reversed by aggressive lipid modification accomplished by partial ileal bypass surgery.

The Lifestyle Heart Trial by Ornish and coworkers was a prospective, randomized control trial to determine whether comprehensive life-style changes could affect coronary atherosclerosis after 1 year.[96] Twenty-eight patients were assigned to an experimental group whose regimen included a low-fat vegetarian diet, smoking cessation, stress management, and moderate exercise. Significantly, no lipid drugs were used in the treatment group. The second group of twenty patients was assigned to usual care and was not asked to make life-style changes although the individuals were free to do so. Initially 195 coronary lesions were analyzed by an independent cardiologist employing quantitative coronary angiography. In the experimental group total cholesterol fell by 24 percent and LDL-cholesterol fell by 37 percent. These declines occurred even though patients had already reduced fat consumption to 31 percent of calories and cholesterol to 213 mg/day on the average before baseline testing. HDL-cholesterol did not change significantly in either group. Patients in the experimental group reported a 91 percent reduction in the frequency of angina, a 42 percent reduction in the duration of angina, and a 28 percent reduction in the severity of angina. In contrast, control group patients described a 165 percent rise in frequency, a 95 percent rise in duration, and a 39 percent rise in severity of angina. Quantitative coronary angiography revealed the average percent diameter stenosis regressed from 40 to 38 percent in the experimental group yet progressed from 43 to 46 percent in controls. When only lesions greater than 50 percent stenosed were analyzed, the average percent diameter stenosis regressed from 62 to 56 percent in the experimental group and progressed from 62 to 64 percent in the control group. Overall, 82 percent of experimental group patients had an average change toward regression. The investigators concluded that comprehensive life-style changes may be able, in highly selected individuals, to bring about regression of even severe coronary atherosclerosis after only 1 year without the use of lipid-lowering drugs.

A Specialized Center of Research Study was initiated by Kane and colleagues to study regression of coronary atherosclerosis during treatment of familial hypercholesterolemia with combined drug regimens.[97] The randomized control trial, which evaluated 31 men and 41 women with heterozygous familial hypercholesterolemia, examined the effect of reduction of LDL-cholesterol levels by diet and combined drug regimens on the regression of coronary lesions. LDL-cholesterol levels were decreased from 283 to 172 mg/dL (7.3 to 4.5 mmol/liter). The mean change in percent area stenosis among male controls was +0.80, indicating progression, while the mean change for men in the treatment group was −1.53, indicating regression. Although analyzed separately, regression among women was also significant. In this study the change in percent area stenosis correlated with changes in LDL-cholesterol during the trial. The investigators concluded that reduction of LDL-cholesterol could induce regression of atherosclerotic lesions of the coronary arteries in patients with familial hypercholesterolemia and that the benefit of the treatment applied to women and men alike. Of interest, most of the subjects in this study had asymptomatic coronary artery atherosclerosis.

The Familial Atherosclerosis Treatment Study (FATS) conducted by Brown and colleagues enrolled 146 men no more than 62 years of age who had apolipoprotein B levels greater than 125 mg/dL, coronary artery disease documented by angiography, and a family history of vascular disease.[98] One-hundred and twenty individuals completed the 2 1/2-year double-blind study that included quantitative arteriography at baseline and after treatment. Patients were given dietary counseling and randomly assigned to one of three treatment groups: lovastatin, 20 mg twice a day, and colestipol, 10 g three times a day; niacin, 1 g four times a day, and colestipol, 10 g three times a day; or conventional therapy with placebo (or colestipol if the LDL-cholesterol was elevated). In the conventional therapy group, levels of LDL- and HDL-cholesterol changed only slightly but changed more substantially among patients treated with lovastatin and colestipol (−46 percent and +15 percent) or with niacin and colestipol (−32 percent and +43 percent). In the conventional therapy group 46 percent of the patients had definite lesion progression and no regression in at least one of nine proximal coronary artery segments; regression was the only change in 11 percent. In comparison, progression as the only change was less frequent among patients who received lovastatin and colestipol (21 percent) than in those who received niacin and colestipol (25 percent), and regression was more frequent [lovastatin and colestipol (32 percent); niacin and colestipol (39 percent)]. Multivariate analysis indicated that a reduction in the level of apolipoprotein B (or LDL-cholesterol) and systolic blood pressure and an increase in HDL-cholesterol correlated independently with regression of coronary lesions. Clinical events (death, myocardial infarction, or revascularization for worsening symptoms) occurred in 10 of 52 patients assigned to conventional therapy as compared with 3 of 46 assigned to receive lovastatin and colestipol and 2 of 48 assigned to receive niacin and colestipol. The conclusions of this study in men with coronary artery disease who were at high risk for cardiovascular events were that intensive lipid-lowering therapy reduced the frequency of progression of coronary lesions, increased the frequency of regression, and reduced dramatically the incidence of cardiovascular events. These results support the hypothesis that lipid-lowering can alter the clinical activity of atheromata (Chap. 55), even without a dramatic decrease in the angiographic size. (See also Chap. 56.)

The St. Thomas Atherosclerosis Regression Study (STARS) was began in 1984 by Watts and co-investigators to investigate diet plus cholestyramine as unifactorial interventions in a randomized controlled trial.[99] Ninety men with symptomatic coronary artery disease not requiring revascularization and with plasma cholesterol levels exceeding 232 mg/dL (6 mmol/liter) were randomized into three groups in a 39-month endpoint blinded trial. The groups received usual care, a lipid-lowering diet plus usual care, or cholestyramine plus lipid-lowering diet plus usual care. Progressive angiographic changes were observed in 54 percent of usual care patients, 19 percent of diet patients, and 17 percent of patients with cholestyramine and diet. Regression was documented in 4 percent of patients with usual care, 42 percent of patients with dietary management, and 38 percent of patients with cholestyramine and dietary management. Thus, dietary changes as the single intervention decreased the number of patients showing net progression and increased the number showing enlarged luminal diameter, while cholestyramine had similar effects on a per patient basis but also achieved a slight net increase in coronary lumen diameter. In this study clinical events paralleled the changes documented in coronary luminal diameter.

The results of a meta-analysis of randomized secondary prevention clinical trials of coronary atherosclerosis progression or regression in patients who had either undergone coronary artery bypass surgery or had suffered an acute myocardial infarction has recently been published.[100] Intensive lipid-modifying therapy in patients with high levels of plasma cholesterol resulted in large reductions in total cholesterol and elevations of HDL-cholesterol. This was associated with slowing or arrest of the coronary arteriosclerosis in a substantial number of patients (27 percent versus 46 percent) but an increase in the incidence of regression in relatively few patients (17 percent versus 7 percent). The effects would be expected to be greater if therapy is continued for a longer period of time, although some progression did occur in 14 to 39 percent after 3 years and in 55 percent after 10 years. These results will likely improve with better lipid-lowering therapy.

ADDITIONAL FACTORS THAT MAY INFLUENCE CHOLESTEROL AND ATHEROSCLEROSIS

Although lipoproteins and the previously discussed risk factors play a major role in the atherogenic process, many other substances have been considered in the mechanism of abnormal coronary vascular reactivity and atherosclerosis.[101,102] Red cells, white cells, and in particular platelets release factors that can influence atherosclerosis or contribute to thrombosis on an existing plaque. Cholesterol levels influence platelet aggregation. Factor VII and fibrinogen are independent risks for ischemic heart disease, and triglycerides enhance factor VII activity.[103,104] Fibrinogen and factor VII levels can be reduced by lipid-lowering therapy. Triglycerides also increase factor X clotting activity. Lipoprotein(a), or LP_a, is composed of an LDL molecule linked by a disulfide bridge to apolipoprotein(a).[31] Lp_a is strikingly similar to plasminogen and competitively inhibits the binding of plasminogen to fibrin, thereby inhibiting fibrinolysis. Cholesterol impairs prostacyclin production that induces coronary vasodilation and inhibits platelet aggregation. However, HDL-cholesterol promotes prostacyclin biosynthesis and release. Prostacyclin stabilizing factor, which prolongs the half-life of prostacyclin, is in fact apolipoprotein A-1, the major component of HDL.

Alcohol can variably raise cholesterol and particularly triglycerides in some individuals but may exert a beneficial role in raising HDL-cholesterol.[105–112] Nine or more cups of coffee per day have been associated with elevated cholesterol values.[113–115] Aspirin exerts a favorable influence on unstable angina and incidence of myocardial infarction.[116] Hyperuricemia has long been associated with lipid abnormalities. Higher levels of homocysteine have been observed in patients with coronary artery disease and associated with lower HDL-cholesterol and higher triglyceride levels.[117–119] Nut consumption can provide a source of unsaturated fatty acids.[120,121] Fish oil supplements can influence thromboxane production, a potent coronary constrictor and platelet aggregator, but lipid levels may rise. Dietary fiber has a modest effect on cholesterol lowering but its benefits have been exaggerated.[122] The observation in Finnish men of the synergistic association of a high stored iron level, as assessed by serum ferritin concentration, and serum LDL-cholesterol with an increased incidence of acute myocardial infarction supports the theory that free iron can induce oxidation of lipids and increase the risk of coronary heart disease.[123]

Clinical studies have suggested that antioxidants may have a role in the reduction of coronary artery disease in men and women.[124–128] Prospective studies are in progress to evaluate the role of vitamins E, C, and beta-carotene, and a coronary regression trial is underway in Sweden to assess the role of probucol, a lipid-lowering drug with antioxidant properties.[129] Although doses have not been established, many people are ingesting antioxidant vitamins since the benefit may exceed the side effects, which have not been reported.

NONCARDIOVASCULAR RISKS AND LOW CHOLESTEROL LEVELS

Meta-analysis of primary prevention trials has revealed higher rates of noncardiac death in men receiving active treatment to lower cholesterol levels.[130] Such increases in mortality with cholesterol levels less than 160 mg/dL (4.1 mmol/liter) were significant for injury and cancer. Middle-aged men with these low levels of cholesterol were at increased risk of dying from a variety of causes, including lung cancer, other noncolon cancers, respiratory disease, digestive disease, trauma, hemorrhagic stroke, and other residual causes. However, these noncardiac conditions were not significantly affected in the secondary prevention trials, that is, in individuals with known coronary heart disease. The patterns of association between low blood cholesterol and increased rates of various causes of noncardiovascular deaths were similar in women with the exception of a smaller cancer mortality. Controversy remains over interpretation of noncardiac death in treated compared to control groups.[131] Long-term follow-up studies of control subjects and patients treated with cholesterol-lowering regimen will be needed to examine the endpoints of coronary heart disease and noncardiac conditions. Nevertheless studies support the decreased risk of coronary heart disease with both primary prevention and secondary intervention.[132]

CHOLESTEROL SCREENING AND TREATMENT CONSIDERATION

Studies have consistently shown a relationship between cholesterol and risk of coronary heart disease. However, some studies have failed to find an association between cholesterol and coronary heart disease in elderly men. Coronary heart disease occurs 7 to 10 years later in women compared to men, but death rates are similar.[133] Low HDL-cholesterol may be a stronger risk factor and high LDL-cholesterol a weaker risk factor in women than in men.[134] However, elevated blood cholesterol remains a risk factor for coronary heart disease recurrence or death among both women and men who already have coronary heart disease.[135]

Although cholesterol screening has properly become widespread as a result of vigorous public health efforts, a lipid profile with cholesterol, HDL-cholesterol, triglyceride, and LDL-cholesterol is specifically indicated in the following groups of patients: (1) Children with relatives having premature coronary heart disease; (2) adult men, women, and elderly people with coronary heart disease; and (3) adults with HDL-cholesterol <35 mg/dL (0.9 mmol/liter) or two or more risk factors. (See Fig. 62-3.)

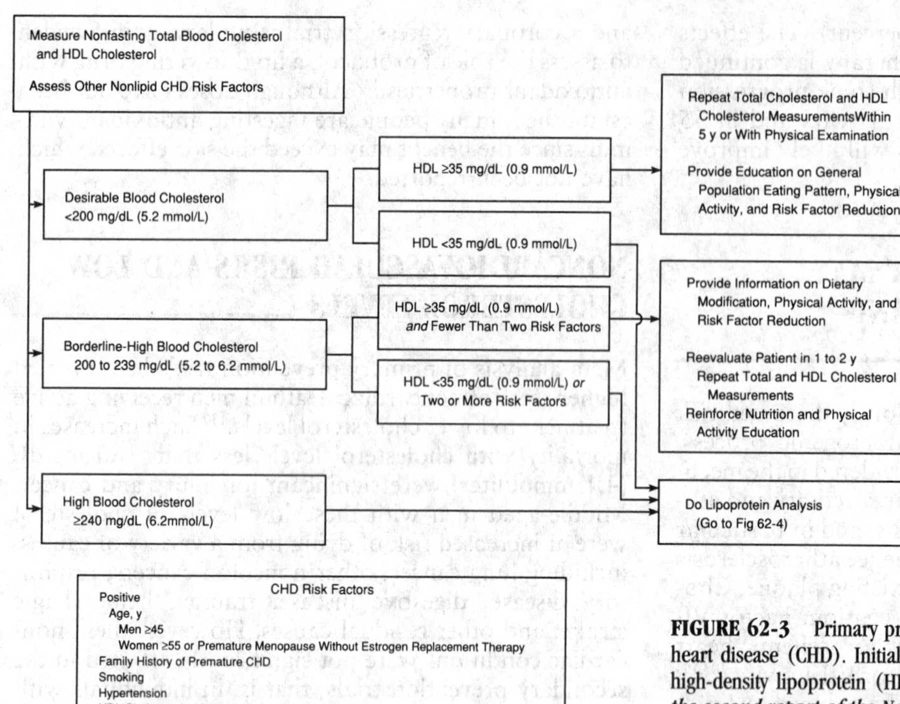

FIGURE 62-3 Primary prevention in adults without evidence of coronary heart disease (CHD). Initial classification is based on total cholesterol and high-density lipoprotein (HDL) cholesterol levels. [*From the Summary of the second report of the National Cholesterol Education Program (NCEP) expert panel on detection, evaluation, and treatment of high blood cholesterol in adults (Adult Treatment Panel II). JAMA 1993; 269:3015–3023. Reproduced with permission from the publisher and authors.*]

Individuals who might be overtreated with lipid-lowering drugs include the following groups: (1) Children with cholesterol between 170 and 200 mg/dL (4.4 and 5.2 mmol/liter); (2) women with HDL-cholesterol greater than 60 mg/dL (1.6 mmol/liter); and (3) elderly patients without coronary heart disease and who are not at high risk.

In 1988, the National Cholesterol Education Program of the NHLBI recommended patients with coronary heart disease or two or more risk factors to lower cholesterol below 200 mg/dL (5.2 mmol/liter) and LDL-cholesterol to less than 130 mg/dL (3.4 mmol/liter).[37] In 1993 the second report of the expert panel on detection, evaluation, and treatment of high blood cholesterol in adults updated the recommendations for cholesterol management.[38,136,137] The second report increased emphasis on coronary heart disease risk status and placed more attention on HDL-cholesterol as a risk factor.[38] Specific findings on risk status were: (1) patients with coronary disease were identified as highest risk with lower target levels for LDL-cholesterol; (2) age as a major risk factor was defined as 45 years or older in men and 55 years or older in women; (3) drug therapy should be delayed in most young adult men and premenopausal women with high HDL-cholesterol who are otherwise at low risk for coronary heart disease; and (4) enhanced recognition for high-risk postmenopausal women and high-risk elderly patients otherwise in good health as candidates for cholesterol-lowering therapy. For HDL-cholesterol, recommendations were: (1) addition of HDL-cholesterol to initial cholesterol screening; (2) designation of high HDL-cholesterol as a negative risk factor; and (3) consideration of HDL-cholesterol levels in choice of drug therapy. The report emphasized physical activity and weight loss as components of the dietary therapy of high blood cholesterol. Screening patterns for primary prevention in adults without evidence of coronary heart disease based on total cholesterol and HDL-cholesterol are shown in Fig. 62-3, and the subsequent classification based on LDL-cholesterol is shown in Fig. 62-4. Secondary prevention in adults with coronary heart disease based on LDL-cholesterol is shown in Fig. 62-5. Finally, treatment decisions for target LDL-cholesterol goals are outlined in Table 62-4. For secondary prevention in patients with coronary heart disease, the goal of therapy is an LDL-cholesterol level of 100 mg/dL (2.6 mmol/liter) or lower. (See also Chaps. 53 and 65.)

FUTURE DIRECTIONS

The initial success in primary and secondary intervention trials plus the demonstration of slowing progression and even regression of some lesions in coronary artery disease will challenge physicians to broaden areas for cholesterol intervention.[138,139] Not only males but also females and elderly and younger patients will be more carefully characterized in terms of cardiovascular risks and indications for risk modification and pharmacologic intervention. Individuals with abnormally low HDL-cholesterol values as well as those with elevated triglycerides will probably become candidates for treatment.

With documentation of retardation of progression and significant regression in clinical trials, all patients with manifest coronary artery disease, even if only reflected by irregularities of or perhaps even abnormal

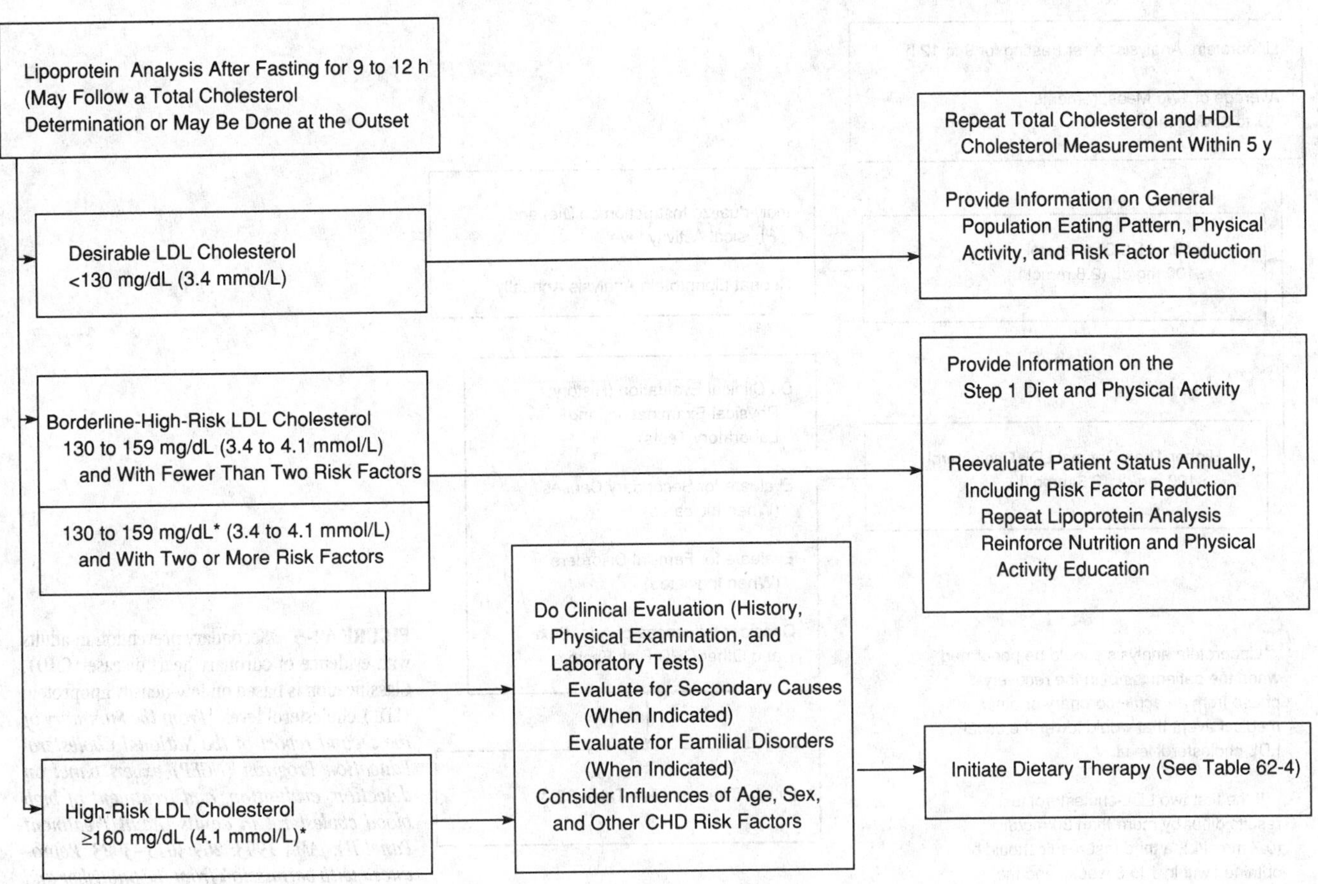

FIGURE 62-4 Primary prevention in adults without evidence of coronary heart disease (CHD). Subsequent classification is based on low-density lipoprotein (LDL) cholesterol level. [*From the Summary of the second report of the National Cholesterol Education Program (NCEP) expert panel on detection, evaluation, and treatment of high blood cholesterol in adults (Adult Treatment Panel II). JAMA 1993; 269:3015–3023. Reproduced with permission from the publisher and authors.*]

TABLE 62-4

Treatment Decisions Based on LDL Cholesterol Level*

Patient Category	Initiation Level	LDL Goal
Dietary Therapy		
Without CHD and with fewer than two risk factors	≥160 mg/dL (4.1 mmol/liter)	<160 mg/dL (4.1 mmol/liter)
Without CHD and with two or more risk factors	≥130 mg/dL (3.4 mmol/liter)	<130 mg/dL (3.4 mmol/liter)
With CHD	>100 mg/dL (2.6 mmol/liter)	≤100 mg/dL (2.6 mmol/liter)
Drug Treatment		
Without CHD and with fewer than two risk factors	≥190 mg/dL (4.9 mmol/liter)	<130 mg/dL (4.1 mmol/liter)
Without CHD and with two or more risk factors	≥160 mg/dL (4.1 mmol/liter)	<130 mg/dL (3.4 mmol/liter)
With CHD	≥130 mg/dL (3.4 mmol/liter)	≤100 mg/dL (2.6 mmol/liter)

* LDL = low-density lipoprotein; CHD = coronary heart disease.

SOURCE: From the Summary of the Second Report of the National Cholesterol Education Program (NCEP) Expert Panel on Detection, Evaluation, and Treatment of High Cholesterol in Adults (Adult Treatment Panel II). JAMA 1993;269:3015–3023. Reproduced with permission from the publisher and authors.

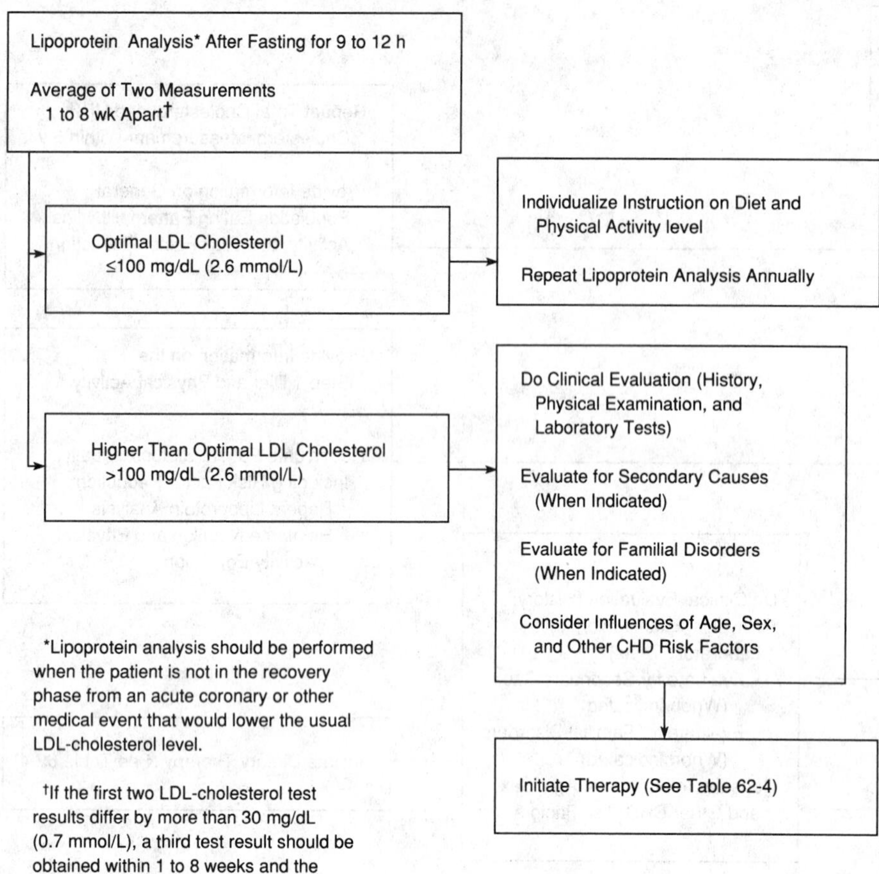

FIGURE 62-5 Secondary prevention in adults with evidence of coronary heart disease (CHD). Classification is based on low-density lipoprotein (LDL) cholesterol level. [*From the Summary of the second report of the National Cholesterol Education Program (NCEP) expert panel on detection, evaluation, and treatment of high blood cholesterol in adults (Adult Treatment Panel II). JAMA 1993; 269:3015–3023. Reproduced with permission from the publisher and authors.*]

vasoreactivity, will become candidates for treatment of blood lipids. Patients with abnormal coronary angiograms, angioplasty, acute infarction, and coronary artery bypass surgery should have major attention paid to their blood lipid values.[38,138–142] More physicians are adopting the view that patients with atherosclerotic vascular disease should be treated even if cholesterol values are "normal." The logic is that a "normal" cholesterol for the population may not be normal for an individual patient's biologic susceptibility. Goals will be to slow progression and induce regression by diet, exercise, and drugs. Symptomatic patients with mild to moderate coronary artery disease may undergo lipid reduction prior to consideration for mechanical revascularization with angioplasty and coronary artery surgery.

The target levels of blood lipids in patients with proven coronary artery disease should be lower than previously recommended by the National Cholesterol Education Program in 1988 (total cholesterol less than 200 mg/dL and LDL-cholesterol less than 130 mg/dL.) Regression trials support the new target values recommended by the adult treatment panel of an LDL-cholesterol less than 100 mg/dL (2.6 mmol/liter). Such efforts will often not only require diet and exercise programs but also one or more lipid-lowering agents.[143] (See Chap. 65.)

Patients with known coronary artery disease require careful follow-up and attention to life-style, diet, exercise, and lipid profiles, with diligent efforts to lower cholesterol, triglycerides, and LDL-cholesterol maximally plus raising HDL-cholesterol. Such interventions should be applied to all patients with documented coronary artery disease who have a reasonable prognosis on the basis of ventricular function and other organ function. In the future such management may also be shown to be cost effective for many other individuals at increased risk.

REFERENCES

1. Schwartz CJ, Valente AJ, Sprague EA: A modern view of atherogenesis. *Am J Cardiol* 1993; 71:9B–14B.
2. Anitschkow N: Experimental atherosclerosis in animals. In: Cowdry EV (ed): *Arteriosclerosis: A Study of the Problem*. New York, MacMillian, 1933; 271–322.
3. Steinberg D, Parthasarathy S, Carew TE, Khoo JC, Witztum JL: Beyond cholesterol: Modification of low-density lipoprotein that increases its atherogenicity. *N Engl J Med* 1989; 320:915–924.
4. Steinberg D: Antioxidants and atherosclerosis: A current assessment. *Circulation* 1992; 84:1420–1425.
5. Bevans M, Davidson JD, Kendall FE: Regression of lesions in canine arteriosclerosis. *Arch Pathol* 1951; 51:288–292.
6. Friedman M, Byers SO: Observations concerning the evolution of atherosclerosis in the rabbit after cessation of cholesterol feeding. *Am J Pathol* 1963; 43:349–354.
7. Clarkson TB, Bond MG, Bullock BC, Marzetta CA: A study of atherosclerosis regression in *Macaca mulatta*: IV. Changes in coronary arteries from animals with atherosclerosis induced for

19 months and then regressed for 24 or 48 months at plasma cholesterol concentration of 300 and 200 mg/dL. *Exp Mol Pathol* 1981; 34:345–368.

8. Armstrong ML, Warner ED, Conner WE: Regression of coronary atherosclerosis in rhesus monkeys. *Circ Res* 1970; 27:59–67.
9. Armstrong ML, Megan MB: Lipid depletion in atheromatous coronary arteries in rhesus monkeys after regression diets. *Circ Res* 1972; 30:675–680.
10. Armstrong ML, Heistad DD, Marcus ML, Piegors OJ, Abboud RM: Hemodynamic sequelae of regression of experimental atherosclerosis. *J Clin Invest* 1983; 71:104–113.
11. Shimokawa H, Vanhoutte PM: Hypercholesterolemia causes generalized impairment of endothelium-dependent relaxation to aggregating platelets in porcine arteries. *J Am Coll Cardiol* 1989; 13:1402–1408.
12. Harrison DH, Armstrong ML, Freiman PC, Heistad DD: Restoration of endothelium-dependent relaxation by dietary treatment of atherosclerosis. *J Clin Invest* 1987; 80:1808–1811.
13. Kuhn FE, Mohler ER, Satler LF, Reagan K, Lu DY, Rackley CE: Effects of high density lipoprotein on acetylcholine-induced coronary vasoreactivity. *Am J Cardiol* 1991; 68:1425–1430.
14. Keys A(ed): Coronary heart disease in seven countries. *Circulation* 1970; 41 (suppl I):I-1–I-211.

14a. Keys A: *Seven Countries: A Multivariate Analysis of Death and Coronary Heart Disease.* Cambridge; MA, Harvard Univ, Press, 1980.

15. Multiple Risk Factor Intervention Trial Research Group: Multiple Risk Factor Intervention Trial. Risk factor changes and mortality results. *JAMA* 1982; 248:1465–1477.
16. Stason WB: Cost and benefits of risk factor reduction for coronary heart disease: Insights from screening and treatment of serum cholesterol. *Am Heart J* 1990; 119:718–724.
17. Martin MJ, Hulley SB, Browner WS, Kuller LH, Wentworth D: Serum cholesterol, blood pressure and mortality: Implications from a cohort of 361,662 men. *Lancet* 1986; 2:933–936.
18. Klein LW, Ambrose J, Pichard A, Holt J, Gorlin R, Teicholz E: Acute coronary hemodynamic response to cigarette smoking in patients with coronary artery disease. *J Am Coll Cardiol* 1984; 3:879–886.
19. Benowitz HL: Pharmacologic aspects of cigarette smoking and nicotine addition. *N Engl J Med* 1988; 319:1318–1330.
20. Garrison RJ, Kannel WB, Feinleib M, Castelli WP, McNamara PM, Padgett SJ: Cigarette smoking and HDL cholesterol. The Framingham Offspring Study. *Atherosclerosis* 1978; 30:17–25.
21. Brischetto CS, Connor WE, Connor SL, Matarazzo JD: Plasma lipid and lipoprotein profiles of cigarette smokers from randomly selected families: Enhancement of hyperlipidemia and depression of high-density lipoprotein. *Am J Cardiol* 1983; 52:675–680.
22. Aberg A, Bergstrand R, Johannson S, Ulvenstam CT, Vedin A, Wedel H, et al: Cessation of smoking after myocardial infarction. Effects on mortality after 10 years. *Br Heart J* 1983; 49:416–422.
23. Galan KM, Deligonul U, Kern MJ, Chaitman BR, Vandormael MG: Increased frequency of restenosis in patients continuing to smoke cigarettes after percutaneous transluminal coronary angioplasty. *Am J Cardiol* 1988; 61:260–263.
24. Assman G, Schulte H: The prospective Cardiovascular Munster Study: Prevalence and prognostic significance of hyperlipidemia in men with systemic hypertension. *Am J Cardiol* 1987; 59:9G–17G.
25. Chobanian AV: The influence of hypertension and other hemodynamic factors in atherogenesis. *Prog Cardiovasc Dis* 1983; 26:177–196.
26. Lardinois CK, Neuman SL: The effects of antihypertensive agents on serum lipids and lipoproteins. *Arch Intern Med* 1988; 148:1280–1288.
27. Anderson KM, Castelli WP, Levy D: Cholesterol and mortality. 30 years of follow-up from the Framingham Study. *JAMA* 1987; 257:2176–2180.
28. Gordon T, Castelli WP, Hjartland MC, Kannel WB, Dawber TR: High density lipoprotein as a protective factor against coronary artery disease. The Framingham Study. *Am J Med* 1977; 62:707–714.
29. Romm PA, Green CE, Reagan K, Rackley CE: Relation of serum lipoprotein cholesterol levels to presence and severity of angiographic coronary artery disease. *Am J Cardiol* 1991; 67:479–483.
30. Scanu AM: Lipoprotein(a). A genetic risk factor for premature coronary heart disease. *JAMA* 1992;267;3326–3329.
31. Schreiner PJ, Morrisett JD, Sharrett AR, Patsch W, Tyroler HA, Wu K, et al: Lipoprotein[a] as a risk factor for preclinical atherosclerosis. *Arterioscler Thromb* 1993; 13:826–833.
32. Edelberg JM, Pizzo SV: Lipoprotein(a) inhibits plasminogen activation in a template-dependent manner. *Blood Coag Fibrinol* 1991; 2:759–764.

32a. Loscalzo J: Lipoprotein(a). A unique risk factor for atherothrombotic disease. *Arteriosclerosis* 1990; 10:672–679.

33. Manninen V, Tenkanen L, Koskinen P, Huttunen JK, Mänttäri M, Heinonen OP, et al: Joint effects of serum triglyceride and LDL cholesterol and HDL cholesterol concentrations on coronary heart disease risk in the Helsinki Heart Study: Implications for treatment. *Circulation* 1992; 85:37–45.
34. Assmann G, Schulte H: Relation of high-density lipoprotein cholesterol and triglycerides to incidence of atherosclerotic coronary artery disease (the PROCAM Experience). *Am J Cardiol* 1992; 70:733–737.
35. Criqui MH, Heiss G, Cohn R, Cowan LD, Suchindran CM, Bangdiwala S, et al: Plasma triglyceride level and mortality from coronary heart disease. *N Engl J Med* 1993; 328:1220–1225.
36. NIH Consensus Development Panel on Triglyceride, High-Density Lipoprotein, and Coronary Heart Disease: Triglyceride, high-density lipoprotein and coronary heart disease. *JAMA* 1993; 269:505–510.
37. The Expert Panel: Report of the National Cholesterol Education Program Expert Panel on Detection, Evaluation and Treatment of High Blood Cholesterol in Adults. *Arch Intern Med* 1988; 148:36–69.
38. Expert Panel on Detection, Evaluation and Treatment of High Blood Cholesterol in Adults: Summary of the Second Report of the National Cholesterol Education Program (NCEP). *JAMA* 1993; 216:3015–3023.
39. Stampfer MS, Sacks FM, Salvini S, Willett WC, Hennekens CH: A prospective study of cholesterol, apolipoproteins and the risk of myocardial infarction. *N Engl J Med* 1991; 325:373–381.
40. Berenson GS, Wattigney WA, Tracy RE, Newman WP III, Srinivasan SR, Webber LS, et al: Atherosclerosis of the aorta and coronary arteries and cardiovascular risk factors in persons aged 6 to 30 years and studied at necropsy (The Bogalusa Heart Study). *Am J Cardiol* 1992; 70:851–858.
41. Klag MJ, Ford DE, Mead LA, He J, Whelton PK, Liang KY, et al: Serum cholesterol in young men and subsequent cardiovascular disease. *N Engl J Med* 1993; 328:313–318.
42. Zimetbaum P, Frishman WH, Ooi WL, Derman MP, Aronson M, Gidez LI, et al: Plasma lipids and lipoproteins and the incidence of cardiovascular disease in the very elderly: The Bronx Aging Study. *Arterioscler Thromb* 1992; 12:416–423.
43. Ettinger WH, Wahl P, Kuller LH, Bush TL, Tracy RP, Manolio TA, et al: Lipoprotein lipids in older people: Results from the Cardiovascular Health Study. *Circulation* 1992; 86:858–869.
44. Donahue RP, Abbott RD, Bloom E, Reed DM, Yano K: Central obesity and coronary heart disease in men. *Lancet* 1987; 1:821–824.
45. Kannel WB: Lipids, diabetes and coronary heart disease: Insights from the Framingham Study. *Am Heart J* 1985; 110:1100–1107.
46. Lyons TJ: Glycation and oxidation: A role in the pathogenesis of atherosclerosis. *Am J Cardiol* 1993; 71:26B–31B
47. Goff DC Jr, Shekelle RB, Katan MB, Gotto AM Jr, Stamler J: Does body fatness modify the association between dietary cholesterol and risk of coronary death? Results from the Chicago Western Electric Study. *Arterioscler Thromb* 1992; 12:755–761.
48. Denke MA, Sempos CT, Grundy SM: Excess body weight: An underrecognized contributor to high blood cholesterol levels in white American men. *Arch Intern Med* 1993; 153:1093–1103.
49. Thompson PD, Cullinane EM, Sady SP, Flynn MM, Chenevert CB, Herbert PN: High density lipoprotein metabolism in endurance athletes and sedentary men. *Circulation* 1991; 84:140–152.
50. Fletcher GF, Blair SN, Bloomenthal J, Caspersen C, Chaitman B, Epstein S, et al: Statement on exercise: Benefits and recommendations for physical activity programs for all Americans. *Circulation* 1992; 86:340–344.
51. Bonaa KH, Arnessan E: Association between heart rate and atherogenic blood lipid fractions in a population: The Tromso Study. *Circulation* 1992; 86:394–405.

52. Curfman GD: The health benefits of exercise: A critical reappraisal (editorial). *N Engl J Med* 1993; 328;574–576.
53. Lesko SM, Rosenberg L, Shapiro S: A case-control study of baldness in relation to myocardial infarction in men. *JAMA* 1993; 269:998–1003.
54. Taylor PA, Ward A: Women, high-density lipoprotein cholesterol, and exercise. *Arch Intern Med* 1993; 153:1178–1184.
55. Sullivan JM, Zwaag RV, Lemp GF, Hughes JP, Maddock V, Groetz FW, et al: Postmenopausal use of estrogen and occlusion of coronary arteries. *Ann Intern Med* 1988; 108:358–363.
56. Stampfer MJ, Colditz GA, Willett WC, Manson JE, Rosner B, Speizer FE, et al: Postmenopausal estrogen therapy and cardiovascular disease: Ten-year follow-up from the nurses health study. *N Engl J Med* 1991; 325:756–762.
57. Grady D, Rubin SM, Petitti DB, Fox CS, Black D, Ettinger B, et al: Hormone therapy to prevent disease and prolong life in postmenopausal women. *Ann Intern Med* 1992; 117:1016–1037.
58. Nabulsi AA, Folsom AR, White A, Patsch W, Heiss G, Wu KK, et al: Association of hormone-replacement therapy with various cardiovascular risk factors in postmenopausal women. *N Engl J Med* 1993; 328:1069–1075.
59. Hong MK, Romm PA, Reagan K, Green C, Rackley CE: Effects of estrogen replacement therapy on serum lipid values and angiographically defined coronary artery disease in postmenopausal women. *Am J Cardiol* 1992; 68:176–178.
60. Costa PT, Krantz DS, Blumenthal JA, Furberg CD, Rosenman RH, Shekelle RB: Psychological risk factors in coronary artery disease. *Circulation* 1987; 76(Suppl I):I-145–I-149.
61. Ornish D, Brown SE, Sherwitz LW, Billings JH, Armstrong WT, Ports TA, et al: Can lifestyle changes reverse coronary heart disease? The Lifestyle Heart Trial. *Lancet* 1990; 336:129–122.
62. Kannel WB, D'Agostino RB, Belanger AJ: Fibrinogen, cigarette smoking and risk fo cardiovascular disease. Insights from the Framingham Study. *Am Heart J* 1987; 113:1006–1010.
63. Smith WM: Treatment of mild hypertension. Results of a ten year intervention trial. U.S. Public Health Service Hospitals Cooperative Study Group. *Circ Res* 1977; 40(suppl I):I-98–I-105.
64. The Hypertension Detection and Follow-up Program Cooperative Group: Effect of stepped care treatment on the incidence of myocardial infarction and angina pectoris. Five year findings of the Hypertension Detection and Follow-up Program. *Hypertension* 1984; 6(suppl I) I-198–I-206.
65. Stamler J, Farinaro E, Mojonnier LM, Hall Y, Moss D, Stamler R: Prevention and control of hypertension by nutritional-hygienic means. Long-term experience of the Chicago Coronary Prevention Evaluation Program. *JAMA* 1980; 243:1819–1823.
66. Patel C, Marmot MG, Terry DJ, Carruthers M, Hunt B, Patel M: Trial of relaxation in reducing coronary risk: Four year follow-up. *Br Med J* 1985; 290:1103–1106.
67. Kannel WB, Wilson P, Blair SN: Epidemiological assessment of the role of physical activity and fitness in development of cardiovascular disease. *Am Heart J* 1985; 109:876–885.
68. Hespel P, Lijnen P, Fagard R, Van Hooj R, Rosseneu M: Changes in plasma lipids and apoproteins associated with physical training in middle-aged sedentary men. *Am Heart J* 1988; 115:786–792.
69. Morris JN, Everitt MG, Pollard R, Chave SP, Semmence AM: Vigorous exercise in leisure time: Protection against coronary heart disease. *Lancet* 1980; 2:1207–1210.
70. Leon AS, Connett J, Jacobs DR Jr, Rauramaa R: Leisure-time physical activity levels and risk of coronary heart disease and death. The Multiple-Risk Factor Intervention Trial. *JAMA* 1987; 258:2388–2295.
71. Gordon T, Kannel WB, Hjortland MC, McNamara PM: Menopause and coronary heart disease. The Framingham Study. *Ann Intern Med* 1978; 89:157–161.
72. Dayton S, Pearce ML, Hashimoto S, Dixon WJ, Tomiyasull: A controlled clinical trial of a diet high in unsaturated fat in preventing complications of atherosclerosis. *Circulation* 1969; 39(suppl II):1-63.
73. Hjermann I, Velve BK, Holme I, Leren P: Effect of diet and smoking intervention on the incidence of coronary heart disease. *Lancet* 1981; 2:1303–1310.
74. Committee of Principal Investigators: Report on a WHO Cooperative trial on primary prevention of ischemic heart disease using clofibrate to lower serum cholesterol mortality follow-up. *Lancet* 1980; 2:379–385.
75. Lipid Research Clinics Program: The Lipid Research Clinics Coronary Primary Prevention Trial results: I. Reduction in incidence of coronary heart disease. *JAMA* 1984; 251:351–364.
76. Frick MH, Elo O, Haapa K, Heinonen OP, Heinsalmi P: Helsinki Heart Study: Primary prevention trial with gemfibrozil in middle-aged men with dyslipidemia: Safety of treatment, changes in risk factors, and incidence of coronary heart disease. *N Engl J Med* 1987; 317:1237–1245.
76a. Manninen V, Tenkanen L, Koskinen P, Huttunen JK, Manttari M, Heinonen OP, et al: Joint effects of serum triglyceride and LDL cholesterol and HDL cholesterol concentrations on coronary risk in the Helsinki Heart Study. Implications for treatment. *Circulation* 1992; 85:37–45.
77. Morrison LM: A nutritional program for prolongation of life in coronary atherosclerosis. *JAMA* 1955; 159:1425–1428.
78. Rose G, Thompson WB, Williams RT: Corn oil treatment of ischemic heart disease. *Br Med J* 1965; 1:1531–1533.
79. Research Committee to the Medical Research Council: Low-fat diet in myocardial infarction—a controlled trial. *Lancet* 1965; 2:501–504.
80. Research Committee to the Medical Research Council: Controlled trial of soya-bean oil in myocardial infarction. *Lancet* 1968; 2:693–699.
81. Leren P: the Oslo Diet Heart Study—11-year report, *Circulation* 1970; 42:935–942.
82. Bierenbaum ML, Fleischman AI, Raichelson RI, Hayton T, Watson PB: Ten-year experience of modified fat diets on younger men with coronary heart disease. *Lancet* 1973; 2:1404–1407.
83. Woodhill JM, Palmer AJ, Leelarthaepin B, McGilchrist C, Blacket RB: Low fat, low cholesterol diet in secondary prevention of coronary heart disease. *Adv Exp Med Biol* 1978; 109:317–330.
84. Schoch HK: The U.S. Veterans Administration Cardiology Drug Lipid Study. An interim report. *Adv Exp Med Biol* 1968; 4:405–420.
85. Physicians of the Newcastle-upon-Tyne Region: Trial of clofibrate in the treatment of ischemic heart disease. *Br Med J* 1971; 4:767–775.
86. Research Committee of the Scottish Society of Physicians: Ischaemia heart disease: A secondary trial using clofibrate. *Br Med J* 1971; 4:775–784.
87. Dorr AE, Gunderson K, Schneider JC, Spencer JC, Martin WB: Colestipol hydrochloride in hypercholesterolemic patients—effect on serum cholesterol and mortality. *J Chron Dis* 1978; 31:5–14.
88. Rosenhamer G, Carlson LA: Effect of combined clofibrate-nicotinic acid treatment in ischaemia heart disease. *Atherosclerosis* 1980; 37:129–142.
89. Coronary Drug Project Research Group: Clofibrate and niacin in coronary heart disease. 1975; *JAMA* 231:360–381.
89a. Canner PL, Berg KG, Wenger NK, et al: Fifteen year mortality in Coronary Drug Project patients: Long-term benefit with niacin. *J Am Coll Cardiol* 1986; 8:1245–1255.
90. Brown BG, Zhao XQ, Sacco DE, Albers JJ: Lipid lowering and plaque regression: New insights into the prevention of plaque disruption and clinical events in coronary disease. *Circulation* 1993; 87:1781–1791.
91. Nikkila EA, Viikinkoski P, Valle M, Frick MH: Prevention of progression of coronary atherosclerosis by treatment of hyperlipidemia. A seven year prospective angiographic study. *Br Med J* 1984; 289:220–223.
92. Arntzenius AC, Kromhout D, Barth JD, Reiber J, Bruschke A, Buis B: Diet lipoproteins and the progression of coronary atherosclerosis: The Leiden Intervention Trial. *N Engl J Med* 1985; 312:805–811.
93. Brensike JF, Levy RI, Kelsey SF, Passamani ER, Richardson JM, Loh IK, et al: Effects of therapy with cholestyramine on progression of coronary arteriosclerosis: Results of the NHLBI Type II Coronary Intervention Study. *Circulation* 1984; 69:313–324.
94. Blankenhorn DH, Nessim SA, Johnson RL, San Marco ME, Azen SP, Cashen-Hemphill L: Beneficial effects of combined colestipol-niacin therapy on coronary atherosclerosis and coronary venous bypass grafts. *JAMA* 1987; 257:3233–3240.
94a. Cashin-Hemphill L, Mack WJ, Pogoda JM, Sanmarco ME, Azen SP, Blankenhorn DH: Beneficial effects of colestipol-niacin on coronary atherosclerosis. A 4-year follow-up. *JAMA* 1990; 264:3013–3017.

95. Buchwald H, Varco RL, Matts JP, Long JM, Fitch LL, Campbell GS, et al: Effect of partial ileal bypass surgery on mortality from coronary heart disease in patients with hypercholesterolemia: Report of the Program on the Surgical Control of the Hyperlipidemias (POSCH). *N Engl J Med* 1990; 323:946–955.
96. Ornish D, Brown SE, Scherwitz LW, Billings JH, Armstrong WT, Ports TA, et al: Can lifestyle changes reverse coronary heart disease? The Lifestyle Heart Trial. *Lancet* 1990; 336:129–133.
97. Kane JP, Malloy MJ, Ports TA, Phillips NR, Diehl JC, Havel RJ: Regression of coronary atherosclerosis during treatment of familial hypercholesterolemia with combined drug regimens. *JAMA* 1990; 264:3007–3012.
98. Brown G, Albers JJ, Fisher LD, Schaefer SM, Lin JT, Kaplan C, et al: Regression of coronary artery disease as a result of intensive lipid-lowering therapy in men with high levels of apolipoprotein B. *N Engl J Med* 1990; 323:1289–1298.
99. Watts GF, Lewis B, Brunt JN, Lewis ES, Coltart DJ, Smith LD, et al: Favorable effects on coronary artery disease of lipid lowering diet or diet and cholestyramine in a unifactorial randomized controlled trial: The STARS study. *Lancet* 1992; 339:563–569.
100. Vos J, de Feyter PJ, Simoons ML, Tijssen JGP, Deckers JW: Retardation and arrest of progression or regression of coronary artery disease: A review. *Prog Cardiovasc Dis* 1993; 25:435–454.
101. Kuhn FE, Mohler ER, Rackley CE: Cholesterol and lipoproteins: Beyond atherogenesis. *Clin Cardiol* 1992; 15:883–890.
102. Krikler DM, Cleland JGF: Modification of atherosclerosis by agents that do not lower cholesterol. *Br Heart J* 1993; 69(suppl):S54–S62.
103. Lee AJ, Lowe GDO, Woodward M, Tunstall-Pedoe H: Fibrinogen in relation to personal history of prevalent hypertension, diabetes, stroke, intermittent claudication, coronary heart disease, and family history: the Scottish Heart Health Study. *Br Heart J* 1993; 69:338–342.
104. Ernst E Resch KL: Fibrinogen as a cardiovascular risk factor: A meta-analysis and review of the literature. *Ann Intern Med* 1993; 118:956–963.
105. Garg R, Wagener DK, Madans JH: Alcohol consumption and risk of ischemic heart disease in women. *Arch Intern Med* 1993; 153:1211–1216.
106. Hein HO, Sorensen H, Suadicani P, Gyntelberg F: Alcohol consumption, lewis phenotypes, and risk of ischaemic heart disease. *Lancet* 1993; 341:392–396.
107. Klatsky AL, Armstrong MA: Alcoholic beverage choice and risk of coronary artery disease mortality: Do red wine drinkers fare best? *Am J Cardiol* 1993; 71:467–469.
108. Renaud S, de Lorgeril M: Wine, alcohol, platelets, and the France paradox for coronary heart disease. *Lancet* 1992; 339:1523–1526.
109. Puddey IB, Parker M, Beilin LJ, Vandongen R, Masarei JRL: Effects of alcohol and caloric restrictions on blood pressure and serum lipids in overweight men. *Hypertension* 1992; 20:533–541.
110. Langer RD, Criqui MH, Reed DM: Lipoproteins and blood pressure as biological pathways for effect of moderate alcohol consumption on coronary heart disease. *Circulation* 1992; 85:910–915.
111. Kupari M, Koskinen P: Comparison of the cardiotoxicity of ethanol in women versus men. *Am J Cardiol* 1992; 70:645–649.
112. Suh I, Shaten BJ, Cutler JA, Kuller LH: Alcohol use and mortality from coronary heart disease: The role of high-density lipoprotein cholesterol. *Am Intern Med* 1992; 116:881–887.
113. Tverdal A, Stensvold I, Solvoll K, Foss OP, Lund-Larsen P, Bjartveit K: Coffee consumption and death from coronary heart disease in middle-aged Norwegian men and women. *Br Med J* 1990; 300:566–569.
114. Fried RE, Levine DM, Kwiterovich PO, Diamond EL, Wilder LB, Moy TF, et al: The effect of filtered-coffee consumption on plasma lipid levels: Results of a randomized clinical trial. *JAMA* 1992; 267:811–815.
115. Myers MG, Basinski A: Coffee and coronary heart disease. *Arch Intern Med* 1992; 152:1767–1772.
116. Yusuf S, Wittes J, Friedman L: Overview of results of randomized clinical trials and heart disease. II. Unstable angina, heart failure, primary prevention with aspirin and risk factor modification. *JAMA* 1988; 260:2259–2263.
117. Genest JJ Jr, McNamara JR, Salem DN, Wilson PWF, Schaefer EJ, Malinow MR: Plasma homocysteine levels in men with premature coronary artery disease. *J Am Coll Cardiol* 1990; 16:1114–1119.
118. Clarke R, Daly L, Robinson K, Naughten E, Cahalane S, Fowler B, et al: Hyperhomocysteinema: An independent risk factor for vascular disease. *N Engl J Med* 1991; 324:1149–1155.
119. Stampfer MJ, Malinow R, Willett WC, Newcomer LM, Upson B, Ullmann D, et al: A prospective study of plasma homocysteine and risk of myocardial infarction in U.S. physicians. *JAMA* 1992; 268:877–881.
120. Fraser GE, Sabaté J, Beeson WL, Strahan M: A possible protective effect of nut consumption on risk of coronary heart disease: The Adventist Health Study. *Arch Intern Med* 1992; 152:1416–1424.
121. Sabaté J, Fraser GE, Burke K, Knutsen SF, Bennett H, Lindsted KD: Effects of walnuts on serum lipid levels and blood pressure in normal men. *E Engl J Med* 1993; 328:603–607.
122. Rispin CM, Keenan JM, Jacobs DR Jr, Elmer PJ, Welch RR, Van Horn L, et al: Oat products and lipid lowering: a meta-analysis.; JAMA 1992; 267:3317–3325.
123. Salonen JT, Nyyssonen K, Korpela H, Tuomilehto J, Seppanen R, Salonen R: High stored iron levels are associated with excess risk of myocardial infarction in eastern Finnish men. *Circulation* 1992; 86:803–811.
124. Steinberg D and Workshop Participants: Antioxidants in the prevention of human atherosclerosis: Summary of the proceedings of a National Heart, Lung, and Blood Institute Workshop: September 5–6, 1991, Bethesda, Maryland. *Circulation* 1992; 85:2338–2344.
125. Steinberg D: Antioxidant vitamins and coronary heart disease (Editorial). *N Engl J Med* 1993; 328:1487–1488.
126. Rimm EB, Stampfer MJ, Ascherio A, Giovannucci E, Colditz GA, Willett WC: Vitamin E consumption and the risk of coronary heart disease in men. *N Engl J Med* 1993; 328:1450–1456.
127. Regnström J, Nilsson J, Tornvall P, Landou C, Hamsten A: Susceptibility to low-density lipoprotein oxidation and coronary atherosclerosis in men. *Lancet* 1992; 339:1183–1186.
128. Stampfer MJ, Hennekens CH, Manson JE, Colditz GA, Rosner B, Willet WC: Vitamin E consumption and the risk of coronary disease in women. *N Engl J Med* 1993; 328:1444–1449.
129. Walldius G, Regnström J, Nilsson J, Johansson J, Schäfer-Elinder L, Moelgaard J, et al: The role of lipids and antioxidative factors for development of atherosclerosis: The Probucol Quantitative Regression Swedish Trial (PQRST). *Am J Cardiol* 1993; 71:15B–19B.
130. Hulley SB, Walsh JMB, Newman TB: Health policy on blood cholesterol: Time to change directions. *Circulation* 1992; 86:1026–1029.
131. Jacobs D, Blackburn H, Higgins M, Reed D, Iso H, McMillan G, et al: Report of the conference on low blood cholesterol: Mortality associations. *Circulation* 1992; 86:1046–1060.
132. Grundy SM: Primary prevention of coronary heart disease with drug therapy: Safety and total mortality issues. *Arch Intern Med* 1992; 152:1369–1371.
133. Castelli WP: Cardiovascular disease in women. *Am J Ob Gyn* 1988; 158:1552–1560.
134. Bush TL, Barrett-Connor B, Cowan LD, Criqui MH, Wallace RB, Suchindran CM, et al: Cardiovascular mortality and noncontraceptive rise of estrogen in women. Results from the Lipid Research Clinics Program Follow-up Study. *Circulation* 1987; 75:1102–1109.
135. Wong ND, Wilson PWF, Kannel WB: Serum cholesterol as a prognostic factor for myocardial infarction: The Framingham Study. *Ann Intern Med* 1991; 115:687–693.
136. Miller M, Seidler A, Kwiterovich PO, Pearson TA: Long-term predictors of subsequent cardiovascular events with coronary artery disease and desirable levels of plasma and total cholesterol. *Circulation* 1992; 86:1165–1170.
137. LaRosa JC, Cleeman JI: Cholesterol lowering as a treatment for established coronary heart disease. *Circulation* 1992; 85:1229–1235.
138. LaRosa JC, Cleeman JI: Cholesterol lowering as a treatment for established coronary heart disease. *Circulation* 1992; 85:1229–1235.
139. International Task Force for Prevention of Coronary Heart Disease: Prevention of Coronary Heart Disease: Scientific background and clinical guidelines. Recommendations of the Euro-

pean Atherosclerosis Society. *Nutr Metabol Cardiovasc Dis* 1992; 2:113–156.

140. Reis GJ, Kuntz RE, Silverman DI, Pasternak RC: Effects of serum lipid levels on restenosis after coronary angioplasty. *Am J Cardiol* 1991; 68:1431–1435.
141. Rossouw JE, Lewis B, Rifkind BM: The value of lowering cholesterol after myocardial infarction. *N Engl J Med* 1990; 323:1112–1119.
142. Sacks FM, Pheffer MA, Moye L, Brown LE, Hamm P, Cole TG, et al: Rationale and design of a secondary prevention trial of lowering normal plasma cholesterol levels after acute myocardial infarction: The Cholesterol and Recurrent Events Trial (CARE). *Am J Cardiol* 1991; 68:1436–1446.
143. Hunninghake DB, Stein EA, Dujovne CA, Harris WS, Feldman EB, Miller VT, et al: The efficacy of intensive dietary therapy alone or combined with lovastatin in outpatients with hypercholesterolemia. *N Engl J Med* 1993; 328:1213–1219.

Chapter 63

Rehabilitation of the Patient with Coronary Heart Disease

Nanette Kass Wenger, M.D.

Changes in rehabilitative care reflect changes in the demography of the coronary population, the time course of coronary care, and the severity and risk of coronary heart disease. In the early years of coronary rehabilitation, most patients in exercise training programs were recovering from uncomplicated myocardial infarction. In subsequent years, patients with a complicated clinical course were considered for more limited and gradual exercise rehabilitation. Currently some patients also receive rehabilitative care after coronary artery bypass surgery or coronary angioplasty. With aging of the U.S. population, coronary rehabilitative care is now provided to more elderly patients, many with severe and complicated coronary illness. Patients once arbitrarily excluded as unsuitable for exercise rehabilitation currently derive benefit from more gradual, protracted, and supervised exercise. There is greater contemporary emphasis on education, using the behavioral approach to assist patients in coronary risk reduction and other cardiovascular health-related goals; on psychosocial assessment and interventions; and on occupational assessment and vocational counseling.

Rehabilitative care aims to reduce the physical and psychosocial impact of disabling and handicapping conditions by efforts to restore and enhance functional status[1,2]; these are designed to help the coronary patient "rapidly resume a normal or preillness lifestyle and return to a productive, active, and satisfying role in society." Rehabilitation is described as "those exercise and counseling services which reduce symptoms or improve cardiac function."[3] Rehabilitative care of the coronary patient involves (1) limitation of adverse physiologic and emotional consequences of the acute illness; (2) identification of patients at increased risk of proximate coronary events—i.e., risk stratification and institution of therapies to lessen risk; (3) control of symptoms by medical and surgical therapies, with consequent improvement in function; (4) institution of measures to retard progression or induce regression of the underlying atherosclerosis; and (5) assessment, maintenance, and enhancement of residual physiologic, psychosocial, and vocational status.

The changing pattern of coronary care has mandated comparable changes and increased diversity in rehabilitative services. A shorter hospital stay for uncomplicated myocardial infarction necessitates early ambulation and an accelerated educational regimen, with deferral of some teaching to the post-hospital phase. Even earlier discharge from the hospital appears feasible in selected patients after myocardial reperfusion by thrombolysis or acute primary angioplasty.[4] Complications of infarction, such as ventricular dysfunction or serious arrhythmias, typically engender a more prolonged hospital stay, more supervision and gradual increases in ambulation, and supplementary education and counseling, often including work assessment and vocational counseling. Many of these patients require further diagnostic assessment. Patients undergoing elective coronary bypass surgery or coronary angioplasty often have had preoperative education and orientation. Patients recovering from coronary artery bypass surgery (CABS) typically undergo rapid ambulation, have a short hospital stay, and constitute an increased percentage of participants in cardiac rehabilitation programs; those without prior myocardial infarction typically have good ventricular function, greater survival, and are at low risk for proximate coronary events. Their potential for physical rehabilitation is excellent, and, although their ability to return to work is substantial, actual work resumption has had limited success. Many postoperative and other low-risk coronary patients are candidates for earlier exercise rehabilitation and prompt return to prior levels of activity, including return to work; however, most of these patients require guidance for coronary risk reduction, and early counseling appears to aid in averting physiologic and psychologic disability. Patients following successful coronary angioplasty have earlier resumption of preillness activity levels, family relationships, sexual activity, and employment,[5] and often require more medication short term (to avert restenosis) than patients following coronary bypass surgery, but may not perceive their illness to be significant or appreciate their need for secondary preventive therapies. Patients with stable angina, without myocardial infarction, constitute almost one fourth of the total coronary population, but are underserved in terms of rehabilitative care. They are often not referred for formal rehabilitative care, commonly due to lack of insurance reimbursement. This population has a substantial loss of productivity, and requires comprehensive surveillance, with needs that may exceed those of patients after uncomplicated infarction.

EXERCISE TRAINING

Alterations in the Response of the Coronary Patient to Exercise

Abnormalities of myocardial perfusion, some evident at rest, typically increase with exercise and may be associated with regional abnormalities of myocardial wall motion. As the intensity of exercise progresses, the stroke volume of coronary patients may decrease and result in exercise-induced hypotension; this inotropic incompetence indicates an adverse prognosis (see also Chap. 16). Many patients with coronary disease do not maintain the normal linear relationship between increased workload intensity and increased heart rate; this chronotropic incompetence is also associated with an unfavorable prognosis. Patients with moderate coronary arterial obstruction and/or a reasonably effective collateral circulation often have a normal cardiac output at rest and at low workloads; however, as the intensity of activity progresses, limitation of cardiac output becomes evident. In patients with symptomatic myocardial ischemia, e.g., angina, the increased myocardial oxygen demand of exercise cannot be met by an increase in coronary blood flow, and evidence of myocardial dysfunction and electrical instability may appear in association with angina. This exercise intensity is closely associated with its resultant rate-pressure product, a well-defined, reproducible threshold for myocardial ischemia in a given patient at a given time.

Appropriate and Inappropriate Expectations of Exercise Training

Although most published controlled clinical trials of exercise training examined reductions in coronary morbidity and mortality, many physicians currently recommend exercise and many coronary patients currently engage in exercise rehabilitation to decrease symptoms, augment functional capability, and enhance their sense of well-being. The major beneficial physiologic effect of exercise training is improvement in functional capacity, averaging 20 percent after recovery from myocardial infarction.[7] This is associated with a reduction in activity-related symptoms: angina, dyspnea, fatigue, and at times claudication. Exercise training improves oxygen transport, evident as an increase in maximal cardiac output and oxygen consumption; a reduction in heart rate, systolic blood pressure, and thereby myocardial oxygen requirement at rest and at submaximal work levels; and more rapid return to normal of the exercise heart rate. Increased muscle strength lessens the percentage of contractile force required for daily tasks, and thus the activity-induced increases in heart rate and blood pressure. This lessened myocardial oxygen demand increases the intensity of exercise at which angina occurs, improving activity tolerance before the onset of ischemic symptoms.

Improvement in functional capacity and decrease in activity-related symptoms following usual moderate-intensity exercise training appear due primarily to peripheral adaptations. These include an increase in oxygen extraction and utilization by trained skeletal muscle, with a decrease in myocardial oxygen demand and requirement for coronary blood flow at a submaximal exercise. The redistribution of cardiac output, decrease in systemic vascular resistance, and autonomic nervous system adaptations (particularly lowering of heart rate) result in a lessened rate-pressure product. High-intensity, long-term endurance exercise training has been reported to effect cardiac (central) adaptations, possibly including improved ventricular contractility and increased maximal stroke volume in selected coronary patients[8–10]; such intensive exercise training is feasible for only a small subset of coronary patients. There is no evidence that exercise training alters angiographic characteristics of coronary lesions, increases coronary blood flow or myocardial oxygen supply, or stimulates the formation of a coronary collateral circulation in humans (although some animal studies suggested favorable morphologic adaptations). No consistent improvement in myocardial perfusion or ventricular systolic function has resulted from exercise training.[11]

No single randomized trial of exercise training demonstrated a reduction in mortality and morbidity in postinfarction patients, although favorable trends occurred in several, in part owing to inadequate sample size and/or duration of follow-up, to high dropout rates, etc.[12–24] A decrease in fatal reinfarction was evident in exercising patients in the National Exercise and Heart Disease Project,[15] without change in total reinfarction. A multifactorial intervention trial[14] showed a reduction in coronary mortality, particularly sudden death, during the initial six months following infarction, but the intervention was both exercise and comprehensive care, including risk reduction; the significantly lower sudden death and coronary mortality at 3 years persisted to 10 years, and low-risk patients benefited most.[25] Metaanalysis[24,26] of pooled data from large prospective randomized exercise trials suggests as much as a 25 percent survival advantage for exercising subjects in the initial years following infarction, as well as lower reinfarction rates in some, although most trials included coronary risk modification as well as exercise.[12-24]

Early coronary thrombolysis and myocardial revascularization for eligible subjects at moderate or high risk have so lessened early coronary mortality that exercise as an isolated intervention is unlikely favorably to affect morbidity and mortality. Exercise, however, is often the mechanism to encourage patients to participate in other aspects of rehabilitation, including risk reduction; and participation in group programs may afford psychosocial support. In future years, it is likely that quality of life attributes will be evaluated as outcome measures of rehabilitation.[27]

The decrease in symptoms and improvement in functional status that result from exercise training often enable a return to remunerative employment, as well as leisure and recreational activities. For more impaired coronary patients, including many elderly ones, even a modest increase in work capacity can help maintain independence.

Guidelines for Prescriptive Exercise Training

Individualized medically prescribed physical activity is the hallmark of rehabilitative exercise training, although exercise may be undertaken individually or in groups and with or without medical supervision. Standards and guidelines have been promulgated by several professional organizations.[3,7,28-33] The prescriptive components of exercise training include its "dosage," determined by the intensity, frequency, and duration of exercise; prescription also addresses types of exercise and rate of progression of intensity. The results of a graded exercise test determine the effective and safe prescription of exercise. It is inappropriate to use age-predicted target heart rates for coronary patients; disease, therapies, and prior levels of training or fitness may influence the heart rate response to exercise. Coronary patients should not exercise at a level higher than that documented to produce an appropriate cardiovascular response during testing. The predischarge (or early post-hospitalization) exercise test, typically performed for risk stratification, can serve as a basis for early exercise recommendations (see Chap. 16).

Although in prior years patients were advised to train to a target heart rate range between 70 and 85 percent of the highest level safely achieved at exercise testing,[34] exercise intensities in the 50 to 70 percent heart rate range have produced comparable improvement in functional capacity, provided greater safety because of the low risk of cardiovascular complications with unsupervised exercise, been effective in developing endurance, and are less likely to engender discomfort that may deter long-term adherence.[35,36] This documented efficacy of lower-intensity exercise to improve aerobic capacity has increased both its applicability and acceptance by coronary patients.[22,36] Particularly in unfit patients or those with low exercise capacities, increased comfort of lower-intensity exercise may encourage adherence, although increased duration of training may be required. An alternate method for calculating target heart rate involves 70 to 85 percent of the difference between peak exercise test heart rate and resting heart rate, added to resting rate.[37] This method may be advantageous in patients whose heart rate is attenuated by β-blocking drugs.

Exercise is recommended two or three times weekly, preferably on nonsuccessive days, although sedentary older or deconditioned patients may improve their physical work capacity by one or two exercise sessions weekly. Exercise sessions are generally 45 to 60 min in duration, including warm-up and cool-down. Although an increased duration or frequency of exercise can compensate for a decreased intensity, excessively long or frequent exercise sessions engender an increase in orthopedic and musculoskeletal injuries, as well as poorer adherence to exercise.

The Role of Exercise Testing in Coronary Rehabilitation

Predischarge Exercise Testing

Low-intensity graded exercise testing, using either a treadmill or a bicycle protocol, is safely performed within the first one or two weeks following myocardial infarction,[38,39] and has been undertaken as early as three days following thrombolytic reperfusion therapy for acute infarction (in whom it predicted the in-hospital clinical outcome).[40] The intensity of exercise testing approximates the level of physical activity recommended during the latter days of hospitalization, 3 to 3.5 metabolic equivalents (METs, one MET = 3.5 mL 02/kg body weight/min); or a workload evoking a heart rate response of 120–140 beats/min or 60 percent of age-predicted maximal heart rate. Most centers currently test patients to a sign- or symptom-limited endpoint, as heart rate limits are often inaccurate because of antianginal therapy. Treadmill testing typically entails serial 3-min stages of walking at 1.2 mi/h, initially on the level, and then at 3 and 6 percent elevation; comparable test protocols are available for a bicycle ergometer. (See Chap. 16.) Arm testing may be undertaken in patients with claudication or musculoskeletal problems that make leg testing not feasible.[41,42]

The results of predischarge exercise tests, performed with or without radionuclide studies, contribute independent prognostic information for risk stratification.[43] Patients identified as at high risk for an early recurrent coronary event may require prompt angiography to evaluate for more intensive medical or surgical therapy. High-risk patients are characterized by a low exercise capacity (peak workload below 4 to 6 METs); occurrence of angina, ischemic ST segment abnormalities, and/or exercise-induced hypotension at low levels of exercise; and occurrence of ventricular arrhythmias at low levels of exercise. Radionuclide evidence of myocardial hypoperfusion with exercise and late reperfusion or of left ventricular dysfunction also indicates an adverse prognosis; exercise two-dimensional echocardiography provides comparable prognostic information.[44] (See Chaps. 132 and 134.) Predischarge exercise testing was initially used predominantly to identify jeopardized myocardium following infarction; however, following coronary angioplasty and bypass surgery, it helps assess the adequacy of revascularization, indicates prognosis, defines exercise tolerance, and defines recommendations for exercise training.

Predischarge exercise testing also helps identify low-risk patients with a favorable prognosis who do not require additional diagnostic testing, are well-suited for accelerated rehabilitation, and for whom early discharge home and prompt resumption of preinfarction activities, including return to work, can be recommended.[43,45] The exercise test can define safe levels of activity and guide the surveillance necessary during exercise rehabilitation. This permits simple, effective, accelerated, and less costly programs for low-risk coronary patients, while reserving financial and personnel resources for high-risk patients who may derive substantial benefit from exercise training. Satisfactory performance of an exercise test, coupled with explanation of its relationship to activities to be undertaken at home, lessens the common fear of postinfarction patients that physical activity may result in reinfarction or death.[46]

Serial Surveillance with Standard Exercise Testing

Exercise testing following a coronary event should be repeated after 6 and 12 months. Repeated testing enables revision of the exercise prescription; defines changes in risk status and need for changes in medication; and may indicate progression to an intermediate or high-risk status that may warrant further diagnostic studies including coronary angiography. Subsequently, serial exercise testing can be undertaken at longer intervals, based on the coronary anatomy and clinical manifestations.

Characteristics of Dynamic and Isometric Exercise Training

Dynamic (aerobic) exercise, rhythmic repetitive movements of large muscle groups, is traditionally prescribed for coronary patients. The physiologic response is an increase in heart rate that parallels the intensity of activity and an increase in stroke volume in young and middle-aged patients. In elderly patients, increase in heart rate predominates, with little increase in stroke volume. Systolic blood pressure increases progressively with intensity of exercise, with maintenance of or a slight decrease in diastolic blood pressure, and widening of the pulse pressure.

In contrast, the increase in heart rate with isometric exercise is modest and the increase in cardiac output is slight. There is a substantial increase in systolic blood pressure with high-intensity isometric activity, particularly in unfit individuals. This may provoke angina, ventricular dysfunction, and/or arrhythmias; and is the basis for limiting isometric activity in patients with a low exercise capacity and recent infarction. Once a reasonable level of aerobic capacity is achieved, however, combined dynamic and isometric exercise may produce substantial training effects and improve strength in coronary patients.[47] The enhanced muscle strength from isometric training aids in improving endurance with dynamic exercise. Caution is necessary since wall motion abnormalities may be accentuated by isometric exercise, even in patients with a reasonable dynamic exercise capacity.[48]

Arm versus Leg Exercise Training

Because exercise training is predominantly muscle-specific, both arm and leg exercise should be included in rehabilitative regimens.[49] The heart rate and blood pressure responses to leg work decrease following leg training with only modest improvement in response to arm work. Following arm training, the predominant decreases in heart rate and blood pressure response occur with arm work. In one study, improvement in exercise performance of the untrained limb was 50 to 75 percent of the trained limb, suggesting that half of the increase in trained limb performance is due to a generalized training effect; the other half reflects predominantly improved oxygen extraction by trained skeletal muscle.

Guidelines for arm training involve a workload approximately 50 percent of that for leg training. Arm work, at a comparable oxygen uptake, evokes a higher heart rate and systolic blood pressure response than leg exercise. Since most occupational and recreational activities entail both arm and leg work (and often predominantly arm work), arm exercise training should be included in rehabilitative exercise.

The Effect of Cardiovascular Drugs on Exercise Training

Exercise training can occur in patients receiving antianginal drugs, which may lessen symptoms and improve the ability to exercise.[50] Although β-blocking drugs decrease heart rate and blood pressure response to exercise, they do not attenuate the improvement in physical work capacity or maximal exercise capacity that results from exercise training. When exercise testing is undertaken to prescribe exercise, it should be performed with patients receiving medications that are planned for their training.

IMPLEMENTATION OF REHABILITATIVE CARE

Inpatient or Hospital Phase (Phase I)

The major components of rehabilitative care for patients hospitalized for a coronary event include progressive resumption of physical activity (early ambulation) and education and counseling of both patient and family.

Early Ambulation

The decrease in physical work capacity that follows hospitalization for a coronary event reflects the underlying disease severity and the deconditioning response to protracted bed rest. Although rarely a problem in low-risk coronary patients, deconditioning commonly complicates the outcome of seriously ill, elderly patients with residual myocardial ischemia and ventricular dysfunction. Early ambulation is designed to limit or avert these detrimental effects: reduced physical work capacity and maximal oxygen uptake; orthostatic intolerance, characterized by orthostatic hypotension and tachycardia (due to both hypovolemia and a lessened cardiovascular reflex response); increase in blood viscosity owing to a decrease in plasma volume disproportionate to the decrease in red blood cell mass; and decrease in pulmonary ventilation. The decrease in muscle mass and muscular contractile strength render muscular contraction inefficient, with more oxygen required for comparable work.

Guidelines[51] for the initiation of physical activity in the coronary or surgical intensive care unit are for low-intensity exercise (1 to 2 METs), with gradual progression in work demand; supervision of progressive ambulation permits detection of inappropriate responses. Patients are encouraged to feed themselves, perform personal care, use a bedside commode, and sit in a bedside chair. Cardiac work is less in the seated than supine position. Sitting in a chair two or three times daily limits the hypovolemia of immobilization and resultant orthostatic hypotension. Exposure to gravitational stress, rather than intensity of physical activity, appears the determinant limiting hypovolemia, cardiac underfilling, and deterioration of oxygen transport capacity with effort intolerance.[52] Postural fluid shifts, rather than inactivity, appear to underlie some of the cardiovascular deconditioning of bed rest.[53] Patients perform selected arm and leg exercises designed to maintain muscle tone and increase flexibility and joint mobility. Incentive spirometry is important for postoperative patients.

Disporportionate responses[51] to low-level activity include chest discomfort, dyspnea, or palpitations; a heart rate > 120 beats per minute or < 50 beats per minute (increase in heart rate of patients receiving β-blocking drugs should not be greater than 15 to 20 beats per minute above resting levels); ST segment displacement on the electrocardiographic monitor; appearance of arrhythmias; or decrease of >10 to 15 mmHg in systolic blood pressure. Although the latter usually indicates ischemic ventricular dysfunction, the vasodilator effect of nitrate or calcium-blocking drugs must also be considered. A systolic blood pressure response to low-level activity >180 mmHg or a diastolic pressure >110 mmHg may be an indication for antihypertensive therapy (see Chap. 77). Appropriate responses to activity indicate that the patient can progress to higher-intensity activity; disproportionate responses require restriction of activity and clinical reassessment for unrecognized cardiac dysfunction.

Progressive physical activity during the remainder of the hospitalization is designed to enable patients to attain a functional level that facilitates self-care and homebound activities at discharge. Most household tasks require a work intensity of 2 to 3 METs. Patients perform personal care, sit in a chair for increasing periods of time, and perform selected dynamic warm-up exercises involving the extremities and trunk. The major prescriptive activity is walking, with stepwise increases in pace and distance. Patients who must climb steps at home should practice this in the hospital. Electrocardiographic telemetry monitoring during ambulation is indicated only for selected patients, e.g., with serious ventricular arrhythmias or asymptomatic myocardial ischemia.

An early ambulation protocol for patients with myocardial infarction delineates prescribed exercises, in-hospital "daily-living" activities, and educational activities of comparable intensity for a series of steps (Table 63–1). The initial two steps encompass the intensive care unit phase; the subsequent five, performed in a general medical care area, include warm-up exercise and progressive increases in walking. This format, with minor modification, is applicable to postoperative coronary patients, or those hospitalized for coronary angioplasty or angina pectoris. (See also Table 60–16.)

Neither early ambulation nor early hospital discharge has adversely affected short- or long-term morbidity or mortality for appropriately selected coronary patients.[4,54] Benefits include prevention of deconditioning, decrease in pulmonary atelectasis and thromboembolic complications, lessened anxiety and depression, and an enhanced sense of well-being, related to improved functional status. Early ambulation encourages attainment of the activity level required on return home, even with the current abbreviated hospital stay, and has effected savings in medical care costs and potentially improved use of hospital beds. Improved functional status of patients at hospital discharge has been associated with an earlier and more complete return to work.

Education and Counseling of Hospitalized Patients and Their Families[55]

The current abbreviated hospital stay limits the ability of health professionals to address informational and learning needs of the patient, spouse, and family; to assist them through recovery; and to adequately prepare them for convalescence. Although accelerated hospital care has economic advantages and appears to be associated with an earlier and increased return to work or preillness activity, it requires instruction and counseling on an ambulatory basis.

The initial education, answering patients' questions or concerns, provides reassurance in a coronary or surgical intensive care unit (or during the preprocedure phase for elective coronary angioplasty or bypass surgery). Elements include a brief explanation of medical or surgical problem(s), events anticipated in subsequent days, and familiarization with regulations, procedures, and equipment; this information helps patients adjust to a perceived life-threatening situation. The temporary nature of most restrictions should be emphasized; citing improved cardiac status with recovery lessens the intensity of surveillance and care.

During the remainder of the hospitalization, more detailed information and planning for discharge are appropriate. Increased knowledge lessens anxiety and unwarranted exercise limitations, improves adherence to recommendations for convalescence, and increases self-confidence.[56] Information about coronary disease and its management enables patients and families to assume responsibility for health care on return home. Although teaching optimally begins during the acute hospital stay, continuity is needed between hospital instruction and

TABLE 63-1

In-Patient Rehabilitation: Seven-Step Myocardial Infarction Program (Revised 1992: Grady Memorial Hospital/Emory University School of Medicine)

Step	Date	M.D. Initials	Nurse/PT Notes	Supervised Exercise	CCU/Ward Activity	Educational Activity
				CCU		
1	—			Active and passive ROM all extremities, in bed Teach patient ankle plantar and dorsiflexion—repeat hourly when awake	Partial self-care Feed self Dangle legs on side of bed Use bedside commode Sit in chair 15 min, 1–2 times/day	Orientation to CCU Personal emergencies, social service aid as needed Bedside teaching (CCU staff)
2	—			Active ROM all extremities, sitting on side of bed	Sit in chair 15–30 min, 2–3 times/day Complete self-care in bed	Orientation to rehabilitation team, program Smoking cessation Educational literature if requested Planning transfer from CCU
				Ward		
3	—			Warm-up exercises, 2 METs: Stretching Calisthenics Walk 50 ft and back at slow pace	Sit in chair ad lib To ward class in wheelchair Walk in room	Normal cardiac anatomy and function Development of atherosclerosis What happens when myocardial infarction occurs
4	—			ROM and calisthenics, 2.5 METs Walk length of hall (75 ft) and back, average pace Teach pulse counting	OOB as tolerated Walk to bathroom Walk to ward class, with supervision	Coronary risk factors and their control
5	—			ROM and calisthenics, 3 METs Check pulse counting Practice walking few stairsteps Walk 300 ft bid	Walk to waiting room or telephone Walk in ward corridor prn	Diet Energy conservation Work simplification techniques (as needed)
6	—			Continue above activities Walk down flight of steps (return by elevator) Walk 500 ft bid Instruct on home exercise	Tepid shower or tub bath, with supervision To cardiac clinic teaching room, with supervision Predischarge exercise test (as appropriate)	Heart attack management: Medications Exercise Surgery Response to symptoms Family, community adjustments on return home
7	—			Continue above activities Walk up flight of steps Walk 500 ft bid Continue home exercise instruction; present information regarding outpatient exercise program	Continue all previous ward activities	Discharge planning Medications, diet, activity Return appointments Scheduled tests Return to work Community resources Educational literature Medication cards

SOURCE: Reprinted with permission of Grady Memorial Hospital/Emory University School of Medicine.

that done during ambulatory care; inclusion of family members in the education is advantageous. There should be a review of the coronary problem initiating hospitalization, with an emphasis on healing. These descriptions provide the basis for subsequent recommendations for care, including coronary risk modification and medical or surgical therapies. Patients should be instructed about medications: purpose, dosage, desired effects, and potential adverse responses to each; many patients have not taken medications prior to a coronary event and may be unfamiliar with problems of taking medications. Patients and family members should be taught appropriate response to new or recurrent symptoms and how to gain access to emergency medical care. Even following what was perceived to be adequate preoperative counseling, patients and spouses describe postoperative needs for additional information about usual physical and emotional responses, return to sexual activity, how to deal with overprotection by family, and changes in the way others respond to them after cardiac surgery.

Outpatient or Ambulatory Phase

For most low-risk coronary patients, particularly following myocardial revascularization, exercise rehabilitation begins shortly after discharge from the hospital; many enter immediately into what has traditionally been considered a Phase III program, without intervening supervision in a Phase II component. These patients usually progress rapidly in increasing the intensity and duration of exercise. The other end of the spectrum are elderly coronary patients, those with significant comorbidity, high-risk patients with continuing ischemia or arrhythmia, with complications of infarction or bypass surgery, or with severe angina; they may require surveillance for protracted periods. Exercise rehabilitation is better divided into hospital and post-hospital components; the outpatient phase can then be described by characteristics of exercise training and requirements, duration, and complexity of surveillance, based on the patient's clinical and risk status; rather than by traditional phases that typically have fixed compositions and durations. This is concordant with responding to an individual patient's needs for exercise training, rather than requiring a patient to conform to program phases or requirements.

Therapeutic Exercise Training

Therapeutic exercise training (Phase II, typically 8 to 12 weeks) can occur in a hospital-based program or a community facility, and ideally involves medical supervision of exercise, at least for the initial sessions following hospital discharge. Even unsupervised exercise may be appropriate for low-risk coronary patients, if it preferably follows a brief period of observation, instruction, and training in a medically supervised setting. This permits instruction in exercise techniques, importance of adhering to recommendations, symptoms of exercise intolerance, and self-monitoring of exercise intensity; provides reassurance; often permits more rapid progression of exercise intensity; and reinforces adherence to diet, medications, and other aspects of risk reduction.

In the early years of outpatient exercise rehabilitation, few patients had continuous ECG monitoring because ECG telemetry was not widely available. In subsequent years, complication rates were described as lower in exercise programs with continuous ECG monitoring[34]; it was not known whether ECG monitoring, closer medical supervision, and/or differences in exercise intensity were the safety determinants. More recently, continuous ECG monitoring has not been shown to provide added safety for low-risk patients during supervised exercise[57]; safety data for non-ECG-monitored exercise have also been reported from Australia.[58] ECG monitoring is currently reserved for high-risk patients and other selected patients with problems in exercising.[43] The uniform success of resuscitation with supervised exercise, despite the rarity of its application, suggests that exercise supervision may be beneficial for selected patients.[57] Patients in supervised exercise programs without continuous ECG monitoring can be taught to check their heart rate response intermittently to ensure that it remains in the prescribed target heart rate range, or to estimate exercise intensity by rating perceived exertion as described by Borg[59]; heart rate response also may be documented by intermittent use of defibrillator paddles as ECG leads.

High-risk coronary patients require supervised and often ECG-monitored exercise. High-risk patients are characterized by a markedly reduced exercise capacity, severely depressed ventricular function, complex ventricular arrhythmias, exercise-induced angina, ischemia, or hypotension at low exercise intensities, and/or inability to self-monitor exercise heart rate. Because of their increased risk for adverse events, exercise training should occur in a medically supervised and, at least initially, ECG-monitored setting.[60] Because exercise-related cardiac complications may not be increased only in proximity to the acute coronary event, the appropriate duration of ECG surveillance of exercise remains uncertain. Another subset at high risk for adverse events, typically 1 or 2 years postinfarction, are patients with above-average exercise performance but with marked, asymptomatic ST depression.[61]

About half of all survivors of myocardial infarction are at low risk; for them, both medically directed home exercise and supervised exercise training result in comparable improvements in functional capacity[35]; this has also been demonstrated for patients recovered from coronary bypass surgery.[62] Although there were no complications of exercise, data are not available as to efficacy of risk factor reduction or long-term compliance with unsupervised exercise, but all training regimens appear to increase functional capacity more than "spontaneous activity." A technique of value in maintaining appropriate exercise intensity in unsupervised settings is the "talk test," wherein patients exercise only to the level that permits continued conversation with an exercising companion, a level below the anaerobic threshold at which respiratory rate accelerates.

Supervision of exercise may not entail an "all or nothing" approach; intermittent supervision may be feasible in a community facility, there may be periodic telephone transmission of the exercise ECG of patients who exercise at home, patients may use inexpensive heart rate monitors during home exercise, or a combination of these approaches may be used. It is not known whether any of these improves adherence to exercise; several studies of independent exercise showed a lack of coronary risk reduction. Patient characteristics[63] help identify individuals likely to do well with unsupervised exercise; they include patients with prior exercise experience and with family and social support. Cigarette smokers, overweight patients, blue collar workers, and those with inactive occupations and leisure time activities are less likely to adhere to independent exercise; this is also the case for patients who perceive their health status as poor.

The goal of prescriptive exercise is enhancement of physical work capacity, termed the training effect. Training-mediated increases of as much as 20 percent in maximal oxygen consumption may occur due primarily to peripheral mechanisms; i.e., increase in oxygen extraction by trained skeletal muscle, combined with redistribution of cardiac output. These adaptations enable a decreased heart rate and systolic blood pressure response to submaximal exertion. Because of lowered rate-pressure product at submaximal work levels, the trained coronary patient may experience less or no angina and have fewer or no ECG abnormalities of myocardial ischemia. The trained individual functions farther from the ischemic threshold in usual daily activities and perceives an improved tolerance for these tasks as they entail a lesser percentage of the improved physical work capacity.

The individualized exercise prescription varies with the needs and goals of each patient—age, health status, exercise capacity, musculoskeletal competence, prior exercise activity and level of fitness, planned occupational and recreational activities, and the patient's skills, likes, and dislikes (as well as accessibility of exercise facilities and equipment). The basic design of an exercise session involves an initial 5 to 10 min of warm-up exercise: stretching and range-of-motion activities that affect musculoskeletal and circulatory readiness for exercise. This is followed by a 30- to 45-min endurance component that initially involves walk-run sequences or exercise on a stationary bicycle or treadmill; in these activities, skill is a minimal component of the intensity of work demand. Prescription of target heart rate range is based on the results of exercise testing; the documented efficacy of low- to moderate-intensity exercise is likely to increase its adoption by larger numbers of patients. Intermittent exercise or alternation of high- and low-intensity activities allows a greater total workload to be imposed at each session without producing inappropriate cardiovascular responses or symptoms. On the other hand, continuous exercise effects more rapid improvement in endurance in patients with a reasonable baseline exercise capacity. Since the activities described train primarily leg muscles, supplementary arm muscle training is accomplished by selected repetitive calisthenics, shoulder wheels, rowing machines, and arm ergometers. When data from leg exercise testing are used to prescribe arm exercise, a reduction of about 10 beats per minute in target heart rate range is appropriate. The workload for arm training is about half that for leg training.[49] When space for exercise is limited, "station" training may be preferable, with participants serially using bicycle ergometry, arm ergometry, rowing machines, and treadmills. When more space is available, gymnasium-type programs can accommodate larger numbers of patients for walk-jog activities and floor exercises; some facilities have indoor or outdoor tracks. A final 5- to 10-min cool-down period entails a gradual decrease in intensity that allows the heart rate to decrease and averts postexercise hypotension. Three exercise sessions weekly appear adequate, and a greater frequency does not significantly improve aerobic capacity. Aerobic games, as recreational component, add variety to an exercise program and improve adherence; they also provide upper body exercise. Because the oxygen cost of these activities varies with each patient's skills and competitiveness, they should be limited early in exercise training.

Addition of isometric (static, resistive) activities to training of low-risk coronary patients who can perform adequate levels of dynamic exercise does not appear to increase risk, and may improve strength and ability to return to active occupational and recreational lifestyles. As the intensity of dynamic exercise increases, isometric exercise, including weight training, is often incorporated.[47,64]

Detailed written instructions should be provided for patients who undertake unsupervised home exercise. Initial home exercise may involve progressive walking and walk-jog sequences or serial increases in intensity and duration of use of a stationary bicycle. Videotapes may help guide and pace home exercise and are available for varying intensities of exercise training. As the level of training increases, recreational activities in which skill often influences intensity of work may add variety to the exercise regimen. Enjoyable, effective endurance activities include rope-skipping, bicycling, skating, swimming, rowing, and aerobic dancing; both rope-skipping and swimming (for unskilled swimmers) impose higher work loads and should be undertaken carefully (see Phase III).

Maintenance Exercise Training (Phase III)

This phase of exercise training is typically undertaken in community recreational facilities or at home. A lifetime pattern of regular physical activity is necessary to maintain adequate fitness. For this to occur, patients must achieve reasonable independence in exercising, and become progressively involved in an exercise regimen that is social, enjoyable, convenient, and appropriate. Most coronary patients with prior exercise restrictions who can safely attain a 7- to 8-MET level of performance can progress to unsupervised exercise. Patients leaving supervised exercise regimens may require counseling as to the selection and initiation of long-term exercise in the community. Serial exercise testing may be warranted to revise exercise recommendations.

Long-term reasonable levels of exercise aid in weight control, favorably affect psychologic status, and appear to help patients renounce the sick role and resume a normal lifestyle, including return to work (Table 63-2).[65,66] Both improved physical work capacity and attitudinal benefits associated with exercise encourage resumption of employment.

Education and Counseling (Phases II and III)

The behavioral approach to coronary risk reduction is increasingly used to encourage coronary patients to

TABLE 63-2

Exercise Training Post CABS: Return to Work

Study			Patient Characteristics				Return to Work, %		
Author	Year	Number of Patients	Gender	Mean Age at Entry	Intervention	Time	E	C	Outcome of Intervention
Waites[65]	1983	22*	M	54	E	6 mo	82	36	Sig ↑ functional capacity, ↑ RTW, ↓ smoke
Ben Ari[66]	1986	96†	M	53	E	5 yr	59	20	Sig ↑ functional capacity, ↑ RTW

E = Exercise; C = Control; RTW = Return to work.
*Nonrandomized, 11E, 11C.
†Nonrandomized, 51E, 45C.

adopt and maintain healthy lifestyles and improve adherence to medications and other regimens.[67,68]

Coronary risk modification, by retarding atherosclerotic progression, has contributed to the decrease in coronary morbidity and mortality; hyperlipidemia, hypertension, and cigarette smoking all adversely affect the outcome of patients recovering from infarction. Postoperative recurrence of coronary symptoms or deterioration of function after saphenous vein coronary bypass surgery also relates predominantly to progression of atherosclerosis, both in the bypass graft vessels and in native circulation. There is no evidence that coronary bypass surgery encourages favorable modification of coronary risk status postoperatively.[69,70] Control of hypertension and diabetes; control of elevated blood lipid levels and obesity; and cessation of cigarette smoking,[71] even at advanced age, are designed to limit progression or induce regression of atherosclerosis and decrease subsequent coronary events (see Chap. 62). Patients should be trained in the skills needed for lifestyle changes, encouraged to practice these new techniques, have benefits measured, and be provided periodic reinforcement and motivation needed to maintain desired changes.[67] Most contemporary approaches to education and counseling of coronary patients are labor intensive and limited in flexibility to meet the diverse learning preferences of individual patients. Also, many books and pamphlets exceed the reading and comprehension abilities of some patients. Technologic advances may extend the availability and variety of instructional components; assure maintenance of a consistent, effective, and high-quality message; enable family members to participate in learning, enable tracking of accomplishments and delivery of timely reinforcements, yet decrease or control costs.

Family counseling should include lifestyle adjustments appropriate during convalescence, focusing on avoiding invaliding the coronary patient. Many patients voice concern about inadequate or ambiguous information, so that tests or procedures planned should be addressed. There should be review of permitted activities and plans for serial resumption of others; as well as attention to return to work and long-term outlook. Many psychosocial outcomes, including return to work, appear related to the patient's perception of personal health status after a coronary event or myocardial revascularization; this may be favorably altered by education and counseling.[55,72] The patient's perception of cardiac limitations determines postinfarction limitations of activity more than treadmill-measured exercise capacity.[73]

Because infarction or coronary surgical procedures often have negative impact on sexuality, related to combinations of fear, anxiety, depression, and adverse effects of medications; resumption of sexual activity should be recommended once other daily activities are reinstituted. Both partners should be counseled about the safety of sexual intercourse. Neither severity of the coronary event nor the patient's functional capacity predicts the occurrence of sexual dysfunction. Although return to sexual activity occurs earlier and to a greater extent in postoperative than postinfarction patients, physician-initiated sexual counseling may favorably affect both populations.[74]

The role of relaxation techniques or biofeedback training in rehabilitation remains to be defined. Although the value of stress management has not been established, favorable responses in a pilot study are encouraging.

Community resources that may be helpful in rehabilitation should be identified: counseling and guidance services, home-care agencies, vocational rehabilitation facilities and services for job training and placement, services for financial aid, outpatient coronary rehabilitation programs and postcoronary groups or clubs. The patient's participation in community heart clubs or educational groups may further facilitate rehabilitation between discharge from the hospital and return to preillness function. Coronary risk reduction and other skills learned and practiced in these settings may encourage health-related behaviors and aid in reinforcing maintenance of these changes. Acquisition of knowledge appears to affect favorably behaviors involving implementing recommendations for care, as well as coping behaviors.[55]

CORONARY POPULATIONS WITH SPECIAL REHABILITATION NEEDS

Elderly Coronary Patients

With aging of the population, elderly patients constitute a progressively larger component of hospital admissions for myocardial infarction, coronary angioplasty, and bypass surgery. Complications of infarction and myocardial revascularization are more frequent in the elderly, with prolongation both of hospitalization and of the period at bed rest, predisposing to deconditioning. Early mobilization can limit functional deterioration and decrease depression, as the aged patient is reassured by performing personal care. In both medical and surgical coronary intensive care settings, the major educational strategy involves concise and repeated explanations, reassurance, and time and place orientation to help avert confusion and delirium. Teaching energy-conserving techniques for self-care and performance of household tasks helps maintain independent living, a valued outcome among elderly patients. Modification of conventional coronary risk factors is feasible and effective in elderly patients, and appears warranted given the greater prevalence and severity of their coronary disease.

Elderly patients in post-hospital exercise regimens can obtain improvements in physical work capacity similar to those of their younger counterparts,[75,76] although they require a longer time to attain a training effect because of the low-intensity training stimulus. In one report, exercise testing was feasible in about half of patients 70 years or older before hospital discharge following infarction; this enabled accurate risk stratification and exercise prescription.[77] Warm-up exercises permit more effective training, and greater time is required between exercise components because of delayed return of the exercise heart rate to normal in an elderly population. Walking provides an adequate training stimulus for many elderly patients because it constitutes a significant percentage of the decreased aerobic capacity of aging.[78] Running, jumping, and other high-impact activities should be limited to avoid orthopedic complications. Walking, bicycle ergometry, and/or walking in a pool in shallow water can favorably modify the decreased joint mobility of aging; enhance neuromuscular coordination, balance, and stability, and lessen propensity for falls; and improve endurance. Elderly individuals should decrease exercise levels in hot and humid environments.

Coronary Patients with Congestive Heart Failure

In the early years of exercise rehabilitation, patients with moderate-to-severe ventricular dysfunction or compensated congestive heart failure were not considered candidates for exercise. These patients typically had a protracted hospital stay and delayed mobilization following infarction. Newer therapies, primarily with vasodilator drugs, have favorably altered both the disabling symptoms and adverse prognosis of patients with heart failure. Data also suggest benefit from exercise training in selected patients with severely impaired ventricular function and a low exercise capacity,[79] reflecting predominant peripheral adaptations to training; i.e., increased oxygen extraction by trained skeletal muscle.[80] The ejection fraction poorly predicts either exercise capacity or potential for improvement of exercise performance with training; indeed, some patients with substantial ventricular dysfunction have a normal exercise capacity.[81]

The impairment of exercise capacity with heart failure appears in part due to inadequate nutritive blood flow to skeletal muscle; factors other than lack of increase in cardiac output with exercise seem important, including the ability to decrease peripheral vascular resistance and possibly the adequacy of right ventricular function. (See Chap. 25.)

Because low-level physical activities constitute a large proportion of the physical work capacity of these impaired patients, even a regimen of slow walking provides an effective training stimulus. Increased duration can compensate for low intensity of activity, yet produce a training effect. Low-intensity physical activity imposed gradually over protracted time has no apparent adverse consequences, although the optimal modes, intensity, and duration of training have yet to be determined. The resultant training effect, with improvement in the physical work capacity, may permit patients to continue at independent living. Although ventricular function does not improve with training, neither does it appear to deteriorate. In a small series of patients with severe ischemic ventricular dysfunction, a 38 percent increase in exercise capacity and > 50 percent return to full-time employment was described.[82] Even small improvements in symptomatic status and physical work capacity exert a substantial favorable impact on the quality of life.

The initial training of patients with ventricular dysfunction was predominantly supervised, typically with continuous ECG monitoring; subsequently, moderate-intensity unsupervised physical activity was safely undertaken by some patients.[82,83] The optimal duration of exercise supervision and duration and need for ECG monitoring of these patients remain uncertain, but should be guided by clinical evidence of ischemia and/or arrhythmia.[79] Current information about exercise rehabilitation of medically complex patients is comparable to the limited information about exercise training of patients with uncomplicated infarction two decades ago.

Additional important components of rehabilitative care for patients with significant activity limitations include teaching work simplification, particularly pacing of daily living activities, working in a seated rather than standing position, and taking frequent rest periods between activity.

Patients with Implanted Pacemakers and Cardioverter Defibrillators

Exercise prescription is determined by the characteristics of the implanted pacemaker. Most patients likely to exercise currently receive rate-responsive pacemakers; exercise testing can ascertain the appropriateness of the sensor response to the exercise intensity.[84] Reprogramming can be undertaken as needed.

The exercise target heart rate range for patients with implanted cardioverter defibrillators (ICDs) should be set at 20 to 30 beats per minute below the threshold rate of the device to fire. This also enables appropriate work-related activities.[85] Coparticipants in the exercise setting should be reassured that they cannot be harmed by physical contact with the patient whose ICD discharges.

PSYCHOLOGIC ASPECTS OF CORONARY REHABILITATION

The major psychologic problems in coronary patients are anxiety, depression, denial, and dependence.[86] (See also Chap. 117.) Denial of presenting symptoms may limit or delay access to care, often with adverse effect. "Appropriate" denial, characterized by confidence of a favorable outcome, is an effective coping strategy of many patients with infarction and is associated with a favorable prognosis. Anxiety is often the initial psychologic manifestation at arrival in the hospital; this is realistic anxiety, related to a fear of dying. Anxiety often progresses to depression as patients contemplate the potential inability to resume former family, occupational, and community roles. Anxiety and depression, the most common psychologic complications of infarction, contribute to the failure to make satisfactory life adjustments, return to work, return to sexual function, and engage in social activities subsequent to the hospital stay. Involving the patient in planning for recovery, teaching self-monitoring of heart rate response to activity, and teaching coronary risk reduction return control to the patient and encourage adherence to recommendations for care.

Many patients with successful physical recovery following infarction or myocardial revascularization often have residual psychologic impairment.[86,87] Depression is also the major emotional problem during convalescence and may be accentuated by family overprotection and exclusion of the patient from prior roles and responsibilities. The characteristics of the family and social support system importantly influence the success of rehabilitation. Depression may mimic organic illness because of the frequent complaints of fatigue, insomnia, memory impairment, headache, and vague chest discomfort.

Two major strategies that appear to limit psychologic complications are education and counseling and initiation of a physical activity regimen. This adoption of behaviors and capacities to meet life demands, i.e., coping abilities, may be enhanced by acquisition of skills, techniques, and knowledge. Many patients remain psychologically disabled because they inappropriately perceive an excessive severity of infarction and vulnerability to sudden death. The demonstration that modest physical activity can be performed with safety provides reassurance and restores self-confidence.[46] Exercising patients in randomized exercise trials more rapidly returned to sexual activity, to work, and to a near-normal lifestyle; and had greater improvements in work capacity, income, and job responsibility.[15,88] Both physical and psychosocial benefits occurred with low-level exercise, once believed to be of "placebo" level, but currently considered to impart benefit, particularly among older and sicker coronary patients. In one randomized controlled trial, muscle relaxation therapy added to the benefits of exercise.[89] Despite the paucity of controlled studies, consistent moderate psychosocial benefit appears to result from combinations of structured exercise education, and counseling[55,72]; although the contribution of peer support in a group program has not been ascertained, it may be helpful given the predictive power of social isolation for coronary mortality.[90]

Controversy remains as to the relationship of type A behavior to increased incidence and prevalence of coronary disease. Although the results of the Recurrent Coronary Prevention Project suggest that modification of type A behavior can reduce cardiac morbidity and mortality in postinfarction patients,[91] these data have not been replicated by others. Contemporary investigation suggests that hostility or suppressed anger may be more related to adverse outcomes than the general time urgency, control, and overcompetitive lifestyle components of type A behavior.

VOCATIONAL ASPECTS OF CORONARY REHABILITATION

A major goal of rehabilitative care for patients recovered from infarction or myocardial revascularization is resumption of gainful employment, a change in occupation if needed, and the resultant economic and psychologic benefits.

In prior years, about 80 percent of patients who recovered from uncomplicated infarction and were younger than age 65 and employed at the time of infarction returned to work within 2 to 3 months, typically resuming former jobs.[92] Despite this favorable early return to work, cessation of employment each year is also high; in one report, although 83 percent of patients had returned to work by 6 months, only 63 percent were gainfully employed at 1 year. Comparable data are not available for patients with complications of infarction or residual functional impairments, although their return to work is estimated as 25 to 33 percent.

These data contrast with work resumption after coronary bypass surgery. Despite substantial decrease in symptoms, improvement in functional capacity, and reported enhancement of life quality and participation in leisure activities, return to work following coronary bypass surgery has been less favorable than anticipated,[93,94] with no difference in employment status at 10 years between patients randomized to medical and surgical treatment in the Coronary Artery Surgery Study (CASS).[95] Return to work following coronary angioplasty is comparable to that following coronary bypass surgery, although angioplasty patients return to work more promptly.[94] In one study coronary angioplasty effected a more favorable return to work than in a historical control population treated medically[96]; however, another report described lack of confidence in ability to resume work following angioplasty, even when physically able to do so.[97]

Most studies involved predominantly or exclusively men; more recent examination of working women with coronary disease showed them to have a longer convalescence and lesser return to work; whether this is a gender issue or reflects older age or greater occurrence of depression among women warrants study.[98]

Many patients younger than age 65 survive myocardial infarction or myocardial revascularization each year. The indirect health care costs of disability, including lessened productivity, loss of income, welfare payments, and unemployment insurance costs must be considered when cost-effectiveness of rehabilitation is ascertained.[45] Coronary heart disease is the leading problem in the United States for which adults receive premature disability benefits under the Social Security system; and almost one-fourth of men and women receiving Social Security disability allowances were considered permanently disabled by coronary disease. In patients following both myocardial infarction and myocardial revascularization, symptomatic and functional improvement correlate poorly with the return to work and the resumption of preillness lifestyle; psychosocial status appears a more important determinant.[93] Since only about 15 percent of the U.S. labor force currently performs manual labor (a percentage that decreases with age), the severity of angina or heart failure in patients with marginal residual cardiac function only rarely precludes or delays return to work. Many nonmedical factors negatively influence resumption of employment: older age, adequate nonwork income, anxiety or depression, activity-induced symptoms, lower social class and less education, jobs involving high-level physical activity (more common among blue-collar workers), and perception of the coronary illness as job-related. Patients who fail to resume employment within 6 months after a coronary event are unlikely ever to do so.[99]

Among the medical reasons for failure to return to work are unwarranted medical restrictions, or even more commonly, lack of professional assurance of the safety of so doing.[99] Exercise testing performed for risk stratification can serve as a component of work evaluation. It permits a relatively precise assessment of function[6] that may help allay apprehensions of the patient,[46] family,[100] physician, and employer about the capability and safety of return to work.[101] In one study, occupational work evaluation within the first month following infarction resulted in identification of low-risk patients; counseling them about appropriateness of prompt return to work effected a 3-week-earlier work resumption than in a control population.[102] The extrapolation of exercise test data to job requirements requires job analysis to be performed; also to be considered are differences in temperature, environment, intellectual demands, relation to meals, travel requirements, and emotional stress, among others. Nevertheless, patients without evidence of ischemia or arrhythmia during a symptom-limited standard exercise test are typically free of these problems when static and dynamic work are combined at work.[103] Arm ergometry may be preferable for occupational assessment of patients who perform predominantly arm work.[49]

Further, since most occupational work is intermittent, with brief periods of strenuous activity and longer intervals of low-level activity or rest, occupational myocardial work demand is lower than for the same level of steady-state exercise; cardiac output, blood pressure, and oxygen uptake do not approach steady state until about 2 minutes after onset of work. This explains the tolerance of patients with modest cardiac impairment and limitation of cardiac output of significant workloads of short duration, provided that adequate rest periods are interspersed. Recommendations for full-time work should be for work levels approximating 30 percent of measured physical work capacity.

Other nonmedical considerations also influence postinfarction or postoperative employment, particularly the financial, social, disability, and compensation benefits of not returning to work. Although appropriate physician and employer attitudes may facilitate reemployment, the viewpoint of the patient appears the major determinant; in a number of studies, the patient's preoperative perception about ability to return to work appeared as the most influential determinant.

REFERENCES

1. World Health Organization, Regional Office for Europe: The rehabilitation of patients with cardiovascular diseases (EURO 0381). Copenhagen, 1969.
2. Report of the WHO Expert Committee on Disability Prevention and Rehabilitation: *Disability Prevention and Rehabilitation.* WHO Tech. Rep. Ser., No. 668. Geneva, World Health Organization, 1981.
3. American College of Cardiology: Position report on cardiac rehabilitation. Recommendations of the American College of Cardiology on cardiovascular rehabilitation. *J Am Coll Cardiol* 1986; 7:451–453.
4. Mark DB, Sigmon K, Topol EJ, Kereiakes DJ, Pryor DB, Candela RJ, et al: Identification of acute myocardial infarction patients suitable for early hospital discharge after aggressive interventional therapy. Results from the Thrombolysis and Angioplasty in Acute Myocardial Infarction Registry. *Circulation* 1991; 83:1186–1193.
5. Raft D, McKee DC, Popio KA, Haggerty JJ: Life adaptation after percutaneous transluminal coronary angioplasty and coronary artery bypass grafting. *Am J Cardiol* 1985; 56:395–398.
6. Bonow RO, Bacharach SL, Green MV, LaFreniere RL, Epstein SE: Prognostic implications of symptomatic versus asymptomatic (silent) myocardial ischemia induced by exercise in mildly symptomatic and in asymptomatic patients with angiographically documented coronary artery disease. *Am J Cardiol* 1987; 60:778–783.
7. Council on Scientific Affairs: Physician-supervised exercise programs in rehabilitation of patients with coronary heart disease. *JAMA* 1981; 245:1463–1466.
8. Ehsani AA, Martin WH III, Heath GW, Coyle EF: Cardiac effects of prolonged and intense exercise training in patients with coronary artery disease. *Am J Cardiol* 1982; 50:246–254.
9. Ehsani AA, Biello DR, Schultz J, Sobel BE, Holloszy JO: Improvement of left ventricular contractile function by exercise training in patients with coronary artery disease. *Circulation* 1986; 74:350–358.
10. Schuler G, Schlierf G, Wirth A, Mautner H-P, Scheurlen H, Thumm M, et al: Low-fat diet and regular, supervised physical exercise in patients with symptomatic coronary artery disease: Reduction of stress-induced myocardial ischemia. *Circulation* 1988; 77:172–181.
11. Hung J, Gordon EP, Houston N, Haskell WL, Goris ML, DeBusk RF: Changes in rest and exercise myocardial perfusion and left ventricular function 3 to 26 weeks after clinically uncomplicated acute myocardial infarction: Effects of exercise training. *Am J Cardiol* 1984; 54:943–950.
12. Kentala E: Physical fitness and feasibility of physical rehabilitation after myocardial infarction in men of working age. *Ann Clin Res* 1972; 4(suppl 9):1–84.
13. Wilhelmsen L, Sanne H, Elmfeldt D, Grimby G, Tibblin G, Wedel

H: A controlled trial of physical training after myocardial infarction. Effects on risk factors, nonfatal reinfarction, and death. *Prev Med* 1975; 4:491–508.
14. Kallio V, Hamalainen H, Hakkila J, Luurila OJ: Reduction in sudden deaths by a multifactorial intervention programme after acute myocardial infarction. *Lancet* 1979; 2:1091–1094.
15. Shaw LW for the Project Staff: Effects of a prescribed supervised exercise program on mortality and cardiovascular morbidity in patients after a myocardial infarction. The National Exercise and Heart Disease Project. *Am J Cardiol* 1981; 48:39–46.
16. Carson P, Phillips R, Lloyd M, Tucker H, Neophytou M, Buch NJ, et al: Exercise after myocardial infarction: A controlled trial. *J R Coll Phys Lond* 1982; 16:147–151.
17. Rechnitzer PA, Cunningham DA, Andrew GM, Buck CW, Jones NL, Kavanagh T, et al: Relation of exercise to the recurrence rate of myocardial infarction in men. Ontario Exercise-Heart Collaborative Study. *Am J Cardiol* 1983; 51:65–69.
18. Roman O, Gutierrez M, Luksic I, Chavez E, Camuzzi AL, Villalon E, et al: Cardiac rehabilitation after acute myocardial infarction. 9-year controlled follow-up study. *Cardiology* 1983; 70:223–231.
19. Vermeulen A, Lie KI, Durrer D: Effects of cardiac rehabilitation after myocardial infarction: Changes in coronary risk factors and long-term prognosis. *Am Heart J* 1983; 105:798–801.
20. Dorossiev D: Rehabilitation and comprehensive secondary prevention after acute myocardial infarction. Report on a study. EURO Reports and Studies 84. Copenhagen, World Health Organization, Regional Office for Europe, 1983.
21. Marra S, Paolillo V, Spadaccini F, Angelino PF: Long-term follow-up after a controlled randomized post-myocardial infarction rehabilitation programme: Effects on morbidity and mortality. *Eur Heart J* 1985; 6:656–663.
22. Goble AJ, Hare DL, Macdonald PS, Oliver RG, Reid MA, Worcester MC: Effect of early programmes of high and low intensity exercise on physical performance after transmural acute myocardial infarction. *Br Heart J* 1991; 65:126–131.
23. P. RE. COR. Group: Comparison of a rehabilitation programme, a counselling programme and usual care after an acute myocardial infarction: Results of a long-term randomized trial. *Eur Heart J* 1991; 12:612–616.
24. Oldridge NB, Guyatt GH, Fischer ME, Rimm AA: Cardiac rehabilitation after myocardial infarction. Combined experience of randomized clinical trials. *JAMA* 1988; 260:945–950.
25. Hamalainen H, Luurila OJ, Kallio V, Knuts L-R, Arstila M, Hakkila J: Long-term reduction in sudden deaths after a multifactorial intervention programme in patients with myocardial infarction: 10-year results of a controlled investigation. *Eur Heart J* 1989; 10:55–62.
26. O'Connor GT, Buring JE, Yusuf S, Goldhaber SZ, Olmstead EM, Paffenbarger RS Jr, et al: An overview of randomized trials of rehabilitation with exercise after myocardial infarction. *Circulation* 1989; 80:234–244.
27. Oldridge N, Guyatt G, Jones N, Crowe J, Singer J, Feeny D, et al: Effects on quality of life with comprehensive rehabilitation after acute myocardial infarction. *Am J Cardiol* 1991; 67:1084–1089.
28. American College of Sports Medicine: *Guidelines for Exercise Testing and Prescription,* 4th ed. Philadelphia, Lea and Febiger, 1991.
29. Fletcher GF, Froelicher VF, Hartley LH, Haskell WL, Pollock ML: Exercise Standards. A Statement for Health Professionals from the American Heart Association. *Circulation* 1990; 82:2286–2322.
30. Health and Public Policy Committee, American College of Physicians: Cardiac rehabilitation services. *Ann Intern Med* 1988; 109:671–673.
31. American Association of Cardiovascular and Pulmonary Rehabilitation: Guidelines for Cardiac Rehabilitation Programs. Champaign, IL, Human Kinetics, 1991.
32. Wenger NK, Balady GJ, Cohn LH, Hartley H, King SB III, Miller HS, et al: Ad Hoc Task Force on Cardiac Rehabilitation: Cardiac rehabilitation services following PTCA and valvular surgery. Guidelines for use. *Cardiology* 1990; 19:4–5.
33. Wenger NK, Haskell WL, Kanter K, Squires RW, Yusuf S: Ad Hoc Task Force on Cardiac Rehabilitation: Cardiac rehabilitation services after cardiac transplantation. Guidelines for use. *Cardiology* 1991; 20:4–5.
34. Haskell WL: Cardiovascular complications during exercise training of cardiac patients. *Circulation* 1978; 57:920–924.
35. DeBusk RF, Haskell WL, Miller NH, Berra K, Taylor CB: Medically directed at-home rehabilitation soon after clinically uncomplicated acute myocardial infarction: A new model for patient care. *Am J Cardiol* 1985; 55:251–257.
36. Blumenthal JA, Rejeski WJ, Walsh-Riddle M, Emery CF, Miller H, Roark S, et al: Comparison of high- and low-intensity exercise training early after acute myocardial infarction. *Am J Cardiol* 1988; 61:26–30.
37. Karvonen MJ, Kentala K, Mustala O: The effects of training on heart rate: A longitudinal study. *Ann Med Exper Bio Fen* 1957; 35:307–315.
38. Hamm LF, Crow RS, Stull GA, Hannan P: Safety and characteristics of exercise testing early after acute myocardial infarction. *Am J Cardiol* 1989; 63:1193–1197.
39. Guidelines for Exercise Testing. A Report of the Joint American College of Cardiology/American Heart Association Task Force on Assessment of Cardiovascular Procedures (Subcommittee on Exercise Testing). *J Am Coll Cardiol* 1986; 8:725–738. *Circulation* 1986; 74:653A–667A.
40. Topol EJ, Juni JE, O'Neill WW, Nicklas JM, Shea MJ, Burek K, et al: Exercise testing three days after onset of acute myocardial infarction. *Am J Cardiol* 1987; 60:958–962.
41. Balady GJ, Weiner DA, Rothendler JA, Ryan TJ, Mangene C, LaGambina J, et al: Arm exercise-thallium imaging testing for the detection of coronary artery disease. *J Am Coll Cardiol* 1987; 9:84–88.
42. Balady GJ, Weiner DA, Rose L, Ryan TJ, Erario M: Physiologic responses to arm ergometry exercise relative to age and gender. *J Am Coll Cardiol* 1990; 16:130–135.
43. DeBusk RF, Blomqvist GC, Kouchoukos NT, Luepker RV, Miller HS, Moss AJ, et al: Identification and treatment of low-risk patients after acute myocardial infarction and coronary-artery bypass graft surgery. *N Engl J Med* 1986; 314:161–166.
44. Ryan T, Armstrong WF, O'Donnell JA, Feigenbaum H: Risk stratification after acute myocardial infarction by means of exercise two-dimensional echocardiography. *Am Heart J* 1987; 114:1305–1316.
45. Picard MH, Dennis C, Schwartz RG, Ahn DK, Kraemer HC, Berger WE III, et al: Cost-benefit analysis of early return to work after uncomplicated acute myocardial infarction. *Am J Cardiol* 1989; 63:1308–1314.
46. Ewart CK, Taylor CB, Reese LB, DeBusk RF: Effects of early postmyocardial infarction exercise testing on self-perception and subsequent physical activity. *Am J Cardiol* 1983; 51:1076–1080.
47. Kelemen MH, Stewart KJ, Gillilan RE, Ewart CK, Valenti SA, Manley JD, et al: Circuit weight training in cardiac patients. *J Am Coll Cardiol* 1986; 7:38–42.
48. Sagiv M, Hanson P, Besozzi M, Nagle F, Zager L: Left ventricular responses to upright isometric handgrip and deadlift in men with coronary artery disease. *Am J Cardiol* 1985; 55:1298–1302.
49. Franklin BA: Exercise testing, training and arm ergometry. *Sports Med* 1985; 2:100–119.
50. Wenger NK: Ischemic heart disease: Exercise training, selected aspects of pharmacologic therapy, and drug-exercise interactions. *Emory J Med* 1989; 3:253–259.
51. Wenger NK: In-hospital exercise rehabilitation after myocardial infarction and myocardial revascularization: Physiologic basis, methodology, and results. In: Wenger NK, Hellerstein HK (eds): *Rehabilitation of the Coronary Patient,* 3d ed. New York, Churchill Livingstone, 1992, pp. 351–365.
52. Hung J, Goldwater D, Convertino VA, McKillop JH, Goris ML, DeBusk RF: Mechanisms for decreased exercise capacity after bed rest in normal middle-aged men. *Am J Cardiol* 1983; 51:344–348.
53. Gaffney FA, Nixon JV, Karlsson ES, Campbell W, Dowdey ABC, Blomqvist CG: Cardiovascular deconditioning produced by 20 hours of bedrest with head-down tilt (−5°) in middle-aged healthy men. *Am J Cardiol* 1985; 56:634–638.
54. Rowe MH, Jelinek MV, Liddell N, Hugens M: Effect of rapid mobilization on ejection fractions and ventricular volumes after acute myocardial infarction. *Am J Cardiol* 1989; 63:1037–1041.
55. Maeland JG, Havik OE: The effects of an in-hospital educational programme for myocardial infarction patients. *Scand J Rehab Med* 1987; 19:57–65.

56. Comoss PM: Education of the coronary patient and family: Principles and practice. In: Wenger NK, Hellerstein HK (eds): *Rehabilitation of the Coronary Patient,* 3d ed. New York, Churchill Livingstone, 1992, pp. 439–460.
57. Van Camp SP, Peterson RA: Cardiovascular complications of outpatient cardiac rehabilitation programs. *JAMA* 1986; 256:1160–1163.
58. Fagan ET, Wayne VS, McConachy DL: Serious ventricular arrhythmias in a cardiac rehabilitation programme. *Med J Aust* 1984; 141:421–424.
59. Borg GA: Psychophysical bases of perceived exertion. *Med Sci Sports Exerc* 1982; 14:377–381.
60. Williams RS, Miller H, Koisch FP, Jr., Ribisl P, Graden H: Guidelines for unsupervised exercise in patients with ischemic heart disease. *J Cardiac Rehabil* 1981; 1:213–219.
61. Hossack KF, Hartwig R: Cardiac arrest associated with supervised cardiac rehabilitation. *J Cardiac Rehabil* 1982; 2:402–408.
62. Stevens R, Hanson P: Comparison of supervised and unsupervised exercise training after coronary bypass surgery. *Am J Cardiol* 1984; 53:1524–1528.
63. Erdman RAM, Duivenvoorden HJ, Verhage F, Kazemier M, Hugenholtz PG: Predictability of beneficial effects in cardiac rehabilitation: A randomized clinical trial of psychosocial variables. *J Cardiopulmonary Rehabil* 1986; 6:206–213.
64. Franklin BA, Bonzheim K, Gordon S, Timmis GC: Resistance training in cardiac rehabilitation. *J Cardiopulmonary Rehabil* 1991; 11:99–107.
65. Waites TF, Watt EW, Fletcher GF: Comparative functional and physiologic status of active and dropout coronary bypass patients of a rehabilitation program. *Am J Cardiol* 1983; 51:1087–1090.
66. Ben-Ari E, Kellermann JJ, Fisman EZ, Pines A, Peled B, Drory Y: Benefits of long-term physical training in patients after coronary artery bypass grafting—a 58-month follow-up and comparison with a nontrained group. *J Cardiopulmonary Rehabil* 1986; 6:165–170.
67. Blumenthal JA, Levenson RM: Behavioral approaches to secondary prevention of coronary heart disease. *Circulation* 1987; 76(suppl I):I-130–I-137.
68. Ornish D, Brown SE, Scherwitz LW, Billings JH, Armstrong WT, Ports TA, et al: Can lifestyle changes reverse coronary heart disease? The Lifestyle Heart Trial. *Lancet* 1990; 336:129–133.
69. CASS Principal Investigators and Their Associates: Coronary Artery Surgery Study (CASS): A randomized trial of coronary artery bypass surgery: Quality of life in patients randomly assigned to treatment groups. *Circulation* 1983; 68:951–960.
70. Leaman DM, Brower RW, Meester GT: Coronary artery bypass surgery: A stimulus to modify existing risk factors? *Chest* 1982; 81:16–19.
71. Kottke TE, Battista RN, DeFriese GH, Brekke ML: Attributes of successful smoking cessation interventions in medical practice. A meta-analysis of 39 controlled trials. *JAMA* 1988; 259:2883–2889.
72. Maeland JG, Havik OE: Psychological predictors for return to work after a myocardial infarction. *J Psychosom Res* 1987; 31:471–481.
73. Neill WA, Branch LG, DeJong G, Smith NE, Hogan CA, Corcoran PJ, et al: Cardiac disability. The impact of coronary heart disease on patients' daily activities. *Arch Intern Med* 1985; 145:1642–1647.
74. Papadopoulos C: Education and counseling of the patient and family: Sexual problems/interventions. In: Wenger NK, Hellerstein HK (eds): *Rehabilitation of the Coronary Patient,* 3d ed. New York, Churchill Livingstone, 1992, pp. 473–481.
75. Williams MA, Maresh CM, Esterbrooks DJ, Harbrecht JJ, Sketch MH: Early exercise training in patients older than age 65 years compared with that in younger patients after acute myocardial infarction or coronary artery bypass grafting. *Am J Cardiol* 1985; 55:263–266.
76. Shephard RJ: The scientific basis of exercise prescribing for the very old. *J Am Geriatr Soc* 1990; 38:62–70.
77. Saunamaki KI: Early post-myocardial infarction exercise testing in subjects 70 years or more of age. Functional and prognostic evaluation. *Eur Heart J* 1984; 5(suppl E):93–96.
78. Bruce RA, Larson EB, Stratton J: Physical fitness, functional aerobic capacity, aging, and responses to physical training or bypass surgery in coronary patients. *J Cardiopulmonary Rehabil* 1989; 9:24–34.
79. Coats AJS, Adamopoulos S, Meyer TE, Conway J, Sleight P: Effects of physical training in chronic heart failure. *Lancet* 1990; 335:63–66.
80. Sullivan MJ, Higginbotham MB, Cobb FR: Exercise training in patients with severe left ventricular dysfunction. Hemodynamic and metabolic effects. *Circulation* 1988; 78:506–515.
81. Litchfield RL, Kerber RE, Benge JW, Mark AL, Sopko J, Bhatnagar RK, et al: Normal exercise capacity in patients with severe left ventricular dysfunction: Compensatory mechanisms. *Circulation* 1982; 66:129–134.
82. Squires RW, Lavie CJ, Brandt TR, Gau GT, Bailey KR: Cardiac rehabilitation in patients with severe ischemic left ventricular dysfunction. *Mayo Clin Proc* 1987; 62:997–1002.
83. Williams RS: Exercise training of patients with ventricular dysfunction and heart failure. In: Wenger NK (ed): *Exercise and the Heart,* 2d ed. Philadelphia, F.A. Davis, 1985:219–231.
84. Tamarisk NK: Enhancing activity levels of patients with permanent cardiac pacemakers. *Heart Lung* 1988; 17:698–707.
85. Kalbfleisch KR, Lehmann MH, Steinman RT, Jackson K, Axtell K, Schuger CD, et al: Reemployment following implantation of the automatic cardioverter defibrillator. *Am J Cardiol* 1989; 64:199–202.
86. Razin AM: Psychosocial intervention in coronary artery disease: A review. *Psychosom Med* 1982; 44:363–387.
87. White PD: *Heart Disease.* New York, Macmillan, 1951.
88. Stern MJ, Cleary P: National Exercise and Heart Disease Project: Psychosocial changes observed during a low-level exercise program. *Arch Intern Med* 1981; 141:1463–1467.
89. van Dixhoorn J, Duivenvoorden HJ, Staal HA, Pool J: Physical training and relaxation therapy in cardiac rehabilitation assessed through a composite criterion for training outcome. *Am Heart J* 1989; 118:545–552.
90. Orth-Gomer K, Unden A-L, Edwards M-E: Social isolation and mortality in ischemic heart disease. A 10-year follow-up study of 150 middle-aged men. *Acta Med Scand* 1988; 224:205–215.
91. Friedman M, Thoresen CE, Gill JJ, Ulmer D, Powell LH, Price VA, et al: Alteration of type A behavior and its effect on cardiac recurrences in post myocardial infarction patients: Summary results of the recurrent coronary prevention project. *Am Heart J* 1986; 112:653–665.
92. Wenger NK, Hellerstein HK, Blackburn H, Castranova SJ: Physician practice in the management of patients with uncomplicated myocardial infarction: Changes in the past decade. *Circulation* 1982; 65:421–427.
93. Walter PJ (ed): *Return to Work after Coronary Artery Bypass Surgery. Psychosocial and Economic Aspects.* Berlin, Springer-Verlag, 1985.
94. Russell RO Jr, Abi-Mansour P, Wenger NK: Return to work after coronary bypass surgery and percutaneous transluminal angioplasty: Issues and potential solutions. *Cardiology* 1986; 73:306–322.
95. Rogers WJ, Coggin CJ, Gersh BJ, Fisher LD, Myers WO, Oberman A, et al: Ten-year follow-up of quality of life in patients randomized to receive medical therapy or coronary artery bypass graft surgery. The Coronary Artery Surgery Study (CASS). *Circulation* 1990; 82:1647–1658.
96. Ellis SG, Fisher L, Dushman-Ellis S, Pettinger M, King SB III, Roubin GS, et al: Comparison of coronary angioplasty with medical treatment for single- and double-vessel coronary disease with left anterior descending coronary involvement: Long-term outcome based upon an Emory-CASS registry study. *Am Heart J* 1989; 118:208–220.
97. Fitzgerald ST, Becker DM, Celentano DD, Swank R, Brinker J: Return to work after percutaneous transluminal coronary angioplasty. *Am J Cardiol* 1989; 64:1108–1112.
98. Walling A, Tremblay GJ, Jobin J, Charest J, Delage F, Leblanc M, et al: Evaluating the rehabilitation potential of a large population of post-myocardial infarction patients: Adverse prognosis for women. *J Cardiopulmonary Rehabil* 1988; 8:99–106.
99. Almeida D, Bradford JM, Wenger NK, King SB, Hurst JW: Return to work after coronary bypass surgery. *Circulation* 1983; 68(suppl II):II-205–II-213.
100. Taylor CB, Bandura A, Ewart CK, Miller NH, DeBusk RF: Exercise testing to enhance wives' confidence in their husbands' cardiac capability soon after clinically uncomplicated acute myocardial infarction. *Am J Cardiol* 1985; 55:635–638.
101. Hellerstein HK: Vocational aspects of rehabilitation: Work eval-

uation. In: Wenger NK, Hellerstein HK (eds): *Rehabilitation of the Coronary Patient,* 3d ed. New York, Churchill Livingstone, 1992, pp. 523–542.

102. Dennis C, Houston-Miller N, Schwartz RG, Ahn DK, Kraemer HC, Gossard D, et al: Early return to work after uncomplicated myocardial infarction. Results of a randomized trial. *JAMA* 1988; 260:214–220.

103. Hung J, McKillip J, Savin W, Magder S, Kraus R, Houston N, et al: Comparison of cardiovascular response to combined static-dynamic effort, postprandial dynamic effort and dynamic effort alone in patients with chronic ischemic heart disease. *Circulation* 1982; 65:1411–1419.

Chapter 64

Nonatherosclerotic Coronary Heart Disease

Bruce F. Waller, M.D.

Although atherosclerotic disease of the coronary arteries is the most common cause of luminal narrowing and coronary heart disease, there are multiple nonatherosclerotic (congenital and acquired) causes of severe luminal narrowing and subsequent clinical coronary events (angina pectoris, acute myocardial infarction, sudden death) (Table 64-1). Various nonatherosclerotic coronary artery diseases can reduce or interrupt coronary blood flow by various mechanisms: (1) *fixed luminal obstructions* (internal narrowing), (2) *encroachment of the lumen by disease of the arterial wall or adjacent tissues* (external narrowing), or *both*.[1] Reduction in coronary arterial blood flow may also result from *dynamic changes in the walls of an otherwise normal artery* (spasm) or from myocardial *oxygen demand-supply disproportion*. In view of current trends toward rapid coronary artery reperfusion to salvage jeopardized myocardium during evolving acute myocardial infarction, the various nonatherosclerotic etiologies of coronary artery disease must be kept in mind.

FREQUENCY OF NONATHEROSCLEROTIC CORONARY NARROWING PRODUCING FATAL MYOCARDIAL INFARCTION

Approximately 4 to 7 percent of all patients with acute myocardial infarction (nearly 4 times this percentage for patients aged <35 years) do not have atherosclerotic coronary artery disease (CAD) as demonstrated by coronary arteriography, at necropsy, or both.[1-5] In view of the fact that coronary angiography simply represents a "lumenogram," the specificity for etiology of the coronary luminal narrowing is extremely low. Review of necropsy studies[1,3,4] suggests that approximately 95 percent of patients with fatal acute myocardial infarction have, at least, one major epicardial coronary artery (left anterior descending, left circumflex, right, left main) with severe luminal narrowing or total occlusion (Fig. 64-1). The remaining 5 percent of patients have normal major epicardial coronary arteries. Of the 95 percent of patients with severe coronary luminal narrowing, 95 percent of these patients have typical atherosclerotic plaque with (85 percent) or without (15 percent) superimposed thrombus. The remaining 5 percent of the patients with severe coronary luminal narrowing have a host of etiologies (Table 64-1), including coronary arteritis, trauma, systemic metabolic disorders, intimal fibrous proliferation, and coronary emboli. (Certain medical centers with large populations of cardiac transplant patients will exceed the 5 percent nonatherosclerotic approximation owing to the high frequency of intimal fibrous proliferation in the coronary arteries late after transplantation.) Of the 5 percent necropsy patients after fatal acute myocardial infarction with normal or nearly normal epicardial coronary arteries, perhaps 50 to 60 percent of these patients represent clinical coronary spasm, but the remaining 40 to 50 percent represent a combination of congenital coronary artery anomalies, spontaneous recanalization, and coronary supply-myocardial demand mismatches (see also Chap. 55).

TABLE 64-1

Nonatherosclerotic Causes of Coronary Artery Disease (Coronary Heart Disease)

Congenital Anomalies	Metabolic Disorders
Anomalous origin from the aorta	Mucopolysaccharidoses (Hurler, Hunter)
Right from left sinus of Valsalva	Homocystinuria
Left from right sinus of Valsalva	Fabry disease
Single coronary artery	Amyloid
Atresia of coronary ostium	Intimal Proliferation
High-takeoff coronary ostium	Irradiation therapy
Ostial ridges	Cardiac transplantation
Anomalous origin from the pulmonary trunk	Fibromuscular hyperplasia (methylsergide therapy)
Fistula	Ostial cannulation
Myocardial bridges ("tunneled" epicardial artery)	Transluminal balloon angioplasty
Embolus	Idiopathic infantile arterial calcification (juvenile internal sclerosis)
Natural	Cocaine
Thrombus	External compression
Tumor	Aortic aneurysm
Calcium	Tumor metastases
Vegetation (infective, noninfective)	Muscle bridges
Iatrogenic	Thrombosis Without Underlying Atherosclerotic Plaque
Cardiac surgery	Polycythemia
Cardiac catheterization	Thrombocytosis
Coronary angioplasty	Hypercoagulability
Prosthetic valves	Substance Abuse
Paradoxical	Cocaine
Dissection	Amphetamines
Coronary artery	Myocardial Oxygen Demand–Supply Disproportion
Aortic	Aortic stenosis
Spasm	Systemic hypotension
Trauma	Carbon monoxide poisoning
Nonpenetrating	Increased myocardial function (thyrotoxicosis)
Penetrating	Intramural coronary artery disease (small vessel disease)
Surgery	Hypertrophic cardiomyopathy
Catheterization	Amyloid
Arteritis	Cardiac transplantation
Takayasu disease	Neuromuscular
Polyarteritis nodosa	Diabetes mellitus
Systemic lupus erythematosus	Normal coronary arteries
Kawasaki syndrome (mucocutaneous lymph node syndrome)	
Syphilis	
Other infections (infective endocarditis, salmonella, parasites)	
Burger's disease	
Giant cell	

SOURCE: Adapted from Waller,[1] Alpert and Braunwald,[2] Cheitlin et al,[4] and Baim and Harrison.[5]

CONGENITAL CORONARY ARTERY ANOMALIES

Variation in the origin, course, or distribution of the epicardial coronary arteries are found in 1 to 2 percent of the population (Table 64-2).[1,6–14] Certain types of these anomalies (ostial lesions, passage of a major artery between the walls of the pulmonary trunk and aorta, origin of a major artery from the pulmonary truck, myocardial "bridges") may be more likely to produce ischemia with subsequent myocardial infarction.[8] (See also Chaps. 97 and 138.)

ORIGIN OF BOTH RIGHT AND LEFT CORONARY ARTERIES FROM THE SAME SINUS OF VALSALVA

When either the right or left coronary artery arises from the left or right sinus of Valsalva, respectively, the anomalous vessel transverses the base of the heart in a course anterior to the pulmonary trunk, posterior to the aorta, or between the aorta and pulmonary trunk (Figs. 64-2, 64-3). At least 43 necropsy patients have been reported with the origin of the left (left main) coronary artery from the right sinus and passage between the aorta and

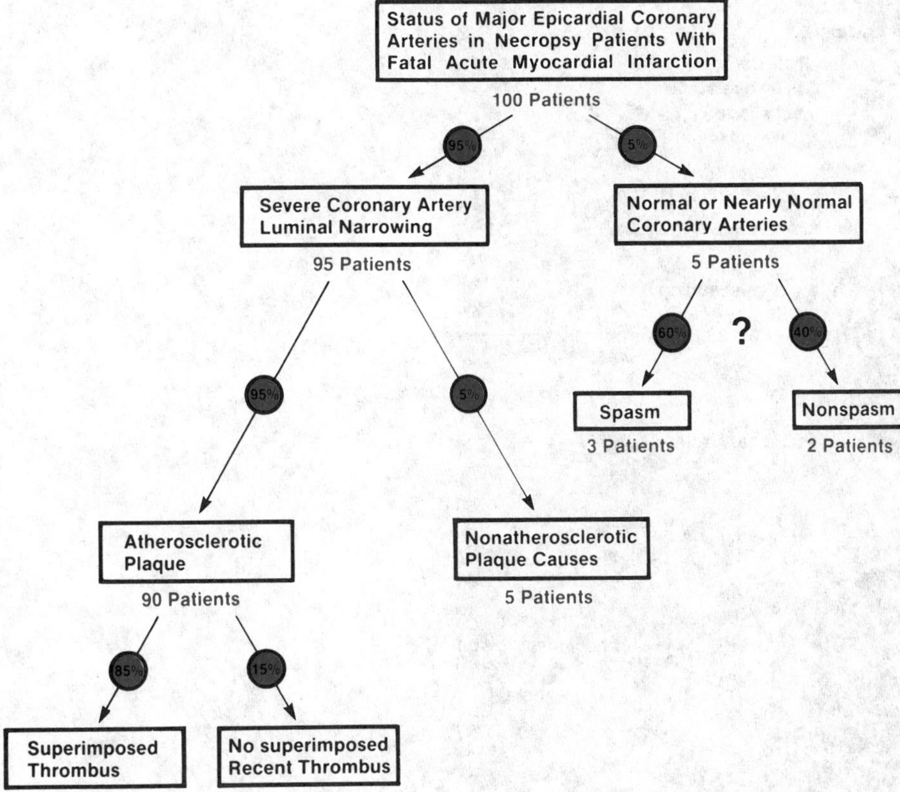

FIGURE 64-1 Diagram displaying the approximate breakdown of status of major epicardial coronary arteries in necropsy patients with fatal acute myocardial infarction. (From Waller.[1] Reproduced with permission from the publisher, editor, and author.)

pulmonary trunk,[7] and, in 34 (79 percent), death was related to the anomaly (sudden death, AMI). At necropsy, 5 of 26 patients age <20 years had myocardial infarcts.[7] Origin of the right coronary artery from the left sinus of Valsalva and passage between the aorta and pulmonary trunk also may be associated with symptoms of myocardial ischemia, infarction, or sudden death.[7] Of 12 necropsy patients with this anomaly reported by Roberts and associates,[9] 3 died suddenly, and 2 had angina or syncope. At necropsy, transmural ventricular scars (healed infarction) were seen in two.

The mechanism of ischemia, infarction, and/or sudden death in this coronary anomaly appears related to the shape of the coronary ostium of the anomalous vessel (Fig. 64-3). Normally, the coronary ostia are round to oval in shape, but, in this anomaly, the coronary artery

TABLE 64-2

Certain Coronary Arterial Anomalies Associated with Clinical Coronary Events or Coronary Artery Narrowing

- Anomalous Origin of One or More Coronary Arteries from the Aorta
  - Origin of both right (R) and left (L) from same sinus of Valsalva
    - R + LM (left main) from right sinus
    - R + LM (left main) from left sinus
- Single Coronary Artery
  - Arising from right sinus
  - Arising from left sinus
  - Arising from posterior sinus
- Anomalous Origin of One or More Coronary Arteries from Pulmonary Trunk (PT)
  - Origin of R from PT
  - Origin of LM from PT
  - Origin of left anterior descending from PT
  - Origin of left circumflex from PT
- Coronary Artery Atresia
  - Atresia of R
  - Atresia of LM
- High-Takeoff Coronary Ostia
- Ostial Narrowing
  - Syphilis
  - Takayasu's disease (pulseless disease)
  - Fibromuscular hyperplasia (drug induced)
  - Aortic valve surgery
  - Fibrous ridges
  - Protruding masses
    - Calcific nodules
    - Supravalvular aortic stenosis
    - Aortic dissection
    - Adhesion of aortic cusp to sinus wall
    - Embolism
    - Fibroelastosis
- Coronary Artery Fistula
- Myocardial Bridges

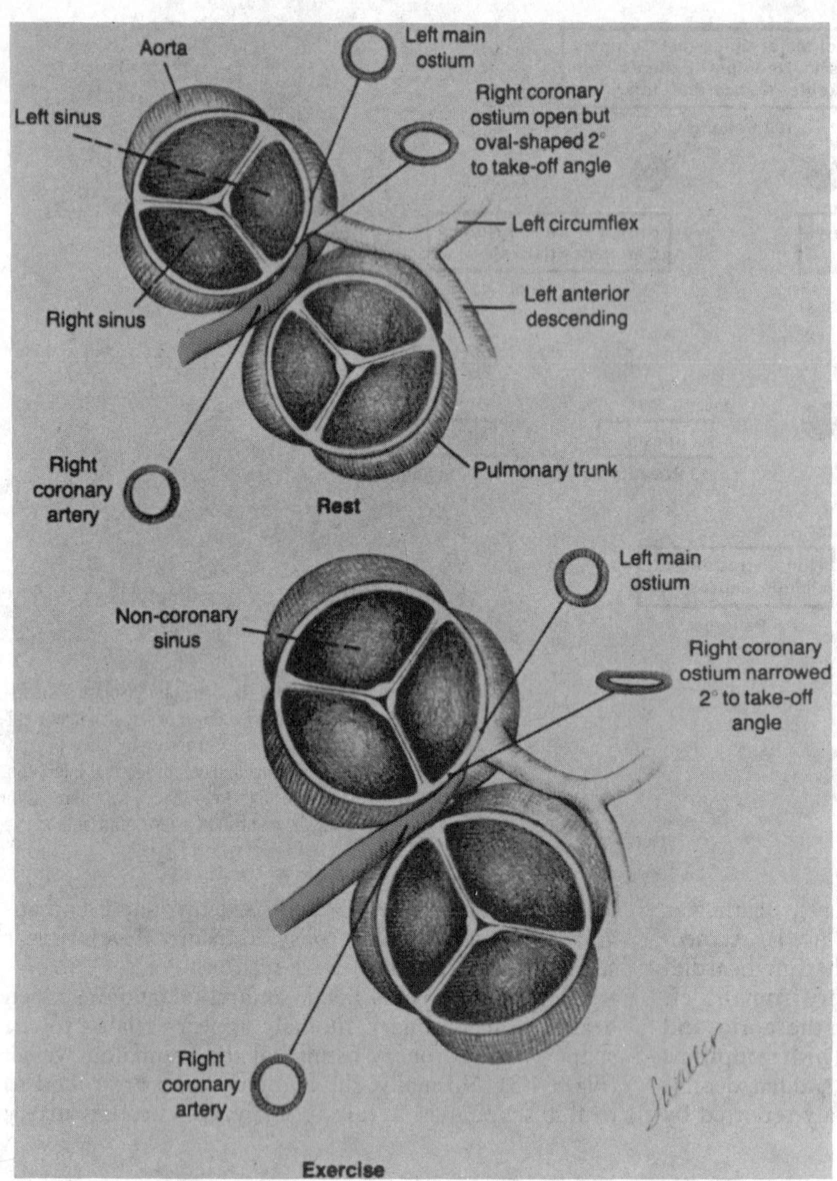

FIGURE 64-2 Diagram showing the proposed mechanism of myocardial ischemia produced by anomalous origin of the right coronary artery from the left sinus of Valsalva. With exercise, the aorta and pulmonary trunk dilate, thereby reducing the already narrowed coronary ostium of the anomalous right coronary. (From Waller.[10] Reproduced with permission from the publisher, editor, and author.)

has an acute takeoff angle that makes the ostium slitlike in shape. With increased cardiac output (e.g., exercise), the aorta dilates and upon aortic wall stretching, this slitlike ostium becomes severely narrowed (Figs. 64-3 to 64-5). It is unlikely that "compression" of the anomalous coronary artery by the aorta and pulmonary trunk occurs, in view of the marked differences in diastolic pressures. At best, there would be an anterior shift of the anomalous vessel rather than a vicelike compression.

SINGLE CORONARY ARTERY

Origin of the entire coronary circulation from a single aortic ostium has been termed "single coronary." This anomaly is rare in the absence of other associated anomalies of the heart. One or more branches of the single artery may cross the base of the heart in a fashion described above and thus may be exposed to the risks of ischemia owing to acute angulation.[5] Angina pectoris and myocardial lactate production have been demonstrated in patients with single coronary arteries in whom coronary atherosclerosis or anomalous coronary artery passage were not present.[13] (See also Chap. 97.)

CORONARY ARTERY ATRESIA

Atresia of one of the two main coronary ostia may be associated with myocardial ischemia/infarction in infancy or childhood.[5] The involved vessel becomes dependent on collateral coronary blood flow from the contralateral coronary artery.

HIGH-TAKEOFF CORONARY OSTIA

Normally, the coronary ostia are located within the sinuses of Valsalva, which permits maximal opportunity for coronary artery diastolic filling. Location of the ostia in the tubular portion of the aorta (i.e., "high-takeoff" position) may be associated with decreased coronary

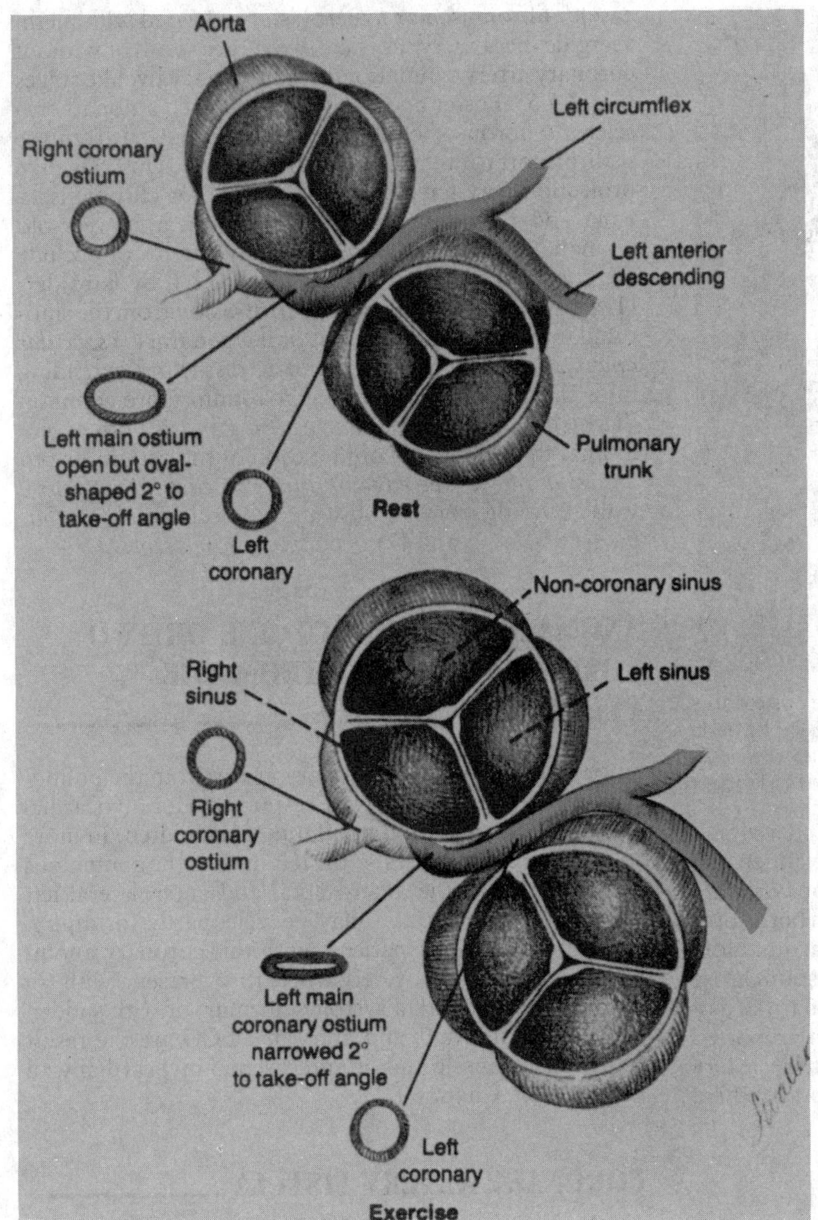

FIGURE 64-3 Diagram showing the proposed mechanism of myocardial ischemia produced by anomalous origin of the left coronary artery from the right sinus of Valsalva. With exercise, the aorta and pulmonary trunk dilate, thereby reducing the already narrowed coronary ostium of the anomalous left coronary. (From Waller.[10] Reproduced with permission from the publisher, editor, and author.)

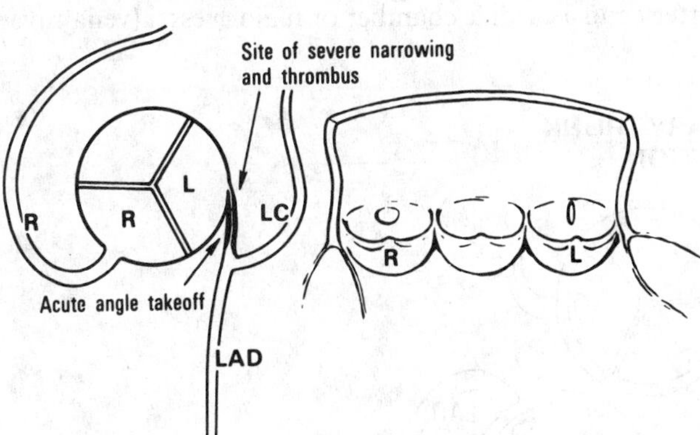

FIGURE 64-4 Diagram showing acute angle takeoff of the left main coronary artery with ostial ridge and slitlike orifice. The proximal left main is occluded by atherosclerotic plaque and thrombus, but the remaining vessels are normal. Accelerated coronary atherosclerosis may result from the acute angle takeoff malformation. Ao = aorta; L = left cusp; L = left main; LC = left circumflex; LAD = left anterior descending; R = right cusp; RC = right coronary. (From Menke.[11] Reproduced with permission from the publisher and author.)

perfusion (Fig. 64-6). Morphologic evidence of chronic ischemia was reported by Menke and associates[14,15] in a patient with a high-takeoff right coronary artery who had right and left ventricular wall scarring. High-takeoff position of the coronary ostium also has been postulated

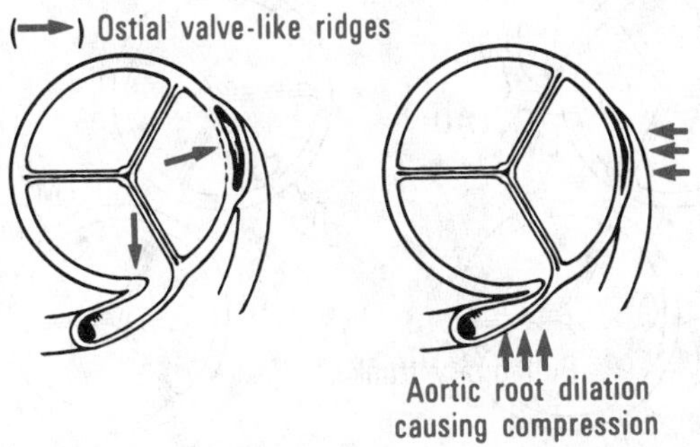

FIGURE 64-5 Diagram illustrating ostial valve-like ridges and the proposed mechanism of ostial compression with aortic root dilation. (From Vermani et al.[12] Reproduced with permission from the publisher, and author.)

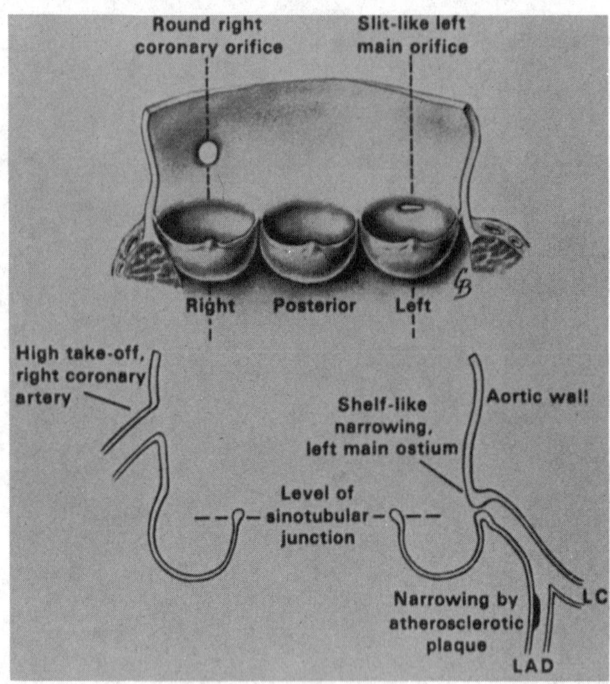

FIGURE 64-6 Diagram showing high takeoff position of the right coronary artery and the nonatherosclerotic fibrous ridge occluding the left main coronary ostium. LAD = left anterior descending; LC = left circumflex. (From Foster et al.[14] Reproduced with permission from the publisher, and author.)

as a cause of sudden coronary death.[16] Alexander and Griffith,[17] in a series of 54 major and minor coronary artery anomalies, found two patients in whom both coronary artery ostia arose above the sinotubular junction, five in whom only the right coronary artery ostium arose high, and three in whom only the left coronary artery ostium was in a high-takeoff position. Burth[18] reported two cases of high origin of the right coronary artery ostium. He attributed ischemia and death in one of these patients to the ostial lesion.

Ostial Fibrous Ridges

Nonatherosclerotic causes of coronary ostial narrowing include syphilis,[19] Takayasu's disease (pulseless disease),[20] fibromuscular hyperplasia associated with methysergide therapy,[21,22] aortic valve surgery with or without coronary artery canulation,[14,23] and ostial valvelike ridges (Fig. 64-5). Foster and Waller[14,15] reported a nonatherosclerotic fibrous shelflike ridge that projected from the wall of aorta into the left main ostium. This ridgelike projection may have been responsible for chronic ischemia and recent myocardial necrosis in a 56-year-old woman. Other rare diseases that may narrow or occlude the coronary ostia have been summarized by Baroldi[24]: (1) a nonatheromatous, *calcific protrusion* from the sinotubular junction into the right or left ostium; (2) *saccular aneurysm* of the aorta; (3) *aortic dissection* extending into the coronary ostium (right ostium more common than left); (4) *supravalvular aortic stenosis* with severe intimal thickening; (5) obliteration of the ostium due to *adhesion of the free edge of an aortic cusp* to the aortic wall above the coronary ostium; (6) occlusion by *embolus* (see below); and (7) occlusive *fibroelastosis*.

ANOMALOUS ORIGIN OF ONE OR TWO CORONARY ARTERIES FROM THE PULMONARY TRUNK

Anomalous origin of a coronary artery from the pulmonary trunk (Fig. 64-7) may be responsible for myocardial ischemia and infarction in infants and children. In more than 90 percent of cases,[5,7] the left main is the anomalous artery, and thus the anteroseptal and anterolateral left ventricular myocardium may be at jeopardy for injury. Asymptomatic older patients with this coronary anomaly usually are discovered when they present with an abnormal ECG, with a systolic murmur, or with sudden death.[7] The murmur and abnormal ECG are the result of papillary muscle and/or anteroseptal myocardial wall damage (see Chap. 60).

CORONARY ARTERY FISTULA

Direct connection between a major epicardial coronary artery and a cardiac chamber or major vessel (vena cava,

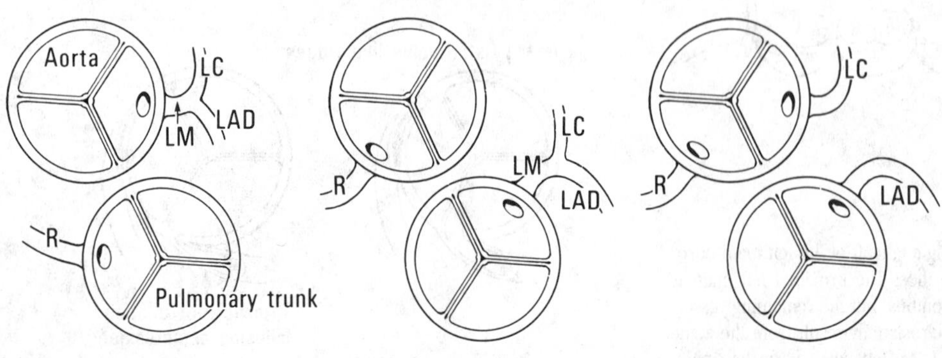

FIGURE 64-7 Anomalous origin of one or two major epicardial coronary arteries from the pulmonary trunk. (From Waller.[1] Reproduced with permission from the publisher, editor, and author.)

coronary sinus, pulmonary artery) is the most common hemodynamically significant coronary artery anomaly.[5] Fistulas from the right coronary artery are more common than from the left. Over 90 percent of the fistulas drain into the venous circulation.[5] Myocardial ischemia has been documented in some patients with coronary artery fistulas who have no evidence of coronary atherosclerosis.[5]

MYOCARDIAL BRIDGES ("TUNNELED" EPICARDIAL CORONARY ARTERY)

The coronary arteries, which normally course over the epicardial surface of the heart, may dip into the myocardium to travel for varying lengths and then reappear on the heart's surface (Figs. 64-8 to 64-16). The muscle overlying the intramyocardial segment of the epicardial coronary artery is termed a "myocardial bridge," and the artery coursing within the myocardium is called a "tunneled" artery (see Figs. 64-8 to 64-10). Tunneled coronary arteries have been recognized anatomically for more than two centuries,[25] but recent reports indicating an association with myocardial ischemia and myocardial bridge have heightened clinical relevance.[26,27] Tunneled coronary arteries have been presumed congenital in origin. Visscher and colleagues[28] reported a tunneled left anterior descending artery in a 42-day-old infant, supporting the presumption that myocardial bridging of coronary arteries existed since birth. At least three factors have been postulated to account for differences between the high frequency of tunneled major coronary arteries observed at necropsy (5 percent[29] to 86 percent[30]), and the lower frequency of tunneled coronary arteries observed angiographically (0.5 percent[26] to 12 percent[31,32]) or associated with symptoms of myocardial ischemia (18 percent[32]): (1) length of the tunneled coronary segment, (2) degree of systolic compression, and (3) heart rate. Isolated reports have suggested that longer tunneled segments of coronary arteries,[27] more severe systolic diameter narrowing of the tunneled segment,[27] and tachycardia[33] are contributing factors in the production of myocardial ischemia in association with myocardial bridging (see Figs. 64-14, 64-15). The length of coronary

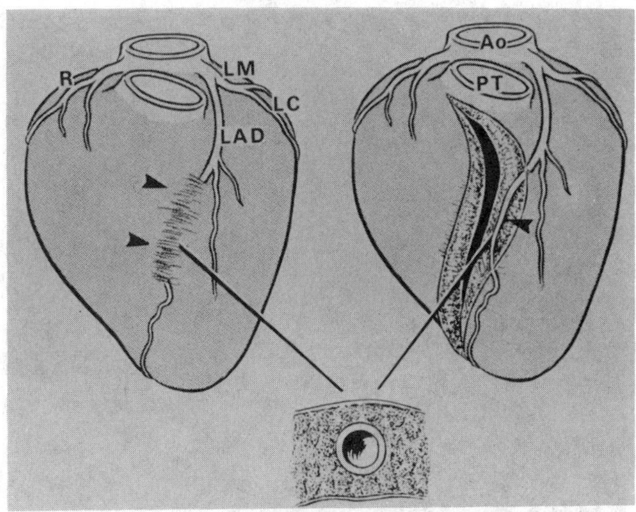

FIGURE 64-8 (Left) Diagram showing tunneled left anterior descending coronary artery (LAD) (arrows). (Right) Opened left ventricle showing intramyocardial segment (arrow). (Below) Transverse section of left ventricular wall showing tunneled coronary artery surrounded by myocardium. (From Waller.[1] Reproduced with permission from the publisher, editor, and author).

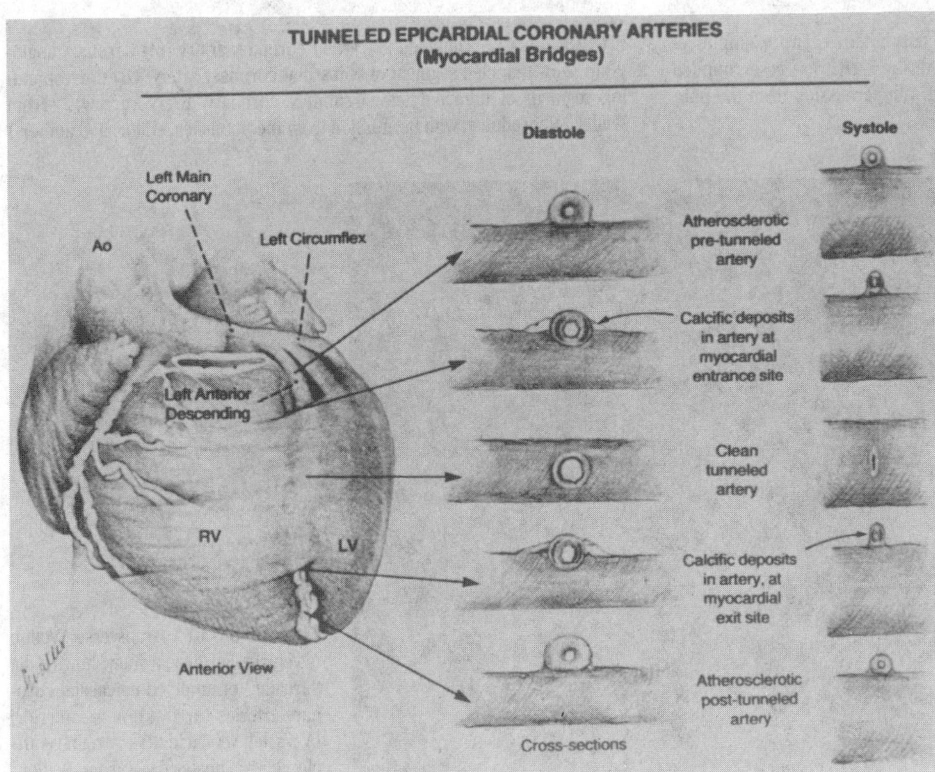

FIGURE 64-9 Diagram showing segments of tunneled and nontunneled epicardial coronary artery with changes during ventricular systole and diastole. Ao = aorta; LV = left ventricle; RV = right ventricle. (From Waller.[10] Reproduced with permission from the publisher, editor, and author.)

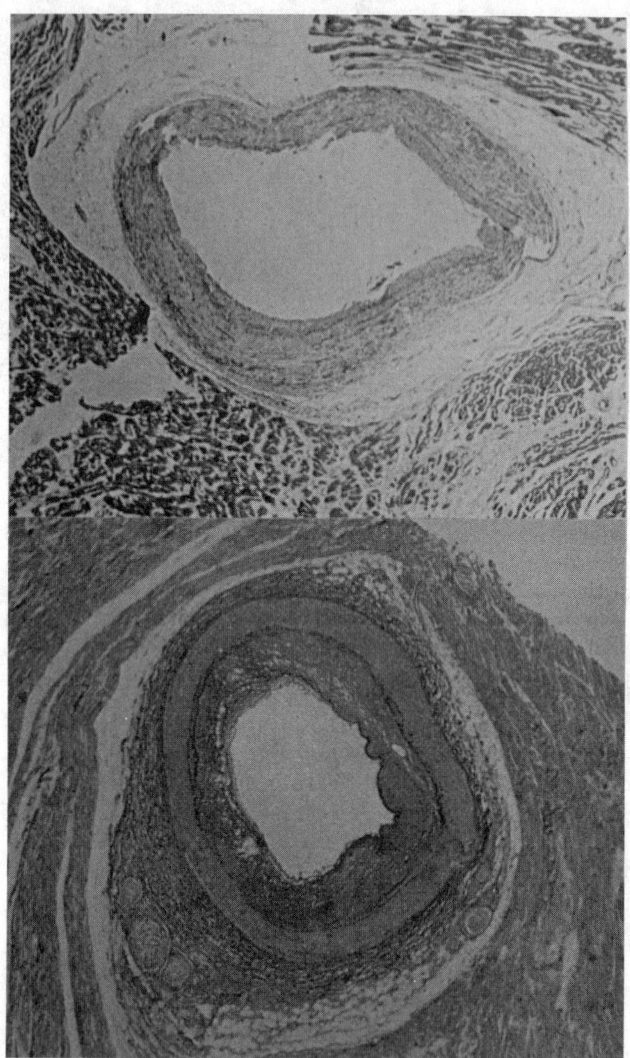

FIGURE 64-10 Tunneled epicardial coronary arteries. Two examples of tunneled left anterior descending coronary arteries. Each artery is surrounded by myocardium. (From Waller.[1] Reproduced with permission from the publisher, editor, and author.)

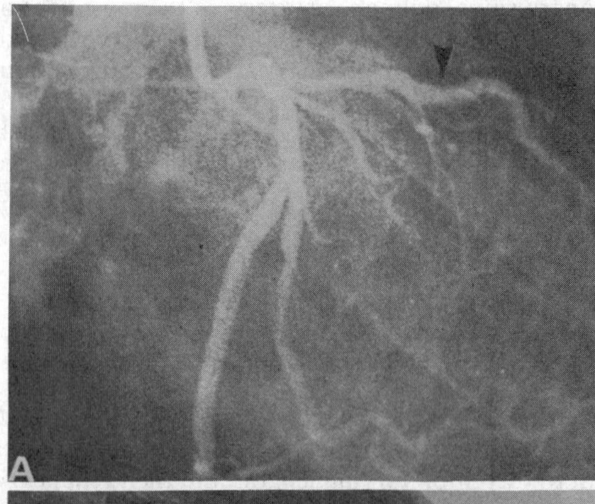

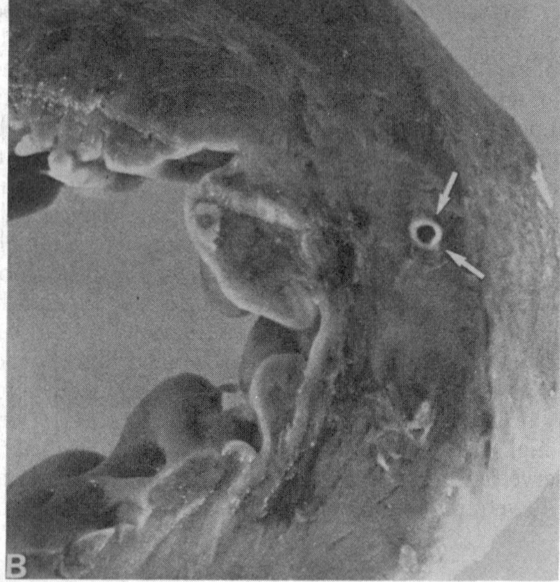

FIGURE 64-12 Tunneled epicardial coronary artery. (*A*) Coronary angiogram show tunneled segment of epicardial coronary artery. (*B*) Corresponding segment of tunneled left circumflex coronary artery (arrow). (From Waller.[1] Reproduced with permission from the publisher, editor, and author.)

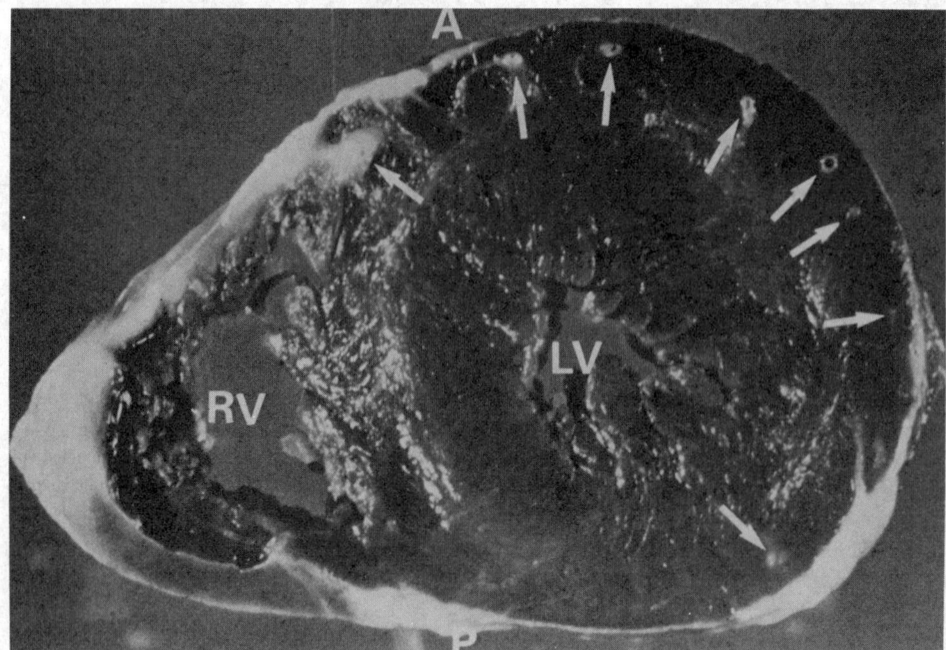

FIGURE 64-11 Transverse section of ventricular myocardium showing the "arcade" of tunneled epicardial coronary arteries (arrows). A = anterior; LV = left ventricle; RV = right ventricle; P = posterior. (From Waller.[1] Reproduced with permission from the publisher, editor, and author.)

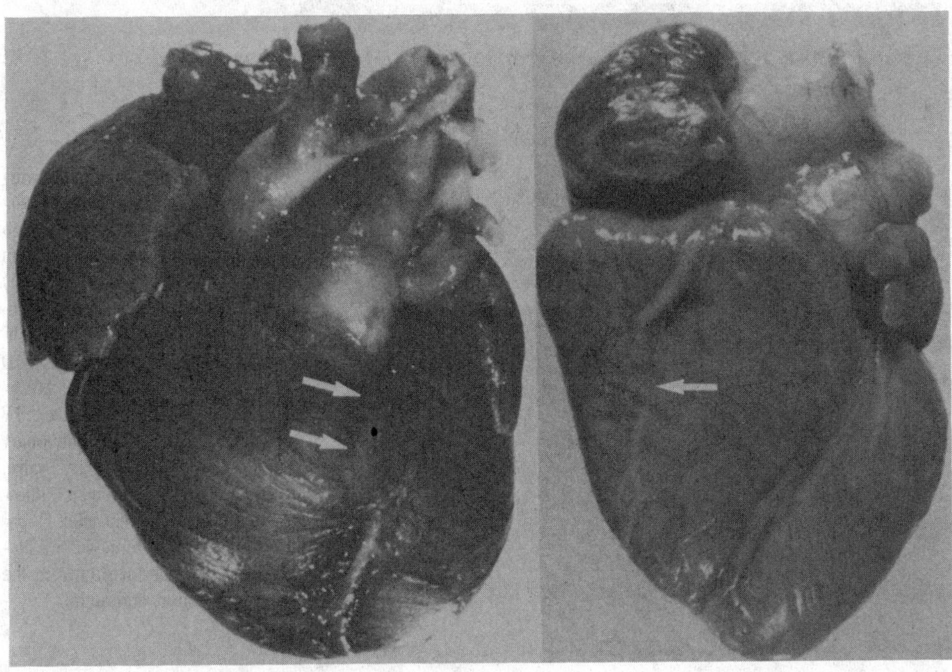

FIGURE 64-13 Tunneled left anterior epicardial coronary arteries from two newborn infants. (Left) Tunneled left anterior descending. (Right) Tunneled marginal branch of right coronary artery. (From Waller.[1] Reproduced with permission from the publisher, editor, and author.)

tunneling may not always be an important factor in causing myocardial ischemia, as evidenced by two recent reports.[34,35] The authors of these reports describe three men with intramyocardial tunneling of greater than 40 mm of the left main coronary artery. Although the left main coronary artery was tunneled, none of the patients had clinical or morphologic evidence of myocardial ischemia (see Fig. 64-16).

CORONARY ANEURYSMS

Congenital coronary artery aneurysms are found most commonly in the right coronary artery.[36] Abnormal flow patterns within the aneurysm may lead to thrombus formation with subsequent vessel occlusion, distal thromboembolization, and myocardial infarction.[37] In general, angina pectoris, or acute myocardial infarction present in young patients (under 20 years of age), should prompt suspicion of a congenital coronary artery anomaly or a congenital coronary artery aneurysm.[36] The incidence of coronary arterial aneurysms is about 1.5 percent of patients studied at necropsy or by coronary arteriography.[37] Aneurysms may be multiple and be acquired or congenital in origin. Causes for coronary arterial aneurysms include congenital, atherosclerosis, trauma, angioplasty, atherectomy and laser procedures, arteritis (including syphilis), mycotic emboli, mucocutaneous lymph node syndrome (Kawasaki's disease), and dissection (spontaneous or secondary) (Table 64-3). Atherosclerotic-induced aneurysms are thought to result from primary thinning and/or destruction of the media and may represent up to 50 percent of the causes (Table 64-3). Angioplasty, atherectomy, vasculitis, and arteritis may also

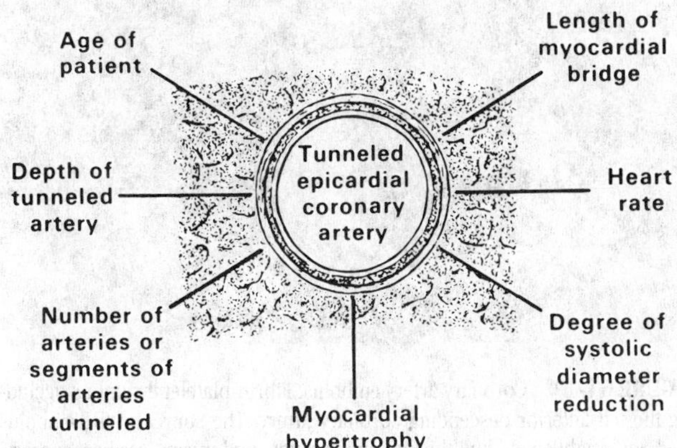

FIGURE 64-14 Diagram shows some of the clinical and anatomic factors in a tunneled epicardial coronary artery. (From Waller.[1] Reproduced with permission from the publisher, editor, and author.)

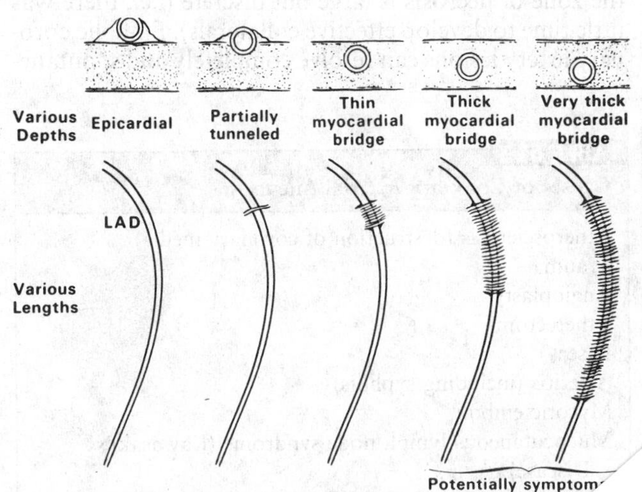

FIGURE 64-15 Diagram showing morphologic variations in (length of tunneled segment, depth of tunneled segment). Reproduced with permission from the publisher, editor,

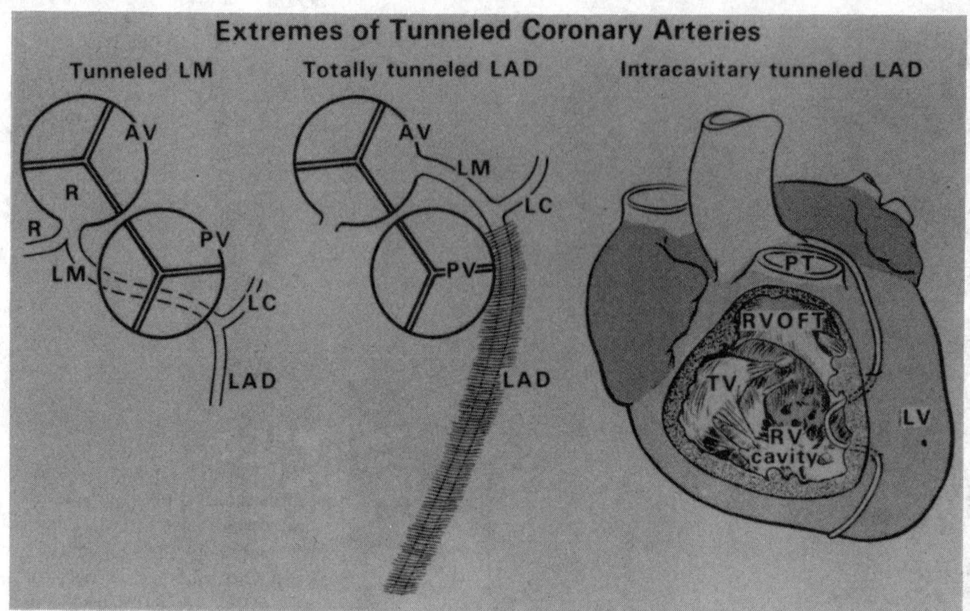

FIGURE 64-16 Diagram showing extremes of tunneled coronary arteries: left main (LM) tunneled through the ventricular septum, total length of the left anterior descending (LAD) located within the myocardium, tunneled segment of LAD becoming intracavitary. AV = aortic valve; LAD = left anterior descending; LC = left circumflex; LM = left main; LV = left ventricular; PT = pulmonary trunk; PV = pulmonary valve; RVOFT = right ventricular outflow tract; RV = right ventricle; TV = tricuspid valve. (From Waller.[1] Reproduced with permission from the publisher, editor, and author.)

damage the arterial wall (media) and cause coronary aneurysms.

CORONARY ARTERY EMBOLI

Coronary arterial emboli (Figs. 64-17 to 64-20) are clinically suspected in patients who develop severe chest pain (acute myocardial infarction) under the following circumstances: in the presence of a prosthetic left-sided valve, active infective endocarditis, native left-sided valve stenosis, atrial fibrillation, left ventricular aneurysm, dilated cardiomyopathy, known cardiac tumor, or during cardiac catheterization or cardiac surgery. The etiology of coronary emboli can be classified as natural causes, iatrogenic causes, and "paradoxical" causes (Tables 64-4 and 64-5) (Figs. 64-17 to 64-19). Coronary embolism most often involves the left anterior descending coronary artery.[36] Coronary embolism is suspected as the cause of acute myocardial infarction when, at necropsy, the zone of necrosis is large but discrete (i.e., there was little time to develop effective collaterals). Embolic coronary artery lesions can resolve completely and spontaneously and are one of the explanations for angiographically normal coronary arteries several months following an acute myocardial infarction.[36]

The consequences of coronary embolism depend on two major factors (see Fig. 64-20): the size of the embolus and the size of the lumen of the artery in which it becomes impacted.[38,39] The smaller the embolus, the greater the chance that it will travel distally to a small coronary arterial segment, and the less the likelihood of myocardial infarction or fatal arrhythmia.[38,39] An embolus so small that it travels distally and impacts in a single intramural vessel is probably clinically silent and observed only at necropsy.[38,39] The status of the coronary lumen before the embolus also determines the subsequent myocardial consequences. An embolus to a previously normal coronary artery is likely to migrate distally and may result in localized myocardial infarction because of ab-

TABLE 64-3

Causes of Coronary Arterial Aneurysms
Atherosclerosis (destruction of coronary media)
Trauma
Angioplasty
Atherectomy
Laser
Arteritis (including syphilis)
Mycotic emboli
Mucocutaneous lymph node syndrome (Kawasaki's Disease)
Congenital
Dissection

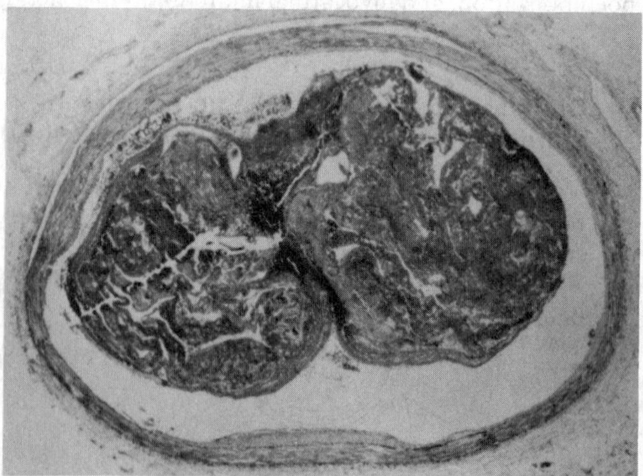

FIGURE 64-17 Coronary artery embolus. Fibrin-platelet thrombus occluding the left anterior descending coronary artery. The source of the embolus was not established, but the patient recently underwent cardiac surgery. (From Waller.[1] Reproduced with permission from the publisher, editor, and author.)

COLOR PLATES*

*The figures in each Plate have been double-numbered in order to indicate the chapter in which they are cited and the order of their citation therein.

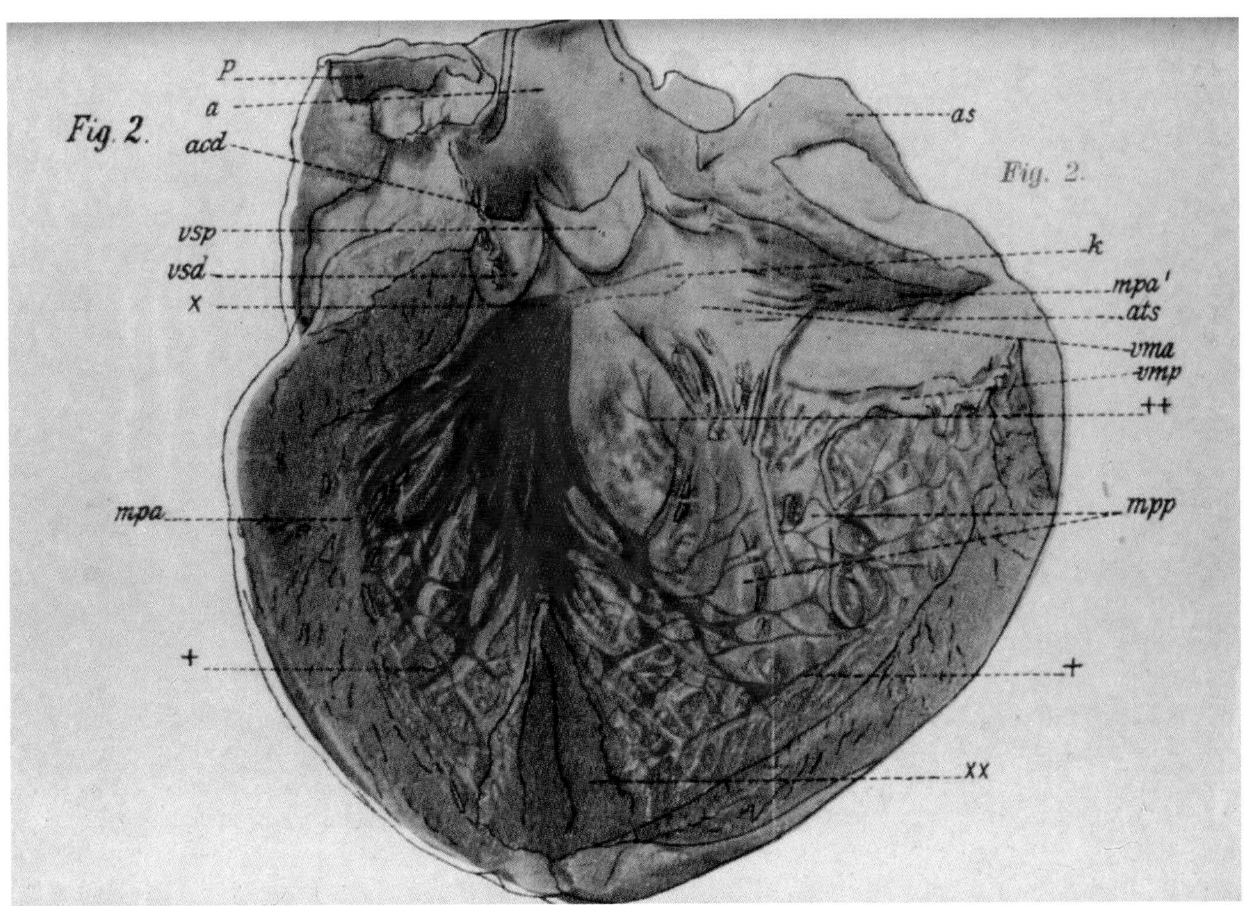

4-1 This diagram is taken from the monograph of Tawara (1906), which established and elucidated the significance of the atrioventricular conduction axis. It shows the fanlike arrangement of the left bundle branch. The clinical value of the so-called concept of hemiblocks should not be extended to presume that the left bundle branch is arranged anatomically in bifascicular fashion. As shown here, it is arranged as a fan, and if it divides at all, it forms three rather than two divisions. [*From Tawara (see Ref. 117 of Chap. 4). Figure provided from Anderson RH, Wilcox BR, Becker AE: Anatomy of the normal heart, in Hurst JW (editor-in-chief): Atlas of the Heart. Gower Medical Publishing, New York, 1988, p. 1.115. Used with permission from the publisher.*]

PLATE II Diagram of the cardiac cycle and related cardiovascular events

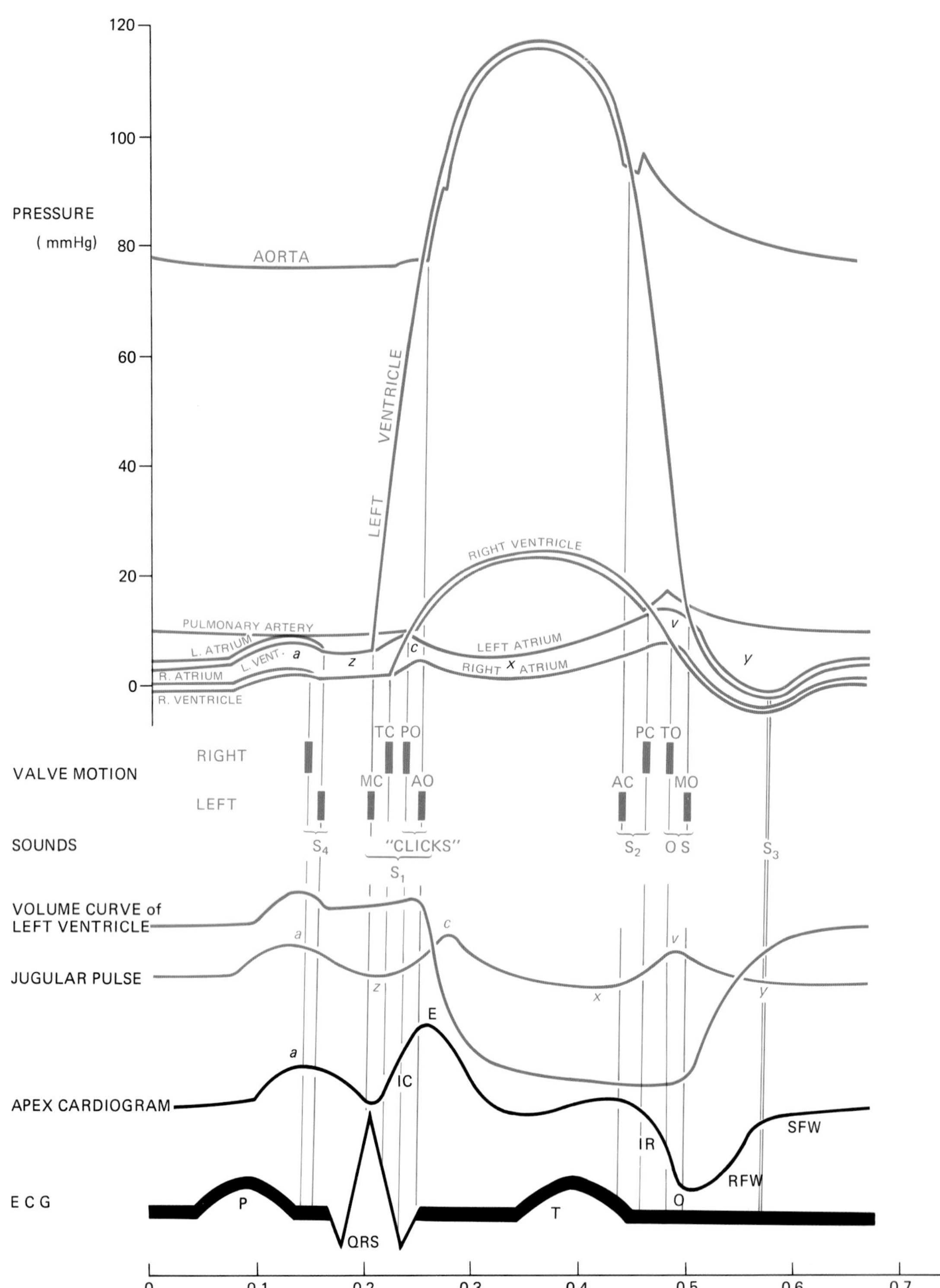

5-1 Diagram of the cardiac cycle, showing the pressure curves of the great vessels and cardiac chambers, valvular events and heart sounds, left ventricular volume curve, jugular pulse wave, apex cardiogram (Sanborn piezo crystal), and the electrocardiogram. For illustrative purposes, the time intervals between the valvular events have been modified and the *z* point has been prolonged. Valve motion: MC = mitral component of the first heart sound; MO = mitral valve opening; TC = tricuspid component of the first heart sound; TO = tricuspid valve opening; AC = aortic component of the second heart sound: AO = aortic valve opening; PC = pulmonic valve component of the second heart sound; PO = pulmonic valve opening; OS = opening snap of atrioventricular valves. Apex cardiogram: IC = isovolumic or isovolumetric (isochoric) contraction wave; IR = isovolumic or isovolumetric (isochoric) relaxation wave; O = opening of mitral valve; RFW = rapid-filling wave; SFW = slow-filling wave.

PLATE V Clubbing of the fingers; Osler's node; dermatomyositis; hemorrhagic telangiectasia under the fingernails; hemorrhagic telangiectasia on the tongue and lips; tuberous sclerosis

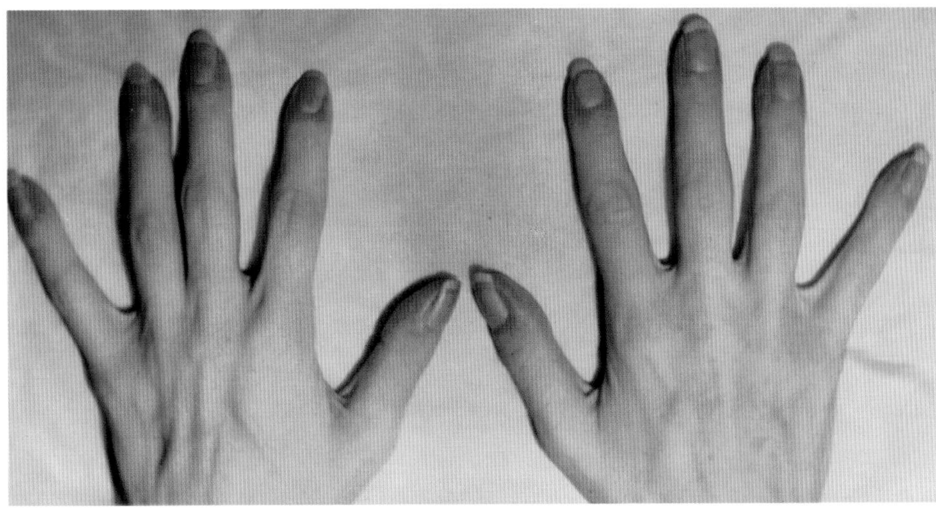

10-5 Clubbing due to bacterial endocarditis.

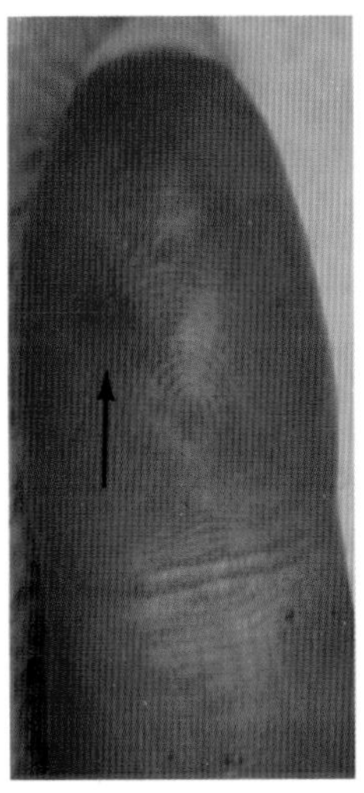

10-6 Osler's node (arrow).

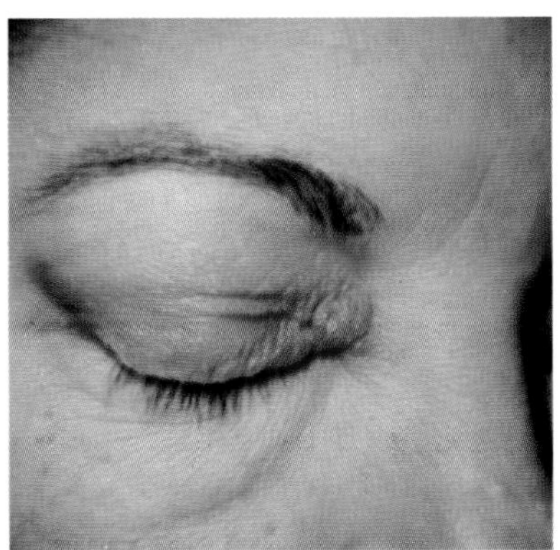

10-7 Dermatomyositis. A violaceous hue and edema of upper eyelid may be associated with myocardial disease.

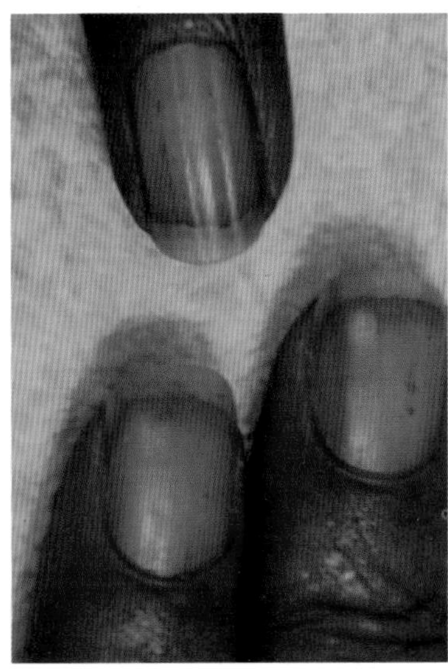

10-8 Hereditary hemorrhagic telangiectasia. Telangiectasia under nails. (*With permission of publisher, from Silverman and Hurst: The hand and the heart. Am J Cardiol 22:609, 1968.*)

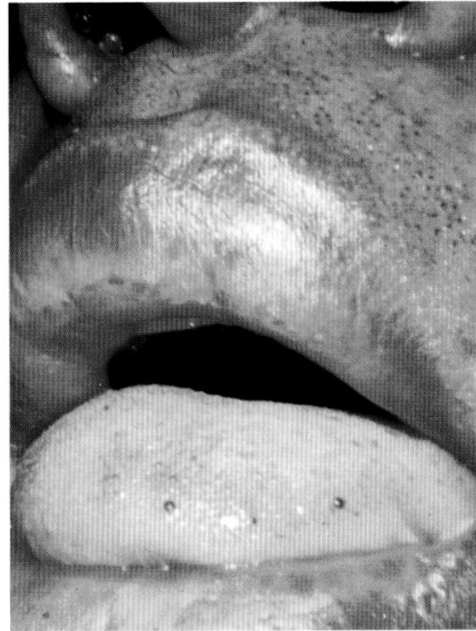

10-9 Hereditary hemorrhagic telangiectasia. Telangiectasia on tongue and lips may be associated with a pulmonary arteriovenous fistula.

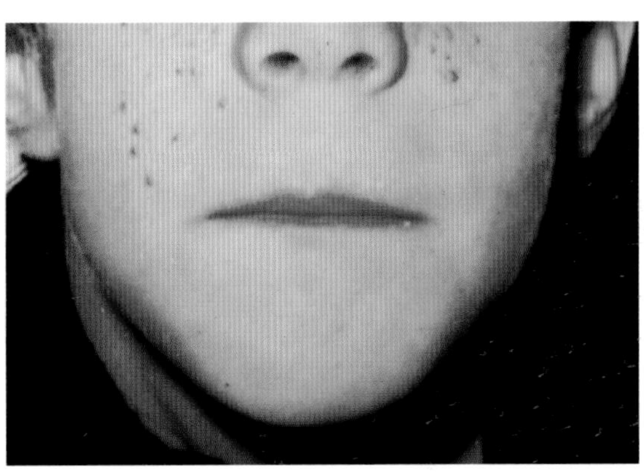

10-10 Tuberous sclerosis. Adenoma sebaceum may be associated with rhabdomyomas of the myocardium.

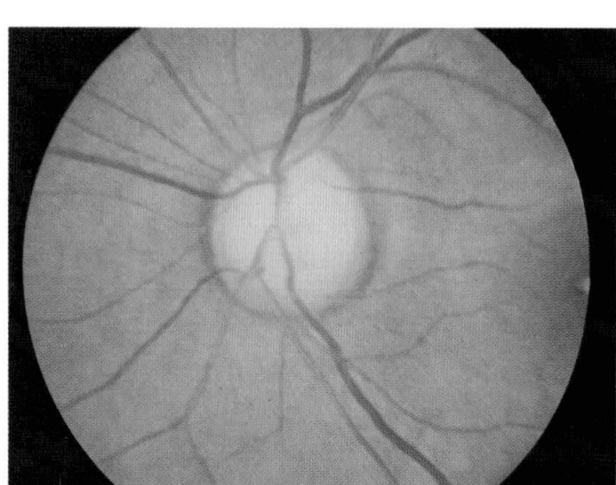

12-1 The retina of a 49-year-old black woman with asymptomatic "essential hypertension" of at least 10 years duration, showing arteriolar narrowing and straightening, increased light reflex, irregular caliber, loss of small arteriolar branches, and early AV crossing changes. (*Courtesy of Dr. Joseph A. Wilber.*)

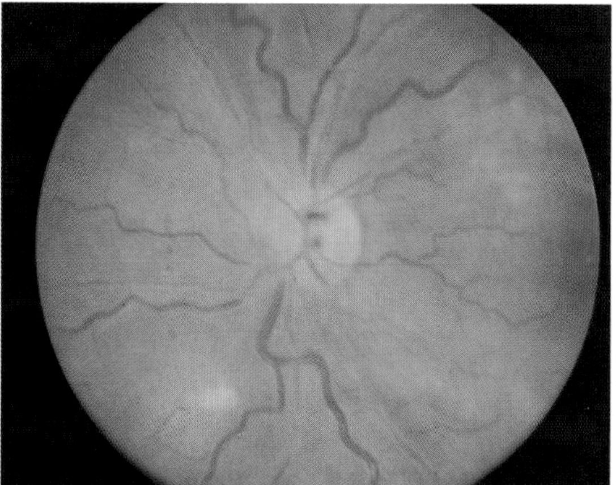

12-2 The retina of a 42-year-old black woman with essential hypertension and blood pressure levels averaging 260/130. She was asymptomatic except for headaches. Note the severe vascular sclerosis seen as marked irregularity of arteriolar caliber, "sheathing," and nearly complete loss of transparency of the arterioles. A "cotton wool" exudate is seen at 7 o'clock. The nasal disk margin is blurred, which may occur normally. (*Courtesy of Dr. Joseph A. Wilber.*)

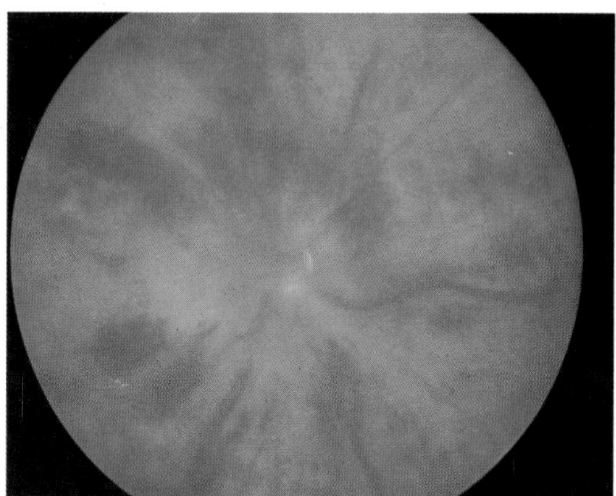

12-3 The retina of a 74-year-old white man with normal blood pressure who complained of sudden loss of vision in one eye. This shows the typical picture of central retinal vein occlusion, probably due to atherosclerosis of its adjacent artery behind the disk. Diffuse edema (loss of retinal detail), massive hemorrhages, and papilledema are present. (*Courtesy of Dr. Joseph A. Wilber.*)

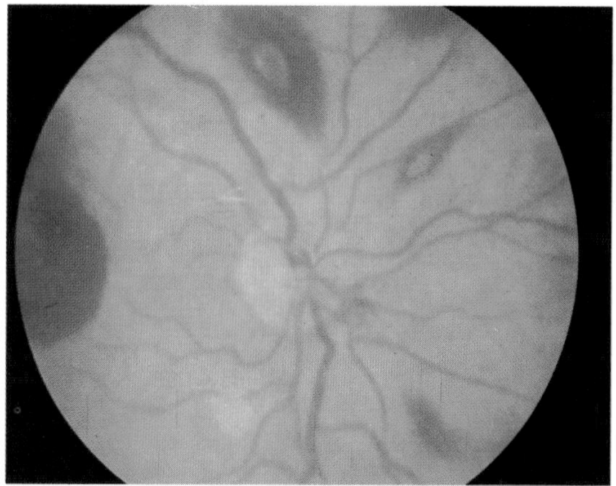

12-4 The retina of a 24-year-old white woman with acute myeloblastic leukemia and severe anemia; the blood pressure was normal. Note the scattered hemorrhages, some with whitish centers (Roth spots) and the portion of the large preretinal hemorrhage at 9 o'clock. The blood vessels are pale but otherwise normal. (*Courtesy of Dr. Joseph A. Wilber.*)

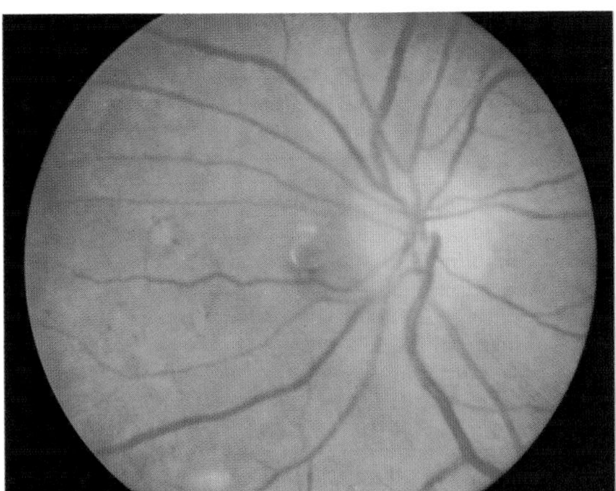

12-5 The retina of a 68-year-old white man with hypertension and mild diabetes mellitus. Note the very small red dots, or capillary aneurysms, scattered between the disk and the macular region. There is also a faint "cotton wool" exudate at 7 o'clock. *(Courtesy of Dr. Joseph A. Wilber.)*

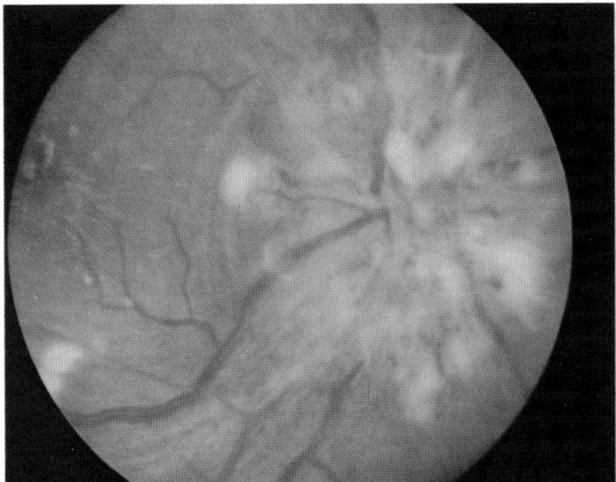

12-6 The retina of a 38-year-old black man with malignant hypertension and with bilateral papilledema and azotemia. There was no visual disturbance. Note the massive edema, hemorrhages, and exudates, completely obscuring the disk and burying the blood vessels. The veins are congested and the arterioles show diffuse thickening ("copper wire"). There are hard exudates (edema residues) forming in the nerve bundle grooves in the macular region at 10 o'clock. *(Courtesy of Dr. Joseph A. Wilber.)*

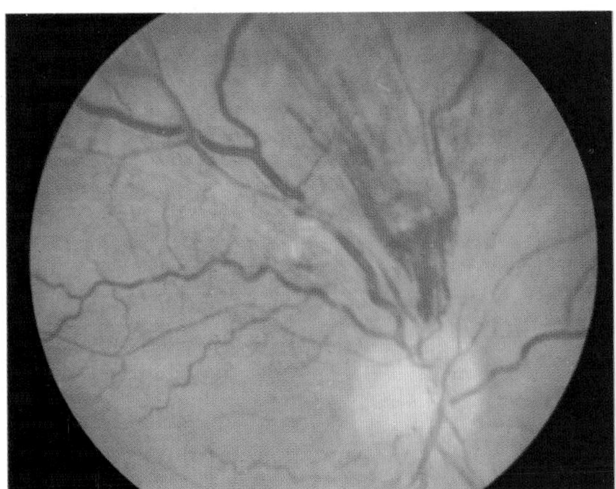

12-7 The retina of a 50-year-old black woman with severe hypertension of 25 years duration. Arteriosclerosis is shown by the marked narrowing, irregular caliber, increased light reflex, and AV crossing changes. Atherosclerosis is suggested by the large fan-shaped superficial hemorrhage, due to occlusion of a branch of the superior temporal vein as it enters the disk region. *(Courtesy of Dr. Joseph A. Wilber.)*

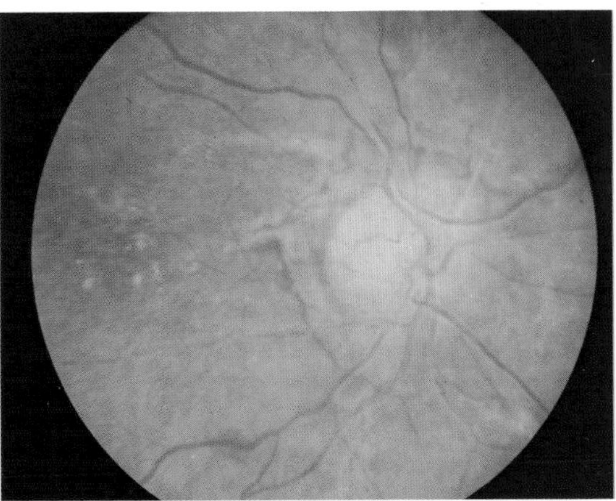

12-8 The retina of a 36-year-old woman with pseudoxanthoma elasticum. Severe hypertension, marked visual disturbance, and renal insufficiency were present. Note the characteristic brownish angioid streaks around the disk and extending toward the macula. Also seen are marked retinal arteriosclerotic changes, sheathing, irregular caliber, occluded vessels, and hard exudates with a "smudge" hemorrhage at 7 o'clock. *(Courtesy of Dr. Joseph A. Wilber.)*

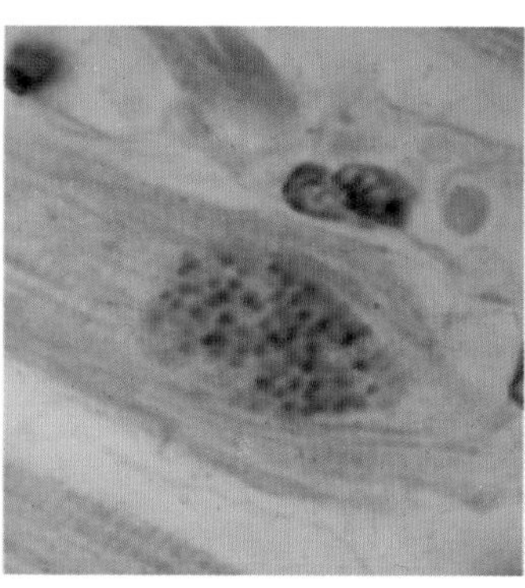

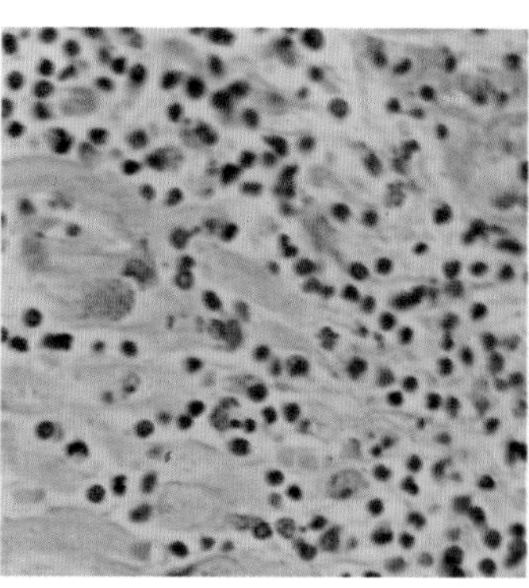

88-1 Toxoplasmosis of the heart in a 27-year-old man with acute lymphocytic leukemia. His illness was characterized by paroxysmal arrhythmias (atrial fibrillation, atrial tachycardia). He died with ventricular fibrillation; *Toxoplasma gondii* organisms were found in myocardial cells. *Right:* Area of focal myocarditis associated with *T. gondii* organisms. *Left:* Close-up view of the encysted organisms. Hematoxylin and eosin stains: × 275 *(right)*, × 915 *(left)*. *(From Roberts WC, Bodey GP, Vertlake PT: The Heart in Acute Leukemia. A Study of 420 Autopsy Cases. Am J Cardiol 21:388, 1968. Reproduced with permission from the publisher and author.)*

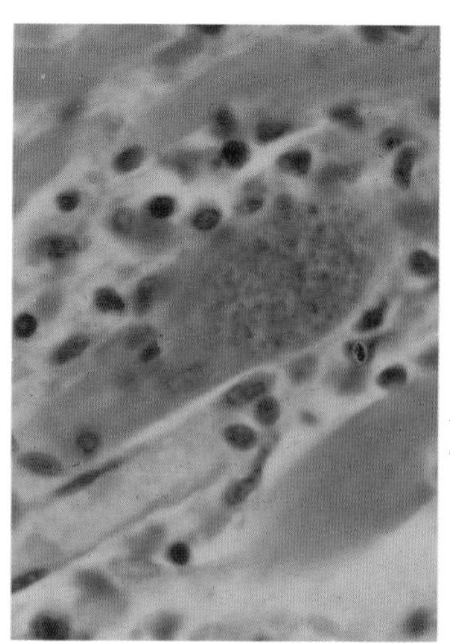

88-4 *Trypanosoma cruzi* in its leishmanial state parasitizing the sarcoplasm of the myocardial cell. The surrounding fiber edema and acute inflammatory reaction are indicative of rupture of the myocardial cell. Hematoxylin and eosin stains: × 125. *(Courtesy of Dr. M. Gravanis, Professor of Pathology, Emory University School of Medicine.)*

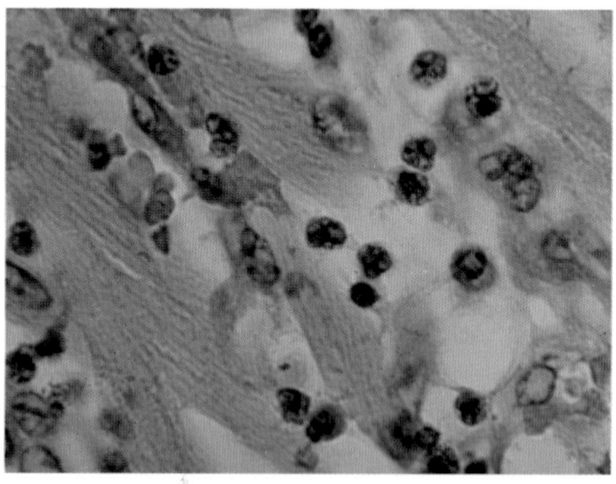

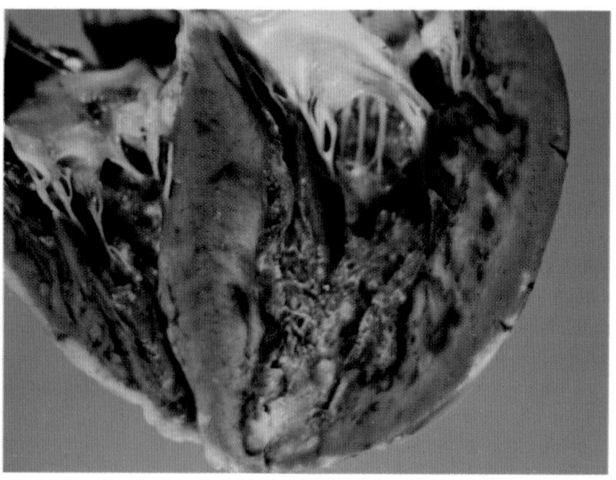

88-2 Trichinosis. Photomicrograph of eosinophilic myocarditis *(upper)* and gross specimen showing left ventricular extensive mural thrombosis *(lower)* in a 46-year-old woman who was well until 13 days before death when she noted fever, headache, neck stiffness, myalgias, dizziness, and pleuritic chest pain. These symptoms worsened, and 3 days before death she was hospitalized. She appeared acutely ill, febrile, and had tachycardia (120 beats per minute). The neck was rigid and the proximal limb muscles very tender. The leukocyte count was 11,000 per cubic millimeter, and the blood smear disclosed 38 percent eosinophils. The ECG was normal except for sinus tachycardia; chest roentgenogram disclosed no abnormalities. She was found dead in bed. After death, it was learned that she often ate raw meat. At necropsy, the heart weighed 260 g; its myocardial walls were filled with extravasated inflammatory cells, mainly eosinophils. Hematoxylin and eosin stain; × 860 *(upper)*. *(From Andy JJ, O'Connell JP, Daddario RC, et al: Trichinosis causing extensive ventricular mural endocarditis with superimposed thrombosis. Evidence that severe eosinophilia damages endocardium. Am J Med, 63:824, 1977. Reproduced with permission from the publisher and author.)*

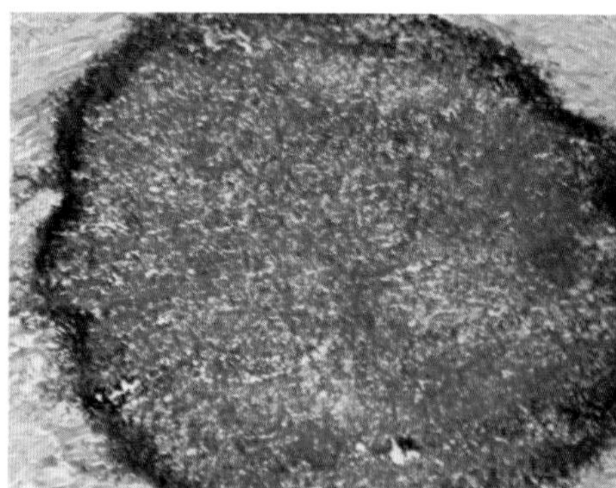

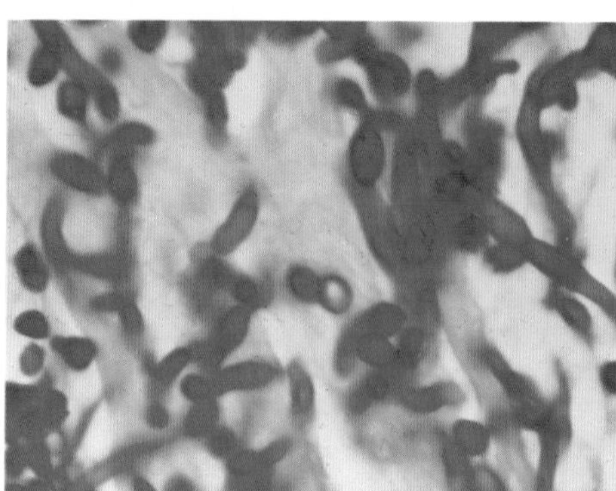

88-3 Cardiac candidiasis in a 20-year-old man with acute myeloblastic leukemia. Gross myocardial abscesses were present in the left and right ventricular free walls, ventricular septum, and papillary muscles. Large myocardial abscess containing massive numbers of *Candida* organisms *(upper)*. Close-up of the *Candida* organisms *(lower)*. Periodic acid Schiff stains: × 12 *(upper)*, × 320 *(lower)*. *(From Ihde DC, Roberts WC, Marr KC, et al: Cardiac Candidiasis in Cancer Patients. Cancer, 41:2364, 1978. Reproduced with permission from the publisher and author.)*

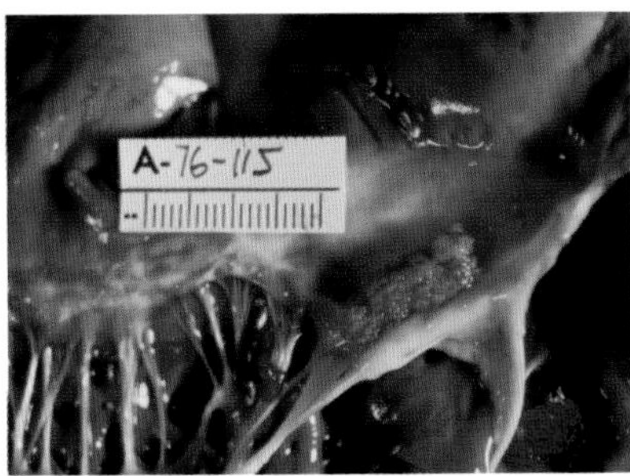

94-1 Typical vegetation of nonbacterial thrombotic endocarditis, found at necropsy in a cachectic patient who died with disseminated lung cancer.

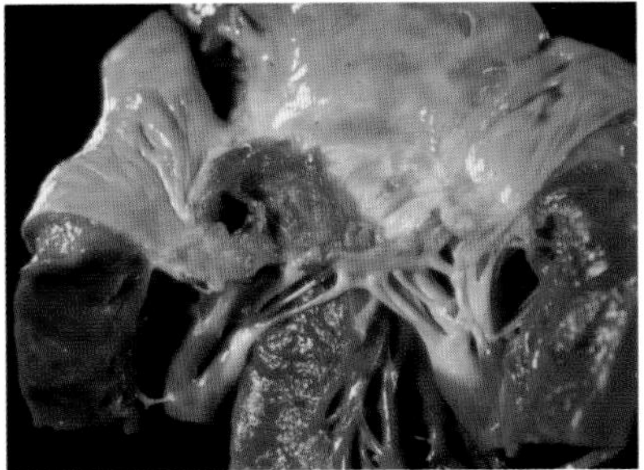

94-2 Typical vegetation of bacterial endocarditis, complicated by perforation of the anterior mitral valve leaflet. Note that the valve shows preexisting chronic rheumatic disease, with thickening, deformity, and fusion of chordae tendineae.

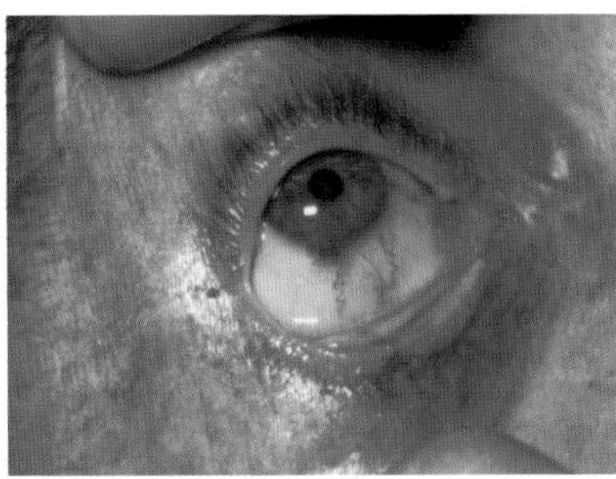

94-3 Typical conjunctival petechia in a patient with SBE due to *Streptococcus sanguis.*

The consequences of embolization from the vegetation shown in a patient with subacute bacterial endocarditis (SBE).

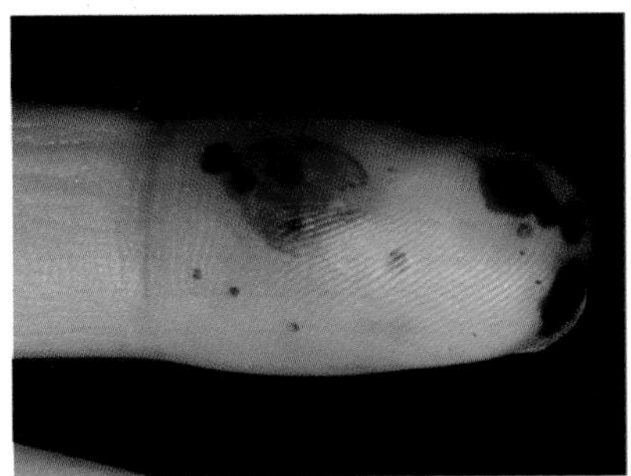

94-4 Ischemic, hemorrhagic, and pustular lesions on the extremities in acute *Staphylococcus aureus* endocarditis.

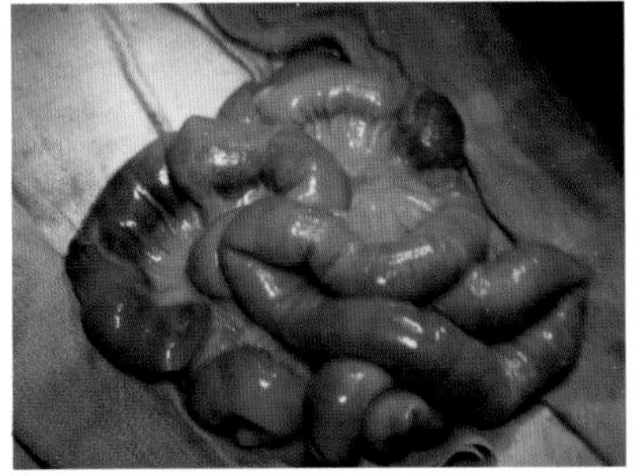

94-5 Segmental ischemia and necrosis in the gut, presenting as acute abdomen.

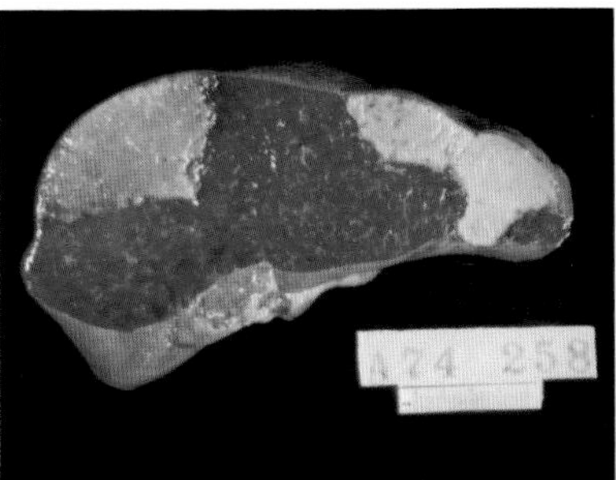

94-6 Infarctions in the spleen.

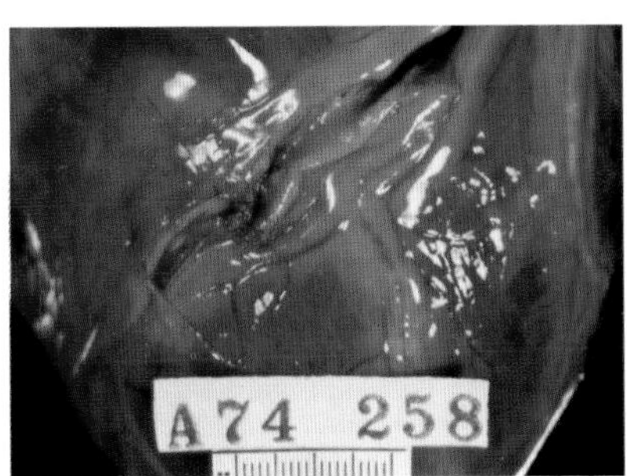

94-7 An infected embolus in a coronary artery.

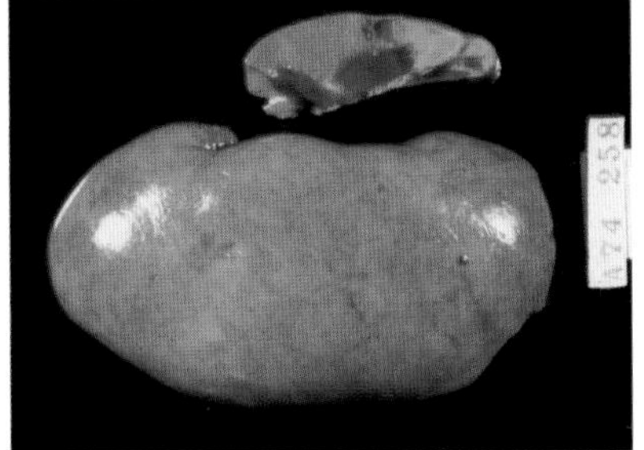

94-8 Kidney from a case of subacute bacterial endocarditis, showing two abnormalities: (1) typical ischemic infarctions due to emboli, and (2) swelling and petechiae ("flea-bitten kidney") due to immune-complex glomerulonephritis.

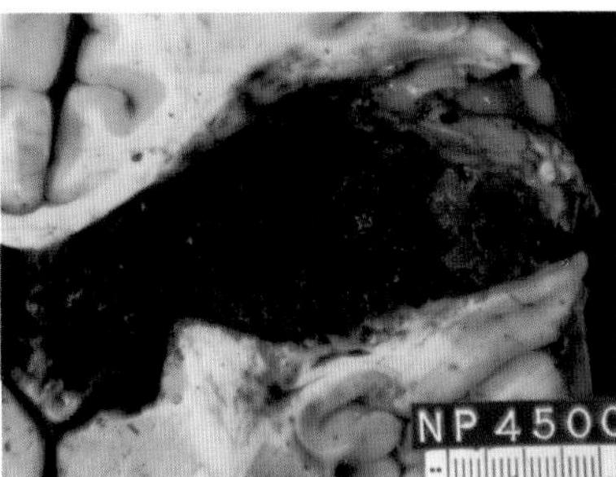

94-9 Massive cerebral hemorrhage with intraventricular extension due to rupture of a small, peripheral mycotic aneurysm (arrowed). The patient had been *bacteriologically* cured of *Staphylococcus epidermidis* endocarditis several weeks previously. Cultures of the blood, valve, and aneurysm taken at necropsy were negative.

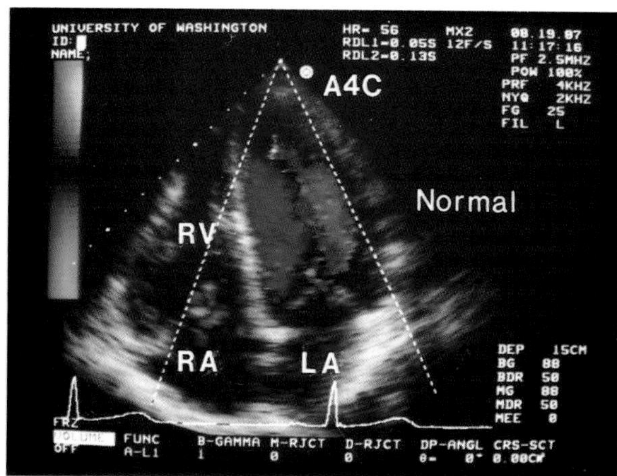

130-1 Normal left ventricular diastolic flow by color Doppler flow imaging, apical four-chamber view. Left ventricular inflow toward the transducer is coded in red. This flow stream passes along the distal lateral wall, rounds the apex, and moves toward the aortic valve. Because of its direction, the resulting vortex (a normal phenomenon) is coded blue. LA, left atrium; RA, right atrium; RV, right ventricle; A4C, apical four-chamber.

130-2 Assessment of aortic regurgitant severity using color Doppler flow imaging.

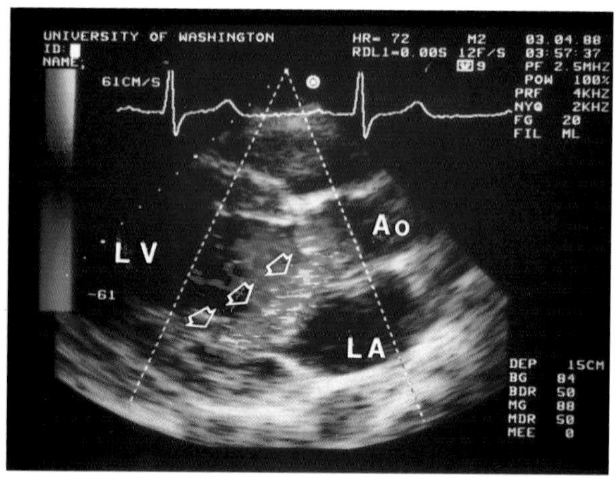

A. Moderately severe aortic regurgitation appears as a moderately broad jet of turquoise, blue, orange, and red pixels (open arrows) that passes obliquely down the anterior mitral leaflet and well into the left ventricular cavity. Apical views showed extension of this jet to the cardiac apex.

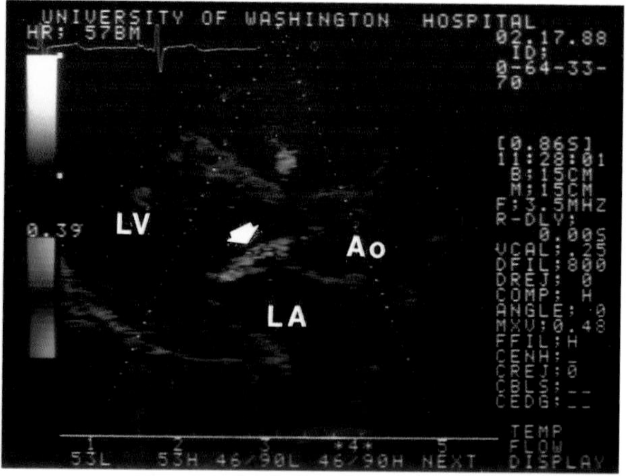

B. Mild aortic regurgitation is denoted by a narrow jet (solid arrow) confined to the outflow tract. LV, left ventricle; Ao, aorta; LA, left atrium.

130-3 Assessment of mitral regurgitant severity by color Doppler flow imaging, intraoperative long-axis images.

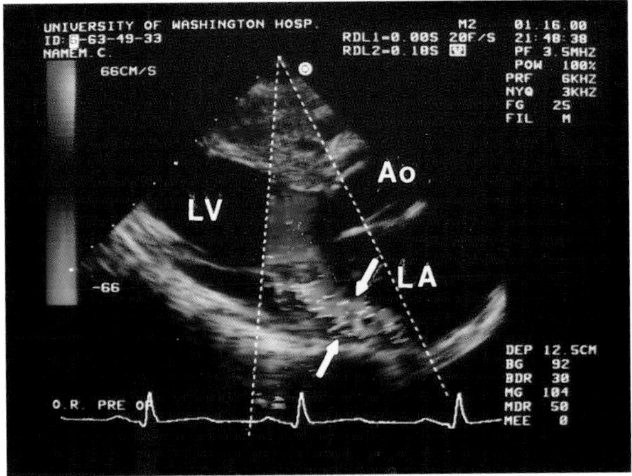

A. In a patient with ischemic left ventricular dysfunction, moderately severe mitral regurgitation appears as a relatively broad mosaic jet (solid arrows) extending well back into the left atrium.

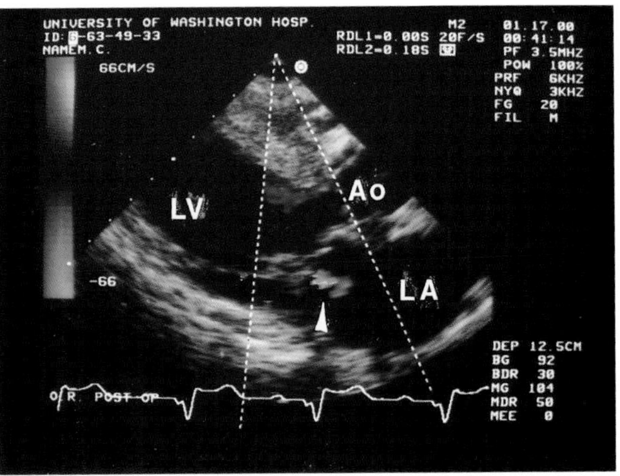

B. After insertion of a mitral annuloplasty ring, the regurgitant jet is localized (arrowhead), indicating only mild residual regurgitation.

130-4 Ostium secundum atrial septal defect, visualized by color Doppler flow imaging in a low parasternal short-axis orientation. *Top.* Anatomic image demonstrating the aorta, left atrium, right atrium, and right ventricle. Although the chambers of the right side of the heart are large, dropout of echoes in the interatrial septum in this view may occur because the atrial septum and the ultrasound beam are nearly parallel. *Bottom.* The color flow jet shows a central aliased portion (coded blue) surrounded by unaliased flow (coded red-orange). This clearly proves the existence of a large secundum defect with left-right shunting. PSAX, parasternal short axis; Ao, aorta; LA, left atrium; RA, right atrium; RV, right ventricle.

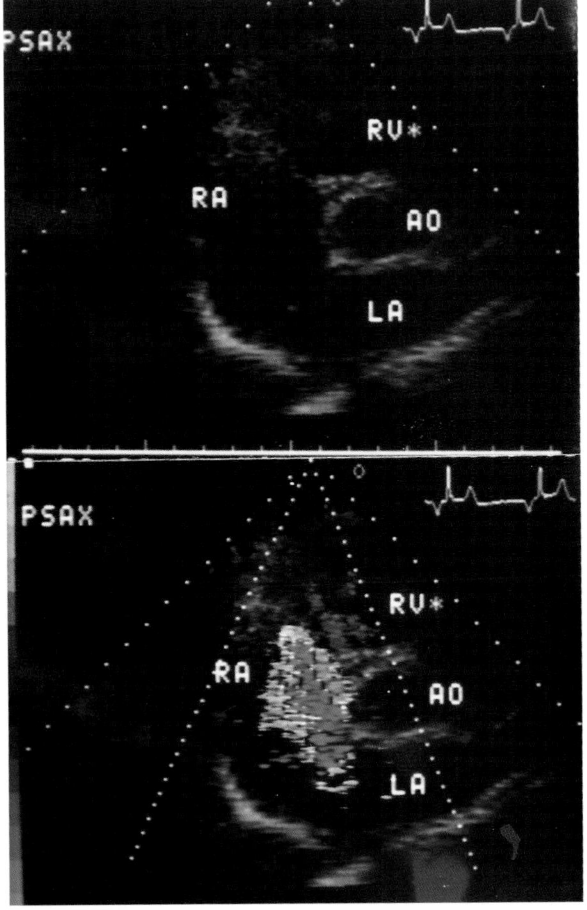

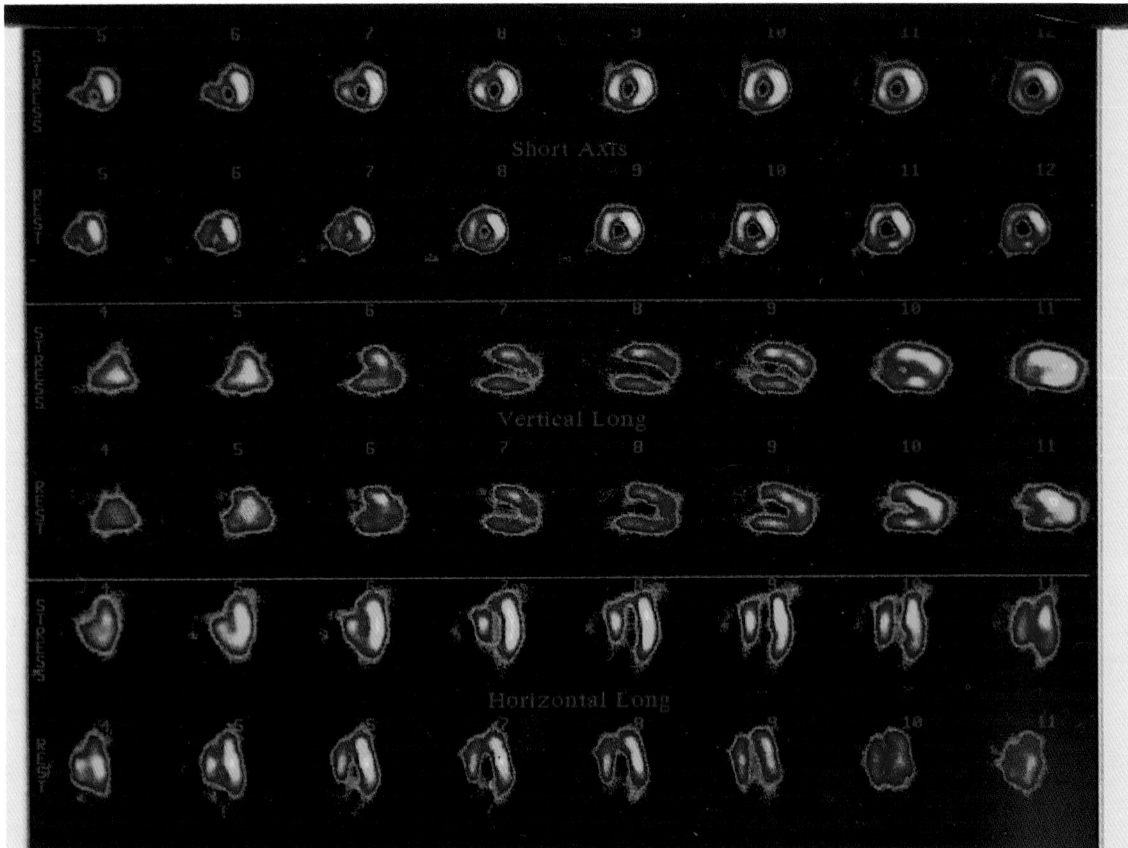

134-1 Tomographic slices two pixels in thickness from a TC-99m sestamibi study in standard display. The top two rows show short axis tomographs from apex to base with stress above, rest below. There is an anteroseptal and apical defect in the exercise stress tomographic slices that fills in partially, but not completely, on the rest injection tomographic slices. Because the patient had no history of prior MI and the defect fill-in was almost complete, except for the apex, the scan was read as showing ischemia in the distribution of the LAD.

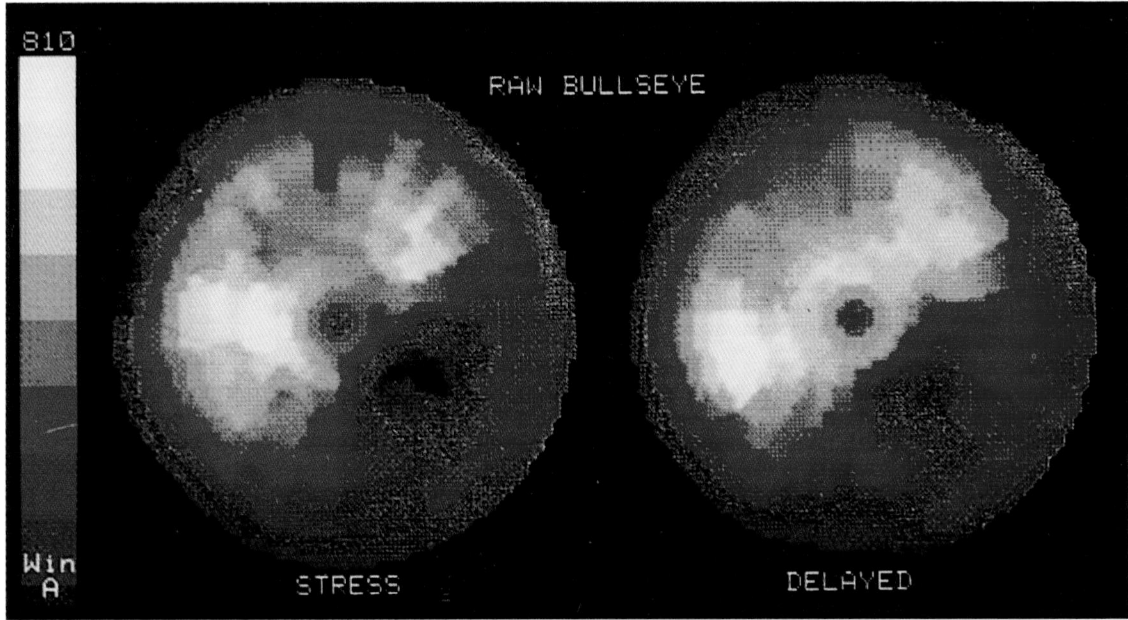

134-2 Polar "bull's-eye" displays of Tc-99m sestamili distribution at stress *(left)* and at rest *(right)*. The short axis tomographic slices are telescoped from the apex at the center to the base at the perimeter. The anterior wall extends from about 10 o'clock to 1 o'clock, the lateral wall from 1 o'clock to 4 o'clock, the inferior wall from 4 o'clock to 7 o'clock, and the septum from 7 o'clock to 10 o'clock. There is an inferolateral defect that shows moderate "fill-in" at the defect edges following tracer injection at rest. *(Courtesy of Dr. Gordon DePuey.)*

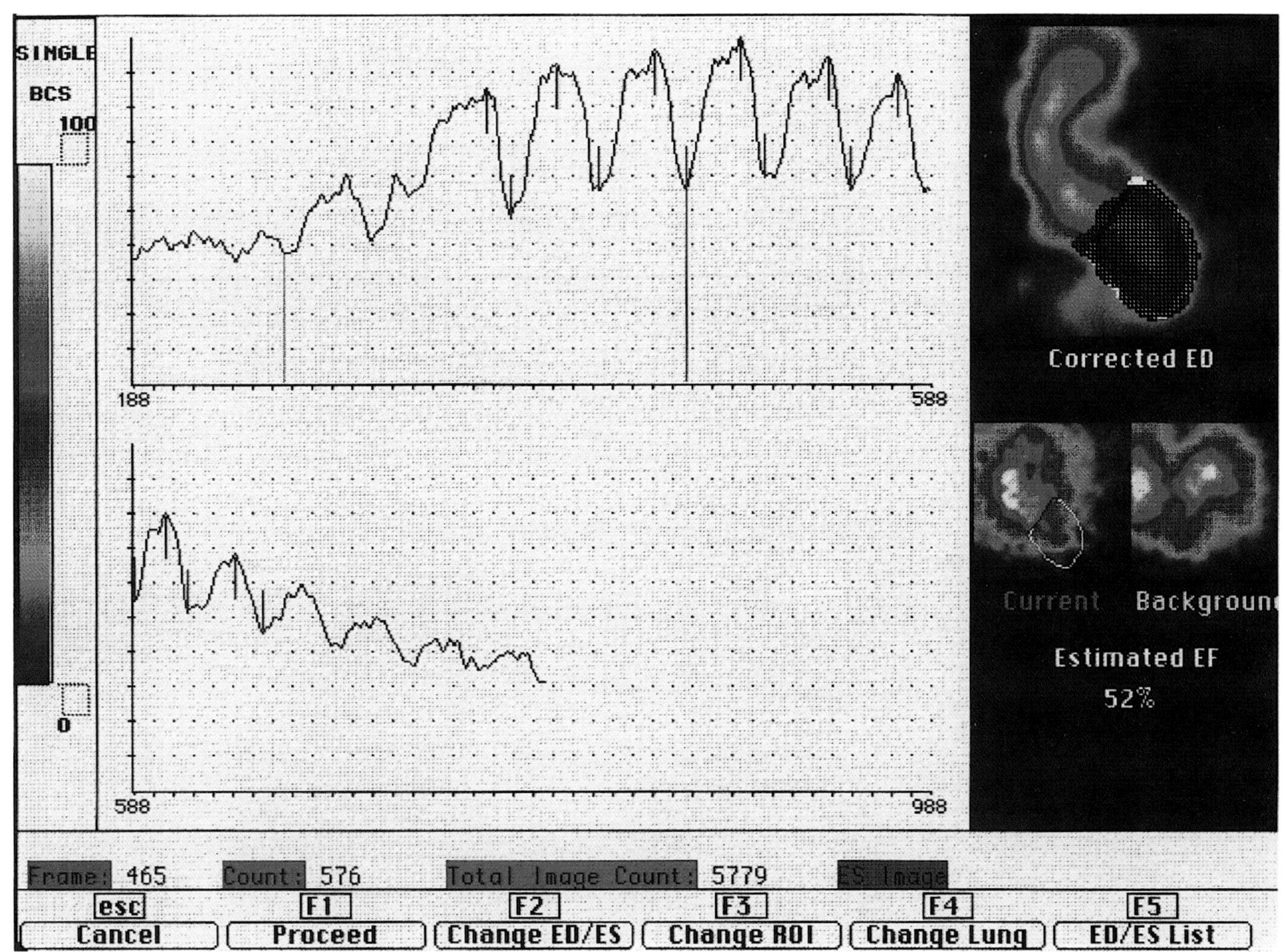

134-3 Method of calculation of the left ventricular ejection fraction using the first pass technique and a multi-crystal camera. The left ventricular time activity curve is displayed in the left panel with vertical markers denoting the background frame and the end-diastoles and end-systoles selected. The images in the right panels show the left ventricular region selected *(top)* and the count distribution in the end-systolic and background frames *(bottom panels)*.

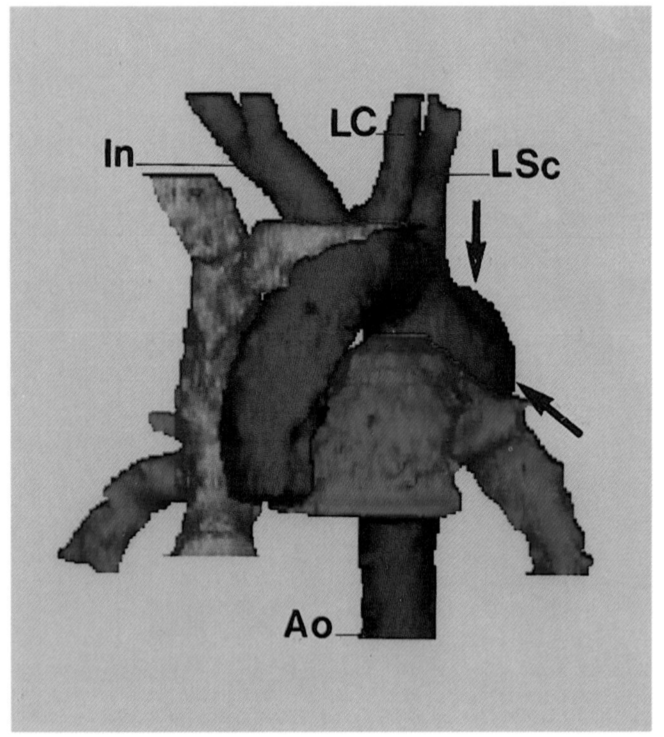

A

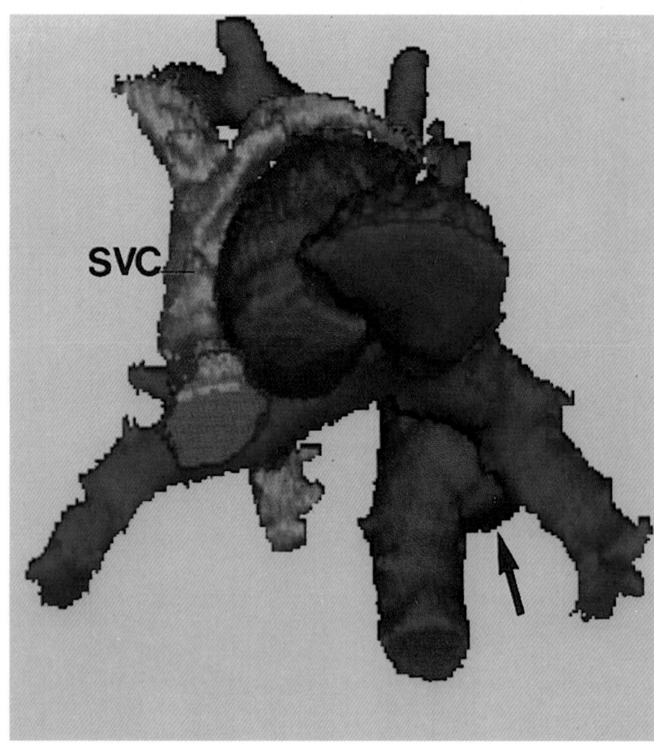

B

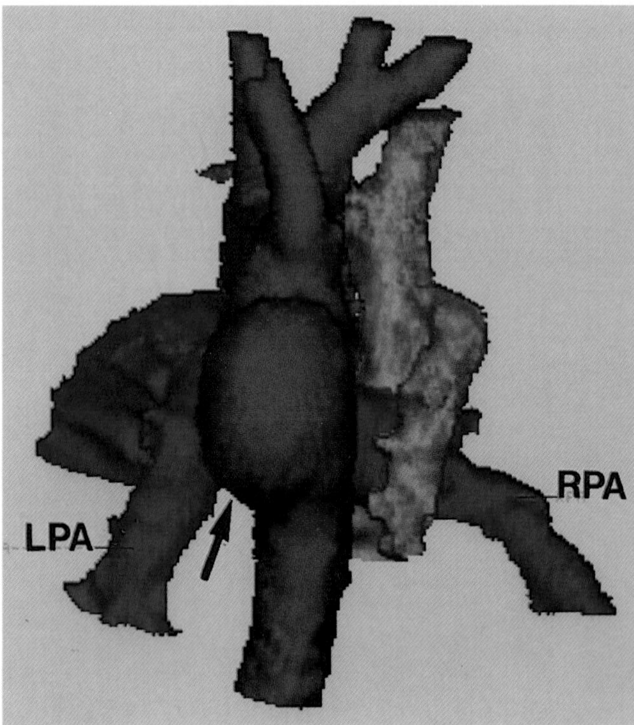

C

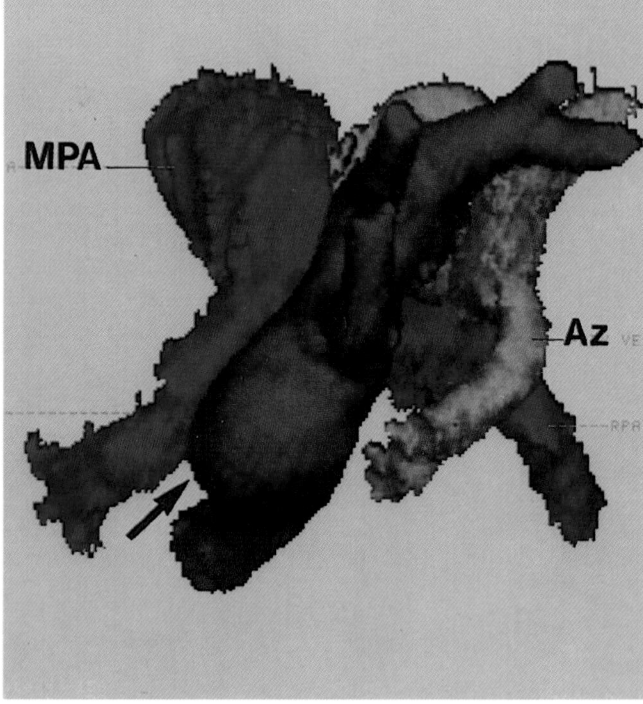

D

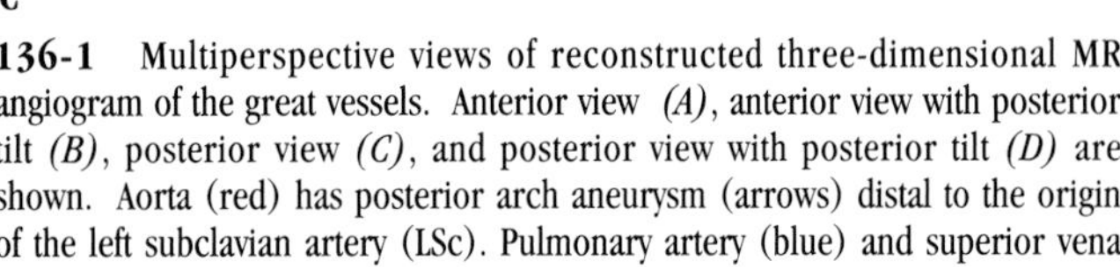

136-1 Multiperspective views of reconstructed three-dimensional MR angiogram of the great vessels. Anterior view *(A)*, anterior view with posterior tilt *(B)*, posterior view *(C)*, and posterior view with posterior tilt *(D)* are shown. Aorta (red) has posterior arch aneurysm (arrows) distal to the origin of the left subclavian artery (LSc). Pulmonary artery (blue) and superior vena cava (gray) are also shown. (Ao = aorta; In = innominate artery; LC = left carotid artery; LSc = left subclavian artery; SVC = superior vena cava; MPA = main pulmonary artery; LPA = left pulmonary artery; RPA = right pulmonary artery; AZ = azygous vein.) *(Courtesy James Parks, M.D., and Scott Sheppard, M.S., Emory University School of Medicine.)*

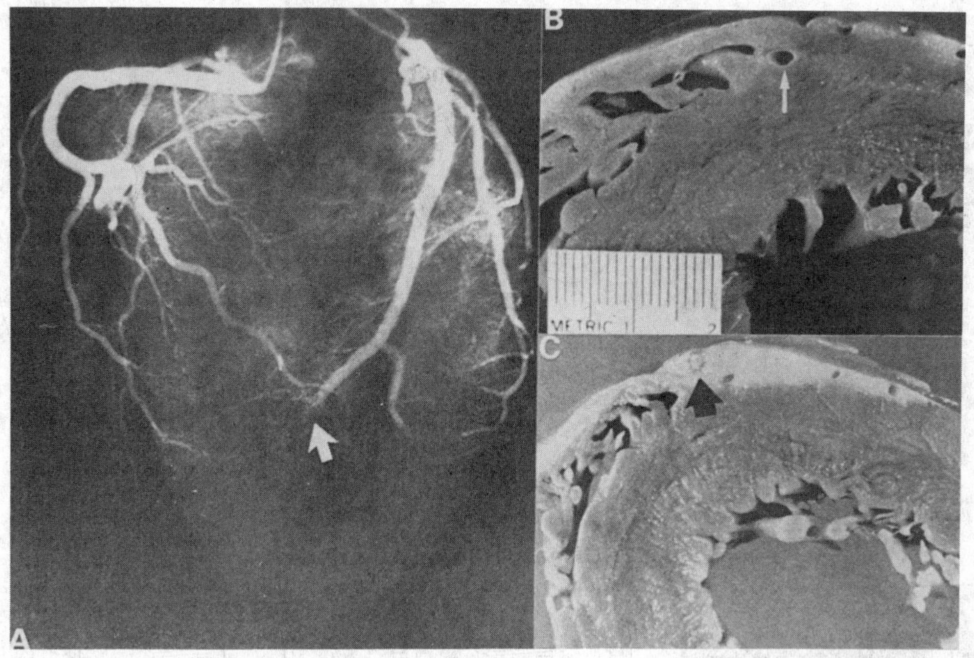

FIGURE 64-18 Coronary artery embolus. (*A*) Postmortem coronary angiogram showing normal epicardial coronary arteries except for sudden cutoff of the distal third of the left anterior coronary artery (arrow). (*B*) Portion of anterior left ventricle and proximal left anterior descending coronary artery showing normal artery. (*C*) Site (arrow) of embolic occlusion of the left anterior descending coronary artery. The remaining distal left anterior descending, right, left circumflex and left main coronary arteries were normal. (From Waller.[1] Reproduced with permission from the publisher, editor, and author.)

sence of collaterals. An embolus traveling to a previously diseased coronary artery is more likely to impact proximally. Emboli to the left main coronary arteries are rare but usually fatal (see Fig. 64-19).[39]

CORONARY ARTERY DISSECTION

Separation of the media by hemorrhage with or without an associated intimal tear is termed "coronary artery dissection." The medial separation forces the intimal-medial layer (wall of true channel) toward the true coronary lumen and produces distal myocardial ischemia/infarction (Figs. 64-21 and 64-22). Coronary artery dissections may be primary or secondary. Secondary coronary artery dissections are more frequent, especially those associated as an extension from aortic root dissection.[5] Primary coronary artery dissections may occur spontaneously or as a consequence of coronary angioplasty or angiography, cardiac surgery, or chest trauma. Most spontaneous coronary artery dissections occur in women (postpartum, commonly) and may be associated with coronary arterial wall eosinophils.[40] The left ante-

TABLE 64-4

Etiology of Coronary Artery Emboli

Natural	Coronary artery
Vegetation	Plaque rupture
Active infective endocarditis (native valve)	Thrombus dislodgement
Active infective endocarditis (prosthetic valve)	Iatrogenic
Mural endocarditis	Cardiac surgery (ostial cannalization, prosthetic valve, patch repair)
Noninfective (marantic) endocarditis	Cardiac catheterization and angiography (catheter thrombus, catheter fragments)
Calcific deposit	Coronary angioplasty and thrombolysis
Aortic valve stenosis	Prosthetic valves (thrombus, vegetation, occluders, leaflets, cloth covering, struts)
Mitral valve stenosis	Cardioversion (left atrial thrombus, left ventricular thrombus)
Intracardiac thrombus	Cardiac resuscitation (thrombus)
Left ventricle (myocardial infarction, cardiomyopathy, fibroelastosis with mural thrombus, ventricular aneurysm)	"Paradoxical"
Left atrium-appendage (low cardiac output states)	Congenital heart disease (atrial septal defect, ventricular septal defect)
Left atrium-body (mitral stenosis, native or prosthetic)	Probe patent foramen ovale defect (thrombophlebitis, right atrial catheters)
Pulmonary veins (mitral stenosis)	Pulmonary hypertension (acquired atrial septal defect)
Intracardiac tumor	
Primary (myxoma)	
Secondary (extension from pulmonary veins, lymphatic extension, direct extension)	

SOURCE: Waller.[1] Reproduced with permission from FA Davis, Philadelphia

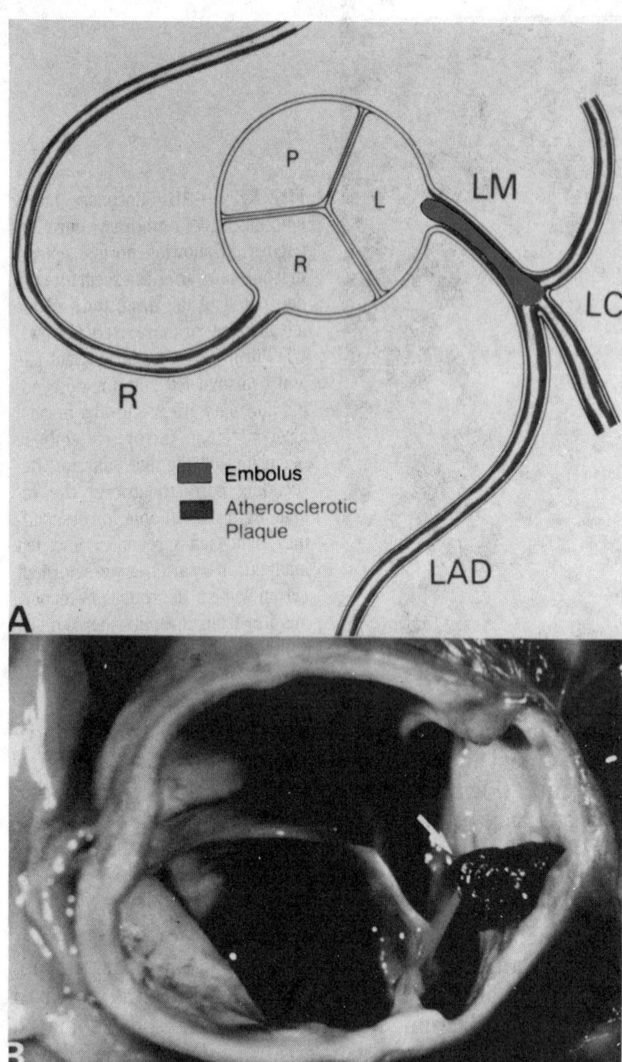

FIGURE 64-19 Coronary artery embolism. (*A*) Diagram showing location and extent of occlusion of the left main (LM) coronary artery by an embolus. (*B*) Photograph of aortic root showing embolus protruding from the LM coronary ostium (arrows). LAD = left anterior descending; LC = left circumflex; R = right. (From Waller et al.[38] Reproduced with permission from the publisher and author.)

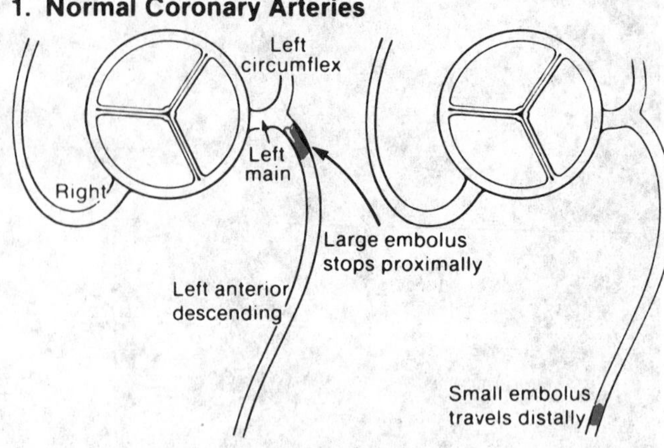

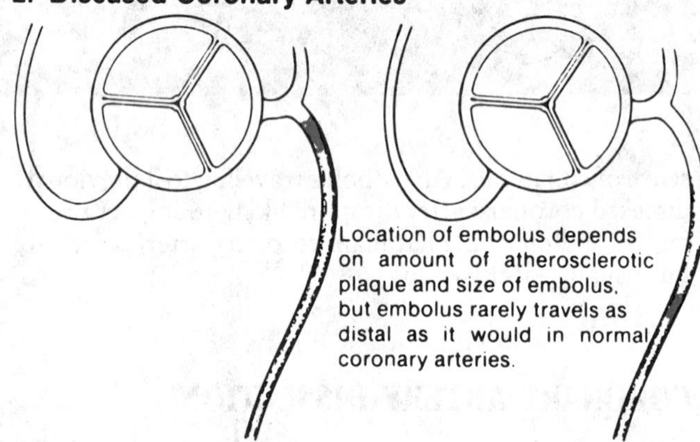

FIGURE 64-20 Coronary emboli in normal and diseased coronary arteries. (From Waller.[1] Reproduced with permission from the publisher, editor, and author.)

rior descending artery is the most frequently involved artery. Systemic hypertension does not appear to be a significant risk factor.[36] Spontaneous coronary artery dissection may result in sudden death or acute myocardial infarction and subsequent death. Parenthetically, localized and limited coronary artery dissection (i.e., intimal-media tear) appears necessary for a clinically successful coronary artery balloon angioplasty procedure.[41,42] (See also Chaps. 70 and 71.)

CORONARY ARTERY SPASM

Coronary artery luminal narrowing produced by spasm has been associated with angina pectoris, acute myocardial infarction, and sudden death (Chap. 59). Despite the extensive clinical information about coronary artery spasm, relatively few necropsy data are available from these patients[43–56] (Table 64-5). Contraction of the smooth-muscle cells in the coronary artery wall may contract in response to various neurologic and pharmacologic stimuli and temporarily reduce the vessel lumen. Various postulates exist as the exact mechanism of spasm, but the specific pathogenesis of this disorder is unknown[54] (see also Chap. 56). Enhanced α-adrenergic tone[57] and various vasoactive substances (histamine, catecholamines, prostaglandins, thromboxane A_2)[58,59] are presently thought to be relevant factors. Roberts and colleagues[54] and Isner[55] have reviewed the necropsy findings in 13 previously reported cases and in 3 new cases (see Table 64-5) (Figs. 64-23, 64-24). Most of the 13 previous patients with clinical evidence of spasm had significant fixed coronary luminal narrowing due to atherosclerotic plaque, although coronary angiograms during life did not recognize these lesions which were later identified at necropsy.[55] In one of the original patients described by Prinzmetal and colleagues,[43] both major epicardial coronary arteries were "markedly sclerotic," and the "posterior coronary artery" was 80 percent narrowed. Of the subsequent 12 necropsy patients, 10 had at least one major artery severely narrowed by artherosclerotic plaque at necropsy (Table 64-5). In the three necropsy patients with clinical spasm described by Rob-

TABLE 64-5

Previous Necropsy Findings in Patients with Coronary Artery Spasm

	Clinical Findings				Necropsy Findings				
			Evidence of Spasm		Coronary Narrowing			Myocardial	
Authors	Sex	Age	ECG	Angio	R	LAD	LC	Necrosis	Fibrosis
Prinzmetal[43]	M	58	I	—	80	—	—	0	0
Petetz[44]	M	50	AS	—	0			?VS	0
Gianelly[45]	F	49	I	0		mild		0	VS
Silverman[46]	M	40	A	—	0	100	0	VS	
Dhurandhar[47]	M	52	IL	R	75	0	0	0	0
Cosby[48]	F	46	I	0	67	0	0	—	—
Cheng[49]	M	60	A	0	0	0	0	0	0
Donsky[50]	F	44	I	0		severe		0	0
Wiener[51]	F	67	I	R	R	0	0	PW	PW
	M	48	A	LAD	0	0	0	AW	0
Bharati[52]	F	33	I	0	R	0	0	0	0
Maseri[53]	M	52	A	LC	0	100	90	0	PW
	M	52	A	0	50	80	40	0	APW
Roberts[54]	F	32	+	LAD	>75	>75	<50	0	0
	M	57	+	LAD	<75	>75	<25	0	0
	M	61	+	R	>75	>75	<75	0	0

A = anterior; Angio = angiography; AS = anteroseptal; AW = anterior free wall; ECG = electrocardiography; F = female; I = inferior; IL = inferolateral; LAD = left anterior descending; LC = left circumflex; M = male; PW = posterior wall; R = right; VS = ventricular septum; O = none.

SOURCE: Isner and Donaldson.[5] Reproduced with permission from the publisher, editor, and author.

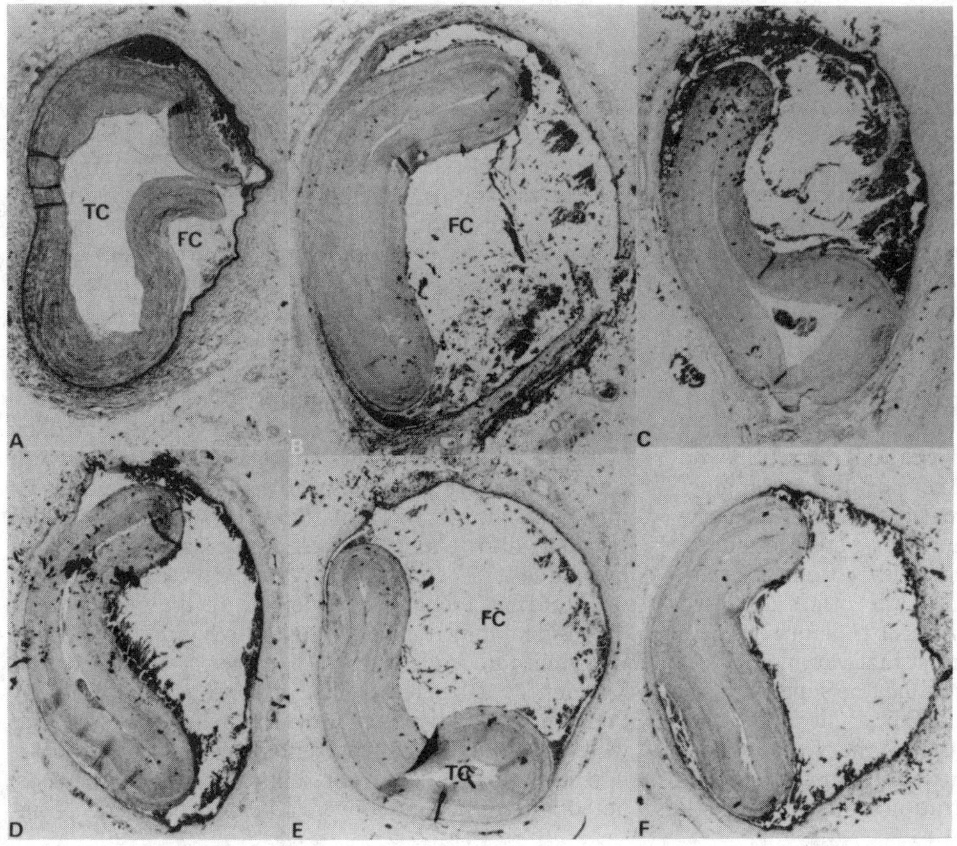

FIGURE 64-21 Coronary artery dissection. Serial cross-section (*A–F*) showing dissection of the left anterior descending coronary artery. The true channel (TL) is severely compromised by external compression from the false channel (FC) ("dissection channel"). (From Waller.[1] Reproduced with permission from the publisher, editor, and author.)

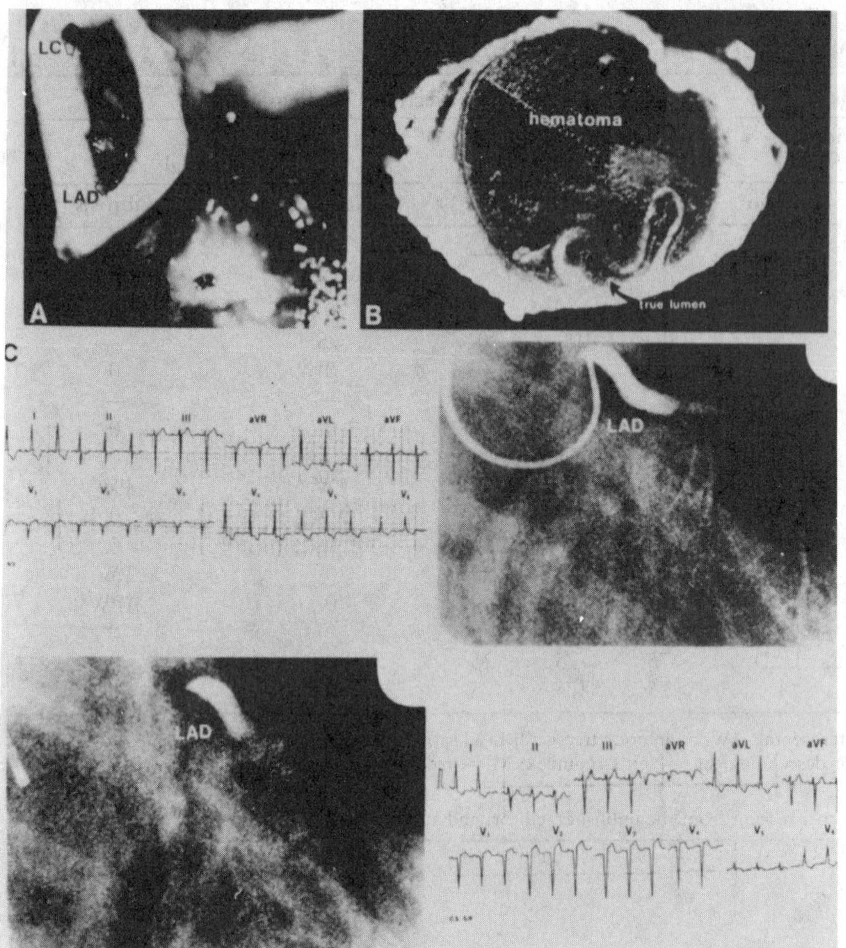

FIGURE 64-22 Coronary artery dissection. Occlusion of the left anterior descending (LAD) artery due to dissection. (*A*) The LAD and left circumflex (LC) are seen through the left main artery. (*B*) Cross-section shows hematoma in false channel severely narrows native (true channel) unobstructed lumen. (*C*) Sequential electrocardiograph and angiographic findings. (From Isner and Donaldson.[53] Reproduced with permission from the publisher, editor, and author.)

erts and colleagues,[54,55] all three had severe luminal coronary narrowing by atherosclerotic plaque at necropsy in at least the artery in which spasm had been demonstrated during life (see Figs. 64-2, 64-3). In two of these patients, the coronary arteries were devoid of calcific deposits. In the remaining patient, histologic sections of the left anterior descending artery at the site of spasm disclosed luminal concentric plaque that had a predominance of smooth muscle cells. These findings suggest that the plaque may have been responsive to pharmacologic and neurologic stimuli compared with "garden-variety" fibrotic and calcified atherosclerotic plaque (Fig. 64-24). El-Maraghi and Sealey[60] reported a patient with normal angiograms and documented myocardial infarction who had "intimal ridges" observed on postmortem angiography. These authors interpreted these ridges as "necropsy evidence of spasm." Isner[61] has observed similar ridges at necropsy in a patient with coronary artery spasm. Histologic examination of the ridges disclosed that they were typical atherosclerotic plaque.[61] These clinical pathologic findings suggest that varying degrees of dynamic muscular contraction may be superimposed upon fixed atherosclerotic lesions. The ability and extent of "dynamic augmentaton" of the coronary wall to contract is presumably related to the amount of smooth muscle present.[55] The demonstration by Isner and colleagues[62] that coronary artery smooth muscle depletion ("medial attenuation") accompanies advanced degrees of luminal narrowing by atherosclerotic plaque suggests that the potential for augmentation of coronary wall tone at the sites of severe luminal narrowing is diminished. Factor and colleagues[63] have recently suggested that medial "contraction" bands may represent a morphologic-histologic marker for arteries that have spasm during life (see also Chap. 57).

Eccentric atherosclerotic plaques have a segment of disease-free wall that has preserved media and presumably has the potential for spasm[62] (see also Chap. 56). This form of stenosis has recently been evaluated by Hangartner and colleagues[65] in relation to patients with clinical coronary spasm, unstable and stable angina pectoris, and episodes of silent myocardial ischemia. Of 448 segments narrowed >75 percent in cross-sectional area by plaques, 15 percent had a variable arc of disease-free wall (normal media) (≥16 percent of the perimeter of the residual lumen). This is similar to figures reported by Quyyumi and colleagues[66] (15 percent), and Hort and associates[67] (20 percent) but in contrast to studies by Freudenberg[68] and Saner[69] in which an arc of disease-free wall was found in 70 percent of cases. This disease-free coronary segment represents a site of "vasospastic potential" and could convert a hemodynamically insig-

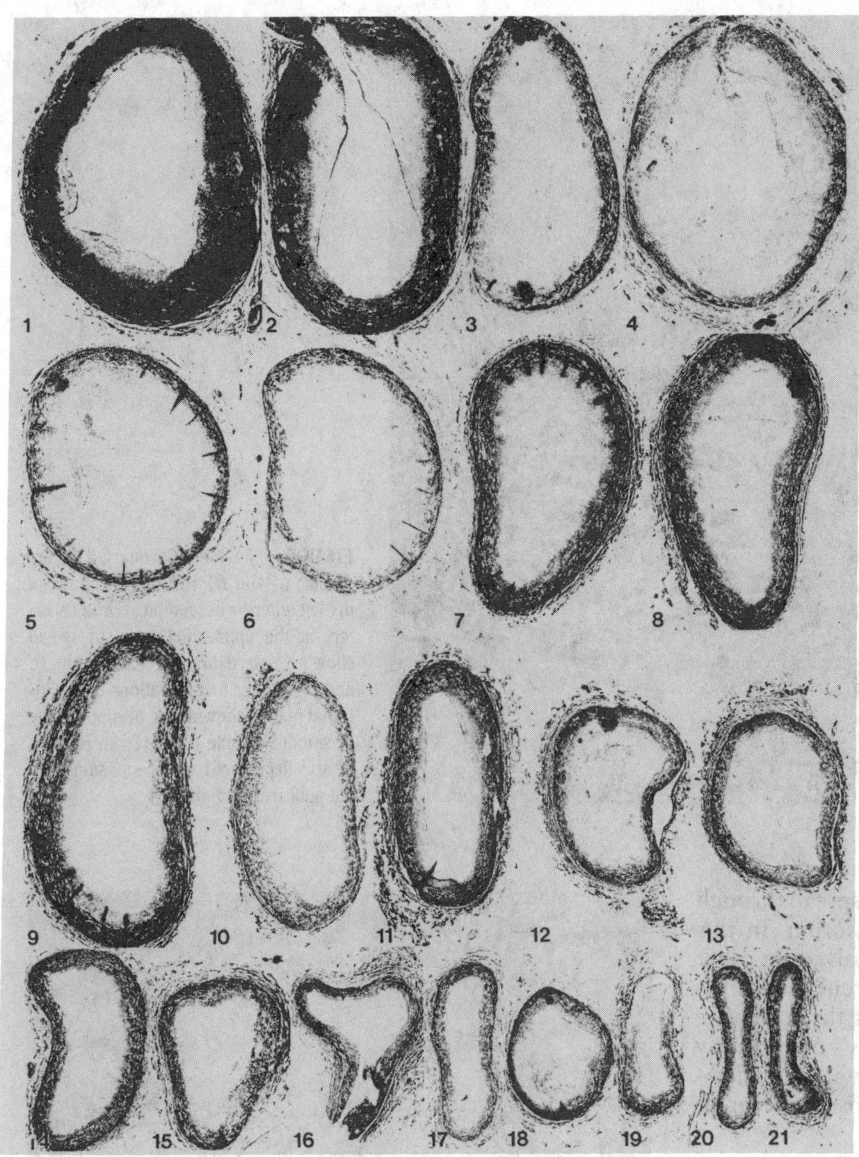

FIGURE 64-23 Coronary artery spasm. Composite of coronary artery cross-sections of a patient with coronary spasm during life. Clinical spasm involved segments 3–7. Severe atherosclerotic plaque is seen in 8 of the 21 segments. (From Roberts et al.[52] Reproduced with permission from the publisher and author.)

nificant (<50 percent cross-sectional area) lesion or borderline significant (70 percent cross-sectional area) lesion to a hemodynamically significant (>75 percent) lesion.

CORONARY ARTERY TRAUMA

Coronary artery trauma may produce myocardial ischemia and/or acute myocardial infarction. Traumatic injury may result from a nonpenetration blunt chest wall injury (e.g., steering wheel injury), penetration trauma (e.g., laceration from stab wound or bullet), or during coronary angiography (e.g., inadvertent ligation, laceration, intimal dissection), or during coronary angiography (e.g., laceration, dissection, embolus). Nonpenetrating trauma may produce coronary injury and subsequent myocardial infarction as a result of coronary dissection, contusion and thrombosis, fistula formation, and/or coronary artery aneurysm formation.[5] Extensive coronary artery dissections appear more likely to occur as the result of catheter or cannula injury in normal or nearly normal arteries as opposed to coronary arteries with severe atherosclerotic plaque (see also Chap. 112).

CORONARY ARTERY ARTERITIS (VASCULITIS)

Epicardial coronary arteries (vasculitis) is a rare event that has been reported in several conditions (Table 64-6) (Figs. 64-2 to 64-5). The resulting coronary injury may directly lead to myocardial ischemia/infarction with or without associated coronary artery thrombosis. Baroldi[24] provides a useful classification of the arteritis conditions based upon type of coronary artery route of entry. Coronary arteritis may result from direct extension from adjacent organ or tissue infections (e.g., epicardial or myocardial abscess from aortic valve endocarditis, pericardial tuberculosis) (Fig. 64-25). In this situation, the coronary artery adventitial layer is initially involved. Coronary

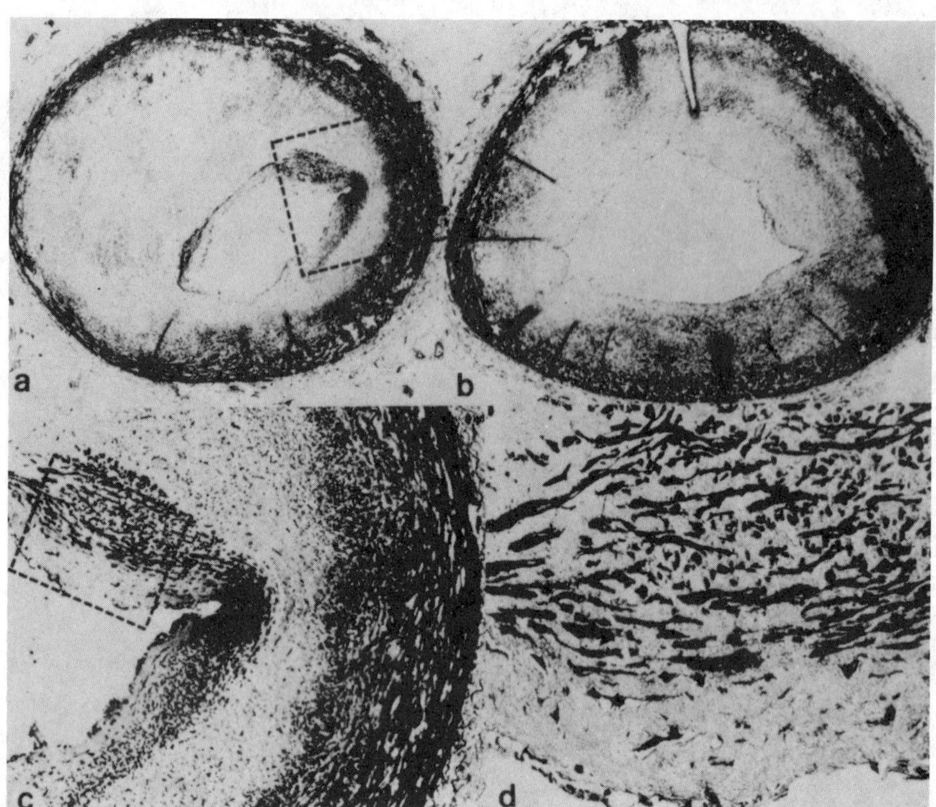

FIGURE 64-24 Coronary artery spasm. (*A* and *B*) Histology sections of the left anterior descending coronary artery at the approximate site of spasm showing severe luminal narrowing. (*C* and *D*) Higher magnifications of the internal plaque showing the predominance of smooth muscle cells. (From Roberts et al.[52] Reproduced with permission from the publisher and author.)

arteritis may result from a hematogenous spread through the coronary lumen or through vasa vasorum. In this situation, the intimal layer is initially involved. In other vasculitides, the exact mechanism of vascular origin is not understood. Baroldi[24] also considers the following morphologic-histologic findings as "signs" of coronary arteritis: (1) focal artery necrosis with or without calcification; (2) acute coronary artery thrombosis or recanal-

TABLE 64-6

Some Conditions Associated with Coronary Artery Arteritis (Vasculitis)
Tuberculosis[24, 4, 71]
Polyarteritis nodosa[24, 74, 4, 5, 72, 73]
Giant cell arteritis[24, 74–76]
Rheumatic fever[24, 77, 80]
Systemic lupus erythematosus[24, 4, 5, 36, 78, 79, 81–83]
Burger's disease (thrombo-angiitis obliterans)[24, 84, 85]
Wegener's granulomatosis[5, 78, 86]
Salmonella[4, 89]
Leprosy[4]
Mucocutaneous lymph node syndrome[93–95]
Takayasu's disease[80, 96, 97]
Typhus[90]
Infective endocarditis[88]
Rheumatoid arthritis[36, 97–99]
Ankylosing spondylitis[100]
Syphilis[5, 36, 87]

SOURCE: Waller.[1] Reproduced with permission from FA Davis, Philadelphia.

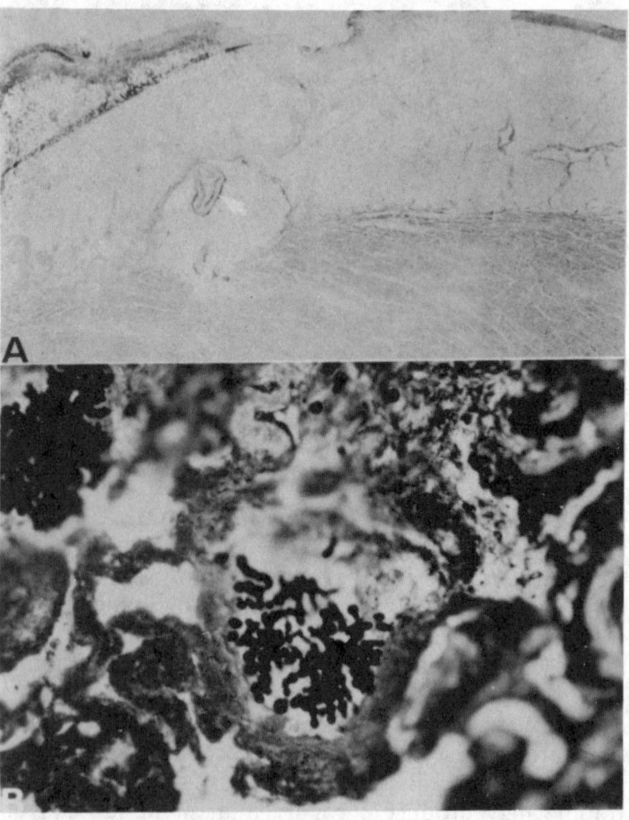

FIGURE 64-25 Coronary arteritis. (*A*) Extensive yeast (Candida) percarditis which involves the adventitial layer of a branch of a major subepicardial coronary artery (arrow). (*B*) Closeup shows the budding yeast organisms (GMS stain). (From Waller.[1] Reproduced with permission from the publisher, editor, and author.)

ized thrombus unassociated with underlying atherosclerotic plaque; (3) rupture of the vessel wall unassociated with trauma or an interventional procedure; (4) coronary artery wall thickening with secondary luminal narrowing; and (5) wall thickening with aneurysm formation.[70] Specific coronary lesions also may be seen in specific systemic diseases (e.g., polyarteritis nodosa) (see also Chap. 103).

Tuberculosis

Tuberculosis arteritis is seen chiefly in patients with pericardial or myocardial lesions. Specific coronary artery granuloma may involve the adventitia, the intima, or the entire wall. [24,71]

POLYARTERITIS NODOSA

Polyarteritis nodosa is probably the most common cause of coronary angiitis. It is a systemic necrotizing vasculitis that affects medium and small vessels. Of 66 cases studied by Holsinger and colleagues,[72] 41 (62 percent) had involvement of the epicardial coronary arteries, and 41 also had myocardial infarcts of varying size. The coronary lesions resemble necrotizing vascular lesions found elsewhere with an acute cellular phase with destruction of the media and internal elastic membrane and subsequent intimal proliferation and scar in the healed phase. The coronary artery may dilate to form small berrylike aneurysms, become occluded by thrombus, or rupture, producing fatal pericardial tamponade[73](see Chap 103).

GIANT CELL ARTERITIS

Giant cell arteritis chiefly affects the temporal and other cranial arteries, but coronary artery involvement and myocardial infarction have been reported by Ainsworth and associates.[74,75] The arterial wall lesion is a granulomatous inflammation with giant cells found along a degenerated internal elastic membrane.[74] The intima becomes greatly thickened, and ultimately the vessel is converted into a fibrous cord. Luminal thrombus may also be present. Of 16 cases of temporal arteritis reported by Harrison,[76] only 1 case involved the epicardial coronary arteries.

SYSTEMIC LUPUS ERYTHEMATOSUS

Pericardial and myocardial involvement are common complications in systemic lupus erythematosus (SLE). Several young patients with SLE and absent coronary atherosclerosis have suffered acute myocardial infarction.[78,79,81,82] Necropsy examination of the coronary arteries in these patients showed intimal fibrous proliferation, which may represent healed arteritis. In a 16-year-old girl with SLE studied by Bonfiglio and colleagues,[81] acute myocardial infarction was associated with recent thrombotic occlusion of all three major arteries. Tsakraklides and colleagues[83] studied a 29-year-old woman with SLE and fatal acute myocardial infarction who had severe coronary atherosclerosis. This case suggested that SLE and other conditions causing arteritis may predispose to premature coronary atherosclerosis. Smaller intramyocardial coronary arteries are involved frequently in the diffuse vasculitis with fibrinoid necrosis and fibrosis.[36] Glucocorticosteroids used in the treatment of SLE may also predispose to premature coronary atherosclerosis (see Chap. 103).

Burger's Disease (Thromboangiitis Obliterans)

In a few patients with Burger's disease, the epicardial coronary arteries have shown focal polymorphonuclear infiltrates, histiocytes, and giant cells with or without coronary artery thrombosis,[84] or with only coronary thrombosis.[85] In 30 cases studied by Saphir,[84] only 1 patient had coronary involvement, whereas in 19 cases studied by Averbuck and Silbert,[85] 6 patients had coronary thrombosis (see also Chap. 124).

WEGENER'S GRANULOMATOSIS

Wegener's granulomatosis is a necrotizing vasculitis commonly affecting renal and pulmonary systems. Fibrinoid necrosis of the small and medium-sized coronary arteries has been reported by Parrillo and Fauci.[78] Larger epicardial coronary artery occlusion and myocardial infarction was reported by Gatenby and colleagues.[86]

INFECTIOUS DISEASES

Various infectious diseases have been associated with coronary arteritis: syphilis,[36,87] infective endocarditis,[88] salmonellosis,[4,89] typhus,[90] and leprosy.[4] Syphilis is stated to be one of the most common infectious diseases affecting the coronary arteries.[5] Up to one quarter of patients with tertiary syphilis may have ostial stenosis.[87] The first 3 to 4 mm of the left and right coronary arteries may be involved with an obliterative arteritis.[36] Rarely does a coronary artery contain a gumma.[36] Angina and acute myocardial infarction may result from syphilitic coronary disease[87] (see Chap. 106). Malarial parasites and parasitized red blood cells also may plug larger coronary arteries.[91] Schistosoma haematobium has been found in a major epicardial coronary artery unassociated with myocardial infarction.[92]

Mucocutaneous Lymph Node Syndrome (Kawasaki's Disease)

This acute febrile illness affects infants and young children. In about 20 percent of patients, a vasculitis of the coronary vasa vasorum leads to coronary arterial aneurysm formation, thrombosis, and myocardial infarction. Death may result from myocardial infarction or ventricular arrhythmia in 1 percent to 2 percent. Late presentation with myocardial infarction secondary to dislodged aneurysmal thrombus may also occur.[93,94] Occasionally, death may result from rupture of a coronary artery aneurysm (see also Chap. 10).

Takayasu's Disease (Pulseless Disease)

This disease results in granulomatous panarteritis and fibrosis of the aorta and its large branches, which, in turn, leads to luminal narrowing.[5] Involvement of the coronary artery ostia and proximal main coronary artery segments has been described in several patients.[80, 96,97] Angina pectoris and acute myocardial infarction may result from these coronary lesions (see also Chap. 124).

Rheumatoid Disease

Rarely, arteritis and intimal thickening associated with rheumatoid disease severely narrow major epicardial coronary arteries. More commonly, diffuse arteritis involves smaller coronary arteries (including conduction system vessels) in 10 to 20 percent of necropsy patients with rheumatoid arthritis.[97–100] Small myocardial vessels may also be narrowed severely in patients with ankylosing spondylitis. Grismer and colleagues have described a patient with ankylosing spondylitis who had occlusion of the left main ostium.[100]

METABOLIC DISORDERS NARROWING CORONARY ARTERIES

Specific metabolic substances may accumulate in the walls of large and small coronary arteries as a result of inborn errors of metabolism. The deposition of this material may severely narrow the coronary artery lumen and produce acute myocardial infarction.[5] Inherited inborn errors of metabolism that are known to affect major epicardial coronary arteries include Hunter's and Hurler's diseases (mucopolysaccharidoses).[100–103] The involvement of the coronary arteries in these disorders may be so severe as to occlude totally the vessel and to produce myocardial ischemia/infarction. Other disorders of metabolism such as primary oxalosis,[104] Fabry's disease,[36] Sandhoff's disease (gangliosidoses),[105] and homocystinuria may affect smaller coronary vessels by severe intimal proliferation[106] (see also Chap. 96).

INTIMAL PROLIFERATION

Fibrous hyperplasia of the coronary arteries may severely narrow the lumen and produce myocardial ischemia/infarction. The process may be associated with mediastinal irradiation,[107] fibromuscular hyperplasia of the renal arteries,[5] the use of methysergide,[22, 108] ostial cannulation during cardiac surgery, or follow aortic valve replacement.[23, 109] Up to 50 percent of patients undergoing cardiac transplantation develop significant epicardial coronary artery luminal narrowing or total occlusion by intimal fibrous proliferation within 3 to 5 years after transplantation.[110] Myocardial infarction and sudden death may result from this "chronic rejection" process. Fibrosis of the intramural vessels may also occur. Intimal damage from immunologic rejection is believed to be the basis for the accelerated intimal fibrous hyperplasia involving the coronary arteries (see also Chap. 32).

A similar histologic picture of intimal fibrous proliferation is seen in epicardial coronary arteries late after undergoing percutaneous balloon angioplasty (Fig. 64-26).[41, 42] Waller and colleagues[111] recently reported intimal fibrous proliferation of the left main coronary artery occurring late after balloon angioplasty of a lesion in the proximal left anterior descending coronary artery. They postulated that the left main intimal reaction (identical to that seen at the left anterior descending coronary artery angioplasty site) resulted from balloon rubbing of the intimal surface and/or extension of the fibrous process from the angioplasty dilation site (see also Chaps.70 and 71).

EXTERNAL COMPRESSION

External compression of the epicardial coronary arteries may result in severe luminal narrowing and progressive myocardial ischemia. External compression of a major epicardial coronary artery has been reported in patients with sinus of Valsalva aneurysms and epicardial tumor metastases.[112, 113] Myocardial bridging (external muscle compression during ventricular systole) has been reviewed earlier.

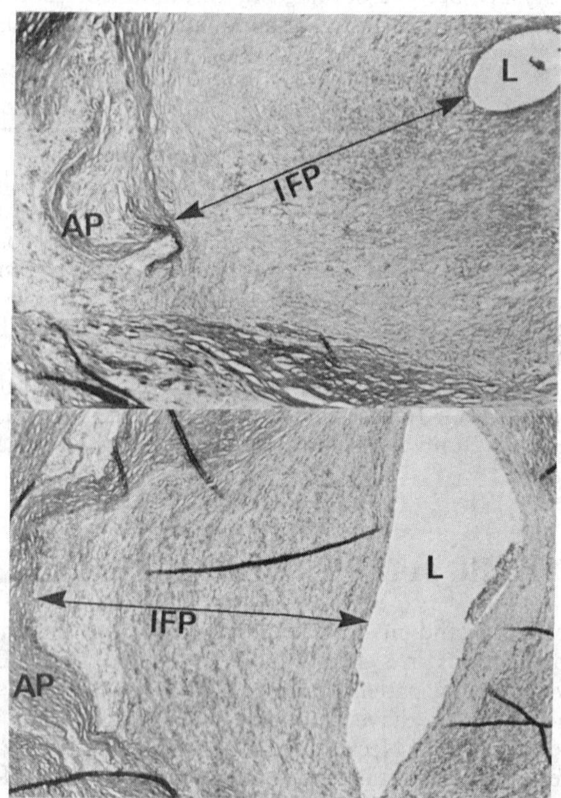

FIGURE 64-26 Intimal fibrous proliferation. Severe luminal narrowing of the left anterior descending coronary artery by intimal fibrous proliferation (IFP) several months after percutaneous balloon angioplasty. The IFP superimposes underlying atherosclerotic plaque (AP). L = lumen. (From Waller.[1] Reproduced with permission from the publisher, editor, and author.)

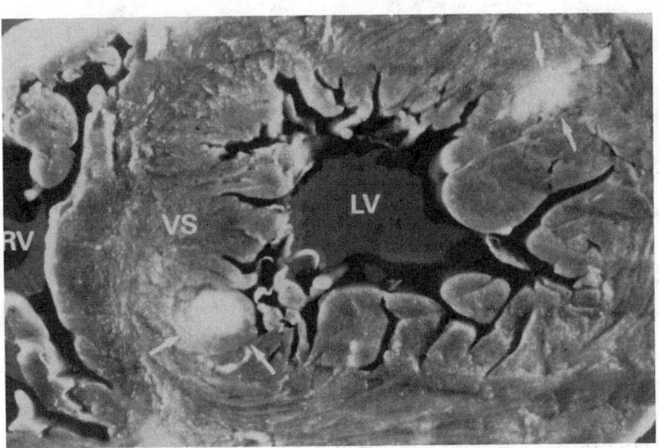

FIGURE 64-27 Metastatic deposits mimicking myocardial infarction. Transverse section of cardiac ventricle showing two discrete myocardial metastatic deposits of lymphoma. These whitish deposits may be mistakenly interpreted as healed myocardial infarctions in a patient with clean epicardial coronary arteries. LV = left ventricle; RV = right ventricle; VS = ventricular septum. (From Waller.[1] Reproduced with permission from the publisher, editor, and author.)

METASTATIC IMPLANTS

Myocardial metastatic lesions from various tumors (carcinomas, sarcomas, lymphomas) may mimic a healed myocardial infarct at necropsy (Fig. 64-27). The discrete location or locations of these metastatic deposits generally are unrelated to specific coronary arterial supply zones, and the lesions are usually surrounded by normal myocardium. These two gross observations suggest the lesions are metastatic tumor implants rather than healed myocardial infarcts (see also Chap. 111).

CORONARY ARTERY THROMBOSIS WITHOUT UNDERLYING ATHEROSCLEROTIC PLAQUE (THROMBOSIS IN SITU)

Thrombotic occlusion of the coronary system that is unassociated with underlying atherosclerotic plaque may be seen with several hematologic diseases: thrombocytopenia purpura,[35] leukemia,[114] polycythemia vera,[113] sickle cell anemia,[36] and primary thrombocytosis.[116] Occasionally, acute myocardial infarction may be the initial manifestation of these hematologic disorders. A main factor responsible for the myocardial ischemia in these conditions is blockage of small intramural coronary vessels by platelet aggregates.[117] These platelet aggregates initially may form in the major coronary arteries, then embolize distally.

SUBSTANCE ABUSE (COCAINE)

Cocaine abuse is now a major health hazard; more than 22 million Americans have tried cocaine at least once, and 5 million are current users.[118] Recent reports have documented that cocaine abuse can result in myocardial ischemia and infarction in the absence of coronary artery disease.[118–124] Cocaine-induced coronary artery vasoconstriction has been reported in patients following intranasal cocaine.[123, 125–128] (See also Chap. 110.)

Several instances of coronary artery thrombosis and spasm have been reported in patients with cocaine abuse. Acute coronary thrombosis in association with cardiac events (angina, acute myocardial infarction, sudden death) has been reported.[118, 121, 126–128] In some instances, there is underlying atherosclerotic plaque; in others, the coronary arteries are normal. Coronary thrombosis occurring in coronary arteries free of atherosclerotic plaque suggests the role of cocaine-induced spasm or possible primary thrombogenicity of cocaine or its metabolites.[125]

Coronary spasm has been associated with cocaine usage and has been postulated as a mechanism of myocardial infarction in those users with clean coronary arteries.[118, 129–134] Simpson and Edwards[135] reported coronary artery narrowing in a young patient without underlying atherosclerotic plaque. The coronary artery was severely narrowed by fibrointimal proliferation that was attributed to underlying coronary artery spasm that caused focal vessel endothelial injury, platelet adherence, and aggregation. Platelets liberate platelet-derived growth factor (PDGF) which can induce intimal proliferative lesions. In patients with underlying coronary plaque, cocaine-induced spasm also may produce endothelial disruption at the surface of the plaque and promote platelet aggregation and further vasoconstriction from the release of platelet prostaglandins.[136] (See also Chap. 110.)

MYOCARDIAL OXYGEN DEMAND–SUPPLY DISPROPORTION[4]

In this category are disease states in which there is failure to deliver adequate oxygen to the myocardium over a prolonged period, or increased myocardial wall tension requiring increased oxygen supply. The classic example of the first situation is carbon monoxide poisoning,[4] which has been associated with extensive nontransmural infarction in the presence of normal epicardial coronary arteries. Prolonged shock (from any cause) can also result in extensive nontransmural necrosis and frequently is associated with transmural necrosis of the papillary muscles. The classic example of the situation in which there is increased myocardial wall tension requiring increased coronary oxygen supply is aortic valve stenosis[4] (Chap. 79). In the face of increased oxygen demand (increased muscle mass), coronary blood supply is limited by poor perfusion resulting from the lower coronary arterial pressure. In addition, poor perfusion results from the high coronary resistance caused by increased wall pressure on the intramural coronary arteries and the high left ventricular end-diastolic pressure from a stiff ventricle.[4] Excessive myocardial oxygen demand exceeding supply (resulting in myocardial ischemia/infarction) may also be seen in thyrotoxicosis.[137]

INTRAMURAL CORONARY ARTERY DISEASE (SMALL VESSEL DISEASE)

Acute myocardial infarction may result from abnormally thickened or totally occluded intramural coronary arteries in the presence of normal extramural (epicardial) coronary arteries. A few of the conditions in this category include: (1) hypertrophic cardiomyopathy; (2) diabetes mellitus; (3) amyloid heart disease; (4) neuromuscular disorders (Friedreich's ataxia, progressive muscular dystrophy); (5) cardiac transplantation; (6) rheumatoid arthritis; (7) collagen-vascular disorders (scleroderma, systemic lupus erythematosus); (8) metabolism abnormalities (mucopolysaccharidoses, gangliosidoses); and (9) polyarteritis nodosa.

NORMAL EPICARDIAL CORONARY ARTERIES

Relatively few necropsy reports have evaluated patients with acute myocardial infarction who had angiographically normal coronary arteries and normal coronary arteries at necropsy.[3, 4,137–143] Of 100 consecutive necropsy cases of acute myocardial infarction (AMI) studied by Baroldi and colleagues,[3] 7 percent had infarcts without evidence of coronary luminal narrowing. Eliot and colleagues[3] studied 10 necropsy patients with a typical picture of AMI who died within 25 days of onset of symptoms. The coronary arterial systems showed minimal or no luminal narrowing by atherosclerosis. No thrombotic material was observed in the coronary arteries despite the fact that the AMI was 2 days old in five patients and 3 to 4 days old in three other patients. Numerous theories have been proposed to explain the occurrence of AMI in these patients: coronary artery spasm; coronary artery disease in vessels too small to be visualized angiographically (i.e., small vessel disease); coronary artery thrombosis, or embolus, with subsequent clot lysis, retraction, or reconciliation; congenital coronary anomalies; and myocardial oxygen supply–demand disproportion.

REFERENCES

1. Waller BF: Atherosclerotic and nonatherosclerotic coronary artery factors in acute myocardial infarction. In: Pepine CJ (ed): *Acute Myocardial Infarction*. Philadelphia, FA Davis, 1989:29–104.
2. Alpert JS, Braunwald E: Acute myocardial infarction: Pathological, pathophysiological and clinical manifestations. In: Braunwald E (ed): *Heart Disease. A Textbook of Cardiovascular Medicine*, Philadelphia, Saunders, 1984:1262–1300.
3. Eliot RS, Baroldi G: Necropsy studies in myocardial infarction with minimal or no coronary luminal reduction due to atherosclerosis. *Circulation* 1974; 49:1127–1131.
4. Cheitlin MD, McAllister HA, deCastro CM: Myocardial infarction without atherosclerosis. *JAMA* 1975; 231:951–959.
5. Baim DS, Harrison DC: Nonatherosclerotic coronary heart disease (including coronary artery spasm). In: Hurst JW, et al (eds): *The Heart*, 5th ed. New York, McGraw-Hill, 1982:1158–1170.
6. Engel HJ, Torres C, Page HL: Major variations in anatomical origin of the coronary arteries: Angiographic observations in 4,250 patients without associated congenital heart disease. *Cathet Cardiovasc Diag* 1975; 1:157–161.
7. Roberts WC: Major anomalies of coronary arterial origin seen in adulthood. *Am Heart J* 1986; 111:941–963.
8. Levin DC, Fellows KE, Abrams HL: Hemodynamically significant primary anomalies of the coronary arteries. Angiographic aspects. *Circulation* 1978; 58:25–34.
9. Roberts WC, Siegel RJ, Zipes DP: Origin of the right coronary artery from the left sinus of Valsalva and its functional consequences: Analysis of 10 necropsy patients. *Am J Cardiol* 1982; 49:863–868.
10. Waller BF: Exercise related sudden death in young (age < 30 years) and old (age > 30 years) conditioned athletes. In: Wenger NK (ed): *Exercise and the Heart* (2d ed). *Cardiovascular Clinics*. Philadelphia, FA Davis, 1985:9–73.
11. Menke DM, Jordan MD, Sut CH, Aust CH, Waller BF: Isolated and severe left main coronary atherosclerosis and thrombosis: A complication of acute angle takeoff of the left main coronary artery. *Am Heart J* 1986; 112:1319–1320.
12. Virmani R, Chun PKC, Goldstein RE, Rabinowitz M, McAllister HA: Acute takeoffs of the coronary arteries along the aortic wall and congenital coronary ostial valve-like ridges. Association with sudden death. *J Am Coll Cardiol* 1984; 3:766–771.
13. Joswig BF, Warren SE, Vieweg WV, Hagan AD: Transmural myocardial infarction in the absence of coronary arterial luminal narrowing in a young man with single coronary arterial anomaly. *Cathet Cardiovasc Diag* 1978; 4:297–301.
14. Foster L, Waller BF, Pless JE: Hypoplastic coronary arteries and high takeoff position of the right coronary artery. *Chest* 1985; 88:299–301.
15. Foster L, Waller BF: Nonatherosclerotic fibrous ridges: A previously unrecognized cause of ostial left main stenosis. *J Indiana Med Assoc* 1983; 76:682–683.
16. Vlodaver Z, Amplatz K, Burchell HB, Edwards JE: *Coronary Heart Disease. Clinical, Angiographic and Pathologic Profiles*. New York, Springer-Verlag, 1976.
17. Alexander RW, Griffith GC: Anomalies of the coronary arteries and their clinical significance. *Circulation* 1956; 14:800–805.
18. Burch HC: Hoher und trichterformiger Ursprung der Herz Kanzarterien. *Beitr Pathol Anal* 1963; 128:139–148.
19. Holt S: Syphilitic ostial occlusion. *Br Heart J* 1977; 39:469–470.
20. Young JA, Sengupta A, Khaja FU: Coronary arterial stenosis, angina pectoris and atypical coarctation of the aorta due to nonspecific arteritis: Treatment, with aortocoronary bypass graft. *Am J Cardiol* 1973; 32:356–361.
21. Rozavi M: Unusual forms of coronary artery disease. In: D Vedt (ed): *Cleveland Clinic Cardiovascular Consultations*. Philadelphia, FA Davis, 1975:25.
22. Hudgson P, Foster JB, Walton JN: Methysergide and coronary artery disease. *Am Heart J* 1967; 74:854–855.
23. Yates JD, Kirsh MM, Sodeman TM, Walton JA, Brymer JF: Coronary ostial stenosis: A complication of aortic valve replacement. *Circulation* 1974; 49:530–534.
24. Baroldi G: Diseases of the coronary arteries. In: Silver MD (ed): *Cardiovascular Pathology*. New York, Churchill Livingstone, 1983:341.
25. Reyman HC: Disertatis de vasis cordis propiis. *Bibl Anat* 1737; 2:366–373.
26. Noble J, Bourassa MG, Petitclerc R, Dyrda I: Myocardial bridging and milking effect of the left anterior descending coronary artery: Normal variant or obstruction? *Am J Cardiol* 1976; 37:933, 993–999.
27. Faruqui AM, AMA, Maloy WC, Felner JM, Schlant RC, Logan WD, Symbas P. Symptomatic myocardial bridging of the coronary artery. *Am J Cardiol* 1978; 41:1305–1310.
28. Visscher DW, Mildes BM, Waller BF: Tunneled ("bridged") left anterior descending coronary artery in a newborn without clinical or morphological evidence of myocardial ischemia. *Cath Cardiovasc Diag* 1983; 9:493–498.
29. Edwards JC, Burnsides C, Swarm RL, Lansing AJ: Arteriosclerosis and extramural portions of coronary arteries in the human heart. *Circulation* 1956; 13:235–241.
30. Polacek P: Relation of myocardial bridges and loops in the coronary arteries to coronary occlusions. *Am Heart J* 1961; 61:44–52.
31. Levin DC, Fellows KE, Abrams HL: Hemodynamically significant primary anomalies of the coronary arteries. Angiographic aspects. *Circulation* 1978; 58:25–34.
32. Kramer JR, Kitazume H, Proudin WI, Sones IM: Clinical signifi-

cance of isolated coronary bridges: Benign and frequent condition involving the left anterior descending artery. *Am Heart J* 1982; 103:283–288.
33. Ishimori T, Raizner AE, Chahine RA, Awdeh M, Luchi RJ. Myocardial bridges in man: Clinical correlations and angiographic accentuation with nitroglycerin. *Cathet Cardiovas Diag* 1977; 3:59–65.
34. Roberts WC, Dicicco BS, Waller BF, Kishel JC, McManus BM, Dawson SL: Origin of the left main from the right coronary artery or from the right aortic sinus with intramyocardial tunneling to the left side of the heart via the ventricular septum: The case against clinical significance of myocardial bridge or coronary tunnel. *Am Heart J* 1982; 104:303–305.
35. Schulte MA, Waller BF, Hull MT, Pless JE: Origin of the left anterior descending artery from the right aortic sinus with intramyocardial tunneling to the left side of the heart via the ventricular septum: A case against clinical and morphologic significance of myocardial bridging. *Am Heart J* 1985; 110:499–501.
36. Wenger NK: Nonatherosclerotic causes of myocardial ischemia and necrosis. In: Hurst JW, et al (eds): *The Heart*, 4th ed. New York, McGraw-Hill, 1978:1345–1362.
37. Glickel SZ, Maggs PR, Ellis FH: Coronary artery aneurysm. *Ann Thorac Surg* 1978; 25:372–376.
38. Roberts WC: Coronary embolism: A review of causes, consequences and diagnostic considerations. *Cardiovasc Med* 1978; 3:699–709.
39. Waller BF, Dixon DS, Kem RW, Roberts WC: Embolus to the left main coronary artery. *Am J Cardiol* 1982; 50:658–660.
40. Rabinowitz M, Virmani R, McAllister HA: Spontaneous coronary artery dissection and eosinophilic infiltration: A cause, and effect relationship? *Am J Med* 1982; 72:923–928.
41. Waller BR: Pathology of transluminal balloon angioplasty used in the treatment of coronary heart disease, *Hum Pathol* 1987; 18:476–484.
42. Waller BF: Crackers, breakers, stretchers, drillers, scrapers, shavers, burners, welders and melters: The future of atherosclerotic coronary artery disease? A clinical-morphologic assessment. *J Am Coll Cardiol* 1989; 13:969–987.
43. Prinzmetal M, Kennamer R, Merliss R, Wada T: Angina pectoris. I. A variant form of angina pectoris. Preliminary report. *Am J Med* 1959; 27:375–388.
44. Peretz DI: Variant angina pectoris of Prinzmetal. *Can Med Assoc J* 1961; 85:1101–1102.
45. Gianelly R, Mugler F, Harrison DC: Prinzmetal's variant of angina pectoris with only slight coronary atherosclerosis. *California Med* 1968; 108:129–132.
46. Silverman ME, Flamm MD: Variant angina pectoris. Anatomic findings and prognostic implications. *Ann Intern Med* 1971; 75:339–343.
47. Dhurandhar RW, Watt DL, Silver MD, Trimble AS, Adelman AS: Prinzmetal's variant form of angina with arteriographic evidence of coronary arterial spasm. *Am J Cardiol* 1972; 30:902–905.
48. Cosby RS, Giddins JA, See JR, Mayo M: Variant angina. Case reports and critique. *Am J Med* 1972; 53:739–742.
49. Cheng TO, Bashour T, Kelser GA, Weiss L, Bacos J: Variant angina of Prinzmetal with normal coronary arteriograms. A variant of the variant. *Circulation* 1973; 47:476–485.
50. Donsky MS, Harris MD, Curry GC, Blomquest CG, Willerson JT, Mullins CB: Variant angina pectoris: A clinical and coronary arteriographic spectrum. *Am Heart J* 1975; 89:571–578.
51. Wiener L, Kasparian H, Duca PR, Walinsky P, Gottlieb RS, Henckel F, et al: Spectrum of coronary arterial spasm. Clinical, angiographic and myocardial metabolic experience in 29 cases. *Am J Cardiol* 1976; 38:945–955.
52. Bharati S, Dhingra RC, Lev M, Towne WD, Rahimtoolash SH, Rosen KM: Conduction system in a patient with Prinzmetal's angina and transient atrioventricular block. *Am J Cardiol* 1977; 39:120–125.
53. Maseri A, L'Abbate A, Baroldi G, Chierchia S, Marzilli M, Ballestra AM, et al: Coronary vasospasm as a possible cause of myocardial infarction. A conclusion derived from the study of "preinfarction" angina. *N Engl J Med* 1978; 299:1271–1277.
54. Roberts WC, Curry RC, Isner JM, Waller BF, McManue BM, Constantine MR, et al: Sudden death in Prinzmetal's angina with coronary spasm documented by angiography. Analysis of 3 necropsy patients. *Am J Cardiol* 1982; 50:203–210.
55. Isner JM, Donaldson RF: Coronary angiographic and morphologic correlation. In: Waller BF (ed): *Cardiac Morphology. Cardiology Clinics.* Philadelphia, Saunders, 1984:571–592.
56. Brown BF: Coronary vasospasm. Observations linking the clinical spectrum of ischemic heart disease to the dynamic pathology of coronary, atherosclerosis. *Arch Intern Med* 1981; 141:716–722.
57. Hillis LD, Braunwald E: Coronary artery spasm. *N Engl J Med* 1978; 299:695–702.
58. Ginsburg R, Birstow MR, Harrison DC, Stinson EB: Studies with isolated human coronary arteries: Some general observations, potential mediators of spasm, role of calcium antagonists. *Chest 1980;* 78:180–186.
59. Maseri A, Severi S, De Nes M, L'Abbate A, Chierchia S, Marzilli M, et al: "Variant" angina. One aspect of a continuous spectrum of vasospastic myocardial ischemia. *Am J Cardiol* 1978; 42:1019–1035.
60. El-Maraghi NRH, Sealey BJ: Recurrent myocardial infarction in a young man with coronary arterial spasm, demonstrated at autopsy. *Circulation* 1980; 61:199–207.
61. Isner JM, Donaldson RF, Katsas GC: Spasm at autopsy: A prospective study. (abstr.) *Circulation* 1983; 68:III-1028.
62. Isner JM, Fortin AH, Fortin RV: Depletion of smooth muscle from the media of atherosclerotic coronary arteries: A potential factor in the pathogenesis of myocardial ischemia and the variable response to anti-anginal therapy (Abstr.). *Clin Res* 1983; 31: 193A.
63. Factor SM, Cho S: Smooth muscle contraction bands in the media of coronary arteries: A postmortem marker of antemortem coronary spasm? *J Am Coll Cardiol* 1985; 6:1329–1337.
64. Waller BF: The eccentric coronary atherosclerotic plaque: Morphologic observations and clinical relevance. *Clin Cardiol* 1988; 12:14–20.
65. Hangartner JRW, Charleston AJ, Davies MJ, Thomas AC: Morphologic characteristics of clinically significant coronary artery stenosis in stable angina. *Br Heart J* 1986; 56:501–508.
66. Quyyumi AA, Al-Rufaii HK, Olsen EGJ, Fox KM: Coronary anatomy in patients with various manifestations of three vessel coronary artery disease. *Br Heart J* 1985; 54:362–366.
67. Hort W, Moosdorf R, Kalbfleisch H, Kohler F, Milzner-Schwarz U, Frenzel H: Postmortale Untersuchungen uber Lokalisation und Form der starksten stenosen inden Koronararterien und ihre Beziehung Zu den Risikofaktoren. *Z Kardiol* 1977; 66:333–340.
68. Freudenberg H, Lichtlen PR: Das Normale Wandsegment bei Koronarstenosen-ein postmortale Studie. *Z Kardiol* 1981; 70:863–869.
69. Saner HE, Gobel FL, Salomonowitz E, Erlich DA, Edwards JE: The disease-free wall in coronary atherosclerosis: Its relation to degree of obstruction. *J Am Coll Cardiol* 1985; 6:1096–1099.
70. Manion WC: Infectious angiitis. In: Orbison JL, Smith DE (eds): *The Peripheral Blood Vessels.* Baltimore, Williams & Wilkins, 1963: 221.
71. Gouley BA, Bellet S, McMillan TM: Tuberculosis of the myocardium: Report of six cases, with observations on involvement of coronary arteries. *Arch Intern Med* 1933; 51:244–263.
72. Holsinger DR, Osmundson PJ, Edwards JE: The heart in periarteritis nodosa. *Circulation* 1962; 25:610–618.
73. Sinclair W, Nitsch E: Polyarteritis nodosa of the coronary arteries. Report of a case with rupture of an aneurysm and intrapericardial hemorrhage. *Am Heart J* 1949; 38:898–904.
74. Crawford T: *Pathology of Ischemic Heart Disease.* London, Buttersworth, 1977.
75. Ainsworth RW, Gresham GA, Balmforth GV: Pathologic changes in temporal arteries removed from unselected cadavers. *J Clin Pathol* 1961; 14:115–119.
76. Harrison CV: Giant-cell or temporal arteritis: A review. *J Clin Pathol* 1948; 1:197–211.
77. Karsner HT, Bayless F: Coronary arteries in rheumatic fever. *Am Heart J* 1934; 9:557–585.
78. Parrillo JE, Fauci AS: Necrotizing vasculitis, coronary angiitis and the cardiologist. *Am Heart J* 1980; 99:547–554.
79. Meller J, Conde CA, Deppisch LM, Donoso E, Dact S: Myocardial infarction due to coronary atherosclerosis in three young adults with systemic lupus erythematosus. *Am J Cardiol* 1975; 35:309–314.
80. Heibel RH, O'Toole JD, Curtiss EI, Medsger TA, Reddy SP,

Shaver JA: Coronary arteritis in systemic lupus erythematosus. *Chest* 1976; 69:700–703.
81. Bonfiglio TA, Botti RE, Hagstrom JWC: Coronary arteritis, occlusion and myocardial infarction due to lupus erythematosus. *Am Heart J* 1972; 83:153–158.
82. Benisch BM, Pervez N: Coronary artery vasculitis and myocardial infarction with systemic lupus erythematosus. *NY State J Med* 1974; 74:873–874.
83. Tsakraklides VG, Blieden LC, Edwards JE: Coronary atherosclerosis and myocardial infarction associated with lupus erythematosus. *Am Heart J* 1974; 87:637–641.
84. Saphir O: Thromboangiitis obliterans of the coronary arteries and its relation to atherosclerosis. *Am Heart J* 1936; 12:521–535.
85. Averbuck SH, Silbert S: Thromboangiitis obliterans: Cause of death. *Arch Intern Med* 1934; 54:436–465.
86. Gatenby PA, Lytton DG, Bulteau VG, O'Reilly B, Basten A: Myocardial infarction in Wegener's granulomatosis. *Aust NZ J Med* 1976; 6:336–340.
87. Holt S: Syphilitic ostial occlusion. *Br Heart J* 1977; 39:469–470.
88. Saphir O, Katz LN, Gore I: The myocardium in subacute bacterial endocarditis. *Circulation* 1950; 1:1155–1167.
89. Hennigar GR, Thabet R, Bundy WE, Sutton LE: Salmonellosis complicated by pancarditis. Report of a case with autopsy findings. *J Pediatr* 1953; 43:524–531.
90. Allen AC, Spitz S: A comparative study of the pathology of scrub typhus (Tsutsugamushi disease) and other rickettsial diseases. *Am J Pathol* 1945; 21:603–682.
91. Merkel WC: Plasmodium falciparum malaria: The coronary and myocardial lesions observed in autopsy in two cases of acute fulminating *P. falciparum* infection. *Arch Pathol* 1946; 41:290–298.
92. Gazayerli M: Unusual site of a schistosome worm in the circumflex branch of the left coronary artery. *J Egypt Med Assoc* 1939; 22:34–39.
93. Fukushige J, Nihill MR, McNamara DG: Spectrum of cardiovascular lesions in mucocutaneous lymph node syndrome. *Am J Cardiol* 1980; 45:98–107.
94. Kitamura S, Kawashima Y, Fujita T, Mori T, Oyama C, Fujino M: Aortocoronary bypass grafting in a child with coronary artery obstruction due to mucocutaneous lymph node syndrome. Report of a case. *Circulation* 1976; 53:1035–1040.
95. Kato H, Koike S, Yamamoto M, Ito Y, Yano E: Coronary aneurysms in infants and young children with acute febrile mucocutaneous lymph node syndrome. *J Pediatr* 1975; 86:892–898.
96. Cipriano PR, Silverman JF, Perlroth MG, Grupp RB, Wexler L: Coronary arterial narrowing in Takayasu's aortitis. *Am J Cardiol* 1977; 39:744–750.
97. Young JA, Sengupta A, Khaja FU: Coronary arterial stenosis, angina pectoris, and atypical coarctation of the aorta due to nonspecific arteritis. Treatment with aortocoronary bypass graft. *Am J Cardiol* 1973; 32:356–360.
98. James TN: De Subitaneis Mortibus. XXIII Rheumatoid arthritis and ankylosing spondylitis. *Circulation* 1977; 55:669–677.
99. Hoffman FG, Leight L: Complete atrioventricular block associated with rheumatoid disease. *Am J Cardiol* 1965; 16:585–592.
100. Grismer JT, Anderson WR, Weiss L: Chronic occlusive rheumatic coronary vasculitis and myocardial dysfunction. *Am J Cardiol* 1976; 20:739–745.
101. Brosius FC, Roberts WC: Coronary artery disease in the Hurler Syndrome. *Am J Cardiol* 1981; 47:649–653.
102. Renteria VG, Ferrans VJ, Roberts WC: The heart in the Hurler syndrome. Gross histologic and ultrastructural observations in five necropsy cases. *Am J Cardiol* 1976; 38:487–501.
103. Lindsay S: The cardiovascular system in gargoylism. *Br Heart J* 1950; 12:17–32.
104. Stauffer M: Oxalosis. Report of a case with a review of the literature and discussion on pathogenesis. *N Engl J Med* 1960; 263:386–390.
105. Blieden LC, Desnick RJ, Carter JB, Krivit W, Moller JH, Sharp HL: Cardiac involvement in Sandhoff's disease. An inborn error of glycosphingolipid metabolism. *Am J Cardiol* 1974; 34:83–88.
106. Blieden LC, Moller JH: Cardiac involvement in inherited disorders of metabolism. *Prog Cardiovasc Dis* 1974; 16:615–631.
107. Brosius FC III, Waller BF, Roberts WC: Radiation heart disease. Analysis of 16 young (aged 15 to 33 years) necropsy patients who received over 3500 rads to the heart. *Am J Med* 1981; 70:519–530.
108. Brill IC, Brodeur MTH, Oyama AA: Myocardial infarction in two sisters less than 20 years old. *JAMA* 1971; 217:1345–1348.
109. Trimble AS, Bigelow WG, Wigle ED: Coronary ostial stenosis: A late complication of coronary perfusion in open-heart surgery. *J Thorac Cardiovasc Surg* 1969; 57:792–795.
110. Billingham M: Personal communication, 1988.
111. Waller BF, Pinkerton CA, Foster LN: Morphologic evidence of accelerated left main coronary artery stenosis: A late complication of percutaneous transluminal angioplasty of the proximal left anterior descending coronary artery. *J Am Coll Cardiol* 1987; 9:1019–1023.
112. Gardia-Rinaldi R, Von Koch L, Howell JF: Aneurysm of the sinus of Valsalva producing obstruction of the left main coronary artery. *J Thorac Cardiovasc Surg* 1976; 72:123–126.
113. Kopelson G, Herwig KJ: The etiologies of coronary artery disease in cancer patients. *Int J Radiat Oncol Biol Phys* 1978; 4:895–906.
114. Fomina LG: A case of myocardial infarct in acute leukemia. *Sov Med* 1960; 24:141–143.
115. Wirth L: Myocardial infarction as the initial manifestation of polycythemia vera. *Milit Med* 1960; 125:544–548.
116. Spach MS, Howell DA, Harris JS: Myocardial infarction and multiple thrombosis in a child with primary thrombocytosis. *Pediatrics* 1963; 31:268–276.
117. James TN: Pathology of the small coronary arteries. *Am J Cardiol* 1963; 20:679–691.
118. Isner JM, Estes NAM III, Thompson PD, Costanzo-Nordin MR, Subramanian R, Miller G, et al: Acute cardiac events temporally related to cocaine abuse. *N Engl J Med* 1986; 315:1438–1443.
119. Simpson RW, Edwards WD: Pathogenesis of cocaine-induced ischemic heart disease. *Arch Pathol Lab Med* 1986; 110:479–484.
120. Zimmerman FH, Gustafson GM, Kemp HG: Recurrent myocardial infarction associated with cocaine abuse in a young man with normal coronary arteries: Evidence for coronary artery spasm culminating in thrombosis. *J Am Coll Cardiol* 1987; 9:964–968.
121. Smith HWB, Liberman HA, Brody SL, Battey LL, Donohue BC, Morris DC: Acute myocardial infarction temporally related to cocaine use. Clinical, angiographic and pathophysiologic observations. *Ann Intern Med* 1987; 107:13–18.
122. Patel R, Haider B, Ahmed S, Regan TJ: Cocaine-related myocardial infarction: High prevalence of occlusive coronary thrombi without significant obstructive atherosclerosis (Abstr.). *Circulation* 1988; 78 (suppl II): II–436.
123. Lange RA, Cigarroa RG, Yancy CW, Willard JE, Popma JJ, Sills MN, et al: Cocaine-induced coronary artery vasoconstriction. *N Engl J Med* 1989; 321:1557–1562.
124. Waller BF: Cocaine and the heart. *Indiana Med* 1988; 81:956–959.
125. Lam D, Goldschlager N: Myocardial injury associated with polysubstance abuse. *Am Heart J* 1988; 115:675–680.
126. Rod JL, Zucker RD: Acute myocardial infarction shortly after cocaine inhalation. *Am J Cardiol* 1987; 59:161.
127. Kossowsky WA, Lyon AF: Cocaine and myocardial infarction: a probable connection. *Chest* 1984; 86:729–731.
128. Hollander JE, Hoffman RS: Cocaine-induced myocardial infarction: An analysis and review of the literature. *J Emerg Med* 1992; 10:169–177.
129. Miller GW: The cocaine habit. *Am Fam Physician* 1985; 31:173–176.
130. Wetli CV, Wright RK: Death caused by recreational cocaine use. *JAMA* 1979; 241:2519–2522.
131. Benchimol A, Bartall H, Desser KB: Acceleration of ventricular rhythm and cocaine abuse. *Ann Intern Med* 1978; 88:519–520.
132. Nanji AA, Filipenko JD: Asystole and ventricular fibrillation associated, with cocaine intoxication. *Chest* 1984; 85:132–133.
133. Schachne JS, Roberts BH, Thompson PD: Coronary artery spasm and myocardial infarction associated with cocaine use. *N Engl J Med* 1984; 310:1665–1666.
134. Howard RE, Hueter DC, Davis GJ: Acute myocardial infarction following cocaine abuse in a young woman with normal coronary arteries. *JAMA* 1985; 254:95–96.
135. Simpson RW, Edwards WD: Pathogenesis of cocaine-induced

ischemic heart disease. Autopsy finding in a 21-year-old man. *Arch Pathol Lab Med* 1986; 110:479–484.
136. Virmani R, Robinowitz M, Smialek JE, Smyth DF: Cardiovascular effects of cocaine: an autopsy study of 40 patients. *Am Heart J* 1988; 115:1068–1076.
137. Gross II, Stenberg WH: Myocardial infarction without significant lesions of coronary arteries. *Arch Intern Med* 1939; 64:249–267.
138. Friedberg CK, Horn H: Acute myocardial infarction not due to coronary artery occlusion. *JAMA* 1939; 112:1675–1679.
139. Baroldi G, Scomazzoni X: Coronary Circulation in the Normal and Pathologic Heart. American Registry of Pathology, Armed Forces Institute of Washington DC, US Government Printing Office, 1967:1–80.

SECTION C

Pharmacology of Drugs Used to Treat Patients with Known or Potential Coronary Artery Disease

Chapter 65

The Pharmacologic Management of Hyperlipidemia

Scott M. Grundy, M.D., Ph.D.

Recent clinical trials showing that treatment of hyperlipidemia with drugs reduces the risk of coronary heart disease (CHD) have rekindled an interest in lipid-lowering drugs and have intensified the search for new agents. In addition, a new class of drugs, the inhibitors of 3-hydroxy-3-methylglutaryl coenzyme A (HMG CoA) reductase, may constitute a breakthrough in the treatment of hypercholesterolemia. Furthermore, several of the older drugs still have utility for treatment of various dyslipidemias. In this chapter, the major drugs for the treatment of dyslipidemia will be reviewed and indications for their use will be discussed. In patients with severe forms of dyslipidemia, the use of a single lipid-lowering drug may not be sufficient to achieve a satisfactory reduction of plasma lipids. In these patients, drugs used in combination may be necessary, and several practical combinations will be considered. To provide an understanding of the mechanisms by which drugs alter plasma lipid levels, it may be helpful to review the basic pathways for lipoprotein transport (Fig. 65-1) and outline the major categories of hyperlipidemia for which these drugs are indicated (Table 65-1). (See also Chap. 53.)

GENERAL CONSIDERATIONS FOR DRUG THERAPY

The National Cholesterol Education Program (NCEP), under the auspices of the National Heart, Lung and Blood Institute, has developed guidelines for treatment of high blood cholesterol.[1,1a] These guidelines focus on the low-density lipoprotein (LDL) cholesterol as the primary target of therapy. The general classification of LDL cholesterol is presented in Table 65-2. An LDL cholesterol level below 130 mg/dL (3.4 mmol/liter) is considered *desirable*. For most people, this corresponds to a total cholesterol of less than 200 mg/dL (5.2 mmol/liter). An LDL cholesterol concentration of 130 to 160 mg/dL (3.4 to 4.1 mmol/liter), generally corresponding to a total cholesterol of 200 to 239 mg/dL (5.2 to 6.2 mmol/liter), is considered *borderline–high* LDL cholesterol. An LDL cholesterol over 160 mg/dL (4.1 mmol/liter) is called *high* LDL cholesterol; and a level over 190 mg/dL (4.9 mmol/liter) was designated a *very high risk* LDL cholesterol.[1] Most individuals with LDL cholesterol levels in the high risk or very high risk category will have some form of primary hypercholesterolemia or mixed hyperlipidemia (Table 65-1). (See also Chaps. 53 and 62.)

Patients without CHD or other forms of atherosclerotic disease who persist with high risk or very high risk LDL cholesterol levels should enter active medical therapy. The same is true for patients with borderline-high-risk LDL cholesterol levels who have two other risk factors for CHD (Table 65-3). The goals for reduction of LDL cholesterol levels depend on the overall risk status of patients (Table 65-4). If patients do not have CHD or two other coronary risk factors, the LDL cholesterol levels should be reduced to 160 mg/dL (4.1 mmol/liter) or less; if two other risk factors are present, LDL-

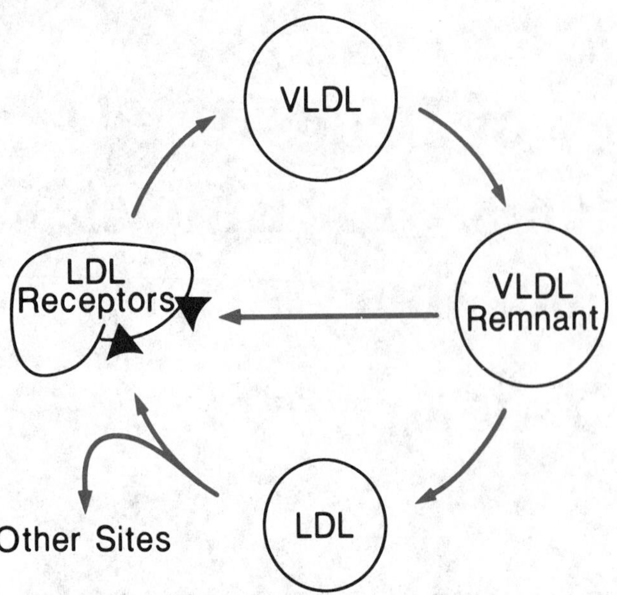

FIGURE 65-1 The liver exports cholesterol in a triglyceride-rich lipoprotein called very low density lipoproteins. VLDL-triglycerides also undergo lipolysis through the action of lipoprotein lipase, leaving VLDL remnants. The remnants can be taken up by the liver or transformed to low-density lipoproteins, the major cholesterol-carrying lipoproteins of the plasma. About one-third of LDL cholesterol is taken up by extrahepatic tissues to be used in cell membrane structure; the remainder of LDL is recycled to the liver. Most LDL is cleared by binding to specific cell surface proteins called LDL receptors; these are located on both hepatic and extrahepatic tissues. A lesser fraction of LDL is removed via nonreceptor pathways.

cholesterol concentrations should be lowered to at least 130 mg/dL (3.4 mmol/liter). Dietary therapy always should be tried first, and a trial of dietary therapy for at least 6 months is justified for patients with hypercholesterolemia. The exceptions are those individuals with severe elevations of LDL cholesterol levels (>220 mg/dL, or 5.7 mmol/liter) and for those with CHD who can be started on drugs sooner. For men under age 35 and for premenopausal women who are otherwise at low risk, drug therapy generally should be delayed until patients are older, except for those with very high cholesterol

TABLE 65-2
Categories of Elevated Cholesterol

Category	LDL Cholesterol mg/dL (mmol/liter)	Total Cholesterol mg/dL (mmol/liter)
Desirable	<130 (3.4)	<200 (5.2)
Borderline-high	130–159 (3.4–4.1)	200–239 (5.2–6.2)
High	≥160 (4.1)	≥240 (6.2)

SOURCE: The Expert Panel. Summary of the second Report of the National Cholesterol Education Program (NCEP) Expert Panel on Detection, Evaluation, and Treatment of High Blood Cholesterol in Adults (Adult Treatment Panel II). *JAMA* 1993; 269:3015–3023. Reproduced with permission from the publisher and authors.

TABLE 65-1
Categories of Hyperlipidemia

Category	Plasma Lipids (mg/dL)	Lipoprotein Abnormality	Major Mechanism	Frequency in Population (%)
Primary severe hypercholesterolemia	TC > 300 TG < 250	↑ LDL-C	Reduced activity of LDL receptors*	1–2
Primary moderate hypercholesterolemia	TC 240–300 TG < 250	↑ LDL-C	Multiple†	15
Primary hypertriglyceridemia	TC < 240 TG > 250	↑ VLDL (± ↓ HDL) ± ↑ Chylomicrons	Overproduction of VLDL-TG‡ or TG lipolytic defect	5–10
Primary mixed hyperlipidemia	TC > 240 TG > 250	↑ VLDL (± ↓ HDL) ± ↑ Chylomicrons (type 5 HLP) ± ↑ LDL (type 2b HLP) ± ↑ β-VLDL (type 3 HLP)	Multiples§	2–3

TC = total cholesterol; TG = triglyceride; LDL-C = low-density lipoprotein cholesterol; VLDL = very low density lipoprotein; HLP = hyperlipoproteinemia; HDL = high-density lipoprotein; ↑ = elevated; ± = unchanged. To convert cholesterol values to mmol/liter, divide by 38.6; to convert triglyceride values to mmol/liter, divide by 88.5.

* Some cases of primary severe hypercholesterolemia are due to heterozygous familial hypercholesterolemia, which is caused by a congenital defect in genes encoding for LDL receptors; this occurs in 0.2% of the population. In other cases, the cause of reduced activity of LDL receptors has not been determined.

† Most cases are due to reduced activity of LDL receptors, but others are the result of defective binding of LDL to receptors or overproduction of LDL.

‡ Hypertriglyceridemia frequently is accentuated by obesity or excessive alcohol intake.

§ Among the mixed hyperlipidemias, about 1% of the population has familial combined hyperlipidemia, which may be due to overproduction of VLDL. However, other abnormalities in lipoprotein metabolism can contribute to hyperlipoproteinemia types 2b, 3, and 5.

TABLE 65-3

Risk Status Based on Presence of CHD Risk Factors Other Than Low-Density Lipoprotein Cholesterol*

Positive Risk Factors
Age, years Male ≥45 Female ≤55 or premature menopause without estrogen replacement therapy Family history of premature CHD (definite myocardial infarction or sudden death before 55 years of age in father or other male first-degree relative, or before 65 years of age in mother or other female first-degree relative) Current cigarette smoking Hypertension (blood pressure ≥140/90 mmHg,† or taking antihypertensive medication) Low HDL cholesterol [<35 mg/dl† (0.9 mmol/liter)] Diabetes mellitus
Negative Risk Factor‡
High HDL cholesterol (≥60 mg/dL [1.6 mmol/liter])

SOURCE: The Expert Panel. Summary of the second Report of the National Cholesterol Education Program (NCEP) Expert Panel on Detection, Evaluation, and Treatment of High Blood Cholesterol in Adults (Adult Treatment Panel II). *JAMA* 1993; 269:3015–3023. Reproduced with permission from the publisher and authors.

* High risk, defined as a net of two or more CHD risk factors, leads to more vigorous intervention, shown in Figs. 62-3 and 62-4. Age (defined differently for men and women) is treated as a risk factor because rates of CHD are higher in the elderly than in the young, and in men than in women of the same age. Obesity is not listed as a risk factor because it operates through other risk factors that are included [hypertension, hyperlipidemia, decreased high-density lipoprotein (HDL) cholesterol, and diabetes mellitus], but it should be considered a target for intervention. Physical inactivity is similarly not listed as a risk factor, but it too should be considered a target for intervention, and physical activity is recommended as desirable for everyone. High risk due to coronary or peripheral atherosclerosis is addressed directly in Fig. 62-5.

† Confirmed by measurements on several occasions.

‡ If the HDL cholesterol level is ≥60 mg/dL (1.6 mmol/liter), subtract one risk factor (because high HDL cholesterol levels decrease CHD risk).

levels (e.g., LDL cholesterol >220 mg/dL, or 5.7 mmol/liter.

If patients have established CHD or other forms of atherosclerotic disease, a more aggressive approach to cholesterol lowering is indicated.[1a–5] In such patients, cholesterol lowering therapy should be initiated if LDL cholesterol levels are greater than 100 mg/dL (2.6 mmol/liter). The goal of therapy is to reduce LDL cholesterol levels to 100 mg/dL (2.6 mmol/liter) or less. For almost all patients with CHD, maximal cholesterol-lowering dietary therapy should be employed. If LDL-cholesterol levels exceed 130 mg/dL (3.4 mmol/liter) or greater despite a short trial of maximal dietary therapy, drug therapy should be considered. If LDL cholesterol levels decline to the range of 100 to 129 mg/dL (2.6 to 3.3 mmol/liter) on dietary therapy alone, however, clinical judgment should be employed as to whether or not cholesterol-lowering drugs are appropriate. Similarly, if LDL cholesterol levels are in this range as a result of one drug, clinical judgment is needed to decide whether or not to add a second drug.

The second adult treatment panel report[1a] classified drugs into two categories: major drugs—bile acid sequestrants, nicotinic acid, and HMG CoA reductase inhibitors (statins)—and other drugs—fibric acids and probucol. Estrogen replacement is listed as a possible alternative or adjunct to drug therapy in postmenopausal women with elevated LDL cholesterol levels. Both bile acid sequestrants[6,7] and niacin[8,9] have proved to be effective for reducing the risk of CHD without producing serious side effects. The HMG CoA reductase inhibitors are drugs of considerable potential and may become the mainstay of therapy. Other drugs include the fibric acids (gemfibrozil and clofibrate) and probucol; these drugs are considered to be alternatives to the drugs of first choice for the treatment of elevated LDL cholesterol levels. Because of the recent results of the Helsinki Heart Study,[10,11] gemfibrozil may reduce the risk of CHD in patients with moderate hypertriglyceridemia, although it probably has little value in patients with an isolated elevation of LDL cholesterol.[11]

The guidelines[1,1a] put hypertriglyceridemia behind hypercholesterolemia as a risk factor for CHD. However, it has become increasingly recognized that a lipoprotein pattern consisting of mild hypertriglyceridemia and reduced HDL cholesterol is found in many patients with CHD.[12] Thus, in hypertriglyceridemic patients who have CHD and/or other risk factors or who have concomitant hypercholesterolemia (mixed hyperlipidemia), drug therapy for hypertriglyceridemia may be indicated. Again, however, drugs should be used in hypertriglyceridemic patients only after appropriate dietary therapy, most notably weight reduction and reduced alcohol intake. The specific drugs or categories of drugs recommended by the NCEP guidelines will be considered in the following sections. (See also Chap. 62.)

BILE ACID SEQUESTRANTS

The bile acid sequestrants are ion exchange resins that bind bile acids in the intestinal tract and thus interfere with their reabsorption. The sequestrants currently available are cholestyramine (Questran) and colestipol (Colestid). By interfering with the reabsorption of bile acids, these drugs decrease the return of bile acids to the liver, which releases the feedback inhibition of bile acids on the conversion of cholesterol in bile acids. This leads to an enhanced degradation of cholesterol into bile acids, and hepatic concentrations of cholesterol fall. The decrease in hepatic cholesterol stimulates the synthesis of LDL receptors, which promotes uptake of plasma LDL by the liver. However, the degree of reduction of LDL levels is limited because of a compensatory increase in hepatic synthesis of cholesterol, which lessens the decline in hepatic cholesterol contents and thus the stimulus to LDL receptor synthesis. Generally, decreases in LDL cholesterol levels are in the range of 15 to 25 percent.[6,7]

Indications

The major indication for bile acid sequestrants is an

isolated increase in LDL cholesterol levels (primary hypercholesterolemia). Most patients with this condition probably have a decreased number of LDL receptors.[13] Patients with primary severe hypercholesterolemia [e.g., heterozygous familial hypercholesterolemia (FH)] usually are responsive to bile acid sequestrants, but these drugs used alone rarely produce the desired lowering of LDL cholesterol levels.[14] Bile acid sequestrants, however, are valuable when used in combination with other cholesterol-lowering drugs (see "Drug Combinations" later in this chapter). For patients with primary moderate hypercholesterolemia (LDL cholesterol 160 to 210 mg/dL, or 4.1 to 5.4 mmol/liter), bile acid sequestrants used alone frequently produce an adequate reduction of LDL cholesterol levels. Certainly many patients with moderate hypercholesterolemia respond sufficiently to dietary therapy alone, and drug treatment is unnecessary; for those who persist with significant hypercholesterolemia in spite of dietary therapy, use of bile acid sequestrants may prove adequate. If a patient has an LDL cholesterol level in the range of 160 to 190 mg/dL (4.1 to 4.9 mmol/liter) but does not have CHD or other risk factors, low-dose bile acid sequestrants can be considered; however, some investigators question whether drug therapy is necessary for LDL levels in this range in otherwise low risk patients. (See also Table 65-4 and Chap. 62.)

Dosage

The full dosage for cholestyramine is 16 g/day (8 g twice daily), and for colestipol it is 20 g/day in divided doses. The sequestrants are best tolerated when started at low dosage with a gradual buildup. In many patients, half the typical dose is sufficient to achieve the desired LDL cholesterol lowering. For patients who develop constipation, a high-fiber diet of a psyllium-containing laxative taken concomitantly may be beneficial.

Side Effects

The major side effects of bile acid sequestrants are gastrointestinal, especially constipation and indigestion. Gastrointestinal complaints generally decrease with continued use.[1] Resins may interfere with absorption of some drugs (e.g., digitoxin, thiazide diuretics, tetracycline, penicillin G, thyroxine, propranolol, and warfarin), and these drugs should be taken an hour before the sequestrant. The sequestrants often raise the triglyceride level,[15] particularly in patients with an underlying mild-to-moderate hypertriglyceridemia, especially those who consume excessive alcohol. Bile acid sequestrants are contraindicated in patients with severe hypertriglyceridemia because they can raise triglyceride levels even more and precipitate acute pancreatitis.[10] (See also Chap. 109.)

NIACIN

Niacin (nicotinic acid) is a drug that has multiple effects on the plasma lipoproteins; these effects appear to be secondary to its action of inhibiting the hepatic secretion of very low density lipoprotein (VLDL).[16] This drug reduces plasma concentrations of both VLDL triglycerides and LDL cholesterol, and it raises HDL cholesterol levels. In the Coronary Drug Project,[8] treatment of patients who had established CHD with niacin resulted in a decrease in recurrence of myocardial infarction; in long-term follow-up total mortality was reduced in patients who had been treated with niacin. This benefit was achieved without serious side effects.

Indications

Niacin is effective in most categories of hyperlipidemia listed in Table 65-1. It reduces LDL cholesterol in pa-

TABLE 65-4

Treatment Decisions Based on LDL Cholesterol Level*

Patient Category	Initiation Level	LDL Goal
	Dietary Therapy	
Without CHD and with fewer than two risk factors	≥160 mg/dL (4.1 mmol/liter)	<160 mg/dL (4.1 mmol/liter)
Without CHD and with two or more risk factors	≥130 mg/dL (3.4 mmol/liter)	<130 mg/dL (3.4 mmol/liter)
With CHD	>100 mg/dL (2.6 mmol/liter)	≤100 mg/dL (2.6 mmol/liter)
	Drug Treatment	
Without CHD and with fewer than two risk factors	≥190 mg/dL (4.9 mmol/liter)	<160 mg/dL (4.1 mmol/liter)
Without CHD and with two or more risk factors	≥160 mg/dL (4.1 mmol/liter)	<130 mg/dL (3.4 mmol/liter)
With CHD	≥130 mg/dL (3.4 mmol/liter)	≤100 mg/dL (2.6 mmol/liter)

*LDL indicates low-density lipoprotein; and CHD, coronary heart disease.

SOURCE: The Expert Panel. Summary of the second Report of the National Cholesterol Education Program (NCEP) Expert Panel on Detection, Evaluation, and Treatment of High Blood Cholesterol in Adults (Adult Treatment Panel II). *JAMA* 1993; 269:3015–3023. Reproduced with permission from the publisher and authors.

tients with hypercholesterolemia and reduces plasma triglycerides in those with hypertriglyceridemia. For both categories of patients, the drug usually raises HDL cholesterol concentrations. Niacin produces an additive lipid lowering when used in combination with other drugs.[17] Degrees of reduction of plasma triglycerides and cholesterol generally are proportional to the dosage level achieved in therapy. However, some patients show substantial lipid lowering at relatively low doses.

Dosage

The usual dose range for niacin required to produce a maximal effect on plasma lipoprotein concentrations is 3 to 6 g/day. This range is best achieved by beginning at a very low dose and gradually increasing it. A common starting dose is 50 mg three times daily, which can be increased by 50 mg at each dose to 500 mg three times daily and then at 100-mg increments to about 1.0 to 2.0 g three times daily. Other means of progressively increasing the dose can be tried depending on the patient's tolerance. Patients should make every effort to take every dose, because missing doses fosters the recurrence of side effects. There is some suggestion that the slow-release forms may be associated with an increased incidence of liver function abnormalities.

Side Effects

Niacin can produce several adverse reactions that limit its usefulness. Some patients are not able to tolerate the drug because of flushing of the skin, itching, or gastrointestinal distress. The presence of peptic ulcer disease is generally a contraindication to its use. Niacin also can produce a variety of biochemical changes, such as abnormalities in liver function tests, worsening of glucose tolerance in diabetics, and hyperuricemia.[1] Rare patients may develop acanthosis nigracans or maculopathy. All these abnormalities are reversed after stopping the drug. Occasional patients may develop hypotension or atrial tachycardia. Starting the drug at low doses will mitigate the flushing and gastrointestinal symptoms, and one 325 mg aspirin per day may help reduce flushing.[12] In spite of the effectiveness of niacin, up to one-third of patients are not able to tolerate the drug because of one or more side effects. Even those who initially tolerate the drug may develop side effects after prolonged usage. (See also Chap. 109.)

HMG CoA REDUCTASE INHIBITORS

This new class of drugs leads to a lowering of plasma cholesterol by competitive inhibition of HMG CoA reductase,[18] the rate-limiting enzyme in the synthesis of cholesterol. These inhibitors act mainly in the liver. Blocking cholesterol synthesis reduces the hepatic content of cholesterol, which stimulates the synthesis of LDL receptors.[19] This leads to increased uptake of circulating VLDL remnants and LDL by the liver, changes that lower the LDL cholesterol levels and also VLDL cholesterol. Through this mechanism, cholesterol levels in both VLDL and LDL fractions are reduced 25 to 40 percent.[20,21]

Indications

The major indication for HMG CoA reductase inhibitors is primary severe hypercholesterolemia (e.g., heterozygous FH). However, in spite of the potency of these drugs, they do not "normalize" LDL cholesterol levels in many patients with heterozygous FH.[21] In most of these patients, combined drug therapy is required (see below). Reductase inhibitors also may be indicated in patients with moderate hypercholesterolemia who have CHD or other risk factors (Tables 65-3 and 65-4). These individuals include not only smokers and hypertensive people but also patients with diabetes mellitus,[22] the nephrotic syndrome,[23] and coexisting hypertriglyceridemia.[24] For patients with moderate hypercholesterolemia who do not have CHD or other risk factors, the role of HMG CoA reductase inhibitors will remain unclear until their effectiveness for prevention of CHD and long-term safety has been proved; until such proof has been obtained, it may be prudent to withhold reductase inhibitors in patients of this type.

Dosage

Three HMG CoA reductase inhibitors are now available in the United States. These are lovastatin (Mevacor), pravastatin (Pravacol), and simvastatin (Zocor). The starting dose for moderate hypercholesterolemia can be 20 mg at night for lovastatin and pravastatin. The starting dose for simvastatin is 10 mg. If the response is inadequate, the dose for each can be doubled. For severe hypercholesterolemia, doubling the dose once again will produce a somewhat greater reduction in LDL cholesterol levels, although the expense is high and chances for side effects are increased.

Side Effects

HMG CoA reductase inhibitors produce indigestion in some individuals. Others may develop mild increases in transaminases of hepatic origin.[25] Patients should be monitored regularly for this effect, but the drug need not be discontinued unless the levels become two or three times normal. These drugs also can produce myopathy and even rhabdomyolysis with renal failure in very rare patients, particularly those with cardiac transplant who are taking cyclosporine.[26,27] More frequently, the combination of an HMG CoA reductase inhibitor and gemfibrozil (or nicotinic acid) can produce the same reactions; therefore, the combinations should be used cautiously. Current data indicate that these agents do not cause cataracts.[28]

FIBRIC ACIDS

Fibric acids currently available in the United States are gemfibrozil (Lopid) and clofibrate (Atromid-S). Two others—fenofibrate and bezafibrate—are used extensively in other countries. The actions of these drugs are complex.[29] They apparently have the following effects on plasma cholesterol and lipoprotein metabolism: (1) enhancement of the activity of lipoprotein lipase, (2) partial inhibition of synthesis of VLDL triglycerides, (3) partial inhibition of synthesis of cholesterol with increased activity of LDL receptors, (4) reduced conversion of cholesterol into bile acids, and (5) the enhanced secretion of cholesterol into bile. As a consequence of 1 and 2, the plasma level of HDL cholesterol may be mildly increased. These drugs are highly effective for lowering plasma triglycerides, but when used in patients with hypertriglyceridemia, they may raise the LDL cholesterol level. For individuals with normal triglycerides, in contrast, they actually lower the LDL cholesterol level in the range of 10 to 20 percent. Both clofibrate[29] and gemfibrozil[10] have been shown to reduce rates of myocardial infarction in hypercholesterolemic patients during clinical trials. Offsetting side effects have been attributed to clofibrate[29] but not to gemfibrozil.[10]

Indications

The fibric acids can be useful in preventing acute pancreatitis in many patients with severe hypertriglyceridemia. Theoretically, they may benefit patients with moderate hypertriglyceridemia who have CHD or other risk factors, although this has not been proved. Finally, as shown in clinical trials,[10,29] they reduce the risk for CHD in patients with moderate hypercholesterolemia, but only if the patients have a concomitant elevation of serum triglycerides.[11] For hypercholesterolemic patients without elevated triglycerides, fibric acids have little or no utility. Also, for patients with isolated low HDL cholesterol they are largely ineffective for raising HDL levels.[30]

Dosage

The typical dose for gemfibrozil is 600 mg twice daily; for clofibrate, it is 1000 mg twice daily.

Side Effects

The major side effects of the fibric acids are gastric distress, indigestion, transient abnormalities in liver function tests, myopathy, weight gain, impotency, neutropenia, and skin rash. All fibric acids apparently increase the risk for cholesterol gallstones. An increased risk for cancer has been attributed to clofibrate,[29] but this adverse effect is questionable. Gemfibrozil seemingly does not raise the risk for cancer.[10]

PROBUCOL

The primary action of probucol (Lorelco) is to reduce the LDL cholesterol level. The drug promotes the clearance of LDL from plasma by unknown mechanisms.[31] It also lowers the HDL cholesterol level. Recent work in laboratory animals has suggested that probucol may interfere with the development of atherosclerosis by blocking the oxidation of LDL within the arterial wall.[32] Neither effectiveness for reducing risk for CHD nor the long-term safety of probucol has been proved in clinical trials. Therefore, it is difficult to assess the risk-benefit ratio of probucol for clinical practice.

Indications

The primary indication for probucol is moderate hypercholesterolemia; however, because of the lack of clinical trial data on efficacy and long-term safety, probucol cannot be considered a drug of first choice (see above). Even so, it has been used widely as an adjunct in therapy for hypercholesterolemia.

Dosage

The usual dose of probucol for adults is 500 mg twice daily.

Side Effects

Probucol can produce various gastrointestinal complaints, particularly diarrhea. It induces ventricular arrhythmias in dogs and should be used with caution in patients with potential ventricular irritability. The long-term effects of reduced HDL cholesterol levels on atherogenesis have not been assessed.

DRUG COMBINATIONS

For patients with severe or mixed hyperlipidemias, the use of lipid-lowering drugs in combination can enhance the response. For example, for heterozygous FH, the combination of bile acid sequestrants and nicotinic acid frequently will "normalize" the LDL cholesterol level,[17] and the same is true for bile acid sequestrants and lovastatin.[33,34] Bile acid sequestrants likewise have been combined with probucol.[35] For patients with mixed hyperlipidemia, the combination of a bile acid sequestrant (or lovastatin) and gemfibrozil can cause a lowering of both cholesterol and triglycerides and at the same time raise the HDL cholesterol level.[35] Future studies may reveal the value of other drug combinations.

REFERENCES

1. The Expert Panel: Report of the National Cholesterol Education Program Expert Panel on Detection, Evaluation, and Treatment of High Blood Cholesterol in Adults. *Arch Intern Med* 1988; 148:36–69.

1a. The Expert Panel. Summary of the second Report of the National Cholesterol Education Program (NCEP) Expert Panel on Detection, Evaluation, and Treatment of High Blood Cholesterol in Adults (Adult Treatment Panel II). *JAMA* 1993; 269:3015–3023.

2. Grundy SM: Management of high blood cholesterol in patients with a history of coronary heart disease: Overview. *Coron Art Dis* 1991; 2:863–869.

3. Rossouw JE, Rifkind BM: Contribution of high serum cholesterol to progression of coronary atherosclerosis and subsequent clinical events in patients with coronary heart disease. *Coron Art Dis* 1991; 2:870–874.

4. Blankenhorn DH: Angiographic trials testing the efficacy of cholesterol lowering in reducing progression or inducing regression of coronary atherosclerosis. *Coron Art Dis* 1991; 2:875–879.

5. Hunninghake DB: Clinical management of dyslipidemia in patients with established coronary disease. *Coron Art Dis* 1991; 2:880–887.
6. Lipid Research Clinics Program: The Lipid Research Clinics Coronary Primary Prevention Trial Results: I, Reduction in incidence of coronary heart disease. *JAMA* 1984; 251:351–364.
7. Lipid Research Clinics Program: The Lipid Research Clinics Primary Prevention Trial Results: II, The relationship of reduction in incidence of coronary heart disease to cholesterol lowering. *JAMA* 1984; 251:365–374.
8. The Coronary Drug Project Research Group: Clofibrate and niacin in coronary heart disease (The Coronary Drug Project). *JAMA* 1975; 231:360–381.
9. Canner PL, Berge KG, Wenger NK, Stamler J, Friedman L, Prineas RJ, et al: Fifteen year mortality in coronary drug project patients: Long-term benefit with niacin. *J Am Coll Cardiol* 1986; 8:1245–1255.
10. Frick MH, Elo O, Haapa K, Heinonen OP, Heinsalmi P, Helo P, et al: Helsinki Heart Study: Primary prevention trial with gemfibrozil in middle-aged men with dyslipidemia: Safety of treatment, changes in risk factors, and incidence of coronary heart disease. *N Engl J Med* 1987; 317:1237–1245.
11. Huttunen JK, Manninen V, Manttari M: The Helsinki Heart Study: Central findings and clinical implications. *Ann Med* 1991; 23:155–159.
12. Castelli WP: The triglyceride issue: A view from Framingham. *Am Heart J* 1986; 112:432–437.
13. Grundy SM, Vega GL: Influence of mevinolin on metabolism of low-density lipoproteins in primary moderate hypercholesterolemia. *J Lipid Res* 1985; 26:1464–1475.
14. Beil U, Crouse JR, Einarsson K: Effects of interruption of the enterohepatic circulation of bile acids on the transport of very low density lipoprotein-triglycerides. *Metabolism* 1982; 31:438–444.
15. Crouse JR III: Hypertriglyceridemia: A contraindication to the use of bile acid binding resins. *Am J Med* 1987; 83:243–248.
16. Grundy SM, Mok HYI, Zech LA: Transport of very low density lipoprotein-triglycerides in varying degrees of obesity and hypertriglyceridemia. *J Clin Invest* 1979; 63:1274–1283.
17. Kane JP, Malloy MJ, Tun P, Phillips NR, Freeman DD, Williams MD, et al: Normalization of low-density-lipoprotein levels in heterozygous familial hypercholesterolemia with combined drug regimen. *N Engl J Med* 1981; 304:251–258.
18. Endo A, Kuroda M, Tsujita Y: JL-236A, ML-236B, and ML-236C, new inhibitors of cholesterogenesis produced by *Penicillium citrinum. J Antibiot (Tokyo)* 1976; 29:1346–1348.
19. Goldstein JL, Brown MS: The LDL receptor defect in familial hypercholesterolemia: Implications for pathogenesis and therapy. *Med Clin North Am* 1982; 66:335–362.
20. The Lovastatin Study Group II: Therapeutic response to lovastatin (mevinolin) in nonfamilial hypercholesterolemia. *JAMA* 1986; 256:2829–2834.
21. Havel RJ, Hunninghake DN, Illingworth DR, Lees RS, Stein EA, Tolbert JA: A multicenter study of lovastatin (mevinolin) in the treatment of heterozygous familial hypercholesterolemia. *Ann Intern Med* 1987; 107:609–615.
22. Garg A, Grundy SM: Lovastatin for lowering cholesterol levels in noninsulin dependent diabetes mellitus. *N Engl J Med* 1988; 318:81–86.
23. Vega GL, Grundy SM: Lovastatin therapy in nephrotic hyperlipidemia: Effects on lipoprotein metabolism. *Kidney Intern* 1988; 33:1160–1168.
24. Arad Y, Ramakrishnan R, Ginsberg HN: Lovastatin therapy reduces low density lipoprotein apo B levels in subjects with combined hyperlipidemia by reducing the production of apo B containing lipoproteins: Implications for the pathophysiology of apo B production. *J Lipid Res* 1990; 31:567–682.
25. Tobert JA: New developments in lipid-lowering therapy: The role of inhibitors of hydroxymethylglutaryl-coenzyme A reductase. *Circulation* 1987; 76:534–538.
26. Norman DJ, Illingworth DR, Munson J: Myolysis and acute renal failure in a heart-transplant recipient receiving lovastatin. *N Engl J Med* 1988; 318:46–47.
27. East C, Alivizatos PA: Rhabdomyolysis in patients receiving lovastatin after cardiac transplantation. *N Engl J Med* 1988; 318:47–48.
28. Tobert JA, Shear CL, Chremos AN, Mantell GE: Clinical experience with lovastatin. *Am J Cardiol* 1990; 65:23F–26F.
29. A co-operative trial in the primary prevention of ischemic heart disease using clofibrate: Report from the Committee of Principal Investigators. *Br Heart J* 1978; 40:1069–1118.
30. Vega GL, Grundy SM: Comparison of lovastatin and gemfibrozil in normolipidemic patients with hypoalphalipoproteinemia. *JAMA* 1989; 262:3148–3153.
31. Kesaniemi VA, Grundy SM: Influence of probucol on cholesterol and lipoprotein metabolism in man. *J Lipid Res* 1984; 25:780–790.
32. Kita T, Nagano Y, Yokode M, Ishii K, Kume N, Ooshima A, et al: Probucol prevents the progression of atherosclerosis in Watanabe heritable hyperlipidemic rabbit, an animal model for familial hypercholesterolemia. *Proc Natl Acad Sci USA* 1987; 84:5928–5931.
33. Illingworth DR: Mevinolin plus colestipol in therapy for severe heterozygous familial hypercholesterolemia. *Ann Intern Med* 1984; 101:598–604.
34. Grundy SM, Vega GL, Bilheimer DW: Influence of combined therapy with mevinolin and interruption of bile acid reabsorption on low density lipoproteins in heterozygous familial hypercholesterolemia. *Ann Intern Med* 1985; 103:339–343.
35. East C, Bilheimer DW, Grundy SM: Combination drug therapy for treatment of familial combined hyperlipidemia. *Ann Intern Med* 1988; 109:25–32.

Chapter 66

Beta-Adrenergic Blocking Drugs

William H. Frishman, M.D. ■ *Edmund H. Sonnenblick, M.D.*

Beta-adrenergic blocking drugs, which constitute a major pharmacotherapeutic advance, were conceived initially for the treatment of patients with angina pectoris and arrhythmias; however, they also have therapeutic effects in many other clinical disorders, including systemic hypertension, hypertrophic cardiomyopathy, mitral valve prolapse, silent myocardial ischemia, migraine, glaucoma, essential tremor, and thyrotoxicosis.[1–3] Beta blockers have been effective in treating unstable angina and for reducing the risk of cardiovascular mortality and nonfatal reinfarction in patients who have survived an acute myocardial infarction.[4,5] Beta blockade is a potential treatment modality, with and without thrombolytic therapy, for reducing the extent of myocardial injury and mortality during the acute phase of myocardial infarction.[6–9]

In this chapter, both the molecular and the clinical pharmacology of β-adrenergic blockers is reviewed. Also summarized are the clinical applications and adverse experiences with these drugs.

THE BETA ADRENOCEPTOR: CHANGING CONCEPTS

Hormonal and Drug Receptors

The effects of an endogenous hormone or exogenous drug depend ultimately on physiochemical interactions with macromolecular structures of cells called receptors (see Chap. 3). Agonists interact with a receptor and elicit a response; antagonists interact with receptors and prevent the action of agonists.

In the case of catecholamine action, the circulating hormone or drug ("first messenger") interacts with its specific receptor on the external surface of the target cells. The drug hormone-receptor complex, mediated by a G protein called Gs, activates the enzyme adenyl cyclase on the internal surface of the plasma membrane of the target cell, which accelerates the intracellular formation of cyclic adenosine monophosphate (cyclic AMP) (see Chap. 5). Cyclic AMP-dependent protein kinase ("second messenger") then stimulates or inhibits various metabolic or physiological processes.[10–13] Catecholamine-induced increases in intracellular cyclic AMP are usually associated with stimulation of β-adrenergic receptors, whereas α-adrenergic receptor stimulation is mediated by a G protein known as Gi and is associated with lower concentrations of cyclic AMP[14] and possibly increased amounts of guanosine-3′5′-monophosphate in the cell. These changes may result in the production of opposing physiologic effects, depending on what adrenergic receptor is activated by catecholamines.

Until recently, most research on receptor action bypassed the initial binding step and the intermediate steps, and examined either the accumulation of cyclic AMP or the end step, the physiological effect. Currently, radioactive agonists or antagonists (radioligands) that attach to and label the receptors have been used to study binding and hormone action.[11–15]

The Beta-Adrenergic Receptor

The catecholamines norepinephrine and epinephrine are important regulators of many physiological and metabolic effects. Norepinephrine acts primarily as a neurotransmitter released from sympathetic nerve terminals, and epinephrine functions as a circulating hormone released from the adrenal medulla.[11] In 1948, Ahlquist[16] characterized the receptors relative to the actions of epinephrine and norepinephrine, and defined two major types of receptors: α and β adrenoceptors. Adrenergic receptors have since been subclassified into discrete β_1 and β_2 as well as α_1 and α_2 subtypes. Radioligand labeling techniques have greatly aided the investigation of adrenoreceptors,[11–15] and molecular pharmacologic techniques have positvely delineated the β-adrenoceptor structure as a polypeptide with a molecular weight of 67,000.[12]

In contrast to the older concept of adrenoreceptors as static entities in cells that simply serve to initiate the chain of events, newer theories hold that the adrenoceptors are subject to a wide variety of controlling influences that result in dynamic regulation of adrenoceptor sites and/or their sensitivity to catecholamines. Changes in tissue concentration of receptor sites are probably involved in mediating important fluctuations in tissue sensitivity to drug action.[13,15,17] These principles may have significant clinical and therapeutic implications. For example, an apparent increase in the number of β adrenoceptors, and thus a supersensitivity to agonists, may be induced by chronic exposure to antagonists.[13,17] With prolonged adrenoceptor-blocker therapy, receptor occupancy by catecholamines can be diminished and the number of available receptors can be increased.[17] When the β-adrenoceptor blocker is withdrawn suddenly, an increased pool of sensitive receptors will be open to endogenous catecholamine stimulation. The resultant adrenergic stimulation could precipitate unstable angina pectoris and/or a myocardial infarction.[18] The concentration of β adrenoceptors in the membrane of mononuclear cells decreases significantly with age.[11]

Using radioligand techniques, a decrease in β-adrenoceptor sites in the myocardium has been demonstrated in patients with chronic congestive heart failure.[19,20] An apparent reduction in β adrenoceptors and/or β-adrenoceptor function has also been associated with the development of refractoriness or desensitization to endogenous and exogenous catecholamines, a phenomenon probably caused by the prolonged exposure of these adrenoceptors to high levels of catecholamines.[19] This desensitization phenonenon is caused, not by a change in receptor formation or degradation, but, rather, by catecholamine-induced changes in the conformation of the receptor sites, thus rendering them ineffective.[21] Beta-adrenoceptor blocking drugs do not induce desensitization or changes in the conformation of receptors but do block the ability of catecholamines to desensitize receptors.[21]

BETA-ADRENOCEPTOR BLOCKING DRUGS: BASIC PHARMACOLOGIC DIFFERENCES

More than 100 β-adrenoceptor blockers have been synthesized during the past 25 years, and over 30 are available worldwide for clinical use.[22] Selectivity for two subgroups of the β adrenoceptor population has also been taken advantage of: β_1 receptors in the heart and β_2 receptors in the peripheral circulation and bronchi.[1,22] More controversial has been the introduction of β-blocking drugs with α-adrenergic blocking actions, varying amounts of selective and nonselective intrinsic sympathomimetic activity (partial agonist activity), calcium-channel blocker activity, and nonspecific membrane-stabilizing effects.[3] There are also pharmacokinetic differences between β-blocking drugs that may be of clinical importance.[1,23]

Thirteen β-adrenoceptor blockers are now marketed in the United States for cardiovascular disorders: propranolol for angina pectoris, arrhythmias, systemic hypertension, migraine prophylaxis, essential tremor, and hypertrophic cardiomyopathy and for reducing the risk of cardiovascular mortality in survivors of an acute myocardial infarction; nadolol for hypertension and angina pectoris; timolol for hypertension, for reducing the risk of cardiovascular mortality and nonfatal reinfarction in survivors of myocardial infarction, and in topical form for glaucoma; atenolol and metoprolol for hypertension and angina and in intravenous and oral formulations for reducing the risk of cardiovascular mortality in survivors of myocardial infarction; penbutolol, carteolol, and pindolol for treating hypertension; betaxolol for hypertension and in topical form for glaucoma; acebutolol for hypertension and ventricular arrhythmias; intravenous esmolol for supraventricular arrhythmias; sotalol for ventricular arrhythmias; and labetalol for hypertension and in intravenous form for hypertensive emergencies.[1,3,24–31] In addition, oxprenolol has been approved for use in hypertension but is not marketed in the United States; bisoprolol, bucindolol, and carvedilol, are either in the process of being approved for clinical use or are being evaluated in clinical trials.

Despite the extensive experience with β blockers in clinical practice, there have been no studies suggesting that any of these agents have major advantages or disadvantages in relation to the others for treatment of cardiovascular diseases. When any available blocker is titrated properly, it can be effective in patients with arrhythmia, hypertension, or angina pectoris.[1,3,23–31] However, one agent may be more effective than other agents in reducing adverse reactions in some patients and for managing specific situations.[30]

Potency

Beta-adrenergic receptor blocking drugs are competitive inhibitors of catecholamine binding at β-adrenergic receptor sites. The dose-response curve of the catecholamine is shifted to the right; that is, a given tissue response requires a higher concentration of agonist in the presence of β-blocking drugs.[2] Beta_1-blocking potency can be assessed by the inhibition of tachycardia produced by isoproterenol or exercise (the more reliable method in the intact organism); the potency varies from compound to compound (Table 66-1).[2] These differences in potency are of no therapeutic relevance; however, they do explain the different drug doses needed to achieve effective β-adrenergic blockade when initiating therapy in patients or when switching from one agent to another.[1,32]

TABLE 66-1
Pharmacodynamic Properties of β-Adrenoceptor Blocking Drugs

Drug	β_1-Blockade Potency Ratio (Propranolol = 1.0)	Relative β_1 Selectivity	Intrinsic Sympathomimetic Activity	Membrane-Stabilizing Activity
Acebutolol	0.3	+	+	+
Atenolol	1.0	++	0	0
Betaxolol	1.0	++	0	+
Bisoprolol	10.0	++	0	0
Carteolol	10.0	0	+	0
Carvedilol*	10.0	0	0	++
Esmolol	0.02	++	0	0
Labetalol†	0.3	0	+	0
Metoprolol	1.0	++	0	0
Nadolol	1.0	0	0	0
Oxprenolol	0.5–1.0	0	+	+
Penbutolol	1.0	0	+	0
Pindolol	6.0	0	++	+
Propranolol	1.0	0	0	++
Sotalol‡	0.3	0	0	0
Timolol	6.0	0	0	0
YM 151§	1.0	++	0	0
Isomer: D-propranolol	—	—	—	++

* Carvedilol has additional α_1-adrenergic blocking activity without peripheral β_2 agonism.
† Labetalol has additional α_1-adrenergic blocking activity and direct vasodilatory actions (β_2 agonism).
‡ Sotalol has an additional type of antiarrhythmic activity.
§ YM 151 has additional dihydropyridine calcium channel blocker activity.
SOURCE: Frishman.[2,3,23]

Structure-Activity Relationships

The chemical structures of most β-adrenergic blockers have several features in common with the agonist isoproterenol (Fig. 66-1): an aromatic ring with a substituted ethanolamine side chain linked to it by an —OCH_2 group.[1,3,33] The β blocker timolol has a catecholamine-mimicking side chain but a more complex ring.

Most β-blocking drugs exist as pairs of optical isomers and are marketed as racemic mixtures. Almost all the β-blocking activity is found in the negative (−) levorotatory stereoisomer. The two stereoisomers of propranolol are useful for differentiating between the pharmacologic effects of β blockade and membrane-stabilizing activity (possessed by both optical forms). The positive (+) dextrorotatory stereoisomers of β-blocking agents have no apparent clinical value,[1,32,33] except for D-sotalol, which appears to have type III antiarrhythmic properties.[34] Penbutolol and timolol are marketed only in the L form.

Membrane-Stabilizing Activity

At concentrations well above therapeutic levels, certain β blockers have a quinidine-like or local anesthetic membrane-stabilizing effect on the cardiac action potential. This property is exhibited equally by the two stereoisomers of the drug and is unrelated to β-adrenergic blockade and major therapeutic antiarrhythmic actions. There is no evidence that membrane-stabilizing activity is responsible for any direct negative inotropic effect of the β blockers, since drugs with and without this property equally depress left ventricular function.[35] However, membrane-stabilizing activity can manifest itself clinically with massive β-blocker intoxications.[2,36,37]

Beta$_1$ Selectivity

Beta-adrenoceptor blockers may be classified as selective or nonselective, according to their relative abilities to antagonize the actions of sympathomimetic amines in some tissues at lower doses than those required in other tissues.[1,24] When used in low doses, β_1-selective blocking agents such as acebutolol, betaxolol, bisoprolol, esmolol, atenolol, and metoprolol inhibit cardiac β_2 receptors but have less influence on bronchial and vascular β adrenoceptors (β_2). In higher doses, however, β_1-selective blocking agents also block β_2-receptors. Accordingly, β_1-selective agents may be safer than nonselective ones in patients with obstructive pulmonary disease, since β_2 receptors remain available to mediate adrenergic bronchodilatation. Even selective β blockers may aggravate bronchospasm in certain patients, however, and these drugs should generally not be used in patients with bronchospastic disease.

A second theoretical advantage is that, unlike nonselective β blockers, β_1-selective blockers in low doses may not block the β_2 receptors that mediate dilatation of arterioles. During infusion of epinephrine, nonselective β blockers can cause a pressor response by blocking β_2-receptor-mediated vasodilatation, since α-adrenergic vasoconstrictor receptors are still operative. Selective β_1

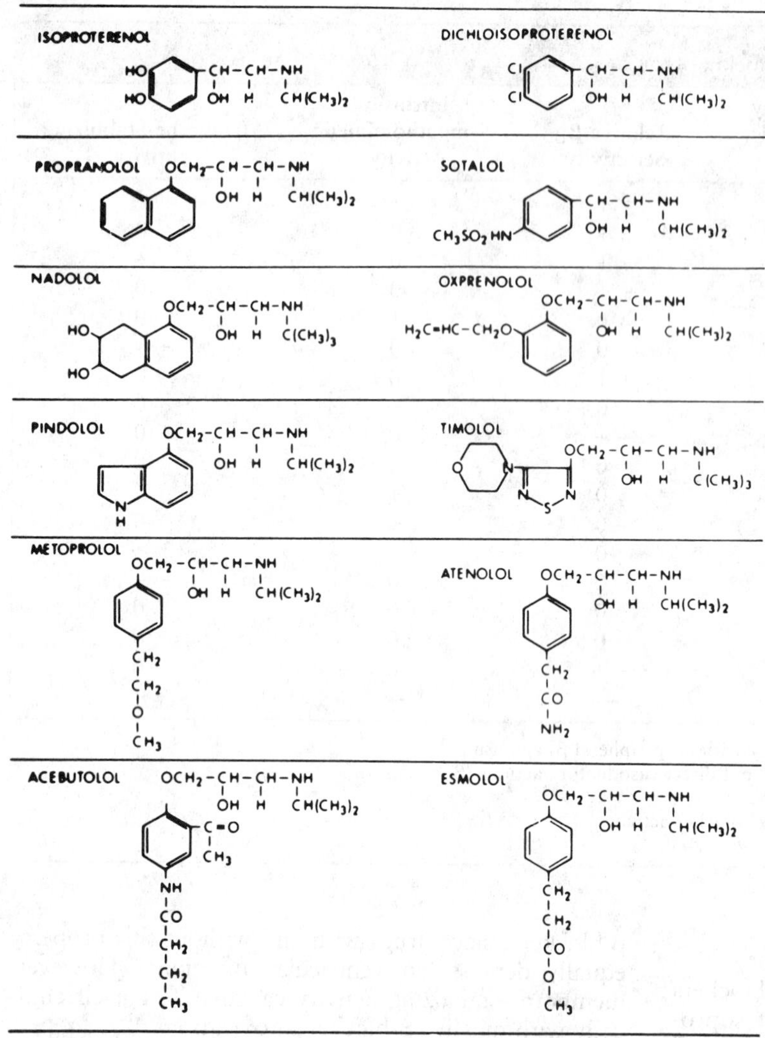

FIGURE 66-1 Molecular structure of the β-adrenergic agonist isoproterenol and some β-adrenergic β-blocking drugs. (*From WH Frishman, Clinical Pharmacology of the β-Adrenoreceptor Blocking Drugs, 2d ed. Norkwalk, CT, Appleton-Century-Crofts, 1984. Reproduced with permission from the publisher and author.*)

antagonists may not induce this pressor effect in the presence of epinephrine and may lessen the impairment of peripheral blood flow. It is possible that leaving the β_2 receptors unblocked and responsive to epinephrine may be functionally important in some patients with asthma, hypoglycemia, hypertension, or peripheral vascular disease treated with β-adrenergic blocking drugs.[1,3,24]

Intrinsic Sympathomimetic Activity (Partial Agonist Activity)

Certain β-adrenoceptor blockers possess intrinsic sympathomimetic activity (partial agonist activity) at β_1-adrenoceptor receptor sites, β_2-adrenoceptor receptor sites, or both. In a β blocker, this property is identified as a slight cardiac stimulation, which can be blocked by propranolol.[1,3,27,28,30] The β blockers with this property slightly activate the β receptor in addition to preventing the access of natural or synthetic catecholamines to the receptor (Fig. 66-2). Dichloroisoprenaline, the first β-adrenoceptor blocking drug synthesized, exerted such marked partial agonist activity that it was unsuitable for clinical use.[30] Compounds with less partial agonist activity, however, are effective β-blocking drugs. The partial agonist effects of β-adrenoceptor blocking drugs such as pindolol differ from those of the agonists epinephrine and isoproterenol in that the maximum pharmacologic response that can be obtained is low, although the affinity for the receptor is high. In the treatment of patients with arrhythmias, angina pectoris of effort, and hypertension, drugs with mild-to-moderate partial agonist activity appear to be as efficacious as are β blockers lacking this property. It is still debated whether the presence of partial agonist activity in a β blocker constitutes an overall advantage or disadvantage in cardiac therapy.[27] Drugs with partial agonist activity cause less slowing of the heart rate at rest than do propranolol and metoprolol, although the increments in heart rate with exercise are similarly blunted. These beta-blocking agents reduce peripheral vascular resistance and may also cause less depression of atrioventricular (AV) con-

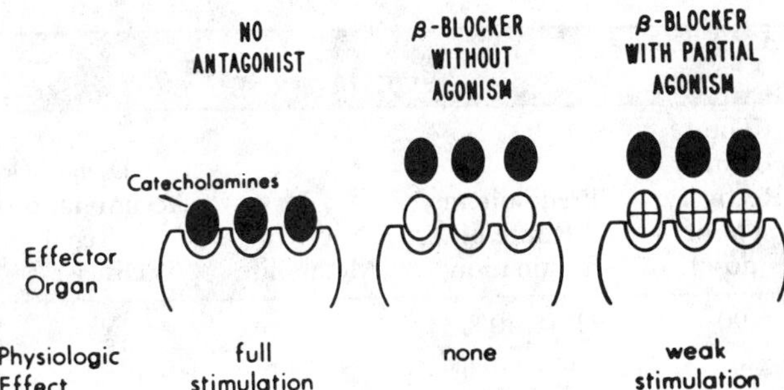

FIGURE 66-2 Physiologic effects of β-adrenergic blocking drugs with and without partial agonist activity in the presence of circulating catecholamines. When circulating catecholamines (●) combine with β-adrenergic receptors, they produce a full physiologic response. When these receptors are occupied by a β blocker lacking partial agonist activity (○), no physiologic effects from catecholamine stimulation can occur. A β-blocking drug with partial agonist activity (⊕) also blocks the binding of catecholamines to β-adrenergic receptors, but the drug also causes a relatively weak stimulation of the receptor. *(From WH Frishman. Pindolol: A new β-adrenoreceptor antagonist with partial agonist activity. N Engl J Med 1983; 308:940–944. Reproduced with permission from the publisher and author.)*

duction compared with drugs lacking these properties.[27,38] Some investigators claim that partial agonist activity in a β blocker protects against myocardial depression, adverse lipid changes, bronchial asthma, and peripheral vascular complications, which are caused by propranolol.[27,38–40] The evidence to support these claims is not conclusive, however, and more definitive clinical trials will be necessary to resolve these issues.

Alpha-Adrenergic Blocking Activity

Labetalol is a β blocker with antagonistic properties at both α and β adrenoceptors, and it has direct vasodilator activity.[2,3,41] Labetalol has been shown to be 6 to 10 times less potent than phentolamine at α-adrenergic receptors and 1.5 to 4 times less potent than propranolol at β-adrenergic receptors, and is itself 4 to 16 times less potent at α than at β adrenoceptors.[2,3,41] Like other β blockers, it is useful in the treatment of hypertension and angina pectoris.[2,42,43] Unlike most β-blocking drugs, however, the additional α-adrenergic blocking actions of labetalol lead to a reduction in peripheral vascular resistance that may maintain cardiac output.[2,41] Whether or not concomitant α-adrenergic blocking activity is actually advantageous in a β blocker remains to be determined.[44,45]

Combined Beta-Adrenergic and Calcium-Entry Blockade

An agent, YM 151, has been developed that demonstrates the pharmacologic properties of a β_1-selective adrenergic blocker and a dihydropyridine-like calcium channel blocker (Table 66-1). This unique compound is now undergoing clinical study in patients with hypertension and angina pectoris.

Pharmacokinetics

Although the β-adrenergic blocking drugs as a group have similar therapeutic effects, their pharmacokinetics are markedly different (Tables 66-2 and 66-3).[3,32,35,46,47]

TABLE 66-2

Pharmacokinetic Properties of Various β-Adrenoceptor Blocking Drugs

Drug	Extent of Absorption (percent of dose)	Extent of Bioavailability (percent of Dose)	Dose-Dependent Bioavailability (Major First-Pass Hepatic Metabolism)	Interpatient Variations in Plasma Levels	β-Blocking Plasma Concentrations	Protein Binding (percent)	Lipid Solubility*
Acebutolol	≈70	≈40	No	7-fold	0.2–2.0 μg/mL	25	Moderate
Atenolol	≈50	≈40	No	4-fold	0.2–5.0 μg/mL	<5	Weak
Betaxolol	>90	≈80	No	2-fold	5–20 ng/mL	50	Moderate
Carteolol	≈90	≈90	No	2-fold	40–160 ng/mL	20–30	Weak
Celiprolol	≈30	≈30	No	3-fold		≈30	Weak
Esmolol†	NA	NA	NA	5-fold	0.15–1.0 μg/mL	55	Weak
Labetalol	>90	≈33	Yes	10-fold	0.7–3.0 μg/mL	≈50	Weak
Metoprolol	>90	≈50	No	7-fold	50–100 ng/mL	12	Moderate
Nadolol	≈30	≈30	No	7-fold	50–100 ng/mL	≈30	Weak
Oxprenolol	≈90	≈40	No	5-fold	80–100 ng/mL	80	Moderate
Penbutolol	>90	≈90	No	4-fold		98	High
Pindolol	>90	≈90	No	4-fold	5–15 ng/mL	57	Moderate
Propranolol	>90	≈30	Yes	20-fold	50–100 ng/mL	93	High
Long-acting propranolol	>90	≈20	Yes	10- to 20-fold	20–100 ng/mL	93	High
Sotalol	≈70	≈60	No	4-fold	0.5–4.0 μg/mL	0	Weak
Timolol	>90	≈75	No	7-fold	5–10 ng/mL	≈10	Weak

* Determined by the distribution ratio between octanol and water.
† Ultra-short-acting β blocker available only in intravenous form.
NOTE: NA = not applicable.
SOURCE: Frishman.[2,3,23]

TABLE 66-3

Elimination Characteristics of β-Adrenoceptor Blocking Drugs

Drug	Elimination Half-Life (h)	Total Body Clearance (mL h/ng)	Urinary Recovery of Unchanged Drug (% of Dose)	Total Urinary Recovery (% of dose)	Predominant Route of Elimination*	Active Metabolites	Drug Accumulation in Renal Disease
Acebutolol	3–4†	6–15	≃40	>90	RE (≃40% unchanged and HM)	Yes	Yes
Atenolol	6–9	130	≃40	>95	RE	No	Yes
Betaxolol	15	350	15	>90	HM	No	Yes
Carteolol	5–6	497	40–68	90	RE	Yes	Yes
Esmolol‡	9 min	27,000	<2	70–90	BE§	No	No
Labetalol	3–4	2700	<1	>90	HM	No	No
Metoprolol	3–4	1100	≃3	>95	HM	No	No
Nadolol	14–24	200	70	70	RE	No	Yes
Oxprenolol	2–3	380	2–5	70–95	HM	No	No
Penbutolol	27	350	50–70	>90	RE	No	No
Pindolol	3–4	400	≃40	>90	RE (≃40% unchanged and HM)	No	No
Propranolol	3–4	1000	<1	>90	HM	Yes	No
Long-acting propranolol	10	1000	<1	>90	HM	Yes	No
Sotalol	9–10	150	≃60	>90	RE	No	Yes
Timolol	4–5	660	≃20	65	RE (≃20% unchanged and HM)	No	No

* RE = renal excretion; HM = hepatic metabolism.
† Acebutolol has an active metabolite with elimination half-life of 8 to 13 h.
‡ Ultra-short-acting β blocker available only in intravenous form.
§ Metabolized by blood esterases.
SOURCE: Frishman.[2,3,23]

Their varied aromatic ring structures lead to differences in completeness of gastrointestinal absorption, amount of first-pass hepatic metabolism, lipid solubility, protein binding, extent of distribution in the body, penetration into the brain, concentration in the heart, rate of hepatic biotransformation, pharmacologic activity of metabolites, and renal clearance of the drug and its metabolites, which may influence the clinical usefulness of these drugs in some patients.[1,3,32,35,47] The desirable pharmacokinetic characteristics in this group of compounds are a lack of major individual differences in bioavailability and in metabolic clearance of the drug and a rate of removal from active tissue sites that is slow enough to allow longer dosing intervals.[1,3,47]

The β blockers can be divided by their pharmacokinetic properties into two broad categories: those eliminated by hepatic metabolism, which tend to have relatively short plasma half-lives, and those eliminated unchanged by the kidney, which tend to have longer half-lives.[1] Propranolol and metoprolol are both lipid-soluble, are almost completely absorbed by the small intestine, and are largely metabolized by the liver. They tend to have highly variable bioavailability and relatively short plasma half-lives.[3,24,32,47] A lack of correlation between the duration of clinical pharmacologic effect and plasma half-life may allow these drugs to be administered once or twice daily.[1]

In contrast, agents such as atenolol and nadolol are more water-soluble, are incompletely absorbed through the gut, and are eliminated unchanged by the kidney.[25,26] They tend to have less variable bioavailability in patients with normal renal function, in addition to longer half-lives, allowing one dose a day.[25,26] The longer half-lives may be useful in patients who find compliance with frequent β-blocker dosing a problem.[25]

A long-acting sustained-release preparation of propranolol is available (Tables 66-2 and 66-3).[48] The propranolol is part of a soluble matrix inside tiny spheroids made of an insoluble membrane. Gastrointestinal fluid enters the spheroids, and propranolol exits via a concentration gradient into the gut lumen and then the bloodstream. The absorption of long-acting propranolol is not dependent on gastric acidity or enzymatic action. Studies have shown that long-acting propranolol provides a much smoother curve of daily plasma levels than do comparable divided doses of conventional propranolol.[48,49] Currently a propranolol nasal spray, which can provide immediate β blockade, is being tested in clinical trials.[50]

Ultra-short-acting β blockers are now available and

may be useful where a short duration of action is desired (e.g., in patients with questionable congestive heart failure). One of these compounds, esmolol, a β_1-selective drug (Tables 66-1, 66-2, and 66-3) has been shown to be useful in the treatment of perioperative hypertension and supraventricular tachycardias (see also Chap. 38).[51] Another drug, flestolol, is under evaluation in clinical trials.[52] The short half-life (approximately 15 min) is related to the rapid metabolism of the drug by blood and hepatic esterases. Metabolism does not seem to be altered by disease states.[53]

The specific pharmacokinetic properties of individual β-adrenergic blockers (for example, first-pass metabolism, active metabolites, lipid solubility, and protein binding) may be clinically important.[3,47,54] When drugs with extensive first-pass metabolism are taken by mouth, they undergo so much hepatic biotransformation that relatively little drug reaches the systemic circulation.[1,3,32,46] Depending on the extent of first-pass effect, an oral dose of β blocker must be larger than an intravenous dose to produce the same clinical effects.[24,32,46] Some β-adrenergic blockers are transformed into pharmacologically active compounds (acebutolol) rather than inactive metabolities.[55] The total pharmacologic effect therefore depends on the amount of the drug administered and its active metabolites.[47] Characteristics of lipid solubility in a β blocker have been associated with the ability of the drug to become concentrated in the brain,[1,3] and many side effects of these drugs that have not been clearly related to β blockade may result from their actions on the central nervous system (for example, lethargy, mental depression, and hallucinations).[1,26] It is still not certain, however, whether drugs that are less lipid-soluble cause fewer of these adverse reactions.[25,26,54,56–59]

Relationship among Dose, Plasma Level, and Efficacy

Attempts have been made to establish a relationship among the oral dose, the plasma level measured by gas chromatography, and the pharmacologic effect of each β-blocking drug.[47] After administration of a certain oral dose, β-blocking drugs that are largely metabolized in the liver show large interindividual variation in circulating plasma levels.[1,3] Many explanations have been proposed to explain the wide individual differences in the relationship between plasma concentrations of β blockers and any associated therapeutic effect. First, patients may have different levels of "sympathetic tone" (circulating catecholamines and active β-adrenoceptor binding sites) and may thus require different drug concentrations to achieve adequate β blockade.[32] Second, many β blockers have flat plasma drug level response curves.[47] Third, active drug isomers and active metabolites are not specifically measured in many plasma assays. Fourth, the clinical effect of a drug may last longer than the period suggested by the drug's half-life in plasma,[32] since recycling of the β blocker between receptor site and neuronal nerve endings may occur. Despite the lack of correlation between plasma levels and therapeutic effect, there is some evidence that a relationship does exist between the logarithm of the plasma level and the β-blocking effect (blockade of exercise- or isoproterenol-induced tachycardia).[24,32,47] Plasma levels have little to offer as therapeutic guides, except for ensuring compliance and for diagnosis of overdose. Pharmacodynamic characteristics of β blockers and clinical response should be used as guides in determining efficacy.

CLINICAL EFFECTS AND THERAPEUTIC APPLICATIONS

The therapeutic efficacy and safety of β-adrenoceptor blocking drugs has been well established in patients with angina pectoris, cardiac arrhythmias, and hypertension and for reducing the risk of mortality and possibly nonfatal reinfarction in survivors of acute myocardial infarction.[1–3,7] These drugs may be useful as a primary protection against cardiovascular morbidity and mortality in hypertensive patients.[60] The drugs are also employed for a multitude of other cardiac (Table 66-4)[2,3,7,61–71] and noncardiac (Table 66-5)[2,3,54,72–80] uses.

Cardiovascular Effects

Effects on Elevated Systemic Blood Pressure

Beta-adrenergic blockers are effective in reducing the blood pressure of many patients with systemic hypertension (Tables 66-6 and 66-7; see also Chap. 77) and were recently cited as a first-line treatment by the fifth report of the Joint National Committee on Detection, Evaluation, and Treatment of High Blood Pressure (JNCV).[81] However, there is no consensus as to the mechanism by

TABLE 66-4

Reported Cardiovascular Indications for β-Adrenoceptor Blocking Drugs

Hypertension (systolic and diastolic)*
Isolated systolic hypertension in elderly patients
Angina pectoris*
"Silent" myocardial ischemia
Supraventricular arrhythmias*
Ventricular arrhythmias*
Reducing the risk of mortality and reinfarction in survivors of acute myocardial infarction*
Hyperacute phase of myocardial infarction*
Dissection of aorta
Hypertrophic cardiomyopathy*
Reversing left ventricular hypertrophy
Digitalis intoxication
Mitral valve prolapse
QT-interval prolongation syndrome
Tetralogy of Fallot
Mitral stenosis
Congestive cardiomyopathy
Fetal tachycardia
Neuocirculatory asthenia

* Indications formally approved by the U.S. Food and Drug Administration.

TABLE 66-5

Some Reported Noncardiovascular Indications for β-Andrenoceptor Blocking Drugs

Neuropsychiatric
- Migraine prophylaxis*
- Essential tremor*
- Situational anxiety
- Alcohol withdrawal (delirium tremens)

Endocrine
- Thyrotoxicosis*
- Hyperparathyroidism

Other
- Glaucoma*
- Portal hypertension and gastrointestinal bleeding

* Indications formally approved by the U.S. Food and Drug Administration.

which these drugs lower blood pressure. It is probable that some or all of the proposed mechanisms discussed below play a part. Beta blockers without vasodilatory activity appear to be more efficacious in white patients and younger patients than they are in black patients and elderly patients.[82]

Negative Chronotropic and Inotropic Effects Slowing of the heart rate and some decrease in myocardial contractility with β blockers lead to a decrease in cardiac output, which in the short term and long term may lead to a reduction in blood pressure.[1] It might be expected that these factors would be of particular importance in the treatment of hypertension related to high cardiac output[81] and increased sympathetic tone.

Differences in Effects on Plasma Renin The relationship between the hypotensive action of β-blocking drugs and their ability to reduce plasma renin activity remains controversial. Some β-blocking drugs antagonize sympathetically mediated renin release,[83] although adrenergic activity is not the only mechanism by which renin release is mediated. Other major determinants are sodium balance, posture, and renal perfusion pressure.

TABLE 66-6

Proposed Mechanisms to Explain the Antihypertensive Actions of β Blockers

- Reduction in cardiac output
- Inhibition of renin
- Central nervous system effects
- Effects on prejunctional β receptors: reductions in norepinephrine release
- Reduction in peripheral vascular resistance
- Reduction in venomotor tone
- Reduction in plasma volume
- Resetting of baroreceptor levels
- Attenuation of pressor response to catecholamines with exercise and stress

SOURCE: Frishman.[2]

The important question remains whether there is a clinical correlation between the effect of the β blocker on the plasma renin activity and the lowering of blood pressure. Investigators[83] have found that "high-renin" patients do not respond or may even show a rise in blood pressure and that "normal-renin" patients have less predictable responses. In high-renin hypertensive patients, it has been suggested that renin may not be the only factor maintaining the high blood pressure state. At present, the role of renin reduction in blood pressure control is not well defined (see also Chap. 75).

Central Nervous System Effects There is now good clinical and experimental evidence to suggest that β blockers cross the blood-brain barrier and enter the central nervous system.[84] Although there is little doubt that β blockers with high lipophilicity (e.g., metoprolol and propranolol) enter the central nervous system in high concentrations, a direct antihypertensive effect mediated by their presence has not been well defined. Also, β blockers that are less lipid-soluble and less likely to concentrate in the brain appear to be as effective in lowering blood pressure as propranolol.[25,26]

Peripheral Resistance Nonselective β blockers have no primary action in lowering peripheral resistance and indeed may cause it to rise by leaving the α-stimulatory mechanisms unopposed.[85] The vasodilating effect of catecholamines on skeletal muscle blood vessels is β_2-mediated, suggesting possible therapeutic advantages in using β_1-selective blockers, agents with partial agonist activity, and drugs with α-blocking activity. Since β_1-selectivity diminishes as the drug dosage is raised and since hypertensive patients generally have to be given far larger doses than are required simply to block the β_1-receptors alone, β_1-selectivity[86] offers the clinician little if any real specific advantage in antihypertensive treatment (see also Chap. 77).[24,86]

Effects on Prejunctional Receptors Apart from their effects on postjunctional tissue β receptors, it is believed that blockade of prejunctional β receptors may be involved in the hemodynamic actions of β-blocking drugs. The stimulation of prejunctional α_2 receptors leads to a reduction in the quantity of norepinephrine released by the postganglionic sympathetic fibers.[87,88] Conversely, stimulation of prejunctional β receptors is followed by an increase in the quantity of norepinephrine released by the postganglionic sympathetic fibers.[89–91] Blockade of prejunctional β receptors should therefore diminish the amount of norepinephrine released, leading to a weaker stimulation of postjunctional α receptors, an effect that would produce less vasoconstriction. Opinions differ, however, on the contributions of presynaptic β blockade to both a reduction in the peripheral vascular resistance and the antihypertensive effects on β-blocking drugs.

Other Proposed Mechanisms Less well-documented effects of β blockers that may contribute to their antihypertensive actions include favorable effects on venous tone and plasma volume,[2] membrane stabilizing activity,[92,93] and resetting of baroreceptors.[94]

TABLE 66-7

Pharamacodynamic Properties and Cardiac Effects of β-Adrenoceptor Blockers

Drug	Relative β_1 Selectivity*	Partial Agonist Activity	Membrane Stabilizing Activity	Resting Heart Rate	Exercise Heart Rate	Resting Myocardial Contractility	Resting Blood Pressure	Exercise Blood Pressure	Resting Atrioventricular Conduction	Antiarrhythmic Effect
Acebutolol	+	+	+	↓↔	↓	↓	↓	↓	↓	+
Atenolol	++	0	0	↓	↓	↓	↓	↓	↓	+
Betaxolol	++	0	+	↓	↓	↓	↓	↓	↓	+
Carteolol	0	+	0	↓↔	↓	↓↔	↓	↓	↓	+
Carvedilol†	0	0	++	↓↔	↓	↓↔	↓	↓	↓↔	+
Esmolol	++	0	0	↓	↓	↓	↓	↓	↓	+
Labetalol‡	0	+	0	↔	↓	↓↔	↓	↓↓	↓↔	+
Metoprolol	++	0	0	↓	↓	↓	↓	↓	↓	+
Nadolol	0	0	0	↓	↓	↓	↓	↓	↓	+
Oxprenolol	0	+	+	↓↔	↓	↓↔	↓	↓	↓↔	+
Penbutolol	0	+	0	↓↔	↓	↓↔	↓	↓	↓↔	+
Pindolol	0	++	0	↓↔	↓	↓↔	↓	↓	↓↔	+
Propranolol	0	0	++	↓	↓	↓	↓	↓	↓	+
Sotalol	0	0	0	↓	↓	↓	↓	↓	↓	+
Timolol	0	0	0	↓	↓	↓	↓	↓	↓	+
Isomer: D-propranolol	0	0	++	↔	↔	↔↓§	↔	↔	↔↓§	+§

* β_1 selectivity is seen only with low therapeutic drug concentrations. With higher concentrations, β_1 selectivity is not seen.
† Carvedilol has peripheral vesodilating activity.
‡ Labetalol has additional α_1-adrenergic blocking properties and direct β_2-adrenergic vasodilator activity.
§ Effects of D-propranolol with doses in human beings well above the therapeutic level. The isomer also lacks β-blocking activity.
SOURCE: Frishman.[2,3,23]
NOTE: ++ = strong effect; + = modest effect; 0 = absent effect; ↑ = elevation; ↓ = reduction; ↔ = no change.

Effects in Angina Pectoris

Ahlquist[16] demonstrated that sympathetic innervation of the heart causes the release of norepinephrine, activating β adrenoreceptors in myocardial cells (Table 66-7). This adrenergic stimulation causes an increment in heart rate, isometric contractile force, and maximal velocity of muscle fiber shortening, all of which lead to an increase in cardiac work and myocardial oxygen consumption.[95] The decrease in intraventricular pressure and volume caused by the sympathetic-mediated enhancement of cardiac contractility tends, on the other hand, to reduce myocardial oxygen consumption by reducing myocardial wall tension (Laplace's law) (see Chap. 5).[96] Although there is a net increase in myocardial oxygen demand, it is normally balanced by an increase in coronary blood flow. Angina pectoris is believed to occur when oxygen demand exceeds supply, that is, when coronary blood flow is restricted by coronary atherosclerosis. Since the conditions that precipitate anginal attacks (exercise, emotional stress, food, etc.) cause an increase in cardiac sympathetic activity, it might be expected that blockade of cardiac β adrenoreceptors would relieve the anginal symptoms. It is on this basis that the early clinical studies with β-blocking drugs in patients with angina pectoris were initiated.[97]

Three main factors—heart rate, ventricular systolic pressure, and the size of the left ventricle—contribute to the myocardial oxygen requirements of the left ventricle. Of these, heart rate and systolic pressure appear to be the most important (the product of heart rate multiplied by the systolic blood pressure is a reliable index for predicting the precipitation of angina in a given patient).[98,99]

The reduction in heart rate effected by β blockade has two favorable consequences: (1) a decrease in blood pressure, thus reducing myocardial oxygen needs, and (2) a longer diastolic filling time associated with a slower heart rate, allowing for increased coronary perfusion. Beta blockade also reduces exercise-induced blood pressure increments, the velocity of cardiac contraction, and oxygen consumption at any patient work load.[98,99]

Studies in dogs have shown that propranolol causes a decrease in coronary blood flow.[100] Subsequent experimental animal studies, however, have demonstrated that β-blocking-induced shunting occurs in the coronary circulation, maintaining blood flow to ischemic areas, especially in the subendocardial region.[101] In human beings, concomitantly with the decrease in myocardial oxygen consumption, β blockers can cause a reduction in coronary blood flow and a rise in coronary vascular resistance.[102] On the basis of coronary autoregulation, the overall reduction in myocardial oxygen needs with β blockers may be sufficient cause for this decrease in coronary blood flow.[98,99]

Virtually all β blockers, whether or not they have partial agonist activity, α-blocking effects, membrane-stabilizing activity, and general or selective β-blocking properties, produce some degree of increased work capacity without pain in patients with angina pectoris. Therefore, it must be concluded that this results from their common property: blockade of cardiac β receptors.[98] Both D- and L-propranolol have membrane-stabilizing activity, but only L-propranolol has significant β-blocking activity. The racemic mixture (D- and L-propranolol) causes a decrease in both heart rate and force of contraction in dogs, while the D-isomer has hardly any effect.[103] In human beings, D-propranolol, which has "membrane" activity but no β-blocking properties, has been found to be ineffective in relieving angina pectoris, even at very high doses.[104]

Although exercise tolerance improves with β blockade, the increments in heart rate and blood pressure with exercise are blunted, and the rate-pressure product (systolic blood pressure × heart rate) achieved when pain occurs is lower than that reached during a control run.[105] The depressed pressure-rate product at the onset of pain (about 20 percent reduction from control) is reported to occur with various β-blocking drugs, probably related to decreased cardiac output. Thus, although there is increased exercise tolerance with β blockade, patients exercise less than might be expected. This may also be related to the action of β blockers in increasing left ventricular size, causing increased left ventricular wall tension and an increase in oxygen consumption at a given blood pressure.[106]

Combined Use of Beta Blockers with Other Antianginal Therapies in Angina Pectoris

Nitrates Combined therapy with nitrates and β blockers may be more efficacious for the treatment of angina pectoris than the use of either drug alone.[98,107] The primary effect of β blockers is to cause a reduction in both resting heart rate and the response of heart rate to exercise. Since nitrates produce a reflex increase in heart rate and contractility secondary to a reduction in arterial pressure, concomitant β-blocker therapy is extremely effective because it blocks this reflex increment in the heart rate. Similarly, the preservation of diastolic coronary flow with a reduced heart rate will also be beneficial.[98] In patients with a propensity for myocardial failure who may have a slight increase in heart size with the β blockers, the nitrates will counteract this tendency by reducing heart size as a result of its peripheral venodilator effects. During the administration of nitrates, the reflex increase in contractility that is mediated through the sympathetic nervous system will be checked by the presence of β blockers. Similarly, the increase in coronary resistance associated with β-blocker administration can be ameliorated by the administration of nitrates.[98]

Calcium-Entry Blockers Calcium-entry blockers are a group of drugs that block transmembrane calcium currents in vascular smooth muscle to cause arterial vasodilatation (see Chap. 67). Some calcium-entry blockers (diltiazem and verapamil) also slow the heart rate and reduce AV conduction. Combined therapy with β-adrenergic and calcium-entry blockers can provide clinical benefits for patients with angina pectoris who remain symptomatic with either agent used alone.[108–110] Because adverse cardiovascular effects can occur, however, patients being considered for such treatment must be carefully selected and observed.[108,109]

Angina at Rest and Vasospastic Angina

Angina pectoris can be caused by multiple mechanisms, including coronary vasospasm and thrombosis, which appear to be responsible for ischemia in a significant proportion of patients with unstable angina and angina at rest.[98–108] Therefore, β blockers that primarily reduce myocardial oxygen consumption but fail to exert vasodilating effects on coronary vasculature may not be totally effective in patients in whom angina is caused or increased by dynamic alterations in coronary luminal diameter.[98,109] Despite potential dangers in rest and vasospatic angina, β blockers have been used successfully as monotherapy and in combination with vasodilating agents in many patients (see also Chap. 59).[98]

Electrophysiological and Antiarrhythmic Effects

Adrenoceptor-blocking drugs have two main effects on the electrophysiological properties of specialized cardiac tissue (Table 66-8).[111] The first effect results from specific blockade of adrenergic stimulation of cardiac pacemaker potentials. In concentrations causing significant inhibition of adrenergic receptors, β blockers produce little change in the transmembrane potentials of cardiac muscle. By competitively inhibiting adrenergic stimulation, however, beta blockers decrease the slope of phase IV depolarization and the spontaneous firing rate of sinus or ectopic pacemakers and thus decrease automaticity. Arrhythmias occurring in the setting of enhanced automaticity, as seen in myocardial infarction, digitalis toxicity, hyperthyroidism, and pheochromocytoma, would therefore be expected to respond well to β blockade.[2,111]

The second electrophysiological effect of β blockers involves membrane-stabilizing action, also known as "quinidine-like" or "local anesthetic" action, which is observed only at very high dose levels. This property is unrelated to inhibition of catecholamine action and is possessed equally by both the D- and L-isomers of the drugs (D-isomers have almost no β-blocking activity).[111] Characteristic of this effect is a reduction in the rate of

TABLE 66-8

Antiarrhythmic Properties of β Blockers

β blockade
- Electrophysiology: depress excitability; depress conduction
- Prevention of ischemia: decrease automaticity; inhibit reentrant mechanisms

Membrane-stabilizing effects
- Local anesthetic, "quinidine-like" properties: depress excitability; prolong refractory period; delay conduction
- Clinically: probably not significant

Special pharmacologic properties (β_1 selectivity, intrinsic sympathomimetic activity) do not appear to contribute to antiarrhythmic effectiveness

SOURCE: Frishman.[2]

rise of the intracardial action potential without an effect on the spike duration of the resting potential.[111] Associated features include an elevated electric threshold of excitability, a delay in conduction velocity, and a significant increase in the effective refractory period. This effect and its attendant changes have been explained by inhibition of the depolarizing inward sodium current.[111]

Sotalol is unique among the β blockers in that it possesses class III antiarrhythmic properties, causing prolongation of the action potential period and thus delaying repolarization.[34] Clinical studies have verified the efficacy of sotalol in control of ventricular arrhythmias,[34] but additional investigation will be required to determine whether its class III antiarrhythmic properties contribute significantly to its efficacy as an antiarrhythmic agent.

The most important mechanism underlying the antiarrhythmic effect of β blockers, with the possible exclusion of sotalol, is believed to be β blockade, with resultant inhibition of pacemaker potentials. The contribution of membrane-stabilizing action does not appear to be clinically significant. In vitro experiments with human ventricular muscle have shown that the concentration of propranolol required for membrane stabilizing is 50 to 100 times the concentration usually associated with inhibition of exercise-induced tachycardia and at which only β-blocking effects occur.[111] Moreover, D-propranolol, which possesses membrane-stabilizing properties but no β-blocking action, is a weak antiarrhythmic even at high doses, while β blockers devoid of membrane-stabilizing action (atenolol, esmolol, metoprolol, nadolol, pindolol, etc.) have been shown to be effective antiarrhythmic drugs.[2,3,51] Differences in overall clinical usefulness are related to their other associated pharmacologic properties (see also Chap. 38).[2,3]

Therapeutic Uses in Cardiac Arrhythmias

Beta-adrenergic blocking drugs have become an important treatment for various cardiac arrhythmias (Table 66-9).[2,3,111] While it has long been believed that β blockers are more effective in treating supraventricular arrhythmias than ventricular arrhythmias, it is now well appreciated that this may not be the case. These agents can be quite useful in the treatment of ventricular tachyarrhythmias in the setting of myocardial ischemia, mitral valve prolapse, and other cardiovascular conditions (see also Chap. 36).[111–114]

Effects in Survivors of Acute Myocardial Infarction

Beta-adrenergic blockers have beneficial effects on many determinants of myocardial ischemia (Table 66-10).[2,99,115] The results of placebo-controlled, long-term treatment trials with some β-adrenergic blocking drugs in survivors of acute myocardial infarction have demonstrated a favorable effect on total mortality; cardiovascular mortality, including sudden and nonsudden cardiac deaths; and the incidence of nonfatal reinfarction.[7,116] These beneficial results with β-blocker therapy can be explained by both the antiarrhythmic (Table 66-9) and the anti-ischemic effects of these drugs.[99,112,117] It has also been proposed that β-adrenergic blockers could reduce the risk of atherosclerotic plaque fissure and subsequent thrombosis.[118] Two nonselective β blockers, propranolol and timolol, have been approved for reducing the risk of mortality in infarct survivors when started 5 to 28 days after an infarction. Metoprolol and atenolol, two β_1-selective blockers, are approved for the same indication, and both can also be used intravenously in the hyperacute phase of a myocardial infarction. Beta blockers

TABLE 66-9

Effects of β Blockers on Various Arrhythmias

Arrhythmia	Comment
Supraventricular	
Sinus tachycardia	Treat underlying disorder; excellent response to β blocker if need to control rate (e.g., ischemia)
Atrial fibrillation	β blockers reduce rate, rarely restore sinus rhythm; may be useful in combination with digoxin
Atrial flutter	β blockers reduce rate, sometimes restore sinus rhythm
Atrial tachycardia	Effective in slowing ventricular rate; may restore sinus rhythm; useful in prophylaxis
Ventricular	
Premature ventricular complexes	Good response to β blockers (as effective as quinidine), especially digitalis-induced, exercise (ischemia)-induced, mitral valve prolapse, or hypertrophic cardiomyopathy
Ventricular tachycardia	As effective as quinidine; most effective in digitalis toxicity or exercise (ischemia)-induced
Ventricular fibrillation	Electric defibrillation is treatment of choice; β blockers can be used to prevent recurrence in cases of excess digitalis or sympathomimetic amines; appear to be effective in reducing incidence of ventricular fibrillation and sudden death after myocardial infarction

SOURCE: Frishman.[2]

TABLE 66-10

Possible Mechanisms by Which β Blockers Protect the Ischemic Myocardium

Reduction in myocardial oxygen consumption, heart rate, blood pressure, and myocardial contractility
Augmentation of coronary blood flow, increase in diastolic perfusion time by reducing heart rate, augmentation of collateral blood flow, and redistribution of blood flow to ischemic areas
Prevention of attenuation of atherosclerotic plaque, rupture, and subsequent coronary thrombosis
Alterations in myocardial substrate utilization
Decrease in microvascular damage
Stabilization of cell and lysosomal membranes
Shift of oxyhemoglobin dissociation curve to the right
Inhibition of platelet aggregation

have also been suggested as a treatment for reducing the extent of myocardial injury[7,119,120] and mortality during the hyperacute phase of myocardial infarction,[8,121] but their role in this situation remains unclear.[122] Intravenous and oral atenolol have been shown to be effective in causing a modest reduction in early mortality when given during the hyperacute phase of acute myocardial infarction.[8] Atenolol and metoprolol reduce early infarct mortality by 15 percent,[8,121] an effect that may be improved upon when β-adrenergic blockade is combined with acute thrombolytic therapy. Metoprolol combined with acute thrombolysis has been evaluated in the TIMI-II study (see also Chap. 60).[9]

"Silent" Myocardial Ischemia

In recent years, investigators have observed that not all myocardial ischemic episodes detected by electrocardiography (ECG) are associated with detectable symptoms.[123] Positron emission imaging techniques have validated that these silent ischemic episodes are indicative of true myocardial ischemia.[124] The prognostic importance of silent myocardial ischemia occurring at rest and/or during exercise has not been determined. Beta-blockers are as successful in reducing the frequency of silent ischemic episodes detected by ambulatory ECG monitoring as in reducing the frequency of painful ischemic events.[123]

Other Cardiovascular Applications

Although β blockers have been studied extensively in patients with angina pectoris, arrhythmias, and hypertension, they have also been shown to be safe and effective for other cardiovascular conditions (Table 66-4). Some of these conditions are described below.

Hypertrophic Cardiomyopathy Beta-adrenergic receptor blocking drugs have been proven effective in therapy for patients with hypertrophic cardiomyopathy and idiopathic hypertrophic subaortic stenosis.[62,125] These drugs are useful in controlling the symptoms: dyspnea, angina, and syncope.[2,3] Beta-blockers have also been shown to lower the intraventricular pressure gradient both at rest and with exercise.

The outflow pressure gradient is not the only abnormality in hypertrophic cardiomyopathy; more important is the loss of ventricular compliance, which impedes normal left ventricular function. It has been shown by invasive and noninvasive methods that propranolol can improve left ventricular function in this condition.[126] The drug also produces favorable changes in ventricular compliance while it relieves symptoms. Propranolol has been approved for this condition and may be combined with the calcium entry blocker verapamil in patients who do not respond to the β blocker alone.

The salutary hemodynamic and symptomatic effects produced by propranolol are derived from its inhibition of sympathetic stimulation of the heart.[127] There is no evidence that the drug alters the primary cardiomyopathic process; many patients remain in or return to their severely symptomatic state, and some die despite it administration (see also Chap. 90).[62,125]

Dilated Cardiomyopathy The ability of intravenously administered sympathomimetic amines to effect an acute increase in myocardial contractility through stimulation of the β adrenoceptor has prompted hope that oral analogues may provide long-term benefit for patients with severe heart failure. Recent observations concerning the regulation of the myocardial adrenoceptor and abnormalities of β-receptor-mediated stimulation in the failing myocardium have caused a critical reappraisal of the scientific validity of sustained β_1-adrenoceptor stimulation, however.[19,20] New evidence suggests that β_1-adrenoceptor blockade may, when tolerated, have a favorable effect on the underlying cardiomyopathic process.[71,128–130]

The excessive catecholamine stimulation of the heart that occurs in chronic congestive heart failure can cause myocardial catecholamine depletion,[131] a direct toxic effect on the heart,[132,133] alterations in the β-adrenergic receptor–adenylate cyclase complex,[134] and down regulation of β-adrenergic receptors.[19,20,135] It appears that β-adrenergic blockade can correct these abnormalities and possibly improve left ventricular function (see also Chap. 25).[129,130]

Preliminary studies with chronic β blockade have demonstrated improvement in left ventricular function in many patients with advanced cardiomyopathy.[136–139] These studies have included patients who showed dramatic improvement in their hemodynamic situations while awaiting cardiac transplantation.[140] A large, prospective, double-blind, multicenter study (Metoprolol in Dilated Cardiomyopathy) is in progress, evaluating the efficacy of B-blocker therapy in patients with idiopathic dilated cardiomyopathy (see also Chaps. 26 and 89).

Mitral Valve Prolapse An auscultatory complex characterized by a nonejection systolic click, a late systolic murmur, or a midsystolic click followed by a late systolic murmur, mitral valve prolapse has been studied extensively over the past 15 years.[141] Atypical chest pain, malignant arrhythmias, and nonspecific ST- and T-wave abnormalities have been observed with this condition. By decreasing sympathetic tone, β-adrenergic blockers have been shown to be useful for relieving the chest pains and palpitations that many of these patients experience and for reducing the incidence of life-threatening arrhythmias and other ECG abnormalities (see Chap. 80).[64]

Dissecting Aneurysms Beta-adrenergic blockade plays a major role in the treatment of patients with acute aortic dissection. During the hyperacute phase, β-blocking agents reduce the force and velocity of myocardial contraction (*dP/dt*) and hence the progression of the dissecting hematoma.[61] Moreover, such administration must be initiated simultaneously with the institution of other antihypertensive therapy that may cause reflex tachycardia and increases in cardiac output, factors that can aggravate the dissection process. Initially, propranolol is administered intravenously to reduce the heart rate to below 60 beats per minute. Once a patient's condition is stabilized and long-term medical management is contemplated, the patient should be maintained on oral β-blocker therapy to prevent recurrence.[61]

Recently, it has been demonstrated that long-term β-blocker therapy may also reduce the risk of dissection in patients prone to developing this complication (e.g., patients with Marfan's syndrome). Systolic time intervals are used to assess the adequacy of β blockade in children with Marfan's syndrome (see also Chap. 123).[67]

Tetralogy of Fallot By reducing the effects of increased adrenergic tone on the right ventricular infundibulum in tetralogy of Fallot, β blockers have been shown to be useful for the treatment of severe hypoxic spells and hypercyanotic attack.[66,67] With chronic use, these drugs have also been shown to prevent prolonged hypoxic spells. These drugs should be looked at only as palliative, and definitive surgical repair of this condition is usually required (see Chap. 97).

QT-Interval Prolongation Syndrome The syndrome of ECG QT-interval prolongation is usually a congenital condition associated with deafness, syncope, and sudden death.[65] Abnormalities in sympathetic nervous system functioning in the heart have been proposed as explanations for the electrophysiological aberrations seen in these patients.[65] Propranolol appears to be the most effective drug for treatment of this syndrome. It reduces the frequency of syncopal episodes in most patients and may prevent sudden death.[65] This drug will reduce the ECG QT interval (see also Chap. 36).

Regression of Left Ventricular Hypertrophy Left ventricular hypertrophy induced by systemic hypertension is an independent risk factor for cardiovascular mortality and morbidity.[142] Regression of left ventricular hypertrophy with drug therapy is feasible and may improve patient outcome.[142] Beta-adrenergic blockers can cause regression of left ventricular hypertrophy, as determined by echocardiography, with or without an associated reduction in blood pressure.[142] (See also Chap. 77.)

Noncardiovascular Applications

Beta-adrenergic receptors are ubiquitous in the human body, and their blockade affects a variety of organ and metabolic systems (Table 66-11).[2,3,54] Some noncardio-

TABLE 66-11

Pharmacodynamic Properties and Noncardiac Effects of β-Adrenoceptor Blockers

Drug	Relative β_1 Selectivity*	Partial Agonist Activity	Membrane-Stabilizing Activity	Bronchial Tone	Platelet Aggregability	Plasma Renin Activity	Peripheral Vascular Resistance	RBF	GFR	HDL-C	LDL-C	VLDL-TRI
Acebutolol	+	+	+	↑↔↓		↓↔	↑↔	↓↔	↓↔	↔	↔	↔
Atenolol	+ +	0	0	↑↔↓		↓↔	↑↔	↓↔	↓↔	↔	↔	↔
Betaxolol	+ +	0	+	↑↔↓		↓↔	↑↔	↑↔	↔	↔	↔	↔
Carteolol	0	+	0	↑↔↓	↓	↓↔	↓↔↑	↓↔	↓↔	↔	↔	↔
Esmolol	+ +	0	0	↑↔↓		↓↔	↑↔	?	?	?	?	?
Labetalol†	0	+	0	↑↔↓	↔	↓↔	↓	↔↑	↔	↔	↔	↔
Metoprolol	+ +	0	0	↑↔↓		↓↔	↑↔	↓↔	↓↔	↔↓	↔	↑↔
Nadolol	0	0	0	↔↓		↓↔	↑	↑	↑↔	?	?	?
Oxprenolol	0	+	+	↑↔↓	↓	↓↔	↑↔	↓↔	↓	?	?	?
Penbutolol	0	+	0	↑↔↓		↓↔	↔↓	?	?	?	?	?
Pindolol	0	+ +	0	↑↔↓	↓	↓↔↑	↔↓	↓↔	↓↔	↔	↔	↔
Propranolol	0	0	+ +	↔↓	↓	↓	↑	↓	↓		↔	↑
Sotalol	0	0	0	↔↓		↓	↑	↓	↓	?	?	?
Timolol	0	0	0	↔↓	↓	↓	↑	↓	↓	?	?	?
Isomer: D-propranolol	0	0	+ +	↔	↓	↔	↔	↔	↔	?	?	?

* β_1 selectivity is seen only with low therapeutic drug concentrations. With higher concentrations, β_1 selectivity is not seen.
† Labetalol has additional α-adrenergic blocking properties and direct vasodilator activity.
SOURCE: Frishman.[2,3]
NOTE: + + = strong effect; + = modest effect; 0 = absent effect; ↑ = elevation; ↓ = reduction; ↔ = no change; RBF = renal blood flow; GFR = glomerular filtration rate; HDL-C = high-density lipoprotein cholesterol; LDL-C = low-density lipoprotein cholesterol; VLDL-TRI = very low-density lipoprotein triglycerides.

vascular uses of β blockers (for glaucoma, migraine headache prophylaxis, and essential tremor) have been approved by the U.S. Food and Drug Administration.[1]

ADVERSE EFFECTS OF BETA-BLOCKERS

Evaluation of adverse effects is complex because of the use of various definitions of side effects, the kinds of patients studied, study design features, and various methods of ascertaining and reporting adverse side effects from study to study.[143–145] Overall, the types and frequencies of adverse effects attributed to various β-blocker compounds appear similar.[144,145] The side effect profiles resemble those seen with concurrent placebo treatments, attesting to the remarkable safety margin of the β blockers (see also Chap. 109).[143]

Adverse effects fall into two categories (1) those from known pharmacologic consequences of β-adrenoceptor blockade, and (2) other reactions apart from β-adrenoceptor blockade.

The first type includes asthma, heart failure, hypoglycemia, bradycardia and heart block, intermittent claudication, and Raynaud's phenomenon. The incidence of these adverse effects varies with the β blocker used.[2,144,145]

Side effects of the second category are rare. They include an unusual oculomucocutaneous reaction and the possibility of carcinogenesis.[2,144,145]

Adverse Cardiac Effects Related to Beta-Adrenoceptor Blockade

Congestive Heart Failure

Blockade of β-receptors may cause congestive heart failure in a patient with an enlarged heart and impaired systolic function where excessive sympathetic drive is essential to maintain the myocardium on a compensated Starling curve and where left ventricular stroke volume is restricted and tachycardia is needed to maintain cardiac output.

Thus, any β-blocking drug may be associated with the development of heart failure. Furthermore, heart failure may also be augmented by increases in peripheral vascular resistance produced by nonselective agents (e.g., propranolol, timolol, and sotalol).[145] It has been claimed that β blockers with intrinsic sympathomimetic activity and α-blocking activity are better in preserving left ventricular function and less likely to precipitate heart failure,[146] but there have been only limited in vivo studies in human beings to support this contention.[40]

In patients with impaired myocardial systolic function who require β-blocking agents, digitalis and diuretics can be used.

Sinus Node Dysfunction and AV Conduction Delay

Slowing of the resting heart rate is a normal response to treatment with β-blocking drugs with and without intrinsic sympathomimetic activity. Healthy persons can sustain a heart rate of 40 to 50 beats per minute without disability unless there is clinical evidence of heart failure.[33] Drugs with intrinsic sympathomimetic activity do not lower the resting heart rate to the same degree as does propranolol,[147] but all β-blocking drugs are contraindicated (unless an artificial pacemaker is present) in patients with sick sinus syndrome.[145]

If there is a partial or complete AV conduction defect, the use of a β-blocking drug may lead to a serious bradyarrhythmia.[145] The risk of AV impairment may be less with β blockers that have intrinsic sympathomimetic activity.[148]

Overdosage

Suicide attempts and accidental overdosing with β blockers are being described with increasing frequency. Since B-adrenergic blockers are competitive pharmacologic antagonists, their life-threatening effects (bradycardia and myocardial and ventilatory failure) can be overcome with an immediate infusion of β-agonist agents, such as isoproterenol and dobutamine.[36] In situations where catecholamines are not effective, intravenously administered glucagon amrinone and milrinone have been used.[36]

Close monitoring of cardiorespiratory function is necessary for at least 24 h after the patient responds to therapy. Patients who recover usually have no long-term sequelae; however, they should be observed for the cardiac signs of sudden β-blocker withdrawal.[36]

Beta-Adrenoceptor Blocker Withdrawal

After abrupt cessation of chronic β-blocker therapy, exacerbation of angina pectoris and, in some cases, acute myocardial infarction and death have been reported.[18] Observations made in multiple double-blind randomized trials have confirmed the reality of a propranolol withdrawal reaction.[18,149] The mechanism for this reaction is unclear. There is some evidence that the withdrawal phenomenon may be due to the generation of additional β adrenoceptors during the period of β-adrenoceptor blockade. When the β-adrenoceptor blocker is then withdrawn, the increased β-receptor population readily results in an excessive β-receptor stimulation that is clinically important when the delivery and use of oxygen are finely balanced, as occurs in ischemic heart disease. Other suggested mechanisms for the withdrawal reaction include heightened platelet aggregability, an elevation in thyroid hormone activity, and an increase in circulating catecholamines.[18]

Adverse Noncardiac Side Effects Related to Beta-Adrenoceptor Blockade

Effect on Ventilatory Function

The bronchodilatory effects of catecholamines on the bronchial β_2 adrenoceptors are inhibited by nonselective β blockers (e.g., propranolol and nadolol).[145] Beta-blocking compounds with partial agonist activity,[27,38] β_1 selectivity,[24,25] and α-adrenergic blocking actions[150] are less likely to increase airway resistance in asthmatics. However, β_1 selectivity, is not absolute and may be lost with high therapeutic doses, as shown with atenolol and metoprolol. It is possible in treating asthma to use a β_2-selective agonist (such as albuterol) in certain patients with concomitant low-dose β_1-selective blocker treatment.[151] In general, all β blockers should be avoided in patients with bronchospastic disease.

Peripheral Vascular Effects (Raynaud's Phenomenon)

Cold extremities and absent pulses have been reported more frequently in patients receiving β blockers for hypertension than in those receiving methyldopa.[46] Among the β blockers, the incidence was highest with propranolol and lower with drugs having β_1 selectivity or intrinsic sympathomimetic activity. In some instances, vascular compromise has been severe enough to cause cyanosis and impending gangrene,[152] probably due to the reduction in cardiac output and blockade of β_2-adrenoceptor-mediated skeletal muscle vasodilation, resulting in unopposed β-adrenoceptor vasoconstriction.[153] Beta-blocking drugs with β_1 selectivity or partial agonist activity will not affect peripheral vessels to the same degree as does propranolol.

Raynaud's phenomenon is one of the more common side effects of propranolol treatment.[154] It is more troublesome with propranolol than with metoprolol, atenolol, or pindolol, probably because of the β_2-blocking properties of propranolol.

Patients with peripheral vascular disease who suffer from intermittent claudication occasionally report worsening of the claudication when treated with β-blocking drugs.[155] Whether or not drugs with β_1 selectivity or partial agonist activity can protect against this adverse reaction has not been determined.[156]

Hypoglycemia and Hyperglycemia

Several authors have described severe hypoglycemic reactions during therapy with β-adrenergic blocking drugs.[157] Some of the patients affected were insulin-dependent diabetics, while others were nondiabetic. Studies of resting normal volunteers have demonstrated that propranolol produces no alteration in blood glucose values,[158] although the hyperglycemic response to exercise is blunted.

The enhancement of insulin-induced hypoglycemia and its hemodynamic consequences may be less with β_1-selective agents (where there is no blocking effect on β_2 receptors) and agents with intrinsic sympathomimetic activity (which may stimulate β_2 receptors).[159]

There is also marked diminution in the clinical manifestations of the catecholamine discharge induced by hypoglycemia (tachycardia).[160] These findings suggest that β blockers interfere with compensatory responses to hypoglycemia and can mask certain "warning signs" of this condition. Other hypoglycemic reactions, such as diaphoresis, are not affected by β-adrenergic blockade.

Central Nervous System Effects

Dreams, hallucinations, insomnia, and depression can occur during therapy with β blockers.[54,76] These symptoms provide evidence of drug entry into the central nervous system (CNS), and may be more common with the highly lipid-soluble β blockers (propranolol and metoprolol), which presumably penetrate the CNS better. It has been claimed that β blockers with less lipid solubility (atenolol and nadolol) cause fewer CNS side effects.[25,26] This claim is intriguing, but its validity has not been corroborated by other extensive clinical experiences.[56,57]

Miscellaneous Side Effects

Diarrhea, nausea, gastric pain, constipation, and flatulence have been noted occasionally with all β blockers (2 to 11 percent of patients).[161] Hematologic reactions are rare. Rare cases of purpura[162] and agranulocytosis[163] have been described with propranolol. A devastating blood pressure rebound effect has been described in patients who discontinued clonidine while being treated with nonselective β-blocking agents. The mechanism of this effect may be related to an increase in circulating catecholamines and an increase in peripheral vascular resistance.[164] Whether or not β_1-selective or partial agonist β blockers have similar effects following clonidine withdrawal has not been determined. Such effects have not been a problem with labetalol.[165]

Adverse Effects Unrelated to Beta-Adrenoceptor Blockade: Oculomucocutaneous Syndrome

A characteristic immune reaction, the oculomucocutaneous syndrome, affecting singly or in combination the eyes, the mucous and serous membranes, and the skin, often in association with a positive antinuclear factor, was reported in patients treated with practolol and led to the curtailment of its clinical use.[145,166] Close attention has been focused on this syndrome because of fears that other β-adrenoceptor blocking drugs may be associated with this syndrome.

Drug-Drug Interactions

Beta blockers are commonly employed, and the list of commonly used drugs with which they interact is extensive (Table 66–12).[2,54,167,168] The majority of the reported interactions have been associated with propranolol, the best studied β blocker, and may not necessarily apply to other drugs in this class. (See also Chap. 109.)

HOW TO CHOOSE A BETA BLOCKER

The various β-blocking compounds given in adequate dosage appear to have comparable antihypertensive, antiarrhythmic, and antianginal effects. Therefore, the β-blocking drug of choice in an individual patient is determined by the pharmacodynamic and pharmacokinetic differences among the drugs, in conjunction with the patient's other medical conditions (Table 66–13).[2,3,27]

TABLE 66-12

Drug-Drug Interactions That May Occur with β-Adrenoceptor Blocking Drugs

Drug	Possible Effects	Precautions
Aluminum hydroxide gel	Decreases β-blocker absorption and therapeutic effect	Avoid β blocker–aluminum hydroxide combination.
Aminophylline	Mutual inhibition	Observe patient's response.
Amiodarone	May induce cardiac arrest	Combination should be used with extreme caution.
Antidiabetic agents	Enhanced hypoglycemia; hypertension	Monitor for altered diabetic response.
Calcium channel inhibitors (verapamil, diltiazem)	Potentiation of bradycardia, myocardial depression, and hypotension	Avoid use, although few patients show ill effects.
Cimetidine	Prolongs half-life of propranolol	Combination should be used with caution.
Clonidine	Hypertension during clonidine withdrawal	Monitor for hypertensive response; withdraw β blocker before withdrawing clonidine.
Digitalis glycosides	Potentiation of bradycardia	Observe patient's response; interactions may benefit angina patients with abnormal ventricular function.
Epinephrine	Hypertension; bradycardia	Administer epinephrine cautiously; cardioselective β blocker may be safer.
Ergot alkaloids	Excessive vasoconstriction	Observe patient's response; few patients show ill effects.
Glucagon	Inhibition of hyperglycemic effect	Monitor for reduced response.
Halofenate	Reduced β-blocking activity; production of propranolol withdrawal rebound syndrome	Observe for impaired response to β blockade.
Indomethacin	Inhibition of antihypertensive response to β blockade	Observe patient's response.
Isoproterenol	Mutual inhibition	Avoid concurrent use, or choose cardiac-selective β blocker.
Levodopa	Antagonism of levodopa's hypotensive and positive inotropic effects	Monitor for altered response; interaction may have favorable results.
Lidocaine	Propranolol pretreatment increases lidocaine blood levels and potential toxicity	Combination should be used with caution; use lower doses of lidocaine.
Methyldopa	Hypertension during stress	Monitor for hypertensive episodes.
Monoamine oxidase inhibitors	Uncertain, theoretical	Manufacturer of propranolol considers concurrent use contraindicated.
Phenothiazines	Additive hypotensive effects	Monitor for altered response, especially with high doses of phenothiazines.
Phenylpropanolamine	Severe hypertensive reaction	Avoid use, especially in hypertension controlled by both methyldopa and β blockers.
Phenytoin	Additive cardiac depressant effects	Administer IV phenytoin with great caution.
Quinidine	Additive cardiac depressant effects	Observe patient's response; few patients show ill effects.
Reserpine	Excessive sympathetic blockade	Observe patient's response.
Rifampin	Increased metabolism of β blockers	Observe patient's response.
Smoking	Increased metabolism of β blockers	Observe patient's response.
Tricyclic antidepressants	Inhibits negative inotropic and chronotropic effects of β blockers	Observe patient's response.
Tubocurarine	Enhanced neuromuscular blockade	Observe response in surgical patients, especially after high doses of propranolol.

SOURCE: Frishman[2] and Missri.[167]

TABLE 66-13
Clinical Situations That Would Influence the Choice of a β-Blocking Drug

Condition	Choice of β Blocker
Asthma, chronic bronchitis with bronchospasm	Avoid all β blockers if possible, but small doses of β_1-selective blockers can be used; β_1 selectivity is lost with higher doses; drugs with partial agonist activity and labetalol with α-adrenergic blocking properties can also be used.
Congestive heart failure	Drugs with partial agonist activity and labetalol may have an advantage, although β blockers are usually contraindicated.
Angina	In patients with angina at low heart rates, drugs with partial agonist activity are probably contraindicated; patients who have angina at high heart rates but who have resting bradycardia may benefit from a drug with partial agonist activity; in vasospastic angina, labetalol may be useful; other β blockers should be used with caution.
Atrioventricular conduction defects	β blockers are generally contraindicated, but drugs with partial agonist activity and labetalol can be tried with caution.
Bradycardia	β blockers with partial agonist activity and labetalol have less of a pulse-slowing effect and are preferable.
Raynaud's phenomenon, intermittent claudication, cold extremities	β_1-selective blocking agents, labetalol, and agents with partial agonist activity may have an advantage.
Depression	Avoid propranolol; substitute a β blocker with partial agonist activity.
Diabetes mellitus	β_1-selective agents and partial agonist drugs are preferable.
Thyrotoxicosis	All agents will control symptoms, but agents without partial agonist activity are preferred.
Pheochromocytoma	Avoid all β blockers unless an α blocker is given; labetalol may be used as a treatment of choice.
Renal failure	Use reduced doses of compounds largely eliminated by renal mechanisms (nadolol, sotalol, and atenolol) and drugs whose bioavailability is increased in uremia (propranolol); also consider possible accumulation of active metabolites (propranolol).
Insulin and sulfonylurea use	There is a danger of hypoglycemia; possibly less using drugs with β_1 selectivity.
Clonidine	Avoid nonselective β blockers; there is a severe rebound effect with clonidine withdrawal.
Oculomucocutaneous syndrome	Stop drug; substitute with any β blocker.
Hyperlipidemia	Avoid nonselective β blockers; use agents with partial agonism or β_1 selectivity, or labetalol.

SOURCE: Frishman.[2,23]

REFERENCES

1. Frishman WH: β-Adrenoceptor antagonists: New drugs and new indications. *N Engl J Med* 1981; 305:500–506.
2. Frishman WH: *Clinical Pharmacology of the β-Adrenoceptor Blocking Drugs*, 2d ed. Norwalk, CT, Appleton-Century-Crofts, 1984.
3. Frishman WH: β-Adrenergic blockers. *Med Clin North Am* 1988; 72:37–81.
4. Norwegian Multicenter Study Group: Timolol induced reduction in mortality and reinfarction in patients surviving acute myocardial infarction. *N Engl J Med* 1981; 304:801–807.
5. Beta-Blocker Heart Attack Trial Research Group: A randomized trial of propranolol in patients with acute myocardial infarction: 1. Mortality results. *JAMA* 1982; 247:1707–1714.
6. Braunwald E: Treatment of the patient after myocardial infarction. *N Engl J Med* 1980; 302:290–293.
7. Frishman WH, Furberg CD, Friedewald WT: β-Adrenergic blockade for survivors of acute myocardial infarction. *N Engl J Med* 1984; 310:830–837.
8. ISIS-I Collaborative Group: Randomized trial of intravenous atenolol among 16,027 cases of suspected acute myocardial infarction: ISIS-I. *Lancet* 1986; 2:57–66.
9. TIMI Study Group: Comparison of invasive and conservative strategies after treatment with intravenous tissue-type plasminogen activator in acute myocardial infarction: Results of the thrombolysis in myocardial infarction (TIMI) trial phase II. *N Engl J Med* 1989; 320:618–627.
10. Sutherland EW, Robinson GA, Butcher RW: Some aspects of the biological role of adenosine 3′5′-monophosphate (cyclic AMP). *Circulation* 1968; 37:279–306.
11. Motulsky HJ, Insel PA: Adrenergic receptors in man: Direct identification, physiologic regulation, and clinical alterations. *N Engl J Med* 1982; 307:18–29.
12. Lefkowitz RJ, Caron MG: Adrenergic receptors: Models for the study of receptors coupled to guanine nucleotide regulatory proteins. *J Biol Chem* 1988; 263:4993–4996.
13. Benovic JL, Bouvier M, Caron MG, Lefkowitz RJ: Regulation of adenyl cyclase-coupled beta-adrenergic receptors. *Annu Rev Cell Biol* 1988; 4:405–428.
14. Limbird LE: Receptors linked to inhibition of adenyl-cyclase: Additional signaling mechanisms. *FASEB J* 1988; 2:2686–2695.
15. Watanabe AM: Recent advances in knowledge about beta-adrenergic receptors: Application to clinical cardiology. *J Am Coll Cardiol* 1983; 1:82–89.
16. Ahlquist RP: A study of adrenotropic receptors. *Am J Physiol* 1948; 153:586–600.
17. Glaubiger G, Lefkowitz RJ: Elevated beta-receptor number after chronic propranolol treatment. *Biochem Biophys Res Commun* 1977; 78:720–725.

18. Frishman WH: Beta-adrenergic blocker withdrawal. *Am J Cardiol* 1987; 59:26F–32F.
19. Bristow MR, Port JD, Sandoval A, Rasmussen R, Ginsburg R, Feldman AM: β-Adrenergic receptor pathways in the failing human heart. *Heart Failure* 1989; 5:77–90.
20. Colucci WS, Alexander RW, Williams GH, et al: Decreased lymphocyte beta-adrenergic receptor density in patients with heart failure and tolerance to the beta-adrenergic agonist pirbuterol. *N Engl J Med* 1981; 305:185–190.
21. Lefkowitz RJ, Caron MG, Stile GL: Mechanisms of membrane-receptor regulation: Biochemical, physiological and clinical insights derived from studies of the adrenergic receptors. *N Engl J Med* 1984; 310:1570–1579.
22. Cruickshank JM, Prichard BNC (eds): *Beta-Blockers in Clinical Practice*. Edinburgh, Churchill Livingstone, 1987: 925.
23. Frishman WH: The beta-adrenoceptor blocking drugs. *Int J Cardiol* 1982; 2:165–178.
24. Koch-Weser J: Metoprolol. *N Engl J Med* 1979; 301:698–703.
25. Frishman WH: Atenolol and timolol: Two new systemic adrenoceptor antagonists. *N Engl J Med* 1982; 306:1456–1462.
26. Frishman WH: Nadolol: A new β-adrenoceptor antagonist. *N Engl J Med* 1981; 305:678–684.
27. Frishman WH: Pindolol: A new β-adrenoceptor antagonist with partial agonist activity. *N Engl J Med* 1983; 308:940–944.
28. Frishman WH, Covey S: Penbutolol and carteolol: Two new beta-adrenergic blockers with partial agonism. *J Clin Pharmacol* 1990; 30:412–421.
29. Frishman WH, Tepper D, Lazar E, Behrmann D: Betaxolol: A new long-acting β_1-selective adrenergic blocker. *J Clin Pharmacol* 1990; 30:669–703.
30. Frishman W, Silverman R: Clinical pharmacology of the new beta-adrenergic blocking drugs: 3. Comparative clinical experience and new therapeutic applications. *Am Heart J* 1979; 98:119–131.
31. Dollery CT, Frishman WH, Cruickshank JM: *Current Cardiovascular Drugs*. Philadelphia, Current Science Press, 1993.
32. Frishman W: Clinical pharmacology of the new beta-adrenergic blocking drugs: 1. Pharmacokinetic and pharmacodynamic properties. *Am Heart J* 1979; 97:663–670.
33. Conolly ME, Kersting F, Dollery CT: The clinical pharmacology of beta-adrenoceptor blocking drugs. *Prog Cardiovasc Dis* 1976; 19:203–234.
34. Singh BN, Deedwania P, Nademanee K, Ward A, Sorkin E: Sotalol: A review of its pharmacodynamic and pharmacokinetic properties and therapeutic use. *Drugs* 1987; 34:311–349.
35. Opie LH: Drugs and the heart: 1. Beta-blocking agents. *Lancet* 1980; 1:693–698.
36. Frishman W, Jacob H, Eisenberg E, Ribner H: Clinical pharmacology of the new beta-adrenergic blocking drugs: 8. Self-poisoning with beta-adrenoceptor blocking drugs: Recognition and management. *Am Heart J* 1979; 98:798–811.
37. Henry JA, Cassidy SL: Membrane stabilizing activity: A major cause of fatal poisoning. *Lancet* 1986; 1:1414–1417.
38. Frishman WH: Clinical perspective on celiprolol. *Am Heart J* 1991; 121:724–729.
39. Johnson BF, Danylchuk MA: The relevance of plasma lipid changes with cardiovascular drug therapy. *Med Clin North Am* 1989; 73:449–474.
40. Taylor SH, Silke B, Lee PS: Intravenous beta-blockade in coronary heart disease: Is cardioselectivity or intrinsic sympathomimetic activity hemodynamically useful? *N Engl J Med* 1982; 306:631–635.
41. Frishman W, Halprin S: Clinical pharmacology of the new beta-adrenergic blocking drugs: 7. New horizons in beta-adrenoceptor blocking therapy: Labetalol. *Am Heart J* 1979; 98:660–665.
42. Frishman WH, Strom J, Kirschner M, et al: Labetalol therapy in patients with systemic hypertension and angina pectoris: Effects of combined alpha- and beta-adrenergic blockade. *Am J Cardiol* 1981; 48:917–928.
43. Frishman WH: Properties of labetalol, a combined β- and α-adrenergic blocking agent relevant to the treatment of myocardial ischemia. *Cardiovasc Drug Ther* 1988; 2:343–353.
44. Van Zwieten A: Pharmacology of antihypertensive agents with multiple actions: *Eur J Clin Pharmacol* 1990; 38:577–581.
45. Gilbert EM, Anderson JL, Deitchman D, Yanowitz FG, O'Connell JB, Renlund DG, et al: Long-term β-blocker vasodilator therapy improves cardiac function in idiopathic dilated cardiomyopathy: A double-blind randomized study of bucindolol versus placebo. *Am J Med* 1990; 88:223–229.
46. Waal Manning HJ: Hypertension: Which beta-blocker? *Drugs* 1976; 12:412–441.
47. Frishman WH, Lazar EJ, Gorodokin G: Pharmacokinetic optimization of therapy with beta-adrenergic blocking agents. *Clin Pharmacokin* 1991; 20:311–318.
48. Halkin H, Vered I, Saginer A, Rabinowitz B: Once-daily administration of sustained release propranolol capsules in the treatment of angina pectoris. *Eur J Clin Pharmacol* 1979; 16:387–391.
49. Parker JO, Porter A, Parker JD: Propranolol in angina pectoris: Comparison of long-acting and standard formulation propranolol. *Circulation* 1982; 65:1351–1355.
50. Landau AJ, Frishman WH, Alturk N, Adjei-Poku M, Fornasser-Bongo M, Furia S: Improvement in exercise tolerance and immediate β-adrenergic blockade with intranasal propranolol in patients with angina pectoris. *Am J Cardiol* 1993; 72, in press.
51. Frishman WH, Murthy VS, Strom JA: Ultra-short acting β-adrenergic blockers. *Med Clin North Am* 1988; 72:359–372.
52. Strom J, Josephson M, Frishman WH: Hemodynamics of flestolol: A titratable short-acting intravenous beta-adrenergic receptor blocker. *J Clin Pharmacol* 1988; 28:1008–1016.
53. Murthy VF, Frishman WH: Controlled beta-receptor blockade with esmolol and flestolol. *Pharmacotherapy* 1988; 8:168–182.
54. Cruickshank JM, Prichard BNC: *Beta-Blockers in Clinical Practice*. Edinburgh, Churchill Livingstone, 1987.
55. Frishman WH: Acebutolol. *Cardivasc Rev Rep* 1985; 6:979–983.
56. Wurzelmann J, Frishman W, Aronson M, Masur D, Ooi, Wee Lock: Neuropsychiatric effects of antihypertensive drugs in the old. *Cardiol Clin* 1987; 5:689–699.
57. Carney RM, Rich MW, te Velde AJE, Saini J, Clark K, Freedland K: Prevalence of major depressive disorders in patients receiving β-blocker therapy versus other medications. *Am J Med* 1987; 83:223–226.
58. Kostis JB, Rosen RC: Central nervous system effects of β-adrenergic blocking drugs: The role of ancillary properties. *Circulation* 1987; 75:204–212.
59. Greenblatt DJ, Scavone JM, Harmatz JS, Engelhardt N, Shaderl: Cognitive effects of β-adrenergic antagonists after single doses: Pharmacokinetics and pharmacodynamics of propranolol, atenolol, lorazepam, and placebo. *Clin Pharmacol Ther* 1993; 53:577–584.
60. Wikstrand J, Warnold I, Olsson G, Tuomilehto J, Elmfeldt D, Berglund G: Primary prevention with metoprolol in patients with hypertension. *JAMA* 1988; 259:1976–1982.
61. Slater EE, DeSanctis RW: Dissection of the aorta. *Med Clin North Am* 1979; 63:141–154.
62. Cohen LS, Braunwald E: Amelioration of angina pectoris in idiopathic hypertrophic subaortic stenosis with beta-adrenergic blockade. *Circulation* 1967; 35:847–851.
63. Turner JRB: Propranolol in the treatment of digitalis-induced and digitalis-resistant tachycardia. *Am J Cardiol* 1966; 18:450–457.
64. Winkle RA, Lopes MG, Goodman DS, Fitzgerald J, Schroeder JS, Harrison DC: Propranolol for patients with mitral valve prolapse. *Am Heart J* 1970; 93:442–427.
65. Schwartz PJ: Idiopathic long QT syndrome: Progress and questions. *Am Heart J* 1985; 109:339–411.
66. Shah PM, Kidd L: Circulatory effects of propranolol in children with Fallot's tetralogy: Observations with isoproterenol infusion, exercise and crying. *Am J Cardiol* 1967; 19:653–657.
67. Kornbluth A, Frishman WH, Ackerman M: Beta-adrenergic blockade in children. *Cardiol Clin* 1987; 5:629–649.
68. Meister SG, Engel TR, Feitosa GS, Helfant RH, Frankl WS: Propranolol in mitral stenosis during sinus rhythm. *Am Heart J* 1977; 94:685–688.
69. Bhatia ML, Shrivastava S, Roy SG: Immediate haemodynamic effects of a beta-adrenergic blocking agent—propranolol—in mitral stenosis at fixed heart rates. *Br Heart J* 1972; 34:638–644.
70. Svedberg K, Hjalmarson A, Waagstein F, Wallentin I: Beneficial effects of long-term beta-blockade in congestive cardiomyopathy. *Br Heart J* 1980; 44:117–133.
71. Sullebarger JT, Liang C-S: Beta-adrenergic receptor stimulation and inhibition in chronic congestive heart failure. *Heart Failure* 1991; 7:154–160.
72. Kraus ML, Gottlieb LD, Horwitz RI, Anscher M: Randomized

clinical trial of atenolol in patients with alcohol withdrawal. *N Engl J Med* 1985; 313:905–909.

73. Weber RB, Reinmuth OM: The treatment of migraine with propranolol. *Neurology (NY)* 1972; 22:366–369.
74. Young RR, Growdon JH, Shahani BT: Beta-adrenergic mechanisms in action tremor. *N Engl J Med* 1975; 293:950–953.
75. Granville-Grossman KL, Turner P: The effect of propranolol on anxiety. *Lancet* 1966; 1:788–790.
76. Frishman WH, Razin A, Swencionis C: Beta-adrenoceptor blockade in anxiety states: A new approach to therapy: 13:8–31. *Cardiovasc Rev Rep* Classics of the Decade Series, 1992; in press.
77. Sellers EM, Degani NC, Zilm DH, Macleod SM: Propranolol decreased noradrenaline secretion and alcohol withdrawal. *Lancet* 1976; 1:94–95.
78. Ingbar SH: The role of antiadrenergic agents in the management of thyrotoxicosis. *Cardiovasc Rev Rep* 1981; 2:683–689.
79. Caro JF, Castro JH, Glennon JA: Effect of long-term propranolol administration on parathyroid hormone and calcium concentration in primary hyperparathyroidism. *Ann Intern Med* 1979; 91:740–741.
80. Lebrec D, Poynard T, Hillon P, Benhamou J-P: Propranolol for prevention of recurrent gastrointestinal bleeding in patients with cirrhosis. *N Engl J Med* 1981; 305:1371–1374.
81. The Fifth Report of The Joint National Committee on Detection, Evaluation, and Treatment of High Blood Pressure (JNCV). *Arch Intern* 1993; 153:154–183.
82. Saunders E, Weir MR, Kong BW, Hollifield J, Gray J, Vertesv, et al: A comparison of the efficacy and safety of a β blocker, a calcium channel blocker, and a converting enzyme inhibitor in hypertensive blacks. *Arch Intern Med* 1990; 150:1707–1713.
83. Laragh JH: Vasoconstriction-volume analysis for understanding and treating hypertension: The use of renin and aldosterone profiles. *Am J Med* 1973; 55:261–274.
84. Myers MG, Lewis PJ, Reid JL, Dollery CT: Brain concentration of propranolol in relation to hypotension effects in the rabbit with observations on brain propranolol levels in man. *J Pharmacol Exp Ther* 1975; 192:327–335.
85. Prichard BNC: Propranolol as an antihypertensive agent. *Am Heart J* 1979; 79:128–133.
86. Imhof PR: Characterization of beta-blockers as antihypertensive agents in the light of human pharmacology studies. In: Schweizer W (ed): *Beta-Blockers: Present Status and Future Prospects.* Bern, Switzerland, Huber, 1974: 40–50.
87. Langer SZ: Presynaptic receptors and their role in the regulation of transmitter release. *Br J Pharmacol* 1977; 60: 481–497.
88. Berthelsen S, Pettinger WA: A functional basis for classification of β-adrenergic receptors. *Life Sci* 1977; 21:596–606.
89. Yamaguchi N, de Champlain J, Nadeau RL: Regulation of norepinephrine release from cardiac sympathetic fibers in the dog by presynaptic α- and β-receptors. *Circ Res* 1976; 41:108–117.
90. Stjarne L, Brundin J: β-Adrenoceptors facilitate noradrenaline secretion from human vasoconstrictor nerves. *Acta Physiol Scand* 1976; 97:88–93.
91. Majewski HJ, McCulloch MW, Rand MJ, Story DF: Adrenaline activation of pre-junctional β-adrenoceptors in guinea pig atria. *Br J Pharmacol* 1980; 71:435–444.
92. Waal HJ: Hypotensive action of propranolol. *Clin Pharmacol Ther* 1966; 7:588–598.
93. Rahn KH, Hawlina A, Kersting F, Peanz G: Studies on the antihypertensive action of the optical isomers of propranolol in man. *Naunyn-Schmiedebergs Arch Pharmacol* 1974; 286:319–323.
94. Pickering TG, Gribbin B, Petersen ES, Cunningham DJC, Sleight P: Effects of autonomic blockade on the baroreflex in man at rest and during exercise. *Circ Res* 1972; 30:177–185.
95. Sonnenblick EH, Ross J Jr, Braunwald E: Oxygen consumption of the heart: Newer concepts of its multifactorial determination. *Am J Cardiol* 1968; 22:328–336.
96. Sonnenblick EH, Skelton CL: Myocardial energetics: Basic principles and clinical implications. *N Engl J Med* 1971; 285:668–675.
97. Black JW, Stephenson JS: Pharmacology of a new adrenergic beta-receptor blocking compound (Nethalide). *Lancet* 1962; 2:311–314.
98. Frishman WH: Beta-adrenergic blockade in the treatment of coronary artery disease. In: Hurst JW (ed): *Clinical Essays on the Heart*, vol 2. New York, McGraw-Hill, 1983: 25–63.
99. Frishman WH: Multifactorial actions of beta-adrenergic blocking drugs in ischemic heart disease: Current concepts. *Circulation* 1983; 67(suppl 1):I11–I18.
100. Parratt JR, Grayson J: Myocardial vascular reactivity after β-adrenergic blockade. *Lancet* 1966; 1:338–340.
101. Becker LC, Fortuin NJ, Pitt B: Effects of ischemia and antianginal drugs on the distribution of radioactive microspheres in the canine left ventricle. *Circ Res* 1971; 28:263–269.
102. Wolfson S, Gorlin R: Cardiovascular pharmacology of propranolol in man. *Circulation* 1969; 40:501–511.
103. Barrett AM: A comparison of the effect of (±) propranolol and (+) propranolol in anesthetized dogs: β-Receptor blocking and hemodynamic action. *J Pharm Pharmacol* 1969; 21:241–247.
104. Bjorntorp P: Treatment of angina pectoris with beta-adrenergic blockade: Mode of action. *Acta Med Scand* 1968; 184:259–262.
105. Frishman WH, Smithen C, Befler B, Kergfield P, Killip T: Non-invasive assessment of clinical response to oral propranolol. *Am J Cardiol* 1975; 35:635–644.
106. Robinson BF: The mode of action of beta-antagonists in angina pectoris. *Postgrad Med J* 1971; 47:41–43.
107. Parmley WW: The combination of beta-adrenergic blocking agents and nitrates in the treatment of stable angina pectoris. *Cardiovasc Rev Rep* 1982; 3:1425–1430.
108. Weiner DA, Klein MD: Calcium antagonists for the treatment of angina pectoris. In: Weiner DA, Frishman WH (eds): *Therapy of Angina Pectoris.* New York, Marcel Dekker, 1986:145–204.
109. Weiner DA: Calcium channel blockers. *Med Clin North Am* 1988; 72:83–115.
110. Frishman WH, Charlap S, Farham J, Sawin HS, Michelson EL, Crawford MH, et al: Combination propranolol and bepridil therapy in stable angina pectoris. *Am J Cardiol* 1985; 55:43C–49C.
111. Miura D, Frishman WH: Class II drugs. In: Dangman DH, Miura D (eds): *Basic and Clinical Electrophysiology and Pharmacology of the Heart.* New York, Marcel Dekker, 1991:665–676.
112. Pratt C, Lichstein E: Ventricular anti-arrhythmic effects of beta-adrenergic blocking drugs: A review of mechanism and clinical studies. *J Clin Pharmacol* 1982; 22:335–347.
113. Ryden L, Ariniego R, Arnman K, Herlitz J, Hjalmarson A, Holmberg S, et al: A double-blind trial of metoprolol in acute myocardial infarction: Effects on ventricular tachyarrhythmias. *N Engl J Med* 1983; 308:614–618.
114. Lichstein E, Morganroth J, Harrist R, Hubble E, for the BHAT Study Group: Effect of propranolol on ventricular arrhythmia: The Beta Blocker Heart Attack Trial experience. *Circulation* 1983; 67:I5–I10.
115. Braunwald E, Muller JE, Kloner RA, Maroko P: Role of beta-adrenergic blockade in the therapy of patients with myocardial infarction. *Am J Med* 1983; 74:113–123.
116. Boissel J-P, Leizorovicz A, Picolet H, Peyrieux J-C, for the APSI Investigators: Secondary prevention after high risk myocardial infarction with low-dose acebutolol. *Am J Cardiol* 1990; 66:251–260.
117. Furberg CD, Hawkins CM, Lichstein E: Effect of propranolol in post-infarction patients with mechanical or electrical complications. *Circulation* 1984; 69:761–765.
118. Frishman WH, Lazar EJ: Reduction of mortality, sudden death and non-fatal reinfarction with beta-adrenergic blockers in survivors of acute myocardial infarction: A new hypothesis regarding the cardioprotective action of beta-adrenergic blockade. *Am J Cardiol* 1990; 66:66G–70G.
119. International Collaborative Study Group: Reduction of infarct size with the early use of timolol in acute myocardial infarction. *N Engl J Med* 1984; 310:9–15.
120. Hjalmarson A, Elmfeldt D, Herlitz J, Holmberg S, Malek I, Nyberg G, et al: Effect of mortality of metoprolol in acute myocardial infarction: A double-blind randomised trial. *Lancet* 1981; 2:823–827.
121. MIAMI Trial Research Group: Metoprolol in acute Myocardial Infarction (MIAMI): A randomized placebo-controlled international trial. *Eur Heart J* 1985; 6:199–226.
122. Muller J, Roberts R, Stone P, Rude R, Raabe D, Gould H, et al: Failure of propranolol administration to limit infarct size in patients with acute myocardial infarction (abstract). *Circulation* 1983; 68:III-294.
123. Frishman WH, Teicher M: Antianginal drug therapy for silent myocardial ischemia. *Med Clin North Am* 1988; 72:185–196.
124. Deanfield JE, Shea MJ, Selwyn AP: Clinical evaluation of tran-

sient myocardial ischemia during daily life. *Am J Med* 1985; 79(suppl 3A):18–24.
125. Swan DA, Bell B, Oakley CM, Goodwin J: Analysis of symptomatic course and prognosis and treatment of hypertrophic obstructive cardiomyopathy. *Br Heart J* 1971; 33:671–685.
126. Hubner PJB, Ziady GM, Lane GK, Hardarson T, Scales B, Oakley CM, et al: Double-blind trial of propranolol and practolol in hypertrophic cardiomyopathy. *Br Heart J* 1973; 35:1116–1123.
127. Epstein SE, Henry WL, Clark CE, Roberts WC, Maron BJ, Ferrans VJ, et al: Asymmetric septal hypertrophy. *Ann Intern Med* 1974; 81:650–680.
128. Bristow MR: The adrenergic nervous system in heart failure. *N Engl J Med* 1984; 311:850–851.
129. Andersson E, Blomstrom-Lundquist C, Hedner T, Waagstein F: Exercise hemodynamics and myocardial metabolism during long-term beta-adrenergic blockade in severe heart failure. *J Am Coll Cardiol* 1991; 18:1059–1066.
130. Lichstein E, Hager WD, Gregory JJ, Fleiss JL, Rolnitzky LM, Bigger JT: Relation between beta-adrenergic blocker use, various correlates of left ventricular function, and the chance of developing congestive heart failure. The Multicenter Diltiazem Post-Infarction Research Group. *J Am Coll Cardiol* 1990; 16:1327–1332.
131. Sole MG, Kamble AB, Hussain MN: A possible change in the rate-limiting step for cardiac norepinephrine synthesis in the cardiomyopathic Syrian hamster. *Circ Res* 1977; 41:814–817.
132. Bloom S, Davis DL: Calcium as mediator of isoproterenol-induced myocardial necrosis. *Am J Pathol* 1972; 69:459–470.
133. Kahn DS, Rona G, Chappel CI: Isoproterenol-induced cardiac necrosis. *Ann NY Acad Sci* 1969; 156:285–293.
134. Gilbert EM, Port JD, Hershberger RI, Bristol MR: Clinical significance of alterations in the β-adrenergic receptor–adenylate cyclase complex in heart failure. *Heart Failure* 1989; 5:91–98.
135. Heinsimer JA, Lefkowitz RJ: The beta-adrenergic receptor in heart failure. *Hosp Pract* 1983; 18:103–125.
136. Eichorn EJ, Bedotto JB, Malloy CR, Hatfield BA, Deitchman D, Brown M, et al: Effect of β-adrenergic blockade of myocardial function and energetics in congestive heart failure: Improvements in hemodynamic, contractile, and diastolic performance with bucindolol. *Circulation* 1990; 82:473–483.
137. Waagstein F, Caidahl K, Wallentin I, Bergh C-H, Hjalmarson A: Long-term β-blockade in dilated cardiomyopathy: Effects of short- and long-term metoprolol treatment followed by withdrawal and readministration of metoprolol. *Circulation* 1989; 80:551–563.
138. Heilbrunn SM, Shah P, Bristow MR, Valentine HA, Ginsburg R, Fowler MB: Increased β-receptor density and improved hemodynamic response to catecholamine stimulation during long-term metoprolol therapy in heart failure from dilated cardiomyopathy. *Circulation* 1989; 79:483–490.
139. Jessup M: Beta-adrenergic blockade in congestive heart failure: Answering the old questions. *J Am Coll Cardiol* 1991; 18:1067–1069.
140. Fowler MB, Bristow MR, Laser JA, Ginsburg R, Scott LB, Schroeder JS: Beta-blocker therapy in severe heart failure: Improvement related to β_1-adrenergic receptor regulation? (abstract). *Circulation* 1984; 70:112.
141. Jeresaty RM: Mitral valve prolapse syndrome. *Prog Cardiovasc Dis* 1973; 15:623–652.
142. Hachamovitch R, Strom JA, Sonnenblick EH, Frishman WH: Left ventricular hypertrophy in hypertension and the efeects of antihypertensive drug therapy. *Curr Probl Cardiol* 1988; 13:371–421.
143. Friedman LM: How do the various beta-blockers compare in type, frequency and severity of their adverse effects? *Circulation* 1983; 67(suppl 1):89–90.
144. Frishman W, Silverman R, Strom J, Elkayam U, Sonnenblick E: Clinical pharmacology of the new beta-adrenoceptor blocking drugs: 4. Adverse effects: Choosing a β-adrenoceptor blocker. *Am Heart J* 1979; 98:256–262.
145. Frishman WH: Beta-adrenergic receptor blockers: Adverse effects and drug interactions. *Hypertension* 1988; 11(suppl II):II21–II29.
146. Frishman WH, Kostis J: The significance of intrinsic sympathomimetic activity in beta-adrenoceptor blocking drugs: Update. *Cardiovasc Rev Rep* Classics of the Decade Series, 1991; 12:46–59.
147. Frishman W, Kostis J, Strom J, Hossler M, Elkayam U, Guidner S, et al: Clinical pharmacology of the new beta-adrenergic blocking drugs: 6. A comparison of pindolol and propranolol in treatment of patients with angina pectoris: The role of intrinsic sympathomimetic activity. *Am Heart J* 1979; 98:526–535.
148. Giudicelli JF, Lhoste F: β-Adrenoceptor blockade and atrioventricular conduction in dogs: Role of intrinsic sympathomimetic activity. *Br J Clin Pharmacol* 1982; 13(suppl 2):167–174.
149. Frishman WH, Klein N, Strom J, Cohen MN, Shamoon H, Willens H, et al: Comparative effects of abrupt propranolol and verapamil withdrawal in angina pectoris. *Am J Cardiol* 1982; 50:1191–1195.
150. George RB, Manocha K, Burford JG, Conrad SA, Kinasewitz GT: Effects of labetalol in hypertensive patients with chronic obstructive pulmonary disease. *Chest* 1983; 83:457–460.
151. Benson MK, Berrill WT, Cruickshank JM, et al: A comparison of four adrenoceptor antagonists in patients with asthma. *Br J Clin Pharmacol* 1978; 5:415–419
152. Frohlich ED, Tarazi RC, Dustan HP: Peripheral arterial insufficiency: A complication of beta-adrenergic blocking therapy. *JAMA* 1969; 208:2471–2472.
153. Lundvall J, Jarhult J: Beta-adrenergic dilator component of the sympathetic vascular response in skeletal muscle. *Acta Physiol Scand* 1976; 96:180–192.
154. Simpson FO: β-Adrenergic receptor blocking drugs in hypertension. *Drugs* 1974; 7:85-1095.
155. Radack K, Deck C: β-Adrenergic blocker therapy does not worsen intermittent claudication in subjects with peripheral arterial disease. *Arch Inern Med* 1991; 151:1769–1776.
156. Hiatt WR, Stoll S, Nies A: Effect of beta-adrenergic blockers on the periphral circulation in patients with peripheral vascular disease. *Circulation* 1985; 72:1226–1231.
157. Reveno WS, Rosenbaum H: Propranolol and hypoglycaemia. (letter). *Lancet* 1968; 1:920.
158. Allison SP, Chamberlain MI, Miller JE: Effects of propranolol on blood sugar, insulin and free fatty acids. *Diabetologia* 1969; 5:339–342.
159. Deacon SP, Barnett D: Comparison of atenolol and propranolol during insulin-induced hypoglycaemia. *Br Med J* 1976; 272–273.
160. Lloyd-Mostyn RH, Oram S: Modification by propranolol of cardiovascular effects of induced hypoglycaemia. *Lancet* 1975; 1:1213–1215.
161. Jacob H, Brandt LJ, Farkas P, Frishman WH: Beta-adrenergic blockade and the gastrointestinal system. *Am J Med* 1983; 74:1042–1051.
162. Stephen SA: Unwanted effects of propranolol. *Am J Cardiol* 1966; 18:463–468.
163. Nawabi IU, Ritz ND: Agranulocytosis due to propranolol. *JAMA* 1973; 223:1376–1377.
164. Bailey R, Neale TJ: Rapid clonidine withdrawal with blood pressure overshoot exaggerated by beta-blockade. *Br Med J* 1976; 1:942–943.
165. Agabiti-Rosei E, Brown JJ, Lever AF, Robertson AS, Robertson JI, Trust PM: Treatment of phaeochromocytoma and clonidine withdrawal hypertension with labetalol. *Br J Clin Pharmacol* 1976; 3(suppl 3): 809–813.
166. Wright P: Untoward effect associated with practolol administration: Oculomucocutaneous syndrome. *Br Med J* 1975; 1:595–598.
167. Missri JC: How do beta-blockers interact with other commonly used drugs? *Cardiovasc Med* 1983; 8:668–673.
168. Hansten P: *Drug Interactions*, 4th ed. Philadelphia, Lea & Febiger, 1979.

Chapter 67

Calcium Channel Blockers

William H. Frishman, M.D. ■ *Edmund H. Sonnenblick, M.D.*

The calcium channel blockers are a heterogeneous group of drugs with widely variable effects on heart muscle, sinus node function, atrioventricular (AV) conduction, peripheral blood vessels, and coronary circulation.[1-3] Nine of these drugs—nifedipine, nicardipine, nimodipine, felodipine, isradipine, amlodipine, verapamil, diltiazem, and bepridil—are approved in the United States for clinical use.

PHYSIOLOGICAL BACKGROUND

The Calcium Channel Blockers: Basic Principles

Calcium ions play a fundamental role in the activation of cells. An influx of calcium ions into the cell through specific ion channels is required for myocardial contraction, for determining peripheral vascular resistance through calcium dependent–regulated tone of vascular smooth muscle, and for helping to initiate the pacemaker tissues of the heart, which are activated largely by the slow calcium current.[2]

The concept of calcium channel inhibition originated in 1960 when it was noted that prenylamine, a newly developed coronary vasodilator, depressed cardiac performance in canine heart-lung preparations.[4] Initial studies with verapamil showed that it also exerted negative inotropic effect on the isolated myocardium, in addition to having vasodilator properties.[5] These potent negative inotropic effects seemed to differentiate these drugs from the classical coronary vasodilators, such as nitroglycerin and papaverine, which have little, if any, myocardial depressant activity. Unlike β-adrenergic antagonists, the calcium antagonists depress cardiac contractility without altering the height or contour of the monophasic action potential and thus interfere with excitation-contraction coupling.[6] Reversible closure of specific calcium ion channels in the membrane of mammalian myocardial cells was suggested as the explanation of these observed effects.[7]

Subsequently, the effects of verapamil on atrial and ventricular intracellular potentials were studied.[8] Antiarrhythmic compounds were classified into local anesthetics which decreased the maximum rate of depolarization, β blockers, and a third class that prolonged the duration of the cardiac action potential.[9] None of these electrophysiologic actions, however, could explain the antiarrhythmic effect of verapamil.[9] Thus, a fourth class of antiarrhythmic drug, typified by verapamil, was proposed, with effects separate from those of sodium channel inhibitors and β blockers.[8] It has been shown that the antiarrhythmic actions and negative inotropic effects of verapamil are mediated predominantly through interference with calcium conductance.[8]

CHEMICAL STRUCTURE AND PHARMACODYNAMICS

Structure of the Calcium Channel Blockers

The structures of some of the available calcium channel blockers are shown in Fig. 67-1. Diltiazem is a benzothiazepine derivative that is structurally unrelated to other vasodilators.[1] Nifedipine is a dihydropyridine derivative unrelated to the nitrates; it is lipophilic and is inactivated by light.[1,10] Nicardipine, amlodipine, felodipine, isradipine, and nimodipine are also dihydropyridine derivatives similar in structure to nifedipine. Verapamil ([±] verapamil) has some structural similarity to papaverine.[1]

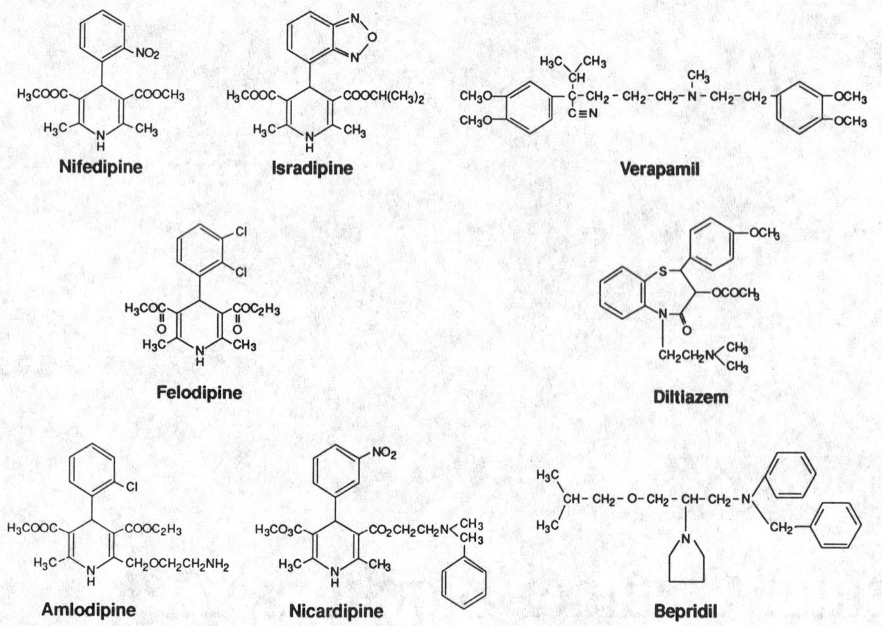

Nifedipine Isradipine Verapamil Felodipine Diltiazem Amlodipine Nicardipine Bepridil

FIGURE 67-1 Chemical structures of diltiazem (a benzothiazepine derivative), nifedipine, felodipine, isradipine, amlodipine, nicardipine (dihydropyridine derivatives), verapamil (structurally similar to papaverine), and bepridil (structure unlike other cardioactive drugs).

Bepridil is not related chemically to other cardioactive drugs.[11]

Differential Effects on Slow Channels

The predominant effect of calcium channel blocking drugs is on the slow channels of the cell membrane. These calcium channels permit the entry of some sodium in addition to calcium and are activated much more slowly than the fast channels through which sodium predominantly enters to cause the initial rapid rise in the action potential.

Nifedipine has been shown to depress the slow inward calcium ion current in a dose-dependent manner in isolated cat papillary muscles under voltage clamp conditions. At concentrations of 10^{-7} to 10^{-5} *M*, there was no effect on the fast inward Na^+ current or on the rates of activation, inactivation, or recovery of the slow currents.[2,12–14] This action of nifedipine is similar to that of tetrodotoxin on the sodium channels, and thus nifedipine is thought to "plug" the Ca^{2+} channels, leaving their control mechanisms unaffected, which explains its dose-dependent effect. Further research is required to define the specific site of action of nifedipine.

Verapamil is a racemic mixture of the (R) (+)-enantiomer and the (S) (−)-enantiomer, with each having different electrophysiologic effects.[1] The (+)-isomer depresses the maximal rate of rise of the action potential and has additional effects on the plateau phase and overall shape of the action potential. The (−)-isomer depresses the plateau phase of the action potential. Both of these effects are frequency-dependent, being much more pronounced at a stimulus rate of 90 per minute than at 15 per minute.[15] These effects are markedly enhanced by increasing the length of exposure to the drug.[16] In contrast to nifedipine, verapamil alters the kinetics of the slow channels, slowing both activation and, more markedly, recovery from inactivation.[17] The effects of verapamil are thus quite complex as it is a mixture of (+)- and (−)-enantiomers, each with different actions. The drug cannot be thought of as just a selective blocker of the slow inward current.[18]

Diltiazem lowers the plateau phase and shortens the duration of the action potential.[19] High concentrations also reduce the maximal rate of rise of the action potential, suggesting that diltiazem is primarily an inhibitor of the slow channel at low concentrations (2.2×10^{-6} *M*) but exerts fast (sodium) channel inhibitory effects at higher concentrations (2.2×10^{-5} *M*). It has been proposed that there are two sets of calcium channels: potential-operated channels and receptor-operated channels (Fig. 67-2).[20] These two sets of channels are believed to exist because of their selective sensitivities to D-600 (a verapamil analogue) and because they are additive. It is also thought that there is a passive influx of calcium into smooth muscle (most noticeable in sodium-free media) that is insensitive to D-600. Diltiazem does not seem to inhibit calcium extrusion from the cell but does inhibit calcium entry through both types of calcium channels.[21]

Bepridil possesses all the characteristics of the traditional calcium antagonists. In addition, the drug appears to affect the sodium channel (fast channel) and possibly the potassium channel, producing a quinidine-like effect. Bepridil specifically inhibits maximal upstroke velocity (*dV/dt* max), that is, the influx of sodium in appropriate load dosages. The effect of bepridil on the maximum rate of depolarization has been examined: The action potential *height* is not changed; however, the action potential *duration* is extended in a quinidine-like manner.[22]

In conclusion, each of the calcium channel blockers differs in apparent mode of action, time course of action, concentration-effect relation, and pharmacologic action in different tissues.[1]

Intracellular Effects

In addition to their effects on the slow channels, calcium channel antagonists can inhibit the availability of calcium ions for excitation coupling at intracellular sites. Such an interaction may take place at the inner surface

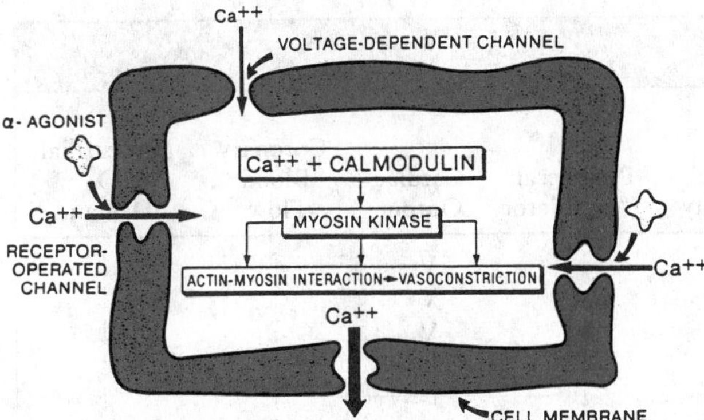

FIGURE 67-2 Calcium ion–dependent regulation of muscle tone in vascular smooth muscle. Calcium ion (Ca^{2+}) entry can occur in response to electric stimulation through the voltage-dependent channel, receptor activation through the adrenergic receptor–mediated channel, or both. On entry into the cell, the cellular free calcium ions bind to the calcium-binding protein, calmodulin. This calmodulin–calcium ion complex in turn activates myosin kinase, which causes phosphorylation of the light chain of myosin. Phosphorylation then activates the binding of actin to myosin and leads to contraction. Intracellular calcium ion levels are reduced through energy-dependent membrane pumps which promote calcium efflux, which involves sodium/calcium countertransport. (*From Frishman WH, Stroh JA, Greenberg SM, et al: Calcium-channel blockers in systemic hypertension. Curr Probl Cardiol 1987; 12:287–364. Reproduced with permission from the publisher and authors.*)

of the sarcolemma, sarcoplasmic reticulum, or mitochondria or at any site where calcium may be made available as an excitation-response messenger.[23]

Cardiovascular Effects

Effects on Muscular Contraction

Calcium is the primary ionic link between neurologic excitation and mechanical contraction of cardiac, smooth, and skeletal muscle.[2] Actin and myosin are the protein filaments that slide past one another in the adenosine triphosphate (ATP)-dependent contractile process of all muscle cells (See Chap. 5). In myocardial cells, the regulatory proteins tropomyosin and troponin inhibit this process. When the myocardial cell membrane repolarizes, calcium enters the cell and triggers the release of additional calcium from internal stores within the sarcoplasmic reticulum. Calcium released from this large intracellular reservoir then initiates contraction by combining with the inhibitors troponin and tropomyosin. Previously hidden active sites on actin molecules are then available for binding by myosin.[2]

Effects on Coronary and Peripheral Arterial Blood Vessels (Table 67-1)

The contraction of vascular smooth muscle, such as that found in the coronary arteries, is slightly different from the contraction of cardiac and skeletal muscles. Myosin must be phosphorylated, and calmodulin is the regulatory protein to which calcium binds.[2] In addition, vascular smooth-muscle cells have significantly less intracellular calcium stores than do myocardial cells and so rely more heavily on the influx of extracellular calcium.[2]

The observation that calcium channel blockers are significantly more effective in inhibiting contraction in coronary and peripheral arterial smooth muscle than in cardiac and skeletal muscle is of great clinical importance. This differential effect is explained by the observation that arterial smooth muscle is more dependent on external calcium entry for contraction, whereas cardiac and skeletal muscle rely on a recirculating internal pool of calcium.[2] Because calcium-entry blockers are membrane-active drugs, they reduce the entry of calcium into cells and therefore exert a much larger effect on vascular wall contraction.[2,24] This preferential effect allows calcium-entry blockers to dilate coronary and peripheral arteries in doses that do not severely affect myocardial contractility or have little, if any, effect on skeletal muscle.

Effects on Veins

The calcium channel blockers seem to be less active in veins than in arteries and are ineffective at therapeutic doses (in contrast to nitrates) for increasing venous capacitance.[21]

Effects on Myocardial Contractility (Table 67-1)

Force generation during cardiac muscle contraction depends, in part, on calcium influx during membrane depolarization.[25] In isolated myocardial preparations, all calcium channel antagonists have been demonstrated to exert potent negative inotropic effects.[26] In guinea pig atria exposed to drug concentration of 10^{-6} *M*, the order of potency for depressing the maximal rate of force development during constant pacing was found to be nifedipine > verapamil > diltiazem.[27] In dog papillary muscle, developed tension was also decreased most markedly by nifedipine; the relative potencies (on a weight basis) of verapamil and diltiazem were 1/15 and 1/40 respectively.[28]

The negative inotropic effects of the calcium channel antagonists are dose-dependent.[17] The excitation-contraction coupling of vascular smooth muscle is three to ten times more sensitive to the action of calcium channel antagonists than is that of myocardial fibers.[17,26] Hence, the relatively low doses of these drugs used in vivo to produce vasodilatation or beneficial antiarrhythmic effects may not produce significant negative inotropic effects.[17,29] Furthermore, in intact animals and human beings, the intrinsic negative inotropic properties of these compounds are greatly modified by a baroreceptor-mediated reflex augmentation of β-adrenergic tone consequent to vasodilatation and a decrease in blood pressure.[30,31] Nifedipine and other dihydropyridines, which exert the greatest vasodilator effects among these agents, accordingly produce the strongest reflex β-adrenergic response and the one most likely to offset the negative inotropic activity of the drugs and lead to enhancement of ventricular performance.[32] While this mechanism plays an important role in patients with normal or nearly normal left ventricular function, it is unlikely to play a similar role in patients with severe congestive heart failure, in whom the baroreceptor sensitivity is markedly attenuated.[29,33]

TABLE 67-1
Pharmacologic Effects of the Calcium Channel Blockers

	Heart Rate		Conduction						
	Acute	Chronic	SA Node	AV Node	Myocardial Contractility	Peripheral Vasodilator	Cardiac Output	Coronary Blood Flow	Myocardial O_2 Demand
Diltiazem	↓	↓	↓	↓	↓	↓	V	↑	↓
Bepridil	↓	↓	↓	↓	V	—	V	↑	↓
Verapamil	↑	↓	↓	↓	↓↓	↓	V	↑	↓
Amlodipine	↑	↑—	—	—	↓	↓↓	↑—	↑	↓
Felodipine	↑	↑—	—	—	—	↓↓	↑—	↑	↓
Isradipine	↑	↑—	—	—	—	↓↓	↑—	↑	↓
Nicardipine	↑	↑—	—	—	—	↓↓	↑—	↑	↓
Nifedipine	↑	↑—	—	—	↓	↓↓	↑—	↑	↓
Nimodipine	↑	↑—	—	—	—	V	↑—	↑	↓

Note: ↑ = increase; ↓ = decrease; — = no change; V = variable; SA = sinoatrial; AV = atrioventricular

SOURCE: Frishman WH et al.[112] Reproduced with permission from the publisher and authors.

Electrophysiological Effects

Although verapamil, nifedipine, diltiazem, and bepridil all depress cardiac contractility with only quantitative differences (Table 67-1), their effects on the electrophysiology of the heart are different qualitatively.[23,34,35] Local anesthetic actions of bepridil, diltiazem, and particularly of verapamil may account for some of these differences.[36] Nifedipine and other dihydropyridines have a more selective action at the slow channels, whereas verapamil and diltiazem, at least at higher doses, also inhibit currents in the fast channels in the manner of the local anesthetics.[37] Bepridil has definite class I antiarrhythmic properties.

Verapamil and diltiazem prolong the conduction and refractoriness in the (AV) node; the AH interval is lengthened more than is the HV interval.[38] In therapeutic concentrations, there are no demonstrable actions on the rate of depolarization or the repolarization phases of the action potentials in atrial, ventricular, and Purkinje fibers.[35] The rate of discharge of the sinus node, which depends on the calcium ion current, is depressed by all calcium channel blockers. In vivo, this effect can be compensated or overcompensated for by activation of baroreceptor reflexes which increase sympathetic nervous activity.[35]

The antiarrhythmic actions of verapamil and diltiazem relate to their effect on nodal cardiac tissues.[35] In sinoatrial (SA) and AV nodal cells, the drugs modify slow-channel electropotentials in three ways: first, there is a decrease in the rate of rise and slope of diastolic slow depolarization and an increase in the membrane threshold potential, which reduces the rate of firing in the cell[39]; second, the action potential upstroke is decreased in amplitude, which slows conduction[40]; and third, the duration of the action potential is increased.[39] These electrophysiological effects are dose related, and above the clinical range electrical standstill may occur in SA and AV nodal cells.[38] These observations and others support the concept that slow-channel activity is important in the generation of pacemaker potential in the SA node. Verapamil and diltiazem also exert a depressant effect on the AV node and in low concentrations prolong the effective refractory period.[40,41] Unlike β-adrenergic blocking drugs and vagomimetic interventions, which depress AV node transmission by altering autonomic impulse traffic, verapamil and diltiazem prolong AV nodal refractoriness directly.[41] Verapamil may have additional vagomimetic effects.[35]

Bepridil has a modest depressant effect on heart rate and intranodal and infranodal conduction, accompanied by a significant increment in the effective and functional refractory periods of the AV node. Unexpected effects that cannot be explained solely on the basis of slow-channel inhibition on the myocardium include lengthening of the QTc interval and significant prolongation of the atrial and ventricular effective refractory periods.

Effects on Nonvascular Tissues

Calcium ions are required for contraction in all smooth muscles, and these drugs can inhibit contractions in the gastrointestinal tract.[42] Calcium is also important in excitation-secretion coupling; however, there is no evidence that these drugs have significant effects on the endocrine glands in clinical doses.[43,44] Although antiadrenergic effects of some calcium-entry blockers have been suggested, further studies are needed.[23,45]

Some calcium-entry blockers may partially inhibit adenosine diphosphate (ADP)- and epinephrine-induced platelet aggregation and thromboxane release from platelets.[46–50]

PHARMACOKINETICS

Although classified together, calcium-entry blockers demonstrate important differences in their pharmacokinetic properties (Tables 67-2, 67-3).[1,51–53] Differences in completeness of gastrointestinal absorption, amount of first-pass hepatic metabolism, protein binding, extent of distribution in the body, and the pharmacologic actions

TABLE 67-2
Pharmacokinetics of the Calcium Channel Blockers and Sustained-Release Preparations

Agent	Trade	Absorption, %	Bioavailability, %*	Protein Binding, %	Volume of Distribution, liters/kg	$t_{1/2}$ β, h	Clearance, mL/min per kg	Time to Peak Plasma Concentration, h
Diltiazem	Cardizem	>90	35–60	78	5.0	4.1–5.6	15	2–3
Diltiazem SR	Cardizem SR	>90	35–60	78	5.0	5–7	15	6–11
Diltiazem IV	Cardizem							
Diltiazem CD	Cardizem CD	>95	40	70–80	5.0	5–8	15	10–14
Diltiazem XR	Dilacor XR	>95	40	70–80	5.0	5–10	15	4–6
Verapamil	Calan, Isoptin	>90	10–20	90	4.3	6 ± 4 IV 8 ± 6 po	13 ± 7	1–2
Verapamil SR	Calan SR, Isoptin SR	>90	10–20	90	4.3	4.5–12	13 ± 7	1–2
	Verelan	>90	20–35	90	162–380 liters	12		7–9
Nifedipine	Procardia	>90	65	90	1.32	≈5	500–600	0.5
Nifedipine GITS	Procardia XL	>90	85	>95	1.32	3.8–16.9	500–600	6 to plateau
Nicardipine	Cardene	>90	≈30	>90	0.66	≈1 IV 1–2 po	14	0.5–2.0
Nicardipine SR	Cardene SR	>90	35	>95		8.6	0.6	1–4 immed
Nicardipine IV	Cardene		100	>90	9.3			
Amlodipine	Norvasc	>90	60–65	>95	21	35–45	7	6–12
Isradipine	Dynacirc	90–95	17	97	2.9	8.8	10	1.5
Felodipine	Plendil	>95	15–25	>99	10	15.1 ± 2.6	12	2.5–5
Bepridil	Vascor	>90	≈60	>95	8.0	33		5.3
Nimodipine	Nimotop	>90	13	>95	0.94	8–9		0.6

* Extraction ratio.
Note: SR = sustained release; IV = intravenous; CD, XR, XL = extended release; po = oral; GITS = Gastrointestinal system.

of different metabolites may influence the clinical usefulness of these drugs in different patients.[1,51]

Dosage and Therapeutic Levels

After administration of a certain oral dose, the calcium-entry blocking drugs, which are largely metabolized in the liver, show large interindividual variation in circulating plasma levels.[51,52,54,55] In angina pectoris and hypertension, wide individual differences also exist in the relation between plasma concentrations of calcium-entry blockers and the associated therapeutic effect.[54,55]

CLINICAL APPLICATIONS

The calcium channel blockers are available in the United States for the treatment of patients with angina pectoris (diltiazem, nifedipine, amlodipine, nicardipine, verapamil, bepridil); for chronic treatment of systemic hypertension (verapamil, isradipine, diltiazem, amlodipine, nicardipine, felodipine); the management of hypertensive emergencies and perioperative hypertension (intravenous nicardipine); treatment and prophylaxis of supraventricular arrhythmias (verapamil and diltiazem); and for reducing morbidity and mortality in patients with subarachnoid hemorrhage (nimodipine). These drugs are also being evaluated for a multitude of other cardiovascular and noncardiovascular conditions.

Angina Pectoris

The antianginal mechanisms of calcium-entry blockers are complex (Table 67-4).[1-3,56-59] The drugs exert vasodilator effects on the coronary and peripheral vessels as well as depressant effects on cardiac contractility and conduction; all these actions may be important in mediating the antianginal effects of the drugs.[2,3,56-59] These drugs are only mild dilators of epicardial vessels not in spasm, but they markedly attenuate sympathetically mediated and ergonovine-induced coronary vasoconstriction; these actions provide a rational basis for effectiveness of the drugs in vasospastic ischemic syndromes.[2,3,58] In patients with exertional angina pectoris, the peripheral vasodilator actions of diltiazem and verapamil and the inhibitory effects on the sinus node serve to attenuate the increases in double product that normally accompany, and serve to limit, exercise.[3,57]

Stable Angina Pectoris

Multiple double-blind placebo-controlled studies have clearly confirmed the efficacy of diltiazem,[55,59-62] nifedi-

TABLE 67-3

Clinical Characteristics of Calcium Channel Blockers

Agent	Dosage: Oral	Dosage: IV	Onset of Action, min: Oral	Onset of Action, min: IV	Therapeutic PC	Site of Metabolism	Active Metab-olites	Excretion, %
Diltiazem	30–90 mg q 6–8 h	75–150 μg/kg 10–20 mg	<30	<10	50–200 ng/mL	Deacetylation *N*-deacetylation *O*-demethylation Major hepatic first-pass effect	Yes	60 (fecal) 2–4 (unchanged in urine)
Diltiazem SR	60–120 mg q 12 h		30–60		50–200 ng/mL		Yes	
Diltiazem IV		0.15–0.25 mg/kg (initial bolus over 2 min)						
Diltiazem CD	180–360 mg q 24 h		30–60		50–200 ng/mL		Yes	
Dilacor XR	180–540 mg q 24 h		30–60		40–200 ng/mL		Yes	
Verapamil	80–120 mg q 6–12 h	0.075–0.15 mg/kg (initial bolus over 2 min)	<30	<5	>100 ng/mL	*N*-dealkylation *O*-demethylation Major hepatic first-pass effect	Yes	15 (fecal) 70 (renal) 3–4 (unchanged in urine)
Verapamil SR	240–480 mg q 12 or 24 h		<30		>50 ng/mL		Yes	15 (fecal) 70 (renal) 3–4 (unchanged in urine)
Verelan	120–480 mg q 24 h						Yes	16 (fecal) 70 (renal) 3–4 (unchanged in urine)
Nifedipine	10–40 mg q 6–8 h	3 SL	<20		25–100 ng/mL	A hydroxy-carbolic acid and a lactone with no known activity. Major hepatic first-pass effect	No	20–40 (fecal) 50–80 (renal) <0.1 (unchanged in urine)
Nifedipine GITS	30–180 mg q 24 h		120				No	
Nicardipine	10–20 mg TID	1.15 mg/h	<20	<5	28–50 ng/mL	Major hepatic first-pass effect	No	35 (fecal) 60 (renal) <1 (unchanged in urine)
Nicardipine SR	30–60 mg BID		20		28–50 ng/mL			35 (fecal) 60 (renal) <1 (unchanged in urine)
Nicardipine IV			5–15 mg/h	<2–3	60–80 ng/mL	Hepatic	No	
Nimodipine	60 mg q 4 h		<30		7 ng/mL	Major hepatic first-pass effect	No	
Amlodipine	5–10 mg q 24 h		90–120 in vitro		6–10 ng/mL	Oxidation Extensive but slow hepatic metabolism	No	20–25 (fecal) 60 (renal) 10 (unchanged in urine)
Isradipine	2.5–10 mg q 12 h		120		nd	Hepatic de-esterification and aromatization	No	30 (fecal) 70 (renal) 0 (unchanged in urine)
Felodipine ER	5–20 mg q 24 h		120–300		2–20 nmol/liter	Hepatic microsomal P-450 system oxidation Major hepatic first-pass effect	No	10 (fecal) 60–70 (renal) <0.5 (unchanged in urine and feces)
Bepridil	200–400 mg q 24 h		30–60		1200–3500 ng/mL			70 (renal) 20 (fecal)

Note: PC = plasma concentration; SR = sustained release; IV = intravenous; CD, XR, ER = extended release; GITS = extended release (gastrointestinal system); SL = sublingual; TID = thrice daily; BID = twice daily; nd = no data.

TABLE 67-4
Hemodynamic Effects of the Calcium-Entry Blockers On Myocardial O_2 Supply and Demand

	Verapamil	Nifedipine	Diltiazem	Bepridil
Demand				
Wall tension	↑ ↔	↔ (reflex)	↔	↔
Systolic BP	↓	↓	↓	↔
Ventricular volume	↑	↔	↔	↔
Heart rate	↓*	↑ (reflex)	↓ ↔	↓ ↔
Contractility	↓ ↓	↓	↓	↓
Supply				
Coronary blood flow	↑	↑ ↑	↑	↑
Coronary vascular resistance	↓	↓ ↓	↓	↓
Spasm	↓	↓	↓	↓
Diastolic perfusion time	↑	↓	↑ ↔	↑ ↔
Collateral blood flow	↔	↑	↑	↔

*Heart rate may increase acutely but decreases with chronic use.
Note: ↑ = increase; ↓ = decrease; ↔ = no apparent effect.

pine,[55,63,64] amlodipine, nicardipine, verapamil,[65–68] and bepridil[69,70] in stable angina pectoris; patients show a reduction in chest pain attacks and nitroglycerin consumption and improved exercise tolerance. Calcium-entry blockers for the most part appear to be as safe and effective as β blockers and nitrates when used as monotherapies in patients.[71–77] They can also be used as single-dose therapies in hypertensive patients with angina.[77,78]

In choosing between a calcium channel antagonist and a β-adrenergic blocking drug in the management of patients with effort-related symptoms, it is apparent that some patients do better with one drug than with the other. Unfortunately, we know little about how to predict with confidence the superior agent in a specific patient without a therapeutic trial. However, verapamil and diltiazem can be used as effective alternatives in patients who remain symptomatic despite therapy with propranolol and as first-time antianginal drugs in patients with contraindications to β blockade. The use of nifedipine as a first-line drug in its original formulation was limited by the reflex tachycardia and potential aggravation of angina that accompanied its use.[55,76,79] However, this is probably not a problem with the new sustained-delivery nifedipine (GITS) formulation.[57] Diltiazem is also approved as a once-daily treatment for angina pectoris in a sustained-delivery formulation.

The usual dose of nicardipine is 10 to 30 mg thrice daily for patients with either hypertension or angina pectoris.

Bepridil is available in doses of 200 to 400 mg once daily for use in patients with angina pectoris who are refractory to other antianginal drug therapy.[70] Close monitoring of patients with this drug is necessary at the onset of therapy because a small percentage of patients can have a prolongation of the QT interval on the electrocardiogram (ECG). Bepridil can be combined with a β blocker if necessary.[80]

The comparative effects of abrupt withdrawal of verapamil and propranolol in patients with angina pectoris have been studied.[45] Ten percent of patients with stable effort-related symptoms experienced a severe clinical exacerbation of the anginal syndrome upon withdrawal of propranolol; no patient experienced rebound symptoms when verapamil was abruptly discontinued.[45] There also appear to be no major withdrawal reactions with nifedipine and diltiazem.[55]

Angina at Rest

Patients with angina at rest have a wide spectrum of disorders, ranging from variant angina (ST elevation) associated with angiographically normal coronary arteries to unstable angina with ST depression or elevation associated with multivessel coronary artery disease.[57,59,78] (See also Chap. 59.) Studies suggest that the coronary vasospasm and/or thrombosis plays a major role in the pathogenesis of ischemia in many patients with angina at rest, regardless of the coronary anatomy.[57] In clinical trials, calcium channel antagonists were effective in this syndrome because of their ability to block spontaneous and drug-induced spasm.[81–88]

The comparative efficacy of verapamil and propranolol was assessed in a randomized blinded crossover trial in angina at rest. Only verapamil reduced symptomatic and asymptomatic episodes of ischemia. These findings are consistent with the concept that coronary vasospasm plays a crucial role in patients with angina at rest; in contrast, rather than providing any benefit, propranolol may exacerbate vasospastic phenomena.[89]

Another study assessed the comparative efficacy of verapamil and nifedipine. Both verapamil and nifedipine proved equally effective, and neither drug depressed ventricular function at rest or during exercise.[90] Accordingly, in the management of patients with variant angina, the choice of a calcium antagonist is likely to be determined not so much by which drug is more effective but by which agent is better tolerated by an individual patient.

The usefulness of calcium channel antagonists in the long-term management of unstable angina was demonstrated in a double-blind randomized clinical trial which showed that giving nifedipine to patients already receiving nitrates and propranolol reduced the number of patients with unstable anginal syndromes requiring surgery for relief of pain; the incidence of sudden death and myocardial infarction was similar in the two groups.[91] However, clinical benefits were largely confined to patients whose pain was accompanied by ST segment elevation. (See Chap. 59.)

Combination Therapy

Combination therapy with nitrates and/or β blockers may be more efficacious for the treatment of angina pectoris than one drug used alone.[57,59,73,80,92,93] The hemodynamic effects of a calcium blocker–β blocker combination are shown in Table 67-5.[73] Because adverse effects can occur from this combination (heart block, severe bradycardia, congestive heart failure), patients need careful selection and observation.[94,95] The hemodynamic effects of combined nitrate–calcium channel blocker therapy are shown in Table 67-6. Hypotension should be avoided. Different calcium blockers may also be combined (nifedipine with verapamil or diltiazem) with added benefit; however, side effects may be prohibitive compared with monotherapy.[55]

Arrhythmias (Table 67-7)

Atrial Fibrillation

Except in rare situations, verapamil is ineffective in converting acute and chronic atrial fibrillation to normal sinus rhythm. However, verapamil (oral and intravenous) is effective for decreasing and controlling ventricular rate during atrial fibrillation by prolonging AV nodal conduction and refractoriness and thereby increasing AV block. Clinical trials with verapamil in patients with atrial fibrillation have shown that its ability to decrease ventricular rate appears to be unrelated to the chronicity of the arrhythmia, its etiology, or the patient's age.[96–99] Verapamil appears to be more effective than digoxin in slowing the rapid ventricular rate in response to physical activity.[100] The drug can be used orally in combination with digoxin in treating acute and chronic atrial fibrillation and flutter.[35]

TABLE 67-5

Hemodynamic Effects of Calcium-Entry Blockers, Beta Blockers, and Combination Treatment

	Calcium Blockers	Beta Blockers	Combination
Heart rate	↓←→↑ (reflex)	↓	↓←→
Contractility	↓←→ (reflex)	↓	↓←→
Wall tension	↓	←→	↓
Systolic blood pressure	↓	↓	↓
Left ventricular volume	↓←→	↑	↑←→
Coronary resistance	↓	↑←→	↓←→

Note: ↓ = decrease; ←→ = no change; ↑ = increase.

SOURCE: Frishman WH: Beta-adrenergic blockade in the treatment of coronary artery disease, in Hurst JW (ed): *Clinical Essays on the Heart*. New York, McGraw-Hill, 1984, vol 2, p 48. Reproduced with permission from the publisher and author.

TABLE 67-6

Hemodynamic Rationale for Combining Nitrates and Calcium-Entry Blockers in Angina Pectoris

	Nitrates	Calcium Blockers	Combination
Heart rate	↑ (reflex)	↓←→↑	↑ (reflex)
Blood pressure	↓	↓	↓↓ ?
Heart size	↓/0	↓←→↑	0
Contractility	↑ (reflex)	↓	0
Venomotor tone	↓	0	↓
Peripheral resistance	↓	↓	↓↓ ?
Coronary resistance	↓	↓	↓↓ ?
Coronary blood flow	↑	↑	↑↑ ?
Collateral blood flow	↑	↑	↑↑ ?

Note: ↑ = increase; ↓ = decrease; ↓↓ = questionable additive effects; ←→ = no change.

SOURCE: Frishman WH: Beta-adrenergic blockade in the treatment of coronary artery disease, in Hurst JW (ed): *Clinical Essays on the Heart*. New York, McGraw-Hill, 1984, vol 2, p 48. Reproduced with permission from the publisher and author.

TABLE 67-7

Effects of Diltiazem and Verapamil in the Treatment of Common Arrhythmias

Effective	Ineffective
Supraventricular tachycardia	Sinus tachycardia
AV nodal reentrant PSVT*	Nonparoxysmal automatic atrial tachycardia
Accessory pathway reentrant PSVT	Atrial fibrillation and flutter in WPW syndrome (ventricular rate may not decrease)
SA nodal reentrant PSVT	Ventricular tachyarrhythmias†
Atrial reentrant PSVT	
Atrial flutter (Ventricular rate decreases but arrhythmia will only occasionally convert)	
Atrial fibrillation (Ventricular rate decreases but arrhythmia will only occasionally convert)	

*PSVT = paroxysmal supraventricular tachycardia.
†Only limited experience in this area.

SOURCE: Frishman.[35] Reproduced with permission from the publisher and authors.

Intravenous diltiazem is also an effective agent for reducing rapid ventricular rates in patients with atrial fibrillation,[101] and the intravenous form is used for this indication by bolus or continuous infusion therapy.

Paroxysmal Supraventricular Tachycardia

Many cases of supraventricular tachycardia due to intranodal reentry and those related to circus movement type of tachycardia in preexcitation respond promptly and predictably to intravenous verapamil or diltiazem, whereas only about two-thirds of ectopic atrial tachycardias convert to sinus rhythm after adequate doses of the drug.[35,102,103] Intravenous verapamil and diltiazem are highly efficacious in treating reentry paroxysmal supraventricular tachycardia, regardless of etiology or the patient's age.[35,103]

The recommended dosage range of verapamil for terminating paroxysmal supraventricular tachycardia in adults is 0.075 to 0.15 mg/kg infused over 1 to 3 min, repeated at 30 min.[35] In patients with myocardial dysfunction, the dose should be reduced. Children have been treated safely with a regimen of 0.075 to 0.15 mg/kg.[35] The recommended dose of diltiazem is 0.25 mg/kg infused over 2 min, repeated at 0.35 mg/kg after 15 min.

There have been few clinical studies comparing intravenous verapamil and diltiazem with other standard regimens in the treatment of paroxysmal supraventricular tachycardia.[104] However, in a number of clinical situations verapamil and diltiazem may offer an advantage over either digitalis preparations or β-adrenergic blockers. For instance, verapamil would be preferable in cases where there is an urgent need to terminate paroxysmal supraventricular tachycardia, as it can produce therapeutic responses within 3 min of infusion, whereas the effects of digoxin are not evident for approximately 30 min.[35] Also, if drug therapy fails to achieve normal sinus rhythm, the short duration of action of verapamil and diltiazem permits earlier cardioversion without some of the dangers that accompany electric cardioversion during digoxin therapy. Verapamil and diltiazem also offer distinct advantages over β-adrenergic blocking drugs in patients whose arrhythmias are associated with chronic obstructive lung disease and/or peripheral vascular disease.[35]

Oral verapamil has been approved for prophylaxis against paroxysmal supraventricular tachycardia in doses of 160 to 480 mg/day, and the treatment experiences have yielded favorable results.[105] Diltiazem is not yet approved in oral form as an antiarrhythmic agent.

Atrial Flutter

The immediate effect of intravenous verapamil and diltiazem in atrial flutter in most patients is an increase in AV block that slows the ventricular response, rarely followed by a return to sinus rhythm.[35,99] In some, the response occurs through the development of atrial fibrillation with a controlled ventricular response.[35] A single intravenous dose of verapamil or diltiazem has been found to be of diagnostic value in differentiating rapid atrial flutter from paroxysmal supraventricular tachycardia when these two arrhythmias are indistinguishable on the ECG. If the rhythm is atrial flutter, the AV block increases immediately, revealing the true nature of the arrhythmia.[97] Oral verapamil has also been used to convert paroxysmal atrial flutter and reduce the rapid ventricular rates associated with this arrhythmia.[105]

Preexcitation

Verapamil and diltiazem have been found to induce reversion of most cases of accessory pathway superventricular tachycardia.[102] Using intracardiac recordings of electric activity during programmed electric stimulation of the heart, data have become available regarding the actions of verapamil on the electrophysiological properties of the accessory pathway in overt cases of the Wolff-Parkinson-White (WPW) syndrome.[106,107] The drug has a minimal effect on the antegrade and retrograde conduction times and on the refractory period.[35,39,108] Verapamil and diltiazem, therefore, terminate accessory pathway paroxysmal supraventricular tachycardia in the same manner as they do AV nodal reentrant paroxysmal supraventricular tachycardia: by slowing AV nodal conduction and increasing refractoriness. The minimal effect of verapamil and diltiazem on the electrophysiological properties of the bypass tract is consistent with the observation that the drug is ineffective in atrial fibrillation complicating WPW syndrome, in which fibrillatory impulses conduct predominantly through the anomalous pathway.[97]

Ventricular Arrhythmias

Intravenous verapamil and diltiazem have no apparent benefit in ventricular arrhythmias except in acute myocardial infarction.[39,109] Oral verapamil has no demonstrated role in the management of ventricular tachyarrhythmias. However, bepridil, with its class I antiarrhythmic activity, has been shown to be effective in the short- and long-term control of ventricular arrhythmias. The drug, however, is not approved in the United States as an antiarrhythmic.

Precautions in Treating Arrhythmias

A diseased SA node is much more sensitive to slow-channel blockers and may be depressed to the point of atrial standstill.[110] Sinus arrest can also occur without overt evidence of "sick-sinus syndrome."[35] Calcium channel blockade may also suppress potential AV nodal escape rhythms that need to arise if atrial standstill occurs.[35] In patients with the "brady-tachy" form of sick-sinus syndrome, probably neither digoxin nor β-adrenoceptor blocking drugs should be combined with verapamil or diltiazem in the prophylaxis of tachyarrhythmias unless a demand ventricular pacemaker is first inserted.[35]

Systemic Hypertension

Calcium channel blockers are effective in the treatment of systemic hypertension and hypertensive emergencies.[52,111,112] Calcium channel blocking drugs can be considered as potential first-line therapy for initiating treatment in patients with chronic hypertension. In the United States experience has accumulated evaluating diltiazem,[113,114] nifedipine,[115,116] amlodipine,[117] nicardipine,[118,119] felodipine,[120] and isradipine[121] in patients with hypertension. Verapamil, nicardipine, nifedipine, felodipine, and diltiazem are available in the United States in both conventional and sustained-release oral formulations, allowing once- and twice-daily dosing. Amlodipine is approved for once-daily use, and isradipine twice daily. (See Chap. 77.)

The calcium blocker drugs reduce both systolic and diastolic pressures with a minimal amount of side effects, including orthostasis.[112] They can cause left ventricular hypertrophy to regress in patients with hypertension.[122,123] These drugs may also exhibit antiadrenergic and natriuretic activities.[124] They can be combined with other antihypertensive drugs if necessary (β blockers, angiotensin-converting enzyme inhibitors, and diuretics).[112,116] They are equally effective both in black and white patients[125] and in the young and the old.[112,125] They do not lower the pressures of normotensive patients.[112] These drugs may be most useful in patients with low-renin, salt-dependent forms of hypertension.[126,127]

Hypertensive Emergencies and Perioperative Hypertension

Some of the calcium channel blockers have also been shown to be beneficial and safe in patients with severe hypertension and hypertensive crises.[112,128–130] Single oral, sublingual, and intravenous doses of these drugs have rapidly and smoothly reduced blood pressure in adults and children without causing significant untoward effects.[112,128–130] The absolute reduction in blood pressure with treatment appears to be inversely correlated with the height of the pretreatment blood pressure level, and few episodes of hypotension have been reported.[128] Continuous hemodynamic monitoring of patients does not seem necessary in most instances.[128] Recently, intravenous nicardipine was approved for clinical use in the treatment of hypertensive emergencies and perioperative hypertension. Its clinical utility compared to other parenteral treatments needs to be determined.[131,132]

"Silent" Myocardial Ischemia

In addition to their favorable effects in relieving painful episodes of myocardial ischemia, the calcium blockers are also effective in relieving transient myocardial ischemic episodes (detected by ECG) that are unrelated to symptoms ("silent" myocardial ischemia).[133,134] Diltiazem,[55] nifedipine (low dose), and verapamil, alone and in combination with β blockers and nitrates, have all been shown to be effective in reducing the number of ischemic episodes and their duration.[135] The prognostic importance of relieving silent myocardial ischemia with calcium blockers and other treatments is now being evaluated in a study sponsored by the National Heart Lung and Blood Institute.[136]

Myocardial Infarction

Several experimental studies have indicated that nifedipine, verapamil, and diltiazem can reduce the size of myocardial necrosis induced in experimental ischemia.[137–139] Ischemia can lead to diminished ATP production, which can eventually affect the sodium and calcium ion pumps with the ultimate consequence of calcium ion accumulation in the cytoplasm and calcium overload in the mitochondria. Calcium channel blockers can diminish myocardial oxygen consumption and inhibit the influx of calcium ions to the myofibrils and thus favorably influence the outcome of experimental coronary occlusion.[23,137] These experimental observations have suggested the use of calcium channel blockers for reducing or containing the extent of myocardial infarction during acute coronary artery occlusions in human beings and as an adjunct to cardioplegia during open heart surgery. However, there have been no adequate studies in human beings to support these approaches.

Compared with the established protective actions of some β-blocking drugs used intravenously or orally in prolonging life and reducing the risk of nonfatal reinfarction in survivors of an acute myocardial infarction,[140] the results with calcium channel blockers (diltiazem, lidoflazine, nifedipine, verapamil) have not been as favorable.[139,141–154] Over 17,000 patients have been studied in 11 randomized controlled trials. Eight of the eleven trials showed a small excess in mortality in the treated group (not statistically significant in any trial). Overall, there were 836 deaths among the 8678 patients randomized to the active treatment group (9.5 percent) compared with 830 deaths among the 8762 controls (9.1 percent).

The plausibility of these mortality results with calcium blockers are supported by a failure to show a beneficial effect on infarct size, development of myocardial infarctions, or reinfarctions in most trials of patients with myocardial infarctions or unstable angina.[152] A trial using diltiazem in patients with non-Q wave infarction reported a reduction in recurrent myocardial infarction in the diltiazem-treated patients but no reduction in mortality.[147] In a larger trial with diltiazem in infarction survivors, no favorable effects on mortality were seen.[151] A subgroup of patients with left ventricular dysfunction did worse with diltiazem therapy than with placebo; however, diltiazem therapy was effective in patients with relatively normal left ventricular function.[151] Similarly, a more recent study did show beneficial effects of verapamil compared to placebo in infarction survivors, with less benefit observed in patients with left ventricular dysfunction.[152] (See Chap. 60.)

Prophylactic use of calcium channel blockers to improve patient survival following Q-wave myocardial infarction cannot be recommended as a first-line therapy unless there are specific indications for using these drugs.[141,153,154] However, in patients with contraindications to β-adrenergic blockade, one can consider using verapamil or diltiazem in survivors of myocardial infarction who have good ventricular function.[154] (See also Chap. 60.)

Hypertrophic Cardiomyopathy

Beta-blockers remain the therapeutic agents of choice for symptomatic patients with hypertrophic cardiomyopathy. The beneficial effects produced derive from blocking the effects of catecholamine stimulation on the heart.[155]

Clinical studies have shown that the administration of verapamil can also improve exercise capacity and symptoms in many patients with hypertrophic cardiomyopathy.[156–159] The exact mechanism by which verapamil produces these beneficial effects is not known. Acute and chronic verapamil administration reduces left ventricular outflow obstruction, but examination of indices of left ventricular systolic function during chronic therapy shows that this effect does not result from a reduction in left ventricular hypercontractility.[156] Because patients with hypertrophic cardiomyopathy also exhibit abnormal diastolic function, it is possible that improvement in diastolic filling may be responsible in part for the benefit conferred by verapamil.[156] Enhanced early diastolic filling and improvement in the diastolic pressure-volume relation might be expected to result in an increase in left ventricular end-diastolic volume; this would decrease the Venturi forces that act to move the anterior mitral valve leaflet across the outflow tract toward the septum.[156] The decrease would cause a diminution of obstuction, reducing left ventricular pressure and myocardial wall stress and thus raising the threshold at which symptoms occur.[156]

In a large study[156] of patients with hypertrophic cardiomyopathy refratory to β blockers, verapamil proved to be effective on a long-term basis with almost 50 percent of patients showing either a significant improvement in exercise tolerance or an improvement in symptoms. Approximately 50 percent of patients who were considered to be candidates for surgery because of moderately severe symptoms unresponsive to propranolol showed significant improvement on verapamil, and surgery was no longer considered necessary.[156]

Other studies have reported that chronic administration of verapamil can not only improve symptoms in patients with hypertrophic cardiomyopathy but can also reduce the left ventricular muscle mass and the ventricular septal thickness measured by echocardiographic and ECG analysis.[157] Verapamil and nifedipine were shown to improve the impaired left ventricular filling characteristics.[160,161] This beneficial effect on left ventricular diastolic relaxation has not occurred after propranolol.[160]

There may be serious and fatal complications of verapamil treatment in patients with hypertrophic cardiomyopathy.[156] These complications result from the accentuated hemodynamic or electrophysiologic effects of the drug. It is not clear whether the fatal complications occur as a result of verapamil-induced reduction in blood pressure with a resultant increase in left ventricular obstruction or from the negative inotropic effects of the drug.[156] Verapamil probably should not be used in patients with clinical congestive heart failure. The loss of sequential atrial ventricular depolarization caused by the electrophysiological effects of the drug could also compromise cardiac function. The adverse electrophysiological effects are often transient; however, they could prevent the use of larger drug doses which might provide better relief.[156]

If the calcium-entry blocking effects of verapamil are responsible for its therapeutic actions in hypertrophic cardiomyopathy, other drugs in this class may also be useful. However, the results of a double-blind trial comparing verapamil with nifedipine indicated that verapamil is more effective than nifedipine in improving exercise tolerance and clinical symptoms.[162] (See also Chap. 90.)

Congestive Heart Failure

The potent systemic vasodilatory actions of nifedipine and other dihydropyridine calcium-entry blockers make them potentially useful as afterload-reducing agents in patients with left ventricular failure.[27,33,163,164] Unlike other vasodilatory drugs, however, nifedipine also exerts a direct negative inotropic effect on the myocardium that is consistent with its ability to block transmembrane calcium transport in cardiac muscle cells.[27,28] The successful use of nifedipine as a vasodilator in patients with left ventricular failure would be dependent on its effect in reducing ventricular afterload exceeding its direct negative inotropic actions, thereby leading to an improvement in hemodynamics and forward flow.[57]

Studies evaluating the effect of nifedipine on hemodynamics in patients with heart failure have uniformly demonstrated significant reductions in systemic vascular resistance, usually associated with increases in cardiac output.[57] Resting left ventricular ejection fraction may also rise with nifedipine therapy.[116] Reflex increases in heart rate have been reported,[165] but most investigators have found heart rate to remain the same[166,167] and, in isolated cases, to fall.[168] Left ventricular filling pressures usually decrease[166,167] or do not change significantly,[168] but there are instances where pulmonary capillary wedge pressures rise with the use of nifedipine in heart failure.[169,170] Patients with left ventricular dysfunction and nearly normal levels of left ventricular afterload, i.e., disproportionately low wall stress, and those with intrinsic fixed mechanical interference to forward flow, such as aortic stenosis, appear most likely to have unfavorable hemodynamic responses to nifedipine therapy.[33,163] Most of the published data have dealt only with the acute hemodynamic effects of the agent after single sublingual dosing, with little work done on the use of nifedipine as chronic oral therapy for left ventricular failure.

Total clinical experience with nifedipine and the new dihydropyridine calcium blockers in chronic heart failure is limited.[33,163,164] Therefore, the evidence at present would not support use of these drugs as a ventricular unloading agent of first choice because there are other vasodilators available which do not have negative inotropic activity.[163] Use of dihydropyridine calcium blockers as acute vasodilator therapy in patients with left ventricular failure should be considered only if additional clinical reasons for its administration exist, i.e., angina pectoris and systemic hypertension, and particularly if these conditions play important contributory roles in the development or exacerbation of left ventricular dysfunction. The drug should be administered only after careful assessment of the clinical situation and preferably with invasive monitoring of pulmonary artery or pulmonary capillary wedge pressure.[33,163] Further clinical experience, including controlled clinical trials, will ultimately help define the precise role of calcium channel antagonists in the acute and chronic treatment of systolic heart failure. There is a suggestion that some calcium antagonists might be beneficial to patients with predominant diastolic ventricular dysfunction, but more data are needed to substantiate this claim.

Primary Pulmonary Hypertension

Primary pulmonary hypertension is an entity characterized by excessive pulmonary vasoconstriction and increased pulmonary vascular resistance induced by unknown stimuli.[171] Typically, the affected patient is a young to middle-aged woman presenting with fatigue, dyspnea, chest discomfort, or syncope. Despite many attempts to develop effective therapy, the results of drug treatment have been generally unsatisfactory, and the syndrome continues to bear a poor prognosis.[171]

Based on the currently available data, it may be concluded that some calcium channel antagonists provide beneficial responses in selected patients with pulmonary hypertension.[171–173] In general, patients with less severe pulmonary hypertension appear to respond better than do those with more advanced disease.[174] Furthermore, early treatment may serve to attenuate progression of the disease. (See Chap. 99.)

Cerebral Arterial Spasm and Stroke

A major complication of subarachnoid hemorrhage is cerebral arterial spasm, which may occur several days after the initial event.[175] Such a spasm may be a focal or diffuse narrowing of one or more of the larger cerebral vessels, which may cause additional ischemic neurologic deficits. Although the exact etiology of this spasm is unknown, a combination of various blood constituents and neurotransmitters has been postulated to produce a milieu that enhances the reactivity of the cerebral vasculature.[175] The final pathway for the vasoconstriction, however, involves an increase in the free intracellular calcium concentration.[176] Accordingly, it is reasonable to postulate that the calcium channel antagonists may have a beneficial effect in reducing cerebral spasm.[177] (See Chap. 122.)

Although verapamil and nifedipine have been shown to prevent cerebral arterial spasm in experimental studies,[178,179] nimodipine, a nifedipine analogue, has demonstrated a preferential cerebrovascular action in this disorder.[180] The lipid solubility of nimodipine enables it to cross the blood-brain barrier; this may account for its more potent cerebrovascular effects. In a multicenter placebo-controlled study involving 116 patients,[175] it was demonstrated that nimodipine significantly reduced the occurrence of severe neurologic deficits following angiographically demonstrated cerebral arterial spasm. All patients had a documented subarachnoid hemorrhage and a normal neurologic status within 96 h of entry into the study. While 8 of the 60 placebo-treated patients developed a severe neurologic deficit, only 1 of 56 nimodipine-treated patients suffered such an outcome. Nimodipine improves neurologic outcome by reducing the incidence and severity of ischemic deficits, and the drug is now approved for patients with subarachnoid hemorrhage from ruptured congenital aneurysms who are in good neurologic condition postictus. The recommended dose is 60 mg by mouth every 4 h for 21 consecutive days.

Subsequent investigations have suggested that increased cellular calcium concentration may be implicated in neuronal death after ischemia.[181] Nimodipine administered to laboratory animals after global cerebral ischemia had a more favorable effect on neurologic outcome than did placebo.[182] The results of a prospective double-blind placebo-controlled trial of oral nimodipine administered to 186 patients within 24 h of an acute ischemic stroke showed a reduction in both mortality and neurologic deficit with active treatment. The benefit was confined predominantly to men.[181] (See also Chap. 122.)

Migraine and Dementia

Classic migraine is characterized by prodromal symptoms with transient neurologic deficits. Cerebral blood flow is reduced during these prodromes and then is increased during the subsequent vasodilatory phase, causing severe headache.[183] Because the entry of calcium ions into the smooth-muscle cells is the final common pathway that controls vasomotor tone, calcium antagonists may prevent or ameliorate the initial focal cerebral vasoconstriction.[184]

Results from controlled studies have demonstrated that 80 to 90 percent of patients with vascular headaches benefit from nimodipine, confirming the selectivity of this agent for the cerebral blood vessels.[185] Verapamil and nifedipine have also been reported to be effective in the prophylaxis of migraine, but they are less selective for the cephalic blood vessels and thus cause more systemic side effects.[185,186] Relief from the migraine prodrome usually began 10 to 14 days after initiation of the drugs but could be delayed 2 to 4 weeks.[187] Cerebral vascular resistance was decreased by all three established calcium antagonists, but only nimodipine reduced the cerebral vasoconstriction induced by inhalation of 100% oxygen.[185] None of the calcium-entry blocking drugs are effective against muscle contraction or tension headaches.

Multiple clinical trials are now being carried out examining the effects of calcium-entry blockers on the progression of dementing illness, both vascular and Alzheimer types. The results have been equivocal to date.

Other Cardiovascular Uses

Calcium channel blockers have been shown to be effective in some patients with Raynaud's phenomenon, mesenteric insufficiency, and intermittent claudication.[177,188] They have also been shown in experimental studies to be effective in arresting the atherosclerotic process.[189] Studies are now in progress to assess whether or not specific calcium channel blockers can retard the progress of atherosclerosis in humans, using noninvasive indices of assessment.[190] A recent report with diltiazem showed its ability to retard the development of coronary artery disease in heart transplant recipients.[191]

It has been shown that coronary artery vasospasm may be an important pathophysiological mechanism in some types of experimental cardiomyopathy.[192] Experimentally, verapamil has been shown to reduce vasospasm in response to myocarditis and, by this mechanism, to prevent the development of cardiomyopathy.[193]

Noncardiovascular Applications

Calcium-entry blockers are being investigated for the treatment of bronchial asthma, nocturnal cramps, esophageal spasm, dysmenorrhea, and premature labor.[177,188] The pathophysiology of these conditions may be influenced in part by abnormalities in calcium ion transport across cell membranes, thus explaining the potential application of calcium channel blockers.

ADVERSE EFFECTS

In addition to their widely varying effects on cardiovascular function, these agents also have differing spectra of adverse effects (Table 67-8).[1,57,194] Nifedipine has a very high incidence of minor adverse effects (approximately 40 percent), but serious adverse effects are uncommon.[195] The most frequent adverse effects reported with nifedipine and other dihypdropyridines include headache, pedal edema, flushing, paresthesias, and dizziness. The most serious adverse effects of this drug include exacerbation of angina, which may occur in up to 10 percent of patients, and occasional hypotension.[55,76,79] These side effects are reduced in number with the long-acting formulation of nifedipine[196] and may also be fewer in number with some of the new dihydropyridine calcium antagonists.

Both diltiazem and verapamil can exacerbate sinus node dysfunction and impair AV nodal conduction, particularly in patients with underlying conduction system disease.[1,57,194] The most frequent adverse effect of verapamil is constipation.[1,57,194] The drug may also worsen congestive heart failure, particularly when used in combination with β blockers or disopyramide.[1,57,194] Most of the adverse effects noted with diltiazem have been cardiovascular, with occasional headache and gastrointestinal complaints.[1,57,194] The side effects of the calcium blockers may increase considerably when these agents are used in combination.[55]

Bepridil, which has class I antiarrhythmic properties, has the potential to induce malignant ventricular arrhythmias. In addition, because of its ability to prolong the QT inteval, bepridil can cause torsades de pointes-type ventricular tachycardia. Because of these properties, bepridil should be reserved for patients in whom other antianginal agents do not offer a satisfactory effect.[197]

Drug Withdrawal

Serious problems have been reported with abrupt withdrawal of long-term β-blocker therapy in patients with angina; the problems appear to be related to heightened adrenergic activity.[45] Clinical experiences with calcium-entry blocker withdrawal suggest that although patients with angina get worse after treatment when a calcium-entry blocker is stopped abruptly, there is no evidence of an "overshoot" in anginal symptoms.[45,55]

Drug Overdose

Calcium-entry blocker overdosage has been described with increasing frequency. The cardiovascular problems associated with this condition are hypotension, left ventricular conduction, bradycardia, nodal blocks, and asystole. Treatment approaches are described in Table 67-9.[198]

Drug-Drug Interactions

There are few data on the interactions of diltiazem with other drugs.[1,55] Rifampin severely reduces the bioavail-

TABLE 67-8

Adverse Effects of the Calcium Channel Blockers

	Overall %	Headache	Dizziness	GI	Flushing	Parasthesia	Decreased SA and/or AV Conduction	CHF	Hypotension	Pedal Edema	Worsening of Angina
Diltiazem	≃5	+	+	+	+	0	3+	+	+	+	0
Diltiazem SR	≃5	+	+	+	+	0	3+	+	+	+	0
Verapamil	8	+	+	3+	0	0	3+	2+	+	+	0
Verapamil SR	≃8	+	+	3+	0	0	3+	2+	+	+	0
Bepridil	15	0	2+	3+	0	0	+	+	0	0	0
Amlodipine	≃15	2+	+	+	+	+	0	0	+	2+	0
Isradipine	≃15	2+	2+	+	+	+	0	0	+	2+	0
Nifedipine	≃20	3+	3+	+	3+	+	0	+	+	2+	+
Nifedipine GITS	≃10	+	+	+	+	+	0	+	+	+	0
Nicardipine	≃20	3+	3+	+	3+	+	0	0	+	2+	+
Nimodipine	15	+	+	+	+	0	0	+	+	+	0
Felodipine	20	2+	2+	+	2+	+	0	0	+	2+	0

Note: GI = gastrointestinal; SA = sinoatrial node; AV = atrioventricular node; CHF = congestive heart failure; 0 = no report; + = rare; 2+ = occasional; 3+ = frequent; SR = sustained release; GITS = gastrointestinal system.

SOURCE: Frishman WH et al.[112] Reproduced with permission of the publisher and authors.

TABLE 67-9

Cardiovascular Toxicity of Calcium Channel Blockers and Recommendations for Treatment

Effects*	Suggested Treatment
Profound hypotension	1. 10% calcium gluconate or calcium chloride 2. Norepinephrine or dopamine
Severe left ventricular dysfunction	1. 10% calcium gluconate or calcium chloride 2. Isoproterenol or dobutamine 3. Glucagon 4. Norepinephrine or dopamine
Profound bradycardia Sinus bradycardia SA node and AV node block Asystole	1. Atropine sulfate (not always effective) 2. 10% calcium gluconate or calcium chloride 3. Isoproterenol or dobutamine 4. External cardiac massage and cardiac pacing (if above measures fail)

* These effects are seen more frequently in patients who have underlying myocardial dysfunction and/or cardiac conduction abnormalities and who are receiving concomitant β-adrenergic blocker treatment.

SOURCE: Frishman WH et al.[198] Reproduced with permission from the publisher, editors, and authors.

ability of oral verapamil by enhancing the first-pass liver metabolism of the drug. Both nifedipine and verapamil increase serum digoxin levels, an observation not made with diltiazem. Verapamil has been reported to increase serum digoxin levels by approximately 70 percent,[199,200] apparently by decreasing renal clearance,[199] nonrenal clearance, and the volume of distribution.[200,201] Studies of the time course of this effect show that it begins with the first dose and reaches steady state within 1 to 4 weeks. Nifedipine has also been reported to increase serum digoxin concentrations in patients but to a lesser extent (about 45 percent).[202] The mechanism for this interaction is not clear. Verapamil[200] and diltiazem[203] have additive effects on AV conduction in combination with digitalis. They can be used with digitalis to help control the ventricular response rate in patients with atrial fibrillation. (See Chaps. 36 and 38.)

Combinations of propranolol with nifedipine or verapamil have been extensively studied for the therapy of angina pectoris.[57,73] Several studies have shown improved efficacy for the combination compared with any of the drugs used alone.[92,93] Hemodynamic studies have shown mild negative inotropic effects of verapamil in patients on a β blocker.[94] There are also slight decreases in heart rate, cardiac output, and left ventricular ejection fraction.[94] Combinations of nifedipine and propranolol or metoprolol and of verapamil and propranolol are well tolerated by patients with normal left ventricular function, but there may be a greater potential for hemodynamic compromise in patients with impaired left ventricular function with combined verapamil-propranolol treatment.[94] Combinations of diltiazem, nifedipine, or verapamil with nitrates are well tolerated and clinically useful.[57] When diltiazem is combined with nifedipine, blood levels of nifedipine increase significantly, which may contribute to an increased frequency of adverse reactions with this combination.[55] The combination of verapamil with dihydropyridines has not been well studied. (See also Chap. 109.)

CONCLUSION

Each of the calcium antagonists exerts its effects through inhibition of slow channel–mediated calcium ion transport. Many of the drugs, however, appear to accomplish this by different mechanisms and with differing effects on various target organs. These differences allow the clinician to select the particular drug most suitable for the specific needs of the patient. In addition, the side effect profiles of these drugs (with little overlap between them) assure that most patients will tolerate at least one of these agents.

REFERENCES

1. Keefe D, Frishman WH: Clinical pharmacology of the calcium-channel blocking drugs. In: Packer M, Frishman WH (eds): *Calcium Channel Antagonists in Cardiovascular Disease.* Norwalk, Appleton-Century-Crofts, 1984:3–19.
2. Braunwald E: Mechanism of action of calcium-channel blocking agents. *N Engl J Med* 1983; 307:1618–1627.
3. Weiner DA: Calcium channel blockers. *Med Clin North Am* 1988; 72:83–115.
4. Lindner E: Phenyl-propyl-diphenyl-prophyl-amine, a new substance with a dilating action in the coronary vessels. *Arzneimittelforschung* 1960; 10:569–576.
5. Haas H, Hartfelder G: α-Isopropyl-α (*N*-methyl-*N*-homoveratryl)-(γ-aminopropyl)-3,4-dimethoxyphenylacetonitrol, a substance with vasodilating properties. *Arzneimittelforschung* 1962; 12:549–558
6. Fleckenstein A, Kammermeier H, Doring H, Freund HJ: On the action mechanism of new coronary dilators with oxygen sparing myocardial effects—Prenylamine and Iproveratril. *Z Kreislaufforschung* 1967; 56:716–744, 839–858.
7. Fleckenstein A: Control of myocardial metabolism by verapamil: Sites of action and therapeutic effects. *Arzneimittelforschung* 1970; 20:1317–1322.
8. Singh BN, Vaughan-Williams EM: A fourth class of antidysrhythmic action? Effect of verapamil on ouabain toxicity, on atrial and ventricular intracellular potentials, and on other features of cardiac function. *Cardiovasc Res* 1972; 6:109–119.
9. Vaughan-Williams EM: Classification of antiarrhythmic drugs. In: Sande E, Flensted-Jensen E, Olsen KH (eds): *Symposium on Cardiac Arrhythmias.* Elsinor, Ab Astra, 1979: 449–501.
10. Ebel VS, Schutz H, Hornitschek A: Studies on the analysis of nifedipine considering in particular transformation products formed by light exposure. *Arzneimittelforschung* 1978; 28:2188–2193.
11. Benet LZ: Pharmacokinetics and metabolism of bepridil. *Am J Cardiol* 1985; 55: 8C–13C.
12. Bayer R, Rodenkirchen R, Kaufman R, Lee JH, Hennekes R: The effects of nifedipine on contraction and monophasic action potential of isolated cat myocardium. *Naunyn Schmiedebergs Arch Pharmacol* 1977; 301:29–37.
13. Bayer R, Ehara T: Comparative studies on calcium antagonists. *Prog Pharmacol* 1978; 2:31.

14. Kolhardt M, Fleckenstein A: Inhibition of the slow inward current by nifedipine in mammalian ventricular myocardium. *Naunyn Schmiedebergs Arch Pharmacol* 1977; 298:267–272.
15. Bayer R, Kalusche D, Kaufmann R, Mannhold R: Inotropic and electrophysiological actions of verapamil and D600 in mammalian myocardium: III. Effects of the optical isomers on transmembrane action potentials. *Naunyn Schmiedbergs Arch Pharmacol* 1975; 290:81–97.
16. Ehara T, Kaufmann R: The voltage and time-dependent effects of (−) verapamil on the slow inward current in isolated cat ventricular myocardium. *J Pharmacol Exp Ther* 1978; 207:49–55.
17. Kohlhardt M, Krause H, Kubler M, Herdey A: Kinetics of inactivation and recovery of the slow inward current in the mammalian ventricular myocardium. *Pflugers Arch* 1975; 355:1–17.
18. Henry PD: Comparative pharmacology of calcium antagonists: Nifedipine, verapamil and diltiazem. *Am J Cardiol* 1980; 46:1047–1058.
19. Saikawa T, Nagamoto Y, Arita M: Electrophysiologic effects of diltiazem, a new slow channel inhibitor, on canine cardiac fibers. *Jpn Heart J* 1977; 18:235–245.
20. Meisheri KD, Hwang O, van Breeman C: Evidence of two separate Ca^{2+} pathways in smooth muscle plasmalemma. *J Membr Biol* 1981; 59:19–25.
21. van Breeman C, Mangel A, Fahim M, Meisheri K: Selectivity of calcium antagonistic action in vascular smooth muscle. *Am J Cardiol* 1982; 49:507–510.
22. Schwartz A, Matlib A, Balwierczak J, Lathrop DA: Pharmacology of calcium antagonists. *Am J Cardiol* 1985; 55:3C–7C.
23. Zsoter TT, Church JG: Calcium antagonists—pharmacodynamic effects and mechanism of action. *Drugs* 1983; 25:93–112.
24. Braunwald E: Calcium-channel blockers: Pharmacologic considerations. *Am Heart J* 1982; 104:665–671.
25. Millard RW, Lathrop DA, Grupp G, Ashraf M, Grupp IL, Schwartz A: Differential cardiovascular effects of calcium channel blocking agents: Potential mechanisms. *Am J Cardiol* 1982; 49:449–506.
26. Fleckenstein A: Specific pharmacology of calcium in myocardium, cardiac pacemakers, and vascular smooth muscle. *Annu Rev Pharmacol Toxicol* 1977; 17:149–166.
27. Henry PD, Borda L, Schuchleib R: Chronotropic and inotropic effects of vasodilators. In: Lichtlen PR, Kmura E, Taira N (eds): *International Adalat Panel Discussion: New Experimental and Clinical Results*. Amsterdam, Exerpta Medica, 1979:14–21.
28. Cohn JN, Franciosa JA: Vasodilatory therapy of cardiac failure. *N Engl J Med* 1977; 297:27–31.
29. Himori N, Ono H, Taira N: Simultaneous assessment of effects of coronary vasodilators on the coronary blood flow and the myocardial contractility by using the blood perfused canine papillary muscle. *Jpn J Pharmacol* 1976; 26:427–435.
30. Singh BN, Hecht HS, Nademanee K, Chew CYC: Electrophysiologic and hemodynamic effects of slow channel blocking drugs. *Prog Cardiovasc Dis* 1982; 25:103–132.
31. Braunwald E, Stone PH, Antman EM, Muller JE: Calcium channel blocking agents in the treatment of cardiovascular disorders: II. Hemodynamic effects and clinical applications. *Ann Intern Med* 1980; 93:886–904.
32. Ellrodt G, Chew CYC, Singh BN: Therapeutic implications of slow-channel blockade in cardiocirculatory disorders. *Circulation* 1980; 62:669–679.
33. Frishman WH, Landau AJ, Charlap S, Lazar EJ: Calcium antagonists and heart failure. *Heart Failure* 1991; VII(4):138–153.
34. Mitchell LB, Schroeder JS, Mason JW: Comparative clinical electrophysiologic effect of diltiazem, verapamil and nifedipine—a review. *Am J Cardiol* 1982; 49:629–635.
35. Frishman WH, LeJemtel T: Electropharmacology of calcium channel antagonists in cardiac arrhythmias. *PACE* 1982; 5:402–413.
36. Singh BN, Nademanee K, Baky S: Calcium antagonists. *Drugs* 1983; 25:125–153.
37. Nayler WG, Poole-Wilson PH: Calcium antagonists: Definition and mode of action. *Basic Res Cardiol* 1981; 76:1–15.
38. Yamaguchi I, Obayashi K, Mandel WJ: Electrophysiologic effects of verapamil. *Cardiovasc Res* 1978; 12:597–608.
39. Singh BN, Collet J, Chew CYC: New perspectives in the pharmacologic therapy of cardiac arrhythmias. *Prog Cardiovasc Dis* 1980; 22:243–301.
40. Wit A, Cranefield P: The effects of verapamil on the sinoatrial and atrioventricular nodes of the rabbit and the mechanisms by which it arrests reentrant AV nodal tachycardia. *Circ Res* 1974; 35:413–425.
41. Zipes DP, Fischer JC: Effects of agents which inhibit the slow channel on sinus node automaticity and atrioventricular conduction in the dog. *Circ Res* 1974; 34:184–192.
42. Triggle CR, Swamy VC, Triggle DJ: Calcium antagonists and contractile responses in rat vas deferens and guinea pig ileal smooth muscle. *Can J Physiol Pharmacol* 1979; 57:804–818.
43. Schoen RE, Frishman WH, Shamoon H: Hormonal and metabolic effects of calcium-channel antagonists in man. *Am J Med* 1988; 84:492–504.
44. Shamoon H, Baylor P, Kamobosos D, Charlap S, Plawes S, Frishman WH: Influence of oral verapamil on glucoregulatory hormones in man. *J Clin Endocrinol Metabol* 1985; 60:536–541.
45. Frishman WH, Klein N, Strom J, Cohen MN, Shamoon H, Willens H, et al: Comparative effects of abrupt withdrawal of propranolol and verapamil in angina pectoris. *Am J Cardiol* 1982; 50:1191–1195.
46. Pumphrey CW, Fuster V, Dewanjee MK, Chesebro JH, Vlieststra RE, Kaye MP, et al: Comparison of the antithrombotic action of calcium antagonist drugs with dipyridamole in dogs. *Am J Cardiol* 1983; 51:591–595.
47. Mehta JL: Influence of calcium-channel blockers on platelet function and arachidonic acid metabolism. *Am J Cardiol* 1985; 55:158B–164B.
48. Burns ER, Frishman WH: The antiplatelet effects of calcium channel blockers add to their antianginal properties. *Int J Cardiol* 1983; 4:372–379.
49. Barnathan ES, Addonizio VP, Shattil SJ: Interaction of verapamil with human platelet α-adrenergic receptors. *Am J Physiol* 1982; 242:H19–H23.
50. Frishman WH, Miller KP: Platelets and antiplatelet therapy in ischemic heart disease. *Curr Probl Cardiol* 1986; 11(2):72–136.
51. McAllister RG: Clinical pharmacology of slow channel blocking agents. *Prog Cardiovasc Dis* 1982; 25:83–102.
52. Kates R: Calcium antagonists—pharmacokinetic properties. *Drugs* 1983; 25:113–124.
53. Frishman WH, Stroh JA, Greenberg SM, Suarez T, Karp A, Peled H, et al: Calcium-channel blockers in systemic hypertension. *Curr Probl Cardiol* 1987; 12:287–346.
54. Frishman WH, Kirstein E, Klein M, Kates R: Clinical relevance of verapamil plasma levels in stable angina pectoris. *Am J Cardiol* 1982; 50:1180–1184.
55. Frishman WH, Charlap S, Kimmel B, Teicher M, Cinnamon J, Allen L, et al: Diltiazem compared to nifedipine and combination treatment in patients with stable angina: Effects on angina, exercise tolerance and the ambulatory ECG. *Circulation* 1988; 77:774–786.
56. Singh BN, Chew CYC, Josephson MA, Packer M: Hemodynamic mechanisms underlying the antianginal actions of verapamil. *Am J Cardiol* 1982; 50:886–893.
57. Frishman WH, Sonnenblick EH: Cardiovascular uses of calcium-channel blockers. In: Messerli F (ed): *Current Cardiovascular Drug Therapy*. Philadelphia, Saunders, 1990:896–909.
58. Weiner DA: Calcium channel blockers. *Med Clin North Am* 1988; 72:93–116.
59. Theroux P, Taeymans Y, Waters D: Calcium antagonists: Clinical use in the treatment of angina. *Drugs* 1983; 25:178–195.
60. Hossack KF, Pool PE, Steele P: Efficacy of diltiazem in angina of effort—a multicenter trial. *Am J Cardiol* 1982; 49:567–572.
61. Straus WE, McIntyre KM, Parisi AR, Shapiro W: Safety and efficacy of diltiazem hydrochloride for the treatment of stable angina pectoris—report of a cooperative trial. *Am J Cardiol* 1982; 49:560–566.
62. Weiner DA, Cutler SS, Klein MD: Efficacy and safety of sustained-release diltiazem in stable angina pectoris. *Am J Cardiol* 1986; 57:6–9.
63. Moskowitz RM, Piccini PA, Nacarelli GV, Zelis R: Nifedipine therapy for stable angina pectoris: Preliminary results of effects on angina frequency and treadmill exercise response. *Am J Cardiol* 1979; 44:811–815.
64. Mueller HS, Chahine RA: Interim report of multicenter double-blind placebo-controlled studies of nifedipine in chronic stable angina. *Am J Med* 1981; 71:645–657.
65. Bala Subramanian V, Parmasivan R, Lahiri A, Raftery EB: Vera-

pamil in chronic stable angina—a controlled study with computerized multistage treadmill exercise. *Lancet* 1980; 1:841–844.
66. Weiner DA, Klein MD: Verapamil therapy for stable exertional angina. *Am J Cardiol* 1982; 50:1153–1157.
67. Weiner DA, Klein MD, Cutler SS: Evaluation of sustained-release verapamil in chronic stable angina pectoris. *Am J Cardiol* 1987; 59:215–218.
68. Scheidt S, Frishman WH, Packer M, Mehta J, Parodi O, Bala Subramanian V: Long-term effectiveness of verapamil in stable and unstable angina pectoris: One year follow-up of patients treated in placebo-controlled double-blind randomized clinical trials. *Am J Cardiol* 1982; 50:1185–1190.
90. Shapiro W, DiBianco R, Thadani U, and other members of the Bepridil Collaborative Study Group: Comparative efficacy of 200, 300 and 400 mg of bepridil for chronic stable angina pectoris. *Am J Cardiol* 1985; 55:36C–42C.
70. Singh BN for the Bepridil Collaborative Study Group: Comparative efficacy and safety of bepridil and diltiazem in chronic stable angina pectoris refractory to diltiazem. *Am J Cardiol* 1991; 68:306–312.
71. Livesley B, Catley PF, Campbell RC, Oram S: Double-blind evaluation of verapamil, propranolol and isosorbide dinitrate against placebo in the treatment of angina pectoris. *Br Med J* 1973; 1:375–378.
72. Frishman WH, Klein NA, Strom JA, Willens H, LeJemtel TH, Jentzer J, et al: Superiority of verapamil to propranolol in stable angina pectoris—a double-blind, randomized crossover trial. *Circulation* 1982; 65(suppl I):I51–I59.
73. Frishman WH: The use of beta-adrenoceptor blockers in cardiac disorders. In: Messerli F (ed): *Current Cardiovascular Drug Therapy*. Philadelphia, Saunders, 1990:394–407.
74. Kenmure ACF, Scruton JH: A double-blind controlled trial of the antianginal efficacy of nifedipine compared with propranolol. *Br J Clin Pract* 1980; 8:49–52.
75. Bala Subramanian V, Bowles MJ, Davies AB, Raftery EB: Comparative effectiveness of verapamil and propranolol in angina of effort. *Am J Cardiol* 1982; 50:1158–1163.
76. Bala Subramanian V, Bowles MJ, Khurmi NS, Davies A, Raftery EB: Comparative effectiveness of verapamil and nifedipine in stable angina pectoris. *Am J Cardiol* 1982; 50:1173–1179.
77. Frishman WH, Klein N, Klein P, Strom JA, Tawil R, Strair R, et al: Comparison of oral propranolol and verapamil for combined systemic hypertension and angina pectoris: A placebo-controlled double-blind randomized crossover trial. *Am J Cardiol* 1982; 50:1164–1172.
78. Frishman WH, Charlap S: Calcium-channel blockers for combined systemic hypertension and myocardial ischemia. *Circulation* 1988; 75:V154–V162.
79. Boden WE, Korr KS, Bough KW: Nifedipine-induced hypotension and myocardial ischemia in refractory angina pectoris. *JAMA* 1985; 253:1131–1135.
80. Frishman WH, Charlap S, Farnham J, Sawin HS, Michelson EL, Crawford MH, et al: Combination propranolol and bepridil therapy in angina pectoris. *Am J Cardiol* 1985; 55:43C–49C.
81. Johnson SM, Mauritson DR, Willerson JT, Hillis LD: A controlled trial of verapamil for Prinzmetal's variant angina. *N Engl J Med* 1981; 304:862–866.
82. Mehta J, Conti CR: Calcium channel antagonists in the treatment of unstable angina. *Am J Cardiol* 1982; 50:919–922.
83. Theroux P, Waters DD, Affaki GS, Crittin J, Bonan R, Mizgala HF: Provocative testing with ergonovine to evaluate the efficacy of treatment with calcium antagonists in variant angina. *Circulation* 1979; 60:504–510.
84. Antman E, Muller JE, Goldberg S, MacAlpin R, Rubenfire M, Tabatznik B, et al: Nifedipine therapy for coronary artery spasm experience in 127 patients. *N Engl J Med* 1980; 302:1269–1273.
85. Schroeder JS, Feldman RL, Giles TD, Friedman MJ, DeMaria AN, Kinney EL, et al: Multiclinic controlled trial of diltiazem for Prinzmetal's angina. *Am J Med* 1982; 72:227–232.
86. Feldman RL, Pepine CJ, Whittle J, Conti R: Short- and long-term responses to diltiazem in patients with variant angina. *Am J Cardiol* 1982; 49:554–559.
87. Goldberg S, Reichek N, Wilson J, Hirshfield JW, Muller J, Kastor JA: Nifedipine in the treatment of Prinzmetal's (variant) angina. *Am J Cardiol* 1979; 44:804–810.
88. Prida XE, Gelman JS, Feldman RL, Hill JA, Pepine CJ, Scott E: Comparison of diltiazem alone and in combination in patients with coronary artery spasm. *J Am Coll Cardiol* 1987; 9:412–419.
89. Parodi O, Simonetti I, L'Abbate A, Maseri A: Comparative effectiveness of verapamil and propranolol in angina at rest. *Am J Cardiol* 1982; 50:923–928.
90. Johnson SM, Mauritson DR, Willerson JT, Hillis LD: Comparison of verapamil and nifedipine in the treatment of variant angina pectoris—preliminary observations in 10 patients. *Am J Cardiol* 1981; 47:1295–1300.
91. Gerstenblith G, Ouyang P, Achuff S, Bulkley BH, Becker LC, Mellits ED, et al: Nifedipine in unstable angina: A double-blind randomized trial. *N Engl J Med* 1982; 306:885–889.
92. Subramanian B, Bowles MK, Davies AB, Raftery EB: Combined therapy with verapamil and propranolol in chronic stable angina. *Am J Cardiol* 1982; 49:125–132.
93. Dargie HJ, Lynch PG, Krikler DM, Harris L, Krikler S: Nifedipine and propranolol: A beneficial drug interaction. *Am J Med* 1981; 71:676–682.
94. Packer M, Leon MB, Bonow RO, Kieval J, Rosing DR, Bala Subramanian V: Hemodynamic and clinical effects of combined therapy with verapamil and propranolol in ischemic heart disease. *Am J Cardiol* 1982; 50:903–912.
95. Packer M, Frishman WH: Calcium channel antagonists in perspective. In: Packer M, Frishman WH (eds): *Calcium Channel Antagonists in Cardiovascular Disease*. Norwalk, Appleton-Century-Crofts, 1984: XVII.
96. Schamroth L, Krikler DM, Garrett C: Immediate effects of intravenous verapamil in cardiac arrhythmias. *Br Med J* 1972; 1:660–662.
97. Heng MK, Singh BN, Roche AHG, Norris RM, Mercer CJ: Effects of intravenous verapamil on cardiac arrhythmias and on the electrocardiogram. *Am Heart J* 1975; 90:487–498.
98. Klein HO, Pauzner H, DiSegni E, David D, Kaplinsky E: The beneficial effects of verapamil in chronic atrial fibrillation. *Arch Intern Med* 1979; 139:747–749.
99. Weiner I: Verapamil therapy for atrial flutter and fibrillation. In: Packer M, Frishman WH (eds): *Calcium Channel Antagonists in Cardiovascular Disease*. Norwalk, Appleton-Century-Crofts, 1984: 257–268.
100. Klein HO, Kaplinsky E: Verapamil and digoxin. Their respective effects on atrial fibrillation and their interaction. *Am J Cardiol* 1982; 50:894–902.
101. Ellenbogen KA, Dias VC, Plumb VJ, Heywood JT, Mirvis DM: A placebo-controlled trial of continuous intravenous diltiazem infusion for 24-hour heart rate control during atrial fibrillation and atrial flutter: A multicenter trial. *J Am Coll Cardiol* 1991; 18:891–897.
102. Krikler DM, Spurrell RAJ: Verapamil in the treatment of paroxysmal supraventricular tachycardia. *Postgrad Med J* 1974; 50(585):447–453.
103. Singh BN, Nademanee D, Baky S: Calcium antagonists: Uses in the treatment of cardiac arrhythmias. *Drugs* 1983; 25:125–153.
104. Hartel G, Hartikainen M: Comparison of verapamil and practolol in paroxysmal supraventricular tachycardia. *Eur J Cardiol* 1976; 4:87–90.
105. Mauritson DR, Winniford MD, Walker WS, Rude RE, Cary JR, Hillis LD: Oral verapamil for paroxysmal supraventricular tachycardia: A long term, double-blind, randomized trial. *Ann Intern Med* 1982; 96:409–412.
106. Spurrell RAJ, Krikler DM, Sowton GE: The effect of verapamil on the electrophysiological properties of the anomalous atrioventricular connections in Wolff-Parkinson-White syndrome. *Br Heart J* 1974; 36:256–264.
107. Matsuyama E, Konishi T, Okazaki H, Matsuda H, Kawai C: Effects of verapamil on accessory pathway properties and induction of circus movement tachycardia in patients with the Wolff-Parkinson-White syndrome. *J Cardiovasc Pharmacol* 1981; 3:11–24.
108. Shigenobu K, Schneider JA, Sperelakis N: Verapamil blockade of slow Na^+ and Ca^{++} responses in myocardial cells. *J Pharmacol Exp Ther* 1974; 190: 280–288.
109. Gotsman M, Lewis B, Bakst A, Mitha AS: Verapamil in life-threatening tachyarrhythmias. *S Afr Med J* 1972; 46:2017–2019.
110. Carrasco HA, Fuenmayor A, Barboza J, Gonzalez G: Effect of verapamil on normal sino-atrial node dysfunction and on sick sinus syndrome. *Am Heart J* 1978; 96:760–771.
111. Cummings DM, Amadio P, Nelson L, Fitzgerald JM: The role of calcium channel blockers in the treatment of systemic hypertension. *Arch Intern Med* 1991; 151:250–259.

112. Frishman WH, Stroh JA, Greenberg SM, Suarez T, Karp A, Peled HB: Calcium-channel blockers in systemic hypertension. *Med Clin North Am* 1988; 72:449–499.
113. Frishmann WH, Zawada ET, Smith LK, Sowers J, Swartz SL, Kirkendall W, et al: A comparative study of diltiazem and hydrochlorothiazide as initial medical therapy for mild to moderate hypertension. *Am J Cardiol* 1987; 59:615–623.
114. Massie B, MacCarthy EP, Ramanathan KB, Weiss RJ, Anderson M, Eidelson BA, et al: Diltiazem and propranolol in mild to moderate essential hypertension as monotherapy or with hydrochlorothiazide. *Ann Intern Med* 1987; 107:150–157.
115. Frishman WH, Garofalo JL, Rothschild A, Rothschild M, Greenberg SM, Soberman J: Multicenter comparison of the nifedipine gastrointestinal system and long-acting propranolol in patients with mild to moderate systemic hypertension receiving diuretics: A preliminary experience. *Am J Med* 1987; 83:15–19.
116. Ferlinz J: Nifedipine in myocardial ischemia, systemic hypertension and other cardiovascular disorders. *Ann Intern Med* 1986; 105:714–729.
117. Johnson BF, Frishman WH, Brobyn R, Brown RD, Reeves RL, Wombolt DG: A randomized placebo-controlled, double-blind comparison of amlodipine and atenolol in patients with essential hypertension. *Am J Hypertens* 1992; 5:727–732.
118. Charlap S, Kimmel B, Laifer L, Weinberg P, Singer M, Saltzberg S, et al: Twice daily nicardipine in the treatment of patients with mild to moderate hypertension. *J Clin Hypertens* 1986; 2:271–277.
119. Taylor SH, Frais MA, Lee P, Verma SP, Jackson N, Reynolds G, et al: A study of the long-term efficacy and tolerability of oral nicardipine in hypertensive patients. *Br J Clin Pharmacol* 1985; 20(suppl 1): 139S–142S.
120. Todd PA, Faulds D: Feldopine: A review of the pharmacology and therapeutic use of the extended-release formulation in cardiovascular disorders. *Drugs* 1992; 44:252–272.
121. Hamilton BP: Treatment of essential hypertension with PN 200-110 (isradipine). *Am J Cardiol* 1987; 59:141–145.
122. Hachamovitch R, Strom JA, Sonnenblick EH, Frishman WH: Left ventricular hypertrophy in hypertension and the effects of antihypertensive drug therapy. *Curr Probl Cardiol* 1988; 13(6):371–421.
123. Frishman WH, Skolnick AE: Effects of calcium blockade on hypertension-induced left ventricular hypertrophy. *Circulation* 1989; 80(suppl IV):151–161.
124. Buhler F, DeLeeuw PW, Doyle A, Fleckenstein A, Fleckenstein-Grun G, Frishman WH, et al: Calcium metabolism and calcium-channel blockers for understanding and treating hypertension. *Am J Med* 1984; 77(6B):1–23.
125. Zing W, Ferguson RK, Vlasses PH: Calcium antagonists in elderly and black hypertensive patients: Therapeutic controversies. *Arch Intern Med* 1991; 151:2154–2162.
126. Buhler FR, Hulthen UL, Kiowski W, Bolli P: Greater antihypertensive efficacy of the calcium channel inhibitor verapamil in older and low renin patients. *Clin Sci* 1982; 63:439S–442S.
127. Erne P, Bolli P, Bertel O, Hulthen UL, Kiowski W, Muller FB, et al: Antihypertensive monotherapy with calcium antagonists relates to older age, liver pretreatment renin and higher blood pressure: Comparison of nifedipine and verapamil. *Hypertension* 1983; 5(suppl II):97–102.
128. Frishman WH, Weinberg P, Peled H, Kimmel B, Charlap S, Beer N: Calcium-entry blockers for the treatment of severe hypertension and hypertensive emergencies. *Am J Med* 1984; 77(2B):35–45.
129. Beer N, Gallegos I, Cohen A, Klein N, Sonnenblick EH, Frishman W, et al: Efficacy of sublingual nifedipine in the acute treatment of systemic hypertension. *Chest* 1981; 79:571–574.
130. Ellrodt AG, Ault M, Riedinger MS, Murata GH: Efficacy of sublingual nifedipine in hypertensive emergencies. *Am J Med* 1985; 79(4A):19–22.
131. Wallin JD, Fletcher E, Ram CVS, Cook E, Cheung DG, MacCarthy EP, et al: Intravenous nicardipine for the treatment of severe hypertension. *Arch Intern Med* 1989; 149(12):2662–2669.
132. IV Nicardipine Study Group: Efficacy and safety of intravenous nicardipine in the control of postoperative hypertension. *Chest* 1991; 99:393–398.
133. Frishman WH, Teicher M: Antianginal drug therapy for silent myocardial ischemia. *Med Clin North Am* 1988; 72:185–196.
134. Deedwania PC, Carbajal EV: Silent myocardial ischemia: A clinical perspective. *Arch Intern Med* 1991; 151:2373–2382.
135. Epstein SE, Quyyumi AA, Bonow RO: Myocardial ischemia—silent or symptomatic. *N Engl J Med* 1988; 318:1038–1043.
136. The ACIP Investigators. Asymptomatic Cardiac Ischemia Pilot Study (ACIP). *Am J Cardiol* 1992; 70:744–747.
137. Nayler WG: Cardioprotective effects of calcium ion antagonists in myocardial ischemia. *Clin Invest Med* 1980; 3:91–99.
138. Melin JA, Becker LC, Hutchins GM: Protective effect of early and late treatment with nifedipine during myocardial infarction in the conscious dog. *Circulation* 1984; 69:131–141.
139. Skolnick AE, Frishman WH: Calcium channel blockers in myocardial infarction. *Arch Intern Med* 1989; 149:1669–1677.
140. Frishman WH, Furberg CD, Friedewald WT: β-Adrenergic blockade in survivors of acute myocardial infarction. *N Engl J Med* 1984; 310:830–837.
141. Messerli FH: "Cardioprotection"—not all calcium antagonists are created equal. *Am J Cardiol* 1990; 66:855–856.
142. Crea F, Deanfield J, Crean P, Sharon M, Davies G, Maseri A: Effects of verapamil in preventing early post infarction angina and reinfarction. *Am J Cardiol* 1985; 55:900–904.
143. Gottlieb SO, Weiss JL, Flaherty JT, Mellits D, Ouyang P, Gottlieb SH, et al: Effect of nifedipine on clinical course and left ventricular function in low risk acute myocardial infarction: A double-blind randomized trial. (Abstract) *Circulation* 1984; 70:II–257.
144. Sirnes PA, Overskeid K, Pedersen TR, Bathen J, Drivenes A, Froland GS, et al: Evolution of infarct size during the early use of nifedipine in patients with acute myocardial infarction: The Norwegian Nifedipine Multicenter Trial. *Circulation* 1984; 70:638–644.
145. Wilcox RG, Hampton JR, Banks DC, Birkhead JS, Brooksby IAB, Burns-Cox CJ, et al: Trial of early nifedipine in acute myocardial infarction: The TRENT Study. *Br Med J* 1986; 293:1204–1208.
146. The Danish Study Group on Verapamil in Myocardial Infarction: Verapamil in acute myocardial infarction. *Eur Heart J* 1984; 5:516–528.
147. Gibson RS, Boden WE, Theroux P, Strauss HD, Pratt CM, Gheorghiade M, et al: Diltiazem and reinfarction in patients with non-Q-wave myocardial infarction. *N Engl J Med* 1986; 315:423–429.
148. Muller JE, Morrison J, Stone PH, Rude RE, Rosner B, Roberts R, et al: Nifedipine therapy for patients with threatened and acute myocardial infarction: A randomized, double-blind, placebo-controlled comparison. *Circulation* 1984; 69:740–747.
149. Neufeld HN: Calcium antagonists in secondary prevention after acute myocardial infarction: The Secondary Prevention Reinfarction Nifedipine Trial (SPRINT). *Eur Heart J* 1986; 7(suppl B):51–52.
150. The Myocardial Infarction Study Group: Secondary prevention of ischemic heart disease: A long-term controlled lidoflazine study. *Acta Cardiol* 1979; 24(suppl):7–46.
151. The Multicenter Diltiazem Postinfarction Trial Research Group: The effect of diltiazem on mortality and reinfarction after myocardial infarction. *N Engl J Med* 1988; 319(7):385–392.
152. The Danish Study on Verapamil in Myocardial Infarction: The effect of verapamil on mortality and major events after myocardial infarction. The Danish Verapamil Infarction Trial II (DAVIT II). *Am J Cardiol* 1990; 66:779–785.
153. Yusuf S, Held P, Furberg CD: Update of effects of calcium antagonists in myocardial infarction or angina in light of the second Danish Verapamil Infarction Trial (DAVIT II) and other recent studies. *Am J Cardiol* 1991; 67:1295–1297.
154. Frishman WH, Skolnick AE, Miller KP: Secondary prevention post infarction: The role of β-adrenergic blockers, calcium-channel blockers and aspirin. In: Gersh BJ, Rahimtoola SH (eds): *Management of Myocardial Infarction.* New York, Elsevier, 1991:469–492.
155. Cohen LS, Braunwald E: Amelioration of angina pectoris in idiopathic hypertrophic subaortic stenosis with beta-adrenergic blockade. *Circulation* 1967; 35:847–851.
156. Rosing DR, Bonow RO, Packer M, et al: Verapamil therapy for the management of hypertrophic cardiomyopathy. In: Packer M, Frishman WH (eds): *Calcium Channel Antagonists in Cardiovascular Disease.* Norwalk, Appleton-Century-Crofts, 1984: 313–342.
157. Kaitenbach M, Hopf R, Kober G, Bussmann W, Keller M, Peterson Y: Treatment of hypertrophic obstructive cardiomyopathy with verapamil. *Br Heart J* 1979; 42:35–42.
158. Rosing DR, Kent KM, Maron BJ, Epstein S: Verapamil therapy—a new approach for the pharmacologic treatment of hypertrophic

cardiomyopathy. II. Effects on exercise capacity and symptomatic status. *Circulation* 1979; 60:1208–1213.
159. Rosing DR, Kent KM, Borer JS, Seides SF, Maron BJ, Epstein SE: Verapamil therapy—a new approach to the pharmacologic treatment of hypertrophic cardiomyopathy: I. Hemodynamic effects. *Circulation* 1979; 60:1201–1207.
160. Bonow RO, Rosing DR, Bacharach SL, Green MV, Kent KM, Lipson LC, et al: Effects of verapamil on left ventricular systolic function and diastolic filling in patients with hypertrophic cardiomyopathy. *Circulation* 1981; 64:787–796.
161. Lorell BH, Paulus WJ, Grossman W, Wynne J, Cohn PF: Modification of abnormal left ventricular diastolic properties by nifedipine in patients with hypertrophic cardiomyopathy. *Circulation* 1982; 65:499–507.
162. Rosing DR, Cannon RO, Watson RM, Kent KM, Lakatos É, Epstein SE, et al: Comparison of verapamil and nifedipine effects on symptoms and exercise capacity in patients with hypertrophic cardiomyopathy. (Abstract) *Circulation* 1982; 66(suppl II):II–24.
163. Frishman WH, Landau AJ, Charlap S, Lazar E: Calcium antagonists and heart failure. *Heart Failure* 1991; 7:138–153.
164. Charlap S, Frishman WH: Calcium antagonists and heart failure. *Med Clin North AM* 1989; 73:339–360.
165. Losardo AA, Klein NA, Beer N, Strom J, Wexler JP, Sonnenblick EH, et al: Beneficial effects of sublingual nifedipine in patients with ischemic heart disease and depressed left ventricular function. *Angiology* 1982; 33:811–817.
166. Klugmann S, Salvi A, Camerini F: Haemodynamic effects of nifedipine in heart failure. *Br Heart J* 1980; 43:440–446.
167. Polese A, Fiorentini C, Olivari MT, Guazzi M: Clinical use of a calcium antagonistic agent (nifedipine) in acute pulmonary edema. *Am J Med* 1979; 66:825–830.
168. Fifer MA, Colucci WS, Lorell BH, Jaski BE, Barry WH: Comparison of hemodynamic responses to nifedipine in heart failure: Comparison with nitroprusside. *J Am Coll Cardiol* 1985; 5:731–737.
169. Packer M, Lee WH, Medina N, Yushak M, Bernstein JL, Kessler PDL: Prognostic importance of the immediate hemodynamic response to nifedipine in patients with severe left ventricular dysfunction. *J Am Coll Cardiol* 1987; 10:1303–1311.
170. Elkayam U, Weber L, McKay C, Rahimtoola S: Spectrum of acute hemodynamic effects of nifedipine in severe congestive heart failure. *Am J Cardiol* 1985; 546:506–566.
171. Fein SA, Frishman WH; The pathophysiology and management of primary pulmonary hypertension. *Cardiol Clin* 1987; 5:563–576.
172. Kambara H, Fujimoto K, Wakabayashi A, Kawai C: Primary pulmonary hypertension: Beneficial therapy with diltiazem. *Am Heart J* 1981; 101:230–231.
173. DeFeyter PJ, Kerkkamp HJJ, deJong JP: Sustained beneficial effect of nifedipine in primary pulmonary hypertension. *Am Heart J* 1983; 105:333–334.
174. Packer M: Vasodilator therapy for primary pulmonary hypertension. Limitations and hazards. *Ann Intern Med* 1985; 103: 258–270.
175. Allen GS, Ahn HS, Preziosi TJ, Battye R, Boone SC, Chou SN, et al: Cerebral arterial spasm—a controlled trial of nimodipine in patients with subarachnoid hemorrhage. *N Engl J Med* 1983; 308:619–632.
176. Towart R: The pathophysiology of cerebral vasospasm and pharmacological approaches to its management. *Acta Neurochir (Wien)* 1982; 62:253–258.
177. Bussey HI, Talbert RL: Promising uses of calcium-channel blocking agents. *Pharmacotherapy* 1984; 4:137–143.
178. Allen GS, Bahr AL: Cerebral arterial spasm: X. Reversal of acute and chronic spasm in dogs with orally administered nifedipine. *Neurosurgery* 1979; 4:43–47.
179. Allen GS, Banghart SB: Cerebral arterial spasm: IX. In vitro effects of nifedipine on serotonin, phenylephrine and potassium-induced contractions of canine basilar and femoral artery. *Neurosurgery* 1979; 4:37–42.
180. Kazda S, Towart R: Nimodipine: A new calcium antagonistic drug with a preferential cerebrovascular action. *Acta Neurochir (Wien)* 1982; 63:259–265.
181. Gelmers HJ, Gorter K, DeWeerdt CJ, Wiezer HJA: A controlled trial of nimodipine in acute ischemic stroke. *N Engl J Med* 1988; 318:203–207.
182. Steen PA, Gisvold SE, Milde JH, Newberg LA, Scheithauer BW, Lanier WL, et al: Nimodipine improves outcome when given after complete cerebral ischemia in primates. *Anesthesiology* 1985; 62:406–414.
183. Edmeads J: Cerebral blood flow in migraine. *Headache* 1977; 17:148–152.
184. Meyer JS: Calcium channel blockers in the prophylactic treatment of vascular headache. *Ann Intern Med* 1985; 102:395–397.
185. Meyer JS, Hardenberg J: Clinical effectiveness of calcium entry blockers in prophylactic treatment of migraine and cluster headaches. *Headache* 1983; 23:266–277.
186. Solomon GD, Steele JG, Spaccavento LJ: Verapamil prophylaxis of migraine: A double-blind placebo-controlled study. *JAMA* 1983; 250:2500–2505.
187. Meyer JS, Dowell R, Mathew NJ, Hardenberg J: Clinical and hemodynamic effects during treatment of vascular headaches with verapamil. *Headache* 1984; 24:313–321.
188. Schwartz ML, Rotmensch HH, Frishman WH, Vlasses P: Potential applications of calcium-channel antagonists in the management of noncardiac disorders. In: Packer M, Frishman WH (eds): *Calcium Channel Antagonists in Cardiovascular Disease*. Norwalk, Appleton-Century-Crofts, 1984:371–382.
189. Ram CV: Antiatherosclerotic and vasculoprotective actions of calcium antagonists. *Am J Cardiol* 1990; 66:29I–32I.
190. Borhani NO, Bond MG, Sowers JR, Canossa-Terris M, Buckalew V, Gibbons ME, et al: The Multicenter Isradipine/Diuretic Atherosclerosis Study: A study of the anti-atherogenic properties of isradipine in hypertensive patients. *J Cardiovasc Pharmacol* 1991; 18(suppl 3):515–519.
191. Schroeder JS, Gao S-Z, Alderman EL, Hunt S, Johnstone I, Boothroyd DB, et al: A preliminary study of diltiazem in the prevention of coronary artery disease in heart transplant recipients. *N Engl J Med* 1993; 328:164–170.
192. Factor SM, Minase T, Cho S, Dominitz R, Sonnenblick E: Microvascular spasm in the cardiomyopathic Syrian hamster: A preventable cause of focal myocardial necrosis. *Circulation* 1982; 66:342–354.
193. Factor SM, Sonnenblick EH; Microvascular spasm as a cause of cardiomyopathies. *Cardiovasc Rev Rep* 1983; 4:1177–1184.
194. Lewis JG: Adverse reactions to calcium antagonists. *Drugs* 1983; 25:196–222.
195. Terry RW: Nifedipine therapy in angina pectoris: Evaluation of safety and side effects. *Am Heart J* 1982; 104:681–689.
196. Vetrovec GW, Parker VE, Cole S, Procacci PM, Tabatznik B, Terry R: Nifedipine gastrointestinal therapeutic system in stable angina pectoris: Results of a multicenter open-label, crossover comparison with nifedipine. *Am J Med* 1987; 83(6B):24–30.
197. Funk-Brentano C, Coudray P, Planellas J, Motte G, Maillon P: Effects of bepridil and diltiazem on ventricular repolarization in angina pectoris. *Am J Cardiol* 1990; 66:812–817.
198. Frishman WH, Klein NA, Charlap S, Klein P, Cohen MN, Rotmensch HH: Recognition and management of verapamil poisoning. In: Packer M, Frishman WH (eds): *Calcium Channel Antagonists in Cardiovascular Disease*. Norwalk, Appleton-Century-Crofts, 1984:365–370.
199. Klein HO, Lang R, Weiss E, DiSegni E, Libhaber C, Guerrero J, et al: The influence of verapamil on serum digoxin concentrations. *Circulation* 1982; 65:998–1003.
200. Schwartz JB, Keefe D, Kates RE, Kirsten E, Harrison DC: Acute and chronic pharmacodynamic interaction of verapamil and digoxin in atrial fibrillation. *Circulation* 1982: 65:1163–1170.
201. Pedersen KE, Dorph-Pedersen A, Hvidt S, Klitgaard NA, Nielsen-Kudsk F: Digoxin-Verapamil interaction. *Clin Pharmacol Ther* 1981; 30:311–316.
202. Belz GG, Aust PE, Munkes R: Digoxin plasma concentrations and nifedipine. *Lancet* 1981; 1:844–845.
203. Mitchell LB, Jutzy KR, Lewis SJ, Schroeder JS, Mason JW: Intracardiac electrophysiologic study of intravenous diltiazem and combined diltiazem-digoxin in patients. *Am Heart J* 1982; 103:57–60.

Chapter 68

Pharmacology of Anticoagulants and Platelet Inhibitor Drugs

Bernardo Stein, M.D. ■ Valentin Fuster, M.D., Ph.D.

Thrombosis within the circulatory system is the principal mechanism responsible for cardiovascular morbidity and mortality. During pathological processes, the coagulation system may be activated via the intrinsic pathway (through contact of blood with damaged endothelium or exposed collagen) or the extrinsic pathway (through the release of tissue factor after vessel damage). This leads to activation of factor X and the prothrombinase complex, resulting in the generation of thrombin. Thrombin plays a fundamental role in the pathogenesis of thromboembolic disorders by initiating potent positive-feedback mechanisms on the coagulation cascade, thus generating more procoagulant factors; by catalyzing the conversion of fibrinogen to fibrin, which provides support to the growing platelet/thrombus mass; and by being a direct and powerful activator of platelets.

Platelets participate with the coagulation and fibrinolytic systems in the maintenance of hemostasis. They do not interact with intact, normal endothelium but rapidly adhere to damaged vascular tissue. Under appropriate stimulation, platelets release the contents of their intracytoplasmic granules, produce thromboxane A_2, and undergo conformational changes that result in the exposure of their membrane receptors to adhesive macromolecules. This leads to the recruitment of additional platelets and the formation of aggregates at sites of vessel wall injury. Platelets also provide a surface for the localization and interaction of coagulation factors and thus enhance the conversion of prothrombin to thrombin. Therefore, platelets and the coagulation system are intimately interrelated in the pathogenesis of thrombosis (Fig. 68-1).

Thrombosis within the coronary arteries involves activation of both platelets and the coagulation system. Thromboembolism in patients with diseases of the cardiac chambers (i.e., atrial fibrillation or ventricular dysfunction) or valves (i.e., prosthetic devices) is primarily related to hemodynamic abnormalities, in which activation of the coagulation system predominates over that of platelets. Finally, thrombosis within the venous system is mostly related to blood stasis and endothelial damage, leading to activation of the clotting system. A systematic approach to the patient with or at risk for a thromboembolic event has been proposed,[1] allowing the selection of the most appropriate antithrombotic therapy based on pathogenetic principles and the risk of thromboembolism. In general, the higher the risk, the more intensive the recommended antithrombotic approach (Table 68-1). (See also Chap. 7.)

In this chapter salient pharmacologic aspects of anticoagulants and platelet inhibitors, their clinical uses, adverse reactions, and new developments are analyzed.

ANTICOAGULANTS

Heparin

Agents inhibiting thrombin can be divided into two broad categories: those, like heparin, that act via the natural coagulation inhibitor antithrombin III and those with a mechanism of action independent of antithrombin III, such as hirudin, argatroban, and tripeptide chloromethyl ketones. Heparin is a naturally occurring sul-

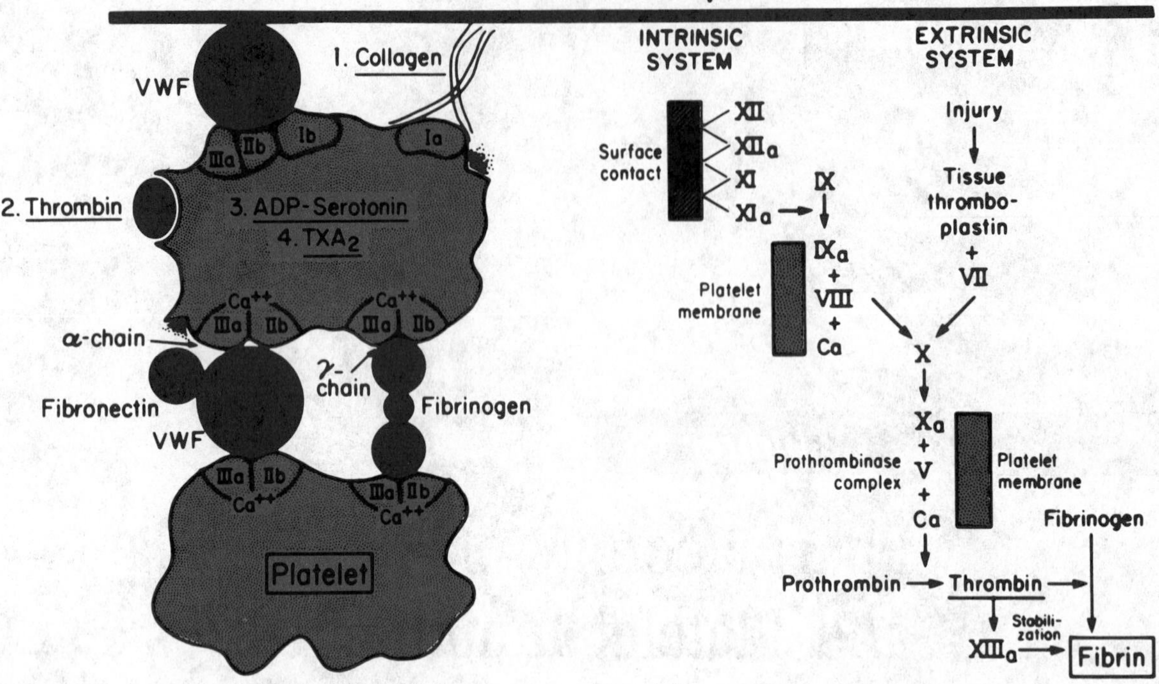

FIGURE 68-1 *Left:* Schematic representation of the interaction of platelet membrane receptors (glycoproteins Ia, Ib, IIb–IIIa), adhesive macromolecules [von Willebrand factor (VWF), fibrinogen, fibronectin], and the disrupted vessel wall. Numbers indicate the different pathways of platelet activation dependent on (1) collagen, (2) thrombin, (3) adenosine diphosphate (ADP) and serotonin, and (4) thromboxane A_2 (TXA_2). *Right:* The coagulation cascade. Note the interaction of clotting factors and the platelet membrane. CA = calcium. (*From B Stein, et al: Platelet inhibitor agents in cardiovascular disease: An update. J Am Coll Cardiol 14:813–836, 1989. By permission of the American College of Cardiology.*)

fated glucosaminoglycan formed by repeating disaccharide units containing glucosamine and uronic acid, which exerts most of its anticoagulant action via the plasma protein antithrombin III. Because thrombin exerts a positive-feedback action on the coagulation cascade (specifically through the activation of factors V and VIII), which would rapidly result in the generation of large concentrations of thrombin, the inhibition of the first traces of this enzyme is important for inhibition of the coagulation process.

Pharmacology

Heparin accelerates the formation of a molecular complex between antithrombin III and several serine proteases including thrombin; coagulation factors XII, XI, IX, and X; plasmin; and kallikrein. It binds to lysine sites on antithrombin III and produces a conformational change on this molecule at the arginine reactive center; this accelerates its inhibitory activity on thrombin and other coagulation factors by approximately 1000-fold.[2] Once the inhibition reaction is completed, heparin is released from the antithrombin III–thrombin complex and can be reused. Because of the amplification process inherent in the coagulation cascade, whereby a single molecule of factor Xa can lead to the generation of multiple molecules of thrombin, inhibition of early steps of the pathway (i.e., inhibition of factor Xa) may produce a better antithrombotic response than inhibition of subsequent steps. There is increasing evidence that heparin's main anticoagulant effect is through the inhibition of thrombin-induced activation of factors V and VIII.[3]

Commercial preparations of heparin are heterogeneous; they are produced from porcine intestine or bovine lung, and their components have molecular weights ranging from 3000 to 30,000. Only about one-third of the heparin molecule binds to antithrombin III; the rest has minimal anticoagulant properties at therapeutic concentrations, but high concentrations catalyze the antithrombin effect of another plasma protein, the heparin cofactor II.[4] The anticoagulant effect of heparin is modified by a number of factors including platelets, fibrin, vascular surfaces, and plasma proteins.[3] Platelets interfere with heparin's activity by binding factor Xa and protecting it from inactivation and by secreting the heparin-neutralizing platelet factor 4. In addition, thrombin bound to fibrin is protected from inactivation by the heparin-antithrombin complex; thus approximately 20 times more heparin is required to inactivate fibrin-bound thrombin than to inactivate free thrombin.[4] This may explain the need for higher heparin doses to prevent the extension of venous thrombi rather than to prevent their formation as well as the significant risk of coronary reocclusion after thrombolysis despite heparin therapy.

Heparin is poorly absorbed from the gastrointestinal tract and must be given parenterally; it circulates bound to plasma proteins. After intravenous injection, a phase of rapid elimination due to equilibrium is followed by a slower disappearance that follows nonlinear kinetics and results from a combination of a saturable mechanism

TABLE 68-1

Approach to Antithrombotic Therapy Based on Pathogenesis and Risk

	Thromboembolic Risk		
Location and Pathogenesis	**High (>6% per year)**	**Medium (2–6% per year)**	**Low (<2% per year)**
Arterial system	Unstable angina Acute MI MI, postthrombolyisis PTCA, early phase SVBG, early phase	Chronic stable angina Chronic phase after MI PTCA, chronic phase SVBG, chronic phase	Primary prevention of cardiovascular disease
Platelets plus coagulation system	Platelet inhibitor plus anticoagulant*	Platelet inhibitor or anticoagulant (INR 2.0–3/0)†	Platelet inhibitor‡
Cardiac chambers	A-fib, prior embolism A-fib, mitral stenosis	A-fib, other forms of organic heart disease Early phase after anterior MI Dilated cardiomyopathy	A-fib, idiopathic§ LV aneurysm (remote)
Coagulation system > platelets	Anticoagulant (INR 2.0–3.5) plus platelet inhibitor¶	Anticoagulant (INR 2.0–3.0)##	Usually no need for therapy
Prosthetic valves	Old mechanical prostheses Mechanical prostheses, prior embolism	Recent mechanical prostheses Bioprostheses, A-fib	Bioprostheses, sinus rhythm
Coagulation system > platelets	Anticoagulant (INR 3.0–4.5) plus platelet inhibitor	Anticoagulant (INR 3.0–4.5 in mechanical valves, or 2.0–3.0 in bioprostheses)#	Usually no need for therapy#

SOURCE: V Fuster, et al: Antithrombotic therapy in cardiac disease: An approach based on pathogenesis and risk stratification. *Am J Cardiol* 1990; 65(suppl): 38C–44C. By permission from the American Journal of Cardiology.

MI = myocardial infarction; PTCA = percutaneous transluminal coronary angioplasty; SVBG = saphenous vein bypass grafting; INR = international normalized ratio of prothrombin suppression; A-fib = atrial fibrillation.

* Heparin may be used in the acute phase (activated thromboplastin time 1.5–2.0 × control); its value in combination with aspirin is emerging.

† Although both beneficial, platelet inhibitor preferred based on lower cost, toxicity, and ease of administration.

‡ Recommended to men over 50 years of age with significant coronary risk factors.

§ Patients over 60 years of age have higher risk of embolism.

¶ Lower anticoagulant dose (INR 2.0–3.0) may suffice in patients with mitral stenosis without prior embolism.

Moderate-intensity anticoagulation (INR 3.0–4.5) recommended to patients with bioprostheses for the first 3 months after surgery.

Aspirin is effective in some patients with nonrheumatic atrial fibrillation.

(uptake by endothelium and mononuclear phagocytes) and a linear, unsaturable mechanism (renal excretion).[3] The dose-response relation to heparin is nonlinear, in which the anticoagulant response increases disproportionately in duration and intensity as the dose increases.[6] Consequently, its biologic half-life can vary from 30 to more than 300 min depending on the dose used. Heparin does not cross the placental barrier and may be given during pregnancy without the risk of producing embryopathy (see below).

When given by continuous intravenous infusion, standard dosing includes a loading dose of 5000 units (occasionally 10,000 units) followed by an infusion of 15 to 20 units/kg per h, which is regulated by the results of the activated partial thromboplastin time (APTT) (see below). Given intermittently (via the intravenous route), the dosing can vary from 5000 to 10,000 units every 4 to 6 h to 15,000 units at 8-h intervals. In most instances, continuous intravenous infusion is favored over intermittent dosing.

Low-dose subcutaneous heparin (5000 units every 8 to 12 h) has been used for prophylaxis for venous thromboembolism, whereas higher doses (12,500 to 17,500 units every 12 h) have been used in the treatment of venous thromboembolism and acute myocardial infarction. Subcutaneous heparin is associated with a slower onset of action; therapeutic levels may not be reached in a substantial proportion of patients or may take a few days to do so. When prompt and reliable anticoagulation is mandatory (i.e., during the acute coronary syndromes), the intravenous route is preferred.[7]

Monitoring of Therapy

The anticoagulant response to heparin varies widely among patients with thromboembolic disease. Clinical efficacy is optimized and bleeding risk is reduced with appropriate monitoring. The most widely used test for this purpose is the APTT. The usual therapeutic goal is to maintain the ratio of the patient's APTT to the control APTT within a range of approximately 1.5 to 2.5. This is equivalent to a heparin level of 0.2 to 0.4 units/mL plasma by protamine titration, or 0.35 to 0.7 units/mL according to the level of antifactor Xa activity, a level of anticoagulation that has been shown to prevent extension in experimental thrombi.[8] The APTT results can be affected by the sensitivity of the commercial thromboplastin used, the technique of blood sampling, the interval from blood drawing to assay, and the number of platelets in plasma. Given the variability of commercial reagents used, it has been proposed that the therapeutic range for any given APTT be established in the clinical laboratory to correspond to a heparin level of 0.2 to 0.4 units/mL by protamine titration.[3]

Clinical Utility

Extensive clinical testing has documented the value of heparin in the prevention and treatment of venous and pulmonary thromboembolism and in the treatment of patients with acute ischemic syndromes. The value of intravenous heparin in patients with *unstable angina* for the prevention of myocardial infarction or recurrent ischemia has been documented[9,10] (Table 68-2). The relative value of heparin versus aspirin is still a matter of controversy.[9,11] However, because patients with unstable angina are at a substantial risk of death or myocardial infarction, there is widespread interest in testing the combination of aspirin plus heparin. Whereas one study[9] found no benefit from this combination, a second trial[11] showed that maximal benefit was derived from combining intravenous heparin plus low-dose aspirin (Fig. 68-2). Recent data[11a] suggest that early reactivation of ischemia and progression to myocardial infarction can occur after discontinuation of heparin, which can be prevented by adding aspirin to heparin therapy. Additional studies are currently underway. (See also Chap. 59.)

The role of heparin in *acute myocardial infarction* prior to the thrombolytic era has been evaluated by numerous trials. Whereas the results of each individual study were not convincing, a metaanalysis of 20 trials[12] suggested that heparin reduces mortality and reinfarction by approximately 20 percent. A recent study[13] showed that subcutaneous heparin at a dose of 12,500 units twice daily reduced mortality in patients with acute infarction whether or not a thrombolytic agent was given. The effectiveness of intravenous heparin in maintaining coronary patency in patients with acute infarction treated with a thrombolytic agent has been recently demonstrated.[14,15] Because these patients are at high risk of reocclusion, particularly in the first few days after thrombolysis, antithrombotic treatment with both intravenous heparin and oral aspirin seems justified. When heparin is given subcutaneously, a therapeutic effect is delayed and may not be reached in one-half of patients. This may explain the marginal benefit from subcutaneous heparin in large thrombolytic trials of patients with acute myocardial infarction.[16–18] The value of adjuvant aspirin plus intravenous heparin for patients receiving thrombolytic therapy is currently being tested. (See also Chap. 69.)

Left ventricular mural thrombosis is a common occurrence in patients with acute anterior myocardial infarction. Two trials[13,19] showed that heparin at a dose of 12,500 units given subcutaneously every 12 h markedly reduced the incidence of mural thrombi by 60 to 70 percent. Because left ventricular thrombi can lead to cerebral or systemic embolism in 3 to 5 percent of patients with anterior myocardial infarction, the importance of preventing mural thrombosis in these patients is obvious. (See also Chap. 60.)

The value of heparin for prophylaxis and treatment of venous and pulmonary thromboembolism has been reviewed.[3,20] It is recommended that medical and surgical patients at *risk for venous thrombosis* receive prophylactic heparin (5000 units every 12 h). Patients undergoing major orthopedic surgery and those at high risk (i.e., previous venous thrombosis) should receive subcutaneous heparin adjusted to the upper normal range of the APTT or low-dose warfarin.[21,22] For patients with *deep venous thrombosis or pulmonary embolism,* high-dose intravenous heparin (5000-unit bolus followed by 30,000 units per 24 h) is recommended and should be continued for 5 to 10 days. Oral anticoagulation should be overlapped with heparin for 4 to 5 days. If subcutaneous heparin is used, the initial dose should be 17,500

TABLE 68-2

Antithrombotic Therapy in Unstable Angina

Trial	Number of Patients	Follow-up	Drug (mg/day)	Reduction Death + MI (%)	*p*
Telford and Wilson[10]	214	7 days	Heparin (20,000 units)	80	<.05
Lewis et al[67]	1266	12 weeks	Aspirin (324)	51	<.001
Cairns et al.[68]	555	18 months	Aspirin (1300)	51	<.01
			Sulfinpyrazone (800)	(−6)	NS
Theroux et al.[9]	479	6 days	Aspirin (650)	72	<.01
			Heparin (24,000 units)	89	<.001
			Aspirin plus heparin	88	.001
RISC Group[11]	796	3 months	Aspirin (75)	58	<.005
			Heparin (20,000 units)	5	NS
			Aspirin plus heparin	68	<.0005
Balsano et al.[107]	652	6 months	Ticlopidine (500)	55	<.01

MI = myocardial infarction; NS = nonsignificant.

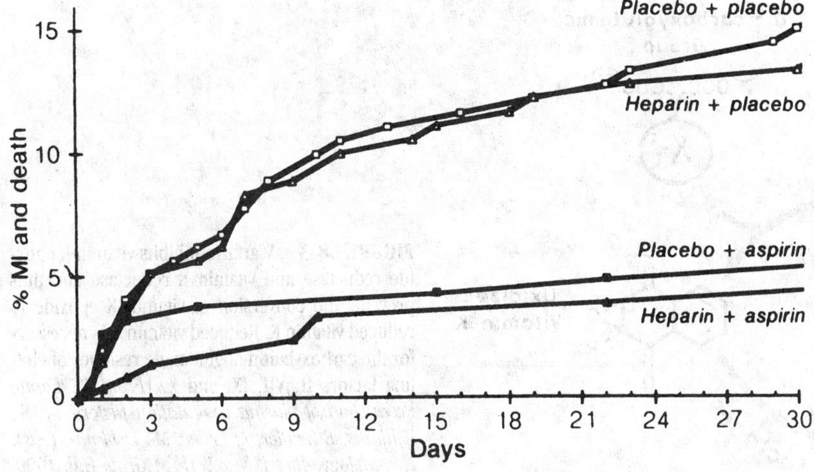

FIGURE 68-2 Efficacy of low-dose aspirin (75 mg/day) for the prevention of myocardial infarction (MI) and death in patients with unstable angina or non-Q-wave MI. Note that maximal benefit was obtained by combining aspirin and intravenous heparin for the first 5 days of the trial. (*From the RISC Group: Risk of myocardial infarction and death during treatment with low dose aspirin and intravenous heparin in men with unstable coronary disease. Lancet 336:827–830, 1990. By permission from L Wallentin and the Lancet, Ltd.*)

units every 12 h, with the dose adjusted to prolong the APTT to a ratio of 1.5 to 2.5.[3] (See also Chap. 100.)

Adverse Effects

The most frequent and important complication of heparin is bleeding. Risk factors for spontaneous bleeding include age older than 60 years, serious concurrent illness, presence of pathological lesions in the gastrointestinal or genitourinary tract, renal dysfunction, chronic alcoholism, and concomitant use of platelet inhibitors. The dose and method of administration influence the rate of bleeding. Intermittent intravenous heparin injections may be more likely to cause bleeding compared to continuous infusion; subcutaneous and continuous intravenous heparin carry a similar risk.

Thrombocytopenia is a well-known and usually asymptomatic complication of heparin.[23] The reported incidence varies widely and may be as high as 20 percent. It is more common with heparin from bovine than porcine source. Two types of interactions have been recognized. The first is an immediate reaction caused by heparin-induced platelet aggregation, which results in a transient drop in the platelet count and prolongation of the bleeding time. The second is a delayed, idiosyncratic reaction that occurs between days 7 and 11 of treatment and may be complicated occasionally by arterial thrombosis. Heparin may act as hapten and induce an immune response against the platelet-heparin complex. This anamnestic response is not dose dependent and may occur after subcutaneous injections and even heparin flushes. In these cases, immediate discontinuation of heparin is mandatory.

Long-term heparin therapy can cause osteoporosis through decreased synthesis and increased resorption of bone. This is not apparent until 6 to 8 weeks of therapy, which exceeds the usual duration of treatment of acute thrombosis but may be a problem when prolonged therapy is required.

Future Developments

Intensive research is focused on the improvement of the safety and efficacy of anticoagulant therapy. The use of low-molecular-weight heparins may provide adequate antithrombotic effect with less disturbance of the hemostatic system and a lower risk of bleeding. Because of their longer half-life compared with standard heparin, these agents can be given subcutaneously once daily. In initial testing these heparins have proved effective and safe for prevention of venous thromboembolism in patients at high risk.[24]

Potent thrombin inhibitors that act independently of antithrombin III include hirudin, hirulog, argatroban, tripeptide-chloromethyl ketones, and activated protein C. Because of their unique thrombin inhibitor properties, these agents have proved very effective in experimental models of deep arterial injury,[25] prosthetic vascular grafting,[26,27] and coronary thrombosis.[28] Arterial thrombosis in these models is particularly resistant to heparin or conventional platelet inhibitors. These novel agents are able to inhibit free and clot-bound thrombin and may prove effective in highly thrombogenic processes in the coronary circulation such as in unstable angina, or during thrombolysis, angioplasty, or placement of intravascular stents. Clinical, dose-finding studies are underway. (See also Chap. 7.)

Oral Anticoagulants

There are two types of oral anticoagulants: coumarins (warfarin, dicumarol, and acenocoumarol) and indanediones (phenindione). Warfarin is a 4-hydroxycoumarin compound and is the most widely used agent in North America because of its predictable pharmacokinetics and excellent bioavailability. Oral anticoagulants act by interfering with the cyclic interconversion of vitamin K and its epoxide (Fig. 68-3).[29] Vitamin K is an essential factor for the posttranslational carboxylation of glutamate residues on the N-terminal regions of vitamin K–dependent proteins. This reaction is catalyzed by a carboxylase that requires the reduced form of quinone vitamin K (hydroquinone). By interfering with two essential enzymes (vitamin K reductase and epoxide reductase), warfarin leads to the accumulation of vitamin K epoxide and the depletion of hydroquinone. Through the inhibition of the gamma-carboxylation reaction, warfarin interferes with the synthesis of several coagu-

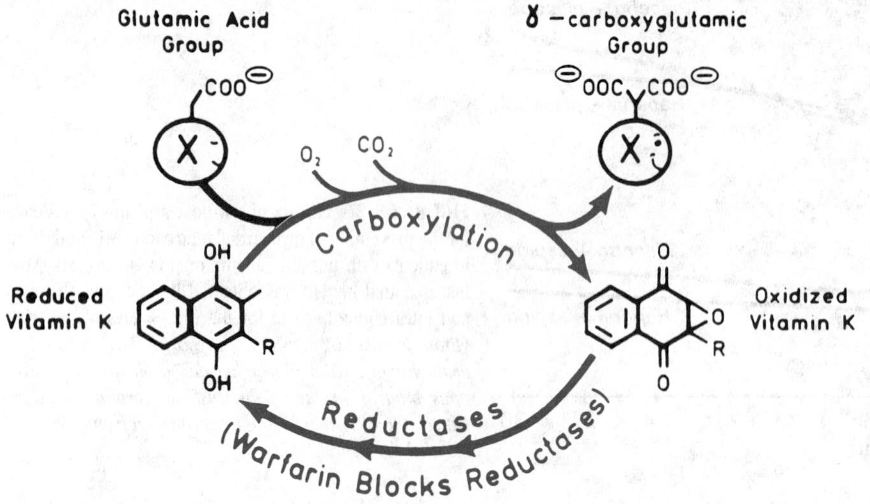

FIGURE 68-3 Warfarin inhibits vitamin K epoxide reductase and vitamin K reductase and thus prevents the conversion of vitamin K epoxide to reduced vitamin K. Reduced vitamin K is necessary for the carboxylation of glutamate residues of clotting factors II, VII, IX, and X. [*From PC Comp: Production of plasma coagulation factors. In: WJ Williams, E Beutler, AJ Erslev, MA Lichtman (eds): Hematology, 4th ed. New York, McGraw-Hill, 1990, 1285–1289. By permission from the publisher.*]

lant proteins (prothrombin, factors VII, IX, and X) and coagulant inhibitors (protein C and S), thus impairing their biologic function.[29]

Pharmacology

Absorption of oral warfarin is rapid and complete, reaching peak blood levels in 90 min; plasma half-life is 36 to 42 h. Warfarin circulates bound to plasma proteins and accumulates in hepatic microsomes. After metabolic transformation, warfarin is eliminated either in urine or bile depending on its optical isomerism. It crosses the placental barrier and is contraindicated during pregnancy. Fortunately, it appears in the milk of nursing mothers in its inactive form and thus is safe for the lactating infant.[30]

The dose of warfarin and the anticoagulant response are directly related in the same subject but are markedly different between subjects. Clinically important variations in response occur during long-term anticoagulant therapy that may be related to availability of vitamin K, levels of vitamin K–dependent coagulation factors, patient compliance, and changes in the pharmacokinetics and pharmacodynamics of warfarin.[31] Hereditary resistance to warfarin has been described[32]; to be effective, these patients require much larger doses of warfarin.

Dietary vitamin K is obtained predominantly from plant phylloquinone. Diets rich in green vegetables and nutritional supplements rich in vitamin K reduce the anticoagulant response to warfarin; in contrast, anticoagulation is potentiated when vitamin K absorption is impaired, as in fat malabsorption states. The response to warfarin may be increased by liver dysfunction and during hypermetabolic states produced by fever or hyperthyroidism.[31]

Numerous drugs can interact with warfarin and alter the prothrombin time (PT) response (Table 68-3). Plasma warfarin levels are lowered and the anticoagulant effect is reduced by drugs that impair its absorption (cholestyramine) or increase its metabolic clearance (barbiturates, rifampin, carbamazepine).

Prolongation of the PT can occur by drugs that inhibit the clearance of warfarin (phenylbutazone, metronidazole, sulfinpyrazone, trimethoprim-sulfamethoxazole, amiodarone), interfere with the synthesis of clotting factors (possibly anabolic steroids and quinidine), increase the metabolism of clotting factors (thyroxine), or alter the availability of vitamin K (broad-spectrum antibiotics, ion exchange resins, colestipol, oil laxatives). Other drugs that prolong the PT through unknown mechanisms are erythromycin and clofibrate. Because the interaction of warfarin with other drugs of common use can result in serious bleeding, these effects need to be anticipated by the physician and frequent monitoring of the PT level done during the initial stages of combined drug therapy (Table 68-3). (See also Chap. 109.)

Monitoring of Therapy

The test most often used to monitor oral anticoagulant therapy is the one-stage PT test, introduced by Quick[33]

TABLE 68-3

Drug Interactions with Oral Anticoagulants

Drugs That Prolong the Prothrombin Time	
Allopurinol	Ketoprofen
Amiodarone	Isoniazid
Anabolic steroids	Metronidazole
Cephalosporins	Naproxen
Chloramphenicol	Omeprazole
Cimetidine	Phenylbutazone
Clofibrate	Piroxicam
Co-trimoxazole	Ouinidine
Disulfiram	Sulfinpyrazone
Erythromycin	Tamoxifen
Fluconazole	Thyroxine
Ketoconazole	Trimethoprim-sulfamethoxazole
Drugs That Reduce the Prothrombin Time	
Barbiturates	Glutethimide
Carbamazepine	Griseofulvin
Cholestyramine	Rifampin
Colestipol	Vitamin K

in 1935. This test, which measures the reduction of factors II, VII, and X by warfarin, is performed by adding calcium and thromboplastin to citrated plasma. Interpretation of the PT results has been complicated by the variability in the preparation and in the responsiveness of currently used thromboplastin reagents.[31] In an effort to standardize anticoagulant therapy, the international normalized ratio (INR) of prothrombin suppression was adopted in 1983. The INR is the PT ratio that reflects the result that would have been obtained with the use of an international reference thromboplastin.[31,34] The INR is derived from the international sensitivity index (ISI) for each thromboplastin. This is obtained by parallel testing of controls and anticoagulated patients with the local reagent and the international reference preparation and comparing their responsiveness (Fig. 68-4). Therefore, an accurate assessment of the anticoagulation level of a particular patient can only be obtained if the sensitivity index of the thromboplastin reagent used is known.

For most indications, a moderate anticoagulant effect with a targeted INR of 2.0 to 3.0 (equivalent PT ratio of 1.3 to 1.6 if a North American rabbit brain thromboplastin with an ISI of 2.3 to 2.4 is used) is appropriate.[34] A higher anticoagulation intensity—an INR of 2.5 to 3.5—is recommended in patients with mechanical valve prostheses.[34,35] If systemic embolism occurs, the recommended INR is 3.0 to 4.5, plus either aspirin, 160 mg/day, or dipyridamole, 400 mg/day.[34] Lower anticoagulant levels are presently being evaluated.

Clinical Utility

Numerous trials of short-and long-term anticoagulant therapy *after acute myocardial infarction* have been conducted. Earlier studies[36–38] showed that short-term anticoagulation (INR 2.0, PT ratio 1.35) was associated with a beneficial trend toward lower mortality or reinfarction and a significant reduction in arterial and pulmonary embolism. A recent large, randomized trial[35] in patients after myocardial infarction showed that warfarin (INR 2.8 to 4.8, PT ratio 1.5 to 2.0) given for 3 years significantly reduced the rates of death, reinfarction, and stroke with a low incidence of major bleeding. Another trial[39] conducted in anticoagulated patients (6 years after infarction) showed that continuing the anticoagulant led to lower mortality and reinfarction rates.

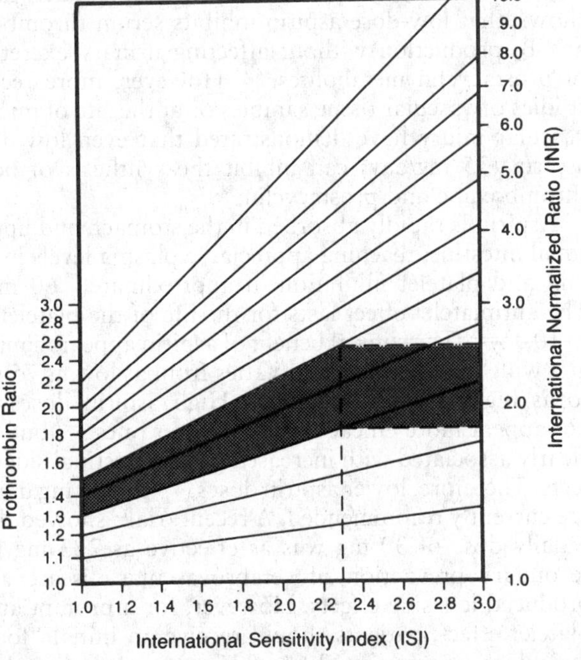

FIGURE 68-4 Relation between the PT ratio and the INR for thromboplastin reagents over a range of international sensitivity index (ISI) values. In the example shown for a reagent with an ISI of 2.3, a PT ratio of 1.3 to 1.5 would correspond to an INR of 1.8 to 2.5. [*From J Hirsh, et al: Optimal therapeutic range for oral anticoagulants. Chest 95(suppl):5S–11S, 1989. By permission from Chest and the American College of Chest Physicians.*]

Patients with a large anterior myocardial infarction are at significant risk for *left ventricular thrombosis.* Anticoagulant therapy reduces the incidence of systemic or cerebral embolism.[35–38] and is recommended for patients with extensive infarctions and for those with documented left ventricular thrombus or concomitant heart failure or atrial fibrillation. The duration of treatment is dependent on the persistence of risk factors for embolism. (See also Chap. 60.) In addition, patients with *dilated cardiomyopathy* may benefit from long-term anticoagulation; these patients have a risk of thromboembolism of 3.5 percent per year, which was eliminated by the use of oral anticoagulants, according to a retrospective study.[40] (See also Chap. 89.)

Patients with *rheumatic atrial fibrillation* are at a very high risk of embolism and should receive chronic anticoagulation therapy, even when support from prospective, randomized trials is lacking. (See Chap. 80.) For patients with *nonrheumatic atrial fibrillation,* warfarin was found extremely effective in preventing embolism in four trials.[41–43,43a] In two trials,[43,43a] a relatively low intensity warfarin regimen (INR 1.5 to 2.5, PT ratio 1.2 to 1.5) reduced the stroke rate by 80 percent and was not associated with clinically important bleeding. (See also Chap. 122.) Aspirin was found beneficial in one trial[41] but not in the other.[42] An ongoing study is comparing the value of warfarin versus aspirin in these patients.

Anticoagulants are essential for prevention of thromboembolism in patients with *mechanical prosthetic heart valves.*[44] Without long-term anticoagulation, the incidence of thromboembolism increases by two- to six-fold. Recent studies[45–46] have shown that less intense regimens of anticoagulation provide protection equal to more intense regimens but carry a much lower risk of bleeding. In patients with mechanical prostheses, an INR of 3.0 to 4.5 (PT ratio 1.6 to 1.9) has been recommended, although lower intensities may be effective. In those with bioprostheses, an INR of 2.0 to 3.0 (PT ratio 1.3 to 1.6) appears sufficient.[47]

Warfarin is effective for prevention of *venous thrombosis* after major abdominal or pelvic surgery at a targeted INR of 1.5 to 3.0 (PT ratio 1.2 to 1.6).[48] Oral anticoagulants should be continued for 3 months in patients with proximal deep-vein thrombosis or symptomatic calf thrombosis. A less intense regimen (INR 2.0 to 2.3, PT ratio 1.3 to 1.4) was as effective as a more intense one (INR 2.5 to 4.1, PT ratio 1.5 to 1.8) but was associated with less bleeding.[49] Long-term warfarin is necessary in patients with persistent risk factors for venous thromboembolism or in those with recurrent thromboembolic events. (See also Chap. 100.)

Adverse Effects

Bleeding is the main complication of oral anticoagulation. The intensity of anticoagulant therapy is probably the most important risk factor for hemorrhage. Clinical trials[45–47,49] that compared high- versus low-intensity anticoagulation showed that whereas efficacy was similar, the higher intensity anticoagulation resulted in a two- to fivefold increase in bleeding. Risk factors for bleeding include age older than 65 years, history of stroke or gastrointestinal bleeding, coexisting morbidity, and concomitant aspirin use. Spontaneous bleeding that occurs when the INR is below 3.0 (PT ratio less than 1.6) is frequently secondary to an occult gastrointestinal or genitourinary lesion.

Coumarin-induced necrosis of the skin and subcutaneous tissues is a rare but striking complication of warfarin therapy. It usually involves areas with abundant subcutaneous fat and occurs 3 to 10 days after drug administration. It is caused by extensive thrombosis of venules and capillaries in the subcutaneous tissue and may be associated with protein C or protein S deficiency.

Warfarin crosses the placenta and can produce a specific *embryopathy* if exposure occurs between the 6th and 12th weeks of gestation. Its incidence has been reported to be as high as 29 percent.[50] Central nervous system abnormalities can occur with exposure to coumarin at any time during pregnancy.[51] Thus, warfarin should be avoided throughout the pregnancy if possible; this is particularly important in the first trimester. Subcutaneous heparin (15,000 units every 12 h, aimed at an APTT of 1.5 × control) should be used instead of warfarin when anticoagulants are indicated, such as in women with mechanical prosthetic heart valves. Heparin therapy in such patients may be associated with some increase in fetal wastage although not embryopathy. Unfortunately, long-term heparin therapy is associated with osteoporosis.

Future Developments

There is substantial interest in the evaluation of lower intensity warfarin therapy. Very low dose warfarin (1 mg/day) was found effective in the prevention of thrombosis in patients with central venous catheters[52] and in those undergoing major pelvic surgery.[48] The combination of low-dose warfarin and low-dose aspirin is undergoing clinical evaluation in patients with unstable angina, after coronary bypass surgery, for primary prevention of myocardial infarction in men at risk, and for secondary prevention after myocardial infarction.

PLATELET INHIBITOR DRUGS

The ideal platelet inhibitor should be effective orally and relatively inexpensive, have adequate antithrombotic properties and sustained action, and be devoid of toxic side effects, particularly bleeding. Although not ideal, aspirin is clearly the most widely used antiplatelet agent. Whereas the mechanisms of action of several different platelet inhibitors have been elucidated (Fig. 68-5), intensive efforts are being focused on defining the appropriate dosing and clinical applications of the currently available agents as well as on developing new and more potent compounds (see below).

Aspirin

The major antithrombotic effect of aspirin is associated with its ability to inhibit platelet thromboxane A_2 synthesis.[53] At physiological shear rates, aspirin has no effect on platelet adhesion and, therefore, does not prevent formation of the initial layer of platelets on the damaged endothelium or subendothelium.[54] Likewise, it does not inhibit the release of serotonin, adenosine diphosphate (ADP), or platelet-derived growth factor from the platelet granules. Aspirin inhibits the secondary wave of aggregation induced by ADP, epinephrine, and low doses of collagen. However, thrombin and high concentrations of collagen can cause a full aggregation response even in the presence of aspirin.[55]

Pharmacology

Aspirin irreversibly inhibits cyclooxygenase by acetylating the serine residue at the active site of the enzyme. Because platelets are unable to generate new enzyme, the inhibition of cyclooxygenase lasts for the lifetime of the cell. In the platelet, cyclooxygenase transforms arachidonic acid to thromboxane A_2 and, in the vascular wall, converts arachidonic acid to prostacyclin and prostaglandin E_1. Thromboxane A_2 has proaggregatory and vasoconstrictive properties, whereas prostacyclin opposes this action through its antiaggregatory and vasodilative effects. The differential effects of various doses of aspirin on platelet and vessel wall prostanoid synthesis have been extensively debated. Several studies have shown that low-dose aspirin inhibits serum thromboxane B_2 production without affecting urinary excretion of prostacyclin metabolites.[56,57] However, more recent studies of vascular tissue samples or at the site of microvascular injury have demonstrated that even low-dose aspirin (35 mg/day) can inhibit the synthesis of both thromboxane and prostacyclin.[58,59]

Aspirin is rapidly absorbed in the stomach and upper small intestine, reaching appreciable plasma levels in 20 min and platelet inhibition in approximately 60 min. The antiplatelet effect lasts for the life of the platelet (9 to 10 days). The clinical benefit of aspirin appears similar at a wide dosage range that varies from as low as 75 mg to as high as 1500 mg daily. High aspirin doses do not appear more efficacious than lower ones[60–62] but are clearly associated with increased gastrointestinal side effects. Therefore, lower aspirin doses (75 to 325 mg daily) are currently recommended. A recent trial[62] showed that a daily dose of 30 mg was as effective as 283 mg for secondary prevention of cerebrovascular disease and produced less side effects. However, for a prompt antiplatelet effect, patients should receive an initial "loading" dose of aspirin (120 to 325 mg) before low-dose therapy is instituted.[62]

Absorption from enteric-coated tablets is sometimes incomplete but may produce less gastrointestinal irritation. Preparations containing alkali or buffer may also be better tolerated. Aspirin does not cause a generalized

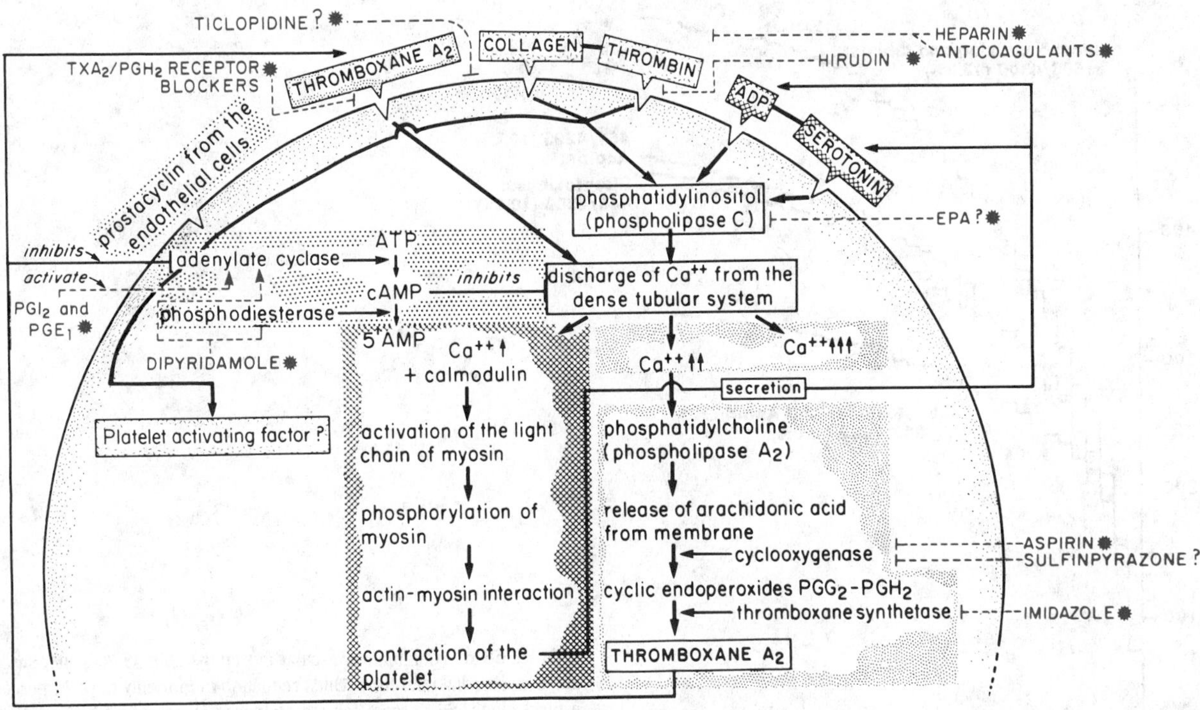

FIGURE 68-5 Mechanisms of platelet activation and presumed sites of action of various platelet inhibitors. Platelet agonists lead to the mobilization of calcium and activation of metabolic pathways dependent on ADP, thromboxane A_2 (TXA_2), thrombin, and collagen. An asterisk indicates a platelet inhibitor. A dashed line indicates a presumed site of drug action. ATP = adenosine triphosphate; cAMP = cyclic adenosine monophosphate; EPA = eicosapentaenoic acid; PG = prostaglandin. (*From B Stein, et al: Platelet inhibitor agents in cardiovascular disease: An update. J Am Coll Cardiol 14:813–836, 1989. By permission from the American College of Cardiology.*)

bleeding diathesis, except when given to patients with an underlying bleeding abnormality or when used in high doses (>500 mg/day) in combination with anticoagulants.[63]

More effective aspirin formulations are being sought. A very low dose of aspirin (20 mg) or of enteric-coated aspirin (325 mg) can inhibit thromboxane B_2 formation before any aspirin is detected in the systemic circulation.[64,65] This suggests that slow administration of low doses of aspirin may inhibit the platelets circulating in the portal system (presystemic inhibition) without reaching the systemic circulation and impairing the endothelial production of prostacyclin. A recent study[66] showed that whereas low-dose aspirin (162 mg/day or 325 mg on alternate days) inhibited both platelet and endothelial prostaglandin synthesis, a controlled-release formulation of 75 mg of aspirin inhibited platelet thromboxane A_2 generation without affecting systemic vascular wall prostacyclin production. This interesting concept is currently being tested in several clinical trials. If this "selective" inhibition of cyclooxygenase can be proved clinically relevant, a controlled-release low-dose aspirin may become the optimal aspirin regimen for antithrombotic therapy.[66]

Clinical Utility

Numerous clinical trials have confirmed the beneficial effects of aspirin in patients with different cardiovascular disorders. For patients with *unstable angina,* aspirin in doses ranging from 75 to 1300 mg/day[9,11,67,68] has been shown clearly to decrease the progression to myocardial infarction or death (Table 68-2). In a recent study,[11] the combination of low-dose aspirin and intravenous heparin for the first 5 days of the trial produced maximal benefit (Fig. 68-2). (See also Chap. 59.)

For patients with *acute myocardial infarction,* the landmark Second International Study of Infarct Survival (ISIS-2),[69] which included more than 17,000 patients, demonstrated that aspirin alone (160 mg/day) reduced vascular mortality at 5 weeks by 21 percent and that this benefit was maintained at the 15-month follow-up. When aspirin was combined with streptokinase, a 40 percent mortality reduction was seen (Fig. 68-6). Aspirin was found to reduce reinfarction and stroke by approximately one-half in this group of patients. Based on these results, aspirin at a dose of 160 to 325 mg daily is recommended to patients with acute myocardial infarction whether or not thrombolytic therapy is used. (See also Chap. 60.)

Multiple trials of aspirin for *secondary prevention of myocardial infarction* have been conducted (Fig 68-7). However, no single study has provided definitive results. The results of an extensive overview of available clinical trials[70] that included more than 18,000 patients after myocardial infarction suggest that platelet inhibitor therapy reduced cardiovascular mortality by 13 percent, nonfatal reinfarction by 31 percent, and nonfatal stroke by 42 percent. Aspirin alone was found as effective in combination with dipyridamole and possibly more effective than sulfinpyrazone. There is no clinical evidence that these more expensive antiplatelet drugs are more effective than aspirin alone for secondary prevention of myocardial infarction.[70,71] This overview also pointed out

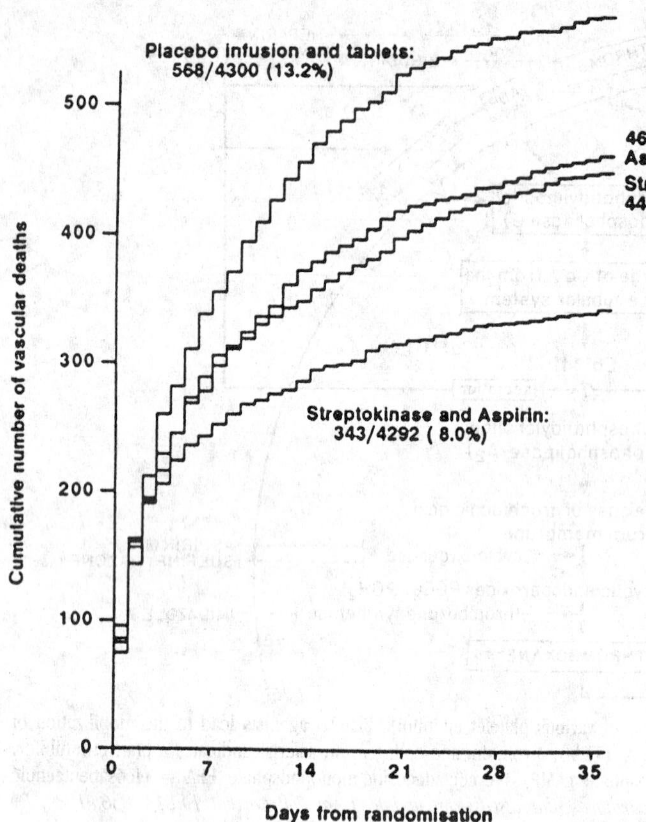

FIGURE 68-6 Cumulative vascular mortality within 35 days after suspected acute myocardial infarction. Odds reduction in mortality were 23 percent for aspirin alone, 25 percent for streptokinase alone, and 42 percent for the combination of aspirin and streptokinase. (*From the ISIS-2 Collaborative Group: Randomized trial of intravenous streptokinase, oral aspirin, both, or neither in 17,187 cases of suspected acute myocardial infarction: ISIS-2. Lancet 2:349–360, 1988. By permission from the Lancet, Ltd.*)

that higher doses of aspirin do not provide more protection than lower ones.[70] Additional studies[72,73] have also found long-term aspirin therapy useful for patients with stable coronary disease. However, a disconcerting increase in the incidence of stroke was found in patients with stable angina treated with aspirin.[73] Further studies are warranted.

The benefit of aspirin for *primary prevention* of cardiovascular morbidity and mortality has raised controversy. The British primary prevention trial[74] did not disclose benefit from aspirin at a dose of 500 mg/day. In contrast, the larger U.S. Physician's Health Study[75] demonstrated that aspirin at a dose of 325 mg on alternate days markedly reduced the occurrence of myocardial infarction in men, albeit at a slight increase in the risk of hemorrhagic stroke. Aspirin did not affect total mortality. At present, aspirin for primary prevention can be recommended to men older than 50 years who have evidence of atherosclerosis or have risk factors for coronary disease.[76] In these patients, the potential benefits of aspirin seem to outweigh its risks. No prospective data of aspirin for primary prevention in women are yet available. (See also Chap. 62.)

Aspirin, with or without dipyridamole, has been found clearly effective for prevention of acute occlusion and myocardial infarction in patients undergoing *percutaneous transluminal coronary angioplasty.*[77–79] Its important antithrombotic role has also been documented in *aortocoronary saphenous vein graft surgery,*[61,80–87] particularly when treatment was started before or immediately after surgery (Table 68-4). One study[61] showed that a single daily dose of 325 mg of aspirin was as effective as aspirin given three times a day. A recent study[82] demonstrated that aspirin at a dose of 325 mg daily started soon after surgery was very effective in reducing early (1-week) and late (1-year) graft occlusion rates. Because aspirin given *before* surgery increases perioperative bleeding and the need for reoperation, in most patients it should be administered immediately *after* surgery, whenever possible.[61,88] (See also Chaps. 71 and 73.)

For patients with *transient ischemic attacks,* low-dose aspirin (300 mg/day) was as effective as high-dose aspirin (1200 mg/day) for reduction of myocardial infarction, stroke, and death but produced less gastrointestinal toxicity.[60] Furthermore, very low aspirin dose (30 mg/day) was shown as effective as and less toxic than a dose 10 times higher.[62] Aspirin combined with dipyridamole was very effective for secondary prevention after stroke.[89] (See Chap. 122.) In addition, aspirin was recently proved beneficial for prevention of stroke in patients younger than 75 years with *nonrheumatic atrial fibrillation*[41] (see above).

Adverse Effects

The most common side effects of aspirin are gastrointestinal and dose related. Low doses (80 to 325 mg/day) are much better tolerated than higher doses (500 to 1500 mg/day), although gastrointestinal toxicity can occur even with low doses.[60] Side effects include epigastric pain or burning, dyspepsia, erosive gastritis or ulceration, bleeding, nausea, vomiting, and constipation. Hypersensitivity reactions may occur in susceptible individuals.

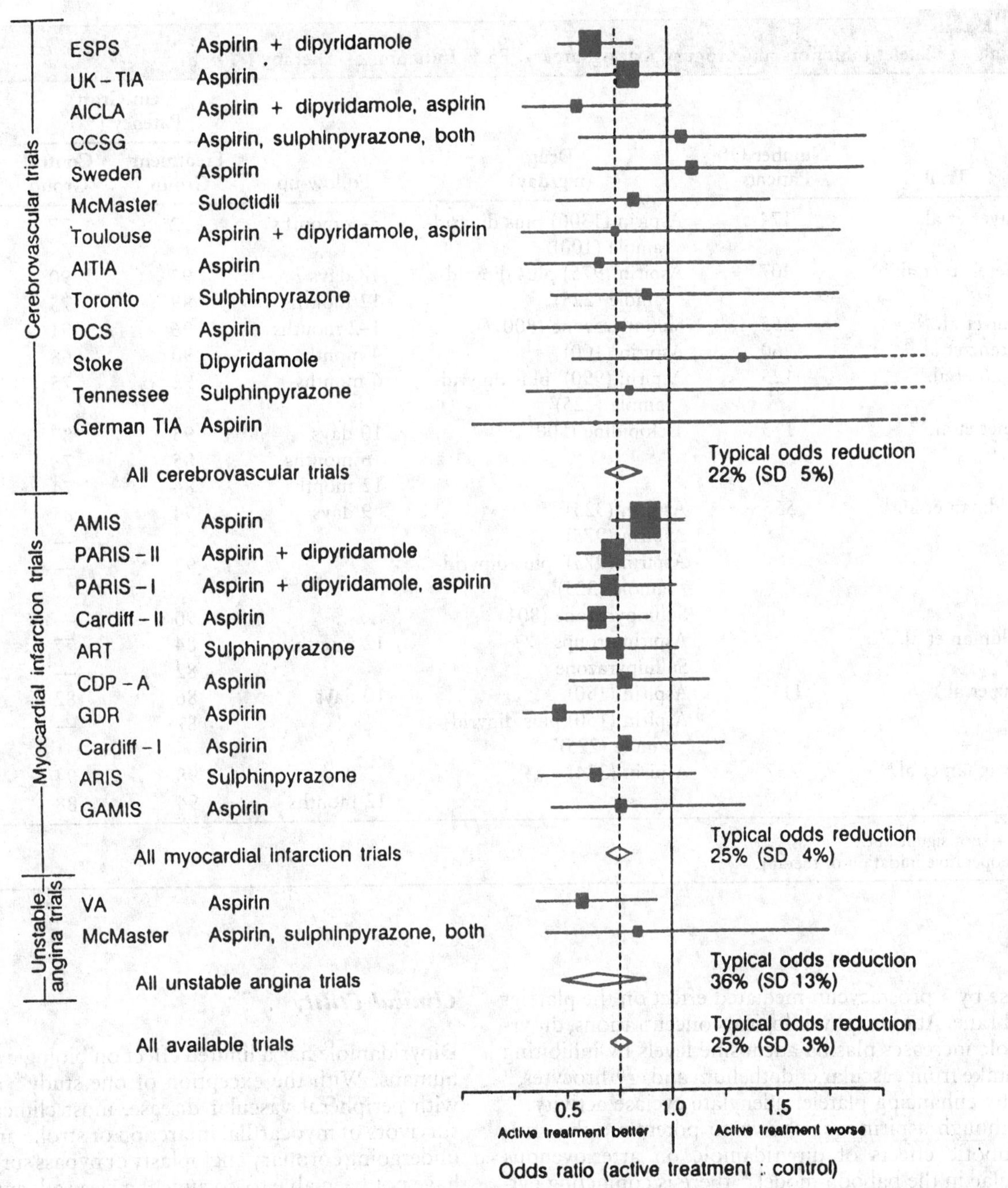

FIGURE 68-7 Results of an extensive overview of the effects of platelet inhibitors in patients with coronary or cerebrovascular disease. Platelet inhibitor therapy was associated with an odds reduction in important vascular events (death, myocardial infarction, or stroke) of 25 percent. (*From Antiplatelet Trialists' Collaboration: Secondary prevention of vascular disease by prolonged antiplatelet treatment. Br Med J 296:320–321, 1988. By permission from the British Medical Journal.*)

Nonsteroidal Anti-Inflammatory Agents

The nonsteroidal anti-inflammatory drugs inhibit cyclooxygenase in a reversible fashion and thus have a reduced effect on platelet function and a shorter duration of action compared to aspirin. The antithrombotic properties of these compounds have not been adequately tested in clinical trials and their use for this purpose cannot be recommended. In addition, one of these agents, indomethacin, increases vascular resistance and may exacerbate ischemia in patients with coronary artery disease.[90]

Dipyridamole

Pharmacology

Dipyridamole is a pyrimidopyrimidine compound with antithrombotic and vasodilating properties. Although the exact mechanism of action remains unknown, in vitro studies have disclosed three mechanisms by which intracellular platelet cyclic adenosine monophosphate (cAMP) is increased. At high concentrations, dipyridamole inhibits phosphodiesterase, which reduces the breakdown of cAMP; it also activates the enzyme adenylate

TABLE 68-4

Trials of Platelet Inhibitors in Coronary Artery Surgery: Early Initiation of Therapy (<48 h)

Trial	Number Of Patients	Drug (mg/day)	Follow-up	Vein Graft Patency (%)		p
				Treatment Group	Control Group	
Mayer et al.[83]	174	Aspirin (1300) plus dipyridamole (100)	3–6 months	92	77	<.02
Chesebro et al.[80,86]	407	Aspirin (975) plus dipyridamole (225)*	8 days	97	90	<.0001
			12 months	89	75	<.0001
Baur et al.[145]	255	Sulfinpyrazone (800)	1–2 months	96	91	<.025
Lorenz et al.[84]	60	Aspirin (100)	4 months	90	68	.012
Rajah et al.[85]	125	Aspirin (990)* plus dipyridamole (225)*	6 months	92	75	<.01
Limet et al.[109]	173	Ticlopidine (500)	10 days	93	87	<.05
			6 months	85	76	<.02
			12 months	84	74	<.01
Goldman et al.[61]	555	Aspirin (325)*	9 days	94	85	<.01
		Aspirin (975)*		92	—	<.05
		Aspirin (975)* plus dipyridamole (225)*		92	—	<.05
		Sulfinpyrazone (801)*		90	—	NS
Goldman et al.[87]		Aspirin groups	12 months	84	77	<.03
		Sulfinpyrazone		82	—	NS
Sanz et al.[81]	1112	Aspirin (150)	10 days	86	82	.058
		Aspirin (150) plus dipyridamole (225)*		87	—	<.02
Gavaghan et al.[82]	237	Aspirin (324)	7 days	98	94	.004
			12 months	94	88	.01

NS = not significant.
* Preoperative initiation of therapy.

cyclase by a prostacyclin-mediated effect on the platelet membrane. At more physiological concentrations, dipyridamole increases plasma adenosine levels by inhibiting its uptake from vascular endothelium and erythrocytes,[91] thereby enhancing platelet adenylate cyclase activity.

Although aspirin was shown to potentiate the antithrombotic effects of dipyridamole on arteriovenous cannulae in the baboon model,[92] there is conflicting evidence regarding the pharmacokinetic interactions between these two agents in humans. More importantly, there are no convincing data indicating that such interaction leads to a synergistic antithrombotic effect.[93] Experimentally, dipyridamole appears more effective in inhibiting platelet deposition on prosthetic materials than on biologic surfaces.[92,94] In human beings dipyridamole prolongs the shortened platelet survival times associated with prosthetic heart valves and prosthetic grafts.[95] Platelet activation associated with cardiopulmonary bypass and postoperative blood loss are reduced by dipyridamole.[96]

Absorption of dipyridamole is variable and greatly reduced when gastric pH is above 4. Peak levels are reached 75 min after ingestion, and the half-life is approximately 40 min. The recommended dose is 75 to 100 mg four times daily.

Clinical Utility

Dipyridamole has a limited effect on biologic surfaces in humans. With the exception of one study[97] in patients with peripheral vascular disease, most clinical trials in survivors of myocardial infarction or stroke and in those undergoing coronary angioplasty or bypass surgery[61,98–102] have not been able to document a clear advantage of the combination of aspirin and dipyridamole over aspirin alone.

Because dipyridamole, as opposed to aspirin, does not increase perioperative bleeding in patients undergoing coronary bypass surgery, its use for 2 days before surgery has been recommended for prevention of platelet activation by the extracorporeal pump.[80] It is not known whether or not this is necessary. More importantly, antiplatelet therapy *with aspirin* should be started in the immediate postoperative period.[82,88] Whereas one study[61] found no advantage of adding dipyridamole to aspirin, a more recent and larger trial[81] disclosed a small advantage from combined therapy.

Patients with *prosthetic mechanical heart valves* are at continuous risk of thromboembolism despite adequate anticoagulation. For patients at risk (i.e., those with prior embolism), the addition of a platelet inhibitor to the anticoagulant regimen has been advocated.[34,63,103,104] Adding dipyridamole reduces the incidence of embolism without increasing the risk of bleeding. At present, the only approved indication for oral dipyridamole is as adjuvant treatment with an oral anticoagulant in patients with prosthetic heart valves.

Adverse Effects

Its main side effects are headache, dizziness, epigastric discomfort, and nausea, which occur in up to 10 percent of patients, are dose related, and often subside with continued use. Dipyridamole does not exacerbate gastroduodenal ulcers and does not increase bleeding, even when combined with an anticoagulant.[63]

Ticlopidine

Pharmacology

Ticlopidine, one of the most potent antiplatelet agents available, has recently been approved for clinical use by the Food and Drug Administration. It is chemically unrelated to other platelet inhibitors and does not inhibit prostaglandin synthesis or cAMP degradation. Ticlopidine may act on the platelet membrane to alter its reactivity and may block the interaction of fibrinogen and von Willebrand factor with platelets. It inhibits ADP-induced platelet aggregation, even at high agonist concentrations.[105] Platelet aggregation induced by low concentrations of thrombin, collagen, thromboxane A_2, and platelet activating factor is also inhibited, but high agonist concentrations may overcome these effects.[105] Ticlopidine prolongs the bleeding time.

Optimal efficacy is reached only after several days of therapy; the inhibition of platelet function may persist for more than 72 h after discontinuation of the drug, with return to baseline values after 4 to 10 days.[105,106] The ex vivo inhibition of ADP-induced aggregation appears proportional to the dose administered, reaching a maximum effect at a dose of 500 mg/day.[106] The dose of ticlopidine used in most clinical trials has been 250 mg twice daily.

Clinical Utility

Ticlopidine was found effective in reducing the occurrence of death and myocardial infarction in patients with *unstable angina.*[107] It prevents abrupt thrombotic occlusion in patients undergoing *coronary angioplasty*[77,108] but is ineffective in reducing late restenosis. Ticlopidine reduced the incidence of vein graft occlusion rate after *coronary bypass surgery.*[109]

In a large trial[110] of patients with *transient ischemic attacks,* ticlopidine was found more effective than aspirin for prevention of death or stroke, although it was associated with a higher incidence of side effects. In another trial[111] of patients with a recent *stroke,* ticlopidine reduced significantly the incidence of vascular death or recurrent stroke in both men and women. (See also Chap. 122.)

In summary, ticlopidine is effective in a variety of clinical disorders, including unstable angina, coronary angioplasty, coronary bypass surgery, and cerebrovascular disease. Its widespread acceptance by the medical community will depend on several issues such as cost, safety, and relative efficacy when compared with aspirin. It may be particularly useful for patients intolerant or allergic to aspirin.

Adverse Effects

The most important side effects are diarrhea (20 percent), rash (12 percent), and neutropenia (less than 1 percent). The neutropenia can be severe but is reversible and resolves promptly upon discontinuation of the drug.[110,111]

Sulfinpyrazone

This agent is structurally related to phenylbutazone but has minimal anti-inflammatory activity. In contrast to aspirin, it is a competitive inhibitor of platelet cyclooxygenase, but the exact mechanism of action remains unknown.[92] It inhibits platelet adhesion to collagen, reduces thrombus formation on subendothelium, and may protect the endothelium from chemical injury.[92] Sulfinpyrazone produces a dose-dependent inhibition in experimental thromboembolism in artificial cannulae,[92] reduces thrombosis of arteriovenous cannulae, and normalizes platelet survival in patients with artificial heart valves.

Like dipyridamole, the beneficial effects of sulfinpyrazone are more consistent on prosthetic than on biologic surfaces. Its clinical benefits have been variable. Some benefit was seen when given to patients after myocardial infarction[112] or aortocoronary bypass surgery.[61] However, no benefit was evident in patients with unstable angina[68] or stroke.[113]

It is well absorbed orally, reaching plasma peak concentrations in 1 to 2 h. It is strongly protein bound and, therefore, may displace other protein-bound drugs such as warfarin and the sulfonylureas, causing potentiation of their effects. Other side effects include exacerbation of peptic ulcer, renal insufficiency, and precipitation of uric acid stones.

Fish Oils

Ingestion of a diet rich in omega-3 fatty acids has been speculated to prevent or delay atherosclerosis and thrombosis. Both eicosapentaenoic acid (20 : 5ω3) and docosahexaenoic acid (22 : 6ω3) are present in high concentration in saltwater fish and may account for the lower incidence of coronary disease in populations that include fish in their diet.[114] These polyunsaturated fatty acids become incorporated into the platelet membrane between 1 and 4 weeks after administration and result in decreased aggregation responses.[115] Eicosapentaenoic acid competes with arachidonic acid for platelet cyclooxygenase. This leads to the formation of two endoperoxidases (prostaglandins G_3 and H_3) and thromboxane A_3, which have minimal biologic activity. In endothelial cells, production of prostacyclin is not markedly inhibited and prostaglandin I_3 is produced, which retains platelet inhibitory properties.[116] The net result is a shift in the hemostatic balance toward an antiaggregatory and vasodilative state.

Fish oils were shown experimentally to suppress thromboxane production and accelerate the response to thrombolysis.[117] In addition to their interference with platelet metabolism, omega-3 fatty acids have multiple other effects including reduced production of leukotriene B_4, platelet-derived growth factor, interleukin-1, tumor necrosis factor, and fibrinogen.[118] They also reduce blood pressure, blood viscosity, triglycerides, and very low density lipoprotein levels and increase the actions of endothelium-derived relaxing factor.[118] Whether or not these actions of fish oils will result in antiatherogenic and antithrombotic effects in human trials remains unknown. The use of omega-3 fatty acids for the prevention of restenosis in patients undergoing angioplasty is still controversial given the conflicting results of available clinical trials.[119–122, 122a] There is some evidence suggesting that high-dose fish oils reduce the rate of restenosis when given 7 to 21 days prior to coronary angioplasty.[119, 122a] Whereas recommending an increased consumption of fish is prudent and may lower the incidence of coronary heart disease,[114] the administration of pharmacologic doses of omega-3 fatty acids is associated with gastrointestinal side effects and potential adverse events such as increased bleeding diathesis and reduced inflammatory and immune responses. (See also Chap. 62.)

Dextran

Intravenous infusion of dextran prolongs the bleeding time. Its mechanism of antiplatelet activity is unclear, perhaps involving an alteration of platelet membrane function or interference with factor VIII–von Willebrand factor complex.[123] Although antithrombotic activity has been demonstrated experimentally, no beneficial effect was found in patients undergoing coronary angioplasty.[124] Based on experimental observations suggesting inhibition of thrombosis in artificial surfaces, dextran infusions are currently being used before and immediately after placement of intravascular coronary stents. Its potential side effects include volume overload and anaphylactoid reactions.

Prostaglandins E_1 and I_2

These prostaglandins increase the concentration of cAMP in platelets and thus are potent inhibitors of platelet metabolism. They are also powerful systemic vasodilators. Intravenous prostaglandin E_1 is commonly used in neonates with congenital heart disease who are dependent on the persistence of a patent ductus arteriosus until surgical correction can be done. In addition, it has been used in patients with acute myocardial infarction complicated by left ventricular dysfunction for its beneficial hemodynamic effects.[125]

Prostacyclin is a potent, naturally occurring platelet inhibitor whose use has been limited by its instability and its propensity to cause significant systemic hypotension at doses required for platelet inhibition. Its pharmacologic effects disappear within 30 min after infusion. Prostacyclin has been shown to limit platelet interaction with artificial surfaces and to preserve the platelet count during cardiopulmonary bypass.[126]

Despite beneficial effects in animal models of myocardial ischemia, small trials in humans have been controversial.[127] Despite favorable effects on platelet aggregation and systemic hemodynamics, prostacyclin administration in patients with acute coronary syndromes did not improve clinical outcome and may even aggravate ischemia.[128] Experimental[129] and clinical[130] studies showed that iloprost, a stable prostacyclin analogue, increases the hepatic degradation of tissue plasminogen activator and thus may reduce its thrombolytic activity. Similarly, the use of these agents in patients undergoing coronary angioplasty is controversial. Given these conflicting data, further animal and clinical research appears necessary before recommendations can be made.

Future Developments

Imidazole analogue thromboxane synthetase inhibitors have been developed with the expectation of not only suppressing thromboxane A_2 biosynthesis but also sparing or even enhancing the production of prostacyclin by the vessel wall. Whereas some of these compounds were shown to reduce platelet-mediated vascular occlusion and reduce infarct size in different experimental models of arterial thrombosis, no consistent benefit occurred in small clinical trials.[131] Because of the difficulties in inhibiting thromboxane synthetase completely, drugs that block the receptor of both thromboxane A_2 and its cyclic endoperoxidase precursors have been developed and successfully tested in animal models.[132] Results from small clinical trials suggest that thromboxane receptor blockers may reduce platelet deposition on Dacron grafts[133] and may decrease the early coronary bypass graft occlusion rate.[134] More effective inhibition of platelet function can be achieved by combining a thromboxane synthetase inhibitor and a receptor antagonist, which not only prevents the action of thromboxane and cyclic endoperoxidases but also reorients endoperoxide metabolism toward the formation of platelet inhibitory prostaglandins. Whereas the antithrombotic activity of the combination of these agents has been demonstrated experimentally,[135,136] their usefulness awaits clinical testing.

In addition to thromboxane A_2, serotonin is secreted by platelets and can activate neighboring platelets, induce vasoconstriction, and play a role in myocardial ischemia.[137,138] Animal studies[139] have shown that the combination of serotonin S_2 and thromboxane A_2 receptor antagonists enhances coronary thrombolysis and prevents reocclusion. Few clinical studies with these agents are available. Ketanserin, a selective serotonin S_2-receptor antagonist, was able to prevent serotonin-induced vasoconstriction in patients with atherosclerosis.[137] However, it did not reduce vascular morbidity and mortality in patients with peripheral vascular disease.[140] This agent is currently being tested for the prevention of restenosis after coronary angioplasty.

Currently available drugs are unable to block all the different pathways of platelet activation and thus are unable to prevent thrombus formation in many situations. Because exposure of receptors in the platelet membrane that bind fibrinogen and von Willebrand factor (the glycoprotein IIb/IIIa) appears to play a pivotal role in the common final stage of platelet aggregation, inhibition of platelet-dependent thrombosis by the use of monoclonal antibodies against these platelet membrane receptors may be a viable antithrombotic strategy. Based on the positive results in experimental models,[141,142] these antibodies are being tested in patients treated with thrombolysis for acute myocardial infarction and in patients undergoing high-risk coronary angioplasty. Polypeptides derived from viper venoms that contain the amino acid sequence Arg-Gly-Asp have also been found to inhibit the platelet glycoprotein IIb/IIIa receptor, increase the rate and extent of thrombolysis, prevent reocclusion, and inhibit platelet aggregation in a canine model of coronary thrombosis.[143] Agents that inhibit adhesive macromolecules such as von Willebrand factor have been shown experimentally to reduce platelet-dependent thrombosis.[144] These powerful agents, as well as the aforementioned direct inhibitors of thrombin, may be effective in the short-term management of patients at very high risk of thrombotic occlusion, such as during thrombolysis for acute myocardial infarction or during coronary intervention. Long-term therapy, however, can be hazardous because of increased risk of bleeding. (See also Chap. 7.)

REFERENCES

1. Stein B, Fuster V, Halperin JL, Chesebro JH: Antithrombotic therapy in cardiac disease. An emerging approach based on pathogenesis and risk. *Circulation* 1989; 80:1501–1513.
2. Rosenberg RD: The heparin-antithrombin system: A natural anticoagulant mechanism. In: Colman RW, Hirsh J, Marder VJ, Salzman EW (eds): *Hemostasis and Thrombosis: Basic Principles and Clinical Practice,* 2d ed. Philadelphia, JB Lippincott, 1987: 1373–1392.
3. Hirsh J: Heparin. *N Engl J Med* 1991; 324:1565–1574.
4. Ofosu FA, Modi GJ, Hirsh J, Buchanan M, Blachman MA: Mechanisms for inhibition of the generation of thrombin activity by sulfated polysaccharides. *Ann NY Acad Sci* 1986; 485:41–55.
5. Weitz JI, Hudoba M, Massel D, Maraganore J, Hirsh J: Clot-bound thrombin is protected from inhibition by heparin–antithrombin III but is susceptible to inactivation by antithrombin III–independent inhibitors. *J Clin Invest* 1990; 86:385–391.
6. de Swart CAM, Nijmeyer B, Roelofs JMM, Sixma JJ: Kinetics of intravenously administered heparin in normal humans. *Blood* 1982; 60:1251–1258.
7. Prins MH, Hirsh J: Heparin as adjunctive treatment after thrombolytic therapy for acute myocardial infarction. *Am J Cardiol* 1991; 67(suppl):3A–11A.
8. Chiu HM, Hirsh J, Yung WL, Regoeczi E, Gent M: Relationship between the anticoagulant and antithrombotic effects of heparin in experimental venous thrombosis. *Blood* 1977; 49:171–184.
9. Théroux P, Ouimet H, McCans J, et al: Aspirin, heparin, or both to treat acute unstable angina. *N Engl J Med* 1988; 319:1105–1111.
10. Telford AM, Wilson C: Trial of heparin versus atenolol in prevention of myocardial infarction in intermediate coronary syndrome. *Lancet* 1981; 1:1225–1228.
11. The RISC Group: Risk of myocardial infarction and death during treatment with low dose aspirin and intravenous heparin in men with unstable coronary artery disease. *Lancet* 1990; 336:827–830.

11a. Théroux P, Waters D, Lam J, Juneau M, McCans J: Reactivation of unstable angina after the discontinuation of heparin. *N Engl J Med* 1992; 327:141–145.

12. MacMahon S, Collins R, Knight C, Yusuf S, Peto R: Reduction of major morbidity and mortality by heparin in acute myocardial infarction (abstr). *Circulation* 1988; 78(suppl II):II-98.
13. The SCATI (Studio sulla Calciparina nell'Angina e nella Trombosi Ventricolare nell'Infarto) Group: Randomised controlled trial of subcutaneous calcium heparin in acute myocardial infarction. *Lancet* 1989; 2:182–186.
14. Hsia J, Hamilton WP, Kleiman N, Roberts R, Cheitman BR, Ross AM: A comparison between heparin and low-dose aspirin as adjunctive therapy with tissue plasminogen activator for acute myocardial infarction. *N Engl J Med* 1990; 323:1433–1437.
15. Bleich SD, Nichols TC, Schumacher RR, Cooke DH, Tate DA, Teichman SL: Effect of heparin on coronary arterial patency after thrombolysis with tissue plasminogen activator in acute myocardial infarction. *Am J Cardiol* 1990; 66:1412–1417.
16. Gruppo Italiano per lo Studio della Sopravvivenza nell'Infarto Miocardico: GISSI-II: A factorial randomised trial of alteplase versus streptokinase and heparin among 12,490 patients with acute myocardial infarction. *Lancet* 1990; 336:65–70.
17. The International Study Group: In-hospital mortality and clinical course of 20,891 patients with suspected acute myocardial infarction randomised between alteplase and streptokinase with or without heparin. *Lancet* 1990; 336:71–75.
18. ISIS-3 (Third International Study of Infarct Survival) Collaborative Group: ISIS-3: A randomised comparison of streptokinase vs. tissue plasminogen activator vs. anistreplase and of aspirin plus heparin vs. aspirin alone among 41,299 cases of suspected acute myocardial infarction. *Lancet* 1992; 339:753–770.
19. Turpie AGG, Robinson JG, Doyle DJ, Mulji AS, Mishkel GU, Sealey BJ, et al: Comparison of high-dose with low-dose subcutaneous heparin to prevent left ventricular mural thrombosis in patients with acute transmural anterior myocardial infarction. *N Engl J Med* 1989; 320:352–357.
20. Collins R, Scrimgeour A, Yusuf S, Peto R: Reduction in fatal pulmonary embolism and venous thrombosis by perioperative administration of subcutaneous heparin: Overview of results of randomized trials in general, orthopedic and urologic surgery. *N Engl J Med* 1988; 318:1162–1173.
21. Leyvraz PF, Richard J, Bachmann F, van Melle G, Treyvaud JM, Livio JJ, et al: Adjusted versus fixed-dose subcutaneous heparin in the prevention of deep-vein thrombosis after total hip replacement. *N Engl J Med* 1983; 309:954–958.
22. Powers PJ, Gent M, Jay RM, Julian DH, Turpie AGG, Levine M, et al: A randomized trial of less intense postoperative warfarin or aspirin in the prevention of venous thromboembolism after surgery for fractured hip. *Arch Intern Med* 1989; 149:771–774.
23. King DJ, Kelton JG: Heparin-associated thrombocytopenia. *Ann Intern Med* 1984; 100:535–540.
24. Levine MN, Hirsh J, Gent M, Leclerc J, Powers PJ, Jay RM, et al: Prevention of deep vein thrombosis after elective hip surgery: A randomized trial comparing low molecular weight heparin with standard unfractionated heparin. *Ann Intern Med* 1991; 114:545–551.
25. Heras M, Chesebro JH, Penny WJ, Bailey KR, Badimon L, Fuster V: Effects of thrombin inhibition on the development of acute platelet thrombus deposition during angioplasty in pigs. *Circulation* 1989; 79:657–665.
26. Hanson SR, Harker LA: Interruption of acute platelet-dependent thrombosis by the synthetic antithrombin D-phenylalanyl-L-prolyl-L-arginyl chloromethyl ketone. *Proc Natl Acad Sci USA* 1988; 85:3184–3188.
27. Gruber A, Griffin JH, Harker LA, Hanson SR: Inhibition of platelet-dependent thrombus formation by human activated protein C in a primate model. *Blood* 1989; 73:639–642.
28. Jang I-K, Gold HK, Ziskind AA, Leinbach RC, Fallon JT, Collen D: Prevention of platelet-rich arterial thrombosis by selective thrombin inhibition. *Circulation* 1990; 81:219–225.
29. Sadowski JA, Bovill EG, Mann KG: Warfarin and the metabolism of vitamin K. In: Poller L (ed): *Recent Advances in Blood Coagulation-5.* Edinburgh, Churchill Livingstone, 1991: 93–118.
30. McKenna R, Cale ER, Vasan U: Is warfarin sodium contraindicated in the lactating mother? *J Pediatr* 1983; 103:325–327.
31. Hirsh J: Oral anticoagulant drugs. *N Engl J Med* 1991; 324:1865–1875.
32. Alving BM, Strickler MP, Knight RD, Barr CF, Berenberg JL, Peck CC: Hereditary warfarin resistance. *Arch Intern Med* 1985; 145:499–501.

33. Quick AJ: The prothrombin time in haemophilia and in obstructive jaundice. *J Biol Chem* 1935; 109:73–74.
34. Dalen JE, Hirsh J: Third ACCP Consensus Conference on Antithrombotic Therapy. *Chest* 1992; 102(suppl):303S–549S.
35. Smith P, Arnesen H, Holme I: The effect of warfarin on mortality and reinfarction after myocardial infarction. *N Engl J Med* 1990; 323:147–152.
36. Report of the Working Party on Anticoagulation Therapy in Coronary Thrombosis to the Medical Research Council: Assessment of short-term anticoagulation administration after cardiac infarction. *Br Med J* 1969; 1:335–342.
37. Drapkin A, Merskey C: Anticoagulation therapy after acute myocardial infarction: Relation of therapeutic benefit to patient's age, sex and severity of infarction. *JAMA* 1972; 222:541–548.
38. Veterans Administration Hospital Investigators: Anticoagulants in acute myocardial infarction: Results of a cooperative clinical trial. *JAMA* 1973; 225:724–729.
39. Report of the Sixty Plus Reinfarction Study Research Group. A double-blind trial to assess long-term anticoagulant therapy in elderly patients after myocardial infarction. *Lancet* 1980; 2:989–993.
40. Fuster V, Gersh BJ, Giuliani ER, Tajik AJ, Brandenburg RO, Frye RL: The natural history of idiopathic dilated cardiomyopathy. *Am J Cardiol* 1981; 47:525–531.
41. Stroke Prevention in Atrial Fibrillation Investigators: Stroke prevention in atrial fibrillation study. Final results. *Circulation* 1991; 84:527–539.
42. Petersen P, Boysen G, Godtfredsen J, Andersen ED, Andersen B: Placebo-controlled, randomised trial of warfarin and aspirin for prevention of thromboembolic complication in chronic atrial fibrillation: The Copenhagen AFASAK study. *Lancet* 1989; 1:175–179.
43. The Boston Area Anticoagulation Trial for Atrial Fibrillation Investigators: The effect of low-dose warfarin on the risk of stroke in patients with nonrheumatic atrial fibrillation. *N Engl J Med* 1990; 323:1505–1511.
43a. Esekowitz MD, Bridgers SL, James KE, Clarliner NH, Colling CL, Gornick GC, et al: Warfarin in the prevention of stroke associated with non-rheumatic atrial fibrillation. *N Engl J Med* 1992; 327:1406–1412.
44. Mok CK, Boey J, Wang R, Chan TK, Cheung KL, Lee PK, et al: Warfarin versus dipyridamole-aspirin and pentoxifylline-aspirin for the prevention of prosthetic heart valve thromboembolism: A prospective clinical trial. *Circulation* 1985; 72:1059–1063.
45. Saour JN, Sieck JO, Mamo LAR, Gallus AS: Trial of different intensities of anticoagulation in patients with prosthetic heart valves. *N Engl J Med* 1990; 322:428–432.
46. Altman R, Rouvier J, Gurfinkel E, D'Ortencio O, Manzanel R, de la Fuenta L, et al: Comparison of two levels of anticoagulant therapy in patients with substitute heart valves. *J Thorac Cardiovasc Surg* 1991; 101:427–441.
47. Turpie AGG, Gunstensen J, Hirsh J, Nelson H, Gent M: Randomised comparison of two intensities of oral anticoagulant therapy after tissue heart valve replacement. *Lancet* 1988; 1:1242–1245.
48. Poller L, McKernan A, Thomson JM, Elstein M, Hirsh PJ, Jones JB: Fixed minidose warfarin: A new approach to prophylaxis against venous thrombosis after major surgery. *Br Med J* 1987; 295:1309–1312.
49. Hull R, Hirsh J, Jay R, Carter C, England C, Gent M, et al: Different intensities of oral anticoagulant therapy in the treatment of proximal-vein thrombosis. *N Engl J Med* 1982; 307:1676–1681.
50. Iturbe-Alessio I, Fonseca MC, Mutchinik O, Santos MA, Zajarias A, Salazar E: Risks of anticoagulant therapy in pregnant women with artificial heart valves. *N Engl J Med* 1986; 315:1390–1393.
51. Hall JG, Pauli RM, Wilson KM: Maternal and fetal sequelae of anticoagulation during pregnancy. *Am J Med* 1980; 68:122–140.
52. Bern MM, Lokich JJ, Wallach SR, Bothe A, Benotti PN, Arkin CF, et al: Very low doses of warfarin can prevent thrombosis in central venous catheters. *Ann Intern Med* 1990; 112:423–428.
53. Moncada S, Vane JR: Arachidonic acid metabolites and the interactions between platelets and blood vessel walls. *N Engl J Med* 1979; 300:1142–1147.
54. Tschopp TB: Aspirin inhibits platelet aggregation, but not adhesion to collagen fibrils: An assessment of platelet adhesion and deposited platelet mass by morphometry and 51-Cr-labeling. *Thromb Res* 1977; 11:619–632.
55. Oates JA, FitzGerald GA, Branch RA, Jackson EK, Knapp HR, Roberts LJ II: Clinical implications of prostaglandin and thromboxane A_2 formation. *N Engl J Med* 1988; 319:689–698.
56. Patrignani P, Filabozzi P, Patrono C: Selective cumulative inhibition of platelet thromboxane production by low-dose aspirin in healthy subjects. *J Clin Invest* 1982; 69:1366–1372.
57. FitzGerald GA, Oates JA, Hawiger J, Mass RL, Roberts LJ II, Lawson JA, et al: Endogenous biosynthesis of prostacyclin and thromboxane and platelet function during chronic administration of aspirin in man. *J Clin Invest* 1983; 71:676–688.
58. Weksler BB, Tack-Goldman K, Subramanian VA, Gay WA: Cumulative inhibitory effect of low-dose aspirin on vascular prostacyclin and platelet thromboxane production in patients with atherosclerosis. *Circulation* 1985; 71:332–340.
59. Kyrle PA, Eichler HG, Jager U, Lechner K: Inhibition of prostacyclin and thromboxane A_2 generation by low-dose aspirin at the site of plug formation in man in vivo. *Circulation* 1987; 75:1025–1029.
60. UK-TIA Study Group: United Kingdom Transient Ischemic Attack (UK-TIA) Aspirin Trial: Interim results. *Br Med J* 1988; 296:316–320.
61. Goldman S, Copeland J, Moritz T, Henderson W, Zadina K, Ovitt T, et al: Improvement in early saphenous vein graft patency after coronary artery bypass surgery with antiplatelet therapy: Results of a Veterans Administration cooperative study. *Circulation* 1988; 77:1324–1332.
62. The Dutch TIA Trial Study Group: A comparison of two doses of aspirin (30 mg vs. 283 mg a day) in patients after a transient ischemic attack or minor stroke. *N Engl J Med* 1991; 325:1261–1266.
63. Chesebro JH, Fuster V, Elveback LR, McGoon DC, Pluth JR, Puga FJ, et al: Trial of combined warfarin plus dipyridamole or aspirin in prosthetic heart valve replacement: Danger of aspirin compared with dipyridamole. *Am J Cardiol* 1983; 51:1537–1541.
64. Pedersen AK, FitzGerald GA: Dose-related kinetics of aspirin. Presystemic acetylation of platelet cyclooxygenase. *N Engl J Med* 1984; 311:1206–1211.
65. Cerletti C, Marchi S, Lauri D, Domanin M, Lorenzi G, Urso R, et al: Pharmacokinetics of enteric-coated aspirin and inhibition of platelet thromboxane A_2 and vascular prostacyclin generation in humans. *Clin Pharmacol Ther* 1987; 42:175–180.
66. Clarke R, Mayo G, Price P, FitzGerald GA: Suppression of thromboxane A_2 but not of systemic prostacyclin by controlled-release aspirin. *N Engl J Med* 1991; 325:1137–1141.
67. Lewis HD, Davis JW, Archibald DG, Steinke WE, Smitherman TC, Doherty JE, et al: Protective effects of aspirin against acute myocardial infarction and death in men with unstable angina: Results of a Veterans Administration Cooperative Study. *N Engl J Med* 1983; 309:396–403.
68. Cairns JA, Gent M, Singer J, Finnie KJ, Froggatt GM, Holder DA, et al: Aspirin, sulfinpyrazone, or both in unstable angina. *N Engl J Med* 1985; 313:1369–1375.
69. ISIS-2 (Second International Study of Infarct Survival) Collaborative Group: Randomized trial of intravenous streptokinase, oral aspirin, both, or neither among 17,187 cases of suspected acute myocardial infarction: ISIS-2. *Lancet* 1988; 2:349–360.
70. Antiplatelet Trialists' Collaboration: Secondary prevention of vascular disease by prolonged antiplatelet treatment. *Br Med J* 1988; 296:320–331.
71. Stein B, Fuster V, Israel DH, Cohen M, Badimon L, Badimon JJ, et al: Platelet inhibitor agents in cardiovascular disease: An update. *J Am Coll Cardiol* 1989; 14:813–836.
72. Chesebro JH, Webster MWI, Smith HC, Frye RL, Holmes DR, Reeder GS, et al: Antiplatelet therapy in coronary disease progression: Reduced infarction and new lesion formation. (abstr). *Circulation* 1989; 80(suppl II):II–266.
73. Ridker PM, Manson JE, Gaziano JM, Buring JE, Hennekens CH: Low-dose aspirin therapy for chronic stable angina. A randomized, placebo-controlled clinical trial. *Ann Intern Med* 1991; 114:835–839.
74. Peto R, Gray R, Collins R, Wheatley K, Hennekens C, Janrozik K, et al: A randomized trial of the effects of prophylactic daily aspirin among British male doctors. *Br Med J* 1989; 299: 1247–1250.
75. The Steering Committee of the Physicians' Health Study Research Group: Final report on the aspirin component of the ongoing Physicians' Health Study. *N Engl J Med* 1989; 321:129–135.

76. Fuster V, Cohen M, Halperin JL: Aspirin in the prevention of coronary disease (editorial). *N Engl J Med* 1989; 321:129–131.
77. White CW, Chaitman B, Lassar TA, Marcus ML, Chisholm RJ, Knudson M, et al: Antiplatelet agents are effective in reducing the immediate complications of PTCA: Results from the ticlopidine multicenter trial (abstr). *Circulation* 1987; 76(suppl IV):IV–400.
78. Schwartz L, Bourassa MG, Lesperance J, Aleridge HE, Kazim F, Salvatori VA, et al: Aspirin and dipyridamole in the prevention of restenosis after percutaneous transluminal coronary angioplasty. *N Engl J Med* 1988; 318:1714–1719.
79. Barnathan ES, Schwartz JS, Taylor L, Laskey WK, Klearsland JP, Kussmaul WG, et al: Aspirin and dipyridamole in the prevention of acute coronary thrombosis complicating coronary angioplasty. *Circulation* 1987; 76:125–134.
80. Chesebro JH, Clements IP, Fuster V, Elveback LR, Smith HC, Bardsley WT, et al: A platelet inhibitor-drug trial in coronary artery bypass operations: Benefit of perioperative dipyridamole and aspirin therapy on early postoperative vein-graft patency. *N Engl J Med* 1982; 307:73–78.
81. Sanz G, Pajaron A, Alegria E, Coello I, Cardona M, Fournier JA, et al: Prevention of early aortocoronary bypass occlusion by low-dose aspirin and dipyridamole. *Circulation* 1990; 82:765–773.
82. Gavaghan TP, Gebski V, Baron DW: Immediate postoperative aspirin improves vein graft patency early and late after coronary artery bypass graft surgery. A placebo-controlled, randomized study. *Circulation* 1991; 83:1526–1533.
83. Mayer JE, Lindsay WG, Castaneda W, Nicoloff DM: Influence of aspirin and dipyridamole on patency of coronary artery bypass grafts. *Ann Thorac Surg* 1981; 31:204–210.
84. Lorenz RL, Weber M, Kotzur J, Theisen K, Schacky CV, Meister W, et al: Improved aortocoronary bypass patency by low-dose aspirin (100 mg/daily): Effects on platelet aggregation and thromboxane formation. *Lancet* 1984; 1:1261–1264.
85. Rajah SM, Salter MCP, Donaldson DR, Rao RS, Boyle RM, Partridge JB, et al: Acetylsalicylic acid and dipyridamole improve the early patency of aorta-coronary bypass grafts: A double-blind, placebo-controlled, randomized trial. *J Thorac Cardiovasc Surg* 1985; 90:373–377.
86. Chesebro JH, Fuster V, Elveback LR, Clements IP, Smith HC, Holmes DR, et al: Effect of dipyridamole and aspirin on late vein-graft patency after coronary bypass operations. *N Engl J Med* 1984; 310:209–214.
87. Goldman S, Copeland JG, Moritz T, Henderson W, Zadina K, Ovitt T, et al: Saphenous vein graft patency 1 year after coronary artery bypass surgery and effects of antiplatelet therapy: Results of a Veterans Administration cooperative study. *Circulation* 1989; 80:1190–1197.
88. Goldman S, Copeland J, Moritz M, Henderson W, Zadina K, Ovitt T, et al: Starting aspirin therapy after operation. Effects on early graft patency. *Circulation* 1991; 84:520–526.
89. The ESPS Group: The European Stroke Prevention Study: Principal endpoints. *Lancet* 1987; 2:1351–1354.
90. Friedman PL, Brown EJ, Gunther S, Alexander RW, Barry WH, Mudge GH, et al: Coronary vasoconstrictor effect of indomethacin in patients with coronary artery disease. *N Engl J Med* 1981; 305:1171–1175.
91. Gresele P, Arnout J, Deckmyn H, Vermylen J: Mechanisms of the antiplatelet action of dipyridamole in whole blood: Modulation of adenosine concentration and activity. *Thromb Haemost* 1986; 55:12–18.
92. Hanson SR, Harker LA, Bjornsson TD: Effect of platelet-modifying drugs on arterial thromboembolism in baboons: Aspiring potentiates the antithrombotic actions of dipyridamole and sulfinpyrazone by mechanism(s) independent of platelet cyclooxygenase inhibition. *J Clin Invest* 1985; 75:1591–1599.
93. FitzGerald GA: Dipyridamole. *N Engl J Med* 1987; 316: 1247–1257.
94. Fujitani RM, Nordestgaard AG, Marcus CS, Wilson SE: Perioperative suppression of platelet adherence to small-diameter polytetrafluoroethylene grafts. *J Surg Res* 1988; 44:455–460.
95. Harker LA, Slichter SJ: Studies of platelet and fibrinogen kinetics in patients with prosthetic heart valves. *N Engl J Med* 1970; 283:534–537.
96. Theo KH, Christakis GT, Weisel RD, Wong PY, Mae AV, Iranov J, et al: Dipyridamole preserved platelets and reduced blood loss after cardiopulmonary bypass. *J Thorac Cardiovasc Surg* 1988; 96:332–341.
97. Hess H, Mietaschk A, Deichsel G: Drug-induced inhibition of platelet function delays progression of peripheral occlusive arterial disease: A prospective double-blind arteriographically controlled trial. *Lancet* 1985; 1:415–419.
98. The Persantin-Aspirin Reinfarction Study Group: Persantine and aspirin in coronary heart disease. *Circulation* 1980; 62:449–461.
99. Bousser MG, Eschwege E, Haugenau M, Lefaucconnier JM, Thibult N, Touboul D, et al: "AICLA" controlled trial of aspirin and dipyridamole in the secondary prevention of atherothrombotic cerebral ischemia. *Stroke* 1983; 14:5–14.
100. American-Canadian Cooperative Study Group: Persantine-aspirin trial in cerebral ischemia. Part II: Endpoint results. *Stroke* 1985; 16:406–415.
101. Brown BG, Cukingnan RA, DeRouen T, Goede LV, Wong M, et al: Improved graft patency in patients treated with platelet-inhibiting therapy after coronary bypass surgery. *Circulation* 1985; 72:138–146.
102. Lembo JN, Black AJ, Roubin GS, Wilentz JR, Mufson LH, Douglas JS, et al: Effect of pretreatment with aspirin versus aspirin plus dipyridamole on frequency and type of acute complications of percutaneous transluminal coronary angioplasty. *Am J Cardiol* 1990; 65:422–426.
103. Sullivan JM, Harken DE, Gorlin R: Pharmacologic control of thromboembolic complications of cardiac-valve replacement. *N Engl J Med* 1971; 284:1391–1394.
104. Kasahara T: Clinical effect of dipyridamole ingestion after prosthetic heart valve replacement—especially on the blood coagulation system. *Nippon Kyobu Geka Gakkai Zarshi* 1977; 25:1007–1021.
105. Defreyn G, Bernat A, Delebassee D, Maffrand J-P: Pharmacology of ticlopidine: A review. *Sem Thromb Hemost* 1989; 15:159–166.
106. McTavish D, Faulds D, Goa KL: Ticlopidine. An updated review of its pharmacology and therapeutic use in platelet-dependent disorders. *Drugs* 1990; 40:238–259.
107. Balsano F, Rizzon P, Violi F, Scrutinio O, Cimminiello D, Aguglia F, et al: Antiplatelet treatment with ticlopidine in unstable angina. A Controlled Multicenter Clinical Trial. *Circulation* 1990; 82:17–26.
108. Bertrand ME, Allain H, Lablanche JM: Results of a randomized trial of ticlopidine versus placebo for prevention of acute closure and restenosis after coronary angioplasty. The TACT study (abstr). *Circulation* 1990; 82(suppl III):III–190.
109. Limet R, David JL, Magotteaux P, Larock MP, Rigo P: Prevention of aorta-coronary bypass graft occlusion. *J Thorac Cardiovasc Surg* 1987; 94:773–783.
110. Hass WK, Easton JD, Adams HP, Pryse-Phillips W, Molony BA, Anderson S, et al: A randomized trial comparing ticlopidine hydrochloride with aspirin for the prevention of stroke in high-risk patients. *N Engl J Med* 1989; 321:501–507.
111. Gent M, Blakely JA, Easton JD, Ellis DJ, Hachinski VC, Harbison JW, et al: The Canadian American Ticlopidine Study in thromboembolic stroke. *Lancet* 1989; 1:1215–1220.
112. Report from the Anturane Reinfarction Italian Study: Sulfinpyrazone in post-myocardial infarction. *Lancet* 1982; 1:237–242.
113. Canadian Cooperative Study Group: A randomized trial of aspirin and sulfinpyrazone in threatened stroke. *N Engl J Med* 1978; 229:53–59.
114. Kromhout D, Bosschieter EB, Coulander CDL: The inverse relation between fish consumption and 20-year mortality from coronary heart disease. *N Engl J Med* 1985; 312:1205–1209.
115. Dyerberg J, Bang HO: Haemostatic function and platelet polyunsaturated fatty acids in Eskimos. *Lancet* 1979; 2:433–435.
116. Von Schacky C: Prophylaxis of atherosclerosis with marine omega-3 fatty acids: A comprehensive strategy. *Ann Intern Med* 1987; 107:890–899.
117. Braden GA, Knapp HR, Fitzgerald DJ, FitzGerald GA: Dietary fish oil accelerates the response to coronary thrombolysis with tissue-type plasminogen activator. Evidence for a modest platelet inhibitory effect in vivo. *Circulation* 1990; 82:178–187.
118. Leaf A: Cardiovascular effects of fish oils. Beyond the platelet. *Circulation* 1990; 82:624–628.
119. Dehmer GJ, Popma JJ, van den Berg EK, Eichhorn EJ, Prewitt JB, Campbell WB, et al: Reduction in the rate of early restenosis after coronary angioplasty by a diet supplemented with N − 3 fatty acids. *N Engl J Med* 1988; 319:733–740.
120. Grigg LE, Kay TWH, Valentine PA, Larkins R, Flower DJ, Manolas EG, et al: Determinants of restenosis and lack of effect of

dietary supplementation with eicosapentaenoic acid on the incidence of coronary restenosis after angioplasty. *J Am Coll Cardiol* 1989; 13:665–672.

121. Reis GJ, Boucher TM, Sipperly ME, Silverman, DI, McCabe CH, Bain DS, et al: Randomised trial of fish oil for prevention of restenosis after coronary angioplasty. *Lancet* 1989; 2:177–181.

122. Milner MR, Gallin RA, Leffingwell A, Pichard AD, Brooks-Robinson S, Rosenberg V, et al: Usefulness of fish oil supplements in preventing clinical evidence of restenosis after percutaneous transluminal coronary angioplasty. *Am J Cardiol* 1989; 64:294–299.

122a. Bairati I, Roy L, Francois M: Double-blind randomized, controlled trial of fish oil supplements in prevention of recurrences of stenosis after coronary angioplasty. *Circulation* 1992; 85:950–956.

123. Oberg M, Hedner U, Bergentz SE: Effect of dextran 70 on factor VIII and platelet function in von Willebrand's disease. *Thromb Res* 1978; 12:629–634.

124. Swanson KT, Vlietstra RE, Holmes DR, Smith HC, Reeder GS, Bresnahan JF, et al: Efficacy of adjunctive dextran during percutaneous transluminal coronary angioplasty. *Am J Cardiol* 1984; 54:447–448.

125. Popat KD, Pitt B: Hemodynamic effect of prostaglandin E infusion in patients with acute myocardial infarction and left ventricular failure. *Am Heart J* 1982; 103:485–489.

126. Coppe D, Sobel M, Seavans L, Levine F, Salzman E: Preservation of platelet function and number by prostacyclin during cardiopulmonary bypass. *J Thorac Cardiovasc Surg* 1981; 81:274–278.

127. Pitt B, Shea MJ, Romson JL, Lucchesi BR: Prostaglandins and prostaglandin inhibitors in ischemic heart disease. *Ann Intern Med* 1983; 99:83–92.

128. Bugiardini R, Galvani M, Ferrini D, Gridelli C, Tallemeto D, Macri N, et al: Myocardial ischemia during intravenous prostacyclin administration: Hemodynamic findings and precautionary measures. *Am Heart J* 1987; 113:234–240.

129. Nicolini FA, Mehta JL, Nichols WW, Saldeen TGP, Grant M: Prostacyclin analogue iloprost decreases thrombolytic potential of tissue-plasminogen activator in canine coronary thrombosis. *Circulation* 1990; 81:1115–1122.

130. Topol EJ, Ellis SG, Califf RM, George BS, Stump DC, Bates ER, et al: Combined tissue-plasminogen activator and prostacyclin therapy for acute myocardial infarction. *J Am Coll Cardiol* 1989; 14:877–884.

131. Fiddler GI, Lumley P: Preliminary clinical studies with thromboxane synthase inhibitors and thromboxane receptor blockers: A review. *Circulation* 1990; 81(suppl I):I69–I78.

132. Ashton JH, Schmitz JM, Campbell WB, Ogletree ML, Raheja S, Taylor AL, et al: Inhibition of cyclic flow variations in stenosed canine coronary arteries by thromboxane A_2/prostaglandin H receptor antagonists. *Circ Res* 1986; 59:568–578.

133. Lane IF, Irwin JTC, Jennings SA, Poskitt KR, Greenhalgh RM, McCollum CM: et al: A specific thromboxane A_2 antagonist evaluated in vascular graft patients (abstr). *Br J Surg* 1984; 71:903.

134. Hacker RW, Torka M, Yuksetan I: Reduction of the vein graft occlusion rate after coronary artery bypass surgery by treatment with a thromboxane receptor antagonist. *Z Kardiol* 1989; 78(suppl 3): 48–49.

135. Yao S-K, Rosolowsky M, Anderson V, Golino P, McNatt JM, deClerck F, et al: Combined thromboxane A_2 synthetase inhibition and receptor blockade are effective in preventing spontaneous and epinephrine-induced canine coronary cyclic flow variations. *J Am Coll Cardiol* 1990; 16:705–713.

136. Hoet B, Arnout J, Van Geet C, Deckmyn H, Verhaeghe R,Vermylen J: Ridogrel, a combined thromboxane synthase inhibitor and receptor blocker, decreases elevated plasma beta-thromboglobulin levels in patients with documented peripheral arterial disease. *Thromb Haemost* 1990; 64:87–90.

137. Golino P, Piscione F, Willerson JT, Capelli-Bigazzi M, Focaccio A, Villari B, et al: Divergent effects of serotonin on coronary-artery dimensions and blood flow in patients with coronary atherosclerosis and control patients. *N Engl J Med* 1991; 324:641–648.

138. McFadden EP, Clarke JG, Davies GJ, Kaski JC, Haider AW, Maseri A: Effect of intracoronary serotonin on coronary vessels in patients with stable angina and patients with variant angina. *N Engl J Med* 1991; 324:648–654.

139. Golino P, Ashton JH, McNatt J, Glas-Greenwalt P, Shang-Kun Y, O'Brien RA, et al: Simultaneous administration of thromboxane A_2– and serotonin S_2–receptor antagonists markedly enhances thrombolysis and prevents or delays reocclusion after tissue-type plasminogen activator in a canine model of coronary thrombosis. *Circulation* 1989; 79:911–919.

140. Prevention of Atherosclerotic Complications with Ketanserin Trial Group: Prevention of atherosclerotic complications: controlled trial of ketanserin. *Br Med J* 1989; 298:424–430.

141. Coller BS, Folts JD, Smith SR, Scudder LE, Jordan R: Abolition of in vivo platelet thrombus formation in primates with monoclonal antibodies to the platelet GPIIb/IIIa receptor. Correlation with bleeding time, platelet aggregation, and blockade of GPIIb/IIIa receptors. *Circulation* 1989; 80:1766–1774.

142. Gold HK, Coller BS, Yasuda T, Saito T, Fallon JT, Guerrero L, et al: Rapid and sustained coronary artery recanalization with combined bolus injection of recombinant tissue-type plasminogen activator and monoclonal antiplatelet GPIIb/IIIa antibody in a canine preparation. *Circulation* 1988; 77:670–677.

143. Shebuski RJ, Stabilito IJ, Sitko GR, Polokoff MH: Acceleration of recombinant tissue-type plasminogen activator–induced thrombolysis and prevention of reocclusion by the combination of heparin and the Arg-Gly-Asp-containing peptide bitistatin in a canine model of coronary thrombosis. *Circulation* 1990; 82:169–177.

144. Badimon L, Badimon JJ, Chesebro JH, Fuster V: Inhibition of thrombus formation: Blockage of adhesive glycoprotein mechanisms versus blockage of the cyclooxygenase pathway (abstr). *J Am Coll Cardiol* 1988; 11(suppl A):30A.

145. Baur HR, Van Tassel RA, Pierach CA, Gobel RL: Effects of sulfinpyrazone early graft closure after myocardial infarction. *Am J Cardiol* 1982; 49:420–424.

Chapter 69

Pharmacology of Thrombolytic Drugs

D. Collen, M.D., Ph.D. ■ M. Verstraete, M.D., Ph.D.

One approach to the treatment of an established thrombosis consists of the pharmacologic dissolution of the blood clot by the intravenous infusion of substances, called plasminogen activators, which activate a blood enzyme system known as the fibrinolytic system.[1] Plasminogen activators have a high specificity for their substrate plasminogen in which a single peptide bond Arg^{561}—Val^{562} is hydrolyzed yielding the active enzyme *plasmin*. Free plasmin is very rapidly neutralized by the serine proteinase inhibitor (serpin), α_2-antiplasmin, whereas fibrin-bound plasmin is protected from rapid inhibition.[1]

Currently, five plasminogen activators are available for thrombolytic therapy: streptokinase, anisoylated plasminogen streptokinase activator complex (APSAC), single-chain urokinase-type plasminogen activator (scu-PA), two-chain urokinase-type plasminogen activator (tcu-PA, urokinase), and tissue-type plasminogen activator (t-PA).

STREPTOKINASE

Physicochemical Properties

Streptokinase is a nonenzyme protein produced by several strains of hemolytic streptococci. It consists of a single polypeptide chain with a molecular weight of 47,000 to 50,000 daltons and contains 414 amino acids.[2] The region comprising amino acids 1 to 230 shows some homology with trypsin-like serine proteinases but lacks an active site serine residue.

Mechanism of Plasminogen Activation

Streptokinase activates plasminogen indirectly, following a three-step mechanism.[3] In the first step, streptokinase forms an equimolar complex with plasminogen, which undergoes a conformational change resulting in the exposure of an active site in the plasminogen moiety. In the second step, this active site catalyzes the activation of plasminogen to plasmin. In a third step, plasminogen-streptokinase molecules are converted to plasmin-streptokinase complexes.[4] The presence of an active site in the plasminogen-streptokinase complex was demonstrated by reaction with an active site titrant, thereby blocking its conversion to the plasmin-streptokinase complex.[3,5] The plasminogen activating potential of the plasminogen-streptokinase complex is two- to threefold higher than that of the plasmin-streptokinase complex.[6] The activation of native plasminogen by the plasminogen-streptokinase complex is enhanced 6.5-fold in the presence of fibrin and twofold in the presence of fibrinogen.[7,8]

The equimolar plasminogen-streptokinase complex converts rapidly to the plasmin-streptokinase complex by proteolytic cleavage of both the plasminogen and the streptokinase moieties. In plasminogen, the Arg^{561}—Val^{562} and the Lys^{77}—Lys^{78} peptide bonds are cleaved[9,10]; four modified forms of streptokinase differing in molecular weight by 4000 to 5000 daltons have been observed depending on the species origin of the plasminogen.[11] With human plasminogen, a major proteolytic derivative with molecular weight of 36,000 daltons is generated.[12]

The plasmin-streptokinase complex can also be formed by mixing plasmin and streptokinase, which react with a rate constant of 5.4×10^7 per *M* per s.[13] The complex has a dissociation constant of 5×10^{-11} *M*; these data indicate that the complex is extremely rapidly formed and that it is very stable. The active site residues in the plasmin-streptokinase complex are the same as those in the plasmin molecule. The main differences between the enzymatic properties of plasmin and the plasmin-streptokinase complex are found in their interaction with plasminogen and with α_2-antiplasmin. Plasmin, in contrast to its complex with streptokinase, is unable to activate plasminogen, and it is rapidly neutralized by α_2-antiplasmin, which does not inhibit the plasmin(ogen)-streptokinase complex.

In addition to its effects on fibrin within the thrombus, plasmin also degrades plasma proteins involved in the maintenance of blood coagulation. Since streptokinase ultimately generates free circulating plasmin, it is associated with a *systemic fibrinolytic state* characterized by plasminogen activation in plasma (hyperplasminemia), diminished α_2-antiplasmin, and breakdown of fibrinogen, factor V, and factor VIII.

Pharmacokinetic Properties

The elimination half-life of streptokinase is approximately 20 min ($t_{\frac{1}{2}\alpha}$ = 4 min; $t_{\frac{1}{2}\beta}$ = 30 min).[14] The level of antistreptokinase antibodies from previous infections with beta-hemolytic streptococci varies greatly among individuals. About 350,000 units of streptokinase is required to neutralize the circulating antibodies in 95 percent of a healthy population, with individual requirements ranging between 25,000 and 3×10^6 units.[15] A few days after streptokinase administration, the antistreptokinase titer rises rapidly to 50 to 100 times the preinfusion value and remains high for at least 4 to 6 months, during which period renewed thrombolytic treatment with streptokinase or compounds containing streptokinase is impracticable since exceedingly high doses are required to overcome the antibodies.

Dosage

The initial dose of streptokinase must be adequate to neutralize the plasma levels of antistreptococcal antibodies: The streptokinase-antibody complex thus formed is rapidly cleared from the circulation. The initial dose for an individual patient can be determined either by the streptokinase resistance test (if laboratory facilities are available) or, more practically, a standard initial intravenous dose ranging from about 500,000 to 750,000 units can be given over 10 to 30 min followed by a continuous intravenous maintenance dose of 100,000 units hourly for one or more days. Such a fixed dosage regimen produces a satisfactory thrombolytic effect in most patients.[15,16] Moreover, laboratory control is simplified and thrombolytic treatment can be started without delay. In the last 15 years, however, high-dose (1.5×10^6 units), short-term (15 to 60 min infusion) streptokinase treatment has been routinely used with great success in patients with acute myocardial infarction.

Adverse Effects

In the larger, detailed trials incidences of transient hypotension as high as 10 percent have been reported.[17] While a hypotensive episode may be dramatic, it is usually halted by cessation of infusion. The more rapidly streptokinase is infused, the more likely a hypotensive reaction will occur; therefore, in order to avoid hypotension, the intravenous infusion should not exceed 500 units/kg per min.

Streptokinase is antigenic in humans and thus is able to provoke serious anaphylactic reactions (urticaria, bronchospasm, angioedema). In practice, however, major allergic reactions are relatively rare. Shivering, pyrexia, or rashes appear in up to 10 percent of patients during or shortly after streptokinase infusion.

Bleeding is the most common complication of streptokinase. Minor bleeding occurs in 3 to 4 percent of patients.[17] These episodes are usually related to puncture or injection sites, but microscopic hematuria and blood-streaked sputum are also noted. Major bleeding (requiring transfusion) occurs in 0.4 to 10 percent of all patients.[17] Heparin and/or aspirin treatment may enhance the frequency of bleeding, as does invasive catheter insertions. The most serious complication is cerebral bleeding, which is reported at an incidence of 0.1 to 0.2 percent, while ischemic stroke occurs in 0.8 percent of patients. In the large trials there is an excess of "early" hemorrhagic or other strokes on the day of streptokinase treatment or the day after. Thereafter, however, there are fewer strokes, and the overall risk of stroke is similar in streptokinase and placebo-treated patients.[17]

If streptokinase infusion is repeated between 5 days and 6 months following the initial infusion, it may be ineffective clinically because of a high titer of circulating antibodies. Recently, it was found that 3 months after streptokinase treatment, antibody titers were high enough to neutralize fully 1.5×10^6 units of streptokinase.[18] At 4 to 8 months, 18 of 20 patients had neutralization titers such that at least 50 percent of a dose of 1.5×10^6 units of streptokinase would have been neutralized. After 8 months, neutralization titers still ranged from 0.4×10^6 to 2.0×10^6 units in 40 percent of the patients. (See also Chap. 60.)

ANISOYLATED PLASMINOGEN STREPTOKINASE ACTIVATOR COMPLEX

Anisoylated plasminogen streptokinase activator complex (APSAC) was constructed with the intention to control the enzymatic activity of the plasmin(ogen)-streptokinase complex by a specific reversible chemical protection of its catalytic center (i.e., by insertion of a *p*-anisoyl group). This approach should prevent premature neutralization of the agent in the bloodstream and enable its activation to proceed in a controlled and sustained manner.[19]

Physicochemical Properties

Anistreplase (APSAC, Eminase) is an equimolar noncovalent complex between human lysine-plasminogen and streptokinase. The catalytic center is located at the carboxyterminal region of plasminogen, whereas the lysine-binding sites are comprised within the aminoterminal region of the molecule. Specific acylation of the catalytic center is achieved by the use of a reversible acylating agent, *p*-amidinophenyl-*p*′-anisate·HCl. The cationic amidino group is positioned to interact with the anionic carboxyl group of Asp^{735} within the catalytic center of plasminogen. The anisoyl head is located at a position near the Ser^{741} residue of the active center, so that the required acyl transfer can take place.[19]

Pharmacokinetic Properties

There is a slow dissociation of streptokinase from the plasminogen-streptokinase complex with a rate constant of less than 10^{-4} per s.[20] The deacylation rate constant of APSAC, however, is greater than 10^{-4} per s,[21] and the activity of the complex is controlled by the deacylation rate rather than by dissociation. The deacylation half-life of anistreplase in human plasma was claimed to be 105 to 120 min,[22] although it was previously reported to be 40 min in buffer.[19] In healthy volunteers, an apparent clearance half-life of 70 min was found for anistreplase, as compared to 25 min for the plasminogen-streptokinase complex formed upon administration of streptokinase alone.[14] In patients with acute myocardial infarction treated with anistreplase, half-lives of 90 to 112 min were reported for the plasma clearance of fibrinolytic activity.[23] This reversible blocking of the catalytic site by acylation delays the formation of the fibrinolytic enzyme plasmin but has no influence on the lysine-binding sites involved in binding of the complex to fibrin, although the affinity of plasminogen for fibrin is very weak. Deacylation starts immediately after dissolution of the lyophilized material and proceeds gradually after intravenous injection. Deacylation uncovers the catalytic center, which converts plasminogen to plasmin. This deacylation of the complex occurs both in the circulation and at the fibrin surface, and the fibrin specificity of thrombolysis by anistreplase is only marginal.

Dosage

The recommended dose of anistreplase in acute myocardial infarction is 30 units (1 mg = 1 unit and 30 mg contains approximately 1,250,000 units of streptokinase) to be given as a bolus injection. In aggregate, comparative studies indicate that the efficacy for coronary thrombolysis (angiographic patency) of anistreplase is comparable or somewhat higher than intravenous streptokinase but lower than intracoronary streptokinase.[24]

Adverse Effects

In trials comparing anistreplase (30 units) versus intravenously infused streptokinase (1.5×10^6 IU over 60 min), the same fall in fibrinogen concentrations and the same incidence of adverse events were noted.[25–28] Since anistreplase contains considerable amounts of streptokinase, it causes immunization. The antibody titer may increase up to 60-fold within 2 to 3 weeks and still be very high after 3 months.[14,18] Repeated administration within a year should be avoided. (See also Chap. 60.)

SINGLE-CHAIN UROKINASE-TYPE PLASMINOGEN ACTIVATOR

Physicochemical Properties

Single-chain urokinase-type plasminogen activator (scu-PA, pro-urokinase) is a single-chain glycoprotein with a molecular weight of 54,000 containing 411 amino acids.[29,30] scu-PA is the native zymogenic precursor of urokinase. Limited hydrolysis by plasmin or kallikrein of the Lys^{158}-Ile^{159} peptide bond converts the molecule to two-chain urokinase-type plasminogen activator (tcu-PA). Specific hydrolysis of the Glu^{143}-Leu^{144} peptide bond in scu-PA yields a low-molecular-weight scu-PA with a molecular weight of 32,000 (scu-PA-32k).[31] Thrombin cleaves the Arg^{156}-Phe^{157} peptide bond in scu-PA, resulting in an inactive tcu-PA molecule.[32] scu-PA is synthesized by epithelial cells, by mononuclear cells, and by the placenta.

Mechanism of Plasminogen Activation

scu-PA has no specific affinity for fibrin.[33] In purified systems, scu-PA has some intrinsic plasminogen activating potential that is, however, less than 1 percent of that of tcu-PA.[34] Conversion of scu-PA to tcu-PA at a fibrin clot apparently causes a significant positive-feedback mechanism for clot lysis in human plasma in vitro.[34,35] This conversion may, however, play a less important role in in vivo thrombolysis due to preferential fibrin-associated activation of plasminogen by scu-PA.

Recombinant scu-PA (rscu-PA, saruplase) is under clinical investigation as a fibrin-specific thrombolytic agent in patients with acute myocardial infarction. Therapeutic doses range between 40 and 80 mg infused over 1 h.[36] These doses were found to cause a systemic activation of the fibrinolytic system and fibrinogen degradation. This may be due, at least in part, to conversion of scu-PA to tcu-PA in the circulation.

One approach to improve the thrombolytic potential and fibrin specificity of scu-PA has consisted in the construction of more stable recombinant molecules by destroying the plasmin cleavage site using site-directed mutagenesis. Such mutations included replacement of Lys^{158} by Glu, Gly, Met, Ala, or Val or replacement of Ile^{159} by Pro or Gly.[37–39] The fibrinolytic potential in a plasma milieu of all these mutants was much lower than that of wild-type rscu-PA. In a rabbit jugular vein thrombosis model, however,[40] rscu-PA-Ala^{158} and rscu-PA-Glu^{158} at a dose of 2 mg/kg produced significant clot lysis (22 to 23 percent, as compared to 45 percent for wild-type rscu-PA). These findings support the hypothesis that scu-PA has intrinsic plasminogen activating potential in vivo. The potency of these plasmin-resistant rscu-PA mutants is, however, three- to fivefold lower than that of wild-type rscu-PA and thus probably too low to allow their use in humans.

Mutants of rscu-PA with impaired cleavage by plasmin have also been constructed by substitution of both Lys^{135} by Gln and Phe^{157} by Asp.[41] This resulted in a molecule that is not cleaved at position 135 and that is converted 10 times slower to tcu-PA due to a negatively charged residue adjacent to Lys^{158}.

Low-molecular-weight scu-PA (scu-PA-32k) purified from the conditioned medium of a human lung adenocarcinoma cell line[31] or prepared by recombinant deoxyribonucleic acid (DNA) technology[42] had a fibrinolytic capacity in a rabbit jugular vein thrombosis model comparable to that of wild-type rscu-PA.[42] The relative fibrin specificity of scu-PA, as compared to tcu-PA, was maintained at thrombolytic doses. Provided this relative fibrin specificity also holds for patients with thromboembolic disease, scu-PA-32k might be a practical alternative molecule for the large-scale production of a fibrin-specific thrombolytic agent by recombinant DNA technology.

Dosage

Saruplase is the generic name for full-length unglycosylated human recombinant scu-PA obtained from *Escherichia coli.* With a preparation containing 160,000 IU/mg, the dose used successfully in patients with acute myocardial infarction was 20 mg given as a bolus and 60 mg over the next 60 min, immediately followed by an intravenous heparin infusion (20 IU/kg per h) for 72 h.[36]

Adverse Effects

In a direct double-blind comparison between intravenous saruplase (80 mg over 60 min) and streptokinase (1.5×10^6 IU over 60 min) in 401 patients with acute myocardial infarction, a somewhat smaller reduction in circulating fibrinogen levels was observed with saruplase.[36] The transfusion requirement was significantly less in the saruplase group versus the streptokinase group (4 vs. 11 percent), and the same holds for the bleeding episodes (14 vs. 25 percent).

TWO-CHAIN UROKINASE-TYPE PLASMINOGEN ACTIVATOR

Physicochemical Properties

Urokinase is a naturally occurring plasminogen activator excreted in human urine, from which it can be extracted; urokinase may also be isolated from tissue cultures of human embryonic kidney cells. It is a trypsin-like enzyme composed of two polypeptide chains (molecular weight 20,000 and 34,000). Urokinase may occur in two molecular forms designated S_1 (molecular weight 31,600, low-molecular-weight urokinase) and S_2 (molecular weight 54,000, high-molecular-weight urokinase), the former being a proteolytic degradation product of the latter.[43] The complete primary structure of high-molecular-weight urokinase has been elucidated[44]; the light chain contains 158 amino acids and the heavy chain 253.

Mechanism of Plasminogen Activation

Urokinase activates plasminogen directly following Michaelis-Menten kinetics. This double-chain molecule has no specific affinity for fibrin and activates fibrin-bound and circulating plasminogen relatively indiscriminately. Extensive plasminogen activation and depletion of α_2-antiplasmin may occur following treatment with urokinase, leading to systemic activation of the fibrinolytic system with low levels of fibrinogen.

Dosage

As the level of inhibitors in plasma is relatively constant, a fixed dosage regimen can readily be used. In acute myocardial infarction, the dose of urokinase is either 2×10^6 units as a bolus or 3×10^6 units over 90 min.[45] For over a decade, an initial intravenous dose of 4000 units/kg body weight over 10 min followed by the same maintenance dose per kilogram hourly has been recommended for the treatment of acute major pulmonary embolism. At present, a bolus dose in the right atrium of 15,000 units/kg of body weight has been recommended in this indication; an intravenous infusion of 3×10^6 units of urokinase (1×10^6 units over 10 min and 2×10^6 units over the next 110 min) is presently being tested.

Adverse Effects

Purified urokinase preparations are nonantigenic and nonpyrogenic and their use is usually associated with a milder coagulation defect than observed with streptokinase but with a similar incidence of bleeding.

TISSUE-TYPE PLASMINOGEN ACTIVATOR

The plasminogen activator in blood is synthesized and secreted by endothelial cells and is called tissue-type plasminogen activator (t-PA). Antigen levels of t-PA in normal plasma are about 5 ng/mL. Tissue-type plasminogen activator has been purified from the tissue culture fluid of stable human melanoma cell lines in sufficient amounts to study its biochemical and biologic properties.[46]

Physicochemical Properties

Tissue-type plasminogen activator is a serine proteinase with a molecular weight of about 70,000 consisting of a single polypeptide chain of 527 amino acids with Ser as the NH_2-terminal amino acid (Fig. 69-1). The complete primary structure has been deduced from the complementary DNA (cDNA) sequence.[47] It was shown subsequently that native t-PA contains an NH_2-terminal extension of three amino acids (Gly-Ala-Arg).[48] Plasmin (but also kallikrein and factor Xa) converts t-PA to a two-chain molecule by hydrolysis of the Arg^{275}-Ile^{276} peptide bond (using a numbering system based on a total of 527 amino acids). The NH_2-terminal region (heavy chain) is composed of multiple structural-functional domains, including a *fingerlike* domain (F) homologous to the finger domains in fibronectin[49]; an *epidermal growth factor–like domain* (E) homologous to that of urokinase, protein C, and coagulation factors IX and X; and two disulfide bond triple-loop structures commonly called

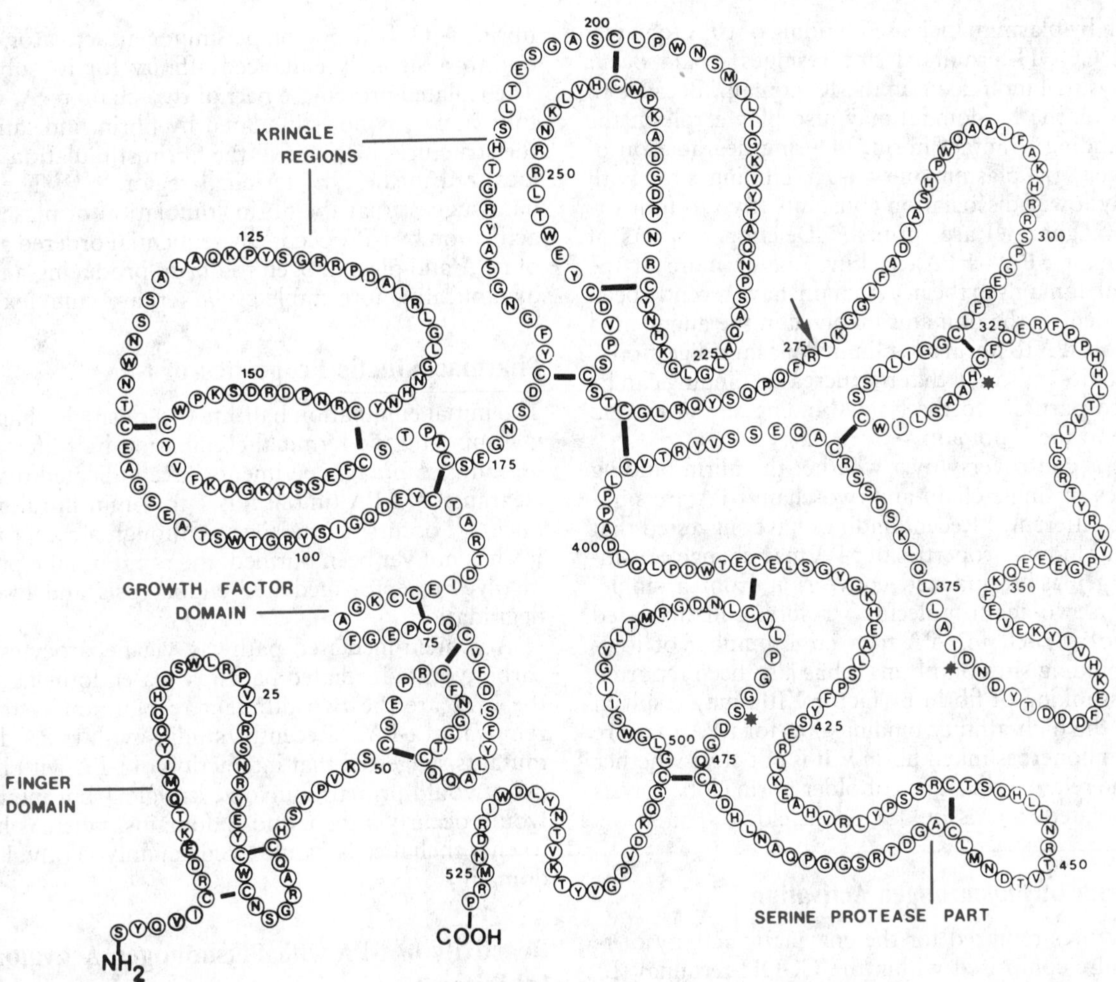

FIGURE 69-1 Schematic representation of the primary structure of tissue-type plasminogen activator. The arrow indicates the cleavage site for plasmin. The active site residues are indicated with an asterisk.

"kringles" (K_1 and K_2), homologous to the kringle regions in plasminogen.[47] The COOH-terminal region (light chain), comprising residues 276 to 527, is homologous to other serine proteinases and contains the catalytic site, which is composed of His^{322}, Asp^{371}, and Ser^{478}.[47]

The assembly of the t-PA gene is an example of the *exon-shuffling* principle; the different structural domains on the heavy chain are encoded by a single exon or by two adjacent exons.[50] Because of the striking correlation between the intron-exon distribution of the gene and the domain structure of the protein,[51] it was suggested that these domains would be autonomous, structural, and/or functional entities (*modules*).[50,52] These structural domains of t-PA are involved in most of its functions and interactions, including its enzymatic activity, binding to fibrin, stimulation of plasminogen activation by fibrin, binding to receptors, and inhibition by plasminogen activator inhibitors. The validity of the exon-shuffling concept for t-PA has been investigated by the construction of mutants with precise domain deletions, insertions, or substitutions and the evaluation of the fibrin affinity, the fibrin specificity, and the pharmacokinetic and thrombolytic properties of such mutants.

Fibrin Affinity of t-PA

The NH_2-terminal (heavy) chain of t-PA comprises the structures involved in its fibrin binding as evidenced by the intact fibrin affinity of the heavy chain isolated after mild reduction of two-chain t-PA.[53,54] Evidence obtained with domain deletion mutants of t-PA indicated that its affinity for fibrin is mediated via the finger domain and mainly via the second kringle domain. A lysine-binding site is involved in the interaction of the kringle-2 domain but not of the finger domain with fibrin.[55] Gething et al.[56] have suggested, however, that the kringle-1 and kringle-2 domains of t-PA would be equivalent in their affinity for fibrin, although the kringle-1 domain contains no lysine-binding site. A weaker lysine-binding site in kringle 2[57] similar to the *AH site* (aminohexyl site) in plasminogen has also been suggested. This AH site would interact with internal lysine residues in the fibrin matrix, whereas the lysine-binding site would interact with COOH-terminal lysine residues.[55]

It has been suggested that in the process of fibrinolysis, binding of t-PA to intact fibrin would be mediated initially by the F domain. Subsequently, upon partial fibrin digestion by plasmin, increased binding of t-PA to newly exposed COOH-terminal lysine residues would occur via the lysine-binding site in the K_2 domain. Because of its AH site, the K_2 domain may also play a role in the initial binding to intact fibrin.[57] During degradation of fibrin(ogen) by plasmin, new t-PA binding sites with markedly lower dissociation constants (two to four orders of magnitude) are formed.[58] Deletion mutants of recombinant t-PA (rt-PA), lacking one or more of the structural domains in the heavy chain, have recently been used to identify the domains involved in the augmented binding of t-PA to fibrin after limited plasmic digestion.[59] These studies indicated that the increased binding can be attributed partially to the lysine-binding site in K_2 and partially to the F domain.

There is controversy over whether the fibrin-binding properties of single-chain and two-chain t-PA are similar[58,60] or different.[61] Recent findings have suggested that the fibrin-binding properties of t-PA may change considerably by plasmin-induced conversion from a single-chain to a two-chain molecule,[62] resulting in enhanced binding of two-chain t-PA to a large number of low-affinity binding sites on fibrin. It has also been reported that crosslinking of fibrin by factor XIIIa may result in masking the high-affinity binding sites for t-PA that are present in noncrosslinked fibrin.[62] It is not clear whether or not the relative resistance of older fibrin clots to lysis may be related to crosslinking of the clot.

Mechanism of Plasminogen Activation

The structures required for the enzymatic activity of t-PA are fully comprised within the COOH-terminal (B) chain, as evidenced by the intact activity of the isolated B chain, separated chemically[53,54] or prepared by recombinant DNA technology.[63] This COOH-terminal region contains the catalytic triad composed of His^{322}, Asp^{371}, and Ser^{478}.[47]

In the absence of fibrin, t-PA is a poor plasminogen activator, mainly because of a low affinity for its substrate.[64] Single-chain t-PA is less active toward low-molecular-weight substrates and inhibitors,[65] but its activity toward plasminogen was shown to be comparable to that of the two-chain form.[60] The intrinsic enzymatic activity of single-chain t-PA was confirmed by the construction of rt-PA mutants in which the plasmin cleavage site for conversion to two-chain t-PA was destroyed by site-specific mutagenesis of Arg^{275} to Glu (ref. 61) or to all other amino acids.[58] Such mutants were demonstrated to have lower activity than two-chain t-PA in the absence of fibrin but full plasminogen activating activity in the presence of fibrin.[61] The catalytic activity of single-chain t-PA was confirmed by Boose et al.[66] using a mutant enzyme with Arg^{275} replaced by Gly. Inhibition by plasminogen activator inhibitor 1 (PAI 1) was also comparable for the wild-type and mutant t-PA. In contrast to other zymogen precursors of serine proteinases, the single-chain form of t-PA thus appears to be an active enzyme. The enzymatic properties of single-chain t-PA may be due to the formation of a salt bridge between the positively charged epsilon amino group in the side chain of Lys^{416} and Asp^{477}, thereby stabilizing the one-chain form in an active conformation.[67] In the presence of fibrin, t-PA is a potent plasminogen activator, mainly due to a strongly enhanced affinity for its substrate.[64] The isolated proteinase part of two-chain t-PA, which is fully active, is not stimulated by fibrin, indicating that the structures involved in the fibrin stimulation are also localized in the NH_2-terminal region.[53,54,63] The kinetic data suggest that the fibrin stimulation of plasminogen activation by t-PA occurs by sequential ordered addition of t-PA and plasminogen to fibrin, producing a thermodynamically more stable cyclic ternary complex.[64]

Pharmacokinetic Properties of t-PA

The initial elimination half-life ($t_{\frac{1}{2}\alpha}$) of single chain rt-PA is 4 min and the terminal elimination half-life $t_{\frac{1}{2}\beta}$ about 46 min.[68] Animal experiments have indicated that rapid clearance of t-PA (initial $t_{\frac{1}{2}}$ is 1 to 4 min in rabbits and mice)[69,70] occurs via the liver. Although a receptor for t-PA has not yet been purified, the rapid uptake probably involves receptor-mediated endocytosis and lysosomal degradation.

A protein-mediated pathway via hepatocytes and a carbohydrate-mediated pathway via endothelial cells in the liver are the two different recognition systems for removal of t-PA.[71] Recently, studies with rt-PA deletion mutants suggested that interaction of t-PA with hepatocytes would primarily involve kringle 1 but in addition would occur via the F and E domains, whereas binding to endothelial cells would occur mainly via the F and E domain.[72]

Reactivity of t-PA with Plasminogen Activator Inhibitor 1

Plasminogen activator inhibitor 1 belongs to the serpin superfamily; it neutralizes very rapidly single-chain t-PA, two-chain t-PA, and urokinase.[73] To design mutants of t-PA that are resistant to inhibition by PAI-1, the interactions between the active site of t-PA and PAI-1 have been modeled based on the known three-dimensional structure of the trypsin-trypsin inhibitor complex.[74,75] Specific amino acids (residues Lys^{296}-His-Arg-Arg-Ser-Pro-Gly^{302} and Arg^{304}) in t-PA have been identified that make contact with PAI-1 but not with the substrate plasminogen. Mutants of rt-PA obtained by site-specific mutagenesis in this region are fully active toward substrates but display significant resistance to inhibition by PAI-1. In view of the large excess of t-PA over PAI-1 achieved during thrombolytic therapy, resistance of t-PA mutants to PAI-1 may not directly constitute a significant advantage over wild-type t-PA. High PAI-1 levels may, however, contribute to the occurrence of reocclusion, and PAI-1-resistant mutants of rt-PA may be useful for maintenance infusion after initial thrombolysis.

Dose of Single-Chain t-PA (Alteplase)

The presently recommended dose of alteplase (Activase, Actilyse) for the treatment of acute myocardial infarction is 100 mg administered as 60 mg in the first hour (of which 6 to 10 mg is administered as a bolus over the first 1 to 2 min), 20 mg over the second hour, and 20 mg over the third hour. More recently it was proposed to give the same total dose of 100 mg but "front loaded," commencing with a bolus of 15 mg followed by 50 mg in the next 30 min and the remaining 35 mg in the following 60 min.[76] Recently, the dose of 15 mg intravenous bolus of alteplase followed by 0.75 mg/kg over 30 min (not to exceed 50 mg) and then 0.50 mg/kg over 60 min (not to exceed 35 mg) was utilized in a large clinical trial (GUSTO). Whichever regimen used, it is important to coadminister intravenous heparin during and after alteplase treatment. (See Chap. 68.) For catheter-directed local thrombolysis with alteplase in patients with recent peripheral arterial occlusion, the dose of 0.05 to 0.10 mg/kg per h over an 8-h period is usually recommended.

Duteplase is the generic name for recombinant tissue-type plasminogen activator produced in its two-chain form. It also differs from recombinant human alteplase due to a substitution of a methionine for a valine in position 245 in the amino acid sequence and is therefore a variant of the naturally occurring human t-PA. The specific activity of duteplase is approximately 300,000 units per milligram of protein, but different production lots may have specific activities that vary as much as ±100,000.[77] For this reason the dosage of duteplase is given in megaunits per kilogram of body weight (0.6 to 1.0 MU/kg over 4 h).[78,79]

Adverse Effects

Bleeding complications are the most common side effects with any thrombolytic agent, including alteplase. The reported rates of bleeding during treatment with any thrombolytic agent depend on the methods of data collection, which can be very elaborate in trials on a limited number of patients or limited in megatrials including thousands of patients. Valid conclusions can only be obtained by direct comparisons between drugs in a given trial. In a recent large trial directly comparing alteplase and streptokinase, the reported incidence of cerebral bleeding (confirmed by computed tomography scan and necropsy) was similar for the two thrombolytic agents, but overall, significantly more strokes were reported in the alteplase group.[80,81] For both agents there was an excess of strokes in patients above 70 years of age (>70: 2.7 percent alteplase, 1.6 percent streptokinase; ≤70: 0.9 percent alteplase, 0.8 percent streptokinase). Significantly more major bleeds occurred in patients allocated to streptokinase. The total number of bleeds (minor plus major), however, was significantly higher with alteplase (4.2 vs. 3.3 percent). More allergic reactions (0.2 vs. 1.7 percent) and hypotension (1.7 vs. 3.8 percent) were seen with streptokinase. (See also Chap. 60.)

PLASMINOGEN ACTIVATOR FROM BAT SALIVA

Physicochemical Properties

The saliva of the vampire bat (*Desmodus rotundus*) contains a single-chain plasminogen activator (Bat-PA) that is about 85 percent homologous to alteplase but lacks the kringle-2 domain and the plasmin-sensitive cleavage site for conversion to a two-chain form.[81] A smaller molecular form additionally lacks the finger domain.[82] In contrast to alteplase, the component present in the vampire bat saliva exhibits a stricter requirement for a fibrin cofactor[81,83] that is not satisfied by fibrinogen.[84] Furthermore, the Bat-PA activity is quiescent in human plasma, but levels of activity similar to alteplase are manifest in the presence of fibrin.[85] Since the molecule lacks the plasmin-sensitive cleavage point, this naturally occurring protein remains stable in the circulation. The protein is now being produced by recombinant DNA technology in a eukaryotic cell line with a specific activity of about 300,000 units/mg as compared to alteplase on fibrin plates.[84]

Pharmacokinetic Properties

The efficacy of bolus injection of Bat-PA was compared to an intravenous bolus of alteplase in a rabbit model of femoral arterial thrombosis.[86] The maximal femoral artery reperfusion flows were equivalent after intravenous injection of 42 nmol of Bat-PA per kilogram or 42 nmol of alteplase per kilogram, but the time to reach maximal flow was approximately one-half that of alteplase. Equipotent thrombolytic doses of Bat-PA and alteplase reduce the plasma fibrinogen concentrations maximally by 14 and 69 percent, respectively from control values.

The clearance of Bat-PA from rabbits is best described by a biphasic profile that exhibits a short α phase (1.5 min) and a longer β phase (17 min) with approximately 80 percent clearance by the relatively slow β elimination phase. The overall clearance rate for Bat-PA is approximately 11 mL/min per kg, which is fourfold less than that of alteplase.

STAPHYLOKINASE

Physicochemical Properties

Staphylokinase, a protein with a molecular weight of 15,500 produced by *Staphylococcus aureus*, was reported to have profibrinolytic properties in 1948.[86] The gene coding for the bacterial protein has now been cloned and expressed in *E. coli*[87,88] and in *Bacillus subtilis*.[89] Staphylokinase, like streptokinase, forms a stoichiometric complex with plasminogen, and this complex then activates plasminogen following Michaelis-Menten kinetics.[90] In the absence of fibrin, α_2-antiplasmin rapidly inhibits the plasminogen-staphylokinase complex but not the plasminogen-streptokinase complex. Addition of 6-aminohexanoic acid induces a concentration-dependent reduction of the inhibition rate of the plasminogen-staphylokinase complex. Staphylokinase induces dose-dependent lysis of a ^{125}I-fibrin-labeled human plasma clot submersed in citrated human plasma without causing fibrinogenolysis.

Mechanism of Plasminogen Activation

The following mechanism may explain the relatively fibrin-specific clot lysis with staphylokinase in a plasma milieu.[90–92] In the absence of fibrin, the plasminogen-staphylokinase complex is rapidly neutralized by α_2-antiplasmin, thus preventing systemic plasminogen activation. In the presence of fibrin, the plasminogen-staphylokinase complex binds to the clot via the lysine-binding sites of the plasminogen moiety. Thus, its inhibition rate by α_2-antiplasmin is markedly reduced, allowing preferential plasminogen activation at the fibrin surface.[90]

Pharmacokinetics

In models of venous thrombosis in hamsters and rabbits, staphylokinase is a potent thrombolytic agent with a thrombolytic potency comparable to that of streptokinase.[93] The plasma clearance following bolus injection of staphylokinase in hamsters and rabbits is rapid (1.1 to 1.4 mL/min and 14 to 15 mL/min, respectively) as a result of short initial half-lives (1.8 to 1.9 min in hamsters and 1.7 to 2.0 min in rabbits).

THROMBUS TARGETED THROMBOLYTIC DRUGS

Thrombi contain both fibrin-rich and platelet-rich material. Plasminogen activators may be targeted to a thrombus by conjugation with monoclonal antibodies directed against specific epitopes in fibrin or against surface proteins on platelets. Furthermore, bispecific monoclonal antibodies containing one site that recognizes the thrombus and one site that binds the plasminogen activator may be used to concentrate the therapeutic agent at the surface of the thrombus.

One approach is to target the thrombolytic agent to a fibrin clot by conjugation with monoclonal antibodies that are fibrin specific and do not cross-react with fibrinogen.[94] Chemical conjugates of two-chain urokinase[94,95] with monoclonal antibodies directed against the NH_2 terminal of the Bβ chain of fibrin were shown to have a threefold enhanced thrombolytic potency in a plasma milieu in vitro.

A chemical conjugate between saruplase and a monoclonal antibody (MA-15C5) with a more than 1000-fold higher affinity for fragment D-dimer of human cross-linked fibrin than for fibrinogen has been prepared.[96,97] This conjugate had a 6.4-fold higher fibrinolytic potency than saruplase in a human plasma milieu in vitro[96] and an eightfold higher thrombolytic efficiency with fourfold slower clearance than unconjugated saruplase in a rabbit jugular vein thrombosis model.[98]

The fibrin selectivity of the saruplase conjugate is superior to that of saruplase. While conjugation per se reduces the thrombolytic potency, its targeting property against the thrombus overcomes the negative effect of conjugation.[99] Experiments in rabbits cannot directly be extrapolated to humans because the monoclonal antibodies used do not interact with rabbit fibrin and fibrinogen, whereas in humans interaction of the conjugate with circulating fibrinogen or fibrin(ogen) degradation products may interfere with its thrombolytic potency.

Chemical conjugates have also been made between single-chain alteplase and a monoclonal antibody specific for the NH_2-terminal part of the Bβ chain of fibrin (MA-59D8).[100–102] This resulted in a 3.2- to 4.5-fold enhancement of clot lysis in human plasma in vitro and a 2.8 to 9.6 times higher potency than t-PA in a rabbit thrombosis model without causing fibrinogenolysis. Schnee and coworkers[103] have engineered a recombinant version of the alteplase MA-59D8 conjugate. The MA-59D8 heavy-chain gene was cloned and combined in an expression vector with sequence coding for a portion of the c2b constant region and for the B chain of alteplase that contains the catalytic site. This construct was transfected into cloned cells derived from the MA-59D8 hybridoma, which had lost the capacity to express the heavy chain. The chimeric proteins indeed had antifibrin antibody activity and retained plasminogen activating potential.[103]

Another approach consists in the production of bifunctional antibodies that contain a fibrin-specific monoclonal antibody and an alteplase-specific monoclonal antibody. Such duplex antibodies have been obtained by chemical coupling[104,105] or by recombinant DNA technology[106] and were indeed shown to concentrate alteplase at a fibrin matrix.

Monoclonal antibodies that recognize epitopes on the surface of activated platelets, but not of resting platelets, represent another targeting vector for thrombolytic agents toward platelet-rich thrombi. Bode et al.[107] have chemically coupled two-chain t-PA to a monoclonal antibody that selectively binds to platelet membrane glycoprotein IIb/IIIa with a significant in vitro enhancement of clot lysis. In addition, saruplase was chemically conjugated to monoclonal antibodies directed against proteins that are expressed on the surface of stimulated platelets but not on the surface of resting platelets.[108] These antibody-saruplase complexes have a significantly increased thrombolytic potency as compared to saruplase.

REFERENCES

1. Collen D: On the regulation and control of fibrinolysis. *Thromb Haemost* 1980; 43:77–89.
2. Jackson KW, Tang J: Complete amino acid sequence of streptokinase and its homology with serine proteases. *Biochemistry* 1982; 21:6620–6625.
3. Reddy KNN: Mechanism of activation of human plasminogen by streptokinase. In: Kline DL, Reddy KNN (eds): *Fibrinolysis*. Boca Raton, FL, CRC Press, 1980: 71–94.
4. Summaria L, Wohl RC, Boreisha IG, Robbins KC: A virgin enzyme derived from human plasminogen. Specific cleavage of the arginyl-560-valyl peptide bond in the diisopropoxyphosphinyl virgin enzyme by plasminogen activators. *Biochemistry* 1982; 21:2056–2059.
5. McClintock DK, Bell PH: The mechanism of activation of human plasminogen by streptokinases. *Biochem Biophys Res Commun* 1971; 43:694–702.
6. Markus G, DePasquale JL, Wissler FC: Quantitative determination of the binding of E-aminocaproic acid to native plasminogen. *J Biol Chem* 1978; 253:727–732.
7. Fears R, Hibbs MJ, Smith RAG: Kinetic studies on the interaction of streptokinase and other plasminogen activators with plasminogen and fibrin. *Biochem J* 1985; 229:555–558.
8. Camiolo SM, Markus G, Evers JL, Hobika GH: Augmentation of streptokinase activator activity by fibrinogen or fibrin. *Thromb Res* 1980; 17:697–706.
9. McClintock DK, Englert ME, Dziobkowski C, Snedeker EH,

Bell PH: Two distinct pathways of the streptokinase-mediated activation of highly purified human plasminogen. *Biochemistry* 1974; 13:5334–5344.
10. Bajaj SP, Castellino FJ: Activation of human plasminogen by equimolar levels of streptokinase. *J Biol Chem* 1977; 252:492–498.
11. Reddy KNN: Kinetics of active center formation in dog plasminogen by streptokinase and activity of a modified streptokinase. *J Biol Chem* 1976; 251:6624–6629.
12. Siefring Jr GE, Castellino FJ: Interaction of streptokinase with plasminogen. Isolation and characterization of a streptokinase degradation product. *J Biol Chem* 1976; 251:3913–3920.
13. Cederholm-Williams SA, De Cock F, Lijnen HR, Collen D: Kinetics of the reactions between streptokinase, plasmin and α_2-antiplasmin. *Eur J Biochem* 1979; 100:125–132.
14. Staniforth DH, Smith RAG, Hibbs M: Streptokinase and anisoylated streptokinase plasminogen complex. Their action on haemostasis in human volunteers. *Eur J Clin Pharmacol* 1983; 24:751–756.
15. Verstraete M, Vermylen J, Amery A, Vermylen C: Thrombolytic therapy with streptokinase using a standard dosage scheme. *Br Med J* 1966; 5485:454–456.
16. Hirsh J, O'Sullivan EF, Martin M: Evaluation of a standard dosage schedule with streptokinase. *Blood* 1970; 35:341–349.
17. Goa KL, Henwood JM, Stolz JF, Langley MS, Clissold SP: Intravenous streptokinase. A reappraisal of its therapeutic use in acute myocardial infarction. *Drugs* 1990; 39:693–719.
18. Jalihal S, Morris GK: Antistreptokinase titres after intravenous streptokinase. *Lancet* 1990; 335:184–185.
19. Smith RAG, Dupe RJ, English PD, Green J: Fibrinolysis with acyl-enzymes: A new approach to thrombolytic therapy. *Nature* 1981; 290:505–508.
20. Törngren S: Optimal regimen of low-dose heparin prophylaxis in gastrointestinal surgery. *Acta Chir Scand* 1979; 145:87–93.
21. Esmail AF, Dupe RJ, English PD, Smith RAG: Pharmacokinetic and pharmacodynamic comparisons of acylated streptokinase, plasminogen complexes with different deacylation rate constants (abstr.). *Haemostasis* 1984; 14:84.
22. Ferres H, Hibbs M, Smith RAG: Deacylation studies in vitro on anisoylated plasminogen streptokinase activator complex. *Drugs* 1987; 33(suppl 3):80–82.
23. Nunn B, Esmail A, Fears R, Ferres H, Strandring R: Pharmacokinetic properties of anisoylated plasminogen streptokinase activator complex and other thrombolytic agents in animals and in humans. *Drugs* 1987; 33(suppl):88–92.
24. Verstraete M: Thrombolytic treatment in acute myocardial infarction. *Circulation* 1990; 82(suppl II):II96–II109.
25. Monnier P, Sigwart U, Vincent A, Bachmann F, Goy JJ, Schaller MD, et al: Anisoylated plasminogen streptokinase activator complex versus streptokinase in acute myocardial infarction. Preliminary results of a randomised study. *Drugs* 1987; 33(suppl 3):175–178.
26. Monassier JP, Hanssen M: Haematological effects of anisoylated plasminogen streptokinase activator complex and streptokinase in patients with acute myocardial infarction. Interim report of the IRS II study. *Drugs* 1987; 33(suppl 3):247–252.
27. Hoffmann JJML, Bonnier JJRM, de Swart JBRM, Custers P, Vijgen M: Systemic effects of anisoylated plasminogen streptokinase activator complex and streptokinase therapy in acute myocardial infarction. Coagulation aspects of the Dutch Invasive Reperfusion Study. *Drugs* 1987; 33(suppl 3):242–246.
28. Prowse CV, Hornsey V, Ruckley CV, Boulton FE: A comparison of acylated streptokinase-plasminogen complex and streptokinase in healthy volunteers. *Thromb Haemost* 1982; 47:132–135.
29. Holmes WE, Pennica D, Blaber M, Rey MW, Guenzler WA, Steffens GJ, et al: Cloning and expression of the gene for prourokinase in *Escherichia coli. Biotechnology* 1985; 3:923–929.
30. Steffens GJ, Günzler WA, Ötting F, Frankus E, Flohé L: The complete amino acid sequence of low molecular mass urokinase from human urine. *Hoppe-Seyler's Z Physiol Chem* 1982; 363:1043–1058.
31. Stump DC, Lijnen HR, Collen D: Purification and characterization of single-chain urokinase-type plasminogen activator from human cell cultures. *J Biol Chem* 1986; 261:1274–1278.
32. Ichinose A, Fujikawa K, Suyama T: The activation of pro-urokinase by plasma kallikrein and its inactivation by thrombin. *J Biol Chem* 1986; 261:3486–3489.
33. Lijnen HR, Zamarron C, Blaber M, Winkler ME, Collen D: Activation of plasminogen by pro-urokinase. I. Mechanism. *J Biol Chem* 1986; 261:1253–1258.
34. Lijnen HR, Van Hoef B, De Cock F, Collen D: The mechanism of plasminogen activation and fibrin dissolution by single chain urokinase-type plasminogen activator in a plasma milieu in vitro. *Blood* 1989; 73:1864–1872.
35. Declerck PJ, Lijnen HR, Verstreken M, Moreau H, Collen D: A monoclonal antibody specific for two-chain urokinase-type plasminogen activator. Application to the study of the mechanism of clot lysis with single-chain urokinase-type plasminogen activator in plasma. *Blood* 1990; 75:1794–1800.
36. PRIMI Trial Study Group: Randomised double-blind trial of recombinant pro-urokinase against streptokinase in acute myocardial infarction. *Lancet* 1989; 1:863–868.
37. Nelles L, Lijnen HR, Collen D, Holmes WE: Characterization of a fusion protein consisting of amino acids 1 to 263 of tissue-type plasminogen activator and amino acids 144 to 411 of urokinase-type plasminogen activator. *J Biol Chem* 1987; 262:10855–10862.
38. Lijnen HR, Nelles L, Van Hoef B, Demarsin E, Collen D: Structural and functional characterization of mutants of recombinant single-chain urokinase-type plasminogen activator obtained by site-specific mutagenesis of Lys^{158}, Ile^{159} and Ile^{160}. *Eur J Biochem* 1988; 177:575–582.
39. Gurewich V, Pannell R, Broeze RJ, Mao J: Characterization of the intrinsic fibrinolytic properties of pro-urokinase through a study of plasmin-resistant mutant forms produced by site-specific mutagenesis of lysine 158. *J Clin Invest* 1988; 82:1956–1962.
40. Collen D, Mao J, Stassen JM, Broeze R, Lijnen HR, Abercrombie D, et al: Thrombolytic properties of Lys^{158} mutants of recombinant single chain urokinase-type plasminogen activator (scu-PA) in rabbits with jugular vein thrombosis. *J Vasc Med Biol* 1989; 1:46–49.
41. Fujitani B, Furuichi M, Okamura H, Komiya M, Karasawa T, Tokemoto H: Thrombolytic properties of recombinant human single chain urokinase type plasminogen activator and its mutants (abstr). *Thromb Haemost* 1989; 62:544.
42. Lijnen HR, Nelles L, Holmes WE, Collen D: Biochemical and thrombolytic properties of a low molecular weight form (comprising Leu^{144} through Leu^{411}) of recombinant single-chain urokinase-type plasminogen activator. *J Biol Chem* 1988; 263:5594–5598.
43. White WF, Barlow GH, Mozen MM: The isolation and characterization of plasminogen activators (urokinase) from human urine. *Biochemistry* 1966; 5:2160–2169.
44. Günzler WA, Steffens GJ, Ötting F, Kim SMA, Frankus E, Flohé L: The primary structure of high molecular mass urokinase from human urine. The complete amino acid sequence of the A chain. *Hoppe-Seyler's Z Physiol Chem* 1982; 363:1155–1165.
45. Mathey DG, Schofer J, Sheehan FH, Becher H, Tilsner V, Dodge HT: Intravenous urokinase in acute myocardial infarction. *Am J Cardiol* 1985; 55:878–882.
46. Collen D, Rijken DC, Van Damme J, Billiau A: Purification of human tissue-type plasminogen activator in centigram quantities from human melanoma cell culture fluid and its conditioning for use in vivo. *Thromb Haemost* 1982; 48:294–296.
47. Pennica D, Nedwin E, Hayflick JS, Seeburg PH, Derynck R, Palladino MA, et al: Human tumour necrosis factor: Precursor structure, expression and homology to lymphotoxin. *Nature* 1984; 312:724–729.
48. Jörnvall H, Pohl G, Bergsdorf N, Wallén P: Differential proteolysis and evidence for a residue exchange in tissue plasminogen activator suggest possible association between two types of protein microheterogeneity. *FEBS Lett* 1983; 156:47–50.
49. Banyai L, Varadi A, Patthy L: Common evolutionary origin of the fibrin-binding structures of fibronectin and tissue-type plasminogen activator. *FEBS Lett* 1983; 163:37–41.
50. Patthy L: Evolution of the proteases of blood coagulation and fibrinolysis by assembly from modules. *Cell* 1985; 41:657–663.
51. Ny T, Elgh F, Lund B: The structure of the human tissue-type plasminogen activator gene: Correlation of intron and exon structures to functional and structural domains. *Proc Natl Acad Sci USA* 1984; 81:5355–5359.
52. Pannekoek H, de Vries C, van Zonneveld AJ: Mutants of human tissue-type plasminogen activator (t-PA): Structural aspects and functional properties. *Fibrinolysis* 1988; 2:123–132.

53. Rijken DC, Groeneveld E: Isolation and functional characterization of the heavy and light chains of human tissue-type plasminogen activator *J Biol Chem* 1986; 261:3098–3102.
54. Holvoet P, Lijnen HR, Collen D: Characterization of functional domains in human tissue-type plasminogen activator with the use of monoclonal antibodies. *Eur J Biochem* 1986; 158:173–177.
55. van Zonneveld AJ, Veerman H, Pannekoek H: On the interaction of the finger and the kringle-2 domain of tissue-type plasminogen activator with fibrin. Inhibition of kringle-2 binding to fibrin by E-amino caproic acid. *J Biol Chem* 1986; 261:14214–14218.
56. Gething MJ, Adler B, Boose JA, Gerard RD, Madison EL, McGoockey D, et al: Variants of human tissue-type plasminogen activator that lack specific structural domains of the heavy chain. *EMBO J* 1988; 7:2731–2740.
57. Verheijen JH, Caspers MPM, de Munk GAW, Enger-Valk BE, Chang GTG, Pouwels PH: Sites in tissue-type plasminogen activator involved in the interaction with fibrin, plasminogen and low molecular weight ligands. *Thromb Haemost* 1987; 58:491 (abstr).
58. Higgins DL, Vehar GA: Interaction of one-chain and two-chain tissue plasminogen activator with intact and plasmin-degraded fibrin. *Biochemistry* 1987; 26:7786–7791.
59. de Vries C, Veerman H, Pannekoek H: Identification of the domains of tissue-type plasminogen activator involved in the augmented binding to fibrin after limited digestion with plasmin. *J Biol Chem* 1989; 264:12604–12610.
60. Rijken DC, Hoylaerts M, Collen D: Fibrinolytic properties of one-chain and two-chain human extrinsic (tissue-type) plasminogen activator. *J Biol Chem* 1982; 257:2920–2925.
61. Tate KM, Higgins DL, Holmes WE, Winkler ME, Heyneker HL, Vehar GA: Functional role of proteolytic cleavage at arginine-275 of human tissue plasminogen activator as assessed by site-directed mutagenesis. *Biochemistry* 1987; 26:338–343.
62. Husain SS, Hasan AAK, Budzynski AZ: Differences between binding of one-chain and two-chain tissue plasminogen activators to non-cross-linked and cross-linked fibrin clots. *Blood* 1989; 74:999–1006.
63. Verheijen JH, Caspers MPM, Chang GTG, De Munk GAW, Pouwels PH, Enger-Valk BE. Involvement of finger domain and kringle 2 domain of tissue-type plasminogen activator in fibrin binding and stimulation of activity by fibrin. *EMBO J* 1986; 5:3525–3530.
64. Hoylaerts M, Rijken DC, Lijnen HR, Collen D: Kinetics of the activation of plasminogen by human tissue plasminogen activator. Role of fibrin. *J Biol Chem* 1982; 257:2912–2919.
65. Wallén P, Bergsdorf N, Rånby M: Purification and identification of two structural variants of porcine tissue plasminogen activator by affinity adsorption on fibrin. *Biochim Biophys Acta* 1982; 719:318–328.
66. Boose JA, Kuismanen E, Gerard R, Sambrook J, Gething MJ: The single-chain form of tissue-type plasminogen activator has catalytic activity: Studies with a mutant enzyme that lacks the cleavage site. *Biochemistry* 1989; 28:635–643.
67. Petersen LC, Boel E, Johannessen M, Foster D: Quenching of the amidolytic activity of one-chain tissue-type plasminogen activator by mutation of lysine-416. *Biochemistry* 1990; 29:3451–3457.
68. Garabedian HD, Gold HK, Leinbach RC, Johns JA, Yasuda T, Kanke M, et al: Comparative properties of two clinical preparations of recombinant human tissue-type plasminogen activator in patients with acute myocardial infarction. *J Am Coll Cardiol* 1987; 9:599–607.
69. Korninger C, Stassen JM, Collen D: Turnover of human extrinsic (tissue-type) plasminogen activator in rabbits. *Thromb Haemost* 1981; 46:658–661.
70. Fuchs HE, Berger H, Pizzo SV: Catabolism of human tissue plasminogen activator in mice. *Blood* 1985; 65:539–544.
71. Kuiper J, Otter M, Rijken DC, van Berkel TJC: Characterization of the interaction in vivo of tissue-type plasminogen activator with liver cells. *J Biol Chem* 1988; 263:18220–18224.
72. Chen SA, Foster DL, Keyt BA, Fendly B, Sinicropi D, Baughman RA, et al: Correlation of hepatocyte uptake with in vivo clearance of recombinant tissue-type plasminogen activator and identification of the domains responsible for clearance (abstr). *Thromb Haemost* 1989; 62:337.
73. Kruithof EKO, Tran-Thang C, Ransijn A, Bachmann F: Demonstration of a fast-acting inhibitor of plasminogen activators in human plasma. *Blood* 1984; 64:907–913.
74. Sambrook J, Hanahan D, Rodgers L, Gething MJ: Expression of human tissue-type plasminogen activator from lytic viral vectors and in established cell lines. *Mol Biol Med* 1986; 3:459–481.
75. Madison EL, Goldsmith EJ, Gerard RD, Gething MJH, Sambrook JF, Bassel-Duby RS: Amino acid residues that affect interaction of tissue-type plasminogen activator with plasminogen activator inhibitor 1. *Proc Natl Acad Sci USA* 1990; 87:3530–3533.
76. Neuhaus KL, Feuerer W, Jeep-Tebbe S, Niederer W, Vogt A, Tebbe U: Improved thrombolysis with a modified dose regimen of recombinant tissue-type plasminogen activator. *J Am Coll Cardiol* 1989; 14:1566–1569.
77. Christodoulides M, Boucher DW: The potency of tissue-type plasminogen activator (TPA) determined with chromogen and clot-lysis assays. *Biologicals* 1990; 18:103–111.
78. Grines CL, for the Burroughs Wellcome Study Group: Efficacy and safety of weight adjusted dosing of a new tissue plasminogen activator preparation in acute myocardial infarction (abstr). *Circulation* 1988; 78(suppl II):127.
79. Grines CL, Nissen SE, Booth DC, Branco MC, Gurley JC, Bennett KA, et al: A new thrombolytic regimen for acute myocardial infarction using combination half dose tissue-type plasminogen activator with full dose streptokinase: A pilot study. *J Am Coll Cardiol* 1989; 14:573–580.
80. The International Study Group: In-hospital mortality and clinical course of 20,891 patients with suspected acute myocardial infarction randomised between alteplase and streptokinase with or without heparin. *Lancet* 1990; 336:71–75.
81. Gardell SJ, Duong LT, Diehl RE, York JD, Hare TR, Register RD, et al: Isolation, characterization, and cDNA cloning of a vampire bat salivary plasminogen activator. *J Biol Chem* 1989; 264:17947–17952.
82. Baldus B, Donner P, Boidal W, Schleuning WD: A novel plasminogen activator from the saliva of the vampire bat *Desmodus rotundus*. 6th GTH-Kongres, Kiel, 1990.
83. Baldus B, Gehrmann G, Bringmann P, Donner P: Kinetics of Glu-plasminogen activation do not explain the fibrinolytic potency of recombinant *Desmodus rotundus* salivary plasminogen activator α_1 (rDSPA$_{\alpha 1}$) (abstr). *Thromb Haemost* 1991; 65:884.
84. Gardell SJ, Hare TR, Bergum PW, Cuca GC, O'Neill-Palladino L, Zavodny SM: Vampire bat salivary plasminogen activator is quiescent in human plasma in the absence of fibrin unlike human tissue plasminogen activator. *Blood* 1990; 76:2560–2564.
85. Gardell SJ, Ramjit T, Stabilito II, Fujita T, Lynch JJ, Cuca GC, et al: Effective thrombolysis without marked plasminemia after bolus intravenous administration of vampire bat salivary plasminogen activator in rabbits. *Circulation* 1991; 84:244–253.
86. Lack CH: Staphylokinase: An activator of plasma protease. *Nature* 1948; 161:559–560.
87. Sako T, Sawaki S, Sakurai T, Ito S, Yoshizawa Y, Kondo I: Cloning and expression of the staphylokinase gene of *Staphylococcus aureus* in *E. coli*. *Mol Gen Genet* 1983; 190:271–277.
88. Sako T: Overproduction of staphylokinase in *Escherichia coli* and its characterization. *Eur J Biochem* 1985; 149:557–563.
89. Behnke D, Gerlach D: Cloning and expression in *Escherichia coli, Bacillus subtilis* and *Streptococcus sanguis* of a gene for staphylokinase—A bacterial plasminogen activator. *Mol Gen Genet* 1987; 210:528–534.
90. Lijnen HR, Van Hoef B, De Cock F, Okada K, Ueshima S, Matsuo O, et al: On the mechanism of fibrin-specific plasminogen activation by staphylokinase. *J Biol Chem* 1991; 226:11826–11832.
91. Matsuo O, Okada K, Fukao H, Tomioka Y, Ueshima S, Watanuki M, et al: Thrombolytic properties of staphylokinase. *Blood* 1990; 76:925–929.
92. Sakai M, Watanuki M, Matsuo O: Mechanism of fibrin-specific fibrinolysis by staphylokinase: Participation of α_2-plasmin inhibitor. *Biochem Biophys Res Commun* 1989; 162:830–837.
93. Lijnen HR, Stassen JM, Vanlinthout I, Fukao H, Okada K, Matsuo O, et al: Comparative fibrinolytic properties of staphylokinase and streptokinase in animal models of venous thrombosis. *Thromb Haemost* 1991; 66:468–473.
94. Bode C, Matsueda GR, Hui KY, Haber E: Antibody-directed

urokinase: A specific fibrinolytic agent. *Science* 1985; 229:765–767.

95. Bode C, Runge MS, Newell JB, Matsueda GR, Hager E: Thrombolysis by a fibrin-specific antibody Fab′-urokinase conjugate. *J Mol Cell Cardiol* 1987; 19:335–341.
96. Dewerchin M, Lijnen HR, Van Hoef B, De Cock F, Collen D: Biochemical properties of conjugates of urokinase-type plasminogen activator with a monoclonal antibody specific for cross-linked fibrin. *Eur J Biochem* 1989; 185:141–149.
97. Declerck PJ, Mombaerts P, Holvoet P, De Mol M, Collen D: Fibrinolytic response and fibrin fragment D-dimer levels in patients with deep vein thrombosis. *Thromb Haemost* 1987; 58:1024–1029.
98. Collen D, Dewerchin M, Stassen JM, Kieckens L, Lijnen HR: Thrombolytic and pharmacokinetic properties of conjugates or urokinase-type plasminogen activator with a monoclonal antibody specific for crosslinked fibrin. *Fibrinolysis* 1989; 3:197–202.
99. Collen D, Dewerchin M, Rapold HJ, Lijnen HR, Stassen JM: Thrombolytic and pharmacokinetic properties of a conjugate of recombinant single-chain urokinase-type plasminogen activator with a monoclonal antibody specific for cross-linked fibrin in a baboon venous thrombosis model. *Circulation* 1990; 82:1744–1753.
100. Runge MS, Bode C, Matsueda GR, Haber E: Conjugation to an antifibrin monoclonal antibody enhances the fibrinolytic potency of tissue plasminogen activator in vitro. *Biochemistry* 1988; 27:1153–1157.
101. Bode C, Runge MS, Matsueda GR, Gold HK, Haber E: Can intrinsic tissue-type plasminogen activator be concentrated at the site of a thrombus? (abstr). *J Am Coll Cardiol* 1987; 9:81A.
102. Runge MS, Bode C, Matsueda GR, Haber E: Antibody-enhanced thrombolysis: Targeting of tissue plasminogen activator in vivo. *Proc Natl Acad Sci USA* 1987; 84:7659–7662.
103. Schnee JM, Runge MS, Matsueda GR, Hudson NW, Seidman JG, Haber E, et al: Construction and expression of a recombinant antibody-targeted plasminogen activator. *Proc Natl Acad Sci USA* 1987; 84:6904–6908.
104. Bode C, Runge MS, Newell JB, Matsueda GR, Haber E: Characterization of an antibody-urokinase conjugate. A plasminogen activator targeted to fibrin. *J Biol Chem* 1987; 262:10819–10823.
105. Charpie JR, Runge MS, Matsueda GR, Collen D, Haber E: Enhancement of fibrinolysis by single chain urokinase (scu-PA) with a bifunctional antibody having both fibrin and scu-PA specificities (abstr). *Clin Res* 1988; 36:436A.
106. Haber E, Quertermous T, Matsueda GR, Runge MS: Innovative approaches to plasminogen activator therapy. *Science* 1989, 243:51–56.
107. Bode C, Meinhardt G, Runge MS, Eberle T, Schuler G, Kübler W, et al: Conjugation of urokinase to an antiplatelet antibody results in a more potent fibrinolytic agent (abstr). *Thromb Haemost* 1989; 52:483.
108. Dewerchin M, Lijnen HR, Stassen JM, et al: Effect of chemical conjugation of recombinant single-chain urokinase-type plasminogen activator with monoclonal antiplatelet antibodies, on platelet aggregation and on plasma clot lysis in vitro and in vivo. *Blood* 1991; 78:1005–1018.

SECTION D

Interventional and Surgical Techniques to Treat Patients with Coronary Artery Disease

Chapter 70

Indications for Percutaneous Transluminal Coronary Angioplasty and Atherectomy

Spencer B. King III, M.D. ■ *John S. Douglas, Jr., M.D.*

Coronary angioplasty was first performed by Andreas Gruentzig in September 1977.[1] The procedure has had a dramatic growth, with an estimated 133,000 procedures performed in 1986,[2] and over 350,000 in 1991. Such growth brings into question the proper role for angioplasty, both as an adjunct to medical therapy for coronary disease and as an alternative to coronary bypass surgery. Although the balloon catheter was the first and is still the predominant method of angioplasty, other techniques such as atherectomy,[3–5] lasers,[6] and stents[7,8] have expanded the capabilities of coronary interventions.[9] (See Chap. 71.) Since the procedure is invasive and carries some risk, the selection of patients for the procedure is of great interest to the patients, physicians, and third-party carriers.

Initially, coronary angioplasty was performed for discrete, proximal, noncalcified, subtotal lesions principally in one coronary artery. Because of the demonstrated early beneficial results and the dramatic improvements in technology, the technique has undergone rapid growth. The use of angioplasty for single-vessel disease continues to predominate, but there is also a significant shift toward angioplasty as a substitute for bypass surgery in multivessel disease. Accordingly, the procedure should be tested against the standards established by surgery.[10] Principal indications for surgery continue to be the relief of angina, and indeed the Veterans Administration (VA) study[11] and the Coronary Artery Surgery Study (CASS)[12] showed the significant superiority of surgery over medical therapy in relief of angina. In addition, several subsets of patients in whom survival has been improved with surgery have been established. These include patients with left main coronary disease,[13] patients with three-vessel coronary disease, and some patients with two-vessel disease when the anterior descending coronary artery is involved and when left ventricular function is impaired.[14–17]

Coronary angioplasty, which has been used since 1977, is only now undergoing controlled randomized trials against surgery and medical therapy. The National Institutes of Health is sponsoring two major trials comparing percutaneous transluminal coronary angioplasty (PTCA) with surgery for multivessel disease.[18] The first, begun in mid-1987 and entry completed in 1990, is the Emory Angioplasty Surgery Trial (EAST), and the other, a multicenter trial, is the Bypass Angioplasty Revascularization Investigation (BARI), in which recruitment was completed in 1991. The results of the Emory trial on 392 randomized patients will be available in mid-1993, and the BARI study involving over 1800 patients will be complete in 1996. Meanwhile, long-term follow-up of the first patients undergoing angioplasty in Zurich has shown encouraging results.[19] One hundred and thirty-three of 169 patients were successfully treated, and with a completed follow-up of 10 years there have been only 8 cardiac deaths with 75 percent of the surviving patients remaining asymptomatic. Repeat angioplasty, required in 29 patients, and subsequent bypass surgery, required in 31, document the reality of restenosis and progression of the disease. Review of the 427 patients undergoing angioplasty at Emory University Hospital in 1981 showed a 5-year survival rate of 97 percent, with 79 percent of the patients remaining free of cardiac events.[20] More recent experience in the National Heart, Lung, and Blood Institute (NHLBI) registry of patients collected in 1985 and 1986 showed the results in patients more typical of current experience. One-half had single-vessel disease, and the other half had multivessel disease. The operative mortality was 1 percent, and the 1-year event-free survival rate was 75 percent.[21] The ACME (Angioplasty Compared to Medicine) trial, sponsored by the VA system, compared angioplasty to medical therapy in single- and some double-vessel patients.[22] Angioplasty patients had a significant improvement in symptoms and exercise performance but more subsequent revascularization procedures.

Restenosis following coronary angioplasty occurs in 25 to 35 percent of patients,[23-25] and the restenosis rate is likely higher in patients with multivessel disease.[26] Repeat angioplasty has often been successful in managing those patients with restenosis.[27] Importantly, since the restenosis usually progresses slowly to a subtotal stenosis, the return of stable symptoms is a common event rather than a sudden, expected infarction. Nevertheless, restenosis contributes significantly to the cost of angioplasty.

Patients with two-vessel disease treated at Emory had a 5-year survival rate of 94 percent, and 71 percent were without myocardial infarction (MI) or coronary artery bypass surgery.[28] The 1-year follow-up of the NHLBI registry of patients treated in 1985 shows that 75 percent of the treated patients with multivessel disease were free from cardiac events.[21] The results of bypass surgery are also improving,[29] but they are moderated by the fact that many lower risk patients currently go for angioplasty, thereby leaving higher risk patients for surgery.

RISK OF ANGIOPLASTY

Despite technical improvements, angioplasty still poses some risk to the patient. At Emory University Hospital emergency bypass surgery is needed in 1.5 to 2.5 percent and MI has occurred in 2 percent of patients treated. Overall mortality among over 10,000 patients treated in the 1980s has been 0.3 percent,[30] with a slight increase in mortality in the past 3 years due to selection of increasing numbers of inoperable patients for salvage angioplasty. The 1985 to 1986 NHLBI registry showed a 3.5 percent incidence of emergency surgery, a 4 percent infarction rate, and a 1 percent mortality rate.[21] Because of the occasional need for emergency surgery, it is felt that surgical backup must be available in every institution performing angioplasty. The American College of Cardiology and the American Heart Association (ACC/AHA) Committee on PTCA in fact stated, "An experienced cardiovascular surgical team should be available within the institution for emergency surgery for all angioplasty procedures."[31] This statement may be reassessed in true emergency settings as angioplasty for acute MI becomes more commonly practiced. (See Chap. 71.)

Certain predictors of successful angioplasty have been identified. Some of these are male gender, single-vessel disease, single-lesion angioplasty, subtotal occlusions, absence of calcification, accessibility of the lesion, and normal left ventricular function. Features identified as being associated with acute, abrupt vessel closure at the time of angioplasty have been female gender, length of lesion, eccentric lesions, bifurcation/side branch lesions, angulation of the segment being dilated, other stenoses in the same vessel, and the presence of thrombus. Following angioplasty, the presence of an intimal tear or dissection and a high residual translesional gradient are strong predictors of abrupt reclosure.[32] If such closure occurs, the mortality risk is increased by advanced age, female gender, a history of hypertension, diabetes, prior MI, prior bypass surgery, multivessel disease, left main coronary disease, a large area of myocardium at risk, impairment of left ventricular function, and collateral vessels that supply significant areas of myocardium and originate distal to the segment to be dilated.[31,33] Restenosis, which may occur in all subsets of patients, has its own set of predictors: recent onset of angina of less than 2 months, unstable angina, variant angina, diabetes mellitus, multivessel disease, right ostial lesions, lesions located at the origin of the left anterior descending (LAD) or in the proximal anastomosis or body of vein grafts, chronic total occlusions, presence of thrombus, severity of the residual lesion, and severity of the residual translesional gradient.[23,24]

New technology has begun to provide solutions to clinical situations where balloon angioplasty has shown weakness.[9] Directional coronary atherectomy has shown definite advantages over balloon angioplasty in opening lesions that are very eccentric or at the origin of the LAD. Although directional atherectomy and excimer laser angioplasty were the only other technologies approved by the Food and Drug Administration (FDA) by 1992, rotoblator may be useful in very hard lesions, and stents may be useful as bailout devices after dissection and acute closure. (See also Chap. 71.) Stents may also improve restenosis rates in some large proximal vessels, but definitive conclusions await comparative trials.

SELECTION OF PATIENTS FOR PTCA

Considering the preceding information, selection for coronary angioplasty should be based on (1) the chance that a successful procedure can be performed without significant major complications, (2) the chance that a successful procedure will result in improvement of the patient's symptoms or avoidance of complications of coronary artery disease, (3) the chance that the procedure will have a sustained benefit, and (4) the relative likelihood that angioplasty will have a greater chance of achieving results equivalent to bypass surgery at a lower morbidity and cost.

CONTRAINDICATIONS

Certain contraindications are considered absolute: (1) absence of significant obstructing lesion, (2) multivessel disease with diffuse atherosclerosis in cases where coronary artery bypass grafting would be unequivocally more efficacious, (3) left main coronary artery disease in which the distal vessels are not protected by at least one completely patent bypass graft, and (4) absence of a formal cardiac surgical program within the institution.[31]

A number of relative contraindications include the following: (1) presence of coagulopathy; (2) no clinical evidence for inducible myocardial ischemia; (3) multivessel angioplasty in which sudden occlusion at any one dilatation site could result in massive left ventricular impairment and cardiogenic shock; (4) lesions in which the anticipated success rate is low; (5) borderline stenotic lesions, because recurrence following angioplasty of such lesions may produce significantly obstructing lesions; (6) angioplasty of the non-infarct-related arteries in patients with multivessel disease who are undergoing catheterization during the acute phase of MI; and (7) vein grafts with large eccentric lesions, which may tend to embolize.

INDICATIONS FOR CORONARY ANGIOPLASTY

Indications have been divided into those generally agreed upon throughout the community of cardiologists and surgeons and those in which there is some controversy at the present time. These categories have been taken from the ACC/AHA report on indications for PTCA.[31]

Single-Vessel Coronary Artery Disease: Asymptomatic or Mildly Symptomatic

Generally agreed-on indications are present in patients who have a significant lesion in a major epicardial coronary artery that subtends a large area of viable myocardium and who (1) show objective evidence of severe myocardial ischemia; (2) have been resuscitated from cardiac arrest or sustained ventricular tachycardia in the absence of acute MI; or (3) must undergo major vascular surgery such as repair of aortic aneurysm, iliofemoral bypass, or carotid surgery and who have angina or objective evidence of ischemia. Asymptomatic patients should have a lesion that would predict a high chance of angioplasty success and have a low risk for mortality should acute vessel closure occur.

There is somewhat more controversy concerning the indications for angioplasty in asymptomatic or minimally asymptomatic patients with lesions subtending at least a moderate-sized area of viable myocardium and who show objective evidence of myocardial ischemia and who have the following additional characteristics: at least a moderate likelihood of successful dilatation based on lesion-specific characteristics; a low risk of abrupt closure of the vessel; and a low risk for mortality and morbidity of the procedure.

Asymptomatic or mildly symptomatic patients who should *not* undergo angioplasty include those who have only a small area of myocardium at risk or do not manifest evidence of ischemia during laboratory testing. Additional characteristics in minimally symptomatic or asymptomatic patients that ordinarily preclude angioplasty include borderline lesions less than 50 percent in diameter, lesions that predict a poor chance of success or a high risk of abrupt closure, or the presence of disease that places them in a high-risk group for mortality and morbidity.

Single-Vessel Coronary Artery Disease: Symptomatic Patients

Patients with significant symptoms can be approached somewhat differently since a principal objective of angioplasty is to alleviate those symptoms. Generally agreed-upon indications include patients with angina pectoris class II, III, or IV and those with unstable angina pectoris with single-vessel disease who have (1) significant lesions in a major epicardial coronary artery subtending at least a moderate-sized area of myocardium and who show evidence of myocardial ischemia during laboratory testing or (2) angina pectoris that has been inadequately responsive to medical treatment or (3) intolerance of medical therapy because of side effects. These patients should have at least a moderate likelihood of successful dilatation and remain in a low-risk group for mortality and morbidity.

There is greater controversy concerning the indications for angioplasty in symptomatic single-vessel patients with lesions in a major epicardial coronary subtending at least a moderate-sized area of myocardium, objective evidence of myocardial ischemia, and a fair likelihood of successful dilatation without significant chance of abrupt closure but who are in a moderate-risk group for procedural morbidity and mortality. There are also differences of opinion concerning indications in patients who have significant angina but no evidence of myocardial ischemia and yet have a moderate likelihood of successful angioplasty and are also in the low-risk group for mortality and morbidity.

Those felt not suitable for angioplasty include patients who have only a small area of viable myocardium at risk in the absence of significant symptoms or who have clinical symptoms not likely indicative of ischemia. Furthermore, those who have lesions that have a very low likelihood of angioplasty success or a very high chance of abrupt closure or who are in a high-risk group for morbidity and mortality should not have angioplasty.

It is important that the chance of a successful procedure be weighed carefully against any risk of morbidity or mortality since the prognosis for survival in these single-vessel patients treated medically has generally been excellent.

Multivessel Coronary Artery Disease: Asymptomatic or Mildly Symptomatic Patients

Generally agreed-upon indications include the presence of a significant lesion in a major epicardial coronary artery that could be dilated and in which nearly complete revascularization would be accomplished because the additional lesion(s) subtend a small viable or nonviable area of myocardium. Patients in this group (1) should have a large area of myocardium at risk, (2) show objective evidence of severe myocardial ischemia while on medical therapy, (3) have been resuscitated from cardiac arrest or from sustained ventricular tachycardia in the absence of infarction, or (4) are undergoing major vascular surgery with objective evidence of ischemia and have lesions that have a high chance of successful dilatation and are in a low-risk group for abrupt closure, morbidity, or mortality.

More controversial indications in minimally symptomatic patients with multivessel disease are a moderate-sized area of myocardium at risk or objective evidence of myocardial ischemia that is not severe while the patient is on medical therapy. Additional features of some patients in this group that elicit controversy with respect to the need for angioplasty include significant lesions in two or more major epicardial coronary arteries, each of which subtends at least a moderate-sized area of myocardium; objective evidence of myocardial ischemia while on medical therapy; and lesions that have at least a moderately good chance of angioplasty success without risk of abrupt closure and have a low risk for mortality and morbidity.

Asymptomatic or mildly symptomatic patients who should *not* undergo angioplasty include those who have (1) only a small area of myocardium at risk, (2) subtotally occluded vessels requiring angioplasty wherein the development of total occlusion would result in severe hemodynamic collapse due to left ventricular dysfunction, (3) more than two major arteries with lesions that would predict either a low chance of angioplasty success or a high chance for abrupt closure and complications, or (4) lesions that place them in a high-risk group for morbidity and mortality.

Multivessel Coronary Artery Disease: Symptomatic Patients

Patients in this category who are generally considered candidates for angioplasty include those who have significant lesions in each of two major epicardial coronary arteries both subtending at least moderate-sized areas of viable myocardium and who (1) show objective evidence of myocardial ischemia while on medical therapy or (2) have angina pectoris that has proved inadequately responsive to medical therapy or (3) are intolerant of medical therapy because of uncontrollable side effects and have lesions that have a moderate or high chance of successful dilatation without undue risk of abrupt closure and if successfully dilated would provide relief of all major regions of ischemia. The latter are in the low-risk group for mortality and morbidity.

More controversial candidates for PTCA are patients with significant lesions in two or more major epicardial coronary arteries that subtend at least a moderate-sized area of myocardium and who are in a moderate-risk group for mortality and morbidity or who have angina pectoris but not necessarily objective evidence of myocardial ischemia while on medical therapy and who have lesions that have at least a moderate chance of successful dilatation and if dilated would provide relief of all major regions of ischemia. These patients are in a moderate-risk group for morbidity and mortality. In addition, this category includes patients who have disabling angina pectoris that has proved inadequately responsive to medical therapy and who are considered poor surgical candidates because of either advanced physiological age or coexisting medical conditions and in whom not all lesions can be successfully dilated and who are in a moderate-risk group for mortality and morbidity. Such so-called salvage patients should be selected only in close coordination with the cardiovascular surgeons to ensure that an attempt at angioplasty can be accomplished with a lower risk to the patient than an attempt at bypass surgery.

Those who should *not* have angioplasty attempted include patients with only a small area of myocardium at risk in the absence of disabling symptoms or who have a subtotally occluded vessel requiring angioplasty wherein the development of total occlusion of that vessel would result in severe hemodynamic collapse due to left ventricular dysfunction or who have lesions that have a very low chance of angioplasty success or a very high risk of abrupt closure of the vessel or those who are in a high-risk group for mortality and morbidity. Some patients totally unsuitable for coronary surgery can have high-risk angioplasty performed successfully, and this should be closely coordinated with surgical colleagues. This category, especially those with multiple prior bypass surgeries, currently represents a fairly frequent indication in some specialized angioplasty centers.

Acute Myocardial Infarction

The role of angioplasty in acute MI is the subject of a great deal of current investigation. The role of thrombolysis in the management of acute MI is now well established.[34–37] (See also Chap. 60.)

Generally agreed-upon indications for angioplasty in the setting of acute MI include those patients who, following infarction, have recurrent episodes of ischemic chest pain, particularly if accompanied by electrocardiographic changes or evidence of severe myocardial ischemia; have recurrent ventricular fibrillation while on intensive antiarrhythmic therapy; and have lesions that have a high chance of angioplasty success, have a low risk of abrupt vessel closure, and are in the low-risk group for mortality and morbidity.

More controversial indications include postinfarct patients with lesions that have a moderate chance of success and likelihood of avoiding abrupt vessel reclosure; those who require multivessel angioplasty; and those who are in a moderate-risk group for morbidity or mortality. There is also some controversy concerning the role of direct angioplasty as opposed to thrombolysis early in the course of MI.[38–40] (See Chap. 60.) Additional categories of patients in which the role of angioplasty is not yet clearly defined include those who have cardiogenic shock within the first few hours of MI or those who survived cardiogenic shock prior to hospital discharge; those who are asymptomatic and yet have a significant residual lesion in the infarct-related artery following thrombolytic therapy; those who show objective evidence of myocardial ischemia during laboratory testing performed prior to hospital discharge; and those who have suffered a non-Q-wave MI and although asymptomatic have a single high-grade lesion that is suitable for angioplasty and who are in the low-risk group for acute closure, morbidity, and/or mortality. (See Chap. 60.)

Angioplasty in the postinfarction patient should not be undertaken in certain situations. For example, dilatation of additional lesions in vessels other than the infarct-related artery within the early hours of infarction should not be attempted nor should angioplasty of residual lesions that are insignificant or borderline. Similarly, extremely complex lesions that have a low chance of angioplasty success or very high chance of abrupt closure should not be dilated. Furthermore, angioplasty in patients who are in a very high risk group for procedure-related mortality or morbidity or are within 48 h of thrombolytic therapy should ordinarily not be treated with angioplasty.[41]

The results at three recent trials comparing immediate angioplasty with thrombolytic treatment have been very encouraging.[38–40] It may be of particular value in patients with a contraindication to thrombolytic therapy. (See Chap. 60.)

THE VALUE OF CORONARY ANGIOPLASTY

Randomized trials are not the only method of establishing value of therapy. The high degree of symptomatic improvement documented in patients with single-vessel coronary artery disease undergoing angioplasty with the avoidance of bypass surgery has spawned the rapid development of coronary angioplasty. Most have agreed that suitable patients with symptomatic single-vessel disease are best treated with angioplasty. There is, however, a significant lack of data concerning the long-term efficacy of angioplasty in multivessel coronary artery disease, vis-à-vis coronary artery bypass surgery. Patients who have historically undergone multivessel angioplasty may differ significantly from those currently undergoing bypass surgery. Nonetheless, it has been claimed that the results of angioplasty can rival bypass surgery in multivessel disease. This is of great importance, not only for patients but also for society.

The National Institutes of Health has funded the two trials of angioplasty in patients with multivessel disease in order to establish whether or not the strategy of initial angioplasty is indeed competitive with the more traditional strategy of bypass surgery. The first of these trials, the EAST, as indicated earlier, has undergone completion of the entry phase in 1990 and follow-up is completed. The EAST is designed to test the strategy of initial angioplasty versus initial bypass surgery in patients in whom (1) it is agreed that revascularization is warranted, (2) multivessel disease is present, (3) prior bypass surgery or angioplasty has not been performed, (4) significant left main disease is absent, (5) left ventricular function shows an ejection fraction greater than 25 percent, and (6) chronic total occlusions that likely have been present for more than 3 months or long lesions exceeding 2 cm and serving viable myocardium are absent. Such patients who are suitable either for angioplasty or bypass surgery were asked to volunteer for this NIH-sponsored trial. In order to obtain useful answers in the shortest period of time, a 3-year duration of the trial was chosen. The endpoint of mortality is unlikely to be significantly different in this size study with a short follow-up. It was therefore decided that a composite endpoint of freedom from death, MI, or a large ischemic burden shown on tomographic stress thallium imaging would be the primary endpoint. All patients in EAST undergo angiography at 1 and 3 years to assess the degree of coronary artery obstruction and the status of the left ventricular function. The patients also undergo thallium tomography at 1 and 3 years in order to evaluate the degree of myocardial ischemia with exercise. Additional endpoints will include mortality, morbidity, cardiac event rates, crossover rates, and the cost of each strategy.

Sixty percent of the patients randomized in the EAST had double-vessel disease and 40 percent had triple-vessel disease. Seventy-two percent had proximal LAD disease and 80 percent had normal left ventricular function. It is hoped that the results of the Emory trial and the BARI investigation as well as a trial being performed by the European Cardiac Society will shed additional light on which groups of patients with multivessel disease should be best served by initial angioplasty or initial bypass surgery.

REFERENCES

1. Gruentzig AR, Senning A, Siegenthaler WE: Nonoperative dilatation at coronary artery stenosis: Percutaneous transluminal coronary angioplasty. *N Engl J Med* 1979; 301:61–68.
2. National Center for Health Statistics: *1986 Summary: National Hospital Discharge Survey. Advance Data from Vital and Health Statistics.* No. 145, DHHS pub no (PHS) 87-1250. Hyattsville, MD, Public Health Service, 1987.
3. Hinohara T, Selmon MR, Robertson GC, Braden L, Simpson JS: Directional atherectomy: New approaches for treatment of obstructive coronary and peripheral vascular disease. *Circulation* 1990; 81(suppl IV):IV-79–IV-91.
4. O'Neill W, Meany TB, Kramer B, Knopf WD, Pichard AD, Sketch MH, Stack MD: The role of atherectomy in the management of saphenous vein graft disease (abstr). *J Am Coll Cardiol* 1991; 17(suppl A):384A.
5. Arbel R, O'Neill W, Auth D, Haude N, Nixdorf U, Rupprecht HJ, et al: High-frequency rotablation of occluded coronary artery during heart catheterization. *Cathet Cardiovasc Diagn* 1989; 17:56–58.
6. Forrester JS, Litvack F, Grundfest WS: Laser angioplasty in cardiovascular disease. *Am J Cardiol* 1986; 5:929–933.
7. Roubin GS, King SB III, Douglas JS Jr, Lembo NJ, Robinson KA: Intracoronary stenting during percutaneous transluminal coronary angioplasty. *Circulation* 1990; 81(suppl IV):IV-92–IV-100.
8. Schatz RA, Baim DS, Leon M, Ellis SG, Goldberg S, Hirshfeld JW, et al: Clinical experience with the Palmaz-Schatz coronary stent: Initial results of a multicenter study. *Circulation* 1991; 83:148–161.
9. King SB III: Role of new technology in balloon angioplasty. *Circulation* 1991; 84:2574–2579.
10. Weintraub WS, Jones EL, King SB III, Craver J, Douglas JS Jr, Guyton R, et al: Changing use of coronary angioplasty and coronary bypass surgery in the treatment of chronic coronary artery disease. *Am J Cardiol* 1990; 65:183–188.
11. Veterans Administration Coronary Artery Bypass Surgery Cooperative Study Group: Eleven-year survival in the Veterans Administration randomized trial of coronary artery bypass surgery. *Circulation* 1985; 72(suppl 5):90–101.

12. CASS principal investigators and their associates: Coronary Artery Surgery Study (CASS). A randomized trial of coronary artery bypass surgery. Quality of life in patients randomly assigned to treatment groups. *Circulation* 1983; 68:951–960.
13. Takaro T, Hultgren HN, Lipton MJ, Detre KM: The VA cooperative randomized study of surgery for coronary arterial occlusive disease, II. Subgroup with significant left main lesions. *Circulation* 1976; 54(suppl 3):107–117.
14. Varnauskas E: The European Coronary Surgery Study Group: Survival, myocardial infarction, and employment status in a prospective randomized study of coronary bypass surgery. *Circulation* 1985; 72(suppl 5):90–101.
15. Killip T, Passamani E, Davis K, and the CASS principal investigators and their associates: Coronary artery surgery study (CASS): A randomized trial of coronary artery bypass surgery. Eight-year follow-up and survival in patients with reduced ejection fraction. *Circulation* 1985; 72(suppl 3):102–109.
16. Kaiser GC, Dais KB, Fisher LD, Myers WO, Foster ED, Passaman ER, et al: Survival following coronary artery bypass grafting in patients with severe angina pectoris (CASS). *J Thorac Cardiovasc Surg* 1985; 89:513–524.
17. Ryan TJ, Weiner DA, McCabe CH, Davis KB, Sheffield LT, Chaitman BR, et al: Exercise testing in the coronary artery surgery study randomized population. *Circulation* 1985; 72(suppl 5):31–38.
18. Lembo NJ, King SB: Randomized trials of percutaneous transluminal coronary angioplasty, coronary artery bypass surgery or medical therapy in patients with coronary artery disease. *Coron Art Dis* 1990; 1:449–454.
19. King SB, Schlumpf M: Ten year completed follow-up of percutaneous transluminal coronary angioplasty—The early Zurich experience. *J Am Coll Cardiol* 1993; 22:353–360.
20. Talley JD, Hurst JW, King SB, Douglas JS, Roubin GS, Gruentzig AR, et al: Clinical outcome 5 years after attempted percutaneous coronary angioplasty in 427 patients. *Circulation* 1988; 77:820–829.
21. Detre K, Holubkov R, Kelsey S, Bourassa M, Williams D, Holmes D Jr, et al: One year follow-up results of the 1985 to 1986 National Heart, Lung, and Blood Institute Percutaneous Transluminal Coronary Angioplasty Registry. *Circulation* 1989; 80:421–428.
22. Folland ED, Hartigan P, Parisi AF: Angioplasty vs medicine for single vessel disease: Initial angiographic results of the randomized VA ACME Trial (abstr). *J Am Coll Cardiol* 1991; 17(2):112A.
23. Holmes DR, Vlietstra RE, Smith HC, Vetrovec GW, Kent KM, Cowley MJ, et al: Restenosis after percutaneous transluminal coronary angioplasty (PTCA): A report from the PTCA Registry of the National Heart, Lung, and Blood Institute. *Am J Cardiol* 1984; 53:77c–81c.
24. Leimgruber PP, Roubin GS, Hollman J, Cotsonis GA, Meier B, Douglas JS, et al: Restenosis after successful coronary angioplasty in patients with single-vessel disease. *Circulation* 1986; 73:710–717.
25. Roubin GS, King SB III, Douglas JS Jr: Restenosis after percutaneous transluminal coronary angioplasty: The Emory University Hospital experience. *Am J Cardiol* 1987; 60:39B–43B.
26. Vandormael M, Deligonul U, Medhirad A, Harper M, Chaitman B: Late angiographic outcome following successful multiple lesion PTCA (abstr). *J Am Coll Cardiol* 1986; 7:62A.
27. Meier B, King SB III, Gruentzig AR, Douglas JS, Hollman J, Ischinger T, et al: Repeat coronary angioplasty. *J Am Coll Cardiol* 1984; 4:463–466.
28. Weintraub WS, King SB III, Jones EL, Douglass SS Jr., Craver JM, Liberman HA, et al: Coronary surgery and coronary angioplasty in patients with two vessel coronary artery disease. *Am J Cardiol* 1993; 71:511–517.
29. Kaiser GC: Institutional variation of coronary artery bypass graft surgery: Emphasis on myocardial protection. *Circulation* 1982; 65:85–89.
30. Weintraub WS, Douglas JS Jr, Liberman HA, Morris DC, King SB III: Prediction models of immediate and longterm outcome after coronary angioplasty (abstr). *J Am Coll Cardiol,* 1993; 19:24A.
31. Ryan TJ, Reeves TJ, Faxon DP, and the ACC/AHA task force on the assessment of diagnostic and therapeutic cardiovascular procedures: Guidelines for percutaneous transluminal coronary angioplasty. *J Am Coll Cardiol* 1988; 12:529–545.
32. Ellis SG, Roubin GS, King SB III, Douglas JS Jr, Weintraub WS, Thomas RG, Cox WR: Angiographic and clinical predictors of acute closure after native vessel coronary angioplasty. *Circulation* 1988; 77:372–379.
33. Ellis, SG, Roubin GS, King SB, Douglas JS, Shaw RE, Steitzer SH, Myler RK: In-hospital cardiac mortality following acute closure after PTCA: Analysis of risk factors from 8207 procedures. *J Am Coll Cardiol* 1988; 11:211–216.
34. Gruppo Italiano per lo studio della streptochinasi nell' Infarto Miocardico (GISSI): Effectiveness of intravenous thrombolytic treatment in acute myocardial infarction. *Lancet* 1986; i:397–401.
35. ISIS-2 (Second International Study of Infarct Survival) Collaborative Group: Randomised trial of intravenous streptokinase, oral aspirin, both, or neither among 17,187 cases of suspected acute myocardial infarction: ISIS-2. *Lancet* 1988; ii:349–360.
36. Wilcox RG, VonderLippe G, Olsson CG, Skene AM, Jensen G, Hampton JR for the ASSET Study Group: Trial of tissue plasminogen activator for mortality reduction in acute myocardial infarction. *Lancet* 1988; ii:525–530.
37. AIMS Trial Study Group: Effect of intravenous APSAC on mortality after acute myocardial infarction: Preliminary report of a placebo-controlled clinic trial. *Lancet* 1988; i:545–549.
38. Grines CL, Browne KF, Marco J, Rothbaum D, Stone GW, O'Keefe J, et al: A comparison of immediate angioplasty with thrombolytic therapy for acute myocardial infarction. *N Engl J Med* 1993; 328:673–679.
39. Zijlstra F, Jan de Boer NM, Hoorntje JCA, Reiffers S, Reiber JHC, Suryapranata H: A comparison of immediate coronary angioplasty with intravenous streptokinase in acute myocardial infarction. *N Engl J Med* 1993; 328:680–684.
40. Gibbons RJ, Holmes DR, Reeder GS, Bailey KR, Hopfenspirger MR, Gersh BJ: Immediate angioplasty compared with the administration of a thrombolytic agent followed by conservative treatment for myocardial infarction. *N Engl J Med* 1993; 328:685–691.
41. The TIMI Study Group: Comparison of invasive and conservative strategies after treatment with intravenous tissue plasminogen activator in acute myocardial infarction. Results of the Thrombolysis in Myocardial Infarction (TIMI) Phase II trial. *N Engl J Med* 1989; 320:618–627.

Chapter 71

Techniques of Percutaneous Transluminal Angioplasty and Atherectomy of the Coronary Arteries

John S. Douglas, Jr., M.D. ■ *Spencer B. King, III, M.D.*

Percutaneous transluminal coronary angioplasty (PTCA) was shepherded into existence, worldwide acceptance, and application by Andreas R. Gruentzig. As with most innovations in medicine, the stage for this contribution was set by the pioneering efforts of others. Gruentzig's ideas were a direct extension of the work of Dotter and Judkins,[1] who in 1964 mechanically dilated femoral arteries with a coaxial double-catheter system, and of Zeitler et al.,[2] who successfully applied this technique in West Germany and introduced it to Gruentzig. After Gruentzig's introduction of a polyvinyl chloride balloon catheter with fixed maximal inflated diameters in 1974, modern balloon angioplasty evolved rapidly. Initially, successful dilatation of iliofemoral artery disease was accomplished and artery patency rates of 70 percent at 2 years were reported. With further balloon catheter miniaturization, Gruentzig succeeded in dilating experimental stenoses first in canine coronary arteries and then in human coronary arteries during bypass surgery, failing to find evidence of distal atheroembolization.[3–5] In September 1977 the first percutaneous transluminal coronary angioplasty was performed in a 37-year-old insurance salesman with severe angina pectoris and high-grade stenosis of the proximal left anterior descending coronary artery.[6] Successful dilatation was accomplished with complete relief of symptoms. On the tenth anniversary of this landmark procedure, the patient remained asymptomatic and had angiographically normal coronary arteries (Fig. 71-1). Following the report of Gruentzig's first five coronary cases in 1978[7] and the subsequent 50 cases in 1979,[8] worldwide interest in the technique was assured. Fabrication of an over-the-wire balloon catheter system by Simpson et al.[9] combined with advances in guide-wire and balloon catheter technology resulted in a steerable balloon catheter system capable of reaching and dilating heretofore unapproachable remote stenoses.

The mechanism by which balloon angioplasty achieved an increase in arterial luminal diameter was mistakenly thought by Gruentzig, Dotter, and Judkins to be primarily a matter of plaque compression. Subsequently, it has become evident that plaque compression is insignificant and that plaque splitting and mural tearing and stretching are the principal mechanisms that lead to an increased luminal diameter.[10–18] Remodeling of softer atheromatous tissue also probably occurs in "younger" lesions. Plaque splitting associated with medial and intimal tearing results in the angiographic appearance of haziness and intramural contrast medium staining. In some lesions, dilatation may occur with inti-

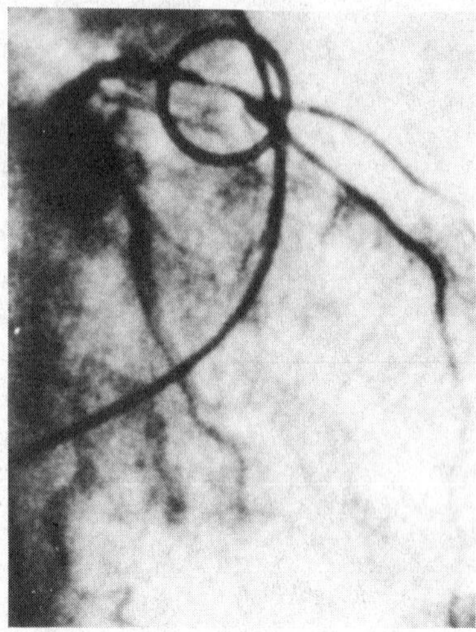

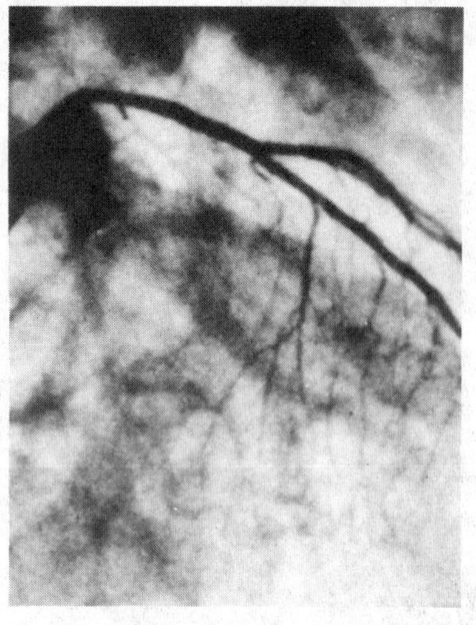

FIGURE 71-1 Right anterior oblique coronary arteriogram of the first patient who underwent transluminal coronary angioplasty on September 16, 1977 (*left*) and on September 16, 1987 (*right*). During this 10-year period, the patient remained completely asymptomatic and the arteriogram at 10 years showed no narrowing in the coronary arteries.

mal and medial tearing not evident angiographically. Intramural hemorrhage and coagulation necrosis, intimal flap formation, platelet aggregation, and thrombus formation may also occur, resulting in acute occlusion, the most common serious complication of the procedure, in about 5 percent of cases. If acute occlusion is avoided, the dilated segment undergoes a healing reaction including phagocytosis of damaged myocytes and cellular debris, retraction, and neoendothelialization, following which the hazy arterial appearance is usually replaced by sharp arterial edges and the luminal diameter is sometimes further increased. The mechanism that results in restenosis in about 30 percent of cases appears to include an excessive fibrocellular response associated with migration and proliferation of smooth-muscle cells and/or organization of mural thrombus results in a marked fibrous thickening of the intima with luminal narrowing.[19–22] Restenosis, if it occurs, usually does so 3 to 4 months following the procedure and rarely after 1 year.[23–25] Embolization of atherosclerotic debris at the time of angioplasty was an initial fear not borne out in early studies but occasionally seen clinically, most often during angioplasty of older vein graft stenoses.[26–29] Multiple attempts to modify the response to injury and thus reduce the incidence of restenosis have been unsuccessful.[30–34] Restenosis rates reported currently are similar to the 30 percent rate reported in early series.[7,25]

The conclusion that angioplasty results in an improved arterial lumen caliber has been based on a number of criteria, including symptom relief and improved angiographic and pressure gradient measurements and relief of ischemia as indicated by stress electrocardiography. More recently, quantitative arteriographic approaches and studies of systolic left ventricular function, coronary flow reserve, coronary flow velocity, myocardial perfusion, intravascular ultrasound, and angioscopy have substantiated the improved blood flow.[35–41]

Many factors have caused an increased use of coronary angioplasty. In his early experience Gruentzig campaigned to limit the procedure to single-vessel disease with proximal, noncalcified, concentric lesions, thereby optimizing the chance for success with the crude equipment available. Success in this narrowly defined patient population stimulated the development of atraumatic steerable guide-wires and ultra-low-profile balloon catheters (Figs. 71-2 and 71-3) capable of dilating the most rigid lesions as well as high-resolution x-ray imaging systems specifically designed for angioplasty. These technological advances improved the safety of the procedure and led to broadened indications.

Directional coronary atherectomy, successfully performed by Simpson in 1987,[42,43] is utilized in selected patients as an alternative or adjunct to balloon angioplasty. Directional coronary atherectomy permits excision and removal of atherosclerotic plaque from proximal and mid-coronary artery sites with acceptable success and complication rates. The mechanisms resulting in improved luminal dimensions remain controversial.[44–47] It appears that less than one-half of the gain in lumen size may be due to tissue removal, with the remaining gain apparently resulting from mechanical dilatation, the so-called Dotter effect, and from inflation of the atherectomy balloon.[48] Directional atherectomy frequently yields a larger, smoother lumen than that obtained by balloon dilatation, and it was hoped that this better initial result would lead to a more favorable outcome with less tendency for early acute occlusion and subsequent restenosis. Although directional atherectomy and balloon angioplasty are being compared in an ongoing randomized trial, reports from single- and multiple-center experience indicate acute occlusion occurs in approximately 4 percent of patients and restenosis in approximately 30 percent, similar to figures reported with balloon dilatation.[42, 49–53] Preliminary observations suggest that aggressive atherectomy strategies aimed at achieving maximal improvement in lumen diameter may result in removal of media and adventitia with a consequent increased risk of perforation and aneurysm formation and, paradoxically, a high rate of restenosis, apparently related to increased vessel injury.[54–56] Fortunately, perforation is infrequent, occurring in approximately 0.7 to 0.9 percent of patients.[49,52] Clinical experiences suggest that atherectomy may have a place in treatment of some lesions that are unfavorable for

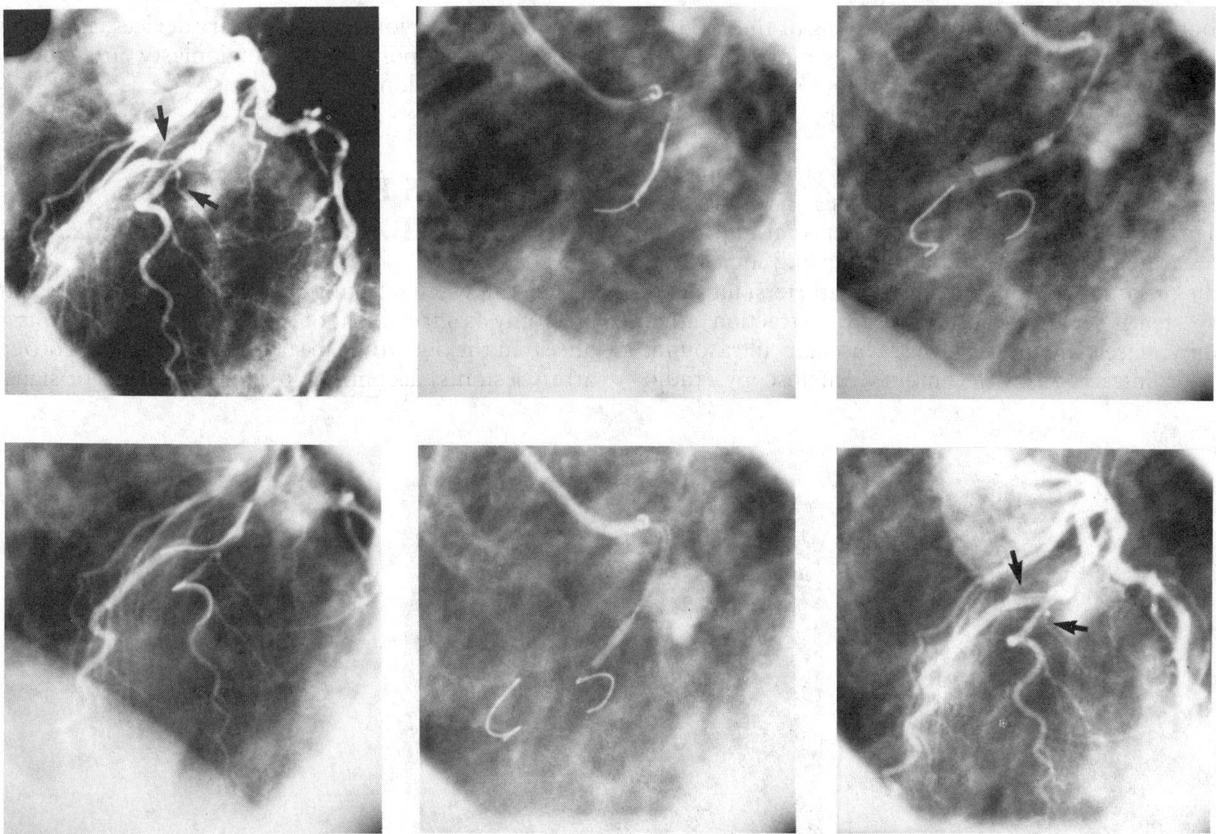

FIGURE 71-2 Angioplasty of high-grade stenoses of the left anterior descending artery diagonal bifurcation (see arrow) using a single guiding catheter through which two dilatation devices (USCI Probe) were passed. The left anterior descending artery was dilated with a 2.5-mm balloon (note "waist" of the balloon produced by the lesion), and the diagonal was dilated with a 2-mm balloon. Note small intimal tear in the left anterior descending artery following the small procedure (left anterior oblique views).

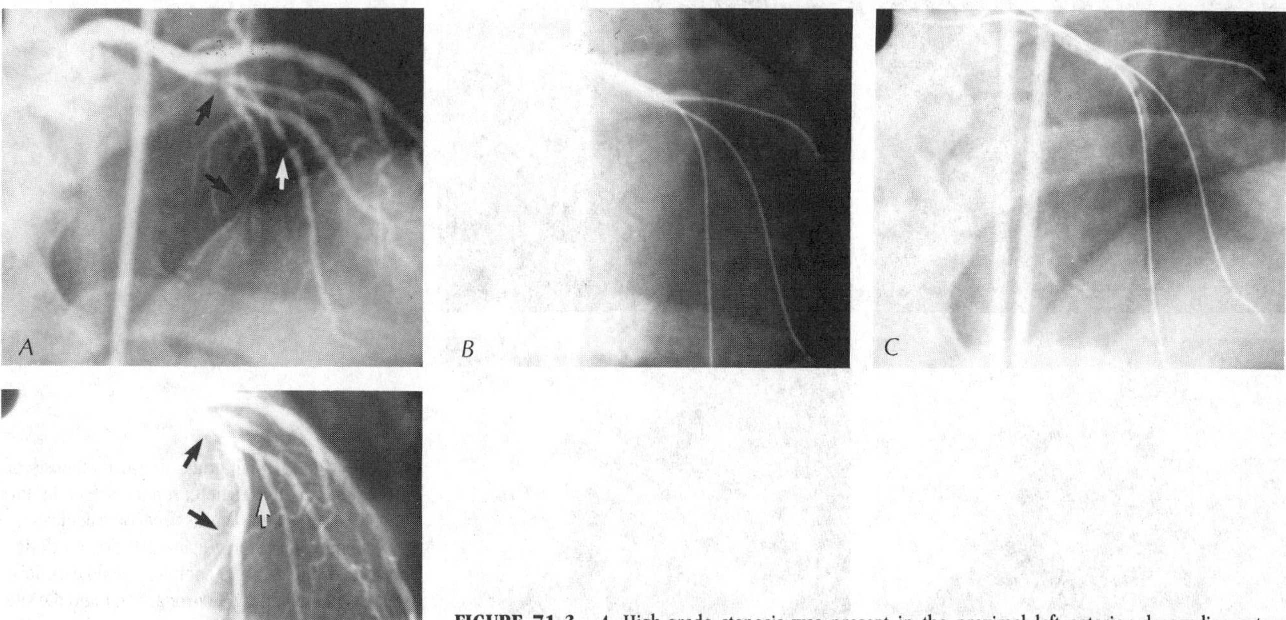

FIGURE 71-3 *A.* High-grade stenosis was present in the proximal left anterior descending artery (black arrow), the distal left anterior descending artery was occluded (black arrow), and severe stenosis was present in a diagonal branch (white arrow). *B.* To protect the side branches involved, steerable wires were placed in the distal left anterior descending artery and in the two diagonal branches. *C.* The left anterior descending artery was dilated with a 2.5-mm balloon and the diagonal with a 2-mm balloon producing revascularization (*D*) of all involved arteries (frontal cranial view).

balloon dilatation. These include lesions of the ostia[57,58] (Fig. 71-4*A* and *B*), lesions of complex morphology[42,59] (Fig. 71-4*C* to *F*), and vein graft sites.[60,61] In these instances, directional atherectomy may be effective when balloon angioplasty fails.[42, 62, 63]

The successes and limitations of coronary angioplasty, especially acute closure and restenosis, have resulted in many new devices and strategies aimed at improving success rates and safety and at broadening indications for the procedure. Perfusion balloon catheters, intracoronary stents, rotational atherectomy, extraction atherectomy, laser angioplasty, intravascular ultrasound, Doppler intracoronary techniques, angioscopy, radio frequency and cryotherapy coronary devices, and cardiopulmonary support during angioplasty are currently under investigation.

INDICATIONS FOR ANGIOPLASTY AND DIRECTIONAL ATHERECTOMY

In general, when selecting angioplasty or directional atherectomy as a treatment of choice, there should be assurance that the operator can successfully treat the coronary artery lesion(s) accounting for the symptoms or signs of

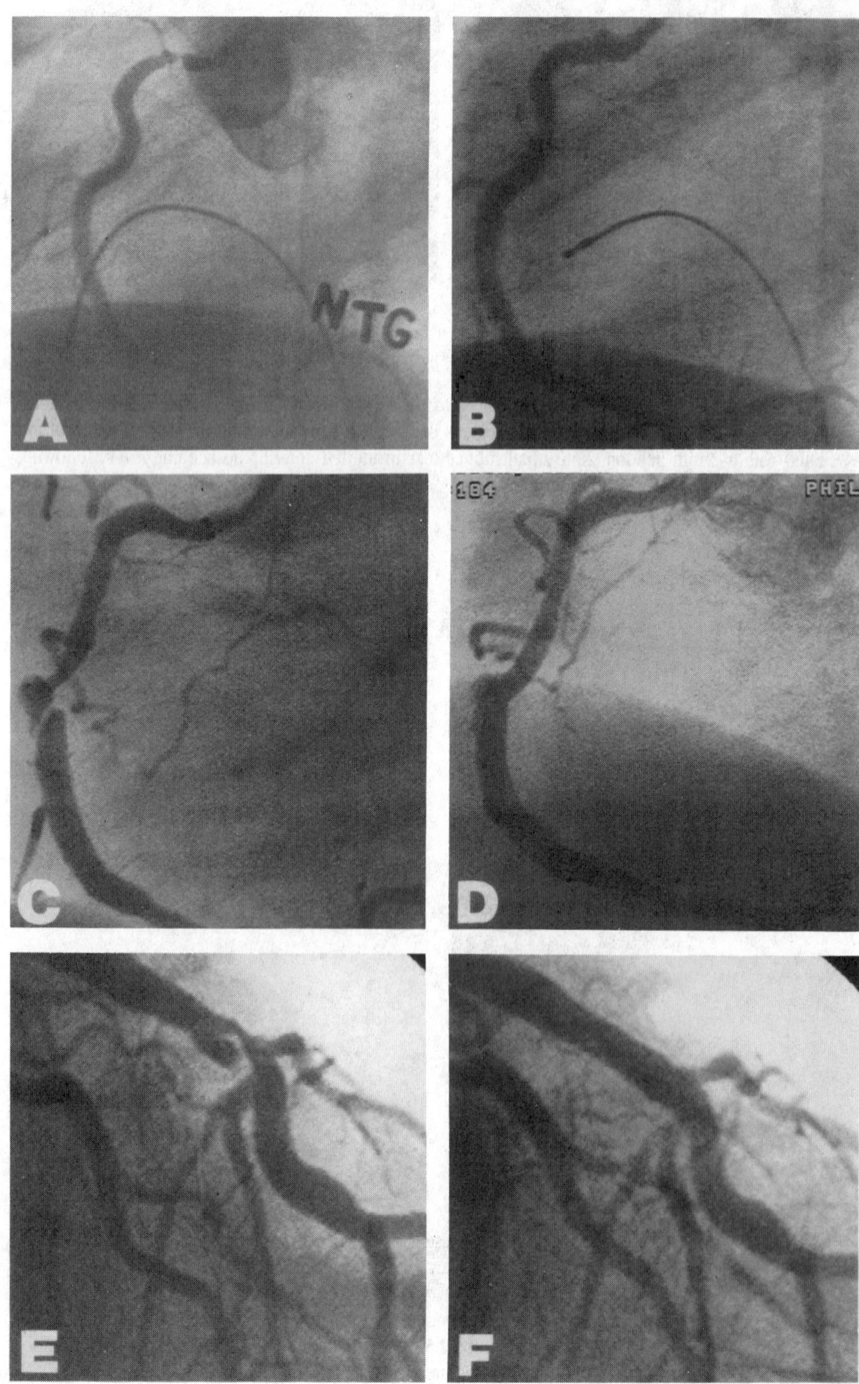

FIGURE 71-4 High-grade de novo stenosis of the ostium of the right coronary artery in the middle-aged male (*A*) was free of calcification. Directional atherectomy using a 6 French device was successful (*B*). Very complex shelflike de novo stenosis in the mid right coronary (*C*) and the site 2 years after successful directional atherectomy (*D*). Histology showed atheroma and organized thrombus. Flaplike de novo stenosis (*E*) was removed with directional atherectomy (*F*). Sites (*A*), (*C*), and (*E*) are poor lesions for conventional PTCA.

TABLE 71-1
ACC/AHA Classification of Lesions

Type A Lesions (high success, >85%; low risk)	
• Discrete (<10 mm length) • Concentric • Readily accessible • Nonangulated segment, <45° • Smooth contour	• Little or no calcification • Less than totally occlusive • Not ostial in location • No major branch involvement • Absence of thrombus
Type B Lesions (moderate success, 60 to 85%; moderate risk)	
• Tubular (10–20 mm length) • Eccentric • Moderate tortuosity of proximal segment • Moderately angulated segment, >45°, <90° • Irregular contour	• Moderate to heavy calcification • Total occlusions <3 months old • Ostial in location • Bifurcation lesions requiring double guide wires • Some thrombus present
Type C Lesions (low success, <60%; high risk)	
• Diffuse (>2 cm length) • Excessive tortuosity of proximal segment • Extremely angulated segments >90°	• Total occlusion >3 months old • Inability to protect major side branches • Degenerated vein grafts with friable lesions

SOURCE: Ryan et al.[66] Reprinted with permission of the authors and the American College of Cardiology.

myocardial ischemia. Further, the associated risk should be equal to or less than that associated with the bypass surgery or medical therapy during both early and long-term follow-up. Factors such as the likelihood of restenosis also assume importance. A number of clinical, angiographic, and procedural variables have been seen to be predictive of the outcome of balloon angioplasty. Since acute coronary occlusion is the most common serious complication of PTCA, most estimates of negative immediate outcome relate to the probability of acute occlusion and its potential adverse consequences. The following factors are associated with increased risk of acute occlusion: unstable angina, lesion length, female gender, bend point or branch point stenosis, thrombus in situ, the presence of multiple stenoses in the vessel dilated, and multivessel disease.[64] Estimates of the consequence of acute occlusion take into account the amount of myocardium in jeopardy, the ventricular function, and the ability rapidly to intervene surgically in the event of acute closure.[65]

The importance of coronary stenosis morphology in predicting PTCA outcome is reflected in the American College of Cardiology/American Heart Association (ACC/AHA) guidelines for PTCA.[66] Lesions were classified as type A for anticipated high-success, low-risk stenoses; type B for moderate-success, moderate-risk stenoses; and type C for anticipated low-success, high-risk lesions (Table 71-1). The validity of this classification in predicting outcome of balloon angioplasty has been affirmed in low-risk patients[67] and in patients with multivessel disease.[68] Similar angiographic lesion characteristics and clinical factors are important predictors of outcome of directional atherectomy.[51,58,69,70] In a multicenter report, success and complication rates for directional atherectomy were 93 and 3 percent for type A lesions, 88 percent success and 6 percent complication rates when one type B characteristic was present, and 75 percent success and 13 percent complication rates when more than one type B characteristic were present.[70] These observations emphasize the importance of case selection in determining the outcome of angioplasty and atherectomy. Operator training and experience also affect outcome,[70–72] and guidelines for training of angioplasty operators have been offered by a ACP/ACC/AHA Task Force.[72]

Given a decision that revascularization is deemed necessary, advanced age, complicating medical problems, pulmonary or renal insufficiency, or malignancy may sway the therapeutic decision toward balloon angioplasty or atherectomy rather than surgery. The patient, however, who is a poor candidate for elective coronary bypass surgery is an even poorer candidate for emergency surgery in case of angioplasty complications. As with any treatment, selection of balloon angioplasty, atherectomy, or bypass surgery involves an analysis of risks and benefits for the individual patient. A complicated patient selected for percutaneous angioplasty or atherectomy in an experienced angioplasty center might be better treated surgically in a facility with good surgical results but only rudimentary angioplasty experience. In many cardiac centers, most patients with proximal single-vessel disease who require revascularization are treated initially with balloon angioplasty or atherectomy, and patients with diffuse triple-vessel disease that is amenable to surgery undergo coronary artery bypass operations. Between these extremes there is currently little standardization of therapy.

In general, patients with unstable angina benefit from a "cooling-off" period of 2 to 3 days, if possible, on intravenous heparin and nitroglycerin prior to coronary intervention. This is especially true when obvious intracoronary thrombi are present.[73] Patients presenting with restenosis lesions in native coronary arteries may undergo repeat angioplasty with extraordinarily low risk, but second recurrences develop in about one-third of patients.[74]

In three randomized trials that compared immediate (direct) angioplasty with thrombolytic therapy in patients with acute myocardial infarction, the results favored immediate PTCA in two studies[75,75a] whereas there was no difference in one study.[75b] Coronary artery bypass surgery[76] has also been used acutely to restore antegrade coronary blood flow in such patients. Because of the difficult logistics of applying either type of mechanical reperfusion rapidly and consistently, however, this strategy is not widely applied. Randomized trials provide evidence that routine adjunctive balloon angioplasty soon after thrombolytic therapy has a higher complication rate than anticipated.[77] Balloon angioplasty (or atherectomy), however, may be indicated in selected patients with evidence of ischemia following thrombolytic therapy, in selected patients with multivessel coronary disease, and in patients presenting a cardiogenic shock, in whom angioplasty may reduce the mortality from the 70 percent rate reported for thrombolytic therapy to about 50 percent. (See Chap. 60.)

One of the largest subgroups of patients undergoing PTCA is comprised of post-bypass surgery patients in whom stenosis of a native vessel, saphenous vein graft, or internal mammary artery may require percutaneous intervention.[78,79] The best results are obtained in patients who develop stenoses at the junction of grafts with native coronary arteries within 6 months of surgery, in which case complication-free dilation is usually possible and restenosis rates are the lowest of any other coronary site. Angioplasty and atherectomy of mid- and proximal vein graft sites are usually complication free when performed within 3 years of surgery, but afterward atheroembolization becomes increasingly frequent, reaching about 25 percent in saphenous vein grafts implanted for over 6 years. Recurrence of stenoses in vein grafts implanted for over 6 years. Recurrences of stenoses in vein grafts following atherectomy and angioplasty remains a significant problem, especially when the site is a restenotic lesion. (See also Chap. 70.)

PERFORMANCE OF CORONARY ANGIOPLASTY AND ATHERECTOMY

Interventional Laboratory

Optimal conditions for performance of coronary angioplasty and atherectomy require sophisticated imaging systems, trained personnel, a large inventory of dilatation and atherectomy hardware and software, and a variety of therapeutic safety nets to protect the patient when angioplasty or atherectomy fails or is complicated. The quality of the video image of the coronary arteries is an important determinant of angioplasty and atherectomy success. A freeze-frame storage and display capability is required for use during the procedure, as is a high-quality video replay with slow motion and stop-frame capability. Since the objective of imaging is lesion and arterial visualization free of overlap and foreshortening, steep cranially and caudally angled views should be easily obtained in oblique projections. The ability to solve specific problems such as lesion eccentricity or rigidity, vessel tortuosity, and unusual position or orientation of coronary ostia is often dependent on specific device characteristics. Consequently, it is necessary to have available dilating catheters, atherectomy devices, guide-wires, and guiding catheters in a variety of shapes and sizes. The cardiac surgery operating room should be no more than a few minutes away.

Dilatation and Atherectomy Equipment

The standard over-the-wire steerable catheter system used most often for coronary angioplasty is illustrated in Fig. 71-5. It consists of a dilatation catheter through which a steerable guide-wire has been placed, a guiding catheter that extends to the coronary ostia, a balloon pressuring device, and manifolds for selection of constant pressure measurement or for injection of contrast medium or heparinized saline.

Guiding catheters for coronary angioplasty are usually 7, 8, or 9 French and serve as semirigid conduits through which contrast medium is injected and dilatation catheters are passed. The most commonly used catheters are the Judkins right and left coronary shapes. Many other catheter shapes, however, are available, for example, Amplatz, multipurpose, Arani, El Gamal, venous bypass, hockey stick, and internal mammary. Ideally, the guiding catheter should sit within the coronary artery ostium without obstructing flow and have the same axial orientation as the coronary artery. Although damage of the arterial intima by the catheter tip is not recognized commonly, manufacturers have softened the catheter tip to reduce further this possibility.

The advantages of the Judkins shape guide catheter for most left anterior descending PTCAs and of the Amplatz catheter for high or posterior left coronary take-off or for PTCA of the circumflex artery are illustrated in Fig. 71-6. Figure 71-7 shows catheter shapes that are useful in superiorly oriented right coronary artery take-offs where the more commonly used Judkins right coronary catheter does not perform well. If the guiding catheter wedges in the right coronary artery and obstructs flow, commercially available catheters with side holes can be used or a hole may be cut by the operator. Inability to find a suitable guiding catheter is one of the more common causes of angioplasty failure. Common anatomic problems and solutions include the following:

1. "shepherd's crook" proximal right coronary: Arani catheter, left venous bypass catheter, left Amplatz catheter, or a multipurpose catheter;
2. abrupt downward circumflex take-off: left Amplatz or short tip left Judkins;
3. anterior right coronary artery take-off: left Amplatz, left venous bypass, anteriorly reshaped left Judkins; and
4. superior vein graft take-off: left Amplatz, left venous bypass.

After good results were obtained in "ideal" patients who had recent onset angina and focal noncalcific lesions, the interest of angioplasty operators moved to more chronic lesions that were often fibrotic, rigid, and

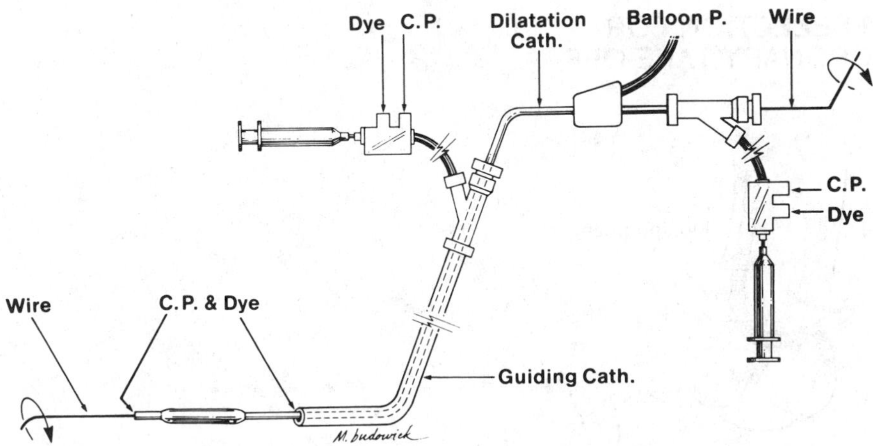

FIGURE 71-5 Diagram of the over-the-wire dilatation catheter with capacity for contract media (dye) injection. The floppy guide wire is steerable. (*From FM Aueron, AR Gruentzig: Percutaneous transluminal coronary angioplasty: Indications and current status. Primary Cardiol 1984; 10:91. Reproduced with permission of the publisher and authors.*)

calcified. The important elements for success were low dilatation catheter profile (diameter of the deflated balloon) to cross the lesion and balloon material strong enough to withstand the high-pressure inflation required to dilate successfully chronic stenoses (greater than 10 atm).

Dilatation catheters are available with an array of balloon lengths (12 to 40 mm), diameters (1.5 to 4.5 cm), and special features. Especially flexible and low-profile balloons have been developed for use in multivessel coronary disease where rigid stenoses are almost the rule. It is important for angioplasty operators to be aware of the inflation characteristics of balloon catheters. Polyethylene teraphthalate balloons reach nominal size at about 5 atm and are noncompliant, i.e., have very little increase in size at higher pressures. On the other hand, polyethylene and polyolefin materials are compliant and stretch at higher pressures, yielding a larger balloon size. Marked differences in balloon sizes after the first inflation have been described for polyolefin balloons.[80]

The steerable guide-wire is a cornerstone upon which current angioplasty techniques evolved. Modern steerable wires have soft flexible tips to avoid arterial trauma with a smooth transition to a stiffer proximal shaft. A floppy-tipped wire, favored for routine use, may be inadequate for total occlusions where a stiffer guide-wire tip is commonly required. Steerable guide-wires are commercially available in diameters ranging from 0.010 to 0.021 in., sizes 0.014 to 0.018 in. being used most frequently.

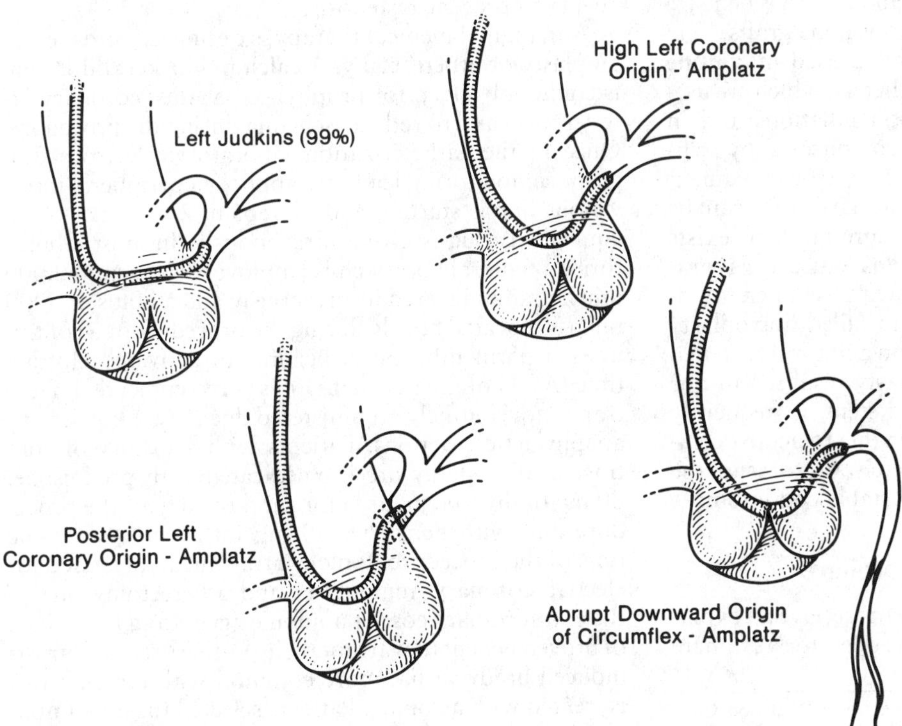

FIGURE 71-6 The most commonly used guide catheters for angioplasty of the left coronary artery.

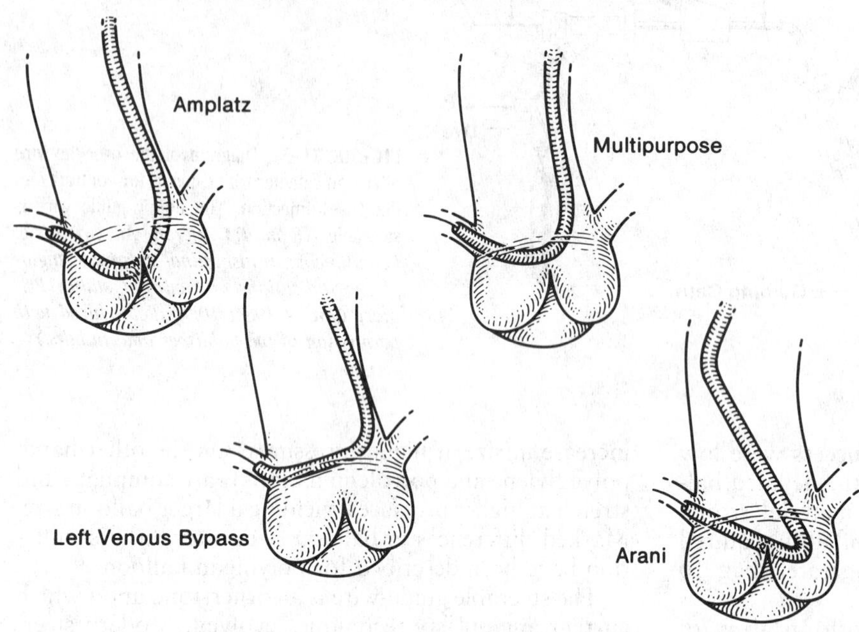

FIGURE 71-7 Guide catheter shapes that are effective when the right coronary artery has a steep upward initial course.

The directional atherectomy catheter* is shown in Fig. 71-8. It is supplied in 5, 6, and 7 French sizes and is advanced over a 0.014-in. steerable guide-wire. The tapered nose cone is reasonably flexible; however, the housing for the cutter is rigid. The housing contains a 10-mm-long window and a supporting balloon on the opposite side. The proximal end of the atherocath has a balloon inflation port, a guide-wire port, a lever for movement of the cutter, and an attachment for the battery-powered motor that spins the cutter at 2000 rpm. Guide catheters are supplied in 10 and 11 French sizes for use in the left coronary artery and a 9.5 French size for right coronary atherectomy and venous grafts.

A variety of adjunctive devices are used in routine practice. Autoperfusion balloon catheters, which are useful in permitting prolonged balloon inflations and in failed angioplasty or atherectomy complicated by ischemia, have multiple side holes over a 10-cm segment through which some antegrade coronary flow can be maintained when a significant pressure gradient exists between the aorta and the distal coronary artery. Favorable results have also been obtained with use of endovascular stents as "bail-out" devices in failed angioplasty complicated by acute vessel occlusion and for threatened closure due to suboptimal angioplasty results.[81] In our experience with a balloon-mounted stent, it frequently has been possible to relieve ischemia due to acute occlusion and to avoid surgery completely or to send the patient to bypass surgery in a very stable condition.[82]

The Angioplasty/Atherectomy Procedure

Prior to coronary intervention, patients receive an explanation of the procedure including the operator's estimate of success, possible complications, risks, and benefits. A booklet and videotape describing the procedure and an explanation by the nursing staff help to reduce anxiety and ensure that both the patient and the family are well informed.

Antiplatelet therapy is used routinely. The therapy most widely used is aspirin, 160 to 325 mg daily. Restenosis trials have failed to show a definite advantage of one antiplatelet regimen over another and have not shown calcium channel-blocking agents, warfarin anticoagulation, steroids, or nonsteroidal anti-inflammatory agents to prevent restenosis.

Antianginal medical therapy is optimized prior to angioplasty or atherectomy. A calcium blocker, diltiazem, is commonly given for prophylaxis against coronary artery spasm and to reduce ischemia during the procedure. Once in the catheterization laboratory, electrocardiographic monitoring leads are applied, a peripheral intravenous line is started, and diazepam, 2 to 5 mg, or an equivalent drug is given intravenously. In most laboratories a femoral approach is employed. Heparin, 10,000 units, is administered intravenously and a bolus of 5000 units is repeated hourly during the procedure or a continuous heparin infusion is begun. An activated clotting time (ACT) of greater than 300 s is recommended. Dextran is not routinely administered due to rare but serious anaphylactic reactions. Patients with a history of contrast media allergy are premedicated with prednisone, 60 mg orally, the night before and the day of the procedure and with benadryl, 50 mg intravenously, at the time of the procedure. Ionic contrast medium is used for elective coronary angioplasty and atherectomy due to the extraordinary cost of nonionic agents and to the lack of proven benefit to warrant their routine use.[83] Contrast-induced bradycardia, more common with ionic agents, is treated with atropine. Patients selected for use of nonionic agents include those with renal insufficiency, diabe-

*Atherocath, Devices For Vascular Interventions, Redwood City, CA.

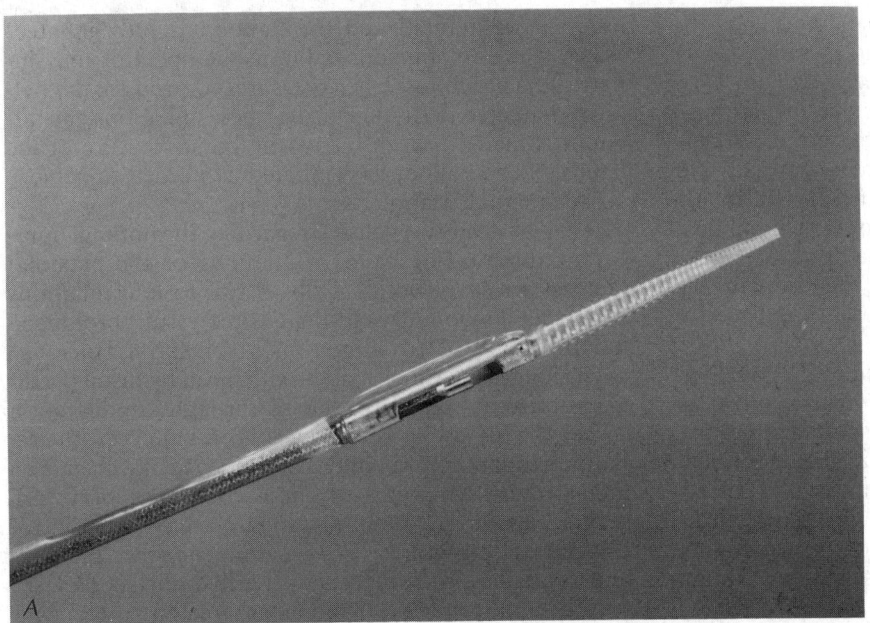

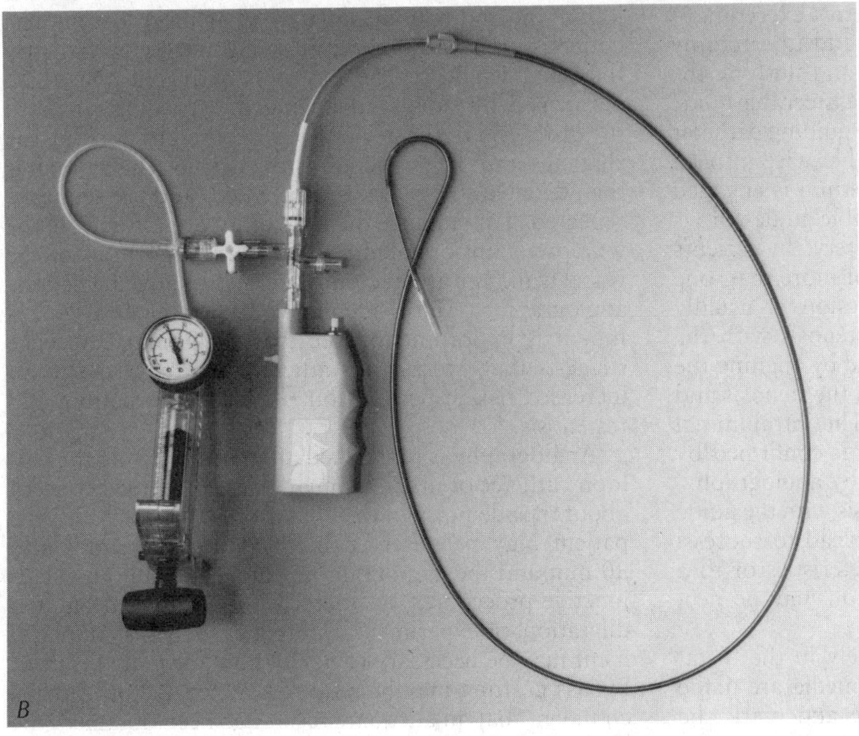

FIGURE 71-8 Directional atherectomy catheter (*top*). The atherectomy catheter is attached to a motor device unit and inflation device and passed through a guide catheter (*bottom*).

tes, severe left ventricular dysfunction, known allergy to the available ionic agents, and previous severe bradycardia with ionic agents.

In selecting a guiding catheter, proper seating of the tip in the coronary ostia and a stable position in the aortic root are required. The choice of catheter external diameter is influenced by the diameter of the femoral artery and the coronary ostia; 8 French (rarely 7 French) is used in most patients for coronary angioplasty. A 9 French catheter size is occasionally selected when there is a need to accommodate multiple balloons or when placement of a large stent may be necessary. A 10 or 11 French coronary guide catheter is currently used for directional atherectomy for left coronary lesions and a 9.5 French for the right coronary artery and bypass grafts.

Coronary arteriograms are performed in two approximately perpendicular views selected to demonstrate the lesion(s) to be treated and the course of the parent artery without overlap by other vessels. The angles chosen are recorded and freeze frames demonstrating the anatomy are stored and displayed during the procedure. A dilatation catheter is selected based on the diameter of the target coronary artery to be dilated and the length of the stenotic segment determined by comparison with the guiding catheter of known diameter. The balloon diameter is chosen to approximate closely the diameter of the normal adjacent vessel since oversizing the angioplasty balloon has been associated with increased complications and no reduction in the rate of restenosis.[84] In general, an over-the-wire dilatation catheter system is preferred because of the ability to exchange easily for alternative balloons or other devices such as a perfusion catheter or stent in the event of angioplasty complications. The operator's impression of the difficulty of the case may influence selection of a particularly low profile catheter to cross severe stenosis, a flexible catheter to negotiate tortuous segments, or a high-pressure balloon capability to dilate fibrotic, calcified lesions. Balloon-on-a-wire devices are especially useful when an ultralow balloon profile is required or when simultaneous use of two balloons is required (Fig. 71-2). In directional atherectomy, the size of the coronary artery also determines the size of the device chosen. A 7 French directional atherectomy catheter is used for vessels 3.5 to 4 mm in diameter, a 6 French for vessels 3 to 3.5 mm, and a 5 French for arteries with a diameter of 2.5 to 3 mm. A 7 French catheter with a 4.5-mm working diameter is available for grafts or arteries exceeding 4 mm in diameter. The dilatation catheter and atherectomy devices are prepared by aspirating air and flushing the lumen with heparinized saline. A flexible, steerable guide wire is selected and introduced into the guiding catheter after shaping the soft tip of the steerable wire into an angle of 45° or more. The coronary ostium is engaged with the guiding catheter and the steerable guide wire is cautiously advanced into the target artery. In patients requiring angioplasty or atherectomy of more than one coronary artery, the most difficult lesion is usually treated first. A clean crossing of the stenosis with the guide wire is critical and is accomplished by aligning the steerable wire tip with the entry point of the stenosis and gently advancing it across the lesion. The intraluminal position of the wire in the distal artery is confirmed by free rotation of the guide-wire tip and by angiography. If there is difficulty in crossing the stenosis with the guide wire, reshaping the tip will commonly lead to success. Shifting to a wire with different characteristics or to a stiffer wire in the case of total occlusion may be necessary.

With the steerable guide wire securely in the distal coronary artery, injections of contrast media are made through the guiding catheter to locate and mark the position of the stenosis to be treated. While fixing the position of the guide wire, the operator advances the balloon catheter or atherectomy device until it is centered on the lesion. If it is not possible to push the balloon or atherectomy device across the stenosis in spite of maneuvers with the guiding catheter and gentle rotation of the atherectomy device, it is wise to exchange it for the lowest profile over-the-wire balloon system available and to exchange this for the proper size device after partially opening the lesion. If it is not possible to cross with the smallest over-the-wire balloon, a balloon-on-a-wire system may be tried. If angioplasty is being performed, the balloon is inflated to an initial pressure of 2 atm. Indentation of the inflated balloon by the lesion confirms proper placement. The balloon is subsequently inflated in 2-atm increments until the "waist" caused by the lesion is obliterated and the balloon is fully inflated. When using a compliant balloon, the operator may inflate the balloon to higher pressures to produce the balloon diameter desired. During these inflations, an attempt is made to keep below the burst pressure of the balloon. The balloon is reinflated as needed to achieve an adequate dilatation.

There is no clear evidence regarding the optimal number or duration of balloon inflations or the maximal balloon pressure. Occasionally, if two to four inflations of 30 to 60 s do not yield the desired result, prolonged inflations up to 5 to 10 min may be helpful. Tolerance of the longer inflations may be enhanced by distal perfusion of arterial or venous blood through the dilatation catheter or by use of an autoperfusion balloon catheter. Balloon inflations are limited by evidence of ischemia as indicated by symptoms of chest discomfort or by ST segment elevation. Some investigators have used intracoronary electrograms (ECGs) from the steerable wire and found these to be more sensitive than surface ECGs.[85]

When performing directional atherectomy, the "window" of the atherectomy device is oriented toward the lesion and the balloon inflated to at most 1 atm. The cutter is then withdrawn, allowing the lesion to enter the open window. The motor is activated and a cut performed by slowly advancing the spinning cutter to the distal end of the device housing, thereby packing the shavings into the nose cone of the device. The balloon is then deflated, the window reoriented, and the sequence repeated. To minimize the possibility of perforation, the window is not oriented toward normal portions of the vessel wall. The atherectomy device is removed when the angiographic result is adequate or when the nose cone is full. It is important to note that preliminary evidence suggests that overzealous atherectomy may lead to an increased risk of perforation, aneurysm formation, and restenosis.[54,56]

Angiography is performed after withdrawing the balloon catheter or atherectomy device. If there is concern about the adequacy of the dilatation or atherectomy, the patient may be observed in the laboratory for 15 to 30 min and the angiogram repeated. In some cases adjunctive procedures of atherectomy, prolonged balloon dilatation, or experimental strategies such as stent placement may be necessary to achieve an adequate result or bypass grafting may be required. When the operator is confident that an adequate result has been obtained, the patient is returned to his or her room where an ECG is obtained and the patient is placed on telemetry. Creatine kinase determinations are performed immediately and every 8 h for three determinations. Because of the dehydrating effect of the osmotic load, most patients receive at least 1 liter of intravenous fluids postprocedure. Sheath removal is performed at 2 to 4 h when the activated clotting time is at most 140 s. If a large intimal tear in the coronary artery has been induced with the procedure, heparin is administered overnight. There is evidence that routine heparin administration following uncomplicated angioplasty is not helpful in reducing acute occlusion or restenosis.[86] Routine postprocedure medications in-hospital include aspirin, a calcium channel-blocking agent, and topical nitrates. Most patients are discharged on the first or second day following the procedure after receiving instructions on a low-fat diet, exercise, and cessation of smoking and a discussion of the follow-up procedure. In selected patients, stress electrocardiography (Chap. 16) and thallium scintigraphy (Chap. 134) are performed prior to discharge.

Results

The results obtained with coronary angioplasty have been significantly influenced by improvements in technology, operator experience, and the difficulty of the cases selected. With crude equipment, Gruentzig was able to dilate successfully 64 percent of the initial 50 patients and 78 percent of the first 169 patients.[8,29] Defining primary success as 20 percent or greater reduction in all stenoses attempted, a final stenosis less than 50 percent of the luminal diameter, and freedom from major complication (myocardial infarction, bypass surgery, or death), we obtained a success rate of 90 percent in over 10,000 patients undergoing elective angioplasty at Emory University Hospital between 1980 and 1989 (Table 71-2). Experienced operators should achieve primary success rates in excess of 95 percent in more ideal proximal lesions compared to a reduced success rate of approximately 75 percent in recent total occlusions and when attempting to treat fibrotic calcified eccentric stenoses located distally in tortuous coronary arteries. Success rates with directional atherectomy in carefully selected patients are comparable to balloon angioplasty. With both techniques, lesion characteristics are a major determinant of outcome of the procedure.[51,58,67–70] For further discussion of results of balloon angioplasty and atherectomy, see Chap. 70.

Complications

Patients undergoing coronary angioplasty or atherectomy are subject to the same complications encountered with the performance of coronary arteriography. In addition, because instrumentation of the atherosclerotic lesion occurs, coronary artery dissection, thrombus formation, and coronary artery spasm may occur, leading to acute occlusion of the coronary artery or of side branches arising from the artery. Acute occlusion of the dilated artery is the most common serious complication of coronary angioplasty and accounts for most of the morbidity and mortality related to the procedure.

In Gruentzig's first 50 patients, 5 experienced an acute deterioration necessitating emergency bypass surgery and 3 patients showed electrocardiographic evidence of myocardial infarction.[8] The results of the first 3500 patients undergoing elective coronary angioplasty at Emory were analyzed and reported in detail.[87] Angioplasty was attempted in 3933 lesions with a success rate of 91 percent. No complications occurred in 89 percent of cases, minor complications occurred in 6.9 percent, and major complications (emergency surgery, myocardial infarction, death) occurred in 4.1 percent of patients. Emergency coronary bypass surgery was performed in 2.7 percent of patients, who had a myocardial infarction rate of 49 percent and a Q-wave infarction rate of 23 percent. In patients sent for emergency surgery, the mortality rate was 2 percent. The overall myocardial infarction rate was 2.6 percent. There were two nonsurgical deaths, giving a total mortality rate of 0.1 percent (4/3500). Five preprocedural predictors of a major complication were identified: multivessel coronary disease, lesion eccentricity, presence of calcium in the lesion, female gender, and lesion length. The strongest predictor of a major complication was the appearance of an intimal dissection during the procedure. Intimal dissection was evident in 29 percent of patients, and its presence resulted in a sixfold increase in the risk of a major complication. Minor complications tabulated in this study included the following: side branch occlusion (1.7 percent), ventricular arrhythmia requiring DC shock (1.5 percent), emergency recatheterization (0.8 percent), femoral artery repair (0.6 percent), transfusion requirement (0.3 percent), coronary embolus (0.1 percent), cardiac tamponade (0.1 percent), and stroke (0.03 percent).

TABLE 71-2

Results of Coronary Angioplasty (Emory University Hospital)*

	1980–1981	1982–1983	1984–1985	1986–1987	1988–1989	Total
Patients	511	1779	2404	2560	2914	10,168
Arterial segments dilated	538	1991	2994	3362	4118	13,011
Initial success,† %	83	93	93	93	92	92
Complication-free success,‡ %	79	91	89	90	90	90
Single-vessel disease, %	87	76	66	55	51	61
Multivessel disease,§ %	13	24	34	45	49	39
Multivessel PTCA,¶ %	0.8	3.8	9	12	13	9.4
Emergency CABG, %	7.2	2.6	3.7	2.8	2.9	3.0
Q-wave AMI, %	2.5	1.1	1.6	1.3	0.8	1.4
In-hospital death, %	0	0.1	0.2	0.3	0.5	0.3

*Patients with evolving myocardial infarction excluded.
†Less than 50% residual stenosis.
‡Less than 50% residual stenosis and freedom from complications.
§At least 50% stenosis of LAD + RCA, LAD + CIRC, CIRC + RCA, or LAD + RCA + CIRC. (LAD = left anterior descending; RCA = right coronary artery; CIRC = circumflex coronary artery.)
¶Dilatation of LAD + RCA, LAD + CIRC, CIRC + RCA, or LAD + CIRC + RCA.

The 1985 to 1986 PTCA Registry of 1801 patients treated in 15 centers with experienced operators revealed that 6.8 percent had acute vessel occlusion.[88] Factors independently associated with increased occlusion rates included unstable angina, triple-vessel disease, complex lesion morphology, thrombus, and intimal tear or dissection. In 49 percent of patients, the artery could be reopened with PTCA, 35 percent had CABG, and 16 percent were treated medically. Fifty-six percent of those treated with immediate surgery had myocardial infarctions, compared to 27 percent when repeat PTCA was utilized and 47 percent when medical therapy was given. Five percent of patients died in each group. Analysis of 4772 patients at Emory revealed a 4.4 percent incidence of acute occlusion[64] and identified four preprocedural risk factors for acute occlusion: bend point location, branch point location, thrombus in the artery, and the presence of other stenoses greater than 50 percent diameter narrowing located elsewhere in the vessel dilated.

The ACC/AHA classification of lesions (Table 71-1) is an imperfect but useful guide that was validated by two recent reports.[67,68] The procedural success and complication rates of PTCA in these two reports were as follows: 92 to 94 and 0 to 2 percent for the A lesions attempted, 84 to 91 and 3 to 7 percent for type B, and 61 to 89 and 9 to 21 percent for type C, respectively. Although these variables indicate the risk of acute occlusion and other complications for coronary angioplasty, of equal or greater importance is the estimate of the consequences if acute occlusion occurs. This estimate is determined in large part by the amount of myocardium that is supplied by the artery that is in jeopardy. Occlusion of a small diagonal branch is of little consequence compared, for example, to the occlusion of a large left anterior descending coronary artery that is also supplying collateral vessels to an occluded right coronary artery. In the first case, a small non-Q-wave infarction is likely, whereas in the latter, occlusion would likely result in abrupt anterior and inferior ischemia and be associated with hypotension and possibly cardiogenic shock. Immediate bypass surgery may be life-saving, but myocardial infarction will occur in at least one-half of patients, and there is a significant risk of mortality in this subgroup of patients.

Analysis of 294 acute occlusions occurring during 8207 consecutive coronary angioplasty procedures performed in two centers revealed 13 cardiac deaths (4.4 percent of acute occlusions) and an overall cardiac mortality of 0.16 percent.[65] Twelve of 13 patients who died were women. Multivariate analysis identified three independent predictors of death: collaterals originating from the dilated vessel, female gender, and multivessel disease. In our analysis of 32 deaths associated with 8052 PTCA procedures in three centers, left ventricular failure due to vessel occlusion, the most common cause of death, was independently correlated with female sex, "jeopardy score," and PTCA of a proximal right coronary artery (RCA) site but not with ejection fraction or presence of multivessel disease.[89] Right ventricular failure due to occlusion of the proximal RCA and left main coronary dissections accounted for the majority of the remaining deaths.

Complications of directional atherectomy, which are quite similar to those experienced with PTCA, have also been reported in detail. In a single-center experience with 382 patients, procedural success occurred in 89 percent, abrupt vessel closure in 4.1 percent, nonobstructive guide catheter-induced dissection in 0.3 percent, vessel perforation in 0.8 percent, Q-wave infarctions in 0.8 percent, non-Q-wave infarction in 4.2 percent, and 3.1 percent required coronary bypass surgery.[90] Atherectomy alone yielded a successful procedure in 80 percent of patients overall but in only 52 percent of de novo lesions with calcification. In a multicenter experience with a similar number of patients, procedural success was achieved in 88 percent of cases, but major complications (death, myocardial infarction, or bypass surgery) occurred in 6.3 percent.[70] Complication rates were 3 percent for type A stenosis attempted, 6 percent if one type B characteristic was present, and 13 percent if more than one type B characteristic was present. Vessel tortuosity, lesion eccentricity, and calcification were multivariate predictors of atherectomy failure.

Patient selection continues to be the primary factor influencing the results and complications of coronary angioplasty and atherectomy. Although the improvements in technology and experience have allowed angioplasty and atherectomy to be performed safely in a majority of patients, the conscious decision of what constitutes an acceptable complication rate is a primary determinant of the complication rate. This is the probable explanation for the wide range of reported annual mortality rates, which vary from 25 per 1000 in some experienced centers[91] to 2 to 10 per 1000 in other equally experienced angioplasty centers and in the National Heart, Lung, and Blood Institute PTCA registry.[92] The diversity in patients undergoing angioplasty and atherectomy makes comparison of patient groups in different centers at different times impossible and emphasizes the need for randomized trials to determine the benefit of coronary angioplasty compared to atherectomy and coronary bypass surgery in the treatment of coronary artery disease.

REFERENCES

1. Dotter CT, Judkins MP: Transluminal treatment of arteriosclerotic obstruction: Description of a new technique and a preliminary report of its application. *Circulation* 1964; 30:654–670.
2. Zeitler EJ, Schmidtke J, Schoop W: Die Perkutane Behandlung von Arteriellen Durchbluteungasstorungen der Estremiaten mit Katheter. *Vasa* 1973; 2:401–404.
3. Gruentzig AR, Turina MI, Schneider JA: Experimental percutaneous dilatation of coronary artery stenosis (abstr). *Circulation* 1976; 54(suppl II):II–81.
4. Gruentzig AR, Kumpe DA: Technique of percutaneous transluminal angioplasty with the Gruentzig balloon catheter. *Am J Roentgenol* 1979; 132:547–552.
5. Hurst JW: Tribute: Andreas Roland Gruentzig (1939–1985) A private perspective. *Circulation* 1986; 73:606–610.
6. Hurst JW: History of cardiac catheterization. In: King SB III, Douglas JS Jr (eds): *Coronary Arteriography and Angioplasty.* New York, McGraw-Hill, 1985: 1–9.
7. Gruentzig A: Transluminal dilatation of coronary artery stenosis. *Lancet* 1978; 1:263.
8. Gruentzig AR, Senning A, Siegenthaler WE: Nonoperative dilatation of coronary artery stenosis: Percutaneous transluminal coronary angioplasty. *N Engl J Med* 1979; 303:61–68.

9. Simpson JB, Baim DS, Robert EW, Harrison DC: A new catheter system for coronary angioplasty. *Am J Cardiol* 1982; 49:1216–1222.
10. Kinney TB, Chin AK, Rurik GW, Finn JC, Shoor PM, Hayden WG, et al: Transluminal angioplasty: A mechanical-pathophysiological correlation of its physical mechanisms. *Radiology* 1984; 153:85–89.
11. Sanborn TA, Faxon DP, Haudenschild C, Gottsman SB, Ryan TJ: The mechanisms of transluminal angioplasty: Evidence for formation of aneurysms in experimental atherosclerosis. *Circulation* 1983; 68:1136–1140.
12. Castaneda-Zuniga WR, Formanek A, Tadavarthy M, Vlodaver Z, Edwards JE, Zollikofer C, et al: The mechanism of balloon angioplasty. *Radiology* 1980; 135:565–571.
13. Block PC: Mechanism of transluminal angioplasty: *Am J Cardiol* 1984; 53:69C.
14. Mizuno K, Kurita A, Imazeki N: Pathological findings after percutaneous transluminal coronary angioplasty. *Br Heart J* 1984; 52:588–590.
15. Soward AL, Essed CE, Serruys PW: Coronary arterial findings after accidental death immediately after successful percutaneous transluminal coronary angioplasty. *Am J Cardiol* 1985; 56:794–795.
16. Farb A, Virmani R, Atkinson JB, Kolodgie FD: Plaque morphology and pathologic changes in arteries from patients dying after coronary balloon angioplasty. *J Am Coll Cardiol* 1990; 16:1421–1429.
17. Fishbein MC: Coronary artery plaque morphology after balloon angioplasty. *J Am Coll Cardiol* 1990; 16:1430–1431.
18. Waller BF: Pathology of coronary balloon angioplasty and related topics. In: Topol EJ (ed): *Textbook of Interventional Cardiology.* Philadelphia, Saunders, 1990: 395–451.
19. Leimgruber PP, Roubin GS, Hollman J, Cotsonis GA, Meier B, Douglas JS, et al: Restenosis after successful coronary angioplasty in patients with single-vessel disease. *Circulation* 1986; 73:710–717.
20. Essed CE, Van den Brand M, Becker AE: Transluminal coronary angioplasty and early restenosis: Fibrocellular occlusion after wall laceration. *Br Heart J* 1983; 49:393–396.
21. Austin GE, Ratliff NB, Hollman J, Tabei S, Phillips DF: Intimal proliferation of smooth muscle cells as an explanation for recurrent coronary artery stenosis after percutaneous transluminal coronary angioplasty. *J Am Coll Cardiol* 1985; 6:369–375.
22. Waller BF, Pinkerton CA, Orr CM, Slack JD, Vantassel JW, Peters T: Restenosis 1 to 24 month after clinically successful coronary balloon angioplasty: A necropsy study of 20 patients. *J Am Coll Cardiol* 1991; 17:58B–70B.
23. Nobuyoshi M, Kimura T, Nosaka H, Mioka S, Ueno K, Yokoi H, et al: Restenosis after successful percutaneous transluminal coronary angioplasty: Serial angiographic follow-up of 229 patients. *J Am Coll Cardiol* 1988; 12:616–623.
24. Califf RM, Fortin DF, Frid DJ, Harlan WR, Ohman EM, Bengtson Jr, et al: Restenosis after coronary angioplasty: An overview. *J Am Coll Cardiol* 1991; 17:2B–13B.
25. Gruentzig AR, King SB III, Schlumpf M, Siegenthaler WE: Long-term follow-up after percutaneous transluminal coronary angioplasty: The early Zurich experience. *N Engl J Med* 1987; 316:1127–1132.
26. Gruentzig AR, Myler RK, Hann EH, Turina MI: Coronary transluminal angioplasty (abstr). *Circulation* 1977; 55(suppl III):III–84.
27. Block PC, Elmer D, Fallon JT: Release of atherosclerotic debris after transluminal angioplasty. *Circulation* 1982; 65:950–952.
28. Douglas JS Jr, Robinson K, Schlumpf M: Percutaneous transluminal angioplasty in aortocoronary venous graft stenoses: Immediate results and complications (abstr). *Circulation* 1986; 74(suppl II):II–363.
29. Aueron F, Gruentzig A: Distal embolization of a coronary artery bypass graft atheroma during percutaneous transluminal coronary angioplasty. *Am J Cardiol* 1984; 53:953–954.
30. Douglas JS Jr, King SB III, Roubin GS: Influence of the methodology of percutaneous transluminal coronary angioplasty on restenosis. *Am J Cardiol* 1987; 60:29B–33B.
31. Whitworth HB, Roubin GS, Hollman J, Meier B, Leimgruber PP, Douglas JS Jr, et al: Effect of nifedipine on recurrent stenosis after percutaneous transluminal coronary angioplasty. *J Am Coll Cardiol* 1986; 8:1271–1276.
32. Thornton MA, Gruentzig AR, Hollman J, King SB, Douglas JS Jr: Coumadin and aspirin in prevention of recurrence after transluminal coronary angioplasty: A randomized study. *Circulation* 1984; 69:721–727.
33. Roubin GS, King SB III, Douglas JS Jr: Restenosis after percutaneous transluminal coronary angioplasty: The Emory University Hospital experience. *Am J Cardiol* 1987; 60:39B–43B.
34. Topol EJ, Faxon DP: Symposium on restenosis: From basic studies to clinical trials. *J Am Coll Cardiol* 1991; 17:1B–199B.
35. O'Neill WW, Walton JA, Bates ER, Colfer HT, Aueron FM, LeFree MT, et al: Criteria for successful coronary angioplasty as assessed by alterations in coronary vasodilatory reserve. *J Am Coll Cardiol* 1984; 3:1382–1390.
36. Hirzel H, Neusch K, Gruentzig A, Leutolf UM: Short and long-term changes in myocardial perfusion after percutaneous transluminal coronary angioplasty assessed by thallium-201 exercise scintigraphy. *Circulation* 1981; 63:1001–1007.
37. Scholl JM, Chaitman BR, David PR, Dupras G, Brevers G, Val PG, et al: Exercise electrocardiography and myocardial scintigraphy in the serial evaluation of the results of percutaneous transluminal coronary angioplasty. *Circulation* 1982; 66:380–390.
38. Kent KM, Bonow RO, Rosing DR, Ewels CJ, Lipson LC, McIntosh CL, et al: Improved myocardial function during exercise after successful percutaneous transluminal coronary angioplasty. *N Engl J Med* 1982; 306:441–446.
39. Mancini J: Quantitative coronary arteriographic methods in the interventional catheterization laboratory: An update and perspective. *J Am Coll Cardiol* 1991; 17:23B–33B.
40. Yock PG, Fitzgerald PJ, Linker DT, Angelsen BAJ: Intravascular ultrasound guidance for catheter-based coronary interventions. *J Am Coll Cardiol* 1991; 17:39B–45B.
41. White CJ, Ramee SR, Mes JE, Collins TJ: Percutaneous coronary angioscopy in patients with restenosis after coronary angioplasty. *J Am Coll Cardiol* 1991; 17:46B–49B.
42. Robertson GC, Hinohara T, Selmon MR, Johnson DE, Simpson JB: Directional coronary atherectomy. In: Topol EJ (ed): *Textbook of Interventional Cardiology.* Philadelphia, Saunders, 1990: 593–579.
43. Robertson GC, Simpson JB, Selmon MR, Vetter JW, Bartzokis TC, Rowe MH, et al: Experience with directional coronary atherectomy over four years. *J Am Coll Cardiol* 1991; 17:384A.
44. Sharaf BL, Williams DO: "Dotter effects" contributes to angiographic improvement following directional coronary atherectomy (abstr). *Circulation* 1990; 82(suppl III)III–310.
45. Safian RD, Gelbfish JS, Erny RE, Schmitt SJ, Baim DS: Coronary atherectomy: Clinical, angiographic, and histologic findings and observations regarding potential mechanisms. *Circulation* 1990; 82:69–79.
46. Garratt KN, Edwards WD, Vlietstra RE, Kaufmann UP, Holmes DR: Coronary morphology after percutaneous directional coronary atherectomy in humans: Autopsy analysis of three patients. *J Am Coll Cardiol* 1990; 16:1432–1436.
47. Penny WF, Schmidt DA, Safian RD, Erny RE, Baim DS: Insights into the mechanism of luminal improvement after directional coronary atherectomy. *Am J Cardiol* 1991; 67:435–437.
48. Rowe MH, Robertson GC, Simpson JB, Selmon MR, Vetter JW, Braden LJ, et al: Amount of tissue removed by directional coronary atherectomy (abstr). *Circulation* 1990; 82(suppl III):III–312.
49. U.S. Directional Coronary Atherectomy Group: Complications of directional coronary atherectomy in a multicenter experience (abstr). *Circulation* 1990; 82(suppl III):II–311.
50. U.S. Directional Coronary Atherectomy Group: Restenosis following directional coronary atherectomy in a multicenter experience (abstr). *Circulation* 1990; 82(suppl III):III–679.
51. Popma JJ, Topol EJ, Pinkerton CA, Whitlow PL, Hartzler GO, Selmon MR, et al: Abrupt closure following directional coronary atherectomy: Clinical, angiographic and procedural outcome (abstr). *J Am Coll Cardiol* 1991; 17:23A.
52. Robertson GC, Simpson JB, Selmon MR, Vetter JW, Bartzokis TC, Rowe MH, et al: Experience of directional coronary atherectomy over four years (abstr). *J Am Coll Cardiol* 1991; 17:384A.
53. Hinohara T, Selmon MR, Robertson GC, Vetter JW, Rowe MH, Bartzokis TC, et al: Angiographic predictors of restenosis following directional coronary atherectomy (abstr). *J Am Coll Cardiol* 1991; 17:385A.
54. Selmon MR, Robertson CF, Simpson JB, Rowe MH, Johnson DE, Leggett JH, et al: Retrieval of media and adventitia by directional coronary atherectomy and angiographic correlation (abstr). *Circulation* 1990; 82(suppl III):III–624.

55. Dick RJ, Kunkel JF, Debowey DL: Does ectasia following directed coronary atherectomy predict the histological depth of excision? (abstr). *Circulation* 1990; 83(suppl III):IIII–623.
56. de Cesare NB, Popma JJ, Whitlow PL, Pinkerton CA, Kereiakes DJ, Garratt KN, et al: Excision beyond the "normal" arterial wall with directional coronary atherectomy—Acute and long-term outcome (abstr). *J Am Coll Cardiol* 1991; 17:384A.
57. Popma J, Dick R, Handenschild C, Topol E, Ellis S: Atherectomy of right coronary ostial stenoses: Initial and long-term results, technical features and histologic findings. *Am J Cardiol* 1991; 67:431–433.
58. Hinohara T, Vetter JW, Rowe MH, Robertson GC, Selmon MR, Doucettet JW, et al: The effect of angiographic risk factors on the outcome of directional coronary atherectomy (abstr). *J Am Coll Cardiol* 1991; 17:23A.
59. Robertson GC, Rowe MH, Selmon MR, Hinohara T, Vetter JW, Braden LJ, et al: Directional coronary atherectomy for lesions with complex morphology (abstr). *Circulation* 1990; 82(suppl III):III–312.
60. Ghazzel ZMB, Douglas JS, Holmes DR, Ellis SG, Keriakes DJ, Simpson JF, et al: Directional coronary atherectomy of saphenous vein grafts: Recent multicenter experience (abstr). *J Am Coll Cardiol* 1991; 17:219A.
61. Selmon MR, Hinohara T, Robertson GC, Rowe MH, Vetter JW, Bartzokis TC, et al: Directional coronary atherectomy for saphenous vein graft stenoses (abstr). *J Am Coll Cardiol* 1991; 17:23A.
62. Vetter JW, Simpson JB, Robertson GC, Selmon MR, Rowe MH, Bartzokis TC, et al: Rescue directional coronary atherectomy for failed balloon angioplasty (abstr). *J Am Coll Cardiol* 1991; 17:384A.
63. Whitlow PL, Robertson GC, Rowe MH, Douglas JS, Cowley MJ, Kereiakes DJ, et al: Directional coronary atherectomy for failed percutaneous transluminal coronary angioplasty (abstr). *Circulation* 1990; 82(suppl III):III–1.
64. Ellis SG, Roubin GS, King SB III, Douglas JS Jr, Weintraub WS, Thomas RG, et al: Angiographic and clinical predictors of acute closure after native vessel coronary angioplasty. *Circulation* 1988; 77:372–379.
65. Ellis SG, Roubin GS, King SB III, Douglas JS Jr, Shaw RE, Stertzer SH, et al: In-hospital cardiac mortality following acute closure after percutaneous transluminal coronary angioplasty–Analysis of risk factors from 8207 procedures. *J Am Coll Cardiol* 1988; 11:211–216.
66. Ryan TJ, Faxon DP, Gunnar RM, Kennedy JW, King SB III, Loop FD, et al: Guidelines for percutaneous transluminal coronary angioplasty. *J Am Coll Cardiol* 1988; 12:529–545.
67. Cragg DR, Friedman HZ, Almany SL, Gangadharan V, Ramos RG, Levine AB, et al: Early hospital discharge after percutaneous transluminal coronary angioplasty. *Am J Cardiol* 1989; 64:1270–1274.
68. Ellis SG, Vandormael MG, Cowley MJ, DiSciascio G, Deligonul U, Topol EJ: Coronary morphologic and clinical determinants of procedural outcome with angioplasty for multivessel coronary disease. *Circulation* 1990; 82:1193–1203.
69. Robertson GC, Selmon MR, Hinohara T, Rowe MH, Leggett JH, Braden LJ, et al: The effect of lesion length on outcome of directional coronary atherectomy (abstr). *Circulation* 1990; 82(suppl III):III–623.
70. Ellis SG, de Cesare NB, Pinkerton CA, Whitlow P, King SB, Ghazzal ZMB: Relation of stenosis morphology and clinical presentation to the procedural results of directional coronary atherectomy. *Circulation* 1991; 84:644–653.
71. Kelsey SF, Mullin SM, Detre KM, Mitchell H, Cowley MJ, Gruentzig AR: Effect of investigator experience on PTCA. *J Am Coll Cardiol* 1984; 53:56C–64C.
72. Ryan TJ, Klocke FJ, Reynolds WA: Clinical competence in percutaneous transluminal coronary angioplasty. *Circulation* 1990; 81:2041–2046.
73. Douglas JS Jr, Lutz JF, Clements SD, Robinson PH, Roubin GS, Lembo NJ, et al: Therapy of large intracoronary thrombi in candidates for percutaneous transluminal coronary angioplasty (abstr). *J Am Coll Cardiol* 1988; 238A.
74. Black AJ, Anderson HV, Roubin GS, Powelson SW, Douglas JS Jr, King SB III: Repeat coronary angioplasty: Correlates of a second restenosis. *J Am Coll Cardiol* 1988; 11:714–718.
75. Grines CL, Browne KF, Marco J, Rothbaum D, Stone GW, O'Keefe J, et al: A comparison of immediate angioplasty with thrombolytic therapy for acute myocardial infarction. *N Engl J Med* 1993; 328:673–679.
75a. Zijlestra F, De Boer MJ, Hoorntje JCA, Reiffers S, Reiber JHC, Suryapranata H: A comparison of immediate coronary angioplasty with intravenous streptokinase in acute myocardial infarction. *N Engl J Med* 1993; 328:680–684.
75b. Gibbons RJ, Holmes DR, Reeder GS, Bailey KR, Hopfenspirger MR, Gersh BJ: Immediate angioplasty compared with the administration of a thrombolytic agent followed by conservative treatment for myocardial infarction. *N Engl J Med* 1993; 328:685–691.
76. DeWood MA, Spores J, Berg R, Kendall RW, Grunwald RP, Selinger SL, et al: Acute myocardial infarction: A decade of experience with surgical reperfusion in 701 patients. *Circulation* 1983; 68(suppl 2):8–16.
77. The TIMI Study Group: Comparison of invasive and conservative strategies after treatment with intravenous tissue-plasminogen activator in acute myocardial infarction. Results of the Thrombolysis in Myocardial Infarction (TIMI) Phase II trial. *N Engl J Med* 1989; 320:618–627.
78. Douglas JS Jr, Gruentzig AR, King SB III, Hollman J, Ischinger T, Meier B, et al: Percutaneous transluminal coronary angioplasty in patients with prior coronary bypass surgery. *J Am Coll Cardiol* 1983; 2:745–754.
79. Douglas JS Jr: Angioplasty of saphenous vein and internal mammary artery bypass grafts. In: Topol EJ (ed): *Textbook of Interventional Cardiology*. Philadelphia, Saunders, Philadelphia, 1990: 327–343.
80. Gray WA, Williams DO: Marked diameter enlargement in polyolefincopolymer angioplasty balloons after first inflation (abstr). *Circulation* 1991; 84(suppl II):II–591.
81. Sigwart U, Puel J, Mirkovitch V, Joffre F, Kappenberger L: Intravascular stents to prevent occlusion and restenosis after transluminal angioplasty. *N Engl J Med* 1987; 316:701–706.
82. Hearn JA, Douglas JS Jr, Roubin GS, Ghazzal ZMB, Scott NA, King SB III: Late outcome in patients receiving a balloon-expandable intracoronary stent for acute closure (abstr). *Circulation* 1991; 84(suppl IV):II–589.
83. Lembo NJ, King SB III, Roubin GS, Black AJ, Douglas JS Jr: Effects of nonionic versus ionic contrast media on complications of percutaneous transluminal coronary angioplasty. *Am J Cardiol* 1991; 67:1046–1050.
84. Roubin GS, Douglas JS Jr, King SB III, Lin S, Hutchinson N, Gruentzig AR: Influence of balloon size in initial success, acute complications and restenosis after percutaneous transluminal coronary angioplasty—A prospective randomized study. *Circulation* 1988; 78:557–565.
85. Meier B, Rutishauser W: Coronary pacing during percutaneous transluminal coronary angioplasty. *Circulation* 1985; 71:557–561.
86. Ellis SG, Roubin GS,. Wilentz J, Lin S, Douglas JS Jr, King SB III: Results of a randomized trial of heparin and aspirin vs. aspirin along for prevention of acute closure and restenosis after angioplasty (abstr). *Circulation* 1987; 76(suppl IV):IV–213.
87. Bredlau CE, Roubin GS, Leimbruger PP, Douglas JS Jr, King SB III, Gruentzig AR: In-hospital morbidity and mortality in patients undergoing elective coronary angioplasty. *Circulation* 1985; 72:1044–1052.
88. Detre KM, Holmes DR Jr, Holubkokv R, Cowley MJ, Bourassa MG, Faxon DP, et al: Incidence and consequences of periprocedural occlusion: The 1985–1986 National Heart, Lung, and Blood Institute Percutaneous Transluminal Coronary Angioplasty Registry. *Circulation* 1990; 82:739–750.
89. Ellis SG, Myler RK, King SB III, Douglas JS Jr, Topol EJ, Shaw RE, et al: Causes and correlates of death after unsupported coronary angioplasty: Implications for use of angioplasty and advanced support techniques in high-risk settings. *Am J Cardiol* 1991; 68:1447–1451.
90. Hinohara T, Rowe MH, Robertson GC, Selmon MR, Braden L, Leggett JH, et al: Effect of lesion characteristics on outcome of directional coronary atherectomy. *J Am Coll Cardiol* 1991; 17:1112–1120.
91. Hartzler GO, Rutherford BD, McConahay DR: Angioplasty in evolution: Six years of changing indications, success and risks (abstr). *J Am Cardiol* 1987; 9:181A.
92. Holmes DR Jr, Vliestra RE, Kelsey S: Comparison of current and earlier complications of angioplasty. NHLBI PTCA registry (abstr). *J Am Coll Cardiol* 1987; 9:19A.

Chapter 72

The Use of the Laser in the Treatment of Coronary and Peripheral Arterial Obstruction

George S. Abela, M.D., M.Sc. ■ *C. Richard Conti, M.D.*

BACKGROUND

The acronym *laser* stands for light amplification by stimulated emission of radiation. The laser is an amplified monochromatic and coherent light that has several properties that allow its use in biology and medicine. These properties include the ability to photocoagulate tissue and to be selectively absorbed, precisely directed, and transmitted through an optical fiber. All of these qualities suggest that the laser, when used appropriately, is a suitable instrument to recanalize obstructed blood vessels and widen channels through partially obstructive lesions within the vascular system. Laser parameters can be varied by changing the medium through which lasing is performed (e.g., blood versus saline solution), the optical fiber through which it is delivered, the pulse duration and power, or the radiation wavelength that is utilized.[1]

Historically, three types of lasers were most frequently used for medical purposes. These included the argon, carbon dioxide, and neodymium-yttrium aluminum garnet (Nd-YAG). Because of their absorption characteristics and transmission through standard optical fibers, the argon and Nd-YAG lasers were preferred to CO_2 lasers for intravascular application.[1–5] Recently, other laser systems have become the lasers of choice for intravascular recanalization. These include the excimer laser, which is the ultraviolet region of the spectrum, and the holmium and erbium YAG lasers in the near infrared region of the spectrum, which also show promise for arterial recanalization. The advantage of these systems is the ability for precise cutting with minimal or no thermal injury to the arterial wall adjacent to the plaque. Also, the high-frequency pulses of the excimer and erbium YAG lasers allow for ablation of calcium more readily than with the continuous-wave lasers. Although a limitation of high-pulse-energy lasers is transmission through standard optical fibers, it has been possible to overcome this difficulty for the 308-nm excimer wavelength that is now being widely used in arterial recanalization. Fibers for the erbium YAG require further development for such applications.

EXPERIMENTAL STUDIES

Investigations indicate that the effectiveness of vaporizing atherosclerotic plaque depends on the total energy delivered over a specific surface area (i.e., energy density).[1,6] Histological and gross examination of continuous-wave laser irradiation shows it is capable of ablating atherosclerotic plaque, resulting in a smooth wall channel that is free of debris and surrounded by zones of thermal and vacuolization injury (Fig. 72-1). Radiation, however, from pulsed lasers results in a smoother surface with minimal or no thermal injury. It has been postulated that the long-term effects might be better with less ther-

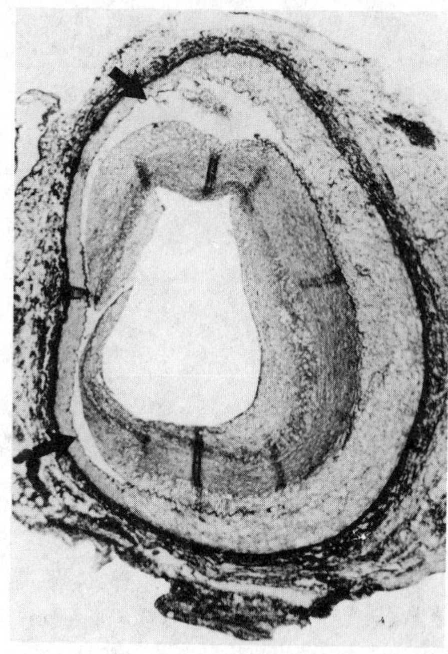

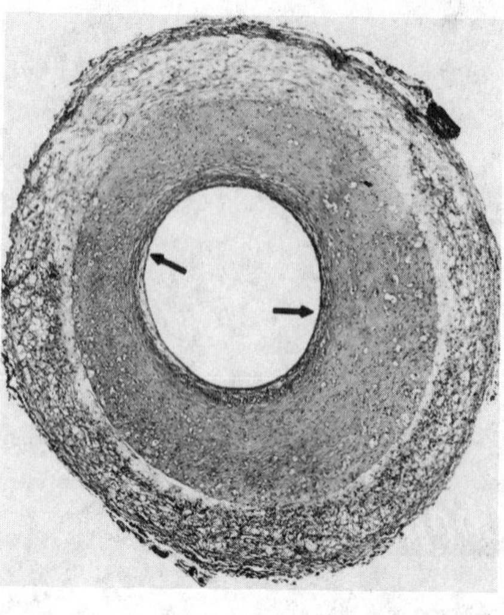

FIGURE 72-1 Cross section of atherosclerotic rabbit iliac arteries after balloon angioplasty (*left panel*) and laser canalization (*right panel*). Both vessels were demonstrated to have high-grade stenoses by angiography prior to treatment. *Left:* Plaque compression and dissection with intimal-medial separation and tearing after balloon inflation. *Right:* Smooth-walled recanalized atheromatous plaque after thermal laser vaporization. There is a thin layer of charring along edges of recanalized channel (arrows) but no evidence of dissection. Hematoxylin and eosin stain; ×50 reduced 15 percent. [*From GS Abela: Other catheter based techniques for treatment of coronary artery disease: In: CJ Pepine (ed): Diagnostic and Therapeutic Cardiac Catheterization. Baltimore, Williams & Wilkins, 1989. Reproduced with permission from the publisher and the author.*]

mal injury; however, severe tissue dissection and explosion may occur with high doses and frequencies of pulsed lasers. A study comparing arterial surfaces treated with a thermally activated probe versus an excimer laser was conducted in vitro and showed that platelet deposition on the thermally treated surface was significantly lower than on the excimer-treated surface and control vessel.[7] In another study using an argon laser to irradiate atherosclerotic plaque in monkeys, irradiated areas did not develop rapid progression of atherosclerosis and thrombi were rare.[8] Other studies have shown extensive thrombus formation at thermally treated surfaces,[9] especially when severe thermal damage was present with full-thickness thermal necrosis of the arterial wall. These disparate results demonstrate the need for a better standard of the energy dose matrix needed for therapeutic plaque ablation. Since different devices used in laser angioplasty may have different energy matrix requirements, this needs to be well defined for each device.

Because of the possibility of laser exposure of the normal portion of the blood vessels, the immediate and long-term effects of laser radiation on normal vascular tissue were examined.[10] Biopsy specimens of lased vascular sites in the dog femoral or carotid arteries taken at 2, 3, 7, 14, and 30 days were examined by light, scanning, and transmission electron microscopy. Results indicated that the artery heals almost completely within 1 month. The initial laser impact site forms a crater that is then filled by a coagulum of blood elements and is subsequently covered by surface endothelium that begins to appear 10 to 14 days after lasing. The same experiments were performed on blood vessels of atherosclerotic monkeys, and similar results were found. Studies have shown similar long-term results with CO_2, argon, and excimer lasers.[6,10]

Arterial homografts of an atrioventricular (AV) shunt model connecting the left carotid artery with the right jugular vein in normal dogs were treated with direct laser, balloon angioplasty, thermal probe, and a thermal probe followed by balloon angioplasty.[11] Radioactive ^{111}indium-labeled platelets were used to assess thrombogenicity of the treated arterial surface. These studies demonstrated that balloon angioplasty resulted in the highest amount of platelet adhesion. Also, it was noted that thermal treatment of the arterial wall prior to balloon angioplasty resulted in a significant reduction in platelet adhesion when compared to balloon angioplasty alone. Other studies support these observations and suggest that these effects are related to the level of temperature achieved.[12] Arterial wall temperatures between 70 and 100°C result in a less thrombogenic surface whereas higher temperatures result in arterial thrombosis. Whether or not these observations will result in less restenosis in the clinical setting has yet to be shown.

FIBER-OPTIC CATHETER DEVELOPMENT

A variety of optical catheter systems have been developed to deliver laser radiation to vaporize intraarterial plaque. Early devices were comprised of a single optical fiber with or without modifications of the fiber tip. One such device, the hot-tip, consisted of a metal cap at the tip of the optical fiber. Other modifications included a metal cap with a recessed lens that allowed 20 percent of the laser beam to exit in a focused fashion. Both the hot-tip and its variation, known as a hybrid probe, were used to recanalize totally occluded vessels in the peripheral circulation. In most instances, however, balloon angioplasty was necessary to further enlarge the arterial lumen.[13]

The majority of current devices are composed of an optical fiber bundle surrounding a central channel. This allows the use of a steerable guide wire passed across a stenotic lesion to maintain a coaxial position within the arterial lumen. The laser catheter system then cores out a channel in the stenotic lesion equal to the size of the

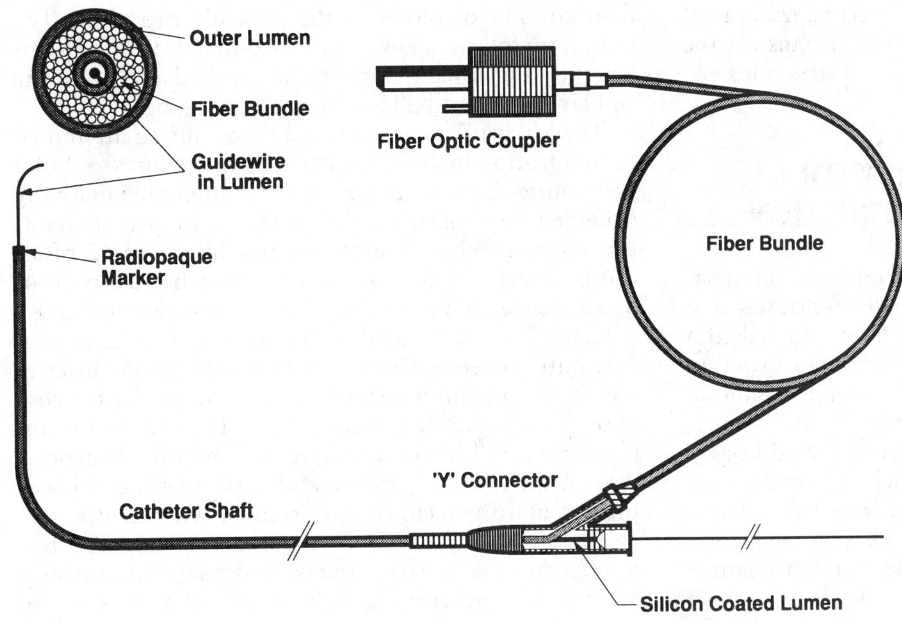

FIGURE 72-2 Laser catheter used to deliver excimer (308 nm) irradiation. Fiber bundle is composed of 100 fibers surrounding a central lumen to allow for normal saline flush and guide wire passage. Coupling to the laser is made via an optical plug system. (*Adapted from Spectranetics Laser Catheter System, Colorado Springs, CO.*)

diameter of the catheter. Thus, these catheter systems function primarily by direct tissue contact. The number of fibers packed into the catheter greatly influences the ability to deliver sufficient energy density at the catheter tip to obtain plaque vaporization with minimal mechanical trauma. Thus, reduction of "dead space" between fibers is essential in reducing the potential for dissection and incomplete vaporization during laser angioplasty (Fig. 72-2).

Other devices have used laser energy for arterial tissue welding purposes. A laser-balloon combination allows for balloon dilation of the stenosis followed by thermal sealing or welding of the cracks and tears resulting from the conventional balloon dilation[14] (Fig. 72-3). This approach has been shown to be effective in treating abrupt closure of the coronary artery by welding the flaps caused by balloon angioplasty. In a multicenter clinical trial both the short- and long-term efficacy of percutaneous coronary application of laser-balloon angioplasty was evaluated. In 55 patients, an Nd-YAG laser dose ranged from 250 to 450 J and was given over 20 s. There were no adverse effects noted in any patient either acutely or over the following 24 h, and minimal lumen diameter was significantly increased. Restenosis by clinical assessment after 6 months showed an overall restenosis rate of 51 percent. Although this device proved to be effective in salvaging abrupt closure of the coronary artery after balloon angioplasty, the high restenosis rate has been a deterrent for its wide application.

Other investigators have developed a system using fluorescence spectroscopy to differentiate atheromatous plaque from normal endothelium and arterial wall.[15] Tissues are analyzed and data are fed into a computer, which then directs laser energy through appropriate optical fibers of a shielded multifiber catheter. With this feedback, fibers that are facing plaque discharge the laser beam, whereas those that are facing the normal wall are inhibited. This approach may result in selective plaque ablation. At present, this has been shown to be a major

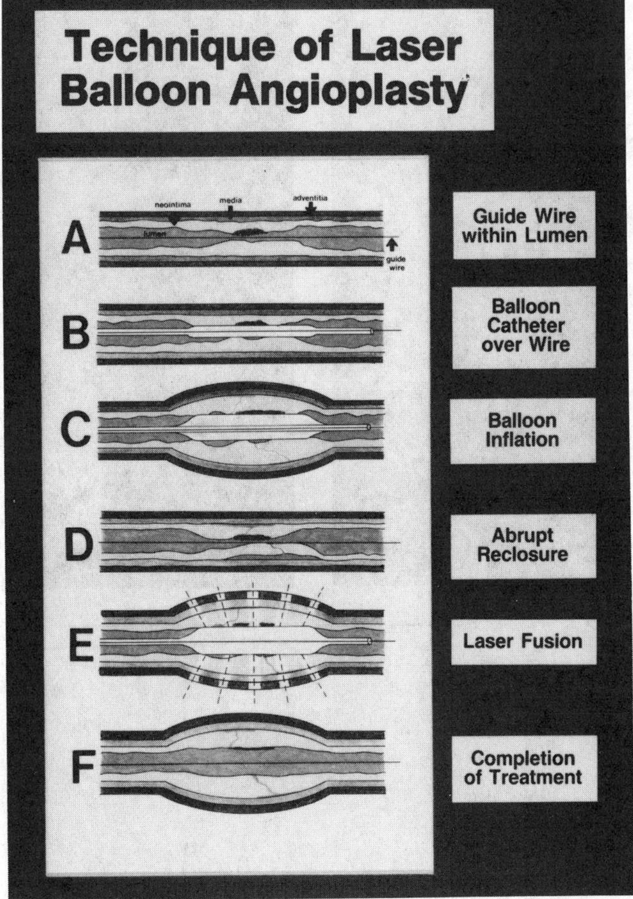

FIGURE 72-3 *A–C.* Conventional balloon angioplasty in which a guide wire is inserted into the arterial lumen. The balloon is threaded over the guide wire to the obstructing plaque and inflated, sometimes producing fracture planes into the arterial wall extending into the media or occasionally even the adventitia. Extensive dissection may cause abrupt reclosure. *D.* In this instance, laser balloon angioplasty (*E*) may be useful in fusing separated layers of arterial wall, resulting in a smooth, dilated lumen (*F*). (*From JF Hiehle et al: Am J Cardiol 56:953–957, 1985.*)

advantage during coronary artery recanalization of stenosed arteries. Also, it may provide a means for the recanalization of total chronic arterial obstructions.

OBSERVATIONS IN PATIENTS WITH PERIPHERAL VASCULAR OBSTRUCTION

In 1984, Geschwind and colleagues[16] reported three patients with obstructed femoral or popliteal arteries that were recanalized using an Nd-YAG laser coupled to a bare optical fiber. Ginsburg et al.[17] reported using an argon laser and a bare optical fiber through a balloon catheter to salvage an ischemic limb.

Cumberland et al.,[18] using the laser-activated hot-tip probe through a percutaneous approach, reported results in 56 patients. They successfully penetrated the plaque in 89 percent of cases. All arteries were subsequently dilated by balloon angioplasty because the initial channel made by the hot-tip probe was too small to serve as the final conduit of blood to the ischemic extremity. The long-term follow-up by physical examination and Doppler study suggested that the technique had a patency rate similar to that of balloon angioplasty alone.

The "hybrid" probe was evaluated during attempted recanalization in 103 patients (115 procedures).[19] In 84 procedures, laser recanalization was attempted in totally occluded superficial or iliac arteries. In percutaneous procedures, technical success was achieved in 42 of 55 (76 percent) and clinical success was achieved in 36 of 55 (65 percent). Balloon angioplasty was required in 87 percent of cases to further enlarge the arterial lumen. Perforations seemed to be increased in calcific arteries where temperatures recorded from the probe tip rose above 250°C during recanalization[20] (Fig. 72-4). On angiographic follow-up at 8.1 ± 5.7 months, restenosis was present in 28 percent and total obstruction was present in 16 percent of laser recanalized patients.

Similar results have been obtained in a prospective multicenter trial in 167 patients using a sapphire-tip laser angioplasty catheter coupled to an Nd-YAG laser to

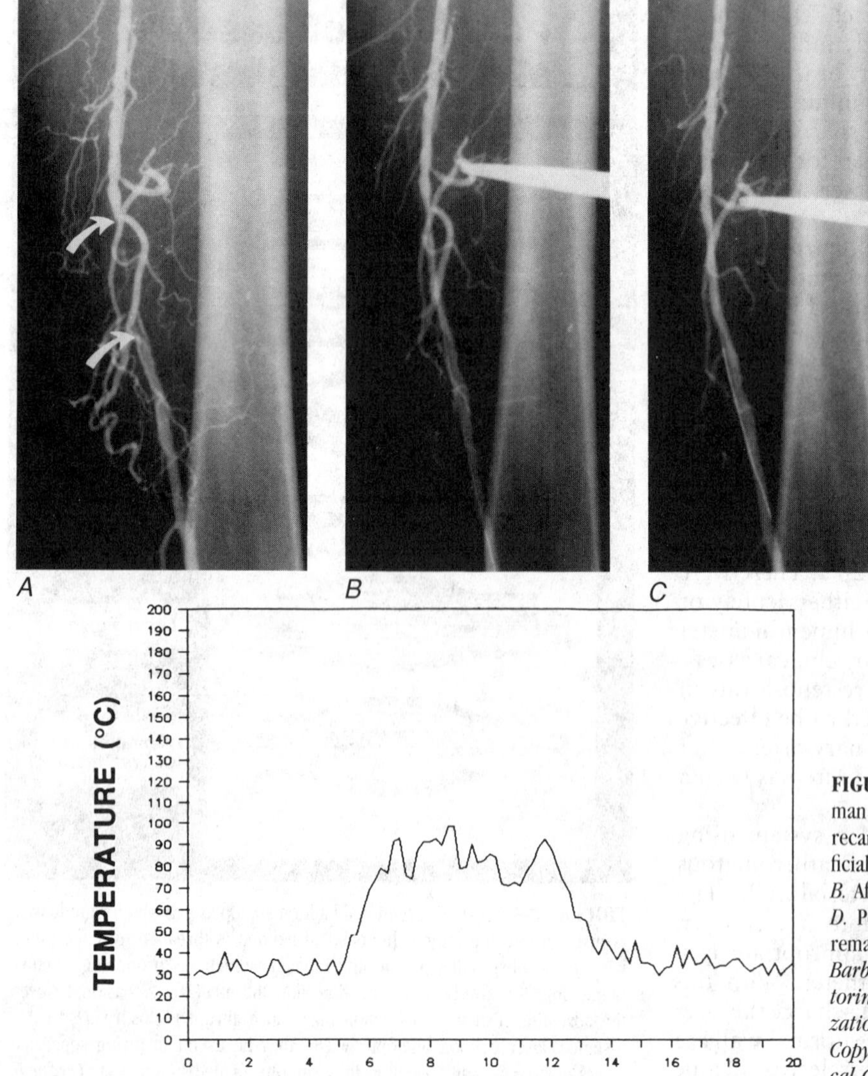

FIGURE 72-4 Sequential angiograms of a 58-year-old man with recent onset of claudication. *A.* Before laser recanalization showing 5-cm occlusion (arrows) of superficial femoral artery with collateral filling of distal segment. *B.* After laser recanalization. *C.* After balloon angioplasty. *D.* Power as well as probe temperature of 95 to 100°C remained constant during recanalization. (*From GR Barbeau, GS Abela, JM Seeger, et al: Temperature monitoring during peripheral thermo-optical laser recanalization in humans. Clin Cardiol 13:690–697, 1990. Copyrighted and reprinted with the permission of Clinical Cardiology Publishing Co. and the Foundation for Advances in Medicine and Science.*)

recanalize totally occluded femoropopliteal occlusions.[21] In 132 of 167 (79 percent) patients, the occluded artery was recanalized and clinical improvement was reported in 126 of 167 (75 percent). At 36 months follow-up, the cumulative patency rate was 63 percent. Patency was significantly lower in patients who were less than 60 years of age and had reduced peripheral runoff.

In all the peripheral clinical studies, complications included burning pain, dissection or perforation, embolization, and groin hematomas. The use of laser technology for treatment of peripheral vascular disease is limited to a select group of patients with total obstructions who cannot be recanalized using standard balloon angioplasty. Otherwise, current lasers do not appear to have a major advantage over balloon angioplasty with respect to restenosis.

LASER RECANALIZATION OF CORONARY ARTERIES

Several investigators have reported experiences with laser recanalization of occluded coronary arteries at the time of surgery using a bare optical fiber coupled to an argon laser or a hand-held CO_2 gun.[22,23] Vessels were subsequently bypassed distal to the recanalized site. At follow-up angiography, many of the laser-treated sites became reoccluded. Competitive flow, small channel size, and perhaps excessive thermal damage could have caused these reocclusions. In two small series of patients with occluded coronary arteries treated with a hot-tip probe catheter device followed by balloon angioplasty, successful recanalization was achieved in only about one-half of the patients.[24,25]

Since these early experiences with continuous-wave lasers and thermal devices, pulsed laser systems have been extensively evaluated in the human coronary circulation. Three commercial excimer laser systems have been tested percutaneously in over 2000 cases in the catheterization laboratory. All of these devices have a similar configuration in that they incorporate a bundle of optical fibers around a central channel used for guide wire placement. The advantages of pulsed lasers over continuous-wave lasers is their ability to create more precise tissue cuts with less thermal damage to the surrounding tissues. However, calcific plaque continues to be extremely difficult to ablate. In addition, arterial spasm and dissections are commonly noted. Although the mechanism of acute closure and spasm is unknown, experimental studies suggest that prolonged irradiation over 10 s in one delivery sequence is likely to result in rapid gas generation in the subintimal layers. This can cause dissection and occasional explosion of the vascular tissues requiring balloon angioplasty to salvage the artery.[26] To limit these effects, energy from pulsed lasers is delivered in short bursts of 5 s on and 5 s off. Despite these limitations, pulsed lasers have been used successfully in certain types of atheromatous lesions not amenable to standard balloon angioplasty.[27] These include ostial lesions and long diffuse stenoses as well as saphenous bypass graft stenoses (Fig. 72-5). (See also Chap. 70.)

Restenosis following laser angioplasty has been difficult to evaluate since most laser procedures are followed by balloon angioplasty in order to obtain a larger vascular lumen. Karsch et al.[28] evaluated 60 patients undergoing laser angioplasty using a 308-nm XeCl excimer laser delivered by concentrically arranged quartz fibers in a 1.4-mm-diameter over-the-wire catheter system. Follow-up angiography at 6 months was performed in 47 of these patients. Overall, 22 patients (47 percent) developed restenosis, defined as loss of at least 50 percent of the gain in the lumen diameter. In 19 patients who had laser angioplasty alone, follow-up angiography showed 6 (32 percent) had restenosis. In 28 of 32 patients who had balloon angioplasty subsequent to laser follow-up angiography showed 16 (57 percent) had developed restenosis. Although this study suggested that restenosis may be lower with laser therapy as stand-alone, further follow-up by this group of investigators has not borne out these preliminary observations. Other studies using excimer lasers have not shown a benefit on restenosis. In a study using a similar device as described above there was no difference in the restenosis rate in patients treated as laser stand-alone (15 of 29, 52 percent) or following balloon angioplasty (12 of 28, 43 percent) at 6 months follow-up.[29] In another study, a reduction of restenosis was noted in those patients who received a higher energy dose.[30] In 189 of 446 patients who underwent follow-up angioplasty, restenosis (lumen diameter reduction below 50 percent) was present in 60 (32 percent). Within this group there was a lower restenosis rate in those patients who received higher energy fluences (50 to 59 mJ/mm^2)

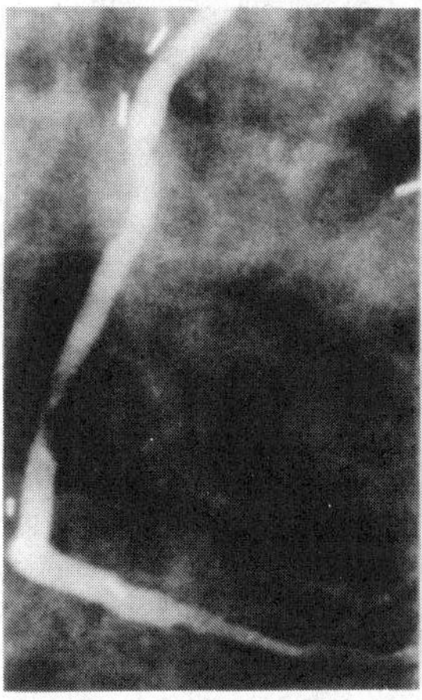
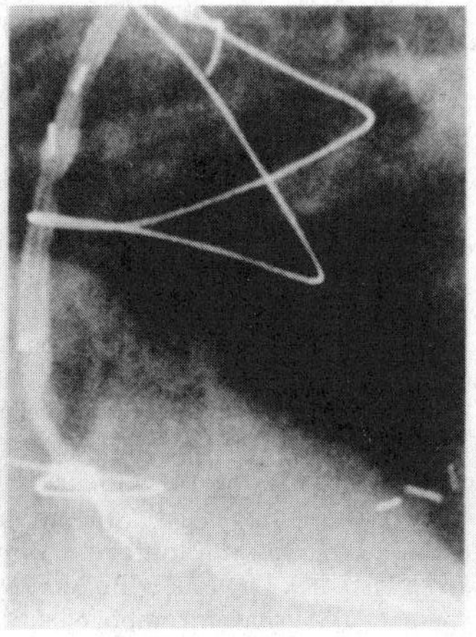
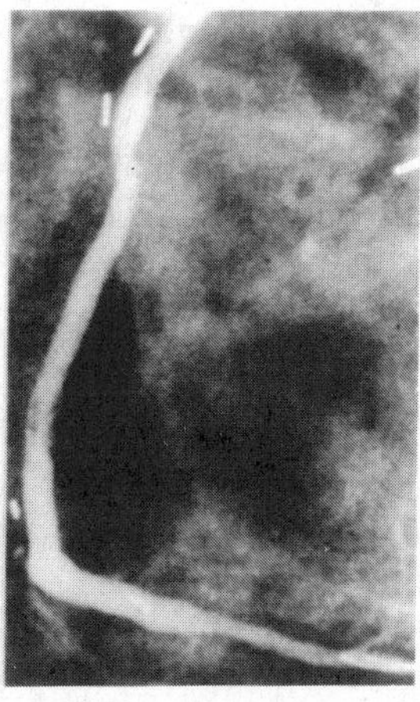

FIGURE 72-5 Angiograms of saphenous bypass graft to the right coronary artery in a 51-year-old man who developed recurrent angina 5 years following coronary bypass surgery. Left panel shows a 90 percent midgraft stenosis. The middle panel shows the stenosis after the first laser treatment using a 2.0-mm-diameter laser catheter as described above. The catheter tip is seen above the lesion site. The right panel shows the final result following completion of laser angioplasty. There is minimal residual stenosis (<20 percent), and this was left as a laser stand-alone result. (*Courtesy GS Abela et al, Deaconess Hospital, Boston, MA.*)

as compared to those who received lower energy fluences (30 to 39 mJ/mm^2 and 40 to 49 mJ/mm^2).

Generally, the technical success (lesion reduction by more than 20 percent) and complication rates of the three currently available excimer laser systems appear to be comparable. In the clinical trials using ELCA (excimer laser coronary artery, Advanced Interventional System, Irvine, CA), the PELCA (percutaneous excimer laser angioplasty, Spectranetics, Colorado Springs, CO, and Technolas, Munich, Germany), the acute technical success rate is reported between 84 and 94 percent depending on the type of lesion treated. On an average, the stenosis is reduced by 30 to 44 percent following laser angioplasty and required balloon angioplasty to obtain an additional 20 to 30 percent improvement. Complications include abrupt closure (3.6 to 20 percent), myocardial infarction (5 percent), and death (1 to 2 percent).[27,31,32] Recently, the Food and Drug Administration has granted premarket approval for clinical use of two excimer systems.

POTENTIAL HAZARDS, COMPLICATIONS, AND MEASURES TO LIMIT THEM

In 1986, three complications were perceived to be the major limitations of the use of lasers in the arterial system: (1) thrombosis, (2) embolization, and (3) perforation of the vessel. Studies have revealed that excessive thermal or shock wave trauma to the arterial wall could result in severe necrosis and disruption of the vascular anatomy leading to acute thrombosis.[33] There seems to be a "temperature window" ranging between 70 and 100°C that results in less platelet adhesion to the arterial surface. With both continuous and pulsed lasers, healing appears to occur with reendothelialization of the blood vessel by 1 month. Distal embolization may occur; however, this is a very rare event in clinical studies performed to date. Perforation during peripheral artery recanalization is serious but has rarely led to any life-threatening complications. In the coronary circulation, on the other hand, perforation of coronary arteries has led to tamponade and, in a rare exception, to death. Although perforation was initially perceived as the major difficulty with laser recanalization, this problem has been greatly curtailed. The use of a steerable guide wire with fiber-optic laser catheters has reduced the chance for perforation considerably. In order to create larger channels and, at the same time, maintain a safe margin to avoid perforation, efforts have been directed toward (1) development of computer-directed feedback mechanisms using fluorescence spectroscopy techniques to differentiate arterial plaque from normal vessel wall, (2) adaptation of ultrasound and/or angioscopy to the tip of the catheter to define the wall thickness and lumen dimension respectively, (3) identification of various energy sources and parameters that are best suited for plaque vaporization, and (4) development of techniques to weld vascular flaps following balloon angioplasty. These approaches have both advantages and certain limitations; however, the variety of catheter delivery systems and techniques for laser recanalization suggests that several systems will probably be effective in arterial recanalization. Perhaps the most pressing issue at present is the use of the laser to create a large enough channel to provide sufficient blood flow to the ischemic tissue. A feedback technique for fine control of the recanalization process appears to provide that capability.

POTENTIAL APPLICATIONS IN HUMANS

Great technological progress toward bringing laser recanalization to clinical application has been made in recent years. This technology, along with other mechanical devices that have appeared recently, has greatly affected the perspectives of arterial recanalization. (See also Chap. 71.) Laser recanalization has the following potential advantages: (1) it can be adapted to treat chronic total arterial obstructions; (2) it can be used for unusual lesions such as ostial and long diffuse stenosis; (3) results are immediate; (4) small distal vessels can be treated; and (5) atherosclerotic plaque is ablated rather than disrupted and dissected. The current clinical experience in the peripheral and coronary circulation reveals that laser recanalization is feasible. However, long-term studies are necessary to substantiate any potential long-term benefit as compared to bypass surgery or balloon angioplasty. The experience with lasers in the peripheral circulation has allowed investigators to understand the potential hazard and the benefits that could be gained from this technique. Also, the current clinical experience has demonstrated that lasers can be used safely and effectively in coronary arteries.

If the laser reaches its full potential application in humans, however, it will likely be used for recanalization in patients who are not candidates for surgical or balloon angioplasty procedures. It is doubtful that laser will replace balloon angioplasty or coronary artery bypass surgery; rather, its major role may be viewed as that of an adjunct to these procedures.

REFERENCES

1. Abela GS, Norman S, Cohen DM, Feldman RL, Geiser EA, Conti CR: Effects of carbon dioxide, Nd:YAG and argon laser radiation on coronary atheromatous plaques. *Am J Cardiol* 1982; 50:1199–1205.
2. Lee G, Ikeda RM, Herman C, Dwyer RM, Bass M, Hussein H, et al: The qualitative effects of laser irradiation on human arteriosclerotic disease. *Am Heart J* 1983; 105:885–889.
3. Eldar M, Battler A, Neufeld HN, Gaton L, Arieli R, Akselrod S, et al: Transluminal carbon dioxide–laser catheter angioplasty for dissolution of atherosclerotic plaques. *J Am Coll Cardiol* 1984; 3:135–137.
4. Choy DSJ, Stertzer S, Rotterdam H, Bruno MS: Laser coronary angioplasty: Experience with nine cadaver hearts. *Am J Cardiol* 1982; 50:1209–1211.
5. Deckelbaum LI, Isner JM, Donaldson RF, Clarke RH, Laliberte SA, Aharon AS, et al: Reduction of laser-induced pathologic tissue injury using pulsed energy delivery. *Am J Cardiol* 1985; 56:662–667.
6. Gerrity RG, Loop FD, Golding LAR, Ehrhart LA, Argenyi ZB: Arterial response to laser operation for removal of atherosclerotic plaques. *J Thorac Cardiovasc Surg* 1983; 85:409–421.
7. Provosti LG, Lawrence JB, Leon MB, Smith PD, Lu DY, Kramer WS, et al: Surface thrombogenicity after excimer laser and hot-tip

thermal ablation of plaque: Morphometric studies using an anular perfusion chamber. *Surg Forum* 1987; 38:330–331.

8. Abela GS, Crea F, Seeger JM, Franzini D, Fenech A, Norman SJ, et al: The healing process in normal canine arteries and in atherosclerotic monkey arteries after transluminal laser irradiation. *Am J Cardiol* 1985; 56:983–988.
9. Sanborn TA, Alexopoulos D, Marmur JD, Kahn H, Badimon JJ, Badimon L, et al: Coronary excimer laser angioplasty: Reduced complications and indium-111 platelet accumulation compared with thermal laser angioplasty. *J Am Coll Cardiol* 1990; 16:502–506.
10. Higgingson LAJ, Farrell EM, Walley VM, Taylor RS, Keon WJ: Arterial response to excimer and argon laser irradiation in the atherosclerotic swine. *Lasers Med Sci* 1989; 4:85–92.
11. Abela GS, Barbeau G, Tomaru T, Franzini D, Seeger J: Thermal coagulation of collagen reduces platelet adhesion following balloon angioplasty (abstr). *J Am Coll Cardiol* 1991; 17:205A.
12. Borst C, Bos AN, Zwaginaga JJ, Rienks R, de Groot PG, Sixma JJ: Loss of platelet adhesion after heating native and cultured human subendothelium to 100 degrees Celsius. *Cardiovasc Res* 1990; 24:665–668.
13. Abela GS, Seeger JM, Barbieri E, Franzini D, Fenech A, Pepine CJ, et al: Laser angioplasty with angioscopic guidance in humans. *J Am Coll Cardiol* 1986; 8:182–194.
14. Spears JR, Reyes VP, Wynne J, Fromm BS, Sinofsky EL, Andrus S, et al: Percutaneous coronary laser balloon angioplasty: Initial results of a multicenter experience. *J Am Coll Cardiol* 1990; 16:293–303.
15. Cothren RM, Hayes GB, Kramer JR, Sacks B, Kittrell C, Feld MS: A multifiber catheter with an optical shield for laser angiosurgery. *Lasers Life Sci* 1986; 1:1–12.
16. Geschwind H, Boussignac G, Teisseire B, Vieilledent C, Gaston A, Becquemin JP, et al: Percutaneous transluminal laser angioplasty in man. *Lancet* 1984; 1:844.
17. Ginsburg R, Wexler L, Mitchell R, Profitt D: Percutaneous transluminal laser angioplasty for treatment of peripheral vascular disease: Clinical experience with sixteen patients. *Radiology* 1985; 155:619–624.
18. Cumberland DC, Sanborn TA, Tayler D, Moore DJ, Welsh CL, Greenfield AJ: Percutaneous laser thermal angioplasty: Initial clinical results with a laser probe in total peripheral artery occlusion. *Lancet* 1986; 28:1457–1459.
19. Abela GS, Seeger JM, Pry RS, Akins EW, Siragusa RJ, Rarbieri E, et al: Percutaneous laser recanalization of totally occluded peripheral arteries: A technical approach. *Dynam Cardiovasc Imag* 1988; 1:302–308.
20. Barbeau GR, Abela GS, Seeger JM, Friedl SE, Tomaru T, Giacomino P: Temperature monitoring during laser peripheral thermo-optical laser recanalization in humans. *Clin Cardiol* 1990; 13:690–697.
21. Pilger E, Lammer J, Bertuch H, Stark G, Decrinis M, Pfeiffer KP, et al: Nd:YAG laser with sapphire tip combined with balloon angioplasty in peripheral arterial occlusions: Long-term results. *Circulation* 1991; 83:141–147.
22. Choy DSJ, Stertzer SH, Myler RK, Marco P, Fourinal G: Human coronary laser recanalization. *Clin Cardiol* 1984; 7:377–381.
23. Livesay JJ, Dewitt R, Leachman R, Hogan PJ, Cooper JR, Sweeney MS: Preliminary report on laser coronary endarterectomy in patients (abstr). *Circulation* 1985; 72 (III):302.
24. Cumberland DC, Oakley GDG, Smith GH, Tayler DI, Starkey IR, Fleming JS, et al: Percutaneous laser-assisted coronary angioplasty (letter to the editor). *Lancet* 1986; 26:214.
25. Sanborn TA, Faxon DP, Kellett MA, Ryan T: Percutaneous coronary laser thermal angioplasty. *J Am Coll Cardiol* 1986; 8:1437–1440.
26. van Leeuwen TG, Motamedi M, Meertens JM, van Erven L, Velema M, Post MJ, et al: In vivo tissue damage by excimer, Ho-Yag, and Th:Yag laser ablation of porcine aorta. *Circulation* 1991; 84(suppl): II-360.
27. Cook SL, Eigler NL, Shefer A, Goldenberg T, Forrester JS, Litvack F: Percutaneous excimer laser coronary angioplasty of lesions not ideal for balloon angioplasty. *Circulation* 1991; 84:632–643.
28. Karsch KR, Haase KK, Voelker W, Baumbach A, Mauser M, Seipel L: Percutaneous coronary excimer laser angioplasty in patients with stable and unstable angina pectoris: Acute results and incidence of restenosis during 6-months follow-up. *Circulation* 1990; 81:1849–1859.
29. Rothbaum D, Linnemeier T, Landin R, Ball M, Hodes Z, Riddell R: Excimer laser coronary angioplasty: Angiographic restenosis rate at six months follow-up (abstr). *J Am Coll Cardiol* 1991; 17:205A.
30. Margolis JR, Krauthamer D, Litvack F, Rauthbaum DA, Untereker WJ, Bresnahan JF, et al: Six month follow-up of excimer laser coronary angioplasty registry patients (abstr). *J Am Coll Cardiol* 1991; 17:218A.
31. Litvack F, Eigler NL, Margolis JR, Grundfest WS, Rothbaum D, Linnemeier T: Percutaneous excimer laser coronary angioplasty. *Am J Cardiol* 1990; 66:1027–1032.
32. Sanborn TA, Sabino TR, Samin KS, Hershman RA, Cohen M, Sherman W, et al: Percutaneous coronary excimer laser-assisted balloon angioplasty: Initial clinical and quantitative angiographic results in 50 patients. *J Am Coll Cardiol* 1991; 17:94–99.
33. Abela GS, Barbieri E, Friedl SE, Normann SJ: Direct laser and laser-thermal irradiation of normal canine coronary arteries: Implication for laser delivery methods. *J Clin Laser Med Surg* 1990; 8:63–71.

Chapter 73

The Surgical Treatment of Atherosclerotic Coronary Heart Disease

Floyd D. Loop, M.D.

In 1957, F. Mason Sones first performed selective cine coronary arteriography. This development opened a new surgical field. For the first time, an arteriogram provided clear visual documentation of coronary arterial pathoanatomy. Coronary arteriography is indicated for patients who have angina or suspected angina, a positive stress electrocardiogram, or other signs of ischemia and selectively for those with previous documented myocardial infarction. (See Chaps. 58 to 60.) In the left coronary system, coronary atherosclerosis tends to occur proximally, and this distribution leaves the distal arterial runoff amenable to bypass surgery. In the right coronary artery, lesions may occur throughout the vessel but are distributed mainly above the major branches.

In the late 1960s, cardiac surgery advanced to the point where surgeons were able to construct autologous venous conduits from the ascending aorta to these distal coronary arteries. Although there were many previous attempts, in May 1967, Favaloro[1] started the first series by performing vein grafts interposed in the right coronary artery and then aortocoronary bypass grafting. Soon afterward the operation was expanded to all major coronary vessels by Johnson and colleagues.[2]

Selection criteria for coronary bypass surgery were hotly debated during the 1970s. Randomized prospective studies of medical and surgical treatment failed to show a significant benefit for surgery, except in the direst subset of patients with three-vessel stenoses and poor left ventricular function. These major trials enrolled patients between 1972 and 1979, a time when angiography did not produce images of optimal clarity and many participating surgeons were inexperienced in small-vessel surgery. As experience widened, relative indications and contraindications for coronary artery bypass grafting were developed (Table 73-1) and benefits in certain subsets documented.[3,4]

INDICATIONS

By the time patients become candidates for operation, coronary atherosclerosis is generally advanced and complicated, affecting all three major coronary arteries. In most surgical series today, between 66 and 80 percent of patients have severe involvement of all three major coronary arteries with complicated atheromatous plaques. Natural history studies have correlated reduced survival with increasing extent of coronary atherosclerosis. The classic natural history studies of Proudfit and colleagues[5] found that survival at 15 years for one-vessel disease was 48 percent; for two-vessel, 28 percent; for three-vessel, 18 percent; and for left main stenosis, 9 percent. Most natural history studies find no appreciable survival difference related to gender. Factors predictive of lower survival include poor left ventricular function,

TABLE 73-1

Current Indications and Contraindications for Coronary Artery Surgery

Indications for coronary artery bypass grafting
Angina interfering with daily activities and/or evidence of severe ischemia by exercise test or resting electrocardiogram
Left main coronary artery stenosis at least 50%
Proximal left anterior descending stenosis at least 70% in conjunction with other major and significant coronary artery stenosis
Proximal three-vessel disease at least 50%
Multivessel stenoses at least 50% combined with moderate-to-severe (left ventricular ejection fraction at most 0.50) left ventricular impairment
Contraindications to coronary artery bypass grafting
Advanced age with marked debility and restricted activity
No angina or ischemia
Poor left ventricular function (ejection fraction below 0.30) and symptoms/signs of heart failure only
Ungraftable coronary arteries
Noncompliance or lack of consent

duration of symptoms, multivessel coronary atherosclerosis, and comorbidity, namely, peripheral vascular disease, diabetes, and hypertension. (See also Chap. 61.)

The rate of coronary atherosclerosis in *women* appears to be increasing, and the number of female surgical candidates has increased. Women have certain characteristics that affect risk and relate to outcome. Exercise testing is not as reliable for detecting severe coronary atherosclerosis in women as in men. Women tend to have a higher fatality rate with first infarction. Some investigations have reported that the severity of angina is greater in women than in men preoperatively; coronary atherosclerosis is equally severe in women, although they tend to have slightly better preoperative left ventricular contraction overall than men. Most studies have shown that the operative mortality is higher in women, and at first glance, gender appears to be a strong indicator of operative risk. When one adjusts the population for physical size, weight, or body surface area, however, gender per se is no longer a significant risk factor for operative mortality.[6,7] Patients of smaller size are at higher risk, probably because of the size of their recipient coronary vessels.

Clinical and Angiographic Indicators

Selection for surgical treatment tends to be based on arteriographic findings and, especially, the perception of myocardial jeopardy. Left main coronary artery narrowing of at least 50 percent in diameter is the most powerful arteriographic indicator of adverse prognosis. Apart from left main coronary artery narrowing, a lesion in the proximal anterior descending coronary artery carries the most prognostic weight. Patients with angina/ischemia and two-vessel disease with anterior descending stenosis or proximal three-vessel disease deserve consideration for bypass surgery, regardless of left ventricular status. When severe ischemia is elicited, referral for revascularization should be contemplated. A delay in diagnosis or treatment may be associated in time with progressive ventricular damage and even loss of life. The severity of left ventricular dysfunction is the single best prognostic indicator, irrespective of the type of treatment. If multivessel disease is identified before left ventricular impairment occurs, longevity, employment, and lifestyle stand to benefit from coronary bypass surgery. Increasing left ventricular dysfunction may show wider survival differences favorable to surgery. As left ventricular performance diminishes, surgery compared with medical treatment may show significant benefit, but with poor ventricular function, overall survival is far less than with normal left ventricular function.

The comparative benefit of coronary bypass surgery increases with the following preoperative characteristics: (1) severity of angina; (2) severity of ischemia documented by perfusion studies, electrocardiogram, and/or exercise testing; (3) number of major coronary vessels with important proximal stenoses, especially with involvement of the left main or proximal anterior descending coronary arteries, or three-vessel disease irrespective of left ventricular function; (4) extent of left ventricular dysfunction; and (5) severity of coronary atherosclerosis combined with peripheral vascular disease, operable valve disorders, and complications of myocardial infarction.

Isolated coronary artery surgery is contraindicated when there are no symptoms or signs of spontaneous or stress-induced ischemia, especially with poor left ventricular function and clinical evidence of heart failure. The very elderly with multiple comorbidities should be evaluated for surgery conservatively. The four *A*s—age, attitude, activity, and associated diseases—may be helpful in judging harm versus benefit.

Asymptomatic Status

Asymptomatic patients and those with no ischemia are only candidates for coronary artery surgery infrequently, such as the unusual circumstances of asymptomatic severe left main disease or severe three-vessel disease with proximal lesions. Only about 4 percent of patients with left main disease of at least 50 percent narrowing are asymptomatic.

Hibernating Myocardium

Hibernating myocardium is a form of painless ischemia caused by chronically reduced myocardial blood flow.[8] (See Chap. 58.) This phenomenon may be confirmed by left ventricular wall improvement after nitroglycerin administration, by positron emission tomography demonstrating metabolism in areas of regional ventricular abnormality, and any other indirect methods that could document reversible exercise-induced ischemia. Coronary artery surgery may be indicated, depending on the pathoanatomy, for its potential to reverse ischemia and improve left ventricular function. Overall, left ventricular segmental wall abnormalities are more often permanent, and contractility is improved in only a minority of cases. In contrast, stunned myocardium is a condition in which coronary blood flow has been restored after a discrete episode of myocardial ischemia but ultrastructural abnormalities persist.[9] Stunned myocardium may occur after myocardial infarction, vasospasm, coronary balloon angioplasty, or coronary bypass surgery performed during acute ischemia. (See also Chaps. 57 and 60.)

Unstable Angina

Unstable angina is a broad but classifiable syndrome and a medical emergency. Approximately 10 percent of these patients experience a myocardial infarction. Stability is the goal, preferably before angiography and referral for revascularization. Continued angina refractory to medical therapy warrants emergency coronary arteriography. Disrupted fissured plaques often associated with mural thrombi are frequently found in unstable angina patients and are thought to acutely narrow the vessel and cause instability of symptoms. Patients with one-vessel disease are most often treated by coronary angioplasty, unless the vessel is not amenable to dilation. The role of acute coronary angioplasty is not settled. Multivessel disease, especially with left ventricular dysfunction, or left main disease is most often treated by coronary artery surgery, preferably when the patient's status is stable. It is important to recognize that preoperative stability lessens the perioperative infarction rate in coronary bypass surgery and is associated with lower operative risk. Necropsy studies have shown that unstable angina is often associated with the most severe forms of coronary atherosclerosis. (See also Chaps. 55 and 59.)

Myocardial Infarction

Myocardial infarction patients are candidates for coronary artery surgery mainly when complications ensue. These complications include ventricular aneurysm, left ventricular rupture, ruptured papillary muscle, and postinfarction ventricular septal defect. (See Chaps. 60 and 74.) Formation of a ventricular aneurysm is treated expectantly. If angina, congestive heart failure, ventricular arrhythmia, or rarely, systemic embolism occurs, consideration is given to aneurysmectomy. These patients frequently have multivessel disease and require combined coronary artery grafting. Left ventricular rupture, ventricular septal defect, and papillary muscle rupture are surgical emergencies. Unless the patient is extremely aged with longstanding multisystem failure, surgical treatment, even with high risk, is better than nonsurgical treatment, which is nearly uniformly fatal.

Surgery has been advocated and achieved with good results in stable myocardial infarction; however, immediate investigation and treatment of every myocardial infarction is generally not practical. Anterior left ventricular infarction is prognostically more dangerous than inferior wall myocardial infarction; however, the latter may be a marker for advanced multivessel coronary atherosclerosis. Some investigators have found that a third of patients with inferior wall infarction had at least 90 percent obstruction of the proximal anterior descending coronary artery and two-thirds had obstruction above 75 percent in the anterior descending coronary artery. Also, when there is evidence of ischemia distant from the site of infarction, the prognosis worsens; these patients should be revascularized, if possible.

Postinfarction Angina

Postinfarction angina is generally regarded as an indication for coronary arteriography. Many reports attest to its low surgical mortality. Poor ventricular function, older age, and cardiogenic shock carry higher risk. Immediate successful revascularization results in an excellent intermediate-term survival rate. (See Chap. 60.)

Sudden Cardiac Death

Sudden cardiac death, defined as death within 1 h, becomes an issue in selection when patients are resuscitated from cardiac arrest. The prognosis is generally better when cardiac arrest occurs with acute myocardial infarction. Survivors should be investigated both by coronary arteriography and electrophysiological studies. It is well known that sudden cardiac death is almost always associated with underlying heart disease, and in this heterogeneous population, approximately half had no ischemic symptoms prior to the event. Referral to surgery depends on the anatomic diagnosis, left ventricular function, and results of electropharmacologic testing. When coronary pathoanatomy is conducive to bypass surgery, surgery appears to reduce the incidence of sudden, unexpected death but may not prevent subsequent myocardial infarction.[10] (See also Chap. 51.)

Peripheral Vascular Disease

Peripheral vascular disease is frequently a marker for coronary atherosclerosis.[11] Abdominal aortic aneurysms are most likely to be associated with severe coronary atherosclerosis. If atherosclerosis is suspected by symptoms or a history of previous myocardial infarction, coronary arteriography should be performed in the workup. In most cases, coronary artery surgery is scheduled first and elective abdominal aneurysmectomy follows, the timing dependent on the size of the aneurysm. If a large abdominal aneurysm is detected and the coronary artery situation is stable, the order may be reversed. Rarely, coronary bypass surgery and aneurysmectomy are performed simultaneously because of unstable angina, left main or three-vessel disease, and an enlarging symptomatic abdominal aneurysm. The risk is considerably less when the procedures are staged. (See also Chaps. 123 to 125.)

Internal carotid narrowing is usually detected first by a bruit and confirmed by ultrasound examination, digital subtraction angiography, or conventional brachiocephalic angiography. Recent evidence confirms that patients with severe (70 to 99 percent) carotid artery stenosis face a significant risk of ipsilateral ischemic stroke within a few years.[12] If the surgical stroke and death rates are within 2 percent, the absolute risk of ipsilateral stroke is reduced significantly in the first 2 years after carotid endarterectomy.[13] If the patient is neurologically asymptomatic and the lesion is unilateral and less than approximately 90 percent stenotic, coronary artery surgery may be staged first and carotid endarterectomy performed electively later. For patients with severe unilateral or bilateral disease and a history of transient ischemic attack or stroke, simultaneous carotid endarterectomy and myocardial revascularization may be considered. In experienced hands, the stroke and mortality rates for combined treatment are less than 5 percent. In most other instances, myocardial revascularization precedes planned and staged carotid endarterectomy, which may occur weeks or years later depending on symptoms. The reverse order may occur when patients are neurologically unstable but have stable angina and coronary pathoanatomy that is not considered dangerous. (See also Chap. 122.)

Concomitant Valve Disease

Concomitant valve disease may be associated with severe coronary atherosclerosis. Aortic stenosis is the most frequently associated form of valve dysfunction, probably because it is a form of atherosclerosis. Combining aortic valve replacement with coronary bypass grafting is routine and, for men, the risk is about the same as that for isolated aortic valve replacement. For elderly women, the risk is still significantly higher. When severe coronary atherosclerosis is present, coronary surgery should be performed simultaneously with all valve operations because survival is significantly improved by coronary bypass grafting compared with valve replacement alone. (See Chap. 79.)

Coronary atherosclerosis is found less frequently in other valvular conditions. Coronary arteriography should be included in the preoperative investigation, except in young patients, because the absence of angina does not exclude coronary atherosclerosis. Valvular aortic regurgitation, mitral stenosis, and mitral regurgitation are frequently repaired today rather than replaced. Mitral valve repair, which is frequently combined with coronary bypass surgery, carries a lower operative risk than mitral valve replacement. (See Chaps. 84 and 85.)

Emergencies

Experience with thrombolytic therapy in acute myocardial infarction indicates that up to 10 percent of patients require immediate surgical treatment because of coronary balloon angioplasty complications, failure of reperfusion, or discovery of dangerous myocardial jeopardy, especially left main coronary artery disease. Modern methods of myocardial protection allow emergency surgery to be undertaken with a hospital mortality rate of approximately 5 percent or less.

Surgical treatment of postinfarction angina may be undertaken when the patient is in stable condition with even lower risk.[14] Early postinfarction angina emanating from a site distant to the infarct carries a poor prognosis,[15] and these patients should be considered for emergency bypass surgery. Controversy about the risk of surgery in acute myocardial infarction has lessened considerably since the advent of thrombolytic therapy. Today, patients with postinfarction angina or dangerous coronary pathoanatomy are recommended for early coronary bypass surgery. Failure of balloon dilatation is infrequent, and the risk of emergent surgery is relatively low; however, the mortality related to emergency reoperation after balloon angioplasty failure is upward of 20 percent. (See also Chaps. 60 and 71.)

CHANGING PRACTICE

In 1990, the median age of patients undergoing coronary artery bypass surgery at the Cleveland Clinic Foundation was 64 years, with 23 percent over age 70 and 2 percent older than age 80; 22 percent were women. Fifty-eight percent had left ventricular dysfunction preoperatively, and 24 percent had undergone open heart surgery previously. In comparing patients operated on in the 1970s and in the 1980s, most investigators have found a significant rise in age, more female surgical candidates, more severe angina, a greater incidence of recent infarction, more patients with three-vessel disease, more left ventricular dysfunction, a greater incidence of emergency operation, and more comorbidity in the form of diabetes, arrhythmias, heart failure, and peripheral vascular disease.[16,17] With advancing age there is a greater prevalence of previous cerebrovascular events and cardiac enlargement and more female patients.[18]

Elderly patients tend to have angina preoperatively more often than younger patients. Operative mortality and perioperative stroke rates rise with advancing age. In the absence of major complications, elderly patients react and recover like younger patients. They have less physiological reserve; consequently, there is less room for error, and seemingly minor events may result in major morbidity. The technology is continuously improving and the safety of surgery in the geriatric age group has improved since the 1970s as a result of improved myocardial protection and better overall management.

THE OPERATION

The objectives of coronary artery surgery are to relieve symptoms, alleviate ischemia, reduce the possibility of subsequent cardiac events, and lengthen life. The first step toward achieving these goals is to perform a complication-free operation. The operation begins with preoperative assessment; risk is lessened by preoperative stability. An experienced anesthesiologist is vital to the team effort. (See also Chap. 140.)

Intraoperatively, skill and judgment combined with technological support and communication are the fundamental elements that determine risk.[19] Risk may also be predicted and stratified by statistical assessment of preoperative characteristics.[20,21] Variables such as emergency status, elevated serum creatinine, advanced age, congestive heart failure, severe peripheral vascular disease, small stature (and low weight), left main coronary artery disease, and severe angina are generally regarded as risk factors. Risk tends to be reduced with each advance in myocardial protection, and the relative position or weight of these variables as risk factors changes. Statistical methodologies can stratify risk based on these and other characteristics, so that high and low probability of mortality and even morbidity may be predicted with more accuracy today and conveyed to patients preoperatively.

The results of use of the various bypass conduits will be discussed later. The conduit of choice is the internal thoracic artery graft. Use of this conduit may be extended in the form of bilateral thoracic artery grafts, free (aortocoronary) arterial grafts,[22] and sequential usage, which involves one or more side-to-side anastomoses, followed by an end-to-side conduit-to-recipient artery anastomosis. The internal thoracic artery may be applied with no increase in morbidity in either young or older patients. The only caveat is that bilateral usage in diabetic patients is fraught with a higher rate of wound infection.

Other arterial conduits that are particularly applicable for patients with diffuse disease and small-sized vessels are the gastroepiploic artery on the greater curvature of the stomach[23] and the inferior epigastric artery,[24,25] which lies behind the rectus muscle. All arterial conduit operations are generally reserved for younger patients with premature onset of coronary atherosclerosis. Generally one or two internal thoracic artery grafts are combined with vein grafts for older patients.

Extensive use of internal thoracic artery grafts would seem applicable in younger patients with premature coronary atherosclerosis; in patients with severe hyperlipidemia, small vessel size, or poor arterial runoff; and in patients whose saphenous veins are unsuitable or absent. Formerly, the saphenous vein graft was the standard conduit. Atherosclerotic deterioration of this graft and the disproportionately large size of the graft to the coronary artery have relegated the vein graft to a secondary role in revascularization of totally obstructed arteries that receive collaterals or for bypass grafting in very elderly patients or in those in whom arterial grafts are unsuitable.

Once considered the mundane aspect of the operation, saphenous vein procurement is recognized today as important to the long-term success of coronary bypass surgery. Veins may be damaged by rough preparation, which results in separation and desquamation of the vascular endothelium.[26] Endothelial trauma can cause platelet adhesion, fibrin deposition, smooth-muscle-cell proliferation, vasospasm, and reduced fibrinolytic activity. Endothelial loss may be accompanied by a reduction in prostacyclin and endothelial-derived relaxing factor release. The delicate vein is best preserved by procurement after heparinization, irrigation with a balanced electrolyte solution and dilute papaverine, low distension pressure, and brief storage.

Endarterectomy is reserved for vessels that are otherwise ungraftable by traditional techniques. Coronary endarterectomy has undergone a resurgence because of improved myocardial protection and greater technical experience in removing all atheromatous material from the individual side branches. Endarterectomy is probably not a satisfactory technique for small vessels that have been occluded for many years.

Myocardial Protection

Myocardial protection may be achieved by (1) either crystalloid or blood cardioplegia, delivered antegrade into the aortic root below the aortic cross-clamp, alone or combined with retrograde (coronary sinus) delivery; (2) continuous ventricular fibrillation under moderate hypothermia without aortic cross-clamping; (3) hypothermic cardiac arrest using continuous intrapericardial cooling with cold saline solution; (4) intermittent occlusion of the ascending aorta preceded by administration of nifedipine, lidoflazine, or similar drugs; and (5) continuous retrograde warm blood cardioplegia delivered under normothermic core conditions.

Cold chemical cardioplegia initiates a potassium arrest that allows the oxygen-deprived heart to be protected for increasingly longer periods of time during complex repairs. Blood cardioplegia[27] with various additives appears advantageous for the following reasons: The heart is oxygenated during arrest and blood cardioplegia provides reoxygenation during reperfusion. Blood cardioplegia may reduce "myocardial stunning" or reperfusion injury and its attendant myocardial necrosis.[28] Less hemodilution occurs with blood cardioplegia. Myocardial recovery is perceptibly stronger than with asanguinous cardioplegia. Longer aortic cross-clamp time is tolerated for complex reconstruction and, in these higher risk cases, myocardial damage appears to be significantly less than with other methods. Significant reductions of perioperative myocardial infarction, stroke, respiratory distress, and wound complications have been noted with substrate-enhanced blood cardioplegia, including use of a warm terminal reperfusate and a single aortic cross-clamp. The reduction in morbid events translates into shorter intensive care unit time, shorter length of hospitalization, and decreases length-of-stay outliers and hospital cost.

Recently, warm blood cardioplegia at normothermic core temperature has been delivered continuously through the coronary sinus.[29] Flow rates of warm blood cardioplegia of approximately 80 mL/min or greater seem to keep the heart aerobic and result in reduced lactate production and improved maintenance of energy stores. If the field is obscured by the installation of blood cardioplegia, the continuous perfusion may be temporarily stopped during anastomotic construction.

The advent of improved myocardial protection has made coronary artery bypass grafting more scientific. Complex arterial grafting, emergency operations, technically arduous reoperations, and combined coronary artery surgery and other cardiac surgery have been made safer by the advances in myocardial protection. Not only have mortality and morbidity lessened over time for both low- and high-risk patients, but more complete revascularization is now possible and with arterial conduits. (See also Chap. 141.)

COMPLICATIONS

The major complications after coronary artery surgery are bleeding requiring reoperation, myocardial infarction, stroke, respiratory distress, wound infection, and renal failure. Patients who experience one or more complications have an 8- to 10-times greater probability of mortality compared with those who sustain no complications.[30] Length of hospital stay and cost are affected by most of these major complications.[31] Important predictors of morbidity include previous cardiac surgery, emergency operation, advanced age, peripheral vascular disease, and preoperative elevated serum creatinine. These indicators affect myocardial and respiratory status but do not predict bleeding or wound infection with the same accuracy.[32]

Bleeding

In our experience, the propensity for bleeding is multifactorial but relates to advanced age, use of antiplatelet drugs preoperatively, prolonged operating time, previous cardiac surgery, and less frequently, preoperative coagulopathy. Aspirin taken within a week to 10 days before coronary bypass surgery has been associated with an increased rate of bleeding, increased use of blood and blood products, and longer intensive care unit hospitalization.[33] Newer products such as fibrin glue and aprotinin are reported to decrease postoperative bleeding. The routine use of preoperative tests in assessing bleeding risk is not justified. Need for transfusions relates to body surface area, preoperative anemia, and advanced age more than any other factors. Erythropoietin has been used to increase red blood cell production after autologous blood donation; however, its role in postoperative anemia is not yet defined.

Myocardial Infarction

In elective coronary bypass surgery, the transmural myocardial infarction rate is approximately 2 percent. The rate of perioperative myocardial infarction is less in low-risk patients and greater in high-risk patients, i.e., reoperations and coronary arterial operations combined with other cardiac surgery. The rate of myocardial infarction has declined in each decade from the 1970s to the 1990s, presumably because of better myocardial protection. The large Q-wave infarctions seen in the early years of coronary bypass surgery are infrequent today. Transient abnormal Q waves may occur as a result of alterations in ventricular depolarization or may be unmasked by improved function of a contiguous ventricular segment. Patients who experience nonfatal perioperative myocardial damage have essentially the same intermediate-term course as patients without myocardial infarction. The exceptions are those who require intraaortic balloon pumping for ischemia/infarction postoperatively. Although postoperative intraaortic balloon pumping is required in only 1 to 2 percent of elective surgeries today, most studies have shown that the requirement for balloon pumping portends a lower survival rate because these patients tend to have complicated perioperative infarctions.

Stroke

The mechanisms of stroke after cardiac surgery include embolization, hypoperfusion, or inflammatory responses stimulated by extracorporeal circulation. Ascending aortic atherosclerosis is a major contributor to brain injury and myocardial complications.[34] Aortic disease is to be suspected in patients with diffuse brachiocephalic disease, documented peripheral vascular disease, or left main coronary narrowing and is demonstrated directly by palpable atheroma or plaque discovered during cannulation or construction of aortic anastomoses. It has been shown recently that aortic atheroemboli occur more frequently in patients undergoing coronary artery surgery than other cardiac procedures.[35] A correlation between increased incidence of atheroembolism, advanced age, and peripheral vascular disease is apparent. The surgeon should anticipate finding aortic atherosclerosis before entering the aorta. The problem may be circumvented by femoral artery or distal arch cannulation. If atherosclerosis is discovered during construction of the bypass grafts, the ascending aorta should be opened and debrided, possibly under deep hypothermia. Obviously, signs of aortic atherosclerosis contraindicate aortic cross-clamping. In situ internal thoracic arteries should be used if the subclavian vessels are widely patent. Vein grafts or other arterial conduits may be anastomosed directly to the internal thoracic arteries.

Respiratory Distress

Respiratory distress has been related to lengthy operating time; increased number of blood transfusions; increased amount of crystalloid fluid infused; suboptimal preoperative nutritional status of the patient; presence of intrinsic pulmonary disease, neurologic deficit, or phrenic nerve dysfunction; and cardiac failure.[36] Congestive heart failure during the operation is the most important risk factor for postoperative pulmonary complications. In our experience, this complication is relatively infrequent in otherwise uncomplicated patients. Nosocomial pneumonia may be related to prolonged intensive care unit stay, presence of chronic obstructive pulmonary disease, administration of gastric acid inhibitor drugs, and prolonged mechanical ventilatory support and may be prevented by keeping long-term intensive care unit patients in the head-up position to avoid aspiration, providing oral hygiene, frequent sterile suctioning, and use of sucralfate for stress ulcer prophylaxis rather than antacids or H_2 antagonists.[37] The role of selective digestive decontamination (SDD)[38] is not fully settled, but we practice it routinely in all high-risk patients.

Wound Infection

Sternal wound infection with mediastinitis occurs in approximately 1 percent of elective coronary bypass patients and is usually detected around the seventh to ninth postoperative day. In unusual cases, this complication may arise several weeks postoperatively. The mortality related to mediastinitis is high—in our experience, 14 percent. Wound infections increase hospital cost more than any other nonfatal complication because of the protracted hospitalization related to chest wall reconstruction. Wound infections are more likely to occur in diabetic patients; however, after comparable operations, the sternal blood supply is not reduced in diabetics compared with nondiabetics. Use of the internal thoracic artery is not a risk factor for wound complications except in bilateral usage in diabetic patients.[39] Treatment is surgical drainage and either primary closure or treatment with rotational muscle flaps.

Renal Failure

Renal failure may be the result of underlying renal disease, especially when coupled with cardiac instability postoperatively. Vasopressor use, intraaortic balloon pumping, excessive bleeding, history of chronic renal disease, and advanced age are predictors of postoperative renal failure. Some studies have supported use of low-dose dopamine to enhance renal blood flow as a protective measure. Renal failure associated with jaundice and intraaortic balloon pump use carries a particularly poor prognosis. (See also Chap. 108.)

Abdominal Complications

Though rare, the most common abdominal complication is gastrointestinal hemorrhage due to esophagitis or gastritis. Pancreatitis is correlated with low cardiac output and multisystem complications. Patients who have a history of pancreatitis and suffer complications postoperatively may be more prone to recurring pancreatitis. Transient elevation of bilirubin is noted with vasopressor and intraaortic balloon pump support.

Atrial Fibrillation

Atrial fibrillation may be a source of emboli postoperatively. Advanced age is related to atrial dysrhythmia. The incidence of atrial fibrillation varies from a low of 4 percent in patients less than 40 years old to more than 50 percent in patients more than 75 years old. The risk of incurring new atrial fibrillation appears to be independent of advanced coronary atherosclerosis or even left ventricular function. A number of factors, such as beta-blocker withdrawal, lengthy operation, and postcardiotomy syndrome, have been implicated but none heralds atrial fibrillation consistently. Electrical conversion to normal sinus rhythm may cause embolization, and prophylactic oral anticoagulation has been advocated. (See also Chap. 36.)

Other Complications

Other infrequent complications include brachial plexus injuries, which may be related to spreading the sternum and compressing the plexus between the clavicle and first rib. This may result in median nerve trauma, which usually resolves over several months. Horner's syndrome may result from a fracture of the first rib near the costotransverse articulation, affecting the cervical sympathetic chain. Asymptomatic deep vein thrombosis of the calf may occur with relative frequency; however, pulmonary embolism is rare. Lower extremity wound complications at the site of saphenous vein procurement are unusual, but cellulitis may occur in diabetic patients with poor circulation.

In the first few months after hospital discharge, the clinician should be vigilant for pericarditis/pleuritis, wound infection, atrial arrhythmias, hepatitis, and recurring angina. Pulmonary embolism is rare but should be suspected in those who had a protracted hospital course or who have a history of pulmonary embolism or phlebitis.

FACTORS AFFECTING LATE GRAFT PATENCY

The fate of the internal thoracic artery graft and perhaps some other arterial conduits is different than that of vein grafts. Ten or more years after surgery, patency for the left internal thoracic artery graft to the anterior descending coronary artery is in the 90th percentile, in contrast with the patency of vein grafts, which tends to deteriorate after the fifth-to-seventh postoperative years.[40] The high patency rate of internal thoracic artery grafts probably relates to vasoactivity, which may forestall the development of atherosclerosis.[41] In this conduit, prostacyclin and endothelial-derived relaxing factor releases are preserved. Other observations that may have bearing on high patency include a uniform internal elastic lamina in this small artery[42] and the fact that it is nourished from the lumen, not the vasa vasorum, as in larger arteries.

Approximately 80 percent of vein grafts remain open 5 years after operation. According to studies from the Montreal Heart Institute,[43] the Cleveland Clinic Foundation,[44] and others, this probability takes into account a 5 to 10 percent graft closure rate in the first month, 10 to 15 percent closure at 1 year, and only slight attrition between years 1 and 5 postoperatively. After the fifth-to-seventh postoperative years, there appears to be a progressive increase of atheromatous disease in coronary bypass vein grafts, so that at 10 to 12 years, only 40 to 60 percent of the grafts are open.[45] Approximately half to three-fourths of those late, patent vein bypass grafts show angiographic evidence of lumen irregularities, presumably atheromatous degeneration. The late occlusion of vein grafts is associated with thrombosis occurring at the site of atherosclerotic lesions. Vein graft atherosclerosis is generally diffuse and has been correlated with elevations of serum cholesterol, low HDL cholesterol levels, high serum triglycerides, and cigarette smoking.[46] Vein and arterial graft patency are comparable in young and elderly patients.

According to Fuster,[47] there are four consecutive phases of aortocoronary vein graft disease. The first is an early postoperative phase of thrombotic occlusion, which may be prevented by platelet inhibitor therapy. The classic study from the Mayo Clinic showed that dipyridamole administered preoperatively followed by aspirin and dipyridamole postoperatively significantly improved the vein graft patency rate in the first year after surgery.[48,49] Subsequently it has been shown that one aspirin tablet or even a low-dose aspirin (81 to 100 mg) may prevent initiation of platelet thrombi, the release of platelet mediators, and the occurrence of platelet damage in vein grafts. Veterans Administration investigators found that aspirin three times a day was as effective as dipyridamole and aspirin.[50] Aspirin started preoperatively offers no additional benefit, nor does aspirin appear to improve internal thoracic artery graft patency.[51] Long-term antiplatelet therapy is preferable to anticoagulation because it incurs less risk of hemorrhage, does not necessitate laboratory monitoring, and costs less. (See also Chap. 68.)

The second phase of vein graft disease involves platelet-related intimal hyperplasia, which is seen within the first postoperative year and is not prevented by platelet inhibitor therapy. The third phase occurs at the end of the first postoperative year, in which further intimal hyperplasia or platelet thrombi are superimposed on intimal hyperplasia and may contribute to occlusion. In this stage, platelet inhibitor therapy is of benefit in preventing thrombotic occlusion. Finally, a phase of atherosclerotic disease occurs after the first postoperative year. It is not yet known whether or not platelet inhibitor therapy affects the formation of vein graft atherosclerosis.

Late stenoses in vein grafts appear to be more dangerous prognostically than late stenoses in any of the three major native coronary vessels.[52] Patients catheterized 5 years or more postoperatively had different survival rates subsequently, depending upon whether a lesion was in the vein graft or in the native coronary circulation. Late stenoses in saphenous vein grafts to the anterior descending coronary artery predict a high rate of death and cardiac events and are an indication for reoperation. This point is to be emphasized: Vein graft atherosclerosis and native vessel coronary atherosclerosis appear to have different prognoses. For patients who undergo catheterization 5 years or more postoperatively, mortality in the subsequent 2 years is 30 percent for patients with a stenotic vein graft to the anterior descending coronary artery compared with 3 percent of those with a stenotic native vessel (Fig. 73-1).

Progression of Native Vessel Coronary Atherosclerosis

Progression of native vessel coronary atherosclerosis has been studied by serial cardiac catheterization.[53] In the first postoperative year, the rate of progression is higher in grafted arteries, irrespective of whether the grafts are open or closed. In the first postoperative year, approximately half of the grafted arteries demonstrated progression compared with only about 10 percent progression in ungrafted vessels. Progression, however, depends on time and is related to the severity of the initial obstruction.[54] The grafted vessels tended to have much more severe obstruction than ungrafted vessels at the time of the initial surgery. At the subsequent five years, progression was found more in previously ungrafted vessels, probably because the proximal lesions in the grafted vessels had progressed to total occlusion. We have found that proximal native vessel occlusion occurs less frequently after internal thoracic artery grafting than with saphenous vein grafting.[55] The most plausible explanation for accelerated proximal closure in bypassed vessels is that graft flow predominates and reduces or eliminates flow across the proximal atherosclerotic narrowing. Surgical error may cause tenting, angulation, or stenosis in the recipient vessel, which may further decrease the flow between the proximal lesion and the distal anastomosis. Any reduction of flow in the proximal native coronary artery may induce local thrombosis.

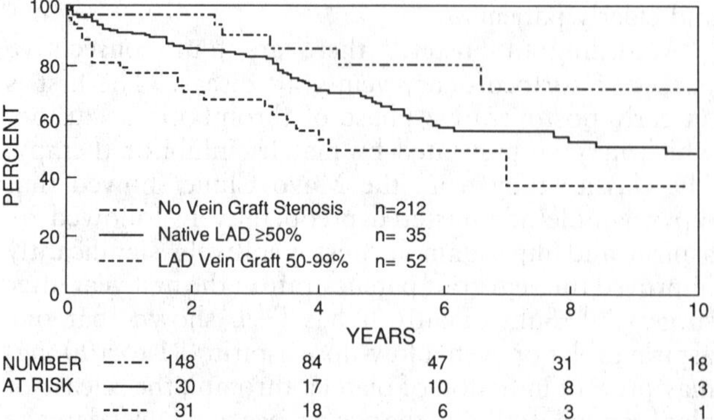

FIGURE 73-1 Patients with stenoses (50 to 99 percent) in left anterior descending (LAD) vein grafts had worse survival than either patients with native vessel LAD stenoses (50 to 99 percent) ($p = 0.002$) or the control group. Patients with stenotic vein grafts to the LAD had survival rates of 70 and 50 percent at two and five postoperative years, compared with 97 and 80 percent for patients with native LAD stenoses. *(From Lytle[52]; reprinted with permission.)*

OUTCOME

The evolution of coronary artery surgery may be traced from the results of medical and surgical therapy reported through the Duke University data bank.[56] These investigators have shown that survival has improved from 1969 through 1984 in both medical and surgical therapy, but that the magnitude of improvement was significantly greater in surgically treated patients. They attribute the improvement in surgical patients to refinements in technology; in medical patients, the higher survival in the more recent experience may occur because of application of medical therapy to patients with milder disease who have lower risk prognostically[57] (Fig. 73-2).

Most of the current information about lifestyle, cardiac events, and survival is confined to the first 10 years after surgery. Some exceptions will be noted. The clinical, angiographic, and surgical variables that predict 10-year survival include age of the patient, left ventricular function, type of conduit used, complete revascularization, continued cigarette smoking, and the presence of hypertension, diabetes, and peripheral vascular disease.[58] Despite a difference in baseline characteristics, the predictors of long-term mortality in men and women are nearly identical and depend mainly on preoperative left ventricular function.

The diabetic patient with documented severe coronary atherosclerosis is thought to have a higher frequency of asymptomatic myocardial ischemia. Surgery improves survival of diabetic patients with silent ischemia, compared with medical therapy, and the greatest impact is in those with three-vessel disease. Whereas diabetes tends to increase the complication rate after bypass surgery, it is generally acknowledged that the intermediate-term survival is not affected by the presence of diabetes mellitus. (See also Chap. 102.)

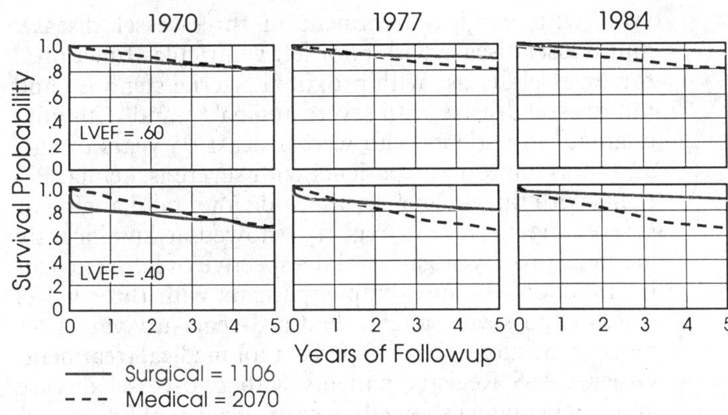

FIGURE 73-2 Survival data from Duke University showing differences in 5-year survival after medical and surgical treatment of three-vessel disease during three time periods. The latest experience in 1984 shows an improved survival for surgical therapy that differs widely from the 5-year results obtained with medical treatment. (*From Pryor*[57]; *reprinted with permission.*)

Complete Revascularization

Complete revascularization is generally defined as bypass grafts constructed to all major epicardial coronary vessels that are at least 1 mm in size with estimated 50 to 70 percent narrowing in lumen diameter. Complete revascularization should not affect hospital mortality, but it is an influential variable over the long term, as it better relates to amelioration of severe angina and preservation of left ventricular function and reduction in the need for reoperation.

Emergency Operations

Emergency operations may be undertaken in the face of acute myocardial infarction. A report from Spokane, Washington, attests to the good long-term survival (10 years or more) in patients with Q-wave myocardial infarction who were deliberately assigned to surgical or nonsurgical treatment.[59] Medical and surgical groups had similar clinical characteristics. Surgery within 4 h resulted in improved long-term survival and better left ventricular function than traditional medical therapy. This improvement did not extend to those who were operated on later in the course of the infarct. The benefit of surgery applied more to the anterior infarction group than to patients with inferior infarction.[60] (See also Chap. 60.)

Recent multicenter trials of thrombolytic therapy have offered another view of emergency myocardial revascularization. As many as one in five patients may undergo emergency or urgent coronary bypass surgery during the initial hospitalization. Despite the fact that many patients were in a high-risk category, the hospital course and 1-year results, event-free survival, angina status, and general health status were similar to those who underwent successful thrombolysis and angioplasty.[61] The number of grafts per patient and more complete revascularization in the surgical group indicate an excellent long-term prognosis.

Patients who have survived an out-of-hospital cardiac arrest generally have a poor natural history. Surgical revascularization may suppress inducible ventricular fibrillation in patients who have reasonably well-preserved left ventricular function.[62] Postoperative electrophysiological testing is essential because bypass surgery suppresses ventricular arrhythmias in only about half the cases. Actuarial 5-year survival, cardiac survival, and arrhythmia-free survival have been reported to be 88, 98, and 88 percent, respectively. Poor preoperative left ventricular function is predictive of death. (See Chaps. 51 and 52.)

Influence of the Conduit

Influence of the type of conduit on long-term results is evident by contrasting survival after left internal thoracic artery grafting with survival following vein grafting. The arterial conduit grafted to the anterior descending coronary artery performed either alone or in combination with vein bypass grafts significantly improves 10-year survival and reduces the incidence of important cardiac events, notably myocardial infarction, rehospitalization for cardiac causes, and reoperation.[63] The 10-year survival of patients who had one internal thoracic artery graft and that of those with vein grafts only were 93.4 and 88 percent, respectively, for one-vessel disease; 90.0 and 79.5 percent for two-vessel disease; and 82.6 and 71.0 percent for three-vessel disease. This difference favored the internal thoracic artery graft over the vein graft irrespective of gender and held true for good and poor ventricular performance. Few 20-year follow-ups of vein grafts are available. Cameron[64] has shown that 20-year survivals were 38 percent for vein graft patients and 50 percent for patients with one internal thoracic artery graft; at 19 years, 63.5 percent of patients with double internal thoracic artery grafts were alive. In the Cleveland Clinic experience, the incremental benefit of two internal thoracic artery grafts seemed to be more pronounced in patients below age 60 compared with older patients.[65]

The graphic description of the difference achieved by one internal thoracic artery graft to the anterior descending coronary artery compared with patients who had vein grafts only is shown in Fig. 73-3. Proudfit and colleagues[66] reported observational data on patients who corresponded clinically and angiographically to the Coronary Artery Surgery Study (CASS) controlled trial. The 10-year survival for patients having only saphenous vein bypass grafts was essentially the same as that of the medical group. In contrast, those who received a left internal thoracic artery graft to the anterior descending coronary artery (some combined with vein grafts to other vessels) had a 10-year survival of 91 percent. The greatest

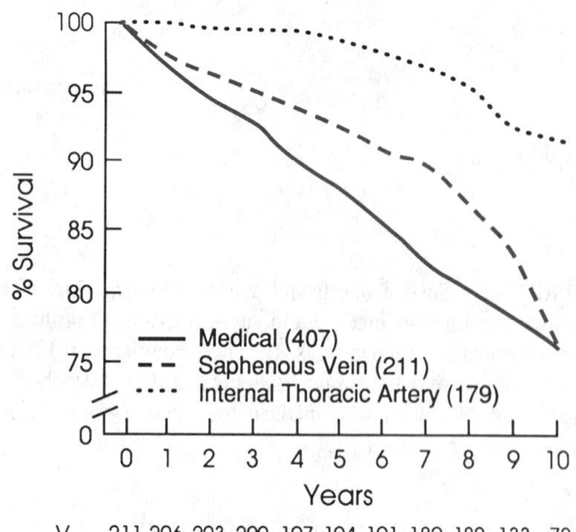

FIGURE 73-3 A retrospective series of patients from the Cleveland Clinic Foundation matched for CASS entry criteria received medical or surgical treatment and were followed for 10 years. The 10-year survival data show that patients who had vein grafts only experienced a relatively sharp attrition after the fifth postoperative year; their survival at 10 years was essentially the same as patients treated medically. In contrast, patients who received a left internal thoracic artery graft to the anterior descending artery alone or combined with vein grafts had a 10-year survival rate of 91 percent, which was significantly higher than either the vein-graft-only or the medically treated group. (*From Proudfit*[66]*; reprinted with permission.*)

problem during the first 10 years after surgery is not progression of disease but deterioration of vein grafts.

Few arterial bypass grafts were constructed during the 1970s, when the three most widely reported randomized trials assigned patients to medical or surgical treatment. These important randomized studies were also undertaken in an era when many of the current cardiac drugs and lipid-lowering therapies were not available, when myocardial protection was not optimal, and when internal thoracic artery grafting was not applied widely. In the European Cooperative Study, there was consistent improvement in 10-year survival for surgical patients with three-vessel disease or two-vessel disease with involvement of the proximal anterior descending coronary artery.[67] In a 12-year follow-up, the study reported results for patients with respect to treatment received as well as the policy of treatment. Interestingly, the survival was 62 percent at 10 to 12 years for patients compliant with medical treatment and 86 percent for those who had crossed over to surgery. The European Coronary Surgery Study Group concluded that "the time-honored advice of medical care until symptoms deteriorate to an unacceptable level is proved invalid . . . [And] surgery was the treatment of choice even when angina pectoris responded adequately to medical management."

The CASS randomized trial of relatively asymptomatic low-risk patients found nearly equal survival between medical and surgical treatment. The exception was the subset of patients with poor ventricular function in whom surgical treatment offered improved intermediate-term survival. The CASS Registry, which followed about 7000 patients operated on at the same time the trial was conducted, found improved 5- to 7-year survival with surgical treatment in three-vessel disease, multivessel disease with poor left ventricular function,[68] three-vessel disease with proximal arterial stenoses, and multivessel disease with severe angina[69,70] and with mild angina,[71] in patients who were at least 65 years of age, and in asymptomatic patients with severe ischemia. Patients with three-vessel disease and either mild angina or severe angina in the registry showed a significantly greater 5- to 7-year survival irrespective of left ventricular function. As an example, patients with three-vessel disease and severe angina had a 6-year survival of 81 percent for surgery and 40 percent for medical treatment. Other CASS Registry patients with two-vessel disease and severe angina showed a 6-year survival of 89 percent after surgery, compared to 76 percent for patients treated medically. In all multivessel disease categories, the spread between survival of medical and surgical therapy widens with increasingly worse left ventricular function.[72]

There are few 15- to 20-year follow-up reports. Given the facts that distribution of coronary atherosclerosis was more benign and left ventricular function was generally good in these early series, these reports, based largely on vein graft surgery, provide an important perspective on the evolution of the surgical candidate and the long-term results. Lawrie et al.[73] report actuarial 20-year survivals of 40 percent for one-vessel disease patients, 26 percent for two-vessel disease, 20 percent for three-vessel disease, and 25 percent for left main coronary artery disease. Approximately two-thirds of patients were asymptomatic at 20 years, and nearly half of the vein bypass grafts were patent 16 to 20 years postoperatively.

Unstable Angina

The Veterans Administration Cooperative Study Group reviewed the management of unstable angina. The 5-year survival for patients with three-vessel disease and all gradations of left ventricular function was better for surgery (89 percent) than for medical treatment (75 percent).[74,75] Surgery yielded fewer hospitalizations for cardiac causes, and the difference in favor of surgery widened considerably in categories of reduced ejection fractions.

ANGINA RELIEF AND LIFESTYLE

Quality of life refers to symptom relief, well-being, return to full activity, and where applicable, return to employment. The randomized controlled studies consistently have shown the effectiveness of coronary bypass surgery in alleviating angina.[76] At about the fifth year, however, the slope of the angina-free patients curve changes so that the dramatic symptom relief is attenuated in the next 5 years. Only about half of the patients originally angina free at year 5 remain so by years 10 to 12.[77] The type of conduit used does not correlate with angina relief. Late angina return does appear to correlate with factors such as hyperlipidemia and hypertension. Sudden death is more related to preoperative left ventricular function than any other factor and fortunately is a rare occurrence in the first 10 years after surgery.

Angina relief is better in the elderly than among their younger counterparts.[78] In fact, successful bypass surgery in the elderly confers consistent angina relief over the intermediate term, and their longevity exceeds that of the U.S. population matched for age and gender.[79,80] Most reports indicate that coronary artery surgery does not cause long-term intellectual or neuropsychological dysfunction. The intellectual defects that are reported immediately after surgery tend to have a short course and generally resolve within 3 months after operation.

According to reports from the CASS Registry, the myocardial infarction–free survival is significantly improved by coronary artery surgery for both severe angina and mild angina cases.[81] Other earlier reports indicate that freedom from late myocardial infarction is no different from medical treatment, but the fatality rate from myocardial infarction is significantly less after surgery compared with those treated conservatively.[82]

Return to work is a complicated subject. Since the median age of coronary bypass patients is approaching 65 years and is older in many communities, return to full activity may be a more realistic expectation. Nonetheless, factors affecting return to work include the status of employment preoperatively, age, income, gender, self-employment, whether white collar or blue collar, college education, relief of symptoms, and preoperative left ventricular function. It is known that the longer the unemployment preoperatively, the less likely the return to full employment. Other factors that adversely affect future employment include comorbidity, physician advice, and disability compensation.

REOPERATION

The incidence of coronary artery *reoperation* tends to increase with time. In our experience, only 3 percent of patients were reoperated on in the first 5 years after their initial bypass surgery, and this rate may be even less today with the advent of balloon angioplasty. At 10 to 12 years postoperatively, the rate rises to 12 to 17 percent, and at 15 years it approaches 30 percent among those who survived this interval. The factors that predispose a patient to a reoperation include young age, incomplete revascularization at the first operation, use of vein grafts only, one- or two-vessel disease at time of first operation, and good left ventricular function.[83]

The use of more internal thoracic artery grafts at the initial procedure has lengthened the mean interval between the operations, which approaches 10 years today. Vein graft atherosclerosis has become the leading indication for reoperation.[84] Angiography underestimates severity of vein graft atherosclerosis.[85] Since atherosclerotic disease progresses at a highly unpredictable rate and is associated with a bad prognosis, especially in anterior descending coronary artery grafts, we recommend replacement of vein grafts in most instances when the reoperation occurs more than 5 years postoperatively. In experienced hands, hospital mortality for second operations range from 2 to 5 percent. The complication rate is approximately twice that of the first procedure.

Of all the variables that may affect 10-year survival after reoperation, advanced age and the presence of left main coronary disease consistently show an impact on 10-year survival. Poor ventricular function is not as big a factor because patients with very poor function generally do not survive long enough to undergo a reoperation. Factors associated with an improved 10-year survival after reoperation include age younger than 65 years, mild angina, no major comorbidity, no left main coronary disease, good left ventricular performance, and performance of an internal thoracic artery graft (Fig. 73-4). In our experience, 5- and 10-year survivals are approximately 90 and 75 percent, respectively, after coronary artery reoperation. Approximately half of the patients are angina free postoperatively and about half survive 10 years event free.

Coronary artery surgery a third time is still infrequent but rising in some referral centers. The risk is about triple that of the second operation, i.e., about 9 percent, according to published reports.

LONG-TERM MANAGEMENT

Patients who undergo coronary artery bypass surgery tend to have partial or complete alleviation of angina for the first 5 years and improved exercise tolerance. It is generally agreed that platelet inhibitor drugs should be continued for at least 1 year postoperatively. Recurrent angina requires investigation, and coronary arteriography is the most definitive test. Early recurring angina is unusual, but angiography may document anastomotic constriction that may be amenable to coronary balloon angioplasty.

Later on, especially after the fifth postoperative year, progression of coronary atherosclerosis and vein graft atherosclerosis become increasingly more frequent. Progression of native vessel disease is more likely to occur proximal to the distal anastomosis rather than affecting the distal arterial runoff. Treatment of late lesions in vein grafts is both risky and fraught with a high restenosis rate. Atherectomy may be a promising treatment, but results are preliminary. On an individual basis, progression of disease in the native coronary arteries may be treated by balloon angioplasty, which may spare the patient a reoperation. (See also Chap. 70.)

Constrictive pericarditis is seen months or years postoperatively and is rare. The etiology is obscure. As the condition worsens, pericardiectomy may be required. Even more rarely, chronic pericardial irritation caused by either a reaction to Teflon felt used in cardiac surgery or by large, loculated, organized intrapericardial hematoma that fail to resolve may require reoperation. (See also Chap. 92.)

Modification of risk factors applies to all but the very elderly. Advice should be given concerning proper weight, strict abstinence from tobacco, exercise consistent with age and lifestyle, and control of hyperlipidemia. Reduction in serum lipids may reduce progression of disease and improve graft patency. Lipid-lowering drug therapy has been correlated with regression of atherosclerosis[86] and has reduced the progression of coronary

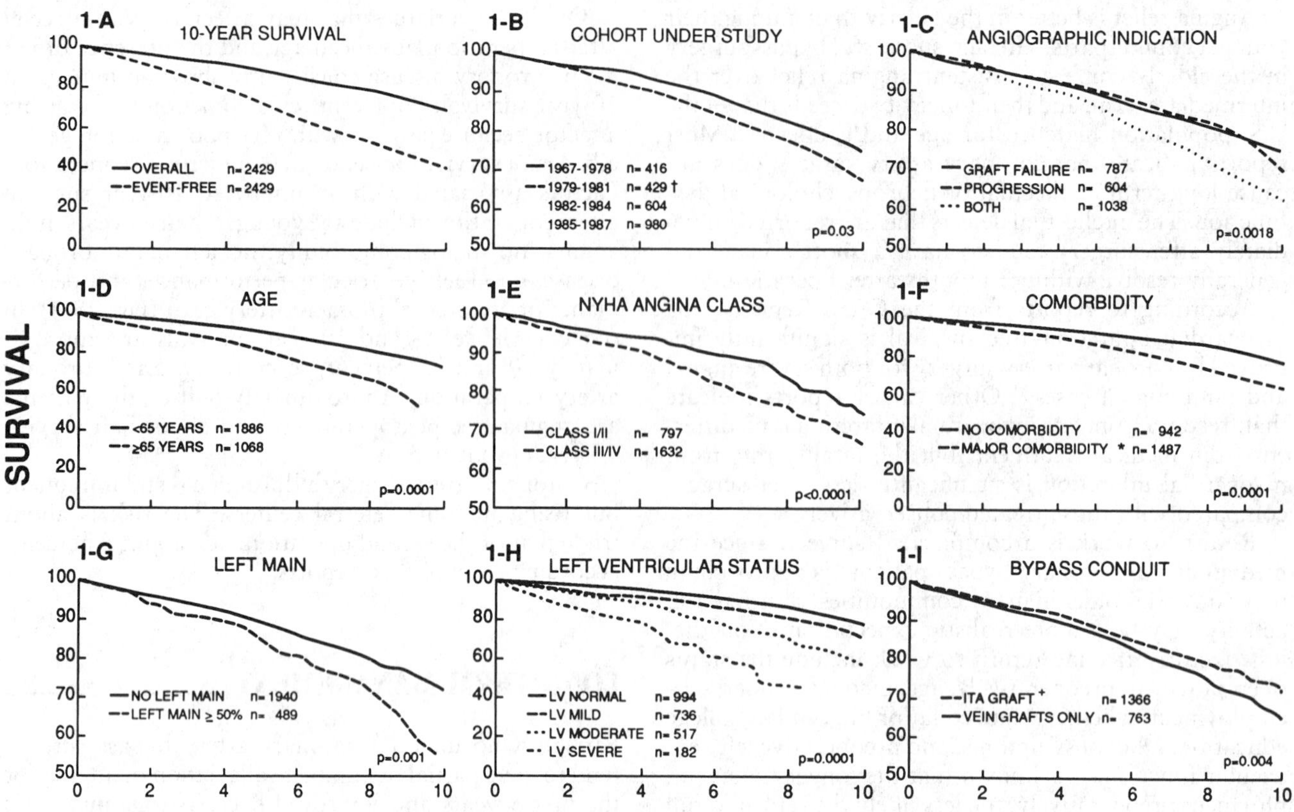

FIGURE 73-4 Overall survival and event-free survival for 2429 patients discharged alive after undergoing coronary artery reoperation. All comparisons are statistically significant. The 10-year survival rate was 69 percent and the event-free survival rate was 41 percent (*A*). The earliest experience, i.e., patients operated on from 1967 through 1978, enjoyed a higher 10-year survival rate (75 percent), than the remainder of the consecutive series compiled through 1987 (67 percent). Risk was lower in the earlier patients (*B*). Analysis of longevity by the angiographic indication group showed that patients operated on for graft failure or progressive atherosclerosis had a significantly better 10-year survival rate than patients who experienced progressive native vessel atherosclerosis and graft failure, 76 and 70 percent vs. 63 percent, respectively (*C*). Patients younger than age 65 before reoperation had a better 10-year survival rate (72 percent) than patients over age 65 (51 percent) (*D*). Survival rate by a New York Heart Association functional class shows that patients with mild angina, classes I and II, had a 69 percent 10-year survival rate while those with more severe angina, classes III and IV, had a 64 percent survival rate (*E*). Comorbidity was defined as diabetes, hypertension, peripheral vascular disease, and cigarette smoking. Patients with no comorbidity had a 10-year survival rate of 77 percent; those with one or all comorbid conditions, 64 percent (*F*). The presence (72 percent) or absence (55 percent) of left main coronary artery narrowing at least 50 percent influenced 10-year survival rate (*G*). Left ventricular status affected 10-year survival, which ranged from 45 percent for those with severe impairment to 77 percent for patients with pre-reoperative normal ventricular function (*H*). Use of internal thoracic artery grafts at either the first or second operation yielded a better 10-year survival rate (73 percent) than use of vein grafts only (66 percent) (*I*). (*From Loop*[84]*; reprinted with permission.*)

lesions in both native vessels and in vein graft atherosclerosis.[87] Blood pressure control and diabetic management affect prognosis and should be attended to regularly. Postoperative management is directed toward prevention of progressive arterial disease and prolongation of vein graft patency. Relentless progression of disease in native arteries and grafts emphasizes the need for yearly surveillance after coronary bypass surgery. Too often, especially after the first year, patients return to their bad habits. They should be instructed that the operation is not curative and that risk factor modification is never-ending. Compliance with a thoughtful program is proven to be beneficial. Failure to observe the guidelines could affect the patient adversely. (See also Chaps. 62, 63, and 65.)

REFERENCES

1. Favaloro RG: Saphenous vein autograft replacement of severe segmental coronary artery occlusion: Operative technique. *Ann Thorac Surg* 1968; 5:334–339.
2. Johnson WD, Flemma RJ, Lepley D Jr, Ellison EH. Extended treatment of severe coronary artery disease: A total surgical approach. *Ann Surg* 1969; 170:460–470.
3. Frye RL, Gibbons RJ, Schaff HV, Vlietstra RE, Gersh BJ, Mock MB: Treatment of coronary artery disease. *J Am Coll Cardiol* 1989; 13:957–968.
4. Kirklin JW, Akins CW, Blackstone EH, Booth RC, Califf RM, Cohen LJ, et al: ACC/AHA Guidelines and Indicators for Coronary Artery Bypass Graft Surgery. *Circulation* 1991; 83:1125–1173.
5. Proudfit WL, Bruschke AVG, MacMillan JP, Williams GW, Sones FM Jr: Fifteen year survival study of patients with obstructive coronary artery disease. *Circulation* 1983; 68:986–997.

6. Fisher LD, Kennedy JW, Davis KB, Maynard C, Fritz JK, Kaiser G, et al: Association of sex, physical size, and operative mortality after coronary artery bypass in the Coronary Artery Surgery Study (CASS). *J Thorac Cardiovasc Surg* 1982; 84:334–341.
7. Loop FD, Golding LR, MacMillan JP, Cosgrove DM, Lytle BW, Sheldon WC: Coronary artery surgery in women compared with men: Analyses of risks and long-term results. *J Am Coll Cardiol* 1983; 1:383–390.
8. Rahimtoola SH: The hibernating myocardium. *Am Heart J* 1989; 117:211–221.
9. Braunwald E, Kloner RA: The stunned myocardium: Prolonged, postischemic ventricular dysfunction. *Circulation* 1982; 66:1146–1149.
10. Brooks R, McGovern BA, Garan H, Ruskin JN: Current treatment of patients surviving out-of-hospital cardiac arrest. *JAMA* 1991; 265:762–768.
11. Hertzer NR, Beven EG, Young JR, O'Hara PJ, Ruschhaupt WF III, Graor RA, et al: Coronary artery disease in peripheral vascular patients: A classification of 1,000 coronary angiograms and results of surgical management. *Ann Surg* 1984; 199:223–233.
12. European Carotid Surgery Trialists' Collaborative Group: MRC European Carotid Surgery Trial: Interim results for symptomatic patients with severe (70–99%) or with mild (0–29%) carotid stenosis. *Lancet* 1991; 337:1235–1243.
13. North American Symptomatic Carotid Endarterectomy Trial Collaborators: Beneficial effect of carotid endarterectomy in symptomatic patients with high-grade carotid stenosis. *N Engl J Med* 1991; 325:445–453.
14. Jones EL, Waites TF, Craver JM, Bradford JM, Douglas JS, King SB, et al: Coronary bypass for relief of persistent pain following acute myocardial infarction. *Ann Thorac Surg* 1981; 32:33–43.
15. Schuster EH, Bulkley BH: Early post-infarction angina: Ischemia at a distance and ischemia in the infarct zone. *N Engl J Med* 1981; 305:1101–1105.
16. Cosgrove DM, Loop FD, Lytle BW, Baillot R, Gill CC, Golding LAR, et al: Primary myocardial revascularization: Trends in surgical mortality. *J Thorac Cardiovasc Surg* 1984; 88:673–684.
17. Miller DC, Stinson EB, Oyer PE, Jamieson SW, Mitchell RS, Reitz BA, et al: Discriminant analysis of the changing risks of coronary artery operations: 1971–1979. *J Thorac Cardiovasc Surg* 1983; 85:197–213.
18. Jones EL, Weintraub WS, Craver JM, Guyton RA, Cohen CL: Coronary bypass surgery: Is the operation different today? *J Thorac Cardiovasc Surg* 1991; 101:108–115.
19. Kirklin JW: Technical and scientific advances in cardiac surgery over the past 25 years. *Ann Thorac Surg* 1990; 49:26–31.
20. Parsonnet V, Dean D, Bernstein AD: A method of uniform stratification of risk for evaluating the results of surgery in acquired adult heart disease. *Circulation* 1989; 79(suppl I):I-3–12.
21. Higgins TL, Estafanous FG, Loop FD, Beck GJ, Blum JM, Paranandi L: Stratification of morbidity and mortality outcome by preoperative risk factors in coronary artery bypass patients. *JAMA* 1992; 267:2344–2348.
22. Loop FD, Lytle BW, Cosgrove DM, Golding LAR, Taylor PC, Stewart RW: Free (aorta-coronary) internal mammary artery graft: Late results. *J Thorac Cardiovasc Surg* 1986; 92:827–831.
23. Pym J, Brown PM, Charrette EJP, Parker JO, West RO: Gastroepiploic-coronary anastomosis: A viable alternative bypass graft. *J Thorac Cardiovasc Surg* 1987; 94:256–259.
24. Puig LB, Ciongolli W, Cividanes GVL, Dontos A, Kopel L, Bittencort D, et al: Inferior epigastric artery as a free graft for myocardial revascularization. *J Thorac Cardiovasc Surg* 1990; 99:251–255.
25. Barner HB, Naunheim KS, Fiore AC, Fischer VW, Harris HH: Use of the inferior epigastric artery as a free graft for myocardial revascularization. *Ann Thorac Surg* 1991; 52:429–437.
26. Baumann FG, Catinella FP, Cunningham JN Jr, Spencer FC: Vein contraction and smooth muscle cell extensions as causes of endothelial damage during graft preparation. *Ann Surg* 1981; 194:199–211.
27. Buckberg GD: Studies of controlled reperfusion after ischemia: A series of experimental and clinical observations from the Division of Thoracic and Cardiovascular Surgery, UCLA School of Medicine. *J Thorac Cardiovasc Surg* 1986; 92:483–648.
28. Beyersdorf F, Sarai K, Maul FD, Wendt T, Satter P: Immediate functional benefits after controlled reperfusion during surgical revascularization for acute coronary occlusion. *J Thorac Cardiovasc Surg* 1991; 102:856–866.
29. Lichtenstein SV, Abel JG, Salerno TA: Warm heart surgery and results of operation for recent myocardial infarction. *Ann Thorac Surg* 1991; 52:455–460.
30. Hammermeister KE, Burchfiel C, Johnson R, Grover FL: Identification of patients at greatest risk for developing major complications at cardiac surgery. *Circulation* 1990; 82(suppl IV):IV-380–389.
31. Taylor GJ, Mikell FL, Moses HW, Dove JT, Katholi RE, Malik SA, et al: Determinants of hospital charges for coronary artery bypass surgery: The economic consequences of postoperative complications. *Am J Cardiol* 1990; 65:309–313.
32. Higgins TL (ed): Postoperative care of cardiothoracic surgery patients. *Semin Thorac Cardiovasc Surg* 1991; 3:1–94.
33. Bashein BG, Nessly ML, Rice AL, Counts RB, Misbach GA: Preoperative aspirin therapy and reoperation for bleeding after coronary artery bypass surgery. *Arch Intern Med* 1991; 151:89–93.
34. Mills NL, Everson CT: Atherosclerosis of the ascending aorta and coronary artery bypass: Pathology, clinical correlates, and operative management. *J Thorac Cardiovasc Surg* 1991; 102:546–553.
35. Blauth CI, Cosgrove DM, Webb BW, Ratliff NB, Boylan M, Piedmonte MR, et al: Atheroembolism from the ascending aorta: An emerging problem in cardiac surgery. *J Thorac Cardiovasc Surg* 1992; 103:1104–1112.
36. Matthay MA, Wiener-Kronish JP: Respiratory management after cardiac surgery. *Chest* 1989; 95:424–432.
37. Gaynes R, Bizek B, Mowry-Hanley J, Kirsh M: Risk factors for nosocomial pneumonia after coronary artery bypass graft operations. *Ann Thorac Surg* 1991: 51:215–218.
38. Ford EG, Baisden CE, Matteson ML, Picone AL: Sepsis after coronary bypass grafting: Evidence for loss of the gut mucosal barrier. *Ann Thorac Surg* 1991; 52:514–517.
39. Loop FD, Lytle BW, Cosgrove DM, Mahfood S, McHenry MC, Goormastic M, et al: Sternal wound complications after isolated coronary artery bypass grafting: Early and late mortality, morbidity, and cost of care. *Ann Thorac Surg* 1990; 49:179–187.
40. Grondin CM, Campeau L, Lesperance J, Enjalbert M, Bourassa MG: Comparison of late changes in internal mammary artery and saphenous vein grafts in two consecutive series of patients 10 years after operation. *Circulation* 1984; 70(suppl I):I-208–212.
41. Johns RA, Peach MJ, Flanagan T, Kron IL: Probing of the canine mammary artery damages endothelium and impairs vasodilation resulting from prostacyclin and endothelium-derived relaxing factor. *J Thorac Cardiovasc Surg* 1989; 97:252–258.
42. Ferro M, Conti M, Novero D, Micca FB, Palestro G: The thin intima of the internal mammary artery as the possible reason for freedom from atherosclerosis and success in coronary bypass. *Am Heart J* 1991; 122:1192–1195.
43. Bourassa MG: Fate of venous grafts: The past, the present and the future. *J Am Coll Cardiol* 1991; 17:1081–1083.
44. Lytle BW, Loop FD, Cosgrove DM, Ratliff NB, Easley K, Taylor PC: Long-term (5 to 12 years) serial studies of internal mammary artery and saphenous vein coronary bypass grafts. *J Thorac Cardiovasc Surg* 1985; 89:248–258.
45. Fitzgibbon GM, Leach AJ, Kafka HP, Keon WJ: Coronary bypass graft fate: Long-term angiographic study. *J Am Coll Cardiol* 1991; 17:1075–1080.
46. Campeau L, Enjalbert M, Lesperance J, Bourassa MG, Kwiterovich P Jr, Wacholder S, et al: The relation of risk factors to the development of atherosclerosis in saphenous-vein bypass grafts and the progression of disease in the native circulation: A study 10 years after aortocoronary bypass surgery. *N Engl J Med* 1984; 311:1329–1332.
47. Fuster V: Drugs interfering with platelet function: Mechanisms and clinical relevance. In: Verstraete M (ed.): *Thrombosis and Haemostasis*. Leuven, Belgium, Leuven University Press, 1987.
48. Chesebro JH, Fuster V, Elveback LR, Clements IP, Smith HC, Holmes DR Jr, et al: Effect of dipyridamole and aspirin on late vein-graft patency after coronary bypass operations. *N Engl J Med* 1984; 310:209–214.
49. Chesebro JH, Clements EP, Fuster V, Elveback LR, Smith HC, Bardsley WT, et al: A platelet-inhibitor-drug trial in coronary-artery bypass operations: Benefit of perioperative dipyridamole and aspirin therapy on early postoperative vein-graft patency. *N Engl J Med* 1982; 307:73–78.

50. Goldman S, Copeland J, Mortiz T, Henderson W, Zadina K, Ovitt T, et al: Saphenous vein graft patency 1 year after coronary artery bypass surgery and effects of antiplatelet therapy. *Circulation* 1989; 80:1190–1197.
51. Goldman S, Copeland J, Moritz T, Henderson W, Zadina K, Ovitt T, et al: Internal mammary artery and saphenous vein graft patency: Effects of aspirin. *Circulation* 1990; 82(suppl IV):IV-237–242.
52. Lytle BW, Loop FD, Taylor PC, Simpfendorfer C, Kramer JC, Ratliff NB, et al: Vein graft disease: The clinical impact of stenoses in saphenous vein bypass grafts to coronary arteries. *J Thorac Cardiovasc Surg* 1992; 103:831–840.
53. Bourassa MG, Lesperance J, Corbara F, Saltiel J, Campeau L: Progression of obstructive coronary artery disease 5 to 7 years after aortocoronary bypass surgery. *Circulation* 1978; 58(suppl I):I-100–106.
54. Bruschke AVG, Kramer JR Jr, Bal ET, Haque IU, Detrano RC, Goormastic M: The dynamics of progression of coronary atherosclerosis studied in 168 medically treated patients who underwent coronary arteriography three times. *Am Heart J* 1989; 117:296–305.
55. Cosgrove DM, Loop FD, Saunders CR, Lytle BW, Kramer JR: Should coronary arteries with less than fifty percent stenosis be bypassed? *J Thorac Cardiovasc Surg* 1981; 82:520–530.
56. Califf RM, Harrell FE Jr, Lee KL, Rankin JS, Hlatky MA, Mark DB, et al: The evolution of medical and surgical therapy for coronary artery disease: A 15-year perspective. *JAMA* 1989; 261:2077–2086.
57. Pryor DB, Harrell FE Jr, Rankin JS, Lee KL, Muhlbaier LH, Oldham HN, et al: The changing survival benefits of coronary revascularization over time. *Circulation* 1987; 76(suppl V):V-13–V-21.
58. Johnson WD, Brenowitz JB, Kayser KL: Factors influencing long-term (10-year to 15-year) survival after a successful coronary artery bypass operation. *Ann Thorac Surg* 1989; 48:19–25.
59. DeWood MA, Notske RN, Berg R Jr, Ganji JH, Simpson CS, Hinnen ML, et al: Medical and surgical management of early Q wave myocardial infarction. I. Effects of surgical reperfusion on survival, recurrent myocardial infarction, sudden death and functional class at 10 or more years of follow-up. *J Am Coll Cardiol* 1989; 14:65–77.
60. DeWood MA, Leonard J, Grunwald RP, Hensley GR, Mouser LT, Burroughs RW, et al: Medical and surgical management of early Q wave myocardial infarction. II. Effects on mortality and global and regional left ventricular function at 10 or more years of follow-up. *J Am Coll Cardiol* 1989; 14:78–90.
61. Kereiakes DJ, Topol EJ, George BS, Abbottsmith CW, Stack RS, Candela RJ, et al: Favorable early and long-term prognosis following coronary bypass surgery therapy for myocardial infarction: Results of a multicenter trial. *Am Heart J* 1989; 118:199–207.
62. Kelly P, Ruskin JN, Vlahakes GJ, Buckley MJ, Freeman CS, Garan H: Surgical coronary revascularization in survivors of prehospital cardiac arrest: Its effect on inducible ventricular arrhythmias and long-term survival. *J Am Coll Cardiol* 1990; 15:267–273.
63. Loop FD, Lytle BW, Cosgrove DM, Stewart RW, Goormastic M, Williams GW, et al: Influence of the internal-mammary-artery graft on 10-year survival and other cardiac events. *N Engl J Med* 1986; 314:1–6.
64. Cameron A, Brogno DA, Green GE: Internal thoracic artery grafts, twenty years clinical follow-up. *Circulation* 1991; 84(suppl II):II-463.
65. Cosgrove DM, Lytle BW, Hill AC, Taylor PC, Stewart RW, Novoa R, et al: Are two internal thoracic arteries better than one? *J Thorac Cardiovasc Surg*, in press.
66. Proudfit WL, Kramer JR, Goormastic M, Loop FD: Ten-year survival of patients with mild angina or myocardial infarction without angina: A comparison of medical and surgical treatment. *Am Heart J* 1990; 119:942–948.
67. European Coronary Surgery Study Group: Long-term results of prospective randomized study of coronary artery bypass surgery in stable angina pectoris. *Lancet* 1982; 2:1173–1180.
68. Alderman EL, Fisher LD, Litwin P, Kaiser GC, Myers WO, Maynard C, et al: Results of coronary artery surgery in patients with poor left ventricular function (CASS). *Circulation* 1983; 68:785–795.
69. Kaiser GC, Davis KB, Fisher LD, Myers WO, Foster ED, Passamani ER, et al: Survival following coronary artery bypass grafting in patients with severe angina pectoris (CASS). *J Thorac Cardiovasc Surg* 1985; 89:513–524.
70. Myers WO, Schaff HV, Gersh BJ, Fisher LD, Kosinski AS, Mock MB, et al: Improved survival of surgically treated patients with triple vessel coronary artery disease and severe angina pectoris: A report from the Coronary Artery Surgery Study (CASS) registry. *J Thorac Cardiovasc Surg* 1989; 97:487–495.
71. Myers WO, Gersh BJ, Fisher LD, Mock MB, Holmes DR, Schaff HV, et al: Medical versus early surgical therapy in patients with triple-vessel disease and mild angina pectoris: A CASS Registry study of survival. *Ann Thorac Surg* 1987; 44:471–486.
72. Alderman EL, Bourassa MG, Cohen LS, Davis KB, Kaiser GG, Killip T, et al: Ten-year follow-up of survival and myocardial infarction in the randomized Coronary Artery Surgery Study. *Circulation* 1990; 82:1629–1646.
73. Lawrie GM, Morris GC Jr, Earle N: Long-term results of coronary bypass surgery: Analysis of 1,698 patients followed 15 to 20 years. *Ann Surg* 1991; 213:377–387.
74. Parisi AF, Khuri S, Deupree RH, Sharma GVRK, Scott SM, Luchi RJ: Medical compared with surgical management of unstable angina: 5-year mortality and morbidity in the Veterans Administration Study. *Circulation* 1989; 80:1176–1189.
75. Booth DC, Deupree RH, Hultgren HN, DeMaria AN, Scott SM, Luchi RJ, et al: Quality of life after bypass surgery for unstable angina: 5-year follow-up results of a Veterans Affairs Cooperative Study. *Circulation* 1991; 83:87–95.
76. Rogers WJ, Coggin CJ, Gersh BJ, Fisher LD, Myers WO, Oberman A, et al: Ten-year follow-up of quality of life in patients randomized to receive medical therapy or coronary artery bypass graft surgery: The Coronary Artery Surgery Study (CASS). *Circulation* 1990; 82:1647–1658.
77. Sergeant P, Lesaffre E, Flameng W, Suy R, Blackstone E: The return of clinically evident ischemia after coronary artery bypass grafting. *Eur J Cardiothorac Surg* 1991; 5:447–457.
78. Gersh BJ, Kronmal RA, Schaff HV, Frye RL, Ryan TJ, Mock MB, et al: Comparison of coronary artery bypass surgery and medical therapy in patients 65 years of age or older: A nonrandomized study from the Coronary Artery Surgery Study (CASS) Registry. *N Engl J Med* 1985; 313:217–224.
79. Johnson WD, Brenowitz JB, Kayser KL: Factors influencing long-term (10-year to 15-year) survival after a successful coronary artery bypass operation. *Ann Thorac Surg* 1989; 48:19–25.
80. Loop FD, Lytle BW, Cosgrove DM, Goormastic M, Taylor PC, Golding LAR, et al: Coronary artery bypass graft surgery in the elderly: Indications and outcome. *Cleve Clin J Med* 1988; 55:23–34.
81. Myers WO, Schaff HV, Fisher LD, Gersh BJ, Mock MB, Holmes DR, et al: Time to first new myocardial infarction in patients with severe angina and three-vessel disease comparing medical and early surgical therapy: A CASS Registry study of survival. *J Thorac Cardiovasc Surg* 1988; 95:382–389.
82. Schaff HV, Gersh BJ, Fisher LD, Frye RL, Mock MB, Ryan TJ, et al: Detrimental effect of perioperative myocardial infarction on late survival after coronary artery bypass. *J Thorac Cardiovasc Surg* 1984; 88:972–981.
83. Lytle BW, Loop FD, Cosgrove DM, Taylor PC, Goormastic M, Peper W, et al: Fifteen hundred coronary reoperations: Results and determinants of early and late survival. *J Thorac Cardiovasc Surg* 1987; 93:847–859.
84. Loop FD, Lytle BW, Cosgrove DM, Woods EL, Stewart RW, Golding LAR, et al: Reoperation for coronary atherosclerosis: Changing practice in 2509 consecutive patients. *Ann Surg* 1990; 212:378–386.
85. Marshall WG Jr, Saffitz J, Kouchoukos NT: Management during reoperation of aortocoronary saphenous vein grafts with minimal atherosclerosis by angiography. *Ann Thorac Surg* 1986; 42:163–167.
86. Brown G, Albers JJ, Fisher LD, Schaefer SM, Lin JT, Kaplan C, et al: Regression of coronary artery disease as a result of intensive lipid-lowering therapy in men with high levels of apolipoprotein B. *N Engl J Med* 1990; 323:1289–1298.
87. Blankenhorn DH, Nessim SA, Johnson RL, Sanmarco ME, Azen SP, Cashin-Hemphill L: Beneficial effects of combined colestipol-niacin therapy on coronary atherosclerosis and coronary venous bypass grafts. *JAMA* 1987; 257:3233–3240.

Chapter 74

Techniques for the Surgical Treatment of Atherosclerotic Coronary Artery Disease and Its Complications

Ellis L. Jones, M.D. ■ *Charles R. Hatcher, Jr., M.D.*

The objective of this chapter, which has been written for physicians who are not cardiac surgeons, is to define the technical factors important in the performance of coronary bypass surgery and to discuss the surgical treatment of ventricular rupture, septal rupture, papillary muscle rupture, and ventricular aneurysm.

PERFORMANCE OF CORONARY BYPASS SURGERY

Techniques of Cardiopulmonary Bypass

So that the surgeon may operate on a quiet bloodless heart, the pumping function of the ventricles is assumed by an external mechanical pump. Systemic and cardiac hypothermia is usually utilized to arrest the heart and reduce myocardial oxygen needs, thereby avoiding ischemic cellular damage. Venous flow is returned to the pump with either separate caval cannulas or a single cannula in the right atrium. Systemic cooling to a nasopharyngeal temperature of 28°C is frequently used in order to reduce myocardial oxygen requirements for complex procedures; for those with poor left ventricular function, systemic temperatures are decreased to 25°C. As the beating heart cools, stroke volume initially increases but then rapidly decreases, so that left ventricular distension and elevation of pulmonary artery pressure may occur in some patients. To avoid ventricular distension and the concomitant increase in myocardial metabolism, the left ventricle may be vented through the right superior pulmonary vein. A significant disadvantage of left ventricular venting is the introduction of air into the cardiac chambers. In spite of every effort to remove air bubbles at the conclusion of the operation, instances of neurologic injury continue to occur. Accordingly, there has been a trend away from the venting technique in recent years. Alternatively, pulmonary artery pressure can be monitored carefully, and if there is no concomitant aortic regurgitation, venting may not be necessary or may be accomplished through the main pulmonary artery.

Choice of Graft for Coronary Bypass Operation

Autogenous veins and arteries have been used to connect the aorta with distal portions of narrowed or occluded coronary arteries.[1] The reversed saphenous vein graft from the calf has been the choice for most vascular arterial conduits (Fig. 74-1). This vein, taken from ankle to

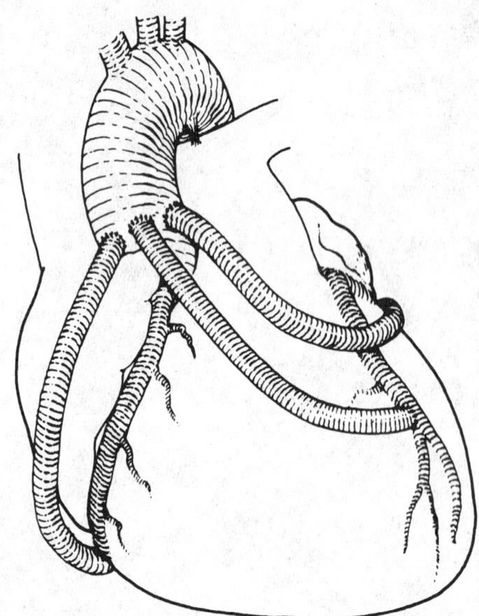

FIGURE 74-1 Reversed autogenous saphenous vein aortocoronary bypass grafts to left anterior descending, marginal circumflex, and right coronary arteries.

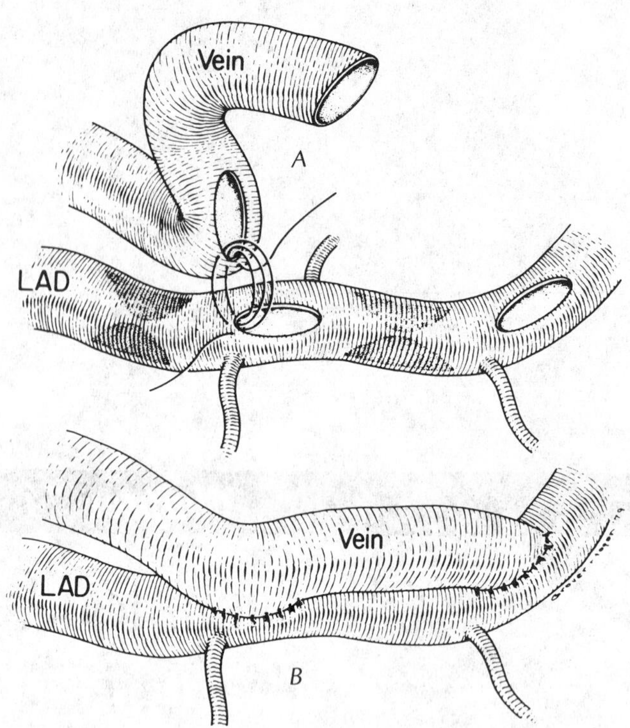

FIGURE 74-2 Sequential grafting for multiple lesions of the anterior descending coronary artery. (*From EL Jones: Coronary artery bypass grafting: Simplification and refinement of surgical technique, Ann Thorac Surg 1980; 30:84. Reproduced with permission from the publisher and author.*)

knee, is usually superior to a vein in the thigh because of its closer approximation in size to that of the coronary arteries. Where there has been prior stripping and ligation, the lesser saphenous vein has usually been found intact and offers a satisfactory alternative. If the lesser saphenous system is inadequate or nonexistent, the cephalic vein from the arm may be used, but unless the arm is positioned very carefully, the combination of upper extremity hypertension and the scissor effect of the clavicle and first rib on the brachial plexus may produce a severe injury while the sternum is retracted. Cryopreserved allograft veins have been used in a limited number of revascularization procedures, but long-term results are not yet known.

Extremes in diameter of the veins used for bypass grafting can present some problems. Varicose segments are excluded whenever possible. Diameters of at least 2.0 mm are necessary to ensure adequate flow through the bypass graft.

Sequential grafting is often performed for multiple lesions of a single artery and branches of other coronary arteries (Fig. 74-2). Rarely should there be more than two distal anastomoses for any single vein segment. The possibility of proximal graft failure due to late atherosclerosis and kinking or angulation of the graft on its way to the aorta generally limits multiple anastomoses using a single vein segment.

The internal mammary (thoracic) artery (IMA) offers an excellent alternative to the saphenous vein as an arterial conduit, particularly for grafting to the left anterior descending coronary artery. The internal mammary (thoracic) artery provides an artery-to-artery graft that results in excellent long-term patency rates that have approximated 95 percent after many years.[1,2] Disadvantages and limitations in the use of the internal mammary graft are that it must have adequate size and flow and require a finite period of time for the retrosternal dissection in its preparation. The latter may limit the use of the internal mammary artery in patients with unstable angina pectoris where operating time is a critical factor. In addition, the mammary artery may frequently be very small in female patients. Recently, surgeons at the Cleveland Clinic have shown that long-term patency of the detached (free) IMA approaches that of the in situ graft. Its use enhances flexibility of artery-to-artery anastomoses to many distant cardiac locations and allows multiple grafting sites to be performed with each IMA. Actuarial patient survival has been significantly increased when the IMA has been used instead of saphenous vein to bypass the left anterior descending artery.[3] Application of such sophisticated grafting techniques is far removed from the humble beginnings of the pioneering work of Alexis Carrel, who received the Nobel Prize for small-vessel arterial anastomoses.

In recent years, an autogenous radial artery has been used as a free graft between the aorta and coronary artery. Poor results have been universally experienced, however, primarily because of proximal stenosis and high early occlusion rates, so that the technique has been largely abandoned.[4]

In the preparation of the venous segment to be employed, autologous heparinized blood or buffered electrolyte solution (Normosol) is injected into the vein at moderate pressure while the venous branches are ligated. It is important to minimize the trauma of distension during the injection and removal of the venous segment from the leg to reduce the incidence of late stenosis of the grafts.

Technique of Myocardial Preservation

Once coronary flow has been interrupted by cross-clamping the aorta, a hyperosmolar potassium solution* or dilute blood (Hct approximately 8%) at 4°C is injected into the ascending aorta to arrest the heart. Asanguineous cardioplegia has been preferred by many because of its greater simplicity and because it affords the ability to operate at lower myocardial temperatures without increased viscosity and provides a coronary vascular bed free of formed elements. However, in recent years oxygenated cold-blood cardioplegia with and without glutamate and aspartate has been employed to prevent depletion of myocardial high-energy phosphate stores in order to improve perioperative left ventricular function.[5] Myocardial temperature is usually lowered to between 15 and 20°C, where metabolic activity is usually reduced well below half that at normothermia. In addition to the protection afforded by reduced myocardial temperature, electromechanical dissociation induced by the high potassium content may aid in the preservation of myocardial glycogen and high-energy phosphate stores. The alkaline nature of the solution combats the deleterious effect of acid metabolites on intracellular enzyme systems, whereas the hyperosmolality reduces both myocardial and endothelial cellular edema induced by the anoxic arrest.[6–9] Cessation of all electrical activity is usually observed after injection of approximately 200 to 300 mL. An additional 700 to 1000 mL of solution reduces the myocardial temperature to approximately 15 to 16°C. Injection of larger volumes or use of solutions with higher concentrations of potassium frequently produces troublesome bradyarrhythmias, consisting of bundle branch block, atrioventricular dissociation, or sinus arrest, in the immediate postoperative period. Failure or difficulty with the cardioplegic technique is usually seen when there is incompetency of the aortic valve or where there is marked left ventricular hypertrophy secondary to long-standing hypertension, hypertrophic subaortic stenosis, or concomitant valve disease. Excessive noncoronary collateral flow may produce difficulties during the operation by rapid clearing of the cardioplegic solution from the coronary arteries with premature resumption of electrical activity or by obscuring vision as a result of the large flow of blood emanating from the open coronary arteries.

Recently, Buckberg[10] has recommended addition of the retrograde administration of cardioplegic solution via the coronary sinus to obtain a more homogeneous distribution of the cold solution when proximal arterial stenoses are severe, thereby reducing the efficacy of the antegrade technique.

Technique of Dissection and Anastomosis

The epicardium is dissected from the coronary artery only in the area to be used for anastomosis. The surrounding epicardial attachments are left intact to prevent angulation and distortion at the area of the anastomosis. Intramyocardial coronary arteries may be difficult to locate at times but often can be identified along the obtuse margin of the heart as a thin, pale pink line just visible beneath the epicardial surface. Intramyocardial left anterior descending arteries may be more difficult to find and usually lie beneath a visible epicardial groove running cephalad from the apex or may be found by tracing the diagonal branch of the left anterior descending artery (LAD) proximally. Intramyocardial arteries lack the usual thickness of vessel walls and may be delicate and fragile when the anastomosis is performed. However, intramyocardial arteries are usually free of atheromatous disease.

Currently, the choice of a coronary anastomotic site has moved to a more distal location since the most extensive obstruction usually occurs proximally. As optical magnification and surgical techniques have improved, access to smaller, more disease-free peripheral arteries has become easier. Patency rates have been very acceptable in arteries 1.25 mm or greater in diameter. Endarterectomy has been employed extensively by some surgeons when the atherosclerotic process has become so severe that usual grafting techniques are not possible.

Conclusion of Operation

Once all distal anastomoses have been completed, rewarming is begun (if systemic hypothermia is used), coronary perfusion is reestablished by removing the aortic clamp, and the heart is electrically defibrillated if spontaneous conversion has not occurred. The proximal ends of the graft are sutured to the aorta using a single application of a large side-biting clamp. As many as six separate grafts may be constructed to the side of the aorta without difficulty (Fig. 74-3). One of the most important aspects of the operation is accurate adjustment of the length of the graft so that there is a symmetrical, graceful curve of the bypass vein. Proper adjustment of the graft length is best performed by transiently retarding the venous line to the oxygenator, thereby distending the pulmonary artery. Air is evacuated from the aorta and vein grafts, and the patient is removed from cardiopulmonary bypass.

Relation of Arteriogram to Gross Findings at Operation

Arteries less than 1 mm in diameter by arteriographic measurements are usually not satisfactory for bypass grafting. Akinesis determined by ventriculographic analysis is not necessarily a contraindication for bypass grafting provided that the distal vessels are suitable in size and quality and ischemic but viable myocardium is present in the region. However, when akinesis of a ventricular segment is present, there is usually a concomitant reduction in the size, quality, and distribution of the arteries supplying this region. Preservation of the artery to a segment of myocardium is usually (but not always) indicative of the existence of viable, but poorly functioning, muscle.

*Contents of the basic solution (concentrations in meq/L): sodium, 120; magnesium, 32; potassium, 16; calcium, 2.4; chloride, 160. Ten mL of 8.4% sodium bicarbonate are added to 1 liter, resulting in 324 mosm and pH 7.8.

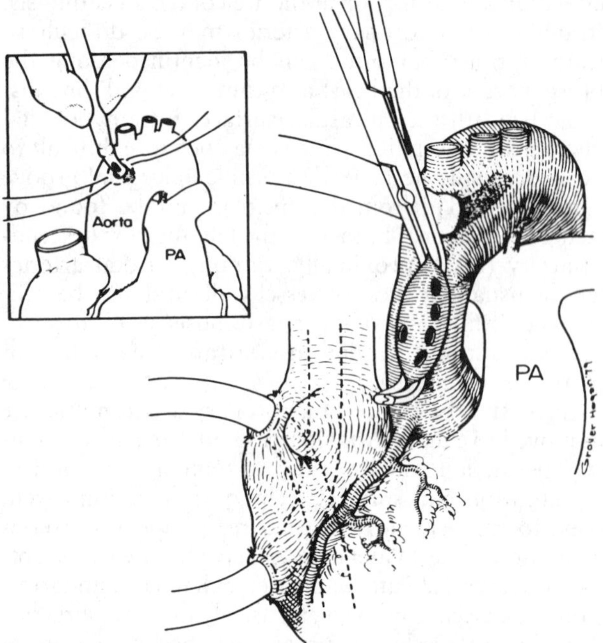

FIGURE 74-3 Construction of multiple graft sites along ascending aorta. (*From EL Jones: Coronary artery bypass grafting: Simplification and refinement of surgical technique. Ann Thorac Surg 1980; 30:84. Reproduced with permission from the publisher and author.*)

Proximally occluded vessels are usually found adequate for bypass grafting if the area they supply has normal or near-normal angiographic wall motion. This is true even when the totally occluded vessel cannot be adequately visualized at the time of catheterization. However, when the artery can be visualized and is shown to be very small, irregular, and diffusely diseased, this has usually been the finding at the time of operation. Arteries that are difficult to revascularize are the circumflex artery in the atrioventricular groove, which frequently lies under the great cardiac vein and is inaccessible, and large septal perforators, which frequently have a long area of obstructive disease at their takeoff from the anterior descending coronary artery. Vigorous exploration to locate septal perforating branches may often lead to extensive bleeding and sometimes entry into the right ventricular cavity. In addition, the origins of the septal perforators are proximal and thus in the area of greatest disease. Another area that may be somewhat difficult to expose is the distal right coronary artery well below the takeoff of the posterior descending branch. This area is frequently buried deep within the fat and becomes intramyocardial toward the crux of the heart.

The decision to revascularize areas demonstrated to be angiographically akinetic may be difficult, but certain guidelines have been helpful. Preservation of adequate size and quality of the artery supplying the akinetic segment usually means that significant distal regional vascular bed and its associated dependent muscle mass remain viable and worthy of bypass grafting. Postoperative angiography in several patients has shown patent grafts into the posterior descending branch of the right coronary artery supplying a large distribution of blood to the posterior one-third of the ventricular septum while the base and inferior segments of the heart remain noncontractile. In patients with totally obstructed anterior descending arteries distal to the first septal perforator, the anterior wall may be noncontractile, while the septum and cardiac base are seen to move satisfactorily. A graft of the proximal LAD may be beneficial in this situation.

Some patients have a profound depression of left ventricular function as determined by the ejection fraction but have little difficulty in the postoperative period after coronary bypass grafting. Such patients may obtain striking relief of angina and heart failure symptoms. Arteriography in such patients usually demonstrates total proximal obstruction of one or more major coronary arteries, with satisfactory distal vessels filling late through collaterals. The ejection fraction represents left ventricular function at only one point in time, and to exclude patients with low calculated values and adequate distal vessels is unjustified. Conversely, if segmental muscle mass has been replaced with scar tissue and little or no viable muscle remains, the size of the artery supplying this area usually diminishes proportionately.

Complications of the Coronary Bypass Operation

Postoperative complications of this operation are similar to those seen in any patients undergoing cardiac surgery with cardiopulmonary bypass. Such problems consist of aortic dissection, cerebral embolus or ischemia, anastomotic bleeding, perioperative infarction, deep mediastinal infection, and requirements for inotropic drugs in order to discontinue cardiopulmonary bypass.

Aortic dissection continues to account for significant mortality in performance of the coronary bypass operation. Patients at increased risk are the elderly, those with a long history of hypertension, and patients with occult medial cystic necrosis or severe atherosclerotic involvement of the ascending aorta. Treatment is difficult, and the problem is most effectively handled by prophylactic maneuvers to avoid this lethal complication. Preventive maneuvers consist of reducing central aortic pressure each time a clamp is applied or removed from the aorta, minimizing the frequency with which clamps are placed on the ascending aorta, meticulous incorporation of all layers of the aorta into the proximal graft suture line, and pharmacologic prevention of wide swings in systemic blood pressure once the operation has been completed.

Central nervous system damage such as strokes or transient postoperative neurologic sequelae has occurred with increasing frequency (2 to 4 percent) as the age and debilitation of the patient population increases. This may be due to particulate embolization from the aorta to the cerebral circulation. Embolization of particulate matter may also occur from left ventricular mural thrombus or calcific debris dislodged at the time of aortic cannulation or when the proximal aortic clamp is released. Platelet-fibrin deposition on the aortic suture line is also a cause of early or late embolization. However, the occurrence of this latter phenomenon is sufficiently infrequent that routine anticoagulation is unjustified. Neurologic deficits secondary to air embolism are usually transient and resolve completely at a variable rate during the postoperative period. Embolization of particulate matter, on the other hand, is usually more devastating, and resolution, if it occurs, requires a more prolonged period of time.

Anastomotic bleeding is usually seen when grafts have been placed to arteries of marginal quality and the vessel wall is friable and thin, particularly where a posterior atherosclerotic plaque terminates anteriorly and laterally. Repairing sutures are frequently necessary, often resulting in compromise of the vessel lumen. For this reason, the ultimate decision of whether to graft questionable coronary arteries must be reserved until the moment of surgery.

The frequency of perioperative myocardial infarction is not statistically related to extent of vessel disease, abnormality of left ventricular function, or inability to achieve complete revascularization.[11] Most perioperative infarction can now be attributed to poor distal reperfusion once grafting of the more proximal arteries has been performed. Since routine employment of better myocardial preservation techniques by most cardiac surgical centers, the incidence of perioperative infarction has diminished significantly but is still a significant complication of the operation.

The prevention of deep mediastinal wound infections requires constant attention to antiseptic detail. Introduction of organisms through intravenous or intraarterial monitoring lines or at the time of operation must be meticulously avoided. *Streptococcus* and *Staphylococcus* are the most frequently offending organisms. Gram-negative infections are more prevalent in patients with chronic obstructive pulmonary disease.

The need for inotropic drugs to permit discontinuation of cardiopulmonary bypass has progressively decreased over the years as techniques of myocardial preservation have improved and technical proficiency has increased. If left ventricular function is abnormal, the need for inotropic drugs is significantly increased.

We use the principles enumerated in this text to manage patients having the coronary bypass operation, and operative mortality, which was 1.3 percent in 1986, has now increased to 4.1 percent (1990). Precise definition and understanding of factors important in the technical performance of this procedure have in the past made it one of the safest major operations in recent surgical history.

MECHANICAL DEFECTS COMPLICATING ACUTE MYOCARDIAL INFARCTION

Mechanical defects occurring as a result of myocardial infarction are usually catastrophic and result in high mortality. Patients in cardiogenic shock following myocardial infarction should be carefully assessed for the presence of such mechanical defects, which include (1) rupture of the ventricular free wall, (2) rupture of the ventricular septum, and (3) rupture of papillary muscle.

Acute Rupture of the Ventricular Free Wall

Rupture of the ventricular free wall is described in more detail in Chap. 60. Cardiac rupture accounts for 10 to 15 percent of deaths from infarction.[12] Of ventricular ruptures, 84 percent occur in the first week, and 33 percent occur within the first 24 h of infarction.[13]

Ventricular rupture is usually abrupt and is difficult to distinguish from postinfarction cardiogenic shock without rupture. The anterior left ventricular wall is three times more likely to be involved than is the inferior wall. Sudden death is usual, but there may be tamponade of an irregular rupture by hematoma, adhesions, or false aneurysm formation, which may allow stabilization of hemodynamic status for a period of time.[14]

Surgical Treatment

When rupture is suspected, prompt pericardiocentesis should be performed to establish the diagnosis and improve hemodynamic status. Continuous drainage through a soft catheter with side holes may allow time for transport of the patient to the operating room. Once the diagnosis is confirmed, the patient should be placed on cardiopulmonary bypass and the defect repaired. If cardiopulmonary bypass is used, infarctectomy and closure of viable ventricular wall is performed. Late deaths have resulted from cardiogenic shock, recurrent rupture, or myocardial infarction.

Rupture of the Ventricular Septum

Chapter 60 describes the clinical features of rupture of the ventricular septum. Septal rupture occurs in approximately 1 percent of patients who die as a result of myocardial infarction. The majority of these ruptures occur within the first week, and 20 to 30 percent develop as early as the first 24 h after the onset of initial symptoms of infarction. Of patients with septal rupture, 50 percent die within the first week, and 85 percent die by the end of the second week following rupture. Because of the inordinately high mortality with medical management, surgical repair should be considered in most patients.

The blood supply to the septum arises from branches of the left anterior descending coronary artery, the posterior descending branch of the right coronary artery, or the circumflex artery when it is dominant. Approximately 60 percent of septal ruptures occur with infarction of the anterior wall and 40 percent with infarction of the posterior or inferior wall.[15]

When septal rupture is recognized, administration of digitalis and intravenous administration of sodium nitroprusside may improve pump function by decreasing afterload, ventricular filling, and regurgitant flow. If hypotension is present, an inotropic drug is also utilized. If there is not prompt hemodynamic stabilization, which is usually the case, an intraaortic balloon assist device should be inserted prior to cardiac catheterization and eventual surgery. The benefit of intraaortic balloon pumping is twofold: (1) reduction in afterload with a decrease in left-to-right shunting and (2) diastolic augmentation with an increase in coronary blood flow resulting in improvement in the oxygen supply-demand ratio. This aggressive approach often results in temporary stabilization of these extremely ill patients, but in general, the benefits achieved are disappointingly brief. Therefore, early diagnostic evaluation and rapid surgical intervention should usually be planned. Only about 15 percent of patients can be controlled by conventional medical measures for the period of 3 to 6 weeks, after which surgery can be performed at a greatly reduced risk.

Surgical Treatment

Surgical repair of postinfarction ventricular septal defect was first reported by Cooley et al. in 1957.[16] The method used at that time was to approach the defect through a right ventriculotomy, much as a congenital defect would be corrected today. Since then, extensive modifications in surgical technique have occurred, and at present the site of ventriculotomy is through the area of infarction.[17] This allows optimal exposure of the defect while minimizing damage to functional myocardium.

Operative mortality is directly related to the interval between infarction and surgical repair. If repair is performed 3 weeks or more after infarction, operative mortality is approximately 20 percent; if surgery is performed prior to this time, mortality approaches 50 percent.[18] The most obvious reason for this is the fact that the greater the myocardial damage and hemodynamic compromise, the more urgent the need for early intervention.

The technique of closure of these defects has resulted in several ingenious procedures. The procedure utilized is determined by the location of the defect. Most defects are anteroapical, and closure utilizes a technique of buttressing the defect with viable muscle from the adjacent anterior left ventricular wall. Small chronic defects located high in the ventricular septum and the larger defects are closed with a Dacron or bovine pericardial patch[19] (see Fig. 74-4).

The less common high posterior septal or inferior defect is approached through the inferior portion of the heart, usually in the distribution of the posterior descending branch of the right coronary artery. The incision is made in the area of maximal infarction, which is usually on the right ventricular side of the septum. A well-proven principle of repair of these defects is synthetic patch closure without tension[20] (see Fig. 74-5).

Papillary Muscle Rupture

Mitral regurgitation following myocardial infarction reflects loss of structural and functional integrity of the papillary muscle apparatus and is said to occur with an autopsy incidence of approximately 1 percent. The anterolateral papillary muscle receives its blood supply from the obtuse marginal branch of the circumflex artery, while the posteromedial papillary muscle is dependent on the right coronary artery. Injury to the posteromedial papillary muscle is significantly more frequent than injury to the anterolateral papillary muscle. Interference with this blood supply may result in frank infarction and rupture or gradual replacement with fibrosis, both of which will impair function of the mitral apparatus. Principles of management include all measures to improve left ventricular function and decrease regurgitant flow. The spectrum of therapeutic intervention may include administration of digitalis, diuretics,

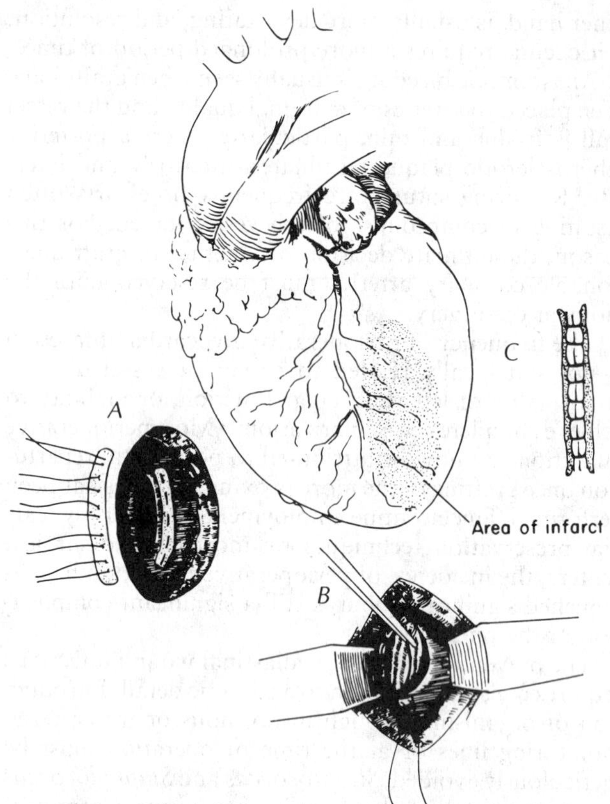

FIGURE 74-4 Repair of anterior ventricular septal defect secondary to anterior myocardial infarction. (*From WM Daggett: Surgery for postmyocardial infarct ventricular septal defect. Ann Surg 1977; 186:260. Reproduced with permission from the publisher and author.*)

and sodium nitroprusside; infusion of inotropic agents; and intraaortic balloon assistance.

Surgical Treatment

At best, the surgical treatment of these patients is difficult and carries with it a mortality of between 10 and 25 percent, depending on the extent of impairment of left ventricular function. Surgical exposure of the mitral valve is often difficult because of the small left atrium uniformly noted in patients with acute mitral regurgitation. The goal of surgical intervention is to provide the patient with a competent, nonstenotic mitral valve, and

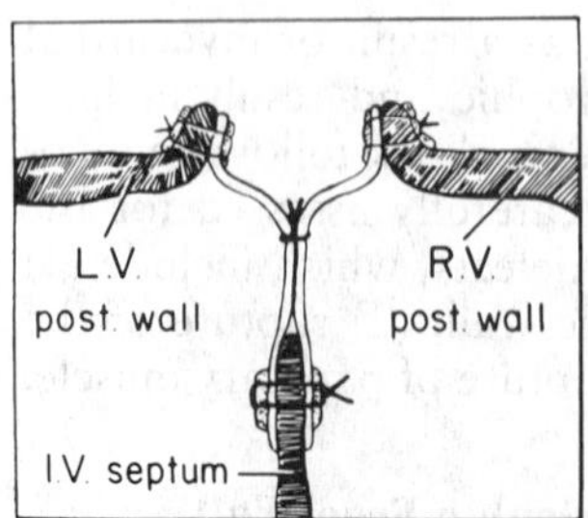

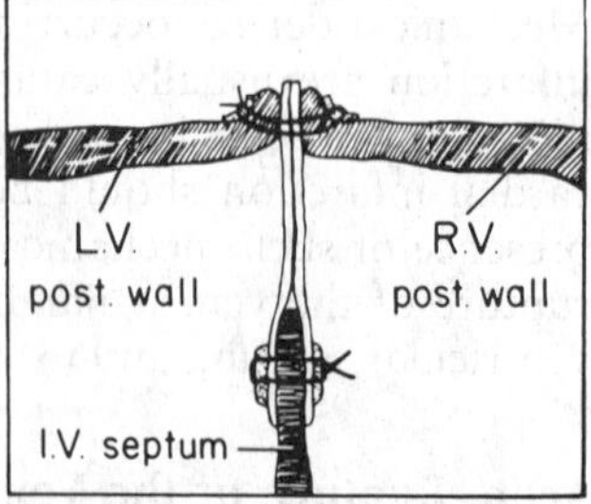

FIGURE 74-5 Synthetic patch repair of postinfarct VSD. (*From WM Dagget: Surgical management of ventricular septal defects complicating myocardial infarction. World J Surg 1978; 2:756. Reproduced with permission from the publisher and author.*)

this can be reliably accomplished with prosthetic valve replacement. Recently, annuloplastic techniques have been used in these emergency situations, but this will depend on the clinical status of the patient and operative findings at the time of surgery.[21-23]

LEFT VENTRICULAR ANEURYSM

Indications for Surgery

Primary indications for surgical treatment of left ventricular aneurysm consist of left ventricular failure, angina pectoris, thromboembolism, and tachyarrhythmias. In recent years the primary indication for resection of left ventricular aneurysm has been angina pectoris associated with prior myocardial infarction and multivessel coronary artery disease. However, the occurrence of complex ventricular arrhythmias with hemodynamic impairment has increased in frequency over the last several years, and the need for proper preoperative evaluation with signal averaging, programmed electrophysiological stimulation, and intraoperative mapping must be considered prior to any surgical intervention. Persistent severe left ventricular failure, as a result of multiple infarctions or a single massive infarction, is less of an indication today.

Endocardial thrombosis frequently accompanies transmural myocardial infarction, and mural thrombus is usually identified at the time of aneurysm resection. One potential complication of left ventricular aneurysm is thromboembolism. However, the occurrence of this complication has probably been overstated in the past and rarely is an indication by itself for aneurysm resection.

Surgical Treatment

Once cardiopulmonary bypass is instituted, the heart is decompressed and cooled. The heart is allowed to cool until it fibrillates. Resection of the aneurysm may then be performed without cross-clamping the aorta and prolonging ventricular ischemic time. At very cold temperatures (25°C) left ventricular fibrillation is probably not injurious to the myocardium. A left ventricular vent is inserted across the right superior pulmonary vein into the left ventricle to minimize distension. In addition, this allows precise delineation of the aneurysmal sac and adjacent viable myocardium. Care should be taken not to embolize thrombus from the left ventricular endocardium by excessive manipulation of the heart prior to fibrillation. A linear incision is made in the collapsed aneurysm and all thrombus removed. The left ventricular endocardium is wiped clean of residual thrombus and the left ventricular cavity irrigated copiously with iced saline solution. The aneurysm has traditionally been closed with multiple layers of running zero and 3-0 monofilament suture reinforced with strips of Teflon felt. More recently, the aneurysm has been isolated from viable muscle within the endocardial cavity by use of a geometric configuration of bovine pericardium according to the technique of Jatene.[24] This latter technique prevents ventricular distortion and compromise of functioning myocardium. Once the aneurysm is closed, coronary bypass can then be performed in routine fashion.[25]

Technical complications of closure primarily involve tearing of the myocardium at the base of the suture line. For this reason an adequate margin of fibrous left ventricular aneurysm, which retains sutures well, should be left. The extent of placement of the initial sutures is determined by vital structures such as epicardial circumflex arteries as well as the muscular components of the mitral valve apparatus.

Aneurysm resection performed with modern techniques can be done with mortalities well below 5 percent at the present time. The risk of operation is determined by the quality of residual left ventricular myocardial function.[26]

REFERENCES

1. Loop FD, Irarrazaval MJ, Bredee JJ, Siegel W, Taylor PC, Sheldon WC: Internal mammary artery graft for ischemic heart disease, effect of revascularization on clinical status and survival. *Am J Cardiol* 1977; 39:516–522..
2. Kay EB, Naraghipour H, Beg RA, DeManey M, Tambe A, Zimmerman HA: Internal mammary artery bypass graft. Long-term patency rate and follow-up. *Ann Thorac Surg* 1974; 18:269–279.
3. Loop FD, Lytle BW, Cosgrove DM, Golding LA, Taylor PC, Stewart RW: Influence of the internal-mammary-artery graft on 10 year survival and other cardiac events. *N Engl J Med* 1986; 314:1–6.
4. Carpentier A, Guermonprez JL, Deloche A, Frechette C, DuBost C: The aorta-to-coronary radial artery bypass graft. *Ann Thorac Surg* 1973; 16:111–121.
5. Allen BS, Buckberg GD, Schwaiger M, Yeatman L, Tillisch J, Kawata N, et al: Studies of controlled reperfusion after ischemia. XVI. Early recovery of regional wall motion in patients following surgical revascularization after eight hours of acute coronary occlusion. *J. Thorac Cardiovasc Surg* 1986; 92:636–648.
6. Leaf A: Cell swelling (editorial) *Circulation* 1973; 48:455–458.
7. Willerson JT, Powell WJ, Guiney T, Stark JJ, Sanders DA, Leaf A: Improvement in myocardial function and coronary blood flow in ischemic myocardium after mannitol. *J Clin Invest* 1972; 51:2989–2998.
8. Leaf A: On the mechanism of fluid exchange of tissues in vitro. *Biochem J* 1956; 62:241–248.
9. Jones EL, Tyras DH, King SB, Logue RB, Hatcher CR Jr: Myocardial revascularization combined with intracoronary infusion of hyperosmolar solution in the early management of post infarction ventricular septal defect. Report of a case. *Circulation* 1975; 52:170–176.
10. Buckberg GD: Antegrade/retrograde blood cardioplegia to ensure cardioplegic distribution: Operative techniques and objectives. *J Cardiac Surg* 1989; 3:216–238.
11. Jones EL, Craver JM, King SB, Douglas JS, Bradford JM, Brown CM, et al: Clinical, anatomic and functional descriptors influencing morbidity, survival and adequacy of revascularization following coronary bypass. *Ann Surg* 1980; 192(3):390–392.
12. Bates RJ, Bentler S, Resnekov L, Anagnostopoulos CE: Cardiac rupture—Challenge in diagnosis and management. *Am J Cardiol* 1977; 40:429–437.
13. Rasmussen S, Leth A, Kjoller E, Pedersen A: Cardiac rupture in acute myocardial infarction. A review of seventy-two consecutive cases. *Acta Med Scand* 1979; 205:11–16.
14. Van Tassel RA, Edwards JE: Rupture of the heart complicating myocardial infarction. *Chest* 1972; 61:104–116.
15. Swithinbank JM: Perforation of the intraventricular septum in myocardial infarction. *Br Heart J* 1959; 21:562–566.
16. Cooley DA, Belmonte BA, Zeis LB, Schnur S: Surgical repair of ruptured inter-ventricular septum following acute myocardial infarction. *Surgery* 1957; 41:930–937.
17. Kitamura S, Mendez A, Kay JH: Ventricular septal defect following myocardial infarction: Experience with surgical repair through a left ventriculotomy and review of the literature. *J Thorac Cardiovasc Surg* 1971; 61:186–199.

18. Daggett WM, Guyton RA, Mundth ED, Buckley MJ, McEnany MT, Gold HK, et al: Surgery for post–myocardial infarct ventricular septal defect. *Ann Surg* 1977; 186:260–271.
19. Daggett WM, Buckley MJ: The surgical treatment of post infarction ventricular septal defect. Indications, techniques and results. In: Moran J, Michaelis LL (eds): *Surgery for the Complications of Myocardial Infarction.* New York, Grune & Stratton, 1980: 211–229.
20. Daggett WM: Surgical technique for early repair of posterior ventricular septal rupture. *J Thorac Cardiovasc Surg* 1982; 84:306–312.
21. Austen WG, Sokol DM, DeSanctis RW, Sanders CA: Surgical treatment of papillary muscle rupture complicating myocardial infarction. *N Engl J Med* 1968; 278:1137–1141.
22. Gerbode FL, Hetzer R, Krebber HJ: Surgical management of papillary muscle rupture. *World J Surg* 1978; 2:791–796.
23. Rankin JS, Hickey MSt J, Smith R, Muhlbaier L, Reves JG, Pryor DB, et al: Ischemic mitral regurgitation. *Circulation* 1989; 79(6 Pt 2):I-116–I-121.
24. Jatene AD: Left ventricular aneurysmectomy. Resection or reconstruction. *J Thorac Cardiovasc Surg* 1985; 89:321–331.
25. Harken AH: Left ventricular aneurysm. In: Sabiston DC Jr, Spencer FC (eds): *Gibbons Surgery of the Chest,* vol 2. Philadelphia, WB Saunders, 1983: 1480–1489.
26. Jones EL, Craver JW, Hurst JW, Bradford JA, Bone DK, Robinson PH, et al: Influence of left ventricular aneurysm on survival following the coronary bypass operation. *Ann Surg* 1981; 193:733–742.

Systemic Arterial Hypertension

Chapter 75

Pathophysiology of Systemic Arterial Hypertension

Edward D. Frohlich, M.D.

PRESSOR MECHANISMS IN HYPERTENSION

To understand the pathophysiological alterations associated with the systemic arterial hypertensive diseases there must first be a clear-cut understanding of the hemodynamic alterations; by definition, hypertension is a hemodynamic derangement.[1–4] The elevated arterial pressure in systemic arterial hypertension (SAH) may be associated with an increased cardiac output or vascular resistance. Any changes in blood viscosity would not result in a major increase in arterial pressure even though they may alter local tissue blood flow in organs. For the most part, however, an increased vascular resistance is the hemodynamic hallmark of the disease; and the mechanisms responsible for this increased vascular smooth-muscle tone are implicit in the multifactorial nature of the disease.[4–6] This chapter considers the factors that may be involved with the elaboration and maintenance of hypertensive diseases in essential hypertension as well as in the other forms of hypertension (Table 75-1). This discussion, however, places a primary emphasis on essential hypertension since this primary form of hypertension occurs in approximately 95 percent of all patients with SAH.[3,4] This pathophysiological discussion is particularly relevant to other (i.e., secondary) clinical forms of hypertension; and they will be cited for comparison with those derangements that occur in patients with essential hypertension.

Hemodynamics

As indicated, all patients with hypertension have an increased arterial pressure that is associated with an increased contractile state or increased mass of vascular smooth muscle in both the arterioles and venules. This luminal narrowing serves to increase the total peripheral resistance but to reduce the total-body venous capacity.[1,3,7] The result of the former is an increase in left ventricular afterload, which serves as the major hemodynamic mechanism responsible for the left ventricular hypertrophy (LVH) associated with the progression in severity of hypertensive vascular disease.[8,9] The reduced venous capacity due to venular constriction has been demonstrated clinically and in experimental forms of hypertension.[10–12] Early in hypertension, this venoconstriction is not associated with contraction in intravascular volume; hence, the venoconstriction serves to redistribute volume to the cardiopulmonary area from the periphery.[10,13,14] With progression of the vascular disease and more intense vasoconstriction, however, intravascular volume contracts progressively.[15,16] This is reflected in a proportionally diminished right atrial venous return, thereby reducing the cardiac output to a more normal level from, frequently, an elevated level.[13,17] As left ventricular hypertrophy becomes more manifest, left ventricular function becomes impaired and the resting cardiac output diminishes.[17,18] With these alterations in systemic blood flow there are proportional changes in organ blood flows; and the reductions in specific organ

TABLE 75-1

Classification of the Various Forms of Systemic Arterial Hypertension Based on Causes

Primary (Essential) Hypertension (Hypertension of Undetermined Cause)
Borderline (labile) essential hypertension
Essential hypertension (sustained diastolic hypertension)
Mild severity: diastolic pressures 90 to 104 mmHg
Moderate severity: diastolic pressures 105 to 114 mmHg
Severe: persistent diastolic pressures greater than 114 mmHg
Isolated systolic hypertension: systolic pressures greater than 140 mmHg with diastolic pressures less than 90 mmHg
Secondary Hypertension
Coarctation of the aorta
Renal arterial disease (renovascular hypertension)
Nonatherosclerotic (fibrosing) renal arterial disease
Atherosclerotic renal arterial disease
Aneurysm(s) of renal artery
Embolic renal arterial disease
Extravascular compression (of renal artery): tumor, fibrosis
Perinephric hull (Page kidney)
Renal parenchymal diseases
Chronic pyelonephritis
Acute glomerulonephritis
Chronic glomerulonephritis
Polycystic renal disease
Diabetic nephropathy
Others: amyloidosis, ureteral obstruction, etc.
Hormonal diseases
Thyroid
Hyperthyroidism
Hypothyroidism
Hashimoto's thyroiditis
Adrenal
Cushing disease or Cushing syndrome
Primary hyperaldosteronism
Adenoma
Bilateral hyperplasia
Adrenal enzyme deficiencies
Pheochromocytoma
Others
Ectopic production of hormones
Growth hormone excess
Hypercalcemic disease states (including hyperparathyroidism)
Drugs, chemicals, and foods
Excessive alcohol intake
Excessive dietary sodium intake
Exogenously administered adrenal steroids: birth control pills; adrenal steroids for asthma, malignancies; anabolic steroids
Licorice excess (imported)
Cold preparations: phenylpropanolamine; nasal decongestants
Milk-alkali syndrome; hypervitaminosis D
Snuff
Complications from specific therapy
Antidepressant therapy (tricyclics; monoamine oxidase inhibitors)
Chronic steroid administration
Cyclosporine (transplantation and certain diseases requiring immunosuppressive therapy)
Beta-adrenergic receptor agonists (e.g., for asthma)
Radiation nephritis, arteritis

flows are in direct relation to the increased organ vascular resistance.[14] Therefore, the organ or regional vascular resistances seem to be more or less uniformly distributed systemically in proportion to the increased total peripheral resistance.[1,2,14]

Thus, the major hemodynamic alteration in hypertensive disease is an increased vascular resistance, which is achieved through an active increase in the state of tone of vascular smooth muscle in both the arterioles and the venules. This state of vessel tone can be achieved whether the myocyte is stimulated by enhanced adrenergic input (elevated circulating levels) of humoral agents (e.g., catecholamines, angiotensin II, serotonin, vasopressin), local vasoactive peptides (e.g., angiotensin II, vasoactive intestinal polypeptide, endothelium), or ions (e.g., calcium); by a reduced amount of vasoconstrictors; or by an increase in vasodilating agents (e.g., acetylcholine, histamine, adenosine, prostaglandins), local vasoactive peptides (e.g., insulin, calcitonin gene–related peptide), or ions (e.g., potassium, magnesium, Krebs intermediate metabolites).[1-4] Whatever the myocyte stimulus, there is a consequent rise in cytoplasmic free calcium ions from the resting state and a resulting enhanced phosphorylation of myosin light chains. This increased calcium ionic milieu may be achieved either through an inflow of calcium ions through calcium or other (e.g., alpha-adrenergic) receptor-activated membrane channels or by a release of calcium ions from intracellular organelles (primarily the sarcoplasmic reticulum) although it also may be released from the mitochondria or from binding with protein substrates. The former receptor-operated channels explain the mechanisms of action of the various membrane receptors of naturally occurring humoral substances or of various antihypertensive agents (e.g., calcium antagonists). The intracytoplasmic calcium release seems to be initiated by the formation of inositol triphosphate (IP_3), which serves as the second messenger mediating the calcium ion release.[19,20] The net effect is the availability of calcium ions for the mechanical coupling that permits the enhanced state of contractility of vascular smooth muscle. As noted, another factor that participates in the increased vascular resistance is an increased wall-to-lumen diameter of the arterial and arteriolar wall. This structural alteration of the vessel wall in hypertension serves to augment vascular responsiveness to constrictor stimuli, thereby serving to perpetuate the hypertension.[21] Recent investigations have suggested that the hemodynamic stress of vessel stretch may not be the sole responsible mechanism accounting for the vessel wall thickening.[22,23] Indeed, numbers of growth factors, such as platelet-derived growth factor, have been shown to participate in this process, some of which are vasoconstrictors (e.g., angiotensin II, endothelin) and are produced within the arteriolar wall.[24-28] Growth factors and vascular smooth-muscle cell growth represent common features of hypertension and atherosclerosis.[29,30]

Fluid Volume Partitions

In general, total-body water is normal in hypertension; it seems to be normally distributed between the extracellular and intracellular fluid compartments.[31] Although there is much epidemiologic evidence for a metabolic derangement in the handling of sodium in patients with hypertension, there is little evidence to indicate that total-body sodium is increased or that it is associated with abnormal total-body water.[32] Nevertheless, there is good clinical evidence that the extracellular fluid volume is maldistributed.[31] Thus, as intravascular (i.e., plasma) volume becomes contracted in patients with essential hypertension[15,16]; it is associated with a greater degree of interstitial fluid volume.[33] The pathophysiological implications of these alterations were extremely important in the earlier days of antihypertensive therapy. Thus, if arterial pressure were reduced by direct-acting smooth-muscle vasodilators or antiadrenergic compounds, capillary hydrostatic and renal arterial perfusion pressures would diminish. As a consequence, interstitial fluid would migrate intravascularly to expand (or "reconstitute") the intravascular compartment.[34,35] The net result was an attenuation of the antihypertensive effectiveness. With addition of a diuretic, however, intravascular volume would again become contracted, thereby restoring the antihypertensive effectiveness. This provides the physiological explanation for the phenomenon of "pseudotolerance."[34,36] In more recent years, with the introduction of the beta-adrenergic receptor, angiotensin converting enzyme, and calcium channel inhibitor therapies, the induced hypotension is not associated with expanded intravascular volume and pseudotolerance has been of less concern.[37,38] In the intensive care setting, when therapies may still include ganglion blocking drugs or sodium nitroprusside, however, pseudotolerance may become a very real problem. Thus, with prolonged pressure reduction using these agents, antihypertensive effectiveness may diminish as a result of intravascular volume expansion and not "tachyphylaxis" (or diminished end-organ pharmacologic effectiveness); by adding a diuretic, the desired hypotensive effect may be anticipated.[37-39]

As indicated, most patients with essential hypertension demonstrate an inverse relationship between height of arterial pressure (or total peripheral resistance) and the magnitude of intravascular volume.[15,16,18] Other forms of hypertension demonstrate a similar inverse relationship, including patients with renal arterial disease and pheochromocytoma.[16] These considerations are of major pathophysiological significance since inordinate intraoperative hypotension may occur if intravascular volume is not expanded prior to excision of a pheochromocytoma (e.g., with prior therapy with alpha-adrenergic receptor inhibiting therapy to lower pressure and expand plasma volume) or with direct intraoperative volume expansion using the patient's own blood (preferably collected prior to surgery).

In contrast, other patients with hypertension may demonstrate a direct relationship between the height of arterial pressure and intravascular volume.[16] These patients may have a steroidal dependent form of hypertension (e.g., primary aldosteronism, Cushing's disease), renal parenchymal disease, or volume-dependent essential hypertension (which includes a small number of patients) (i.e., also with low plasma renin activity that is suppressed by this volume expansion).[16,40-42] In this respect, even in patients with parenchymal renal disease who have normal renal function tests (e.g., serum creatinine and glomerular filtration rate), intravascular volume is expanded.[41] These considerations have important clinical and therapeutic considerations. For example, studies have shown that patients with low plasma renin and essential hypertension are particularly responsive to diuretic therapy.[43] (See Chap. 77.)

Sodium Metabolism

Epidemiologic studies have repeatedly demonstrated a high direct correlation between dietary sodium intake of populations and the prevalence of hypertension.[44] Further, studies have shown that those societies with daily sodium intakes of less than 60 mmol (1.38 g sodium or 3.51 g sodium chloride) also fail to show a rise in arterial pressure with aging. Other studies have demonstrated that there may be genetically determined alterations in sodium transport across cell membranes in different population groups of patients with essential hypertension.[45] Notwithstanding the massive epidemiologic data supporting an important role for the sodium ion in essential hypertension, there is a paucity of pathophysiological data that have demonstrated this in clinical studies.[37] It remains a major problem to identify which patients with essential hypertension are sodium sensitive and which are not. At this point, therefore, the subject still remains one of great controversy.

Hormonal Alterations

Because of the foregoing issue concerning the role of the sodium ion in essential hypertension, many studies have focused upon the role of adrenal corticosteroids. For the most part, these studies have failed to demonstrate any specific abnormality in the metabolism of the adrenal steroidal hormones. Aldosterone seems to be synthesized, released, and excreted in proportion to the levels of stimulation of the renin-angiotensin system.[46] No clear-cut derangement in adrenal steroid biosynthesis has been demonstrated in patients with essential hypertension. Patients with abnormal levels of steroidal biosynthesis and release have specific adrenal diseases (Cushing's syndrome and disease, primary hyperaldosteronism, hydroxylase deficiencies, etc.).[47]

States of hormonal alteration have been associated with hypertension. There is a high prevalence of hypertension in patients with both hyperthyroidism and hypothyroidism; there also is an increased incidence of hypertension among patients with hypercalcemic diseases (including hyperparathyroidism). Furthermore, recent studies have suggested an abnormality in parathyroid hormone in patients with essential hypertension[48]; this observation requires further confirmation and study. Other hormonal diseases associated with hypertension include acromegaly and gigantism, ectopically produced hormones associated with tumors and, of course, with exogenously administered hormones (e.g., oral contraceptives, androgens).

Neural Mechanisms

The autonomic nervous system participates importantly in the normal control of arterial pressure and may be altered in patients with essential hypertension. One would normally expect that the higher the arterial pressure, the slower the heart rate. On the other hand, most patients with essential hypertension (no matter what the severity) demonstrate a relatively rapid heart rate, even if frank tachycardia is not present.[49] This is but one manifestation of the altered baroreceptor sensitivity in hypertension.[50] In addition, increased release of, sensitivity to, and excretion of norepinephrine have been demonstrated in many patients with essential hypertension, more frequently in patients with borderline or mild degrees of severity.[51] In addition, other studies have related increased levels of serum catecholamines in proportion to the altered hemodynamics.[52] On the other hand, no abnormalities have been demonstrated in patients with essential hypertension with respect to catecholamine biosynthesis.

A variety of studies have demonstrated increased responsiveness of blood vessels to catecholamine stimulation and stressful stimuli (including cold and physiological interventions); several studies involving patients with essential hypertension have related alterations in response to upright tilting, Valsalva maneuver, and tyramine stimulation of norepinephrine release from nerve endings.[53,54] Thus, patients with milder forms of hypertension may demonstrate orthostatic hypertension and a greater degree of diastolic pressure overshoot during the Valsalva maneuver, suggesting a greater neural component in this group. By contrast, patients with severe hypertension (e.g., malignant hypertension) may demonstrate orthostatic hypotension and a lesser degree of pressure/overshoot after the Valsalva maneuver, indicating a significant neural contribution in the late stages of the disease.[53] Furthermore, patients with essential hypertension who have higher than normal levels of plasma catecholamines will demonstrate an appropriate suppression of these levels with clonidine administration in contrast to patients with pheochromocytoma.[55] In these latter patients, because the catecholamines are produced by the adrenal tumor, suppression of catecholamine levels does not occur.

Renin is released from the juxtaglomerular (JG) apparatus of the kidney upon stimulation by intravascular volume contraction, decreases in dietary sodium intake, beta adrenergically mediated neural input to the JG apparatus, reduced plasma levels of aldosterone, posture, certain drugs, and other causes.[3,46] (See also Chap. 25.) The released renal enzyme, renin, acts on a circulating peptide-protein substrate complex (produced in the liver), angiotensinogen; the result is the liberation of the decapeptide angiotensin I. Angiotensin I is transformed especially in the pulmonary circulation by the angiotensin converting enzyme, which cleaves off a terminal dipeptide to form the powerful pressor octapeptide angiotensin II. Angiotensin II then acts on multiple target sites: vascular smooth muscle to produce vasoconstriction; adrenal cortex to release aldosterone; adrenal medulla to release catecholamines; certain medullary centers of the brain to initiate adrenergic outflow; and certain thirst centers in the brain. It also stimulates myocyte hypertrophy and has some inotropic effect.

Angiotensin II, however, may be produced by means other than this classical endocrine mechanism. Recently, alternative means of angiotensin II generation have been demonstrated in the heart.[56] Furthermore, it is now clear that the entire renin-angiotensin system has been shown to be present locally in a number of cellular systems of brain, ovary, salivary gland, uterus, liver, vascular smooth muscle, and cardiac myocytes. The precise roles for these local systems are not yet known clearly, but much has been written about the role of the intracellular generation of angiotensin II on muscle protein synthesis and its role in the development and regression of vascular and ventricular hypertrophy.[57–62] (See also Chap. 6B.) This locally generated angiotensin II may be of particular importance: (1) in the function of the cell that produced the peptide (intracrine action), (2) on neighboring cells (paracrine action), or (3) in association (autocrine) with other hormones (e.g., kinins, catecholamines, the atrial natriuretic hormone).

Measurement of plasma renin activity has important clinical implications not only in the classification of patients with essential hypertension[43,46] but also in other hypertensive states. Thus, if an adrenal steroidal form of hypertension is suspected (e.g., primary aldosteronism), plasma renin activity will be suppressed and will be associated with an expanded plasma volume, hypokalemic alkalosis, and increased urinary (or plasma levels of) aldosterone.[47] Moreover, if there are inordinately elevated levels of plasma renin activity and renal arterial disease is suspected, collection of blood from both renal veins with a vena cava sample below the level of the kidneys will be useful in the diagnosis of functionally significant renal arterial disease with hypertension. (See also Chaps. 76 and 108.)

Renopressor System

Much interest and excitement has been engendered in recent years with the role of the renin-angiotensin system in patients with essential hypertension. Sealey and Laragh[46] have suggested that patients with essential hypertension may be classified (or "profiled") according to the levels of plasma renin activity. This categorization has been suggested to be useful not only conceptually with respect to the pathophysiological alterations producing the disease but also for selecting antihypertensive therapy.[43] In general, the levels of plasma renin activity are directly related to the generated angiotensin II and to the production and release and excretion of the adrenal cortical hormone aldosterone. In order to classify these patients reproducibly, however, one must carefully determine their daily sodium intake. The higher the sodium intake, the lower the plasma renin activity and vice versa; for a given sodium intake patients with higher, normal, and lower plasma renin activity may be identified. These investigators have also suggested that the patients with high plasma renin activity are more likely to develop myocardial infarction.[63] Although no precise physiological mechanism was offered to explain this association, by employing these physiological concepts, one mechanism might be suggested. Thus, since the higher the arterial pressure or the greater the total peripheral resistance, the more contracted the intravascular volume,[16,31] and the more contracted the intravascular volume, the higher the plasma renin activity,[64] it may be argued that patients with high plasma renin activity have a circulation with greater blood and plasma viscosity.[65] These intravascular changes might, in association with potential effects of angiotensin II on atherosclerotic lesions, lead to an increased likelihood of clot formation.

Modulatory Considerations

It is particularly pertinent to consider that hormones, vasoactive substances, and growth factors not only act at their own "classical" target organs but also may modify the actions of other blood or neurally borne or local substances. Thus, certain agents may exert their physiological actions very subtly by acting with other substances. As already suggested, angiotensin II is known to amplify adrenergic function by its interaction in certain brain centers as well as at peripheral ganglionic or postganglionic areas.[66,67] Additionally, angiotensin II may interact with kinins and prostaglandins in kidney, with the atrial peptides at nerve endings or on vascular smooth-muscle membrane, and with these or other peptides (e.g., endothelin, neuropeptide Y, or substance P) at the vascular smooth-muscle membrane or intracellularly. Another possible example of this modulatory cardiovascular action occurs at the endothelial level to alter local hemodynamic functions. (See also Chap. 2.)

COMPLICATIONS OF HYPERTENSIVE DISEASE

Cardiac Complications

A number of cardiac disorders may complicate systemic arterial hypertension. The following discussion concerns primarily those that are directly attributable to the natural history of essential hypertension. Other cardiac abnormalities that complicate hypertension belong to the natural history of other diseases. For example, myocardial infarction results from occlusion of epicardial coronary arteries as a consequence of atherosclerosis, a disease with its own natural history. Nevertheless, SAH accelerates and aggravates the progression of atherosclerosis[68,69] (see also Chaps. 54 and 55) and is a major independent risk factor favoring the development of coronary artery disease.[70] (See also Chap. 62.) Diabetes mellitus is another disease that may be associated with specific cardiac complications; and it also accelerates and aggravates the development of atherosclerotic cardiovascular disease.[71,72] (See also Chap. 102.) Still another example is exogenous obesity, another independent risk factor underlying atherosclerotic coronary arterial disease,[73] which exacerbates hypertensive heart disease.[74] (See also Chap. 104.)

Left Ventricular Hypertrophy

Left ventricular hypertrophy is the major cardiac alteration associated with hypertension accounting for a risk that is independent of the elevated arterial pressure.[75] As already indicated, the left ventricle increases its mass and wall thickness progressively as a direct result of the progressive overload and increased left ventricular wall stress imposed by the increasing arterial pressure and total peripheral resistance.[8,9,17,18] The adaptive structural changes of concentric ventricular hypertrophy that occur in response to this overload[76] serve as an efficient means for the chamber to provide the forces necessary to maintain stable contractile function and to slow the development of left ventricular failure.[6,9,77] (See also Chap. 23.) Although Meerson[78] suggested that the functional sequence in this pressure overload hypertrophy is one of ventricular hyperfunction followed by a stable function and eventually failure, this does not necessarily occur in sequence. Recent studies have supported the concept that simultaneously with the increased functional performance of pressure overload hypertrophy, there is a concurrent biological response of the cardiac myocytes to increase protein synthesis and cellular hypertrophy.[79,80] These studies have demonstrated that the myocytic stretch stimulus provokes initiation of the growth program, one manifestation of which is the cellular protooncogene (c-*myc*). (See also Chap. 6B.) This hypertrophic response is also associated with functional changes. One of the earlier changes related to the development of LVH is impaired diastolic function. These changes are identified clinically and electrocardiographically by the presence of an atrial diastolic gallop rhythm (fourth heart sound) that is highly concordant with left atrial abnormality on the electrocardiogram (ECG) and an increased prevalence of cardiac dysrhythmias.[81,82] Subsequent echocardiographic studies confirmed atrial enlargement in association with diminished distensibility of the hypertrophied left ventricle[18] and impaired left atrial emptying index.[83] Subsequent studies have also confirmed left ventricular diastolic dysfunction by nuclear scintigraphy and other means.[84,85] Diastolic dysfunction, therefore, is an early manifestation of impaired ventricular function that is associated with hypertrophy. Moreover, cardiac failure associated with diastolic dysfunction in the absence of systolic functional impairment has been described, especially in elderly but also in other patients with hypertension.[86] (See Chaps. 25, 26, and 115.) Eventually, left ventricular systolic function becomes impaired following the development of diastolic dysfunction[17,18]; ultimately, if arterial pressure and ventricular afterload are not reduced, cardiac failure will supervene.[78] Prior to the advent of antihypertensive therapy, hypertension was by far the most common cause of cardiac failure[87]; recently, other diseases complicating hypertension (e.g., coronary artery disease) have also become common.

Hemodynamic mechanisms, however, are not the sole cause of the development of LVH, and additional contributing factors have been identified, including the following: the stage of hypertensive heart disease; the age, race, and gender of the patient; the presence of coexisting diseases that frequently complicate hypertensive heart disease (e.g., atherosclerosis, diabetes mellitus, exogenous obesity); vasoactive or humoral substances; growth factors; and whether or not antihypertensive or other therapy has been prescribed.[6,8,9,88-90] While it is generally appreciated that if any type of antihypertensive medication program is utilized for a long enough period of time there will be a reversal of hypertrophy and a decrease in the development of heart failure, certain types of antihypertensive agents have the ability to reverse LVH, at times independently of the hemodynamic effects of the drugs.[9,91-94] This may be demonstrated best following short-term (i.e., 3 to 8 weeks) antihypertensive therapy (clinically or experimentally) with certain centrally acting adrenergic inhibitors, beta-adrenergic blocking agents, calcium antagonists, or the angiotensin converting enzyme inhibitors.[6,8,9,75,88,90] Ongoing clinical studies may answer whether or not reversal of ventricular hypertrophy will be associated with reversal of the risk of cardiovascular morbidity and mortality that is associated with LVH.[91] To date, however, this has not been demonstrated. If this is shown, it will be necessary to know whether or not that reduction in risk is associated with the reduced arterial pressure, improved coronary blood flow, possible antiarrhythmic effects of the drugs employed, or the reversal of LVH itself. For the time being, the best means of decreasing the increased morbidity and mortality is to prevent the development of LVH. This requires early and continuous antihypertensive therapy, even before the hypertrophy becomes clinically manifest.[93] (See also Chap. 77.)

LVH: An Independent Risk Factor

A review of the pathophysiological mechanisms associated with the risk from LVH[95,96] is appropriate. Although the precise mechanisms imparting that risk are not known, they are suggested in part from the clinical diagnoses offered for the deaths that have been associated with LVH. It is reasonable to suggest that the diagnosis of sudden cardiac death, which may have been attributed to coronary heart disease, may actually be related to hypertensive heart disease. Patients with LVH have an increased prevalence of unifocal and multifocal ventricular premature beats as well as ventricular tachycardia.[95-99] Thus, sudden death may be produced by lethal ventricular arrhythmias even if arterial occlusive disease is not present. There is also abundant evidence that coronary blood flow per gram of tissue is reduced in LVH and that this is associated with an increased minimal coronary vascular resistance and a diminished coronary blood flow reserve.[100-103] Each of these factors may be attributable to the coronary arteriolar disease that is associated with hypertension per se; each may provide a reasonable pathophysiological mechanism for acute myocardial ischemia and sudden death. In addition, since LVH provides an adaptive and functional protection against increased myocardial demands (e.g., by physiological or other interventions), acute left ventricular failure may also provide another pathophysiological explanation for death.[96] Finally, atherosclerotic coronary artery disease may be present in patients with LVH and hypertension and may provide a precipitating cause of death.

Myocardial Ischemia and Myocardial Infarction

There are several mechanisms that may explain the presence of angina pectoris or myocardial infarction in the hypertensive patient with LVH. Chest pain may occur in these patients even in the absence of atherosclerotic coronary artery disease. A major determinant of myocardial oxygen demand is systolic wall stress, which is dependent on two factors: left ventricular systolic pressure

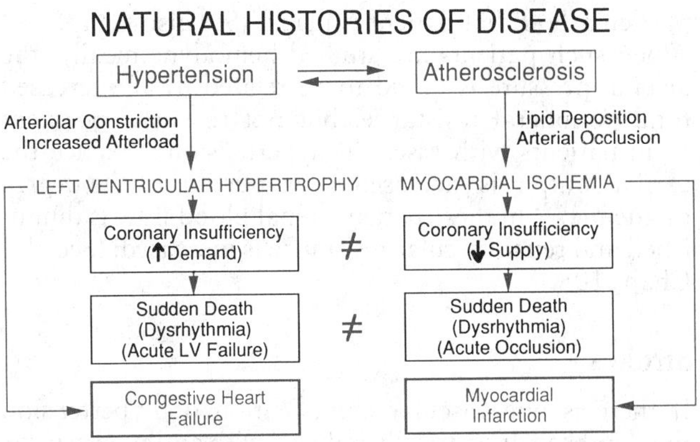

NATURAL HISTORIES OF DISEASE

Hypertension ⇄ Atherosclerosis

Arteriolar Constriction
Increased Afterload

Lipid Deposition
Arterial Occlusion

LEFT VENTRICULAR HYPERTROPHY — MYOCARDIAL ISCHEMIA

Coronary Insufficiency (↑Demand) ≠ Coronary Insufficiency (↓Supply)

Sudden Death (Dysrhythmia) (Acute LV Failure) ≠ Sudden Death (Dysrhythmia) (Acute Occlusion)

Congestive Heart Failure — Myocardial Infarction

FIGURE 75-1 The natural histories of hypertensive and atherosclerotic disease are independent, but the two diseases also interact with one another to facilitate and exacerbate ischemic heart disease.

and the left ventricular chamber diameter.[104] (See Chap. 5.) Both of these functions are increased in the hypertensive patient with LVH; hence, myocardial ischemia often occurs in pure hypertensive heart disease.[17,102,103] Myocardial infarction, especially subendocardial, may also occur. Moreover, since hypertension is an important accelerating factor for the development of atherosclerotic coronary artery disease,[68,69,105,106] this always remains as an important consideration (Fig. 75-1). Finally, since both hypertension and atherosclerosis may be associated with alterations in the endothelium of the coronary arteries, it is possible that local coronary arterial factors may be associated with impaired coronary blood flow. (See also Chap. 56.) Of course, other factors or a combination of mechanisms may also account for these changes.

In recent years several explanations have been offered to explain why the incidence of myocardial infarction has not been decreased to the extent that stroke has been diminished in studies of antihypertensive therapy. In part, this discrepancy might be explained on the basis that many of the cardiac deaths in patients with hypertension (in the large number of multicenter clinical studies) may have been due to hypertensive heart disease rather than to what has been typically termed "coronary heart disease." Another possible explanation is that most of these studies have been conducted with agents (e.g., diuretics) that may have increased serum lipids, a factor that may have offset the antihypertensive benefits and favored atherogenesis and, hence, occlusive epicardial coronary artery disease.[107] Alternatively, the deaths in these patients could also be attributable to hypokalemia or some other factor discussed above. Finally, since hypertensive and atherosclerotic heart diseases each have their own natural history, it may require a longer treatment period to reduce the cardiac atherosclerotic complications compared to other complications (e.g., stroke).[108]

J-Shaped Curves Phenomenon

Another controversy is the possibility that mildly hypertensive patients (i.e., those whose pretreatment diastolic pressures ranged from 90 through 94 mmHg) may have the potential of an increased incidence of death coincident with antihypertensive therapy.[109–111] In these patients and in more severe hypertensives excessive lowering of blood pressure has been speculated to increase mortality. (See also Chap. 77.) Although the mechanisms of this so-called J-shaped mortality curve are unknown, several possibilities include the following: impaired autoregulatory flow responses in the hypertensive heart; impaired coronary perfusion during diastole due to excessively vigorous reduction of diastolic pressure; or a combination. This issue must be resolved by prospective studies. Recently, three multicenter studies were conducted in elderly hypertensive and normotensive patients with symptomatic or asymptomatic ischemic heart disease. In those elderly patients having isolated systolic hypertension, deaths from stroke and myocardial infarction were significantly reduced in association with a reduction in diastolic pressure.[112] Moreover, normotensive patients of the SAVE and SOLVD studies having ischemic heart disease were also treated with angiotensin converting enzyme inhibiting agents that reduced diastolic pressure.[113,114] These patients also demonstrated a significant reduction in myocardial infarction. At present, however, it is reasonable to suggest that in patients with hypertension and coexisting coronary artery disease particular caution should be exercised in reducing arterial pressure and that diastolic pressure reduction be confined to levels above 75 to 80 mmHg. (See also Chap. 77.)

Aortic Dissection

Dissecting aneurysms of the thoracic and abdominal aorta were frequent complications of hypertension in the past. In recent years, the prevalence of this complication has diminished with antihypertensive therapy. Indeed, such therapy has been advocated for these patients even if they are normotensive. The elevated arterial pressure and the increased force of left ventricular ejection and flow may favor the shearing flow forces that aggravate aortic or other arterial dissection.[115] It is for this reason that agents with some negative inotropic action (i.e., beta-adrenergic receptor blocking drugs) are useful in this condition. (See also Chap. 123.)

Malignant and Accelerated Hypertension

These forms of hypertension have become less common with the widespread use of antihypertensive therapy. It represents a sudden acceleration in the vascular disease associated with essential hypertension. It is always wise to evaluate the affected patient for a secondary form of hypertension such as occlusive renal arterial disease (fibrosing or atherosclerotic). (See Chap. 76.) The clinical course is rapidly progressive with over 97 percent of the patients dying within 1 year if not treated.[116] Pathologically, there is an onion-skinned appearance of the arterioles throughout the body that is associated with a necrotizing arteriolitis, round cell infiltration in the media of the vessel wall, deposition of protein and complement within the muscle layer, and severe arteriolar spasm. Physiologically, these changes are associated with diminished blood flow, particularly to the kidney, which provokes a state of secondary hyperaldosteronism manifested by hyperreninemia and hyperaldosteronism, hypokalemic alkalosis, and microangiopathic hemolytic anemia. Vigorous antihypertensive therapy will reverse this seemingly positive feedback mechanism that produces a "vicious cycle" toward death. (See also Chap. 123.)

End-Stage Renal Disease and Nephrosclerosis

More frequently, essential hypertension is associated with renal arteriolar thickening, fibrinoid deposition in the glomeruli, and proteinuria (usually less than 0.5 g daily).[117] Hyperuricemia that is independent of abnormal purine metabolism or a personal or familial history of gout frequently is associated with untreated hypertension,[118] and the height of serum uric acid levels in these untreated patients is directly related to a decrement in renal blood flow and an increase in renal vascular resistance.[119] These renal changes usually follow the development of echocardiographically demonstrable LVH.[120] Nephrologists have become increasingly concerned with the dramatic increase in end-stage renal failure, particularly in patients with hypertension and even more so in those who are black.[121] For any level of arterial pressure, black patients have lesser renal blood flow and higher renal vascular resistance[122,123]; they are also at greater risk for end-stage renal disease.[121] (See also Chap. 108.)

There have been few renal hemodynamic studies of patients with nephrosclerosis. Some have demonstrated a reduction in renal blood flow that may or may not be associated with a reduction in glomerular filtration rate.[117] Most intrarenal hemodynamic studies of experimental hypertension have been concerned with renal micropuncture of an experimental model with a remnant kidney.[124,125] In these studies, reduction in renal blood flow and glomerular filtration rate have been associated with increased renal filtration fraction and proteinuria. These findings suggested that renal functional impairment associated with more advanced nephrosclerosis may be related to glomerular ultrafiltration, proteinuria, and consequent glomerulosclerosis. Renal micropuncture was also accomplished in the spontaneously hypertensive rat (without remnant kidney), and hemodynamics were determined before and after further increase in arterial pressure produced by phenylephrine (an alpha-adrenergic receptor agonist). Pressure elevation was associated with reduction in renal blood flow, efferent arteriolar constriction, increased glomerular hydrostatic pressure, and increased renal filtration fraction.[126,127] Each of these changes was reversed by an alpha-adrenergic receptor inhibitor. Further studies in patients with essential hypertension are necessary to unravel the pathophysiological alterations involved and to determine whether or not the intrarenal hemodynamic alterations progress to end-stage renal disease.

Parenchymal Renal Disease

Hypertension is a frequent complication of most renal diseases, whether glomerulonephritis, polycystic renal disease, or others. Hypertension associated with parenchymal disease of the kidney should be considered in any hypertensive patient with anemia of undetermined cause, particularly if that patient is black. (See also Chap. 76.) When such patients are studied hemodynamically, the arterial pressure is found to be related to an increased total peripheral resistance, but not to such an extent as in patients with essential hypertension[1,2,41] since the cardiac output is increased in proportion to the degree of anemia.[128] In these patients renal blood flow is diminished and renal vascular resistance is increased. (See also Chap. 108.)

Strokes

If there is one vascular complication of hypertension that has been dramatically reduced with antihypertensive therapy, it is that due to stroke, whether hemorrhagic, thrombotic, or rupture of small Charcot-Beauchard aneurysms.[129] (See also Chap. 122.) Since the advent of widespread, effective antihypertensive therapy, there has been at least a 50 percent reduction in fatal strokes, which are also common in the majority of the population who do not have systemic arterial hypertension. Other common complications are the so-called small strokes. These may also be the result of embolic disease from the major great vessels or left side of the heart; paradoxic emboli, or rupture of small Charcot-Beauchard cerebral artery aneurysms. They should be considered in any patient with hypertension with unexplained, transient signs and symptoms of sensory, motor, or speech deficits.

REFERENCES

1. Frohlich ED: Hemodynamics of hypertension. In: Genest J, Koiw E, Kuchel O (eds): *Hypertension: Physiopathology and Treatment.* New York, McGraw-Hill, 1977: 15–49.
2. Frohlich ED: Hemodynamic factors in the pathogenesis and maintenance of hypertension. *Fed Proc* 1982; 41:2400–2408.
3. Frohlich ED, Messerli FH, Re RN, Dunn FG: Mechanisms controlling arterial pressure. In: Frohlich ED (ed): *Pathophysiology: Altered Regulatory Mechanisms in Disease,* 3d ed. Philadelphia, Lippincott, 1984: 45–81.
4. Frohlich ED: Mechanisms contributing to high blood pressure. *Ann Intern Med* 1983; 98:709–714.
5. Page IH: The mosaic theory of arterial hypertension—its interpretation. *Perspect Biol Med* 1967; 10:325–333.
6. Frohlich ED: (State of the Art): The first Irvine H. Page lecture: The mosaic of hypertension: Past, present, and future. *J Hypertens* 1988; 6(suppl 4):S2–S11.
7. Freis ED: Hemodynamics of hypertension. *Physiol Rev* 1960; 40:27–54.
8. Frohlich ED: The heart in hypertension. In: Genest J, Kuchel O, Hamet P, Cantin M (eds): *Hypertension: Physiopathology and Treatment,* 2d ed. New York, McGraw-Hill, 1983: 791–810.
9. Frohlich ED: The heart in hypertension: A 1991 overview. *Hypertension* 1991; 18(III):62–68.
10. Ulrych M, Frohlich ED, Dustan HP, Page IH: Cardiac output and distribution of blood volume in central and peripheral circulations in hypertensive and normotensive man. *Br Heart J* 1969; 31:570–574.
11. Trippodo NC, Yamamoto J, Frohlich ED: Whole-body venous capacity and effective total tissue compliance in SHR. *Hypertension* 1981; 3:104–112.
12. Yamamoto J, Trippodo NC, MacPhee AA, Frohlich ED: Decreased total venous capacity in Goldblatt hypertensive rats. *Am J Physiol* 1981; 240:H487–H492.
13. Frohlich ED, Kozul VJ, Tarazi RC, Dustan HP: Physiological comparison of labile and essential hypertension. *Circ Res* 1970; 27:55–69.
14. Messerli FH, de Carvalho JGR, Christie B, Frohlich ED: Systemic

and regional hemodynamics in low, normal, and high cardiac output in borderline hypertension. *Circulation* 1978; 58:441–448.

15. Tarazi RC, Frohlich ED, Dustan HP: Plasma volume in men with essential hypertension. *N Engl J Med* 1968; 278:762–765.
16. Tarazi RC, Dustan HP, Frohlich ED, Gifford RW Jr, Hoffman GC: Plasma volume and chronic hypertension. Relationship to arterial pressure levels in different hypertensive diseases. *Arch Intern Med* 1970; 125:835–842.
17. Frohlich ED, Tarazi RC, Dustan HP: Clinical-physiological correlations in the development of hypertensive heart disease. *Circulation* 1971; 44:446–455.
18. Dunn FG, Chandraratna P, de Carvalho JGR, Basta LL, Frohlich ED: Pathophysiologic assessment of hypertensive heart disease with echocardiography. *Am J Cardiol* 1977; 39:789–795.
19. Bond M, Somlyo AP: Calcium regulation of contraction of arterial smooth muscle. In: Aoki K, Frohlich ED (eds): *Calcium in Essential Hypertension.* Tokyo, Academic, 1989: 39–64.
20. Nishimura J, van Breeman C: Regulation of the Ca^{2+}-sensitivity of vascular smooth muscle contractile elements. *Adv Exper Med Biol* 1991; 308:9–25.
21. Folköw B: The fourth Volhard lecture. Cardiovascular structural adaptation: Its role in the initiation and maintenance of primary hypertension. *Clin Sci Mol Med* 1978; 55:3–225.
22. Berk BC, Corson MA: Autocrine/paracrine growth mechanisms in vascular smooth muscle. *Curr Opin Cardiol* 1992; 7:739–744.
23. Owens GK: Influence of blood pressure on the development of medial smooth muscle hypertrophy in spontaneously hypertensive rats. *Hypertension* 1987; 9:178–187.
24. Dzau VJ, Gibbons GH: Endothelium and growth factors in vascular remodeling of hypertension. *Hypertension* 1991; 18(suppl III):III-115–III-121.
25. Murphy TJ, Alexander RW, Griendling KK, Runge MS, Bernstein KE: Isolation of a cDNA encoding the vascular type-1 angiotensin II receptor. *Nature* 1991; 351:233–235.
26. Hahn AW, Resink TJ, Scott BT, Powell J, Dohi Y, Buhler FR: Stimulation of endothelin mRNA and secretion in rat vascular smooth muscle cells: A novel autocrine function. *Cell Regul* 1990; 1:649–659.
27. Sarzani R, Arnaldi G, Takasaki I, Brecher P, Chobanian AV: Effects of hypertension and aging on platelet-derived growth factor and platelet-derived growth factor receptor expression in rat aorta and heart. *Hypertension* 1991; 18(suppl III):III-93–III-99.
28. Battegay EJ, Raines EW, Seifert RA, Bowen PDF, Ross R: TGF-beta induces bimodal proliferation of connective tissue cells via complex control of an autocrine PDGF loop. *Cell* 1990; 63:515–524.
29. Ross RC, Bowen-Pope DP, Raines EW: Platelets, macrophages, endothelium, and growth factors. Their effects upon cells and their possible roles in atherogenesis. *Ann NY Acad Sci* 1985; 454:254–260.
30. Libby P, Warner SJC, Salomon RN, Birinyi LK: Production of platelet-derived growth factor–like mitogen by smooth-muscle cells from human atheroma. *N Engl J Med* 1988; 318:1493–1498.
31. Tarazi RC: Hemodynamic role of extracellular fluid. *Circ Res* 1976; 38(suppl II):73–83.
32. Frohlich ED, Messerli FH: Sodium and hypertension. In: Papper S (ed): *Cations of Biologic Significance,* vol 2: *Sodium.* Boca Raton, FL, CRC Press, 1982: 144–174.
33. Tarazi RC, Dustan HP, Frohlich ED: Relation of plasma to interstitial fluid volume in essential hypertension. *Circulation* 1969; 40:357–365.
34. Weil JV, Chidsey CA: Plasma volume expansion resulting from interference with adrenergic functions in normal man. *Circulation* 1968; 37:54–61.
35. Dustan HP, Tarazi RC, Bravo EL: Dependence of arterial pressure on intravascular volume in treated hypertensive patients. *N Engl J Med* 1972; 286:861–866.
36. Dustan HP, Tarazi RC, Bravo EL: Diuretic and diet treatment of hypertension. *Arch Intern Med* 1974; 133:1007–1013.
37. The Joint National Committee on the Detection, Evaluation, and Treatment of High Blood Pressure: The 1988 Report of the Joint National Committee on Detection, Evaluation, and Treatment of High Blood Pressure. *Arch Intern Med* 1988; 148:1023–1038.
38. Frohlich ED: Hypertension: Essential. In: Hurst JW (ed): *Current Therapy in Cardiovascular Disease,* 3d ed. Philadelphia, BC Decker, 1991: 297–304.
39. Frohlich ED: Hypertension. In: Rakel RE (ed): *Conn's Current Therapy 1989.* Philadelphia, BC Decker, 1989: 225–241.
40. Bravo EL, Dustan HP, Tarazi RC: Spironolactone as a nonspecific treatment for primary aldosteronism. *Circulation* 1973; 48:491–498.
41. Frohlich ED, Tarazi RC, Dustan HP: Hemodynamic and functional mechanisms in two renal hypertension: Arterial and pyelonephritis. *Am J Med Sci* 1971; 261:189–195.
42. Dustan HP, Bravo EL, Tarazi RC: Volume-dependent essential and steroid hypertension. *Am J Cardiol* 1973; 31:606–615.
43. Bühler FR, Laragh JH, Baer L, Vaughan ED Jr, Brunner HR: Propranolol inhibition of renin secretion: A specific approach to diagnosis and treatment of renin-dependent hypertensive diseases. *N Engl J Med* 1972; 287:1209–1214.
44. Page LB: Hypertension and atherosclerosis in primitive and accelerating societies. In: Hunt JC, Cooper T, Frohlich ED, Gifford RW Jr, Kaplan NM, Laragh JH, Maxwell MH, Strong CG (eds): *Hypertension Update: Mechanisms, Epidemiology, Evaluation, Management.* Bloomfield, NJ, Health Learning Systems, 1980: 1–12.
45. Ives H: Ion transport defects and hypertension. Where's the link. *Hypertension* 1989; 14:590–597.
46. Sealey JE, Laragh JH: The renin-angiotensin-aldosterone system for normal regulation of blood pressure and sodium and potassium homeostasis. In: Laragh JH, Brenner BM (eds): *Hypertension: Pathophysiology, Diagnosis and Management.* New York, Raven Press, 1990: 1287–1317.
47. Bravo EL: Clinical aspects of endocrine hypertension. *Med Clin NA* 1987; 71:907–920.
48. Resnick LM: Calciotropic hormones in human and experimental hypertension. *Am J Hypertens* 1990; 3:171S–178S.
49. Frohlich ED, Tarazi RC, Dustan HP: Re-examination of the hemodynamics of hypertension. *Am J Med Sci* 1969; 257:9–23.
50. McCubbin JW, Green JH, Page IH: Baroreceptor function in chronic renal hypertension. *Circ Res* 1956; 4:205–210.
51. DeQuattro V, Miura Y: Neurogenic factors in human hypertension: Mechanism or myth? *Am J Med* 1971; 55:362–378.
52. Messerli FH, Frohlich ED, Suarez DH, Reisin E, Dreslinski GR, Dunn FG, et al: Borderline hypertension: Relationship between age, hemodynamics, and circulating catecholamines. *Circulation* 1981; 64:760–764.
53. Frohlich ED, Tarazi RC, Ulrych M, Dustan HP, Page IH: Tilt test for investigation of a neural component in hypertension and its correlation with clinical characteristics. *Circulation* 1967; 36:387–393.
54. Ferrario CM, Averill DB: Do primary dysfunctions in neural control of arterial pressure contribute to hypertension? *Hypertension* 1991; 18(I):38–51.
55. Bravo EL, Tarazi RC, Fouad FM, Vidt DG, Gifford RW Jr: Clonidine-suppression test: A useful aid in the diagnosis of pheochromocytoma. *N Engl J Med* 1981; 305:623–626.
56. Santos RAS, Brum JM, Brosnihan KB, Ferrario CM: The renin angiotensin system during acute myocardial ischemia in dogs. *Hypertension* 1990; 15(I):121–127.
57. Dzau VJ, Re RN: Evidence for the existence of renin in the heart. *Circulation* 1987; 75(suppl I):I-134–I-136.
58. Dzau VJ, Bart DW, Piatt RE: Molecular biology of the renin-angiotensin system. *Am J Physiol* 1988; 255:F563–573.
59. Re RN, Dzau VJ, Fallon JT, Quay S, Haber E: Renin synthesis by cultured arterial smooth muscle cells. *Life Sci* 1982; 30:99–106.
60. Dzau VJ: Significance of vascular renin-angiotensin pathways. *Hypertension* 1986; 89:544–548.
61. Frohlich ED, Iwata T, Sasaki O: Clinical and physiological significance of local tissue renin-angiotensin systems. *Am J Med* 1989; 87(I):19–23.
62. Unger T, Gohlke P: Tissue renin-angiotensin systems in the heart and vasculature: Possible involvement in the cardiovascular enzyme inhibitions. *Am J Cardiol* 1990; 65(I):3–10.
63. Alderman MH, Madhavan S, Ooi WL, Cohan H, Sealey JE, Laragh JH: Association of the renin sodium profile with the risk of myocardial infarction in patients with hypertension. *N Engl J Med* 1991; 324:1098–1104.
64. Dustan HP, Tarazi RC, Frohlich ED: Functional correlates of

plasma renin activity in hypertensive patients. *Circulation* 1970; 41:555–567.

65. Chrysant SG, Frohlich ED, Adamopoulos PN, Stein PD, Whitcomb WH, Allen EW, et al: Pathophysiologic significance of "stress" or relative polycythemia in essential hypertension. *Am J Cardiol* 1976; 37:1069–1072.
66. Joy MD, Lowe RD: Site of cardiovascular action of angiotensin II in the brain. *Clin Sci* 1970; 39:327–336.
67. McCubbin JW, Page IH: Neurogenic component of chronic renal hypertension. *Science* 1963; 139:210–215.
68. Dustan HP: George Lyman Duff Lecture. Atherosclerosis complicating chronic hypertension. *Circulation* 1974; 50:871–879.
69. Wittels EW, Gotto AM Jr: Atherogenic mechanisms. In: Frohlich ED (ed): *Pathophysiology: Altered Regulatory Mechanisms in Disease,* 3d ed. Philadelphia, Lippincott, 1984: 107–118.
70. Kannel WB, Dawber TR, Kagan A, Revotskie N, Stokes J III: Factors of risk in the development of coronary heart disease. Six years' follow-up experience. *Ann Intern Med* 1961; 55:33–50.
71. Ostrander LD Jr, Francis T Jr, Hayer NS, Kjelsberg MD, Epstein FH: The relationship of cardiovascular disease in hyperglycemia. *Ann Intern Med* 1965; 62:1188–1198.
72. Grossman E, Shemesh J, Shemiss A, Thaler M, Carroll J, Rosenthal T: Left ventricular mass in diabetes/hypertension. *Arch Intern Med* 1992; 152(5):1001–1004.
73. Kannel WB, Brand N, Skinner J, Dawber T, McNamara P: Relation of adiposity to blood pressure and development of hypertension: The Framingham Study. *Ann Intern Med* 1967; 67:48–59.
74. Frohlich ED, Reisin E: Hemodynamics in patients with overweight and hypertension. In: Safar ME, Fouad-Tarazi FM (eds): *The Heart in Hypertension.* The Netherlands, Kluwer Academic Publishers, 1989: 105–122.
75. Frohlich ED, Apstein C, Chobanian AV, Devereux RB, Dustan HP, Dzau V, et al: The heart in hypertension. *N Engl J Med* (in press).
76. Linzbach AJ: Heart failure from the point of view of quantitative anatomy. *Am J Cardiol* 1960; 5:370–382.
77. Grossman W: Cardiac hypertrophy: Useful adaptation or pathologic process? *Am J Med* 1980; 69:576–584.
78. Meerson FZ: Compensatory hyperfunction, hyperadaptation, and insufficiency of the heart. In: Katz AM (ed): *The Failing Heart: Adaptation and Deadaptation.* New York, Raven, 1983: 47–66.
79. Komuro I, Kaida T, Shibazaki Y, Kurabayashi M, Katoch Y, Hoh E, et al: Stretching cardiac myocytes stimulates proto-oncogene expression. *J Biol Chem* 1990; 265:3595–3598.
80. Kumuro I, Sibazaki Y, Kurabayashi M, Takaku F, Yazaki Y: Molecular cloning of gene sequences from rat heart rapidly responsive to pressure overload. *Circ Res* 1990; 66:979–985.
81. Tarazi RC, Miller A, Frohlich ED, Dustan HP: Electrocardiographic changes reflecting left atrial abnormality in hypertension. *Circulation* 1966; 34:818–822.
82. Tarazi RC, Frohlich ED, Dustan HP: Left atrial abnormality and ventricular pre-ejection period in hypertension. *Dis Chest* 1969; 55:214–218.
83. Dreslinski GR, Frohlich ED, Dunn FG, Messerli FG, Suarez DH, Reisin E: Echocardiographic diastolic ventricular abnormality in hypertensive heart disease: Atrial emptying index. *Am J Cardiol* 1981; 47:1087–1090.
84. Inouye I, Massie B, Loge D, Topic N, Silverstein D, Simpson P, Tabau J: Abnormal left ventricular filling: An early finding in mild to moderate systemic hypertension. *Am J Cardiol* 1984; 53:120–126.
85. Fouad FM, Slominski JM, Tarazi RC: Left ventricular diastolic function in hypertension: Relation to left ventricular mass and systolic function. *J Am Coll Cardiol* 1984; 3:1500–1506.
86. Topol EJ, Traill TA, Fortulin NJ: Hypertensive hypertrophic cardiomyopathy of the elderly. *N Engl J Med* 1985; 312:377–383.
87. Kannel WB, Castelli WP, McNamara PM, McKee PA, Feinlieb M: Role of blood pressure in the development of congestive heart failure. The Framingham Study. *N Engl J Med* 1972; 287:781–787.
88. Frohlich ED: Hemodynamics and other determinants in development of left ventricular hypertrophy: Conflicting factors in its regression. *Fed Proc* 1983; 42:2709–2715.
89. Frohlich ED, Tarazi RC: Is arterial pressure the sole factor responsible for hypertensive cardiac hypertrophy? *Am J Cardiol* 1979; 44:959–963.
90. Frohlich ED: Overview of hemodynamic and non-hemodynamic factors associated with LVH. *J Mol Cell Cardiol* 1989; 21:3–10.
91. Frohlich ED: Is reversal of left ventricular hypertrophy in hypertension beneficial? *Hypertension* 1991; 18(I):133–138.
92. Pfeffer JM, Pfeffer MA, Weiss AK, Frohlich ED: Development of SHR hypertension and cardiac hypertrophy during prolonged beta blockage. *Am J Physiol* 1977; 232:H639–H644.
93. Frohlich ED: Regression of cardiac hypertrophy and left ventricular pumping ability post-regression. *J Cardiovasc Pharmacol* 1991; 17(suppl 2):81–86.
94. Frohlich ED, Horinaka S: Cardiac and aortic effects of angiotensin in converting enzyme inhibitors. *Hypertension* 1991; 18(II):2–7.
95. Kannel WB, Gordon T, Castelli WP, Margolia JR: Electrocardiographic left ventricular hypertrophy and risk of coronary heart disease. The Framingham Study. *Ann Intern Med* 1970; 72:813–822.
96. Frohlich ED: Left ventricular hypertrophy: An independent factor of risk. In: Frohlich Ed (ed): *Preventative Aspects of Coronary Heart Disease.* Philadelphia, FA Davis, 1990: 297–304.
97. Messerli FH, Ventura HO, Elizardi DJ, Dunn FG, Frohlich ED: Hypertension and sudden death: Increased ventricular ectopic activity in left ventricular hypertrophy. *Am J Med* 1984; 77:18–22.
98. Levy D, Anderson KM, Savage DD, Balkus SA, Kannel WB, Castelli WP: Risk of ventricular arrhythmias in left ventricular hypertrophy: The Framingham Heart Study. *Am J Cardiol* 1987; 60:560–565.
99. MeLenachan JM, Henderson E, Morris KI, Dargie HJ: Ventricular arrhythmias in patients with hypertensive left ventricular hypertrophy. *N Engl J Med* 1987; 317:787–792.
100. Harrison DG, Barnes DH, Diratzka LF, Eastham CL, Kerber RE, Marcus ML: The effect of cardiac hypertrophy on the coronary collateral circulation. *Circulation* 1985; 71:1135–1145.
101. Harrison DG, Florentine MS, Brooks LA, Cooper SM, Marcus ML: The effect of hypertension and left ventricular hypertrophy on the lower range of coronary autoregulation. *Circulation* 1988; 77:1108–1115.
102. Brush JE Jr, Cannon RO, Schenke WH, Bonow RO, Leon MB, Maron BJ, Epstein SE: Angina due to coronary microvascular disease in hypertensive patients without left ventricular hypertrophy. *N Engl J Med* 1988; 319:1302–1307.
103. Houghton JL, Frank MJ, Carr AA, vonDohlen TW, Prisant LM: Relations among impaired coronary flow reserve, left ventricular hypertrophy and thallium perfusion defects in hypertensive patients without obstructive coronary artery disease. *J Am Coll Cardiol* 1991; 15:43–51.
104. Sarnoff SJ, Braunwald E, Welch GH Jr, et al: Hemodynamic determinants of oxygen consumption of the heart with special reference to the tension-time index. *Am J Physiol* 1958; 192:148–156.
105. MacMahon S, Peto R, Cutler J, Collins R, Sorlie P, Neaton J, et al: Blood pressure, stroke, and coronary heart disease. part I: Prolonged differences in blood pressure: Prospective observational studies corrected for the regression dilution bias. *Lancet* 1990; 335:765–774.
106. Neaton JD, Wentworth D: Serum cholesterol, blood pressure, cigarette smoking, and death from coronary heart disease. Overall findings and differences by age for 316 099 white men. *Arch Int Med* 1992; 152:56–64.
107. Weinberger MH: Influence of an angiotensin converting enzyme inhibitor on diuretic-induced metabolic effects in hypertension. *Hypertension* 1983; 5(suppl III):132–138.
108. Frohlich ED: Current issues in hypertension: Old questions with new answers and new questions. *Med Clin N Am* 1992; 76:1043–1056.
109. Cruickshank JM, Thorp JM, Zacharias FJ: Benefits and potential harm of lowering blood pressure. *Lancet* 1987; 1:581–584.
110. Alderman MH, Ooi WL, Madharsn S: Treatment induced blood pressure reduction and the risk of myocardial infarction. *JAMA* 1989; 262:920–924.
111. Farnett L, Mulrow CD, Linn WD, Lucey CR, Tuley MR: The J-curve phenomenon and the treatment of hypertension. *JAMA* 1991; 265:489–495.
112. SHEP Cooperative Research Group: Prevention of stroke by antihypertensive drug treatment in older persons with isolated systolic hypertension. Final results of the Systolic Hypertension

in the Elderly Program (SHEP). *JAMA* 1991; 265:3255–3264.

113. Pfeffer MA, Braunwald E, Moye LA, Basta L, Brown EJ Jr, Cuddy TE, et al: Effect of captopril on mortality and morbidity in patients with left ventricular dysfunction after myocardial infarction. Results of the survival and ventricular enlargement trial. *N Engl J Med* 1992; 327:669–677.
114. Effect of enalapril on survival in patients with reduced left ventricular ejection fractions and CHF, SOLVD Trial Investigators. *N Engl J Med* 1991; 325:293–302.
115. Bhatia S, Frohlich ED: Hemodynamic comparison of agents useful in hypertensive emergencies. *Am Heart J* 1973; 85:367–373.
116. Frohlich ED: Hypertensive Emergencies. In: Chung EK (ed): *Cardiac Emergency Care.* Philadelphia, Lea & Febiger, 1991: 304–319.
117. Schwartz GL, Strong CG: Renal parenchymal involvement in essential hypertension. *Med Clin N Am* 1987; 71:843–858.
118. Stanton JR, Freis ED: The serum uric acid concentration in essential hypertension. *Proc Soc Exp Biol Med* 1947; 66:193–194.
119. Messerli FH, Frohlich ED, Dreslinski GR, Suarez DH, Aristimuno GG: Serum uric acid in essential hypertension: An indicator of renal vascular involvement. *Ann Intern Med* 1980; 93:817–821.
120. Kobrin I, Frohlich ED, Ventura HO, Messerli FH: Renal involvement follows cardiac enlargement in essential hypertension. *Arch Intern Med* 1986; 146:272–276.
121. Luke RG: Can renal failure due to hypertension be prevented. *Hypertension* 1991; 18(I):139–142.
122. Frohlich ED, Messerli FH, Dunn FG, Oigman W, Ventura HO, Sundgaard-Riise K: Greater renal vascular involvement in the black patient with essential hypertension. A comparison of systemic and renal hemodynamics in black and white patients. *Miner Electrolyte Metab* 1984; 10:173–177.
123. Dustan HP, Curtis JJ, Luke RG, Rostand SG: Systemic hypertension and the kidney in black patients. *Am J Cardiol* 1987; 60(I):73–77.
124. Brenner BM, Meyer TW, Hostetter TH: Dietary protein intake and the progressive nature of kidney disease: The role of hemodynamically mediated glomerular injury in pathogenesis of progressive glomerular sclerosis in aging, renal ablation, and intrinsic renal disease. *N Engl J Med* 1982; 307:652–659.
125. Hostetter TH, Olson JL, Rennke HG, Venkatachalam MA, Brenner BM: Hyperfiltration in remnant nephrons: A potentially adverse response to renal ablation. *Am J Physiol* 1981; 241:F85–F93.
126. Kobrin I, Pegram BL, Frohlich ED: Acute pressure increase and intrarenal hemodynamics in conscious WKY and SHR rats. *Am J Physiol* 1985; 249:H1114–H1118.
127. Uchino K, Frohlich ED, Nishikimi T, Isshiki T, Kardon MB: Spontaneously hypertensive rats demonstrate increased renal vascular alpha$_1$-adrenergic receptor responsiveness. *Am J Physiol* 1991; 260(Regulatory, Integrative Comp Physiol 29):R889–R893.
128. Neff MS, Kim KE, Persoff M, Onesti G, Swarz C: Hemodynamics of uremic anemia. *Circulation* 1971; 43:876–883.
129. Roccella EJ, Boroler AE, Horan M: Epidemiologic considerations in defining hypertension. *Med Clin N Am* 1987; 71:785–802.

Chapter 76

Diagnostic Evaluation of the Patient with Systemic Arterial Hypertension

W. Dallas Hall, M.D. ■ Gary L. Wollam, M.D.
Elbert P. Tuttle, Jr., M.D.

BLOOD PRESSURE MEASUREMENT

The measurement of blood pressure requires precision and consideration of a number of factors to avoid erroneous labeling of a normotensive patient as hypertensive.[1-3] False elevations occur often if regular-size blood pressure cuffs are used in adult patients whose midarm circumference exceeds 33 cm.[4,5] Auscultatory measurements can also overestimate intraarterial pressure in some elderly patients, presumably because of "pipe-stem" arteries due to extensive peripheral arteriosclerosis. The frequency of pseudohypertension in the elderly is not established.[6] Cuff measurements of systolic or diastolic blood pressure have been reported to exceed intraarterial levels by more than 20 mmHg in as few as 2 percent to as many as 9 percent of relatively healthy elderly normotensive or hypertensive patients.[7-9]

An "auscultatory gap" is not uncommon in elderly patients with arteriosclerosis; it can cause either an underestimation of systolic pressure or an overestimation of diastolic pressure.[10] It occurs most often in the sitting or standing positions and in elderly patients with high systolic pressures. The auscultatory gap is detected by first estimating systolic pressure by palpation and continuing to listen over the artery until the manometer falls 20 to 30 mm below the disappearance of the Korotkov sounds.

Blood pressure should initially be measured in both arms, and all subsequent determinations should be performed in the arm with the highest pressure. If measurements are made simultaneously with deflation of the cuff at a rate less than 1 mmHg per second, differences greater than 10 mmHg are unusual in the absence of advanced arteriosclerosis.[11]

The position of the arm during the blood pressure measurement can be a source of variation in readings. When blood pressure is measured in the sitting or standing position, lowering the arm from a near-horizontal (i.e., "heart level") to a near-vertical position results in an increase in both the systolic and diastolic blood pressure readings. This increase in the measured blood pressure with vertical arm displacement has been attributed to changes in hydrostatic pressure.[12,13]

Blood pressure should always be measured in the standing as well as the supine or sitting position in patients with hypertension. This is because orthostatic hypotension, especially common in diabetic and elderly patients, can influence the choice of antihypertensive therapy. The normal blood pressure response to standing is a slight decrease in systolic and a slight increase in diastolic pressure, with little change in mean arterial pressure.[14] Standing reductions in systolic pressure of 20 mmHg or more, or mean arterial pressure of 10 percent or more, are often used as criteria for orthostatic hypotension. In general, marked orthostatic decreases in the pretreatment blood pressure indicate a poor prognosis[15] and are more common in hypertensive patients with target organ complications such as cardiomegaly, congestive heart failure, and associated vascular disease.[16]

Orthostatic hypertension (i.e., an increase in diastolic pressure exceeding 8 to 10 mmHg upon standing) has been associated with elevated norepinephrine levels and evidence of increased neurogenic tone[16,17]; it may also predict the response to adrenergic blocking drugs such as clonidine.

BLOOD PRESSURE VARIABILITY

The variability of blood pressure increases with age and with the level of the blood pressure; it is more striking with systolic than with diastolic pressure.[18,19] Some studies have found that the magnitude of variability in systolic and mean arterial pressure is related inversely to baroreceptor sensitivity.[20]

Even for normotensive individuals, however, blood pressure varies considerably throughout a 24-h period; isolated intermittent elevations of systolic pressure to levels above 150 mmHg and diastolic pressure to levels above 90 mmHg are not uncommon.[21] Blood pressure follows a circadian rhythm and is highest in the early morning hours and lowest at night.[22] When two or three consecutive blood pressure readings are taken, the first systolic reading is usually 2 to 4 mmHg higher than the second or third readings.[23] Diastolic pressure follows a similar pattern but to a lesser degree.

Souchek et al.[24] found that the mean of two or three consecutive readings at one visit provided a more accurate prediction of blood pressure over an 8-year follow-up period than did a single reading. In the Framingham Study, the mean, maximum, and minimum of three blood pressure measurements obtained during a 1-h examination were equally predictive of subsequent cardiovascular disease.[25] The lowest or more "basal" of the three blood pressures was no better predictor of cardiovascular disease than the average or the highest of the blood pressure measurements.

Blood pressure is more variable between days than within days.[26] Decreases in systolic pressure of 10 to 30 mmHg and diastolic pressure of 5 to 10 mmHg between the first and subsequent follow-up clinic visits are common.[27] In the Hypertension Detection and Follow-Up Program, over 30 percent of untreated subjects with average diastolic pressures of 95 mmHg or greater on the initial home screening had diastolic pressures below 90 mmHg approximately 1 week later.[28] In the Systolic Hypertension in the Elderly Program (SHEP), 36 percent of elderly individuals with isolated systolic hypertension at the initial visit (i.e., systolic blood pressure of 160 mmHg or more and diastolic blood pressure below 90 mmHg on the average of the last two of three readings) did not qualify at the follow-up visit within a few weeks.[29] Of those who did confirm for the second visit, an additional 30 percent did not qualify for randomization at the third visit. Ninety percent of the reason for nonrandomization was spontaneous reduction in the level of systolic blood pressure. Thus, the time of day, the number of measurements during the visit, the variability between visits, and regression toward the mean are all important considerations in making a diagnosis of hypertension.[30] In uncomplicated cases with mild or moderate elevation of blood pressure, a minimum of two measurements on each of three different days is recommended for a diagnosis of hypertension. In patients with labile or borderline elevations of blood pressure, additional visits are frequently required to accurately assess blood pressure status.[27,31]

Home blood pressure measurement and ambulatory monitoring of daytime pressure can assist in evaluation of the patient with mild or borderline hypertension.[32–35] Perloff and associates[36] demonstrated that patients whose ambulatory blood pressures remained high (as compared with the average of three initial office visit pressures) had more target organ complications and an increased number of cardiovascular events over 5 years than did a group of patients with similar average office pressures but lower ambulatory home pressures. Home blood pressure monitoring can also assist in evaluation of the response to antihypertensive therapy and in the detection of "white coat" hypertension where blood pressure is elevated when measured by the physician in an office setting but is normal during usual daytime activities.[37]

Automated ambulatory blood pressure monitoring with computerized recordings and graphic displays can be useful for the diagnosis, prognosis, and treatment of hypertension.[38,39] Current devices use either auscultatory or oscillometric methods and are relatively accurate and reproducible when used properly.[40,41] The most appropriate indication for diagnostic use is the patient with labile or borderline office readings. Figure 76-1 illustrates hourly average blood pressures in a 69-year-old male with borderline office readings (i.e., 140/88 mmHg). Blood pressure levels rose markedly while driving to work on the expressway; definite hypertension [(160–170)/(100–114) mmHg] persisted throughout the workday, but blood pressure fell dramatically during a late afternoon nap and subsequently during sleep. The results suggested that treatment was indicated and that a drug with a 12-h duration of action would be sufficient to reduce the persistent daytime hypertension. Ambulatory blood pressure measurement is more predictive than casual office pressure as an indicator of the presence of target organ damage, including echocardiographic left ventricular hypertrophy (LVH),[42–44] impaired diastolic cardiac filling,[45] microalbuminuria,[46] and the presence of lacunae and periventricular hyperintense central nervous system lesions on magnetic resonance imaging (MRI).[47]

DIAGNOSTIC EVALUATION

The Patient with Mild or Moderate Hypertension

Important considerations in the history and our recommended evaluation procedures and diagnostic tests for mild to moderate hypertension are summarized in Tables 76-1 and 76-2.[48–50] Mild to moderate hypertension is widely held to be an asymptomatic disease. However, Bulpitt et al.[51] compared symptoms in 99 untreated hypertensive subjects with those of 78 normotensive subjects of similar age; unsteadiness, waking headaches, blurred vision, depression, and nocturia were more frequent in untreated hypertensives. In addition to these

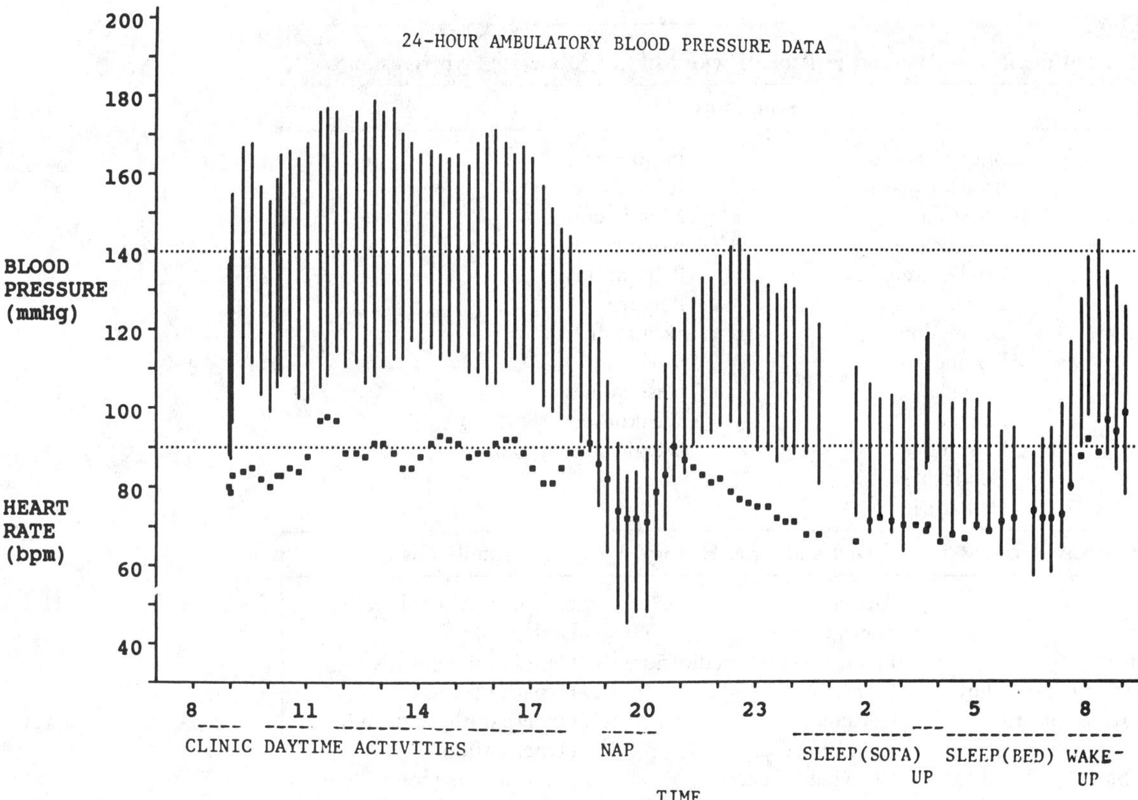

FIGURE 76-1 Ambulatory blood pressure monitoring graph of a 69-year-old untreated male with borderline office readings.

five symptoms, the clinician should also ask about other items listed in Table 76-1.

In the initial evaluation, efforts should be made to detect clinical clues to reversible causes of hypertension. For example, coarctation of the aorta is suggested by diminished leg pulses, a delay in the femoral pulse when palpated simultaneously with the radial pulse, a reduced blood pressure in the leg, a coarse systolic murmur at the left sternal border, or rib notching on the chest x-ray. Renovascular hypertension, aldosteronism, renoparenchymal hypertension, and pheochromocytoma are discussed later in this chapter. Acromegaly, hyperthyroidism, hypothyroidism, Cushing's syndrome, and alcoholism should be suspected from the history and general appearance of the patient.

In the baseline evaluation, the clinician should search for target organ damage and assess risk factors for cardiovascular disease. A careful history must be included for angina, past myocardial infarction, transient ischemic attacks, stroke, claudication, cigarette smoking, and a family history of cardiovascular events before age 55. The clinician must listen carefully for bruits over the carotid, renal, and femoral arteries and grade the amplitude of arterial pulsations in the limbs. He or she should also inspect the electrocardiogram (ECG) for evidence of ischemia and measure cholesterol levels[52] as well as perform the other recommended laboratory tests listed in Table 76-2.

Hypertension is the most common cause of congestive heart failure, which, in the Framingham Study, was associated with a 5-year mortality of 43 to 62 percent.[53] Hence, the examiner should search for LVH, rales, ventricular gallop, distended neck veins, edema, and other clinical signs of congestive heart failure.

The initial evaluation is also important for the selection of drug therapy, which may be modified if there is a history of diabetes, gout, nephrolithiasis, peptic ulcer, breast disease, severe depression, bronchospasm, edema, or a variety of other illnesses. Also, the likelihood must be estimated of proper adherence to medications and compliance in keeping appointments, because long-term control of hypertension depends on good cooperation by the patient. Choice of dosage schedules and cost of medications also influence the choice of therapy.[54–56]

The Patient with Severe, Accelerated, or Malignant Hypertension

Diagnostic criteria for "malignant hypertension" include severe hypertension, generally with diastolic pressure of 125 mmHg or more, in conjunction with target organ damage and physiological abnormalities.[57] Target organ damage includes retinal hemorrhages and exudates, papilledema, heart failure, encephalopathy, and renal insufficiency. Physiological abnormalities include impaired renal perfusion, elevated plasma renin and aldosterone levels, and increased sympathetic tone.

Because of the infrequent occurrence and the morbid prognosis of either accelerated or malignant hypertension,[58] an aggressive diagnostic approach is indicated. In addition to the items listed in Tables 76-1 and 76-2, plasma renin activity can be helpful in planning therapy. Diagnostic studies for renal artery stenosis (i.e., arterial digital subtraction angiography or renal arteriography)

TABLE 76-1
Key Items of the Baseline History in Patients with Mild or Moderate Hypertension

Symptoms	
Blurred vision	Impotence
Bronchospasm	Joint pains
Chest pain	Muscle cramps
Claudication	Nocturia
Cold extremities	Palpitations
Cough	Polyuria
Depression	Skin rash
Dizziness	Sweating
Dyspnea	Unsteadiness
Fatigue	Weakness
Flushing	Weight loss or gain
Headaches	
Hematuria	

Past Disease History	Diet and Drug History	Family History
Angina	Alcohol	Coronary heart disease
Asthma	Aspirin	Diabetes
Diabetes	Blood pressure medications	Hereditary nephritis
Congestive heart failure	Cigarettes	Hyperlipidemia
Glomerulonephritis	Cocaine	Hyperparathyroidism
Gout	Cold remedies	Hypertension
Heart block	Chewing tobacco	Pheochromocytoma
Hepatitis	Cyclosporine	Polycystic kidney disease
Hypertension	Licorice	Renovascular hypertension
Lupus erythematosus	Nasal sprays	Thyroid disorders
Myocardial infarction	Nonsteroidal anti-inflammatory agents	
Peptic ulcer	Oral contraceptives	
Pyelonephritis	Potassium (dietary)	
Toxemia	Salt (dietary)	
Transient ischemic attacks	Tricyclic antidepressants	

are indicated in severely hypertensive patients who are candidates for surgical correction or angioplasty. Davis et al.[59] identified anatomic renal artery stenosis in 7 percent of black and 42 percent of white patients who presented with a diastolic blood pressure of 125 mmHg plus retinal flame hemorrhages, cotton-wool exudates, or papilledema. Pheochromocytoma can also present with severe or resistant hypertension and can usually be excluded by obtaining plasma or urinary tests for catecholamines or their metabolites. Quantitative estimates of left ventricular anatomy and function, symmetry of renal perfusion, and ultrasonic kidney size should be considered. Appropriate studies to rule out correctable causes of hypertension are discussed in later sections of this chapter.

The Patient with Labile Hypertension

Examination of patients with labile hypertension should be much the same as that for mild and moderate hypertension because labile hypertension is associated with an increased risk of cardiovascular disease.[60] Special attention should be given to symptoms suggestive of pheochromocytoma or the abuse of alcohol,[61] diet pills,[62] cocaine,[63–69] chewing tobacco,[70] and nasal decongestants or cold remedies containing stimulants such as phenylpropanolamine.[71] The clinician should inquire about recent stressful events because emotional stress can be associated with intermittent elevations of blood pressure. Rapid pulse, dilated pupils, and sweating suggest hyperactivity of the sympathetic nervous system.

There should be no evidence of target organ damage, and the biochemical profile and urinalysis should be normal in patients with labile hypertension. The presence of any abnormality should be a cause for concern and may indicate that the seemingly intermittent elevations of blood pressure may be more persistent, of longer duration, and/or of greater magnitude than previously appreciated.

The Patient with Isolated Systolic Hypertension

Guidelines for evaluation of mild and moderate hypertension also apply to patients with isolated systolic hypertension,[72] because the cardiovascular risks associated with elevated systolic pressure are as great or even greater than those of elevated diastolic pressure.[73,74] This is particularly appropriate since the recently published SHEP

TABLE 76-2

Key Items of the Baseline Physical and Laboratory Examinations in Patients with Mild or Moderate Hypertension

Physical Examination					
General	**HEENT**†	**Chest**	**Abdomen**	**Extremities**	**Neurologic**
Appearance Blood pressure (supine or sitting; standing; both arms) Heart rate (supine or sitting; standing)	Carotid bruit Fundi Neck veins Temporal arteries Thyroid gland	Aortic regurgitation Apex impulse Breast Rales S_3; S_4 Systolic murmur Wheezes	Bruit Palpable kidneys	Edema Peripheral pulses Peripheral bruits	Focal signs Proximal muscle strength

Laboratory Examination			
General	**Kidney**	**Metabolic**	**Miscellaneous**
Hemoglobin Hematocrit White blood cell count	Blood urea nitrogen Creatinine Urine dipstick Urine sediment	Calcium Cholesterol* Glucose (fasting) Potassium Uric acid	Chest x-ray ECG Echocardiogram

* Also obtain fasting triglyceride and high-density lipoprotein cholesterol levels if the serum cholesterol level is 200 mg/dL or more in patients with other cardiovascular risk factors or 240 mg/dL or more in patients without other cardiovascular risk factors.
† HEENT = Head, Eyes, Ears, Nose, and Throat.

trial results documented that pharmacologic treatment of isolated systolic hypertension reduced the 5-year incidence of stroke by 36 percent.[29] (See Chap. 77.)

Isolated systolic hypertension is associated with an increased prevalence of diabetes mellitus, and particular note should be made of symptoms and laboratory values suggestive of glucose intolerance. Elevation of the systolic blood pressure can also be the first clue to large-vessel atherosclerosis, as can be more unusual etiologies such as coarctation of the aorta, aortic regurgitation, hyperthyroidism, arteriovenous fistulas, Paget's disease, or heavy alcohol intake.[75]

The Athlete with Hypertension

Athletes often present to the clinician for evaluation of an elevated blood pressure detected on a routine screening examination.[76] The usual story is that a physician's clearance is needed before the patient can compete in athletic events. The trained athlete's ECG can show evidence of increased vagal tone (sinus bradycardia, first- or second-degree atrioventricular block, junctional rhythm), which sometimes reverts to normal in the standing position. Other changes include high-amplitude R waves, a semivertical QRS axis in asthenic runners, or elevation of the ST segments or inversion of the T waves suggestive of ischemia.[77,78] An S_3 gallop may be heard,[76] and borderline cardiomegaly is often present on the chest x-ray. Isolated systolic hypertension in an unusually tall basketball player can be the first clue to Marfan's syndrome with aortic regurgitation. (See also Chap. 114.)

Echocardiography frequently reveals increased left ventricular posterior wall and septal wall thickness as well as increased left ventricular mass index (LVMI) in highly trained athletes participating in certain types of isometric exercise such as wrestling, shot-putting, or weight lifting. In contrast, an increase in left ventricular end-diastolic internal dimension and volume are characteristic findings in professional athletes participating primarily in isotonic exercises such as competitive running, swimming, or basketball.[79,80]

Almost all of these changes can occur in athletes with normal left-sided heart catheterization and patent coronary arteries.[81] Great caution, however, must be taken in the evaluation of such patients because almost 75 percent of reported sudden deaths in young athletes have occurred during major exertion, especially in athletes with previously undiagnosed hypertrophic cardiomyopathy.[82] Thus, in addition to the usual evaluation, consideration should be given to diagnostic procedures not generally done in the usual asymptomatic patient with hypertension. For example, echocardiography should be considered in athletes who have abnormal ST- and T-wave changes, findings suggestive of left LVH on the ECG, and/or clinical findings or a family history suggestive of hypertrophic cardiomyopathy. Echocardiography often reveals physiological LVH in athletes, although septal or posterior wall thicknesses of 13 mm or more are uncommon.[83] Diastolic left ventricular function is usually normal in athletes with physiological LVH.[84]

Monitoring of blood pressure during a treadmill test can sometimes reveal a marked increase, rather than the expected decrease, in diastolic blood pressure. These particular patients should be advised not to resume their usual exercise activities until blood pressure is well controlled. Blood pressure monitoring can also be conducted under circumstances that simulate the patient's usual exercise setting (e.g., weight lifting). The blood pressure response to the same exercise can then be reevaluated following institution of selected antihypertensive therapy.

THE DIAGNOSIS OF TARGET ORGAN DAMAGE

Hypertensive Retinopathy

The fundoscopic examination helps assess the prognosis and severity of hypertension. Keith, Wagener, and Barker[85] first noted that patients with group I (constriction), II (sclerosis, arteriovenous nicking), III (hemorrhages and exudates), and IV (papilledema) retinopathy had untreated 5-year survivals of 85, 50, 13, and 0 percent, respectively. Recent studies suggest that grade III as well as grade IV hypertensive retinopathy is also associated with a poor long-term prognosis.[58] Advanced hypertensive retinopathy (i.e., groups III and IV) is found in less than 10 percent of all hypertensive patients and is an indication for aggressive diagnostic evaluation and treatment. (See also Chap. 12.)

Arteriovenous nicking and a copper- or silver-wire appearance of the arterioles often occur in older patients and generally indicate arteriosclerosis.[86] Large inter- and intraobserver variability limits the value of fine distinctions between group I and II retinopathy, although most agree that both focal and generalized arteriolar narrowing are retinal vascular signs of hypertension.[87]

Hypertensive Cardiovascular Disease

Two major forms of heart disease occur in the patient with hypertension: coronary heart disease and hypertensive heart disease. Criteria for the diagnosis of coronary heart disease are described elsewhere. Criteria for the diagnosis of hypertensive heart disease include the presence of hypertension plus LVH when other causes of LVH are reasonably excluded. Hypertension is the most common cause of LVH.[88] Neither a long duration nor any particular level of severity of blood pressure elevation are necessary prerequisites for LVH because factors other than blood pressure elevation are important for its development. Occasional patients will develop a form of hypertensive hypertrophic cardiomyopathy characterized by dyspnea and congestive heart failure with normal systolic but impaired diastolic function of the left ventricle.[89,90]

Syndrome X is the occurrence of angina-type chest pain (often with a positive exercise test) but with normal coronary angiography and no evidence of vasospasm.[91] Cannon and Epstein[92] have presented evidence for myocardial ischemia related to microvascular angina. A similar syndrome has also been noted in hypertensive patients, especially those with LVH. Patients with syndrome X typically demonstrate ischemic ST-segment depression with dipyridamole infusion. Picano and associates[93] noted similar ischemic ST-segment changes in 10 of 28 asymptomatic patients with essential hypertension, especially those with higher left ventricular mass indices (LVMIs) and longer durations of hypertension. Opherk et al.[94] had earlier shown that in patients with longstanding essential hypertension and LVH, the coronary blood flow response was impaired following coronary vasodilation with dipyridamole. Hence, patients with hypertension and LVH are susceptible to episodes of myocardial ischemia, even in the absence of visible coronary atherosclerosis at catheterization. These observations may help explain the frequently noted ischemic T-wave changes following marked or sudden reductions of blood pressure with minoxidil,[95,] nifedipine,[96–98] or sodium nitroprusside.[97–99] (See also Chap. 58.)

Noninvasive diagnostic techniques that provide assessment of LVH include the physical examination, chest x-ray, ECG, and echocardiogram (ECHO). Detection of LVH by physical examination depends on palpation of an enlarged and sustained left ventricular impulse at the apex.[100] An enlarged apical impulse is defined as one with a diameter greater than that of a quarter (i.e., more than 2.4 cm); a sustained apical impulse has an outward thrust that lasts one-half to two-thirds or more of the duration of systole. Evaluation is maximized by examining the patient in the left lateral decubitus position where an apical impulse diameter greater than 3 cm is a more sensitive and specific finding of left ventricular enlargement than is the location of the apex impulse 10 cm or more from the midsternal line or lateral to the midclavicular line.[101,102] (See also Chap. 10.)

Detection of LVH by chest x-ray is fraught with the problems of defining which portions of the cardiac silhouette belong specifically to the left ventricle. In general, the cardiothoracic ratio should not exceed 0.5 in adults and is usually below 0.45.[103] (See also Chap. 14.)

Table 76-3 lists the criteria of Romhilt and Estes[104] for the electrocardiographic diagnosis of definite LVH (five points) or probable LVH (four points). Left ventricular hypertrophy was detected by the ECG point-score system in 58 percent of hearts hypertrophied at autopsy, but false-positive results occurred in 3 percent. A number of criteria for summed precordial voltage are as sensitive

TABLE 76-3

Estes Point-Score System for the Electrocardiographic Diagnosis of Left Ventricular Hypertrophy

	Points*
Amplitude R or S wave in limb lead ≥ 20 mm, or S wave in V_1 or V_2 ≥ 30 mm, or R wave in V_5 or V_6 ≥ 30 mm	3
Terminal negativity of the P wave in V_1 of 1 mm or more in depth and ≥ 0.04 s duration	3
ST-T segment vector opposite to QRS vector	3†
QRS axis of −30° or more	2
QRS duration ≥ 0.09 s	1
Intrinsicoid defection (ventricular activation time) ≥ 0.05 s in V_5 or V_6	1

* Five or more points equals LVH; four points equals probable LVH.

†Reduced to one point if the patient is receiving digitalis.

SOURCE: Romhilt and Estes.[104]

as the point-score system but are less specific and lead to false-positive readings of LVH in as many as 15 percent of cases.[105] As defined originally, the "typical" ST-segment shift (i.e., "strain pattern") requires more than 0.5 mm depression of the ST segment and 0.5 mm or more inversion of the T wave in the limb or left precordial leads; the resultant ST segments and T-wave vectors are opposite to the direction of the main QRS vector.[106] Refinements in the Romhilt-Estes point-score system have improved the specificity of the electrocardiographic diagnosis of LVH.[107] (See also Chap. 13.)

Electrocardiographic evidence of left atrial abnormality often precedes that of left ventricular abnormality in patients with hypertension. One set of criteria for left atrial abnormality requires two of the following four findings: terminal (negative) atrial forces in V_1 above 0.04 mm-s, bipeak interval greater than 0.04 s in deeply notched P waves in any lead, ratio of P-wave duration to PR segment exceeding 1.6 in lead II, and P wave above 0.3 mV height or above 0.12 duration in lead II.[108]

Echocardiography has revolutionized the diagnosis of LVH because echocardiographic evidence of LVH occurs in 30 to 40 percent of hypertensive patients whose ECG and chest x-ray appear normal. In fact, Savage et al.,[109,110] in a study of 234 hypertensive patients, found cardiomegaly on chest x-ray or LVH by electrocardiography in less than 10 percent of patients who had an abnormal echocardiographic left ventricular mass. Echocardiographic parameters that assess left ventricular muscle anatomy include the interventricular septal thickness (IVST), posterior wall thickness (PWT), and LVMI. Two-dimensional guided M-mode echocardiography is satisfactory for the assessment of LVH provided that there are no regional wall motion abnormalities.[111]

Devereaux and associates[112] correlated LVMI with left ventricular weight at postmortem examination of 55 adult patients. Echocardiographic estimates of left ventricular mass, using both the Penn and American Society of Echocardiography conventions, correlated strongly with anatomic left ventricular mass. Thus, ECHO is a sensitive and early indicator of anatomic abnormality of the left ventricle in patients with hypertension.[113–116] Echocardiographic LVH is an important clinical finding because of its association with an excess risk of complex ventricular arrhythmias, coronary heart disease, and sudden death.[117–121] Echocardiography is also useful to demonstrate changes in left ventricular anatomy and function following therapy for hypertension.[122–124] However, the current cost of echocardiography is about fivefold that of electrocardiography and must be considered in context of the diagnostic and therapeutic yields in individual patients with hypertension.[125]

Hypertensive Cerebrovascular Disease

Cerebrovascular Accidents

Hypertension is the most important risk factor for the development of hemorrhagic or atheroembolic stroke. The incidence of stroke increases with each higher stratum of blood pressure.[126]

Microhemorrhage or occlusion of small vessels can result in small areas of infarction, most often in the putamen, thalamus, caudate nucleus, pons, or posterior limb of the internal capsule. These "lacunar" infarcts are usually associated with neurologic deficits that clear over days to weeks. Four distinct clinical syndromes have been identified: (1) pure motor hemiparesis (weakness of the face, arm, and leg), (2) pure sensory stroke (numbness and sensory loss over the face, arm, trunk, and leg), (3) homolateral ataxia and crural paresis (ataxia of the arm and leg and weakness of the leg), and (4) dysarthria and clumsy hand (dysarthria, central facial weakness, deviation of the tongue, and weakness and ataxia of the arm).[127,128] Multiple lacunas can lead to multi-infarct dementia, characterized by lability of affect, dementia, abnormal gait, dysarthria, incontinence, and bilateral long-tract signs. (See also Chap. 122.)

Cerebrovascular accidents of the hemorrhagic and infarctive types are diagnosed on the basis of the neurologic examination, supplemented by the computerized axial tomography (CT) scan. In cerebral infarction, the CT scan may show a sharply marginated, homogeneous, low-density lesion in a specific vascular territory. In intracerebral hemorrhage, the scan usually shows an irregularly shaped, consolidated, high-density mass.[129] The differentiation between a transient ischemic attack (TIA) and a small lacunar infarct is often difficult; the CT scan is usually normal in both conditions, but lacunar infarction may be apparent by MRI. Also, TIAs tend to recur in a repetitive pattern, whereas lacunar infarcts by definition cannot. Evanescent neurologic symptoms or findings in conjunction with a carotid artery bruit justify carotid duplex ultrasonography and/or angiography in an operable patient, with attention to the potential nephrotoxicity of radiographic contrast material.[130]

Hypertensive Encephalopathy

Hypertensive encephalopathy is a syndrome characterized by acute or subacute alterations in neurologic status that occur as the result of elevated arterial pressure and are reversed by lowering the blood pressure.[131] It usually occurs in the setting of accelerated malignant hypertension, although advanced hypertensive retinopathy can occasionally be absent. This syndrome can occur with almost any variety of hypertension, but it is rare with primary aldosteronism and coarctation of the aorta.

Hypertensive encephalopathy usually presents with severe headache, confusion, and lethargy, frequently accompanied by nausea, vomiting, and visual disturbances. The symptoms generally worsen over 12 to 48 h and seizures, myoclonus, obtundation, and in some instances, blindness can develop. (See Chap. 122.)

Hypertensive encephalopathy must be differentiated from other disorders that also present with diffuse neurologic findings in patients with hypertension.[132] For example, uremic encephalopathy can also present with hypertension, confusion, lethargy, and seizures. However, severe headache and retinal hemorrhages, exudates, or papilledema are more characteristic of hypertensive encephalopathy, whereas uremic encephalopathy is often accompanied by myoclonic jerking. Moreover, the symptoms of hypertensive encephalopathy are usually reversed within 12 to 72 h by effective antihypertensive therapy. In malignant hypertension with renal insufficiency, the encephalopathy may well be due to both. Other causes of encephalopathy (e.g., hyponatremia, meningitis, drug intoxication, and collagen vascular diseases) should be considered and evaluated as indicated by other signs and symptoms.

Focal seizures and other focal neurologic signs can occur in patients who appear clinically to have hypertensive encephalopathy. However, in an autopsy study of patients with the clinical diagnosis of hypertensive encephalopathy, Chester et al.[132] found that focal neurologic deficits were almost invariably attributable to structural lesions such as cerebral hemorrhage or infarction. Patients who appear to have hypertensive encephalopathy and exhibit focal neurologic signs should undergo further diagnostic evaluation. The CT scan and MRI are the procedures most likely to identify focal areas of intracerebral hemorrhage or infarction.

Severe hypertension can occur in previously normotensive patients who develop intracranial hemorrhage or a wide variety of other primary neurologic disorders. In these settings, considerable caution must be taken to avoid the erroneous diagnosis of hypertensive encephalopathy. In general, such patients have neither advanced hypertensive retinopathy nor LVH.

Hypertensive Nephrosclerosis

The urinalysis, creatinine clearance, kidney size, pyelogram, angiogram, renal scan, and renogram are usually normal in patients with primary hypertension. More specific diagnostic tests, however, often reveal malfunction of the kidney, including a reduced renal blood flow[133] and an increased fractional excretion of sodium.[134,135] These special tests are not justified for the prognosis or treatment of hypertension when the usual clinical tests of kidney function are within the normal range. If the urine sediment, blood urea nitrogen (BUN), and creatinine are normal and proteinuria does not exceed 500 mg daily, it can usually be assumed that the hypertension is not secondary to primary renal parenchymal disease.

Both glomerular hyperfiltration[136,137] and microalbuminuria[138–141] may be early markers of hypertensive nephropathy. Microalbuminuria is defined as a urinary albumin excretion of 15 to 200 μg/min without detectable abnormality on the usual clinical dipstick tests for proteinuria. Its presence in patients with uncomplicated essential hypertension may predict subsequent cardiovascular disease.[139,140]

Benign Nephrosclerosis

Abnormalities of standard kidney function tests in patients with long-standing, poorly controlled hypertension in the absence of intercurrent primary disease of the kidneys are attributable to benign nephrosclerosis. Under these circumstances low-grade proteinuria (less than 0.5 to 1 g/day) and granular casts may appear, creatinine clearance may fall, and kidneys may shrink slightly. Pyelograms may show poor visualization of the kidneys or delayed excretion of contrast without distortion of the renal contour or collecting system. Renal scans and renal ultrasonography provide information on the symmetry, size, vascularization, and function of the kidneys. Advanced nephrosclerosis is characterized by a symmetrical reduction in kidney size and increased echogenicity on renal ultrasonography. Although not required for the diagnosis of benign nephrosclerosis, renal angiography will show moderately constricted and tortuous renal blood vessels with "corkscrewing" of the renal arterioles but a normal ratio of parenchyma to vascularity of the kidney (Fig. 76-2). Kidney biopsy is not indicated unless hematuria, red blood cell casts, heavy proteinuria, or systemic evidence of collagen vascular or neoplastic disease are found.

An appreciable number of patients, especially blacks, develop renal failure as a consequence of long-standing, poorly controlled hypertension causing nephrosclerosis.[142,143] In patients with end-stage renal disease, a diagnosis of benign hypertensive nephrosclerosis depends on multiple lines of evidence: that hypertension preceded renal disease by a number of years, that glucose tolerance has been normal prior to renal failure, that proteinuria is low grade and microscopic hematuria is absent, that no other intercurrent primary renal disease occurred, that the hypertension was at least moderately severe and poorly controlled, or that kidney biopsy shows only advanced arteriolar intimal and medial changes with interstitial fibrosis and glomerular atrophy and fibrosis.

Malignant Nephrosclerosis

The renal disease associated with malignant essential hypertension differs in pathology, physiology, and natural history from benign nephrosclerosis. Renal failure from malignant hypertension is usually seen in a clinical context of multiple-target-organ decompensation (i.e., retinopathy, encephalopathy, and congestive heart failure) in association with elevated plasma renin, elevated aldosterone, and increased sympathetic outflow.

If renal arteriography is performed in patients with malignant nephrosclerosis, only small amounts of contrast material should be used because larger doses can further impair the already marginal renal function. "Pruning" of the vascular tree with relatively large, poorly perfused kidneys is indicative of malignant nephrosclerosis (Fig. 76-3).

The urinalysis in malignant nephrosclerosis can range from negative in patients whose lesion is confined to the arterioles to 4+ proteinuria, hematuria, and red blood cell or pigmented casts in those with associated glomerulitis or interstitial bleeding. Low-grade proteinuria occurs in about one-third of patients,[144] but nephrotic-range proteinuria occurs in less than 5 percent of patients and usually responds rapidly to the lowering of blood pressure.

Quantitation of plasma renin activity may be desirable in cases of malignant nephrosclerosis with renal failure. It is of clinical value in interpretation of the pathological physiology of the renal failure, in planning for renal transplantation, in titrating beta blocker or angiotensin converting enzyme (ACE) inhibitor therapy, and in prescription for sodium intake and ultrafiltration if hemodialysis is required. Elevated levels of renin occur in approximately 80 percent of cases and therefore do not provide specific evidence for renal artery stenosis as a cause of the malignant nephrosclerosis. Serum aldoste-

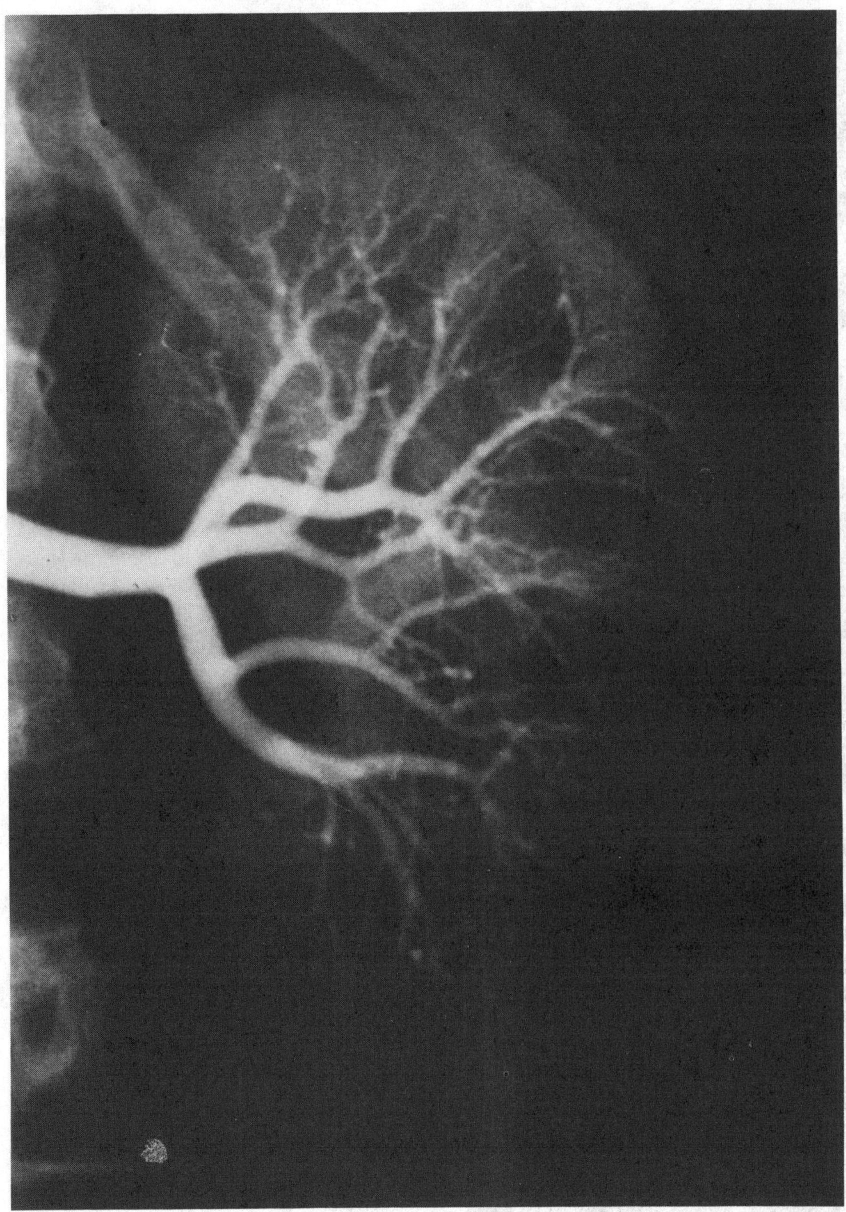

FIGURE 76-2 Benign nephrosclerosis. Tortuosity and corkscrewing of the vessels (represented by white dots in the vascular tree) with preservation of renal mass and good cortical nephrogram.

rone concentrations are elevated in the majority of cases. This secondary aldosteronism probably accounts for the disproportionately low serum potassium concentrations in the setting of mild to moderate renal failure.

THE DIAGNOSIS OF SECONDARY CAUSES OF HYPERTENSION

Estimates of the prevalence of hypertension secondary to identifiable cause vary considerably (Table 76-4).[145–149] In the largest series from the Cleveland Clinic, the prevalence of secondary hypertension was 11 percent.[145] In unselected populations, the best estimate of the prevalence of secondary hypertension would appear to be 5 to 10 percent. Curable etiologies are even less frequent, emphasizing the importance of limiting extensive evaluations to patients in whom the diagnostic yield is likely to be increased.[50,145,150]

Renovascular Hypertension

Prevalence

Renal artery stenosis is the most common curable cause of hypertension, but it probably occurs in 3 percent or less of hypertensive patients (Table 76-4). The prevalence depends in part on the demographic characteristics of the hypertensive population. For example, below the age of 40, renovascular hypertension is more frequent in women than men.[151] Renovascular hypertension is less common in black patients with hypertension.[152]

Clinical Findings

The likelihood of renovascular hypertension is increased when hypertension begins before age 30 or after age 50 (Table 76-5). In addition, an abdominal bruit is heard six to nine times more often in renovascular hypertensive patients than in essential hypertensive patients. The presence of severe hypertensive retinopathy (hemorrhages,

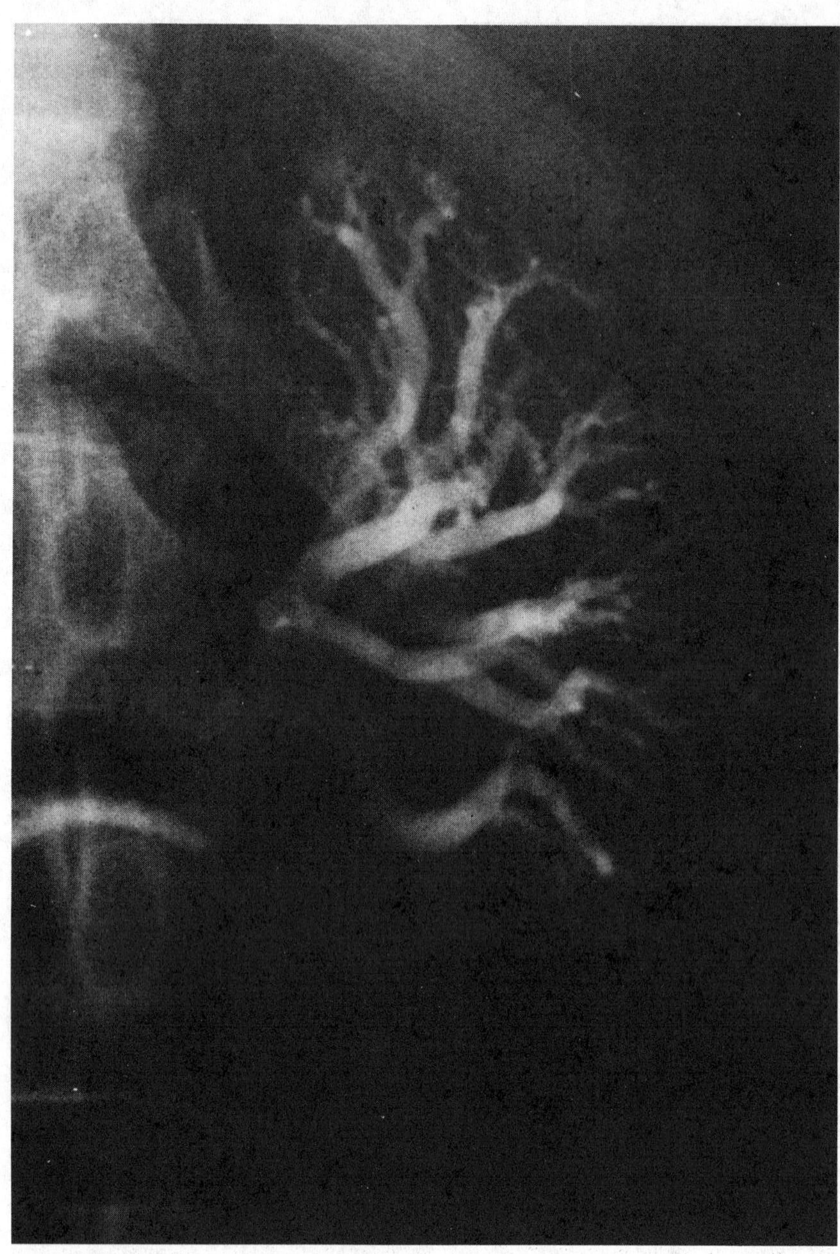

FIGURE 76-3 Malignant nephrosclerosis. Distended main branches with pruning of small arteries and minimal opacification of the cortical nephrogram despite preservation of renal mass.

TABLE 76-4

Secondary Hypertension in Adults: Results of Five Major Studies (%)

	Gifford[145]	Kennedy[146]	Ferguson[147]	Bech[148]	Berglund[149]
Essential hypertension	89	73	89	79	94
Chronic renal disease	5	17	2	13	4
Renovascular disease	4	6	3	5	0.6
Primary aldosteronism	0.4	0.3	0.4	0.4	0.1
Coarctation	0.6	—	—	0	0.1
Cushing's syndrome	0.2	—	—	—	—
Pheochromocytoma	0.2	0.1	—	0.2	—
Miscellaneous*	—	4	4	3	1

*Includes oral contraceptive hypertension as well as patients not thoroughly investigated for secondary causes.

NOTE: In the Gifford study,[145] the patient population was 4939, partly referred; in Kennedy,[146] patient population was 750, partly referred; in Ferguson,[147] patient population was 246; partly referred; in Bech,[148] patient population was 482, partly referred; and in Berglund,[149] patient population was 689, randomly selected men between the ages of 47 and 54 years with blood pressure ≥ 175/115.

exudates, or papilledema) also increases its likelihood. The sudden onset of severe hypertension or the onset of uncontrolled hypertension in a patient whose blood pressure was previously well controlled are the usual clues to renovascular disease. In addition, obesity is less common among renovascular hypertensive patients than essential hypertensive patients.[153]

Pathological Types of Renal Artery Stenosis

Fibrous dysplasia and atherosclerosis of the renal artery account for almost all cases of renovascular hypertension. Table 76-5 contrasts the clinical features of these two types of renovascular hypertension with those of essential hypertension.

Fibrous Dysplasia With fibrous dysplasia, hypertension generally presents before age 35, most often in women. Fibrous dysplasia can involve either or both renal arteries but is usually unilateral when initially diagnosed.[151] An upper abdominal bruit is audible in about 60 percent of patients. Bruits originating from the renal artery are heard best in the midepigastrium; they radiate toward one or both upper quadrants, unlike benign epigastric bruits that radiate vertically but not laterally. The bruit is high pitched, often intermittent, and occasionally systolic-diastolic in character. If combined with hypertension of less than 3 years duration, the presence of a systolic-diastolic bruit is predictive of a favorable response to surgery in patients with fibrous dysplasia.[154]

Atherosclerotic Renovascular Disease Atherosclerotic disease accounts for two-thirds or more of patients with renovascular hypertension. In contrast to fibrous dysplasia, atherosclerotic renovascular disease occurs predominantly in men over age 45. At least one-third of patients with atherosclerotic renovascular disease have bilateral lesions at the time of initial diagnosis.[151] Diabetes mellitus is more prevalent in patients with atherosclerotic renal artery disease[155] and should increase the clinician's suspicion of renal artery stenosis. Abdominal bruits are a less specific finding than in fibrous dysplasia because the atherosclerotic process often generates bruits from other abdominal arteries. The general approach to the detection, evaluation, and treatment of renovascular hypertension is discussed in an excellent report of the Working Group on Renovascular Hypertension.[156]

Special Diagnostic Tests

General When renovascular hypertension is suspected, diagnostic evaluation should generally be conducted in younger patients (below age 35), the group with the highest prevalence of fibrous dysplasia of the renal artery. This is particularly true in those patients with moderate or severe hypertension of less than 3 years duration or when blood pressure is inadequately controlled on three or more antihypertensive drugs. Evaluation should also be considered in selected older patients who may have atherosclerotic renovascular disease and are judged to be good candidates for either surgical intervention or angioplasty.[157] Diagnostic testing is not usually indicated in patients with advanced renal failure and bilateral small kidneys, although improvement or preservation of renal function following revascularization has been observed in selected patients who generally have at least one relatively normal-size kidney.[158–160]

TABLE 76-5

Clinical Characteristics of Patients with Essential Hypertension Versus Surgically Cured Renovascular Hypertension

		Renovascular Hypertension	
Clinical Characteristics	Essential Hypertension (N = 339)	Atherosclerosis (N = 91)	Fibrous Dysplasia (N = 84)
History			
Age of onset, years	35	46*	33
Duration, years	3.1	1.9*	2.0*
Sex, % female	40	34	81*
Race, % black	29	7*	10*
Family history of hypertension, %	67	58	41*
Physical			
Obese, %	38	17*	11*
Thin, %	6	13	30*
Systolic BP, mmHg	169	181*	174
Diastolic BP, mmHg	109	108	108
Fundi grade 3 or 4, %	12	26*	10
Abdominal bruit, %	7	41*	57*
Laboratory			
Cardiomegaly (chest x-ray), %	26	26	8*
Serum creatinine > 1.5 mg/dl, %	11	15	2*
Serum potassium < 3.4 meq/l, %	7	14	17*

*Indicates significant difference ($p < .05$) when compared with the group with essential hypertension.

SOURCE: Adapted from Simon et al.[153]

Radioactive Renograms and Differential Estimates of Renal Plasma Flow Semiquantitative estimate of kidney size and position, combined with visualization of homogeneity of intrarenal perfusion, and the symmetry and rate of isotope excretion by the kidney and its appearance in the bladder can be obtained from the combination of ^{131}I-hippuran radioactive renograms and ^{99m}Tc-diethylenetriamine pentaacetic acid (DTPA) scintigrams of the kidneys and measurement of the disappearance rates of ^{131}I-hippuran from the plasma. These anatomic and physiological measurements can be made with minimal risk in patients with advanced renal and vascular disease. If plasma flow is symmetric, homogeneous, and markedly reduced in small kidneys, the likelihood of correctable renovascular hypertension is low. Conversely, asymmetry of flow greater than 40 to 60 percent or unilateral delayed isotope appearance but good bilateral renal concentration and excretion is strongly suggestive of large renal artery vascular occlusive disease.

Captopril Renography Isotope renography detects the acute reductions of glomerular filtration rate (GFR) following the administration of captopril to patients with functionally significant renal artery stenosis and is often an effective screening procedure for renovascular hypertension.[161] Isotope renography, generally using ^{99m}Tc-DTPA (which largely reflects GFR), is performed immediately before and 60 to 90 min after the administration of a single 25-mg dose of captopril. Following converting enzyme inhibition, both the uptake and excretion of DTPA on the stenotic side are usually decreased from baseline (i.e., pre-captopril) in patients with unilateral renal arterial disease, whereas no consistent decrease is generally observed in the contralateral uninvolved kidney. In contrast, the total uptake of ^{131}I-hippuran [which predominantly reflects renal blood flow (RBF)] by the stenotic kidney is frequently unchanged (although excretion is delayed), suggesting that RBF may not be significantly altered by captopril in most cases.[162] This acute reduction in filtration fraction (i.e., the ratio of GFR/RBF) that occurs in the stenotic kidney following converting enzyme inhibition may be due to interruption of angiotensin II–mediated vasoconstriction of the postglomerular efferent arteriole. Efferent arteriolar vasoconstriction appears to develop initially as a compensatory adaptation to help preserve glomerular capillary filtration pressure in settings, such as renal artery stenosis, that are associated with a reduced renal arterial perfusion pressure.

Digital Subtraction Angiography or Aortography Vascular anatomic evaluation usually begins with either digital subtraction angiography (DSA) or aortography. The rapid-sequence intravenous urogram (IVP) has been abandoned as a screening test because the sensitivity of the test is 80 percent at best.[163–165] Venous DSA combines intravenous urography with angiotomography to create subtraction images of the abdominal arteries following rapid injection of a large bolus of contrast material into the central venous circulation.[166–168] Lesions of the main renal artery can be detected in up to 90 percent or more of cases if adequate visualization is achieved,[166,168] although DSA is less reliable for detecting segmental renal artery lesions.[167] When the index of clinical suspicion is high or when the risk of complications seems excessive, it is usually more expedient to proceed directly to arterial DSA or renal arteriography. If the serum creatinine is greater than 2 mg/dL, the total amount of contrast material should be limited with adequate hydration and volume expansion.[169]

Renal Vein Renin Ratio Once the presence of renal arterial disease has been established, the functional significance of the stenosis can be evaluated to help determine if the renal artery lesion is the cause of the hypertension. This is done by measuring the "renal vein renin ratio," i.e., the ratio of plasma renin activity in blood samples obtained from the venous effluent of each kidney. Blood samples for renal vein renin activity are often obtained following sodium depletion (e.g., the administration of oral furosemide, 40 mg bid for 24 to 48 h in conjunction with a low-sodium diet). In general, to enhance differential secretion, patients should be free of beta blocker and central antisympathetic drugs. However, administration of a single oral dose of captopril 30 min prior to obtaining renal vein renin studies can enhance lateralization in patients with unilateral renal artery disease, even when other drug therapy is continued.[170–172] However, ACE inhibitors such as captopril, enalapril, or lisinopril should be used with caution in this setting because acute renal insufficiency (usually reversible following discontinuation of the drug) occurs in many patients with severe bilateral renal artery stenosis or renal artery stenosis in a solitary kidney.[173,174] A single dose of captopril just prior to the split renin testing is usually tolerated well and can also be useful in improving control of blood pressure during the procedure.

A renal vein renin ratio of 1.5 or greater favoring the stenotic side is abnormal and is generally indicative of a functionally significant renal artery stenosis.[175] Lateralization has additional significance if the peripheral plasma renin activity is also elevated and renin secretion from the unaffected kidney is suppressed; i.e., the renal venous renin activity from the unaffected side is similar to or no more than 30 percent above the renin activity of a sample obtained from the inferior vena cava below the renal veins.[176,177] In general, when renal vein renins reveal a stenotic-to-nonstenotic ratio of at least 1.5, approximately 90 percent of patients will be improved or relieved of hypertension following successful angioplasty, surgical revascularization, or nephrectomy. However, up to 50 percent of selected patients with nonlateralizing renal vein renin ratios below 1.5 also have a favorable response to surgery.[178–181] Hence, a lateralizing renal vein renin ratio predicts improvement of hypertension with a high degree of accuracy in patients with unilateral renal arterial disease, whereas a nonlateralizing value is not necessarily a reliable predictor of lack of improvement of hypertension following technically successful surgery or angioplasty.[176,181] The renal vein renin ratio is frequently not reliable for predicting surgical response in patients with bilateral renovascular disease.

Post-Captopril Plasma Renin Activity The unstimulated peripheral vein renin activity is not a very useful test for renovascular hypertension because up to 50 percent of patients have values within the normal range.[182] This is most likely because renin secretion from the uninvolved kidney is suppressed in patients with unilateral renal artery stenosis or because renin can sometimes be normalized by the sodium retention that occurs with bilateral renovascular disease. In contrast, the peripheral renin response 60 min following a 25- or 50-mg dosage of oral captopril is a useful and noninvasive screening test for renovascular hypertension.[183] A positive test is when the post-captopril renin level is above 12 ng/mL per h, increases 10 ng/mL per h or more, and is at least 150 percent above the baseline value (400 percent if the baseline renin is below 3 ng/mL per h). Optimal interpretation of the test requires that the patient is not receiving antihypertensive medications, especially diuretics. False-positive and false-negative results are not infrequent in patients with serum creatinine levels of 2.0 mg/dL or more.

Duplex ultrasound combines β-mode imaging and pulsed Doppler flow analysis. Preliminary data are promising with regard to the diagnosis of renal artery stenosis, although the procedure is limited technically by obesity and excess bowel gas and anatomically by the presence of either multiple renal arteries or stenosis of branch vessels.[184,185]

Renoparenchymal Hypertension

Two types of renoparenchymal hypertension are (1) the acute form associated with glomerulitis and (2) the chronic form associated with loss of viable nephrons. In neither of these is plasma renin activity usually very elevated. In contrast to essential hypertension associated with nephrosclerosis, the urinalysis is typically abnormal in patients with hypertension due to renal parenchymal disease.[186]

Hypertension in Acute Renal Disease

Hematuria with dysmorphic red blood cells, red blood cell casts, proteinuria, periorbital and/or pedal edema, and elevation of the BUN-to-creatinine ratio to above 15:1 are diagnostic of acute diffuse glomerulitis. The reduction of single-nephron urine flow with acute glomerulitis results in a greater reduction of urea clearance (by virtue of its avid reabsorption) than of creatinine clearance. This gives a serum BUN-to-creatinine clearance ratio similar to that which is often called "prerenal azotemia." A more accurate term for the setting of acute glomerulitis would be "intact nephron azotemia." If plasma renin is measured, it is often normal or slightly depressed,[187] but it may be considered elevated relative to the increased blood volume and pressure.

Radiographic examination in hypertensive acute glomerulitis usually shows the kidneys to be enlarged or at the upper limit of normal size. Sometimes retrograde pyelography, done because of gross hematuria, reveals large kidneys with a delicate or filigree pattern of the calyces resulting from intracapsular swelling of the kidney and compression of the collecting system.

Other laboratory tests may confirm the etiologic diagnosis: bacteriologic or serologic evidence of streptococcal infection, antinuclear antibodies, or reduced serum complement. If 1+ or more proteinuria is present repeatedly on qualitative testing, 24-h urine protein and creatinine clearances should be determined to ascertain whether a nephrotic type of protein leak is present.[188] Meltzer and coworkers[189] noted that hypotensive idiopathic nephrotics often have high plasma renins, whereas hypertensive nephrotics usually have low plasma renins.

If nephrotic syndrome is diagnosed or if renal function remains severely depressed after 2 weeks of treatment with appropriate antibiotics, antihypertensive agents, and diuretics, a renal biopsy should be performed. Immunologic and ultrastructural classification of the disease will modify diagnosis, prognosis, and therapy.

Hypertension in Chronic Renal Disease

The second major category of renal disease associated with hypertension is that related to loss of nephron population in chronic nephritis. In this type of renoparenchymal hypertension, creatinine clearances and urea clearances are reduced proportionately and the BUN-to-creatinine ratio is usually normal, approximately 10:1. Urinalysis usually shows moderate proteinuria (0.5 to 2 g/day), moderate numbers of red blood cells, and frequent granular casts with glomerulonephritis. Pyuria, bacteriuria, and white blood cell casts are present with pyelonephritis. Pyuria can also occur with abacterial forms of interstitial nephritis such as analgesic nephropathy.

X-ray and ultrasound studies in chronic nephritis usually show variable degrees of reduction in kidney size, often to 10 cm or less. The kidneys are symmetric and smooth in chronic glomerulonephritis, whereas they are asymmetric and irregular in chronic pyelonephritis and polycystic kidney disease. With uremia, small kidneys indicate irreversibility of the underlying disease. Shrunken kidneys are not optimal to biopsy because tissue is difficult to obtain and the end-stage histologic pattern is hard to interpret.

If arteriograms are done in advanced parenchymal nephritis, the small kidney shows relatively profuse blood vessels extending almost to the capsule with no cortical tissue remaining (Fig. 76-4). The caliber of the vessels is small, but the number is normal. This angiographic pattern differs from that described for benign or malignant nephrosclerosis.

When chronic renal failure occurs in conjunction with diabetes mellitus, the pathological lesion can be intercapillary glomerulosclerosis, large- or medium-vessel atherosclerotic disease, or atrophy with interstitial fibrosis. Ultrasonography usually shows smooth and symmetrical kidneys, often of normal or even increased size. Asymmetry of renal size can be a tip-off to coexistent renal artery occlusive disease.

The hypertension of most patients with end-stage renal disease on maintenance hemodialysis is volume dependent, but about 10 percent of cases are renin mediated. When hypertension is difficult to control in dialysis patients, plasma renin determinations are of value. The renin level can also be important if kidney transplantation is planned because posttransplant hypertension can

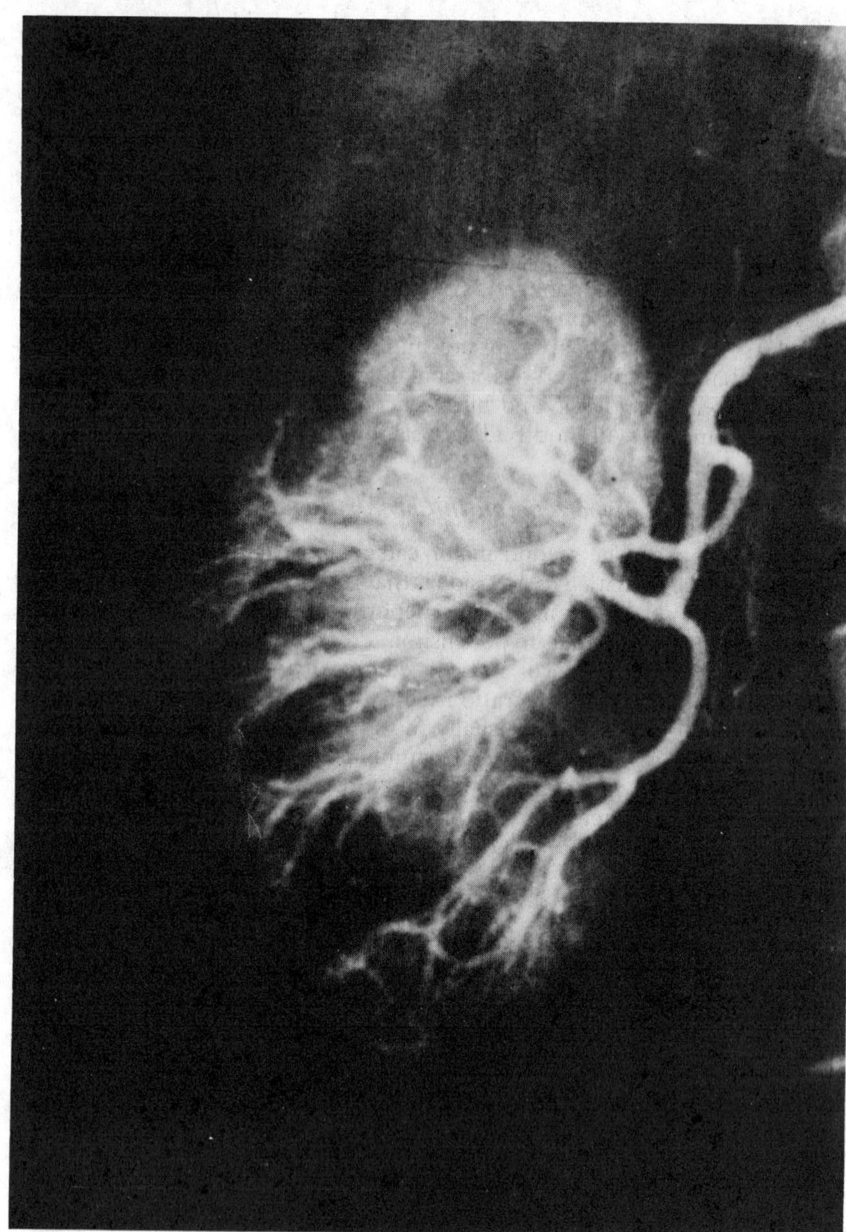

FIGURE 76-4 Chronic parenchymatous nephritis. Disproportionately profuse vasculature of small caliber running out to the capsule of the small kidney with an atrophic cortex.

be caused by renin secretion from the native kidneys as well as acquired stenosis of the implanted renal artery.

Primary Aldosteronism

Prevalence

Primary aldosteronism (Conn's syndrome) is an uncommon but potentially curable cause of hypertension. In centers where patients are referred and extensively investigated for primary aldosteronism, this diagnosis has been confirmed in up to 12 percent of patients.[190] In most studies of secondary causes of hypertension, however, primary aldosteronism is found in 0.5 to 1 percent of patients (Table 76-4).

Clinical Findings

The majority of cases of primary aldosteronism are diagnosed between the ages of 30 and 50 years.[191] The hypertension is usually of mild or moderate severity, although severe hypertension has been observed.[192] Except for hypokalemia, primary aldosteronism does not usually present with clinical manifestations that readily suggest the diagnosis. Occasionally, the presenting feature is nocturia, polyuria, polydipsia, proximal muscle weakness, intermittent paralysis, rhabdomyolysis, paresthesias, or tetany resulting from severe potassium depletion. The manifestations of primary aldosteronism can temporarily ameliorate during pregnancy because of the antimineralocorticoid effect of high levels of progesterone.[193,194]

Hypokalemia Hypokalemia is the most common manifestation of primary aldosteronism and is often associated with metabolic alkalosis and mild hypernatremia. Hypomagnesemia can also occur.[195]

Primary aldosteronism can present with either unprovoked or diuretic-induced hypokalemia. Unprovoked hypokalemia occurs in the absence of diuretics, vomiting, diarrhea, alcoholism, or abuse of laxatives or chewing tobacco. It is particularly suggestive of primary aldosteronism because *spontaneous* hypokalemia is observed in such a small percentage of otherwise healthy patients with uncomplicated essential hypertension. Hence, the likelihood of primary aldosteronism is increased markedly in untreated hypertensive patients who present with unexplained hypokalemia.[196,197]

The presence of a normal serum potassium concentration (i.e., "normokalemic primary aldosteronism") has been observed in patients who otherwise have the characteristic features of primary aldosteronism.[198] However, when unselected normokalemic hypertensive patients have been screened by measuring renin and aldosterone levels, in general, relatively few cases of aldosteronism have been found.[196] In addition, most patients with normokalemic primary aldosteronism appear to have bilateral hyperplasia. Of those with adenomas (i.e., the surgically remediable group), few are persistently normokalemic if the serum potassium is checked on multiple occasions.[192]

Other Varieties of Mineralocorticoid Hypertension

A number of infrequently encountered varieties of mineralocorticoid hypertension can cause hypertension and hypokalemia.[199,200] In most instances, they can be identified by their clinical and laboratory characteristics.[199–201]

Chronic excessive ingestion of licorice-containing candy or chewing tobacco can induce mineralocorticoid hypertension[70] with elevation of blood pressure caused by glycyrrhizinic acid, a component of licorice extract. Glycyrrhizinic acid directly inhibits the kidney enzyme 11β-hydroxydehydrogenase necessary for the intrarenal inactivation of steroids with an 11-hydroxy group, primarily cortisol and corticosterone.[202] Cases of "pseudoaldosteronism" have also been reported following the chronic use of nasal sprays containing 9-alpha-fluoroprednisolone.[203]

Confirming the Diagnosis of Primary Aldosteronism

Plasma Renin Activity The major criterion for the diagnosis of primary aldosteronism is autonomous overproduction of aldosterone, usually in conjunction with a low plasma renin activity. Typically, the plasma renin activity is suppressed to low levels and remains subnormal despite volume depletion and upright posture. Most methods to test renin responsiveness examine the response to 2 to 4 h of upright posture following the administration of 40 to 160 mg furosemide over 12 to 24 h. Some also use a 10- to 15-meq/day low-sodium diet for 3 to 5 days in conjunction with diuretics and upright posture. Under these conditions, a threefold or more increase in baseline plasma renin activity is generally considered normal. The renin levels of patients with primary aldosteronism are usually stimulated minimally or not at all by sodium restriction or diuretic therapy.

Use of the plasma renin activity as a screening test for primary aldosteronism is nonspecific because approximately 30 percent of essential hypertensive patients (i.e., the subgroup with "low renin" essential hypertension) also have subnormal plasma renin activity. Furthermore, a random plasma renin activity, obtained without appropriate stimulation, may not be suppressed in 10 percent or more of patients with primary aldosteronism[192,204] and can even be increased in patients receiving spironolactone.

Aldosterone Suppression Tests The diagnosis of primary aldosteronism is confirmed by plasma or 24-h urinary levels of aldosterone that are increased relative to sodium intake and excretion and that fail to suppress normally with volume expansion. Several methods have been used to test aldosterone suppressibility. These include volume expansion by administration of intravenous saline or oral salt loads. The lack of suppression of aldosterone is a critical diagnostic feature because considerable overlap exists in the plasma and urinary aldosterone levels of patients with essential hypertension and primary aldosteronism, particularly when sodium intake has not been controlled. In patients with primary aldosteronism, the plasma aldosterone level usually fails to suppress below 5 to 10 ng/dL following the intravenous administration of 2 liters of normal saline solution over 4 h.[205]

Ratio of Plasma Aldosterone to Plasma Renin Activity The ratio of plasma aldosterone to plasma renin activity can also be useful in the diagnosis of primary aldosteronism. Hiramatsu et al.[206] found the ratio of plasma aldosterone concentration (in picograms per deciliter) to plasma renin activity (in nanograms per milliliter per hour) to be below 200 in patients with essential hypertension and above 400 in patients with aldosterone-secreting adenomas. Lyons et al.[207] reported that the ratio of plasma aldosterone concentration to plasma renin activity in blood samples obtained 2 h following the administration of a single 25-mg oral dose of captopril provided better discrimination between essential hypertension and primary aldosteronism than did the baseline values.

Differential Diagnosis of Types of Primary Aldosteronism

There are two major pathological varieties of primary aldosteronism: *adrenocortical adenomas* (*aldosteronomas*, or aldosterone-producing adenomas, APAs) and *bilateral adrenocortical (zona glomerulosa) hyperplasia.* Aldosterone-producing adenomas account for approximately 60 percent of cases. They are almost invariably benign, and women are affected more commonly than men.[191,192] Aldosteronomas are usually associated with higher levels of aldosterone and more pronounced hypokalemia and hyporeninemia than bilateral hyperplasia.

Bilateral hyperplasia is sometimes referred to as *idiopathic hyperaldosteronism* (IHA) or *pseudoprimary aldosteronism.* In contrast to aldosteronomas, bilateral hyperplasia affects men and women with approximately equal frequency.[192] In addition, some studies have found that patients with hyperplasia, as a group, tend to be older than those with adenoma.[192,204] Most patients with aldosterone-secreting adenomas exhibit a fall in plasma aldosterone levels after 2 to 4 h of upright posture in the morning, whereas those with bilateral hyperplasia usually demonstrate an increase.[208,209] These findings have led to speculation that bilateral hyperplasia may be due to excessive secretion of an anterior pituitary hormone, aldosterone-stimulating factor (ASF).[210–212] Carey and associates[213] reported elevated plasma and urine levels of ASF in seven patients with idiopathic hyperaldosteronism. Franco-Saenz et al.[210] described a patient with bilateral adrenal hyperplasia due to nodular basophilic hyperplasia of the intermediate lobe of the pituitary. Cases of unilateral adrenal hyperplasia have also been described.[200,214,215] These are referred to as the primary adrenal hyperplasia (PAH) type of primary aldosteronism, and the associated hypertension responds to unilateral adrenalectomy.

A number of patients have been described with the typical features of primary aldosteronism but whose clinical and laboratory abnormalities were reversed with dexamethasone administration, suggesting supersensitivity to adrenocorticotropic hormone (ACTH).[200,216,217] This variety has been termed *dexamethasone-suppressible hyperaldosteronism.* A specific biochemical defect has not been identified and the etiology is unknown; large amounts of 18-hydroxycortisol are secreted. Bilateral adrenal hyperplasia is the only reported histologic abnormality. Such cases are rare and appear to be familial, with autosomal dominant inheritance. Some authors advocate excluding this possibility by administering a 2-week course of 1 to 2 mg/day of dexamethasone to patients with the presumptive diagnosis of bilateral hyperplasia.

Localization Methods

General Once the diagnosis of primary aldosteronism is established, further tests are indicated in patients judged to be operative candidates. Evaluation must include efforts to distinguish between adenoma and bilateral hyperplasia and to localize the side of any tumor-bearing gland. Adrenal venography is unreliable for identifying bilateral hyperplasia or the 20 percent of adenomas that are smaller than 1 cm in diameter.

Adrenal Vein Aldosterone Levels A sensitive localization method is that of measuring the aldosterone levels of the venous effluent from each adrenal. Regardless of size, aldosteronomas can be localized with about 90 percent accuracy. The aldosterone levels of venous blood from tumor-bearing glands are often increased 10-fold or more above those from the contralateral uninvolved gland. Bilateral elevation of aldosterone levels suggests bilateral hyperplasia or the rare circumstance of bilateral adenomas. Adrenal vein epinephrine levels above 1500 pg/mL assure that the sample was indeed from the adrenal vein.[218]

CT and Isotopic Scans Adenomas larger than 1 cm in diameter can be identified in 60 to 75 percent of cases with the CT scan.[209,219,220] Adrenal scintillation scanning with ^{131}I-6-iodomethyl-19-norcholesterol (NP-59) is a technique based on the uptake of cholesterol by the adrenal gland. Several reports suggest that adenomas are identified with reasonably good accuracy,[219,220] but this procedure is not available everywhere for routine clinical use. Dexamethasone in a dose of 0.5 to 1.0 mg every 6 h suppresses the uptake in glands with bilateral hyperplasia, but not those with adenoma.

Plasma 18-Hydroxycorticosterone Levels The plasma concentration of 18-hydroxycorticosterone, a precursor of aldosterone, can help distinguish between patients with aldosteronomas and bilateral hyperplasia. Levels are generally higher in patients with aldosterone-secreting adenomas than in those with bilateral hyperplasia.[221]

Pheochromocytoma

Clinical Findings

The initial clinical suspicion of pheochromocytoma usually occurs because the patient complains of severe headaches (often of the vascular type), inappropriate sweating, or palpitations.[222] The first hint can occur, however, when the patient has hypertension that is difficult to control; when the patient has neurofibromatosis, café-au-lait spots, von Hipple–Lindau disease, Sturge-Weber disease, or tuberous sclerosis; when the patient exhibits a pressor response to beta blockers; or when the family history reveals hypertension plus either thyroid carcinoma or hyperparathyroidism. These clinical clues are summarized in Table 76-6.

Urinary Screening Tests

The urinary excretion of total catecholamines, metanephrine, and vanillylmandelic acid are the most commonly used screening tests for pheochromocytoma. Table 76-7 provides data on the sensitivity of these tests found in three large series of hypertensive patients.[223–225] All these studies indicate that the excretion of metanephrine is the most sensitive of the three urinary screening tests. Hence, a 24-h urine measurement of metanephrine and creatinine is an excellent screening test for pheochromocytoma.

Gitlow et al.[226] reported that the ratio of urinary metanephrine (expressed in micrograms) to creatinine (expressed in milligrams) was above 2.2 in 90 of 92 patients with pheochromocytoma but only 2 percent in control subjects without pheochromocytoma. Kaplan et al.[227]

TABLE 76-6

Clinical Clues to the Diagnosis of Pheochromocytoma

1. Classic symptom triad of headaches, sweating, and palpitations
2. Hypertension difficult to control
3. Inappropriate sinus tachycardia
4. Orthostatic hypotension
5. Recurrent arrhythmias
6. Neurofibromatosis, café-au-lait spots, von Hippel–Lindau disease, Sturge–Weber disease, tuberous sclerosis
7. Previously catastrophic anesthesia or surgery
8. Pressor response to beta blockers
9. Family history of pheochromocytoma, medullary thyroid carcinoma, or hyperparathyroidism

TABLE 76-7

Sensitivity of Urinary Total Catecholamines, Vanillylmandelic Acid, and Metanephrines as Screening Tests in Patients with Pheochromocytoma

	Total Catecholamines	Vanillylmandelic Acid	Metanephrines
Mayo Clinic[223]	47/60 (79%)	37/52 (71%)	50/52 (96%)
Cleveland Clinic[224]	18/27 (67%)	27/33 (82%)	25/25 (100%)
NIH[225]	60/62 (97%)	59/62 (95%)	60/62 (97%)

documented the usefulness of the metanephrine-to-creatinine ratio on single-voided urine specimens. The ratio ranged between 0.20 and 0.56 in 10 untreated adult hypertensive patients without pheochromocytoma, whereas the lowest ratio was 2.8 in multiple urine samples from seven adult patients with pheochromocytoma. A ratio above 1 is strongly suggestive of pheochromocytoma in an untreated and otherwise uncomplicated hypertensive patient over 15 years of age.

Elevated urinary metanephrine levels have been noted in patients with coma and increased intracranial pressure[226] as well as in patients with ruptured intracranial aneurysms.[228] False-negative urinary metanephrine levels can occur for 24 to 72 h following the use of methylglucamine contrast media for angiography or intravenous pyelography.[229,230]

Plasma Catecholamine Levels

Radioenzymatic measurements of plasma catecholamines, usually both norepinephrine and epinephrine, in the supine and rested state are abnormally elevated in 90 to 96 percent of patients with pheochromocytoma.[231–233] Levels may even be abnormal in occasional patients with normal urinary screening tests or when blood pressure is not elevated. In general, there is minimal overlap between catecholamine levels of patients with pheochromocytoma and the highest catecholamine levels of either normotensive subjects or uncomplicated patients with essential hypertension. A common clinical dilemma occurs, however, when samples are drawn from patients with essential hypertension who are undergoing acute stress. For example, marked elevations of plasma catecholamines can accompany acute myocardial infarction[234,235] as well as subarachnoid hemorrhage,[236] clonidine withdrawal syndrome,[237] volume depletion, and other stressful clinical settings. Less striking but still abnormally elevated plasma catecholamines can also be a consequence of antihypertensive drug therapy including diuretics,[238] hydralazine,[239,240] calcium channel blockers,[239,241] labetalol,[242] and prazosin.[243,244]

To reduce the effects of stress or ambulation, an indwelling intravenous catheter or heparin lock should be placed with the patient rested in a quiet area in the supine position for at least 20 min before obtaining the blood sample for plasma catecholamines. Plasma levels of dopamine should be obtained along with the norepinephrine and epinephrine levels, because malignant pheochromocytomas occasionally secrete only dopamine.[245] In addition, rare patients with essential hypertension have episodic surges of dopamine with hypertensive episodes that can mimic pheochromocytoma.[246]

Clonidine Suppression Test

The clonidine suppression test is very useful to differentiate pheochromocytoma from essential hypertension in patients with elevated plasma catecholamines.[247] It is often expedient to proceed directly to this test when plasma catecholamines are first measured. A dose of 0.3 mg of clonidine is given and plasma catecholamine levels are drawn immediately before and 3 h later. Blood pressure and heart rate are reduced similarly in hypertensive pheochromocytoma and nonpheochromocytoma patients. However, plasma norepinephrine (and to a lesser extent epinephrine) is essentially unchanged in patients with pheochromocytoma but is reduced markedly (i.e., by at least 50 percent and to a level below 500 pg/mL) in patients with essential hypertension. This is because the central action of clonidine does not block peripheral production of catecholamines. Elevated plasma catecholamines occur in some patients with autonomic epilepsy, but these are also suppressed by clonidine.[248]

Suppression of plasma norepinephrine by clonidine in patients with pheochromocytoma (i.e., a false-negative test) has been noted rarely in metastatic, epinephrine-secreting, and otherwise uncomplicated pheochromocytoma.[249,250] Moreover, false-negative clonidine suppression tests are not uncommon in patients with pheochromocytoma whose baseline plasma catecholamine levels are not elevated at the time of testing.[251] For optimal interpretation, the clonidine suppression test should be performed under controlled environmental conditions when the patient is not receiving concomitant antihypertensive therapy.

Localizaton of the Tumor

The intravenous pyelogram with tomography is a relatively insensitive procedure for localization of adrenal pheochromocytomas. Adrenal arteriography detects 80 to 85 percent of tumors, and adrenal venography will occasionally identify small or hypovascular tumors. Noninvasive axial CT scans, however, have replaced angiography as the primary localization procedure, particularly since the average tumor size is approximately 4.5 cm.[224] The CT scan is effective in localizing intraabdominal pheochromocytomas in 90 percent or more of cases.[252,253] Scintigraphic imaging with ^{131}*meta*-iodobenzylguanidine (^{131}I-MIBG), a radiolabeled analogue of

TABLE 76-8

Results of Diagnostic Tests and Scan Procedures in 19 Patients with Pheochromocytoma

	Positive	Negative
Urine metanephrine	17	1
Plasma norepinephrine	17	2
MIBG scan	17	2
CT scan	16	3
MRI scan	12	2

SOURCE: Adapted from Velchik et al.[256]

guanethidine that is concentrated in adrenergic tissue, has demonstrated pheochromocytoma tumors in occasional patients in whom the CT scan was negative.[254,255]

Magnetic resonance imaging is another sometimes useful procedure for the identification of pheochromocytoma, which produces a high signal intensity on T_2-weighted images, often described as a light bulb appearance.[256] However, false-negative tests can occur with either the CT, MRI, or MIBG scans (Table 76-8).

REFERENCES

1. Kaplan, NA (ed): *Clinical Hypertension*, 5th ed. Baltimore, Williams and Wilkins, 1990: 9–10.
2. Frohlich ED, Grim C, Labarthe DR, Maxwell MH, Perloff D, Weidman WH: Recommendations for human blood pressure determination by sphygmomanometers. Report of a Special Task Force Appointed by the Steering Committee, American Heart Association. *Circulation* 1988; 77(2):501A–514A.
3. Kaplan NM: Misdiagnosis of systemic hypertension and recommendations for improvement. *Am J Cardiol* 1987; 60:1383–1386.
4. Nielsen PE, Janniche H: The accuracy of auscultatory measurement of arm blood pressure in very obese subjects. *Acta Med Scand* 1974; 195:403–409.
5. Beevers DG: Sphygmomanometer cuff sizes—new recommendations. *J Human Hypertens* 1990; 4:587–588.
6. Oster JR, Materson BJ: Pseudohypertension: A diagnostic dilemma. *J Clin Hypertens* 1986; 4:307–313.
7. Messerli FH, Ventura HO, Amodeo C: Osler's maneuver and pseudohypertension. *N Engl J Med* 1985; 312:1548–1551.
8. Vardan S, Mookherjee S, Warner R, Smulyan H: Systolic hypertension: Direct and indirect BP measurements. *Arch Intern Med* 1983; 143:935–938.
9. Kuwajima I, Hoh E, Suzuki Y, Matsushita S, Kuramoto K: Pseudohypertension in the elderly. *J Hypertens* 1990; 8:429–432.
10. Rodbard S, Margolis J: The auscultatory gap in arteriosclerotic heart disease. *Circulation* 1957; 15:850–854.
11. Goldhill DR: Bilateral simultaneous indirect systolic blood pressure measurements. *Cardivasc Res* 1986; 20:774–777.
12. Mitchell PL, Parlin RW, Blackburn H: Effect of vertical displacement of the arm on indirect blood-pressure measurement. *N Engl J Med* 1964; 271:72–74.
13. Kahn HS, Bain RP: Vertex-corrected blood pressure in black girls. *Hypertension* 1987; 9:390–397.
14. Currens JH: A comparison of the blood pressure in the lying and standing positions: A study of five hundred men and five hundred women. *Am Heart J* 1948; 35:646–654.
15. Davis BR, Langford HG, Blaufox MD, Curb JD, Polk BF, Shulman NB: The association of postural changes in systolic blood pressure and mortality in persons with hypertension: The Hypertension Detection and Follow-up Program Experience. *Circulation* 1987; 75:340–346.
16. Frohlich ED, Tarazi RC, Ulrych M, Dustan HP, Page IH: Tilt test for investigating a neural component in hypertension. Its correlation with clinical characteristics. *Circulation* 1967; 36:387–393.
17. Esler MD, Nestel PJ: Sympathetic responsiveness to head-up tilt in essential hypertension. *Clin Sci* 1973; 44:213–216.
18. Gordon T, Sorlie P, Kannel WB: Problems in the assessment of blood pressure: The Framingham Study. *Int J Epidemiol* 1976; 5:327–334.
19. Conway J: Blood pressure and heart rate variability. *J Hypertens* 1986; 4:261–263.
20. Mancia G, Ferrari A, Gregorini L, Parati G, Pomidossi G, Bertinieri G, et al: Blood pressure variability in man: Its relation to high blood pressure, age and baroreflex sensitivity. *Clin Sci* 1980; 59(suppl 6):401–404.
21. Bevan AT, Honour AJ, Scott FH: Direct arterial pressure recording in unrestricted man. *Clin Sci* 1969; 36:329–334.
22. Drayer JIM, Weber MA, DeYoung JL, Wyle FA: Circadian blood pressure patterns in ambulatory hypertensive patients. Effects of age. *Am J Med* 1982; 73:493–499.
23. Armitage P, Fox W, Rose GA, Tinker CM: The variability of measurements of casual blood pressure. II. Survey experience. *Clin Sci* 1966; 30:337–344.
24. Souchek J, Stamler J, Dyer AR, Paul O, Lepper MH: The value of two or three versus a single reading of blood pressure at a first visit. *J Chronic Dis* 1979; 32:197–210.
25. Kannel WB, Sorlie P, Gordon T: Labile hypertension: A faulty concept? The Framingham Study. *Circulation* 1980; 61:1183–1187.
26. Glock CY, Vought RL, Clark EG, Schweitzer MD: Studies in hypertension. II. Variability of daily blood pressure measurements in the same individuals over a three-week period. *J Chronic Dis* 1956; 4:469–476.
27. Watson RDS, Lumb R, Young MA, Stallard TJ, Davies P, Littler WA: Variation in cuff blood pressure in untreated outpatients with mild hypertension—implications for initiating antihypertensive treatment. *J Hypertens* 1987; 5:207–211.
28. Hypertension Detection and Follow-up Program Cooperative Group: Blood pressure studies in 14 communities. A two-stage screen for hypertension. *JAMA* 1977; 237:2385–2391.
29. SHEP Cooperative Research Group: Prevention of stroke by antihypertensive drug treatment in older persons with isolated systolic hypertension. Final results of the Systolic Hypertension in the Elderly Program. *JAMA* 1991; 265:3255–3264.
30. Rosner B, Polk BF: The implications of blood pressure variability for clinical and screening purposes. *J Chronic Dis* 1979; 32:451–461.
31. Rosner B, Polk BF: Predictive values of routine blood pressure measurements in screening for hypertension. *Am J Epidemiol* 1983; 117:429–442.
32. Julius S, Ellis CN, Pascual AV, Matice M, Hansson L, Hunyor SN, et al: Home blood pressure determination. Value in borderline ("labile") hypertension. *JAMA* 1974; 229:663–666.
33. White WB: Assessment of patients with office hypertension by 24-hour noninvasive ambulatory blood pressure monitoring. *Arch Intern Med* 1986; 146:2196–2199.
34. Weber MA, Drayer JIM: Role of blood pressure monitoring in the diagnosis of hypertension. *J Hypertens* 1986; 4(suppl 5):S325–S327.
35. National High Blood Pressure Education Program Coordinating Committee: National High Blood Pressure Education Program Working Group Report on Ambulatory Blood Pressure Monitoring. *Arch Intern Med* 1990; 150:2270–2280.
36. Perloff D, Sokolow M, Cowan R: The prognostic value of ambulatory blood pressures. *JAMA* 1983; 249:2792–2798.
37. Pickering TG, James GD, Boddie JC, Harshfield GA, Blank S, Laragh J: How common is white coat hypertension? *JAMA* 1988; 259:225–228.
38. Zachariah PK, Krier JD: Clinical uses of ambulatory blood pressure monitoring. *J Hypertens* 1991; 9(suppl 1):S7–S12.
39. Cox J, O'Malley K, Atkins N, O'Brien E: A comparison of the twenty-four-hour blood pressure profile in normotensive and hypertensive subjects. *J Hypertens* 1991; 9(suppl 1):S3–S6.
40. White WB, Lund-Johansen P, McCabe E, Omvik P: Clinical evaluation of the Accutracker II ambulatory blood pressure monitor: Assessment of performance in two countries and comparison with sphygmomanometry and intra-arterial blood pressure at rest and during exercise. *J Hypertens* 1989; 7:967–975.
41. Santucci S, Cates EM, James GD, Schussel YR, Steiner D, Picker-

ing TG: A comparison of two ambulatory blood pressure monitors, the Del Mar Avionics Pressurometer IV and the Spacelabs 90202. *Am J Hypertens* 1989; 2:797–799.

42. Gosse P, Roudaut R, Reynaud P, Jullien E, Dallocchio M: Relationship between left ventricular mass and noninvasive monitoring of blood pressure. *Am J Hypertens* 1989; 2:631–633.
43. Verdecchia P, Schillaci G, Boldrini F, Guerrieri M, Gatteschi C, Benemio G, et al: Risk stratification of left ventricular hypertrophy in systemic hypertension using noninvasive ambulatory blood pressure monitoring. *Am J Cardiol* 1990; 66:583–590.
44. Prisant LM, Carr AA: Ambulatory blood pressure monitoring and echocardiographic left ventricular wall thickness and mass. *Am J Hypertens* 1990; 3:81–89.
45. White WB, Schulman P, Dey HM, Katz AM: Rapid left ventricular filling is more dependent on age and twenty-four-hour blood pressure than on cardiac size. *J Hypertens* 1989; 7(suppl 6):S102–S103.
46. Giaconi S, Levanti C, Fommei E, Innocenti F, Seghieri G, Palla L, et al: Microalbuminuria and casual and ambulatory blood pressure monitoring in normotensives and in patients with borderline and mild essential hypertension. *Am J Hypertens* 1989; 2:259–261.
47. Shimada K, Kawamoto A, Matsubayashi K, Ozawa T: Silent cerebrovascular disease in the elderly. Correlation with ambulatory pressure. *Hypertension* 1990; 16:692–699.
48. 1988 Joint National Committee: The 1988 report of the Joint National Committee on detection, evaluation, and treatment of high blood pressure. *Arch Intern Med* 1988; 148:1023–1038.
49. Hall WD: Initial evaluation of the patient with hypertension. In: Wollam GL, Hall WD (eds): *Hypertension Management: Clinical Practice and Therapeutic Dilemmas*. Chicago, Year Book Medical Publishers, 1988: 145–163.
50. Gifford RW Jr, Kirkendall W, O'Conner DT, Weidman W: Office evaluation of hypertension. A statement for health professionals by a writing group of the Council for High Blood Pressure Research, American Heart Association. *Hypertension* 1989; 13:283–293.
51. Bulpitt CJ, Dollery CT, Carne S: Changes in symptoms of hypertensive patients after referral to hospital clinic. *Br Heart J* 1976; 38:121–128.
52. Working Group on Management of Patients with Hypertension and High Blood Cholesterol: National Education Programs Working Group Report on the Management of Patients with Hypertension and High Blood Cholesterol. *Ann Intern Med* 1991; 114:224–237.
53. Kannel WB, Castelli WP, McNamara PM, McKee PA, Feinleib M: Role of blood pressure in the development of congestive heart failure. *N Engl J Med* 1972; 287:781–787.
54. Shulman NB, Martinez B, Brogan D, Carr AA, Miles CG: Financial cost as an obstacle to hypertension therapy. *Am J Public Health* 1986; 76:1105–1108.
55. Roccella EJ: Cost of hypertensive medications: Is it a barrier to hypertension control? *Geriatrics* 1989; 44(suppl B):49–55.
56. Stason WB: Cost and quality trade-offs in the treatment of hypertension. *Hypertension* 1989; 13(suppl I):I145–I148.
57. Kincaid-Smith P, McMichael J, Murphy EA: The clinical course and pathology of hypertension with papilledema (malignant hypertension). *Q J Med* 1958; 105:117–153.
58. Ahmed MEK, Walker JM, Beevers DG, Beevers M: Lack of difference between malignant and accelerated hypertension. *Br Med J* 1986; 292:235–237.
59. Davis BA, Crook JE, Vestal RE, Oates JA: Prevalence of renovascular hypertension in patients with grade III or IV hypertensive retinopathy. *N Engl J Med* 1979; 301:1273–1276.
60. Julius S, Schork NA: Borderline hypertension—a critical review. *J Chronic Dis* 1971; 23:723–754.
61. Klatsky AL, Friedman GD, Siegelaub AB, Gerard MJ: Alcohol consumption and blood pressure. Kaiser-Permanente multiphasic health examination data. *N Engl J Med* 1977; 296:1194–1200.
62. Messerli FH, Frohlich ED: High blood pressure. A side effect of drugs, poisons, and food. *Arch Intern Med* 1979; 139:682–687.
63. Lichtenfeld PJ, Rubin DB, Feldman RS: Subarachnoid hemorrhage precipitated by cocaine snorting. *Arch Neurol* 1984; 41:223–224.
64. Isner JM, Estes NAM III, Thompson PD, Costanzo-Nordin MR, Subramanian R, Miller G, et al: Acute cardiac events temporally related to cocaine abuse. *N Engl J Med* 1986; 315:1438–1443.
65. Brody SL: Cocaine. Actions, abuse, and emergencies. *Emory Univ J Med* 1988; 2:257–271.
66. Virmani R, Robinowitz M, Smialek JE, Smyth DF: Cardiovascular effects of cocaine: An autopsy study of 40 patients. *Am Heart J* 1988; 115:1068–1076.
67. Lange RA, Cigarroa RG, Yancy CW Jr, Willard JE, Popma JJ, Sills MN, et al: Cocaine-induced coronary-artery vasoconstriction. *N Engl J Med* 1989; 321:1557–1562.
68. Nademanee K, Gorelick DA, Josephson MA, Ryan MA, Wilkins JN, Robertson HA, et al: Myocardial ischemia during cocaine withdrawal. *Ann Intern Med* 1989; 111:876–880.
69. Brody SL, Slovis CM, Wrenn KD: Cocaine-related medical problems: Consecutive series of 233 patients. *Am J Med* 1990; 88:325–331.
70. Blachley JD, Knochel JP: Tobacco chewer's hypokalemia: Licorice revisited. *N Engl J Med* 1980; 302:784–785.
71. Dietz AJ Jr: Amphetamine-like reactions to phenylpropanolamine. *JAMA* 1981; 245:601–602.
72. Hall WD: Isolated systolic hypertension in the elderly. *Mod Concepts Cardiovasc Dis* 1987; 56:29–33.
73. Wollam GL, Hall WD: Systolic hypertension. In: Hurst JW (ed): *The Heart*, 4th ed. New York, McGraw-Hill, 1981: 135–152.
74. Hall WD, Wollam GL: Systolic hypertension. In: Harvey WP (ed): *Current Problems in Cardiology*, vol 7 (no 6). Chicago, Year Book Medical Publishers, 1982: 1–40.
75. Sobocinski KA, Gruchow HW, Anderson AJ, Barboriak JJ: Associations of aerobic exercise and alcohol consumption with systolic blood pressure in employed males. *J Hypertens* 1986; 4(suppl 5):358–360.
76. Walther RJ, Tifft CP: High blood pressure in the competitive athlete: Guidelines and recommendations. *Phys Sports Med* 1985; 113:93–114.
77. Lichtman J, O'Rourke RA, Klein A, Karliner JS: Electrocardiogram of the athlete. Alterations simulating those of organic heart disease. *Arch Intern Med* 1973; 132:763–770.
78. Huston TP, Puffer JC, Rodney WM: The athletic heart syndrome. *N Engl J Med* 1985; 313:24–32.
79. Roeske WP, O'Rourke RA, Klein A, Leopold G, Karliner JS: Noninvasive evaluation of ventricular hypertrophy in professional athletes. *Circulation* 1976; 52:286–292.
80. Morganroth J, Maron BJ, Henry WL, Epstein SE: Comparative left ventricular dimensions in trained athletes. *Ann Intern Med* 1975; 82:521–524.
81. Oakley DG, Oakley CM: Significance of abnormal electrocardiograms in highly trained athletes. *Am J Cardiol* 1982; 50:985–989.
82. Maron BT, Roberts WC, McAllister HA, Rosing DR, Epstein SE: Sudden death in young athletes. *Circulation* 1980; 62:218–229.
83. Pelliccia A, Maron BJ, Spataro A, Proschan MA, Spirito P: The upper limit of physiologic cardiac hypertrophy in highly trained elite athletes. *N Engl J Med* 1991; 324:295–301.
84. Colan SD, Sanders SP, MacPherson D, Borow KU: Left ventricular diastolic function in elite athletes with physiologic cardiac hypertrophy. *J Am Coll Cardiol* 1985; 6:545–549.
85. Keith NM, Wagener HP, Barker ND: Some different types of essential hypertension: Their course and prognosis. *Am J Med Sci* 1939; 197:332–343.
86. van Buchem FSP, Heuvel-Aghina JWM, Heuvel JEA: Hypertension and changes in the fundus oculi. *Acta Med Scand* 1964; 176:539–548.
87. Kagan A, Aurell E, Dobree J, Hara K, McKendrick C, Michaelson I, et al: A note on signs in the fundus oculi and arterial hypertension: Conventional assessment and significance. *Bull WHO* 1966; 34:955–960.
88. Kannel WB, Gordon T, Offutt D: Left ventricular hypertrophy by electrocardiogram. Prevalence, incidence, and mortality in the Framingham Study. *Ann Intern Med* 1969; 71:89–105.
89. Dougherty AH, Naccarelli GV, Gray EL, Hicks CH, Goldstein RA: Congestive heart failure with normal systolic function. *Am J Cardiol* 1984; 54:778–782.
90. Topol EJ, Traill TA, Fortuin NJ: Hypertensive hypertrophic cardiomyopathy of the elderly. *N Engl J Med* 1985; 312:277–283.
91. Levy RD, Shapiro LM, Wright C, Mockus L, Fox KM: Syndrome X: The hemodynamic significance of ST segment depression. *Br Heart J* 1986; 56:353–357.

92. Cannon RO III, Epstein SE: "Microvascular angina" as a cause of chest pain with angiographically normal coronary arteries. *Am J Cardiol* 1988; 61:1338–1343.
93. Picano E, Lucarini AR, Lattanzi F, Marini C, Distante A, Salvetti A, et al: ST segment depression elicited by dipyrimadole infusion in asymptomatic hypertensive patients. *Hypertension* 1990; 16:19–25.
94. Opherk D, Mall G, Zebe H, Schwarz F, Weihe E, Manthey J, et al: Reduction of coronary reserve: A mechanism for angina pectoris in patients with arterial hypertension and normal coronary arteries. *Circulation* 1984; 69:1–7.
95. Hall D, Charocopos F, Froer K-L, Rudolph W: ECG changes during long-term minoxidil therapy for severe hypertension. *Arch Intern Med* 1979; 139:790–794.
96. O'Mailia JJ, Sander GE, Giles TD: Nifedipine-associated myocardial ischemia or infarction in the treatment of hypertensive urgencies. *Ann Intern Med* 1987; 107:185–186.
97. Pepi M, Alimento M, Maltagliata A, Guazzi MD: Cardiac hypertrophy in hypertension. Repolarization abnormalities elicited by rapid lowering of pressure. *Hypertension* 1988; 11:84–91.
98. Phillips RA, Goldman ME, Ardeljan M, Eison HB, Shimabukuro S, Krakoff LR: Isolated T-wave abnormalities and evaluation of left ventricular wall motion after nifedipine for severe hypertension. *Am J Hypertens* 1991; 4:432–437.
99. Guazzi MD, Alimento M, Guazzi M, Maltagliati A, Pepi M: Acute blood pressure reduction in the presence of hypertensive cardiac hypertrophy: Any interference with coronary circulation? *Scand J Clin Lab Inv* 1989; 196(suppl):53–61.
100. Davie JC, Langley JO, Dodson WH, Eddleman EE Jr: Clinical and kinetocardiographic studies of paradoxical precordial motion. *Am Heart J* 1962; 63:775–807.
101. Burchell HB: Clinical recognition of cardiac hypertrophy. *Circ Res* 1974; 35(suppl 2):116–121.
102. Eilen SD, Crawford MH, O'Rourke RA: Accuracy of precordial palpation for detecting increased left ventricular volume. *Ann Intern Med* 1983; 99:628–630.
103. Lusted LB, Keats TE: *Atlas of Roentgenographic Measurement*, 4th ed. Chicago, Year Book Medical Publishers, 1978: 225.
104. Romhilt DW, Estes EH Jr: A point-score system for the ECG diagnosis of left ventricular hypertrophy. *Am Heart J* 1968; 75:752–758.
105. Romhilt DW, Bove KE, Norris RJ, Conyers E, Conradi S, Rowlands DT, et al: A critical appraisal of the electrocardiographic criteria for the diagnosis of left ventricular hypertrophy. *Circulation* 1969; 40:185–195.
106. Carter WA, Estes EH Jr: Electrocardiographic manifestations of ventricular hypertrophy; a computer study of ECG-anatomic correlations in 319 cases. *Am Heart J* 1964; 68:173–182.
107. Murphy ML, Thenabadu PN, Soyza ND, Doherty JE, Meade J, Baker BJ, et al: Reevaluation of electrocardiographic criteria for left, right and combined cardiac ventricular hypertrophy. *Am J Cardiol* 1984; 53:1140–1147.
108. Tarazi RC, Miller A, Frohlich ED, et al: Electrocardiographic changes reflecting left atrial abnormality in hypertension. *Circulation* 1966; 34:818–822.
109. Savage DD, Drayer JIM, Henry WL, Mathews EC Jr, Ware JH, Gardin JM, et al: Echocardiographic assessment of cardiac anatomy and function in hypertensive subjects. *Circulation* 1979; 59:623–632.
110. Savage DD, Garrison RJ, Kannel WB, Levy D, Anderson SJ, Stokes J III, et al: The spectrum of left ventricular hypertrophy in a general population sample: The Framingham Study. *Circulation* 1987; 75(suppl I):I26–I33.
111. Woythaler JN, Singer SL, Kwan OL, Meltzer RS, Reubner B, Bommer W, et al: Accuracy of echocardiography in detecting left ventricular hypertrophy: Comparison with postmortem mass measurements. *J Am Coll Cardiol* 1983; 2:305–311.
112. Devereaux RB, Alonso DR, Lutas EM, Gottlieb GJ, Campo E, Sachs I, et al: Echocardiographic assessment of left ventricular hypertrophy: Comparison to necropsy findings. *Am J Cardiol* 1986; 57:450–458.
113. Dunn FG, Chandraratna P, de Carvalho JGR, Basta LL, Frohlich ED: Pathophysiologic assessment of hypertensive heart disease with echocardiography. *Am J Cardiol* 1977; 39:789–795.
114. Safar ME, Lehner JP, Vincent MI, Plainfosse MT, Simon ACh: Echocardiographic dimensions in borderline and sustained hypertension. *Am J Cardiol* 1979; 44:930–935.
115. Baker BJ, Bass KM, Scovil JA, Kane JJ, Murphy ML: M-mode echocardiographic correlates of left ventricular mass: An anatomic correlation. *J Cardiovasc Ultrasonogr* 1982; 1:263–266.
116. Levy D, Anderson KM, Savage DD, Kannel WB, Christiansen JC, Castelli WP: Echocardiographically detected left ventricular hypertrophy: Prevalence and risk factors. The Framingham Heart Study. *Ann Intern Med* 1988; 108:7–13.
117. McLenachan JM, Henderson E, Morris KI, Dargie HJ: Ventricular arrhythmias in patients with hypertensive left ventricular hypertrophy. *N Engl J Med* 1987; 317:787–792.
118. Devereux RB: Importance of left ventricular mass as a predictor of cardiovascular morbidity in hypertension. *Am J Hypertens* 1989; 2:650–654.
119. Devereux RB: Echocardiographic insights into the pathophysiology and prognostic significance of hypertensive cardiac hypertrophy. *Am J Hypertens* 1989; 2(6 Pt 2):186S–195S.
120. Levy D, Garrison RJ, Savage DD, Kannel WB, Castelli WP: Prognostic implications of echocardiography determined left ventricular mass in the Framingham Heart Study. *N Engl J Med* 1990; 322:1561–1566.
121. Koren MJ, Devereux RB, Casale PN, Savage DD, Laragh JH: Relation of left ventricular mass and geometry to morbidity and mortality in uncomplicated essential hypertension. *Ann Intern Med* 1991; 114:345–352.
122. Wollam GL, Hall WD, Porter VD, Douglas MB, Unger DJ, Blumenstein BA, et al: Time course of regression of left ventricular hypertrophy in treated hypertensive patients. *Am J Med* 1983; 75(suppl 3A):100–110.
123. Wollam GL, Schlant RC, Hall WD: Hypertensive heart disease. In: Wollam GL, Hall WD (eds): *Hypertension Management: Clinical Practice and Therapeutic Dilemmas*. Chicago, Year Book Medical Publishers, 1988: 164–199.
124. Liebson PR: Clinical studies of drug reversal of hypertensive left ventricular hypertrophy. *Am J Hypertens* 1990; 3:512–517.
125. Moser M: "Cost containment" in the management of hypertension. *Ann Intern Med* 1987; 107:107–108.
126. Kannel WB, Wolf PA, Verter J, McNamara PM: Epidemiologic assessment of the role of blood pressure in stroke. The Framingham Study. *JAMA* 1970; 214:301–310.
127. Cuneo RH, Caronna JJ: The neurologic complications of hypertension. *Med Clin North Am* 1977; 61:565–580.
128. Tuszynski MH, Petito CK, Levy DE: Risk factors and clinical manifestations of pathologically verified lacunar infarctions. *Stroke* 1989; 20:990–999.
129. Weisberg LA: Computed tomography in the diagnosis of intracranial disease. *Ann Intern Med* 1979; 91:87–105.
130. Cramer BC, Parfrey PS, Hutchinson TA, Baran D, Melanson DM, Ethier RE, et al: Renal function following infusion of radiologic contrast material. A prospective controlled study. *Arch Intern Med* 1985; 145:87–89.
131. Ram CVS: Hypertensive encephalopathy. Recognition and management. *Arch Intern Med* 1978; 138:1851–1853.
132. Chester EM, Agamanolis DP, Banker BQ, Victor M: Hypertensive encephalopathy: A clinicopathologic study of 20 cases. *Neurology (NY)* 1978; 28:928–939.
133. Goldring W, Chasis H, Ranges HA, Smith HW: Effective renal blood flow in subjects with essential hypertension. *J Clin Invest* 1941; 20:637–653.
134. Schalekamp MADH, Krauss XH, Schalekamp-Kuyken MPA, Kolster SG, Birkenhager WH: Studies on the mechanism of hypernatriuresis in essential hypertension in relation to measurements of plasma renin concentration, body fluid compartments, and renal function. *Clin Sci* 1971; 41:219–231.
135. Firth JD, Raine AEG, Ledingham JGG: The mechanism of pressure natriuresis. *J Hypertens* 1990; 8:97–103.
136. Schmieder RE, Messerli FH, Garavaglia G, Nunez B: Glomerular hyperfiltration indicates early target organ damage in essential hypertension. *JAMA* 1990; 264:2775–2780.
137. Odutola TA, Ositelu SB, D'Almeida EA, Okeiyi JC: Supra-normal creatinine clearance in black mild hypertensive patients in Nigeria. *J Human Hypertens* 1988; 2:133–134.
138. Pedersen EB, Mogensen CE: Effect of antihypertensive treatment on urinary albumin excretion, glomerular filtration rate and renal plasma flow in patients with essential hypertension. *Scand J Clin Lab Invest* 1976; 36:231–237.
139. Cerasola G, Cottone S, D'Ignoto G, Grasso L, Mangano MT, Carapelle E, et al: Micro-albuminuria as a predictor of cardiovas-

cular damage in essential hypertension. *J Hypertens* 1989; 7(suppl 6):S332–S333.
140. Ljungman S: Microalbuminuria in essential hypertension. *Am J Hypertens* 1990; 3:956–960.
141. Bianchi S, Bigazzi R, Baldari G, Campese VM: Microalbuminuria in patients with essential hypertension. Effects of an angiotensin converting enzyme inhibitor and of a calcium channel blocker. *Am J Hypertens* 1991; 4:291–296.
142. Tobian L: Does essential hypertension lead to renal failure? *Am J Cardiol* 1987; 60:42I–46I.
143. National High Blood Pressure Working Group: Report on Hypertension and Chronic Renal Failure. U.S. Department of Health and Human Services, NIH Publication No. 90-3032, August 1990: 1–20.
144. Battey LL, Felner JM, Hall WD: Clinical manifestations of 104 patients with diastolic blood pressure ≥ 140 mmHg. *Emory Univ J Med* 1988; 2:102–105.
145. Gifford RW Jr: Evaluation of the hypertensive patient with emphasis on detecting curable causes. *Milbank Mem Fund Q* 1969; 47:170–186.
146. Kennedy AC, Luke RG, Briggs JD, Barr Sterling W: Detection of renovascular hypertension. *Lancet* 1965; 2:963–968.
147. Ferguson RK: Cost and yield of the hypertensive evaluation: Experience of a community-based referral clinic. *Ann Intern Med* 1975; 82:761–765.
148. Bech K, Hilden T: The frequency of secondary hypertension. *Acta Med Scand* 1975; 197:65–69.
149. Berglund G, Andersson O, Wilhelmsen L: Prevalence of primary and secondary hypertension: Studies in a random population sample. *Br Med J* 1976; 2:554–556.
150. Tucker RM, Labarthe DR: Frequency of surgical treatment for hypertension in adults at the Mayo Clinic from 1973 through 1975. *Mayo Clin Proc* 1977; 52:549–555.
151. Maxwell MH, Bleifer KH, Franklin SS, Varady PD: Cooperative study of renovascular hypertension. Demographic analysis of the study. *JAMA* 1972; 220:1195–1204.
152. Hall WD: Secondary causes of hypertension in blacks. In: Hall WD, Saunders E, Shulman NB (eds): *Hypertension in Blacks: Epidemiology, Pathophysiology and Treatment.* Chicago, Year Book Medical Publishers, 1985: 144–155.
153. Simon N, Franklin SS, Bleifer KH, Maxwell MH: Clinical characteristics of renovascular hypertension. *JAMA* 1972; 220:1209–1216.
154. Eipper DF, Gifford RW, Jr, Stewart BH, Alfidi RJ, McCormack LJ, Vidt DG: Abdominal bruits in renovascular hypertension. *Am J Cardiol* 1976; 37:48–52.
155. Shapiro AP, Perez-Stable E, Moutsos SE: Coexistence of renal arterial hypertension and diabetes mellitus. *JAMA* 1965; 192:813–816.
156. Working Group on Renovascular Hypertension: Detection, evaluation, and treatment of renovascular hypertension. Final report. *Arch Intern Med* 1987; 147:820–829.
157. Olin JW, Vidt DG, Gifford RW Jr, Novick AC: Renovascular disease in the elderly: An analysis of 50 patients. *J Am Coll Cardiol* 1985; 5:1232–1238.
158. Novick AC, Pohl MA, Schreiber M, Gifford RW Jr, Vidt DG: Revascularization for preservation of renal function in patients with atherosclerotic renovascular disease. *J Urol* 1983; 129:907–911.
159. Sos TA, Pickering TG, Sniderman K, Saddenki S, Case DB, Silane MF, et al: Percutaneous transluminal renal angioplasty in renovascular hypertension due to atheroma or fibromuscular dysplasia. *N Engl J Med* 1983; 309:274–279.
160. Ying CY, Tifft CP, Gavras H, Chobanian AV: Renal revascularization in the azotemic hypertensive patient resistant to therapy. *N Engl J Med* 1984; 311:1070–1075.
161. Frommei E, Ghione S, Palla L, Mesca F, Ferrari M, Palombo C, et al: Renal scintigraphic captopril test in the diagnosis of renovascular hypertension. *Hypertension* 1987; 10:212–220.
162. Geyskes GG, Oei HY, Puylaert CBAJ, Dorhout Mees EJ: Renovascular hypertension identified by captopril-induced changes in the renogram. *Hypertension* 1987; 9:451–458.
163. Bookstein JJ, Abrams HL, Buenger RE, Lecky J, Franklin SS, Reiss MD, et al: Radiologic aspects of renovascular hypertension. Part 2. The role of urography in unilateral renovascular disease. *JAMA* 1972; 220:1225–1230.
164. Pollack HM, Banner MP: Current status of excretory urography. A premature epitaph? *Urol Clin North Am* 1985; 12:585–601.
165. Mushlin AI, Thornbury JR: Intravenous pyelography: The case against its routine use. *Ann Intern Med* 1989; 111:58–70.
166. Buonocore E, Meaney TF, Borkowski GP, Pavlicek W, Gallagher J: Digital subtraction angiography of the abdominal aorta and renal arteries. Comparison with conventional aortography. *Radiology* 1981; 139:281–286.
167. Smith CW, Winfield AC, Price RR, Harding DR, Tucker SW, Witt WS, et al: Evaluation of digital venous angiography for the diagnosis of renovascular hypertension. *Radiology* 1982; 144:51–54.
168. Fiedler V, Peters PE: Digital subtraction angiography of renal arteries—pitfalls and benefits. *Cardiology* 1985; 72(suppl 1):10–12.
169. Berkseth RO, Kjellstrand CM: Radiologic contrast-induced nephropathy. *Med Clin North Am* 1984; 65:351–370.
170. Lyons DF, Streck WF, Kem DC, Brown RD, Galloway DC, Williams GR, et al: Captopril stimulation of differential renins in renovascular hypertension. *Hypertension* 1983; 5:615–622.
171. Thibonnier M, Joseph A, Sassano P, Guyenne TT, Corvol P, Raynaud A, et al: Improved diagnosis of unilateral renal artery lesions after captopril administration. *JAMA* 1984; 251:56–60.
172. Tomoda F, Takata M, Ohashi S, Veno H, Ikeda K, Yasumoto K, et al: Captopril-stimulated renal vein renin in hypertensive patients with or without renal artery stenosis. *Am J Hypertens* 1990; 3:918–926.
173. Hricik DE, Browning PJ, Kopelman R, Goorno WE, Madias NE, Dzau VJ: Captopril-induced functional renal insufficiency in patients with bilateral renal-artery stenosis or renal-artery stenosis in a solitary kidney. *N Engl J Med* 1983; 308:373–376.
174. Fotino S, Sporn P: Nonoliguric acute renal failure after captopril therapy. *Arch Intern Med* 1983; 143:1252–1253.
175. Strong CG, Hunt JC, Sheps SG, Tucker RM, Bernatz PE: Renal venous renin activity: Enhancement of sensitivity of lateralization by sodium depletion. *Am J Cardiol* 1971; 27:602–611.
176. Maxwell MH, Marks LS, Lupu AN, Cahill PJ, Franklin SS, Kaufman JJ: Predictive value of renin determinations in renal artery stenosis. *JAMA* 1977; 238:2617–2620.
177. Vaughan ED Jr, Buhler FR, Laragh JH, Sealey JE, Baer L, Bard RH: Renovascular hypertension: Renin measurements to indicate hypersecretion and contralateral suppression, estimate renal plasma flow, and score for surgical curability. *Am J Med* 1973; 55:402–414.
178. Marks LS, Maxwell MH, Varady PD, Lupu AN, Kaufman JJ: Renovascular hypertension: Does the renal vein renin ratio predict operative results? *J Urol* 1976; 115:365–368.
179. Sellars L, Siamopoulos K, Hacking PM, Proud G, Taylor RMR, Essenhigh DM, et al: Renovascular hypertension: Ten years' experience in a regional center. *Q J Med* 1985; 56:403–416.
180. Lüscher TF, Greminger P, Kuhlmann U, Siegenthaler W, Largiader F, Vetter W: Renal venous renin determinations in renovascular hypertension. *Nephron* 1986; 44(suppl 1):17–24.
181. Wollam GL: Renovascular hypertension. In: Wollam GL, Hall WD (eds): *Hypertension Management: Clinical Practice and Therapeutic Dilemmas.* Chicago, Year Book Medical Publishers, 1988: 228–259.
182. Grim CE, Luft FC, Weinberger MH, Grim CM: Sensitivity and specificity of screening tests for renal vascular hypertension. *Ann Intern Med* 1979; 91:617–622.
183. Muller FB, Sealey JE, Case DB, Atlas SA, Pickering TG, Pecker MS, et al: The captopril test for identifying renovascular disease in hypertensive patients. *Am J Med* 1986; 80:633–644.
184. Hawkins PG, McKnoulty LM, Gordon RD, Klemm SA, Tunny TJ: Noninvasive renal artery duplex ultrasound and computerized nuclear renography to screen for and follow progress in renal artery stenosis. *J Hypertens* 1989; 7(suppl 6):S184–S185.
185. Taylor DC: Duplex ultrasound in the assessment of vascular disease in clinical hypertension. *Am J Hypertens* 1991; 4:550–556.
186. Lemann J Jr: Diagnostic value of urinalysis in patients with hypertension. *Am J Surg* 1964; 107:38–42.
187. Birkenhäger WH, Schalekamp MADH, Schalekamp-Kuyken MPA, Kolsters G, Krauss XH: Interrelations between arterial pressure, fluid-volumes, and plasma renin concentration in the course of acute glomerulonephritis. *Lancet* 1970; 1:1086–1087.

188. Abuelo JG: Proteinuria: Diagnostic principles and procedures. *Ann Intern Med* 1983; 98:186–191.
189. Meltzer JS, Keim HJ, Laragh JH, Sealey JE, Jan K-M, Chien S: Nephrotic syndrome: Vasoconstriction and hypervolemic types indicated by renin-sodium profiling. *Ann Intern Med* 1979; 91:688–696.
190. Conn JW: Primary aldosteronism and primary reninism. *Hosp Pract* 1974; 9:131–140.
191. Conn JW, Knopf RF, Nesbit RM: Clinical characteristics of primary aldosteronism from an analysis of 145 cases. *Am J Surg* 1964; 107:159–172.
192. Ferriss JB, Beevers DG, Brown JJ, Davies DL, Fraser R, Lever AF, et al: Clinical, biochemical and pathological features of low-renin ("primary") hyperaldosteronism. *Am Heart J* 1978; 95:375–388.
193. Biglieri EG, Slaton PE Jr: Pregnancy and primary aldosteronism. *J Clin Endocrinol Metab* 1967; 27:1628–1632.
194. Drucker WD, Hendrikx A, Laragh JH, Christy NP, Vande Wiele RL: Effect of administered aldosterone upon electrolyte excretion during and after pregnancy in two women with adrenal cortical insufficiency. *J Clin Endocrinol Metab* 1963; 23:1247–1255.
195. Mader IJ, Iseri LT: Spontaneous hypopotassemia, hypomagnesemia, alkalosis and tetany due to hypersecretion of corticosterone-like mineralocorticoid. *Am J Med* 1955; 19:976–988.
196. Fishman LM, Kuchel O, Liddle GW, Michelakis AM, Gordon RD, Chick WT: Incidence of primary aldosteronism uncomplicated "essential" hypertension. A prospective study with elevated aldosterone secretion and suppressed plasma renin activity used as diagnostic criteria. *JAMA* 1968; 205:497–502.
197. Kaplan NM: Hypokalemia in the hypertensive patient: With observations on the incidence of primary aldosteronism. *Ann Intern Med* 1967; 66:1079–1090.
198. Conn JW, Cohen EL, Rovner DR, Nesbit RM: Normokalemic primary aldosteronism. A detectable cause of curable "essential" hypertension. *JAMA* 1965; 193:200–206.
199. Kaplan NM: Primary aldosteronism. In: Kaplan NM (ed): *Clinical Hypertension*, 5th ed. Baltimore, Williams and Wilkins, 1990: 368–385.
200. Biglieri EG: Spectrum of mineralocorticoid hypertension. *Hypertension* 1991; 17:251–261.
201. Biglieri EG, Stockigt JR, Schambelan M: Adrenal mineralocorticoids causing hypertension. *Am J Med* 1972; 52:623–632.
202. Stewart PM, Wallace AM, Valentino R, Burt D, Shackleton CHL, Edwards CRW: Mineralocorticoid activity in licorice: 11-Beta-hydroxysteroid dehydrogenase deficiency comes of age. *Lancet* 1987; 2:821–824.
203. Mantero F, Armanini D, Opocher G, Fallo F, Sampier L, Cuspidi B, et al: Mineralocorticoid hypertension due to a nasal spray containing 9α-fluoroprednisolone. *Am J Med* 1981; 71:352–357.
204. Weinberger MH, Grim CE, Hollifield JW, Kem DC, Ganguly A, Kramer NJ, et al: Primary aldosteronism. Diagnosis, localization, treatment. *Ann Intern Med* 1979; 90:386–395.
205. Weinberger MH: Primary aldosteronism: Diagnosis and differentiation of subtypes. *Ann Intern Med* 1984; 100:300–302.
206. Hiramatsu K, Yamada T, Yukimura Y, Komiya I, Ichikawa K, Ishihara M, et al: A screening test to identify aldosterone-producing adenoma by measuring plasma renin activity. Results in hypertensive patients. *Arch Intern Med* 1981; 141:1589–1593.
207. Lyons DF, Kem DC, Brown RD, Hanson CS, Carollo ML: Single dose captopril as a diagnostic test for primary aldosteronism. *J Clin Endocrinol Metab* 1983; 57:892–896.
208. Ganguly A, Melada GA, Luetscher JA, Dowdy AJ: Control of plasma aldosterone in primary aldosteronism: Distinction between adenoma and hyperplasia. *J Clin Endocrinol Metab* 1973; 37:765–775.
209. Bravo EL: The syndrome of primary aldosteronism and pheochromocytoma. In: Schrier RW, Gottschalk CW (eds): *Diseases of the Kidney*, 4th ed. Boston, Little, Brown, 1988: 1623–1651.
210. Franco-Saenz R, Mulrow PJ, Kim K: Idiopathic aldosteronism. A possible disease of the intermediate lobe of the pituitary. *JAMA* 1984; 251:2555–2558.
211. Sen S, Valenzuela R, Smeby R, Bravo EL, Bumpus FM: Localization, purification, and biological activity of a new aldosterone-stimulating factor. *Hypertension* 1981; 3(suppl 1):81–86.
212. Saito I, Saruta T: Regulation of aldosterone secretion by a new aldosterone stimulating factor. *Jpn Circ J* 1982; 46:523–530.
213. Carey RM, Sen S, Dolan LM, Malchoff CD, Bumpus FM: Idiopathic hyperaldosteronism. A possible role for aldosterone-stimulating factor. *N Engl J Med* 1984; 311:94–100.
214. Oberfield SE, Levine LS, Firpo A, Lawrence D, Stoner E, Levy DJ, et al: Primary aldosteronism in childhood due to unilateral macronodular hyperplasia. *Hypertension* 1984; 6:75–84.
215. Irony I, Kater CE, Biglieri EG, Shackleton CHL: Correctable subsets of primary aldosteronism. Primary adrenal hyperplasia and renin responsive adenoma. *Am J Hypertens* 1990; 3:576–582.
216. Giebink GS, Gotlin RW, Biglieri EG, Katz FH: A kindred with familial glucocorticoid-suppressible aldosteronism. *J Clin Endocrinol Metab* 1973; 36:715–723.
217. Ganguly A: Glucocorticoid-suppressible hyperaldosteronism: An update. *Am J Med* 1990; 88:321–324.
218. Levinson PD, Zadik Z, Hamilton BPM, Mersey JH, White RI, Kowarski AA: Adrenal vein epinephrine levels: A useful aid in venous sampling for primary aldosteronism. *Ann Intern Med* 1982; 97:690–693.
219. Gross MD, Shapiro B, Grekin RJ, Freitas JE, Glazer G, Beierwaltes WH, et al: Scintigraphic localization of adrenal lesions in primary aldosteronism. *Am J Med* 1984; 77:839–844.
220. Gross MD, Shapiro B: Scintigraphic studies in adrenal hypertension. *Semin Nuc Med* 1989; 19:122–143.
221. Biglieri EG, Schambelan M: The significance of elevated levels of plasma 18-hydroxycorticosterone in patients with primary aldosteronism. *J Clin Endocrinol Metab* 1979; 49:87–91.
222. Manger WM, Gifford RW Jr: *Pheochromocytoma.* New York, Springer-Verlag, 1977.
223. Remine WH, Chong GC, van Heerden JA, Sheps SG, Harrison EG Jr: Current management of pheochromocytoma. *Ann Surg* 1974; 179:740–748.
224. DeOreo GA Jr, Stewart BH, Tarazi RC, Gifford RW Jr: Preoperative blood transfusion in the safe surgical management of pheochromocytoma: A review of 46 cases. *J Urol* 1974; 111:715–721.
225. Sjoerdsma A, Engelman K, Waldmann TA, Cooperman LH, Hammond WG: Pheochromocytoma: Current concepts of diagnosis and treatment. *Ann Intern Med* 1966; 65:1302–1326.
226. Gitlow SE, Mendlowitz M, Bertani LM: The biochemical techniques for detecting and establishing the presence of a pheochromocytoma: A review of ten years' experience. *Am J Cardiol* 1970; 26:270–278.
227. Kaplan NM, Kramer NJ, Holland OB, Sheps SG, Gomez-Sanchez C: Single-voided urine metanephrine assays in screening for pheochromocytoma. *Arch Intern Med* 1977; 137:190–193.
228. Miller R, Stark DCC, Gitlow SE: Paroxysmal hyperadrenergic state. A case during surgery for intracranial aneurysm. *Anaesthesia* 1976; 31:743–749.
229. Sheps S, Van Heerden J, Sheedy P II: Current approach to the diagnosis of pheochromocytoma. In: Blaufox MD, Bianchi C (eds): *Secondary Forms of Hypertension. Current Diagnosis and Management.* New York, Grune & Stratton, 1981: 11–18.
230. Gifford RW Jr, Manger WM, Bravo EL: Pheochromocytoma. In: Wollam GL, Hall WD (eds): *Hypertension Management: Clinical Practice and Therapeutic Dilemmas.* Chicago, Year Book Medical Publishers, 1988: 291–302.
231. Engelman K, Portnoy B, Sjoerdsma A: Plasma catecholamine concentrations in patients with hypertension. *Circ Res* 1970; 27(suppl 1):141–146.
232. Bravo EL, Tarazi RC, Gifford RW, Stewart BH: Circulating and urinary catecholamines in pheochromocytoma. Diagnostic and pathophysiologic implications. *N Engl J Med* 1979; 301:682–686.
233. Bravo EL: Diagnosis of pheochromocytoma. Reflections on a controversy. *Hypertension* 1991; 17:742–744.
234. Karlsberg RP, Cryer PE, Roberts R: Serial plasma catecholamine response early in the course of clinical acute myocardial infarction: Relationship to infarct extent and mortality. *Am Heart J* 1981; 102:24–29.
235. Mueller HS, Ayres SM: Propranolol decreases sympathetic nervous activity reflected by plasma catecholamines during evolution of myocardial infarction in man. *J Clin Invest* 1980; 65:338–346.
236. Benedict CR, Loach AB: Sympathetic nervous system activity in patients with subarachnoid hemorrhage. *Stroke* 1978; 9:237–244.

237. Hansson L, Hunyor SN, Julius S, Hoobler SW: Blood pressure crisis following withdrawal of clonidine (Catapres, Catapresan), with special reference to arterial and urinary catecholamine levels, and suggestions for acute management. *Am Heart J* 1973; 85:605–610.
238. Weidmann P, Beretta-Piccoli C, Meier A, Kuesch G, Gluck Z, Ziegler WH: Antihypertensive mechanism of diuretic treatment with chlorthalidone. Complementary roles of sympathetic axis and sodium. *Kidney Int* 1983; 23:320–326.
239. Murphy MB, Scriven AJ, Brown MJ, Causon R, Dollery CT: The effects of nifedipine and hydralazine induced hypotension on sympathetic activity. *Eur J Clin Pharmacol* 1982; 23:479–482.
240. Lin M-S, McNay JL, Shepherd AMM, Musgrave GE, Keeton TK: Increased plasma norepinephrine accompanies persistent tachycardia after hydralazine. *Hypertension* 1983; 5:257–263.
241. Klein W, Brandt D, Vrecko K, Haaringer M: Role of calcium antagonists in the treatment of essential hypertension. *Circ Res* 1983; 52(suppl 1):174–181.
242. Richards DA: Labetalol and urinary catecholamines (letter). *Br Med J* 1979; 1:165.
243. Izzo JL Jr, Horwitz D, Keiser HR: Physiologic mechanisms opposing the hemodynamic effects of prazosin. *Clin Pharmacol Ther* 1981; 29:7–11.
244. Inouye I, Massie B, Benowitz N, Simpson P, Loge D, Topic N: Monotherapy in mild to moderate hypertension: Comparison of hydrochlorothiazide, propranolol and prazosin. *Am J Cardiol* 1984; 53 (Proceedings of a symposium):24A–28A.
245. Proye C, Fossati P, Fontaine P, Lefebvre J, Decoulx M, Wemeau JL, et al: Dopamine-secreting pheochromocytoma: An unrecognized entity? Classification of pheochromocytomas according to their type of secretion. *Surgery* 1986; 100:1154–1162.
246. Kuchel O, Buu NT, Larochelle P, Hamet P, Genest J Jr: Episodic dopamine discharge in paroxysmal hypertension. Page's syndrome revisited. *Arch Intern Med* 1986; 146:1315–1320.
247. Bravo EL, Tarazi RC, Fouad FM, Vidt DG, Gifford RW Jr: Clonidine-suppression test. A useful aid in the diagnosis of pheochromocytoma. *N Engl J Med* 1981; 305:623–626.
248. Metz SA, Halter JB, Porte D Jr, Robertson RP: Autonomic epilepsy: Clonidine blockade of paroxysmal catecholamine release and flushing. *Ann Intern Med* 1978; 88:189–193.
249. Halter JB, Beard JC, Pfeifer MA, Metz SA: Clonidine-suppression test for diagnosis of pheochromocytoma (letter). *N Engl J Med* 1982; 306:49–50.
250. Dupont AG, Velkeniers B, Somers G, Gerlo E, Vanhaelst L: Unusual clonidine-suppression test in an epinephrine-secreting pheochromocytoma (letter). *N Engl J Med* 1984; 310:266.
251. Elliott WJ, Murphy MB: Reduced specificity of the clonidine suppression test in patients with normal plasma catecholamine levels. *Am J Med* 1988; 84:419–424.
252. Stewart BH, Bravo EL, Haaga J, Meaney TF, Tarazi R: Localization of pheochromocytoma by computed tomography. *N Engl J Med* 1978; 299:460–461.
253. Ganguly A, Henry DP, Yune HY, Pratt JH, Grim CE, Donohue JP, et al: Diagnosis and localization of pheochromocytoma. Detection by measurement of urinary norepinephrine excretion during sleep, plasma norepinephrine concentration and computerized axial tomography (CT-scan). *Am J Med* 1979; 67:21–26.
254. Sisson JC, Frager MS, Valk TW, Gross MD, Swanson DP, Wieland DM, et al: Scintigraphic localization of pheochromocytoma. *N Engl J Med* 1981; 305:12–17.
255. Swensen SJ, Brown ML, Sheps SG, Sizemore GW, Gharib H, Grant CS, et al: Use of ^{131}I-MIBG scintigraphy in the evaluation of suspected pheochromocytoma. *Mayo Clin Proc* 1985; 60:299–304.
256. Velchik MG, Alavi A, Kressel HY, Engelman K: Localization of pheochromocytoma: MIBG, CT, and MRI correlation. *J Nucl Med* 1989; 30:328–336.

Chapter 77

Treatment of Patients with Systemic Arterial Hypertension

Ray W. Gifford, Jr., M.D.

Identifying and managing patients with hypertension and other risk factors are important to prevent or postpone morbidity and mortality from cardiovascular disease, including stroke, atherosclerotic heart disease, congestive heart failure, and end-stage renal disease.

Many hypertensive patients have additional risk factors such as hyperlipoproteinemia, glucose intolerance, cigarette smoking, and obesity that should also be treated.

Appropriate management of hypertension requires knowledge of the pharmacology and side effects of the drugs, the severity of hypertension, and the presence or absence of target organ disease. In addition, the physician and the therapeutic team must foster adherence to life-long regimens by being sympathetic, understanding, patient, and persuasive; office visits must be opportunities not only to reinforce the importance of adherence but also to measure the blood pressure, elicit symptoms of target organ involvement, and inquire about side effects.

Although effective treatment of hypertension will reduce cardiovascular morbidity and mortality,[1,2] only 21 percent of the 50 million hypertensive patients in the United States have their blood pressures controlled to less than 140/90 mmHg.[3]

WHEN TO START TREATMENT

Not all hypertensive patients require drug therapy. Recommendations from the fourth and fifth Joint National Committee reports[3,4] suggest that a 3- to 6-month trial of life-style modifications be prescribed for patients whose diastolic blood pressure averages 90 to 94 mmHg and who have no evidence of target organ disease (Table 77-1). If the diastolic blood pressure can be controlled (<90 mmHg) on a hygienic regimen, drug treatment is unnecessary but close follow-up is required. If diastolic pressure is unaffected by life-style modifications, the addition of an appropriate antihypertensive drug should be considered. In making this decision, the older the patient, the higher the systolic blood pressure, and the greater the burden of additional risk factors (including male gender, Black race, and family history of premature cardiovascular disease), the stronger the case for prescribing drugs.

Some authorities do not recommend pharmacologic treatment for patients with diastolic blood pressure of 90 to 94 mmHg in the absence of target organ disease or other risk factors. The Hypertension Detection and Follow-up Program (HDFP) showed a 22 percent reduction in all-cause 5-year mortality comparing the stepped care or intensively treated group to the referred care or control group when pretreatment diastolic blood pressure was 90 to 94 mmHg.[5] Furthermore, it is perilous to wait for evidence of target organ disease before starting drug treatment for patients with mild (stage 1) hypertension because the 5-year mortality rate was more than three times higher for HDFP participants who had evidence of target organ disease before medical treatment was started than it was for those who did not, even in the stepped care or intensively treated group.[5]

TABLE 77-1
Indications for Drug Treatment of Hypertension

Diastolic Blood Pressure (mmHg)	Target Organ Damage		Other Major Risk Factors	
	Present	Absent	Present	Absent
85–89	No	No	No	No
90–94*	Yes	?	Yes	?
95–100	Yes	Yes*	Yes	Yes*
> 100	Yes	Yes	Yes	Yes

No = no pharmacologic treatment indicated; yes = pharmacologic treatment indicated.
*Three- to 6-month trial of nonpharmacologic therapy indicated first.

If the decision is made not to prescribe drug treatment for patients with diastolic blood pressure of 90 to 94 mmHg, the physician is obligated to follow them just as closely as if they were on medication because they are at considerable risk of blood pressure rising to higher levels.

There is consensus that drug treatment is indicated for most hypertensive patients whose diastolic blood pressure averages 95 to 99 mmHg even in the absence of other risk factors or evidence of target organ disease if a 3- to 6-month trial of nonpharmacologic intervention has failed. When diastolic blood pressure averages 100 mmHg or more, drug treatment along with life-style modifications should be prescribed from the outset.

Persons whose diastolic blood pressure averages 85 to 89 mmHg and systolic blood pressure averages less than 140 mmHg are in a "high-normal" category and should be under closer surveillance than people with diastolic blood pressure below 85 mmHg because they are at higher risk for cardiovascular complications and they are more likely to develop higher diastolic blood pressures that will require drug treatment. There is some evidence that life-style modifications such as dietary sodium restriction, weight reduction when appropriate, reduction of alcohol intake, and aerobic exercise may delay or prevent the onset of diastolic hypertension for some people in this group,[3,6,7] but drug treatment is not indicated.

Elderly patients with isolated systolic hypertension (≥160/<90 mmHg) also benefit from pharmacologic treatment.[8] Nonpharmacologic treatment may be tried initially for those with systolic blood pressure of 160 to 180 mmHg with no cardiovascular complications and no other risk factors, but if it fails to reduce systolic blood pressure to less than 150 mmHg within 6 months, drugs should be introduced (see the section on hypertension in the elderly).

LIFE-STYLE MODIFICATIONS

Although it will have little or no effect on blood pressure, cessation of cigarette smoking will have a proximate and significant impact to reduce risk of cardiovascular disease, especially for the hypertensive patient.

Mild hypertension can sometimes be controlled with dietary sodium restriction, weight reduction for the obese, modification of alcohol intake to no more than the equivalent of 1 oz of ethanol daily, and regular exercise.[3,9–14]

In the Treatment of Mild Hypertension Study (TOMHS), a nonpharmacologic approach reduced average blood pressure from 141/91 mmHg to 130/83 mmHg for 234 participants after 1 year.[10] Drug treatment plus the hygienic regimen was more effective in reducing blood pressure and in achieving normotension than was the hygienic regimen plus placebo. The background of nonpharmacologic treatment seemed to make control of hypertension possible with smaller than expected doses of drugs. In the Trial of Antihypertensive Interventions and Management (TAIM) Study, weight loss enhanced the antihypertensive response to both chlorthalidone and atenolol, but dietary sodium restriction did not.[13] Weight reduction in excess of 4.5 kg or sodium restriction to less than 70 meq daily was equally effective to drug treatment without dietary modification.[13] Weight reduction, dietary sodium restriction, and increased physical activity have been effective in reducing systolic and diastolic blood pressure for elderly patients with stage 1 hypertension.[14]

Perhaps 50 to 60 percent of hypertensive patients will not respond to dietary sodium control. Nevertheless, a trial of low-sodium diet (<2 g sodium or <5 g sodium chloride) is worthwhile for most patients with hypertension; for responders with mild hypertension it may obviate the need for drug therapy.[9,15] If diastolic blood pressure is not reduced after 8 to 12 weeks, adherence to the diet should be verified by measuring 24-h urinary sodium excretion. If urinary sodium is below 90 meq/24 h, it suggests that the patient is indeed adhering to the diet and that the hypertension is not sodium sensitive. On the other hand, if the patient appears to be noncompliant, this should be discussed and further instructions may be helpful.

Weight reduction for obese patients is effective in reducing blood pressure even if dietary sodium is not restricted.[16–19] The beneficial effect on blood pressure is realized before ideal body weight is achieved.[19,20] Behavioral modification is often necessary to motivate patients to reduce their weight, and it is even more important in maintaining weight reduction once achieved.

Increasing the intake of potassium has been shown to have a modest effect to reduce blood pressure in some patients.[21] It seems to enhance the antihypertensive effect of dietary sodium restriction, perhaps by promoting natriuresis.

Although calcium supplementation has been advocated as part of a nonpharmacologic approach to control hypertension, the effectiveness of this cation has not been documented as well as has reduction of dietary sodium.[9]

Excessive alcohol intake tends to raise blood pressure and to counteract the antihypertensive effect of drugs, even for patients who are not alcoholics.[22,23] Furthermore, alcoholic patients are often noncompliant with treatment regimens. The effect on blood pressure is reversible, so that excessive alcohol intake is potentially a curable cause of hypertension. Alcohol intake should be restricted to no more than 30 mL (1 oz) of ethanol daily, which is equivalent to 60 mL (2 oz) of 100-proof whiskey, 240 mL (8 oz) of wine, or 720 mL (24 oz) of beer.[4]

While some studies have shown that regular aerobic exercise has a modest effect in reducing blood pressure,[24] this is lost if training is not maintained. Exercise is an important adjunct to diet for weight control.

Control of stress by hypnosis, biofeedback, relaxation response, and similar modalities has not been shown to have a lasting or important beneficial effect on blood pressure, but well-controlled studies are lacking.[3,9,12]

In the Trial of Hypertension Prevention, a low-sodium diet and weight reduction were effective in reducing blood pressure while stress management and supplementation with calcium, potassium, magnesium, and fish oil were not.[7]

A major disadvantage of the nonpharmacologic approaches to management of hypertension is nonadherence to regimens that require life-style changes. Most patients would rather take medication than alter their diets. Behavior modification is difficult to achieve and maintain, which greatly limits the effectiveness of nonpharmacologic/hygienic management.

PHARMACOLOGIC TREATMENT

The concept of *stepped care* in managing hypertension was introduced in the "Database for Effective Antihypertensive Therapy,"[25] which was the first publication by the National High Blood Pressure Education Program offering guidelines to physicians for treatment of hypertension. It was the forerunner of the Joint National Committee (JNC) reports on detection, evaluation, and treatment. At that time the only available choices among antihypertensive drugs were ganglion-blocking agents, guanethidine, hydralazine, methyldopa, reserpine, and thiazide diuretics. Given the limited choices, it is not difficult to understand that a thiazide diuretic was selected as the step 1 drug of choice. Unfortunately, those not familiar with the genesis of the stepped care approach have come to equate stepped care with "diuretic-based" treatment. Nothing is farther from the truth. The "Database Task Force" clearly defined stepped care in the original publication as follows: "It calls for beginning therapy with a small dose of an antihypertensive drug, increasing the dose of that drug, and then adding, one after another, additional drugs as needed."[25] This generic definition permits building a regimen, the ingredients of which will change as new agents are introduced and older ones are discarded.

With the advent of new classes of drugs, such as the beta-adrenergic blockers, calcium antagonists, and angiotensin converting enzyme (ACE) inhibitors, none of which were available and/or approved for hypertension in 1973, subsequent JNC reports[3,4] have broadened the selection for step 1 to include not only the diuretics but also the beta blockers, including the alpha and beta blocker labetalol, the ACE inhibitors, the calcium antagonists, and the alpha$_1$-adrenergic blockers. Furthermore, subsequent JNC reports have also made stepped care more flexible by offering the option of *substituting* another step 1 drug if the first choice fails to control hypertension or causes troublesome side effects.[3,4]

The reports of JNC IV,[4] JNC V,[3] and the Veterans Administration (VA) cooperative trial on monotherapy of hypertension[26] have suggested guidelines for selecting the appropriate step 1 drug for a given patient, and these are included in the tables that list the drugs, their doses, and the common side effects for each category of antihypertensive agents. Basically, in making the choice, preference should be given to agents that have been demonstrated to reduce cardiovascular morbidity and mortality in controlled clinical trials.[3,27] Presently, these include only the diuretics and beta blockers. Consideration should also be given to age and race as well as preexisting symptoms and conditions that might be benefited or aggravated by a given class of drugs (e.g., angina pectoris, myocardial infarction, migraine headache, diabetes mellitus, cardiac arrhythmias, congestive heart failure, constipation, etc.). These guidelines are imprecise, are subject to revision as new data become available, and should not contravene the physician's best judgment in selecting the appropriate agent to initiate therapy.

The reliability of measurements of hemodynamic or biochemical parameters such as plasma catecholamines or plasma renin activity has not been great enough to justify their routine use in selecting the appropriate step 1 drug.

While the 1988 JNC report promulgated the concept of "individualized stepped care,"[4] the truth is that our desire to select, prospectively, the appropriate drug for a given patient exceeds our ability to do so.

To enhance adherence, it is preferable to select a long-acting drug that can be given once daily, usually in the morning. The more tablets and the more times a day they are administered, the less likely that a patient will adhere to the regimen.

The TOMHS trial[10] compared in a parallel design as monotherapy a diuretic (chlorthalidone), a beta-adrenergic blocker (acebutolol), a calcium antagonist (amlodipine), an ACE inhibitor (enalapril), and an alpha$_1$-adrenergic blocker (doxazosin). Their effects on blood pressure after 1 year were remarkably similar, the only difference being that the average systolic blood pressure reduction was significantly greater for the diuretic (21.8 mmHg) than it was for doxazosin (16.1 mmHg) ($p = .007$). The systolic reduction fell between these two extremes for the other agents. There was no statistically significant difference in diastolic blood pressure reductions comparing the five drugs.

Diuretics

For many years the diuretics were the mainstay of antihypertensive therapy and the only logical choice for step 1 (Tables 77-2 and 29-1).

All of the controlled clinical trials that have shown a reduction in cardiovascular morbidity and mortality have used diuretics or beta-adrenergic blockers as step 1.[1,8,28-31] Nevertheless, it has been postulated that atherogenic and arrhythmogenic metabolic side effects of diuretic therapy (hyperlipoproteinemia, hyperglycemia, and hypokalemia) may be responsible for the observation that coronary events have not been reduced as much as anticipated or as dramatically as stroke events have.[1] It is interesting that in three prospective clinical trials in elderly patients in which a low-dose diuretic was employed, coronary events were reduced to the anticipated level.[8,30,31]

The metabolic side effects of diuretics are now well recognized and should be monitored. They are minimized but not eliminated by employing small doses (equivalent to 12.5 to 25 mg of hydrochlorothiazide or chlorthalidone).

Many patients are not susceptible to the hyperlipidemic effects of diuretics, which include a rise in serum cholesterol concentration of 5 to 10 mg/dL, mostly in the low-density lipoprotein (LDL) fraction, and a rise in triglyceride concentration. This can be minimized, if not eliminated, by a low-fat, low-cholesterol diet.[10,32] It has been recommended by the National Education Programs on High Blood Pressure and High Cholesterol that when hypertensive patients receiving diuretics or certain beta blockers present with elevated LDL cholesterol that cannot be controlled with diet, consideration should be given to cautiously discontinuing these antihypertensive medications temporarily unless otherwise contraindicated and closely observing the effects of

TABLE 77-2
Diuretics

Agent	Usual Daily Dose (mg)*	Precautions and Special Considerations	Side Effects
Thiazides and related sulfonamide diuretics			
Bendroflumethiazide (Naturetin) Benzthiazide (Exna) Chlorothiazide (Diuril) Chlorthalidone (Hygroton) Hydrochlorothiazide (HydroDiuril, Esidrix) Hydroflumethiazide (Saluron, Diucardin) Indapamide (Lozol) Methylchlothiazide (Enduron) Metolazone (Zaroxolyn) Metolazone (Mykrox) Polythiazide (Renese) Quinethazone (Hydromox) Trichlormethiazide	2.5–5 12.5–50 125–500† 12.5–50 12.5–50 12.5–50 2.5–5 2.5–5 2.5–5 0.5–1 1–4 25–100 1–4	May be ineffective in renal failure except for indapamide and metolazone; hypokalemia increases digitalis toxicity; may cause an increase in blood levels of lithium. Decrease in urinary calcium excretion. May precipitate acute gout.	Hypokalemia, hypomagnesemia, hyperuricemia, glucose intolerance, insulin resistance, hypercholesterolemia, increased low-density lipoprotein cholesterol, hypertriglyceridemia, hypercalcemia, sexual dysfunction, weakness, photosensitivity (except for ethacrynic acid), leukopenia, allergic skin rash.
Loop diuretics‡			
Bumetanide (Bumex) Ethacrynic acid (Edecrin) Furosemide (Lasix)	0.5–5† 25–100† 20–320†	Effective in chronic renal failure. Increase urinary calcium excretion.	As above, except for hypercalcemia.
Potassium-sparing agents			
Amiloride (Midamor) Spironolactone (Aldactone) Triamterene (Dyrenium)	5–10 25–100† 50–150†	Danger of hyperkalemia in patients receiving a potassium supplement, a potassium-containing salt substitute or an ACE inhibitor, and in patients with renal failure; can cause renal failure in patients treated with a nonsteroidal anti-inflammatory drug (indomethacin and triamterene). May increase blood levels of lithium. Spironolactone interferes with digoxin immunoassay. Danger of renal calculi (triamterene).	Hyperkalemia for all three agents. For spironolactone only: gynecomastia, mastodynia, gastrointestinal irritation, drowsiness, lethargy, irregular menses or postmenopausal bleeding, hirsutism.

TABLE 77-2

Diuretics *(continued)*

Agent	Usual Daily Dose (mg)*	Precautions and Special Considerations	Side Effects

Combination Thiazide and Potassium-Sparing Diuretic Preparations

Product	Dose (tablets or capsules/day)	Product	Dose (tablets or capsules/day)
Hydrochlorothiazide 25 mg + triamterene 37.5 mg (Maxzide 25)	½–2	Hydrochlorothiazide 50 mg + triamterene 75 mg (Maxzide 50)	½–1
Hydrochlorothiazide 25 mg + triamterene 50 mg (Dyazide)	1–2	Hydrochlorothiazide 50 mg + amiloride 5 mg (Moduretic)	½–1
Hydrochlorothiazide 25 mg + spironolactone 25 mg (Aldactazide 25)	1–2	Hydrochlorothiazide 50 mg + spironolactone 50 mg (Aldactazide 50)	½–1

Special indications: Diuretics or beta blockers should be agents of choice for most patients with uncomplicated hypertension unless contraindicated, ineffective, unacceptable, or there are special indications for other agents (see text); especially indicated for black patients, elderly patients, obese patients, congestive heart failure, chronic renal failure (loop diuretics), resistant hypertension, recurrent renal calculi (calcium) (non–loop diuretics).

Contraindications: History of hypersensitivity to diuretics, hypovolemia, hyponatremia, hypochloremia, hypomagnesemia, uncontrolled gout, severe hypertrophic cardiomyopathy, asymmetric septal hypertrophy (idiopathic hypertrophic subaortic stenosis), preeclampsia, and eclampsia.

Advantages: ***Effective in reducing cardiovascular morbidity and mortality***, effective in ≥50% of mild hypertensives, inexpensive, one dose daily, easy to titrate, well tolerated, enhance potency of all other agents, no pseudotolerance, reduce total peripheral resistance.

Disadvantages: Metabolic side effects: (K^+ ↓, Mg^{2+} ↓, urate ↑, Ca^{2+} ↑, Na^+ ↓, Cl^- ↓, glucose ↑, lipids ↑).

*The dosage range may differ slightly from recommended dosage in *Physicians' Desk Reference* or package insert. Given once daily unless otherwise indicated.

†This drug is usually given in divided doses twice daily.

‡Larger doses of loop diuretics may be required in patients with renal failure.

withdrawal on blood cholesterol and blood pressure levels.[33]

Because the rise in serum cholesterol and triglyceride concentrations usually occurs in the first 6 weeks, the patients who are going to respond adversely can easily and quickly be identified by measuring serum lipids and glucose before and 6 to 8 weeks after initiating diuretic therapy. If no adverse effect has occurred by 6 months, frequent measurement of lipids can be discontinued, although serum potassium and glucose should be monitored every 6 months.

In the TOMHS trial[10] in which all participants were asked to follow low-fat, low-cholesterol diets, average serum total cholesterol rose only 1 mg/dL during the first year for the 125 subjects treated with chlorthalidone compared to a decrease of 5.2 mg/dL for 221 subjects on diet and placebo ($p < .01$). The LDL and high-density lipoprotein (HDL) cholesterol fractions and triglyceride levels did not change significantly for the diuretic-treated group compared to the group on placebo.

Several long-term studies have shown that the hyperlipidemic effect of diuretics becomes less evident or subsides after the first year of therapy.[34–37] Moreover, it is important to recognize that the rise in cholesterol induced by diuretic therapy is inversely proportional to the pretreatment level of serum cholesterol,[35,38] and Jeunemaitre et al.[39] have demonstrated a "regression to the mean" phenomenon for both cholesterol and glucose in hypertensive patients treated with diuretics, so that those patients with the highest serum cholesterol and glucose concentrations actually had the largest decreases when diuretics were administered, whereas those with normal pretreatment values had the largest increases. The clinical implication is that diuretics are not de facto contraindicated for patients with hyperlipoproteinemia or diabetes.

For patients who have left ventricular hypertrophy or other resting electrocardiographic abnormalities or who have a history of tachyarrythmias, it is sometimes preferable to use a combination potassium-sparing/thiazide type diuretic unless there is a contraindication to the potassium-sparing drug (Tables 77-2 and 29-1). (See also Chap. 29.)

Diuretics are the least expensive of the step 1 drugs, and this is an important consideration because the cost of therapy can detract from compliance to lifelong treatment for many patients.[40] Moreover the diuretics have an additive, if not synergistic, antihypertensive effect with all of the other classes of drugs for hypertension. Failure to incorporate a diuretic in the regimen is sometimes the cause for suboptimal control of hypertension, and it is inappropriate to classify hypertension as resistant to treatment unless a diuretic has been included in a multidrug regimen.[41]

The Canadian Hypertension Society Consensus Conference on Pharmacologic Treatment of Hypertension[42] and the 1993 JNC report[3] have recommended that either a beta blocker or low-dose thiazide diuretic be prescribed as initial therapy for patients with uncomplicated essential hypertension. This recommendation is supported by editorial comment from the British Isles[43–45] and the United States[27] that diuretics and beta-adrenergic blockers have been subjected to long-term clinical trials that have demonstrated a reduction in cardiovascular morbidity and mortality, whereas the newer and more expensive agents have not.

Beta-Adrenergic Blocking Agents

Beta-adrenergic blockers were first recommended as an alternative to diuretics for initial therapy of hypertension in the 1984 report of the JNC (Tables 77-3 and 66-1).[46] These agents have been shown to reduce cardiovascular events in the placebo-controlled MRC[29] and STOP[28] trials. Beta blockers have demonstrated a distinct cardioprotective effect compared to placebo following myocardial infarctions in randomized studies.[47–49] Compared to placebo, the beta blockers reduced recurrent nonfatal infarctions, sudden death, and total mortality for up to 6 years following myocardial infarction,[47] but without clear benefit following non-Q-wave infarction.[50] (See Chap. 60.) The beta blockers with intrinsic sympathomimetic activity (ISA) have been less effective than those without ISA.[49] No other classes of antihypertensive drugs have demonstrated this effect so convincingly; *consequently, a non-ISA beta blocker is the drug of first choice*

TABLE 77-3

Beta-adrenergic Blocking Agents

Agent	Usual Daily Dose (mg)*	Precautions and Special Considerations	Side Effects
Cardioselective, with ISA		Should not be used in patients with asthma, chronic obstructive pulmonary disease (COPD) with bronchospasm, congestive heart failure, heart block (greater than first degree), sick sinus syndrome. Use with caution in insulin-dependent diabetics and patients with peripheral vascular disease. Should not be discontinued abruptly in patients with ischemic heart disease.	Bronchospasm, peripheral arterial insufficiency, fatigue, insomnia, sexual dysfunction, exacerbation of congestive heart failure, may mask symptoms of hypoglycemia; hyperglycemia; hypertriglyceridemia, decreased high-density lipoprotein (HDL) cholesterol (except for drugs with ISA and labetalol)
Acebutolol (Sectral)†	200–1200‡		
Cardioselective, without ISA			
Atenolol (Tenormin)†	25–100		
Betaxolol (Kerlone)	5–40		
Metoprolol (Lopressor)	50–200		
Metoprolol XL (Toprol XL)	50–200		
Noncardioselective, with ISA			
Carteolol (Cartrol)†	2.5–10		
Penbutolol (Levatol)†	20–80		
Pindolol (Visken)†	10–60‡		
Noncardioselective, without ISA			
Labetalol¶ (Normodyne, Trandate)	200–1200‡		
Nadolol (Corgard)†	40–320		
Propranolol (Inderal)	40–240‡		
Propranolol LA (Inderal LA)	60–240		
Timolol (Blocadren)	20–40‡		
Bisoprolol	5–20		

ISA = intrinsic sympathomimetic activity

Special indications: Diuretics or beta blockers should be agents of choice for most patients with uncomplicated hypertension unless contraindicated, ineffective, unacceptable, or there are special indications for other agents (see text); especially indicated for patients who have had myocardial infarction because of cardioprotective effect (non-ISA, non-alpha-blocking agents), white patients, hyperkinetic circulation, angina pectoris, migraine headache, senile tremor; severe hypertrophic cardiomyopathy of the elderly, severe asymmetric septal hypetrophy with outflow obstruction (idopathic hypertrophic subaortic stenosis), atrial fibrillation to control ventricular rate, paroxysmal supraventricular tachycardia (non-ISA, non-alpha-blocking agents preferred).

Contraindications: History of hypersensitivity reaction to beta-adrenergic blockers, more than first-degree heart block, sick sinus syndrome, left ventricular failure, asthma, chronic obstructive pulmonary disease with bronchospasm. Relative contraindications (see text): insulin-dependent diabetes, remote history of bronchial asthma, intermittent claudication, Raynaud's disease.

Advantages: Effective in reducing cardiovascular morbidity and mortality; cardioprotective after myocardial infarction, antianginal drug, relatively inexpensive, effective in ~50% of mild hypertensives, reduce CO in hyperkinetic circulation, one dose daily (for most agents), no pseudotolerance, migraine prophylaxis (propranolol), reduce senile tremor (propranolol).

Disadvantages: Many do not reduce total peripheral resistance; central nervous system side effects; metabolic side effects (HDL cholesterol ↓, triglycerides ↑ (except for ISA beta blockers, see text), glucose ↑, insulin resistance ↑. Multiple contraindications and precautions.

*The dosage range may differ slightly from recommended dosage in *Physicians' Desk Reference* or package insert. Given once daily unless otherwise indicated.

†Drug is excreted by kidney; may require dosage reduction in patients with renal insufficiency.

‡This drug is usually given in divided doses twice daily.

¶Combined alpha and beta blocker.

for hypertensive patients following a myocardial infarction.

Although beta blockers can be classified according to the presence or absence of cardioselectivity and the presence or absence of ISA (Table 77-3), they are all equipotent in reducing blood pressure when given in effective doses. Cardioselectivity is lost as dose is increased, and in average antihypertensive doses the cardioselective $beta_1$ blockers may also block $beta_2$ receptors similar to nonselective agents (Table 66-1).

Cardioselective agents have marginal advantages over nonselective agents for patients with occlusive arterial disease and intermittent claudication, patients with chronic obstructive pulmonary disease with minimal or no bronchospasm, and insulin-dependent diabetics who are predisposed to hypoglycemic reactions. The recovery from hypoglycemia is prolonged less by cardioselective beta blockers than by nonselective ones. (See also Chap. 66.)

Beta-adrenergic blockers of any type are contraindicated for asthmatic patients unless the asthma has been inactive for years, in which case a cardioselective beta-adrenergic blocker may be given cautiously if the indication is strong. One of the disadvantages of beta-adrenergic blockers is the long list of precautions and contraindications noted in Tables 77-3 and 66-7.

The nonselective, non-ISA beta-adrenergic blockers are the only antihypertensive agents that reduce blood pressure primarily by decreasing cardiac output rather than total peripheral resistance. For most patients with primary (essential) hypertension, this is unphysiological, but nevertheless these drugs have been effective over long periods of time and have reduced cardiovascular mortality. These agents are particularly useful in managing hypertension associated with the hyperdynamic beta-adrenergic circulatory state,[51] which is characterized by an increase in cardiac output and cardiac rate with relatively normal total peripheral resistance (TPR), and is sometimes encountered in adolescents and young adults.

The ISA beta-adrenergic blockers are less likely than non-ISA agents to produce excessive bradycardia and to cause serum lipid abnormalities (hypertriglyceridemia and depressed HDL cholesterol). Nevertheless, ISA beta blockers have not been shown to have as great a cardioprotective effect after a myocardial infarction as non-ISA beta blockers even though the latter can have an adverse effect on lipid profile.

In TOMHS, the cardioselective, ISA beta-adrenergic blocker acebutolol reduced average total serum cholesterol by 12.7 mg/dL during the first 12 months of the trial for 124 participants compared to 5.2 mg/dL for the placebo; LDL cholesterol was reduced by 10.2 mg/dL compared to 2 mg/dL for the placebo ($p < .01$), and HDL cholesterol was reduced by 0.4 mg/dL compared to an increase of 1.6 mg/dL for placebo.[10]

While beta-adrenergic blockers can impair glucose tolerance by inhibiting insulin release[52] or by causing insulin resistance,[52,53] they do not often interfere with control of diabetes clinically. Certainly one would not want to convert a non-insulin-dependent diabetic to insulin dependency, and if this becomes a problem, a drug from an alternative class of antihypertensive agents should be selected. (See also Chap. 66.)

Calcium Antagonists

The 1988 and 1993 reports of the JNC[3,4] included calcium antagonists as candidates for initial monotherapy of hypertension (step 1) (Tables 77-4, 67-4, and 67-5).

The calcium antagonists differ in their action on various vascular beds. Verapamil and to a lesser extent diltiazem act on the heart to reduce rate, slow atrioventricular (AV) conduction, and depress contractility. On the other hand, the dihydropyridine calcium antagonists have very little effect on the myocardium in the normal intact person but are excellent peripheral vasodilators reducing TPR.[54] (See Chap. 67.)

In general, the long-acting preparations are preferred, not only to enhance adherence but also because they seem to produce fewer side effects than the shorter acting formulations.

There is controversy about whether or not diuretics and calcium antagonists are additive in their antihypertensive effects, but most reports suggest that they are.[54] Because of their negative inotropic effects, beta blockers should not be prescribed with either verapamil or diltiazem for patients who have significant left ventricular dysfunction. They do have additive effects on blood pressure, however, and can be used together safely when left ventricular function and cardiac conduction are normal.

Long-term studies have not demonstrated a convincing cardioprotective effect for the calcium antagonists after myocardial infarction similar to that shown for beta blockers, and in the case of the dihydropyridine group there is some evidence that they may have a deleterious effect.[55] (See also Chap. 60.)

Because of their negative inotropic effect, verapamil and diltiazem are contraindicated in patients with left ventricular systolic dysfunction or failure.[56,57] Nifedipine, which may have little or no negative inotropic effect because of reflex sympathetic stimulation, also tends to worsen left ventricular failure,[58] even though it reduces afterload. (See also Chap. 67.)

Like the diuretics, calcium antagonists appear to be especially effective in elderly patients and Black patients,[26] although there are many exceptions to this rule. Like the beta-adrenergic blockers, the calcium antagonists are effective antianginal drugs and should be considered for step 1 therapy in hypertensive patients who have angina pectoris. The calcium antagonists do not have known metabolic side effects.

Angiotensin Converting Enzyme Inhibitors

Although ACE inhibitors (Table 77-5) specifically block the conversion of angiotensin I to angiotensin II, they are effective in reducing blood pressure for a wide spectrum of antihypertensive patients, even when angiotensin II does not seem to be playing a role. Perhaps this is because they also block the degradation of bradykinin, which is a potent vasodilator and also increases the production of prostacyclin and prostaglandin E_2.[59]

The ACE inhibitors listed in Table 77-5 are equally effective and have similar side effect profiles. In antihypertensive potency it does not make a difference whether they are prodrugs or directly active or whether or not they have a sulfhydryl group.[59]

TABLE 77-4
Calcium Antagonists

Agent	Usual Daily Dose (mg)*	Special Precautions and Considerations	Side Effects
Benzothiazepine derivative			
Diltiazem (Cardizem)	90–360†	Contraindicated for congestive heart failure, sick sinus syndrome, or greater than first-degree heart block. Can increase blood levels of cyclosporine.	Constipation, rash, headache, flushing, ankle edema, liver dysfunction.
Diltiazem SR (Cardizem SR)	120–360‡		
Diltiazem CD (Cardizem CD)	120–360		
Diltiazem XR (Dilacor XR)	180–480		
Diphenylalkylamine derivative			
Verapamil (Calan, Isoptin)	80–480†	As above.	As above.
Verapamil (Verelan)	120–480		
Verapamil SR (Calan SR, Isoptin SR)	180–480		
Dihydropyridines			
Nifedipine (Procardia, Adalat)	30–120†	Short-acting forms rapidly lower blood pressure; use cautiously when hypertension is severe. Nifedipine GITS capsules should not be broken or punctured. Use with caution in patients with congestive heart failure, may aggravate angina and myocardial ischemia.	Headache, palpitations, tachycardia, ankle edema, flushing, gastrointestinal symptoms, gingival hyperplasia.
Nifedipine GITS (Procardia XL)	30–90		
Nicardipine (Cardene)	60–120†		
Nicardipine XL (Cardene XL)	60–120‡		
Isradipine (DynaCirc)	2.5–10‡		
Amlodipine (Norvasc)	2.5–10		
Felodipine (Plendil)	2.5–10		

Special indications: Elderly patient, black patient, angina pectoris, hypertension induced by cyclosporine; paroxysmal supraventricular tachycardia (verapamil); migraine, atrial fibrillation to slow atrioventricular conduction (verapamil, diltiazem).
Contraindications: History of hypersensitivity reaction to calcium antagonists, severe left ventricular dysfunction with or without congestive heart failure; greater than first-degree heart block, sick sinus syndrome, Wolff-Parkinson-White and Lown-Genong-Levine syndromes (verapamil, diltiazem).
Advantages: Long-acting (verapamil SR, Verelan, nifedipine GITS, felodipine), reduce TPR, effective, no pseudotolerance, antianginal, no metabolic side effects, easy to titrate (sustained-release preparations).
Disadvantages: Expensive, no trials to demonstrate long-term efficacy in reducing cardiovascular events.
* The dosage range may differ slightly from recommended dosage in *Physicians' Desk Reference* or package insert.
† This drug is usually given in divided doses three or four times daily.
‡ This drug is usually given in divided doses twice daily.

Diuretics enhance the hypotensive potency of ACE inhibitors[60] probably more than for any other class of drugs with the possible exception of the adrenergic neuroeffector blockers (reserpine, guanethidine, and guanadrel). While ACE inhibitors alone seem to be more effective for young and white patients than they are for old and black patients,[26] these age and race differences in blood pressure response are obliterated by adding a diuretic to the regimen.

The ACE inhibitors are not direct venodilators, but they do reduce filling pressure of the failing left ventricle and dilate arterioles, thereby reducing preload and afterload. Because of this, they are particularly effective in managing hypertension complicated by left ventricular systolic failure. In fact, *the regimen of choice for hypertensive patients with congestive heart failure includes an ACE inhibitor and a diuretic.* Even in the absence of hypertension, ACE inhibitors have been shown to prolong life in patients with moderate to severe congestive heart failure when added to conventional regimens.[61,62] (See also Chap. 30.) Although only captopril and enalapril have been approved for treatment of congestive heart failure, it is reasonable to assume that other ACE inhibitors will be equally effective, because all appear to have similar hemodynamic effects.

The ACE inhibitors have a unique effect on renal hemodynamics because they selectively dilate the efferent (postglomerular) arteriole, thus reducing pressure within the glomerular capillaries usually without reducing glomerular filtration rate (GFR). Theoretically, this tends to reduce the rate of progression of glomerulosclerosis in various types of glomerulopathies according to the theory promulgated by Brenner and others.[63] This may not always be beneficial because renal function can deteriorate abruptly when GFR is being maintained by angiotensin II–mediated constriction of the efferent arteriole, as is the case when renal blood flow is jeopardized by renal artery stenosis, congestive heart failure, hypovo-

TABLE 77-5
Angiotensin Converting Enzyme Inhibitors

Agent	Usual Daily Dose (mg)*	Special Precautions and Considerations	Side Effects
Captopril (Capoten)[†]	12.5–150	Can cause reversible, acute renal failure in patients with bilateral renal arterial stenosis or unilateral stenosis in an artery to a solitary kidney and in patients with preexisting renal insufficiency or congestive heart failure. Excreted by kidney; may require dosage reduction in patients with renal insufficiency. Hypotension has been observed with initiation of ACE inhibitors, especially in patients with high plasma renin activity or hypovolemia (e.g., in those receiving diuretic therapy).	Cough, angioedema (rare), hyperkalemia (especially when given to patients with renal failure and/or with a potassium-sparing diuretic or a nonsteroidal anti-inflammatory drug), dysgeusia, neutropenia (rare), proteinuria (rare at recommended doses), rash.
Cilazapril[‡]	2.5–5		
Enalapril (Vasotec)	2.5–40		
Lisinopril (Prinivil, Zestril)	5–40		
Benazepril (Lotensin)	10–40		
Fosinipril (Monopril)[¶]	10–40		
Quinapril (Accupril)	5–80		
Perindopril[‡]	1–16		
Ramipril (Altace)	1.25–20		
Spirapril[‡]	12.5–50		

Special indications: Congestive heart failure, young patient, white patient, heavy proteinuria, diabetes mellitus with or without renal disease, impotence from other drugs.
Contraindications: History of hypersensitivity to these agents or history of angioedema; bilateral renal artery stenosis or severe stenosis in an artery to a solitary kidney; hyperkalemia; advanced renal failure; pregnancy.
Advantages: Beneficial for congestive heart failure, no metabolic side effects (except for hyperkalemia as noted), low side effect profile, effective, long-acting (except captopril), no pseudotolerance, easy to titrate, reduce TPR.
Disadvantages: Expensive, risk of acute renal failure and/or hyperkalemia (see above), no long-term trials to demonstrate reduction in cardiovascular morbidity or mortality.
*The dosage range may differ slightly from recommended dosage in *Physicians' Desk Reference* or package insert. Given once daily unless otherwise indicated.
¶Fosinopril is excreted by the liver as well as by the kidney; may require dosage reduction in patients with hepatic insufficiency.
†This drug is usually given in divided doses two or three times daily.
‡Pending approval by the Food and Drug Administration.

lemia, and hypotension.[64–67] It is in these situations that ACE inhibitors can cause an abrupt increase in serum creatinine concentration, if not acute renal failure. (See also Chap. 29.)

After extensive renal ablation in rats, ACE inhibitors have been shown to protect animals against hypertension, heavy proteinuria, glomerulosclerosis, and progressive renal failure.[68] This is also true in rats made diabetic by streptozotocin.[69] Angiotensin converting enzyme inhibition with captopril reduced albuminuria in 16 insulin dependent hypertensive patients with overt diabetic glomerulosclerosis[70] as well as microalbuminuria in insulin dependent diabetic patients with normal blood pressure.[71] During a 4-year period of observation, 7 of 23 diabetic patients who did not receive ACE inhibitors developed overt diabetic nephropathy with heavy proteinuria compared to none of 21 patients who were treated with captopril.[71] Before the advent of ACE inhibitors and calcium antagonists, Parving et al.[72] demonstrated that blood pressure reduction by a variety of agents including diuretics and beta-adrenergic blockers would slow the rate of increase of serum creatinine in hypertensive patients with diabetic renal disease. It has not yet been shown conclusively that ACE inhibitors will have any greater effect than other antihypertensive agents to retard progression of renal failure in patients with diabetic glomerulosclerosis.

Nevertheless, it is tempting to recommend ACE inhibitors for hypertensive insulin-dependent diabetic patients in an effort to prevent or retard glomerulosclerosis, provided that renal failure is not far advanced (serum creatinine below 3 mg/dL). This must be done cautiously with close observation because ACE inhibitor therapy can cause hyperkalemia and abrupt worsening of renal function in patients with renal insufficiency. In some patients with nephrosclerosis[73] or polycystic disease,[74] ACE inhibition has been associated with sudden increases in serum creatinine that are not always predictable. Consequently, serum creatinine and potassium should be measured within 48 h of initiating ACE inhibitor therapy for patients with chronic renal disease and at least once a week for 2 to 3 weeks thereafter. Moreover, it is important to continue to monitor serum creatinine and potassium at regular intervals for any patient who has chronic renal disease and is receiving an ACE inhibitor.[73]

Angiotensin converting enzyme inhibitors do not have

adverse effects on lipid or glucose metabolism and, in fact, may favorably affect insulin resistance.[75]

Except for a troublesome, dry irritative cough that occurs in 5 to 10 percent of patients,[59,76] ACE inhibitors are relatively free of symptomatic side effects and are the least likely of all antihypertensive drugs to cause sexual dysfunction in the male. Unfortunately, they are considerably more expensive than diuretics and many of the beta-adrenergic blockers.

Alpha-Adrenergic Blocking Drugs

The nonselective alpha-adrenergic blockers block both the $alpha_1$ receptor on vascular smooth-muscle wall, activation of which causes vasoconstriction, and the $alpha_2$ or presynaptic receptor that mediates a negative feedback to inhibit the release of norepinephrine from the sympathetic nerve terminal (Tables 77-6 and 30-3). The nonselective adrenergic blockers, phentolamine and dibenzyline, therefore permit release of excessive norepinephrine by blocking the presynaptic alpha receptor located on the nerve terminal, and this causes palpitations and tachycardia among other side effects. They are used primarily in the management of hypertension secondary to pheochromocytoma.

Drugs that selectively block the $alpha_1$-adrenergic receptor usually do not produce tachycardia and palpitations because they do not interfere with the negative-feedback mechanism that controls the release of norepinephrine. The 1993 report of the Joint National Committee (JNC V) included the selective $alpha_1$-adrenergic receptor blockers as candidates for initial (step 1) monotherapy.[3]

These are the only antihypertensive agents that have a beneficial effect on serum lipids, including reductions in total cholesterol, triglycerides, and LDL cholesterol and an increase in HDL cholesterol.[10,77–79] In the TOMHS trial, doxazosin was the only drug that produced a statistically significant increase in HDL/total cholesterol ratio compared to placebo.[10]

While the magnitude of these beneficial changes in serum lipids is not great, they are particularly useful in patients who have only modest abnormalities in their lipid profiles for whom a drug of this class might control hypertension and hyperlipoproteinemia simultaneously.[33] For patients who have major elevations in serum lipids, treatment directed at that risk factor will be necessary in addition to whatever antihypertensive drugs are selected.

Selective $alpha_1$-adrenergic blockers also have a favorable effect on glucose metabolism by reducing insulin resistance,[77,78,80] which is frequently found in hypertensive patients, especially the obese.

There are no contraindications to the use of selective $alpha_1$-adrenergic blocking agents, provided that appropriate caution is exercised in warning patients, particularly the elderly, about the possibility of an orthostatic hypotensive response to the first dose ("first-dose effect"). This is more likely to occur when an $alpha_1$-blocking agent is added to an existing regimen, especially a diuretic, than when it is given as monotherapy. It is less likely to occur with the long-acting drugs terazosin and doxazosin than with prazosin. Obviously, treatment should be started with the smallest possible "test dose" of whichever drug is selected.

$Alpha_1$-adrenergic blockade has been reported to reduce the obstructive symptoms of prostatic hyperplasia.[81]

A rather high incidence of adverse effects requiring

TABLE 77-6

$Alpha_1$-Adrenergic Blockers

Agent	Usual Daily Dose mg*	Precautions and Special Considerations	Side Effects
Nonselective		Use cautiously in elderly patients because of orthostatic hypotension. Phentolamine, phenoxybenzamine, and prazosin are more likely to produce orthostatic hypotension than are terazosin and doxazosin.	First-dose syncope, orthostatic hypotension, dizziness, headache, drowsiness, weakness, palpitations, nausea.
Phentolamine (Regitine)	—†		
Phenoxybenzamine (Dibenzyline)	20–80‡		
Selective			
Prazosin (Minipress)	1–20‡		
Terazosin (Hytrin)	1–20		
Doxazosin (Cardura)	1–16		

Special indications: Phentolamine and phenoxybenzamine are used almost exclusively for management of patients with pheochromocytoma; the selective $alpha_1$ blockers may also be prescribed as initial therapy for any patient with primary hypertension; especially useful for those with diabetes, lipid abnormalities, or benign prostatic hyperplasia.
Contraindications: History of hypersensitivity to these agents.
Advantages: No absolute contraindications; beneficial effects on serum lipids and insulin resistance; reduce total peripheral resistance.
Disadvantages: Moderately expensive; hypotensive effect after first dose and high side effect profile (especially phentolamine, phenoxybenzamine, and prazosin); no trials to demonstrate long-term efficacy in reducing cardiovascular events; can produce pseudoresistance (fluid retention).
*The dosage range may differ slightly from recommended dosage in *Physicians' Desk Reference* or package insert. Given once daily unless otherwise indicated.
†Phentolamine is used only parenterally for pre- and intraoperative management of patients with pheochromocytoma.
‡This drug is usually given in divided doses two or three times a day.

TABLE 77-7
Centrally Acting Alpha$_2$-Adrenoreceptor Agonists

Agent	Usual Daily Dose mg*	Precautions and Special Considerations	Side Effects
Methyldopa (Aldomet) Clonidine (Catapres) Clonidine TTS (patch) (Catapres TTS) Guanabenz (Wytensin) Guanfacine (Tenex)	250–2000† 0.1–1.2† 0.1–0.3‡ 4–64† 1–3	Rebound hypertension may occur with abrupt discontinuation (especially oral clonidine), particularly with prior administration of high doses or with continuation of concomitant beta-blocker therapy. Methyldopa interferes with fluorometric measurements of urinary catecholamine levels.	Drowsiness, sedation, lethargy, dry mouth, fatigue, depression, sexual dysfunction. Drug fever, hepatotoxicity, abnormal liver function tests ± hepatitis, positive Coomb's test with or without hemolytic anemia (methyldopa).

Special indications: Elderly patients, usually with a diuretic. Methyldopa: preeclampsia.
Contraindications: History of hypersensitivity reaction to these agents. Hepatic dysfunction (methyldopa).
Advantages: Reduce total peripheral resistance, relatively inexpensive, no metabolic side effects.
Disadvantages: High side effect profile, rebound hypertension after sudden withdrawal, especially oral clonidine. Potential to cause fluid retention and pseudotolerance. No trials to demonstrate long-term efficacy in reducing cardiovascular events.
*The dosage range may differ slightly from recommended dosage in *Physicians' Desk Reference* or package insert. Given once daily unless otherwise indicated.
†This drug is usually given in divided doses twice daily.
‡This drug is administered as a skin patch once weekly.

discontinuation of the drug has been attributed to prazosin in two controlled trials.[26,79] The longer acting agents seem to be better tolerated.

Alpha$_1$-blocking agents are particularly effective in managing hypertension associated with pheochromocytoma.

Alpha$_2$-Adrenoreceptor Agonists

The centrally acting sympathetic inhibitors have not been recommended for monotherapy because of their high side effect profile and their propensity to cause fluid retention and pseudoresistance (Table 77-7). Usually they are prescribed as step 2 drugs, added to a diuretic so that they do not cause fluid retention. Rebound hypertension has been described after sudden withdrawal of these agents, especially for oral clonidine.[82]

To enhance adherence, the long-acting drug guanfacine is preferred. The transdermal preparation of clonidine has a duration of action of 7 days, but surprisingly it has not been popular with patients, even though it appears to cause fewer side effects than the oral preparation.

Methyldopa, given as monotherapy, is the drug of choice for managing hypertension associated with preeclampsia.[83]

Neuroeffector Adrenergic Blocking Drugs

Reserpine and guanethidine were among the first antihypertensive drugs introduced more than 30 years ago (Table 77-8). Guanadrel was introduced more recently but shares many of the undesirable side effects of guanethidine, including orthostatic hypotension and sexual dysfunction. None is widely used because more effective agents with fewer side effects have been marketed.

Reserpine in small doses (0.05 to 0.125 mg daily) combined with a diuretic to prevent pseudotolerance is the least expensive antihypertensive regimen available and was effective and well tolerated in a VA controlled clinical trial.[84] This combination is still widely used in large inner city clinics where cost is an important consideration.

Direct Vasodilators

Hydralazine and minoxidil are direct vasodilators whose mechanism of action is not well understood (Table 77-9). They both cause reflex tachycardia and fluid retention, which can be profound with minoxidil. For this reason they are usually prescribed with both a sympathetic inhibitor, frequently a beta-adrenergic blocker, to control cardiac rate and a diuretic to control fluid retention. In the case of minoxidil large doses of a loop diuretic are often required.

Methyldopa, given as monotherapy, is the preferred drug in managing the hypertension associated with eclampsia.[83]

Minoxidil is almost exclusively reserved to manage hypertension that is resistant to multidrug regimens and is particularly effective when renal failure is present.[85,86] Since the advent of ACE inhibitors and calcium antagonists, minoxidil is seldom needed.

TABLE 77-8
Neuroeffector Adrenergic Inhibitors

Agent	Usual Daily Dose mg*	Precautions and Special Considerations	Side Effects
Guanadrel (Hylorel) Guanethidine (Ismelin)	10–75† 10–50	Use cautiously because of orthostatic hypotension.	Diarrhea (especially guanethidine), sexual dysfunction including retrograde ejaculation, orthostatic hypotension (especially in the morning or after exercise).
Rauwolfia alkaloids			
Reserpine (generic)	0.1 every other day to 0.25 daily	Use with caution in patients with history of peptic ulcer.	Lassitude, lethargy, sedation, depression, sexual dysfunction, loss of libido, nasal congestion, aggravation of peptic ulcer, Parkinson-like syndrome.

Special indications: Should be used with a diuretic to minimize dosage.
Contraindications: Reserpine: history of depression or peptic ulcer; Parkinson's disease. Guanethidine and guanadrel: elderly patients, patients with diabetic autonomic neuropathy and patients on dialysis (because of the propensity of these drugs to produce orthostatic hypotension).
Advantages: Inexpensive; reduce total peripheral resistance; no metabolic side effects.
Disadvantages: High side effect profile. Can cause fluid retention and pseudotolerance. No trials to demonstrate long-term efficacy in reducing cardiovascular events. Guanethidine and guanadrel: Reduction in blood pressure is primarily orthostatic.
*The dosage range may differ slightly from recommended dosage in *Physicians' Desk Reference* or package insert. Given once daily unless otherwise indicated.
†This drug is usually given in divided doses twice daily.

TABLE 77-9
Direct Vasodilators

Agent	Usual Daily Dose mg*	Precautions and Special Considerations	Side Effects
Hydralazine (Apresoline) Minoxidil (Loniten)	100–300† 2.5–80	Minoxidil may cause or aggravate pleural and pericardial effusions. Both precipitate angina pectoris in patients with coronary disease. Hydralazine: lupus syndrome. Should be administered with a diuretic to prevent fluid retention and an adrenergic inhibitor (usually a beta-adrenergic blocker) to prevent reflex tachycardia.	Headache, anorexia, nausea and vomiting, diarrhea, palpitations, reflex tachycardia, fluid retention, aggravation of angina. Hydralazine: positive antinuclear antibody test, positive lupus erythematosus test, lupus-like reactions. Minoxidil: hirsutism.

Special indications: Hydralazine: eclampsia or preeclampsia (usually given intravenously). Minoxidil: severe and resistant hypertension.
Contraindications: Atherosclerotic heart disease; lupus erythematosus (hydralazine).
Advantages: Minoxidil is one of the most potent antihypertensive agents available. Relatively inexpensive. Reduce total peripheral resistance, no metabolic side effects.
Disadvantages: Must be prescribed with a diuretic to prevent fluid retention and a sympathetic inhibiting drug to prevent reflex tachycardia. High side effect profile. No trials to demonstrate long-term efficacy in reducing cardiovascular events.
*The dosage range may differ slightly from recommended dosage in *Physicians' Desk Reference* or package insert. Given once daily unless otherwise indicated.
†This drug is usually given in divided doses two to four times daily.

J-CURVE

Farnett et al.[87] have summarized 13 publications, nine of which demonstrated that reducing diastolic blood pressure below 85 to 90 mmHg may paradoxically increase the risk of coronary mortality for hypertensive patients and two of which showed a flattening of coronary mortality at the lower end of diastolic blood pressure achieved by treatment, but not actually an upswing. In one of the original reports Cruickshank et al.[88] stated that the J-curve phenomenon was observed only in those hypertensive patients who had clinical evidence of ischemic heart disease, but others have reported that excess mortality was not limited to patients with ischemic heart disease when the diastolic blood pressure was reduced below 85 to 90 mmHg.[87,89–97] Some authors report that the J-curve is limited to diastolic blood pressure only,[88–90,92,96] while others have found it for systolic blood pressure as well (less than 150 to 155 mmHg).[93,97]

Stroke mortality seems to decrease with diastolic blood pressure without a J-curve phenomenon, and there is evidence that maximal protection from end-stage renal failure is achieved when blood pressure is reduced to 130/85 or below.[98]

The J-curve phenomenon is not confined to hypertensive patients on antihypertensive therapy but has also been observed in the Framingham observational study,[99,100] in the placebo group in the European Working Party on Hypertension in the Elderly (EWPHE),[97] and in an untreated group of elderly hypertensive patients.[95] In the EWPHE trial the participants who had the lowest systolic and diastolic blood pressures also had the most pronounced decreases in body weight and hemoglobin concentration, suggesting that they were ill.[97] Noncardiovascular mortality was also highest in patients who were in the lowest third of diastolic pressure.[97] Low blood pressure, with or without therapy, may simply be a marker for chronic illness.

A metaanalysis of observational studies[101] and the large MRC trial[29] failed to show a J-curve. In the Systolic Hypertension in the Elderly (SHEP) trial, the 5-year average diastolic blood pressure was 68 mmHg for the treated group and 72 mmHg for the placebo group, yet the treated group had significantly fewer coronary and stroke events than did the participants in the placebo group.[8]

Fletcher and Bulpitt[102] have concluded a very thoughtful and comprehensive review of this subject with this recommendation: "In conclusion, it appears reasonable to lower diastolic blood pressure to below 85 mmHg. This gives maximal benefit in reducing the risk of stroke, and the risk of myocardial infarction is reduced compared with that at pressures over 100 mmHg. On balance, we consider the J-curve is probably a consequence, not a cause of coronary heart disease. Systolic blood pressure should be lowered to below 125 mmHg, since there is no indication that doing so has any adverse effects." Most patients are not having their blood pressures controlled to this level at the present time.[3,103]

It is equally important to control systolic blood pressure as noted by Fletcher and Bulpitt.[102] Oxygen consumption of the myocardium is more dependent on systolic blood pressure than it is on diastolic blood pressure, whereas coronary flow (oxygen supply) is dependent on diastolic blood pressure. A disparity, therefore, between oxygen demand and supply might explain the J-curve phenomenon, if indeed there is one.

The J-curve has been a retrospective observation in nonrandomized clinical trials or randomized trials that were not designed to test this hypothesis. A prospective, controlled, randomized trial is needed to settle this issue.

DIABETES AND/OR INSULIN RESISTANCE

Many hypertensive patients, obese and nonobese, have insulin resistance manifested by higher than normal fasting and post–glucose load plasma insulin levels, even if they are not frankly diabetic.[104–106] A direct relationship between diastolic blood pressure and fasting insulin levels has been demonstrated.[104] Although it has been postulated that insulin may increase blood pressure by promoting sodium retention and increasing sympathetic nervous activity, there is evidence that insulin resistance may be the result of and not the cause for the heightened adrenergic outflow.[107] Lipid abnormalities, including high triglyceride and low HDL cholesterol levels in the blood, are often associated with hyperinsulinemia. Indeed, this combination of risk factors has been designated "Syndrome X"[105] or the "Deadly Quartet,"[108] which includes upper body obesity, hypertension, insulin resistance (glucose intolerance), and hypertriglyceridemia. (See also Chap. 102.)

Reducing the blood pressure with medication does not necessarily improve insulin resistance,[105] although a short-term study did show that the ACE inhibitor captopril reduced insulin resistance whereas a diuretic made it worse.[75] Alpha$_1$-adrenergic blocking agents have also been shown to improve insulin resistance.[77,78,80] The long-term implications of this are not clear. Weight reduction and physical exercise decrease insulin resistance.[105]

In addition to diuretics, beta blockers[52,53] can increase insulin resistance and raise blood glucose in some patients. Diuretic therapy has been associated with increased mortality in diabetic patients with retinopathy in nonrandomized observations in which there was no attempt to allocate treatment regimens prospectively.[109,110]

It should be noted that diuretic-based therapy was used in several of the large prospective randomized trials in which diabetics were not excluded (EWPHE,[30] HDFP,[111] SHEP[8]), and no adverse effects were reported. Indeed, in the HDFP trial, diabetic patients had higher mortality rates than nondiabetic patients in both the stepped care and referred care groups, but the benefit of stepped care, although less for diabetic than for nondiabetic patients, was not statistically significantly different between the two groups.[111]

Diuretics and beta blockers usually do not adversely affect glucose control and are not contraindicated in patients with diabetes provided that blood glucose and lipids are carefully monitored. Randomized trials are needed to determine if drugs that do not have an adverse effect on insulin resistance (calcium antagonists) or that may actually improve it (ACE inhibitors, alpha$_1$-adrenergic blocking agents) will be more effective than diuretics in reducing cardiovascular morbidity and mortality for diabetic patients.

Nonselective beta blockers (as well as selective beta blockers in large doses) should be used with caution in patients with type I diabetes mellitus, especially those who are subject to insulin reactions because they can prolong recovery from insulin-induced hypoglycemia.

The putative benefit of ACE inhibitors in patients with diabetic glomerulosclerosis was described previously.

MANAGEMENT OF HYPERTENSION IN SPECIAL POPULATIONS

Black Patients

In the United States hypertension occurs more frequently, tends to be more severe, and is accompanied by a higher mortality rate in blacks than in whites, irrespective of age.[3,4,112] For comparable levels of blood pressure blacks have echo-LVH and/or evidence of renal disease more often than do whites.[4,112]

The HDFP trial showed that the overall mortality rate was reduced more for blacks than for whites by stepped care therapy compared to referred care.[111]

Black hypertensive patients seem to respond better to diuretics[13] or calcium antagonists[26] than they do to beta blockers or ACE inhibitors, although there are many exceptions to this. Because of the obvious racial differences in vulnerability to the complications of hypertension, therapy should be initiated early and should be pursued aggressively for black patients, especially young males.

Women

While there is no evidence that women respond any differently than men to the hypotensive effects of antihypertensive drugs, the long-term effect of reducing blood pressure on cardiovascular events for white women has been questioned.[113] It is true that women were not included in the major VA trials showing efficacy of treatment. It is also true that premenopausal hypertensive women have a lower incidence of cardiovascular disease than do hypertensive men of the same age. When hypertensive women are compared to normotensive women of the same age, however, the *relative risk* of cardiovascular morbidity and mortality is about the same for women as it is for men, especially as it relates to systolic blood pressure.[114]

In the HDFP trial the 5-year mortality rate for 908 white women in the stepped care (SC) group with mild hypertension (stratum I; diastolic blood pressure 90 to 104 mmHg) was 27.1 percent lower than for the 917 white women in referred care (RC). This was second only to a 29 percent reduction in mortality enjoyed by black women in stepped care. For white men the reduction was 17.6 percent and for black men it was 6.8 percent.[111] In the groups with more severe hypertension (diastolic blood pressure $\geq$ 105 mmHg) the white women in stepped care did not fare as well as those in referred care, but this is not necessarily the result of pharmacologic treatment because both groups received antihypertensive agents. The numbers of white women were so small in these groups (SC = 272, RC = 233) that this difference was not statistically significant.

More worrisome is the observation that in the placebo-controlled MRC trial all-cause mortality was *increased* by 26 percent for white women on active treatment compared to those on placebo, whereas there was a 15 percent reduction in mortality for men on active treatment.[29]

In the HDFP trial total strokes were reduced by 30.4 percent for white women.[115] In the SHEP trial white women on active treatment had 27 percent fewer strokes than those on placebo.[8]

As yet there is no justification from available evidence that treatment guidelines should be different for the genders, except that ACE inhibitors are contraindicated for pregnant women.[83]

Elderly

The prevalence of hypertension, both diastolic and isolated systolic, increases with age. If one uses at least 140 mmHg systolic and/or at least 90 mmHg diastolic as the criterion, the prevalence of hypertension is 63 percent for whites and 76 percent for blacks ages 65 to 74 years, determined by the National Health and Nutrition Examination Survey (NHANES II) of 1976 to 1980.[116] These data were derived by averaging three blood pressure measurements on a single occasion. The prevalence of isolated systolic hypertension was 10.9 percent in a survey of individuals 75 years of age or older.[117] Most elderly hypertensive patients have primary hypertension that started in middle life or earlier.

There is good evidence from prospective controlled trials that treating diastolic hypertension[28,30,31,94,118,119] as well as isolated systolic hypertension[8,31] is beneficial in reducing morbidity and mortality for elderly patients. These trials have shown that elderly patients tolerate antihypertensive drugs well and are as adherent to regimens as younger patients are.

It is advisable to initiate therapy with smaller than average doses and to increase doses or to add new drugs very gradually to avoid reducing blood pressure rapidly and to minimize the risk of orthostatic hypotension. (See also Chap. 116.)

The drug of choice for most elderly patients is a thiazide-type diuretic in low dose, simply because all the clinical trials that have demonstrated the benefit of treatment have used diuretic-based stepped care. Beta-adrenergic blocking agents were also found to be effective in the STOP[28] and the Hypertension in Elderly Patients trials.[94] Moreover, a VA trial showed that a diuretic as step 1 followed by hydralazine, methyldopa, metoprolol, or reserpine, if needed for step 2, was effective and well tolerated and did not have an adverse effect on cognitive or behavioral function in elderly patients compared to placebo administered in the pretreatment control period.[120,121] Similarly, in the SHEP Feasibility Trial, participants on diuretic therapy did not have changes in cognitive function or level of depression compared to those on placebo.[122]

MANAGING PATIENTS WITH COMPLICATIONS OF HYPERTENSION

Cerebrovascular Disease

Controlling diastolic as well as isolated systolic hypertension has had a profound effect on reducing morbidity and mortality from stroke in randomized clinical trials.[1,2,8,28,31,115]

Several small trials have shown that control of blood pressure for patients who have already had one stroke will reduce the risk of recurrent stroke, including fatal ones,[123–125] although one large multicenter trial failed to confirm this.[126]

Management of hypertension during acute stroke is discussed in the section on hypertensive crises. Once a patient has recovered from the acute phase of cerebral infarction or hemorrhage, the neurologic deficit has stabilized and the patient is ambulatory (usually 3 or 4 weeks after the stroke), hypertension should be treated with the same regimens that would be used for hypertensive patients who have never had a stroke. The goal should be to normalize blood pressure gradually (<140/90 mmHg). (See also Chap. 122.)

Surprisingly, these patients usually tolerate normotension quite well, including inadvertent orthostatic hypotension, although this is not desirable and should be avoided if at all possible. While none of the antihypertensive agents are absolutely contraindicated, agents that have a proclivity for producing disproportionate orthostatic decreases in blood pressure (e.g., $alpha_1$-adrenergic blockers, guanadrel, guanethidine) should be used with extra caution, and patients should be warned about rising from the seated or recumbent positions rapidly.

If treatment produces symptoms of global cerebral ischemia unrelated to measurable hypotension, the clinician should suspect that the patient has severe occlusive disease in both carotid arteries and/or the vertebral basilar system. Monitoring blood pressure in the standing as well as seated (or supine) positions is particularly important for patients with cerebrovascular disease.

In patients with transient ischemic attacks the treatment of systemic arterial hypertension will not only reduce the frequency of the ischemic episodes but will also lessen the risk of subsequent stroke.[127] Blood pressure should be reduced gradually with special attention devoted to avoiding orthostatic hypotension. Aspirin should be prescribed in a dose of 325 mg daily. Obviously, a surgically approachable lesion in the extracranial carotid arteries should be sought. (See Chap. 122.)

Cardiac Complications

Atherosclerotic Heart Disease

The management of hypertension with unstable angina or acute myocardial infarction is discussed in the section on hypertensive crises.

Angina Pectoris There is a special indication for beta-adrenergic blockers or calcium antagonists in the management of hypertension in patients with angina pectoris because both classes of drugs are beneficial for relieving angina and controlling hypertension. Their mechanisms for relieving angina pectoris are different so that there is sometimes an advantage to using these two classes of drugs together when angina is resistant to one, although this must be done judiciously because both the beta-adrenergic blockers and the calcium antagonists verapamil and diltiazem slow conduction and have negative inotropic effects that might lead to heart block or left ventricular failure in patients who already have a conduction defect or left ventricular dysfunction.

Drugs that can cause reflexive tachycardia, such as hydralazine and minoxidil, can aggravate angina pectoris and should not be used without an adrenergic inhibitor in the regimen, usually a beta blocker, to prevent tachycardia.

Post–Myocardial Infarction Only the non-ISA beta blockers have been shown conclusively to have a cardioprotective effect following myocardial infarction[49] and are the agents of choice for treating hypertension in patients who have had a myocardial infarction, unless there is a bona fide contraindication to their use. The evidence of a cardioprotective effect for verapamil is less impressive than for the beta-adrenergic blockers, and in patients with significant left ventricular dysfunction, diltiazem had an adverse effect on survival after myocardial infarction.[57] The dihydropyridine calcium antagonists have failed to show any cardioprotective effect following myocardial infarction and in some studies have been detrimental.[55] (See also Chaps. 60, 66, and 67.)

Left Ventricular Hypertrophy

While left ventricular hypertrophy (LVH) is an adaptive mechanism to handle the increased workload imposed by high systemic arterial pressure, it nevertheless is an independent risk factor for arrhythmias, myocardial infarction, and sudden death.[128] Because there is as yet no convincing evidence that reversing LVH will eliminate or mitigate this risk, the goal should be to prevent LVH in the first place by treating hypertension before LVH develops. The concept that only certain classes of antihypertensive drugs reverse LVH is being questioned as long-term studies become available.[129–131] All of the major classes of antihypertensive agents with the possible exception of the direct vasodilators (hydralazine, minoxidil) will eventually reduce left ventricular mass when it is increased.[132] The central $alpha_2$ agonists, beta-adrenergic blockers, ACE inhibitors, and calcium antagonists seem to reduce mass sooner than do the diuretics, but this is not an obvious advantage, especially when it has not been convincingly shown that reversal of LVH will reduce the risk that it imposes and might even leave the left ventricle vulnerable to recurrent hypertension.[128]

Consequently, LVH does not present a special indication or contraindication for any of the antihypertensive drugs recommended for initial therapy. If a diuretic is selected, however, hypokalemia should be avoided as it could enhance the arrhythmogenic potential of LVH. The use of a combination thiazide/potassium-sparing agent is recommended under these circumstances.

Congestive Heart Failure

Agents of choice for hypertensive patients with congestive heart failure due to systolic dysfunction are diuretics and ACE inhibitors, which reduce preload by decreasing venous return and afterload by dilating arterioles. The ACE inhibitors have been shown to improve survival in patients with chronic congestive heart failure with or without hypertension.[61,62] They are just as effective as conventional vasodilator therapy with hydralazine and isosorbide dinitrate[62] but are more reliable antihypertensive agents. Beta-adrenergic blockers and calcium antagonists are relatively contraindicated in patients with congestive heart failure due to left ventricular systolic dysfunction and low ejection fraction. (See also Chaps. 66 and 67.)

Occasionally, recurrent episodes of left ventricular failure, sometimes with pulmonary edema, are due to *diastolic* rather than systolic dysfunction, especially in elderly patients. This is characterized by severe concentric left ventricular hypertrophy that may nearly obliterate the left ventricular cavity, compromising diastolic filling of the ventricle, which relaxes poorly during diastole. Ejection fraction is high but cardiac index is low in spite of vigorous systolic contractions. (See also Chaps. 25 and 26.) In this situation, diuretics and vasodilators such as ACE inhibitors, the dihydropyridine calcium antagonists, $alpha_1$-adrenergic blockers, and the direct vasodilators can have an adverse effect by causing hypotension.[133] Drugs of choice are the beta-adrenergic blockers and the calcium antagonists, verapamil or diltiazem, because they may improve relaxation of the left ventricle, thereby enhancing diastolic filling. (See also Chaps. 25, 26, and 67.)

Cardiac Arrhythmias and Conduction Disturbances

Certain antihypertensive drugs may be especially indicated or relatively contraindicated when hypertension is complicated by cardiac arrhythmias or conduction disturbances.

Non-ISA beta blockers may be helpful in controlling paroxysmal supraventricular tachycardia and premature ventricular contractions due to adrenergic hyperactivity. On the other hand, by slowing the heart rate, they can actually increase premature ventricular contractions arising from an irritable focus.

Verapamil is even more effective than beta blockers in treating and preventing recurrences of paroxysmal supraventricular tachycardia. Intravenous verapamil or diltiazem is recommended for terminating an acute episode of paroxysmal supraventricular tachycardia. (See also Chaps. 36 and 38.)

Beta-adrenergic blockers, verapamil, and diltiazem slow AV conduction and therefore are often effective in controlling the ventricular rate in patients with atrial fibrillation or flutter. For the same reason, however, they are contraindicated in the presence of greater than first-degree AV block but may be used in patients with intraventricular block and bundle branch block. All are contraindicated for patients with "sick sinus syndrome" unless a functioning ventricular pacemaker is in place. Special precautions must be observed in using verapamil, diltiazem, or beta-adrenergic blockers in patients with an accessory bypass tract (Wolff-Parkinson-White or Lown-Genong-Levine syndromes). Verapamil and diltiazem can convert atrial flutter or atrial fibrillation to ventricular tachyarrhythmias including ventricular fibrillation when administered to patients with accessory bypass tracts. Rare instances of severe bradycardia requiring a demand pacemaker have been reported when beta blockers have been given to patients with paroxysmal atrial tachycardia in the presence of Wolff-Parkinson-White syndrome. (See also Chap. 36.)

Valvular Heart Disease

Arteriolar vasodilating agents such as calcium antagonists and ACE inhibitors are helpful in minimizing the regurgitant flow in patients with either mitral or aortic regurgitation.[134]

Chronic Renal Failure

Treatment of hypertension may prevent or retard progression of renal failure.[98,135] The dramatic increase in the number of patients with diabetes and hypertension coming to end-stage renal failure and requiring dialysis is therefore disturbing.

It was the consensus of the Working Group on Hypertension and Chronic Renal Failure of the National High Blood Pressure Education Program that efforts to treat hypertension have not been vigorous enough and that reducing blood pressure to 130/85 or lower may be beneficial for patients with established renal insufficiency.[98] (See also Chap. 108.)

The potential advantage and risks of ACE inhibitors for patients with diabetic glomerulosclerosis have already been discussed in the section on ACE inhibitors.

Calcium antagonists, selective $alpha_1$-adrenergic blocking agents, beta-adrenergic blocking agents, $alpha_2$ agonists, and loop diuretics have all been used in managing hypertension in patients with renal failure. Loop diuretics are particularly important when fluid retention seems to be causing or aggravating the hypertension. Minoxidil is especially effective in patients with renal failure and severe hypertension.[86]

Appropriate adjustments in dosage of antihypertensive agents that are excreted by the kidney must be made when renal failure is present (see Tables 77-3 and 77-5).

A low-protein diet (40 to 50 g daily) may have a renal protective effect and should be prescribed for most patients with chronic renal failure. Dietary sodium restriction is also important as an adjunct to prevent fluid retention. (See also Chaps. 29 and 108.)

SEVERE AND REFRACTORY HYPERTENSION

The more severe the hypertension, the less likely that monotherapy will control it and the greater the urgency for reducing it. Consequently, in the absence of complications that would require immediate reduction of blood pressure (see the section on hypertensive crises), it is usually advisable to initiate therapy with two drugs simultaneously when diastolic blood pressure is at least 115 mmHg and with three drugs simultaneously when diastolic blood pressure is at least 125 mmHg. The selection of drugs should be made on an individualized basis using criteria listed in the tables. Hospitalization is not necessary in the absence of complications, but patients should be seen in the office or clinic at frequent intervals until the blood pressure is controlled. Monitoring blood pressure at home is almost mandatory in this situation.

Not all severe hypertension is refractory to treatment, and not all refractory hypertension is severe.[41] When hypertension does not respond to a rational triple-drug regimen that includes a diuretic, the physician should suspect nonadherence to the regimen as the most likely cause. This may be manifested by failure to take drugs as prescribed or by consuming too much sodium or both. Drug-drug interactions should be suspected. Leading the list of drugs that can interfere with an otherwise effective regimen are nonsteroidal anti-inflammatory drugs and oral contraceptives. Pseudohypertension[136] and white coat hypertension[137] should be ruled out. Finally, the physician should reconsider the possibility that a secondary form of hypertension has been overlooked. These include pheochromocytoma, renovascular hypertension, and primary aldosteronism. (See Chap. 76.)

When it is apparent that the hypertension is truly resistant, changes in the regimen can be made empirically.[138] Doses of all the drugs in this regimen should be maximized. Consideration should be given to adding a fourth drug with a different mechanism of action. Minoxidil is one of the most potent agents available.

Sometimes it is necessary to evaluate the mechanism of the hypertension while patients are on their regimen to see which drug or drugs are failing. This would include measurements of plasma renin activity, catecholamines, aldosterone, plasma volume, cardiac output, and total peripheral resistance.

HYPERTENSIVE CRISES

Table 77-10 lists some of the hypertensive emergencies and urgencies that require prompt antihypertensive therapy. True emergencies require immediate reduction of blood pressure to prevent or to ameliorate target organ damage.

Rapid reduction of blood pressure to or toward normal is recommended for patients with acute hypertensive encephalopathy, acute left ventricular failure with pulmonary edema, and acute aortic dissection. It is not desirable to reduce blood pressure rapidly or to normotensive levels for patients with cerebral hemorrhage, subarachnoid hemorrhage, or acute brain infarction.[139–141] (See Chap. 122.)

The availability of drugs such as nifedipine (not sustained release), captopril, and clonidine, which can reduce blood pressure within minutes to 1 h when given by mouth or sublingually, has blurred the distinction between hypertensive emergencies and urgencies.[142] Sometimes, oral medication will suffice for some emergencies, and parenteral drugs are used for other urgencies, especially when patients are unable to take medication by mouth (e.g., postoperative state).

Patients with *hypertensive emergencies* present with evidence of target organ involvement or are in immediate danger of developing it, whereas patients with *hypertensive urgencies* have no evidence of target organ involvement, and it is only the height of the blood pressure that is of concern. Usually, reduction of blood pressure to a safer, though not necessarily normotensive, level over a period of 12 to 24 h is sufficient in managing urgencies. Hospitalization may not even be required, or if it is, monitoring in an intensive care unit is not necessary. Most patients with hypertensive urgencies can be managed on an outpatient basis if they can be seen frequently

TABLE 77-10

Hypertensive Emergencies and Urgencies

Emergencies

A. Require immediate blood pressure reduction, not necessarily to normal:
   - Hypertensive encephalopathy
   - Acute left ventricular failure
   - Acute aortic dissection
   - Eclampsia
   - Post–coronary artery bypass
   - Some cases of hypertension associated with increased circulating catecholamines (pheochromocytoma, clonidine withdrawal hypertension, food or drug interactions with monoamine oxidase inhibitors, ingestion or injection of sympathomimetic agents including cocaine)

B. Require immediate reduction of blood pressure only when it is excessively high (see text):
   - Hypertensive intracerebral bleeding
   - Acute subarachnoid hemorrhage
   - Some acute brain infarcts
   - Unstable angina or acute myocardial infarction

Urgencies

Require blood pressure reduction within 12–24 h
   - Severe diastolic hypertension (≥140 mmHg) without complications
   - Malignant hypertension without complications
   - Perioperative hypertension
   - Some cases of hypertension associated with increased circulating catecholamines (pheochromocytoma, clonidine withdrawal hypertension, food or drug interactions with monoamine oxidase inhibitors, ingestion or injection of sympathomimetic agents including cocaine)

SOURCE: Reprinted from RW Gifford Jr: Management of hypertensive crises. *JAMA*, 266:829–835, 1991. Copyright 1991, American Medical Association. With permission from the publisher and author.

in the clinic or office for both diagnostic evaluation and therapeutic follow-up.

The drugs that can be given parenterally for managing hypertensive emergencies and urgencies are listed in Table 77-11. Sodium nitroprusside is recommended for most of the emergencies listed in Table 77-10 except for eclampsia, acute myocardial ischemia, and post–coronary bypass hypertension.[142] Methyldopa, given intravenously, is the drug of choice for eclampsia,[83] while intravenous nitroglycerin is recommended for patients with acute myocardial ischemia and post–coronary bypass hypertension.[142] A beta-adrenergic blocker must be given orally or parenterally with sodium nitroprusside for managing patients with acute dissecting aneurysm, and the goal of treatment is to maintain systolic blood pressure within the range of 100 to 120 mmHg. (See also Chap. 123.) Trimethaphan camsylate may also be used for managing acute dissection of the aorta.

Continuous intravenous infusion of antihypertensive drugs (nitroprusside, nitroglycerin, trimethaphan) re-

TABLE 77-11

Parenteral Drugs for Treatment of Hypertensive Emergencies

Drug	Dose	Onset of Action	Adverse Reactions	Special Indications
			Vasodilators	
Sodium nitroprusside	0.3–10 μg/kg per min as IV infusion, maximal dose for no more than 10 min	Instantaneous	Nausea, vomiting, muscle twitching, thiocyanate intoxication, methemoglobinemia, cyanide toxicity, hypotension	Hypertensive encephalopathy, acute intracranial hemorrhage, acute cerebral infarction, acute left ventricular failure, acute coronary insufficiency, dissecting aneurysm, catecholamine crisis, head injury, extensive body burns, malignant hypertension, postoperative hypertension
Nitroglycerin	5–100 μg/min as IV infusion	2–5 min	Headache, tachycardia, vomiting, methemoglobinemia	Acute left ventricular failure, acute coronary insufficiency, postoperative hypertension (especially coronary bypass)
Diazoxide	50–150 mg IV bolus, repeated, or 15–30 mg/min by IV infusion	1–2 min	Hypotension, tachycardia, acute MI or stroke, aggravation of angina pectoris, hyperglycemia, fluid retention	Hypertensive encephalopathy, eclampsia, extensive body burns, malignant hypertension, postoperative hypertension
Hydralazine	10–20 mg IV 10–50 mg IM	10 min 20–30 min	Tachycardia, headache, vomiting, aggravation of angina pectoris, fluid retention	Eclampsia, extensive body burns, malignant hypertension, postoperative hypertension
Enalaprilat	0.625–1.25 mg q 6 h IV slowly over 5 min	15–30 min	Hypotension, headache, nausea, fatigue, dizziness, acute MI	Congestive heart failure and when oral administration is not feasible
Verapamil	5–10 mg IV repeated, or 0.005 mg/kg per min by infusion	2–3 min	Hypotension, bradycardia, asystole, heart failure, rapid ventricular rate due to antegrade conduction in flutter/fibrillation with Wolff-Parkinson-White and Lown-Ganong-Levine syndromes	Paroxysmal supraventricular tachycardia

TABLE 77-11
Parenteral Drugs for Treatment of Hypertensive Emergencies *(continued)*

Drug	Dose	Onset of Action	Adverse Reactions	Special Indications
		Adrenergic Inhibitors		
Phentolamine	5–15 mg IV	1–2 min	Tachycardia, orthostatic hypotension	Catecholamine crisis
Trimethaphan camsylate	1–4 mg/min as IV infusion	1–5 min	Paresis of bowel and bladder, orthostatic hypotension, blurred vision, dry mouth	Dissecting aneurysm
Labetalol	20–80 mg IV bolus every 10 min, 2 mg/min IV infusion	5–10 min	Bronchoconstriction, heart block, orthostatic hypotension, LV dysfunction, sick sinus syndrome	Hypertensive encephalopathy, acute coronary insufficiency, extensive body burns, malignant hypertension, postoperative hypertension
Methyldopa	250–500 mg IV infusion	30–60 min	Drowsiness	Eclampsia, perioperative hypertension

MI = myocardial infarction, LV = left ventricular.
SOURCE: Reprinted from RW Gifford Jr: Management of hypertensive crises. *JAMA* 266:829–835, 1991. Copyright 1991, American Medical Association. With permission from the publisher and author.

quires close observation in an intensive care environment, whereas intermittent intravenous administration of drugs (diazoxide, labetalol) can be accomplished on a regular nursing floor or even in the emergency room.

Although it is unusual, administration of antihypertensive agents orally or sublingually can precipitate a rapid and excessive decrease in blood pressure, sometimes to hypotensive levels. This is particularly deleterious for patients who have severe atherosclerotic disease, especially in the cerebral or coronary circulation. Before administering one of these agents orally, the physician should assure that effective antidotes to raise the blood pressure under these circumstances are available.

The availability of potent antihypertensive drugs that can be given orally to control severe hypertension invites their indiscriminate use for any patient whose blood pressure seems inordinately high, without adequate evaluation of the clinical situation.[143,144]

ACKNOWLEDGMENT

The author gratefully acknowledges the technical assistance of Ray Borazanian in the preparation of this manuscript and Alan Bakst, Pharm.D., for reviewing the tables.

REFERENCES

1. Collins R, Peto R, MacMahon S, Hebert P, Fiebach NH, Eberlein KA, et al: Blood pressure, stroke, and coronary heart disease. Part 2, Short-term reductions in blood pressure: Overview of randomised drug trials in their epidemiological context. *Lancet* 1990; 335:827–838.
2. Gifford RW Jr: Review of the long-term controlled trials of usefulness of therapy for systemic hypertension. *Am J Cardiol* 1989; 63:8B–16B.
3. Joint National Committee on Detection, Evaluation, and Treatment of High Blood Pressure: The fifth report of the Joint Natural Committee on Detection, Evaluation, and Treatment of High Blood Pressure (JNCU) *Arch Int Med* 1993; 153:154–183.
4. The 1988 report of the Joint National Committee on Detection, Evaluation, and Treatment of High Blood Pressure. *Arch Intern Med* 1988; 148:1023–1038.
5. Hypertension Detection and Follow-up Program Cooperative Group: Results of the Hypertension Detection and Follow-up Program. The effect of treatment on mortality in "mild" hypertension. *N Engl J Med* 1982; 307:976–980.
6. Stamler R, Stamler J, Gosch FC, Civinelli J, Fishman J, McKeever P, et al: Primary prevention of hypertension by nutritional-hygienic means. Final report of a randomized, controlled trial. *JAMA* 1989; 262:1801–1807.
7. The Trials of Hypertension Prevention Collaborative Research Group: The effects of nonpharmacologic interventions on blood pressure of persons with high normal levels. *JAMA* 1992; 267:1213–1220.
8. SHEP Cooperative Research Group: Prevention of stroke by antihypertensive drug treatment in older persons with isolated systolic hypertension. Final results of the Systolic Hypertension in the Elderly Program (SHEP). *JAMA* 1991; 265:3255–3264.
9. Nonpharmacological approaches to the control of high blood pressure. Final report of the Subcommittee on Nonpharmacological Therapy of the 1984 Joint National Committee on Detection, Evaluation, and Treatment of High Blood Pressure. *Hypertension* 1986; 8:444–467.
10. The Treatment of Mild Hypertension Research Group: The Treatment of Mild Hypertension Study. *Arch Intern Med* 1991; 151:1413–1423.
11. Stamler R, Stamler J, Grimm R, Gosch FC, Elmer P, Dyer A, et al: Nutritional therapy for high blood pressure. Final report of a four-year randomized controlled trial—The Hypertension Control Program. *JAMA* 1987; 257:1484–1491.
12. Chockalingam A, Abbott D, Bass M, Battista R, Cameron R, de Champlain J, et al: Recommendations of the Canadian Consensus Conference on Non-pharmacological Approaches to the Management of High Blood Pressure, March 21–23, 1989, Halifax, Nova Scotia. *Can Med Assoc J* 1990; 142:1397–1409.

13. Wassertheil-Smoller S, Oberman A, Blaufox MD, Davis BR, Langford H: The Trial of Antihypertensive Interventions and Management (TAIM) study. Final results with regard to blood pressure, cardiovascular risk, and quality of life. *Am J Hypertens* 1992; 5:37–42.
14. Applegate WB, Miller ST, Elam JT, Cushman WC, El Derwi D, Brewer A, et al: Nonpharmacologic intervention to reduce blood pressure in older patients with mild hypertension. *Arch Intern Med* 1992; 152:1162–1166.
15. Elmer PJ, Grimm RH Jr, Flack J, Laing B: Dietary sodium reduction for hypertension prevention and treatment. *Hypertension* 1991; 17(suppl I):I-182–I-189.
16. Reisin E, Abel R, Modan M, Silverberg DS, Eliahou HE, Modan B: Effect of weight loss without salt restriction on the reduction of blood pressure in overweight hypertensive patients. *N Engl J Med* 1978; 298:1–6.
17. Schotte DE, Stunkard AJ: The effects of weight reduction on blood pressure in 301 obese patients. *Arch Intern Med* 1990; 150:1701–1704.
18. Langford HG, Davis BR, Blaufox D, Oberman A, Wassertheil-Smoller S, Hawkins M, et al, for the TAIM Research Group: Effect of drug and diet treatment of mild hypertension on diastolic blood pressure. *Hypertension* 1991; 17:210–217.
19. Eliahou HE, Iaina A, Gaon T, Shochat J, Modan M: Body weight reduction necessary to obtain normotension in the overweight hypertensive patient. *Int J Obes* 1981; 5(suppl 1):157–163.
20. Cohen N, Flamenbaum W: Obesity and hypertension. Demonstration of a "floor effect." *Am J Med* 1986; 80:177–181.
21. Cappuccio FP, MacGregor GA: Does potassium supplementation lower blood pressure? A meta-analysis of published trials. *J Hypertens* 1991; 9:465–473.
22. Larbi ER, Cooper RS, Stamler J: Alcohol and hypertension. *Arch Intern Med* 1983; 143:28–29.
23. World Hypertension League: Alcohol and hypertension—implications for management. A consensus statement by the World Hypertension League. *J Hum Hypertens* 1991; 5:227–232.
24. Physical exercise in the management of hypertension: A consensus statement by the World Hypertension League. *J Hypertens* 1991; 9:283–287.
25. National High Blood Pressure Education Program: Report to the Hypertension Information and Education Advisory Committee. Task Force I. Data Base. Recommendations for a national high blood pressure program data base for effective antihypertensive therapy. DHEW Publication No. (NIH) 75-593, September 1, 1973.
26. Materson, BJ, Reda DJ, Cushman, WC, Massie, BM, Freis ED, Kochar, MS, et al: Single-drug therapy for hypertension in men. A comparison of six antihypertensive agents with placebo. *N Engl J Med* 1993; 328:914–921.
27. Alderman MH: Which antihypertensive drugs first—and why! *JAMA* 1992; 267:2786–2787.
28. Dahlöf B, Lindholm LH, Hansson L, Schersten B, Ekbom T, Wester PO: Morbidity and mortality in the Swedish Trial in Old Patients with Hypertension (STOP-Hypertension). *Lancet* 1991; 338:1281–1284.
29. Medical Research Council Working Party: MRC trial of treatment of mild hypertension: Principal results. *Br Med J* 1985; 291:97–104.
30. Amery A, Birkenhager W, Brixko P, Bulpitt C, Clement D, Deruyterre M, et al: Mortality and morbidity results from the European Working Party on High Blood Pressure in the Elderly Trial. *Lancet* 1985; 1:1349–1354.
31. MRC Working Party: Medical Research Council trial of treatment in older adults: Principal results. *Br Med J* 1992; 304:405–412.
32. Grimm RH, Leon AS, Hunninghake DB, Lenz K, Hannan P, Blackburn H: Effects of thiazide diuretics on plasma lipids and lipoproteins in mildly hypertensive patients. A double-blind study. *Ann Intern Med* 1981; 94:7–11.
33. National High Blood Pressure Education Program (NHBPEP) and National Cholesterol Education Program (NCEP) Working Group report on management of patients with hypertension and high blood cholesterol. *Ann Intern Med* 1991; 114:224–237.
34. Veterans Administration Cooperative Study Group on Antihypertensive Agents: Comparison of propranolol and hydrochlorothiazide for the initial treatment of hypertension. II. Results of long-term therapy. *JAMA* 1982; 248:2004–2011.
35. Williams WR, Schneider KA, Borhani NO, Schnaper HW, Slotkoff LM, Ellefson RD: The relationship between diuretics and serum cholesterol in Hypertension Detection and Follow-up Program participants. *Am J Prev Med* 1986; 2:248–255.
36. Berglund G, Andersson O: Beta-blockers or diuretics in hypertension? A six-year follow-up of blood pressure and metabolic side effects. *Lancet* 1981; 1:744–747.
37. Hulley SB, Furberg CD, Gurland B, McDonald R, Perry HM, Schnaper HW, et al: Systolic Hypertension in the Elderly Program (SHEP): Antihypertensive efficacy of chlorthalidone. *Am J Cardiol* 1985; 56:913–920.
38. Goldman AI, Steele BW, Schnaper HW, Fritz AE, Frohlich ED, Perry HM: Serum lipoprotein levels during chlorthalidone therapy. A Veterans Administration–National Heart, Lung, and Blood Institute cooperative study on antihypertensive therapy: Mild hypertension. *JAMA* 1980; 244:1691–1695.
39. Jeunemaitre X, Charru A, Chatellier G, Degoulet P, Julien J, Plouin PF, et al: Long-term effects of spironolactone and thiazides combined with potassium-sparing agents for treatment of essential hypertension. *Am J Cardiol* 1988; 62:1072–1977.
40. Roccella EJ: Cost of hypertension medications: Is it a barrier to hypertension control? *Geriatrics* 1989; 44(suppl B):49–55.
41. Gifford RW Jr: Resistant hypertension. Introduction and definitions. *Hypertension* 1989; 11(suppl II):II-65–II66.
42. Myers MG, Carruthers SG, Leenen FHH, Haynes RB: Recommendations from the Canadian Hypertension Society Consensus Conference on the Pharmacologic Treatment of Hypertension. *Can Med Assoc J* 1989; 140:1141–1146.
43. New trials in older hypertensives (editorial). *Lancet* 1991; 338:1299–1300.
44. McMurray J, McLenachan J, Dargie HJ: Angiotensin converting enzyme inhibitors (reply). *J Hypertens* 1991; 9:1075–1076.
45. Swales JD, Ramsay LE, Coope JR, Pocock SJ, Robertson JIS, Sever PS, et al: Treating mild hypertension. Agreement from the large trials. Report of the British Hypertension Society working party. *Br Med J* 1989; 298:694–698.
46. The 1984 report of the Joint National Committee on Detection, Evaluation, and Treatment of High Blood Pressure. *Arch Intern Med* 1984; 144:1045–1057.
47. Pedersen TR, for the Norwegian Multicenter Study Group: Six-year follow-up of the Norwegian Multicenter Study on Timolol After Acute Myocardial Infarction. *N Engl J Med* 1985; 313:1055–1058.
48. Beta Blocker Heart Attack Trial Research Group: A randomized trial of propranolol in patients with acute myocardial infarction: I. Mortality results. *JAMA* 1982; 247:1707–1714.
49. Yusuf S, Peto R, Lewis J, Collins R, Sleight P: Beta blockade during and after myocardial infarction: An overview of the randomized trials. *Prog Cardiovasc Dis* 1985; 27:335–371.
50. Yusuf S, Wittes J, Probstfield J: Evaluating effects of treatment in subgroups of patients within a clinical trial: The case of non-Q-wave myocardial infarction and beta blockers. *Am J Cardiol* 1990; 66:220–222.
51. Frohlich ED, Tarazi RC, Dustan HP: Hyperdynamic β-adrenergic circulatory state: Increased β-receptor responsiveness. *Arch Intern Med* 1969; 123:1–7.
52. Pollare T, Lithell H, Selinus I, Berne C: Sensitivity to insulin during treatment with atenolol and metoprolol: A randomised, double blind study of effects on carbohydrate and lipoprotein metabolism in hypertensive patients. *Br Med J* 1989; 298:1152–1157.
53. Cressman MD, Vidt DG, Mohler H, Gifford RW Jr: Glucose tolerance during chronic propranolol treatment. *J Clin Hypertens* 1985; 2:138–144.
54. Kaplan NM: Calcium entry blockers in the treatment of hypertension. Current status and future prospects. *JAMA* 1989; 262:817–823.
55. Yusuf S, Held P, Furberg C: Update of effects of calcium antagonists in myocardial infarction or angina in light of the second Danish Verapamil Infarction Trial (DAVIT-II) and other recent studies. *Am J Cardiol* 1991; 67:1295–1297.
56. Packer M, Kessler PD, Lee WH: Calcium-channel blockade in the management of severe chronic congestive heart failure: A bridge too far. *Circulation* 1987; 75(suppl V):V-56–V-64.
57. Goldstein RE, Boccuzzi SJ, Cruess D, Nattel S: Diltiazem increases late-onset congestive heart failure in postinfarction pa-

tients with early reduction in ejection fraction. *Circulation* 1991; 83:52–60.

58. Elkayam U, Amin J, Mehra A, Vasquez J, Weber L, Rahimtoola SH: A prospective, randomized, double-blind crossover study to compare the efficacy and safety of chronic nifedipine therapy with that of isosorbide dinitrate and their combination in the treatment of chronic congestive heart failure. *Circulation* 1990; 82:1954–1961.
59. Williams GH: Converting-enzyme inhibitors in the treatment of hypertension. *N Engl J Med* 1988; 319:1517–1525.
60. Townsend RR, Holland OB: Combination of converting enzyme inhibitor with diuretic for the treatment of hypertension. *Arch Intern Med* 1990; 150:1175–1183.
61. The SOLVD Investigators: Effect of enalapril on survival in patients with reduced left ventricular ejection fractions and congestive heart failure. *N Engl J Med* 1991; 325:293–302.
62. Cohn JN, Johnson G, Ziesche S, Cobb F, Francis G, Tristani F, et al: A comparison of enalapril with hydralazine–isosorbide dinitrate in the treatment of chronic congestive heart failure. *N Engl J Med* 1991; 325:303–310.
63. Brenner BM, Meyer TW, Hostetter TH: Dietary protein and the progressive nature of kidney disease: The role of hemodynamically mediated glomerular injury in the pathogenesis of progessive glomerular sclerosis in aging, renal ablation, and intrinsic renal disease. *N Engl J Med* 1982; 307:652–660.
64. Hricik DE, Browning PJ, Kopelman R, Goorno WE, Madias NE, Dzau VJ: Captopril-induced functional renal insufficiency in patients with bilateral renal artery stenosis or renal artery stenosis in a solitary kidney. *N Engl J Med* 1983; 308:373–376.
65. Coulie P, De Plaen JF, van Ypersele de Strihou C: Captopril-induced acute reversible renal failure. *Nephron* 1983; 35:108–111.
66. Hollenberg NK: Angiotensin-converting enzyme inhibition: Renal aspects. *J Cardiovasc Pharmacol* 1985; 7(suppl 1):S40–S44.
67. Suki WN: Renal hemodynamic consequences of angiotensin-converting enzyme inhibition in congestive heart failure. *Arch Intern Med* 1989; 149:669–673.
68. Meyer TW, Anderson S, Rennke HG, Brenner BM: Converting enzyme inhibitor therapy limits progressive glomerular injury in rats with renal insufficiency. *Am J Med* 1985; 79:31–36.
69. Zatz R, Dunn BR, Meyer TW, Anderson S, Rennke HG, Brenner BM: Prevention of diabetic glomerulopathy by pharmacological amelioration of glomerular capillary hypertension. *J Clin Invest* 1986; 77:1925–1930.
70. Hommel E, Parving HH, Mathiesen E, Edsberg B, Nielsen MD, Giese J: Effect of captopril on kidney function in insulin-dependent diabetic patients with nephropathy. *Br Med J* 1986; 293:467–470.
71. Mathiesen ER, Hommel E, Giese J, Parving HH: Efficacy of captopril in postponing nephropathy in normotensive insulin dependent diabetic patients with microalbuminuria. *Br Med J* 1991; 303:81–87.
72. Parving HH, Andersen AR, Smidt U, Hommel E, Mathiesen ER, Svendsen PA: Antihypertensive treatment postpones end stage renal failure in diabetic nephropathy. *Br Med J* 1987; 294:1443–1447.
73. Toto RD, Mitchell HC, Lee HC, Milam C, Pettinger WA: Reversible renal insufficiency due to angiotensin converting enzyme inhibitors in hypertensive nephrosclerosis. *Ann Intern Med* 1991; 115:513–519.
74. Chapman AB, Gabow PA, Schrier RW: Reversible renal failure associated with angiotensin-converting enzyme inhibitors in polycystic kidney disease. *Ann Intern Med* 1991; 115:769–773.
75. Pollare T, Lithell H, Berne C: A comparison of the effects of hydrochlorothiazide and captopril on glucose and lipid metabolism in patients with hypertension. *N Engl J Med* 1989; 321:868–873.
76. Sebastian JL, McKinney WP, Kaufman J, Young MJ: Angiotensin-converting enzyme inhibitors and cough. Prevalence in an outpatient medical clinic population. *Chest* 1991; 99:36–39.
77. Khoury AF, Kaplan NM: α-Blocker therapy of hypertension. An unfulfilled promise. *JAMA* 1991; 266:394–398.
78. Waite MA: Alpha$_1$ blockers: Antihypertensives whose positive metabolic profile with regard to hyperinsulinaemia and lipid metabolism cannot be ignored. *J Intern Med* 1991; 29(suppl 2):113–117.
79. Stamler R, Stamler J, Gosch FC, Berkson DM, Dyer AR, Hershinow P: Initial antihypertensive drug therapy. Final report of a randomized, controlled trial comparing α-blocker and diuretic. *Hypertension* 1988; 12:574–581.
80. Pollare T, Lithell H, Selinus I, Berne C: Application of prazosin is associated with an increase of insulin sensitivity in obese patients with hypertension. *Diabetoligia* 1988; 31:415–420.
81. Caine M: Alpha-adrenergic blockers for the treatment of benign prostatic hyperplasia. *Urol Clin North Am* 1990; 17:641–649.
82. Oster JR, Epstein M: Use of centrally acting sympatholytic agents in the management of hypertension. *Arch Intern Med* 1991; 151:1638–1644.
83. Gifford RW Jr, August P, Chesley LC, Cunningham G, Ferris TF, Lenfant C, et al: National High Blood Pressure Education Program Working Group report on high blood pressure in pregnancy. *Am J Obstet Gynecol* 1990; 163:1689–1712.
84. Participating Veterans Administration Medical Centers: Low doses v standard dose of reserpine. A randomized, double-blind, multiclinic trial in patients taking chlorthalidone. *JAMA* 1982; 248:2471–2477.
85. Pettinger WA: Minoxidil and the treatment of severe hypertension. *N Engl J Med* 1980; 303:922–926.
86. Mitchell HC, Graham RM, Pettinger WA: Renal function during long-term treatment of hypertension with minoxidil. Comparison of benign and malignant hypertension. *Ann Intern Med* 1980; 93:676–681.
87. Farnett L, Mulrow CD, Linn WD, Lucey CR, Tuley MR: The J-curve phenomenon and the treatment of hypertension. Is there a point beyond which pressure reduction is dangerous? *JAMA* 1991; 265:489–495.
88. Cruickshank JM, Thorpe JM, Zacharias FJ: Benefits and potential harm of lowering high blood pressure. *Lancet* 1987; 1:581–584.
89. Fletcher AE, Beevers DG, Bulpitt CJ, Butler A, Coles EC, Hunt D, et al: The relationship between a low treated blood pressure and IHD mortality: A report from the DHSS Hypertension Care Computing Project. *J Human Hypertens* 1988; 2:11–15.
90. Waller PC, Isles CG, Lever AF, Murray GD, McInnes GT: Does therapeutic reduction of diastolic blood pressure cause death from coronary heart disease? *J Human Hypertens* 1988; 2:7–10.
91. Stewart IMcDG: Relationship of reduction in pressure to first myocardial infarction in patients receiving treatment for severe hypertension. *Lancet* 1979; 1:861–865.
92. Alderman MH, Ooi WL, Madharan S: Treatment induced blood pressure reduction and the risk of myocardial infarction. *JAMA* 1989; 262:920–924.
93. Samuelsson O, Wilhelmsen L, Anderson OK, Pennert K, Berglund G: Cardiovascular morbidity in relation to change in blood pressure and serum cholesterol levels in treated hypertension: Results from the Primary Prevention Trial in Goteborg, Sweden. *JAMA* 1987; 258:1768–1776.
94. Coope J, Warrender TS: Randomized trial of treatment of hypertension in elderly patients in primary care. *Br Med J* 1986; 293:1145–1151.
95. Coope J, Warrender TS: Lowering blood pressure (letter). *Lancet* 1987; 1:1380.
96. Cooper SP, Hardy RJ, Labarthe DR, Hawkins CM, Smith EO, Blaufox MD, et al: The relation between degree of blood pressure reduction and mortality among hypertensives in the Hypertension Detection and Follow-up Program. *Am J Epidemiol* 1988; 127:387–402.
97. Staessen J, Bulpitt C, Clement D, De Leeuw P, Fagard R, Fletcher A, et al: Relation between mortality and treated blood pressure in elderly patients with hypertension: Report of the European Working Party on High Blood Pressure in the Elderly. *Br Med J* 1989; 298:1552–1556.
98. National High Blood Pressure Education Program Working Group report on hypertension and chronic renal failure. *Arch Intern Med* 1991; 151:1280–1287.
99. Anderson TW: Re-examination of some of the Framingham blood pressure data. *Lancet* 1978; 2:1139–1141.
100. D'Agostino RB, Belanger AJ, Kannel WB, Cruickshank JM: Relation of low diastolic blood pressure to coronary heart disease death in presence of myocardial infarction: The Framingham Study. *Br Med J* 1991; 303:385–389.
101. MacMahon S, Peto R, Cutler J, Collins R, Sorlie P, Neaton J, et al: Blood pressure, stroke, and coronary heart disease. Part 1,

Prolonged difference in blood pressure: Prospective observational studies corrected for the regression dilution bias. *Lancet* 1990; 335:765–774.
102. Fletcher AE, Bulpitt CJ: How far should blood pressure be lowered? *N Engl J Med* 1992; 326:251–254.
103. Roccella EJ, Horan MJ: The National High Blood Pressure Education Program: Measuring progress and assessing its impact. *Health Psychol* 1988; 7(suppl):297–303.
104. Rocchini AP: Insulin resistance and blood pressure regulation in obese and nonobese subjects. *Hypertension* 1991; 17:837–842.
105. Reaven GM: Role of insulin resistance in human disease. *Diabetes* 1988; 37:1595–1607.
106. Epstein M, Sowers JR Jr: Diabetes mellitus and hypertension. *Hypertension* 1992; 19:403–418.
107. Julius S, Gudbrandsson T, Jamerson K, Shahab ST, Andersson O: The hemodynamic link between insulin resistance and hypertension. *J Hypertens* 1991; 9:983–986.
108. Kaplan NM: The deadly quartet. Upper-body obesity, glucose intolerance, hypertriglyceridemia, and hypertension. *Arch Intern Med* 1989; 149:1514–1520.
109. Warram JH, Laffel LMB, Valsania P, Christlieb AR, Krolewski AS: Excess mortality associated with diuretic therapy in diabetes mellitus. *Arch Intern Med* 1991; 151:1350–1356.
110. Klein R, Moss SE, Klein BEK, DeMets DL: Relation of ocular and systemic factors to survival in diabetes. *Arch Intern Med* 1989; 149:266–272.
111. Langford HG, Stamler J, Wassertheil-Smoller S, Prineas RJ: All-cause mortality in the Hypertension Detection and Follow-up Program: Findings for the whole cohort and for persons with less severe hypertension, with and without other traits related to risk of mortality. *Prog Cardiovasc Dis* 1986; 14:29–54.
112. Saunders E: Hypertension in African Americans. *Circulation* 1991; 83:1465–1467.
113. Anastos K, Charney P, Charon RA, Cohen E, Jones CY, Marte C, et al: Hypertension in women: What is really known? The Women's Caucus, Working Group on Women's Health of the Society of General Internal Medicine. *Ann Intern Med* 1991; 115:287–293.
114. Vokonas PS, Kannel WB, Cupples LA: Epidemiology and risk of hypertension in the elderly: The Framingham Study. *J Hypertens* 1988; 6:S3–S9.
115. Hypertension Detection and Follow-up Program Cooperative Group: Five-year findings of the Hypertension Detection and Follow-up Program. III, Reduction in stroke incidence among persons with high blood pressure. *JAMA* 1982; 247:633–638.
116. The Working Group on Hypertension in the Elderly: Statement on hypertension in the elderly. *JAMA* 1986; 256:70–74.
117. Garland C, Barrett-Connor E, Suarez L, Criqui MH: Isolated systolic hypertension and mortality after age 60 years. A prospective population-based study. *Am J Epidemiol* 1983; 118:365–376.
118. Hypertension Detection and Follow-up Program Cooperative Group: Five-year findings of the Hypertension Detection and Follow-up Program. II. Mortality by race-sex and age. *JAMA* 1979; 242:2572–2577.
119. National Heart Foundation of Australia: Treatment of mild hypertension in the elderly. *Med J Aust* 1981; 2:398–402.
120. Materson BJ, Cushman WC, Goldstein G, Reda DJ, Freis ED, Ramirez EA, Talmers FN, et al: Treatment of hypertension in the elderly: I. Blood pressure and clinical changes. Results of a Department of Veterans Affairs Cooperative Study. *Hypertension* 1990; 15:348–360.
121. Goldstein G, Materson BJ, Cushman WC, Reda DJ, Freis ED, Ramirez EA, Talmers FN, et al: Treatment of hypertension in the elderly: II. Cognitive and behavioral function. Results of a Department of Veterans Affairs cooperative study. *Hypertension* 1990; 15:361–369.
122. Gurland BJ, Teresi J, Smith WM, Black D, Hutches G, Edlavitch S: Effects of treatment for isolated systolic hypertension on cognitive status and depression in the elderly. *J Am Geriat Soc* 188; 36:1015–1022.
123. Beevers DG, Fairman MJ, Hamilton M, Harpur JE: Antihypertensive treatment and the course of established cerebral vascular disease. *Lancet* 1973; 1:1407–1409.
124. Carter AB: Hypotensive therapy in stroke survivors. *Lancet* 1970; 1:485–489.
125. Marshall J: A trial of long-term hypotensive therapy in cerebrovascular disease. *Lancet* 1964; 1:10–12.
126. Hypertension-Stroke Cooperative Study Group: Effect of antihypertensive treatment on stroke recurrence. *JAMA* 1974; 229:409–418.
127. Whisnant JP, Cartlidge NEF, Elveback LR: Carotid and vertebral-basilar transient ischemic attacks: Effect of anticoagulants, hypertension, and cardiac disorders on survival and stroke occurrence—a population study. *Ann Neurol* 1978; 3:107–115.
128. Frohlich ED: The heart in hypertension: A 1991 overview. *Hypertension* 1991; 18(suppl III):III-62–III-68.
129. Moser M, Setaro JF: Antihypertensive drug therapy and regression of left ventricular hypertrophy: A review with a focus on diuretics. *Eur Heart J* 1991; 12:1034–1039.
130. Frohlich ED, Apstein C, Chobanian AV, Devereux RB, Dustan HP, Dzau V, et al: The heart in hypertension. National High Blood Pressure Education Program Coordinating Committee working group report. *N Engl J Med* 1992; 327:998–1008.
131. Ofili EO, Uy ND, Castello R, St. Vrain J, Martin TJ, Lewis B, et al: Effectiveness of treatment on left ventricular mass reduction in elderly subjects with isolated systolic hypertension (abstr). *Circulation* 1991; 84(suppl II):II-137.
132. Dalhöf B, Pennert K, Hansson L: Reversal of left ventricular hypertrophy in hypertensive patients. A metaanalysis of 109 treatment studies. *Am J Hypertens* 1992; 5:95–110.
133. Topol EJ, Traill TA, Fortuin NJ: Hypertensive hypertrophic cardiomyopathy of the elderly. *N Engl J Med* 1985; 312: 277–283.
134. Abrams J: Vasodilator therapy for chronic congestive heart failure. *JAMA* 1985; 254:3070–3074.
135. Pettinger WA, Lee HC, Reisch J, Mitchell HC: Long-term improvement in renal function after short-term strict blood pressure control in hypertensive nephrosclerosis. *Hypertension* 1989; 13:766–772.
136. Messerli FH, Ventura HO, Amodeo C: Osler's maneuver and pseudohypertension. *N Engl J Med* 1985; 312:1548–1551.
137. Pickering TG, James CD, Boddie C, Harshfield GA, Blank S, Laragh JH: How common is white coat hypertension? *JAMA* 1988; 259:225–228.
138. Gifford RW Jr: An algorithm for the management of resistant hypertension. *Hypertension* 1988; 11(suppl II):II-101–II-105.
139. Biller J, Godersky JC, Adams HP: Management of aneurysmal subarachnoid hemorrhage. *Stroke* 1988; 20:694–697.
140. Brott T, Reed R: Intensive care for acute stroke in the community hospital setting: The first 24 hours. *Stroke* 1989; 20:694–697.
141. Phillips SJ, Whisnant JP: Hypertension and the brain. *Arch Intern Med* 1992; 152:938–945.
142. Gifford RW Jr: Management of hypertensive crises. *JAMA* 1991; 266:829–835.
143. Fagan TC: Acute reduction of blood pressure in asymptomatic patients with severe hypertension: An idea whose time has come and gone. *Arch Intern Med* 1989; 149:2169–2170.
144. Ferguson RK, Vlasses PH: How urgent is 'urgent' hypertension? *Arch Intern Med* 1989; 149:257–258.

PART IX

Valvular Heart Disease

Chapter 78

Acute Rheumatic Fever

Edward L. Kaplan, M.D.

Acute rheumatic fever, a sequel to group A streptococcal upper respiratory tract infection, ranks among the leading causes of cardiovascular disease in the world today. In the developing countries, which account for approximately two-thirds of the world's population, rheumatic fever is responsible for almost half of cardiovascular disease in all age groups and is the leading cause of cardiovascular death in the first five decades of life.[1] The importance of this disease is further emphasized by the mid-1980s resurgence of rheumatic fever in the United States. Available evidence suggests increases in the numbers of cases in many different states in the United States.[2]

ETIOLOGIC AGENT AND EPIDEMIOLOGY

The epidemiology of acute rheumatic fever is that of an infectious disease, group A streptococcal infection of the upper respiratory tract. Since Lancefield, more than five decades ago, described a method of differentiating the hemolytic streptococci into serologic groups,[3] the association between group A beta-hemolytic streptococci and acute rheumatic fever has been recognized. Although a possible role for other etiologic agents, such as viruses, has been considered, the evidence is not supportive.[4]

Rheumatic fever follows only group A streptococcal upper respiratory tract infection, not streptococcal pyoderma or impetigo. Group A streptococcal pharyngitis is primarily, but not exclusively, a disease of children. Just as the highest incidence of group A streptococcal sore throat occurs in children between the ages of 5 and 15, the peak age for attacks of acute rheumatic fever is in this same age range. Although attacks of rheumatic fever are concentrated in children, it is not uncommon for outbreaks of streptococcal pharyngitis (and rheumatic fever) also to occur in adults, for example, in military recruits.[5]

It has been shown that 3 percent of individuals with true streptococcal infection of the upper respiratory tract develop acute rheumatic fever. There are data suggesting that, in some instances, the attack rate may be less than 3 percent in children. These data probably describe a large percentage of streptococcal carriers, individuals who harbor the organism in their upper respiratory tract but appear to be at minimal danger to themselves of developing rheumatic fever and do not appear to readily spread the organism to close family or school contacts.[6]

In the 1940s, 1950s, and early 1960s, acute rheumatic fever was common in the United States. Reliable incidence rates of 20 to 50 per 100,000 population per year were reported from various sources in this country.[7]

Beginning in the mid-1960s, the incidence of acute rheumatic fever in the United States decreased to very low levels, reaching rates of less than 1 per 100,000 population per year by the late 1970s.[8,9] In contrast, the incidence of acute rheumatic fever remains alarmingly high in many developing countries.[10] It has been suggested that incidence rates in some of these countries have increased with trends toward urbanization; this is not very different from what is thought to have happened at the time of the industrial revolution in Great Britain and the United States. Data collected during the 1970s and 1980s from various areas of the world, particularly developing countries, continue to show incidence rates of over 20 per 100,000 population per year.[10] Furthermore, prevalence rates for rheumatic heart disease among children in many developing countries remain high; figures of over 30 per 1000 schoolchildren have been reported.[11] The economic impact on these countries is significant.

Although the incidence of acute rheumatic fever fell to very low levels in the United States by the late 1970s, in the mid-1980s a resurgence occurred in geographically separated areas of the country.[2,12–14] The reasons for the resurgence are as yet unexplained. One possible explanation is the appearance of more virulent strains of group A streptococci in the population.[15] In fact, published data suggest that multiple serotypes were involved in the late-1980s resurgence. Of special interest is that rheumatic fever has always been considered a disease associated with poverty, but the 1980s resurgence in the United States primarily affected middle-class families with ready access to medical care.[12,16]

PATHOGENESIS

Although clearly related to the antecedent group A streptococcal upper respiratory tract infection, the pathogenetic mechanism or mechanisms responsible for the development of acute rheumatic fever after a latent period of several weeks remain unknown. Numerous theories have been proposed. The failure to provide a satisfactory explanation for the pathogenesis of rheumatic fever is related to a lack of experimental or clinical evidence of a specific role for any known somatic or extracellular antigen of the group A streptococci. Furthermore, the lack of a suitable experimental animal model for laboratory study has been an important impediment to study of this disease. Because of this, epidemiological approaches can add significant information.[17]

Early hypotheses centered around the organism itself; there was enthusiasm in the late 1930s for implicating direct infection by the group A beta-hemolytic streptococcus of the heart, valves, and tissues. This hypothesis could not be proved, however, and is no longer seriously considered.[18]

A second major group of hypotheses to explain the pathogenesis of rheumatic fever involves toxins produced by the group A streptococcus. Among the most frequently considered toxins is the oxygen-labile streptolysin O. This antigen is known to be directly cardiotoxic in experimental animals and in tissue culture.[19] Numerous other toxins and enzymes produced by group A streptococci have been implicated. Injection of many of these antigens into experimental animals has produced tissue damage, but never a clinical syndrome identical to rheumatic fever. At the present time, there is no suitable experimental animal model for the laboratory study of rheumatic fever.

Perhaps the most widely held group of hypotheses to explain the pathogenesis of rheumatic fever is that which includes a qualitatively and/or quantitatively abnormal immunologic response to either extracellular or somatic antigens of the group A streptococcus. For example, it has been shown that the group-specific carbohydrate of the group A streptococcal cell wall is antigenically similar to glycoprotein found in bovine and human heart valves.[20] It has been hypothesized that, with exposure to group A streptococci during infection, "antigenic mimicry" leads to an autoimmune-like reaction by the human host and results in valvulitis, ultimately leading to rheumatic valvular heart disease. In support of the existence of this unusual immune response are studies showing that antibodies to the group A carbohydrate moiety of the streptococcal cell wall appear to persist longer in individuals with rheumatic valvular heart disease than in individuals with only uncomplicated streptococcal pharyngitis or even acute poststreptococcal glomerulonephritis.[21] There even have been intriguing reports that group A streptococcal carbohydrate antibodies have decreased after surgical removal of the rheumatic mitral valve in individuals with chronic rheumatic heart disease, providing further support for this concept.[22]

Among the other antigens proposed to play a role in the abnormal immune response in the pathogenesis of rheumatic fever are the streptococcal cell membranes, which have been shown to cross-react with myocardial sarcolemma.[23] This cross-reactive or heart-reactive antibody was originally described in the early 1960s as being related to the cell wall, but later studies suggest that the cross-reaction is due to the cell membrane. This hypothesis suggests that an "autoimmune" reaction following a streptococcal infection results in the carditis seen in patients with rheumatic fever. Similarly, a cross-reactive antigen in the brain has been reported, and antibodies to caudate nucleus have been reported in persons with Sydenham's chorea.

Genetic predisposition to the development of rheumatic fever has been very important among the hypotheses proposed to explain this mysterious illness. Numerous investigators have shown that rheumatic fever tends to be found in multiple members of some families, but the actual genetics have never been fully explained. Recently, a marker on the surface of non-T lymphocytes has been shown to be present in a majority of patients with rheumatic fever or rheumatic heart disease (when compared with control patients).[24,25] Several studies have shown that 75 percent or more of patients with rheumatic fever and/or rheumatic heart disease have lymphocytes that test positive for this marker when a monoclonal antibody is used. Furthermore, family studies have indicated a higher prevalence of positivity in families with rheumatic fever patients than in control families. It has been suggested that these markers may assist in identifying individuals who process streptococcal antigens in an abnormal, but as yet incompletely defined, fashion. These findings require further confirmation in a variety of populations and ethnic groups.

In summary, although many hypotheses have been suggested to explain how the group A streptococcus triggers the pathologic processes of rheumatic fever, the pathogenetic mechanisms responsible for the development of this disease remain unexplained.

DIAGNOSIS OF ACUTE RHEUMATIC FEVER

The diagnosis of acute rheumatic fever is a clinical one, but requires supporting laboratory confirmation. Although Aschoff bodies have been considered to be pathognomonic of rheumatic heart disease, controversy does exist. They are seldom observed today because deaths during acute rheumatic fever are extremely rare. It is important to note again that there is no specific laboratory test that can confirm the diagnosis. This fact is often overlooked.

In 1944, T. Duckett Jones published the Jones Criteria, describing a constellation of clinical and laboratory findings frequently found in association with rheumatic fever. Revisions and modifications of the Jones Criteria have been made periodically since the original publication in 1944. The most significant changes were published in 1965 by the American Heart Association, modified slightly in 1984,[26] and most recently updated in 1992.[27] These changes are referred to as the Revised Jones Criteria and are shown in Table 78-1. It should be noted that former guidelines included previous rheumatic fever or rheumatic heart disease as major or minor manifestations. The current (1992) guidelines are intended only for the diagnosis of initial attacks of acute rheumatic fever; therefore, previous rheumatic fever and rheumatic heart disease are not included as manifestations.

TABLE 78-1

Guidelines for the Diagnosis of Initial Attack of Rheumatic Fever (Jones Criteria, 1992 Update)*

Major Manifestations
Carditis Polyarthritis Chorea Erythema marginatum Subcutaneous nodules
Minor Manifestations

Clinical findings
  Arthralgia
  Fever
Laboratory findings
  Elevated levels of acute-phase reactants
    Erythrocyte sedimentation rate
    C-reactive protein
  Prolonged PR interval

Supporting Evidence of Antecedent Group A Streptococcal Infection
Positive throat culture or rapid streptococcal antigen test results Elevated or rising streptococcal antibody titer

*If supported by evidence of preceding group A streptococcal infection, the presence of two major manifestations or of one major and two minor manifestations indicates a high probability of acute rheumatic fever. See text for details.

SOURCE: The Special Writing Group of the Committee on Rheumatic Fever, Endocarditis, and Kawasaki Disease of the Council on Cardiovascular Disease in the Young of the American Heart Association.[27] Reproduced with permission from the Journal of the American Medical Association and the American Heart Association.

There are five major criteria and a number of minor criteria. In addition, there is the requirement that supporting evidence of an *antecedent group A beta-hemolytic streptococcal infection must be present.* The presence of one major and two minor criteria *or* two major criteria is necessary for the diagnosis of acute rheumatic fever. It must be remembered, however, that there are many diseases that can fulfill the Jones Criteria and yet do not represent acute rheumatic fever. Illnesses such as infective endocarditis, serum sickness, connective tissue diseases, and rheumatoid arthritis are only a few of the many diseases that may mimic rheumatic fever and even fulfill the Jones Criteria unless very carefully applied. It is beyond the scope of this chapter to discuss the Jones Criteria in detail, but several specific points should be made. Of special interest is the fact that rheumatic fever may present in unusual ways, and therefore a modification of the Jones Criteria by the World Health Organization may prove clinically helpful.[10] Three categories of patients have been singled out for special consideration: patients in whom chorea is the sole manifestation, those with insidious or late-onset carditis, and those experiencing rheumatic recurrences.

Rheumatic fever produces a *pancarditis,* affecting pericardium, epicardium, myocardium, and endocardium. In very fulminant cases, the cardiac manifestations may mimic viral myocarditis, but often the manifestations may be very subtle. A transient murmur of mitral regurgitation and/or a pericardial friction rub may be all that is evident. Among the more frequent cardiac findings is mitral regurgitation; isolated aortic regurgitation is unusual in first attacks of acute rheumatic fever. Hemodynamically significant stenotic lesions of the aortic or mitral valves also are not seen in first attacks. In contrast, in individuals who have had several previous attacks of rheumatic fever and have chronic rheumatic heart disease, both stenosis and regurgitation may be seen. The valves of the right side of the heart are not infrequently involved in patients who have had multiple recurrent attacks. In the patient with previous attacks of rheumatic fever the differentiation between acute carditis and congestive cardiac failure may be very difficult. Echocardiography may be helpful for such patients.

The *arthritis* associated with acute rheumatic fever is almost always an exquisitely painful migratory polyarthritis, most often affecting the larger joints such as ankles, knees, elbows, shoulders, and wrists. It is important to recognize the migratory nature. The arthritis may or may not be symmetrical. Involvement of a single joint is rare in acute rheumatic fever. Occasionally, the small joints of the hands or feet may be affected. In the latter instances, other diagnoses should be considered. The arthritis of rheumatic fever does not lead to chronic joint involvement (see "Natural History," below).

Perhaps the most common error made by physicians during the process of establishing a diagnosis of acute rheumatic fever is the administration of salicylates early in the course of the disease, before there is sufficient time for the arthritis to manifest itself completely. Salicylates should be withheld from patients until the diagnosis is clarified. (Some physicians feel that all anti-inflammatory drugs should be withheld.) If the joints are very painful, codeine or a similar drug can relieve the pain without influencing the progression of the disease. The possible beneficial effects of acetaminophen and the nonsteroidal anti-inflammatory agents have not been carefully studied in patients with rheumatic fever.

Erythema marginatum, an unusual rash seen primarily on the trunk, is evident in less than 10 percent of cases of rheumatic fever. Early in its development, erythema marginatum may look like pink macules, but with time, the rash shows blanching in its center with the outer borders forming an irregular pattern. It may be evanescent and can be accentuated or elicited by application of heat. The lesions are not pruritic, and there is no induration. Although unusual, erythema marginatum may be isolated as a major manifestation of acute rheumatic fever. It is not difficult to confuse erythema marginatum with the skin manifestations of Lyme disease.

Subcutaneous nodules are small, pea-size nodules, appearing over extensor surfaces of joints such as wrists and elbows, and even on the spine (Fig. 78-1). These are painless and nonfixed. These are rare (less than 5 percent of cases) and generally are seen only in persons with significant long-standing rheumatic carditis.

Sydenham's chorea is an unusual manifestation of rheumatic fever. There is a long latent period of perhaps several months following the streptococcal infection before this becomes evident. Chorea is often associated with emotional lability, and it may be either bilateral or unilateral. The diagnosis of Sydenham's chorea is one of exclusion. It is imperative that the physician, often in consultation with a neurologist, actively eliminate other causes of chorea. Since there is a prolonged latent period, the evidence of a preceding streptococcal infection is frequently not present, making the diagnosis even more difficult.

The *minor manifestations of an initial attack of acute rheumatic fever* include arthralgia, fever, a prolonged PR interval on the electrocardiogram, and elevated levels of acute-phase reactants (such as the erythrocyte sedimentation rate or C-reactive protein). In the 1984 guidelines,[26] which did not differentiate between initial and recurrent attacks of rheumatic fever, a history of rheumatic fever or rheumatic heart disease was also considered a minor criterion. In the 1992 guidelines,[27] which update guidelines only for an initial attack, this is obviously not included.

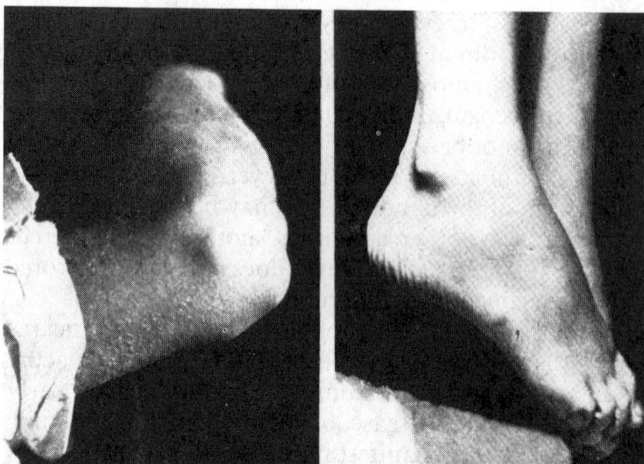

FIGURE 78-1 Photograph showing joints of a child with rheumatic nodules of the elbow, ankle, and foot. Note the nodule on the Achilles tendon. (*From PD White: Heart Disease. Boston, Macmillan, 1931: facing p 336. Reproduced with permission from the publisher and author*).

Minor manifestations are so named because of their lack of specificity. They are included as a part of many clinical syndromes and illnesses. Of particular importance is the differentiation between arthritis and arthralgia. It must be remembered that if arthritis is included as a major criterion, arthralgia cannot be included among the minor criteria in the patient. A prolonged PR interval is very nonspecific and has been associated with many disorders; the same is true for the sedimentation rate and C-reactive protein. In evaluating a patient for rheumatic fever, the minor criteria must be used with caution.

The presence of one major and two minor or two major criteria should make the physician very suspicious of the diagnosis of rheumatic fever. Unless there is *evidence of a preceding group A streptococcal infection*, however, the diagnosis should be entertained with great suspicion.

Evidence of a preceding streptococcal infection may be obtained by means of a positive throat culture for group A streptococci or a history of scarlet fever. Most reliable, however, is elevation of the streptococcal antibody titers such as antistreptolysin O (ASO) titer, antistreptokinase, and antideoxyribonuclease B titer (anti-DNase B). Interpretation of streptococcal antibody titers is not always simple. Although a single elevated antibody titer is helpful, a rise between an acute and a convalescent titer is far more reliable. Furthermore, the clinician must remember that "normal" antibody titers vary with the age of the patient, as well as with the population. The latter variations are another reason why both acute and convalescent titers (usually obtained 2 to 4 weeks apart) are more desirable. Other antibodies may be studied. The antihyaluronidase (AH) antibody test is also commercially available. A rapid agglutination test that tests for antibodies to more than one streptococcal antigen is also used, but results using this test alone must be interpreted with caution because of reported standardization problems with reagents.

No laboratory test is specific for rheumatic fever, so the clinician must carefully interpret laboratory studies. For example, presence of a murmur of mitral regurgitation plus an elevated antistreptolysin O test might be compatible with rheumatic fever but also is compatible with presence of mitral valve prolapse in a patient who has had a recent uncomplicated streptococcal infection. In addition to laboratory studies to confirm the presence of a previous streptococcal infection and studies of acute-phase reactants, other blood studies may prove useful in some cases to eliminate other infectious diseases, collagen vascular diseases, and similar disorders.

The echocardiogram can be a valuable addition to the laboratory studies often requested in the work-up of a patient suspected of having acute rheumatic fever if it is carefully evaluated. For example, it has been reported that patients with isolated manifestations of rheumatic fever such as arthritis or chorea may have "subclinical" carditis.[12] Stretching of the chordae tendineae with "prolapse" of the anterior leaflet of the mitral valve has been reported. This possibility is intriguing, since it may explain those patients without clinical evidence of carditis at the initial attack who later are found to have rheumatic heart disease. Some authorities now feel that patients with acute rheumatic fever in whom there is any question of carditis should undergo echocardiographic examination.

TREATMENT OF ACUTE RHEUMATIC FEVER

The medical therapy for acute rheumatic fever has three objectives: to treat the group A streptococcal infection, to reduce inflammation, and to treat congestive heart failure (when present). Note that therapy is *not* directed toward prevention of development of rheumatic valvular heart disease. Numerous studies have shown that the anti-inflammatory therapy used for an acute attack of rheumatic fever does not prevent development of valvular heart disease.

Patients with arthritis as a major component of the clinical syndrome are usually treated and promptly helped with salicylates. Relief is dramatic. Dosage sufficient to give serum salicylate levels of 15 to 20 mg/dL causes the arthritis of rheumatic fever to disappear, usually within 12 to 24 h. In patients with arthritis who do not promptly respond to salicylates, another diagnosis should be seriously considered. As mentioned previously, however, salicylates or corticosteroids should *not* be started until the clinical picture has fully evolved. Withholding anti-inflammatory therapy until the diagnosis is confirmed poses no danger to the patient with acute rheumatic fever. The use of the newer nonsteroidal anti-inflammatory drugs has not been studied in a systematic fashion for use in acute rheumatic fever.

Most physicians do not administer corticosteroids in patients with only arthritis. Corticosteroids are used in patients with carditis, especially when there is evidence of congestive heart failure. It is generally agreed that, although corticosteroids may be clinically helpful during the acute phases of the attack, they have no effect in preventing the development of rheumatic valvular heart disease. The dose of corticosteroids is usually in the range of 2 to 4 mg/kg per day of prednisone and divided into two doses. Short courses of 2 weeks, with a relatively rapid taper of the steroid, are most frequently used. Careful clinical and laboratory monitoring must be performed. If there is clinical relapse, a longer course may be required. Patients who are receiving corticosteroids are frequently given salicylate (aspirin) concomitantly. Maintaining adequate salicylate levels as one is reducing corticosteroid dosage usually prevents rebound.

The treatment of Sydenham's chorea has been helped considerably by the addition of two agents. Diazepam, a benzodiazepine derivative, is now the initial treatment of choice for Sydenham's chorea. Haloperidol, a butyrophenone, has been used with encouraging results but must be monitored very carefully because of potential toxicity.[27]

An essential part of the therapy for acute rheumatic fever is the treatment of the preceding group A streptococcal pharyngitis. Even though group A streptococci often cannot be cultured at the time of the onset of acute rheumatic fever, all patients should be treated for streptococcal pharyngitis, and secondary long-term rheumatic fever prophylaxis should be initiated. Penicillin is the antimicrobial agent of choice for both treatment of the acute streptococcal pharyngitis and long-term secondary prophylaxis. Intramuscular injection of 1,200,000 units of benzathine penicillin G once a month has been recommended for many years by the American Heart Association.[29] Because this is painful and because of a largely unjustified fear of untoward reactions, however, oral secondary prophylaxis is widely used in the United States. Administration of penicillin V, 250 mg twice daily, is the most frequently used method of secondary rheumatic fever prophylaxis. For those allergic to penicillin, oral sulfadiazine, 1 g daily, is an effective substitute. In persons allergic to penicillin and to sulfadiazine, oral erythromycin, 250 mg twice daily, is recommended. The reader is referred to the American Heart Association recommendations for a more complete discussion of this aspect.[29]

In patients who develop congestive heart failure, the usual anticongestive measures, including cardiac glycosides and diuretics, have been effective (see also Chap. 26). Of course, in persons with congestive heart failure, bed rest is necessary. In the past, patients with acute rheumatic fever were put to bed for several months, but this is no longer considered necessary unless there is evidence of significant carditis. The purpose of bed rest is to reduce the cardiac work. The arthritis of rheumatic fever does not necessitate bed rest except during the first day or two after the diagnosis is made. Shortly thereafter, aspirin controls the arthritis.

For patients with rheumatic valvular heart disease, bacterial endocarditis prophylaxis is necessary at the time of dental procedures or surgery on infected or contaminated tissues. In contrast, patients who have had rheumatic fever but who do not have rheumatic heart disease do not require endocarditis prophylaxis. A discussion of current recommendations for bacterial endocarditis prophylaxis is provided in Chap. 94.[30]

NATURAL HISTORY

The natural history of individuals who have had documented acute rheumatic fever varies considerably from patient to patient. Continuous antimicrobial secondary prophylaxis generally protects patients from recurrent attacks and therefore from a worsening cardiac status. Thompkins and colleagues demonstrated that if secondary prophylaxis is reliably followed, approximately 70 percent of individuals developing the murmur of mitral regurgitation at the time of the acute attack lose that murmur over the next 5 years.[31]

For this reason, continuous secondary prophylaxis is very important. Patients who have had one episode of rheumatic fever are likely to experience a second attack with a recurrent streptococcal infection. The duration of secondary prophylaxis varies. Some authorities feel that if there is no evidence of rheumatic heart disease, 5 years of secondary prophylaxis may often be sufficient. Most, however, continue secondary prophylaxis until at least the eighteenth birthday. If there is evidence of rheumatic heart disease, prolonged secondary prophylaxis is indicated; some authorities recommend lifelong secondary prophylaxis for these patients. In addition, one must take into consideration the patient's risk of streptococcal infection. Individuals at higher risk of developing streptococcal infection (e.g., schoolteachers, health care workers, and individuals in the military) often are given secondary prophylaxis for longer periods of time.

The prognosis for the arthritis of rheumatic fever is excellent. There is no residual arthritis or deformity. Rarely, a patient may have *Jaccoud's arthritis*, with increased ulnar deviation of the fourth and fifth fingers and flexion at the metacarpophalangeal joints. Sydenham's chorea may recur, but this is rare.

Patients with severe valvular heart disease often require cardiovascular surgery, many during the third or fourth decade of life. In some parts of the world, however, an entity known as juvenile or malignant mitral stenosis occurs[32] and results in the need for surgery much earlier, often late in the first or early in the second decade.

Although methods of prevention are imperfect, the beneficial effects of consistent secondary prophylaxis cannot be too strongly emphasized (see earlier discussion). It is probably the single most effective measure that the physician has to offer patients who have had a previous documented episode of rheumatic fever. Because of the complex nature of the group A streptococcus, efforts to produce a safe and effective vaccine against group A streptococcal infections have been hampered. Recent advances in molecular biological techniques have provided new knowledge in this regard, and progress is being made in the first and most important aspect of development in this vaccine, the understanding of the antigenicity and cross-reactivity of the M protein of the group A streptococcus. Although experimental vaccines have been tried in animals, they are still in a relatively early stage of development, and sizable human trials have not yet been undertaken.

REFERENCES

1. Markowitz M, Taranta A: *Rheumatic Fever: A Guide to Its Recognition, Prevention and Cure, with Special Reference to Developing Countries.* Boston, MTP Press, 1981: 16
2. Kavey RW, Kaplan EL: Resurgence of rheumatic fever. *Pediatrics* 1989; 84: 585–586.
3. Lancefield RC: A serologic differentiation of human and other groups of hemolytic streptococci. *J Exp Med* 1933; 57:571.
4. Limson BM, Chan VR, Guzman SU, Maaba MR, Mendoza MT: Occurrence of infection with group B coxsackie virus in rheumatic and nonrheumatic Filipino children. *J Infect Dis* 1979; 140:415.
5. Papadimas T, Escamilla J, Garst P, Oldfield E, Counihan C, Schiffer S, et al: Acute rheumatic fever at a Navy Training Center—San Diego, California. *MMWR* 1988; 37:101–104.
6. Kaplan EL: The group A streptococci upper respiratory tract carrier state: An enigma *J Pediatr* 1980; 97:337.
7. Markowitz M, Gordis L: *Rheumatic Fever.* Philadelphia, Saunders, 1972:110
8. Land MA, Bisno AL: Acute rheumatic fever: A vanishing disease in suburbia. *JAMA* 1983; 249:895.
9. Odio A: The incidence of acute rheumatic fever in a suburban area of Los Angeles: A ten-year study. *West J Med* 1986; 144:179.
10. World Health Organization: *Rheumatic Fever.* Geneva, Switzerland, Technical Report Series, No. 764, 1988.
11. De Oliviera A, de Souza MJ, Benchetrit LC: Rheumatic heart disease and streptococcal carriage in Brazilian children. In: Doyle E, Engle M, Gersony W, Rashkind W, Talner N (eds): *Pediatric Cardiology.* New York, Springer-Verlag, 1986: 998.
12. Veasy LG, Wiedmeier SE, Orsmond G, Ruttenberg HD, Boucek MM, Roth SJ: Resurgence of acute rheumatic fever in the intermountain area of the United States. *N Engl J Med* 1987; 316:421–427.
13. Hosier D, Craenen J, Teske DW, Wheller JJ: Resurgence of rheumatic fever. *N Engl J Med* 316:421, 1987.
14. Congeni B, Rizzo C, Congeni J, Sreenivasan VV: Outbreak of acute rheumatic fever in southeast Ohio. *J Pediatr* 1987; 119:176–179.
15. Kaplan EL, Johnson DR, Cleary PP: Group A streptococcal serotypes isolated from patients and sibling contacts during the resurgence of rheumatic fever in the United States in the mid-1980s. *J Infect Dis* 1989; 159:101–103.
16. Markowitz MM, Kaplan EL: Reappearance of rheumatic fever. In: Barness LA (ed): *Advances in Pediatrics,* vol 3. Chicago, Year Book Medical, 1989; 3:39–66.
17. Kaplan EL: Epidemiologic approaches to understanding the pathogenesis of rheumatic fever. *Int J Epidemiol* 1985; 14:499.
18. Watson RF, Hirst GK, Lancefield RC: Bacteriological studies of cardiac tissues obtained at autopsy from 11 patients dying with rheumatic fever. *Arthritis Rheum* 1961; 4:74.
19. Ginsburg I: Mechanism of cell and tissue injury induced by group A streptococci: Relation to past streptococcal sequelae. *J Infect Dis* 1972; 126:294.
20. Goldstein I, Halpern B, Robert L: Immunologic relationship between streptococcus A polysaccharide and the structural glycoproteins of heart valve. *Nature* 1967; 213:44.
21. Dudding BA, Ayoub EM: Persistence of streptococcal group A antibody in patients with rheumatic valvular disease. *J Exp Med* 1968; 128:1081.
22. Shulman ST, Ayoub EM, Victorica BC, Gessner IH, Tamer DF, Hernandez FA: Differences in antibody response to streptococcal antigens in children with rheumatic and nonrheumatic valve disease. *Circulation* 1974; 50:1244–1251.
23. Zabriskie JB, Freimer EH: The immunological relationship between the group A streptococcus and mammalian muscle. *J Exp Med* 1966; 124:661.
24. Patarroyo ME, Winchester RJ, Vejerano A, Gibofsky A, Chalem F, Zabriskie JB, et al: Association of a B-cell antigen with susceptibility to rheumatic fever. *Nature* 1979; 278:173–174.
25. Gray ED, Regelmann WR, Abdin Z, el-Kholy A, Zahers S, Kamel R, et al: Compartmentalization of cells bearing "rheumatic" cell surface antigens in peripheral blood and tonsils in rheumatic heart disease. *J Infect Dis* 1987; 155:242–247.
26. Committee on the Prevention of Rheumatic Fever and Bacterial Endocarditis of the American Heart Association: The Jones Criteria (revised). *Circulation* 1984; 70:893A.
27. Special Writing Group of the Committee on Rheumatic Fever, Endocarditis, and Kawasaki Disease of the Council on Cardiovascular Disease in the Young of the American Heart Association: Guidelines for the diagnosis of rheumatic fever: Jones Criteria, 1992 update. *JAMA* 1992; 268:2069–2073.
28. Shield WD, Bray PF: A danger of haloperidol therapy in children. *J Pediatr* 1976; 88:301.
29. Committee on the Prevention of Rheumatic Fever and Bacterial Endocarditis of the American Heart Association: Prevention of rheumatic fever. *Circulation* 1988; 78:1082.
30. Committee on Rheumatic Fever, Endocarditis, and Kawasaki Disease of the Council on Cardiovascular Disease in the Young of the American Heart Association: Prevention of bacterial endocarditis. *JAMA* 1990; 264:2919–2922.
31. Thompkins DG, Boxerbaum B, Liebman J: Long-term prognosis of rheumatic fever patients receiving regular intramuscular benzathine penicillin. *Circulation* 1972; 45:543.
32. Ilyas M, Haidry JG: Juvenile mitral stenosis: A pathogenic puzzle. *J Pak Med Assoc* 1980; 30:254.

Chapter 79

Aortic Valve Disease

Elliot Rapaport, M.D. ■ *Charles E. Rackley, M.D.* ■
Lawrence H. Cohn, M.D.

AORTIC STENOSIS

Definition, Etiology, and Pathology

Aortic stenosis is the obstruction of flow across the aortic valve during left ventricular systolic ejection. Aortic stenosis can be caused by a congenital unicuspid or bicuspid valve, rheumatic fever, or degenerative calcification of the valve in the elderly. The incidence and prevalence of aortic stenosis have been modified by observations of the cardiac surgeon, reexamination of pathological studies, a significant decline in the incidence of rheumatic fever, and an increase in the life span of the adult population. Early pathological studies during the early part of the century attributed aortic stenosis to inflammation or valvular sclerosis, and a series in 1947 suggested rheumatic valvulitis as the major cause.[1,2] Subsequent studies confirmed congenital valvular stenosis as the most common cause, with the recognition of a bicuspid valve as a major cause of aortic stenosis.[3,4]

Detection of aortic stenosis in a patient under the age of 30 suggests a congenitally stenotic aortic valve as the etiology.[5] Between the ages of 30 to 60 or 70 years, rheumatic disease may still play a role, although calcification of a congenital bicuspid valve is increasingly responsible. Beyond 70 years, degenerative calcification of the aortic valve is the most common cause.[6,7] If aortic stenosis is the only valvular lesion clinically apparent, 6 to 24 percent of affected individuals may have a rheumatic basis, while aortic stenosis in combination with mitral valve disease increases the likelihood of a rheumatic etiology.[8,9] The growing elderly population has resulted in an increased incidence of calcific or degenerative aortic stenosis. If the patient is over 65 years of age and the aortic murmur has been noted only relatively recently, 90 percent will be degenerative in etiology.[10] In a significant proportion of these patients, concomitant mitral annular calcification is present.

Acquired stenosis of the aortic valve results either from commissural fusion, yielding the fibrous type of stenosis, or from calcification of the cusps of the valve. Although rheumatic fever can result in aortic stenosis from either of these processes, calcific stenosis more often results from changes in a congenitally bicuspid valve or, especially in patients over 60 years of age, a tricuspid valve.

In the fibrous type of aortic stenosis, recurrent rheumatic carditis causes fibrous contracture with shortening of the cusps and a tendency for fusion of adjacent cusps at the commissures. If commissural adhesion occurs on one aortic commissure, the valve becomes bicuspid (acquired bicuspid valve). In such a valve the orifice is somewhat reduced, but usually not measurably. Such valves create, as do congenital bicuspid valves, a tendency for acquired calcification of the cusp.

If there is fusion at two or three commissures, the cusp is sufficiently restrained to cause obstruction at the valve level. The stenotic valve created by commissural fusion may exhibit varying degrees of calcification, but the primary basis for the stenosis resides in adhesions of one cusp to another.[11] This fibrous type of aortic stenosis is usually of rheumatic origin (Fig. 79-1). Due to associated shortening of the cusp, this form of aortic stenosis is generally accompanied by some degree of aortic regurgitation. Furthermore, if the disease is rheumatic, some evidence of rheumatic involvement is present in the mitral valve and, rarely, in the tricuspid valve.

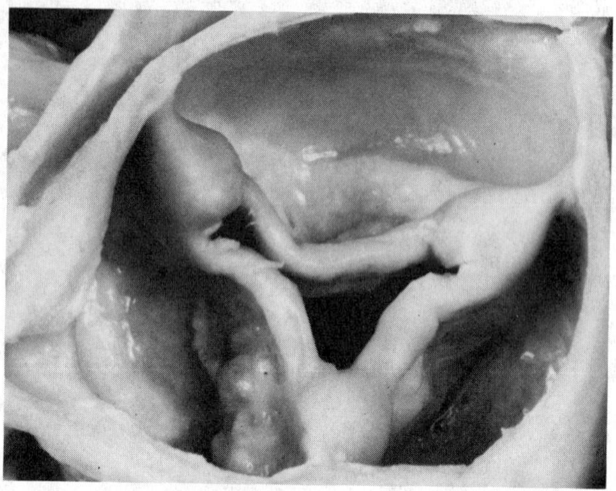

FIGURE 79-1 Fibrous (rheumatic) aortic stenosis. There is fusion of all three commissures. *(From JE Edwards: Pathology of acquired valvular disease of the heart. Semin Roentgenol 14:96, 1979. Reproduced with permission from the publisher and author.)*

In calcific aortic stenosis, rigidity of cuspid tissue occurs due to calcification usually in a bicuspid or tricuspid aortic valve.[6,12] There are two etiologies for the bicuspid state: acquired through rheumatic disease or congenital (Fig. 79-2*A* and *B*). In the calcific type of aortic stenosis the congenital bicuspid valve is more common than the acquired bicuspid valve by a ratio of about 4 to 1. Classically, the aortic valve is competent and, in instances of the congenital bicuspid valve, no other valve of the heart is diseased. In the congenital bicuspid valve the large conjoined cusp usually lies anteriorly, and the two coronary arteries arise from its sinus. In an acquired bicuspid valve, the conjoined cusp may occupy the same position or may be oriented toward the right or left. It is noteworthy that congenital bicuspid aortic valve disease is the most common form of congenital aortic regurgitation. (See also Chap. 97.)

Some degree of fibrosis and calcification commonly appears in the normal aortic valves of persons 70 years of age and older.[13] Usually the calcification is not sufficient to cause significant stenosis, although it may be responsible for a systolic murmur. In some patients each of the three cusps becomes highly calcific, making the valve stenotic. This condition is referred to as degenerative, or Mönckeberg's senile, calcific aortic stenosis. It is recognized with increasing frequency in the aging population (Fig. 79-2*C*).

In addition to the fibrous and calcific types of aortic stenosis, there are several less common miscellaneous types. Aortic stenosis observed from infancy to adolescence can result from a congenital unicommissural unicuspid aortic valve. Sometimes individuals with such valves may reach adulthood before significant signs of aortic stenosis are displayed. This phenomenon may result in calcification with secondary incompetence or in a congenitally deformed but mildly stenotic valve (Fig. 79-2*D*). The resulting aortic regurgitation then may serve to bring the stenosis into clinical recognition.

Secondary anatomical effects of aortic stenosis include left ventricular hypertrophy and poststenotic dilatation of the ascending aorta. Both aortic stenosis and aortic regurgitation can produce downward enlargement of the left ventricle and restrain the mitral chordae with resulting secondary mitral regurgitation.[14] Mitral regurgitation can also result in congenital aortic stenosis from fibrosis of the papillary muscles to the left ventricular free wall.[15] Although some earlier studies contended that aortic stenosis affords some protection against coronary atherosclerosis, the incidence of coronary atherosclerosis among patients with aortic stenosis is not significantly different from that in persons with a normal aortic valve.[16]

Pathophysiology

Stenosis of the aortic valve creates resistance to ejection, and a systolic pressure gradient develops between the left ventricle and the ascending aorta. The aortic orifice area is normally 2 to 3 cm^2, and a reduction in orifice is accompanied by a progressive increase in left ventricular systolic pressure. Elevation of the systolic pressure imposes a pressure overload on the left ventricle, which compensates by an increase in ventricular wall thickness and mass.[17] This concentric hypertrophy without chamber dilatation normalizes systolic wall stress and preserves ventricular function as evidenced by a normal cardiac output and ejection fraction.[18] At this stage, abnormalities in diastolic filling or compliance (diastolic dysfunction) can be found in the concentrically hypertrophied left ventricle even though systolic function is preserved. Eventually, the systolic contractile state becomes depressed and the left ventricle dilates, further increasing the systolic and diastolic wall stress.[19] (See Chaps. 23 and 25.)

The decreased compliance in the hypertrophied left ventricle in aortic stenosis is associated with an elevation of the left ventricular end-diastolic pressure, which is further raised by an increase in the vigor of atrial systole. Atrial systole contributes significantly to the percent of systolic volume ejected in aortic stenosis, as compared to the normal ventricle.[20] Although the Frank-Starling mechanism has been proposed to explain the contribution of atrial systole in aortic stenosis, end-diastolic wall stress or preload may be normal in the hypertrophied left ventricle of aortic stenosis.[21]

A sustained pressure overload on the myocardium in chronic aortic stenosis eventually results in depression of the contractile properties of the myocardium.[22] With declining contractility, the adaptive mechanisms of dilatation and hypertrophy are ultimately unable to maintain normal forward cardiac output. While systolic wall stress remains within the normal range during the compensated concentric hypertrophy phase of aortic stenosis, chamber dilatation and impaired contractility abnormally elevate systolic wall stress (preload-afterload mismatch), which produces an elevation of left ventricular end-diastolic pressure, corresponding elevations in pulmonary capillary arterial pressures, a decline in ejection fraction, decreased cardiac output, and eventual congestive heart failure. It is important to note that the ventricle with marked concentric hypertrophy does not develop marked ventricular dilatation.

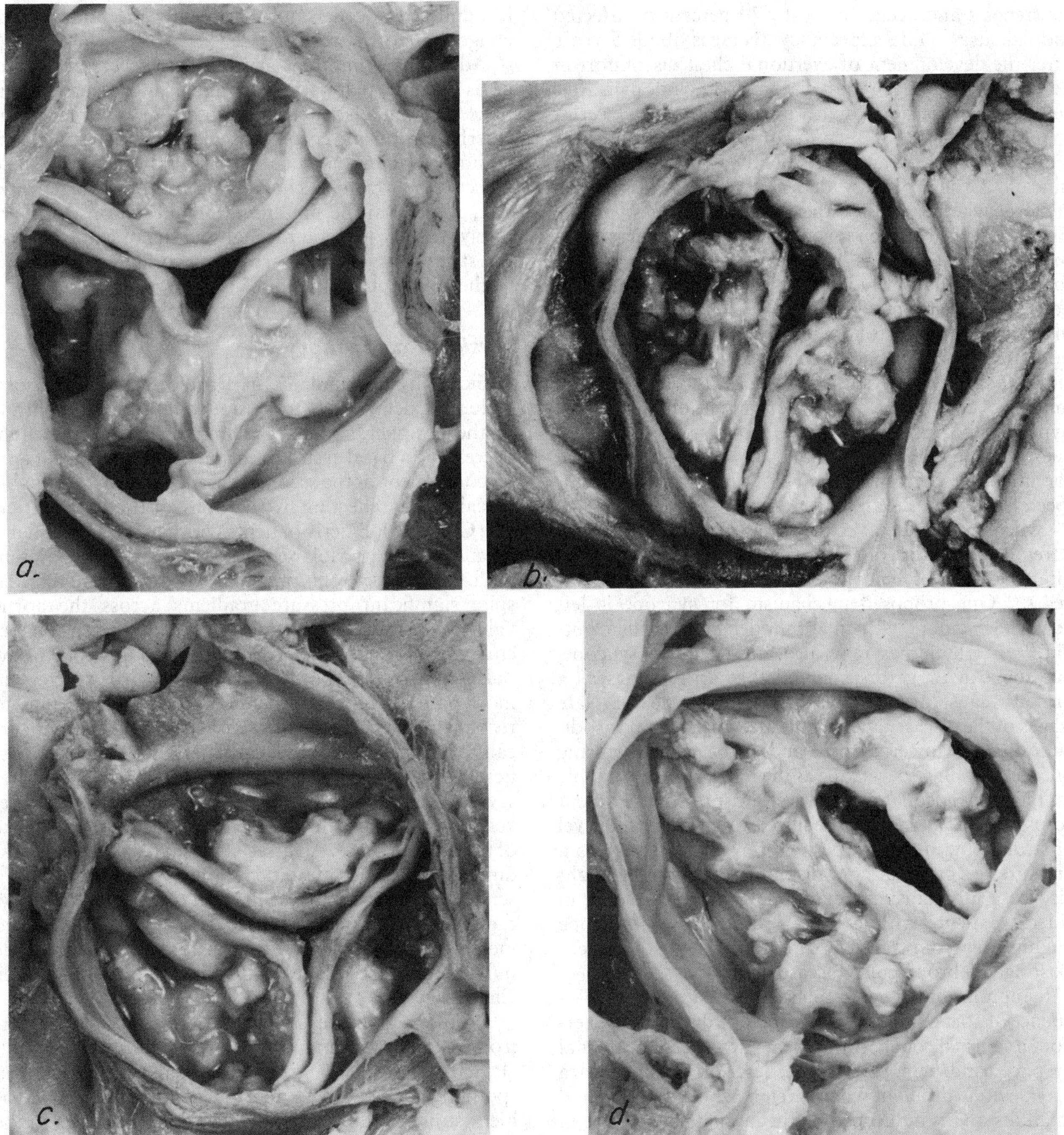

FIGURE 79-2 Four types of calcific aortic stenosis. In each, the unopened aortic valve is viewed from above. *A.* Acquired bicuspid aortic valve with secondary calcification. At the center of the conjoined cusp (*lower center*) are elements of two preexisting cusps, now fused. *B.* Congenital bicuspid valve. The characteristic raphe of the congenital bicuspid aortic valve appears at the lower portion of the figure. *C.* Senile type. None of the commissures is fused, but there is a major intrinsic calcification of the three cusps. *D.* Unicuspid, unicommissural congenital aortic stenosis with secondary calcification. (*From JE Edwards: Pathology of acquired valvular disease of the heart. Semin Roentgenol 14:96, 1979. Reproduced with permission from the publisher and author.*)

Clinical Manifestations

History

The classic triad of clinical manifestations of aortic stenosis are chest pain, heart failure, and syncope. Sudden death may also occur.[23] The patient's age at the time of the recognition of the murmur and the presence or absence of other valvular disease can be helpful in attributing the lesion to a congenital, rheumatic, or degenerative etiology. Symptoms of aortic stenosis occur only when critical reduction of valve size has developed, usually at an orifice area of 1.0 cm^2 or smaller. In adults, presentation of the usual manifestations of aortic stenosis may be complicated by underlying coronary artery disease. In some patients, both congenital and calcific aortic stenosis may progress rapidly over a few years' period of observation.

Angina pectoris is the most frequent symptom of aortic stenosis and occurs in 50 to 70 percent of affected individuals.[24,25] Life expectancy averages about 5 years after the development of exertional chest discomfort in adults. Features of the chest discomfort include pain after physical exertion and a higher incidence of nitroglycerin-induced syncope than seen in coronary artery disease.[26] Coronary arteriography frequently demonstrates significant coronary artery disease in adults with aortic stenosis whether or not they experience chest pain.[27] The difference between myocardial oxygen demand and oxygen availability has been proposed as a mechanism for the chest pain. Myocardial oxygen consumption in aortic stenosis is greater than normal due to an increase in left ventricular systolic wall tension and mass, with the potential for inadequate oxygenation of the vulnerable subendocardium.[28] Systolic wall stress is a major determinant of myocardial oxygen consumption, and in the hypertrophied myocardium the highest stress value develops in the subendocardial layer.[29] A rare mechanism for impaired coronary blood flow is calcific emboli.[30] (See also Chaps. 23 and 26.)

Syncope that often occurs during physical exertion is a frequent symptom of aortic stenosis.[24] Average survival after the onset of syncope has been estimated at 3 to 4 years.[23] One proposed mechanism for syncope is left ventricular failure with an abrupt decline in cardiac output.[31,32] Arrhythmias may also contribute to syncope, but some investigators contend that arrhythmias as a primary cause are features primarily of the very late stages of the disease. Exercise-induced peripheral vasodilatation may lower carotid and myocardial perfusing pressure, leading to syncope as the left ventricle is unable to increase adequately the systolic pressure gradient across the stenotic orifice required to augment the level of stroke output. Reflex peripheral vasodilatation from pressure receptors in the walls of the left ventricle might also be a mechanism of exertional syncope. Finally, in elderly patients with calcific aortic stenosis, syncope might result from transient cerebral ischemia due to coexisting cerebrovascular disease.

Symptoms of left ventricular failure are a third consequence of aortic stenosis. These include dyspnea on exertion, nocturnal cough, orthopnea, paroxysmal nocturnal dyspnea, and hemoptysis. The description of dyspnea may be quite different when given by children compared to adults and is influenced by the amount of exercise in the different age groups.[33] In adults with aortic stenosis, survival has been estimated at 2 years after symptoms of heart failure develop.[23,33] Since patients with aortic stenosis develop concentric left ventricular hypertrophy, they have dyspnea on exertion on the basis of diastolic dysfunction for a much longer period of time. Studies of survival based primarily on subjective symptoms of dyspnea on exertion are often very inexact, particularly since everyone has dyspnea with sufficient exertion to some degree.

Sudden death may occur in 15 to 20 percent of symptomatic patients with aortic stenosis and has been attributed to arrhythmias and myocardial ischemia.[34] Although most patients examined at autopsy have had symptoms, approximately 15 percent of patients with aortic stenosis at autopsy have died suddenly without documented previous symptoms. This is very uncommon in adults but occurs more frequently in children with congenital aortic stenosis (see Chap. 97).

Additional symptoms attributed to severe aortic stenosis include palpitations, fatigue, and visual disturbances. Fatigue is an early symptom in children. In the elderly, carotid and cerebrovascular disease may produce additional central nervous system symptoms. Visual field defects result from calcific emboli from the aortic valve and, rarely, can be presenting manifestations.[30,35] Very rarely, the jet of blood through the stenotic aortic valve can strike the wall of the ascending aorta and predispose to the development of aortic dissection.

Physical Examination

Typical physical findings in significant aortic stenosis include a delayed upstroke and diminished amplitude of the peripheral pulse, a diamond-shaped crescendo, decrescendo basal systolic murmur, a soft or absent aortic component of the second heart sound, and a palpable apical thrust reflecting hypertrophy of the left ventricle (see Chap. 10). Elderly patients with calcific aortic stenosis and loss of arteriolar elasticity can sometimes present with systemic systolic pressures above 180 mmHg despite significant pressure gradients across the aortic valve.[24,36] Although systemic arterial hypertension occurs, it is distinctly uncommon. Delayed upstroke of the pulse contour can be detected in the carotid artery in most patients under the age of 70. It is important to recognize that carotid sinus sensitivity in elderly patients can result in sudden bradycardia and loss of consciousness. An anacrotic notch in the arterial pulse indicates severe stenosis;[24] and as the stenosis becomes more severe, the notch is detected earlier on the initial upstroke of the arterial pulse. An arterial pulse with delayed peak, diminished amplitude, and gradual downslope is described by the term *pulsus parvus et tardus*. In the elderly, the decreased elasticity of the arteries with the associated increase in pulse pressure can distort the characteristic pulse contour and make the diagnosis more difficult (see Chap. 10).

Despite significant concentric left ventricular hypertrophy, the apical impulse may remain within the midclavicular line. There may be a palpable *a* wave, corresponding to an audible S_4 or atrial gallop sound. A palpable systolic thrill may be felt over the aortic area in the second right intercostal space. This may radiate into the carotid arteries, especially on the right side. (See Chap. 10.)

Auscultatory findings include an ejection click, a diamond-shaped crescendo-decrescendo systolic murmur, and a soft and delayed aortic component of the second heart sound (see Chap. 11). The ejection click is high-pitched and is usually audible at the apex or along the left sternal border shortly after the first sound.[37] The ejection sound occurs with systolic elevation of the central aortic pulse and probably originates from the aortic valve leaflets. It is most common in bicuspid valves. The ejection click is related to the mobility of the valve and not necessarily to the severity of the gradient; it may disappear with increasing severity of the stenosis.

The systolic murmur is characteristically a harsh crescendo-decrescendo or diamond-shaped (spindle-shaped) pattern of vibrations heard loudest at the base and transmitted into the neck. An interval can be recognized between the first heart sound and the onset of the murmur. The murmur terminates before the aortic component of the second heart sound (see Chap. 11). The aortic second sound, if audible, is often delayed in severe stenosis, and there may be a paradoxical splitting of the second sound. With expiration, the pulmonic sound will migrate toward the first sound, and the delayed aortic second sound may produce the paradoxical splitting. With calcification, the valve loses mobility and the intensity of the aortic component of the second heart sound diminishes. With severe stenosis, the aortic component is absent, and the systolic murmur may extend through and obliterate the pulmonic component of the second heart sound. One-third to one-half of individuals with aortic stenosis have a high-pitched diastolic blow of accompanying aortic regurgitation.[38]

In the elderly, calcific aortic stenosis with calcification in the aortic cusps and lack of commissural fusion can produce distinct and characteristic auscultatory features.[39] The murmur may be musical, higher pitched, and prominent at the apex as well as along the left sternal border. Occasionally, it is louder at the apex. Detection of the murmur at the apex may raise the possibility of associated mitral annular calcification and mitral regurgitation. The murmur of aortic stenosis is often higher pitched and spindle-shaped, and rarely radiates into the axillary area. It may be louder in the beat following a premature ventricular beat, unlike the murmur of mitral regurgitation, which does not increase in loudness.

Laboratory Tests

Electrocardiogram

Electrocardiographic abnormalities in aortic stenosis are produced by left ventricular hypertrophy, which increases the amplitude of the QRS complex with ST and T wave alterations,[24,40] with increased amplitude of the S waves in right precordial leads, increased amplitude of the R waves in the left precordial leads, depression of the ST segment, and inversion of the T wave. A superior axis shift in the frontal plane leads may be seen, resulting in tall R waves in I and aV_L and deep S waves in II, III, and aV_F. Conduction defects are frequent and range from first-degree heart block to left bundle branch block in about 13 percent of patients (see Chap. 13).

Chest Roentgenogram

Since the pressure overload of aortic stenosis initially produces concentric hypertrophy of the left ventricle without dilatation, radiographically determined heart size is often within normal limits.[41] Prominent curvature of the apex may suggest concentric hypertrophy. Poststenotic dilatation of the ascending aorta is a common feature of long-standing aortic stenosis. Calcification in the aortic valve often cannot be confidently identified on plain films and is usually identified with overpenetrated films or by fluoroscopy. Calcification of the aortic valve is best seen on lateral or oblique views. It is commonly observed in patients over the age of 40 years with significant aortic stenosis. Enlargement of the left atrium can occur secondarily to decreased compliance of the left ventricle, but excessive dilatation of the atrium should raise other possibilities, such as mitral valve disease or idiopathic dilated cardiomyopathy (see Chaps. 14 and 89).

Echocardiogram

Echocardiography can delineate structure and mobility in valvular as well as nonvalvular forms of aortic stenosis (see Chaps. 15 and 130).[42] Thickening, calcification, and reduced mobility of the aortic leaflet are characteristic echocardiographic changes (see Fig. 15-29).[43] Measurements of septal and left ventricular wall thickness permit estimation of the extent of left ventricular hypertrophy as well as the detection of asymmetrical septal hypertrophy in hypertrophic obstructive cardiomyopathy (Chap. 90). Chamber dimensions, estimates of end-diastolic and end-systolic volumes, fractional shortening rate, and ejection fraction provide information on left ventricular function. A bicuspid aortic valve can be recognized by the asymmetry of the two leaflets (see Fig. 15-30).[44] Aortic cusp separation measured at less than 8 mm in the long axis by two-dimensional echocardiographic technique is highly predictive of severe aortic stenosis.[45] In severe calcific aortic stenosis, movement of the valve leaflets frequently cannot be detected.

Echo-Doppler techniques for measuring the velocity across the aortic valve provide good estimates of the systolic gradient.[46–49] With additional estimations of aortic flow using the continuity equation, the aortic valve area can be calculated from the echo-Doppler pressure gradient (see Figs. 79-3, 130-9, and 130-10).[50,51] Concomitant mitral or aortic regurgitation can also be detected and its severity estimated by echo-Doppler techniques (see Chap. 130).

Cardiac Catheterization

Cardiac catheterization in aortic stenosis can record the gradient across the valve, estimate the stenotic area, evaluate left ventricular function, recognize coexistent valve involvement, and detect coronary artery disease. The normal aortic valve area is 2 to 3 cm^2, and calculations indicate that reduction of the orifice size to less than 0.8 cm^2 significantly impedes systolic flow.[52] A valvular gradient exceeding 50 mmHg usually accompanies this degree of stenosis. It is important to note that a decline in the cardiac output can dramatically reduce the gradient across the valve even though the valve area is severely stenotic. Thus, it is important always to calculate the aortic valve area (see also Chap. 138).[53]

Quantitative angiographic studies can provide measurements of chamber volume and ejection fraction (Fig. 79-3), but these indexes can also be obtained noninvasively using echocardiographic techniques.[54] Left ventricular wall thickness can be measured and estimates of left ventricular mass, preload, and afterload derived.

The need for coronary arteriography is frequently the major indication for catheterization in aortic stenosis in patients over the age of 40. In such patients there is a 50 percent incidence of underlying coronary artery disease,

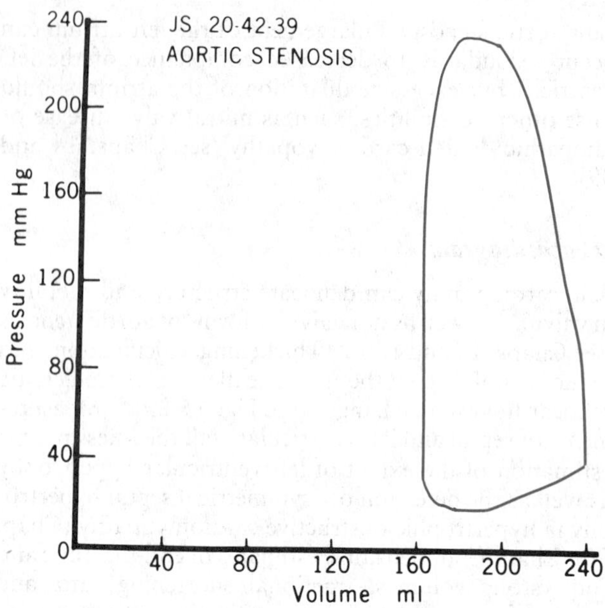

FIGURE 79-3 Left ventricular pressure-volume diagram in decompensated aortic stenosis. The systolic pressure remains abnormally elevated, but left ventricular stroke volume is maintained by abnormal increases in end-diastolic and end-systolic volume. The left ventricular end-diastolic pressure is also abnormally elevated. *(From CE Rackley, WP Hood Jr: Aortic valve disease. In: HJ Levine, ed: Clinical Cardiovascular Physiology. New York, Grune & Stratton, 1976. Reproduced with permission from the publisher and author.)*

whether or not the patient has experienced exertional chest pain.[27] It is essential to delineate coronary anatomy, since any necessary coronary artery bypass surgery should be performed at the time of aortic valve replacement.

Radionuclide Studies

Radionuclide scans can evaluate ventricular function and myocardial perfusion both at rest and during exertion.[55] Perfusion abnormalities in the hypertrophied ventricle, however, can be similar to those seen in coronary artery disease (see Chap. 134).

Exercise Studies

Exercise should be performed cautiously in patients with aortic stenosis, particularly if there is a history of syncope. In general, symptomatic aortic stenosis is a relative contraindication to exercise testing. Exercise testing occasionally may be carefully performed to ascertain that a patient who has evidence of aortic stenosis but who claims to be asymptomatic has indeed maintained exercise capacity without symptoms. Symptoms, exercise tolerance, blood pressure, and ventricular function can be assessed during exercise (see also Chap. 16).[55]

Usual Strategy of Workup

After the initial history for documentation of symptoms and observation of the physical findings of aortic stenosis, a standard 12-lead electrocardiogram and chest films are indicated. Echocardiography can accurately estimate the valve gradient as well as delineate the underlying anatomy and document the presence and extent of accompanying aortic regurgitation or other valvular lesions. Asymptomatic patients should be followed every 3 to 6 months with history and physical examination, be educated about prophylaxis against endocarditis (Chap. 94), have a Doppler echocardiogram about once a year, and be warned to watch for the development of any symptoms. Should aortic stenosis be judged to be hemodynamically very severe, however, surgery should be considered even in the absence of symptoms. The onset of symptoms warrants definitive studies, including delineation of the coronary anatomy in patients over 40 years of age or with angina pectoris, in preparation for aortic valve surgery.

Natural History and Prognosis

The incidence of bicuspid aortic valve has been estimated at 4 in 1000 live births, with males predominating over females at 4:1.[3] Leaflets often thicken by age 40, and almost invariably by age 50, but calcium deposits are rarely detected before 40 years of age. Although symptoms generally occur late in the course of aortic stenosis, 3 to 5 percent of patients may die suddenly during an otherwise asymptomatic period, presumably due to an arrhythmia.[23,56] Any symptom of angina pectoris, syncope, or heart failure presages a significant reduction in life expectancy. Adults with aortic stenosis have an average mortality of 9 percent per year. In one study, the average age at clinical presentation was 48 years, whereas the average age of death was 63 years.[57] Once symptoms develop, the survival is often less than 5 years, and the incidence of sudden death in symptomatic patients increases to 15 to 20 percent.[34] Exertional chest discomfort is associated with an average life expectancy of five years; fewer than 5 percent of patients with angina survive 10 to 20 years.[24] The prognosis after syncope is usually 3 to 4 years, but patients survive a mean of less than 2 years after left ventricular failure develops.[23,33] Aortic stenosis may progress more rapidly in elderly patients with a degenerative etiology than in patients with congenital or rheumatic disease.[58–60] Symptoms in aortic stenosis indicate a much worse long-term prognosis than any other lesion affecting the aortic or mitral valve.

Medical Therapy

It is important to establish whether or not a patient with clinical evidence of aortic stenosis is asymptomatic. Thorough questioning of the patient and occasionally a spouse or close friend about current activity levels and symptoms is appropriate. It is well known that some patients decrease their activity levels to prevent the occurrence of symptoms.

Medical management of aortic stenosis in the asymptomatic state requires prophylactic antibiotics to prevent bacterial endocarditis (see Chap. 94). In patients with a suspected rheumatic basis for the aortic stenosis, rheumatic prophylaxis should be continued until adulthood. In the management of exertional chest discomfort, nitrates should be used with extreme caution, and patients should be fully informed about the complications of orthostatic hypotension and possible syncope. Even though digitalis and diuretics are indicated in left ventricular failure, the mechanical obstruction to left ventricular outflow will not be altered by medical therapy. In general, symptoms warrant mechanical improvement of flow across the stenotic valve.

Since depression of the contractile state and reduction of forward cardiac output will diminish intensity of the systolic murmur, the patient with aortic stenosis may rarely present in advanced heart failure or cardiogenic shock without an audible systolic murmur. Echocardiography can detect calcium and immobilization of the aortic valve and suggest a valvular basis for the heart failure. This scenario is most common in the elderly with senile, degenerative Mönckeberg's calcific aortic stenosis. Similarly in the elderly, an acute myocardial infarction may be the first clinical event in a patient with underlying aortic stenosis, and the basal midsystolic murmur may not be initially appreciated due to a low stroke output.

Criteria for valve replacement in the asymptomatic patient have not been established, but a gradient greater than 80 mmHg or an orifice size less than 0.6 cm^2 warrants serious consideration for intervention. Echocardiography can be used to follow the valve gradient as well as the chamber dimensions, but left ventricular dilatation may not occur until significant depression of left ventricular contractility has developed. The potential for sudden death as well as the increased operative mortality once myocardial failure has developed underscore the need to proceed with mechanical efforts to improve valve flow based on hemodynamic measurements.

Unlike the results of balloon mitral valvuloplasty, results with catheter balloon aortic valvotomy have been disappointing. The procedure has been applied primarily to the elderly with degenerative calcific aortic stenosis in whom the risks of aortic valve replacement have been felt to be unacceptably high or in whom valve replacement has been contraindicated because of other life-threatening illnesses. Generally, these patients have been highly symptomatic and exhibited tight aortic stenosis. In-hospital morbidity has been significant, and mortality has been disturbingly high.[61–64] Long-term results have also been poor.[61–65] Cumulative probability of survival at 12 months in 125 patients with a mean age of 76 ± 13 years who underwent catheter balloon valvotomy ("valvuloplasty") was only 62 ± 6 percent.[61] Balloon valvotomy, when successful, can produce distinct hemodynamic benefit with approximately a 50 to 70 percent increase in aortic valve area.[64] The rate of restenosis, however, is high. Grollier and associates[66] have shown that the immediate benefits of decreased aortic valve gradient and increased valve area may return significantly toward the prevalvotomy values as soon as 8 days after catheter balloon valvotomy.

Elderly patients with tight aortic stenosis tolerate aortic valve replacement significantly better than mitral valve replacement. Age per se is not a contraindication to aortic valve replacement, and, as noted below, the procedure can be performed on octogenarians. Because of the generally poor results with balloon aortic valvotomy, this procedure should primarily be used to manage the patient who presents with tight aortic stenosis and hemodynamic collapse, such as severe failure or systemic hypotension, as a bridge to subsequent surgery. It may also be appropriate in the pregnant patient with tight congenital aortic stenosis. Another use is in the patient who requires urgent noncardiac surgery. Finally, it can be used as a palliative measure in the very elderly patient in whom surgery is contraindicated because of either other organ-system disease or an additional life-threatening illness (see also Chap. 86).

Patient preparation for aortic valve replacement should include elective surgical or dental work to reduce the postoperative incidence of endocarditis. In older patients carotid flow studies should be considered to detect significant underlying cerebrovascular disease. Symptomatic carotid lesions can be corrected at the same time as aortic valve replacement (see also Chap. 122).

Surgical Therapy

As with any surgical procedure, the natural history of the disease must be weighed against the results achieved by surgical intervention. Longitudinal studies of patients with valvular heart disease are limited to studies carried out before the widespread use of valve replacement and, in many instances, before the availability of objective means of assessing the degree of severity of the disease. Natural history studies provide some information on the outcome of patients with mitral and aortic valve disease and indicate that patients with aortic stenosis have the poorest prognosis.[67] Approximately 50 percent of patients diagnosed clinically as having severe stenosis with or without symptoms will die within 5 years of the time of diagnosis. If only those patients who are symptomatic are considered, the prognosis is much worse. The majority of patients with aortic stenosis develop symptoms of congestive heart failure, angina, or syncope. Sudden death, usually due to arrhythmia, may occur in 3 to 5 percent of asymptomatic patients and in a significantly higher percentage of symptomatic patients.[23,56] Successful aortic valve replacement results in a marked reduction in the subsequent likelihood of sudden death.[68]

Aortic stenosis, which is a ventricular pressure-overload condition, as opposed to aortic regurgitation, which is a volume-overload condition, usually results in well-maintained ventricular function except in far-advanced situations. Thus, significant improvement in the patient's clinical status and longevity usually follows surgery.

Indications for Operation

Patients with congestive heart failure, angina, or exertional syncope in the presence of significant aortic valvular stenosis should undergo aortic valve replacement promptly (see below). Asymptomatic patients with extremely tight aortic valvular stenosis should also be advised to have surgery. Although clinical assessment, including the presence of left ventricular hypertrophy and strain as seen on the electrocardiogram, will identify most patients with severe aortic valvular stenosis, certain patients may be missed by clinical assessment alone. Echo-Doppler examination should be carried out in all patients with suspected aortic stenosis. The measurement of a Doppler-derived peak systolic gradient across a stenotic aortic valve requires a well-trained technician who will persist in attempting to maximize the actual velocity signal, including use of a dedicated continuous-wave Doppler probe to record the gradient accurately. Recorded systolic flow velocities decrease as the angle of the probe deviates from the longitudinal axis of the blood flow and can result in a significant underestimation of the severity of the stenosis. If a gradient greater than about 50 mmHg is estimated by Doppler echocardiographic examination, cardiac catheterization should be undertaken. If a lesser gradient is recorded but the clinical features suggest the possibility of significant aortic stenosis, cardiac catheterization should also be carried out. Coronary arteriography should be performed at the time the aortic stenosis is being evaluated for aortic valve replacement in all postmenopausal women and in men over the age of 35.[69] If significant lesions are found in the coronary arteries, they should be bypassed at the time of valve replacement.

The decision to operate is particularly difficult in certain patients with aortic stenosis. One group consists of those who are extremely ill with terminal aortic stenosis and severe depression of left ventricular function.[70] In such patients, the heart may dilate modestly in association with depression of both left ventricular systolic and diastolic function. Unless severe coexisting morbid conditions make operation a prohibitive risk, however, most patients with terminal aortic stenosis should be candidates for operation. Many of these patients have a relatively low mean transvalvar gradient (20 to 30 mmHg) but a calculated valve area that suggests severe aortic valve stenosis.[70] In these patients, the cardiac output may be reduced by several mechanisms, including the long-term effects of aortic stenosis, coronary artery disease, or heart muscle disease of other etiology. If the decrease in ventricular function is due to aortic stenosis, there is a very good likelihood that it will improve significantly following aortic valve replacement, whereas it is much less likely to improve if due to a different cause. Most such patients should be treated surgically, however. In a few, highly selected patients there may be a place for catheter balloon valvotomy, with valve replacement indicated if there is evidence of improved ventricular performance after relief of the stenosis.

The elderly now account for a large fraction of patients requiring aortic valve surgery; in one recent series the mean age for aortic valve replacement was 65 years, and 30 percent of patients were over 70 years.[71] The pathologic deformation of the aortic valves in these patients is such that catheter balloon dilatation ("valvotomy," "valvuloplasty," or "commissurotomy") is ineffective in providing long-term relief and far less effective than aortic valve replacement.[72] (See Chap. 86.) Thus, an increasing number of septuagenarians and octogenarians with satisfactory mental acuity are candidates for surgery and can be operated on with excellent results provided that there are no serious coexisting morbid conditions, such as renal failure.[73,74] Other elderly patients undergoing coronary artery bypass grafting may have a moderate aortic valve gradient due to moderate, noncritical aortic stenosis. Since it is known that stenosis of the native valve may progress within 2 to 4 years from a relatively modest gradient to a very significant gradient,[58–60] some such patients should be considered for aortic valve replacement at the time of coronary artery bypass surgery even if the calculated valve area is not critical.

Operation

There are a number of surgical alternatives. In young patients with congenital aortic stenosis, commissurotomy of the noncalcified valve may be possible. Even in some adult patients with rheumatic aortic stenosis, commissurotomy and removal of fibrous tissue may open the valve adequately and provide symptomatic relief.[75] Occasionally, mechanical calcium debridement for mild aortic stenosis of the valve leaflets may be possible, although in general the results of either mechanical[76] or ultrasonic[77] debridement are not long lasting.

In general, the vast majority of patients with aortic stenosis will require valve replacement. The choice of valve prostheses in the aortic area is now quite variable due to the development of new prosthetic and bioprosthetic valves. The currently available (FDA-approved) prosthetic heart valves for use in the United States are the St. Jude valve, the Medtronic–Hall valve, the Starr-Edwards ball valve, and the Omniscience valve. All have excellent durability. Three (St. Jude, Medtronic-Hall, and Omniscience) are low-profile valves with excellent hemodynamic performance. All mechanical prosthetic valves require lifetime anticoagulation. The currently available FDA-approved tissue valves are the Hancock modified orifice and the Carpentier-Edwards porcine bioprosthetic valves, and the Carpentier-Edwards pericardial valve. Patients with biologic valves do not require anticoagulation, but the long-term durability of these devices is finite. The selection of an individual device depends on patient age, life-style, avoidance of or contraindication to anticoagulation, etiology of aortic disease, and anatomic limitations of the aortic annulus and ascending aorta.

The cryopreserved allograft is the current allograft valve, which began as chemically preserved or as fresh grafts about 30 years ago with implantation of the first subcoronary homograft aortic valves in London[78] and New Zealand.[79] Current homograft valves may have better preservation of the collagen durability than valves preserved by previous techniques, and they have been very effective in patients who desire the best hemodynamics and lowest thromboembolic rate.[80] Long-term durability, however, is uncertain, since all previous tissue preservation techniques have not yielded significant durability beyond 15 years.

The pulmonary autotransplant operation has been advocated for the young patient (<25 years) who requires aortic valve replacement.[81] The patient's own pulmonic valve is removed en bloc and used to replace the irreparably damaged native aortic valve. A homograft aortic valve is then inserted into the patient's pulmonary artery. The advantage of transplanting the patient's own tissue is that it may have the best durability of any tissue valve, since it has been documented that the valve will grow with the patient.[81] The disadvantages include the removal of the pulmonic valve, with possible damage to a septal artery branch of the left anterior descending coronary and the much lengthier operation required.

Aortic valve replacement is performed through a median sternotomy using cardiopulmonary bypass, with venting of the right superior pulmonary vein or the pulmonary artery. After the aorta is cross-clamped, antegrade and retrograde coronary sinus blood or crystalloid cardioplegic solution is administered. The valve is excised and the calcium carefully debrided from the valve annulus. When all the calcium is removed, the valve annulus should be quite pliable. The probability of a perivalvar leak is diminished significantly by this maneuver. Everting mattress sutures are usually used for both prosthetic and bioprosthetic valves. Homograft valve implantation requires two layers of monofilament suture for implanting both the lower and the upper aspect of the donor valve and aorta in the recipient annulus and ascending aorta. Careful attention is paid to sutures near the Bundle of His at the confluence of the right and noncoronary commissure to prevent heart block. Concomitant coronary bypass grafts are usually performed before the implantation of the valve to permit the infusion of cardioplegic solution through the grafts distal to the coronary artery obstructions. After closure of the aortotomy, proximal coronary bypass anastomoses are performed before removing the aortic cross-clamp. Air is evacuated from the heart and cardiopulmonary bypass is terminated when the patent is normothermic. Special problems exist with a very small aortic root. Several procedures may be utilized to increase annular size and allow a valve size consistent with patient size and cardiac output demands. These procedures include making an aortic outflow gusset, incision of anterior leaflet mitral valve, homograft root replacement, and, rarely, aortoventriculoplasty.[82]

Postoperative Management

During the postoperative period, careful monitoring of left ventricular filling pressures by pulmonary artery catheter or by a left atrial catheter via the right superior pulmonary vein is important. Systemic hypertension is a frequent complication of aortic valve replacement, and sodium nitroprusside or nitroglycerin is infused to reduce the blood pressure. This decreases afterload, improves myocardial performance, and has the practical advantage of preventing suture line leakage in the previously heparinized patient. After aortic valve replacement, the atrial contribution to cardiac output is very important; for this reason, pacing wires are placed in both the right atrium and right ventricle in order to be able to optimize the atrioventricular contraction sequence. If there is bradycardia, atrial or atrioventricular pacing is especially critical, since stroke volume is relatively fixed in the perioperative period. This is particularly important in the hypertrophied heart, in which atrial contraction provides an important contribution to cardiac output.

Operative Results

The current operative mortality for isolated primary aortic valve replacement is less than 3 percent, and in the younger patient with no coexisting morbid condition it is less than 1 percent.[83] Complicating coronary artery disease despite complete revascularization by coronary bypass increases operative risk.[84] The results of aortic valve replacement in the elderly indicate that there appears to be only an insignificantly increased risk in septuagenarian and octogenarian patients. In these elderly age groups, only women who require concomitant coronary artery bypass plus aortic valve replacement have a significantly higher operative risk.[85] In larger series, operative mortality was 7 percent for patients older than 70, 7 percent for patients 80 or older, but 10 percent for women 70 or older who required concomitant coronary grafting.[85,86]

Late Results

Late morbidity and mortality in patients after aortic valve replacement are generally quite satisfactory. Actuarial survival at 5 years with various types of valve prostheses is about 80 percent (Fig. 79-4).[87–91] The degree of left ventricular dysfunction, as well as concomitant coronary disease and coexisting morbid conditions are significant determinants of late mortality. Late deaths are most often due to chronic congestive failure, thromboembolic stroke, myocardial infarction in those with coronary disease, and cardiac arrhythmias leading to sudden death, especially in those with an enlarged dilated heart.[83,87–89]

Sudden death after aortic valve replacement is most commonly thought to be due to ventricular arrhyth-

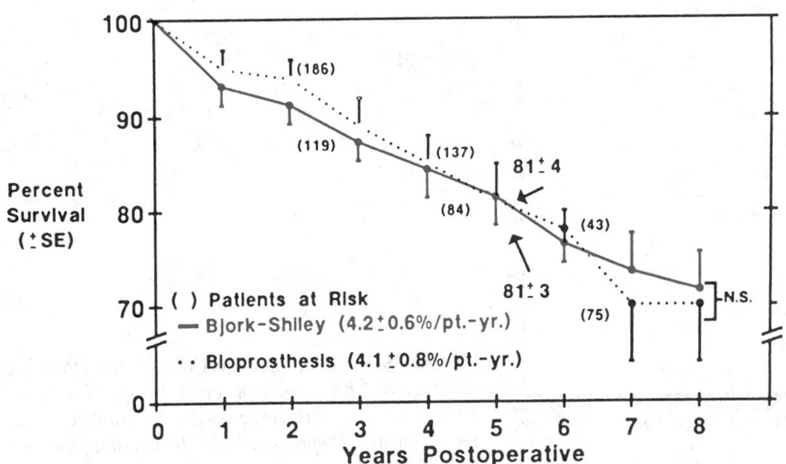

FIGURE 79-4 Actuarial survival depicted for hospital survivors of prosthetic and bioprosthetic valves. NS, not significant; SE, standard error.[91] *(Reproduced with permission from the publisher and author.)*

mias,[68,92] but it may also result from thromboemboli. The risk of thromboembolism is much less after aortic valve replacement than after mitral valve replacement because most patients are in sinus rhythm. The thromboembolic risk is lowest after a homograft or pulmonary autograft valve replacement, following which it is virtually zero.[79] Patients with porcine or pericardial valves have a risk of about 1.5 events per 100 patient years, and in patients with prosthetic valves the risk is 1.5 and 2.5 events per 100 patient years.[93] Thrombosis of prosthetic valves was a more frequent complication with previous prosthetic valves, but it now occurs rarely and only when anticoagulation is stopped for a long period of time. In previous decades, a major morbidity after prosthetic valve replacement was anticoagulation hemorrhage. With newer, low-profile, more hemodynamically efficient valves, this morbidity has decreased, and warfarin anticoagulation provides excellent protection from thromboemboli for most patients.[94] It is recommended that patients with mechanical prosthetic heart valves be maintained on levels of warfarin that prolong the INR to 2.5 to 3.5.[95]

Patients with biologic aortic valves, of course, have the risk of late structural valve degeneration. The probability of freedom from valve reoperation at 10 years in patients with a cryopreserved homograft is about 90 percent; this is somewhat better than with the porcine bioprostheses, where the freedom from structural valve degeneration is about 90 percent at 8 years and 40 percent at 15 years.[96] In the aortic position, a bioprosthetic valve is the valve of choice in most elderly patients[90,96] because the rate of valve tissue degeneration is considerably lower than in younger age groups and the probability of tissue valve failure in patients over 70 is 20 percent at 10 years (Fig. 79-5).[90] The use of tissue valves in the elderly obviates the use of anticoagulation, which is very advantageous. In the younger age group, mechanical prosthetic valves tend to be used because most patients wish to minimize the probability of reoperation due to valve dysfunction and because of accelerated fibrosis-calcification in biologic prosthetic valves in children and young adults. An exception is the child-bearing-age female, who should not risk anticoagulation during pregnancy because of the teratogenic potential of warfarin in the first trimester,[97] and who should receive a biologic valve if replacement is indicated.

AORTIC REGURGITATION

Definition, Etiology, and Pathology

Aortic regurgitation is the diastolic flow of blood from the aorta into the left ventricle. Although regurgitation is due to incompetence of the aortic valve, it can be caused by any disturbance of the valvular appartus from the leaflets to the annulus of the aorta.

Aortic regurgitation was one of the earliest recognized cardiac abnormalities, but the disease mechanisms that affect competence of the aortic valve have changed with time. In the past, rheumatic fever and syphilis were major causes of aortic regurgitation, but these diseases have diminished in frequency in recent years due to effective antimicrobials.[98-100] As these two infectious conditions have diminished, diseases of the connective tissue and anatomic abnormalities of the ascending aorta and of the valve have become more frequent causes. Annuloectasia of the ascending aorta is one of the more common causes of severe aortic regurgitation. Marfan's syndrome and the associated aortic dilatation often result in incompetence of the aortic valve; myxomatous changes in the leaflets may further exaggerate the condition.[101] Ankylosing spondylitis, systemic lupus erythematosus, the primary antiphospholipid syndrome, Reiter's syndrome, osteogenesis imperfecta, and rheumatoid arthritis are connective tissue disorders that can be associated with aortic regurgitation (see Chap. 103).[101-105] Congenital abnormalities include the bicuspid valve and a ventricular septal defect associated with a sinus of Valsalva aneurysm.[106] Long-standing vascular disorders such as hypertension and atherosclerosis can also produce incompetence of the aortic valve.[107] Finally, any primary cause of aortic stenosis frequently results in regurgitation across the fixed stenotic leaflets during diastole.

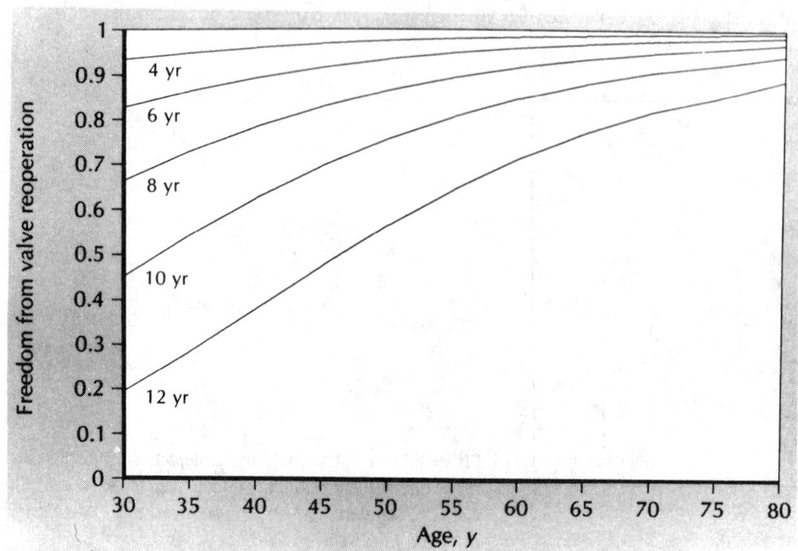

FIGURE 79-5 Cox proportional hazards model to evaluate freedom from valve reoperation by age at 4, 6, 8, 10, and 12 years after aortic porcine bioprosthetic valve replacements.[96] (*Reproduced with permission from the publisher and author.*)

TABLE 79-1

Etiology of Chronic and Acute Aortic Regurgitation

Chronic aortic regurgitation
- Rheumatic heart disease
- Syphilis
- Aortitis (Takayasu)
- Annuloaortic ectasia
- Heritable disorders of connective tissue
  - Marfan's syndrome
  - Ehlers-Danlos syndrome
  - Osteogenesis imperfecta
- Congenital heart disease
  - Bicuspid aortic valve
  - Interventricular septal defect
  - Sinus of Valsalva aneurysm
- Connective tissue disorders
  - Ankylosing spondylitis
  - Reiter's syndrome
  - Rheumatoid arthritis
  - Systemic lupus erythematosus
  - Primary antiphospholipid syndrome
- Cystic medial necrosis of aorta
- Hypertension
- Arteriosclerosis
- Myxomatous degeneration
- Infective endocarditis
- Following prosthetic valve surgery
- Associated with aortic stenosis

Acute aortic regurgitation
- Rheumatic fever
- Infective endocarditis
- Congenital (rupture of sinus of Valsalva)
- Acute aortic dissection
- Following prosthetic valve surgery
- Trauma

NOTE: Certain disorders are capable of producing acute and chronic aortic regurgitation.

Acute disturbances can produce sudden aortic regurgitation involving a normal or a diseased valve apparatus. Aortic dissection, infective endocarditis, and acute rheumatic fever can create sudden regurgitation across the valve.[108,109] Aortic dissection can disturb the competence of the annulus support for the valve. Infective endocarditis can lead to leaflet perforation or cause paravalvular regurgitation, and any other inflammatory condition involving the leaflet can create prolapse or eversion of an aortic cusp.

The major etiologies of chronic and acute aortic regurgitation are shown in Table 79-1.

Incompetent closure of the aortic valve can result from intrinsic disease of the cusp or from diseases affecting the aorta. Acquired intrinsic diseases of the aortic valve are most commonly the result of either rheumatic fever or bacterial infection. In Marfan's syndrome the primary basis for aortic regurgitation usually resides in the aorta, but there may be prolapse of the aortic cusps due to myxomatous changes. Infrequent etiologies include rheumatoid arthritis, systemic lupus erythematosus, and trauma.[110] (See also Chaps. 103 and 112.)

Rheumatic fever can cause either pure aortic regurgitation or regurgitation associated with some degree of stenosis. An incompetent valve results from fibrosis and contractions of the margins of the cusp, which become shorter than normal (Fig. 79-6).[107] The process may affect all three cusps to the same degree of severity, or there may be unequal involvement so that one cusp undergoes greater contracture than the remaining two. This malalignment of the cusp creates incompetence of the valve. In pure rheumatic aortic regurgitation commissural fusion is either absent or minimal. If the contracture of the leaflet is associated with fusion of two or three commissures, the result is a combination of aortic stenosis and regurgitation.

Aortic regurgitation may occur in patients with ankylosing spondylitis, and complete heart block also can be associated with this condition (see Chap. 102).[111]

Infective endocarditis may involve a normal tricuspid aortic valve, but frequently the valve is bicuspid from congenital or acquired mechanisms. Incompetence is produced through destruction of cusp tissue, perforation of one or more cusps, or detachment of a cusp at its aortic insertion (Fig. 79-7). If the infectious process extends to the nearby conducting system, atrioventricular conduction defects may develop with the aortic regurgitation.[112] (See also Chap. 94.)

Deceleration external blunt trauma may rarely cause rupture of a cusp. A more common basis for posttraumatic aortic regurgitation is laceration of the aorta (see Chap. 112).[113]

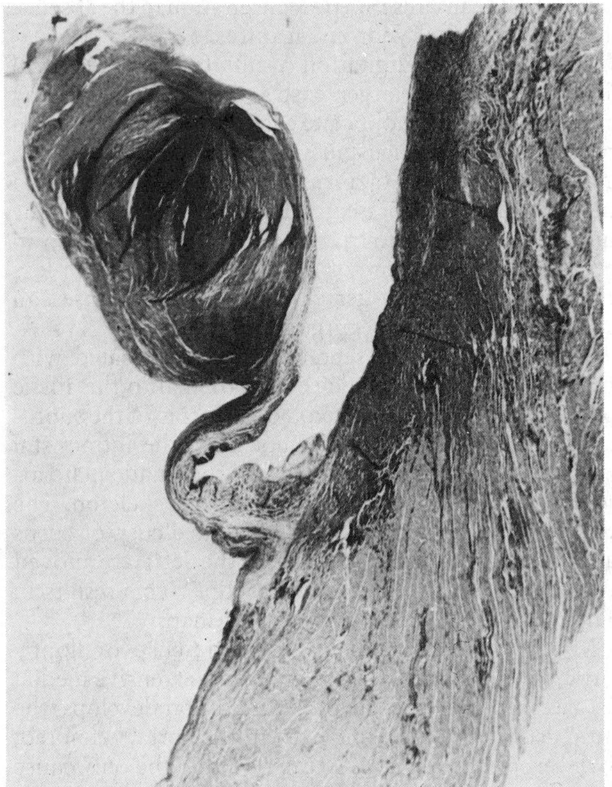

FIGURE 79-6 Low-power photomicrograph of an aortic cusp in chronic rheumatic aortic insufficiency. The distal half of the cusp is grossly thickened by fibrous tissue. Elastic tissue stain; ×5.

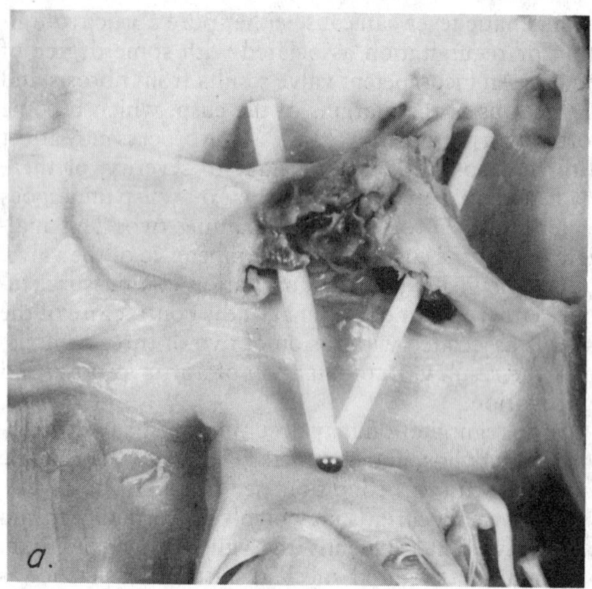

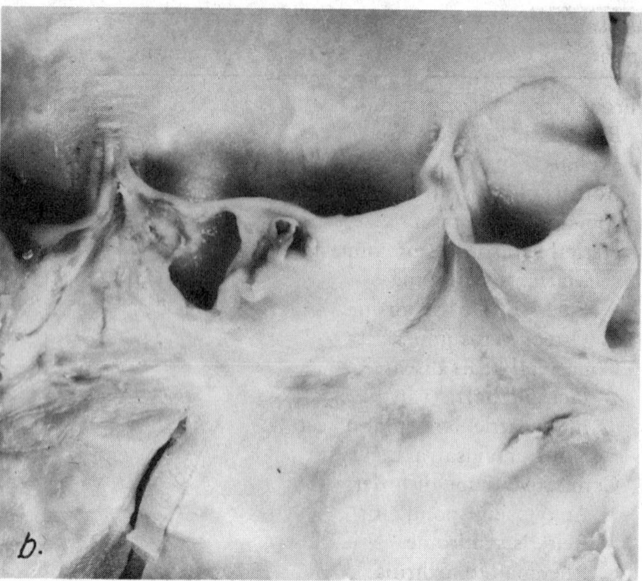

FIGURE 79-7 Bacterial endocarditis. *A.* Each of two cusps of the aortic valve shows perforation (probes) as part of active bacterial endocarditis. *B.* Perforation in an aortic cusp as a manifestation of bacteriologically healed bacterial endocarditis. (*From JE Edwards: Lesions causing or simulating aortic insufficiency. Cardiovasc Clin 5:128, 1973. Reproduced with permission from the publisher and author.*)

The two principal congenital causes of aortic regurgitation are a bicuspid aortic valve and a ventricular septal defect. Fenestration of aortic cusps is common but rarely produces significant aortic regurgitation.[114] Such small congenital abnormalities, however, might predispose to bacterial endocarditis. Myxomatous changes within the valve leaflets can cause aortic regurgitation in the absence of other Marfan's syndrome features.

When aortic regurgitation results from a congenital bicuspid valve, the larger cusp is redundant and may prolapse beyond the opposite cusp. Aortic regurgitation from a congenital bicuspid valve is often not detected until early adult life. In a less common type of bicuspid valve the raphe is represented by a thin strand of tissue running from near the free aspect of the larger cusp to the aortic wall. Rupture of the strand will result in loss and support of the larger cusp, and this prolapse can produce major aortic regurgitation.[115]

When a ventricular septal defect is associated with aortic regurgitation, the defect is proximal to the aortic root and valve. The more common defect is of the supracristal type, and the less common is of the infracristal type.[116] Aortic regurgitation results from inadequate attachment of the aortic root to the cardiac skeleton. The aorta deviates to the right and the related cusp or cusps (usually the right, less commonly the left) are moved laterally with the displaced aorta "tip." This results in malalignment of the cusp. (See also Chap. 97.)

Myxomatous changes in the aortic cusp or floppy aortic valve are usually associated with extensive medial disease of the aorta. If aortic regurgitation develops, the cause usually resides principally in the aorta. As noted, however, prolapse of a cusp can be either the only cause or a contributing factor.

Primary disease of the aorta leading to aortic regurgitation may be manifest either as dilatation or dissection of the vessel. Dilatation of the ascending aorta creates tension on the individual cusps, causing them to be relatively too short for competent closure of the dilated aortic root. Syphilitic aortitis is the classic example of this condition (Fig. 79-8).[117] Similar changes may be observed with aortic annuloectasia or rheumatoid spondylitis.[118] In rheumatoid arthritis the root of the aorta may be affected with associated inflammatory and fibrotic changes of the valve cusps.[103] In the aging individual the process of aortic dilatation may infrequently reach such proportions as to create significant aortic regurgitation.

Cystic medial necrosis of the aorta, whether idiopathic or associated with Marfan's syndrome, is another cause of aortic regurgitation even in the absence of dissection of the aorta (Fig. 79-9). In this condition the intrinsic changes of the cusps can result in prolapse or, rarely, rupture of the leaflets (Fig. 79-10).[101]

Disruption of the intima of the ascending aorta may develop with hypertension, extensive cystic medial necrosis, external blunt trauma, or aortitis. The process may be localized or lead to a dissecting aneurysm.[119] When the primary intimal disruption occurs near a commissural attachment of two cusps, the secondary retraction of aortic tissue causes prolapse of the cusps at the related commissure (Fig. 79-11*A* and *B*).[120] The resulting malalignment of the cusps produces aortic regurgitation, which can appear suddenly. In some instances, the disruption of the intima is below the upper aspect of a commissure and there is the chance of tearing related cusps by retraction of the edges of the laceration (Fig. 79-11*C*).[120]

Pathophysiology

Regurgitation of diastolic flow across the incompetent aortic valve increases filling of the left ventricle and imposes a volume overload. The size of the regurgitant area, the diastolic pressure gradient across the valve, and

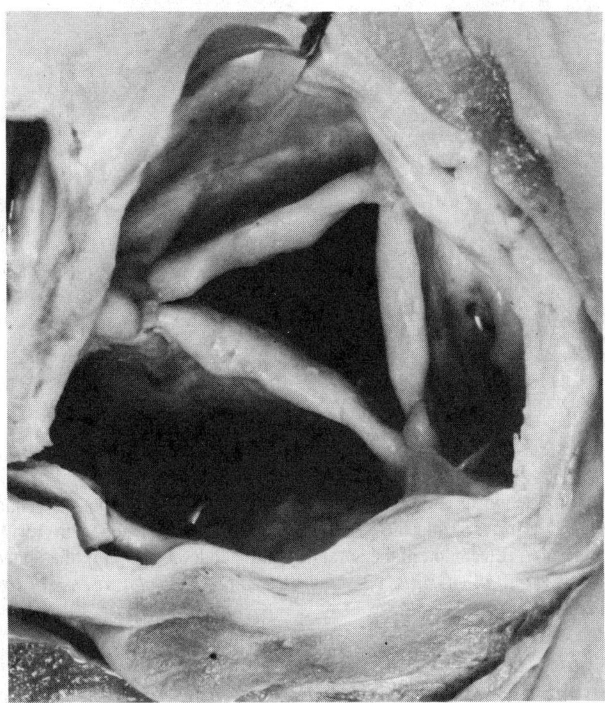

FIGURE 79-8 Aortic valve viewed from above in aortitis. Bowing of the cusps incident to dilatation of the aorta leaves a triangular defect through which regurgitation occurs. The commissures are not fused.

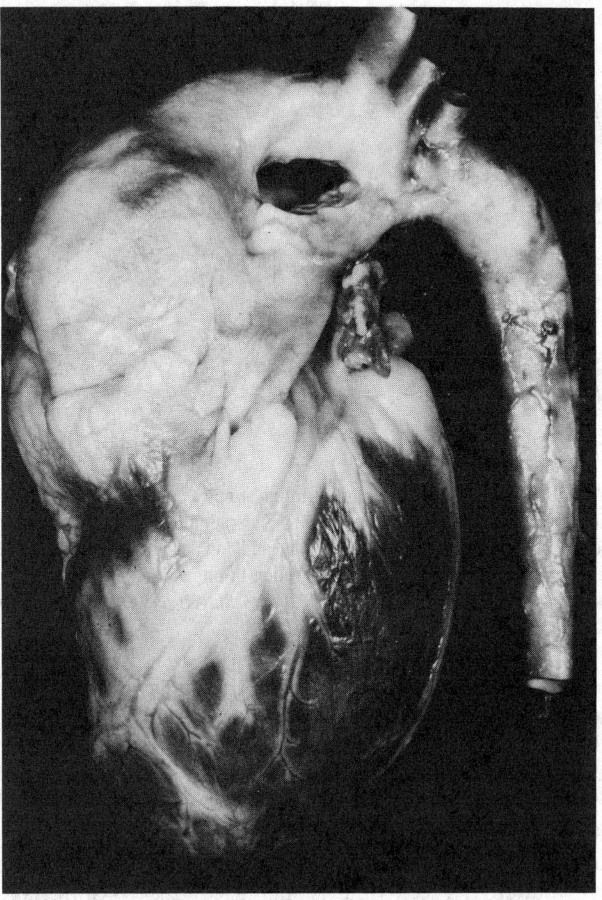

FIGURE 79-9 Cystic medial necrosis of the aorta in Marfan's syndrome. Exterior view of heart and aorta viewed from the left side. Note marked dilatation of the ascending aorta. *(From JE Edwards: Lesions causing or simulating aortic insufficiency. Cardiovasc Clin 5:128, 1973. Reproduced with permission from the publisher and author.)*

the duration of systole influence the regurgitant volume (Fig. 79-12).[121,122] Marked decreases in heart rate, which are associated with a significant prolongation of diastole, can increase the regurgitant flow. A small incompetent area of the valve can lead to significant aortic regurgitation over a period of time.[123]

Chronic aortic regurgitation gradually increases left ventricular end-diastolic volume, since the chamber re-

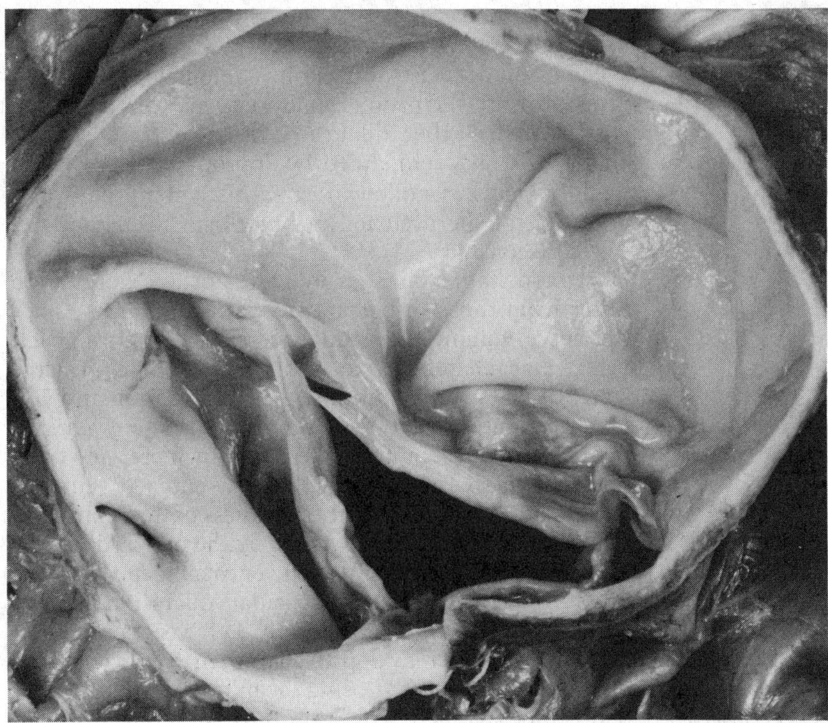

FIGURE 79-10 Interior of ascending aorta and aortic valve viewed from above in a case with extensive cystic medial necrosis of the aorta. Note marked dilatation of aorta. The aortic cusps have been stretched and also show some features of prolapse. *(From JE Edwards: Lesions causing or simulating aortic insufficiency. Cardiovasc Clin 5:128, 1973. Reproduced with permission from the publisher and author.)*

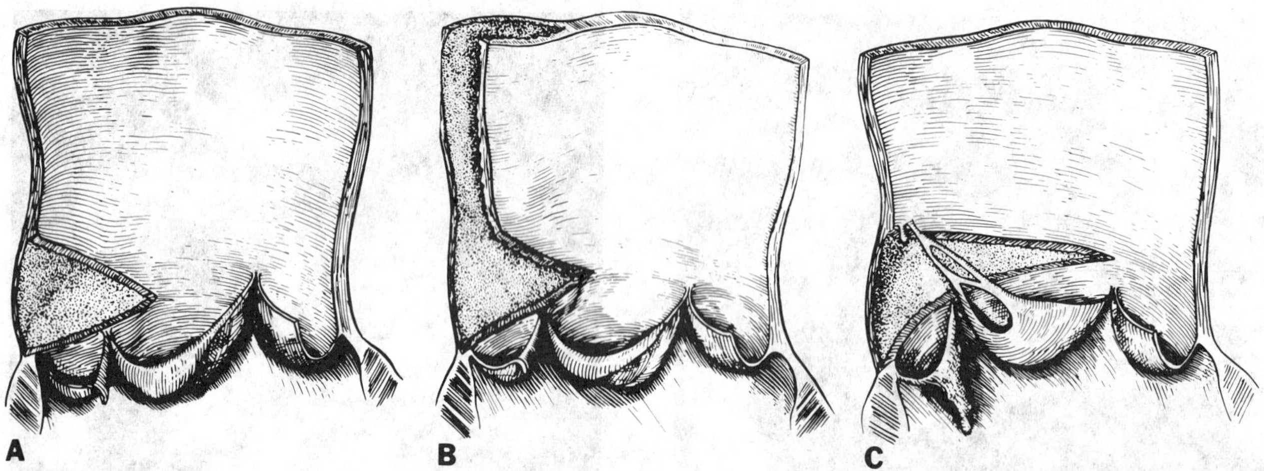

FIGURE 79-11 Diagrammatic portrayal of consequences of laceration of the aorta in relation to an aortic commissure. *A.* Laceration without dissecting aneurysm. Retraction of the edges of the laceration allows for commissural prolapse and aortic incompetence. *B.* The process is the same shown in *A* with regard to the aortic valve, but there is the additional feature of classical dissecting aneurysm. *C.* Laceration of the aorta has been at a level just below the upper level of the commissure causing attenuation of one aortic cusp and rupture of the other. (*From JE Edwards: Pathology of acquired valvular disease of the heart. Semin Roentgenol 14:96, 1979. Reproduced with permission from the publisher and author.*)

ceives blood from the left atrium and the systemic circulation. Total left ventricular stroke volume is appropriately increased to maintain the forward or effective stroke volume to the systemic circulation. Compensatory dilatation of the left ventricle may be accompanied by minimal or no elevation of the left ventricular end-diastolic pressure.[21] Diastolic compliance of the volume overloaded left ventricle is increased due to splippage and reorientation of myocardial fibers and other mechanisms, including stress relaxation and creep.[124] Forces within the ventricular wall or systolic wall stress are maintained within the normal range by appropriate increase in left ventricular wall thickness and ventricular mass or hypertrophy.[18] (See also Chap. 23.)

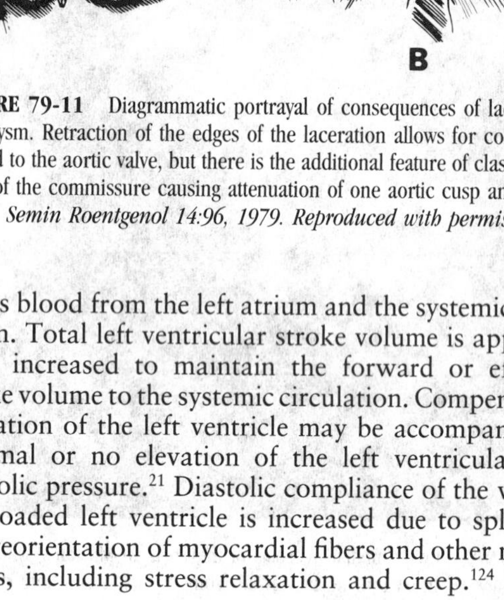

During the early stage of chronic aortic regurgitation, left ventricular stroke volume increases to maintain normal forward cardiac output both at rest and with exercise. The ratio of the total left ventricular stroke volume to the end-diastolic volume or ejection fraction remains within the normal range or even greater than normal. In the late stage of chronic aortic regurgitation, a decrease in myocardial contractility or ischemia due to underlying coronary artery disease can lead to an increase in the end-systolic volume in association with a decline in ejection fraction (Fig. 79-12). As the compliant properties or elasticity of the ventricle decline, the left ventricular end-diastolic pressure increases. The increased end-systolic volume and decrease in diastolic compliance elevate left atrial pressure and produce pulmonary venous hypertension. When further dilatation of the left ventricular chamber is unaccompanied by appropriate increases in wall thickness, systolic wall stress rises abnormally as a reflection of the preload and afterload mismatch (Fig. 79-13) (see Chap. 23).[18,125]

Hemodynamic changes in acute aortic regurgitation differ from those of chronic aortic regurgitation, since the acute volume overload occurs with a normal left ventricular chamber size and myocardial contractile state. Under such conditions, the regurgitation and volume overload are suddenly imposed on a left ventricle unable to dilate acutely and to adapt by increasing compliance to increased diastolic filling. Acute left ventricular dilatation is limited by the thickness of the ventricular myocardium and to some extent by the pericardium. As a result, marked elevation of left ventricular end-diastolic pressure with minimal ventricular dilatation accompanies acute aortic regurgitation. Left ventricular end-diastolic pressure may approach or even exceed left atrial pressure, prematurely closing the mitral valve. Such sudden hemodynamic changes produce pulmonary venous hypertension and acute pulmonary edema. Should an

EW 19-02-38
AORTIC REGURGITATION
Pressure mm Hg
0
20
40
60
80
100
120
100 200 300 400 500
Volume ml

FIGURE 79-12 Left ventricular pressure-volume diagram in decompensated aortic regurgitation. The abnormal features of the loop are extreme displacement to the right due to an increase in end-diastolic volume and increased end-systolic volume indicative of depression of myocardial contractility. The isovolumic relaxation phase on the left-hand side of the pressure-volume loop is shortened due to early diastolic filling of the left ventricle from the aorta. The end-diastolic pressure is also abnormally elevated. [*From CE Rackley, WP Hood Jr: Aortic valve disease. In: HJ Levine (ed.): Clinical Cardiovascular Physiology. New York, Grune & Stratton, 1976. Reproduced with permission from the publisher and author.*]

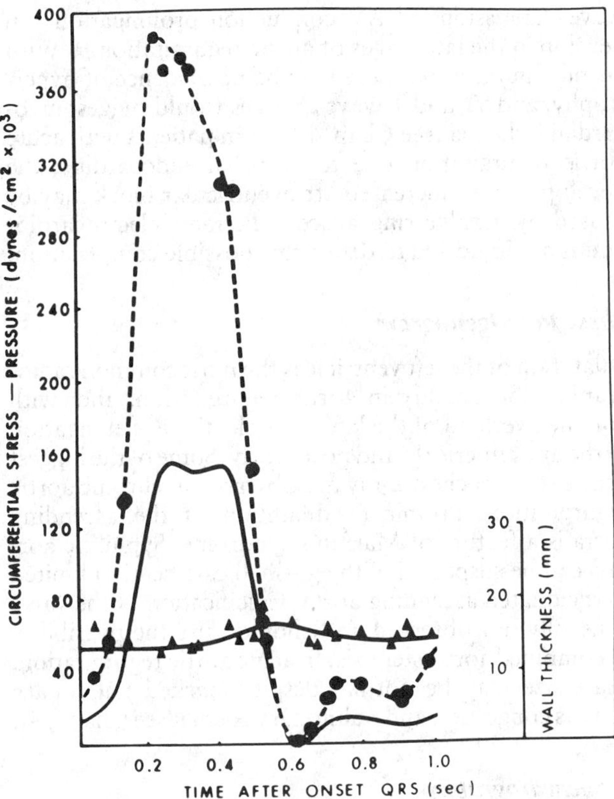

FIGURE 79-13 Left ventricular pressure, wall stress, and wall thickness in decompensated aortic regurgitation. Although the diastolic wall thickness is increased, there is a marked decrease in systolic wall thickening. This results in sustained elevation of the systolic wall stress, even though the left ventricular systolic pressure remains within the normal range (- - - , stress; ——, pressure; ▲——▲, wall thickness.) [*From CE Rackley, WP Hood Jr: Aortic valve disease. In: HJ Levine (ed.): Clinical Cardiovascular Physiology. New York, Grune & Stratton, 1976. Reproduced with permission from the publisher and author.*]

acute increase in aortic regurgitation be superimposed on a chronically diseased and incompetent aortic valve, the magnitude of the hemodynamic changes will be determined by the extent of preexisting left ventricular dilatation and the compliance properties of the left ventricle.

Chronic aortic regurgitation with severe chamber enlargement can produce the largest left ventricular stroke volume of any disease affecting the left ventricle.[126] The large left ventricular stroke volume will greatly increase the mechanical pressure-volume work of the ventricle and, along with the compensatory hypertrophy, will significantly elevate myocardial oxygen consumption.

Clinical Manifestations

History

Compensatory mechanisms of the volume-overloaded left ventricle enable the patient to remain asymptomatic for many years with aortic regurgitation. When symptoms develop, common clinical manifestations are the symptoms of left ventricular failure, including fatigue, dyspnea, and edema. Before experiencing symptoms of limited exercise performance, patients may notice palpitations and experience circulatory sensations due to the large left ventricular stroke volume with rapid diastolic runoff. These sensations can be appreciated as prominent pulsations in the neck as well as an awareness of the heartbeat when the patient turns onto the left side.[98] Patients may also experience exertional chest pain, but angina pectoris seems to be less frequent than reported in some studies.[102,127] Such chest discomfort is atypical compared to angina pectoris and can occur at rest as well as persist for longer durations than in coronary artery disease. Flushing, sweating, and palpitations may accompany chest pain in aortic regurgitation.[128] In patients with severe aortic regurgitation, pain at rest or during the night has been attributed to the deleterious effects of bradycardia, which increase ventricular filling and wall stress while coronary perfusion pressure during diastole is decreased.

Other unusual cardiac symptoms in severe aortic regurgitation include neck and abdominal pain, postural dizziness, and excessive sweating on the trunk.[128] Stretching of the carotid sheath by the large left ventricular stroke volume may contribute to neck discomfort, and a similar mechanism could explain the abdominal pain. Dizziness is attributed to disturbances in cerebral circulation with marked pressure changes during the rapid diastolic runoff.[100]

Physical Examination

Physical findings in aortic regurgitation are caused by the large left ventricular stroke volume and rapid diastolic runoff. The peripheral pulse is quick, with a rapid rise in upstroke followed by a peripheral collapse known as Corrigan's pulse or water-hammer pulse. The arterial pulse may also have a bisferiens character. Systolic blood pressure is increased and attended by an abnormally low diastolic pressure. If the pulse pressure does not exceed 50 percent of the peak systolic pressure or if the diastolic pressure is above 70 mmHg, aortic regurgitation is usually not hemodynamically severe unless left ventricular failure has developed.[129]

Physical abnormalities may include asthenic body habitus, long extremities, and the arachnodactyly of Marfan's syndrome. Bluish discoloration of the sclera is seen with osteogenesis imperfecta, and subluxation of the lens occurs in Marfan's syndrome. Retinal artery pulsations suggest significant hemodynamic aortic regurgitation. Head bobbing with each cardiac pulsation was described by DeMusset. Carotid arterial pulsations are likewise exaggerated and, if aneurysmal dilatation of the aortic arch is present, a tracheal tug with each heartbeat can be palpated.

If the heart size and apical impulse are normal, aortic regurgitation is usually mild.[99] Severe regurgitation with dilatation of the ventricle will displace the apical impulse inferiorly and laterally.[130] A systolic ejection click is sometimes audible along the left sternal border and is produced by a large stroke volume ejecting into a dilated aorta. A systolic murmur is invariably audible along the left sternal border as well as at the apex and in the primary aortic area in significant aortic regurgitation.[98,99] A systolic thrill can also sometimes be felt in the second right intercostal space, even in pure aortic regurgitation. Scarring of the aortic leaflet margins may diminish the aortic component of the second sound.

The high-pitched diastolic blow along the left sternal border is the characteristic auscultatory finding, and the duration of the diastolic blowing murmur correlates with the hemodynamic abnormality.[100] The murmur is typically high-pitched, decrescendo, and blowing in quality, but eversion of a cusp can give a musical or cooing quality to the murmur.[131] A ventricular (S_3) gallop is frequently heard and may reflect exaggerated early diastolic filling, an increase in the end-diastolic volume, or a decrease in the contractile state as evidence of left ventricular dysfunction.[132,133] A rumbling diastolic murmur may be heard at the apex, as described by Austin Flint. This murmur can be presystolic, middiastolic, or holodiastolic.[100] The mechanism of the murmur is impingement of the aortic regurgitation flow on the anterior leaflet of the mitral valve, which both produces functional mitral stenosis and vibrates. The mid-diastolic component of the murmur occurs when the valve closes quickly after rapid ventricular filling from the aorta and left atrium.[134] The Austin Flint murmur suggests more severe aortic regurgitations, since this murmur is not present with mild regurgitation. (See also Chap. 11.)

In acute aortic regurgitation with a normal left ventricle, the diastolic blow may have musical or coarse, vibrating qualities.[135] These vibrations suggest leaflet laceration, eversion, or separation from the aortic annulus. The mitral leaflet may close prematurely, and the first heart sound may be diminished or absent. The diastolic murmur may extend into early systole, since diastolic filling from the aorta continues after initiation of electrical depolarization of the ventricle.

The peripheral manifestations of a large stroke volume and rapid diastolic runoff in chronic aortic regurgitation include Corrigan's pulse, which is abruptly rising and collapsing, Müller's sign, which is a rhythmic pulsation of the uvula, and Quincke's sign of arterial pulsation of the nail beds. Duroziez' murmur is the systolic and diastolic murmur over the femoral artery, and a disproportionate elevation in femoral artery systolic pressure has been designated Hill's sign.

The classic peripheral manifestations of chronic aortic regurgitation may be absent or significantly attenuated in acute regurgitation. The systolic pressure may not rise, since acute left ventricular dilation is limited and forward stroke output may fall. Although diastolic pressure usually does decrease, it cannot fall below the usually markedly elevated left ventricular diastolic pressure. Thus, aortic diastolic pressures in the range of 40 to 60 mmHg are not uncommon. Consequently, the pulse pressure may not reflect the severity of the acute regurgitation. The classic picture of bounding peripheral and capillary pulses may also be absent. Taken together with the fact that the aortic diastolic murmur can be quite soft under these circumstances, the diagnosis may be overlooked or the severity underestimated. Echo-Doppler examination is quite helpful in clarifying the issue. (See Chaps. 15 and 130.)

Laboratory Tests

Electrocardiogram

The electrocardiogram changes reflect left ventricular hypertrophy with increased QRS amplitude and ST-T wave depression.[79,81] AV conduction prolongation can develop in the late stages of aortic regurgitation.[136] With aortic regurgitation there may be no evidence of hypertrophy, and ST and T wave changes would suggest myocardial ischemia (see Chap. 13).[137] In patients with acute aortic regurgitation due to bacterial endocarditis, the development of increased atrioventricular block may be caused by a valve ring abscess. Periodic electrocardiograms are indicated to detect this possible complication.

Chest Roentgenogram

Dilatation of the left ventricle is the most common radiographic abnormality in aortic regurgitation, and, with volume overload of the left ventricle, there is elongation of the apex inferiorly and posteriorly. Some of the biggest hearts seen on chest x-ray are observed in chronic aortic regurgitation. Prominent dilatation of the ascending aorta is a feature of Marfan's syndrome. Syphilitic aortitis can be suspected with egg-shell calcification limited to the dilated ascending aorta. Calcification of the valve is usually not observed and should raise the possibility of combined aortic stenosis. In acute aortic regurgitation, heart size may be normal despite marked pulmonary venous congestion and pulmonary edema (see Chap. 14).

Echocardiography

The echocardiogram can provide anatomical information on the aortic valve apparatus, the aortic root, the etiology of the regurgitation, measurements of ventricular function, and estimates of the severity of regurgitation (see Chap. 15). Disturbances in mitral valve function due to the regurgitant flow across the aortic valve can also be recognized.[138,139] Vegetations of endocarditis can sometimes be identified on the aortic leaflets (Fig. 15-31).[140,141] Valve ring abscesses may be identified, particularly by transesophageal echocardiography. Increased aortic dimensions suggest a chronic basis for the regurgitation.[142] Left ventricular chamber dimensions and wall thickness permit calculation of chamber volume, stroke volume, shortening fraction, left ventricular mass, and end-diastolic and end-systolic wall stress, preload, and afterload, respectively.[143–145] Mitral valve abnormalities include diastolic fluttering of the anterior leaflet, rapid diastolic closure rate of the mitral leaflet, premature closure of the mitral valve before onset of the QRS complex, and thickening of the leaflets.[138,139] Echo-Doppler (Figs. 130-13, 130-14) with various mapping techniques, along with color Doppler (Color plate X, 130-2), can aid in the quantification of the regurgitation (see Chap. 130).[146–150]

In acute aortic regurgitation diastolic oscillations in the aortic root or ventricular outflow track can be observed with a flail leaflet.[151] Aortic dissection can be diagnosed by a double lumen in the ascending aorta. Transesopheal echocardiography (see Chap. 131) is especially valuable in the evaluation of patients with suspected aortic dissection.

Echocardiographic studies before and after valve replacement have suggested that a left ventricular end-systolic dimension greater than 55 mm can identify a high-risk group for surgery, congestive heart failure, or failure in significant reduction in heart size.[152,153] Others have questioned the value of preoperative M-mode echocardiographic measurements as predictors of postoperative outcome.[154,155]

Cardiac Catheterization

Cardiac catheterization in aortic regurgitation can document aortic regurgitation and estimate its severity, evaluate left ventricular function, and identify other abnormalities in the aorta, mitral valve, and coronary anatomy. Aortic root injection of a contrast medium during cineangiographic studies has been the traditional method of assessing regurgitation, but inconsistencies have been found between visual estimates and the results of quantitative angiocardiographic studies.[156] With the latter, left ventricular stroke volume can be compared to the forward stroke volume measured by Fick or indicator dilution technique to quantitate the regurgitant flow per beat across the aortic valve.[157] A dilated left ventricular chamber may dilute the regurgitant contrast material and render an impression of mild aortic regurgitation, whereas regurgitation of the same volume into a normal-size left ventricular chamber can create an impression of severe aortic regurgitation.

Left ventricular end-diastolic pressure may remain normal in chronic aortic regurgitation due to the increased compliant properties of the volume-overloaded ventricle.[154] As left ventricular end-diastolic pressure becomes elevated with time, compensatory increases in wall thickness will maintain a near normal end-diastolic wall stress or preload (see Chap. 23). The ejection fraction remains an index of mechanical performance but is spuriously preserved in the volume-overloaded condition of aortic regurgitation, since systolic ejection is initiated at a lower left ventricular pressure than normal. End-systolic pressure-volume wall stress indexes reflect the contractile state and may become depressed before the clinical appearance of congestive heart failure.[157a]

Coronary arteriography is indicated in adults over 40 years of age whether or not chest pain is present.[69] Coronary disease can contribute to abnormal left ventricular function and, if severe, should be corrected at the time of valve replacement.

In acute aortic regurgitation, marked elevation of the left ventricular end-diastolic pressure is a major hemodynamic abnormality, since the end-diastolic volume can remain normal or only slightly increased.[135] The diastolic pressure may attain a level that prematurely closes the mitral valve and abnormally elevates left atrial and pulmonary capillary pressures.

Radionuclide Studies

Ventricular function at rest and during exercise can be evaluated with radionuclide angiography.[158–160] Decline of exercise ejection fraction in aortic regurgitation suggests myocardial impairment, whereas preservation of the contractile state is associated with a normal increase in ejection fraction with exercise. Perfusion defects in the myocardium can be identified with thallium scintigraphy and raise the possibility of coronary artery disease.[161,162] Exercise-induced wall motion abnormalities may not be reliable for detection of underlying coronary disease in aortic regurgitation, since such abnormalities can be seen with normal coronary anatomy.[163] Radionuclide exercise testing can be used to detect and follow early deterioration of left ventricular function (see Chap. 134).[164]

Usual Strategy of Workup

A patient initially seen with aortic regurgitation requires the taking of a careful history, a physical examination, and noninvasive studies to develop a base for follow-up, as well as for discerning the etiology. Echocardiography can provide information on the aortic valve, aorta, and left ventricle. Echo-Doppler studies (see Chap. 130) provide similar quantitative information on the amount of regurgitation. An exercise nuclear or echocardiographic study can recognize deterioration in exercise ejection fraction. These measures can be followed at periodic intervals. Significant progression in the left ventricular end-systolic volume (>200 mL) or end-diastolic volume (>300 mL) and the echo-Doppler and color Doppler estimates of regurgitation, and a decline in the exercise ejection fraction at rest (<55 percent) or a progressive decrease in the normal increase during exercise may lead to a recommendation for surgery before severe symptoms develop.

Natural History and Prognosis

Aortic regurgitation is usually well-tolerated for a long period before development of heart failure.[165] Echo-Doppler studies suggest that aortic regurgitation increases in prevalence with advancing age; and there is Doppler echocardiographic evidence of aortic regurgitation without auscultatory confirmation in the vast majority of patients over age 80.[166] Eighty-five to 95 percent of patients with mild-to-moderate regurgitation will survive for 10 years. Once a patient has become symptomatic, there is fairly rapid deterioration. Survival after onset of congestive heart failure is often less than 2 years, whereas patients may survive for 5 years after the onset of angina. Three-fourths of patients with significant aortic regurgitation survive 5 years, and 50 percent have been shown to live for 10 years after diagnosis.[67]

Optimal Time for Valve Replacement

Selecting the optimal time for valve replacement in chronic aortic regurgitation has been an important clinical issue. Obviously, in light of the good long-term prognosis of many patients with severe aortic regurgitation, one would like to postpone aortic valve replacement until it is clearly indicated. Asymptomatic patients with normal left ventricular systolic performance have an excellent prognosis despite considerable cardiac enlargement.[167,167a] For this reason, one should not use the echocardiographic end-systolic dimension as a sole arbitrary criterion to judge that a patient is either an immediate candidate for valve replacement or that valve replacement carried out in a patient with an end-systolic dimension greater than 55 mm will necessarily result in a poor outcome. The presence of significant left ventricular dilatation in the presence of excellent systolic pump function is generally associated with a good outcome. In contrast, once significant left ventricular systolic dysfunction is apparent, the surgical outcome is less satisfactory. Subsequent mortality and morbidity are greater than in those patients in whom left ventricular dysfunction is absent.[168,169] Many such patients will still demonstrate a postoperative improvement in left ventricular systolic function. This is particularly likely in those patients in whom an early postoperative reduction in left ventricular volume is observed.[170] The overwhelming majority of patients whose left ventricular dimensions diminish postoperatively will show evidence of it within 2 weeks.[171] It has been noted that the patients with left ventricular dysfunction who are most likely to improve after surgery are those in whom preoperative left ventricular dysfunction has been of a relatively brief duration.[170,171] This emphasizes the importance of closely following asymptomatic patients either for rapid increases in ventricular size or for the development of significant symptoms. The development of left ventricular dysfunction in the absence of symptoms is relatively uncommon. In a longitudinal study of asymptomatic patients, only 4 out of 104 developed asymptomatic left ventricular dysfunction over a mean follow-up period of 8 years.[172] In general, therefore, the timing of aortic valve replacement may be generally delayed in the asymptomatic patient until the onset of significant symptoms, significant left ventricular dysfunction, or both. When such an onset does occur, aortic valve replacement will generally be associated with an excellent postoperative survival rate with substantial improvement in left ventricular dilatation and left ventricular function and regression of left ventricular hypertrophy. One cannot be as certain regarding timing in asymptomatic patients who demonstrate left ventricular dysfunction only with exercise, as evidenced by a decrease in ejection fraction. If the left ventricle is quite dilated and the end-systolic left ventricular dimension is greater than 55 mm on M-mode echocardiography, surgery should probably be undertaken if other causes are eliminated. If heart size is relatively small, however, close follow-up with serial measurements is appropriate until either progressive enlargement and/or further deterioration in left ventricular systolic pump function is demonstrable. Patients with chronic, severe aortic regurgitation who have marked left ventricular dilatation and an ejection fraction less than about 15 to 20 percent have a high operative mortality rate and a poor recovery of ventricular function postoperatively.

Medical Therapy

Prophylaxis against bacterial endocarditis remains a primary responsibility in the care of the asymptomatic patient with aortic regurgitation. Coverage is indicated not only for dental care, but also for surgical instrumentation of the gastrointestinal or genitourinary tract. (See Chap. 94.) Studies using oral hydralazine have shown that it improves cardiac performance both at rest and during exercise in patients with chronic, severe aortic regurgitation.[173,174] These beneficial responses from short-term hemodynamic studies are supported by the results of a double-blind, placebo-controlled trial of hydralazine in which left ventricular volumes and functions were followed up to 24 months.[175] Significant reductions at the end of 2 years in end-diastolic and end-systolic volume indexes and a significant improvement in ejection fraction were seen among those receiving hydralazine compared to those given placebo. Other studies also suggest that progression of left ventricular dilatation in asymptomatic cases can be delayed with long-term use of hydralazine.[176] Although it has not been demonstrated to date that patients receiving afterload reduction with hydralazine have either reduced mortality or a delay in the time from initial evaluation to aortic valve replacement, it would appear desirable to institute long-term arteriolar vasodilator therapy in patients with chronic, stable aortic regurgitation who are not considered immediate surgical candidates. The choice of vasodilator is uncertain. Although most of the data on long-term benefit have involved the use of hydralazine, nifedipine produced significant reductions in left ventricular volumes and wall stress at the end of 1 year in a randomized trial in 72 asymptomatic patients with chronic severe aortic regurgitation.[177] Beneficial short-term effects have also been demonstrated with prazosin and captopril.[178] When heart failure is present, digitalis and diuretics can be added to the vasodilator being used (see Chap. 26). One must always keep in mind, however, that the primary defect is mechanical and that medical therapy alone cannot modify the impaired or defective valve.

Prior to aortic valve surgery, ventricular function should be stabilized, arrhythmias controlled, and electrolyte abnormalities corrected. Elective dental repair and other minor surgical procedures should be performed prior to cardiac surgery in order to reduce the potential for endocarditis.

Acute aortic regurgitation is often a surgical emergency. Patients who present in acute pulmonary edema, peripheral vascular collapse, or both require aortic valve replacement as soon as it is feasible. In the interim, medical therapy should be started. The patient should be hospitalized on an intensive care ward and a Swan-Ganz catheter should be inserted into the pulmonary circulation (see Chap. 18). Interarterial pressure should be monitored and intravenous sodium nitroprusside begun. Nitroprusside should be titrated with a view toward lowering the pulmonary artery wedge pressure, which will generally be markedly elevated, to under 15 mmHg. If the patient demonstrates significant hypotension, one may have to lessen the nitroprusside infusion in order to maintain a reasonable systemic perfusing pressure. Unfortunately, in the presence of wide-open aortic regurgitation, an intraaortic balloon pump is contraindicated and cannot be used to maintain adequate perfusion even when severe hypotension is present. These measures are utilized only to stabilize the patient while emergency surgery is being arranged. Infective endocarditis is usually the etiology. If that is the case, immediate intensive antibiotic therapy should be instituted (after blood for at least three sets of blood cultures has been drawn), and it should be continued throughout surgery and postoperatively (see Chap. 94). If the patient is free of acute hypotension or pulmonary edema at the onset, one may temporize with medical management while attempting to get the infective process under control. Most of these patients, however, will require valve replacement within days to weeks.

Surgical Therapy

Chronic aortic regurgitation may be well tolerated for several years, as indicated by the natural history of this lesion (reviewed earlier), before causing left ventricular dysfunction and symptoms.[98] Patients with chronic aortic regurgitation may develop left ventricular dysfunction in the absence of any symptoms. Such dysfunction may be irreversible and may compromise both early and late results of valve replacement.[152] It is therefore important that asymptomatic patients be identified before the onset of left ventricular dysfunction. Serial assessment of left ventricular function, both at rest and with exercise, is increasingly important in determining the appropriate time for surgical intervention in asymptomatic patients with chronic aortic regurgitation.

On the other hand, aortic regurgitation from dissection, trauma, or endocarditis is a true cardiac surgical emergency. This wide variation in the presentation of the etiology makes the surgical treatment of aortic regurgitation extremely challenging. The timing of aortic valve surgery for aortic regurgitation is often a difficult clinical decision similar to that for mitral regurgitation and requires serial clinical noninvasive study of the dimensions and function of the left ventricle. It is important that the asymptomatic or mildly symptomatic patients be followed carefully so that aortic valve surgery is performed before there has been irreversible left ventricular dysfunction. Similarly, surgery for acute aortic regurgitation, especially in conjunction with endocarditis, must also be exquisitely timed before irreversible left ventricular dysfunction occurs.

Indications for Operation

As noted above, patients with chronic aortic regurgitation who are functionally compromised and significantly symptomatic on therapy should be operated upon on a relatively urgent basis before there is significant deterioration of left ventricular function. Although it is uncommon, asymptomatic patients with severe chronic aortic regurgitation may have normal physical activity despite increasing left ventricular systolic and diastolic dimensions and overall left ventricular dysfunction.[152,172] Serial echocardiographic indexes of systolic and diastolic function at rest and during exercise aid in timing an aortic valve replacement. Asymptomatic patients who have normal dimensions at exercise and at rest are not considered for operation, but surgery should be considered if they have significantly decreased left ventricular function on stress scintigraphy or echocardiography or develop hypotension or arrhythmia on exercise testing.[179] Patients who have an end-systolic left ventricular diameter greater than 55 mm by echocardiographic study, have worse longevity and left ventricular function than patients operated upon with smaller ventricles.[180] This single measurement must, however, be interpreted in light of all tests of left ventricular function and should not exclude any patient from operative consideration. Other criteria for surgery are discussed above.

In patients who have acute aortic regurgitation, including those with acute bacterial endocarditis or rare cases of traumatic injury to the aortic valve and those who have sustained acute aortic dissection of the ascending aorta, acute left ventricular dysfunction may occur that will often reverse after valve replacement. In patients with endocarditis with concomitant heart failure and sepsis, particularly with nonstreptococcal organisms, the surgical indication is often quite urgent to prevent irreversible ventricular dysfunction and to prevent further damage to the myocardium and cardiac skeleton by the spread of sepsis.[181] Aortic regurgitation from acute ascending aortic dissection is also absolutely an emergency indication for surgery. This indicates proximal compression and distortion of the aortic valve by the dissecting hematoma and requires emergency surgery before the aorta ruptures, severs a coronary artery, or produces pericardial tamponade. Surgical treatment of ascending aortic dissection is the treatment of choice, and aortic regurgitation indicates an even higher degree of urgency. Transesophageal echocardiogram or computerized tomographic scanning may often make aortographic studies unnecessary if the site of the tear can be exactly localized, since the mortality is correlated with the time interval from onset to the time of repair (see also Chap. 123).[182]

Operation

The type of operation and the valve device used depend on the local cardiac pathology, the etiology of the disease, and the age of the patient. In most cases of chronic aortic regurgitation with the disease limited to the valve and where there is no possibility of reconstruction because of calcification and/or distortion of the leaflets, valve replacement is indicated. A mechanical prosthetic valve may be indicated for those who wish to minimize the risk of reoperation, particularly in the younger and middle-aged groups, while a homograft valve is also an excellent substitute for the younger patient who wishes a relatively morbidity-free existence.[183] Bioprosthetic valves (porcine and pericardial) are used very successfully in the elderly age group, who may not outlive their valves and in whom anticoagulation is difficult.[184,185]

Reparative procedures for valvar aortic regurgitation are also possible when calcium has not been deposited on the valve. In cases of endocarditis when there is an isolated perforation of a leaflet, a pericardial patch may be used to close the hole. Debridement of mild calcification and incision of commissures for rheumatic valvulitis will allow better coaptation of the leaflets. Recently, techniques to primarily reconstruct the valve leaflets in aortic regurgitation, either by pericardial leaflet advancement[186] or by resection and suturing of the valve leaflets, have been advocated.[187] Considerably more long-term follow-up will be necessary to validate these techniques, but early results are encouraging.

In cases of acute aortic dissection producing aortic regurgitation because of distortion of the ascending aorta and aortic root with normal valve leaflets, simple resuspension of leaflets may restore valvular competence (see Chap. 123).[188] Patients with annuloaortic ectasia usually require aortic valve replacement, and in patients with Marfan's syndrome, complete replacement of the aortic root with a combined low-profile prosthetic valve synthetic graft conduit or an intact homograft root including

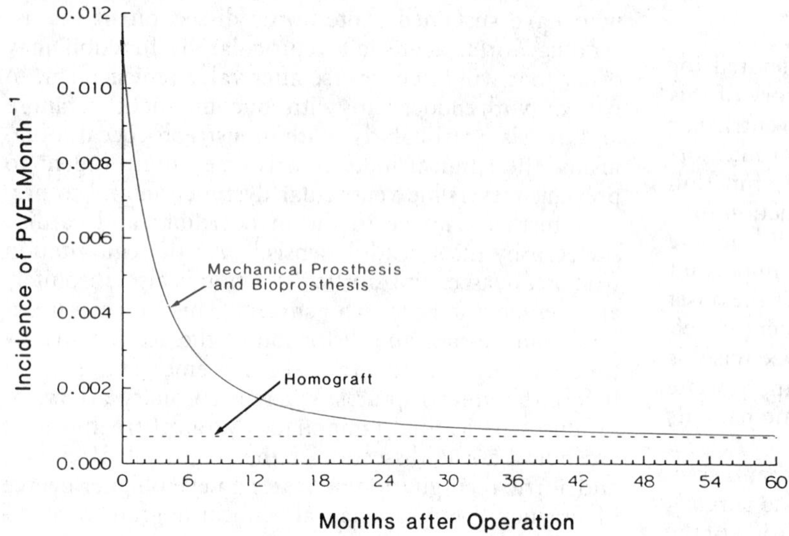

FIGURE 79-14 Hazard function analysis of prosthetic valve endocarditis (PVE). The patients are stratified into those receiving homografts versus those receiving mechanical prostheses and bioprostheses.[196] *(Reproduced with permission from the publisher and author.)*

all of the aortic sinus tissue is imperative to prevent recurrence of the dissection. In order to exclude all the diseased aortic sinus tissue in this operation, the coronary ostia are attached to the Dacron ascending aorta by a button incorporated into the aortic wall by the Bentall technique[189] or by using a Dacron tube to anastomose to both coronary arteries and then to the body of the ascending aortic graft.[190]

The homograft is particularly valuable for the replacement of an infected aortic valve because there is no prosthetic material in an active or potentially septic area. Endocarditis surgery may be extremely difficult because of annular abscesses, perforations of the ventricular septum, and destruction of the cardiac exoskeleton. The surgical procedure must eradicate all sepsis, separately and completely close and repair all defects, and adequately fixate whatever type of valve is inserted.[191] Violation of these three precepts will result in recurrent aortic regurgitation requiring reoperation. The use of total biologic tissue replacement, even with contiguous mitral endocarditis, has yielded excellent results in this setting.[192]

Postoperative Care

Immediate postoperative management is similar to that described for aortic stenosis. Anticoagulation is determined by the patient's valve type and the presence of chronic atrial fibrillation. The newest models of prosthetic valves, the low-profile disc or bileaflet valves, all require warfarin anticoagulation. (See above.) Prophylactic antibiotics are indicated for procedures associated with bacteremia, especially dental work (see also Chap. 94). If an ascending graft has been placed, patients should be followed with periodic noninvasive echocardiographic studies indefinitely to assess valve function and root abnormalities. Arrhythmias should be diagnosed and appropriately treated (see Chap. 36). The extent of ventricular remodeling can also be evaluated by echocardiographic and clinical examination. Patients should be immunized against pneumococcal pneumonia unless contraindicated and be immunized against influenza each year.

Operative Results

The results of surgery for aortic regurgitation have changed dramatically in the past several years. Earlier reports of patients with severe aortic regurgitation and left ventricular dysfunction undergoing aortic valve replacement documented high operative mortality rates and poor long-term results.[193] Currently, as a result of improved myocardial protection, especially retrograde cardioplegia, patients with aortic regurgitation, regardless of the degree of left ventricular dysfunction, have a low risk for operation.[194,195] Operative risk in the nondysfunctional ventricle is about 1 percent but increases with age and concomitant coronary disease, as well as in a severely compromised ventricle. Operative mortality rates for endocarditis of the aortic valve may vary from 1 to 15 percent[190] depending on the extent of annular destruction and acuity of regurgitation. The homograft valve is especially resistent to postoperative infection when used for endocarditis (Fig. 79-14).[196] Repair of ascending aortic dissection has a risk of about 5 percent in patients operated upon prior to sustaining a major aortic complication such as perforation, tamponade, or stroke.[197]

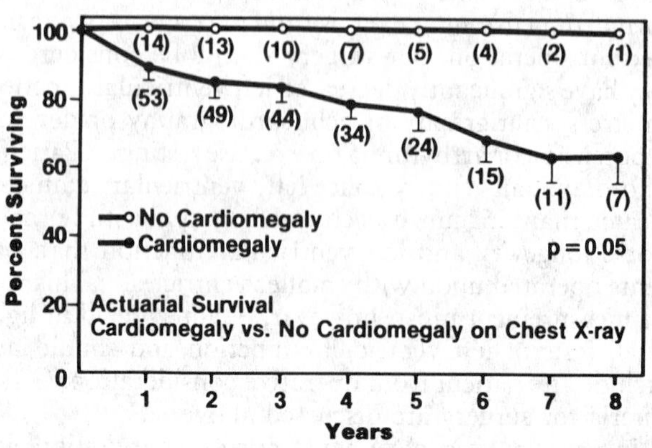

FIGURE 79-15 Aortic valve replacement for aortic regurgitation. Effect of cardiomegaly on long-term survival.

Late Results

Long-term results of patients who have valve replacement for chronic aortic regurgitation are negatively affected by preoperative left ventricular dysfunction and cardiomegaly, presumably from chronic heart failure, fatal arrhythmias, or thromboemboli (Fig. 79-15). Patients operated on with preoperative left ventricular end-systolic dimensions greater than 55 mm have lower long-term survival rates and increased morbidity.[198] Remodeling of the left ventricle will take place up to 3 years after valve replacement, and improvement is related to the extent of preoperative left ventricular dysfunction.[198-200]

REFERENCES

1. Mönckeberg JG: Der normale histologische Bau und die sklerose der Aorenklappen. *Virchows Arch (Pathol Anat)* 1904; 176:472–514.
2. Karsner HT, Koletsky S: *Calcific Disease of Aortic Valves.* Philadelphia, JB Lippincott, 1947.
3. Campbell M, Kauntze R: Congenital aortic valvular stenosis. *Br Heart J* 1953; 15:179–194.
4. Roberts WC: The congenitally bicuspid aortic valve stenosis. *Am J Cardiol* 1970; 26:72–93.
5. Glancy DL, Epstein SE: Differential diagnosis of type and severity of obstruction to left ventricular outflow. *Prog Cardiovasc Dis* 1971; 14:153–191.
6. Roberts WC: The structure of the aortic valve in clinically isolated aortic stenosis: An autopsy study of 162 patients over 15 years of age. *Circulation* 1970; 42:91–97.
7. Roberts WC, Perloff JK, Costantino T: Severe valvular aortic stenosis in patients over 65 years of age: A clinicopathologic study. *Am J Cardiol* 1971; 27:497–506.
8. Roberts WC: Anatomically isolated aortic valvular disease: The case against its being of rheumatic etiology. *Am J Med* 1970; 49:151–159.
9. Pomerance A: Pathogenesis of aortic stenosis and its relation to age. *Br Heart J* 1972; 34:569–574.
10. Waller BF, Dorros G, Lewin RF, King JF, McKay C, Van Tassel JW: Catheter balloon valvuloplasty of stenotic aortic valves. Part II: Balloon valvuloplasty during life subsequent tissue examination. *Clin Cardiol* 1991; 14:924–930.
11. Edwards JE: Pathology of acquired valvular disease of the heart. *Semin Roentgenol* 1979; 14:96–115.
12. Edwards JE: On the etiology of calcific aortic stenosis. *Circulation* 1962; 26:817–818.
13. Promerance A: Cardiac pathology and systolic murmurs in the elderly. *Br Heart J* 1968; 30:687–689.
14. Levy MJ, Edwards JE: Anatomy of mitral insufficiency. *Prog Cardiovasc Dis* 1962; 5:119–144.
15. Moller JH, Nakib A, Edwards JE: Infarction of papillary muscles and mitral insufficiency associated with congenital aortic stenosis. *Circulation* 1966; 34:87–91.
16. Nakib A, Lillehei CE, Edwards JE: The degree of coronary atherosclerosis in aortic valvular disease. *Arch Pathol* 1965; 80:517–520.
17. Kennedy JW, Twiss RD, Blackmon JR, Dodge HT: Quantitative angiocardiography: III. Relationships of left ventricular pressure, volume and mass in aortic valve disease. *Circulation* 1968; 38:838–845.
18. Hood WP Jr, Rackley CE, Rolett EL: Wall stress in the normal and hypertrophied human left ventricle. *Am J Cardiol* 1968; 22:550–558.
19. Rackley CE, Hood WP Jr: Aortic valve disease. In: Levin HJ (ed): *Clinical Cardiovascular Physiology.* New York, Grune & Stratton, 1976:493–521.
20. Stott DK, Marpole DG, Bristow JD, Kloster FE, Griswold HE: The role of left atrial transport in aortic and mitral stenosis. *Circulation* 1970; 41:1031–1041.
21. Rackley CE, Hood WP Jr, Rolett EL, Young DT: Left ventricular end-diastolic pressure in chronic heart disease. *Am J Med* 1970; 48:310–319.
22. Dodge HT, Baxley WA: Left ventricular volume and mass and their significance in heart disease. *Am J Cardiol* 1969; 23:528–534.
23. Ross J Jr, Braunwald E: Aortic Stenosis. *Circulation* 1968; 38(suppl 5):61–67.
24. Wood P: Aortic stenosis. *Am J Cardiol* 1958; 1:553–571.
25. Rotman M, Morris JJ, Behar VS, Peter RH, Kong Y: Aortic valvular disease: Comparison of types and their medical and surgical management. *Am J Med* 1971; 51:241–257.
26. Kumpe CW, Bean WB: Aortic stenosis: Study of the clinical and pathological aspects of 107 proved cases. *Medicine (Baltimore)* 1948; 27:139–168.
27. Moraski RE, Russell RO Jr, Mantle JA, Rackley CE: Aortic stenosis, angina pectoris, coronary artery disease. *Cathet Cardiovasc Diagn* 1976; 2:157–164.
28. Baxley WA, Dodge HT, Rackley CE, Sandler H, Pugh D: Left ventricular mechanical efficiency in man with heart disease. *Circulation* 1977; 55:564–568.
29. Hood WP Jr, Thompson WJ, Rackley CE, Rolett EL: Comparison of calculations of left ventricular wall stress in man from thin-walled and thick-walled ellipsoidal models. *Circ Res* 1969; 24:575–582.
30. Holley KE, Bahn RC, McGoon DC, Mankin HT: Spontaneous calcific embolization associated with calcific aortic stenosis. *Circulation* 1963; 27:197–202.
31. Flamm MD, Braiff BA, Kimball R, Hancock EW: Mechanism of effort syncope in aortic stenosis (abstract). *Circulation* 1967; 36(suppl 2):II–109.
32. Schwartz LS, Goldfischer J, Sprague GJ, Schwartz SP: Syncope and sudden death in aortic stenosis. *Am J Cardiol* 1969; 23:647–658.
33. Baker C, Somerville J: Clinical features and surgical treatment of fifty patients with severe aortic stenosis. *Guys Hosp Rep* 1959; 108:101–125.
34. Frank S, Johnson A, Ross J Jr: Natural history of valvular aortic stenosis. *Br Heart J* 1973; 35:41–46.
35. Brockmeier LB, Adolph RJ, Gustin BW, Holmes JC, Sacks, JG: Calcium emboli to the retinal artery in calcific aortic stenosis. *Am Heart J* 1981; 101:32–37.
36. Andersen JA, Hansen BF, Lyngborg K: Isolated valvular aortic stenosis. *Acta Med Scand* 1975; 197:61–64.
37. Hancock EW: The ejection sound in aortic stenosis. *Am J Med* 1966; 40:569–577.
38. Crawley IS, Morris DC, Silverman BD: Valvular heart disease. In: Hurst JW, Logue RB, Schlant RC, Wenger NK (eds): *The Heart,* 4th ed. New York, McGraw-Hill, 1978:922–1080.
39. Davison ET, Friedman SA: Significance of systolic murmurs in the aged. *N Engl J Med* 1968; 279:225–230.
40. Myler RK, Sanders CA: Aortic valve disease and atrial fibrillation: Report of 122 patients with electrographic, radiographic and hemodynamic observations. *Arch Intern Med* 1968; 121:530–533.
41. Klatte EC, Tampas JP, Campbell JA, Lurie PR: The roentgenographic manifestations of aortic stenosis and aortic valvular insufficiency. *Am J Roentgenol Radium Ther Nucl Med* 1962; 88:57–69.
42. Feigenbaum H: *Echocardiography.* Philadelphia, Lea & Febiger, 1976.
43. Johnson ML, Kisslo J, Habersberger PG, Wallace AG: The echocardiographic evaluation of aortic valvular disease (abstract). *Circulation* 1973; 48(suppl 4):IV–46.
44. Radford DJ, Bloom KR, Izukawa T, Moes CA, Rowe RD: Echocardiographic assessment of biscuspid aortic valves: Angiographic and pathological correlates. *Circulation* 1976; 53:80–85.
45. Godley RW, Green D, Dillon JC, Rogers EW, Feigenbaum H, Weyman AE: Reliability of two-dimensional echocardiography in assessing the severity of valvular aortic stenosis. *Chest* 1981; 79:657–662.
46. Reichek N, Devereux RB: Reliable estimation of peak left ventricular systolic pressure by M-mode echographic-determined end-diastolic relative wall-thickness: Identification of severe aortic stenosis in adult patients. *Am Heart J* 1982; 103:202–203.

47. Teien D, Eriksson P: Quantification of transvalvular pressure differences in aortic stenosis by Doppler ultrasound. *Int J Cardiol* 1985; 7:121–128.
48. Teirstein P, Yeager M, Yock PG, Popp RL: Doppler echocardiographic measurement of aortic valve area in aortic stenosis: A noninvasive application of the Gorlin formula. *J Am Coll Cardiol* 1986; 8:1059–1065.
49. Yeager M, Yock PG, Popp RL: Comparison of Doppler-derived pressure gradient to that determined at cardiac catheterization in adults with aortic valve stenosis: Implication for management. *Am J Cardiol* 1986; 57:644–648.
50. Richards KL, Cannon SR, Miller JF, Crawford MH: Calculation of aortic valve area by Doppler echocardiography: A direct application of the continuity equation. *Circulation* 1986; 73:964–969.
51. Neumann A, Lang RM, Borow KM: Doppler echo in aortic stenosis. *Cardiology* 1988; 5:120–125.
52. Hancock EW, Fleming PR: Aortic stenosis. *Q J Med* 1960; 29:209–234.
53. Braunwald E, Goldblatt A, Aygen MM, Rockoff SD, Morrow AG: Congenital aortic stenosis: I. Clinical and hemodynamic findings in 100 patients; Morrow AG, Goldblatt A, Braunwald E: Congenital aortic stenosis: II. Surgical treatment and the results of operation. *Circulation* 1963; 27:426–462.
54. Rackley CE: Quantitative evaluation of left ventricular function by radiographic technique. *Circulation* 1976; 54:862–879.
55. Borer JS, Bacharach SL, Green MV, Kent KM, Rosing DR, Seides SF et al: Left ventricular function in aortic stenosis: Response to exercise and effects of operation (abstract). *Am J Cardiol* 1978; 41:382.
56. Takeda J, Warren R, Holzman D: Prognosis of aortic stenosis. *Arch Surg* 1963; 87:931–936.
57. Dexter L: Evaluation of the results of cardiac surgery. In: Jones AM (ed): *Modern Trends in Cardiology* vol 2. New York, Appleton-Century-Crofts, 1969: 311–333.
58. Wagner S, Selzer A: Patterns of progression of aortic stenosis: A longitudinal hemodynamic study. *Circulation* 1982; 65:709–712.
59. Selzer A: Changing aspects of the natural history of valvular aortic stenosis. *N Engl J Med* 1987; 317:91–98.
60. Kennedy KD, Nishimura RA, Holmes DR Jr, Bailey KR: Natural history of moderate aortic stenosis. *J Am Coll Cardiol* 1991; 17:313–319.
61. Lewin RF, Dorros G, King JF, Mathiak L: Percutaneous transluminal aortic valvuloplasty: Acute outcome and follow-up of 125 patients. *J Am Coll Cardiol* 1989; 14:1210–1217.
62. Dorros G, Lewin RF, Stertzer SH, King JF, Waller BF, Myler RK, et al: Percutaneous transluminal aortic valvuloplasty—the acute outcome and follow-up of 149 patients who underwent the double balloon technique. *Eur Heart J* 1990; 11:429–440.
63. Acar J, Vahanian A, Slama M, Cormier B, Michel PL, Luxereau P, et al: Treatment of calcified aortic stenosis: Surgery or percutaneous transluminal aortic valvuloplasty? *Eur Heart J* 1988; 9:163–168.
64. Safian RD, Kuntz RE, Berman AD: Aortic valvuloplasty. *Cardiol Clin* 1991; 9:289–299.
65. Litvack F, Jakubowski AT, Buchbinder NA, Eigler N: Lack of sustained clinical improvement in an elderly population after percutaneous aortic valvuloplasty. *Am J Cardiol* 1988; 62:270–275.
66. Grollier G, Commeau P, Sesboüé B, Huret B, Potier JC, Foucault JP: Short-term clinical and haemodynamic assessment of balloon aortic valvuloplasty in 30 elderly patients. Discrepancy between immediate and eighth-day haemodynamic values. *Eur Heart J* 1988; 9:155–162.
67. Rapaport E: Natural history of aortic and mitral valve disease. *Am J Cardiol* 1975; 35:221–227.
68. Gohlke-Bärwolf C, Peters K, Petersen J, Samek L, Eschenbruch E, Birnbaum D, et al: Influence of aortic valve replacement on sudden death in patients with pure aortic stenosis. *Eur Heart J* 1988; 9(Suppl E), 139–141.
69. Ross J Jr, Brandenburg RO, Dinsmore RE, Friesinger GC II, Hultgren HH, Pepine CJ, et al: Guidelines for coronary angiography. A report of the American College of Cardiology/American Heart Association Task Force on Assessment of Diagnostic and Therapeutic Cardiovascular Procedures (Subcommittee on Coronary Angiography). *J Am Coll Cardiol* 1987; 10:935–950.
70. Carabello BA, Green LH, Grossman W, Cohn LH, Koster JK, Collins JJ Jr: Hemodynamic determinants of prognosis of aortic valve replacement in critical aortic stenosis and advanced congestive heart failure. *Circulation* 1980; 62:42–48.
71. Cohn LH: Valvular surgery. *Curr Opinion Cardiol* 1991; 6:235–245.
72. Bernard Y, Etievent J, Mourand J-L, Anguenot T, Schiele F, Guseibat M, Bassand J-P: Long term results of percutaneous aortic valvuloplasty compared with aortic valve replacement in patients more than 75 years old. *J Am Coll Cardiol* 1992; 20:796–801.
73. Fremes SE, Goldman BS, Ivanov J, Weisel RD, David TE, Salerno T, et al: Valvular surgery in the elderly. *Circulation* 1990; 80(suppl I):I-77–I-90.
74. Galloway AC, Colvin SB, Grossi EA, Baumann FG, Sabban YP, Esposito R, et al: Ten year experience with aortic valve replacement in 482 patients 70 years of age or older: operative risk and long term results. *Ann Thorac Surg* 1990; 49:84–93.
75. Duran C, Kumar N, Gometza B, Halees ZAL: Indications and limitations of aortic valve reconstruction. *Ann Thorac Surg* 1991; 52:447–454.
76. King RM, Pluth JR, Giuliani ER, Piehler JM: Mechanical decalcification of the aortic valve. *Ann Thorac Surg* 1986; 42:269–272.
77. McBirde LR, Naunheim KS, Fiore AC, Harris HH, Willman VL, Kaiser GC et al: Aortic valve decalcification. *J Thorac Cardiovasc Surg* 1990; 100:36–43.
78. Ross DN: Homograft replacement of the aortic valve. *Lancet* 1962; 2:487–490.
79. Barratt-Boyes BG, Roche MB, Subramanyan R, Pemberton JR, Whitlock RML: Long term followup of patients with the antibiotic-sterilized aortic homograft valve inserted freehand in the aortic position. *Circulation* 1987; 75:768–777.
80. O'Brien MF, Stafford EG, Gardner MAH, Pohlner PG, McGiffin DC: A comparison of aortic valve replacement with viable cryopreserved and fresh allograft valves, with a note on chromosomal studies. *J Thorac Cardiovasc Surg* 1987; 94:812–823.
81. Ross D, Jackson M, Davies J: Pulmonary autograft aortic valve replacement: Long term results. *J Cardiovasc Surg* 1991; 6(suppl 4):529–533.
82. Konno S, Imai Y, Lida Y, Nakajima M, Tatsuno K: A new method for prosthetic valve replacement in congenital aortic stenosis associated with hypoplasia of the aortic valve ring. *J Thorac Cardiovasc Surg* 1975; 70:909–916.
83. Lindblom D, Lindblom U, Qvist J, Lundstrom H: Long term relative survival rates after heart valve replacement. *J Am Coll Cardiol* 1990; 15:566–573.
84. Mullany CJ, Elveback LR, Frye RL, Pluth JR, Edwards WD, Orszulak TA, et al: Coronary artery disease and its management: Influence on survival in patients undergoing aortic valve replacement. *J Am Coll Cardiol* 1987; 10:66–72.
85. Aranki SF, Rizzo RJ, Couper GS, Adams DH, Collins JJ Jr, Gildea JS: Aortic valve replacement in the elderly: Effect of gender and coronary artery disease on operative mortality. *Circulation* (submitted) 1992.
86. Culliford AT, Galloway AC, Colvin SB, Grossi EA, Baumann G, Esposito R, et al: Aortic valve replacement for aortic stenosis in persons ages 80 years and over. *Am J Cardiol* 1991; 67:1256–1260.
87. Cohn LH, Allred EN, DiSesa VJ, Sawtelle K, Shemin RJ, Collins JJ Jr: Early and late risk of aortic valve replacement: A 12-year concomitant comparison of the porcine bioprosthetic and tilting disc prosthetic aortic valves. *J Thorac Cardiovasc Surg* 1984; 88:695–705.
88. Nair CK, Mohiuddin SM, Hilleman DE, Schultz R, Bailey RT, Cook CT, et al: Ten year results with the St. Jude medical prosthesis. *Am J Cardiol* 1990; 65:217–225.
89. Nitter-Hauge S, Abdelnoor M: Ten year experience with the Medtronic Hall valvular prosthesis. A study of 1104 patients. *Circulation* 1989; 8(suppl I):I-43–48.
90. Jones EL, Weintraub WS, Craver JM, Guyton RA, Cohen CL, Corrigan VE, et al: Ten year experience with porcine bioprosthetic valve: interrelationship of valve survival and patients survival in 1050 valve replacements. *Ann Thorac Surg* 1990; 49:370–384.
91. Borkon AM, Soule LM, Baughman KL, Aoun H, Baumgartner WA, Gardner TJ, et al: Comparative analysis of mechanical and bioprosthetic valves after aortic valve replacement. *J Thorac Cardiovasc Surg* 1987; 94:20–33.
92. Michel P-L, Mandagout O, Vahanian A, Cormier B, Iung B,

Luxereau P: Ventricular arrhythmias in aortic valve disease before and after surgery. *J Heart Valve Dis* 1992; 1:72–79.
93. Grunkemeier GL, Rahimtoola SH: Artificial heart valves. *Annu Rev Med* 1990; 41:251–263.
94. DiSesa VJ, Collins JJ Jr, Cohn LH: Hematologic complications with the St. Jude valve and reduced dose coumadin. *Ann Thorac Surg* 1989; 48:280–283.
95. Stein PD, Alpert JS, Copeland J, Dalen JE, Goldman S, Turpie AGG: Antithrombotic therapy in patients with mechanical and biological prosthetic heart valves. *Chest* 1992; 102(suppl.):445S–455S.
96. Cohn LH, Collins JJ Jr, DiSesa VJ, Couper GS, Peigh PS, Kowalker W, Allred E: Fifteen year experience with 1678 Hancock porcine bioprosthetic heart valve replacements. *Ann Surgery* 1989; 210:435–443.
97. Larrea JL, Nunez L, Reque JA, Aguado MG, Matarros R, Minguez JA: Pregnancy and mechanical valve prostheses: A high-risk situation for the mother and the fetus. *Ann Thorac Surg* 1983; 36:459–463.
98. Segal J, Harvey WP, Hufnagel CL: A clinical study of one hundred cases of severe aortic insufficiency. *Am J Med* 1956; 21:200–210.
99. Stapleton JF, Harvey WP: A clinical analysis of aortic incompetence. *Postgrad Med* 1969; 46:156–165.
100. Enghoff E: Aortic incompetence. Clinical, haemodynamic and angiocardiographic evaluation. *Acta Med Scand* 1972; 193(suppl 538):3–143.
101. Read RC, Thal AP, Wendt VE: Symptomatic valvular myxomatous transformation (the floppy valve syndrome): A possible forme fruste of the Marfan syndrome. *Circulation* 1965; 32:897–910.
102. Roberts WC, Hollingsworth JF, Bulkley BH, Jaffe RB, Epstein SE, Stinson EB: Combined mitral and aortic regurgitation in ankylosing spondylitis: Angiographic and anatomic features. *Am J Med* 1974; 56:237–243.
103. Bulkley BH, Roberts WC: Ankylosing spondylitis and aortic regurgitation: Description of the characteristic cardiovascular lesion from study of eight necropsy patients. *Circulation* 1973; 48:1014–1027.
104. Paulus HE, Pearson CM, Pitts W Jr: Aortic insufficiency in five patients with Reiter's syndrome: A detailed clinical and pathologic study. *Am J Med* 1972; 53:464–472.
105. Roberts WC, Kehoe JA, Carpenter DF, Golden A: Cardiovascular valvular lesions in rheumatoid arthritis. *Arch Intern Med* 1968; 122:141–146.
106. Sakakibara S, Konno S: Congenital aneurysm of the sinus of Valsalva anatomy and classification. *Am Heart J* 1962; 63:405–424.
107. Puchner TC, Huston JH, Hellmuth GA: Aortic valve insufficiency in arterial hypertension. *Am J Cardiol* 1960; 5:758–760.
108. Karp RB, Carlson DE: *Dissection of Aorta.* Philadelphia, FA Davis, Cardiovascular Clinics, 1981:209–219.
109. Wilcox BR, Proctor HJ, Rackley CE, Peters RM: Early surgical treatment of valvular endocarditis. *JAMA* 1967; 200:820–827.
110. Oh WMC, Taylor TR, Olsen EGJ: Aortic regurgitation in systemic lupus erythematosus requiring aortic valve replacement. *Br Heart J* 1974; 36:413–416.
111. Roberts WC, Hollingsworth JF, Bulkley BH, Golden A: Combined mitral and aortic regurgitation in ankylosing spondylitis: Angiographic and anatomic features. *Am J Med* 1974; 56:237–243.
112. Wang K, Gobel F, Gleason DF, Edwards JE: Complete heart block complicating bacterial endocarditis. *Circulation* 1972; 46:939–947.
113. Spurny OM, Hara M: Rupture of the aortic valve due to strain. *Am J Cardiol* 1961; 8:125–129.
114. Symbas PN, Walter PF, Hurst JW, Schlant RC: Fenestration of aortic cusps causing aortic regurgitation. *J Thorac Cardiovasc Dis* 1969; 57:464–470.
115. Carter JB, Sethi S, Lee GB, Edwards JE: Prolapse of semilunar cusps as causes of aortic insufficiency. *Circulation* 1971; 43:922–932.
116. Tatsuno K, Konno S, Sakakibara S: Ventricular septal defect with aortic insufficiency. *Am Heart J* 1973; 85:13–21.
117. Heggtveit HA: Syphilitic aortitis. A clinicopathologic autopsy study of 100 cases, 1950 to 1960. *Circulation* 1964; 29:346–355.
118. Eversmeyer WH, Rosenstock D, Biundo JJ Jr: Aortic insufficiency with mild ankylosing spondylitis in black men. *JAMA* 1978; 240:2652–2653.
119. Murray CA, Edwards JE: Spontaneous laceration of ascending aorta. *Circulation* 1973; 47:848–858.
120. Edwards JE: Lesions causing or simulating aortic insufficiency. *Cardiovasc Clin* 1973; 5:127–148.
121. Brawley RK, Morrow AG: Direct determination of aortic blood flow in patients with aortic regurgitation: Effects of alterations in afterload, and Isoproterenol. *Circulation* 1967; 35:32–45.
122. Judge TP, Kennedy JW, Bennett LJ, Wills RE, Murray JA, Blackman JR: Quantitative hemodynamic effects of heart rate in aortic regurgitation. *Circulation* 1971; 44:355–372.
123. Morrow AG, Brawley RK, Braunwald E: Effects of aortic regurgitation on left ventricular performance: Direct determination of aortic blood flow before and after valve replacement. *Circulation* 1965; 31(suppl 1):80–95.
124. Linsbach AJ: Heart failure from the point of view of quantitative anatomy. *Am J Cardiol* 1960; 5:370–382.
125. Ross J Jr: Afterload mismatch and preload reserve: A conceptual framework for the analysis of ventricular function. *Prog Cardiovasc Dis* 1976; 18:255–264.
126. Dodge HT, Kennedy JW, Petersen J: Quantitative angiographic methods in the evaluation of valvular heart disease. *Prog Cardiovasc Dis* 1973; 16:1–23.
127. Basta LL, Raines D, Najjar S, Kioschos JM: Clinical, hemodynamic, and coronary angiographic correlates of angina pectoris in patients with severe aortic valve disease. *Br Heart J* 1975; 37:150–157.
128. Harvey WP, Segal JP, Hufnagel CA: Unusual clinical features associated with severe aortic insufficiency. *Ann Intern Med* 1957; 47:27–38.
129. Cohn LH, Mason DT, Ross J Jr, Morrow AG, Braunwald E: Preoperative assessment of aortic regurgitation in patients with mitral valve disease. *Am J Cardiol* 1967; 19:177–182.
130. Conn RD, Cole JS: The cardiac apex impulse: Clinical and angiographic correlations. *Ann Intern Med* 1971; 75:185–191.
131. Groom D, Boone JA: The dove-coo murmur and murmurs heard at a distance from the chest wall. *Ann Intern Med* 1955; 42:1214–1226.
132. Porter CM, Baxley WA, Eddleman EE Jr, Frimer M, Rackley CE: Left ventricular dimensions and dynamics of filling in patients with gallop heart sounds. *Am J Med* 1971; 50:721–727.
133. Abdulla AM, Frank MJ, Erdin RA, Canedo MI: Clinical significance and hemodynamic correlates of the third heart sound gallop in aortic regurgitation: A guide to optimal timing of cardiac catheterization. *Circulation* 1981; 64:464–471.
134. Fortuin NJ, Craige E: On the mechanism of the Austin Flint murmur. *Circulation* 1972; 45:558–570.
135. Wigle ED, Labross CJ: Sudden, severe aortic insufficiency. *Circulation* 1965; 32:708–720.
136. Herbert WA: Prolonged atrioventricular conduction and aortic insufficiency. *Thorax* 1970; 25:577–580.
137. Selzer A, Naruse DY, York E, Kahn KA, Matthews HB: Electrocardiographic findings in concentric and eccentric left ventricular hypertrophy. *Am Heart J* 1962; 63:320–328.
138. Winsberg F, Gabor GE, Hernberg JG, Weiss B: Fluttering of the mitral valve in aortic insufficiency. *Circulation* 1970; 41:225–231.
139. Pridie RB, Benhan MB, Oakley CM: Echocardiography of the mitral valve in aortic valve disease. *Br Heart J* 1971; 33:296–304.
140. Wray TM: The variable echocardiographic features in aortic valve endocarditis. *Circulation* 1975; 52:658–663.
141. Stewart JA, Silimperi D, Harris P, Wise NK, Fraker TD Jr, Kisslo JA: Echocardiographic documentation of vegetative lesions in infective endocarditis: Clinical implications. *Circulation* 1980; 61:374–380.
142. Gramiak R, Shah PM: Echocardiography of the normal and diseased aortic valve. *Radiology* 1970; 96:1–8.
143. Pombo JF, Troy BL, Russell RO Jr: Left ventricular volumes and ejection fraction of echocardiography. *Circulation* 1971; 43:480–490.
144. Troy BL, Pombo J, Rackley CE: Measurement of left ventricular wall thickness and mass by echocardiography. *Circulation* 1972; 45:602–611.
145. Ratshin RA, Rackley CE, Russell RO Jr: Determination of left ventricular preload and afterload using quantitative echocardiog-

raphy in man: Calibration of the method. *Circ Res* 1974; 34:711–718.

146. Diebold B, Peronneau P, Blanchard D, Colonna G, Guermonprez JL, Forman J, et al: Noninvasive quantification of aortic regurgitation by Doppler echocardiography. *Br Heart J* 1983; 49:167–173.
147. Veyrat C, Lessana H, Abitbo G, Ameur A, Benaim R, Kalmanson D: New indexes for assessing aortic regurgitation with two-dimensional Doppler echocardiographic measurement of the regurgitant aortic valvular area. *Circulation* 1983; 68:998–1005.
148. Grayburn PA, Smith MD, Handshoe R, Friedman BJ, DeMaria AN: Detection of aortic insufficiency by standard echocardiography, pulsed Doppler echocardiography, and auscultation: A comparison of accuracies. *Ann Intern Med* 1986; 104:599–605.
149. Hoffmann AP, Pfisterer M, Stulz P, Schmitt HE, Burkhart F, Burkhart D: Noninvasive grading of aortic regurgitation by Doppler ultrasonography. *Br. Heart J* 1986; 55:283–285.
150. Perry GJ, Helmcke F, Nanda NC, Byard C, Soto B: Evaluation of aortic insufficiency by Doppler color flow mapping. *J Am Coll Cardiol* 1987; 9:952–959.
151. Whipple RL, Morris DC, Felner JM, Merrill AJ Jr, Miller JI: Echocardiographic manifestations of the flail aortic valve leaflet syndrome. *J Clin Ultrasound* 1977; 5:417–422.
152. Henry WL, Bonow RO, Borer JS, Ware JH, Kent KM, Redwood DR, et al: Observations on the optimum time for operative intervention for aortic regurgitation: I. Evaluation of the results of aortic valve replacement in symptomatic patients. *Circulation* 1980; 61:471–483.
153. Nishimura RA, McGoon MD, Schaff HV, Giuliani ER: Chronic aortic regurgitation: Indications for operation—1988. *Mayo Clin Proc* 1988; 63:270–280.
154. Daniel WG, Hood WP Jr, Siart A, Hausmann D, Nellessen U, Oelert H, et al: Chronic aortic regurgitation: Reassessment of the prognostic value of preoperative left ventricular end-systolic dimension and fractional shortening. *Circulation* 1985; 71:669–680.

154a Rackley CE, Dalldorf FG, Hood WP Jr, Wilcox BR: Sarcomere length and left ventricular function in chronic heart disease. *Am J Med Sci* 1970; 259:90–96.

155. Fioretti P, Roelandt J, Sclavo M, Domenicucci S, Haalaebos M, Bos E, et al: Postoperative regression of left ventricular dimensions in aortic insufficiency: A long-term echocardiographic study. *J Am Coll Cardiol* 1985; 5:856–861.
156. Hunt D, Baxley WA, Kennedy JW, Judge TP, Williams JE, Dodge HT: Quantitative evaluation of cineaortography in the assessment of aortic regurgitation. *Am J Cardiol* 1973; 31:696–703.
157. Sandler H, Dodge HT, Hay RE, Rackley CE: Quantitation of valvular insufficiency in man by angiocardiography. *Am Heart J* 1963; 65:501–513.

157a Osbakken M, Bove AA, Spann JF: Left ventricular function in chronic aortic regurgitation with reference to end-systolic pressure, volume and stress relations. *Am J Cardiol* 1981; 47:193–198.

158. Borer JS, Bacharach SL, Green MV: Exercise-induced left ventricular dysfunction in symptomatic and asymptomatic patients with aortic regurgitation: Assessment with radionuclide cineangiography. *Am J Cardiol* 1978; 42:351–357.
159. Borer JS, Bacharach SL, Green MV: Radionuclide cineangiography at rest and during exercise in the evaluation of patients with heart disease. *Cardiovasc Rev Rep* 1980; 1(3):31ff.
160. Baxter RH, Becker LC, Alderson PO, Rigo P, Wagner HN Jr, Weisfeldt ML: Quantification of aortic valvular regurgitation in dogs by nuclear imaging. *Circulation* 1980; 61:404–410.
161. Ritchie JL, Zaret BL, Strauss HW, Pitt B, Berman DS, Schelbert HR, et al: Myocardial infarction. *Am J Cardiol* 1978; 42:345–350.
162. Turner JD, Schwartz KM, Logic JR, Sheffield LT, Kansal S, Roitman DI, et al: Detection of residual jeopardized myocardium three weeks after myocardial infarction by exercise testing with thallium-201 myocardial scintiography. *Circulation* 1980; 61:729–737.
163. Hecht HS, Hopkins JM: Exercise-induced regional wall motion abnormalities in the presence of valvular heart disease. *Am J Cardiol* 1981; 47:861–865.
164. Sheffield LT, Roitman DI: Stress testing methodology. *Prog Cardiovasc Dis* 1976; 19:33–49.
165. Goldschlager N, Pfeifer J, Cohn K, Popper R, Selzer A: The natural history of aortic regurgitation: A clinical and hemodynamic study. *Am J Med* 1973; 54:577–588.
166. Akasaka T, Yoshikawa J, Yoshida K, Okumachi F, Koizumi K, Shiratori K, et al: Age-related valvular regurgitation: A study by pulsed Doppler echocardiography. *Circulation* 1987; 76:262–265.
167. Errichetti A, Greenberg JM, Gaasch WM: Is valve replacement indicated in asymptomatic patients with aortic stenosis or aortic regurgitation? In: AN Brest, (ed): *Cardiovascular Clinics*, vol. III. Philadelphia, FA Davis, 1990, pp 199–210.

167a Zile MR: Chronic aortic and mitral regurgitation. Choosing the optimal time for surgical correction. *Cardiol Clin* 1991; 9:239–253.

168. Bonow RO, Epstein SE: Is preoperative left ventricular function predictive of survival and functional results after aortic valve replacement for chronic aortic regurgitation? *J Am Coll Cardiol* 1987; 10:713–716.
169. Bonow RO, Dodd JT, Maron BJ, O'Gara PT, White GG, McIntosh CL, et al: Long-term serial changes in left ventricular function and reversal of ventricular dilatation after valve replacement for chronic aortic regurgitation. *Circulation* 1988; 78:1108–1120.
170. Gaasch WH, Andrias CW, Levine HJ: Chronic aortic regurgitation: The effect of aortic valve replacement on left ventricular volume, mass, and function. *Circulation* 1978; 58:825–836.
171. Levine HJ: Left ventricular function after correction of chronic aortic regurgitation. *Circulation* 1988; 78:1319–1321.
172. Bonow RO, Lakatos E, Maron BJ, Epstein SE: Serial long-term assessment of the natural history of asymptomatic patients with chronic aortic regurgitation and normal left ventricular systolic function. *Circulation* 1991; 84:1625–1635.
173. Greenberg BH, DeMots H, Murphy E, Rahimtoola S: Beneficial effects of hydralazine on rest and exercise hemodynamics in patients with chronic severe aortic insufficiency. *Circulation* 1980; 62:49–55.
174. Elkayam U, McKay CR, Weber L, Eisenberg D, Rahimtoola SH: Favorable effects of hydralazine on the hemodynamic response to isometric exercise in chronic severe aortic regurgitation. *Am J Cardiol* 1984; 53:1603–1607.
175. Greenberg B, Massie B, Bristow JD, Cheitlin M, Siemienczuk D, Topic N, et al: Long-term vasodilator therapy of chronic aortic insufficiency: A randomized double-blinded, placebo-controlled clinical trial. *Circulation* 1988; 78:92–103.
176. Dumesnil JG, Tran K, Dagenais GR: Beneficial long-term effects of hydralazine in aortic regurgitation. *Arch Intern Med* 1990; 150:757–760.
177. Scognamiglio R, Fasoli G, Ponchia A, Dalla-Volta S: Long-term nifedipine unloading therapy in asymptomatic patients with chronic severe aortic regurgitation. *J Am Coll Cardiol* 1990; 16:424–429.
178. Greenberg BH: Medical therapy for patients with aortic insufficiency. *Cardiol Clin* 1991; 9:255–270.
179. Boucher CA, Wilson RA, Kanarek DJ, Hutter AM Jr, Okada RD, Liberthson RR, et al: Exercise testing in asymptomatic or minimally symptomatic aortic regurgitation: Relationship of left ventricular ejection fraction to left ventricular filling pressure during exercise. *Circulation* 1983; 67:1091–1100.
180. Bonow RO, Rosing DR, Kent KM, Epstein SE: The timing of operation for chronic aortic regurgitation. *Am J Cardiol* 1982; 50:325–36.
181. Larbalestier RI, Kinchla NM, Aranki SF, Couper GS, Collins JJ Jr, Cohn LH: Acute bacterial endocarditis: Optimizing surgical results. *Circulation* 1992; 86(suppl II):II-68–74.
182. Ballal RS, Nanda NC, Gatewood R, D'Arcy B, Samdarshi TE, Holman WL, et al: Usefulness of transesophageal echocardiography in assessment of aortic dissection. *Circulation* 1991; 84:1903–1914.
183. O'Brien MF, McGiffin DC, Stafford EG, Gardner MAH, Pohlner PF, McLachlan GJ, et al: Allograft aortic valve replacement: Long term comparative clinical analysis of the viable cryopreserved and antibiotic 4° C stored valves. *J Cardiac Surg* 1991; 6(4 suppl):534–543.
184. Frater RWM, Salomon NW, Rainer WG, Cosgrove DM, Wickham E: The Carpentier-Edwards pericardial aortic valve: Intermediate results. *Ann Thorac Surg* 1992; 53:764–771.
185. Cohn LH, DiSesa VJ, Collins JJ Jr: The Hancock modified-orifice

porcine bioprosthetic valve: 1976–88. *Ann Thorac Surg* 1989; 48:S-81–S-82.

186. Duran C, Kumar N, Gometza, Halees ZA: Indications and limitations of aortic valve reconstruction. *Ann Thorac Surg* 1991; 52:447–454.
187. Cosgrove DM, Rosenkranz ER, Hendren WG, Barlett JC, Stewart WJ: Valvuloplasty for aortic insufficiency. *J Thorac Cardiovasc Surg* 1991; 102:571–577.
188. Koster KJ, Cohn LH, Mee RB, Collins JJ Jr: Late results of operation for acute aortic dissection producing aortic insufficiency. *Ann Thorac Surg* 1978; 26:461–467.
189. Bentall A, DeBono A: A technique for complete replacement of the ascending aorta. *Thorax* 1968; 23:338–339.
190. Cabrol C, Pavie A, Mesnildrey P, Gandjbakhch I, Laughlin L, Bors V, et al: Long term results with total replacement of the ascending aorta and reimplantation of the coronary arteries. *J Thorac Cardiovasc Surg* 1986; 91:17–25.
191. Cohn LH, Birjiniuk V: Therapy of acute aortic regurgitation. *Cardiol Clin* 1991; 9:339–352.
192. Haydock D, Barratt-Boyes B, Macedo T, Kirklin JW, Blackstone E: Aortic valve replacement for active infectious endocarditis in 108 patients: a comparison of freehand allograft valves with mechanical prostheses and bioprostheses. *J Thorac Cardiovasc Surg* 1992; 103:130–139.
193. Bonow RO, Borer JS, Rosing DR, Henry WL, Pearlman AS, McIntosh CL, et al: Preoperative exercise capacity in symptomatic patients with aortic regurgitation as a predictor of postoperative left ventricular function and long term prognosis. *Circulation* 1980; 62:1280–1290.
194. Turina J, Turina M, Rothlin M, Krayenbuehl HP: Improved late survival in patients with chronic aortic regurgitation by earlier operation. *Circulation* 1984; 70(suppl I): I-147–I-152.
195. Fioretti P, Roelandt J, Bos RJ, Meltzer RS, van Hoogenhuijze D, Serruys PW, et al: Echocardiography in chronic aortic insufficiency. Is valve replacement too late when left ventricular end-systolic dimension reaches 55 mm? *Circulation* 1983; 67:216–224.
196. Kirklin JW, Barratt-Boyes BG: Aortic valve disease. In: Kirklin JW, Barratt-Boyes BG (eds): *Cardiac Surgery*. New York, Wiley, 1986; 373–429.
197. Cohn LH: Thoracic aortic aneurysms and aortic dissections. In: Sabiston DC Jr, Spencer FC (eds): *Gibbon's Surgery of the Chest*, 5th ed. Philadelphia, WB Saunders, 1990, vol. 2, pp 1182–1209.
198. Borer JS, Herrold EM, Hochreiter C, Roman M, Supino P, Devereux RB, et al: Natural history of left ventricular performance at rest and during exercise after aortic valve replacement for aortic regurgitation. *Circulation* 1991; 84(suppl III):III-133–III-139.
199. Roman MJ, Klein L, Devereux RB, Kligfield P, Niles NW, Hochreiter C, et al: Reversal of left ventricular dilatation, hypertrophy, and dysfunction by valve replacement in aortic regurgitation. *Am Heart J* 1989; 118:553–63.
200. Schuler G, Peterson KL, Johnson AD, Francis G, Ashburn W, Dennish G, et al: Serial noninvasive assessment of left ventricular hypertrophy and function after surgical correction of aortic regurgitation. *Am J Cardiol* 1979; 44:585–594.

Chapter 80

Mitral Valve Disease

William H. Gaasch, M.D. ■ *Robert A. O'Rourke, M.D.* ■
Lawrence H. Cohn, M.D. ■ *Charles E. Rackley, M.D.*

MITRAL STENOSIS

Definition, Etiology, and Pathology

Mitral stenosis develops when scarring or another pathologic process obstructs flow through the mitral valve; it eventually leads to left atrial enlargement, episodic pulmonary edema, pulmonary hypertension, and right heart failure.

Rheumatic endocarditis is the most common cause of mitral stenosis. Rare causes are congenital mitral stenosis, the parachute mitral valve deformity, atrial myxoma, thrombus, vegetations, and calcification of the mitral annulus and leaflets.[1-11] Calcification is often seen in elderly patients, is more common in females than males, and is quite prevalent in patients with chronic renal failure. Although such calcification is usually not important from a functional standpoint, it can produce stenosis and regurgitation.[12,13] When mitral stenosis develops in association with an atrial septal defect, it is called *Lutenbacher syndrome.* This combination may also occur when an atrial septal defect occurs during mitral catheter balloon valvotomy (CBV) (see Chap. 86).

In rheumatic mitral endocarditis the leaflets and chordae tendineae are scarred and contracted (Fig. 80-1). Adhesions and fusion of the commissures restrict motion of the two leaflets. The process of scarring and contraction, along with shortening of the chordae, causes the thickened leaflets to be tethered in a downward position. This results in a funnel-shaped leaflet structure with the inlet at the level of the atrial floor and the narrow apex in the ventricular cavity.

Normally, blood flows from the atrium through the principal orifice and into the ventricle through that part of the opening that lies between the papillary muscles; blood also enters the ventricle through multiple secondary orifices. In rheumatic mitral stenosis, these secondary orifices or spaces between the chordae are narrowed or obliterated by interchordal and commissural fusion. The anterior leaflet is deformed, and the principal orifice is reduced in size. In systole the leaflet is convex toward the left atrium. In early diastole the deformity buckles in

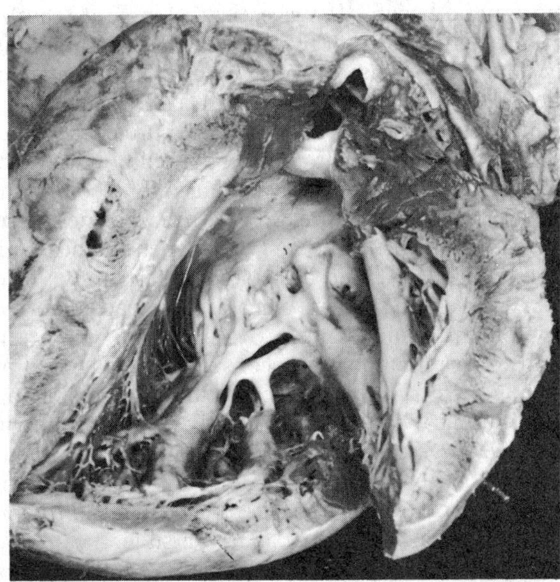

FIGURE 80-1 Rheumatic mitral stenosis viewed from the left ventricle. The leaflets and chordae tendineae are thickened, scarred, and contracted; the valve becomes funnel-shaped with its narrow apex in the left ventricle.

the opposite direction; this contributes to the opening snap that is heard on auscultation and the diastolic doming that is seen on echocardiography.

Secondary changes in the valve include calcification and fragmentation of leaflet tissue with thrombus formation on the valve surface. Thrombus commonly occurs in the atrial appendage and other areas of the atrium. Eventually embolization of calcific or thrombotic material may occur.

Pathophysiology

In the normal adult, the mitral orifice area is approximately 4 to 6 cm². A decrease in the orifice area causes left atrial hypertension and a diastolic pressure gradient between the left atrium and the left ventricle. This pressure gradient is determined by the effective orifice area and the flow through the valve. When the orifice area exceeds 2 cm², the left atrial pressure and the transvalvular pressure gradient are only minimally elevated; the patient is usually asymptomatic. By contrast, an orifice area of 1 cm² is usually associated with a significant pressure gradient across the valve and a pressure overload of the left atrium, the pulmonary vasculature, and the right ventricle.[14]

Although a decrease in the effective area of the valve is the primary factor responsible for left atrial hypertension, the hemodynamics of mitral stenosis are critically dependent on cardiac output and the heart rate. As heart rate increases, the diastolic filling period decreases and (at any given orifice area and output) the transvalvular pressure gradient increases. Thus, the development of atrial fibrillation with a rapid ventricular response is generally associated with an increase in left atrial pressure and symptoms of pulmonary venous hypertension and congestion. Dynamic exercise, by increasing the transvalvular flow *and* reducing the diastolic filling period, can produce a marked elevation of the left atrial pressure. If atrial fibrillation is present, digitalization can limit the ventricular rate and produce a dramatic symptomatic benefit. If the patient is in sinus rhythm, beta-adrenergic receptor blockers or calcium antagonists may improve exercise capacity by blunting the increase in heart rate that occurs during exercise.

Chronic elevation of left atrial pressure causes structural and functional alterations in the pulmonary vasculature that eventually lead to a reduced lung compliance and increased work of breathing. Thus, dyspnea at rest can be a prominent complaint even when the heart rate is well controlled. Hyperplasia and hypertrophy of pulmonary vessels, in concert with a passive transmission of the pulmonary venous pressure to the pulmonary artery, and an active pulmonary vasoconstriction lead to pulmonary hypertension. Such changes can be reversible and thus pulmonary hypertension largely resolves following corrective surgery or CBV.[15–17] By contrast, pulmonary hypertension due to in situ thrombosis, chronic pulmonary embolism, or other obliterative changes in the pulmonary vasculature tend to be irreversible.

A variety of changes in right and left ventricular function may be seen in mitral stenosis.[18–21] Early in the course of the disease, right ventricular function may remain normal, even in the presence of moderate pulmonary hypertension.[22] Eventually, right ventricular afterload excess and decreased contractility lead to right heart failure. Functional tricuspid regurgitation is generally present at this stage.

Left ventricular size and function remain within the wide range of normal in most patients with pure mitral stenosis. There are, however, several mechanisms, peculiar to mitral stenosis, that contribute to ventricular dysfunction.[23,24] Immobilization and atrophy of the posterobasal wall related to scarring and thickening of the mitral apparatus and a tethering or restriction of the adjacent myocardium can produce a regional dysfunction and a decline in the ejection fraction (EF). This process, especially if annular and subvalvular fibrosis and calcification are prominent, tends to restrict or limit ventricular distensibility and, as a result, left ventricular chamber size may be low-normal or small. Left ventricular size and function may also be influenced by an overloaded right ventricle. Such ventricular interaction, modulated by the pericardium, is especially important when right heart pressures are elevated. Thus, a minimally depressed or borderline ejection fraction produces a low stroke volume if the end-diastolic volume is sufficiently small. Catheter balloon valvotomy and even surgical commissurotomy may have little effect on the scarring and immobilization of the annulus, subvalvular apparatus, and adjacent myocardium; this likely explains the suboptimal clinical result that is occasionally seen after mechanical treatment of severe mitral stenosis. In most patients, however, CBV relieves the mitral obstruction and favorably influences ventricular distensibility.[24] As a result, ventricular filling is increased in the presence of a lower filling pressure.

Clinical Manifestations

History

Many, if not most, patients with rheumatic mitral stenosis do not recall a history of acute rheumatic fever (see Chap. 78). The most frequent and prominent complaint is dyspnea.[25–27] Conditions that suddenly increase cardiac output and transmitral flow such as physical exertion, fever, emotional upset, and pregnancy can elevate the left atrial and pulmonary venous pressures and produce acute dyspnea or even pulmonary edema.[27,28] The loss of atrial contraction and especially the rapid ventricular response that accompany atrial fibrillation contribute to dyspnea as well as palpitations and fatigue. Hemoptysis can occasionally be massive,[29] but it usually consists merely of pink or blood-tinged sputum that occurs with pulmonary edema and rupture of capillaries or other thin-walled vessels. In the absence of coronary disease or pulmonary embolism, chest pain may be related to pulmonary hypertension and right ventricular ischemia.[30] Hoarseness can result from enlargement of the left atrium and compression of the recurrent laryngeal nerve. Emboli to the central nervous system can cause a stroke or seizure.[31] (See Chap. 122.)

Physical Examination

The typical auscultatory findings of mitral stenosis are an accentuated first heart sound, a mitral opening snap, and a low-frequency diastolic murmur (rumble) that is best heard at the cardiac apex (see Chap. 11). In the early stages of mitral stenosis, the characteristic apical murmur may not be detected on routine cardiac examination unless the patient is examined in the left lateral decubitus position after exercise (see Chap. 11). If pulmonary hypertension and right ventricular hypertrophy have developed, a right ventricular lift can be palpated along the left sternal border (see Chap. 10).[18] With more advanced disease the patient may display mitral facies with a malar flush and peripheral cyanosis. The neck veins will be distended if right ventricular failure is present. Systolic pulsation of the jugular veins indicates tricuspid regurgitation, and a prominent *a* wave suggests tricuspid stenosis.

With severe mitral stenosis, it is often possible to palpate an accentuated first heart sound and the vibrations of the diastolic rumble at the cardiac apex.[32] Accentuation of the first sound in mitral stenosis is due to sudden cessation of the upward motion of the valve that has been depressed in the left ventricular chamber during diastole.[33–35] The mobility of the valve leaflets, the diastolic gradient across the valve, the PR interval, and the contractile state of the left ventricle all contribute to the intensity of the first sound.[36] Shortening of the PR interval by tachycardia, fever, or thyrotoxicosis can accentuate the first heart sound. When mitral valve mobility is diminished due to calcification of the leaflets or if mitral regurgitation is present, the first sound diminishes in intensity.

The opening snap is perhaps the most important physical sign of mitral stenosis. It is produced during maximum excursion of anterior leaflet of the mitral valve (Fig. 80-2).[26] The opening snap occurs 0.03 to 0.14 s after the second heart sound.[37] The higher the left atrial pressure, the shorter the interval between aortic closure and the opening snap (2-OS time). Critical mitral stenosis produces a 2-OS time of less than 0.08 s. The time from the onset of the QRS complex on the electrocardiogram to the first heart sound (Q-S1) is delayed in mitral stenosis. This interval and its relation to the 2-OS time has been used to estimate the severity of mitral stenosis.[38] Interpretation of these intervals is clouded by the fact that other factors, such as valve mobility, calcification, cardiac output, left ventricular systolic pressure, and relaxation of the left ventricle, can influence the (Q-1)-(2-OS) time.[39,40] Opening snaps, however, are not specific for mitral stenosis. They may also be heard in patients with mitral regurgitation, ventricular septal defect, second and third degree heart block, tricuspid atresia with a large atrial septal defect, and tetralogy of Fallot after a Blalock-Taussig procedure.[41,42] An early diastolic sound similar to the opening snap can be heard in the presence of an atrial myxoma. Finally, a tricuspid origin should be considered in the differential diagnosis of an opening snap, since these sounds can be generated by the tricuspid valve in tricuspid stenosis, atrial septal defect, or Ebstein's anomaly.[43–45]

The opening snap is usually detected at the cardiac apex, but it is audible along the left sternal border, at the base of the heart, and rarely, in the suprasternal notch.[46] The opening snap must be differentiated from the second (pulmonic) component of the second heart sound as well as from a ventricular protodiastolic (S_3)

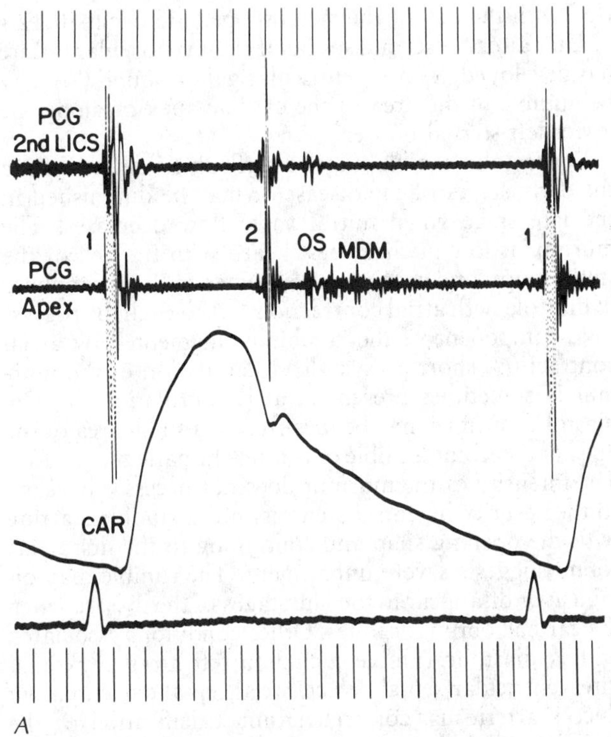

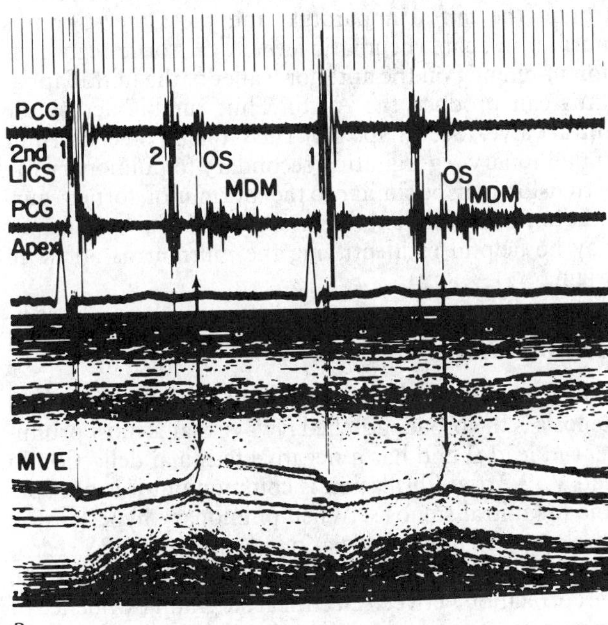

FIGURE 80-2 Phonocardiogram with carotid pulse tracing and M-mode echocardiogram in mitral stenosis. *A.* The first heart sound is loud; an opening snap (OS) occurs 0.11 s after the second heart sound; the snap is followed by a low-frequency mid-diastolic murmur (MDM). *B.* The echophonocardiogram (slower paper speed: 50mm/s) illustrates the relation between mitral closure and the first heart sound; the opening snap occurs at the termination of the opening movement of the leaflets. (*Courtesy of Dr. Ernest Craige.*)

gallop. Inspiration may separate the aortic and pulmonic components of the second heart sound. The time from the aortic second sound to the opening snap will increase with standing, which decreases venous return and lowers left atrial pressure.[47] Exercise will shorten the 2-OS time by elevating left atrial pressure. In contrast to the opening snap, the ventricular gallop sound is low-pitched, heard best with the bell of the stethoscope, and occurs 0.12 s or later after the second sound. If right ventricular failure has developed, a right ventricular gallop sound (S_3) may be audible in the area of the cardiac apex or along the lower left sternal border.

A diastolic rumble may be difficult to detect during the early stages of the disease or may be diminished in the late stage when mitral valve flow decreases. The murmur is low-pitched, best heard with the bell of the stethoscope, and becomes accentuated in the latter phase of diastole with atrial contraction.[48] Although the presystolic component of the rumble is augmented by atrial contraction, short presystolic accentuation of the murmur is sometimes present in atrial fibrillation.[49,50] The diastolic murmur may be localized to a small area of the apex and become audible only after the patient exercises. The intensity of the murmur does not necessarily relate to the severity of mitral stenosis, but a rumble starting with the opening snap and continuing to the first heart sound suggests severe impairment. The rumble may diminish or disappear in the late stages of the disease when the cardiac output declines. Other conditions associated with a diastolic rumble include a left atrial myxoma, interventricular septal defect, atrial septal defect, patent ductus arteriosus, cor triatriatum, calcification of the mitral annulus, pericardial constriction of the *av* groove around the mitral apparatus, and the Carey-Coombs murmur in acute rheumatic fever.[2,51–53] Aortic regurgitation impinging on the anterior leaflet of the mitral apparatus can produce the Austin Flint rumble across the mitral valve. (See Chap. 11.) The Graham Steel murmur of pulmonary regurgitation secondary to pulmonary hypertension may be similar to the murmur of aortic regurgitation, but peripheral signs of rapid diastolic runoff may be helpful in identifying the murmur as aortic in origin.[54]

Electrocardiogram

The characteristic electrocardiographic finding in mitral stenosis is the broad, notched P wave that is most prominent in lead II and has a negative terminal deflection in lead V_1.[55] Atrial fibrillation is common but it is not specific for mitral stenosis. When pulmonary hypertension develops, a rightward deviation of the mean QRS vector may reflect right ventricular hypertrophy. Unfortunately, the correlation between electrocardiographic evidence of right ventricular hypertrophy is not predictive of the degree of pulmonary hypertension.[56,57]

Chest Roentgenogram

The radiographic changes of mitral stenosis (see Chap. 14) are produced by left atrial hypertension which results in left atrial enlargement, alterations in the pulmonary venous pattern, prominence of the pulmonary arteries, and right ventricular enlargement (Fig. 80-3). Since the left atrial appendage occupies a position between the pulmonary artery and the left ventricle, left atrial enlargement appears as a straightening of the left cardiac border on the standard posteroanterior chest film.[58] This finding may not be present in postoperative films if the appendage has been removed. The left atrium enlarges to the right of the spine and can often be recognized as a larger than normal double density through the cardiac silhouette on a slightly overexposed chest film. The large left atrium may elevate the left main-stem bronchus and produce posterior deviation of the barium-filled esophagus.

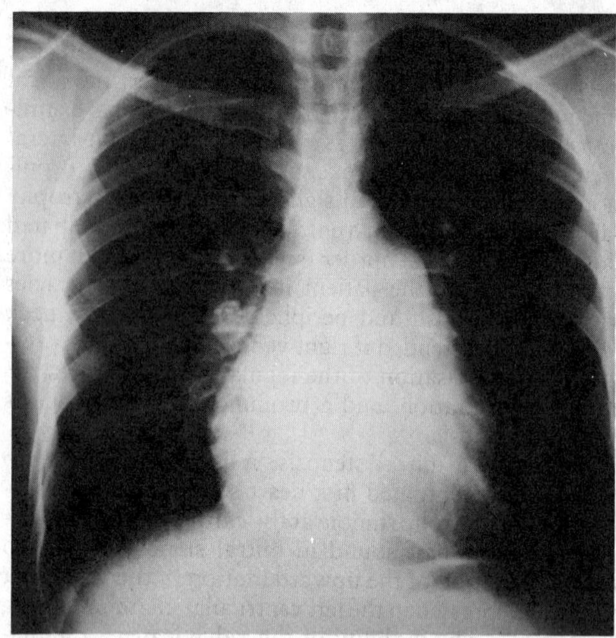

FIGURE 80-3 Chest roentgenogram of a patient with mitral stenosis (valve area 0.7 cm²) and pulmonary hypertension. The main pulmonary artery is large, and the left atrial appendage is seen along the left cardiac border. The modest increase in the size of the cardiac silhouette is due to right and left atrial enlargement. (*Courtesy of Dr. I. Sylvia Crawley.*)

In chronic pulmonary venous hypertension, not only do the vessels appear prominent, but the flow redistributes from the bases to the apices of the lung. This redistribution of pulmonary blood flow is typical of any condition that causes left atrial hypertension. When the pulmonary capillary pressure exceeds the oncotic pressure of plasma proteins (approximately 20 to 25 mmHg), fluid will accumulate in the interstitial space of the lungs.[59] The interlobular septal changes and the linear shadows that are perpendicular to the pleura at the bases of the lungs were described by Kerley.[60] Kerley B lines are due to fibrosis and lymphatic engorgement and are frequently identified with elevated capillary pressure. Acute elevation of the pulmonary venous pressure will cause the typical radiographic picture of pulmonary edema with interstitial and alveolar extravasation of fluid.[61,62] Changes in right ventricular size are best evaluated on the lateral chest roentgenogram.

Echocardiography

Echocardiography (see Chap. 15) is the most useful and reliable noninvasive technique for the detection and evaluation of mitral stenosis.[63–65] The characteristic M-mode finding is a decrease in the EF slope of the anterior leaflet, concordant posterior leaflet motion, decreased excursions, and dense echoes suggesting calcification (see Fig. 15-21). Two-dimensional echocardiography reveals a typical diastolic doming and restriction of leaflet motion. The orifice size can be visualized and measured.[66] The extent of disease can be assessed, and an echocardiographic score can be used to select patients for mitral CBV. Doppler echocardiography can be used to evaluate the diastolic pressure gradient and to calculate the mitral valve area (see Fig. 130-11).[67-69] Color Doppler techniques yield additional information on flow patterns and associated mitral regurgitation (see Plate XI, 130-3). (See Chap. 130.)

Transesophageal echocardiography can provide detailed anatomic and functional information that may not be available from transthoracic echocardiography. This technique can be particularly useful for the detection of atrial thrombus or vegetations, especially when transthoracic visualization of the left atrium is obscured by dense calcification or prosthetic valve echoes (Figs. 131-7 and 131-9). (See Chap. 131.)

Information on left atrial dimensions, right ventricular size, and left ventricular size and function can be obtained. Nonrheumatic causes of mitral valve obstruction such as atrial myxoma (Chap. 111) or, on occasion, thrombus or vegetation can be detected.[70-73] The characteristic picture of an atrial myxoma consists of multiple tumor echoes and displacement of the anterior mitral leaflet (Fig. 80-4), but small tumor masses may not produce these typical findings.

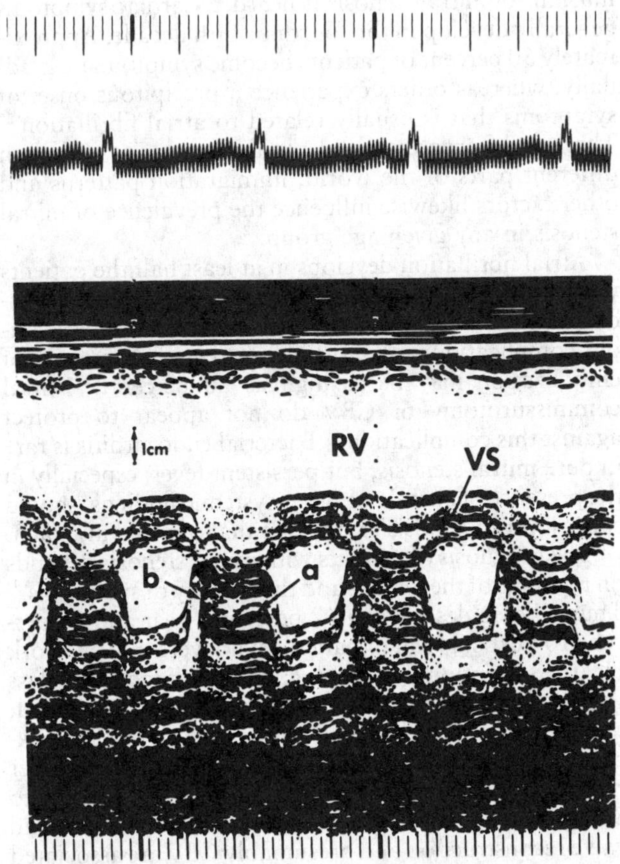

FIGURE 80-4 M-mode echocardiogram of a left atrial myxoma. Arrow *a* indicates echoes originating from the tumor. Arrow *b* points to a clear space which represents the time between mitral valve opening and movement of the tumor from the left atrium to the left ventricle. RV = right ventricle; VS = ventricular septum. (*Courtesy of Dr. Joel M. Felner.*)

Cardiac Catheterization

Cardiac catheterization (see Chap. 138) can be used to determine the pressure gradient across the mitral valve, provide data for calculation of the valve area, measure the pulmonary artery pressure and other parameters during exercise, identify other valvular lesions, assess ventricular function, and define the anatomy and patency of the coronary arteries (Fig. 80-5).

The transmitral pressure gradient is obtained by simultaneously recording the pulmonary capillary wedge pressure (or left atrial pressure) and the left ventricular pressure. Cardiac output is determined, and the Gorlin hydraulic formula is used to calculate the effective mitral orifice area.[74-76] This formula indicates that the orifice area is directly proportional to the diastolic flow across the valve and inversely related to the square root of the transmitral pressure gradient (see Chap. 138). Hemodynamic abnormalities begin to develop when the area is 2 cm^2. The term *critical mitral stenosis* refers to hemodynamic pressure-flow relations; when the orifice area is 1 cm^2, little additional flow can be achieved by increasing the pressure gradient across the stenotic valve.[77] At this stage dyspnea, fatigue, and pulmonary hypertension are generally present.

Symptomatic patients usually exhibit a pulmonary capillary wedge pressure that exceeds 15 to 20 mmHg. If the wedge pressure does not exceed this level, exercise should be performed during the catheterization. On occasion, a marked increase in pulmonary artery pressure may occur with little change in cardiac output. An important clue to the presence of pulmonary vascular disease is the presence of an end-diastolic pressure gradient across the pulmonary vasculature. Thus, if the pulmonary artery diastolic pressure exceeds the pulmonary capillary wedge pressure by more than 5 mmHg, significant pulmonary arteriolar disease is present. With severe stenosis, the pulmonary artery pressures can approach systemic levels.[78] Such marked elevation of pulmonary artery pressure is usually associated with a reduced cardiac output.

In pure mitral stenosis, the left ventricular end-diastolic pressure is almost always normal. In the absence of coronary disease, significant depression of left ventricular function is uncommon. Angiographic studies, however, may indicate a variety of segmental and global abnormalities.[18,19,23,79-81] Coronary arteriography should be performed to identify underlying coronary artery disease.[82]

Radionuclide Techniques

Nuclear techniques (see Chap. 134) can be used to assess right and left ventricular volumes and ejection fractions at rest and during exercise.[83] Serial postoperative studies can be used to evaluate the results of CBV or corrective surgery. These methods can supply information about right ventricular function that is not provided by cardiac catheterization. Improvement in the right ventricular ejection fraction following such treatment is to a large extent related to the fall in right ventricular afterload that occurs as a consequence of a reduction in pulmonary artery pressure.

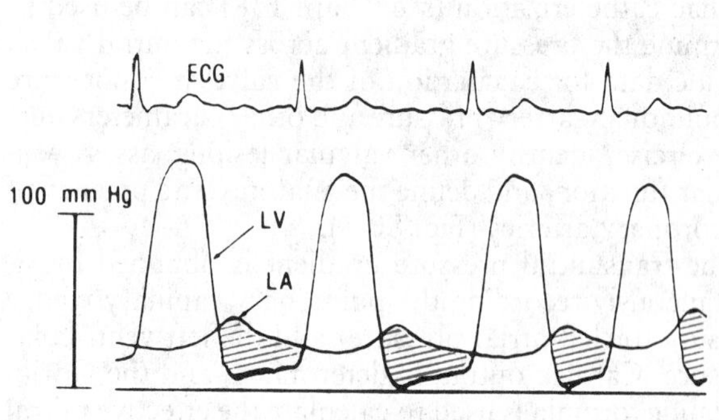

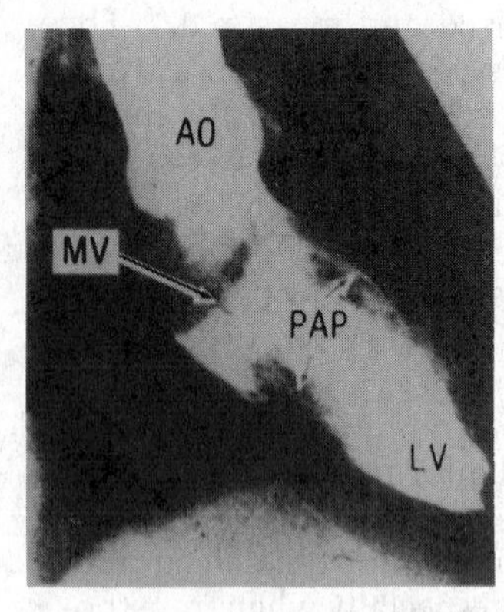

FIGURE 80-5 Pressure records and a left ventricular angiogram from a patient with rheumatic mitral stenosis. The left ventricular (LV) and left atrial (LA) pressures illustrate a diastolic pressure gradient across the mitral valve. The left ventricular angiogram shows a thickened mitral valve (MV) and a small left ventricle with prominent papillary muscles (PAP). ECG = electrocardiogram; AO = aorta. (*From WH Gaasch, JP Murgo: Cardiac catheterization and angiography. In: JH Stein (ed): Internal Medicine, 3d ed. Boston, Little, Brown, 1990. Reproduced with permission from the publisher and authors.*)

Exercise Testing

In the early phases of mitral stenosis, noninvasive exercise testing can be helpful in evaluating symptoms and assessing functional capacity. (See Chap. 16.) Such testing can also be used to assess the effects of drugs that are used to control atrial fibrillation or other tacharrhythmias.[84–86] A hemodynamic hallmark of mitral stenosis is a limited cardiac output during exercise.[78] Pulmonary artery pressure may increase substantially during exercise, even if the pressure is only modestly elevated at rest. Indeed, exercise can be especially useful in uncovering hemodynamic abnormalities that are not apparent at rest.

Usual Strategy of Workup

After the initial examination and radiographic and electrocardiographic studies, an echocardiogram should be obtained. Echocardiography is the most effective noninvasive method for assessing and evaluating the severity of mitral stenosis and its consequences. Despite the remarkable utility of an echocardiogram, cardiac catheterization is used to measure the pulmonary artery and intracardiac pressures, and to define the coronary anatomy. If the diagnosis is well established in younger patients, however, catheterization before surgery is not always necessary. A major consideration is given to the presence of pulmonary hypertension and its severity. Exercise testing can be used to evaluate symptoms and functional limitations. If the hemodynamic and functional abnormalities are not severe, the patient may be managed medically. Periodic echocardiographic and exercise studies may be used to follow changes in the mitral orifice area, left atrial size, and the functional consequences. When critical mitral stenosis is present in a symptomatic patient, CBV (Chap. 86) can provide remarkable hemodynamic and symptomatic benefits.[17,87,88] Surgical valvotomy or valvuloplasty may likewise be effective.

On occasion, there may be a discrepancy between the calculated effective mitral orifice area and the patient's symptoms. This is most common when mitral regurgitation or other disorder coexists with mitral stenosis. Under such circumstances, hemodynamic studies at rest and during exercise, in conjunction with good clinical judgment, generally provide a firm rationale on which to base a therapeutic decision.

Natural History and Prognosis

Rheumatic fever remains the most common cause of mitral stenosis. The average age at the time of the initial attack of rheumatic fever is 12 years; thereafter there is a latent period of approximately 19 years before the murmur of mitral stenosis is heard.[26] Cardiac symptoms generally develop in the fourth or fifth decade. Approximately 50 percent of patients become symptomatic gradually, whereas others experience a precipitous onset of symptoms that is usually related to atrial fibrillation.[27] The rate of progression of the disease varies widely in different parts of the world; immigration patterns and other factors likewise influence the prevalence of mitral stenosis in any given age group.[88]

Atrial fibrillation develops in at least half the patients with mitral stenosis. Aside from the hemodynamic burden of atrial fibrillation, systemic embolization is a serious complication with morbid sequelae; the incidence of embolization may be as high as 20 percent.[89] Mitral commissurotomy or CBV do not appear to protect against this complication.[90] Bacterial endocarditis is rare in pure mitral stenosis, but persistent fever, especially in the presence of anemia or other systemic findings, should suggest this diagnosis or perhaps that of atrial myxoma.

The prognosis of patients with mitral stenosis depends on the stage of the disease and the severity of symptoms.[91] Thus, Olesen described a 62 percent 5-year and 38 percent 10-year survival in patients who were in New York Heart Association functional class III; in functional class IV, the 5-year survival rate was 15 percent.[92] By contrast, the 10-year survival rate in asymptomatic patients exceeds 60 percent.[93] These data are consonant with other reports of 5-year survival ranging from 45 percent to 80 percent (Fig. 80-6).[91,94] Mitral commissurotomy and valve reconstruction and presumably CBV are associated with improved survival. Medical therapy is primarily directed at the acute management of atrial fibrillation and its consequences; this, too, may have a beneficial effect on survival.[95] The introduction of these surgical and balloon techniques and medical therapies has limited

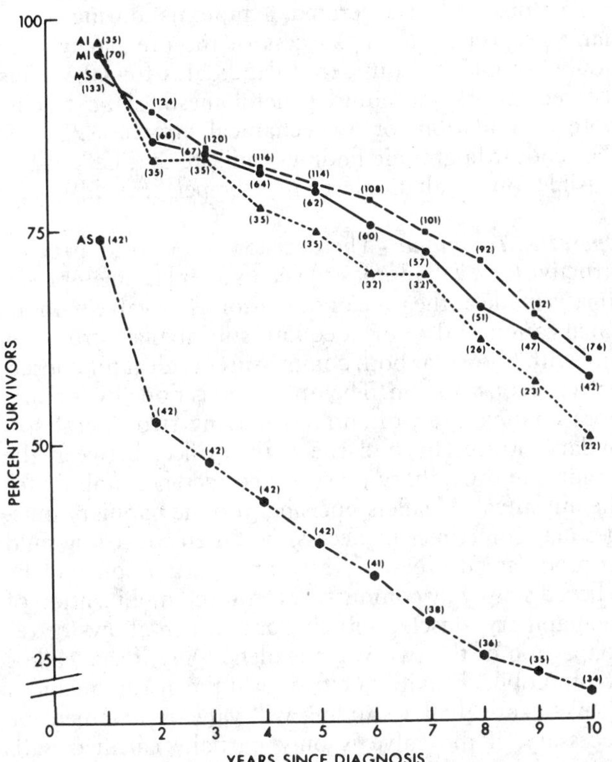

FIGURE 80-6 Actuarial survival in valvular heart disease treated medically. The prognosis of mitral stenosis (MS), mitral insufficiency (MI), and aortic insufficiency (AI) are similar. AS = aortic stenosis. (*From E Rapaport.*[91] *Reproduced with permission from the publisher and author.*)

modern descriptions of the "natural history" of mitral stenosis.

Medical Management

Because the medical management of mitral stenosis cannot reduce the mechanical obstruction, efforts are directed at prevention of recurrent rheumatic fever (see Chap. 78) and bacterial endocarditis (see Chap. 94), as well as correction of some of the consequences of the obstruction.

Digitalis, alone or in combination with quinidine, can be useful in preventing paroxysmal atrial fibrillation or the recurrence of atrial fibrillation after cardioversion. Digitalis has little, if any, benefit in patients with mitral stenosis and sinus rhythm, but it is very effective in the treatment of patients with atrial fibrillation and a rapid ventricular response, especially if pulmonary edema or right heart failure is present. In an emergency situation, electrical cardioversion may be used. Chronic atrial fibrillation is best treated with digitalis. If it is not possible to achieve a ventricular rate of 60 to 70 beats per minute, a beta-adrenergic blocking agent should be added; this combination therapy is especially effective in blunting exercise-induced tachycardia. In this regard beta-adrenergic blocking agents can be beneficial even in patients with sinus rhythm. The calcium antagonist, diltiazem, can also be used intravenously to control the ventricular rate as well as orally in patients who are not able to tolerate beta-adrenergic blocking drugs.

In chronic atrial fibrillation, digitalis and quinidine or other antiarrhythmic agents are unlikely to restore normal sinus rhythm. Electrical cardioversion, however, can be effective if the duration of the arrhythmia is less than 12 months and the atrial size does not exceed 5 cm. If cardioversion is to be performed, the patient should be adequately digitalized and quinidine or other antiarrhythmic therapy should be instituted. Elective cardioversion should be preceded by at least 3 to 4 weeks of anticoagulation to reduce the risk of arterial embolization. If an echocardiogram indicates the presence of thrombus, the duration of anticoagulation should be at least twice as long. If sinus rhythm is restored, anticoagulation should be continued for another 3 to 4 weeks or until atrial mechanical activity has returned. Then, if the patient is at low risk for embolization and has not had an embolus in the past, anticoagulants may be discontinued.

Catheter Balloon Valvotomy

The technique of percutaneous transvenous valvotomy incorporates balloon catheters that can be advanced across the atrial septum and across the stenotic mitral valve to enlarge its orifice area (see Chap. 86). First used for pulmonic stenosis,[96] this procedure has been applied to all four native valves as well as biologic prosthetic valves. While CBV may be the treatment of choice for many, if not most, patients with rheumatic mitral stenosis,[97,98] the relative merits of CBV versus surgical correction must be considered for each patient.[88]

The procedure involves advancement of a balloon catheter (or two catheters) from the femoral vein and right atrium, through the interatrial septum to the mitral valve. The balloon is guided across the valve and, with transient inflation, produces an increase in the stenotic orifice area. The mechanism underlying relief of the stenosis is largely a simple separation of the fused commissures that is similar to that produced by the closed mitral commissurotomy (surgical) technique. Fracture of leaflet and adjacent calcification may also contribute to enhanced leaflet motility and improved valve function.

Selection of patients for CBV relies heavily on two-dimensional and Doppler echocardiography; transesophageal echocardiography can provide information that is not available from transthoracic echocardiography. The presence and severity of stenosis can be confirmed, associated disease and the presence of mitral regurgitation can be assessed, and significant left atrial thrombus may be excluded. With rare exception, thrombus is considered a contraindication to balloon valvotomy. Echocardiographic scoring of the disease severity provides a guideline as to the likelihood of a successful valvotomy; such scoring incorporates an assessment of leaflet thickness, calcification, and rigidity, as well as the degree of subvalvular disease.

Balloon valvotomy has been used only since 1984. There are, therefore, no data on the long-term results of this procedure. (See Chap. 86.) The immediate results and those from medium-term follow-up, however, are very gratifying.[99–102] Valve area generally increases from critical or near critical stenosis to approximately 2 cm^2, the left atrial pressure declines substantially, and most patients exhibit a prominent and sustained symptomatic improvement. These results of mitral CBV are comparable to those formerly obtained with closed (surgical) commissurotomy. CBV has also been performed retrogradely through the aortic valve and left ventricle into the left atrium.[103]

An atrial septal occurs in as many as one-third of patients undergoing CBV across the atrial septum, but it is rarely of clinical consequence. Other complications of CBV include embolic events, mitral regurgitation, and cardiac perforation.[104] As the technique is further developed and refined, the complication rate will undoubtedly fall. Patient selection likewise needs better definition. In this regard, the use of CBV appears to be the treatment of choice in the pregnant female. The decision between CBV and surgery is more difficult in the patient with multivalvular disease in whom the mitral stenosis appears to be dominant; correction of the mitral stenosis may allow a postponement of aortic or other surgery. The indications for CBV in patients with heart failure or severe pulmonary hypertension remain to be defined, but it is likely that the procedure may at least provide temporary relief so that later surgery can be offered at a lower risk.

Surgical Management

The prevalence of mitral stenosis in North America has decreased over the past several decades. With the surge in immigration from countries where rheumatic fever is epidemic, however, increased numbers of patients with mitral stenosis are expected.[88] Symptomatic patients with hemodynamically significant mitral stenosis should undergo mechanical relief of the obstruction. The introduction of percutaneous CBV has provided an alternative to surgical valvuloplasty in selected patients (Chap. 86), but the relative merits of these two modalities are still under investigation.[105]

The decision to perform open surgical valvuloplasty rather than balloon dilatation of the stenotic mitral valve depends on preoperative echocardiographic assessment. The ideal valve for both CBV and open surgical valvuloplasty exhibits pliability of the leaflets and minimal subvalvular malformation or calcification. Although open valvuloplasty has been done with great precision and excellent long-term results,[106] CBV is being used with increasing frequency.[107] Attempts to dilate calcified valves with the percutaneous catheter balloon technique have been associated with excessive morbidity and poor hemodynamic results.[108] (See Chap. 86.) The calcified valve will usually need to be replaced.

Severe pulmonary hypertension in patients with longstanding mitral stenosis has been considered a relative contraindication for mitral valve surgery, especially in the elderly.[109] However, pulmonary venous pressure generally declines after the mitral obstruction has been relieved, and, as a result, pulmonary arterial pressure falls in almost all patients regardless of the degree of pulmonary hypertension.[110] Thus, relatively few patients with mitral stenosis and pulmonary hypertension need be deferred from surgical intervention. Modern surgical techniques and postoperative care allow the vast majority of patients to survive operation, to exhibit normal hemodynamics, and to experience improved functional status.[111,112]

Patients with accelerated symptoms during pregnancy, especially if the success of the pregnancy is in doubt, should be considered candidates for CBV; this technique does not require general anesthesia, extracorporeal circulation, or a mechanical prosthesis.[113,114] If the echocardiographic findings indicate that CBV is not feasible, open valvuloplasty may be performed.[115]

Operative Technique The decision to perform a reconstructive (i.e., valvuloplasty) versus a replacement procedure is made at the time of operation. The valve without calcification and with adequate subvalvular structures and with fibrosis at both commissures is ideal for conservative reconstruction. The operation is done by incising both commissures, oftentimes making two lateral secondary orifices beyond the main orifice, between the annulus and papillary muscles. To increase mobility of the mitral valve leaflets, incising into the papillary muscles may sometimes be necessary. Often coexisting mild to moderate degrees of valvular regurgitation will be relieved simply by commissurotomy and mobilization of the papillary muscles and chordae, which allows better coaptation of the two valve leaflets. Only if the leaflets are immobile, heavily calcified, or if the disease includes a severe subvalvular scarring will valve replacement be necessary; if the valve is only partially calcified with superficial nodules, and can be debrided, reconstruction may be possible.[116] Thrombi in the left atrium are meticulously removed, and the left atrial appendage is obliterated or removed. If thrombus is present, postoperative anticoagulation is utilized regardless of procedure or valve type.

The technique of mitral valve replacement has changed considerably since the first artificial valve, the Starr-Edwards ball valve, was implanted in 1960.[117] With more hemodynamically efficient low-profile prosthetic valves and the central flow bioprosthetic valve, there is little need to utilize oversized valves. The anterior leaflet of the native valve is usually excised, but the posterior leaflet is left intact with the chordae tendineae attached to the papillary muscle; this protects against posterior rupture of the left ventricle, and provides an improved postoperative ventricular function that is related to preservation of annular-papillary muscle continuity.[118] In selected cases, the anterior leaflet with annular papillary muscle continuity may be left in situ; interrupted horizontal mattress sutures must be everting (atrial to ventricle) to prevent subvalvular leaflet entrapment if a bileaflet valve is used. If chronic atrial fibrillation is present and refractory to cardioversion, a prosthetic heart valve is generally used, since the requirement for anticoagulation obviates the advantages of porcine or pericardial valves. Biologic prosthetic valves should be considered when valve replacement is required in a woman of childbearing age[119] or in the older patient in sinus rhythm; thus, it may be possible to avoid long-term anticoagulation. If patients are in atrial fibrillation but cannot tolerate anticoagulation, a porcine valve should be used; under these circumstances, aspirin (325 mg/day) is administered.

Postoperative Care Direct left atrial pressure measurements are used to optimize cardiac output. In patients with severe pulmonary hypertension, the use of pulmonary artery and left atrial catheters provides pressure data that allows precise calculation of pulmonary vascular resistance during the potentially unstable early postoperative period. It can be particularly important to utilize diuretic therapy to attenuate the accumulation of lung water which aggravates a high pulmonary vascular resistance. Nitrates and especially inotropic agents such as milrinone, isoproterenol, or dobutamine are used to augment cardiac output without increasing pulmonary vascular resistance. (See Chap. 28.) Digitalis is especially useful in patients with atrial fibrillation.

Anticoagulation is utilized in all patients who have undergone mitral valve replacement, whether or not they are exhibiting normal sinus rhythm and whether or not they have a bioprosthetic valve. Anticoagulation is continued for at least 6 weeks; if a bioprosthetic valve has been used and the patient remains in sinus rhythm, anticoagulation may be discontinued. Patients having open mitral valvuloplasty are not maintained on long-term anticoagulant therapy if they remain in sinus rhythm. If atrial fibrillation can be converted to sinus rhythm after surgery, approximately 50 percent of patients will maintain a normal rhythm for 7 years.[120]

Results The operative mortality of patients undergoing open mitral valvuloplasty varies from essentially 0 to 5 percent.[106] Freedom from reoperation, thromboembolism, and death at 10 years is 84 percent, 91 percent, and 95 percent, respectively (Fig. 80-7). When extensive decalcification and reconstruction of the subvalvular apparatus is attempted during radical valvuloplasty, the probability for reoperation within 3 years is at least 50 percent.

The results of mitral valve replacement for nonreparable mitral stenosis have also been satisfactory, no matter what type of prosthetic or bioprosthetic valve has been used. Operative risk factors include coronary artery disease, poor left ventricular function, increasing age, a reoperation, and extreme pulmonary hypertension. Current operative mortality for mitral valve replacement ranges from 3 to 10 percent.[121–123] This depends on whether or not concomitant coronary artery bypass is performed. Even with coronary artery bypass, however, mitral valve replacement mortality can be as low as 3 percent.[124] The late mortality is approximately 30 percent at 5 years.[111]

Thromboembolic rates for the various types of prostheses used in the mitral area vary from about 2 events per 100 patient-years for porcine, St. Jude, or Medtronic-Hall valves to about 4 events per 100 patient years for the Starr-Edwards Ball valve (Fig. 80-8).[125] These results, of course, may be different depending on the presence or absence of fibrillation. Other late complications, such as prosthetic valve dysfunction, occur somewhat less frequently (Chap. 83).

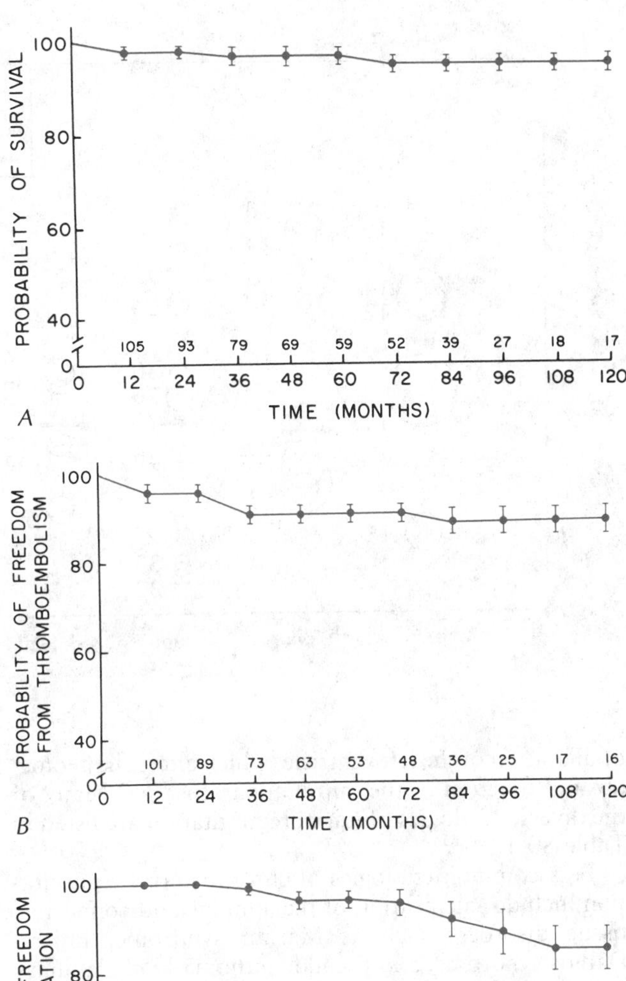

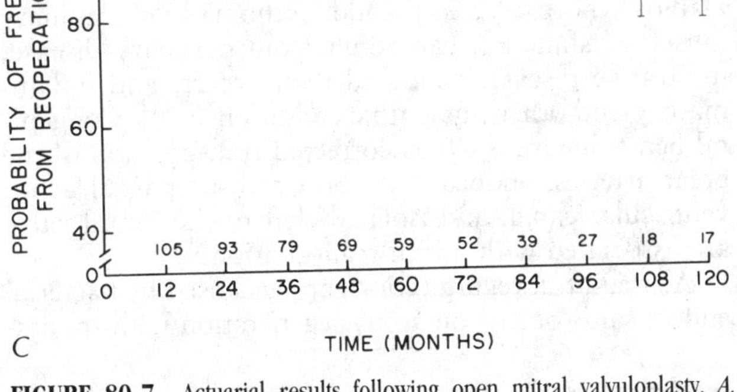

FIGURE 80-7 Actuarial results following open mitral valvuloplasty. *A.* Probability of long-term survival. *B.* Probability of freedom from thromboembolism. *C.* Probability of freedom from reoperation for recurrent mitral valve disease. In all three parts, numbers on the bottom indicate the number of patients at risk at each time period. (*From LH Cohn et al.*[106] *Reproduced with permission from the publisher and authors.*)

MITRAL REGURGITATION

Definition, Etiology, and Pathology

Mitral regurgitation develops when inadequate closure of the mitral leaflets allows retrograde blood flow into the left atrium. This can be caused by abnormalities of one or more of the functional components of the mitral valve; these components include the mitral annulus, the leaflets, chordae tendineae, papillary muscles, and the adjacent atrial and ventricular myocardium. As a result of inadequate mitral closure, a portion of the total left ventricular stroke volume is ejected into the left atrium and, unless compensatory mechanisms ensue, the forward stroke volume falls.

For many years rheumatic fever was considered the most common etiology of mitral regurgitation, but in the United States mitral valve prolapse and coronary heart disease are now the predominant mechanisms underlying functional incompetence of the mitral valve.[126,127] Functional mitral regurgitation also occurs as a consequence

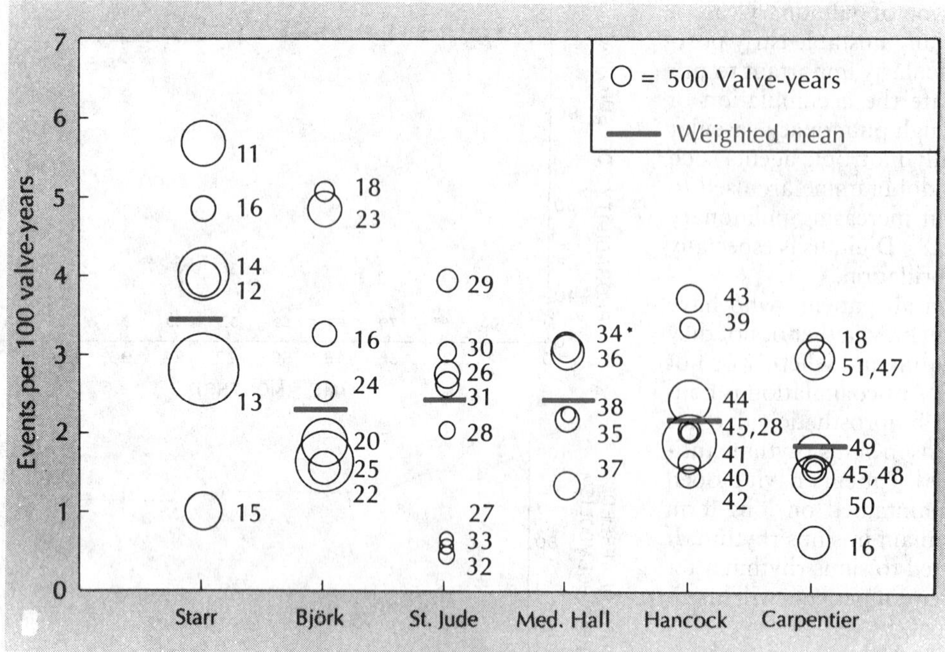

FIGURE 80-8 Thromboembolism rates with mitral valve prostheses. (*From GL Grunkemeier, SH Rahimtoola.*[125] *Reproduced with permission from the publisher and authors.*)

of dilatation of the left ventricle, which alters the geometry and function of the mitral apparatus.[128,129] Many of the diverse etiologies of mitral regurgitation are listed in Table 80-1.[126–155]

Less common etiologies of chronic mitral regurgitation include calcification of the annulus and connective tissue disorders such as Marfan syndrome, Ehlers-Danlos syndrome, and pseudoxanthoma.[130–132] Papillary muscle dysfunction can result from coronary disease, infiltrative disease, endocardial disorders, and inflammatory and other myopathic conditions.[133–135] Congenital heart disease, such as corrected transposition of the great arteries, endocardial fibroelastosis, partial atrioventricular canal, and isolated cleft of the mitral valve are associated with mitral regurgitation.[136]

Acute mitral regurgitation can be caused by bacterial endocarditis or myxomatous degeneration with spontaneous or traumatic rupture of the chordae.[137,138] More commonly, ischemic injury or rupture of a papillary muscle is produced by acute myocardial infarction.

TABLE 80-1

Etiology of Mitral Regurgitation

Chronic regurgitation
Mitral leaflet prolapse (myxomatous, inflammatory)
Coronary heart disease
Left ventricular dilatation (of any cause)
Rheumatic fever
Calcified mitral annulus
Heritable disorders of connective tissue (Marfan, Ehlers-Danlos, osteogenesis imperfecta)
Papillary muscle dysfunction (infarction or ischemia)
Congenital heart disease
Systemic lupus erythematosus
Primary antiphospholipid syndrome
Acute regurgitation
Rupture of chordae tendineae (myxomatous, trauma, endocarditis)
Rupture of papillary muscle (infarction, trauma)
Papillary muscle dysfunction (ischemia)
Valve perforation (endocarditis)

In rheumatic endocarditis the inflammatory process that results in mitral stenosis may similarly cause mitral regurgitation. The differences depend on fortuitous changes in physical orientation of the leaflets. The following structural patterns are found in mitral regurgitation of rheumatic origin: (1) fibrous fusion and calcification of commissures; (2) fibrous contracture of leaflet tissue; and (3) minor intrinsic leaflet shortening with secondary distortion of the valve by the enlarged left atrium (Fig. 80-9).[141,142] Calcification that causes mitral regurgitation extends from one leaflet into the other across one or both of the commissures, thus distorting and preventing normal leaflet coaptation. Fibrous contracture as a cause of mitral regurgitation is usually dominant at one commissure; without fusion, shortening of valvular tissue is so great that the two leaflets cannot make complete contact.

Secondary distortion of the valvular tissue as a cause of mitral regurgitation results from progressive enlargement of the left atrium. As the left atrium enlarges the posterior leaflet is restrained in the opposite direction by the tensor apparatus. The result is that the posterior leaflet loses its capacity to move as it becomes hamstrung over the base of the left ventricular wall. In this manner "mitral regurgitation begets mitral regurgitation."[143]

Myocardial infarction as a result of coronary artery disease may cause mitral regurgitation in several ways: (1) dilatation of the left ventricle; (2) rupture of a papillary muscle; and (3) dysfunction of a nonruptured papillary muscle.

Rupture of the papillary muscle involves the posteromedial muscles more commonly than the anterior by a ratio of 4:1.[144] Severity of mitral regurgitation resulting from such rupture depends upon whether or not an entire set or only isolated heads of a muscle are involved.[145]

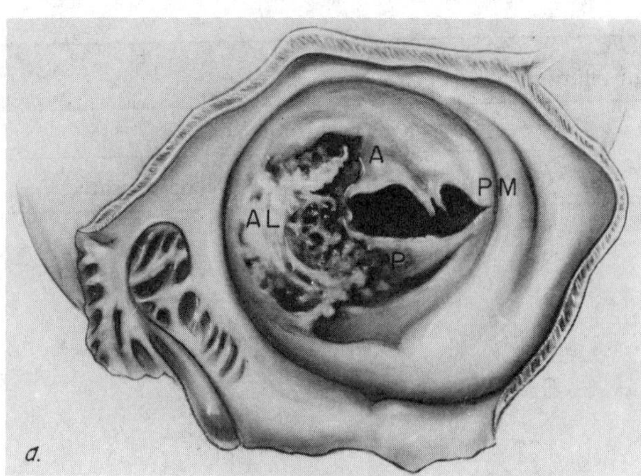

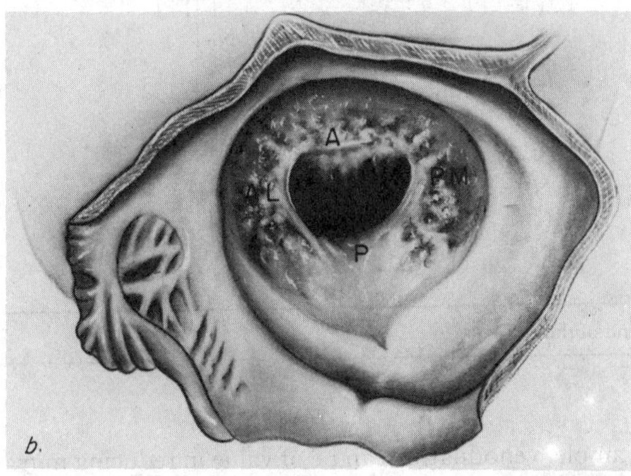

FIGURE 80-9 Anatomic variants of rheumatic mitral regurgitation. The valve leaflets are viewed from the left atrial side. *A.* Calcification and fusion of the anterolateral commissure give rise to the teardrop shape of the orifice. *B.* Calcification of the leaflets and commissures in continuity produces a round ("wedding-ring") orifice. Some restriction of the orifice is present but the dominant hemodynamic lesion is mitral regurgitation. (*From JE Edwards: Pathology of mitral incompetence. In: Silver MD (ed): Cardiovascular Pathology. Churchill Livingstone, New York, 1983. Reproduced with permission from the publisher, editor, and author.*)

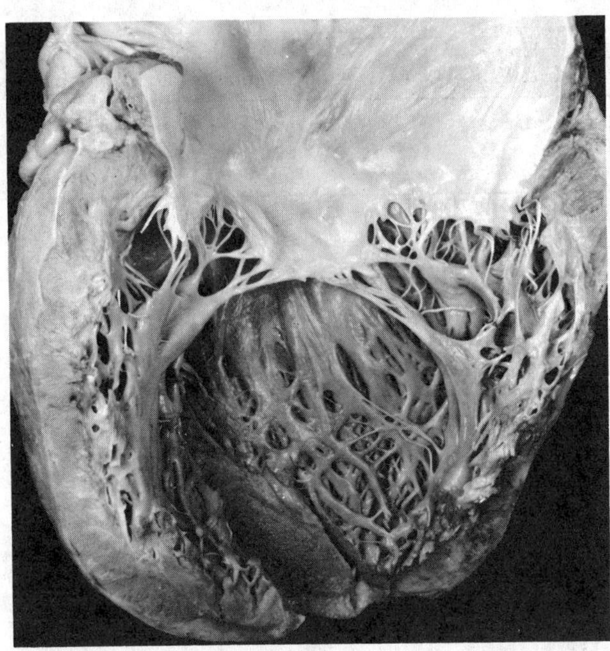

FIGURE 80-10 Healed myocardial infarction involving the inferior wall of the left ventricle and the adjacent papillary muscle. The inferior wall of the ventricle is thinned, and the papillary muscle is atrophic. Subvalvular mitral regurgitation is more commonly seen with infarction involving the inferior wall than with infarction at other sites.

Abnormal function of a nonruptured papillary muscle with mitral regurgitation is usually associated with infarction of the adjacent free wall of the left ventricle (Fig. 80-10). According to clinical and experimental evidence, regurgitation of the valve depends not only on intrinsic dysfunction of the papillary muscle, but also on geometric distortion of the papillary muscle by asynergic contraction of the wall of the ventricle.[146,156,157]

Even in the presence of a structurally normal mitral valve, regurgitation may result from left ventricular failure or dilatation for any reason including idiopathic dilated cardiomyopathy. Mechanical factors leading to valvular malfunction include enlargement of the valvular orifice and distortion of the alignment of the tensor apparatus.[143] The primary form of dilated endocardial fibroelastosis is comparable to the other dilated cardiomyopathies in regard to its cause of mitral regurgitation.[147]

Hypertrophic obstructive cardiomyopathy may be associated with mitral regurgitation, which is probably caused by the systolic anterior motion of the anterior mitral valve leaflet. The anatomic counterpart is fibrous thickening of the mural endocardium of the septal wall of the left ventricular outflow tract. Such thickening results from contact of the anterior mitral leaflet with the mural endocardium. This form of mitral regurgitation is especially dynamic and sensitive to alterations in left ventricular load and contractility. (See Chap. 90.)

Calcification of the mitral ring is commonly found in older patients, particularly in elderly females.[148] In the majority of instances the calcification does not cause recognized valvular dysfunction. When valvular malfunction results, it may take the form of regurgitation due to adhesions of the posterior mitral leaflet to the calcific mass.

Bacterial endocarditis causes mitral regurgitation usually through destructive effects of erosion or perforation of leaflets and/or rupture of chordae. Rupture of chordae can produce a "flail" mitral leaflet recognized on echocardiography. These processes may result from primary infection of the mitral valve or secondarily from primary infective endocarditis of the aortic valve.[149] A less common cause of regurgitation from infective endocarditis is through healing of those vegetations in the angle between the posterior leaflet and the left ventricular wall. This process results in immobilization of the posterior leaflet.[139]

Loeffler's endomyocardial fibrosis (Chap. 91) and systemic lupus erythematosus (Chap. 103) may produce a restraint or tethering of the leaflets and chordae and thereby lead to mitral regurgitation.[150,151] In these conditions the posterior mitral leaflet can become immobilized by adhesions to the adjacent left ventricular myocardium.

Traumatic rupture of a papillary muscle, as an isolated lesion, only rarely causes mitral regurgitation. It is usually associated with contusion or rupture of the

TABLE 80-2

Left Ventricular (LV) and Circulatory Dynamics in Mitral Regurgitation (MR)

	Acute MR	Chronic MR	
		Compensated	Decompensated
Heart rate	↑	N	↑
Effective cardiac output	↓	N	N–↓
Systemic vascular resistance	↑	N	↑
LV end-diastolic pressure	↑↑↑	N–↑	↑–↑↑↑
LV end-diastolic volume (EDV)	↑	↑↑	↑↑–↑↑↑
LV end-systolic volume	N–↓	↑	↑↑
Ejection fraction	↑	N	↓–↓↓
Total stroke volume (TSV)	↑	↑↑↑	↑↑
Regurgitant volume (RgV)	↑↑	↑↑–↑↑↑	↑↑–↑↑↑
Forward stroke volume	↓	N	N–↓
Ratio of RgV/TSV	↑↑↑	↑	↑↑
Ratio of RgV/EDV	↑↑↑	↑↑	↑
LV mass	N	↑–↑↑	↑↑
Ratio of EDV/LV mass	↑	N–↑	↑↑
LV systolic stress	↓	N	↑–↑↑
LV chamber stiffness	N	N–↓	↓
Myocardial stiffness	N	N	↑–↑↑
LV oxygen consumption	N–↑	↑–↑↑	↑↑–↑↑↑

SOURCE: Modified from Gaasch et al.[166] with permission of the publisher and authors.

ventricular septum or free wall. Traumatic or even spontaneous rupture of chordae tendineae can likewise cause mitral regurgitation. Spontaneous chordal rupture is usually related to myxomatous degeneration of leaflet and chordal tissue.[152–155]

The mitral prolapse syndrome is discussed below.

Pathophysiology

Mitral regurgitation develops as a result of slow relentless disease processes or as a result of one or more abrupt decrements in valve function. The eventual result may be quite similar, but the differences between acute and chronic mitral regurgitation are profound (Table 80-2). The major burden and threat of acute mitral regurgitation is to the pulmonary venous circulation and the lungs, whereas in chronic mitral regurgitation, the major burden is carried by the left ventricle.[158–165]

The volume of mitral regurgitant flow is determined hydraulically by the size of the regurgitant orifice and the magnitude and duration of the systolic pressure gradient across the valve.[166] Thus, by rearranging the factors in the Gorlin formula for valve orifice area, the equation representing mitral regurgitant volume (MRV) is:

$$\text{MRV} = \text{MROA} \cdot \sqrt{\text{LVP}_S - \text{LAP}_S} \cdot T_S \cdot C$$

where MROA = mitral regurgitant orifice area, LVP_S and LAP_S = left ventricular and left atrial mean systolic pressures, T_S = time of duration of systole, and C = constant. Recognizing that the pressure gradient across the valve is variable and that the regurgitant orifice area in some forms of mitral regurgitation is dynamic, one may explain the effects of a variety of hemodynamic interventions and therapies on regurgitant volume. For example, venodilators can be of value in reducing mitral regurgitant flow in patients with ventricular enlargement and papillary muscle dysfunction by reducing ventricular size and the functional mitral regurgitant orifice area.[167,168] In some patients with mitral valve prolapse or hypertrophic cardiomyopathy, however, venodilators may augment mitral regurgitant flow through an influence on ventricular size and mitral leaflet coaptation. In patients with fixed-orifice mitral regurgitation (i.e., those with chronic rheumatic disease or annular and valvular calcification), venodilation might reduce pulmonary venous hypertension and congestion in association with an increased regurgitant volume; this could occur if the fall in left atrial pressure were greater than the reduction in left ventricular systolic pressure. By contrast, a pure reduction in left ventricular systolic pressure would reduce mitral regurgitation, particularly in the hypertensive patient. These considerations of the dynamic determinants of the mitral regurgitant volume are especially relevant to the development of a rational therapeutic strategy.

The etiology of mitral disease has an important effect on the magnitude of regurgitation and its reversibility. In coronary heart disease, for example, the development of significant mitral regurgitation requires a critical combination of papillary muscle dysfunction and abnormal wall motion; the extent of the wall dysfunction and its location interact as important determinants of the regurgitant volume.[128,169] In idiopathic dilated cardiomyopathy, mitral regurgitation is determined by altered leaflet function and annular size. In such patients annular dilatation does not develop in direct proportion to the degree of left ventricular enlargement;[170,171] ventricular volume appears to be less important than annulus size. Changes in ventricular geometry (i.e., a more spherical shape) also affect competence of the valve. These and other nonrheumatic alterations in the functional components of the mitral valve influence the severity, operability, and prognosis.[172] This is especially the case in patients with mitral valve prolapse where a variety of pathophysiologic mechanisms contribute to the hemodynamic lesion and its consequences.[173–181]

In acute mitral regurgitation, a large regurgitant, or *v*, wave is seen in the left atrial pressure tracing. This systolic pressure wave is transmitted to the pulmonary veins, capillaries, and on occasion to the pulmonary arteries. Thus, the regurgitant lesion produces an acute pressure load on the pulmonary vasculature; the result can be acute pulmonary edema. These events are rapidly followed by several myocardial and circulatory compensatory adjustments. With the acute volume overload, the left ventricle uses its preload reserve and the total stroke volume increases via the Frank-Starling mechanism. In addition, the low resistance runoff into the left atrium contributes to an early reduction in left ventricular size; thus, according to the law of Laplace, left ventricular systolic load (i.e., afterload) declines. The reduction in left ventricular afterload leads to an increase in the extent and velocity of myocardial fiber shortening and, at least initially, the ejection fraction increases. Thus, in acute mitral regurgitation, an increased ejection fraction occurs as a result of an increase in preload in combination with a decrease in afterload.[158]

The alterations in left ventricular size and function and other circulatory changes that occur in acute and chronic mitral regurgitation are summarized in Table 80-2. The major change that occurs during the transition from acute to chronic mitral regurgitation is enlargement of the ventricle. This comes about through a rearrangement and slippage of myocardial fibers in association with the addition of new sarcomeres and the development of eccentric hypertrophy. (See also Chap. 25.) As a result, preload at the sarcomere level returns to normal. Moreover, the systolic unloading that is characteristic of acute mitral regurgitation is reversed and calculated values for stress return to normal.[182,183] Thus, the enhancement of pump function (i.e., stroke volume) is "mediated through a normal performance of each unit of an enlarged circumference."[184] As this new steady state develops, hypertrophy and geometric changes convert the small hyperkinetic chamber of acute mitral regurgitation to a large, compliant ventricle that is well suited to deliver a large stroke volume.[185] The left atrium enlarges and atrial compliance increases to accommodate a large atrial volume with only a small increment in pressure. Therefore, in chronic compensated mitral regurgitation, the left ventricular end-diastolic volume, mass, and stroke volume are substantially increased and there is little or no increase in ventricular diastolic or pulmonary venous pressure (Fig. 80-11). This new compensated steady state may be maintained for years with few or no cardiorespiratory symptoms.

The most elusive and poorly understood aspect of the pathophysiology of mitral regurgitation is the nature of the transition from the compensated to the decompensated state. While this may be heralded by the development of congestive symptoms, an insidious deterioration of ventricular function can develop without major clinical signs; this may occur to an extent that may preclude the full benefit of surgical correction of the regurgitant lesion.

Compensated mitral regurgitation is characterized by left ventricular chamber dilatation, appropriate myocardial hypertrophy, a normal end-diastolic volume/mass ratio, normal end-diastolic pressure, and normal contractility. As a consequence, systolic wall stress (afterload) is normal, the ejection fraction is normal, and the patient remains asymptomatic (Figs. 80-11 and 80-12). With progression to the decompensated state, substantial left ventricular enlargement, inadequate hypertrophy, high wall stress, increase in end-diastolic pressure, and depressed fiber shortening are seen; such a

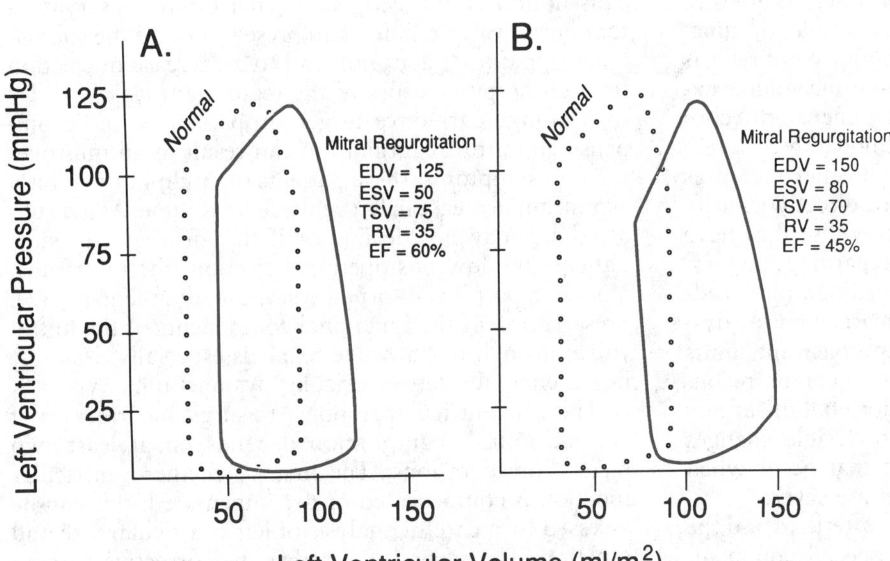

FIGURE 80-11 Left ventricular pressure-volume loops in chronic mitral regurgitation; normal loops are shown for comparison. *A.* In compensated mitral regurgitation the end-diastolic volume (EDV) is increased, the ejection fraction (EF) is normal, and the total stroke volume (TSV) is increased. In this example the regurgitant volume (RV) is 35 mL/m^2 and the effective stroke volume is 40 mL/m^2; the regurgitant fraction is 47 percent. *B.* In decompensated mitral regurgitation the end-diastolic volume is substantially increased, the ejection fraction is depressed, and the total stroke volume remains high. In this example the regurgitant volume is 35 mL/m^2 and the effective stroke volume is 35 mL/m^2; the regurgitant fraction is 50 percent. The regurgitant volume and regurgitant fraction are essentially the same in these two distinctly different hearts. The consequences of the regurgitant lesion are better described in terms of ventricular volume, the ratio of regurgitant volume to end-diastolic volume, and the ejection fraction.

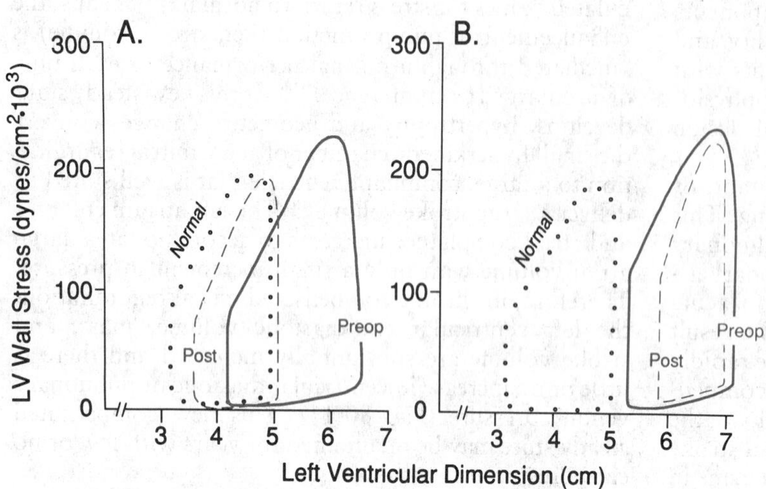

FIGURE 80-12 Left ventricular stress-dimension loops in chronic mitral regurgitation. These echocardiographic data were obtained before (Preop) and after (Post) mitral valve replacement; normal loops are shown for comparison. *A.* In compensated mitral regurgitation the chamber is moderately enlarged; peak systolic stress is increased but late systolic stress is normal; fractional shortening is normal (35 percent). After corrective surgery, end-diastolic dimension and systolic wall stresses are normal but fractional shortening is mildly depressed (28 percent). *B.* In decompensated mitral regurgitation the chamber is markedly enlarged; peak systolic and late systolic stresses are increased; fractional shortening is low (25 percent). After corrective surgery there is no change in end-diastolic dimension and little change in systolic wall stress; fractional shortening is only 16 percent. Ideally, corrective surgery should be performed before this decompensated condition develops. (*Modified with permission from MR Zile, WH Gaasch, HJ Levine: Left ventricular stress-dimension-shortening relations before and after correction of chronic aortic or mitral regurgitation. Am J Cardiol 56:99–105, 1985.*)

condition may occur as a consequence of a progressive increase in the regurgitant volume and/or chamber size.

Guidelines that separate patients with compensated mitral regurgitation from those with decompensated disease have been difficult to develop. For example, mitral regurgitation by its very nature results in ventricular enlargement. Therefore, the mere presence of a dilated ventricle can not be used as evidence of ventricular dysfunction or decompensation. However, gross left ventricular enlargement (i.e., an end-diastolic volume approaching 200 mL/m^2 or an echocardiographic dimension approaching 70 mm) usually indicates severe dysfunction.[166,186–188] The left ventricular ejection fraction may also be difficult to interpret. The systolic unloading and high ejection fraction that are seen early in the course of mitral regurgitation are reversed as contractility falls and the chamber dilates; thus, afterload tends to increase and the ejection fraction declines. Therefore, an ejection fraction approaching 50 percent generally signals mildly impaired contractility. As the decompensated state evolves, there is a progressive increase in afterload and a decrease in contractility. An ejection fraction of 40 to 50 percent indicates moderate left ventricular dysfunction, while an ejection fraction below 40 percent reflects severe dysfunction. Likewise, an end-systolic volume exceeding 60 mL/m^2 or an end-systolic dimension (echo) of 50 mm can be taken as evidence for moderate to severe left ventricular dysfunction. These and other measures of ventricular size and function do not directly identify an optimal time for mitral valve surgery, but they have a strong influence on the decision regarding surgery. Thus, if serial hemodynamic or echocardiographic studies indicate progressive ventricular enlargement or dysfunction, especially if such changes approach the limits discussed above, elective valve replacement or reconstruction should be performed. A major goal of surgery is to prevent the development of irreversible changes in myocardial structure and function that occur when ventricular dilatation and dysfunction are severe.

Traditional views of left ventricular afterload and the effects of corrective surgery deserve special comment. First, detailed studies of left ventricular size and function indicate that systolic wall stress in chronic mitral regurgitation tends to be normal in compensated hearts and to be increased in decompensated hearts[182,183]; only in acute mitral regurgitation is afterload low. Thus, the notion that afterload is always low in mitral regurgitation is an oversimplification. Second, corrective surgery in patients with compensated ventricular function usually results in a decrease in ventricular volume; diastolic dimensions decline more than systolic dimensions. As a result, there may be a decline in systolic stress (Fig. 80-12); in patients with compensated mitral regurgitation, afterload commonly falls after corrective surgery.[182] Therefore, afterload mismatch is not an acceptable explanation for the reduced ejection fraction that is commonly present after mitral valve replacement. A more likely explanation is that valve replacement (with loss of integrity of papillary muscles and chordae, and a tethering of posterobasal wall motion by the prosthesis) produces a change in geometry and a reduction in long-axis shortening, and that this results in a decreased ejection fraction.[182,189,190] This notion is indirectly supported by the observation that mitral valve repair (with preservation of the subvalvular apparatus) does not lead to a decrease in ejection fraction despite closure of the regurgitant leak.[166,190,191]

Although corrective surgery in patients with decompensated mitral regurgitation can result in an improvement in symptoms, these patients often do not exhibit a significant decrease in left ventricular volume. As a result, afterload may not decline or it may increase; in such patients the low postoperative ejection fraction is due, at least in part, to abnormal systolic loading (Fig. 80-12). Preservation of the functional components of the mitral valve through mitral valve repair is especially desirable in patients with left ventricular dysfunction.

The left ventricular response to surgical correction of chronic mitral regurgitation depends on at least two major considerations. The first is whether ventricular function is compensated or decompensated; this can be assessed by a careful analysis of left ventricular size and function. The second is whether the corrective surgery consists of a replacement or repair procedure; systolic function is better preserved with mitral valve repair.

Clinical Manifestations

Symptoms

Chronic mitral regurgitation may be tolerated for many years without clinical evidence of a reduction in cardiac reserve.[192] Fatigue and dyspnea are common symptoms. Eventually, orthopnea, paroxysmal nocturnal dyspnea, and peripheral edema develop.[193,194] Angina pectoris and dyspnea can be especially prominent in patients with coronary disease and mitral regurgitation.[135,195] The combination of coronary disease and mitral regurgitation can lead to refractory symptoms of heart failure; this has sometimes been referred to as *ischemic cardiomyopathy* (see Chap. 61). At this stage systemic emboli can cause vascular or neurologic symptoms, but angina pectoris may be minimal or absent.

Acute mitral regurgitation in the United States is now most commonly a complication of coronary disease. Moderate to severe symptoms of congestive failure occur in patients with ischemic ventricular dysfunction or infarction of papillary muscles. In this setting, acute pulmonary edema is common. Another cause of acute mitral regurgitation is chordal rupture.[196] In general, most patients with mitral valve prolapse experience few or no symptoms; less than half complain of palpitations, chest discomfort, anxiety and fatigue, or symptoms related to autonomic dysfunction[197,198] (see below).

Physical Examination

The cardiac examination in chronic mitral regurgitation reveals lateral displacement of the apical impulse and a diffuse hyperdynamic motion that reflects left ventricular enlargement. Right ventricular enlargement may be palpable along the lower left sternal border. A lifting impulse of the lower sternum or along the lower left sternal border may occur due to systolic left atrial expansion from regurgitation into that chamber.[199] Anterior motion of the heart from the posterior regurgitant jet may also contribute.

The characteristic auscultatory finding is a high-pitched holosystolic murmur that is best heard at the apex. The murmur begins with the first heart sound and extends up to or slightly past the aortic component of the second heart sound.[200] Its intensity is usually constant throughout systole, but there may be late systolic accentuation in mitral valve prolapse or coronary disease with papillary muscle dysfunction. By contrast, in acute mitral regurgitation the murmur occurs in early and midsystole; this is due to the late-peaking left atrial *v* (regurgitant) wave and the decrease in the transmitral pressure gradient and flow during late systole. There is little correlation between the intensity of the murmur and the severity of the regurgitation. Respiration has little effect on the intensity of the murmur, and there is usually no significant variation in the murmur with variations in cycle length when atrial fibrillation is present.[201] The murmur is characteristically not louder in the beat following a premature ventricular contraction. Exceptions to this are seen in dynamic forms of mitral regurgitation such as mitral valve prolapse and hypertrophic cardiomyopathy. (See also Chap. 11.)

In chronic mitral regurgitation mitral leaflet closure is altered and the intensity of the first heart sound is diminished. The duration of left ventricular ejection is shortened, the aortic valve closes early, and as a result there is increased splitting of the second heart sound.[202,203]

Hemodynamically significant mitral regurgitation is usually associated with an audible protodiastolic gallop(S_3) or filling sound.[204] These sounds occur later and exhibit a lower frequency than an opening snap, which is rare in pure mitral regurgitation.[202] If the protodiastolic filling sound (S_3) is accompanied by a harsh mitral systolic murmur, ventricular function tends to be preserved; this is often the case in acute or subacute mitral regurgitation. By contrast, when an S_3 accompanies a soft systolic murmur, ventricular function is usually depressed.[164] The intensity of these gallop sounds may be attenuated during vasodilator or diuretic therapy. By contrast, they may be quite loud in severe mitral regurgitation, especially if the sound merges with a diastolic rumble that is caused by a large transmitral flow in early diastole.[204a] (See also Chap. 11.)

In coronary disease, mitral regurgitation may develop during angina pectoris, with myocardial infarction, and in severe left ventricular failure.[128,134,195] The murmur may be holosystolic or it may occur in early, middle, or late systole[205,206]; the murmur of dynamic papillary muscle dysfunction is especially labile. An atrial gallop (S_4), which is very rare in isolated chronic mitral regurgitation, may be heard, particularly during acute myocardial ischemia. A ventricular gallop (S_3) usually indicates significant depression of ventricular function in this situation.

In acute mitral regurgitation, the physical findings are often those of acute pulmonary edema and heart failure.[207,208] The heart size may be normal, the apical impulse is hyperdynamic, and a systolic thrill can sometimes be detected at the apex.[209] If the posterior leaflet has prolapsed, the thrill may radiate up to the base of the heart due to the anterior direction of the regurgitant jet. In acute regurgitation the harsh systolic murmur radiates over the precordium, to the axilla, and even to the back of the neck, vertebrae, and sacrum.[210] Atrial gallops (S_4) and ventricular protodiastolic filling sounds (S_3) are common; at rapid heart rates a summation gallop may be heard.

Thus, the characteristic auscultatory findings of mitral regurgitation are: (1) a holosystolic murmur at the cardiac apex, (2) a widely split second heart sound, and (3) a ventricular gallop (S_3) or filling sound. An atrial gallop (S_4) is heard in acute mitral regurgitation, especially if due to coronary disease, but not in chronic mitral regurgitation. In mitral valve prolapse, the dynamic nature of the disorder results in remarkable variations in the click-murmur.[211–216]

Electrocardiogram

Chronic mitral regurgitation produces left atrial and left ventricular enlargement which can alter the amplitude and morphology of the P waves and QRS complex.[217] If atrial fibrillation has developed, atrial enlargement may be suggested by a coarse fibrillatory pattern.[218] Although ST segment changes have been attributed to papillary muscle dysfunction, these are nonspecific and can occur due to left ventricular hypertrophy, conduction defects, and digitalis.[156] When regurgitation is caused by left ventricular dilatation, as occurs in idiopathic dilated cardiomyopathy, there will usually be voltage criteria for hypertrophy and secondary ST-T wave changes. If an infiltrative cardiomyopathy is present, loss of precordial R waves may be indistinguishable from a previous myocardial infarction. When mitral regurgitation develops as a consequence of myocardial infarction, electrocardiographic changes are observed more frequently in the inferior leads than in the anterior leads.[134]

In mitral valve prolapse, nonspecific electrocardiographic abnormalities, ST-T wave changes, QT prolongation, and rhythm disturbances may be present.[173,197,200,219]

Chest Roentgenogram

In long-standing mitral regurgitation, the left atrium can achieve enormous proportions with radiographic evidence of an elevated left main stem bronchus and a double density along the right cardiac border.[220] (See Chap. 14.) Cardiac fluoroscopy may reveal calcification in the region of the mitral valve and systolic pulsations can sometimes be detected in the left atrium. When regurgitation is secondary to calcification of the annulus, there may be prominence of the calcification on the plain chest film and fluoroscopy will reveal conspicuous motion of the atrioventricular calcified groove.

Most patients with chronic mitral regurgitation exhibit substantial left ventricular enlargement, but if the etiology is coronary disease, the heart size may range from markedly enlarged to near normal. Acute mitral regurgitation due to disruption of the mitral apparatus can manifest with pulmonary edema and a normal cardiac size.[134,135] In mitral valve prolapse, the cardiac silhouette is often normal, and abnormalities, such as a narrow anteroposterior diameter or pectus excavatum, may be confined to the chest wall.[221,222]

Echocardiogram

The echocardiogram (see Chap. 15) can be useful in defining the etiology of mitral regurgitation and describing its consequences. Thus, thickening and calcification of the mitral apparatus, mitral valve prolapse and ruptured chordae, vegetations, and left ventricular wall motion abnormalities may be useful diagnostic findings. Left ventricular and left atrial enlargement are important consequences that can be assessed in a quantitative fashion. The echo Doppler technique (Chap. 130) provides an estimate of the severity of the regurgitation by assessing the velocity, width, and length of the regurgitant jet (Plate XI, 130-3).[223,224]

The presence of wall motion abnormalities, color Doppler patterns that localize the site of regurgitation, annular calcification, and especially leaflet and subvalvular disease are of considerable importance when consideration is being given to surgical repair of the valve.[225-227]

In acute mitral regurgitation, the echocardiogram can be used to detect abnormalities of the chordae, tendineae, papillary muscles, perforated leaflets, and vegetation.[228,229] Often the transesophageal echocardiogram (Chap. 131) provides diagnostic information that is not available or cannot be detected with transthoracic echocardiography, such as decreased pulmonary venous systolic/diastolic flow ratio and reversed pulmonary venous systolic flow.[230] Associated findings in acute mitral regurgitation include exaggerated left ventricular wall motion, increased excursions of the mitral valve, and a normal left atrial size; in the absence of other disease the left ventricular chamber may not be enlarged in acute mitral regurgitation.

Echocardiography has made major contributions in the description and diagnosis of mitral valve prolapse and its complications (see below).[231-234]

Radionuclide Studies

Radionuclide techniques (see Chap. 134) can be used to determine the ejection fraction of both the right and left ventricles. Ventricular volumes can be measured, and differences in the output of the two ventricles can be used to estimate the regurgitant volume or fraction.[235-237] Such measurements provide data that are important to our understanding of the consequences of the regurgitation. Radionuclide studies can also be used to evaluate regional wall motion. Myocardial perfusion studies can be especially useful in the assessment of the coronary circulation during basal or exercise conditions.

Cardiac Catheterization

Cardiac catheterization with angiography (see Chap. 138) is used to confirm the diagnosis of mitral regurgitation and assess its severity (Fig. 80-13). Catheterization techniques are also used to measure pulmonary artery pressure, assess ventricular function, clarify etiologic mechanisms, identify other cardiac lesions, and define the anatomy and patency of the coronary arteries.

Measurement of right and left heart pressures are an important step in the evaluation of mitral valve disease. In chronic mitral regurgitation, the pulmonary capillary wedge pressure recording commonly reveals a prominent systolic regurgitant wave (v wave). However, alterations in left atrial and pulmonary venous compliance, central blood volume, and other factors in concert with the regurgitant volume determine the magnitude of a v wave.[238,239] Thus, a large compliant left atrium may be responsible for a normal left atrial pressure in the presence of advanced mitral regurgitation. By contrast, large v waves may be seen in patients with heart failure and increased central blood volume, despite the presence of only modest mitral regurgitation. On occasion, a large v wave may be transmitted to the pulmonary artery.[240-242]

Left ventricular cineangiography is used to assess the severity of mitral regurgitation and evaluate left ventricular function.[161] Quantitative angiographic techniques provide data that can be used to determine the left ven-

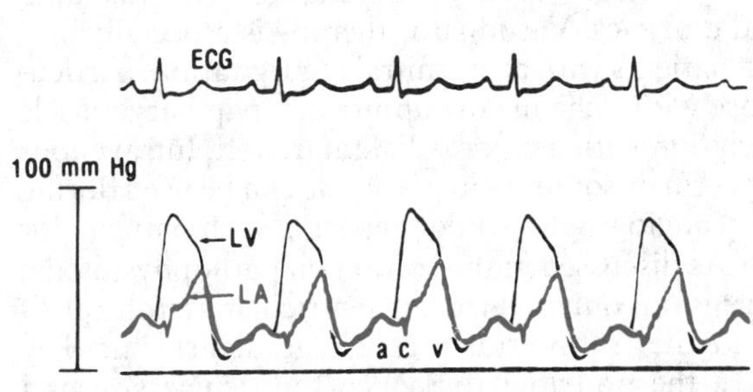

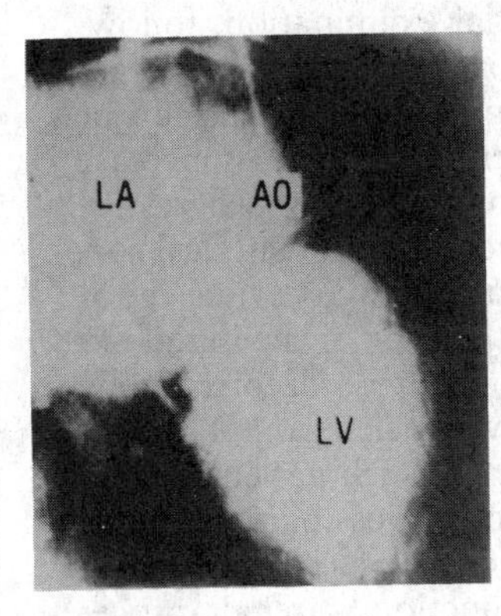

FIGURE 80-13 Pressure records and a left ventricular angiogram from patients with mitral regurgitation. Left ventricular and left atrial pressures from a patient with acute mitral regurgitation; there is a prominent regurgitant (*v*) wave in the left atrium. Left ventricular angiogram from a different patient with chronic mitral regurgitation; the left ventricle is moderately enlarged and there is regurgitation into a very large left atrium (*From WH Gaasch, JP Murgo: Cardiac catheterization and angiography. In: JH Stein (ed) Internal Medicine, 3d ed. Boston, Little, Brown, 1990. Reproduced with permission from the publisher, editor, and authors.*)

tricular end-diastolic and end-systolic volumes, the total stroke volume, and the ejection fraction. The forward (i.e., systemic) stroke volume is determined with indicator dilution techniques or by using the Fick principle for oxygen. Thus, the difference between total stroke volume and forward stroke volume yields the mitral regurgitant volume.[241] The ratio of the regurgitant volume to the total stroke volume (i.e., the regurgitant fraction) and the ratio of the regurgitant volume to the end-diastolic volume reflect the impact of the lesion on systemic blood flow and left ventricular chamber size, respectively.

Quantitative angiography may also be used to define left ventricular wall thickness and mass.[243] Thus, the ratio of end-diastolic volume to mass or of radius to thickness can be determined and used as a relative index of hypertrophy.[244] Using the Laplace relationship and measurements of chamber pressure, dimensions, and wall thickness, one can calculate left ventricular wall stress throughout the cardiac cycle, and systolic stress-shortening relations can be used to assess ventricular (myocardial) function. The ratio of end-systolic wall stress to end-systolic volume has also been used as a functional and prognostic index.[245-247] In chronic mitral regurgitation, however, this index does not provide more prognostic information than is contained in end-systolic volume alone.

In patients with coronary heart disease and mitral regurgitation, coronary arteriography and an assessment of regional wall motion are performed. Wall motion abnormalities, particularly at the base of the inferior papillary muscle, play an important role in the development of mitral regurgitation.

In acute mitral regurgitation, left ventricular angiography demonstrates a vigorous contraction with prominent regurgitation of contrast material into the left atrium.[172,248] Occasionally, ruptured interventricular septum simulates the clinical findings of mitral regurgitation in acute myocardial infarction. This possibility is evaluated by measuring the right heart pressures (including pulmonary capillary wedge pressure) and oxygen saturation and by confirming the presence and location of the shunt with left ventricular angiography. Echocardiography provides very useful, usually diagnostic, information when this differential diagnosis is considered.

In patients with uncomplicated mitral valve prolapse, hemodynamic measurements are often normal and regurgitation is minimal.[174,249] Although cardiac catheterization is not usually performed in such patients, older patients with chest pain, arrhythmias, and heart failure may require coronary angiography to confirm or rule out the presence of coronary disease (see below).[250]

Usual Strategy of Workup

The medical history, physical examination, electrocardiogram, chest x-ray, and Doppler echocardiogram are essential ingredients in an initial evaluation. The echocardiogram allows a confirmation of the diagnosis and an assessment of the severity of regurgitation and its consequences; this should include a detailed assessment of left ventricular size and function. Acute mitral regurgitation may require urgent medical therapy and surgical intervention. If the regurgitation is not severe and a conservative course is to be followed, however, the patient should undergo periodic evaluations to detect progressive regurgitation and/or deterioration of ventricular function; it may be necessary to examine the patient as frequently as every 3 to 4 months, at least initially. If the hemodynamic lesion remains stable and the patient remains free of major symptoms on medical therapy, less frequent evaluations can be performed.

If the diagnosis of chronic mitral regurgitation is apparent at the time of the initial evaluation and the left ventricle remains compensated, a confirmatory echocardiogram is usually performed within a few months. On occasion, cardiac catheterization with quantitative angiography may be necessary to confirm or clarify the diagnosis. Likewise, an exercise test (Chap. 16) may be used to evaluate symptoms. Thereafter, the patient is examined every 4 to 6 months; under most circumstances it is not necessary to repeat the echocardiogram more frequently than annually.

If the left ventricle is moderately enlarged (i.e., end-diastolic dimension is 60 to 65 mm) and/or the systolic function is borderline (i.e., ejection fraction is 50 to 55 percent) at the time of the initial examination, follow-up examinations should be more frequent. In such patients, the development of even mild symptoms can be taken as an indication for surgery; certainly, an increase in symptoms, especially if accompanied by progressive ventricular dysfunction, is an indication for surgical correction of the regurgitant lesion. If there is evidence for left ventricular dysfunction at the time of the initial examination, surgery is usually indicated. Unfortunately, patients with decompensated ventricles cannot expect an optimal postoperative result. In such patients, every consideration should be given to the possibility of mitral valve repair. (See Chap. 85.) Because of a salutary effect on postoperative ventricular function,[118] repair procedures can benefit patients with mitral regurgitation and depressed ventricular function[118], especially those whose regurgitation is due to coronary heart disease.

Natural History and Prognosis

The prognosis of patients with mitral regurgitation depends on the underlying etiology, the severity of regurgitation, and the state of left ventricular function.[192] Many patients with significant mitral regurgitation tolerate the left ventricular volume overload for decades, but eventually symptoms of heart failure develop. Left atrial enlargement and atrial fibrillation may be complicated by systemic arterial embolization; the incidence of this complication can be as high as 10 to 20 percent. Systemic emboli are less frequent in mitral regurgitation than in mitral stenosis.[192,194] Infective endocarditis can also have a negative impact on the natural history. A survival analysis of patients with valvular heart disease indicates that 80 percent of patients with mitral regurgitation were alive at 5 years; 60 percent were alive at 10 years (see Fig. 80-6).[91] Whether or not medical therapy, especially vasodilator therapy, has contributed to an improvement in these statistics is not known.

The natural history and the surgical mortality of valve replacement or repair is substantially higher in patients with coronary artery disease than in those with rheumatic or degenerative disease.[251] When coronary disease results in mitral regurgitation, the extent of the coronary disease and the severity of ventricular dysfunction are the primary determinants of prognosis.

Medical Treatment

Endocarditis prophylaxis is indicated in all patients with mitral regurgitation. (See Chap. 94.) In those with rheumatic valve disease, attempts should also be made to prevent recurrent rheumatic fever (see Chap. 78). Although atrial fibrillation is generally managed by administering digitalis to slow the ventricular response, this traditional treatment does not always control the ventricular rate; the addition of beta-adrenergic receptor blocking drugs or a calcium antagonist such as diltiazem can be very useful for this purpose. Because of the high incidence of systemic arterial embolism with atrial fibrillation, anticoagulation with warfarin is almost always indicated. (See Chap. 68.)

Digitalis is used not only in the management of atrial fibrillation, but it is also indicated in symptomatic patients with left ventricular dysfunction. In such patients, digitalis is generally used in combination with vasodilators and diuretics. Vasodilator therapy is especially dramatic in patients with acute mitral regurgitation, particulary those with ischemia or rupture of a papillary muscle in association with a myocardial infarction. Intravenous nitroglycerin or sodium nitroprusside can be used during coronary angiography while preparing such patients for surgery. As discussed in the section on pathophysiology, these drugs not only reduce left ventricular systolic pressure (and the transmitral pressure gradient), but they also have the potential to reduce ventricular size and the mitral regurgitant orifice area (Fig. 80-14). In this fashion, vasodilator therapy can reduce the regurgitant volume and the left atrial and pulmonary venous pressures. In chronic mitral regurgitation, oral vasodilator therapy with hydralazine, nitrates, prazosin, or angiotensin-converting enzyme inhibitors, may have similar effects.[252–254] (See Chap. 30.) Unfortunately, it is not known whether or not these agents slow the progressive deterioration of left ventricular function or delay the time until surgical correction of the regurgitant lesion is necessary. Patients with severe ventricular dysfunction who are not candidates for surgery benefit from digitalis, diuretics, vasodilator therapy, and other measures that are used in the treatment of heart failure (see Chap. 26).

Surgical Treatment

Mitral valve replacement has been widely applied in symptomatic patients with hemodynamically significant mitral regurgitation for almost three decades. An important problem that has limited successful mitral valve replacement has been a decline in the left ventricular ejection fraction after such surgery. This has generally been thought to be mediated through an increase in ventricular afterload,[255] but as noted above, the functional state of the ventricle before surgery and the type

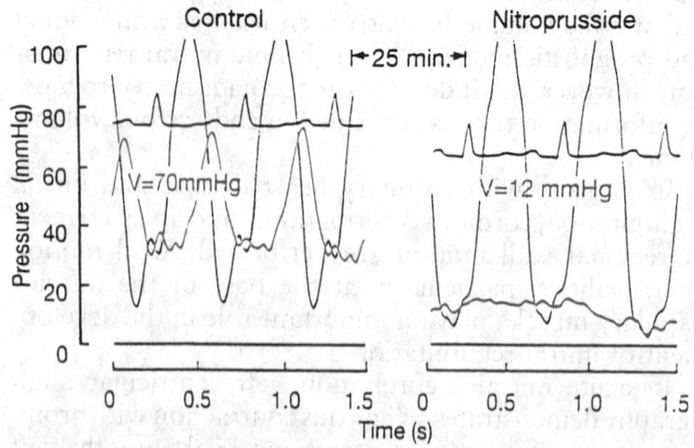

FIGURE 80-14 Effect of vasodilator therapy (nitroprusside) in mitral regurgitation. During nitroprusside infusion the pulmonary wedge regurgitant wave (*v* wave) decreased from 70 to 12 mmHg; the left ventricular diastolic pressure also fell but there was no change in systolic pressure. Thus, there was an increase in the systolic pressure gradient between the left ventricle and the pulmonary wedge. This suggests a decrease in the effective regurgitant orifice area. (*From K Chatterjee et al: Circulation 58:684–690, 1973. Reproduced with permission from the American Heart Association and the authors.*)

of surgical procedure have a substantial impact on postoperative ventricular function. Indeed, these two factors have a greater impact on postoperative ventricular function than closure of the regurgitant leak per se. A large body of clinical and laboratory data supports the concept that maintenance of the papillary muscle–chordae-annular continuity preserves left ventricular function after repair or replacement of the mitral valve.[256–259] For these reasons, mitral valve reparative procedures are being utilized with greater frequency; when valve replacement is performed, attempts are made to preserve at least some of the subvalvular continuity.[118]

Chronic atrial fibrillation contributes to morbidity and mortality in large populations of patients without valvular heart disease,[260,261] and it is likely that the arrhythmia underlies some of the morbidity seen after surgical correction of mitral regurgitation. For this reason, corrective surgery should be considered before atrial fibrillation is established, just as surgery is considered before irreversible changes in left ventricular size and function are present. These considerations, especially when coupled with surgical techniques that preserve the papillary muscle–annular continuity, contribute to improved functional results and survival after restoration of a competent mitral valve (Fig. 80-15). As a result, clinicians are considering earlier surgery than was recommended in the past, especially when a reparative rather than replacement procedure is feasible.[262–264]

Operative Technique Interest in reparative procedures for mitral regurgitation has surfaced since the development of uniform annuloplasty rings, standardization of valvuloplasty procedures, and documentation of long-term durability of these techniques.[265–268] Reparability of a valve will depend on valve pathology and the experience of the surgeon. Patients with a noncalcified regurgitant mitral valve with appropriate volume of leaflet tissue, regardless of etiology, will have a high degree of probability of successful repair. Reparative procedures are most commonly performed in patients who have degenerative myxomatous disease; regurgitation secondary to coronary disease is the next most common, followed by rheumatic and infectious etiologies. A variety of reparative techniques are frequently used alone and in combination (see Chap. 85). These include resection of leaflets, chordal shortening, commissuroplasty, and artificial chordae replacement with Gortex.[269,270] Resection of the posterior leaflet middle scallop of a myxomatous valve is by far the most commonly employed technique.[271] A rigid Carpentier-Edwards or a flexible Duran annuloplasty ring is used to stabilize the annulus. Some controversy exists as to the optimal annuloplasty ring for myxomatous degeneration; some favor the flexible Duran ring because of the better postoperative ventricular performance.[272] For patients with mitral valve endocarditis, reparative procedures are possible either by pericardial patch techniques or by leaflet resections. In most instances, however, valve replacement is necessary.[273]

The use of intraoperative transesophageal echocardiography (Chap. 131) has been extremely important in the assessment of postrepair valve competence, evaluating functional changes, and in assessing left ventricular outflow tract obstruction.[274–277]

Mitral valve replacement is indicated when the valve is irreversibly damaged by scar, calcification, or infection, and coaptation of the two mitral leaflets by reparative procedures is not possible. Comparison of patients in whom the papillary muscle–annular continuity has been preserved with patients in whom it has been removed in valve replacement operations indicates that there is improved cardiac output in the former group.[257,258] At the very least, mitral valve replacement should incorporate some preservation of the posterior leaflet papillary muscle–chordal continuity; this has contributed to a decrease in the incidence of midventricular rupture after mitral valve replacement.[278] If necessary, the anterior leaflet can also be preserved with its chordae, but special reefing techniques must be used so as not to interfere with the opening and closing of mechanical disc valves.[279] As noted above, postoperative monitoring should include both pulmonary artery pressure and direct left atrial pressure measurements to determine the

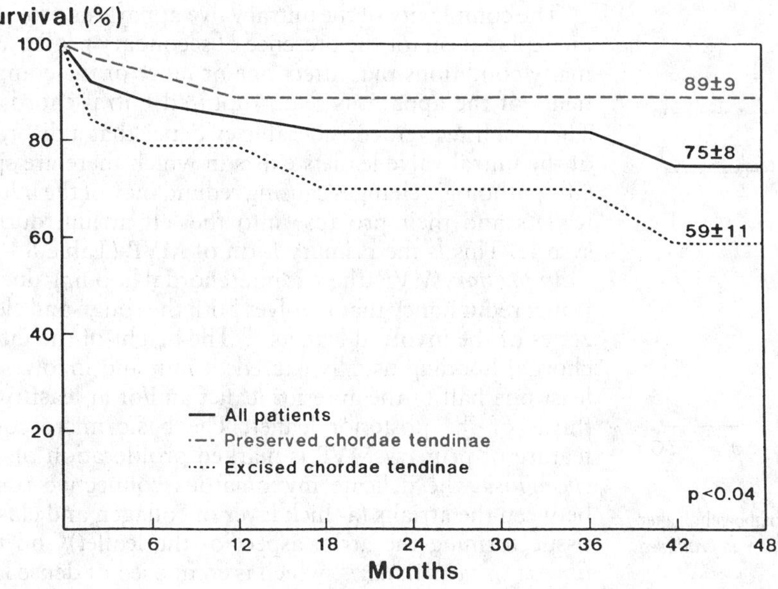

FIGURE 80-15 Actuarial survival curves of all patients and of those who had mitral valve replacement with and without preservation of chordae tendineae. (*From TE David, WC Ho: The effect of preservation of chordae tendineae on mitral valve replacement for postinfarction mitral regurgitation. Circulation 1986; 74(suppl I):I-116–I-120. Reproduced with permission from the American Heart Association and the authors.*)

pulmonary vascular resistance and more precise measurements of left ventricular filling.

If a valve replacement is needed, the type of replacement device is again determined by clinical and anatomic indications. If the patient is in chronic atrial fibrillation, a mechanical valve is used since chronic anticoagulation will be required. In young females who wish to bear children, a biologic valve should be used with the knowledge that a reoperation will be necessary. If patients are over 70 years and in sinus rhythm, a porcine valve is indicated as suggested previously.

Results The operative risk for repair procedures is 2 to 5 percent versus 2 to 7 percent for replacement. Coronary artery disease effects mortality, particularly with valve replacement.[280–285] The operative risk of mitral valve surgery is also related to the functional class of the patient prior to surgery, the function of the left ventricle, comorbidities, and age of the patient.[286–288] Recent improvements in myocardial protection, better patient selection with optimal timing of surgery, and preservation of the papillary muscle–annular continuity have all contributed to operative results that are now as low as in aortic valve surgery, even in reoperated patients.[289]

Long-term mortality is better after repair than after replacement. The incidence of thromboembolism is dramatically less than after any form of valve replacement (Fig. 80-16).[280–284] However, reoperation for structural valve degeneration after mitral repair is necessary in 2 to 10 percent; this is highest in patients with rheumatic valve disease.[265–268] Ischemic mitral regurgitation is associated with a higher early and late mortality due to the concomitant underlying coronary artery disease.[285]

The major morbidity in mitral valve disease is thromboembolism and its sequelae. Better survival after valve repair is probably due in part to the decreased incidence of emboli as well as a beneficial effect on left ventricular function. The presence of atrial fibrillation accounts for the majority of the thromboembolic problems in patients with mitral valve replacement; the incidence of thromboembolism is distinctly lower in patients after mitral valve repair, even in those with atrial fibrillation. The difference here is probably related to the preservation of the native valve and subvalvular structures, improved cardiac output, and the avoidance of bulky prosthetic material in the left atrium. Late survival is dependent upon preoperative left ventricular function; if left ventricular dysfunction is severe, the long-term results will be poor.[280–288] Patients in functional class IV, patients with severe endocarditis of the mitral valve, and those undergoing a reoperation also have decreased long-term survival.[289]

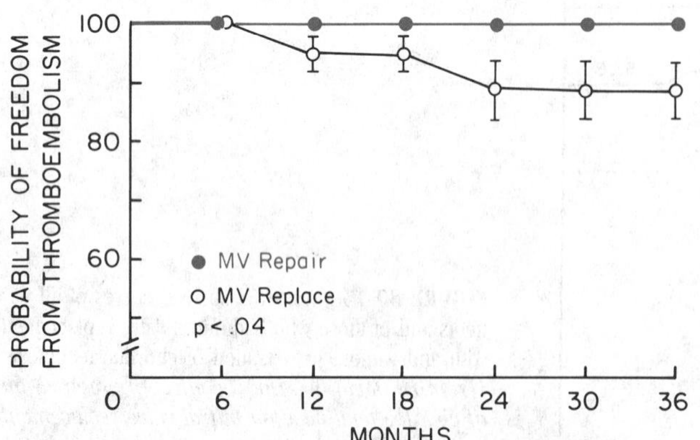

FIGURE 80-16 Actuarial probability of freedom from thromboemboli after mitral valve (MV) repair or replacement. (*From LH Cohn et al.*[282] *Reproduced with permission from the publisher and authors.*)

Elderly patients undergoing repair of the mitral valve do remarkably well; even patients age 70 or older should have repair if valve calcification is not present.[290,291] Late left ventricular outflow tract obstruction has been documented with the use of the Carpentier annuloplasty ring after mitral valve repair (Fig. 80-17).[292–295] The incidence varies from 4 to 6 percent and has been variably associated with systolic anterior motion of the mitral valve; the obstruction has been stable, not requiring reoperation in most cases.

MITRAL VALVE PROLAPSE SYNDROME

Definition, Etiology, and Pathology

Mitral valve prolapse (MVP) refers to the systolic billowing of one or both mitral leaflets into the left atrium, with or without mitral regurgitation. It is the most common form of valvular heart disease, occurring in 3 to 8 percent of the population.[296–303] MVP often occurs as a clinical entity with no or only mild mitral regurgitation, and frequently it is associated with unique clinical characteristics when compared to other causes of mitral regurgitation.[214,296–303]

As noted above, the mitral valve apparatus is a complex structure composed of the mitral annulus, valve leaflets, chordae tendineae, papillary muscles, and the supporting left ventricular, left atrial, and aortic walls.[129] Disease processes involving any one or more of these components may result in dysfunction of the valvular apparatus and prolapse of the mitral leaflets toward the left atrium during systole when left ventricular pressure exceeds left atrial pressure.

The complexity of the mitral valve apparatus provides an explanation for the presence of secondary prolapse in many conditions that affect one or more of the components of the apparatus (e.g., ruptured mitral chordae). There is, however, considerable evidence that a disorder of the mitral valve leaflets exists in which there are specific pathologic changes causing redundancy of the mitral leaflets and their prolapse into the left atrium during systole. This is the primary form of MVP (Table 80-3).

In *primary MVP*, there is interchordal hooding due to leaflet redundancy that involves both the rough and clear zones of the involved leaflets.[301] The height of the interchordal hooding usually exceeds 4 mm and involves at least one-half of the anterior leaflet and/or at least two-thirds of the posterior leaflet. The basic microscopic feature of primary MVP is marked proliferation of the *spongiosa*, the delicate myxomatous connective tissue between the atrialis (a thick layer of collagen and elastic tissue forming the atrial aspect of the leaflet) and the *fibrosa* or *ventricularis*, which is composed of dense lay-

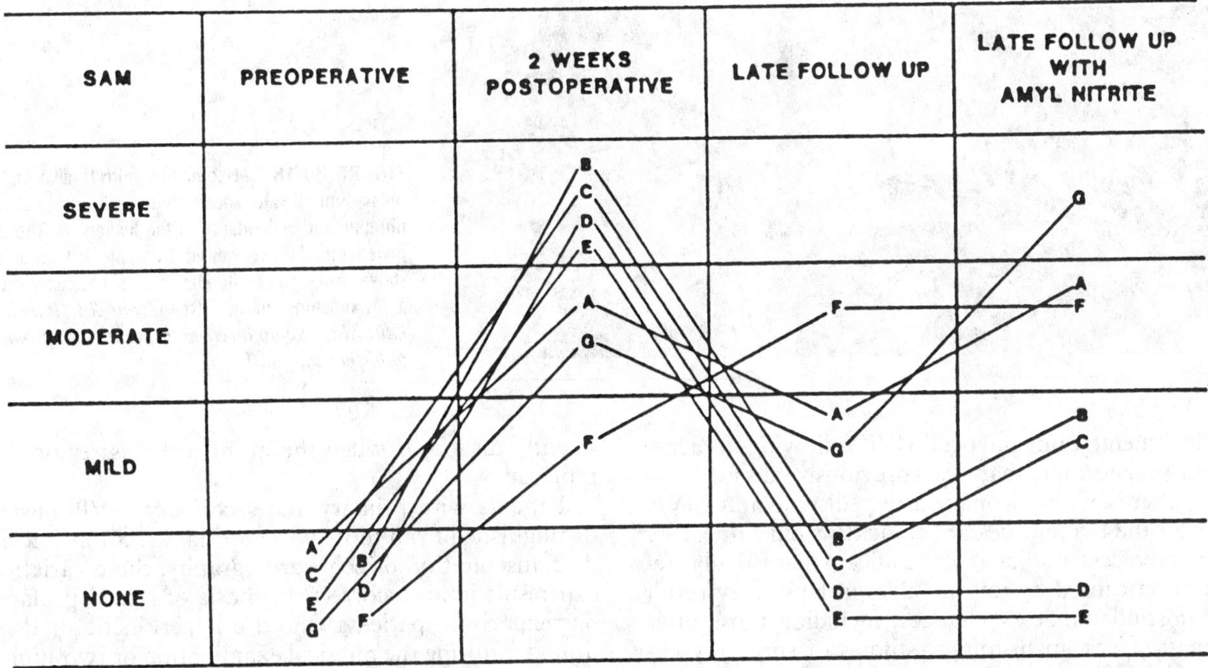

FIGURE 80-17 Left ventricular outflow tract obstruction after mitral valve repair and insertion of a carpentier annuloplasty ring. Systolic anterior motion (SAM) of the mitral valve was graded for patients A through G as none, mild, moderate, or severe; preoperatively, 2 weeks postoperatively, at late follow-up, and at late follow-up with amyl nitrite inhalation. (*From WA Schiavone et al.*[295] *Reproduced with permission from the publisher and authors.*)

ers of collagen and forms the basic support of the leaflet.[301] In primary MVP, myxomatous proliferation of the acid mucopolysaccharide-containing spongiosa tissue causes focal interruption of the fibrosa.[301] Secondary effects of the primary MVP syndrome include fibrosis of the surfaces of the mitral valve leaflets, thinning and/or elongation of chordae tendineae, and ventricular friction lesions. Fibrin deposits often form at the mitral valve–left atrial angle (Figs. 80-18 and 80-19).

The primary form of MVP may occur in families where it is inherited as an autosomal dominant trait with varying penetrance.[304,305] It also often occurs in isolated cases.[306,307] Primary MVP has been found with increasing frequency in patients with Marfan's syndrome,[301] where it is almost always present, and in other connective tissue diseases such as Ehlers-Danlos syndrome,[308] pseudoxanthoma elasticum,[309] and osteogenesis imperfecta.[310] Marfan's syndrome also has an autosomal dominant mode of inheritance. (See also Chap. 96.)

TABLE 80-3
Classification of Mitral Valve Prolapse

- Primary mitral valve prolapse
  - Familial
  - Nonfamilial
  - Marfan's syndrome
  - Other connective tissue diseases
- Secondary mitral valve prolapse
  - Coronary artery disease
  - Rheumatic heart disease
  - Cardiomyopathies
  - "Flail" mitral valve leaflet(s)
- Normal variant
  - Inaccurate auscultation
  - "Echocardiographic heart disease"

Several clinical observations have led to the speculation that primary MVP syndrome represents a generalized disorder of connective tissue. Thoracic skeletal abnormalities such as straight thoracic spine and pectus excavatum are commonly associated with this syndrome.[311,312] The mitral valve undergoes differentiation between the thirty-fifth and forty-second days of fetal life, when the vertebrae and thoracic cage are beginning chondrification and ossification.[313] Any adverse factors in this period might affect both the mitral valve and the bones of the thoracic cage. Of possible relevance, rats fed a diet containing large amounts of peas of the genus *Lathyrus* develop both bony abnormalities and myxomatous changes in their valve leaflets.[314] Therefore, it has been postulated that the MVP syndrome is a connective tissue disorder resulting from fetal exposure to toxic agents during the early part of pregnancy.[314]

Others have suggested that MVP is a result of defective embryogenesis of cell lines of mesenchymal origin. The association of the primary MVP with an increased incidence in patients with von Willebrand disease and other coagulopathies, primary hypomastia, and various connective tissue diseases has been used to support this concept.[315,316]

A *secondary form* of MVP (Table 80-1) occurs in which myxomatous proliferation of the spongiosa portion of the mitral valve leaflet is absent. Tei and associates[317] were able to produce de novo echocardiographic evidence of MVP, often with mitral regurgitation, in closed chest dogs undergoing transient coronary artery occlusion; MVP was attributed to relative displacement of ischemic papillary muscles. Also, serial studies in patients with known ischemic heart disease have occasion-

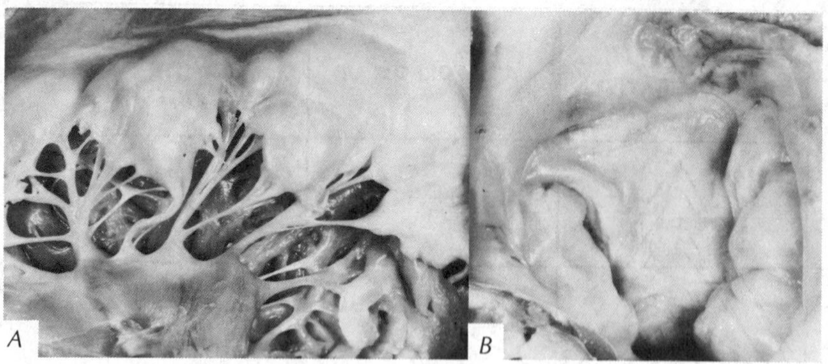

FIGURE 80-18 Myxomatous mitral valve. *A.* The opened mitral valve shows characteristic interchordal hooding and redundancy of the leaflets. *B.* The unopened mitral valve viewed from the left atrial side shows extensive scalloping that is characteristic of a myxomatous mitral valve. (*From RB Guthrie, JE Edwards.*[152] *Reproduced with permission from the publisher and authors.*)

ally documented unequivocal MVP following an acute coronary syndrome that was previously absent.[318] In most patients with coronary artery disease and MVP, however, the two entities are coincident but unrelated.

Several recent studies[155,319,320] indicate that valvular regurgitation caused by mitral valve prolapse may result from postinflammatory changes, including those after rheumatic fever. In histologic studies of surgically excised valves, fibrosis with vascularization and scattered infiltration of round cells, including lymphocytes and plasmacytes, were found without myxomatous proliferation of the spongiosa.[155] With rheumatic carditis the anterior mitral leaflet is more likely to prolapse.[320]

Mitral valve prolapse has been observed in patients with hypertrophic cardiomyopathy in whom posterior MVP may result from a disproportionally small left ventricular cavity, altered papillary muscle alignment, or a combination of factors.[321] The mitral valve leaflet is usually normal. Since left ventricular segmental wall motion abnormalities and sometimes depressed global left ventricular function occur in certain patients with echocardiographic and auscultatory evidence of MVP and regurgitation, nonhypertrophic cardiomyopathy has been listed as a cause of mitral prolapse.[321] This likely is not the case; the ventricular wall motion abnormalities frequently disappear when the mitral valve is repaired or replaced.

Patients with primary and secondary MVP must be distinguished from those with normal variations on cardiac auscultation or echocardiography; these variations can result in an incorrect diagnosis of mitral prolapse, particularly in patients who are hyperkinetic or dehydrated[322] during the physical examination or two-dimensional echocardiography. Other auscultatory findings may be misinterpreted as midsystolic clicks or late systolic murmurs (Chap. 11). Patients with mild to moderate billowing of one or more nonthickened leaflets toward the left atrium with the leaflet coaptation point on the ventricular side of the mitral annulus and no or minimal mitral regurgitation by Doppler echocardiography are probably normal. Unfortunately, many such patients with neither a nonejection click nor murmur of mitral regurgitation are frequently overdiagnosed as having the MVP syndrome.[323]

Pathophysiology

In patients with MVP, there is frequently left atrial enlargement and left ventricular enlargement depending upon the presence and severity of mitral regurgitation.

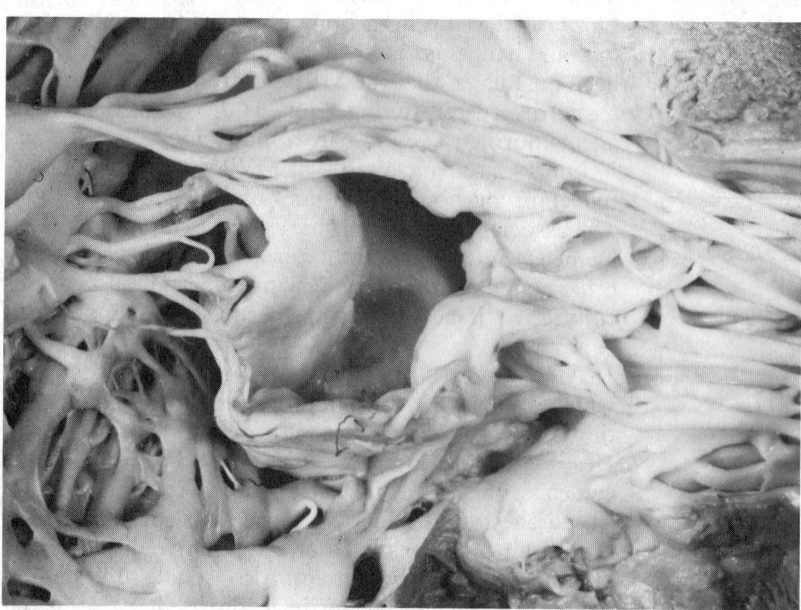

FIGURE 80-19 Myxomatous mitral valve with ruptured posterior leaflet chordae. The central part of the posterior leaflet (lower center) shows fragments of ruptured chordae. The intact chordae are elongated and the leaflets show redundancy and fibrous thickening. (*From JE Edwards: Pathology of mitral incompetence. In: MD Silver (ed): Cardiovascular Pathology. New York, Churchill Livingstone, 1983. Reproduced with permission from the publisher and authors.*)

The supporting apparatus is often involved, and in patients with connective tissue syndromes such as Marfan's syndrome, the mitral annulus is usually dilated, sometimes calcified, and does not decrease its circumference by the usual 30 percent during left ventricular systole. The effects of mild to moderate mitral regurgitation on cardiac function are similar to those from other causes of mitral regurgitation.

Many studies suggest the increased likelihood of autonomic nervous system dysfunction in patients with primary MVP.[325–330] In 1979, Gaffney and associates[325] reported a reduced heart rate slowing with intravenous phenylephrine and an abnormal diving reflex heart rate response in patients with MVP as compared to age-matched controls. They also showed a lesser lower extremity pooling of blood in response to lower body negative pressure in patients with MVP. There is a higher incidence of increased vagal tone and of prolonged QT interval on the electrocardiogram in patients with MVP. In several studies, measurements of serum and 24-h urine epinephrine and norepinephrine levels were increased in patients with symptomatic MVP as compared to age-matched controls.[326,327] Patients with MVP often have an increased heart rate and contractility response to intravenous isoproterenol.[327,330] An increased incidence of high-affinity beta receptors in the lymphocytes of patients with MVP has been reported as well as an augmented increase in cyclic AMP with isoproterenol stimulation as compared to normal individuals.[330] Patients with MVP often have postural phenomena such as orthostatic tachycardia and hypotension. Low intravascular volume and/or an abnormality in the renin-aldosterone axis may contribute to the orthostatic changes.[212,303,331]

Associated Conditions

Tricuspid valve prolapse, with similar interchordal hooding and histologic evidence of mucopolysaccharide proliferation and collagen dissolution, occurs in about 40 percent of patients with MVP.[301] Pulmonic valve prolapse and aortic valve prolapse occur in approximately 10 percent and 2 percent of patients with MVP, respectively.[301] The frequent findings of thoracic skeletal abnormalities in patients with MVP have been noted above. There is an increased incidence of secundum atrial septal defect in patients with MVP and an increased incidence of MVP in patients with atrial septal defects that cannot be explained by a chance occurrence and does not represent only stretching of a patent fossa ovalis.[301,324] (See also Chap. 97.) An increased incidence of left-sided atrioventricular bypass tracts and supraventricular tachycardias also occurs in patients with MVP.[332]

Clinical Manifestations

Symptoms

The diagnosis of MVP is most commonly made by cardiac auscultation in asymptomatic patients or by echocardiography being performed for some other purpose. The patient may be evaluated because of a family history of cardiac disease or occasionally may be referred because of an abnormal resting electrocardiogram.

Some patients consult their physicians because of one or more of the common symptoms that occur in patients with this syndrome. The most common presenting complaint is *palpitation*. The source of palpitation is usually ventricular premature beats, but various supraventricular arrhythmias are also frequent and the most common sustained tachycardia is paroxysmal reentry supraventricular tachycardia. (See Chap. 36.) Ventricular tachycardia has been observed in some patients, and others have had symptomatic bradyarrhythmias. Palpitation often is reported by patients at a time when continuous ambulatory electrocardiographic recordings show no arrhythmias.

Chest pain is a frequent complaint in patients with MVP. It is atypical in most patients without coexistent ischemic heart disease and rarely resembles classic angina pectoris. Occasionally, it is recurrent and can be incapacitating. The etiology of the chest pain is unknown; sometimes it may represent true myocardial ischemia produced by abnormal tension on the papillary muscles and supporting ventricular wall by the prolapsing mitral leaflets. In one study, it could be reproduced by elevating the systemic arterial pressure with intravenous phenylephrine.[333] Coronary artery spasm has been reported in patients with MVP, but it is unlikely to be the cause of most episodes of atypical chest pain.

Dyspnea and fatigue are frequent symptoms in patients with MVP including many without severe mitral regurgitation. Objective exercise testing often fails to show an impairment in exercise tolerance, and some patients exhibit distinct episodes of hyperventilation. Neuropsychiatric complaints are not uncommon in patients with MVP. Some patients have panic attacks (Chap. 118), and others frank manic-depressive syndromes. Perhaps, small platelet emboli from the mitral valve may lead to abnormal behavior secondary to central nervous system damage. Transient cerebral ischemic episodes occur with increased incidence in patients with MVP, and some patients develop stroke syndromes.[334–338] Reports of amaurosis fugax, homonymous field loss, and retinal artery occlusion have been described; occasionally the visual loss persists.[339] These signs likely are due to embolization of platelets and fibrin deposits which occur on the atrial side of the mitral valve leaflets.[301,340] (See also Chap. 122.)

Physical Examination

The presence of thoracic skeletal abnormalities may suggest the diagnosis of MVP, the most common being scoliosis, pectus excavatum, straightened thoracic spine, and narrowed anterior-posterior diameter of the chest.[303] Some patients with mitral valve prolapse may show signs such as arachnodactyly, more typical of Marfan's syndrome.

The principal cardiac auscultatory feature of this syndrome is the midsystolic click, a high-pitched sound of short duration (Chap. 11). The click may vary considerably in intensity and location in systole according to left ventricular loading conditions and contractility. It results from the sudden tensing of the mitral valve apparatus as

TABLE 80-4

Response of the Murmur of Mitral Valve Prolapse to Interventions

	Mitral	Mitral Valve Prolapse	
Intervention	Intensity	Timing	Intensity
Standing upright	↓	←	↑
Recumbent	±	→	↓ or 0
Squatting	↑	→	↓ or 0
Handgrip	↑	←	±
Valsalva	↓	←	±
Amyl nitrite	↓	±	↑

Note: ↑ = increase; ↓ = decrease; 0 = no change; ± = variable; ← = earlier; → = later.

SOURCE: Modified with permission of publisher and authors from MH Crawford, RA O'Rourke[314] and from JA Paraskos: Combined valvular disease. In: JE Dalen, JS Alpert (eds). *Valvular Heart Disease*. Boston, Little, Brown, 1987:365–371.

the leaflets prolapse into the left atrium during systole. Multiple systolic clicks may be generated by different portions of the mitral leaflet prolapsing at varying times during systole. The major differentiating feature of the midsystolic click of mitral prolapse from that due to other causes (e.g., aneurysm of the ventricular septum, atrial myxomas, pericarditis) is that its timing during systole may be altered by maneuvers that change hemodynamic conditions (Table 80-4).

The midsystolic click is frequently followed by a late systolic murmur, usually medium- to high-pitched and most audible at the apex. Occasionally, the murmur has a musical or honking quality. The character and intensity of the murmur also vary under certain conditions, from brief and almost inaudible to holosystolic and loud (Fig. 80-20).

Dynamic auscultation is often useful for establishing the clinical diagnosis of the MVP syndrome.[214,314] Changes in the left ventricular end-diastolic volume lead to changes in the timing of the midsystolic click and murmur. When end-diastolic volume is decreased, the critical volume is achieved earlier in systole and the click-murmur complex occurs shortly after the first heart sound (Fig. 80-21).

In general, any maneuver that decreases the end-diastolic left ventricular volume, increases the rate of ventricular contraction, or decreases the resistance to left ventricular ejection of blood causes the MVP to occur early in systole and the systolic click and murmur to move toward the first heart sound (Table 80-4). By contrast, any maneuver that augments the volume of blood in the ventricle, reduces myocardial contractility, or increases left ventricular afterload, lengthens the time from the onset of systole to the initiation of MVP, and the systolic click and/or murmur move toward the second heart sound. Maneuvers causing the click and/or murmur to occur earlier in systole include standing from the supine position, submaximal isometric handgrip exercise, the Valsalve maneuver, and amyl nitrite inhalation. Those that cause the click and murmur to move toward the second heart sound include squatting from the upright position and maneuvers that slow the heart rate.

Electrocardiogram

The electrocardiogram is usually normal in patients with MVP. The most common abnormality in the MVP syndrome is the presence of ST-T wave depression and inversion in the inferior leads (III, aVF).[341] These changes may reflect ischemia of the inferior wall due to traction on the posteromedial papillary muscle by the prolapsing mitral leaflets. Occasionally, ST-T wave changes are present only during interventions that induce MVP earlier in systole as discussed above. More unusual electrocardiographic changes include prominent U waves, peaked T waves in the midprecordial leads, and prolongation of the QT interval.

Mitral valve prolapse is associated with an increased incidence of false-positive exercise electrocardiographic results in patients with normal coronary arteries, especially females. Myocardial perfusion imaging (Chap. 134) has been useful for differentiating false from true abnormal exercise electrocardiographic findings in patients with MVP.

Although arrhythmias may be observed on the resting electrocardiogram or during treadmill or bicycle exercise, they are detected more reliably by continuous ambulatory electrocardiographic recordings (Chap. 45). The reported incidence of documented arrhythmias is higher in patients with MVP, ranging from 40 to 75 percent.[314] Most of the arrhythmias detected, however, are not life-threatening. Patients with ST-T wave changes in the inferior electrocardiographic leads appear to have a higher incidence of serious ventricular arrhythmias on ambulatory recordings.[314]

Echocardiography

Echocardiography is the most useful noninvasive test for defining MVP (Chap. 15). The M-mode echocardiographic definition of MVP includes ⩾2 mm posterior displacement of one or both leaflets or holosystolic posterior "hammocking" >3 mm.[303] On two-dimensional echocardiography, systolic displacement of one or both mitral leaflets, particularly when they coapt on the left atrial side of the annular plane, in the parasternal long-

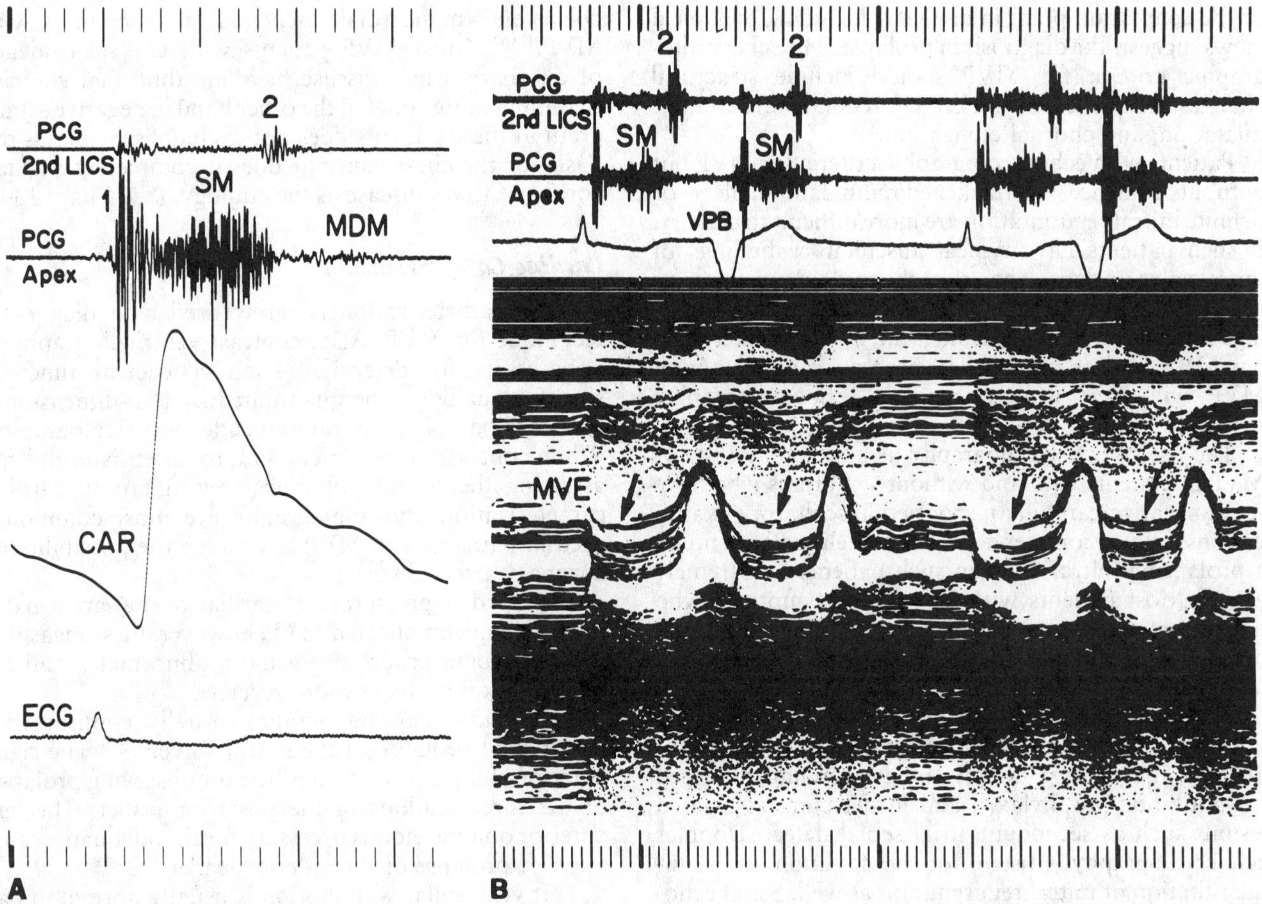

FIGURE 80-20 Phonocardiogram and echocardiogram in mitral valve prolapse. *A.* The phonocardiogram shows a high-frequency holoysystolic murmur (SM) with late systolic accentuation. A low-frequency mid-diastolic murmur (MDM) is present at the apex. *B.* The echocardiogram demonstrates a hammock-shaped systolic motion of the valve leaflets. The rhythm is atrial fibrillation with bigeminy. 1 = first heart sound; 2 = second heart sound; MVE = mitral valve echogram. (*Courtesy of Dr. Ernest Craige.*)

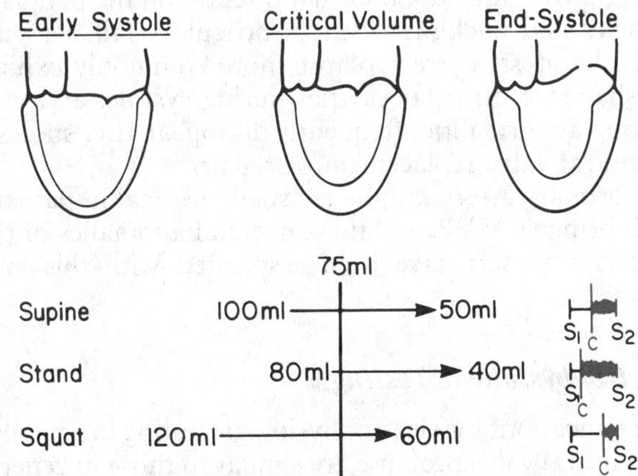

FIGURE 80-21 The effect of left ventricular volume on the timing of mitral valve prolapse and the accompanying murmur. In the upper panels, three phases of left ventricular systole are illustrated. In early systole, there is coaptation of the leaflets and no prolapse; when a critical ventricle volume of 75 mL is reached, valve prolapse commences and progresses until the end of systole. In the lower panel, three body positions are indicated; the corresponding change in volume and timing of the click-murmur are shown. The critical volume for prolapse remains constant. When the critical volume occurs earlier, the onset of click-murmur is earlier. When the critical volume occurs later, the onset of the click murmur is later. (*From MH Crawford, RA O'Rourke: In: KJ Isselbacher et al (eds): Harrison's Principles of Internal Medicine, 9th ed. New York, McGraw-Hill, 1980: 91–105. Reproduced with permission from the publisher, editors, and authors.*)

axis view indicates a high likelihood of mitral valve prolapse (Figs. 15-21 and 15-28).[342] There is disagreement concerning the reliability of an echocardiographic diagnosis of MVP when observed only in the apical four-chamber view.[323,342] The diagnosis of MVP is even more certain when the leaflet thickness is >5 mm during ventricular diastole. Leaflet redundancy is often associated with an elongated mitral annulus and elongated chordae tendineae.[303] On Doppler velocity recordings, the presence or absence of mitral regurgitation is an important consideration, and MVP is more likely when the mitral regurgitation is detected as a high-velocity jet midway or more posterior in the left atrium.[323]

At present, there is no consensus on the two-dimensional echocardiographic criteria for MVP. Since echocardiography is a tomographic cross-sectional technique, no single view should be considered diagnostic.[343] The parasternal long-axis view permits visualization of the medial aspect of the anterior mitral leaflet and middle scallop of the posterior leaflet. If the findings of prolapse are localized to the lateral scallop in the posterior leaflet, they would be best visualized by the apical four-chamber view.[343] All available echocardiographic views should be utilized with the provision that *anterior leaflet billowing alone* in the four-chamber apical view is not evidence of prolapse; however, a displacement of the posterior leaflet or the coaptation point in any view including the apical views suggests the diagnosis of prolapse. The echocardiographic criteria for MVP should include structural changes such as leaflet thickening, redundancy, annular dilatation, and chordal elongation.[343]

Patients with echocardiographic criteria for MVP but without evidence of thickened/redundant leaflets or definite mitral regurgitation are more difficult to classify. If such patients have typical auscultatory findings of mitral valve prolapse, then the echocardiogram confirms the diagnosis. A patient with typical auscultatory findings and a negative echocardiogram, however, likely also has MVP, and as many as 10 percent of patients with MVP will have a nondiagnostic echocardiographic study.

The use of echocardiography as a screening test for MVP in patients with and without symptoms who have serial negative carefully performed auscultatory examinations is not recommended.[303] The likelihood of finding a prolapsing mitral valve in such patients is extremely low.[303] Most patients with or without symptoms who have negative dynamic cardiac auscultation and "mild mitral valve prolapse" by echocardiography should not be diagnosed as having MVP.

The echocardiogram is the confirmatory test for diagnosing MVP but is not always abnormal. It is helpful for defining the natural history, in determining the need for antibiotic prophylaxis, and in detecting associated lesions such as secundum atrial septal defect. Doppler echocardiography is useful for the detection and semiquantitation of mitral regurgitation as well. Serial echocardiograms are useful for following patients with murmurs, especially holosystolic murmurs where quantitation of mitral regurgitation by examination is more difficult. In a carefully performed study comparing auscultatory findings with echocardiographic results in patients with clinical evidence of MVP, the amount of billowing of one or both mitral leaflets into the left atrium, the level of the leaflets coaptation point, and the presence or absence of moderate or severe mitral regurgitation were each important considerations in deciding on the likelihood of MVP.[323]

Chest Roentgenogram

Posterior-anterior and lateral chest x-ray films usually show normal cardiopulmonary findings. The skeletal abnormalities described above can be seen.[313] When severe mitral regurgitation is present, both left atrial and ventricular enlargement often result. Various degrees of pulmonary venous congestion are evident when left heart failure results. Acute chordal rupture with a sudden increase in the amount of mitral regurgitation may present as pulmonary edema without obvious left ventricular or left atrial dilatation. Calcification of the mitral annulus may be seen, particularly in adults with Marfan's syndrome. (See Chap. 14.)

Myocardial Perfusion Scintigraphy

Exercise thallium 201 myocardial perfusion imaging has been recommended as an adjunct to exercise electrocardiography for determining the presence or absence of coexistent myocardial ischemia in patients with MVP.[314,344] Most MVP patients with clinical evidence of coronary artery disease have an abnormal exercise thallium scintigram. On the other hand, a negative scintigram in these patients does not exclude ischemia as the basis for the chest pain nor does it completely exclude coronary artery disease as the etiology. (See Chap. 134.)

Cardiac Catheterization

Cardiac catheterization is rarely used as a diagnostic technique for MVP. Also, contrast ventriculography is unnecessary for determining left ventricular function since it usually can be quantitated by two-dimensional echocardiography or radionuclide ventriculography. While contrast cineventriculography often is useful for assessing the severity of mitral regurgitation, cardiac catheterization and angiography are most commonly used in patients with MVP to exclude the possibility of coronary artery disease.

Intracardiac pressures and cardiac output are usually normal in uncomplicated MVP; however, these measurements become progressively more abnormal as mitral regurgitation becomes more severe.

Left ventricular angiography usually confirms the presence of prolapse of the mitral valve.[214,303] The right anterior oblique projection is best for observing prolapse of the three scallops of the posterior leaflet. The left anterior oblique view is necessary for the adequate evaluation of prolapse of the anterior leaflet.

Left ventricular wall motion is usually normal in patients with primary MVP, but some patients show abnormal contraction patterns in the absence of coronary artery disease.[214,321] These contraction abnormalities usually represent indentation of the left ventricle at the point of attachment of the papillary muscles that is thought to be due to abnormal traction on the papillary muscles and buckling of the ventricular wall. Patients with the most severe prolapse more commonly exhibit misshapen ventricular cavities during systole, and wall motion abnormalities frequently disappear after successful mitral valve replacement or repair.[321]

Coronary arteriography is usually normal in patients with primary MVP, and no congenital anomalies of the coronary vessels have been associated with this syndrome.

Electrophysiologic Testing

The indications for electrophysiologic testing in a patient with mitral valve prolapse are similar to those in general practice (i.e., recurrent unexplained syncope, sudden death survivors, symptomatic complex ventricular ectopy, and the presence of the preexcitation syndromes).[303] (See Chap. 46.) Upright tilt studies with monitoring of blood pressure and rhythm may be valuable in patients with lightheadedness or syncope and in diagnosing autonomic dysfunction.[303] (See Chap. 50.)

Natural History, Prognosis, and Complications

In most patient studies, the MVP syndrome is associated with a benign prognosis (Fig. 80-22).[301,345-348] The age-

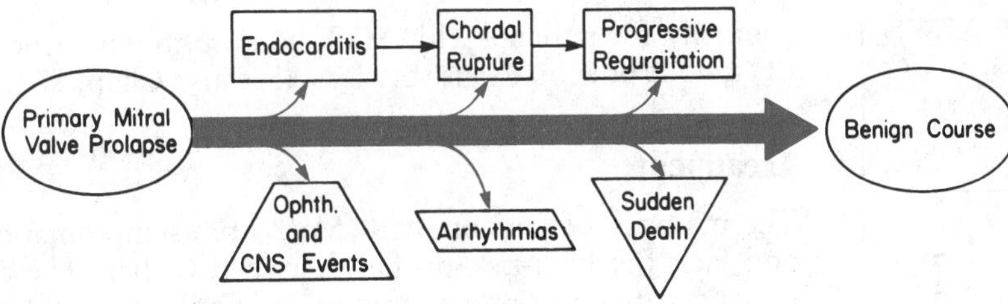

FIGURE 80-22 The course and possible complications of mitral valve prolapse. In most patients the mitral valve prolapse syndrome is associated with a benign prognosis. CNS = central nervous system; Ophth = ophthalmologic. *(From MH Crawford, RA O'Rourke: In: KJ Isselbacher et al (eds): Harrison's Principles of Internal Medicine, 9th ed. New York, McGraw-Hill, 1980: 91–105. Reproduced with permission from the publisher, editors, and authors.)*

adjusted survival rate for both males and females with MVP is similar to that in patients without this common clinical entity. The gradual progression of mitral regurgitation in patients with mitral prolapse, however, may result in progressive dilatation of the left atrium and ventricle. Left atrial dilatation often results in atrial fibrillation, and moderate to severe mitral regurgitation eventually results in left ventricular dysfunction and the development of congestive heart failure.[303] Pulmonary hypertension may occur with associated right ventricular dysfunction. In some patients, with an initially prolonged asymptomatic interval, the entire process may enter an accelerated phase as a result of left atrial and left ventricular dysfunction, atrial fibrillation, and in certain instances ruptured mitral valve chordae.[303] The latter occurs more commonly in males and with increasing age.[301,303]

Several long-term prognostic studies suggest that complications occur most commonly in patients with a mitral systolic murmur, in patients with thickened redundant mitral valve leaflets, and in patients with increased left ventricular or left atrial size (Fig. 80-23).

In a prospective follow-up study of 237 asymptomatic or minimally symptomatic patients with MVP documented by echocardiography, sudden death occurred in 6 patients.[347] In a multivariant analysis of the echocardiographic findings, the presence or absence of redundant mitral valve leaflets by M-mode echocardiography was the only variable associated with sudden death. Ten patients sustained a cerebral embolic event, six of whom were in atrial fibrillation with left atrial enlargement.

Marks et al.[342] confirmed these data in a retrospective two-dimensional echocardiographic study from 456 patients with MVP. Two groups of patients were compared: those with thickening and redundancy of the mitral valve leaflet and those without leaflet thickening. Complications, or a history of complications, were more prevalent in those with leaflet thickening and redundancy compared to those without leaflet thickening. The incidence of stroke, however, was similar in the two groups.

Long-term follow-up studies in patients with MVP associated with a floppy, myxomatous mitral valve permit several conclusions.[303] Serious complications occur in some patients with MVP, predominantly in those with diagnostic auscultatory findings. Also, redundant mitral valve leaflets and increased left ventricular size are associated with a high frequency of serious complications. Finally, men and those over 50 years of age are at increased risk of complications, including severe mitral regurgitation requiring surgery.[303]

Sudden death is the least common but obviously the most severe complication of mitral valve prolapse (Table 80-5). While infrequent, the highest incidence of sudden death has been reported in the familial form of MVP. Some of these patients have been noted to have QT-prolongation. Also, patients with MVP with severe autonomic dysfunction and excessive vagotonia resulting in bradyarrhythmias and asystole have been reported.[176,303,349] Therefore, arrhythmias likely are the usual cause of sudden death in patients with MVP, so it seems prudent to limit ambulatory electrocardiographic recordings to those patients at highest risk. Many believe

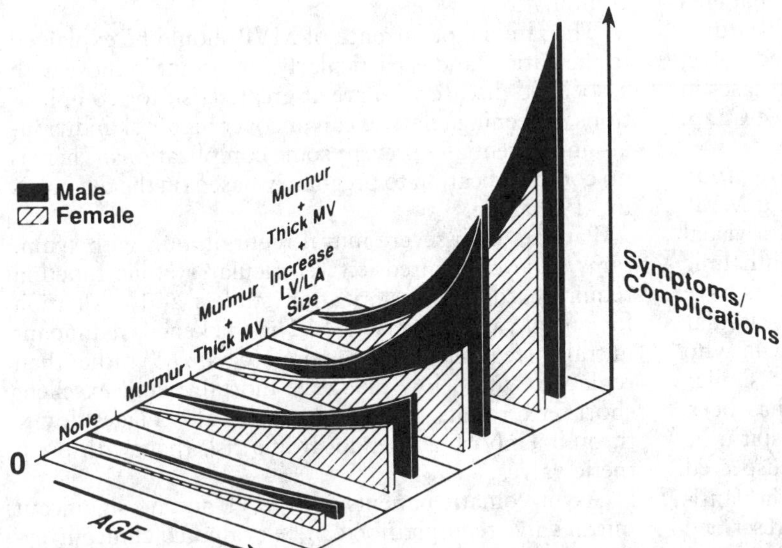

FIGURE 80-23 The relations between cardiac structure, age, and complications in the mitral valve (MV) prolapse syndrome. Patients with mitral valve prolapse, typical auscultatory findings, thickening of the valve leaflets, and left ventricular (LV) or left atrial (LA) enlargement are at risk of developing complications. When two or more of these findings are present, the likelihood of complications is highest. By contrast, the absence of these features can be used to identify patients with mitral valve prolapse who have an exceedingly low risk. In general, complications increase with age and are more common in males than in females. *(From BH Kolibash, CF Wooley: Primary Cardiology, in press. Reproduced with permission from the publisher and authors.)*

TABLE 80-5

Mitral Valve Complications in 102 Hearts with Mitral Valve Prolapse

	No.	%
Sudden death	0	0
Primary rupture of chordae	7	7
Bacterial endocarditis	7	7
Mitral valve regurgitation	18	18
Primary rupture of chordae	(7)	—
Bacterial endocarditis	(4)	—
Severe prolapse	(4)	—
Entrapped chordae	(3)	—
Fibrin deposits	4	4

SOURCE: Modified from RV Lucas Jr, JE Edwards: The floppy mitral valve. *Curr Probl Cardiol* 1982;1:1–60.

that patients with electrocardiographic ST-T wave changes are more likely to have complex ventricular arrhythmias.[301,303] Certainly, any patients with symptoms suggestive of arrhythmias or who have arrhythmias noted during physical examination or on the resting electrocardiogram should be evaluated further. (See Chap. 36.)

Infective endocarditis is a serious complication of MVP,[301,303,350] and MVP is the leading predisposing cardiovascular diagnosis in most series of patients reported with endocarditis. Since the absolute incidence of endocarditis is extremely low for the entire MVP population, there has been much discussion concerning the risk of endocarditis in MVP.[350] While there is general agreement that MVP patients with murmurs and/or thickened redundant valves confirmed by echocardiography or cineangiography should receive antibiotic prophylaxis, some authorities state that the patients with isolated systolic clicks and no murmurs do not need antibiotic prophylaxis for endocarditis.[351] The dynamic nature of MVP, with variable physical findings on different examinations, makes it difficult to make judgments on the basis of the presence or absence of a systolic murmur. With the increasing use of color-flow echo-Doppler studies, mitral regurgitation often has been observed in patients in whom no murmur is heard.[352,353] Since endocarditis can cause destruction of even a mildly affected valve, prophylaxis would seem warranted in nearly all cases in which the diagnosis of MVP seems certain. (See Chap. 94.)

As indicated above, *progressive mitral regurgitation* occurs frequently in patients with long-standing MVP. *Fibrin emboli* are responsible in some patients for visual problems consistent with involvement of the ophthalmic or posterior cerebral circulation.[339] Several studies have indicated an increased likelihood of cerebral vascular accidents of various types in patients under age 45 who have MVP than would have been expected in a similar population without MVP.[334–338] Therefore, it has been recommended that antiplatelet drugs such as aspirin be administered to patients who have MVP and suspected cerebral nervous system emboli. However, neither antiplatelet drugs nor anticoagulants should be prescribed routinely for patients with MVP because the incidence of embolic phenomena is very low. (See also Chap. 122.)

Treatment

The majority of patients with MVP are asymptomatic and lack the high-risk profile described earlier. These patients with mild or no symptoms and findings of milder forms of prolapse should be reassured of a benign prognosis. A normal life-style and regular exercise is encouraged.[214,303]

We recommend antibiotic prophylaxis for the prevention of infective endocarditis while undergoing procedures associated with bacteremia for most patients in whom the diagnosis of MVP is definite.[214] Patients with MVP and palpitation associated with sinus tachycardia or mild tachyarrhythmias and those with chest pain, anxiety, or fatigue often respond to therapy with beta blockers.[214,303,354] In many cases, however, the cessation of catecholamine stimulants such as caffeine, alcohol, cigarettes, and certain drugs[303] may be sufficient to control symptoms.

Orthostatic symptoms are best treated with volume expansion, preferably by liberalizing fluid and salt intake. Mineralcorticoid therapy may be needed in severe cases, and wearing support stockings may be beneficial.[303] In sudden death survivors and those patients with symptomatic complex arrhythmias, specific antiarrhythmic therapy should be guided by monitoring techniques, including electrophysiologic testing when indicated (Chap. 46).[303]

Daily aspirin therapy (80 to 325 mg/day) is recommended for MVP patients with documented focal neurologic events. Such patients also should avoid cigarettes and oral contraceptives. Some clinicians utilize long-term anticoagulant therapy with warfarin in poststroke patients with prolapse, particularly when symptoms occur on aspirin therapy. (See also Chap. 122.)

Restriction from competitive sports is recommended when moderate left ventricular enlargement, left ventricular dysfunction, uncontrolled tachyarrhythmias, long QT interval, unexplained syncope, prior sudden death, or aortic root enlargement is present, individually or in combination.[303]

The familial occurrence of MVP should be explained to the patient and is particularly important in those with associated disease who are at greater risk for complications. Screening relatives can uncover high-risk individuals and potentially prevent some complications. There is no contraindication to pregnancy based on the diagnosis of MVP alone.

Patients with severe mitral regurgitation with symptoms and/or impaired left ventricular systolic function require cardiac catheterization studies and evaluation for mitral valve surgery.[355–358] The thickened, redundant mitral valve often can be repaired (Chap. 85) rather than replaced, with a low operative mortality and excellent short-term results. Follow-up studies also suggest lower thromboembolic and endocarditis risk than with prosthetic valves.

Asymptomatic patients with MVP and no significant mitral valve regurgitation can be evaluated clinically every 2 to 3 years. Echocardiography has been suggested every 5 years in such patients to help determine the natural history and the likelihood of complications.[303] Patients with MVP who have high-risk characteristics, including those with moderate to severe regurgitation, should be followed more frequently, even if no symptoms are present.

REFERENCES

1. Perloff JK, Roberts WC: The mitral apparatus. Functional anatomy of mitral regurgitation. *Circulation* 1972; 46:227–239.
2. Nasser WK, Davis RH, Dillon JC, Tavel ME, Helmen CH, Feigenbuam H, et al: Atrial myxoma: Clinical and pathological features in nine cases. *Am Heart J* 1972; 83:694–704.
3. Buchbinder NA, Roberts WC: Left-sided valvular active infective endocarditis: A study of forty-five necropsy patients. *Am J Med* 1972; 53:20–35.
4. Hammer WJ, Roberts WC, de Leon AC Jr: "Mitral stenosis" secondary to combined "massive" mitral annular calcific deposits and small, hypertrophied left ventricles: Hemodynamic documentation in four patients. *Am J Med* 1978; 64:371–376.
5. Osterberger LE, Goldstein S, Khaja F, Lakier JB: Functional mitral stenosis in patients with massive mitral annular calcification. *Circulation* 1981; 64:472–476.
6. Bonnabeau RV Jr, Stevenson JE, Edwards JE: Obliteration of the principal orifice of the stenotic mitral valve: A rare form of "Re-Stenosis." *J Thorac Cardiovasc Surg* 1965; 49:264–268.
7. Wooley CF, Baba N, Kilman JW, Ryan JM: Thrombotic calcific mitral stenosis: Morphology of the calcific mitral valve. *Circulation* 1974; 49:1167–1174.
8. Jordon RA, Scheifley CH, Edwards JE: Mural thrombosis and arterial embolism in mitral stenosis: A clinicopathologic study of fifty-one cases. *Circulation* 1951; 3:363–367.
9. Shone JD, Sellers RD, Anderson RC, Adams P Jr, Lillehei CW: The developmental complex of "parachute mitral valve," supravalvular ring of left atrium, subaortic stenosis and coarctation of aorta. *Am J Cardiol* 1963; 11:714–725.
10. da Silva CL, Edwards JE: Parachute mitral valve in an adult. *Arq Bras Cardiol* 1973; 26:149.
11. Olson LJ, Subramanian R, Ackermann DM: Surgical pathology of the mitral valve: A study of 712 cases spanning 21 years. *Mayo Clin Proc* 1987; 62:22–29.
12. Nestico PF, DePace NL, Kotler MN, Rose LI, Brezin JH, Swartz C, et al: Calcium phosphorus metabolism in dialysis patients with and without mitral annular calcium: Analysis of 30 patients. *Am J Cardiol* 1983; 51:497–500.
13. Labovitz AJ, Nelson JG, Windhurst DM, Kennedy HL, Williams GA: Frequency of mitral valve dysfunction from mitral annular calcium as detected by Doppler echocardiography. *Am J Cardiol* 1985; 55:133–137.
14. Kennedy JW, Yarnall SR, Murray JA, Figley MM: Quantitative angiocardiography: IV. Relationships of left atrial and ventricular pressure and volume in mitral valve disease. *Circulation* 1970; 41:817–824.
15. Braunwald E, Braunwald NS, Ross J Jr, Morrow AG: Effects of mitral valve replacement on the pulmonary vascular dynamics of patients with pulmonary hypertension. *N Engl J Med* 1965; 273:509–514.
16. Dalen JE, Matloff JM, Evans GL, Hoppin FG Jr, Bhardwaj P, Harken DE, et al: Early reduction of pulmonary vascular resistance after mitral valve replacement. *N Engl J Med* 1967; 277:387–394.
17. Levine MJ, Weinstein JS, Diver DJ, Berman AD, Wyman RM, Cunningham MJ, et al: Progressive improvement in pulmonary vascular resistance after percutaneous mitral valvuloplasty. *Circulation* 1989; 79:1061–1067.
18. Curry GC, Elliott LP, Ramsey HW: Quantitative left ventricular angiocardiographic findings in mitral stenosis: Detailed analysis of the anterolateral wall of the left ventricle. *Am J Cardiol* 1972; 29:621–627.
19. Silverstein DM, Hansen DP, Ojiambo HP, Griswold HE: Left ventricular function in severe pure mitral stenosis as seen at the Kenyatta National Hospital. *Am Heart J* 1980; 99:727–733.
20. Wroblewski E, Spann JF, Bove AA: Right ventricular performance in mitral stenosis. *Am J Cardiol* 1981; 47:51–57.
21. Thompson CR, Kingma I, MacDonald RPR: Transseptal pressure gradient and diastolic ventricular septal motion in patients with mitral stenosis. *Circulation* 1987; 76:974–980.
22. Wroblewski E, Spann JF, Bove AA: Right ventricular performance in mitral stenosis. *Am J Cardiol* 1981; 47:51–55.
23. Gaasch WH, Folland ED: Left ventricular function in rheumatic mitral stenosis. *Eur Heart J* 1991: 12(suppl B): 66–69.
24. Liu C, Ting C, Yang T, Chen J, Chang M, Maughan WL, et al: Reduced left ventricular compliance in human mitral stenosis: Role of reversible internal constraint. *Circulation* 1992; 85:1447–1456.
25. Rowe JC, Bland EF, Sprague HB, White PD: The course of mitral stenosis without surgery: Ten and twenty year perspectives. *Ann Intern Med* 1960; 52:741–749.
26. Wood P: An appreciation of mitral stenosis. *Br Med J* 1954; 1:1051–1063.
27. Selzer A, Cohn KE: Natural history of mitral stenosis: A review. *Circulation* 1972; 45:878–890.
28. Szekely P, Turner R, Snaith L: Pregnancy and the changing pattern of rheumatic heart disease. *Br Heart J* 1973; 35:1293–1303.
29. Schwartz R, Meyerson RM, Lawrence LT, Nichols HT: Mitral stenosis, massive pulmonary hemorrhage and emergency valve replacement. *N Engl J Med* 1966; 272:755–758.
30. Ross RS: Right ventricular hypertension as a cause of precordial pain. *Am Heart J* 1961; 61:134–137.
31. Baker CG, Finnegan TRL: Epilepsy and mitral stenosis. *Br Heart J* 1957; 19:159–163.
32. Mounsey JP: Inspection and palpation of the cardiac impulse. *Prog Cardiovasc Dis* 1967; 10:187–206.
33. Thompson ME, Shaver JA, Heidenreich FP, Leon DF, Leonard JJ: Sound, pressure and motion correlates in mitral stenosis. *Am J Med* 1970; 49:436–450.
34. Luisada AA, MacCanon DM, Kumar S, Feigen LP: Changing views on the mechanism of the first and second heart sounds. *Am Heart J* 1974; 88:503–514.
35. Wooley CF, Klassen KP, Leighton RF, Goodwin RS, Ryan JM: Left atrial and left ventricular sound and pressure in mitral stenosis. *Circulation* 1968; 38:295–307.
36. Dack S, Bleifer S, Grishman A, et al: Mitral stenosis: Auscultatory and phonocardiographic findings. *Am J Cardiol* 1960; 5:815–835.
37. Mounsey P: The opening snap of mitral stenosis. *Br Heart J* 1953; 15:135–142.
38. Wells B: The assessment of mitral stenosis by phonocardiography. *Br Heart J* 1954; 16:261–266.
39. Rackley CE, Craig RJ, McIntosh HD, Orgain ES: Phonocardiographic discrepancies in the assessment of mitral stenosis. *Arch Intern Med* 1968; 121:50–53.
40. Ebringer R, Pitt A, Anderson ST: Haemodynamic factors influencing opening snap interval in mitral stenosis. *Br Heart J* 1970; 32:350–354.
41. Nixon PG, Wooler GH, Radigan LR: The opening snap in mitral incompetence. *Br Heart J* 1960; 22:395–402.
42. Millward DK, McLaurin LP, Craige E: Echocardiographic studies to explain opening snaps in presence of non-stenotic mitral valves. *Am J Cardiol* 1973; 31:64–70.
43. Leatham A, Gray I: Auscultatory and phonocardiographic signs of atrial septal defect. *Br Heart J* 1956; 18:193–225.
44. Vacca JB, Bussman DW, Mudd JG: Ebstein's anomaly: Complete review of 108 cases. *Am J Cardiol* 1958; 2:210–226.
45. Perloff JK, Harvey WP: Clinical recognition of tricuspid stenosis. *Circulation* 1960; 22:346.
46. Crawley IS, Morris DC, Silverman BD: Valvular heart disease. In: Hurst JW, Logue RB, Schlant RC, Wenger NK (eds): *The Heart,* 4th ed. New York, McGraw-Hill, 1978, 992–1081.
47. Surawicz B: Effect of respiration and upright position on the interval between the two components of the second heart sound and that between the second sound and mitral opening snap. *Circulation* 1957; 16:422–424.
48. Fortuin NJ, Craige E: Echocardiographic studies of genesis of mitral diastolic murmurs. *Br Heart J* 1973; 35:75–81.
49. Lakier JB, Pocock WA, Gale GE, Barlow JB: Haemodynamic and

sound event preceding first heart sound in mitral stenosis. *Br Heart J* 1972; 34:1152–1155.
50. Bonner AJ Jr, Stewart J, Travel ME: "Presystolic" augmentation of diastolic heart sounds in atrial fibrillation. *Am J Cardiol* 1976; 37:427–431.
51. McGuire LB, Nolan TB, Reeve R, et al: Cor triatriatum as a problem of heart disease. *Circulation* 1965; 31:263.
52. Korn D, DeSanctis RW, Sell S: Massive calcification of the mitral annulus. *N Engl J Med* 1962; 267:900–909.
53. Spodick DH: *Chronic and Constrictive Pericarditis.* New York, Grune & Stratton, 1964.
54. McArthur JD, Sukumar IP, Munsi SC, et al: Reassessment of Graham Steell murmur using platinum electrode technique. *Br Heart J* 1974; 36:1023–1027.
55. Saunders JL, Calatayud JB, Schultz KJ, Maranhao V, Gooch AS, Goldberg H: Evaluation of ECG criteria for P-wave abnormalities. *Am Heart J* 74:757–765.
56. Lee YC, Scherlis L, Singleton RT: Mitral stenosis: Hemodynamic, electrocardiographic and vector cardiographic studies. *Am Heart J* 1965: 69:559–566.
57. Walston A, Harley A, Pipberger HV: Computer analysis of the orthogonal electrocardiogram and vectorcardiogram in mitral stenosis. *Circulation* 1974; 50:472–478.
58. Chen JT, Behar VS, Morris JJ Jr, McIntosh J, Lester RG: Correlation of roentgen findings with hemodynamic data in pure mitral stenosis. *Am J Roentgenol Radium Ther Nucl Med* 1968; 102:280–292.
59. Grainger RG: Interstitial pulmonary edema and its radiographic diagnosis: Signs of pulmonary edema and its radiographic diagnosis: Signs of pulmonary venous and capillary hypertension. *Br J Radiol* 1958; 31:301–217.
60. Felson B: *Chest Roentgenology.* Philadelphia, Saunders, 1973.
61. Chait A: Interstitial pulmonary edema. *Circulation* 1972; 45:1323–1330.
62. Meszaros WT: Lung changes in left heart failure. *Circulation* 1973; 47:859–871.
63. Duchak JM, Chang S, Feigenbaum H: The posterior mitral valve echo and the echocardiographic diagnosis of mitral stenosis. *Am J Cardill* 1972; 29:628–632.
64. Teichholz E: Echocardiography in valvular heart disease. *Prog Cardiovasc Dis* 1975; 17:283–302.
65. Cope GD, Kisslo JA, Johnson ML, Behar VS: A reassessment of the echocardiogram in mitral stenosis. *Circulation* 1975; 52:664–678.
66. Lutas EM, Devereux RB, Borer JS, Goldstein JE: Echocardiographic evaluation of mitral stenosis: A critical appraisal of its clinical value in detection of severe stenosis and valvular calcification. *J Cardiovasc Ultrasonog* 1983; 2:131–139.
67. Yang SS, Goldberg H: Simplied Doppler estimate of mitral valve area. *Am J Cardiol* 1985; 56:488–489.
68. Smith MD, Handshoe R, Handshoe S, Kwan OL, DeMaria AN: Comparative accuracy of two-dimensional echocardiography and Doppler pressure half-time methods in assessing severity of mitral stenosis in patients with and without prior commissurotomy. *Circulation* 1986; 73:100–107.
69. Pearlman JD, Gibson RS: Doppler measurement of left atrial depressurization and mitral valve area in patients with suspected mitral stenosis: Validation of a new method. *Am Heart J* 1987; 113:868–873.
70. Wolfe SB, Popp RL, Feigenbaum H: Diagnosis of atrial tumors by ultrasound. *Circulation* 1969; 39:615–622.
71. McLauriny LP, Gibson TC, Waider W, Grossman W, Craige E: An appraisal of mitral valve echocardiograms mimicking mitral stenosis in conditions with right ventricular pressure overload. *Circulation* 1973; 48:801–809.
72. Quinones MA, Gaasch WH, Waisser E, Alexander JK: Reduction in the rate of diastolic descent of the mitral valve echogram in patients with altered left ventricular diastolic pressure-volume. *Circulation* 1974; 49:246–254.
73. Stewart JA, Silimperi D, Harris P, Wise NK, Fraker TD Jr, Kisslo JA: Echocardiographic documentation of vegetative lesions in infective endocarditis: Clinical implications. *Circulation* 1980; 61:374–380.
74. Gorlin R, Gorlin SG: Hydraulic formula for calculation of the area of the stenotic mitral valve, other cardiac valves and central circulatory shunts. *Am Heart J* 1951; 41:1–29.
75. Cohen MV, Gorlin R: Modified orifice equation for the calculation of mitral valve area. *Am Heart J* 1972; 84:839–840.
76. Hakki A, Iskandrian AS, Bemis CE, Hakki AH, Kimbiris D, Mintz GS, et al: A simplified valve formula for the calculation of stenotic valve areas. *Circulation* 1981; 63:1050–1055.
77. Carabello BA, Grossman W: Calculation of stenotic valve orifice area. In: Grossman W (ed): *Cardiac Catheterization and Angiography,* 3d ed. Philadelphia, Lea & Febiger, 1986:143–154.
78. Hungenholtz PG, Ryan TJ, Stein SW, Abelmann WH: The spectrum of pure mitral stenosis: Hemodynamic studies in relation to clinical disability. *Am J Cardiol* 1962; 10:773–784.
79. Bolen JL, Lopes MG, Harrison DC, Alderman EL: Analysis of left ventricular function in response to afterload changes in patients with mitral stenosis. *Circulation* 1975; 52:894.
80. Heller SJ, Carleton RA: Abnormal left ventricular contraction in patients with mitral stenosis. *Circulation* 1970; 42:1099–1110.
81. Hildner FJ, Javier RP, Cohen LS, Samet P, Nathan MJ, Yahr WZ, et al: Myocardial dysfunction associated with valvular heart disease. *Am J Cardiol* 1972; 30:319–326.
82. Chun PK, Gertz E, Davia JE, Cheitlin MD: Coronary atherosclerosis in mitral stenosis. *Chest* 1982; 81:36–41.
83. Newman GE, Bounous PW, Jones RH, Rerych SK, Bounous PE, Upton MT: Noninvasive assessment of hemodynamic effects of mitral valve commissurotomy during rest and exercise in patients with mitral stenosis. *J Thorac Cardiovasc Surg* 1979; 78:750–756.
84. Bhathia ML, Shriuastava S, Roy SB: Immediate haemodynamic effects of a beta adrenergic blocking agent, propranolol in mitral stenosis at fixed heart rates. *Br Heart J* 1972; 34:638.
85. Meister SG, Engel TR, Feitosa GS, Helfant RH, Frankl WS: Propranolol in mitral stenosis during stress rhythm. *Am Heart J* 1977; 94:685–688.
86. Giuffrida G, Bonzani G, Betocchi S, Piscione F, Guiduice P, Miccli D, et al: Hemodynamic response to exercise after propranolol in patients with mitral stenosis. *Am J Cardiol* 1979; 44:1076–1082.
87. Reid CL, McKay CR, Chandraratna PA, Kawanishi DT, Rahimtoola SH: Mechanisms of increase in mitral valve area and influence of anatomic features in double-balloon, catheter balloon valvuloplasty in adults with rheumatic mitral stenosis: A Doppler and two-dimensional echocardiographic study. *Circulation* 1987; 76:628–636.
88. Carroll JD, Feldman T: The new face of mitral stenosis in the 1990's: Demographics and percutaneous mitral balloon valvotomy. *JAMA* 1993, (in press).
89. Abernathy WS, Willis PW III: Thromboembolic complications of rheumatic heart disease. *Cardiovasc Clin* 1973; 5:131–175.
90. Kellogg F, Lui CK, Fishman W, Larson R: Systemic and pulmonary emboli before and after mitral commissurotomy. *Circulation* 1961; 24:263–266.
91. Rapaport E: Natural history of aortic and mitral valve disease. *Am J Cardiol* 1975; 35:221–227.
92. Olesen KH: The natural history of 271 patients with mitral stenosis under medical treatment. *Br Heart J* 1962; 24:349–357.
93. Rowe JC, Bland EF, Sprague HB, White PD: The course of mitral stenosis without surgery: Ten and twenty year perspectives. *Ann Intern Med* 1975; 35:234-242.
94. Munoz S, Gallardo J, Diaz-Gorrin JR, Medina O: Influence of surgery on the natural history of rheumatic mitral and aortic valve disease. *Am J Cardiol* 1975; 35:234–242.
95. Rackley CE: Valvular heart disease. In *Cecil's Textbook of Medicine* 18th ed. Wyngaarden JB, Smith LH, (eds.) Philadelphia, Saunders, 1988: 340–352.
96. Kan JS, White RI, Mitchell SE, Gardner TJ: Percutaneous balloon valvuloplasty: A new method for treating congenital pulmonary valve stenosis. *N Engl J Med* 1982; 307:540–542.
97. Patel JJ, Shama D, Mitha AS, Blyth D, Hassan F, LeRoux BT, et al: Balloon valvuloplasty versus closed commissurotomy for pliable mitral stenosis: A prospective hemodynamic study *J Am Coll Cardiol* 1991; 18:1318–1322.
98. Turi ZG, Reyes VP, Raju BS, Raju AR, Kumar DN, Rajagopal P, et al: Percutaneous balloon versus surgical closed commissurotomy for mitral stenosis. A prospective randomized trial. *Circulation* 1991; 83:1179–1185.
99. The National Heart, Lung, and Blood Institute Balloon Valvuloplasty Registry Participants: Multicenter experience with balloon mitral commissurotomy. NHLBI balloon valvuloplasty reg-

istry report on immediate and 30-day follow-up results. *Circulation* 1992; 85:448–461.

100. Cohen DJ, Kuntz RE, Gordon SPF, Piana RN, Safian RD, McKay RG, et al: Predictors of long-term outcome after percutaneous balloon mitral valvuloplasty. *N Engl J Med* 1992; 327:1329–1335.
101. Block PC, Palacios IF, Block EH, Tuzcu EM, Griffin B: Late (two-year) follow-up after percutaneous balloon mitral valvotomy. *Am J Cardiol* 1992; 69:537–541.
102. Desideri A, Vanderperren O, Serra A, Barraud P, Petitclerc R, Lespérance J, et al: Long-term (9 to 33 months) echocardiographic follow-up after successful percutaneous mitral commissurotomy. *Am J Cardiol* 1992; 69:1602–1606.
103. Stefanadis C, Stratos C, Pitsavos C, Kallikazaros I, Triposkiadis F, Trikas A, et al: Retrograde nontransseptal balloon mitral valvuloplasty. Immediate results and long-term follow-up. *Circulation* 1992; 85:1760–1767.
104. National Heart, Lung, and Blood Institute Balloon Valvuloplasty Registry: Complications and mortality of percutaneous balloon mitral commissurotomy. *Circulation* 1992; 85:2014–2024.
105. Hickley MSJ, Blackstone EH, Kirklin JW, Dean LS: Outcome probabilities and life history after surgical mitral commissurotomy: Implications for balloon commissurotomy. *J Am Coll Cardiol* 1991; 17:29–42.
106. Cohn LH, Allred EN, Cohn LA, DiSesa VJ, Shemin RJ, Collins JJ Jr: Long term results of open mitral valve reconstruction for mitral stenosis. *Am J Cardiol* 1985; 55:731–734.
107. Cohen DJ, Kuntz RE, Gordon SPF, Piana RN, Safian RD, McKay RG, et al: Predictors of long-term outcome after percutaneous balloon mitral valvuloplasty. *N Engl J Med* 1992; 327:1329–1335.
108. Lefevre T, Bonan R, Serra A, Crepeau J, Dyrda I, Petitclerc R, et al: Percutaneous mitral valvuloplasty in surgical high risk patients. *J Am Coll Cardiol* 1991; 17:348–354.
109. Ward C, Hancock BW: Extreme pulmonary hypertension caused by mitral valve disease. Natural history and results of surgery. *Br Heart J* 1975; 37:74–78.
110. Braunwald E, Braunwald NS, Ross J Jr, Morrow AG: Effects of mitral valve replacement on the pulmonary vascular dynamics of patients with pulmonary hypertension. *N Engl J Med* 1965; 273:509–514.
111. Cohn LH, Allred EN, Cohn LA, Austin J, Sabik J, DiSesa VJ, et al: Early and late risk of mitral valve replacement: A 12-year concomitant comparison of porcine bioprosthetic and prosthetic disc mitral valves. *J Thorac Cardiovasc Surg* 1985; 90:872–881.
112. Zener JC, Hancock EW, Shumway NE, Harrison DC: Regression of extreme pulmonary hypertension after mitral valve surgery. *Am J Cardiol* 1972; 30:820–826.
113. Larrea JL, Nunez L, Reque A, Aguado MG, Matarros R, Minguez JA: Pregnancy and mechanical valve prostheses: A high-risk situation for the mother and the fetus. *Ann Thorac Surg* 1983; 36:459–463.
114. Esteves CA, Ramos AIO, Braga SLN, Harrison JK, Sousa JEMR: Effectiveness of percutaneous balloon mitral valvotomy during pregnancy. *Am J Cardiol* 1991; 68:930–934.
115. Becker RM: Intracardiac surgery in pregnant women. *Ann Thorac Surg* 1983; 36:453–458.
116. Eguaras MG, Luque I, Montero A, Garcia MA, Calleja F, Roman M, et al: A comparison of repair and replacement for mitral stenosis with partially calcified valve. *J Thorac Cardiovasc Surg* 1990; 100:161–166.
117. Starr A: Total mitral valve replacement, fixation, and thrombosis. *Surg Forum* 1960; 11:258–259.
118. Rozich JD, Carabello BA, Usher BW, Kratz JM, Bell AE, Zile MR: Mitral valve replacement with and without chordal preservation in patients with chronic mitral regurgitation: Mechanisms for differences in postoperative ejection performance. *Circulation* 1992; 86:1718–1726.
119. Salazar E, Zajarias A, Gutierrez N, Iturbe I: The problem of cardiac prostheses, anticoagulants, and pregnancy. *Circulation* 1984; 70(suppl I):I-169–I-177.
120. Sato S, Kawashima Y, Hirose H, Nakano S, Matsuda H, Shirakura R: Long-term results of direct-current cardioversion after open commissurotomy for mitral stenosis. *Am J Cardiol* 1986; 57:629–633.
121. He G-W, Hughes CF, McCaughan B, Thomson DS, Leckie BD, Yang C-Q, et al: Mitral valve replacement combined with coronary artery operation: Determinants of early and late results. *Ann Thorac Surg* 1991; 51:916–923.
122. Scott WC, Miller DC, Haverich A, Mitchell RS, Oyer PE, Stinson EB, et al: Operative risk of mitral valve replacement: Discriminant analysis of 1329 procedures. *Circulation* 1985; 72(suppl II):II-108–II-119.
123. Teoh KH, Ivanov J, Weisel RD: Determinants of survival and valve failure after mitral valve replacement. *Ann Thorac Surg* 1990; 49:643–648.
124. Cohn LH, Couper GS, Kinchla NM, Collins JJ Jr: Decreased operative risk of surgical treatment of mitral regurgitation with or without coronary artery disease. *J Am Coll Cardiol* 1990; 16:1575–1578.
125. Grunkemeier GL, Rahimtoola SH: Artificial heart valves. *Annu Rev Med* 1990; 41:251–263.
126. Silverman ME, Hurst JW: The mitral complex. *Am Heart J* 1968; 76:399–418.
127. Barlow JB, Pocock WA: The problem of nonejection systolic clicks and associated mitral systolic murmurs: Emphasis on the billowing mitral leaflet syndrome. *Am Heart J* 1975; 90:636–655.
128. Rackley CE, Dear HD, Baxley WA, Jones WB, Dodge HT: Left ventricular chamber volume, mass and function in severe coronary artery disease. *Circulation* 1970; 41:605–613.
129. Perloff JK, Roberts WC: The mitral apparatus: Functional anatomy of mitral regurgitation. *Circulation* 1972; 46:227–239.
130. Rytand DA, Lipsitch LS: Clinical aspects of calcification of the mitral annulus fibrosus. *Arch Intern Med* 1946; 78:544–564.
131. Roberts WC, Dangel JC, Bulkley BH: Nonrheumatic valvular cardiac disease: A clinicopathologic survey of 27 different conditions causing valvular dysfunction, in Likoff W (guest ed): *Valvular Heart Disease. Cardiovasc Clin* 1973; 5(2):333–446.
132. McKusick VA: *Heritable Disorders of Connective Tissue.* St. Louis, Mosby, 1972.
133. Burch GE, DePasquale NP, Phillips JH: Clinical manifestation of papillary muscle dysfunction. *Arch Intern Med* 1963; 112:112–117.
134. Heikkila J: Mitral incompetence complicating acute myocardial infarction. *Br Heart J* 1967; 29:162–169.
135. DeBusk RF, Harrison DC: The clinical spectrum of papillary-muscle disease. *N Engl J Med* 1969; 281:1458–1467.
136. Fowler NO, Van der Mel-Kahn JM: Indications for surgical replacement of the mitral valve; with particular reference to common and uncommon causes of mitral regurgitation. *Am J Cardiol* 1979; 44:148–157.
137. Selzer A, Kelly JJ Jr, Vannitamby M, Walker P, Gerbode F, Kerth WJ: The syndrome of mitral insufficiency due to isolated rupture of the chordae tendineae. *Am J Med* 1967; 43:822–836.
138. Sanders CA, Armstrong PW, Willerson JT, Dinsmore RE: Etiology and differential diagnosis of acute mitral regurgitation. *Prog Cardiovasc Dis* 1971; 14:129–152.
139. Edwards JE: Pathology of acquired valvular disease of the heart. *Semin Roentgenol* 1979; 14:96–115.
140. Perloff JK, Roberts WC: The mitral apparatus: Functional anatomy of mitral regurgitation. *Circulation* 1972; 46:227–239.
141. Burchell HB, Edwards JE: Rheumatic mitral insufficiency. *Circulation* 1953; 7:747–756.
142. Levy MJ, Edwards JE: Anatomy of mitral insufficiency. *Prog Cardiovasc Dis* 1962; 5:119–144.
143. Edwards JE, Burchell HB: Pathologic anatomy of mitral insufficiency. *Proc Mayo Clin* 1958; 33:497–509.
144. Vlodaver Z, Edwards JE: Rupture of ventricular septum or papillary muscle complicating myocardial infarction. *Circulation* 1977; 55:815–822.
145. Lee KS, Johnson T, Karnegis JN, Quattlebaum FW, Edwards JE: Acute myocardial infarction with long-term survival following papillary muscle rupture. *Am Heart J* 1970; 79:258–264.
146. Tsakiris AG, Rastelli GC, Amorim D, Amorin Ddes, Titus JL, Wood EH: Effect of experimental papillary muscle damage on mitral valve closure in intact anesthetized dogs. *Proc Mayo Clin* 1970; 45:275–285.
147. Moller JH, Lucas RV Jr, Adams P Jr, Anderson RC, Jorgens J, Edwards JE: Endocardial fibroelastosis: A clinical and anatomic study of 47 patients with emphasis on its relationship to mitral insufficiency. *Circulation* 1964; 30:759–782.

148. Pomerance A: Pathological and clinical study of calcification of the mitral valve ring. *Br J Clin Pathol* 1970; 23:354–361.
149. Edwards JE: Mitral insufficiency secondary to aortic valvular bacterial endocarditis. *Circulation* 1972; 46:623–626.
150. Hall SW Jr, Theologides A, From AHL, From AH, Gobel FL, Fortuny IE, et al: Hyperosinophilic syndrome with biventricular involvement. *Circulation* 1977; 55:217–222.
151. Bulkley BH, Roberts WC: Systemic lupus erythematosus as a cause of severe mitral regurgitation: New problem in an old disease. *Am J Cardiol* 1975; 35:305–308.
152. Guthrie RG, Edwards JE: Pathology of the myxomatous mitral valve: Its nature, secondary changes and complications. *Minnesota Med* 1976; 59:637–647.
153. Ranganathan N, Silver MD, Robinson TI, Kostuk WJ, Felderhof CH, Patt NL: Angiographic morphologic correlation in patients with severe mitral regurgitation due to prolapse of the posterior mitral leaflet. *Circulation* 1973; 48:514–518.
154. Salazar AE, Edwards JE: Friction lesions of ventricular endocardium: Relation to chordae tendineae of mitral valve. *Arch Pathol* 1970; 90:364–376.
155. Tomaru T, Uchida Y, Mohri N: Post-inflammatory mitral and aortic valve prolapse: A clinical and pathological study. *Circulation* 1987; 76:68–76.
156. Burch GI, DePasquale NP, Phillips JH: The syndrome of papillary muscle dysfunction. *Am Heart J* 1968; 75:399–415.
157. Hickey MStJ, Smith LR, Muhlbaier LV, Harrell FE Jr, Reves JG, Hinohara T, et al: Current prognosis of ischemic mitral regurgitation: Implications for future management. *Circulation* 1988; 78(3 Pt 2): 151–159.
158. Braunwald E: Mitral regurgitation: Physiologic, clinical and surgical considerations. *N Engl J Med* 1969; 281:425–433.
159. Ross J Jr, Braunwald E, Morrow AG: Clinical and hemodynamic observations in pure mitral insufficiency. *Am J Cardiol* 1958; 2:11.
160. Dodge HT, Baxley WA: Left ventricular volume and mass and their significance in heart disease. *Am J Cardiol* 1969; 23:528–537.
161. Rackley CE, Hood WP Jr: Quantitative angiographic evaluation and pathophysiologic mechanisms in valvular heart disease. In: Sonnenblick EJ, Lesch M (eds): *Valvular Heart Disease.* New York, Grune & Stratton, 1974: 109–129.
162. Hood WP Jr, Rackley CE, Rotlett EL: Wall stress in the normal and hypertrophied human left ventricle. *Am J Cardiol* 1968; 22:550–558.
163. Rackley CE: Value of ventriculography in cardiac function and diagnosis, in Brest AN (ed): *Diagnostic Methods in cardiology. Cardiovasc Clin* 1975; 6(3):283–296.
164. Porter CM, Baxley WA, Eddleman EE Jr, et al: Left ventricular dimensions and dynamics of filling in patients with gallop heart sounds. *Am J Med* 1971; 50:721–727.
165. Rackley CE, Hood WP Jr, Rolett EL, Young DT: Left ventricular end-diastolic pressure in chronic heart disease. *Am J Med* 1970; 48:310–319.
166. Gaasch WH, Levine HJ, Zile MR: Chronic aortic and mitral regurgitation: Mechanical consequences of the lesion and the results of surgical correction. In: Levine HJ, Gaasch WH (eds): *The Ventricle.* Boston, Martinus Nijhoff, 1985:237–258.
167. Borgenhagen DM, Serur JR, Gorlin R, Adams D, Sonnenblick EH: The effects of left ventricular load and contractility on mitral regurgitation orifice size and flow in the dog. *Circulation* 1977; 56:106–113.
168. Keren G, Katz S, Strom J, Sonnenblick EH, LeJemtel TH: Dynamic mitral regurgitation: An important determinant of the hemodynamic response to load alterations and inotropic therapy in severe heart failure. *Circulation* 1989; 80:306–313.
169. Rackley CE, Russell RO Jr, Mantle JA, et al: Modern approach to the patient with acute myocardial infarction. In Harvey WP (ed): *Current Problems in Cardiology,* vol 1. Chicago, Yearbook Medical, 1977, p 10.
170. Boltwood CM, Tei C, Wong M, et al: Quantitative echocardiography of the mitral complex in dilated cardiomyopathy: The mechanism of functional mitral regurgitation. *Circulation* 1983; 68:498–508.
171. Chandraratna PAN, Aronow WS: Mitral valve ring in normal vs dilated left ventricle: Cross-sectional echocardiography study. *Chest* 1981; 79:151–154.
172. Klughaupt M, Flamm MD, Hancock EW, et al: Nonrheumatic mitral insufficiency: Determination of operability and prognosis. *Circulation* 1969; 39:307–316.
173. Jeresaty RM: Mitral valve prolapse-click syndrome. *Prog Cardiovasc Dis* 1973; 15:623–652.
174. Nutter DO, Wickliffe C, Gilbert CA, et al: The pathophysiology of idiopathic mitral valve prolapse. *Circulation* 1975; 52:297–305.
175. Bulkley BH, Roberts WC: Dilatation of the mitral annulus. *Am J Med* 1975; 59:457–463.
176. Gooch AS, Vicencio F, Maranbao V, Goldberg H: Arrhythmias and left ventricle asynergy in the prolapsing mitral leaflet. *Am J Cardiol* 1972; 29:611–620.
177. Newman GE, Gibbons RJ, Jones RH: Cardiac function during rest and exercise in patients with mitral valve prolapse. *Am J Cardiol* 1981; 47:14–19.
178. Aranda JM, Befeler B, Lazzara R, Embi A, Machado H: Mitral valve prolapse and coronary artery disease. *Circulation* 1975; 52:245–253.
179. Verani MS, Carroll RJ, Falsetti HL: Mitral valve prolapse in coronary disease. *Am J Cardiol* 1976; 37:1–6.
180. Sabom MB, Curry RC Jr, Pepine CJ, Christie LG, Conti CR: Ergonovine testing for coronary artery spasm in patients with angiographic mitral valve prolapse. *Cath Cardiovasc Diag* 1978; 4:265–274.
181. Pasternac A, Tubau JF, Puddu PE, Krol RB, de Champlain J: Increased plasma catecholamine levels in patients with symptomatic mitral valve prolapse. *Am J Med* 1982; 73:783–790.
182. Zile MR, Gaasch WH, Levine HJ: Left ventricular stress-shortening relations before and after correction of chronic mitral and aortic regurgitation. *Am J Cardiol* 1985; 56:99–105.
183. Corin WJ, Monrad ES, Murakami T, Nonogi H, Hess OM, Krayenbuehl HP: The relationship of afterload to ejection performance in chronic mitral regurgitation. *Circulation* 1987; 76:59–67.
184. Ross J Jr: Adaptations of the left ventricle to chronic volume overload. *Circ Res* 1974; 35(II):64–70.
185. Corin WJ, Murakami T, Monrad ES, Hess OM, Krayenbuehl HP: Left ventricular passive diastolic properties in chronic mitral regurgitation. *Circulation* 1991; 83:797–807.
186. Vokonas PS, Gorlin R, Cohn PF, Herman MV, Sonnenblick EH: Dynamic geometry of the left ventricle in mitral regurgitation. *Circulation* 1973; 48:786–796.
187. Schuler G, Peterson KL, Johnson A, Francis G, Dennish G, Utley J, et al: Temporal response of left ventricular performance to mitral valve surgery. *Circulation* 1979; 59:1218–1231.
188. Zile MR, Gaasch WH, Carroll JD, Levine HJ: Chronic mitral regurgitation: Predictive value of preoperative echocardiographic indexes of left ventricular function and wall stress. *J Am Coll Cardiol* 1984; 3:235–242.
189. Gaasch WH, Zile MR: Left ventricular function after surgical correction of chronic mitral regurgitation. *Eur Heart J* 1991; 12(suppl B):48–51.
190. Rozich JD, Carabello BA, Usher BW, Kratz JM, Bell AE, Zile MR: Mitral valve replacement with and without chordal preservation in patients with chronic mitral regurgitation. *Circulation* 1992; 86:1718–1726.
191. Krayenbuehl HP: Surgery for mitral regurgitation: Repair versus valve replacement. *Eur Heart J* 1986; 7:638–643.
192. Selzer A, Katayama F: Mitral regurgitation: Clinical patterns, pathophysiology and natural history. *Medicine (Baltimore)* 1972; 51:337–366.
193. Bentivoglio L, Urichio J, Goldberg H: Clinical and hemodynamic features of advanced rheumatic mitral regurgitation. *Am J Med* 1961; 30:372–381.
194. Ellis LB, Ramirez A: The clinical course of patients with severe "rheumatic" mitral insufficiency. *Am Heart J* 1969; 78:406.
195. Brody W, Criley JM: Intermittent severe mitral regurgitation. *N Engl J Med* 1970; 283:673–676.
196. Grenadier E, Pan GA, Keidar S, Alpan G, Palant P: The prevalence of ruptured chordae tendineae in the mitral valve prolapse syndrome. *Am Heart J* 1983; 105:603–610.
197. Winkle RA, Lopes MG, Fitzgerald JW, Goodman DJ: Arrhythmias in patients with mitral valve prolapse. *Circulation* 1975; 52:73–81.

198. Coghlan HC, Phares P, Cowley M, Copley D, James TN: Dysautonomia in mitral valve prolapse. *Am J.Med* 1979; 67:236–244.
199. Basta LL, Wolfson P, Eckberg DL, Abboud FM: The value of left parasternal impulse recordings in the assessment of mitral regurgitation. *Circulation* 1973; 48:1055–1065.
200. Reichek N, Shelburne JC, Perloff JK: Clinical aspects of rheumatic valvular disease. *Prog Cardiovasc Dis* 1973; 15:491–537.
201. Karliner JS, O'Rourke RA, Kearney DJ, Shabetai R: Haemodynamic explanation of why the murmur of mitral regurgitation is independent of cycle length. *Br Heart J* 1973; 35:397–401.
202. Perloff JK, Harvey WP: Auscultatory and phonocardiographic manifestations of pure mitral regurgitation. *Prog Cardiovasc Dis* 1962; 5:172–194.
203. Perloff JK, Harvey WP: Mechanisms of fixed splitting of the second heart sound. *Circulation* 1958; 18:998–1009.
204. Folland ED, Kriegel BJ, Henderson WG, Hammermeister KE, Sethi GK: Implications of third heart sounds in patients with valvular heart disease. *N Engl J Med* 1992; 327:458–462.
204a. Bleifer S, Dack S, Grishman A, et al: The auscultatory and phonocardiographic findings in mitral regurgitation. *Am J Cardiol* 1960; 5:836.
205. Shelburne JC, Rubenstein D, Gorlin R: A reappraisal of papillary muscle dysfunction. *Am J Med* 1969; 46:862–871.
206. Holmes AM, Logan WF, Winterbottom T: Transient systolic murmurs in angina pectoris. *Am Heart J* 1968; 76:680–684.
207. Sanders CA, Austen WG, Harthorne JW, Dinsmore RE, Scannel JG: Diagnosis and surgical treatment of mitral regurgitation secondary to ruptured chordae tendineae. *N Engl J Med* 1967; 276:943–949.
208. Ronan JA Jr, Steelman RB, de Leon AC Jr, Waters TJ, Perloff JK, Harvey WP: The clinical diagnosis of acute severe mitral insufficiency. *Am J Cardiol* 1971; 27:284–290.
209. Sleeper JC, Orgain ES, McIntosh HD: Mitral insufficiency simulating aortic stenosis. *Circulation* 1962; 26:428–433.
210. Goodman D, Kimbiris D, Linhart JW: Chordae tendineae rupture complicating the systolic click-late systolic murmur syndrome. *Am J Cardiol* 1974; 33:681–684.
211. Devereux RB, Perloff JK, Reichek N, Josephson ME: Mitral valve prolapse. *Circulation* 1976; 54:3–14.
212. Santos AD, Puthenpurakal MK, Ahmad H, Wallace WA, Mathew PK, Hilal A: Orthostatic hypotension: A commonly unrecognized cause of symptoms in mitral valve prolapse. *Am J Med* 1981; 71:746–750.
213. Epstein EJ, Coulshed N: Phonocardiogram and apex cardiogram in systolic click-late systolic murmur syndrome. *Br Heart J* 1973; 35:260–275.
214. O'Rourke RA, Crawford MH: The systolic click-murmur syndrome: Clinical recognition and management. *Curr Probl Cardiol* 1976; 1(1):1.
215. Wei J, Fortuin NJ: Diastolic sounds and murmurs associated with mitral valve prolapse. *Circulation* 1981; 63:559–564.
216. Fontana ME, Wooley CG, Leighton RF, Lewis RP: Postural changes in left ventricular and mitral valvular dynamics in the systolic click-late systolic murmur syndrome. *Circulation* 1975; 51:165–173.
217. Bentivoglis LG, Uricchio JF, Waldow A, Likoff W, Goldberg H: An electrocardiographic analysis of mitral regurgitation. *Circulation* 1956; 18:572–580.
218. Peter RH, Morris JJ Jr, McIntosh HD: Relationship of fibrillatory waves and P waves in the electrocardiogram. *Circulation* 1966; 33:599–606.
219. DeMaria AN, Amsterdam EA, Vismara LA, Neumann A, Mason DT: Arrhythmias in the mitral valve prolapse syndrome. *Ann Intern Med* 1976; 84:656–660.
220. Priest EA, Finlayson JK, Short DS: The x-ray manifestations in the heart and lungs of mitral regurgitation. *Prog Cardiovasc Dis* 1962; 5:219–229.
221. BonTempo CP, Ronan JA, de Leon AC, Twigg HL: Radiographic appearance of the thorax in systolic click, late systolic murmur syndrome. *Am J Cardiol* 1975; 36:27–31.
222. Solomon J, Shab PM, Heinkle RA: Thoracic skeletal abnormalities in idiopathic mitral valve prolapse. *Am J Cardiol* 1975; 36:32–36.
223. Blumlein S, Bouchard A, Schiller NB: Quantitation of mitral regurgitation by Doppler echocardiography. *Circulation* 1986; 74:306–314.
224. Dang TY, Gardin JM, Clark S: Redefining the criteria for pulsed Doppler diagnosis of mitral regurgitation by comparison with left ventricular angiography. *Am J Cardiol* 1987; 60:663–666.
225. Rackley CE, Russell RO Jr, Ratshin RA: Hemodynamics of acute myocardial infarction: Invasive and noninvasive studies. Proceedings of the William Likoff Symposium, New York, Dec 14–16, 1973. In Russek HI (ed): *New Horizons in Cardiovascular Practice.* Baltimore, University Park Press, 1975:197–207.
226. Helmcke F, Nanda NC, Hsuing MC: Color Doppler assessment of mitral regurgitation with orthogonal planes. *Circulation* 1987; 75:175–183.
227. Mellino M, Salcedo EE, Lever HM, Vasudevan G, Kramer JR: Echographic quantified severity of mitral annulus calcification: Prognostic correlation to related hemodynamic valvular, rhythm and conduction abnormalities. *Am Heart J* 1982; 103:222–225.
228. Sweatman T, Selzer A, Kamageki M, Kamigaki M, Cohn K: Echocardiographic diagnosis of mitral regurgitation due to ruptured chordae tendineae. *Circulation* 1972; 46:580–586.
229. Izumi S, Miyatake K, Beppu S: Mechanism of mitral regurgitation in patients with myocardial infarction: A study using real-time two-dimensional Doppler flow imaging and echocardiography. *Circulation* 1987; 76:777–785.
230. Klein AL, Stewart WJ, Bartlett J, Cohen GI, Kahan F, Pearce G, et al: Effects of mitral regurgitation on pulmonary venous flow and left atrial pressure: An intraoperative transesophageal echocardiographic study. *J Am Coll Cardiol* 1992; 20:1345–1352.
231. Popp RL, Brown OR, Silverman JF, Harrison DC: Echocardiographic abnormalities in the mitral valve prolapse syndrome. *Circulation.* 1974; 49:428–433.
232. Burgess J, Clark R, Kamigaki M, Cohn K: Echocardiographic findings in different types of mitral regurgitation. *Circulation* 1973; 48:97–106.
233. DeMaria AN, King JF, Bogren HG, Lies JE, Mason DT: The variable spectrum of echocardiographic manifestations of the mitral valve prolapse syndrome. *Circulation* 1974; 50:33–41.
234. Goldstein JA, Tiefenbruna AJ: Myxomatous mitral apparatus and flail leaflet. *Cardiology* 1988; 5:80–86.
235. Slutsky R, Karliner J, Ricci D, Kaiser R, Pfisterer M, Gordon D, et al: Left ventricular volumes by gated equilibrium radionuclide angiography: A new method. *Circulation* 1979; 60:556–564.
236. Dehmer GJ, Lewis SE, Hillis LD, Twieq D, Falkoff M, Parkey RW: Nongeometric determination of left ventricular volumes from equilibrium blood pool scans. *Am J Cardiol* 1980; 45:293–300.
237. Gottdiener JS, Borer JS, Bacharach SL, Green MV, Epstein SE: Left ventricular function in mitral valve prolapse: Assessment with radionuclide cineangiography. *Am J Cardiol* 1981; 47: 7–13.
238. Fuchs RM, Heuser RR, Yin FCP, Brinker JA: Limitations of pulmonary wedge *v* waves in diagnosing mitral regurgitation. *Am J Cardiol* 1982; 49:849–854.
239. Pichard AD, Kay R, Smith H, Rentrop P, Holt J, Gorlin R: Large *v* waves in the pulmonary wedge pressure tracing in the absence of mitral regurgitation. *Am J Cardiol* 1982; 50:1044–1050.
240. Grose R, Strain J, Cohen MV: Pulmonary arterial *v* waves in mitral regurgitation: Clinical and experimental observations. *Circulation* 1984; 69:214–222.
241. Sandler H, Dodge HT, Hay RE, Rackley CE: Quantitation of valvular insufficiency in man by angiocardiography. *Am Heart J* 1963; 65:501–513.
242. Braunwald E, Awe WC: The syndrome of severe mitral regurgitation with normal left atrial pressure. *Circulation* 1963; 27: 29–35.
243. Rackley CE, Dodge HT, Coble YD, Hay RE: A method for determining left ventricular mass in man. *Circulation* 1964; 29:666–671.
244. Gaasch WH: The left ventricular radius/wall thickness ratio. *Am J Cardiol* 1979; 433:1189–1193.
245. Mantle JA, Russell RO Jr, Rogers WJ, et al: Advances in the treatment of heart failure. In: Russell RO Jr, Rackley CE (eds): *Hemodynamic Monitoring in a Coronary Intensive Care Unit.* Mt. Kisco, NY, Futura Publishing, 1981; 279–289.
246. Carabello BA, Spann JF: The uses and limitations of end-systolic indexes of left ventricular function. *Circulation* 1984; 69: 1058–1060.
247. Wisenbaugh T: Does normal pump function relieve muscle dys-

function inpatients with chronic severe mitral regurgitation? *Circulation* 1988; 77:515–525.
248. Rackley CE, Russell RO Jr, Mantle JA: Recognition of acute myocardial infarction. In: Rackley CE, Russell RO Jr (eds): *Coronary Artery Disease: Recognition and Management.* Mt Kisco, NY, Futura Publishing, 1979; 315–370.
249. Scampardonis G, Yang SS, Maranhao V, Goldberg H, Gooch AS: Left ventricular abnormalities in prolapsed mitral leaflet syndrome. *Circulation* 1973; 48:287–297.
250. Kokibash AJ, Bush CA, Fontana MB, Ryan JM, Kilman J, Woosley CF: Mitral valve prolapse syndrome: Analysis of 62 patients aged 60 years and older. *Am J Cardiol* 1983; 52:534–539.
251. Cosgrove DM, Stewart WJ: Mitral valvuloplasty. *Curr Prob Cardiol* 1989; 14:359–363.
252. Greenberg BH, Masie BM, Brundage BH, Batvinick EH, Parmley WW, Chatterjee K: Beneficial effects of hydralazine in severe mitral regurgitation. *Circulation* 1978; 58:273–279.
253. Miller RR, Awan NA, Maxwell KS, Mason DT: Sustained reduction of cardiac impedance and preload in congestive heart failure with the antihypertensive vasodilator prazosin. *N Engl J Med* 1977; 297:303–307.
254. Hoit BD: Medical treatment of valvular disease. *Current Opin Cardiol* 1991; 6:207–212.
255. Kirklin JW: Replacement of mitral valve for mitral incompetence. *Surgery* 1972; 72:827–833.
256. Gams E, Hagl S, Schad H, Heimisch W, Mendler N, Sebening F: Importance of the mitral apparatus for left ventricular function: An experimental approach. *Eur J Cardiothorac Surg* 1992; 6(suppl 1):S17–24.
257. David TE, Uden DE, Strauss HD: The importance of the mitral apparatus in left ventricular function after correction of mitral regurgitation. *Circulation* 1983; 68(suppl II):II-76–II-82.
258. Rozich JD, Carabello BA, Usher BW, Kratz JM, Bell AE, Zile MR: Mitral valve replacement with and without chordal preservation in patients with chronic mitral regurgitation. Mechanisms for differences in postoperative ejection performance. *Circulation* 1992; 86:1718–1726.
259. Pitarys CJ, Forman MB, Panayiotou H, Hansen DE: Long-term effects of excision of the mitral apparatus on global and regional ventricular function in humans. *J Am Coll Cardiol* 1990; 15:557–563.
260. Kannel WB, Abbott RD, Savage DO, McNamara PM: Epidemiologic features of chronic atrial fibrillation: The Framingham study. *N Engl J Med* 1982; 306:1018–1022.
261. Gajewski J, Singer RD: Mortality in an insured population with atrial fibrillation. *JAMA* 1981; 245:1540–1544.
262. Schuler G, Peterson KL, Johnson A, Francis G, Dennish G, Utley J, et al: Temporal response of left ventricular performance to mitral valve surgery. *Circulation* 1979; 59:1218–1231.
263. Phillips HR, Levine FH, Carter JE, Boucher CA, Osbakken MD, Okada RD, et al: Mitral valve replacement for isolated mitral regurgitation: Analysis of clinical course and late postoperative left ventricular ejection fraction. *Am J Cardiol* 1981; 48: 647–654.
264. Boudoulas H, Wooley CF: Mitral valve disorders. *Curr Opin Cardiol* 1990; 5:162–170.
265. Duran CG, Revuelta JM, Gaite L, Alonso C, Fleitas MG: Stability of mitral reconstructive surgery at 10–12 years for predominantly rheumatic valvular disease. *Circulation* 1988; 78(suppl I): I-91–I-96.
266. Chavez AM, Cosgrove DM, Lytle BW, Gill CC, Loop FD, Stewart RW, et al: Applicability of mitral valvuloplasty techniques in a North American population. *Am J Cardiol* 1988; 62:253–256.
267. Deloche A, Jebara VA, Relland JYM, Chauvaud S, Fabiani J-N, Perier P, et al: Valve repair with Carpentier techniques. The second decade. *J Thorac Cardiovasc Surg* 1990; 99:990–1002.
268. Cohn LH: Surgery for mitral regurgitation. *JAMA* 1988; 260:2883–2887.
269. Zussa C, Frater RWM, Polesel E, Galloni M, Valfre C: Artificial mitral valve chordae: Experimental and clinical experience. *Ann Thorac Surg* 1990; 50:367–373.
270. Kawashima Y, Kawazoe K, Eishi K, Sasako Y, Kosakai Y, Kitoh Y, Nakajima N: Clinical experience of mitral valve reconstruction with artificial chordae implantation. *Eur J Cardiothorac Surg* 1992; 6:297–301.
271. Cohn LH, DiSesa VJ, Couper GS, Peigh PS, Kowalker W, Collins JJ Jr: Mitral valve repair for myxomatous degeneration and prolapse of the mitral valve. *J Thorac Cardiovasc Surg* 1989; 98:987–993.
272. David TE, Komeda M, Pollick C, Burns RJ: Mitral valve annuloplasty: The effect of the type on left ventricular function. *Ann Thorac Surg* 1989; 47:524–528.
273. Cachera J-P, Loisance D, Mourtada A, Castanie JB, Heurtematte Y: Surgical techniques for treatment of bacterial endocarditis of the mitral valve. *J Cardiac Surg* 1987; 2:265–274.
274. Kenny J, Cohn LH, Shemin R, Collins JJ Jr, Plappert M, St. John Sutton MG: Doppler echocardiographic evaluation of ring mitral valvuloplasty for pure mitral regurgitation. *Am J Cardiol* 1987; 59:341–345.
275. Czer LSC, Maurer G, Bolger AF, De Robertis M, Resser KJ, Kass RM, et al: Intraoperative evaluation of mitral regurgitation by Doppler color flow mapping. *Circulation* 1987; 76(suppl III):III-108–III-116.
276. Freeman WK, Schaff HV, Khandheria BK, Oh JK, Orszulak TA, Abel MD, et al: Intraoperative evaluation of mitral valve regurgitation and repair by transesophageal echocardiography: Incidence and significance of systolic anterior motion. *J Am Coll Cardiol* 1992; 20:599–609.
277. Goldman ME, Mora F, Guarino T, Fuster V, Mindich BP: Mitral valvuloplasty is superior to valve replacement for preservation of left ventricular function: An intraoperative two-dimensional echocardiographic study. *J Am Coll Cardiol* 1987; 10:568–575.
278. Miller DW Jr, Johnson DD, Ivey TD: Does preservation of the posterior chordae tendineae enhance survival during mitral valve replacement? *Ann Thorac Surg* 1978; 28:22–27.
279. David TE: Mitral valve replacement with preservation of chordae tendinae: Rationale and technical considerations. *Ann Thorac Surg* 1986; 41:680–682.
280. Craver JM, Cohen C, Weintraub WS: Case-matched comparison of mitral valve replacement and repair. *Ann Thorac Surg* 1990; 49:964–969.
281. Rankin JS, Feneley MP, St. John Hickey M, Muhlbaier LH, Wechsler AS, Floyd RD, et al: A clinical comparison of mitral valve repair versus valve replacement in ischemic mitral regurgitation. *J Thorac Cardiovasc Surg* 1988; 95:165–177.
282. Cohn LH, Kowalker W, Bhatia S, DiSesa VJ, St. John-Sutton M, Shemin RJ, et al: Comparative morbidity of mitral valve repair versus replacement for mitral regurgitation with and without coronary artery disease. *Ann Thorac Surg* 1988; 45:284–290.
283. Galloway AC, Colvin SB, Baumann FG, Grossi EA, Ribakove GH, Harty S, et al: A comparison of mitral valve reconstruction with mitral valve replacement: Intermediate term results. *Ann Thorac Surg* 1989; 47:655–662.
284. Sand ME, Naftel DC, Blackstone EH, Kirklin JW, Karp RB: A comparison of repair and replacement for mitral valve incompetence. *J Thorac Cardiovasc Surg* 1987; 94:208–219.
285. Henderson WG, Nemec JJ, Lytle BW, Loop FD, Taylor PC, Stewart RW, et al: Mitral valve repair for ischemic mitral insufficiency. *Ann Thorac Surg* 1991; 52:1246–1252.
286. Bonchek LI, Olinger GN, Siegel R, Tresch DD, Keelan MH Jr: Left ventricular performance after mitral reconstruction for mitral regurgitation. *J Thorac Cardiovasc Surg* 1984; 88: 122–127.
287. Kontos GJ Jr, Schaff HV, Gersh BJ, Bove AA: Left ventricular function in subacute and chronic mitral regurgitation. Effect on function early postoperatively. *J Thorac Cardiovasc Surg* 1989; 98:163–169.
288. Phillips HR, Levine FH, Carter JE, Boucher CA, Osbakken MD, Okada RD, et al: Mitral valve replacement for isolated mitral regurgitation: Analysis of clinical course and late postoperative left ventricular ejection fraction. *Am J Cardiol* 1981; 48: 647–654.
289. Cohn LH, Aranki SF, Rizzo RJ, Cogswell K, Couper GS, Collins JJ Jr: Decrease in operative risk of reoperative valve surgery. *Ann Thorac Surg* 1993; 56:15–20.
290. Scott ML, Stowe CL, Nunnally LC, Spector SD, Moseley PW, Schumacher PD, et al: Mitral valve reconstruction in the elderly population. *Ann Thorac Surg* 1989; 48:213–217.
291. Cohn LH, Couper GS, Kinchla KM, Collins JJ Jr: Decreased operative risk of surgical treatment of mitral regurgitation with or without coronary artery disease. *J Am Coll Cardiol* 1990; 16:1575–1578.

292. Mihaileanu S, Marino JP, Chauvaud S, Perier P, Forman J, Vissoat J, et al: Left ventricular outflow obstruction after mitral valve repair (Carpentier's technique). Proposed mechanisms of disease. *Circulation* 1988; 78(suppl I):I-78–I-84.
293. Grossi EA, Galloway AC, Parish MA, Asai T, Gindea AJ, Harty S, et al: Experience with 28 cases of systolic anterior motion after mitral valve reconstruction by the Carpentier technique. *J Thorac Cardiovasc Surg* 1992; 103:466–470.
294. Kreindel MS, Schiavone WA, Lever HM, Cosgrove D: Systolic anterior motion of the mitral valve after Carpentier ring valvuloplasty for mitral valve prolapse. *Am J Cardiol* 1986; 57:408–412.
295. Schiavone WA, Cosgrove DM, Lever HM, Stewart WJ, Salcedo EE: Long-term followup of patients with left ventricular outflow tract obstruction after Carpentier ring mitral valvuloplasty. *Circulation* 1988; 78(suppl I): I-60–I-65.
296. Barlow JB, Pocock WA, Marchand P, Denny M: The significance of late systolic murmurs. *Am Heart J* 1963; 66:443–452.
297. Read RC, Thal AP, Wendt VE: Symptomatic valvular myxomatous transformation (the floppy valve syndrome). *Circulation* 1965; 32:897–910.
298. Criley JM, Lewis KB, Humphries JO, Ross RS: Prolapse of the mitral valve: Clinical and cine-angiocardiographic findings. *Br Heart J* 1966; 28:488–496.
299. Barlow JB, Bosman CK, Pocock WA, Marchland P: Late systolic murmurs and non-ejection ("mid-late") systolic clicks: An analysis of 90 patients. *Br Heart J* 1968; 30:203–218.
300. Pomerance A: Ballooning deformity (mucoid degeneration) of atrioventricular valves. *Br Heart J* 1969; 31:343–351.
301. Lucas RV Jr, Edwards JE: The floppy mitral valve. *Curr Probl Cardiol* 1982; 7:1–48.
302. Cheitlin MD, Byrd RC: Prolapsed mitral valve: The commonest disease? *Curr Probl Cardiol* 1984; 8:1–54.
303. Fontana ME, Sparks EA, Boudoulas H, Wooley CF: Mitral valve prolapse in the mitral valve prolapse syndrome. *Curr Probl Cardiol* 1991; 16:315–375.
304. Devereux RB, Brown WT, Kramer-Fox R, Sachs I: Inheritance of mitral valve prolapse: Effect of age and sex on gene expression. *Ann Intern Med* 1982; 97:826–832.
305. Shell WE, Walton JA, Clifford ME, Willis PW III: The familial occurrence of the syndrome of mid-late systolic click and late systolic murmur. *Circulation* 1969; 39:327–338.
306. Savage DD, Garrison RJ, Devereux RB, Castelli WP, Anderson SJ, Levy D, et al: Mitral valve prolapse in the general population. I: Epidemiologic features: The Framingham study. *Am Heart J* 1983; 106:571–576.
307. Procacci PM, Savran SV, Schreiter SL, Bryson AL: Prevalence of clinical mitral valve prolapse in 1169 young women. *N Engl J Med* 1976; 294:1086–1088.
308. Leier CV, Call TD, Fulkerson PK, Wooley CF: The spectrum of cardiac defects in the Ehlers-Danlos syndrome, types I & III. *Ann Intern Med* 1980; 92:171–178.
309. Lebwohl MG, Distefano D, Prioleau PG, Uram M, Yannuzzi LA, Fleischmajer R: Pseudoxanthoma elasticum and mitral valve prolapse. *N Engl J Med* 1982; 307:228–231.
310. Schwartz T, Gotsman MS: Mitral valve prolapse in osteogenesis imperfecta. *Isr J Med Sci* 1981; 17:1087–1088.
311. Udoshi MB, Shah A, Fisher VJ, Dolgin M: Incidence of mitral valve prolapse in subjects with thoracic skeletal abnormalities—a prospective study. *Am Heart J* 1979; 97:303–311.
312. Salomon J, Shah PM, Heinle RA: Thoracic skeletal abnormalities in idiopathic mitral valve prolapse. *Am J Cardiol* 1875; 36: 32–36.
313. BonTempo CP, Ronan JA Jr: Radiographic appearance of the thorax in systolic click–late systolic murmur syndrome. *Am J Cardiol* 1975; 36:27–31.
314. Crawford MH, O'Rourke RA: Mitral valve prolapse syndrome. In: Isselbacher KJ, Adams RD, Braunwald E, et al (eds): *Update I. Harrison's Principles of Internal Medicine.* New York, McGraw Hill, 1981:91–152.
315. Pickering NJ, Brody JI, Barrett MJ: von Willebrand syndromes and mitral valve prolapse. *N Engl J Med* 1981; 305:131–134.
316. Rosenberg CA, Derman GH, Grabb WC, Buda AJ: Hypomastia and mitral valve prolapse. Evidence of a linked embryologic and mesenchymal dysplasia. *N Engl J Med* 1983; 309:1230–1232.
317. Tei C, Sakamaki T, Shah PM, Meerbaum S, Kondo S, Shimoura K, et al: Mitral valve prolapse in short-term experimental coronary occlusion: A possible mechanism of ischemic mitral regurgitation. *Circulation* 1983; 68:183–189.
318. Crawford MH: Mitral valve prolapse due to coronary artery disease. *Am J Med c*1977; 62:447–451.
319. Lembo NJ, Dell'Italia LJ, Crawford MH, Miller JF, Richards KL, O'Rourke RA: Mitral valve prolapse in patients with prior rheumatic fever. *Circulation* 1988; 77:830–836.
320. Marcus RH, Sareli P, Pocock WA, Meyer TE, Magalhaes MP, Grieve T, et al: Functional anatomy of severe mitral regurgitation in active rheumatic carditis. *Am J Cardiol* 1986; 63:577–584.
321. Crawford MH, O'Rourke RA: Mitral valve prolapse: A cardiomyopathic state? *Prog Cardiovasc Dis* 1984; 27:133–139.
322. Lax D, Eicher M, Goldberg SJ: Mild dehydration induces echocardiographic signs of mitral valve prolapse in healthy females with prior normal cardiac findings. *Am Heart J* 1992; 124: 1533–1540.
323. Krivokapich J, Child JS, Dadourian BJ, Perloff JK: Reassessment of echocardiographic criteria for the diagnosis of mitral valve prolapse. *Am J Cardiol* 1988; 61:131–135.
324. Betriu A, Wigle ED, Felderhof CH, McLoughlin MJ: Prolapse of the posterior leaflet of the mitral valve associated with secundum atrial septal defect. *Am J Cardiol* 1975; 35:363–369.
325. Gaffney FA, Karlsson ES, Campbell W, Schutte JE, Nixon JV, Willerson JT, et al: Autonomic dysfunction in women with mitral valve prolapse. *Circulation* 1979; 59:894–899.
326. Boudoulas H, Reynolds JC, Mazzaferri E, Wooley CF: Metabolic studies in mitral valve prolapse syndrome. *Circulation* 1980; 61:1200–1205.
327. Boudoulas H, Reynolds JC, Mazzaferri E, Wooley CF: Mitral valve prolapse syndrome: The effect of adrenergic stimulation. *J Am Coll Cardiol* 1983; 2:638–644.
328. Davies AO, Mares A, Pool JL, Taylor AA: Mitral valve prolapse with symptoms of beta adrenergic hypersensitivity. Beta$_2$ adrenergic receptor supercoupling with desensitization of isoproterenol exposure. *Am J Med* 1987; 82:193–201.
329. Gaffney FA, Bastian BC, Lane LB, Taylor WF, Horton J, Schutte JE, et al. Abnormal cardiovascular regulation in the mitral valve prolapse syndrome. *Am J Cardiol* 1983; 52:316–320.
330. Anwar A, Kohn SR, Dunn JF, Hymer TK, Kennedy GT, Crawford MH, O'Rourke RA, Katz MS: Altered beta-adreneregic receptor function in subjects with symptomatic mitral valve prolapse. *Am J Med Sci* 1991; 302(2):89–97.
331. Fontana ME, Pence HL, Leighton RF, Wooley CF: The varying clinical spectrum of the systolic click–late systolic murmur syndrome. *Circulation* 1970; 41:807–816.
332. Josephson ME, Horowitz LM, Kastor JA: Paroxysmal supraventricular tachycardia in patients with mitral valve prolapse. *Circulation* 1978; 57:111–119.
333. LeWinter MM, Hoffman JR, Shell WE, Karliner JS, O'Rourke RA: Phenylephrine-induced atypical chest pain in patients with prolapsing mitral valve leaflets. *Am J Cardiol* 1974; 34:12–18.
334. Barnett HJM, Jones MW, Boughner DR, Kostuk WJ: Cerebral ischemic events associated with prolapsing mitral valve. *Arch Neurol* 1976; 33:777–782.
335. Boughner DR, Barnett HJM: The enigma of the risk of stroke in mitral valve prolapse. *Stroke* 1985; 16:175–177.
336. Barletta GA, Gagliardi R, Benvenuti L, Fantini F: Cerebral ischemic attacks as a complication of aortic and mitral valve prolapse. *Stroke* 1985; 16:219–223.
337. Jones HR Jr, Nagger CZ, Seljan MP, Downing LL: Mitral valve prolapse and cerebral ischemic events. A comparison between a neurology population with stroke and a cardiology population with mitral valve prolapse observed for five years. *Stroke* 1982; 13:451–453.
338. Barnett HJM, Boughner DR, Taylor DW, Cooper PE, Kostuk VJ, Nichol PM: Further evidence relating mitral valve prolapse to cerebral ischemic event. *N Engl J Med* 1980; 302:139–144.
339. Wilson LA, Keeling PW, Malcolm AD, Russel RW, Webb-Peploe MM: Visual complications of mitral leaflet prolapse. *Br Med J* 1977; 2:86–88.
340. Chesler E, King RA, Edwards JE: The myxomatous mitral valve and sudden death. *Circulation* 1983; 67:632–639.
341. Bhutto ZR, Barron JT, Liebson PR, Uretz EF, Parrillo JE: Electrocardiographic abnormalities in mitral valve prolapse. *Am J Cardiol* 1992; 70:265–266.

342. Marks AR, Choong CY, Sanfilippo AJ, Ferre M, Weyman AE: Identification of high-risk and low-risk subgroups of patients with mitral valve prolapse. *N Engl J Med* 1989; 320:1031–1036.
343. Shah PM: Personal communication.
344. Klein GJ, Kostuk WJ, Bougher DR, Chamberlain MJ: Stress myocardial imaging in mitral leaflet prolapse syndrome. *Am J Cardiol* 1978; 42:746–750.
345. Allen H, Harris A, Leatham A: Significance and prognosis of an isolated late systolic murmur: A 9 to 22 year follow-up. *Br Heart J* 1974; 36:525–532.
346. Mills P, Rose J, Hollingsworth J, Amara I, Craige E: Long-term prognosis of mitral valve prolapse. *N Engl J Med* 1977; 297: 13–18.
347. Nishimura RA, McGood MD, Shub C, Miller FA Jr, Ilstrup DM, Tajik AJ: Echocardiographically documented mitral-valve prolapse: Long-term follow-up of 237 patients. *N Engl J Med* 1985; 313:1305–1309.
348. Düren DR, Becker AE, Dunning AJ: Long-term follow-up of idiopathic mitral valve prolapse in 300 patients: A prospective study. *J Am Coll Cardiol* 1988; 11:42–47.
349. Marshall CE, Shappel SD: Sudden death and the ballooning posterior leaflet syndrome: Detailed anatomic and histochemical investigation. *Arch Pathol* 1974; 98:134–138.
350. Clemens JD, Horwitz RI, Jaffe CC, Feinstein AR, Stanton BF: A controlled evaluation of the risk of bacterial endocarditis in persons with mitral valve prolapse. *N Engl J Med* 1982; 307: 776–781.
351. Dajani AS, Bisno AL, Chung KJ, Durack DT, Freed M, Gerber MA, et al: Prevention of bacterial endocarditis. Recommendations by the American Heart Association. *JAMA* 1990; 264:2919–2922.
352. Bansal RC, Shah PM: Usefulness of echo-Doppler in management of patients with valvular heart disease. *Curr Probl Cardiol* 1989; 14:287–350.
353. Panidis IP, McAllister M, Ross J, Mintz GS: Prevalence and severity of mitral regurgitation in the mitral valve prolapse syndrome; a Doppler echocardiographic study of 80 patients. *J Am Coll Cardiol* 1986; 7:975–981.
354. Winkle RA, Lopes MG, Goodman DJ, Fitzgerald JW, Schroeder JS, Harrison DC: Propranolol for patients with mitral valve prolapse. *Am Heart J* 1977; 93:422–427.
355. Galloway AC, Colvin SB, Baumann FG, Harty S, Spencer FC: Current concepts of mitral valve reconstruction for mitral insufficiency. *Circulation* 1988; 78:1087–1098.
356. Cheitlin MD: The timing of surgery in mitral and aortic valve disease. *Curr Probl Cardiol* 1987; 12:75–149.
357. Cosgrove DM, Stewart WJ: Mitral valvuloplasty. *Curr Probl Cardiol* 1989; 14:359–415.
358. Kirklin JW: Mitral valve repair for mitral incompetence. *Mod Concepts Cardiovasc Dis* 1987; 56:7–11.

Chapter 81

Tricuspid and Pulmonary Valve Disease

Charles E. Rackley, M.D. ■ *Robert B. Wallace, M.D.*
Jesse E. Edwards, M.D. ■ *Nevin M. Katz, M.D.*

DEFINITION, ETIOLOGY, AND PATHOLOGY

Tricuspid Valve

Tricuspid regurgitation develops when the tricuspid valve allows blood to enter the right atrium during right ventricular contraction. Tricuspid stenosis represents obstruction to diastolic flow across the valve during diastolic filling of the right ventricle.

The most common cause of tricuspid stenosis is rheumatic fever (Fig. 81-1). This is usually associated with concomitant mitral stenosis. Isolated stenosis of the tricuspid valve can be seen with the carcinoid syndrome, endocardial fibroelastosis, endomyocardial fibrosis, and systemic lupus erythematosus. Mechanical obstruction of the valve can occur with a right atrial myxoma, tumor metastases, and thrombi in the right atrium that produce the hemodynamic abnormalities of tricuspid stenosis.[1,2]

Regurgitation of the tricuspid valve is due most commonly to right ventricular dilatation and failure.[3] Left ventricular failure and/or pulmonary hypertension can result in tricuspid regurgitation. The most common etiology of isolated tricuspid regurgitation is infectious endocarditis in drug addiction.[4] (See Chap. 94.) Less common causes include myocardial infarction; trauma; carcinoid, prolapsed leaflet; and congenital abnormalities, such as atrial septal defect and Ebstein's anomaly.

As previously noted, rheumatic disease is the most common cause of tricuspid stenosis.[5] Alterations in the valve are characterized by fibrosis with contracture of the leaflets and commissural fusion; the former leads to tricuspid regurgitation and the latter to senosis. The stenotic component of rheumatic tricuspid valve disease is often minor and would go undetected were it not for the high flow across the valve caused by the coexistent regurgitation. Whenever the tricuspid valve is involved by rheumatic disease, there is always involvement of left-

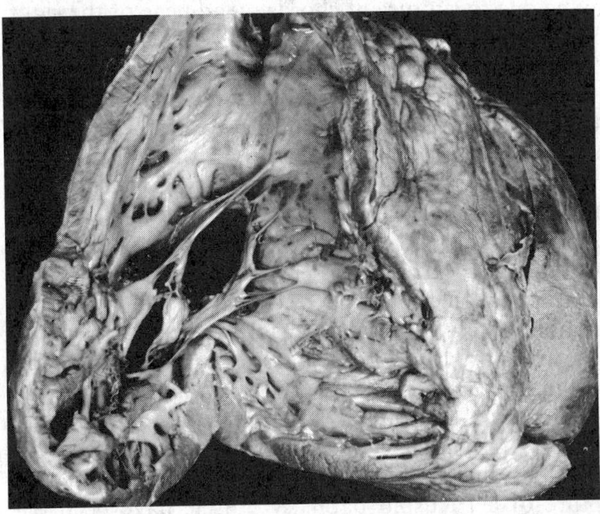

FIGURE 81-1 Tricuspid valves seen from below in chronic rheumatic endocarditis. Although the chordae are relatively uninvolved, there is fusion of the leaflets at the commissures creating a narrow and fixed orifice. The valve is both stenotic and incompetent.

sided valves, an observation in agreement with that of Clawson.[6]

Flammang and associates observed that 9.5 percent of cases requiring surgical replacement of both the mitral and aortic valves exhibited rheumatic involvement of the tricuspid valve.[7] Among cases undergoing mitral commissurotomy, the incidence of clinically evident tricuspid disease was 3 percent. Cooke and White found 47 cases (22 percent) in a series of 217 autopsied cases of rheumatic heart disease where the tricuspid valve was also involved by rheumatic disease.[8]

In about 10 percent of cases of malignant carcinoid tumor (usually originating in the ileum) with extensive metastases, the tricuspid and pulmonary valves may be affected. Changes include deposits of fibrous tissue on the surfaces of these valves. Fibrous plaques can also develop on the endocardial surfaces of the right atrium and ventricle as well as on the intima of the coronary sinus and pulmonary artery.[9] The hemodynamic effects result from the rigidity and contracture of the fibrous tissues deposited on the valves. Although tricuspid stenosis may result, the major functional effect is usually regurgitation.

Atrial myxomas represent a common cause of mechanical obstruction of the tricuspid valve, which can produce the clinical and hemodynamic effects of stenosis. Right atrial thrombi from systemic sources as well as metastatic tumors can also lead to involvement of the tricuspid valve and right atrium, producing mechanical obstruction across the valve. (See also Chap. 111.)

The most common type of tricuspid regurgitation is the secondary type resulting from enlargement of the orifice and annulus secondary to congestive cardiac failure with right ventricular dilatation due to left ventricular disease. Tricuspid regurgitation may diminish when the heart failure is treated successfully but can be permanent with long-standing dilatation of the right ventricle.[10,11]

In infective endocarditis the tricuspid regurgitation results from improper apposition of the leaflets because of interposed vegetations. Major degrees of regurgitation may be due to rupture of chordae tendineae of the right ventricle or perforation of the valve leaflets.

Myocardial infarction has not been considered a common cause of tricuspid regurgitation in earlier studies except when secondary to chronic congestive failure.[12] Rare cases were described from rupture of a right ventricular papillary muscle.[12–15] In recent years, however, right ventricular infarction has been recognized clinically together with tricuspid regurgitation documented by echocardiography.

Various degrees of prolapse of the tricuspid valve are commonly present, usually in association with prolapse of the mitral valve. Reported instances of severe tricuspid regurgitation from prolapse have been uncommon.[16]

External blunt trauma has been a classic cause of traumatic tricuspid regurgitation, most commonly occurring in automobile accidents. Isolated instances of rupture of a tricuspid papillary muscle have been described from external cardiopulmonary resuscitation.[17] The main cause of traumatic tricuspid regurgitation is rupture of one or more of the elements of the tensor apparatus, with disruption of the papillary muscle occurring more often than rupture of the chordae. Less frequently, there is laceration of leaflet tissue, and occasionally, more than one of the anatomic elements of the valve are affected.[18,19] In an unusual case, traumatic tricuspid regurgitation and ruptured ventricular septum coexisted.[20] (See also Chap. 112.)

Tolerance of traumatic tricuspid regurgitation varies, with up to 39 years of survival reported.[21–24] Patients with rupture of a papillary muscle tend to tolerate the tricuspid regurgitation less well than those in which the trauma resulted in rupture of chordae.[22] Among reported cases of tricuspid regurgitation resulting from rupture of the chordae, a traumatic etiology is more common than that due to bacterial endocarditis.[25]

Primary congenital lesions of the tricuspid valve that cause incompetence are Ebstein's malformation and valvular dysplasia (Chap. 97).

Pulmonic Valve

Pulmonary stenosis is created by obstruction to systolic flow across the valve and is most commonly congenital (Chap. 97). Acquired lesions of the pulmonary valve generally lead to regurgitation. On rare occasions, an inflammatory process can create stenosis and regurgitation of the valve. Pulmonary hypertension from any cause, such as mitral stenosis, chronic lung disease, or pulmonary emboli, can produce pulmonary incompetence. Inflammatory diseases such as endocarditis, rheumatic fever, and on rare occasions, tuberculosis can result in pulmonary regurgitation.[26,27] Sarcomas and myxomas can sometimes extend to the pulmonic valve.[28] Previous cardiac surgery on a congenital pulmonary valvular lesion can result in pulmonary incompetence. Carcinoid syndrome with cardiac involvement can create slight pulmonic stenosis and associated regurgitation[29] (Fig. 81-2). Compression of the pulmonary artery can simulate valvular stenosis and is rarely produced by tumor, aneurysm, or even constrictive pericarditis.

PATHOPHYSIOLOGY

Tricuspid valve stenosis decreases diastolic flow across the valve, elevates the right atrial pressure, and reduces the cardiac output.[30,31] The normal area of the tricuspid valve is 7 cm^2, and impairment of right ventricular filling occurs when the valve area is reduced to less than 1.5 cm^2. Elevation of the mean right atrial pressure above 10 mmHg usually produces peripheral edema. Development of atrial fibrillation produces a higher right atrial pressure in tricuspid stenosis than when sinus rhythm and normal atrial contraction are present. Hemodynamic abnormalities in tricuspid stenosis can be further influenced by the frequently coexistent mitral stenosis. Reduced right ventricular flow in tricuspid valve obstruction has been proposed as a mechanism for protection against severe pulmonary hypertension.

In tricuspid incompetence the systolic regurgitation into the right atrium elevates the mean right atrial pressure.[32] The regurgitant flow produces a prominent *cv* wave reflected throughout the venous system.

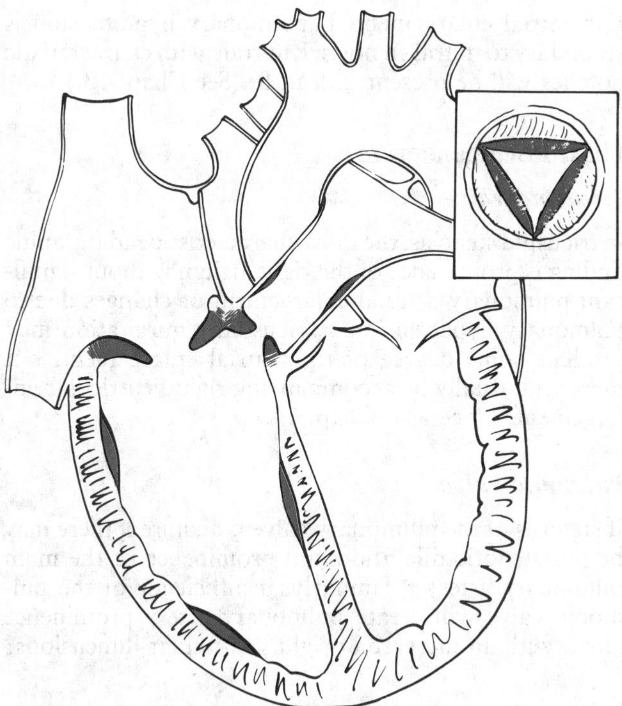

FIGURE 81-2 Carcinoid heart disease. Insert shows pulmonary stenosis. The leaflets of the tricuspid valve are thickened. The valve is predominantly incompetent and causes pulmonary regurgitation. Fibrous plaques are deposited on the lining of the right ventricle and pulmonary trunk. *(From JE Edwards: Effects of malignant noncardiac tumors upon the cardiovascular system. Cardiovasc Clin 4:282, 1971. Reproduced with permission from the publisher and the author.)*

Pulmonary regurgitation is the most frequently acquired lesion of the valve (Table 81-1). Incompetence may be secondary to pulmonary hypertension or it may be caused by primary abnormality in the leaflets. Pulmonary regurgitation imposes a volume overload on the right ventricle, and if pulmonary hypertension preexists, the overload is superimposed on hypertrophied myocardium. Isolated pulmonary valvular regurgitation can be tolerated for a long time without cardiac decompensation.[33]

TABLE 81-1

Acquired Lesions of the Pulmonary Valve
Pulmonary hypertension with pulmonary regurgitation
Mitral stenosis
Chronic lung disease
Pulmonary emboli
Inflammatory lesions
Endocarditis
Rheumatic fever
Tuberculosis
Tumors
Sarcoma
Myxoma
Previous surgery of angioplasty for congenital lesions
Mediastinal lesions
Tumor
Aneurysm
Constrictive pericarditis
Miscellaneous
Carcinoid syndrome

CLINICAL MANIFESTATIONS

Symptoms

The most frequent symptoms in tricuspid stenosis are dyspnea and fatigue. When mitral stenosis coexists, the development of significant tricuspid stenosis can diminish the paroxysmal symptoms of dyspnea, pulmonary congestion, and hypertension.[1,2] Occasionally, patients with tricuspid stenosis complain of prominent pulsations in the neck veins which may precede the development of peripheral edema.

Since tricuspid regurgitation generally accompanies left ventricular failure or mitral stenosis, symptoms are dyspnea, orthopnea, and peripheral edema.[34] Paroxysmal nocturnal dyspnea may be surprisingly infrequent. Tricuspid regurgitation under these conditions may occasionally ameliorate the pulmonary symptoms and provide a physiological basis for the alleviation of left-sided heart failure by the development of right-sided heart failure. Some patients also have less pulmonary edema due to the development of pulmonary arteriolar disease. If the tricuspid regurgitation is produced by bacterial endocarditis, symptoms of febrile illness may be accompanied by fatigue and peripheral edema.

Clinical manifestation of acquired pulmonary valvular lesions depend on severity of the impairment as well as extent of the underlying disease. Isolated pulmonary regurgitation can be tolerated without symptoms. Severe pulmonary hypertension may cause not only dyspnea and fatigue but also syncope. With inflammatory lesions of the valve, febrile manifestations and pulmonary infections may be present. Carcinoid syndrome is characterized by episodes of facial flushing, increased intestinal activity, diarrhea, and bronchospasm. Tumors involving the pulmonary valve may exert pressure from expansion and metastases which affect the heart and lungs.

Physical Examination

Tricuspid Valve

Tricuspid stenosis is frequently associated with lesions of the mitral and aortic valves. Internal jugular veins will display the prominent *a* wave indicative of impaired right ventricular diastolic filling with atrial systole. The *a* wave in the neck may be of moderate height and sometimes reach the mandible.[1,2] Auscultation of the heart is required to confirm that the rise of the venous *a* wave is simultaneous with the first heart sound. The *cv* wave is small, and the *y* descent is slow and insignificant. (See also Chaps. 10 and 11.)

Right ventricular hypertrophy, detected on physical examination, renders tricuspid stenosis less likely. Respiratory variation in splitting of the second heart sound may be absent in tricuspid stenosis, since right ventricular filling remains fairly constant throughout the respiratory cycle. The characteristic auscultatory finding in tricuspid stenosis is the diastolic rumble, heard best at the left lower sternal border.[1,2,35] With sinus rhythm, the murmur is presystolic; with atrial fibrillation, the murmur may be early or middiastolic. The influence of respiration is the most effective differentiation of the murmur from that of mitral stenosis since the diastolic rumble of tricuspid stenosis is markedly accentuated during the inspiratory phase. Augmentation of the rumble of tricuspid stenosis with inspiration is designated Carvallo's sign and is due to the augmented venous return to the right atrium as well as to the increase in right ventricular filling.[36] An opening snap in tricuspid stenosis is rarely detected with auscultation but sometimes can be recorded with intracardiac phonocardiography.

Atrial fibrillation is common in tricuspid regurgitation, and the internal jugular veins display a prominent *cv* wave produced by the regurgitant flow into the right atrium.[34] The *cv* wave and the jugular pulse are more gradual in upstroke than the contrasted sharp rise of the *a* wave. Simultaneous auscultation of the heart remains the best method for timing venous pulsations. A characteristic auscultatory finding of tricuspid regurgitation is a holosystolic murmur at the left sternal border that increases during inspiration. Although the murmur of mitral regurgitation may also be present, respiration exerts a predominant influence on tricuspid regurgitation with little alteration in the intensity of a mitral regurgitation murmur. (See also Chap. 11.)

Pulmonic Valve

If right ventricular failure and tricuspid regurgitation have developed as a result of pulmonary regurgitation, a prominent *cv* wave will be present in the jugular pulse. Increased right ventricular activity may be visible and palpable along the left sternal border. If pulmonary hypertension is present, the pulmonic second sound will be accentuated over the pulmonary area. The murmur of acquired pulmonary regurgitation is a high-pitched diastolic blow along the left sternal border. This murmur may be difficult to differentiate from the murmur of aortic regurgitation, but the absence of peripheral findings of aortic regurgitation can be useful in identifying an incompetent pulmonary valve as the source of the diastolic blow. Congenital pulmonary regurgitation characteristically is associated with a low-pitched, decrescendo murmur along the left sternal border.

ELECTROCARDIOGRAM

Tricuspid Valve

The characteristic electrocardiographic finding in tricuspid stenosis is a large P wave of right atrial enlargement in the absence of right ventricular hypertrophy.[1,30] Atrial fibrillation is quite common in patients with tricuspid regurgitation.[34] In myocardial infarction, acute or chronic changes will be seen in the inferior leads. (See Chaps. 13 and 60.)

Pulmonic Valve

Although there are no characteristic changes with pulmonary valvular lesions, preexisting pulmonary hypertension will produce right ventricular hypertrophy, right-axis deviation, and changes in the P wave, suggesting right atrial enlargement. If pulmonary hypertension is secondary to mitral stenosis, P mitrale with characteristic notches will be present in lead II. (See Chap. 13.)

Chest Roentgenogram

Tricuspid Valve

In tricuspid stenosis, the most characteristic radiographic finding is prominence of the right atrium without significant pulmonary arterial enlargement or changes due to pulmonary hypertension.[1] Tricuspid regurgitation may produce some degree of right atrial enlargement, but there will usually be accompanying right ventricular enlargement.[34] (See also Chap. 14.)

Pulmonic Valve

If stenosis of the pulmonary valve is acquired, there may be poststenotic dilatation and prominence of the main pulmonary artery.[33] Similarly, insufficiency of the pulmonic valve will create pulmonary artery prominence along with an increase in right ventricular dimensions.

Echocardiogram

A characteristic pattern of stenosis of the tricuspid valve can often be recorded with the echocardiogram. Fibrosis and calcification of the valve can be identified. Obstructive lesions such as myxoma, thrombus, or other tumors can be recognized echocardiographically. The echo Doppler technique can be used to estimate the diastolic gradient across the valve with generally good accuracy. (See Chaps. 15 and 130.)

With tricuspid regurgitation one may recognize systolic prolapse, rupture of the chordae or papillary muscle, as well as vegetative lesions on the valve.[37] Increased right ventricular dimensions indicate impaired right ventricular function and the likelihood of secondary tricuspid regurgitation. Contrast echocardiography with peripheral venous injection can identify the back-and-forth flow across the tricuspid valve.[38] Echo Doppler technique can estimate the severity of the regurgitation and the systolic pressure in the right ventricle[39] (Fig. 81-3). Color Doppler technique can delineate the patterns and sites of regurgitation across the valve apparatus.[40]

Echocardiography can delineate the anatomy of the pulmonary valve as well as intrinsic or extrinsic lesions impinging on the valve apparatus (Fig. 81-4). Sometimes a vegetative lesion or tumor can be detected in the pulmonary valve area. The echo Doppler technique can estimate both the severity of the regurgitation as well as stenosis of the valve,[41] and analysis of echo Doppler recordings can provide estimates of pulmonary artery pressure[42–44] (Fig. 81-5). Color Doppler can further confirm the patterns of regurgitation in the right ventricular outflow track. (See Chap. 130.)

Nuclear Scans

Nuclear scans can delineate dimensions of the right atrium and right ventricle, which may help differentiate between stenosis and incompetence of the tricuspid valve. (See Chap. 134.) Perfusion techniques are useful in detecting right ventricular infarction as a cause of

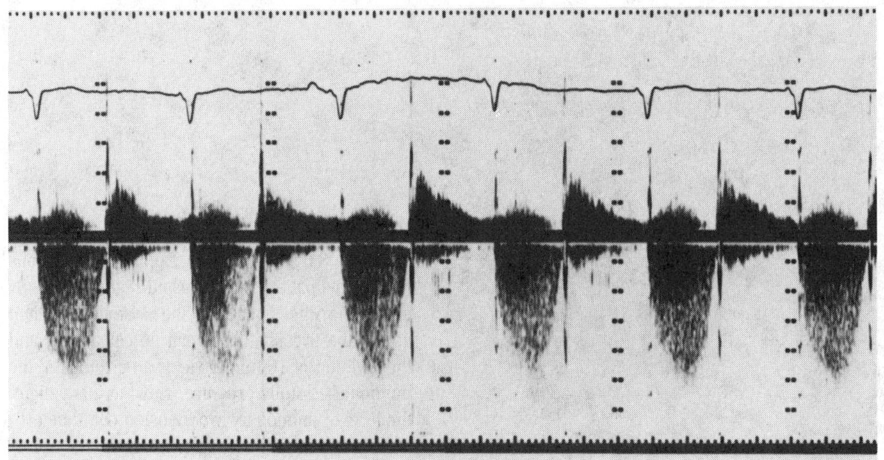

FIGURE 81-3 A continuous echo Doppler recording in a patient with tricuspid valve disease illustrates tricuspid regurgitation in the lower portion and tricuspid stenosis in the upper portion of the tracing. *(Reproduced with permission from and courtesy of Dr. Pamela Sears-Rogan.)*

tricuspid regurgitation as well as providing estimates on right ventricular function.

Right ventricular size and function can be evaluated in stenotic and regurgitant lesions of the pulmonary valve.

Cardiac Catheterization

If tricuspid stenosis is clinically suspected, simultaneous pressures should be recorded in the right atrium and in the right ventricle in order to measure accurately the gradient across the valve.[30] Since the normal gradient across the tricuspid valve is less than 1 mmHg, small gradients may not be detected if pullback pressure is recorded from the right ventricle to the right atrium. The area of the tricuspid valve in significant stenosis is usually less than 1.5 cm^2; in severe stenosis it is less than 1 cm^2.

Angiographic documentation of tricuspid regurgitation is difficult to secure because the catheter overrides the tricuspid valve and ventricular irritability with a right ventricular injection can induce tricuspid regurgitation. A prominent *cv* wave in the right atrium suggests tricuspid regurgitation, and an intracardiac phonocardiogram may record a regurgitation murmur in the absence of Carvallo's sign.[45]

Pulmonic regurgitation is not easily demonstrated angiographically, but a right-sided injection can outline the pulmonary valve as well as poststenotic dilatation. An aortic root injection can be helpful in the elimination of aortic regurgitation as the etiology of a diastolic murmur along the left sternal border, although this distinction is usually best made by echo Doppler studies. Intracardiac phonocardiography has been employed to detect the diastolic murmur in the right ventricular outflow track.

USUAL STRATEGY OF WORKUP

The history should document underlying conditions such as rheumatic fever, systemic disorders, and left-sided heart failure as etiologies for tricuspid valve disease (Table 81-2). The physical examination should carefully document patterns in the jugular veins. The auscultatory changes of systolic and diastolic murmurs at the left lower sternal border should be carefully observed. In addition, physical findings of left-sided valvular abnormalities, particularly mitral stenosis and/or evidence of left-sided failure, should be observed. Peripheral edema as evidence of impaired right-sided filling should be noted.

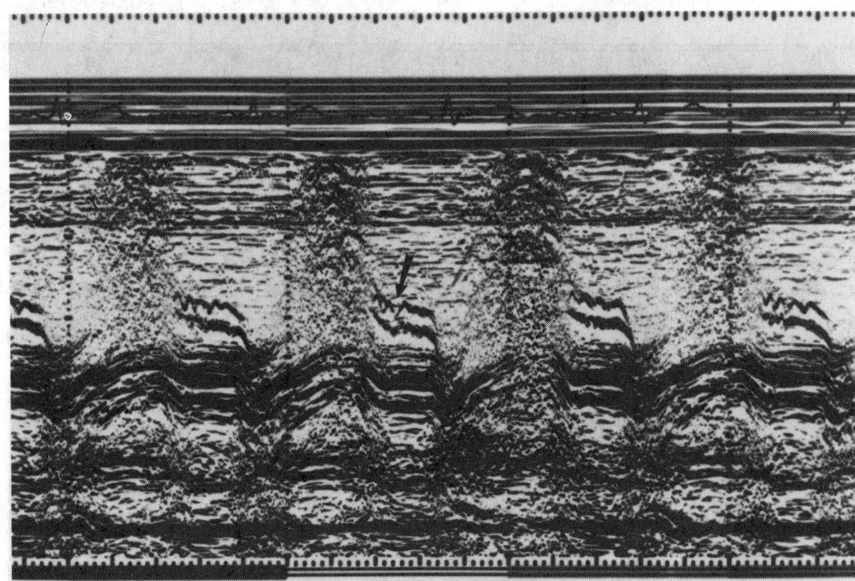

FIGURE 81-4 M-mode echocardiogram in a patient with pulmonary insufficiency illustrates thickening and fluttering of the pulmonic valve, as indicated by the arrow. *(Reproduced with permission from Dr. Pamela Sears-Rogan.)*

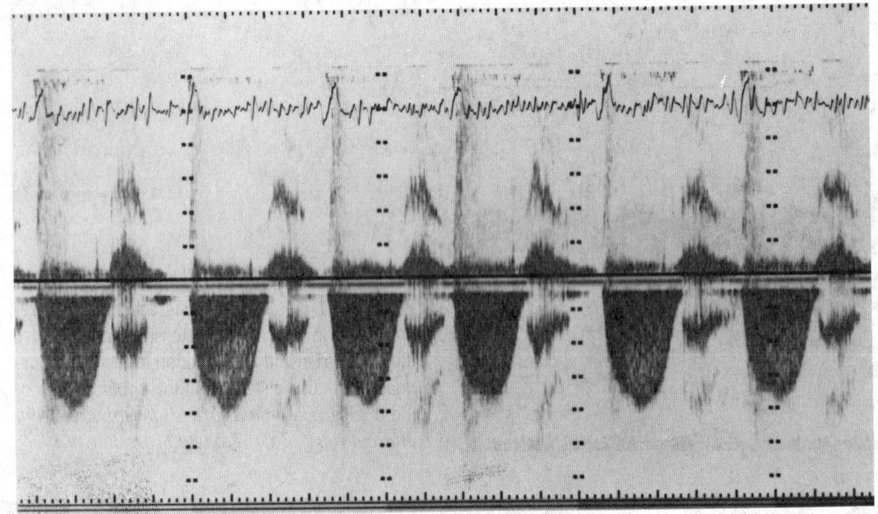

FIGURE 81-5 An echo Doppler continuous tracing in a patient with tricuspid regurgitation. By employing the equation, the systolic gradient across the tricuspid valve can be calculated, and the addition of 10 mmHg yields an estimate of the pulmonary systolic pressure. Thus, in this patient, the level of pulmonary hypertension could be estimated from the echo Doppler tracing of the tricuspid regurgitation. *(Reproduced with permission from Dr. Pamela Sears-Rogan.)*

Although an electrocardiogram and chest film should accompany the most recent examination, echocardiography is the most helpful noninvasive technique for identifying the presence, severity, and potential etiologies of stenosis and/or regurgitation of the tricuspid valve (Chaps. 15 and 130). Should the patient undergo cardiac catheterization for assessment of left-sided heart disease, right-sided hemodynamics should be recorded and, if clinically indicated, simultaneous pressures recorded in the right atrium and the right ventricle (Chap. 138).

The clinical history is important in delineating causes of left-sided heart failure that can lead to pulmonary hypertension and incompetence of the pulmonic valve. Symptoms of the carcinoid syndrome, tumors, or infectious etiologies involving the pulmonic valve should be ascertained. The physical examination is important in evaluating the venous pulsations in the neck veins as well as the pulmonic murmurs. Right ventricular activity should be carefully evaluated as well as concomitant left-sided valve lesions and evidence of heart failure. Although an electrocardiogram and chest film should be obtained to assess the pulmonary artery, right ventricular outflow area, and body of the right ventricle, the major noninvasive tool is the echocardiograph. The anatomy, competence of the valve, extent of the regurgitation, and stenosis can be recognized and assessed by echo Doppler. In addition, other valve lesions involving the left side of the heart can be documented. Since pulmonic regurgitation can be relatively well tolerated, this individual lesion does not require as frequent follow-up, but underlying mechanisms for pulmonary hypertension or left-sided heart failure should be monitored closely.

NATURAL HISTORY AND PROGNOSIS

With tricuspid stenosis the symptoms are usually those of mitral stenosis, but absence of pulmonary congestion in the presence of peripheral edema should raise the possibility of underlying stenosis of the tricuspid valve. Significant tricuspid stenosis may slow the development of characteristic symptoms of mitral stenosis and result in underestimation of the severity of mitral valve obstruction.

With tricuspid regurgitation the symptoms and clinical course are primarily related to the left-sided heart

TABLE 81-2
Tricuspid Valve Disease

Etiology	Physiology	Symptoms	Physical Examination	Electrocardiogram	Chest Film	Echocardiogram	Nuclear Scan	Catheterization	Medical Therapy	Surgical Therapy
Rheumatic Myxoma Endocarditis Right ventricular dilatation Trauma	Pressure and volume overload right atrium Systemic venous congestion	Dyspnea Fatigue Edema	A wave or *cv* wave in neck Systolic or diastolic murmur left sternal border Accentuated by inspiration	Tall P wave Inferior myocardial infarction	Right atrial prominence	Valve anatomy Myxoma Vegetations Diastolic gradient Estimate of right ventricular systolic pressure regurgitation	Right ventricular function Myocardial perfusion	Gradient across valve Pressure recordings	Antibiotics Diuretics Vasodilators	Myxoma Combined with other valve procedures

conditions that produce a pressure-volume overload on the right ventricle. Tricuspid regurgitation virtually always develops with severe right ventricular failure. In bacterial endocarditis of the tricuspid valve the type of organism may significantly influence the course and the response to antibiotics. (See Chap. 94.)

TREATMENT

Medical

In tricuspid stenosis the usual precautionary measures of antibiotic coverage and prevention of endocarditis apply. Peripheral edema may not respond well to administration of digitalis, diuretics, and preload and afterload reduction, which emphasizes the clinical importance of detecting underlying tricuspid stenosis.

With tricuspid regurgitation, treatment of right ventricular failure requires digitalis, diuretics, or vasodilating agents for management of left ventricular failure. If failure of the right side of the heart is caused by mitral stenosis, early intervention to enlarge or replace the mitral valve is appropriate. Patients with congenital pulmonary valve stenosis are usually best treated by catheter balloon valvotomy. (See Chaps. 86, 97, and 98.)

Antibiotic prophylaxis against endocarditis (Chap. 94) is appropriate for patients with either tricuspid or pulmonary valve lesions. If pulmonary emboli contribute to the pulmonary hypertension, anticoagulation is indicated (Chap. 100). Further treatment of pulmonary hypertension may require management of failure of the left side of the heart, correction of mitral stenosis, or the use of vasodilating agents that can lower pulmonary artery pressure. Vasodilating agents may not be effective in treating primary pulmonary hypertension.

Surgical

The decision to proceed with valvular heart surgery is usually based on the severity of the aortic and mitral valve disease, rather than on the severity of the disease of the tricuspid valve. The usual decisions to be made regarding the tricuspid valve are (1) whether or not a procedure should be added to the mitral and/or aortic valve procedures and, if so, (2) which procedures—annuloplasty or valve replacement—should be performed. Patients may present with mild mitral valve disease but severe tricuspid dysfunction. Such patients may require an operation on the tricuspid valve.

Pulmonary valve surgery for acquired disease is performed infrequently. Pulmonary valve stenosis on an acquired basis is rare. Though there are a variety of causes of pulmonary valve regurgitation, this hemodynamic condition is relatively well tolerated if pulmonary vascular resistance is normal. Pulmonary valve replacement may be performed for acquired conditions such as carcinoid heart disease and infective endocarditis, but it generally has been limited to cases where right ventricular dysfunction has become severe after congenital heart disease surgery.[46,47] Although pulmonary regurgitation is generally well tolerated for several years after correction of malformations such as tetralogy of Fallot, the regurgitation may become hemodynamically significant, especially if pulmonary artery hypertension is present or develops. In such a case the placement of a pulmonary valve prosthesis may significantly improve the patient's functional status. In general, bioprosthetic valves have been preferred because of the tendency for mechanical valve thrombosis in this position. In the future, pulmonary valve surgery probably will be performed earlier and more frequently, as studies indicate right ventricular dysfunction may be present in asymptomatic postoperative patients with pulmonary regurgitation.[48]

Infective endocarditis involves the pulmonary valve in about 1 percent of cases seen at autopsy.[13] Isolated pulmonary valve infective endocarditis is even rarer but may be the cause of metastatic pulmonary infections. In a review of 28 cases of this entity, overall mortality was 24 percent, with all those treated by operation surviving.[50] Valvulectomy in combination with antibiotic therapy is sometimes the most effective treatment. (See also Chap. 94.)

Indications for Surgery

The severity of the symptoms and clinical signs of tricuspid valve disease are used to determine whether or not to perform tricuspid valve surgery. If there are signs of tricuspid stenosis and, particularly, if stenosis is demonstrated by cardiac catheterization and two-dimensional echocardiography, the tricuspid valve is directly visualized at operation with the anticipation of performing commissurotomy or valve replacement.

When there are signs of significant tricuspid regurgitation secondary to mitral stenosis, it is important to document the duration of the regurgitation and the severity and duration of pulmonary artery hypertension. These features of the condition are helpful in planning tricuspid valve surgery. If the tricuspid regurgitation is severe and long-standing and if there is chronic pulmonary artery hypertension, it is unlikely that the tricuspid regurgitation will resolve in the early postoperative period after mitral valve surgery alone. In this circumstance, tricuspid valve surgery is usually indicated. In contrast, if the tricuspid regurgitation and pulmonary artery hypertension are of short duration, mitral valve replacement usually will reduce pulmonary artery pressure in the early postoperative period, and this will be followed by a decrease in the tricuspid valve regurgitation. In this circumstance we prefer to wait until discontinuation of bypass following mitral valve surgery to decide whether or not a procedure to reduce tricuspid regurgitation is indicated. Occasionally, severe tricuspid regurgitation will be present with only modest elevation of pulmonary artery pressure. In this circumstance the tricuspid valve leaflets are usually deformed and valve replacement is necessary.

The appearance of the heart at the time of surgery is helpful in assessing the severity of tricuspid valve disease. A thinned-out right atrial wall together with moderate to marked enlargement of the right atrium and venae cavae are indications of significant disease. The degree of stenosis and regurgitation can be estimated by palpation through the right atrial appendage. If tricuspid valve surgery is not performed as the initial surgical approach, examination through the right atrial appendage can be performed after discontinuation of bypass for mitral valve surgery to assess residual tricuspid regurgitation. Intraoperative transesophageal echocardiography

(Chap. 131) provides more precise information as to the degree of residual valvular regurgitation after repair.

Tricuspid Valve Surgery

Tricuspid stenosis may be successfully treated by commissurotomy. This is usually performed under direct vision. The procedure may be combined with annuloplasty to correct valve regurgitation. Valve replacement occasionally is necessary if the changes in the leaflets and subvalvular mechanism are advanced or if severe regurgitation cannot be relieved by annuloplasty. For tricuspid regurgitation, three basic reconstructive techniques have been described (Fig. 81-6). The first procedure is used widely and consists of plication of the posterior leaflet.[51,52] This technique, which can be accomplished quickly, converts the tricuspid valve into a functionally bicuspid valve. De Vega described a second type of annuloplasty that narrows the annulus along the anterior and posterior leaflets with a purse string suture.[53] Carpentier described the third major technique: Placement of a carefully sized semiflexible ring along the anterior and posterior aspects of the annulus.[54] It draws in and supports the tissue evenly. Studies have shown that annular dilatation occurs in these areas rather than along the septal leaflet.[55]

When the leaflets and subvalvular mechanism are deformed as a result of rheumatic fever, reconstruction may not be feasible. In such a case, replacement is performed with either a mechanical or tissue valve. Anticoagulation with warfarin (Coumadin) (Chap. 68) is generally advisable in patients with tricuspid valve replacement, and therefore the major advantage of a bioprosthetic valve is negated. Nevertheless, the bioprosthetic valve has been the prosthesis of first choice of a number of surgeons. If a mechanical valve is preferred and the cavity of the right ventricle is not capacious, a low-profile, tilting disk-type prosthesis seems advisable. Usually, however, if tricuspid regurgitation is severe, a ball-cage prosthesis functions better.

Surgical Results

Mild tricuspid regurgitation does not seem to increase the risk of surgery involving the mitral valve or both aortic and mitral valves. When the tricuspid disease is moderate to severe, however, the risk of operation is significantly increased. Though long-term improvement in tricuspid regurgitation after mitral valve replacement alone had been documented, a tricuspid procedure is generally employed in the setting of moderate to severe tricuspid regurgitation to enhance cardiac function in the critical early days after operation.[56] Mitral valve replacement alone does not invariably decrease tricuspid regurgitation even several months after operation.[57]

In general, the early and late results of tricuspid annuloplasty have been superior to those of valve replacement, and therefore the trend of surgical practice has been to avoid valve replacement when possible. There is a significant incidence of thrombosis with tricuspid prostheses, and the long-term functional results have been less favorable than those of aortic and mitral valve replacements.[58] The less favorable results may be related to more advanced disease in these patients but also may be a function of the less favorable position of the prosthesis in relation to the ventricular outflow tract. The risk of annuloplasty in combination with aortic and mitral valve surgery is about 10 percent. Good early results have been obtained with all three methods of annuloplasty.[59-64] Ring annulosplasty probably gives the best long-term results. When tricuspid valve replacement is necessary, the 30-day operation risk increases 15 to 20 percent. A study of long-term results after tricuspid valve surgery identified two preoperative factors—severity of edema and mean pulmonary artery pressure—as important predictors of long-term survival.[65] A variety of prostheses have been used for tricuspid valve replacement with variable results.[66-69] The valve of choice remains a topic of controversy. Experience with the St. Jude prosthesis in the tricuspid position has generally been favorable.[70]

Tricuspid Valve Surgery for Infective Endocarditis

Infective endocarditis of the tricuspid valve is seen much more frequently today because of drug abuse. In general, the treatment of tricuspid valve endocarditis is medical. When septic pulmonary embolization occurs despite intensive antibiotic treatment, tricuspid valve surgery is indicated. Excision of the valve without replacement has been recommended, particularly since most cases seem related to drug abuse and reinfection of the new valve is an important risk.[71] Nevertheless, since valvulectomy alone carries an important risk of heart failure, tricuspid valve replacement has been recommended by others.[72] It is recognized that continued drug abuse will ultimately result in fatal reinfection, but a good result will likely occur if there is abstinence from drug abuse.

Postoperative Management for Tricuspid Valve Surgery

It is relatively common for the cardiac output to be marginal after tricuspid valve surgery. This is usually a reflection of persistent pulmonary arterial hypertension and long-standing right ventricular dysfunction. Measurements of cardiac output and pulmonary artery pressure are used to guide postoperative care. If annuloplasty is performed, a Swan-Ganz catheter can be used for such measurements. (See Chap. 18.) Nitroglycerin infused via a central venous catheter is a valuable adjunct in reducing pulmonary artery pressure. Prostaglandin E, in combination with pressor agents, may also be employed to treat severe postoperative pulmonary hypertension.[73] Intravenous dopamine and dobutamine may be used to enhance myocardial contractility. If cardiac output remains marginal, an intraaortic balloon pump may be used to reduce left-sided pressures (see Chap. 31). Pulmonary artery balloon counterpulsation has been employed for acute right ventricular failure.[74] Use of a temporary circulatory assist device, such as a centrifugal pump, to bypass the right ventricle may sustain adequate circulation when right ventricular failure is unresponsive to other measures.[75]

Digitalis and diuretics are usually employed for several months after tricuspid valve surgery. For patients

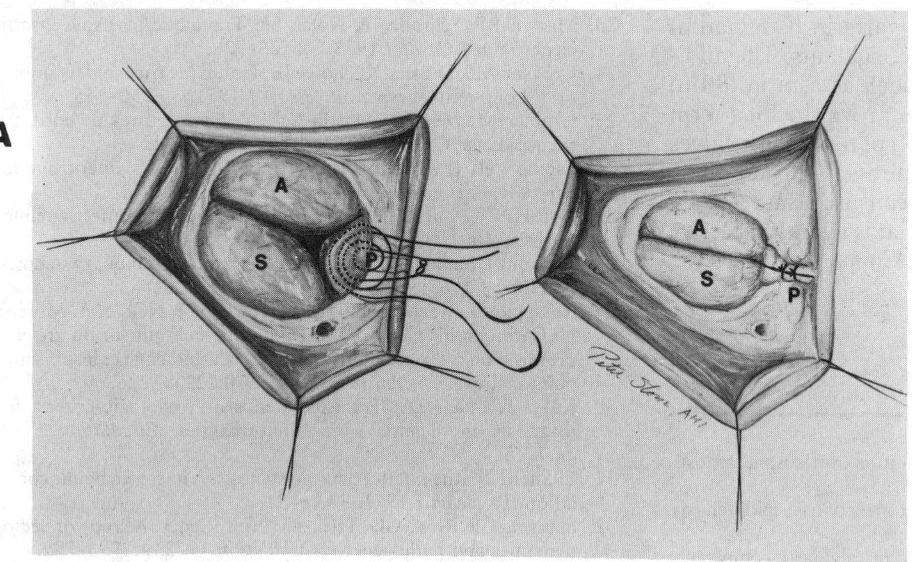

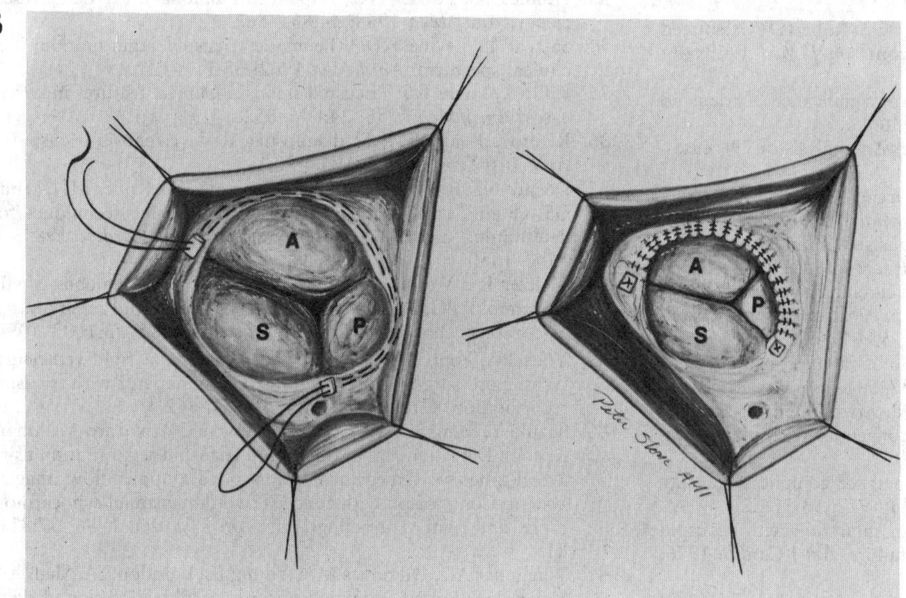

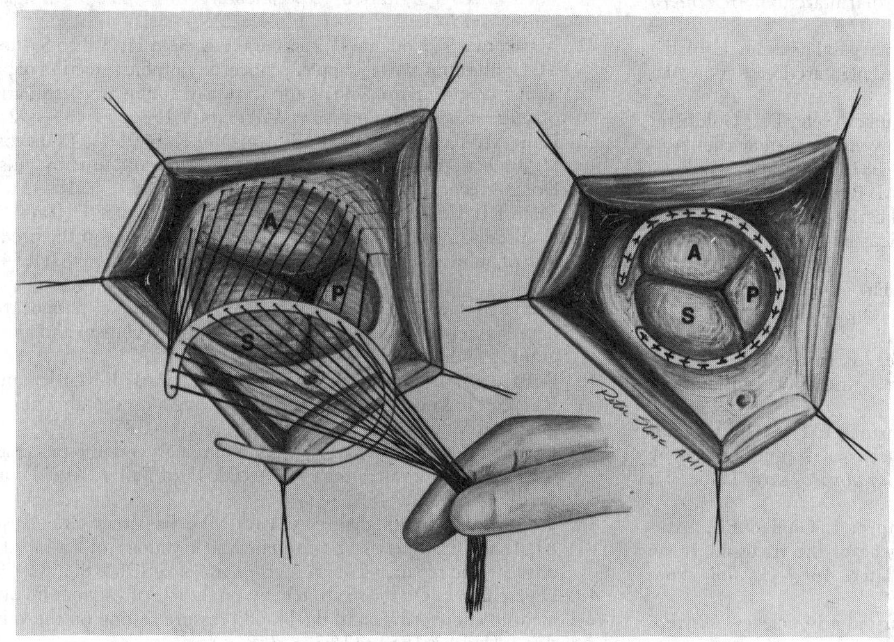

FIGURE 81-6 Three major types of tricuspid annuloplasty have been used. *A.* The posterior leaflet may be placated with production with a bileaflet valve, as described by Kay.[51] *B.* The annulus may be narrowed by a purse string suture, as described by De Vega.[53] *C.* The annulus may also be narrowed by a prosthetic ring, as described by Carpentier.[54] ***(Drawings by Peter Stone, medical illustrator, Georgetown University Medical Center, Washington, DC.)***

with tricuspid valve replacement, warfarin (Coumadin) and dipyridamole are used as anticoagulants. The additional use of antiplatelet agents (such as aspirin, 80 to 160 mg/day) in this setting may improve the long-term results.[75] A serious late complication of tilting disk valves in the tricuspid position is thrombosis. Thrombolytic therapy with streptokinase has been used successfully to restore valve function.[76] Prophylaxis against infective endocarditis is also required. (See Chap. 94.)

REFERENCES

1. Perloff JK, Harvey WP: Clinical recognition of tricuspid stenosis. *Circulation* 1960; 22:346–364.
2. Kitchin A, Turner R: Diagnosis and treatment of tricuspid stenosis. *Br Heart J* 1964; 26:354–379.
3. McMichael J, Shillingford JP: The role of valvular incompetence in heart failure. *Br Med J* 1957; 1:537–541.
4. Glancy DL, Marcus FI, Cuadra M, Ewy GA, Roberts WC: Isolated organic tricuspid valvular regurgitation. *Am J Med* 1969; 46: 989–996.
5. Edwards JE: The specturm and clinical significance of tricuspid regurgitation. *Practical Cardiol* 1980; 6:86.
6. Clawson BJ: Rheumatic heart disease: An analysis of 796 cases. *Am Heart J* 1940; 20:454–474.
7. Flammang D, Jaumin P, Kremer R: Organic tricuspid pathology in rheumatic valvulopathics. *Acta Cardiol* 1975: 30:155–170.
8. Cooke WT, White PD: Tricuspid stenosis: With particualr reference to diagnosis and prognosis. *Br Heart J* 1941; 3:147–165.
9. Ludwig J: Cardiac vein involvement in carcinoid syndrome: Possible evidence of retrograde blood flow in cardiac veins in tricuspid insufficiency. *Am J Clin Pathol* 1971; 55:617–623.
10. McMichael J, Shillingford JP: The role of valvular incompetence in heart failure. *Br Med J* 1957; 1:537–541.
11. Boucek RJ Jr, Graham TP, Morgan JP, Atwood GF, Boerth RC: Spontaneous resolution of massive congential tricuspid insufficiency. *Circulation* 1976; 54:795–800.
12. Collins R, Daly JJ: Tricuspid incompetence complicating acute myocardial infarction. *Postgrad Med J* 1977; 53:51–52.
13. Zone DD, Botti RE: Right ventricular infarction with tricuspid insufficiency and chronic right heart failure. *Am J Cardiol* 1976; 37:445–448.
14. McAllister RG Jr, Friesinger GC, Sinclair-Smith BC: Tricuspid regurgitation following inferior myocardial infarction. *Arch Intern Med* 1976; 95:95–99.
15. Eisenberg S, Suyemoto J: Rupture of a papillary muscle of the tricuspid valve following acute myocardial infarction: Report of a case. *Circulation* 1964; 30:588–591.
16. Maranhao V, Gooch AS, Yang SS, Sumathisena DR, Goldberg: Prolapse of the tricuspid leaflets in the systolic murmur-click syndrome. *Cath Cardiovasc Diag* 1975; 1:81–90.
17. Gerry JL Jr, Bulkley BH, Hutchins GM: Rupture of the papillary muscle of the tricuspid valve: A complication of cardiopulmonary resuscitation and a rare cause of tricuspid insufficiency. *Am J Cardiol* 1977; 40:825–828.
18. Jahnke EJ Jr, Nelson WP, Aaby GV, FitzGibbon GM: Tricuspid insufficiency: The result of nonpenetrating cardiac trauma. *Arch Surg* 1967; 95:880–886.
19. VanGilder JE, Jain AC, Weiss RB, Boyer AF, Tarney TJ: Traumatic right ventricular aneurysm presenting as tricuspid regurgitation. *W Va Med J* 1979; 75:93–98.
20. Stephenson LW, MacVaugh H III, Kastor JA: Tricuspid valvular incomptence and rupture of the ventreicular septum caused by nonpenetrating trauma. *J Thorac Cardiovasc Surg* 1979; 77: 768–772.
21. Brandenburg RO, McGoon DC, Campeau L, Giuliani ER: Traumatic rupture of the chordae tendineae of the tricuspid valve: Successful repair twenty-four years later. *Am J Cardiol* 1966; 18:911–915.
22. Morgan JR, Forker AD: Isolated tricuspid insufficiency. *Circulation* 1971; 43:559–564.
23. Marvin RF, Schrank JP, Nolan SP: Traumatic tricuspid insufficiency. *Am J Cardiol* 1973; 32:723–726.
24. Croxson MS, O'Brien KP, Lowe JB: Traumatic tricuspid regurgitation: Long-term survival. *Br Heart J* 1971; 33:750–755.
25. Grubier M, Denis B, Martin-Noël P: Les ruptures de cordages tricuspidiens. *Coeur Med Int* 1976; 15:215–222.
26. Espino Vela J, Contreras R, Rustrian Rosa F: Rheumatic pulmonary valve disease. *Am J Cardiol* 1969; 23:12–18.
27. Roberts WC, Buchbinder NA: Right-sided valvular infective endocarditis. *Am J Med* 1972; 53:7–19.
28. Seymour J, Emanuel R, Patterson N: Acquired pulmonary stenosis. *Br Heart J* 1968; 30:776–785.
29. Rossignol B, Machecourt J, Denis B, Roche J, NGolet A, Morena H: Cardiopathie carcinoide secondaire à une tumeur du grêle: A propos d'un cas associat insuffisance tricuspidienne et insuffisance pulmonaire. *Arch Mal Coeur* 1977; 70:1221–1226.
30. Killip T, Lukas DS: Tricuspid stenosis: Physiologic criteria for diagnosis and hemodynamic abnormalities. *Circulation* 1957; 16:3–13.
31. El-Sherif N: Rheumatic tricuspid stenosis: A haemodynamic correlation. *Br Heart J* 1971; 33:16–31.
32. Hansing CE, Rowe GG: Tricuspid insufficiency: A study of hemodynamics and pathogenesis. *Circulation* 1972; 45:793–799.
33. Holmes JC, Fowler NO, Kaplan S: Pulmonary valvular insufficiency. *Am J Med* 1968; 44:851–862.
34. Salazar E, Levine HD: Rheumatic tricuspid regurgitation: The clinical specturm. *Am J Med* 1962; 33:111–129.
35. Killip T, Lukas DS: Tricuspid stenosis: Clinical features in twelve cases. *Am J Med* 1958; 24:836–852.
36. Rivero-Carvallo JM: El diagnostica de la estenosis tricuspides. *Arch Inst Cardiol Mex* 1950; 20:1–11
37. DePace NL, Ross J, Ashandrian AS, Nestico PF, Kotler MN, Mintz GS, et al: Tricuspid regurgitation: Noninvasive techniques for determining causes and severity. *J Am Coll Cardiol* 1984; 3: 1540–1550.
38. Meltzer RS, VanHoogenhuyze D, Serruys PW, Haalebos MMP, Hugenholtz PG, Roelandt J: Diagnosis of tricuspid regurgitation by contrast echocardiography. *Circulation* 1981; 63:1093–1099.
39. Yock PG, Popp RL: Noninvasive estimation of right ventricular systolic pressure by Doppler ultrasound in patients with tricuspid regurgitation. *Circulation* 1984; 70:657–662.
40. Suzuki Y, Kambara N, Kadota K, Tamaki S, Yamazato A, Nohara R, et al: Detection and evaluation of tricuspid regurgitation using a real-time two-dimensional color-coded Doppler flow imaging system: Comparison with contrast two-dimensional echocardiography and right ventriculography. *Am J Cardiol* 1986; 57:811–815.
41. Waggoner AD, Quinones MA, Young JB, Brandon TA, Shah AA, Verani MS: Pulsed Doppler echocardiographic detection of right-sided valve regurgitation: Experimental results and clinical significance. *Am J Cardiol* 1981; 47:279–286.
42. Masuyama T, Kodama K, Kitabatake A, Sato H, Nanto S, Inoue M: Continuous-wave Doppler echocardiographic detection of pulmonary regurgitation and its application to noninvasive estimation of pulmonary artery pressure. *Circulation* 1986; 74:484–492.
43. Isobe M, Yazaki Y, Takaku F, Koizumi K, Hara K, Tsuneyoshi H: Prediction of pulmonary arterial pressure in adults by pulsed Doppler echocardiography. *Am J Cardiol* 1986; 57:316–321.
44. Chan KL, Currie PJ, Seward JB, Hagler DJ, Mair DD, Tajik AJ: Comparison of three Doppler ultrasound methods in the prediction of pulmonary artery pressure. *J Am Coll Cardiol* 1987; 9:549–554.
45. Cha SD, Gooch AS, Maranhao V: Intracardiac phonocardiography in tricuspid regurgitation: Relation to clinical and angiographic findings. *Am J Cardiol* 1981; 48:573–583.
46. DePace NL, Iskandrian AS, Morganroth J, Ross J, Mattleman S, Nestico PF: Infective endocarditis involving a presumably normal pulmonic valve. *Am J Cardiol* 1984; 53:385–387.
47. Misbach GA, Turley K, Ebert PA: Pulmonary valve replacement for regurgitation after repair of tetralogy of Fallot. *Ann Thorac Surg* 1983; 36:684–691.
48. Wessel HU, Cunningham WJ, Paul MH, Bastanier CK, Muster AJ, Idriss FS: Exercise performance in tetralogy of Fallot after intracardiac repair. *J Thorac Cardiovasc Surg* 1980; 80:582–593.
49. Lepeschkin E: On the relation between the site of valvular involvement in endocarditis and the blood pressure resting on the valve. *Am J Med Sci* 1952; 224:318–319.

50. Cassling R, Rogler W, McManus B: Isolated pulmonic valve infective endocarditis: A diagnostically elusive study. *Am Heart J* 1985; 109:558–567.
51. Kay JH, Maselli-Campagna G, Tsuji HK: Surgical treatment of tricuspid insufficiency. *Ann Surg* 1965; 162:53–58.
52. Boyd AD, Engelman RM, Isom OW, Reed GE, Spencer FC: Tricuspid annuloplasty: Five and one-half years' experience with 78 patients. *J Thorac Cardiovasc Surg* 1974; 68:344–351.
53. DeVega NF: La annuloplastia selectiva: Reguable y permanente. *Rev Esp Cardiol* 1972; 25:555–556.
54. Carpentier A, Deloche A, Hanania G, Forman J, Sellier P, Piwnica A: Surgical management of acquired tricuspid valve disease. *J Thorac Cardiovasc Surg* 1974; 67:53–65.
55. Deloche A, Guerino J, Fabiani JN, Morillo F, Caramanian M, Carpentier A, et al: Étude anatomique des valvulopathies rheumatismales tricuspidiennes. *Ann Chir Thorac Cardiovasc* 1973; 44:343–349.
56. Braunwald NS, Ross J, Morrow AG: Conservative management of tricuspid regurgitation in patients undergoing mitral valve replacement. *Circulation* 1967; 35(suppl. 1):163–169.
57. Simon R, Oelert H, Borst HG, Lichtlen PR: Influence of mitral valve surgery on tricuspid incompetence concomitant with mitral valve disease. *Circulation* 1980; 62:1152–1157.
58. Thorburn CW, Morgan JJ, Shanahan MX, Chang VP: Long-term results of tricuspid valve replacement and the problem of prosthetic valve thrombosis. *Am J Cardiol* 1983; 51:1128–1132.
59. Carpentier A, Deloche A, Hanania G, Forman J, Sellier P, Piwnica A, et al: Surgical management of acquired tricuspid valve disease. *J Thorac Cardiovasc Surg* 1974; 67:53–65.
60. Grondin P, Meere C, Limet R, Lopez-Bescos L, Delcan JL, Rivera R: Carpentier's annulus and De Vega's annuloplasty: The end of the tricuspid challenge. *J Thorac Cardivoasc Surg* 1975; 70:852–861.
61. Kay JH, Mendez AM, Zubiate P: A further look at tricuspid annuloplasty. *Ann Thorac Surg* 1976; 22:498–500.
62. Peterffy A, Jonasson R, Szamosi A, Henze A: Comparison of Kay's and De Vega's annuloplasty in surgical treatment of tricuspid incompetence. *Scand J Thorac Cardivoasc Surg* 1980; 14:249–255.
63. Rabago G, De Vega NG, Castillon L, Moreno T, Fraile J, Azpitarte J, et al: The new De Vega technique in tricuspid annuloplasty: Results in 150 patients. *J Cardiovasc Surgery* 1980; 21:231–238.
64. Reed GE, Boyd AD, Spencer FC, Engelman RM, Isom OW, Cunningham JN Jr; Operative management of tricuspid regurgitation. *Circulation* 1976; 54(suppl 3): III-96–III-98.
65. Baughman K, Kallman C, Yurchak P, Daggett WM, Buckley MJ: Predictors of survival after tricuspid surgery. *Am J Cardiol* 1984; 54:137–141.
66. Breyer RH, McClenathan JH, Michaelis LL, McIntosh CL, Morrow AG: Tricuspid regurgitation: A comparison of nonoperative management, tricuspid annuloplasty, and tricuspid valve replacement. *J Thorac Cardiovasc Surg* 1976; 72:867–874.
67. Jugdutt BI, Fraser RS, Lee SJK, Rossall RE, Callaghan JC: Long-term survival after tricuspid valve replacement: Results with seven different prostheses. *J Thorac Cardiovasc Surg* 1977; 74:20–27.
68. Kouchoukos NT, Stephenson LW: Indications for and results of tricuspid valve replacement. *Adv Cardiol* 1976; 17:199–206.
69. Sanfelippo PM, Giuliani ER, Danielson GK, Wallace RB, Pluth JR, McGoon DC: Tricuspid valve prosthetic replacement: Early and late results with the Starr-Edwards prosthesis. *J Thorac Cardovasc Surg* 1976; 71:441–445.
70. Singh AK, Christian FD, Williams DO, Georas CS, Riley RR, Nanian KB, et al: Follow-up assessment of St. Jude medical prosthetic valve in the tricuspid position: Clinical and hemodynamic results. *Ann Thorac Surg* 1984; 37:324–327.
71. Arbulu A, Asfaw I: Tricuspid valvulectomy without prosthetic replacement: Ten years of clinical experience. *J Thorac Cardiovasc Surg* 1981; 82:684–691.
72. Stern H, Sisto D, Strom J, Soeiro R, Jones SR, Frater WM: Immediate tricuspid valve replacement for endocarditis. *J Thorac Cardiovasc Surg* 1986; 91:163–167.
73. D'Ambra M, LaRaia P, Philbin D, Watkins WD, Hilgenberg AD, Buckley MJ: Prostanglandin E_1-A: New therapy for refractory right heart failure and pulmonary hypertension after mitral valve replacement. *J Thorac Cardiovasc Surg* 1985; 89:567–572.
74. Miller DD, Moreno-Cabral RJ, Stinson EB, Shinn, JA, Shumway NE: Pulmonary artery balloon counterpulsation for acute right ventricular failure. *J Thorac Cardiovasc Surg* 1980; 80:760–763.
75. Chesebro JH, Fuster V, Elveback LR, McGoon, DC, Pluth JR, Puga FJ, et al: Trial of combined warfarin plus dipyridamole or aspirin therapy in prosthetic heart valve replacement: Danger of aspirin compared with dipyridamole. *Am J Cardiol* 1983; 51:1537–1541.
76. Boskovic D, Elezovic I, Boskovic D, Simin N, Rolovic Z, Josipoulc V: Late thrombosis of the Bjork-Shiley tilting disc valve in the tricuspid position. *J Thorac Cardiovasc Surg* 1986; 91:1–8.

Chapter 82

Multivalvular Disease

Charles E. Rackley, M.D. ■ *Jesse E. Edwards, M.D.*
Robert B. Karp, M.D.

DEFINITION, ETIOLOGY, AND PATHOLOGY

Multivalvular disease indicates obstruction and/or incompetence of the aortic, mitral, and triscuspid valves.

Rheumatic fever remains an important cause in combined disease of the mitral and aortic valves. The tricuspid valve is rarely involved in the rheumatic process but more commonly is affected by right ventricular failure secondary to left ventricular decompensation in valvular heart disease. Roberts reported a high incidence of anatomic lesions involving two or more valves when the characteristic Aschoff body was observed at necropsy.[1] Connective tissue diseases (Chap. 103.) can involve not only the aortic but also the mitral valve. In the Marfan syndrome the mitral valve apparatus can be rendered incompetent along with the frequently observed changes in the aortic valve and ascending aorta. In the aging patient, calcification can develop in the aortic valve and the mitral valve apparatus as well as the mitral annulus. Finally, bacterial endocarditis of the aortic or mitral valve can extend to the adjacent valve apparatus.

Combined aortic and mitral valve disease was observed in 32 percent of 996 patients with rheumatic fever in an autopsy series.[2,3] In the follow-up of 1042 children with a history of rheumatic fever over a 30-year period, multiple valve involvement became apparent in 50 percent of the individuals.[4] Of 699 patients with cardiac involvement due to rheumatic fever followed for 20 years by Bland and Jones,[5] 99 percent eventually exhibited aortic and mitral valve involvement.

Pathology

Conditions that impair both the aortic and mitral valves include rheumatic fever, myxomatous degeneration and prolapse, calcification in the aged, and endocarditis. The inflammatory process of rheumatic fever thickens and scars valve leaflets, which leads to fusion, fibrosis, and calcification (Fig. 82-1). Earlier pathological series described one-third of rheumatic hearts exhibiting involvement of mitral and aortic valves, but Roberts and Virmani[1] later reported that histologic evidence of rheumatic fever confirmed by the Aschoff body was frequently associated with anatomic lesions in two or more cardiac valves.

Myxomatous degeneration in valvular prolapse occurs in the aortic as well as the mitral valve (Fig. 82-2). Fusiform aneurysms of the aortic sinus and ascending aorta can develop in the Marfan syndrome, while changes of dilated annulus, prolapse, ruptured chordae, and annular calcification can be seen in the mitral valve (Fig. 82-3). Annular dilatation, with or without prolapse, is a major cause of mitral regurgitation in the Marfan syndrome.[6]

In aging patients calcification can involve the aortic and mitral valves. Stenosis of the aortic valve is common, whereas mitral annular calcification usually creates regurgitation (Fig. 82-4).

Infective endocarditis can extend from either the aortic or mitral valve to the adjacent valve through the inflammatory process (Fig. 82-5).

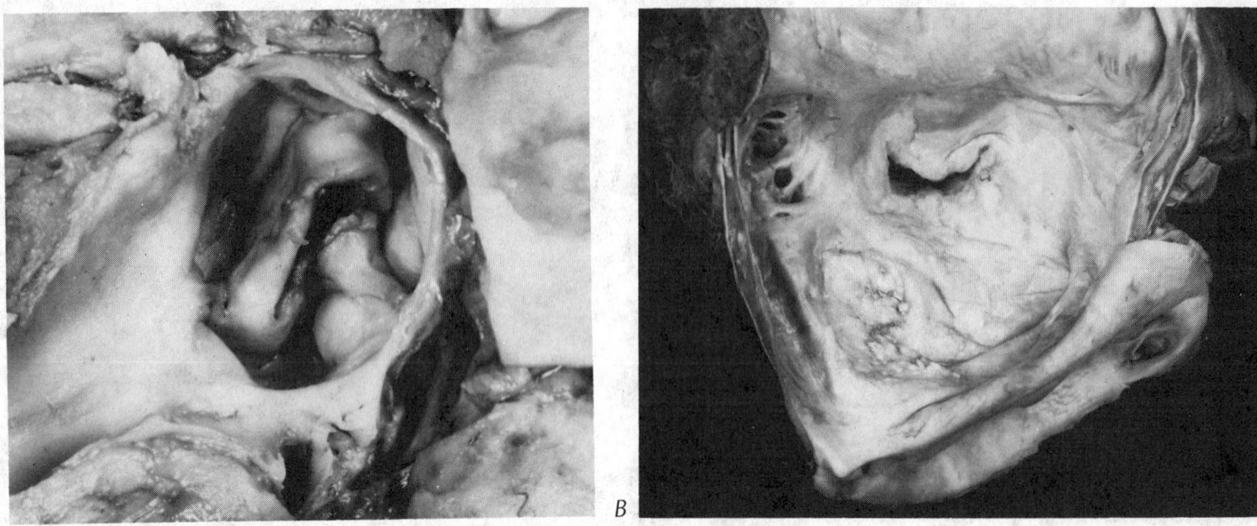

FIGURE 82-1 Rheumatic aortic stenosis and regurgitation and rheumatic mitral stenosis specimens from a 57-year-old woman. *A.* Aortic valve, unopened and viewed from above. Fusion of each of the three-aortic valvular commissures, causing reduction in caliber of the orifice of the aortic valve, is apparent. The associated shortening of the cusps results in aortic regurgitation. *B.* Mitral valve, unopened and viewed from above, and opened left atrium. The mitral valve shows fusion at each of the commissures. The orifice is reduced in caliber. The left atrium is large, and calcification of the posterior part of the left atrial wall is present (lower part of figure).

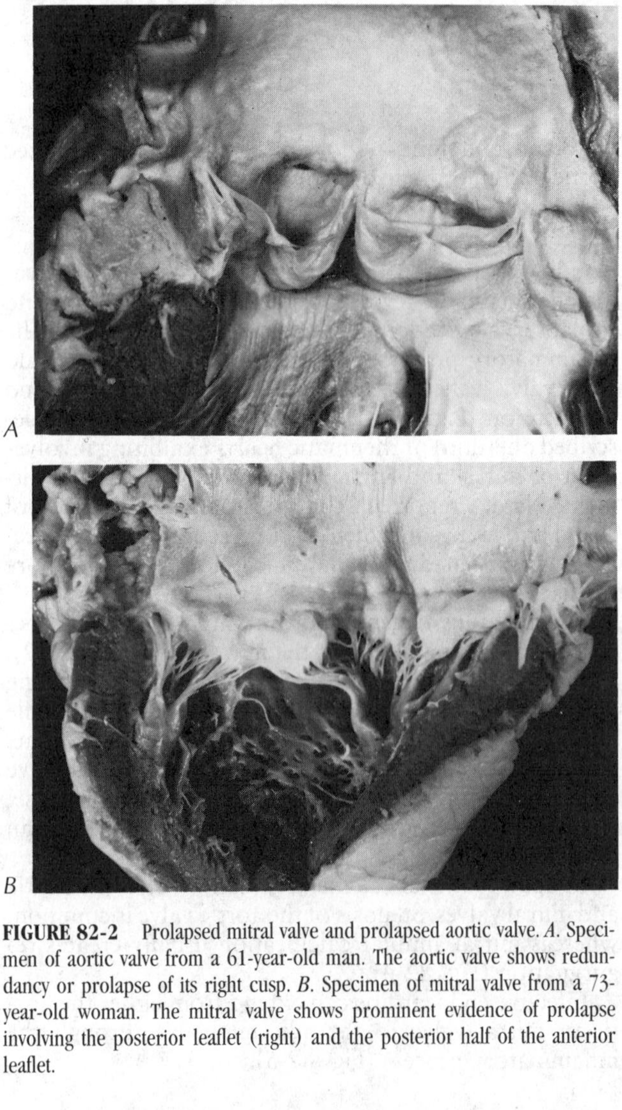

FIGURE 82-2 Prolapsed mitral valve and prolapsed aortic valve. *A.* Specimen of aortic valve from a 61-year-old man. The aortic valve shows redundancy or prolapse of its right cusp. *B.* Specimen of mitral valve from a 73-year-old woman. The mitral valve shows prominent evidence of prolapse involving the posterior leaflet (right) and the posterior half of the anterior leaflet.

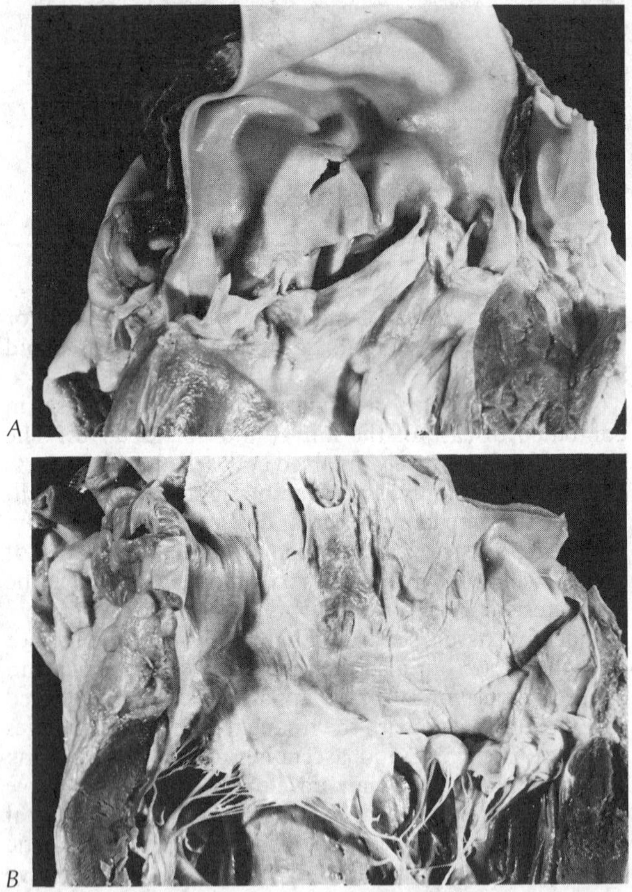

FIGURE 82-3 Floppy mitral valve and limited dissecting aneurysm of ascending aorta leading to aortic regurgitation—specimen from a 60-year-old man. *A.* Ascending aorta and aortic valve. The ascending aorta exhibits a laceration leading to a false channel within the aortic wall in which a hematoma is present (seen on each side of the opened aorta). Secondary distortion of the aortic valvular mechanism caused aortic insufficiency. *B.* Mitral valve, left atrium, and a portion of the left ventricle. The posterior leaflet of the mitral valve (right) shows several areas of prolapse.

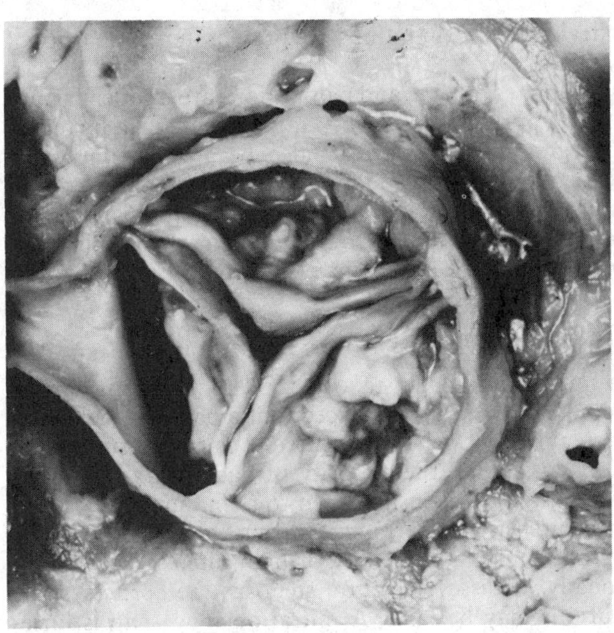

A

B

FIGURE 82-4 Senile calcific aortic stenosis and calcification of the mitral ring—specimens from two different individuals. *A*. Aortic valve. Classic example of senile calcific aortic stenosis in unopened aortic valve viewed from above. *B*. Left atrium, mitral valve, and lateral wall of left ventricle. Sagital section through left atrial and left ventricular walls reveals a calcified mass at the junction of the atrium, the left ventricle, and the posterior mitral leaflet.

PATHOPHYSIOLOGY

Depending on the hemodynamic abnormality, disturbances of the mitral and aortic valves can produce a pressure overload, a volume overload, or combinations of the two.[7] In the presence of combined valvular lesions the pressure overload will cause concentric hypertrophy of the left ventricle even if myocardial failure develops.[8] A left ventricular volume overload will result from aortic and mitral regurgitation, and further dilatation will follow with development of heart failure.[9] The combination of mitral stenosis and aortic regurgitation usually results in a volume overload on the left ventricle with chamber dilatation. Pressure and volume overloads with aortic

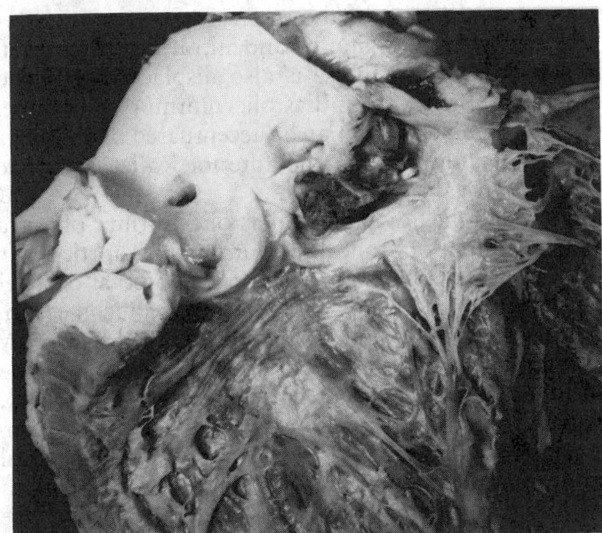

A

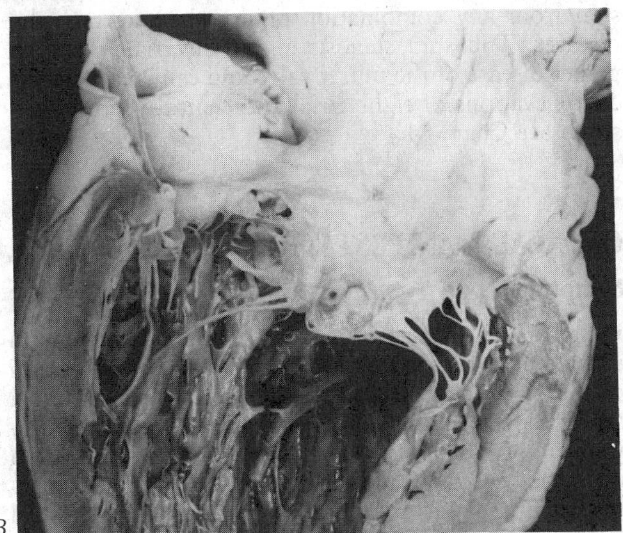

B

FIGURE 82-5 Bacterial endocarditis—specimens from a 36-year-old man. *A*. Aortic valve. The base of the aortic valve shows major destruction of a cusp with extension of inflammation onto the subjacent mitral valve. Near the free edge of the mitral valve, its ventricular aspect shows an ostium of a nonruptured mycotic aneurysm. *B*. Mitral valve, left atrium, and left ventricle. The lobulated mycotic aneurysm of the mitral valve lies near its free edge.

and mitral valve diseases increase left ventricular pressure-volume work and myocardial oxygen consumption.[10,11] Impaired contractility with the development of heart failure decreases the mechanical efficiency of the left ventricle.

An important physiological consideration in combined valvular disease is the dominance of a single valve on altered hemodynamics and potential concealment of the second abnormal valve. Mitral stenosis produces left atrial and pulmonary venous hypertension with eventual pulmonary hypertension and right ventricular failure even though aortic stenosis may also be present. Despite the presence of mitral stenosis, concomitant aortic stenosis can create a pressure overload and hypertrophy of the left ventricle. When mitral regurgitation accompanies aortic stenosis, the pressure and volume overloads create both dilatation and hypertrophy of the left ventricle. Left atrial enlargement and elevation of pulmonary artery pressure eventually accompany this condition. In regurgitation of both mitral and aortic valves, severe dilatation of the left ventricle develops, accompanied by compensatory hypertrophy.[12] Compliant properties of the ventricular myocardium in mitral and aortic regurgitation increase and result in smaller elevations of end-diastolic pressure in the left ventricle and left atrium for larger end-diastolic volumes.[13] Abnormalities in early as well as late diastolic filling can accompany valvular regurgitation.[14] Significant left ventricular hypertrophy can impair filling in both the early and late phases of diastole.

In all combinations of aortic and mitral valve lesions, pulmonary congestion and elevated capillary pressure usually follow significant depression of the contractile state of the left ventricle. Left atrial enlargement produced by either stenosis or insufficiency of the mitral valve often is associated with atrial fibrillation. Changes in pulmonary blood flow and cardiac rhythm frequently accompany the left ventricle pressure-volume overload in combined mitral and aortic valve disease. (See also Chap. 23.)

Tricuspid regurgitation usually accompanies right ventricular dilatation secondary to pulmonary hypertension from any combination of mitral or aortic valve diseases. Tricuspid stenosis almost invariably accompanies disease of the mitral valve and can create significant elevations of right atrial and central venous pressure. (See Chap. 81.)

CLINICAL MANIFESTATIONS

Symptoms

Dyspnea is the most frequent complaint of patients with mitral and aortic valve disease.[15] With the combination of mitral and aortic stenosis, chest pain, palpitations, and syncope are frequent clinical manifestations. Symptoms of heart failure result from pulmonary congestion and usually include fluid retention. Although angina pectoris is infrequent in patients with predominant mitral regurgitation, this symptom is more frequent with incompetence of both aortic and mitral valves. Similarly, syncope is rare in predominant mitral regurgitation but may develop when regurgitation involves both aortic and mitral valves. Palpitations are present in the majority of patients.

Angina, syncope, and palpitations are frequent symptoms in aortic stenosis when it is accompanied by mitral regurgitation. Angina may also be a complaint when aortic regurgitation and mitral stenosis are the predominant lesions; but the more frequent symptoms, dyspnea and fatigue, are attributed to pulmonary congestion and heart failure. (See also Chaps. 79 and 80.)

Physical Examination

In mitral and aortic stenosis the left ventricular apical impulse may not be displaced, but a palpable right ventricular heave can be appreciated. A mitral diastolic rumble is audible in the majority of patients and can vary from grade III intensity down to a minimum of grade I to II intensity (scale ranging from I to VI). The aortic systolic murmur is usually of high intensity, but occasionally, with severe mitral stenosis, the aortic systolic murmur may be faint. A mitral opening snap is infrequently audible, and in a small percentage of patients the diastolic rumble of mitral stenosis cannot be heard.

In regurgitant lesions of the aortic and mitral valves diastolic arterial blood pressure is usually less than 70 mmHg. However, as many as 40 percent of patients with combined regurgitant lesions may exhibit diastolic blood pressures above 70 mmHg. A majority of patients have a loud holosystolic mitral murmur. If aortic regurgitation is the dominant lesion, the early diastolic murmur is usually prominent, whereas when mitral regurgitation prevails, the aortic murmur becomes less intense. A diastolic "flow murmur" across the mitral valve is heard in the majority of individuals with combined mitral and aortic regurgitation. If aortic regurgitation is significant, a systolic murmur produced by the large forward flow across the aortic valve is present. (See also Chap. 11.)

When aortic stenosis and mitral regurgitation occur concomitantly, the apex impulse is displaced, enlarged, forceful, and sustained. A loud mitral holosystolic murmur is heard in most patients, and a diastolic flow murmur across the mitral valve is present.

When aortic regurgitation and mitral stenosis are both present, the apex impulse is also displaced, sustained, and forceful. The early diastolic murmur at the apex may be prominent and may be accentuated by the aortic regurgitant flow striking the anterior leaflet of the stenotic mitral valve.

Although the low-pitched diastolic murmur of mitral stenosis and the diastolic flow murmur with aortic regurgitation are usually reliable diagnostic observations, neither murmur correlates with hemodynamic measurements when the two lesions coexist. As noted previously, when mitral and aortic regurgitation occur simultaneously, as many as 40 percent of patients may have a diastolic blood pressure above 70 mmHg despite severe aortic regurgitation. Mitral regurgitation may diminish the aortic regurgitation due to the increased left ventricular diastolic filling from the enlarged left atrium. Depending on the contractile state of the myocardium, loud regurgitant murmurs may accompany mild regurgitation, while faint murmurs may accompany severe valvular regurgitation if myocardial failure has developed.

Similarly, when regurgitation is present in both the mitral and aortic valves, an aortic systolic murmur or a mitral diastolic murmur does not necessarily indicate stenosis but can be caused by relative "stenosis" secondary to the large blood flow across the valve.

In the presence of aortic stenosis and possible mitral regurgitation, an apical holosystolic murmur is reasonable evidence for associated mitral regurgitation, but the intensity of the murmur is not a reliable indicator in estimating severity. When aortic regurgitation is combined with mitral stenosis, the systemic pulse pressure may be useful, but not necessarily indicative of the severity of aortic regurgitation. A prominent apex impulse in pure mitral stenosis suggests the possibility of associated aortic regurgitation but may not indicate severity. Finally, the intensity of the aortic diastolic murmur is of little value in predicting the severity of aortic regurgitation in the presence of mitral stenosis. (See also Chap. 11.)

While the murmur of tricuspid regurgitation is often accentuated with inspiration (Carvallo's sign), distinction from a concomitant mitral regurgitant murmur can be difficult. Recognition of the rumble of tricuspid stenosis requires careful auscultation during inspiration at the left lower sternal border. Detection by auscultation is rendered difficult by the frequent association of mitral and tricuspid stenosis.

Electrocardiogram

In stenosis of mitral and aortic valves electrocardiographic evidence of left ventricular hypertrophy, left atrial enlargement, and atrial fibrillation is often present. Similar findings are observed in mitral and aortic regurgitation, with a high incidence of left atrial and left ventricular enlargement along with atrial fibrillation. With aortic stenosis and mitral regurgitation, left ventricular hypertrophy is accompanied by a moderate incidence of atrial fibrillation. Mitral stenosis with significant aortic regurgitation similarly produces left ventricular hypertrophy.

Chest Roentgenogram

With mitral stenosis and aortic stenosis the left atrium is always enlarged. Left ventricular chamber size may not be significantly enlarged, but prominent right ventricular dimensions are usually present. Often, both the mitral and aortic valves are calcified. In regurgitation of both mitral and aortic valves, marked cardiomegaly and left atrial and left ventricular enlargement are present. Valvular calcification at either site is relatively infrequent. In aortic stenosis with mitral regurgitation, heart size is increased with both left ventricular and left atrial enlargement. In mitral stenosis with aortic regurgitation, marked left ventricular enlargement is often present.

Echocardiogram

Echocardiography (Chaps. 15 and 130) provides information on valve anatomy, chamber dimensions, pressure gradients, valve size, patterns of regurgitation, and estimates of ventricular function. Stenosis of the mitral (Fig. 15-27) and aortic (Fig. 15-29) valves produces characteristic echoes. Prolapse of mitral, aortic, and tricuspid valves can be characteristically recognized with echocardiography (Fig. 82-6). The number of aortic cusps can be identified (Fig. 15-30) as well as the presence of calcium in either the aortic or the mitral valve apparatus. Dimensions of the left atrium, left ventricle, and right ventricle along with left ventricular wall thickness measurements and mass are useful in estimating the extent of volume and pressure overload. Echocardiography and echo Doppler techniques can assess the orifice size of the

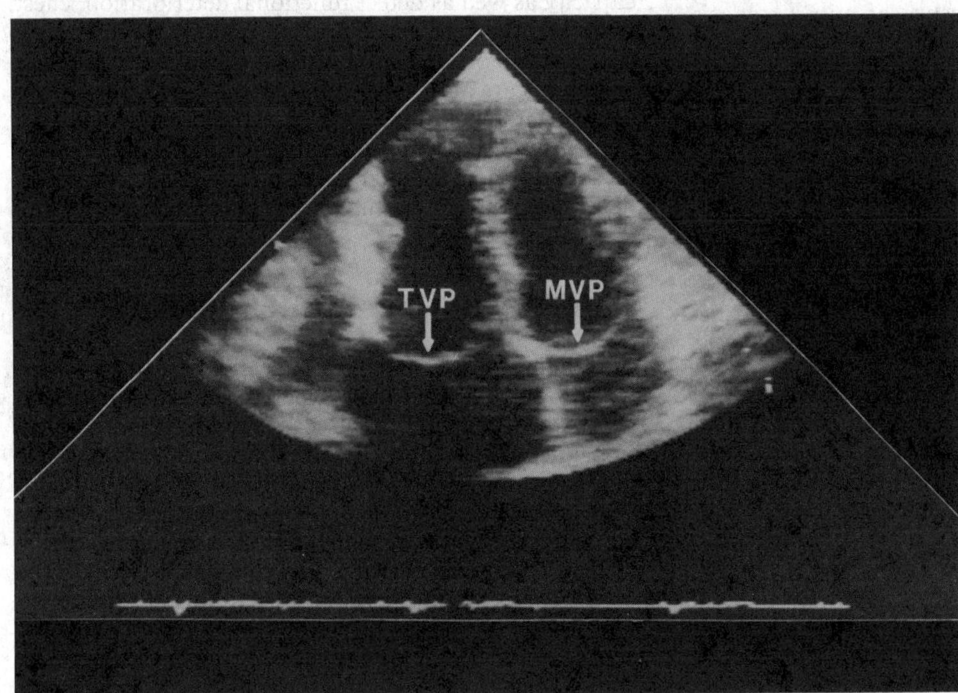

FIGURE 82-6 A four-chamber echocardiograph demonstrates prolapse of both the mitral valve on the right (MVP) and the tricuspid valve on the left (TVP). (*Reproduced with permission from Dr. Pamela Sears-Rogan.*)

aortic and mitral valves and accurately estimate the valve gradients.[17,18] (Figs. 130–10 and 130–11.) Even with the presence of aortic regurgitation, appropriate modifications in the mathematical analysis of the pressure gradient can yield reasonably accurate estimates of aortic valve gradients. Color echo Doppler readings can identify patterns and sites of valvular regurgitation across the aortic and mitral valves.[19,20] In addition, thrombus formation in the left atrium and left ventricle can be detected with various echocardiographic methods. Transesophageal echocardiography can accurately assess prosthetic valve function and valvular repair during the operative procedure.

Nuclear Scan

Information on left ventricular function at rest and during exercise can be provided by radioisotopic techniques. Segmental wall motion can be examined at rest and during exercise and will assist in the recognition of underlying coronary artery disease. Since combined lesions of the aortic and mitral valves often create pulmonary hypertension and right ventricular dysfunction, radionuclide techniques can estimate right ventricular ejection fraction and performance.[21] (See Chap. 134.)

Cardiac Catheterization

Cardiac catheterization is warranted in most patients with combined vulvular disease to calculate the stenotic and regurgitant status of each valve as well as to identify the predominant valvular lesion. Delineation of coronary anatomy is also important because underlying coronary disease should be taken into account in planning the operative approach. Gradients across the valve can be measured with precision and the valve area calculated. Pulmonary hypertension is frequently present in these patients, and left ventricular end-diastolic pressure is often elevated despite the presence of mitral stenosis. (See Chap. 138.)

In mitral and aortic regurgitation, the left ventricular end-diastolic pressure is elevated in the majority of patients, and the central aortic pressure will generally be greater than 40 mmHg. As noted, however, in 30 to 40 percent of these individuals the central aortic diastolic pressure may be above 70 mmHg. A *v* wave of mitral regurgitation can be recorded in the wedge position, and capillary and pulmonary arterial pressures are abnormally elevated in most of these individuals.

In aortic stenosis with mitral regurgitation, left ventricular end-diastolic and pulmonary pressures are elevated, but the extent of the elevation does not necessarily reflect the severity of the mitral incompetence. When mitral regurgitation is significant, forward cardiac output may be reduced; thus, a spuriously small pressure gradient may be recorded across a significantly stenotic aortic valve.

In mitral stenosis with aortic regurgitation, the left ventricular end-diastolic pressure is abnormal and the central aortic diastolic pressure is usually less than 70 mmHg.

In combined valvular lesions, measurement of total angiographic left ventricular stroke volume is useful in calculating the regurgitant volume across each valve.[9] When both valves are incompetent, however, it is more difficult to calculate regurgitant volume across each valve.

Assessment of ventricular function (Chap. 23) is important in combined valve lesions; yet the ejection fraction may be spuriously elevated in regurgitation across the mitral valve and, to a lesser extent, in aortic regurgitation. Measurements of left ventricular end-systolic pressure, volume, and wall thickness permit calculation of end-systolic wall stress.[22] This value has been particularly helpful in pressure and volume overload conditions since the end-systolic pressure-volume wall stress calculation is relatively independent of loading conditions.

Finally, coronary arteriography should be performed at the time of cardiac catheterization in patients above the age of 35 since coronary artery disease may be present without symptoms and may contribute to left ventricular dysfunction.

USUAL STRATEGY OF WORKUP

The clinical history should document symptoms of dyspnea, exercise intolerance, chest discomfort, or syncope. On physical examination, attention should focus on peripheral, arterial, and venous waveforms. Cardiac size, precordial movements, and auscultatory findings should be recorded. A standard 12-lead electrocardiogram and posterioranterior and lateral chest films should be obtained. Echocardiography is indicated to delineate valve anatomy, measure valve gradients, recognize regurgitant pattern, calculate orifice size, and estimate ventricular function and wall motion. A limited exercise test with or without radionuclide studies may help establish exercise capacity as well as detect functional deterioration, chest pain, arrhythmias, or deterioration of ventricular ejection fraction or segmental wall motion abnormalities. If symptoms are atypical and the extent of valvular or left ventricular function cannot be satisfactorily evaluated by noninvasive techniques, cardiac catheterization is indicated. Patients should be seen on a 3- to 6-month basis depending on their status on initial examination.

NATURAL HISTORY AND PROGNOSIS

In combined aortic and mitral valve disease due to rheumatic fever, patients may experience a 10-year period before development of significant murmurs and an additional decade (or more) before symptoms become manifest. If lesions of the aortic and mitral valves are due to degenerative collagen changes, symptoms may develop later in life. When combined lesions are due to calcific changes in the aortic valve and annulus as well as the mitral valve annulus, symptoms develop much later in life. There may, however, be rapid progression of degenerative aortic calcific stenosis over 2- or 3-year periods.

TREATMENT

Medical

If rheumatic fever is believed to be a cause of combined aortic and mitral valve disease, prophylactic penicillin should usually be continued until age 35 years. (See Chap. 78.) Dental prophylaxis with antibiotic coverage, using either amoxicillin or erythromycin, should be provided in all patient groups prior to dental procedures. For genitourinary or other abdominal procedures, gram-negative antibiotic coverage should be provided. (See Chap. 94.)

The development of atrial fibrillation warrants chronic anticoagulation with low-dose warfarin [international normalized ratio (INR) 2.0 to 3.0] since the accompanying incidence of systemic and cerebral emboli is estimated at 10 to 20 percent.

Early development of atrial fibrillation associated with hemodynamic deterioration warrants an initial attempt at electrical cardioversion. If this is sucessful, digitalis as well as antiarrhythmic preparations should be administered thereafter for prophylaxis. Chronic atrial fibrillation should be controlled with digitalis. The development of symptoms, particularly dyspnea, limitations of exercise activity, chest pain, syncope, and class III symptoms, warrants consideration for surgery.

Surgical

A number of patients with severe and progressive symptoms exhibit evidence of disease at both the mitral and aortic valves.[23] Our experience indicates that both valves can be replaced with a hospital mortality that is now between 5 and 10 percent—considerably less than the 22 percent reported for an earlier period.

Frequently in the presence of aortic and mitral valve disease, repair, rather than replacement, of the stenotic or regurgitant mitral valve can be accomplished (Chap. 85). Damage to the aortic valve usually demands replacement. The combination of aortic valve replacement with mitral valve repair probably decreases early mortality and improves long-term survival. There has been marked subjective and objective improvement in surviving patients. When tricuspid replacement is added, the risk of the operation has been higher (about 20 percent), but even here the long-term results are considerably better than the life history of surgically untreated patients with triple valve disease. The use, when possible, of tricuspid annuloplasty rather than replacement has greatly improved the early results of operation in this group of patients.

Indications for Operation

Indication for operation in patients with involvement of aortic and mitral valves is usually the New York Heart Association (NYHA) class III status, but a number of patients are diagnosed at a later stage of their disease. Atrial fibrillation is usually present, and tricuspid involvement is somewhat more frequent than it is in left-sided, isolated valvular disease.

There may be a place for surgical intervention in patients who have volume overload of the left ventricle when they remain in functional class II. Thus, in severe aortic regurgitation with moderate mitral valve involvement, or in important mitral regurgitation together with moderate aortic stenosis and regurgitation, surgery may be advised to avert progressive and poorly reversible left ventricular dysfunction associated with dilatation. (See also Chaps. 79 and 80.)

Operation

Techniques of valvular surgery are described in Chaps. 84 and 85. When hemodynamic derangement is significant at both valves, the decision to repair both is easily made, and the principles of surgical treatment are the same as they are when one valve alone requires attention.

Median sternotomy is performed. With current techniques of myocardial preservation, using cold potassium cardioplegia, the operation can be done in an unhurried, precise manner with the expectation of optimal cardiac performance. On cardiopulmonary bypass, the heart is cooled by the perfusate and by external cardiac cooling. The aorta is cross-clamped. The aorta is opened, and cardioplegic solution is infused into each coronary orifice to attain a myocardial temperature of between 10 and 15°C (50 to 59°F). Reinfusion of the cardioplegic solution is done every 20 to 30 min or when the myocardial temperature reaches 19 or 20°C (66 or 68°F). The aortic valve is resected and attention is then turned to the mitral valve. The left atrium is opened from the right side and the mitral valve is assessed and resected, if necessary, or repaired. The mitral prosthesis is inserted, and the left atrium is left open while the aortic valve is then sutured into place. If there is also tricuspid valve disease, the right attrium is opened at this time and either annuloplasty or replacement is done. The aortotomy is then closed and reperfusion with the perfusate is done while the left atriotomy and right atriotomy are closed. The usual procedures are followed for removing all air from the heart and preventing air embolization as the heart begins to eject.

Occasionally, when the aortic valve is severely diseased and only class II mitral regurgitation (on a scale of I to VI) is evident, it is not necessary to replace the mitral valve. This is true even if left atrial pressure preoperatively was very high, since such pressure can result solely from severe pressure or volume overload of the left ventricle. After repair of the aortic valve disease, incompetence of the mitral valve usually regresses. When there is class II regurgitation of the aortic valve in the presence of severe disease at the mitral valve, however, the aortic valve incompetence often appears to be of greater magnitude after repair of the mitral valve and may contribute to poor postoperative performance. In these situations, therefore, replacement of both the mitral and aortic valves seems indicated.

Results

Long-term survival after replacement of either the aortic or the mitral valve or both is only partially related to factors having to do with the device.[24,25] Other factors, related to the preoperative condition of the patient, intraoperative events, and early postoperative events, also are statistically significant with regard to late mortality. In particular, patients having had previous valve replacement who need a second replacement, because of xenograft degeneration, paraprosthetic leak, or other complications, do less well than patients having primary valve replacement. Patients who have left ventricular aneurysmectomy along with valve replacement have less satisfactory long-term survival rates. There is, however, no deleterious influence of ischemic heart disease in general, as suggested by the lack of any negative effect on long-term survival associated with coronary artery bypass grafting. Finally, patients in whom treatment of ventricular arrhythmias is necessary in the early postoperative course have less satisfactory survival rates.

REFERENCES

1. Roberts WC, Virmani R: Aschoff bodies at necropsy in valvular heart disease. *Circulation* 1978; 57:803–815.
2. Clausen BJ: Rheumatic heart disease: An analysis of 796 cases. *Am Heart J* 1940; 20:454–474.
3. Cooke WT, White PD: Tricuspid stenosis: With particular reference to diagnosis and prognosis. *Br Heart J* 1940; 3:147–165.
4. Wilson MG, Lubschez R: Longevity in rheumatic fever. *JAMA* 1948; 138:794–798.
5. Bland EF, Jones TD: Rheumatic fever and rheumatic heart disease: A twenty year report on 1000 patients followed since childhood. *Circulation* 1951; 4:836–843.
6. Roberts WC, Honig HS: The spectrum of cardiovascular disease in the Marfan's syndrome: A clinico-pathologic study of 18 necropsy patients and comparison to 151 previously reported patients. *Am Heart J* 1982; 104:115–135.
7. Rackley CE, Hood WP Jr, Rolett EL, Young DT: Left ventricular end-diastolic pressure in chronic heart disease. *Am J Med* 1970; 48:310.
8. Hood WP Jr, Rackley CE, Rolett EL: Wall stress in the normal and hypertrophied left ventricle. *Am J Cardiol* 1968; 22:550–558.
9. Sandler H, Dodge HT, Hay RE, Rackley CE: Quantitation of valvular insufficiency in man by angiocardiography. *Am Heart J* 1963; 65:501–513.
10. Rackley CE, Bechar VS, Whalen RE, McIntosh HD: Biplane cineangiographic determinations of left ventricular function: Pressure-volume relationships. *Am Heart J* 1967; 74:766–779.
11. Baxley WA, Dodge HT, Rackley CE, Sandler H, Pua LD: Left ventricular mechanical efficiency in man with heart disease. *Circulation* 1977; 55:564–568.
12. Jones JW, Rackley CE, Bruce RA, Dodge HT, Cobb LA, Sander H: Left ventricular volumes in valvular heart disease. *Circulation* 1964; 29:887–891.
13. Dodge HT, Hay RE, Sandler H: Pressure-volume characteristics of the diastolic left ventricle in man with heart disease. *Ann Heart J* 1962; 64:503–511.
14. Rousseau MF, Pouleur H, Charlier AA, Bruseur LA: Assessment of left ventricular relaxation in patients with valvular regurgitation. *Am J Cardiol* 1982; 50:1028–1036.
15. Terzaki AK, Cokkinos DV, Leachman RD, Merde JB, Hallman GL, Cooley DA: Combined mitral and aortic valve disease. *Am J Cardiol* 1970; 25:588–601.
16. Ogawa S, Hayashi J, Sasaki H, Tani M, Akaishi M, Mitamura H, et al: Evaluation of combined valvular prolapse syndrome by two-dimensional echocardiography. *Circulation* 1982; 65:174–180.
17. Otto CM, Pearlman AS, Comens KA, Reamer RP, Janko CL, Huntzman LL: Determination of the stenotic aortic valve area in adults using Doppler echocardiography. *J Am Coll Cardiol* 1986; 7:509–517.
18. Smith MD, Handshoe R, Handshoe S, Kwan OL, DeMaria AN: Comparative accuracy of two-dimensional echocardiography and Doppler pressure half-time methods in assessing severity of mitral stenosis in patients with and without prior commissurotomy. *Circulation* 1986; 78:100–107.
19. Perry GJ, Helmcke F, Nanda NC, Byard C, Soto B: Evaluation of aortic insufficiency by Doppler color flow mapping. *J Am Coll Cardiol* 1987; 9:952–959.
20. Enriquez-Serano M, Bailey KP, Seward JB, Tajik AJ, Krohn MJ, Mays JM: Quantitative Doppler assessment of valvular regurgitation. *Circulation* 1993; 87:841–848.
21. Winzelberg GG, Boucher CA, Pohost GM, McKusick KA, Bingham JB, Okada RD, et al: Right ventricular function in aortic and mitral valve disease. Relation of gated first-pass radionuclide angiography to clinical and hemodynamic findings. *Chest* 1981; 79:520–528.
22. Rackley CE: Quantitative evaluation of left ventricular function by radiographic techniques. *Circulation* 1976; 54:862–879.
23. Stephenson LW, Edic RN, Harken AH, Edmunds H Jr: Combined aortic and mitral valve replacement: Changes in practice and prognosis. *Circulation* 1984; 69:640–644.
24. Blackstone EH, Kirklin JW: Death and other time-related events after valve replacement. *Circulation* 1985; 72:753–767.
25. Kirklin JW, Barratt-Boyes BG: Combined aortic and mitral valve disease with and without tricuspid valve disease. In: *Cardiac Surgery*. 2d ed. New York, John Wiley, 1993:573–587.

Chapter 83

Artificial Valve Disease

E. William Hancock, M.D.

INTRODUCTION

Artificial heart valves that are implanted surgically to correct diseases of the natural valves are subject to a variety of disorders that may be grouped together as artificial valve diseases. These disorders include those that are similar to the disorders of native valves, such as valvular stenosis, valvular regurgitation, thromboembolism, and infective endocarditis, as well as those that are virtually unique to artificial valves, such as mechanical breakdown, thrombotic obstruction, and hemolytic anemia.

Artificial heart valves are implanted in approximately 40,000 patients in the United States each year.[1] Approximately 80 different models have been used since the first successful implantations were performed in 1960.[2] Artificial valves can be classified broadly as mechanical prosthetic devices or tissue valves. The mechanical devices in common use include caged-ball prostheses, tilting disc prostheses, and bileaflet hinged disc prostheses. Tissue valves are usually porcine aortic valves that are mounted on struts of prosthetic materials (bioprostheses). Smaller numbers of freely sewn human tissue valves, bioprosthetic devices using human valves, or devices fashioned from pericardial or other tissue have also been used.[1] (See also Chaps. 79 and 80.)

Patients with artificial heart valves have an annual mortality rate of approximately 5 percent per year for the first 15 to 20 years after the operation. Most of the late deaths are due to heart disease, but only about 20 percent are caused by disorders of the artificial valve itself.[3] Late mortality is higher after mitral valve replacement than after aortic valve replacement. In addition to the increased risk of death, patients with artificial valves require reoperations for valvular complications at the rate of about 1 percent per year for the first 5 years, and more often after that, especially in tissue valves, where the rate of reoperation rises to approximately 4 percent per year after the first 5 years.

Complications of artificial valves are more frequent in patients who had more advanced heart disease, as manifested by cardiac enlargement, congestive heart failure, and cardiac arrhythmia, prior to the operation. Artificial valve disorders would be less frequent if valve replacement were performed routinely in a prophylactic manner before the development of symptoms and other cardiac complications. Those patients who have isolated aortic valve replacement in the absence of such adverse preoperative factors have been estimated to have a long-term mortality risk that is equivalent to that of the general age-matched population.[3,4] (See also Chap. 79.) This approach would be appropriate for valvular heart disease in general if the artificial valves performed as well as natural human valves. Until such an ideal valve can be developed, however, the problem of artificial valve disease will continue to be a frequent one.[5]

HEMODYNAMIC DYSFUNCTION

Valve-Prosthesis/Patient Mismatch

Placement of an artificial valve that is either too small or too large for the patient may result in a valve prosthesis/patient mismatch. Too large a valve, usually a mitral caged-ball mechanical prosthesis in a patient with mitral stenosis and a small left ventricle, can impede the filling and emptying of the left ventricle and cause a fatal low cardiac output state in the early postoperative period.[6,7]

Too small a valve, a much more frequent problem, results in a condition that is equivalent to valvular stenosis even though the device is intact and functioning according to its specifications.[8]

In general, artificial valves are somewhat stenotic and often have abnormal pressure gradients.[9] As in naturally occurring valvular stenosis, the size of the gradient varies with the rate of blood flow. The smaller aortic prostheses may have mean systolic gradients ranging up to 50 mmHg at rest, and as high as 100 mmHg after exercise. Mitral prostheses often have diastolic gradients in the range of 3 to 10 mmHg at rest, rising to 6 to 25 mmHg after exercise.[9,10] Calculation of the orifice area of a prosthetic valve by either the Gorlin formula or the continuity equation is not as reliable as it is for stenotic native valves.[11,12] Measurement of the gradient may also be technically difficult, requiring demonstration of a representative jet with the Doppler method or requiring pressure measurements in a location very close to the valve in the case of the cardiac catheterization method.[13–15] (See also Chap. 130.)

Arrhythmias such as atrial fibrillation with a rapid ventricular rate may be unusually detrimental in the presence of an artificial mitral valve with an opening time that is delayed; the shortening of diastole is excessive and the mitral transvalvular pressure gradient may rise markedly.

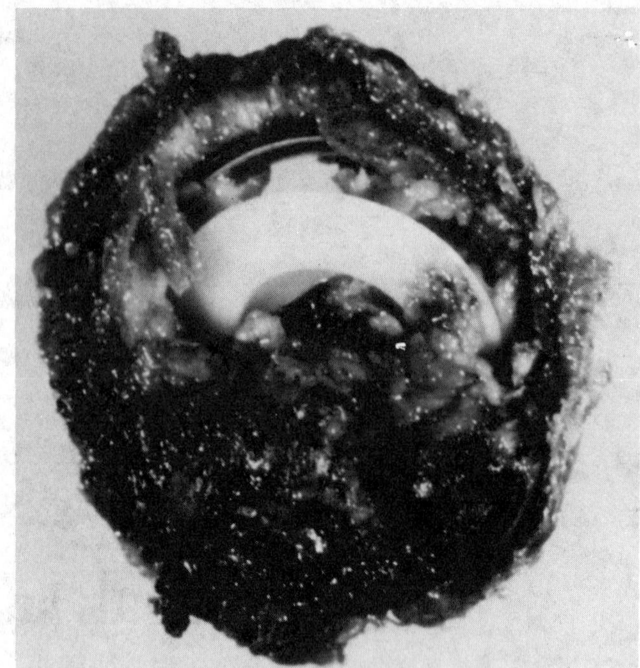

FIGURE 83-1 Thrombosis causing obstruction of an aortic Bjork-Shiley tilting disc valve in a 63-year-old woman who had discontinued anticoagulation several years earlier. *(Courtesy of Dr. Nevin M. Katz.)*

Structural Failure of Mechanical Prostheses

Structural Failure of the Orifice Occluder

This was an important problem in the earliest caged-ball prostheses from 1960 to 1965; swelling, deformation, and fracture of the silastic rubber ball occurred due to absorption of serum lipids. The problem disappeared with changes in the manufacturing process. Structural changes in various occluding balls and discs now occur very rarely. A worn disc may lock in a partially closed position, resulting in acute valvular dysfunction with both stenosis and regurgitation.[1]

Fracture of the Cage

This has occurred with escape of the ball or disc occluder at least occasionally in most mechanical valve models. The most important examples are the Bjork-Shiley 60° and 70° convexo-concave models, used in approximately 86,000 patients from 1976 to 1986; these models experienced an excessive incidence of fracture of the struts due to a defect in the welding process.[16,17]

Mechanical failures tend to produce sudden clinical deterioration. If the valve occluder, or the whole valve, escapes from its normal position in the heart, the condition is often fatal before corrective surgical therapy can be applied. Successful operations have been reported, however.[18,20] Other mechanical faults may present in a more gradual manner; they may be suspected by changes in the heart sounds and documented by characteristic findings in the chest radiograph.

Thrombotic Obstruction

Thrombi that form on artificial heart valves may be large enough to obstruct the valve orifice and produce a significant stenosis (Fig. 83-1). The obstruction may develop acutely, subacutely, or chronically; occasionally, it may be found in a routine examination in the absence of symptoms. This complication occurs with about equal frequency in aortic and mitral mechanical valves. Failure to maintain an adequate level of anticoagulation is often a factor, but this is not uniformly the case.[21–23]

Thrombotic obstruction often presents as a sudden emergency, but symptoms may develop gradually over as long as 6 months.[24] Less than one-half have associated systemic embolism. The prosthetic heart sounds are abnormal in the majority. In most instances the thrombus is a sizable mass that is detected by echocardiography (see Fig. 15-32). In some instances the obstructing tissue is a flat pannus of mainly fibrous tissue that may not be appreciated by echocardiography.

Thrombolytic therapy has been used successfully in the treatment of thrombotic obstruction of artificial valves, but the frequency of such successes is not well established.[21] Thrombolytic therapy may be particularly suitable for those unusual situations in which thrombi obstruct right-sided valves that have been implanted during surgical repairs of congenital heart disease.[25,26] Recurrent thrombus after thrombolytic therapy has been observed, and in some cases, such as those with a fibrous pannus, it is clear that thrombolytic therapy has a very low chance of success. Surgical treatment is probably preferable in those instances in which the patient's condition is sufficiently stable to tolerate the operation.[27] The operation may consist of debridement of the obstructing tissue or replacement of the entire prosthesis.

Tissue Degeneration with Stenosis

Prosthetic valve stenosis develops in tissue valves by a process of fibrosis and calcification of the leaflets. This complication is especially likely to occur prematurely in porcine mitral valves in children and young adults, but it also occurs occasionally in older patients, especially those with chronic renal failure (see Chap. 108), and in aortic valves.[28] The clinical features are generally similar to those of naturally occurring valve stenosis. Some cases, especially in children, present in a more rapid, even catastrophic manner.[29]

Catheter balloon valvotomy can be used successfully in mitral bioprosthetic stenosis, but its use should be carefully restricted to valves that are free of thrombosis, regurgitation, or subvalvular tissue ingrowth.[30] (See Chap. 86.)

Tissue Degeneration With Regurgitation

Tissue degeneration with regurgitation is the most frequent and important hemodynamic form of artificial valve disease. The valve leaflets undergo gradual thinning and stiffening, and ultimately develop linear tears, usually near the base of the leaflets where there is a hingelike action (Fig. 83-2). Microscopic deposits of calcium appear to underly this process in most instances; there may also be fraying and disruption of the collagen fibers.[1]

This complication is rare in the first 3 years after implantation, but after 3 years it occurs in 2 to 3 percent per year and, after 10 years, in about 5 percent per year.[31] The rate is higher in mitral than in aortic valves and higher in young and middle-aged patients than in the elderly. More than 90 percent of aortic, and more than 75 percent of mitral porcine, bioprostheses that are placed in patients older than 65 years are still intact after 12 years of follow-up. Corresponding figures for patients under 35 years of age are approximately 55 and 20 percent.[32] The reasons for the more rapid degeneration of porcine bioprostheses in younger patients are unknown.

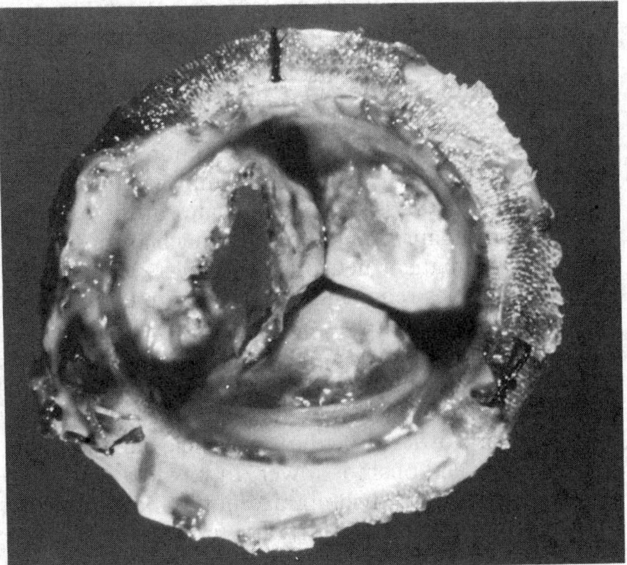

FIGURE 83-2 Calcific degeneration and leaflet rupture, causing severe regurgitation in a mitral bioprosthesis in a 72-year-old woman. The patient had been taking dietary calcium supplements. *(From Moront MG, Katz NM: Early degeneration of a porcine aortic valve bioprosthesis in the mitral valve position in an elderly woman and its association with long-term calcium carbonate therapy. Am J Cardiol 59:1006, 1987. Reproduced with permission from the publisher and author.)*

Valvular regurgitation due to structural valvular degeneration usually develops gradually, and is first discovered by the appearance of a regurgitant murmur on a routine examination. Occasionally, the appearance of a loud musical murmur is noted by the patient, with dyspnea on exertion and congestive heart failure developing later.[33] Some patients, however, have a much more precipitous clinical course. When the original valve disease is aortic stenosis, with a hypertrophied, fibrotic, nondilated left ventricle, the advent of prosthetic aortic regurgitation may lead to a clinical syndrome similar to that of acute severe aortic regurgitation, with pulmonary edema as an early manifestation. Some patients with mitral bioprosthetic regurgitation also develop pulmonary edema relatively quickly, probably because an entire leaflet becomes nonfunctional due to a large tear.

Aortic and mitral bioprosthetic regurgitation can usually be assessed accurately by the same clinical features that are used in naturally occurring valvular regurgitation, including the typical aortic and mitral regurgitant murmurs. (See Chaps. 79 and 80.) For aortic regurgitation, standard transthoracic echo-Doppler examination (Chap. 130) offers the same confirmation that it does in naturally occurring aortic regurgitation. For bioprosthetic mitral regurgitation, however, transthoracic echocardiography is not nearly so reliable, because the prosthesis deflects most of the ultrasound and prevents an adequate imaging of the regurgitant jet in the left atrium. Transesophageal echocardiographic imaging with color-Doppler examination is especially valuable in the study of prosthetic mitral regurgitation.[9,34] (See Chap. 131.)

Patients with valve regurgitation due to structural degeneration may often be managed medically for months or years, with the appropriate time for reoperation selected on the basis of the patients' symptoms as well as the apparent severity of regurgitation. The appearance of a loud regurgitant murmur or the development of new or increasing symptoms indicates the need for surgery relatively soon in most patients. These events reflect advanced pathological changes in the valve, and clinical deterioration is predictable.

Paravalvular Regurgitation

Paravalvular regurgitation occurs when one or more of the sutures that secure the valve to the annulus becomes disrupted, creating a fistula at the periphery of the valve. The incidence of this complication diminished after it was shown that the use of larger individual mattress sutures gave a lower incidence of fistulae than did the older technique of continuous suturing with fine material.[35] Paravalvular leaks which may be first noted many years after the valve implantation, are equally common in aortic and mitral valves and in mechanical and bioprosthetic models. Predisposing factors include past infective endocarditis, calcific changes in the valve annulus, mitral regurgitation as the original valve disease, and the presence of Marfan's syndrome.

Small fistulae can often be detected by transesophageal color-Doppler examination or, at autopsy, as probe-patent fistulae.[36,37] These do not require surgical correction. Large leaks usually present with congestive heart failure, often severe and rapidly progressive. The mitral leaks are often difficult to detect clinically, since they may produce atypical or inconspicuous murmurs. The regurgitant jets tend to course along the wall of the upstream chamber rather than mixing freely in the cavity. A paravalvular leak should be considered in any patient who develops congestive heart failure after mitral valve replacement, even if the clinical examination is not particularly suggestive. Hemodynamic and angiographic data are often a better guide to the severity of the leak than is the color-Doppler image.[38] Abnormal motion of the valve in chest radiography, cinefluoroscopy, or echocardiography is also a helpful clue in some cases.

Rarely, the valve may become partially detached, but without regurgitation, because it falls into place when regurgitant flow begins. This problem can be detected by showing abnormal motion of the valve during the cardiac cycle. It is best displayed by cinefluoroscopy.[39]

Surgical correction of paravalvular leaks can usually be accomplished by simply adding the necessary additional sutures, rather than replacing the entire valve.

Surveillance and Early Recognition

Patients who have artificial heart valves need regular and expert follow-up to detect early disorders of the artificial valve as well to regulate anticoagulation and to maintain surveillance of their other cardiac and noncardiac medical problems. Many patients have persistent dyspnea and reduced effort tolerance after successful mitral valve replacement because of the mild stenosis of the artificial valve, residual myocardial dysfunction, atrial fibrillation, etc. New or progressive symptoms may suggest an artificial valve disorder.

Examination of the heart provides clues to many of the artificial valve disorders, but its interpretation requires knowledge of the heart sounds and murmurs that are present in normally functioning artificial valves of various types.[40,41] Mechanical valves generally create very loud metallic-sounding closing sounds (S1 for the mitral, S2 for the aortic). Similar loud sounds are created by the opening of the caged-ball models (early systolic opening click for the aortic, early diastolic opening click for the mitral), but not of the tilting disc or the bileaflet models. The caged-ball models may also cause a volley of sounds (during systole for the aortic, diastole for the mitral) as blood flow through the orifice causes the ball to bounce between the struts of the cage. Systolic murmurs are generally present in both aortic and mitral mechanical models, because of turbulent flow through or around the cage. Diastolic murmurs are not present in normally functioning mechanical prosthetic valves except in rare instances. The absence of a rumbling diastolic murmur, even in small-sized mitral mechanical prosthetic valves in which a substantial diastolic pressure gradient may be present, indicates that the mitral stenosis murmur found in natural valves is caused, in part, by vibration of the stenotic valvular structure, not simply by turbulent flow caused by a narrow orifice. A faint aortic diastolic murmur may occur in certain aortic tilting disc models, in which the disc requires a longer than usual time to become seated.

The closing sounds of mechanical valves are often loud enough to be heard by the patient, and may be a source of complaints, particularly in young people.[42]

Patients with bioprostheses have essentially normal S1 and S2, with no abnormal opening sounds. The aortic bioprosthesis is usually associated with a short- to medium-length midsystolic murmur of grade 2 to 3 intensity, but a diastolic murmur is abnormal. The mitral bioprosthesis is not necessarily associated with any systolic murmur, but a soft, short- or medium-length diastolic rumble is sometimes present. An unusually loud diastolic rumble in a mitral bioprosthesis is more likely to represent significant mitral regurgitation than mitral stenosis; the regurgitant flow leads to increased forward flow in diastole, with increased turbulence because of the mild inherent stenosis of the valve.

A baseline transthoracic echocardiogram is very useful, but serial echocardiography need not be done routinely in follow-up. It is very useful if artificial valve dysfunction is suspected and as a method of evaluating left ventricular function. Serial echocardiograms in patients with bioprostheses often show the gradual development of structural abnormalities that predict the eventual development of clinical deterioration.[42] When new, or changed, symptoms or signs are noted, echocardiography and chest radiographs are indicated; cinefluoroscopy, phonocardiography, and cardiac catheterization with angiocardiography may also be considered for selected indications. Transesophageal echocardiography should especially be considered if a strong suspicion of mitral regurgitation is present.

THROMBOEMBOLISM

Systemic embolism, originating in thrombus formation on the artificial valve, is the most important complication of mechanical models, but also occurs with bioprostheses. The rate is constant over a 10- to 15-year follow-up and usually ranges from 1 to 2 percent per year in aortic valves and from 2 to 3 percent per year in mitral valves.[44] Many embolic episodes are minor, causing such events as transient neurological symptoms, amaurosis fugax, or self-limited ischemic episodes in the extremities, or other organs. Major episodes, such as those causing death, permanent neurological defects, or ischemia of the extremities requiring surgical treatment occur at the rate of approximately 1 percent per year.[44–46] Because it is usually impossible to distinguish embolic episodes that originate from thrombosis on the artificial valve from those originating in the left atrium, the left ventricular cavity, or aortic wall, the true incidence of valve-related major embolism is lower. In most patients who have had embolism, thrombi are not demonstrable on the valve by echocardiography. This reflects the fact that some thrombi form and then disappear, as well as the fact that both thrombi and vegetations are difficult to recognize specifically because of the high reflectivity for ultrasound by the prosthesis itself.

Major bleeding episodes, such as those serious enough to require hospitalization or transfusion, occur at the rate of 1 to 3 percent per year[47] in patients taking long-term anticoagulation, compared with about 0.5 percent per year in those patients with bioprostheses who do not take anticoagulation. All mechanical valves require long-term anticoagulation with warfarin to prolong the INR prothrombin time (PT) to 2.5 to 3.5, which corresponds to a PT prolongation of approximately 1.5 to 2.0 times normal.[48] Patients who have a mitral bioprosthesis inserted should be maintained on warfarin to prolong the INR to 2.0 to 3.0 (1.3 to 1.5 control using North American thromboplastin). This may be discontinued after 3 months if the rhythm is normal sinus, the left atrium not markedly enlarged, and there is no history of systemic embolism.

INFECTIVE ENDOCARDITIS

Infective endocarditis occurs on artificial valves at the rate of approximately 0.5 percent per year. It affects aortic and mitral valves, and mechanical and bioprosthetic models about equally. The incidence is higher in the first 6 months after the operation. These early cases are presumed to result from contamination at the time of the operation; staphylococci are the most frequent organisms, and gram-negative bacilli and fungi are also notable etiologies. Late infective endocarditis is presumably acquired in the same manner as infection involving native valves, with *Streptococcus viridans* the most frequent organism (Fig. 83-3). (See Chap. 94.)

Prosthetic infective endocarditis has a high incidence of complications, such as valve ring abscess, valvular obstruction, paravalvular regurgitation, and regurgitation due to leaflet degeneration in tissue valves. The mortality is approximately 50 percent, even when surgery is used aggressively. Relatively few patients can be expected to be cured by antibiotic therapy alone.[49,50] The preserved human aortic valve is favored by several surgeons as the artificial valve of choice when patients with prosthetic endocarditis require replacement of the valve.[51,52]

Whenever such complications as embolism, thrombotic obstruction, paravalvular leak, or tissue degeneration with regurgitation occur in patients with artificial valves, infective endocarditis should be considered as a possible cause.

HEMOLYTIC ANEMIA

An increased rate of intravascular destruction of red blood cells is produced frequently by artificial valves, particularly the mechanical models. In most instances, the increased rate of destruction is mild and is readily compensated for by increased production in the bone marrow, so anemia is not present.[53] Elevated serum levels of lactic dehydrogenase (LDH) (≥500 units), reduced levels of haptoglobin, and schistocytosis (≥1 percent) are the principal features of low-grade hemolysis. Occasionally, the rate of red blood cell destruction is much greater, and a hemolytic anemia results. If the hemolysis is mild, there may be hemosiderinuria, but hemoglobinuria is absent and reticulocytosis is less than 5 percent.

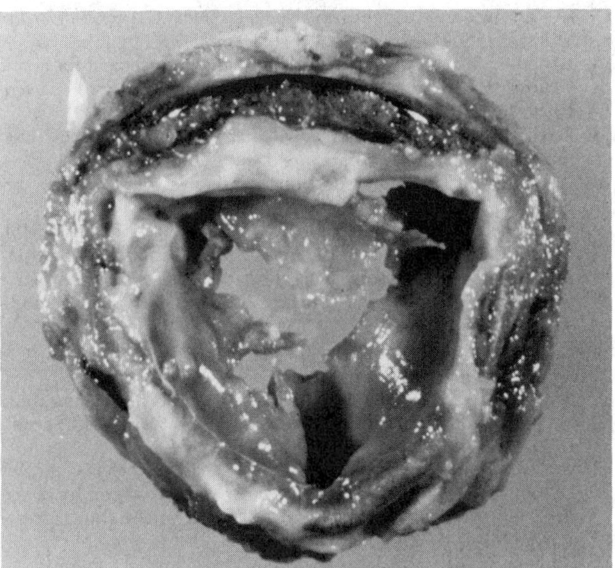

FIGURE 83-3 Streptococcus viridans infection of a degenerated aortic bioprosthesis in a 20-year-old patient. *(Courtesy of Dr. Nevin M. Katz.)*

With moderate hemolysis, levels of LDH are greater than 500 units, haptoglobins are absent, schistocytosis is >1 percent, reticulocytosis is <5 percent, hemosiderinuria is present, but hemoglobinuria is absent. In severe hemolysis, the LDH level is much greater than 500, haptoglobin is absent, reticulocytosis is much more than 5 percent, schistocytosis is much more than 1 percent, hemosiderinuria is marked, and hemoglobinuria is present.[53]

Deficiencies of iron and folic acid may develop. When severe anemia develops there is usually an additional abnormality, such as a paravalvular leak, that plays a major contributing role in the exaggerated hemolysis. Hemolytic anemia has occurred in normally functioning valves, however.

Hemolysis is more likely to occur in men than women, in patients with dilated hypokinetic left ventricles, and in patients with some degree of congestive heart failure. It is particularly likely to occur with caged-ball prostheses that have prosthetic cloth covering the struts, and with the low-profile caged-disc model.[4,54,55]

Mild or moderate degrees of increased hemolysis can usually be treated successfully with oral iron supplemented by folic acid, if necessary. It may be necessary to restrict physical activity. The presence of hemolytic anemia often plays a role in the decision to perform a reoperation in a patient with a paravalvular leak. Rarely, the hemolytic anemia alone may be the indication for reoperation.

REFERENCES

1. Schoen FJ: Cardiac valve prostheses: Pathological and bioengineering considerations. *J Cardiovasc Surg* 1987; 2:65–108.
2. Mehlman DJ: A pictorial and radiographic guide for identification of prosthetic heart valve devices. *Prog Cardiovasc Dis* 1988; 30:441–464.
3. Lindblom D, Lindblom U, Qvist J, Lundstrom H: Long-term rela-

tive survival rates after heart valve replacement. *J Am Coll Cardiol* 1990; 15:566–573.
4. Lund O: Late chronic hemolysis after valve replacement for aortic stenosis. Relation to residual hypertrophy and impaired left ventricular function. *Angiology* 1990; 41:836–847.
5. Davila JC: Where is the ideal valve substitute? What has frustrated its realization? *Ann Thorac Surg* 1989; 48 (Suppl):S20-3.
6. Roberts W: Choosing a substitute cardiac valve; type, size, surgeon. *Am J Cardiol* 1976; 38:633–644.
7. Waggoner AD, Perez JE, Barzilai B, Rosenbloom M, Eaton MH, Cox JL: Left ventricular outflow obstruction resulting from insertion of mitral prostheses leaving the native leaflets intact: Adverse clinical outcome in seven patients. *Am Heart J* 1991; 122:483–488.
8. Rahimtoola SH: The problem of valve prosthesis–patient mismatch. *Circulation* 1978; 58:20–25.
9. Nanda NC, Cooper JW, Mahan EF 3d, Fan P: Echocardiographic assessment of prosthetic valves. *Circulation* 1991; 84 (3 Suppl): I-228–I-239.
10. van den Brink RBA, Verheul HA, Visser CA, Koelemay MJW, Dunning AJ: Value of exercise Doppler echocardiography in patients with prosthetic or bioprosthetic cardiac valves. *Am J Cardiol* 1992; 69:367–372.
11. Cannon SR, Richards KL, Cawford MH, Folland ED, Pierpont G, Sethi GK, et al: Inadequacy of the Gorlin formula for predicting prosthetic valve area. *Am J Cardiol* 1988; 62:113–116.
12. Chambers JB, Sprigings DC, Cochrane T, Allen J, Morris R, Black MM, et al: Continuity equation and Gorlin formula compared with directly observed orifice area in native and prosthetic aortic valves. *Br Heart J* 1992; 67:193–199.
13. Baumgartner H, Khan S, DeRobertis M, Czer L, Maurer G: Effect of prosthetic aortic valve design on the Doppler-catheter gradient correlation; an in vitro study of normal St. Jude, Medtronic-Hall, Starr-Edwards and Hancock valves. *J Am Coll Cardiol* 1992; 19:324–332.
14. Burstow DJ, Nishimura RA, Bailey KR, Reeder GS, Holmes DR Jr, Seward JB, et al: Continuous wave Doppler echocardiographic measurement of prosthetic valve gradients. A simultaneous Doppler-catheter correlative study. *Circulation* 1989; 80:504–514.
15. Stewart SFC, Nast EP, Arabia FA, Talbot TL, Proschan M, Clark RE: Errors in pressure gradient measurement by continuous wave Doppler ultrasound: Type, size and age effects in bioprosthetic aortic valves. *J Am Coll Cardiol* 1991; 18:769–779.
16. Treasure T: Management of patients with Bjork-Shiley prosthetic valves. *Br Heart J* 1991; 66:333–334.
17. van der Graef Y, de Waard F, van Herwerden LA, Defauw J: Risk of strut fracture of Bjork-Shiley valves. *Lancet* 1992; 339:257–261.
18. Hendel PN: Bjork-Shiley strut fracture and disc escape; literature review and a method of disc retrieval. *Ann Thorac Surg* 1989; 47:436–440.
19. Kumar N, Balasundaram S, Rickard M, al Halees Z, Duran CMG: Leaflet embolisation from Duromedics valves; a report of two cases. *Thorac Cardiovasc Surg* 1991; 39:382–383.
20. Stoneburner JM Jr, Tucker BL, Hurvitz RJ: Survival after embolization of a complete prosthetic aortic valve to the aortic arch. *Ann Thorac Surg* 1990; 49:140–142.
21. Deviri E, Sarell P, Wisenbaugh T, Cronje SL: Obstruction of mechanical heart valve prostheses; clinical aspects and surgical management. *J Am Coll Cardiol* 1991; 17:646–650.
22. Pansini S, Ottino G, Forsennati PG, Serpieri G, Zattera G, Casabona R, et al: Reoperation on heart valve prostheses; an analysis of operative risks and late results. *Ann Thorac Surg* 1990; 50:590–596.
23. Kontos GJ, Schaff HV, Orszulak TA, Puga FJ, Pluth JR, Danielson GK: Thrombotic obstruction of disc valves: Clinical recognition and surgical management. *Ann Thorac Surg* 1989; 48:60–65.
24. Chen HJ, Schlaifer JD, Guentzel SM, Conti CR: Documentation of successful treatment of prosthetic mitral valve thrombosis with intravenous urokinase infusion for twenty-four hours. *Clin Cardiol* 1992; 15:127–133.
25. Fyfe DA, Taylor AB, Kline CH, Sade RM, Gillette PC: Doppler echocardiographic evaluation of streptokinase lysis of thrombosed right-sided St. Jude Medical valves in patients with congenital heart defects. *Am Heart J* 1991; 121:1156–1160.
26. Marti V, Subirana MT, Ballester M, Obrador D, Auge JM, Font-cuberta J, et al: Successful thrombolytic therapy for prosthetic pulmonary valve thrombosis evaluated by Doppler echocardiography. *Am Heart J* 1992; 123:1065–1067.
27. Martinell J, Jimenez A, Rabago G, Artiz V, Fraile J, Farre J: Mechanical cardiac valve thrombosis. Is thrombectomy justified? *Circulation* 1991; 84 (Suppl III):III70–75.
28. Solymar L, Rao PS, Mardini MK, Fawzy ME, Guinn G: Prosthetic valves in children and adolescents. *Am Heart J* 1991; 121:557–568.
29. Kopf GS, Geha AS, Hellenbrand WE, Kleinman CS: Fate of left-sided cardiac bioprosthesis valves in children. *Arch Surg* 1986; 121:488–490.
30. Waller BF, McKay C, VanTassel J, Allen M: Catheter balloon valvuloplasty of stenotic porcine bioprosthetic valves: Part II: Mechanisms, complications, and recommendations for clinical use. *Clin Cardiol* 1991; 14:764–772.
31. Jamieson WRE, Janusz MT, Miyagishima RT, Munro AI, Gerein AN, Allen P, et al: The Carpentier-Edwards standard porcine bioprosthesis: long-term evaluation of the high pressure glutaraldehyde fixed prosthesis. *J Cardiovasc Surg* 1988; 3 (3 Suppl):321–363.
32. Jamieson WRE, Tyers GFO, Janusz MT, Miyagishima RT, Munro AI, Ling H, et al: Age as a determinant for selection of porcine bioprothesis for cardiac valve replacement: Experience with Carpentier-Edwards standard bioprosthesis. *Can J Cardiol* 1991; 7:181–188.
33. Errington M, Bloomfield P, Starkey IR, Shaw TR: Patients' observations of bioprosthetic valve failure: "My heart is honking, doctor." *Br Heart J* 1990; 64:393–394.
34. Khanderia BK, Seward JB, Oh JK, Freeman WK, Nichols BA, Sinak LJ, et al: Value and limitations of transesophageal echocardiography in assessment of mitral valve prostheses. *Circulation* 1991; 83:1956–1968.
35. Dhasmana JP, Blackstone EH, Kirklin JW, Kouchoukos NT: Factors associated with periprosthetic leakage following primary mitral valve replacement; with special consideration of the suture technique. *Ann Thorac Surg* 1983; 35:170–178.
36. Jindani A, Neville EM, Venn G, Williams BT: Paraprosthetic leak: A complication of cardiac valve replacement. *J Cardiovasc Surg* 1991; 32:503–508.
37. Zeien LB, Klatt EC: Cardiac valve prostheses at autopsy. *Arch Pathol Lab Med* 1990; 114:933–937.
38. Baumgartner H, Khan S, DeRobertis M, Czer L, Maurer G: Color Doppler regurgitant characteristics of normal mechanical mitral valve prostheses in vitro. *Circulation* 1992; 85:323–332.
39. Sands MJ Jr, Lachman AS, O'Reilly DJ, Leach CN Jr, Sappington JB, Katz AM: Diagnostic value of cinefluoroscopy in the evaluation of prosthetic heart valve dysfunction. *Am Heart J* 1982; 104:622–627.
40. Smith ND, Raizada V, Abrams J: Auscultation of the normally functioning prosthetic valve. *Ann Intern Med* 1981; 95: 594–598.
41. DePace NL, Kotler MN, Mintz GS, Lichtenberg R, Goel IP, Segal BL: Echocardiographic and phonocardiographic assessment of the St. Jude cardiac valve prosthesis. *Chest* 1981; 80:272–277.
42. Moritz A, Steinseifer U, Kobina G, Neuwirth-Reidl K, Wolters H, Ruel H, et al: Closing click of St. Jude Medical and Duromedics Edwards bileaflet valves: Complaints created by valve noise and their relation to sound pressure and hearing level. *Eur Heart J* 1991; 12:673–679.
43. Teoh KH, Ivanov J, Weisel RD, Daniel LB, Darcel IC, Rakowski H: Clinical and Doppler echocardiographic evaluation of bioprosthetic valve failure after 10 years. *Circulation* 1990; 82 (Suppl IV):IV-110–116.
44. Grunkemeier, GL, Rahimtoola SH: Artificial heart valves. *Ann Rev Med* 1990; 41:251–263.
45. Bloomfield P, Wheatley DJ, Prescott RJ, Miller HC: Twelve-year comparison of Bjork-Shiley mechanical heart valve with porcine bioprostheses. *N Engl J Med* 1991; 324:573–579.
46. Myers ML, Lawrie GM, Crawford ES, Howell JF, Morris GC Jr, Glaeser DH, et al: The St. Jude valve prosthesis: Analysis of the clinical results in 815 implants and the need for systemic anticoagulation. *J Am Coll Cardiol* 1989; 13:57–62.
47. Wilson DB, Dunn MI, Hassanein K: Low-intensity anticoagulation in mechanical cardiac prosthetic valves. *Chest* 1991; 100:1553–1557.
48. Stein PD, Alpert JS, Copeland J, Dalen JE, Goldman S, Turpie AGG: Antithrombotic therapy in patients with mechanical and

biologic prosthetic heart valves. *Chest* 1992; 102(Suppl):445S–455S.
49. Cowgill LD, Addonizio VP, Hopeman AR, Harken AH: Prosthetic valve endocarditis. *Curr Prob Cardiol* 1986; 11:618–664.
50. Watanakunakor C: Prosthetic valve infective endocarditis. *Prog Cardiovasc Dis* 1979; 22:181–192.
51. Haydock D, Barratt-Boyes B, Macedo T, Kirklin JW, Blackstone E: Aortic valve replacement for active infectious endocarditis in 108 patients. A comparison of freehand allograft valves with mechanical prostheses and bioprostheses. *J Thorac Cardiovasc Surg* 1992; 103:130–139.
52. Miller DC: Predictors of outcome in patients with prosthetic valve endocarditis (PVE) and potential advantages of homograft aortic root replacement for prosthetic ascending aortic valve-graft infections. *J Cardiovasc Surg* 1990; 5:53–62.
53. Kloster FE: Diagnosis and management of complications of prosthetic heart valves. *Am J Cardiol* 1975; 35:872–875.
54. Saad RM, Wolfe MW: Progressive hemolytic anemia due to delayed recognition of a Beall mitral valve prosthesis. *Chest* 1991; 99:496–498.
55. Smith RE, Berg D: Occult paravalvular leak in a clinically normal St. Jude's mitral valve presenting with life-threatening microangiopathic hemolytic anemia. *J Cardiovasc Surg* 1991; 32:56–58.

Chapter 84

Techniques of Valvular Surgery

John Parker Gott, M.D. ■ *Robert A. Guyton, M.D.*

HISTORICAL PERSPECTIVE

The forbidden territory inside the heart was first explored in 1923 with a bold attempt at mitral valvotomy by Cutler and Levine.[1] After an initial success, failure followed, and the field of endeavor lay dormant until after World War II. Harken et al.[2] and Bailey[3] in the late 1940s proved digital mitral commissurotomy to be safe and effective. The development of the Tubbs dilator in the 1950s led to a more reliable technique of closed mitral commissurotomy.[4]

Effective intracardiac operation awaited the development of cardiopulmonary bypass in the mid-1950s. As early as 1953, however, Hufnagel and Harvey[5] placed a ball valve into the descending aorta that allowed some improvements in patients with aortic regurgitation. Open debridement of the aortic valve with partial replacement of leaflets was performed in the late 1950s. Prosthetic replacement of the aortic valve was accomplished in 1960 by Harken et al.[6] and in 1961 by Lillehei et al.[7] and by Muller et al.[8] The mitral valve was first replaced successfully with the ball valve of Starr and Edwards in 1961. Prosthetic replacement of the tricuspid valve was accomplished in 1963 by Starr and colleagues.[9]

THE AORTIC VALVE

Preoperative Evaluation

Careful review of preoperative data is essential (see Chap. 79). Particular attention is given to peripheral and cerebral vascular disease, examining femoral vessels for potential cardiopulmonary bypass access or intraaortic balloon pump insertion and the carotid vessels for cerebrovascular disease, the signs and symptoms of which may be masked by aortic valve disease. The chest film aids assessment of cardiac chamber enlargement and dilation or calcification of the ascending aorta. A cineangiogram reveals further information about the ascending aortic size and calcification. One can also determine proximity of the ascending aorta to the posterior table of the sternum and possible fixation of the aorta to the sternum, a serious hazard at the time of sternotomy. Coronary angiography is performed for patients over the age of 40 and in all patients with angina pectoris. Right-sided heart catheterization should be performed in selected patients to evaluate the possibility of pulmonary vascular disease and right ventricular dysfunction. When retrograde catheter passage across the aortic valve is impossible, echocardiographic assessment of the mitral valve should be performed. If subaortic stenosis is suspected, the subaortic region should be examined preoperatively by both angiography and echocardiography. Echocardiography can also be useful in determining the size of the ascending aorta.

The Operative Technique

Median sternotomy provides excellent exposure of the ascending aorta and aortic valve. Enlargement of the ascending aorta secondary to intrinsic disease of the aorta, aortic stenosis, or aortic regurgitation often places the ascending aorta very close to the posterior table of the sternum, and erosion of the posterior table can indeed occur. In such cases, the sternum is carefully opened with an oscillating saw after the femoral artery is exposed for possible cannulation should inadvertent, premature entry into the aorta occur. After the pericardium has been opened, the aorta is carefully examined and palpated. The enlarged aorta is often thin in the area midway between the aortic valve and the brachiocephalic artery. The aorta is usually thicker and of normal diameter near the brachiocephalic artery. Cannulation is therefore accomplished just proximal or medial to the brachiocephalic artery. If ascending aortic cannulation is hazardous, the common femoral artery is an option for inflow from the heart-lung machine. Venous cannulation is usually accomplished through the right atrium using inferior vena cava and superior vena cava cannulae. This allows effective isolation of the heart if an extensive procedure is anticipated. Alternatively, a single venous cannula with an atrial and an inferior vena cava opening may be used. (See also Chap. 141.)

The patient is placed on cardiopulmonary bypass, and depending on the carefully individualized myocardial protection technique, the patient undergoes systemic cooling or maintenance of normothermia using the heat exchanger. (See Chap. 141.) If cold myocardial protection is used, intravenous propranolol is administered, both as an adjunct to myocardial protection and as a means to delay ventricular fibrillation. For patients with aortic regurgitation, it is particularly important that the heart continue ejecting during cooling because fibrillation of the heart may lead to rapid ventricular distension and consequent subendocardial ischemia. The heart is better protected if it has been cooled to 25° or 23°C prior to aortic cross-clamping; with aortic regurgitation, it is usually several minutes after the clamp is placed before protective solutions can be infused antegrade into the coronary circulation and cold cardioplegic arrest accomplished. While cooling proceeds, the aortic root is mobilized, but it is important not to manipulate the ventricle and thereby induce ventricular fibrillation. To minimize the chance for systemic air embolism, the left ventricular vent is not introduced through the right superior pulmonary vein until effective ejection has ceased. After ventricular fibrillation has occurred, cooling can continue if aortic regurgitation is minimal and the left ventricular vent can maintain a low intraventricular pressure. If the heart cannot be decompressed by venting due to a high regurgitant flow, the aortic clamp is placed at once and antegrade delivery of cardioplegic solution accomplished by infusion directly into the coronary ostia. The volume of infusion is based on knowledge of the coronary anatomy in each particular patient, so that a volume proportional to the amount of muscle supplied by that vessel is infused. If aortic regurgitation is minimal, cardioplegic solution can be infused into the aortic root after placement of the aortic clamp. Depending on the surgeon's chosen protection technique, additional cardioplegia infusions may be given in a retrograde fashion using a special coronary sinus catheter placed through the right atrium. (See Chap. 141.)

Warm myocardial protection techniques[10,11] are based on continuous delivery of warm, oxygenated, hyperkalemic, blood cardioplegia to the myocardium either antegrade through the coronary arteries or retrograde via the coronary sinus. The underlying goal of this new protective technique is operation on a quiet, electromechanically arrested heart with its basal metabolic energy requirements met by a more or less constant supply of substrate and oxygen. Shortly after establishment of normothermic cardiopulmonary bypass the aorta may be clamped, the heart arrested with the warm aerobic technique, and valve replacement commenced.

An oblique aortotomy, beginning about 1 cm cephalad to the commissure between the right and left coronary cusps and spiraling down into the noncoronary sinus, is standard. Proper excision of the valve is crucial. Excision is begun at the commissure between the right and noncoronary cusps. If this region is heavily calcified, however, a different beginning site should be chosen lest the surgeon cut too deeply and damage the bundle of His in the top of the septum (Fig. 84-1). Calcification in the right coronary cusp can usually be peeled away from the annulus using scissor tips to elevate the calcium as the valve is excised. This is also true for the leftward half of the left coronary cusp. Calcium in the noncoronary cusp and the rightward half of the left coronary cusp is often continuous with calcium in the anterior mitral leaflet, and it may be necessary to cut across calcified deposits in this region. The loose calcium deposits should be debrided carefully to prevent subsequent systemic emboli. The ventricle and the annulus are then rinsed with balanced electrolyte solution, while the left coronary ostium is protected from debris with a sucker tip or a cardioplegia infusion cannula.

Sutures are next placed around the aortic annulus. Sutures may be positioned in a simple horizontal mattress or figure-of-eight fashion. The use of horizontal mattress sutures reinforced with Teflon pledgets virtually eliminates perivalvar leaks. Sutures should not be placed into muscle underneath the right coronary cusp since complete heart block may result (Fig. 84-1). The sutures are passed through the sewing ring of the prosthesis. After the valve is lowered into place and the sutures are tied, both coronary ostia are again inspected to be certain that they are not obstructed by the prosthesis. At this point, the valve may be tested for a perivalvar leak by filling the aortic root with an irrigating solution while negative pressure is exerted within the ventricular cavity with the ventricular vent. If a significant perivalvar leak is present, it is easily detected as the irrigating solution is quickly sucked into the ventricle.

Closure of the aortotomy is accomplished by one of several methods. If the aorta is particularly fibrous and tough as during reoperation, it may be securely closed with a single-layer closure by using a running monofilament suture. For the typical aorta, a two-layer running monofilament closure often is used with a horizontal mattress suture reinforced with a simple over-and-over suture. Occasionally if the aorta is particularly tenuous, the suture line must be reinforced with a strip of Teflon felt along either side. Ventricular venting is stopped and the ascending aorta is allowed to fill with blood as the suture line is completed. A vent hole for air evacuation is placed in the most superior aspect of the aorta. At this point particular attention is given to the evacuation of air from the heart prior to removal of the aortic cross-clamp. The lungs are inflated and the heart is massaged as air and blood are sucked from the aortic vent hole. The cross-clamp is then removed and the heart allowed to recover. Rewarming is completed now if a cold protec-

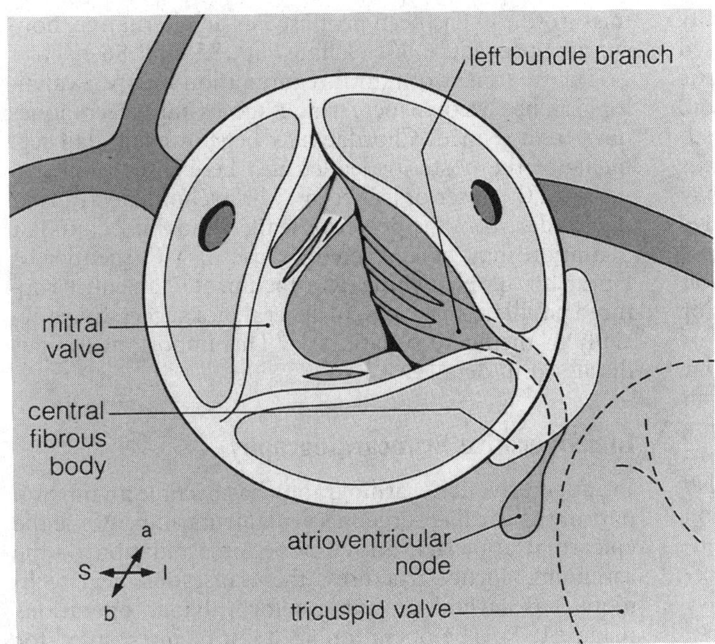

FIGURE 84-1 Surgeon's view of important anatomic relationships for aortic valve operation.

tive technique was chosen. After an effective and stable rhythm has been established, the ventricular vent is removed and air is further evacuated through the large vent hole in the ascending aorta by rotating the operating table from side to side while the ventricle is ejecting and the heart is vigorously massaged.

After removal from cardiopulmonary bypass, the patient often requires an elevated end-diastolic pressure because of the hypertrophied, noncompliant left ventricle. Systolic ventricular function is usually excellent.

Operative Management of the Small Aortic Annulus

Preoperative evaluation should alert the surgeon that the aortic annulus may be too small for placement of an adequate prosthesis. In an average man, a No. 23 bioprosthesis or a No. 21 tilting disc prosthesis is the smallest that can be inserted without a significant postoperative gradient. The problem of a small aortic annulus is even more common in children, since the largest possible prosthesis is used to allow for growth. There are three major techniques for insertion of a prosthesis larger than the annulus of the original valve. First, the prosthetic valve may be tilted in order to place a larger device in the root without enlargement of the annulus. Usually, the valve is sewn to the original annulus beneath the left and right coronary ostia and is placed several millimeters above the annulus in the noncoronary cusp.[12] The second technique involves extension of the aortotomy down to or into the annulus in the region of the noncoronary cusp and enlargement of the aorta with a patch of pericardium or cloth. This incision can be extended down into the anterior leaflet of the mitral valve if the annulus is unusually small. The valve is then sewn to the annulus underneath the right and left coronary ostia and to the aorta and the new patch above the noncoronary cusp. This allows placement of a valve two or three sizes larger than that originally measured.[13] Finally, in a few situations, it is necessary to perform an extensive operation to enlarge a small aortic annulus. The Konno or Rastan operation involves incision of the aorta between the left and right coronary ostia and cutting into the ventricular septum and the right ventricle. The newly created ventricular septal defect is repaired with a cloth patch and the annulus enlarged by three to four valve sizes as the left coronary ostium is moved away from the right coronary ostium. This technique requires a vertical aortic incision and should therefore be planned prior to aortotomy.[14,15] Most techniques of aortic annular enlargement require a more lengthy period of cardiopulmonary bypass and myocardial protection. A compromise must sometimes be reached between placement of a large prosthesis and the need to avoid prolonged cardioplegic arrest and the damaging systemic effects of a long period of cardiopulmonary bypass.

Efforts to extend the success of valve-conserving reconstructive techniques that have been achieved for the atrioventricular valves to the aortic valve continue to have variable results. Reparative operation (primarily calcium debridement and commissurotomy) for *stenotic* aortic valves carries a high risk for early recurrent stenosis and subsequent valve replacement. Shapira et al.[16] demonstrated good early reduction of gradient and increase in orifice area, but by 36 months the values had deteriorated to preoperative levels. Valvuloplastic repair of *regurgitant* aortic valves has recently yielded excellent early results, but enthusiasm must be tempered by the current lack of long-term assessment of the durability of these repairs.[17,18] (See also Chap. 79.)

Postoperative Care

Left ventricular function after aortic valve replacement is usually predictable by preoperative evaluation of left ventricular size, ejection fraction, and end-diastolic pressures. Replacement of the stenotic aortic valve generally leads to improved cardiac function when it is depressed before operation; replacement of the regurgitant aortic valve usually leads to a lesser improvement in function. The hypertrophied heart is particularly susceptible to damage during ischemic arrest, and attention to details of myocardial protection is important. Cardioplegia may be infused directly into the coronary ostia during valve replacement. Possible catastrophic events include dissection of the left or right coronary ostium or infusion of cardioplegia selectively down either the left anterior descending or circumflex coronary artery in the case of a short left main artery. Calcific debris is a particular threat to the left coronary system, while air embolism during reperfusion is a particular complication involving the right coronary system. Obstruction of either coronary ostium with the stent of a bioprosthesis may also lead to ischemic complications. If myocardial protection is globally rather than regionally inadequate, a concentric subendocardial infarction may occur. This may result in poor left-sided heart function in the postoperative interval or in ventricular arrhythmias.

Surgical bleeding after aortic valve replacement is a special problem because of the often encountered thin ascending aorta. Brief periods of hypertension in the intensive care unit may lead to torn suture lines and catastrophic bleeding. This may require emergency reentry to the mediastinum in the intensive care unit to allow digital control of bleeding as the patient is returned to the operating room.

THE MITRAL VALVE

Mitral Commissurotomy and Repair

Closed mitral commissurotomy was the first effective intervention in valvular heart disease. Although closed mitral commissurotomy is now an uncommon operation in the United States, it remains a life-saving procedure in other countries for large numbers of carefully selected patients (Chap. 80). The ideal patient for closed mitral commissurotomy is a young woman with no calcium in a purely stenotic mitral valve. Closed mitral commissurotomy is usually performed through the left side of the chest, placing a finger in the left atrium through a purse string suture and a dilator through the apex of the ventricle. The dilator is guided with the finger into the center of the valve and expanded, enlarging the orifice to a predetermined size.

Open mitral valvuloplasty permits more precise direct visual reconstruction of the mitral valve than either closed or percutaneous techniques. With the use of cardiopulmonary bypass and cardioplegic myocardial protection, the mitral valve is exposed and the commissures examined and carefully incised. Fused chordae can be split, as can papillary muscles. Results of open mitral valvuloplasty have been excellent, with freedom from reoperation at 1, 5, 10, and 15 years of 97, 95, 91, and 85 percent.[19] Open mitral valvuloplasty is the surgical procedure of choice in most U.S. centers for any patient in whom the valve is not heavily calcified and subvalvar chordal fusion is not extensive.[20] For some patients with mitral stenosis, mitral valve balloon valvuloplasty (commissurotomy) has been proposed as an alternative, nonsurgical procedure. (See Chaps. 80, 85, and 86.)

The treatment of mitral regurgitation by open valvuloplasty has become increasingly successful as techniques have been refined. Chordae may be shortened, flail segments of the posterior leaflet may be excised, flail segments of the anterior leaflets may be anchored by transfer of chordae from the posterior leaflet, and mitral annular dilatation may be corrected by use of a Carpentier or Duran annuloplasty ring. Reattachment of an entire ruptured papillary muscle is, in general, not successful, especially in the acute situation.[21,22] This important topic is discussed in detail in Chap. 85.

Intraoperative Echocardiography

Intraoperative echocardiography has become an integral part of the cardiac surgeon's armamentarium. While the epicardial approach allows superior evaluation of the ascending aortic structures, the transesophageal technique has several advantages for valvular operations (Chap. 131). The operation need not be interrupted for positioning of the probe, sterility of the operative field is not broken, and there is freedom from arrhythmia associated with epicardial manipulation. The greatest impact to date has been on intraoperative assessment of the quality of valvular reconstructive operations with a lesser role for the assessment of prosthetic function, notably intraoperative evaluation of periprosthetic leak.[23] (See also Chap. 131.)

Mitral Valve Replacement

Replacement of the mitral valve is best performed through a median sternotomy, but it can be accomplished through the right or left side of the chest in unusual circumstances. Dissection of the superior vena cava up to the level of the azygos vein and dissection of the inferior vena cava toward the hepatic veins allow greater mobility of the right side of the heart and facilitates exposure of the left atrium. Dual atrial cannulation is used for isolation of the heart and allows retraction of the right side of the heart without compromising venous return. The usual exposure of the mitral valve is through an incision on the right side of the heart anterior and parallel to Waterston's groove (see Fig. 84-2). Exposure may be improved in the setting of a small or normal-sized atrium by an approach that opens the right atrium and interatrial septum or through the roof of the left atrium between the superior vena cava and aorta.[24-26] Cardiopulmonary bypass is begun and the perfusate temperature regulated depending on the method of myocardial protection selected, and the aorta is cross-clamped; cardioplegic solution is infused to protect the myocardium and to facilitate exposure of the valve. If an atrial thrombus is present, it is carefully dissected away from the atrium, establishing a smooth plane just beneath the endocardium. The atrial appendage may be sutured closed from the atrial cavity in order to minimize postoperative thromboembolism. The anterior leaflet is pulled upward into the wound and is excised, leaving a 3-mm rim of valve tissue attached to the annulus. It is desirable to leave the posterior leaflet and its chordal

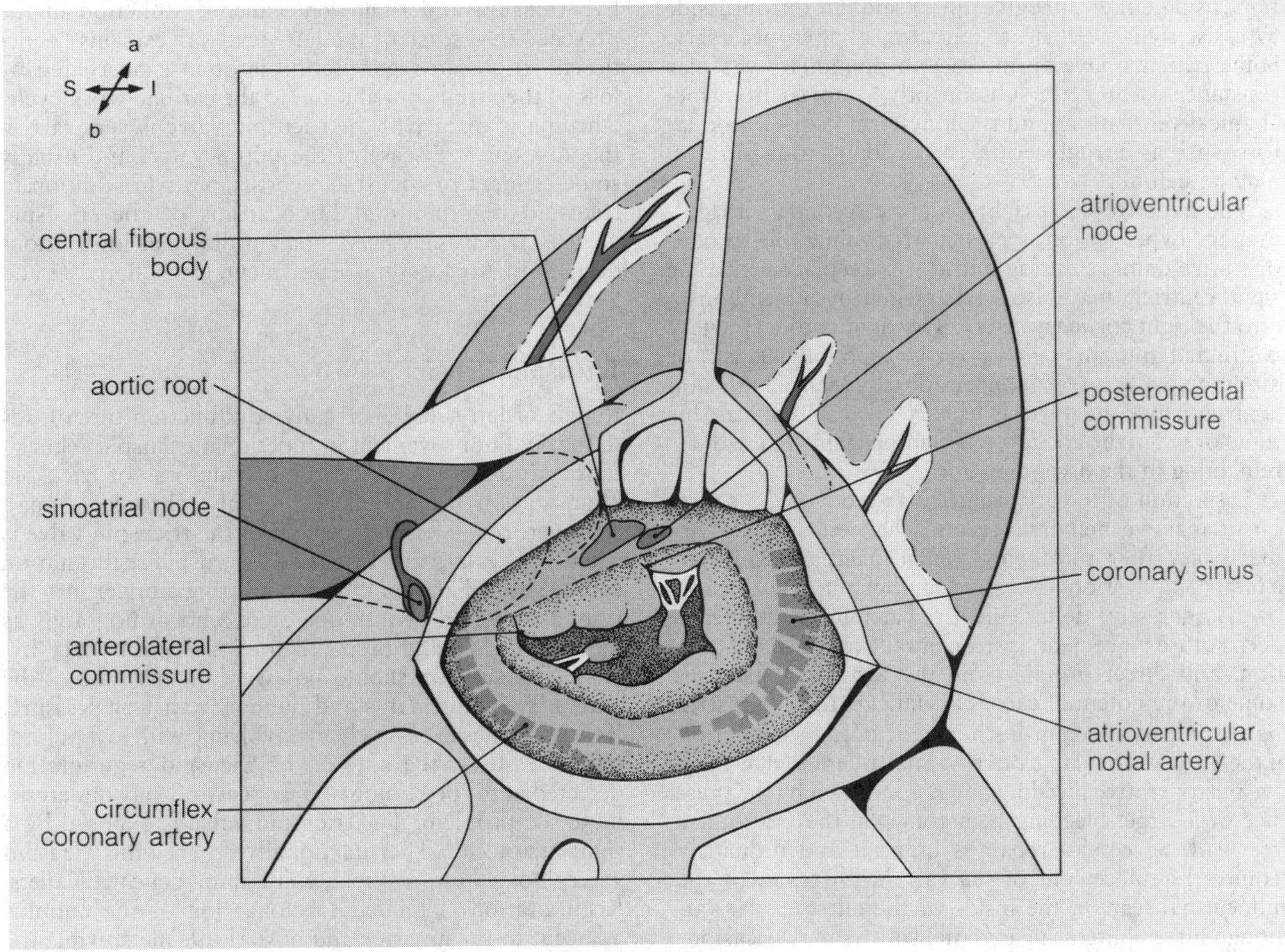

FIGURE 84-2 Typical operative exposure of mitral valve demonstrating the major surgical landmarks.

attachments in place. There is increasing evidence that ventriculoannular continuity provided by the chordae and their papillary muscle attachments has a beneficial effect on left ventricular function.[27,28] The preservation of the posterior leaflet also has a protective effect against potentially lethal atrioventricular groove dissection. Heavy calcification is often encountered in the commissures and can usually be removed. If the mitral annulus adjacent to the posterior leaflet is heavily calcified, some calcium may be left in place and the valve sewn directly to the supraannular atrial muscle. Alternatively, the entire mitral apparatus may be left in situ and a valve inserted within the mitral orifice, secured to leaflet tissue, thus avoiding disturbance of the calcified annulus and injury of surrounding structures.[29]

Interrupted, nonabsorbable sutures are placed around the annulus, usually reinforced with Teflon felt pledgets placed on the atrial side of the annulus. If felt pledgets are placed on the ventricular side of the annulus, subsequent removal of the valve may be very difficult, a factor particularly important with bioprosthetic valves. There are several potential dangers in valve excision and suture placement. As illustrated from the surgeon's perspective in Fig. 84-2, the potential for conduction system damage and subsequent heart block is evident. An errant suture may tear or tether the noncoronary cusp of the aortic valve with resultant aortic regurgitation. Injury to the circumflex coronary artery may result in ischemia or infarct. Excessive debridement of calcium or a deep muscular suture along the atrioventricular groove may lead to lethal hemorrhage.[30–33]

After the valve is secured, the aortic cross-clamp is removed while air is vented from the ascending aorta. The right coronary artery is occluded by the surgeon's finger as the cross-clamp is removed to prevent air embolism into the right coronary artery. The mitral valve is kept incompetent. In the case of a porcine valve, a chest tube or vent is temporarily placed across the valve into the ventricle, and in the case of a mechanical valve, a small Foley catheter prevents seating of the disc or ball. The left atriotomy is then closed as the heart begins to recover. Air is carefully evacuated from the heart as the vent or Foley catheter is removed and the ventricle begins to eject. The patient is rewarmed if a hypothermic technique was employed and tapered from cardiopulmonary bypass.

Postoperative Care

In patients with pulmonary hypertension consequent to mitral valve disease, special difficulties may arise in the postoperative period. Pulmonary end-diastolic pressure may not accurately reflect left atrial pressure. Therefore, a left atrial catheter is often useful. Pulmonary vasodilation, using either nitroglycerin or sodium nitroprusside to assist right-sided heart function, is often necessary. Some patients have an increase in pulmonary vascular resistance as they are subsequently removed from mechanical ventilation; and the long-term use of vasodilators (such as nitroglycerin paste or long-acting nitrates) may be helpful.

The hypertrophied right ventricle secondary to pulmonary hypertension is particularly vulnerable to perioperative damage during mitral valve replacement. The right ventricle may also be damaged by air embolism into the right coronary artery. The right coronary artery is situated anteriorly, in a position especially at risk for air embolism if a repeat antegrade cardioplegia infusion is given (since the aorta is usually filled with air at this time) or when the aortic cross-clamp is removed with air remaining in the ascending aorta.

Dissection of the atrioventricular groove with subsequent massive hemorrhage into the pericardial cavity may occur after mitral valve replacement and is usually a fatal complication. Excessive papillary muscle excision, overly aggressive debridement of calcium, inadvertently deep suture placement, instrumental endocardial laceration, and direct trauma from the prosthesis itself are some of the potential causes of damage to the ventricle that may lead to a rent in the endocardium. Dissection of the atrioventricular groove is usually heralded by massive postoperative bleeding and is confirmed by the presence of a large, bleeding hematoma on the ventricular free wall. Successful repair is unusual and ordinarily requires rereplacement of the valve with repair of the endocardial tear on the inside of the left ventricle (although huge obliterating external sutures may occasionally be successful).[30,33]

After mitral valve replacement, left ventricular function is usually less vigorous than expected. In mitral stenosis, this may be related to a left ventricle that has been protected from volume loading by the stenotic valve. In mitral regurgitation, left ventricular function is usually worse than one might expect from the preoperative angiogram because the preoperative ventricle is ejecting both into the aorta and into the low-pressure left atrium (Chaps. 23, 25, and 80). Elimination of the "pop-off" into the left atrium may lead to a lower ejection fraction postoperatively. Postoperative left atrial pressures of 18 to 20 mmHg are often needed, and temporary inotropic support may be necessary.

Urine production is usually decreased after mitral valve replacement as filling pressures in both the left and right atria are generally decreased from preoperative values. This decrease in urine flow represents a physiological response of the body to decreased atrial pressures mediated by atrial volume receptors and elevation of antidiuretic hormone (ADH) secretion. Treatment by diuretic administration, after confirmation that cardiac output is adequate, is usually effective.

THE TRICUSPID VALVE

Organic versus Functional Disease

The most common cause of tricuspid regurgitation is dilation of the tricuspid annulus secondary to pulmonary hypertension and right ventricular dysfunction in the presence of disease of the left-sided valves. This "functional" tricuspid regurgitation is often exacerbated by loss of the atrial contribution to the cardiac work cycle. Rheumatic disease of the tricuspid valve is very rare in the absence of disease of the mitral valve, and usually some element of tricuspid stenosis exists in addition to tricuspid regurgitation. Endocarditis of the tricuspid valve is increasingly becoming a problem as intravenous drug abuse becomes more prevalent. (See Chaps. 81 and 94.)

Tricuspid Repair

Repair of left-sided heart valve dysfunction often leads to marked improvement in functional tricuspid regurgitation. If a patient has chronic symptoms of tricuspid regurgitation (ascites, hepatomegaly, chronic edema), however, repair or replacement of the tricuspid valve is usually necessary and beneficial. Tricuspid regurgitation can be gauged at operation by inserting a finger into the right atrium and by intraoperative echocardiography as the patient is being prepared for cardiopulmonary bypass. The surgeon should be aware at this time of the patient's volume status and pulmonary artery pressure. If the patient is excessively hypovolemic with low pulmonary pressures, the amount of tricuspid regurgitation detected at the beginning of the operation may underestimate the problem. The tricuspid valve is exposed by a right atriotomy. The functionally regurgitant tricuspid valve looks quite normal, with thin, delicate leaflets. Regurgitation is related to elongation of the annulus adjacent to the anterior and posterior leaflets, while the septal portion of the annulus is unchanged.[34] The Carpentier tricuspid annuloplasty ring may also be used to shorten the tricuspid annulus and to reshape the tricuspid valve into an oval configuration. By remodeling the annulus, the Carpentier ring may achieve a competent tricuspid valve with a large effective residual orifice. Palpation of the valve or 2-D and Doppler echocardiography after operation permits an evaluation of the success of the procedure; again, the surgeon must take into account the fluid status and pulmonary artery pressure. If the patient derives substantial and sustained relief from correction of left-sided heart valve dysfunction, further problems with the tricuspid valve are unusual.

Tricuspid Replacement

The need for tricuspid valve replacement is unusual but can arise due to bacterial endocarditis, organic tricuspid regurgitation, or severe functional tricuspid regurgitation. Mechanical prostheses have not functioned well in this position, and the porcine or pericardial bioprosthesis is usually used. Along the septal portion of the annulus, the surgeon sutures the valve to the septal leaflet of the tricuspid valve, taking care not to place sutures into the ventricular septum because of proximity of atrioventricular (AV) conduction tissue. Insertion of a large mitral prosthesis and a large tricuspid prosthesis can compress the AV conduction system between the valves and cause complete heart block. If the patient is in third-degree block at the end of the operation, permanent epicardial pacing wires should be placed before the sternum is closed to preclude the necessity of positioning transvenous pacing wires across the prosthetic tricuspid valve.

RESULTS OF VALVE SURGERY

Aortic Valve Replacement

Replacement of the aortic valve as an isolated procedure has a 2 to 5 percent surgical mortality rate and an 80 to 85 percent 5-year survival rate. Major determinants of the results of aortic valve replacement include the age of the patient, the predominant aortic valve lesion (aortic regurgitation has a worse prognosis), and left ventricular function. Minimal impairment of left ventricular function often is reversed after valve replacement for either aortic stenosis or aortic regurgitation, but more severe deterioration of left ventricular function may not be reversible particularly with aortic regurgitation and may compromise long-term survival. Coexisting coronary artery disease usually is not an incremental risk factor for operative mortality if coronary revascularization is accomplished simultaneously.[35-37] (See also Chaps. 73 and 79.)

Mitral Valve Replacement

The surgical survival rate for isolated mitral valve replacement ranges between 3 and 8 percent, and the 5-year survival rate is 70 to 85 percent. Major determinants of surgical survival are the age of the patient, the left ventricular function, and the coexistence of coronary artery disease. The type of mitral valve lesion (stenosis or regurgitation) ordinarily does not alter postoperative or long-term survival.[38] The presence of pulmonary hypertension importantly influences postoperative survival rate, long-term survival rate, and postoperative relief of symptoms.[37,39,40] (See also Chap. 80.)

Multiple-Valve Replacement

Combined replacement of the aortic and mitral valves has an operative mortality rate slightly higher than that of replacement of the mitral valve alone, ranging from 5 to 15 percent. The 5-year survival rate, however, is considerably reduced to approximately 50 to 60 percent. Concomitant disease of the tricuspid valve or stenoses of coronary arteries further increases postoperative and long-term mortality rates.[41,42]

In general, when multiple-valve replacement is necessary, the replacement valves should be exclusively mechanical or bioprosthetic. Combinations of the two types of valves should be avoided in the same patient due to the expected and documented loss of the advantages of each device.[43,44] The important exception to this principle is the advantage of a bioprosthesis as opposed to a mechanical valve in the tricuspid position when repair is not feasible.[45] (See also Chap. 82.)

Choice of the Prosthetic Valve

Each type of prosthetic valve has deficiencies and advantages. The choice must be carefully individualized. Bioprostheses have a low thromboembolism rate in both the aortic and mitral positions, but long-term durability of the valve remains in question. Effective bioprosthetic valve duration averages about 7 years in young adults (less than 35 years old) and 10 years in older patients, although some reports are more encouraging. In children, deterioration of the porcine valve is further accelerated. Anticoagulation is not necessary for patients in sinus rhythm.[46-52]

In the United States mechanical valves account for approximately 60 percent of valve replacements.[53] There are four mechanical valve designs currently approved for implantation. The Starr-Edwards ball-valve models 1260 and 6120 have been available since 1965, and the newer tilting disc valves were introduced in the late 1970s after design efforts focused on reduction of thromboembolic complications and improved hemodynamic characteristics. The Medtronic-Hall and the Omniscience are single-tilting-disc valves, and the St. Jude Medical has a bileaflet design. The Starr-Edwards ball valve prosthesis offers excellent long-term durability and a moderately low rate of valve thrombosis or thromboembolism (aortic, 5 per 100 patient-years; mitral, 4 to 9 per 100 patient-years). In the mitral position, however, it requires a large ventricle, and in the aortic position, there is a larger transvalvular pressure gradient than with a disc valve or bioprosthesis of similar size.[47,54] New tilting disc prostheses offer a low thromboembolism rate (approximately 1.5 per 100 patient-years in the aortic position and 2 per 100 patient-years in the mitral position) and possibilities for superior hemodynamic performance.[46,47,54,55,56] An ongoing prospective randomized comparison of mechanical valves does not demonstrate any difference in rest and exercise hemodynamic performance between the Medtronic-Hall and the St. Jude Medical valves in the aortic or mitral positions.[57]

Anticoagulation is reliably accomplished with warfarin anticoagulants. Platelet inhibitors are poor substitutes for anticoagulation with warfarin compounds. The risk of a hemorrhagic complication during warfarin anticoagulation is approximately 2 per 100 patient-years. This risk must be added to the above-mentioned thromboembolism rate when considering the use of a mechanical valve in either the aortic or the mitral position or when considering use of a bioprosthetic valve in a patient for whom a large left atrium or chronic atrial fibrillation dictates chronic anticoagulation.[46] (See also Chap. 68.)

The use of cryopreserved human homografts in the aortic position has been strongly advocated because of low incidence of reoperation and freedom from thromboembolism and anticoagulation.[58] Impediments to widespread use have been the limited availability of the homografts and the learning curve associated with the increased technical demands for placement.[59] The homograft may also be used as an aortic root replacement and is invaluable in the reconstruction of native or prosthetic aortic valve endocarditis complicated by aortic root or annular abscess.[60,61]

The choice of a valve prosthesis should be a joint decision of the patient, the surgeon, the patient's cardiologist, and the patient's primary physician. Difficulty with anticoagulation is a strong argument against a mechanical prosthesis. Patients under the age of 55, in general, should receive a mechanical prosthesis because of rapid deterioration of bioprostheses. In young women who are eager to bear children, a bioprosthesis is appropriate to avoid the potential teratogenic and perinatal hemorrhagic dangers of warfarin. (See also Chaps. 68 and 113.) When considering placement of a bioprosthesis in a young person, one must evaluate the subsequent risk of reoperation. The risk is generally low when surgery is carried out under elective circumstances but becomes as high as 50 percent when reoperation is emergent.[62,63] Porcine valves deteriorate slowly, and if the patient and physician are vigilant, reoperation can usually be done electively. In some cases, however, clinical and echocardiographic evidence of accelerated structural deterioration of certain bioprostheses may warrant prophylactic replacement even before symptoms occur.[64] Mechanical valve dysfunction is more frequently catastrophic, often necessitating emergency valve reoperation.

REFERENCES

1. Cutler EC, Levine SA: Cardiotomy and valvulotomy for mitral stenosis. *Boston Med Surg J* 1923; 188:1023–1027.
2. Harken DE, Ellis LB, Ware PF, Norman LR: The surgical treatment of mitral stenosis. *N Engl J Med* 1948; 239:801–809.
3. Bailey CP: The surgical treatment of mitral stenosis (mitral commissurotomy). *Dis Chest* 1949; 15:377–393.
4. Logan A, Turner R: Surgical treatment of mitral stenosis with particular reference to the transventricular approach with a mechanical dilator. *Lancet* 1959; 2:874–880.
5. Hufnagel CA, Harvey WP: The surgical correction of aortic regurgitation: Preliminary report. *Bull Georgetown Univ Med Ctr* 1953; 6:60–61.
6. Harken DE, Soroff HS, Taylor WJ, Lefemine AA, Gupta SK, Lunzer S: Partial and complete prostheses in aortic insufficiency. *J Thorac Cardiovasc Surg* 1960; 40:744–762.
7. Lillehei CW, Barnard CN, Long DM: Aortic valve reconstruction and replacement by total valve prosthesis. In: Merendino KA (ed): *Prosthetic Heart Valves for Cardiac Surgery*. Springfield, IL, Charles C Thomas, 1961: 527–575.
8. Muller WH Jr, Littlefield JB, Dammann JF: Subcoronary prosthetic replacement of the aortic valve. In: Merendino KA (ed): *Prosthetic Heart Valves for Cardiac Surgery*. Springfield, IL, Charles C Thomas, 1961: 493–526.
9. Starr A, McCord CW, Wood J: Surgery for multiple valve disease. *Ann Surg* 1964; 160:596–613.
10. Lichtenstein SV, Ashe KA, El Dalati H, Cusimano RJ, Panos A, Slutsky AS: Warm heart surgery. *J Thorac Cardiovasc Surg* 1991; 101:269–274.
11. Lichtenstein SV, Fremes SE, Abel JG, Christakis GT, Salerno TA: Technical aspects of warm heart surgery. *J Cardiac Surg* 1991; 6:278–285.
12. David TE, Uden DE: Aortic valve replacement in adult patients with small aortic annuli. *Ann Thorac Surg* 1983; 36:577–583.
13. Manouguian S, Seybold-Epting W: Patch enlargement of the aortic valve ring by extending the aortic incision into the anterior mitral leaflet: New operative technique. *J Thorac Cardiovasc Surg* 1979; 78:402–412.
14. Rastan H, Koncz J: Aortoventriculoplasty: A new technique for the treatment of left ventricular outflow tract obstruction. *J Thorac Cardiovasc Surg* 1976; 71:920–927.
15. Misbach GA, Turley K, Ullyot DJ, Ebert PA: Left ventricular outflow enlargement by the Konno procedure. *J Thorac Cardiovasc Surg* 1982; 84:696–703.
16. Shapira N, Lemole GM, Fernandez J, Dailey PO, Dembitsky WP, O'Yek V, et al: Aortic valve repair for stenosis in adults. *Ann Thorac Surg* 1990; 50:110–120.
17. Duran C, Kumar N, Gometza B, Al Halees ZA: Indications and limitations of aortic valve reconstruction. *Ann Thorac Surg* 1991; 52:447–454.
18. Cosgrove DM, Rosenkranz ER, Hendren WG, Bartlett JC, Stewart WJ: Valvuloplasty for aortic insufficiency. *J Thorac Cardiovasc Surg* 1991; 102:571–577.
19. Legget ME, Jaffe WM, Ellis CJ, Kerr AR, Neutze JM: Low mortality and morbidity with open mitral valvotomy: Implications for those performing balloon valvuloplasty. *Circulation* 1991; 84(suppl II):II-640.
20. Laschinger JC, Cunningham JN Jr, Baumann FG, Isom OW, Catinella FP, Mendelsohn A, et al: Early open radical commissurotomy: Surgical treatment of choice for mitral stenosis. *Ann Thorac Surg* 1982; 34:287–298.
21. Carpentier A: Cardiac valve surgery—the "French correction." *J Thorac Cardiovasc Surg* 1983; 86:323–337.
22. Galloway AC, Colvin SB, Baumann FG, Grossi EA, Ribakove GH, Harty S, et al: A comparison of mitral valve reconstruction with mitral valve replacement: Intermediate term results. *Ann Thorac Surg* 1989; 47:655–662.
23. Lazar HL, Plehn J: Intraoperative echocardiography. *Ann Thorac Surg* 1990; 50:1010–1018.
24. Campanella C, Cameron E, Feilberg VL: Mitral prosthetic replacement in small left atria. *Ann Thorac Surg* 1990; 50:836–837.
25. Brawley RK: Improved exposure of the mitral valve in patients with a small left atrium. *Ann Thorac Surg* 1980; 29:179–181.
26. Balasundarum SG, Duran C: Surgical approaches to the mitral valve. *J Cardiac Surg* 1990; 5:163–169.
27. Hansen DE, Cahill PD, Derby GC, Miller DC: Relative contributions of the anterior and posterior mitral chordae tendinae to canine global left ventricular systolic function. *J Thorac Cardiovasc Surg* 1987; 93:45–55.
28. Miki S, Kusuhara K, Ueda Y, Komeda M, Ohkita Y: Mitral valve replacement with preservation of chordae tendineae and papillary muscles. *Ann Thorac Surg* 1988; 45:28–34.
29. Coselli JS, Crawford ES: Calcified mitral valve annulus: Prosthesis insertion. *Ann Thorac Surg* 1988; 46:584–586.
30. Cobbs BW, Hatcher CR Jr, Craver JM, Jones EL, Sewell CW: Transverse midventricular disruption after mitral valve replacement. *Am Heart J* 1980; 99:33–50.
31. Gosalbez F, de Linera FA, Cofiño JL, Naya JL, Rodríguez J, Ortuna A: Isolated mitral valve replacement and ventricular rupture: Presentation of 6 patients. *Ann Thorac Surg* 1981; 31:105–110.
32. Virmani R, Chun PKC, Parker J, McAllister HA: Suture obliteration of the circumflex coronary artery in three patients undergoing mitral valve operation. *J Thorac Cardiovasc Surg* 1982; 84:773–778.
33. Craver JM, Jones EL, Guyton RA, Cobbs BW, Hatcher CR Jr: Avoidance of transverse midventricular disruption following mitral valve replacement. *Ann Thorac Surg* 1985; 40:163–171.
34. Grondin P, Meere C, Limet R, Lopez-Bescos L, Delcan J-L, Rivera R: Carpentier's annulus and DeVega's annuloplasty: The end of the tricuspid challenge. *J Thorac Cardiovasc Surg* 1975; 70:852–861.
35. Kirklin JW, Barratt-Boyes BG: *Cardiac Surgery*. New York, Wiley, 1986: 373–430.
36. Jacobs ML, Austen WG: Acquired aortic valve disease. In: Sabiston DC Jr, Spencer FC (eds): *Surgery of the Chest*, 5th ed. Philadelphia, Saunders, 1990: 1566–1596.
37. Sethi GK, Miller DC, Souchek J, Oprian C, Henderson WG, ul Hassan Z, et al: Clinical, hemodynamic, and angiographic predictors of operative mortality in patients undergoing single valve replacement. *J Thorac Cardiovasc Surg* 1987; 93:884–897.
38. He GW, Hughes CF, McCaughan B, Thomson DS, Leckie BD, Yang C-Q, et al: Mitral valve replacement combined with coronary artery operation: Determinants of early and late results. *Ann Thorac Surg* 1991; 51:916–922.
39. Kirklin JW, Barratt-Boyes BG: *Cardiac Surgery*. New York, Wiley, 1986: 323–372.
40. Spencer FC: Acquired disease of the mitral valve. In: Sabiston DC Jr, Spencer FC (eds): *Surgery of the Chest*, 5th ed. Philadelphia, Saunders, 1990: 1511–1538.
41. Teoh KH, Christakis GT, Weisel RD, Tong CP, Mickleborough LL, Seully HE, et al: The determinants of mortality and morbidity after multiple valve operations. *Ann Thorac Surg* 1987; 43:353–358.
42. Gersh BJ, Schaff HV, Vatterott PJ, Danielson GK, Orzulak TA,

Piehler JM, et al: Results of triple valve replacement in 91 patients: Perioperative mortality and long-term follow-up. *Circulation* 1985; 72:130–137.

43. Bortolotti U, Milano A, Testolin L, Tursi V, Mazzucco A, Gallucci V: Influence of type of prosthesis on late results after combined mitral-aortic valve replacement. *Ann Thorac Surg* 1991; 52:84–91.
44. Roberts WC: The logic of using either two mechanical or two bioprosthetic valves for replacement of both mitral and aortic valves. *Am J Cardiol* 1988; 61:871.
45. Kawachi Y, Masuda M, Tominaga R, Tokunaga K: Comparative study between St. Jude Medical and bioprosthetic valves for replacement of both mitral and aortic valves. *Jpn Circ J* 1991; 55:553–562.
46. Edmunds LH: Thrombotic and bleeding complications of prosthetic heart valves. *Ann Thorac Surg* 1987; 44:430–445.
47. Crawford FA Jr (ed): Current heart valve prostheses. *Cardiac Surgery: State of the Art Rev* 1987; 1:143–158.
48. Foster AH, Greenberg GJ, Underhill DJ, McIntosh CL, Clark RE: Intrinsic failure of Hancock mitral bioprostheses: 10 to 15 year experience. *Ann Thorac Surg* 1987; 44:568–577.
49. Bortolotti U, Milano A, Thiene G, Guerra F, Mazzucco A, Talenti E, et al: Long-term durability of the Hancock porcine bioprosthesis following combined mitral and aortic valve replacement: An 11 year experience. *Ann Thorac Surg* 1987; 44:139–144.
50. Milano A, Vouhé PR, Baillot-Vernant F, Donzeau-Gouge P, Trinquer F, Roux P-M, et al: Late results after left-sided cardiac valve replacement in children. *J Thorac Cardiovasc Surg* 1986; 92:218–225.
51. Ilbawi MN, Idriss FS, DeLeon SY, Muster AJ, Duffy CE, Gidding SS, et al: Valve replacement in children: Guidelines for selection of prosthesis and timing of surgical intervention. *Ann Thorac Surg* 1987; 44:398–403.
52. Angell WW, Angell JD, Kosek JC: Twelve-year experience with gluteraldehyde-preserved porcine xenografts. *J Thorac Cardiovasc Surg* 1982; 83:493–502.
53. Akins CW: Mechanical cardiac valve prostheses. *Ann Thorac Surg* 1991; 52:161–172.
54. Fessatidis I, Hackett D, Oakley CM, Sapsford RN, Bentall HH: Ten-year clinical evaluation of isolated mitral valve and double valve replacement with the Starr-Edwards prostheses. *Ann Thorac Surg* 1987; 43:368–372.
55. Arom KV, Nicoloff DM, Kersten TE, Lindsay WG, Northrup WF: St. Jude Medical prosthesis: Valve-related deaths and complications. *Ann Thorac Surg* 1987; 43:591–598.
56. Nitter-Hauge S, Semb B, Abdelnoor M, et al: A five year experience with the Medtronic-Hall disc valve prosthesis. *Circulation* 1983; (suppl 2)68:169–174.
57. Tatineni S, Barner HB, Pearson AC, Halbe D, Woodruff R, Labovitz AJ: Rest and exercise evaluation of St. Jude Medical and Medtronic Hall prostheses. *Circulation* 1989; 80(suppl I):16–23.
58. O'Brien MF, Stafford EG, Gardner MAH, Pohlner PG, McGiffin DC: A comparison of aortic valve replacement with viable cryopreserved and fresh allograft valves, with a note on chromosomal studies. *J Thorac Cardiovasc Surg* 1987; 94:812–823.
59. Jones EL: Freehand homograft aortic valve replacement—the learning curve: A technical analysis of the first 31 patients. *Ann Thorac Surg* 1989; 48:26–32.
60. Bodnar E, Ross DN: Valvular homografts. In: Bodnar E, Frater R (eds): *Replacement Cardiac Valves*. New York, Pergamon, 1991: 287–306.
61. Kirklin JK, Pacifico AD, Kirklin JW: Surgical treatment of aortic valve endocarditis with homograft aortic valve replacement. *J Cardiac Surg* 1989; 4:340–347.
62. Huseby DG, Pluth JR, Piehler JM, Schaff HV, Orszylak TA, Puga FJ, et al: Reoperation on prosthetic heart valves: An analysis of risk factors in 552 patients. *J Thorac Cardiovasc Surg* 1983; 86:543–552.
63. Lytle BW, Cosgrove DM, Taylor PC, Gill CC, Goormasricm, Golding LR, et al: Reoperations for valve surgery: Perioperative mortality and determinants of risk for 1,000 patients, 1958–1984. *Ann Thorac Surg* 1986; 42:632–643.
64. Bortolotti U, Milano A, Guerra F, Mazzucco A, Mossuto E, Thiene G, et al: Failure of Hancock pericardial xenografts: Is prophylactic bioprosthetic replacement justified? *Ann Thorac Surg* 1991; 51:430–437.

Chapter 85

Surgical Reconstruction for Regurgitant Lesions of the Mitral Valve

Joseph M. Craver, M.D.

Dissatisfaction with the results of existing therapeutic methods has often been the stimulus to innovation, especially in surgery. The early recurrence of regurgitation, production of mitral stenosis, high operation mortality, or failure to maintain the initial improvement caused such dissatisfaction with the early repair or plication techniques used to surgically treat mitral regurgitation.[1,2] Those problems along with the desire to avoid prosthetic valve replacement led Carpentier in Paris in 1968 to study the causes and mechanisms that underlie regurgitation of this valve.[3,4] His study reduced the problem of mitral regurgitation to three basic physiological mechanisms (Fig. 85-1): type I, annular dilatation with normal leaflet motion; type II, excessive motion (prolapse) of one or both leaflets; and type III, restrictive leaflet motion. Combinations of these mechanisms were also found to exist, for example, annular dilatation (type I) and leaflet prolapse (type II); therefore, types I and II (Fig. 85-2).

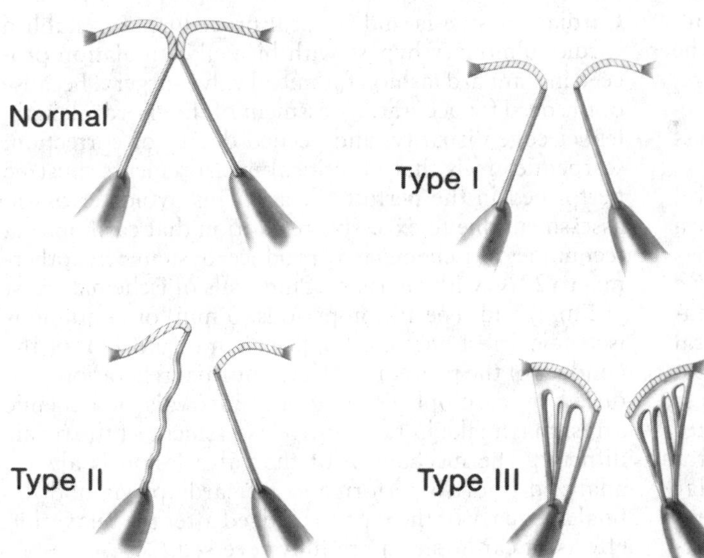

FIGURE 85-1 Basic physiological mechanisms producing mitral insufficiency: types I, II, III.

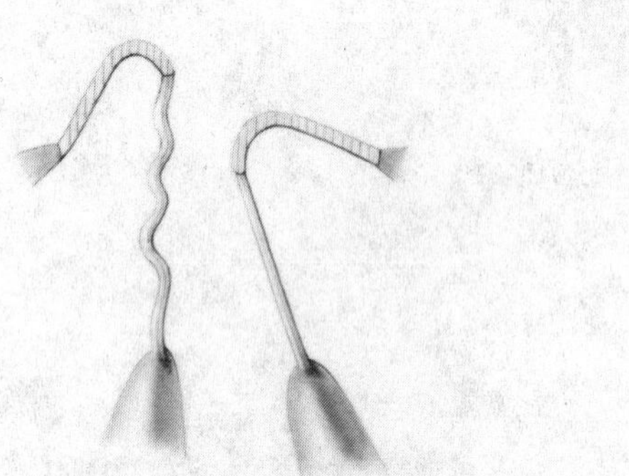

Type I, II
Prolapse with Annular Dilatation

FIGURE 85-2 Physiological mechanisms can be multiple and therefore types I and II.

He established a set of principles that defined the objective of successful valvular reconstruction to be as follows: (1) restoring leaflet pliability, (2) returning valve edges to the same level, and (3) obtaining a surface of leaflet coaptation. Restoration of leaflet pliability involved removal of restrictive bands, secondary leaflet chordae, and adhesions between adjacent leaflets—most often secondary to rheumatic disease. Excessive leaflet motion produces a disparity of the level of the leaflet edges and most commonly results from conditions that produce elongation or rupture of the leaflet chordae or papillary muscles. Correcting the level of the leaflet edges would not prevent flow regurgitation if there were not an adequate area of leaflet coaptation. Correction of annular dilatation and/or deformity to restore leaflet coaptation is essential as the third component to complete successful mitral repair. Surgical techniques to accomplish these three principles were developed by Carpentier and form the foundation of the surgical correction of regurgitation of the mitral valve.[3–5] He also introduced the implantation of a rigid annuloplasty ring, which serves to maintain the surface area of the anterior mitral leaflet while reducing the mitral annular size by compressing the annulus related to the posterior leaflet. The ring annuloplasty is felt essential in maintaining the geometry of the mitral annulus and in preventing subsequent annular dilatation, which could place new stress on the repaired valve.

While use of a ring annuloplasty has been a central element in mitral valve repair, the decision to employ a rigid ring (Carpentier's) or a flexible ring (Duran's) has not been settled. David et al.[6] reported a prospective randomized study of the effect of rigid or flexible annuloplasty rings on left ventricular function after mitral valve repair for mitral regurgitation. At 1 year most patients had normal left ventricular function regardless of the type of annuloplasty and at surgery.[7] Advocates of the rigid-ring annuloplasty maintain that its long-term advantages of larger orifice area, reduced transvalvular gradient, lower incidence of thromboembolism, and stronger fixation far outweigh a slightly greater short-term improvement in ventricular systolic function that is noted when a completely flexible annuloplasty ring is used.[8] The controversy is not yet resolved.

RESULTS OF VALVE RECONSTRUCTION

Mitral valve repair utilizing the techniques developed by Carpentier has resulted in excellent early results, long-term durability, expanding application, and freedom from reoperation that compare favorably with corresponding series of patients who undergo mitral valve replacement with mechanical, biologic, or bioprosthetic valve.[9–15] A series of 400 patients having mitral valve operations at the Hospital Broussais was reported in 1984 by Perier.[15] Four groups of 100 patients each received nonrandomly elective mitral valve repair, Bjork-Shiley prostheses, Starr-Edwards prostheses, or Carpentier-Edwards bioprostheses. The procedures were concurrently performed with all patients having mitral regurgitation or mixed mitral stenosis and regurgitation and followed for 7 years. Those patients who received mitral valve reconstruction had a lower operative mortality rate, an improved long-term survival rate, the same need for reoperation as that of the other valves, and a lower incidence of thromboembolic events. Since the valve repair patients experienced a low rate of thromboembolic events (96 ± 1.2 percent embolism free at 7 years), they were not maintained on long-term warfarin anticoagulation.

The immediate and long-term superiority of mitral valve repair to mitral valve replacement has been emphasized by other series.[10,16,17] These reports confirm a lower operative mortality, low incidence of reoperations after valve repair, low incidence of late thromboembolism, and excellent long-term survival free of valve-related problems or complications of anticoagulation.

SURGICAL PROCEDURE

Cardiac anesthesia and surgical procedures to establish cardiopulmonary bypass with bicaval cannulation proceed in standard fashion for mitral valve surgery. Because of the need for accurate assessment of the chordal length, leaflet edge disparity, and needed degree of correction, Carpentier feels that all critical measurements must be performed in the perfused heart. This avoids errors in assessment due to excessive relaxation that cardioplegia techniques or ischemia may produce. Systemic hypothermia to 22°C with alternating intervals of ischemic arrest (12 min) and reperfusion periods (3 min) or continuous ischemic arrest with cardioplegia can be utilized for the conduct of the procedure. The abnormal relaxation produced by cardioplegia or longer intervals of ischemic arrest may make intraoperative assessment of the repair difficult. The mechanism of the valve lesion is always analyzed prior to performance of cardioplegia and the final adequacy of the repair is judged after the relaxation effects of cardioplegia are fully reversed.[5]

Surgical Exposure

The mitral valve apparatus is exposed by opening the right side of the left atrium with the atrial incision extended well under the superior vena cava and vertically to the left of the inferior vena cava. This allows a fuller rotation of the heart to the left and improves exposure when the atrium is small. Exposure through alternate routes can also be employed. Because of the extended duration of time that may be needed, retraction of the atrial wall with a fixed rather than a hand-held retractor is advisable.

Assessment of Mechanism of Regurgitation

Once the patient has gradually cooled systemically, the left atrium is opened, proper exposure gained, and visual inspection of the mitral apparatus carried out. Jet lesions may be present as scarring or deposits on the wall of the atrium or annulus opposite sites of severe regurgitant flow. Chordal or papillary muscle rupture as well as presence of annular dilatation or deformity are often readily evident. The aortic cross-clamp is then applied, and detailed evaluation is carried out.

Prolapse evaluation is carried out by locating a point of valve edge, usually in the mural leaflet, that is not prolapsed. This is termed the *reference point* by Carpentier. It should remain in the plane of the annulus when lightly tugged by a nerve hook. The remaining margins of the mitral leaflets are then compared to this reference point, and any prolapse and its degree and location are noted. The leaflets, chordae, and muscles are then further examined. Elongation or rupture of papillary muscles or chordae or a combination of problems may be present to varying degrees in different areas of the valve. Excessive leaflet tissue may also be present with or without prolapse.

Restrictive mechanisms are also determined and commissural fusion is relieved. Thickening, shrinkage, and destruction of leaflet and chordal tissue may indicate that valve repair is not possible. However, restriction is often produced by retraction of chordae that attach to the ventricular surface of the leaflet (secondary and basal chordae) rather than to the leaflet edge (marginal chordae). Removal of these fibrous and thickened secondary chordal groups may unfurl what appeared to be a rolled and retracted leaflet and restore leaflet pliability.

Annular dilatation and deformity of the mitral annulus are assessed by visual inspection. Annular dilatation is usually secondary to ventricular decompensation, volume overload, or both. Annular deformity may be produced when the effects of the disease process are present unequally around the annulus.

Surgical Correction Techniques

Leaflet Prolapse without Rupture

The surgical repair of leaflet prolapse depends on the degree of prolapse and its location (anterior or posterior leaflet) and on whether the underlying problem is chordal elongation, papillary muscle elongation, or both. The surgical repair for prolapse involves two components: (1) correcting the abnormal chordal length and (2) remodeling the dilated and often deformed mitral annulus. Whether the prolapse involves the anterior or posterior leaflet, which parts of either or both are affected, and the degree of prolapse determine which repair techniques will be applied.

Because of the major contribution made to the mitral valve orifice area by the anterior leaflet, efforts to preserve this leaflet while correcting prolapse are essential. The abnormally long chordae are identified and grouped according to their attachment on the valve margin. It is noted whether all chordae within a group are elongated or whether the problem involves only one or two. If all are involved, the group can be repaired as a unit. If individual chordae are normal, however, inclusion of these in a group shortening plasty would result in excessive tension and hence retraction and might produce persistent regurgitation. Once the chordal groups are analyzed and isolated, the shortening techniques to be applied are determined by the amount of shortening required and the anatomic characteristics of the papillary muscles.

Generally, prolapse of the posterior leaflet can be repaired by performing a quadrangular resection of the prolapsed segment. This technique is discussed in the section on posterior leaflet rupture. Resection of more than one scallop of the leaflet may be needed if an area of intervening valve is normally supported and not prolapsed. When it is determined that the prolapsed posterior leaflet tissue must be retained, the chordae shortening techniques are the same as described below.

Chordoplasty

Three surgical techniques are generally employed to correct abnormal chordal length, depending on the degree of shortening needed: (1) trench chordoplasty, (2) sliding chordoplasty, and (3) cylindrical chordoplasty (shortening of papillary muscle).

Trench Chordoplasty A deep trench is created in the head of the papillary muscle, starting at the point of attachment of the chord or group of chordae that needs shortening. The trench is extended into the papillary muscle to one-half the amount of chordal shortening required since the chord is doubled on itself when it is pulled into and secured into the trench (Fig. 85-3). A double-armed suture is passed around the chord and the needle passed into the depth of the trench and brought out farther down the papillary muscle body. This suture is then tied under the appropriate tension to result in the correct degree of shortening. Tying this suture too tightly may result in its cutting through the papillary muscle tissue. The trench is closed with other sutures. This method is most useful when long degrees (4 to 8 mm) of shortening are needed.

Sliding Chordoplasty This technique differs in that the papillary head supporting the elongated chordae to be shortened is folded down and sutured to an adjacent papillary head or bundle (Fig. 85-4). It is used to correct moderate degrees of prolapse. This technique has also

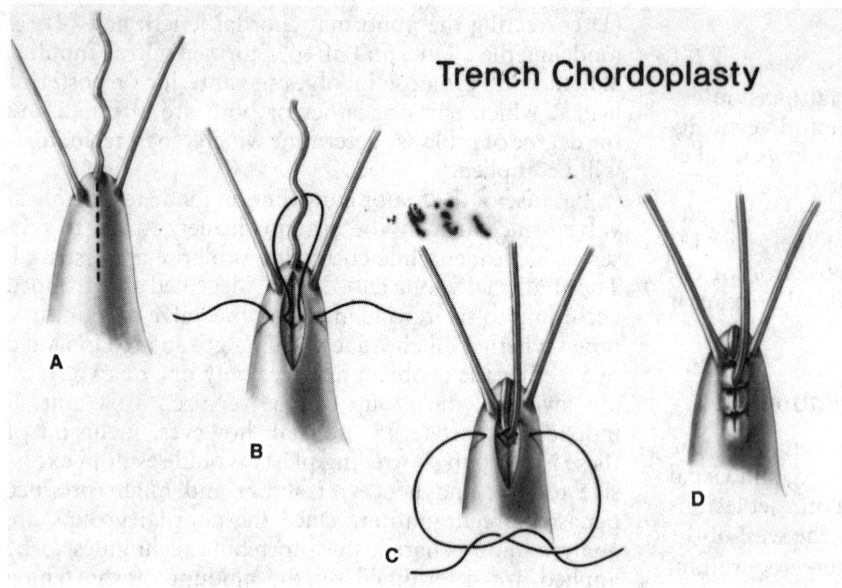

FIGURE 85-3 Trench chordoplasty shortens chordae by embricating the elongated chordae into a trench in the body of the papillary muscle.

proved valuable when elongated chordae are attached to a papillary muscle too thinned to permit a trench chordoplasty. In this case the entire papillary muscle can be folded on itself and attached to an adjacent papillary muscle body (Fig. 85-5) or buried in a trench in the ventricular wall (Fig. 85-6).

Cylindrical Chordoplasty The cylindrical chordoplasty procedure on the papillary muscle is utilized when only a minimal degree of shortening (2 mm) is required or when a larger shortening procedure in which there was a slight degree of residual prolapse is "fine-tuned." It is performed by placing three or four sutures circumferentially in the body of the papillary muscle in its long axis and gently tying them down. This achieves an "accordion" effect that produces a lesser, fine degree of shortening.

The Annular Ring

Reduction of the dilated annulus, correction of deformity, and prevention of future dilatation by insertion of the annular ring are the components of the second stage of correcting valve prolapse (Fig. 85-7). In remodeling the annulus, the ring also serves to reduce tension on the leaflets and chordae caused by the dilatation. It thereby reduces tension on the repaired areas and contributes to durability of the valve and its repair.

Selection of the appropriate size ring is made by obtaining a ring that corresponds to the area of the anterior leaflet. The anterior-posterior dimension is most important and must be correctly evaluated by placing gentle tension on the leaflet. This is easily done by placing a clamp under the anterior chordae and pulling the leaflet forward. Usually the posterior leaflet serves as a coaptation surface and contributes little to the functional area of the repaired valve.

Ring implantation is performed with interrupted sutures placed deeply into the mitral valve annulus 2 mm behind the flexion point of the leaflets (Fig. 85-7). Strong deep bites in the annulus must be secured as ring dehiscence is a major cause of failure of the repair. Four sutures are equally spaced across the base of the anterior leaflet, which compromises the mitral-aortic fibrous tri-

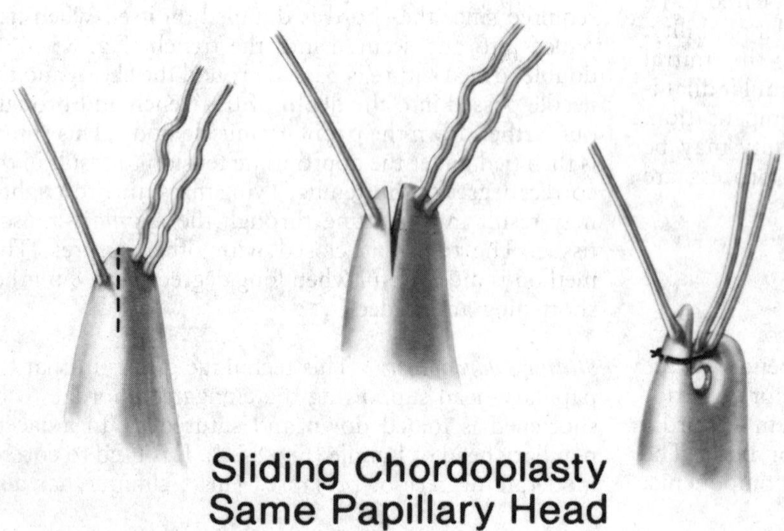

FIGURE 85-4 Sliding chordoplasty attaches the papillary tip at a deeper level in the ventricular musculature.

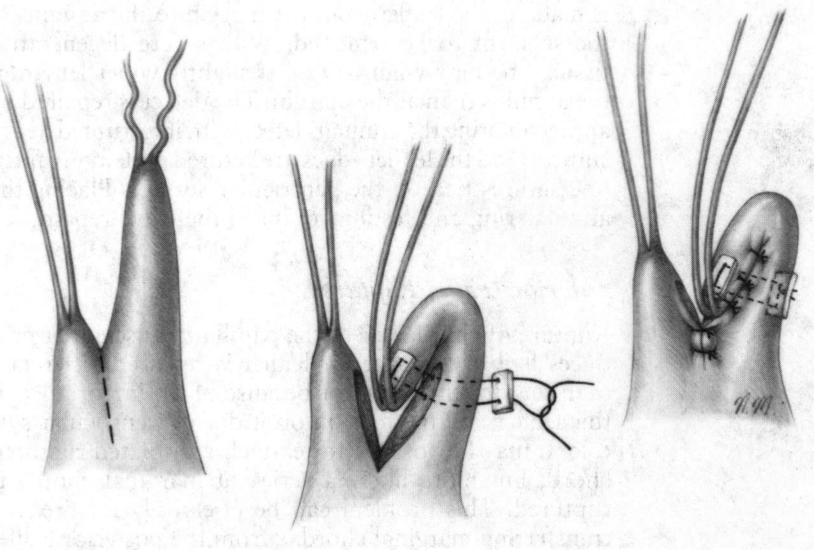

FIGURE 85-5 Folding an elongated papillary muscle on itself.

gone. The width of the base of the anterior leaflet is carefully maintained; therefore, all reduction is carried out on the mural and septal components of the annulus. Equally important is the correct location of the midpoint of the posterior annular suture line. Proportional adjustment in the remaining sutures of the posterior annulus into the prosthetic ring corrects deformity of the mitral orifice and reduces its dilatation to fit the reconstruction.

Once the sutures have all been placed into the ring, the ring is lowered into place and secured to the annulus. The competency of the valve repair is tested before tying the sutures. This allows any recorrection or adjustment to be made without removal of a tied-in ring. A bulb syringe with rubber extension infuses saline to fill the ventricular cavity to test competency of the repair and to detect any persistent prolapse. This is performed in the reperfused nonischemic and non-cardioplegia-relaxed heart. Ideally, there should be no prolapse and a coaptation surface of 3 mm with a natural curve to the orifice that parallels the posterior edge of the ring. Very slight degrees of regurgitation with normal coaptation surfaces often are corrected when the papillary muscles regain their tone and all remaining induced relaxation is eliminated. If the chordae are overly shortened, restoration of papillary tone can produce severe regurgitation by leaflet retraction as the coaptation surfaces are separated in systole. Therefore, the degree of relaxation that may still be present in the myocardium must be carefully considered in evaluating the status of the valve repair. If the repair is felt to be satisfactory, the ring sutures are tied and cut and the valve is again tested for competency.

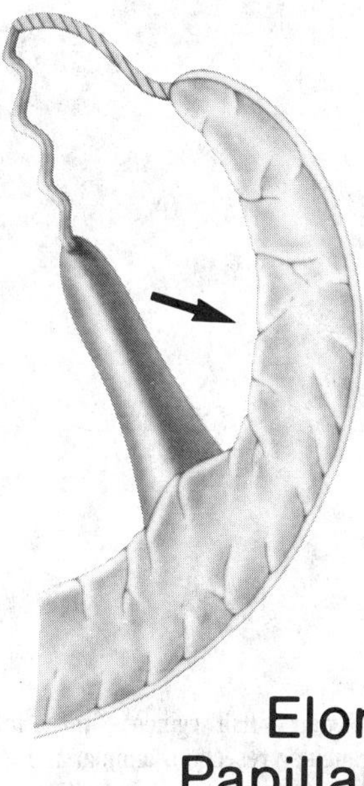

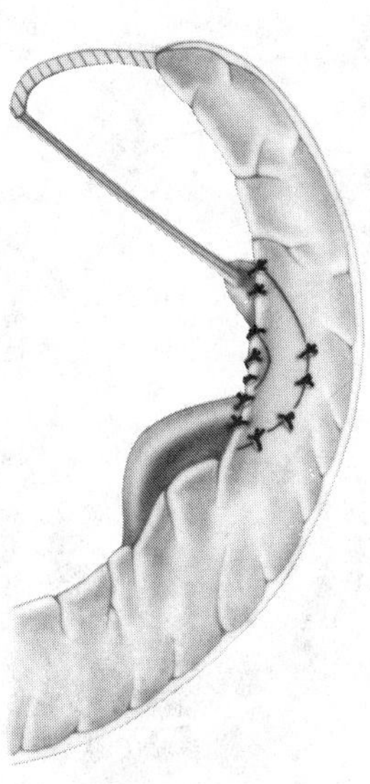

FIGURE 85-6 Burying an elongated papillary muscle into ventricular wall trench.

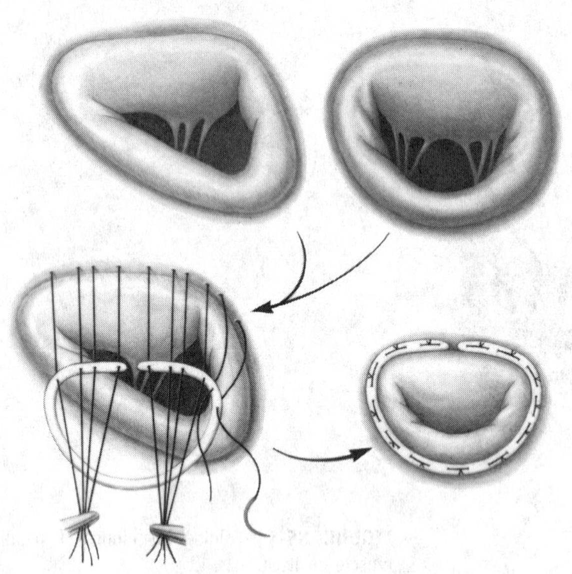

FIGURE 85-7 Annuloplasty ring insertion corrects annular deformities, reduces annular dimension, and prevents future dilatation.

Posterior Leaflet Rupture

Posterior leaflet rupture most often involves rupture of several chords to a given segment and less often an isolated major chord. When the latter problem exists, it may be possible to repair the prolapse by suturing the ruptured major chord to an intact secondary chord in the same area or to an adjacent healthy chord. Insertion of a ring is necessary since annular dilatation is usually present and a hazard to future durability of the valve repair even when only a small segment is involved.

When a more extensive area of the posterior leaflet is prolapsed or is flail as a result of multiple ruptured chordae or isolated rupture of the papillary muscle, it is repaired by performing a quadrangular resection of the affected leaflet area (Fig. 85-8). This is done by isolating the chordae involved from those to be saved. An incision is made in the leaflet from the margin to the annulus in the segment to be removed. With severe degenerative tissue, one may want to take a slightly wider length at the annulus than at the margin. The defect is repaired by approximating the annular defect with interrupted heavy sutures, and the leaflet edges are sutured with interrupted fine sutures tied on the ventricular surface. Placing the annular ring and testing complete the valve repair.

Anterior Leaflet Rupture

Rupture of chordae or of the papillary muscle that produces flail of the anterior leaflet is repaired differently than that for the posterior because of the importance of this leaflet and the tension on it during ventricular systole. It may be possible to reattach an isolated ruptured chord, but more likely a series of marginal chords is ruptured. This problem can be effectively repaired by transferring marginal chordae from the posterior leaflet to resupport the anterior leaflet (Fig. 85-9). This is accomplished exactly as it sounds: A thin margin of the posterior leaflet is transferred to the corresponding anterior flailed segment. The segment of posterior leaflet edge margin is excised and securely fixed to the margin of the anterior leaflet with multiple fine interrupted sutures. This transfer not only resupports the anterior leaflet but also brings it back into proper length and coaptation. A small wedge of tissue is resected in the margin of the posterior leaflet where the marginal was removed, and this defect is closed with fine interrupted sutures. With placement of the ring and testing of the valve, the repair is completed. If the rupture involves a majority of the anterior leaflet, one should consider translocation of two segments of posterior leaflet margin. By placing these in an area corresponding to the posterior papillary muscles, support may be achieved and the anterior valve leaflet saved. By using the "indentations" in the posterior leaflet between the three scallops, a wider edge of leaflet can be

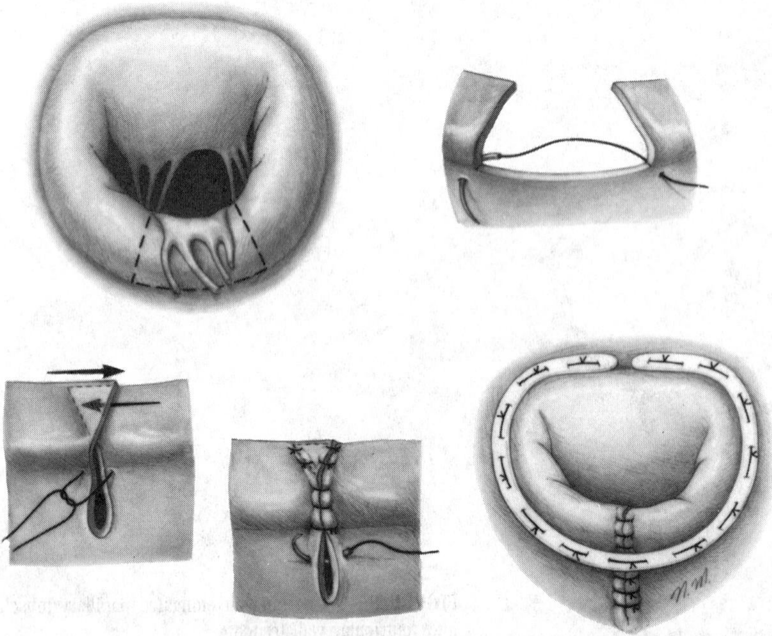

FIGURE 85-8 Repair of flail segment of posterior leaflet by quandrangular resection, annular reduction, and primary leaflet resuture.

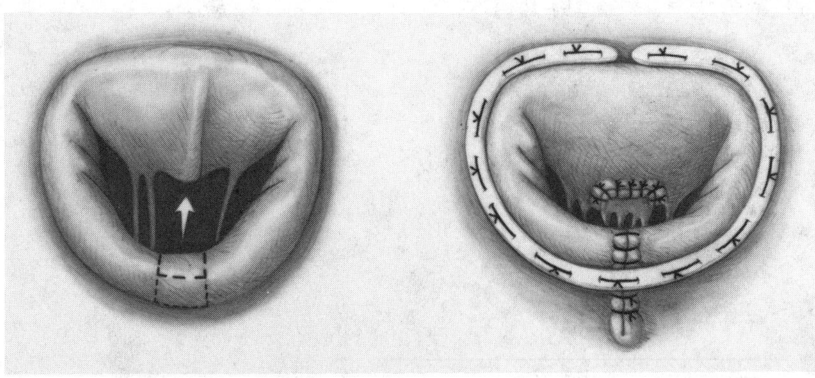

FIGURE 85-9 Transfer of posterior leaflet margin to anterior leaflet to correct flail of anterior leaflet with annular ring implanted.

obtained with marginal chordae attached with minimal loss of posterior leaflet.

When a flail anterior leaflet is due to a rupture of the papillary muscle with a fragment of muscle still attached, one can implant the residual fragment into a trench in the ventricular wall or into a healthy papillary bundle (Fig. 85-10). An area proximal to the remaining papillary stem is selected to give the proper chordal length. A suture is placed through the fibrous tip of the residual head where the chordae attach. Both needles of this suture are then passed deeply into the trench. Tying the suture pulls the papillary tip into the trench, which is closed with interrupted sutures. Completion of this anterior rupture repair is accomplished by inserting the ring and testing the repair.

Endocarditis-Induced Regurgitation

Whether or not mitral regurgitation secondary to leaflet injury by endocarditis can be repaired depends on the activity of the infection, the extent of the valve injury, and the experience of the operating surgeon. Active infection on a valve precludes attempts to save the valve. On the other hand, chronic defects, such as fenestration of a leaflet or loss of chordal support, can be repaired with confidence. Excision of the area of leaflet fenestration and repair with a glutaraldehyde-stabilized pericardial patch can effectively replace destroyed leaflet tissue (Fig. 85-11). Loss of marginal support chordae can be repaired by techniques noted above for prolapse or leaflet rupture. Ring annuloplasty may not be needed in correcting regurgitation due to endocarditis if the annulus is normal and leaflet resection is not required.

Testing the Repair by Echo Doppler

Initial testing of the repair is accomplished by filling the ventricular cavity by a flush of saline from a bulb syringe as noted above. More objective testing can be attained by utilization of an intraoperative transesophageal echo color flow Doppler. This provides an excellent and accurate method of assessment of the completed repair.[18] The echo of the repaired valve is compared to its preoperative status and evaluated in terms of leaflet motion; the color flow shows any degree of persistent regurgitation. Transesophageal or direct epicardial echo probes have proved most accurate in this evaluation. This procedure is performed after the patient has been separated from cardiopulmonary bypass when cardiac output and afterload pressures have been optimized. This evaluation allows any necessary recorrection to be carried out before the patient leaves the operating room and may prevent a needed reoperation or unsatisfactory result of reconstruction. (See also Chap. 131.)

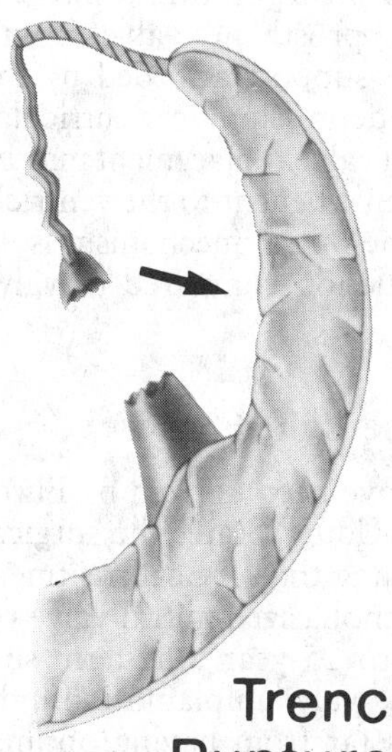

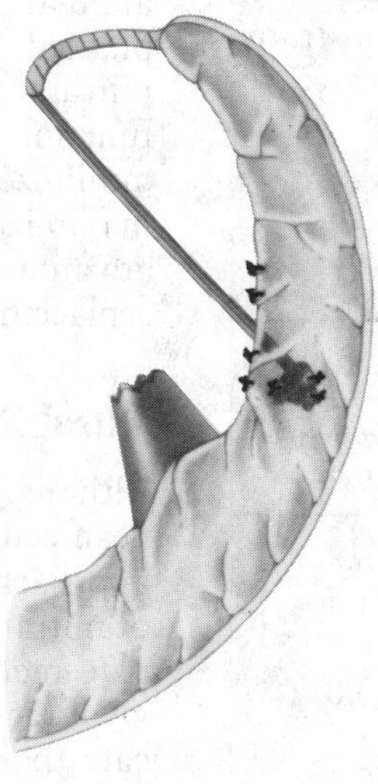

FIGURE 85-10 Reattachment of ruptured papillary tip to ventricular wall.

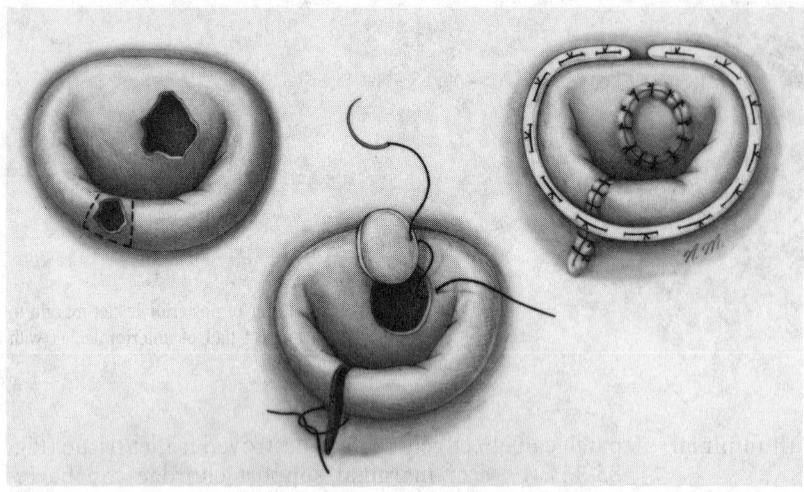

FIGURE 85-11 Repair of leaflet lesion due to endocarditis—patch of fenestration and resection of area of chordal destruction.

Operative Mortality and Ventricular Function after Valve Repair

Five series have been reported in which comparable but nonrandomized patient groups received either mitral replacement or repair.[10–14] The operation mortality rate was lower for mitral valve repair: 1.9 percent versus 10.3 percent for mitral valve replacement ($P < .0001$) (Table 85-1).

The improved operative mortality, ventricular function, and long-term survival rate after mitral valve repair likely were influenced by patient selection but also have been attributed in part to the preservation of the mitral valve–papillary muscle apparatus.[19–21] This has focused renewed attention on the importance that the "mitral valve loop" may have in maintaining ventricular performance. The mitral leaflets and chordae tendinae are parts of a continuous fibrous unit that includes the papillary muscles, endocardium, and over the epicardial surface of the left ventricle.[22] The continuity of this "mitral loop" is felt to play an important role in left ventricular function, especially during isometric contraction. Interruption of this continuous loop by excision of the mitral valve results in the loss of this support and in an "untethering" of the ventricle. The loss of intrinsic support by this mitral loop has also been proposed as the mechanism whereby distention of the ventricle can result in transverse midventricular disruption after mitral valve replacement.[20,23] Experimental and clinical studies have supported the value of maintaining the mitral loop intact.[19,21,24] David and collaborators compared three groups of patients who underwent mitral valve surgery: (1) mitral valve surgery with the removal of the entire valve apparatus, (2) mitral valve replacement with preservation of the valve apparatus, and (3) mitral valve reconstruction with preservation of the valve apparatus. Those patients in whom the valve apparatus was preserved, whether they had a prosthetic valve implanted or a valve reconstruction procedure, had significantly better postoperative ventricular function than those whose valve apparatus was removed.[21] Bonchek et al.[19] have reported similar findings in a series of 18 patients who were studied after mitral reconstruction.

Knowledge of the importance of the mitral valve apparatus in maintaining the continuity of the "mitral loop" has led surgeons to retain the posterior leaflet when implanting a mitral prosthesis.[19,23,25] It is of particular importance for the patient with chronic mitral regurgitation whose left ventricle confronts significantly higher ventricular afterload after the loss of decompression into the left atrium. David and associates have advocated retaining the margin of the anterior mitral leaflet with its attached chordae and incorporating it into the annular suture line when a prosthetic valve is implanted.[26] By maintaining the support afforded by the mitral valve apparatus, the depression in ventricular function often seen after mitral valve replacement may be minimized and the hemodynamic benefit to the ventricle maximized. Preservation of the mitral mechanism is an advantage of mitral reconstruction compared to valve replacement.

TABLE 85-1
Comparison of Operative Mortality Rates ($P < .0001$)

Reference	Repair N	Repair *Mortality, %*	Replacement N	Replacement *Mortality, %*
Adebo and Ross[14]	21	0	44	6.8
Duran et al.[10]	255	1.8	307	11.4
Oliveira et al.[11]	84	4.9	101	5.0
Oury et al.[12]	34	0	46	13.0
Yacoub et al.[13]	86	5.0	46	11.0
Total	480	1.9	544	10.3

Mitral Reconstruction in the United States

Although repair techniques have been utilized by European centers for years, in the United States the surgical approach and teaching regarding the surgical treatment of mitral regurgitation have emphasized mitral valve replacement. However, the 5- to 15-year long-term survival rate data after prosthetic valve implantation indicate that the United States is far from having optimal valve substitutes.[15,27–30] Mechanical valves, whether ball-in-cage, tilting disk, or leaflet valves, continue to have significant incidence of thromboembolism, valve thrombosis, structural failure, and anticoagulant-related complications. Similarly, long-term data on bioprosthetic valves show significant deterioration, primarily thrombosis or tissue fracture occurring after 8 to 10 years. The limitations of mitral valve replacement coupled with the excellent results and durability of repair techniques have led to an expanding interest in application of mitral valve reconstruction techniques. Whether or not the results obtained in the European series would be attainable in the U.S. patient population has been questioned. Mitral regurgitation in the European series is usually due to rheumatic heart disease, whereas valve degenerative disorders form the majority in the United States.[16,17] Despite a difference in underlying disease process, several reported series from the United States indicate that mitral reconstruction can be applied effectively with low operative mortality and freedom from recurrence of significant mitral regurgitation.[12,19,31,32] Cosgrove,[31] in a study of 247 patients having mitral valve surgery, found that degeneration disease was the most common cause of mitral regurgitation and that in 60 percent of the subjects studied this was successfully corrected by valve repair techniques. The late survival of his 112 hospital survivors of mitral valve reconstruction was 90.6 percent at 2 years. Only 2 patients sustained a thromboembolic event within 2 years (freedom from thromboembolism 99.1 percent at 2 years). Two of his patients required reoperation (2.5 percent per year rate). Of his 104 survivors, 96.2 percent are New York Heart Association Function class I or II (old classification).

A report by Craver et al.[33] demonstrated that the results after 3 years when mitral repair was used to correct mitral regurgitation were the same as in a matched population who underwent mitral valve replacement with a porcine bioprosthesis. There was an equally low incidence (<3 percent) of need for reoperation in both groups despite a preponderance of degenerative disease (80 percent) or ischemic disease as the etiology for mitral regurgitation in both study groups. These favorable early data suggest that the long-term durability of mitral valve repair seen in European series,[8–10,15] where rheumatic disease was the principal etiology, can also be anticipated in our North American population.

With these data suggesting that the early risks and results may be the same, one can speculate that the long-term benefits of mitral repair may exceed those of mitral replacement because of enhanced ventricular function by maintaining fully the intrinsic support mechanism, freedom from anticoagulation, freedom from morbidity associated with valve substitutes, and possibly improved durability.

TIMING FOR REFERRAL FOR MITRAL VALVE RECONSTRUCTION

Patients who must undergo mitral valve replacement for chronic mitral valve regurgitation have, as a group, the highest morbidity and mortality rates of any group undergoing elective cardiac surgery. This is especially true if the etiology of the mitral valve lesion is coronary artery disease. The postoperative problems with ventricular decompensation are reflected by depressed hemodynamic function, elevation of intracardiac pressures and volumes, and increased dependence on inotropic or mechanical ventricular support. The ventricular dysfunction often improves slowly but may persist long into the follow-up interval. If optimal functional results are to be obtained by correcting mitral regurgitation, surgery should be performed before deterioration of left ventricular function or development of pulmonary hypertension occurs. The development of atrial fibrillation appears to be a marker that the problems of deterioration may be beginning and should raise the question of mitral valve surgery.[34,35] Successful cardioversion of the atrial fibrillation into sinus rhythm can be accomplished when it has been present either transiently preoperatively or for less than 1 year. This freedom from chronic atrial fibrillation improves long-term functional results and lessens the hazards of thromboembolism. In general, patients should be referred for surgical correction at earlier stages when there is objective evidence of significant deterioration of ventricular function. (See Chap. 80.)

REFERENCES

1. Ellis FH Jr, Callahan JA, McGoon DC, Kirklin JW: Results of open operation for acquired mitral valve disease. *N Engl J Med* 1965; 272:869–874.
2. Bigelow WG, Kuypers PJ, Heimbecker RO, Gunton RW: Clinical assessment of the efficiency and durability of direct vision annuloplasty. *Ann Surg* 1961; 154:320–329.
3. Carpentier A, DeLoche A, Dauptain, J, Soyer R, Blondeau P, Piwnica A, et al: A new reconstructive operation for correction of mitral and tricuspid insufficiency. *J Thorac Cardiovasc Surg* 1971; 61:1–13.
4. Carpentier A, Relland J, DeLoche A, Fabiani JN, D'Allaines C, Blondeau P, et al: Conservative management of the prolapsed mitral valve. *Ann Thorac Surg* 1978; 26:294–309.
5. Carpentier A: Cardiac valve surgery—the "French Correction." *J Thorac Cardiovasc Surg* 1983; 86:323–337.
6. David TE, Komeda M, Pollick C, Burns RJ: Mitral valve annuloplasty. The effect of the type on left ventricular function. *Ann Thorac Surg* 1989; 47:524–528.
7. David TE: The effect of the type annuloplasty ring on left ventricular function. *Newslett Club Mitrale* 1989; 1(6):16.
8. Deloche A, Jebara VA, Relland JYM, Chauvaud S, Fabiani JN, Perier P, et al: Valve repair with Carpentier techniques. The second decade. *J Thorac Cardiovasc Surg* 1990; 99:990–1002.
9. Carpentier A, Chauvaud S, Fabiani JN: Reconstructive surgery of mitral valve incompetence—ten year appraisal. *J Thorac Cardiovasc Surg* 1980; 79:338–348.
10. Duran CG, Pomar JL, Revuelta JM, Gallo I, Poveda J, Ochoteco A, et al: Conservative operation for mitral insufficiency—critical analysis supported by postoperative hemodynamic studies of 72 patients. *J Thorac Cardiovasc Surg* 1980; 79:326–337.
11. Oliveira DB, Kawkins KD, Kay PH, Paneth, M: Chordal rupture II: Comparison between repair and replacement. *Br Heart J* 1983; 50:318–324.
12. Oury JH, Peterson KL, Folkerth TL, Daily PO: Mitral valve replacement versus reconstruction. *J Thorac Surg* 1977; 73:824–835.
13. Yacoub M, Halim M, Radley-Smith R, McKay R, Nijveld A, Towers M, et al: Surgical treatment of mitral regurgitation caused by floppy valves: Repair versus replacement. *Circulation* 1981; 64(suppl 2):210–216.
14. Adebo OA, Ross JK: Surgical treatment of ruptured mitral valve chordae: A comparison between mitral valve replacement and valve repair. *Thorac Cardiovasc Surg* 1984; 32:139–142.

15. Perier P, DeLoche A, Chauvaud S, Fabiani JN, Rossant P, Bessou JP, et al: Comparative evaluation of mitral valve repair and replacement with Starr, Bjork, and porcine valve prostheses. *Circulation* 1984; 70(suppl 1):187–192.
16. Spencer FC, Colvin SB, Culliford AT, Isom OW: Experiences with the Carpentier techniques of mitral valve reconstruction in 103 patients (1980–1985). *J Thorac Cardiovasc Surg* 1985; 90:341–350.
17. Cosgrove DM, Altagracia M, Chavez MD, Lytle BW, Gill CC, Stewart RW, et al: Results of mitral valve reconstruction. *Circulation* 1986; 74(suppl 1):82–87.
18. Czer LSC, Mauer G, Bolger AF, Robertis MD, Resser KJ, Kass RM, et al: Intra operative evaluation of mitral regurgitation by Doppler color flow mapping. *Circulation* 1987; 76(suppl 3):108–116.
19. Bonchek LI, Olinger GN, Siegle R, Tresch DD, Keelan MH: Left ventricular performance after mitral reconstruction for mitral regurgitation. *J Thorac Cardiovasc Surg* 1984; 88:122–127.
20. Cobbs BW Jr, Hatcher CR, Craver JM, Jones EL, Sewell CW: Transverse midventricular disruption after mitral valve replacement. *Am Heart J* 1980; 99:33–49.
21. David TE, Uden DE, Strauss HD: The importance of the mitral apparatus in left ventricular function after correction of mitral regurgitation. *Circulation* 1983; 68(suppl 2):76–82.
22. Armour JA, Randall WC: Structural basis for cardiac function. *Am J Physiol* 1970; 218:1517.
23. Craver JM, Jones EL, Guyton RA, Cobbs BW, Hatcher CR: Avoidance of transverse midventricular disruption following mitral valve replacement. *Ann Thorac Surg* 1985; 40:163–171.
24. David TE, Strauss HD, Mesher E, Anderson MJ, MacDonald IL, Buda AJ: Is it important to preserve the chordae tendinae and papillary muscles during mitral valve replacement? *Can J Surg* 1981; 24:236–239.
25. Lillehei CW, Levy MU, Bonnabeau RC Jr: Mitral valve replacement with preservation of papillary muscles and chordae. *J Thorac Cardiovasc Surg* 1964; 47:532–543.
26. David TE: Mitral valve replacement with preservation of chordae tendinae: Rationale and technical considerations. *Ann Thorac Surg* 1980; 41:680–682.
27. Oyer PE, Stinson EB, Reitz BA: Long term evaluation of the porcine xenograft bioprosthesis. *J Thorac Cardiovasc Surg* 1979; 73:343–350.
28. Horstkotte D, Korfer R, Seipel, Bircks W, Loogen F: Late complications with Bjork-Shiley and St. Jude Medical heart valve replacement. *Circulation* 1983; 68(suppl 2):175–184.
29. Metzdorff MI, Grunkelmeier GL, Pinson W, Starr A: Thrombosis of mechanical heart valves: A quantitative comparison of the silastic ball and the tilting disc. *J Am Coll Cardiol* 1984; 4:50–53.
30. Schoen FJ, Collins JJ Jr, Cohn LH: Long term failure rate and morphologic correlations in porcine bioprosthetic heart valves. *Am J Cardiol* 1983; 51:957–964.
31. Cosgrove DM: Valve construction versus valve replacement. In: Crawford FA Jr (ed): *Cardiac Surgery: Current Heart Valve Prostheses*, vols 1 and 2. Philadelphia, Hanley and Belfus, 1987: 143–158.
32. Nunley DL, Starr A: The evolution of reparative techniques for the mitral valve. *Ann Thorac Surg* 1984; 37:393–397.
33. Craver JM, Cohen C, Weintraub WS: Case-matched comparison of mitral valve replacement and repair. *Ann Thorac Surg* 1990; 49:964–969.
34. Betriu A, Chaitman BR, Almazan A, Guiteras Val P, Pelletier C: Preoperative determinations of return to sinus rhythm after valve replacement. In: Cohn LH, Galucci V (eds): *Cardiac Bioprosthesis*. New York, Yorke Medical Books, 1982: 184–191.
35. Gajewski J, Singer RB: Mortality in an insured population with atrial fibrillation. *JAMA* 1981; 245:1540–1544.

Chapter 86

Percutaneous Balloon Valvotomy

Peter C. Block, M.D.

PERCUTANEOUS BALLOON MITRAL VALVOTOMY

Percutaneous mitral balloon valvotomy (PMV) using dilating balloon catheters has become a therapeutic alternative to surgical mitral commissurotomy for some patients with mitral stenosis.[1-14] The procedure can be done in a cardiac catheterization laboratory, percutaneously, without general anesthesia, and with relatively low risk. Patients usually leave the hospital 24 h after the procedure.

Technique of PMV

PMV can be performed using multiple techniques, including a retrograde arterial technique combined with transseptal puncture,[5] single-balloon, bifoil, and double-balloon techniques. The degree of success is similar for all techniques. The most common technique involves a transseptal approach to the mitral valve.

A transseptal puncture is performed first, using the standard technique from the right femoral vein. A Mullin's sheath* is advanced with a dilator over a modified Brockenbrough needle into the left atrium. Left arial position is confirmed by oximetry, pressure measurements, and/or contrast injection. The dilator is removed, and the sheath is left in the left atrium. Heparinization is performed with 100 units/kg given intravenously.

In the double-balloon technique, a No. 7 French "floating" balloon† catheter is advanced through the Mullin's sheath across the stenotic mitral valve. Pressure across the mitral valve can be measured simultaneously from the tip of the floating balloon catheter and from the Mullin's sheath or from the Mullin's sheath and a retrogradely placed pigtail catheter in the left ventricle. Cardiac output is measured by thermodilution, green dye, or Fick techniques. The floating balloon catheter is advanced with the help of a guide wire out the aortic valve and into the ascending aorta. A 0.038-in transfer guide wire is then advanced through the floating balloon catheter into the transverse and descending aorta (Fig. 86-1*A* and *B*). If it is not easy to pass the floating balloon catheter out the aortic valve, the 0.038-in transfer guide wire tip can be placed at the left ventricular apex with a large loop so as to minimize the chance of left ventricular apical injury. The floating balloon catheter and Mullin's sheath are removed, leaving the guide wire behind. In order to pass larger dilating balloon catheters across the atrial septum and stenotic mitral valve, the hole in the atrial septum may need to be dilated. If so, a 5-mm dilating balloon catheter is advanced over the transfer guide wire until it traverses the atrial septum. Two or three dilations are performed to enlarge the opening in the atrial septum, and the 5-mm dilating balloon catheter is removed (Fig. 86-1*C* and *D*). With the use of a double-lumen catheter,* a second 0.038-in transfer guide wire is advanced across the stenotic valve. The tip is left either at the left ventricular apex or is advanced down the descending aorta parallel to the first transfer guide wire.

There are a number of variations on where the tips of the guide wires can be placed. Both 0.038-in transfer guide wires can be placed at the left ventricular apex,

*United States Catheter and Instrument Co., Billerica, MA.
†Arrow International, Reading, PA.

‡United States Catheter and Instrument Co., Billerica, MA.

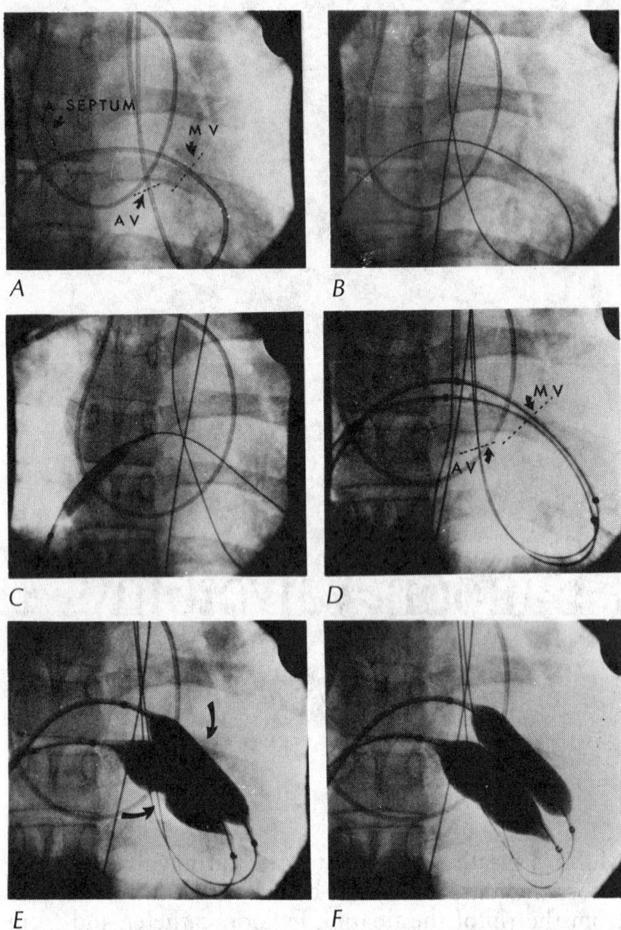

FIGURE 86-1 Sequence of percutaneous mitral valvotomy. *A.* Floating balloon catheter in position across the atrial septum through the mitral and aortic valves. The tip is in the ascending aorta. *B.* The 0.038-in transfer guide wire has been passed through the floating balloon catheter. The floating balloon catheter has been removed. *C.* An 8-mm dilating balloon catheter enlarging the atrial septal puncture site. *D.* Two 20-mm dilating balloon catheters advanced into position across the stenotic mitral valve over two separate 0.038-in transfer guide wires. *E.* Partially inflated dilating balloon catheters across the mitral valve. Note the "waist" produced by the stenotic valve (*arrows*). *F.* Fully inflated dilating balloon catheters in position across the mitral valve. (A. septum = atrial septum; AV = aortic valve; MV = mitral valve.)

one tip may be placed at the apex and one in the descending aorta, or both tips may be placed in the aorta. The appropriately sized dilating balloon catheters are then advanced over the guide wires and placed across the mitral valve (Fig. 86-1). The balloons are positioned to straddle the mitral valve, and one or two simultaneous inflations are performed. A "waist" can frequently be seen with the first inflation as the stenotic mitral valve impinges upon the expanding balloon catheters (Fig. 86-1*E* and *F*). Full inflation causes the "waist" to disappear as the commissures split. Transient hypotension always occurs as left ventricular inflow decreases. After the inflations, the balloon catheters are removed. The Mullin's sheath and floating balloon catheter are advanced over one of the two guide wires left behind. Repeat simultaneous pressure measurements are made across the mitral valve. Cardiac output is measured to permit accurate determinations of mitral valve area. Left atrial pressure should be lowered to less than a mean of 14 mmHg (alternatively, the gradient across the mitral valve should be 6 mmHg or less). PMV should not be considered satisfactory unless these values are achieved. If the gradient is not satisfactorily reduced or left atrial pressure remains high, slightly larger dilating balloons can be advanced across the stenotic valve and repeated dilations performed.

In the single-balloon technique, a single guide wire is first placed through the transseptal sheath-dilator into the left atrium. A single Inoue balloon* is then advanced over the guide wire into the left atrium. The balloon is partially inflated and advanced across the stenotic mitral valve. Partial further inflation allows anchoring of the distal portion of the balloon just below the stenotic valve orifice. The dumbbell balloon is then fully inflated to the appropriate size. After deflation, the balloon is withdrawn to the left atrium and left atrial pressure is measured. The degree of mitral regurgitation can be evaluated by Doppler echocardiographic studies. If left atrial pressure is still high and the degree of mitral regurgitation has not increased, repeated dilations using larger inflation volumes are performed.

Selection of Patients for PMV

Experience with closed mitral commissurotomy for mitral stenosis has shown that the best results of surgical commissurotomy have been in patients with minimally calcified, mobile valves.[15–18] The presence of an opening snap is clinically a predictor of a good mitral split. The mechanism of successful PMV is splitting of fused mitral commissures by the expanding balloons, as in closed or open surgical commissurotomy.[2] One would therefore anticipate that the best results of PMV would be in patients with mobile valves, little calcium, and little subvalvular disease and without valvular calcification.[19,20]

The prediction of the results of PMV can be made by careful echocardiographic evaluation of the mitral valve before the procedure. Four factors should be evaluated echocardiographically: valvular rigidity, valvular calcification, valvular thickening, and the amount of subvalvular disease. These four factors can be graded from 0 to 4+, depending on the severity of the abnormality. For example, a valve with minimal rigidity, trace calcification, minimal thickening, and evidence of only mild subvalvular fibrosis would receive a 1 for each of the four factors; the total echocardiograph score would be 4. In contrast, a valve with severe rigidity, calcification, severe thickening, and considerable subvalvular thickening would receive a score of 4 for each of the four factors; the total echocardiograph score would be 16 (Table 86-1). In general, patients who have mitral valves with echo scores of 8 or less have the best results with PMV. Patients with an echocardiograph score of 8 to 10 may have reasonable initial results from PMV but have a greater incidence of recurrent narrowing of the mitral valve within 1 year. Patients with echocardiograph scores of 11 or more have poor results and probably are better served by surgery. Hence, the best candidates for PMV are those with echocardiograph scores of less than 8.

*Toray Industries, Inc., Tokyo, Japan.

TABLE 86-1

Grading of Characteristics of Mitral Valve Morphology from Echocardiographic Examination

Leaflet Mobility	
Grade 1.	Highly mobile valve with restriction of only leaflet tips
Grade 2.	Reduced mobility of mid-portion and base of leaflets
Grade 3.	Forward movement of valve leaflets in diastole mainly at the base
Grade 4.	No or minimal forward movement of leaflets in diastole
Valvular Thickening	
Grade 1.	Leaflets near normal (4–5 mm)
Grade 2.	Mid-leaflet thickening, marked thickening of the margins
Grade 3.	Thickening extending through entire leaflets (5–8 mm)
Grade 4.	Marked thickening of all leaflet tissue (>8–10 mm)
Subvalvular Thickening	
Grade 1.	Minimal thickening of chordal structures just below the valve
Grade 2.	Thickening of chordae extending up to one-third of chordal length
Grade 3.	Thickening to the distal third of the chordae
Grade 4.	Extensive thickening and shortening of all chordae extending down to the papillary muscle
Valvular Calcification	
Grade 1.	Single area of increased echocardiograph brightness
Grade 2.	Scattered areas of brightness confined to leaflet margins
Grade 3.	Brightness extending into the midportion of the leaflets
Grade 4.	Extensive brightness through most of leaflet tissue

Additional factors that contribute to good results are the presence of sinus rhythm, young age, and a relatively short history of the symptoms of mitral stenosis (Table 86-2).

There are several contraindications of PMV. Severe mitral valve calcification and/or severe subvalvular mitral fibrosis and/or thickening are relative contraindications. Results of PMV will not be good in these patients. There are several *absolute* contraindications. Some patients should not undergo attempted transseptal puncture. These are patients who have evidence of left atrial thrombus, severe dilation of the aortic root, or other anatomic abnormalities, such as thoracolumbar scoliosis or a rotational anomaly of the heart or great vessels. Thickening of the atrial septum to more than 4 to 5 mm should raise the possibility of laminated atrial thrombus

TABLE 86-2

Percutaneous Balloon Mitral Valvotomy (PMV)

Percutaneous Balloon Mitral Valvotomy (PMV)
Factors Favorable for PMV
1. Echocardiographic score of 8 or less
2. Young age
3. Presence of opening snap
4. No calcification of valve
Factors Unfavorable for PMV
1. Echocardiograph score of 11 or more
2. Age > 70
3. No opening snap
4. Atrial fibrillation (long-standing)
5. Calcification of valve
6. Subvalvular fibrosis
7. Thickened atrial septum (>3 mm)
Contraindications to PMV
1. Left atrial thrombus
2. Recent (3 months) thromboembolic event
3. 2+ or more mitral regurgitation
4. Left ventricular thrombus
5. Associated surgical coronary or other valve disease

and is also a contraindication of PMV. Other contraindications are recent (within 3 months) thromboembolic events, 2+ or more mitral regurgitation, left ventricular apical thrombus, and associated surgical coronary or other valvular disease (Table 86-3).

Results

Although the initial results with PMV included patients with a range of morphologic conditions and of severity of mitral valve stenosis, better selection of patients has resulted in larger valve areas and better outcome.[2–14,19,20] The results from the National Heart, Lung, and Blood Institute Registry, and centers are shown in Table 86-4.

TABLE 86-3

Contraindications of PMV

Contraindications of PMV
Anatomic
1. Giant right atrium
2. Rotational anomaly of heart or great vessels
3. Severe dilation of aortic root
4. Thoracolumbar scoliosis
Pathophysiologic
1. Left atrial thrombus
2. Thickening of atrial septum to >4 mm (laminated left atrial thrombus?)
3. Recent (3 months) thromboembolic event
4. 2+ or more mitral regurgitation
5. Left ventricular thrombus
6. Associated surgical coronary or other valve disease

TABLE 86-4
Results of Mitral Valvotomy in Three Centers

Number of Patients	Age (Years)	Gradient (mmHg)		Valve Area (cm^2)	
		Before	After	Before	After
737 (NHLBI Registry)*	54	14	6	1.0	2.0
727 (Paris, France)†	43	16	6	1.1	2.2
510 (Boston)‡	56	15	5	0.9	2.0

*National Heart, Lung, and Blood Institute Registry.
†Personal communication, A. Vahanian, Hôpital Tenon, Paris.
‡Unpublished, Massachusetts General Hospital, Boston, MA.

In general, mitral valve area should increase from 0.8 ± 0.1 cm^2 to about 2 cm^2. The mitral valve gradient can be expected to fall from about 18 to 6 mmHg. Cardiac output may rise slightly or remain unchanged after successful PMV. Pulmonary artery pressure drops significantly, as does pulmonary vascular resistance (Fig. 86-2). Changes in pulmonary vascular resistance occur rapidly, although there may be a further drop later after successful PMV.[21]

When patients are grouped with regard to their echocardiograph score, patients with "echo scores" of 8 or less have increases in mitral valve area from 0.9 ± 0.1 cm^2 to 2.0 ± 0.1 cm^2 or more. If the echo score is less than 8, a good result should be achieved in more than 90 percent of the patients. If, however, the echo score is more than 8, up to 40 percent of those patients may have a less than optimal result. Overall, the increase in valve area in patients with scores of 8 or less is considerably greater than that in patients with scores greater than 8 (Fig. 86-3). In the Massachusetts General Hospital experience, patients with lower scores have a better result than those with high scores (Fig. 86-4). Grouping of patients into those with scores greater than or less than 8 is arbitrary. The echo score represents a continuum of increasing mitral valve disease and should be used only as a guideline for the chances of successful PMV.

Patients with Calcified Mitral Valves on Fluoroscopy

Patients with calcification of the mitral valve that can be seen fluoroscopically are older than patients without calcium, have a higher New York Heart Association classification, commonly have atrial fibrillation, and may have a history of previous surgical commissurotomy. Patients with calcium in the mitral valve have a mean echo score of 8.9 (compared to 6.8 in the uncalcified group).[22] A final mitral valve area of greater than 1.5 cm^2 can be achieved in about 65 percent of patients who have calcification of the mitral valve, compared to approximately 85 percent of patients who do not have calcification on fluoroscopy. Development of left-to-right shunting and significant mitral regurgitation is more common, and post-PMV mitral valve replacement is re-

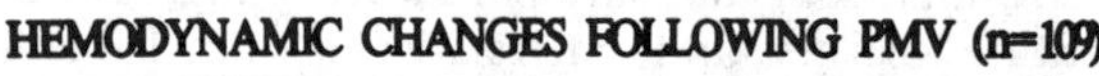

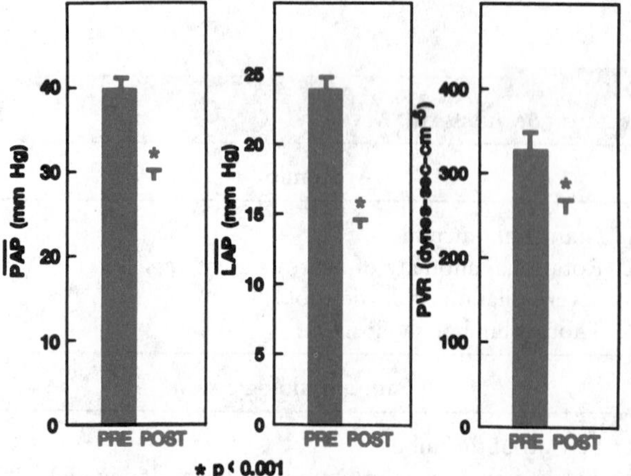

FIGURE 86-2 Changes in mean pulmonary artery pressure, mean left atrial pressure, and pulmonary vascular resistance produced by percutaneous mitral valvotomy. Pulmonary artery and left atrial mean pressures both fall immediately after successful PMV. Similarly, pulmonary vascular resistance drops rapidly. (LAP = mean left atrial pressure; PAP = mean pulmonary pressure; PVR = pulmonary vascular resistance.)

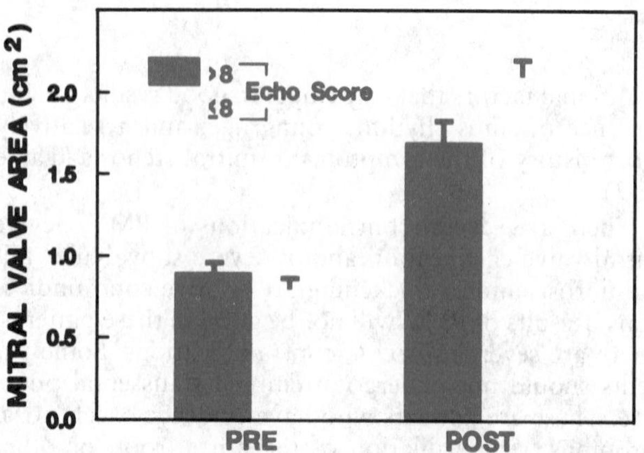

FIGURE 86-3 Changes in mitral valve area after successful percutaneous mitral valvotomy in patients with echo scores greater than 8 (black bars) and less than 8 (light bars). Patients with echo scores less than 8 have greater improvement immediately after PMV.

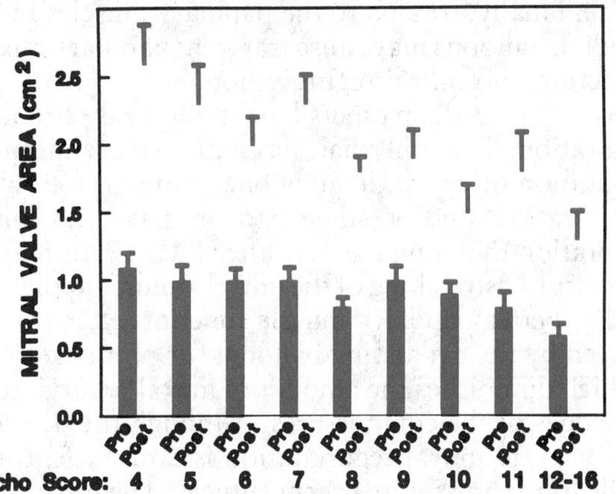

FIGURE 86-4 Changes in mitral valve area in patients undergoing successful percutaneous mitral valvotomy in relation to their echo scores. Patients with low echo scores have the greatest improvement in mitral valve area. Patients with higher echo scores have less improvement in mitral valve area.

quired more frequently in patients who have calcified mitral valves, especially in patients with heavily calcified (3+ or 4+) mitral valves. Thus, in patients with heavily calcified valves, strong consideration should be given to surgical treatment with mitral valve replacement (see Chap. 84).

Patients 65 Years of Age and Older

PMV can be performed in patients who are older than 65 years with a low morbidity and mortality; however, good immediate and long-term outcomes occur in only about 50 percent of patients. Careful patient selection with clinical evaluation, together with echocardiographic evaluation of mitral valve morphology and assessment of valvular calcification fluoroscopically, help identify those patients who are good candidates in this subgroup. The low success rate probably reflects the severity and longstanding nature of mitral stenosis in this age group. A high New York Heart Association classification, atrial fibrillation, a high echo score, mitral valve calcification, and disease of other organ systems occur more commonly in the elderly population. Since many patients in this age group are not ideal candidates for PMV, the risk of perioperative mortality with mitral valve replacement must be weighed against the risks and benefits of PMV. Patients with symptomatic mitral stenosis and low echo scores, no fluoroscopically visible valvular calcification, and otherwise reasonably good health are likely to have a successful result from PMV. Surgical therapy is a better option for patients with high echo scores and/or calcified valves. If the surgical risk is prohibitively high because of comorbidities, PMV may provide palliation of symptoms, since PMV increases the mitral valve area by approximately 50 percent in three-fourths of elderly patients. It is important to note that the final mitral valve area may only relieve symptoms moderately and that the incidence of restenosis is higher in elderly patients. Older patients who are not suitable candidates for PMV are generally referred for surgical treatment. With open mitral commissurotomy, surgical mortality in many centers is less than 2 percent.[23-25] Many patients referred for open mitral commissurotomy require mitral valve replacement because valvular morphology unsuitable for commissurotomy is found at operation. Morbidity and mortality in elderly patients who have valve replacement is considerably higher than in younger patients (see Chap. 80). In deciding between PMV and surgical therapy, one should consider not only the factors affecting the outcome of the procedure but also the relative risks. Valvular morphology and risk factors should be reviewed, and the outcome can be predicted from these factors. Surgical treatment is a better option for patients who have severely deformed valves and calcified valves. If the valve is mobile and has little calcification, the result of PMV is usually adequate as a palliative measure. If the surgical risk is prohibitively high because of comorbidities and it appears that mitral valve replacement would be a likely surgical outcome, PMV may provide palliation.

Previous Surgical Mitral Commissurotomy

An increase in mitral valve area after PMV is inversely related to the presence of a previous surgical mitral commissurotomy. PMV can produce a good outcome in this group of patients, however, and overall a mean mitral valve area of approximately 1.8 ± 0.1 cm^2 should be expected. This area is slightly less than one would expect in patients without previous commissurotomy, in whom the final valve area should be approximately 2.0 cm^2. As in patients without previous commissurotomy, the amount of mitral valve thickening, calcification, rigidity, and subvalvular disease are predictors of the immediate outcome.

In all groups of patients undergoing PMV, the immediate outcome is related to patient selection and operator experience. Recent improvements in the technique have decreased left-to-right shunting and the incidence of significant mitral regurgitation after PMV and have been associated with a trend toward lower mortality while maintaining the high success rate of the procedure.

Follow-up Results

Follow-up data on patients who have had PMV is limited, since the procedure is relatively new. Actuarial survival rates without mitral valve replacement and without New York Heart Association functional ratings of class III or IV for a group of patients over 65 years of age at 1, 2, and 3 years were 72 ± 5 percent, 53 ± 6 percent, and 46 ± 7 percent, respectively. Patients who had a successful outcome were significantly better, with an actuarial survival rate at 3 years of 54 ± 12 percent.

In a follow-up study of 41 patients who had cardiac catheterization, echocardiographic studies, and clinical evaluation as close to 2 years after PMV as possible, 41 percent of patients were New York Heart Association class I, 49 percent were class II, and 10 percent were class III. Cardiac catheterization data indicated that mitral valve area rose significantly from immediately before to immediately after PMV but that there was a decrease in the calculated mitral valve area at 2-year follow-up transseptal catheterization. Analysis by both two-dimensional planimetric and echocardiographic Doppler studies, however, did not show as large an increase in the immediate post-PMV mitral valve area. In addition, there was no significant decrease in mitral valve area at 2 years (pre-PMV planimetric results 1.1 ± 0.1 cm^2, immediate post-PMV planimetric results, 1.8 ± 0.1 cm^2; follow-up valve area, 1.6 ± 0.1 cm^2. Doppler half-time measurements were similar.

Echocardiography appears to be the most reliable method of measuring mitral valve area in the post-PMV follow-up. Cardiac catheterization data calculated by the Gorlin formula should be relied upon only if there is no evidence of left-to-right shunting. The presence of a left-to-right shunt in the immediate post-PMV evaluation lowers left atrial pressure and produces an increased right ventricular output when measured by right-sided thermodilation techniques. This flow does not represent the actual flow across the mitral valve or the cardiac output.

PMV is effective therapy, with good mid-term results for selected patients with mitral stenosis. Restenosis is more likely in patients who have high echo scores and who initially are not as good candidates for PMV. Patients with higher echo scores have a tendency to develop earlier restenosis, which will probably become more apparent at longer follow-up periods.

Complications of PMV

Mitral Regurgitation

There are a number of potential mechanisms for the development of mitral regurgitation after PMV. Since the commissures are split by the expanding balloons (Fig. 86-5),[9,27,28] unless the valve is relatively flexible, regurgitation at the edges of the commissures may occur.[26–28] The mitral annulus or mitral valve (usually the anterior leaflet) also can be directly damaged by the balloons.[29] Rupture of the chordae tendineae by the expanding balloons may occur if the balloons are not placed through the central mitral orifice but instead lie between the chordae. Finally, trauma to the papillary muscles by the expanding balloons may cause transient papillary muscle dysfunction and mitral regurgitation.

About half of the patients have no increase in mitral regurgitation. The other half have an increase in mitral regurgitation of approximately one grade. In follow-up catheterization studies, some patients have less mitral regurgitation than immediately after PMV. This may be due to a loss of stretching of the mitral annulus at the time of PMV, better papillary muscle function after trauma produced by the expanding balloons, or partial restenosis, which diminishes the amount of mitral regurgitation at the edges of the commissures. Although the development of severe mitral regurgitation is a rare event, this complication can require urgent surgery. The use of "unloading" agents such as intravenously administered nitroprusside or nitroglycerine, hemodynamic support by using the intraaortic balloon pump, and pressor agents (preferably beta-inotropic) may all be needed in order to stabilize the patient's condition before transfer to the operating room.

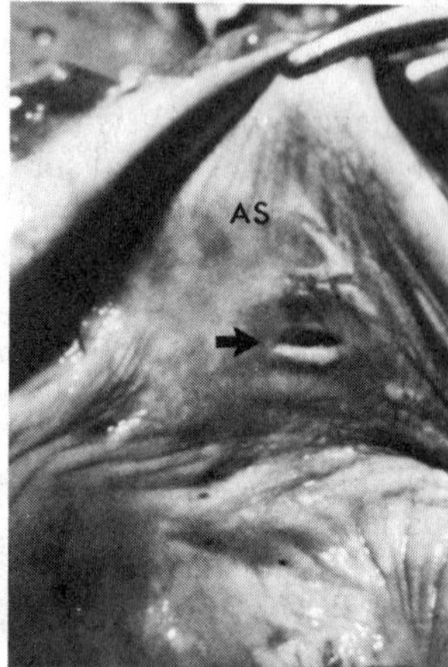

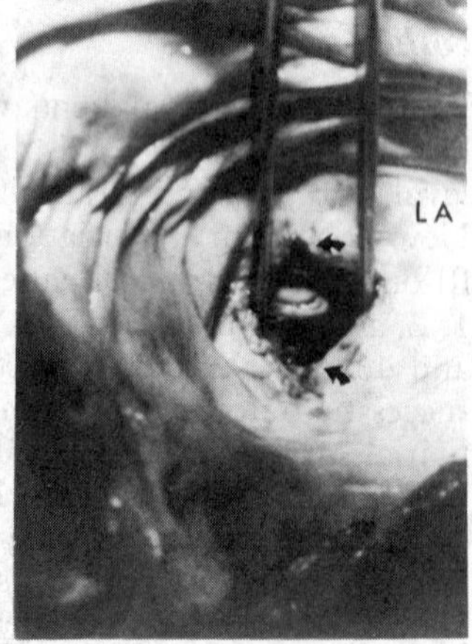

A *B*

FIGURE 86-5 Anatomic changes produced by percutaneous mitral valvotomy. *A.* A hole measuring 1 × 6 mm in the atrial septum (*arrow*) caused by passage of the dilating balloon catheters. *B.* Mitral valve after PMV viewed from the left atrium. There is splitting of the commissures toward the mitral annulus (*arrows*). (AS = atrial septum; LA = left atrium.)

Complications Associated with Transseptal Puncture

Complications include the development of cardiac tamponade, rhythm disturbances, and left to right shunt (Fig. 86-5). Occasionally, vagal tone is increased by transseptal puncture and bradycardia, and/or heart block may occur. These developments are usually transient. Tamponade can be relieved in the catheterization laboratory by placement of a pericardial drainage catheter percutaneously.

Left-to-right shunts may be produced if the atrial septal hole is large (due to tearing of the septum, inflation of the septum with a portion of the dilating balloons, removal of balloons without complete deflation, or use of large-diameter balloons). Hemodynamically significant left-to-right shunting could be measured immediately after PMV in 20 percent of the patients in the Massachusetts General Hospital series. At follow-up in 6 months, however, only one-third had shunting. Shunting is greater if left atrial hypertension is not relieved by adequate valvotomy. The atrial septal defect produced by PMV can lower left atrial pressure. As noted above, the left-to-right shunt increases the pulmonary blood flow; and if this flow is measured by thermodilution methods and the value is used for cardiac output in the Gorlin formula, a falsely high valve area is calculated. The discrepancies can be corrected if the septal defect is occluded.[30]

Systemic Embolism

Embolism usually occurs due to dislodgment of a left atrial thrombus or disruption of a laminated clot that lies against the atrial septum. It is possible that calcific debris may be dislodged from the mitral valve by the expanding balloons, although this appears to be a rare event. Transesophageal echocardiographic studies are especially useful in ruling out left atrial thrombi prior to PMV.

Mortality

Death can occur from right heart failure secondary to pulmonary hypertension (which may be increased by the stress of the procedure), unrecognized pericardial tamponade produced at the time of the transseptal puncture, perforation of the left ventricular apex by the balloons or guide wires, or associated coronary artery disease. A careful watch should be kept for tamponade during the procedure. Tamponade may be insidious and may not be apparent clinically until the end of the procedure. Tamponade associated with apical perforation of the balloon may be catastrophic and require urgent surgery. If the diagnosis of apical perforation is suspected, urgent surgery should be undertaken even if the patient's condition can be stabilized with pericardiocentesis, and the apical perforation should be repaired at the time of mitral valve surgery.

Medications Given before, during, and after PMV

Before PMV, it is preferable to administer anticoagulant therapy (with warfarin) for at least 2 to 3 months. The usefulness of anticoagulant therapy in preventing the development of left atrial thrombi and arterial emboli is not established in patients with sinus rhythm. All patients with mitral stenosis in atrial fibrillation should be maintained on low-dose warfarin International Normalized Ratio (INR 2.0 to 3.0) indefinitely. Warfarin should be discontinued several days prior to transseptal PMV. Although beta blockers may be useful to help control the ventricular response to atrial fibrillation before PMV, high-dose beta blockers may produce bradycardia and hypotension during the procedure and should be used with caution in the days before PMV.

During PMV, all patients are given intravenous heparin (100 units/kg) immediately after the transseptal puncture is completed successfully. Heparin does not need to be reversed at the end of the procedure. Since PMV is usually done using a femoral vein, bleeding is rarely a problem. Compression of the right femoral vein after the procedure usually leads to prompt hemostasis.

Warfarin administration is begun the day after PMV, when patients are placed back on their standard pre-PMV anticoagulation dosage. Even though the mitral stenosis is relieved by PMV, if the patient is in atrial fibrillation or has a history of paroxysmal atrial fibrillation or systemic embolism, anticoagulation with warfarin (INR 2.0 to 3.0) should be continued indefinitely. If the patient is in sinus rhythm, the efficacy of warfarin or "antiplatelet" agents such as aspirin is unknown. If the left atrial diameter is in excess of 55 mm, there is an increased likelihood of developing atrial fibrillation, and long-term warfarin therapy should be considered. If warfarin is not used, aspirin (160 to 324 mg/day) would be appropriate (see also Chaps. 68 and 80).

Summary

PMV is an excellent alternative to surgery for the palliative relief of mitral stenosis. Patients with mobile, minimally calcified, minimally thickened valves without severe subvalvular fibrosis are the best candidates. Follow-up studies show little evidence of restenosis at 2 years. Analysis of 36-month clinical follow-up indicates that patients with low echo scores have an excellent clinical outcome. Patients with more thickened, calcified valves have a higher incidence of restenosis and recurrence of symptoms. It appears likely that the long-term results of PMV will be similar to the results of closed surgical mitral commissurotomy.

PERCUTANEOUS AORTIC VALVOTOMY

Percutaneous aortic valvotomy (PAV) is performed in a cardiac catheterization laboratory and can be done using a retrograde approach from a femoral (or brachial) artery or using a transseptal antegrade approach from the right femoral vein. Patients usually leave the hospital 36 to 48 h after the procedure.[31–35]

Description of Techniques of PAV

Retrograde Approach

A right or left femoral puncture is made using standard Seldinger technique, or a cutdown is made from the right or left brachial artery if the artery is large enough to accommodate the balloon catheters. After heparinization (100 units/kg intravenously), a retrograde catheter (pigtail catheter, retrograde catheter, multipurpose catheter, etc.) is advanced to the level of the ascending aorta. Careful measurements are taken of the ascending aortic pressure, and they are balanced either against radial artery pressure monitored through an indwelling catheter or through a "side-port" pressure monitor through a femoral artery sheath. The aortic valve is then traversed retrogradely, most commonly using a guide wire. The catheter is placed in the body of the left ventricle, and left ventricular pressure measurements are made, with simultaneous measurement of the pressure in the radial or femoral arteries. The gradient across the aortic valve is documented, and cardiac output is measured to calculate the aortic valve area.

A 0.038-in exchange guide wire is then advanced through the catheter. The tip of the exchange wire should be performed to make a large loop that can nestle in the apex of the left ventricle without fear of perforation (Fig. 86-6). Care should be taken to maintain hemostasis at either the femoral or the brachial puncture site. The arterial opening is enlarged by using progressively larger arterial dilators, and a No. 12 French introducer is placed. A 15- or 20-mm diameter dilating balloon catheter is advanced over the transfer guide wire until it straddles the stenotic aortic valve. The size of the dilating balloon catheter is chosen to avoid overdistension of the aortic annulus; usually a 20-mm dilating balloon catheter is used first. If a previous aortic root or left ventricular cine angiogram is available, the annulus can be measured directly, and a balloon no larger than the annular size can be chosen. Alternatively, echocardiography can be used to measure aortic annulus size. The balloon is large enough if full inflation produces systemic hypotension due to obstruction of the aortic annulus. Two or three inflations are performed. Measurements

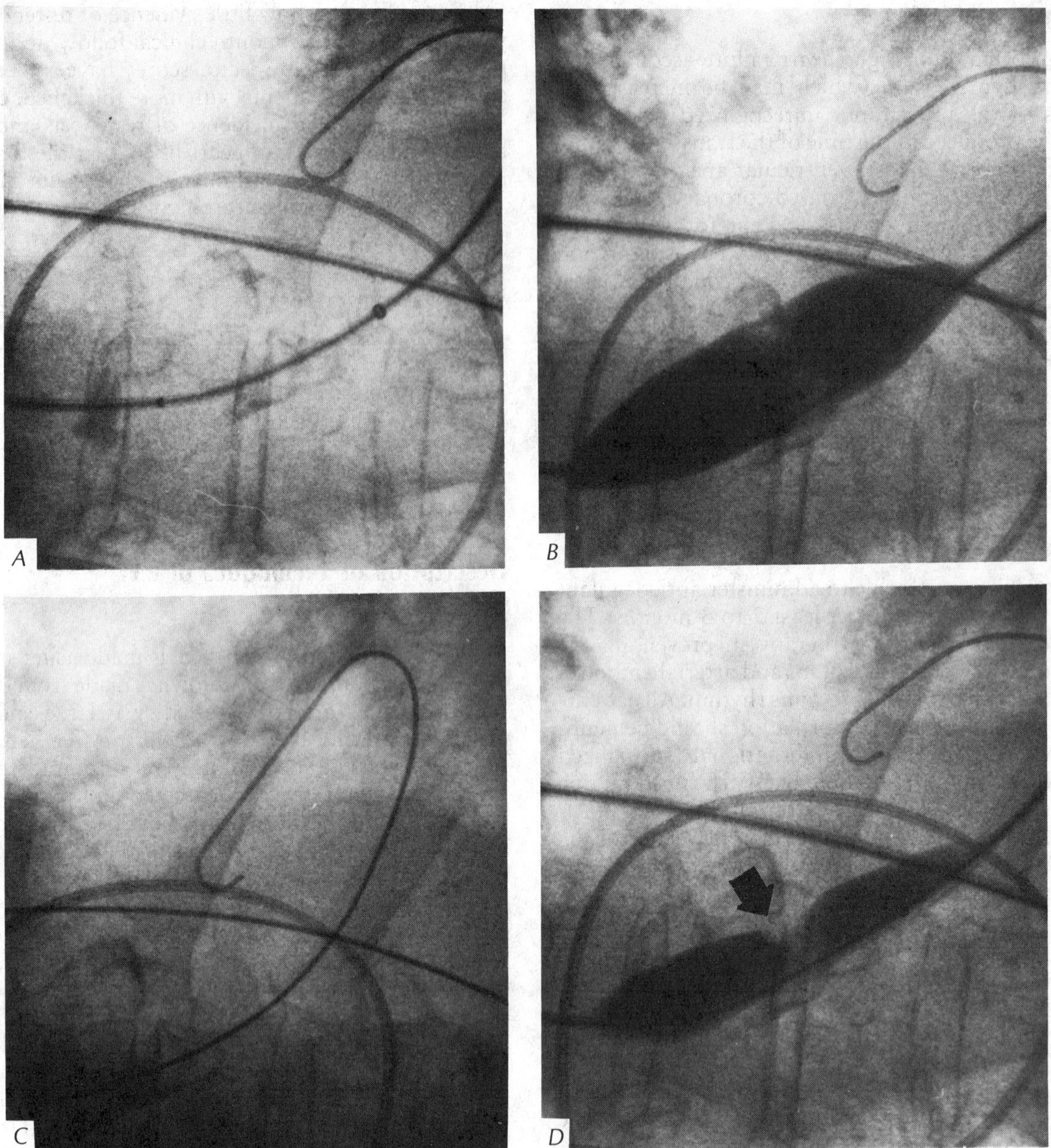

FIGURE 86-6 Sequence of retrograde percutaneous aortic valvuloplasty. *A.* A 0.038-in transfer guide wire placed across the stenotic aortic valve with the loop at the left ventricular apex. *B.* Deflated dilating balloon catheter across the stenotic aortic valve over the guide wire. *C.* Partially inflated 20-mm dilating balloon catheter in position across the aortic valve. Note the indentation caused by the stenotic aortic valve (*arrow*). *D.* Fully inflated 20-mm dilating balloon catheter across the aortic valve.

are then repeated by removing the dilating balloon catheter and replacing it with a pigtail catheter. Pressure can also be measured through the empty lumen of a double-lumen catheter,* which can be advanced over the transfer guide wire. This eliminates the necessity of removing the guide wire. If the gradient has been reduced to less than 20 to 30 mmHg, cardiac output is measured and a rough calculation of the aortic valve area is undertaken. If the reduction in pressure gradient is not adequate and the aortic valve area remains less than 0.7 cm^2, a larger dilating balloon catheter (23 mm in diameter) or two dilating balloon catheters can be advanced and repeated dilations undertaken. Attempts should be made to increase the aortic valve area to at least 0.9 to 1 cm^2 (Fig. 86-7).

If the aortic gradient is still high after the use of a 23-mm balloon, a second femoral puncture can be made using the contralateral femoral artery, and a second guide wire can be placed through the aortic valve from that artery. Two 15-mm or two 18-mm dilating balloon catheters can be passed over the transfer guide wires and simultaneous inflations undertaken. After satisfactory reduction of the gradient across the aortic valve, the catheters are withdrawn, and heparinization is reversed with protamine. Hemostasis is achieved by pressure over the arterial puncture site or repair of the brachial arteriotomy site.

*Mansfield, Watertown, MA.

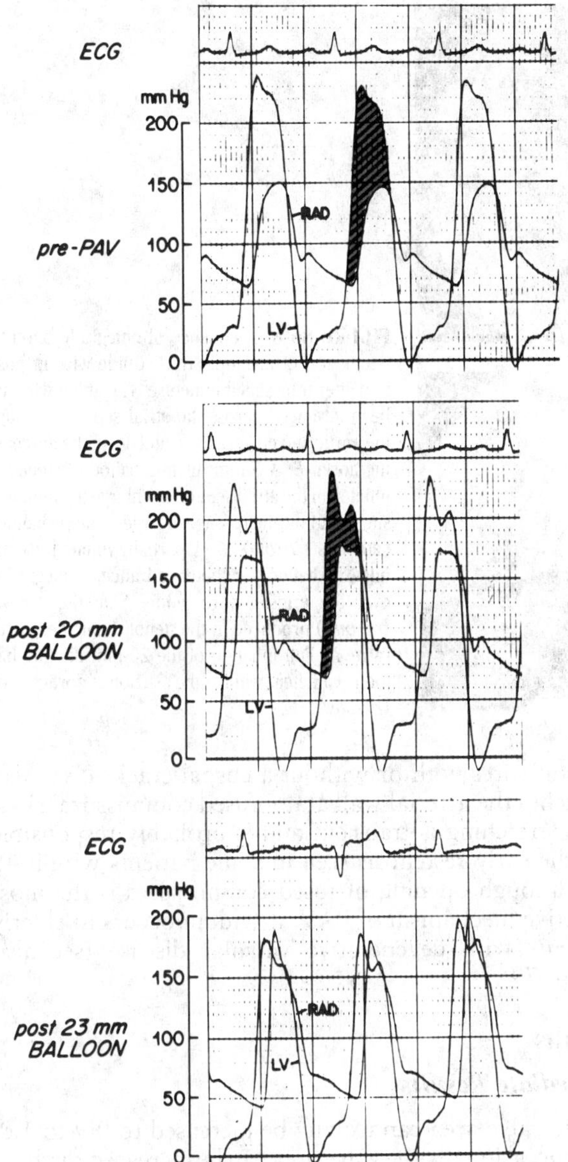

FIGURE 86-7 Hemodynamic changes before and after successful percutaneous aortic valvuloplasty. (*Top*) Simultaneous radial artery and left ventricular pressure before PAV. The peak gradient across the aortic valve is approximately 80 mmHg. (*Middle*) After PAV with a 20-mm balloon, the gradient is decreased to approximately 35 mmHg. (*Bottom*) After PAV using a 23-mm balloon in the same patient, the gradient across the aortic valve is abolished. (LV = left ventricular pressure; RAD = radial artery pressure.)

Antegrade Approach

A transseptal puncture is performed using standard technique from the right femoral vein. A floating balloon catheter is advanced across the mitral valve and, with the help of a guide wire, is advanced out of the stenotic aortic valve and into the ascending aorta. A 0.038-in transfer guide wire is advanced through the floating balloon catheter into the descending aorta. The floating balloon catheter and Mullin's sheath are removed, leaving the single transfer guide wire behind.

A 5-mm dilating catheter is advanced over the wire to straddle and dilate the atrial septum. One or two inflations are performed to allow passage of larger dilating balloon catheters. A 15- or 20-mm dilating balloon catheter is then advanced over the guide wire and placed in position to straddle the stenotic aortic valve (Fig. 86-8). Care must be taken to assure that the body of the dilating balloon does not lie within the chordae tendineae of the mitral valve, since inflation in that position might damage the mitral supporting apparatus. Multiple inflations of the dilating balloon catheter are made within the stenotic aortic valve. Repeated measurements are made after the dilating balloon catheter is removed. If the aortic gradient has not been satisfactorily diminished, a 23- or 25-mm dilating balloon catheter can be advanced antegradely across the aortic valve, or, alternatively, two 15- or two 18-mm dilating balloon catheters can be placed over two guide wires. Larger catheters or double-balloon catheters should be chosen with care in order not to overdistend the aortic annulus and possibly cause damage to the aortic outflow tract. In one series of over 100 patients who have undergone aortic valvuloplasty, 64 percent had the procedure done retrogradely and 36 percent antegradely.[34] There were no demographic differences in the patient population, and the results of PAV using either the retrograde of the antegrade approach were the same.

Selection of Patients for PAV

Although PAV diminishes the aortic valve gradient and increases the aortic valve area, the results are not as striking as the increase in valve area produced by balloon mitral valvotomy.[36] One would expect, therefore, that the rate of restenosis would be higher and that the benefit would be transient. The best candidates appear to fall into four groups.

Nonoperative Candidates

Patients may not be candidates for valve replacement because of their age, frailty, or the presence of severe associated noncardiac disease, such as chronic obstructive lung disease, renal failure, neoplasms, and so on, which make them unsuitable candidates for cardiac surgery.

Patients with Aortic Stenosis and Other Acute Surgical Problems

If there are other surgical problems requiring intervention, severe aortic stenosis may need treatment first. Examples include patients with a bleeding ulcer, with a carcinoma that can be cured by resection, or with a fractured hip. Percutaneous aortic valvotomy can be performed to relieve the aortic stenosis, and the other surgical procedure can then be undertaken at a diminished risk.[37]

Patients with Cardiogenic Shock Due to Aortic Stenosis

Patients with hemodynamic embarrassment due to heart failure and aortic stenosis frequently need intubation and intravenous pressor support to maintain blood pressure. Urgent PAV can relieve aortic stenosis and allow wean-

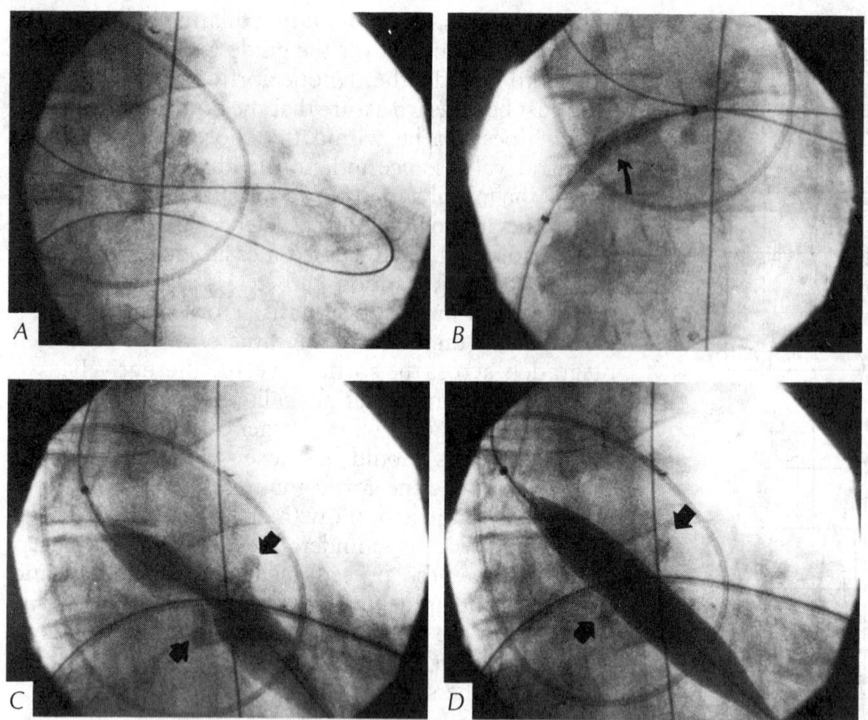

FIGURE 86-8 Sequence of antegrade percutaneous aortic valvuloplasty. *A.* Guide wire in position after transseptal puncture. The guide wire has been advanced across the atrial septum, through the aortic and mitral valves, and down the descending aorta. *B.* A 5-mm dilating balloon catheter is inflated in the atrial septum to enlarge the puncture site and allow the passage of larger dilating balloon catheters (*arrow*). *C.* A partially inflated 20-mm dilating balloon catheter advanced antegradely over the transfer wire guide. Note the "waist" (*arrows*) produced by the stenotic, calcified aortic valve. *D.* Full inflation of the 20-mm dilating balloon catheter within the stenotic aortic valve (*arrows*).

ing of pressors within hours. Extubation can frequently be accomplished as well. These patients can then be considered candidates for more elective aortic valve replacement at a lower risk.

Patients with Poor Left Ventricular Function, Low Cardiac Output, and a Low Gradient (Less Than 35 mmHg) across the Aortic Valve

Whether such patients have significant aortic stenosis that accounts for their heart failure or whether there is underlying heart muscle disease that diminishes left ventricular function frequently cannot be ascertained by currently available diagnostic methods. If the aortic valve is stenotic and responsible for poor left ventricular function, relief of the stenosis by PAV may improve left ventricular function.[38–40] Sequential left ventricular function can be measured by noninvasive means, such as echocardiography or gated cardiac blood pool scanning. If left ventricular function improves and aortic stenosis recurs, these patients can be considered candidates for aortic valve replacement. If, however, no improvement occurs despite an increase in valve area by PAV, it is likely that there is underlying irreversible heart muscle disease. Aortic valve replacement in such patients has high mortality and should not be considered. Prognosis after PAV is also poor.[39]

Mechanism of PAV

Postmortem studies of patients with degenerative calcific aortic stenosis show that commissural fusion is minimal and that the increase in aortic valve area following PAV is a result of the fracture of calcium deposits in the aortic leaflets.[40,41] In patients with commissural fusion (e.g., with rheumatic aortic stenosis or noncalcified bicuspid aortic valve stenosis), PAV may result in splitting of the commissures with or without a cuspal crack. PAV also stretches the arterial wall at nonfused commissural sites. This stretching is transient and is probably responsible for the early restenosis seen in some patients within 48 h. Although opening of fused commissures is the most effective mechanism of PAV, it seldom occurs in elderly patients with degenerative valvular disease (see also Chap. 79).

Results

Immediate Results

Aortic valve area can usually be increased to 0.9 to 1.0 cm^2. Occasionally the valve area can be increased further, although this is not possible in all patients, especially in elderly patients with severely calcified aortic valves. Table 86-5 shows the results of PAV in a French study (Rouen), in studies at Beth Israel Hospital and Massachusetts General Hospital in Boston, and in the combined center results in the Mansfield Registry. Immediate results are similar in the three institutions. Of note is the fact that, with increasing experience and improved technology, the percentage of patients in whom aortic valve area is increased to 1 cm^2 or more is greater. For example, early in the French experience, only 25 percent of 85 patients undergoing PAV had final aortic valve areas greater than 1 cm^2 (patients number 51 to number 135). In patients number 136 to number 218, 44 percent had final valve areas greater than 1 cm^2, and in patients number 219 to number 275, 60 percent had valve areas greater than 1 cm^2.[42]

The age of patients undergoing PAV is also related to the outcome. In patients 80 years or older, aortic valve area increases from 0.48 to 0.90 cm^2, compared to patients younger than 70 years, in whom aortic valve area increases from 0.6 to 1.0 cm^2.[42] The rate of restenosis may not be related to the final aortic valve area produced

TABLE 86-5
Results of Percutaneous Aortic Valvotomy

Number of Patients	Gradient (mmHg) Before	After	Valve Area (cm^2) Before	After
334 (Rouen, France)	72	29	0.52	0.93
205 (Beth Israel Hospital, Boston)	09	33	0.6	1.0
308 (Massachusetts General Hospital, Boston)	61	30	0.5	0.8
492 (Mansfield Registry)	60 ± 23	30 ± 13	0.5 ± 0.2	0.8 ± 0.3

by PAV. Rather, restenosis may be related to the mechanism of aortic valve enlargement. The increase in aortic valve area produced by disruption of calcium nodules in the valve may be relatively short-lived because of recurrent fibrous ingrowth. Release of commissural fusion (if present) may produce a better long-term result.[32,36,41]

Long-Term Results

Mortality within the first year after PAV is 24.5 percent and 28 percent in the French and Massachusetts General Hospital experiences, respectively. Most of the patients were not operative candidates, however, and comparable groups of patients who had symptomatic aortic stenosis and only medical therapy may have mortality rates of more than 40 percent.[37,43] Clinical follow-up shows that cardiac mortality and clinical restenosis (defined as either cardiac mortality or patients who return to their pre-PAV New York Heart Association functional class) is high. Mortality is greater in patients with an aortic valve area less than 0.7 cm^2 after PAV than in patients with valve areas greater than 0.7 cm^2. Overall, the impact of PAV on the natural history of aortic stenosis treated medically is small. Poor left ventricular function and the presence of associated coronary artery disease adversely affect the post-PAV prognosis. Although the difference is not great, clinical restenosis at 1 year is higher in patients whose aortic valve area is less than 0.7 cm^2 after PAV than in those whose aortic valve area is larger (Fig. 86-9).

Advantages

The advantages of PAV are that it can be done in a cardiac catheterization laboratory, percutaneously, without general anesthesia. Patients usually leave the hospital within 36 to 48 h after the procedure and can return to full activity immediately, assuming that their aortic stenosis is relieved.

Disadvantages

The disadvantages of PAV are that the restenosis rate is high and the mortality rate is unaffected. Symptoms of heart failure, however, may improve until restenosis occurs. Dilation of the aortic valve using balloon techniques produces either separation of fused commissures or fractures of the calcific deposits within the valve. Both effects would improve aortic leaflet flexibility and allow better opening of the aortic valve. The reparative process after aortic valvotomy, particularly in patients with

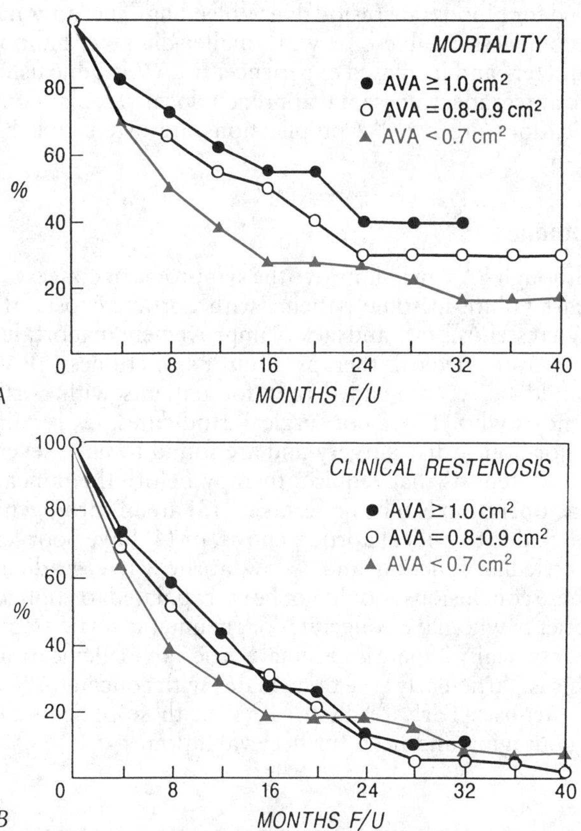

FIGURE 86-9 *A.* Survival (mortality) curves for patients with severe aortic stenosis treated with balloon valvuloplasty. Survival curves are shown for three different post-PAV valve areas. *B.* Curves for clinical restenosis for patients with severe aortic stenosis treated with balloon valvuloplasty. Curves for three different post-PAV aortic valve areas are shown. (AVA = aortic valve area post-PAV.) (*Palacios IG: Aortic balloon valvuloplasty. Cardiac surgery: State of the Art Reviews 1991; 5:267–274. Reproduced with permission from the publisher and author.*)

TABLE 86-6
Complications of Percutaneous Aortic Valvuloplasty

	%
Severe aortic regurgitation	1.3
Cerebrovascular accident/embolism	1.5
Tamponade (perforation)	1.1
Arrhythmia (ventricular fibrillation, heart block)	2.1
Vascular (hematoma, bleeding)	10.7
Death	4.6

SOURCE: Pooled data from Rouen, France; Beth Israel Hospital, Boston; Massachusetts General Hospital, Boston; and the Mansfield Registry.

calcified, degenerative aortic stenosis, probably lead to recurrence of aortic valve rigidity within months. If splitting of commissures is produced, it may account for patients with better long-term results.

Complications of PAV

Local vascular complications are the most common. They include vascular problems such as thrombosis or laceration, production of a large hematoma, and the need for blood transfusion due to bleeding. The latter has become less troublesome with smaller-diameter balloon catheters and increased experience. If PAV is done using the antegrade, transseptal approach, local vascular complications are rare.[34] Complications are listed in Table 86-6.

Summary

Although PAV may improve the symptoms of congestive heart failure in some patients with aortic stenosis, the high restenosis rate and lack of improvement in mortality rate over medical therapy limit its usefulness. PAV should be recommended only for patients with aortic stenosis who (1) are *not* surgical candidates, (2) require major noncardiac surgery and are found to have severe aortic stenosis that requires therapy before the noncardiac operation can be undertaken, (3) are in cardiogenic shock due to critical aortic stenosis, or (4) have poor left ventricular function and a low aortic valve gradient. These conclusions should not be extrapolated to younger patients who have congenital or rheumatic aortic stenosis, especially if there is minimal aortic valve calcification. This is particularly true of neonates with congenital aortic stenosis. Early results of PAV in these patients are encouraging and need further evaluation.

PERCUTANEOUS BALLOON VALVOTOMY FOR PULMONIC STENOSIS

Percutaneous balloon catheter dilation has been used in the treatment of a variety of stenotic lesions of congenital origin, particularly coarctation of the aorta and pulmonic stenosis (see Chap. 97). The most commonly treated lesion has been pulmonary valve stenosis.[44-49] The immediate and long-term results of balloon valvotomy have been well documented. The reported average gradient reduction ranges from 53 to 68 percent, somewhat less than that provided by standard surgical procedures. Early attempts at balloon valvotomy of the pulmonic valve were done with relatively small balloons; the use of oversized balloons or of the double-balloon technique provides adequate relief of pulmonic stenosis in most patients and prevents the need for cardiac surgery.[46,47,50]

Technique of Percutaneous Balloon Valvotomy

Operative Procedure

Right heart catheterization is performed using the femoral vein approach and standard percutaneous Seldinger techniques. Both groins are prepared and draped, and a No. 7 French sheath is introduced into the right femoral vein. Heparin (100 units/kg) is administered intravenously. Cardiac output is measured by the thermodilution technique. Right ventricular and pulmonary artery pressures are recorded, as is cardiac output. Femoral arterial pressure is usually monitored continuously throughout the procedure. A No. 7 French balloon-tipped wedge pressure catheter is advanced from the right femoral vein into the left pulmonary artery. A 0.035- or 0.038-in transfer guide wire (J tip) is introduced into the catheter and positioned with its soft tip well into the left lower-lobe pulmonary artery if possible. The No. 7 French catheter and introducing sheaths are removed, leaving the guide wire in place in the left pulmonary artery. The right femoral vein is dilated with a No. 9 French dilator. Catheters used for valvotomy are No. 8 or No. 9 French.* The diameter of the balloons is carefully selected according to pulmonary annular size (see below). The valvotomy catheter is advanced over the exchange wire and positioned across the stenotic pulmonary valve, leaving the guide wire in place in the left pulmonary artery. Rapid inflation and deflation are undertaken to minimize the time of occlusion of the right ventricular outflow tract. Disappearance of the "waist" caused by the stenotic pulmonic valve usually occurs suddenly as the valve is opened. The balloon is reinflated once or twice subsequently to document that there is no further constriction by the valve in the early phase of inflation. The dilating balloon catheter is deflated and removed, and repeated pressure and cardiac output measurements are obtained.

Selection of Balloon Size

The balloon diameter should be selected according to an estimate of annular size made from the lateral angiocardiogram. Correction for magnification must be made. The annulus is defined by the leaflet attachment points. Although it may be necessary to undertake an initial valvotomy with a small balloon to reduce the risk of hemodynamic compromise, the final balloon diameter should be 20 to 40 percent larger than the pulmonary annulus. If a double-balloon technique is used, the "ef-

*Mansfield, Watertown, MA.

fective dilating diameter" should be determined by calculating the cross-sectional area of the oval enveloping the two balloons and then calculating the diameter of the circle with the same area.[47]

If the femoral vein is too small to easily accommodate a large balloon, a double-balloon technique can be used, with smaller-diameter balloons inserted into each femoral vein. Two transfer guide wires are needed. The double-balloon technique may have several advantages: (1) it reduces trauma at the time of insertion into the femoral vein; (2) it extends the range of patients treated with balloon dilation because of small-sized femoral vessels; and (3) since double-balloon catheters may not completely occlude the stenotic orifice during balloon inflation, hemodynamic deterioration does not occur during inflation, and the ventricle is "vented" because some blood continues to flow past the balloons.

Selection of Patients

Critical pulmonic stenosis in the newborn may be a medical emergency. Infants who have suprasystemic right ventricular pressure (measured at cardiac catheterization), cardiomegaly, heart failure, and cyanosis fall into this category. In general, they have a tiny pulmonary orifice with severely compromised hemodynamic status (see Chap. 97).

More elective balloon valvotomy for pulmonic stenosis should be undertaken in children or adults who meet the following criteria:

- Right ventricular pressure is three-quarters or more of systemic pressure.
- The pulmonic valve gradient is 50 mmHg or more.
- Mild-to-moderate pulmonic stenosis (gradient, 25 to 50 mmHg) is a *questionable* indication. The natural history of unoperated patients in this group shows good survival without symptoms. Issues of right ventricular dysfunction in adulthood, however, have not been clarified in patients with mild-to-moderate pulmonic stenosis who are not treated. Further evaluation and long-term follow-up data are necessary before any final recommendations can be made (see also Chap. 98).
- Pulmonary valve dysplasia is present. A few patients (some with Noonan's syndrome) have thicker valves with less doming and little valve mobility. The annulus may be small, and there may be supravalular hypoplasia. Most of these patients cannot be effectively treated with balloon valvotomy, which produces poor results and should not be undertaken unless there are no good alternatives.

Results

Gradient reduction should be in the range of 60 to 75 percent. A summary of the results from three major centers undertaking balloon pulmonic valvotomy is shown in Table 86-7. In general, the gradient is reduced less than 50 percent (from 74 ± 30 to 42 ± 30 mmHg without Noonan's syndrome; from 79 ± 35 to 49 ± 20 mmHg with Noonan's syndrome,[51] although occasionally patients may have better results.[52] Using oversized balloons improves gradient reduction and achieves results more equivalent to those of surgery.[47] The advantage of the procedure is that it can be done without significant morbidity and with a tolerable incidence of pulmonary regurgitation. Long-term follow-up studies also show that the reduction in gradient persists, indicating that relief of pulmonary valve obstruction may well be similar to the long-term results of surgical pulmonary valvotomy (Fig. 86-10).

The disadvantages of the technique are that care must be taken in choosing balloon size. Too small a balloon size will not effectively open the pulmonary valve; too large a balloon size may cause a hematoma of the pulmonary outflow tract and overdilation of the pulmonary annulus. Balloon valvotomy may not be possible in all patients due to a very small size of the femoral vein or due to abnormalities of the inferior vena cava. In such instances, a jugular vein or brachial vein must be used, although the procedure is more difficult to undertake using that approach.

Complications of Pulmonic Valvotomy

Major complications of pulmonic valvotomy are listed in Table 86-8. They include infundibular reaction, arrhythmias (transient bradycardia and ventricular ectopy), blood loss (transfusion), venous damage, and death. Pulmonary regurgitation after balloon valvotomy

TABLE 86-7
Pulmonic Valvotomy

Number of Patients	Mean Age	Age Range	Gradient (mmHg) Before	After
173 (Saudi Arabia)*	46 months	1–12 years	100	28
100 (Brazil)†	10 years	1–59 years	98	15
72 (Houston, Texas)‡	48 months	3 days–75 years	72	17
(VACA Registry)§			71 ± 33	16 ± 15

*Personal communication, M.A. Ali Khan, M.D., Riyadh Military Hospital, Riyadh, Saudi Arabia.
†Personal communication, Cesar Esteves, M.D., Instituto (Dante Pazzanese) de Cardiologia, Sao Paulo, Brazil.
‡Personal communication, Charles Mullins, M.D., Texas Children's Hospital, Houston, TX.
§Valvuloplasty and Angioplasty of Congenital Anomalies Registry.

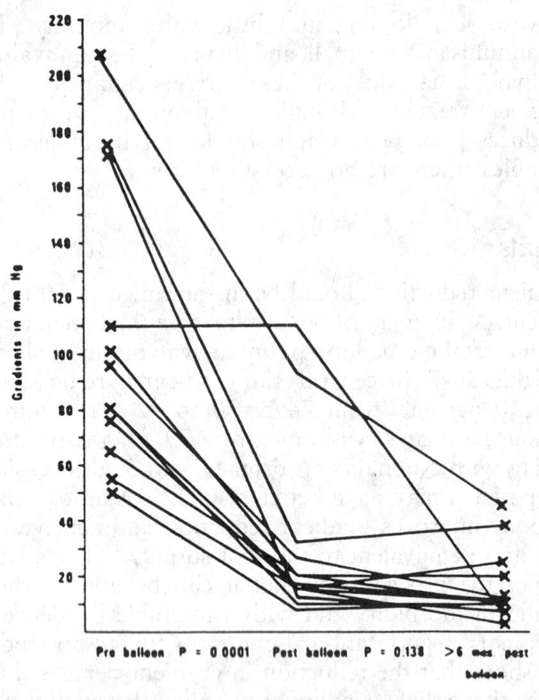

FIGURE 86-10 Hemodynamic measurements before, immediately after, and 6 months after successful percutaneous balloon pulmonary valvuloplasty. At follow-up catheterization, there is no evidence of restenosis. (*From MA Ali Khan, SA Yousef, CE Mullins: Percutaneous transluminal balloon pulmonary valvuloplasty for the relief of pulmonary valve stenosis with special reference to double-balloon technique. Am Heart J 112:158–166, 1986. Reproduced with permission from the publisher and authors.*)

is common, and frequency varies from 20 percent[46] to more than 75 percent.[51] It is usually mild and of little hemodynamic significance. Infundibular reaction is not uncommon after balloon dilation of the pulmonic valve. Right ventricular pressure may not drop immediately after valvotomy due to hypercontractility of the hypertrophied outflow tract. Patients with severe infundibular hypertrophy may need treatment with beta blockers, although whether or not this is effective in avoiding a "suicidal" right ventricle immediately after the procedure or in promoting regression of infundibular stenosis is unknown. Infundibular stenosis regresses over weeks to months after the procedure, just as it does after surgical relief of pulmonic stenosis. Bradycardia is not uncommon during balloon inflation, and atropine can be administered just prior to balloon dilation if the heart rate slows or if bradycardia is anticipated. Right bundle branch block may occur and may be related to stretching of the infundibular region at the time of valvotomy. Other rare complications that have been reported are avulsion of a valve cusp,[53] pulmonary artery tears,[54] balloon rupture,[55] cerebrovascular accident (CVA),[55] and heart block.[56]

TABLE 86-8

Complications of Pulmonic Valvotomy*

Infundibular reaction	37
Arrhythmia	12
Blood loss (transfusion)	25
Venous damage	2
Death	1

*Number of patients = 173.

SOURCE: Personal communication, M.A. Ali Khan, M.D., Riyadh Military Hospital, Riyadh, Saudi Arabia.

PERCUTANEOUS BALLOON VALVOTOMY IN TRICUSPID STENOSIS

Rheumatic tricuspid stenosis can be treated using percutaneous balloon valvotomy techniques. Experience using balloon valvotomy for tricuspid stenosis is limited, but early reports show that the pressure gradient can be reduced by approximately 70 percent and the valve area can be doubled.[57–59]

Description of Technique

Both femoral regions are prepared and draped in the usual fashion. If thermodilution cardiac output is to be measured, a Swan-Ganz catheter can be placed from a right internal jugular vein. The presence of tricuspid regurgitation, however, may make measurements of cardiac output by thermodilution unreliable. The Fick technique should be used in most patients. A No. 7 French introducer is placed in the right femoral vein, and a floating balloon (No. 7 French) catheter is passed across the tricuspid valve. Simultaneous measurement of pressure in the right atrium and the right ventricle can be made from the Swan-Ganz line placed in the right atrium or from the second floating balloon catheter passed from the contralateral femoral vein or inserted into the same femoral vein via a separate sheath. Care must be taken to calibrate identical simultaneous right atrial pressure tracings from both catheters, and then one catheter is advanced to the right ventricular cavity. The gradient across the tricuspid valve and cardiac output are measured simultaneously.

A 0.038-in Teflon-coated exchange wire with a curved J tip is advanced through the floating balloon catheters. The curved end of each guide wire can be positioned at the apex of the right ventricle or, if possible, can be passed antegradely out the pulmonary valve into the distal left or right pulmonary artery. Placement of the guide wire tip in the pulmonary circulation provides better stability. Dilating balloon catheters* of 20-mm or 15-mm diameter are advanced percutaneously over each guide wire and positioned across the tricuspid valve under fluoroscopic control. The balloons are fully inflated. It may be difficult to align the balloons properly across the tricuspid valve, since the valve plane may be difficult to establish with certainty by fluoroscopy. In addition, the relatively small size of the right ventricle makes alignment of the balloons toward the ventricular apex difficult. A "waist" is seen if the balloons are in the proper position during inflation. With full inflation, the "waist" should disappear, and subsequent inflations

*Mansfield, Watertown, MA; USCI, Billerica, MA.

should not show any indentation by the valve. Inflation should last for 10 to 15 s. After two or three dilations, the balloon catheters are deflated and removed; repeated pressure measurements are carefully made across the tricuspid valve, and repeated cardiac output measurements are made simultaneously.

Selection of Patients

Isolated tricuspid stenosis is a relatively rare phenomenon. If it does occur, percutaneous valvotomy is an alternative to surgical therapy. If tricuspid stenosis is found in association with mitral stenosis, both lesions can be treated by percutaneous balloon valvotomy. On the other hand, if there is associated regurgitant valvular disease that requires surgery of the mitral, aortic, or tricuspid valve, balloon valvotomy is probably not indicated, since the tricuspid valve can be repaired surgically at operation.

Results

Since there has been relatively little experience with tricuspid valvotomy using balloon techniques, results are still preliminary. The experience from Saudi Arabia has shown a mean decrease in tricuspid valve gradient from 6 ± 1 to 1.8 ± 0.06 mmHg ($p < 0.01$). There was no increase in the degree of tricuspid regurgitation produced by balloon valvotomy. Tricuspid valve area increased from 0.75 ± 1 to 1.8 ± 0.6 cm^2 ($p < 0.05$). As with percutaneous mitral valvotomy, cardiac output rises after relief of tricuspid stenosis by approximately 1 L/min.

REFERENCES

1. Lock JE, Khalilullah N, Shrivasta S, Bahl V, Keane JF: Percutaneous catheter commissurotomy in rheumatic mitral stenosis. *N Engl J Med* 1985; 313:1515–1518.
2. Palacios I, Block PC, Brandi S, Blanco P, Casal H, Pulido JI, et al: Percutaneous balloon valvotomy for patients with severe mitral stenosis. *Circulation* 1987; 75:778–784.
3. Al Zaibag M, Ribeiro PA, Al Kassab SA, Al-Fagig MR: Percutaneous double-balloon mitral valvotomy for rheumatic mitral stenosis. *Lancet* 1986; 1:757–761.
4. Vahanian A, Michel PL, Cormier B, Vitoux B, Michel X, Enriquez M, et al: Results of percutaneous mitral commissurotomy in 200 patients. *Am J Cardiol* 1989; 63:847–852.
5. Babic UU, Pejcic P, Dgurisiz Z, Vucinic M, Grujicic SM: Percutaneous transarterial balloon valvuloplasty for mitral valve stenosis. *Am J Cardiol* 1986; 57:1101–1104.
6. Ribeiro PA, Fawzy ME, Arafat MA, Dunn B, Sriram R, Mercer E, et al: Comparison of mitral valve area results of balloon mitral valvotomy using the Inoue and double-balloon techniques. *Am J Cardiol* 1991; 68:687–688.
7. Shim WH, Jang YS, Cho SY, Chung N, Kim SS, Lee WK: Comparison of outcome among double, bifoil, and Inoue balloon techniques for percutaneous mitral valvuloplasty and severe mitral stenosis. (abstr.) *Circulation* 1990; 82(suppl 3):498.
8. McKay CR, Otto C, Block P, Bonan R, Mickel M, David K, et al: Immediate results of mitral balloon commissurotomy in 737 patients. *Circulation* 1990; 82(suppl 3):545.
9. McKay RG, Lock JE, Safian RD, Come PC, Diver DJ, Baim DS, et al: Balloon dilation of mitral stenosis in adult patients: Postmortem and percutaneous mitral valvuloplasty studies. *J Am Coll Cardiol* 1977; 9:723–731.
10. Rediker DE, Block PC, Abascal VM, Palacios IF: Mitral balloon valvuloplasty for mitral stenosis after surgical commissurotomy. *J Am Coll Cardiol* 1988; 11:252–256.
11. Palacios IF, Lock JE, Keane JF, Block PC: Percutaneous transvenous balloon valvotomy in patient with severe calcific mitral stenosis. *J Am Coll Cardiol* 1986; 7:1416–1419.
12. Inoue K, Owaki T, Nakamura T, Kitamura F, Miyamota N: Clinical application of transvenous mitral commissurotomy by a new balloon catheter. *J Thorac Cardiovasc Surg* 1984; 87:394–402.
13. Al Zaibag M, Ribeiro PA, Al Kasab S, Al-Fagih MR: Percutaneous double-balloon mitral valvotomy for rheumatic mitral valve stenosis. *Lancet*: 1986; 1:757–761.
14. McKay CR, Kawanishi DT, Rahimtoola SH: Catheter balloon valvuloplasty of the mitral valve in adults using a double-balloon technique. *JAMA* 1987; 1753–1761.
15. Hoeksema TD, Wallace RB, Kirklin JW: Closed mitral commissurotomy: Recent results in 291 cases. *Am J Cardiol* 1966; 17:825–828.
16. Scannel JG, Burke JF, Saidi F, Turner JD: Five-year follow-up study of closed mitral valvulotomy. *J Thorac Cardiovasc Surg* 1960; 40:723–727.
17. Nathaniels EK, Moncoure AC, Scannel JG: A 15 year follow-up study of closed mitral valvuloplasty. *Ann Thorac Surg* 1970; 10:27–36.
18. Grantham RN, Daggett WM, Cosimi AB, Buckley MJ, Mundth ED, McEnany T, et al: Transventricular mitral valvotomy: Analysis of factors influencing operative and late results. *Circulation* 1974; 50(suppl 2):200–212.
19. Herrmann HC, Wilkins GT, Abascal VM, Weyman AE, Block PC, Palacios IF: Percutaneous balloon mitral valvotomy for patients with mitral stenosis: Analysis of factors influencing early results. *J Thorac Cardiovasc Surg* 1988; 96:33–38.
20. Block PC: Who is suitable for percutaneous balloon mitral valvotomy? (editorial). *Int J Cardiol* 1988; 20:9–16.
21. Block PC, Palacios IF: Pulmonary vascular dynamics after percutaneous mitral valvotomy. *J Thorac Cardiovasc Surg* 1988; 96:39–43.
22. Block PC, Palacios LF, Block EH, Tuzcu EM, Griffin B: Late (two-year) follow-up after percutaneous balloon mitral valvotomy. Am J Cardiol 1992; 69:537–541.
23. Housman LB, Bonchek L, Labert L, Grunkemeier G, Starr A: Prognosis of patients after open mitral commisurotomy: Actuarial analysis of late results in 100 patients. *J Thorac Cardiovasc Surg* 1977; 73:742–745.
24. Smith WM, Neutze JM, Barrat-Boyes BG, Lowe JB: Open mitral valvotomy: Effect of preoperative factors on result. *J Thorac Cardiovasc Surg* 1981; 82:738–751.
25. Laschinger JC, Cunningham JN, Baumann FG, Isom OW, Catinella FP, Mendelshon A, et al: Early open radical commisurotomy: Surgical treatment of choice for mitral stenosis. *Ann Thorac Surg* 1982; 34:287–298.
26. Abascal VM, Wilkins GT, Choong CY, Block PC, Palacios IF, Weyman AE: Mitral regurgitation after percutaneous balloon mitral valvuloplasty in adults: Evaluation by pulsed Doppler echocardiography. *J Am Coll Cardiol* 1988; 11:257–263.
27. Reid CL, Chandraratna PAN, Kawanishi DT, Kotlewski A, Rahirebilemtoola SH: Influence of mitral valve morphology on double-balloon catheter balloon valvuloplasty in patients with mitral stenosis: Analysis of factors predicting immediate and 3-month results. *Circulation* 1989; 80:515–524.
28. Block PC, Palacios IF, Jacobs M, Fallon JT: The mechanism of successful mitral valvotomy in humans. *Am J Cardiol* 1987; 59:178–179.
29. Rediker DE, Guerrero JL, Block DS, Southern JF, Fallon JT, Block PC: Limits of mitral valve apparatus distensibility: Observations from balloon mitral valvotomy in a canine model. *Am Heart J* 1987; 114:1513–1515.
30. Petrossian GA, Tuzcu EM, Ziskind AA, Block PC, Palacios IF: Atrial septal occlusion improves the accuracy of mitral valve area determination following percutaneous mitral balloon valvotomy. *Cath Cardiovasc Diag* 1991; 22:21–24.
31. Cribier A, Savin T, Berland J, Rocha P, Mechmeche R, Saoudi N, et al: Percutaneous balloon valvuloplasty of adult aortic stenosis: Report of 92 cases. *J Am Coll Cardiol* 1987; 9:381–386.
32. McKay RG, Safian RD, Lock JE, Mandell VS, Thurer RL, Schmitt SJ: Balloon dilatation of calcific aortic stenosis in elderly patients: Postmortem, perioperative, and percutaneous valvuloplasty studies. *Circulation* 1986; 74:119–125.
33. Cribier A, Savin T, Saoudi N, Rocha P, Berland J, Letac B: Percutaneous transluminal valvuloplasty of acquired aortic stenosis in

elderly patients: An alternative to valve replacement? *Lancet:* 1986; 1:63–67.
34. Block PC, Palacios IF: Comparison of hemodynamic results from anterograde versus retrograde percutaneous balloon aortic valvuloplasty. *Am J Cardiol* 1987; 60:659–662.
35. Isner JM, Salem DW, Desmoyers MR: Treatment of calcific aortic stenosis by balloon valvuloplasty. *Am J Cardiol* 1987; 59:313–317.
36. Robicsek F, Harbold NB: Limited value of balloon dilatation in calcified aortic stenosis in adults: Direct observations during open heart surgery. *Am J Cardiol* 1987; 60:857–864.
37. Schneider JF, Wilson M, Gallant TE: Percutaneous balloon aortic valvuloplasty for aortic stenosis in elderly patients at high risk for surgery. *Ann Intern Med* 1987; 106:696–700.
38. McKay RG, Safian RD, Lock JE, Diver DJ, Berman AD: Assessment of left ventricular and aortic valve function after aortic balloon valvuloplasty in adult patients with critical aortic stenosis. *Circulation* 1987; 75:192–203.
39. Davidson CJ, Harrison KJ, Pieper KS, Kisslo K, Harding MJ, Bashore TM: Balloon aortic valvuloplasty: What constitutes a successful one year outcome? (abstr.) *Circulation* 1990; 82(suppl 3):80.
40. Safian RD, Mandell VS, Thurer RE: Postmortem and intraoperative balloon valvuloplasty of calcific aortic stenosis in elderly patients. *J Am Coll Cardiol* 1987; 9:655–660.
41. Safian RD, Mandell VS, Thurer RE: Postmortem and intraoperative balloon valvuloplasty of calcific aortic stenosis in elderly patients: Mechanisms of successful dilatation. *J Am Coll Cardiol* 1987; 9:655–660.
42. Personal communication.
43. O'Keefe JH Jr, Vlietstra RE, Bailey KR, Holmes DR Jr: Natural history of candidates for balloon aortic valvuloplasty. *Mayo Clin Proc* 1987; 62:986–991.
44. Kan JS, White RI, Mitchell SE, Anderson JH, Gardner TJ: Percutaneous transluminal balloon valvuloplasty for pulmonary valve stenosis. *Circulation* 1984; 69:554–560.
45. Mullins CE, Nihill MR, Vick GW, Ludomirsky A: Double balloon technique for dilation of valvular or vessel stenosis in congenital and acquired heart disease. *J Am Coll Cardiol* 1987; 10:107–114.
46. Ali Khan MA, Yousef SA, Mullins CE: Percutaneous transluminal balloon pulmonary valvuloplasty for the relief of pulmonary valve stenosis with special reference to double-balloon technique. *Am Heart J* 1986; 112:158–166.
47. Radtke W, Keane JF, Fellows KE, Lang P, Lock JE: Percutaneous balloon valvotomy of congenital pulmonary stenosis using oversized balloons. *J Am Coll Cardiol* 1986; 4:909–915.
48. Walls JT, Lababidi Z, Curtis JJ: Operative balloon pulmonary valvuloplasty. *J Thorac Cardiovasc Surg* 1987; 93:792–793.
49. Locke JE, Keane JF, Fellows KE: The use of catheter invention procedures for congenital heart disease. *J Am Coll Cardiol* 1986; 7:1420–1423.
50. Rao PS, Fauzi ME, Solymar L, Marchini MK: Long-term results of balloon pulmonary valvuloplasty of valvar pulmonary stenosis. *Am Heart J* 1988; 115:1291–1296.
51. Rothman A, Locke J: Percutaneous balloon valvotomy in pediatric congenital and acquired heart disease: *Cardiac Surgery, State of the Art Reviews* 1991; 5(2):197–219.
52. Rao PS: Balloon pulmonary valvuloplasty: A review. *Clin Cardiol* 1989; 12:55–74.
53. Walls JT, Lababidi Z, Curtis JJ: Morphologic effects of percutaneous balloon pulmonary valvuloplasty. *South Med J* 1987; 80:475–478.
54. Burrows PE, Benson LN, Moes CAF, Freedom R: Pulmonary artery tears following balloon valvotomy for pulmonary stenosis. *Cardiovasc Intervent Radiol* 1989; 12:38–42.
55. Rey C, Morache P, Francart C, Dupuys C: Percutaneous transluminal balloon valvuloplasty of congenital pulmonary valve stenosis, with a special report on infants and neonates. *J Am Coll Cardiol* 1988; 11:815–820.
56. Lo RNS, Lau KC, Leung MP: Complete heart block after balloon dilatation for congenital pulmonary stenosis. *Br Heart J* 1988; 59:384–386.
57. Al Zaibag M, Ribeiro P, Kasab SA: Percutaneous balloon valvotomy in tricuspid stenosis. *Br Heart J* 1987; 57:51–53.
58. Goldenberg IF, Pedersen W, Olson J, Madison JD, Mooney MR, Gobel FL: Percutaneous double balloon valvuloplasty for severe tricuspid stenosis. *Am Heart J* 1989; 118:417–419.
59. Khalilullah M, Tyagi S, Yadav BS, Jain P, Choudhry A, Lochan R: Double-balloon valvuloplasty of tricuspid stenosis. *Am Heart J* 1987; 114:1232–1233.

PART X

Myocardial, Pericardial and Endocardial Disease

Chapter 87

Classification of Cardiomyopathy

Jay W. Mason, M.D.

Despite controversy in classifying the cardiomyopathies, there is general agreement on the definition. *Cardiomyopathy* is a primary disorder of the heart muscle that causes abnormal myocardial performance and is not the result of disease or dysfunction of other cardiac structures. Thus, the term cardiomyopathy excludes cases of myocardial failure due to myocardial infarction (so-called ischemic cardiomyopathy, a misnomer), systemic arterial hypertension, and valvular stenosis or regurgitation. Although cardiomyopathy is easily defined, classification of its various forms is difficult. This difficulty results because the great majority of cases of cardiomyopathy are associated with generalized cardiac dilatation and ventricular systolic dysfunction, in which the etiology is unknown. Although there is evidence that many insults, deficiencies, and defects may result in this final common pathway known as congestive, idiopathic, or dilated cardiomyopathy, the cause in most cases is still unknown.

CLASSIFICATION SCIENCE

Physicians and biomedical scientists use classification schemes to draw relationships and distinctions between diseases. This process promotes understanding and aids recollection. Even disorders we know little about can be understood if appropriately placed in a class with other disorders we do know about.

The science of classification requires that all items within the domain being classified be included and that each item appear in only one class. Inability to make clear distinctions between biologic systems makes this latter requirement the most demanding. Classification must be based on those features of the individual units within the domain that are understood or recognizable and that permit a useful distinction between groups.

Thus, the classification of cardiomyopathies should be based on an extensive, current category of knowledge about heart muscle diseases and should be as useful as possible to physicians and scientists.

CATEGORIES OF KNOWLEDGE ABOUT CARDIOMYOPATHIES

Our knowledge about cardiomyopathies falls into several categories: Etiology, gross anatomy, histology, genetics, biochemistry, immunology, hemodynamic function, prognosis, treatment, and others. No single classification scheme can utilize all of these areas of knowledge because there is so much overlap between them.[1]

The best classifications use a single category of knowledge with which to separate items in the domain. On the other hand, the most useful knowledge category differs among users of the classification. A histological classification will be useful to the pathologist, while a functional categorization is more valuable to the treating physician. If only one classification is to be used by both clinicians and scientists, etiologic categorization seems to be most successful. It must be recognized, however, that no single classification can serve all users and all purposes.

Several commonly employed classifications of cardiomyopathy are discussed below. For clarity, the primary categories of each classification are displayed in the accompanying tables (87-1 to 87-6), but only a few representative diseases are mentioned within each category.

The one exception is the etiologic classification (Table 87-3), in which a more nearly complete listing is provided.

THE WORLD HEALTH ORGANIZATION CLASSIFICATION

The only currently used classification of cardiomyopathy that was developed by consensus is that of the World Health Organization (WHO) and the International Society and Federation of Cardiology.[2] This scheme is outlined in Table 87-1. Because it was developed by a panel of experts and has the implied backing of the WHO, it is widely recognized and frequently used. Although it has been in existence since 1980, it has not gained general acceptance.

The 1980 WHO committee reserved the term cardiomyopathy for myocardial disease of *unknown* cause. This somewhat restricted usage has not been adopted widely and is not fully adhered to in this text. The more common usage includes all forms of heart disease in which the myocardium is *primarily* involved, as defined at the start of this chapter, but excluding valvular heart disease, systemic arterial hypertension, and coronary atherosclerosis.

Examination of the 1980 WHO classification reveals that it is, in fact, a somewhat awkward scheme that employs two separate categorizations in series, one based primarily on left ventricular cavitary morphology and the other based on etiology. The WHO classification does deal realistically with the fact that we know so little about the etiology of most cardiomyopathies. Its disadvantage is that diseases are placed in two schema that overlap.

FUNCTIONAL CLASSIFICATION OF CARDIOMYOPATHY

The most widely used functional classification of cardiomyopathy recognizes three disturbances of function: dilatation, hypertrophy, and restriction (Table 87-2). Dilatation is dominated by left ventricular cavity enlargement and systolic failure. Hypertrophy includes both obstructive and nonobstructive forms. Restriction is characterized by inadequate compliance causing restriction of diastolic filling. The value of this scheme is that virtually all cardiomyopathies are readily placed in one of the three categories and the therapeutic approaches to each category are distinctly different. For example, left ventricular afterload reduction is a cornerstone of therapy for dilated cardiomyopathies with systolic failure but of little benefit in the restrictive forms.

TABLE 87-1

World Health Organization Classification of Cardiomyopathy

I. Cardiomyopathy of unknown cause
  - Dilated cardiomyopathy
  - Hypertrophic cardiomyopathy
  - Restrictive cardiomyopathy
  - Unclassified cardiomyopathy

II. Specific heart muscle disease
  - Infective
  - Metabolic
  - General systems diseases
  - Heredofamilial
  - Sensitivity and toxic reactions

From a report of the WHO/ISFC task force.[2] This is a listing of major categories only; specific disorders are not listed.

TABLE 87-2

Functional Classification of Cardiomyopathy

I. Cardiac dilatation
  - A. With systolic failure
    - Idiopathic dilated cardiomyopathy
    - Late cardiac amyloidosis
  - B. Without systolic failure
    - High cardiac output state
    - Tachycardia-induced congestive failure

II. Cardiac hypertrophy
  - A. With obstruction
    - Hypertrophic obstructive cardiomyopathy
  - B. Without obstruction
    - Hypertrophic cardiomyopathy
    - Left ventricular hypertrophy due to systemic hypertension

III. Cardiac restriction
  - Early cardiac amyloidosis
  - Endomyocardial fibrosis

This is a complete listing of primary categories, but only a few specific examples are provided for illustration.

There are, however, some shortcomings of the functional classification. Many diseases are physiologically heterogeneous. Almost all hypertrophic conditions have an element of diastolic restriction. Most dilated ventricles display myocyte hypertrophy. Some diseases change from one category to another during their course; the best example is cardiac amyloidosis, which initially exhibits diastolic stiffness, with complete preservation of systolic performance, followed years later by dilatation and systolic failure.

The functional scheme also associates diseases that have vastly different causes, some of which require special therapeutic interventions. For example, the primary therapy for cardiac hemochromatosis, often an initially restrictive disease, is removal of excessive iron stores; this would not, of course, be effective treatment for any coclassified diseases. Despite its shortcomings, the functional classification of cardiomyopathy remains the most popular among clinicians because it is based on easily understood physiology and is relevant to therapy.

ETIOLOGIC CLASSIFICATION

This scheme utilizes our knowledge about cardiomyopathies more extensively than all the others. It has the most primary categories as a result of the fact that there are numerous known causes that are not interrelated. The table included here (Table 87-3) categorizes the diseases covered in Chaps. 24, 88 to 91, 96, 101 to 108, 110, 111, and 113. The general outline established by the WHO is followed roughly. In many cases the etiologic agent is poorly understood (e.g., uremic "cardiomyopathy") or the cardiomyopathy is associated with another

TABLE 87-3

Etiologic Classification of Cardiomyopathy

I. Infective/inflammatory
  Idiopathic lymphocytic myocarditis
  Peripartum myocarditis
  Eosinophilic myocarditis
  Giant-cell myocarditis
  Viral myocarditis
  Rickettsial myocarditis
  Bacterial myocarditis
  Mycobacterial heart disease
  Spirochetal heart disease
  Fungal myocarditis
  Protozoal myocarditis
  Metazoal myocarditis
II. Metabolic
  A. Endocrine
    1. Thyroid disease
      Thyrotoxicosis
      Hypothyroidism
    2. Pheochromocytoma
    3. Acromegaly
    4. Diabetes mellitus
    5. Carcinoid heart disease
  B. Uremia
  C. Hyperoxaluria
  D. Gout
  E. Storage diseases and infiltrative processes
    1. Lysosomal storage diseases
      GM1 gangliosidosis
      Tay-Sachs disease and variants
      Sandhoff's disease
      Niemann-Pick disease
      Gaucher's disease
      Fabry's disease
      Farber's disease
      Fucosidosis
      Hurler's syndrome
      Scheie's syndrome
      Hunter's syndrome
      Sanfilippo
      Morquio
      Moroteaux-Lamy
    2. Glycogen storage diseases
      Pompe's disease
      Cori's disease
      Andersen's disease
      Dominantly inherited cardioskeletal myopathy with lysosomal glycogen storage and normal acid maltase levels
    3. Refsum's syndrome
    4. Hand-Schuller-Christian
    5. Adipositos cordis
    6. Hemochromatosis

TABLE 87-3

Etiologic Classification of Cardiomyopathy *(continued)*

  F. Deficiencies
    1. Electrolyte
      Hypocalcemia
      Hypophosphatemia
    2. Nutritional
      Kwashiorkor
      Beriberi
      Pellagra
      Scurvy
      Selenium
      Carnitine
III. Amyloid
  AL (primary amyloid, myeloma-associated amyloid)
  AA (secondary amyloid, familial Mediterranean fever–associated amyloid)
  AF (familial amyloid)
  SSA (senile cardiac amyloid, senile systemic amyloid)
  IAA (atrial amyloid)
IV. General system disorders
  A. Collagen vascular (connective tissue)
    Systemic lupus erythematosus
    Polyarteritis nodosa
    Rheumatoid arthritis
    Scleroderma
    Dermatomyositis
    Whipple's disease
    Kawasaki's disease
  B. Sarcoidosis
  C. Neoplastic
V. Muscular dystrophies, myopathies, and neuromuscular disorders
  A. Muscular dystrophies
    Duchenne muscular dystrophy
    Becker's muscular dystrophy
    Myotonic dystrophy
    Facioscapulohumeral muscular dystrophy
    Limb girdle dystrophy
    Scapuloperoneal dystrophy, including Emery-Driefuss
    Congenital muscular dystrophy
    Distal muscular dystrophy
  B. Congenital myopathies
    Central-core disease
    Nemaline myopathy
    Myotubular myopathy (centronuclear)
    Congenital fiber-type disproportion
  C. Mitochondrial myopathies, including Kearns-Sayre syndrome
  D. Neuromuscular disorders, Fredreich's ataxia
VI. Toxicity, hypersensitivity, and physical agent effects
  A. Toxic effects
    1. Caused by drugs, heavy metals, and chemical agents
      Alcohol (ethyl)
      Amphetamine/methamphetamine
      Anthracyclines
      Antidepressants
      Antimony
      Arsenic

TABLE 87-3
Etiologic Classification of Cardiomyopathy *(continued)*

Arsine gas
Carbon monoxide
Catecholamines
Chloroquine
Cobalt
Cocaine
Cyclophosphamide
Emetine
5-Fluorouracil
Hydrocarbons
Interferon
Lead
Lithium
Mercury
Methysergide
Paracetamol
Phenothiazines
Phosphorus
Reserpine
2. Caused by scorpions, spiders, arthropods, and snakes
Scorpions
Arthropods
Black widow spider
Snakes

B. Hypersensitivity reactions
Acetazolamide
Amitriptyline
Amphotericin B
Ampicillin
Carbamazepine
Chlorthalidone
Hydrochlorothiazide
Indomethacin
Isoniazid
Methyldopa
Oxyphenbutazone
para-Aminosalicylic acid
Penicillin
phenindione
Phenylbutazone
Phenytoin
Streptomycin
Sulfadiazine
Sulfisoxazole
Sulfonylureas
Tetracycline

C. Physical agents
Heat
Hypothermia
Radiation

VII. Miscellaneous
Peripartum heart disease
Tachycardia-induced cardiomyopathy
Ectodermal dysplasia-associated cardiomyopathy
Idiopathic endocardial fibrosis
Endocardial fibroelastosis
Infantile cardiomyopathy

This is an essentially complete listing of cardiomyopathies of known cause.

disease, but the mechanism responsible for heart failure is not known (e.g., cardiomyopathy of systemic neoplasia).

While this classification has the advantage of being inclusive, it has the disadvantage of being awkwardly long. It has 7 primary and 40 secondary categories. In addition, most coclassified disorders are anatomically, physiologically, and therapeutically unrelated. Thus, this classification is not used routinely by clinicians. It has been used most frequently as an organizational scheme in textbooks and reviews concerning heart muscle disease and cardiomyopathy.

ENDOMYOCARDIAL BIOPSY CLASSIFICATION

Because the heart can be safely biopsied, antemortem histological diagnosis can be used to classify cardiomy-

TABLE 87-4
Endomyocardial Biopsy Histology Classification of Cardiomyopathy

I. Inflammatory/immune cardiomyopathy
Lymphocytic myocarditis
Rheumatic carditis
Sarcoidosis
Giant-cell myocarditis
Cardiac allograft rejection
Chagas' cardiomyopathy
Hypersensitivity myocarditis

II. Infectious cardiomyopathy
Toxoplasmosis
Lyme carditis
Cytomegalovirus

III. Infiltrative cardiomyopathy
Glycogen storage
Hemochromatosis
Right ventricular lipomatosis
Amyloidosis

IV. Cardiac tumors
Cardiac origin
Noncardiac origin

V. Miscellaneous specific cardiomyopathies
Anthracycline cardiotoxicity
Endocardial fibrosis
Endocardial fibroelastosis
Fabry's disease
Carcinoid disease
Irradiation injury
Kearns-Sayre syndrome
Henoch-Schonlein purpura
Chloroquine cardiomyopathy
Carnitine deficiency
Hypereosinophilic syndrome

VI. Nonspecific abnormalities
Idiopathic dilated cardiomyopathy
Other cardiomyopathies of unknown cause

VII. No histological abnormality

This represents a relatively complete listing of diagnoses that have been made by endomyocardial biopsy and reported in the literature.

TABLE 87-5
Reported Analyses of Endomyocardial Biopsy Tissue

Histology	Mitochondrial deoxyribonucleic acid deletion analysis
Electron microscopy	Beta-receptor quantitation
Quantitative morphometry	Adenine nucleotide/metabolite quantitation
Immunofluorescence	Adenylate cyclase activity
Immunohistochemistry	Norepinephrine content
Sarcoplasmic reticulum function analysis	Metabolic pathway activities
Lymphocyte subtyping with monoclonal antibodies	Enzyme activities
Major histocompatibility complex antigen detection with monoclonal antibodies	Culture of lymphocytes
Actin, myosin, and other polypeptide quantitation	Messenger ribonucleic acid quantitation
Isolation of single myocardial cells	Culture for organisms
Viral genome detection using in vitro hybridization and polymerase chain reaction	

opathies. Dozens of specific myocardial diseases can be detected by biopsy (Table 87-4). The great strength of histological diagnosis is that it is definitive and unequivocal when a specific disease is observed. On the other hand, numerous deficiencies make this method of classification relatively restricted in use. The foremost problem is that although the number of specific histological diagnoses is large, they represent a small proportion of all cases—certainly less than 15 percent. The histology in most patients with cardiomyopathy is nonspecific and nondiagnostic. Hypertrophy, or fiber attenuation, and fibrosis may be seen in varying degrees in almost any disorder and are the only findings in most cases of idiopathic dilated cardiomyopathy and hypertrophic cardiomyopathy (as well as in many instances of heart failure due to myocardial infarction and valvular dysfunction). Furthermore, completely normal histology may occasionally be seen on biopsy in cases of severe dilatation and systolic failure.

Myocardial biopsy samples can be subjected to several additional analytic techniques (Table 87-5). These techniques expand the potential for classification using endomyocardial biopsy. While at present these analyses are only investigational and none can be generally applied, it is likely that one or more of them will become clinically useful in the future and could form the basis of a classification with wide appeal.

TABLE 87-6
Therapeutic Classification of Cardiomyopathy

I. Reduce ventricular afterload
   - Idiopathic dilated cardiomyopathy
   - Late cardiac amyloidosis

II. Reduce ventricular preload
   - Endocardial fibrosis
   - Early cardiac amyloidosis

III. Increase ventricular compliance
   - Hypertrophic cardiomyopathy

IV. Relieve ventricular outflow obstruction
   - Hypertrophic obstructive cardiomyopathy

V. Improve cardiac rhythm
   - Cardiomyopathy of persistent tachycardia

VI. Specific therapy
   - A. Replace deficiency
     - Carnitine deficiency cardiomyopathy
   - B. Remove toxic agent
     - Hemochromatosis
     - Hypersensitivity
   - C. Immunosuppression
     - Giant-cell myocarditis
     - Lymphocytic myocarditis (?)
   - D. Correct systemic disease
     - Uremic cardiomyopathy
     - Cardiomyopathy of cancer
     - Systemic lupus erythematosus

This is a complete listing of primary categories with a few specific examples for illustration.

THERAPEUTIC CLASSIFICATION

A classification based on specific therapies borrows heavily from the functional and the etiologic classifications of cardiomyopathy. This classification adds information regarding treatment that is not available in other schemes and therefore may be useful to clinicians.

Nevertheless, this classification has several shortcomings. First, often more than one class of therapy is appropriate for a disease. Therefore, the classification must categorize diseases on the basis of their primary therapy. This introduces some instability to the classification, since therapeutic preferences are subject to variance in opinion and to change with new research. The greatest fault of therapeutic categorization is that when new therapies are introduced, the existing classification becomes obsolete. The therapeutic classification shown in Table 87-6 illustrates the sensitivity of this approach to opinion. Some might argue, for example, that diuretic therapy remains the primary treatment for dilated cardiomyopathy.

Note that some commonly employed therapies, such as inotropic agents and cardiac transplantation, do not appear in Table 87-6 because they are often not the initial or primary therapies.

SUMMARY

No single classification of cardiomyopathy is generally accepted within the biomedical community. An attempt to gain a consensus for one of the many classifications in current use is not likely to succeed because we are unable to subdivide meaningfully cases of idiopathic dilated cardiomyopathy, which constitute the large majority of all cases. At present, it seems best for the individual health practitioner or scientist to use the classification scheme that best serves his or her purpose. For clinicians, often this will be the functional classification.

In the future a widely acceptable classification may develop that is based on the molecular genetics of myocardial disease. Although this field is only beginning to develop, it is the discipline most likely to contribute to our understanding of causes and our development of new treatments for myocardial disease.

REFERENCES

1. Abelmann WH: Classification and natural history of primary myocardial disease. *Prog Cardiovasc Dis* 1984; 27:73–94.
2. Report of the WHO/ISFC task force on the definition and classification of cardiomyopathies. *Br Heart J* 1980; 44:672–673.

Chapter 88

Myocarditis and Specific Myocardial Diseases

John B. O'Connell, M.D. ■ *Dale G. Renlund, M.D.*

Specific myocardial diseases (also known as secondary cardiomyopathies; see Chap. 87 and Table 87-3) are heart muscle disorders in which either the etiology is known or the myocardial dysfunction is associated with disorders of other systems. Excluded from consideration are heart disorders caused by systemic or pulmonary hypertension, coronary artery disease, valvular heart disease, and congenital cardiac anomalies. The specific heart muscle diseases nonetheless represent a fascinating array of diseases with widely divergent pathogenetic mechanisms. While more than 70 specific heart muscle diseases have been described, when considered as a group, they are infrequent, and when considered individually, they are rare.

MYOCARDITIS

Since myocarditis was initially defined by autopsy as any inflammation or degeneration of the heart,[1] unexplained heart diseases were commonly mistaken as myocarditis in the nineteenth and early twentieth centuries. While a relationship between infection and chronic heart disease (diphtheria) was postulated as early as 1806, the diagnosis of myocarditis could not be established during life because of lack of precise diagnostic tools until the 1970s. Even though the use of endomyocardial biopsy in patients with symptomatic heart disease of unknown etiology has provided greater insights into the pathogenesis, etiology, and treatment of myocarditis (Chap. 33), the majority of patients with active myocarditis will likely remain unsuspected because the cardiac dysfunction is subclinical, asymptomatic, and self-limited.

Etiology

Multiple infectious agents have been associated with myocarditis.[2–34] (See Table 88-1.) The most commonly identified cause of myocarditis is Coxsackie B virus infection. Neutralizing antibody against two serotypes of Coxsackie B virus was detected in 86 percent of sera from normal adults,[35] indicating that most adults have been infected by cardiotropic viruses. Electrocardiographic abnormalities were identified in 9 to 13 percent of those with symptoms due to influenza infection of sufficient severity to require attention by a physician during two separate epidemics.[36,37] Histologic evidence of myocarditis following traumatic death was identified in 1 to 3 percent of autopsies,[38,39] suggesting that the frequency of myocarditis is underestimated by analyzing data only from symptomatic patients.

Pathogenesis

The association of cardiac disease with infection by cardiotropic viruses prompted the hypothesis that the viral infection was responsible for the myocardial injury. Corvisart, as early as 1806, noted that a smoldering inflammatory process could result in progressive abnormalities in cardiac function after all evidence of the infective agent had disappeared.[40] Woodroff[41] noted that histo-

TABLE 88-1
Important Causes of Myocarditis

I. Infection
  A. Viral
    Coxsackie (A, B)
    ECHO
    Influenza (A, B)
    Polio
    Herpes simplex
    Varicella-zoster virus
    Epstein-Barr virus
    Cytomegalovirus
    Mumps
    Rubella
    Rubeola
    Vaccinia
    Coronavirus
    Rabies
    Hepatitis B
    Arbovirus
    Junin virus
    Human immunodeficiency virus
  B. Bacterial, rickettsial, spirochetal
    Corynebacterium diphtheriae
    Salmonella typhi
    Beta-hemolytic streptococci
    Neisseria meningitidis
    Legionella pneumophila
    Listeria monocytogenes
    Campylobacter jejuni
    Coxiella burnetii (Q fever)
    Chlamydia trachomatis
    Mycoplasma pneumoniae
    Chlamydia psittaci (psittacosis)
    Rickettsia rickettsii (Rocky Mountain spotted fever)
    Borrelia burgdorferi (Lyme disease)
    Mycobacterium tuberculosis
  C. Protozoal
    Trypanosoma cruzi (Chagas' disease)
    Toxoplasma gondii
  D. Metazoal
    Trichinosis
    Echinococcosis
  E. Fungal
    Aspergillosis
    Blastomycosis
    Candidiasis
    Coccidioidomycosis
    Cryptococcosis
    Histoplasmosis
    Mucormycosis
II. Toxic
  Anthracyclines
  Catecholamines
  Interleukin-2
  $Alpha_2$ interferon
III. Hypersensitivity

logic evidence of cardiac injury in Coxsackie B virus–induced murine myocarditis only developed after virus was no longer detected in the myocardium. Furthermore, elimination of T-cell-mediated immune responses by antithymocyte serum or bone marrow irradiation with reconstitution following viral clearance attenuated inflammation with improved survival, less cellular infiltrate, and less necrosis. These observations led to the proposal that infective agents induce adverse immunologic responses that persist despite the eradication of the infective agent.

The specific immune responses that lead to the myocardial injury are incompletely defined. When serial sections of murine myocardium following infection with Coxsackie B3 virus were analyzed, macrophages were present in the infiltrate until day 8.[42] After macrophage activity decreased, both effector (CD8) and helper (CD4) T cells were identified within myocardial lesions. At peak infiltration, some murine strains showed a predominance of CD8 positive cells while in others CD4 cells predominated, suggesting participation of both humoral- and cell-mediated immune responses.[43] In human subjects, T-lymphocyte and macrophage infiltration characterizes the immunohistochemical picture, whereas B lymphocytes and natural killer cells are absent.[44] T-lymphocyte subset analysis of human serum does not demonstrate consistency in dominance of CD4 or CD8 cells.

The mechanism of injury when lymphocytes infiltrate the myocardium is unknown. Cardiac function improves in most patients as myocarditis resolves histologically. Cytotoxic injury alone cannot explain these reversible abnormalities. In the murine model, messenger ribonucleic acid (m-RNA) of perforin, the pore-forming protein mediating cytotoxicity, was identified in cytoplasmic granules of infiltrating cells by in situ hybridization.[45] Biopsy samples from patients with active myocarditis contain perforin granules in infiltrating cells.[46] Interleukin-1 and other cytokines may cause reversible depression of myocardial contractility without resulting in cell death. Whole-mount preparations and beating heart cell cultures of cardiac myocytes verify reversible depression of cardiac function when these mediators are infused in physiological concentrations.[47] The effect of T-cell-mediated immune injury, therefore, may be either irreversible as a result of cell death through cytotoxicity (perforin) or reversible as a result of injury mediated by cytokines.

Observations before endomyocardial biopsy techniques were developed suggested that antiheart antibodies in serum are common but nonspecifically reflect myocardial damage.[48] The addition of vital adult cardiocytes as a target in vitro has improved the specificity by identification of antimyolemmal antibodies in heart muscle disease.[49] When serum from patients with myocarditis was screened for autoantibodies, high-titer immunoglobulin G (IgG) with cardiac specificity was detected in 59 percent of patients with myocarditis compared to none of the normal samples.[50] Antibodies with specificity for contractile and energy transport proteins have recently been identified. Cardiac myosin antibodies develop in select murine strains following Coxsackie B virus infection.[51] Injection of cardiac myosin alone in these strains without infection results in myocarditis that is histologically similar to that seen following Coxsackie B3 virus infection.[52] In sera from patients with active myocarditis, Western blotting demonstrated reactivity of the 190- to 199-kDa fraction, which includes antibody to the heavy chain of cardiac myosin.[50] Autoantibodies against the beta receptor with a strong association to human leukocyte antigen (HLA) DR4 and DR1 phenotype have been detected in patients with dilated cardiomyopathy.[53] Antibodies to the adenine nucleotide translocator and branch chain alpha ketoacid dehydrogenase have been identified.[54,55] Additionally, the anti–adenine nucleotide translocator protein antibody cross-reacts with calcium channel proteins in the plasma membrane of normal cardiac myocytes. By blocking the calcium channel and interrupting high-energy phosphate transport,[56] these autoantibodies may impair cardiac function, providing an attractive hypothesis to explain the reversibility of functional abnormalities following resolution of myocarditis.

The precise role of the virus is unclear. Attempts to culture virus from human myocardial tissue have been frustrating. Coxsackie virus has been identified in a myocardial biopsy specimen obtained during life in a single adult case report.[57] While the role of the virus had been deemphasized following the introduction of the immune injury hypothesis, the identification of viral genomic fragments in 18 to 50 percent of myocardial samples from patients with myocarditis and dilated cardiomyopathy by in situ hybridization and polymerase chain reaction has caused reassessment of the role of the virus.[58] The viral genome localization does not correlate with the intensity or the presence of the inflammatory infiltrate. These genomic fragments may not necessarily be capable of replicating as intact virus but may serve as a persistent source of antigen to drive the adverse immune responses.

While infection of the heart with cardiotropic virus is likely common, progressive cardiac disease is unusual. In addition to the tropism of the virus, host immune responses play an important role in determining the severity of the clinical disease. When quantitative peripheral T- and B-lymphocyte populations were analyzed in patients with dilated cardiomyopathy and myocarditis, no consistent changes were detected.[59,60] However, immunoregulatory assays demonstrate reduction in natural killer cell, antibody-dependent cellular cytotoxicity, and suppressor cell functions.[61,62] These immunoregulatory defects may predispose a host with a high antigenic load to develop immune responses that are not modulated by the natural inhibitory immunoregulatory mechanisms.

Clinical Manifestations

The clinical manifestations of myocarditis are variable and reflect abnormalities in left ventricular function, systolic or diastolic, and/or electrical activation with arrhythmias and heart block. In most instances, however, active myocarditis is clinically silent with neither symptoms nor physical findings to suggest the diagnosis.

The most obvious symptom suggesting myocarditis is an antecedent viral syndrome. Flulike symptoms occur in approximately 60 percent of patients with active myocarditis.[63] Chest pain may occur and be typically ischemic, somewhat atypical, or pericardial in character. Approximately 35 percent of patients with myocarditis and congestive heart failure will have chest discomfort.[63] Occasionally patients will present with a clinical syndrome identical to an acute myocardial infarction with left ventricular asynergy, electrocardiographic evidence of injury or Q waves, and ischemic cardiac pain.[64] In this syndrome at autopsy, the coronary arteries are widely patent, although viral coronary arteritis has been reported.[65,66] Coronary vasospasm has also been associated with acute myocarditis.[67] The clinical presentation in a large series of subjects with active myocarditis is summarized in Table 88-2.

Left ventricular dysfunction and a syndrome compatible with dilated cardiomyopathy identify a significant proportion of patients with active myocarditis.[68] These patients, who may or may not have an antecedent viral syndrome, have no clinical signs or symptoms specific for active myocarditis.

Patients may present with syncope or palpitations with atrioventricular (AV) block or ventricular arrhythmia. Myocarditis is a known cause of sudden death. In a 20-year review of sudden death among Air Force recruits, 20 percent had myocarditis documented at autopsy.[69]

Systemic or pulmonary thromboembolic disease is associated with myocarditis.[70,71] Myocarditis may be identified in multiple family members, and in one report a suppressor cell defect was detected predisposing to development of active myocarditis.[72] Patients with peripartum cardiomyopathy have a high frequency of myocarditis on endomyocardial biopsy.[73] The immunoregulatory changes during and following pregnancy may heighten susceptibility to viral myocarditis, and exposure to trophoblastic antigens may predispose to immune-mediated myocardial injury.

Laboratory Evaluation

Blood Studies

An elevated erythrocyte sedimentation rate occurs in 60 percent of patients with active myocarditis and an elevated white blood cell count in 25 percent.[63] While elevated titers to enteroviruses or other cardiotropic viruses

TABLE 88-2

Clinical Characteristics of Patients with Active Myocarditis ($n=111$)

Age	42 ± 14 years
Sex	62% male
Ejection fraction	0.24 ± 0.10
Chest pain	35%
Increased MB fraction of creatine kinase (MB-CK)	12%
Flulike symptoms	59%
Increased erythrocyte sedimentation rate (ESR)	61%
Elevated white blood cell count	24%
Fever	18%

SOURCE: From the Myocarditis Treatment Trial.[63]
NOTE: Data are expressed as mean ± SD.

may be present, a fourfold rise in IgG titer over a 4- to 6-week period is required to document acute infection. Elevated IgM antibody titer to enterovirus may denote an acute infection more specifically than a rise in IgG antibody titer. Unfortunately, a rise in antibody titer documents only the reaction to a recent viral infection and does not indicate active myocarditis.

Abnormalities in peripheral T- and B-lymphocyte counts have been reported. The T helper-suppressor ratio (CD4/CD8) may be abnormal in some patients with active myocarditis. Peripheral lymphocyte subpopulations vary and the abnormalities lack specificity. While functional abnormalities in antibody-dependent cytotoxicity, natural killer cells, and T-suppressor cells have been noted, these findings have not been consistent and cannot be used as diagnostic adjuncts. Heart-specific antibody may occur in peripheral blood with myocarditis but also occurs in many patients with dilated cardiomyopathy in the absence of myocarditis.

Creatine kinase MB release occurs in approximately 12 percent of patients.[63] Abnormalities in other cardiac enzymes such as serum aspartate transaminase and lactic dehydrogenase (LDH) may also be present, but superimposed mild viral hepatitis or myositis may cloud the interpretation of these abnormalities.[74] In patients with acute pericarditis, elevation of creatine kinase MB fraction may be helpful in suggesting myocardial involvement.

Cardiac Studies

Electrocardiogram The most common electrocardiographic abnormality is sinus tachycardia. The 12-lead electrocardiogram (ECG) may suggest myocarditis when diffuse ST-T-wave changes occur in the setting of a viral syndrome.[75] The possibility of a superimposed pericarditis complicates the interpretation of electrocardiographic abnormalities. Prolongation of the QTc interval and/or low voltage has been noted in patients with myocarditis compared to controls. A myocardial infarction pattern may occur in some patients (Fig. 88-1). Conduction delay is common,[76] and left bundle branch block is identified in at least 20 percent of patients. Complete AV block is also common, particularly in Japan, where acute myocarditis often presents with Stokes-Adams attacks from complete heart block. The complete heart block is generally transient and rarely requires a permanent pacemaker.[77]

Supraventricular arrhythmias are common, particularly when myocarditis presents with congestive heart failure or when pericardial inflammation is present. Ventricular arrhythmias may occur in all patients with active myocarditis.[78] While the frequency is unknown, sudden cardiac death occurs in myocarditis. The cause of death in most cases is unclear, but both complete heart block and ventricular tachycardia have been postulated. Patients with recurrent uncontrolled ventricular tachycardia in whom no other etiology has been identified may have myocarditis when careful diagnostic analysis is completed.

Echocardiography Echocardiography is a useful tool in managing patients with active myocarditis. Left ventricular systolic dysfunction is common in patients with congestive heart failure. Segmental wall motion abnormalities occur, and left ventricular asynergy simulating a myocardial infarction may be identified.[79] Left ventricular cavity size is typically normal to only mildly dilated. Wall thickness may be increased, particularly if the diagnosis is established early in the course of the disease and inflammation is fulminant.[80] Ventricular thrombi are detected in 15 percent of those studied.[81] Digital image analysis techniques may help differentiate the image texture alterations in active myocarditis from pure fibrosis.[82] These textural changes, however, are distinctly uncommon. Therefore, the echocardiographic findings in active myocarditis may mimic restrictive, hypertrophic or dilated cardiomyopathy and coronary artery disease. Following resolution of inflammation, these abnormalities may persist.

Cardiac Catheterization and Hemodynamic Analysis The left ventricular end-diastolic pressure may be elevated in association with depression of cardiac output. In some

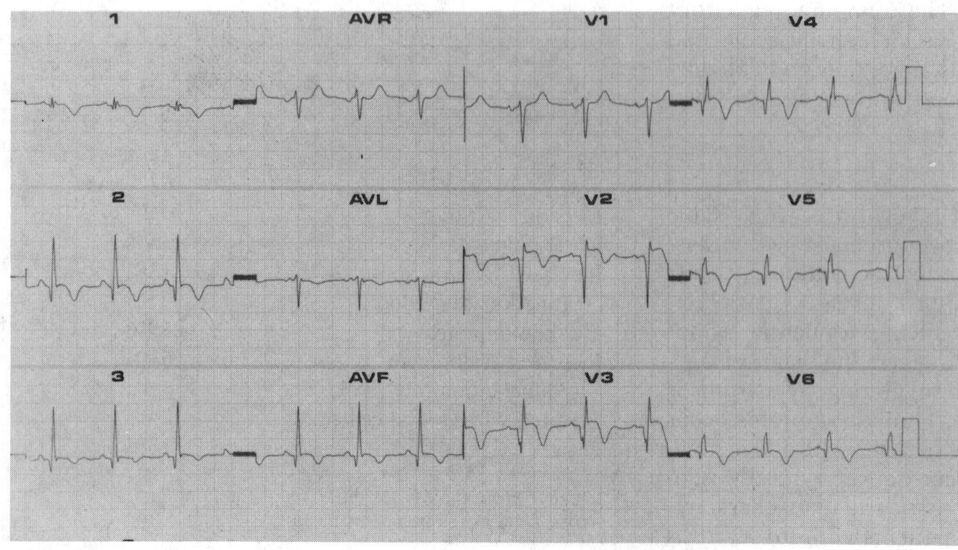

FIGURE 88-1 Twelve-lead ECG suggesting acute anterior myocardial infarction in a patient with active myocarditis (*From MR Costanzo-Nordin et al.*[64] *Reproduced with permission.*)

patients a restrictive hemodynamic pattern may occur early in the disease. Left ventriculographic studies confirm the segmental wall motion abnormalities detected on noninvasive analysis. Left ventricular angioscopy demonstrates white, light yellow, and reddish patches of the endocardium.[83] The angioscopy-guided biopsy is most apt to demonstrate the characteristic histologic change of active myocarditis in portions of the myocardium that appear red on visual analysis.

Endomyocardial Biopsy The development and refinement of percutaneous, intravascular endomyocardial biopsy techniques enable the repetitive sampling of the human myocardium during life with minimal discomfort and minor morbidity (Chap. 33).[68,84,85] Essentially two techniques are available to sample right ventricular myocardium involving access through the right internal jugular or femoral vein. Intravascular biopsy of the left ventricle may also be employed, but its potential morbidity limits its use. The right ventricular bioptome is positioned under fluoroscopy or echocardiography so that the interventricular septum is sampled.[86] A minimum of four to six fragments are obtained. Using the Stanford bioptome, typical samples are 2 to 3 mm in maximal diameter and 5 mg wet weight. Samples are processed, paraffin imbedded, sectioned, and stained with hematoxylin-eosin and trichrome (Fig. 88-2). Special stains are employed if other diagnoses are considered, such as amyloidosis (Chap. 33). The cardiac pathologist is careful to examine several levels of all fragments removed.

A number of investigators have applied endomyocardial biopsy to patients with unexplained congestive heart failure and/or ventricular arrhythmia.[68,87–117] As demonstrated in Table 88-3, the percentage of biopsies interpreted as myocarditis varies widely. A major reason for the variability is the different diagnostic criteria for active myocarditis. The number of lymphocytes necessary and the intensity of the infiltrate before the diagnosis is established are also a source of confusion. Leukocytic infiltrates are common in explanted hearts with dilated cardiomyopathy; i.e., more than 50 percent of these hearts have small foci not characteristic of myocarditis.[118] The variability of endomyocardial biopsy interpretation prompted a consensus panel of cardiac pathologists to propose a working standard, the *Dallas criteria*, to define *active* myocarditis as "an inflammatory infiltrate of the myocardium with necrosis and/or degeneration of adjacent myocytes not typical of the ischemic damage associated with coronary artery disease."[119] A sample is technically adequate only when four to six fragments are available for interpretation. "Borderline" myocarditis is applied when the inflammatory infiltrate is too sparse or myocyte injury is not demonstrated. Repeat biopsy is suggested. Dec et al.[120] demonstrated a high frequency (four of six) of active myocarditis confirmed by repeat biopsy in patients whose initial histologic samples demonstrated borderline myocarditis. Critics of this definition have expressed concern that the criteria are too

TABLE 88-3
Incidence of Biopsy-Proven Myocarditis

Investigators	Year	Patients Biopsied	Myocarditis (%)
Unexplained Congestive Heart Failure			
Mason et al.[68]	1980	400	2
Noda[87]	1980	52	1
Baandrup and Olsen[88]	1981	201	4
Das et al.[89]	1981	12	8
Nippoldt et al.[90]	1982	34	12
Fenoglio et al.[91]	1983	135	25
Unverferth et al.[92]	1983	42	9
Parillo et al.[93]	1984	74	26
Zee-Cheng et al.[94]	1984	35	63
O'Connell et al.[95]	1984	68	7
Daly et al.[96]	1984	69	17
Rose et al.[97]	1984	76	0
Regitz et al.[98]	1985	150	27
Dec et al.[99]	1985	27	67
Salvi et al.[100]	1985	74	18
Mortensen et al.[101]	1985	65	18
Hosenpud et al.[102]	1985	38	16
Cassling et al.[103]	1985	80	2
French et al.[104]	1986	25	0
Hammond et al.[105]	1987	52	19
Maisch et al.[106]	1988	123	8
Chow et al.[107]	1988	90	4
Leatherbury et al.[108]	1988	20	25
Hobbs et al.[109]	1989	148	21
Latham et al.[110]	1989	52	13
Popma et al.[111]	1989	61	13
Vasiljevic et al.[112]	1990	85	12
Lieberman et al.[113]	1991	348	10
Unexplained Ventricular Arrhythmias			
Strain et al.[114]	1983	18	17
Vignola et al.[115]	1984	12	50
Sugrue et al.[116]	1984	12	8
Hosenpud et al.[117]	1986	12	33

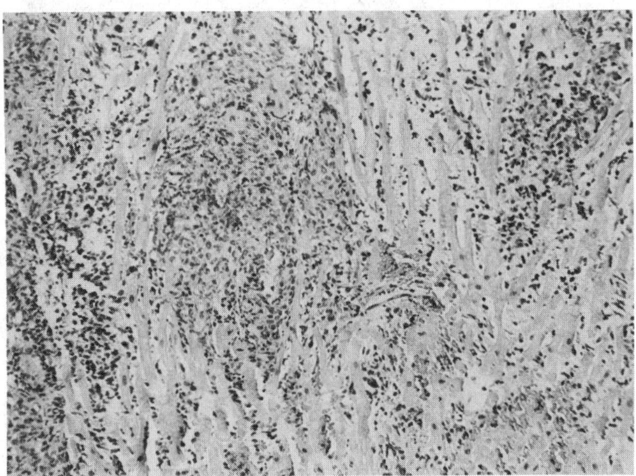

FIGURE 88-2 Photomicrograph showing the extensive lymphocytic infiltrates and myocyte necrosis of active myocarditis (H&E, ×20). (*From JB O'Connell, JW Mason: Immunosuppressive therapy in experimental and clinical myocarditis. Pathol Immunopathol Res 7:292–304, 1988. Reproduced with permission.*)

stringent and that myocyte necrosis is not necessary to establish the diagnosis.

Endomyocardial biopsy samples primarily the right side of the ventricular septum. Myocarditis may be focal or patchy. In cardiac allograft rejection, sampling error is less than 5 percent when four to six samples are analyzed.[121] Reports defining the sampling error of myocarditis have used autopsy hearts that are not comparable to the state of the myocardium at the time of endomyocardial biopsy during life.[122,123] When right ventricular endomyocardial biopsy has failed to establish the diagnosis, sampling the left ventricle may improve diagnostic yield. Myocarditis cannot be ruled out with complete certainty by biopsy but can be ruled in by morphologic features. (See Chap. 33.)

Endomyocardial biopsy must be applied as quickly as possible to maximize the diagnostic yield. Patients with peripartum cardiomyopathy have the highest yield when biopsy is performed early after onset of symptoms.[73] Resolution of active myocarditis has been documented within 4 days of initial biopsy with progressive clearing over several weeks on serial biopsy.[124] Progression of active myocarditis to dilated cardiomyopathy has been documented when serial biopsies are performed.[125]

Noninvasive Studies

While technetium 99m pyrophosphate, thallium 201 myocardial imaging, and gated blood pool scanning have not shown diagnostic potential in myocarditis, imaging with gallium 67, an inflammation avid radioisotope, showed promise as a screening method for active myocarditis.[95] Technical variations in imaging have precluded its application to a large population. Indium 111–antimyosin monoclonal antibody is an isotope that is avid for the injured myocardium. Application of this technique to patients with suspected myocarditis demonstrated a sensitivity of 83 percent, a specificity of 53 percent, and a positive predictive value of a normal scan of 92 percent.[126] In those patients who were antimyosin antibody positive and biopsy negative, the possibility of inflammation undetected by biopsy has been considered. Antimyosin imaging, however, detects myocyte injury independent of etiology, and multiple causes of heart muscle injury in young patients may cause false-positive scans. (See also Chap. 134.)

Tissue alterations associated with myocarditis may be identifiable using magnetic resonance imaging.[127] Preliminary results suggest that myocardial inflammation may induce abnormal signal intensity of the myocardial walls. Analysis in a large patient population has not been reported, and consequently the reliability cannot be judged. Despite the promise of noninvasive techniques, endomyocardial biopsy remains the diagnostic standard.

Natural History

In all likelihood the majority of patients have a self-limited disease that is asymptomatic at onset and has no residual evidence of cardiac functional impairment. Some patients, however, will die suddenly and unpredictably. Before the widespread application of endomyocardial biopsy, it was recognized that approximately one-third of patients who recover from active myocarditis will have residual functional abnormalities ranging from minor electrocardiographic changes to congestive heart failure. Histologic and clinical findings of progression from active myocarditis to dilated cardiomyopathy have been documented in patients who undergo endomyocardial biopsy to document myocarditis, presumably those with a more severe form of the disease.[128] Because endomyocardial biopsy has only been applied to a small percentage of the patients with this disease, however, the frequency of progression cannot be ascertained and is probably overestimated.

Treatment

If the patient presents with left ventricular dysfunction, the management is similar to other forms of congestive heart failure (Chap. 26). Sodium restriction, digitalis glycosides, diuretics, and vasodilators should be administered. In profound hemodynamic compromise, an aggressive approach to the management of shock should be employed, including intravenous inotropic and vasodilator agents, intraaortic balloon pump, and mechanical left ventricular assistance. Spontaneous improvement may occur despite rather profound abnormalities of hemodynamic function; therefore, cardiac transplantation should only be considered when aggressive left ventricular support has been attempted and an adequate time for recovery allowed. Cardiac transplantation in patients with active immune-mediated myocardial injury is associated with a high early postoperative mortality due to rejection (Fig. 88-3).[129] The immunologic milieu of activated T lymphocytes and humoral antibodies committed to myocyte antigens offers a donor heart an aggressive immune system from the very onset.

Laboratory animals forced to perform regular physical exercise following infection with cardiotropic viruses

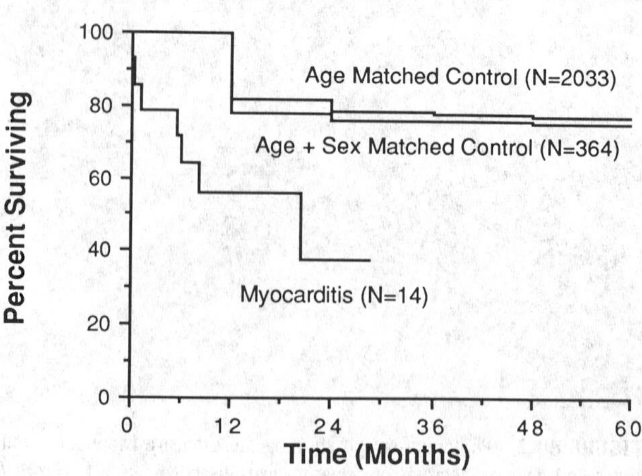

FIGURE 88-3 Actuarial survival of 14 patients with active myocarditis following cardiac transplantation (*From O'Connell et al.*[129] *Reproduced with permission.*)

experienced an increased intensity of the inflammatory response with increased necrosis and higher mortality.[130] In vitro study of the infected hearts demonstrated cardiac dilatation, deposition of antiheart antibody, and lymphocyte activation to heart-specific antigen.[131] Either augmented immune responses or intensification of virus-mediated injury is thought to account for this phenomenon. It is prudent, therefore, to suggest that patients with active myocarditis restrict their physical activity until documentation of resolution of inflammatory infiltrate.

A higher risk of mural thrombosis with subsequent thromboemboli has been observed in the animal model and isolated human reports.[70,71] It has been suggested that patients with active myocarditis receive anticoagulant therapy even when left ventricular dysfunction is only mild and that patients with histologically proved active myocarditis should receive oral anticoagulation (warfarin) until resolution of myocarditis.

Twenty-four-hour ambulatory monitoring demonstrates runs of nonsustained ventricular tachycardia in 25 percent of patients with even mild myocarditis.[78] Myocarditis may present with recurrent episodes of ventricular tachycardia and syncope or even sudden death. Although antiarrhythmic therapy has not been studied carefully in this population, controlling ventricular arrhythmia temporarily until the myocardial inflammation subsides may be warranted. Antiarrhythmic agents that adversely affect left ventricular function should be avoided, and long-term treatment of the ventricular arrhythmia by amiodarone or the automatic implantable cardioverter defibrillator (AICD) should be applied only after all other attempts at controlling arrhythmia have failed and adequate time for improvement in the histology has passed. A temporary pacemaker should be considered for complete AV block. (See Chaps. 39 and 42.)

Following the initial demonstration that 5 of 10 patients with biopsy-proven myocarditis responded when treated with prednisone and azathioprine,[68] a number of uncontrolled and nonrandomized investigations (Table 88-4) suggested a possible role for immunosuppression.[68,91,94,96,99,101,102,109,115,132–137] Unfortunately, most of these reports antedated the Dallas criteria, the histologic standards for entry were inconsistent, and immunosuppressive therapy was not standardized within or among the trials. A prospective randomized trial of prednisone in patients with dilated cardiomyopathy who did not meet Dallas criteria for active myocarditis identified early improvement in a "reactive" group that was not sustained by 6 months.[138] The natural history of active myocarditis is unknown, and the reported improvement rates could conceivably only reflect the natural history of the disease. Unfortunately, the significant morbidity associated with immunosuppression was not emphasized in these reports. To determine prospectively whether or not immunosuppression is beneficial in myocarditis, a multicenter Myocarditis Treatment Trial was organized.[139] The initial results of this study indicate that there was no apparent benefit of immunosuppressive therapy upon clinical course, rate of resolution of histologic evidence of myocarditis, or mortality. Other more aggressive forms of immunosuppression such as interferon and anti-CD3 monoclonal antibodies have been administered to patients with myocarditis.[140,141]

TABLE 88-4

Uncontrolled Reports of Immunosuppression in Biopsy-Proven Myocarditis

Investigators	Year	Total *n*	Improved *n*	Therapy
Mason et al.[68]	1980	10	5	CS,AZA
Sekiguchi et al.[132]	1980	3	2	CS
Edwards et al.[133]	1982	4	2	CS
Fenoglio et al.[91]	1983	19	8	CS,AZA
Zee-Cheng et al.[94]	1984	11	5	CS,AZA, ATG
Daly et al.[96]	1984	9	7	CS,AZA
Vignola et al.[115]	1984	6	5	CS,AZA
Fenely et al.[134]	1984	2	2	CS,AZA
Dec et al.[99]	1985	9	4	CS,AZA
Mortensen et al.[101]	1985	12	8	CS,AZA, CYA
Hosenpud et al.[102]	1985	6	0	CS,AZA
Salvi et al.[135]	1989	14	8	CS,AZA
Hobbs et al.[109]	1989	34	25	CS,AZA
Chan et al.[136]	1990	13	6	CS,AZA
Jones et al.[137]	1991	9	4	CS,AZA
Total		161	91 (56%)	

CS = corticosteroids; AZA = azathioprine; ATG = antithymocyte globulin; CYA = cyclosporine

SPECIFIC CAUSES OF MYOCARDITIS

Chagas' Disease

American trypanosomiasis, or Chagas' disease, is the most common cause of congestive heart failure in the world.[29] This condition results from infection with *Trypanosoma cruzi* and is endemic to rural South and Central America. In the chronic form of the illness the autonomic ganglia of the gastrointestinal tract are affected, leading to megacolon and megaesophagus. The characteristics of the cardiac disease include congestive heart failure, heart block, and arrhythmia.

Although the presence of the trypanosomes can be documented, cellular and humoral immune responses may be responsible for the myocardial injury.[142] Various antiheart antibodies have also been detected in high frequency in patients with Chagas' disease. Endomyocardial biopsy may show active myocarditis using the Dallas criteria.[143] Noninvasive assessment commonly shows segmental wall motion abnormalities, specifically apical aneurysms. The ECG may show complete heart block, AV block, or right bundle branch block with or without fascicular block in 11 percent of infected individuals.[144] Elevated antibody titers to *T. cruzi* may lead to suspicion of the diagnosis. Ventricular arrhythmias may require antiarrhythmic drugs, including amiodarone.[145]

The treatment of Chagas' disease includes a pacemaker if warranted for complete heart block and standard therapy for congestive heart failure as outlined for other forms of myocarditis. Nifurtimox should be administered if the disease has not previously been treated and may be used as prophylaxis if there is a high likelihood of recurrence such as following immunosuppressive therapy. The role of immunosuppression therapy for Chagasic myocarditis is controversial.

Toxoplasmosis

Acute infection by *Toxoplasma gondii* may result in active myocarditis, particularly following cardiac transplantation when the infection may be transmitted by the donor heart. The diagnosis is established by identification of toxoplasma cysts in areas of focal myocyte necrosis, edema, and a mixed inflammatory infiltrate including plasma cells, macrophages, lymphocytes, and eosinophils.[146] The organisms are ordinarily seen within the myocytes. A rise in antibody titer to *T. gondii* is commonly detected. Treatment is pyrimethamine and sulfadizaine. Toxoplasmosis is a curable form of myocarditis when it is discovered and treated early.

Cytomegalovirus

Cytomegalovirus may lead to myocarditis in the general population, but ordinarily the myocarditis is self-limited and asymptomatic. In the cardiac transplant recipient, however, cytomegalovirus myocarditis may become a more serious disease resulting in cardiac dysfunction.[147] The treatment of cytomegalovirus myocarditis is intravenous ganciclovir, which effectively eradicates the virus. Early cytomegalovirus infection correlates with the development of allograft coronary artery disease, the major cause of death beyond the first year after cardiac transplantation. It is proposed that infection of either subintimal fibroblasts or endothelial cells results in immunologic injury that predisposes to this potentially fatal condition.

Lyme Disease

Infection with the spirochete *Borrelia bergdorferi* introduced by a tick bite may result in Lyme disease, which is characterized by erythema chronica migrans, myalgias, arthralgias, headache, fever, lymphadenopathy, and fatigue. The treatment of choice is tetracycline during the early phase. Occasionally the disease may progress to Lyme carditis, which presents with complete heart block.[27,148] Left ventricular dysfunction is unusual. Endomyocardial biopsy may reveal active myocarditis, and in one report spirochetes were identified in the myocardium. Administration of corticosteroids has been successful in treating Lyme carditis following therapy with tetracycline.[149]

Acquired Immunodeficiency Syndrome

See Chap. 107.

Eosinophilic Myocarditis

The diagnosis of eosinophilic myocarditis is established when the dominant cells infiltrating the myocardial interstitium are eosinophils. The major basic protein of the eosinophil granule may be detected in the presence of acute necrotizing myocarditis, suggesting toxicity of the contents of these granules.[150] Although endocardial thickening and restrictive myocardial disease are associated with peripheral eosinophilia, eosinophilic myocarditis may occur in the absence of elevations in the total eosinophil count. The cardiac dysfunction in this condition is similar to that of active myocarditis with a predominance of lymphocytes infiltrating the biopsy. Prompt improvement in cardiac function and resolution of histologic abnormalities have been reported following administration of corticosteroids in uncontrolled trials.[151]

Giant-Cell Myocarditis

Giant cells in endomyocardial biopsies identify a particularly aggressive form of myocarditis (Fig. 88-4). This histologic abnormality may be associated with autoimmune disease such as myasthenia gravis, autoimmune hemolytic anemia, or polymyositis. Brady- and tachyarrhythmias are common manifestations and may precede left ventricular dysfunction in giant-cell myocarditis.[152] Although isolated reports have been optimistic toward response to immunosuppression, the overall experience is that of progressive disease unabated by medical therapy. Giant-cell myocarditis has recurred in the allograft following cardiac transplantation.

THE HEART AND ENDOCRINE DISEASE

See Chap. 102.

PHEOCHROMOCYTOMA AND THE HEART

Pheochromocytomas, usually found in the adrenal medulla or in association with sympathetic ganglia, produce, store, and secrete catecholamines,[153-155] which cause a variety of clinical presentations including signs and symptoms of ventricular dysfunction. (See Chaps. 76 and 102.) Hypertension, while common, may be sustained or intermittent, and orthostatic hypotension can be present due to abnormal neural control of vascular tone. Sinus tachycardia, sinus bradycardia, supraventricular arrhythmias, and premature ventricular depolarizations are seen. Ischemic manifestations may occur even in the absence of coronary artery disease. When congestive heart failure occurs, ventricular dilatation and systolic dysfunction are present, usually associated with spotty myocardial fibrosis. Occasionally concentric or asymmetric hypertrophy is seen. The catecholamine-induced myocardial damage is multifactorial (see Chaps. 109 and 110), but medical therapy to decrease circulating catecholamine levels and tumor removal are associated with hemodynamic, electrocardiographic, and clinical improvement in the cardiomyopathy.[154,155]

CARCINOID HEART DISEASE

Carcinoid tumors usually arise from argentaffin cells in the gastrointestinal tract and may secrete large amounts

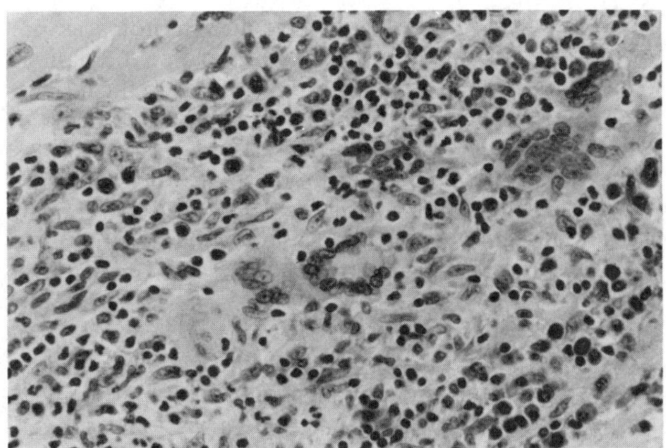

FIGURE 88-4 Photomicrograph showing mixed cellular infiltrate and giant cells characteristic of giant cell myocarditis (H&E, ×50). (*From W Gries et al: Giant cell myocarditis: First report of recurrence in the transplanted heart. J Heart Lung Transplant, 1992; 11:370–374. Reproduced with permission.*)

of serotonin (5-hydroxytryptamine), which is subsequently metabolized to 5-hydroxyindoleacetic acid (5-HIAA) by monoamine oxidase in the vascular endothelium of the lungs and the liver. The carcinoid syndrome, which is characterized by flushing, telangiectasias, diarrhea, and bronchoconstriction, occurs with less than 10 percent of carcinoid tumors. The primary tumors are generally located in the ileum but may infrequently be found in a bronchus and rarely in the jejunum, rectum, a Meckel's diverticulum, or ovary.[156–158]

Carcinoid heart disease occurs in approximately half of the patients with a classic carcinoid syndrome. The myofibromatous cardiac lesions usually involve the right side of the heart, causing dysfunction of the tricuspid and pulmonary valves. Severe tricuspid regurgitation (Chap. 81) with right-sided volume overload can predominate the presentation. The tricuspid valve may be thickened with the valve leaflets fixed in a partially open position. Extensive involvement of the mural endocardium may cause restrictive physiology in some affected individuals. The superficial and right-sided cardiac location of the valvular and endocardial lesions lead to the suggestion that a blood-borne product of the tumor is responsible for the cardiac disease.

Although the severity of right-sided involvement correlates with plasma levels of serotonin and the tachykinins, neuropeptide K, and substance P, as well as higher urinary excretion of the serotonin metabolite 5-HIAA, it does not correlate with disease duration. The major causes of death include hepatic failure, right ventricular failure, bowel obstruction, and bowel perforation; 5-year survival rates of 70 to 80 percent have been achieved using interferon and somatostatin analogues. Surgical management of the abnormal right-sided heart valves is encouraging.

THE HEART AND KIDNEY DISEASE

See Chap. 108.

HYPEROXALURIA

Both primary oxalosis, a rare autosomal recessive disorder, and secondary hyperoxaluria are characterized by calcium oxalate deposition in body tissues, including the myocardium.[159–161] Primary oxalosis is caused by an abnormality in alanine glyoxylate aminotransferase activity, the enzyme that converts glyoxylate to glycine in the liver. In the setting of normal renal function, primary oxalosis manifests itself as relatively benign hyperoxaluria. Unfortunately, nephrolithiasis and nephrocalcinosis may occur, producing renal insufficiency. As renal function deteriorates, urinary excretion of oxalate decreases, causing further renal deposition of calcium oxalate and destroying remaining renal function. The progressive disease that subsequently develops is associated with painful arthropathy, peripheral neuropathy, retinopathy, osteodystrophy, and ischemic vasculopathy with digital and limb necrosis frequently requiring amputation. The causes of secondary oxalosis include chronic renal failure, ingestion of oxalates or of substances metabolized to oxalates (including ethylene glycol, intravenous feeding with xylitol, anesthesia with methoxyflurane), and enteric hyperoxaluria occurring in patients with extensive disease of the small bowel and pyridoxine deficiency.

In all types of oxalosis, oxalate crystals frequently deposit in the conducting system of the heart, causing heart block, and occasionally in the myocardium and the coronary arteries. Calcium oxalate crystals appear in H&E staining as a light brown, strongly birefringent crystal and cause variable degrees of cellular reaction, including necrosis, fibrosis, and mononuclear cell infiltration. Foreign-body giant cells and myocardial granulomas can occur. Congestive heart failure and cardiac arrhythmias may occur. Interestingly, the cardiac dysfunction seen in primary oxalosis has been reported to reverse after combined kidney-liver transplantation.[161]

GOUT

While atherosclerosis and coronary artery disease is the most common cardiovascular manifestation associated with gout, cardiovascular lesions can be found in gout and include uric acid crystals in the walls of blood vessels, myocardial interstitium, pericardium, conducting system, mitral annulus, and mitral, aortic, and tricuspid valve leaflets. Such deposits can calcify and cause a foreign-body type of granulomatous response, including the formation of multinucleated giant cells.[162,163]

LYSOSOMAL STORAGE DISEASES

See Chap. 96.

GLYCOGEN STORAGE DISEASES

See Chap. 96.

REFSUM'S SYNDROME

See Chap. 96.

CARNITINE DEFICIENCY

See Chap. 96.

HEMOCHROMATOSIS

Hemochromatosis is the progressive overload of iron in tissues leading to cirrhosis, diabetes, hyperpigmentation, and cardiac dysfunction (Fig. 88-5).[164–170] (See also Chap. 96.) Hemochromatosis may be inherited (genetic) or occur secondary to another process associated with iron loading (acquired). In genetic hemochromatosis, the metabolic defect is associated with an abnormal gene tightly linked to the A locus of the HLA complex on chromosome 6 and may affect the relationship between ferritin mRNA and transferrin receptor mRNA expression in the intestinal mucosa cell.[169,170] Inherited as an autosomal recessive disease, homozygotes usually develop severe iron overload whereas heterozygotes show either no abnormalities or develop only minor abnormalities in iron metabolism. Determination of both transferrin saturation and ferritin concentration in serum detects genetic hemochromatosis with 95 percent specificity and sensitivity.

Congestive heart failure is the leading cause of death in genetic hemochromatosis. About 15 percent of hemochromatosis patients have cardiac symptoms as presenting complaints and about one-third of the patients subsequently develop symptoms referable to the heart.[170]

Acquired hemochromatosis occurs primarily in chronic disorders of erythropoiesis, such as in sideroblastic anemia and thalassemia. In these disorders, not only is the absorption of iron increased, but iron and transfusions are commonly administered. Acquired hemochromatosis may also result from excessive iron ingestion over many years.

The ECG in hemochromatosis may show low voltage and nonspecific ST-T changes. The most common disturbances in rhythm are supraventricular arrhythmias, although premature ventricular depolarizations and ventricular tachycardia can be seen. The heart muscle disease associated with hemochromatosis usually produces dilated ventricles with impaired systolic function, although less commonly a restrictive physiology may occur. Patients with hemochromatosis may initially only have increased left ventricular mass and normal function, but progressive dilatation and dysfunction ensues. A transition from a restrictive heart muscle disease to a dilated, poorly contracting ventricle may occur.

Although the iron deposition causes fibrosis in a majority of patients, the fibrosis tends to be mild. Iron deposits are most prominent in the ventricles, more epicardial than endocardial in location. The atria tend to be less involved and the conducting system least involved with iron deposition. Even in the conducting system, differences exist since the sinus node is usually less involved than the AV node and His bundle. Since cardiac iron deposition tends to be greater in the subepicardial than in the subendocardial regions, endomyocardial bi-

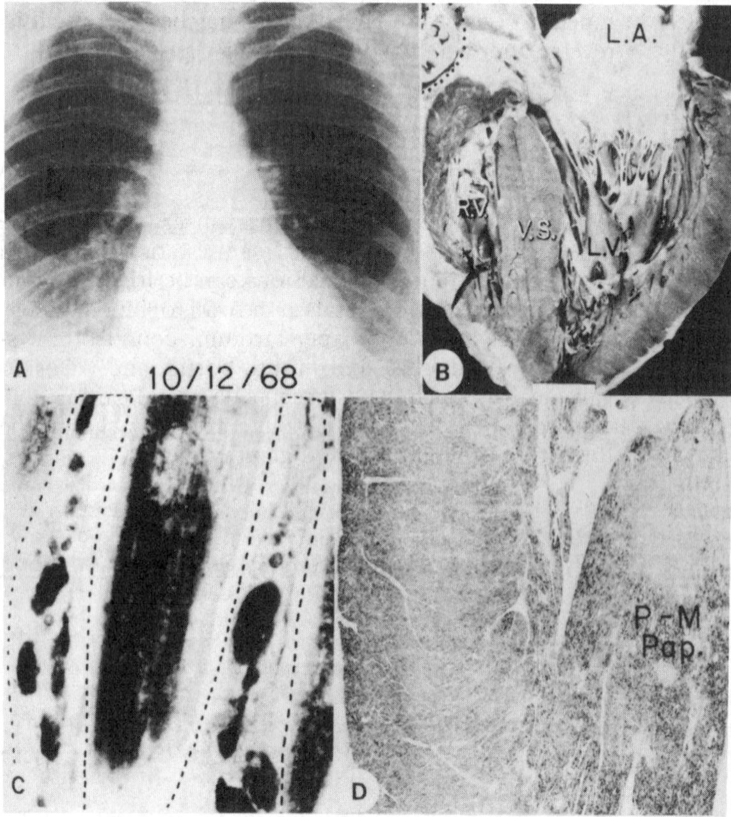

FIGURE 88-5 Cardiac hemosiderosis in a 42-year-old woman with sickle cell anemia. She had received 260 units of blood when congestive heart failure developed 6 years before death. *A.* Chest roentgenogram showed cardiomegaly. By the time of death she had received 359 units of blood (90 g iron). *B.* At necropsy, the walls of the right and left ventricles and left atrium were rusty brown due to extensive iron deposits. In contrast, the right atrial wall was tan and only minute particles of iron were detected in it by histologic examination. *C.* Photomicrograph of several myocardial cells showing huge deposits of iron in them. Despite large deposits of iron in the working myocardium, no iron deposits were observed in conducting myocardium. *D.* Longitudinal section of left ventricular wall including posteromedial (P-M) papillary muscle. Foci of necrosis and fibrosis are present. The necrotic and fibrotic areas probably are anatomic indicators of chronic myocardial hypoxia, a result of the chronic anemia. Prussian blue iron stains; ×628 (*C*), ×3 (*D*). (*From Wenger et al.*[162] *Reproduced with permission.*)

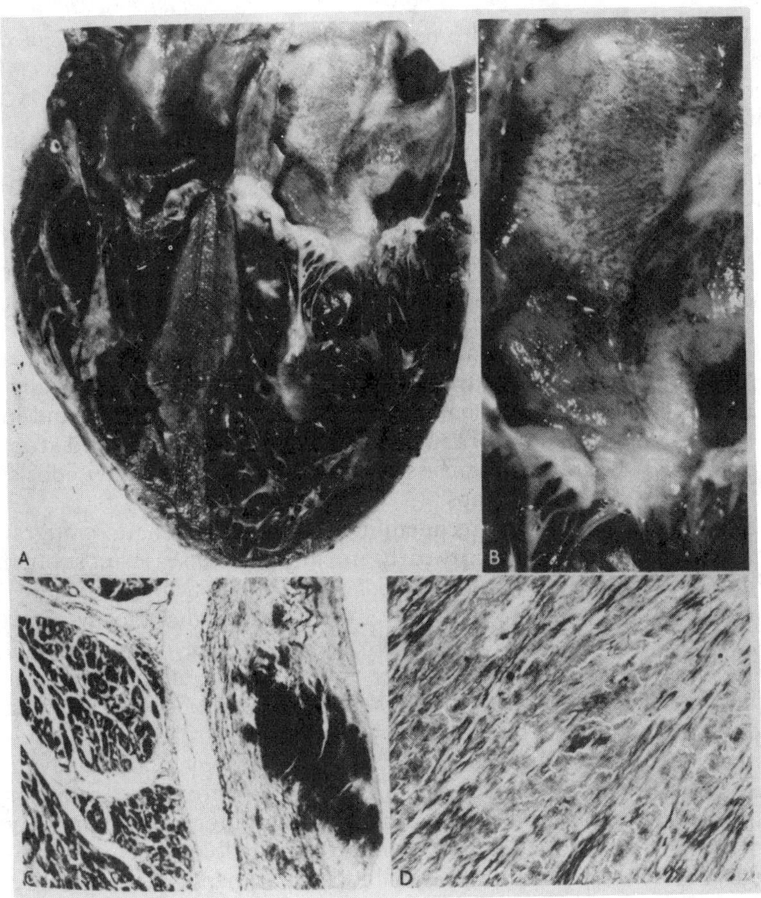

FIGURE 88-6 Cardiac amyloidosis. *A.* Posterior half of the heart in an 86-year-old man who had angina pectoris and healed myocardial infarction as well as large amyloid deposits. *B.* Close-up of left atrial endocardium. The waxy lesions on this endocardium represent amyloid deposits and are indicative of extensive ventricular amyloid deposits. *C.* Photomicrograph of left atrial endocardial amyloid deposit, ×107. *D.* Amyloid has infiltrated extensively a left ventricular papillary muscle, ×32. *C, D.* Crystal violet stain. (*From Wenger et al.*[162] *Reproduced with permission.*)

opsy may underestimate myocardial iron overload. Although endomyocardial biopsy has been shown to be an insensitive method for the determination of early myocardial iron deposition in transfusion-related hemochromatosis associated with thalassemia major, one study suggests that histologically demonstrable myocardial iron is a consistent finding in endomyocardial biopsy tissue from patients with nontransfusional iron overload and associated cardiac dysfunction.[167]

Treatment of genetic hemochromatosis involves removal of the excess body iron and supportive treatment for the damaged organs. While removal of iron is cheaply done by phlebotomy, chelation therapy with deferoxamine can also be used. After iron removal by either phlebotomy or chelation, cardiac dysfunction may normalize, left ventricular dimensions decrease, and resting and exercise left ventricular function improve.

NUTRITIONAL DISEASE AND THE HEART

See Chap. 105.

SELENIUM DEFICIENCY AND KESHAN'S DISEASE

See Chap. 105.

AMYLOID HEART DISEASE

Amyloid cardiomyopathy is caused by the deposition of abnormal protein in the interstitium of the myocardium, resulting in increased ventricular wall thickness and the eventual development of congestive signs and symptoms (see Fig. 88-6). (See also Chap. 91.) Systolic left ventricular function is usually preserved until late in the disease; and once cardiomegaly, pulmonary edema, or systolic dysfunction has occurred, marked amyloid deposition in the myocardium is usually present.[162,171–178]

Amyloid AL (Myeloma-Associated and Primary Systemic Amyloid)

The amyloid protein subunit of amyloid AL is the ammonia terminal portion of an immunoglobulin light chain (kappa or lambda).[171] Of patients with amyloid AL, one-third to one-half have cardiac involvement, and more than one-fourth have symptomatic heart failure. The median survival in individuals with any cardiac involvement is less than 1 year, and the 5-year survival rate is less than 10 percent. In patients presenting with cardiac involvement, the majority have a monoclonal protein spike in the serum or in the urine.[171]

Amyloid AA (Secondary Amyloidosis and Familial Mediterranean Fever)

Amyloid AA results from the deposition of amyloid A protein and is seen in chronic inflammatory disorders (rheumatoid arthritis, juvenile rheumatoid arthritis, ankylosing spondylitis, Crohn's disease, paraplegia associated with decubitus ulcers, cystic fibrosis, and heroin use with chronically infected cutaneous injection sites) and in familial Mediterranean fever, an autosomal recessively inherited disease of Sephardic Jews, Armenians, and other Mediterranean peoples. In general, aside from amyloid A protein deposition in the intima and media of arterioles, the heart is not involved.

Amyloid AF (Familial Amyloidosis)

Familial amyloidosis can be manifest initially with progressive neuropathy, cardiomyopathy, or renal involvement. The abnormal protein deposited is designated amyloid AF and is a variant of prealbumin known as transthyretin. The familial amyloidosis diseases are inherited as autosomal dominant disorders, unlike familial Mediterranean fever, which is inherited in an autosomal recessive fashion. All known variant forms of transthyretin can be produced by the alteration of a single nucleotide in the deoxyribonucleic acid (DNA) sequence that codes for the protein. The heart disease in amyloid AF is variable. In some families, cardiac amyloidosis is not even symptomatic, while in other families cardiac symptoms predominate. Although ventricular function can appear normal in most members of some families with familial amyloid polyneuropathy, many affected individuals have detectable reductions in peak filling rates and in time to peak filling by radionuclide scanning, suggesting myocardial amyloid deposition.

Amyloid SSA (Senile Cardiac Amyloid and Senile Systemic Amyloid)

Amyloid SSA, like amyloid AF, is also related to the deposition of an abnormal transthyretin, albeit in older individuals. One form of amyloid SSA appears to affect only the atria; another form affects only the aorta; and a third form, commonly known as senile systemic amyloidosis, may involve the lungs, liver, kidneys, and myocardium. It should be noted that amyloid deposition is seen in one-fourth of individuals older than 70 years of age. While amyloid SSA has not been felt to be a frequent cause of cardiac symptoms, senile cardiac amyloid has been retrospectively associated with antemortem congestive heart failure and cardiac arrhythmias. While it appears that those with senile amyloidosis have a much better prognosis than those with immunoglobulin derived amyloidosis, cardiac involvement by senile systemic amyloidosis may be an important, although uncommon, cause of cardiovascular morbidity.

Amyloid IAA (Isolated Atrial Amyloid)

Amyloid IAA has been found to be derived from atrial naturetic polypeptide, the clinical consequences of which are unknown.

Amyloid CAA (Cerebral Amyloid Angiopathy)

Amyloid CAA is seen in the cerebral vessels and neurofibrillatory tangles of patients with senile dementia and Down's syndrome. The subunit protein has been called A4 or beta.

Laboratory Evaluation

Echocardiography is probably the most effective noninvasive screening tool for amyloid heart disease. Echocardiography can demonstrate symmetrical thickening of the left ventricular wall. It is not certain that qualitative (diffuse hyperrefractile, granular sparkling appearance of the myocardium) or even quantitative texture analysis can identify amyloid and distinguish it from hypertrophic cardiomyopathy. Abnormal left ventricular diastolic filling manifested by reduction in the rate and in the volume of rapid diastolic filling with enhanced atrial contraction can be seen very early in cardiac amyloidosis. (See also Chaps. 15 and 91.)

Although technetium 99m–pyrophosphate scintigraphy may identify early amyloid heart disease, most often in patients with familial amyloid polyneuropathy, amyloid is detected easily in endomyocardial biopsy specimens. Amyloid may be deposited in the interstitium in a pericellular or nodular pattern, in the endocardium, or in myocardial blood vessels. Since Congo red staining may not be satisfactory in endomyocardial biopsy specimens, sulfated alcian blue, methyl violet, and thioflavine T stains may be required. Immunoperoxidase stains for kappa and lambda light chains and for prealbumin may categorize the type of cardiac amyloid. Electronmicroscopic examination of biopsy specimens is likely the most sensitive method of recognizing amyloidosis.

COLLAGEN VASCULAR AND CONNECTIVE TISSUE DISORDERS

See Chap. 103.

WHIPPLE'S DISEASE

Whipple's disease, a rare disorder characterized by arthritis, prolonged diarrhea, malabsorption, and weight loss, is thought to be caused by an undefined microbe. Cardiac involvement is common, resulting from a pancarditis that causes fibrous thickening of cardiac valves with thickening and fusion of the chordae tendineae. The mitral valve is more commonly affected than the tricuspid valve, and aortic valve involvement is sometimes seen. Microscopically, large macrophages with Periodic Acid-Schiff PAS-positive granules are present. Scattered rod-shaped bacteria may be seen in affected valves, myocardium, and pericardium.[162,179–181]

SARCOIDOSIS

Sarcoidosis, a systemic granulomatous disease of undetermined etiology, will most commonly involve lymph nodes, lung, liver, spleen, eyes, phalangeal bones, and parotid glands but may also affect other organs and tissues including the heart and pericardium.[162,182,183]

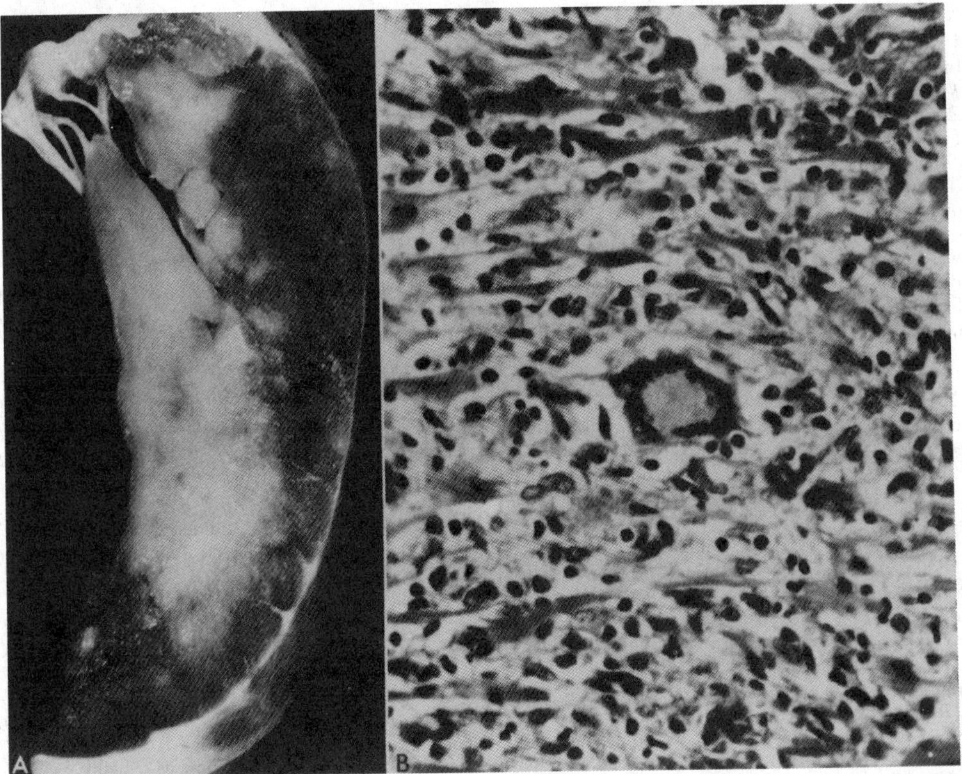

FIGURE 88-7 Cardiac sarcoidosis. *A*. Longitudinal section through anterolateral papillary muscle in a 26-year-old woman who had been asymptomatic until 10 days before her death, when dyspnea appeared. The dyspnea rapidly worsened, and when hospitalized on the day of death, she was in acute pulmonary edema. The blood pressure was 80/80 mmHg, heart rate 160 beats per minute, and a grade 3 to 4/6 holosystolic blowing murmur, which radiated to the axilla, was audible. Chest roentgenogram showed congested lungs, cardiomegaly, and prominent hilar adenopathy. The ECG showed nonspecific ST-T-wave changes and atrial hypertrophy. She developed complete heart block and died shortly thereafter. *A*. At necropsy, large, firm white deposits were present in the walls of all four cardiac chambers and completely replaced both left ventricular papillary muscles. *B*. On histologic section, the firm white areas represented hard granulomas typical of sarcoidosis. H&E, ×400. Similar hard granulomas were present in lymph nodes, liver, spleen, and lung. Stains for acid-fast organisms, other bacteria, and fungi did not show evidence of infection. (*From Wenger et al.*[162] *Reproduced with permission.*)

While only 5 percent of patients with sarcoid have symptoms referable to the cardiovascular system, approximately one-fifth of patients have myocardial sarcoid at autopsy.[184]

In myocardial sarcoid, portions of the myocardial wall are replaced by sarcoid granulomas (Fig. 88-7), and sarcoid granulomas are invariably found in noncardiac tissue as well. The sarcoid granulomas are not distributed randomly in the heart but involve preferentially the ventricular septum (cephalad portion) or the left ventricular papillary muscles adjacent to free walls. Granulomas can also affect the right or left ventricular free walls.

Because of the location of the myocardial granulomas, conduction system abnormalities, mitral regurgitation, and wall motion abnormalities are frequently seen. Aneurysm formation can occur. Ventricular tachyarrhythmias are frequent and sudden death may occur. Myocardial involvement is much more common than pericardial involvement.[162,185–188]

MUSCULAR DYSTROPHIES, MYOPATHIES, AND NEUROMUSCULAR DISORDERS

See Chap. 96.

TOXICITY, HYPERSENSITIVITY, AND PHYSICAL AGENT EFFECTS

See Chaps. 105, 110, and 120.

ALCOHOL

See Chap. 105.

PERIPARTUM HEART DISEASE

See Chap. 113.

REFERENCES

1. Olsen EGJ: Myocarditis—a case of mistaken identity? *Br Heart J* 1983; 50:303–311.
2. O'Connell JB, Robinson JA: Coxsackie viral myocarditis. *Postgrad Med J* 1985; 61:1127–1131.
3. Sainani GS, Krompotic E, Slodki SJ: Adult heart disease due to the Coxsackie virus B infection. *Medicine* 1968; 47:133–147.

4. Proby CM, Hackett S, Gupta S, Cox TM: Acute myopericarditis in influenza A infection. *Q J Med* 1986; 60:887–892.
5. Bell RW, Murphy WM: Myocarditis in young military personnel. *Am Heart J* 1967; 74:309–323.
6. Lorber A, Zonis A, Maisuls E, Dembo L, Palant A, Iancu TC: The scale of myocardial involvement in varicella myocarditis. *Int J Cardiol* 1988; 20:257–262.
7. Millett R, Tomita T, Marshall HE, Cohen L, Hannah III H: Cytomegalovirus endomyocarditis in a transplanted heart. *Arch Pathol Lab Med* 1991; 115:511–515.
8. Frishman W, Kraus ME, Zabkar J, Brooks V, Alonso D, Dixon LM: Infectious mononucleosis and fatal myocarditis. *Chest* 1977; 72:535–538.
9. Chaudary S, Jaski BE: Fulminant mumps myocarditis. *Ann Intern Med* 1989; 110:569–570.
10. Ainger LE, Lawyer NG, Fitch CW: Neonatal rubella myocarditis. *Br Heart J* 1966; 28:691–697.
11. Datta D, Zaidi A, Brendan DH: Carditis associated with coronavirus infection (letter). *Lancet* 1980; 2:100–101.
12. Raman GV, Prosser A, Spreadbury PL, Cockcroft PM, Okubadejo OA: Rabies presenting with myocarditis and encephalitis. *J Infect* 1988; 17:155–158.
13. Ursell PC, Habib A, Sharma P, Mesa-Tejada R, Lefkowitch JH, Fenoglio Jr JJ: Hepatitis B virus and myocarditis. *Human Pathol* 1984; 15:481–484.
14. Obeyesekere I, Hermon Y: Arbovirus heart disease: Myocarditis and cardiomyopathy following dengue and chikungunya fever—A follow-up study. *Am Heart J* 1973; 85:186–194.
15. Milei J, Bolomo NJ: Myocardial damage in viral hemorrhagic fevers. *Am Heart J* 1982; 104:1385–1391.
16. Burch GE, Sun S-C, Sohal RS, Chu K-C, Colcolough HL: Diphtheritic myocarditis. *Am J Cardiol* 1968; 21:261–268.
17. Shalit M, Braverman AJ, Eliakim M: Congestive heart failure in the course of typhoid fever. *J Infect* 1982; 4:81–84.
18. Karjalainen J: Streptococcal tonsillitis and acute nonrheumatic myopericarditis. *Chest* 1989; 95:359–363.
19. Brasier AR, Macklis JD, Vaughan D, Warner L, Kirshenbaum JM: Myopericarditis as an initial presentation of meningococcemia. *Am J Med* 1987; 82:641–644.
20. Gross D, Willens H, Zeldis SM: Myocarditis in Legionnaires' Disease. *Chest* 1981; 79:232–234.
21. McCue MJ, Moore EE: Myocarditis with microabscess formation caused by *Listeria* monocytogenes associated with myocardial infarct. *Human Pathol* 1979; 10:469–472.
22. Florkowski CM, Ikram RB, Crozier IM, Ikram H, Berry ME: Campylobacter jejuni myocarditis. *Clin Cardiol* 1984; 7:558–559.
23. Willey RF, Matthews MB, Peutherer JF, Marmion BP: Chronic cryptic Q-fever infection of the heart. *Lancet* 1979; 2:270–272.
24. Ringel RE, Brenner JI, Rennels MB, Huang S-W, Wang S, Grayston T, et al: Serologic evidence for *Chlamydia tachomatis* myocarditis. *Pediatrics* 1982; 70:54–56.
25. Lewes D, Rainford DJ, Lane WF: Symptomless myocarditis and myalgia in viral and *Mycoplasma pneumoniae* infections. *Br Heart J* 1974; 36:924–932.
26. Marin-Garcia J, Barrett FF: Myocardial function in Rocky Mountain Spotted Fever: Echocardiographic assessment. *Am J Cardiol* 1983; 51:341–343.
27. McAlister HF, Klementowicz PT, Andrews C, Fisher JD, Feld M, Furman S: Lyme carditis: An important cause of reversible heart block. *Ann Intern Med* 1989; 110:339–345.
28. Horn H, Saphir O: The involvement of the myocardium in tuberculosis. *Am Rev Tub* 1935; 32:492–506.
29. Marsden PD: South American trypanosomiasis (Chagas' Disease). *Int Rev Trop Med* 1971; 4:97–121.
30. Leak D, Meghji M: Toxoplasmic infection in cardiac disease. *Am J Cardiol* 1979; 43:841–849.
31. Bessoudo R, Marrie TJ, Smith ER: Cardiac involvement in trichinosis. *Chest* 1981; 79:698–699.
32. Perez-Gomez F, Duran H, Tamames S, Perrote JL, Blanes A: Cardiac echinococcosis: Clinical picture and complications. *Br Heart J* 1973; 35:1326–1331.
33. Samlowski WE, Ward JH, Craven CM, Freedman RA: Severe myocarditis following high-dose interleukin-2 administration. *Arch Pathol Lab Med* 1989; 113:838–841.
34. Cohen MC, Huberman MS, Nesto RW: Recombinant alpha$_2$ interferon-related cardiomyopathy. *Am J Med* 1988; 85:549–551.
35. Eggers HJ, Mertens Th: Viruses and myocardium: Notes of a virologist. *Eur Heart J* 1987; 8(suppl J):129–133.
36. Gibson TC, Arnold J, Craige E, Curnen E: Electrocardiographic studies in Asian influenza. *Am Heart J* 1959; 57:661–668.
37. Karjalainen J, Nieminen MS, Heikkila J: Influenza A1 myocarditis in conscripts. *Acta Med Scand* 1980; 207:27–30.
38. Stevens PJ, Underwood Ground KE: Occurrence and significance of myocarditis in trauma. *Aerospace Med* 1970; 41:776–780.
39. Gravanis MB, Sternby NH: Incidence of myocarditis. *Arch Pathol Lab Med* 1991; 115:390–392.
40. Wenger NK, Abelmann WH, Roberts WC: Myocardial disease. In: Hurst JW, Logue RB, Rackley CE, Schlant RC, Sonnenblick EH, Wallace AG, et al. (eds): *Diseases of the Heart and Blood Vessels*, 5th ed. New York, McGraw-Hill, 1982: 1278–1299.
41. Woodruff JF: Viral myocarditis: A review. *Am J Pathol* 1980; 101:427–479.
42. Godeny EK, Gauntt CJ: In situ immune autoradiographic identification of cells in heart tissues of mice with coxsackievirus B3–induced myocarditis. *Am J Pathol* 1987; 129:267–276.
43. Lodge PA, Herzum M, Olszewski J, Huber SA: Coxsackievirus B3 myocarditis. *Am J Pathol* 1987; 128:455–463.
44. Chow LH, Ye Y, Linder J, McManus BM: Phenotypic analysis of infiltrating cells in human myocarditis. *Arch Pathol Lab Med* 1989; 113:1357–1362.
45. Seko Y, Shinkai Y, Kawasaki A, Yagita H, Okumura K, Takaku F, et al: Expression of perforin in infiltrating cells in murine hearts with acute myocarditis caused by Coxsackie-virus B3. *Circulation* 1991; 84:788–795.
46. Young LHY, Joag SV, Zheng L-M, Lee C-P, Lee Y-S, Young JD: Perforin-mediated myocardial damage in acute myocarditis. *Lancet* 1990; 336:1019–1021.
47. Woodley SL, McMillan M, Shelby J, Lynch DH, Roberts LK, Ensley RD, et al: Myocyte injury and contraction abnormalities produced by cytotoxic T lymphocytes. *Circulation* 1991; 83:1410–1418.
48. Camp TF, Hess EV, Conway G, Fowler NO: Immunologic findings in idiopathic cardiomyopathy. *Am Heart J* 1969; 77:610–618.
49. Maisch B, Trostel-Soeder R, Stechemesser E, Berg PA, Kochstek K: Diagnostic relevance of humoral and cell-mediated immune reactions in patients with acute viral myocarditis. *Clin Exp Immunol* 1982; 48:533–545.
50. Neumann DA, Burek CL, Baughman KL, Rose NR, Herskowitz A: Circulating heart-reactive antibodies in patients with myocarditis or cardiomyopathy. *J Am Coll Cardiol* 1990; 16:839–846.
51. Neu N, Craig SW, Rose NR, Alvarez F, Beisel KW: Coxsackievirus induced myocarditis in mice: Cardiac myosin autoantibodies do not cross-react with the virus. *Clin Exp Immunol* 1987; 69:566–574.
52. Neu N, Rose NR, Beisel KW, Herskowitz A, Gurri-Glass G, Craig SW: Cardiac myosin induces myocarditis in genetically predisposed mice. *J Immunol* 1987; 139:3630–3636.
53. Limas CJ, Goldenberg IF, Limas C: Influence of anti-beta-receptor antibodies on cardiac adenylate cyclase in patients with idiopathic dilated cardiomyopathy. *Am Heart J* 1990; 119(6):1322–1328.
54. Schulze K, Becker BF, Schauer R, Schultheiss HP: Antibodies to ADP-ATP carrier—An autoantigen in myocarditis and dilated cardiomyopathy—Impair cardiac function. *Circulation* 1990; 81:959–968.
55. Ansari AA, Wang Y-C, Danner EJ, Gravanis MB, Mayne A, Neckelmann N, et al: Abnormal expression of histocompatibility and mitochondrial antigens by cardiac tissue from patients with myocarditis and dilated cardiomyopathy. *Am J Pathol* 1991; 139:337–354.
56. Schulze K, Becker BF, Schultheiss HP: Antibodies to the ADP-ATP carrier, an autoantigen in myocarditis and dilated cardiomyopathy, penetrate into myocardial cells and disturb energy metabolism in vivo. *Circ Res* 1989; 64:179–191.
57. Sutton GC, Harding HB, Truehart LRP, Clark HP: Coxsackie B4 myocarditis in an adult: Successful isolation of virus from ventricular myocardium. *Aerospace Med* 1967; 38:66–69.
58. Tracy S, Wiegand V, McManus B, Gauntt C, Pallansch M, Beck M, et al: Molecular approaches to enteroviral diagnosis in idiopathic cardiomyopathy and myocarditis. *J Am Coll Cardiol* 1990; 15:1688–1694.
59. Gerli R, Rambotti P, Spinozzi F, Bertotto A, Chiodini V, Solinas P, et al: Immunologic studies of peripheral blood from patients

with idiopathic dilated cardiomyopathy. *Am Heart J* 1986; 112:350–355.

60. Huber KC, Gersh BJ, Sugrue DD, Frye RL, Bailey KR, Ritts RE Jr: T-lymphocyte subsets in patients with idiopathic dilated cardiomyopathy. *Int J Cardiol* 1989; 22:59–66.
61. Fowles RE, Bieber CP, Stinson EB: Defective in vitro suppressor cell function in idiopathic congestive cardiomyopathy. *Circulation* 1979; 59:483–491.
62. Anderson JL, Fowles RE, Bieber CP, Stinson EB: Idiopathic cardiomyopathy, age, and suppressor-cell dysfunction as risk determinants of lymphoma after cardiac transplantation. *Lancet* 1978; 2:1174–1177.
63. Myocarditis Treatment Trial Investigators: Incidence and clinical characteristics of myocarditis (abstr). *Circulation* 1991; 84(suppl II):II-2.
64. Costanzo-Nordin MR, O'Connell JB, Subramanian R, Robinson JA, Scanlon PJ: Myocarditis confirmed by biopsy presenting as acute myocardial infarction. *Br Heart J* 1985; 53:25–29.
65. Saffitz JE, Schwartz DJ, Southworth W, Murphree S, Rodriguez ER, Ferrans VJ, et al: Coxsackie viral myocarditis causing transmural right and left ventricular infarction without coronary narrowing. *Am J Cardiol* 1983; 52:644–647.
66. Burch GE, Shewey LL: Viral coronary arteritis and myocardial infarction. *Am Heart J* 1976; 92:11–14.
67. Ferguson DW, Farwell AP, Bradley WA, Rollings RC: Coronary artery vasospasm complicating acute myocarditis. *West J Med* 1988; 148:664–669.
68. Mason JW, Billingham ME, Ricci DR: Treatment of acute inflammatory myocarditis assisted by endomyocardial biopsy. *Am J Cardiol* 1980; 45:1037–1044.
69. Phillips M, Robinowitz M, Higgins JR, Boran KJ, Reed T, Virmani R: Sudden cardiac death in Air Force recruits. A 20-year review. *JAMA* 1986; 256:2696–2699.
70. Tomioka N, Kishimoto C, Matsumori A, Kawai C: Mural thrombus in experimental viral myocarditis in mice: Relation between thrombosis and congestive heart failure. *Cardiovasc Res* 1986; 20:665–671.
71. Kojima J, Miyazaki S, Fujiwara H, Kumada T, Kawai C: Recurrent left ventricular mural thrombi in a patient with acute myocarditis. *Heart Vessels* 1988; 4:120–122.
72. O'Connell JB, Fowles RE, Robinson JA, Subramanian R, Henkin RE, Gunnar RM: Clinical and pathologic findings of myocarditis in two families with dilated cardiomyopathy. *Am Heart J* 1984; 107:127–135.
73. O'Connell JB, Costanzo-Nordin MR, Subramanian R, Robinson JA, Wallis DE, Scanlon PJ, et al: Peripartum cardiomyopathy: Clinical, hemodynamic, histologic and prognostic characteristics. *J Am Coll Cardiol* 1986; 8:52–56.
74. Karjalainen J, Heikkila J: Acute pericarditis: Myocardial enzyme release as evidence for myocarditis. *Am Heart J* 1986; 111:546–552.
75. Karjalainen J: Functional and myocarditis-induced T-wave abnormalities. *Chest* 1983; 83:868–864.
76. Toshima H, Ohkita Y, Shingu M: Clinical features of acute coxsackie B viral myocarditis. *Jpn Circ J* 1979; 43:441–444.
77. Kimby AG, Sodermark T, Volpe U, Zetterquist S: Stokes-Adams attacks requiring pacemaker treatment in three patients with acute nonspecific myocarditis. *Acta Med Scand* 1980; 207:177–181.
78. Karjalainen J, Viitasalo M, Kala R, Heikkila J: 24-Hour electrocardiographic recordings in mild acute infectious myocarditis. *Ann Clin Res* 1984; 16:34–39.
79. Chandraratna PAN, Nimalasuriya A, Reid CL, Cohn S, Rahimtoola SH: Left ventricular asynergy in acute myocarditis. *JAMA* 1983; 250:1428–1430.
80. Arvan S, Manalo E: Sudden increase in left ventricular mass secondary to acute myocarditis. *Am Heart J* 1988; 116:200–202.
81. Pinamonti B, Alberti E, Cigalotto A, Dreas L, Salvi A, Silvestri F, et al: Echocardiographic findings in myocarditis. *Am J Cardiol* 1988; 62:285–291.
82. Ferdeghini EM, Pinamonti B, Picano E, Lattanzi F, Bussani R, Slavich G, et al: Quantitative texture analysis in echocardiography: Application to the diagnosis of myocarditis. *J Clin Ultrasound* 1991; 19:263–270.
83. Uchida Y, Nakamura F, Oshima T, Fujimori Y, Hirose J: Percutaneous fiberoptic angioscopy of the left ventricle in patients with dilated cardiomyopathy and acute myocarditis. *Am Heart J* 1990; 120:677–687.
84. Konno S, Sakakibara S: Endomyocardial biopsy. *Chest* 1963; 44:345–350.
85. Caves PK, Schulz WP, Dong E Jr, Stinson EB, Shumway NE: New instrument for transvenous cardiac biopsy. *Am J Cardiol* 1974; 33:264–267.
86. Miller LW, Labovitz AJ, McBride LA, Pennington DG, Kanter K: Echocardiography-guided endomyocardial biopsy. *Circulation* 1988; 78(suppl III):III-99–III-102.
87. Noda S: Histopathology of endomyocardial biopsies from patients with idiopathic cardiomyopathy; quantitative evaluation based on multivariate statistical analysis. *Jpn Circ J* 1980; 44:95–116.
88 Baandrup V, Olsen EGJ: Critical analysis of endomyocardial biopsies from patients suspected of having cardiomyopathy. I: Morphological and morphometric aspects. *Br Heart J* 1981; 45:475–486.
89. Das JP, Rath B, Das S, Sarangi A: Study of endomyocardial biopsies in cardiomyopathy. *Indian Heart J* 1981; 33(1):18–26.
90. Nippoldt TB, Edwards WD, Holmes DR Jr, Reeder GS, Hartzler GO, Smith HC: Right ventricular endomyocardial biopsy. *Mayo Clin Proc* 1982; 57:407–418.
91. Fenoglio JJ Jr, Ursell PC, Kellogg CF, Drusin RE, Weiss MB: Diagnosis and classification of myocarditis by endomyocardial biopsy. *N Engl J Med* 1983; 308:12–18.
92. Unverferth DV, Fetters JK, Unverferth BJ, Leier CV, Magorien RD, Arn AR, et al: Human myocardial histologic characteristics in congestive heart failure. *Circulation* 1983; 68:1194–1200.
93. Parrillo JE, Aretz HT, Palacios I, Fallon JT, Block PC: The results of transvenous endomyocardial biopsy can frequently be used to diagnose myocardial diseases in patients with idiopathic heart failure. *Circulation* 1984; 69:93–101.
94. Zee-Cheng C-S, Tsai CC, Palmer DC, Codd JE, Pennington DG, Williams GA: High incidence of myocarditis by endomyocardial biopsy in patients with idiopathic congestive cardiomyopathy. *J Am Coll Cardiol* 1984; 3:63–70.
95. O'Connell JB, Henkin RE, Robinson JA, Subramanian R, Scanlon PJ, Gunnar RM: Gallium-67 imaging in patients with dilated cardiomyopathy and biopsy-proven myocarditis. *Circulation* 1984; 70:58–62.
96. Daly K, Richardson PJ, Olsen EGJ, Morgan-Capner P, McSorley C, Jackson G, et al: Acute myocarditis. Role of histological and virological examination in the diagnosis and assessment of immunosuppressive treatment. *Br Heart J* 1984; 51:30–35.
97. Rose AG, Fraser RC, Beck W: Absence of evidence of myocarditis in endomyocardial biopsy specimens from patients with dilated (congestive) cardiomyopathy. *S Afr Med J* 1984; 66:871–874.
98. Regitz V, Olsen EGJ, Rudolph W: Histologisch nachweisbare Myokarditis bei Patienten mit eingeschrankter linksventrikularer Funktion. *Herz* 1985; 10:27–35.
99. Dec GW Jr, Palacios IF, Fallon JT, Aretz HT, Mills J, Lee DC-S, et al: Active myocarditis in the spectrum of acute dilated cardiomyopathies. *N Engl J Med* 1985; 312:885–890.
100. Salvi A, Silvestri F, Gori D, Klugmann S, Tanganelli P, Camerini F: La biopsia endomiocardica: un'esperienza relativa a 156 pazienti. *G Ital Cardiol* 1985; 15:251–259.
101. Mortensen SA, Baandrup U, Buch J, Bendtzen K, Hvid-Jacobsen K: Immunosuppressive therapy of biopsy proven myocarditis: Experiences with corticosteroids and cyclosporin. *Int J Immunother* 1985; 1:35–45.
102. Hosenpud JD, McAnulty JH, Niles NR: Lack of objective improvement in ventricular systolic function in patients with myocarditis treated with azathioprine and prednisone. *J Am Coll Cardiol* 1985; 6:797–801.
103. Cassling RS, Linder J, Sears TD, Waller BF, Rogler WC, Wilson JE, et al: Quantitative evaluation of inflammation in biopsy specimens from idiopathically failing or irritable hearts: Experience in 80 pediatric and adult patients. *Am Heart J* 1985; 110:713–720.
104. French WJ, Siegel RJ, Cohen AH, Laks MM: Yield of endomyocardial biopsy in patients with biventricular failure. *Chest* 1986; 90:181–184.
105. Hammond EH, Menlove RL, Anderson JL: Predictive value of immunofluorescence and electron microscopic evaluation of endomyocardial biopsies in the diagnosis and prognosis of myocarditis and idiopathic dilated cardiomyopathy. *Am Heart J* 1987; 114:1055–1065.
106. Maisch B, Bauer E, Hufnagel G, Pfeifer U, Rohkamm R: The use

of endomyocardial biopsy in heart failure. *Eur Heart J* 1988; 9(suppl H):59–71.
107. Chow LC, Dittrich HC, Shabetai R: Endomyocardial biopsy in patients with unexplained congestive heart failure. *Ann Intern Med* 1988; 109:535–539.
108. Leatherbury L, Chandra RS, Shapiro SR, Perry LW: Value of endomyocardial biopsy in infants, children and adolescents with dilated or hypertrophic cardiomyopathy and myocarditis. *J Am Coll Cardiol* 1988; 12:1547–1554.
109. Hobs RE, Pelegrin D, Ratliff NB, Bott-Silverman C, Rincon G, Sterba R, et al: Lymphocytic myocarditis and dilated cardiomyopathy: Treatment with immunosuppressive agents. *Cleve Clin J Med* 1989; 56:628–635.
110. Latham RD, Mulrow JP, Virmani R, Robinowitz M, Moody JM: Recently diagnosed idiopathic dilated cardiomyopathy: Incidence of myocarditis and efficacy of prednisone therapy. *Am Heart J* 1989; 117:876–882.
111. Popma JJ, Cigarroa RG, Buja LM, Hillis LD: Diagnostic and prognostic utility of right-sided catheterization and endomyocardial biopsy in idiopathic dilated cardiomyopathy. *Am J Cardiol* 1989; 63:955–958.
112. Vasiljevic JD, Kanjuh V, Seferovic P, Sesto M, Stojsic D, Olsen EGJ: The incidence of myocarditis in endomyocardial biopsy samples from patients with congestive heart failure. *Am Heart J* 1990; 120:1370–1381.
113. Lieberman EB, Hutchins GM, Herskowitz A, Rose NR, Baughman KL: Clinicopathologic description of myocarditis. *J Am Coll Cardiol* 1991; 18:1617–1626.
114. Strain JE, Grose RM, Factor SM, Fisher JD: Results of endomyocardial biopsy in patients with spontaneous ventricular tachycardia but without apparent structural heart disease. *Circulation* 1983; 68:1171–1181.
115. Vignola PA, Aonuma K, Swaye PS, Rozanski JJ, Blankstein RL, Benson J, et al: Lymphocytic myocarditis presenting as unexplained ventricular arrhythmias: Diagnosis with endomyocardial biopsy and response to immunosuppression. *J Am Coll Cardiol* 1984; 4:812–819.
116. Sugrue DD, Holmes DR Jr, Gersh BJ, Edwards WD, McLaran CJ, Wood DL, et al: Cardiac histologic findings in patients with life-threatening ventricular arrhythmias of unknown origin. *J Am Coll Cardiol* 1984; 4:952–957.
117. Hosenpud JD, McAnulty JH, Niles NR: Unexpected myocardial disease in patients with life threatening arrhythmias. *Br Heart J* 1986; 56:55–61.
118. Tazelaar HD, Billingham ME: Leukocytic infiltrates in idiopathic dilated cardiomyopathy. *Am J Surg Pathol* 1986; 10:405–412.
119. Aretz HT, Billingham ME, Edwards WD, Factor SM, Fallon JT, Fenoglio JJ Jr, et al: Myocarditis. *Am J Cardiovasc Pathol* 1986; 1:3–14.
120. Dec GW, Fallon JT, Southern JF, Palacios I: "Borderline" myocarditis: An indication for repeat endomyocardial biopsy. *J Am Coll Cardiol* 1990; 15:283–289.
121. Spiegelhelter DJ, Stovin TGI: An analysis of repeated biopsies following cardiac transplantation. *Stat Med* 1983; 2:33–40.
122. Chow LH, Radio SJ, Sears TD, McManus BM: Insensitivity of right ventricular endomyocardial biopsy in the diagnosis of myocarditis. *J Am Coll Cardiol* 1989; 14:915–920.
123. Hauck AJ, Kearney DL, Edwards WD: Evaluation of postmortem endomyocardial biopsy specimens from 38 patients with lymphocytic myocarditis: Implications for role of sampling error. *Mayo Clin Proc* 1989; 64:1235–1245.
124. Keogh AM, Billingham ME, Schroeder JS: Rapid histological changes in endomyocardial biopsy specimens after myocarditis. *Br Heart J* 1990; 64:406–408.
125. Billingham ME, Tazelaar HD: The morphological progression of viral myocarditis. *Postgrad Med J* 1986; 62:581–584.
126. Dec GW, Palacios I, Yasuda T, Fallon JT, Khaw BA, Strauss HW, et al: Antimyosin antibody cardiac imaging: Its role in the diagnosis of myocarditis. *J Am Coll Cardiol* 1990; 16:97–104.
127. Gagliardi MG, Bevilacqua M, Di Renzi P, Picardo S, Passariello R, Marcelletti C: Usefulness of magnetic resonance imaging for diagnosis of acute myocarditis in infants and children, and comparison with endomyocardial biopsy. *Am J Cardiol* 1991; 68:1089–1094.
128. Quigley PJ, Richardson PJ, Meany BT, Olsen EGJ, Monaghan MJ, Jackson G, et al: Long-term follow-up of acute myocarditis. Correlation of ventricular function and outcome. *Eur Heart J* 1987; 8(suppl J):39–42.
129. O'Connell JB, Dec GW, Goldenberg IF, Starling RC, Mudge GH, Augustine SM, et al: Results of heart transplantation for active lymphocytic myocarditis. *J Heart Transplant* 1990; 9:351–356.
130. Ilback N-G, Fohlman J, Friman G: Exercise in Coxsackie B3 myocarditis: Effects on heart lymphocyte subpopulations and the inflammatory reaction. *Am Heart J* 1989; 117:1298–1302.
131. Hosenpud JD, Campbell SM, Niles NR, Lee J, Mendelson D, Hart MV: Exercise induced augmentation of cellular and humoral autoimmunity associated with increased cardiac dilatation in experimental autoimmune myocarditis. *Cardiovasc Res* 1987; 21:217–222.
132. Sekiguchi M, Hiroe M, Take M, Hirosawa K: Clinical and histopathological profile of sarcoidosis of the heart and acute idiopathic myocarditis. Concepts through a study employing endomyocardial biopsy. II. Myocarditis. *Jpn Circ J* 1980; 44:264–273.
133. Edwards WD, Holmes DR Jr, Reeder GS: Diagnosis of active lymphocytic myocarditis by endomyocardial biopsy. Quantitative criteria for light microscopy. *Mayo Clin Proc* 1982; 57:419–425.
134. Feneley MP, Gavaghan TP, Ralston M, Hickie JB, Baron DW: Diagnosis and management of acute myocarditis aided by serial myocardial biopsy. *Aust NZ J Med* 1984; 14:826–830.
135. Salvi A, Di Lenarda A, Dreas L, Silvestri F, Camerini F: Immunosuppressive treatment in myocarditis. *Int J Cardiol* 1989; 22:329–338.
136. Chan KY, Iwahara M, Benson LN, Wilson GJ, Freedom RM: Immunosuppressive therapy in the management of acute myocarditis in children: A clinical trial. *J Am Coll Cardiol* 1991; 17:458–460.
137. Jones SR, Herskowitz A, Hutchins GM, Baughman KL: Effects of immunosuppressive therapy in biopsy-proved myocarditis and borderline myocarditis on left ventricular function. *Am J Cardiol* 1991; 68:370–376.
138. Parrillo JE, Cunnion RE, Epstein SE, Parker MM, Suffredini AF, Brenner M, et al: A prospective, randomized, controlled trial of prednisone for dilated cardiomyopathy. *N Engl J Med* 1989; 321:1061–1068.
139. O'Connell JB, Mason JW: The applicability of results of streamlined trials to clinical practice: The Myocarditis Treatment Trial. *Stat Med* 1990; 9:193–197.
140. Miric M, Brkic S, Vircburger M, Keserovic N, Vuckovic S, Kdravkovic M, et al: The effects of interferon-alpha administration on lymphocyte subsets and clinical findings in coxsackie-virus B induced myocarditis. *Iugoslav Physiol Pharmacol Acta* 1988; 24:257–263.
141. Gilbert EM, O'Connell JB, Hammond ME, Renlund DG, Watson FS, Bristow MR: Treatment of myocarditis with OKT3 monoclonal antibody (letter). *Lancet* 1988; 1:759.
142. Sadigursky M, von Kreuter BF, Ling P-Y, Santos-Buch CA: Association of elevated anti-sarcolemma, anti-idiotype antibody levels with the clinical and pathologic expression of chronic Chagas myocarditis. *Circulation* 1989; 80:1269–1276.
143. Higuchi MDL, De Morais CF, Barreto ACP, Lopes EA, Stolf N, Bellotti G, et al: The role of active myocarditis in the development of heart failure in chronic Chagas' disease: A study based on endomyocardial biopsies. *Clin Cardiol* 1987; 10:665–670.
144. Maguire JH, Mott KE, Lehman JS, Hoff R, Muniz TM, Guimaraes AC, et al: Relationship of electrocardiographic abnormalities and seropositivity to *Trypanosoma cruzi* within a rural community in northeast Brazil. *Am Heart J* 1983; 105:287–294.
145. Chiale PA, Halpern MS, Nau GJ, Tambussi AM, Przybylski J, Lazzari JO, et al: Efficacy of amiodarone during long-term treatment of malignant ventricular arrhythmias in patients with chronic chagasic myocarditis. *Am Heart J* 1984; 107:656–665.
146. Luft BJ, Billingham M, Remington JS: Endomyocardial biopsy in the diagnosis of toxoplasmic myocarditis. *Transplant Proc* 1986; 18:1871–1873.
147. Gonwa TA, Capehart JE, Pilcher JW, Alivizatos PA: Cytomegalovirus myocarditis as a cause of cardiac dysfunction in a heart transplant recipient. *Transplantation* 1989; 47:197–199.
148. Steere AC, Batsford WP, Weinberg M, Alexander J, Berger HJ, Wolfson S, et al: Lyme carditis: Cardiac abnormalities of Lyme disease. *Ann Intern Med* 1980; 93(1):8–16.
149. Olson LJ, Okafor EC, Clements IP: Cardiac involement in Lyme disease: Manifestations and management. *Mayo Clin Proc* 1986; 61:745–749.

150. Spry CJF, Tai P-C: The eosinophil in myocardial disease. *Eur Heart J* 1987; 8(suppl J):81–84.
151. Kim CH, Vlietstra RE, Edwards WD, Reeder GS, Gleich GJ: Steroid-responsive eosinophilic myocarditis: Diagnosis by endomyocardial biopsy. *Am J Cardiol* 1984; 53:1472–1473.
152. Davidoff R, Palacios I, Southern J, Fallon JT, Newell J, Dec GW: Giant cell versus lymphocytic myocarditis. A comparison of their clinical features and long-term outcomes. *Circulation* 1991; 83:953–961.
153. Scully RE, Mark EJ, McNeely WF, McNeely BU, Samuel MA: Case records of the Massachusetts General Hospital. *N Engl J Med* 1988; 970–981.
154. Wood R, Commerford PJ, Rose AG, Tooke A: Reversible catecholamine-induced cardiomyopathy. *Am Heart J* 1991; 610–613.
155. Imperato-McGinley J, Gautier T, Ehlers K, Zullo MA, Goldstein DS, Vaughan ED Jr: Reversibility of catecholamine-induced dilated cardiomyopathy in a child with a pheochromocytoma. *N Engl J Med* 1987; 316:793–797.
156. Lundin L. Norheim I, Landelius J, Oberg K, Theodorsson-Norheim E: Carcinoid heart disease: Relationship of circulating vasoactive substances to ultrasound detectable cardiac abnormalities. *Circulation* 1988; 77:264–269.
157. Himelman RB, Schiller NB: Clinical and echocardiographic comparison of patients with the carcinoid syndrome with and without carcinoid heart disease. *Am J Cardiol* 1989; 63:347–352.
158. Lundin L, Obert K, Landelius J, Hansson HE, Wilander E, Theodorsson E: Plasma atrial natriuretic peptide in carcinoid heart disease. *Am J Cardiol* 1989; 63:969–972.
159. Danpure CJ: Recent advances in the understanding, diagnosis, and treatment of primary hyperoxaluria type 1. *J Inherited Metab Dis* 1989; 12:210–224.
160. Boquist L, Lindqvist B, Ostberg Y, Steen L: Primary oxalosis. *Am J Med* 1973; 54:673–681.
161. Rodby RA, Tyszka TS, Williams JW: Reversal of cardiac dysfunction secondary to type 1 primary hyperoxaluria after combined liver-kidney transplantation. *Am J Med* 1991; 90:498–504.
162. Wenger NK, Abelmann WH, Roberts WC: Cardiomyopathy and specific heart muscle disease. In: Hurst JW, Schland RC, Rackley CE, Sonnenblick EH, Wenger NK (eds): *The Heart*, 7th ed. New York, McGraw-Hill, 1990: 1278–1347.
163. Mavrikakis ME, Sfikakis PP, Kontoyannis DA, Antoniades LG, Tsankanikas C: Gout and neurological abnormalities associated with cardiomyopathy in a young man. *Ann Rheum Dis* 1990; 49:942–943.
164. Dabestani A, Child JS, Perloff JK, Figueroa WG, Schelbert HR, Engel TR: Cardiac abnormalities in primary hemochromatosis. *Ann NY Acad Sci* 1988; 526:234–243.
165. Strohmeyer G, Niederau C, Stremmel W: Survival and causes of death in hemochromatosis. *Ann NY Acad Sci* 1988; 526:245–257.
166. Barosi G, Arbustini E, Gavazzi A, Grasso M, Pucci A: Myocardial iron grading by endomyocardial biopsy. A clinicopathologic study on iron overloaded patients. *Eur J Haematol* 1989; 42:382–388.
167. Olson LJ, Edwards WD, Holmes DR, Miller FA, Nordstrom LA, Baldus WP: Endomyocardial biopsy in hemochromatosis: Clinicopathologic correlates in six cases. *J Am Coll Cardiol* 1989; 13:116–120.
168. Weintraub LR, Edwards CQ, Krikker M (eds): *Hemochromatosis: Proceedings of the First International Conference*, vol 526. New York, New York Academy of Sciences, 1988.
169. Edwards CQ, Griffen LM, Goldgar D, Drummond C, Skolnick MH, Kushner JP: Prevalence of hemochromatosis among 11,065 presumably healthy blood donors. *N Engl J Med* 1988; 318:1355–1362.
170. Powell LW, Isselbacher KJ: Hemochromatosis. In: Wilson JD, Braunwald E, Isselbacher KJ, Petersdorf RG, Martin JB, Fauci AS, et al (eds): *Harrison's Principles of Internal Medicine*, 12th ed. New York, McGraw-Hill, 1991: 1825–1829.
171. Cohen AS: Amyloidosis. In: Wilson JD, Braunwald E, Isselbacher KJ, Petersdorf RG, Martin JB, Fauci AS, et al. (eds): *Harrison's Principles of Internal Medicine*, 12th ed. New York, McGraw-Hill, 1991: 1417–1421.
172. Cohen AS: Amyloidosis. *N Engl J Med* 1967; 277:522–530.
173. Kyle RA, Greipp PR: Amyloidosis (AL): Clinical and laboratory features in 229 cases. *Mayo Clin Proc* 1983; 58:665–683.
174. Roberts WC, Waller BF: Cardiac amyloidosis causing cardiac dysfunction: Analysis of 54 necropsy patients. *Am J Cardiol* 1983; 52:137–146.
175. Olson LJ, Gertz MA, Edwards WD, Li Cy, Pellika PA, Holmes DR Jr, et al: Senile cardiac amyloidosis with myocardial dysfunction: Diagnosis by endomyocardial biopsy and immunohistochemistry. *N Engl J Med* 1987; 317:738–742.
176. Nichols WC, Liepnieks JJ, Snyder EL, Benson MD: Senile cardiac amyloidosis associated with homozygosity for a transthyretin variant (ILE-122). *J Lab Clin Med* 1990; 117:175–180.
177. Nordlie M, Sletten K, Husby G, Ranlov PJ: A new prealbumin variant in familial amyloid cardiomyopathy of Danish origin. *Scand J Immunol* 1988; 27:119–122.
178. Gertz MA, Kyle RA, Greipp PR: Response rates and survival in primary systemic amyloidosis. *Blood* 1991; 77:257–262.
179. Pelech T, Fric P, Huslarova A, Jirasek A: Interstitial lymphocytic myocarditis in Whipple's disease. *Lancet* 1991; 337:553–554.
180. McAllister HA Jr, Fenoglio JJ Jr: Cardiac involvement in Whipple's disease. *Circulation* 1975; 52:152–156.
181. Southern JF, Moscicki RA, Margo C, Dickersin GR, Fallot JT, Block KJ: Lymphedema, lymphocytic myocarditis, and sarcoid-like granulomatosis: Manifestation of Whipple's disease. *JAMA* 1989; 261:1467–1470.
182. Roberts WC, McAllister HA, Ferrans VJ: Sarcoidosis of the heart: A clinicopathologic study of 35 necropsy patients and review of 78 previously described necropsy patients. *Am J Med* 1977; 63:86–106.
183. Silverman KJ, Hutchins GM, Bulkley BH: Cardiac sarcoid: A clinicopathologic study of 84 unselected patients with systemic sarcoidosis. *Circulation* 1978; 58:1204–1211.
184. Valantine H, McKenna WJ, Nihoyannopoulos P, Mitchell A, Foale RA, Davies MJ, et al: Sarcoidosis, a pattern of clinical and morphological presentation. *Br Heart J* 1987; 57:256–263.
185. Stein E, Stimmel B, Siltzbach LE: Clinical course of cardiac sarcoidosis. *Ann NY Acad Sci* 1976; 278:470–474.
186. Matsui Y, Iwai K, Tackibana T, Frrie T, Shigematsu N, Izumi T, et al: Clinicopathologic study of fatal cardiac sarcoidosis. *Ann NY Acad Sci* 1976; 278:455–469.
187. Burstow DJ, Tajik J, Bailey KR, DeRemee RA, Taliercio CP: Two-dimensional echocardiographic findings in systemic sarcoidosis. *Am J Cardiol* 1989; 63:478–482.
188. Johns CJ (ed): Tenth International Conference on Sarcoidosis and Other Granulomatous Disorders, New York, vol 465. New York Academy of Sciences, 1986.

Chapter 89

Idiopathic Dilated Cardiomyopathy

Edward M. Gilbert, M.D. ■ *Michael R. Bristow, M.D., Ph.D.*

DEFINITION

Idiopathic dilated cardiomyopathy (IDC) is a disease of unknown etiology that principally affects the myocardium.[1,2] *The diagnosis of IDC is established by the presence of left ventricular dilatation and systolic dysfunction in the absence of congenital, coronary, valvular, hypertensive, or pericardial heart disease.* In some patients the development of IDC is associated with clinical factors such as alcoholism, pregnancy, or a family history of cardiomyopathy.[1,2] However, IDC is distinct from "secondary myocardial diseases" that occur with a specific systemic disorder that may be metabolic, collagen-vascular, infiltrative, neuromuscular, inflammatory, toxic, genetic, or neoplastic in origin (see Chaps. 87, 88, 90, 91, and 96.) There are currently no specific gross anatomic, histologic, or ultrastructural morphologic features that can unequivocally differentiate IDC from other causes of heart failure.[3] Since IDC is defined clinically, it is likely that several specific etiologies are responsible for this condition.

PATHOLOGY

The major morphologic feature of IDC on postmortem examination is dilatation of the cardiac chambers.[3,4] One ventricle (usually the left) may be more dilated than the other ventricle. The weight of the heart is increased in IDC with a mean cardiac weight of 551 g for women and 632 g for men.[4] Although there is an increase in muscle mass and myocyte cell volume in IDC, left ventricular wall thickness is usually not increased because of the marked dilatation of the ventricular cavities. Grossly visible scars may be present in either ventricle. While most scars are small, some may be large and transmural. Scarring occurs in the absence of significant narrowing of the epicardial coronary arteries. In most cases, the degree of fibrosis does not appear to be extensive enough to cause changes in systolic or diastolic function. Intracardiac thrombi and mural endocardial plaques (from the organization of thrombi) are present at necropsy in more than 50 percent of patients with IDC.[3,4] The effect of anticoagulation on the incidence of thrombi has not been carefully studied, but systemic and pulmonary emboli are more frequent in patients with ventricular thrombi or plaques.[4]

The characteristic findings of IDC on microscopy are marked myocyte hypertrophy and very large, bizarre-shaped nuclei[4–7] (Fig. 89-1). Myocyte atrophy and myofilament loss are also seen.[4,8] Myocyte width in IDC is increased compared to normal hearts, but not when compared to valvular heart disease.[5,7] Average myocyte nuclear area is higher in IDC than in either nonfailing controls or valvular heart disease. These morphometric changes in IDC do not correlate with the severity of illness.[7,8] Ultrastructural abnormalities such as mitochondrial changes, T-tubular dilatation, and intracellular lipid droplets may be observed in IDC but can also be observed in other forms of heart disease.[7] There may be interstitial parenchymal and perivascular focal infil-

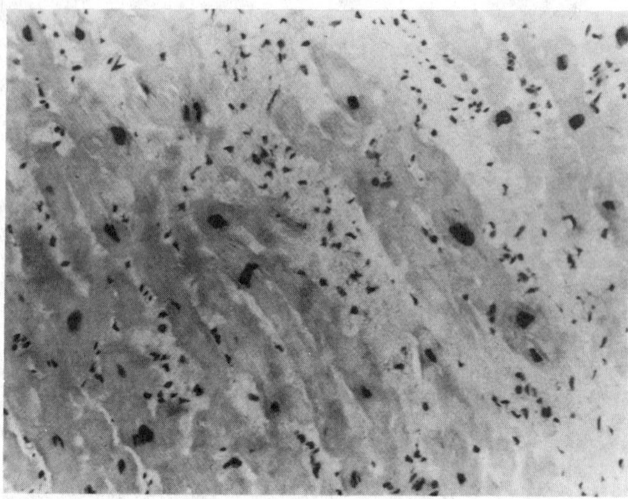

FIGURE 89-1 Endomyocardial biopsy from a patient with IDC (H&E × 200). There is marked myocyte hypertrophy, interstitial fibrosis, and lymphocytic infiltrate. *(From ME Billingham: Histopathological diagnosis of acute myocarditis and dilated cardiomyopathy. In: G Baroldi, F Camerini, Goodwin JF (eds): Advances in Cardiomyopathies. Berlin, Springer-Verlag, 1990. Reproduced with permission from the publisher and author.)*

trates of small lymphocytes.[6–10] The lymphocytic infiltrates present on histologic examination in IDC are not associated with adjacent myocyte damage, in contrast to myocarditis, where adjacent myocyte necrosis is observed. Fibrosis is nearly always present in IDC,[4–10] and its pattern is quite variable from a fine perimyocytic distribution to coarse scars indistinguishable from those present in chronic ischemia. Small intramural arteries and capillaries, however, are normal in IDC.[7]

IMMUNOLOGY

A number of immune regulatory abnormalities have been identified in IDC, including humoral and cellular autoimmune reactivity against myocytes,[11] decreased natural killer cell activity,[12] and abnormal suppressor cell activity.[13,14] These abnormalities suggest that immune defects may be important etiologic factors in the development of IDC. These findings, however, are not universally present in patients with IDC, and some abnormalities are also present in other heart diseases. For example, an increase in the cardioselective M7 antimitochondrial antibodies is found in both IDC and hypertrophic cardiomyopathy but not in heart failure from coronary artery disease.[15] The incidence of some autoreactive antibodies, such as antinuclear and antifibrillary antibodies, increases with the severity of heart failure.[16] It is likely that many of the antibodies detected in IDC and other myocardial diseases do not have pathogenetic relevance. Other antibodies present in IDC may have important functional implications. For example, anti-β_1-adrenergic receptor antibodies could modify β-adrenergic receptor activity.[17]

There has been great interest in histocompatibility locus antigens (HLAs) in IDC since these antigens are known to be associated with immune regulatory functions and many autoimmune diseases are found to have positive HLA antigenic associations. HLA associations have also been identified in IDC; the frequency of HLA-B27, HLA-A2, HLA-DR4, and HLA-DQ4 is increased compared to controls, and the frequency of HLA-DRw6 is decreased compared to controls.[18] Genetic abnormalities in the HLA region could potentially alter immune response and thereby increase disease susceptibility to infectious agents such as enteroviruses. Thus, the association in IDC with specific HLAs suggest a possible immunologic etiology for this disease. These specific HLAs, however, are present in less than 50 percent of patients with IDC, and the heterogeneity of these antigens does not point to a unique site for a putative disease-associated gene. Further investigation will be necessary to understand the significance of these findings.

A clinical and pathologic syndrome that is similar to IDC may develop after resolution of viral myocarditis in animal models and biopsy-proven myocarditis in human subjects.[19] This has led to speculation that IDC may develop in some individuals as a result of subclinical viral myocarditis. Theoretically, an episode of myocarditis could initiate a variety of autoimmune reactions that injure the myocardium and ultimately result in the development of IDC. The abnormalities in immune regulation and the variety of antimyocardial antibodies present in IDC are consistent with this hypothesis. However, it is generally not possible to isolate an infectious virus or to demonstrate the presence of viral antigens in the myocardium of patients with IDC.[20] Enteroviral ribonucleic acid (RNA) sequences are found in heart biopsy samples in IDC, but only in approximately one-third of patients.[21] Furthermore, active myocardial inflammation is usually not detected in IDC.[9,10] Finally, corticosteroid therapy of patients with IDC does not result in significant clinical improvements.[22] Thus, while the viral infection–autoimmune hypothesis is an attractive candidate for the etiology of some cases of IDC, it remains unproven.

THE β-ADRENERGIC PATHWAY IN IDC

There is activation of the adrenergic nervous system in chronic heart failure.[23,23] The changes in adrenergic activity are regional, with increased activity in the heart and kidney but not in the lung or skeletal muscle.[24,25] Direct peripheral nerve recordings have also shown an increase in adrenergic activity in heart failure.[26] Cardiac tissue norepinephrine[27,28] and cardiac adrenergic nerve density[29] are reduced in the failing human heart. Although total cardiac norepinephrine uptake is decreased in failing heart,[25,30,31] norepinephrine "spillover" is increased in the failing human heart.[24] This can occur as a consequence of increased norepinephrine release of individual adrenergic neurons and/or decreased neuronal norepinephrine uptake.[31,32] As a result of these changes, the failing heart becomes a net producer of norepinephrine,[24,31,32] and myocyte exposure to norepinephrine is increased. The signal for this increase in cardiac adrenergic activity is not yet established. (See also Chap. 35.)

Significant alterations in the receptor-G protein-adenylate cyclase (RGC) complex occur in IDC. In severe heart failure, there is a 60 to 70 percent reduction in β_1-receptor density.[33-35] Myocardial β_2-receptor density is not changed in IDC, but β_2-agonist responsiveness is mildly reduced (approximately 30 percent) due to β_2-receptor uncoupling.[33] A 30 to 40 percent increase in the activity of the inhibitory G_i protein is also present in heart failure.[35] Preliminary observations suggest that β_2-receptor uncoupling may be related to the increase in G_i activity. The vasoactive intestinal peptide (VIP) receptor is decreased by approximately 60 percent, but it exhibits increased affinity for VIP, which tends to counteract the effects of VIP receptor down-regulation.[36] The G_s protein function,[35] H_2-histamine receptor,[37] M_2-muscarinic receptor, α-receptor,[34,38] and adenylate cyclase[39] are not significantly altered in IDC. Other mechanisms related to contractility are also entirely normal in end-stage IDC, including the density of calcium antagonist binding sites,[40] maximal tension response to calcium in vitro[41] or in vivo,[42] levels of contractile protein,[43] and creatine kinase activity.[44]

Recent data suggest that abnormalities of the RGC complex vary with the etiology of heart failure.[45] Total β-receptor and β_2-receptor down-regulation are greater in IDC than in postinfarction heart muscle disease, while β-receptor uncoupling is greater in postinfarction heart muscle disease. Although the causes for these differences are not known, one potential explanation is that cardiac adrenergic activity (and therefore myocardial norepinephrine exposure) may be greater in IDC than in postinfarction cardiomyopathy. It also should be emphasized, however, that dysfunction of adrenergic neuroeffector mechanisms is across various types of cardiomyopathy and heart muscle disease. For example, β_1-receptor down-regulation, β_2-receptor uncoupling, and tissue norepinephrine depletion are present in IDC, postinfarction heart muscle disease, and heart failure secondary to pressure overload.[45]

Since the human heart does not appear to have "spare" β-adrenergic receptors,[46,47] the reductions in β_1-receptor density and β_2-receptor affinity in IDC could account for a 50 percent decrease in the response to exogenously administered β agonists.[42,43,47] In contrast, the inotropic response to calcium administration is unchanged[41,42] (Fig. 89-2). While these changes may theoretically serve a "cardioprotective" function, they compromise the ability of the RGC system to support cardiac function in times when increased contractility is desirable. Because of the importance of these changes, the RGC system is a potential target for therapeutic intervention with drugs that modify the β-adrenergic pathway.

INCIDENCE AND PROGNOSIS

The incidence of IDC is estimated at 3 to 10 cases per 100,00, and approximately 20,000 new cases are diagnosed annually in the United States.[48,49] Patients with IDC usually develop progressive deterioration of ventricular function resulting in death from either pump failure or arrhythmia.[49-61] Currently, the 5-year mortality is estimated at 40 to 80 percent.[49-52] A representative survival curve is shown in Fig. 89-3. In the majority of reports, 1-year mortality is about 25 percent and 2-year mortality is about 35 to 40 percent. Some authors have reported, however, that patients who survive more than 2 or 3 years have a relatively good long-term prognosis, and survival curves of such long-term survivors may even parallel survival curves of the general population.[52,54] Stabilization and even spontaneous improvement has been observed in 20 to 50 percent of patients,[50,52,54,61] but complete recovery of cardiac function is rare.

What accounts for the large variability in patient survival in IDC reported by these different authors? Several potential factors can be suggested, including differences in underlying pathogenic mechanism for IDC, differences in duration or severity of disease, as well as differences in medical therapy. Currently, patients with IDC

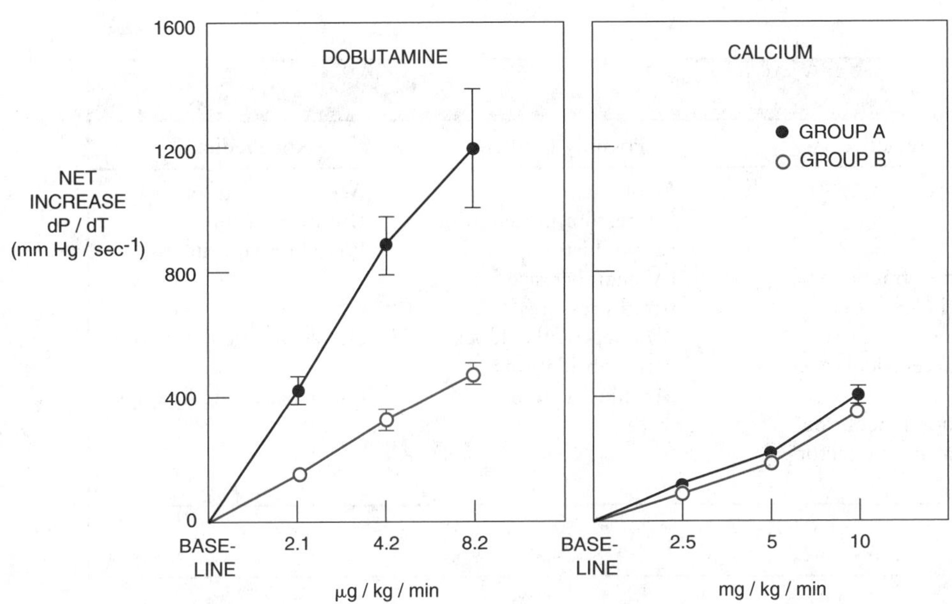

FIGURE 89-2 Peak *dP/dt* responses to dobutamine and to calcium in control subjects with left ventricular ejection fraction above 40 percent (group A) and in patients with IDC and left ventricular ejection fraction below 20 percent and a 50 percent reduction in β-receptor density (group B). *(From MB Fowler, JA Laser, GL Hopkins, et al: Assessment of the β-adrenergic receptor pathway in the intact failing human heart: Progressive receptor down-regulation and subsensitivity to agonist response. Circulation 74:1290, 1986. Reproduced with permission from the publisher and author.)*

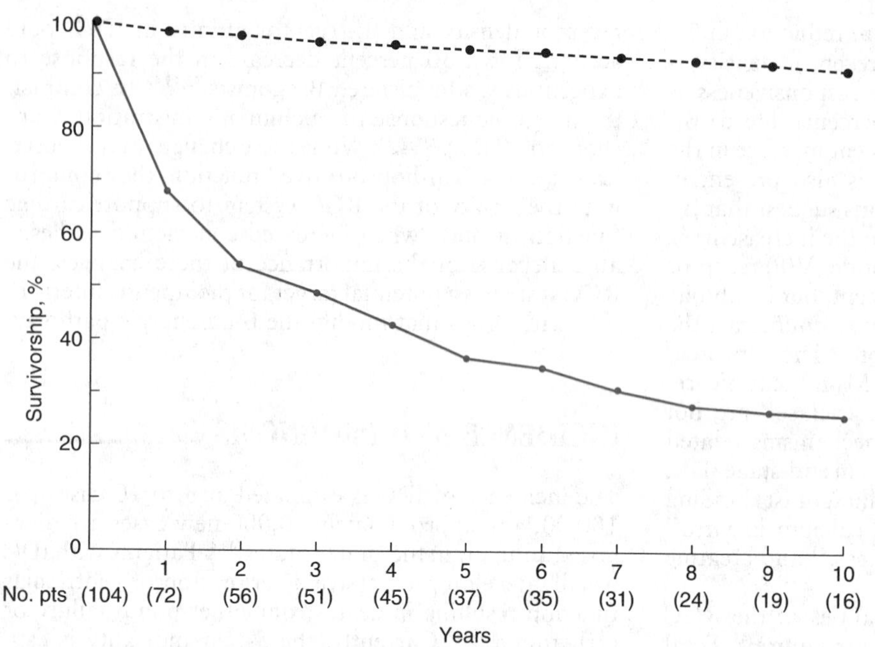

FIGURE 89-3 Observed survival of 104 patients (pts.) with IDC *(solid line)* and their expected survival based on age and sex distribution according to the death rates of the Minnesota 1970 White Population Life Table *(dashed line)*. The number of surviving patients under observation at each follow-up interval is indicated in parentheses. *(From V Fuster, BJ Gersh, ER Giuliani, et al: The natural history of idiopathic dilated cardiomyopathy. Am J Cardiol 47:525, 1981. Reproduced with permission from the publisher and author.)*

are being identified earlier in the course of their disease due to technologic advances in noninvasive cardiac imaging and a greater awareness of the disease among clinicians. Recent advances in medical therapy may also produce a favorable-effect on long-term outcome. Thus, the patient with IDC in the 1990s may have a better prognosis than patients reported in the literature. An understanding of factors that affect prognosis in IDC is important for proper patient management and may also improve our understanding of the pathophysiological processes involved in the progression of disease. Several authors have analyzed the impact of several clinical, hemodynamic, laboratory, and histologic parameters on survival in IDC. The prognostic significance of these parameters is summarized in Table 89-1.

Some cases of "idiopathic" dilated cardiomyopathy are familial and presumably genetic in etiology.[2,3] (See Chap. 96.) Several authors have reported that the survival of patients with familial cardiomyopathy does not differ from other patients with IDC.[50,54,55] Although spontaneous improvements have been reported for patients with biopsy-proven myocarditis,[62] preceding viral illness does not appear to affect overall survival in patients with IDC.[54,55] Prognosis in peripartum cardiomyopathy is good when there is early improvement in cardiomegaly and heart failure and poor when spontaneous improvement is not observed.[52,54,55,60,63] (See also Chap. 113.)

Heart muscle disease has been associated with alcoholism,[1,2,64] but the presence of alcohol abuse does not appear to influence survival in many studies.[50,52,54] Abstention from alcohol has been associated with a more favorable clinical course in some reports.[8,60,64] (See Chap. 105.) Age[50,54,55,61,65] or the duration of symptoms of heart failure[54–56,65] have not been found to predict survival in the majority of reports. Most investigators using univariate analysis have observed that patients with more severe

TABLE 89-1
Predicting Prognosis in IDC

	Predictive	Possibly Predictive	Not Predictive
Clinical factors	Symptoms	Alcoholism Peripartum presentation Family history	Age Duration of illness Preceding viral illness
Hemodynamic factors	LV ejection fraction Cardiac index	LV chamber size Atrial pressures	
Dysrrhythmia	LV conduction delay Complex ventricular ectopy	Atrioventricular block Atrial fibrillation	Simple ventricular ectopy
Histologic morphology		Myofibril volume	Other histologic findings
Neuroendocrine factors	Plasma norepinephrine* Atrial natriuretic factor* Hyponatremia*		

LV = left ventricular.
*Identified as prognostic factors for all causes of heart failure.

functional impairment have a higher mortality risk.[50,56,67,65] This finding was confirmed using multivariate analysis by Costanzo-Nordin et al.[65] but not by Unverferth et al.[55]

Left ventricular enlargement has been reported to correlate with poor prognosis in IDC by most authors using univariate analysis,[50,52–54,58,59] but not by authors using multivariate analysis.[53,55,61,65] The severity of left ventricular dysfunction appears to be a better predictor of prognosis. Left ventricular ejection fraction is significantly lower in patients who die from IDC,[50,53–55,57,59,61,65] and it has been found to be an independent predictor of survival by multivariate analysis by Hofmann et al.[53] and Keogh et al.[61] but not by Unverferth et al.[55] or Costanzo-Nordin et al.[65] Cardiac index, another measure of left ventricular function, has also been shown to correlate with clinical outcome in IDC in the majority of reports.[50,52,53,58,60,65] Multivariate analysis identified cardiac index as an independent prognostic factor in the studies of Hofmann et al.[53] and Costanzo-Nordin et al.[65] but not in studies of Unverferth et al.[55] or Keogh et al.[61] The impact of left ventricular diastolic function on survival has been indirectly assessed using left ventricular end-diastolic pressure or pulmonary artery wedge pressure. Higher filling pressures have been observed in patients who died from IDC in the majority of reports.[50,52,54,55,57,58,65] Patients who die from IDC also have higher right atrial and pulmonary artery pressures than survivors.[55,59]

Atrioventricular and intraventricular conduction abnormalities are frequently observed in IDC. Convert et al.[57] observed an increase in mortality in patients with atrioventricular conduction abnormalities (43 versus 23 percent), but others have not confirmed their findings. Intraventricular conduction abnormalities, in particular left bundle branch block, have frequently been identified as predicting a poor prognosis[50,53,57,66] but has not been a significant factor in all reports.[65] Unverferth et al.[55] found that the presence of left-sided conduction abnormalities were the most prominent factor for predicting 1-year mortality by multivariate analyses. The impact of atrial fibrillation on survival is controversial. Many authors[53,55,59] have reported that patients with atrial fibrillation have a worse prognosis, but others have not found this association,[50,65] and Convert et al.[57] observed that patients with sinus rhythm had a worse prognosis than patients with atrial fibrillation.

It is well recognized that ventricular arrhythmias are common in patients with IDC,[58] but their significance remains controversial. Many authors have reported that the incidence of sudden death is increased in patients with ventricular arrhythmias.[58,67] Patients with both complex ventricular arrhythmias and a reduced left ventricular ejection fraction appear to have the greatest risk for sudden death.[58] Patients with complex ventricular arrhythmias also have an increased incidence of deaths from heart failure.[53,55,59,67] Using multivariate analysis, Olshauser et al.[66] found that complex ventricular arrhythmias were an independent risk factor for death from heart failure but not for sudden death. Programmed electrical ventricular stimulation has been evaluated in IDC in an attempt to define better which patients are at risk for sudden death.[68,69] Ventricular tachycardia or fibrillation can be induced in approximately 40 percent of patients without symptomatic ventricular arrhythmias.[68] Inducibility of polymorphic ventricular tachycardia or ventricular fibrillation does not correlate with clinical or hemodynamic variables or with the risk of sudden death.[68] The induction of unimorphic ventricular tachycardia, however, does appear to predict the later occurrence of spontaneous unimorphic ventricular tachycardia.[68] Sustained, uniform ventricular tachycardia can be induced in most patients presenting with this arrhythmia, but it is unusual to induce ventricular tachycardia in patients who presented with cardiac arrest or nonsustained ventricular tachycardia.[69] Patients who have inducible ventricular tachycardia that is suppressed by antiarrhythmic therapy have a good prognosis, while patients with inducible ventricular tachycardia that is not suppressed by therapy are likely to die suddenly.[69]

The prognostic significance of morphologic features on endomyocardial biopsy have also been evaluated by several authors.[6,55,61,70,71] Unverferth et al.[55] reported that cell diameter, endocardial thickness, and percent fibrosis were not significantly different between survivors and nonsurvivors. Baandrup and Olsen[6] studied morphologic variations in biopsy materials from 125 patients with IDC and found that neither the severity nor the prognosis of patients with IDC could be assessed from histologic changes. Keogh et al.[61] also found no significant histologic differences in the endomyocardial biopsy specimens of survivors and nonsurvivors. Figulla et al.[70] found no relationship between hemodynamic status and myofibril volume fraction using light microscopy. A 60 percent reduction in myofibril volume fraction, however, predicted the occurrence of both hemodynamic deterioration and death. Using electron microscopy, Hammond et al.[71] graded myofilament loss and found an increase in mortality at 18 months for patients with extensive myofilament loss. Confirmation by other investigators will be necessary to establish the clinical usefulness of estimates of myofibril loss on endomyocardial biopsy. Moreover, endomyocardial biopsy yields only a limited amount of tissue that may not be representative of the whole heart.

Neuroendocrine activation occurs in patients with left ventricular dysfunction and congestive heart failure.[72,73] Patients with heart failure who have the most marked elevation of plasma catecholamines have the most unfavorable long-term prognosis.[73,74] Patients with heart failure who die within 6 months of evaluation have significantly higher venous plasma concentrations of angiotensin II, aldosterone, atrial natriuretic factor, norepinephrine, and epinephrine than patients who survive beyond 6 months.[74] The presence of hyponatremia is also a powerful predictor of cardiovascular mortality.[75] It is likely that hyponatremia is related to the marked elevation in plasma renin activity observed in these patients. Such abnormalities may also be viewed as a marker per se of the severity of the heart failure. The poor prognosis of heart failure patients with elevated neuroendocrine hormones or hyponatremia is improved somewhat with the administration of angiotensin converting enzyme (ACE) inhibitors.[73,74] (See Chap. 26.)

CLINICAL MANIFESTATIONS

Patients of all ages may develop IDC with the highest incidence found in middle age.[4] Symptoms often develop gradually in IDC, and some patients may be asymptomatic for months or years. Other patients with IDC present with a sudden onset of symptoms, frequently after some clinical event that has increased cardiac demands such as surgery or systemic infection. In young adults this initial acute presentation may be incorrectly diagnosed as "pneumonia" since heart disease is usually not expected in this age group. While it is attractive to attribute the rapid onset of heart failure to an acute process such as myocarditis, it is uncommon to find specific myocardial diseases on endomyocardial biopsy.[19]

History and Physical Examination

Most symptoms of IDC are caused by heart failure (see Chaps. 25 and 26). These include symptoms from pulmonary congestion (e.g., dyspnea on exertion, orthopnea, paroxysmal nocturnal dyspnea, and dyspnea at rest), systemic congestion (e.g., peripheral edema, nausea and abdominal pain from hepatic congestion, and nocturia), and low cardiac output (e.g., fatigue and weakness). Angina pectoris may be present even though coronary arteries are normal. Symptoms of lightheadedness, dizziness, or syncope may occur from arrhythmias or drug-related orthostatic hypotension. Some patients with severely reduced left ventricular ejection fraction may have very few symptoms of congestive failure.

The findings on physical examination are nonspecific and are related to the hemodynamic abnormalities of heart failure (see Chap. 26). Blood pressure may be normal when heart failure is well compensated, but with progression of left ventricular dysfunction the pulse pressure narrows, pulsus alternans appears, and hypotension develops. Resting tachycardia is common. Peripheral edema develops in the presence of salt and water retention. Cool, pale, or cyanotic extremities with delayed capillary refill and constricted peripheral veins suggest poor peripheral perfusion. Although less impressive to the novice observer than edema, physical signs of poor peripheral perfusion are of greater clinical importance since such findings indicate that cardiac output is severely reduced. When pulmonary congestion is present, patients may develop tachypnea, breathlessness, pulmonary rales, wheezing, and physical signs of pleural effusion. Jugular venous distension and hepatomegaly are found when right-sided heart pressures are elevated. (Chap. 10). The left ventricular impulse may be laterally displaced and a right ventricular impulse may be present on palpation. Gallop sounds and the murmurs of mitral and tricuspid regurgitation are frequently audible (Chap. 11).

Laboratory Examination

Cardiomegaly is the typical feature of IDC on chest roentgenogram. With the development of pulmonary venous hypertension, there may be pulmonary venous redistribution, interstitial edema, and alveolar edema. Dilation of the azygos vein and superior vena cava may be observed with the development of systemic venous hypertension. Pleural effusions may also be present (Chap. 14). There are no "typical" electrocardiographic findings in IDC.[76] Sinus tachycardia is common, and atrial and ventricular arrhythmias or atrioventricular conduction abnormalities may be observed. Intraventricular conduction abnormalities (including bundle branch blocks) and ST-segment and T-wave changes are common. Some patients will present with poor precordial R-wave progression and even with Q waves that mimic old myocardial infarction. As discussed above, arrhythmias are frequently recorded on ambulatory electrocardiogram.

The echocardiogram is an excellent tool for the evaluation of IDC.[77] Two-dimensional study may show left-sided or four-chamber dilatation. Mitral and tricuspid regurgitation are frequently seen with Doppler evaluation. Left ventricular and septal wall thickness are usually normal. A pericardial effusion may be present. In most cases of IDC there is global left ventricular hypokinesis, but some individuals will have segmental wall motion abnormalities. (See Chap. 15.) These findings can also be observed with radionuclide ventriculography[78] and left ventricular angiography. Hemodynamic findings are typical for left ventricular or biventricular failure (see Chap. 23). Coronary arteriography generally shows normal coronary arteries, but older patients may have "incidental" coronary artery lesions (stenosis below 50 percent of luminal diameter). The diagnosis of IDC, however, cannot be made in the presence of significant coronary artery disease.

MANAGEMENT OF IDC

Diagnostic Studies

Diagnostic studies can be used to establish the diagnosis of IDC, evaluate prognosis, and direct medical therapy. All patients should be evaluated with a complete history and physical examination, chest x-ray, electrocardiogram, and echocardiogram with Doppler. These studies will identify most known causes of heart failure. Patients older than 40 years of age or who have a history suggestive of ischemia or a high coronary risk profile should also undergo coronary angiography to exclude coronary disease. A 24-h ambulatory electrocardiogram should be considered when patients complain of lightheadedness or palpitations. Exercise tolerance testing is useful in selected patients for assessment of functional capacity.

Endomyocardial biopsy is frequently performed in patients with unexplained heart failure since this procedure is the only accurate technique for the diagnosis of myocarditis and infiltrative cardiomyopathies. (See also Chap. 33.) This interest in diagnosing myocarditis is based on anecdotal reports that patients with biopsy-proven myocarditis may respond to immunosuppressive therapy.[19] Until clinical trails have established that immunosuppression is effective for the treatment of myocarditis, however, the role of endomyocardial biopsy in the evaluation of IDC remains undefined. Although infiltrative cardiomyopathies such as sarcoidosis or hemosiderosis may respond to specific treatment, the results from endomyocardial biopsy will alter therapy in only 10 percent of cases of unexplained dilated cardiomyopathy.

Medical Therapy

Medical therapy of IDC is directed at controlling the heart failure state. This is accomplished by controlling salt and water retention, reducing the workload on the heart, and improving its pumping performance. Patients should be counseled to limit their physical activities based on their functional capacity and to reduce their dietary intake of sodium. Most patients with congestive symptoms will need the salt restriction of a 2-g Na (5g Na Cl) diet. Patients with significant hyponatremia should also restrict fluid intake. (See also Chap. 26.)

Diuretic therapy must be individualized to account for variations in intravascular volume and renal function. Inadequate diuretic therapy will result in symptomatic pulmonary and systemic venous congestion. Excess diuresis will result in azotemia and electrolyte disorders and will ultimately decrease cardiac output. While the physical examination is usually adequate for the assessment of a patient's intravascular volume, right-sided heart catheterization may occasionally be necessary to guide therapy. Patients should be instructed to record their weights daily so that diuretic doses can be changed in response to weight changes that usually occur prior to the development of frank symptoms. Serum electrolytes, including magnesium, should be carefully monitored with diuretic therapy.

Loop diuretics such as furosemide or bumetanide are the agents of choice when dietary measures are not adequate for controlling congestive failure.[78] Thiazide diuretics are frequently ineffective at the low glomerular filtration rates that occur with heart failure.[79] Most patients receiving diuretics will also require potassium supplementation and/or the addition of a potassium-sparing diuretic such as amiloride to maintain serum potassium above 4.5 meq/dl. (See also Chap. 29.) When patients are refractory to loop diuretic therapy alone, the addition of metolazone can result in marked diuresis. Metolazone is a potent long-acting diuretic whose site of action is primarily the cortical diluting segment and secondarily the proximal tubule.[79,80] Metolazone is unique among the thiazide class of diuretics because it is the only thiazide diuretic that is effective when the glomerular filtration rate is less than 25 mL/min. Combined therapy with furosemide and metolazone therapy should be initiated with caution because of the potential for excessive diuresis and electrolyte loss. Very careful follow-up and monitoring are necessary because of the hazards of electrolyte imbalance and excessive volume contraction with this regimen. (See also Chap. 26.)

Vasodilator therapy reduces the workload of the heart and improves pumping performance. The ACE inhibitors and the combination of hydralazine and isosorbide dinitrate are the two established effective vasodilator regimens. (See also Chaps. 26 and 30.) Therapy with ACE inhibitors[81] or the combination of hydralazine and isosorbide dinitrate[82] also improves survival in heart failure. The ACE inhibitors also have important neuroendocrine effects in addition to their vasodilator activity. Treatment of heart failure with ACE inhibitors reduces circulating norepinephrine.[83] In addition, patients experience less hypokalemia and less hyponatremia on ACE inhibitor therapy.[84] Vasodilator therapy should be initiated at low dose and titrated upward with careful observation for orthostatic hypotension. Hypotension is most frequently observed in volume-depleted patients. Therefore, it is necessary to assess carefully intravascular volume status and, when necessary, to correct relative hypovolemia prior to initiation of vasodilator therapy. Downward adjustment of a diuretic dose is frequently required.

Digitalis is a complex drug, and observed beneficial clinical responses in heart failure may be related to a variety of properties, not just its positive inotropic effects. Digitalis is the undisputed drug of choice for the control of ventricular rate in atrial fibrillation. In the presence of atrial flutter, relatively large amounts of digitalis may be needed to control the ventricular rate if the rhythm does not change to atrial fibrillation. The use of digoxin in heart failure with sinus rhythm has been more controversial. (See Chap. 27.) Three recent randomized drug trials[85–87] have shown that digitalis improves ejection fraction, exercise tolerance, and clinical symptoms compared to placebo. Digitalis therapy is also associated with arrhythmias, however, particularly in patients with hypokalemia or hypomagnesemia. It is our practice to use digoxin in sinus rhythm when cardiomegaly and left ventricular systolic dysfunction are present and heart failure symptoms have not been readily controlled with diuretics and vasodilators. It is important to follow digoxin and serum electrolyte concentrations to avoid lethal arrhythmias of digitalis toxicity.

Because of the risk for pulmonary and systemic emboli, it is our practice to initiate warfarin anticoagulation in patients with left ventricular mural thrombi, atrial fibrillation, left ventricular ejection fraction below 20 percent, New York Heart Association (NYHA) functional class IV symptoms, or history of systemic embolic disease. Anticoagulant therapy must be carefully monitored, with warfarin dose adjusted to maintain the international normalized ratio (INR) at 2 to 3. (See also Chap. 68.)

Treatment of arrhythmias in IDC is a difficult problem, and the roles for antiarrhythmic drugs, use of electrophysiological testing to guide therapy, and use of the automatic implantable defibrillator still need to be defined. The most important steps in the management of arrhythmia are to correct hypoxia, electrolyte, and acid-base abnormalities and to treat heart failure. Antiarrhythmic medications have not been shown to improve survival in IDC. Virtually all antiarrhythmic drugs have at least some negative inotropic effects. In addition, most antiarrhythmic drugs are also potentially proarrhythmic, particular in patients with severe heart failure. Because of these problems, it is our practice to reserve antiarrhythmic therapy to patients with sustained ventricular tachycardia, syncope, or sudden death. Therapy for these patients is guided by electrophysiological study. An automatic implantable defibrillator should be considered in such patients if they do not have inducible sustained ventricular tachycardia or if they have sustained ventricular tachycardia that is not suppressed with antiarrhythmic therapy.

β-Adrenergic Blockade

The morbidity and mortality of IDC remains very high despite the therapeutic interventions described above. Thus, alternative therapeutic approaches must be developed to improve the natural history of IDC. One promising new, but still investigational, approach to therapy of IDC is β-adrenergic blockade.[88] The potential mechanisms for benefit from β blockade include protection from catecholamine toxicity, up-regulation of myocardial β-adrenergic receptors, reduction in sudden death, reduction in heart rate, improved ventricular diastolic function, and reduction in afterload via indirect mechanisms such as a reduction in renin.

Beginning with the report by Waagstein et al. in 1975,[89] several investigators have suggested that long-term β blockade may improve hemodynamic function, clinical symptoms, and survival in patients with IDC. Although data from controlled trials are limited and some reports have been negative, recent studies of β-adrenergic blockade have been very encouraging. In a placebo-controlled study, Engelmeier et al.[90] administered metoprolol to 21 patients with IDC. Metoprolol-treated patients had significant improvements in exercise capacity, NYHA functional classification, and left ventricular ejection fraction. These changes were not observed in control patients receiving placebo. Gilbert et al.[91] reported on a controlled study of the β-blocker/vasodilator bucindolol. Patients treated with bucindolol had significant improvements in resting hemodynamic function and rest and exercise left ventricular ejection fraction and a reduction in questionnaire-measured symptoms and NYHA functional class (Fig. 89-4).

Therapy with β-adrenergic blockers can be successfully initiated in most patients with IDC and heart failure (95 percent of patients tolerated β blockade in the metoprolol and bucindolol studies cited above). Clinical experience suggests that β_1-selective antagonists (such as metoprolol) or β-antagonists with vasodilator properties (such as bucindolol or carvedilol) are better tolerated than nonselective β antagonists such as propranolol. In our experience, significant improvement in left ventricular ejection fraction and clinical symptoms occur in greater than 50 percent of patients treated with β-blocking agents.[92] However, β-blocker therapy must be initiated at very low doses, and the dose must be tritrated upward very slowly.

The mechanisms for these improvements are still under investigation. Protection from the cardiotoxic effects of chronic adrenergic stimulation appears to be an important factor. This is supported by the observation that systemic norepinephrine, which is a marker of systemic adrenergic activity, is significantly higher in responders than in nonresponders to β-blocker therapy.[92] Chronic β blockade can increase myocardial β-adrenergic receptor density and β-agonist responsiveness and thus improve maximal exercise tolerance;[42] however, improvements in left ventricular function can occur in the absence of β-receptor up-regulation.[92] Reduction in resting heart rate may not be a major mechanism for the observed improvement in hemodynamic function, since neither baseline heart rate nor the change in heart rate with β blockade differentiates responders from nonresponders.[92] Further study is needed to define the mechanisms responsible for the observed improvements.

There is also suggestive evidence that survival may increase with chronic β-blocker therapy. Swedberg et al.[94] reported that the survival of IDC patients treated with β blockers was significantly greater than retrospective controls. Anderson et al.[95] randomized 50 patients with IDC in pairs to receive standard therapy alone or

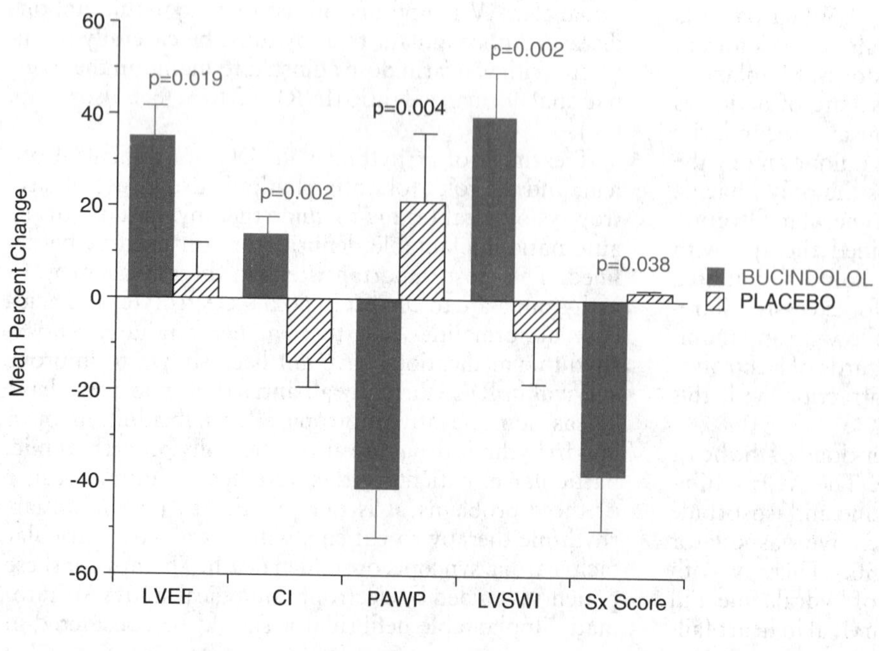

FIGURE 89-4 Mean percent change from baseline in selected functional measures in patients treated with bucindolol *(solid bars)* and placebo *(hatched bar)*. LVEF = resting radionuclide left ventricular ejection fraction; CI = cardiac index; PAWP = pulmonary artery wedge pressure; LVSWI = left ventricular stroke work index; Sx Score = heart failure symptom score (negative value = improvement). Values are given as mean ± SEM. *(From EM Gilbert, JL Anderson, D Deitchman, et al: Long-term β-blocker vasodilator therapy improves cardiac function in idiopathic dilated cardiomyopathy. Am J Med 88:223, 1990. Reproduced with permission from the publisher and author.)*

therapy including metoprolol. A trend toward improved survival was noted for metoprolol-treated patients, but the differences were not significant. These initial reports are encouraging, but results from large randomized trials are needed. The β blockers have not been approved for the treatment of IDC by the Food and Drug Administration. Therefore, the use of β blockers for this purpose cannot be recommended outside the context of controlled clinical trials.

Cardiac Transplantation

With improved understanding of donor and recipient selection, the establishment of an aggressive approach to the treatment of infections, the development of endomyocardial biopsy to diagnose accurately acute cardiac allograft rejection, and improved immunosuppression, 1-year survival for cardiac transplant recipients now exceeds 85 percent.[96] The survival of carefully selected transplant recipients far exceeds the survival of similar patients who are not transplanted. Transplantation is an important option in the management of IDC since so many patients are young or middle-age adults, and patients with advanced NYHA class III or class IV symptoms refractory to medical management should be considered for transplantation (see Chap. 32).

REFERENCES

1. Shabetal R: Cardiomyopathy: How far have we come in 25 years, how far yet to go? *J Am Coll Cardiol* 1983; 1:252–263.
2. Johnson RA, Palacios I: Dilated cardiomyopathies of the adult. *N Engl J Med* 1982; 307:1051–1058.
3. Silver MA: Anatomy of the failing heart in dilated cardiomyopathy. In: Engelmeier RS, I'Connel JB (eds): *Drug Therapy in Dilated Cardiomyopathy and Myocarditis.* New York, Marcel Dekker, 1988: 1–12.
4. Roberts WC, Siegel RJ, McManus BM. Idiopathic dilated cardiomyopathy: Analysis of 152 necropsy patients. *Am J Cardiol* 1987; 60:1340–1355.
5. Rowan R, Maesk MA, Billingham ME: Ultrastructural morphometric analysis of endomyocardial biopsies. *Am J Cardiovasc Pathol* 1988; 2:137–144.
6. Baandrup U, Olsen EG: Critical analysis of endomyocardial biopsies from patients suspected of having cardiomyopathy. *Br Heart J* 1981; 45:475–486.
7. Arbustini E, Pucci R, Pozzi R, Grasso M. Graziano G, Campani C: Ultrastructural changes in myocarditis and dilated cardiomyopathy. In: Baroldi G, Camerini F, Goodwin JF (eds): *Advances in Cardiomyopathies.* Berlin, Springer-Verlag, 1990: 274–289.
8. Schwaetz F, Mall G, Zebe H, et al: Determinants of survival in patients with congestive cardiomyopathy: Quantitative morphologic findings and left ventricular hemodynamics. *Circulation* 1984; 70:923–928.
9. Tazelaar HD, Billingham ME: Leukocytic infiltrates in idiopathic dilated cardiomyopathy. *Am J Surg Pathol* 1986; 10:405–412.
10. Hammond EH, Anderson JL, Menlove RL: Diagnostic and prognostic value of immunofluorescence and electron-microscopic findings in idiopathic dilated cardiomyopathy. In: Bavoldi G, Camerini F, Goodwin JF (eds): *Advances in Cardiomyopathies*, 1st ed. Berlin, Springer-Verlag, 1990: 290–301.
11. Kawai C, Takatsu T: Clinical and experimental studies on cardomyopathy. *N Engl J Med* 1975; 293:592–597.
12. Anderson JL, Carlquist JF, Hammond EH: Deficient natural killer cell activity in patients with idiopathic dilated cardiomyopathy. *Lancet* 1982; 2:1124–1127.
13. Fowles RE, Bieker CP, Stinson EB: Defective in vitro suppressor cell function in idiopathic congestive cardiomyopathy. *Circulation* 1979; 59:483–491.
14. Gerli R, Rambotti P, Spinozzi F, et al. Immunologic studies of peripheral blood from patients with idiopathic dilated cardiomyopathy. *Am Heart J* 1986; 112:350–355.
15. Klein R, Maisch B, Kochsiek K, Berg PA: Demonstration of organ specific antibodies against heart mitochondria (anti-M) in sera from patients with some forms of heart disease. *Clin Exp Immunol* 1984; 58:283–292.
16. Maisch B, Deeg P, Liebau G, Kichsiek K: Diagnostic relevance of humoral and cytotoxic immune reactions in primary and secondary dilated cardiomyopathy. *Am J Cardiol* 1983; 52:1071–1078.
17. Limas CJ, Goldenberg IF, Limas C: Autoantibodies against B-adrenoreceptors in human idiopathic dilated cardiomyopathy. *Circ Res* 1989; 64:97–103.
18. Anderson JL, Carlquist JF, Lutz JR, et al: HLA A, B, and DR typing in idiopathic dilated cardiomyopathy: A search for immune response function. *Am J Cardiol* 1984; 33:1326–1330.
19. Gilbert EM, Mason JW: Immunosuppressive therapy of myocarditis. In: Engelmeier RS, O'Connell JB (eds): *Drug Therapy in Dilated Cardiomyopathy and Myocarditis.* New York, Marcel Dekker, 1987; 233–263.
20. Archard LC, Freeke CA, Richardson PJ, Olsen EGJ: Persistence of enterovirus RNA in dilated cardiomyopathy: A progression from myocarditis. In: Shultheis HP (ed): *New Concepts in Viral Heart Disease.* Berlin, Springer-Verlag, 1989: 347–359.
21. Bowles NE, Richardson PJ, Olsen ECJ, Archard LC: Detection of Coxsackie-B virus specific RNA sequences in myocardial biopsy samples from patients with myocarditis and dilated cardiomyopathy. *Lancet* 1986; 1:1120–1128.
22. Parrillo JE, Cunnion RE, Epstein SE, Parker MF, Suffredini AF, Brenner M, et al: A prospective, randomized, controlled trial of prednisone for dilated cardiomyopathy. *N Engl J Med* 1989; 321:1061–1067.
23. Swedberg K, Viquerat C, Fouleau JL, Reizen M, Atherton B, Parmley WW, et al: Comparison of myocardial catecholamine balance in chronic congestive heart failure and in angina pectoris without failure. *Am J Cardiol* 1984; 54:783–786.
24. Hasking GJ, Esler MD, Jennings GL, Burton D, Johns JA, Mark AL: Norepinephrine spill-over to plasma in patients with congestive heart failure. *Circulation* 1986; 73:615–621.
25. Rose CP, Burgess JH, Cousineau D: Reduced aortocoronary sinus extraction of epinephrine in patients with left ventricular failure secondary to long-term pressure or volume overload. *Circulation* 1983; 68:241–244.
26. Leimbach WN, Wallin BG, Victor RG, Aylward PE, Schedlöf G. Mark AL: Direct evidence from intraneural recordings for increased central sympathetic outflow in patients with heart failure. *Circulation* 1986; 73:913–919.
27. Braunwald D, Harrison DC, Chidsey CA: The heart as an endocrine organ. *Am J Med* 1964; 36:1–4.
28. Pierpont GL, Francis GS, DeMaster EG, et al: Heterogeneous myocardial catecholamine concentrations in patients with congestive heart failure. *Am J Cardiol* 1987; 60:316–321.
29. Pickrell J, Hammond E, Larrabee P, et al: Comparison of sympathetic innervation of failing and nonfailing human hearts by quantitative evaluation of catecholamine fluorescence (abstract). *J Am Coll Cardiol* 1991; 17:220A.
30. Petch MC, Nayler WG: Uptake of catecholamines by human cardiac muscle in vitro. *Br Heart J* 1979; 41:336–339.
31. Rose CP, Buargess JH, Cousineau D: Tracer norepinephrine kinetics in coronary circulation of patients with heart failure secondary to chronic pressure and volume overload. *J Clin Invest* 1985; 76:1740–1747.
32. Sandoval AB, Gilbert EM, Rose CP, Bristow MR: Cardiac norepinephrine uptake and release is decreased in dilated cardiomyopathy (abstract). *Circulation* 1989; 80:II–393A.
33. Bristow MR, Ginsburg R, Fowler M, Umans V, Minobe W, Rasmussen R, et al: β_1 and β_2-adrenergic receptor subpopulations in normal and failing human ventricular myocardium. *Circ Res* 1986; 59:297–309.
34. Brodde OE, Schuler S, Kretsch R, et al: Regional distribution of β-adrenoceptors in the human heart. *J Cardiovasc Pharmacol* 1986; 8:1235–1242.
35. Feldman AM, Cates AE, Veazey WB, Hershberger RE, Bristow MR, Baughman KL: Increase of the 40,000-mol wt pertussis toxin substrate (G protein) in the failing human heart. *J Clin Invest* 1988; 82:189–197.

36. Hershberger RE, Anderson FL, Bristow MR: Vasoactive intestinal peptide receptor in failing human ventricular myocardium exhibits increased affinity and decreased density. *Circ Res* 1989; 65:283–294.
37. Bristow MR, Cubicciotti R, Ginsburg R, Stinson EB, Johnson C: Histamine mediated adenylate cyclase stimulation in human myocardium. *Mol Pharmacol* 1982; 21:671–679.
38. Bohm M, Diet F, Feiler G, Kemkes B, Erdmann E: α-Adrenoceptors and α-adrenoceptors-mediated positive inotropic effects in failing human myocardium. *J Cardiovasc Pharmacol* 1988; 12:357–364.
39. Kessler PD, Van Dop C, Feldman AM: G Proteins: Transmembrane signal processors in the heart. *Heart Failure* 1988; 3:239–247.
40. Rasmussen RP, Minobe W, Bristow MR: Calcium antagonist binding sites in failing and nonfailing human ventricular myocardium. *Biochem Pharmacol* 1990; 39(4):691–696.
41. Ginsburg R, Bristow MR, Billingham ME, Stinson EB, Schroeder JS, Harrison DC: Study of the normal and failing isolated human heart: Decreased response of failing heart to isoproterenol. *Am Heart J* 1983; 106:535–540.
42. Fowler MB, Laser JA, Hopkins GL, Minobe W. Bristow M: Assessment of the β-adrenergic receptor pathway in the intact failing human heart: Progressive receptor down-regulation and subsensitivity to agonist response. *Circulation* 1986; 74:1290–1302.
43. Bristow MR, Ginsburg R, Minobe WA, Cubicciotti RS, Sageman WS, Lucie R: Decreased catecholamine sensitivity and β-adrenergic receptor density in failing human hearts. *N Engl J Med* 1982; 307:205–211.
44. Brodde EO, Miches MC, Gordon EP, Sandoval A, Gilbert EM, Bristow MR: β-adrenoceptor regulation in the human heart: Can it be monitored in circulating lymphocytes. *Eur Heart J* 1989; 10:2–10.
45. Bristow MR, Anderson FL, Port D, Skerl L, Hershberger RE, Larrabe P: Differences in β-adrenergic neuroeffector mechanisms in ischemic versus idiopathic dilated cardiomyopathy. *Circulation* 1991; 84:1024–1039.
46. Port JD, Bristow MR: Lack of spare β-adrenergic receptors in the human heart (abstract). *FASEB J* 1988; 2:A602.
47. Colucci WS, Denniss AR, Leatherman GF, Quigg RJ, Ludmer PL, Marsh JD: Intracoronary infusion of dobutamine to patients with and without severe congestive heart failure. *J Clin Invest* 1988; 81:1103–1110.
48. McKee PA, Castelli UP, McNamara PM, et al: The natural history of congestive heart failure: The Framingham study. *N Engl J Med* 1971; 285;1441–1446.
49. Torp A: Incidence of congestive cardiomyopathy. *Postgrad Med J* 1978; 54:435–437.
50. Gavazzi A, Lanzarini L, Cornalba C, Desperati M, Raisaro A, Angoli L: Dilated (congestive) cardiomyopathy. *G Ital Cardiol* 1984; 14:492–498.
51. Gorlin R: Incidence, etiology and prognosis of heart failure. *Cardiovasc Rev Rep* 1983; 4:765–761.
52. Fuster V, Gersh BJ, Giuliani ER, Tajik AJ, Brandenburg RD, Frye RL: The natural history of idiopathic dilated cardiomyopathy. *Am J Cardiol* 1981; 47:525–531.
53. Hofmann T, Meinertz T, Kasper W, Geibel A, Zehender M. Hohnloser S: Mode of death in idiopathic dilated cardiomyopathy: A multivariate analysis of prognostic determinants. *Am Heart J* 1988; 116:1455–1463.
54. Diaz RA, Obasohan A, Oakley CM: Prediction of outcome in dilated cardiomyopathy. *Br Heart J* 1987; 58:393–399.
55. Unverferth DV, Magorien RD, Moeschberger ML, Baker PB, Fetters JK, Leier CV: Factors influencing the one-year mortality of dilated cardiomyopathy. *Am J Cardiol* 1984; 54:147–152.
56. Franciosa JA, Wilen M, Ziesche S, Cohn JN: Survival in men with severe chronic left ventricular failure due to either coronary heart disease or idiopathic dilated cardiomyopathy. *Am J Cardiol* 1983; 51:831–836.
57. Convert G, Delaye J, Beaune J, Biron A, Gonin A: Etude pronostique des myocardiopathies primitives non obstructives. *Arch Mal Coeur* 1980; 27:227–237.
58. Meinertz T, Hofmann T, Kasper W, Treese N, Bechtold H, Stienen U: Significance of ventricular arrhythmias in idiopathic dilated cardiomyopathy. *Am J Cardiol* 1984; 53:902–907.
59. Romeo F, Pelliccia F, Cianfrocca C, Cristofani R, Reale A: Predictors of sudden death in idiopathic dilated cardiomyopathy. *Am J Cardiol* 1989; 63:138–140.
60. Koide T, Kato A, Takabatake Y, Iizuka M, Uchida Y, Ozeki K: Variable prognosis in congestive cardiomyopathy. Role of left ventricular function, alcoholism, and pulmonary thrombosis. *Jpn Heart J* 1980; 21:451–463.
61. Keogh AM, Freund J, Baron DW, Hickie JB: Timing of cardiac transplantation in idiopathic dilated cardiomyopathy. *Am J Cardiol* 1988; 61:418–422.
62. Quigley PJ, Richardson PJ, Meany BT, Olsen EGJ, Monaghan M: Long-term follow-up in biopsy proven myocarditis (abstr). *Br Heart J* 1987; 57:71.
63. Demakis JG, Rahimtoola SH, Sutton GC, Meadows R, Szanto PB, Jolsin JR: Natural course of peripartum cardiomyopathy. *Circulation* 1971; 44:1053–1061.
64. Demakis JG, Proskey A, Rahimtola SH, et al: The natural course of alcoholic cardiomyopathy. *An Intern Med* 1974; 80:293–297.
65. Costanzo-Nordin MR, O'Connell JB, Engelmeier RS, Moran JF, Scanlon PJ: Dilated cardiomyopathy: Functional status, hemodynamics, arrhythmias, and prognosis. *Cathet Cardiovasc Diag* 1985; 11:445–453.
66. Olshausen AV, Stienen U, Schwarz F, Kubler W, Meyer J: Long-term prognostic significance of ventricular arrhythmias in idiopathic dilated cardiomyopathy. *Am J Cardiol* 1988; 61:146–151.
67. Holmes J, Kubo SH, Cody RJ: Arrhythmias in ischemic and non-ischemic dilated cardiomyopathy. *Am J Cardiol* 1985; 55:146–151.
68. Das SK, Mordy F, DiCarlo L, Baerman J, Krol R, De Buitleir M: Prognostic usefulness of programmed ventricular stimulation in idiopathic dilated cardiomyopathy without symptomatic ventricular arrhythmias. *Am J Cardiol* 1986; 58:998–1000.
69. Poll DS, Marchlinski FE, Buston AE, Josephson ME: Usefulness of programmed stimulation in idiopathic dilated cardiomyopathy. *Am J Cardiol* 1986; 58:992–997.
70. Figulla HR, Rahlf G, Nieger M, Luig H, Kreuzer H: Spontaneous hemodynamic improvement or stabilization and associated biopsy findings in patients with congestive cardiomyopathy. *Circulation* 1985; 71:1095–1104.
71. Hammond EH, Menlove RL, Anderson JL: Predictive value of immunofluorescence and electron microscopic evaluation of endomyocardial biopsies in the diagnosis and prognosis of myocarditis and idiopathic dilated cardiomyopathy. *Am Heart J* 1987; 114:1055–1065.
72. Maisel AS, Scott NA, Motulsky HG, Michel MC, Boublik JN, Rivier JB: Elevation of plasma neuropeptide Y levels in congestive heart failure. *Am J Med* 1989; 86:43–48.
73. Cohn N, Levine TB, Olivare MT, Garberg V, Lora D, Francis GS: Plasma norepinephrine as a guide to prognosis in patients with chronic congestive heart failure. *N Engl J Med* 1984; 311:819–823.
74. Swedberg K, Eneroth P, Kjekshus J, Wilhelmsen L: Hormones regulating cardiovascular function in patients with severe congestive heart failure and their relation to mortality. *Circulation* 1990; 82:1730–1736.
75. Lee WH, Packer M: Prognostic importance of serum sodium concentration and its modification by converting-enzyme inhibition in patients with severe chronic heart failure. *Circulation* 1986; 73:257–267.
76. Wilensky RL, Yudelman P, Cohen AI, Fletcher RD, Atkinson J, Virmani R: Severe electrocardiographic changes in idiopathic dilated cardiomyopathy confirmed at necropsy. *Am J Cardiol* 1988; 62:276–283.
77. Wallis DE, O'Connell JB, Henkin RE, Costanzo-Nordin MR, Scanlon PJ: Segmental wall motion abnormalities in dilated cardiomyopathy: A common finding and good prognostic sign. *J Am Coll Cardiol* 1984; 4:674–679.
78. Doherty JE: Use of digitalis and diuretics in the treatment of heart failure. In: Cohn JN (ed): *Drug Treatment of Heart Failure*. Secausus, NJ, Advanced Therapeutics Communications International. 1988: 147–178.
79. Renlin FC: the actions and use of diuretics in renal disease. In: Friedkey CD (ed): *Heart, Kidney and Electrolytes*. New York, Grune & Stratton, 169–193.
80. Craswell PW, Ezzati E, Kopstein J, et al: Use of metolazone, a new diuretic, in patients with renal disease. *Nephron* 1973; 12:63–73.
81. CONSENSUS Trial Study Group: Effect of enalapril on mortality in severe congestive heart failure; results of the Cooperative North Scandinavian Enalapril Survival Study (CONSENSUS). *N Engl J Med* 1987; 316:1429–1435.

82. Cohn JN, Archibald DG, Ziesche S, et al: Effect of vasodilator therapy on mortality in chronic congestive heart failure. *N Engl J Med* 1986; 314:1547–1552.
83. Cody RJ, Franklin KW, Kluger J, Laragh JH, Tristani F: Sympathetic responsiveness and plasma norepinephrine during therapy of chronic congestive heart failure with captopril. *Am J Med* 1982; 72:791–797.
84. Cleland JGF, Dangic H, Horsman GP, Ball SG, Robertson JIS, Morton JJ: Captopril in heart failure, a double blind controlled trial. *Br Heart J* 1984; 52:530–535.
85. Captopril-Digoxin Multicenter Research Group: Comparative effects of therapy with captopril and digoxin in patients with mild to moderate heart failure. *JAMA* 1988; 259:539–554.
86. DiBianco R, Shabetai R, Kostuk W, Moran J, Schlant RC, Wright R: A comparison of oral milrinone, digoxin and their combination in the treatment of patients with chronic heart failure. *N Engl J Med* 1989; 320:677–683.
87. Packer M. Gheorghiade M, Young JB, Costantini PJ, Adams KF, et al: Withdrawal of digoxin from patients with chronic heart failure treated with angiotensin-converting-enzyme inhibitors. *N Engl J Med* 1993; 329:1–7.
88. Gilbert EM, O'Connell JB, Bristow MR: Therapy of idiopathic dilated cardiomyopathy with chronic β-adrenergic blockade. *Heart Vessels* 1991(suppl 6):33–43.
89. Waagstein F, Hjalmmarson A, Varnauskas E, Wuallentin I: Effect of chronic beta-adrenergic receptor blockade in congestive cardiomyopathy. *Br Heart J* 1975; 37:1022–1036.
90. Engelmeier RS, O'Connell JB, Walsh R, Rod N, Scanlon PJ, Civanar RM: Improvement in symptoms and exercise tolerance by metoprolol in patients with dilated cardiomyopathy. *Circulation* 1985; 72:526–546.
91. Gilbert EM, Anderson JL, Deitchman D, Yanowitz F, O'Connell JB, Renlund DO: Long-term β-blocker vasodilator therapy improves cardiac function in idiopathic dilated cardiomyopathy. *Am J Med* 1990; 88:223–229.
92. Gilbert EM, Mestroni L, Anderso JL, Woodley SL, Bristow MR: Can response to β-blocker therapy in idiopathic dilated cardiomyopathy be predicted by baseline parameters? *Circulation* 1989; 80:II–428.
93. Gilbert EM, Olsen SL, Mealey P, Volkman K. Larrabee P, Bristow MR: Is β-receptor up-regulation necessary for improved LV function in dilated cardiomyopathy? *Circulation* 1991; 84:II-469.
94. Swedberg K, Waagstein F, Hjalmarson S, Wuellentin I: Prolongation of survival in congestive cardiomyopathy by beta receptor blockade. *Lancet* 1979; 1:1374–1376.
95. Anderson JL, Lutz JR, Gilbert EM, Sorenson SG, Yanowitz F, Mealove RL: A randomized trial of low dose β-blockade therapy for idiopathic dilated cardiomyopathy. *Am J Cardiol* 1985; 55:471–475.
96. O'Connell JB, Renlund DG, Bristow MR: Cadiac transplantation: Emerging role of the internist/cardiologist. *J Intern Med* 1989; 225:147–156.

Chapter 90

Hypertrophic Cardiomyopathy

Barry J. Maron, M.D. ■ **William C. Roberts, M.D.**

Hypertrophic cardiomyopathy (HCM) is a primary cardiac disease that is frequently genetically transmitted.[1-9] Although relatively uncommon, this disease has nevertheless been of great interest to clinicians and scientists due to its particularly diverse clinical, morphologic, and pathophysiological manifestations.[10-43] Also, because of this broad clinical spectrum and complexity, a certain degree of confusion and uncertainty persists regarding HCM.[2,5,44]

HISTORICAL CONSIDERATIONS

There is some controversy as to who should be credited with the first gross anatomic description of HCM. Around 1900, French and German authors described four patients with cardiac disease and findings at autopsy that in retrospect may have represented early examples of HCM.[45-47] These reports described hearts characterized by striking hypertrophy involving the ventricular septum that appeared to the authors to be responsible for obstruction to left ventricular ejection.

The first unequivocal description of HCM was in the detailed anatomic report of Teare,[48] which ultimately stimulated widespread interest in this "new" disease among cardiologists, pathologists, and surgeons. Teare described a condition in eight patients (seven of whom died suddenly) characterized by an asymmetric pattern of left ventricular hypertrophy and nondilated ventricular cavities. The striking ventricular septal hypertrophy present in these patients was thought to represent a benign tumor; a bizarre arrangement of muscle bundles and variability in cardiac muscle cell size were described as prominent histologic features.

DEFINITION AND NOMENCLATURE

The most characteristic morphologic abnormality of HCM is a hypertrophied and nondilated left ventricle in the absence of another cardiac or systemic disease that itself is capable of producing left ventricular hypertrophy (such as systemic hypertension or aortic stenosis)[6] (Fig. 90-1). Over the past three decades, numerous investigations have led to a dramatic evolution of our concepts concerning the clinical and pathological spectrum of HCM; in the process, the disease has acquired myriad names (more than 75) (Fig. 90-2). This multiplicity of descriptive terms given to HCM seems largely related to the enormous clinical, functional, and morphologic diversity characteristic of this disease and institutional referral patterns in which only a few selected tertiary centers evaluate large numbers of patients with this particular condition. Many of the terms that have been used to describe HCM are somewhat misleading in emphasizing the presence of left ventricular outflow obstruction, a clinical feature that we now know occurs in only a minority of patients with HCM referred to major centers. The precise prevalence of HCM in the general population is not known, although the disease appears to be uncommon (estimated occurrence of about 0.1 to 0.2 percent). It is possible, however, that many individuals with HCM go undetected in the community because they manifest no or only mild symptoms and do not have echocardiographic studies.[49,50] Reports from a large number of diverse geographical areas suggest that HCM occurs worldwide; there is some suggestion that the precise morphologic expression of the disease may differ in certain ethnic or racial groups (such as the Japanese).[12,16,26,41]

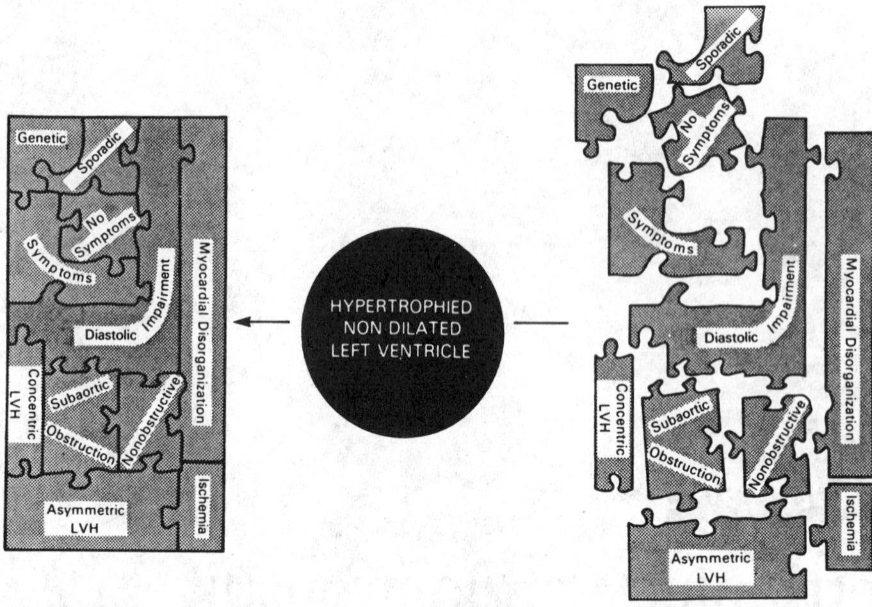

FIGURE 90-1 Diagrammatic representation of the basic morphologic definition of HCM (dark circle) as it unifies the clinical and morphologic diversity characteristic of the disease spectrum.

MORPHOLOGIC CHARACTERISTICS

Gross Features

Hypertrophy is the gross anatomical marker and likely a determinant of many of the clinical features of HCM in most patients with this disease[2,5,6] (Fig. 90-3 to 90-6). Since the left ventricular cavity is usually small or normal in size, the increased left ventricular mass is due almost entirely to an increase in ventricular wall thickness. Although a symmetric (concentric) pattern of left ventricular hypertrophy may occur,[10,25] the distribution of hypertrophy is almost always asymmetric; i.e., all segments of the left ventricular wall are not thickened to a similar degree, and the ventricular septum usually shows the greatest magnitude of hypertrophy.[2,4,10,27] Gross observations at necropsy in patients with HCM typically show, in addition to asymmetric hypertrophy without ventricular dilatation, enlargement of the atria, thickening of the mitral valve leaflets, and areas of fibrosis in the ventricular wall.[18,24] In addition, about 75 percent of hearts show a characteristic fibrous plaque on the mural endocardium of the left ventricle in apposition to the anterior mitral leaflet, presumably resulting from systolic (as well as diastolic) contact between mitral valve and septum[18] (Fig. 90-3).

Based on echocardiographic analyses in large numbers of patients, it is apparent that HCM is characterized by structural heterogeneity with regard to the patterns and extent of left ventricular hypertrophy[10] (Fig. 90-4 and 90-5). Thickness of the left ventricular wall is greatly increased in many patients, including some who have the most severe hypertrophy observed in any cardiac disease.[27] For example, not uncommonly we have evaluated patients with maximal wall thickness of 35 to 45 mm (usually the ventricular septum) with the most extreme dimension observed to date being 52 mm. Often the pattern of wall thickening is strikingly heterogeneous, involving noncontiguous segments of left ventri-

Asymmetrical hypertrophic cardiomyopathy
Asymmetrical hypertrophy of the heart
Asymmetrical septal hypertrophy
Brock's disease
Diffuse muscular subaortic stenosis
Diffuse subvalvular aortic stenosis
Dynamic hypertrophic subaortic stenosis
Dynamic muscular subaortic stenosis
Familial hypertrophic subaortic stenosis
Familial muscular subaortic stenosis
Familial myocardial disease
Functional aortic stenosis
Functional hypertrophic subaortic stenosis
Functional obstructive cardiomyopathy
Functional obstruction of the left ventricle
Functional obstructive subvalvular aortic stenosis
Functional subaortic stenosis
Hereditary cardiovascular dysplasia
HYPERTROPHIC CARDIOMYOPATHY
Hypertrophic constrictive cardiomyopathy
Hypertrophic hyperkinetic cardiomyopathy
Hypertrophic infundibular aortic stenosis
Hypertrophic nonobstructive cardiomyopathy
Hypertrophic obstructive cardiomyopathy
Hypertrophic stenosing cardiomyopathy
Hypertrophic subaortic stenosis
Idiopathic hypertrophic cardiomyopathy
Idiopathic hypertrophic obstructive cardiomyopathy
Idiopathic hypertrophic subaortic stenosis
Idiopathic hypertrophic subvalvular stenosis
Idiopathic muscular hypertrophic subaortic stenosis
Idiopathic muscular stenosis of the left ventricle
Idiopathic myocardial hypertrophy
Idiopathic stenosis of the flushing chamber of the left ventricle
Idiopathic ventricular septal hypertrophy
Irregular hypertrophic cardiomyopathy
Left ventricular muscular stenosis
Low subvalvular aortic stenosis
Muscular aortic stenosis
Muscular hypertrophic stenosis of the left ventricle
Muscular stenosis of the left ventricle
Muscular subaortic stenosis
Muscular subvalvular aortic stenosis
Non-dilated cardiomyopathy
Nonobstructive hypertrophic cardiomyopathy
Obstructive cardiomyopathy
Obstructive hypertrophic aortic stenosis
Obstructive hypertrophic cardiomyopathy
Obstructive hypertrophic myocardiopathy
Obstructive myocardiopathy
Pseudoaortic stenosis
Stenosing hypertrophy of the left ventricle
Stenosis of the ejection chamber of the left ventricle
Subaortic hypertrophic stenosis
Subaortic idiopathic stenosis
Subaortic muscular stenosis
Subvalvular aortic stenosis of the muscular type
Teare's disease

FIGURE 90-2 Terms used to describe HCM.

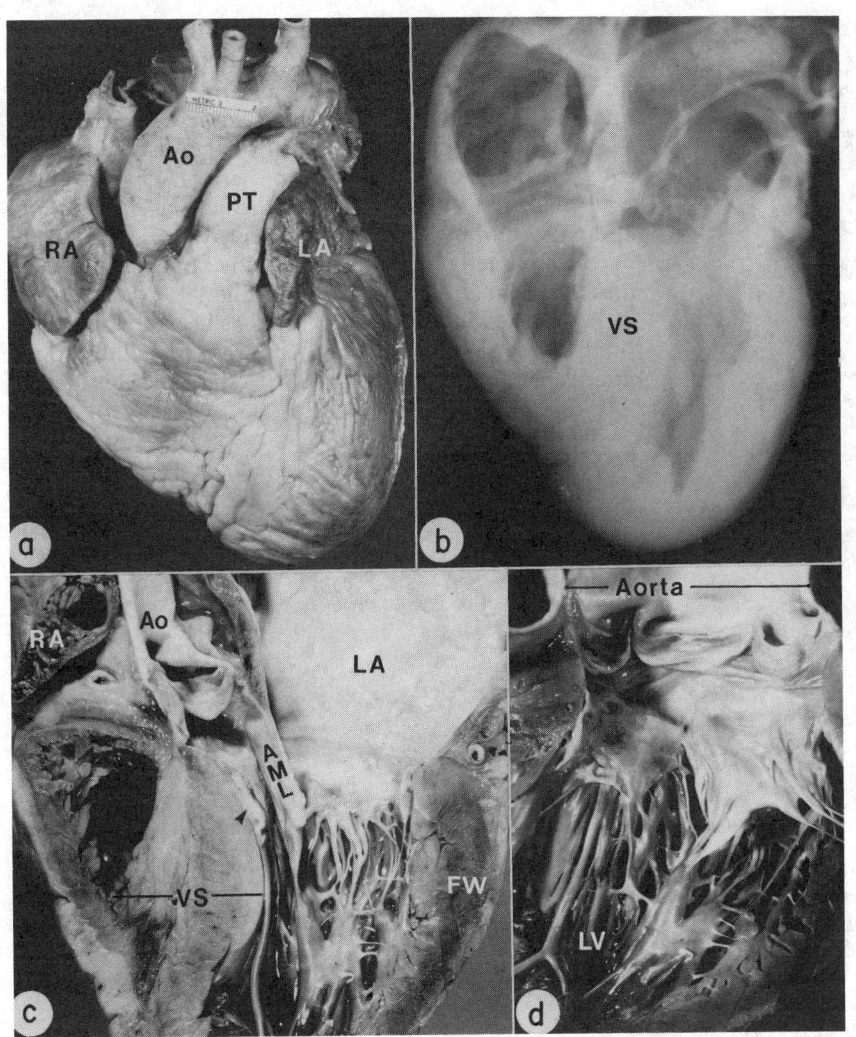

FIGURE 90-3 Anatomic features of HCM are demonstrated in the heart of a 26-year-old man. *A.* Exterior view; both right atrium (RA) and left atrium (LA) are dilated. Ao = aorta; PT = pulmonary trunk. *B.* Radiograph of specimen showing asymmetric thickening of ventricular septum (VS). *C.* Coronal section; the septum is clearly thicker than left ventricular free wall (FW); an endocardial mural contact plaque (arrow) is present in the left ventricular outflow tract in apposition to the anterior mitral leaflet (AML). *D.* Closer view of plaque and thickened anterior leaflet. *(From WC Roberts, VJ Ferrans: Hum Pathol 6:287–342, 1975. Reproduced with permission from the publisher and authors.)*

cle (with areas of normal thickness evident in between) or marked differences in wall thickness in contiguous segments. The transition between regions of the wall that are thickened and regions of normal thickness is often sharp and abrupt, not infrequently creating right-angled contours of the ventricular wall. Characteristic echocardiographic findings are shown in Fig. 15-25.

In the majority of patients (about 55 percent), the pattern of hypertrophy is diffuse and involves both the septum and substantial portions of the anterolateral free wall, with the posterior segment of free wall the least affected by the hypertrophic process.[10] In other patients, hypertrophy involves only the ventricular septum while the free wall is spared. In still other patients, the wall thickening may be relatively mild and localized to a single segment of myocardium. Such segmental hypertrophy may be confined to the anterior or posterior septum, the anterolateral free wall,[10] the posterobasal free wall,[28] or even the most apical portion of the left ventricle[12–15,17,26]; the latter morphologic form has been described most commonly in Japan.[12,16,26] Japanese investigators[12,16,26] have reported a subgroup of patients with a form of HCM that appears to be clinically benign and to differ in several important respects from the more typical clinical and morphologic expressions of the disease. Based primarily on angiographic studies, it has been suggested

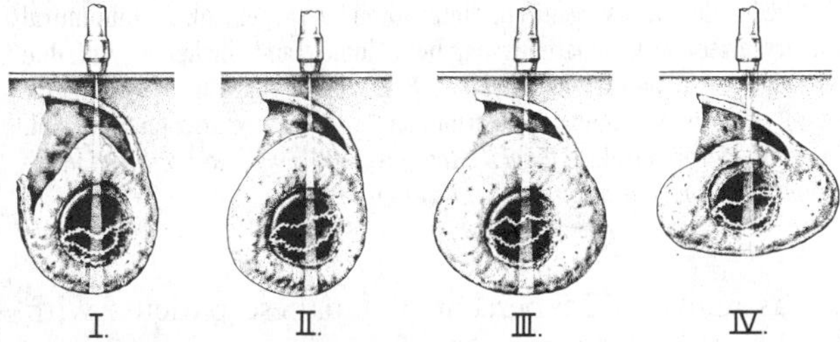

FIGURE 90-4 Morphologic variability in HCM, based on observations made from two-dimensional echocardiography. All images are drawn in the short-axis cross-sectional plane at mitral valve level. *I.* Relatively mild left ventricular hypertrophy confined to anterior portion of ventricular septum (VS). *II.* Hypertrophy of anterior and posterior septum in the absence of free-wall thickening. *III.* Diffuse hypertrophy of substantial portions of both ventricular septum and anterolateral free wall (ALFW). *IV.* Includes more unusual patterns of hypertrophy in which M-mode echo beam (M) does *not* traverse the thickened portions of left ventricle in posterior septum or anterolateral free wall (as shown here) or the left ventricular apex. AML = anterior mitral leaflet; A or ANT = anterior; L = (patient's) left; LVFW = LV free wall; P or POST = posterior; PML = posterior mitral leaflet; R = (patient's) right; RV = right ventricle. *(From BJ Maron: Am J Cardiol 55:835–838, 1985. Reproduced with permission from the American Journal of Cardiology and authors.)*

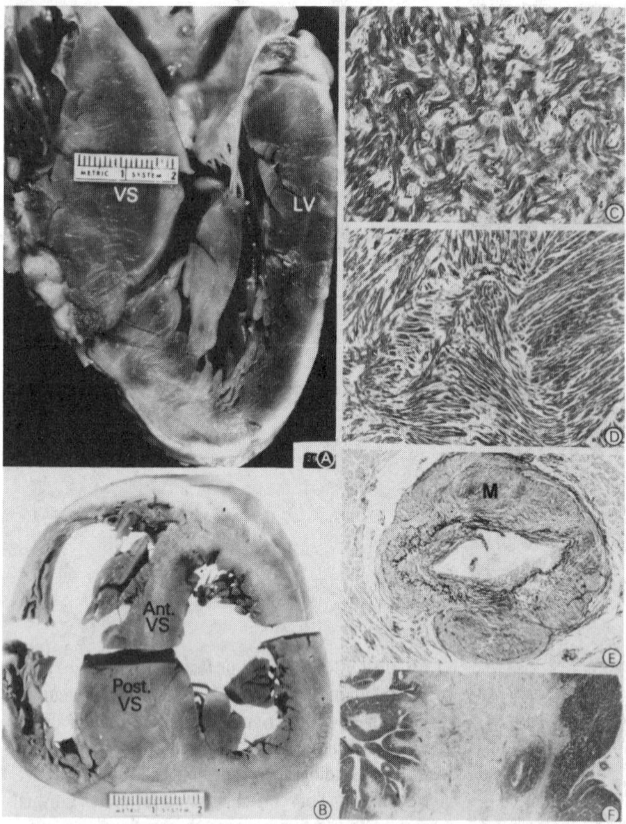

FIGURE 90-5 Morphologic components of the underlying disease process in HCM. *A.* Gross heart specimen sectioned in a cross-sectional plane similar to that of the echocardiographic (parasternal) long axis. The pattern of left ventricular hypertrophy is asymmetrical, with wall thickening confined primarily to the anterior ventricular septum (VS), which bulges into the left ventricular outflow tract. *B.* Heart specimen illustrating a different pattern of hypertrophy in which marked left ventricular wall thickening is localized to the posterior portion of the ventricular septum (Post. VS), while the anterior septum (Ant. VS) is only mildly thickened. *C, D.* Histology characteristic of the left ventricle in HCM. In *C*, septal myocardium shows markedly disordered architecture with adjacent hypertrophied cardiac muscle cells arranged at perpendicular and oblique angles to each other. In *D*, bundles of hypertrophied cells show a disorganized, "interwoven" arrangement. *E.* Intramural coronary artery with apparently narrowed lumen and thickened wall due primarily to medial (M) hypertrophy. *F.* Extensive scarring of ventricular septum which is transmural in distribution. LV = left ventricular free wall. *(From BJ Maron* et al: *N Engl J Med 316:780, 1987. Reproduced with permission from the publisher and authors.)*

that as many as 25 percent of Japanese patients with HCM have hypertrophy confined to the true left ventricular apex (below the level of the papillary muscles).[16] This distribution of hypertrophy characteristically creates a "spade" deformity of the left ventricular cavity and is also associated with a distinctive electrocardiographic pattern of deep ("giant") T-wave inversion. Similar to the Japanese experience, patients with localized apical hypertrophy and/or giant T-wave inversions reported in North America and Europe have been described as generally (but not exclusively) having benign natural history.[13,14,16,17] In addition, some young asymptomatic individuals may show segmental hypertrophy involving the ventricular septum (with wall thicknesses of 13 to 14 mm) suggestive of a relatively mild morphologic expression of HCM that may often be difficult to distinguish from the "physiologic" form of left ventricular hypertrophy induced by chronic athletic training.[51]

The variability in morphologic expression of HCM is underlined by the fact that even first-degree relatives with the genetically transmitted form of the disease usually show great dissimilarities in the pattern of left ventricular wall thickening.[4] In fact, variability in the distribution and pattern of hypertrophy appears to be as substantial between related members of the same family as between unrelated patients in different families.

Hypertrophic cardiomyopathy has been reported in a small number of very young children, including a few infants under 6 months of age.[52–54] When HCM is identi-

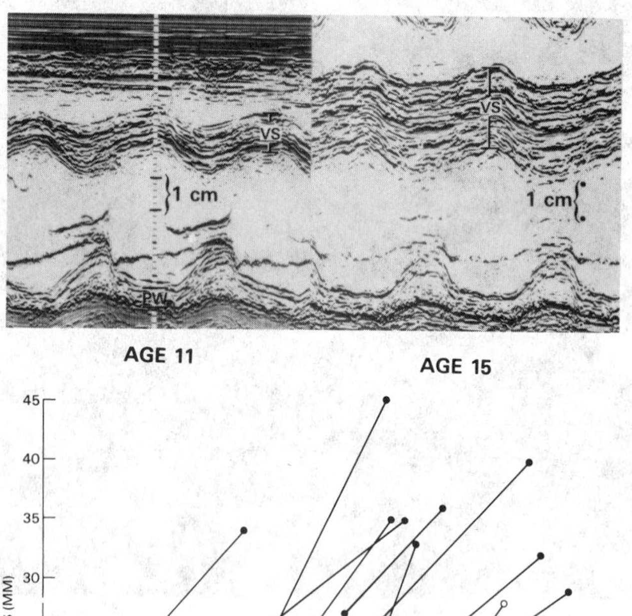

FIGURE 90-6 Development and progression of left ventricular hypertrophy in children with HCM. *Upper panel:* Development of marked hypertrophy of the anterior basal ventricular septum (VS). M-mode echocardiograms shown here were obtained at the same cross-sectional level in a girl with a family history of HCM. At age 11, ventricular septal thickness was at upper limit of normal (10 mm); at age 15, septal thickness had increased markedly (to 33 mm), and appearance of the echocardiogram is typical of HCM. The patient remained asymptomatic throughout this period of time but died suddenly and unexpectedly at age 17. PW = posterior left ventricular free wall. *Lower panel:* Dynamic, striking changes in left ventricular wall thickness with age in 22 children; each patient is represented by the left ventricular segment that showed the greatest change in wall thickness. Open symbols denote five patients who had no evidence of hypertrophy in any segment of the left ventricle at the initial evaluation but subsequently developed de novo hypertrophy typical of HCM. *(From BJ Maron et al: N Engl J Med 315:610, 1986. Reproduced with permission from the publisher and authors.)*

fied in infancy, the disease is usually associated with marked septal hypertrophy, severe progressive congestive heart failure, and often, biventricular outflow obstruction. Thus, HCM can represent a congenital heart malformation in which left ventricular wall thickening begins during fetal development and is evident shortly after birth.

Serial echocardiographic investigations have shown the "dynamic" nature of the left ventricular hypertrophy in HCM. For example, the morphologic expression of HCM may not be complete until adulthood.[30] Patients often show striking spontaneous increases in wall thicknesses (i.e., of 33 to 250 percent, mean 100 percent) and more extensive distribution of hypertrophy with increasing age during childhood, including de novo development during adolescence when body growth and maturation are most accelerated (Fig. 90-6). In children with evolving left ventricular hypertrophy, abnormalities on the 12-lead electrocardiogram (ECG) may be the initial clinical manifestation of the disease, preceding both the onset of symptoms and appearance of hypertrophy on echocardiogram.[55] Of note, these dynamic changes in hypertrophy appear to be part of the predetermined morphologic evolution of the disease and are not at that time usually associated with development or progression of symptoms or sudden death; once patients with HCM achieve full growth and maturation (at about age 18), further progression in left ventricular hypertrophy does not usually occur.[56] Progression of hypertrophy during childhood may, however, be associated with the development of mitral valve systolic anterior motion and outflow obstruction.[57]

Of note, in a population of symptomatic patients with HCM, left ventricular hypertrophy is considerably more severe in younger than in older patients. Furthermore, an inverse relation between left ventricular wall thickness and age is evident[58]; indeed, particularly marked degrees of hypertrophy (e.g., wall thickness exceeding 30 mm) appear to be limited largely to patients under age 40, while more elderly patients over age 55 to 60 generally have more modest degrees of hypertrophy and rarely show wall thickness greater than 25 mm. The explanation for this inverse relation between age and magnitude of hypertrophy is not known for certain but could be due to a higher rate of premature death in younger patients with severe left ventricular hypertrophy or, alternatively, to a process of gradual wall thinning (perhaps due to progressive fibrosis) occurring in many patients with HCM.[38,64]

The extent and distribution of left ventricular hypertrophy also appear to be determinants of clinical features and course in patients with HCM.[10,59] For example, in a population of patients with HCM, more marked and diffuse patterns of hypertrophy confer a predisposition not only for congestive cardiac symptoms and subaortic obstruction but also for sudden death and potentially lethal arrhythmias such as nonsustained ventricular tachycardia on ambulatory ECG or induced by programmed electrical stimulation. Indeed, we have found it to be less common for adult patients with HCM and a mild degree of left ventricular hypertrophy to die suddenly[60]; furthermore, we[61] and others[29] have only rarely encountered young patients with sudden cardiac death who appeared to have HCM in the *absence* of left ventricular hypertrophy. The relation between the echocardiographic assessment of left ventricular wall thickness and mass and clinical findings in HCM are nevertheless not strong enough to permit prospective prediction of clinical course for individual patients.

Histologic Features

Certain histologic features of left ventricular myocardium are components of the cardiomyopathic muscle and the underlying disease process in HCM[31–37,62]: (1) cardiac muscle cell disorganization; (2) replacement fibrosis; and (3) abnormalities of the small intramural coronary arteries (Fig. 90-5). Distorted cellular architecture, described by Teare in his initial report of HCM, [48] is a characteristic feature of the left ventricle in this disease.[34–37] Many cardiac muscle cells in both the ventricular septum and left ventricular free wall show increased transverse diameter, have bizarre shapes, maintain intercellular connections with several adjacent cells, and are arranged in a disorganized pattern at oblique and perpendicular angles to each other. This cellular disarray is present in about 95 percent of patients dying of HCM and usually occupies substantial portions of left ventricular myocardium (about 33 percent of septum and 25 percent of free wall). (See Fig. 90-5*D*.) Although the potential clinical significance of disordered myocardial architecture has not been precisely defined, it may well contribute importantly to impaired diastolic or systolic function,[5] or possibly even serve as a substrate for ventricular arrhythmias.[63,64]

Patients with HCM (but without atherosclerotic coronary artery disease) studied at necropsy often exhibit fibrous tissue formation in the left ventricle.[31–33,65] A spectrum in severity and distribution is observed ranging from patchy interstitial and perivascular matrix connective tissue to grossly visible replacement scarring that may be extensive[66] or even transmural.[65] Such fibrous tissue formation probably results from prior episodes of myocardial ischemia[67,68] (or is due in some other way to the underlying cardiomyopathic disease process), is identifiable during life as thallium-201 myocardial perfusion abnormalities,[69] and may well be largely responsible for the increased ventricular chamber stiffness and impaired relaxation[66] identifiable in most patients with HCM.[2,5,70–74]

Abnormal intramural coronary arteries are present in about 80 percent of those patients with HCM studied at necropsy, most commonly in the ventricular septum.[33] The walls of these intramural vessels are thickened (due to increased smooth-muscle cells, collagen, elastic fibers, and mucoid deposits in the intima and/or media), and frequently the lumen appears substantially narrowed. Increased numbers or clusters of abnormal intramural arteries are often observed within or at the margins of sizeable areas of fibrosis, including large regions of transmural infarction.[65] This observed association between abnormal intramural coronary arteries and scarring implies a causal relation between the two and suggests that "small-vessel disease" in HCM may be responsible for myocardial ischemia and necrosis.

Mitral Valve Abnormalities

Recent evidence supports the concept that structural abnormalities of the mitral valve are also characteristic of many patients with this disease[21,22] (Fig. 90-7). In a morphometric analysis of almost 100 mitral valves removed at operation or necropsy from patients with HCM, about two-thirds showed alterations in size, shape, and morphology.[22] These abnormalities included increased overall mitral valve area ranging up to twice normal that was due primarily to elongation of the leaflets (but without evidence of "floppy" mitral valve). The enlarged and elongated mitral valves from patients with HCM show considerable variability with regard to structure, including increased size of both anterior and posterior leaflets or asymmetric and segmental enlargement of either the anterior leaflet or a posterior leaflet scallop.

In addition, other patients with virtually normal-sized mitral valves show anomalous insertion of papillary muscle directly into anterior mitral leaflet (without interposition of chordae tendineae)[21] (Fig. 90-8). This constellation of structural malformations of the mitral apparatus expands the morphologic definition of HCM by demonstrating the disease process is not confined to cardiac muscle.

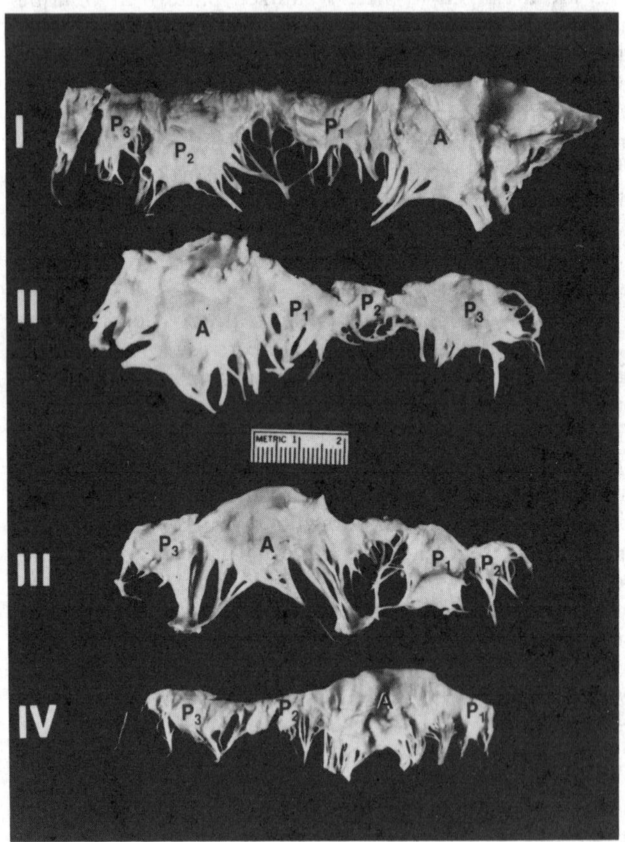

FIGURE 90-7 Mitral valves from three patients with obstructive HCM, aged 31, 29, and 60 years (*I, II,* and *III*) and from a normal control patient without cardiovascular disease (*IV*), showing variation in valvular size and structure present in HCM. Valves are opened with the circumference displayed in a horizontal orientation, exposing the atrial surface, with anular margin to top and chordal attachments to bottom. *I.* Large valve (area 22 cm^2) in which both the anterior (A) and posterior (P) leaflets are greatly elongated and increased in area. *II.* Large valve in which increased valve size (area 18 cm^2) is due primarily to elongation and enlargement of the anterior leaflet (A). *III.* Segmental elongation and increased area confined to a scallop of posterior mitral leaflet. *(From HG Klues et al: Circulation 85:1651, 1992. Reproduced with permission of the American Heart Association and authors.)*

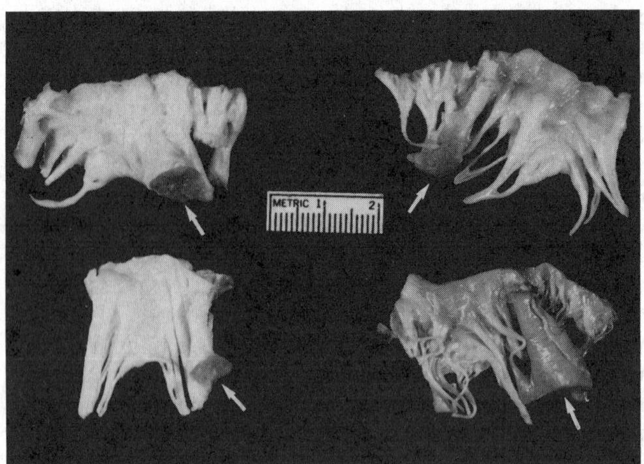

FIGURE 90-8 Mitral valve specimens (with ventricular aspect exposed) excised at operation from four patients with obstructive HCM showing anomalous papillary muscle insertion directly into anterior mitral leaflet (arrows). Papillary muscles are of various sizes and insert into the region of either the posteromedial (valve at upper right) or anterolateral commissure (the other three valves). *(From HG Klues et al: Circulation 84:1188, 1991. Reproduced with permission of the American Heart Association and authors.)*

PATHOPHYSIOLOGY

The symptoms of HCM are varied and include pulmonary congestion (exertional dyspnea, orthopnea, paroxysmal nocturnal dyspnea), fatigue, chest pain that may be typical or atypical of angina pectoris, palpitations, and impaired consciousness.

A number of pathophysiological components of the disease process have been identified at present[2]: (1) left ventricular outflow obstruction,[5,75–78] (2) diastolic dysfunction,[70–74] (3) myocardial ischemia,[67,68] and (4) arrhythmias.[2,5] Other pathophysiological mechanisms may exist that have not yet been clearly identified. Cardiac symptoms in patients with HCM do not always show a direct (one-to-one) correlation with a particular pathophysiological mechanism in a given patient, however, and the relative contributions of each component to symptoms appear to vary among patients.

Left Ventricular Outflow Obstruction

The dynamic type of obstruction to left ventricular outflow exhibited by patients with HCM (due to systolic anterior motion of the mitral valve and midsystolic contact with ventricular septum[2,5,19,20,40,75–78]) often shows spontaneous variability.[1] Interventions or circumstances that decrease myocardial contractility (beta-blocking drugs) or increase ventricular volume or arterial pressure (squatting or vasoconstrictor agents) reduce or abolish the obstruction. Interventions or circumstances that increase contractility (exercise or isoproterenol) or that decrease arterial pressure or ventricular volume (Valsalva maneuver or administration of an agent producing hypotension) will increase the degree of obstruction. Some patients with little or no obstruction to left ventricular outflow under basal conditions are capable of generating substantial "labile" gradients with physiological or pharmacologic provocations, and often such gradients may be evident only after the cessation of exercise.[79]

The increase in systolic intraventricular pressure (and thereby in myocardial wall stress) caused by outflow obstruction may augment myocardial oxygen demand. This abnormal hemodynamic state may have long-term detrimental effects on the left ventricle and be responsible for the genesis of symptoms. The magnitude of the peak systolic pressure gradient can be estimated noninvasively by the degree of mitral valve systolic anterior motion on M-mode echocardiogram[77] or by continuous-wave Doppler.[80,81]

Mechanisms by which subaortic gradients are produced in patients with HCM have been scrutinized,[2,5,22,76–78,82] and numerous studies have focused on defining the contributions of several morphologic and hemodynamic factors, including (1) reduced diastolic outflow tract dimension, (2) substantial hypertrophy involving the anterior basal ventricular septum, (3) anterior displacement of mitral valve and papillary muscles within the ventricular cavity, (4) increased size and length of the mitral leaflets, (5) hyperdynamic left ventricular ejection producing a high-velocity jet that streams through a narrowed outflow tract pulling the mitral leaflets toward the septum (i.e., Venturi effect), and (6) primary geometric abnormalities of the papillary muscle–mitral valve apparatus responsible for altered distribution of tension to the mitral leaflets. In addition, malposition of the mitral valve during midsystole (due to anterior systolic motion) almost invariably interferes with normal valve closure, thereby causing mitral regurgitation[83]; while usually mild in HCM, mitral regurgitation may be more marked when associated with large subaortic gradients. Mitral regurgitation may also occur because of a primary intrinsic abnormality of the valve (e.g., primary floppy valve with prolapse), in which case the degree of incompetence is likely to be severe.[84]

Although outflow obstruction is due to mitral systolic anterior motion in the vast majority of patients with HCM (about 95 percent), occasional patients may demonstrate a peak systolic outflow gradient due to muscular midcavity obstruction (in the absence of systolic anterior motion)[21,43]; such gradients may result from anomalous papillary muscle insertion directly into anterior mitral leaflet[21] (Fig. 90-8) or in some instances are associated with segmental apical or more generalized ventricular hypokinesia.[39]

Diastolic Dysfunction

Echocardiographic, Doppler, contrast or radionuclide angiographic, and hemodynamic studies of left ventricular diastolic function have identified abnormalities in relaxation and filling that are characteristic features of HCM, are present in about 80 percent of patients with this disease,[2,5,70–74] and are presumed to be responsible for symptoms of fatigue, exertional dyspnea, and angina pectoris. These investigations have shown that the rapid filling phase of diastole is significantly prolonged and associated with a decreased rate and volume of rapid filling compared to normal. Consequently, there is an apparent compensatory increase in the contribution of atrial systole to overall left ventricular filling. Also, diastolic dysfunction may occur in the absence of symptoms or in the presence of outflow obstruction[71] and is usually unrelated to the severity or distribution of ventricular hypertrophy.[85]

Altered left ventricular filling dynamics and increased diastolic chamber stiffness or reduced left ventricular distensibility are associated with reduced stroke volume, increased filling pressures, and compressive effects on the intramural coronary vasculature. Reduced distensibility results both from those factors determining the passive elastic properties of the ventricular chamber (including severity of hypertrophy, myocardial fibrosis, and cardiac muscle cell disorganization) and from those influencing the rate and extent of active left ventricular relaxation.

Myocardial Ischemia

There is abundant evidence that myocardial ischemia occurs in HCM.[31–33,65–69] Patients with this disease may have angina and ECG abnormalities consistent with ischemia and infarction. When a patient with HCM and anginal chest pain undergoes right atrial pacing, the characteristic chest pain usually develops, the increase in coronary flow induced by pacing is less than that observed in normal subjects, and lactate is often produced.[67] Also, such patients usually have exercise-induced reversible thallium defects indistinguishable from those in patients with myocardial ischemia due to coronary artery disease.[69]

There are several potential mechanisms responsible for myocardial ischemia in HCM: (1) excessive myocardial oxygen demand that exceeds the capacity of the coronary system to deliver oxygen, (2) compromised coronary blood flow to the myocardium due to abnormal (narrowed) intramural coronary arteries, and (3) prolonged diastolic relaxation resulting in elevated myocardial wall tension.

GENETICS

Hypertrophic cardiomyopathy commonly demonstrates genetic transmission with an autosomal pattern of inheritance.[2–4,7–9] Mutations in the gene that encodes for β-cardiac myosin heavy chain (localized to chromosome 14) have been identified in several affected kindreds (in relatives with and without clinical or morphologic expression of the disease), suggesting that such defects are the cause of HCM.[7–9,86–90] Hypertrophic cardiomyopathy has also been shown to be genetically heterogeneous with defects in at least two gene loci[8,90]; at present one of a total of ten myosin mutations have been identified in about 50 percent of patients.[91] (See also Chap. 96.) Recently, it has also been suggested that particular disease-producing mutations may be associated with a more or less favorable natural history and clinical course in certain families.[91] Prior clinical studies based on extensive echocardiographic surveys of pedigrees[3] showed that about 60 percent of families (in which there is an index case with HCM) had at least one other first-degree relative with clinical and/or morphologic evidence of HCM. In such studies a genetic etiology for HCM could not be documented in about 40 percent of families, even after systematic echocardiographic pedigree surveys. Undoubtedly, some patients previously considered to have sporadic (nongenetic) forms of HCM on the basis of echocardiographic surveys[3] may in reality have had affected relatives with subtle or subclinical expressions.[87]

Occurrence of premature sudden cardiac death in a family should dictate a genetic and echocardiographic evaluation in surviving relatives, since the clinical expression of HCM may be particularly virulent in certain families (e.g., "malignant" HCM).[92,93] Also, because HCM appears to be the leading cause of sudden unexpected death in young competitive athletes,[94] young family members should be screened for HCM prior to participation in competitive athletic training. Because the morphologic expression of HCM may not be complete until adulthood,[30] however, a single screening echocardiogram may not definitively exclude HCM. Therefore, children suspected or shown to harbor the genetic defect of HCM (but without left ventricular hypertrophy on echocardiogram) should continue to have periodic echocardiographic examinations until achieving full growth and maturation. At present, it is unresolved as to whether or not children with HCM identified by genetic analysis to have mutations in the cardiac myosin heavy-chain gene prior to the appearance of left ventricular hypertrophy should be disqualified from competitive athletics.[95]

NATURAL HISTORY AND SUDDEN CARDIAC DEATH

Predicting the clinical course and outcome for individual patients with HCM has proved to be difficult because of variability in natural history and the complexity in disease expression.[96-110] The annual mortality rate due to premature sudden cardiac death in a hospital-based population with HCM has been reported to be about 2 to 4 percent.[99,101] On the other hand, estimates of the frequency of sudden death have been derived only from those patients with HCM evaluated at major centers (usually because they are symptomatic or judged to be at enhanced risk).[49] Therefore, because of such biases resulting from highly selective referral patterns for patients with HCM, the reported mortality figures probably represent an overestimation of the risk for premature death.

Sudden death is most common in children and young adults 15 to 35 years of age,[53,54,64,92,94,99-103,106,107] but it may also occur later, even in patients who have remained asymptomatic through midlife[98] (Fig. 90-9). Most patients are asymptomatic (or only mildly asymptomatic) prior to sudden death; such catastrophes are often the first clinical manifestation of HCM.[92] Most patients die while sedentary or performing mild exertion. A substantial number (about one-third) die during or just after

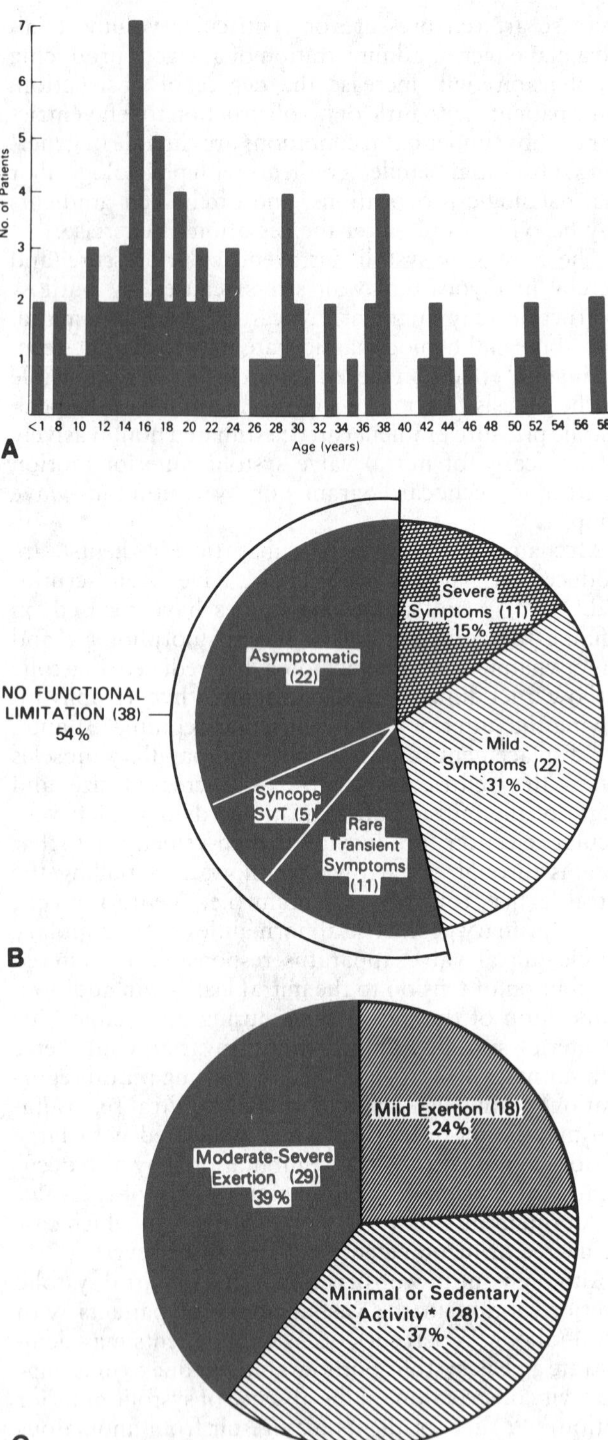

FIGURE 90-9 Clinical profile of patients with HCM and sudden death. *A.* Age distribution for 78 patients who died suddenly or experienced cardiac arrest; of note, the true incidence of sudden death by age is not defined because the frequency with which HCM occurs in each age group is not known. *B.* Functional state before sudden death or cardiac arrest; SVT = supraventricular tachycardia. *C.* Activity at time of sudden death or arrest; * includes four patients who died during sleep. *(From BJ Maron et al: Circulation 67:1388, 1982. Reproduced with permission of the American Heart Association and authors.)*

vigorous physical activity,[92,94] however, a finding that supports the generally accepted recommendation to disqualify such patients from competitive athletics.[95]

No particular symptom complex has been shown to be reliably associated with subsequent sudden death, with the possible exception of syncope.[100] The magnitude of the outflow gradient has not been associated with increased risk for sudden death, which may occur in patients with or without subaortic obstruction.[2,5,93,94] However, other disease variables that are associated with sudden death and have previously been proposed as "risk factors"[53,54,59,60,63,64,93,99–101,107,108,110] include the following: young age, markedly increased left ventricular wall thickness, "malignant" family history of sudden death, and nonsustained ventricular tachycardia on ambulatory ECG. The latter abnormality has previously been linked to sudden cardiac death independently by two institutions[107,108] with risk reported as high as 8 percent per year compared to only 1 percent per year in the absence of ventricular tachycardia.[107] On the other hand, there are several reasons to doubt the predictability of nonsustained ventricular tachycardia in the overall population of patients with HCM. First, the predictive accuracy of ventricular tachycardia in the general HCM population is low. Second, paradoxically, the link between nonsustained ventricular tachycardia and sudden cardiac death has proved to be weakest in those young patients who are of the age when the risk for premature death is perceived to be greatest.[106] Third, the prognostic significance of ventricular tachycardia in HCM may be greatest in those patients experiencing impaired consciousness, and it would appear most prudent to view ventricular tachycardia in the context of symptoms such as syncope. Therefore, it is probably desirable to investigate with invasive testing those patients with both ventricular tachycardia and syncope to define the precise pathophysiological mechanisms that are operative and develop a treatment strategy accordingly. Empiric treatment with antiarrhythmic agents in such patients may not reliably produce clinical benefit and can also be fraught with risk due to proarrhythmic effects.

Substantial progress has been achieved in defining risk stratification profiles for patients with HCM.[63,64,110,111] The probable mechanisms by which sudden death occurs in HCM, defined largely by combined hemodynamic and electrophysiological laboratory studies, involve (1) ventricular tachyarrhythmias, (2) bradyarrhythmias (sinus or conduction related), (3) a variety of supraventricular tachycardias, (4) myocardial ischemia, (5) left ventricular outflow tract obstruction, (6) diastolic dysfunction, (7) exercise-induced hypotension,[97] and (8) activation of a ventricular baroreflex with hypotension (with or without bradycardia).[112] In the largest electrophysiological investigation reported to date,[110] which attempted to define abnormalities in a heterogeneous population with a variety of clinical presentations, about 60 percent had sinus node disease and one-third had conduction abnormalities. Also, an association was evident between inducible sustained ventricular arrhythmias and unfavorable clinical events such as cardiac arrest and syncope, suggesting that electrophysiological testing has potential value in the risk stratification of these patients (Fig. 90-10). Thus, about 75 percent of cardiac arrest survivors and 50 percent of patients with syncope had an inducible ventricular tachycardia compared to less than 20 percent of HCM patients with nonsustained ventricular tachycardia on Holter in whom symptoms of impaired consciousness were absent. While the ultimate prognostic significance of such inducible ventricular arrhythmias is not yet known with absolute certainty, diagnostic and therapeutic strategies designed with electrophysiological guidance may prove to be of value for patients with HCM.

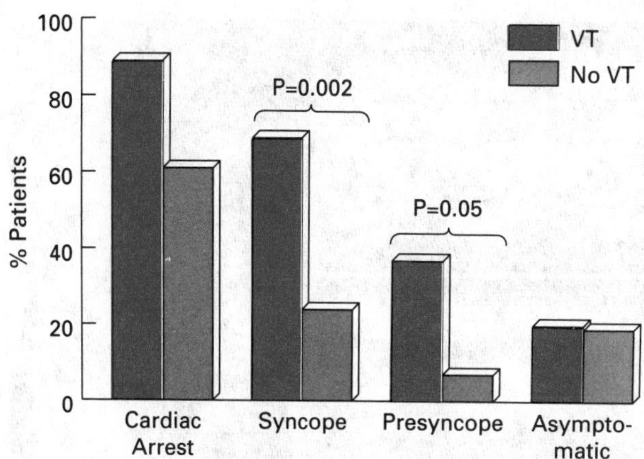

FIGURE 90-10 Bar graph showing relation of ventricular tachycardia induced at electrophysiologic study to clinical profile in patients with HCM. Data are shown separately for patients with and without ventricular tachycardia (VT) on ambulatory electrocardiographic monitoring. *(From L Fananapazir et al: Circulation 80:1259, 1989. Reproduced with permission of the American Heart Association and authors.)*

END-STAGE PHASE

A distinctive final phase of disease evolution has been observed in approximately 10 to 15 percent of symptomatic patients with HCM[2,11,38,42,65,113] (Fig. 90-11). This particular clinical course is characterized by thinning of portions of the left ventricular wall, enlarging cavity size (usually without marked absolute ventricular dilatation), impaired left ventricular contractile function (as manifested by reduced ejection fraction), and occasionally spontaneous reduction of the subaortic gradient. Such "end-stage" patients are thereby transformed from the typical morphologic and functional appearance of HCM (hyperdynamic, hypertrophied, and nondilated left ventricle) to a clinical state that is more suggestive of an idiopathic dilated form of cardiomyopathy (Chap. 89), in which left ventricular wall thickness is normal or mildly increased. Many of these patients with a hypocontractile left ventricle exhibit irreversible thallium-201 myocardial perfusion abnormalities, which undoubtedly reflect extensive myocardial scarring.[33,65] It is possible that these morphologic and functional changes, resulting in end-stage depression of left ventricular contractile function, either are due to underlying myocardial ischemia and infarction resulting from impaired coronary blood flow or represent a primary component of the disease process. Patients who develop the end-stage

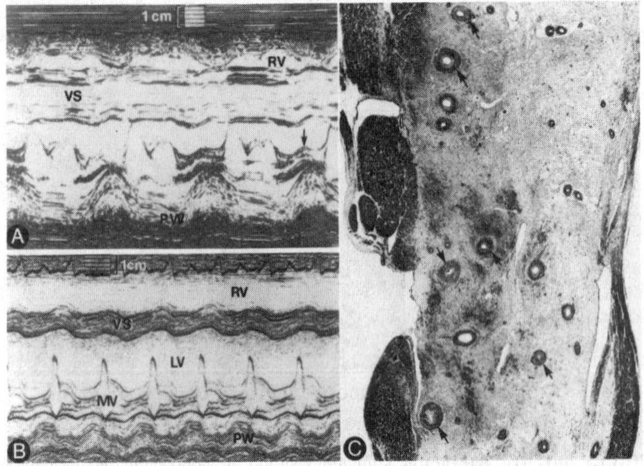

FIGURE 90-11 Studies in patients with HCM and normal extramural coronary arteries showing changes occurring concomitantly with progressive congestive cardiac failure and transmural myocardial infarction ("end-stage" phase). *A*. Echocardiographic study from a 26-year-old patient with exertional chest pain and dyspnea. Ventricular septum (VS) is markedly thickened (23 mm), and pattern of hypertrophy is asymmetric. Left ventricular end-diastolic dimension is reduced (38 mm), and there is a trivial degree of mitral systolic anterior motion (arrow). PW = posterior wall; RV = right ventricle. *B*. From same patient at 30 years of age (9 months before death) after clinical deterioration with progressive cardiac failure, pulmonary edema associated with chronic atrial fibrillation, and cardiopulmonary collapse. Appearance of left ventricle has changed dramatically. Septum has thinned considerably (to 13 mm) and is about as thick as the posterior wall; left ventricular (LV) and right ventricular cavities have enlarged substantially. MV = mitral valve. *C*. Low-power photomicrograph of a specimen from a patient with a clinical course similar to that of the patient in *A* and *B* showing transmural scarring of the septum and numerous abnormal intramural coronary arteries, some with thickened walls and a narrowed lumen (arrows). (Magnification × 6.) *(From BJ Maron et al: N Engl J Med 316:780, 1987. Reproduced with permission from the publisher and authors.)*

phase of HCM may be closely related to (and share the same genetic substrate) as patients experiencing sudden cardiac death.[42]

ATRIAL FIBRILLATION

Atrial fibrillation occurs in a minority (about 10 percent) of patients with HCM[2,5,113,114] and is usually associated with substantial left atrial enlargement but relatively mild left ventricular hypertrophy.[113] This arrhythmia may importantly impair clinical course since the loss of the atrial systolic contribution to ventricular filling is critical to patients with HCM with their poorly compliant ventricles. In many patients, however, atrial fibrillation is well tolerated with long-term consequences similar to those patients remaining in sinus rhythm.[114] Nevertheless, atrial fibrillation can be a challenging arrhythmia to manage in HCM. Its onset may precipitate congestive heart failure, and the restoration of sinus rhythm is best achieved with electrical cardioversion. For chronic atrial fibrillation, verapamil (or a beta blocker) can be utilized to control ventricular rate. Because of the risk for systemic embolism and stroke, anticoagulant therapy should be administered (and continued indefinitely) once atrial fibrillation has been documented.

HCM IN THE ELDERLY

Elderly patients with morphologic and clinical features consistent with HCM have been reported.[23,115-117] In these patients important symptoms are not usually present early in life, and severe functional limitation and heart failure may intervene abruptly for the first time after age 60. The prolonged period of symptomatic latency demonstrated by these patients is, perhaps, surprising for a disease that is expressed morphologically by age 20 and in which symptoms are usually expressed by age 40 to 50. Also, elderly patients with HCM have relatively small hearts with only modest increases in left ventricular wall thickness (usually below 22 mm)[23]; ventricular morphology is severely distorted as evidenced by the greatly reduced outflow tract size and exaggerated anterior displacement of the normal-sized anterior mitral valve leaflet within the cavity. Substantial deposits of calcium in the mitral annular region (posterior to the mitral valve) are frequently present and may contribute to anterior displacement of the valve. In elderly patients with HCM, outflow obstruction is often produced by restricted systolic anterior motion of the anterior mitral valve leaflet (with little or no leaflet bending) with mitral valve–septal contact produced by both mitral valve excursion toward the ventricular septum and posterior excursion of the septum toward the mitral valve.[23] Because older patients who appear to have HCM differ in certain clinical and echocardiographic respects from many younger patients with more "typical" expressions of this disease,[2,5,23] it is uncertain whether such patients harbor the same or similar genetic defects described in other patients within the clinical spectrum of HCM,[91] or, alternatively, represent a phenotypically similar but acquired cardiac abnormality.

MEDICAL TREATMENT

Asymptomatic or Mildly Symptomatic Patients

Therapeutic strategy for asymptomatic (or minimally symptomatic) patients with HCM is unresolved and remains controversial. Some investigators favor prophylactic administration of either beta-adrenergic blocking drugs or calcium channel blockers (such as verapamil) in an effort to prevent or delay progression of the disease process or the occurrence of sudden death. It has also been suggested that such prophylactic drug therapy be limited to those patients perceived to be at risk for premature sudden death.[92,93] On the other hand, evidence that beta-adrenergic or calcium channel blockers either alter left ventricular hypertrophy or reduce the risk of sudden cardiac death in HCM is lacking. Amiodarone has been administered to asymptomatic or mildly symptomatic patients with nonsustained ventricular tachycardia, and it has been suggested that this drug enhances survival and diminishes risk for sudden death compared to standard antiarrhythmic therapy.[118] The administration of amiodarone to severely symptomatic HCM patients with congestive symptoms, however, may be fraught with risk.[119]

Alleviation of Moderate and Severe Symptoms

Historically, beta-adrenergic blocking drugs have been utilized extensively to treat symptomatic patients with the obstructive or nonobstructive forms of HCM and have been shown to have benefit.[2,5,120,121] Calcium channel blockers (principally verapamil) have also become important therapeutic agents in the management of symptomatic patients with HCM.[122,123] Oral verapamil provides improvement in cardiac symptoms and exercise capacity for many patients with HCM who fail to benefit from beta blockers, and it has been suggested that the beneficial effects of verapamil in symptomatic patients exceed those of propranolol.[121] The positive actions that verapamil exerts on left ventricular diastolic filling appear to contribute importantly to this symptomatic improvement.[73,74] When patients fail to achieve improvement in symptoms with beta blockers and calcium antagonists (or diuretic therapy), a trial of disopyramide may be useful.[124,125]

These therapeutic considerations apply to those patients with HCM in whom symptoms occur in the presence of normal or hyperdynamic systolic performance. In patients experiencing congestive symptoms secondary to impaired systolic function (i.e., "end stage" of HCM),[2,11,38,42,65,113] therapeutic strategy is similar to that utilized for heart failure in other diseases, including consideration for cardiac transplantation. (See Chap. 26.)

SURGICAL TREATMENT

Operation in HCM is performed to relieve the subaortic obstruction and to normalize the markedly increased systolic intraventricular pressures.[126–132] Surgery is reserved for those patients with severe symptoms that prove to be refractory to standard medical therapy and in whom obstruction to left ventricular outflow is present (gradient at least 50 mmHg under basal conditions or with provocation). Although ventricular septal myotomy-myectomy (Morrow operation)[126] (Fig. 90-12) is the operative procedure of choice, mitral valve replacement has been employed[132] in selected patients in whom the basal anterior ventricular septum is relatively thin ($\leq$ 18 mm), the distribution of hypertrophy is atypical, or the outflow gradient is due to midcavity muscular obstruction.[21,43] Suture plication of the anterior mitral leaflet has also been suggested (in combination with myotomy-myectomy) to decrease the likelihood that mitral valve systolic anterior motion will persist postoperatively in selected patients in whom it is desirable to avoid mitral valve replacement.[133]

Intraoperative echocardiography may be utilized to map the distribution and magnitude of septal hypertrophy, using a sterile transducer placed directly on the right ventricle.[132] Information obtained is useful in determining whether myotomy-myectomy can be performed safely (without incurring undue risk for iatrogenic ventricular septal defect) and in what manner the standard resection may be tailored to the individual patient's distribution of septal hypertrophy in order to achieve the desired hemodynamic result. Transesophageal echocardiography (Chap. 131) may also be useful during surgery.

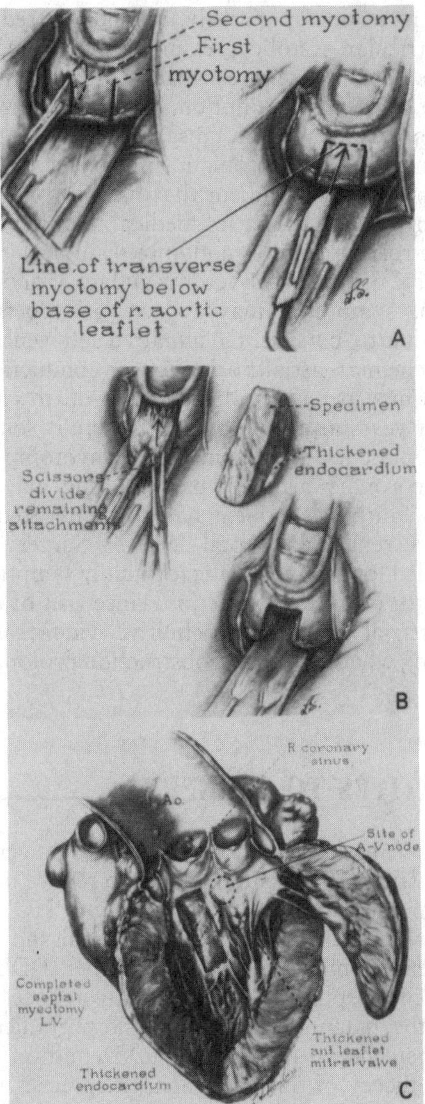

FIGURE 90-12 Illustration of ventricular septal myotomy-myectomy operation (Morrow procedure). *A.* Two vertical parallel myotomies are made in the cephalad portion of the septum about 1 cm apart. A transverse incision is then made, connecting the two parallel myotomies. *B.* Attachments of the muscle bar to the septum are divided, and this segment of muscle is isolated and then excised. *C.* After completion of the myotomy-myectomy, a rectangular channel about 4 cm long and 2 cm wide is evident extending from the aortic annulus to a point just distal to the caudal margins of the mitral leaflets. *[From BJ Maron et al: Eur Heart J 4(suppl F):175, 1983. Reproduced with permission from the publisher and authors.]*

Results from several medical centers employing primarily septal myotomy-myectomy over the past 25 years have demonstrated salutary symptomatic as well as hemodynamic effects.[126–132,134] Operative mortality has been about 5 percent (range 2 to 10 percent). Basically, three important effects of operation in obstructive HCM have been defined. First, in most patients, surgery consistently abolishes or substantially reduces the basal subaortic gradient and mitral systolic anterior motion without importantly compromising left ventricular function[126–131]; the gradient and marked systolic anterior motion only very rarely recur postoperatively. Second, the reduction in left ventricular systolic pressure is associated with an improvement in exercise capacity,[135] a decrease in myocardial oxygen consumption, and improvement in lactate metabolism.[136] Third, most operated patients experience long-lasting symptomatic improvement after relief of their subaortic gradient that has been judged to be more beneficial than that of medical treatment alone (albeit in retrospective, nonrandomized studies).[121] Even with adequate myotomy-myectomy and relief of outflow obstruction, symptoms may reoccur postoperatively (probably due to persistently impaired left ventricular filling or ischemia), atrial fibrillation or conduction abnormalities may persist, and premature death can still ensue many years after operation.[127] There is some evidence that patients undergoing both myotomy-myectomy and coronary artery bypass grafting may be at enhanced operative risk, due in part to greater frequency of iatrogenic ventricular septal defect.[137] Surgery is not recommended for asymptomatic (or mildly symptomatic patients) with outflow obstruction, since risk of operation is not trivial and because definitive evidence is lacking regarding whether relief of obstruction prolongs survival.

ALTERNATIVES TO SURGERY

Recently, there has also been an interest in right ventricular atrioventricular sequential pacing to relieve outflow obstruction and symptoms in patients with HCM who are refractory to drug therapy.[138–140] Initial short-term results appear promising with dual-chamber (DDD) permanent pacing reported to significantly reduce symptoms and the magnitude of the outflow gradient (by about 50 percent) in many patients. Definition of the long-term efficacy of this approach, the precise mechanism by which the gradient is altered, and the role of permanent pacing in the therapeutic management of patients with the obstructive form of HCM will require further follow-up studies.

REFERENCES

1. Braunwald E, Lambrew CT, Rockoff SD, Ross J Jr, Morrow AG: Idiopathic hypertrophic subaortic stenosis. I. A description of the disease based upon an analysis of 64 patients. *Circulation* 1964; 30 (suppl IV): 3–217.
2. Maron BJ, Bonow RO, Cannon RO, Leon MB, Epstein SE: Hypertrophic cardiomyopathy: Interrelation of clinical manifestations, pathophysiology, and therapy. *N Engl J Med* 1987; 316:780–789, 844–852.
3. Maron BJ, Nichols PF, Pickle LW, Wesley YE, Mulvihill JJ: Patterns of inheritance in hypertrophic cardiomyopathy. Assessment by M-mode and two-dimensional echocardiography. *Am J Cardiol* 1984; 53:1087–1094.
4. Cirò E, Nichols PF, Maron BJ: Heterogeneous morphologic expression of genetically transmitted hypertrophic cardiomyopathy: Two-dimensional echocardiographic analysis. *Circulation* 1983; 67:1227–1233.
5. Wigle ED, Sasson Z, Henderson MA, Ruddy TD, Fulop J, Rakowski H, et al: Hypertrophic cardiomyopathy. The importance of the site and extent of hypertrophy. A review. *Prog Cardiovasc Dis* 1985; 28:1–83.
6. Maron BJ, Epstein SE: Hypertrophic cardiomyopathy: A discussion of nomenclature. *Am J Cardiol* 1979; 43:1242–1244.
7. Geisterfer-Lowrance AA, Kass S, Tanigawa G, Vosberg HP, McKenna WJ, Seidman CE, et al: A molecular basis for familial hypertrophic cardiomyopathy: A beta cardiac myosin heavy chain gene missense mutation. *Cell* 1990; 62:999–1006.
8. Solomon SD, Jarcho JA, McKenna WJ, Geisterfer-Lowrance A, Germain R, Salerni R, et al: Familial hypertrophic cardiomyopathy is a genetically heterogeneous disease. *J Clin Invest* 1990; 86:993–999.
9. Jarcho JA, McKenna WJ, Pare JAP, Solomon SD, Holcombe RF, Dickie S, et al: Mapping a gene for familial hypertrophic cardiomyopathy to chromosome 14ql. *N Engl J Med* 1989; 321:1372–1377.
10. Maron BJ, Gottdiener JS, Epstein SE: Patterns and significance of distribution of left ventricular hypertrophy in hypertrophic cardiomyopathy. A wide-angle, two-dimensional echocardiographic study of 125 patients. *Am J Cardiol* 1981; 48:418–428.
11. Spirito P, Maron BJ, Bonow RO, Epstein SE: Severe functional limitation in patients with hypertrophic cardiomyopathy and only mild localized left ventricular hypertrophy. *J Am Coll Cardiol* 1986; 8:537–544.
12. Yamaguchi H, Ishimura T, Nishiyama S, Nagasaki F, Nakanishi S, Takatsu F, et al: Hypertrophic nonobstructive cardiomyopathy with giant negative T waves (apical hypertrophy): Ventriculographic and echocardiographic features in 30 patients. *Am J Cardiol* 1979; 44:401–412.
13. Louie EK, Maron BJ: Apical hypertrophic cardiomyopathy: Clinical and two-dimensional echocardiographic assessment. *Ann Intern Med* 1987; 106:663–670.
14. Keren G, Belhassen B, Sherez J, Miller HI, Megidish R, Berenfeld D, et al: Apical hypertrophic cardiomyopathy: Evaluation by noninvasive and invasive techniques in 23 patients. *Circulation* 1975; 71:45–56.
15. Alfonso F, Nihoyannopoulos P, Stewart J, Dickie S, Lemery R, McKenna WJ: Clinical significance of giant negative T waves in hypertrophic cardiomyopathy. *J Am Coll Cardiol* 1990; 15:965–971.
16. Koga Y, Itaya K-I, Toshima H: Prognosis in hypertrophic cardiomyopathy. *Am Heart J* 1984; 108:351–359.
17. Webb JG, Sasson Z, Rakowski H, Liu P, Wigle ED: Apical hypertrophic cardiomyopathy: Clinical follow-up and diagnostic correlates. *J Am Coll Cardiol* 1990; 15:83–90.
18. Roberts CS, Roberts WC: Morphologic features. In: Zipes DP, Rowlands DJ (eds): *Progress in Cardiology 2/2*. Philadelphia, Lea & Febiger, 1989: 3–22.
19. Maron BJ, Harding AM, Spirito P, Roberts WC, Waller BF: Systolic anterior motion of the posterior mitral leaflet: A previously unrecognized cause of dynamic subaortic obstruction in patients with hypertrophic cardiomyopathy. *Circulation* 1983; 68:282–293.
20. Gilbert BW, Pollick C, Adelman AG, Wigle ED: Hypertrophic cardiomyopathy: Subclassification by M-mode echocardiography. *Am J Cardiol* 1980; 45:861–872.
21. Klues HG, Roberts WC, Maron BJ: Anomalous insertion of papillary muscle directly into anterior mitral leaflet in hypertrophic cardiomyopathy: Significance in producing left ventricular outflow obstruction. *Circulation* 1991; 84:1188–1197.
22. Klues HG, Maron BJ, Dollar AL, Roberts WC: Diversity of structural mitral valve alterations in hypertrophic cardiomyopathy. *Circulation* 1992; 85:1651–1660.
23. Lewis JF, Maron BJ: Elderly patients with hypertrophic cardiomyopathy: A subset with distinctive left ventricular morphology and progressive clinical course late in life. *J Am Coll Cardiol* 1989; 13:36–45.
24. Olsen EG: Anatomic and light microscopic characterization of hypertrophic obstructive and non obstructive cardiomyopathy. *Eur Heart J* 1983; 4(suppl F):1–8.
25. Shapiro LM, McKenna WJ: Distribution of left ventricular hypertrophy in hypertrophic cardiomyopathy: A two-dimensional echocardiographic study. *J Am Coll Cardiol* 1983; 2:437–444.
26. Sakamoto T, Tei C, Murayama J, Ichiyasu H, Hada Y, Hayashi T, et al: Giant T wave inversion as a manifestation of asymmetrical apical hypertrophy (AAH) of the left ventricle: Echocardiographic and ultrasono-cardiotomographic study. *Jpn Heart J* 1976; 17:611–629.
27. Louie EK, Maron BJ: Hypertrophic cardiomyopathy with ex-

treme increase in left ventricular wall thickness: Functional and morphologic features and clinical significance. *J Am Coll Cardiol* 1986; 8:57–65.

28. Lewis JF, Maron BJ: Hypertrophic cardiomyopathy characterized by marked hypertrophy of the posterior left ventricular free wall: Significance and clinical implications. *J Am Coll Cardiol* 1991; 18:421–428.
29. McKenna WJ, Stewart JT, Nihoyannopoulos P, McGinty F, Davies MJ: Hypertrophic cardiomyopathy without hypertrophy: Two families with myocardial disarray in the absence of increased myocardial mass. *Br Heart J* 1990; 63:287–290.
30. Maron BJ, Spirito P, Wesley Y, Arce J: Development and progression of left ventricular hypertrophy in children with hypertrophic cardiomyopathy. *N Engl J Med* 1986; 315:610–614.
31. Tanaka M, Fujiwara H, Onodera T, Wu D-J, Hamashima Y, Kawai C: Quantitative analysis of myocardial fibrosis in normals, hypertensive hearts, and hypertrophic cardiomyopathy. *Br Heart J* 1986; 55:575–581.
32. St John Sutton MG, Lie JT, Anderson KR, O'Brien PC, Frye RL: Histopathological specificity of hypertrophic obstructive cardiomyopathy. *Br Heart J* 1980; 44:433–443.
33. Maron BJ, Wolfson JK, Epstein SE, Roberts WC: Intramural ("small vessel") coronary artery disease in hypertrophic cardiomyopathy. *J Am Coll Cardiol* 1986; 8:545–557.
34. Ferrans VJ, Morrow AG, Roberts WC: Myocardial ultrastructure in idiopathic hypertrophic subaortic stenosis: A study of operatively excised left ventricular outflow tract muscle in 14 patients. *Circulation* 1972; 45:769–792.
35. Maron BJ, Roberts WC: Quantitative analysis of cardiac muscle cell disorganization in the ventricular septum of patients with hypertrophic cardiomyopathy. *Circulation* 1979; 59:689–706.
36. Maron BJ, Anan TJ, Roberts WC: Quantitative analysis of the distribution of cardiac muscle cell disorganization in the left ventricular wall of patients with hypertrophic cardiomyopathy. *Circulation* 1981; 63:882–894.
37. Fujiwara H, Kawai C, Hamashima Y: Myocardial fascicle and fiber disarray in 25 μ-thick sections. *Circulation* 1979; 59:1293–1298.
38. Spirito P, Maron BJ, Bonow RO, Epstein SE: Occurrence and significance of progressive left ventricular wall thinning and relative cavity dilatation in patients with hypertrophic cardiomyopathy. *Am J Cardiol* 1987; 60:123–129.
39. Fighali S, Krajcer Z, Edelman S, Leachman RD: Progression of hypertrophic cardiomyopathy into a hypokinetic left ventricle: Higher incidence in patients with midventricular obstruction. *J Am Coll Cardiol* 1987; 9:288–294.
40. Spirito P, Maron BJ: Patterns of systolic anterior motion of the mitral valve in hypertrophic cardiomyopathy: Assessment by two-dimensional echocardiography. *Am J Cardiol* 1984; 54:1039–1046.
41. Ando H, Imaizumi T, Urabe Y, Takeshita A, Nakamura M: Apical segmental dysfunction in hypertrophic cardiomyopathy: Subgroup with unique clinical features. *J Am Coll Cardiol* 1990; 16:1579–1588.
42. Hecht GM, Maron BJ: Coexistence of sudden death and "end-stage" heart failure within pedigrees with genetically transmitted hypertrophic cardiomyopathy (abstr). *Circulation* 1990; 82(suppl III):332.
43. Falicov R, Resnekov L, Bharati S, Lev M: Mid-zone ventricular obstruction: A variant of obstructive cardiomyopathy. *Am J Cardiol* 1976; 37:432–437.
44. Abelmann WH, Lorell BH: The challenge of cardiomyopathy. *J Am Coll Cardiol* 1989; 13:1219–1239.
45. Schmincke A: Ueber linkseitige muskulöse Conusstenosen. *Dtsch Med Wochenschr* 1907; 33:2082.
46. Liouville H: Rètrècissement cardiaque sous aortique. *Gazette Med Paris* 1869; 24:161–163.
47. Hallopeau M: Rètrècissement ventriculo-aortique. *Gazette Med Paris* 1869; 24:683–684.
48. Teare D: Asymmetrical hypertrophy of the heart in young adults. *Br Heart J* 1958; 20:1–18.
49. Spirito P, Chiarella F, Carratino L, Zoni-Berisso M, Bellotti P, Vecchio C: Clinical course and prognosis of hypertrophic cardiomyopathy in an outpatient population. *N Engl J Med* 1989; 320:749–755.
50. Shapiro LM, Zezulka A: Hypertrophic cardiomyopathy: A common disease with a good prognosis. Five year experience of a district general hospital. *Br Heart J* 1983; 50:530–533.
51. Maron BJ: Structural features of the athlete's heart as defined by echocardiography. *J Am Coll Cardiol* 1986; 7:190–203.
52. Maron BJ, Tajik AJ, Ruttenberg HD, Graham TP, Atwood GF, Victorica BE, et al: Hypertrophic cardiomyopathy in infants: Clinical features and natural history. *Circulation* 1982; 65:7–17.
53. Fiddler GI, Tajik AJ, Weidman WH, McGoon DC, Ritter DG, Giuliani ER: Idiopathic hypertrophic subaortic stenosis in the young. *Am J Cardiol* 1978; 42:793–799.
54. Maron BJ, Henry WL, Clark CE, Redwood DR, Roberts WC, Epstein SE: Asymmetric septal hypertrophy in childhood. *Circulation* 1976; 53:9–19.
55. Panza JA, Maron BJ: Relation of electrocardiographic abnormalities to evolving left ventricular hypertrophy in hypertrophic cardiomyopathy. *Am J Cardiol* 1989; 63:1258–1265.
56. Spirito P, Maron BJ: Absence of progression of left ventricular hypertrophy in adult patients with hypertrophic cardiomyopathy. *J Am Coll Cardiol* 1987; 9:1013–1017.
57. Panza JA, Maris TJ, Maron BJ: Development and determinants of dynamic obstruction to left ventricular outflow in young patients with hypertrophic cardiomyopathy. *Circulation* 1992; 85:1398–1405.
58. Spirito P, Maron BJ: Relation between extent of left ventricular hypertrophy and age in patients with hypertrophic cardiomyopathy. *J Am Coll Cardiol* 1989; 13:820–823.
59. Spirito P, Watson RM, Maron BJ: Relation between extent of left ventricular hypertrophy and occurrence of ventricular tachycardia in hypertrophic cardiomyopathy. *Am J Cardiol* 1987; 60:1137–1142.
60. Spirito P, Maron BJ: Relation between extent of left ventricular hypertrophy and occurrence of sudden cardiac death in hypertrophic cardiomyopathy. *J Am Coll Cardiol* 1990; 15:1521–1526.
61. Maron BJ, Kragel AH, Roberts WC: Sudden death due to hypertrophic cardiomyopathy in the absence of increased left ventricular mass. *Br Heart J* 1990; 63:308–310.
62. Tanaka M, Fujiwara H, Onodera T, Wu D-J, Matsuda M, Hamashima Y, et al: Quantitative analysis of narrowings of intramyocardial small arteries in normal hearts, hypertensive hearts, and hearts with hypertrophic cardiomyopathy. *Circulation* 1987; 75:1130–1139.
63. Maron BJ, Fananapazir L: Sudden cardiac death in hypertrophic cardiomyopathy. *Circulation* 1992; 85(suppl I):I-57–63.
64. McKenna WJ, Camm AJ: Sudden death in hypertrophic cardiomyopathy: Assessment of patients at high risk. *Circulation* 1989; 80:1489–1492.
65. Maron BJ, Epstein SE, Roberts WC: Hypertrophic cardiomyopathy and transmural myocardial infarction without significant atherosclerosis of the extramural coronary arteries. *Am J Cardiol* 1979; 43:1086–1102.
66. Factor SM, Butany J, Sole MJ, Wigle ED, Williams WC, Rojkind M: Pathologic fibrosis and matrix connective tissue in the subaortic myocardium of patients with hypertrophic cardiomyopathy. *J Am Coll Cardiol* 1991; 17:1343–1351.
67. Cannon RO, Rosing DR, Maron BJ, et al: Myocardial ischemia in hypertrophic cardiomyopathy: Contribution of inadequate vasodilator reserve and elevated left ventricular filling pressures. *Circulation* 1985; 71:234–243.
68. Pasternac A, Noble J, Streulens Y, Elie R, Henschke C, Bourassa MG: Pathophysiology of chest pain in patients with cardiomyopathies and normal coronary arteries. *Circulation* 1982; 65:778–789.
69. O'Gara PT, Bonow RO, Maron BJ, et al: Myocardial perfusion abnormalities in patients with hypertrophic cardiomyopathy: Assessment with thallium-201 emission computed tomography. *Circulation* 1987; 76:1214–1223.
70. Sanderson JE, Gibson DG, Brown DJ, Goodwin JF: Left ventricular filling in hypertrophic cardiomyopathy. An angiographic study. *Br Heart J* 1977; 39:661–670.
71. Maron BJ, Spirito P, Green KJ, Wesley YE, Bonow RO, Arce J: Noninvasive assessment of left ventricular diastolic function by pulsed Doppler echocardiography in patients with hypertrophic cardiomyopathy. *J Am Coll Cardiol* 1987; 10:733–742.
72. Hanrath P, Mathey DG, Siegert R, Biefield W: Left ventricular relaxation and filling patterns in different forms of left ventricular hypertrophy: An echocardiographic study. *Am J Cardiol* 1980; 45:15–23.

73. Bonow RO, Frederick TM, Bacharach SL, Green MV, Goose PW, Maron BJ, et al: Atrial systole and left ventricular filling in patients with hypertrophic cardiomyopathy: Effect of verapamil. *Am J Cardiol* 1983; 51:1386–1391.
74. Hanrath P, Mathey DG, Kremer P, Sonntag F, Bleifeld W: Effect of verapamil on left ventricular isovolumic relaxation time and regional left ventricular filling in hypertrophic cardiomyopathy. *Am J Cardiol* 1980; 45:1258–1264.
75. Shah PM, Gramiak R, Kramer DH: Ultrasound location of left ventricular outflow obstruction in hypertrophic obstructive cardiomyopathy. *Circulation* 1969; 40:3–11.
76. Spirito P, Maron BJ: Significance of left ventricular outflow tract cross-sectional area in hypertrophic cardiomyopathy: A two-dimensional echocardiographic assessment. *Circulation* 1983; 67:1100–1108.
77. Pollick C, Rakowski H, Wigle ED: Muscular subaortic stenosis: The quantitative relationship between systolic anterior motion and pressure gradient. *Circulation* 1984; 69:43–49.
78. Maron BJ, Epstein SE: Clinical significance and therapeutic implications of the left ventricular outflow tract pressure gradient in hypertrophic cardiomyopathy. *Am J Cardiol* 1986; 58:1093–1096.
79. Klues HG, Leuner C, Kuhn H: Hypertrophic obstructive cardiomyopathy: No increase of the gradient during exercise. *J Am Coll Cardiol* 1991; 19:527–533.
80. Sasson Z, Yock PG, Hatle LK, Aldermann EL, Popp RL: Doppler echocardiographic determination of the pressure gradient in hypertrophic cardiomyopathy. *J Am Coll Cardiol* 1988; 11:752–756.
81. Panza JA, Petrone RK, Fananapazir L, Maron BJ: Utility of continuous wave Doppler in noninvasive assessment of the left ventricular outflow tract pressure gradient in patients with hypertrophic cardiomyopathy. *J Am Coll Cardiol* 1992; 19:91–99.
82. Cape EG, Simons D, Jimoh A, Weyman AE, Yoganathan AP, Levin RA: Chordal geometry determines the shape and extent of systolic anterior motion. *J Am Coll Cardiol* 1989; 13:1438–1448.
83. Wigle ED, Adelman AG, Auger P, Marquis Y: Mitral regurgitation in muscular subaortic stenosis. *Am J Cardiol* 1969; 24:698–706.
84. Petrone RK, Klues HG, Panza JA, Peterson EE, Maron BJ: Significance of the occurrence of mitral valve prolapse in patients with hypertrophic cardiomyopathy *J Am Coll Cardiol* 1992; 20:55–61.
85. Spirito P, Maron BJ: Relation between extent of left ventricular hypertrophy and diastolic filling abnormalities in hypertrophic cardiomyopathy. *J Am Coll Cardiol* 1990; 15:808–813.
86. Solomon SD, Geisterfer-Lowrance AA, Vosberg HP, et al: A locus for familial hypertrophic cardiomyopathy is closely linked to the cardiac myosin heavy chain genes, CRI-L436 and CRI-L329 on chromosome 14 at q11–q12. *Am J Hum Genet* 1990; 47:389–394.
87. Rosenzweig A, Watkins H, Hwang D-S, et al: Preclinical diagnosis of familial hypertrophic cardiomyopathy by genetic analysis of blood lymphocytes. *N Engl J Med* 1991; 325:1753–1760.
88. Hejtmancik JF, Brink PA, Towbin J, Hill R, Brink L, Tapscott T, et al: Localization of the gene for familial hypertrophic cardiomyopathy to chromosome 14q1 in a diverse US population. *Circulation* 1991; 83:1592–1597.
89. Watkins H, Seidman CE, MacRae C, Seidman JG, McKenna W: Progress in familial hypertrophic cardiomyopathy: Molecular genetic analyses in the original family studied by Teare. *Br Heart J* 1992; 67:34–38.
90. Epstein ND, Fananapazir L, Lin HJ, White R, Lalouel JM, Nienhuis A, et al: Evidence of genetic heterogeneity in five kindreds with familial hypertrophic cardiomyopathy. *Circulation* 1992; 85:635–648.
91. Watkins H, Rosenzweig A, Hwang D-S, Levi T, McKenna WJ, Seidman CE, et al: Characteristics and prognostic implications of myosin missense mutations in familial hypertrophic cardiomyopathy. *N Engl J Med* 1992; 326:1108–1114.
92. Maron BJ, Roberts WC, Epstein SE: Sudden death in hypertrophic cardiomyopathy: A profile of 78 patients. *Circulation* 1982; 67:1388–1394.
93. Maron BJ, Lipson LC, Roberts WC, Savage DD, Epstein SE: "Malignant" hypertrophic cardiomyopathy: Identification of a subgroup of families with unusually frequent premature death. *Am J Cardiol* 1978; 41:1133–1140.
94. Maron BJ, Roberts WC, McAllister HA, Rosing DR, Epstein SE: Sudden death in young athletes. *Circulation* 1980; 62:218–229.
95. Maron BJ, Gaffney FA, Jeresaty RM, McKenna WJ, Miller WW: Task Force III. Hypertrophic cardiomyopathy, other myopericardial diseases and mitral valve prolapse. Bethesda Conference 16: Cardiovascular abnormalities in the athlete: Recommendations regarding eligibility for competition. *J Am Coll Cardiol* 1985; 6:1215–1217.
96. Newman H, Sugrue DD, Oakley CM, Goodwin JF, McKenna WJ: Relation of left ventricular function and prognosis in hypertrophic cardiomyopathy: An angiographic study. *J Am Coll Cardiol* 1985; 5:1064–1074.
97. Frenneaux MP, Counihan PJ, Caforio ALP, Chikamori T, McKenna WJ: Abnormal blood pressure response during exercise in hypertrophic cardiomyopathy. *Circulation* 1991; 82:1995–2002.
98. Hecht GM, Panza JA, Maron BJ: Clinical course of middle-aged asymptomatic patients with hypertrophic cardiomyopathy. *Am J Cardiol* 1992; 69:935–940.
99. Adelman AG, Wigle ED, Ranganathan N, Webb GD, Kidd BSL, Bigelow WG, et al: The clinical course in muscular subaortic stenosis. A retrospective and prospective study of 60 hemodynamically proved cases. *Ann Intern Med* 1972; 77:515–525.
100. McKenna WJ, Deanfield JE, Faroqui A, England D, Oakley C, Goodwin JF: Prognosis in hypertrophic cardiomyopathy: Role of age and clinical, electrocardiographic and hemodynamic features. *Am J Cardiol* 1981; 47:532–538.
101. Shah PM, Adelman AG, Wigle ED, Gobel FL, Burchell HB, Hardarson T, et al: The natural (and unnatural) history of hypertrophic obstructive cardiomyopathy. *Circ Res* 1973; 34,35(suppl II):II-179–195.
102. Nicod P, Polikar R, Peterson KL: Hypertrophic cardiomyopathy and sudden death. *N Engl J Med* 1988; 318:1255–1257.
103. Cecchi F, Maron BJ, Epstein SE: Long-term outcome of patients with hypertrophic cardiomyopathy successfully resuscitated after cardiac arrest. *J Am Coll Cardiol* 1989; 13:1283–1288.
104. Stafford WJ, Trohman RG, Bilsker M, Zaman L, Catellanos A, Myerburg RJ: Cardiac arrest in an adolescent with atrial fibrillation and hypertrophic cardiomyopathy. *J Am Coll Cardiol* 1986; 7:701–704.
105. Krikler DM, Davies MJ, Rowland E, Goodwin JF, Evans RC, Shaw DB: Sudden death in hypertrophic cardiomyopathy: Associated accessory atrioventricular pathways. *Br Heart J* 1980; 43:245–251.
106. McKenna WJ, Franklin RCG, Nihoyannopoulos P, Robinson KC, Deanfield JE: Arrhythmia and prognosis in infants, children and adolescents with hypertrophic cardiomyopathy. *J Am Coll Cardiol* 1988; 11:147–153.
107. Maron BJ, Savage DD, Wolfson JK, Epstein SE: Prognostic significance of 24-hour ambulatory monitoring in patients with hypertrophic cardiomyopathy: A prospective study. *Am J Cardiol* 1981; 48:252–257.
108. McKenna WJ, England D, Doi JL, Deanfield JE, Oakley CM, Goodwin JF: Arrhythmia in hypertrophic cardiomyopathy. I. Influence on prognosis. *Br Heart J* 1981; 46:168–172.
109. Kuck K-H, Kunze KP, Schlueter M, Nienaber CA, Costard A: Programmed electrical stimulation in hypertrophic cardiomyopathy: Results in patients with and without cardiac arrest or syncope. *Eur Heart J* 1988; 9:177–185.
110. Fananapazir L, Tracy CM, Leon MB, Winkler JB, Cannon RO, Bonow RO, et al: Electrophysiologic abnormalities in patients with hypertrophic cardiomyopathy: A consecutive analysis in 155 patients. *Circulation* 1989; 80:1259–1268.
111. Hecht GM, Klues HG, Roberts WC, Maron, BJ: Coexistence of sudden cardiac death and end-stage heart failure in familial hypertrophic cardiomyopathy. *J Am Coll Cardiol* 1993; 22:489–497.
112. Gilligan DM, Nihoyannopoulas P, Chan WL, Oakley CM: Investigation of a hemodynamic basis for syncope in hypertrophic cardiomyopathy. Use of a head-up tilt test. *Circulation* 1992; 85:2140–2148.
113. Spirito P, Lakatos E, Maron BJ: Degree of left ventricular hypertrophy in chronic atrial fibrillation in hypertrophic cardiomyopathy. *Am J Cardiol* 1992; 69:1217–1222.
114. Robinson KC, Frenneaux MP, Stockins B, Karatasakis G, Poloniecki JD, McKenna WJ: Atrial fibrillation in hypertrophic cardiomyopathy: A longitudinal study. *J Am Coll Cardiol* 1990; 15:1279–1285.

115. Fay WP, Taliercio CP, Ilstrup DM, Tajik AJ, Gersh BJ: Natural history of hypertrophic cardiomyopathy in the elderly. *J Am Coll Cardiol* 1990; 16:821–826.
116. Chikamori T, Doi YL, Yonezawa Y, Dickie S, Ozawa T, McKenna WJ: Comparison of clinical features in patients ≥60 years of age to those ≤40 years of age with hypertrophic cardiomyopathy. *Am J Cardiol* 1990; 66:875–877.
117. Lever HM, Kuram RF, Currie PH, Healy BP: Hypertrophic cardiomyopathy in the elderly. Distinctions from the young based on cardiac shape. *Circulation* 1989; 79:580–589.
118. McKenna WJ, Oakley CM, Krikler DM, Goodwin JF: Improved survival with amiodarone in patients with hypertrophic cardiomyopathy and ventricular tachycardia. *Br Heart J* 1985; 53:412–416.
119. Fananapazir L, Leon MB, Cannon RO, Bonow RO, Winkler J, Epstein SE: Sudden death during empiric amiodarone therapy in symptomatic patients with hypertrophic cardiomyopathy. *Am J Cardiol* 1991; 67:169–174.
120. Adelman AG, Shah PM, Gramiak R, Wigle ED: Long-term propranolol therapy in muscular subaortic stenosis. *Br Heart* 1970; 32:804–811.
121. Seiler C, Hess OM, Schoenbeck M, Turina J, Jenni R, Turina M, et al: Long-term follow-up of medical versus surgical therapy for hypertrophic cardiomyopathy: A retrospective study. *J Am Coll Cardiol* 1991; 17:634–642.
122. Kaltenbach M, Hopf R, Kober G, Bussman W-D, Keller M, Petersen Y: Treatment of hypertrophic obstructive cardiomyopathy with verapamil. *Br Heart J* 1979; 42:35–42.
123. Rosing DR, Condit JR Maron BJ, Kent KM, Leon MB, Bonow RO, et al: Verapamil therapy: A new approach to the pharmacologic treatment of hypertrophic cardiomyopathy. III. Effects of long-term administration. *Am J Cardiol* 1981; 48:545–553.
124. Sherrid M, Delia E, Dwyer E: Oral disopyramide therapy for obstructive hypertrophic cardiomyopathy. *Am J Cardiol* 1988; 62:1085–1088.
125. Pollick C: Muscular subaortic stenosis: Hemodynamic and clinical improvement after disopyramide. *N Engl J Med* 1982; 307:997–999.
126. Morrow AG, Reitz BA, Epstein SE, Henry WL, Conkle DM, Itscoitz SB, et al: Operative treatment in hypertrophic subaortic stenosis: Techniques and the results of pre- and postoperative assessments in 83 patients. *Circulation* 1975; 52:88–102.
127. Maron BJ, Epstein SE, Morrow AG: Symptomatic status and prognosis of patients after operation for hypertrophic obstructive cardiomyopathy: Efficacy of ventricular septal myotomy and myectomy. *Eur Heart J* 1983; 4(suppl F):175–185.
128. Williams WG, Wigle ED, Rakowski H, Smallhorn J, LeBlanc J, Trusler GA: Results of surgery for hypertrophic obstructive cardiomyopathy. *Circulation* 1987; 76(suppl V):104–108.
129. Krajcer Z, Leachman RD, Cooley DA, Coronado R: Septal myotomy-myectomy versus mitral valve replacement in hypertrophic cardiomyopathy. Ten-year follow-up in 185 patients. *Circulation* 1989; 80(suppl I):I-57–64.
130. Bircks W, Schulte, HD: Surgical treatment of hypertrophic obstructive cardiomyopathy with special reference to complications and to atypical hypertrophic obstructive cardiomyopathy. *Eur Heart J* 1983;4(suppl F):187–190.
131. Beahrs MM, Tajik AJ, Seward JB, Giuliani ER, McGoon DC: Hypertrophic obstructive cardiomyopathy: Ten to 21-year follow-up after partial septal myectomy. *Am J Cardiol* 1983; 51:1160–1166.
132. McIntosh CL, Maron BJ: Current operative treatment of obstructive hypertrophic cardiomyopathy. *Circulation* 1988; 78:487–495.
133. McIntosh CL, Maron BJ, Cannon RO, Klues HG: Initial results of combined anterior mitral leaflet plication and ventricular septal myotomy-myectomy for relief of left ventricular outflow tract obstruction in patients with hypertrophic cardiomyopathy. *Circulation* 1992; 86:II-60–II-67.
134. Cohn LH, Trehan H, Collins JJ: Long-term follow-up of patients undergoing myotomy-myectomy for obstructive hypertrophic cardiomyopathy. *Am J Cardiol* 1992; 70:657–660.
135. Lösse B, Kuhn H, Loogen F, Schulte HD: Exercise performance in hypertrophic cardiomyopathies. *Eur Heart J* 1983; 4 (suppl F):197–208.
136. Cannon RO, McIntosh CL, Schenke WH, Maron BJ, Bonow RO, Epstein SE: Effect of surgical reduction of left ventricular outflow obstruction on hemodynamics, coronary flow, and myocardial metabolism in hypertrophic cardiomyopathy. *Circulation* 1989; 79:766–775.
137. Siegman IL, Maron BJ, Permut LC, McIntosh CL, Clark RE: Results of operation for coexistent obstructive hypertrophic cardiomyopathy and coronary artery disease. *J Am Coll Cardiol* 1989; 13:1527–1533.
138. McDonald KM, Maurer B: Permanent pacing as treatment for hypertrophic cardiomyopathy. *Am J Cardiol* 1991; 68:108–110.
139. Fananapazir L, Cannon RO, Tripodi D, Panza JA: Impact of dual-chamber permanent pacing in patients with obstructive hypertrophic cardiomyopathy with symptoms refractory to verapamil and β-adrenergic blocker therapy. *Circulation* 1992; 85:2149–2161.
140. Jeanrenaud X, Goy J-J, Kappenberger L: Effects of dual-chamber pacing in hypertrophic obstructive cardiomyopathy. *Lancet* 1992; 339:1318–1323.

Chapter 91

Restrictive Cardiomyopathy

Ralph Shabetai, M.D.

DEFINITION

Restrictive cardiomyopathy is considerably less common than classical congestive heart failure. Its importance therefore lies primarily in properly distinguishing it from constrictive pericarditis, because of the dire consequences of mistakenly treating a case of constrictive pericarditis as though it were inoperable.

Restrictive cardiomyopathy must be considered within the broader spectrum of diastolic dysfunction. (See Chaps. 5, 23, and 25.) Diastolic dysfunction of some degree and of one or other type is common to many disorders of the heart.[1] Congestive heart failure may be produced by systolic dysfunction, diastolic dysfunction, or combined systolic and diastolic ventricular dysfunction that may affect one or both ventricles, in the latter instance either symmetrically or asymmetrically. The principal hemodynamic manifestations of ventricular systolic dysfunction are reduction of cardiac output and failure of cardiac output to respond normally to the increased demand of exercise. (See Chap. 25.)

The principal clinical and hemodynamic manifestations of diastolic dysfunction are congestion and increased diastolic pressure. In some cases of heart failure, ventricular systolic function is normal or nearly so, whereas diastolic dysfunction is prominent, a syndrome that has been called diastolic heart failure.[2]

Diastolic dysfunction may also occur because the loading conditions of the heart are abnormal. The ventricles are unloaded when there is severe mitral or tricuspid stenosis. Perhaps the most dramatic clinical picture of unloading the heart is that of constrictive pericarditis or cardiac tamponade in which the basic pathophysiology is an impediment to diastolic filling. Severe diastolic dysfunction can also occur when the ventricles hypertrophy in the face of severe increase in their afterload, as in outflow obstruction or hypertension of the systemic or pulmonary circulation. Diastolic dysfunction is also an important component of hypertrophic cardiomyopathy. Details concerning the pathophysiology, quantification, classification, and clinical manifestations of diastolic dysfunction are to be found in Chaps. 23 to 26.

In the past, erroneous concepts regarding restrictive cardiomyopathy have arisen and spurious claims have been made that restrictive cardiomyopathy can easily be distinguished from constrictive pericarditis. Thus, it is necessary to define restrictive cardiomyopathy quite specifically, albeit somewhat arbitrarily.[3]

A workable definition of restrictive cardiomyopathy is a systemic or idiopathic disorder of the myocardium manifest by a clinical and hemodynamic picture that simulates constrictive pericarditis. To meet the criteria, there should be increased jugular venous pressure with prominent *x* and *y* descents, a small or normal-sized heart, pulmonary congestion, and the absence of ventricular hypertrophy or dilatation. Ventricular systolic function should be normal, and there cannot be a stenotic valvular lesion or outflow tract obstruction. Although it is generally unwise to define clinical entities by rigid numbers, patients with a left ventricular end-diastolic dimension of 7 cm or more, true myocardial wall thickness of 1.7 cm or more, left ventricular end-diastolic volume of 150 mL/m^2 or more, or an ejection fraction below 20 percent cannot be considered to have restrictive cardiomyopathy. The closer these values are to normal, the more likely is the diagnosis of restrictive cardiomyopathy to be correct. As a rough guideline, left ventricular end-diastolic volume should not be more than 110 mL/

m² per min and left ventricular end-diastolic dimension certainly should not exceed 6 cm.

RESTRICTIVE CARDIOMYOPATHY

Etiology

Restrictive cardiomyopathy may be either idiopathic and thus be a true cardiomyopathy in the strict sense of the term[4] or secondary to an infiltrative disease of the myocardium, in which case it actually is a systemic myocardial disorder or heart muscle disease rather than a primary cardiomyopathy. Unfortunately, these cases are usually referred to as restrictive cardiomyopathy, the advice of the World Health Organization[4] report notwithstanding. Idiopathic cases may be manifest by extensive fibrosis, but in some cases no pathological substrate for the abnormal diastolic behavior of the heart is apparent.[5] Cardiac amyloidosis is the most common systemic cause, but not all cases of cardiac amyloidosis present as restrictive cardiomyopathy; some have a diastolic abnormality that differs from that of classical restrictive cardiomyopathy and also have major impairment of systolic function. Hemochromatosis can also produce restrictive cardiomyopathy,[6] although more commonly the cardiac manifestation of hemochromatosis is dilated cardiomyopathy,[7] which is often reversible when the iron load has been removed or decreased. Typical pathophysiology of restrictive cardiomyopathy is usual in the transplanted heart soon after operation and in 15 percent persists for at least a year.[8] Late occurrence or recurrence is thought to be evidence of rejection. (See Chap. 32.) Restrictive physiology characterizes a minority of cases of acute myocarditis. Other less common causes of restrictive cardiomyopathy have been reviewed recently.[9] They include scleroderma, in which the cardiopulmonary-pericardial hemodynamic abnormalities are complex (see Chap. 103); carcinoid, in which the restrictive pattern may be due to subacute tricuspid regurgitation causing the heart to engage the pericardium (see Chaps. 88 and 111); and sarcoidosis, which usually presents with arrhythmia or conduction disturbances (see also Chap. 88). The infiltrative cardiomyopathies and endomyocardial disorders are discussed later in this chapter.

History

Unfortunately, many patients present when the disease process is far advanced and when they already have pronounced symptoms of pulmonary and systemic congestion. The leading complaints usually include dyspnea, orthopnea, nocturnal dyspnea, or pulmonary edema, together with ankle swelling, abdominal discomfort, and increase in abdominal girth. In patients in whom the restrictive cardiomyopathy is secondary to a systemic disease, symptoms of other organ involvement may be elicited, but the heart may be the only organ involved even in what is more commonly a systemic disorder.

Clinical Examination

On examination the patients have the classical findings of raised filling pressure on the two sides of the heart. Right-sided heart filling pressure judged from the jugular venous pulse is strikingly elevated. Commonly, neither the A nor V wave is particularly prominent but the *x* and *y* descents are often dramatic. Which of these two inward motions of the jugular pulse predominates varies among patients, but more commonly it is the *y* descent. The central venous pressure can be assessed at the bedside by skilled analysis of the jugular venous pulse (Chap. 10). The patient's thorax must be placed at an angle from the horizontal that optimizes the jugular pulsation. The *x* and *y* descents appear as sharp inward movements, the *x* synchronous and the *y* out of phase with the carotid pulse. In severe cases the peripheral arterial pulses reflect the tachycardia and the low stroke volume with diminished pulse pressure and, occasionally, a prominent dicrotic wave. The apex impulse is usually in a normal location and is of normal character, without left or right ventricular heave. In most cases there is no systolic murmur, but sometimes there is a systolic murmur of mitral or tricuspid regurgitation. A third heart sound marking the abrupt cessation of early rapid filling may be present.

When restrictive cardiomyopathy is secondary to a systemic disorder such as amyloidosis, extracardiac manifestations may be detected upon careful general physical examination, although one frequently has to rely upon abnormal laboratory findings.

Electrocardiogram

The electrocardiogram is almost always abnormal. Left bundle branch block is common, but some patients may have right bundle branch block. When restrictive cardiomyopathy is secondary to amyloidosis, generalized low voltage characteristically is present in the electrocardiogram, a finding that is in contrast to the apparent increase of wall thickness of the left ventricle demonstrated by the echocardiogram[10] (Fig. 91-1). In this instance, much of the increased wall thickness of the left ventricle represents infiltration with amyloid rather than hypertrophy. In idiopathic restrictive cardiomyopathy sinus rhythm is often maintained until the end stages of the disorder, whereas a variety of major arrhythmias commonly occur in patients with cardiac amyloidosis.[11]

Chest Radiogram

Two major features that characterize the chest radiogram are an absence of cardiomegaly and the presence of the various manifestations of pulmonary venous hypertension and pulmonary congestion (Chap. 14).

Echo-Doppler Cardiography

Echo-Doppler cardiography can provide crucial information pertinent to both the anatomic and the physiological abnormalities of restrictive cardiomyopathy. The study should show that neither the left nor the right ventricle is severely dilated and there should be no apparent thickening of the pericardium. Pericardial effusion may be detected, however, either as a manifestation of severe systemic congestion or because of pericardial involvement in some cases of cardiac amyloidosis. There should be no severe valvular abnormality, although some

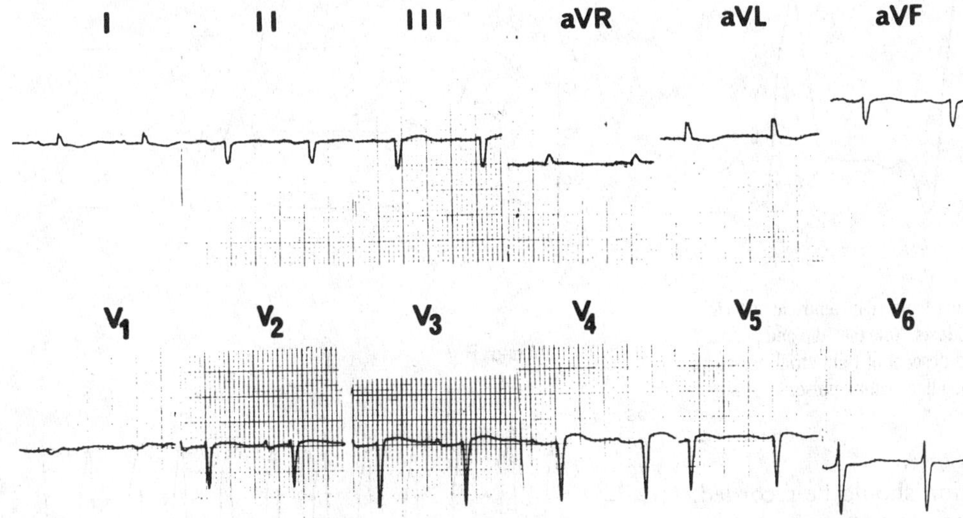

FIGURE 91-1 Electrocardiogram of a 62-year-old woman with cardiac amyloidosis. Portions of the echo Doppler study of the same patient are shown in Fig. 91-4. Note the low voltage, which is in striking contrast to the increased left ventricular wall thickness shown echocardiographically. There is also a ventricular conduction disturbance.

thickening of the mitral or aortic valve or minor calcification, presumably unrelated to the restrictive cardiomyopathy, may be found in older patients. When restrictive cardiomyopathy is secondary to an infiltrative disorder, the walls of the heart may appear grossly thickened, but in the idiopathic cases ventricular wall thickness is well within normal limits. Frequently, both atria are moderately enlarged, and this enlargement usually exceeds that observed in constrictive pericarditis.[12] Careful observation of the image throughout diastole or, better yet, computer-assisted analysis shows a restrictive pattern of filling, in which early rapid filling is even more rapid than normal, but little or no further increase in ventricular size occurs throughout the latter two-thirds of diastole. This filling pattern is also characteristic of constrictive pericarditis. It has been proposed that restrictive cardiomyopathy can be distinguished from constrictive pericarditis because in the former early rapid filling is slower than normal, whereas in the latter it is more rapid.[13–15] While this observation is true of some cases, especially those least typical of restrictive cardiomyopathy, it is not true in many cases of restrictive cardiomyopathy in whom the filling pattern is indistinguishable from that of constrictive pericarditis.[16]

Typically, the Doppler echo signal at the tips of the mitral or tricuspid valve shows a very prominent E wave reflecting the abnormally rapid filling in early diastole. The E wave also has a severely reduced deceleration time, indicating elevated left atrial pressure. Details of Doppler ventricular inflow and outflow signals have also been used to help differentiate constrictive pericarditis from restrictive cardiomyopathy (Chap. 130). This subject is discussed in Chap. 92.

Other Imaging Modalities

Computerized tomography[17] and nuclear magnetic resonance images[18] are frequently obtained in these patients to help differentiate from constrictive pericarditis. Obvious thickening of the pericardium greatly favors constrictive pericarditis, or at least a major contribution by the pericardium. Conversely, the demonstration that the pericardial image by these techniques appears normal strongly favors restrictive cardiomyopathy rather than constrictive pericarditis. In some cases of pericardial constriction produced by a thin tight epicardium,[19] however, the pericardial abnormality may not be detected by these imaging techniques.

Cardiac Catheterization

Almost all patients in whom restrictive cardiomyopathy is a serious consideration should undergo right- and left-sided heart cardiac catheterization to document that the diagnosis is correct, to assess its severity, to distinguish it from constrictive pericarditis if possible, and in some patients, to establish the etiology by means of endomyocardial biopsy (Chap. 33). As in patients with constrictive pericarditis, extra care must be taken to obtain high-quality pressure recordings particularly during diastole. If conventional fluid-filled catheter-transducer systems are employed, care must be taken to create optimal damping conditions as close as possible to critical. The catheters should be short, the stopcocks and other interconnections as few as possible, and the connecting tubing as rigid, short, and relatively large bore as possible. Transducer height and system calibration should be carefully double checked to ensure that simultaneously recorded pressures are strictly comparable.

When the catheter is introduced into the right atrium, the abnormalities of venous pressure detectable at the bedside are confirmed and can be more precisely quantified. Typically, the venous pressure is elevated, frequently to the high teens or even low twenties. The deep and steep nature of the *y* descent in the right atrium is the most striking feature of the tracing (Fig. 91-2). Since tachycardia is frequent, the record may need to be obtained at higher than normal chart speed. Ideally, an

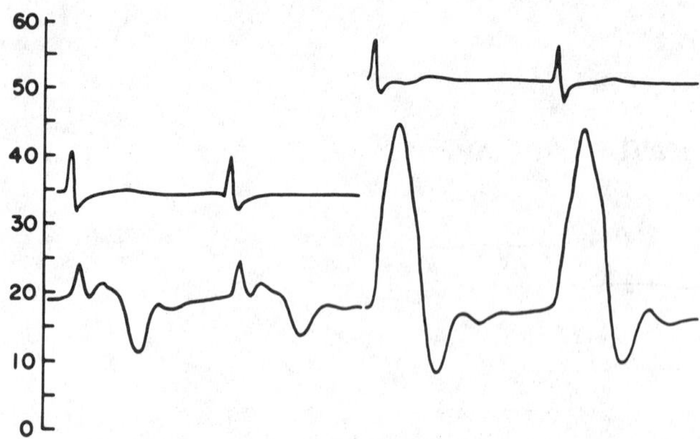

FIGURE 91-2 High-fidelity pressure tracing from right ventricle and right atrium in a case of restrictive cardiac amyloidosis. Note the "dip and plateau" of right ventricular pressure and the deep *y* descent of right atrial pressure. The *y* descent was easily observed in the jugular venous pulse.

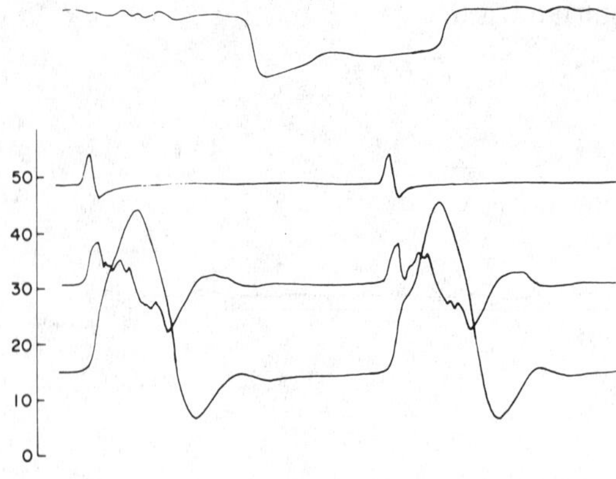

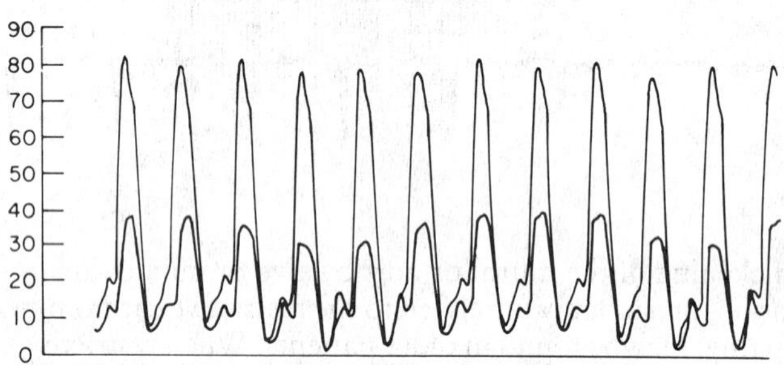

FIGURE 91-3 *Top:* Right-sided heart hemodynamic data from a patient with typical restrictive amyloid cardiomyopathy recorded with a high-fidelity catheter. Tracings from above down, the phase of respiration, the electrocardiogram, and right ventricular pressure with superimposed first derivative of right ventricular pressure. Note the characteristic dip and plateau configuration. The patient displayed a prominent *y* descent of venous pressure corresponding with the early diastolic dip of right ventricular pressure. *Bottom:* Simultaneous right and left ventricular pressure tracings from another patient with cardiac amyloidosis. In this patient, the typical restrictive dip and plateau pattern was not present, but diastolic pressure rose steeply throughout diastole and culminated in a prominent *a* wave reflecting atrial systole. Note also that during inspiration left and right ventricular diastolic pressures are equal, making differentiation from constrictive pericarditis more difficult.

independent marker of respiration should be recorded. This can be either through a separate transducer system or by simultaneously recording the pulmonary wedge pressure, which should track the respiratory cycle faithfully. During inspiration the descent of the *y*-wave in the right atrium becomes deeper, steeper, and more pointed,[20] whereas the other waves of the venous pulse and the mean atrial pressure do not vary throughout the respiratory cycle.[21]

When the catheter is advanced through the tricuspid valve into the right ventricle, a highly characteristic pressure emerges. The right ventricular systolic pressure is within the range of 35 to 45 mmHg. The early portion of diastole is characterized by a deep, sharp dip followed by a plateau during which no further increase in right ventricular pressure occurs[22] (Fig. 91-2). When right ventricular and right atrial pressures are recorded simultaneously, the early diastolic dip of ventricular diastolic pressure is seen to correspond with the *y* descent of right atrial pressure, marking early rapid filling. Also, the plateau of right ventricular diastolic pressure is equal to the right atrial pressure throughout the remainder of diastole. Characteristically, these pressures are elevated considerably above the upper limits of normal for right atrial pressure. These features are identical to those of constrictive pericarditis (Chap. 92). Most authors concur, although one report has stated that the dip and plateau do not occur in restrictive cardiomyopathy.[23]

There is usually modest pulmonary hypertension with no pressure difference in systole across the pulmonary valve. Pulmonary arterial diastolic pressure is a few millimeters higher than the pulmonary wedge pressure, indicating a normal transpulmonary pressure gradient. The pulmonary wedge pressure is elevated, often to extreme levels. Contrary to earlier publications,[24] it is not uncommon for the pulmonary wedge and the right atrial pressures to be identical. The finding of equal filling pressures in the left and right ventricles, therefore, does not necessarily indicate that a patient has constrictive pericarditis (Fig. 91-3). On the other hand, a left ventricular filling pressure appreciably above right-sided heart filling pressure strongly favors the diagnosis of restrictive cardiomyopathy rather than constrictive pericarditis.[25] Left ventricular systolic pressure is normal, while the left ventricular diastolic pressure tracing shows the same abnormalities as those of the right ventricle. Severe pulmonary hypertension, in contrast to some earlier reports, does not occur in restrictive cardiomyopathy.[16,25] Because of suboptimal damping characteristics of the pressure recording systems, catheter motion, and different levels of intracardiac catheters, the *y* descent of atrial pressure and the early diastolic dip of the corresponding ventricular diastolic pressures are frequently not exactly equal. On the other hand, right atrial and right ventricular pressures equilibrate in mid and late diastole, as do the pulmonary wedge and left ventricular diastolic pressures. In those cases that most closely simulate constrictive pericarditis, all four pressures equilibrate during this phase of the cardiac cycle.

Left ventriculography usually shows a normal ejection fraction[16,17] and the absence of major regional wall motion abnormalities. In the most characteristic cases, frame-by-frame analysis of the left ventriculogram shows unduly rapid filling in early diastole followed by little if any additional filling after middiastole. In some atypical cases the early rapid filling is slow,[14] and many of these patients do not have the typical clinical picture of restrictive cardiomyopathy.

Endomyocardial biopsy is an integral part of the workup of many patients with restrictive cardiomyopathy.[25] In cases where distinction from constrictive pericarditis is particularly difficult, the biopsy may furnish proof of myocardial disease or by absence of such proof lend support to the diagnosis of constrictive pericarditis. The biopsy may establish the cause of restrictive cardiomyopathy, for instance, cardiac amyloidosis. (See also Chaps. 33 and 88.)

DISTINGUISHING RESTRICTIVE CARDIOMYOPATHY FROM PERICARDITIS

(See also Chap. 92.)

History

The history can provide important clues to this often difficult differential diagnosis. A history of tuberculosis, trauma, previous episodes of pericarditis or systemic diseases that frequently involve the pericardium, particularly collagen vascular disorders, favor constrictive pericarditis. A history of prior radiation lends more weight to constrictive pericarditis, but in many cases there is considerable myocardial radiation damage as well. Indeed, after extensive mediastinal radiation, as for treatment of lymphoma or in preparation for bone marrow transplantation, some patients subsequently develop combined constrictive pericarditis and restrictive cardiomyopathy.[26] A history of prior cardiac surgery favors constrictive pericarditis, but impaired myocardial preservation during cardiopulmonary bypass can result in restrictive cardiomyopathy. A history of disorders that involve the heart, such as amyloidosis or hemochromatosis, strongly favor restrictive cardiomyopathy. Hypertension and ischemic heart disease usually give rise to diastolic heart failure that does not particularly simulate constrictive pericarditis. (See also Chaps. 25, 26, 58, and 75.)

Clinical Examination

The clinical examination described above is the same as that found in patients with constrictive pericarditis and is therefore not helpful in differentiating these two conditions. Some authorities claim that the third heart sound is usually not present in restrictive cardiomyopathy[27] but that a fourth heart sound is fairly frequent. Nevertheless, some typical cases of restrictive cardiomyopathy have a third heart sound, which may be difficult to distinguish from a pericardial knock.

Electrocardiography

Left and right bundle branch blocks strongly favor restrictive cardiomyopathy over constrictive pericarditis. The same is true for left or right ventricular hypertrophy and atrioventricular conduction disturbances, although the latter is rare even in restrictive cardiomyopathy. Atrial fibrillation may supervene in either condition. Complex arrhythmias, however, are more common in restrictive cardiomyopathy than in constrictive pericarditis. Chronic, especially calcific, constrictive pericarditis can involve the epicardial coronary arteries and produce electrocardiographic changes that are otherwise more frequently found in patients with restrictive cardiomyopathy.[28]

Chest Radiogram

In both conditions the cardiac silhouette is usually of normal size, although the heart may sometimes be somewhat enlarged. Atrial enlargement sufficient to be recognizable by plain chest radiography is more in favor of restrictive cardiomyopathy than constrictive pericarditis. In either condition, pulmonary congestion is a feature of either condition, although often this is less pronounced than in classical congestive heart failure. A heavy, large ring of calcification is obviously much more likely to be present in patients with constrictive pericarditis. Intracardiac calcification should be absent in both conditions unless the patient is old, in which case incidental calcification of the aortic valve or the mitral valve ring may be present. Calcification is best assessed by cardiac fluoroscopy. Striking radiographic left or right ventricular enlargement is not a feature of either condition.

The contributions made by computerized tomography and nuclear magnetic resonance have already been mentioned. Echocardiography is a relatively insensitive means of detecting constrictive pericarditis. Restricted motion of the coronary arteries is a feature of constrictive pericarditis but not of restrictive cardiomyopathy.[29] Furthermore, when the pericardium is greatly thickened, the epicardial coronary arteries are never on the border of the cardiac shadow.[30]

Cardiac Catheterization

The important features detectable by hemodynamic and angiographic studies and their relative frequency in constrictive pericarditis and restrictive cardiomyopathy have already been described. (See also Chap. 92.) It should be reemphasized that the demonstration that left and right ventricular diastolic pressures are equal does not rule out restrictive cardiomyopathy nor does it prove that a patient has constrictive pericarditis.[25] When all clinical imaging and hemodynamic data fail to make a clear distinction between these two conditions, endomyocardial biopsy may be the crucial test. The result may be obvious myocardial disease or an entirely normal biopsy. In the latter circumstance, surgical exploration should be carried out even if imaging techniques fail to show a thickened pericardium. As in the interpretation of most laboratory tests, however, clinical judgment is still of prime importance; nowhere is this more true than when the studies yield data compatible with mixed constrictive pericarditis and restrictive cardiomyopathy. In these patients, the clinician must make a decision whether to explore or treat conservatively on the basis of the hemodynamic findings and the morphologic abnormalities found on biopsy. It is important to appreciate that in many cases, except for cardiac transplantation, there is no satisfactory treatment for restrictive cardiomyopathy.

Treatment

The clinician diagnoses restrictive cardiomyopathy with reluctance, since there is no satisfactory medical treatment. It is difficult to understand the pathophysiological basis of the diastolic disorder characterizing restrictive cardiomyopathy. Not surprisingly, therefore, it is difficult to devise logical therapy. By comparison, the pathophysiology of constrictive pericarditis is simple (Chap. 92). The scarred, noncompliant, shrunken pericardium limits cardiac size from the end of early rapid filling until the end of diastole, thereby producing a marked increase in ventricular diastolic pressures and limiting ventricular end diastolic volumes. In consequence, stroke volume falls, compensatory tachycardia appears, and a picture simulating right-sided heart failure emerges. In patients with diastolic heart failure, it is also easy to conjecture the pathophysiology. In most patients, the ventricles are significantly hypertrophied and therefore stiff and less compliant. If there is also slow diastolic relaxation and an enhanced atrial contribution to filling, one has the rudiments of diastolic heart failure. (See also Chap. 25.) Since the hemodynamics and ventricular filling characteristics in restrictive cardiomyopathy are the same as those found in constrictive pericarditis, it is necessary to postulate that the myocardial disorder allows normal or even increased ventricular diastolic compliance in early diastole but a virtually infinitely stiff ventricle in mid and late diastole. Since the structural basis for this behavior of the myocardium, be it in the myocytes or the collagen, is not known, treatment is empirical.

When the filling pressures are extremely high with systemic and pulmonary congestion, significant benefit can be obtained from the use of diuretics. More caution in the diuretic dosage is advised when treating restrictive cardiomyopathy than when treating conventional heart failure, because in restrictive cardiomyopathy a relatively high level of ventricular filling pressure must be maintained if ventricular filling is to be sustained. Digitalis and other agents with positive inotropic activity are not indicated if systolic pump function and contractility are not impaired. Vasodilatation should also be applied very cautiously, lest it further decreases ventricular filling and causes deterioration of the clinical condition. There is some evidence that in patients with hypertrophic cardiomyopathy diastolic compliance may be increased by administration of calcium channel-blocking agents[31] (Chap. 90). Extrapolation of these data from hypertrophic cardiomyopathy to restrictive cardiomyopathy is fraught with hazards. Nevertheless, attempts to treat the restrictive cardiomyopathy with these agents in the hope of improving diastolic compliance can be justified. On the whole, however, the results have been disappointing, and it remains extremely difficult to obtain a therapeutic benefit with the combined use of low-dose diuretics and agents such as verapamil.

The Infiltrative Cardiomyopathies

Amyloid Heart Disease

The most commonly encountered infiltrative cardiomyopathy is amyloid, the biochemical features of which have recently been reviewed.[32] Electron microscopy identifies amyloid as rigid, nonbranching fibrils. In primary amyloidosis there is no coexisting disease except, in some cases, multiple myeloma; on the other hand, in secondary amyloidosis a chronic disease such as tuberculosis or rheumatoid arthritis may be present. The pathological counterpart of reduced compliance is a stiff, rubbery heart that does not collapse when placed on the autopsy table. Although the coronary vessels and cardiac valves may be involved, this involvement seldom produces clinical manifestations. So-called senile cardiac amyloidosis is common in the very elderly[33] but is often not detected until a postmortem examination is performed. When the amyloid is deposited between myocytes, classic restrictive cardiomyopathy results, but systolic failure may supervene if there is extensive myocardial replacement.[34] (See Chap. 25.)

The clinical and hemodynamic findings have been described above. The echocardiogram shows thickening of both left and right ventricular myocardium (Fig. 91-4). In the earlier literature, the "sparkling" appearance of the myocardium was said to be diagnostic of amyloidosis,[35] but this finding has very poor specificity and should not be relied upon for diagnosis.[36] (See also Chap. 15.) In general, the prognosis is poor and treatment, for the most part, is ineffective. Many cardiologists believe that the amyloid heart is highly sensitive to digitalis, which should therefore be employed with caution when systolic failure or atrial fibrillation supervene. Chemotherapy with melthalan[37] has been tried, but its place in therapy has not yet been established.

Carcinoid Heart Disease

The picture of restrictive cardiomyopathy may develop in carcinoid heart disease due to infiltration of the myocardium by carcinoid. In some cases the restrictive pattern is produced by subacute tricuspid regurgitation with consequent dilatation of the right ventricle and engagement of enlarged heart against the normal pericardium. (See also Chaps. 88 and 111.)

Hemochromatosis

Primary hemochromatosis is an inborn error of metabolism associated with HLA-A3 and HLA-B14. (See Chap. 96.) Large amounts of iron are deposited in the reticuloendothelial system, where they are harmless, as well as in the liver, heart, and pancreas, where they cause bronzed diabetes and heart disease. In addition to iron deposition in the heart, secondary myocardial fibrosis may also develop. Dilated heart failure is far more common than restrictive cardiomyopathy[7] although the latter has been reported on several occasions[38] and may precede the advent of frank systolic heart failure. Unlike the situation in amyloid cardiomyopathy, excellent results can be expected from appropriate treatment (Fig. 91-5) even

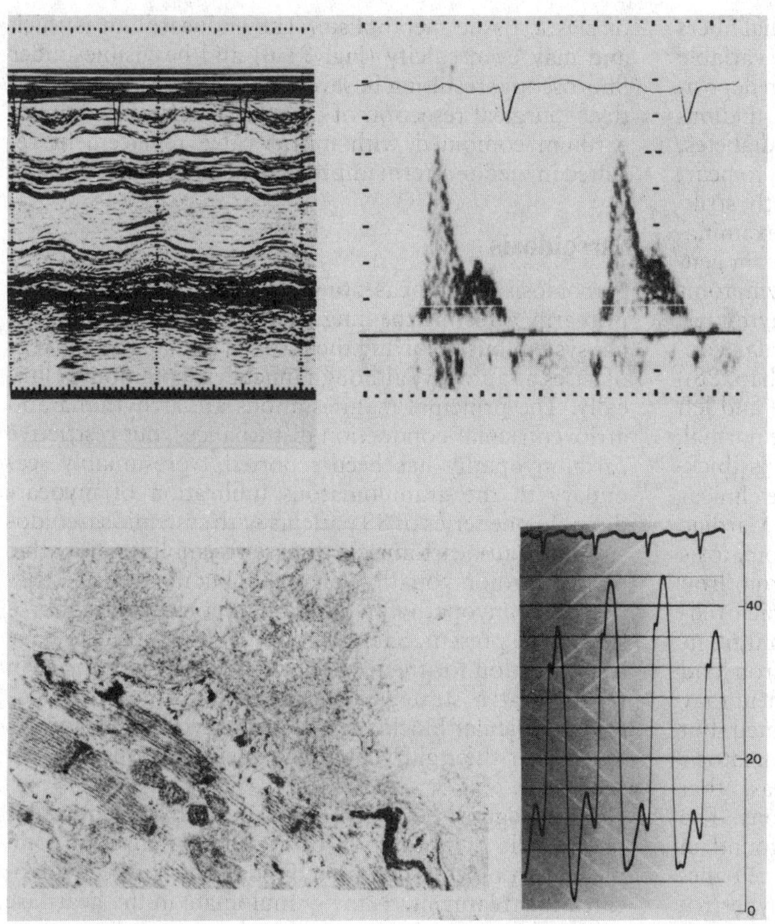

FIGURE 91-4 Data from the patient whose electrocardiogram is illustrated in Fig. 91-1. *Top left:* M-mode echocardiogram showing increased thickness of the left ventricular myocardium, which ordinarily would have suggested left ventricular hypertrophy. Calibration marks 1 cm. *Top right:* Doppler tracing of mitral inflow velocity. Note that velocity is maximum at middiastole. The atrial contribution to mitral blood flow velocity is considerably reduced. Calibration: single mark, 0.2 m; double mark, 1 m/s. *Bottom left:* Electromicrograph showing extensive replacement of myocardium by amyloid. *Bottom right:* Right ventricular pressure tracing. Note the early diastolic dip and plateau of amyloid restrictive cardiomyopathy is not present.

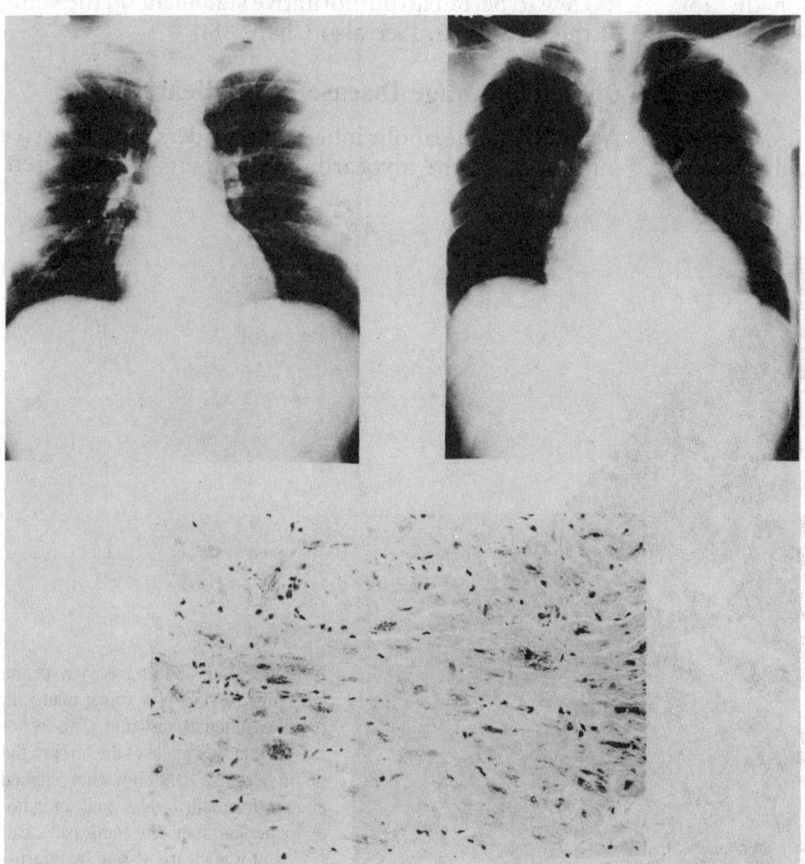

FIGURE 91-5 Chest radiograph of a patient with cardiac hemochromatosis. *Top left:* Before treatment. *Top right:* After several months of regular venesection. *Bottom:* Endomyocardial biopsy that established the diagnosis of cardiac hemochromatosis.

though the iron is deposited within the myocardial fibers themselves. The degree of interstitial fibrosis is variable and apparently is not related to the extent of iron deposition. The patient usually manifests the typical findings of hemochromatosis—hepatic dysfunction, diabetes, and brown pigmentation of the skin in addition to heart failure. In advanced cases, the heart is frequently strikingly enlarged to both clinical and radiologic examination. Left ventricular function tests show significant generalized dilatation and hypokinesis. Typical symptoms of congestive heart failure supervene, and arrhythmias, particularly atrial fibrillation and atrioventricular conduction disturbances, are common. (See also Chap. 88.)

In cases detected early, the overall heart size and left ventricular dimensions and systolic function are normal. At this stage, the left ventricular myocardium is thickened, the dysfunction is mainly diastolic and the clinical picture simulates that of cardiac amyloidosis. Cardiac dysfunction in the presence of possible hemochromatosis should lead to determination of the level of serum iron and ferritin and to endomyocardial biopsy, which reliably shows the typical findings. The fundamental treatment is repeated venesection until the excessive iron load has been removed. Two or more years of treatment may be required. Chelation therapy has been advocated, but its role remains dubious. Secondary hemochromatosis may result from disorders such as a blood dyscrasia that require enormous numbers of blood transfusions. The cardiac manifestations are identical to those found in primary hemochromatosis. Patients with sickle cell anemia may have preexisting cardiac dilation and hypertrophy prior to the development of hemochromatosis. In such patients, treatment consists of chelation therapy rather than phlebotomy.

Pseudoxanthoma Elasticum

Endocardial fibroelastosis is one of the many lesions that may be found in this rare but striking inherited disorder of elastic tissue metabolism. The endocardium is thick and may even calcify (Fig. 91-6) and be visible under fluoroscopy, resulting in severe restrictive cardiomyopathy.[39] Surgical resection of calcified bands of endomyocardium combined with mitral valve replacement resulted in medium-term improvement in a reported case.[40]

Sarcoidosis

Sarcoidosis is a noncaseating granulomatous infiltration primarily affecting the lungs, skin, and reticuloendothelial system but involving the heart in perhaps 25 percent of cases at autopsy, although much less commonly clinically. The principal manifestations are arrhythmia and atrioventricular conduction disturbances, but restrictive cardiomyopathy has been reported,[41] presumably secondary to the granulomatous infiltration of myocardium. In one series of 88 patients with systemic sarcoidosis, nine had heart muscle disease resembling idiopathic dilated cardiomyopathy (Chap. 88) but none had restrictive cardiomyopathy. In addition to granulomata, fibrosis may be present. Sarcoid granulomata appear to have a predilection for the basal myocardium[42] with the twin results that a strategically placed lesion may produce atrioventricular block and that endomyocardial biopsies taken near the right ventricular apex may fail to reveal the lesion.

The prognosis is poor. Sudden death from ventricular tachycardia or fibrillation or the sudden onset of complete heart block is common. Prednisone has been advocated for treatment, as the granulomata in the heart are said to be sensitive. At present, the reported cases are too few to permit an authoritative statement on the value of this treatment. (See also Chap. 88.)

Glycogen Storage Disease of the Heart

A number of metabolic inherited disorders cause massive infiltration of the myocardium in infants and children.

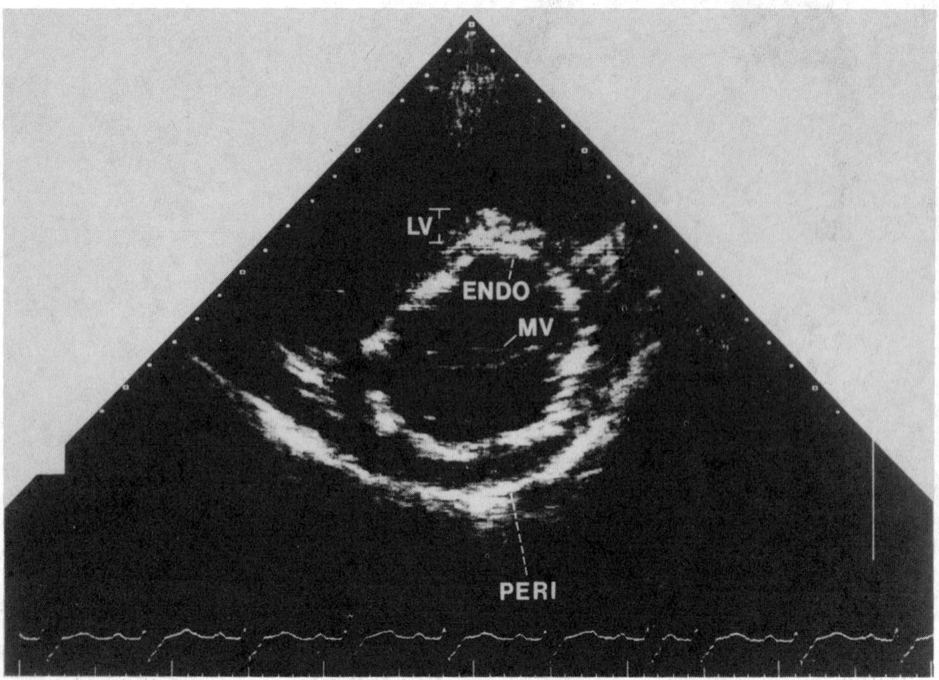

FIGURE 91-6 Short-axis view of the left ventricle (LV) of a young man with pseudoxanthoma elasticum. This echocardiogram was made at the level of the mitral valve (MV) and shows the calcified endomyocardium (endo) and an echo-dense pericardium. The endocardial calcification was clearly visible by fluoroscopy. (*Courtesy Brian Hoit, M.D.*)

The best known is Pompe's disease, otherwise known as Type II glycogenesis, which is an autosomal recessive disorder caused by a deficiency of acid maltase. In this disorder, absence of the enzyme alpha-glucosidase causes glycogen to be deposited in massive amounts in the cardiac and skeletal musculature. Manifestations appear in the first few months of life and almost invariably before the age of $1\frac{1}{2}$ years. Failure to thrive, weakness, and hyperreflexia are observed early in infancy.[43] The myocardium may become so infiltrated that the pathophysiology may resemble that of hypertrophic cardiomyopathy. Usually, however, the heart is massively dilated.[44] In either case, in spite of the heavy infiltration, the picture of restrictive cardiomyopathy does not appear. The diagnosis can be made from a skeletal muscle biopsy, which confirms the absence of alpha-glucosidase activity. The electrocardiogram shows left ventricular hypertrophy, at times with extremely high voltage, and the massively thickened ventricular myocardium is obvious on echocardiography. Regrettably, no satisfactory treatment has been developed and most patients die in the first year of life. (See also Chap. 88.)

A number of other rare abnormalities of glycogen metabolism may affect the heart. Nodular glycogenic infiltration occurs in the pediatric age group and is associated with tuberous sclerosis in half of the cases.[45] (See Chaps. 88 and 96.)

Endomyocardial Fibrosis: Hypereosinophilic Syndrome

Two forms of the eosinophilic syndrome are recognized: tropical eosinophilic endomyocardial fibrosis and nontropical eosinophilic endomyocardial disease, sometimes referred to as Löffler's disease. The major characteristics of the syndrome are eosinophilia in the peripheral blood and an endocardial disease consisting of eosinophilic infiltration,[46] fibrosis, and eventually virtual occlusion of the ventricular cavity by scar and thrombus formation. This results in a very severe form of restrictive myocardial disease, sometimes referred to as obliterative myocardial disease.[47]

It should be noted that the eosinophil responsible for endomyocardial disease is itself an abnormal cell. When compared with the normal eosinophil, the cells appear to have fewer granules and to contain vacuoles. Adjacent to the abnormal eosinophil, myocardial necrosis is intense, indicating that the cells are toxic to the myocardium. Thus, Löffler's endomyocardial disease is considered to be an immunologic disorder caused by clones of abnormal eosinophils.[48] Endomyocardial fibrosis may affect either one or both ventricles. There does not appear to be a clear distinction between Löffler's syndrome and endomyocardial involvement in eosinophilic leukemia. In the acute stage, the endomyocardium is infiltrated with eosinophils and shows severe adjacent necrosis. This stage is followed by a thrombotic stage and, finally, the fibrosis stage with virtual elimination of the ventricular cavity. As in many other restrictive diseases of the ventricle, the atria become greatly enlarged and the mitral and tricuspid valves frequently are incompetent.

Hemodynamic studies reveal the typical findings of restrictive cardiomyopathy, with pressures in the left and right ventricles characterized by an early diastolic dip followed by a plateau occupying the last two-thirds of diastole. The reduction in ventricular end-diastolic volume is responsible for a reduction in cardiac stroke volume, even when systolic function remains normal. Sinus tachycardia, a frequent finding in these patients, is presumably a compensatory mechanism that partially restores cardiac output. Atrial fibrillation is common, an observation that is expected in disease characterized by significant left atrial dilatation.

The differential diagnosis from constrictive pericarditis follows the paradigm applicable to any other syndrome of restrictive cardiomyopathy. In the earlier stages, the diagnosis is readily made by endomyocardial biopsy, which reveals eosinophils and the typical pathological changes described above. As in other restrictive cardiomyopathies, atrial enlargement is more prominent than in constrictive pericarditis. The clinical findings are those of diastolic heart failure characterized by pulmonary congestion, dyspnea, edema, and eventually anasarca, often with a large pericardial effusion. The murmurs of mitral and tricuspid regurgitation are usually present, and enlargement of the heart on chest radiography is principally produced by biatrial rather than ventricular enlargement. Pleural effusions are frequently visible on the chest radiogram.

Two-dimensional echocardiography shows the diminished volume of the ventricles, frequently associated with complete obliteration of the apices of both ventricles. The ventricular diastolic filling pattern is that of restrictive cardiomyopathy with early rapid filling predominating. In some cases, the endocardium, as in pseudoxanthoma elasticum, may show a speckled appearance on echocardiography.

Nontropical eosinophilic endomyocardial fibrosis is not a common disease. Even though the author has a special interest in cardiomyopathy, and particularly restrictive cardiomyopathy, he has personally encountered only two or three well-documented cases. Most of the information concerning the syndrome therefore derives from major referral centers at which the staff has a particular interest in this syndrome. The work of Olson has been particularly useful to cardiologists encountering sporadic cases.[49] The prognosis is poor, perhaps justifying resection of the endocardium, which has been performed in a few cases with some degree of success.[50]

REFERENCES

1. Grossman W: Diastolic dysfunction in congestive heart failure. *New Engl J Med* 1991; 325:1557–1564.
2. Soufer, R, Wohlgelernter D, Vita NA, Amuchestegui M, Sostman HD, Berger HJ, et al: Intact systolic left ventricular function in clinical congestive heart failure. *Am J Cardiol* 1985; 55:1032–1036.
3. Goodwin JF, Oakley CM: The cardiomyopathies. *Br Heart J* 1972; 34:545–552.
4. WHO/ISFC Task Force: Report of the WHO/ISFC Task Force on the definition and classification of cardiomyopathies. *Br Heart J* 1980; 44:672–673.
5. McManus BM, Bren GB, Robertson EA: Hemodynamic cardiac constriction without anatomic myocardial restriction or pericardial constriction. *Am Heart J* 1981; 102:134–136.
6. Cutler DJ, Isner JM, Bracey AW, Hufnagel CA, Conrad PW, Roberts WC, et al: Hemochromatosis heart disease: An unempha-

sized cause of potentially reversible restrictive cardiomyopathy. *Am J Med* 1980; 69:923–928.

7. Skinner C, Kenmure CF: Hemochromatosis presenting as congestive cardiomyopathy and responding to venesection. *Br Heart J* 1973; 35:466–468.
8. Valentine HA, Fowler MB, Hunt SA, Naasz C, Hatle LK, Billingham ME, et al: Changes in Doppler echocardiographic indexes of left ventricular function as potential markers of acute cardiac rejection. *Circulation* 1987; 76(suppl V):V86–V92.
9. Child JS, Perloff JK: The echo-Doppler and color restrictive cardiomyopathies. *Cardiol Clin* 1988; 6:289–316.
10. Carrol JD, Gaasch WH, McAdam KPWJ: Amyloid cardiomyopathy: Characterization by a distinctive volume/mass relation. *Am J Cardiol* 1982; 49:9–13.
11. Eriksson P, Karp K, Bjerle P, Olofsson BO: Disturbances of cardiac rhythm and conduction in familial amyloidosis and polyneuropathy. *Br Heart J* 1984; 51:658–662.
12. Borer JS, Henry WL, Epstein SE: Echocardiographic observations in patients with systemic infiltrative disease involving the heart. *Am J Cardiol* 1977; 39:184–188.
13. Tyberg TI, Goodyer AV, Hurst VW III, Alexander J, Langou RA: Left ventricular filling in differentiating restrictive amyloid cardiomyopathy and constrictive pericarditis. *Am J Cardiol* 1981; 47:791–796.
14. Janos GG, Arjunan K, Meyer RA, Engel P, Kaplan S: Differentiation of constrictive pericarditis and restrictive cardiomyopathy using digitized echocardiography. *J Am Coll Cardiol* 1983; 1:541–549.
15. Gerson MC, Colthar MS, Fowler NO: Differentiation of constrictive pericarditis and restrictive cardiomyopathy by radionuclide ventriculography. *Am Heart J* 1989; 118:1124–120.
16. Meaney E, Shabetai R, Bhargava V, Shearer M, Weidner C, Mangiardi LM: Cardiac amyloidosis, constrictive pericarditis and restrictive cardiomyopathy. *Am J Cardiol* 1976; 38:547–556.
17. Isner JM, Carter BL, Bankoff MS, Pastore JO, Ramaswamy K, McAdam KP, et al: Differentiation of constrictive pericarditis from restrictive cardiomyopathy by computed tomographic imaging. *Am Heart J* 1983; 105:1019–1025.
18. Sechtem U, Higgins CB, Sommerhoff BA, Lipton MJ, Huycke EC: Magnetic resonance imaging of restrictive cardiomyopathy. *Am J Cardiol* 1987; 59:480–482.
19. Tuna IC, Danielson GK: Surgical management of pericardial diseases. *Cardiol Clin* 1990; 8:683–696.
20. Reddy PS, Curtiss EI, O'Toole JD, Shaver JA: Cardiac tamponade: Hemodynamic observations in man. *Circulation* 78; 58:265–272.
21. Shabetai R, Fowler NO, Gunheroth WG: The hemodynamics of cardiac tamponade and constrictive pericarditis. *Am J Cardiol* 1970; 26:480–489.
22. Hansen AT, Eskildsen P, Gotzsche H: Pressure curves from the right auricle and right ventricle in chronic constrictive pericarditis. *Circulation* 1951; 3:881–885.
23. Hirota Y, Kohriyama T, Hayashi T, Kaku K, Nishimura H, Saito T, et al: Idiopathic restrictive cardiomyopathy; differences of left ventricular relaxation and diastolic wave forms from constrictive pericarditis. *Am J Cardiol* 1983; 52:421–423.
24. Wood P: Chronic constrictive pericarditis. *Am J Cardiol* 1961; 7:48–61.
25. Schonfeld MH, Supple EW, Dec EW, Fallon JT, Palacios IF: Restrictive cardiomyopathy versus constrictive pericarditis: Role of endomyocardial biopsy in avoiding unnecessary thoracotomy. *Circulation* 1987; 75:1012–1017.
26. Applefield M, Wiernik PH: Cardiac disease after radiation therapy for Hodgkin's disease: Analysis of 48 patients. *Am J Cardiol* 1983; 51:1679–1681.
27. Chen C, Ziadi GM, Raphael MJ, Oakley CM: The functional defect in amyloid heart disease. The "stiff heart syndrome." *Am J Cardiol* 1975; 36:438–444.
28. Levine HO: Myocardial fibrosis in constrictive pericarditis: Electrocardiographic and pathologic observations. *Circulation* 1973; 48:1268–1281.
29. Alexander J, Kelley MHJ, Cohen LS, Cohen LS, Langou RA: The angiographic appearance of coronary arteries in constrictive pericarditis. *Radiology* 1979; 131:609–617.
30. Ramsay HW, Sbar S, Elliott LP, Eliot RS: The differential diagnosis of restrictive myocardiopathy and chronic constrictive pericardia without calcification: Value of coronary arteriography. *Am J Cardiol* 1970; 25:635–638.
31. Bonow RO, Ostrow HG, Rosing DR, Cannon RO 3d, Lipson LC, Maron BJ, et al: Effects of verapamil on left ventricular systolic and diastolic function in patients with hypertrophic cardiomyopathy: Pressure-volume analysis with a non-imaging scintillation probe. *Circulation* 1983; 68:1062–1073.
32. Hawkins PM, Lavender JP, Pepys MB: Evaluation of systemic amyloidosis by scintigraphy with labelled serum amyloid P component. *N Engl J Med* 1990; 323:508–513.
33. Hodkinson HM, Pomerance A: The clinical significance of senile cardiac amyloidosis: A prospective clinico-pathological study. *Q J Med* 1977: 46:381–387.
34. Swanton RH, Brooksby IAB, Davies MJ, Coltarte JD, Jenkins SB, Webb-Peploe MM: Systolic and diastolic ventricular function in cardiac amyloidosis: Studies in six cases diagnosed with endomyocardial biopsies. *Am J Cardiol* 1977; 39:658–664.
35. Bhandari AK, Nanda NC: Myocardial texture characterization by two dimensional echocardiography. *Am J Cardiogr* 1982; 51:817–825.
36. Falk RH, Plehn JF, Deering T, Shick EC, Boinay P, Rubinow A, et al: Sensitivity and specificity of the echocardiographic features of cardiac amyloidosis. *Am J Cardiol* 1987; 59:418–422.
37. Kyle RA, Bayrd ED: Amyloidosis: Review of 236 cases. *Medicine* 1975; 54:271–299.
38. Short EM, Winkle RA, Billingham ME: Myocardial involvement in idiopathic hemochromatosis, morphological and clinical improvement following venesection. *Am J Med* 1981; 70:1275.
39. Navarro-Lopez F, Lorian A, Ferrer-Roca O, Betrio A, Sanz G: Restrictive cardiomyopathy in pseudoxanthoma elasticum. *Chest* 1980; 78:113–115.
40. Challenor VF, Conway N, Monro JL: The surgical treatment of restrictive cardiomyopathy in pseudoxanthoma elasticum. *Br Heart J* 1988; 59:266–269.
41. Tan LB, Dickie S, McKenna WJ: Left ventricular diastolic characteristics of cardiac sarcoidosis. *Am J Cardiol* 1986; 58:1126–1127.
42. Fawcett FJ, Goldberg MJ: Heart block resulting from myocardial sarcoidosis. *Br Heart J* 1974; 36:220–223.
43. Bordiuk JM, Legato MJ, Lovelace RE, Blumenthal S: Pompe's disease: Electromyographic, electron microscopic, and cardiovascular aspects. *Arch Neurol* 1970; 23:113–119.
44. Hwang B, Meng CC, Lin CY, Hsu HC: Clinical analysis of five infants with glycogen storage disease of the heart—Pompe's disease. *Jpn Heart J* 1986; 27:25–34.
45. Wenger NK, Abelman WH, Roberts WC: Cardiomyopathy and specific heart muscle disease. In: Hurst JW, Schlant RC, Rackley CE, Sonnenblick EH, Wenger NK (eds.): *The Heart,* 7th ed. New York, McGraw-Hill, 1990:1278–1347.
46. Davies J, Spry CJ, Sapsford R, Olsen EG, de Perez G, Oakley CM, et al: Cardiovascular features of 11 patients with eosinophilic endomyocardial disease. *Q J Med* 1983; 52(New Series LII):23–39.
47. Acquatella H, Schiller NB, Puigbo JJ, Gomez-Mancebo JR, Suarez C, et al: Value of two dimensional echocardiography in endomyocardial disease with and without eosinophilia. A clinical and pathologic study. *Circulation* 1983; 67:1219–1226.
48. Spry CJ, Tai PC: Studies on blood eosinophilia: 11 patients with Loeffler's cardiomyopathy. *Clin Exp Immunol* 1976; 24:423–434.
49. Olsen EGJ: Morphologic overview and pathogenetic mechanism in endomyocardial fibrosis associated with eosinophilia in restrictive cardiomyopathy and arrhythmias. In: Olsen EGJ, Sekiguchi M (eds): *Restrictive Cardiomyopathy and Arrhythmias.* Tokyo, University of Tokyo Press, 1990:1–8.
50. Davies J, Sapsford R, Brooksby I, Olsen EGJ, Spry CJF, Oakley CM, et al: Successful surgical treatment of two patients with eosinophilic endomyocardial disease. *Br Heart J* 1981; 46:438–445.

Chapter 92

Diseases of the Pericardium

Ralph Shabetai, M.D.

ANATOMY OF THE PERICARDIUM

The pericardium consists of a tough, fibrous outer coat with discrete attachments to the sternum, great vessels, and diaphragm and an inner membranous coat. The fibrous coat is lined by a serosal layer of cuboidal cells one layer thick. Together, the fibrous pericardium and its serosal membrane make up the parietal pericardium. The serosal membrane is reflected over the epicardial surface of the heart, together with which it forms the visceral pericardium. The pericardial cavity is enclosed between these two serosal layers and normally contains from 15 to 50 mL of clear fluid,[1] which is an ultrafiltrate of blood plasma.[2] The parietal pericardium contacts the flat ventricular surfaces so as to leave only a potential space. Where the cardiac surfaces are more curved—especially in the grooves—a true fluid-filled pericardial space exists.[3] The pericardium has a number of recesses, the most important of which is the oblique sinus. The left atrium lies anterior to the oblique sinus and is, strictly speaking, largely an extrapericardial chamber. This relationship explains why pericardial effusion behind the posterior wall of the left ventricle is usually not seen also behind the left atrium.

The phrenic nerves are embedded in the parietal pericardium; this relationship is the reason why diaphragmatic paralysis may complicate pericardial resection.

The superior and inferior pericardiosternal ligaments attach the pericardium to the sternum. Ligaments also attach the pericardium firmly to the diaphragm. The connective tissue of the pericardium becomes contiguous with the adventitia of the great vessels to provide the superior tether. These attachments maintain the heart in its normal position and are so arranged that external forces exerted on the pericardium by respiration or changes in body posture tend to cancel each other and maintain a constant heart position.[3]

Histology

The major constituent of the parietal pericardium is the fibrosa, the chief ingredient of which is compactly arranged collagen fibers disposed in three layers oriented approximately at equal angles to each other.[4] The collagen bundles have an accordion-like appearance. The elastin fibers are much less numerous, do not occur in dense bundles, and tend to be oriented at right angles to adjacent collagen fibers. The predominance of collagen and its anatomic configuration are important to the viscoelastic properties of pericardium.

Ultrastructure

Scanning electron micrographs disclose that the pericardium is far from being an inert mass of connective tissue, but rather is highly organized, with microvilli and cilia for production and absorption of fluid and facilitation of movement of the serosal surfaces over each other.[5]

MECHANICAL (VISCOELASTIC) PROPERTIES OF THE PERICARDIUM

The pressure-volume curve of the pericardium is characterized by an initial flat portion during which volume is increased with little or no change in pressure, followed by a "knee" leading to the final portion, during which

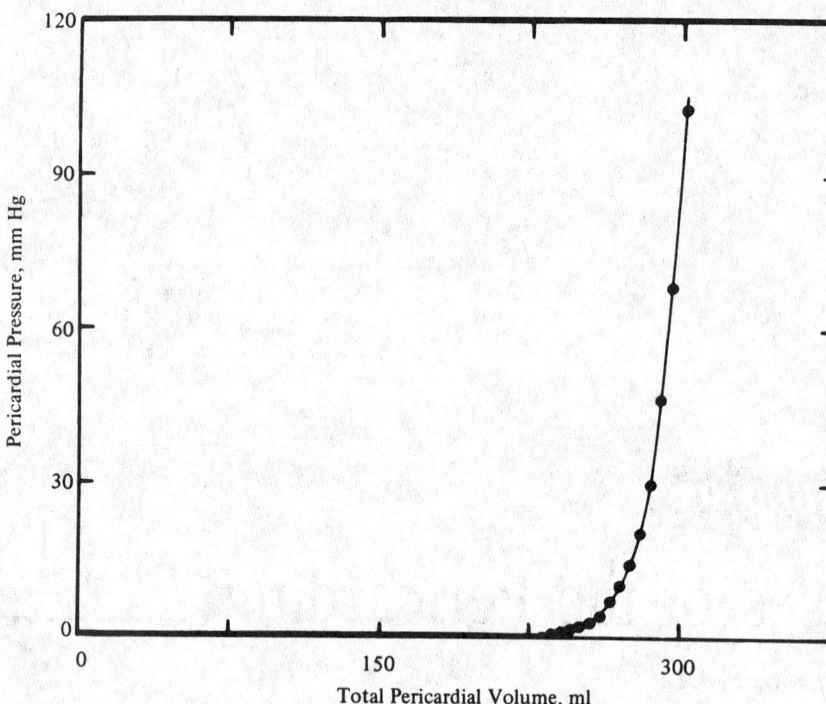

FIGURE 92-1 Pericardial pressure-volume curve (canine). (*From JP Holt: The normal pericardium. Am J Cardiol 26:455, 1970. Reproduced with permission from the publisher and author.*)

pressure rapidly increases with little or no increase in volume[6] (Fig. 92-1). Normally, conventionally measured pericardial pressure is subatmospheric and thus several millimeters of mercury lower than the pressure in the atria and the ventricular diastolic pressures, indicating that although the pericardium appears to fit the heart quite snugly, the heart is not normally engaged by the pericardium. There is appreciable day-to-day and moment-to-moment variation in cardiac volume, but the pericardial volume exceeds cardiac volume by perhaps 10 to 20 percent, the difference constituting the pericardial reserve volume, which allows physiological changes in cardiac volume to occur without restriction by the pericardium.

The pericardium limits or prevents acute pathological distension of the heart once the pericardial reserve volume has been used up and the pericardium is stretched. The pericardium has then reached the steep portion of its pressure-volume relation and the wavy bundles of pericardium have straightened out and become inextensible. The stress-strain curve of excised pericardium is similar to the pressure-volume curve of the whole pericardium.[7] Most observers consider the pericardium anisotropic, a finding that can be explained by the directionality of the collagen bundles. The pericardium stretches more in the short than in the long axis of the heart, and the anisotropy persists after the pericardial attachments are cut.

When the pericardium is subjected to constant stretching over a period of time, the tension in it drops slightly. This *stress relaxation* allows for slight relief of pericardial pressure in acute cardiac tamponade. It has been suggested that with growth of the heart, the collagen fibers are rearranged within the intracellular substance, allowing the pericardium to creep (increase its volume while stretch remains constant) and so adapt to the increased cardiac size,[8] but the magnitude of creep is unlikely to be sufficient to account for this adaptation. Instead, in response to chronic cardiac enlargement, the pericardium undergoes hypertrophy and becomes more compliant.[9]

Pericardial Pressure

Pericardial pressure measured by a catheter in the pericardial cavity is subatmospheric and essentially equal to pleural pressure throughout the respiratory cycle.[10] Superimposed on the large respiratory fluctuations of pericardial pressure are smaller fluctuations related to the events of the cardiac cycle, pericardial pressure being lowest during ventricular ejection. Liquid pressure within the pericardial cavity is lower than pericardial surface pressure measured by an intrapericardial balloon, which may give a more accurate estimate of pericardial restraint on the heart.[11]

Normal Pericardial Fluid: Amount and Turnover

As little as 15 mL of pericardial fluid can be detected by echocardiography.[12] On the other hand, the average amount of pericardial fluid found routinely at autopsy of patients free from pericardial and cardiac disease is 50 mL.[13]

There are no published data on the turnover of normal human pericardial fluid, but in patients with pericardial effusion, it was noted that losses of albumin from the pericardial cavity averaged 1.86 g/day. The albumin disappeared from the pericardial cavity exponentially and accumulated in corresponding concentration in the blood.[14] The membrane characteristics of the pericardium favor removal, rather than accumulation, of fluid.[15] Erythrocytes labeled with a radiopharmaceutical can be detected in the peripheral blood within a few hours, but it may take several days for all the cells to be absorbed.

FUNCTIONS OF THE PERICARDIUM

Numerous experiments have demonstrated that the pericardium restrains cardiac volume; yet no adverse consequences follow congenital absence or surgical removal of the pericardium. The thin-walled right ventricle and atrium are more subject to the influence of the pericardium than the more resistant, thick-walled, left ventricle.[16] Interactions among the cardiac chambers, especially in diastole but also in systole, are more pronounced with the pericardium intact.[17]

The pericardium exerts a powerful restraining effect on the size of the heart in situations of acute volume overload, particularly those that involve all four cardiac chambers, but the role of the pericardium in normal physiology and in chronic cardiac enlargement remains controversial. Conventional *liquid* pressure within the pericardium suggests that pericardial influence on the heart in these circumstances is small[18]; but pericardial *surface* pressure, measured by an intrapericardial balloon, suggests that pericardial restraint may be important in chronic heart failure, in which right atrial pressure may closely approximate intrapericardial pressure.[11] The few attempts to treat congestive heart failure by pericardiectomy, however, have not met with resounding success.

Pericardial pressure is strongly influenced by the intrathoracic pressure, which must be kept normal or itself be measured during the measuring of ventricular diastolic compliance.

Other Pericardial Functions

The pericardium maintains the heart in a relatively fixed position and functionally optimal shape within the mediastinum. The thin layer of pericardial fluid reduces friction on the epicardium and is thought to equalize gravitational forces over the surface of the heart; transmural cardiac pressures, therefore, do not change during acceleration or differ regionally within cardiac chambers.[19] Negative pressure in the pericardium augments atrial filling during ventricular systole. These concepts were developed using conventionally measured liquid pressure in the pericardium and do not hold for surface contact pressure, which may vary in different locations on the heart's surface.[11] The pericardium acts as a barrier to inflammation from contiguous structures and may buttress the thinner portions of the myocardium. The pericardium synthesizes and metabolizes prostaglandins.

ACUTE VIRAL AND IDIOPATHIC PERICARDITIS

> **Like the squeak of leather on a new saddle under a rider, or grating in the knee joint on moving the patella over the femoral condyles.**
>
> **V. Collin, 1955**[20]

Acute fibrinous or dry pericarditis is a syndrome associated with characteristic chest pain, pericardial friction rub, and specific electrocardiographic changes. A great variety of conditions are associated with acute pericarditis (Table 92-1). The following description refers to viral and idiopathic pericarditis without significant effusion. Viral infection is often presumed rather than proven, many cases being classified as idiopathic. Common viral infections causing acute pericarditis are those due to echovirus and Coxsackie virus.

Pathology

The acute fibrinous deposits give rise to the characteristic bread-and-butter appearance of the pericardium described by Laennec: "The knobbed appearance of this exudation is very like what would result from the sudden separation of two pieces of slab joined by a pretty thick layer of butter." In addition to fibrin deposition the usual changes of acute inflammation are found.[21]

History

There may be a prodromal phase characterized by fever and myalgia. The characteristic symptom is chest pain, the nature of which varies appreciably among patients and perhaps with etiology as well. In some cases the pain is indistinguishable from that of myocardial infarction; in others it strongly simulates pleurisy. Often the pain of acute pericarditis lies between the extremes, being retrosternal without radiation to the arms but exacerbated by respiration. Characteristically, pericardial pain is relieved by sitting up, and a typical, although not common, radiation is to the trapezius ridge.

Physical Examination

The characteristic physical finding of acute pericarditis is the pericardial friction rub, which is superficial, scratchy, or creaky and is heard anywhere or everywhere over the precordium but most commonly between the lower left sternal edge and the cardiac apex. Pericardial friction rubs are usually best appreciated with the diaphragm of the stethoscope applied firmly and with respiration suspended. In some patients they are best heard in the sitting position. Most pericardial friction rubs are independent of the respiratory cycle, but on occasion they are louder during inspiration. The classic pericardial friction rub is triphasic, with components in atrial systole, ventricular systole, and ventricular diastole[22] but frequently the rub is biphasic, and occasionally there is only a single component. Pericardial friction, especially when of uremic origin, may be palpable. The triphasic pericardial friction rub is virtually unmistakable, but biphasic rubs must be distinguished from the to-and-fro murmur of aortic valve disease, and monophasic rubs are often mistaken for systolic murmurs. In the differential diagnosis one must consider, in addition to cardiac murmurs, mediastinal crunch and artifacts produced by rubbing of the skin against the stethoscope.

Pericardial friction rubs vary in intensity from hour to hour and from day to day, sometimes transiently disappearing altogether. Pericardial fluid does not prevent the rub.

Depending on etiology, there may be fever and other signs of inflammation or systemic illness. Atrial arrhythmias, perhaps owing to the subepicardial location of the

TABLE 92-1

Etiology of Pericarditis

I. Trauma
- A. Pericardiotomy
- B. Indirect trauma to chest
- C. Transseptal catheterization
- D. Pressure injection of contrast media
- E. Perforation of right ventricle by indwelling catheter
- F. Implantation of epicardial pacemaker
- G. Blow to chest
- H. Perforation of right ventricle with catheter for parenteral nutrition

II. Viral infections
- A. Coxsackie B5, B6
- B. Echovirus
- C. Adenovirus
- D. Infectious mononucleosis
- E. Influenza
- F. Lymphogranuloma venereum
- G. Chickenpox
- H. *Mycoplasma pneumoniae*
- I. AIDS

III. Bacterial infections
- A. Staphylococcus
- B. Pneumococcus
- C. Meningococcus
- D. Streptococcus
- E. *Hemophilus influenzae*
- F. Psittacosis
- G. Salmonella
- H. Tuberculosis

IV. Amebiasis

V. Echinococcus cysts

VI. Fungus infections—histoplasmosis, aspergillosis, blastomycosis, coccidioidomycosis

VII. Rickettsia

VIII. Radiation

IX. Amyloidosis

X. Tumors
- A. Primary
  - 1. Mesothelioma
    - a. Rhabdomyosarcoma
    - b. Teratoma
    - c. Fibroma
    - d. Leiomyofibroma
    - e. Lipoma
    - f. Angioma
  - 2. Metastatic
    - a. Bronchogenic carcinoma
    - b. Carcinoma of breast
    - c. Lymphoma
    - d. Leukemia
    - e. Melanoma
- B. Sarcoid
  - 1. Collagen disease
    - a. Rheumatic fever
    - b. Lupus erythematosus
    - c. Rheumatoid arthritis
    - d. Vasculitis
    - e. Polyarteritis nodosa
    - f. Scleroderma
    - g. Dermatomyositis

XI. Anticoagulants
- A. Heparin
- B. Warfarin

XII. Myocardial infarction—post–myocardial infarction pericarditis (Dressler's syndrome)

XIII. Idiopathic thrombocytopenic purpura

XIV. Drugs
- A. Procainamide
- B. Cromolyn sodium
- C. Hydralazine
- D. Dantrolene
- E. Methysergide

XV. Dissecting aneurysm

XVI. Infective endocarditis with valve ring abscess

XVII. Thymic cyst

Principal causes of pericardial disease and pericardial heart disease. Most can cause pericardial effusion, cardiac tamponade, and/or constrictive pericarditis. The more common causes of these syndromes are mentioned under the syndromes and under specific disorders.

sinus node,[23] may be observed, but they are rare in the absence of concomitant heart disease.[24]

Electrocardiogram

Electrocardiographic changes of acute pericarditis evolve through four stages.[25] In the first, which occurs within hours or days of the onset of pericarditis, there is widespread ST-segment elevation, commonly involving all three standard limb leads and most of the precordial leads. Reciprocal depression is usually found in leads aV_R and V_1. ST-segment elevation seldom reaches 5 mm, and monophasic patterns are seldom if ever seen. In some cases the PR segment is depressed[26] (Fig. 92-2); this is a useful sign in differentiating acute pericarditis from early repolarization variants.[27] During the succeeding several days the ST and PR segments return toward isoelectric status and the electrocardiogram (ECG) becomes normal (stage 2). There may be no further progression, but the T waves may become inverted (stage 3). Abnormal T waves may be permanent or the ECG may revert to normal for a second time (stage 4).

The ST-segment elevation seen in acute pericarditis can usually be distinguished from that of acute myocardial infarction by the absence of Q waves, the upwardly concave ST segments, and the absence of associated T-wave inversion. During evolution, the ECG of acute myocardial infarction does not pass through a normal pattern before T-wave inversion occurs. The acute ST-segment elevation of Prinzmetal's variant of angina is more transitory and is associated with transient ischemic pain. The early repolarization variant common in young

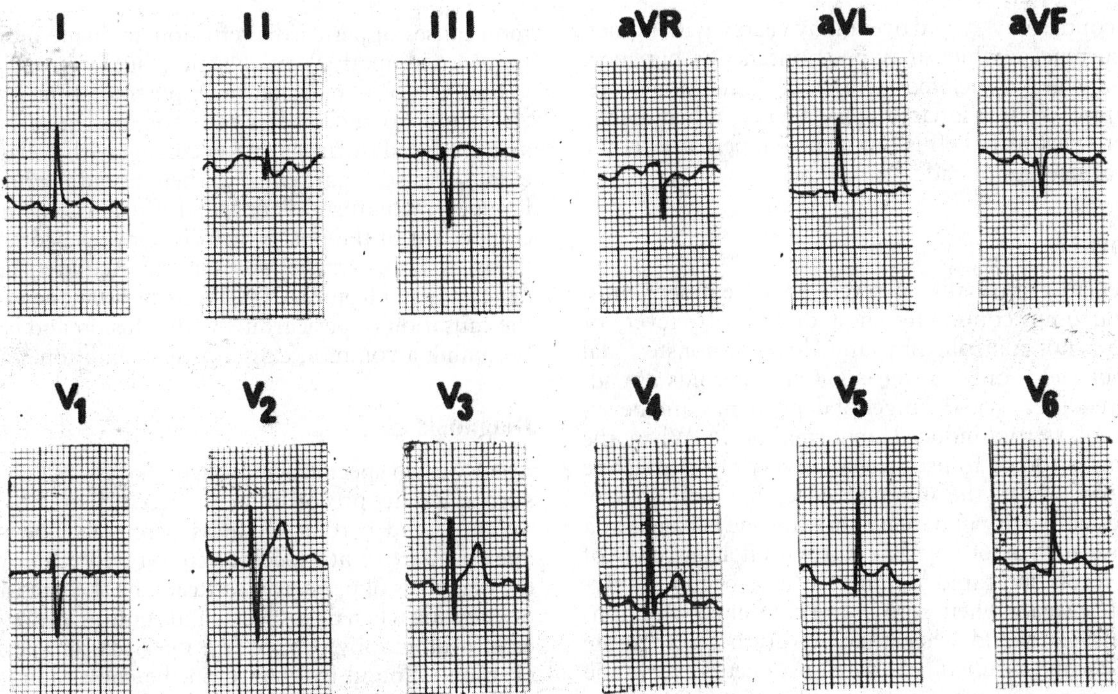

FIGURE 92-2 Electrocardiogram in acute pericarditis showing PR-segment depression and ST-segment elevation. (*From R Shabetai: The Pericardium. New York, Grune & Stratton, 1981: 359. Reproduced with permission from the publisher.*)

individuals, especially blacks and athletes and among patients in psychiatric institutions, may simulate the ECG of acute pericarditis. In these cases PR-segment depression is not seen and the electrocardiographic pattern does not evolve in a manner consistent with pericarditis. (See also Chap. 13.)

Other Laboratory Findings

The erythrocyte sedimentation rate is almost always elevated. Leukocytosis is present early but, depending on etiology, may give way to lymphocytosis. Cardiac enzyme levels are usually normal but may be elevated when there is extensive epicarditis. The results of pyrophosphate and gallium scintigrams may be positive when there is associated myocarditis.[28]

Electrocardiographic changes in acute pericarditis imply inflammation of the epicardium. The epicardium is frequently spared in uremic pericarditis, in which fibrin deposition may be extensive while inflammatory changes are minimal. In these cases electrocardiographic signs of pericarditis do not occur. The occurrence of first-degree heart block or bundle branch block suggests more widespread myocarditis.

In the absence of pericardial effusion or severe myocarditis the ECG and the chest radiograph remain normal. Computed tomography is seldom resorted to, but in difficult cases it can be relied on to demonstrate the thickened and inflamed pericardium.[29]

Differential Diagnosis

The early stages of acute pericarditis may be confused with acute myocardial infarction. In cases of doubt the issue is clarified over the subsequent 24 to 36 h by the clinical course and by serial changes in the ECG and the plasma level of cardiac enzymes. Aortic dissection may be misdiagnosed as pericarditis or may cause pericarditis. (See Chap. 123.)

Treatment

When acute pericarditis is of known etiology, it may respond to treatment of the underlying cause. For viral and idiopathic pericarditis, the patients should be given an analgesic and, if the pain is severe, should be confined to bed. The patient should be observed for pericardial effusion and cardiac tamponade. Usually aspirin suffices for the control of pain, but it may have to be given every 3 or 4 h for the first 48 h. The pain of acute pericarditis usually responds to 25 to 100 mg of indomethacin given every 4 h. Ibuprofen (Motrin), 400 mg four times a day, is also effective. Corticosteroids should not be given unless it is clear that nonsteroidal treatment has failed; when resorted to, they must be tapered and discontinued as rapidly as the clinical course will allow.

RECURRENT PERICARDITIS

One of the most troublesome disorders of the pericardium is relapsing or recurrent acute pericarditis. This syndrome may occur with or without pericardial effusion and occasionally is associated with pleural effusions or parenchymal pulmonary lesions. Why acute pericarditis may be a single illness in some patients and may recur in others is not known, but this phenomenon suggests that in some instances, at least, acute pericarditis is or sets up an autoimmune process.

The course may extend over many years[30] with numerous recurrences, which may be spontaneous but more commonly are associated with discontinuation or reduced doses of anti-inflammatory agents. When associated with pericardial effusion, relapsing pericarditis can cause cardiac tamponade.

Treatment

Recurrences are usually so severe that treatment must be given; quite commonly chest discomfort, fever, or dyspnea is not controlled by large doses of nonsteroidal drugs but yields only to steroids. Once steroids are administered, there is real danger of dependency and development of steroid-induced abnormalities.[31] When the physician is forced to use steroids, every effort must be made to establish the minimal dose that will control pericarditis. In very ill patients, prednisone is begun at a high dose such as 60 mg/day, but within a few days of clinical resolution rapid tapering must be begun. Tapering may be easier when steroids are combined with nonsteroidal agents and when they are given on alternate days. In the most difficult cases, relapse occurs every time the dose of prednisone is reduced below 5 to 10 mg/day. When this occurs, the patient should be maintained for several weeks on the lowest suppressive dose. Occasionally, steroid-resistant cases respond to other immunosuppressive treatment, but this too is undesirable and should be avoided except as a last resort. Colchicine, 1 to 2 mg/dL has been advocated,[32] but its effectiveness remains to be proven. When treatment with steroids and perhaps azathioprine has failed, after several years, to produce permanent remission (there are no reports of cyclosporine treatment), when serious side effects such as osteoporosis with spinal compression or fractures develop, or when severe mental changes appear, pericardiectomy may be considered. It must, however, be recognized that pericardiectomy may abbreviate, rather than end, the course of relapsing pericarditis and may be followed by troublesome pleural and pulmonary manifestations that require vigorous treatment. Pericardiectomy therefore should be considered when repeated attempts at medical treatment have clearly failed or when there is evidence or well-grounded suspicion of steroid-induced complications. Recently encouraging results have been reported in a series of patients who underwent pericardiectomy for recurrent pericarditis.[33] (See Chap. 93.)

PERICARDIAL EFFUSION

There are several syndromes of pericardial effusion. At one extreme, pericardial effusion is discovered only during routine laboratory investigation; at the other, it may cause cardiac tamponade. Effusion may be the principal manifestation of pericardial disease or may be an incidental finding in acute pericarditis or it may complicate constrictive pericarditis.

Etiology

The etiology of pericardial disease—and, by inference, of pericardial effusion—is given in Table 92-1. The common causes of pericardial effusion are acute pericarditis (viral or idiopathic), neoplastic (usually bronchogenic, mammary, or lymphomatous), postradiation, and posttraumatic. Somewhat less common are pericardial effusions induced by drugs and occurring with collagen vascular diseases, particularly rheumatoid arthritis and lupus erythematosus. Pericardial effusion is an important component of the postpericardiotomy syndrome and of many cases of Dressler's syndrome. Acquired immunodeficiency syndrome (AIDS) is an important newcomer in the causation of pericarditis with effusion and is rapidly becoming a common cause of this condition.[34]

Diagnosis

There are no specific symptoms. Likewise, clinical signs such as a quiet precordium, an increased area of cardiac dullness, and cardiac dullness percussible beyond the apex beat are so nonspecific and so rarely employed that the diagnosis of pericardial effusion has become a matter of knowing when to suspect it and confirm its presence by echocardiography (Chap. 15). On occasion, pericardial effusion is found by chance on the chest radiograph, a radionucleotide ventriculogram, an echocardiogram, or an abdominal ultrasound examination or during cardiac catheterization.

Pericardial effusion must be kept in mind whenever a patient with a disorder that may affect the pericardium is encountered, and it should be strongly suspected in such patients when there is evidence of pericardial involvement. Particularly suspect are patients with cancer of the lung or breast, patients undergoing hemodialysis, patients with unexplained enlargement of the cardiopericardial silhouette, patients with unexplained increased venous pressure, and patients with AIDS.

The most specific and sensitive test is echocardiography,[35] which should be performed whenever there is reasonable suspicion of a pericardial effusion. (See Chap. 15.) Pericardial liquid appears on the M-mode echocardiogram as an echo-free space. In smaller effusions the echo-free space is behind the left ventricle, but larger effusions are associated with an additional space in front of the right ventricle (Fig. 92-3). Two-dimensional echocardiography serves to quantify further the amount and distribution of pericardial effusion[36] and also may demonstrate fibrinous adhesions.[37] Echocardiography may also indicate whether the pericardium is thickened. When analyzing the echocardiogram of a patient with pericardial effusion, one can estimate, by determining the dimensions of the cardiac chambers, whether apparent enlargement of the heart can be entirely accounted for by pericardial effusion or whether there is underlying enlargement of the heart itself. By assessing wall motion, one can determine whether or not there is underlying heart failure or cardiac tamponade.

Silent Pericardial Effusion

Routine echocardiography[38] has shown that silent pericardial effusions are quite common,[39] especially in hemodialysis patients. Similarly, echocardiography reveals pericardial effusion in a significant proportion of patients with clinically dry pericarditis. Silent pericardial effusion also occurs during pregnancy.

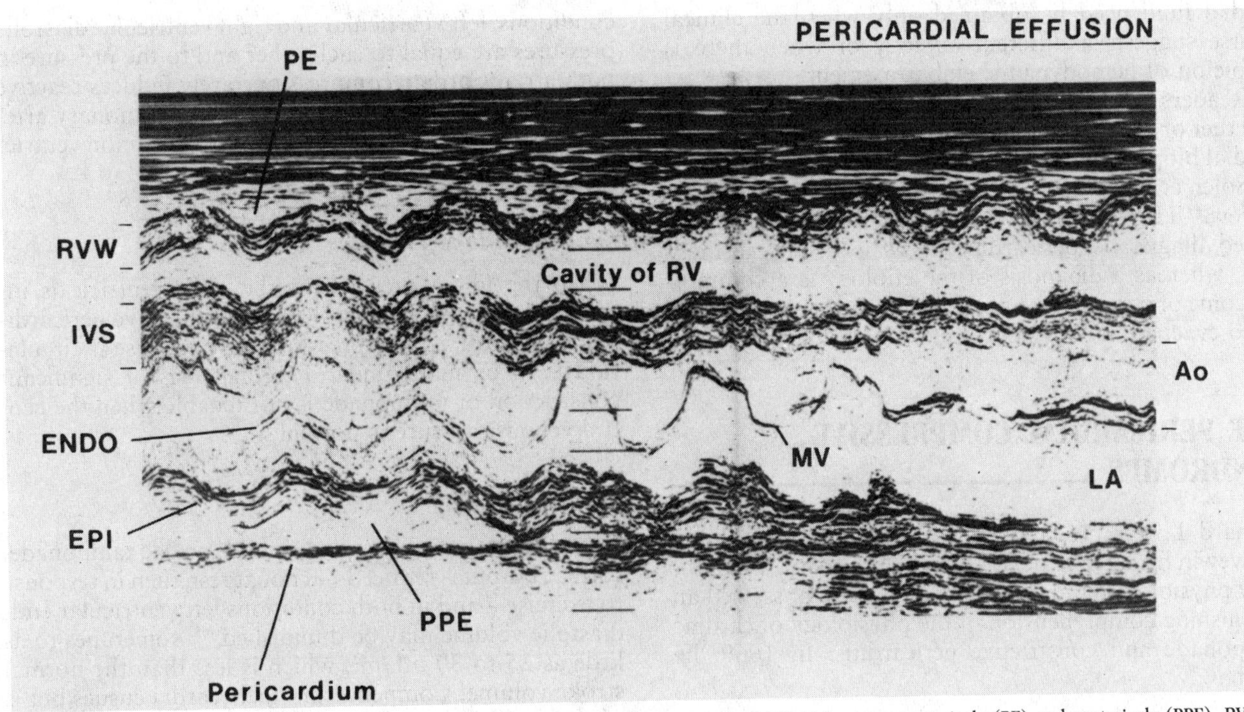

FIGURE 92-3 M-mode echocardiogram showing moderate pericardial effusion. Pericardial fluid is present anteriorly (PE) and posteriorly (PPE). RVW = right ventricular wall; IVS = interventricular septum; endo = endocardium; epi = epicardium; MV = mitral valve; LA = left atrium. (*From R Shabetai: The Pericardium. New York, Grune & Stratton, 1981. Reproduced with permission from the publisher.*)

It is possible to estimate the size of a pericardial effusion by echocardiography,[40] but for clinical purposes it is only necessary to separate small, moderate, and large effusions. Small effusions are detected by an echo-free space confined to the area behind the left ventricle and are not associated with an anterior clear space or enlargement of the radiographic cardiac silhouette. Moderate effusions are characterized by a posterior echo-free space larger than a centimeter and with an anterior space, especially during systole. Cardiac enlargement may not be apparent with chest radiography unless earlier films are available for comparison. Massive effusions are associated with great enlargement of the cardiopericardial silhouette and large echo-free spaces around the heart throughout the cardiac cycle. Radiographs show lung fields as disproportionately clear in relation to apparent cardiomegaly.

Technique

To identify pericardial effusion by M mode, the controls are adjusted to damp out all cardiac structures except the pericardium and are then adjusted to display, in addition, the epicardium, myocardium, and endocardium.[41] Normal structures and spaces may mimic pericardial effusion[42,43]; these include the space between vertebrae and myocardium, the gap between papillary muscle and free wall, pleural effusion,[44] cyst, hematoma (especially postoperative), giant left atrium,[44] calcified mitral valve annulus,[45] and tumors.[46] Two-dimensional echocardiography allows better identification of normal and abnormal structures with corresponding reduction of false-positive diagnosis[47] (Chap. 15).

Chest radiography is not specific. There is overall enlargement of the cardiac silhouette, and the lung fields are less congested than in cardiac failure. This combination, however, is difficult to distinguish from four-chamber cardiac enlargement with tricuspid regurgitation. Rarely, the pericardium and cardiac edge can be distinguished as separate shadows along the left border of the heart.[48]

Nature of the Fluid

In certain situations it is mandatory to determine the nature of the pericardial fluid. In patients with neoplastic disease it is necessary to determine whether pericardial effusion indicates invasion of the pericardium or a postradiation phenomenon. Cytologic examination of the fluid is important in cases in which the primary tumor has not been clearly identified. In cases of bacterial or other nonviral infections it becomes necessary to discover whether the pericardial effusion is an exudate and to culture pericardial fluid; suspected tuberculous pericarditis is a case in point. The presence of blood in pericardial fluid is less ominous than in pleural or peritoneal fluid, since it may be found in pericardial effusions of almost any etiology, including viral and idiopathic pericarditis. Magnetic resonance imaging may prove useful for characterizing pericardial fluid.[49]

There are clinical situations in which it is unnecessary to obtain pericardial fluid for analysis; for example, when pericardial effusion is found in a patient with typical viral or idiopathic pericarditis, pericardiocentesis should not be considered unless the effusion fails to respond to anti-inflammatory treatment or cardiac tamponade develops. Likewise, when a patient undergoing chronic hemodialysis develops pericardial effusion, pericardial fluid need be obtained only when the clinical course suggests a different etiology or when there is suspicion of hemodynamic embarrassment.

Readers who wish to employ a paradigm regarding whether or not to recommend pericardiocentesis or pericardial biopsy are referred to the numerous publications of Soler et al. which are well summarized in a recent review.[49] Here it is emphasized that the yield from so-called diagnostic pericardiocentesis is disappointingly low, whereas a diagnosis of the etiology is a common outcome of pericardiocentesis performed for tamponade or to evacuate an effusion thought to be purulent.

THE PERICARDIAL COMPRESSIVE SYNDROMES

Richard Lower (1631–1691), a colleague of William Harvey in his later years at Oxford University, a pulmonary physiologist and practicing physician, possessed an astonishing comprehension of the physiology of cardiac tamponade and constrictive pericarditis. In 1669, he wrote:

> It sometimes happens that a profuse effusion oppresses and inundates the heart. The envelope becomes filled in hydrops of the heart; the walls of the heart are compressed by the fluid circling everywhere, so that the heart cannot dilate sufficiently to receive the blood; then the pulse becomes exceedingly small, until finally it becomes utterly suppressed by the great inundation of fluid, thence succeed syncope and death itself.[50]

Norman Chevers, in 1842, described constrictive pericarditis:

> The principal cause of dangerous symptoms appears to arise from the occurrence of gradual contraction in the layers of adhesive matter which have been deposited around the heart, compressing its muscular tissue and embarrassing its systolic and diastolic movements, *but more particularly the latter** . . . The patient becomes incapable of continued muscular exertion and always liable to suffer from dropsy and other serous effusions.[51]

Pathophysiology of Compression of the Heart by the Pericardium

Constrictive pericarditis, cardiac tamponade, and restrictive cardiomyopathy are three conditions that restrict diastolic filling. Impaired cardiac filling is manifested by reduced ventricular volumes, elevated ventricular diastolic pressure, and reduced diastolic compliance. Secondarily, cardiac output is reduced.[52]

In cardiac tamponade and constrictive pericarditis, the heart is surrounded either by pericardial fluid under increased pressure or by a noncompliant scar that prevents the heart from attaining its normal diastolic dimensions. The generalized nature of compression by constrictive pericarditis or cardiac tamponade equilibrates the filling pressures of the two sides of the heart. In both conditions, left ventricular and right ventricular diastolic pressures are equal to each other and to the pressure in both atria. Cardiac compression rarely induces reactive pulmonary hypertension; therefore the pulmonary arterial diastolic pressure is the same as the common ventricular filling pressure.

Central Venous Pressure

When the filling pressure of the right ventricle is increased by the pericardial fluid or constrictive pericarditis, the central venous pressure must increase if circulation is to be maintained. The diagnosis of significant constriction or tamponade is not tenable when the central venous pressure is normal.

Cardiac Output

In both constrictive pericarditis and cardiac tamponade, cardiac output is reduced—if not at rest, then in response to exercise—and in both conditions left ventricular end-diastolic volume may be diminished,[6,53] sometimes to as little as 25 to 30 mL/m^2, which is less than the normal stroke volume. Compensatory tachycardia ensues but is often insufficient to maintain cardiac output at rest, and almost invariably cardiac output cannot be adequately increased during exercise. Tachycardia and elevated vascular resistance[54] are mediated by increased sympathetic tone.[55]

The syndrome of raised ventricular diastolic pressure, low cardiac output, and increased systemic vascular resistance mimics cardiac failure. In cardiac failure, however, raised ventricular diastolic pressure is a manifestation of myocardial insufficiency, whereas in constrictive pericarditis and cardiac tamponade it is an expression of increased external restraint.[52] Likewise, decreased cardiac output in the pericardial compressive disorders reflects not systolic pump failure but reduced preload.[52] Cardiac tamponade and constrictive pericarditis thus greatly impair the diastolic function of the heart, but impairment of systolic performance, when it occurs, is a late manifestation.

The Differing Pathophysiologies of Constrictive Pericarditis and Cardiac Tamponade

Knowledge of the similarities between constrictive pericarditis and cardiac tamponade is fundamental to understanding compressive disorders of the heart, but distinction between their pathophysiologies is crucial in understanding their respective clinical and laboratory findings.

In cardiac tamponade intrapericardial pressure is elevated and can be reliably measured. The elevated intrapericardial pressure is exerted on the heart throughout the cardiac cycle with slight momentary relief during ventricular ejection, when intrapericardial pressure falls a little as cardiac volume diminishes. In severe cardiac tamponade venous return is halted in diastole, when cardiac volume and intrapericardial pressure are maximal (Fig. 92-4).

Normal cardiac filling is bimodal. A surge of venous return occurs at the onset of ventricular ejection marked

*Emphasis added.

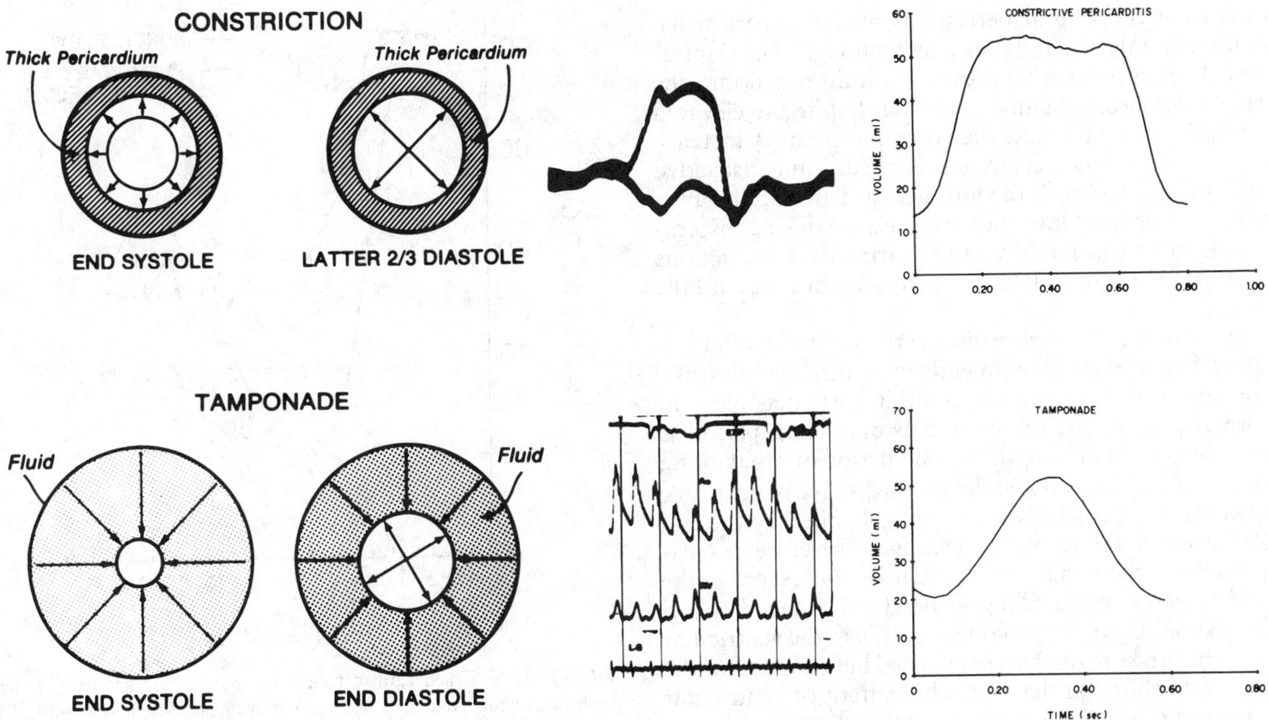

FIGURE 92-4 Diagram illustrating differences between constrictive pericarditis and cardiac tamponade. In constrictive pericarditis the heart is not restricted at end systole, so the heart fills rapidly during early diastole, creating the dip of ventricular pressure and the *y* descent of atrial pressure. When cardiac volume reaches the limit set by the diseased pericardium, further filling cannot take place; thus is created the late plateau of ventricular diastolic pressure. Atrial filling is bimodal, so atrial pressure displays sharp *x* and *y* descents. In cardiac tamponade the heart is compressed throughout the cardiac cycle by the pressure of pericardial fluid. Pulsus paradoxus occurs, and the early diastolic dip of ventricular pressure and the *y* descent of atrial pressure are absent. In constrictive pericarditis early diastolic filling is abnormally rapid, but no filling occurs in mid- and late diastole.

by the x descent of venous pressure and a small drop in intrapericardial pressure; a second surge occurs in diastole when the tricuspid valve opens and the y descent is inscribed.[56] The venous return in cardiac tamponade is unimodal and confined to ventricular systole and corresponds with the x descent of venous pressure[57] (Fig. 92-5).

The waveform of venous pressure in constrictive pericarditis differs from that of cardiac tamponade. In constrictive pericarditis, cardiac volume is set by the pericardial scar and under no circumstances can the heart exceed this set volume, which is attained near the end of the first third of diastole (Fig. 92-4). During ejection there is little impediment to venous return, and therefore the normal systolic surge of venous return and the x descent of venous pressure are preserved. Cardiac compression is still insignificant at end systole, so that when the tricuspid valve opens, blood rushes into the ventricles at a supranormal rate, registering a precipitous y descent of venous pressure. Thus, as in normal physiology, in constrictive pericarditis venous return is bimodal, but the diastolic surge and y descent are equal to or greater than the x descent and the systolic surge[57] (Fig. 92-4).

Respiratory Variation and Central Venous Pressure In cardiac tamponade, the inspiratory fall in intrathoracic pressure is transmitted to the pericardial space. Thus, although intrapericardial pressure is elevated, it falls during inspiration almost as much as the pleural pressure,

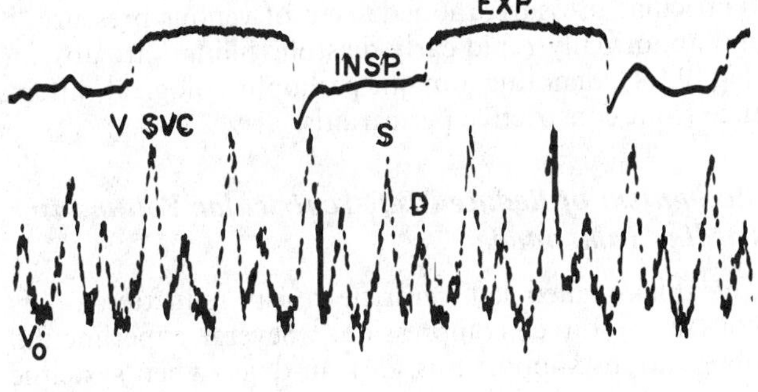

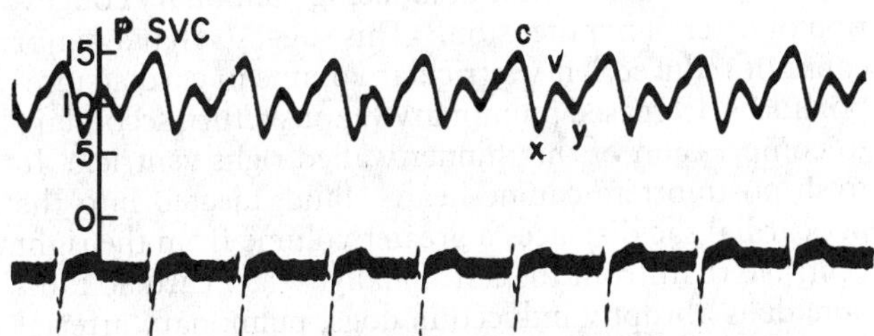

FIGURE 92-5 Normal pericardial filling is bimodal, as shown by this tracing of superior vena cava velocity (V SVC) and pressure (P SVC) obtained during cardiac catheterization of a patient without valvular or pericardial disease. A large surge of venous return (S) accompanies ventricular systole. A second peak (D) occurs during ventricular diastole. (*From R Shabetai: The Pericardium. New York, Grune & Stratton, 1981: 69. Reproduced with permission from the publisher.*)

increasing transmural pericardial pressure (pericardial minus pleural pressure) only 1 or 2 mmHg.[58] The inspiratory drop in pericardial pressure is transmitted into the right-sided heart chambers, so that despite the elevated intrapericardial pressure the normal inspiratory increase in systemic venous return is preserved.[58] In constrictive pericarditis, however, the intrapericardial space is obliterated. Decreased intrathoracic pressure during inspiration is not transmitted to the heart; therefore, venous pressure does not fall, and systemic venous return fails to rise.

In constrictive pericarditis early diastolic filling is faster than normal; consequently the ventricular diastolic pressure is characterized by a dip in early diastole.[59] In normal physiology, the early diastolic filling period is followed by diastasis and a second period of rapid filling associated with atrial systole. In constrictive pericarditis, however, the ventricles are completely filled by the end of the rapid filling phase. Diastasis therefore persists throughout the remainder of diastole, and except in the mildest cases, rapid filling in presystole cannot occur. Corresponding to the prolonged diastasis, the ventricular diastolic pressure remains unchanged but elevated for the latter two-thirds of diastole. The pattern of ventricular diastolic pressure in constrictive pericarditis is frequently referred to as the "dip-and-plateau pattern" or the "square-root sign."

Small ventricles and impeded venous return favor filling by suction.[60] In constrictive pericarditis, the end-systolic volumes of the ventricles are reduced[57] and their recoil is rapid. The prominent early diastolic pressure dip may indicate increased suction during early diastole.

In cardiac tamponade, ventricular diastolic filling is reduced throughout diastole; an early diastolic dip in ventricular pressure, the *y* descent of venous pressure,[61] and abnormally rapid early diastolic filling[57] are absent (Fig. 92-4), denoting a major pathophysiological difference from constrictive pericarditis.

Mechanism of Reduced Left Ventricular Volume in Cardiac Tamponade

The thick-walled left ventricle resists reduction of its volume by direct compression.[62] Several experimental observations support this idea. In dogs, when systemic venous return is diverted and returned by a pump at a slow rate to the right atrium, pericardial pressure can be raised to 20 mmHg without inducing pulmonary congestion or arterial hypotension.[58] This suggests that a major cause of reduced left ventricular volume in cardiac tamponade is decreased pulmonary venous return secondary to compression of the thinner walled right ventricle. In fresh postmortem canine hearts, fluid injected into the pericardial sac displaces a greater volume from the right ventricle than from the left. Finally, when cardiac tamponade is abruptly induced in dogs, pulmonary arterial flow declines immediately, but aortic flow remains normal for several cardiac cycles[62] (Fig. 92-6). Clinicians must recognize that pericardial effusion located behind the heart may cause echocardiographic left ventricular, not right ventricular, diastolic collapse. This circumstance is particularly relevant to postoperative cardiac tamponade.[63]

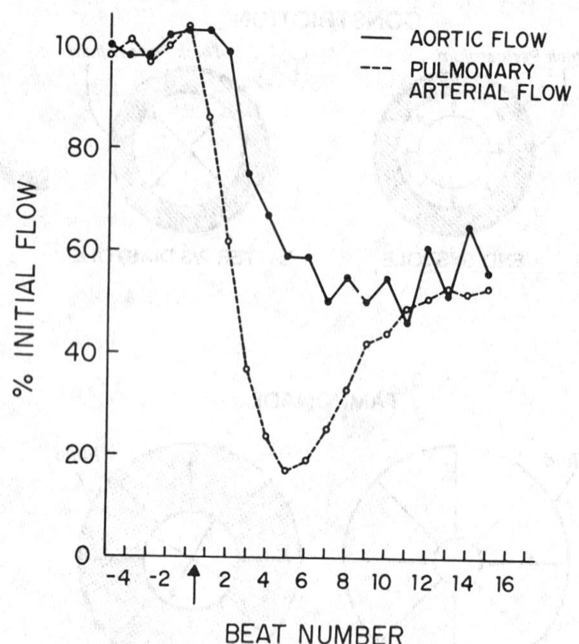

FIGURE 92-6 When cardiac tamponade is induced abruptly (↑), left ventricular stroke volume (solid line) is maintained until left ventricular filling is diminished because of reduced right ventricular stroke volume, which commences at the instant that tamponade is created. (*From R Ditchey et al: The role of the right heart in acute cardiac tamponade in dogs. Circ Res 48:701, 1981. Reproduced with permission from the American Heart Association and the author.*)

Pulsus Paradoxus

Pulsus paradoxus is an abnormally large inspiratory decline in systemic arterial systolic pressure and pulse pressure (Fig. 92-4). Normally, systolic blood pressure declines by as much as 10 mmHg during quiet inspiration. A number of normal and abnormal mechanisms combine to create pulsus paradoxus in cardiac tamponade.

In cardiac tamponade, systemic arterial pressure and left ventricular stroke volume fall during inspiration when pulmonary arterial pressure and right ventricular stroke volume increase.[64] However, minimal aortic pressure and flow do not exactly correspond with maximal pulmonary arterial pressure and flow. Rather, maximal pulmonary arterial pressure and flow precede maximal aortic pressure and flow by one to three beats.[65] This observation is not compatible with the hypothesis that competition between the two sides of the heart for fixed pericardial space is the sole cause of pulsus paradoxus in cardiac tamponade.[58] In normal dogs intrapleural and intrapericardial pressures fall equally during inspiration. However, in tamponade transmural pericardial pressure rises slightly with inspiration[58] (Fig. 92-7). Inspiratory augmentation of systemic venous return in cardiac tamponade increases the volume of the right side of the heart at the expense of the left side. The volume of the left side of the heart may be decreased in part by bulging of the intraventricular septum from right to left[66] and in part by increased transmural pericardial pressure.

The hemodynamic effect of inspiration has been simulated by rapidly adding a small volume of blood to the venous return of dogs studied during apnea while the

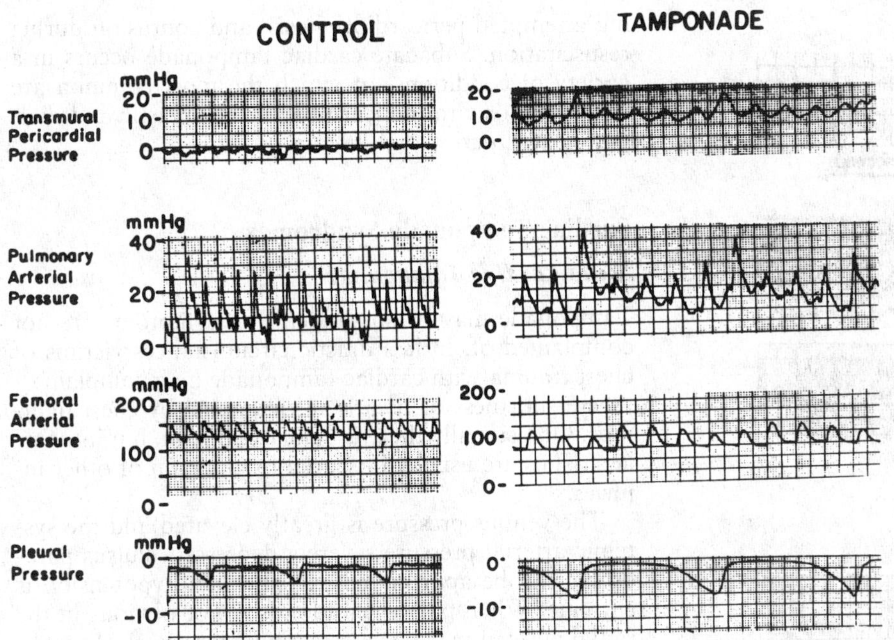

FIGURE 92-7 Tracings made during a study of experimental cardiac tamponade. The top panel shows that during inspiration transmural pericardial pressure increases when tamponade exists, but not otherwise. The third column shows the appearance of pulsus paradoxus with tamponade. Note also that during tamponade, pulmonary arterial pressure is neither exactly in phase nor 180 degrees out of phase with aortic pressure. (*From R Shabetai et al: Pulsus paradoxus. J Clin Invest 44:1898, 1965. Reproduced with permission from the publisher.*)

right side of the heart was supported by a constant-flow pump.[58] When intrapericardial pressure was normal, the addition of blood to the venous return caused an immediate increase in pulmonary arterial pressure. There was no immediate change in aortic pressure, but later there was an increase. Pericardial pressure did not increase. When the experiment was repeated in the presence of cardiac tamponade, the sudden increase in systemic venous return was again followed by an early increase in pulmonary arterial pressure, but now there was a simultaneous increase in intrapericardial pressure and a drop in aortic pressure. Aortic pressure rose two or three beats later (Fig. 92-8). This experiment confirms the importance of inspiratory expansion of the volume of the right side of the heart in the genesis of pulsus paradoxus when pericardial pressure is elevated.

In cardiac tamponade, pulsus paradoxus appears when both ventricles fill against a common resistance. Therefore, when left ventricular diastolic pressure is elevated by coexisting left ventricular disease, pulsus paradoxus does not develop in cardiac tamponade.[67] Atrial septal defect prevents reciprocal inspiratory changes in the filling of the two sides of the heart; therefore, in this condition too, cardiac tamponade can occur without pulsus paradoxus.[68] In patients with aortic regurgitation cardiac tamponade may occur without pulsus paradoxus.

The increased volume of the right side of the heart in inspiration, occurring when the pericardium is overstretched, causes the ventricular septum to bulge to the left. This decreases left ventricular compliance at the same time that transmural pericardial pressure is increased. Pulmonary venous return is diminished and negative thoracic pressure is transmitted to the aorta, increasing left ventricular afterload. Two or three cardiac cycles after the inspiratory augmentation of right ventricular stroke volume, the augmented volume appears in the aorta, but by this time the respiratory phase has shifted to expiration. Finally, left ventricular stroke volume falls more sharply than normal in response to decreased ventricular filling in cardiac tamponade because the small ventricle is operating on the steep ascending limb of the Starling curve.[69] Additional factors, including inspiratory traction by the diaphragm on the already taut pericardium,[70] reflex changes in vascular resistances and cardiac contractility,[71] and increased respiratory effort owing to pulmonary congestion, modify the already complex effect of inspiration on aortic pressure in cardiac tamponade.

Pulsus paradoxus is much less common in constrictive pericarditis than in cardiac tamponade. This may be because in the former, inspiratory increases in venous return[58] and in the volume of the right side of the heart seldom occur. When pulsus paradoxus does occur in constrictive pericarditis, it may be because there is pericardial effusion in addition[72] or because its mechanism differs, inasmuch as the intrapericardial space is obliterated and the position of the ventricular septum relative to the two ventricles is not altered by respiration.[73]

Ventricular Function and Coronary Blood Flow

In constrictive pericarditis and cardiac tamponade systolic function usually is unimpaired.[52] Long-standing calcific constrictive pericarditis may invade the myocardium and coronary vessels, leading to conduction disturbances and impaired ventricular function.[74]

In cardiac tamponade ventricular function remains normal and is often supranormal. Unrelieved extreme tamponade is fatal because circulation ceases when venous pressure cannot increase to equal the pericardial pressure. Diminution of myocardial perfusion in these cases is aggravated by direct compression of the major coronary arteries[75] and abnormal transmyocardial distribution.[76]

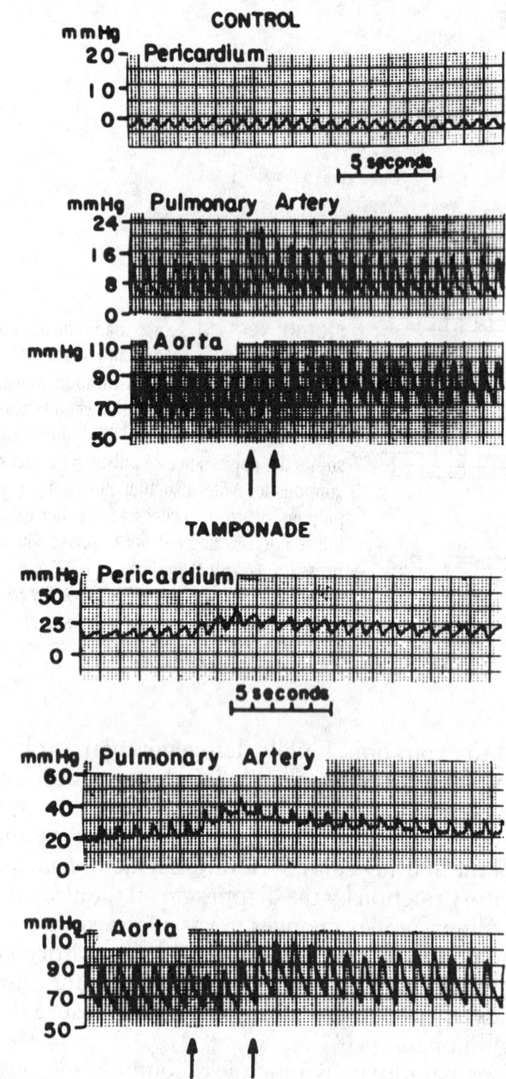

FIGURE 92-8 Tracings made to demonstrate the effects of a transient increase in systemic venous return (arrows) on pericardial, pulmonary arterial, and aortic pressures in control and tamponade in a canine model with right-sided heart bypass. In control, the increase does not influence pericardial pressure. The pulmonary arterial pressure and, subsequently, the aortic pressure rise when the flow increments arrive at these vessels. In tamponade, increased right-sided heart volume also raises pericardial pressure and lowers aortic pressure. (*From R Shabetai et al: Pulsus paradoxus. J Clin Invest 44:1898, 1965. Reproduced with permission from the publisher.*)

Clinical Features of Cardiac Tamponade

Etiology

Virtually any disease that can affect the pericardium may cause pericardial effusion, and tamponade may complicate virtually any pericardial effusion; however, the common causes are few.

Acute tamponade is usually caused by trauma, which may be iatrogenic, or by rupture of the heart or aorta. The trauma may be penetrating or blunt. Rupture of the heart may occur during acute myocardial infarction, and rupture of the aorta may complicate aneurysm or aortic dissection. Iatrogenic injuries include perforation during cardiac catheterization or pacing, cardiac laceration during attempted pericardiocentesis, and contusion during resuscitation. Subacute cardiac tamponade occurs in a variety of conditions, of which the most common are idiopathic or viral pericarditis and neoplastic and dialysis-related pericardial disease.

Cardiac Tamponade Syndromes

Acute Cardiac Tamponade

Tamponade may be so sudden that symptoms are not complained of. In less drastic circumstances victims of chest trauma with cardiac tamponade may complain of severe shortness of breath accompanied by chest tightness. Occasionally there is pericardial pain, but its characteristics are usually obscured by the pain of other injuries.

The venous pressure is greatly elevated and the systemic arterial pressure severely depressed. Pulsus paradoxus can be appreciated except when hypotension is extreme. When pulsus paradoxus is not obvious in the radial pulse, it may be detected in larger vessels. In striking contrast to these abnormalities of venous and arterial pressure, the precordium is quiet, cardiac activity often being impalpable (Beck's triad).[76] In the most severe cases, consciousness may be impaired; but for the raised venous pressure, such patients appear to be in shock.

When cardiac tamponade complicates a diagnostic procedure, the patient complains of discomfort, generalized uneasiness, and precordial pain. Systemic arterial pressure falls, pulsus paradoxus appears, venous pressure rises, and severe tissue hypoperfusion appears. Fluoroscopy shows that the cardiac silhouette has increased and that its pulsations have diminished or disappeared.

Cardiac tamponade should be suspected in any likely victim of recent chest trauma who appears in apparent shock. The suspicion is increased when venous pressure is high and pulsus paradoxus is present. When circumstances are at their most pressing, an immediate therapeutic trial of rapid infusion of fluid and diagnostic pericardiocentesis should be carried out. If the threat of death is more remote, pericardiocentesis should be delayed until the presence of pericardial fluid can be demonstrated by prompt echocardiography; but when tamponade occurs in the diagnostic laboratory, where pressures are being monitored and fluoroscopy is on hand, one can safely establish the diagnosis without waiting for echocardiography.

Another cause of acute cardiac tamponade is cardiac rupture complicating acute myocardial infarction. This catastrophe must be differentiated from cardiogenic shock (see "Specific Pericardial Disorders," below).

Subacute Cardiac Tamponade

A disconcertingly large number of diseases can cause cardiac tamponade. The common ones, however, are idiopathic or viral pericarditis, neoplastic invasion of the pericardium, and nephrogenic pericardial disease.

Symptoms Symptoms may be divided into three categories: those of the underlying illness, those of the accompanying pericardial disease, and those of cardiac compression. Many patients with inflammatory pericarditis give a history of prodromal fever, myalgia, and arthralgia. Patients with neoplastic disease may have symptoms associated with the neoplasm itself and its treatment. In some patients there is pericardial pain similar to that of acute pericarditis, but more often this is absent. The symptoms of cardiac compression include rapidly progressive dyspnea accompanied by fullness or tightness in the chest, occasionally with dysphagia. The course may be less rapid, allowing time for increase in weight and abdominal girth, and the rapid onset and progression of edema.

Physical Examination The examination shows raised venous pressure and lowered systemic arterial pressure with pulsus paradoxus.[77] When there is underlying cardiac disease, the precordium is not necessarily unusually quiet, the apex beat may be palpated, and even cardiac enlargement is not uncommon.[78] (See Chap. 10.)

The abnormalities of venous pressure described under "Pathophysiology of Compression of the Heart by the Pericardium," above, can often be recognized at the bedside. The mean pressure is elevated. When the patient's thorax and neck are placed at the elevation that maximizes the jugular venous pulsations, inspiratory decline in the height of pulsations can be appreciated. The x descent is recognized as an inward pulsation of the internal jugular pulse coincident with the carotid pulse. These abnormalities, together with equal diastolic pressure on the two sides of the heart and reduced ventricular volumes, can also be demonstrated by cardiac catheterization (Fig. 92-9). Catheterization, at least of the right side of the heart, with comparisons of right atrial and pulmonary wedge pressures, should be carried out if there is doubt about the diagnosis or if underlying heart disease is suspected. In the latter instance a full cardiac catheterization and angiographic procedure are required.[78]

Severe pulsus paradoxus is recognized as disappearance of the arterial pulse at the height of inspiration. Less severe pulsus paradoxus is felt as a decrease in pulse amplitude during inspiration. Pulsus paradoxus is difficult to evaluate or may be absent when there is shock,[79] and its identification is also confounded by labored rapid breathing, atrial fibrillation, and frequent extrasystoles. The severity of pulsus paradoxus can be estimated with the sphygmomanometer. The cuff must be deflated evenly and slowly while the patient's respirations are observed. In pulsus paradoxus, the first Korotkov sound is initially heard only during expiration. As the cuff pressure falls, this sound becomes audible throughout the respiratory cycle. The difference in systolic pressure between these events is an estimate of pulsus paradoxus. The "paradox" of pulsus paradoxus is that the arterial pulse weakens or may disappear while the loudness of the heart sounds does not vary.

In some cases it is necessary to document venous and arterial pressure by intravascular recordings. In all cases direct measurement of central venous pressure and systemic arterial pressure should precede and accompany pericardiocentesis whenever possible. The inspiratory drop in systemic arterial systolic and pulse pressure can then be accurately quantified, and the initial portion of the x descent of venous pressure can be identified as coinciding with the QRS complex. The tracing verifies the inspiratory decline in venous or right atrial pressure and the absence or severe attenuation of the y descent.

Echocardiogram in Cardiac Tamponade The diagnosis of cardiac tamponade is seldom secure without echocardiographic demonstration of pericardial effusion. Only under exceptional circumstances should pericardial

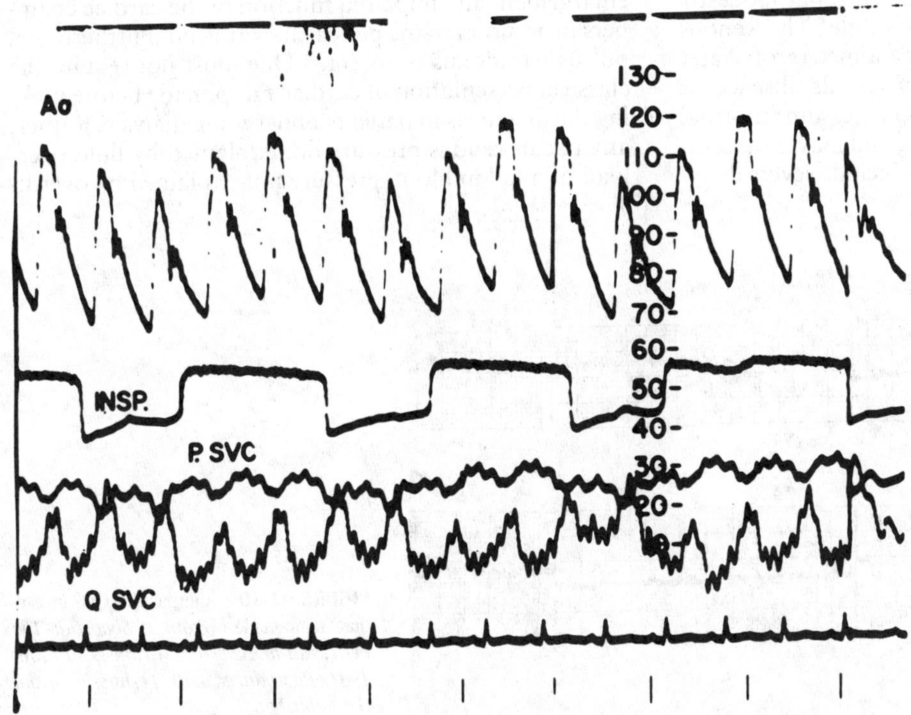

FIGURE 92-9 Cardiac catheterization of a patient with tamponade. From above, aortic pressure showing pulsus paradoxus, respiration, superior vena cava pressure (P SVC), and blood flow velocity (Q SVC). During inspiration (insp.) pressure declines and flow increases in the SVC. The SVC pressure shows a sharp x but no y descent. The SVC flow is monophasic, peaking at the x descent. SVC pressure (and pericardial pressure, not shown) were 27 mmHg.

drainage be undertaken without prior echocardiography to document the effusion and perhaps corroborate tamponade. Two-dimensional echocardiography has proven the value of compression of the right atrium[80] and diastolic collapse of the right ventricle[81] as highly reliable evidence of cardiac tamponade. These two echocardiographic signs appear when cardiac tamponade is hemodynamically significant but before the advent of pulsus paradoxus or profound hypotension, which mark decompensated cardiac tamponade.[82] Less specific signs include exaggerated respiratory variation in ventricular dimensions[66] and the E-F slope of mitral valve closure[83] and pseudoprolapse of the mitral valve. More specific but less common is pendular swinging of the heart within the pericardial fluid.[84] This phenomenon can be recognized by M-mode studies but is dramatically demonstrated by two-dimensional echocardiography and is frequently associated with electrical alternans.[85]

Doppler echocardiography in patients with cardiac tamponade confirms abnormal inspiratory increase in tricuspid inflow and pulmonary outflow velocities and abnormal inspiratory decrease in mitral and aortic blood flow velocities.[86,87] Pulmonary venous return becomes predominantly systolic, much like superior vena cava blood flow velocity in tamponade.[87]

Electrocardiogram in Cardiac Tamponade Frequently, there are no diagnostic electrocardiographic findings. Electrical alternans of the P wave, QRS complex, and T wave is virtually specific for cardiac tamponade but is uncommon. Alternation of the QRS complex alone is more common but less specific.[88] Pericardial fluid tends to lower QRS voltage, and there may be associated abnormalities of the T waves[89] (Fig. 92-10).

Less Common Syndromes of Cardiac Tamponade

Low-Pressure Cardiac Tamponade Cardiac tamponade may develop when pericardial pressure is but modestly increased.[90] The clinical picture is subtle. The venous pressure is increased only a few centimeters of water above normal, although inspection reveals absence or diminution of the *y* descent. The blood pressure is normal and pulsus paradoxus is not striking and may be absent. There may be no symptoms. Causes include severe dehydration, overly vigorous diuresis, and massive extrapericardial blood loss.

One makes the diagnosis by keeping in mind the possibility of pericardial effusion in diseases that may reasonably involve the pericardium. Echocardiography can then confirm the effusion and sometimes tamponade and leads to examination of the neck veins. The diagnosis is established when catheterization of the right atrium and pericardial sac shows equal pressures, and hemodynamic improvement follows removal of pericardial fluid (Fig. 92-11).

Effusive Constrictive Pericarditis When the pericardium is scarred but also contains fluid under pressure, cardiac tamponade results. When the fluid is aspirated, the features of constrictive pericarditis are unmasked.[72] This syndrome may occur in tuberculous pericarditis and in patients undergoing hemodialysis (see "Constrictive Pericarditis," below). If right atrial pressure fails to return to a normal value and shows normal cardiac and respiratory generated contours, the differential diagnosis is between effusive-constrictive pericarditis, right-sided heart failure, and tricuspid valve disease.

Cardiac Tamponade and Preexisting Heart Disease A commonly encountered example of cardiac tamponade modified by preexisting cardiac abnormalities is furnished by the population undergoing hemodialysis, in whom hypertrophy, fibrosis, and decreased compliance of the left ventricle are common.[91] The venous pressure may be affected by abnormalities unrelated to the pericardium; hypertension is common and cardiac output may be elevated by anemia and the access shunt. A third or fourth heart sound, cardiac murmurs, cardiac enlargement, and a left ventricular heave may be found in spite of cardiac tamponade. The ECG frequently suggests ischemic or hypertensive myocardial disease, which obscures the findings of pericardial disease. The ECG discloses enlargement and impaired function of the cardiac chambers in addition to the pericardial effusion. Furthermore, pulsus paradoxus is absent.[67] One must not require the classical presentation of cardiac tamponade before making the diagnosis in patients undergoing dialysis. Rather, any rise in venous pressure not explained by fluid overload or a fall in blood pressure not explained by overdi-

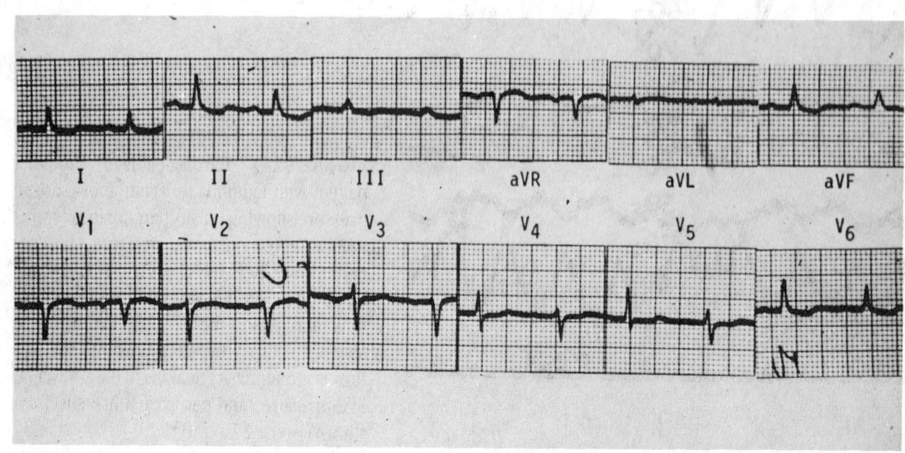

FIGURE 92-10 Alternans of QRS in cardiac tamponade. (*From R Shabetai: The Pericardium. New York, Grune & Stratton, 1981. Reproduced with permission from the publisher.*)

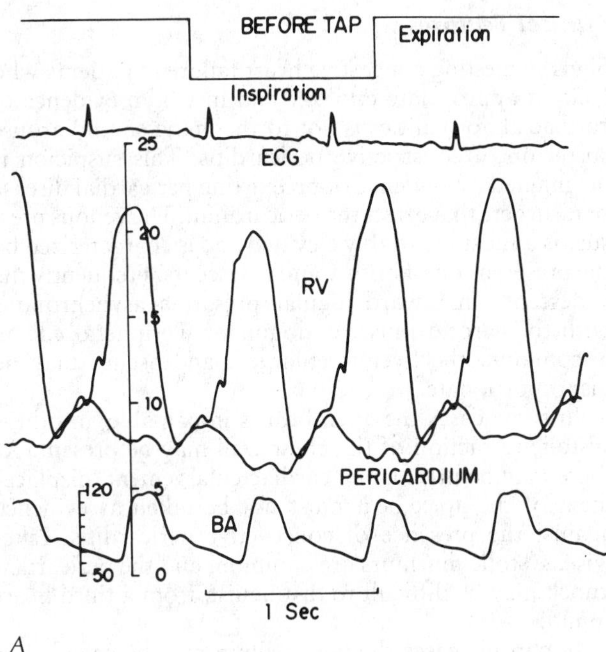

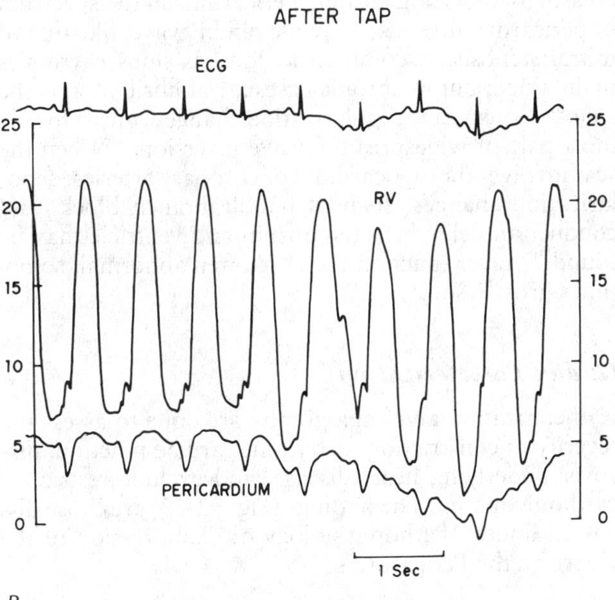

FIGURE 92-11 *A.* Low-pressure cardiac tamponade; tracing obtained during cardiac catheterization. Right ventricular diastolic pressure is only slightly elevated but is equal to pericardial pressure. Hypotension and pulsus paradoxus are absent. *B.* After pericardial pressure is consistently lower than ventricular diastolic pressure. RV = right ventricle.

alysis should lead to the suspicion of cardiac tamponade, especially when there is unexplained enlargement of the heart by chest radiography (see "Specific Pericardial Disorders," below).

Cardiac tamponade is difficult to recognize in patients with severe right ventricular hypertrophy or right-sided heart failure, because the cardiac abnormality and the raised pericardial pressure both contribute to the increase in jugular venous pressure and both modify its waveform. Increased right ventricular diastolic pressure prevents diastolic collapse of the free wall of the right ventricle and compression of the right atrium.[81] Specific criteria for the diagnosis have not been published.

Atypical Cardiac Tamponade Fluid in the pericardial space or mediastinum may be localized, compressing one side of the heart or one cardiac chamber.[92] Selective compression of the right side is more common; but localized left-sided compression has been reported[93] and can be associated with left atrial compression or left ventricular diastolic collapse. Localized cardiac tamponade from blood clots occurs after surgical operations on the heart.[94] Recognition may be difficult, and echocardiography may be inconclusive. In cases of clinical doubt, surgical exploration is fully justified and, when it confirms the diagnosis, produces dramatic relief.

Differential Diagnosis of Cardiac Tamponade

The differential diagnosis depends to a great extent on associated abnormalities. Many cases are confused with cardiac failure, since the two conditions both produce raised venous pressure, low cardiac output, and apparent cardiac enlargement. Abnormalities of jugular venous pressure in such cases may be attributed to cardiac failure and tricuspid regurgitation. The correct diagnosis can be arrived at by echocardiography and analysis of the jugular pulsations. Many cases are confused with shock, particularly after acute myocardial infarction; indeed, both may be present. The superior vena cava syndrome may be mistaken for cardiac tamponade, especially when the obstructing mass is mistaken for pericardial effusion, but in this case, although venous pressure is increased, pulsations are absent.

Treatment of Cardiac Tamponade

> **He had . . . in a case which was believed to be one of pericardial effusion, once inserted a trochar and cannula somewhat boldly, and the withdrawal of the trochar had been followed by a jet of blood which gave him great anxiety, but happily relieved the patient.**
>
> **S. West, 1883[95]**

Pericardiocentesis versus Open Drainage

Most often, the only effective treatment is to drain the fluid. Early cardiac tamponade complicating idiopathic or viral pericarditis may remit with anti-inflammatory treatment. The pericardium may be drained via pericardiocentesis or by limited pericardiectomy.[96] The choice depends on the cause of effusion, the general health of the patient, the experience and preference of the physician, and the facilities available. Pericardiocentesis permits exact hemodynamic diagnosis and evaluation of the effects of pericardial drainage.[97] Simultaneous pressure recordings from the pericardial space, the right atrium, and a systemic artery, before and after removal of pericardial fluid, are the most effective way of diagnosing effusive-constrictive pericarditis. Pericardiocentesis is less expensive and consumes fewer resources than surgical drainage procedures. On the other hand, even in good hands, pericardiocentesis is associated with morbidity and occasional mortality.[98] The risk is reduced by echocardiographic localization of the fluid or echocardiographic guidance.[99]

Surgical drainage is performed under direct vision in a more controlled environment and permits pericardial biopsy. If it is done from the subxiphoid route, local anesthesia may suffice, but general anesthesia is usually preferred. If a more extensive procedure is needed, the incision can be extended cephalad for pericardiectomy. Intraoperative hemodynamic measurements are seldom satisfactory, although when fluid spurts from a pericardiotomy, cardiac tamponade is a reasonable supposition. Recently pericardiotomy has been performed percutaneously using a balloon.[100] It is too early to know how applicable this technique will prove to be.

The need for repeated pericardiocentesis is an indication for open drainage. In effusive-constrictive pericarditis, fluid drainage alone does not suffice but must be followed by pericardiectomy if venous pressure is to be returned to normal. However, in cases of neoplastic pericardial disease, the benefits of pericardiectomy must be considered in the light of the total clinical picture. (See also Chap. 93.)

Pharmacologic Interventions

Experimental studies[54] to the contrary notwithstanding, pharmacologic treatment of cardiac tamponade should not be thought of as anything but a temporizing measure. The most important step is to expand the intravascular volume with blood, plasma, dextran, or even saline solution. Agents such as isoproterenol may be given to sustain venous and arterial pressures, and a vasodilator such as nitroprusside can be given to overcome the intense arterial vasoconstriction.[54]

Constrictive Pericarditis

Etiology

Constrictive pericarditis may follow almost any pericardial reaction and should be suspected should any patient who has had pericardial disease develop increased central venous pressure. Again, a few causes account for the vast majority of cases. Many are idiopathic and some are posttraumatic. There is a small but definite incidence of constrictive pericarditis complicating operations on the heart and pericardium.[101] Neoplasia may invade the pericardium and is an important cause of constrictive pericarditis, effusive-constrictive pericarditis, and cardiac tamponade. Constrictive pericarditis may appear months or years after mediastinal radiation.[102] In the United States, tuberculosis is progressively less important in the etiology of constrictive pericarditis,[103] but cases following tuberculosis and other infections of the pericardium are still encountered.

Symptoms

The usual symptoms are indistinguishable from those of congestive heart failure, but there may have been prior pericarditis. Dyspnea and fatigue[101] are common, and in long-standing cases weight gain, edema, and ascites make their appearance.

Clinical Features

Signs suggesting congestive heart failure in patients who lack an appropriate etiology and in whom evidence of cardiac abnormalities is not forthcoming should arouse suspicion of constrictive pericarditis. This suspicion is heightened by evidence of preexisting pericardial disease or disorders that affect the pericardium. The venous pressure is almost invariably elevated and is characterized by the preservation of both x and y descents. Frequently the y descent, an inward jugular pulsation asynchronous with the carotid pulse, is dominant. Peripheral edema is common, the liver is enlarged, and ascites may be disproportionate.

In some cases the apex beat is impalpable; in others systolic retraction of the chest wall may be present. As there may be preexisting cardiac enlargement, displacement of the apex beat must not be taken as evidence against the presence of constrictive pericarditis. Likewise, systolic murmurs are common, and the pericardial knock may be difficult to distinguish from a third heart sound.

In chronic cases the pericardium may be calcified,[102] but it may not be in subacute pericarditis, which is increasingly replacing chronic pericarditis in the spectrum of pericardial disease.[103] A wide bifid P wave, like that of mitral stenosis, is common as long as sinus rhythm is maintained, but in chronic cases atrial fibrillation is the rule.[104] Nonspecific repolarization changes consist for the most part of widespread T-wave inversion.[25] When the scar involves the myocardium or coronary arteries, depolarization changes, such as bundle branch block, and conduction delay between atrium and ventricle may be found.[105] Liver function tests are often abnormal, sometimes grossly so.

Cardiac Catheterization

Catheterization and angiography are done to assess the severity of constriction, determine cardiac function, discover underlying heart disease, and exclude restrictive cardiomyopathy. The findings (Fig. 92-12) are those discussed under "Pathophysiology of Compression of the Heart by the Pericardium."

Differential Diagnosis

The most commonly encountered erroneous diagnosis is cirrhosis of the liver. However, in cirrhosis the central venous pressure is not much increased. Differentiation from right-sided heart failure with tricuspid regurgitation can be difficult; systemic congestion characterizes both disorders, and both are characterized by a prominent y descent of venous pressure. Furthermore, severe tricuspid regurgitation can be present without a loud murmur, and the v wave may not be impressive when the atrium is greatly enlarged and highly compliant. Tricuspid regurgitation mitigates pulmonary congestion, leading to further confusion with constrictive pericarditis. In right-sided heart failure, the etiology is usually apparent and there is right ventricular hypertrophy and enlargement. The ECG may show tall narrow P waves in the right precordial leads and limb lead 2, right axis

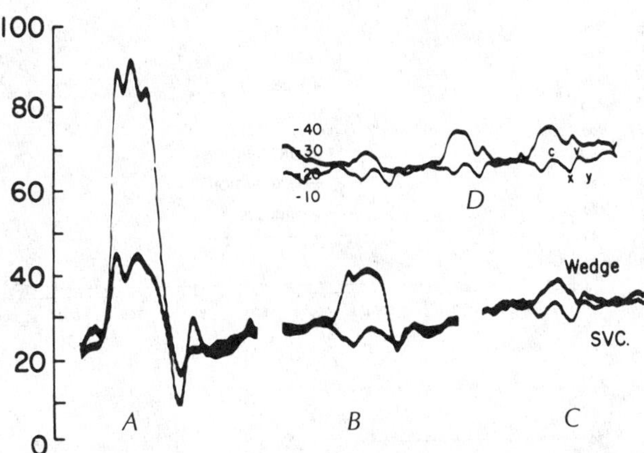

FIGURE 92-12 Cardiac catheterization tracings from a patient with constrictive pericarditis. *A.* Pressures recorded simultaneously from both ventricles. *B.* Simultaneous right atrial and ventricular pressures showing early diastolic dip and *x* and *y* descents. *C.* Simultaneous pulmonary wedged and superior vena cava (SVC) pressures. *D.* Simultaneous pulmonary arterial and SVC pressures. [*From R Shabetai, W Grossman: Profiles in constrictive pericarditis, restrictive cardiomyopathy and cardiac tamponade. In: W Grossman (ed): Cardiac Catheterization and Angiography, 2d ed. Philadelphia, Lea & Febiger, 1980: 360. Reproduced with permission from the publisher and editor.*]

deviation, and right ventricular hypertrophy. Echocardiography or other imaging techniques show enlargement and dysfunction of the right side of the heart.

Right ventricular infarction may produce a hemodynamic picture indistinguishable from constrictive pericarditis, with prominent *y* descent and absent respiratory variation in central venous pressure, early diastolic dip of ventricular pressure, and equal diastolic pressures on the two sides of the heart.[106] This differential diagnosis is particularly difficult when it arises in patients who have undergone saphenous vein bypass grafting operations, because they are at risk for both postoperative constrictive pericarditis and right ventricular infarction. Severe lesions of arteries supplying the right ventricle and evidence found by imaging techniques of right ventricular dysfunction are good clues to right ventricular infarction.

Restrictive cardiomyopathy may also reproduce the hemodynamic picture of constrictive pericarditis. Restrictive cardiomyopathy is not common but may characterize some cases of amyloid heart disease,[107] idiopathic myocardial disease, and other storage diseases.[108] When left ventricular diastolic pressure greatly exceeds right ventricular diastolic pressure, the diagnosis usually is not in doubt,[104] but exceptional cases of localized constrictive pericarditis occur.[109] It is when restrictive cardiomyopathy with equal left and right ventricular diastolic pressure must be distinguished from constrictive pericarditis without pericardial calcification that the real difficulty arises. This situation is considerably more common than was previously thought. Exercise,[110] pharmacologic interventions,[111] and fluid challenge may be used to try to induce separation between left and right ventricular diastolic pressures, but experience is so limited that neither the specificity nor the sensitivity of these tests is known. The same reservation applies to the observation that the rate of early diastolic filling is abnormally rapid in constrictive pericarditis but abnormally slow in restrictive pericarditis.[112] Another major difficulty is that entities such as mediastinal radiation may affect both the pericardium and the myocardium.

The correct diagnosis can sometimes be arrived at by discovery of a systemic disease with a predilection for either the myocardium (amyloidosis) or the pericardium (tuberculosis). Major conduction disturbances and depolarization abnormalities, while possible in constrictive pericarditis,[105] favor the diagnosis of cardiomyopathy.

The thickened parietal pericardium may be visualized by echocardiography[113] or by computed tomography,[114] but imaging techniques are of no help when constriction is from a thin, tight visceral pericardium. The analogue of the hemodynamic early diastolic dip of pericardial pressure may be recognized echocardiographically by rapid expansion of ventricular dimensions in early diastole followed by a long period during which there is little or no change. This abnormality is present in both restrictive cardiomyopathy and constrictive pericarditis, but preservation of motion of the interventricular septum and notching of the motion of the septum in patients with P mitral[73] favor the diagnosis of constrictive pericarditis.

Attention to the preceding points usually serves to distinguish constrictive pericarditis from restrictive cardiomyopathy. In summary, the history often points to the pericardium or myocardium, the examination by definition is not helpful, and calcification of the pericardium and ECG depolarization abnormalities favor myocardial disease, but their absence is nondiagnostic. Grossly different filling pressures on the left and right sides of the heart favor myocardial disease, but equal filling pressures are nondiagnostic. This problem is addressed in more detail in Chap. 91. When doubt remains, endomyocardial biopsy may disclose myocardial disease.[115] When an experienced cardiologist remains in doubt after full investigation, exploratory thoracotomy with a view to possible pericardiectomy is fully justified, though fortunately seldom required.

Syndromes of Constrictive Pericarditis

Chronic Calcific Constrictive Pericarditis This is the classic constrictive pericarditis that is now becoming less common. The clinical picture is striking, with severe cachexia, anasarca, massively increased venous pressure, and atrial fibrillation. Calcium frequently surrounds the whole pericardium and is best seen in lateral or oblique projections of the chest radiograph. Liver dysfunction is severe, amounting to failure, with spider angiomata, bilirubin retention, and even altered states of consciousness.

Subacute Constrictive Pericarditis This form of constrictive pericarditis is becoming more common at the expense of chronic constrictive pericarditis. Frequently, the pericardium is not calcified and the course may be a matter of weeks or months to 2 or 3 years. Subacute constrictive pericarditis may follow upon rheumatoid arthritis.[116] and *Hemophilus influenzae* infections, especially in children. Diagnosis depends on careful evaluation of venous pressure in patients with systemic diseases that may involve the pericardium.

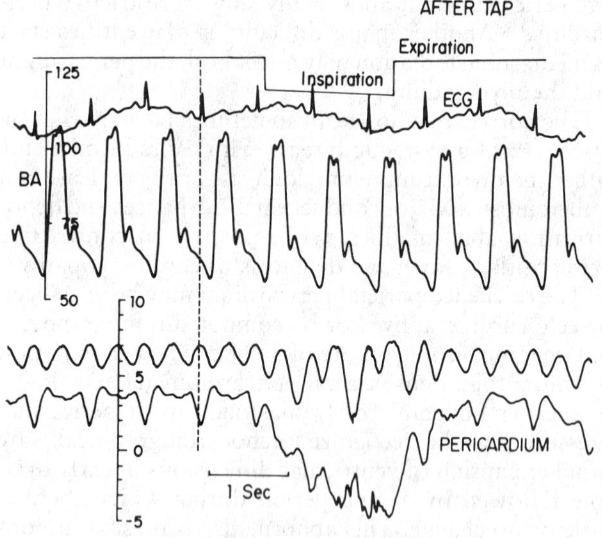

A

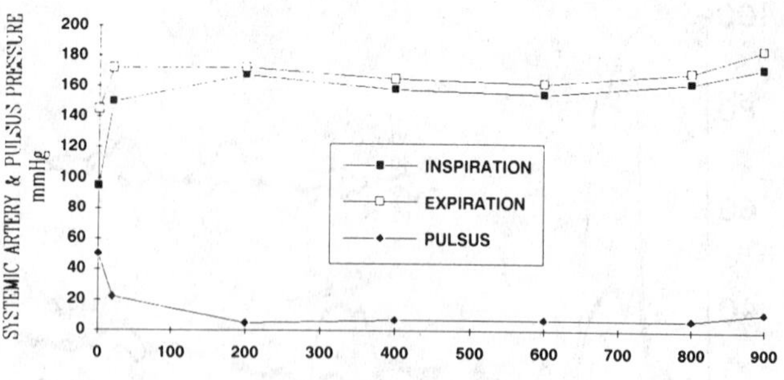

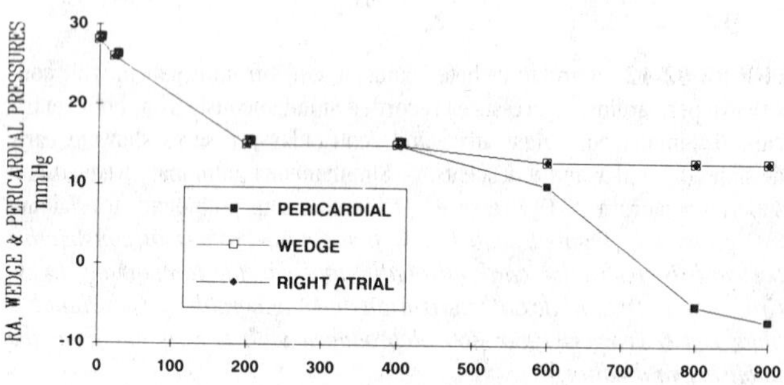

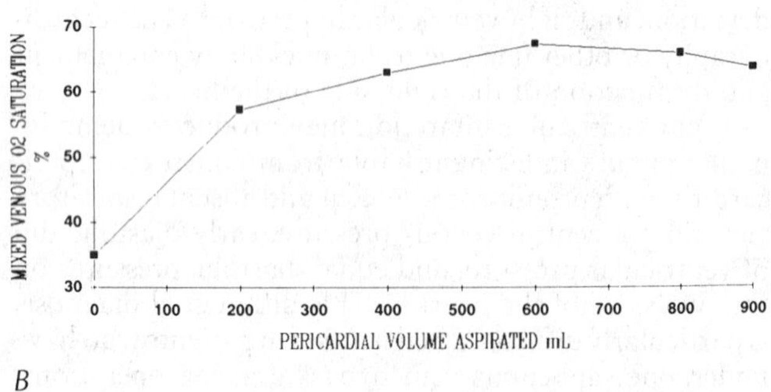

B

FIGURE 92-13 *A.* Recording made during cardiac catheterization of a patient with effusive-constrictive pericarditis due to bronchogenic carcinoma. The tracings were obtained during the pericardiocentesis, which has lowered pericardial pressure; however, right atrial pressure elevation persists and the tracing shows prominent x and y descents and absent respiratory variation. (*From R Shabetai: The Pericardium. New York, Grune & Stratton, 1981: 273. Reproduced with permission from the publisher.*) *B.* Hemodynamic variables recorded from a 62-year-old man with metastatic far advanced bronchogenic carcinoma who presented with ankle swelling, abdominal distension, and shortness of breath. Pericardiocentesis yielded bloody effusion and abundant malignant cells. When the needle was introduced, pulsus paradoxus (upper panel, closed circles) was 50 mmHg and the pericardial, right atrial and pulmonary wedge pressures were 29 mmHg. During aspiration of the first 400 mL via a catheter, the three pressures fell equally, and the mixed venous oxygen saturation rose from 35 to 60 volumes percent. During aspiration of the next 500 mL, pericardial pressure fell to subambient, but right atrial and pulmonary wedge pressures continued to be equal and elevated to 14 mmHg. Mixed venous oxygen saturation failed to reach normal. These findings indicated effusive-constrictive pericarditis, which was confirmed at necropsy.

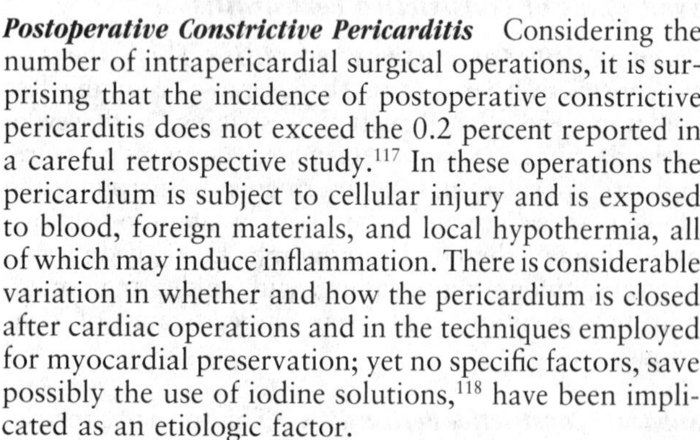

Postoperative Constrictive Pericarditis Considering the number of intrapericardial surgical operations, it is surprising that the incidence of postoperative constrictive pericarditis does not exceed the 0.2 percent reported in a careful retrospective study.[117] In these operations the pericardium is subject to cellular injury and is exposed to blood, foreign materials, and local hypothermia, all of which may induce inflammation. There is considerable variation in whether and how the pericardium is closed after cardiac operations and in the techniques employed for myocardial preservation; yet no specific factors, save possibly the use of iodine solutions,[118] have been implicated as an etiologic factor.

Occult Constrictive Pericarditis This is defined as constrictive pericarditis so mild that it is not detectable without fluid challenge.[119] In the first series reported the patients complained of nondescript chest pain, for which they underwent cardiac catheterization and coronary arteriography. Many reported previous acute pericarditis. Hemodynamic studies revealed normal atrial and ventricular pressures, but following the infusion of approximately a liter of saline solution in roughly 10 min, the right atrial pressure waveform assumed the characteristics of constrictive pericarditis and the diastolic pressures in the two ventricles became equal. At subsequent operation, the pericardium was thickened and fibrosed—findings that were confirmed by histological examination.

This form of constrictive pericarditis must be rare, and its existence, though frequently sought, is seldom found. Caution is advised in applying rapid, large fluid challenges to patients undergoing cardiac catheterization; furthermore, the induction of hemodynamic changes suggesting constrictive pericarditis by this technique should seldom, if ever, be taken alone as an indication for pericardiectomy.[120]

Effusive Constrictive Pericarditis This condition results from combined cardiac tamponade and constrictive pericarditis[72] and may occur in tuberculous pericarditis and in neoplastic or postradiation pericardiopathy. The clinical and hemodynamic presentation is that of cardiac tamponade. Pericardiocentesis, however, reveals persistence of raised venous pressure, absent respiratory varia-

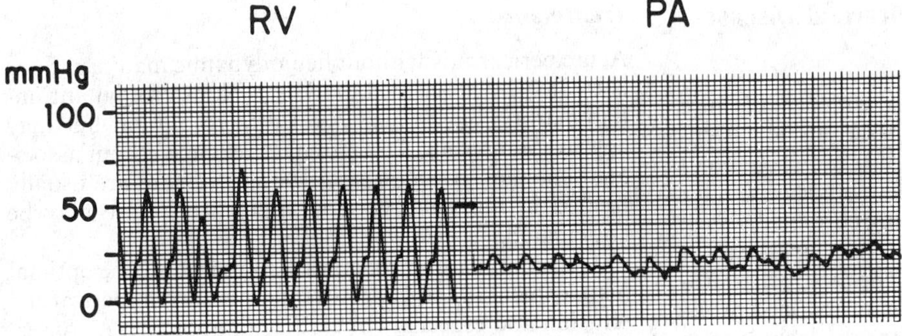

FIGURE 92-14 Pressure tracing from the pulmonary artery (PA) and right ventricle (RV) of a patient with extrinsic pulmonary stenosis caused by a localized band of pericardial constriction that developed after rupture of the esophagus. (*From R Shabetai: The Pericardium. New York, Grune & Stratton, 1981: 208. Reproduced with permission from the publisher.*)

tion of the venous pulse that shows a prominent *y* descent that was not present before pericardiocentesis, and a prominent *y* descent (Fig. 92-13).

Localized Constrictive Pericarditis Localized constrictive pericarditis is rare, but occasionally a localized band constricts the inflow or outflow region of one or more of the cardiac chambers. The clinical picture then simulates valve disease or venous obstruction[121] (Fig. 92-14).

Transient Cardiac Constriction In a series of 117 patients with acute effusive pericarditis, evidence of constriction developed in 16 but disappeared spontaneously. This syndrome appears to be a variant of effusive-constrictive and elastic constrictive pericarditis.[122]

Treatment

The treatment of constrictive pericarditis is usually surgical pericardiectomy. The mildest cases can be followed without surgical treatment, but when jugular venous pressure is consistently raised beyond 7 or 8 mmHg or requires medical treatment for its control, pericardiectomy should be carried out. In the most extreme cases of severe long-standing constrictive pericarditis with profound cachexia and liver dysfunction, it has been argued that treatment with a diuretic and digitalis should suffice,[120] but many surgeons disagree.

Pericardiectomy is commonly carried out via a median sternotomy, although some surgeons prefer thoracotomy. The risk of mortality has declined but is still in the range of 5 to 15 percent.[123,124] The risk is increased by heavy calcification, especially involving the epicardium, and by possible need for removal of the visceral pericardium. Recovery of normal venous pressure and cardiac performance may be delayed for weeks or months; it is more rapid when the operation is carried out before the disease is too chronic and when the pericardiectomy is almost complete and all constricting bands have been resected.[125]

SPECIFIC PERICARDIAL DISORDERS

Congenital Malformations

Absence of the Pericardium

The most important congenital malformation of the pericardium is partial absence of the left pericardium; complete absence is less common. This anomaly may be associated with congenital malformations of the heart,[126] including patent arterial duct, atrial septal defect, mitral stenosis, tetralogy of Fallot, tricuspid regurgitation, and Eisenmenger physiology. Association with mitral valve prolapse has also been reported.

Diagnosis Most cases come to light because of an abnormality on the chest roentgenogram. The heart tends to be shifted to the left, and its left border is elongated, showing prominent separation between the aorta and pulmonary artery. Lucencies caused by interposition of lung may be seen between the pulmonary artery segment and the aortic knob and between the left hemidiaphragm and the base of the heart.

Most patients are symptomless, but chest pain is reported by a significant proportion, perhaps in part because of torsion of the great vessels. Recurrent pulmonary infections may be a significant feature. Physical findings are not often helpful, but a conspicuous left ventricular heave in the anterior or midaxillary line may be found when the deficiency is substantial. A systolic murmur may be present; on occasion diastolic murmurs have been described.

Laboratory Findings The ECG in patients with complete absence of the left side of the pericardium usually shows incomplete right bundle branch block. In the presence of induced or spontaneous pneumothorax, air enters the pericardial space and outlines the pericardium.

Clinical Course and Treatment Total and very small deficiencies are not associated with pathophysiological changes. Medium-size defects may allow herniation of the left atrium, which may then strangulate and require surgical closure or enlargement of the defect to reduce the herniation and prevent recurrence.

Pericardial Cysts

Pericardial cysts vary greatly in size, are smooth and rounded, and most commonly are found in the right cardiophrenic angle. They are benign and produce no local or general symptoms. Their importance lies in differentiation from neoplasm. The roentgenographic appearance of pericardial cysts is highly characteristic, and the nature of the lesion can be confirmed by computed tomography.

Dialysis-Related and Uremic Pericardial Disease

Etiology

The association of pericardial disease with renal failure has been widely recognized since its description by Richard Bright.[127] Bright's report referred to end-stage renal disease in which pericarditis still occurs, but of greater importance is pericarditis complicating chronic dialysis. The mechanism, in spite of considerable investigation and speculation, remains unknown. The theory that uremic pericarditis is a chemical reaction to retained products of metabolism fails to account for the lack of relationship between the level of blood urea nitrogen or other nitrogenous metabolites and the frequency of pericarditis. Pericarditis is less common in patients undergoing peritoneal dialysis than in those undergoing hemodialysis. This suggests a possible role for "middle molecules." The hemorrhagic diathesis, an important component of the uremic syndrome, may predispose to pericarditis, a predisposition that may be aggravated by even regional heparinization. Nephrogenic pericarditis is highly vascular; consequently, uremia or dialysis-related pericardial effusion is usually bloody. The clinical manifestation may be acute fibrinous pericarditis, pericardial effusion, or cardiac tamponade. Classic constrictive pericarditis is a rare sequel. (See also Chap. 108.)

The etiology in dialyzed patients may be different from that in end-stage renal failure. It is possible that some cases are caused by living agents introduced into the bloodstream during hemodialysis or that pericarditis is an immune response to a component of the hemodialysis equipment or fluid.[128] Renal insufficiency is associated with increased susceptibility to infection; therefore the possibility of viral, tuberculous, or even bacterial pericarditis must not be neglected. Since neoplasia, ischemic heart disease, and thyroid disease occur in this population, it is wise to consider the differential diagnosis in general terms before making a presumptive diagnosis of dialysis-related pericarditis.

Diagnosis

Fibrinous pericarditis is manifested by a pericardial friction rub, which may be coarse and sometimes is palpable. Chest pain occurs in about two-thirds of patients and fever in the vast majority.[128] The ECG is of little value since the classic ST-segment elevation may not be present, reflecting sparing of the epicardium.[129]

Pericardial effusion should be suspected whenever there is a sudden unexplained increase in the apparent size of the heart, but differentiation from fluid overload or congestive heart failure is important. Unexplained cardiac enlargement or hemodynamic deterioration suggests either cardiac tamponade, fluid imbalance, or heart failure. Physicians caring for patients undergoing hemodialysis must be constantly on the alert for cardiac tamponade, especially as the clinical manifestations may be atypical and are difficult to distinguish from cardiac and cardiovascular deterioration. Recognition and good treatment are essential, as cardiac tamponade remains one of the principal causes of hemodialysis-associated morbidity and in 20 percent of cases terminates fatally.[130]

Treatment

Acute pericarditis without hemodynamic manifestations is treated by intensified dialysis.[91] Nonsteroidal anti-inflammatory agents may accelerate resolution but may aggravate bleeding. Pericardial effusions without associated changes in venous or arterial pressure are usually treated in the same way; a salutary response may be anticipated.

Considerable controversy exists regarding the optimal management of large, persistent, or recurrent pericardial effusion and especially of cardiac tamponade. A conservative approach to early cardiac tamponade is intensification of hemodialysis combined with either nonsteroidal agents or prednisone. More severe tamponade is an indication for pericardial drainage. The instillation of nonabsorbable steroids directly into the pericardial space has been advocated,[131] but experience with this technique is small.

The Pericardium and Myocardial Infarction

Pericardial Friction Rub in Acute Myocardial Infarction

A pericardial friction rub occurs in approximately 10 percent of patients with acute myocardial infarction[132] and perhaps more commonly, since it is often transitory. Shaggy fibrinous pericarditis may be found overlying Q-wave infarctions. However, pericarditis can occur in non-Q-wave infarctions, and sometimes pericardial friction rubs are audible in patients with inferior-wall myocardial infarction, suggesting that pericarditis may sometimes be an immune reaction to myocardial damage.

The pain is difficult or impossible to distinguish from angina, extension of infarction, or pulmonary embolism. Similarly, it is often impossible to recognize pericarditis on the ECG during evolution of an acute myocardial infarction. Echocardiography has demonstrated that silent pericardial effusion may accompany myocardial infarction.

The most important practical aspect of acute pericarditis in myocardial infarction is the extent to which it contraindicates or modifies treatment with anticoagulants. A pericardial friction rub occurring in the first 2 or 3 days and not accompanied by pericardial effusion or evidence suggesting cardiac tamponade need not modify standard practice, which in any case is variable. Pericarditis occurring later in the course or accompanied by pericardial effusion or tamponade is a contraindication. Thrombolytic therapy is almost always begun before pericarditis develops. Acute pericarditis does not of itself alter the prognosis but tends to be associated with larger infarctions and hence with a higher incidence of arrhythmia and a higher mortality.[133] In a recent study,[134] echocardiography disclosed pericardial effusion in 28 percent of 138 patients with acute myocardial infarction. There was no association between pericardial effusion and early pericarditis. Resorption was surprisingly slow, persistence of effusion up to 6 months being found by serial study in 8 of 98 patients. (See Chap. 60.)

Dressler's Syndrome

Dressler described a syndrome following myocardial infarction, comprising chest pain, pleurisy, pericardial friction rub, fever, and leukocytosis, sometimes associated with pulmonary infiltrate.[135] This complication, described almost in its entirety in the title of the original description,[135] usually occurs weeks or months after the causative infarction but may occur while the patient is still in the hospital. Most authorities consider it a separate entity from acute pericarditis occurring within the first 48 h,[136] but pericarditis associated with myocardial infarction may be an immune reaction to myocardial damage.[137] The post–myocardial infarction syndrome may be caused by a combination of viral activation and myocardial antibodies,[138] bringing it into line with the clinically similar postpericardiotomy syndrome, for which there is strong evidence supporting this dual etiology.[139]

Diagnosis is scarcely tenable without a pericardial friction rub and is strengthened by the presence of pericardial effusion. When Dressler's syndrome occurs soon after infarction, the differential diagnosis must include extension of the infarction, or pulmonary embolism. Later cases must be distinguished from a second infarction and unstable angina. Symptoms and signs usually subside rapidly with treatment with nonsteroidal anti-inflammatory drugs, but more resistant cases need prednisone or a comparable corticosteroid. Over succeeding months or years there may be several recurrences that require treatment. (See also Chap. 60.)

The post–myocardial infarction syndrome appears to be decreasing in prevalence,[138] possibly reflecting the decreased use of warfarin in acute myocardial infarction.

Postpericardiotomy Syndrome

This is a syndrome, with features indistinguishable from those of acute idiopathic pericarditis or Dressler's syndrome, occurring after operations in which the pericardium is opened. The syndrome occurs in children and adults and is not more common in those undergoing operation for rheumatic heart disease. Epidemiologic studies have shown high levels of both antiheart antibody and viral titers.[139] Differential diagnosis is from overt postoperative complications associated with pleurisy, pleural effusion, pericardial effusion, chest pain, and fever.

Treatment

Treatment is with corticosteroids or nonsteroidal anti-inflammatory agents. Recurrences may require reinitiation of treatment.

Posttraumatic Pericardial Syndrome

A virtually indistinguishable syndrome may follow blunt and sharp chest trauma. Common to all these conditions are injury to the pericardial mesothelium, myocardial injury, and blood in the pericardial space. Treatment is with anti-inflammatory drugs.

Neoplastic Pericardial Disease

A number of primary and secondary neoplasms may involve the myocardium and pericardium. Secondary neoplasia of the pericardium is more common than primary, the leading offenders being carcinoma of the breast and lung, lymphoma, and leukemia. Mesothelioma is the most common primary pericardial neoplasm and may respond to treatment with doxorubicin and cyclophosphamide.[140] Melanoma may involve the myocardium extensively yet seldom produces clinical findings except when the pericardium is involved.

Uncommon Neoplasms

Rare metastatic neoplasms of the pericardium include carcinomas of the colon, esophagus, kidney, ovary, prostate, and stomach and sarcoma.[141] Rare primary neoplasms include lymphangioma, hemangioma,[142] and teratoma.[143]

Clinical Features The most common manifestation is pericardial effusion; indeed, the most common cause of cardiac tamponade observed on medical wards is neoplasm. Occasionally tamponade is the initial finding, but more commonly patients are already known to have cancer. The differential diagnosis of the combination of a proven pericardial effusion and an intrathoracic mass lies between cardiac tamponade and the superior vena cava syndrome. In the former the characteristic pulsations of the jugular veins can be observed, whereas in the latter the distended neck veins do not pulsate. Respiratory distress, pulsus alternans, and tachycardia may obscure pulsus paradoxus, which otherwise occurs in cardiac tamponade but not in the superior vena cava syndrome. A pericardial friction rub may be present, but electrocardiographic signs of pericarditis usually are lacking. The pericardial fluid is almost always bloody.

The pericardium itself is frequently normal in gross appearance but may be thickened, sometimes sufficiently to encase the heart. Uncommonly, effusive-constrictive pericarditis is found. Neoplastic cells can be recovered from the pericardial fluid in many of cases, especially when the services of a skilled exfoliative cytologist are available.[144] Rarely, sympathetic pericardial effusion occurs in thoracic neoplasms that do not involve the pericardium.

Treatment Metastatic pericardial effusion almost invariably indicates an inoperable lesion. Treatment is therefore palliative, with the goals being to ameliorate symptoms and prevent death from cardiac tamponade, except in otherwise terminal individuals. Procedures should be as limited as possible and yet meet these goals. There is considerable controversy over the relative merits of pericardiocentesis and open drainage with biopsy. In the latter, the less extensive subxiphoid incision should be used whenever possible. The need for frequently repeated pericardiocenteses can be reduced by draining the fluid via an intrapericardial catheter for several hours. Malignant pericardial effusion may be paliated satisfactorily by balloon pericardiotomy.[100] The ultimate choice depends upon the extent of neoplasia, the general condition of the patient, and local preferences. The decision is best made jointly by the patient's physician, an oncologist, and a cardiologist or cardiac surgeon. Tetracycline or other sclerosing agents can be instilled via an intrapericardial catheter and may succeed in preventing recurrences of pericardial effusion or cardiac tamponade.[145] This is usually followed by transient pain and fever, but, surprisingly, not by constrictive pericarditis. Few controlled trials of instilling chemotherapeutic agents are available because this strategy is not commonly used and because of varied clinical presentation and frequent need for emergency treatment.

Radiation-Induced Pericardial Disease

Exposure of the mediastinum to radiation involves the risk of pericardial and myocardial damage. By far the greatest experience has been in patients treated for Hodgkin's disease. The acute reaction of the pericardium to radiation is fibrinous inflammation, often accompanied by effusion. The less common chronic response usually takes the form of constrictive pericarditis, sometimes effusive-constrictive pericarditis. The latency between exposure and constriction is often remarkably long. In one series of seven patients the lesion developed between 51 and 268 months after radiotherapy.[146]

The pathophysiology is unknown. The acute lesion has been studied mainly in experimental animals[147] but only occasionally in humans.[148] The myocardial, and by inference the pericardial, microcirculation is extensively damaged, resulting in ischemic injury to the tissue. The common opinion that the chronic lesion occurs only after 4000 rad has been delivered is not backed by statistical evidence. The incidence increases when anteriorly weighted thoracic mantle field techniques are employed. It has been suggested that reactivation of a latent virus in the pericardium[147] may occur and that radiation may damage the pericardial lymphatics.[147] The lesion appears to be more common in patients who have also received adjunctive chemotherapy.[147]

The acute lesion usually subsides within 2 years without sequel. The chronic lesion produces the typical picture of constrictive pericarditis or effusive-constrictive pericarditis. In the effusive stage the differential diagnosis is recurrence of the neoplasm. Examination of pericardial fluid is then helpful, as the fluid is positive in about 30 percent of cases.[149] Cytological examination of pericardial fluid is reliable in breast and lung cancer but less so in lymphoma and leukemia, in which pericardial biopsy may be needed.[150] Acute radiation-induced pericarditis can be managed symptomatically along the same lines as acute idiopathic pericarditis; the response is usually gratifying. Pericardial effusions, when not causing tamponade, can also be managed conservatively. Constrictive pericarditis requires pericardiectomy unless biopsy discloses prohibitive associated endomyocardial fibrosis. Significant impairment of left ventricular systolic function indicates severe myocardial damage, but frequently systolic function is preserved in spite of extensive myocardial fibrosis. In case of doubt, endomyocardial biopsy may be helpful, but good results may accrue from pericardiectomy when the biopsy shows mild endomyocardial fibrosis.[150] (See also Chap. 91.)

Hypersensitivity and Collagen-Vascular Pericardial Disease

Rheumatoid Arthritis

Necropsy studies yield an overall incidence of pericardial disease associated with rheumatoid disease of about 30 percent,[151] a prevalence that was known to Charcot.[152] The clinical incidence is appreciably lower, except when ECGs are performed on patients with rheumatoid arthritis who have no symptoms of pericardial disease.[153] Rheumatoid pericardial disease is usually self-limiting but may lead to acute or chronic pericardial effusion, subacute or chronic constrictive pericarditis, or cardiac tamponade.

Rheumatoid pericardial disease appears to be more common in middle-aged males in whom the arthritis was of acute onset. Serological tests for rheumatoid disease are usually positive, and typical rheumatoid nodules are common.

Associated cardiac abnormalities, including mitral valve involvement[142] and heart block,[154] are important but less common.

Constrictive pericarditis is usually subacute and seldom calcified. Pericardiectomy may be required within months of the first diagnosis of acute pericarditis[155] and almost always is required within 5 years.

Systemic Lupus Erythematosus

Pericardial disease develops in nearly all patients when life is prolonged by steroid treatment. The usual lesion is fibrinous pericarditis, but large pericardial effusions may develop.[156] Both cardiac tamponade[157] and constrictive pericarditis[158] have been described. Rarely, pericarditis is the initial manifestation. The pericardial fluid usually has a high content of protein and a normal or slightly reduced glucose content. As in rheumatoid arthritis, the complement level is low, and lupus erythematosus cells may be found. (See also Chap. 103.)

Other Connective Tissue Diseases

Pericardial involvement may be found in systemic sclerosis (scleroderma); often there is an association with cardiomyopathy. The pericardial fluid does not contain antibodies, immune complexes, or low levels of complement. There may be associated cardiac disease, and in some of the cases pericardial involvement is secondary to uremia.[159]

Drug-Induced Pericardial Disease

Pericardial abnormalities may develop in response to a number of drugs, of which the more important are hydralazine, procainamide, and daunorubicin.[160] Pericardial abnormalities have also been reported with psicofuranine, isonicotinic acid, and isoniazid. Pericarditis induced by penicillin presumably is a hypersensitivity reaction. Cardiac tamponade has been reported after administration of cromolyn sodium[161] and methysergide.[162] In patients with lupus nephritis treated with hydralazine it may be difficult to known whether pericarditis is drug induced or is a manifestation of the disease. Minoxidil may cause pericardial effusion.[163]

Infectious (Nonviral) Pericarditis

Tuberculous Pericarditis

The pericardium is infected via lymphatic spread; frequently no other lesion, especially pulmonary, is detectable. Tuberculosis of the pericardium is now rare in the Western Hemisphere. In a series of 72 pericardiectomies performed between 1974 and 1980, none was for tuberculous constrictive pericarditis.[164] Likewise, in two reviews of pericardiocentesis tuberculosis was proven in only 3 of 173[97] and 4 of 52 cases.[98]

Most of the detailed descriptions antedate chemotherapy. Furthermore, the features emphasized in those years of plentiful clinical material, such as insidious onset, lack of constitutional symptoms, thick pericardium found by air contrast, and bloody pericardial effusion, are not sufficiently specific to be of use to the modern clinician.[165] On the other hand, when untreated, tamponade, effusive-constrictive pericarditis, and chronic calcific constriction are common sequels.[166] Consequently, in spite of its rarity, the possibility of tuberculosis must be considered in virtually every case of acute pericarditis, pericardial effusion, cardiac tamponade, or constrictive pericarditis, especially in patients with AIDS (Chap. 107).

The dire consequences of missing the diagnosis have led to the practice of presumptive diagnosis based on such indirect evidence as contact with individuals known to be infectious, skin tests, chronicity, and therapeutic trial. It is now quite impossible to tell either from personal experience or from literature review how many patients treated for tuberculous pericarditis really had the disease or what would have been the consequences of withholding treatment until Koch's postulates were fulfilled. Tubercle bacilli may fail to grow from the pericardial fluid of patients subsequently proven to have had tuberculous pericarditis,[167] and even pericardial biopsy can be negative in such patients.[168] Adenosine deaminase activity in pericardial fluid is elevated,[169] but information on the utility of this enzyme determination is limited.

Treatment A potent triple-drug regimen—such as rifampin, 600 mg; isoniazid, 300 mg; and ethambutol, 15 mg/kg—should be prescribed. After several months isoniazid should be discontinued, but the other two drugs are given for 18 months after activity has subsided. Concurrent treatment with corticosteroids has been proposed,[170] but its role remains unsettled. In southern Africa tuberculosis remains a common cause of pericarditis. In a series of 240 patients with tuberculous pericardial effusion studied in Transkei, quadruple antituberculous chemotherapy was given for only 6 months. The patients were randomized to receive prednisolone or placebo for the first 11 weeks. The investigators concluded that the shorter regimen was effective and that prednisolone improved survival and lessened the need for pericardiectomy.[171]

Histoplasmosis

Most cases of histoplasmosis of the pericardium occur in the Ohio and Mississippi Valleys and western Appalachia.[172] Rarely, *Histoplasma* can be recovered from pericardial fluid,[173] but more commonly diagnosis depends on serology, which must be tested before it is modified by intradermal injections of histoplasmin. A titer exceeding 1 : 32 suggests recent or active infection. Distinction from tuberculosis can be difficult using clinical criteria. Furthermore, neither organism is easy to culture, but adenopathy favors histoplasmosis. Calcific constrictive pericarditis is a documented outcome.[174]

Treatment

Proven active disease, especially with tamponade, should be treated with a total course of 35 to 40 mg/kg of amphotericin B.[175]

Tuberculosis may occur in association with histoplasmosis.[176] When disseminated, these diseases may cause adrenal insufficiency.[177]

Other Organisms

The pericardium may also be infected by *Blastomyces* and by *Candida albicans,* the latter usually after immunosuppressive or broad-spectrum antibiotic treatment. *Actinomyces israelii* and *Nocardia asteroides* may also affect the pericardium and can cause constriction.[178] Purulent pericarditis may complicate pulmonary aspergillosis. Sporotrichosis and mucormycosis were not included in a review[179] to which the reader is referred for references regarding specific pericardial infections.

Treatment

Unlike histoplasmosis, these infections do not remit spontaneously; therefore pericardiectomy should be carried out whenever possible.

Bacterial and Other Pyogenic Infections of the Pericardium

Purulent pericarditis has decreased in frequency because of effective antibiotics, but when it occurs, it is serious, carrying a high risk of mortality. The combination of pericarditis and septicemia demands a relentless search for the causative organism. It is most important to obtain at least four blood cultures, which should be tested on a wide range of media so that fastidious organisms as well as the more common pyrogens will grow. Immunologic studies for tuberculosis, *H. influenzae, Streptococcus, Toxoplasma,* and *Entamoeba histolytica* should be done.

The antibiotic control of common infections has led to a change in the spectrum of bacterial pericarditis. The previously common pneumococcal pericarditis, a direct consequence of pneumococcal pneumonia and streptococcal pericarditis, has given way to infections caused by resistant *Staphylococcus,* anaerobes, fungi, and commensal organisms. Consequently, the population at risk has shifted to the extremes of age, the debilitated, and the immunosuppressed.[180]

Treatment

Infections due to penicillin-sensitive organisms can be brought under control by large doses of penicillin, which achieve therapeutic concentration in the pericardial fluid.[181]

The definitive treatment of purulent pericarditis is surgical drainage. Meningococcal pericarditis is a metastatic infection, usually from the nasopharynx. Meningococcal pericarditis may occur in the absence of meningitis,[182] and frequently the purulent serosanguineous pericardial exudate is sterile because of previous antibiotic treatment; but in some cases sterile pericardial effusion is thought to be an immune reaction.[183] The disease should yield to penicillin, but surgical drainage is often required, and constrictive pericarditis needing pericardiectomy may occur acutely.[184]

Staphylococcal pericarditis is an extremely serious illness and frequently fatal, especially when it is a complication of cardiac surgery or staphylococcal endocarditis. Systemic illness is profound and the pericardial exudate tenacious and loculated. Vigorous and aggressive treatment must be directed at every aspect of the disease, including control of the primary infection, removal of infected venous and arterial catheters, administration of appropriate antibiotics, and surgical drainage. Pericardiocentesis never suffices; surgical decompression must be carried out.[185]

Gram-negative organisms such as *Pseudomonas aeruginosa, Klebsiella pneumoniae,* and *Escherichia coli* produce pericarditis by hematogenous spread in the gravely debilitated.[186] Antibiotic treatment is beset with difficulties in selection and toxicity, and surgical drainage may be required. Pericarditis may result from hematogenous spread or by direct extension of anaerobic infections.[187] Treatment must include drainage of both the primary focus and the pericardium.

Purulent pericarditis in children carries a high mortality and may lead rapidly to constrictive pericarditis.[187] *Hemophilus influenzae* and meningococci are the most common offenders, but pneumococcal pericarditis still occurs in infants and children. Prognosis remains poor despite modern treatment.

Miscellaneous Diseases of the Pericardium

Myxedematous Pericardial Disease

Pericardial effusion occurs in about one-third of patients with myxedema. There is no correlation between pericardial effusion and the level of thyroid activity. Cardiomegaly is often the first clue but may be due to coexisting heart disease. The pericardial effusion rarely causes symptoms, although tamponade has been reported.[188] The pericardial fluid is usually clear but may be myxomatous and is high in cholesterol until restoration of the euthyroid state.

Cholesterol Pericarditis

Cholesterol pericarditis may be idiopathic but more commonly is found in myxedema, tuberculosis, or rheumatoid disease. The effusions are often large, but because they develop slowly, tamponade is uncommon. The associated inflammation may provoke constrictive pericarditis.[189] The cholesterol may be liberated from injured pericardial cells or lysed from red corpuscles or may develop as a consequence of lymphatic obstruction.[190]

Chylopericardium

Chylopericardium is usually idiopathic but may be associated with surgical or traumatic injury of the thoracic duct or neoplastic obstruction of the lymphatic drainage. The diagnosis is established by examination of the pericardial fluid, which is milky-white when allowed to stand and contains fat globules and increased levels of cholesterol and triglycerides. The milky appearance clears promptly after the addition of ether. Treatment is by drainage, and if the thoracic duct is injured, it must be ligated. Lymphopericardium is less common than chylopericardium and is usually secondary to lymphangioma. Pericardial involvement has also been reported in echinococcosis,[191] Degos' disease,[192] and pseudomyxoma peritonei.[193]

Uncommon Causes

There are a number of syndromes associated with pericardial effusion, although the mechanism is unclear. These include Reiter's syndrome,[194] ulcerative colitis,[195] Whipple's disease,[196] thalassemia,[197] atrial septal defect,[198] and Sipple's syndrome.[199] Pericardiopathy may also occur as part of mechanical disorders such as the chylous reflux syndrome,[200] inversion of the diaphragm, and pancreatic fistula[201,202] and in diabetic ketoacidosis.[203]

Constrictive pericarditis is a component of mulibrey nanism. *Mulibrey* is an acronym for *mu*scle-*li*ver-*br*ain-*ey*e, the organs principally affected by this autosomal recessive disorder found mainly in Finland.[204] Other features include yellow dots on the ocular fundi, fibrous dysplasia of the long bones, and an abnormally shaped skull and sella turcica.

A patient with Behçet's syndrome with pericardial effusion and mixed cryoglobulinemia who responded to treatment with indomethacin has been reported.[205] There is also a report of pericardial perforation of a gastric ulcer into the pericardium secondary to a phytobezoar in an oligophrenic man.[206] Increasingly, pericardial involvement in AIDS is being recognized.[34]

REFERENCES

1. Roberts WC, Spray TL: Pericardial heart disease: A study of its causes, consequences, and morphologic features. In: Spodick DH (ed): *Pericardial Diseases.* Philadelphia, FA Davis, 1976; 11–65.
2. Gibson AT, Segal MB: A study of the composition of pericardial fluid with special reference to the probable mechanism of fluid formation. *J Physiol (Lond)* 1978; 277:367–377.
3. Santamore WP, Constantinescu MS, Bogen D, Johnston WE: Non uniform distribution of normal pericardial fluid. *Basic Res Cardiol* 1990; 85:541–549.
4. Elias H, Boyd LJ: Notes on the anatomy, embryology and histology of the pericardium. *J New York Med Coll* 1960; 2:50–75.
5. Ishihara T, Ferrans VJ, Jones M, Boyce SW, Kawanami O, Roberts WC: Histologic and ultrastructural features of the normal human parietal pericardium. *Am J Cardiol* 1980; 46:744–753.
6. Holt JP: The normal pericardium. *Am J Cardiol* 1970; 26:455–465.
7. Rabkin SW, Hsu PH: Mathematical and mechanical modeling of stress-strain relationship of pericardium. *Am J Physiol* 1975; 229:896–900.
8. Lee JM, Boughner DR: Tissue mechanics of canine pericardium in different test environments. *Circ Res* 1981; 49:533–544.
9. Freeman GL, LeWinter MM: Pericardial adaptations during cardiac dilatation in dogs. *Circ Res* 1984; 54:294–300.

10. Morgan BC, Guntheroth WG, Dillard DH: The relationship of pericardial to pleural pressure during quiet respiration and cardiac tamponade. *Circ Res* 1965; 16:493–498.
11. Shabetai R: Pericardial and cardiac pressure. *Circulation* 1988; 77:1–5.
12. Horowitz MS, Schultz CS, Stinson EB, Harrison DC, Popp RL: Sensitivity and specificity of echocardiographic diagnosis of pericardial effusion. *Circulation* 1974; 50:239–247.
13. Holt JP, Rhode EA, Kines H: Pericardial and ventricular pressure. *Circ Res* 1960; 8:1171–1181.
14. Hollenberg M, Dougherty J: Lymph flow and ^{131}I-albumin resorption from pericardial effusions in man. *Am J Cardiol* 1969; 24:514–522.
15. Pegram BL, Bishop VS: An evaluation of the pericardial sac as a safety factor during tamponade. *Cardiovasc Res* 1975; 9:715–721.
16. Ditchey R, Engler RL, LeWinter MM, Pavelec R, Bhargava V, Couell J, et al: The role of the right heart in acute cardiac tamponade in dogs. *Circ Res* 1981; 48:701–710.
17. Janicki JS, Weber KT: The pericardium and ventricular interaction distensibility and function. *Am J Physiol* 1980; 238:H494–H503.
18. Tyson GS, Maier GW, Olsen CO, Davis JW, Rankin JS: Pericardial influences on ventricular filling in the conscious dog. An analysis based on pericardial pressure. *Circ Res* 1984; 54:173–184.
19. Banchero N, Rutishauser WJ, Tsakiris AG, Wood EH: Pericardial pressure during transverse acceleration in dogs without thoracotomy. *Circ Res* 1967; 20:65–77.
20. Collin V, quoted in Boyd LJ, Elias H: Contributions to diseases of the heart and pericardium. I. Historical introduction. *Bull NY Med Coll* 1955; 18:1–37.
21. Laennec RTH: *A Treatise on Diseases of the Chest* (trans Forbes J). London, T and G Underwood, 1821: 264.
22. Spodick DH: Acoustic phenomena in pericardial disease. *Am Heart J* 1971; 81:114–124.
23. James TN: Pericarditis and the sinus node. *Arch Intern Med* 1962; 110:305–311.
24. Spodick DH: Frequency of arrhythmias in acute pericarditis determined by holter monitoring. *Am J Cardiol* 1984; 53:842–845.
25. Surawicz B, Lasseter KC: Electrocardiogram in pericarditis. *Am J Cardiol* 1970; 26:471–474.
26. Spodick DH: Diagnostic electrocardiographic sequences in acute pericarditis: Significance of PR segment and PR vector changes. *Circulation* 1973; 48:575–580.
27. Wanner WR, Schaal SF, Bashore TM, Norton VJ, Lewis RP, Fulkerson PK: Repolarization variant versus acute pericarditis: A prospective electrocardiographic and echocardiographic evaluation. *Chest* 1983; 83:180–184.
28. O'Connell JB, Robinson JA, Henkin RE, Gunnar RM: Gallium-67 citrate scanning for noninvasive detection of inflammation in pericardial diseases. *Am J Cardiol* 1980; 46:879–884.
29. Hackney D, Slutsky R, Mattrey R, Peck WW, Abraham JL, Shabetai R, et al: Experimental pericardial effusion evaluated by computed tomography. *Radiology* 1984; 151:145–148.
30. Burchell HB: Problems in the recognition and treatment of pericarditis. *Lancet* 1954; 74:465–470.
31. Connolly DC, Burchell HB: Pericarditis: A ten year survey. *Am J Cardiol* 1961; 7:7–14.
32. Guindo J, de la Serna AR, Ramió J, de Miguel Diaz MA, Subirana MT, Perez Ayuso MJ, et al: Recurrent pericarditis: Relief with colchicine. *Circulation* 1990; 82:1117–1120.
33. Tuna IC, Danielson GK: Surgical management of pericardial diseases. *Cardiol Clin* 1990; 8:683–696.
34. Dacso CC: Pericarditis in AIDS. *Cardiol Clin* 1990; 8:697–699.
35. Teicholz LE: Echocardiographic evaluation of pericardial diseases. *Prog Cardiovasc Dis* 1978; 21:133–140.
36. Haaz WS, Mintz GS, Kotler MN, Parry W, Segal BL: Two dimensional echocardiographic recognition of the descending thoracic aorta: Value in differentiating pericardial from pleural effusions. *Am J Cardiol* 1980; 46:739–743.
37. Martin RP, Bowden R, Filly K, Popp RL: Intrapericardial abnormalities in patients with pericardial effusion. Findings by two-dimensional echocardiography. *Circulation* 1980; 61:568–572.
38. Riba AL, Morganroth J: Unsuspected substantial pericardial effusions detected by echocardiography. *JAMA* 1976; 236:2623–2625.
39. Goldstein DH, Nagar C, Srivastava N, Schacht RA, Ferris FZ, Flowers NC: Clinically silent pericardial effusions in patients on long term hemodialysis. *Chest* 1977; 72:744–747.
40. Horowitz MS, Schultz CS, Stinson EB, Harrison DC, Popp RL: Sensitivity and specificity of echocardiographic diagnosis of pericardial effusion. *Circulation* 1974; 50:239–247.
41. Feigenbaum H: Echocardiographic diagnosis of pericardial effusion. *Am J Cardiol* 1970; 26:475–479.
42. Hagan AD: Evaluation of pericardial diseases by M mode and two dimensional echocardiography. In: Mason DT (ed): *Advances in Heart Disease,* vol 3. New York, Grune & Stratton, 1980: 699–702.
43. Come PC, Riley MF, Fortuin NJ: Echocardiographic mimicry of pericardial effusion. *Am J Cardiol* 1981; 47:365–370.
44. Shah PM: Echocardiography in pericardial diseases. In: Reddy PS, Leon DF, Shaver JA (eds): *Pericardial Disease.* New York, Raven, 1982: 127–136.
45. Hirschfield DS, Emilson BB: Echocardiogram in calcified mitral anulus. *Am J Cardiol* 1975; 36:354–356.
46. Foote WC, Jefferson CM, Price HL: False positive echocardiographic diagnosis of pericardial effusion: Result of tumor encasement of the heart simulating constrictive pericarditis. *Chest* 1977; 71:546–549.
47. Martin RP, Rakowski H, French J, Popp RL: Localization of pericardial effusion with wide angle phased array echocardiography. *Am J Cardiol* 1978; 42:904–912.
48. Tehranzadeh J, Kelley MJ: The differential density sign of pericardial effusion. *Radiology* 1979; 133:23–30.
49. Permanyer-Miralda G, Sagrista-Sauleda J, Soler-Soler J: Primary acute pericardial disease: A prospective series of 231 consecutive patients. *Am J Cardiol* 1985; 56:623–630.
50. Lower R: *Tractatus de Corde, Item de Motu et Colare Sanguinis et Chyli in Sum Transiti r.* London, J Allestry, 1969.
51. Chevers N: Observations of diseases of the orifice and valves of the aorta. *Guy's Hosp Rep* 1842; 7:387–439.
52. Gaasch WH, Peterson KL, Shabetai R: Left ventricular function in chronic constrictive pericarditis. *Am J Cardiol* 1974; 34:107–110.
53. Craig RJ, Whalen RE, Behar VS, McIntosh HD: Pressure and volume changes of the left ventricle in acute pericardial tamponade. *Am J Cardiol* 1968; 22:65–74.
54. Fowler NO, Gabel M, Holmes JC: Hemodynamic effects of nitroprusside and hydralazine in experimental cardiac tamponade. *Circulation* 1978; 57:563–567.
55. Pegram BL, Kardon MB, Bishop VS: Changes in left ventricular internal diameter with increasing pericardial pressure. *Cardiovasc Res* 1975; 9:707–714.
56. Brecher GA: *Venous Return.* New York, Grune & Stratton, 1956: 111.
57. Shabetai R, Fowler NO, Guntheroth WG: The hemodynamics of cardiac tamponade and constrictive pericarditis. *Am J Cardiol* 1970; 26:480–489.
58. Shabetai R, Fowler NO, Fenton JC, Masangkay M: Pulsus paradoxus. *J Clin Invest* 1965; 44:1882–1898.
59. Hansen AT, Eskildsen P, Gotzsche H: Pressure curves from the right auricle and the right ventricle in chronic constrictive pericarditis. *Circulation* 1951; 3:881–888.
60. Brecher GA: Critical review of recent work on ventricular diastolic suction. *Circ Res* 1958; 6:554–566.
61. DeCristofaro D, Liu CK: The hemodynamics of cardiac tamponade and blood volume overload in dogs. *Cardiovasc Res* 1969; 3:292–298.
62. Ditchey R, Engler RL, LeWinter MM, Pavelec R, Bhargava V, Couell J, et al: The role of the right heart in acute cardiac tamponade in dogs. *Circ Res* 1981; 48:701–710.
63. D'Cruz IA, Kensey K, Campbell C, Replogle R, Jain M: Two-dimensional echocardiography in cardiac tamponade occurring after cardiac surgery. *J Am Coll Cardiol* 1985; 5:1250–1252.
64. Shabetai R, Fowler NO, Gueron M: The effects of respiration on aortic pressure and flow. *Am Heart J* 1963; 65:525–533.
65. Shabetai R, Fowler NO, Braunstein JR, Gueron M: Transmural ventricular pressures and pulsus paradoxus in experimental cardiac tamponade. *Dis Chest* 1961; 39:557–568.
66. Settle HP, Adolph RJ, Fowler NO, Engel P, Agruss NS, Levenson NI: Echocardiographic study of cardiac tamponade. *Circulation* 1977; 56:951–959.
67. Reddy PS, Curtiss EI, O'Toole JD, Shaver JA: Cardiac tampon-

ade: Hemodynamic observations in man. *Circulation* 1978; 58:265–272.
68. Kronzon I, Winer HE: Absence of paradoxical pulse in patients with atrial septal defect and cardiac tamponade (abstr). *Am J Cardiol* 1978; 41:446.
69. Friedman HS, Sakurai H, Choe S-S, Lajam F, Celis A: Pulsus paradoxus: A manifestation of marked reduction of left ventricular end-diastolic volume in cardiac tamponade. *J Thorac Cardiovasc Surg* 1980; 79:74–82.
70. Dock W: Inspiratory traction on the pericardium. *Arch Intern Med* 1961; 108:837–840.
71. Friedman HS, Lajam F, Zaman Q, Gomes JA, Calderon J, Marino ND, et al: Effect of autonomic blockade on the hemodynamic findings in acute cardiac tamponade. *Am J Physiol* 1977; 232:H5–H11.
72. Hancock EW: Subacute effusive-constrictive pericarditis. *Circulation* 1971; 43:183–192.
73. Tei C, Child JS, Tanaka H, Shah PM: Atrial systolic notch on the interventricular septal echogram: An echocardiographic sign of constrictive pericarditis. *J Am Coll Cardiol* 1983; 1:907–912.
74. Jarmakani JMM, McHale PA, Greenfield JC: The effect of cardiac tamponade on coronary hemodynamics in the awake dog. *Cardiovasc Res* 1975; 9:112–117.
75. Wechsler AS, Auerbach BJ, Graham TC, Sabiston DC: Distribution of intramyocardial blood flow during pericardial tamponade: Correlation with microscopic anatomy and intrinsic myocardial contractility. *J Thorac Cardiovasc Surg* 1974; 68:847–856.
76. Beck CS: Two cardiac compression triads. *JAMA* 1935; 104:714–716.
77. Katz LN, Gauchat HW: Observations on pulsus paradoxus (with special reference to pericardial effusions). *Arch Intern Med* 1924; 33:371–393.
78. Guberman BA, Fowler NO, Engel PJ, Gueron M, Allen JM: Cardiac tamponade in medical patients. *Circulation* 1981; 64:633–640.
79. Cohn JN, Pinkerson AL, Tristani FE: Mechanism of pulsus paradoxus in clinical shock. *J Clin Invest* 1967; 46:1744–1755.
80. Gillam LD, Guyer DE, Gibson TC, King ME, Marshall JE, Weyman AE: Hydrodynamic compression of the right atrium: a new echocardiographic sign of cardiac tamponade. *Circulation* 1983; 68:294–301.
81. Leimgruber PP, Klopfenstein HS, Wann LS, Brooks HL: The hemodynamic derangement associated with right ventricular diastolic collapse in cardiac tamponade: An experimental echocardiographic study. *Circulation* 1983; 68:612–620.
82. Klopfenstein HS, Schuchard GH, Wann LS, Palmer TE, Hartz AJ, Gross CM, et al: The relative merits of pulsus paradoxus and right ventricular diastolic collapse in the early detection of cardiac tamponade: An experimental echocardiographic study. *Circulation* 1985; 71:829–833.
83. D'Cruz IA, Cohen HC, Prabhu R, Glick G: Diagnosis of cardiac tamponade by echocardiography. Changes in mitral valve motion and ventricular dimensions, with special reference to paradoxical pulse. *Circulation* 1975; 52:460–465.
84. Feigenbaum H, Zaky A, Grabhorn LL: Cardiac motion in patients with pericardial effusion: A study using reflected ultrasound. *Circulation* 1966; 34:611–619.
85. Price EC, Dennis EW: Electrical alternans, its mechanism demonstrated (abstr). *Circulation* 1969; 39/40(suppl 3):165.
86. Appleton CK, Hatle LA, Popp RL: Cardiac tamponade and pericardial effusion; respiratory variation in transvalvular flow velocities studied by Doppler echocardiography. *J Am Coll Cardiol* 1988; 11:1020-1030.
87. Hoit B: Imaging the pericardium. *Cardiol Clin* 1990; 8:587–600.
88. Littman D, Spodick DH: Total electrical alternation in pericardial disease. *Circulation* 1958; 17:912–917.
89. Toney JC, Kolmen SN: Cardiac tamponade: Fluid and pressure effects on electrocardiographic changes. *Proc Soc Exp Biol Med* 1966; 121:642–648.
90. Antman EM, Gargill V, Grossman W: Low pressure cardiac tamponade. *Ann Intern Med* 1979; 91:403–406.
91. Shabetai R, Rostand SG: Nephrogenic pericardial disease. Contemporary issues in nephrology, 13. In: O'Rourke RA, Brenner BM, Stein JH (eds): *The Heart and Renal Disease.* New York, Churchill Livingstone, 1984: 89–125.
92. Hardesty RL: Delayed postoperative cardiac tamponade: Diagnosis and management. In: Reddy PS, Leon DF, Shaver JS (eds): *Pericardial Disease.* New York, Raven, 1981: 341.
93. Yacoub MH, Cleland WP, Deal CW: Left atrial tamponade, *Thorax* 1966; 21:305–309.
94. Engleman RM, Spencer FC, Reed GE, Tice DA: Cardiac tamponade following open heart surgery. *Circulation* 1970; 41(suppl 2):II-165–II-171.
95. West S: Purulent pericarditis treated by paracentesis and free incision with recovery. *Br Med J* 1883; 1:814.
96. Naunheim KS, Flore AC, Turrentine M, Hammell LM, Brown JW, Kesler KA, et al: Pericardial drainage subxiphoid vs. transthoracic approach. *Eur J Cardiol Thorac Surg* 1991; 5:99–104.
97. Krikorian JG, Hancock EW: Pericardiocentesis. *Am J Med* 1978; 65:808–814.
98. Wong B, Murphy J, Chang CJ, Hassenein K, Dunn M: The risk of pericardiocentesis. *Am J Cardiol* 1979; 44:1110–1114.
99. Clarke DP, Cosgrove DO: Real-time ultrasound scanning in the planning and guidance of pericardiocentesis. *Clin Radiol* 1987; 38:119–122.
100. Palacios IF, Tuzcu EM, Ziskind AA, Younger J, Block PC: Percutaneous balloon pericardial window for patients with malignant pericardial effusion and tamponade. *Cathet Cardiovasc Diag* 1991; 22:244–249.
101. Paul O, Castleman B, White PD: Chronic constrictive pericarditis: A study of 53 cases. *Am J Med Sci* 1948; 216:361–377.
102. Andrews GWS, Pickering GW, Sellors TH: The aetiology of constrictive pericarditis with special reference to tuberculous pericarditis, together with a note on polyserositis. *Q J Med* 1948; 17:291–321.
103. Shabetai R: The pericardium: An essay on some recent developments. *Am J Cardiol* 1978; 42:1036–1043.
104. Wood P: Chronic constrictive pericarditis. *Am J Cardiol* 1961; 7:48–61.
105. Levine HD: Myocardial fibrosis in constrictive pericarditis: Electrocardiographic and pathologic observations. *Circulation* 1973; 48:1268–1281.
106. Lorel B, Leinbach RC, Pohost GM, Gold HR, Dinsmore RE, Hutter AM: Right ventricular infarction. Clinical diagnosis and differentiation from cardiac tamponade and pericardial constriction. *Am J Cardiol* 1979; 43:465–471.
107. Meany E, Shabetai R, Bhargava V, Shearer M, Weidner C, Mangiardi LM, et al: Cardiac amyloidosis, constrictive pericarditis and restrictive cardiomyopathy. *Am J Cardiol* 1976; 38:547–556.
108. Goodwin JP, Oakley CM: The cardiomyopathies. *Br Heart J* 1972; 34:545–552.
109. Schrire V, Gotsman MS, Beck W: Unusual diastolic murmurs in constrictive pericarditis and constrictive endocarditis. *Am Heart J* 1968; 76:4–12.
110. McHenry MM, Ord JW, Johnson RR, Shoener JA: Exercise performance and stroke volume changes in two patients with constrictive pericarditis. *Am Heart J* 1965; 70:180–185.
111. Nakhjavan FK, Goldberg H: Hemodynamic effects of catecholamine stimulation in constrictive pericarditis. *Circulation* 1970; 42:487–490.
112. Tyberg TI, Goodyer AVN, Hurst VW, Alexander J, Langou RA: Left ventricular filling in differentiating restrictive amyloid cardiomyopathy and constrictive pericarditis. *Am J Cardiol* 1981; 47:791–796.
113. Candell-Riera J, del Castillo G, Permanyer-Miralda G, Soler-Soler J: Echocardiographic features of the interventricular septum in chronic constrictive pericarditis. *Circulation* 1978; 57:1154–1158.
114. Doppman JL, Rienmuller R, Lissner J, Cyran J, Boh HD, Strauer BE, et al: Computed tomography in constrictive pericardial disease. *J Comput Assist Tomogr* 1981; 5:1–11.
115. Schoenfeld MH, Supple EW, Dec GW, Fallon JT, Palacios IF: Restrictive cardiomyopathy versus constrictive pericarditis: Role of endomyocardial biopsy in avoiding unnecessary thoracotomy. *Circulation* 1987; 75:1012–1017.
116. Keith TA: Chronic constrictive pericarditis in association with rheumatoid disease. *Circulation* 1962; 25:477–483.
117. Kutcher MA, King SB III, Alimurung BN, Craver JM, Logue RB: Constrictive pericarditis as a complication of cardiac surgery: Recognition of an entity. *Am J Cardiol* 1982; 50:742–748.
118. Marsa R, Mehta S, Willis W, Bailey L: Constrictive pericarditis

after myocardial revascularization. *Am J Cardiol* 1979; 44:177–183.

119. Bush CA, Stang JM, Wooley CF, Kilman JW: Occult constrictive pericardial disease. Diagnosis by rapid volume expansion and correction by pericardiectomy. *Circulation* 1977; 56:924–930.
120. Fowler NO: Constrictive pericarditis: New aspects. *Am J Cardiol* 1982; 50:1014–1017.
121. Shabetai R: *The Pericardium.* New York, Grune & Stratton, 1981: 206–208.
122. Sagrista-Sauleda J, Permanyer-Miralda G, Candell RJ, Angel J, Soler-Soler J: Transient cardiac constriction: An unrecognized pattern of evolution in effusive acute idiopathic pericarditis. *Am J Cardiol* 1987; 59:961–966.
123. Culliford AT, Lipton M, Spencer FC: Operation for chronic constrictive pericarditis: Do the surgical approach and degree of pericardial resection influence the outcome significantly? *Ann Thorac Surg* 1980; 29:146–152.
124. DeValeria PA, Baumgartner WA, Casale AS, Greene PS, Cameron DE, Gardner TJ, et al: Current indications, risks and outcome after pericardiectomy. *Ann Thorac Surg* 1991; 52:219–224.
125. Somerville W: Constrictive pericarditis with special reference to the change in natural history brought about by surgical intervention. *Circulation* 1968; 37 [/] 38(suppl 5):V-102–V-111.
126. Nasser WK: Congenital absence of the left pericardium. *Am J Cardiol* 1970; 26:466–470.
127. Bright R: Tabular view of the morbid appearances in a hundred cases connected with albuminous urine. *Guy's Hosp Rep* 1836; 1:380–400.
128. Comty CM, Cohen SL, Shapiro FL: Pericarditis in chronic uremia and its sequels. *Ann Intern Med* 1971; 75:173–183.
129. Beaudry C, Nakamoto S, Kolff WJ: Uremic pericarditis and cardiac tamponade in chronic renal failure. *Ann Intern Med* 1966; 64:990–995.
130. Comty CM, Wathen RL, Shapiro FL: Uremic pericarditis. In: Spodick DH (ed): *Pericardial Diseases.* Philadelphia, FA Davis, 1976: 219–235.
131. Buselmeier TJ, Simmons RL, Najarian JS, Mauer SM, Matas AJ, Kjellstrand CM: Uremic pericardial effusion. *Nephron* 1976; 16:371–380.
132. Parkinson J, Bedford DE: Cardiac infarction and coronary thrombosis. *Lancet* 1928; 1:4–11.
133. Khan AH: Pericarditis of myocardial infarction: Review of the literature with case presentation. *Am Heart J* 1975; 90:788–794.
134. Galve E, Garcia-del-Castillo H, Evangelista A, Batlle J, Permanyer-Miralda G, Soler-Soler J: Pericardial effusion in the course of myocardial infarction: Incidence, natural history, and clinical relevance. *Circulation* 1986; 73:294–299.
135. Dressler W: A post-myocardial-infarction syndrome. Preliminary report of a complication resembling idiopathic recurrent, benign pericarditis. *JAMA* 1956; 160:1379–1383.
136. Lichstein E, Arsura E, Hollander G, Greengart A, Sanders M: Current incidence of postmyocardial infarction (Dressler's) syndrome. *Am J Cardiol* 1982; 50:1269–1271.
137. Kossowsky WA, Lyon AF, Spain DM: Reappraisal of the postmyocardial infarction Dressler's syndrome. *Am Heart J* 1981; 102:954–956.
138. Burch GE, Colcolough HL: Postcardiotomy and postinfarction syndromes—a theory. *Am Heart J* 1970; 80:290–291.
139. Engle MA, Zabriskie JB, Senterfit LB, Gay WA, O'Loughlin JE, Ehlers KH: Viral illness and the postpericardiotomy syndrome. A prospective study in children. *Circulation* 1980; 62:1151–1158.
140. Antman KH: Current concepts: Malignant mesothelioma. *N Engl J Med* 1980; 303:200–202.
141. Applefeld MM, Pollock SH: Cardiac disease in patients who have malignancies. *Curr Probl Cardiol* 1980; 4:11:5–37.
142. Syed S, Jung RT: Cardiac tamponade caused by metastasising haemangioendothelial sarcoma of the liver. *Br Heart J* 1978; 40:697–699.
143. Arciniegas E, Hakimi M, Farooki ZQ, Green EW: Intrapericardial teratoma in infancy. *J Thorac Cardiovasc Surg* 1980; 79:306–311.
144. Wiener HG, Kristensen IB, Haubek A, Kristensen B, Baandrup U: The diagnostic value of pericardial cytology: An analysis of 95 cases. *Acta Cytol* 1991; 35:149–153.
145. Davis S, Sharma SM, Blumberg ED, Kim CS: Intrapericardial tetracycline for the management of cardiac tamponade secondary to malignant pericardial effusion. *N Engl J Med* 1978; 299:1113–1114.
146. Applefeld MM, Slawson RG, Hall-Craigs M, Green DC, Singleton RT, Wiernik PH: Delayed pericardial disease after radiotherapy. *Am J Cardiol* 1981; 47:210–213.
147. Ruckdeschel JC, Chang P, Martin RG, Byhardt RW, O'Connell MJ, Sutherland JC, et al: Radiation-related pericardial effusions in patients with Hodgkin's disease. *Medicine* 1975; 54:245–259.
148. Schneider JS, Edwards JE: Irradiation induced pericarditis. *Chest* 1979; 75:560–564.
149. King DT, Nieberg RK: The use of cytology to evaluate pericardial effusions. *Ann Clin Lab Sci* 1979; 9:18–23.
150. Hancock EW: Pericardial disease in patients with neoplasm. In: Reddy PS, Leon DF, Shaver JA (eds): *Pericardial Disease.* New York, Raven, 1982: 325.
151. Bywaters EGL: The relation between heart and joint disease including "rheumatoid heart disease" and chronic post-rheumatic arthritis (type Jaccoud). *Br Heart J* 1950; 12:101–131.
152. Charcot JM: *Clinical Lectures on Senile and Chronic Diseases* (trans Tuke NS). London, New Sydenham Society, 95, 1881: 172–175.
153. Prakash R, Atassi A, Poske R, Rosen KM: Prevalence of pericardial effusion and mitral valve involvement in patients with rheumatoid arthritis without cardiac symptoms. An echocardiographic evaluation. *N Engl J Med* 1973; 289:597–600.
154. Gelson A, Sanderson JM, Carson P: Rheumatoid pericardial effusion with heart block treated by pericardiectomy and implantation of permanent pacemaker. *Br Heart J* 1977; 39:113–115.
155. Burney DP, Martin CE, Thomas CS, Fisher RD, Bender HW: Rheumatoid pericarditis. *J Thorac Cardiovasc Surg* 1979; 77:511–515.
156. Brigden W, Bywaters EGL, Lessof MH, Ross IP: The heart in systemic lupus erythematosus. *Br Heart J* 1960; 22:1–16.
157. Bergen SS Jr: Pericardial effusion, a manifestation of systemic lupus erythematosus. *Circulation* 1960; 22:144–150.
158. Bulkley BH, Roberts WC: The heart in systemic lupus erythematosus and the changes induced in it by corticosteroid therapy. A study of 36 necropsy patients. *Am J Med* 1975; 58:243–264.
159. Sackner MA, Heinz ER, Steinberg AJ: The heart in scleroderma. *Am J Cardiol* 1966; 17:542–559.
160. Fowler NO: *Cardiac Diagnosis and Treatment,* 3d ed. Hagerstown, Harper & Row, 1980: 978.
161. Slater EE: Cardiac tamponade and peripheral eosinophilia in a patient receiving cromolyn sodium. *Chest* 1978; 73:878–879.
162. Orlando RC, Moyer P, Barnett TB: Methysergide therapy and constrictive pericarditis. *Ann Intern Med* 1978; 88:213–214.
163. Houston MC, McChesney JA, Chatergee K: Pericardial effusion associated with minoxidil therapy. *Arch Intern Med* 1981; 141:69–71.
164. Logue RB: Etiology, recognition and management of pericardial disease. In: Hurst JW (ed): *The Heart,* 5th ed. New York, McGraw-Hill, 1982: 1371–1393.
165. Gleckman RA: Nonviral infectious pericarditis. In: Spodick DH (ed): *Pericardial Diseases.* Philadelphia, FA Davis, 1976: 159–175.
166. Sagrista-Sauleda J, Permanyer-Miralda G, Soler-Soler J: Tuberculous pericarditis: Ten year experience with a prospective protocol for diagnosis and treatment. *J Am Coll Cardiol* 1988; 11:724–728.
167. Suzman S: Tuberculous perisardial effusion. *Br Heart J* 1943; 5:19–23.
168. Cheitlin MD, Serfas LJ, Sbar SS, Glasser SP: Tuberculous pericarditis: Is limited pericardial biopsy sufficient for diagnosis? *Am Rev Respir Dis* 1968; 98:287–291.
169. Telenti M, Fdez J, de Quiros B, Susano R, Torrico AM: Pericardite tuberculeuse: Valeur diagnostique de l'adenosine desaminase. *Presse Med* 1991; 20:637–640.
170. Lyons HA, Rooney JJ, Crocco JA: Tuberculous pericarditis. *Ann Intern Med* 1968; 68:1175.
171. Strang JIG, Gibson DG, Mitchison DA, Girling DJ, Kakaza HHS, Allen BW, et al: Controlled clinical trial of complete open surgical drainage and of prednisone in treatment of tuberculous pericardial effusion in Transkei. *Lancet* 1988; 2:759–764.
172. Kirchner SG, Heller RM, Sell SH, Altemeier WA: The radiologi-

cal features of *Histoplasma* pericarditis. *Pediatr Radiol* 1978; 7:7–9.
173. Young EJ, Vainrub B, Musher DM: Pericarditis due to histoplasmosis. *JAMA* 1978; 240:1750–1751.
174. Wooley CF, Hosier DM: Constrictive pericarditis due to *Histoplasma capsulatum. N Engl J Med* 1961; 264:1230–1232.
175. Bennett JE: Chemotherapy of systemic mycoses. *N Engl J Med* 1974; 290:30–32.
176. Goodwin RA Jr, Snell JD Jr, Hubbard WW, Terry RT:: Relationships in combined pulmonary infections with *Histoplasma capsulatum* and *Mycobacterium tuberculosis. Am Rev Respir Dis* 1967; 96:990–997.
177. Sarosi GA, Voth DW, Dahl BA, Doto IL, Tosh FE: Disseminated histoplasmosis: Results of long-term follow-up. *Ann Intern Med* 1971; 75:511–516.
178. Chavez CM, Causey WA, Conn JH: Constrictive pericarditis due to infection with *Nocardia asteroides. Chest* 1972; 61:79–81.
179. Fowler NO, Manitsas GT: Infectious pericarditis. *Prog Cardiovasc Dis* 1973; 16:323–336.
180. Klacsmann PG, Bulkley BH, Hutchins GM: The changed spectrum of purulent pericarditis: An 86 year autopsy experience in 200 patients. *Am J Med* 1977; 63:666–673.
181. Tan JS, Holmes JC, Fowler NO, Manitas GT, Phair JP: Antibiotic levels in pericardial fluid. *J Clin Invest* 1974; 53:7–12.
182. Miller HI: Acute pericarditis as a presenting feature of meningococcal septicemia. *Isr J Med Sci* 1973; 9(11):1570–1573.
183. Pierce HI, Cooper EB: Meningococcal pericarditis. *Arch Intern Med* 1972; 129:918–922.
184. Scott LP, Knox D, Perry LW, Pineros-Torres FJ: Meningococcal pericarditis. Report of 2 cases, 1 complicated by acute constrictive pericarditis. *Am J Cardiol* 1972; 29:104–108.
185. Symbas PN, Ware RE, DiOrio DA, Hatcher CR: Purulent pericarditis. A review of diagnostic and surgical principles. *South Med J* 1974; 67:46–48.
186. Gould K, Barnett JA, Sanford JP: Purulent pericarditis in the antibiotic era. *Arch Intern Med* 1974; 134:923–927.
187. Caird R, Conway N, McMillan IKR: Purulent pericarditis followed by early constriction in young children. *Br Heart J* 1973; 35:201–203.
188. Smolar EN, Rubin JE, Avramides A, Carter AC: Cardiac tamponade in primary myxedema and review of the literature. *Am J Med Sci* 1976; 272:345–352.
189. Stanley RJ, Subramanian R, Lie JT: Cholesterol pericarditis terminating as constrictive calcific pericarditis. *Am J Cardiol* 1980; 46:511–514.
190. Brawley RK, Vasko JS, Morrow AG: Cholesterol pericarditis. Considerations of its pathogenesis and treatment. *Am J Med* 1966; 41:235–248.
191. Shojaee S, Hutchins GM: Echinococcosis complicated by purulent pericarditis. *Chest* 1978; 73:512–514.
192. Pierce RN, Walker Smith GJ: Intrathoracic manifestations of Degos' disease (malignant atrophic papulosis). *Chest* 1978; 73:79–84.
193. Mets T, Van Hove W, Louis H: Pseudomyxoma peritonei: Report of a case with extraperitoneal metastasis and invasion of the spleen. *Chest* 1977; 72:792–794.
194. Csonka GW, Oates JK: Pericarditis and electrocardiographic changes in Reiter's syndrome. *Br Med J* 1957; 1:866–869.
195. Mihas AA, Dasher CA: Pericarditis associated with granulomatous colitis. *Am J Gastroenterol* 1977; 68:494–497.
196. Vlietstra RE, Lie JT, Kuhl WE, Danielson GK, Roberts MK: Whipple's disease involving the pericardium. Pathological confirmation during life. *Aust NZ J Med* 1978; 8:649–651.
197. Engle MA: Cardiac involvement in Cooley's anemia. *Ann NY Acad Sci* 1964; 119:694–704.
198. Just H, Mattingly TW: Interatrial septal defect and pericardial disease. *Am Heart J* 1968; 76:157–167.
199. Westfried M, Mandel D, Alderete MN, Groopman J, Minkowitz S: Sipple's syndrome with a malignant pheochromocytoma presenting as a pericardial effusion. *Cardiology* 1978; 63:305–311.
200. Toltzis RJ, Rosenthal A, Fellows K, Castaneda AR, Nadas AS: Chylous reflux syndrome involving the pericardium and lung. *Chest* 1978; 74:457–458.
201. Rogers CI, Meredith HC: Osler revisited: An unusual cause of inversion of the diaphragm. *Radiology* 1977; 125:596.
202. Davidson ED, Horney JT, Salter PP III: Internal pancreatic fistula to the pericardium and pleura. *Surgery* 1979; 85:478–480.
203. McNicholl B, Murray JP, Egan B, McHugh P: Pneumomediastinum and diabetic hyperpnoea. *Br Med J* 1968; 4:493–494.
204. Cumming GR, Kerr D, Ferguson CC: Constrictive pericarditis with dwarfism in two siblings (mulibrey nanism). *J Pediatr* 1976; 88:569–572.
205. Scarlett JA, Kistner ML, Yang LC: Behçet's syndrome. Report of a case associated with pericardial effusion and cryoglobulinemia treated with indomethacin. *Am J Med* 1979; 66:146–148.
206. Bianchi C, DiBonito L, Fonda F, Sauli G: Pericardial perforation of a gastric ulcer secondary to phytobezoar. *Panminerva Med* 1977; 19:353–356.

Chapter 93

Surgical Management of Pericardial Disease

Joseph I. Miller, Jr., M.D.

HISTORICAL ASPECTS OF PERICARDIAL SURGERY

Riolan first suggested performing pericardiotomy for an effusion compressing the heart by practicing a trephining procedure in 1649, although this technique was not utilized until two centuries later.[1] In 1840, Karaneff performed pericardiocentesis for relief of hemorrhagic effusion in 30 patients, 7 of whom survived.[2] In 1913, Rehn and Sauerbruch independently introduced pericardial resection.[3,4] In 1929, Churchill performed the first successful pericardiectomy for constrictive pericarditis in the United States.[5] In 1960, Mannix and Dennis advocated pericardiectomy for chronic effusion producing symptoms of tamponade and for relapsing types of pericarditis with effusion.[6] Radical pericardiectomy was advocated by Shumaker and Roshe in 1960 as the only means by which recurrence of pericardial constriction requiring secondary operations could be prevented.[7]

SURGICAL THERAPY FOR THE PERICARDIUM

There are four operative procedures on the pericardium: (1) pericardiocentesis; (2) pericardiotomy for biopsy, exploration, and drainage; and (3) pericardiectomy; and (4) thoracoscopic pericardial resection.

Pericardiocentesis

Indications for pericardiocentesis are: (1) to establish the diagnosis of pericardial disease by diagnostic studies of pericardial fluid; (2) to relieve acute cardiac tamponade; (3) to evaluate physiologic elevation of the central venous pressure; and (4) to aid in the preoperative management of the decompensated patient requiring pericardiectomy.[8]

Ideally, pericardiocentesis should be performed in the cardiac catheterization laboratory, where appropriate physiologic monitoring is available. Monitoring is especially important in cases of small posterior lobulated effusions or in loculated anterior effusions. In patients with a massive pericardial effusion, the procedure can be safely performed at the bedside by experienced personnel with electrocardiographic or, preferably, two-dimensional echocardiographic monitoring. Individuals performing pericardiocentesis should have knowledge of the surgical anatomy of the heart and the pericardium, as well as of the location of the coronary arteries, the technique of the procedure, and its complications.

The anatomic approach of choice for pericardiocentesis is the subxiphoid approach. Not only is this considered the easiest approach, but it is also the safest because there is a smaller chance of damaging the coronary arteries. In some patients, the echocardiogram may determine that other positions, often anterior, are preferable.

The patient is premedicated with atropine (0.5 to 1 mg) in order to prevent vasovagal reaction. Ideally, the

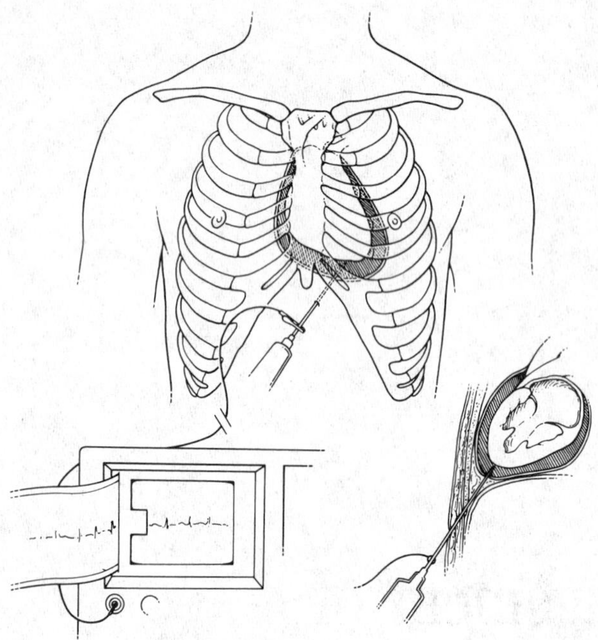

FIGURE 93-1 Technique of subxiphoid pericardiocentesis. A 6-in spinal needle is inserted and directed toward the left shoulder at a 45° angle. Electrocardiography or echocardiography is utilized.

patient receives nothing orally for 3 to 4 h prior to the procedure in case emergency surgery is required.

The classic technique of the subxiphoid approach is as follows (Fig. 93-1). The patient is placed in a semi-Fowler's position at a 45° angle so that a majority of the pericardial fluid is in the most dependent position. A point inferior to the tip of the xiphoid process and just to the left of the midline is anesthetized with a small amount of local anesthetic solution. A 21-gauge spinal needle, at least 6 in long and filled with anesthetic solution, is introduced under cardiographic monitoring and is slowly advanced to the left shoulder. This maneuver can also be performed under two-dimensional echocardiographic monitoring. The technique of two-dimensional echocardiographically directed pericardiocentesis was originally developed and described by the Mayo Clinic. It is the method most frequently employed for pericardiocentesis in the United States. The site of needle puncture is determined by echocardiographic monitoring. The most ideal site is one in which the fluid is closest to the transducer and from which the needle tract avoids the heart and underlying structures.[9] There is some resistance to the needle as it passes through the diaphragm and into the pericardium. If the needle touches the right ventricular epicardium, the V lead connected to the needle shows ST-segment elevation.[10] Rarely, the right atrium is contacted, and PR-segment elevation is recorded. The individual performing the pericardiocentesis may feel a scratch sensation as the needle touches the epicardium. The distance from the skin to the heart is 6 to 8 cm in an adult and 5 cm or less in a child.[11] If the fluid obtained is grossly bloody, it should be tested to see whether it clots. If the aspirated blood clots, the right ventricle has been entered and the fluid is not from the pericardial aspiration. If the pericardial space is easily identified and the effusion is large, a No. 18 spinal needle with a catheter can be introduced into the pericardial space. All fluid is aspirated and sent for appropriate studies. The accurate diagnosis of malignancy or infections, such as tuberculosis, involving the pericardial space is often not possible from pericardial fluid and frequently requires microscopic examination of pericardial tissue (see also Chap. 92).

If the fluid removed is for diagnosis, it may be helpful to inject air into the pericardium at the completion of the procedure. Serial chest films then indicate the thickness of the pericardium, the presence of myocardial masses, the size of the heart, and the amount of residual fluid present.[8]

If malignancy or recurrent effusion is suspected, it may be helpful to leave an intrapericardial catheter plastic intracath in the pericardial space to allow further drainage and instillation of glucocorticosteroids, depending on the definitive diagnosis and as indicated by the underlying condition.

Complications that may arise with pericardiocentesis include laceration of a coronary artery or right ventricle, perforation of the right atrium or ventricle, perforation of the stomach or colon, pneumothorax, arrhythmias, tamponade, and hypotension, with or without ventricular fibrillation.

Subxiphoid Pericardiotomy, Biopsy, and Drainage

In patients in whom pericardiocentesis is not feasible or is associated with increased risk, or when a definitive diagnosis has not been determined, direct open biopsy of the pericardium for tissue biopsy and fluid removal can be safely performed to establish a diagnosis of pericardial disease. It is often utilized in patients with recurrent effusion in whom previous studies have not revealed a definitive diagnosis. The subxiphoid approach allows resection of 3 to 4 cm^2 of pericardial tissue and drainage of the pericardium. For most patients, this is the procedure of choice for the diagnosis of pericardial disease unless a pericardiectomy is indicated on the basis of the suspected underlying process. When constrictive pericarditis or primary idiopathic dilated cardiomyopathy rather than pericarditis is suspected, an approach through the left fourth or fifth intercostal space is preferred. When only pericardial fluid is present and total pericardiectomy is not required, videoendoscopic thoracic resection of the pericardium may be performed.

Technique of Subxiphoid Pericardiotomy

General anesthesia is preferred, but subxiphoid pericardiotomy may be performed under local anesthesia with adequate sedation if the clinical situation so dictates. A small upper midline incision 6 to 8 cm in length is made, beginning at the top of the xiphoid process and extending inferiorly for 3 cm below the tip of the xiphoid process. The linea alba is divided in the midline, and the cleavage plane between the posterior wall of the sternum and the anterior pericardium is developed by blunt finger dissection. The correct plane is identified by the smooth, silky plane of the fascia on the posterior aspect of the sternum. The xiphoid process is then resected in toto with the electric cautery. By blunt dissection and inferior traction on the diaphragm, the fat is swept away with a sponge stick and the lower anterior pericardium and diaphragm are identified. With downward traction and two Kocher forceps utilized on the diaphragm, the pericardium is easily brought into view. It is incised with a No. 15 knife blade. A 4- to 6-cm^2 area of pericardium can be removed for tissue examination and culture. Appropriate drainage catheters may be inserted into the pericardial space and brought out through separate stab wounds. The incision is closed in layers.

If it is desirable to remove a larger amount of pericardium, a left thoracic approach through the fourth or fifth intercostal space is preferred.

Pericardiectomy

Surgical resection of the pericardium is referred to as pericardiectomy. Pericardiectomy may be of two types: (1) parietal pericardiectomy, which is the procedure performed in patients with recurrent pericardial effusion, and (2) visceral pericardiectomy, which is required together with parietal pericardiectomy in patients with constrictive pericarditis. The surgical indications for pericardiectomy are listed in Table 93-1.

The five operative approaches to the pericardium are (1) the subxiphoid, (2) the bilateral anterior thoracotomy, (3) the left anterior thoracotomy, (4) the median sternotomy, and (5) the videoendoscopic thoracic approach.

The subxiphoid approach is generally indicated for diagnostic purposes, in life-threatening situations, or for extremely debilitated patients. Its advantages are that it is quick and easy to perform and is associated with a low morbidity rate. The potential disadvantages include problems with subsequent recurrent effusions and the possibility of future constriction. It is contraindicated for patients with constrictive pericarditis.

Bilateral anterior thoracotomy is the least utilized of the five approaches because of a higher morbidity rate. It is generally indicated when a patient has had a previous operative procedure on the pericardium and repeated median sternotomy is not feasible.

A left anterior thoracotomy is the most common approach utilized in the treatment of effusive pericardial disease. It is the approach of choice when the predominent underlying disease process is an effusive process rather than constrictive pericarditis. It has the advantages of being quick to perform, providing good exposure, having minimal morbidity, and allowing removal of approximately 60 to 65 percent of the parietal pericardium. It is the approach of choice except in constrictive pericarditis.

Median sternotomy is the approach of choice in constrictive pericarditis. When constriction is present, open heart pump standby should always be available, but it is seldom needed.

In the videoendoscopic thoracic approach, three small ports are required, and a 6- to 10-cm area of pericardium can be resected. It is contraindicated in patients with constrictive pericarditis.

TABLE 93-1
Surgical Indications for Pericardiectomy

Surgical Indications for Pericardiectomy
Congenital Problems
Congenital anomalies and defects
Cysts and diverticula
Acute and Chronic Pericarditis
Predominant effusion with and without tamponade
Idiopathic recurrent
Uremic
Infectious
Pyogenic (purulent)
Tuberculosis
Viral
Neoplastic
Associated with systemic disease (connective tissue disease)
Traumatic
Radiation-caused
Predominant constriction with and without effusion
Idiopathic (nonspecific)
Infectious
Following cardiac surgery

SOURCE: Miller.[12]

Types of Pericardiectomy

As mentioned earlier, pericardiectomy can be divided into two types: (1) parietal pericardiectomy, which is required when there is only effusion but no constriction, and (2) visceral pericardiectomy, which is necessary "in all cases of constrictive pericarditis, both in patients whose visceral and parietal layers are fused and in those who retain pericardial effusion associated with constriction by the visceral layers only."[8]

Parietal Pericardiectomy Appropriate cardiovascular monitoring techniques are utilized, including the measurement of radial artery pressures and the use of Swan-Ganz catheters. The patient is placed in the anterior thoracotomy position, with the left chest elevated at 30° by rolled sheets under the left flank with the left arm supported on an ether screen. A 10-cm left anterior thoracotomy incision is made into the inframammary fourth or fifth intercostal space, beginning at the sternal border and extending laterally to the anterior axillary line. The chest is entered, and the appropriate chest retractor placed. The lung is packed off and held with a lung retractor. The pericardium can be removed easily from the anterior to the left phrenic bundle and to the right mediastinal pleural reflection; with further retraction, it can be removed all the way to the right phrenic bundle. The pericardium posterior to the left phrenic bundle is removed to a level of the pulmonary vasculature. A 1-in bridge of tissue containing the phrenic nerve, artery, and vein is preserved (Fig. 93-2). All pericardium is removed with the coagulation mode of the electric cautery, which provides good hemostatis and results in minimal postoperative bleeding. Care must be taken to preserve the phrenic nerve as it leaves the pericardium and branches out into the diaphragm.

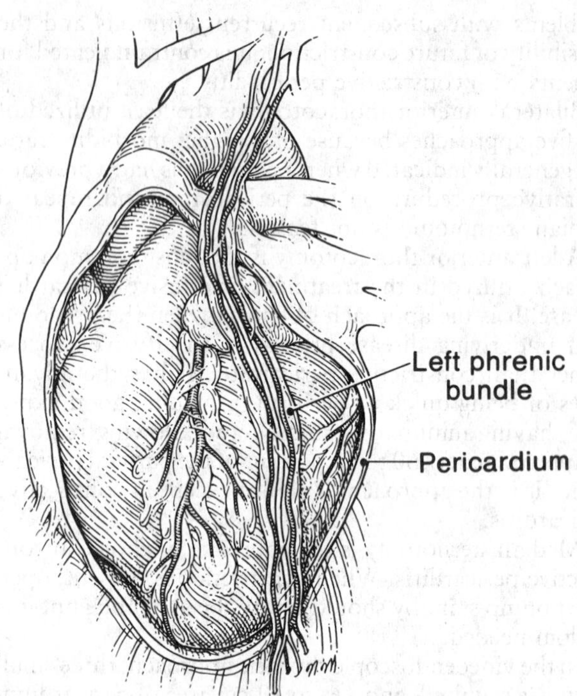

FIGURE 93-2 A heart following anterior pericardiectomy. All anterior pericardium is removed, with a 1-in phrenic bridge remaining.

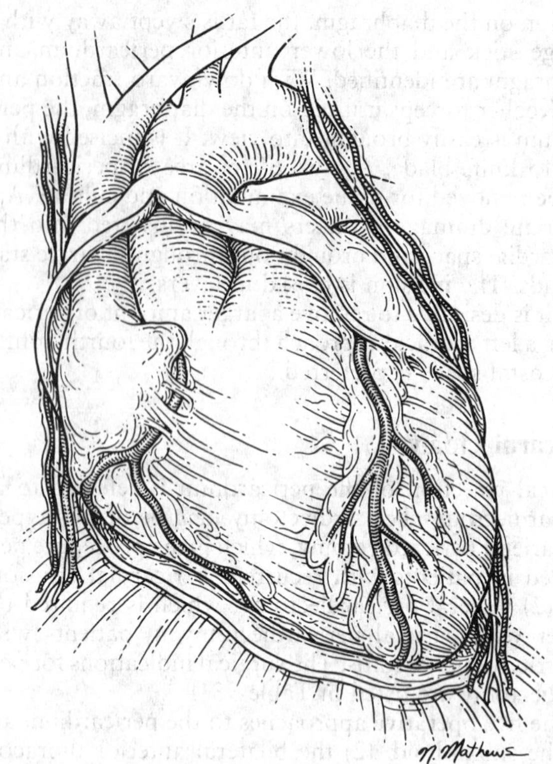

FIGURE 93-3 A median sternotomy with the initial view of the constricted pericardium.

By the use of this technique, 50 to 75 percent of the parietal pericardium can be removed. Two suction catheters are left in the chest, and the incision is closed in layers. The heart after parietal pericardiectomy is shown in Fig. 93-2.

Visceral Pericardiectomy Visceral pericardiectomy is necessary in all cases of constrictive pericarditis. Because of the risk of myocardial tear and excessive blood loss, the procedure is always performed with standby cardiopulmonary bypass. It is our preference not to utilize cardiopulmonary bypass unless absolutely necessary, but to have it immediately available when necessary. Other groups prefer to perform the procedure routinely on cardiopulmonary bypass.[12]

A median sternotomy is made, revealing the constrictive pericardium (Fig. 93-3). The initial point of exposure is around the apex of the left ventricle. There is generally an area of pericardium around the apex of the heart that is not overly adherent or calcified and that allows one to establish exposure in the area. Traction sutures of No. 2-0 silk are then taken 1 cm apart over the anterior wall of the left ventricular pericardium. An incision is then made with a No. 15 knife blade through the thickened pericardium down to the myocardium, where the muscle fibers can be recognized. A plane can generally be developed between the epicardium and the myocardium. By use of a combination of traction on the flaps of the pericardium and retraction on the heart, combined with sharp and blunt dissection, the constrictive pericardium can be removed. It is extremely important that the pericardium overlying the left ventricle be removed before the right ventricle is freed; otherwise, the increased flow of blood to the constrictive left ventricle can result in acute pulmonary edema. An area of calcification embedded in the myocardium and not easily removed should be left alone as long as there is not a sizable area of involvement over either ventricle. The pericardium is removed over both left and right ventricles to the phrenic bundle (Fig. 93-4). If dissection permits, a phrenic bridge of tissue containing artery, nerve, and vein is left, and the pericardium is removed to the pulmonary hilus. Usually, no attempt is made to remove the pericardium from the atrioventricular groove or left atrium. The pericardium is removed from the pulmonary outflow tract, but removal is usually not carried out into the pulmonary

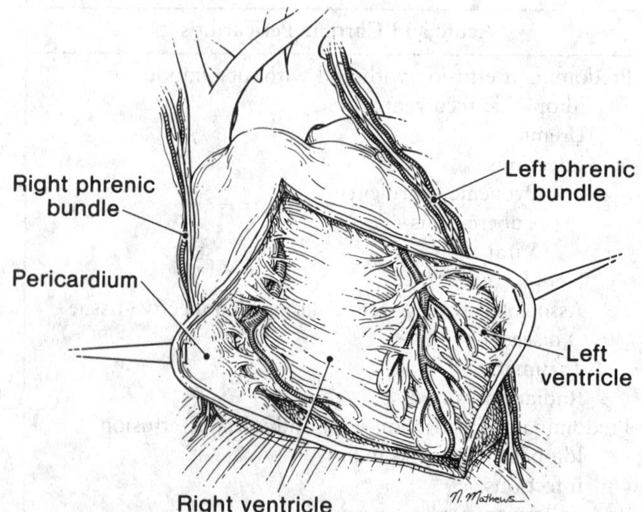

FIGURE 93-4 The initial approach in constrictive pericarditis resection is freeing of left ventricle and then the right ventricle.

artery. The diaphragmatic pericardium is removed and the right ventricle decorticated. If the right ventricle is entered, it is repaired with felt-pledgeted (Teflon) sutures. The right atrioventricular groove is not decorticated. If the superior vena cava and inferior vena cava are involved, they are decorticated. If there is no involvement of the venae cavae, they are left alone. If significant ascites is present, decortication of the inferior vena cava at its entrance into the right atrium is often necessary. One must be extremely careful with areas of calcification in the right atrium. Such areas are best left alone unless the area of involvement is significant. It is extremely important that no constricting epicardium be left behind (Fig. 93-5). At the completion of the procedure, good muscular contraction from both ventricles should be evident.[11] If any significant constricting pericardium is left, the result may be inadequate, and recurrence may result. Adequate hemostasis is achieved, and drainage tubes are inserted and connected to suction.

Thoracoscopic Pericardial Resection Thoracoscopic resection of the pericardium has been performed for several years. Utilizing videoendoscopic techniques, one can remove a 6- to 8-cm piece of pericardium. A three port technique is utilized. The advantage of the thoracoscopic approach is that it can be performed through the right or left chest.

Postoperative Complications

The most common complications of pericardiectomy are congestive heart failure, which occurs in 30 to 35 percent of patients undergoing pericardiectomy for constrictive pericarditis; arrhythmias in 15 to 20 percent; infection in 1 to 3 percent; significant bleeding in less than 1 percent; and postpericardiotomy syndrome.

Emory University Experience With Pericardiectomy

Table 93-2 reflects the author's experience with pericardiectomy at Emory University Affiliated Hospitals during the 19-year period from 1974 to 1993. The majority of procedures were performed for recurrent effusions with tamponade due to neoplastic pericarditis. Idiopathic pericarditis has been the second most common indication for pericardiectomy. In general, a left thoracotomy is employed for benign or malignant effusion due to breast tumor or lymphoma, as the expected outcome is quite good. When the malignant effusion is due to a lung tumor, a subxiphoid approach is used, as the prognosis is limited. Chronic constrictive pericarditis continues to account for approximately 25 to 30 percent of patients undergoing pericardiectomy. The most common cause of constrictive pericarditis in our center continues to be previous open heart surgery (see also Chaps. 92 and 111).

For technical reasons, cases of predominant effusive pericarditis are approached through a left anterior thoracotomy, and cases of constrictive pericarditis are approached through a median sternotomy with cardiopulmonary bypass standby.

TABLE 93-2
Indications for Pericardiectomy, 1974–1993

Cause	Constrictive	Effusive	Number
Neoplastic	0	52	52
Uremic	0	42	42
Idiopathic	12	28	40
Tuberculosis	5	13	18
Infectious	1	12	13
Radiation	4	4	8
Rheumatoid	3	1	4
After open heart surgery	38*	0	38
Traumatic	0	3	3
Drug induced	0	1	1
Totals	63	156	210

* Includes figures of four Emory University Affiliated Hospitals surgeons.

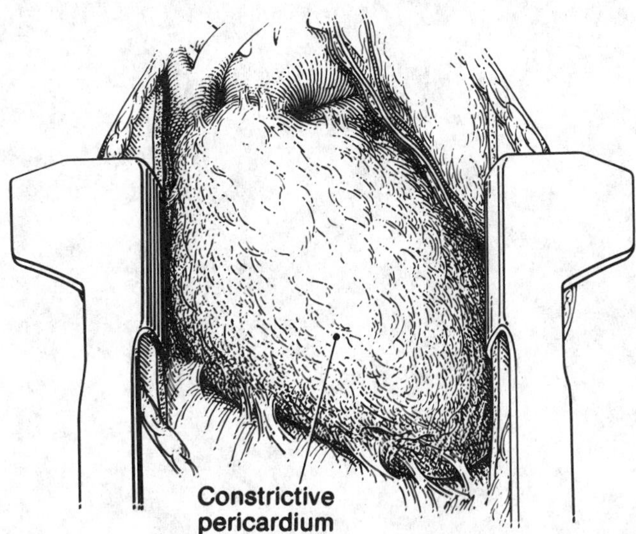

FIGURE 93-5 A heart at the completion of parietal and visceral pericardiectomy.

REFERENCES

1. Riolan J: *Encheiridium Anatomicum et Pathologicum.* Lugdunum, Batavorum, Adriani Wyngaerden, 1649: 206–212.
2. Karawajew W: Paracentese des Brustkastens und des Pericardiums. *Medztg Berl* 1840; 9:251.
3. Rehn L: Zurexperimentellen Pathologie des Herzbeutels. *Verh Dtsch Ges Chir* 1913; 42:339–341.
4. Sauerbruch F: *Die Chirurgie der Brustorgane*, vol. 2. Berlin, Springer-Verlag, 1925:17.
5. Churchill ED: Decortication of the heart for adhesive pericarditis. *AMA Arch Surg* 1929; 19:1457–1469.
6. Mannix EP Jr, Dennis C: The surgical treatment of chronic pericardial effusion and cardiac tamponade. *J Thorac Surg* 1955; 29:381–397.
7. Shumacker HB Jr, Roshe J: Pericardiectomy. *J Cardiovasc Surg* 1960; 1:65–73.
8. Hancock EW: Management of pericardial disease. *Mod Concepts Cardiovasc Dis* 1979; 47:1–6.
9. Callahan JA, Seward JB, Nishimura RA, Miller FA Jr, Reeder GS, Shub C, et al: Two dimensional echocardiographically guided

pericardiocentesis: Experience in 117 consecutive patients. *Am J Cardiol* 1985; 55:476–479.
10. Bishop LH Jr, Estes EH Jr, McIntosh HD: Electrocardiograms as a safeguard in pericardiocentesis. *JAMA* 1956; 162:264–265.
11. Baue AE, Blakemore WS: The pericardium. *Ann Thorac Surg* 1972; 143:81–106.
12. Copeland JG, Stinson EB, Griepp RB, Shumway NE: Surgical treatment of chronic constrictive pericarditis using cardiopulmonary bypass. *J Thorac Cardiovasc Surg* 1975; 69:236–238.
13. Miller JI: Pericardiectomy. In: Hurst JW (ed): *The Heart, Update III*, 4th ed. New York, McGraw-Hill, 1980:147–158.
14. Miller JI, Mansour KA, Hatcher CH Jr: Pericardiectomy: Current indications, concepts, and results in a university center. *Ann Thorac Surg* 1982; 34:40–45.

Chapter 94

Infective and Noninfective Endocarditis

David T. Durack, M.B., Ph.D.

DEFINITIONS AND TERMINOLOGY

Infective endocarditis is the disease caused by microbial infection of the endothelial lining of the heart. Its characteristic lesion is a *vegetation*, which usually develops on a heart valve but occasionally appears elsewhere on the endocardium or on the lining of a large artery. The latter case, more accurately termed *infective endarteritis*, produces a clinical syndrome closely resembling infective endocarditis. Among the many acronyms and abbreviations to be found in the literature on endocarditis, these few are convenient and useful enough to deserve perpetuation:

SBE: subacute bacterial endocarditis

ABE: acute bacterial endocarditis

NVE: native valve endocarditis

PVE: prosthetic valve endocarditis

NBTE: nonbacterial thrombotic endocarditis

The terms *subacute* and *acute bacterial endocarditis* (SBE and ABE) remain in common use and have descriptive value. SBE evolves over several weeks or months; it is usually caused by organisms of low virulence, such as viridans streptococci, which possess limited ability to infect other tissues.[1–4] In contrast, ABE evolves over days to weeks; the progress is hectic, complications develop earlier, and the diagnosis is usually made in less than 2 weeks.[4–7] ABE is most often caused by primary pathogens such as *Staphylococcus aureus*, which are capable of causing invasive infection at other sites in the body.

Infection engrafted upon a heart valve that was either previously normal or damaged by congenital or acquired disease is termed *native valve endocarditis* (NVE). Infection of an artificial valve is termed *prosthetic valve endocarditis* (PVE). This infection is arbitrarily defined as *early PVE* when it occurs within the first 2 months after surgery and as *late PVE* thereafter.[8–10]

The term *noninfective endocarditis* refers to sterile vegetations within the heart. *Endocarditis* is a partial misnomer in this context, because the lesions are thrombotic rather than inflammatory in nature. The central importance of thrombosis in this condition is emphasized appropriately by the term *nonbacterial thrombotic endocarditis* (NBTE), which is broadly defined here to describe any sterile vegetation. This category includes a spectrum of lesions ranging from microscopic aggregates of platelets to the large vegetations of marantic endocarditis, which develop in some patients with terminal malignancy and some other chronic diseases.[11–13]

Infective endocarditis is designated best by naming the infecting organism, for example, *Staph. aureus* endocarditis or *Aspergillus* PVE. This terminology is both specific and informative, allowing useful inferences about natural history, prognosis, and treatment of the case in question.

HISTORICAL NOTE

Riviere, in 1646, Lancisi, in 1706, and Morgagni, in 1761, described patients who died with endocarditis in the seventeenth and eighteenth centuries.[14] Jean-Baptiste

Bouillaud introduced the terms *endocardium* and *endocarditis* between 1824 and 1835. By 1846, Virchow was familiar with the appearance of valvular vegetations at necropsy, but the microbial etiology of infective endocarditis was not fully appreciated until Virchow, Winge, and Heiberg independently demonstrated bacteria in vegetations between 1869 and 1872.[14]

Osler studied the disease extensively.[15] He chose infective endocarditis as the subject for his Goulstonian lectures of 1885.[16] Further major contributions to the knowledge of the natural history, pathogenesis, and pathology of the disease were made by Lenharz, Harbitz, and Schottmuller[14] in Germany; by Horder[17] in England; and by Blumer,[1] Thayer,[2] Allen,[18] Libman and Friedberg,[19] and Beeson[20] in the United States. The technique of blood culture was introduced in Europe and the United States between 1900 and 1910.[3] In 1955, Kerr published a classic monograph summarizing the state of knowledge on subacute bacterial endocarditis to that date.[3]

Attempts to cure endocarditis before the advent of antimicrobial drugs were unsuccessful. The chronicle of the first successes in treatment is closely linked to the history of penicillin. The first patient to receive parenteral penicillin was a young man with streptococcal endocarditis who was treated by Dawson in October 1940 at Columbia University in New York.[21] Although the patient received far too little penicillin to effect a cure, his treatment antedated the first administration of penicillin to a patient by Florey's team in Oxford[22] by several months.[23] After initial failures, by 1944 it had been established that penicillin,[24] unlike sulfonamides,[25] could cure most cases of streptococcal endocarditis. Subsequently, Bloomfield,[26] Hunter,[27] Finland,[28] Geraci,[29] Weinstein,[30] and their colleagues contributed important early studies on the antibiotic treatment of endocarditis.

After the antibiotics, the greatest advance in treatment was the introduction of cardiac valve replacement for endocarditis, first reported from Duke University in 1965.[31]

EPIDEMIOLOGY

The Evolution of Endocarditis

Infective endocarditis today is a different disease from that seen in the preantibiotic era, when its salient clinical features were exhaustively described.[1-3] Since 1961, treatises on the "changing face" of "modern endocarditis" [32-41] have identified the following trends:

- The median age of patients has increased.
- The ratio of males to females has risen.
- The proportion of acute cases has risen.
- Fewer patients develop the classic physical signs of advanced SBE, such as Osler's nodes, finger clubbing, or Roth's spots (see Chap. 10).
- The proportion of cases due to streptococci has fallen slightly.
- The proportion of cases caused by gram-negative bacilli, fungi, and miscellaneous unusual microbes has increased.
- The number of cases in injected drug users has greatly increased.
- Prosthetic valve infections have become more numerous.

These striking changes in the clinical features and epidemiology of infective endocarditis cannot be explained by alterations in the virulence of the infecting microorganisms. Rather, they are due to changes in the susceptible population, to earlier diagnosis and treatment of patients with subacute disease before advanced manifestations develop, and to the impact of antibiotic therapy.[36,37]

The Susceptible Host

Changes in the population at risk are the most important factors responsible for the evolution of the clinical spectrum of endocarditis.[37] The prevalence of rheumatic valvular disease, formerly the most common substrate for endocarditis, has steadily decreased in developed countries; meanwhile, the number of children with congenital heart disease surviving palliative or corrective surgery has increased. The proportion of elderly people in the populations of developed countries has increased, and endocarditis in the elderly has become more common, even though degenerative valvular disease seems to present a relatively low risk for infection.[42] The median age of patients with endocarditis has risen steadily for three decades, from about 30 to about 50 years of age. At present, approximately one-fourth of all patients are over 60 years of age. Over the same period the proportion of males with endocarditis has increased. Male patients now outnumber females by approximately 1.5:1 overall and by as much as 4:1 among patients over 60 years of age.[36-44] In addition, the number of individuals illegally using intravenous drugs has markedly increased in the United States since the early 1960s.

Preexisting Heart Disease

Some patients develop endocarditis even though they have no known heart disease. This phenomenon is most common in cases of ABE, especially in children less than 2 years of age[45-47] and in narcotic addicts.[48-52] However, most patients who develop infective endocarditis have a preexisting cardiac condition. Approximate figures for the frequency of the main predisposing factors[34-54] in children, adults, and injected drug users are given in Table 94-1.

The relative propensity of various cardiac lesions to become infected can be estimated by noting their frequency in published series of cases of infective endocarditis, even though there is wide variation among individual studies. Table 94-2 ranks cardiac abnormalities according to the risk they seem to carry for development of infective endocarditis.

Mitral valve prolapse (MVP) occupies an interesting position in the spectrum of heart lesions that can predispose to endocarditis.[55-61] This common condition, when associated with regurgitation, increases an individual's risk for infective endocarditis by five- to eightfold.[56,57] MVP is now known to underlie a significant proportion

TABLE 94-1

Approximate Frequency of Major Preexisting Cardiac Lesions in Patients with Infective Endocarditis in the United States

Lesion	Children under 2 years, %	Children 2–15 Years, %	Adults 15–50 Years, %	Adults >50 Years, %	Adults Who Are IV Drug Abusers, %
No known heart disease	50–70	10–15	10–20	10	50–60
Congenital heart disease*	30–50	70–80	25–35	15–25	10
Rheumatic heart disease	Rare	10	10–15	10–15	10
Degenerative heart disease	0	0	Rare	10–20	Rare
Previous cardiac surgery	5	10–15	10–20	10–20	10–20
Previous endocarditis	Rare	5	5–10	5–10	10–20

* Includes mitral valve prolapse.
SOURCE: Adapted from Refs. 34–62.

of cases of infective endocarditis: about 15 to 30 percent of subacute cases.[56-59] In the past, many such cases must have been wrongly attributed to chronic rheumatic disease of the mitral valve. Although MVP is common, infective endocarditis is rare; thus, the risk that any individual with MVP will develop infective endocarditis during his or her lifetime remains low (see also Chap. 80).[56,57]

Endocarditis in Parenteral Drug Abusers

Injected drug users are at high risk for infective endocarditis.[48-52] Bacteremias related to parenteral drug abuse are common, either from direct intravenous injection of bacteria or arising secondarily from local infections at injection sites (cellulitis, abscesses, or suppurative thrombophlebitis). Addicts seldom use sterile injection technique, sometimes even taking water from toilet bowls to dissolve their drugs. Nevertheless, the organisms that cause drug-related endocarditis are more often derived from the addict's skin and mucosal bacterial flora than from the drug itself or its solvent.[63] Strains of *Staph. aureus* cause more cases of endocarditis among parenteral drug abusers than any other species (about 50 percent of all cases), but infections with gram-negative bacilli, especially *Pseudomonas* species[64,65] (10 to 15 percent) or fungi[66,67] (5 percent) are notably more common than in nonaddicts (Table 94-3). *Candida parapsilosis* and other *Candida* species are the most common fungi causing drug-related endocarditis, but occasionally infections with a wide range of other fungal species have been recorded.[66,67] Polymicrobial and culture-negative cases of endocarditis occur occasionally in injected drug users but account for only about 5 percent of cases.[48,49,52]

The disease in addicts frequently follows an acute course,[5,48-52] reflecting the high frequency of *Staph. aureus* infection. This finding partly explains the overall modest increase in the proportion of acute to subacute cases that has been observed over the past 25 years.[37]

The incidence of right-sided valvular infection is much higher among parenteral drug abusers (especially those infected by *Staph. aureus*) than among any other group of patients with endocarditis. In various series of patients, the tricuspid valve has been involved in 40 to 70 percent, and the aortic and/or mitral valve in 30 to 48 percent.[48-52] Tricuspid vegetations commonly embolize to the lungs, causing multiple small radiological opacities due to septic pulmonary infarcts. This finding is highly characteristic in addicts with acute right-sided infection.[5,48-52] Nevertheless, it should be remembered that infection is limited to the left-sided valves in about half of addicts with endocarditis.[49,52] More than one valve on either side may be infected simultaneously. Pulmonary

TABLE 94-2

Estimates of the Relative Risk of Infective Endocarditis Posed by Various Cardiac Lesions

Relatively High Risk	Intermediate Risk	Very Low or Negligible Risk
Prosthetic heart valves	Mitral valve prolapse with regurgitation	Mitral valve prolapse without regurgitation
Previous infective endocarditis	Pure mitral stenosis	Atrial septal defects, secundum type
Aortic valve disease	Tricuspid valve disease	Arteriosclerotic plaques
Mitral regurgitation	Pulmonary valve disease	Coronary artery disease
Patent ductus arteriosus	Asymmetrical septal hypertrophy	Syphilitic aortitis
Ventricular septal defect	Calcific aortic sclerosis	Cardiac pacemakers
Coarctation of the aorta	Hyperalimentation or pressure-monitoring lines that reach the right atrium	Surgically corrected cardiac lesions (without prosthetic implants, more than 6 months after operation)
Marfan's syndrome	Nonvalvular intracardiac prosthetic implants	

SOURCE: Adapted from Refs. 34, 43, 53–62.

TABLE 94-3

Frequency of Various Organisms Causing Infective Endocarditis*

Organism	NVE, %	IV Drug Abusers, %	Early PVE, %	Late PVE, %
Streptococci	65	15	5	35
Viridans, alpha-hemolytic	35	5	<5	25
Strep. bovis (group D)	15	<5	<5	<5
Strep. faecalis (group D)	10	8	<5	<5
Other streptococci	<5	<5	<5	<5
Staphylococci	25	50	50	30
Coagulase-positive	23	50	20	10
Coagulase-negative	<5	<5	30	20
Gram-negative aerobic bacilli	<5	5	20	10
Fungi	<5	5	10	5
Miscellaneous bacteria	<5	5	5	5
Diphtheroids, propionibacteria	<1	<5	5	<5
Other anaerobes	<1	<1	<1	<1
Rickettsia	<1	<1	<1	<1
Chlamydia	<1	<1	<1	<1
Polymicrobial infection	<1	5	5	5
Culture-negative endocarditis	5–10	<5	<5	<5

* These are representative figures collated from the literature; wide local variations in frequency are to be expected. NVE = native valve endocarditis; PVE = prosthetic valve endocarditis.
SOURCE: Adapted from Refs. 34, 36, 43, 48–51, 66–71.

valve infection is unusual even among narcotic addicts, occurring in only some 2 percent of cases.

Endocarditis after Cardiac Surgery

Cardiac surgery has created a new population of patients at high risk for infective endocarditis. The number and variety of cases of postcardiotomy endocarditis have increased steadily since the 1950s, when surgeons first noted that *Staphylococcus epidermidis* endocarditis occurred fairly frequently after operations to split stenotic mitral valves.[72] It is probable that these organisms were sometimes inoculated directly onto the endocardium through minor rents in the surgeon's glove, made during palpation of rough, calcified valves. Subsequently, *Staph. epidermidis*, which rarely infects native valves, has become a common cause of both early and late PVE (Table 94-3).[8–10,73,74] Contamination of blood circulating through pump oxygenators with *Staph. epidermidis* or other organisms can initiate infection at the time of operation, resulting in early PVE.[75] In late PVE, the source of bacteremia causing infection is usually unknown but is presumed to be the normal flora of the skin or gastrointestinal tract in most cases.

Gram-negative bacilli and fungi infect prosthetic valves much more frequently than native valves, especially in early postoperative cases.[74] The spectrum of organisms causing late PVE more nearly resembles that of subacute native valve infection (Table 94-3).

The incidence of postcardiotomy endocarditis has decreased over the past 25 years due to improved techniques and possibly to the use of prophylactic antibiotics, although this is unproven. Figure 94-1 shows the curve for incidence of PVE per month after valve replacement. The peak time of onset is 3 to 6 weeks after operation; the patient's risk quickly falls to a much lower level thereafter.[10] This important curve emphasizes the fact that *Staph. epidermidis* and certain other organisms are often inoculated during or immediately after surgery, while streptococci infect the prosthesis during bacteremias that may occur at any time, unrelated to surgery. Review of the literature indicates that in recent years a rate of about 0.5 percent for early PVE is representative, although this varies quite widely among hospitals.[8–10,74] Clearly, an incidence of early PVE that is *persistently* 2 to 3 percent or higher is unacceptable and should lead to a review of surgical and infection-control techniques in that unit.

Reported experience with late PVE has gradually increased,[8–10,76] reflecting longer follow-up of patients who escape early PVE but remain at higher risk for infective endocarditis than are people with native valves each year

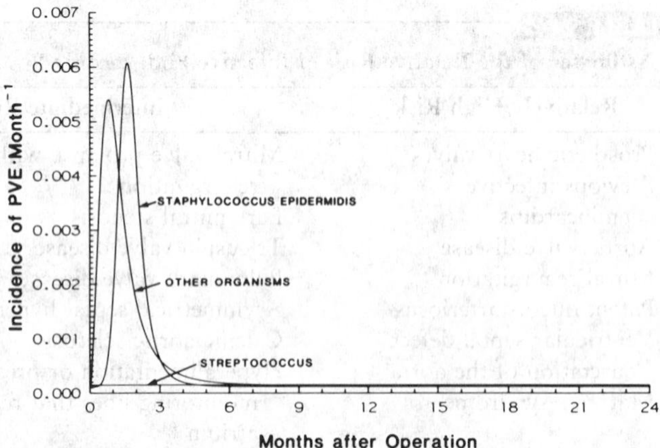

FIGURE 94-1 Incidence of prosthetic valve endocarditis (PVE) over 24 months after valve replacement. The hazard function has been stratified according to the infecting organisms. *(From TSA Ivert, WE Dismukes, CG Cobbs et al: Prosthetic valve endocarditis. Circulation 69:223, 1984. Reproduced with permission from the publisher and authors.)*

thereafter. Late PVE occurs at a rate of about 0.5 percent per year.[74,77] Aortic valve prostheses are two to four times more likely to be infected than are mitral prostheses (1 to 1.5 percent per year versus 0.4 percent).[9,62] It is interesting to note that these figures suggest that the annual risk for late infection of a mitral valve prosthesis may be no higher than that for chronic rheumatic disease affecting a native mitral valve.

Fortunately, coronary artery bypass surgery, which is one of the most common operations performed today in the United States, carries a negligible risk of infective endocarditis because the endocardium is not breached.

Endocarditis in Children

Infective endocarditis occurs at all ages but is relatively uncommon during childhood and rare during infancy.[45–47,78] Reviews of clinical experience indicate that endocardial infection in infants and very young children most often develops in association with obvious infection elsewhere. Thus, infective endocarditis should be considered as a rare complication of septicemia caused by staphylococci or group B streptococci, or of pneumonia, other respiratory tract infections, osteomyelitis, and severe burns.[45,46] Endocarditis in these settings is likely to be caused by invasive pathogens, therefore following an acute course. In older children, subacute disease without an obvious portal of entry for the organisms is more common. *Hemophilus influenzae* type b endocarditis is very rare, even though this organism is a common cause of bacteremia in children.

The leading underlying cardiac lesions are tetralogy of Fallot and other forms of cyanotic congenital heart disease, aortic stenosis, patent ductus arteriosus, ventricular septal defect, pulmonary stenosis, and coarctation of the aorta. Fifty percent or more of cases of endocarditis in children today follow palliative or corrective surgery for congenital cardiac defects.[54] Atrial septal defects of the ostium secundum type very rarely become infected. In developed countries, preexisting rheumatic heart disease is now much less common than congenital disease. No underlying cardiac disease is found in about 15 percent of children with endocarditis, but the proportion is higher in those less than 1 year of age (Table 94-1).

The diagnosis of infective endocarditis is more difficult in children, especially infants. Since the physician's attention is frequently focused on a serious primary bacteremic infection, endocarditis may be an unexpected finding at necropsy. The clinical manifestations of acute rheumatic fever may mimic endocarditis (and vice versa), but fortunately the two conditions rarely coexist. The choice of antibiotic treatment for children should be governed by the same principles as for adults, with appropriate dose adjustment for age. As in adults, valve replacement or other potentially curative surgical treatment[79,80] should not be delayed "until the infection is eradicated" if the child has heart failure that does not respond well to medical therapy.

Endocarditis in Gynecologic and Obstetric Patients

When endocarditis occurs as a complication of pregnancy, it is most likely to develop at the time of delivery, or in the puerperium.[81] Normal delivery presents a low risk of endocarditis, even in the presence of preexisting valvular disease,[82] but bacteremias associated with perinatal infective complications such as endometritis, parametritis, septic thrombophlebitis in pelvic veins, or urinary tract infection can seed the endocardium.[81] Septic abortion or pelvic infection related to intrauterine contraceptive devices can also provide the portal of entry for bacteremia resulting in endocarditis.[83] The organisms most often involved are *Enterococcus fecalis*, group B streptococci, *Staph. aureus*, and occasionally *Bacteroides* or gram-negative enteric bacilli.

Nosocomial Endocarditis

Hospital-acquired infective endocarditis has become more common.[53,84] The highest rate was reported by Pelletier and Petersdorf,[53] who found no fewer than 35 examples of probable nosocomial endocarditis among 125 cases (28 percent). This is not surprising, because intensive medical care can predispose to endocarditis in many ways. Iatrogenic endocardial damage can be produced by surgery, by intracardiac pressure-monitoring catheters, by ventriculoatrial shunts, and by hyperalimentation lines if they reach into the right atrium. Portals of entry for microorganisms are provided by wounds, biopsy sites, pacemakers, intravenous and arterial catheters, urinary catheters, and intratracheal airways. Nosocomial bacteremias arising from local infections are common in seriously ill patients; infected solutions are sometimes accidentally infused intravenously.

Many of the abovementioned factors coexist in severely burned patients. Ehrie and his colleagues[85] found either NBTE or infective endocarditis at autopsy in all of six burned patients who sustained repeated episodes of bacteremia while a pressure-monitoring catheter was maintained in the right side of the heart. This important observation has been confirmed in another necropsy study of patients with flow-directed pulmonary artery catheters.[86] Of 55 patients, 29 had one or more right-sided endocardial lesions, including 13 with thrombi and 4 with infective endocarditis.[86] On the other hand, catheterization of the right side of the heart for brief periods in patients without bacteremia, as in a coronary care unit, presents a very low risk of causing infective endocarditis.

Infective endocarditis is rare in patients with leukemia but has been observed in other immunocompromised patients, for example, after bone marrow transplantation,[87] and heart transplantation.[88]

The leading organisms causing nosocomial endocarditis are staphylococci, *Candida* species, and gram-negative bacilli. *Staph. aureus* is especially associated with wound infections, cellulitis, and cannula infections; *Staph. epidermidis* with ventriculoatrial shunts; and *Candida albicans* with parenteral alimentation.

Nosocomial endocarditis can involve native or prosthetic valves. The prognosis for nosocomial native valve endocarditis is worse than for other forms of native valve infection. These patients usually have serious underlying diseases that may delay diagnosis of endocarditis by obscuring the symptoms and signs, while the organisms most commonly involved are more difficult to eradicate than streptococci.

Hemodialysis and Endocarditis

Creation of an arteriovenous shunt for hemodialysis may predispose patients to infective endocarditis in two ways: by providing a ready portal of entry for bacteremia and by increasing cardiac output. Lillehei[89] showed that dogs with high cardiac output due to surgically created arteriovenous fistulas were predisposed to develop not only infective *endarteritis* at the site of the shunt but *endocarditis* as well. Therefore, it is not surprising that endocarditis has been reported in 2 to 6 percent of patients on long-term hemodialysis via either arteriovenous fistulas or cannulas. In a review of 35 cases, *Staph. aureus* was the most common etiologic organism, followed by viridans streptococci and *E. fecalis*[90] The diagnosis of endocarditis was difficult to make in this group of patients, partly because coexisting intravascular infection at the shunt site often confused the clinical picture. Mortality was high (53 percent). Early recognition and aggressive treatment of both shunt infections and endocarditis in dialysis patients are necessary to improve this rate.[90]

Infective Endarteritis

Intravascular infection outside the heart itself can mimic most of the clinical manifestations of endocarditis, including vascular and immunologic phenomena.[71] In the past, about one-quarter of all patients with an uncorrected patent ductus arteriosus developed bacterial endarteritis.[3] Infections located at coarctations of the aorta, while well known, were less frequent; endocarditis of an associated bicuspid aortic valve was three times more common than endarteritis with vegetations located in the coarctation. Endarteritis occasionally complicates traumatic arteriovenous fistulas, but arteriosclerotic aneurysms rarely become infected.[71] When bacterial endarteritis does occur within an aneurysm, the organisms usually grow in a multilayered thrombus in the lumen of the aneurysm rather than in vegetations.

The spectrum of organisms causing infective endarteritis is similar to that found in endocarditis except for a higher frequency of gram-negative bacillary infection (especially salmonellae) in arteriosclerotic aneurysms.[71] The pattern of embolization observed differs according to the site of infection; thus, petechiae may occur on the skin of the lower extremities in a patient with an infected abdominal aneurysm, and infarctions in the lungs of a patient with an infected dialysis fistula in the forearm.

Because many of the congenital and acquired vascular lesions that predispose to endarteritis can be corrected by modern surgery, endarteritis is uncommon today in developed countries, except in arteriovenous shunts constructed for hemodialysis (see "Nosocomial Endocarditis").

THE ETIOLOGIC ORGANISMS

The range of microbial species that can cause infective endocarditis is extraordinarily wide, yet only a few species account for the great majority of infections. On native valves, streptococci and staphylococci together cause more than 80 percent of infections.[34,43,53] Native valve infections caused by *Staph. epidermidis*, enteric bacilli, and fungi are uncommon. Among intravenous drug abusers and patients with prosthetic valves, however, the incidence of infection due to these organisms is higher. Table 94-3 offers representative figures culled from the literature on the relative frequency of the major etiologic organisms on native valves, in drug addicts, and on prosthetic valves. It should be emphasized that the relative frequency with which various organisms cause endocarditis can vary widely among medical centers.

Streptococci cause more cases of endocarditis than any other group of organisms.[43,53,54,91] Alpha-hemolytic or viridans streptococci account for the majority of these cases. The viridans streptococci are ubiquitous (although outnumbered by anaerobes) in the oropharyngeal and gastrointestinal flora. They are low-grade pathogens, often recovered from clinical specimens in mixed culture with other organisms but seldom themselves causing disease. Their strong association with SBE is therefore determined by the frequency with which they enter the bloodstream and by their ability to adhere to endocardium, rather than by their virulence. In order of frequency, the following species cause SBE most often: *Strep. sanguis, Strep. mutans, Strep. intermedius*, and *Strep. mitis*.[91–94] A few cases are caused by nutritionally dependent strains that require media supplemented with L-cysteine or pyridoxine for growth.[95–97] These strains are harder to isolate from blood[98] and seem to be harder to eradicate with antibiotic treatment than the other viridans streptococci.

Group D streptococci are next in frequency among the streptococci as the cause of endocarditis.[99–101] The nonenterococcal group D species, *Strep. bovis*, accounts for about one-fifth of streptococcal cases. Gastrointestinal lesions, especially colonic polyps and cancers, are commonly present in patients who develop *Strep. bovis* bacteremia and/or endocarditis[102–104] Hence, recovery of this species from blood cultures should prompt an early investigation for colonic disease, whether or not the patient has gastrointestinal symptoms.

Strains of *E. fecalis* (enterococci) cause about 10 percent of streptococcal cases. It is said that this species causes endocarditis "in young women and old men," because it is found in association with infections of the genital and urinary tract in women of childbearing age and of the urinary tract in older men with prostatic enlargement.[100,102] Enterococci commonly cause urinary tract, wound, and intravenous line infections, which often give rise to nosocomial bacteremias.[105,106] Fewer than 5 percent of such patients have endocarditis, but if enterococcal bacteremia is community-acquired, one-third will have infective endocarditis.[105]

Strep. pneumoniae endocarditis has become rather uncommon since the advent of antibiotics. This species causes acute endocarditis.[107,108] In debilitated alcoholics, coexisting pneumococcal pneumonia and pneumococcal meningitis may be present. This triad, known as Austrian's syndrome, carries an extremely poor prognosis.[107,108]

Many other species and strains of streptococci occasionally cause endocarditis, but they are rare compared with the viridans and group D organisms.

Staph. aureus is the leading cause of acute bacterial endocarditis. It is the predominant etiologic organism in intravenous drug users with endocarditis[39–42] and frequently causes PVE.[58] Because it is an invasive primary pathogen, patients with staphylococcal ABE often develop disseminated disease with metastatic infections in skin, bone, joints, eye, or brain.[109–111]

Only a minority of all patients with *Staph. aureus* bacteremia have endocarditis, and it is often difficult to identify this subgroup. Factors that increase the probability that such a patient has endocarditis are (1) community-acquired bacteremia, (2) absence of a primary focus of infection, and (3) presence of metastatic foci of staphylococcal infection. Up to two-thirds of patients with all three of these characteristics have endocarditis.[111]

Staph. epidermidis is a rare cause of native valve infection, usually associated with an indolent subacute or chronic course.[69] In striking contrast, it is a common cause of PVE, which may follow either an acute or subacute clinical course.[69,112]

Although most of the species of gram-negative bacilli that colonize and/or infect humans have been reported to cause endocarditis in at least a few cases, they account for a very small proportion of cases of native valve endocarditis. For example, cases of endocarditis caused by *Escherichia coli* and *Klebsiella* are rare,[65] even though these two species are by far the most frequent cause of gram-negative bacteremias. The reasons for this striking disparity are probably multiple, including low adhesiveness of gram-negative enteric bacilli to heart valves[114,115] and fibrin,[116] and susceptibility to complement-mediated bacteriolysis.[117] Despite these factors, two special populations are at increased risk of gram-negative endocarditis: injected drug users and patients with prosthetic valves. Gram-negative bacilli account for 13 to 20 percent of endocarditis in intravenous drug abusers.[48–52] *Pseudomonas* species, *Serratia*, and *Enterobacter* species predominate. Gram-negative bacilli cause about 20 percent of early PVE and about 10 percent of late PVE.[73–74]

Interesting but unusual cases caused by species of *Salmonella, Brucella, Acinetobacter,* and other gram-negative bacilli have been reviewed by Cohen et al.[65] *Brucella* endocarditis is well-known in the Mediterranean basin[118] but rare in most other regions. Endocarditis caused by anaerobic bacteria is rare (1 percent or less of cases),[70] perhaps because the oxygen tension in heart blood is too high to favor growth of these species on the endocardium.

Among the less common forms of infective endocarditis, a significant number of cases are caused by the HACEK group of organisms (*Hemophilus, Actinobacillus, Cardiobacterium, Eikenella,* and *Kingella*).[119–121] Cases caused by *Hemophilus* predominate in this group. Endocarditis caused by this genus is usually due to *Hemophilus aphrophilus, Hemophilus paraphrophilus,* or *Hemophilus parainfluenzae*[119–121] and very rarely to *Hemophilus influenzae*, even though *Hemophilus influenzae* is more virulent and more frequently found in the blood than the other species.

Neisseria gonorrhoeae causes an acute form of the disease,[2] often involving the right side of the heart. Like the pneumococcus, *N. gonorrhoeae* has become uncommon as a cause of endocarditis since the introduction of penicillin.[7,43,119]

Although many species of fungi can infect the endocardium, only two genera account for the great majority: *Candida* and *Aspergillus*.[66,122,123] *Candida* causes native valve infections in injected drug users and in patients receiving parenteral alimentation, while *Aspergillus* species often involve prosthetic valves. Fungal infection of native valves in nonaddicts is rare (Table 94-3).

Culture-Negative Endocarditis

Culture-negative endocarditis is the term used when a patient has infective endocarditis but the results of *blood* cultures are persistently negative.[124–126] In these cases, a working diagnosis based on clinical manifestations can sometimes be confirmed by the progress of the disease and response to empirical treatment. If blood culture results remain negative, an etiologic diagnosis can be made only by detecting organisms in an infected embolus or in vegetations excised during surgery or at necropsy.

The reported incidence of culture-negative endocarditis varies widely. Among large unselected series of cases collected from several hospitals, 15 to 20 percent of cases may be culture-negative.[43,124–126] Smaller series of patients studied by a single clinical and laboratory team that is highly experienced in evaluation of endocarditis usually show only 5 percent or fewer culture-negative cases.[84] This low figure carries an important clinical implication: *diagnoses other than endocarditis should be meticulously excluded before a diagnosis of culture-negative endocarditis is accepted.*

Negative blood culture results should be expected from about one-third of patients with *Candida* NVE or PVE[66] and from most patients with *Aspergillus* endocarditis.[123] The incidence of negative blood culture results is slightly higher in SBE of long duration. Recent antibiotic therapy may transiently render blood culture results negative without achieving cure, but in most cases organisms will reappear in the blood within a few days of discontinuing antibiotics. The blood of a few patients with active bacterial endocarditis remains persistently culture-negative after receiving a short course of antibiotics.[53]

Rare causes of infective endocarditis with negative blood culture results include mycobacteria,[127] *Coxiella burnetti* (Q fever),[128–132] and chlamydia.[133,134] Q fever endocarditis is a chronic, febrile systemic illness with prominent hepatic as well as cardiac valvular involvement.[128–132] Chlamydial endocarditis is even more rare; a few cases have been reported in bird fanciers.[133,134] In such cases, the etiologic diagnosis can be established only by specialized culture techniques, serologic studies, or examination of vegetations using immunofluorescent antibodies.

Many unusual species occasionally infect prosthetic valves, including *Mycoplasma hominis*[135] and *Legionella* species.[136]

The Influence of Antibiotics

Although the advent of antibiotics revolutionized treatment of endocarditis, the overall incidence of the disease has neither fallen nor risen strikingly during the antibiotic era. It is true that the availability of rapidly effective treatments for pneumococcal pneumonia and gonorrhea has probably been responsible for the striking decrease in the incidence of endocarditis caused by *Strep. pneumoniae* and *N. gonorrhoeae* since 1944 and that the incidence of endocarditis caused by miscellaneous unusual antibiotic-resistant organisms has increased slightly during the antibiotic era.[7,36,43,44,135,136] Apart from these special cases, the widespread use of antimicrobial agents seems to have exerted considerably less influence than have alterations in the populations at risk (described above) on the changing epidemiology of endocarditis.[37] Prophylactic use of antibiotics before medical procedures that cause bacteremia has not reduced the incidence of endocarditis significantly; this is not surprising because only a small proportion of all cases can be attributed to such procedures.[38,137]

PATHOGENESIS AND PATHOLOGY

A general concept of the pathogenesis of NBTE and SBE is presented in Fig. 94-2.

Noninfective Endocarditis

Sterile thrombotic lesions (NBTE) may develop on heart valves in a wide variety of clinical conditions.[138] Small aggregates of platelets have been found occasionally on normal valves, but they occur frequently on the surfaces of valves damaged by congenital or rheumatic disease[139] or by infective endocarditis. Marantic endocarditis occurs most often in patients with advanced malignancy[11-13] but may also complicate other chronic wasting diseases, such as tuberculosis, or uremia. The initiating factor in the pathogenesis of NBTE is not known. Endothelial damage caused by circulating cytokines such as tumor necrosis factor or interleukin-1, which can be increased in patients with malignancy or chronic wasting disease, might trigger platelet deposition.

Sterile vegetations (termed *Libman-Sacks endocarditis*, (see Chap. 103) sometimes develop in patients with systemic lupus erythematosus. Typically, Libman-Sacks vegetations are small, sessile masses located on the ventricular surfaces of the mitral valve leaflets.

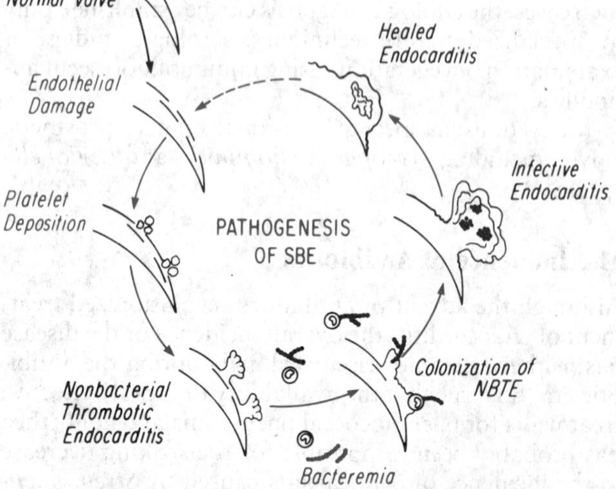

FIGURE 94-2 The main events in the pathogenesis of nonbacterial thrombotic endocarditis (NBTE) and subacute bacterial endocarditis (SBE).

The common factor leading to platelet deposition is endothelial damage. This exposes subendothelial connective tissue containing collagen fibers, which in turn causes platelets to aggregate at the site. These microscopic platelet thrombi may embolize away harmlessly, or they may be stabilized by fibrin to form larger vegetations of NBTE. This process can be duplicated experimentally by passing a catheter into the heart of an animal; NBTE forms at sites of endothelial damage.[140] In humans, intracardiac pressure-monitoring catheters produce identical lesions.[85,87] Both experimental[141] and human[86,138] NBTE can be colonized by circulating bacteria, resulting in infective endocarditis.

The vegetations of NBTE are friable white or tan masses, usually situated along the lines of valve closure. These masses vary greatly in size, being sometimes microscopic but frequently rather large and exuberant, with a corresponding tendency to cause extensive infarctions when they break off and are carried to arteries supplying the myocardium, spleen, kidney, brain, mesentery, or extremities. Since there is little inflammatory reaction at the site of attachment, fresh vegetations often can be picked off easily with forceps, leaving a valve surface that may look normal to the naked eye.[138] It is not surprising that such easily dislodged vegetations embolize frequently (Plate IX, 94-1).

Histologically, the vegetations of NBTE consist of degenerating platelets interwoven with strands of fibrin forming a bland, eosinophilic mass, featureless except for a few trapped leukocytes.[138,140]

Infective Endocarditis

The essential event leading to the development of infective endocarditis is the attachment of microorganisms circulating in the bloodstream to an endocardial surface. If the microbes persist and multiply there, infective endocarditis results. In the case of SBE, which usually develops on previously abnormal valves, the circulating bacteria probably colonize preexisting NBTE.[138] It is not known whether ABE, which often affects apparently normal valves, develops in a like manner by colonization of microscopic sterile vegetations or by direct invasion of normal endothelium.

Once lodged on NBTE, bacteria multiply rapidly, soon reaching high numbers and then entering a resting phase.[141] The vegetation provides an ideal supporting stroma for the growth of microbial colonies, into which essential nutrients can diffuse from the blood. The presence of bacteria is a powerful stimulus for further thrombosis, possibly mediated by thromboplastin generated by leukocytes when they are exposed to fibrin.[142] New layers of fibrin are deposited around growing bacteria, causing the vegetations to enlarge.[140]

Knowledge of the usual location of vegetations is important to both the understanding and the management of endocarditis. Approximate figures for the incidence with which vegetations are found at various sites are given in Table 94-3.

The frequency of involvement of each valve is directly proportional to the mean blood pressure upon it[143]; thus, the left side of the heart is involved much more often

TABLE 94-4

Approximate Frequency of Anatomic Location of Vegetations in SBE, ABE, and Endocarditis Associated with IV Drug Abuse

Location	SBE, %	ABE, %	Endocarditis in IV Drug Abusers, %
Left-sided valves	85	65	40
Aortic	15–26	18–25	25–30
Mitral	38–45	30–35	15–20
Aortic and mitral	23–30	15–20	13–20
Right-sided valves	5	20	50
Tricuspid	1–5	15	45–55
Pulmonary	1	Rare	2
Tricuspid and pulmonary	Rare	Rare	3
Left- and right-sided sites	Rare	5–10	5–10
Other sites (patent ductus, ventricular septal defect, coarctation, jet lesions)	10	5	5

SOURCE: Adapted from Refs. 43, 46–54, 109, 143.

than the right. This rule is reliable for SBE but does not hold true for acute endocarditis in injected drug users. In that group, tricuspid infection predominates due to invasion of the valve by primary pathogens, especially *Staph. aureus* (Table 94-4).

Vegetations are usually located on the downstream side of anatomic abnormalities in the heart or great vessels. This observation is explained by the work of Rodbard, who developed the unifying concept that endocarditis usually occurs where blood flows from a high-pressure source (e.g., the left ventricle) through a narrow orifice (e.g., a stenotic aortic valve) into a low-pressure sink (e.g., the aorta).[144] Illustrative examples from human disease include aortic stenosis, ventricular septal defect, coarctation, and mitral regurgitation. Experimentally, Rodbard showed that bacteria carried in an aerosol flowing through a constricted tube into an area of low pressure were deposited on the walls of the tube immediately beyond the constriction due to Venturi pressure effects and turbulence.[144] These observations fit well with the actual location of vegetations found at necropsy in cases of endocarditis (Fig. 94-3). Vegetations also may develop on *jet lesions*, which are areas of endothelial roughening and reactive fibrosis at sites where a swift, turbulent regurgitant stream of blood strikes the endothelium.[145] MacCallum's patch on the wall of the left atrium in some patients with mitral regurgitation is an example of a jet lesion; an infected vegetation occasionally develops at this site (Fig. 94-3).

The vegetations of infective endocarditis vary greatly in morphology, from small, warty nodules to large, cauliflower-like polypoid masses (Plate IX, 94-2). Vegetations vary in size from less than a millimeter to several centimeters, large enough to cause functional stenosis of valve orifices. The average diameter of vegetations found on the tricuspid valve is greater than on left-sided valves. Fungal vegetations often are larger than bacterial ones, but otherwise the etiologic species does not correlate reliably with vegetation size. Their color also varies widely, from white to tan to greenish-gray.[52,146,147] Histologically, colonies of microorganisms are found embedded in a fibrin-platelet matrix.[140,141,147] Although the inflammatory reaction at the site of attachment may be extensive, even progressing to form a frank abscess, the vegetations themselves characteristically contain relatively few leukocytes. Those few phagocytes present are

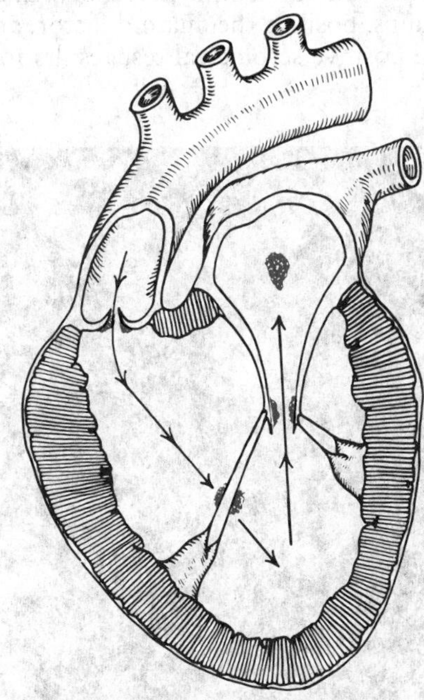

FIGURE 94-3 The sites where endocarditis occurs in aortic and mitral regurgitation. The arrows on the left indicate a high-velocity regurgitant stream passing through the orifice of an incompetent aortic valve into a low-pressure sink (left ventricle in diastole). Vegetations appear on the ventricular surface of the aortic valve. The regurgitant stream may cause a jet lesion on the chordae tendineae of the anterior leaflet of the mitral valve. The arrow on the right shows regurgitation from the high-pressure source of the left ventricle during systole into the left atrium, with vegetations developing on the atrial surface of the mitral valve. Vegetations also can occur on the jet lesion where the regurgitant stream through the mitral valve strikes the atrial endocardium, an area known as MacCallum's patch. *(From S Rodbard: Blood velocity and endocarditis. Circulation 27:8, 1963. Reproduced with permission from the publisher and author.)*

prevented from reaching bacteria by layers of fibrin, which form protective barriers around colonies (Fig. 94-4).

Formation of an abscess is one of the most important complications of valvular infection.[146,147] Abscesses often develop by direct extension of active infection into the fibrous cardiac skeleton, that is, the ring of supporting connective tissue around the valves. From there, abscesses can extend further into the adjacent myocardium. Hematogenous spread occasionally leads to development of abscesses elsewhere in the myocardium.

Abscesses develop more often during the course of ABE because this form of endocarditis is caused by primary pathogens that are adapted to invade tissues. They are less common in SBE, unless a valvular prosthesis is present. Abscesses are found in the majority of patients who die with active prosthetic valve infection, often spreading around the sewing ring of the prosthesis and causing partial dehiscence of the prosthetic valve.[147] Because these valve ring abscesses are located close to the conduction system, conduction disturbances are common clinical manifestations.

The Role of Immunity in Endocarditis

Presence of bacteria in endocardial vegetations stimulates the humoral immune system to produce nonspecific antibodies. This can result in a polyclonal increase in gamma globulins, positive rheumatoid factor, and occasionally, false-positive serological test results for syphilis.[148] Rheumatoid factor develops in about half of patients with SBE and can provide a useful diagnostic clue in culture-negative cases; it reverts to negative after eradication of the organisms.[149-151] Antiendocardial and antisarcolemmal antibodies have been detected in 60 to 100 percent of cases[152]; they are more commonly found in SBE than in ABE.

Specific antibodies to many of the commensal organisms that cause SBE may be present in low titer before infection. Titers rise during active infection[3] and fall after treatment. Obviously, specific antibody prevents neither infection nor reinfection of the endocardium because reinfections with the same species have been reported. It has been claimed that preexisting humoral immunity actually *predisposes* to endocarditis[3,153] and that a "high titer of agglutinating antibody for the infecting organism" is a prime factor in pathogenesis.[153] However, this hypothesis is based only upon theoretical considerations and uncontrolled observations in animals.[154,155] It is unlikely that high titers of agglutinating antibody could exist for all the myriad organisms that may cause endocarditis, while controlled animal experiments suggest that high titers of specific antistreptococcal antibodies actually protect against streptococcal endocarditis.[156] Thus, the reality of the humoral response to endocardial infection is undisputed, but the evidence that preexisting antibody promotes development of endocarditis remains unconvincing.[157]

Hemolytic complement levels are low in about 30 percent of patients early in the course of endocarditis, rising later and returning to normal after treatment.[158,159]

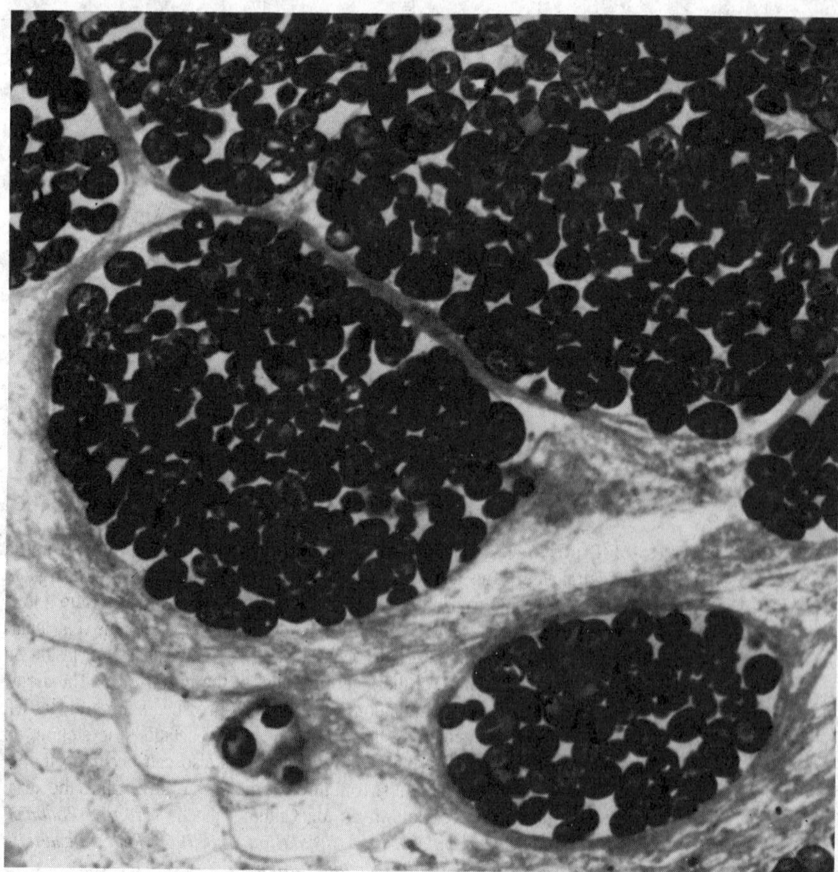

FIGURE 94-4 Electron micrograph of a vegetation of experimental streptococcal endocarditis (×7800). Note the very large number of cocci, the protective layers of fibrin, and the absence of leukocytes—all factors that influence the results of therapy. *(From DT Durack: Experimental bacterial endocarditis: 4. Structure and evolution of very early lesions. J Pathol 115:81, 1975. Reproduced with permission from the publisher and author.)*

The lowest levels are found in patients with immune-complex glomerulonephritis.

Circulating immune complexes have been detected in 82 to 97 percent of patients with either ABE or SBE.[158-161] Higher concentrations correlated with the presence of extracardiac manifestations such as arthritis, splenomegaly, and glomerulonephritis; with longer duration of illness; and with hypocomplementemia. Several studies confirm that glomerulonephritis in patients with endocarditis is mediated by immune complexes.[162-164] It seems likely that arthritis and tenosynovitis—and possibly pericarditis, Osler's nodes, and Roth spots[158,160,161]—also may represent inflammatory responses involving immune complexes, but this has not been proved.

Antibodies to teichoic acids were found in the serum of 14 of 15 patients with *Staph. aureus* endocarditis.[165] Because these antibodies were seldom found in patients who did not have staphylococcal endocarditis, their detection may occasionally be useful in the diagnosis of uncertain cases.[165,166] This test is unnecessary in the diagnosis and management of most cases of endocarditis.

Healed Endocarditis

Even in active, untreated endocarditis, evidence of healing can be found.[147,157] Histiocytes slowly advance into the base of vegetations, while endothelium begins to cover the surface from the periphery. This attempt at healing fails in untreated cases but progresses to completion during and after successful treatment. Macrophages ingest bacterial debris and fibrin, while fibroblasts organize the lesions by laying down collagen fibers. Endocardium gradually covers the surface of the shrinking vegetations. Calcium is often deposited at the site of old bacterial colonies. Dead, but still recognizable, gram-positive cocci can sometimes be found in sections of valves resected at operation or necropsy, months after infection has been eradicated by antibiotic treatment. The healed valve is often scarred and thickened by new collagen; it may be perforated or ruptured, and the supporting structures may be damaged. Therefore, residual functional valvular abnormalities, varying from insignificant to severe, are common. Valvular function often continues to deteriorate at an unpredictable rate after infection is eradicated, due to mechanical stresses. Whether or not adequate hemodynamic function is preserved, the scarred valve surface remains susceptible to reinfection.

Experimental Endocarditis

Because the primary cardiac lesions are inaccessible to direct study in living patients, investigators long ago turned to animal models.[157,167] Bacterial infections of the endocardium in laboratory animals were successfully produced as early as the 1880s. Subsequent studies have contributed significantly to our understanding of the disease; for example, the crucial importance of endothelial damage in pathogenesis was established in animals before 1890, at a time when human investigations were limited to clinical case studies.[157]

Later studies in animals demonstrated that arteriovenous fistulas and other high-output states predispose to endocarditis,[89] confirmed the hypothesis (derived from human necropsy observations) that the lesion of NBTE is a receptive nidus upon which circulating bacteria readily lodge,[141] and permitted study of the earliest stages of vegetative growth.[140] Experiments showing that most bacteria in vegetations are in a metabolically inactive, resting phase helped to explain why antibiotic treatment must be continued longer than for other infections to cure endocarditis. Other experiments demonstrated the reduced propensity of gram-negative bacilli and anaerobes to colonize vegetations when compared with gram-positive cocci, the role of complement in protecting against *E. coli* endocarditis,[117] and the protective effect of humoral immunity against oral streptococci.[156] The immune response to endocardial infection, including demonstration of immune complexes in serum, healing, the effect of anticoagulants, and the comparative efficacy of preventive and therapeutic antibiotics all have been examined in animals with endocarditis.[147,157,168]

For obvious reasons, most of these studies could not have been performed in human beings. Thus, an appreciation of the contribution of experimental studies is essential for a full understanding of this protean disease.

CLINICAL MANIFESTATIONS

The clinical and laboratory manifestations of infective endocarditis can be conveniently grouped under three headings (Table 94-5):

- Evidence of a systemic infection
- Evidence of an intravascular lesion
- Evidence of an immunologic reaction to infection

History

The symptoms of subacute endocarditis develop insidiously and with great variability.[3,34,43,53,169] Fevers, chills, rigors, and night sweats provide evidence of systemic infection. General malaise with anorexia, fatigue, and weakness is typical. The patient often loses weight. Headaches and musculoskeletal complaints, including myalgias, arthralgias, and back pains, are common.[171] This symptom complex is often described by the patient or physician as a "flu-like illness."

Evidence of an intravascular lesion is provided by symptoms of left- or right-sided heart failure and by manifestations of embolization, such as focal neurological injury, chest pain, flank pain, left upper quadrant pain, hematuria, or ischemia of an extremity. Symptoms usually persist and worsen intermittently over 4 to 8 weeks before the diagnosis is made.[172]

In the acute form of infective endocarditis, the symptoms are both accelerated and accentuated in severity. Patients experience hectic fevers, rigors, and prostration, usually leading to admission to hospital within a few days.[5,109,110]

Symptoms of cardiac failure may develop or worsen suddenly in either acute or subacute disease, due to mechanical complications such as perforation of a valve leaflet, rupture of one of the chordae tendineae, or development of functional stenosis from obstruction of blood

TABLE 94-5

Summary of the Major Clinical Manifestations of Infective Endocarditis

Manifestation	History	Examination	Investigations
Systemic infection	Fever, chills, rigors, sweats, malaise, weakness, lethargy, delirium, headache, anorexia, weight loss, backache, arthralgia, myalgia Portal of entry: oropharynx, skin, urinary tract, drug addiction, nosocomial bacteremia	Fever, pallor, weight loss, asthenia, splenomegaly	Anemia, leukocytosis (variable), raised erythrocyte sedimentation rate, blood culture, results positive, abnormal cerebrospinal fluid
Intravascular lesion	Dyspnea, chest pain, focal weakness, stroke, abdominal pain, cold and painful extremities	Murmurs, signs of cardiac failure, petechiae (skin, eye, mucosae), Roth's spots, Osler's nodes, Janeway lesions, splinter hemorrhages, stroke, mycotic aneurysm, ischemia or infarction of viscera or extremities	Blood in urine, chest roentgenogram, echocardiography, arteriography, liver-spleen scan, lung scan, brain scan, CT scan, histology, culture of emboli
Immunologic reactions	Arthralgia, myalgia, tenosynovitis	Arthritis, signs of uremia, vascular phenomena, finger clubbing	Proteinuria, hematuria, casts, uremia, acidosis, polyclonal increases in gamma globulins, rheumatoid factor, decreased complement, immune complexes in serum, antistaphylococcal teichoic acid antibodies

SOURCE: Adapted from Refs. 34, 43, 53, 169.

flow by large vegetations.[173,174] Alternatively, heart failure may develop insidiously, or preexisting chronic heart failure may worsen due to progressive damage to the valves or associated structures. Myocarditis or myocardial infarction due to coronary artery embolism may contribute to heart failure.

Physical Examination

General Appearance

Patients with endocarditis may appear acutely or chronically ill. Evidence of systemic infection is provided by chills, rigors, and sweating. Asthenia and recent weight loss often are notable. Mild or severe anemia is common in all forms of endocarditis; thus, many patients are pallid. The skin of some patients with long-standing SBE will exhibit the sallow hue of uremia.[3]

Vascular Phenomena

Patients with endocarditis may exhibit a variety of striking physical findings arising from vascular abnormalities. Such phenomena are diagnostically useful, even though all have been found at times in conditions other than endocarditis.

Petechiae In both SBE and ABE petechiae are common; they are rare in NBTE. In a few cases, the petechiae have a pale central spot. Most are due to microembolization to small vessels in the skin or mucous membranes. Capillary fragility, evidence by positive tourniquet test results, accounts for the petechiae in some cases, while patients with ABE caused by a virulent bacterial pathogen may develop petechiae due to disseminated intravascular coagulation.

Splinter Hemorrhages Linear subungual hemorrhages, resembling tiny splinters of wood under the nail but not reaching the nail margin, are found in about 20 percent of patients with SBE. Because splinter hemorrhages are found in some 5 to 8 percent of patients admitted to hospital who do not have endocarditis, they are of limited diagnostic value.[175] They are probably caused by microembolization to linear capillaries under the nail.

Osler's Nodes

Osler's nodes occur in 10 to 20 percent of patients with SBE and in fewer than 10 percent of patients with ABE.[176] They are painful, tender erythematous nodules in the skin of the extremities, usually in the pulp of the fingers (Fig. 10-12; Plate V, 10-6). Occasionally, the center of these pea-sized, red lesions is pale, but necrosis does not occur. They are probably caused by inflammation around the site of lodgment of small, infected emboli in distal arterioles, because the etiologic organism can be recovered from the lesions, at least in acute cases.[177] Possibly some of these lesions are caused by inflammation at the site of an immunologic reaction, especially in subacute cases.[161]

Janeway Lesions

Janeway lesions are small (less than 5 mm), flat, nontender red spots, irregular in outline, found on the palms and soles of a few patients with SBE and ABE. Unlike petechiae, they are not hemorrhagic, and blanch on pressure.[3,35]

Eye Lesions

Conjunctival petechiae show up as small, bright-red hemorrhages that are easily seen if the upper and lower eyelids are everted. These petechiae are not specific for endocarditis, being found after cardiac surgery and occasionally in septicemia (Plate IX, 94-3). Nevertheless, the discovery of conjunctival hemorrhages in a patient with unexplained fever and heart murmur makes the diagnosis of endocarditis highly likely.

Retinal hemorrhages are found in 10 to 25 percent of cases of both SBE and ABE. They are quite variable in appearance. Some simply represent petechiae in the retina; their round or flame-shaped outline is determined by the layer of the retina in which they develop. Those with a white or yellow center surrounded by a bright-red, irregular halo are known as Roth spots (Plate VI, 12-4). They probably represent cytoid bodies and associated hemorrhage caused by microinfarction of retinal vessels.

Loss of vision during the course of endocarditis can occur from embolization to the brain or to the retinal artery, from optic neuritis, or from ophthalmitis. *Endophthalmitis* may occur in patients with *Candida* endocarditis and fungemia. The typical retinal lesions are rounded, white, cotton-like exudates with extension into the vitreous and overlying vitreous haze.[178] *Panophthalmitis* occurs in some patients with ABE due to hematogenous spread of virulent pathogens. This phenomenon occurs most often in injected drug users infected with *Staph. aureus*, *Pseudomonas*, or fungi.

Clubbing of the Fingers

Previously common in SBE, finger clubbing is now found in less than 10 percent of cases (Plate V, 10-5). The pathogenesis of this reaction, which usually resolves after eradication of the infecting organism, is not understood.

Embolization

Decreased or absent arterial pulses in an extremity may signal occlusion of a large artery by a fragment of vegetation. Focal neurological signs may develop transiently or progress to a completed stroke due to embolization of a cerebral artery (see "Complications"). Infarctions of the spleen, kidney, or bowel can present with pain and tenderness on palpation of the abdomen, mimicking an acute abdominal event such as bowel obstruction or peritonitis. Myocardial infarction due to obstruction of a coronary artery can cause heart failure or death and is sometimes an unexpected finding at necropsy in patients who die with active disease. These complications are illustrated in Plate IX, 94-4 through 94-9.

Splenomegaly

Development of moderate splenomegaly is common, occurring in about one-third of patients with ABE and one-half of those with SBE. The spleen is usually soft and only slightly tender except in the case of recent embolic infarction, when palpation may be very painful. Radionuclide scanning may reveal infarction or, occasionally, a splenic abscess.

Cardiac Examination

The pulse is often rapid as a result of fever or congestive failure. Irregularities of rhythm may indicate the presence of an abscess near the conducting system. Underlying or newly developed aortic regurgitation associated with infective endocarditis may result in a collapsing pulse (Chaps. 10 and 79). Peripheral arteries should be palpated for evidence of occlusion by emboli or for the pulsatile swelling of a mycotic aneurysm.

One or more *murmurs* are present in virtually all patients at some stage of the disease. Even though some of the classic findings of infective endocarditis are less often seen today than formerly, the classic triad of *fever, anemia, and murmur* should still suggest this disease, provided that one remembers that these manifestations are nonspecific. They may be absent initially. Up to 15 percent of patients do not have a murmur when first seen. These patients are more likely to be individuals with right-sided or acute endocarditis than patients with left-sided SBE.

Murmurs present during the course of endocarditis may be due to preexisting cardiac disease, to the infection itself, or to both. Active endocarditis often causes structural damage to the valve, including deformities, tears, perforations, and rupture of chordae tendineae. Since these changes often lead to valvular insufficiency, the murmurs most often heard in association with endocarditis are those of mitral, aortic, or tricuspid regurgitation. Pure mitral stenosis is complicated by SBE much less often than mitral incompetence with or without associated stenosis (see also Chap. 80). Development of a new aortic regurgitation murmur during a febrile illness strongly suggests the diagnosis of endocarditis, because this finding is seldom associated nonspecifically with increased blood flow due to fever and anemia.

"Changing murmurs" are not a common finding in SBE, despite a persistent misconception to the contrary. This error is partly based upon misreading of Osler's words in which he pointed out that murmurs usually do *not* change much during SBE: "a very slight change in the character of the heart murmur in spite of the . . . most extensive vegetations and alterations in the valve."[179] It is true that appearance of *new* murmurs is not rare in

SBE, as noted above. New murmurs and changing murmurs are common in patients with ABE.

COMPLICATIONS

Heart Failure

Heart failure is the single most important complication of infective endocarditis.[43,53,180,181] No other factor exerts such a critical influence on prognosis. In 1951, Cates and Christie[181] reported a death rate of 37 percent among 314 patients with SBE who had no heart failure and 85 percent in 94 who had moderate or severe failure. In a more recent series,[180] congestive failure occurred in 55 percent but was much more common in patients with aortic valve disease (75 percent) than in those with mitral valve (50 percent) or tricuspid valve disease (19 percent).

Sudden onset or worsening of left ventricular failure is common during the course of ABE because of perforation or destruction of a valve leaflet or rupture of chordae tendineae, but it also occurs in some patients with SBE for the same reasons. Occasionally, bulky vegetations occlude the valve orifice, causing functional stenosis; this phenomenon is most likely to occur during fungal infection of prosthetic valves.[173,174]

Embolization

This complication is recognized in 12 to 35 percent of patients during the course of SBE and in 50 to 60 percent with ABE, but necropsy findings indicate that many arterial emboli go undetected. Pelletier and Petersdorf[53] reported a 50 percent incidence of major arterial emboli in 125 cases, affecting brain (25 cases), lung (17 cases), coronary artery (8 cases), spleen (8 cases), extremities (8 cases), gut (4 cases), and eye (3 cases).

Neurological Manifestations

Involvement of the nervous system during the course of endocarditis is both common and clinically important.[182–186] Jones[182] found neurological abnormalities in 110 of 385 patients (29 percent); Ziment[183] reviewed 21 studies and concluded that the nervous system was involved in 40 to 50 percent of patients with endocarditis. A wide range of syndromes occurs, including toxic confusional states, psychiatric symptoms, minor or major strokes (Plate IX, 94-9), meningoencephalitis, and cranial or peripheral nerve lesions. It is important to know that the presenting complaint involves the nervous system in 10 to 15 percent of patients with endocarditis.

Of 55 patients with cerebrovascular complications of endocarditis, four-fifths suffered infarction and one-fifth hemorrhage.[182] Infarction is usually due to embolism, most often to the middle cerebral arteries; hemorrhage can be a complication of either emboli or mycotic aneurysms.[53,182–189]

A *meningeal reaction* occurs in 7 to 15 percent of patients, especially those with staphylococcal ABE.[34,182–184] This reaction may be mistakenly diagnosed as being due to acute bacterial meningitis because the cerebrospinal fluid (CSF) contains polymorphonuclear leukocytes and slightly raised protein concentration. However, the glucose level is usually normal, and the results of CSF culture are usually negative; the other abnormalities are resolved during treatment of the underlying disease. True bacterial meningitis occurs in some patients with pneumococcal endocarditis[107,108] and occasionally in staphylococcal ABE.

Cerebritis may develop in brain tissue surrounding small infected emboli lodged in cerebral vessels in both SBE and ABE, often with associated meningoencephalitis.[186] Computerized tomography often reveals multiple areas of cerebritis, especially in acute staphylococcal endocarditis. In patients with ABE, this inflammatory reaction in the brain may progress to form a brain abscess, but more often cerebritis will resolve uneventfully during antibiotic treatment of the underlying disease. Brain abscesses are uncommon in patients with SBE.[186]

Mycotic Aneurysm

This complication develops in only 3 to 15 percent of patients with infective endocarditis, but the local consequences of expansion and rupture can be very serious, especially in the brain (Plate IX, 94-9). In order of frequency, the sites most often involved are the proximal aorta, including the sinuses of Valsalva (25 percent of cases), arteries to the viscera (24 percent), arteries to the extremities (22 percent), and arteries to the brain (15 percent).[187–189] Unfortunately, intracerebral aneurysms are often multiple.[188,189]

Mycotic aneurysms develop when the wall of an artery is damaged by the inflammatory response to microbes.[157] These microbes reach the arterial wall via microemboli to the vasa vasorum or by impaction of a larger infected embolus in the lumen. The arterial wall is apparently a poorer culture medium for bacteria than for a valvular vegetation, because the organisms responsible for weakening the vessel often die out spontaneously, even if untreated. The mycotic aneurysm may continue to enlarge even when living organisms are no longer present, due to the physical effects of arterial blood pressure (Plate IX, 94-9).[187–189]

DIFFERENTIAL DIAGNOSIS

Because the clinical manifestations of endocarditis are numerous and often nonspecific, the differential diagnosis of this disease is very wide.[3,34,43,53,169] Of the many conditions that may be considered, only a few leading examples are listed here.

ABE shares many clinical features with nonendocarditic septicemias due to *Staph. aureus, Neisseria*, pneumococci, and gram-negative bacilli. Pneumonia, meningitis, brain abscess, stroke, malaria, acute pericarditis, vasculitis, and disseminated intravascular coagulation may cause diagnostic confusion.

SBE must be considered during the workup of every patient with fever of unknown origin. Its manifestations can mimic those of rheumatic fever, osteomyelitis, tuberculosis, meningitis, intraabdominal infections, salmonellosis, brucellosis, glomerulonephritis, myocardial infarction, stroke, endocardial thrombi, atrial myxoma, connective tissue diseases, vasculitis, occult malignancy (especially lymphomas), chronic cardiac failure, pericarditis, and even psychoneurosis.

Diagnostic Criteria

Infective endocarditis can be surprisingly difficult to diagnose with certainty.[84] As mentioned above, this is because the presenting symptoms and signs can be highly variable and consistent with many other possible diagnoses. Furthermore, the essential lesion of endocarditis (the vegetation) is inaccessible to direct inspection except at surgery or autopsy. To avoid overdiagnosis of doubtful cases, in 1981 von Reyn and colleagues[84] proposed strict case definitions, which have been widely used. These definitions, however, require modification because they make no use of echocardiographic findings, which have since become an essential element in the diagnosis of infective endocarditis. The following diagnostic criteria are suggested:

1. *Pathologic criteria* for infective endocarditis
   - A. Microorganisms: demonstrated by culture *or* histologic studies in a vegetation, a vegetation that has embolized, or an intracardiac abscess *or*
   - B. Pathologic lesions: presence of vegetation or intracardiac abscess confirmed by histologic studies showing active endocarditis
2. *Clinical criteria* for infective endocarditis
   - A. Two major criteria *or*
   - B. One major and three minor criteria *or*
   - C. Five minor criteria using specific definitions for these criteria as listed below
3. *Possible* infective endocarditis: findings consistent with infective endocarditis that fall short of the criteria listed above

Definition of Terms Used in Diagnostic Criteria

The major criteria are defined as follows:

1. Positive blood culture results for infective endocarditis
   - A. Typical microorganisms for infective endocarditis: viridans streptococci, HACEK group, *Strep. bovis, Staph. aureus,* or enterococci, recovered from two or more blood cultures, community-acquired, in the absence of a primary focus of infection elsewhere *or*
   - B. Persistently positive blood culture results: microorganism consistent with infective endocarditis recovered from
     - (1) One or more blood cultures drawn more than 12 h apart *or*
     - (2) All of three or majority of four or more separate blood cultures, with first and last drawn at least 1 h apart
2. *Either* positive echocardiographic study results for infective endocarditis
   - A. Oscillating intracardiac target: on valve or supporting structures, in the path of regurgitant jets, or on iatrogenic devices, in the absence of an alternative anatomic explanation *or*
   - B. Abscess *or*
   - C. New dehiscence of prosthetic valve *or* new valvular regurgitation: must be new; worsening or changing of preexisting murmur not sufficient

The minor criteria are defined as follows:

1. Predisposition: predisposing heart condition *or* injected drug user
2. Febrile syndrome: *either* subacute (classical fever of undetermined origin) *or* acute febrile illness without alternative diagnosis in noninjected drug user
3. Vascular phenomena: arterial embolism, septic pulmonary infarcts, mycotic aneurysm, central nervous system hemorrhage, Osler's nodes, or Roth spots
4. Immunologic phenomena: immune-complex glomerulonephritis, rheumatoid factor, false-positive VDRL test results
5. Echocardiogram: suggestive of infective endocarditis but not positive for major criterion for infective endocarditis as defined above
6. Microbiologic evidence: positive blood culture results but not positive for major criterion for infective endocarditis as defined above, with organism consistent with infective endocarditis and not likely to be a contaminant, *or* serologic evidence of active infection with organism consistent with infective endocarditis

INVESTIGATIONS

Routine Laboratory Tests

Anemia is usual in SBE and fairly common in ABE. It is most often of the hypoproliferative type, with a normochromic, normocytic smear, but may be hemolytic in ABE. Chronic low-grade hemolysis due to a prosthetic valve may confuse interpretation of the blood picture.

Leukocytosis is an unreliable manifestation of SBE. A low-grade, variable elevation of the leukocyte count with some immature forms is characteristic, but in many cases the leukocyte count is normal. A high granulocyte count with an increase in band forms is commonly found in patients with ABE. These neutrophils may show toxic granulation, and in a few cases of ABE staphylococci can be identified inside them on examination of a Gram-stained smear of the buffy coat of the peripheral blood.[190] Abnormal histiocytes may be found in smears of peripheral blood in one-third of patients with SBE.[191]

The erythrocyte sedimentation rate is almost always elevated. A fall of greater than 50 mm/h is common in SBE; the rate of fall is variable in ABE.

Urinalysis shows microscopic hematuria and/or slight proteinuria in about 50 percent of cases, even in the absence of specific renal complications.[3,43,169] Red blood cell casts and heavy proteinuria are found in those patients who develop immune-complex glomerulonephritis, often in association with decreased total serum complement.[162] Gross hematuria suggests that renal infarction has occurred. A positive test result for rheumatoid factor is found in 40 to 50 percent of cases of SBE[149–151] but rarely in ABE. A polyclonal increase in gamma globulins is characteristic. Occasional false-positive serological test results for syphilis occur.[148]

Blood Cultures

Isolation of an organism from the blood is the most important step in the diagnosis of endocarditis. Blood cultures should be drawn from *all patients with fever and heart murmur*, unless their illness is clearly due to another disease or the fever resolves within a few days without treatment. Cultures should also be taken from susceptible patients with other nonspecific symptoms or signs consistent with endocarditis, to help rule out that diagnosis.

Beeson, Brannon, and Warren showed that bacteremia in SBE is usually continuous.[20] The number of organisms per mililiter of blood varies widely but is usually between 1 and 100 organisms per milliliter in subacute cases. Therefore, most blood culture results are positive, and it is usually not necessary to take a large number of cultures.[97,192] Pelletier and Petersdorf[53] found that *all* blood culture results were positive in 68 percent of 125 patients. Similarly, Werner noted that the etiologic organism was recovered from cultures taken on the first day of admission in 93 percent of patients with culture-positive endocarditis.[193]

Katsu[194] found that arterial culture results were positive slightly more often than venous culture results (72 percent versus 64 percent, respectively, in 313 cases) and reported 40 cases in which arterial but not venous culture results were positive. Although this difference was significant, it seems too small to justify obtaining arterial cultures in every case. The following practical approach is suggested: for SBE, draw three separate venous blood cultures on the first day, with at least 1 h between the first and last venipuncture. If all results are negative on the second or third day *but the diagnosis of endocarditis still seems likely*, draw two more venous cultures and one arterial culture. If the patient had received previous antibiotic therapy, three more venous samples may be taken over the following week, to identify any late recrudescence of bacteremia after partial treatment. For ABE, draw three venous blood cultures and begin empirical antibiotic therapy at once, because treatment should not be delayed until culture results are available in patients with acute endocarditis.

Because *Staph. epidermidis*[19] and diphtheroids[195] can cause endocarditis, special care must be taken during venipuncture to avoid contamination of the specimen with these common skin organisms, which could result in diagnostic confusion. For each culture, 10 to 20 mL of blood should be drawn and divided equally between one unvented anaerobic bottle of medium and one vented bottle. Media should be adequately supplemented to allow growth of fastidious, nutritionally variant bacteria.[95–97] Cultures should be incubated for at least 3 weeks, and Gram stains made at intervals even if no growth is apparent on inspection. Pour plates can help to distinguish contaminants from true positive cultures.

Electrocardiography

Electrocardiographic studies should be performed on the patient's admission to the hospital and repeated at intervals according to progress during treatment. Such studies may reveal evidence of otherwise silent myocardial infarction due to embolization of a vegetation to a coronary artery. A disturbance of conduction that develops during the course of endocarditis suggests extension of infection into the myocardium. Such extension may be due to focal myocarditis or to an abscess located close to the conduction system.[76] Thus, development of a prolonged PR interval, if due to an abscess, can have major implications: a probable need for valve replacement and a worse prognosis.[80]

Echocardiography

Echocardiographic studies are vitally important in the diagnosis of infective endocarditis.[196–203] Positive echocardiographic findings, properly defined, constitute a major criterion for the clinical diagnosis of endocarditis, second only to blood cultures in practical importance (see "Diagnostic Criteria"). Transthoracic two-dimensional echocardiography (Chap. 15) combined with color-flow Doppler imaging (Chap. 130) provides a wealth of information for both the diagnosis and the management of endocarditis, including the detection of vegetations, other valvular abnormalities, abscesses, and pericarditis and the assessment of ventricular function (Figs. 15-31 and 94-5).[201–203] Sensitivity for detection of vegetations is 50 to 75 percent, but this can be improved to better than 95 percent by use of transesophageal imaging (Chap. 131) in selected cases (Fig. 131-7).[201] Transesophageal studies also detect abscesses and valve perforation with much greater sensitivity.[203]

Echocardiography has some limitations.[196,197,200] To realize its full value, experienced technicians and expert interpretation are necessary. A negative study result has some negative predictive value[170] (especially if transesophageal studies have been performed) but does not exclude the diagnosis of endocarditis.[196,197] Sensitivity is somewhat lower on the right side; for example, Andy and colleagues detected vegetations in all of three patients with aortic infection but in only 12 of 20 with tricuspid involvement.[170] The presence of a prosthetic valve sometimes interferes with detection of vegetations, but even in these patients the findings usually are informative.

Occasionally, the specificity of echocardiography is limited by false-positive readings for "vegetations" that do not exist. Such readings are particularly common in patients with myxomatous degeneration of the mitral valve.[197]

Sequential echocardiograms performed during treatment can assist materially in making decisions on the necessity for and timing of surgery by providing objective assessments of cardiac function. For example, premature mitral valve closure due to raised end-diastolic pressure is a useful echocardiographic sign indicating severe aortic regurgitation, usually requiring valve replacement (see also Chap. 15).[199] However, sequential echocardiographic studies intended to document the disappearance of vegetations during and after treatment are not reliable criteria for success or failure of antibiotic therapy.[200]

Roentgenography

The most important contribution of the chest x-ray in assessment of endocarditis is to provide evidence of early

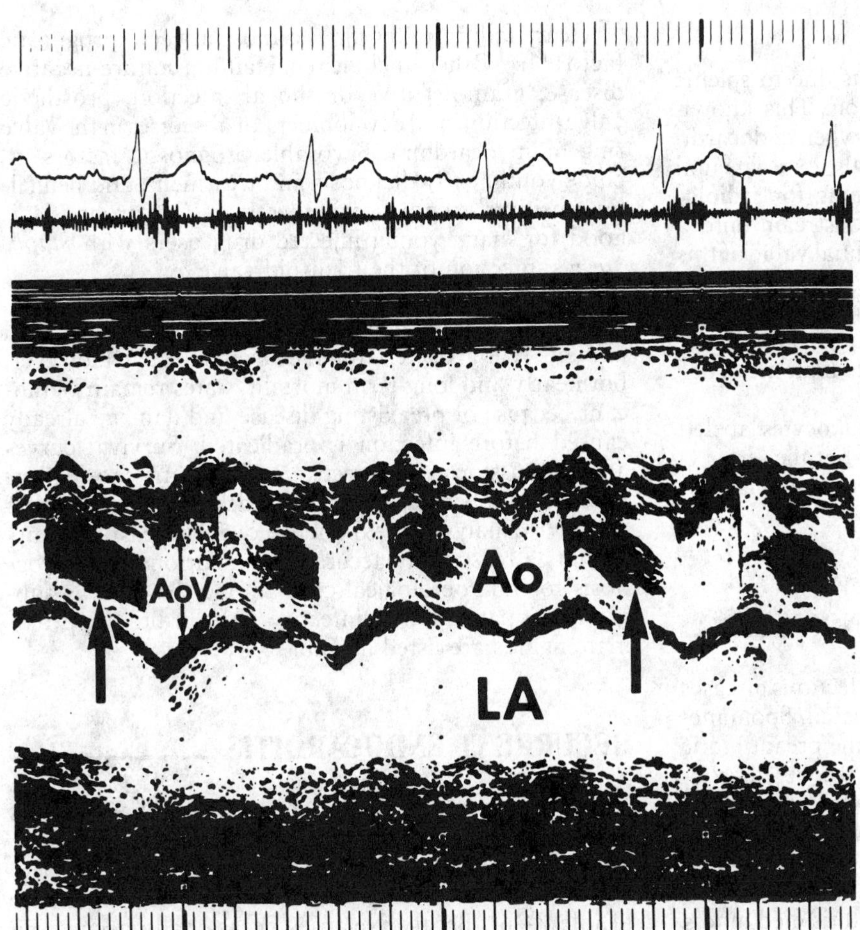

FIGURE 94-5 The echocardiogram shows dense, fuzzy echoes on the diastolic portion of the aortic valve (*arrows*) that are virtually diagnostic of valvular vegetations. Ao = aortic; AoV = aortic valve; LA = left atrium. (*Courtesy of Dr. Joel Felner.*)

congestive heart failure, because this complication carries such important implications for both prognosis and management (see "Complications").

The presence of multiple small, patchy infiltrates in the lungs of an injected drug user with fever strongly suggests the diagnosis of septic emboli arising from right-sided infective endocarditis.[48–52] Valvular calcification may identify a previously abnormal valve, thus aiding the localization of presumed intravascular infection. Widening of the aorta may be caused by a mycotic aneurysm.

Fluoroscopy can demonstrate abnormal motion of a prosthetic valve, indicating presence of a vegetation or partial dehiscence of the valve from the aortic root. This information often helps to decide whether or not valve replacement is needed during management of PVE.

Computerized axial tomography and magnetic resonance imaging (Chap. 136)[186] can be helpful in defining the cause of focal neurological lesions in patients with endocarditis, especially infarction, hemorrhage from a mycotic aneurysm, and brain abscess. Angiographic studies may be necessary to demonstrate mycotic aneurysms in the brain or elsewhere.[188,189]

Cardiac Catheterization and Cineangiography

This investigation is usually not necessary for patients who respond well to antimicrobial therapy without developing cardiac failure. When treatment seems to be failing and/or operation is considered, cardiac catheterization and cineangiography (Chap. 138) can provide vital information. Anatomic abnormalities such as valvular lesions, congenital defects, coronary artery disease, asymmetrical septal hypertrophy, coarctation of the aorta, or mycotic aneurysm can be defined. Occasionally, a previously unsuspected diagnosis, such as the presence of a sinus of Valsalva aneurysm, will be made. Physiologcal measurements including cardiac output, pressures on the left and right sides of the heart, and the degree of aortic regurgitation may help to decide whether or not valve replacement is indicated and influence the timing of the operation. Welton and colleagues reviewed 35 patients who underwent cardiac catheterization during active endocarditis.[204] The clinical assessment was materially modified by catheterization in 23 patients, the diagnosis of the site of valve involvement was altered in 14, and 6 valve ring abscesses were revealed. Surgery was postponed or canceled in 6 patients when catheterization revealed only mild hemodynamic abnormalities. There were no serious complications, indicating that catheterization should not be avoided for fear of dislodging emboli when a proper indication exists. In summary, catheterization and cineangiography should be performed in most patients with infective endocarditis when operation is being considered or treatment seems to be failing.

Radionuclide Imaging

Liver-spleen imaging may reveal defects due to splenic infarction, thus confirming embolization. This knowledge is sometimes useful diagnostically when endocarditis is suspected but unproved. In animals, experimental vegetations have been located by scanning for radiolabeled platelets deposited from the bloodstream onto a growing endocardial lesion.[205] The potential value of this test for diagnosis of human endocarditis has not yet been proved. Gallium-67 scans have shown increased uptake in the heart in cases of endocarditis, but this technique is currently of little value because of the high incidence of false positive results.[206]

Scintigraphic following injection of leukocytes labeled with indium 111 can detect abscesses,[207] but the sensitivity and cost-effectiveness of this new technique has not been documented.

NATURAL HISTORY AND PROGNOSIS

Infective endocarditis is one of the few infectious diseases that are almost universally fatal if untreated. Spontaneous recovery did occur occasionally in the preantibiotic era,[3] but most patients reported to have recovered probably had illnesses other than infective endocarditis. The interval between the onset of symptoms and death in patients with untreated subacute disease varied widely, with a median time to death of about 6 months.[3] Almost all patients with acute infective endocarditis died in less than 4 weeks.

Heart failure is by far the most adverse prognostic factor.[180,181] Others include renal failure, culture-negative disease, gram-negative or fungal infection, prosthetic valve infection, and development of abscesses in the valve ring or myocardium. Favorable prognostic factors include youth, early diagnosis and treatment, and penicillin-sensitive streptococcal infection. The prognosis is good for many young injected drug users with *Staph. aureus* infection of the tricuspid valve.[5,208]

Eradication of the etiologic organisms ("microbiological cure") can be achieved in a high proportion of all patients with bacterial endocarditis.[7,209-212] However, both early and long-term mortality rates remain significant because of preexisting disease and damage already caused before infection is eradicated. Survival curves after admission with infective endocarditis show a significant number of late deaths despite microbiologic cure.[10,213] Analysis of experience over the past 20 years permits a reasonably accurate formulation of the prognosis for microbiological cure among the various subgroups of patients with infective endocarditis. Approximate figures are listed in Table 94-6.

RECURRENT ENDOCARDITIS

Recurrent endocarditis is a general term that includes both *relapses* and *reinfections*. The frequency of relapse after treatment for each of the various forms of infective endocarditis can be predicted from published experience (Table 94-6). Because relapses occasionally occur even after an optimal treatment regimen has been used, fol-

TABLE 94-6

Estimate of Microbiologic Cure Rates for Various Forms of Endocarditis*

Native Valve Endocarditis	Antimicrobial Therapy Alone		Antimicrobial Therapy Plus Surgery	
Viridans streptococci, group A streptococci, *Strep. bovis*, pneumococci, gonococci	98		98	
Enterococcus faecalis	90		>90	
Staph. aureus (in young injected drug users)	90		>90	
Staph. aureus (in elderly patients with chronic underlying diseases)	50		70	
Gram-negative aerobic bacilli†	40		65	
Fungi	<5		50	
Prosthetic Valve Endocarditis	**Early PVE**	**Late PVE**	**Early PVE**	**Late PVE**
Viridans streptococci, group A streptococci, *Strep. bovis*, pneumococci, gonococci	‡	80	‡	90
Enterococcus faecalis	‡	60	‡	75
Staph. aureus	25	40	50	60
Staph. epidermidis	20	40	60	70
Gram-negative aerobic bacilli†	<10	20	40	50
Fungi	<1	<1	30	40

* Morbidity and mortality are significantly greater than these figures for microbiologic cure indicate.
† Excluding *Hemophilus* species.
‡ Insufficient data to estimate rate.
SOURCE: Adapted from Refs. 10, 29, 30, 36, 53, 76, 213, 214, 227–229.

low-up clinical evaluation including blood cultures should be meticulously performed during the first 2 months after treatment. Most relapses occur within a few weeks of ending treatment, but living organisms can persist in seemingly healed vegetations for many months and may occasionally cause late relapse.

The term *reinfection* refers to a new episode of endocarditis occurring after the cure of a previous episode.[214,215] Usually a different etiologic organism is involved, but if it appears identical to the previous organism, one cannot be certain whether an episode of recurrent endocarditis represents a true reinfection or a relapse. Molecular typing techniques may be used to resolve this issue.

Patients remain permanently at risk of reinfection after cure of infective endocarditis because of residual valve scarring (Tables 94-1 and 94-2). Further episodes are fairly common, being recorded in from 2 to 31 percent of cases.[3,36,41,213,215] This wide variation in reported incidence is partly due to variable duration of follow-up. Injected drug users and patients with severe periodontitis are at highest risk for reinfection. Occasionally, a patient may suffer three or more separate episodes of infective endocarditis.[215] Patients who have previously had native-valve endocarditis are at higher risk for prosthetic valve infection (often with a different organism) for reasons that are not yet understood.[10]

TREATMENT OF INFECTIVE ENDOCARDITIS

General Principles

The chief aims of management are to eradicate the infecting organism as soon as possible, to operate with correct timing if surgical intervention should be required, and to treat complications. Because infective endocarditis carries a significant risk of death even when well managed, it is important that treatment be continued long enough to ensure that relapse will not occur. On the other hand, patients with the more easily cured forms of endocarditis should not be subjected to unnecessarily long and expensive treatment in a hospital. This can happen when physicians exercise excessive caution based on outdated rules of thumb such as "all cases of endocarditis should be treated for at least 6 weeks." In fact, some patients with endocarditis require treatment for much longer than 6 weeks, while many can be cured in only 2 weeks.[210,216]

Antimicrobial Therapy

Microbiological Tests

To choose and regulate antibiotic therapy correctly, certain basic microbiological information on the infecting organism is required.[97] For group A streptococcal and pneumococcal endocarditis, nothing more than positive identification of the organism is necessary because these organisms are still sensitive to low concentrations of penicillin, with very rare exceptions. For other species of streptococci, for staphylococci, and for most other bacteria, both the minimal inhibitory concentration (MIC) and minimal bactericidal concentration (MBC) of relevant antibiotics should be determined. Some of these organisms are resistant to intermediate or high concentrations of penicillin[217,218]; others may be tolerant, that is, inhibited but not killed, by antibiotic levels achievable in serum.[219,220]

The serum bactericidal titer (SBT or Schlichter test) is frequently used to monitor the treatment of endocarditis.[30,71,97,221] In this test, the infecting organism is exposed in vitro to the patient's serum, which is drawn while the patient is receiving antibiotic treatment, to determine the maximal dilution of serum that will inhibit and kill the organism. On the basis of empirical clinical experience, it is often said that the SBT should be 1:8 or higher at intervals during each day of treatment. However, the interpretation and clinical relevance of this test remain controversial.[221] Proof that the patient's serum is actually capable of killing the infecting organism reassures the clinician, but for streptococcal and staphylococcal endocarditis this can usually be achieved without difficulty, and SBTs are often very high (e.g., 1:128 to 1:1024). Therefore, SBTs need not be measured repeatedly during management of most patients with endocarditis. Measurement of the SBT is most likely to be clinically helpful when treating unusual organisms, when using unusual antibiotics, when using unusual regimens (such as oral treatment), or when treatment appears to be failing.

Intermittent dosage regimens that result in widely fluctuating SBTs are traditionally employed for treatment of endocarditis and are usually effective. Whether or not maintenance of continuously high SBTs would offer any therapeutic benefit over intermittent dosing regimens is not known; perhaps continuous infusion of antibiotic would be desirable for treatment of gram-negative organisms, which regrow more rapidly than gram-positive organisms when antibiotic levels fall below the minimal inhibitory concentration.

Choice of Antibiotic

Bactericidal antibiotics should be chosen for treatment of endocarditis whenever possible.[30,71] Although cases have occasionally been cured with bacteriostatic drugs such as tetracycline and chloramphenicol, results of treatment with these agents are usually poor.[222] This is because host defense mechanisms are inadequate in the vegetation. Relatively few phagocytes are present, and they are hampered by protective layers of fibrin around the colonies of bacteria (Fig. 94-2, 94-4). To effect a cure, antibiotic therapy must eradicate organisms completely, without the help of phagocytes to eliminate the subpopulation of microbes that are relatively resistant to antibiotics because they are in the resting phase. In this important respect, infective endocarditis differs strikingly from bacterial pneumonia in normal hosts, where phagocytes are plentiful and bacteriostatic antibiotics are usually effective. Nevertheless, it may occasionally be necessary when treating unusual organisms to use a bacteriostatic antibiotic in combination with other drugs to achieve the optimal antibacterial effect. When treatment with unusual combinations of antibiotics is needed, in vitro laboratory tests should be performed to find out whether synergism, indifference, or antagonism exists between them.

For the common forms of bacterial endocarditis caused by gram-positive organisms, published experience is so extensive that specific therapeutic regimens can be recommended with confidence.[208,210] Standard regimens for streptococcal and staphylococcal endocarditis are listed in Table 94-7.

Staph. epidermidis PVE is difficult to eradicate with antibiotics alone.[112,113] These staphylococci are frequently resistant to semisynthetic penicillins and other antibiotics. A regimen combining vancomycin, rifampin, and an aminoglycoside chosen according to sensitivity tests is most likely to succeed, but results are unpredictable. The organism may develop resistance to rifampin during treatment.

Treatment of endocarditis due to less common organisms must be chosen on the basis of more limited published experience,[65,120,223] together with the results of tests performed upon the infecting organism in the microbiology laboratory. Treatment often must be individualized. In general, one of the beta-lactam antibiotics should be included in the regimen whenever possible. Combinations of two or more antibiotics are often employed. The list of potentially useful regimens for these rarer forms of infective endocarditis is too long to detail here.

TABLE 94-7

Treatment Regimens for Infective Endocarditis Caused by Gram-Positive Cocci

Organism	Regimen	Duration, weeks	Comments
Alphahemolytic (viridans) streptococci, *Strep. bovis*	1. Penicillin G 4 million units IV every 6 h *plus* gentamicin 1.0 mg/kg every 12 h IV *or*	2	Standard regimen, for patients less than 65 years old without renal failure, eighth-nerve defects, or serious complications
	2. Penicillin G 4 million units IV every 6 h *plus* gentamicin 1.0 mg/kg every 12 h IV (for first 2 weeks only) *or*	4	For patients with complicated disease, e.g., central nervous system involvement, shock, moderately penicillin-resistant streptococci, failed previous treatment
	3. Penicillin G 4 million units every 6 h IV, *or*	4	For patients more than 65 years old, with renal failure or eighth-nerve defects
	4. Ceftriaxone 2 g IV once daily *or*	4	For patients allergic to penicillins
	5. Vancomycin 10 mg/kg IV every 12 h	4	For patients allergic to penicillins and cephalosporins
E. faecalis and other penicillin-resistant streptococci	1. Ampicillin 2 g IV every 4 h *plus* gentamicin 1.0 mg/kg IV every 8 h, *or*	4–6	4 weeks should be adequate for most cases with symptoms present for less than 3 months
	2. Vancomycin 15 mg/kg IV every 12 h IV *plus* gentamicin 1.0 mg/kg IV (not to exceed 80 mg) every 8 h	4–6	For patients allergic to penicillin; 4 weeks should be adequate for most cases; serum levels should be monitored
Staph. aureus	1. Nafcillin 2 g IV every 4 h, *or*	4 or longer	Standard regimen
	2. Nafcillin as above, *plus* gentamicin 1.0 mg/kg IV every 8 h for the first 3–5 days only, *or*	4 or longer	For patients with severe disseminated staphylococcal disease, synergy may be advantageous during early stages of treatment
	3. Cefazolin 2 g IV every 8 h, *or*	4 or longer	For patients allergic to penicillins
	4. Vancomycin 15 mg/kg IV every 12 h	4 or longer	For patients allergic to penicillins and cephalosporins; for methicillin-resistant strains
Group A streptococci, *Strep. pneumoniae*	1. Penicillin G 2 million units IV every 6 h, *or*	2–4	Organisms usually highly sensitive to penicillin; 2 weeks should be adequate for many patients
	2. Cefazolin 1 g IV every 8 h	2–4	

SOURCE: Adapted with modifications from AL Bisno et al: Antimicrobial treatment of infective endocarditis due to viridans streptococci, enterococci, and staphylococci. *JAMA* 261:1471–1477, 1989.

Empirical Therapy

When the etiologic organism is not known, the choice of empirical therapy should depend on whether the patient has acute or subacute disease. ABE requires broad-spectrum therapy that covers *Staph. aureus* as well as many species of streptococci and gram-negative bacilli. SBE requires a regimen that treats most streptococci, including *E. faecalis*. To meet these requirements, the following suggestions are offered:

For ABE: nafcillin 2.0 g IV every 4 h plus ampicillin 2.0 g IV every 4 h plus gentamicin 1.5 mg/kg IV every 8 h

For SBE: ampicillin 2.0 g IV every 4 h plus gentamicin 1.5 mg/kg IV every 8 h

Treatment should be adjusted when the etiologic organism is identified. In those few cases where empirical therapy is administered as a therapeutic trial to help confirm a diagnosis, treatment should be continued without interruption or unnecessary changes for at least 2 weeks; otherwise, no useful diagnostic information will be gained.

Duration of Therapy

Extensive experience with treatment of the common forms of endocarditis provides sufficient grounds for recommendations[210] on adequate duration of therapy (Table 94-7). An exception to this is *Staph. aureus* endocarditis. The natural history of this disease is highly variable; some patients recover swiftly without complications, especially young injected drug users, who often can be cured within 2 weeks.[5,216] In contrast, some patients remain febrile for several weeks, often with extracardiac manifestations of disseminated staphylococcal disease. Although 4 weeks of therapy is adequate in most cases, this must not be regarded as a rigid rule because some patients with *Staph. aureus* endocarditis require treatment for 6 weeks or longer to achieve a cure. For *E. faecalis* endocarditis, 4 weeks' treatment is usually adequate. However, the relapse rate seems to be higher in patients with mitral valve infection and in those who have had symptoms for more than 3 months.[101] These patients should be treated for 6 weeks.

Parenteral treatment can be completed in the patient's home in carefully selected cases. Availability of antibiotics with long half-lives (such as vancomycin or ceftriaxone), permitting once-daily administration by a home therapy service, has made this feasible. The option of parenteral treatment at home offers obvious benefits for the patient and for cost containment and should be fully effective in achieving a microbiological cure.[211,212] However, the risks posed by a possible late complication such as an embolic stroke or the sudden onset of heart failure must be considered before selecting candidates for home parenteral therapy. Further trials are needed to determine the optimal applications for therapy for endocarditis at home.[212]

In general, the less extensive the published experience with a particular infective agent, the more one should lean toward prolonging treatment in order to provide a reasonable margin of safety. Guidelines for the duration of treatment for gram-positive organisms are listed in Table 94-7. For other organisms, the optimal duration of treatment required varies greatly according to individual circumstances in each patient.[223]

Anticoagulant Therapy and Endocarditis

Can anticoagulant therapy be started or continued safely during treatment of endocarditis? This is a common and vexing question. Even though the infected vegetation is essentially a thrombotic lesion, there is no evidence that anticoagulation has any useful therapeutic effect on the course of the endocarditis itself. On the contrary, early experience showed that simultaneous treatment with penicillin and heparin carried a higher risk of fatal intracerebral hemorrhage from mycotic aneurysm or infarction than treatment with penicillin alone.[224] For this reason, anticoagulation was considered to be strongly contraindicated in patients with endocarditis, until more recent experience showed that warfarin could be given safely during the treatment of patients with prosthetic valve infections.[225,226] Currently available information suggests the following simple guidelines for patients with infective endocarditis:

- Avoid use of heparin entirely (except for immediate treatment of massive pulmonary embolism).
- Discontinue or avoid anticoagulation if possible, especially in patients with intracranial complications.
- Anticoagulate with warfarin if there is a clear-cut indication, such as a mechanical prosthetic heart valve, taking care to regulate the prothrombin time between INR 2.5 and 3.5.
- Choose an antibiotic treatment regimen that does not require intramuscular injections, if anticoagulation is instituted.

Role of Surgery

Optimal management requires operative intervention during treatment of certain patients with endocarditis.[79,80,227,228] The surgery most often involves replacement of a valve to reverse cardiac failure due to newly developed or worsening valvular lesions. Because prosthetic valve infection is more difficult to eradicate with antibiotics than native valve infection, replacement of an infected prosthesis is often necessary for cure. Repeated major emboli constitute a relative indication for valve replacement (see "Management of Complications"). Occasionally, a patient remains "septic" despite antibiotic therapy; surgery may then be required to control infection itself, rather than its hemodynamic consequences. Operation to close a patent ductus arteriosus or septal defect, to excise a coarctation of the aorta, or to relieve asymmetrical septal hypertrophy may be required as part of treatment of endocarditis engrafted upon these lesions. Other indications for surgery are considered under "Management of Complications."

Correct timing is the essence of good surgical management of endocarditis.[79,80,227] If surgery is undertaken too soon, the risks of operative mortality and the early and late morbidity associated with valve replacement may be inflicted on the patient unnecessarily, because some patients respond to medical therapy so well that operation can be postponed indefinitely. If surgery can be delayed safely, antibiotic therapy should eradicate or at least greatly reduce the population of organisms on the valve, thus increasing the chance of a successful outcome if surgery becomes necessary. If time is available for effective treatment of complications such as septicemia, renal failure, pneumonia, myocarditis, and neurologic complications before surgery, ventricular function may improve, lowering the operative risk. On the other hand, if surgery is delayed too long, patients may die suddenly, or their hemodynamic status may deteriorate so seriously that surgery is no longer feasible. This is a tragic error because many such patients can be saved by earlier surgery.[80,227–230] Thus, both the decision to operate and the timing of surgery are of critical importance.

Careful, frequent reexamination of the patient, together with echocardiographic studies and sometimes cardiac catheterization to confirm the clinical findings, is indicated in every case where operation may be needed. The decision to operate should also be influenced by knowledge of the natural history of the type of endocarditis being treated. For example, penicillin-sensitive streptococcal endocarditis almost always can be cured bacteriologically (Table 94-6), and the immediate prognosis is good, provided that cardiac failure does not supervene. Thus, surgery should usually be considered only for those patients with cardiac failure that does not respond well to medical treatment. Similarly, since youthful injected drug users with acute staphylococcal endocarditis have a good prognosis,[5,176,216] surgery usually should be reserved for those who develop serious heart failure. At the other end of the spectrum, the likelihood that fungal prosthetic valve endocarditis can be eradicated with antifungal drugs alone is negligible, even in the absence of heart failure (Table 94-6). Such patients usually should undergo valve debridement or replacement early, without waiting to test the remote possibility that antifungal treatment could eradicate the infection. Other examples of patients who are highly likely to require operation are those with gram-negative infection of prosthetic valves and those with valve ring abscesses. Aortic valve involvement, staphylococcal infection in a non-drug addict, and gram-negative bacillary infection should be regarded as other relative indications favoring early valve replacement.[76,79,80,229]

In addition to valve replacement, several other surgical procedures may be available for the treatment of endocarditis.[512] Debridement of vegetations (vegetectomy), often combined with valvuloplasty or valve repair, can cure the infection while sparing the native valve in carefully selected patients.[173,174,512] This can be especially beneficial for young patients, women who wish to have children, and patients who cannot or will not take anticoagulant therapy reliably. Replacement of the proximal aorta and aortic valve with a homograft or heterograft can be used to salvage patients with abscesses extending into the myocardium from the aortic valve.[231]

Because of the possible need for surgery during the course of any case of endocarditis, it is desirable that patients be managed in consultation with a thoracic surgical service. Such consultation should be obtained early so that an operation can be performed without delay if it becomes necessary during the course of treatment. Sudden onset of aortic or mitral regurgitation with consequent acute left ventricular failure can occur without warning, even in the most favorable forms of endocarditis.

Management of Complications

Heart Failure

Development of moderate or severe cardiac failure due to structural valvular damage indicates the need for immediate surgery in most patients with endocarditis, even if the intracardiac infection is still active.[76,79,80,229,230] In patients with milder heart failure, the decision should be individualized, always remembering that lives may be lost unnecessarily if cardiac function suddenly worsens and operation is either very hazardous or no longer possible.

Emboli

The occurrence of one or more significant arterial emboli during the treatment of endocarditis is a relative indication for surgery. However, the predictable early and long-term mortality and morbidity rates of valve replacement must be weighed against the fact that the likelihood of further emboli is highly unpredictable. For this reason, embolization is much less satisfactory as an indication for valve replacement than is cardiac failure.[230] In the author's opinion, operative intervention during antibiotic treatment should seldom be undertaken solely "to prevent further emboli," unless the patient has suffered more than one or two proven major emboli.

Renal Failure

Patients who died with SBE before 1955 frequently had developed chronic renal failure.[3] Subsequently, both the incidence of renal failure and its importance as a cause of death have greatly diminished. Earlier diagnosis and antibiotic treatment have forestalled the development of immune-complex glomerulonephritis in many patients. In those few (about 5 percent) who still develop this complication of SBE, timely dialysis can maintain the patient until antibiotic treatment results in disappearance of the bacterial antigens that triggered immune-complex nephritis. Renal function usually normalizes smoothly once infection has been controlled, but recovery may take weeks or months. In a few cases creatinine clearance worsens for a time despite effective antibacterial treatment, perhaps reflecting persistence of bacterial antigen in vegetations after bacteriologic cure. Some patients with septicemia, shock, or disseminated intravascular coagulation associated with ABE develop acute renal failure and require dialysis as part of their intensive care.

Mycotic Aneurysm

This complication is diagnosed in less than 5 percent of patients with infective endocarditis, but the local consequences of expansion and rupture can be very serious, especially in the brain (see also Chap. 122).[187–189]

Small aneurysms sometimes will resolve spontaneously after antibiotic therapy. Once they grow larger than 1 to 2 cm in diameter, resolution is unlikely; the aneurysm enlarges and eventually ruptures despite eradication of the etiologic bacteria. Surgery is indicated for accessible aneurysms before this can occur.

Intracerebral aneurysms pose a much more difficult therapeutic dilemma because they are often multiple and relatively inaccessible. Large aneurysms or aneurysms that have bled intracranially should be clipped if possible. An individualized decision must be made on whether or not to operate for smaller aneurysms that have not leaked or ruptured.

THE PROBLEM OF PROPHYLAXIS

Because bacteremias occur during dental or other surgical procedures,[233–235] prophylactic antibiotics are frequently given to susceptible patients in an attempt to prevent bacterial endocarditis. Although prevention of such a serious infection is obviously desirable, many relevant questions remain unanswered. These include:

- Is antibiotic prophylaxis effective?
- What is the risk of developing bacterial endocarditis after an episode of bacteremia?
- Which operations and diagnostic procedures should be covered?
- Which patients should receive antibiotics?
- What antibiotic regimens will be most effective?

Although the risk of infection has not been quantitated, it is sufficiently low that most of these questions probably cannot be answered by clinical trials; the number of susceptible patients required to provide significant results would be far too large.[230]

Less than one in five cases of SBE and even fewer cases of ABE follow identifiable medical procedures that cause transient bacteremias[38,233,234]; therefore, the proportion of cases that is potentially preventable by antibiotics is small. However, because endocarditis causes serious morbidity and mortality, prevention of even a few cases could be worthwhile. For this reason, currently accepted standards of practice require that an antibiotic regimen be administered before certain dental and surgical procedures to patients with known heart lesions that pose a significant risk of endocarditis.

Since several hundred cases of streptococcal endocarditis following dental and genitourinary tract procedures have been recorded, the causative role of these procedures may be regarded as fairly well established.[233,234] A rather short "incubation period" for endocarditis is typical, in that most of these patients noticed symptoms within 2 weeks of the procedure.[172] However, it should be emphasized that the link between a case of endocarditis and a recent procedure causing bacteremia cannot be proved, because the infection could have been caused by one of the transient, asymptomatic, low-grade bacteremias which occur very commonly, induced by everyday events such as chewing and cleaning the teeth.[233]

In the absence of specific information, empirical recommendations[137,236,237] for prophylasix of bacterial endocarditis must be made on the basis of indirect information. This information includes the reported frequency of bacteremia after various procedures (Table 94-8); the relative risk posed by the patient's cardiac lesion (Table 94-2); case reports of prophylaxis failures[58]; in vitro susceptibility studies on the relevant organisms, especially streptococci; and experimental studies in laboratory animals.[168]

For the individual patient, the decision to administer prophylaxis should be made by assessing two main factors: the risk posed by the preexisting cardiac lesion and the risk posed by the procedure that might cause bacteremia. For example, if a patient with a prosthetic valve undergoes prostatic resection, antibiotic prophylaxis should be given because both factors present a significant risk of endocarditis. On the other hand, if a patient with mitral valve prolapse is scheduled for gastroscopy, prophylaxis is not necessary because the risk for endocarditis in this setting is very low.[235] Obviously, such risk assessments may be inaccurate; in many situations undertainties inevitably will remain. To meet a reasonable standard of care, the health care professional should (1) know of the patient's cardiac lesion, (2) inform the patient or guardian that a small risk of endocarditis exists, and (3) then make a reasoned decision as to whether or not to give prophylaxis along the lines described above. The patient's and the physician's preferences may influence the final decision.

Attempted prophylaxis does not always succeed. Of 52 cases of apparent prophylaxis failure in one series, 42 involved patients with heart disease who received oral

TABLE 94-8

Incidence of Transient Bacteremia after Various Dental, Surgical, or Diagnostic Procedures

Procedure	%
Extraction of one or more teeth	82
Periodontal surgery	88
Brushing teeth	40
Tonsillectomy	38
Esophageal dilatation	45
Catheter removal after urologic surgery	50
Prostatectomy (sterile urine)	11
Prostatectomy (infected urine)	57
Normal delivery	4–11
Diagnostic procedures	
Bronchoscopy	15
Barium enema	10
Liver biopsy	10
Upper gastrointestinal endoscopy	4
Sigmoidoscopy	0–5
Colonoscopy	5

SOURCE: Adapted from Refs. 233–235 and from DT Durack: Prophylaxis of infective endocarditis. In: GL Mandell, RG Douglas, JE Bennett (eds): *Principles and Practice of Infectious Diseases*. New York, Wiley, 1979: 701. Copyright 1979, John Wiley & Sons. Reproduced with permission from John Wiley & Sons, editor, and author.

TABLE 94-9

Suggested Regimens for Prophylaxis of Infective Endocarditis*

Standard Regimen	
For dental procedures and oral or upper respiratory tract surgery	Amoxicillin 3.0 g orally 1 h before, then 1.5 g 6 h later†
Special Regimens	
Parenteral regimen for high-risk patients; also for gastrointestinal (GI) or genitourinary (GU) tract procedures	Ampicillin 2.0 g IM or IV *plus* gentamicin 1.5 mg/kg IM or IV, 0.5 h before†
Parenteral regimen for penicillin-allergic patients	Vancomycin 1.0 g IV *slowly* over 1 h, starting 1 h before; *add* gentamicin 1.5 mg/kg IM or IV if GI or GU tract involved†
Oral regimen for penicillin-allergic patients (oral and respiratory tract only)	Erythromycin 1.0 g orally 1 h before, then 0.5 g 6 h later†
Oral regimen for minor GI or GU tract procedures	Amoxicillin 3.0 g orally 1 h before, then 1.5 g 6 h later†
Parenteral regimen for cardiac surgery including valve replacement	Cefazolin 2.0 g IV on induction of anesthesia, repeated 8 and 16 h later‡ *or* Vancomycin 1.0 g IV *slowly* over 1 h starting on induction of anesthesia, then 0.5 g IV 8 and 16 h later‡

* Note that (1) these regimens are empirical suggestions, no regimen has been proved effective for prevention of endocarditis, and prevention failures may occur with any regimen; (2) these regimens are not intended to cover all clinical situations, and the practitioner should use his or her own judgment on safety and cost-benefit issues in each individual case; (3) one or two additional doses may be given if the period of risk for bacteremia is prolonged.

† Pediatric dosages: ampicillin 50 mg/kg; erythromycin 20 mg/kg for first dose, then 10 mg/kg; gentamicin 2 mg/kg; amoxicillin: for children who weigh more than 60 lb, use same as for adults; for children less than 60 lb, use one-half the adult dose; vancomycin 20 mg/kg.

‡ Vancomycin is preferred if *Staph. epidermidis* is an important cause of postoperative infection in that hospital. Gentamicin 1.5 mg/kg IV or IM may be added to each dose, only if postoperative gram-negative infections have occurred with significant frequency.

SOURCE: DT Durack: Nine controversies in the management of infective endocarditis. In RG Petersdorf et al. (eds): *Update V: Harrison's Principles of Internal Medicine*, New York, McGraw-Hill, 1984: 35; and Committee on Rheumatic Fever, Endocarditis, and Kawasaki Disease of the Council on Cardiovascular Disease in the Young of the American Heart Association: Prevention of bacterial endocarditis. *JAMA* 264:2919–2922, 1990. Adapted and reproduced with permission of the publisher and author.

penicillin or erythromycin, usually to cover dental procedures.[58]

Common errors in attempted prevention of endocarditis are starting antibiotics too early, continuing too long, using low doses, covering tooth extractions but not lesser dental procedures, and confusing prevention of rheumatic fever (requiring long-term, low-dose antimicrobial drugs) with prevention of endocarditis (short-term, high-dose).[137]

On the basis of present information, prophylaxis is probably *not* necessary for minor dental procedures that do not involve the gums, such as simple fillings above the gum line and adjustment of orthodontic appliances. When a dentist cleans and scales the teeth, however, the gums are always involved, and susceptible patients should receive a prophylactic antibiotic regimen.[236]

In the absence of pelvic infection, prophylaxis for endocarditis in patients with heart lesions is probably not required to cover normal delivery, therapeutic abortion, dilation and curettage, and insertion or removal of intrauterine contraceptive devices. Similarly, antibiotics need not be given before many common procedures, such as cardiac catheterization, insertion of temporary pacemakers, endotracheal intubation, bronchoscopy, endoscopy, or radiographic contrast studies of the upper and lower gastrointestinal tract. However, some physicians choose to cover even these low-risk procedures in patients with prosthetic valves because they are at higher risk for endocarditis than patients with native valves. Specific regimens suggested for prophylaxis of endocarditis are listed in Table 94-9.

Cardiac surgeons currently administer antibiotics to virtually all patients undergoing cardiac surgery, attempting to prevent both wound infections and endocarditis. This practice is rational and traditional, but as with prophylaxis of endocarditis in other settings, its efficacy has not been conclusively proved.[137,238,239] Current recommendations call for parenteral administration of an antistaphylococcal antibiotic just prior to operation and continuation for one or two further doses (Table 94-9). The regimen may be modified if local experience shows that cases of early PVE caused by *Staph. epidermidis* or gram-negative bacilli have occurred with significant frequency (Table 94-9).

REFERENCES

1. Blumer G: Subacute bacterial endocarditis. *Medicine* 1923; 2:105–170.
2. Thayer WS: Studies on bacterial (infective) endocarditis. *Johns Hopkins Hosp Rep* 1926; 22:1–185.
3. Kerr A Jr: *Subacute Bacterial Endocarditis*. Springfield, IL, Charles C Thomas, 1955.

4. Hermans PE: The clinical manifestations of infective endocarditis. *Mayo Clin Proc* 1982; 57:15–21.
5. Chambers HF, Korzeniowski OM, Sande MA, National Collaborative Endocarditis Study Group: *Staphylococcus aureus* endocarditis: Clinical manifestations in addicts and nonaddicts. *Medicine* 1983; 62:170–177.
6. Arnett EN, Roberts WC: Pathology of active infective endocarditis: A necropsy analysis of 192 patients. *Thorac Cardiovasc Surg* 1982; 30:327–335.
7. Korzeniowski OM, Kaye D: Infective endocarditis. In: Braunwald E (ed): *Heart Disease: A Textbook of Cardiovascular Medicine*. Philadelphia, Saunders, 1992:1078–1105.
8. Baumgartner WA, Miller DC, Reitz BA, Oyer PE, Jamieson SW, Stinson EB, et al: Surgical treatment of prosthetic valve endocarditis. *Ann Thorac Surg* 1983; 35:87–104.
9. Wilson WR. Danielson GK, Guiliani ER, Geraci JE: Prosthetic valve endocarditis. *Mayo Clin Proc* 1982; 57:155–161.
10. Ivert TSA, Dismukes WE, Cobbs CG, Blackstone EH, Kirklin JW, Bergdahl LA: Prosthetic valve endocarditis. *Circulation* 1984; 69:223–232.
11. MacDonald RA, Robbins SL: The significance of nonbacterial thrombotic endocarditis: An autopsy and clinical study of 78 cases. *Ann Intern Med* 1957; 46:255–273.
12. Barry WE, Scarpelli D: Nonbacterial thrombotic endocarditis. *Arch Intern Med* 1962; 109:151–156.
13. Bryan CS: Nonbacterial thrombotic endocarditis in patients with malignant tumors. *Am J Med* 1969; 46:787–793.
14. Major RH: Notes on the history of endocarditis. *Bull Hist Med* 1945; 17:351–359.
15. Pruitt RD: William Osler and his Goulstonian lectures on malignant endocarditis. *Mayo Clin Proc* 1982; 57:4–9.
16. Osler W: The Goulstonian lectures on malignant endocarditis. *Br Med J* 1985; 1:467–470, 522–526, 577–579.
17. Horder T: Infective endocarditis, with an analysis of 150 cases and with special reference to the chronic form of the disease. *Q J Med* 1909; 2:289–329.
18. Allen A: Nature of vegetations of bacterial endocarditis. *Arch Pathol* 1939; 27:661–671.
19. Libman E, Friedberg CK: *Subacute Bacterial Endocarditis*. Oxford, Oxford University Press, 1941.
20. Beeson PB, Brannon ES, Warren JV: Observations on the sites of removal of bacteria from the blood in patients with bacterial endocarditis. *J Exp Med* 1945; 81:9–23.
21. Dawson MH, Hunter TH: The treatment of subacute bacterial endocarditis with penicillin. *JAMA* 1945; 127:129–137.
22. Abraham EP, Chain E, Fletcher CM, et al: further observations on penicillin. *Lancet* 1941; 2:177–189.
23. Durack DT: Review of early experience in treatment of bacterial endocarditis, 1940–1955. In: Bisno AL (ed): *Infective Endocarditis*. New York, Grune & Stratton, 1981: 1–14.
24. Loewe L, Rosenblatt P, Greene H, et al: Combined penicillin and heparin therapy of subacute bacterial endocarditis: Report of seven consecutive successfully treated patients. *JAMA* 1944; 124:144–149.
25. Galbreath WR, Hull E: Sulfonamide therapy of bacterial endocarditis. *Ann Intern Med* 1943; 18:201–203.
26. Bloomfield AL, Armstrong CD, Kirby WMM: the treatment of subacute bacterial endocarditis with penicillin. *J Clin Invest* 24:251–267.
27. Hunter TH: the treatment of some bacterial infections of the heart and pericardium. *Bull N Y Acad Med* 1952; 28:213–228.
28. Finland M: Treatment of bacterial endocarditis. *N Engl J Med* 1954; 250:372–383.
29. Geraci JE: The antibiotic therapy of bacterial endocarditis: Therapeutic data on 172 patients seen from 1951 through 1957: Additional observations on short-term therapy (two weeks) for penicillin-sensitive streptococcal endocarditis. *Med Clin North Am* 1958; 42:1101–1148.
30. Weinstein L, Schlesinger J: Treatment of infective endocarditis. *Prog Cardiovasc Dis* 1973; 16:275–296.
31. Wallace AG, Young G Jr, Osterhout S: Treatment of acute bacterial endocarditis by valve excision and replacement. *Circulation* 1965; 31:450–453.
32. Kaye D, McCormack RC, Hook EW: Bacterial endocarditis: The changing pattern since the introduction of penicillin therapy. *Antimicrob Agents Chemother* 1961; 37–46.
33. Uwaydah MM, Weinberg AN: Bacterial endocarditis: A changing pattern. *N Engl J Med* 1965; 273:1231–1234.
34. Lerner PI, Weinstein L: Infective endocarditis in the antibiotic era. *N Engl J Med* 1966; 274:199–206; 259–266; 323–331; 388–393.
35. Finland M, Barnes NW: Changing etiology of bacterial endocarditis in the antibacterial era: Experiences at Boston City Hospital. *Ann Intern Med* 1970; 72:341–348.
36. Garvey GJ, Neu HC: Infective endocarditis—an evolving disease: A review of endocarditis at the Columbia-Presbyterian Medical Center, 1968–1973. *Medicine* 1978; 57:105–127.
37. Durack DT, Petersdorf RG: Changes in the epidemiology of endocarditis. In: Kaplan EL, Taranta AV (eds): *Infective Endocarditis*. AHA Monograph no. 52. Dallas, American Heart Association, 1977: 3–8.
38. Bayliss R, Clarke C, Oakley C, Somerville W, Whitfield AG: The teeth and infective endocarditis. *Br Heart J* 1983; 50:506–512.
39. Bayliss R, Clarke C, Oakley CM, Somerville W, Whitfield AG, Young SE: The microbiology and pathogenesis of infective endocarditis. *Br Heart J*. 1983; 50:513–519.
40. Bayliss R, Clarke C, Oakley C, Somerville W: The bowel, the genitourinary tract, and infective endocarditis. *Br Heart J* 1983; 51:339–345.
41. Baddour LM: Twelve-year review of recurrent native-valve infective endocarditis: A disease of the modern antibiotic era. *Rev Infect Dis* 1988; 10:1163–1170.
42. Ries K: Endocarditis in the elderly. In: Kaye D (ed): *Infective Endocarditis*. Baltimore, University Park Press, 1977: 143–154.
43. Weinstein L, Rubin RH: Infective endocarditis: 1973. *Prog Cardiovasc Dis* 1973; 16:239–274.
44. Kaye D: Definitions and demographic characteristics. In: Kaye D (ed): *Infective Endocarditis*. Baltimore, University Park Press, 1977:1–8.
45. Johnson DH, Rosenthal A, Nadas AS: A forty-year review of bacterial endocarditis in infancy and childhood. *Circulation* 1975; 51:581–587.
46. Rosenthal A, Nadas AS: Infective endocarditis in infancy and childhood. In: Rahimtoola SH (ed): *Infective Endocarditis*. New York, Grune & Stratton, 1978: 149–178.
47. Johnson CM, Rhodes KH: Pediatric endocarditis. *Mayo Clin Proc* 1982; 57:86–94.
48. El-Khatib MR, Wilson FM, Lerner AM: Characteristics of bacterial endocarditis in heroin addicts in Detroit. *Am J Med Sci* 1976; 271:197–201.
49. Stimmel B, Dack S: Infective endocarditis in narcotic addicts. In: Rahimtoola SH (ed): *Infective Endocarditis*. New York, Grune & Stratton, 1978: 195–209.
50. Reisberg BE: Infective endocarditis in the narcotic addict. *Prog Cardiovasc Dis* 1979; 22:193–204.
51. Cannon NJ, Cobbs CG: Infective endocarditis in drug addicts. in: Kaye D (ed): *Infective Endocarditis*. Baltimore, University Park Press, 1977: 111–127.
52. Dressler FA, Roberts WC: Infective endocarditis in opiate addicts: Analysis of 80 cases studied at necropsy. *Am J Cardiol* 1989; 63:1240–1257.
53. Pelletier LL, Petersdorf RG: Infective endocarditis: A review of 125 cases from the University of Washington Hospitals, 1963–72. *Medicine* 1977; 56:287–313.
54. Kaplan EL, Rich H, Gersony W, Manning J: A collaborative study of infective endocarditis in the 1970s: Emphasis on infections in patients who have undergone cardiovascular surgery. *Circulation* 1979; 59:327–335.
55. Corrigall D, Bolen J, Hancock EW, Popp RL: Mitral valve prolapse and infective endocarditis. *Am J Med* 1977; 63:215–222.
56. Clemens JD, Horwitz RI, Jaffe CC, Feinstein AR, Stanton BF: A controlled evaluation of the risk of bacterial endocarditis in persons with mitral-valve prolapse. *N Engl J Med* 1982; 307:776–781.
57. Beton DC, Brear SG, Edwards JD, Leonard JC: Mitral valve prolapse: An assessment of clinical features, associated conditions and prognosis. *Q J Med* 1983; 52:150–164.
58. Durack DT, Kaplan EL, Bisno AL: Apparent failure of endocarditis prophylaxis: Analysis of 52 cases submitted to a national registry. *JAMA* 1983; 250:2318–2322.
59. Clemens JD, Ransohoff DF: A quantitative assessment of predental antibiotic prophylaxis for patients with mitral-valve prolapse. *J Chronic Dis* 1984; 37:531–544.
60. Devereux RB, Hawkins I, Kramer-Fox R, Lutas EM, Hammond IW, Spitzer MD, et al: Complications of mitral valve prolapse:

Disproportionate occurrence in men and older patients. *Am J Med* 1986; 81:751–758.
61. MacMahon SW, Hickey AJ, Wilcken DEL, Wittes JT, Feneley MP, Hickie JB: Risk of infective endocarditis in mitral valve prolapse with and without precordial systolic murmurs. *Am J Cardiol* 1986; 58:105–108.
62. Wang K, Gobel FL, Gleason DF: Bacterial endocarditis in idiopathic hypertrophic subaortic stenosis. *Am Heart* 1975; 89:359–365.
63. Tuazon CU, Sheagren JN: Increased rate of carriage of *Staphylococcus aureus* among narcotic addicts. *J Infect Dis* 1974; 129:725–727.
64. Reyes MP, Lerner AM: Current problems in the treatment of infective endocarditis due to *Pseudomonas aeruginosa. Rev Infect Dis* 1983; 5:314–321.
65. Cohen PS, Maguire HJ, Weinstein L: Infective endocarditis caused by gram-negative bacteria: A review of the literature, 1945–1977. *Prog Cardiovasc Dis* 1980; 22:205–242.
66. McLeod R, Remington JS: Fungal endocarditis. In: Rahimtoola SH (ed): *Infective Endocarditis.* New York, Grune & Stratton, 1978: 211–290.
67. Rubinstein E, Noriega ER, Simberkoff MS, Holzman R, Rahal JJ: Fungal endocarditis: Analysis of 24 cases and review of the literature. *Medicine* 1975; 54:331–344.
68. Saravolatz LD, Burch KH, Quinn EL, Cox F, Madhavan T, Fisher E: Polymicrobial infective endocarditis: An increasing clinical entity. *Am Heart J* 1978; 95:163–168.
69. Keys TF, Hewitt WL: Endocarditis due to micrococci and *Staphylococcus epidermidis. Arch Intern Med* 1973; 132:216–220.
70. Felner JM, Dowell VR: Anacrobic bacterial endocarditis. *N Engl J Med* 1970; 283: 1188–1192.
71. Scheld WM, Sande MA: Endocarditis and intravascular infections. In: Mandell GL, Douglas RG, Bennett JE (eds): *Principles and Practice of Infectious Diseases.* 3d ed. New York, Wiley, 1990: 670–706.
72. Resnekov L: Staphylococcal endocarditis following mitral valvotomy, with special reference to coagulase-negative *Staphylococcus albus. Lancet* 1959; 2:597–600.
73. Kloster FE: Infective prosthetic valve endocarditis. In: Rahimtoola SH (ed): *Infective Endocarditis.* New York, Grune & Stratton, 1978: 291–305.
74. Watanakunakorn C: Prosthetic valve infective endocarditis. *Prog Cardiovasc Dis* 1979; 22:181–192.
75. Frater RWM, Santos GH: Sources of infection in open heart surgery. *NY State J Med* 1974; 74:2386.
76. Karchmer AW, Dismukes WE, Buckley MJ, Austen WG: Late prosthetic valve endocarditis: Clinical features influencing therapy. *Am J Med* 1978; 64:199–206.
77. Rossiter SJ, Stinson EB, Oyer PE, Miller DC, Schapira JN, Martin RP et al: Prosthetic valve endocarditis: Comparison of heterograft tissue valves and mechanical valves. *J Thorac Cardiovasc Surg* 1978; 76:795–803.
78. Mendelsohn G, Hutchins GM: Infective endocarditis during the first decade of life. *Am J Dis Child* 1979; 133:619–622.
79. Stinson EB: Surgical treatment of infective endocarditis. *Prog Cardiovasc Dis* 1979; 22:145–168.
80. Jung JY, Saab SB, Almond CH: The case for early surgical treatment of left-sided primary infective endocarditis: A collective review. *J Thorac Cardiovasc Surg* 1975; 70:509–518.
81. Seaworth BJ, Durack DT: Infective endocarditis in obstetric and gynecologic practice. *Am J Obstet Gynecol* 1986; 154:180–188.
82. Sugrue D, Blake S, Troy P, MacDonald D: Antibiotic prophylaxis against infective endocarditis after normal delivery: Is it necessary? *Br Heart* 1980; 44:499–502.
83. Cobbs CG: IUD and endocarditis. *Ann Intern Med* 1973; 78:451.
84. von Reyn CF, Levy BS, Arbeit RD, Friedland G, Crumpacker CS: Infective endocarditis: An analysis based on strict case definitions. *Ann Intern Med* 1981; 94:505–518.
85. Ehric M, Morgan AP, Moore FD, O'Connor NE: Endocarditis with the indwelling balloon-tipped pulmonary artery catheter in burn patients. *J Trauma* 1978; 18:664–666.
86. Rowley KM, Clubb KS, Walker Smith GJ, Cabin HS: Right-sided infective endocarditis as a consequence of flow-directed pulmonary-artery catheterization: A clinicopathologic study of 55 autopsied patients. *N Engl J Med* 1984; 311:1152–1156.
87. Martino P, Micozzi A, Venditti M, Gentile G, Girmenia C, Raccah R et al: Catheter-related right-sided endocarditis in bone marrow transplant recipients. *Rev Infect Dis* 1990; 12:250–257.
88. Khoo DE, Zebro TJ, English TAH: Bacterial endocarditis in a transplanted heart. *Pathol Res Pract* 1989; 185:445–447.
89. Lillehei CW, Bobb JRR, Visscher MB: The occurrence of endocarditis with valvular deformities in dogs with arteriovenous fistulas. *Ann Surg* 1950; 132:577–590.
90. Cross AS, Steigbigel RT: Infective endocarditis and access site infections in patients on hemodialysis. *Medicine* 1976; 55:453–466.
91. Brennan RO, Durack DT: The viridans streptococci in perspective. In: Remington JS, Swartz MN (eds): *Current Clinical Topics in Infectious Diseases*, vol 5. New York, McGraw-Hill, 1984: 253–289.
92. Facklam RR: Physiological differentiation of viridans streptococci. *J Clin Microbiol* 1977; 5:184–201.
93. Harder EJ, Wilkowske CJ, Washington JA III, Geraci JE: *Streptococcus mutans* endocarditis. *Ann Intern Med* 1974; 80:364–368.
94. Malacoff RF, Frank E, Andriole VT: Streptococcal endocarditis (nonenterococcal, non-group A). *JAMA* 1979; 241:1807–1810.
95. Carey RB, Gross KC, Roberts RB: Vitamin B_6-dependent *Streptococcus mitior (mitis)* isolated from patients with systemic infections. *J Infect Dis* 1975; 131:722–726.
96. Ellner JJ, Rosenthal MS, Lerner PI, McHenry MC: Infective endocarditis caused by slow-growing, fastidious, gram-negative bacteria. *Medicine* 1979; 58:145–158.
97. Washington JA II: the role of the microbiology laboratory in the diagnosis and antimicrobial treatment of infective endocarditis. *Mayo Clin Proc* 1982; 57:22–32.
98. Roberts WC: Characteristics and consequences of infective endocarditis (active or healed or both) learned from morphologic studies. In: Rahimtoola SH (ed): *Infective Endocarditis.* New York, Grune & Stratton, 1978: 55–123.
99. Moellering RC Jr, Watson BK, Kunz LJ: Endocarditis due to group D streptococci: Comparison of disease caused by *Streptococcus bovis* with that produced by the enterococci. *Am J Med* 1974; 57:239–250.
100. Mandell GL: Enterococcal endocarditis. In: Kaye D (ed): *Infective Endocarditis.* Baltimore, University Park Press, 1977: 101–110.
101. Wilson WR, Wilkowske CJ, Wright AJ, Sande MA, Geraci JE: Treatment of streptomycin-susceptible and streptomycin-resistant enterococcal endocarditis. *Ann Intern Med* 1984; 100:816–823.
102. Levy BS, von Reyn CF, Arbeit RD, Friedland J, Crumpacker C: More on *S. bovis* and bowel carcinoma. *N Engl J Med* 1978; 298:572–573.
103. Murray HW, Roberts RB: *Streptococcus bovis* bacteremia and underlying gastrointestinal disease. *Arch Intern Med* 1978; 138:1097–1099.
104. Klein RS, Catalano MT, Edberg SC, Casey JI, Steigbigel NH: *Streptococcus bovis* septicemia and carcinoma of the colon. *Ann Intern Med* 1979; 91:560–562.
105. Maki DG, Agger WA: Enterococcal bacteremia: Clinical features, the risk of endocarditis, and management. *Medicine* 1988; 67:248–269.
106. Murray BE: The life and times of the enterococcus. *Clin Microbiol Rev* 1990; 3:46–65.
107. Strauss AL, Hamburger M: Pneumococcal endocarditis in the penicillin era. *Arch Intern Med* 1966; 118:190–198.
108. Bruyn GAW, Thompson J, Van Der Meer JWM: Pneumococcal endocarditis in adult patients: A report of five cases and review of the literature. *Q J Med* 1990; 74:33–40.
109. Pankey GA: Acute bacterial endocarditis at the University of Minnesota Hospitals, 1939–1959. *Am Heart J* 1962; 64:583–591.
110. Watanakunakorn C, Tan JS, Phair JP: Some salient features of *Staphylococcus aureus* endocarditis. *Am J Med* 1973; 54:473–481.
111. Bayer AS, Lam K, Gintzon L, Norman DC, Chiu C-Y, Ward JI: *Staphylococcus aureus* bacteremia: Clinical, serologic, and echocardiographic findings in patients with and without endocarditis. *Arch Intern Med* 1987; 147:457–462.
112. Karchmer AW, Archer GL, Dismukes WE: *Staphylococcus epidermidis* causing prosthetic valve endocarditis: Microbiologic and clinical observations as guides to therapy. *Ann Intern Med* 1984; 98:447–455.
113. Levine DP, Fromm BS, Reddy BR: Slow response to vancomycin or vancomycin plus rifampin in methicillin-resistant *Staphylococcus aureus* endocarditis. *Ann Intern Med* 1991; 115: 674–741.

114. Gould K, Ramirez-Ronda CH, Holmes RK, Sanford JP: Adherence of bacteria to heart valves *in vitro*. *J Clin Invest* 1975; 56:1364–1370.
115. Holmes RK, Ramirez-Ronda CH: Adherence of bacteria to the endothelium of heart valves. In: Kaplan EL, Taranta AV (eds): *Infective Endocarditis*. AHA Monograph no. 52. Dallas, American Heart Association, 1977: 12–13.
116. Scheld WM, Valone JA, Sande MA: Bacterial adherence in the pathogenesis of endocarditis: Interaction of bacterial dextran, platelets and fibrin. *J Clin Invest* 1978; 61:1394–1404.
117. Durack DT, Beeson PB: Protective role of complement in experimental *E coli* endocarditis. *Infect Immun* 1977; 16:213–217.
118. Al-Kasab S, Al-Fagih MR, Al-Yousef S, Ali Khan MA, Ribeiro PA, Nazzal S, et al: *Brucella* infective endocarditis: Successful combined medical and surgical therapy. *J Thorac Cardiovasc Surg* 1988; 95:862–867.
119. Kaye D: Infecting microorganisms. In: Kaye D (ed): *Infective Endocarditis* Baltimore, University Park Press, 1977: 43–54.
120. Geraci JE, Wilson WR: Endocarditis due to gram-negative bacteria: Report of 56 cases. *Mayo Clin Proc* 1982; 57:145–148.
121. Jemsek JG, Greenberg SB, Gentry LO, Welton DE, Mattox KL: *Haemophilus parainfluenzae* endocarditis: Two cases and review of the literature in the past decade. *Am J Med* 1979; 66:51–57.
122. Rubinstein E, Noriega ER, Simberkoff MS, Holzman R, Rahal JJ Jr: Fungal endocarditis: Analysis of 24 cases and review of the literature. *Medicine* 1975; 54:331–344.
123. Kammer RB, Utz JP: *Aspergillus* species endocarditis: The new face of a not so rare disease. *Am J Med* 1974; 56:506–521.
124. Cannady PB Jr, Sanford JP: Negative blood cultures in infective endocarditis: A review. *South Med J* 1976; 69:1420–1424.
125. Pesanti EL, Smith IB: Infective endocarditis with negative blood cultures: An analysis of 52 cases. *Am J Med* 1979; 66:43–50.
126. Van Scoy RE: Culture-negative endocarditis. *Mayo Clin Proc* 1982; 57:149–154.
127. Wainwright J: Tuberculous endocarditis: A report of 2 cases. *S Afri Med J* 1979; 56:731–733.
128. Turck WPG, Howitt G, Turnberg LA, Fox H, Longson M, Matthews MB et al: Chronic Q fever. *Q J Med* 1976; 45:193–217.
129. Wilson HG, Neilson GH, Galea EG, Stafford G, O'Brien MF: Q Fever endocarditis in Queensland. *Circulation* 1976; 53:680–684.
130. Kimbrough RC, Ormsbee RA, Peacock M, Rogers WR, Bennetts RW, Raaf J et al: Q Fever endocarditis in the United States. *Ann Intern Med* 1979; 91:400–402.
131. Spelman DW: Q fever: A study of 111 consecutive cases. *Med J Aust* 1982; 1:547–553.
132. Varma MPS, Adgey AAJ, Connolly JH: Chronic Q fever endocarditis. *Br Heart J* 1980; 43:695–699.
133. Ward C, Ward AM: Acquired valvular heart-disease in patients who keep pet birds. *Lancet* 1974; 2:734–736.
134. Van der Bel-Kahn JM, Watanakunakorn C, Menefee MG, Long HO, Dicter R: *Chlamydia trachomatis* endocarditis. *Am Heart J* 1978; 95:627–636.
135. Cohen JI, Sloss LJ, Kundsin R, Golightly L: Prosthetic valve endocarditis caused by *Mycoplasma hominis*. *Am J Med* 1989; 86:819–821.
136. Tompkins LS, Roessler BJ, Redd SC: *Legionella* prosthetic-valve endocarditis. *N Engl J Med* 1988; 318:530–534.
137. Durack DT: Prophylaxis of infective endocarditis. In: Mandell GL, Douglas RG, Bennett JE (eds): *Principles and Practice of Infectious Diseases*. 3d ed. New York, Wiley, 1984: 716–721.
138. Angrist A, Oka M, Nakao K: Vegetative endocarditis. *Pathol Ann* 1967; 2:155–212.
139. Grant RT, Wood JE Jr, Jones TD: Heart valve irregularities in relation to subacute bacterial endocarditis. *Heart* 1927; 14:247–261.
140. Durack DT: Experimental bacterial endocarditis: 4. Structure and evolution of very early lesions. *J Pathol* 1975; 115:81–89.
141. Durack DT, Beeson PB: Experimental bacterial endocarditis: 1. Colonization of a sterile vegetation. *Br J Exp Pathol* 1972; 53:44–49.
142. Van Ginkel CJW, Thorig L, Thompson J, Oh JI, van Aken WG: Enhancement of generation of monocyte tissue thromboplastin by bacterial phagocytosis: Possible pathway for fibrin formation on infected vegetations in bacterial endocarditis. *Infect Immun* 1979; 5:388–395.
143. Lepeschkin E: On the relation between the site of valvular involvement in endocarditis and the blood pressure resting on the valve. *Am J Med Sci* 1952; 224:318–319.
144. Rodbard S: Blood velocity and endocarditis. *Circulation* 1963; 27:18–28.
145. Edwards JE Jr, Burchell HB: Endocardial and intimal lesions (jet impact) as possible sites of origin of murmurs. *Circulation* 1958; 18:946–960.
146. Buchbinder NA, Roberts WC: Left-sided valvular active infective endocarditis: A study of forty-five necropsy patients. *Am J Med* 1972; 53:20–35.
147. Roberts WC: Characteristics and consequences of infective endocarditis (active or healed or both) learned from morphologic studies. In: Rahimtoola SH (ed): *Infective Endocarditis*. New York, Grune & Stratton, 1978: 55–123.
148. Phair JP, Clarke J: Immunology of infective endocarditis. *Prog Cardiovasc Dis* 1977; 22:137–144.
149. Williams RC, Kunkel HG: Rheumatoid factor, complement and conglutinin aberrations in patients with subacute bacterial endocarditis. *J Clin Invest* 1962; 41:666–675.
150. Messner RP, Laxdal T, Quie PG, Williams RC Jr: Rheumatoid factor in subacute bacterial endocarditis: Bacterium, duration of disease or genetic predisposition? *Ann Intern Med* 1968; 68: 746–756.
151. Sheagren JN, Tuazon CU, Griffin C, Padmore N: Rheumatoid factor in acute bacterial endocarditis. *Arthritis Rheum* 1976; 19:887–890.
152. Maisch B, Eichstadt H, Kochsick K: Immune reactions in infective endocarditis: 1. Clinical data and diagnostic relevance of antimyocardial antibodies. *Am Heart J* 1984; 106:329–337.
153. Weinstein L, Schlesinger JJ: Pathoanatomic, pathophysiologic, and clinical correlations in endocarditis. *N Engl J Med* 1974; 291:832–837.
154. Wadsworth AB: A study of the endocardial lesions developing during pneumococcus infection in horses. *J Med Res* 1919; 34:279–291.
155. Mair W: Pneumococcal endocarditis in rabbits. *J Pathol Bacteriol* 1923; 26:426–428.
156. Durack DT, Gilliland BG, Petersdorf RG: Effect of immunization on susceptibility to experimental *Streptococcus mutans* and *Streptococcus sanguis* endocarditis. *Infect Immun* 1978; 22: 52–56.
157. Durack DT, Beeson PB: Pathogenesis of infective endocarditis. In: Rahimtoola SH (ed): *Infective Endocarditis*. New York, Grune & Stratton, 1978: 1–53.
158. Bayer AS, Theofilopoulos AN, Eisenberg R, Dixon FJ, Guze LB: Circulating immune complexes in infective endocarditis. *N Engl J Med* 1976; 295:1500–1505.
159. Bayer AS, Theofilopoulos AN, Tillman DB, Dixon FJ, Guze LB: Use of circulating immune complex levels in the serodifferentiation of endocarditis and nonendocarditis septicemias. *Am J Med* 1979; 66:58–62.
160. Maisch B, Mayer E, Schubert U, Berg PA, Kochsiek K: Immune reactions in infective endocarditis: 2. Relevance of circulating immune complexes, serum inhibition factors, lymphocytotoxic reactions, and antibody-dependent cellular cytotoxicity in endocarditis. *Am Heart J* 1984; 106:338–344.
161. Cabane J, Godeau P, Hereeman A, Acar J, Digeon M, Bach JF: Fate of circulating immune complexes in infective endocarditis. *Am J Med* 1979; 66:277–282.
162. Gutman RA, Striker GE, Gilliland BC, Cutler RE: The immune complex glomerulonephritis of bacterial endocarditis. *Medicine* 1972; 51:1–25.
163. Levy RL, Hong R: The immune nature of subacute bacterial endocarditis (SBE) nephritis. *Am J Med* 1973; 64:645–652.
164. Wilson JW, Houghton DC, Bennett WM, Porter GA: The kidney and infective endocarditis. In: Rahimtoola SH (ed): *Infective Endocarditis*. New York, Grune & Stratton, 1978: 179–194.
165. Crowder JG, White A: Teichoic acid antibodies in staphylococcal and nonstaphylococcal endocarditis. *Ann Intern Med* 1972; 77:87–90.
166. Nagel JG, Tuazon CU, Cardella TA: Teichoic acid serologic diagnosis of staphylococcal endocarditis: Use of gel diffusion and counter-immunoelectrophoretic methods. *Ann Intern Med* 1975; 82:13–17.
167. Freedman LR, Valone J Jr: Experimental infective endocarditis. *Prog Cardiovasc Dis* 1979; 22:169–180.
168. Durack DT: Experience with prevention of experimental endocarditis. In: Kaplan EL, Taranta AV (eds): *Infective Endocarditis*.

AHA Monograph no 52. Dallas, American Heart Association, 1977: 28–32.

169. McAnulty JH, Rahimtoola SH, Demots H, Griswold HE: Clinical features of infective endocarditis. In: Rahimtoola SH (ed): *Infective Endocarditis*. New York, Grune & Stratton, 1978: 125–148.
170. Sussman JI, Baron EJ, Tenenbaum MJ, Kaplan MH, Greenspan J, Facklam RR, et al: Viridans streptococcal endocarditis: Clinical, microbiological, and echocardiographic correlations. *J Infect Dis* 1986; 154:597–603.
171. Churchill MA, Geraci JE, Hunder GG: Musculoskeletal manifestations of bacterial endocarditis. *Ann Intern Med* 1977; 87:754–759.
172. Starkebaum M, Durack D, Beeson P: The "incubation period" of subacute bacterial endocarditis. *Yale J Biol Med* 1977; 50:49–58.
173. Tanaka M, Abe T, Hosokawa S, Suenaga Y, Hikosaka H: Tricuspid valve *Candida* endocarditis cured by valve-sparing debridement. *Ann Thorac Surg* 1989; 48:857–858.
174. Pruett TL, Rotstein OD, Anderson RW, Simmons RL: Tricuspid valve endocarditis: Successful treatment with valve-sparing debridement and antifungal chemotherapy in a multiorgan transplant recipient. *Ann J Med* 1986; 80:116–118.
175. Kilpatrick ZM, Greenberg PA, Sanford JP: Splinter hemorrhages: Their clinical significance. *Arch Intern Med* 1965; 115:730–735.
176. Howard EJ: Osler's nodes. *Am Heart J* 1960; 59:633–634.
177. Alpert JS, Krous HF, Dalen JE, O'Rourke RA, Bloor CM: Pathogenesis of Osler's nodes. *Ann Intern Med* 1976; 85: 471–473.
178. Edwards JE Jr, Foos RY, Montgomerie JZ, Guze LB: Ocular manifestations of *Candida* septicemia: Review of seventy-six cases of hematogenous *Candida* endophthalmitis. *Medicine* 1974; 53:47–75.
179. Osler W: Chronic infectious endocarditis. *Q J Med* 1909; 2:219–230.
180. Mills J, Utley J, Abbott J: Heart failure in infective endocarditis: Predisposing factors, course and treatment. *Chest* 1974; 66:151–159.
181. Cates JE, Christie RV: Subacute bacterial endocarditis: A review of 442 patients treated in 14 centres appointed by the Penicillin Trials Committee of the Medical Research Council. *Q J Med* 1951; 20:93–130.
182. Jones HR, Siekert RG, Geraci JE: Neurologic manifestations of bacterial endocarditis. *Ann Intern Med* 1969; 71:21–28.
183. Ziment I: Nervous system complications in bacterial endocarditis. *Am J Med* 1968: 47:593–607.
184. Pruitt AA, Rubin RH, Karchmer AW, Duncan GW: Neurologic complications of bacterial endocarditis. *Medicine* 1978; 57:329–343.
185. Jones HR Jr, Siekert RG: Neurological manifestations of infective endocarditis: Review of clinical and therapeutic challenges. *Brain* 1989; 112:1295–1315.
186. Francioli P: Central nervous system complications of infective endocarditis. In: Scheld WM, Whitley RJ, Durack DT (eds): *Infections of the Central Nervous System*. New York, Raven, 1991: 515–559.
187. Stengel A, Wolferth CC: Mycotic (bacterial) aneurysms of intravascular origin. *Arch Intern Med* 1923; 31:527–554.
188. Brust JCM, Dickinson PCT, Hughes JEO, Holtzman RNN: The diagnosis and treatment of cerebral mycotic aneurysms. *Ann Neurol* 1990; 27:238–246.
189. Salgado AV, Furlan AJ, Keys TF: Mycotic aneurysm, subarachnoid hemorrhage, and indications for cerebral angiography in infective endocarditis. *Stroke* 1987; 18:1057–1060.
190. Powers DL, Mandell GL: Intraleukocytic bacteria in endocarditis patients. *JAMA* 1974; 227:312–313.
191. Engle RL, Koprowska I: The appearance of histiocytes in the blood in subacute bacterial endocarditis. *Am J Med* 1959; 26:965–972.
192. Belli J, Waisbren BA: The number of blood cultures necessary to diagnose most cases of bacterial endocarditis. *Am J Med Sci* 1956; 232:284–288.
193. Werner AS, Cobbs CG, Kaye D, Hook EW: Studies on the bacteremia of bacterial endocarditis. *JAMA* 1967; 202:199–203.
194. Katsu M: *Spectrum of Endocarditis in Japan and Current Treatment*, Proceedings, 8th World Congress of Cardiology, Tokyo, 1978: 536–537.
195. Gerry JL, Greenough WB: Diphtheroid endocarditis: Report of nine cases and review of the literature. *Johns Hopkins Med J* 1976; 139:61–68.
196. Mintz GS, Morris MD, Kotler N: Clinical value and limitations of echocardiography. *Arch Intern Med* 1980; 140:1022–1027.
197. Chandraratna PAN, Langevin DO: Limitations of the echocardiogram in diagnosing valvular vegetations in patients with mitral valve prolapse. *Circulation* 1978; 56:436–438.
198. Andy JJ, Sheikh MM, Ali N, Barnes BO, Fox LM, Curry CL: Echocardiographic observations in opiate addicts with active infective endocarditis. *Am J Cardiol* 1977; 40:17–23.
199. DeMaria AN, King JF, Salel AE, Caudill CC, Miller RR, Mason DT: Echography and phonography of acute aortic regurgitation in bacterial endocarditis. *Ann Intern Med* 1975; 82:329–335.
200. Stewart JA, Silimperi D, Harris P, Wise NK, Fraker TD Jr, Kisslo JA: Echocardiographic documentation of vegetative lesions in infective endocarditis: Clinical implications. *Circulation* 1980; 61:374–380.
201. Mugge A, Daniel WG, Frank G, Lichtlen PR: Echocardiography in infective endocarditis: Reassessment of prognostic implications of vegetation size determined by the transthoracic and transesophageal approach. *J Am Coll Cardiol* 1989; 14:631–638.
202. Pavlides GS, Hauser AM, Stewart JR, O'Neill WW, Timmis GC: Contribution of transesophageal echocardiography to patient diagnosis and treatment: A prospective analysis. *Am Heart J* 1990; 120:910–914.
203. Daniel WG, Mugge A, Martin RP, Lindert O, Hausmann D, Nonnast-Daniel B, et al: Improvement in the diagnosis of abscesses associated with endocarditis by transesophageal echocardiography. *N Engl J Med* 1991; 324:795–800.
204. Welton DE, Young JB, Raizner AE, Ishimori T, Adyanthaya A, Mattox KL, et al: Value and safety of cardiac catheterization during active infective endocarditis. *Am J Cardiol* 1979; 44:1306–1310.
205. Riba AL, Thakur ML, Gottschalk A, Adriole VT, Zaret BL: Imaging experimental infective endocarditis with indium-111—labeled blood cellular components. *Circulation* 1979; 59:336–343.
206. Miller MH, Casey JI: Infective endocarditis: New diagnostic techniques. *Am Heart J* 1978; 96:123–128.
207. Cerqueira MD, Jacobson AF: Indium-111 leukocyte scintigraphic detection of myocardial abscess formation in patients with endocarditis. *J Nucl Med* 1989; 30:703–706.
208. Korzeniowski O, Sande MA, National Collaborative Endocarditis Study Group: Combination antimicrobial therapy for *Staphylococcus aureus* endocarditis in patients addicted to parenteral drugs and in nonaddicts: A prospective study. *Ann Intern Med* 1982; 97:496–503.
209. Wilson WR, Wilkowske CI, Wright AJ, Sande MA, Geraci JE: Treatment of streptomycin-susceptible and streptomycin-resistant enterococcal endocarditis. *Ann Intern Med* 1984; 100:816–823.
210. Bisno AL, Dismukes WE, Durack DT, Kaplan EL, Karchmer AW, Kaye D, et al: Antimicrobial treatment of infective endocarditis due to viridans streptococci, enterococci and staphylococci. *JAMA* 1989; 261:1471–1477.
211. Francioli P, Etienne J, Hoigne R, Thys J-P, Gerber A: Treatment of streptococcal endocarditis with a single daily dose of ceftriaxone sodium for 4 weeks: Efficacy and outpatient treatment feasibility. *JAMA* 1992; 267:264–267.
212. Stamboulian D, Bonyehi P, Arevalo C, Bologna R, Cassetti I, Scilingo V, et al: Antibiotic management of outpatients with endocarditis due to penicillin-susceptible streptococci. *Rev Infect Dis* 1991; 13:S160–S163.
213. Ormiston JA, Neutze JM, Agnew T, Lowe JB, Kerr AR: Infective endocarditis: A lethal disease. *Aust N Z J Med* 1981; 11:620–630.
214. Kaye D: Cure rates and long-term prognosis. In: Kaye D (ed): *Infective Endocarditis*. Baltimore, University Park Press, 1977: 201–211.
215. Welton DE, Young JB, Gentry WO, Raizner AE, Alexander JK, Chahine RA, et al: Recurrent infective endocarditis: Analysis of predisposing factors and clinical features. *Am J Med* 1979; 66:932–938.
216. Chambers HF, Miller RT, Newman MD: Right-sided *Staphylococcus aureus* endocarditis in intravenous drug abusers: Two-

week combination therapy. *Ann Intern Med* 1988; 109:619–624.
217. Blount JG: Bacterial endocarditis. *Am J Med* 1965; 38:909–922.
218. Pulliam L, Hadley WK: Resistance of viridans streptococci to penicillin. *N Engl J Med* 1979; 300:1442.
219. Denny AE, Peterson LR, Gerding DN, Hall WH: Serious staphylococcal infections with strains tolerant to bactericidal antibiotics. *Arch Intern Med* 1979; 139:1026–1031.
220. Brennan RO, Durack DT: Therapeutic significance of penicillin tolerance in experimental streptococcal endocarditis. *Antimicrob Agents Chemother* 1983; 23:273–277.
221. Reller LB: The serum bacterocidal test. *Rev Infect Dis* 1986; 8:803–808.
222. Kane LW, Finn JJ Jr: the treatment of subacute bacterial endocarditis with aureomycin and chloromycetin. *N Engl J Med* 1951; 244:623–628.
223. Watanakunakorn C: Antimicrobial therapy of endocarditis due to less common bacteria. In: Bisno AL (ed): *Treatment of Infective Endocarditis*. New York, Grune & Stratton, 1981: 123–133.
224. Katz LN, Elek SR: Combined heparin and chemotherapy in subacute bacterial endocarditis. *JAMA* 1944; 124:149–152.
225. Kanis JA: The use of anticoagulants in bacterial endocarditis. *Postgrad Med J* 1974; 50:312–313.
226. Wilson WR, Geraci JE, Danielson GK, Thompson RL, Spittell JA Jr, Washington JA II et al: Anticoagulant therapy and central nervous system complications in patients with prosthetic valve endocarditis. *Circulation* 1978; 57:1004–1007.
227. McAnulty JH, Rahimtoola SH: Surgery for infective endocarditis. *JAMA* 1979; 242:77–79.
228. Wilson WR, Danielson GK, Giuliami ER, Washington JA II, Jaumin PM, Geraci JE: Valve replacement in patients with active infective endocarditis. *Circulation* 1978; 58:585–588.
229. Richardson JV, Karp RB, Kirklin JW, Dismukes WE: Treatment of infective endocarditis: A 10-year comparative analysis. *Circulation* 1978; 58:589–597.
230. Durack DT: Nine controversies in the management of endocarditis. In: Petersdorf RG (ed): *Harrison's Principles of Internal Medicine Update*. New York, McGraw-Hill, 1984: 35–45.
231. Hughes CF, Noble N: Vegetectomy: An alternative surgical treatment for infective endocarditis of the atrioventricular valves in drug addicts. *J Thorac Cardiovasc Surg* 1988; 95:857–861.
232. Glazier JJ, Verwilghen J, Donaldson RM, Ross DN: Treatment of complicated prosthetic aortic valve endocarditis with annular abscess formation by homograft aortic root replacement. *J Am Coll Cardiol* 1991; 17:1177–1182.
233. Everett ED, Hirschmann JV: Transient bacteremia and endocarditis prophylaxis: A review. *Medicine* 1977; 56:61–77.
234. Sullivan NM, Sutter VL, Mims MM, Marsh VH, Finegold SM: Clinical aspects of bacteremia after manipulation of the genitourinary tract. *J Infect Dis* 1973; 127:49–55.
235. Shorvon PJ, Eykyn SJ, Cotton PB: Gastrointestinal instrumentation, bacteraemia and endocarditis. *Gut* 1983; 24:1078–1093.
236. American Heart Association Committee on Prevention of Bacterial Endocarditis: Prevention of bacterial endocarditis. *JAMA* 1990; 264:2919–2922.
237. Prevention of bacterial endocarditis. *Med Lett* 1984; 26:3–4.
238. Goodman JS, Schaffner W, Collins HA, Battersby EJ, Koenig MG: Infection after cardiovascular surgery: Clinical study including examination of antimicrobial prophylaxis. *N Engl J Med* 1968; 278:117–123.
239. Schaffner W: Antibiotic prophylaxis in valvular replacement surgery. In: Duma RJ (ed): *Infections of Prosthetic Heart Valves and Vascular Grafts*. Baltimore, University Park Press, 1977: 313–321.

PART XI

Congenital Heart Disease

Chapter 95

Embryology of the Heart

L.H.S. Van Mierop, M.D. ■ Lynn M. Kutsche, M.D.

Interest in the developing heart dates back to Aristotelian times and perhaps even earlier. Because the heart is bright red and moving and the early chick embryo itself is translucent and nearly invisible, early observers concluded that the heart was the first organ formed during development. However, little progress was made toward the understanding of how precisely it is transformed from a single convoluted tube into the four-chambered, four-valved adult organ. A significant step forward was made when the great systematist and physiologist Albrecht von Haller in 1758 published a monograph devoted exclusively to the development of the heart.[1]

Interest in cardiovascular embryology has recently received added impetus, not only among embryologists and anatomists but also among clinicians, by the spectacular advances made in the diagnosis and surgical treatment of congenital heart disease.

The study of cardiovascular development has expanded greatly, involving many disciplines, and its focus has changed from "classical" embryology to cellular and subcellular levels. A discussion of these modalities of study, however, falls beyond the scope of this chapter, and we will limit our discussion largely to the "gross" development of the heart and large blood vessels.

There are many different cardiac anomalies, some of great complexity, and embryology of the heart, rather than being a difficult subject having little relevance to clinical medicine, has proved to be of enormous value in the understanding of the pathology and pathogenesis of these anomalies.

DEVELOPMENT OF THE HEART

The Heart Prior to Septation

Formation of the Heart Tube

Initially the embryonic cardiovascular system is bilaterally symmetrical.[2] At the cephalic end of the embryo (on each side of the midsagittal plane) a section of main vascular channel specializes, acquiring contractile elements within its wall, thus producing a pair of heart tubes that come to lie parallel and close to each other within the cephalic part of the developing body cavity (intraembryonic coelom), ventral to the foregut.

Fusion of the heart tubes results in the formation of a single tube (Fig. 95-1), the wall of which consists of an external myocardial mantle one to two cell layers thick and a single layer of endothelial cells internally, separated from each other by a relatively thick, acellular, and almost structureless third layer called *cardiac jelly*.[3,4] From this tube will develop initially the embryonic ventricle and bulbus cordis (hence the term *bulboventricular* tube) and later the ventricles and their outflow tracts.[5,6]

Formation of the Heart Loop

At the beginning of the next phase of development the embryo is about 2 mm long and 23 days old. From the dilated cephalic, extrapericardial portion of the bulboventricular tube—the aortic sac—originates the first pair of aortic arches and later also the second, third, fourth, and sixth arches (the fifth pair of aortic arches does not

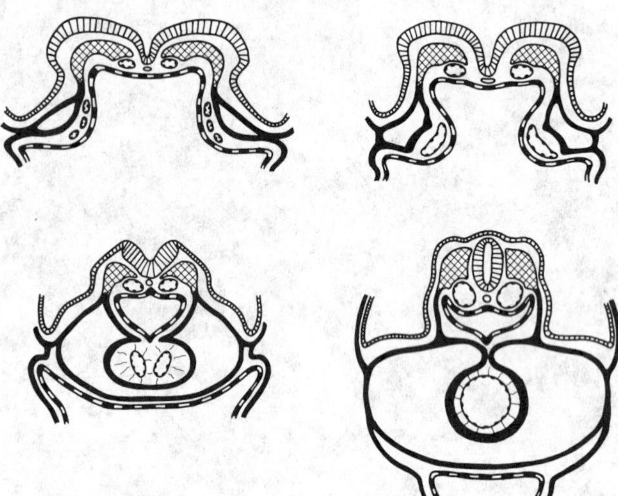

FIGURE 95-1 Schematic transverse sections through embryos of different ages, showing formation of the single heart tube.

normally develop in mammals or is very rudimentary). The caudal part of the bulboventricular tube expands to form the early embryonic ventricle. It receives the paired confluence of veins that lie extrapericardially, caudal to the embryonic ventricles, embedded in mesenchyme.

The growing bulboventricular tube bends to the right and anteriorly into a compound sigmoid structure: the bulboventricular loop (Fig. 95-2). The deepening concavity on the left side of the bulboventricular loop is referred to as the bulbo-(cono-)ventricular *groove* or *sulcus*. Internally, the bulboventricular sulcus corresponds to a fold, the bulbo-(cono-)*ventricular fold.* At this stage the descending limb of the loop is called the *embryonic ventricle,* the ascending limb the *bulbus cordis*.

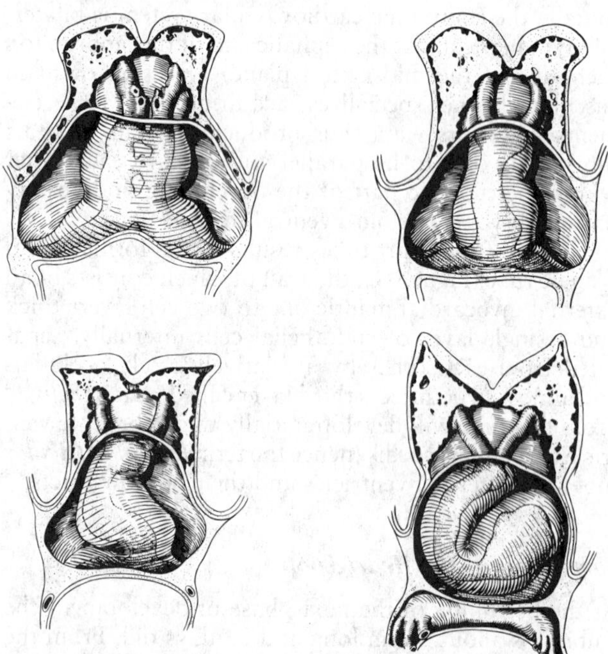

FIGURE 95-2 Schematic ventral dissections of human embryos of different ages, showing formation of the heart loop. *(Adapted from CL Davis: Development of the human heart from its first appearance to the state found in embryos of 20 paired somites. Contrib Embryol 1927; 19:245. Reproduced with permission from the Carnegie Institution)*.

Cardiac looping appears to be due to a fundamental property of the myocardium[7–10] rather than being a passive phenomenon brought about by the necessity for the rapidly lengthening bulboventricular loop to accommodate itself to the smaller available space in the coelomic (pleuropericardial) cavity as was thought previously.[11,12]

Since the arterial and venous poles of the heart tube are fixed, bending of the tube imparts to it a certain amount of torsion that is at least in part responsible for the spiral disposition of the later developing truncoconal septum. The atrioventricular (AV) junction, which at first lies in the midline, is crowded laterally to the left. The embryonic ventricle moves to the left side of the pericardial cavity, and the right side of this cavity is now occupied by the rapidly enlarging bulbus cordis.

Initial changes within the endocardial tube are concerned mainly with the development of local expansions throughout its length (Fig. 95-3). The originally paired venous confluences fuse and dilate to form a large common atrium. The AV junction, the AV canal, remains relatively narrow and shifts cephalad and mesiad. The ventricle and the proximal one-third of the bulbus cordis expand, while the junction between them, the primary interventricular foramen (also referred to as the bulboventricular foramen), remains narrow and comes to lie approximately in the midsagittal plane[12] (Figs. 95-2 and 95-3).

Anomalies *Ventricular Inversion with Transposition of the Great Arteries* If the cardiac loop is formed to the left and anterior, rather than to the right and anterior, then all structures derived from the bulboventricular loop, i.e., the AV valves, the ventricles, and the arterial roots, will develop in an inverted position. Since the truncoaortic sac, the atria, and the sinus venosus all lie extrapericardially, these parts of the heart will be normally located. The aorticopulmonary septum also develops in a normal fashion, but since partitioning of the inverted truncus arteriosus takes place in mirror image, the end result is transposition of the great arteries with the aorta arising anteriorly from a left-sided, morphologically right (arterial) ventricle and the pulmonary trunk arising posteriorly from a right-sided left (venous) ventricle—hence the term *corrected transposition* commonly used for this anomaly.

Primitive Ventricles, Conus Cordis, and Truncus Arteriosus At the close of the previous phase of development, diverticula appear in two sharply defined areas along the right and left ventrolateral borders of the endocardial tube[13] (Fig. 95-3). These diverticula develop initially at the expense of the cardiac jelly and later also penetrate the myocardium as the latter increases in thickness, producing a spongy mass of trabeculae. The capacity of the heart is increased by the added intertrabecular spaces.

The now-trabeculated, embryonic ventricular space is called the *primitive left ventricle,* since it will contribute the major portion of the definitive left ventricle (Fig. 95-3). Similarly, the proximal one-third of the bulbus cordis, also trabeculated, may be called the *primitive right ventricle.*[14]

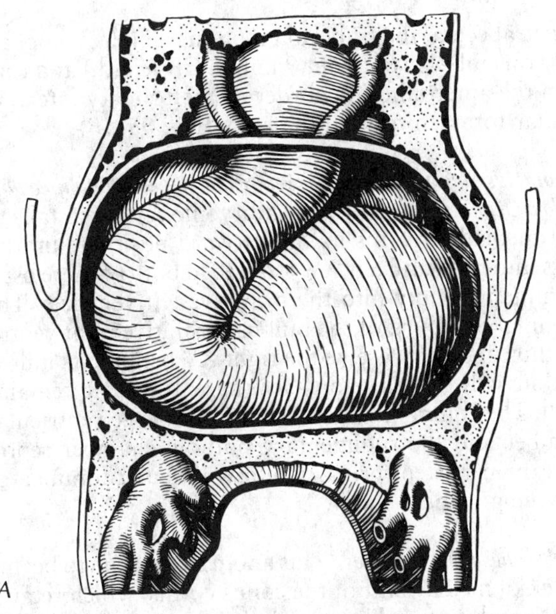

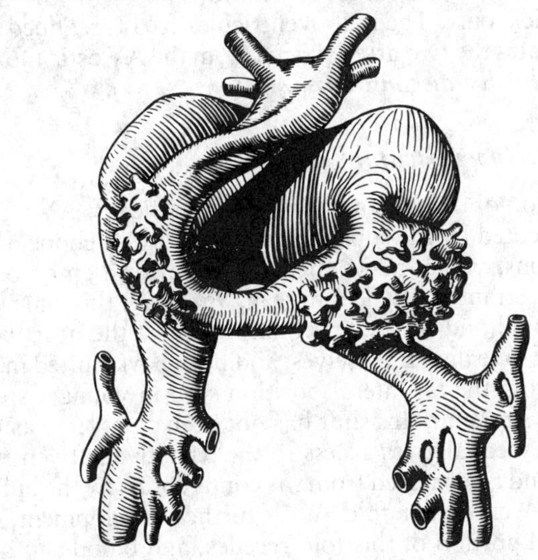

FIGURE 95-3 Twenty-somite human embryo, ovulation age about 25 days. *A.* Ventral dissection. *B.* Reconstruction of cardiac lumen. *(Adapted from CL Davis: Development of the human heart from its first appearance to the state found in embryos of 20 paired somites. Contrib Embryol 1927; 19:245. Reproduced with permission from the Carnegie Institution. Artwork adapted from © 1969 CIBA-GEIGY. Reproduced with permission from Clinical Symposia, by Frank H. Netter, MD. All rights reserved.)*

At this stage of development the embryo is approximately 3 mm long and has an ovulation age of about 25 days.[3] Because of future developments, it is helpful to distinguish three sections in the bulbus cordis, of which the proximal trabeculated one-third is the primitive right ventricle. From the adjacent middle one-third of the bulbus, the conus cordis, the outflow portions of both ventricles will be derived. The terminal one-third of the bulbus, after partitioning, develops into the aortic and pulmonary roots and hence is called the *truncus arteriosus*. The distalmost portion of the truncus arteriosus, together with the adjoining aortic sac from which the aortic arches arise, is called the *truncoaortic sac*.

The rapid growth and expansion of the primitive atria cause the truncoconal section of the bulbus cordis to shift from its initial far lateral position to a more medial location. The result is that the truncus arteriosus comes to lie in a midsagittal position, in a depression of the atrial roof between the primitive right and left atria; the conus cordis assumes an oblique position and lies between the roof of the primitive left ventricle and the anteromedial wall of the right atrium. In an embryo of approximately 4 to 5 mm in crown-rump (CR) length (ovulation age of approximately 27 days), the external shape of the heart already suggests its future four-chambered condition.

Because of rapid growth and continually changing curvature of the embryo during the following period of growth and development, it becomes difficult to continue to appreciate spatial relationships. In the following discussion on cardiac septation, therefore, the diaphragm (septum transversum) is assumed to maintain an approximately horizontal position as in the adult, standing person. The terms *anterior, posterior, superior,* and *inferior* are employed accordingly.

The formation of the various cardiac septa takes place more or less simultaneously; for descriptive purposes, however, it is necessary to consider their development separately.

Septation of the Heart

Mechanisms of Cardiac Septation

There are three ways in which a septum can be formed in a hollow organ such as a heart[6]:

- A short segment increases in diameter only slowly or not at all, while on either side of the segment rapid and expansive growth takes place (Fig. 95-4*A* and *B*). The portions of the walls of the expanded regions on either side of the narrow intervening segment come to face each other, appose, and fuse. Usually, expansive growth takes place mainly in one direction, resulting in the formation of a septum with an eccentrically placed communication between the two adjoining chambers. A septum formed in this fashion is simply a reduplication of the wall of the organ and can never be complete: there is always an opening in it somewhere.
- A different mechanism of septum formation is seen in portions of the heart that possess a well-developed layer of cardiac mesenchyme (*endocardial cushion tissue*) between the myocardium and the endocardium (e.g., the AV canal, the conus cordis, and the truncus arteriosus). This tissue is derived from the earlier cardiac jelly. Local elaborations of such cardiac mesenchyme form two apposing masses of tissue that grow toward each other and fuse. Because of their appearance, these masses of mesenchymal tissue are called *cushions*. Septa developed in this manner are complete, and their thickness characteristically equals or exceeds their height in the early phases of their development (Fig. 95-4C).
- Occasionally a septum in its initial phases of development is formed passively but is completed by actively growing cushion tissue present along its free edge (Fig. 95-4*D*).

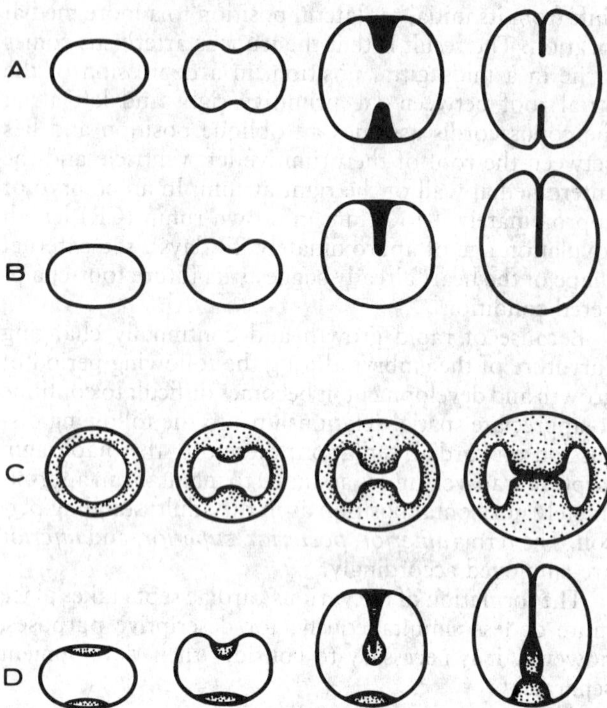

FIGURE 95-4 Mechanism of cardiac septation. *A, B.* Passively formed septum. *C.* Actively formed septum. *D.* Combination of *B* and *C.* *[From LHS Van Mierop: Morphological development of the heart. In RM Berne (ed): Hardbook of Physiology, sec 2: The Cardiovascular System, vol 1: The Heart. Bethesda, MD, American Physiological Society, 1979: 1. Reproduced with permission from the American Physiological Society.]*

Partitioning of the embryonic heart is accomplished by the formation of seven septa. Of these, three are formed passively (septum secundum of the atrium, muscular portion of the ventricular septum, and aorticopulmonary septum), three are formed actively (septum of the AV canal, conal septum, and truncal septum). One, the atrial septum primum, starts out as a passively formed septum, but it is completed by actively growing tissue along its border.

The Ventricles

In an embryo of about 5 mm in CR length, the AV canal leads exclusively into the primitive left ventricle, and blood can reach the primitive right ventricle only by way of the primary interventricular foramen, the borders of which are formed by the developing muscular interventricular septum inferiorly and anteriorly and by the bulbo-(cono-)ventricular fold superiorly and posteriorly (Fig. 95-5*A*) The interventricular septum and the conoventricular fold are continuous with each other anterosuperiorly.

The ventricles enlarge by centrifugal growth of the myocardium, closely followed by increasing diverticulation and formation of trabeculae internally to prevent the compact out layer of the myocardium from becoming too thick.

The medial walls of the growing and expanding ventricles appose and fuse, forming the major portion of the muscular ventricular septum.[12,15–18] On the right side, a large trabecula, the trabecula septomarginalis,[19] appears early (in embryos of about 9 mm in CR length) and runs from the anteroinferior border of the primary interventricular foramen toward the apex (Fig. 95-5*B*).

Anomalies *Single Ventricle, Left Ventricular Type with Rudimentary Outflow Chamber* If the early embryonic AV canal fails to shift medially, retains its far leftward position, and divides into right and left AV ostia, then both of these ostia continue to empty into the primitive left ventricle. The proximal one-third of the bulbus (primitive right ventricle) thus does not receive the right AV ostium, its inflow portion will not develop, and as a result, it remains small. The communication between the large ventricular chamber and the rudimentary outflow chamber represents the persistent primary interventricular foramen of the young embryo heart.

Double-Outlet Right Ventricle This anomaly appears to be due to lack of medial shift of the conus cordis, which retains its original embryological relationships with the right ventricle only. The bulboventricular fold is retained and separates the two arterial ostia from the AV ostia (*aortic-mitral valve discontinuity*).

The Atrioventricular Canal

Division of the AV canal into a right and left AV orifice is executed by the superior and inferior AV endocardial cushions, which make their appearance in embryos of about 6 mm in CR length (Fig. 95-5). At this time, the AV canal and the truncoconal region of the heart have begun to realign themselves, and both have shifted medially from the far lateral position seen in younger specimens. At 6 mm, this shift has not been completed as yet: The AV canal gives access to the primitive left ventricle only and is separated from the conus cordis by the bulbo-(cono-)ventricular fold. With further development, the central portion of this fold recedes, and blood can now enter the primitive right ventricle directly from the atrium (Fig. 95-5). In embryos of about 9 mm in CR length, the left-sided portion of the fold is seen to terminate almost midway along the base of the superior endocardial cushion and is much less prominent (Fig. 95-5*B*), and the right-sided portion becomes part of the parietal band. In older embryos, both the medial shift of the truncoconus and the effacement of the central part of the conoventricular fold continue until this portion eventually becomes unrecognizable as such. As a result, the plane of the primary interventricular foramen inclines more and more to the left from an originally vertical position. As a further result, direct access is gained from the primitive left ventricle to the posteromedial portion of the conus cordis and the aorta. The primary interventricular foramen never closes but actually enlarges, and in the fully developed heart it gives access to the aortic infundibulum or vestibule.[12,17,19]

Meanwhile, the AV canal has enlarged to the right while the growing endocardial cushions project into the lumen (Fig. 95-5*B*). Smaller cushions appear on the lateral borders of the AV canal.

In embryos of about 10 mm in CR length, the major cushions reach each other and fuse, resulting in a com-

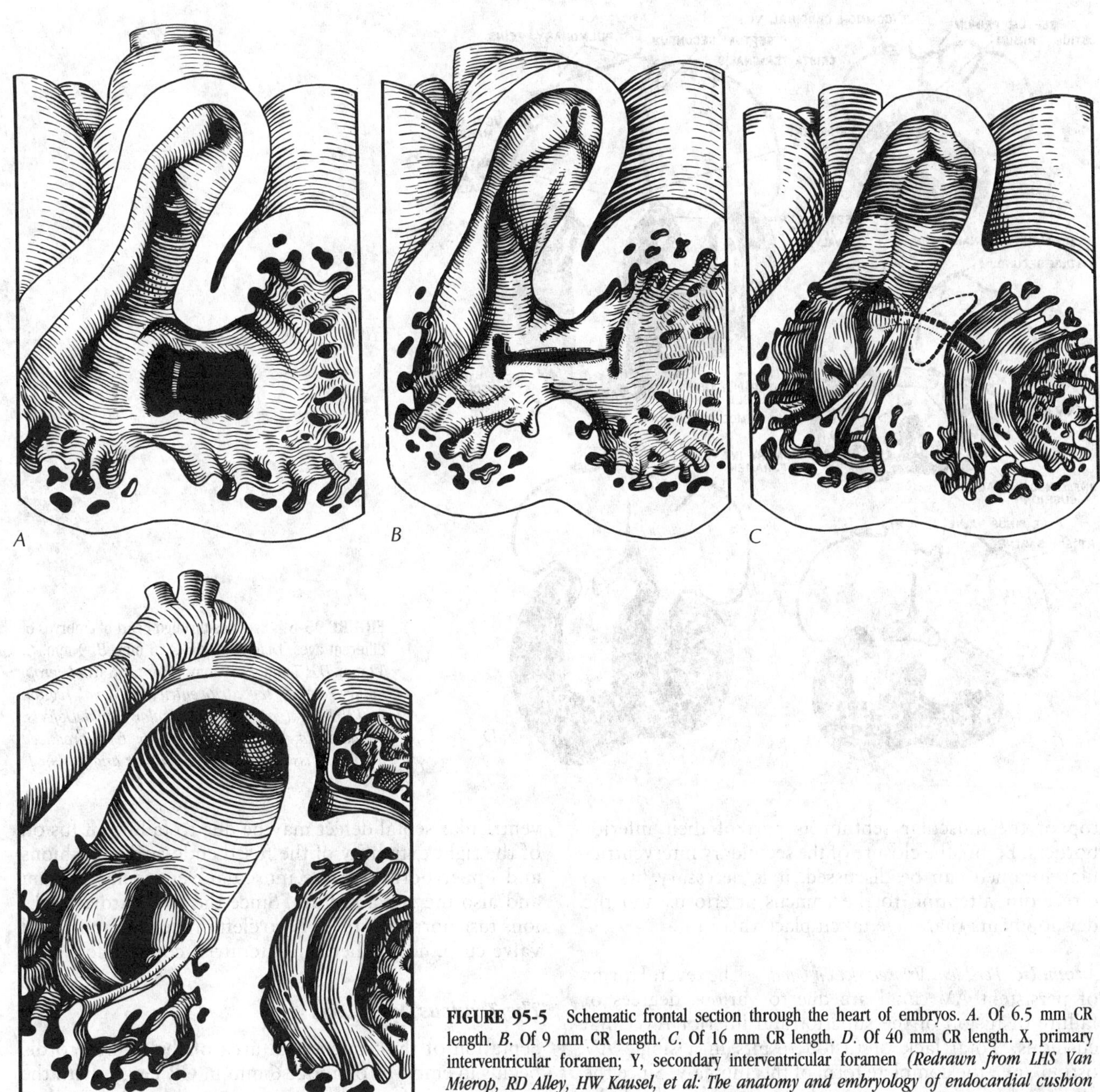

FIGURE 95-5 Schematic frontal section through the heart of embryos. *A.* Of 6.5 mm CR length. *B.* Of 9 mm CR length. *C.* Of 16 mm CR length. *D.* Of 40 mm CR length. X, primary interventricular foramen; Y, secondary interventricular foramen *(Redrawn from LHS Van Mierop, RD Alley, HW Kausel, et al: The anatomy and embryology of endocardial cushion defects. J Thorac Cardiovasc Surg 1962; 43:71. Reproduced with permission from the publisher and author.)*

plete division of the canal into right and left AV orifices. At the same time the cushions also bend, and after fusion they eventually form an arch that has its concavity directed anteriorly and toward the left ventricle[12,20] and its convexity directed anteriorly and toward the atria (Figs. 95-5C and 95-6). The free margin of the atrial septum primum meets the convex atrial side of the fused endocardial cushions about midway between their extremities and fuses with them (Fig. 95-6C). That portion of the endocardial cushions to the left of the septum primum, i.e., the left limb of the arch, eventually becomes incorporated into the anterior or aortic cusp of the mitral valve and therefore does not participate in the formation of the cardiac septum.

With deepening of the endocardial arch or bay, the right half of the fused endocardial cushions comes to lie more and more in a sagittal plane, i.e., in about the same plane but somewhat to the right of the muscular interventricular septum. The communication still remaining between right and left ventricles, the secondary interventricular foramen, is bordered at this point by the muscular ventricular septum inferiorly and anteriorly, the right extremity of the fused endocardial cushions posteriorly, and the conal septum superiorly (Fig. 95-5C). The plane of the secondary interventricular foramen, therefore, inclines somewhat to the right; that of the primary interventricular foramen, as we have seen, has come to deviate to the left. They share, however, the

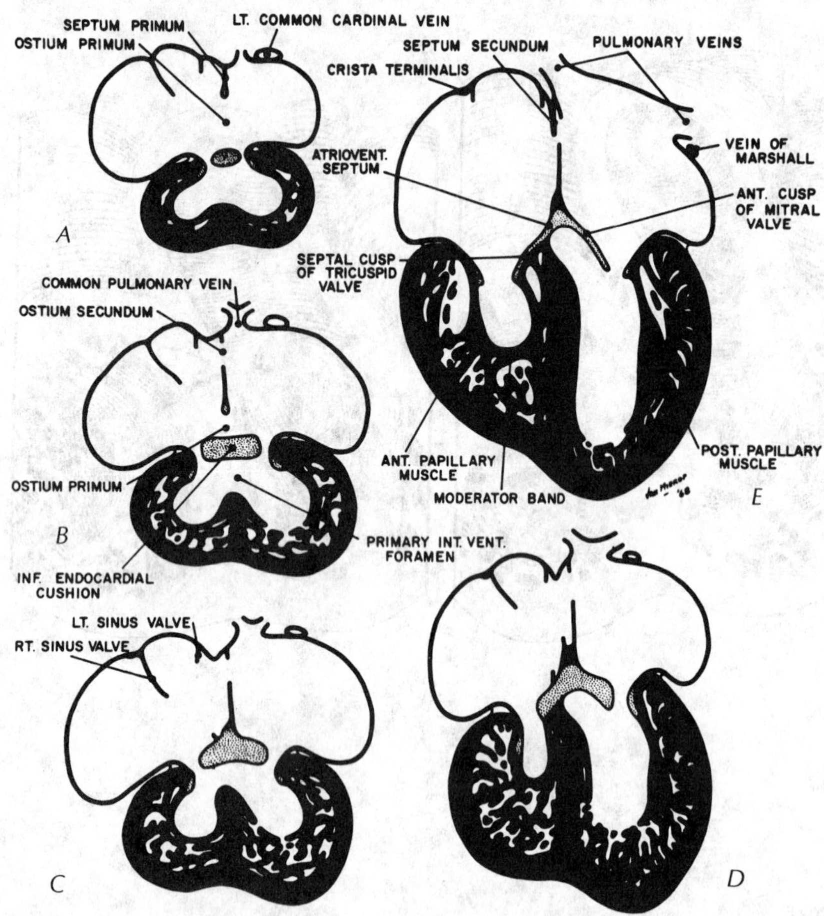

FIGURE 95-6 Sections through heart of embryos of different ages. Diagrammatic. *A*. 6 mm. *B*. 9 mm. *C*. 12 mm. *D*. 17 mm. *E*. 40 mm. *[From LHS Van Mierop: Embryology of the atrioventricular canal region. In RH Feldt (ed): Atrioventricular Canal Defects. Philadelphia, WB Saunders, 1976: 6. Reproduced with permission from the publisher and author.]*

top of the muscular septum as part of their inferior borders. Before the closure of the secondary interventricular foramen can be discussed, it is necessary first to direct our attention to the truncus arteriosus and the developments that have taken place there.

Anomalies *Persistent Atrioventricular Canal* The several forms of persistent AV canal are due to various degrees of failure of fusion of the superior and inferior AV canal cushions. Total lack of fusion results in a single AV ostium, i.e., the complete form of the anomaly. Since the arch or bay normally formed after the fusion of the endocardial cushions fails to develop, the lower border of the atrial septum cannot fuse with the endocardial cushions. The result is a low-lying, large interatrial communication, and the AV part of the cardiac septum is absent. The upperpart of the ventricular septum remains deficient to a greater or lesser degree, and there is an interventricular communication.

In the partial forms the endocardial cushions fuse centrally only, and the arch is generally not formed. The result is an interatrial communication or so-called ostium primum–type atrial septal defect. The upper part of the muscular ventricular septum remains deficient, but this area of the ventricular septum is closed by fibrous tissue. Because the left side of the endocardial cushions does not fuse, the anterior or aortic cusp of the mitral valve is cleft.

Ventricular Septal Defect Some forms of perimembranous ventricular septal defect may be due to failure of fusion of the right extremity of the fused endocardial cushions and upper border of the muscular ventricular septum and also the conal septum. Since the endocardial cushions fuse normally, there is no cleft in the anterior mitral valve cusp, nor is there an interatrial communication.

The Truncus Arteriosus

Septation of the truncoconal area of the bulbus cordis begins in embryos of about 6 mm in CR length with the appearance of two opposing truncal cushions (Fig. 95-5). One of these is located on the dextrosuperior wall of the truncus (dextrosuperior truncal cushion), the other on the sinistroinferior wall (sinistroinferior truncal cushion).

The cushions rapidly enlarge and fuse to form the truncal septum, thus dividing the truncus into aortic and pulmonary channels. The truncus is the first part of the heart to become partitioned (embryos of about 7 mm in CR length). The truncal cushions (and therefore the truncal septum) are large and bulky, and to accommodate them, the initially slender truncal area of the heart expands.

Meanwhile, truncal cushions proximally meet the distal extremities of a similar pair of mesenchymal masses developing in the conus cordis: the conal cushions. With further growth, the distal surface of the fused truncal cushions presents a front that faces the origin of the sixth aortic arches (Fig. 95-5). The distal, still undivided portion of the truncus, together with the adjacent aortic sac, dilates to form the truncoaortic sac. At the same time, the sixth arches move closer together and to the left, their most proximal portions probably fusing for a short distance. The origins of the fourth aortic arches (from the roof of the truncoaortic sac) shift somewhat to the right. As a result, the sixth arches become aligned with the pulmonary channel and the fourth arches with the aortic channel. At the same time, the dorsal wall of the truncoaortic sac between the origins of the fourth and sixth arches invaginates to form a vertical septum, the aorticopulmonary septum, the leading edge of which approaches the distal face of the truncal septum with which it fuses.[12,14,21,22] Partitioning of the truncoaortic area is complete in embryos of about 9 mm in CR length.

Anomalies *Persistent Truncus Arteriosus* If the truncal cushions remain hypoplastic and fail to fuse, partitioning of the truncus arteriosus does not take place. If, in addition to the hypoplastic truncal cushions, both intercalated valve cushions are present, these may each form a valve cusp, and the result is a quadricuspid truncal valve. Fusion between adjacent valve anlagen may produce an apparent tricuspid truncal valve of which one of the cusps is larger than the others and contains a raphe, the most commonly seen condition. In the great majority of cases, the aorticopulmonary septum does develop, and a short common pulmonary trunk arises from the persistent trunk. The ductus arteriosus is almost always absent, except when interruption of the aortic arch is associated.

Aorticopulmonary Septal Defect This anomaly appears to be due to malalignment and/or failure of fusion between the distal extremity of the truncal septum and the aorticopulmonary septum. Both arterial valves are present, but there is a communication of varying size between the ascending aorta and the pulmonary trunk.

The Conus Cordis

The conal cushions make their appearance at about the same time as do the truncal cushions (Fig. 95-5). One is located on the dextrodorsal wall, the other on the sinistroventral wall of the conus cordis. The dextrodorsal conal cushion becomes continuous with the dextrosuperior truncal cushion and the sinistroventral conal cushion with the sinistroinferior truncal cushion. Fusion of the conal cushion begins proximally, progressing rapidly in a distal direction to complete the partition of the truncoconal part of the heart in embryos of about 14 to 15 mm in CR length.

With completion of the conal septum, the originally large interventricular communication becomes much reduced in size, and in a 15- to 16-mm embryo the remaining small secondary interventricular foramen, bordered by the conal septum, the top of the muscular ventricular septum, and the right extremities of the fused endocardial cushions is closed. That part of the endocardial cushion arch or bay between the junction with septum primum and the ventricular septum becomes the AV portion of the membranous septum (Fig. 95-6).

Anomalies *Ventricular Septal Defect, Eisenmenger Type* Hypoplasia or absence of the conal cushions results in a large basilar septal defect, dextroposition of the aortic valve, and a hypoplastic or absent infundibular septum.

Ventricular Septal Defect, Supracristal Type The supracristal type of ventricular septal defect is a form of interventricular communication due to either simple failure of fusion of truncal and conal septa or to malalignment between these septa, which makes fusion impossible. Of interest is that this type of defect appears to be much more common in the Far East than in Western countries.

Tetralogy of Fallot The basic anomaly in tetralogy of Fallot probably is an anterior displacement of varying degree of the conal septum, which leads to unequal partitioning of the conus at the expense of the right ventricular infundibulum—hence the infundibular stenosis. The displaced conal septum cannot participate in the closure of the interventricular foramen. There are, therefore, a very large basilar ventricular septal defect and dextroposition of the aortic valve. Pulmonary valvar anomalies, although commonly associated, are not an essential feature of tetralogy of Fallot.

The Sinus Venosus

In a 4-mm embryo, the sinus venosus consists of a central unpaired part, the transverse portion of the sinus venosus, and the right and left sinus horns (Figs. 95-3 and 95-7). It receives three pairs of veins: the omphalomesenteric (vitelline) veins, the umbilical (allantoic) veins, and the common cardinal veins. At first, the sinus venosus is not well demarcated from the atrium; later it becomes separated from the atrium by the development of a deep fold (Fig. 95-7*B* and *D*). The proximal portions of the umbilical veins soon disappear. As a result of the development of anastomotic channels between right and left systemic veins and preferential flow of blood to the right side, the right sinus horn and proximal cardinal and vitelline veins gain in size and importance, while their left counterparts become attenuated. The right sinus horn attains a vertical position; it becomes incorporated into the right atrium to form the smooth-walled, intercaval part of the atrium; and the communication between the sinus venosus and the atrium is now limited to this horn. The transverse portion and the proximal left sinus horn become the coronary sinus; the distal left sinus horn and left common cardinal vein normally obliterate (fold of Marshall).

On the right side, the infolded cardiac wall at the sinoatrial junction forms the right sinus valve (Figs. 95-3 and 95-6). Another, smaller fold, the left sinus valve, appears somewhat later on the left side of the sinoatrial junction, so that in a 4- to 6-mm embryo the vertical sinoatrial orifice is flanked on each side by a valvelike structure (Fig. 95-6). Superiorly, the sinus valves join to form the septum spurium. The sinus valves, particularly the right sinus valve, are relatively very large in a 16-mm embryo, but later they usually disappear almost completely. The left sinus valve fuses with the atrial septum. The inferior part of the right sinus valve is divided into a larger inferior vena caval (eustachian) valve and a smaller coronary sinus (thebesian) valve; the remainder usually disappears.

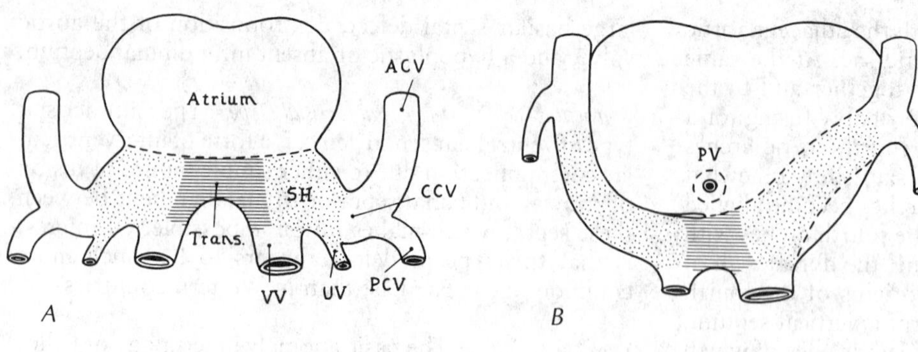

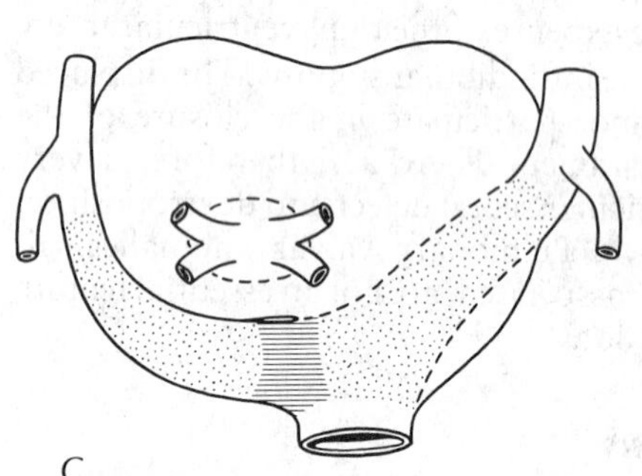

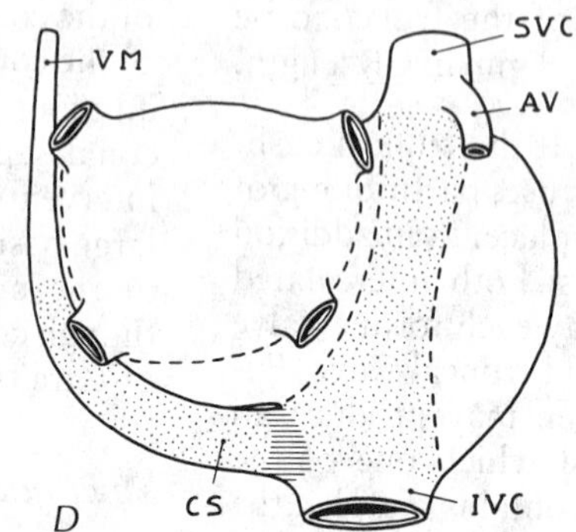

FIGURE 95-7 Posterior view of the atria and sinus venosus in embryos. *A.* Of 3 mm CR length. *B.* Of 5 mm CR length. *C.* Of 12 mm CR length. Diagrammatic. A(C)CV, anterior (common) cardinal vein; AV, azygos vein; CS, coronary sinus; IVC, inferior vena cava; PCV, posterior cardinal vein; PV, pulmonary vein; SH, sinus horn; UV, umbilical vein; VM, vein of Marshall; W, viteline vein. *(From LHS Van Mierop, FW Wigglesworth: Isomerism of the cardiac atria in the aplenia syndrome. Lab Invest 1962; 11:1303. Copyright by U.S. and Canadian Academy of Pathology.)*

Anomalies *Cor Triatriatum Dexter* Total persistence of the right sinus valve of the embryonic heart produces a septum in the right atrium separating the intercaval part of the right atrium from the atrial body. The remaining opening may be quite small and restrictive.

Persistent Left Superior Vena Cava Persistence of the left sinus horn and left common cardinal vein results in a left superior vena cava entering the coronary sinus.

The Atria, Atrial Septum, and Pulmonary Veins

In a 3-mm embryo expansion of the atrial portion of the heart is well under way (Fig. 95-3). Because of the presence of the truncus arteriosus, a depression is formed in the roof of the common atrium. This depression deepens, corresponding internally to a sickle-shaped crest. This is the first indication of the septum primum. Its free edge is directed toward the AV canal, and the opening between the left and right primitive atria that it borders is the ostium primum (Fig. 95-6). Extensions from the superior and inferior endocardial cushions grow along the edge of the septum primum. Proliferation of this tissue with the concomitant fusion of the endocardial cushions brings about closure of the ostium primum, a process that is completed in embryos of about 10 to 11 mm in CR length. Meanwhile, perforations have appeared in septum primum posterosuperiorly. These rapidly coalesce to form the ostium secundum, thus ensuring continued free communication between the right and left primitive atria. Expansive growth of the atria and infolding of the atrial wall between the left sinus valve and septum produce the posterosuperior part of the septum secundum. The anteroinferior part of the septum secundum is believed to have a different origin.[23–25] The opening bordered by the free edge of the septum secundum is the foramen ovale. Postnatally, after fusion of the septum primum and the septum secundum, the foramen ovale becomes the fossa ovalis, and the free edge of the septum secundum is then called the *limbus fossae ovalis.*

Until recently the single embryonic pulmonary vein, already well developed in a 5- to 6-mm embryo (Figs. 95-6 and 95-7) was thought to develop as an outgrowth of the posterior left atrial wall near the atrial floor just to the left of the septum primum and to gain connections with the splanchnic plexus of veins in the region of the developing lung buds.[26–28] In a recent study, however, we have found support for the concept that the common pulmonary vein initially enters the sinus venosus and secondarily, in the process of atrial septation, is transferred to the left atrium.[29] Later in development, the vein itself and parts of its first four branches expand and become incorporated into the embryonic left atrium to form the larger smooth part of the adult left atrium. In the fully developed heart, the original embryonic left atrium is represented by little more than the trabeculated atrial appendage. The intrapulmonary part of the splanchnic venous plexus ultimately loses its connections with the systemic veins and drains exclusively by way of the pulmonary veins.

Atrial Septal Defect at the Fossa Ovalis Atrial septal defect at the fossa ovalis, also often referred to as *secundum-type atrial septal defect,* is due to overresorption of septum primum, producing a very large ostium secundum that cannot be guarded adequately by septum secundum. Frequently, septum secundum is also hypoplastic, further enlarging the atrial septal defect. In some cases ostium secundum is normal but septum secundum is absent. Total absence of both septum primum and septum secundum (common atrium) is rare and almost always associated with a form of persistent AV canal.

Anomalous Pulmonary Venous Connection The total form of anomalous pulmonary venous connection presumably is due either to lack of development or to early involution of the embryonic common pulmonary vein. One or more of the early embryonic channels connecting the pulmonary venous bed to the systemic venous circulation is retained. Depending on which of these channels drains the pulmonary vascular bed, a number of types of total anomalous pulmonary venous connection are recognized. Partial anomalous pulmonary venous return is due to retention of a connection between part of the pulmonary venous system with the systemic venous circulation.

Cor Triatriatum Sinister If incorporation of the common pulmonary vein into the left atrium does not take place and the common pulmonary venous ostium remains narrow, the result is a septumlike structure that divides the left atrium into two components: one receives the pulmonary veins and the other gives access to the mitral valve and left atrial appendage.

DEVELOPMENT OF THE HEART VALVES

The Atrioventricular Valves

In an embryo of about 10 to 12 mm in CR length, both AV orifices are surrounded by mesenchymal endocardial cushion-type tissue that has a provisional valve function.

The definitive AV valves, however, are derived only in very small part from this tissue. Nearly all the material contributing to the AV valve cusps is elaborated from the (muscular) ventricular wall, the internal layer of which is liberated by a process of diverticulation and undermining described earlier (Fig. 95-6).[6] All AV valve cusps are therefore initially thick and fleshy, and only later in development are they transformed into thin and fibrous cusps.[14]

Anomalies *Tricuspid Valve Atresia, Mitral Valve Atresia* Tricuspid and mitral valve atresias are anomalies that probably are due to fusion of endocardial cushion tissue that borders the AV canal in very young embryos, during or shortly after partitioning of the AV canal.

Ebstein's Anomaly of the Tricuspid Valve Ebstein's anomaly of the tricuspid valve is very likely due to an abnormality of the process of undermining of the myocardium.

The Arterial Valves

The primordia of the semilunar valves are already visible as small tubercles in a 9-mm embryo, just after partitioning of the truncus has been completed. Each truncal cushion carries a tubercle on the extremity of its distal

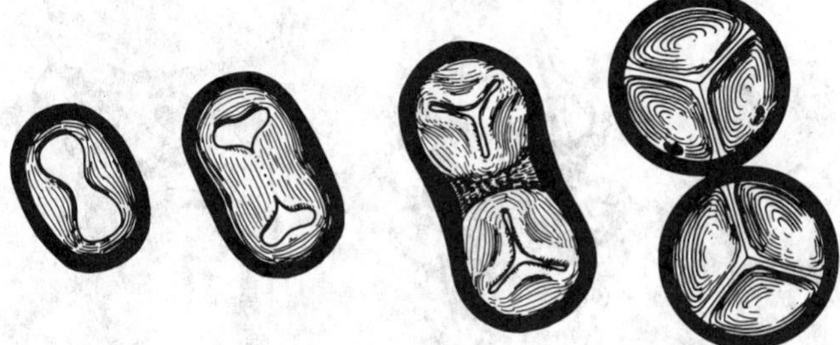

FIGURE 95-8 Development of the arterial valves. Diagrammatic.

face. One of each pair is assigned to pulmonary and aortic channels, respectively. On the walls of both aortic and pulmonary channels, opposite the fused truncus cushions, a third small cushion appears. These two intercalated valve cushions[21] form the third member of each arterial valve primordium (Figs. 95-5 and 95-8). Beginning at the tubercles, the semilunar valve cusps and sinuses of Valsalva are probably formed by a process of excavation of the truncal and intercalated valve cushions in a proximal direction. This process appears well advanced in a 16-mm embryo and is virtually completed in a 40-mm embryo. Both the aortic and pulmonary roots, therefore, consisting of the sinuses of Valsalva and the semilunar valves, are derived from the truncus arteriosus and the truncal and intercalated valve cushions.

Anomalies *Bicuspid Arterial Valves* A bicuspid aortic or pulmonary valve is due either to a failure of development of an intercalated valve cushion, resulting in a valve with two approximately equal-size cusps, neither containing a raphe, or, more commonly, to fusion of adjacent valve anlagen, in which case the cusps are generally unequal in size with the larger containing a raphe of varying height.

ARTERIAL VALVE STENOSIS OR ATRESIA

Fusion of two or all three of the arterial valve anlagen produces stenosis or atresia of the valve.

Absent arterial valves. Absence of the pulmonary or aortic valve is a rare anomaly, particularly the latter, and presumably is due to failure of development of arterial valve anlagen.

DEVELOPMENT OF THE AORTIC ARCH SYSTEM

In an embryo of about 3 mm the first pair of aortic arches is large and the second pair is just forming (Figs. 95-3 and 95-9*A*). A true ventral aorta is not present in mammalian embryos. Caudally the dorsal aortae fuse to form a single vessel; this fusion progresses craniad.

In a 4-mm embryo the first and second arches have largely disappeared. The third aortic arch is well devel-

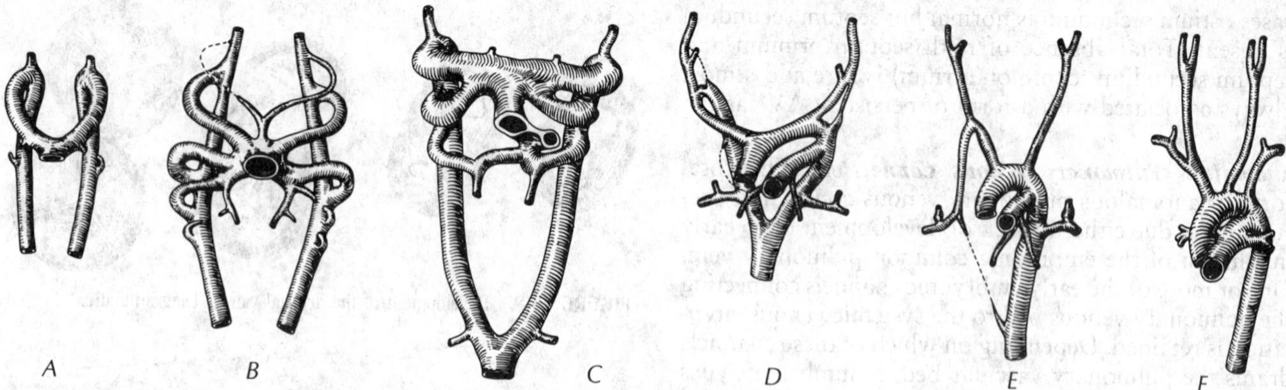

FIGURE 95-9 Development of the aortic arch system. Embryos of (*A*) 3 mm; (*B*) 4 mm; (*C*) 10 mm; (*D*) 14 mm; (*E*) 17 mm; and (*F*) neonate. *(After ED Congdon: Contrib Embryol 1922; 14:47).*

oped, and the fourth and sixth arches are being formed as ventral and dorsal sprouts of the aortic sac and dorsal aorta, respectively. The ventral portion of the sixth arch already has as its major branch the primitive pulmonary artery, even though the arch itself has not yet been completed. The fifth aortic arch in mammals is rudimentary and transient.

In a 10-mm embryo the first two aortic arches are no longer present as such, and the third, fourth, and sixth are large (Fig. 95-9C). The truncoaortic sac has been divided by the formation of the aorticopulmonary septum so that the sixth arches are now continuous with the pulmonary trunk. Of the cervical intersegmental arteries the seventh pair will play an important role in the formation of the subclavian arteries. They are located at about the level where the dorsal aortae join each other.

In a 14-mm embryo the aortic arch system has largely lost its original symmetrical pattern (Fig. 95-9*D*). The segments of the dorsal aortae between the third and fourth arches, the carotid ducts, have disappeared and the third arches begin to elongate as the heart descends further into the thorax. This descent has also caused a relative shortening of the paired portion of the dorsal aorta. The dorsal portion of the right sixth arch has disappeared; its counterpart on the left persists until birth as the ductus arteriosus. The seventh intersegmental arteries have migrated craniad. The aortic sac has been "pulled out" on both sides: on the right it forms the brachiocephalic (innominate) trunk; on the left it becomes part of the definitive arch of the aorta up to the origin of the left third arch (common carotid artery).

In a 17-mm embryo the right dorsal aorta between its junction with the left dorsal aorta and the origin of the right seventh intersegmental artery has become attenuated and later disappears (Fig. 95-9*E*). The remainder of the right dorsal aorta persists and, with the right fourth aortic arch, forms the proximal subclavian artery.

After birth the distal part of the left sixth aortic arch, the ductus arteriosus, normally also obliterates and is converted to the ligamentum arteriosum. Thus the adult aortic system is established. See Table 95-1 for the ultimate fate of the various components of the embryonic aortic arch system.

Anomalies

Most aortic arch anomalies can be explained as being due to abnormal retention or disappearance of various segments.

Double Aortic Arch

Double aortic arch is the result of persistence and continued patency of the segment of the right dorsal aorta between the origin of the right seventh intersegmental artery and its junction with the left dorsal aorta.

Right Aortic Arch

In the right aortic arch anomaly the right rather than the left dorsal aorta is maintained in its entirety. The branching pattern of the aortic arch, therefore, will be the mirror image of normal with the brachiocephalic (innominate) artery arising as the first vessel on the left, rather than the right, side.

Anomalous Subclavian Artery

If the right fourth arch disappears the right dorsal aorta between the origin of the right seventh intersegmental artery and the junction with the left dorsal aorta is maintained to form the proximal portion of the right subclavian artery. Because of its genesis, such a subclavian artery will arise from the aortic arch distal to the left subclavian artery and always run behind the esophagus to enter the right arm.

Interrupted Aortic Arch

In type B of the interrupted aortic arch anomaly (type A is a form of coarctation of the aorta) the left fourth arch disappears. The ascending aorta terminates as brachiocephalic and left common carotid arteries and has no connection with the descending aorta, which receives its blood from the pulmonary trunk by way of a patent

TABLE 95-1
Fate of Embryonic Aortic Arches

Embryonic Vessel	What It Becomes
1. Truncus arteriosus	Aortic and pulmonary roots
2. Aortic sac	Ascending aorta, brachiocephalic artery, and aortic arch up to the origin of the left common carotid artery
3. First arches	Parts persist as components of the maxillary arteries
4. Second arches	Parts persist as the stapedial arteries
5. Third arches	Common carotid arteries and proximal segment of the internal carotid arteries
6. Fourth arches	
a. Right	Most proximal segment of the right subclavian artery
b. Left	Aortic arch segment between the left common carotid and left subclavian arteries
7. Fifth arches	No known derivations; transient and never well developed
8. Sixth arches	
a. Right	Proximal part becomes proximal segment of the right pulmonary artery; distal part disappears early
b. Left	Proximal part becomes proximal segment of the left pulmonary artery; distal part persists, until birth, as ductus arteriosus
9. Right dorsal aorta	Cranial portion becomes part of the right subclavian artery; remainder disappears
10. Left dorsal aorta	Distal aortic arch
11. Right seventh intersegmental artery	Part of the right subclavian artery
12. Left seventh intersegmental artery	Left subclavian artery

ductus arteriosus. If both fourth arches disappear, the right subclavian artery will arise anomalously, usually from the descending aorta, and the ascending aorta terminates into the two carotid arteries.[30]

Absent Left Pulmonary Artery

The left pulmonary artery almost always is absent only in the sense that it arises from a left-sided ductus arteriosus (or ligamentum arteriosum). The anomaly is the result of disappearance of the proximal left sixth arch. If, in this anomaly, the aortic arch is on the left side, the ductus arteriosus that feeds the intrapulmonary part of the left pulmonary artery arises from the usual position on the underside of the arch. If the aortic arch is on the right, the ductus arteriosus usually arises from the brachiocephalic trunk with the left common carotid and left subclavian arteries as a trifurcation or, rarely, from a diverticulum of the descending aorta. Usually the left subclavian artery in such cases also arises from the diverticulum.

REFERENCES

1. Von Haller A: Sur la formation du coeur dans le poulet. Lausanne, 1758.
2. Davis CL: Development of the human heart from its first appearance to the state found in embryos of 20 paired somites. *Contrib Embryol* 1927; 19:245–284.
3. Davis CL: Description of a human embryo having 20 paired somites. *Contrib Embryol* 1923; 15:1–52.
4. Davis CL: The cardiac jelly of the chick embryo. *Anat Rec* 1924; 27:201–202.
5. Van Mierop LHS: Embryology of the heart. In: Netter FH (ed): *The CIBA Collection of Medical Illustrations*, vol 5, pt 1. Summit, NJ, CIBA Pharmaceutical Co, 1969: 112–130.
6. Van Mierop LHS: Morphological development of the heart. In: Berne RM (ed): *Handbook of Physiology*, sec 2: *The Cardiovascular System*, vol 1: *The Heart*. Bethesda, MD, American Physiological Society, 1979: 1–28.
7. Castro-Quezada A, Nadal-Ginard B, de la Cruz MV: Experimental study of the formation of the bulboventricular loop in the chick. *J Embryol Exp Morphol* 1972; 27:623–637.
8. Manasek FJ, Burnside MB, Waterman RE: Myocardial cell shape change as a mechanism of embryonic heart looping. *Dev Biol* 1972; 29:349–371.
9. Stalsberg H: Origin of heart asymmetry: Right and left contributions to the early chick embryo heart. *Dev Biol* 1969; 19: 109–127.
10. Stalsberg H: Mechanism of dextral looping of the embryonic heart. *Am J Cardiol* 1970; 25:265–271.
11. Patten BM: The formation of the cardiac loop in the chick. *Am J Anat* 1922; 30:373–397.
12. Van Mierop LHS, Alley RD, Kausel HW, Stranahan A: Pathogenesis of transposition complexes: I. Embryology of the ventricles and great arteries. *Am J Cardiol* 1963; 12:216–225.
13. Streeter GL: Developmental horizons in human embryos: Description of age groups XI, 13–20 somites, and age group XII, 21–29 somites. *Contrib Embryol* 1942; 30:211–246.
14. Van Mierop LHS, Alley RD, Kausel HW, Stranahan A: The anatomy and embryology of endocardial cushion defects. *J Thorac Cardiovasc Surg* 1962; 43:71–83.
15. Streeter GL: Developmental horizons in human embryos: Description of age groups XV, XVI, XVII, XVIII, being the third issue of a survey of the Carnegie Collection. *Contrib Embryol* 1948; 32:133–204.
16. Mall FP: On the development of the human heart. *Am J Anat* 1912; 13:249–298.
17. Keith A: The Hunterian Lectures on malformation of the heart. *Lancet* 1909; 2:359–363, 433–435, 519–525.
18. Tandler J: Anatomie des Herzens. In: von Bardeleben (ed): *Handbuch der Anatomie des Menschen*, vol 3. Jena, Gustav Fischer Verlag, 1913: 1–292.
19. Grant RP: Embryology of ventricular flow pathways in man. *Circulation* 1962; 25:756–779.
20. Los JA: Embryology. In: Watson H (ed): *Paediatric Cardiology*. St. Louis, Mosby, 1968: 1–23.
21. Kramer TC: The partitioning of the truncus and conus and the formation of the membranous portion of the interventricular septum in the human heart. *Am J Anat* 1942; 71:343–370.
22. Shaner RF: Anomalies of the heart bulbus. *J Pediatr* 1962; 61:233–241.

23. Asami I: Beitrag zur Entwicklungsgeschichte des Vorhofseptums im menschlichen Herzen, eine lupenpraparatorisch-photographische Darstellung. *Z. Anat Entwicklungsgesch* 1972; 139:55–70.
24. Christie GA: Development of the limbus fossae ovalis in the human heart—A new septum. *J Anat* 1963; 97:45–54.
25. Odgers RNB: The formation of the venous valves, the foramen secundum and the septum secundum in the human heart. *J Anat* 1935; 69:412–422.
26. Auer J: The development of the human pulmonary veins and its major variations. *Anat Rec* 1948; 101:581–594.
27. Los JA: The development of the human pulmonary vein and the coronary sinus in the human embryo. Thesis, University of Leiden, 1958.
28. Neill CA: Development of the pulmonary veins. *Pediatrics* 1956; 18:880–887.
29. Kutsche LM, Van Mierop LHS: Development of the pulmonary vein in the American alligator (*Alligator mississippiensis*). *Anat Rec* 1988; 222:170–176.
30. Kutsche LM, Van Mierop LHS: Cervical origin of the right subclavian artery in aortic arch interruption: Pathogenesis and significance. *Am J Cardiol* 1984; 53:892–895.

Chapter 96

Cardiovascular Diseases Due to Genetic Abnormalities

Jeffrey A. Towbin, M.D. ■ *Robert Roberts, M.D.*

Deoxyribonucleic acid (DNA), which forms the chromosomes and their genes, encodes the hereditary information defining structure and function for each individual. When genetic abnormalities occur, they can lead to adverse functional or structural defects in any organ, including the heart. During the past decade, it has become increasingly clear that genetic factors play a significant role in the pathogenesis of most cardiovascular disorders. Although some disorders, such as Romano-Ward Long QT syndrome (LQTS), familial hypertrophic cardiomyopathy (FHCM), and Marfan's syndrome,[1,2,3] have had obvious genetic defects defined, other diseases have a less clear-cut relationship to hereditary factors. The latter group includes congenital cardiac disease and infectious disorders of the heart.

Molecular genetics and cytogenetics (the study of chromosomes and their abnormalities) provide the potential to understand the etiology and pathogenesis of cardiovascular diseases due to genetic abnormalities. Isolation of disease-causing genes has led to the discovery of the protein abnormalities underlying the development of disease and, in some cases, has provided improved genetic counseling through prenatal and postnatal diagnostic capability. Ultimately, it is hoped that the application of molecular genetics and other techniques of recombinant DNA will lead to definitive gene transfer and replacement therapy. In addition, the techniques of molecular genetics provide unique knowledge fundamental to our understanding of the molecular basis for the influence of environmental stimuli upon the adaptive mechanisms of the cardiovascular system.

The aim of this chapter is to review the general principles of hereditary disease and discuss those disorders of the heart and great vessels for which a genetic etiology has been defined.

BASIC MOLECULAR BIOLOGY

All hereditary information is transmitted from parent to offspring through the inheritance of DNA, which determines the base sequence of messenger ribonucleic acid (mRNA) that is transcribed, and the mRNA then directs translation of proteins of unique amino acid sequence (see Chap. 1). Each gene (a segment of DNA) contains the coding information (i.e., base sequences in DNA) specifying the amino acid sequence in a single polypeptide chain; it has been estimated that the total number of human genes is in the range of 50,000. Two copies of each gene—called *alleles*—are localized in linear sequence along 23 pairs of *chromosomes*, the rod-shaped bodies derived from the parents of each individual. Each parent contributes one member of each chromosome pair and thus one copy of each gene. The site at which a gene is located on a particular chromosome is called the *genetic locus*. A given gene always resides at the same specific genetic locus on a particular chromosome. When both genes at the same genetic locus are identical, the individual is homozygous. When the two genes differ (i.e., two different alleles are present at that locus), the individual is heterozygous at that locus. Each individual is homozygous at some loci and heterozygous at others.

The 23 chromosome pairs include 22 pairs of autosomes (chromosomes 1 through 22) and 1 pair of the sex chromosomes, X and Y. Females have two X chromosomes, while males carry an X and a Y chromosome. Both autosomal alleles are *potentially* active in specifying RNA copies of their DNA sequences, but their activity depends on the cell type, developmental stage, and regulatory molecules that interact with promoter and enhancer sequences that control gene transcription. In cells that carry two X chromosomes, whether they are derived from normal females or XXY individuals with Klinefelter's syndrome, only one X is active early after embryogenesis.

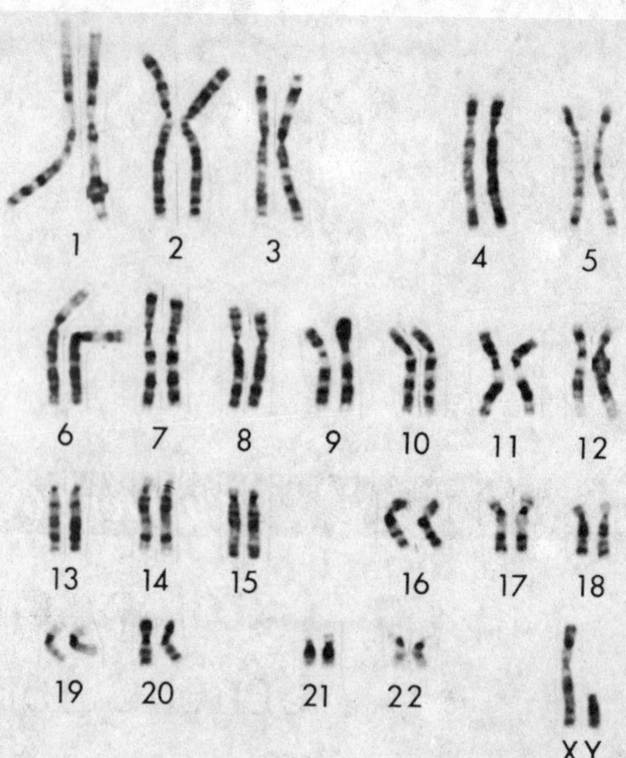

FIGURE 96-1 Normal male chromosome karyotype (22 pairs of autosomes, 1 pair of sex chromosomes). (*Courtesy of David Ledbetter, Ph.D., Kleberg Cytogenetics Laboratory, Baylor College of Medicine.*)

BASIS OF HEREDITARY AND CONGENITAL DISEASE

Hereditary and congenital diseases may be due to chromosomal abnormalities or mutations that may involve one or several genes. Chromosomes can be studied in a variety of dividing cells obtained from a peripheral blood sample. The cell most commonly utilized for genetic diagnosis is the lymphocyte, but other white blood cells, fibroblasts, or cells from chorionic villi or amnion may also be used. Chromosomes are distinguished from each other by their size, characteristic banding pattern (as demonstrated by various staining methods), and shape, as determined by the position of the centromere (the centralized constriction that functions as the attachment of the mitotic apparatus and divides the chromosome into arms of equal or unequal length; Fig. 96-1). Chromosome alterations, especially those involving too many or too few chromosomes (called aneuploidy), are quite common in human development. Chromosome aberrations most commonly cause structural defects of the cardiovascular system and typically are evident at birth. Approximately 50 percent of all fetuses conceived are spontaneously aborted (usually in the first trimester), with one-half of these being aneuploid. Among live-born infants, about 1 in 200 (0.5 percent) have a chromosome abnormality. The frequency of chromosome abnormalities among live-born children with congenital heart defects is in the range of 5 to 13 percent.[4,5,6] Hence, the vast majority of chromosomal aberrations are lost in early fetal life and, in most instances, occur as new mutations. For this reason, with both parents being normal, the risk of recurrence to relatives is usually low.

CARDIOVASCULAR DISORDERS ASSOCIATED WITH CHROMOSOME ABNORMALITIES

Classification of Chromosomal Abnormalities

Aneuploidy

The presence of too many or too few chromosomes is called aneuploidy[7] and occurs most commonly by nondisjunction (failure of a homologous pair of chromosomes to separate). Nondisjunction occurs during meiosis in one parent (i.e., in spermatogenesis or oogenesis) or in the first mitotic cleavage of the zygote. In meiotic nondisjunction, when a pair of chromosomes does not normally separate, it results in both members of the pair (or neither member of the pair) of chromosomes passing into one gamete. When an additional copy of the chromosome is added during fertilization, three copies of the same chromosome (or only one copy) are found in the new zygote instead of the chromosome pair found in normal persons. The two most common chromosomal disorders causing heart disease, Down's syndrome (trisomy 21) and Turner's syndrome (XO), are usually due to nondisjunction. The presence of three chromosomes is called *trisomy,* as seen in Down's syndrome (Fig. 96-2), while the presence of an entire extra set of chromosomes (i.e., a total of 69 chromosomes) is known as *triploidy.* Absence of one chromosome is called *monosomy;* all autosomal monosomies, as well as those containing only a Y sex chromosome, are embryonic lethals.

Chromosomal Rearrangements

Chromosomal rearrangements occur when a chromosome breaks and rejoins in a new configuration and can potentially result in an *inversion* of genetic material. Typically there is no apparent phenotypic effect in persons carrying an inversion, but their offspring may have severe abnormalities due to the disruption in chromosome pairing that can take place during meiosis.

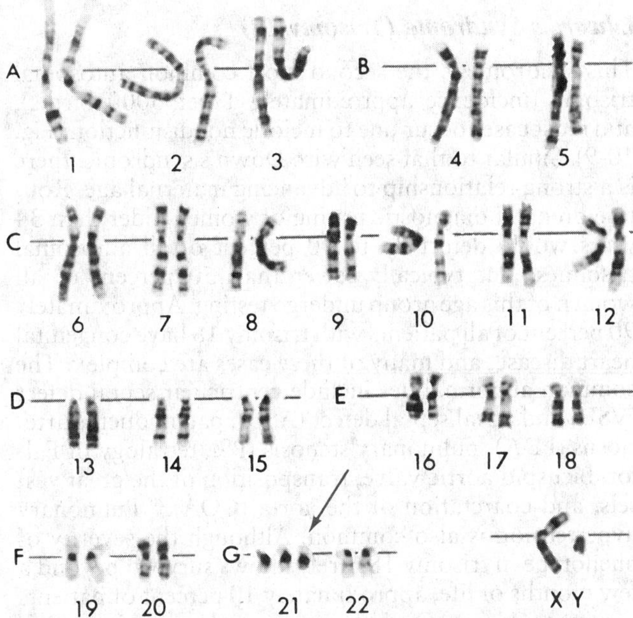

FIGURE 96-2 Chromosomal karyotyping indicative of trisomy 21 (*arrow*) causing Down's syndrome. (*Courtesy of David Ledbetter Ph.D., Kleberg Cytogenetics Laboratory, Baylor College of Medicine.*)

Chromosome Deletions

Loss of chromosomal material may be seen by light microscopy, but the smallest deletion seen by this technique is usually associated with the loss of a large amount of DNA, upwards of 10^6 base pairs. With the loss of this large amount of DNA, more than one gene may be affected (disrupted or lost); a series of abnormalities in a single individual may result due to interruptions in a series of genes within the loci of a single chromosome. These *contiguous gene deletion syndromes*[8] may be heritable (i.e., glycerol kinase deficiency), and the occurrence of the disorder in a family may behave as a dominant disorder (X-linked or autosomal dominant). These deletions are best detected at the DNA level by Southern analysis or polymerase chain reaction (PCR) analysis (see Chap. 1).

Chromosome Duplications

A gain of extra chromosomal material may also be associated with phenotypic abnormality but most commonly causes no obvious aberration.

Cytogenetics: Detection of Chromosomal Abnormalities

High-resolution cytogenetic techniques allow unambiguous identification of each human chromosome and detection of most structural abnormalities, including translocations, deletions, and duplications. High-resolution chromosome analysis involves synchronization of lymphocyte cultures in order to accumulate all cells at one point in the cell cycle.[9] Enrichment of this cell population in prophase and prometaphase rather than the middle-to-late stages of metaphase, which is characteristic of conventional harvesting techniques, allows improved visualization of the subbanding patterns of chromosomes (Fig. 96-1). Each band seen at metaphase actually represents multiple subbands in earlier stages that fused as the chromosome contracted. Whereas a typical metaphase cell contains 300 to 400 bands per haploid genome, synchronized chromosome preparations make it possible to visualize 500 to 1000 bands per haploid set.[10] The primary application of high-resolution analysis is allowing a particular chromosomal region to be studied in greater detail. This technique produces an improved determination of the specific chromosome band or subbands involved in a disorder after routine methods are initially used to detect abnormalities. Prior to the use of chromosome banding techniques, most cytogenetic abnormalities described were aneuploid conditions representing either gain or loss of entire chromosomes. Since there are 3×10^9 base pairs of DNA in the human genome, an average chromosome represents approximately 150×10^6 base pairs. Deletions large enough to be reliably detected by these methods were probably on the order of 10 to 30×10^6 base pairs. With the development of banding methods, the human karyotype could be divided into 300 to 400 discrete bands, or approximately 7 to 10×10^6 base pairs per band, and a much greater number of deletions, duplications, and translocations can be detected at this level of resolution. High-resolution techniques allow visualization of from 500 to 2000 bands per haploid genome, providing a resolution of approximately 1 to 5×10^6 base pairs per band; therefore, the smallest deletion visible on light microscopy is generally considered to be on the order of 1×10^6 base pairs. High-resolution cytogenetic techniques have enabled the delineation of a number of microdeletion or microduplication syndromes (i.e., contiguous gene syndromes)[8] including the DiGeorge syndrome[11] and the Beckwith-Wiedemann syndrome.[12] Cytogenetics may provide the crucial first step for positional cloning strategies (i.e., cloning of a gene of unknown function by its location in the genome) by identifying the physical localization of a gene. For example, sporadically, females are found with full clinical manifestations of an X-linked disorder. This is frequently due to an X autosome translocation in which the break point on the X chromosome disrupts a locus, and the resulting nonrandom pattern of lyonization causes the allele of the normal X chromosome to be inactivated. Duchenne's muscular dystrophy (DMD) was first mapped to the short arm of the X chromosome (Xp21) by this method.[13]

Diseases Due to Chromosomal Abnormalities

Down Syndrome (Trisomy 21)

Chromosome 21 is the smallest of all human chromosomes, containing less than two percent of the genomic DNA. Down's syndrome, however, is the most common phenotype caused by a human chromosome abnormality, occurring approximately once every 500 to 600 births. Down's syndrome is due either to the presence of an extra chromosome 21 (Fig. 96-2) or the presence of only the distal one-half of chromosome 21, band q22 (i.e., 21q22): the "Down's syndrome critical region," so-called due to the presence of a subset of major phenotypic features of Down's syndrome (Fig. 96-3), including men-

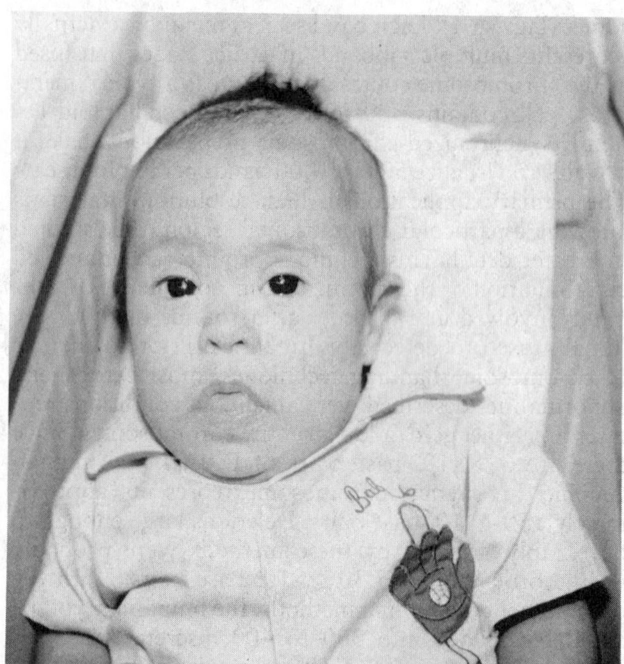

FIGURE 96-3 Child with the characteristic features of Down's syndrome. Phenotypic features of Down's syndrome include mental retardation, congenital heart disease, characteristic facial appearance, and hand and dermatoglyphic changes.

tal retardation, congenital heart disease, characteristic facial appearance, and hand and dermatoglyphic changes. In order to produce this syndrome, then, distal 21q22 must be triplicated.[14] This region has been noted to contain the genes for the enzymes superoxide dismutase, phosphoribosyl glycineamide synthetase, and phosphofructokinase, as well as that for the proto-oncogene ETS-2 sequence. The gene or genes responsible for manifesting Down's syndrome are unknown, but the severity of the disease is believed to depend on the extent of the region q22, and beyond, that is triplicated.[15]

The typical trisomy 21 occurs in 95 percent of cases of Down's syndrome and results from chromosomal nondisjunction.[16] The majority of these events appear to occur at the first maternal meiotic division. Two to 3 percent of Down's syndrome cases are mosaics, and the remainder are due to the translocation of an extra copy of all or part of the long arm of chromosome 21 to another chromosome. The risk of trisomy 21 is exponentially related to maternal age, with the lowest risk for young women, rising steeply after age 35 years, and reaching four percent for women older than 45 years. In mothers under the age of 30 years, Down's syndrome occurs due to translocation more commonly than at older maternal age. Rudd and associates[17] performed molecular analysis on 20 couples and could determine the parental origin of the extra number 21 chromosome in 45 percent of the cases. The risk of recurrence is generally believed to be 1 to 2 percent.[18]

Forty to 50 percent of patients with Down's syndrome have congenital heart disease, most characteristically the endocardial cushion defect or atrioventricular (AV) canal defect, and recently the region of chromosome 21 related to heart disease has been localized (see also Chap. 10).[19]

Edward's Syndrome (Trisomy 18)

This syndrome is the second most common autosomal trisomy (incidence approximately 1 per 3000 births), and most cases occur due to meiotic nondisjunction (Fig. 10-9). Similar to that seen with Down's syndrome, there is a strong relationship to advancing maternal age. Routine prenatal diagnostic testing of women older than 34 years would detect 35 to 40 percent of all autosomal trisomies, but typically fewer than 50 percent of all women of this age group undergo testing. Approximately 90 percent of all patients with trisomy 18 have congenital heart disease, and many of these cases are complex. The common abnormalities include ventricular septal defect (VSD) and atrial septal defect (ASD), patent ductus arteriosus (PDA), pulmonary stenosis (PS), tetralogy of Fallot, bicuspid aortic valve, transposition of the great vessels, and coarctation of the aorta (COA).[20] Pulmonary hypertension is also common. Although the severity of phenotype in trisomy 18 rarely allows survival beyond a few months of life, approximately 10 percent of patients survive to 1 year. On rare occasion, these patients may survive to near adulthood, probably secondary to mosaicism (<1 percent). The diagnosis of this trisomic lesion is generally made by bedside analysis of the phenotype and by routine chromosomal analysis. A 1 to 2 percent risk of recurrence is thought to exist (see also Chap. 10).

Patau Syndrome (Trisomy 13)

Approximately 80 percent of cases of trisomy 13 are due to nondisjunction causing complete trisomy, with the remaining 20 percent due to mosaicism or translocations. The most common translocation is the 13;14 translocation (60 percent are *de novo* rearrangements). Approximately 80 percent of these individuals have associated congenital heart disease, and in the majority of cases these congenital heart defects are complex. These defects include VSD, ASD, PS, COA, PDA, and dextrocardia.[20] This syndrome occurs in approximately 0.01 percent of live births (incidence 1 per 8000) and in progressively higher frequencies in stillbirths and spontaneous abortions. The phenotypic appearance of these patients is usually severe and includes midface hypoplasia-dysplasia; between 60 to 80 percent will have cleft lip and/or palate. The diagnosis of this chromosomal trisomy is made by bedside examination and routine chromosome analysis. The risk of recurrence of full trisomy 13 is 1 to 2 percent, with the risk for inherited translocations closer to 5 percent.

Turner's Syndrome

This disorder of gonadal dysgenesis, which is due to meiotic dysjunction resulting in a single X chromosome in females (i.e., XO genotype), occurs in approximately 1 female in 2500.[21] The frequency of nonmosaic XO karyotypes is significantly higher in spontaneous abortuses than in live-borns, with less than 2 percent of such conceptuses reaching term. Clinically, there is a variable and often mild phenotype, and the diagnosis may go unsuspected until a child's short stature is evaluated or a woman complains of amenorrhea. The clinical findings[22] of patients with Turner's syndrome include lymphedema of hands and feet, inguinal hernias, short stature, primary amenorrhea, facial features including a slightly triangular face with downslated palpebral fissures, epicanthal folds, and ptosis. Ears are frequently low set and posteriorly rotated, and the mandible is commonly micrognathic. The neck is typically short with marked webbing and the posterior hairline may be low, extending to the upper shoulders (Fig. 10-10). A broad thorax with widely spaced nipples is common, as is cubitus valgus and shortening of the fourth and fifth metacarpals. Abnormalities of sexual development are usually associated, including hypogonadotropic hypogonadism with ovarian dysgenesis. Intelligence is normal (see also Chap. 10). Many cases are mosaic for cell lines with the normal 46XX or 46XY makeup. The frequency of congenital cardiac disease varies from 20 to 50 percent, with at least one-half of these having COA.[23] A variety of other cardiac defects may also occur either singly or in combination with COA. The majority of these include other left heart abnormalities, including bicuspid aortic valve, aortic stenosis, dilated ascending aorta,[24] and hypoplastic left heart syndrome.[25] ASD and VSD, as well as partial anomalous pulmonary venous return,[26] have also been reported. Postmortem examination of midtrimester abortuses with cytogenetic evidence of Turner's syndrome demonstrates a higher incidence of left-sided flow lesions than found at birth, and speculation has been forwarded that association between the pathogenesis of the cardiovascular abnormalities and lymphatic obstruction may be important.

DiGeorge Syndrome (DGS)

Initially described by DiGeorge in 1965,[27] these patients frequently present due to problems referable to the cardiovascular system,[28] especially conotruncal abnormalities, including truncus arteriosus and interrupted aortic arch (type B), as well as tetralogy of Fallot. The typical clinical features of patients with DGS include dysmorphic facial features (e.g., hypertelorism, cleft lip and palate, bifid uvula and low-set ears), thymic aplasia, parathyroid hypoplasia, dysplastic kidneys, and lung abnormalities. Mild to moderate mental retardation may occur. Most cases of DGS occur sporadically, although a number of familial cases have been reported. The etiology may be heterogeneous, with chromosomal abnormalities accounting for a significant minority of cases. Approximately 5 to 10 percent of infants with features of DGS have an abnormality of chromosome 22 with monosomy for the proximal portion of the long arm[29]; numerous other chromosomal aberrations have also been reported (e.g., distal 10p deletions)[30] in association with these third and fourth brachial arch defects. De la Chapelle and colleagues[11] were the first to report a specific association of deleted proximal portion of 22q, with subsequent reports of complete and partial monosomy of chromosome 22 involving 22q11, most typically due to unbalanced translocation. The critical region for DGS appears to be mapped between the centromere and 22q11.[31]

Other Chromosome Aberrations with Associated Cardiovascular Disease

A significant number of other chromosome abnormalities are associated with cardiovascular disease (Table 96-1). These abnormalities include triploidy, aneuploidy (other than trisomy 21, trisomy 18, trisomy 13, and Turner's syndrome), deletions, and duplications. The triploidy syndromes, which include 69,XXX, 69,XXY, and 69,XYY, have a greater than 50 percent incidence of congenital heart disease, the vast majority of which are septal defects (ASD or VSD). The aneuploidy syndromes, not discussed thus far, are varied and uncommon. They include mosaicism of chromosome 8[32] and chromosome 9,[33] which present clinically with VSDs with or without other associated complex defects. Aortic root dilatation and mitral valve prolapse (MVP) occur with partial monosomy of chromosome 22.[34] Other cardiovascular abnormalities associated with partial trisomy of chromosome 7q include VSD, PS, PDA, COA, and L-transposition of the great vessels.[35] Partial trisomy of chromosome 7p is most commonly associated with VSD, PS, or AV canal.[36]

Chromosome deletion and duplication syndromes are commonly associated with cardiovascular defects. The 4p- (Wolf-Hirschhorn)[32,33] and 5p- (cri du chat)[37] deletion disorders are associated with septal defects, PDA, and PS. The 4p- syndrome is usually complex, while the 5p- syndrome is associated with similar defects but usually is not complex. The duplication disorders have a variety of abnormalities. Gelb and colleagues recently described the association of tetralogy of Fallot with the San Luis Valley recombinant chromosome 8.[38] The frequency of tetralogy of Fallot among patients with this syndrome is approximately 40 percent, significantly higher than seen in other patients with congenital heart disease. The clinical data on patients with structural aberrations of chromosome 8 permit phenotypic mapping of these patients and suggest locations for the putative cardiogenic genes on chromosome 8.

SINGLE-GENE DISORDERS OF THE CARDIOVASCULAR SYSTEM

Inherited disorders due to a single abnormal gene that is transmitted in a predictable fashion are often referred to as Mendelian disorders. Mendelian inheritance produces phenotypes inherited according to the principles outlined by Mendel. Each gene exists in two alternate forms, or alleles, one each obtained from the mother and father. Mendel's first law states that each allele segregates independently and thus passes unchanged into different gametes at the formation of the next generation. His second law states that the genes sort themselves independently. Single-gene mutations account for most of the defined genetic disorders, such as hypertrophic cardiomyopathy (HCM) or sex-linked cardiomyopathy. The same disease may be due to a single or to multiple mutations in the same gene. Within any one family, however, the mutation responsible for a disease is always the same. Sometimes, however, different genes induce the same phenotype, a phenomenon referred to as genetic heterogeneity.

TABLE 96-1

Cardiovascular Disease Associated with Chromosome Abnormalities

Chromosome Abnormality (Eponym)	%CHD	Cardiovascular Disease
Tripoly		
69,XXX	>50	ASD, VSD
69,XXY	>50	ASD, VSD
69,XYY	>50	ASD, VSD
Aneuploidy		
Trisomy 13 (Patau's)	80–90	Usually complex; VSD, ASD, PDA, TGV, CoA, AS, dextrocardia
Trisomy 18 (Edward's)	90–99	Usually complex; VSD, ASD, PDA, bicuspid semilunar valves, CoA
Trisomy 21 (Down's)	50	Includes VSD, AVC, TOF, AI
Trisomy 11; 22	>50	Usually complex
Trisomy 8, Mosaic	25	VSD, PDA, CoA, PS, CM
Trisomy 8, Mosaic	70	Usually complex; VSD, PD, persistent LSVC
45, XO (Turner's)	10	50% have CoA; AS, aortic root dilation, VSD, ASD, dextrocardia, HLHS
Deletions		
4p- (Wolf-Hirschhorn)	50	Usually complex; VSD, PDA, ASD, PS, LSVC
5p- (cri du chat)	20–30	VSD, PDA, ASD, PS
7q-	20	Usually complex
8p-	85	VSD, TOF, DORV, PS, ASD
9p-	50	VSD, PDA, PS
13q-	25	VSD, ASD
17p- (Miller-Dieker)	60–80	VSD, ASD
18q-	25	VSD, PDA, ASD, PS
ring 18	20	CoA, PA, HLHS, LSVC
Duplications		
4p Trisomy	10	Variable
8q Duplication	45	TOF, DORV, VSD
10p Trisomy	30	Includes dextrocardia, CoA; usually severe
10q24-qter Trisomy	50	Usually complex; AVC, VSD, TOF
22pter-q11 Trisomy (cat eye)	50	Usually complex; TAPVR, VSD, TOF
Miscellaneous		
Fragile X	50	Aortic root dilation, MVP
San Luis Valley recombinant chromosome 8	90–95	TOF, DORV, VSD/PS, PS, TRUNCUS, ASD, HLHS

NOTE: AI = Aortic insufficiency; AS = aortic stenosis; ASD = atrial septal defect; AVC = atrio-ventricular canal defect; CM = cardiomyopathy; CoA = coarctation of the aorta; DORV = double outlet right ventricle; HLHS = hypoplastic left heart syndrome; LSVC = left superior vena cava; MVP = mitral valve prolapse; PA = pulmonary atresia; PDA = patent ductus arteriosus; PS = pulmonary stenosis; TAPVR = total anomalous pulmonary venous return; TGV = transposition of the great vessels; TOF = tetralogy of Fallot; Truncus = truncus arteriosus; VSD = ventricular septal defect.

In HCM, several mutations have been recognized in the β-myosin heavy chain (β-MHC) gene, most of which are missense mutations. In some families with HCM, however, linkage studies show the disease-related gene is not localized to chromosome 14, indicating that the disease is due to a gene at some yet unknown chromosomal locus (see Chap. 90). Thus, HCM is a disease of genetic heterogeneity, which is to be distinguished from a polygenic disorder, in which a trait or disease is due to the interaction of several genes (e.g., in the genetic predisposition for hypertension).

Mutations are stable, heritable alterations in DNA that occur spontaneously by lack of fidelity in sequence transfer or are induced by factors such as radiation, chemicals, and viruses. Base sequence changes, however, can occur. As noted, mutations can involve a visible alteration, such as deletion or translocation of a portion of a chromosome, or a change in as little as one base of a gene. Mutations of a single nucleotide are *point mutations.* A point mutation may substitute one nucleotide for another, resulting in the encoding of a different (*missense mutation*) amino acid; or it may change a codon for an amino acid to a stop-codon (*truncated mutant*) or to eliminate a stop-codon (*elongated mutant*). Furthermore, a nucleotide may be deleted or added, resulting in a frameshift, and the gene is read entirely differently (*nonsense mutation*), resulting in a nonfunctioning protein. There may be a deletion or addition of nucleotides. An example of the latter is the mutation responsible for myotonic dystrophy, where a triplet repeat of several thousand nucleotides is inserted into the 3′ end of the candidate gene from chromosome 19 that makes the mRNA unstable and presumably leads to the disease. Mutations exert their effects via alteration of enzymes or regulatory or structural proteins. Only mutations occurring in the gametes are transmitted.

"Dominant" and "recessive" inheritance of mutant genes refer to characteristics of the phenotype and are *not* characteristics of the gene, per se. Dominant inheritance of a mutant gene is defined as the clinical manifestation of that gene when it is present as only one of the two alleles, a condition known as *heterozygosity*. Recessive traits, on the other hand, imply that a double dose of the mutant allele at the locus is required for clinical detection. Those individuals carrying two identical mutant alleles are called *homozygous*.

Identification of the disease-causing gene when the defective protein is unknown has until recently been nearly impossible. In contrast, in genetic diseases where the protein abnormality is known one can deduce mRNA (and cDNA) sequences and construct probes to identify the approximate chromosomal location and ultimately to clone and sequence the gene and thus define the mutatin. Familial hypercholesterolemia and some of the thalassemias are disorders whose genes have been isolated and cloned using this classic approach. For most diseases, however, the protein defect is unknown, thus limiting this approach. Two techniques have now made it possible to determine the chromosomal locus of the disease-related gene without knowing the protein involved: (1) computerized linkage analysis and (2) the development of DNA markers detected as restriction fragment length polymorphisms (RFLPs), variable number of tandem repeats (VNTRS) or microsatellite variable repeats.[39]

Overview of Chromosomal Mapping, Isolation, and Identification of a Disease-Related Gene

Determining the chromosomal location and isolation of a disease-related gene encoding an unknown protein is virtually impossible without known chromosomal landmarks. Identification of a particular locus is possible by linking the gene of interest to a marker of known chromosomal position (locus). The known marker is usually identified as an RFLP by Southern blot analysis or as variable repeat sequences by PCR. The known marker must cosegregate (be inherited) with the disease so that affected individuals will have the marker at a frequency of greater than chance alone. This will occur when the chromosomal marker and the disease-related gene responsible are in such close physical proximity that they do not segregate separately as frequently as they would if they were either on separate chromosomes or far apart on the same chromosome. Thus, the marker and the disease gene are said to be genetically linked, identifying its chromosomal locus.

Mathematical determination of genetic linkage requires computer programs in order to calculate the likelihood that a marker is linked (or not linked). Using the logarithm of the odds for linkage, also called the lod score, linkage of marker and disease may be established in antosomal disorders a lod score > 3 is required (i.e., odds of 10^3:1 for linkage), while lod score < -2 excludes linkage. A lod score > 2 provides evidence for linkage in X-linked diseases. The distance between a marker and a linked gene varies from 1000 to 50,000 kilobase pairs (kbp) but is usually within 10,000 kbp. On the basis of linkage analysis, it is possible to construct a chromosomal map in which the appropriate distances between various markers are estimated in units referred to as centimorgans (cM), or approximately 1 million base pairs (bp). Even after genetic linkage is established, it is a considerable task to clone, isolate, and identify the gene of interest and its protein product and to identify the pathophysiology of the disease. Huntington's disease and myotonic dystrophy exemplified this problem.

The overall approach[40] to chromosomal mapping of hereditary diseases by linkage analysis and subsequent isolation of the gene may be summarized as follows: (1) collection of data from families through two or three generations having individuals affected by the specific disease; (2) clinical assessment to provide an accurate diagnosis using a consistent and objective criterion to separate normal individuals from those affected, indeterminate, or unknown; (3) collection of blood samples for immediate DNA analysis and to develop lymphoblastoid cell lines for a renewable source of DNA; (4) development of a pedigree analysis of the family; (5) DNA analysis for markers of known chromosomal loci that span the human genome in an attempt to find a known locus that is linked to the disease; (6) development of flanking markers around the region containing the disease locus; (7) isolation and cloning of the region of DNA containing the gene; (8) identification of the gene; (9) sequence analysis of the gene to precisely identify the mutation or mutations causing the disease; (10) demonstration of a causal relationship between the defective protein and the disease; and (11) development of a convenient test to screen for the mutations.

Concept of Genetic Linkage

Over 15,000 chromosomal regions (loci) of DNA can be recognized by appropriate DNA markers.[41,42] Given that there are 3 billion base pairs and 15,000 markers, there should be about 200,000 bp between any two markers; thus, the chances of linking a gene of interest to one of these markers should be rather easy. While it is now conceivable that with the necessary resources and expertise one could map practically any disease, it is still very tedious (Figs. 96-4, 96-5, 96-6, and 96-7). Markers are not evenly distributed, and some chromosomes have areas of up to 50 million bp without a known marker. Since humans inherit two sets of homologous chromosomes (diploid), all the genes carried by the autosomal chromosomes have two forms (alleles), one on the chromosome from the mother and the other on the one from the father. In a Mendelian-dominant disease, individuals affected with the disease will have one defective allele that is responsible for the disease and one normal allele. In some individuals, despite having the disease-related gene, there is no clinical evidence of the disease. The genotype refers to the person's genes or genetic composition, while the phenotype refers to the clinical manifestations. The percentage of individuals with the disease-related gene who do have one or more features of the disease is referred to as *penetrance*. This is to be distinguished from *expressivity*, which refers to the variable nature of the clinical features.

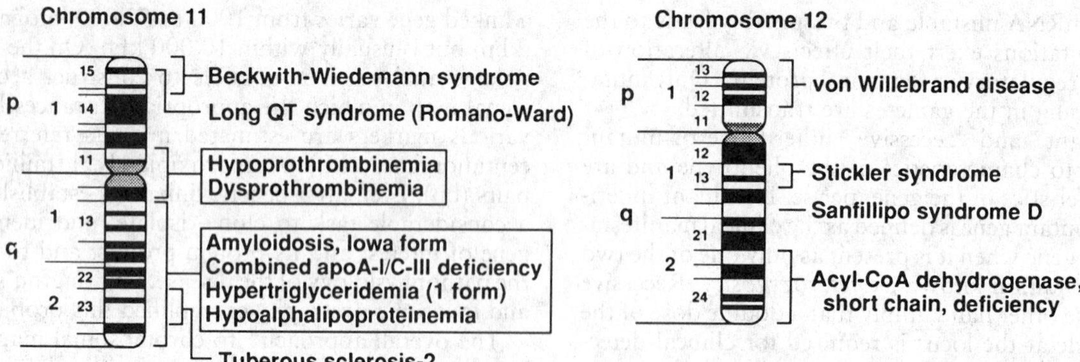

FIGURE 96-4 Ideograms of chromosomes 11 and 12 showing locations of cardiovascular disorders mapped to these chromosomes. Note 11p15, the localization of Beckwith-Wiedemann syndrome and long QT syndrome (Romano-Ward).

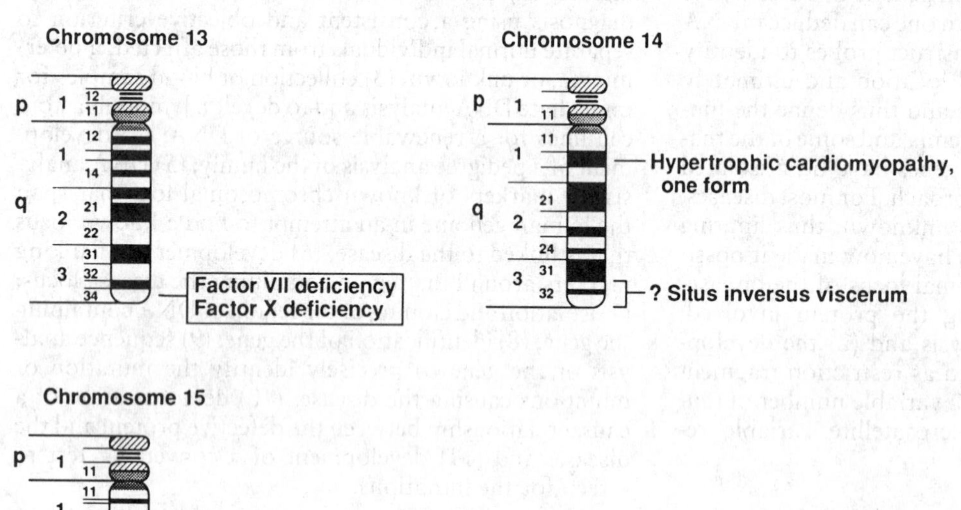

FIGURE 96-5 Ideograms of chromosomes 13, 14, and 15. Note map positions of hypertrophic cardiomyopathy to 14q11 and Marfan's syndrome to 15q21.

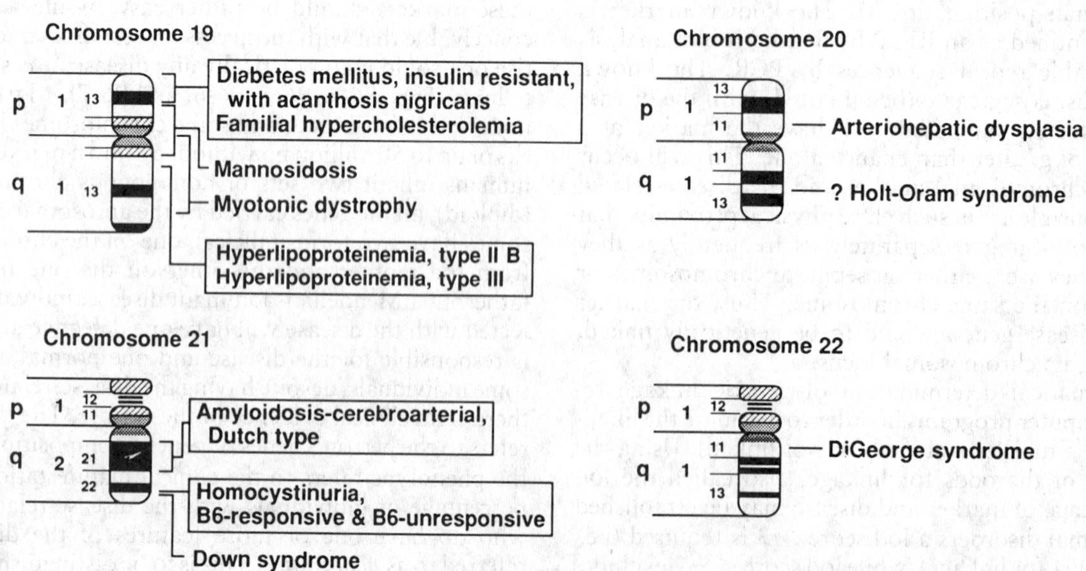

FIGURE 96-6 Ideograms of chromosomes 19, 20, 21, and 22. Specific localized disorders described in the text include myotonic dystrophy (19q1), Holt-Oram syndrome (20q13), Down's syndrome (21q22), and DiGeorge syndrome (22q11).

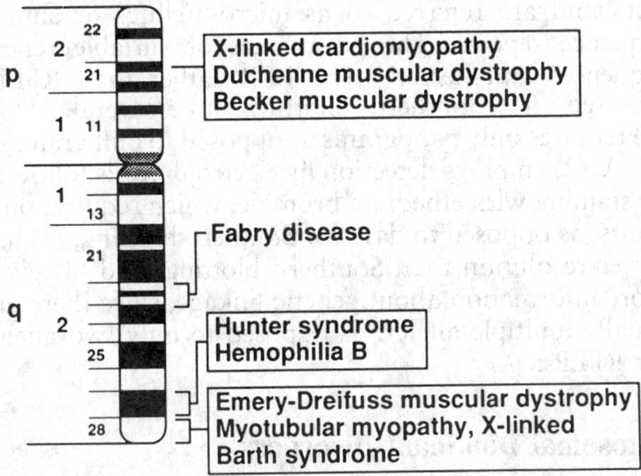

FIGURE 96-7 Ideograms of sex chromosomes X and Y. Positional mapping of X-linked cardiomyopathy, Duchenne's and Becker's muscular dystrophy (Xp21), Emery-Dreifuss muscular dystrophy, and Barth syndrome (Xq28) are shown.

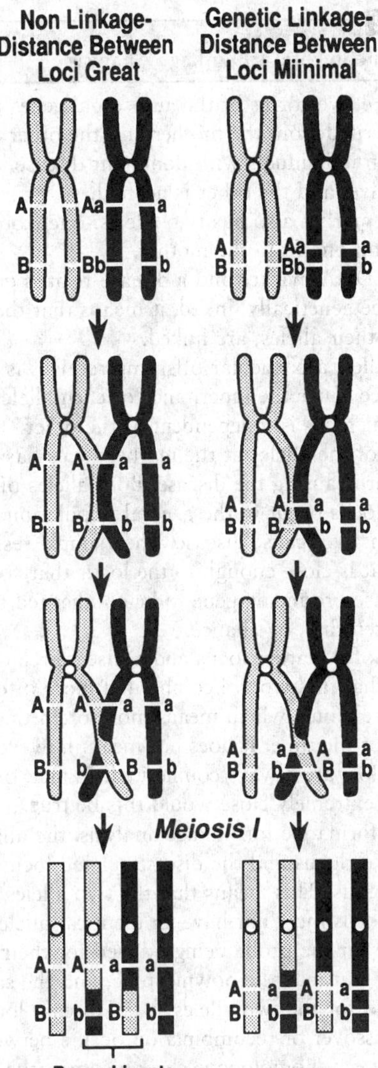

FIGURE 96-8 Comparison of nonlinked genes (*left*) and linked genes (*right*). In nonlinkage the distance between loci is large, allowing crossing over to occur, resulting in recombinants after meiosis. The distance between linked genes is comparatively small, thereby minimizing the chance for recombinants.

The concept of linkage analysis is illustrated in Fig. 96-8. On the left is an illustration of genetic linkage between a locus for a DNA marker and that of a disease that is Mendelian-dominant. The locus designated "A" carries the disease-associated allele. The corresponding locus "a" on the homologous chromosome has the normal allele. The loci designated "B" and the other "b" represent alleles of a DNA marker of known location and unrelated to the disease. In the panel on the right, the disease and the marker loci are so close that they tend to be coinherited, whereas in the lefthand panel the DNA marker is so far from the locus carrying the disease allele that it is far less likely that they will be coinherited. Prior to meioses, homologous chromosomes come together and form bridges (chiasmata) such that segments of equal proportion are exchanged between them, giving rise to crossover of various genes and separating gene loci that otherwise would have been coinherited. The loci occupy the same position on the homologous chromosome to which they recombined as they did on the chromosome from which they separated. This crossing over is referred to as recombination. The recombination frequency or fraction (Θ) between two marker loci is the ratio of the number of crossover events to the total number of meioses and reflects roughly the physical distance between them. The lower Θ between the locus of a marker and that of a disease-related gene, the closer the two must be in physical distance on the chromosome. Theoretically, if two loci are coinherited more than 50 percent of the time they are said to be linked. Θ is used to develop a means of estimating the genetic distance between the linked loci in centimorgans (cM), with 1 cM equivalent to a 1 percent Θ and roughly 1 million bp in physical distance, as noted earlier. This correlation, however, is variable from chromosome to chromosome and from region to region even on the same chromosome.

It is evident from the axioms stated in Table 96-2 that the linkage is not necessarily between the defective allele causing the disease and any one specific allele at the chromosomal marker locus. While the alleles of two genetically linked markers tend to be coinherited, either allele (or both in equal proportions) can occur with the disease allele, even within a single family. Thus, the disease allele, either in a particular family or in the general population, can be coinherited with any of the alleles at the marker locus.

Chromosomal Markers and Their Identification

Until recently, the most common chromosomal marker was that of RFLP, identified by Southern blotting. Hu-

TABLE 96-2

Axioms Fundamental to Linkage Analysis

1. There are two forms of the autosomal genes (alleles), one inherited from the mother and the other from the father. In individuals with dominant disease, one allele is defective, and the other is normal.
2. A DNA marker also has two alleles, one from the father and one from the mother.
3. When a DNA marker and a disease-related gene are said to be genetically linked, it means that the two loci not their alleles, are linked.
4. Which allele a particular offspring receives is totally by chance, since the inheritance of each allele at a particular locus is independent of the other.
5. Neither of the alleles at the marker locus has anything to do with causing the disease. Both alleles of the marker locus occur in the general population and do not themselves cause disease. They simply reside at a locus that is close enough to the locus that contains the disease-producing gene to be coinherited together more often than by chance.
6. Linkage of a marker locus and a disease-related locus implies that the two are coinherited more often than by chance alone, which means more often than 50 percent of the time. It does not mean, however, that the two loci are always coinherited; in fact, only if they are extremely close would this be true.
7. To be informative for linkage analysis, the alleles of the marker locus and the disease-related locus must be heterozygous. This means that the two alleles at the marker locus must not have an identical nucleotide sequence for the probe being utilized for their detection but must be polymorphic, and the same must hold for the two alleles at the disease locus.
8. Since crossover or recombination occurs between, and only between, homologous chromosomes, the alleles that cross over or recombine occupy the same locus on the new chromosome as they did on the previous chromosome.

man DNA shows a difference in individuals in the nucleotide sequence (polymorphism) every 300 to 500 bp. Polymorphisms occur more frequently in the sequence of the unexpressed DNA (intron) than in DNA coding for proteins (exon). Restriction endonucleases cleave foreign DNA by recognizing specific DNA sequences three to eight bases long. Consequently, digestion of human DNA by a restriction endonuclease results in a specific pattern of number and length of fragments. These DNA fragments can be separated by size using agarose gel electrophoresis and detected by hybridization to labeled DNA probes (Southern blotting). If a base change altered the recognition site of a restriction endonuclease or created an additional recognition site in one allele but not in the other, the pattern exhibited by the DNA on gel electrophoresis after restriction enzyme digestion would be distinctly different for the two alleles. This approach provides a means of detecting the minor sequence differences referred to as RFLPs. These polymorphisms between two alleles of the same homologous loci can be localized to provide a landmark along the chromosomal DNA to which other genetic markers, including disease loci, can be linked. These alterations are the basis of RFLP and the use of Southern blotting identifies polymorphic markers of known chromosomal location for linkage analysis.[43,44]

More convenient polymorphic markers are being recognized today due to tandem repeat sequences in which the number of base pairs repeated varies and provides for polymorphism that can be detected by PCR rather than Southern blotting. If the sequences are 15 to 20 bp or more in length, they are referred to as VNTRs, but the repeats may include only dinucleotides or trinucleotides and are referred to as microsatellites or simple sequence repeats. The advantages of variable repeat sequences and detection by PCR rather than RFLPs detected by Southern blotting are several. PCR (1) requires only nanograms as opposed to milligrams of DNA; (2) employs detection by electrophoresis followed by staining with ethedium bromide, which requires only hours, as opposed to days for Southern blotting; (3) has better resolution than Southern blotting; and (4) gives more information about genetic linkage, since there are usually multiple alleles, as opposed to only two alleles for RFLPs.

Autosomal Dominant Disorders

In autosomal dominant disorders, phenotypic manifestation occurs in heterozygous individuals carrying only one abnormal gene, although the corresponding allele on the homologous chromosome is normal. Both males and females can be affected, and since alleles segregate independently at meiosis, there is a 50 percent chance that the offspring of an affected heterozygote will inherit the mutant allele. Some affected individuals may not have an affected parent, since in all autosomal dominant diseases, sporadic occurrence may be due to a new mutation. The parent whose germ cells contain only the new mutation will be clinically normal, as will siblings. This heterozygotic parent, however, will transmit the disease-causing allele to half of the children. Autosomal dominant inheritance of human disease can be misdiagnosed as sporadic if there is incomplete penetrance in the phenotypically normal parent carrying the mutant allele or if extramarital paternity has occurred. The features characteristic of autosomal dominant inheritance are shown in Fig. 96-9. As previously noted, penetrance refers to the proportion of the individuals carrying the mutation that have the phenotype (disease). Expressivity refers to the variable expression of the clinical features (phenotype).

Autosomal Recessive Disorders

Autosomal recessive phenotypes are clinically apparent when the patient carries two mutant alleles (i.e., is homozygous) at the locus responsible for the disease state. Men and women are equally affected. Clinical uniformity is typical and, in contrast to dominant disorders, disease-onset and diagnosis generally occurs early in life. When both parents are heterozygous for a trait, only one in four children (25 percent) on average will be affected. The features characteristic of autosomal recessive disorders are shown in Fig. 96-9.

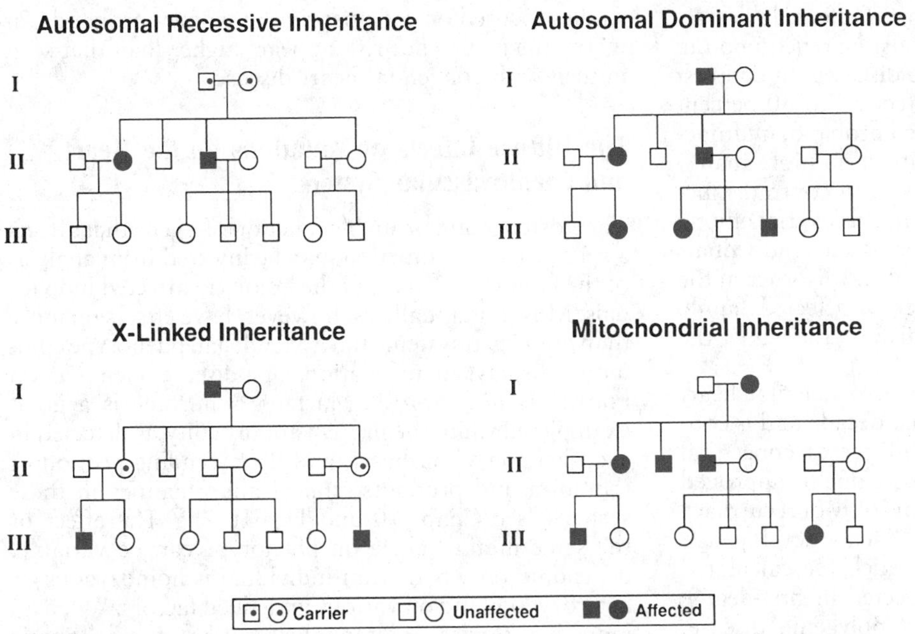

Autosomal Recessive Inheritance

Autosomal Dominant Inheritance

X-Linked Inheritance

Mitochondrial Inheritance

Carrier Unaffected Affected

FIGURE 96-9 Inheritance patterns of disorders described as autosomal recessive (*top left*), autosomal dominant (*top right*), X-linked (*bottom left*), and mitochondrial (*bottom right*).

X-Linked Disorders

Since X-linked disorders are caused by genes located on the X chromosome, the clinical risk and severity of the disease differs between the sexes. Since a woman has two X chromosomes, she may carry either one mutant allele (heterozygote) or two mutant alleles (homozygote); the trait may therefore display dominant or recessive expression. Since men have a single X chromosome (and one Y chromosome), they are expected to display the full syndrome whenever they inherit the gene, regardless of whether the gene behaves as a recessive or a dominant trait in carrier females. Hence, the terms *X-linked dominant* and *X-linked recessive* apply only to the expression of the gene in women. Since men must pass on their Y chromosome to all male offspring, they cannot pass on mutant X alleles to their sons, and therefore no male-to-male transmission of X-linked disorders may occur. On the other hand, males must contribute their one X chromosome to all daughters conceived. All females receiving a mutant X chromosome are known as carriers, and those individuals that become affected clinically with the disease are known as manifesting female carriers. The characteristic features of X-linked inheritance are shown in Fig. 96-9. Two other important points concerning X-linked inheritance should be noted. First, female carriers who express the disorder probably do so because of X inactivation, described by the Lyon hypothesis. Second, some mothers of affected males are not carriers but may have more affected sons if germinal mosaicism occurs. Such an occurrence is uncommon, however.

Mitochondrial Inheritance

Inheritance through the mitochondrial genome has been described recently, and abnormalities in these genes can manifest cardiovascular abnormalities. Energy generation in mitochondria is dependent on oxidative phosphorylation. Each mitochondrion has a single chromosome that encodes for a number of the required enzymes. Mitochondrial genome defects cause diseases that do not behave as Mendelian traits.[45,46] Since the spermatocyte contributes few or no mitochondria to the zygote, the entire mitochondrial complement present in a fetus must therefore be derived from the mitochondria present in the cytoplasm of the oocyte. Thus, phenotypes due to mitochondrial mutations demonstrate maternal inheritance only. The characteristic features of mitochondrial inheritance of disease are shown in Fig. 96-9.

Multifactorial Inheritance of Cardiac Disease

This type of inheritance has been proposed to explain the hereditary component of a number of disorders, including hypertension, coronary artery disease, and congenital heart disease. In multifactorial genetic diseases, there is a polygenic component that consists of multiple genes interacting in a cumulative fashion.[47,48] A combination of genes that interact to create a risk potential above threshold is presumably dependent on environmental factors that become instrumental in determining whether and to what extent the individual is clinically affected. Thus, in a family with multifactorial genetic diseases, other family members must possess the common genetic-environmental combinations to express the same disorder. Since all first-degree relatives of affected individuals (i.e., parents, siblings, and offspring) share one-half of that individual's genes, they are at increased risk of exhibiting the same disorder. Second-degree relatives, such as uncles, aunts, and grandparents, share an average of one-fourth of the affected individual's genes [i.e., $(1/2)^2$], while third-degree relatives (i.e., cousins) share one-eighth [i.e., $(1/2)^3$] of the genes, and so on. Therefore, as the relationship to the affected individual becomes increasingly distant, the likelihood of inheriting the disease decreases significantly. Since the number of genes responsible for polygenic traits is not precisely known, the risk of inheritance cannot be precisely determined.

Empiric risk figures—the proportion of affected relatives in previously reported families—must be relied upon in counseling families with polygenic diseases. In contrast to single-gene disorders, which affect 25 to 50 percent of first-degree relatives of an affected proband, multifactorial genetic disorders generally affect no more than 5 to 10 percent of first-degree relatives. In contradistinction to Mendelian traits, the recurrence risk varies among families depending on the number of affected individuals already diagnosed and the severity of the disorder in the index case. The larger the number of affected family members and the more severe the disease, the higher the risk to other relatives.

The empiric risk of recurrence of congenital heart disease has increased during the past decade and is consistent with the overall higher incidence of congenital heart disease now seen, which may be due to improved detection and reporting. The original study of recurrence risk was performed by Edwards,[49] who developed a method of testing the polygenic model. He calculated the incidence of disease to be expected in first-degree relatives of subjects affected with polygenic disease. Nora and coworkers[50] first undertook family studies in 1970 to determine whether the actual incidence of congenital heart disease in first-degree relatives corresponded to the prediction made by this model. The recurrence risk published for first-degree relatives is in the range of 1 to 5 percent and is in good agreement with the figures predicted by Edwards' theory. For this reason, the concept of polygenic inheritance of congenital heart disease gained wide acceptance. In addition, he observed a sex distribution of congenital heart disease that appeared to conform to that predicted by this model. Recent evidence suggests that different anatomic defects may be the result of the same pathogenic mechanisms. Clark[51] suggested that the majority of congenital cardiovascular defects are due to six disordered developmental mechanisms: (1) abnormal ectomesenchymal tissue migration, (2) abnormal intracardiac blood flow, (3) abnormal targeted growth, (4) extracellular matrix abnormalities, (5) endocardial cushion defects, and (6) looping defects.

This classification was utilized to study the familial aggregation of congenital cardiovascular malformations, and results of two separate studies[52,53] indicated an increased aggregation within families of probands with congenital heart defects that are due to altered embryonic blood flow. Using regressive logistic models, Maestri and colleagues[54] suggested that an autosomal recessive gene may be controlling the risk of congenital heart disease in families with hypoplastic left heart syndrome. In addition, they noted familial aggregation of congenital heart disease in families of probands with VSDs that were more likely to be black, while right heart defects were more closely associated with caucasians. Rose and coworkers[5] and Whittemore and associates[55] showed that the incidence of congenital heart disease in the children of probands with congenital heart disease have a significantly higher risk than the 1 to 5 percent risks described by Nora and colleagues.[47] Their studies demonstrated a risk of 8 to 12 percent, and they felt that these increased risks were associated with environmental factors. These conclusions have been criticized, however, because the studies focused on the offspring of women probands, in whom the recurrence risk appears higher than that seen in men with congenital heart disease.

The Diffuse Effects of Mutations on the Heart and Cardiovascular System

The existence and probable function of a gene that affects a specific cardiac function may be inferred from analysis of the family pedigree and the lesions in affected individuals. Most mutant alleles, however, have effects on more than one organ system, and a Mendelian phenotype commonly displays manifestations of a disease phenomenon known as *pleiotropy*.[56] Marfan's syndrome is a good example; fibrillin, the protein abnormality, is detected in eye, skeleton, skin, heart, and the ascending portion of the aorta and produces clinical abnormalities in these systems (see Chap. 10 and Fig. 10-7).[57] The effect of the same mutant allele on phenotype can be variable, depending on whether an individual is homozygous or heterozygous and on various undefined factors. When an individual carries a mutant allele but has no phenotypic abnormality, the trait is nonpenetrant. This description, however, relies heavily on the sensitivity of the technique utilized for detection. For instance, the diagnosis of familial HCM by bedside examination is significantly less sensitive than that by echocardiography.

SPECIFIC DISORDERS

Hypertrophic Cardiomyopathies

Until recently, the accumulated knowledge of cardiomyopathies was mainly clinical and descriptive, since the cause was unknown. They are classified as hypertrophic (Chap. 90), dilated (Chap. 89), or restrictive (Chap. 91) in form. Myocardial hypertrophy and development of cardiac failure commonly occur, but the molecular basis has remained elusive. The new technology of recombinant DNA and molecular biology has permitted new understanding of some of these disorders. Many may be caused by mutations in single genes.

Familial Hypertrophic Cardiomyopathy (FHCM)

FHCM is characterized by myocardial hypertrophy (Figs. 90-3 and 90-5), a wide spectrum of symptoms, including dyspnea, chest pain, and syncope; and an annual death rate of 2 to 4 percent due to sudden death, which can occur even in asymptomatic individuals (see Chap. 90). This disorder is the leading cause of sudden death in the young and in athletes.[58] The left ventricular hypertrophy is most commonly asymmetric, being predominantly of the septum, but may affect most of the ventricle or be localized. Outflow tract obstruction may or may not occur. Anatomically and histologically, the phenotype is most clearly defined by myocardial hypertrophy without obvious cause, showing cellular and myofiber disarray, myocardial fibrosis, and mediointimal proliferation of small coronary arteries. None of these features is pathognomonic. For example, myofiber disarray is present normally during embryogenesis and in congenital heart defects that place a strain on the right-sided circulation, such as pulmonary atresia with intact ventricular septum.[59,60] The diagnosis of HCM is based on typical clinical features and the demonstration of unexplained left ventricular, right ventricular, or biventricular hypertrophy on two-dimensional echocardiography (see Chap. 90).[61] The genetics of this disorder is consistent with that of an autosomal dominant pattern of inheritance. There is wide variability of expression of the clinical features, and penetrance is age-dependent.

Initially it was claimed that the gene for FHCM was on chromosome 6 in the human leukocyte antigen complex (HLA) region.[62] Others suggested linkage to chromosome 16[63] or 18.[64] Towbin and associates[65] provided molecular genetic data excluding the HLA region as the locus of HCM. Jarcho and colleagues[2] demonstrated linkage to chromosome 14q1 in a large French Canadian family, and Hejtmancik and colleagues[66] confirmed linkage in 8 unrelated families with FHCM from regions distributed throughout North America. Thus, 14q1 is apparently a major locus for this disease. The putative gene for FHCM was shown to be beta-myosin heavy chain (β-MHC).[67] Alpha and beta cardiac MHC genes, arranged in tandem within approximately 4.5 kb of each other on chromosome 14q11-13, are part of a multigene family that encodes at least 10 different myosin heavy-chain isozymes. These genes are highly homologous, with each being composed of 40 exons of approximately 25 kb and transcribing a 6-kb mRNA encoding a polypeptide of 220,000 daltons. Distinctive MHC isoenzymes are present in the heart and skeletal muscle fibers, and play an important role in muscle physiology (see Chap. 1). Several mutations[68,69,70,71,72,73] have now been identified in the β-MHC gene that follow Mendelian inheritance and appear responsible for FHCM. The first was a fusion of the α- and β-MHC gene[68] followed by identification of a missense mutation[69] in exon 13 of the β-MHC consisting of the substitution of adenine for guanine, resulting in a highly conserved arginine being replaced by glutamine. Marian and colleagues identified a mutation that consists of a major deletion in the 3′ end of the gene, consisting of exons 39 and 40 together with the 3′ sequences that contain the poly-A recognition site.[70] All other mutations described are of the missense type. In fact, the hybrid mutation has a missense mutation that may be responsible for the disease rather than the α/β hybrid. The missense mutation in exon 13 is interesting in that it introduced an extra recognition site for the restriction enzyme DdeI that can be used to provide a rapid genetic diagnosis following amplification of exon 13 of β-MHC gene with PCR.[74]

It is clear that β-MHC, with its multiple mutations, is a major locus of FHCM. It is also evident that there are many more mutations to be detected in the β-MHC gene, since it appears that each new family seems to be due to a new mutation. It is of interest that to date all of the missense mutations have been in that portion of the gene that encodes for the globular head of myosin. While this region has several well-recognized domains, such as the domains for binding ATP and binding actin, none of these regions appears to be involved, although it is highly likely that such mutations would be lethal, since they are so essential. The only mutation found to date, other than in the globular region of the myosin, is that of the deletion mutation, which is in the tail of the myosin and is of considerable interest, since it contains the amino acids that are essential to the binding of the protein molecules that form the thick myofilament. It is also of interest that the region that contains the poly-A recognition site is also deleted, which would be expected, to prohibit the mRNA from being transported out of the nucleus for translation. It is for this reason that structure-function analysis of this particular mutation should provide important information fundamental not only to the function of myosin but also to molecular genetics in terms of the exit and transport of mRNA from the nucleus to the cytoplasm. While several mutations have been identified and there appears to be little doubt that they are responsible for the disease, the absolute proof is yet to be obtained.

The evidence indicating that mutations in the β-MHC gene are responsible for this disease in those families linked to chromosome 14 are as follows: (1) linkage analysis in these families has shown that the locus is clearly on chromosome 14 with the strongest Lod score in the region of β-MHC; (2) mutations in β-MHC are observed only in those members of the family who are affected with the disease and not in the normal individuals; (3) in at least one mutation, the mRNA extracted from biopsies of the myocardium was shown to have the mutation,[75] and recently the same mutation was also shown to be present in the mRNA of the β-MHC of skeletal muscle;[76] and (4) a recently described family with sporadic disease was shown to have a mutation in the β-MHC gene that was not present in the unaffected parents.[77] Ultimate documentation of the causality of these mutations for the disease will probably require in vivo structure function analysis through the development of a transgenic animal or in knockout experiments such as homologous recombination. Unfortunately, this has been very difficult for all of the isolated genes but appears to be extremely difficult in the case of β-MHC, since in the mouse, the adult form of myosin is α-myosin heavy chain, with the β-MHC being only the fetal form. The complexity of FHCM has been further compounded by several recent reports showing the HCM in several families is due, not to β-MHC gene locus, but to some other locus not yet determined.[78,79,80] The clinical features, however, of those families that do not link to chromosome 14 appear to be virtually identical to those manifested by families due to β-MHC gene, and thus it will significantly accelerate our understanding of this disease if more loci are found to be responsible for the same clinical phenotype.

The genetic information acquired on FHCM is already of some importance in the overall diagnosis and management of this disorder. In those families with FHCM linked to the chromosome 14 locus, it is possible now to make a genetic diagnosis early in life and to determine whether or not they have the abnormal gene. Second, it is already evident that, despite the general similar clinical phenotype of patients with FHCM, certain mutations appear to be predictive of certain clinical features. Five families have now been described with disease due to the exon 13 missense mutation in which glutamate substitutes for arginine, and in each of these families, premature sudden death occurs in the second or third decade of life.[71,81] Thus, families with FHCM should be screened for known mutations, and any children with the missense mutation exon 13 should be counseled against combatant sports, since this is the most likely precipitant of sudden death in this group of FHCM. A genetic diagnosis of FHCM for known mutations is relatively easy to perform, since DNA can be obtained from white blood cells, or, using PCR, one can convert the mRNA to a cDNA from cells such as lymphocytes.[73,74] It is easy to detect exon 13 missense mutation, since it introduces an additional restriction enzyme site. In families with FHCM due to known mutations, since within a family it is always due to the same mutation, one can separate those with the genetic disorder from those who do not have the gene; this may be important for subsequent marital relationships. Ultimate comprehensive genetic diagnosis of FHCM will require, even for those families in which the disease is due to β-MHC, that all of the mutations be identified so that the genetic assay will include most of the mutations and that when an individual is excluded, one can feel certain the individual does not have FHCM. The identification of other loci and other genes will play a role in excluding this disease in families that do not link to β-MHC.

Pompe's Disease (Type II Glycogen Storage Disease) Genetic deficiency of acid α-1,4 glucosidase results in a wide clinical spectrum ranging from the rapidly fatal infantile-onset of type II glycogen storage disease (GSD), to a slowly progressive adult-onset myopathy. The infantile-onset form (Pompe disease) typically manifests during the first months of life, and patients usually die before their second year.[82] This rare inborn error of glycogen metabolism occurs in less than 1 per 100,000 persons. Massive glycogen accumulation occurs, leading to the clinical findings of enlarged tongue, striking hepatomegaly, hypotonia with decreased deep tendon reflexes, and cardiomyopathy with congestive heart failure. The diagnosis may be predicted from the pathognomonic electrocardiogram with enormous increases in voltage. The disease has autosomal recessive inheritance, and the gene coding for the lysosomal enzyme has been mapped to chromosome 17[83] at subband 17q23-q25. Allelic variation at the acid α-glucosidase locus is presumed to be the most important factor in diversity of type II GSD.[84]

Beckwith-Wiedemann Syndrome The combination of macroglosia, exomphalos, and visceromegaly has been designated the Beckwith-Wiedemann syndrome (BWS). Multiple other abnormalities have also been described, including fetal adrenocortical cytomegaly, hypoglycemia due to pancreatic islet hyperplasia, transverse linear creases of the ear lobules, hemihypertrophy, and accelerated osseous maturation. Infants with this syndrome are at particularly high risk, cumulatively estimated at between 5 and 20 percent, for development of Wilms' tumor, adrenocortical carcinomas, hepatoblastomas, and rhabdomyosarcomas.[85] The cardiovascular system is also commonly affected with the development of hypertrophic cardiomyopathy. In general, cases are sporadic, but familial disease has been described. Most of these familial cases have apparent autosomal dominant inheritance,[86] albeit with variable penetrance and variable expressivity. A variety of structural abnormalities of chromosome 11, reminiscent of alterations seen in Wilms' tumor, have been found.

LEOPARD Syndrome This rare autosomal dominant disorder is characterized by the cardinal features lending to the mnemonic *L* (lentigenes), *E* (ECG conduction defects), *O* (ocular hypertelorism), *P* (pulmonic valve stenosis), *A* (abnormalities of genitals), *R* (retardation of growth), and *D* (deafness, sensorineural). Anatomically, pulmonic stenosis is the most frequent abnormality, followed by hypertrophy and endocardial fibroelastosis. The most common electrocardiographic defects include first-degree AV block, left anterior hemiblock, and complete heart block. At present, no cytogenetic or molecular genetic abnormalities have been associated with this disorder.

Friedreich's Ataxia Friedreich's ataxia is the most common of the hereditary ataxias. This disorder, with an incidence of 1 in 50,000 and a carrier frequency of 1 in 110, is inherited as an autosomal recessive trait in which neurologic and cardiac abnormalities coexist. It is characterized by progressive degeneration of the central and peripheral nervous systems, and has onset before puberty. Typically, the initial abnormality is that of ataxia, with HCM presenting later.[87,88,89] (See also Chap. 10 and Fig. 10-20.) Recently, localization of the Friedreich ataxia-causing locus to chromosome 9q13-21.1 has been reported by demonstration of tight linkage to two anonymous DNA markers, D9S15 (MCT112) and D9S5 (DR47), by Chamberlain and associates[90,91] and Fujita and associates,[92] respectively. Although absence of recombination between these two markers and the gene locus has prevented resolution of the gene-probe order in this region, the strength of linkage (MCT112 Lod score >80, R = 0; DR47 Lod score >50, R = 0) with these probes suggested that they are within 1 mega bp of each other and the Friedreich ataxia locus. More recently, Fujita and colleagues[93] established a 1 million bp (megabase pair, mb) map around these probes and found them to be less than 260 kbp apart. Since no translocations, deletions, or recombination in patients with Friedreich's ataxia has been found—and therefore no indicators of more exact locus position seen—the search for this locus position remains elusive. Furthermore, no differences in gene localization have been seen differentiating individuals affected with HCM and those without cardiac involvement.

Dilated Cardiomyopathies

Idiopathic Dilated Cardiomyopathy

Idiopathic dilated cardiomyopathy (IDCM) is a disease of unknown cause characterized by increased ventricular size and impaired ventricular function; it is sometimes believed to be genetic. (See also Chap. 89). The prevalence of IDCM has been estimated to be approximately 40 cases per 100,000 in the population,[94] and most cases are believed to be sporadic.[95] The diagnosis of IDCM is typically supported by echocardiographic studies, and symptoms usually are those of congestive heart failure (see Chap. 89). Familial IDCM has usually been considered a rare and distinct disorder, causing an estimated 6 to 9 percent of cases of DCM.[96] Michels and coworkers[97] recently studied 315 relatives of 59 index patients with IDCM. They estimated that approximately 20 percent of the index patients had familial disease, an estimate much higher than previously reported. For this reason, molecular genetic analyses of families with IDCM could improve the understanding of the mechanisms of the pathogenesis in these disorders. In addition, once the pathogenesis is known, improved therapy could potentially be developed. It is likely that this disease exhibits genetic heterogeneity (see Chap. 89).

Specific Heart Muscle Diseases

The Muscular Dystrophies

The muscular dystrophies are a heterogeneous group of diseases the primary manifestations of which include progressive muscle wasting secondary to intrinsic defects of the muscle fiber. These defects have a wide spectrum of clinical expression and include Duchenne's muscular dystrophy (DMD), Becker's muscular dystrophy (BMD), Emery-Dreifuss' muscular dystrophy (EDMD), and myotonic dystrophy (MMD). The predominant cardiac lesion is a dilated ventricle, which is central to the associated morbidity and mortality.

Duchenne's Muscular Dystrophy DMD is an X-linked recessive genetic disorder that affects approximately 1 in 3500 males, one-third of whom have new mutations. Progressive muscle wasting and loss of muscle strength generally result in affected boys requiring wheelchairs by 11 years of age and death, usually by age 30 years.[98] The cardiac abnormality is most typically a dilated cardiomyopathy, with the posterobasal left ventricle most affected.[99] The age of onset of the cardiomyopathy varies and may be associated with cardiac arrhythmias.[100] Recently, the gene for DMD was cloned[101] and its protein product (dystrophin)[102] determined. The dystrophin gene was first localized to the Xp21 band in the midportion of the short arm of the X chromosome (Fig. 96-7). DNA cloned from this region was used as probes in skeletal muscle libraries to find the mRNA transcribed. Sequence data from the RNA transcript provided the information needed to determine the amino acid sequence of the protein dystrophin. Mutations in the dystrophin gene may cause either low-level production of a nonfunctional protein or complete absence of dystrophin in the heart and skeletal muscle of affected patients. The dystrophin gene is among the largest discovered thus far, comprising approximately 2.5 mb transcribing a 14 kb mRNA molecule. The gene is normally expressed in striated and smooth muscle, as well as in brain.[104] In muscle tissue, the dystrophin protein has been localized to the cytoplasmic surface of the sarcolemma, and it is believed to be a cytoskeletal protein that is associated with several integral membrane glycoproteins.[105] This glycoprotein-dystrophin complex may be involved in the regulation of intracellular calcium, since dystrophin-deficient muscle has abnormally high levels of intracellular calcium, and increased calcium channel leak activity has been observed at the cell membrane.[106]

The dystrophin mRNA transcripts in muscle and brain tissue are different in sequence. The mRNA transcript is alternatively spliced to encode multiple isoforms of the dystrophin protein in a developmentally and tissue-specific manner. Several of these isoforms appear to be unique to the heart.[107] This posttranscriptional modification may result in a functional diversity for the dystrophin protein. The fact that human cardiac Purkinje fibers express[108] dystrophin isoforms may be important in the development of cardiac arrhythmias in this disorder. The dystrophin mRNA sequence that predominates in skeletal muscle has been cloned as a full-length cDNA, and the recombinant dystrophin protein has been introduced and expressed in tissue culture.[109] This first step toward developing gene therapy strategies to correct the molecular defect in DMD lends hope to the possibility of future molecular-based therapeutic strategies. The precise means whereby dystrophin induces this disorder remains unknown. At present, the diagnosis of DMD is made, not by histologic examination, but by either Southern blotting and PCR analysis of deletion mutations[110,111] from blood or immunoblots of biopsies.[112]

Becker's Muscular Dystrophy (BMD) BMD is a less severe form of X-linked muscle-wasting disorder that is similar to DMD, but more benign, occurring approximately 10 percent as frequently as DMD.[100] Cardiac disease, in the form of dilated cardiomyopathy, may occur, but it is less frequent, and typically less severe. Occasionally, patients demonstrate moderate to severe cardiomyopathy. The BMD-causing gene is located at Xp21 (Fig. 96-7) and represents a different mutation of the same gene causing DMD (i.e., it is allelic with DMD). As with DMD, more than 30 percent of patients with BMD have no family history of the disease, an indication that they represent spontaneous mutations that are probably due to the large size of the dystrophin gene. The phenotypic difference between DMD and BMD patients has been speculated to be due to frameshift mutations leading to more severe disease (Duchenne's).[113] This issue remains controversial, however.

Emery-Dreifuss Muscular Dystrophy (EDMD) This X-linked recessive muscular dystrophy is a rare disease characterized by contractures and severe cardiac manifestations, including dilated cardiomyopathy and complete heart block often requiring pacemaker implantation early in adolescence.[114] EDMD carriers are also at risk of cardiac abnormalities and sudden death but typically do not have significant skeletal disease.

The gene responsible for EDMD is located on the long arm of the X chromosome (Xq27-qter; Fig. 96-7) and is linked to the factor VIII gene but has not yet been cloned.[115] Recently, EDMD was mapped to distal Xq28 in two multigeneration families; tight linkage between proximal Xq28 and EDMD was excluded by finding several recombinations between the more proximal Xq28 loci and the EDMD locus.[116]

Myotonic Dystrophy (Steinert's Disease) MMD, or Steinert's disease, is the most prevalent form of inherited muscular dystrophy in adults and is second only to Duchenne's muscular dystrophy in the incidence of new cases.[117] MMD is an autosomal dominant trait with incomplete penetrance and variable expressivity that is clinically characterized by a unique pattern of muscular weakness and wasting, myotonia, cataracts, ptosis, and frontal balding. Testicular atrophy and infertility are also seen. MMD has a high incidence of serious cardiac involvement varying between 20 and 90 percent of affected patients. A predominant abnormality is a dilated cardiomyopathy, and pathologic studies have also shown replacement of the Purkinje system by fatty and fibrous tissue similar to the involvement in the cardiac muscle. The conduction abnormalities include first-degree AV block, interventricular conduction defects, and bundle branch block. MVP is also fairly common, and sudden death is commonly seen.

The responsible gene was localized to chromosome 19q13.2-13.3 (Fig. 96-6), flanked by the M creatine kinase (MCK)[118] gene and an anonymous DNA marker,[119] but not until 1992 was the gene isolated, cloned, and subsequently sequenced.[120,121] Elucidation of the gene structure was accomplished after noting that a CTG triplet nucleotide repeat undergoes expansion in the 3′ region of the gene and cosegregates with the disease. It is believed that the most likely product of the gene is a protein kinase with a region that spans the cell membrane, indicating that the molecule is probably connected to a receptor from which signals are transduced.

X-Linked Cardiomyopathy (XLCM)

Berko and Swift[122] reported a 5-generation, 63-member family with dilated cardiomyopathy and no clinical evidence of skeletal myopathy. Males presented in the teens or early twenties with clinical evidence of mitral regurgitation and an echocardiographic diagnosis of dilated cardiomyopathy. Ventricular tachycardia was noted in several patients. The males progressed rapidly (within 1 year) to death or cardiac transplantation. Female carriers manifesting the disease developed mild cardiomyopathy in the fourth or fifth decade and progressed slowly. The only abnormality was elevated creatine kinase activity in affected males and carrier females expressing the milder form of the disease. Right ventricular endomyocardial biopsy revealed minimal interstitial fibrosis, while postmortem evaluation showed marked ventricular dilatation, widespread patchy fibrosis that was worse in the posterior wall, and normal mitochondria on electron microscopy. There were no pathognomonic findings differentiating this cardiomyopathy from other dilated forms, except for the apparent X-linked inheritance. (See also Chap. 89).

Towbin and colleagues[123,124] demonstrated linkage of XLCM to the dystrophin locus at Xp21 (Fig. 96-7) in the family described above, as well as in a second family. The tightest linkage occurred in the 5′ portion of this gene locus. No deletions were found. Evaluation of the protein defect in XLCM using antiserum against total cardiac protein showed absence (or low abundance) of the N-terminal dystrophin protein, whereas antiserum to the C-terminal demonstrated normal staining of cardiac dystrophin. The 156-kDa dystrophin-associated glycoprotein[107] was also decreased in cardiac tissue from all affected individuals. Evaluation of the RNA transcript from heart was also consistent with low-abundance message using a 5′ dystrophin cDNA probe; 3′ cDNA probes produced a band consistent with a smaller-than-normal transcript. While the actual mutation has not yet been located, this work allows prenatal and presymptomatic diagnosis in family members, as well as potentially leading to the diagnosis in unrelated sporadic cases of dilated cardiomyopathy.

X-Linked Cardioskeletal Myopathy (Barth's Syndrome)

Barth and coworkers[125] described an X-linked recessive disease in one large family characterized by the triad of dilated cardiomyopathy or endocardial fibroelastosis, neutropenia, and skeletal myopathy. All affected males died in infancy or early childhood from cardiac decompensation or septicemia. There were no affected females. Ultrastructural abnormalities were detected in mitochondria from cardiac and skeletal muscle, as well as in neutrophil bone marrow cells. Furthermore, respiratory chain abnormalities were observed, and isolated skeletal muscle mitochondria demonstrated diminished cytochrome concentrations. Lactic acidemia not provoked by prolonged fasting, increased plasma and muscle carnitine concentrations, growth retardation, and increased levels of urinary 3-methylglutaconic acid and 2-ethyl-hydracrylic acid have been seen.[126]

Molecular mapping of the locus demonstrated linkage to Xq28 (Fig. 96-7), the distal portion of the long arm of the X chromosome.[127] No candidate gene has been found thus far, although two disorders, EDMD and X-linked myotubular myopathy, have both clinical overlap and map to this region. It is possible that Barth's syndrome and EDMD are related in a manner similar to XLCM and DMD.

Idiopathic Hemochromatosis

This is a disease of iron overload with cardiac abnormalities in about 20 percent of cases varying from conduction disturbance to heart failure. The phenotypic expression of hemochromatosis is highly variable and greatly influenced by age, sex (10 times more common in men than women), and environmental factors. This disorder is believed to have autosomal recessive inheritance,[128] with the gene causing hemochromatosis believed to be close to the HLA-A locus on the short arm of chromosome 6 (6p21).[129] The gene is present in the heterozygous state in 8 to 10 percent of caucasians, with 1 in 333 individuals in the population being homozygotes. Molecular genetic confirmation of this linkage has not yet occurred. (See also Chap. 91.)

Restrictive Cardiomyopathy

Restrictive cardiomyopathy is the least common of the three major functional categories of cardiomyopathy in the western countries. Pathogenesis of the majority of cases of restrictive cardiomyopathy involves infiltration or replacement of the myocardium (or both). The causes are varied and can be either genetic or nongenetic. Genetic causes are most commonly due to metabolic diseases with secondary effects on the heart. The hallmark of the restrictive cardiomyopathies is abnormal diastolic function;[130] that is, the ventricular walls are excessively rigid and impede ventricular filling. A variety of specific pathological processes may result in restrictive cardiomyopathy, although the actual cause often remains unknown. Myocardial involvement with amyloid is one common cause of secondary restrictive cardiomyopathy, although restriction may also be seen with endocardial fibroelastosis, glycogen deposition, and hemochromatosis. (See Chap. 91.)

Systemic Amyloidosis

Amyloidosis that is either primary or secondary to chronic infection or malignancies may involve the heart. There is infiltration of the myocardium and coronary arteries and arterioles with either immunoglobulins in the secondary forms or prealbumin (transthyretin) in the primary forms. In either case decreased contractility and restrictive physiology develop. Patients may present initially with congestive heart failure or may manifest chest pain (from coronary artery involvement). Arrhythmias may also be a major manifestation of the disease. Atrial standstill has been described.[131] Various types of autosomal dominant familial amyloidosis have been described.[132] Heart muscle disease is a common feature and may be associated with neuropathy, nephropathy, or ophthalmopathy. These manifestations are associated with various amino acid substitu- tions in prealbumin due frequently to single base changes in the gene.[133] (See also Chaps. 88 and 91 and Fig. 10-23.)

Endocardial Fibroelastosis (EFE)

Endocardial thickening, which leads to decreased compliance and impaired diastolic function, characterizes endocardial fibroelastosis (EFE). Primary forms are typically unassociated with other cardiac anomalies. Most commonly, this disease presents in infancy and early childhood with signs and symptoms of congestive heart failure. The incidence of primary EFE in the United States in the past was relatively high—approximately 1 case in 5000 live births.[134] During the past decade, however, this incidence has decreased markedly for unknown reasons. Three inherited forms of EFE have been described: autosomal recessive,[136] autosomal dominant,[135] and X-linked recessive.[136] The majority of cases occur sporadically, however. In the X-linked forms, electron microscopy commonly demonstrates mitochondrial abnormalities. In many ways this disorder appears similar to Barth's syndrome,[127] except that EFE patients demonstrate endocardial scarring. (See also Chap. 91.)

Inborn Errors of Metabolism Causing Cardiomyopathy

Carnitine Deficiency

Carnitine is important in the shuttling of long-chain fatty acids and activated acetate across the mitochondrial membrane for terminal oxidation. Carnitine deficiency results in myocardial energy deprivation and thus cardiomyopathy, which may be either hypertrophic or dilated. Carnitine deficiency may be inherited recessively in two forms. There may be systemic deficiency characterized by low tissue and serum levels or normal serum and low muscle levels of carnitine due to deficient uptake. A severe skeletal myopathy may also be present. Secondary carnitine deficiency may be due to renal loss. Oral administration of carnitine has been reported to reverse cardiomyopathy in carnitine deficiency.[137]

Phytanic Acid Storage Disease (Refsum's Disease)

Refsum's disease is characterized by retinitis pigmentosa, cerebellar ataxia, and peripheral neuropathy and is inherited as an autosomal recessive trait. It is due to the absence of an α-hydroxylase metabolizing dietary phytol and phytanic acid, leading to the accumulation of tissue phytanic acid. The disease is occasionally associated with cardiomyopathy, which may be dilated and/or hypertrophic. Conduction disturbances and sudden death may occur. Cardiomyopathy preceding development of the neuropathy has been reported.[138] Plasmapheresis acutely or dietary modification may improve function.

The Mucopolysaccharidoses

The mucopolysaccharidoses (MPS) are a group of diseases caused by deficiency of lysosomal enzymes involved in the degradation of glycosaminoglycans (mucapolysaccharides).[139] Undegraded glycosaminoglycans accumulate in lysosomes and affect tissue function. MPS is classified (I, II, III, IV, VI, and VII) according to the deficient enzyme, and includes diseases with eponyms such as Hurler, Scheie, Hurler-Scheie, Hunter, Sanfilippo, Marquio, Maroteaux-Lamy, and Sly. These diseases share many clinical features, such as a chronic and progressive course involving multiple systems, organomegaly, dystosis, multiplex, and facial abnormalities. Hearing, vision, and joint mobility are commonly involved. Mental retardation is a feature of Hurler's syndrome, severe Hunter's syndrome, and all forms of the Sanfilippo's syndrome, but intellect is normal in other forms of MPS. Cardiac disease is common in most MPS patients with moderate-to-severe generalized disease. Myocardial hypertrophy, pulmonary and systemic hypertension, valvular disease, and coronary occlusion may lead to congestive heart failure or sudden death. Both aortic and mitral valve disease occur, and valve replacement has been reported. Cardiac function is monitored serially by echocardiography. Anesthesia may represent a very significant risk because of the skeletal, as well as cardiac, abnormalities. The potential for treating various MPS with gene therapy is being investigated in animal models.

Medium-Chain Acyl CoA Dehydrogenase (MCAD) Deficiency

First described in 1982,[140] MCAD deficiency appears to be the most common inborn error of fatty acid oxidation. It is characterized by recurrent episodes of illness, provoked by fasting for more than 12 h, with the first episode generally occurring between 6 and 24 months. The most common symptoms include vomiting and severe lethargy that can progress to coma, muscle weakness, and exercise intolerance. Hypoglycemia is often present between episodes, when patients appear normal. Hepatomegaly and dilated cardiomyopathy are also seen.[141] Liver biopsy can show marked fatty infiltrate ranging from a predominantly microvesicular to a macrovesicular pattern. This autosomal recessive disorder has recently been localized to 1p31. Cloning and further molecular characterization are in progress.

Long-Chain Acyl CoA Dehydrogenase (LCAD) Deficiency

First described in 1985,[142] LCAD deficiency exhibits recurrent episodes of coma, vomiting, and hypoglycemia triggered by fasting. Both dilated and hypertrophic cardiomyopathies have been seen. The gene locus for this disorder has been localized to chromosome 7.

Other Inborn Errors of Metabolism

Heart muscle disease is a common accompaniment in syndromes due to inborn errors of metabolism, including certain glycogen storage diseases (GSD) such as Forbes-debrancher-enzyme deficiency;[143] amylo-1,6-glucosidase deficiency, which causes hypertrophy and cardiac failure; phosphorylase kinase deficiency, which has associated dilated or hypertrophic cardiomyopathy;[144] and branching enzyme deficiency (type IV GSD) or Andersen's disease.[145]

Mitochondrial Cardiomyopathies

The human mitochondrial genome[46] is a small circular DNA molecule that is maternally inherited. Mitochondrial DNA (mtDNA) encodes 13 of the 69 proteins required for oxidative metabolism, and the 22 transfer RNAs (tRNAs) and 2 ribosomal RNAs (rRNAs) required for their translation. mtDNA has much less redundancy than the nuclear genome (in which essentially identical information is received from both parents), and the mitochondrial genome has been associated with mutations giving rise to disease.[45] The 13 mtDNA genes that code for proteins in the respiratory chain[146] must be coordinated with nuclear genomes to permit assembly of the complex holoenzymes. The DNA contained in each of the numerous mitochondria derives exclusively from the female gamete, and any mutation must be passed from female parent to all progeny, male and female. The replicative segregation of mutant mtDNA during embryogenesis determines phenotype, and the number of mutant mtDNA copies within the cell determines whether this biological disadvantage is expressed. In most mitochondrial disorders, patients carry a mix of mutant and normal mitochondria—a condition known as heteroplasmy, with the proportions varying from tissue to tissue and individual to individual within a pedigree, in a manner correlating with severity of phenotype.[147] Most of the genetic disorders exhibit abnormalities in the muscle, brain, and heart. Some of the better delineated syndromes are discussed below.

Kearns-Sayre Syndrome

KSS is a mitochondrial myopathy characterized by ptosis, chronic progressive external ophthalmoplegia, abnormal retinal pigmentation, and cardiac conduction defects, as well as cardiac dilatation.

MERRF Syndrome

This syndrome is characterized by *M*yoclonic *E*pilepsy with *R*agged *R*ed muscle *F*ibers (MERRF)and is caused by a single nucleotide substitution in tRNA LYS that apparently interferes with mitochondrial translation. Shoffner and coworkers[148] showed an A to G transition mutation as the cause of the disease. It is associated with defects in complexes I and IV of the respiratory chain. This abnormality causes decline in ATP-generating capacity, with onset of disease that includes cardiomyopathy.

Hypoxemia, mtDNA Damage, and Cardiac Disease Since cardiac tissue relies on the mitochondria for energy production, it has been believed that deficiency of portions of this system or its end product can cause cardiac abnormalities. Hypoxemia or ischemia has been shown to increase oxygen radical production, which is thought to result in elevated mtDNA damage and altered oxidative-phosphorylation gene expression. In addition, these enzymes have been shown to decline with age, while mtDNA deletions increase with age. Corral-Debrinski and associates[149] hypothesized that ischemic hearts would be likely to have increased chances of mtDNA deletion due to this effect of hypoxemia. Using PCR amplification across the deletion break points of the common mtDNA[149], they showed mtDNA damage was increased in chronically ischemic hearts as well as in some hearts with other forms of chronic cardiac disease (i.e., dilated or hypertrophic cardiomyopathy). It is possible that mitochondrial gene induction is part of a general response to chronic cardiac failure.

Structural Defects

Familial Atrial Septal Defect (ASD)

Two Mendelian forms of ASD exist as autosomal dominant traits. The first form has no other associated abnormalities; it has been speculated that the gene for this form of secundum ASD is on chromosome 6p, linked to the HLA complex.[150] No molecular genetic analysis of these families has thus far been carried out. The more common form of familial secundum ASD is associated with AV conduction delay.[151] These patients have, on rare occasion, had progression of heart block to a high-grade form. In these patients, attention should be directed to the upper limbs, particularly the thumbs, to rule out the Holt-Oram syndrome, described below. Another form of ASD has been described and is thought to have mitochondrial inheritance.[152] None of these forms of ASD has thus far had molecular analysis, and hence there has been no confirmation of gene localization. (See also Chap. 97.)

Holt-Oram Syndrome

The cardinal manifestations[153] of the autosomal dominant Holt-Oram syndrome include upper limb dysplasia, ASD, and marked variability within families. The abnormalities of the arm are typically bilateral and range from undetectable to distally placed thumbs and hypoplastic thenar eminences, triphylangeal thumbs, anomalies of the carpus, and radial aplasia, to phocamelia and hypoplasia of the clavicles and shoulders. In addition to ASD, VSD or AV node, conduction disturbance has been noted. Recent unconfirmed evidence has placed the disease-causing locus on chromosome 20q13 (see Fig. 10-2 and Chap. 10).

Ellis-Van Creveld Syndrome

The cardinal manifestations of this rare autosomal recessive chondrodysplasia include congenital heart disease, short stature, metaphyseal dysplasia, dysplastic nails and teeth, and postaxial polydactyly (see Fig. 10-1 and Chap. 10). Congenital heart disease is present in more than 50 percent of homozygotes and mostly affects the atrial septum, primarily involving the endocardial cushion, with defects such as ostium primum ASD and single atrium. Other associated abnormalities include COA, hypoplastic left heart syndrome, and PDA, which occur in approximately 20 percent of individuals. A significant number of individuals with this syndrome are born to consanguineous parents. No molecular genetic analyses have been reported.

Supravalvular Aortic Stenosis (SVAS)

SVAS is seen in three situations, most commonly with Williams' syndrome.[154] This disorder is usually sporadic but may be a highly variable autosomal dominant condition. The full spectrum of Williams' syndrome[152,155,156] includes dysmorphic facies, often called "elfin" facies, infantile hy- percalcemia, mental retardation, short stature, SVAS, and multiple peripheral pulmonic stenoses (see Fig. 10-25 and Chap. 10). Occasionally, there are other manifestations, including MVP, bicuspid aortic valve, and hypertension. Many of these individuals have robust personalities that have been called "cocktail party" personalities. Late-onset problems may include progressive joint contractures, gastrointestinal dysfunction, and genitourinary dysfunction. Since hypercalcemia is a typical feature of Williams' syndrome, calcitonin has been considered a likely candidate gene for SVAS but has been excluded.[157] No other linkage or cytogenetic data have been reported.

A second type of SVAS is the autosomal dominant entity that is distinct from that of Williams' syndrome. Mental retardation and abnormal facies are not found in this disorder. They present with clinical evidence of SVAS and/or peripheral pulmonary artery stenoses[158] and the diagnosis relies on echocardiography. Recently, Ewart and colleagues demonstrated linkage to chromosome 7 near the elastin gene (7q11) in 2 families with this disorder.[159]

Mitral Valve Prolapse (MVP)

This heterogeneous cardiac finding appears to be the most common abnormality of the human heart and occurs in association with various syndromes, especially connective tissue disorders such as Marfan's syndrome and Ehlers-Danlos syndrome (see Chap. 80). In the majority of other cases, MVP is noted sporadically as an auscultatory or echocardiographic finding. On occasion, however, familial inheritance of MVP in an autosomal dominant pattern is found and develops in an age- and sex-dependent manner.[160] At present, no molecular genetic studies have been reported on MVP syndrome. The recent discovery on chromosome 15 of fibrillin causing Marfan's syndrome offers some hope. There are several fibrillin proteins with similar structure and function on other chromosomes. If the locus for Marfan's syndrome is not associated with autosomal dominant MVP, it would be reasonable to consider one of the other fibrillin genes as a possible candidate.

Noonan's Syndrome

In 1963, a syndrome characterized by short stature, mild mental retardation, characteristic facies, webbed neck, delayed sexual maturity, chest wall deformity, and intracardiac abnormalities including valvular pulmonary stenosis was described by Noonan and Ehmke.[161] (See Fig. 10-13 and Chap. 10.) Hypertrophic cardiomyopathy is also a common feature. This syndrome is sometimes confused with Turner's syndrome but is distinct, not simply because both men and women are affected, but also because no cytogenetic abnormality is known to occur. They have an unexplained tendency to bleed, and an autosomal dominant inheritance pattern has been described.[162] The entire phenotype of Noonan syndrome, however, is highly variable, and affected people may be asymptomatic. Despite the relatively high frequency of Noonan's syndrome, estimated to be 1 per 1000 population, neither its cause nor its pathogenesis is clear. The gene has not been mapped. Kitchens and Alexander have reported a partial deficiency of coagulation factor XI in four patients with this syndrome,[163] later confirmed by deHaan and colleagues.[164] Factor XI has been mapped to chromosome 15 at the 15q11 locus and could help in locating the gene causing Noonan's syndrome.

Connective Tissue Disorders

The composition, structure, and function of normal and abnormal connective tissue is gradually being elucidated. Until recently, however, little attention has been paid to the biochemistry and molecular genetics of connective tissues relating to the cardiovascular system.[165] Histologically, the fibrous elements of the heart are composed largely of connective tissue structural proteins, which provide the framework for muscle contraction as well as support for the valves and major blood vessels. Collagen and elastin fibrils underlie the endothelial cells and extend into the subendothelial layer of the vasculature. The anuli fibrosi that separate the atria and ventricles and support the two AV valves are largely type I collagen fiber bundles. The major structural components of blood vessel walls are elastin and collagen types I and III, with lesser contributions from types IV, V, and VI. Approximately 50 percent of the total collagen in this tissue is type III collagen. Many of these components have been localized to specific chromosomes.[166] For instance, elastin is found on the long arm of chromosome 7 (7q11); and several collagen genes have been located, such as COL1A1 on the long arm of chromosome 17 (17q21.13-q22.05), COL1A2 on the long arm of chromosome 7 (7q21.3-7q22.1), COL2A1 on the long arm of chromosome 12 (12q13.1-12q13.3), COL3A1 on the long arm of chromosome 2 (2q31), and COL5A2 on the long arm

TABLE 96-3
Heritable Connective Tissue Disorders Associated With Cardiovascular Disease

Disorder	Cardiovascular Manifestation	Genetic Localization	Protein Abnormality
Curtis laxa	PS, PPS, MVP	Unknown	Unknown
Ehlers-Danlos			
I	MVP	Unknown	Unknown
II	MVP	Unknown	Unknown
III	MVP	Unknown	Unknown
IV	MVP, aortic rupture	2q31	Type III procollagen (COL3A1)
VI	MVP	Unknown	Unknown
VIII	MVP	Unknown	Type I procollagen (COL1A1),
X	MVP, aortic root dilation	2q34-36	? Fibronectin deficiency
Osteogenesis imperfecta			
I	MVP	17q21.31–22.05	Type I procollagen (COL1A1)
II	Arterial calcification	17q21.31–22.05	Type I procollagen (COL1A1)
		7q21.3–22.01	Type I procollagen (COL1A2)
III	MVP	17q21.31–22.05	Type I procollagen (COL1A1)
		7q21.3–22.01	Type I procollagen (COL1A2)
IV	Aortic root dilation	17q21.31–22.05	Type I procollagen (COL1A1)
		7q21.3–22.01	Type I procollagen (COL1A2)
Marfan's	MVP, aortic root dilation, aortic dissection	15q15–21.3	Fibrillin
Pseudoxanthoma elasticum	MVP, arteriosclerosis, EFE, MI	Unknown	Unknown

NOTE: EFE = endocardial fibroelastosis; MI = myocardial infarction; MVP = mitral value prolapse; PPS = peripheral pulmonary stenosis; PS = pulmonary stenosis.

of chromosome 2 (2q31). A variety of human disorders are due to abnormalities of these loci, and a few are described below (Table 96-3).

Marfan's Syndrome

This autosomal dominant disease demonstrates complete penetrance but widely variable expression. Approximately 5 percent of all cases are new mutations, and the prevalence appears to be 1 per 10,000.[163] The frequency of Marfan's syndrome is equal in males and females. Clinically, this connective tissue disorder is characterized by abnormalities affecting the bony skeleton, the eyes, and the cardiovascular system. The skeletal features include tall stature, arachnodactyly, dolichostenomelia, anterior chest deformity (i.e., pectus excavatum), high arched palate, and vertebral column deformities such as scoliosis and thoracic lordosis. (See Fig. 10-7 and Chap. 10.) The joints may be hypermobile or, in severe cases, congenitally contracted. Ocular features may include ectopia lentis (50 to 60 percent), myopia, retinal detachment, and corneal flattening. Loss of vision occurs in a significant number of patients. The cardiovascular features most often seen include progressive dilation of the ascending aorta with potential aortic dissection and sudden death, as well as mitral valve prolapse. Aortic and mitral valve regurgitation is a common accompaniment. The clinical phenotype is often apparent in infancy, and the diagnosis may be made if suspected. Most cases, however, are not diagnosed until the teenage years or later (second or third decade). Cardiovascular system involvement is typically diagnosed by echocardiography.

The follow-up and management of the cardiovascular abnormalities in Marfan's syndrome is controversial. Children without aortic valve regurgitation or aortic dilation are usually seen yearly, with echocardiographic evaluation advisable. In patients with mitral valve prolapse, mitral regurgitation, or aortic regurgitation, antibiotic prophylaxis to prevent subacute bacterial endocarditis (SBE) is recommended. Dilation of the ascending aorta, the most troubling abnormality, has been treated by many clinicians with beta-adrenergic blocking agents (i.e., propranolol or atenolol) in an attempt to retard the rate of aortic dilation and the occurrence of aortic dissection (see Chap. 123). Initiation of therapy and restriction of physical activity have been recommended when aortic dilatation is detected. Replacement of the aortic root with a valved conduit is generally performed when the ascending aorta reaches a diameter of 60 mm in adults regardless of symptoms or in patients undergoing aortic dissection. Also important is the screening of family members. Since this disease is inherited as an autosomal dominant trait, other family members have a relatively high risk of having this disorder. Therefore, clinical screening studies, such as history, physical examination, and echocardiography, are appropriate. Genetic counseling should be given to inform families of the autosomal dominant inheritance pattern with 50 percent recurrence in offspring.

In 1990, Marfan's syndrome was mapped to the long arm of chromosome 15 (15q15-21; Fig. 96-5),[3,167] and immunohistological studies have shown a new connective tissue protein[168] to be defective or deficient in patients suffering from Marfan's syndrome.[57] Since fibrillin is an element of elastic tissue and is abundant in tissues affected in Marfan's syndrome, including the aorta, the suspensory ligament of the lens, and the periosteum, it became a candidate gene. A probe from a partially cloned fibrillin gene (FBN1) was mapped to the same region (15q21.1),[169] followed by a description of a DNA polymorphism in the fibrillin gene clone that was tightly linked to the Marfan's phenotype.[170,171] Using clones of the fibrillin gene, de novo point mutations were seen in patients with sporadic Marfan's syndrome.

Fibrillin, a large glycoprotein with a molecular weight of 350 kDa, is a component of the microfibrils that are ubiquitous in the connective tissue space. Cloning and partial sequencing of the FBN1[172] cDNA, followed by hybridization to a single mRNA of approximately 10 kb, was performed. A second fibrillin gene (FBN2), located on chromosome 5 (5q23-31), was discovered and cloned in patients with congenital contractual arachnodactyly (CCA).[168] The chromosome 5 linkage for CCA and that of chromosome 15 for Marfan's syndrome is interesting, since both disorders include arterial dissection, MVP, and annuloaortic ectasia.

Ehlers-Danlos Syndrome (EDS)

EDS includes a heterogeneous group of diseases of at least 11 types characterized primarily by looseness of joints and variable involvement of skin and other connective tissues (see Figs. 10-5*A* and *B*).[173] Soft papules and nodules (pseudotumors) occur on the knees and elbows. The central feature of this autosomal dominant disease with respect to the heart is an abnormality of type III collagen, which causes aortic rupture and sudden death in many patients. The gene was localized to chromosome 2, and defined mutations appear that are similar to those seen in type I procollagen (COL1A1, COL1A2) genes found in many probands with osteogenesis imperfecta. Both point mutations and large deletions have been shown for probands with EDS type IV.

Familial Aneurysms

Procollagen gene defects have been described recently[174] in families with a relatively high frequency of arterial aneurysms. They have a defect in type III procollagen (COL3A1) similar to defects that have been reported in EDS type IV.[175] Familial incidence of aneurysms is fairly common (7 to 15 percent of aneurysms).[176] Since EDS is relatively rare, many of the more common familial aneurysms that have been identified with the type III procollagen abnormality may represent phenotypic overlap. These findings have resulted in a reassessment of the traditional teaching that most aortic aneurysms result from atherosclerosis. Family history should be carefully assessed in all patients with aortic or cerebral aneurysms, and, if it is positive, other family members should be assessed. Many should be followed with noninvasive evaluation in a fashion similar to that described for Marfan's syndrome.

Pseudoxanthoma Elasticum (PXE)

PXE is a genetic disorder of the elastic tissue that involves the skin, eyes, and cardiovascular system. Skin findings are a hallmark of this disease. Soft yellowish papules and polygonal plaques are most often found on the neck, below the clavicle, and in the axillas, antecubital fossae, periumbilical area, and perineum. The lesions vary in appearance and may resemble the skin of an orange (Fig. 10-6). Ophthalmological findings, when present, are characteristic. They include slate-gray to brown linear bands (angioid streaks) due to fibrosis in 50 to 70 percent of patients. Central vision loss can also occur. The heart in this condition is affected in a number of ways, including coronary artery disease with associated myocardial ischemia and infarction, which is the major cause of morbidity and mortality. EFE and MVP are also common.[177,178] Two clinical variants with autosomal dominant inheritance and two with autosomal recessive inheritance occur. The basic genetic defect is unknown.

Cutis Laxa This designation refers not only to a specific dermatologic sign, but to a variety of Mendelian and non-Mendelian, congenital and acquired syndromes sharing the characteristic feature of lax, nonresilient skin. Two varieties of autosomal recessive cutis laxa exist. Death from pulmonary complications may occur in the first months of life, and most patients die by the third year. Signs of right-sided heart failure are often seen in infancy and are generally due to pulmonary disease, although pulmonary artery stenosis also occurs.[179] Histopathologically, the pulmonary artery lesions are due to medioelastic fiber paucity. MVP has also been notable. The gene or genes that cause this spectrum of disease have remained elusive.

Primary Disorders of Rhythm and Conduction

Familial occurrence of virtually all rhythm and conduction abnormalities has been reported. However, since most families have been small, the mode of inheritance (or even whether the inheritance is Mendelian) is uncertain. In many cases, these conduction defects have been associated with other cardiac and systemic disorders. However, since there does appear to be genetic control of normal electrical conduction, it would not be surprising to find mutations in single genes that produce clinically important abnormalities. Recently, molecular genetic studies have allowed some progress to be made in this area.

Romano-Ward Long QT Syndrome (LQTS)

Independently, Romano[180] and Ward[181] described stress-induced syncope, sudden death, and ventricular arrhythmia in association with prolongation of the QT interval and abnormal T waves on electrocardiographic examination. Subsequent investigations demonstrated autosomal dominant inheritance in association with torsade de pointes as well as bradycardia and T-wave alternans.[182–185] Initial linkage analysis by HLA typing suggested that the gene causing Romano-Ward LQTS was localized to the HLA region at 6p21,[186] but molecular genetic analysis subsequently refuted the HLA linkage.[187] In 1991, Keating and coworkers[1] provided definitive evidence of tight molecular genetic linkage to chromosome 11p (Fig. 96-4) in a large Mormon kindred and subsequently in 6 other unrelated families.[188] Towbin and colleagues[189] have recently demonstrated genetic heterogeneity in families with Romano-Ward LQTS. In 11 families, they noted that only 7 were linked to 11p, while the remaining 4 families were clearly unlinked. The search for other gene loci associated with LQTS continues in earnest, as do efforts directed toward cloning the chromosome 11p gene. (See Chap. 36.)

Jervell and Lange-Nielsen Long QT Syndrome

This syndrome, described in 1957, is characterized by congenital deafness, syncope, prolonged QT interval, sudden death, and autosomal recessive inheritance.[190] Affected individuals are usually diagnosed in childhood with congenital, severe bilateral high-tone perceptive deafness; fainting spells precipitated by exertion, rage, or fright; and electrocardiographic evidence of QT interval prolongation and T-wave abnormalities. As would be expected for rare autosomal recessive traits, the parents of affected individuals are more likely than usual to be consanguineous. Although heterozygotes are clinically normal, their ECGs may have mild prolongation of the QT interval. At present, neither the cause nor the pathogenesis is known. No linkage data are available, and hence the chromosomal location of the culprit gene is unknown. The cardiac and hearing abnormalities appear to represent a pleiotropic expression of a single-gene abnormality. An interesting possibility is that those families thought to be unlinked to Romano-Ward are actually heterozygotes with Jervell and Lange-Nielsen syndrome, manifesting long QT interval without deafness. Studies of these families could possibly lead to localization of this locus instead of other Romano-Ward LQTS loci. Since the overall incidence of homozygous-affected individuals among all deaf children (i.e., the frequency of prolonged QT interval among deaf children) is approximately 1 per 100 individuals, routine electrocardiographic screening in this population could be warranted. In the general population, however, approximately 1 individual in 300,000 is expected to have QT interval prolongation, and generalized screening is not likely to be effective in this group. (See Chap. 36.)

Wolff-Parkinson-White Syndrome (WPW)

The preexcitation syndromes, including WPW, have been considered to be congenital, but only a small number of patients demonstrate familial occurrence; the majority of cases are sporadic. Vidaillet and colleagues[191] reported an autosomal dominant pattern of inheritance of accessory pathways based on the first-degree relatives of 383 patients with preexcitation. Gillette and colleagues[192] previously proposed autosomal dominant inheritance in children with WPW and SVT. No molecular genetic or cytologic studies have thus far established the genetic location or cause of WPW. Linkage to the HLA region of chromosome 6p has been speculated but has not been supported thus far. (See Chap. 36.)

Familial Heart Block

This disorder demonstrates adult onset and an autosomal dominant pattern of inheritance with variable expressivity. Although disease onset in its subtle form probably appears by age 20 years, affected individuals typically are seen between ages 30 to 50 years. The common presentations of this familial conduction abnormality include one of the following: (1) right bundle branch block (RBBB) alone, (2) left axis deviation (LAD) alone, (3) RBBB plus LAD, or (4) complete heart block. Affected individuals in the same kindred may manifest different electrocardiographic patterns. Graber and coworkers[193] described a six-generation family with this disorder associated with late-onset dilated cardiomyopathy. No pathognomonic, histologic, or biochemical abnormalities were found.

GENETIC FACTORS PREDISPOSING TO ATHEROSCLEROSIS

It has been established that elevated plasma cholesterol levels are associated with an increased risk of developing accelerated cardiovascular atherosclerosis. Both the environment and genetics are involved in determining the level of plasma cholesterol in various populations, and these two forces typically interact collectively to determine the plasma cholesterol concentration of each individual. At the highest levels of plasma cholesterol, however, genetic abnormalities are predominantly at fault. The following section outlines these genetic causes of accelerated atherosclerotic heart disease and provides a brief description of normal lipid metabolism. (See also Chap. 53.)

Hyperlipidemias

The hyperlipidemias are a group of metabolic disorders characterized by an abnormal accumulation of various lipids in plasma. Cholesterol and triglycerides are the major lipids. These are transported to the tissues via the plasma lipoproteins, which vary greatly with regard to lipid composition, peptide content, and size. Each particle is a complex macromolecular aggregate formed by a predominantly nonpolar lipid core surrounded by surface components of peptides and phospholipids. (See Chap. 53.)

Biochemistry of Lipid Metabolism

Lipoproteins[194,195] are composed of a fatty core of cholesterol esters and triglycerides surrounded by a monolayer of phospholipid and cholesterol in which apoproteins are embedded. The triglyceride-rich lipoproteins are synthesized and secreted from the small intestine and liver as chylomicrons and very low-density lipoproteins (VLDL), respectively. Certain proteins on the surface of lipoprotein particles (apolipoproteins B and E) are responsible for mediating the binding of cholesterol-rich particles to specific lipoprotein receptors on the surface of cells and represent a major pathway controlling blood cholesterol levels. Both lipoproteins (chylomicrons and VLDL) contain apolipoprotein B (apoB), which is essential for assembly of the hydrophobic core. It is interesting to note that the intestinal and hepatic forms of apoB differ in size.[195] The hepatic form, found in VLDL, is large, containing 4563 amino acids, and is called apoB-100.[196,197]

The intestinal form, found in chylomicrons, contains only the amino-terminal 2152 amino acids of apoB-100 and is called apoB-48, since it is 48 percent of the size of apoB-100. A variety of lipolytic enzymes, including lipoprotein lipase and hepatic lipase, act on these lipoproteins after they circulate to the peripheral tissues (heart, muscle, and adipose) and create smaller particles by delipidation. These smaller particles (intermediate-density lipoproteins, or IDLs) are further catabolized to form low-density lipoprotein (LDL) and chylomicron remnants. During the catabolism of the triglyceride-rich plasma lipoproteins, the C-apoproteins are lost from the particle, along with some surface phospholipids. These may associate with high-density lipoproteins (HDLs) for recycling into newly formed VLDL. Hepatic and peripheral tissue degradation of LDL ensues after LDL binding to specific cell-surface receptors. After conversion to LDL, these particles are cleared from the circulation when the carboxyl-terminal domain of apoB-100 binds to LDL receptors.[198] ApoB-48, which lacks the carboxyl-terminal domain, does not bind the LDL receptors. Chylomicron remnants bind receptors via apoE and apoB-48. Endocytosis[199] is stimulated, and lysosomal breakdown on the particle occurs, leading to inhibition of the intracellular pathways of cholesterol biosynthesis via the repression of the enzyme 3-hydroxy-3-methylglutaryl coenzyme A reductase (HMG-CoA reductase). An increase in intracellular esterification of cholesterol by induction of lecithin:cholesterol acetyltransferase (LCAT) follows. HDL is mainly synthesized in the small intestine and liver, with the former containing mainly apoprotein A and the hepatic form containing predominantly apoprotein E. In addition, there are at least two major classes of mature HDL particles, HDL_2 and HDL_3, with an overall diameter of 9.5 to 10 mn and 7 to 7.5 nm, respectively. During the breakdown of VLDL to LDL, some surface components, such as phospholipids and peptides, may associate with HDL_3, causing conversion into a particle similar to HDL_2. (See Chap. 53.)

No fewer than eight apoproteins (and up to 10) are found distributed throughout the lipoprotein system.[200–209] The amino acid sequences of most of them have been determined. The apoproteins initially were thought to serve a structural role in the formation and stabilization of the lipoprotein particle. It is now known, however, that many of them have a functional role in regulation of enzymes or interact with receptors involved in the catabolic pathways of lipoproteins in peripheral tissues. These include ApoA-I, ApoB, ApoC-II, ApoC-III, and ApoE.

Classification of Hyperlipidemias

Hyperlipidemias may be classified on the basis of which specific class of lipoprotein accumulates in plasma.[210,211] The diagnosis of a hyperlipidemia relies on the identification of the elevated plasma lipid and the lipoprotein on which it is transported. After the type of hyperlipidemia is discerned, further characterization of the lipid disorder may include whether it is primary (monogenic or polygenic) or secondary to systemic disease, nutrition, or alcohol abuse. Laboratory analysis of the lipids and lipoproteins[212] will distinguish among the six major forms of hyperlipidemia described below.

Type I Hyperlipidemia

Fasting chylomicronemia occurs while the patient is receiving a normal diet. Two major molecular deficiencies have been identified in this form of hyperlipidemia. The classic defect is extrahepatic lipoprotein lipase deficiency.[213] A second defect is due to the absence of the cofactor for lipoprotein lipase, ApoC-II,[214,215] and has also been identified as a cause of type I hyperlipoproteinemia. Despite the fact that type I disease is generally familial, with autosomal recessive inheritance, this same lipoprotein pattern may be produced as a result of other systemic disorders, such as systemic lupus erythematosus (SLE), diabetes mellitus, and the macroglobulinemias. The primary form usually presents in childhood and clinically demonstrates hepatosplenomegaly, eruptive xanthomas, lipemia retinalis, and recurrent pancreatitis. Despite extreme elevations of chylomicron triglycerides, little evidence of increased incidence of premature vascular disease has been accumulated. (See also Chap. 53.)

Type II Hyperlipidemia (Familial Hypercholesterolemia, or FH)

This defect is characterized by a striking elevation of LDL levels (two- to threefold) with normal VLDL levels, elevated plasma cholesterol levels, normal triglyceride levels, and clear plasma.[216,217] It is the second most common form of inherited hyperlipidemia, affecting 1 out of every 500 people in most countries of the world. The disease is caused by a mutation in the gene that encodes the cell surface receptor for LDL, which normally removes LDL from the blood. Transmission is an autosomal dominant trait and the gene for the LDL receptor is located on chromosome 19(19p13.2-p13.1). Heterozygous FH patients inherit one copy of the mutant LDL receptor gene on chromosome 19 from one parent and a normal copy of the gene from the other parent. Each offspring has a 50 percent chance of inheriting the mutant gene.

The genetic defect in the LDL receptor causes impaired LDL metabolism, with subsequent LDL accumulation in the plasma. Since the LDL receptors play a dual role in LDL metabolism (i.e., clearance and feedback inhibition of HmG-CoA reductase, as previously noted), deficiency of these receptors leads to two abnormalities. First, there is overproduction of LDL; second, there is a decline in LDL catabolism. The combination of overproduction and decreased catabolism leads to sharp elevations of plasma LDL levels.

Clinically, these patients demonstrate tendon xanthomas (Fig. 10-24) by the fourth or fifth decade, arcus corneae, and xanthelasma. Coronary atherosclerosis is common and may lead to early myocardial infarction. (See Chap. 53.)

Familial hypercholesterolemia occurs when two familial hypercholesterolemic heterozygotes have children. In mating of two heterozygotes (1 in every 250,000 matings), one-fourth of the offspring will inherit two mutant LDL receptor genes, one from each parent. Some of the patients have trace LDL receptor activity because at least one or their mutant genes can produce a slightly functional receptor. Clinically, homozygotes have a devastating syndrome with very high blood cholesterol levels from the time of birth and unique planar cutaneous xanthomata on the interdigital webs, as well as other sites.[218] They tend to develop severe atherosclerosis in childhood and usually have myocardial infarctions before 10 years of age. Aortic stenosis secondary to cholesterol deposition in the aortic valve and aortic root may also occur.

Type IIb Hyperlipidemia (Familial Combined Hyperlipoproteinemia, or FCH)

This disease, first described by Goldstein and coworkers,[219] is associated with increased LDL cholesterol and increased triglyceride levels. Plasma triglyceride levels are moderately elevated in the absence of a floating IDL. This disease is the most common inherited disorder of lipoprotein metabolism, and it is an autosomal dominant disorder[220] affecting 1 out of every 250 people. A large fraction of these patients are obese and diabetic; children are generally left unaffected. However, there appears to be gradual expression of the gene throughout the first two decades of life, with laboratory manifestation by the third decade. Although lipid levels may be only moderately elevated, risk of premature cardiac disease is considerable, with 25 to 50 percent of patients suffering a myocardial infarction by age 50. Although the molecular defect is not precisely known, it has been established that VLDL overproduction plays a significant role. (See Chap. 53.)

Type III Hyperlipidemia

This disorder is characterized by hypercholesterolemia and hypertriglyceridemia due to an abnormal β-VLDL particle (cholesterol-rich remnants of chylomicrons and VLDL) in plasma. This abnormal lipoprotein, β-VLDL, is seen as a broad β band on electrophoresis, composed of chylomicron remnants (containing apoB-48 and apoE) and VDL remnants (containing apoB-100 and apoE). ApoE binds to two distinct high-affinity receptors that mediate internalization and catabolism of lipoprotein particles. Accurate diagnosis depends on the following: (1) the presence of floating β-lipoprotein after ultracentrifugation and (2) apoE isoform analysis. The metabolic defect in this disease is related to defective removal of chylomicron remnants and the presence of a particular apoE polymorphic variant. The E-apoproteins exist as three major polymorphic variants (E-2, E-3, and E-4) characterized by differing isoelectric focusing patterns due to cysteine-arginine substitutions at three residues in the peptide.[221,222] The major variant of apoE is the homozygous E-2/E-2 variant, in which cysteine residues are found at each of these sites (substitution of cysteine for arginine at position 158). This phenotype occurs in approximately 1 percent of the population, but more than 90 percent of patients with type III disease have this phenotype. The mutation that alters the structure of apoE decreases the binding of apoE-containing lipoproteins to the hepatic receptor, thus retarding uptake of both chylomicron and VLDL remnants. Heterozygosity for apoE-2 has also been reported. The variant apoE-2 is not sufficient to cause type III disease, however, since less than 2 percent of all ApoE-2 homozygotes have the disease. Type III disease is currently thought to derive from two gene defects, one in the apoE structure gene and the other in a gene causing hyperlipidemia, probably FCH.[223,224]

Clinically, these patients have the virtually pathognomonic sign of planar xanthomas along the palmar creases of the hands and tendoeruptive xanthomas. Peripheral vascular disease and coronary artery disease are common. (See Chap. 53.)

Type IV Hyperlipidemia

Elevations of plasma triglyceride and VLDL levels characterize this disease and often occur as a result of a wide variety of diseases and dietary habits.[225] In addition, several different genetic forms may express as a type IV phenotype, including familial hypertriglyceridemia and FCH. The most common causes of secondary type IV disease include hypothyroidism, diabetes mellitus, and excessive alcohol intake. Studies of the pathophysiology have implicated increased VLDL production by the liver and/or a defective clearance of VLDL from the plasma. The molecular defect is not precisely known but is likely to be polygenic. Expression of this disorder is influenced strongly by environmental factors. (See Chap. 53.)

Type V Hyperlipidemia

This disorder is characterized by elevated plasma triglyceride levels caused by elevations of VLDL and chylomicrons, with normal cholesterol and HDL levels.[226] The plasma is generally opaque, and a floating creamy layer may be seen above the turbid plasma. As with type IV, this disorder often occurs as a result of a wide variety of diseases and life-styles. The chylomicronemia suggests a partial defect in the peripheral lipolytic mechanisms, which delay chylomicron and VLDL clearance. Clinically, there is often a history of recurrent abdominal pain, hepatosplenomegaly, eruptive xanthomas, and lipemia retinalis. (See Chap. 53.)

The Apoprotein Genes

Apoliproteins are the protein components of the lipoprotein particles transporting lipids in the blood and act as ligands for cellular lipoprotein receptors or interact with lipid metabolizing enzymes.[227] Defects in apolipoprotein structure or regulation result in disorders of lipid metabolism and in cardiovascular disease.[228] The genes coding for six of the apolipoproteins are located within two clusters in humans. Those coding for apoA-I, apoA-IV, and apoC-III are close together on chromosome 11,[229,230,231] whereas the genes for apoC-I, apoC-II, and apoE cluster on chromosome 19.[232,233]

There appear to be at least eight apolipoproteins, and the amino acid sequences of six of these have been elucidated (Table 96-4). In addition, synthetic oligonucleotide probes have been used to identify five cDNA clones coding for these peptides. This cloning was performed by screening a human cDNA liver library that contained an abundance of mRNA coding for apolipoproteins. This approach was successful in the isolation of cDNA clones coding for apoA-I, apoA-II, and apoE. It appears that some of the lipoprotein genes arose by duplication from a common ancestral gene. In addition, at least two types of polymorphisms have occurred in the apolipo-

TABLE 96-4

Summary of Apolipoproteins: The Plasma Apolipoproteins

Name	Lipoprotein	Molecular Weight	Function
apoA-I	HDL, chylomicrons*	28,000	Structural; activator of LCAT enzyme
apoA-II	HDL, chylomicrons	16,000	Structural
apoA-IV	HDL, chylomicrons,* VLDL	46,000	Unknown
apoB-100	LDL, VLDL	550,000	Structural; synthesis and secretion of VLDL; binds to LDL receptor (BE)
apoB-48	Chylomicrons	250,000	Structural; synthesis and secretion from intestine
apoC-1	HDL, chylomicrons, VLDL	6,000	Activator of LCAT
apoC-II	HDL, chylomicrons	7,000	Activator of lipoprotein lipase
apoC-III	HDL, chylomicrons, VLDL	7,000	Stabilizes surface; provides negative charge
apoD	HDL, chylomicrons*	21,000	Cholesteryl ester exchange
apoE	HDL, VLDL, chylomicrons*	34,000	Binds to receptor on cell membrane of liver (E and BE) and macrophage

*Only in nascent chylomicrons.

protein system. There is an amino acid polymorphism exemplified by the E-apoprotein variants differing at two main sites in the peptide producing three common variants, E-2, E-3, and E4; posttranslational variation is also found.

As previously noted, the genes coding for apoA-I, apoA-IV, and apoC-III are found clustered on chromosome 11, while the genes for apoC-I, apoC-II, and apoE are close together on chromosome 19. In the latter cluster, one of the two genes for apoC-I (apoC-I-a) is located 4.3 kb from the apoE gene, while the other (apoC-I-b) is found nearly 15 kb further away. On the other hand, apoC-II has been shown to be linked closely to apoE only in family studies. Myklebost and Rogne[234] used pulse field gel electrophoresis (PFGE) to show that this gene cluster extends for 50 kb on chromosome 19. The order from 5′ to 3′ is apoE, apoC-I-a, apoC-I-b, and apoC-II.

ApoC

Posttranslational variation is best seen in apoC-III,[204,229,235–238] a single-chain peptide of 79 residues and a molecular weight of 8.76 kd. This peptide can occur in three isoforms, which are dependent on the number of sialic acid residues attached to threonine 74. These isoforms include apoC-III-0 (0 residues), apoC-III-1 (1 residue), and apoC-III-2 (2 residues). It has been considered that these isoforms serve slightly different functional roles in the process of lipid transport among tissues, since variation in the percentage of these isoforms can be associated with a hyperlipidemia.

ApoA-IV

ApoA-IV, first described in humans by Weisgraber and coworkers,[236] is found in association with chylomicrons, HDL, and in the lipoprotein-free fraction of human plasma. It is synthesized by the intestine as pre-apoA-IV and contains a 20-amino acid prepetide that is cotranslationally cleaved to the mature apolipoprotein. Reduced levels of apoA-IV had been observed in abetalipoproteinemia and Tangier disease, but no established metabolic function has been proven. However, in vitro evidence suggests that it may be involved either as an activator for the plasma enzyme LCAT or in reverse cholesterol transport. Kamboh and Ferrell[239] demonstrated considerable molecular and genetic variation in this apolipoprotein, and they suggested that the multiple isoforms resulted from posttranslational changes in the polypeptide chains.

ApoB

ApoB, one of the largest protein species described (the full-length form is a single polypeptide composed of 4536 amino acids), is an obligatory component of chylomicrons, VLDL, IDL, and LDL, and it is heterogeneous. It has been shown to be located on chromosome 2, at the 2p24 locus, and exists mainly in two forms: the large apoB-100 (the hepatic form) and apoB-48 (the intestinal form). The apoB-100 form is the major protein constituent of VLDL, IDL, and LDL; its nucleotide sequence was deduced from the sequence of overlapping liver cDNAs. The apoB-48 is found in chylomicrons and, as previously mentioned, is 48 percent as large as apoB-100. In the bloodstream, VLDLs and chylomicrons are acted on by lipoprotein lipase (LPL), which removes the triglyceride, converting VLDLs to LDLs. These are then cleared from the circulation when the carboxyl-terminal domain of apoB-100 binds to LDL receptors. ApoB-48, which lacks the carboxyl-terminal domain, does not bind to LDL receptors. In chylomicron remnants, receptor binding is mediated by another protein, apoE, together with apoB-48. In the rare recessive disease abetalipoproteinemia, apoB-48 and apoB-100 are absent from the blood, suggesting that production of both proteins is from the same gene, perhaps through alternative splicing of the mRNA. The cloned gene encoding apoB-100, however, shows no evidence of alternative splicing. Instead, a posttranscriptional base substitution results in early translation termination. This causes the carboxyl-terminal segment to be lost, and LDL receptor binding cannot occur. Dependence on apoE[240] for chylomicron catabolism results, thus allowing these dietary particles to be diverted to a different receptor from that which clears LDL.

ApoE

In normal plasma, apoE is equally divided between VLDL and HDL. It makes up 10 to 20 percent of VLDL protein and approximately 2 percent of HDL protein. Human apoE concentrations are in the range of 25 to 50 mg/mL in plasma. ApoE is synthesized and secreted as sialo-apoE and later is desialated in plasma. It can serve as a ligand for the LDL receptor present on hepatic and extrahepatic tissues. The majority of apoE is synthesized in the liver.

Mature apoE[233,240] is a 299-amino acid polypeptide, and the receptor binding region is in the middle portion of the polypeptide (between residues 140 and 150; residue 158 is important for the conformation of the binding domain). ApoE cDNA sequences have been shown to code for mRNA of 1163 bp in length. Comparison of apoA-I and apoA-IV with apoE suggest a common ancestral origin of these three apolipoprotein genes. The apoE gene has been shown to reside on chromosome 19, within 2 cM of apoC-II and adjacent to apoC-I.

Six common apoE phenotypes are found in the population, apparently the result of a single apoE gene locus with three common alleles (E4, E3, and E2) whose gene products are designated E4, E3, and E2. There are three homozygous phenotypes (E4/4, E3/3, and E2/2) and three heterozygous phenotypes (E4/3, E3/2, and E4/2). This common apoE polymorphism, as noted, plays a role in type III hyperlipoproteinemia, since over 90 percent of individuals with this disorder have the E2/2 phenotype (E2/2 occurs in approximately 1 percent of normal subjects). An increased frequency of the apoE4 allele has been seen in patients with coronary artery disease.[241]

Lp(a)

A variant of LDL,[242] Lp(a) was discovered as an antigen in the blood of certain persons, carries one copy (or perhaps two) of a protein called apo(a), joined to apoB-100 by a disulfide linkage. The amount of Lp(a) in plasma varies from undetectable to 100 mg/dL. High levels of Lp(a) are strongly associated with atherosclerosis,[240] especially when associated with elevated blood LDL levels. (See Chap. 53.)

McLean and associates[202] recently studied Lp(a), and through protein sequencing and cDNA cloning, they showed that apo(a) is related to plasminogen, the precursor of plamin used to dissolve fibrin clots. In addition, apo(a) is encoded by a single locus with multiple alleles, which produce a variety of different-sized proteins. This apparent link between the clotting system and lipoproteins is an important relationship, the full understanding of which should improve our knowledge of atherosclerosis.

ApoA-I

ApoA-I is the major apoprotein of HDL and functionally is an activator of LCAT. The genes for apoA-I and apoC-III are known to have been derived by gene duplication from a common evolutionary precursor. A family with premature atherosclerosis demonstrated a 6.5-kb insert in the apoA-I gene that correlated with a deficiency of both apoA-I and apoC-III, thus providing evidence of linkage between these genes. A cDNA probe was subsequently used to show strong homology between these genes. DNA sequencing of regions flanking the apoA-I gene confirmed the presence of the gene coding for apoC-III to be located 2.6 kb downstream from the 3′ end of the apoA-I gene. These genes appear to be coordinately regulated, and this apoA-I/C-III gene cluster is located on the long arm of chromosome 11.[231]

LDL Receptor Gene

A glycoprotein synthesized in the endoplasmic reticulum, the LDL receptor gene contains 839 amino acids (with many cysteine-rich repeats) and is located on the cell membrane surface. It is initially synthesized as a 120-kDa precursor before undergoing processing in the Golgi complex to form a 160-kDa protein. Lipoprotein levels in the plasma are regulated by this lipoprotein receptor. Cholesterol-carrying LDL and the β-migrating VLDL are bound by this receptor, and then the receptor carries these lipoproteins into cells in coated pits. The LDL receptor interacts preferentially with lipoproteins containing apoE or apoB and is present on the surface of most cells, particularly liver parenchymal cells. The ligand-binding domain consists of seven cysteine-rich repeats of 40 amino acids that are encoded by exons 2 to 6 of the LDL receptor gene.

Mutations in the LDL receptor gene occur in patients with autosomal dominant familial hypercholesterolemia.[243–245] Heterozygotes contain one mutant LDL receptor gene and produce one-half the normal number of functional receptors. Homozygotes have two abnormal receptor genes. Mutations include deletions, nonsense and missense mutations, and exon duplications. These mutations disrupt the biosynthesis of the receptor, its transport from endoplasmic reticulum to Golgi complex, the binding of LDL, or the internalizaton of the receptor in coated pits.

OTHER CAUSES OF PREMATURE CORONARY ARTERY DISEASE

In addition to the familial hyperlipidemias, several inborn errors of metabolism predispose to coronary artery narrowing and occlusion (Table 96-5).

Hunter's Syndrome (Mucopolysaccharidosis II)

This X-linked recessive disorder has been mapped to the Xq26-Xq28 region and is found in approximately 1 in 30,000 live births. The disorder is caused by a deficiency in the enzyme iduronate sulfatase, a lysosomal hydrolase that participates in the catabolism of mucopolysaccharides, and results in abnormally excessive urinary excretion of dermatan and heparan sulfate, as well as accumulation of mucopolysaccharides. The end result is coronary artery obstruction and subsequent childhood myocardial infarction.[246] Most affected individuals die before the third decade.

Phenotypically, these males have coarse faces, skeletal changes, and short stature and have a strong resemblance

TABLE 96-5
Single-Gene Disorders that Predispose to Premature Coronary Artery Disease

Disorder	Typical Age for Myocardial Infarction	Primary Biochemical Defect	Mechanism of Inheritance	Estimated Population Frequency
Familial hypercholesterolemia				
Heterozygous form	Adult	Defective cell-surface receptor for plasma LDL	Dominant	1 in 500
Homozygous form*	Childhood			1 in 1,000,000
Multiple lipoprotein-type hypolipidemia (familial combined hyperlipidemia)	Adult	Not known	Dominant	1 in 250
Familial hypertriglyceridemia	Adult	Not known	Dominant	1 in 300
Familial dysbetalipoproteinemia	Adult	Abnormal apoE-2	Recessive	1 in 40,000
Hurler's syndrome, type I–H	Childhood	Deficiency of α-L-iduronidase	Recessive	1 in 40,000
Hunter's syndrome, type II mucopolysaccharidosis*	Childhood	Deficiency of sulfoiduronide sulfatase	X-linked	1 in 30,000
Homocystinuria*	Young adult	Deficiency of cystathionine β-synthase	Recessive	1 in 75,000
Pseudoxanthoma elasticum	Young adult	Not known	Dominant and recessive	1 in 100,000
Alkaptonuria	Adult	Deficiency of homogentistic acid oxidase	Recessive	1 in 100,000
Werner's syndrome	Adult	Not known	Recessive	1 in 500,000
Fabry's disease*	Young adult	Deficiency of α-galactosidase A	X-linked	1 in 40,000
Cholesterol ester storage	Young adult	Deficiency of lysosomal acid lipase	Recessive	1 in 1,000,000
Arterial calcification of infancy	Neonates	Not known	Recessive	1 in 1,000,000

*Prenatal diagnosis is possible.

to patients with Hurler's syndrome but without corneal clouding.[247] Cardiac disease is common and, in addition to coronary artery involvement, includes mitral and aortic regurgitation as well as myocardial dysfunction. The pathologic findings within the heart are extensive. Gross examination demonstrates endocardial thickening and valve involvement. The valve thickening is usually nodular, with the greatest thickening at the free margins. Thickening of the mitral valve is greater than that seen in the aortic valve; the right heart valves are much less involved. Short, thickened chordae tendineae and mitral annular calcification also occur. Multifocal narrowing of the coronary arteries is also evident, with the intima most involved, and, on light microscopy, contains mucopolysaccharide and increased collagen. Electron microscopy demonstrates inclusions that are clear or lamellar-delimited by a membrane. No specific therapy exists for this disorder. Management consists of supportive therapy for cardiac failure and valvular regurgitation.

Hurler's Syndrome (Mucopolysaccharidosis IH)

This autosomal recessive trait has been mapped to chromosome 22 (22qII) and occurs in approximately 1 in 40,000 live births. This disease is the result of α-L-iduronidase deficiency and causes accumulation of heparan sulfate and dermatan sulfate, which are found in high concentrations in the urine. The major clinical features[247] of this disorder include relentless progression to death (usually prior to the tenth birthday), dwarfism, characteristic coarse facies, central nervous system deterioration, skeletal changes, corneal clouding, and cardiac disease. The most common cardiovascular abnormalities[246] include mitral regurgitation and, less commonly, aortic regurgitation, as well as hypertension and congestive heart failure. Involvement of the coronary arteries is similar to that described for Hunter's syndrome and may result in angina and myocardial infarction. Nearly half of the patients die from chronic heart failure or sudden cardiac decompensation. The pathologic condition of the heart is similar to that seen in Hunter's syndrome. No specific therapy is available.

Homocystinuria

This autosomal recessive disorder occurs in approximately 1 in 75,000 live births and is caused by deficiency of the enzyme cystathionine β-synthase. The defect has been mapped to the subtelomeric region of chromosome 21 at 21q22.3 using in situ hybridization[248] and has been cloned.[249] The results of this enzyme deficiency are elevations of blood methionine and urinary homocystine and methionine levels. Clinically, these patients have a marfanoid habitus with a tall, thin body build and arachnodactyly, kyphoscoliosis, osteoporosis, and pectus excavatum. Subluxation of the lens frequently occurs by age 10 years, and myopia is common. Nearly 60 percent of affected individuals are mentally retarded. The cardiovascular abnormalities[250] include arterial and venous thrombosis,[251] medial degeneration of the aorta and large arteries, and intimal hyperplasia and fibrosis. Myocardial infarctions are also seen. Therapy includes pyridoxine supplementation, which has good response in up to half of all patients.

Fabry's Disease

An X-linked recessive disorder with complete penetrance and variable clinical expressivity, Fabry's disease is due to a deficiency of the enzyme α-galactosidase A, a lysosomal enzyme that participates in the catabolism of neutral glycosphingolipids and is found in 1 in 40,000 live births. The disease usually has its onset in adolescence and typically manifests with sensations of burning pain in the hands and feet. These sensations tend to be associated with fever, heat, cold, and exercise. Multiple angiokeratomas are noticeable with increasing age, with the umbilical area and genitalia most commonly affected. Progressive renal failure develops with age, and central nervous system manifestations commonly include seizures, headaches, hemiplegia, and stroke. Corneal opacities are also frequently seen.

The cardiac manifestations of Fabry's disease[252,253] generally appear in young adulthood. Aortic root dilation, hypertrophy of the left ventricular posterior wall, dilated or hypertrophic cardiomyopathy,[254] valve dysfunction (especially mitral valve), and myocardial infarctions occur in these patients. Electrocardiographic abnormalities commonly include atrial fibrillation, intraventricular conduction delay, right bundle branch block, ST-T wave changes, short PR interval, and left ventricular hypertrophy. The short PR interval can progressively lengthen over time, probably secondary to lipid deposition in the atrioventricular node. Pathologically, chamber thickness and mitral valve prolapse are seen grossly, while light microscopy reveals lipid accumulation in nearly all cardiac tissue. Concentric lamellae are seen within cells and contain the neutral glycophospholipid.

The disease-causing gene is localized to X121.3-Xq22, and full-length cDNA has been isolated and sequenced.[255] Antenatal and postnatal diagnosis is available. Therapy is symptomatic at present, but enzyme replacement therapy is likely to be used in the future.

Cholesterol Ester Storage Disease (CESD)

This lysosomal storage disorder results from a deficiency of the lysosomal enzyme acid lipase.[256] This enzyme deficiency causes progressive accumulation of cholesteryl esters and triglycerides. The disease typically presents with short stature; hepatomgaly, with demonstration of this finding possible at birth; cor pulmonale; hyperlipidemia; and ischemic heart disease due to focal concentric intimal deposits within the coronary arteries. These deposits contain foam cells, extracellular lipid, and fibrosis. The disease is inherited as an autosomal recessive trait, occurring in 1 in 1 million live births. The gene has been localized to chromosome 10 at 10q24-10q25.[257]

CARDIOVASCULAR INVOLVEMENT IN OTHER METABOLIC DISORDERS

G(M2) Gangliosidosis with Hexosaminidase A Deficiency (Tay-Sachs Disease)

This disorder is characterized clinically by visual inattention and developmental retardation beginning within the initial 6 months of life in a physically normal-appearing child. These individuals are typically hypotonic and demonstrate poor head control. The child fails to reach appropriate developmental milestones such as turning over and sitting, and becomes increasingly unresponsive to external stimuli, eventually reaching a vegetative state. Blindness occurs in the latter part of the first year of life, and fundoscopic examination reveals a white halo in the macula region of the eye, which accentuates the normal red color of the fovea, the so-called cherry red macula. Seizures are a later manifestation, usually occurring at the end of the first year of life. Results of the cardiovascular examination and chest X-ray are usually normal, but the electrocardiogram may reveal a prolonged QT interval and abnormal T-wave morphology.[258]

Tay-Sachs disease is an autosomal recessive inherited trait with a high gene frequency in Ashkenazi Jews, approximately 1 in 37. In these Jewish families, the theoretical incidence is of 1 in 3800 live births. The disease occurs due to a failure to degrade the G(M2)-ganglioside, resulting from deficiency of hexosaminidase A. This enzyme deficiency is caused by absence or defective synthesis of the A-chain of hexasaminidase A and results in storage of G(M2)-ganglioside in neurons throughout the body. The neuronal cell body accumulates ganglioside with lipids complexed to it and causes the cell body to balloon out; the neurons eventually die, being replaced by gliosis. The ganglioside accumulations form membranous cytoplasmic bodies that are distinguished under the electron microscope as membrane-bound concentrically laminated structures. The diagnosis may be made by demonstrating a deficiency of hexosaminidase A in serum or tissues. Heterozygotes can be detected by enzymatic assay of serum leukocytes or cultured skin fibroblasts, which usually have 40 to 60 percent of the activity of control patients. The hexosaminidase A A-chain (HEXA) has been mapped to chromosome 15 at 15q23-q24. Prenatal diagnosis is available.[259,260]

G(M2) Gangliosidosis with Hexosaminidase A and B Deficiency (Sandhoff's Disease)

This autosomal recessive disorder is similar to Tay-Sachs disease clinically but has additional signs of systemic lipid storage, including foam cells within the bone marrow. Onset of disease is within the initial 6 months of life, and most patients succumb by age 3 years. Psychomotor retardation, cherry-red macula, hypotonia, and exaggerated startle response dominate the early course. Failure to attain milestones and seizures, blindness, and loss of contact with the environment may be seen by 12 to 15 months. The cardiovascular system is involved early, with cardiomyopathic changes including dilation and hypertrophy of the left ventricle and notable mitral regurgitation.[261] Gross examination of the heart reveals endocardial sclerosis and thickening of the valves and chordae tendiniae. Lipid accumulation in lysosomes can be seen by electron microscopy, along with excess collagen and elastic fibers in the endocardium and valves. Multiple areas of coronary artery narrowing are found secondary to intimal proliferation of fibroblasts engorged with lipid material.

This disorder occurs from defective synthesis of the B-chain of hexosaminidase, leading to deficiency of hexosaminidase A (which is needed for G(M2)-ganglioside hydrolysis) and hexosaminidase B (which is necessary for globoside degradation). Nerve cell enlargement occurs due to G(M2)-ganglioside accumulation, leading ultimately to gliosis. Globoside accumulates in visceral tissues, including the endothelium. The diagnosis relies on enzyme determination in serum, white blood cells, or skin fibroblasts, and prenatal diagnosis can be performed by amniocentesis. The hexosaminidase B B-chain (HEXB) has been mapped to chromosome 5q13.[262]

G(M1) Gangliosidosis, Type I

This metabolic disorder is caused by deficiency of the enzyme β-galactosidase,[263] a lysosomal enzyme in the catabolic pathway of gangliosides, which are glycosphingolipids containing sialic acid. Gangliosides are in the highest concentration in neurons but are found in most cells, including cardiac myocytes. Deficiency of β-galactosidase results in accumulation of G(M1) and numerous other oligosaccharides.

Clinically[264] these patients present with early and severe mental and motor retardation in infancy and unusual facies that includes a flat nose, a full forehead, and widely spaced eyes. Characteristic X-ray changes in long bones include periosteal cloaking leading to hypoplasia and breaking of vertebral bodies. Hepatosplenomegaly, gingeval hyperplasia, generalized edema, and cherry-red macula may be noted. Cardiac involvement may include dilated cardiomyopathy with heart failure.[265] Electrocardiographic studies may reveal left or right ventricular hypertrophy and a short PR interval. Necropsy findings include cardiac hypertrophy and endocardial fibroelastosis. Foamy histiocytes filled with gangliosides are seen on histologic examination in the myocardium and the aortic and mitral valves, and coronary obstruction by lipid-laden cells has also been reported. Death typically occurs by 2 years of age.

The disease has autosomal recessive inheritance, and the gene, galactosidase β-1, has been mapped to the pter-3p21 region of chromosome 3. Prenatal diagnosis is possible, and therapy is supportive.

Gaucher's Disease, Type I

This is the most common sphingolipid disorder and is inherited as an autosomal recessive trait. The metabolic defect leading to the clinical disorder is deficiency of glucocerebrosidase, a firmly membrane-bound member of an enzyme system that acts as the cerebroside-cleaving enzyme. Onset of disease varies from infancy to late adulthood, with a slowly progressive course.[266] The skeletal, reticuloendothelial, and hematologic systems are commonly involved. The presenting features usually include abdominal enlargement due to hepatosplenomegaly, and orthopedic problems, such as pain, pathologic fractures, and aseptic necrosis, result from greatly expanded medullary cavity volume. Yellow patches on the sclerae occur in one-fourth of adults, and abnormal pigmentation of the face, neck, hands, or shins can also be seen. The cardiovascular involvement[267] usually includes restrictive cardiomyopathy, pericarditis (hemorrhagic or constrictive), valvular disease, and cor pulmonale. The cardiomyopathy is attributed to interstitial infiltrate with Gaucher cells, large hisiocytic elements with a "wrinkled-appearing" cytoplasm.

The β-glucosidase gene (GBA) has been mapped to chromosome one at 1q21 and mutations seen.[268,269] Prenatal diagnosis is possible in cell culture from amniotic fluid. Therapy includes splenectomy when necessary. Otherwise, supportive care is given. A normal life expectancy may occur in this disorder.

Fucosidosis, Type I

This disorder occurs due to deficiency of the enzyme A-fucosidase, an enzyme in the catabolic pathway of glycoproteins. Clinical symptoms are first noted at 1 year of age, with onset of coarsened facial features, neurologic determination, and muscular skeletal changes, including weakness hypotonia and spastic quadriplegia prior to muscle contractures.[270] Sweat chloride levels are markedly elevated. The cardiac manifestations include cardiomegaly and incomplete right bundle branch block. A gradual increase in the levels of fucose-containing oligosaccharides and glycolipids occurs in most tissues, including brain. Death usually occurs by 5 years of age due to severe neurologic deterioration. Therapy is symptomatic.

The α-fucosidase-1 gene (FUCA1) has been mapped to chromosome 1p35-1p34, and mutations have been noted.[271] Prenatal diagnosis is feasible.

REFERENCES

1. Keating M, Atkinson D, Dunn C, Timothy K, Vincent GM, Leppert M: Linkage of a cardiac arrhythmia, the long QT syndrome, and the Harvey ras-1 gene. *Science* 1991; 252:704–706.
2. Jarcho JA, McKenna W, Pare JAP, Solomon SD, Holcombe RF, Dickie S, et al: Mapping a gene for familial hypertrophic cardiomyopathy to chromosome 14q1. *N Engl J Med* 1989; 321:1372–1378.
3. Kainulainen K, Pulkkinen L, Savolainen A, Kaitila I, Peltonen L: The gene defect causing Marfan syndrome is located on chromosome 15. *N Engl J Med* 1990; 323:935–939.
4. Nora JJ, Nora AH: Recurrence risks in children having one parent with congenital heart disease. *Circulation* 1976; 53:701–702.
5. Rose VR, Gold RJM, Lindsay G, Allen M: A possible increase in the incidence of congenital heart defects among the offspring of affected parents. *J Am Coll Cardiol* 1985; 6:376–382.
6. Ferencz C, Neill CA, Boughman JA, Rubin JD, Brenner JI, Perry LW: Congenital cardiovascular malformations associated with chromosome abnormalities: An epidemiologic study. *J Pediatr* 1989; 114:79–86.
7. Gardner RJ, Sutherland GR (eds): *Chromosome Abnormalities and Genetic Counseling.* New York, Oxford University Press, 1989.
8. Schmickel RD: Contiguous gene syndromes: A component of recognizable syndromes. *J Pediatr* 1986; 109:231–241.
9. Yunis JJ: High resolution of human chromosomes. *Science* 1976; 191:1268–1270.

10. Yunis JJ: Mid-prophase human chromosomes: The attainment of 2000 bands. *Hum Genet* 1981; 56:293–298.
11. de la Chapelle A, Herva R, Koivisto M, Aula P: A deletion in chromosome 22 can cause DiGeorge syndrome. *Hum Genet* 1981; 57:253–256.
12. Waziri M, Patil SR, Hanson JW, Bartley JA: Abnormality of chromosome 11 in patients with features of Beckwith-Wiedemann syndrome. *J Pediatr* 1983; 102:873–876.
13. Lindenbaum RH, Clarke G, Patel C, Moncrieff M, Hughes JT: Muscular distrophy in an X;1 translocation female suggests that Duchenne locus is on X chromosome short arm. *J Med Genet* 1979; 16:389–392.
14. Korenberg JR, Kawashima H, Pulst S-M, Ikeuchi T, Ogasawara N, Yamamoto K, et al: Molecular definition of a region of chromosome 21 that causes features of the Down syndrome phenotype. *Am J Hum Genet* 1990; 47:236–246.
15. McCormick MK, Schinzel A, Petersen MB, Stetten G, Driscoll D, Cantu ES, et al: Molecular genetics approach to the characterization of the "Down syndrome region" of chromosome 21. *Genomics* 1989; 5:325–331.
16. Licznerski G, Lindsten J: Trisomy 21 in man due to maternal nondisjunction during the first meiotic division. *Hereditas* 1970; 70:153–154.
17. Rudd NL, Dimnik LS, Greentree C, Mendes-Crabb K, Hoar DI: The use of DNA probes to establish parental origin in Down syndrome. *Hum Genet* 1988; 78:175–178.
18. Mikkelsen M, Stene J: Genetic counseling in Down's syndrome. *Hum Hered* 1970; 20:457–464.
19. Greenwood RD, Nadas AS: The clinical course of cardiac disease in Down's syndrome. *Pediatrics* 1976; 58:893–897.
20. Van Praagh S, Truman T, Firpo A, Bano-Rodrigo A, Fried R, McManus B, et al: Cardiac malformations in trisomy-18: A study of 41 postmortem cases. *J Am Coll Cardiol* 189; 13:1586–1597.
21. Gerald PS: Sex chromosome disorders. *N Engl J Med* 1976; 294:706–710.
22. Palmer CG, Reichmann A: Chromosomal and clinical findings in 110 females with Turner syndrome. *Hum Genet* 1976; 35:35–49.
23. Van der Hauwaert LG, Fryns JM, Dumoulin M, Logghe N: Cardiovascular malformations in Turner's and Noonan's syndrome. *Br Heart J* 1978; 40:500–509.
24. Allen DB, Hendricks SA, Levy JM: Aortic dilation in Turner syndrome. *J Pediatr* 1986; 109:302–305.
25. Natowicz M, Kelley RI: Association of Turner syndrome with hypoplastic left-heart syndrome. *Am J Dis Child* 1987; 141:218–220.
26. Moore JW, Kirby WC, Rogers WM, Poth MA: Partial anomalous pulmonary venous drainage associated with 45, X Turner's syndrome. *Pediatrics* 1990; 86:273–276.
27. Di George AM: Discussions on a new concept of the cellular base of immunology. *J Pediatr* 1965; 67:907–908.
28. Conley ME, Beckwith JB, Mancer JFK, Tenckhoff L: The spectrum of the DiGeorge syndrome. *J Pediatr* 1979; 94:883–890.
29. Kelley RI, Zackai EH, Emanuel BS: The association of the DiGeorge anomalad with partial monosomy of chromosome 22. *J Pediatr* 1982; 101:197–200.
30. Greenberg F, Elder FFB, Haffner P, Northrup H, Ledbetter DH: Cytogenetic findings in a prospective series of patients with DiGeorge anomaly. *Am J Hum Genet* 1988; 43:605–611.
31. Fibison WJ, Emanuel BS: Molecular mapping of DiGeorge syndrome. *Am J Hum Genet* 1987; 41:A119.
32. de Grouchy J, Turleau C: *Clinical Atlas of Human Chromosome*, 2d ed. New York, Wiley, 1984.
33. Schinzel AP: *Catalogue of Unbalanced Chromosome Aberrations in Man.* New York, Walter de Gruyter, 1984.
34. Roche KB, Moore JW, Surana RB, Wilson BE: Aortic root dilatation associated with partial trisomy 7 (q31.2-qter). *Pediatr Cardiol* 1989; 10:53–55.
35. Tiller GE, Watson MS, Duncan LM, Dowton SB: Congenital heart defect in a patient with deletion of chromosome 7q. *Am J Med Genet* 1988; 29:283–287.
36. Talley JD, Dooley KJ, Tuboku-Metzger A, Burgess GH, Wilcox WD, Click LA, et al: The cardiovascular abnormalities associated with duplicated segments of chromosome 7. *Clin Cardiol* 1989; 12:227–232.
37. Niebuhr E: The cri-du-chat syndrome: Epidemiology, cytogenetics and clinical features. *Hum Genet* 1978; 44:227–275.
38. Gelb BD, Towbin JA, McCabe ERB, Sujansky E: San Luis Valley recombinant chromosome 8 and tetralogy of Fallot: A review of chromosome 8 anomalies and congenital heart disease. *Am J Med Genet* 1991; 40:471–476.
39. Emanuel BS: Molecular cytogenetics: Toward dissection of the contiguous gene syndromes. *Am J Hum Genet* 1988; 43: 575–578.
40. Roberts R (ed): *Molecular Biology of the Cardiovascular System.* In: Caskey CT (ed): *Molecular Biology Series* Hamden, CT, Blackwell Scientific, 1992.
41. Roberts R (ed): *A Primer of Molecular Biology.* New York, Elsevier, 1992: 103–128.
42. Mares A Jr, Towbin J, Bies RD, Roberts R: Molecular biology for the cardiologist. In: O'Rourke RA (ed): *Current Problems in Cardiology,* vol 17, Mosby-Year Book, St. Louis, 1992.
43. Conference proceedings: Human gene mapping. *Cytogenet Cell Genet* 1988; 49:46–47.
44. Wells RA: DNA fingerprinting. In: Rickwood D, Hames BD (eds): *Genome Analysis: A Practical Approach.* Oxford, IRL Press, 1988: 153–170.
45. Wallace DC: Mitochondrial DNA mutations and neuromuscular disease. *Tends Genet* 1989; 5:9–13.
46. Clarke A: Mitochondrial genome: Defects, disease, and evolution. *J Med Genet* 1990; 27:451–456.
47. Nora JJ: Multifactorial inheritance hypothesis for the etiology of congenital heart diseases: The genetic-environmental interaction. *Circulation* 1968; 18:604–617.
48. Nora JJ, Nora AH: Maternal transmission of congenital heart diseases: New recurrence risk figures and the questions of cytoplasmic inheritance and vulnerability to teratogens. *Am J Cardiol* 1987; 59:459–463.
49. Edwards JG: Familial predisposition in man. *Br Med Bull* 1969; 25:58–64.
50. Nora JJ, McGill CW, McNamara DG: Empiric recurrence risks in common and uncommon congenital heart lesions. *Teratology* 1970; 3:325–330.
51. Clark EB: Mechanisms in the pathogenesis of congenital heart defects. In: Pierpont ME, Moller JM (eds): *The Genetics of Cardiovascular Disease.* Boston, Martinus-Nijhoff, 1985: 3.
52. Maestri NE, Beaty TH, Liang K-Y, Boughman JA, Ferencz C: Familial aggregation of congenital cardiovascular malformations assessed in case-control studies. *Genet Epidemiol* 1988; 5: 343–354.
53. Boughman JA, Berg KA, Astemborski JA, Clark EB, McCarter RJ, Rubin JD, et al: Familial risks of congenital heart defects assessed in a population-based epidemiologic study. *Am J Hum Genet* 1987; 26:839–849.
54. Maestri NE, Beaty TH, Boughman JA: Etiologic heterogeneity in the familial aggregation of congenital cardiovascular malformations. *Am J Hum Genet* 1989; 45:556–564.
55. Whittemore R, Hobbins JC, Engle MA: Pregnancy and its outcome in women with and without surgical treatment of congenital heart disease. *Am J Cardiol* 1982; 50:641–651.
56. Pyeritz RE: Pleiotropy revisited: Molecular explanations of a classic concept. *Am J Med Genet* 1989; 34:124–134.
57. Hollister DW, Godfrey M, Sakai LY: Marfan syndrome: Immunohistologic abnormalities of the elastin-associated microfibrillar fiber system. *N Engl J Med* 1990; 323:152–159.
58. Maron BJ, Roberts WC, Edwards JE, McAllister HA Jr, Foley DD, Epstein SE: Sudden death in patients with hypertrophic cardiomyopathy: Characterization of 26 patients without functional limitation. *Am J Cardiol* 1978; 41:803–810.
59. Becker AE, Caruso G: Myocardial disarray: A critical review. *Br Heart J* 1982; 47:527–538.
60. Bulkley BH, D'Amico B, Taylor AL: Extensive myocardial fiber disarray in aortic and pulmonary atresia: Relevance to hypertrophic cardiomyopathy. *Circulation* 1983; 67:191–198.
61. Gardin JM, Dabestani A, Glasgow GA, Butman S, Burn CS, Henry WL: Echocardiographic and Doppler flow observations in obstructed and nonobstructed hypertrophic cardiomyopathy. *Am J Cardiol* 1985; 56:614–621.
62. Fiorito S, Autore C, Fragola PV, Purpura M, Cannata D, Sangiorgi M: HLA-DR3 antigen linkage in patients with hypertrophic obstructive cardiomyopathy. *Am Heart J* 1986; 111:91–94.
63. Ferraro M, Scarton G, Ambrosini M: Cosegregation of hypertrophic cardiomyopathy and a fragile site on chromosome 16 in a large Italian family. *J Med Genet* 1990; 27:363–366.
64. Nishi H, Kimura A, Sasaki M, Wakisaka A, Matsuyama K, Koga

Y, et al: Localization of the gene for hypertrophic cardiomyopathy to chromosome 18q. *Circulation* 1989; 80:1818A.

65. Towbin JA, Brink PA, Fink D, Hill R, Hejtmancik JF, Roberts R: Hypertrophic cardiomyopathy: Molecular genetic exclusion of HLA linkage. *Clin Res* 1989; 37:302A.
66. Hejtmancik JF, Brink PA, Towbin J, Hill R, Brink L, Tapscott T, et al: Localization of the gene for familial hypertrophic cardiomyopathy to chromosome 14ql in a diverse American population. *Circulation* 1991; 83:2007–2012.
67. Solomon SD, Geisterfer-Lowrance MT, Vosberg H-P, Hiller G, Jarcho JA, Morton CC, et al: A locus for familial hypertrophic cardiomyopathy is closely linked to the cardiac myosin heavy chain genes, CRI-L436 and CRI-L329 on chromosome 14 at q11-q12. *Am J Hum Genet* 1990; 47:389–394.
68. Tanigawa G, Jarcho JA, Kass S, Solomon SD, Vosberg H-P, Seidman JG, et al: A molecular basis for familial hypertrophic cardiomyopathy: An α/β cardiac myosin heavy chain hybrid gene. *Cell* 1990; 62:991–998.
69. Geisterfer-Lowrance MT, Kass S, Tanigawa G, Vosberg H-P, McKenna W, Seidman CE, et al: A molecular basis for familial hypertrophic cardiomyopathy: A β cardiac myosin heavy chain gene missense mutation. *Cell* 1990; 62:999–1006.
70. Marian AJ, Yu Q-T, Mares A, Hill R, Roberts R, Perryman MB: Detection of a new mutation in the β-myosin heavy chain gene in a family with hypertrophic cardiomyopathy. *J Clin Invest* 1992; 90:2156–2165.
71. Epstein N, Cohen G, Cryan F, Zhu WS, Fanapanpazir L: Identification of two mutations in the beta myosin heavy chain gene in hypertrophic cardiomyopathy: A $403^{Arg \rightarrow Glu}$ mutation associated with a high incidence of sudden death and a $908^{Leu \rightarrow Val}$ mutation in a family with infrequent sudden death. *J Am Coll Cardiol* 1992; 12:271A.
72. Watkins H, Rosenzweig A, Hwang D-S, Levi T, McKenna W, Seidman CE, et al: Characterization and prognostic implications of myosin missense mutations in familial hypertrophic cardiomyopathy. *N Engl J Med* 1992; 36:1108–1114.
73. Mares A, Marian AJ, Yu Q-T, Czernuszewicz GZ, Gooch G, Tapscott T, et al: Genetic screening of 75 families with hypertrophic cardiomyopathy show missense mutations the most common genetic defect. *Circulation* 1992; 86:1–228.
74. Rosenzweig A, Watkins H, Hwang D-S, Miri M, McKenna W, Traill TA, et al: Preclinical diagnosis of familial hypertrophic cardiomyopathy by genetic analysis of blood lymphocytes. *N Engl J Med* 1991; 325:1753–1760.
75. Perryman MB, Yu Q-T, Marian AJ, Mares A, Czernuszewicz G, Ifegwu J, et al: Expression of a missense mutation in the mRNA for β-myosin heavy chain in myocardial tissue in hypertrophic cardiomyopathy. *J Clin Invest* 1992; 90:271–277.
76. Yu Q-T, Ifeqwu J, Marian AJ, Mares A, Hill R, Perryman MB, et al: Hypertrophic cardiomyopathy mutation is expressed in mRNA of skeletal as well as cardiac muscle. *Circulation* 1993; 87:406–412.
77. Watkins H, Thierfelder L, McKenna W, Seidman JG, Seidman CE: Sporadic hypertrohic cardiomyopathy due to de novo myosin mutations. *Circulation* 1992; 86:1–228.
78. Bachinski LL, Czernuszewicz GZ, Elstein E, Webber S, Hill R, Schwartz K, et al: Identification of a Canadian family with hypertrophic cardiomyopathy that is not genetically linked to chromosome 14 locus using polymorphic satellite markers. *Circulation* 1992; 86:1–230.
79. Solomon SD, Jarcho JA, McKenna W, Geisterfer-Lowrence A, Germain R, Salerni R, et al: Familial hypertrophic cardiomyopathy is a genetically heterogeneous disease. *J Clin Invest* 1990; 86:993–999.
80. Epstein ND, Fananpazir L, Lin HJ, Lifton RP, Mulvihill J, White R, et al: Evidence of genetic heterogeneity in five kindreds with familial hypertrophic cardiomyopathy. *Circulation* 1992; 85:635–647.
81. Marian AJ, Kelly D, Mares A, Tapscott T, Yu Q-T, Gooch G, et al: The missense mutation in exon 13 of the beta-myosin heavy chain gene, a genetic marker for sudden cardiac death in patients with familial hypertrophic cardiomyopathy. *Circulation* 1992; 86:116.
82. Hers HG, Van Hoof F, de Barsy T: Glycogen storage diseases. In: Scriber CR, Beaudet AL, Sly WS, Valle D (eds): *The Metabolic Basis of Inherited Disease*, 6th ed. New York, McGraw-Hill, 1989: 425.
83. D'Ancona GG, Wurm J, Croce CM: Genetics of type 11 glycogenosis: Assignment of the human gene for acid α-glucosidase to chromosome 17. *Proc Natl Acad Sci U S A* 1979; 76:4526–4529.
84. Zhong N, Martiniuk F, Tzall S, Hirschhorn R: Identification of a missense mutation in one allele of a patient with Pompe disease, and use of endonuclease digestion of PCR-amplified RNA to demonstrate lack of mRNA expression from the second allele. *Am J Hum Genet* 1991; 49:635–645.
85. Sotelo-Avila C, Gonzalez-Crussi F, Fowler JW: Complete and incomplete forms of Beckwith-Wiedemann syndrome: Their oncogenic potential. *J Pediatr* 1980; 96:47–50.
86. Best LG, Hoekstra RE: Wiedemann-Beckwith syndrome: Autosomal dominant inheritance in a family. *Am J Med Genet* 1981; 9:291–299.
87. Geoffrey G, Barbeau A, Breton G, Lemieux B, Aube M, Lepert C, et al: Clinical description and roentgenologic evaluation of patients with Friedreich's ataxia. *Can J Neurol Sci* 1976; 3: 279–287.
88. Maione S, Giunta A, Mansi D, Filla A, Serino A, Teti G, et al: Cardiac abnormalities in Friedreich's ataxia patients and first-degree relatives: Evidence of hypertrophic cardiomyopathy in obligate heterozygotes. *Acta Neurol (Naples)* 1980; 35:354–356.
89. Harding AE, Hewer RL: The heart disease of Friedreich's ataxia: A clinical and electrocardiographic study of 115 patients with an analysis of serial electrocardiographic changes in 30 cases. *Q J Med* 1983; 52:489–502.
90. Chamberlain S, Shaw J, Rowland A, Wallis J, South S, Nakamura Y, et al: Mapping of mutation causing Friedreich's ataxia to human chromosome 9. *Nature* 1988; 334:248–250.
91. Wallis J, Williamson R, Chamberlain S: Identification of a hypervariable microsatellite polymorphisms within D9S15 tightly linked to Friedreich's ataxia. *Hum Genet* 1990; 85:98–100.
92. Fuita R, Agid Y, Trouillas P, Seck A, Tommasi-Davenas C, Driesel AJ, et al: Confirmation of linkage of Friedreich ataxia to chromosome 9 and identification of a new closely linked marker. *Genomics* 1989; 4:110–111.
93. Fujita R, Hanauer A, Vincent A, Mandel J-L, Koenig M: Physical mapping of 2 loci (D9S5 and D9S15) tightly linked to Friedreich ataxia locus (FRDA) and identification of nearby CpG islands by pulse-field gel electrophoresis. *Genomics* 1991; 10:915–920.
94. Codd MB, Sugrue DD, Gersh BJ, Melton LJ: Epidemiology of idiopathic dilated and hypertrophic cardiomyopathy: A population-based study in Olmsted County, Minnesota, 1975–1984. *Circulation* 1989; 80:564–572.
95. Schmidt MA, Michels W, Edwards WD, Miller FA: Familial dilated cardiomyopathy. *Am J Med Genet* 1988; 31:135–143.
96. Michels W, Driscoll DJ, Miller FA Jr: Familial aggregation of idiopathic dilated cardiomyopathy. *Am J Cardiol* 1985; 55:1232–1233.
97. Michels W, Mill PP, Miller FA, Tajik AJ, Chu JS, Driscoll DJ, et al: The frequency of familial dilated cardiomyopathy in a series of patients with idiopathic dilated cardiomyopathy. *N Engl J Med* 1992; 326:77–82.
98. Emery AEH: Duchenne Muscular Dystrophy, Oxford Monographs on Medical Genetics, No. 15, Oxford, Oxford University Press, 1987.
99. Perloff JK, DeLeon AC, O'Doherty D: The cardiomyopathy of progressive muscular dystrophy. *Circulation* 1966; 33:625–648.
100. Perloff JK: Cardiac rhythm and conduction in Duchenne's muscular dystrophy: A prospective study of 20 patients. *J Am Coll Cardiol* 1984; 3:1263–1268.
101. Koenig M, Hoffman EP, Bertelson CJ, Monaco AP, Feener C, Kunkel LM: Complete cloning of the Duchenne muscular dystrophy (DMD) cDNA and preliminary genomic organization of the DMD gene in normal and affected individuals. *Cell* 1987; 50:509–517.
102. Hoffman EP, Brown RH Jr, Kunkel LM: Dystrophin: The protein product of the Duchenne muscular dystrophy locus. *Cell* 1987; 51:919–928.
103. Davies KE, Pearson PL, Harper PS, Murray JM, O'Brien T, Sarfarazi M, et al: Linkage analysis of two cloned DNA sequences flanking the Duchenne muscular dystrophy locus on the short arm of the human X chromosome. *Nucl Acids Res* 1983; 11:2303–2312.
104. Chamberlain JS, Pearlman JA, Muzny DM, Gibbs RA, Ranier JE, Reeves M, et al: Expression of the murine Duchenne muscular dystrophy gene in muscle and brain. *Science* 1988; 239:1416–1418.

105. Campbell KP, Kahl SD: Association of dystrophin and an integral membrane glycoprotein. *Nature* 1989; 388:259–262.
106. Fong P, Turner PR, Denatclau WF, Steinhardt RA: Increased activity of calcium leak channels in myotubes of Duchenne human and mdx mouse origin. *Science* 1990; 250:673–676.
107. Bies RD, Friedman D, Roberts R, Perryman MB, Caskey CT: Expression and localization of dystrophin in human cardiac Purkinje fibers. *Circulation* 1992; 86:147–153.
108. Bies RD, Phelps SF, Cortez MD, Roberts R, Caskey CT, Chamberlain JS: Human and murine dystrophin mRNA transcripts are differentially expressed during skeletal muscle, heart, and brain development. *Nucl Acids Res* 1992; 20:1725–1731.
109. Lee CC, Pearlman JA, Chamberlain JS, Caskey CT: Expression of recombinant dystrophin and its localization to the cell membrane. *Nature* 1991; 349:334–336.
110. Chamberlain JS, Gibbs RA, Ranier JE, Nguyen PN, Caskey CT: Deletion screening of the DMD locus via multiplex DNA amplification. *Nucl Acids Res* 1988; 16:11141–11156.
111. Beggs AH, Koenig M, Boyce FM, Kunkel LM: Detection of 98% of DMD/BMD deletions by PCR. *Hum Genet* 1990; 86:45–48.
112. Bulman DE, Murphy EG, Zubrzycka-Gaarn EE, Worton RG, Ray PN: Differentiation of Duchenne and Becker muscular dystrophy phenotypes with amino- and carboxy-terminal antisera specific for dystrophin. *Am J Hum Genet* 1991; 48:295–304.
113. Malhotra SB, Hart KA, Klamut HJ, Thomas NST, Bodrug SE, Burghes AHM, et al: Frameshift deletions in patients with Duchenne and Becker muscular dystrophy. *Science* 1988; 242: 755–759.
114. Emery AE: X-linked muscular dystrophy with early contractures and cardiomyopathy (Emery-Dreifuss type). *Clin Genet* 1987; 32:360–367.
115. Yates JRW, Affara NA, Jamieson DM, Ferguson-Smith MA, Hausmanowa-Petrusewicz I, Zaremba J, et al: Emery-Dreifuss muscular dystrophy: Localization to Xq27.3-qter confirmed by linkage to the factor VIII gene. *J Med Genet* 1986; 23:587–590.
116. Consalez GG, Thomas NST, Stayton CL, Knight SJL, Johnson M, Hopkins LC, et al: Assignment of Emery-Dreifuss muscular dystrophy to the distal region of Xq28: The results of a collaborative study. *Am J Hum Genet* 1991; 48:468–480.
117. Harper P: *Myotonic Dystrophy*. Philadelphia, Saunders, 1989.
118. Brunner H, Korneluk R, Coerwinkel-Driessen M, Mackenzie A, Smeets H, Lambermon HM, et al: Myotonic dystrophy is closely linked to the gene for muscle type creatine kinase (CKMM). *Hum Genet* 1989; 81:308–310.
119. Johnson K, Shelbourne P, Davies J, Buxton J, Nimmo E, Siciliano MJ, et al: A new polymorphic probe which defines the region of chromosome 19 containing the myotonic dystrophy locus. *Am J Hum Genet* 1990; 46:1073–1081.
120. Brook JD, McCurrack ME, Harley HG, Buckler AJ, Church D, Aburatani H, et al: Molecular basis of myotonic dystrophy: Expansion of a trinucleotide (CTG) repeat at the 3′ end of a transcript encoding a protein kinase family member. *Cell* 1992; 68:799–808.
121. Fu Y-H, Pizzuti A, Fenwick RG Jr, King J, Rajnarayan S, Dunne PW, et al: An unstable triplet repeat in a gene related to myotonic muscular dystrophy. *Science* 255:1256–1258.
122. Berko BA, Swift M: X-linked dilated cardiomyopathy. *N Engl J Med* 1987; 316:1186–1191.
123. Towbin JA, Hejtmancik JF, Brink P, Gelb B, Zhu XM, Chamberlain JS, McCabe ERB, Swift M: X-linked dilated cardiomyopathy. Molecular genetic evidence of linkage to the Duchenne muscular dystrophy (dystrophin) gene at the Xp21 locus. *Circulation* 1993; 87:1854–1865.
124. Towbin JA, Zhu XM, Gelb BD, Bies R, McCabe ERB, Chamberlain JS, et al: X-linked dilated cardiomyopathy (XLCM): Molecular pathogenesis. *Pediatr Res* 1991; 29:25A.
125. Barth PG, Scholte HR, Berden JA, Van der Klei-Van Moorsel JM, Luyt-Houwen IEM, Van 'T VeerKorthof ETH, et al: An X-linked mitochondrial disease affecting cardiac muscle, skeletal muscle and neutrophil leukocytes. *J Neurol Sci* 1983; 62: 327–355.
126. Kelley RI, Cheatham JP, Clark BJ, Nigro MA, Powell BR, Sherwood GW, et al: X-linked dilated cardiomyopathy with neutropenia, growth retardation, and 3-methylglutaconic aciduria. *J Pediatr* 1991; 119:738–747.
127. Bolhuis PA, Hensels GW, Hulsebos TJM, Baas F, Barth PG: Mapping of the locus for X-linked cardioskeletal myopathy with neutropenia and abnormal mitochondria (Barth syndrome) to Xq28. *Am J Hum Genet* 1991; 48:481–485.
128. Saddi R, Feingold J: Idiopathic hemochromatosis: An autosomal recessive disease. *Clin Genet* 1974; 5:234–247.
129. Simon M, Bourel M, Fauchet R, Genetet B: Association of HLA-A3 and HLA-B14 antigens with idiopathic hemochromatosis. *Gut* 1976; 17:332–334.
130. Hosenpud JD, Niles NR: Clinical, hemodynamic and endomyocardial biopsy findings in idiopathic restrictive cardiomyopathy. *West J Med* 1986; 144:303–306.
131. Allensworth DC, Rice GJ, Lowe GW: Persistent atrial standstill in a family with myocardial disease. *Am J Med* 1969; 47:775–784.
132. Benson MD, Wallace MR, Tekada E, et al: Hereditary amyloidosis: Description of a new American kindred with late onset cardiomyopathy, Appalachian amyloid. *Arthritis Rheum* 1987; 30:195–200.
133. Saraiva MJ, Almeida M, Sherman W, Gawinowicz M, Costa P, Costa PP, et al: A new transthyretin mutation associated with amyloid cardiomyopathy. *Am J Hum Genet* 1992; 50: 1027–1030.
134. Opitz JM: Genetic aspects of endocardial fibroelastosis. *Am J Med Genet* 1982; 11:92–96.
135. Ross RS, Bulkley BH, Hutchins GM, Harshey JS, Jones RA, Kraus H, et al: Idiopathic familial myocardiopathy in three generations: A clinical and pathologic study. *Am Heart J* 1978; 96:170–179.
136. Hodgson S, Child A, Dyson M: Endocardial fibroelastosis: Possible X-linked inheritance. *J Med Genet* 1987; 24:210–214.
137. Pepine CJ: The therapeutic potential of carnitine in cardiovascular disorders. *Clin Ther* 1991; 13:2–21.
138. Leys D, Petit H, Bonte-Adnet C, Millaire A, Fourrier F, Dubois F, Rosseaux M, Ducloux G: Refsum's disease revealed by cardiac disorders (letter). *Lancet* 1989; 1:621.
139. Neufeld EF, Muenzer J: The mucopolysaccharidoses. In: Scriver CR, Beaudet AL, Sly NS, Valle D (eds): *The Metabolic Basis of Inherited Disease*, 6th ed. New York, McGraw-Hill, 1989: 1565–1587.
140. Kduraa S, Gregersen N, Christensen E, et al: In vitro fibroblast studies in a patient with C6-C10 dicarboxylic aciduria: Evidence for a defect in general acyl-CoA dehydrogenase. *Clin Chim Acta* 1982; 126:53–67.
141. Roe CR, Coates PM: Acyl-CoA dehydrogenase deficiencies. In: Scriver CR, Beaudet AL, Sly WS, Valle D (eds) *The Metabolic Basis of Inherited Disease*, 6th ed. New York, McGraw-Hill, 1989: 2869.
142. Hale DE, Batshaw ML, Coates PM, et al: Long-chain acyl coenzyme A dehydrogenase deficiency: An inherited cause of nonketotic hypoglycemia. *Pediatr Res* 1985; 19:666–671.
143. Cornelio F, DiDonato S: Myopathies due to enzyme deficiencies. *J Neurol* 1985; 232:329–340.
144. Servidei S, Metlay LA, Chodosh J, DiMauro S: Fatal infantile cardiopathy caused by phosphorylase b kinase deficiency. *J Pediatr* 1988; 113:82–85.
145. Servidei S, Riepe RE, Langston C, Tani LY, Bricker JT, Crisp-Lindgren N, et al: Severe cardiopathy in branching enzyme deficiency. *J Pediatr* 1987; 111:51–56.
146. Grivell LA: Small, beautiful and essential. *Nature* 1989; 341:569–571.
147. Wallace DC, Zheng X, Lott MT, Shoffner JM, Hodge JA, Kelley RI, et al: Familial mitochondrial encephalomyopathy (MERRF): Genetic, pathophysiological, and biochemical characterization of a mitochondrial DNA disease. *Cell* 1988; 55:601–610.
148. Shoffner JM, Lott MI, Lezza AMS, Seibel P, Ballinger SW, Wallace DC: Myotonic epilepsy and ragged-red fiber disease (MERRF) is associated with a mitochondrial DNA $tRNA^{LYS}$ mutation. *Cell* 1990; 61:931–937.
149. Corral-Debrinski M, Stepien G, Shoffner JM, Lott MT, Kanter K, Wallace DC: Hypoxemia is associated with mitochondrial DNA damage and gene induction implications for cardiac disease. *JAMA* 1991; 266:1812–1816.
150. Mohl W, Mayr WR: Atrial septal defect of the secundum type and HLA. *Tissue Antigens* 1977; 10:121–122.
151. Pease WE, Nordenberg A, Ladda RL: Genetic counseling in familial atrial septal defect with prolonged atrioventricular conduction. *Circulation* 1976; 53:759–762.
152. Sherman J, Angulo M, Boxer RA, Gluck R: Possible mitochon-

drial inheritance of congenital cardiac septal defects. *N Engl J Med* 1985; 313:186–187.

153. Smith AT, Sack GH, Taylor GJ: Holt-Oram syndrome. *J Pediatr* 1979; 95:538–543.
154. Preus M: The Williams syndrome: Objective definition and diagnosis. *Clin Genet* 1984; 25:422–428.
155. Becroft DMO, Chambers D: Supravalvular aortic stenosis-infantile hypercalcaemia syndrome: In vitro hypersensitivity to vitamin D52 and calcium. *J Med Genet* 1976; 13:223–228.
156. Hallidie-Smith KA, Karas S: Cardiac anomalies in Williams-Beuren syndrome. *Arch Dis Child* 1988; 63:809–813.
157. Bennett CP, Burn J, Moore GE, Chambers J, Williamson R, Wilkinson J: Exclusion of calcitonin as a candidate gene for the basic defect in a family with autosomal dominant supravalvular aortic stenosis. *J Med Genet* 1988; 25:311–312.
158. Schmidt MA, Ensing GJ, Carter GA, Hagler DJ, Feldt RH: Autosomal dominant supravalvular aortic stenosis: Large three-generation family. *Am J Med Genet* 1989; 32:384–389.
159. Ewart AK, Morris CA, Ensing GJ, Loker J, Moore C, Leppert M, Keating M: A human vascular disorder, supravalvular aortic stenosis, maps to chromosome 7. *Proc Natl Acad Sci USA* 1993; 90:3226–3230.
160. Devereux RB, Kramer-Fox R: Inheritance and phenotypic features of mitral valve prolapse. In: Boudoulas H, Wooley FC (eds): *Mitral Valve Prolapse and the Mitral Valve Prolapse Syndrome.* Mt. Kisco, NY, Futura, 1988: 109.
161. Noonan JA, Ehmke DA: Associated noncardiac malformations in children with congenital heart disease. *J Pediatr* 1963; 63: 468–470.
162. Mendez HMM, Opitz JM: Noonan syndrome: A review. *Am J Med Genet* 1985; 21:493–506.
163. Kitchens CS, Alexander JA: Partial deficiency of coagulation factor XI as a newly recognized feature of Noonan syndrome. *J Pediatr* 1983; 102:224–227.
164. de Haan M, Kamp JJPvd, Briet E, Dubbeldam J: Noonan syndrome: Partial factor XI deficiency. *Am J Med Genet* 1988; 29:277–282.
165. Pyeritz RE: Heritable disorders of connective tissue. In: Pierpont ME, Moller JH (eds): *The Genetics of Cardiovascular Disease.* Boston, Martinus-Nijhoff, 1987: 265.
166. Byers PH: Brittle bones, fragile molecules: Disorders of collagen gene structure and expression. *Trends Genet* 1990; 6:293–300.
167. Dietz HC, Pyeritz RE, Hall BD, Cadle RG, Hamosh A, Schwartz J, et al: The Marfan syndrome locus: Confirmation of assignment to chromosome 15 and identification of tightly linked markers at 15q15-q21.3. *Genomics* 1991; 9:355–361.
168. Sakai LY, Keene DR, Engvall E: Fibrillin, a new 250-kD glycoprotein, is a component of extracellular microfibrils. *J Cell Biol* 1986; 103:2499–2509.
169. Magenis RE, Maslen CL, Smith L, Allen L, Sakai L: Localization of the fibrillin gene to chromosome 15, band 15q21.1. *Genomics* 1991; 11:346–351.
170. Lee B, Godfrey M, Vitale E, Hori H, Mattei M-G, Sarfarazi M, et al: Linkage of Marfan syndrome and phenotypically related disorder to two different fibrillin genes. *Nature* 1991; 352:330–334.
171. Dietz HC, Cutting GR, Pyeritz RE, Maslen CL, Sakai LY, Corson GM, et al: Marfan syndrome caused by a recurrent de novo missense mutation in the fibrillin gene. *Nature* 1991; 352:337–339.
172. Maslen CL, Corson GM, Maddox BK, Glanville RW, Sakai LY: Partial sequence of a candidate gene for the Marfan syndrome. *Nature* 1991; 352:334–337.
173. Kontusaari S, Tromp G, Kuivaniemi H, Ladda RL, Prockop DJ: Inheritance of an RNA splicing mutation ($G^{+1\ IVS20}$) in the type III procollagen gene (COL3A) in a family having aortic aneurysms and Ehlers-Danlos syndrome type IV. *Am J Hum Genet* 1990; 47:112–120.
174. Kontusaari S, Tromp G, Kuivaniemi H, Romanic AM, Prockop DJ: A mutation in the gene for type III procollagen (COL3AI) in a family with aortic aneurysms. *J Clin Invest* 1990; 86:1465–1473.
175. Kuivaniemi H, Tromp G, Prockop DJ: Genetic causes of aortic aneurysms: Unlearning at least part of what the textbooks say. *J Clin Invest* 1991; 88:1441–1444.
176. Kuivaniemi H, Kontusaari S, Stolle C, Pope FM, Prockop DJ: Identical G^{+1} to A mutations in three different introns of the type III procollagen gene (COL3A1) produce different patterns of RNA splicing in three variants of Ehlers-Danlos syndrome IV: An explanation for exon skipping with some mutations and not others. *J Biol Chem* 1990; 265:12067–12074.
177. Challenor VF, Conway N, Munro JL: The surgical treatment of restrictive cardiomyopathy in pseudoxanthoma elasticum. *Br Heart J* 1988; 59:266–269.
178. Pyeritz RE, Weiss JL, Renie WE, Fine SL: Pseudoxanthoma elasticum and mitral-valve prolapse. *N Engl J Med* 1982; 307:1451–1452.
179. Weir EK, Joffe HS, Blaufuss AH, Beighton P: Cardiovascular abnormalities in cutis laxa. *Eur J Cardiol* 1977; 5:255–261.
180. Romano C: Congenital cardiac arrhythmia. *Lancet* 1965; 1:658–659.
181. Ward OC: A new familial cardiac syndrome in children. *J Ir Med Assoc* 1964; 54:103–106.
182. Schwartz PJ, Periti M, Malliani A: The long QT syndrome. *Am Heart J* 1975; 89:378–390.
183. Moss AJ, Schwartz PJ: Sudden death and the idiopathic long QT syndrome. *Am J Ed* 1979; 66:6–7.
184. Moss AJ: Prolonged QT interval syndrome. *JAMA* 1986; 256:2985–2987.
185. Schwartz PJ, Bonazzi O, Locati E, Napditano C, Sala S: Pathogenesis and therapy of the idiopathic long QT syndrome. In: Hashiba K, Moss AJ, Schwartz PJ (eds): QT prolongation and ventricular arrhythmias. *Ann N Y Acad Sci*, 1992.
186. Itoh S, Munemura S, Satoh H: A study of the inheritance pattern of Romano-Ward syndrome. *Clin Pediatr* 1982; 21:20–24.
187. Giuffre RM, Hejtmancik JF, McCabe ERB, Towbin JA: Long QT (Romano-Ward) syndrome: Molecular genetic evidence against tight HLA linkage. *Am J Hum Genet* 1990; 47:A0704.
188. Keating M, Dunn C, Atkinson D, Timothy K, Vincent GM, Leppert M: Consistent linkage of the long QT syndrome to the Harvey ras-1 locus in chromosome 11. *Am J Hum Genet* 1991; 49:1335–1339.
189. Towbin JA, Pagotto L, Siu B, Robinson J, Moss A, McCabe ERB, et al: Romano-Ward Long QT syndrome (RWLQTS): Evidence of genetic heterogeneity. *Pediatr Res* 1992; 31:23A.
190. Fraser GR, Froggatt P, Murphy T: Genetical aspects of the cardio-auditory syndrome of Jervell and Lange-Nielsen (congenital deafness and electrocardiographic abnormalities). *Am Hum Genet* 1964; 28:133–156.
191. Vadaillet HJ Jr, Pressley JC, Henke E, Harrell FE Jr, German LD: Familial occurrence of accessory atrioventricular pathways (preexcitation syndrome). *N Engl J Med* 1987; 317:65–69.
192. Gillette PC, Freed D, McNamara DG: A proposed autosomal dominant method of inheritance of the Wolff-Parkinson-White syndrome and supraventricular tachycardia. *J Pediatr* 1978; 93:257–258.
193. Graber HL, Unverferth DV, Baker PB, Ryan JM, Baba N, Wooley CF: Evolution of a hereditary cardiac conduction and muscle disorder: A study involving a family with six generations affected. *Circulation* 1986; 74:21–35.
194. Brown MS, Goldstein JL: A receptor-mediated pathway for cholesterol homeostasis. *Science* 1986; 232:34–47.
195. Brown MS, Goldstein JL: Plasma lipoproteins: teaching old dogmas new tricks. *Nature* 1987; 330:113–114.
196. Kane JP: Apolipoprotein B: Structural and metabolic heterogeneity. *Annu Rev Physiol* 1983; 45:637–650.
197. Powell LM, Wallis SC, Pease RJ, Edwards YH, Knott TJ, Scott J: A novel form of tissue-specific RNA processing produces apolipoprotein-B48 in intestine. *Cell* 1987; 50:831–840.
198. Milne RW, Marcel YL: The use of monoclonal antibodies to probe human apolipoprotein B structure and function. *Can J Biochem Cell Biol* 1985; 63:906–912.
199. Goldstein JL, Basu SK, Brown MS: Receptor-mediated endocytosis of low-density lipoprotein in cultured cells. *Methods Enzymol* 1983; 98:241–260.
200. Seilhamer JJ, Protter M, Frossard P, Levy Wilson B: Isolation and DNA sequence of full-length cDNA and of the entire gene for human apolipoprotein AI: discovery of a new genetic polymorphism in the apo AI gene. *DNA* 1984; 3:309–317.
201. Wei CF, Tsao YK, Robberson DL, Gotto AM Jr., Brown K, Chan L: The structure of the human apolipoprotein C-II gene: Electron microscopic analysis of RNA:DNA hybrids, complete nucleotide sequence, and identification of 5′ homologous sequences among apolipoprotein genes. *J Biol Chem* 1985; 260:15211–15221.

202. McLean JW, Elshourbagy NA, Chang DJ, Mahley RW, Taylor JM: Human apolipoprotein E mRNA: cDNA cloning and nucleotide sequencing of a new variant. *J Biol Chem* 1984; 259:6498–6504.
203. Chen SH, Yang CY, Chen PF, Setzer D, Tanimura M, Li WH, et al: The complete cDNA and amino acid sequence of human apolipoprotein B-100. *J Biol Chem* 1986; 261:12918–12921.
204. Knott TJ, Rall SC Jr, Innerarity TL, Jacobson SF, Urdea MS, Levy Wilson B, et al: Human apolipoprotein B: Structure of carboxyl-terminal domains, sites of gene expression, and chromosomal localization. *Science* 1985; 230:37–43.
205. Protter M, Levy Wilson B, Miller J, Bencen G, White T, Seilhamer JJ: Isolation and sequence analysis of the human apolipoprotein CIII gene and the intergenic region between the apo AI and apo CIII genes. *DNA* 1984; 3:449–456.
206. McLean JW, Tomlinson JE, Kuang WJ, Eaton DL, Chen EY, Fless GM, et al: cDNA sequence of human apolipoprotein(a) is homologous to plasminogen. *Nature* 1987; 330:132–137.
207. Chen SH, Habib G, Yang CY, Gu ZW, Lee BR, Weng SA, et al: Apolipoprotein B-48 is the product of a messenger RNA with an organ-specific in-frame stop codon. *Science* 1987; 238:363–366.
208. Blackhart BD, Ludwig EM, Pierotti VR, Caiati L, Onasch MA, Wallis SC, et al: Structure of the human apolipoprotein B gene. *J Biol Chem* 1986; 261:15364–15367.
209. Sharpe CR, Sidoli A, Shelley CS, Lucero MA, Shoulders CC, Baralle FE: Human apolipoproteins AI, AII, CII and CIII: cDNA sequences and mRNA abundance. *Nucl Acids Res* 1984; 12:3917–3932.
210. Motulsky AG: Current concepts in genetics: The genetic hyperlipidemias. *N Engl J Med* 1976; 294:823–827.
211. Fredrickson DS, Lees RS: System for phenotyping hyperlipoproteinemia. *Circulation* 1965; 31:321–323.
212. Mahley RW, Weisgraber KH, Innerarity TL, Rall SC Jr: Genetic defects in lipoprotein metabolism: Elevation of atherogenic lipoproteins caused by impaired catabolism. *JAMA* 1991; 265:78–83.
213. Schaefer EJ, Levy R: Pathogenesis and management of lipoprotein disorders. *N Engl J Med* 1985; 312:1300–1310.
214. Gotto AM Jr, Farmer JA: Risk factors for coronary artery disease. In: Braunwald E (ed): *Heart Disease: A Textbook of Cardiovascular Medicine*, 3d ed. Philadelphia, Saunders, 1988: 1153–1190.
215. Breckenridge WC, Little JA, Steiner G, Chow A, Poapst M: Hypertriglyceridemia associated with deficiency of apolipoprotein C-II. *N Engl J Med* 1978; 298:1265–1273.
216. Brown MS, Goldstein JL: Expression of the familial hypercholesterolemia gene in heterozygotes: Mechanism for a dominant disorder in man. *Science* 1974; 185:61–63.
217. Goldstein JL, Brown MS: Familial hypercholesterolemia: A genetic receptor disease. *Hosp Pract* 1985; 20:35–41, 45–6.
218. Brown MS, Kovanen PT, Goldstein JL, Eeckels R, Vandenberghe K, van den Berghe H, et al: Prenatal diagnosis of homozygous familial hypercholesterolaemia: Expression of a genetic receptor disease in utero. *Lancet* 1978; 1:526–529.
219. Goldstein JL, Schrott HG, Hazzard WR, Bierman EL, Motulsky AG: Hyperlipidemia in coronary heart disease: II. Genetic analysis of lipid levels in 176 families and delineation of a new inherited disorder, combined hyperlipidemia. *J Clin Invest* 1973; 52:1544–1568.
220. Rose HG, Kranz P, Weinstock M, Juliano J, Haft J: Inheritance of combined hyperlipoproteinemia: Evidence for a new lipoprotein phenotype. *Am J Med* 1973; 54:148–160.
221. Brewer HB Jr, Zech LA, Gregg RE, Schwartz D, Schaefer EJ: NIH conference: Type III hyperlipoproteinemia: Diagnosis, molecular defects, pathology, and treatment. *Ann Intern Med* 1983; 98:623–640.
222. Utermann G, Jaeschke M, Menzel J: Familial hyperlipoproteinemia type III: Deficiency of a specific apolipoprotein (apo E-III) in the very-low-density lipoproteins. *FEBS Lett* 1975; 56:352–355.
223. Utermann G, Pruin N, Steinmetz A: Polymorphism of apolipoprotein E.III. Effect of a single polymorphic gene locus on plasma lipid levels in man. *Clin Genet* 1979; 15:63–72.
224. Hazzard WR, Warnick GR, Utermann G, Albers JJ: Genetic transmission of isoapolipoprotein E phenotypes in a large kindred: Relationship to dysbetalipoproteinemia and hyperlipidemia. *Metabolism* 1981; 30:79–88.
225. Sniderman AD, Wolfson C, Teng B, Franklin FA, Bachorik PS, Kwiterovich PO Jr: Association of hyperapobetalipoproteinemia with endogenous hypertriglyceridemia and atherosclerosis. *Ann Intern Med* 1982; 97:833–839.
226. Fallat RW, Glueck CJ: Familial and acquired type V hyperlipoproteinemia. *Atherosclerosis* 1976; 23:41–62.
227. Breslow JL: Human apolipoprotein molecular biology and genetic variation. *Annu Rev Biochem* 1985; 54:699–727.
228. Zannis V, Breslow JL: Genetic mutations affecting human lipoprotein metabolism. *Adv Hum Genet* 1985; 14:125–215, 383–386.
229. Karathanasis SK, Oettgen P, Haddad IA, Antonarakis SE: Structure, evolution, and polymorphisms of the human apolipoprotein A4 gene (APOA4). *Proc Natl Acad Sci U S A* 1986; 83:8457–8461.
230. Rogne S, Myklebost O, Olaisen B, Gedde Dahl T Jr, Prydz H: Confirmation of the close linkage between the loci for human apolipoproteins AI and AIV by the use of a cloned cDNA probe and two restriction site polymorphisms. *Hum Genet* 1986; 72:68–71.
231. Karathanasis SK, McPherson J, Zannis VI, Breslow JL: Linkage of human apolipoproteins A-I and C-III genes. *Nature* 1983; 304:371–373.
232. Scott J, Knott TJ, Shaw DJ, Brook JD: Localization of genes encoding apolipoproteins CI, CII, and E to the p13—cen region of human chromosome 19. *Hum Genet* 1985; 71:144–146.
233. Das HK, McPherson J, Bruns GA, Karathanasis SK, Breslow JL: Isolation, characterization, and mapping to chromosome 19 of the human apolipoprotein E gene. *J Biol Chem* 1985; 260:6240–6247.
234. Myklebost O, Rogne S: A physical map of the apolipoprotein gene cluster on human chromosome 19. *Hum Genet* 1988; 78:244–247.
235. Scott J, Knott TJ, Priestley LM, Robertson ME, Mann DV, Kostner G, et al: High-density lipoprotein composition is altered by a common DNA polymorphism adjacent to apoprotein AII gene in man. *Lancet* 1985; 1:771–773.
236. Weisgraber KH, Bersot TP, Mahley RW: Isolation and characterization of an apoprotein from the d less than 1.006 lipoproteins of human and canine lymph homologous with the rat A-IV apoprotein. *Biochem Biophys Res Commun* 1978; 85: 287–292.
237. Karathanasis SK, Zannis VI, Breslow JL: Isolation and characterization of cDNA clones corresponding to two different human apoC-III alleles. *J Lipid Res* 1985; 26:451–456.
238. Stocks J, Paul H, Galton D: Haplotypes identified by DNA restriction-fragment-length polymorphisms in the A-I C-III A-IV gene region and hypertriglyceridemia. *Am J Hum Genet* 1987; 41:106–118.
239. Kamboh M, Ferrell RE: Genetic studies of human apolipoproteins: I. Polymorphism of apolipoprotein A-IV. *Am J Hum Genet* 1987; 41:119–127.
240. Zannis V, Breslow JL, Utermann G, Mahley RW, Weisgraber KH, Havel RJ, et al: Proposed nomenclature of apoE isoproteins, apoE genotypes, and phenotypes. *J Lipid Res* 1982; 23:911–914.
241. Nieminen MS, Mattila KJ, Aalto-Setala K, Kuusi T, Kontula K, Kauppinen-Makelin R, et al: Lipoproteins and their genetic variation in subjects with and without angiographically verified coronary artery disease. *Arterioscler Thromb* 1992; 12: 58–69.
242. Armstrong VW, Cremer P, Eberle E, Manke A, Schulze F, Wieland H, et al: The association between serum Lp(a) concentrations and angiographically assessed coronary atherosclerosis: Dependence on serum LDL levels. *Atherosclerosis* 1986; 62: 249–257.
243. Horsthemke B, Dunning A, Humphries S: Identification of deletions in the human low density lipoprotein receptor gene. *J Med Genet* 1987; 24:144–147.
244. Lehrman MA, Goldstein JL, Russell DW, Brown MS: Duplication of seven exons in LDL receptor gene caused by Alu-Alu recombination in a subject with familial hypercholesterolemia. *Cell* 1987; 48:827–835.
245. Goldstein JL, Brown MS: The LDL receptor defect in familial hypercholesterolemia: Implications for pathogenesis and therapy. *Med Clin North Am* 1982; 66:335–362.

246. Schieken RM, Kerber RE, Ionasescu W, Zellweger H: Cardiac manifestations of the mucopolysaccharidoses. *Circulation* 1975; 52:700–705.
247. Pinnell SR, McKusick VA: Heritable disorders of connective tissue with skin changes. In: Fitzpatrick TB (ed): *Dermatology in General Medicine*, 3d ed. New York, McGraw-Hill, 1987: 1775–1791.
248. Munke M, Kraus JP, Ohura T, Francke U: The gene for cystathionine beta-synthase (CBS) maps to the subtelomeric region on human chromosome 21q and to proximal mouse chromosome 17. *Am J Hum Genet* 1988; 42:550–559.
249. Kraus JP, Williamson CL, Firgaira FA, Yang Feng TL, Munke M, Francke U, et al: Cloning and screening with nanogram amounts of immunopurified mRNAs: cDNA cloning and chromosomal mapping of cystathionine beta-synthase and the beta subunit of propionyl-CoA carboxylase. *Proc Natl Acad Sci U S A* 1986; 83:2047–2051.
250. Mudd SH, Havlik R, Levy HL, McKusick VA, Feinleib M: A study of cardiovascular risk in heterozygotes for homocystinuria. *Am J Hum Genet* 1981; 33:883–893.
251. Boers GH, Smals AG, Trijbels FJ, Fowler B, Bakkeren JA, Schoonderwaldt HC, et al: Heterozygosity for homocystinuria in premature peripheral and cerebral occlusive arterial disease. *N Engl J Med* 1985; 313:709–715.
252. Becker AE, Schoorl R, Balk AG, van der Heide RM: Cardiac manifestations of Fabry's disease: Report of a case with mitral insufficiency and electrocardiographic evidence of myocardial infarction. *Am J Cardiol* 1975; 36:829–835.
253. Goldman ME, Cantor R, Schwartz MF, Baker M, Desnick RJ: Echocardiographic abnormalities and disease severity in Fabry's disease. *J Am Coll Cardiol* 1986; 7:1157–1161.
254. Broadbent JC, Edwards WD, Gordon H, Hartzler GO, Krawisz JE: Fabry cardiomyopathy in the female confirmed by endomyocardial biopsy. *Mayo Clin Proc* 1981; 56:623–628.
255. Bishop DF, Calhoun DH, Bernstein HS, Hantzopoulos P, Quinn M, Desnick RJ: Human alpha galactosidase A: nucleotide sequence of a cDNA clone encoding the mature enzyme. *Proc Natl Acad Sci U S A* 1986; 83:4859–4863.
256. Beaudet AL, Ferry GD, Nichols BL Jr, Rosenberg HS: Cholesterol ester storage disease: Clinical, biochemical, and pathological studies. *J Pediatr* 1977; 90:910–914.
257. Koch G, Lalley PA, McAvoy M, Shows TB: Assignment of LIPA, associated with human acid lipase deficiency, to human chromosome 10 and comparative assignment to mouse chromosome 19. *Somat Cell Genet* 1981; 7:345–358.
258. Rosenberg H, Frewen TC, Li MD, Gordon BL, Jung JH, Finlay JP, et al: Cardiac involvement in diseases characterized by beta-galactosidase deficiency. *J Pediatr* 1985; 106:78–80.
259. Myerowitz R, Costigan FC: The major defect in Ashkenazi Jews with Tay-Sachs disease is an insertion in the gene for the alpha-chain of beta-hexosaminidase. *J Biol Chem* 1988; 263:18587–18589.
260. Myerowitz R, Hogikyan ND: Different mutations in Ashkenazi Jewish and non-Jewish French Canadians with Tay-Sachs disease. *Science* 1986; 232:1646–1648.
261. Blieden LC, Desnick RJ, Carter JB, Krivit W, Moller JH, Sharp HL: Cardiac involvement in Sandhoff's disease: Inborn error of glycosphingolipid metabolism. *Am J Cardiol* 1974; 34:83–88.
262. O'Dowd BF, Klavins MH, Willard HF, Gravel R, Lowden JA, Mahuran DJ: Molecular heterogeneity in the infantile and juvenile forms of Sandhoff disease (O-variant GM2 gangliosidosis). *J Biol Chem* 1986; 261:12680–12685.
263. Okada S, OBrien JS: Generalized gangliosidosis: Beta-galactosidase deficiency. *Science* 1968; 160:1002–1004.
264. Giugliani R, Dutra JC, Pereira ML, Rotta N, Drachler M, Ohlweiller L, et al: GM1 gangliosidosis: Clinical and laboratory findings in eight families. *Hum Genet* 1985; 70:347–354.
265. Charrow J, Hvizd MG: Cardiomyopathy and skeletal myopathy in an unusual variant of GM1 gangliosidosis. *J Pediatr* 1986; 108:729–732.
266. Desnick RJ (ed): *Gaucher Disease: A Century of Delineation and Research*. New York, Alan R. Liss, 1982.
267. Casta A, Hayden K, Wolf WJ: Calcification of the ascending aorta and aortic and mitral valves in Gaucher's disease. *Am J Cardiol* 1984; 54:1390–1391.
268. Fabbro D, Desnick RJ, Grabowski GA: Gaucher disease: Genetic heterogeneity within and among the subtypes detected by immunoblotting. *Am J Hum Genet* 1987; 40:15–31.
269. Zimran A, Sorge J, Gross E, Kubitz M, West C, Beutler E: Prediction of severity of Gaucher's disease by identification of mutations at DNA level. *Lancet* 1989; 2:349–352.
270. Durand P, Borrone C, Della Cella G: Fucosidosis. *J Pediatr* 1969; 75:665–674.
271. Johnson K, Dawson G: Molecular defect in processing alpha-fucosidase in fucosidosis. *Biochem Biophys Res Commun* 1985; 133:90–97.

Chapter 97

The Pathology, Pathophysiology, Recognition, and Treatment of Congenital Heart Disease

Elizabeth W. Nugent, M.D. ■ *William H. Plauth, M.D.*
Jesse E. Edwards, M.D. ■ *Willis H. Williams, M.D.*

INCIDENCE AND ETIOLOGY

The incidence of congenital heart disease in the United States is approximately 8 per 1000 live births.[1,2] Most of the infants born alive with cardiac defects have anomalies that do not represent a threat to life, at least during infancy. Almost one-third, or 2.6 per 1000 live births, however, have *critical disease,* defined as a malformation severe enough to result in cardiac catheterization, cardiac surgery, or death within the first year of life.[3] Today, with early detection and proper management, the majority of infants with critical disease can be expected to survive the first year of life.[3]

Estimates of the incidence of specific lesions vary, depending on whether the data are drawn from infants or older children and whether the diagnosis is based on clinical, catheterization, surgical, or postmortem studies (Table 97-1).[1-5] The incidence in other countries is remarkably similar to that reported for the United States.[6]

Despite these differences in case material, except for bicuspid aortic valve (when older patients are included) and mitral valve prolapse, it is apparent that ventricular septal defect is the most common malformation, occurring in 28 percent of all patients with congenital heart disease (Table 97-1).

Of 2251 infants with critical congenital heart disease in the New England Regional Infant Cardiac Program,[3] 53.7 percent were male. Certain defects, however, are considerably more common in one sex than in the other.

The most popular concept regarding etiology is that cardiac defects are of multifactorial etiology requiring a genetic predisposition, probably polygenic, and an environmental teratogen to which the susceptible fetus is exposed in a critical or vulnerable period.[7] Offspring of parents with certain types of congenital heart disease are at much greater risk,[8] and counseling for these families is important.[7,9] There is exciting work on the role of the neural crest in the pathogenesis of congenital heart disease.[10]

Some examples of congenital heart disease have a primarily genetic basis. An increased incidence of cardiac defects is associated with major chromosomal abnormalities such as trisomy, deletion, and mosaicism.[11] Down syndrome is a well-known example. Mendelian inheritance can be demonstrated in a few families with repeated occurrences of specific cardiac abnormalities. (See also Chap. 96.)

Environmental factors such as maternal cocaine use[12] and high altitude[13] clearly can play a role. On the other hand, the aggressive management of very small premature infants, with a resultant increase in survival, has led to serious problems with patent ductus arteriosus.

TABLE 97-1
Incidence of Specific Congenital Heart Defects

Defect	Percentage of Cases* Averaged
Ventricular septal defect	28.3
Pulmonary stenosis	9.5
Patent ductus arteriosus	8.7
Ventricular septal defect with pulmonary stenosis†	6.8
Atrial septal defect, secundum	6.7
Aortic stenosis	4.4
Coarctation of aorta	4.2
Atrioventricular canal‡	3.5
Transposition of great arteries	3.4
Aortic atresia	2.4
Truncus arteriosus	1.6
Tricuspid atresia	1.2
Total anomalous pulmonary venous connection	1.1
Double outlet right ventricle	0.8
Pulmonary atresia without ventricular septal defect	0.3

* Total number of cases = 103,590.
† Includes tetralogy of Fallot.
‡ Includes partial and complete.
SOURCE: Refs. 1–4, 6.

FETAL CIRCULATION AND THE TRANSITION TO NEONATAL AND ADULT CIRCULATION[14–20]

The fetus obtains all its nutritional requirements, including oxygen, via the placental circulation. Consequently, there is a need for a high blood flow to the placenta, but there is no need to pass most of the blood through the uninflated fetal lungs. The fetal circulation accomplishes its special function with the aid of three vascular channels: (1) the *foramen ovale* in the atrial septum allows blood to pass from the right to the left atrium; (2) the *ductus arteriosus* connects the pulmonary artery to the aorta distal to the origin of the left subclavian artery and enables most of the blood reaching the pulmonary artery to bypass the uninflated lungs; and (3) the *ductus venosus* shunts blood returning from the placenta through the umbilical cord to the inferior vena cava to bypass the liver.

In the developed fetus, the total return of blood to the heart by the inferior vena cava is equal to 65 to 70 percent of the combined ventricular output (CVO); of this volume an amount equal to 25 to 28 percent of CVO passes through the foramen ovale to the left atrium, where it is joined by 5 to 10 percent of CVO returning from the lungs. The left ventricle thus receives and ejects only 33 percent of the CVO of the fetal heart. The remaining 38 to 42 percent of CVO returning in the inferior vena cava mixes with most of the 22 to 25 percent of CVO that returns in the superior vena cava and goes into the right ventricle, which thus receives and ejects about 66 percent of the CVO of the fetal heart. About 85 to 90 percent of the blood ejected by the right ventricle, or about 60 percent of the CVO, is diverted from the lungs through the ductus arteriosus to the aorta; the remainder passes through the pulmonary circulation.[20] About 40 to 50 percent of the CVO goes to the placenta for the exchange of carbon dioxide, oxygen, and other metabolites.

Umbilical venous blood has a P_{O_2} of about 30 to 35 mmHg and an oxygen saturation of about 80 percent. As the result of the various mechanisms described above, fetal arterial blood in the ascending aorta has a P_{O_2} of about 26 to 28 mmHg and an oxygen saturation of 55 to 60 percent.

During the delivery of the fetus, the umbilical cord is usually somewhat compressed and the placenta may begin to separate. Simultaneously, the newborn baby is suddenly exposed to a cold, strange environment. Both asphyxia and cold are strong respiratory stimuli. Within seconds after expansion of the lungs with air, the tremendous increase in blood flow to the lungs takes over the function of gas exchange from the placental circulation. The removal of the placenta from the circulation markedly increases systemic arterial resistance and decreases blood return from the inferior vena cava.

The initial fall in pulmonary vascular resistance after birth is produced by two mechanisms. The first of these is a mechanical reduction due to the physical expansion of the lungs with air, with a resultant decrease in the kinking and compression of the pulmonary vessels. The second and main mechanism is a marked diminution in the pulmonary arterial vasoconstriction related to the increased alveolar and interstitial P_{O_2}.

The pulmonary vascular resistance falls very rapidly after birth and reaches adult levels by about 6 to 8 weeks of age. During this time, there is a rapid regression of the medial muscle layer of the pulmonary arteries and arterioles. There is a further decrease in total pulmonary vascular resistance associated with growth of the lungs for several years.

Prior to birth the foramen ovale is held open by the large flow of blood from the inferior vena cava to the left atrium. After birth, the left atrial pressure increases because of the increase in pulmonary flow and the increase in systemic arterial resistance; the right atrial pressure decreases. These changes in left and right atrial pressures produce functional closure of the foramen ovale by the apposition of the valve of the foramen ovale, the septum primum, against the edge of the crista dividens. The septum primum usually becomes adherent, with permanent closure, in several months. In 15 to 20 percent of normal adults, however, a small opening or potential opening may persist.

Prior to delivery, patency of the ductus arteriosus is probably an active condition produced by a prostaglandin formed intramurally. A likely candidate for this role is PGE_2, which is mainly degraded in the lungs; its action may be complemented by that of prostacycline.

The ductus arteriosus usually is functionally closed 10 to 15 h after birth in a normal full-term infant, with complete closure within 10 to 21 days. The trigger for closure of the ductus arteriosus after birth is the postnatal rise in arterial P_{O_2} or oxygen tension. It is not clear, however, whether the effect of oxygen is exerted directly on the smooth-muscle cells of the ductus or whether other vasoactive agents are involved. Prostaglandins are probably involved, although the exact mechanism is not known. Several possible mechanisms have been suggested.

Prior to birth, the pulmonary and systemic circuits are in communication through the relatively large ductus arteriosus. Consequently, the systolic pressures in both of the ventricles, the aorta, and the pulmonary artery are almost identical. In association with the abrupt fall in pulmonary vascular resistance shortly after birth and the closure of the ductus arteriosus, the pulmonary artery pressure decreases, at first rather abruptly; thereafter it decreases more slowly until it reaches normal childhood values in a few weeks.[15]

Although the right and left ventricles are about the same thickness at birth, the markedly increased load on the left ventricle after birth causes it to increase rapidly in thickness and weight during the first few weeks. The increase in left ventricular mass at this age is predominantly due to hyperplasia, with an increase in the number of cells, rather than to hypertrophy of individual cells. The right ventricular mass remains stable during this period.

Persistence of Fetal Circulation

Persistent fetal circulation,[21,22] or persistent pulmonary hypertension, in the newborn results in right-to-left shunting through the patent foramen ovale and/or patent ductus arteriosus. It most commonly occurs in full-term infants. Severe hypoxia is usually manifested in the first few hours of life with tachypnea, acidosis, and a chest roentgenogram that shows diminished vascular flow but no evidence of pulmonary parenchymal disease. Physical examination may reveal a parasternal heave, a loud second heart sound, and a systolic murmur.

Polycythemia, transient myocardial ischemia from hypoglycemia, and cyanotic congenital cardiac defects must be excluded. A greater oxygen level in the right radial artery than in the umbilical artery confirms right-to-left shunting through the ductus. Echocardiography and Doppler evaluation are of utmost importance.

Initial treatment[22] includes an increase in the inspired oxygen level and correction of acidosis with sodium bicarbonate. Frequently, artificial ventilation is required. Hyperventilation to diminish the partial pressure of carbon dioxide is often successful in lowering the pulmonary pressure and diminishing the right-to-left shunt. Intravenous infusion of tolazoline either into the upper segment of the body to enhance flow to the lungs or directly into the pulmonary artery may be beneficial. Treatment of severe disease with an extracorporeal membrane oxygenator is successful in a significant number of patients.[23] Similar hemodynamic alterations may also be seen in newborns with parenchymal lung disease.

COMPLICATIONS OF CONGENITAL HEART DISEASE

Congestive Heart Failure

Congestive heart failure occurs in one child in five with congenital heart disease and in over 80 percent of infants who have malformations severe enough to require cardiac catheterization or surgery within the first year of life.[24] Its onset usually is a phenomenon of the first 6 months of life. Onset after 1 year of age is rare without a serious intercurrent problem such as infective endocarditis, pneumonia, or anemia.

Heart failure within the first 12 to 18 h of life is usually due to malformations that involve volume overload independent of pulmonary flow, as occurs with severe valvular regurgitation. Rarely, endocardial fibroelastosis or myocarditis may produce failure from the time of birth, as may congenital complete heart block or supraventricular tachycardia. Other causes in this age group include primary cardiac disease, volume overload from a systemic arteriovenous fistula, severe polycythemia, or depressed myocardial contractility from neonatal asphyxia, hypocalcemia, hypoglycemia, anemia, or sepsis.

The majority of full-term infants presenting with severe heart failure during the remainder of the first week have critical obstruction to systemic arterial flow which, in many cases, has been unmasked by narrowing or closure of the ductus arteriosus. Examples are aortic atresia, coarctation of the aorta, interruption of the aortic arch, and critical aortic stenosis. During the second week of life, aortic atresia and coarctation remain the most common causes of heart failure, but ventricular septal defect, transposition of the great arteries with a ventricular septal defect, and truncus arteriosus make their appearance. These malformations require a pulmonary vascular bed with a reduced vascular resistance for full expression of their severity. Thereafter ventricular septal defect is the primary cause of congestive failure, followed by transposition, coarctation, complete atrioventricular canal, and patent ductus arteriosus.

The most common symptom of congestive heart failure is difficulty in breathing, with rapid, grunting, or gasping breathing or breathlessness with feeding, except in those rare instances of isolated right ventricular failure. Observation of the undisturbed infant reveals dyspnea, the signs of which are nasal flaring and subcostal or intercostal retractions. A respiratory rate consistently above 60 is to be expected, and rates in the range of 90 to 100 are not uncommon. Poor weight gain is the rule. Cool, moist skin; a subdued and rapid arterial pulse; and hepatic enlargement are common accompanying signs. A gallop rhythm, pulmonary rales, and expiratory wheezes may be present. It may be difficult to distinguish the pulmonary findings of heart failure from those of pneumonia or bronchiolitis; indeed, many infants have both heart failure and pulmonary infection. Edema, if present, usually is found in the periorbital area and on the dorsa of the feet and hands. Cardiac enlargement is confirmed by chest roentgenogram. Infants with malformations such as coarctation of the aorta and total anomalous pulmonary venous connection, abnormalities usually not characterized by an impressive murmur, sometimes are referred only after weeks of tachypnea and failure to thrive, when a chest roentgenogram, taken to explore the possibility of lung disease, has revealed cardiac enlargement.

When a sizable systemic-to-pulmonary communication exists in a premature infant, usually due to a patent ductus, signs of heart failure usually are associated with signs of ventilatory failure.

Hospitalization is recommended for all infants with heart failure. Elevation of the head and chest to an angle of approximately 30° and administration of humidified oxygen by techniques that do not disturb the infant help relieve dyspnea and cyanosis. Arterial P_{O_2} levels should be monitored in the newborn, particularly the premature, to avoid the risk of retrolental fibroplasia. Rest, aided by sedation, is beneficial. With severe failure, oral feedings should be temporarily suspended and fluid intake restricted to 65 mL/kg per day intravenously for at least the first 24 h. Anemia, acidosis, hypoxia, hypercarbia, hypoglycemia, or hypocalcemia should be corrected; serum sodium, potassium, blood urea nitrogen, and creatinine concentrations should be monitored. A low threshold for the administration of antibiotics is appropriate.

Digoxin is recommended for the management of congestive failure in infants and children because of its excellent absorption when given orally, rapid onset of action, relatively rapid excretion, and convenience of administration. The recommended oral maintenance doses of digoxin for the different age ranges of children, expressed as μg/kg per day, are as follows: for the premature, 5; for the neonate, 10; for the infant between 4 and 24 months of age, 15; for the older child, 10; and for the adolescent, 5. The daily maintenance dose is usually given in two divided doses approximately 12 h apart. The total digitalizing dose is three times the daily maintenance dose. The parenteral doses of digoxin are approximately 75 percent of the oral doses for digitalization and maintenance. Half of the digitalizing dose may be given initially, followed by the remaining two quarter-doses at 4-, 8-, or 12-h intervals, depending upon the desired speed of total digitalization. Maintenance therapy should be started 8 to 12 h after the last digitalizing dose. In the severely ill infant, with decreased perfusion and unpredictable absorption, digitalization by the intravenous route is recommended. Impaired renal function leads to digoxin accumulation and toxicity, so the initial and maintenance doses should be adjusted accordingly. Toxicity, if it is to occur, usually appears within the first week of therapy. If anorexia, nausea or vomiting, or electrocardiographic evidence of either atrial or ventricular ectopy or atrioventricular block appears, digoxin should be stopped and the serum digoxin level determined. Toxicity is probable if the level exceeds 3.0 ng/mL in the infant below 6 months of age or 2.0 ng/mL in the older infant or child. If the need for digoxin continues, the dose is adjusted as the patient grows and gains weight. (See also Chap. 27.)

The diuretic furosemide, used intravenously in doses of 1.0 to 2.0 mg/kg or orally in doses of 2.0 mg/kg, is very effective in the acute management of congestive heart failure. With severe failure, the dose may be increased by increments of 1.0 mg/kg intravenously if no urinary response has been achieved after 45 min. For long-term oral diuretic therapy, 2.0 mg/kg once daily or, if necessary, twice daily is recommended. The diuretic response to furosemide may be very significantly enhanced by the addition of metolazone given orally 30 min prior to furosemide. The dose of metolazone is 0.2 to 0.4 mg/kg every 24 h. Very careful attention to fluid balance and electrolytes is essential with this powerful combination. Chlorothiazide, a slightly less potent diuretic but one with a longer duration of action, may be given orally in a dose of 20 to 50 mg/kg per day. Hypokalemia and hypochloremia can be induced with these potent diuretics, and a daily oral supplement of potassium chloride in the range of 1.0 to 1.5 meq/kg, with adjustment depending on the serum level, is recommended. Spironolactone, an aldosterone antagonist, has proved useful in supplementing the diuresis and in preventing the hypokalemia induced by the diuretics described above. It may be given orally in a single daily dose of 2 to 3 mg/kg. A regimen of spironolactone, 2 mg/kg given every day, and chlorothiazide, 20 mg/kg given on alternate days, usually is adequate for long-term diuretic therapy of mild to moderate heart failure and does not require potassium supplementation. With more severe heart failure, chlorothiazide may be given daily, the dose of both diuretics may be increased, or furosemide may be substituted for chlorothiazide. Under these circumstances, potassium supplementation may be necessary. (See also Chap. 29.)

In emergency situations it may be necessary to provide an immediate inotropic stimulus in the form of intravenous sympathomimetic amines administered by constant infusion pump. Isoproterenol, in a dose of 0.1 μg/kg per min, exerts a powerful inotropic effect, but its usefulness may be limited by induced tachycardia and peripheral vasodilation, sometimes to the detriment of renal perfusion. Epinephrine, in a dose of 0.1 to 1.0 μg/kg per min, or dobutamine or dopamine, in a dose of 5 to 15 μg/kg per min, generally has been more helpful, with dopamine providing more adequate renal flow. The systemic arterial blood pressure, urinary output, and electrocardiogram should be monitored continuously. Vasodilator therapy in the form of intravenous sodium nitroprusside may be of considerable help in patients with severe congestive failure not associated with large left-to-right shunts. The infusion rate at the start should be no greater than 0.5 μg/kg per min, but it may be increased gradually to 4.0 μg/kg per min to achieve the desired effect. Systemic arterial pressure should be monitored continuously to detect serious hypotension. Two oral vasodilators, hydralazine, in a dose of 0.25 to 0.50 mg/kg four times daily for children with normal or only mildly elevated ventricular filling pressure, or prazosin, in a dose of 0.05 to 0.10 mg/kg four times daily if ventricular filling pressures are elevated, have proved beneficial in selected patients. The angiotensin-converting enzyme inhibitors captopril and enalopril have proven effective in selected patients, captopril starting at doses of 0.1 to 0.4 mg/kg per dose in the neonate and 0.3 to 0.6 mg/kg per dose in the older child given one to four times per day or enalopril 0.16 to 0.25 mg/kg per day in two divided doses.[25] (See also Chaps. 28 and 30.)

Infants with potentially exhausting respiratory effort or with hypoxia or hypercapnea secondary to pulmonary edema or respiratory failure benefit from endotracheal intubation and ventilation on a volume-controlled, positive pressure respirator, usually with the addition of positive end-expiratory pressure. These measures may permit additional therapy, cardiac catheterization, and surgical intervention with a much greater margin of safety.

In newborns who have failure as the result of narrowing or closure of the ductus arteriosus in the presence of critical obstruction to flow from the left side of the heart, dramatic and lifesaving relief can be expected with reopening of the ductus by infusion of PGE_1 at a dose of 0.1 μg/kg per min.

Finally, infants or children in whom medical therapy is clearly inadequate or only temporarily successful may require prompt surgical intervention for control of their heart failure. As a rule, the earlier the onset of congestive failure, the more likely will be the need for surgery.

Retardation of Growth and Development

Children having severe cardiac malformations frequently exhibit retardation of growth and development, with height and weight near or below the third percentile or weight 20 percentile points below the percentile for height.

Growth retardation is most severe among those children with overt cyanosis and those with large left-to-right shunts causing heart failure. Cyanosis tends to produce a parallel retardation of both height and weight, while heart failure tends to cause a greater retardation of weight than height. Skeletal retardation, reflected by bone age, usually occurs with height and weight retardation and, among children with cyanotic heart disease, correlates with the severity of hypoxemia.

Other factors contribute to growth retardation including insufficient caloric intake, dyspnea, frequent infections, psychological disturbances, malabsorption, or hypermetabolism.[26] Among infants with severe congenital heart disease recognized within the first year of life, there is a significantly increased incidence of subnormal birth weight, intrauterine growth retardation (6.1 percent), and major extracardiac anomalies (19.9 percent).[27] Finally, a relatively small number of children will have associated syndromes known to be characterized by growth retardation, such as rubella and Noonan, Turner, and Down syndromes.

Growth retardation related primarily to congenital heart disease usually responds to surgical correction or palliation, with an impressive acceleration of growth and a return to or toward normal.

While cardiac surgery seldom is recommended on the basis of growth failure alone, this undesirable trend should be recognized early and, until proved otherwise, considered an index of the severity of the heart disease. In general, the earlier and the more successful the surgery, the less will be the retardation of growth and development, with its sequelae of physical, psychological, and intellectual problems.[28]

Cyanosis

Cyanosis is one of the more frequent initial signs of congenital heart disease in the infant, but it may also be an early sign of pulmonary, central nervous system, or metabolic disease or of methemoglobinemia. Nonsurgical palliation with prostaglandin, as well as the rapid development of surgical techniques, particularly for infants, makes prompt distinction between cardiac and noncardiac cyanosis extremely important. Echocardiography (Chap. 15) and Doppler echocardiography (Chap. 130) are helpful in distinguishing cyanotic heart disease from other causes of cyanosis.

Cyanosis in congenital heart disease may be due to heart failure with pulmonary edema rather than to intracardiac right-to-left shunting. Low cardiac output and peripheral vasoconstriction can cause a grayish discoloration due to the underlying pallor, rather than typical cyanosis. Hypoxia due to heart failure or lung disease with intrapulmonary shunting usually responds dramatically to oxygen administration, whereas that due to cyanotic defects does not.

The normal full-term newborn infant has a hemoglobin concentration of 17 to 21 g/dL. This drops to 10.4 to 12.2 g/dL by 3 months of age and then slowly rises to 12 to 14 g/dL by 2 years.[29] Systemic arterial desaturation results in polycythemia after the newborn period.

When cyanosis is present for several months, clubbing (initially noted as fullness at the base of the thumbnail with obliteration of the normal concavity) occurs. Tachypnea and dyspnea may be due to desaturation and are exaggerated with exercise. Paroxysms of increased cyanosis and squatting may be seen with tetralogy of Fallot.

To a large extent, the complications of cyanosis result from polycythemia and paradoxical embolism. In patients with prolonged polycythemia, the resultant hyperuricemia can precipitate a secondary form of gout.[30] More frequently, the central nervous system is the target organ, with cerebrovascular accidents and brain abscesses occurring[6] as a result of the effects of polycythemia and paradoxical embolism, especially in the setting of dehydration or febrile states. Paradoxical embolism is a potential complication whenever a right-to-left shunt exists. An infected venous thrombus or unfiltered blood during a bacteremia can cause a cerebral abscess, but this is rare under 2 years of age. The incidence and mortality are directly related to the degree of hypoxia.[31] Thrombosis, embolism, and hemorrhage can cause cerebrovascular accidents. (See also Chap. 122.) Venous thrombosis is a common finding at autopsy, particularly in tetralogy of Fallot or transposition of the great arteries. A majority of instances occur in infants up to 1 year of age, with relatively few after 4 or 5 years of age. The younger patients very frequently have iron-deficiency anemia relative to the degree of desaturation, whereas the older patients have polycythemia.[32] Acutely increasing hemoglobin concentration in those with relative anemia has significant hemodynamic benefits[33] as well as an effect on tissue oxygen delivery.[34]

Disturbances in hemostasis also occur with polycythemia.[6] Coagulation factors are commonly abnormal in patients with hematocrits in excess of 60 percent.[35] Actual platelet counts may be normal, but they can be increased initially in some patients, with subsequent decreases related to persistent and worsening desaturation. There is evidence of shortened platelet survival time in patients with cyanotic heart disease.[36] Laboratory evaluation of coagulation status requires that correction be made for the diminished volume of plasma and for the volume of anticoagulant used in the blood samples to avoid false results. Hematologic management of adults with cyanotic congenital heart disease requires special experience and knowledge.[37]

The major consequences of cyanosis can be avoided in many instances, although there have been differences in intelligence demonstrated between cyanotic and acyanotic children.[38] Prevention of iron deficiency by dietary supplementation in infants and of excessive polycythemia by surgical intervention should decrease the number of cerebrovascular accidents and help prevent the occurrence of brain abscess.

Pulmonary Arterial Hypertension and Pulmonary Vascular Obstructive Disease

Pulmonary arterial hypertension (PAH) and pulmonary vascular obstructive disease (PVOD) are serious complications of congenital heart disease. PAH usually is the result of direct transmission of systemic arterial pressure to the right ventricle or pulmonary arteries via a large communication. Less frequently, it is due to severe obstruction to blood flow through the left side of the heart at the pulmonary venous level or beyond. PVOD refers to a process involving structural and developmental changes in the smaller muscular arteries and arterioles of the lung that gradually diminishes and eventually destroys the ability of the pulmonary vascular bed to transport blood from the larger pulmonary arteries to the pulmonary veins without an abnormal elevation of proximal pulmonary arterial pressure.

Pulmonary resistance (R_p) may be as high as 8 to 10 Wood units immediately after birth but falls rapidly throughout the first week. Indexed Wood units, as a measure of resistance to flow across either the pulmonary or systemic vascular beds, are obtained by dividing the mean pressure difference (in mmHg) across the pulmonary or systemic vascular beds by the blood flow *index*, expressed in liters/min per m^2, across those respective beds. By 6 to 8 weeks it usually has reached the normal adult level (1 to 3 Wood units).[4] These changes are accompanied by a gradual dilatation of first the smaller and then the larger muscular pulmonary arteries and then, in the weeks and months that follow, a thinning of their muscular walls, growth of existing arteries, and the development of new arteries and arterioles. The latter process contributes over 90 percent of the smaller or intraacinar pulmonary arterial vessels present in the older child and adult.[39]

Increased pulmonary arterial pressure has an adverse effect on the normal maturation of the pulmonary vascular bed. Such pressure encourages a persistence of the thick muscular medial layer present in the smaller pulmonary arteries of the term newborn, stimulates an extension of smooth muscle into smaller and more peripheral arteries than normal for age, and, lastly, retards the growth of existing and the development of new acinar arteries.

In the presence of a large systemic-to-pulmonary communication, pulmonary arterial pressures tend to remain at or near systemic levels, with the result that the diminution in pulmonary muscle mass and pulmonary resistance is less rapid and of less magnitude than it is in the normal infant. Nevertheless, the diminution is usually sufficient to permit a large pulmonary blood flow and, as a result, congestive failure by the end of the first month. Exceptions are found among those infants with a large systemic-to-pulmonary communication but with alveolar hypoxia, a stimulus for pulmonary vasoconstriction, in whom there is less than normal involution of the medial musculature and diminution in pulmonary vascular resistance. Clinically, this is expressed by the lower incidence of congestive failure observed among infants with large ventricular septal defects born and living at high altitude.[40] Rarely, an infant will maintain a very high pulmonary vascular resistance in the face of an anatomically large systemic-to-pulmonary communication, without evidence of significant hypoxemia or acidemia, and remain free of the signs and symptoms of congestive failure. In the premature infant, in whom the medial muscle mass is less at birth than it is in the full-term infant, the fall in pulmonary vascular resistance usually is much more rapid than normal.

Chronic PAH or increased flow, or both, produces a characteristic series of histologic changes originally described and graded by Heath and Edwards (grades I through VI below)[41] and, later, by Rabinovitch and coworkers[42] (grades A through C below):

- Grade I—medial hypertrophy in the small pulmonary arteries.
- Grade II—concentric or eccentric cellular intimal proliferation and thickening within the smaller pulmonary arteries and arterioles. Increased shearing stresses resulting in endothelial injury and smooth muscle proliferation are considered to play a role in the production of these lesions.[43]
- Grade III—relatively acellular intimal fibrosis with accumulation of concentric or eccentric masses of fibrous tissue leading to widespread occlusion of the smaller pulmonary arteries and arterioles. Grade III changes may be seen as early as 2 months of age in patients with transposition of the great arteries along with a large ventricular septal defect or patent ductus arteriosus and as early as 10 to 12 months of age in patients with complete atrioventricular canal.[41]
- Grade IV—progressive, generalized dilatation of the muscular arteries and the appearance of plexiform lesions, complex vascular structures compose of a network or plexus of proliferating endothelial tissue, frequently accompanied by thrombus, within a dilated thin-walled sac. Whether these are the result of aneurysms of the media, of vasculitis, or of thrombosis is unclear, but their appearance signifies very severe PVOD. Grade IV changes may be seen as early as 2 to 4 months among patients having transposition with ventricular septal defect and by 10 to 12 months among infants with complete atrioventricular canal.
- Grade V—thinning and fibrosis of the media superimposed upon the formation of numerous complex dilatation lesions.
- Grade VI—necrotizing arteritis within the media with surrounding areas of inflammatory reaction and granulation tissue. This is found most commonly among patients with primary pulmonary hypertension.
- Grade A—an extension of muscle into normally non-

muscular peripheral arteries with or without a mild increase in medial wall thickness of normally muscular arteries to between 10 and 15 percent of the arteries' external diameter. The former appears related to increased flow rather than pressure and may be noted as early as 4 to 6 weeks of age among infants with a ventricular septal defect.

- Grade B—extension of muscle as above with an even greater increase in medial wall thickness of normally muscular arteries. Grade B is subdivided into: *mild,* in which the medial wall thickness makes up between 15 and 20 percent of external arterial diameter, and *severe,* in which medial wall thickness makes up 20 percent or more of the external arterial diameter.
- Grade C—changes seen in grade B (severe) but with a decreased arterial concentration relative to alveoli. Grade C is also subdivided into: *mild,* in which the arterial number is still half or more than half the normal number, and *severe,* in which less than half the normal number is present.

Grades A and B are partitions of grade I. Grade C criteria may be found with grades I and II, are invariable with grade III, and usually preclude a complete return to normal of pulmonary arterial pressures and resistance despite successful surgical correction of the systemic-to-pulmonary communication.

Estimation of pulmonary vascular resistance from data obtained at cardiac catheterization remains the most widely used means of assessing the state of the pulmonary vascular bed. Hypoxemia from oversedation, atelectasis, or pneumonitis at the time of study should be scrupulously avoided. If pulmonary vascular resistance is elevated, its responsiveness to vasodilation induced by the inhalation of 100% oxygen or the intravenous administration of tolazoline, or both, should be tested.

Values of R_p of 3 Wood units or less are considered normal. The status of the pulmonary vasculature can also be expressed as a ratio of pulmonary vascular resistance to systemic vascular resistance (R_p/R_s). Pulmonary/systemic resistance ratios of less than 0.2:1 are considered normal.

As pulmonary vascular resistance increases, pulmonary blood flow generally decreases. Eventually, a point is reached where surgical closure of the defect will produce only a small diminution of blood flow, a proportionately small decrease in pulmonary arterial pressure, and no significant change in the factors contributing to the progression of the vascular disease. Patients in this category are considered prohibitive risks for surgery because of the increased mortality associated with the procedure in the early postoperative period. An R_p/R_s ratio $\geq 0.7{:}1$ or an $R_p \geq 11$ Wood units with a pulmonary/systemic blood flow ratio $<1.5{:}1$ are the criteria generally used to define this situation. Without surgery, these patients survive as examples of the *Eisenmenger syndrome,* in which pulmonary vascular resistance is equal to or greater than systemic vascular resistance and at least some right-to-left shunting occurs at rest or with exercise. Some of these patients can survive for several decades and lead productive lives, with relatively mild symptoms and few limitations.[44]

The decision regarding surgery for patients with less severe PVOD is a clinical one. The higher the calculated resistance and the greater the structural changes in the pulmonary vasculature, as judged by lung biopsy or quantitative pulmonary angiography,[39] and the older the patient with any given level of elevated resistance or grade of structural change, the less likely it is that the outcome will be satisfactory.[45]

The prevention of PVOD requires the identification of those patients at risk, namely, all patients with a systemic-to-pulmonary communication and a pulmonary arterial systolic pressure greater than half the systemic arterial systolic pressure. Also included would be all patients with transposition, regardless of pressure or flow, with the possible exception of those with severe pulmonary stenosis. Ideally, all patients at risk should undergo correction or pulmonary arterial banding unless there is proof that the pulmonary arterial systolic pressure has fallen to or is less than half the systemic systolic pressure before the end of the first year of life among those with normally related great arteries. Among patients with transposition with a large ventricular septal defect, action must be taken within the first 6 months of life.

Long-Term Problems with Surgically Corrected Defects

With the advances that have occurred in the surgical treatment of congenital heart defects, more of these patients are becoming adults. This discussion of potential long-term problems is intended for those who follow these children after surgery and through adult life.[46] (See also Chap. 98.)

First, there are residua, sequelae, and complications that result from most surgical procedures for congenital heart defects. A residual part of the original defects, such as those with mitral prolapse and repaired atrial septal defect, may purposefully not have been approached surgically. Sequelae are unavoidable consequences of the surgery, such as pulmonary regurgitation after pulmonary valvotomy. There are also complications that occur as unexpected, but related, events after successful surgery, such as late complete heart block. When viewed with these possibilities in mind, only surgical correction of patent ductus is likely to have no long-term problems.

At the simplest level, most patients have residual murmurs after surgery for congenital heart defects. Proper interpretation of the origin of these murmurs and the evaluation of the severity of the hemodynamic abnormalities that they represent are important. Noninvasive diagnostic tools, especially Doppler and two-dimensional echocardiography, are often useful.

In general, the risk of infective endocarditis to patients is not diminished after surgery, with the exception of those who have undergone ductus ligation or repair of ventricular septal defect or secundum atrial septal defect in whom there is no residual shunt. Those patients with artificial valves are at increased risk.[47]

There are specific problems related to some of the more common defects. For those with repaired atrial, ventricular, and atrioventricular (canal) septal defects, a residual shunt may be present but ordinarily it is small and not of hemodynamic significance. Those with repaired atrioventricular canal defects may have important atrioventricular valvular regurgitation. Repaired coarctation of the aorta can gradually become narrowed again, or patients may develop idiopathic hypertension. Surgery for valvular pulmonary stenosis usually results in mild residual stenosis and regurgitation that are well tolerated and have little tendency to progress with time. The natural history of valvular aortic stenosis after surgery is not so benign. Because significant regurgitation must be avoided, initial results may not be as good in terms of the severity of residual stenosis. In addition, aortic stenosis tends to worsen with time; thus, proper follow-up is mandatory for these patients.

Few patients enter adulthood with the continued problem of cyanosis. Since those with residual defects amenable to surgical correction should have had surgery well before this time, only patients with complex and uncorrectable defects or those with pulmonary vascular disease should have problems of cyanosis during the adult years. Particularly important among these patients is management of any attendant psychosocial problems (employment, insurability,[48] and learning disabilities) and difficulties related to pregnancy.

Those who have had surgery for cyanotic defects are more likely to have sequelae and complications.[49] Some degree of exercise intolerance is not unusual in this group of patients, and exercise stress testing aids in their management.[50,51]

Dysrhythmias are also particularly frequent among these patients. In those who have had intraventricular repairs, most commonly for tetralogy of Fallot, late complete heart block and serious ventricular arrhythmias can occur and may result in sudden death.[52] This risk is highest in those who had transient complete heart block at the time of surgery and who develop right bundle branch block with left anterior hemiblock after surgery.[53] Extensive interatrial surgical procedures for transposition of the great arteries also frequently lead to dysrhythmias, most commonly sick-sinus syndrome with bradytachyarrhythmias. Ambulatory 24-h electrocardiographic monitoring (Chap. 45) and stress testing (Chap. 16) are important in following patients who have had complex repairs.

Serious ventricular dysfunction[54] and venous obstructions may also occur, usually in those who had severe defects. Interatrial repairs for transposition of the great arteries leave the anatomic right ventricle to do the work of the systemic ventricle.[55] In addition, these repairs may lead to pulmonary and/or systemic venous obstruction. Atriopulmonary connections for repair of tricuspid atresia[56] and many types of univentricular hearts frequently leave an anatomically abnormal ventricle as the systemic ventricle. Also, the right atrium has become the "pulmonary ventricle," with an elevated right atrial pressure that may lead to problems from systemic venous hypertension.

Finally, some children have had repairs utilizing synthetic prostheses. Artificial valves do not grow as the child does, and they must be much more durable in view of the life expectancy. There are also some surgical procedures that require placement of conduits, with or without valves, that can degenerate and become obstructive with time. Bioprosthetic valves undergo accelerated fibrosis and calcification in patients less than about 30 to 35 years of age.

The majority of patients who reach adulthood after surgical repair of congenital defects are relatively asymptomatic; they can and do lead productive lives.

INTRACARDIAC COMMUNICATIONS BETWEEN THE SYSTEMIC AND PULMONARY CIRCULATIONS, USUALLY WITHOUT CYANOSIS

Ventricular Septal Defect

Definition

Ventricular septal defect represents an opening in that part of the ventricular septum that separates the two ventricles.

Pathology

A defect of the ventricular septum represents the most common alteration among malformed hearts. In some this is the only condition, whereas in others it is part of a complex malformation.

Anatomic Types Three-fourths of all defects are paramembranous but may extend into the inlet, trabecular, or outlet sections of the muscular septum. Less common (except among Asians) are the conal septal or subarterial doubly committed defects (8 percent), posterior defects lying beneath the septal leaflet of the tricuspid valve in the region of the atrioventricular canal (8 percent), and finally, defects in the muscular septum whether they lie in the inlet, trabecular, or outlet areas (15 percent).[57] (See Fig. 97-1.) Multiplicity of muscular defects is characteristic.

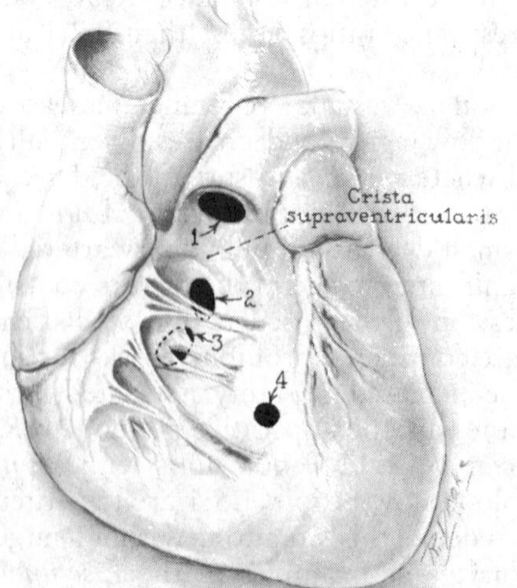

FIGURE 97-1 Types of ventricular septal defects. *1.* A high defect immediately under the pulmonary valve. *2.* The typical high ventricular septal defect. *3.* The atrioventricular canal type of ventricular septal defect. *4.* A defect in the muscular portion of the septum. (*From Kirklin JW, Harshbarger HG, Donald DE, et al: Surgical correction of ventricular septal defect: Anatomic and technical considerations. J Thorac Cardiovasc Surg 33:45, 1957. Reproduced with permission from the publisher and authors.*)

The major conduction tissue is most closely related to the paramembranous defects where it lies along the posteroinferior quadrant of the defect and favors the left ventricular side of the septum.

Associated Conditions Cardiac malformations associated with ventricular septal defect are, in order of decreasing frequency, (1) coarctation of the aorta; (2) additional shunts, most commonly atrial septal defect and patent ductus arteriosus, and other ventricular septal defects; (3) intracardiac obstructions such as subpulmonary or subaortic stenosis, mitral stenosis, and anomalous muscle bundle of the right ventricle; and (4) incompetent atrioventricular valves.

Abnormal Physiology

The consequences of a ventricular septal defect depend upon the size of the defect and the pulmonary vascular resistance. A small defect offers a large resistance to flow. There is no elevation of right ventricular or pulmonary arterial pressures, and the left-to-right shunt may be so small that it can be detected only by selective left ventricular angiography or two-dimensional imaging with Doppler color flow.[58] This type of defect imposes little burden on the heart except for the danger of infective endocarditis.

A defect of moderate size still permits a separation of right and left ventricular systolic pressures with the right ventricular systolic pressure generally being 80 percent or less of the left ventricular systolic pressure, but a large left-to-right shunt may be present with resulting left atrial hypertension and dilatation and left ventricular volume overload. The development of pulmonary vascular disease among these patients is unusual but possible.

When the effective area of the defect is large, approximately equal to or greater than the aortic valve orifice, the defect offers virtually no resistance to flow and the systolic pressures in both ventricles, the aorta, and the pulmonary artery are essentially the same. The relative proportion of blood going to the two circulations is directly governed by the relative resistance of the two vascular beds.

At birth, pulmonary vascular resistance is high and there is little if any left-to-right shunt despite the presence of a large defect. This resistance to flow gradually falls over the first few weeks of life, permitting a progressively greater amount of blood to flow through the defect, the lungs, and back to the left atrium and left ventricle. The left ventricular volume overload eventually leads, in most infants, to left ventricular "failure" with, in many, markedly elevated left ventricular end-diastolic and left atrial pressures and pulmonary edema.

In term infants born at sea level with a large ventricular septal defect, clinical deterioration may occur at any time from about 3 to 12 weeks after birth. In premature infants, in whom the less well developed pulmonary vasculature hypertrophy regresses more rapidly, failure is frequently noted at 1 to 4 weeks.

Clinical Manifestations

Ventricular septal defect is a common form of congenital heart disease, second only to a bicuspid aortic valve and mitral valve prolapse (Chap. 80). It occurs as an isolated defect in approximately 23 percent of infants with congenital heart disease and occurs in combination with other malformations in an additional 26 percent.[6] Its incidence is 2 per 1000 live births, its prevalence among school-age children has been estimated as 1 per 1000,[59] and it constitutes about 10 percent of the congenital cardiac malformations found among adults.[60] Males and females are affected equally. It is the most common defect found among infants with chromosomal abnormalities, with the notable exceptions being Down syndrome (trisomy 21) and Turner syndrome (XO genotype), where it ranks second. (See Chap. 96.)

History Infants or children with a small isolated defect are asymptomatic. The murmur of a small defect may be detected within the first 24 to 36 h of life, since they very restrictive opening permits the normal rapid fall in pulmonary arterial resistance and pressures. Infants with larger defects usually present between 3 and 12 weeks of age with congestive failure, frequently with associated lower respiratory tract infections. Parents describe tachypnea, grunting respirations, and fatigue, particularly with feedings. Weight gain is slow, and excessive sweating is common.

Physical Examination The child with a small defect is comfortable. A systolic thrill at the lower left sternal border is common, although with very small defects this may not be present. The second heart sound is normal. The systolic murmur along the lower left sternal border is characteristically holosystolic, but may be decrescendo and limited to early or midsystole. These latter features suggest a defect in the muscular rather than the membranous septum.

Infants with large defects, large flow, and pulmonary arterial hypertension tend to be restless, irritable, and underweight. Moderate respiratory distress may be present. Both the right and left ventricular systolic impulses are impressively hyperdynamic to palpation. A thrill at the lower left sternal border is the rule. The second heart sound is narrowly split, with a loud, frequently palpable pulmonary component. Third heart sound gallops at the apex are common. Characteristically, the systolic murmur is holosystolic at the lower left sternal border and is accompanied by a middiastolic rumble of grade 2 to 3 intensity at the apex, the latter indicating a pulmonary/systemic blood flow ratio (Q_p/Q_s) of 2:1 or greater. Hepatic enlargement can be identified below the right costal margin. Pulmonary rales are common with severe failure.

With the passage of time, one may observe signs of a diminishing left-to-right shunt with an improved rate of weight gain, less dyspnea, a diminution of the precordial hyperactivity, and disappearance of the apical diastolic flow rumble. This clinical improvement may be the result of the defect becoming smaller, the development of subvalvular pulmonary stenosis with little or no appreciable change in the size of the defect, or, most worrisome, the development of PVOD with continued severe PAH. With developing subpulmonary stenosis, the systolic murmur radiates more and more impressively to the upper left sternal border and the second heart sound becomes more widely split, with a progressive diminution in the intensity of the pulmonary component. Decreased flow due to pulmonary vascular disease is characterized by a gradual reduction in the intensity and duration of the systolic murmur, more narrow splitting of the second heart sound and marked accentuation of the pulmonary component.

The clinical picture of advanced pulmonary vascular disease secondary to a congenital left-to-right shunt, or *Eisenmenger syndrome,* is that of a relatively comfortable older child, adolescent, or young adult with mild cyanosis and clubbing in whom one finds a prominent *a* wave in the jugular venous pulse, a mild right ventricular lift, and a second heart sound which is narrowly split or virtually single with a very loud, usually palatable pulmonary component. An early pulmonary systolic ejection sound, reflecting dilatation of the main pulmonary artery, may be heard, and there may be no systolic murmur at all. In older adolescents and adults, an early diastolic murmur of pulmonary regurgitation or a holosystolic murmur of tricuspid regurgitation may appear.

Chest Roentgenogram In the presence of a small defect, the heart size and shape and the pulmonary blood flow are barely altered. With large defects, there will be moderate to marked enlargement of the heart with prominence of the main pulmonary arterial segment and impressive overcirculation in the peripheral lung fields. The left atrium is dilated in the absence of an associated atrial septal defect. With increasing pulmonary vascular disease, there is diminution in heart size toward normal while the central pulmonary arteries remain dilated. The peripheral pulmonary arterial markings become attenuated and a "pruned" effect is produced in the outer third of the lung fields. (See also Chap. 14.)

Electrocardiogram With a small defect, one can expect the normal progression of the mean QRS axis from right to left and the normal gradual diminution of the prominent right ventricular voltages characteristic of the newborn. The left ventricular forces will either remain within normal limits or become slightly augmented as a reflection of the mild left ventricular volume overload. With large defects, the mean QRS axis tends to remain oriented to the right and there is little or no regression in right ventricular voltage. The left ventricular forces gradually increase, resulting in a pattern of biventricular hypertrophy within the first few weeks of life. Left atrial hypertrophy is usually present, and frequently right atrial hypertrophy as well. With the development of pulmonary vascular disease or significant pulmonary stenosis, the mean QRS axis tends to remain oriented to the right, there is no regression in right ventricular voltage, and the evidence of left ventricular and left atrial hypertrophy lessens or disappears.

Echocardiogram Two-dimensional imaging can distinguish the uncomplicated ventricular septal defect from more complex malformations and is capable of imaging most defects directly when multiple transducer positions are used.[61] The addition of pulsed-wave Doppler with color flow permits identification of small, multiple, muscular, and other less easily visualized defects.[62] Continuous-wave Doppler echocardiography (Fig. 97-2) can predict right ventricular systolic pressure in the absence of aortic stenosis by estimating the interventricular pressure gradient across the defect.[63]

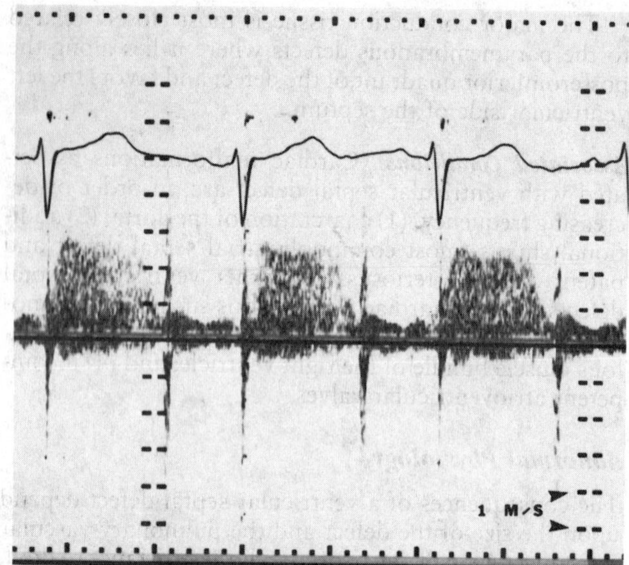

FIGURE 97-2 Continuous-wave Doppler with spectral display from the left lower sternal border of child with a ventricular septal defect that demonstrates holosystolic turbulence with peak velocity = 2.8 m/s across the defect.

Cardiac Catheterization An increase in oxygen saturation at the right ventricular level reflects the left-to-right shunt via the ventricular septal defect. With small defects, the right ventricular and pulmonary arterial systolic pressures are normal. With large defects, these pressures are at or near systemic levels and the mean left atrial pressure may be elevated to the 10- to 15-mmHg range.

Selective left ventricular angiography in the anteroposterior, lateral, and oblique views with craniocaudal angulation is recommended to establish the spatial relations of the great arteries to each other and to the ventricles and also to determine the exact site, size, and number of septal defects (Figs. 97-3 and 138-18). Aortography is also recommended to eliminate the possibility of an associated ductus arteriosus or unsuspected coarctation of the aorta.

Natural History and Prognosis

Fortunately, the majority of ventricular septal defects are small and do not present a serious clinical problem. Approximately 24 percent of these small defects close spontaneously by 18 months, 50 percent by 4 years, and 75 percent by 10 years.[64] A spontaneous closure rate approaching 45 percent within the first 12 to 14 months has been observed among infants with an uncomplicated paramembranous or muscular ventricular septal defect in the neonatal period.[58,65] Even large defects tend to become smaller, but the likelihood of eventual spontaneous closure is much less (probably in the range of 60 percent if judged large at 3 months of age and only 50 percent if still large at 6 months).[64]

Congestive failure is a threatening and almost inevitable complication of a large ventricular septal defect. Al-

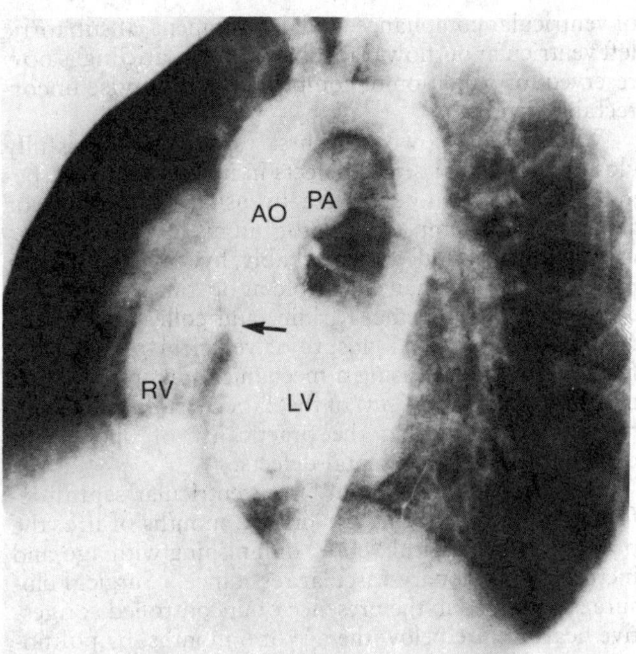

FIGURE 97-3 Left anterior oblique view of the left ventricular angiogram from a 5-year-old child with a small, membranous ventricular septal defect (*arrow*). RV = right ventricle; LV = left ventricle; AO = ascending aorta; PA = pulmonary artery.

most 80 percent of infants with large defects require hospitalization by the age of 4 months.[3] The risk of death with congestive failure is in the range of 11 percent. Significant subvalvular pulmonary stenosis develops in approximately 3 percent of these individuals and may progress to the point of severe tetralogy of Fallot. PVOD is seldom severe and rarely irreversible in the first 12 months of life, but thereafter it becomes progressively more common and less likely to regress. At risk of this complication are those infants and children with a pulmonary systolic pressure in excess of 50 percent of the systemic arterial systolic pressure beyond the first year of life.[66] A very small number of the infants with large ventricular septal defects maintain a high level of pulmonary vascular resistance throughout the first year of life and remain almost entirely free of symptoms and congestive heart failure. In these patients irreversible pulmonary vascular disease may develop without the usual and expected clinical signs and symptoms described above.[40]

A small number of children, 0.6 percent in a large group of carefully followed patients, will develop aortic regurgitation as a result of prolapse of the right, the posterior, or both aortic valve leaflets into the defect.[67] This complication is more prevalent among males, in a ratio of 2:1, and seems particularly likely to occur with defects of the subarterial type. Shunt size appears unrelated to the development of this complication. The characteristic aortic diastolic murmur may appear at any time between the ages of 6 months and 20 years. Regurgitation is usually progressive, sometimes rapidly so, and predisposes these individuals to infective endocarditis.

The risk of infective endocarditis in patients with an uncomplicated ventricular septal defect managed medically is approximately 10 percent for the first 30 years of life.[68]

Medical Management

It is important to identify as early as possible those patients in whom the defect is moderate or large, since these are the patients at special risk of developing congestive failure, pulmonary vascular disease, or serious pulmonary stenosis. Careful and complete two-dimensional Doppler echocardiographic assessment should define the site, size, and number of defects as well as the presence of additional anomalies. The electrocardiogram is helpful in identifying those infants in whom the right ventricular systolic pressure is remaining at or near systemic levels and this can be supported by periodic Doppler reestimation of the interventricular gradient.[63] Heart failure is treated with digoxin and, if necessary, oral diuretics. Anemia is prevented or corrected, and respiratory infections are treated promptly. Cardiac catheterization is performed on all infants who develop overt congestive heart failure, retain impressive right ventricular or biventricular voltage in the electrocardiogram, or who fail to thrive despite intensive treatment. If the pulmonary arterial systolic pressure is greater than half the systemic systolic pressure and congestive failure is difficult to manage medically, the defect should be closed surgically. If congestive failure is not severe, medical management is continued with the hope that spontaneous narrowing of the defect will occur. This trial of medical management is limited to no longer than 6 months at which point, with or without clinical improvement, the patient undergoes repeat cardiac catheterization. Recatheterization may be postponed in selected patients if clinical improvement during this period has been matched by electrocardiographic evidence of decreasing right ventricular voltages, convincing two-dimensional echocardiographic evidence of a smaller defect, and Doppler estimate of an interventricular pressure gradient of greater than one-half the systemic arterial systolic pressure. If, at restudy, the pulmonary arterial systolic pressure is still greater than half of the systemic systolic pressure, the defect should be closed without delay. If, by the second birthday, the pulmonary arterial pressure has not returned to normal (a mean pulmonary arterial pressure of less than 20 mmHg), as judged by persistent right or biventricular hypertrophy or direct measurement at catheterization, the defect should be closed. A few children will remain symptomatic or continue to have cardiac enlargement beyond the second year of life due to a large left-to-right shunt (pulmonary/systemic blood flow ratio >1.8:1) despite a normal pulmonary arterial pressure. Surgical closure is recommended in these children as well. Finally, closure of a defect in an adult is usually recommended if the flow ratio is >1.4:1 and severe pulmonary vascular disease is not present. (See Chap. 98.)

Unfortunately, not all patients with a large defect are encountered during the first or second year of life, when it would be possible to prevent injury to the pulmonary vascular bed. If significant PAH is allowed to persist, one can expect progression to irreversible pulmonary obstructive disease. For this reason, prompt surgical closure of defects is recommended in all individuals beyond the age of 2 years if the pulmonary arterial systolic pressure is greater than half the systemic arterial systolic pressure, the mean pulmonary pressure exceeds 20 mmHg, or the pulmonary/systemic vascular resistance ratio >0.2:1. With severe pulmonary vascular disease, a point is eventually reached where the risk of death at operation or in the months or years immediately following operation due to progressive vascular disease more than offsets the possible benefits from surgical closure. At present, surgery is recommended if the calculated pulmonary vascular resistance is ≤10 Wood units/m^2 or if the ratio of the pulmonary/systemic vascular resistance is <0.7:1, provided the Q_p/Q_s ratio is still ≥1.5:1. In adults, the upper limit of pulmonary vascular resistance for surgery is approximately 800 dynes·sec·cm^{-5} (Wood units × 80). (See Chap. 98.)

Those patients in whom the defect is judged clinically to be small at 6 months of age may be reexamined at 1- or 2-year intervals to reassure the patient and family, to reemphasize the importance of antibiotic protection against infective endocarditis, to document the further narrowing or closure of the defect, and (in a very small number of patients) to detect the first signs of aortic valve prolapse.

In patients with Eisenmenger complex,[44] stamina is limited by systemic arterial hypoxemia and, in some, right-sided heart failure. Complications to be anticipated include syncope, hemoptysis, brain abscess, hyperuricemia, and congestive failure. Pregnancy, with a maternal mortality of 30 to 60 percent, and oral contraceptives are contraindicated. Transient symptomatic relief from extreme polycythemia may be achieved by careful erythropheresis. Travel to or living at high altitudes is poorly tolerated, and supplemental oxygen should be provided and used in commercial airlines. The average age of death for individuals with Eisenmenger complex is 33 years, with sudden death the mode of exit in the majority.[44]

Postoperative cardiac catheterization is recommended for individuals with preoperative elevated pulmonary vascular resistance, a persistent loud murmur, unexplained cardiac enlargement, or congestive failure. Following surgical repair, precautions against infective endocarditis are continued indefinitely, if there is a residual shunt, and for 6 months in those without a shunt. Symptoms suggesting an arrhythmia should be evaluated at least by 24-h ambulatory monitoring of the electrocardiogram. (See Chap. 45.)

The risk of congenital heart disease for a subsequent sibling of a single affected child is in the order of 3 to 4 percent. The risk to the newborn having one parent with ventricular septal defect is probably 10 to 12 percent, particularly if the affected parent is the mother.[69] Pregnancy in the presence of a small defect and normal pulmonary vascular resistance does not appear to carry an increased risk to the patient or infant, although precautions against infective endocarditis should be observed.

Surgical Management

Reduction of pulmonary blood flow by pulmonary arterial banding played an important role in management of congestive heart failure and prevention of PVOD associated with ventricular septal defect prior to the era of predictably successful open-heart surgery in infants. Complications of pulmonary arterial banding include deformity of the pulmonary arteries and the pulmonary valve, progressive right ventricular hypertrophy and loss of ventricular compliance, and development of subaortic left ventricular outflow tract obstruction. Banding is now reserved for palliation of complex and otherwise uncorrectable defects.[70,71]

Warden and coworkers first reported successfully closing ventricular septal defects in infants in 1954, beginning the "open-heart" era by using the mother or father as the "pump-oxygenator" in his low-flow cross-circulation technique.[72] Remarkably, five of his first eight patients were less than 1 year old at operation; only two of them died. DuShane, Kirklin, and colleagues at the Mayo Clinic reported closure of ventricular septal defects in 20 patients using a mechanical pump-oxygenator.[73] Sixteen (80 percent) of the patients survived hospitalization, establishing the practicality of open-heart closure of ventricular septal defects.

Primary patch closure of large ventricular septal defects is advisable during the first 12 months of life, the probability of surgical "cure" diminishing with age and increasing pulmonary vascular resistance.[74] Surgical closure is indicated in the presence of uncontrolled congestive heart failure below the age of 6 months, by pulmonary arterial hypertension or symptoms below the age of 24 months, and by a pulmonary-to-systemic blood flow ratio of 2:1 after 24 months.[75]

Ventricular septal defects are closed during total cardiopulmonary bypass with cardioplegic arrest and moderate systemic hypothermia. Total circulatory arrest or minimal perfusion with profound hypothermia (18°C) facilitates closure of defects in infants weighing less than 5 kg.

Paramembranous ventricular septal defects are exposed through the right atrium and tricuspid valve orifice.[76] The septal leaflet of the tricuspid valve can be incised near and parallel to the annulus for improved visualization of high subaortic outlet defects. A transverse or longitudinal right ventriculotomy avoiding major coronary arterial branches is preferred for closure of high conal septal defects associated with aortic valve leaflet prolapse.[77]

Care is required to prevent injury to the atrioventricular node near the ostium of the coronary sinus and to the bundle of His as it courses inferiorly, passing on the left side of the ventricular septum near the posterocaudal margin of the septal defect. A Dacron patch is secured over the defect using either a continuous monofilament suture or a series of Teflon felt-buttressed mattress sutures placed well away from and parallel to the inferior rim of the defect septum to avoid the conduction system. The portion of the patch adjacent to the tricuspid valve is anchored to the fibrous tricuspid annulus.

Defects of the muscular septum are frequently multiple—the so-called "Swiss cheese septum." They are usually small but difficult to define through the tricuspid valve orifice or the right ventricle. Exposure is facilitated by an apical or posterior left ventriculotomy, although left ventricular function may be compromised. Care is required to prevent injury to coronary arteries, papillary muscles, and the conduction system.[78,79]

Results from primary closure of ventricular septal defects are generally excellent when surgery is performed during the early months of life prior to the evolution of PVOD. Operative risk is between 1 and 2 percent in older children if the pulmonary vascular resistance remains low. The pulmonary vascular bed responds favorably when the systemic-to-pulmonary shunt is eliminated prior to the age of 2 years. Normal life expectancy and functional capabilities should be anticipated postoperatively.[74] Survival 25 years after closure of ventricular septal defect is approximately 95 percent.[80] Mortality is unquestionably higher among patients operated upon after the age of 5 years, those having a pulmonary vascular resistance greater than 7 Wood units, and those developing complete heart block after repair.[81]

Suboptimal postoperative results are due in large part to preexisting PVOD, technical error producing complete heart block or leaving a significant residual shunt,[81] development of left ventricular outflow tract obstruction or persistent right ventricular outflow tract obstruction in those patients who have had a pulmonary arterial band, or presence of anatomically complex or multiple ventricular septal defects.[82]

Atrial Septal Defect

Definition

An atrial septal defect is a through-and-through communication between the atria at the septal level. This is to be distinguished from the valvular-competent foramen ovale, which may persist into adulthood.[83]

Pathology

Atrial septal defects are usually sufficiently large to allow free communication between the atria. They may be subdivided according to anatomic location (Fig. 97-4).[84]

Anatomic Types *Defect at the Fossa Ovalis (Ostium Secundum).* This defect classically involves the region of the fossa ovalis and is the most common type (70 percent)[85] (Figs. 97-4*A* and 97-4*C*).[84,86] Atrial septal tissue separates the inferior edge of the defect from the atrioventricular valves. Associated partial anomalous pulmonary venous connections are not uncommon with one or more of the right pulmonary veins draining into the right atrium or one of its tributaries.[87] Mitral valve prolapse is present in some.

Partial Atrioventricular Canal Defects. Defects of the atrioventricular septum, which lies inferior to the fossa ovalis, constitute approximately 20 percent of atrial septal defects and are part of a complex malformation known as common atrioventricular canal defects considered later (Fig. 97-4*D*).

Sinus Venosus Defects. Such defects, approximately 6 percent of the total, appear to represent a biatrial connection of the superior vena cava (or in rare instances inferior vena cava) which straddles the otherwise normal intact atrial septum. Also involved is an anomalous termination of one or more of the right-sided pulmonary veins, either into the vena cava or into the right atrium near its junction with the vena cava[88] (Fig. 97-4*B*).[84]

Coronary Sinus Defects. This is an uncommon type of atrial septal defect located in the position normally occupied by the ostium of the coronary sinus. This defect is part of a developmental complex consisting of the absence of the coronary sinus and entry of the left superior vena cava directly into the left atrium.[89]

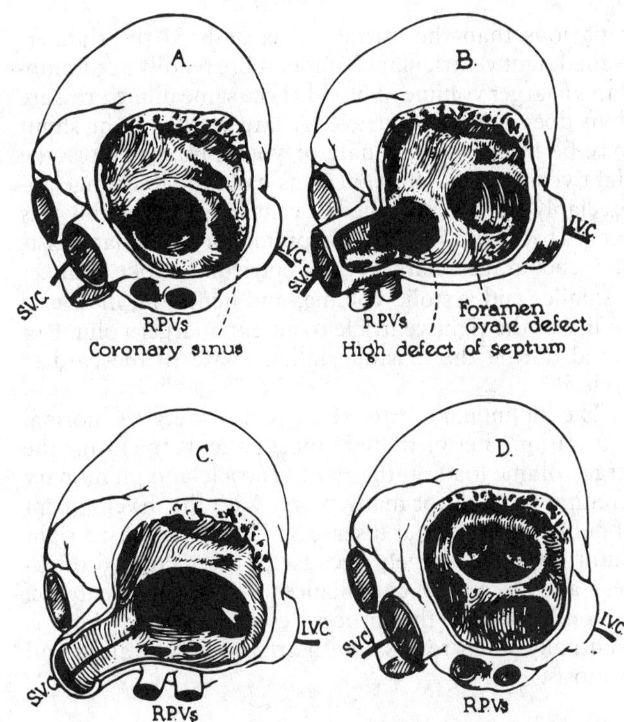

FIGURE 97-4 Types of interatrial communications. *A.* Large ostium secundum type of atrial septal defect. *B.* So-called sinus venosus type of defect—one high in the atrial septum associated with anomalous connection of the right superior pulmonary vein to the junctional area of the superior vena cava and right atrium. *C.* Very large ostium secundum type of atrial septal defect with absence of the posterior rim. *D.* Partial form of common atrioventricular canal with cleft mitral valve. SVC = superior vena cava; RPVs = right pulmonary veins; IVC = inferior vena cava. (*From FW Lewis et al.[84] Copyright 1957, American Medical Association. Reproduced with permission from the publisher and authors.*)

Conditions Common to All Anatomic Types The right atrial and ventricular chambers as well as the central pulmonary arteries become enlarged. When pulmonary hypertension intervenes, the right ventricular wall hypertrophies and atherosclerosis may occur in the major pulmonary arteries. Saccular aneurysm and thrombosis with dissecting aneurysm or rupture may occur.

Pulmonary hypertension may develop, but usually not before the third decade. The earliest lesion is cellular fibrous intimal thickening in the proximal segments of arterioles. The pulmonary arterial pressure then rises followed by the development of medial hypertrophy of muscular arteries and the appearance of plexiform lesions. In the final state, the pulmonary vascular bed may be difficult to distinguish from that in ventricular septal defect with PVOD.[41]

Abnormal Physiology

Usually there is no resistance to blood flow across the defect and no significant pressure difference between the two atria. A left-to-right shunt of blood occurs (Fig. 97-5) because (1) the right atrial system is more distensible than the left, (2) the tricuspid valve is normally more capacious than the mitral valve, and (3) the thinner-walled right ventricular chamber more readily accommodates a larger volume of blood at the same filling pressure than does the left ventricle. A large left-to-right shunt may be found in a neonate or young infant before the right ventricular compliance has had time to change appreciably from that of the left ventricle. Presumably this occurs because a rapid fall in pulmonary vascular resistance encourages a larger right ventricular stroke volume, a smaller end-systolic volume, and hence, an increased ability of the right ventricle to accept a larger volume of blood during the diastolic filling phase of the cardiac cycle.[90]

The pulmonary arterial system undergoes normal maturation after birth, with most patients tolerating the large volume load on the right ventricle and pulmonary circuit quite well for many years. With the development of pulmonary vascular disease and PAH, the left-to-right shunt decreases, largely because of the increased thickness and decreased compliance of the right ventricle. In some patients this process continues until there is eventually shunt reversal with arterial desaturation and cyanosis.

Clinical Manifestations

Atrial septal defect is found in approximately 10 percent of children surviving beyond the first year of life with congenital heart disease.[4] If one excludes mitral valve prolapse and the congenitally bicuspid aortic valve, it is the most common form of congenital heart disease among adults.

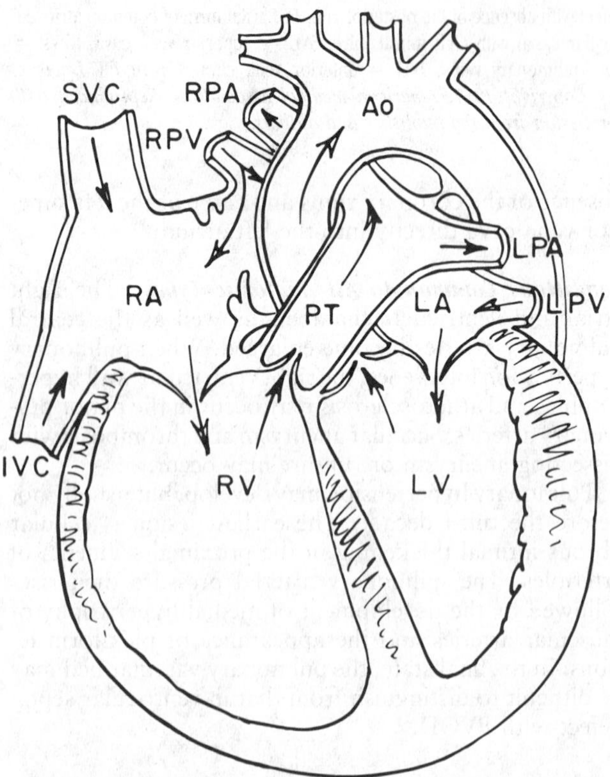

FIGURE 97-5 Atrial septal defect at fossa ovalis, with left-to-right shunt. SVC = superior vena cava; IVC = inferior vena cava; RA = right atrium; RV = right ventricle; PT = main pulmonary arterial trunk; RPA = right pulmonary artery; LPA = left pulmonary artery; RPV = right pulmonary vein; LPV = left pulmonary vein; LA = left atrium; LV = left ventricle; Ao = aorta. (*From JE Edwards.*[86] *Reproduced with permission from the publisher, editor, and author.*)

Atrial septal defects are more common among females, with a female/male ratio of approximately 2:1. The mode of transmission is best explained in most instances on a multifactorial basis, where the risk would be approximately 2.5 percent for first-degree relatives of a single affected family member. However, examples of autosomal dominant transmission are recognized either as an isolated entity, associated with severe atrioventricular conduction disturbances, or with upper extremity malformations as in the Holt-Oram syndrome (Fig. 10-2). Examples of Mendelian autosomal recessive transmission are found in the Ellis-van Creveld (Fig. 10-1) and thrombocytopenia–absent radius syndromes.[91]

History The majority of children are considered asymptomatic, but probably most have some mild diminution of stamina, since it is not unusual for the patient or the parents to comment on the increased endurance that follows surgical correction. Symptoms of mild fatigue and dyspnea tend to be recognized in the late teens and early twenties, and at least three-quarters of individuals will be definitely symptomatic as adults. Congestive heart failure is rare in childhood, but a few infants, perhaps 5 percent, will have heart failure in the first year of life. Failure becomes more common again in the fourth and fifth decades, usually associated with the onset of arrhythmias.[92]

Physical Examination Many children have a slender habitus, but normal growth and development are the rule. Prominence of the left anterior chest is common, and a hyperdynamic right ventricular systolic lift can usually be felt. The first heart sound may be slightly accentuated at the lower left sternal border. The two components of the second heart sound are characteristically widely split, with the interval of splitting fixed despite expiration or the Valsalva maneuver. The pulmonary component of the second heart sound may be accentuated, even in the absence of PAH. With increasing pulmonary arterial pressure and resistance, the interval between the aortic and pulmonary components of the second heart sound narrows and the pulmonary component becomes louder, but the lack of respiratory influence on the interval between the two components persists. A midsystolic spindle-shaped murmur of grade 2 to 3 intensity at the left upper sternal border, reflecting increased right ventricular stroke volume, is to be expected. A low- to medium-pitched early diastolic murmur over the lower left sternal border, denoting increased diastolic flow across the tricuspid valve, is present in most individuals with large shunts. (See also Chap. 11.) Cyanosis and clubbing reflect right-to-left shunting. In this setting, the murmurs of tricuspid and pulmonary regurgitation are not uncommon.

Chest Roentgenogram Mild-to-moderate cardiac enlargement and prominence of the main and branch pulmonary arteries are characteristic (Fig. 14-2*B*). The absence of left atrial displacement of the barium-filled

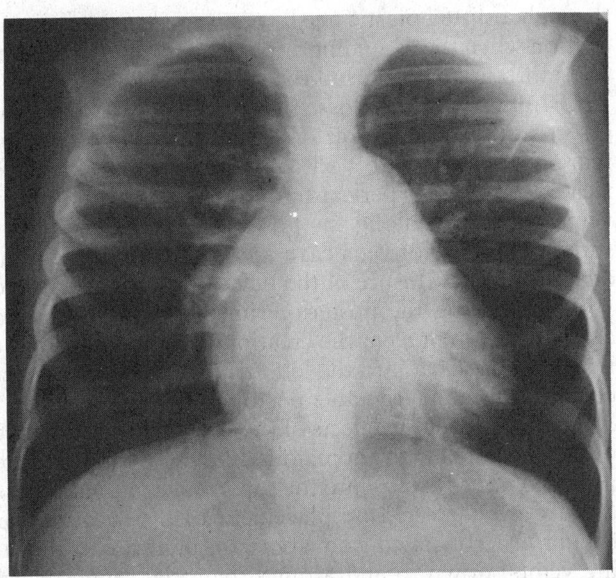

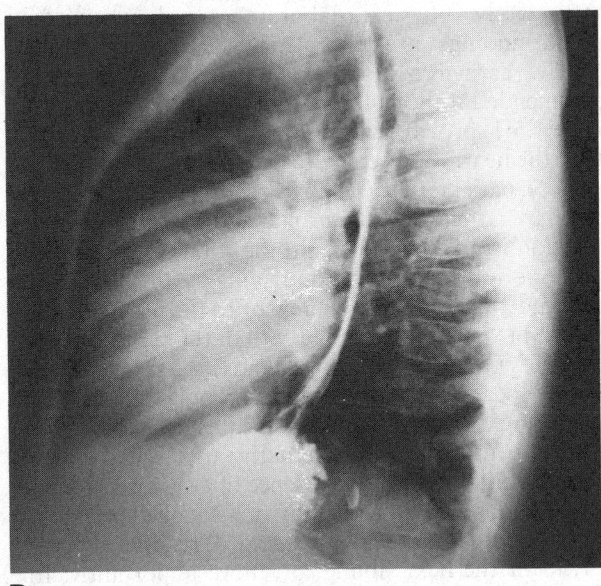

FIGURE 97-6 Chest roentgenograms of a 4-year-old child with a secundum atrial septal defect, a large left-to-right shunt, and normal pulmonary arterial pressures. *A.* Frontal. *B.* Lateral. Right ventricular enlargement (seen in the lateral view) accompanies prominence of the main pulmonary arterial segment and increased blood flow. No left atrial dilatation is present.

esophagus in the lateral view helps to distinguish atrial septal defect from large left-to-right shunts at other levels (Fig. 97-6).

Electrocardiogram An rsR′ pattern over the right precordium, indicating mild right ventricular conduction delay or mild right ventricular hypertrophy, is characteristic. The mean QRS axis in the frontal plane is 90° or greater in 60 percent of patients. Serious arrhythmias are usually, though not invariably, limited to adults; atrial fibrillation and atrial flutter are the most common.

Echocardiogram M-mode studies reflect volume overload of the right side of the heart with increased right atrial and right ventricular dimensions and paradoxical ventricular septal motion. Two-dimensional and Doppler echocardiography with color flow mapping (Chap. 130) permit identification and visualization of virtually all secundum and atrioventricular canal defects.[93] (See Plate XI, 130-4.) Visualization of sinus venosus defects is slightly more difficult.[88] Quantitative assessment of flow and pulmonary arterial pressure is also possible.[94] The transesophageal approach (Chap. 131) offers excellent images for those patients in whom the transthoracic approach is inadequate.[95]

Cardiac Catheterization There is a significant increase in oxygen saturation in the blood samples drawn from the right atrium, right ventricle, and pulmonary artery compared with those from the superior or inferior venae cavae. Pulmonary arterial and right ventricular systolic pressures are normal or only slightly elevated. A systolic pressure gradient of up to 20 mmHg across the right ventricular outflow tract is accepted as secondary to flow rather than to organic obstruction. The right and left atrial mean and phasic pressures will be virtually identical, with little if any elevation above normal (mean pressure gradient < 3 mmHg) unless there are associated abnormalities.[87] (See also Chap. 138.)

Natural History and Prognosis

Defects of the secundum type usually go undetected in the first year or two of life because of the lack of symptoms and unimpressive auscultatory findings. A soft systolic murmur is the usual reason for referral. In the late teens and twenties symptoms become more common, and by age 40 the majority of individuals are symptomatic, some severely so.[96] Pulmonary vascular disease with serious pulmonary hypertension begins to make its appearance in the early twenties. It affects approximately 15 percent of young adults, particularly women, and may be rapidly progressive, especially with pregnancy. The incidence of atrial fibrillation or flutter also increases with each decade and is closely linked to the onset of congestive failure. Spontaneous closure of secundum defects is rare beyond the first 2 years of life. The passage of time is associated with a higher mortality and morbidity with and following corrective surgery.[92] Congestive heart failure is the most common cause of death among unoperated patients. Other causes of death include pulmonary embolism or thrombosis, paradoxical emboli, brain abscess, and infection.

Medical Management

Those few infants presenting with symptoms of congestive failure are treated with digoxin and, if necessary, diuretics, and are studied by cardiac catheterization. If the defect is uncomplicated and the symptoms persist despite a trial of therapy, surgical closure is advised without further delay. For asymptomatic infants and children, closure is recommended just prior to their entry into school. Restrictions of activity or exercise are unnecessary. If the physical, laboratory, and echocardiographic findings are completely characteristic, preoperative catheterization is not necessary. Surgery is recommended if the pulmonary/systemic blood flow ratio is ≥1.5:1, provided no serious malfunction of the left side of the heart is present. Closure is also recommended for those patients with ratios ≥1.5:1 if PAH is documented by catheterization, provided the systemic arterial saturation is ≥92 percent, and the total pulmonary resistance is less than 15 Wood units.[97] Closure would seem prudent prior to pregnancy or to the use of contraceptives, in view of the tendency to develop rapidly progressive PVOD in this setting. Transcatheter closure of centrally located defects in older infants, children, and adults using a double-umbrella ("clamshell") device appears to be an acceptable alternative to surgical closure in selected patients.[98] In the absence of a syndrome transmitted dominantly or recessively in a Mendelian pattern and if the patient is the only first-degree relative affected, the risk for the next sibling, or, more importantly, for the patient's parents, is on the order of 2.5 percent.[96] The risk for the child of an affected parent is probably in the 10 percent range, particularly if that parent is the mother.[69] Infective endocarditis is rare, but antibiotic coverage at times of possible bacteremia is recommended if associated mitral valve disease is suspected.

Surgical Management

Defects of the interatrial septum are exposed through the lateral wall of the right atrium and are either sutured or obliterated with a pericardial or Dacron patch, the choice being determined by the location and size of the defect, integrity of the margins, and the surgeons' preference. The patient is supported on total cardiopulmonary bypass at normothermia. Hemodilution allows operation without blood transfusion even in small children. Risk of cerebral or coronary air embolization is minimized by cardioplegic cardiac arrest and continuous aspiration of blood and air from the ascending aorta through a slitted plastic needle connected to cardiotomy suction when the ascending aorta is not clamped. Operative mortality and morbidity are nil.

Ostium secundum (fossa ovalis) defects are closed by direct suture; a very large defect or one having tenuous margins is closed with a patch—usually glutaraldehyde-treated autologous pericardium. Anomalous pulmonary veins are sought along the posterolateral aspect of the superior or inferior vena cava and from within the right atrium prior to closure of the defect. Sutures are placed with care along the posterior rim of the inferior vena caval orifice to prevent the creation of a tunnel from the inferior vena cava into the left atrium, which would, of course, cause unacceptable postoperative hypoxemia.[99]

High atrial septal defects of the sinus venosus type are often associated with anomalous drainage of one or more right pulmonary veins into the superior vena cava. These defects are corrected by placement of a pericardial or tubular Dacron patch from above the abnormally draining vein(s) down to and around the atrial septal defect (Fig. 97-7). Pulmonary venous blood is thus diverted through the atrial septal defect into the left atrium.[100] Pericardial gusset enlargement of the superior vena cava at the cavoatrial junction may be required. Alternatively, the superior vena cava can be divided cephalad to the orifice(s) of high anomalous pulmonary vein(s), after which it is anastomosed to the right atrial appendage. A patch in the right atrium diverts pulmonary venous blood through the atrial septal defect into the left atrium.[101] Anomalous right pulmonary veins draining to the right atrium are diverted into the left atrium by placement of a patch baffle well anterior and to the right of the pulmonary vein orifices.

Although clinical benefit following closure of atrial septal defects can be anticipated even in adults having significant physiological compromise, mortality is higher than in the young and the magnitude of improvement is uncertain.[102] Mortality in patients over 40 years old approaches 5 percent.[103] (See Chap. 98.) Nonetheless, surgical closure of atrial septal defects is advised even

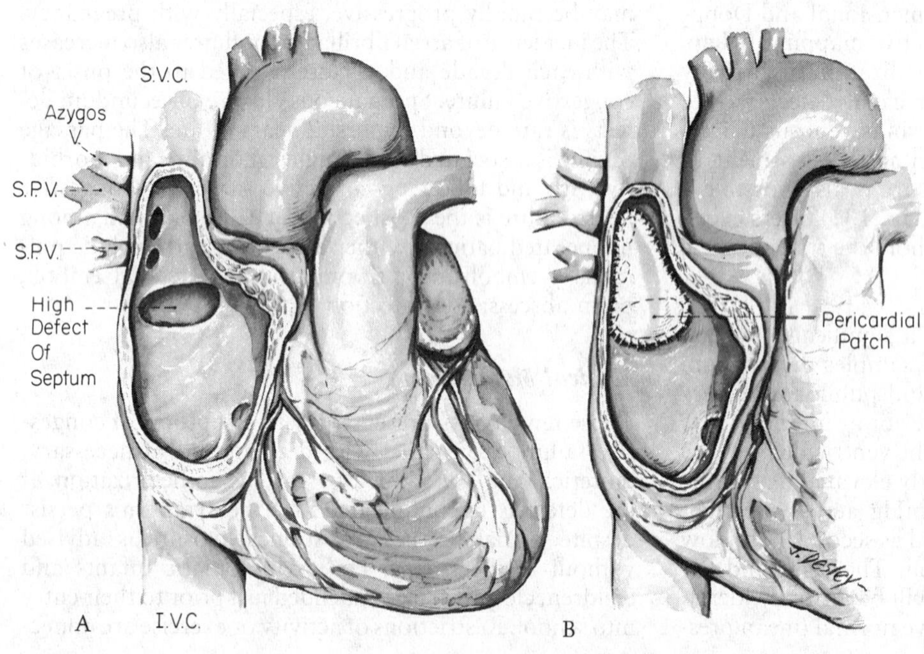

FIGURE 97-7 *A.* Sinus venosus type of atrial septal defect, with its constantly accompanying anomalous pulmonary venous connection of superior pulmonary vein (SPV) to superior vena cava (SVC). *B.* Repair is effected with a pericardial patch, so placed as to divert pulmonary venous blood across the defect into the left atrium and to divert superior vena caval blood to the right atrium. (*This illustration appeared originally in the first edition of The Heart, in 1966, and in all subsequent editions. It is reproduced here by courtesy of Dr. John W. Kirklin, Birmingham, Alabama.*)

when the pulmonary vascular resistance approaches 15 Wood units, because of the excessive morbidity and mortality associated with a persistent interatrial communication.[97] Morbidity in adults and the low risk of surgical closure in young children mandate surgery in the preschool or preadolescent years.[104]

Although life-threatening complications following closure of atrial septal defects in children are rare, transient postoperative atrial arrhythmias and postoperative pericarditis are relatively common. Long-term prognosis for a normal life expectancy and functional capability is excellent for patients having closure of an uncomplicated atrial septal defect during the first two decades of life.

Partial Anomalous Pulmonary Venous Connection

Pathology

In partial anomalous pulmonary venous connection one or more, but not all, of the pulmonary veins enter the right atrium or its venous tributaries. The atrial septum may be intact, but an atrial septal defect is usually present. There are many patterns of anomalous pulmonary venous connection, but the four most common, in order of decreasing frequency, are: (1) pulmonary veins from the right upper and/or middle lobe to the superior vena cava, usually with a sinus venosus atrial septal defect; (2) all of the right pulmonary veins to the right atrium, usually in the polysplenia syndrome; (3) all of the right pulmonary veins to the inferior vena cava, entering this systemic vein just above or below the diaphragm; and (4) the left upper or both left pulmonary veins to an anomalous vertical vein draining to the left brachiocephalic vein.

When the right pulmonary veins are connected to the inferior vena cava, the atrial septum may be intact. This venous anomaly may be isolated or may be part of the *scimitar syndrome.* The latter includes hypoplasia of the right lung, bronchial abnormalities, anomalous systemic pulmonary arterial supply to the right lung from branches of the descending thoracic and/or the abdominal aorta, and dextroposition of the heart.

Clinical Manifestations

This malformation occurs in approximately 1 in every 160 individuals, or 0.6 percent of the population.[87] There is no sex predilection. Approximately 15 percent of all atrial septal defects have this coexisting anomaly; however, in the case of the sinus venosus type of defect the association is in the range of 85 percent.

History When partial anomalous pulmonary venous connection coexists with an atrial septal defect, the symptoms, as well as the other clinical manifestations, are indistinguishable from those of an isolated atrial septal defect. Isolated, uncomplicated anomalous connection of a single pulmonary vein usually goes undetected clinically, since in this circumstance only about 20 percent of the pulmonary venous flow returns to the right atrium or its tributaries. When the entire venous return from one lung or two pulmonary veins are connected anomalously, approximately 65 percent of the pulmonary venous flow returns to the right side of the heart and symptoms are similar to those of an atrial septal defect with a comparable increase in pulmonary blood flow.

Physical Examination The findings are the same as those in patients with an atrial septal defect with the exception that the two components of the second heart sound, though usually widely split, move normally with respiration if the atrial septum is intact.

Chest Roentgenogram Right ventricular enlargement, pulmonary arterial dilatation, and increased pulmonary blood flow are characteristic when more than one pulmonary vein connects anomalously. With anomalous connection of the right pulmonary veins to the inferior vena cava, the pulmonary venous pattern may assume a crescent-shaped or scimitar curve in the right lower lung field along the right lower heart border.

Electrocardiogram The electrocardiogram is either normal (in the case of anomalous connection of a single pulmonary vein) or reflects volume overload of the right side of the heart.

Echocardiogram If more than one pulmonary vein drains anomalously, the volume usually is sufficient to produce the characteristic pattern of right ventricular diastolic overload (Chap. 15). Failure to visualize an atrial septal opening with two-dimensional imaging should arouse suspicion of an intact atrial septum.

Cardiac Catheterization Anomalously connected pulmonary veins may be entered directly with the venous catheter. Selective biplane angiograms in these vessels will document their site of connection (Fig. 138-19). Left-to-right shunting with partial anomalous pulmonary venous connection and an intact atrial septum is usually small or moderate and may go undetected by oximetry techniques. Selective indicator dilution curves in the right and left pulmonary arteries with systemic arterial sampling can detect the lung with the anomalous pulmonary venous connection, and selective biplane angiograms in the pulmonary arterial branches will visualize these connections.

Natural History and Prognosis

Patients with partial anomalous pulmonary venous connection with atrial septal defect appear to follow a course similar to, if not identical with, that of patients with an isolated atrial septal defect. When the atrial septum is intact, the course depends primarily on the volume of pulmonary venous blood returning to the right side of the heart. Rarely, PVOD may be found even in the presence of a single anomalously connected pulmonary vein and an intact atrial septum.[105] Finally, increasing left atrial pressure, due either to mitral valve disease or diminishing left ventricular compliance, will, in the course of time, encourage a greater redistribution of pulmonary arterial blood flow to that portion of the lung drained by the more compliant right atrium. Thus, patients who were initially asymptomatic and had a very modest volume of anomalous pulmonary venous return in youth may become symptomatic and even develop congestive failure in adult life.

Medical Management

Asymptomatic patients with small shunts require no treatment. Those with symptoms, larger pulmonary blood flows, congestive failure, or PAH require surgical correction. With an intact atrial septum, precise preoperative identification of the site of the anomalous venous connection is essential. Long-term follow-up in patients who have not had surgery is indicated to detect increasing flow or the appearance of PAH.

Surgical Management

Anomalous connection of right pulmonary vein(s) to the superior vena cava is usually associated with a sinus venosus atrial septal defect (Fig. 97-7). See "Atrial Septal Defect, Surgical Management." Partial anomalous pulmonary veins draining to the superior vena cava, inferior vena cava, or right atrium are repaired by diverting them through the atrial septal defect into the left atrium using an appropriately placed patch baffle. Isolated left-sided anomalous pulmonary veins draining to the left ascending vertical vein or the left superior vena cava are detached and anastomosed directly to the left atrial appendage. Long-term morbidity and mortality are minimal, equivalent to that observed after closure of atrial septal defect.

Common Atrioventricular Canal Defects

Definition

The condition called atrioventricular (AV) canal is characterized by an atrial septal defect in the lowermost part of the atrial septum, a cleft condition of the mitral valve (either alone or in combination with cleft of the tricuspid valve), and deficiency of ventricular septal tissue. The condition appears to result from incomplete growth of the AV endocardial cushions and atrioventricular septum.

Pathology

The *ostium primum type* of atrial septal defect is characterized by a crescent-shaped upper border and no septal tissue forming the lower border. The lower aspect of the defect is bounded by the atrial surfaces of the AV valves and, in the complete type (see below), in part by the upper edge of the ventricular septum. A small amount of septal tissue separates the defect from the posterior atrial wall.

Anatomic Types Variations occur with respect to the nature of the AV valves. The terms *partial* and *complete* were first introduced to describe these types.[106]

Partial Type. The ostium primum atrial septal defect is associated with a "cleft" in the anterior mitral leaflet or, probably more accurately, a septal commissure between the superior and the inferior leaflets of the left AV valve (Figs. 97-4*D* and 97-8).[86] The tricuspid valve either is not cleft or shows minor central deficiency. The ventricular aspects of the anterior mitral valve elements are fused to the upper edge of the deficient ventricular septum, precluding an interventricular communication. If there is no atrial septal tissue or if the atrial septum is so rudimentary as to produce a common chamber involving both atria, the term *common* or *single atrium* is applied.

Complete Type. The complete type of common AV canal is characterized by failure of partitioning of the primitive canal into separate AV orifices. The orifice between the atria and the ventricles is guarded by a common valve, of which the anterior leaflet is derived from the ventral AV endocardial cushion and represents the anterior halves of the anterior mitral and septal tricuspid leaflets. The posterior leaflet is derived from the dorsal AV endocardial cushion and represents the posterior halves of the anterior mitral and septal tricuspid leaflets.

Usually, considerable space exists between the anterior and posterior leaflets, above, and the ventricular septum, below, so that in most cases of the complete type there is free communication between the ventricles.

Rastelli and associates subdivided the complete variety into three subgroups—types A, B, and C (Fig.

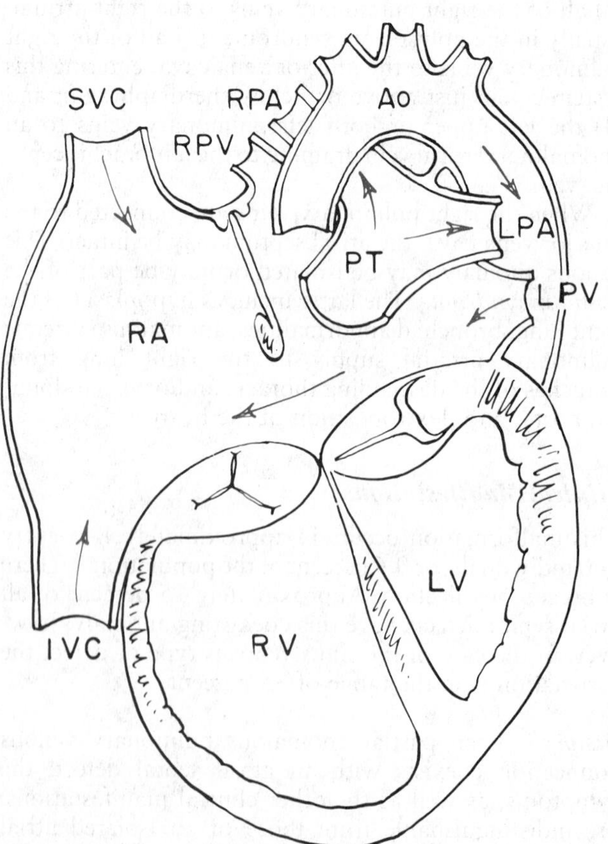

FIGURE 97-8 Common AV canal of the partial type. The mitral valve shows a cleft in its anterior leaflet, while the tricuspid valve is undisturbed. SVC = superior vena cava; IVC = inferior vena cava; RA = right atrium; RV = right ventricle; PT = main pulmonary arterial trunk; RPA = right pulmonary artery; LPA = left pulmonary artery; RPV = right pulmonary vein; LPV = left pulmonary vein; LV = left ventricle; AO = aorta. (*From JE Edwards.*[86] *Reproduced with permission from the publisher, editor, and author.*)

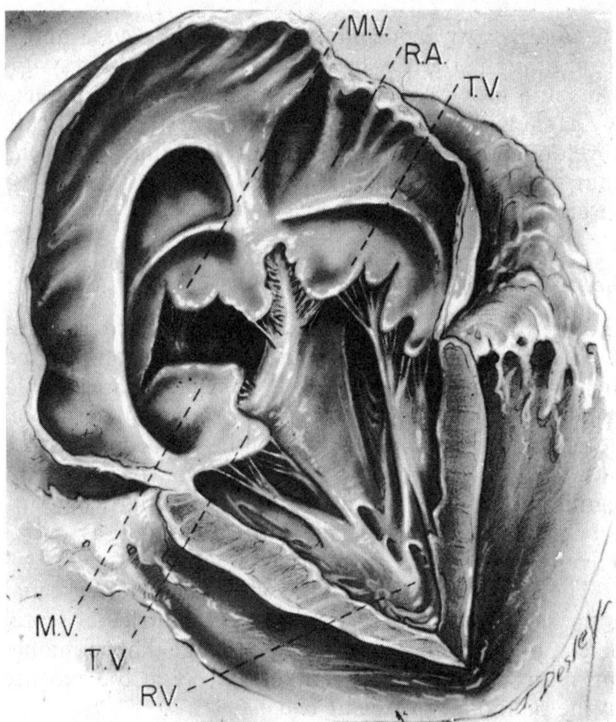

FIGURE 97-9 Complete form of common AV canal, type A. The common anterior leaflet has a recognizable mitral component, MV, and tricuspid component, TV. In Type B, not illustrated, those components are attached by chordae to a papillary muscle in the right ventricle. In type C, not illustrated, the common anterior leaflet is a single unit without any attachment to the underlying ventricular septum. Type A is most amenable to repair. RV = right ventricle; RA = right atrium. (*From GC Rastelli et al.*[107] *Reproduced with permission from the publisher and authors.*)

97-9)[107]—on the basis of the structure of the common anterior leaflet and its chordal attachments to the ventricular septum and/or papillary muscles. With regard to the posterior common leaflet, there is variation among the three types as to presence or absence of subdivision, and as to whether the posterior leaflet is attached to the ventricular septum by chordae or by an imperforate membrane.

Variations from the classic types of AV canal defects are recognized, the most frequent being the AV canal type of isolated ventricular septal defect, isolated ostium primum atrial septal defect without malformed AV valves, and isolated cleft of the anterior mitral or septal tricuspid valve leaflets.

Associated Conditions In the *asplenia syndrome,* the complete variety is almost universal; with polysplenia it occurs in about one-quarter of cases.[108] An atrial septal defect of the secundum type is present in about half of the cases. Double orifice of the mitral valve may be associated with the incomplete type,[109] and tetralogy of Fallot may be associated with the complete type.[110]

Abnormal Physiology

If the communication at the ventricular level is large, the right ventricular and pulmonary artery pressures will be elevated. These patients are similar to those with large ventricular septal defects. Patients with a communication at the atrial level only usually have normal pressures in the right side of the heart and a large pulmonary blood flow, as in the secundum type of atrial septal defect. Defects in the tricuspid or mitral valve, or both, may result in severe regurgitation or direct shunting of blood from the left ventricle to the right atrium.

Clinical Manifestations

Approximately 3 percent of infants and children with congenital heart disease have AV canal defects. The majority, some 60 to 70 percent, have the partial, or incomplete, form.[4] The female/male ratio is approximately 1.3:1. Well over half of the patients with the complete form have associated Down syndrome.[3] Among children with Down syndrome, 45 percent have some form of congenital heart disease. Malformations of the AV canal type, usually of the complete variety, comprise 25 to 36 percent of these abnormalities.[91] (See also Chaps. 10 and 96.)

History Only if the mitral valve is incompetent do the symptoms of patients with partial AV canal differ from those associated with a secundum type of atrial septal defect. Mitral regurgitation may be associated with poor weight gain, easy fatigue, dyspnea, repeated respiratory infections, and congestive heart failure. Patients with complete AV canal are almost invariably very sick.

Examination The findings with a partial defect are those of an atrial septal defect. If the cleft anterior mitral leaflet is incompetent, the findings of mitral regurgitation will also be present.

The physical findings with the complete canal are those of a very large ventricular septal defect usually with full-blown congestive failure, but the second heart sound is split and fixed. The murmur of mitral regurgitation may not be heard or recognized as such.

Chest Roentgenogram Overall cardiac enlargement, out of proportion to the degree of pulmonary plethora, or a cardiac silhouette suggesting combined ventricular dilatation may serve to distinguish the uncomplicated secundum atrial septal defect from the primum defect with significant mitral regurgitation. Marked cardiac enlargement with severe pulmonary overcirculation are features of the complete canal.

Electrocardiogram One of the most helpful diagnostic features in distinguishing individuals with AV canal defects from those with isolated atrial or ventricular septal defects is the characteristic superior orientation of the mean QRS axis in the frontal plane with a right bundle branch delay in the precordial leads. Between 92 and 95 percent of both types of canal have a QRS axis lying between 0 and $-150°$.[111] The patterns of atrial and ventricular hypertrophy reflect the underlying hemodynamic abnormalities.

Echocardiogram Two-dimensional sector scanning is capable of visualizing the extent of septal defects and, with Doppler study, left-to-right shunting at atrial and/or ventricular level and associated mitral and/or tricuspid valvular regurgitation (Fig. 97-10). The anatomic features of the anterior AV leaflet and its connections may be visualized with sufficient clarity to permit subdivision of complete AV canal defects into types A, B, and C (Fig. 97-9).[107,112] Straddling AV valves, double-orifice mitral valve, single papillary muscles, and hypoplasia or outflow obstruction of the right or left ventricles can also be determined with this technique.[113]

Cardiac Catheterization A significant increase in oxygen saturation between the superior vena cava and the right atrium is present. A right ventricular or pulmonary arterial systolic pressure in excess of 60 percent of the systemic systolic pressure favors the presence of a complete canal. With a large communication between the two ventricles below the AV valves, the right ventricular, pulmonary arterial, and systemic arterial systolic pressures are virtually identical. Left ventricular angiography in the frontal view demonstrates the "gooseneck deformity" of the left ventricular outflow tract characteristic of AV canal malformations (Fig. 138-20) and allows a semiquantitative assessment of the degree of mitral regurgitation and shunting from left ventricle to right atrium. The left anterior oblique view with craniocaudal angulation is recommended for visualizing the interventricular defect and judging the extent of ventricular septal deficiency. Aortography is essential to eliminate the possibility of a patent ductus arteriosus.

Natural History and Prognosis

Partial defects without significant mitral regurgitation follow a course similar to that described for the secundum type of septal defects. An exception would be the greater likelihood of infective endocarditis because of the mitral valve deformity. Moderate or severe mitral regurgitation produces heart failure with resulting symptoms and growth retardation. Infants with a complete AV canal without protective pulmonary stenosis quickly develop and continue in congestive failure until the course is altered by death, the development of PVOD, or surgical intervention.

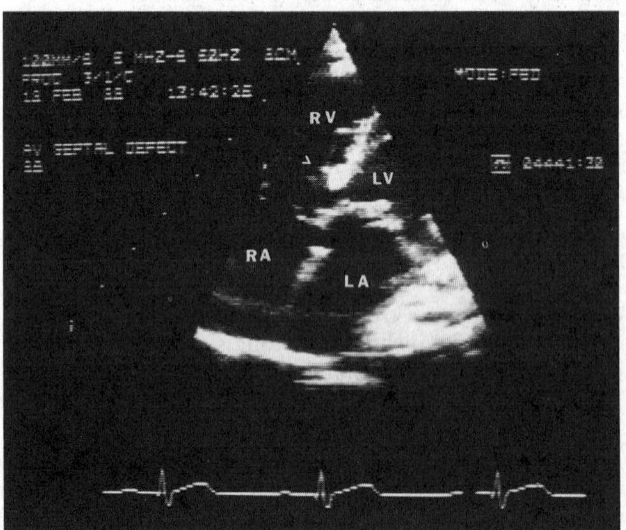

FIGURE 97-10 Two-dimensional echocardiogram in the apical view in a child with atrioventricular canal defect. The defects of the atrial and ventricular septae are clearly outlined. There are attachments from the tricuspid portion of the atrioventricular valve to the interventricular septum (*arrow*). RV = right ventricle; LV = left ventricle; RA = right atrium; LA = left atrium.

Medical Management

Children with an uncomplicated partial defect are managed in the same manner as children with uncomplicated atrial septal defect. Those who are symptomatic should undergo surgical closure of their primum atrial septal defect and, if possible, plication of the septal commissure of the left AV ("mitral") valve. Those few patients with significant residual mitral regurgitation following surgery are managed medically until such time as mitral valve replacement is appropriate.

The approach to the infant with complete AV canal is the same as for infants with a large ventricular septal defect, but is tempered by the knowledge that spontaneous improvement is very unlikely except at the expense of the pulmonary vascular bed.

Antibiotic coverage at times of special risk of bacteremia is indicated indefinitely for all forms of AV canal, with or without surgery.

With regard to genetic counseling, the risk of a subsequent sibling having heart disease in the presence of a single affected family member is in the range of 2 percent; it is probably higher, perhaps as high as 10 percent, for the offspring of an affected parent, particularly if the affected parent is the mother.[114] Concordance for AV canal defects among affected siblings or offspring is much higher than with other forms of congenital heart disease and approaches 90 percent.

Surgical Management

The remarkable clinical improvement following anatomic repair of complete common AV septal defects in infancy encourages early correction within the first year of life.[115-118] Banding of the pulmonary artery deserves consideration in the critically ill infant having a large interventricular communication, increased pulmonary blood flow, and contraindications to cardiopulmonary bypass.[118]

Specifics of repair are dictated by anatomic detail; individual variation is considerable (Figs. 97-9 and 97-11). The defect is exposed through a right atriotomy during hypothermic cardiopulmonary bypass. Total circulatory arrest with profound hypothermia (18°C) permits precise repair in the infant weighing less than 5 kg, but most operations can be accomplished with low-flow perfusion and moderate hypothermia (22 to 28°C). Creation of a competent left-sided AV ("mitral") valve is essential for acceptable early and long-term prognosis.[119]

A Dacron patch is sutured to the right side of the ventricular septum to obliterate the interventricular communication. The anterior and posterior components of the mitral valve are sutured to the Dacron patch at an appropriate level. Mitral valve competence is assessed by gentle distension of the left ventricle with cold saline.

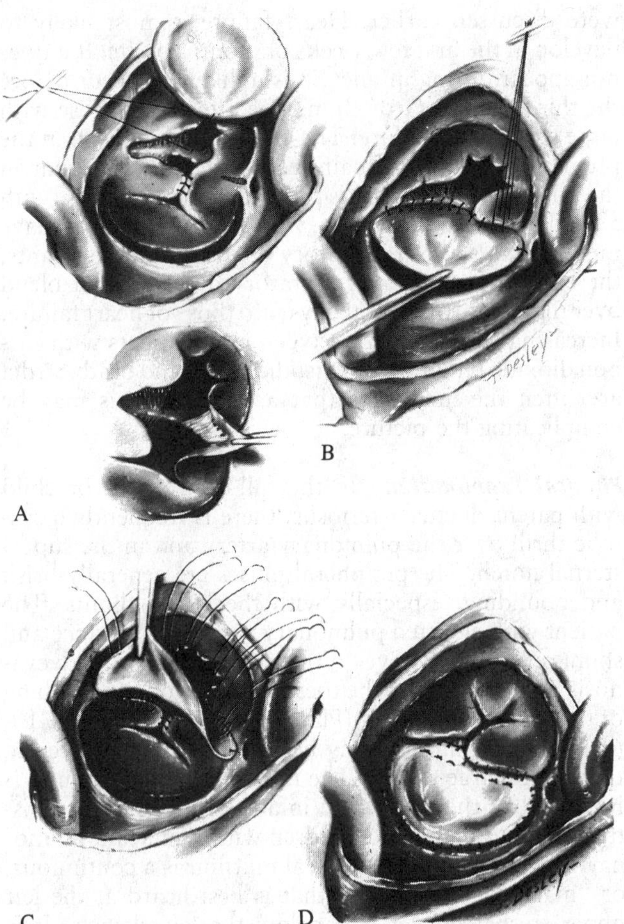

FIGURE 97-11 Steps in the repair of the complete form of common AV canal, type A, *A, B.* A pericardial patch is sutured to the ventricular septum. *C, D.* The anterior leaflet of the mitral valve is reconstructed and attached to the patch. A portion of the tricuspid leaflet is attached to the patch. (*From GC Rastelli et al.*[107] *Reproduced with permission from the publisher and authors*).

The "cleft" created between the left anterior and left posterior leaflets should be closed by suture if approximation of these edges appears to increase competence without creation of stenosis. Prosthetic valve implantation is rarely required during primary anatomic repair.[120] The right-sided AV ("tricuspid") apparatus, although less critical to survival, is repaired using the same principles. The interatrial communication is closed with a separate piece of pericardium to minimize hemolysis in the presence of residual mitral regurgitation.

Hospital mortality following correction of complete AV canal in infancy ranges from 0 to 27 percent,[121,122] the highest mortality being encountered during the first few months of life and in those infants having severe AV valve regurgitation, elevated pulmonary vascular resistance, hypoplasia of the left or right ventricle, or other cardiac malformations.[123] Five-year survival of 91 percent for patients discharged from the hospital after total correction has been reported.[124] Successful corrections of complete AV canal associated with common ventricle,[125] tetralogy of Fallot,[110] double-outlet ventricle,[126,127] and other complex anomalies[128–130] have been reported.

Partial AV canal is repaired through a right atriotomy. The cleft is closed with a few simple interrupted sutures to encourage inversion and coaptation of the leaflet margins. The atrial septal defect is closed with a pericardial patch. McMullan and associates at the Mayo Clinic[131] reviewed 232 patients between the ages of 3 months and 50 years operated upon between 1955 and 1972. Hospital mortality was 6 percent; risk of death was greater in patients having severe preoperative disability, those having a cardiothoracic ratio exceeding 0.60, and infants under 1 year of age. Of 210 patients for whom follow-up data were available, 8 (3.8 percent) required mitral valve replacement 3 months to 14 years after the initial operation. Electrical instability remains threatening.[132] Permanent complete heart block contributed substantially to early mortality and morbidity but is now rare. Patients undergoing repair of partial AV canal should be observed for the possible development of subaortic left ventricular outflow tract obstruction caused by redundant or residual endocardial cushion tissue.

EXTRACARDIAC COMMUNICATIONS BETWEEN THE SYSTEMIC AND PULMONARY CIRCULATIONS, USUALLY WITHOUT CYANOSIS

Patent Ductus Arteriosus

Definition

Patent ductus arteriosus, the most common type of extracardiac shunt, represents persistent patency of the vessel that normally connects the pulmonary arterial system and the aorta in the fetus (Fig. 97-12).[86]

Pathology

The ductus arteriosus usually closes within 2 or 3 weeks after birth and becomes the *ligamentum arteriosum,* but it may remain patent as long as 8 weeks postnatally.[133] It runs from the origin of the left pulmonary artery, below, to the lower aspect of the aortic arch just beyond the level of origin of the left subclavian artery, above. The recurrent branch of the left vagus nerve hooks around its lateral and inferior aspects.

Abnormal Physiology[134,135]

Patients with patent ductus arteriosus may be divided into groups according to whether the vascular resistance through the ductus itself is small, moderate, or large. The resistance of the ductus is related not only to its cross-sectional area but also to its length. In patients with a ductus of high resistance, the flow across the ductus is relatively small. The extra volume of work on the left ventricle is small, and the pulmonary pressure and resistance are not elevated. Patients with only moderate resistance in the ductus have some increase in pulmonary artery pressure with a moderately greater volume of shunting across the ductus.

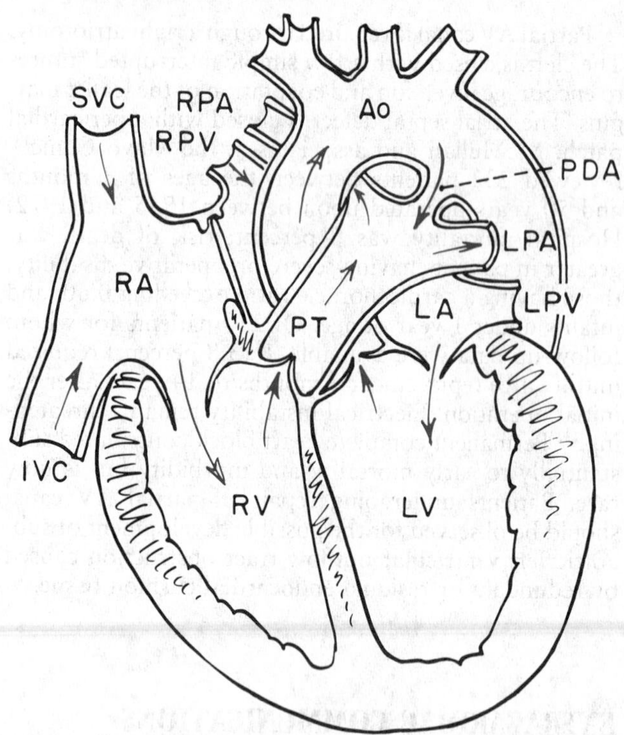

FIGURE 97-12 Patent ductus arteriosus (PDA). SVC = superior vena cava; IVC = inferior vena cava; RA = right atrium; RV = right ventricle; PT = main pulmonary arterial trunk; RPA = right pulmonary artery; LPA = left pulmonary artery; RPV = right pulmonary vein; LPV = left pulmonary vein; LA = left atrium; LV = left ventricle; Ao = aorta. (From *JE Edwards.*[86] *Reproduced with permission from the publisher, editor, and author.*)

In patients with a large patent ductus, the aorta and pulmonary artery are essentially in free communication; the systolic pressure in the pulmonary artery will be equal to that in the aorta. The volume load is on the left ventricle with pulmonary congestion resulting from left ventricular failure. With time, the left ventricle compensates with dilation and hypertrophy to carry the volume load, and the pulmonary vasculature responds to the high pressure. (See preceding section on PAH and PVOD.) The right ventricle is burdened mainly by a pressure load.

If the pulmonary resistance equals or exceeds the resistance of the systemic circulation, there is shunting of unsaturated blood from pulmonary artery to aorta.

Clinical Manifestations

History The history of the mother's pregnancy and of perinatal events may provide clues that are associated with a high incidence of patent ductus arteriosus,[6] such as exposure to rubella in the first trimester by a nonimmunized mother. Patent ductus is also more common in the premature infant, especially those with birth asphyxia or respiratory distress syndrome.[135-137] There is a much higher incidence in females, except in rubella syndrome where the sexes are affected equally.[138]

Symptoms are usually restricted to patients with large shunts that produce heart failure or with other complicating problems, such as respiratory distress in the premature infant. The symptoms related to heart failure were discussed earlier. Heart failure is most likely to develop in the first few weeks or months of life. If it does not appear during infancy, it is unlikely to occur before the third decade. Growth may be affected in those with large shunts and failure. The clinical presentation in the premature infant is usually very different from that in the full-term infant. This is particularly true in those with a birth weight under 1.5 kg, who are more likely to have moderate to severe respiratory distress. In these infants, the clinical features of respiratory distress often blend over the course of several days into those of heart failure. Increasing ventilatory or oxygen requirements with carbon dioxide retention or episodic apnea and bradycardia are often the first signs that a patent ductus may be complicating the picture.

Physical Examination In the full-term infant or child with patent ductus arteriosus, there is frequently a systolic thrill over the pulmonary artery and in the suprasternal notch. The peripheral pulses are generally brisk and bounding, especially with the larger shunts. The patient with elevated pulmonary vascular resistance and shunt reversal will have "differential cyanosis" with cyanosis and clubbing of the toes and occasionally clubbing of the fingers on the left (Plate IV, 10-5 and plate V, 10-6). The apex impulse may be increased or displaced in those with large shunts. The right ventricular impulse is increased in the premature infant with respiratory distress and in infants and children with significant pulmonary hypertension. The typical murmur is a continuous, or "machinery," murmur that is best heard at the left upper sternal border and below the left clavicle. It is usually a rough murmur with eddy sounds, which are helpful in making the diagnosis, and it peaks at or near the second heart sound. In patients with at least a moderate shunt, there is a middiastolic rumble at the apex. The second heart sound may be difficult to hear due to the continuous murmur, but it is usually normal. The pulmonary component will be accentuated in those with pulmonary hypertension. (See also Chap. 11.)

Chest Roentgenogram Findings on chest roentgenogram are also dependent on the magnitude of the shunt. In patients with a small shunt, the chest roentgenogram is normal. With larger shunts, the left atrium and left ventricle are enlarged. Increases in pulmonary arterial flow parallel the magnitude of the shunt. In the presence of heart failure, there are signs of pulmonary edema. In older patients who have developed Eisenmenger physiology, the only abnormality may be marked prominence of the central pulmonary arteries with rapid tapering to the periphery of the lung fields.

Electrocardiogram With a small shunt, the electrocardiogram is normal. Left atrial hypertrophy is probably the most common abnormality found, but left ventricular hypertrophy of the volume overload type, with deep Q waves and increased R-wave voltage in the left precordial leads, is also common. Right ventricular hypertrophy is seen with pulmonary hypertension.

Echocardiogram There is left atrial enlargement, and the left ventricular end-diastolic dimension and mean

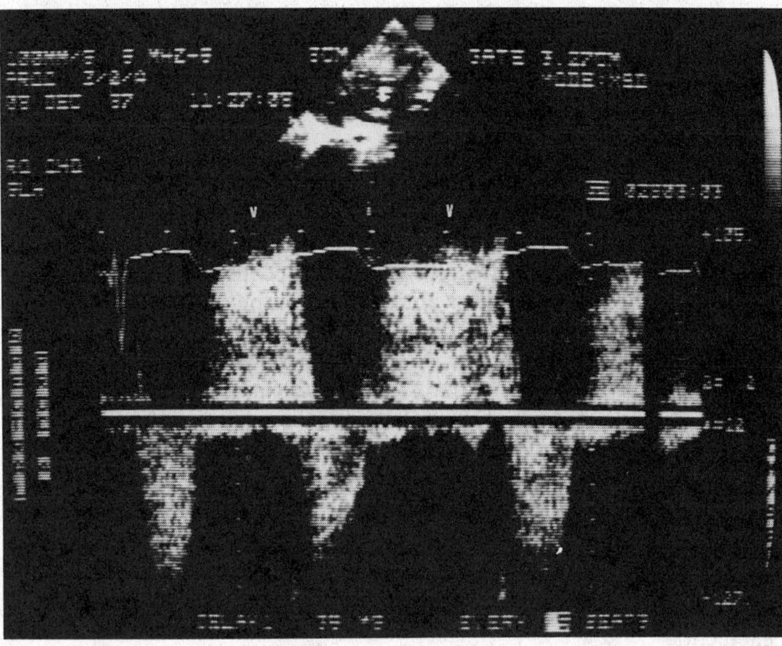

FIGURE 97-13 Pulsed-wave Doppler with spectral display and sampling volume in the pulmonary artery in a patient with a patent ductus arteriosus outlines pandiastolic reversal (*arrows*) of flow with spectral broadening.

velocity of circumferential fiber shortening are significantly increased.[139] Small shunts can be detected with color Doppler imaging[140] with a typical spectral flow pattern (Fig. 97-13), while a larger ductus can be visualized with two-dimensional echocardiography.

Cardiac Catheterization In those with typical, uncomplicated patent ductus, cardiac catheterization is not necessary for diagnosis. When catheterization is performed, the catheter usually passes quite easily from the pulmonary artery to the descending aorta, except when the ductus is too small. The saturation will be increased in the pulmonary artery to a degree relative to the size of the shunt. The pulmonary arterial and right ventricular pressures are elevated in those with a large ductus. The pulmonary vascular resistance will be elevated in older patients who have developed changes in the pulmonary vascular bed. These patients will also have diminished saturation in the descending aorta once the pulmonary resistance reaches a level that will reverse the shunt. Aortography will opacify the ductus and pulmonary arteries.

Natural History and Prognosis[6,134]

The complications related to patent ductus include infective endarteritis, heart failure, and pulmonary hypertension with vascular damage. Infection of the ductus is a risk regardless of its size. The risk increases with length of survival. This can lead to development of a mycotic aneurysm with the potential of compressing the recurrent laryngeal nerve, embolizing septic material to the lungs, or rupturing. Calcification of the ductal wall is common in adults.

In patients with large shunts, heart failure can cause significant morbidity and mortality, particularly in the premature and young infant, and sudden death can occur. Progressive damage to the pulmonary vascular bed can occur in some, but it rarely occurs to an irreversible degree in the first year or two of life. Once irreversible damage occurs, premature death in late adolescence or early adulthood can be anticipated.

Medical Management

Primary prevention results from obstetric measures that decrease the incidence of prematurity and from widespread immunization of children to reduce the number of those born with rubella syndrome. Medical management centers around the symptomatic patients and the prevention of infection of the ductus. The latter is important regardless of the size of the ductus and can be accomplished most effectively in the older infant and child by surgical ligation.

For symptomatic patients, standard medical measures for treatment of heart failure are initiated. Management will be more successful if anemia is also prevented. In the premature infant, attempts to improve oxygenation can promote spontaneous ductus closure. A relation of volume of fluid administration to the incidence of ductus in premature infants has been demonstrated.[141,142]

For those who do not respond to this type of management, alternatives to surgery have been sought, particularly for the higher-risk patients. Transfemoral catheter closure[143,144] has been used successfully. Pharmacologic closure of the ductus in premature infants using inhibitors of prostaglandin synthesis, aspirin and indomethacin, was first reported in 1976.[145,146] Since anatomic closure is delayed beyond functional closure, the ductus may be a recurrent problem in these infants. From a national collaborative study of newborns with birth weights under 1750 g, administration of indomethacin appears to be indicated when other medical treatment fails.[147] Surgical ligation and/or division remains the treatment of choice in many instances since accumulated experience here is great.[148,149]

The current indications for surgery include uncontrollable heart failure in the newborn and young infant, failure to grow properly in association with signs of a significant shunt in the infant, and continued patency with any size of shunt beyond the first 6 months of life. The recommended age for elective surgical ligation is usually 1 to 2 years of age. The tendency in the premature has been toward earlier intervention in attempts to decrease incidence of chronic pulmonary disease. The presence of irreversible pulmonary vascular disease is a contraindication to surgery.

Surgical Management

The patent ductus arteriosus is exposed and mobilized through a small left thoracotomy in the fourth intercostal space.[99] Ductus obliteration is accomplished by division or ligation. A short, broad, or thin-walled ductus is divided between vascular clamps. The ends are closed with continuous suture. A long, narrow, thick-walled ductus can be divided or ligated with two or three sutures spaced a few millimeters apart. The suture ligatures at each end are anchored superficially in the ductus wall to prevent migration and to assure thrombosis and obliteration.

The fragile and thin-walled patent ductus arteriosus of the premature infant is obliterated by gentle ligation with a thick suture to minimize disruption or, if small, by occlusion using metallic surgical clips.[150] Extrapleural exposure is preferred by some surgeons. Ligation in the neonatal intensive care unit, avoiding transport to the operating room, is common. Transport from a remote intensive care unit to a cardiac surgical unit for ductus ligation on a "day-stay" basis is also efficacious.[151] Ductus obliteration offers clinical improvement in infants weighing as little as 500 g, with minimal operative risk, reduced incidence of necrotizing enterocolitis, reduced duration of intubation, and improvement in late survival.[152]

Closure of a patent ductus arteriosus in an adult requires particular caution; calcification and rigidity of the ductus wall complicate clamping. Placement of a Dacron patch over the aortic orifice of the ductus from within the aorta is advisable.[153] (See Chap. 98.)

Mortality for elective closure of uncomplicated patent ductus arteriosus by experienced surgeons is nil. Hemodynamics improve immediately; stroke volume and heart rate fall to nearly normal. Long-term results are excellent, 25-year survival after ductus obliteration exceeding 99 percent.[80] The risk of ductus closure remains somewhat higher in adults; in those patients having an elevated pulmonary vascular resistance the risk may be prohibitive. Death after closure of the ductus is likely within 1 or 2 years in those patients having severe PVOD.[154,155] Single lung transplantation with patent ductus arteriosus ligation offers hope in these otherwise irreversible situations.[156]

Nonsurgical transcatheter closure of patent ductus remains experimental, but the results in the most experienced hands compare favorably with the low mortality and minimal morbidity expected from direct surgical closure.[143–157] Embolization of the occluding device, requiring surgical retrieval in 4 of 190 patients, and a 38 percent incidence of persistent shunting at 1 year indicate that prudence is indicated prior to universal application of transcatheter ductus closure.[158]

Sinus of Valsalva Fistula

Pathology

Sinus of Valsalva fistula is uncommon; it is also referred to as *aortic sinus aneurysm.* Because of an assumed intrinsic weakness at the union of the aorta with the heart, the aortic media may separate from the aortic annulus and retract upward. The structure that lies between becomes aneurysmal and may rupture to form a fistula. The usual sites of the defects are the posterior (noncoronary) sinus aneurysms that rupture through the atrial septal wall into the right atrium (Fig. 97-14*A*) and those of the right sinus that rupture into the right ventricular infundibulum (Fig. 97-14*B*).[86,159,160] The aneurysm is represented by a gray pouch with multiple perforations in the wall. The principal associated condition is a supracristal ventricular septal defect in cases with aneurysms of the right sinus (about 50 percent).

Clinical Manifestations[161]

Sinus of Valsalva fistulas are most common in adults. When the rupture is secondary to bacterial endocarditis,[162] evidence of preceding infection is found. If the rupture occurs slowly, a small fistulous tract into the right atrium or ventricle develops and presents recent-onset findings of a small left-to-right shunt. With sudden rupture, there is usually a tearing pain in the midchest associated with dramatically rapid development of pulmonary congestion due to the sudden onset of a large shunt. Characteristically, the murmur is loud and continuous but heard lower on the chest than the murmur of patent ductus. A to-and-fro murmur rather than a continuous one may be heard at times. The apex impulse is hyperdynamic and the pulse pressure is widened. Ventricular septal defect may complicate the clinical picture.

Cardiac catheterization will confirm the level of the shunt. A pressure difference across the right ventricular outflow tract may be present if the right sinus is involved. Aortography or Doppler echocardiography[163] will confirm the diagnosis.

Natural History and Prognosis

With slow rupture and a small shunt, the major risk is infective endocarditis or extension of the rupture with an increasing shunt. With a large shunt, the heart failure is usually rapidly progressive and may result in death very quickly. A few patients seem to stabilize in this situation.[164]

Medical Management

Appropriate cultures should be drawn and antibiotics begun if endocarditis is suspected. Treatment of heart failure should be instituted rapidly. Because of the natural history, all patients should be corrected surgically.[165]

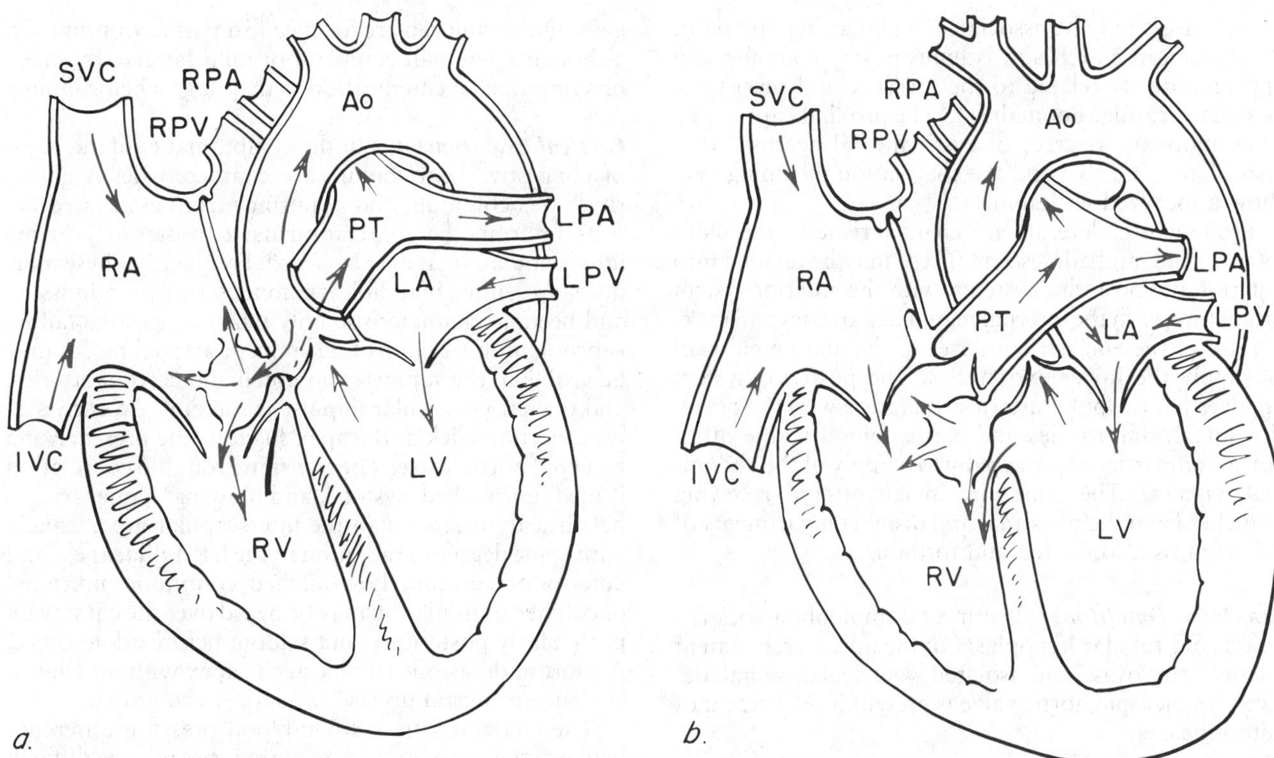

FIGURE 97-14 Sinus of Valsalva fistula. *A.* Aneurysm involves the posterior sinus and ruptures into the right atrium. *B.* Aneurysm involves right aortic sinus and ruptures into the right ventricle. A ventricular septal defect is commonly associated, as illustrated. SVC = superior vena cava; IVC = inferior vena cava; RA = right atrium; RV = right ventricle; PT = main pulmonary arterial trunk; RPA = right pulmonary artery; LPA = left pulmonary artery; RPV = right pulmonary vein; LPV = left pulmonary vein; LA = left atrium; LV = left ventricle; Ao = aorta. (*From JE Edwards.*[86] *Reproduced with permission from the publisher, editor, and author.*)

Surgical Management

Aneurysms or fistulae from the noncoronary or right coronary sinuses are repaired through the aortic root while the patient is supported on total cardiopulmonary bypass with moderate hypothermia using techniques similar to those employed for aortic valve replacement. The aortic valve leaflets, the margins of the aneurysm, and the coronary arterial orifices must be precisely visualized. Aneurysms of the noncoronary sinus can be repaired through the right atrium; those arising from the right coronary sinus are accessible through the right ventricle. In most cases, the orifice of the aneurysmal fistula is surgically obliterated using a Dacron patch.[166]

A conal, or supracristal (type I), ventricular septal defect must be sought and closed through either the aortic valve or the right ventricular outflow tract when an aneurysm of the right coronary sinus extends into the right ventricle. Aortic valve replacement was required to correct associated aortic regurgitation in 24 of 45 patients.[165]

In a review of 176 cases of aortic fistula to the heart, 126 were repaired with success in 108 (86 percent).[167] In another series, correction of ruptured aneurysm of the aortic sinuses was accomplished in 51 patients by exposure through the cardiac chamber into which rupture occurred; survival rate was 88 percent.[168] Improved survival can probably be anticipated on the basis of the 21 patients operated upon at the Mayo Clinic and reviewed in 1971,[169] all of whom survived even though 3 patients required secondary operations to repair dehiscence of the repair.

VALVULAR AND VASCULAR MALFORMATIONS OF THE LEFT SIDE OF THE HEART WITH RIGHT-TO-LEFT, BIDIRECTIONAL, OR NO SHUNT

Coarctation of the Aorta

Pathology

Coarctation of the aorta is a discrete narrowing of the distal segment of the aortic arch. The characteristic lesion is a deformity of the media of the aorta involving the anterior, superior, and posterior walls and is represented by a curtain-like infolding of the wall which causes the lumen to be narrowed and eccentric.[170]

In infants, the lesion lies either opposite the ductus or in a preductal location. In adolescents and adults, it is usually distal to the ligamentum arteriosum. Aberrant right subclavian artery may be associated. In about one-half of such cases the vessel arises proximal to the coarctation and is distal to the coarctation in the other half.[171] In rare cases, the lesion lies proximal to the origin of the left common carotid artery or involves a segment of the abdominal aorta.[172]

The principal cardiac abnormality is left ventricular hypertrophy. In some infants left ventricular endocardial fibroelastosis may be associated. Tubular hypoplasia of the distal aortic arch and isthmus is very common and appears directly related to the presence and severity of associated cardiac anomalies.[173] The proximal aorta may show moderate degrees of cystic medial necrosis. (See also Chap. 123.) Beyond the coarctation the lining may show a localized jet lesion.

Prominent collaterals are characteristic in the older infant, child, and adolescent. These may be divided into anterior and posterior systems, with the anterior system originating with the internal mammary arteries and making use of the epigastric arteries in the abdominal wall to supply the lower extremities. The posterior system involves parascapular arteries connected with the posterior intercostal arteries and carries blood to the distal aortic compartment principally for supply of the abdominal viscera. The anterior spinal artery, receiving branches from the proximal and distal compartments of the aorta, is also dilated and tortuous.

Associated Conditions The most commonly associated defects are tubular hypoplasia of the aortic arch, patent ductus arteriosus, and isolated ventricular septal defect.[174] A bicuspid aortic valve is present in 46 percent of autopsy cases.[171]

Abnormal Physiology

In most instances both the systolic and the diastolic arterial pressures above the coarctation are elevated above normal levels. Below the coarctation, the systolic pressure is lower than that in the upper extremities, and the diastolic pressure usually is near or only slightly below the normal range. The mechanism of upper extremity hypertension appears to involve the increased resistance to aortic flow produced by the coarctation itself, the decreased capacity and distensibility of the vessels into which the left ventricle ejects, and humoral factors.[175]

Clinical Manifestations

This malformation accounts for approximately 8 percent of congenital heart disease in infants and children, ranking behind only ventricular septal defect and patent ductus arteriosus in frequency.[4] Of all individuals born with the coarctation, approximately half present within the first month or two of life with heart failure. About 22 percent of infants so admitted have uncomplicated coarctation, and a similar proportion have a patent ductus. Almost half will have an associated ventricular septal defect.[3] The timing of ductal tissue constriction, both in terms of ductal closure and, perhaps, aortic constriction as well, appears to play a decisive role in the onset or worsening symptoms in most of these patients.[176] The male/female ratio is approximately 3:1 for isolated coarctation but is only 1.1:1 for complicated coarctation. Approximately 45 percent of children with Turner syndrome (Fig. 10-10) have coarctation. Familial occurrence has been described.[176]

History The clinical picture in the symptomatic infant is one of dyspnea, difficulty in feeding, and poor weight gain. Older children are for the most part asymptomatic, although a few will complain of mild fatigue, dyspnea, or symptoms of claudication in their legs when running.

Physical Examination In the symptomatic infant, signs of congestive heart failure are characteristic. A gallop rhythm is common, and a murmur from associated defects or from the coarctation itself (posteriorly in the interscapular area) may be heard. Frequently, these murmurs are either inaudible or nondescript on admission and become characteristic only when congestive failure is brought under control. Prominent arterial pulses may be visible in the suprasternal notch and carotid arteries, and the left ventricular impulse is forceful. An early systolic ejection click at the apex suggests the presence of a bicuspid aortic valve. The murmur from the coarctation is medium-pitched, systolic, and blowing in quality. It is best heard posteriorly in the interscapular area, usually with some degree of radiation to the left axilla, apex, and anterior precordium. Low-pitched, continuous murmurs of collateral circulation may be heard over the chest wall, particularly posteriorly, but seldom before adolescence. A short middiastolic rumble at the apex without clinical evidence of mitral disease is relatively common.

The characteristic systolic blood pressure difference between the upper and lower extremities may be difficult to appreciate or measure in infants with severe congestive failure or with a large ventricular septal defect or ductus. With improved compensation, pulses in the upper extremities become readily palpable. The femoral pulses remain weak, delayed, or absent. In these very young infants, it is important that the pulses in both brachial and carotid arteries be assessed. Weak or absent pulses in all sites are characteristic of critical aortic stenosis or aortic atresia.

In older children and adults, the radial arterial pulses typically are strong; those in the femoral arteries are either diminished, delayed, or absent. A measured systolic pressure difference between the upper and lower extremities is diagnostic. The pulse pressure in the leg is reduced, and in some patients no pressure can be measured by auscultation. Approximately one-third will have mild to severe hypertension, with the latter defined as a systolic pressure above 150 mmHg, a diastolic pressure above 100 mmHg, or both. Some patients have only a mild pressure difference between the arms and legs at rest, but a much larger difference during treadmill exercise. A systolic pressure difference between the two arms suggests that the origin of one subclavian artery is at or below the obstruction.

Chest Roentgenogram For the symptomatic infant, the pattern is one of impressive cardiac enlargement and venous congestion. In the older and asymptomatic child, the heart size is generally at the upper limits of normal with a left ventricular prominence. A figure-three configuration of the left margin of the aorta at the level of the coarctation may be seen in overpenetrated films, with the upper curve formed by the slightly dilated aorta just above the coarctation, the central indentation by the coarctation itself, and the lower curve by the poststenotic dilatation below the coarctation (Fig. 14-1*B*). Notching of the inferior margin of the ribs by tortuous intercostal arteries acting as collaterals is seldom present before 7 or 8 years of age.

Electrocardiogram The electrocardiogram of the symptomatic infant reflects right or biventricular hypertrophy during the first 3 months of life. T-wave inversion in the left precordial leads is common. In older children, the electrocardiogram is usually normal or may indicate mild left ventricular and left atrial hypertrophy.

Echocardiogram Echocardiography is useful in assessing left ventricular function. Two-dimensional echocardiographic imaging of the aortic arch from the suprasternal notch permits visualization of the coarctation and detection of anatomic variations such as isthmic hypoplasia. The precordial and subxiphoid views are of great value in assessing the presence and severity of associated defects. Doppler flow studies are helpful for diagnostic confirmation.[177]

Cardiac Catheterization Study of symptomatic infants characteristically reveals left atrial and left ventricular hypertension and a significant systolic pressure difference between the left ventricle and the femoral artery, particularly if the coarctation is isolated. In the presence of a large ventricular septal defect or patent ductus, the left ventricular hypertension and the systolic pressure difference between the left ventricle and femoral artery is less impressive and may not exist at all. Every attempt should be made to define the nature and severity of associated defects. Aortography is recommended in older children to demonstrate the exact site and length of the coarctation as well as to show unusual features of the collateral circulation that may be of importance to the surgeon. Magnetic resonance imaging (Chap. 136) is an alternative to angiography for demonstrating the site and length of the coarctation (Fig. 97-15).

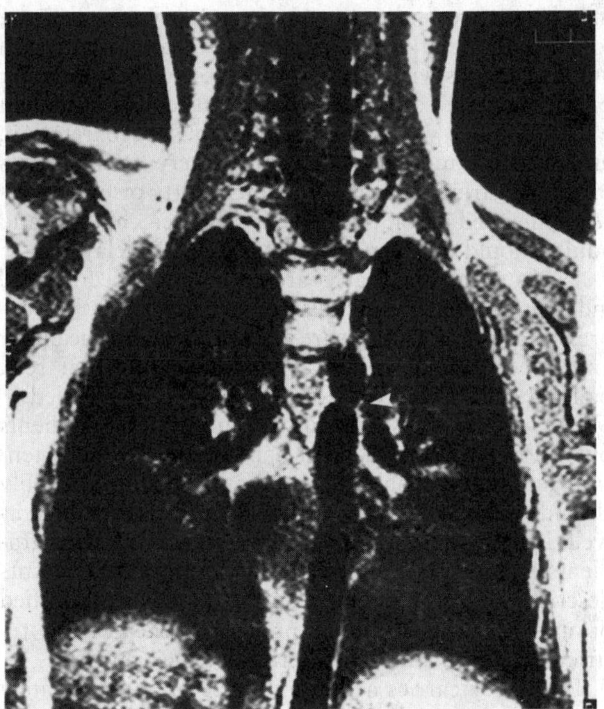

FIGURE 97-15 Selected frame from magnetic resonance imaging study in coronal plane in child with coarctation of the aorta. The proximal aorta is not in the imaging plane, but the isthmus and descending thoracic aorta are clearly imaged with a discrete coarctation (*arrow*) in the common position.

Natural History and Prognosis

Approximately one-fifth of infants admitted with heart failure within the first weeks of life will have coarctation without significant associated defects. The majority of these infants will respond well to medical management and, usually, reach a stage at 2 or 3 years of age where they are indistinguishable from those asymptomatic children of the same age whose coarctation is first detected on a routine physical examination. Upper-extremity hypertension usually increases during the first several months of life and then tends to diminish again as collateral circulation improves, while signs of failure diminish at the same time. For infants with severe failure and any serious associated defects, surgery provides virtually the only chance of survival.

The consequences of persistent hypertension in the individual who has not undergone surgery appear in the second and third decades in the form of aortic rupture or intracranial hemorrhage from an aneurysm of the circle of Willis. Congestive heart failure often complicated by mitral or aortic valve disease, dissecting aneurysm of the aorta, or atherosclerosis is seen in the fourth decade. The risk of endocarditis on the aortic or mitral valves or endarteritis at the site of coarctation appears spread relatively evenly over the years. The average age of death of patients surviving childhood with coarctation without surgery is 34 years.[175] (See Chap. 98.)

Medical Management

Vigorous medical treatment is indicated for infants with severe heart failure. The newborn with severe failure may experience dramatic relief with the intravenous infusion of PGE_1 to reopen the closing ductus.[178] Prompt surgical correction of the coarctation is recommended for all infants in whom there is one or more associated defects and for infants with isolated coarctation unless the response to medical management has been dramatic and sustained. Balloon dilation angioplasty of unoperated coarctation is not currently recommended.[179] The incidence of recoarctation in infants undergoing end-to-end anastomosis or subclavian flap angioplasty of the aorta in the first year of life is in the order of 30 percent.[180] Infants not requiring surgery generally improve steadily despite impressive hypertension in the first months of life.

Residual or recurrent hypertension among patients without demonstrable recurrent coarctation, renal disease, or significant aortic regurgitation appears related to the duration of hypertension prior to surgery. This complication seems rare among individuals operated upon before the age of 6 years but becomes progressively more common as surgery is delayed and may be present in from 45 to 50 percent of individuals operated upon at 20 years of age or beyond.[181]

Elective correction of coarctation is now recommended between the ages of 1 and 4 years in order to avoid the relatively high rate of recoarctation found among patients with coarctation corrected before 1 year of age and the complication of persistent or recurrent hypertension, without demonstrable recoarctation, among those individuals having surgery after 6 years of age. Restriction from strenuous sports or exercise is recommended prior to correction. Older children and adults should undergo correction without delay.

Patients who have had coarctation should be followed indefinitely. For those with significant recoarctation, expressed as a systolic pressure gradient between the upper and lower extremities of 20 mmHg or more at rest, balloon angioplasty or reoperation is recommended.[182] Those who have insignificant or small resting gradients but who manifest abnormal upper-extremity hypertension and significant gradients with exercise probably should undergo balloon angioplasty or reoperation as well. Patients with persistent hypertension without gradients either at rest or with exercise and those patients described above in whom reoperation seems unjustified or unduly hazardous will probably benefit from restricted activity and antihypertensive medication.

Pregnancy carries a mortality rate of approximately 10 percent and a complication rate of 90 percent among women with uncorrected coarctation. After correction, the mortality rate does not differ significantly from the normal, while complications are on the order of 15 percent.[183] The risk of congenital heart disease in the offspring of one affected parent or in a sibling of a single affected family member is estimated at 2 percent, with about a 50 percent chance of the defect being coarctation.[184]

Surgical Management

Coarctation of the aorta should be eliminated in all symptomatic infants and in asymptomatic children by the age of 4 years.[185,186] If the patient does not come to medical attention until later in life, relief of obstruction is still advisable, but long-term outcome is less favorable.[187] Repair by subclavian flap aortoplasty in the first year of life probably offers the greatest likelihood of cure, although the choice of specific operation in infancy remains controversial.[180,188]

The coarctation is exposed and mobilized through a left thoracotomy. It is usually possible to resect the narrow segment and restore continuity by direct end-to-end anastomosis (Fig. 97-16). Occasionally a tubular vascular prosthesis is required to bridge the gap between the two ends of the aorta when the coarctation is unusually long, the aortic isthmus is hypoplastic, or there is an associated aneurysm. In adults with a relatively nonelastic or calcified aorta and in secondary repairs, a tubular vascular prosthesis can be used to bypass the unresected coarctation or the previous repair.[189] The child having Turner syndrome (Fig. 10-10) appears to be at greater risk of perioperative hemorrhage and suture-line compli-

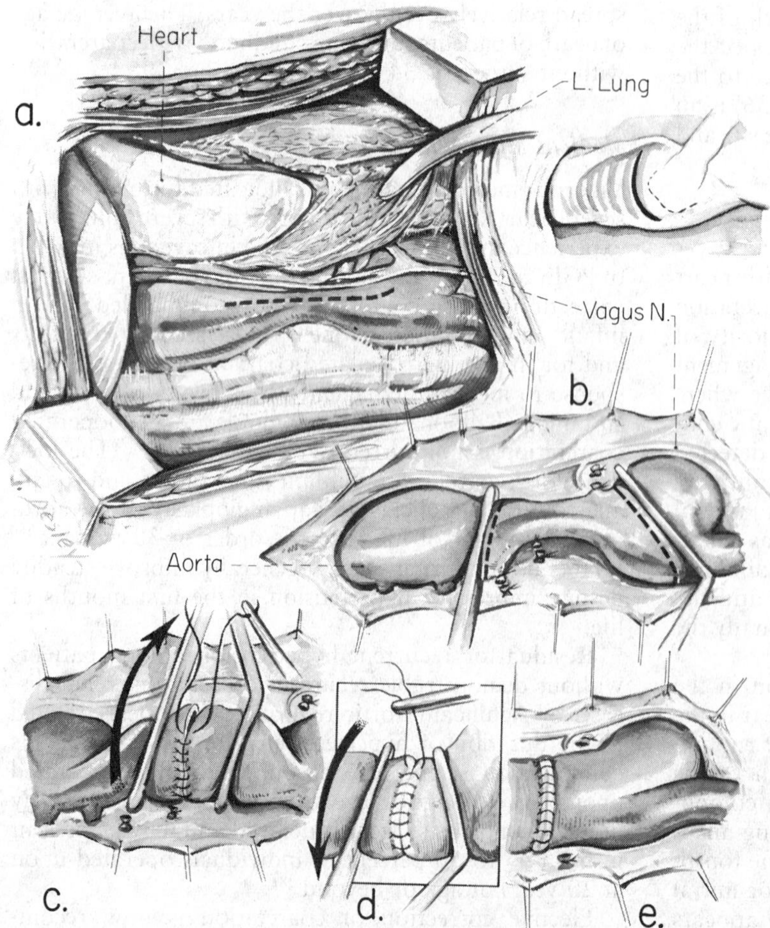

FIGURE 97-16 Steps in operative repair of coarctation of aorta. *A.* Mediastinal pleura is opened over the upper part of the descending thoracic aorta. *B.* After appropriate mobilization of the coarctate area and division of ligamentum arteriosum, appropriate clamps are placed above and below the stricture. At times the distal clamp must be placed farther downstream than is shown here, and then the intercostal arteries are temporarily controlled with bulldog clamps. *C, D,* and *E.* End-to-end anastomosis is made with interrupted simple suture of no. 5-0 silk. (*This illustration appeared originally in the first edition of The Heart, in 1966, and in all subsequent editions. It is reproduced here by courtesy of Dr. John W. Kirklin, Birmingham, Alabama.*)

cations because of friability of the thin-walled aorta.[190] Tension-free suture lines are essential. Postoperative bleeding, chylothorax, paraplegia, and injury to the phrenic and recurrent laryngeal nerves remain potential complications.

The infant and small child with coarctation pose unique problems. Although early repair is desirable, growth of a circular suture line at the site of an end-to-end anastomosis will probably not be adequate. The use of the subclavian arterial flap aortoplasty[191] or Dacron patch aortoplasty[192] (Fig. 97-17) and absorbable sutures[193] is anticipated to reduce the incidence of recoarctation but not to eliminate it. Dacron patch repair of coarctation in older children has an unacceptably high incidence of late aneurysm formation and is no longer advised.[191] Transluminal balloon angioplasty has been applied in the management of coarctation and restenosis.[194–196]

If a significant ventricular septal defect is also present, a pulmonary arterial band is placed at the time of coarctation repair during infancy. The ventricular septal defect is then repaired electively during the following several months when the child's congestive heart failure is well controlled. Alternatively, ventricular septal defect closure following shortly after [197,198] or simultaneously with coarctation repair has been advocated.[199]

Adequacy of collateral circulation is crucial for safe repair of coarctation. A rise in proximal systemic arterial pressure of more than 20 mmHg when the aorta is clamped above the coarctation suggests a marginal collateral circulation. Pressure in the descending aorta can be measured, and, if necessary, cardiopulmonary bypass or a shunt can be used to provide adequate distal perfusion.[200,201] Mild systemic hypothermia is a simple and useful adjunct for spinal cord preservation. Aortic occlusion time should obviously be kept to a minimum, but neurologic sequelae have occurred regardless of the methods used to maintain distal perfusion. Monitoring of somatosensory cortical evoked potentials may warn of impending ischemic insult to the spinal cord.[202]

Postoperative paradoxical hypertension is common between the 2d and 10th postoperative days and may contribute to the postcoarctation syndrome in which ileus, abdominal pain, mesenteric vasculitis, and even visceral infarction can occur. This syndrome is not encountered if the postoperative diastolic blood pressure is maintained within normal range for age with sodium nitroprusside, propranolol, or captopril and if nasogastric tube decompression of the gastrointestinal tract is maintained postoperatively for 48 h. Preoperative treatment with propranolol appears to prevent paradoxical hypertension following repair of coarctation.[203]

Operative mortality was 4 percent for infants with isolated coarctation and 25 percent when other cardiovascular defects were present in 191 infants undergoing coarctation repair before the age of 1 year.[204] There were no subsequent deaths in hospital survivors with isolated coarctation, but the 5-year mortality rate for those having other associated cardiac anomalies was an additional 25 percent. Recurrent coarctation occurred in 54 percent of survivors within 7 years. Hypertension was present in 27 percent of children followed more than 5 years after repair. Very small size of infant, presence of major associ-

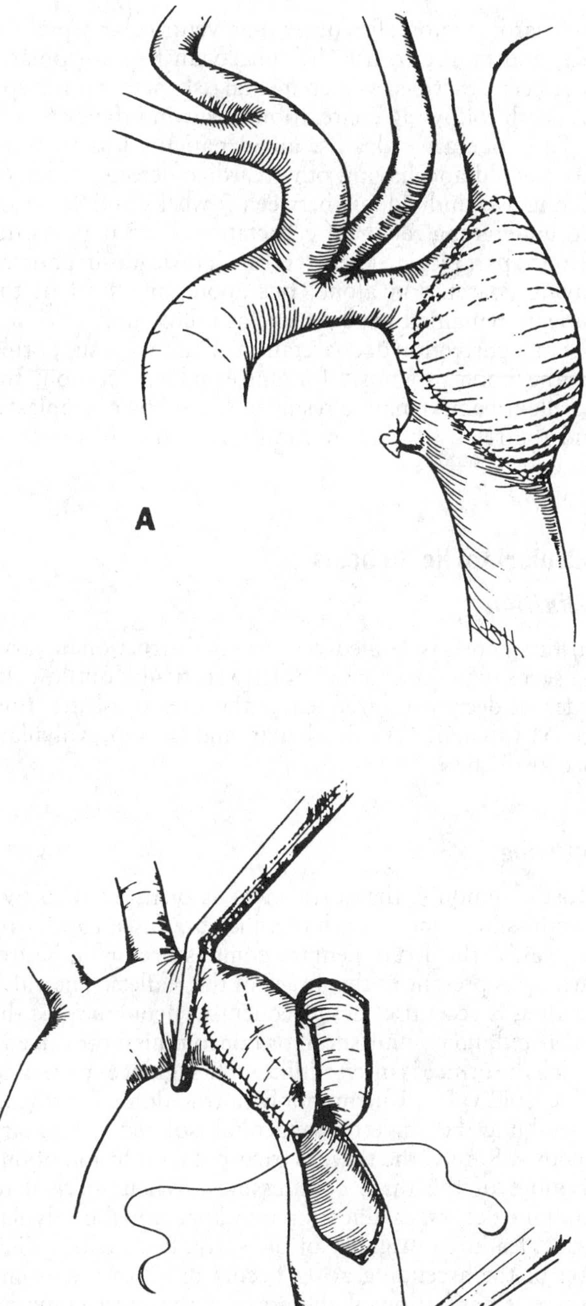

FIGURE 97-17 *A.* Coarctation repair using Dacron patch angioplasty. A longitudinal incision extends from the normal aorta below the coarctation to a point well above the coarctation on the subclavian artery. A relatively large patch is cut from a Dacron tube graft and is sutured across the coarctation after excision of any intraluminal membrane. Circular suture lines are thus avoided. The patch is large, allowing for growth. *B.* Repair of coarctation of the aorta by subclavian arterial flap angioplasty. The subclavian artery is divided in the apex of the left pleural cavity. The lateral wall of the artery is incised downward, the incision continuing across the coarctation onto normal aorta below. The flap thus created is sutured across the coarctation, after excision of intraluminal membrane, using fine, continuous monofilament suture. Circular suture lines are avoided. The viable flap should grow as the child and aorta grow, minimizing recurrent coarctation. (*From Herrmann VM, Laks H, Fagan L, et al: Repair of aortic coarctation in the first year of life. Ann Thorac Surg 25:57, 1978. Reproduced with permission of the publisher and authors.*)

ated cardiac anomalies other than ventricular septal defect, and failure to use the subclavian flap aortoplasty have been described as incremental risk factors for hospital death following coarctation repair in infancy.[205]

Four operative deaths, all in patients less than 14 months old and having other cardiac defects, occurred among 182 individuals between 3 weeks and 60 years old undergoing repair of coarctation. Two patients developed paraplegia. There were no late deaths in patients having coarctation alone, but about one-third of the patients remained hypertensive at follow-up.[185]

Early correction of coarctation in infancy is supported by the poor prognosis for untreated coarctation, the excellent hemodynamic results achieved by aortoplasty, and the relatively low mortality rate and incidence of restenosis.[180]

Valvular Aortic Stenosis

Definition

Aortic stenosis is defined as subtotal obstruction of varying severity in the channel of left ventricular outflow. In order of decreasing frequency, the sites of obstruction are (1) valvular, (2) subvalvular, and (3) supravalvular. (See also Chap. 79.)

Pathology

Most commonly, the aortic valve is bicuspid with two commissures, one or both of which are fused to varying degrees. A third rudimentary commissure or raphe frequently is present in the larger of the leaflets. The valve opening is eccentric. Less frequently encountered is the unicuspid, unicommissural, or noncommissural valve in which the orifice is often slitlike, at first glance suggesting a bicuspid valve. Uncommonly, a true dome is present, resembling the valve of congenital isolated pulmonary stenosis. Rarely, the valve is tricuspid with fusion of one or more of the three commissures. When survival to adult life occurs, calcification may appear in the valvular tissue, leading to rigidity of the valve. Poststenotic dilation of the ascending aorta occurs in all case to some degree. Coarctation of the aorta is the most common associated anomaly.

Abnormal Physiology

The hemodynamics of congenital valvular aortic stenosis are similar to those of acquired aortic stenosis (Chap. 79) except that a persistent ductus arteriosus or stretched foramen ovale in the immediate postnatal period may lessen the severity of pulmonary edema by diverting blood away from the left ventricle.

Severity usually is judged by the peak systolic pressure gradient across the aortic valve, determined at cardiac catheterization, and the calculated aortic valve area. In the presence of a normal cardiac output, a peak systolic gradient of 75 mmHg or more or an aortic valve area of less than 0.5 cm^2/m^2 is considered severe; a gradient between 50 and 75 mmHg or a valve area between 0.5 and 0.8 cm^2/m^2 is considered moderate; a gradient of less than 50 mmHg or a valve area greater than 0.9 cm^2/m^2 is considered mild.[206] (See also Chaps. 79 and 98.)

Clinical Manifestations

About 7 percent of infants and children with congenital heart disease have aortic stenosis in one of its several forms, and approximately 80 percent of these patients have valvular aortic stenosis. Valvular stenosis is much more common among males than females, in a ratio of 4:1.

History The detection of a systolic murmur leads to the discovery of this malformation in most patients, the vast majority of whom are asymptomatic. Easy fatigue, dyspnea, syncope, or angina suggest severe obstruction, but severe obstruction may exist in the absence of any symptoms. Sudden death may occur from this malformation, but in most such cases death is preceded by either symptoms or electrocardiographic changes. Infants with critical stenosis from birth present with congestive failure within the first week or two of life and represent true emergencies. A similar small number of patients with less critical but still very severe obstruction are detected over the course of the next 4 to 6 months.

Physical Examination The arterial blood pressure and the quality of the peripheral arterial pulses of the older infant and child usually are normal. A measured pulse pressure of less than 20 mmHg suggests severe stenosis. The cardiac apex impulse may be forceful and sustained, and a systolic thrill along the upper sternal border and over the carotid arteries is present in about 90 percent of patients. The absence of such a thrill at the right upper sternal border suggests a systolic pressure gradient of 30 mmHg or less. Paradoxical splitting of the second heart sound is rare and is associated either with very severe obstruction or with coexisting myocardial disease. An early systolic ejection click at the apex is characteristic and serves to distinguish valvular aortic stenosis from other forms of left ventricular outflow tract obstruction. The classic auscultatory finding is a harsh systolic spindle-shaped murmur, loudest at the right upper sternal border with radiation into the carotid arteries and down the left sternal border to the apex. (See also Chap. 11.) Among infants with critical obstruction there may be no palpable peripheral pulses and no distinctive murmur, with a return of weak pulses and typical murmur only after decongestive therapy.

Chest Roentgenogram The overall heart size is normal, but infants with failure will have generalized cardiac enlargement and varying degrees of pulmonary edema. Poststenotic dilatation of the ascending aorta is characteristic.

Electrocardiogram Left ventricular hypertrophy, as indicated by voltage criteria in the left precordial leads, seldom is helpful in distinguishing those patients with severe obstruction from those with mild to moderate obstruction. On the other hand, diminished anterior forces in the right precordial leads and a deep SV_1 of 30 mm or more suggests severe stenosis, as does absence of the Q wave in V_6. Fifty percent of patients with severe obstruction have a flat, biphasic, or inverted T wave in V_6 (Fig. 97-18). Severe and even critical obstruction may be present with none of the electrocardiographic abnormalities mentioned above. Monitoring of the ST segment in leads V_5 through V_7 during cautious exercise testing appears to be a reliable method of detecting those children in whom a significant pressure gradient (greater than 50 mmHg) has developed and in whom that gradient might represent a threat of sudden death.[207] Symptomatic infants may show right, left, or biventricular hypertrophy, frequently with T-wave inversion over the left precordium.

Echocardiogram Continuous wave Doppler echocardiography guided by two-dimensional echocardiographic imaging predicts very accurately the systolic pressure gradient across discrete forms of left ventricular outflow tract obstruction. (Chaps. 15 and 130.) Two-dimensional echocardiography can distinguish valvular from supravalvular or subvalvular obstruction and identify those critically ill infants in whom the size of the left ventricle, mitral valve annulus, or aortic root is hypoplastic to a degree that would preclude survival.[208]

Cardiac Catheterization Infants symptomatic with severe aortic obstruction often have a left-to-right shunt through a stretched foramen ovale, PAH, and a right-to-left shunt through a patent ductus arteriosus. A marked increase in left ventricular end-diastolic pressure usually is present. The systolic pressure gradient between the left ventricle and the central aorta artery should be documented whenever possible. If left ventricular output is markedly diminished, this gradient may be relatively small, even in the presence of severe obstruction. Left ventricular angiography will confirm the site of obstruction and outline the size of the left ventricular cavity.

In older infants and children pressures on the right side of the heart usually are normal. Simultaneous recording of central aortic and left ventricular pressures or a pressure tracing upon catheter withdrawal from the left ventricle to the aorta, coupled with an accurate estimate of cardiac output, are necessary for reliable assessment of severity. Left ventricular angiography will document the site of obstruction. The aortic leaflets typically will be thickened and domed, with a central or eccentric jet of contrast material entering the ascending aorta. Poststenotic dilatation is characteristic. Supravalvular aortography is recommended to assess the presence and severity of aortic regurgitation.

Natural History and Prognosis

About half the infants born with severe valvular aortic stenosis are symptomatic enough to require hospitalization within the first week of life. The remainder develop congestive failure over the course of the next 6 months. Not uncommonly, the murmur is mistaken for that of a ventricular septal defect. Failure beyond infancy and before adolescence is not usually seen without the presence of complicating factors. Symptomatic infants require prompt relief of obstruction, either by balloon or surgical valvotomy, but the mortality remains significant. Endocardial fibroelastosis, papillary muscle necrosis, associated intra- and extracardiac deformities, and a small left ventricular cavity contribute to this mortality. Survivors may have significant aortic regurgitation, but the majority can be managed medically until such time as valve replacement is feasible.

Most infants and children with milder degrees of aortic valvular stenosis will demonstrate a gradual progression in the severity of the systolic pressure gradient during childhood. The appearance of symptoms or the development of a left ventricular "strain" pattern in the

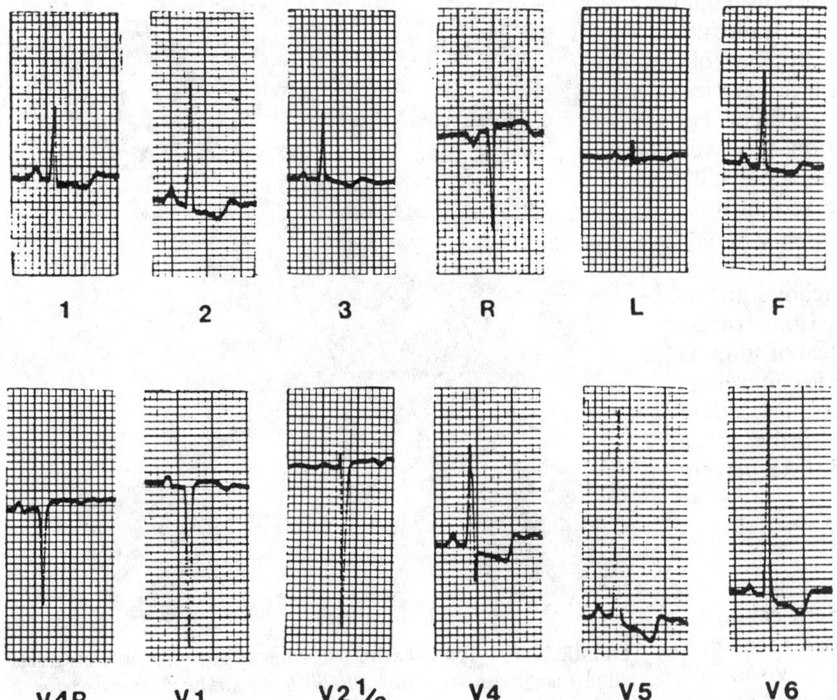

FIGURE 97-18 Electrocardiogram from an 8-year-old boy with valvular aortic stenosis and a 94-mmHg peak systolic pressure gradient. The small anterior QRS forces, abnormally large posterior forces, absent Q waves in leads V_5 and V_6, and abnormal T waves and ST segments reflect severe left ventricular systolic pressure overload with ischemia.

electrocardiogram can be expected in about 40 percent of children followed over a 4- to 8-year period, including some with mild gradients at the outset. Sudden death is a very uncommon but definite threat to those with at least a moderate gradient.[206] Infective endocarditis on the aortic valve (Chap. 94) poses an extremely serious complication in the form of systemic arterial emboli and the production of serious, sometimes catastrophic, aortic regurgitation with congestive failure, shock, and death.

Medical Management

Infants with the characteristic murmur detected in the first weeks of life should be evaluated very carefully to be certain the obstruction is not severe. Those who develop heart failure should be operated upon or undergo balloon valvuloplasty without delay. In the critically ill neonate, intravenous PGE_1 infusion to open the ductus may provide temporary relief of pulmonary edema en route to the operating room or the catheterization laboratory. Beyond infancy, a plan of reexamination with careful questioning regarding symptoms and an electrocardiogram each year, an echocardiogram with Doppler assessment of the pressure gradient every 2 years, and exercise testing about every 3 years should suffice to prevent progression from going unrecognized. Indications for cardiac catheterization include the appearance of symptoms or syncope, an arterial pulse pressure of less than 20 mmHg on physical examination, cardiac enlargement by chest roentgenogram, small anterior forces with an SV_1 of 30 mm or more or flattening or inversion of the T wave in V_6 in the resting electrocardiogram, abnormal ST-T segments on exercise testing, or an estimated systolic pressure gradient of 50 mmHg or a mean pressure gradient of 27 mmHg or more by echocardiographic Doppler techniques.[209] Transluminal catheter balloon valvuloplasty (CBV) has become an alternative to surgery. In skilled hands, it can provide effective reduction of the transvalvular gradient while producing only a mild increment in aortic regurgitation in most instances.[210] Elective balloon dilation is recommended if the systolic pressure gradient is greater than 50 mmHg at catheterization and aortic regurgitation is mild or nonexistent. For the neonate with critical valvular obstruction, however, we continue to rely on surgical intervention, but CBV has become a very competitive alternative and, in some institutions, the procedure of choice for these very sick infants.

Children with more than mild aortic stenosis are restricted from strenuous organized athletics, isometric exercises, and activities that require a good deal of stamina and produce shortness of breath. For genetic counseling, the risk of congenital heart disease is estimated at 3 percent for a subsequent sibling and offspring of an affected father, but it may be as high as 13 to 18 percent for the offspring of an affected mother.[114]

Surgical Management[211]

When surgical intervention is required for critical aortic stenosis during infancy, the heart is exposed through a median sternotomy and the aortic valve is visualized through the ascending aorta during a brief period of low-flow perfusion with moderate hypothermia.[212,213] Standard cardiopulmonary bypass, mild hypothermia, and cardioplegia are used in older children.[214,215] The surgeon must discriminate between true commissures and abortive raphes, incision of the latter producing intolerable aortic valvular regurgitation. Relief of aortic valvular stenosis is accomplished by a carefully placed incision in the middle of each fused but well-supported true commissure (Fig. 97-19).[216]

A conservative attitude is essential during operation for aortic stenosis in the infant or small child. Moderate residual stenosis is preferred to intolerable aortic valvular regurgitation in infants, in whom prosthetic aortic valve implantation is technically difficult; reoperation will be required in a short while since the small prosthesis obviously does not grow with the infant. Mild valvular regurgitation almost always occurs consequent to commissurotomy but is usually well tolerated. In fact, the left ventricular cavity may develop somewhat more normally in the presence of slight valvular regurgitation.

Secondary valvotomy for recurrent or residual stenosis can be attempted,[217] but calcification and restenosis eventually force aortic valve replacement in almost all those requiring surgery on the aortic valve in infancy or childhood.[218] We prefer to salvage the child's own valve for as long as possible since an ideal valve substitute for pediatric use does not exist.[219] Reconstruction using a cryopreserved valve-containing aortic homograft with implantation of the coronary arteries as buttons when valve replacement is necessary is preferred in the small infant. A larger effective orifice can be achieved and anticoagulation is not required.

The risk of surgery is high in critically ill infants, particularly those having a low ejection fraction, high left ventricular end-diastolic pressure, endocardial fi-

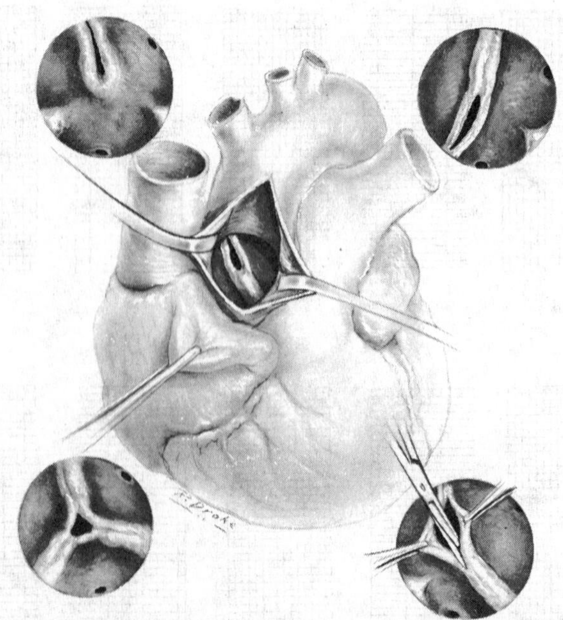

FIGURE 97-19 Types of valvular deformities in patients with congenital valvular aortic stenosis. (*From FH Ellis Jr, JW Kirklin.*[216] *Reproduced with permission from the publisher and authors.*)

broelastosis, marked congestive heart failure, systemic acidosis, and associated small mitral valve.[220,221] Survival in these infants is minimally influenced by choice of surgical approach—visualization directly through the aorta or indirectly by transventricular dilatation with instrument or balloon catheter.[222]

Survival and eventual outcome depend upon the degree to which stenosis can be relieved without creation of intolerable valvular regurgitation and the size of the left ventricle. If the aortic valve has a tricuspid configuration, a good result can be anticipated. Satisfactory results with some reduction in left ventricular pressure are usually obtained even when the valve is bicuspid, but moderate aortic regurgitation is usually present postoperatively. A unicommissural valve orifice cannot be surgically enlarged without creation of severe valvular regurgitation.

A small aortic annulus severely limits the degree to which left ventricular hypertension can be relieved without resorting to Konno's operation, in which the annulus is divided, a ventricular septal defect is created and patched with prosthetic material, a prosthetic or homograft aortic valve is implanted,[223,224] and the ascending aorta and anterior right ventricular wall are reconstructed using a prosthetic graft.

Morbidity following aortic valvotomy in the older child is rare, and the likelihood for relief of left ventricular outflow tract obstruction and survival is good, even after secondary operations.[225,226] Aortic valvotomy, however, must be considered palliation, with only 92 percent of 59 patients remaining free of a serious event (death, reoperation, or endocarditis) 5 years after operation and only 39 percent remaining free of such an event 22 years after surgery.[227]

Subvalvular Aortic Stenosis

Pathology

Three classic varieties of subvalvular aortic stenosis involve the left ventricular outflow tract. These are the discrete, the tunnel, and the muscular types. The *discrete type* is characterized by a localized fibrous encirclement of the left ventricular outflow tract a short distance below the aortic valve. The fibromuscular tissue usually extends onto the mitral leaflet and may also attach to the aortic cusps.[228] The *tunnel type* involves hypoplasia of the aortic annulus and a channel with a fibrous lining in the subjacent left ventricular outflow tract.[229] The *muscular type* is also known as hypertrophic cardiomyopathy (or idiopathic hypertrophic subaortic stenosis) and is discussed in Chap. 90.

More than half the patients have associated malformations, of which patent ductus, ventricular septal defect, or coarctation are most common.[230]

Clinical Manifestations

Discrete stenosis is more frequent among males, with a male/female ratio of approximately 2.5:1. In the isolated forms, the majority of patients are referred because of the detection of a murmur which, not uncommonly, is mistaken initially for that of a ventricular septal defect. Symptoms have the same implications as they do for valvular aortic stenosis.

The physical examination is similar to that of valvular aortic stenosis with two exceptions: an early systolic ejection click is not heard and an early diastolic murmur of aortic regurgitation is present in approximately one-half of these patients.

The roentgenographic features and electrocardiogram are also similar to those of valvular aortic stenosis except for absence of poststenotic dilatation of the ascending aorta. Two-dimensional echocardiography permits excellent visualization of the anatomy of the obstruction.[112] Estimation of the systolic pressure gradient can be obtained from Doppler echocardiographic studies.

At catheterization, a careful pullback pressure tracing across the left ventricular outflow tract will document the severity of the gradient and establish the site of the obstruction. Left ventricular biplane angiography will outline the nature of the obstruction.[231] Aortography is recommended to evaluate the degree of aortic regurgitation.

Natural History and Prognosis

Severe congestive failure in infancy is unusual and, if present, is almost invariably associated with complicating defects.[229] The obstruction is progressive in most instances, sometimes rapidly so. Associated aortic regurgitation also tends to be progressive and appears to result from damage from the jet of blood through the obstruction with secondary thickening and deformity of the valve leaflets. Results of surgery depend on the extent of involvement of the left ventricular outflow tract, with the best results being obtained in patients with a thin, discrete subvalvular membrane. The least satisfactory results occur in patients with tunnel obstruction.

Medical Management

Medical management is similar to that of patients with valvular aortic stenosis, but surgery for the discrete type usually is recommended for pressure gradients of 30 mmHg or more because of the possibility of rapid progression of obstruction, the likelihood of progressive aortic valvular deformity and regurgitation, and the likelihood of complete and lasting relief if the membrane can be removed in its entirety. The role, if any, of percutaneous catheter balloon dilation for this lesion is unclear.[232]

Continued follow-up for assessment of reobstruction and progression of aortic regurgitation and for reemphasis of the precautions against infective endocarditis is essential in all patients.

Surgical Management[211]

Subvalvular fibromuscular (membranous) left ventricular outflow tract obstruction is exposed through the aortic root as described for aortic valvular stenosis (Fig. 97-20).[233] A nasal speculum, a transparent glass ear speculum, and small flat retractors protect the aortic valve leaflets. Small half-circle needles and sutures or hooks are placed into the abnormal fibromuscular tissue, pulling it into view for precise excision from the underlying

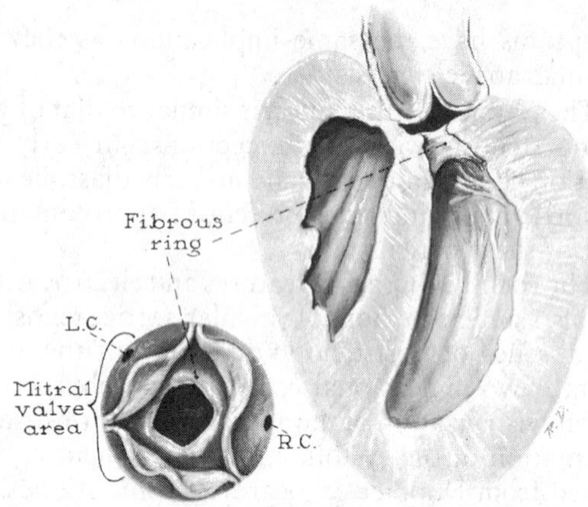

FIGURE 97-20 Localized subvalvular aortic stenosis. Obstruction is immediately upstream from the aortic valve. (*From JW Kirklin, FH Ellis Jr.*[233] *Reproduced by permission of the American Heart Association, Inc., and the authors.*)

ventricular septum and the anterior mitral valve leaflet. The area of the bundle of His, usually just beneath the anterior commissure between the right and noncoronary leaflets, is avoided.[234,235] An additional septal myectomy or myotomy beneath and to the left of the commissure between the right and left leaflets may be required if secondary hypertrophy is significant. An associated ventricular septal defect, if present, is closed with a small patch secured with continuous suture to prevent secondary obstruction from pledgets.[236] Immediate and early operative outcome is generally good, but residual, recurrent, and progressive subaortic obstruction occurs in up to 25 percent of patients,[211] demanding long-term follow-up.[229,237]

Diffuse tunnel obstruction in the left ventricular outflow tract poses a difficult technical problem requiring aortoseptoplasty (Konno's operation or a modification thereof), reconstruction of the left ventricular outflow tract using a cryopreserved valve-containing aortic homograft, or insertion of a valve-containing conduit from the apex of the left ventricle to the lower thoracic or abdominal aorta.[238,239]

Supravalvular Aortic Stenosis

Pathology

The obstruction in the ascending aorta includes the following three types: (1) hourglass, (2) hypoplastic, and (3) membranous. Associated obstructions in the pulmonary trunk, peripheral pulmonary artiers, and branches of the aortic arch are common. Hypertrophy of the coronary arterial walls and premature coronary atherosclerosis have been described.

Clinical Manifestations

Supravalvular stenosis may be familial, associated with characteristic facies and mental retardation, sporadic, or (rarely) the result of congenital rubella. All forms may be, and usually are, associated with varying degrees of peripheral or branch pulmonary arterial stenosis. The familial form is transmitted as an autosomal dominant trait with variable expression. Mental retardation is not present, and there are no characteristic facial features.[240] Supravalvular aortic stenosis associated with mental retardation, frequently called *Williams syndrome,* is sporadic and associated with a high and prominent forehead, epicanthal folds, underdevelopment of the bridge of the nose and mandible, and a broad, overhanging upper lip (Fig. 10-25). It has been linked with idiopathic hypercalcemia of infancy, but in the majority of patients recognized beyond infancy hypercalcemia is not present.[241]

The symptoms of supravalvular aortic stenosis are similar to those of subvalvular aortic stenosis. Patients with the familial form usually have a distinctive family history, but one which seldom emerges in its entirety on initial questioning. The physical findings are also similar to subvalvular aortic stenosis, although a systolic blood pressure difference may be recorded between the two arms on occasion, with the right arm pressure being greater than the left. Chest roentgenogram and electrocardiogram are not distinctive unless associated pulmonary arterial stenosis leads to right ventricular hypertrophy. Echocardiography can identify the narrowed aortic lumen just above the aortic valve and provide an estimate of the severity of the obstruction in terms of the Doppler-derived instantaneous pressure gradient.[240]

At cardiac catheterization, a systolic pressure gradient can be demonstrated just above the aortic valve by careful pullback. Supravalvular aortography or left ventricular angiography will visualize the supravalvular narrowing. Pressure recordings in the branch pulmonary arteries should be obtained, and pulmonary arterial angiography performed in the presence of any significant stenoses.

Natural History and Prognosis

The sequence of progressive obstruction, the appearance of symptoms and electrocardiographic changes, and the possibility of sudden death appears to apply for supravalvular aortic stenosis as well as for valvular aortic stenosis. Infective endocarditis represents a threat to these patients throughout life.

Medical Management

The indications for cardiac catheterization and surgery are the same as for valvular aortic stenosis.

Surgical Management[211]

Discrete supravalvular aortic stenosis is relieved by one or more incisions through the narrow segment of the ascending aorta, usually at the level of the sinotubular ridge at the top of the commissures. Incisions are extended well down into the aortic sinuses (Fig. 97-21).[242] Ridges of obstructing fibrous tissue are excised. The aorta is enlarged by the insertion of a gusset of prosthetic vascular graft material or pericardium to increase the circumference.[243] Rigidity and fibrous thickening of the aortic wall may prevent the aorta from opening up adequately even after insertion of the usual oval gusset in the noncoronary sinus of Valsalva. In this situation, an

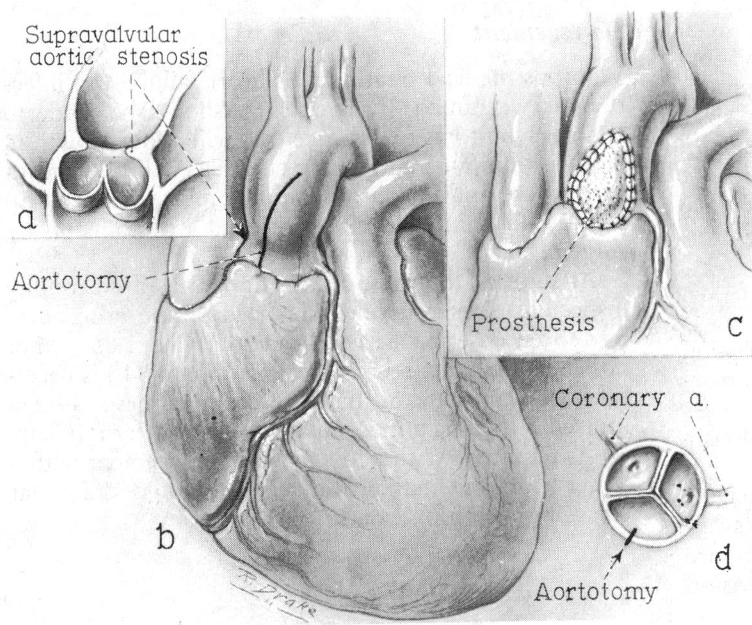

FIGURE 97-21 *A* to *D*. Supravalvular aortic stenosis and its repair. Obstruction is almost diaphragmatic in nature (*A*) and is not easily recognized externally (*B*). The complete repair is shown (*C*). (*From DC McGoon et al.*[242] *Reproduced with permission from the publisher and authors.*)

extended aortoplasty in which the fibrous ring is incised at two points and the aorta augmented with a pants-shaped tailored Dacron prosthesis is used.[244] A favorable outcome can be anticipated postoperatively in most patients having supravalvular aortic stenosis if the arterial wall abnormality is localized.

Diffuse tubular hypoplasia of the ascending aorta is a technically challenging problem associated with a high mortality and poor postoperative hemodynamic results.[245,246] Use of a conduit from the apex of the left ventricle to the descending or abdominal aorta is appealing,[247] although most attempts at repair have used an extensive prosthetic or homograft enlargement of the ascending aorta.[248] Intimal obstruction of the coronary arterial ostia may require debridement, dilatation, or even saphenous vein bypass grafting.[246]

Bicuspid Aortic Valve

Pathology

Classically, the two cusps are oriented anteriorly and posteriorly, the anterior or conjoined cusp being the larger. A raphe, or ridge, is present along the aortic aspect of the larger cusp running from the aortic wall to the free edge of the cusp. The most common associated condition of significance is coarctation of the aorta. The most common complication is calcification of the valve. In about 85 percent of cases of calcific aortic stenosis below the age of 70, the fundamental valve is congenitally bicuspid. Aortic regurgitation from prolapse of the larger cusp is a less common complication and usually is not evident until adolescence or adult life.

Clinical Manifestations

The incidence in the general population approaches 2 percent; therefore it is the most common congenital abnormality of the heart or great vessels except for mitral valve prolapse (Chap. 80). Its importance lies in its frequent association with other forms of congenital heart disease, the predisposition of the valve to become stenotic as a result of fibrosis and deposition of calcium over the course of years, the tendency of the valve to become regurgitant, and, finally, in the susceptibility of the valve to infective endocarditis.[249] It is found in 60 percent of patients with valvular aortic stenosis between the ages of 15 and 65 years.[249] It is also common among patients with isolated or dominant aortic regurgitation, patients with infective endocarditis with or without a history of predisposing heart disease, and, probably most frequently, among otherwise normal individuals who come to the physician's attention because of unrelated illnesses. Patients with uncomplicated bicuspid aortic valve are asymptomatic. The incidence among males in approximately 2.5 times that among females. (See also Chap. 79.)

The characteristic feature is auscultatory and consists of an early systolic ejection click which is best heard at the apex and which does not vary with respiration. A soft, early, or midsystolic murmur frequently is present at the right upper sternal border. Less commonly, a soft murmur of aortic regurgitation may be heard.[250] Two-dimensional echocardiography, with adequate images, can identify the bicuspid valve with a sensitivity of 78 percent and a diagnostic accuracy of 96 percent[251] (Fig. 15-30).

Natural History and Prognosis

The majority of congenitally bicuspid aortic valves are nonobstructive at birth, but with the passage of time a few of these valves will become fibrotic, stiffer, and more obstructive and will eventually be the site of calcium deposition, primarily among individuals between the ages of 15 and 65. Important calcium deposition is unusual before the age of 30, whereas grossly visible deposits of calcium are present in the valves of virtually all patients with severe stenosis beyond that age. A much smaller number of individuals born with a bicuspid aortic valve develop isolated aortic regurgitation. In approximately one-third, this is the result of fibrosis, prolapse, or retraction of one or both of the leaflets; in the remainder, regurgitation results from infective endocarditis on an apparently functionally normal bicuspid valve. (See also Chaps. 79 and 98.)

Right Aortic Arch

Right aortic arch is characterized by the arch passing over the right, rather than the left, bronchus. Mirror-image branching is the most common arrangement. Less commonly, the left subclavian artery arises anomalously as the fourth branch from the aortic arch. In combination with a ductus or its ligament, tracheal and esophageal compression can occur (Figs. 14-9*C*, 9*D*). Barium swallow will demonstrate the typical filling defects that are confirmed by bronchoscopy. This is relieved by division of the ductus or its ligament surgically.

Aberrant Right Subclavian Artery

The right subclavian artery may arise anomalously as the fourth branch of a normal left aortic arch. It runs posterior to the esophagus to assume its normal course thereafter. Posterior indentation on a barium-filled esophagus is diagnostic.

Congenital Mitral Regurgitation

Pathology

Mitral regurgitation may be due to a primary valve abnormality or secondary to a more complex defect. (See "Common Atrioventricular Canal Defects.") There are a variety of rare primary malformations including isolated cleft, fenestration, and double orifice. Mitral regurgitation also occurs frequently with conditions which cause left ventricular dilatation and failure.

Clinical Manifestations

Poor growth, frequent respiratory infections, and failure occur with significant mitral regurgitation. Physical findings are generally similar to those with mitral regurgitation of other causes. (See Chap. 80.) There may be a prominent left precordial bulge if cardiomegaly has been present from infancy. The systolic murmur may radiate to the base of the heart. Left atrial and left ventricular enlargement correlate with the degree of volume overload. Echocardiography with Doppler color flow mapping will demonstrate these as well as left ventricular function and the severity of regurgitation. The specific defect may be outlined, such as an isolated cleft or double orifice valve. Findings at cardiac catheterization substantiate the hemodynamic alterations. (See also Chap. 80.)

Natural History and Prognosis

Mild and even moderate mitral regurgitation may be well tolerated, but severe regurgitation leads to progressive deterioration. Endocarditis is a risk.

Management

Vigorous medical treatment of heart failure and infections is warranted. Every attempt should be made to control symptoms to a degree that will allow growth in infants. In infants and young children, only those with very severe and uncontrollable failure are subjected to surgery. In the adolescent, continued symptoms justify surgery.

At surgery, the valve and its apparatus are carefully inspected. Numerous individualized plastic procedures have been described. Reconstruction (Chap. 85) is not possible in many, and replacement (Chap. 84.) is necessary. Currently, the St. Jude Medical prosthesis is often utilized. Life-long anticoagulation with warfarin (Chap. 80) is required. With body growth, replacement with a larger prosthesis may be difficult, and no good annular enlarging operation exists.

VALVULAR AND VASCULAR MALFORMATIONS OF THE RIGHT SIDE OF THE HEART WITH RIGHT-TO-LEFT, BIDIRECTIONAL, OR NO SHUNT

Pulmonary Stenosis with Intact Ventricular Septum

Pathology

Valvular pulmonary stenosis with intact ventricular septum is usually characterized by the so-called dome-shaped stenosis of the pulmonary valve and less commonly by dysplasia of the valve. The valve may be unicuspid, bicuspid, or tricuspid. The annulus may also be narrow. The pulmonary trunk exhibits poststenotic dilatation. In adult patients, calcification of the valve may appear.[252]

In pulmonary valvular dysplasia, the annulus of the valve may be abnormally narrow, but the most dramatic changes are related to the cusps, of which three are identifiable. The cusps are exceedingly thickened by mucoid and dense connective tissue.[253]

Concentric hypertrophy of the right ventricle is present, its degree reflecting the degree of obstruction at valve level. The hypertrophy of the infundibular musculature may cause secondary infundibular stenosis.

Less commonly, there may be isolated subvalvular pulmonary stenosis due to infundibular narrowing or an anomalous muscle bundle across the middle of the right ventricle.[254] Both types are usually associated with a ventricular septal defect.

Isolated supravalvular pulmonary stenosis, or pulmonary arterial coarctations, may also occur. From angiographic studies, these are classified into four types: (1) localized stenosis with poststenotic dilatation, (2) segmental stenosis, (3) diffuse hypoplasia, and (4) multiple peripheral stenoses.[255] The stenosis may be localized to any segment of the pulmonary arterial system. The process is unilateral in about one-third of cases and bilateral in two-thirds. Pulmonary arterial stenosis is commonly (about 75 percent), *though not universally,* associated with other cardiovascular anomalies. Pulmonary arterial stenosis is a sequela of maternal rubella.[256]

Abnormal Physiology[257–259]

There is a pressure difference during systole between the main right ventricular cavity and the pulmonary artery. The area of the pulmonary valve orifice is normally 2 cm^2/m^2; it is about 0.5 cm^2 at birth and increases in size with body growth. In general, the effective valve area must be decreased by about 60 percent before there is hemodynamically significant obstruction flow.

The peak systolic pressure difference may reach 150 to 240 mmHg. The degree of obstruction is assessed by the peak and mean systolic pressure gradients and the amount of flow across the valve. Severe stenosis can be associated with a relatively small pressure difference if the flow is very low as a result of right ventricular failure. If pulmonary flow is normal, most patients with peak pressure differences at rest of less than 50 mmHg have mild stenosis, and patients with a pressure difference over 100 mmHg have severe stenosis.

When the pulmonary stenosis is severe, the right ventricle may fail and the cardiac output may be decreased, even at rest; this is associated with elevation of both the right ventricular end-diastolic pressure and the right atrial mean pressure. This may cause the foramen ovale to open and allow shunting of blood from the right to the left atrium. Arterial oxygen desaturation and cyanosis result.

In most adolescent or adult patients with significant pulmonary stenosis, the resting cardiac output is within normal limits but usually does not increase normally during exercise. In contrast, children may be able to increase cardiac output during exercise.[257]

Clinical Manifestations

Pulmonary stenosis is one of the most common congenital heart defects and accounts for about 10 percent of patients in most large study populations (Table 97-1). The stenosis is at the level of the pulmonary valve in most instances, but it can occur within the right ventricle, in the pulmonary arteries, or in combination. Approximately one-quarter of patients with stenosis of the pulmonary valve also have an atrial shunt,[260] but this frequency may be dependent on the age group studied.

History Most infants and children are asymptomatic, but a small percentage with very severe obstruction will manifest symptoms. The most common symptoms are mild fatigue or shortness of breath with exertion. Young infants with critical obstruction present with symptoms related to heart failure and may have cyanosis if there is a patent foramen ovale or atrial septal defect. Squatting and syncope are rare in childhood.

Physical Examination Patients with a dysplastic valve and occasional supravalvular stenosis have consistent noncardiac abnormalities in a familial syndrome described by Noonan. They frequently have short stature, hypertelorism, ptosis, low-set ears, and mental retardation.[261] (See Fig. 10-13.) Patients with rubella syndrome[256] have supravalvular stenoses and patent ductus along with cataracts, sensorineural deafness, and microcephaly. Supravalvular stenoses can occur in Williams syndrome, or idiopathic hypercalcemia of infancy. These patients have characteristic facies, dental anomalies, mental retardation, and supravalvular aortic stenoses. (See Fig. 10-25.) There is also a familial occurrence of supravalvular pulmonary and aortic stenosis without these other features.

In patients with valvular pulmonary stenosis, cyanosis is uncommon, except with severe obstruction and an atrial communication. Tachypnea, hepatomegaly, and the murmur of tricuspid regurgitation may be present in infants with severe obstruction. In those with at least moderate obstruction, a prominent *a* wave is seen on examination of the jugular venous pulse. A systolic thrill in the suprasternal notch and at the left upper sternal border is present unless there is isolated subvalvular stenosis. The right ventricular parasternal impulse becomes increasingly forceful with more severe obstruction. An early systolic click, accentuated with expiration, at the left upper sternal border is the hallmark of valvular stenosis unless the obstruction is severe or the valve is dysplastic. A click is not present with isolated stenosis at other levels. As the obstruction increases in severity, the pulmonary component of the second heart sound becomes progressively softer and more delayed. When the right ventricular pressure reaches systemic levels or greater, it becomes inaudible. The second heart sound is normal with supravalvular stenosis. A fourth heart sound is heard if obstruction is severe. The characteristic systolic murmur is harsh, crescendo-decrescendo in shape, and best heard at the left upper sternal border with radiation toward the left clavicle. The murmur radiates more to the axillae and back with supravalvular stenosis. The duration of the murmur and the timing of peak intensity correlate well with the severity of obstruction. With mild to moderate stenosis, the murmur peaks in midsystole and ends at or before the aortic component of the second heart sound. In patients with severe stenosis, the murmur peaks late in systole and extends beyond the aortic component (A_2) of the second heart sound. (See also Chap. 11.)

Chest Roentgenogram Most patients have a normal or only slightly increased heart size. Significant enlargement is seen with critical obstruction and is an ominous sign. Characteristically, the main and proximal left pulmonary arteries are prominent as a result of poststenotic dilatation when the stenosis is valvular. This finding may be absent with very severe obstructions, with a dysplastic valve, in very young infants, or with stenosis above or below the valve. The pulmonary vascular pattern is normal in most but is diminished in those with right-to-left shunt at atrial level.

Electrocardiogram Right ventricular forces in the anterior precordial leads correlate reasonably well with the degree of obstruction.[262] They are normal or demonstrate mild hypertrophy with an rsR′ pattern if there is mild obstruction. With severe stenosis, there are right axis deviation, right atrial hypertrophy, and very tall R waves in the anterior precordial leads. The presence of a qR pattern in these leads is almost always a sign of very severe obstruction. Those with a dysplastic valve frequently have a superior QRS axis.[253]

Echocardiogram Two-dimensional imaging allows identification of the level of obstruction, and Doppler studies provide an excellent measure of severity.[263] Shunting at the atrial level can also be evaluated.

Cardiac Catheterization There is an elevated right ventricular systolic pressure with a distinct systolic pressure difference across the narrowed segment, which can be shown by slow withdrawal of the catheter from the distal pulmonary arterial branches to the proximal right ventricle. If critical obstruction is suspected, it may be wise not to attempt to advance the catheter into the pulmonary artery because of the risk of compromising an already marginal opening. Simultaneous measurement of systemic arterial and right ventricular pressures with measurement of flow is necessary to assess severity accurately. The right ventricular end-diastolic pressure and right atrial *a* wave may be elevated. Systemic oxygen saturation is diminished only in those with more severe obstruction and a patent foramen ovale or, less commonly, a true atrial septal defect. A left-to-right shunt at atrial level is detected in some patients with mild to moderate obstruction.[260] With valvular stenosis, right ventricular angiography demonstrates thickened and doming valve leaflets and a jet of contrast material entering the dilated pulmonary artery (Figs. 97-22 and 138-17). Doming is not characteristic of the dysplastic valve.[253] Infundibular subvalvular narrowing due to muscular hypertrophy may occur secondary to the valvular stenosis or rarely as an isolated anomaly. Isolated anomalous muscle bundles in the right ventricle may also be seen. Pulmonary arterial angiography best demonstrates the sites of obstruction with supravalvular stenoses. Ventricular volume studies have demonstrated depressed ventricular function in patients with right-to-left shunts.[264] Percutaneous transluminal CBV is discussed later under "Medical Management."

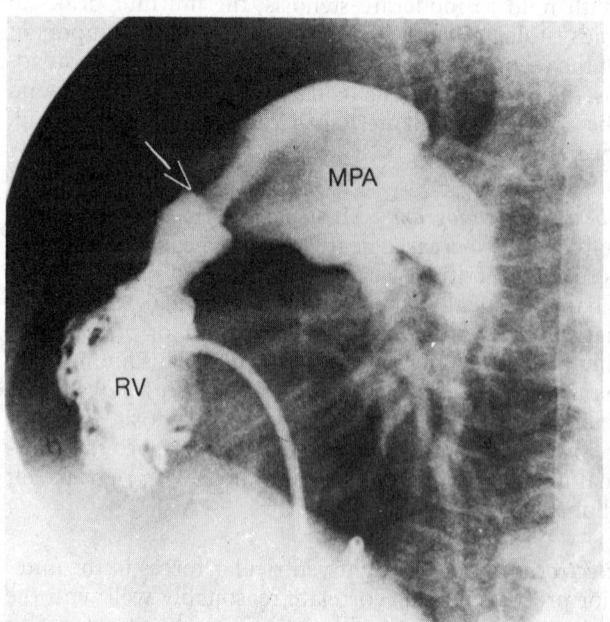

FIGURE 97-22 Lateral view of a right ventricular (RV) angiogram demonstrating the typical features of valvular pulmonary stenosis with doming of the pulmonary valve (*arrow*) and a narrow jet of contrast entering the dilated main pulmonary artery (MPA).

Natural History and Prognosis

The clinical course of valvular stenosis is favorable in most patients with mild to moderate obstruction. In a national cooperative study,[265] 86 percent of patients had no significant increase in their pressure gradients over a 4- to 8-year interval. Those with a significant increase were less than 4 years of age and had at least moderate stenosis initially. Progression during the period of growth seems the likely explanation for most of the increases, but a few patients developed subvalvular muscular hypertrophy, which increased the obstruction. Even mild obstruction may progress significantly in some infants during the first year of life.[259] The prognosis of those with severe obstruction is poor, especially for infants with critical obstruction. With severe obstruction, right ventricular damage and dysfunction can ensue over the years, and heart failure or arrhythmias can cause premature death in adults.[259] Tricuspid regurgitation may also result. Obstruction of the subvalvular type frequently increases with time, while supravalvular stenosis does not usually progress. Brain abscess can occur if a right-to-left shunt is present. Infective endocarditis with vegetations on the valve, pulmonary arterial wall, or infundibular region is also a risk.

Medical Management

Management obviously depends on the severity of obstruction. For those with mild to moderate valvular pulmonary stenosis, periodic reexamination is indicated to detect any evidence of progression, with more frequent evaluation for those under 1 year of age. Measures to treat heart failure should be instituted in the infant with critical stenosis, but prompt intervention is mandatory. Cyanosis or a right ventricular systolic pressure well above systemic levels also is an indication for prompt intervention. Asymptomatic older infants and children should have elective intervention when the right ventricular systolic pressure is near 70 mmHg or the gradient is near 50 mmHg. CBV is a commonly used surgical alternative for valvular and supravalvular pulmonary stenosis. The best results are obtained with valvular stenosis.[266] Although results with dysplastic valves and pulmonary arterial stenosis are less impressive,[267,268] attempts at CBV appear to be justified. For those in whom there is isolated subvalvular stenosis or associated defects or in whom balloon dilatation has failed, surgical intervention is recommended.

Exercise studies[257] during catheterization have demonstrated that altered cardiac function observed in some children is reversible by surgery. This does not appear to be true for adults, so intervention should be carried out relatively early in childhood. Prophylaxis against infective endocarditis is recommended for all patients, whether or not surgery is performed.

Surgical Management

Operation is rarely indicated for isolated pulmonary valvular stenosis; CBV is virtually always successful in eliminating clinically significant obstruction. A thickened, immobile, dysplastic pulmonary valve, however, is best treated by complete surgical excision (valvectomy). A small annulus is augmented with a pericardial or Dacron gusset.[269]

In infants with life-threatening valvular pulmonary stenosis and hypoxemia, valvotomy or valvectomy can be accomplished during about 90 s of venous inflow occlusion and circulatory arrest. Resuscitation usually requires only the restoration of cardiac filling by release of caval tourniquets.[270,271] Closed transventricular valvotomy using a valvulotome without inflow occlusion is preferred by others.[272] Further valve resection or annular augmentation may be required as the child grows, prompting us to consider transannular patch. The noncompliant right ventricle may limit antegrade pulmonary blood flow and cause persistent hypoxemia if a significant right-to-left shunt persists through an interatrial communication (patent foramen ovale or atrial septal defect). Continued infusion of PGE_1 is useful in maintaining patency of the ductus arteriosus in the newborn with such persistent postoperative hypoxemia and acidosis. Gradual weaning from PGE_1 is usually possible, but occasionally a surgically created systemic arterial-to-pulmonary arterial shunt is required.

Subvalvular pulmonary stenosis is relieved through a right ventriculotomy, a main pulmonary arteriotomy, or a right atriotomy. Hypertrophic parietal and septal muscle bands constituting the fibrous orifice of the os infundibulum and obstructing moderator bands or muscle bundles within the body of the right ventricle are excised. Care is exercised to avoid injury to major coronary arterial branches. The right ventriculotomy can usually be closed by direct suture, but a small oval patch of pericardium or Dacron can be used to prevent constriction of the outflow tract. Right ventricular function is minimally compromised by a small patch that does not extend across the annulus; larger patches to the pulmonary arterial bifurcation probably impair ventricular performance but may be necessary when there is associated annular or main pulmonary arterial hypoplasia. When possible, excision from the pulmonary artery or the right atrium is preferred to avoid ventricular injury.

Excellent relief of right ventricular outflow tract obstruction can be expected following resection. Mortality and significant morbidity are rare. Repair during childhood reduces the likelihood of complications related to severe right ventricular hypertrophy, diminished ventricular compliance and function, subendocardial ischemia, tricuspid regurgitation, and supraventricular dysrhythmias associated with right atrial hypertrophy.

Stenoses of main or extraparenchymal branch pulmonary arteries can be relieved by pericardial, synthetic, or homograft aortic or pulmonary arterial patches if poststenotic dilatation is present. Proximal coarctations in the larger portion of the arterial tree are more readily corrected than those located in small distal branches beyond the bifurcation of either the right or left pulmonary artery, where results are poor.[273] Tubular conduits can be placed to bypass obstructions, but these are generally not needed unless there is absence of confluence of the arteries centrally.[274] An artery treated by excision of a discrete stenosis with repair by primary anastomosis is subject to restenosis as the child grows and may result in moving the gradient distally as stenoses remote from the mediastinum are revealed.

Catheter-balloon angioplasty, although certainly not without risk, offers nonsurgical relief of obstruction even in the small pulmonary arterial branches and is the procedure of choice for distal pulmonary arterial stenoses, unless other major cardiac reconstruction is also required.[275,276]

Tetralogy of Fallot

Pathology

Tetralogy of Fallot is characterized by biventricular origin of the aorta above a large ventricular septal defect (Fig. 97-23),[86] obstruction to pulmonary blood flow, and right ventricular hypertrophy. Fibrous continuity of the aortic origin and the anterior mitral valve is maintained.

The right ventricular infundibulum lies anterior to the position of the ventricular septal defect and is bounded by the anterior and septal walls anteriorly and medially; the posterior wall is said to be a vertical crista supraven-

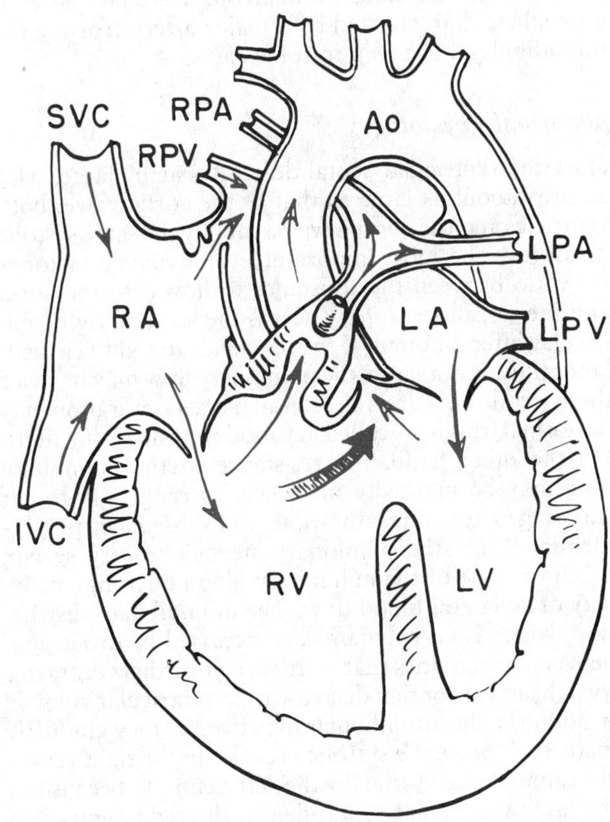

FIGURE 97-23 Classic tetralogy of Fallot. There are infundibular and pulmonary valvular stenoses. SVC = superior vena cava; IVC = inferior vena cava; RA = right atrium; RV = right ventricle; RPA = right pulmonary artery; LPA = left pulmonary artery; RPV = right pulmonary vein; LPV = left pulmonary vein; LA = left atrium; LV = left ventricle; Ao = aorta. *(From JE Edwards.[86] Reproduced with permission from the publisher, editor, and author.)*

tricularis or displaced conus septum.[277] The right ventricular infundibulum is a distinctive channel, but the caliber varies widely from only mild obstruction to atresia. Usually, it exhibits a significant degree of stenosis and is the dominant site of the obstruction to pulmonary flow characteristic of tetralogy.

The pulmonary valve is often malformed, usually being either bicuspid or unicuspid. The valve may contribute to pulmonary stenosis, but only uncommonly will it be the only site of significant obstruction to pulmonary flow.[278] Characteristically, the pulmonary trunk is thin-walled and its lumen is more narrow than normal, but usually it is wider than either the right ventricular infundibulum or the orifice of the pulmonary valve. The aorta is wider than normal, its change in caliber roughly opposite to that of the pulmonary trunk. The foramen ovale is frequently patent in patients of all ages. In all cases of tetralogy with significant pulmonary obstruction, collateral branches to the lungs arise from the aorta.

Associated Conditions The condition most commonly associated with tetralogy of Fallot is right aortic arch (about 30 percent).[278] A persistent left superior vena cava has been described in 10.6 percent of cases. When an associated atrial septal defect exists, this anomaly is referred to as *pentalogy (pentad) of Fallot*. The ductus arteriosus may be absent, present unilaterally on either the right or left side, or bilateral. Coronary arterial anomalies, characterized by a major artery crossing the infundibulum, are seen in some cases.

Abnormal Physiology[279–282]

Since the ventricular septal defect is usually large, with an area about as large as that of the aortic valve, both ventricles and the aorta have essentially the same systolic pressures. The most important hemodynamic factor is the ratio between the resistance to flow into the aorta and the resistance to flow across the stenotic right ventricular infundibulum. If the resistance to right ventricular outflow is not large, the pulmonary flow may be twice the systemic flow and the arterial oxygen saturation may be normal (this is so-called acyanotic tetralogy of Fallot). On the other hand, the resistance to the pulmonary flow may be markedly increased, causing right-to-left shunting, arterial unsaturation, and subsequent polycythemia. When the pulmonary stenosis is very severe, much or most of the pulmonary blood flow may be by way of collateral blood flow. The infundibular obstruction, which is very dynamic, is increased by drugs, maneuvers, or activities that increase myocardial contractility or heart rate or that decrease right ventricular volume. In addition, the infundibular hypertrophy may gradually increase.[283] Since the systolic pressure in the right ventricle cannot exceed that in the left ventricle because of the large ventricular septal defect, the right ventricle is "protected" from excessive pressure-work.

The precise mechanism by which squatting relieves breathlessness and faintness after exercise in patients with tetralogy of Fallot is complex. It is known that the arterial saturation returns to its resting value more rapidly if the patient squats after exercise. In normal subjects, squatting produces an increase in systemic arterial blood pressure and resistance and an increase in venous return to the heart and in systemic cardiac output. In patients with tetralogy, the increase in arterial saturation produced by squatting is largely related to an increase in peripheral resistance by compression and kinking of the femoral arteries. Squatting also usually increases venous return from the abdomen to the heart with increases in right ventricular stroke volume, pressure, and pulmonary blood flow.

Hypercyanotic episodes in patients with tetralogy are of uncertain origin. It is likely that some episodes are caused by unusual hyperactivity of muscular fibers in the right ventricular outflow tract producing, or exaggerating, the infundibular stenosis. Some spells may be caused by a decrease in peripheral resistance and in systemic arterial pressure, which causes the right ventricular pressure and pulmonary blood flow to decrease.

Clinical Manifestations

Tetralogy of Fallot is one of the most common congenital cardiac defects causing cyanosis. Of cyanotic patients over age 2 years and not yet requiring surgery, approximately three-fourths have tetralogy of Fallot.[6] Tetralogy with an associated atrial septal defect, or *pentalogy of Fallot,* is not distinguishable clinically. See the section on cyanosis and its complications earlier in this chapter.

History The majority of patients are first seen by 6 months of age because of cyanosis. If the right ventricular outflow obstruction is very severe, marked cyanosis is present at birth or as soon as the ductus closes. Other patients slowly develop progressively more severe obstruction and cyanosis and present later in infancy, childhood, or even in adulthood. Some patients with a large ventricular septal defect and left-to-right shunt in early infancy may acquire infundibular pulmonary stenosis and become clinically indistinguishable from the usual patient with tetralogy of Fallot. Dyspnea with exertion occurs commonly. Attacks of suddenly increasing cyanosis associated with hyperpnea, or hypoxic spells,[284,285] are common between the ages of 2 months and 2 years. There are many precipitating events, including infection, exertion, and summer heat. They occur most often in the morning, and the infant is usually irritable. Frequency and duration vary widely, but prolonged episodes can lead to syncope, seizures, and death. Squatting with exercise is common from $1\frac{1}{2}$ to 10 years of age and is almost pathognomonic of this diagnosis.

Physical Examination Growth is usually normal unless cyanosis is extreme.[286] Clubbing occurs after 3 months of age and is proportional to the level of cyanosis. Signs of congestive heart failure do not appear in tetralogy of Fallot during childhood unless there is a superimposed illness such as anemia or infective endocarditis.

Increased right ventricular activity is observed. A systolic thrill is frequently palpable at the left midsternal border, with a harsh midsystolic murmur in this location. Softer murmurs signal more severe obstruction and are common when presentation is in the newborn period or during hypoxic spells. The murmur ends before the second heart sound, which is characteristically single. A continuous murmur is heard if a patent ductus or large bronchial collateral vessels are present. An early systolic ejection sound at the left sternal border and apex is common.

Chest Roentgenogram The total heart size is usually normal on chest roentgenogram, but right ventricular enlargement is present in the lateral view. The aorta arches to the right frequently. Pulmonary flow is diminished. The pulmonary segment is concave and the apex elevated, giving the *coeur en sabot* (boot-shaped) contour (Figs. 14-2C, 9A, and 9B). The very young infant may have only diminished pulmonary flow.

Electrocardiogram In tetralogy of Fallot, the mean QRS axis of the electrocardiogram is usually to the right, between +90° and +210°. There is right ventricular hypertrophy with a tall R wave in the right precordial leads and a deep S wave in the left. Some patients have right atrial hypertrophy.

Echocardiogram Two-dimensional echocardiography can delineate the anatomic components of tetralogy.[287] (See Fig. 15-18.) Anomalies of the coronary arteries may be difficult to demonstrate, but associated defects can be excluded.

Hematologic and Other Laboratory Studies Measurement of hemoglobin and hematocrit and pulse oximetry should be done in all patients at initial evaluation and periodically thereafter, both for determination of the degree of polycythemia and the early detection of anemia relative to the degree of cyanosis. The latter is common, especially in those under 2 years of age and in those in this age group with cerebrovascular accidents. Platelet counts and clotting studies may be advisable in patients with marked polycythemia, particularly if a surgical procedure is planned. Serum uric acid levels should be measured if polycythemia is severe and longstanding.

Cardiac Catheterization The right ventricular systolic pressure is equal to that in the left ventricle and aorta. If the pulmonary artery can be entered, the pressure will be normal or low. The level(s) of obstruction can be evaluated by careful pullback to the right ventricle. Caution should be observed if the pulmonary artery is entered, as the catheter may critically reduce the pulmonary flow and cause a hypoxic episode. It is unnecessary to attempt to enter the pulmonary artery in patients with severe cyanosis or with a history of severe hypoxic spells. Systemic arterial oxygen saturation is low because of right-to-left shunting from the right ventricle. If a patent foramen ovale or atrial septal defect is present, there will an additional right-to-left or bidirectional shunt at the atrial level. Selective biplane right ventricular angiography is extremely valuable to demonstrate levels of obstruction, continuity and size of the pulmonary arteries, and size and position of the ventricular defect. Aortography or selective coronary arteriography should be performed on all patients preoperatively to demonstrate the coronary arterial pattern.[288,289]

Natural History and Prognosis

Prognosis is poorest in very young infants who present with severe cyanosis because of the severity of obstruction and the size of the pulmonary arteries, which are usually very small.[280] Hypoxic spells offer a poor prognosis if they are allowed to continue untreated. Obstruction to pulmonary flow tends to progress even to atresia[283] with increasing cyanosis and polycythemia. The complications of polycythemia, including cerebrovascular accident and brain abscess, were discussed in "Cyanosis" earlier in the chapter. The risk of infective endocarditis is high. Without surgery, approximately one-third of patients die by age 1 year, one-half by age 3 years, and three-quarters by age 10 years, with less than 5 percent surviving beyond age 30 years.[290]

Medical Management

The medical management in tetralogy of Fallot is directed primarily toward prevention and treatment of complications. Iron-deficiency anemia should be promptly treated with iron supplementation. Fever or other illness that would lead to dehydration and possible thrombotic complications should also be treated promptly. Hypoxic spells in infants should be treated initially by placing the infant in the knee-chest position. Further treatment of hypoxic spells includes administration of a high concentration of oxygen and morphine sulfate. If acidosis is present and does not correct spontaneously and promptly, intravenous sodium bicarbonate should be given. Propranolol is useful in the acute treatment and prevention of prolonged hypoxic spells.[291] Propranolol, a beta-adrenergic blocker, should be given orally for prevention and intravenously only for severe hypoxic spells. If for some reason the hematocrit should reach a level of 70 to 75 percent, erythropheresis is recommended, using fresh frozen plasma or a colloid equivalent. This will temporarily diminish viscosity, but more definitive surgical treatment is indicated. Early and vigorous treatment should be given for intercurrent infections. Prophylactic antibiotics are recommended for prevention of infective endocarditis. (See Chap. 94.)

For the severely cyanotic newborn, prostaglandin administration is of benefit[292] to open the ductus until surgery can be done. Prompt surgical intervention is indicated. Surgical correction is recommended in children for progressive symptoms or polycythemia with hematocrit approaching 65 percent. Elective surgical correction should be done in early childhood, since further delay offers no advantage and the continuing risks of complications of cyanosis are significant.

The infant who is symptomatic may be treated in one of three ways: palliation with propranolol and delayed correction, palliation with a shunt from systemic artery to pulmonary artery and delayed correction, or early correction. Clearly, certain anatomic variables, such as tiny pulmonary arteries or a coronary arterial abnormality, make early correction less attractive. Otherwise, early correction seems desirable if risk is no more than the total risk of other choices and outcome is equally favorable. Early correction is probably best at centers where early operative mortality is 10 percent or less.[293,294]

Surgical Management[295]

"Ideally, the surgical treatment of the tetralogy of Fallot is primary repair, done whenever signs and symptoms become important or in any event in the first several years of life, performed so that the ventricular septal defect (VSD) is completely closed, sinus rhythm is preserved, no residual right ventricular outflow obstruction is present, and the patient's pulmonary valve remains competent."[296] The presence of small pulmonary arteries or pulmonary atresia in the symptomatic infant with tetralogy of Fallot encourages two-stage management, a Blalock-Taussig shunt (anastomosis of the subclavian artery on the side opposite the aortic arch to the ipsilateral pulmonary artery), or modification thereof,[297,298] followed by secondary repair by the age of 2 years.[299,300]

Determination of the need for transannular patch augmentation of the right ventricular outflow tract at the time of repair is based on measurement of pulmonary annular diameter and the ratio of right ventricular to left ventricular systolic pressure after closure of the ventricular septal defect and excision of obstructive muscle bundles. This ratio should be less the 0.7:1 for optimum outcome[296] and can be predicted with reasonable accuracy by preoperative angiography and intraoperative annular measurements.[296,301] Relief of right ventricular outflow tract obstruction without right ventriculotomy is advocated to preserve right ventricular function.[302]

Long-term prognosis of patients benefiting from correction of tetralogy of Fallot is quite good; there is no adverse effect on life expectancy up to 10 to 22 years after surgery,[303] and near-normal exercise tolerance can be anticipated in those free of significant residual abnormalities.[304] Preliminary data suggest that early primary repair in infancy yields excellent survival[305] and improved long-term left ventricular function.[306] Residual ventricular septal defects, distal pulmonary stenoses, and pulmonary regurgitation significantly impair right ventricular function and maximum exercise potential.[307,308]

Ebstein's Anomaly

Pathology

In Ebstein's anomaly, the anterior leaflet of the tricuspid valve is attached normally to the annulus, while varying portions of the posterior and septal leaflets are displaced downward, being attached to the ventricular wall below the annulus. The proximal part of the right ventricle is thin-walled and continuous with the right atrium. The functional right ventricle is small and made up of the apical and infundibular portions of the right ventricle.[309] An additional common finding is that the papillary muscles and chordae are highly malformed, with great variation in the manner of attachment of the two involved leaflets to the right ventricular wall. Commonly, multiple direct attachments of valvular tissue to the right ventricular mural endocardium occur.[310]

An interatrial communication is present in most cases, usually taking the form of a patent foramen ovale. Continuity of right atrial and right ventricular myocardial tissues, in addition to the usual connections by way of the main conduction pathways, has been observed.

Abnormal Physiology[311]

Ebstein's anomaly results in obstruction to the right ventricular filling because of a decrease in size of the right ventricle, part of which is incorporated into the huge right atrium. The deformed tricuspid valve also frequently allows tricuspid regurgitation with a right-to-left shunt through the foramen ovale.

Clinical Manifestations

History Approximately one-half of reported cases develop symptoms of cyanosis and right-sided heart failure in early infancy. The remainder present because of a murmur or abnormal chest roentgenogram with no symptoms in early childhood or because of gradual progression of symptoms through late childhood or adult life.[312] The most common symptom is dyspnea on exertion at all ages,[312] and the spectrum of exercise intolerance has been described.[313] Palpitations due to supraventricular tachyarrhythmias occur.[311] Occasionally, syncope occurs due to arrhythmia or low cardiac output if the atrial septum is intact.

Physical Examination The newborn with elevated pulmonary vascular resistance has severe cyanosis. In older infants and children, cyanosis and clubbing are mild. Only a small percentage do not have an atrial septal defect or patent foramen ovale and thus are not cyanotic. The precordium is generally quiet, even in those with striking cardiomegaly. The liver is enlarged, and the jugular venous pulse may be elevated. The holosystolic murmur of tricuspid regurgitation is heard at the lower left sternal border and may be accompanied by a "scratchy" diastolic murmur of tricuspid stenosis. The first heart sound is split and loud, and the second heart sound is widely and persistently split. Loud third and fourth heart sounds are usual, especially in older patients.

Chest Roentgenogram Heart size by chest roentgenogram varies but is ordinarily very large, predominantly owing to a very dilated right atrium. In those with cyanosis, pulmonary blood flow is diminished correspondingly (Fig. 14-6C).

Electrocardiogram Giant, peaked P waves are common, along with a prolonged PQ interval and right ventricular conduction delay or complete right bundle branch block. Electrophysiologic correlates of these abnormalities have been reported.[314] In approximately 10 percent, the pattern of Wolff-Parkinson-White syndrome (with a short PQ interval and delayed conduction of initial QRS forces, or a delta wave) is seen.[312] (See also Chap. 13.)

Echocardiogram Two-dimensional echocardiography is very helpful in diagnosis (Fig. 97-24). Studies in the fetus and neonates have identified features associated with high risk.[315]

Cardiac Catheterization There is higher risk than usual associated with cardiac catheterization because of the

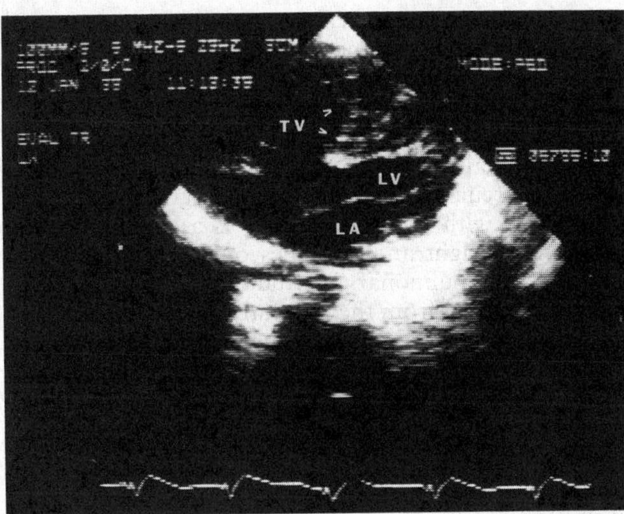

FIGURE 97-24 Two-dimensional echocardiogram in parasternal view in a patient with Ebstein's anomaly of the tricuspid valve (TV). Numerous attachments of the tricuspid valve (arrows) to the interventricular septum and right ventricular apex are seen. LV = left ventricle; LA = left atrium.

frequency of rhythm disturbances. Proper precautions and prompt use of cardioversion when necessary minimize this risk. In most cases, echocardiography and color Doppler evaluation are sufficient. There is usually right-to-left shunting at atrial level. Right atrial hypertension is present. The characteristic right ventricular pressure recording is not obtained until the catheter is advanced to the apex or outflow tract. An intracardiac electrocardiogram[316] demonstrates, on pullback from the right ventricle, an area where the electrocardiogram is ventricular but the pressure is atrial in contour (Fig. 138-11). This method is not infallible, but it is good evidence of tricuspid displacement with an "atrialized" portion of the right ventricle. The pulmonary artery may be difficult to enter, but it is very important in the cyanotic newborn to exclude associated pulmonary atresia.

Natural History and Prognosis

Natural history varies greatly with the severity of the abnormality. Fifty percent of those diagnosed in infancy die early, whereas late survival is reported into the ninth decade.[317] Significant associated cardiac defects lead to a worse prognosis; almost one-half of an autopsy series fell into this group.[309]

Symptomatically, most patients tend to progress. Mortality has been correlated with one or more of these factors: severe symptoms, cardiothoracic ratio greater than 0.65 by chest roentgenogram, cyanosis, and diagnosis in infancy.[317] Premature death can result from heart failure, complications of cyanosis, arrhythmias, and low cardiac output if the atrial septum is intact.

Medical Management

Medical management involves treatment of heart failure and arrhythmias and prevention and treatment of complications of cyanosis and endocarditis. Extracorporeal membrane oxygenation has been used successfully in critically ill neonates.[318] Surgical success has varied, so a conservative approach toward surgery is recommended. Surgical results may offer lower morbidity and mortality for older patients with severe disease.[317] (See also Chap. 98.)

Surgical Management

Reconstruction or replacement of the tricuspid valve is effective management of symptomatic patients with Ebstein's anomaly or those having significant cyanosis, paradoxical emboli, or associated right ventricular outflow tract obstruction.[319,320] The case for plication of the atrialized portion of the right ventricle remains unsettled, but the procedure seems desirable when this chamber contracts poorly or paradoxically (Fig. 97-25).[321] Quaegebeur and colleagues[322] recently reported their experience with vertical plication of the right ventricle and reimplanatation of the tricuspid valve leaflet. There were no deaths among 10 consecutive patients ranging in age from 4 to 44 years. Tricuspid valvular regurgitation was diminished in eight of the patients at late follow-up, but one patient required a tricuspid valve replacement during the first operation after intraoperative echocardiography revealed severe tricuspid regurgitation. All showed significant clinical improvement and, remarkably, all were in normal sinus rhythm at late follow-up.

Accessory conduction pathways associated with the Wolff-Parkinson-White syndrome can be interrupted surgically at the time of repair and atrial septal defects should be closed. Repair does not necessarily free the patient of atrial arrhythmias, a common occurrence in this anomaly.[323]

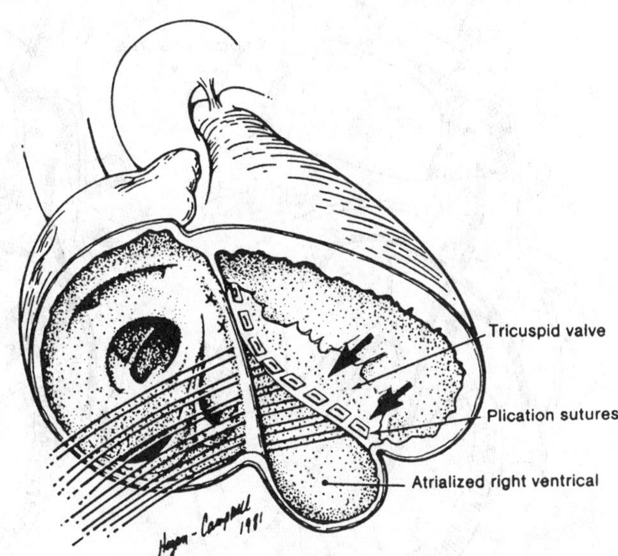

FIGURE 97-25 Plication for Ebstein's malformation. The atrialized aneurysmal portion of right ventricle is obliterated by the placement of Teflon felt–reinforced mattress sutures between the spiral line attachment of the inferiorly displaced tricuspid valve and the true annulus fibrosus. Tricuspid valve replacement may be required. Associated atrial septal defects are closed.

ABNORMALITIES OF THE PULMONARY VENOUS CONNECTIONS

Total Anomalous Pulmonary Venous Connection

Pathology

When all pulmonary veins terminate in a systemic vein or the right atrium, the term *total anomalous pulmonary venous connection* or *return* is applied (Fig. 97-26). The usual veins leave the lung and then join a chamberlike confluence. From the confluence of veins, one vessel leads to the anomalous termination. Less commonly, two or more vessels lead to multiple sites of termination.

Sites of supradiaphragmatic termination, in order of decreasing frequency, are the left brachiocephalic vein, the coronary sinus, the right atrium, the superior vena cava, and the azygous vein.[324] Supradiaphragmatic termination is not always associated with pulmonary venous obstruction.[325]

The site of termination may also be infradiaphragmatic, with connection to the portal venous system. The anomalous vein leaves the confluence of pulmonary veins and descends into the abdomen along the esophagus to join the ductus venosus, the portal vein, or the left gastric vein. Pulmonary venous obstruction characteristically is manifested in all cases of infradiaphragmatic connection.[325,326]

In all cases of total anomalous pulmonary venous connection, there is a patent foramen ovale. The atrium and ventricle of the left side are small in comparison with the right-sided chambers but are within normal limits as to absolute size.

In the absence of asplenia or polysplenia, associated anomalies are not common.

Abnormal Physiology[327]

In this anomaly all the blood from both pulmonary and systemic circulations returns to the right atrium. It is compatible with life only if there is a communication between the right and left sides of the heart. In most situations the pulmonary resistance is low, and a large volume of blood from the right atrium flows to the pulmonary circuit. Consequently, the systemic arterial saturation may remain high. It will be low if pulmonary blood flow is decreased because of either increased pulmonary vascular resistance or obstruction to pulmonary venous flow.

Clinical Manifestations[327]

History Male predominance, particularly of the subdiaphragmatic type, has been noted in some reports. Almost all patients are cyanotic, with over one-half presenting with cyanosis in the first month of life. Most also have congestive heart failure, including all of those with and two-thirds of those without pulmonary hypertension. The symptoms of congestive heart failure occur in almost two-thirds before 3 months of age.

Physical Examination These infants are dusky, tachypneic, and diaphoretic. The jugular venous pulse is elevated, and hepatomegaly appears early. There is a diffuse and hyperdynamic right ventricular impulse. The second

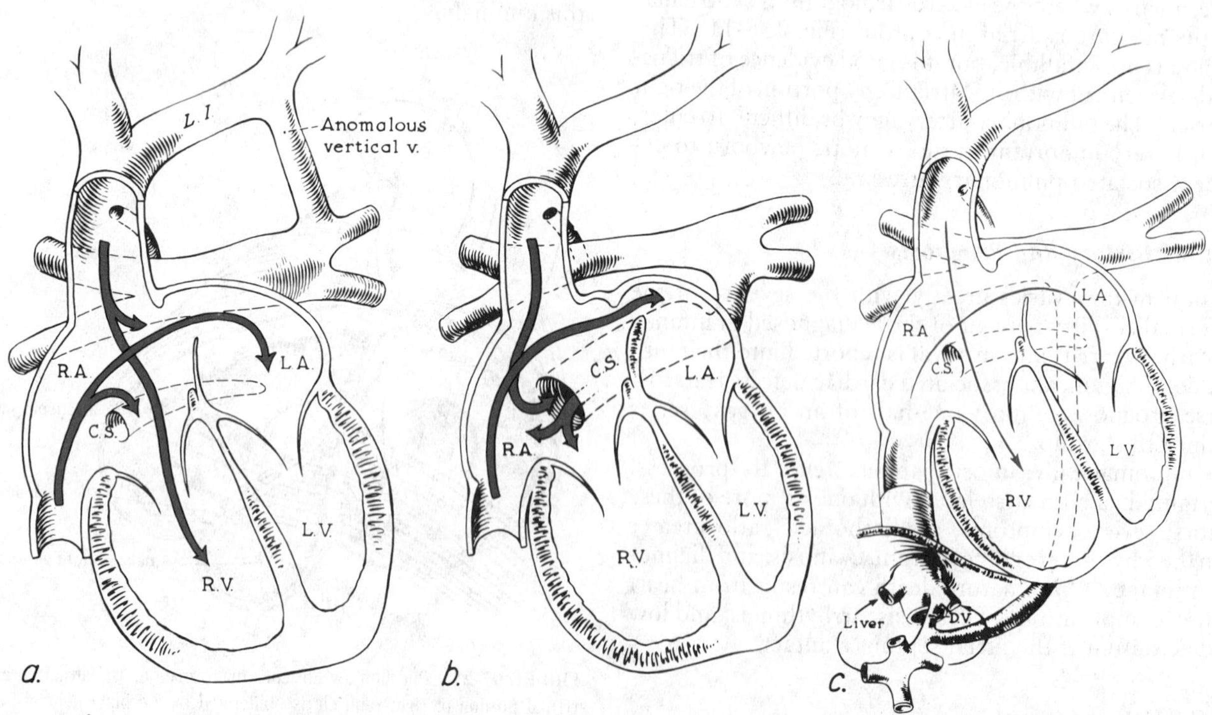

FIGURE 97-26 Three common types of total anomalous pulmonary venous connection. *A.* Total anomalous pulmonary venous connection to the left brachiocephalic (innominate) vein (L.I.). *B.* Total anomalous pulmonary venous connection to the coronary sinus (C.S.). *C.* Total anomalous pulmonary venous connection of the infradiaphragmatic type to the ductus venosus (D.V.). R.A. = right atrium; R.V. = right ventricle; L.A. = left atrium; L.V. = left ventricle.

heart sound is split and relatively fixed; the loudness of the pulmonary component is usually increased. There is usually a grade 2 or 3 midsystolic murmur at the left sternal border. At the lower sternal border, there are a middiastolic rumble and prominent third and fourth heart sounds. Rales may be heard over the lung fields, and periorbital edema is frequent. A continuous murmur may be heard over the common venous channel.

If there is significant obstruction to pulmonary venous flow, the cyanosis is more marked. The heart is not as hyperkinetic, and auscultation may reveal little or no murmur with a very loud second heart sound.

Chest Roentgenogram With the unobstructed types, the heart is enlarged and the pulmonary flow is increased. Pulmonary edema may be seen. In those patients with return to the left innominate vein, there may be a characteristic bulging of the superior mediastinum bilaterally, producing a "snowman," or figure-of-eight, contour.[6] With obstructed types, the heart size is near normal; there is very marked pulmonary edema, which may give a granular appearance to the lungs.

Electrocardiogram There is right axis deviation and right atrial and right ventricular hypertrophy. Commonly, there is a qR pattern in the right precordial leads.

Echocardiogram Echocardiography with color Doppler is specific in defining the anomaly and the site of drainage.[328]

Cardiac Catheterization If echocardiography is inconclusive, catheterization may be necessary. There is an increase in oxygen saturation at the level of the abnormal connection, with similar saturations in the remainder of the chambers on both sides of the heart. Pulmonary arterial pressure is elevated to a variable degree, but it may be above systemic pressure if there is marked pulmonary venous or pulmonary vascular obstruction. Pulmonary capillary wedge pressures are elevated in proportion to the degree of venous obstruction. The atrial communication may be rarely be obstructive,[327] and balloon atrial septostomy may be helpful.[329] Pulmonary arteriography will usually show the anomalous venous connection. Angiography directly in the common venous channel, if it is entered, will outline its course and any sites of obstruction optimally.

Natural History and Prognosis

The clinical course is commonly that of progressive congestive heart failure, with death in the first year of life.[327] There are significant differences among patients with varying degrees of pulmonary hypertension. The majority of those with severe pulmonary hypertension and pulmonary venous obstruction die by the age of 3 months, whereas those with significant pulmonary hypertension alone may survive to 1 year of age. The best clinical course is seen in those with pulmonary pressures lower than one-half of systemic pressure. The majority of patients survive to 1 year, and some do not develop congestive heart failure. Severe growth failure occurs in all but a few of this latter group. At postmortem examination, structural changes in the pulmonary vascular bed are present to some degree at all ages, but changes are more severe in those with venous obstruction.[330]

Medical Management

Medical management involves vigorous treatment of congestive heart failure and intercurrent respiratory infections and prevention of endocarditis.

Because of the poor outlook with medical management alone, surgery is being recommended at even younger ages. Any newborn or young infant with severe obstruction or pulmonary edema should have prompt surgical correction. Failure to grow is also an indication for surgery. For infants with less than one-half systemic pressure in the pulmonary artery who grow, surgery may be deferred for a few months.

Surgical Management

Correction of total anomalous pulmonary venous connection requires: (1) creation of a large communication between the left atrium and the pulmonary venous system, (2) obliteration of the anomalous pulmonary venous connection to the systemic circulation, and (3) closure of the associated interatrial communications,[331,332]

Supracardiac anomalous connection to the left brachiocephalic (vertical) vein and infracardiac connections to the portal venous system or the inferior vena cava are corrected by the creation of a wide anastomosis between the posterior aspect of the left atrium and the common transverse pulmonary venous sinus.[332] The stretched foramen ovale is closed. The ascending or descending anomalous pulmonary venous connection to the systemic circulation is ligated, as is the patent ductus arteriosus.

Anomalous pulmonary venous connection to the coronary sinus is repaired by creation of a large fenestration in the common wall between the coronary sinus and the left atrium. The coronary sinus is diverted into the left atrium by placement of an intracardiac patch which also closes the interatrial communication.

Total anomalous pulmonary venous connection to the right atrium is repaired by excision of the atrial septum and placement of a patch diverting the opening of the anomalous pulmonary venous connection into the left atrium.

Mixed forms of total anomalous pulmonary venous connection pose particular technical difficulties requiring individualized operations. Mortality is high after early repair of the symptomatic neonate having mixed types of total anomalous pulmonary venous connections.

Katz and associates reviewed 51 cases of repair of total anomalous pulmonary venous connection,[333] with 14 percent mortality and excellent late results. Operative survival is poor in infants having significant pulmonary venous obstruction, particularly those with infradiaphragmatic drainage,[334] with prolonged ventilatory support frequently required. A review of 75 patients treated surgically between 1975 and 1986 demonstrated a 9.3 percent operative mortality and an additional 6.7 percent late mortality rate. Determinants of mortality included the type of anomalous connection, degree of pulmonary venous obstruction, presence of associated intracardiac defects, and residual pulmonary venous obstruction.[335]

Operative survival ranges from 87 to 92 percent for unobstructed supracardiac or cardiac types of total anomalous pulmonary venous connections; unfortunately, a 50 percent mortality can still be expected with the infracardiac type, which are usually obstructed, or when there are other associated complex anomalies.[336] Long-term outlook is good for patients surviving hospitalization after the corrective operation.

MALPOSITIONS OF THE CARDIAC STRUCTURES

Definition and Terminology

The segmental approach to the diagnosis of complex congenital heart disease[337] provides an orderly, effective method for determining the anatomic and hemodynamic interrelationships of the cardiac chambers, valves, and great vessels. In order for this approach to be better understood, certain definitions will be helpful.

Positioning of viscera is described as situs solitus, inversus, or ambiguous. In *situs solitus* (S), distribution of all the organs is recognized as normal, as, for example, a left-sided stomach and spleen, a predominantly right-sided liver, a trilobed right lung, and a bilobed left lung. In *situs inversus (totalis)* (I), the organs show a perfect mirror image, as regarding left and right, to that of situs solitus. Anteroposterior relations are not disturbed. When neither situs solitus nor situs inversus can be identified, *situs ambiguous* (A) is said to be present. This usually applies in cases of asplenia or polysplenia.

With the rarest of exceptions, the atria follow the body situs and are so designated (morphologic right atrium to the right of the left atrium in atrial situs solitus and to the left of the left atrium in atrial situs inversus).

The *atrioventricular canal* consists of the tricuspid valve, the mitral valve, and the septum of the atrioventricular canal and connects the atrial with the ventricular portion of the heart. As a rule each atrioventricular valve is part of the specific ventricle into which it leads. The valve situs may be solitus, inversus, or ambiguous.

The *alignment* or *type of atrioventricular* (AV) or *ventriculoarterial* (VA) *connection* addresses the issue of what flows into what. The connection may be described at the AV or VA level as *concordant* (e.g., right atrium to right ventricle, left ventricle to aorta), *discordant* (e.g., right atrium to left ventricle, left ventricle to pulmonary artery), or an arrangement that requires a special description. In the case of AV alignment where the atria are not lateralized, the alignment would be *ambiguous*. In the univentricular heart, the designation would be double-inlet, absent right or absent left AV connection. Special descriptions in the case of VA alignment or type of VA connection include double-outlet or single-outlet VA connection. The *mode* of connections, either AV or VA, on the other hand, addresses the structural makeup of the connecting segments, namely the AV canal and the infundibulum or conus. The *mode of AV connection* may be normal, common, stenotic, imperforate, atretic, double-orifice, overriding, straddling, or unguarded. The *mode of VA connection* may be expressed in terms of the position and development of the conus or infundibulum which, although normally incorporated into the right ventricle, is not an intrinsic part of the true right ventricle. It may be described as subpulmonary, subaortic, very deficient, or bilaterally present or absent.[338]

The position of the ventricles may be described by the terms *d loop* and *l loop*. When the morphologic right ventricle lies to the right of the morphologic left ventricle, the ventricular portion of the heart is said to exhibit a *d loop* (D). The ventricles are said to be *noninverted* or in the solitus position. When the ventricular relations are reversed, *l loop* (L) is said to be present. The ventricles are inverted or in the inversus position. These relationships are independent of visceral or atrial situs as well as position of the heart or its chambers within the chest.

The great arteries may deviate from the usual with respect to both their anteroposterior and their lateral (left to right) relationships.

In *solitus* (S) or *normally related great arteries* (NRGA), the aortic origin lies to the right of and posterior to the position of the pulmonary valve. In the *inversus* (I) relationship, the anteroposterior relationships are not disturbed but the aortic origin lies to the left of the pulmonary arterial origin. In *transposition of the great arteries* (TGA), the aorta arises from the anatomic right ventricle, the pulmonary artery from the anatomic left ventricle, and, usually, the aortic origin is more anterior than that of the pulmonary artery.

When the aortic origin lies to the right of the pulmonary origin, the transposition is called *dextro* or *d transposition* (D-TGA) (see discussion of complete transposition of great arteries below). When the aortic origin lies to the left of the pulmonary origin, *levo transposition* (L-TGA) is said to be present (see the section on congenitally corrected transposition below).

When the abnormal relationship of the great arteries is neither complete nor corrected transposition, the term *malposition of the great arteries* (MGA) may be used. Malpositions are designated as D-MGA or L-MGA, depending on the laterality in the relation between the origins of the two great arteries.[338] Within this group will be found examples of the abnormal VA alignment where one great artery arises from the appropriate ventricle and the other great artery also arises from the same (or inappropriate) ventricle. These will be examples of double-outlet right ventricle (DORV) or double-outlet left ventricle (DOLV). Also included will be the arterial malposition termed *anatomically corrected malposition* (ACM). This is characterized by the great arteries having a normal VA alignment (concordant), but with the aorta anterior to the pulmonary artery by virtue of an abnormal mode of VA connection, namely, the presence of a well-developed conus lying beneath both the aorta and the pulmonary artery or only beneath the aorta. The route for the flow of blood in ACMs may be normal or abnormal, depending on the atrioventricular alignment.[338]

The Segmental Approach to Diagnosis

The segmental or step-by-step approach is a valuable tool for arriving at the correct diagnosis in patients with complex congenital heart disease and is independent of cardiac position. In order, one determines: (1) the locations of the right and left atria and their venous connections; (2) the location of the right and left ventricles and their alignment with the atria; (3) the mode of connection of the atrioventricular valves to the ventricles; (4) the position of the great arteries and their alignment with the ventricles; and (5) the location and status of the infundibulum. In addition, one must search for associated malformations between and within each of these segments.

Determining atrial situs can be accomplished in most instances by taking advantage of the high degree of abdominal visceroatrial concordance. With abdominal situs solitus (S), the liver is on the right and the right atrium will almost invariably be on the right as well; with abdominal situs inversus (I), the liver is on the left and the right atrium will almost invariably be on the left. With abdominal situs ambiguous (A), the liver may be almost symmetrically placed across the midline and the atria may be normally located or inverted or both atria may have morphologic characteristics of either the right or the left atrium (Fig. 14-4). A symmetrical liver is found in approximately 60 percent of patients with situs ambiguous. Lateralization of the liver, evident in the remainder, may simulate either situs solitus or situs inversus.

When both atria have characteristics of a right atrium,[339] *dextroisomerism,* or "bilateral right-sidedness," is said to be present. This situation is usually, though not invariably, accompanied by asplenia. When both atria have characteristics of a left atrium,[339] *levoisomerism,* or "bilateral left-sidedness," is said to exist. This usually, but again not invariably, is accompanied by polysplenia.

Bronchial situs, determined by overpenetrated chest roentgenogram or bronchial tomography, is an excellent predictor of atrial situs, but the most accurate technique appears to be two-dimensional echocardiography with Doppler color flow mapping. The hepatic portion of the inferior vena cava, which almost always enters the morphologic right atrium, usually can be easily identified as can the connections and structural details of the superior vena cava, coronary sinus, pulmonary veins, atrial septum, and atrial appendages.[339]

Additional clinical clues to atrial situs may obtained from the electrocardiogram, where a superior and leftward orientation of the P-wave vector suggests levoisomerism and polysplenia. Howell-Heinz and Howell-Jolly bodies in the peripheral blood smear are characteristic of dextroisomerism or asplenia.

For determination of the atrioventricular, ventricular, and ventriculoarterial relationships, high-quality, selective biplane angiography supplemented by equally high quality two-dimensional echocardiography with Doppler color flow mapping are essential.[339]

Symbols used to designate the combination or sequence of segments are arranged in order as follows: (1) the visceroatrial or bronchoatrial situs, (2) the ventricular loop, and (3) the relations of the great arteries. These may be included within parentheses and preceded by abbreviations which indicate the ventriculoarterial alignment, for example, TGA, DORV, or single ventricle (SV). Associated malformations such as ventricular septal defect, pulmonary stenosis, and straddling tricuspid valve may be listed after the parentheses. Thus, the typical or usual transposition of the great arteries with situs solitus, d-ventricular loop, and aorta arising from the right ventricle and to the right of the pulmonary artery, with an intact ventricular septum (IVS), would be designated TGA (SDD) IVS. The designation for typical corrected transposition (TGA) with situs solitus (S), l-ventricular loop (L), aorta arising from the morphologic right ventricle and lying to the left of the pulmonary artery (L), with ventricular septal defect (VSD) and pulmonary stenosis (PS), would be TGA (SLL), VSD, PS. This designation would apply to transposition with situs solitus, whether the heart lay in the right or left chest (dextrocardia or levocardia, respectively). It should be noted that the description of the position of the heart within the chest would offer no additional information referable to the intracardiac anatomy or great-vessel alignment.[337]

Levocardia, Dextrocardia, and Mesocardia

The position of the cardiac apex indicates a condition of levocardia, dextrocardia, or mesocardia.

The trend today is to discard the terms *dextroposition, dextroversion, mirror-image dextrocardia,* and *isolated dextrocardia* because they do not provide any significant information beyond what is already known, namely, that the cardiac apex is in the right chest, and to use the broad term *dextrocardia* for all right-sided hearts, followed by a description of the visceroatrial situs. In the case of those patients in whom the heart appears to have been pulled or pushed into the right chest by massive atelectasis or hypoplasia of the right lung, diaphragmatic hernia, eventration of the diaphragm, pleural effusion, obstructive emphysema, or pneumothorax, an appropriate descriptive phrase should be added. The term *isolated levocardia* is applied to all left-sided hearts with situs inversus or situs ambiguous, and a description of the visceroatrial situs should follow.

Dextrocardia with complete situs inversus occurs in approximately 2 per 10,000 live births. The incidence of congenital heart disease is relatively low among these individuals and is estimated to be about 3 percent. *Dextrocardia with situs solitus* or *situs ambiguous* is considerably less common and occurs in perhaps 1 per 20,000 live births. The incidence of congenital heart disease is extremely high in this situation, however, and is probably in the range of 90 percent or greater. From these figures, one could project that approximately 12 percent of individuals found to have dextrocardia and congenital heart disease would have complete situs inversus. This estimate compares favorably with the figure of 18 percent observed in large autopsy series. About 50 percent of patients with dextrocardia and heart disease have situs solitus, and the remainder, perhaps 30 percent, have situs ambiguous.[337] An l-ventricular loop is found in the majority of patients with dextrocardia regardless of situs but is most common, as one might expect, among those patients with situs inversus, where it approaches 80 percent. Cardiac malformations usually, although not invariably, are severe and complex. The most common lesions and their approximate frequency are as follows:

transposition of the great arteries, 50 to 75 percent; double-outlet right ventricle, 10 to 18 percent; ventricular septal defect, 60 to 80 percent; single ventricle, 15 to 40 percent; and pulmonary stenosis or atresia, 70 to 80 percent.[337] Approximately three-quarters of the transposed great arteries will have the segmental arrangement of corrected transposition. Tetralogy of Fallot is distinctly uncommon. Polysplenia or asplenia is found in about one-third of patients with dextrocardia and almost invariably with situs ambiguous. *Kartagener's syndrome,* the triad of situs inversus, sinusitis, and bronchiectasis, results from impaired ciliary movement. It is present in approximately 20 percent of patients with dextrocardia and situs inversus totalis.[340] The incidence of *isolated levocardia* is estimated at approximately 0.6 per 10,000 live births. It is estimated that over 90 percent of affected individuals will have associated heart disease.[337] Situs inversus is present in approximately 15 percent, while the remainder have situs ambiguous, with the ratio of asplenia to polysplenia or accessory spleens being from 2.5:1 to 1.5:1. The associated defects are comparable in complexity and severity to those associated with dextrocardia. *Mesocardia* may exist either as a variant position of the normal heart or as a variant position of dextrocardia or isolated levocardia.

Medical and Surgical Management

Medical management of patients with cardiac malposition is similar to that of patients with normally located hearts, with the exceptions of continuous daily antibiotic coverage and pneumococcal vaccine for patients with asplenia and the particular attention to detail that is necessary to establish the correct diagnosis in those individuals with unusual and complex malformations.

Surgical management differs in the technical considerations imposed by the malposition of the heart itself, the frequency of occurrence of the l-ventricular loop, and the variability of the intracardiac conduction system.

Dextro Transposition of the Great Arteries

Definition

In this condition, the aorta and the pulmonary artery are misplaced in relation to the ventricular septum, with the aorta arising from the right ventricle and the pulmonary artery arising from the left ventricle (discordant ventriculoarterial connection).

Pathology

In the majority of cases there are situs solitus of the atria and viscera (S) and concordance of the atrioventricular connection and the right ventricle lies to the right of the left ventricle (d loop, D) (Fig. 97-27). The aorta lies to the right of the pulmonary arterial origin (d transposition, D) and is anterior. Of the communications between the two sides of the circulation, a narrow patent foramen and patent ductus are common in very young infants. The ventricular septum is intact in approximately half the patients, and another 10 percent will have only a very small ventricular septal defect. The remainder will have a large or multiple ventricular septal defects.[341]

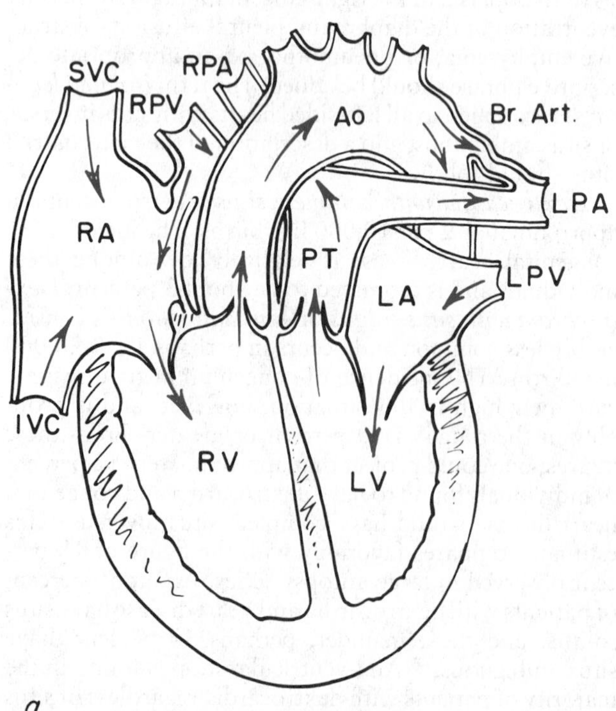

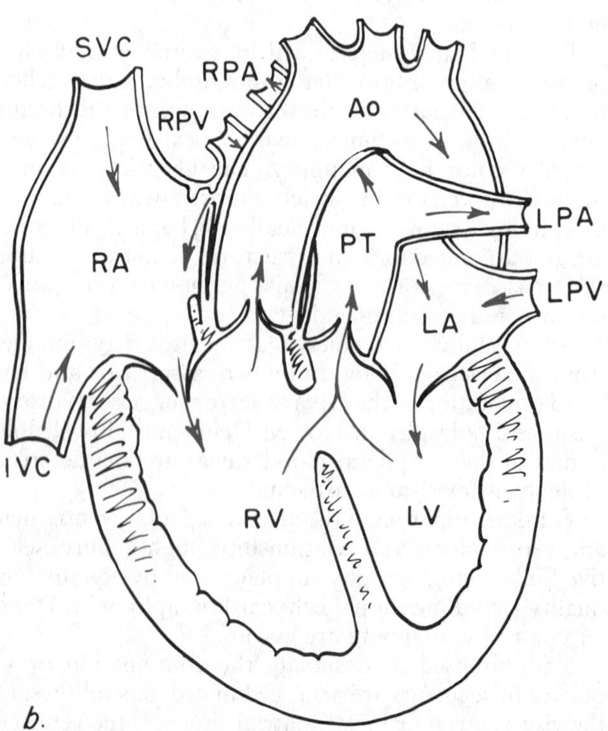

FIGURE 97-27 Complete transposition of the great arteries. *A.* With intact ventricular septum. A patent foramen ovale and enlarged bronchial arteries (Br. Art.) are present. *B.* With ventricular septal defect and without pulmonary stenosis. SVC = superior vena cava; IVC = inferior vena cava; RA = right atrium; RV = right ventricle; Ao = aorta; LA = left atrium; LV = left ventricle; TP = main pulmonary arterial trunk; RPA = right pulmonary artery; LPA = left pulmonary artery; RPV = right pulmonary vein; LPV = left pulmonary vein.

Pulmonary stenosis of significance is very uncommon among neonates with intact ventricular septum but develops with the passage of time in approximately one-third of those patients in whom the right ventricle continues as the systemic ventricle. In most cases it is mild and usually, though not invariably, is the result of a bulging of the ventricular septum into the left ventricular outflow area. Approximately one-third of patients with a large ventricular septal defect will have significant left ventricular outflow tract obstruction. Causes of this obstruction include leftward malalignment of the infundibular septum, presence of a membranous collar or ridge encircling the left ventricular outflow tract, anomalous adhesion of the anterior mitral leaflet to the ventricular septum, stenotic deformity of the pulmonary valve, and, rarely, an aneurysm of endocardial tissue related to the ventricular septal defect.

The coronary arteries usually arise from the two aortic sinuses adjacent to the pulmonary trunk, the "facing sinuses," with the most common arrangement being the right coronary artery arising from the rightward sinus and the left coronary artery, with its anterior descending and circumflex branches, arising from the leftward sinus.

Hypertensive pulmonary vascular disease may occur at an inordinately early age and may occur even in patients with an intact ventricular septum and initially low left ventricular pressures. Three-quarters or more of patients with d transposition, situs solitus, and d loop [TGA (SDD)], either have no significant associated cardiac defects or have relatively simple malformations in the form of ventricular septal defect, atrial septal defect, patent ductus arteriosus, or pulmonary stenosis. The remainder have more complicated lesions and will not be discussed in this section.

Abnormal Physiology

The systemic and pulmonary circulations are arranged so that the systemic venous return is conducted back to the systemic arterial system and the pulmonary venous return back to the pulmonary arterial system, with no obligatory mixing or interchange. For survival, there must be communication between the two circulations in the form of a patent foramen ovale, a patent ductus arteriosus, or a ventricular septal defect. The hemodynamics are dependent on the combination of defects present and particularly on the amount of mixing between the systemic and pulmonary circulations. The right ventricle is the systemic ventricle and its systolic pressure will be the same as systemic arterial pressure.

Clinical Manifestations

Approximately 9 percent of children with recognized congenital heart disease have transposition of the great arteries.[342] Males are more commonly afflicted than females in a ratio between 2:1 and 3:1.

History Among infants with intact ventricular septum, very early, severe, and progressive cyanosis is the presenting symptom or sign. In a very few, a persistent patent ductus in combination with an incompetent foramen ovale or a small ventricular septal defect permits survival for several weeks, but narrowing or closure of any of the three communications produces critical hypoxemia. Infants with a sizable ventricular septal defect present with severe congestive failure and only mild or barely detectable cyanosis toward the middle or latter part of the first month of life. Infants with a large ventricular septal defect and significant pulmonary stenosis may present within the first days of life with cyanosis if stenosis is severe; with more moderate stenosis, they may present with cyanosis and little if any congestive failure somewhat later within the first year.

Physical Examination Among infants with an intact ventricular septum, the most prominent feature is intense cyanosis. Tachypnea and mild dyspnea are present. The right ventricular lift is forceful, and the first sound is usually loud at the lower left sternal border. In most patients the second heart sound may be heard to be split narrowly, confirming the presence of two semilunar valves. Murmurs are seldom impressive or distinctive. Signs of congestive failure are uncommon unless the infant is beyond the first week of life and a large ductus is present. Among infants with a large ventricular septal defect, slenderness and mild cyanosis or a grayish pallor are apparent. Breathing is labored, and both right and left ventricular impulses are hyperactive. A thrill is uncommon. A systolic murmur at the lower left sternal border usually is present, but it is seldom loud or completely holosystolic. A gallop rhythm and a diastolic flow rumble at the apex are typical. Infants and children with ventricular septal defect and significant pulmonary stenosis generally are severely cyanotic.

Chest Roentgenogram With an intact ventricular septum, the heart size and pulmonary vascularity appear normal or at the upper limits of normal during the first week. A narrow base due to the displaced pulmonary artery may give rise to the characteristic "egg-on-side" contour. Impressive cardiomegaly, pulmonary plethora, and this characteristic contour are more common during the second week and beyond. With a large ventricular septal defect, marked cardiac enlargement involving all chambers, impressive pulmonary plethora, and the egg-on-side contour are present. With significant pulmonary stenosis, the heart resembles that of tetralogy of Fallot, but it usually slightly larger and the pulmonary vascularity less diminished than one would expect for a comparable degree of clinical cyanosis. A right aortic arch is present in 4 to 16 percent of patients.

Electrocardiogram If the ventricular septum is intact, the electrocardiogram may reveal tall or peaked P waves by the second or third day of life; however, clearly abnormal right ventricular forces are not usually apparent until the latter part of the first week. The persistence of an upright T wave in leads V_1 and V_3R beyond 4 days of age would provide an early clue that the right ventricular systolic pressure is at systemic levels. The older infant will have abnormal right axis deviation and marked right ventricular hypertrophy. A large ventricular septal defect with a large pulmonary blood flow usually will produce biatrial and biventricular hypertrophy. If pulmonary blood flow is reduced toward normal, whether by significant pulmonary stenosis, pulmonary arterial banding, or severe PVOD, the pattern becomes one of right ventricular and right atrial hypertrophy.

Echocardiogram Two-dimensional study with Doppler color flow mapping is the diagnostic procedure of choice. The pulmonary artery can be seen arising from the left ventricle and the aorta from the right ventricle. The presence or absence of ventricular septal defects, anomalies of the atrioventricular connections, status of the left ventricular outflow tract, and, in very skilled hands, the coronary arterial pattern can be identified.[343]

Cardiac Catheterization Systemic arterial oxygen desaturation will be present in all patients. The pulmonary arterial oxygen saturation invariably is higher than the systemic arterial saturation. The right ventricular systolic pressure will be at systemic levels; the left ventricular pressure will also be at systemic levels if a large ventricular septal defect, ductus arteriosus, or significant pulmonary stenosis is present. A wide pressure difference between the two ventricles or between the two atria indicates an intact or virtually intact ventricular or atrial septum, but the lack of such a gradient certainly does not guarantee the presence of an adequate opening at either level. Selective ventricular angiography will document the diagnosis and associated defects. The pulmonary artery can and should be entered using a balloon-guided catheter in all patients with transposition, with the possible exception of very small infants with critical hypoxemia and those with extremely severe pulmonary stenosis. The coronary arterial pattern should be established.[344] All newborns with transposition will benefit from balloon atrial septostomy at initial catheterization by virtue of the increased mixing of the pulmonary and systemic venous circulations and the decompression of the left atrium.

Natural History and Prognosis

Without balloon septostomy or surgical intervention, 50 percent of infants with transposition will die within the first month and 90 percent within the first year of life. Those with an intact ventricular septum die very early from hypoxemia. Those with a large ventricular septal defect usually live somewhat longer, but the majority die in the first months of congestive failure, while the few survivors will have severe PVOD. Those with a large ventricular septal defect and pulmonary stenosis have the best outlook, but the average life expectancy is barely 5 years even with this combination of defects. With an adequate interatrial opening, whether it be natural, balloon-induced, or surgically created, infants with an intact ventricular septum do relatively well during the first year. Increasing cyanosis during the first year in these patients may be due to a gradual diminution of the size of the atrial septal opening, narrowing or closure of a persistent patent ductus or small ventricular septal defect, the gradual development of subvalvular pulmonary stenosis, or the development of PVOD. Below the age of 2 years, cerebrovascular accidents are a hazard to these hypoxemic infants and occur, almost invariably, in a setting of relative anemia rather than extreme polycythemia. The appearance of PVOD is unusual, but can occur within the first 12 months of life. It becomes more frequent, approaching 40 percent, in the second year of life and thereafter. Infants with a large ventricular septal defect and no significant pulmonary stenosis will develop PVOD and become prohibitive risks for corrective surgery by the end of the first year of life. Those with a ventricular septal defect and severe pulmonary stenosis usually become progressively more cyanotic.

Palliative and subsequent corrective operations have enabled a relatively large group of patients to survive beyond infancy and early childhood. Among the survivors of the atrial inversion operations, such as the Mustard and Senning procedures, will be found such residual abnormalities as pulmonary stenosis or PVOD, as well as complications that are the result of surgery. Late sudden death has been described in about 3 percent of survivors and is very possibly the result of arrhythmias.[342] Finally, right ventricular dysfunction, with or without progressive tricuspid regurgitation, has been documented in many of the somewhat older survivors of the atrial inversion operations and raises the question of whether or not the right ventricle can function adequately as the systemic arterial ventricle beyond adolescence and early adult life. Survivors of the arterial switch operation may develop supravalvular pulmonary or aortic stenosis at the site of the anastomoses, but these are usually mild and amenable to balloon dilatation.

Medical Management

The first step in treatment of infants with intact ventricular septum is to provide without delay an adequate systemic arterial oxygen saturation. This can be achieved by balloon atrial septostomy, establishing an adequate interatrial opening by using intravenous PGE_1 infusion, supplemented by endotracheal intubation to compensate for prostaglandin-related apnea. The adequacy of the atrial septostomy opening can be determined by a sustained increase in the systemic arterial oxygen saturation to above 60 percent or P_{O_2} above 30 mmHg and verified by direct visualization with two-dimensional echocardiography. If the relief of hypoxemia is unsatisfactory, if the interatrial opening is judged by echocardiography to be small, or if an unacceptable systemic arterial oxygen saturation returns upon withdrawal of the prostaglandin infusion, the alternatives are to perform a surgical atrial septectomy without delay in those infants in whom an atrial inversion repair is planned at 4 to 8 months of age, or to proceed directly with corrective surgery in the form of the arterial switch operation. Today, if the infant were less than 2 weeks of age or the left ventricular systolic pressure was known to be 60 percent or more of the systemic arterial or left ventricular systolic pressure, we would recommend the arterial switch operation.

Once an adequate atrial septal defect has been created, infants with transposition, an intact septum, or a very small ventricular septal defect in whom an atrial inversion repair is anticipated should be followed carefully over the intervening 4 to 8 months. Care is taken to prevent anemia or infective endocarditis. Increasing hypoxemia or a suspicion of increasing pulmonary arterial pressure is an indication for prompt recatheterization.

Even if the course is uncomplicated, these infants are recatheterized electively at 3 to 7 months of age and the defect repaired shortly thereafter using either the Senning or Mustard operation or the two-stage arterial switch operation.

Arterial switch repair is now the preferred surgical alternative to the atrial inversion procedures for the neonate with an intact ventricular septum and for the slightly older infant with a large ventricular septal defect and without significant structural pulmonary stenosis. Arterial switching should be performed within the first 2 weeks of life, before left ventricular systolic pressure falls significantly below that of the right ventricle. For infants beyond 2 weeks of age, if the ratio of left ventricular to right ventricular pressure has fallen below 0.60, a pulmonary arterial band may be applied with or without a systemic-to-pulmonary arterial shunt and the arterial switch operation performed approximately 1 week later.[345] Most patterns of coronary arterial origin and course appear to be amenable to the operation, and infants as small as 2.5 kg may be successfully repaired. Repair usually is preceded by cardiac catheterization, balloon atrial septostomy, and infusion of PGE_1 to keep the ductus open and the left ventricular systolic pressure at or near systemic levels until the switch can be accomplished. Expert echocardiography and immediate surgery may make catheterization and septostomy unnecessary.

For infants with transposition, a large ventricular septal defect, and PAH, the arterial switch technique with ventricular septal defect closure or banding of the pulmonary artery must be carried out within the first 2 months of life if severe PVOD is to be prevented. Our current preference is for repair. Infants with a large ventricular septal defect and severe pulmonary stenosis usually are palliated with a systemic-to-pulmonary arterial shunt and repaired in later infancy or as young children. Finally, the severe hypoxemia present in those children with a large ventricular septal defect and severe PVOD may be reduced, in selected patients, by an intraatrial repair performed as a palliative procedure with no attempt at closure of the ventricular septal defect.[342]

Surgical Management

Initial successful physiologic repair of transposition of the great arteries was accomplished using either the Senning operation[346,347] (employing virtually no prosthetic material) or the Mustard operation[347,348] (in which pericardium or prosthetic material is used) to create a baffle positioned to divert systemic venous blood from the venae cavae into the left atrium, mitral orifice, left ventricle, and posterior pulmonary artery. Complications included pulmonary and systemic venous obstruction, loss of sinus rhythm, troublesome arrhythmias, tricuspid valve regurgitation, and right ventricular failure.[347,349] Although technically demanding, neonatal anatomic repair by the arterial switch operation of Jatene,[350–353] as modified by LeCompte and others, is now preferred. Operation is performed during the first 2 weeks of life while the left ventricle is still sufficiently hypertrophic to function in the presence of normal systemic vascular resistance. When discovered late, older infants and children can be anatomically repaired by a staged arterial switch repair, a pulmonary arterial band being placed first to "prepare" the left ventricle, with a systemic arterial–to–pulmonary arterial shunt placed just distal to the band to maintain adequate pulmonary blood flow.[347,354,355] One to two weeks later, the band is removed, the shunt is eliminated, and an arterial switch operation is performed. Both early and late survival rates are excellent, actually approaching that of the normal neonate.[354,356–358]

Repairs of complex forms of transposition of the great arteries, including those with associated ventricular septal defect[359] and subpulmonic left ventricular outflow tract obstruction[360] or double-outlet right ventricle (the Taussig-Bing heart),[361] are beyond the scope of this discussion.[362] Initial management of infants having these complex defects consists of provision of adequate intracardiac mixing of systemic and pulmonary venous blood by atrial septostomy or surgical septectomy and the adjustment of pulmonary blood flow by pulmonary arterial banding or the creation of a systemic arterial–to–pulmonary arterial shunt. Complex anatomic repairs are accomplished later, when risk of injury to the conduction system and growth-related problems imposed by the repair are less significant.

Double-Outlet Right Ventricle

Pathology

In this malformation more than 50 percent of the semilunar valve orifices of both great arteries arise from the morphologic right ventricle. In most cases the ventricles display a d loop, and the pulmonary arterial origin is normally positioned, arising from a conus above the right ventricle. The aorta also arises from the right ventricle above conal tissue. The two semilunar valves are at about the same level, and there is no fibrous continuity between the semilunar and mitral valves (Fig. 97-28).

In most cases the aortic origin is to the right (d malposition) of the pulmonary arterial origin, the two vessels usually displaying a side-by-side relationship. Uncommonly, the aortic origin is distinctly anterior to the pulmonary origin or the aorta arises to the left (l malposition) of the pulmonary artery.[363]

With rare exceptions, there is a ventricular septal defect. The condition may be further subdivided on the basis of the relation of the ventricular septal defect to the origin of the great arteries. The ventricular septal defect will be subaortic in approximately two-thirds of patients, subpulmonary (*Taussig-Bing heart*) in 20 percent, related to both great arteries (*doubly committed*) in 3 percent, and remote or unrelated to either great artery in about 7 percent.[363]

Associated Conditions Pulmonary stenosis occurs in over half of cases, the condition usually resulting from a narrow subpulmonary conus. Atrial septal defect, subaortic stenosis, and coarctation of the aorta are also relatively common, with the latter particularly associated with the subpulmonary defect. Obstruction at the mitral valve may be observed in about one-fifth of cases of double-outlet right ventricle. Mitral valve straddling of

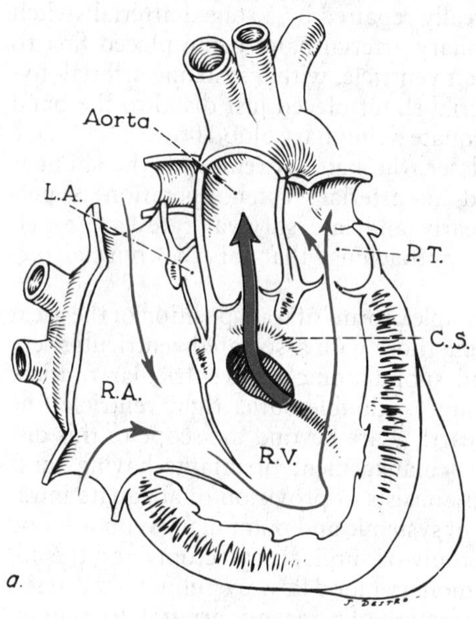

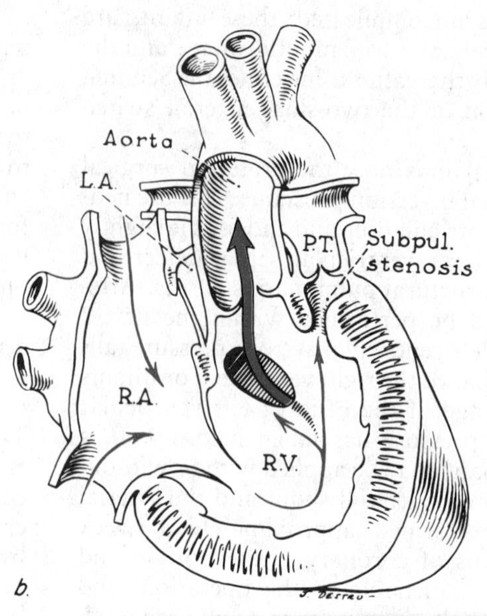

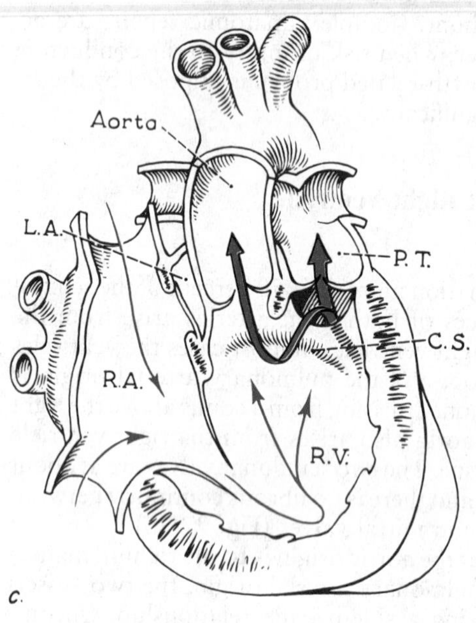

FIGURE 97-28 Double-outlet right ventricle. *A.* With subaortic ventricular septal defect without pulmonary stenosis. *B.* With subaortic ventricular septal defect and subpulmonary stenosis (Subpul. stenosis). *C.* With subpulmonary ventricular septal defect, the sos-called Taussig-Bing complex. R.A. = right atrium; R.V. = right ventricle; C.S. = crista supraventricularis; L.A. = left atrium; P.T. = main pulmonary arterial trunk.

the ventricular septal defect and varying degrees of left ventricular hypoplasia also are encountered.

Clinical Manifestations

Double-outlet right ventricle, or origin of both great arteries from the right ventricle, is a relatively rare malformation found in only 0.5 percent of patients with congenital heart disease.[6] It is of considerable importance, however, because its clinical and laboratory features frequently resemble those of more common and more easily correctable malformations.

History and Physical Examination Patients with a subaortic ventricular septal defect without pulmonary stenosis (Fig. 97-28*A*) have the same findings on examination as do patients with a large isolated ventricular septal defect. Congestive failure appears within a few weeks of birth, and cyanosis is seldom described. Those with a subaortic ventricular septal defect and pulmonary stenosis (Fig. 97-28*B*) usually present after the newborn period and follow a course similar to patients with tetralogy of Fallot. Patients with a subpulmonary defect without pulmonary stenosis (Fig. 97-28*C*), the Taussig-Bing malformation, resemble patients with transposition of the great arteries and a large ventricular septal defect without pulmonary stenosis. The findings are those of severe congestive failure and impressive cyanosis.

Chest Roentgenogram Cardiomegaly with pulmonary overperfusion is characteristic of all types of this anomaly without pulmonary stenosis. Double-outlet right ventricle with subaortic ventricular septal defect and pulmonary stenosis resembles tetralogy of Fallot. In the case of subpulmonary ventricular septal defect without pulmonary stenosis, the pulmonary artery usually lies beside rather than posterior to the aorta; this clearly visible, dilated main pulmonary artery may permit distinction of this malformation from transposition, which it mimics so closely.

Electrocardiogram Right axis deviation and right atrial and right ventricular hypertrophy are characteristic of double-outlet right ventricle.

Echocardiogram Two-dimensional echocardiography is capable of demonstrating the anatomic components and associated defects.[364]

Cardiac Catheterization There is an increase in oxygen saturation at the right ventricular level. The pulmonary arterial saturation is lower than that of the aorta in patients with a subaortic ventricular septal defect and is invariably higher than that of the aorta in those with a subpulmonary septal defect. Left ventricular systolic pressure may be higher than the right if the ventricular septal defect is small and restrictive. Selective right and left ventricular biplane angiography as well as an aortogram are recommended.

Natural History and Prognosis

The clinical course of each variety of double-outlet right ventricle is determined by the associated defects. Without surgical intervention, those with an unguarded pulmonary artery either die in infancy with congestive failure or develop PVOD. Spontaneous narrowing or closure of the ventricular septal defect may occur and is life-threatening. Increasing dyspnea, increasing intensity of the systolic murmur, and progressive left ventricular hypertrophy suggest this complication. Patients with pulmonary stenosis tend to have progressive obstruction and cyanosis.

Medical Management

Vigorous treatment of heart failure is required for those without pulmonary stenosis. Essentially all cases are best treated with surgical palliation or correction in infancy. If there is pulmonary hypertension, banding or correction should be done by 3 to 4 months of age. Whether or not corrective surgery has been performed, all patients in whom the left ventricular output must pass through the ventricular septal defect should be observed continuously for the possibility of spontaneous narrowing and obstruction at that site.

Surgical Management

Great variability exists in the morphologic spectrum of double-outlet right ventricle.[365–367] Although primary total repair of most forms of double-outlet right ventricle is now performed and preferred in infancy, palliation (pulmonary arterial banding, atrial septal excision, and creation of systemic arterial–to–pulmonary arterial or systemic venous–to–pulmonary arterial shunts) to adjust pulmonary blood flow and preserve ventricular function, the pulmonary vascular bed, and AV valve competence should be considered in complex variants or in the critically ill neonate.[365]

In all forms of double-outlet ventricle, the relation of the ventricular septal defect to the great arteries and the magnitude of ventricular outflow tract obstruction dictate management.[368] Surgical correction requires (1) closure of the ventricular septal defect, (2) relief of pulmonary stenosis when present, (3) diversion of oxygenated pulmonary venous blood to the aorta, and (4) diversion of hypoxemic systemic venous blood to the pulmonary artery.[367] When the ventricular septal defect is committed to the aorta, a Dacron semiconduit or tunnel-shaped patch is placed to obliterate the interventricular communication while diverting the left ventricular blood through the ventricular septal defect to the aorta.[369] Pulmonary stenosis is corrected by a valvotomy with excision of obstructive muscle bundles and placement of a transannular patch when necessary. Otherwise, an extracardiac conduit is placed between the right ventricle and the pulmonary artery.[365,370]

When the great arteries are transposed or the ventricular septal defect is not committed to the aorta, the arterial switch operation using the concepts of Jatene and LeCompte permits patch closure of the ventricular septal defect, directing left ventricular blood into the neo-aorta.[362] Further consideration of repair of double-outlet right ventricle associated with more complex defects is beyond the scope of this discussion.[365–367,371,372] Patients having ventricular hypoplasia, mitral stenosis, or straddling of AV valves are usually not candidates for biventricular repair; initial palliation should prepare the child for a modification of Fontan's operation.[373]

In a 10-year review of repair of classic double-outlet right ventricle in 62 patients,[371] early mortality was 15 percent with 21 percent of late deaths attributable to arrhythmias. All but one of the surviving patients were in New York Heart Association class I or II.

Risks and protocols for operations for double-outlet right ventricle, summarized by Kirklin and colleagues,[374] describe an overall actuarial survival rate of 38 percent at 12 years, but suggest recent improvement such that current expectations for 10-year survival are 97 percent for repair in the 6-month-old infant.

Corrected Transposition of the Great Arteries

Definition

Atrioventricular discordance and ventriculoarterial discordance form the characteristics of corrected transposition.

Pathology

Usually situs solitus is present, but the ventricles are inverted (an l loop). The great arteries are transposed and in the l position so that the pulmonary artery arises posteriorly from the right-sided morphologic left ventricle and the l-transposed aorta arises anteriorly from the left-sided right ventricle (Fig. 97-29). If situs inversus is present, the segmental pattern is IDD. Along with the ventricular inversion there is AV valvar inversion. The two coronary arteries arise from the right and left (posteriorly positioned) sinuses with the right giving off the anterior descending and the circumflex branches.

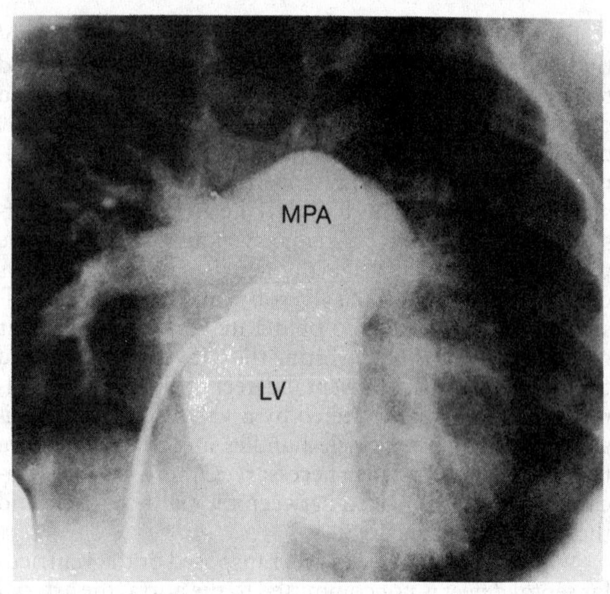

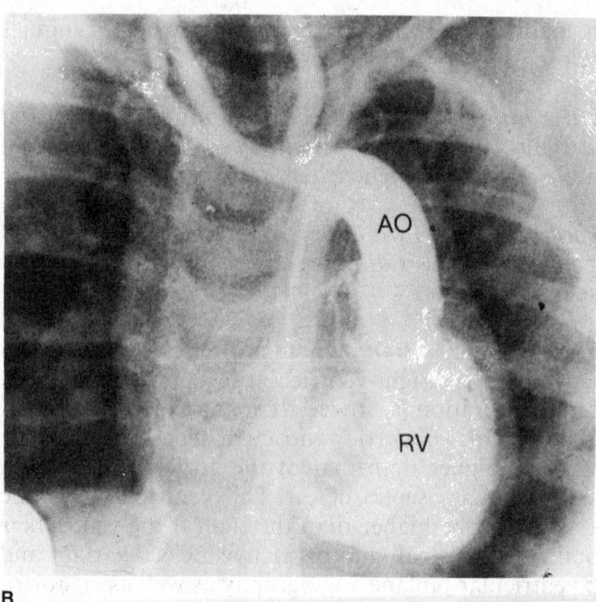

FIGURE 97-29 *A.* Posteroanterior view of the left ventricular (LV) angiogram in a child with corrected transposition of the great arteries. The main pulmonary artery (MPA) arises from the smooth-walled left ventricle, which receives the systemic venous blood. *B.* Posteroanterior view of the right ventricular angiogram (RV). The ascending aorta (AO) arises to the left of the pulmonary artery from the more heavily trabeculated right ventricle, which receives the pulmonary venous blood. The ventricular septum, seen here perpendicular to the frontal plane, is intact.

Associated Conditions Rarely, no associated conditions are present and the circulation is normal. In the majority of cases (about 80 percent), a ventricular septal defect is present. It may be in any location, but a perimembranous subpulmonary defect is most common.

The inverted left-sided systemic tricuspid valve frequently shows some degree of abnormality, usually leading to incompetence. The most common abnormality is an Ebstein-like displacement of the septal and posterior leaflets, but dysplasia, clefts, and straddling of the ventricular septum are also described.

Pulmonary atresia or stenosis is present in about 70 percent of cases.[375] This obstruction is usually subvalvular, rarely only valvular, and may result from attachments of accessory mitral valve tissue.

Clinical Manifestations

Corrected transposition is an uncommon malformation, occurring in slightly less than 1 percent of children with congenital heart disease. The importance of this anomaly lies in its frequent association with serious AV conduction disturbances, the intracardiac malformations, and in the medical and surgical implications of the ventricular inversion. The clinical picture is determined primarily by the associated anomalies. Approximately half of patients can be expected to develop complete AV block if followed for a 20-year period.[376]

History A slow, irregular heart rate is often detected in utero, and 10 percent of patients with congenital complete block prove to have corrected transposition. Those patients with a large ventricular septal defect without pulmonary stenosis usually present within the first month or so of life with symptoms indistinguishable from those of infants with a large septal defect alone. Patients with ventricular septal defect and pulmonary stenosis may present with symptoms of cyanosis and resemble patients with tetralogy of Fallot.

Physical Examination The murmur of left AV valve regurgitation may be best heard either at the apex or at the lower left sternal border. Most cases have a murmur of ventricular septal defect or pulmonary stenosis. Occasionally an inordinately accentuated second heart sound at the upper left sternal border suggests the presence of PAH, although in reality it represents the sound of aortic valve closure augmented to auscultation by the anterior and superior displacement of the aorta.

Chest Roentgenogram A straight or gently curved convex upper left heart border, representing the contour of the transposed ascending aorta, is characteristic and is most easily recognized in those patients with a ventricular septal defect and pulmonary stenosis, in whom there is a mild dilatation of the ascending aorta.

Electrocardiogram Varying degrees of AV conduction delay are present in almost a third of patients. The initial forces of ventricular depolarization characteristically are oriented anteriorly and to the left, with Q waves in the right precordial leads and not in leads I, V_5, and V_6. With normal or near-normal pressure in the systemic venous or morphologic left ventricle, a QS pattern in the right and an RS pattern in the left precordial leads are usual.

Echocardiogram Two-dimensional echocardiography permits identification of the anatomic components and associated defects.[377]

Cardiac Catheterization From the right atrium the morphologic left ventricle is entered, and, in the presence of a ventricular septal defect, the catheter may cross the defect, traverse the morphologic right ventricle, and enter the ascending aorta in the position normally occupied by the pulmonary artery. Entry into the medially placed pulmonary artery may be much more difficult, but the use of flow-guided catheters will permit successful entry for measurement of pressure in most instances. Selective angiography in both ventricles will outline the defects. The ventricular septum usually lies in the anteroposterior plane, and frequently a ventricular septal defect may be imaged best angiographically in the frontal view (Fig. 97-29). Gentle manipulation of the catheter within the heart is indicated, since the production of varying degrees of transient AV block is not uncommon and, in a rare instance, the block may prove permanent.

Natural History and Prognosis

The clinical course is determined primarily by the severity of the associated defects. It is estimated that only about 1 percent of individuals with corrected transposition have an otherwise normal heart. Even with complicating anomalies, survival to adulthood is possible. Congestive heart failure associated with a large ventricular septal defect has been the most common cause of death, with most fatalities occurring within the first year of life. AV conduction abnormalities tend to be progressive, and complete AV block may appear at any age. Similarly, left AV valve regurgitation may present at any age and significantly alters long-term outcome.[378] Finally, the morphologic right ventricle may not be capable of sustaining adequate cardiac output over a normal life span.

Medical Management

Management of corrected transposition includes the treatment of congestive failure, cyanosis, and AV block and the prevention of infective endocarditis. Patients with severe pulmonary hypertension or congestive heart failure should undergo early banding of the pulmonary artery or repair of the defect. Similarly those patients with a ventricular septal defect, severe pulmonary stenosis, and cyanosis benefit from systemic-to-pulmonary artery shunting procedures or total correction. The vulnerability of the ventricular conduction system and the difficulty in visualization of the septal defect in the subpulmonary region of the morphologic left ventricle have influenced us to recommend the palliative approach in both groups of patients, especially during infancy. Those with congenital block require pacemaker therapy if they are symptomatic. Patients with significant left AV valve regurgitation require valve replacement. Regularly scheduled follow-up examinations are recommended for all patients to detect progressive AV conduction disorders and the late appearance of left AV valve incompetence.

Surgical Management

Ventricular septal defect closure, relief of pulmonary stenosis, and correction of systemic AV valve regurgitation are sometimes required in patients having corrected transposition of the great arteries.[379–381] The specialized electrical conduction system is particularly at risk in these patients because of its right-sided location and abnormal anatomic course. Approach to the ventricular septal defect through an incision in the left-sided ventricle[382] or aorta[383] or a combined right atrial–mitral valve and aortic approach,[384] placement of sutures through the septal defect on the left side of the septum, and the use of intracardiac mapping[379] appear to reduce the incidence of complete heart block. Nonetheless, the high morbidity and mortality associated with operation demand a conservative surgical attitude.[385]

Relief of pulmonary stenosis is technically complicated by the fact that obstruction is usually subvalvar, lying posteriorly and to the right of the right ventricle while the mitral valve apparatus obscures exposure from the right side. Again, the conduction system is vulnerable. Left ventricular–to–pulmonary arterial conduits have been advised when subvalvular pulmonary stenosis is severe.[386]

Of 17 patients undergoing intracardiac repair,[380] all had large ventricular septal defects requiring closure; 8 had associated pulmonary stenosis for which surgical intervention was required. A valve-containing extracardiac conduit was implanted in four of the patients having obstruction to pulmonary blood flow. Left AV valve incompetence required tricuspid valve replacement in three. There were four hospital deaths (23.5 percent), two late deaths (11.8 percent), six instances of AV dissociation (37.5 percent), and six cases of postoperative tricuspid valvular incompetence. A more recent review of 18 patients[379] revealed similar outcomes.

Univentricular Heart

Definition

The univentricular heart, or *single ventricle,*[387] is characterized by the entire flow from the two atria being carried directly through the mitral and tricuspid valves into the same ventricular chamber (Fig. 97-30). This *double-inlet* type of AV connection may take the form of either one common or two separate AV valves.[388] Straddling of one AV valve is sometimes included. The ventriculoarterial connections may be *concordant* (pulmonary artery from the right ventricle and aorta from the left ventricle), *discordant* (pulmonary artery from the left ventricle and aorta from the right ventricle), *double-outlet* (both great arteries from either the left or right ventricle), or *single-outlet* (atresia of one great artery). By this definition, cases of *mitral* or *tricuspid atresia* are excluded as are those of *pulmonary* or *aortic atresia* with an intact ventricular septum.

Pathology

The most common type of univentricular heart (65 to 75 percent of cases)[389] is that in which the dominant ventricular chamber has the trabecular pattern of a left ventricle and communicates through an opening, the bulboventricular foramen, with a rudimentary right ventricle. The ventriculoarterial connection is discordant (transposition of the great arteries) in about 90 percent of patients.[388] In about 20 percent of cases the dominant

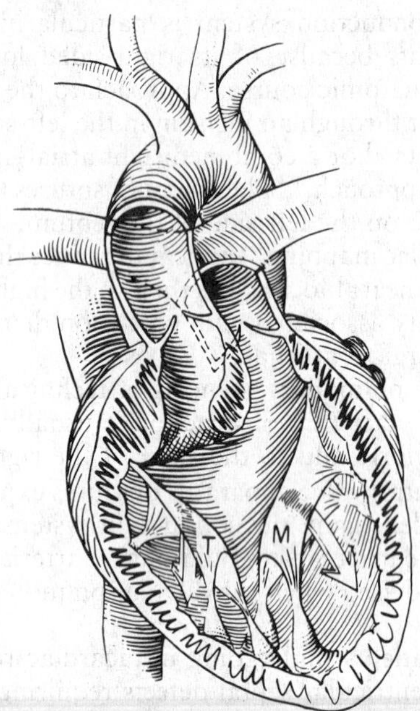

FIGURE 97-30 Common ventricle with dextro-malposition and without pulmonary stenosis. T = tricuspid valve; M = mitral valve.

ventricle shows the trabecular features of a right ventricle and the rudimentary chamber those of a left ventricle. The majority of these patients have a double-outlet ventriculoarterial connection from the main chamber, and a smaller number have a single-outlet connection, with pulmonary atresia.[390] In 10 to 14 percent neither ventricular sinus can be identified; this is the so-called primitive ventricle.[388,389]

Associated Conditions Pulmonary stenosis or atresia is common. Subaortic stenosis may result from a narrow bulboventricular foramen.[391]

Clinical Manifestations

This complex and challenging malformation is relatively rare. The clinical picture is determined largely by the associated defects of which pulmonary stenosis, present in a little over half of the patients, and obstruction to aortic flow are the most important.

History All patients will have some degree of systemic arterial oxygen desaturation, although cyanosis, appreciated clinically, may range from barely detectable to severe. Congestive failure is common. The majority will require hospitalization in the first month of life.

Physical Examination The findings on palpation and auscultation are quite variable and not distinctive.

Chest Roentgenogram Almost all patients have at least some degree of cardiac enlargement. Those with little or no pulmonary stenosis generally have very large hearts with marked pulmonary plethora. Only those patients with very severe pulmonary stenosis or atresia show a near-normal heart size and diminished pulmonary arterial blood flow.

Electrocardiogram Evidence of right or left ventricular hypertrophy is common.

Echocardiography Two-dimensional echocardiography with Doppler color flow studies can identify virtually all of the morphologic and functional features of this malformation necessary to establish the diagnosis and make a plan for clinical management.[112,392]

Cardiac Catheterization A degree of systemic arterial oxygen desaturation is present in all patients, although the severity appears to be related mainly to the volume of pulmonary blood flow. Careful recording of intracardiac and arterial pressures is essential in order to detect significant or potentially significant obstruction to blood flow across either AV valve, across the atrial septum, or between the ventricle and the aorta or pulmonary artery. The morphologic features of the ventricle, relation of the aorta and pulmonary artery, and other features can be established by high-quality selective ventricular angiography using specially angled views to supplement conventional views.[231]

Natural History and Prognosis

Patients usually present as newborns with cyanosis, congestive failure, or a combination of both. Those in whom the pulmonary arterial pressure and blood flow are increased require surgery to prevent death from congestive heart failure or progressive PVOD. Patients with severe pulmonary stenosis or atresia require systemic-to-pulmonary arterial shunting procedures. Among patients with univentricular heart, there is a propensity for the development of subaortic obstruction[392] and AV valve regurgitation.[393] Both threaten ventricular compliance and diminish the likelihood of successful long-term palliation.[394] Survivors are subject to the threats of infective endocarditis, brain abscess, and progressive PVOD.

Medical Management

Early recognition and identification of patients with these complex defects are important if successful palliative surgical procedures are to be carried out for the relief of congestive failure or cyanosis. Prostaglandin E_1 is useful in neonates with ductal-dependent defects. Digitalis and diuretics may be necessary for those patients with continuing heart failure. Care should be taken that anemia or severe polycythemia does not develop and that these patients are adequately protected against infective endocarditis. If more definitive procedures are to be considered, the pulmonary vascular bed must be protected and ventricular function and compliance must be carefully preserved. The long-term outlook for the survivors has yet to be determined.

Surgical Management

Palliation for patients with univentricular AV connections requires adjustment of pulmonary blood flow with a pulmonary arterial band when excessive or, when pulmonary blood flow is diminished, creation of a shunt. The modified Blalock-Taussig shunt is preferred in the neonate. An adequate interatrial communication is essential. Prognosis deteriorates with a single ventricle of the right ventricular type[395] and the evolution of AV valvular regurgitation[393] or subaortic obstruction.[396,397] Ventricular function and AV valvular competence are preserved by early creation of a bidirectional modified Glenn anastomasis (superior vena cava–to–undivided pulmonary artery).[398] Subaortic stenosis or obstruction at the bulboventricular foramen can be palliated by anastomosis of the proximal pulmonary artery to the lateral aspect of the ascending aorta while pulmonary blood flow is delivered to the distal pulmonary arterial tree through a systemic arterial or systemic venous shunt. Palliation by arterial switch operation has also been advocated, but experience is limited.[399]

In the past, physiologic or orthoterminal correction was accomplished in a small number of patients by septation of the single ventricle using a woven Dacron patch.[400,401] Commonly, this is now accomplished by exclusion of the pulmonary circulation from the systemic ventricular outflow using modifications of Fontan's operation to direct systemic venous blood directly to the pulmonary arteries.[402] The single ventricle is thus relieved of the burden of the pulmonary circulation and is required only to deliver systemic cardiac output. Repair by Fontan's concepts early in life, usually between the age of 2 and 4 years, minimizes the development of PVOD, AV valvular regurgitation, and congestive heart failure and relieves the child of the burden of hypoxemia. Experience with atresia of the aortic tract (the hypoplastic left heart syndrome) has encouraged earlier orthoterminal repair using cavopulmonary connection and staged modifications of Fontan's operation.[398]

Timing and patient selection have yielded improved and far more optimistic survival in more recently corrected patients.[399,403] Quality and length of life are clearly improved, but persistent problems include AV valvular regurgitation, limitation of exercise tolerance, protein-losing enteropathy, atrial or supraventricular arrhythmias, and deterioration of ventricular function.[398,399]

CONGENITAL ABNORMALITIES OF THE CORONARY ARTERIAL CIRCULATION

Coronary Arteriovenous Fistula

Pathology

A coronary arteriovenous fistula is represented by a gross communication between a coronary artery and a cardiac chamber, the coronary sinus, or the pulmonary trunk (Fig. 97-31).

The site of origin may involve any of the epicardial coronary arteries. The right coronary artery is the site of origin in somewhat over half the cases, and the two most common sites into which the fistula feeds are a cardiac vein (usually the coronary sinus) and the right ventricle. Although solitary communication is the rule, there may be multiple sites of termination.[404] A fistula into the pulmonary trunk is usually characterized by one or more vessels opening into the pulmonary trunk and connecting with branches of each of the two main coronary arteries. The artery or arteries feeding the fistula are grossly enlarged and tortuous. Saccular aneurysms may develop in segments of dilated vessels; such aneurysms are usually observed in the adult and frequently show calcification of the wall.

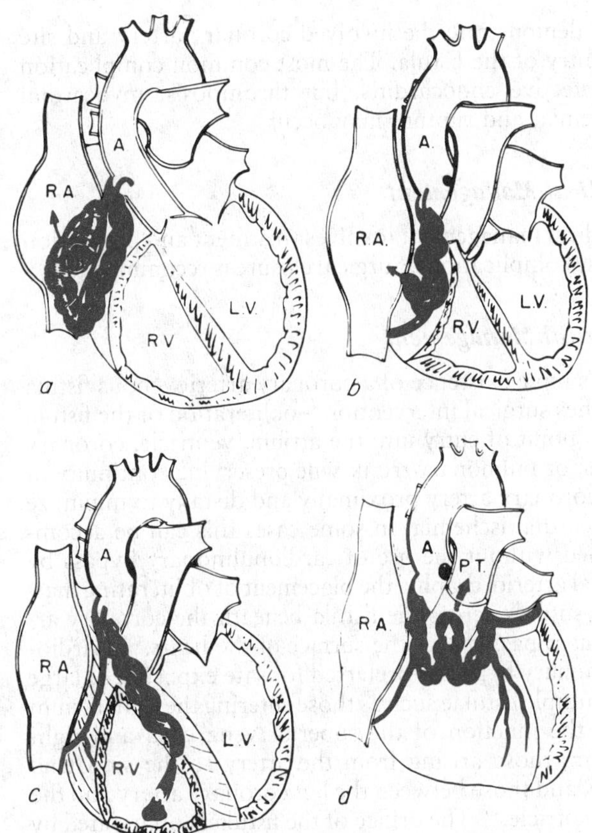

FIGURE 97-31 Anomalous communications of coronary arteries. *A.* Right coronary artery communicates with coronary sinus. *B.* Right coronary artery communicates with right atrium (RA). *C.* Anomalous communication of right coronary artery with right ventricle (RV). *D.* Two coronary arteries arise from the aorta (A) and make collateral communication with accessory coronary artery arising from pulmonary trunk (PT). LV = left ventricle.

Clinical Manifestations[405,406]

Many patients with a coronary arteriovenous fistula are asymptomatic. In some, the magnitude of the shunt into the right side of the heart is great enough to cause congestive heart failure, with a tendency for this to occur in early infancy or after 40 years of age. The classic finding is that of continuous murmur with an unusual location, since it is loudest over the fistula. It may have a louder diastolic component, especially if communication is with the right ventricle. In those with large shunts, there may be cardiomegaly and increased pulmonary flow shown by chest roentgenogram and right ventricular hypertrophy shown by electrocardiogram. At cardiac catheterization, an increase in oxygen saturation may be encountered, usually in the right atrium or right ventricle, if the shunt is large enough. Selective coronary arteriography[288] will demonstrate the involved coronary artery and site of entry of the fistula. The most common complication is infective endocarditis, but thrombosis, myocardial ischemia, and rupture may occur.

Medical Management

Medical management involves treatment and prevention of the complications. Surgical closure is recommended.[407]

Surgical Management

The simple existence of a coronary arteriovenous fistula justifies surgical intervention—obliteration of the fistula at its point of entry into the atrium, ventricle, coronary sinus, or pulmonary trunk wile preserving continuity of the coronary artery proximally and distally to minimize myocardial ischemia. In some cases this can be accomplished without the use of cardiopulmonary bypass by lateral arteriorrhaphy, the placement of obliterating mattress sutures across the fistula beneath the coronary artery as it passes over the surface of the heart.[408] Cardiopulmonary bypass is preferred for safe exposure of large or multiple fistulae such as those entering the right atrium near the junction of the superior vena cava and right atrium, those arising from the artery to the sinoatrial node, and those between the left coronary artery and the left ventricle.[409] The orifice of the fistula is obliterated by direct suture or placement of a Dacron or pericardial patch. Fistulae have been closed from within the opened coronary artery; the artery is then repaired by direct suture.

Only 4 deaths occurred in 116 reported cases of coronary arteriovenous fistulas that were closed surgically.[407] Operation is safe, relatively simple, and effectively eliminates symptoms and prevents subsequent complications.

Origin of the Left Coronary Artery from the Pulmonary Artery

In this anomaly, the right coronary artery arises from the aorta, while the left coronary artery arises from the pulmonary artery (Fig. 97-32). This is also known as the Bland-White-Garland syndrome. The course and branching of the vessel are normal. In the young, the coronary arteries are of normal size, but if the patient survives beyond infancy, there is noticeable dilatation of these vessels. In cases of infant death from this condition, the left ventricle is dilated and may show sites of infarction with calcification of affected myocardium. In subjects surviving infancy, there is often scarring of the left ventricular papillary muscles and of the left ventricular wall, particularly in the distribution of the left coronary artery. The left ventricular cavity is dilated and the chamber shows endocardial fibroelastosis. The mitral valve may become incompetent.[410] Associated conditions are uncommon. (See also Chaps. 64 and 138.)

The clinical spectrum and mode of presentation in patients with this abnormality vary.[411,412] The majority of patients present at a few months of age. Acute episodes of irritability, profuse cold sweating, pallor, and respiratory distress occur, with evidence of heart failure. Less often, the patients present at any age with mitral regurgitation and heart failure. A few reach adolescence or adulthood with relatively few symptoms other than occasional exertional angina or palpitations. Sudden death may be the first and only sign of this diagnosis.

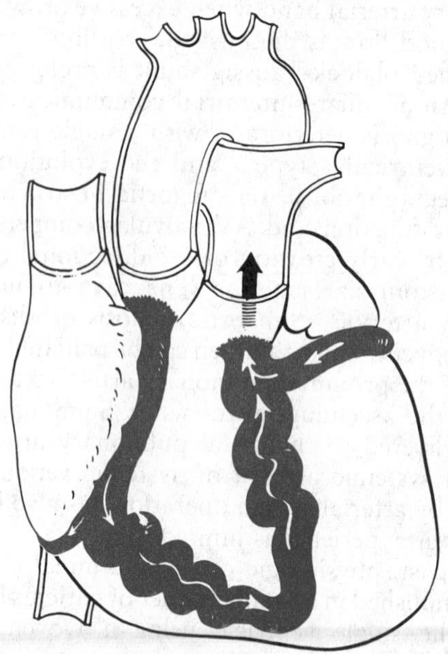

FIGURE 97-32 Anomalous origin of the left coronary artery from the pulmonary trunk. With time, wide collaterals develop between the two coronary systems, so that right coronary arterial blood is shunted into the left coronary system and thence into the pulmonary trunk.

On physical examination, the heart is enlarged with an abnormal left ventricular apex impulse. Other signs of failure are usually present. Pallor and clammy skin are common. In some, a soft continuous murmur is heard at the upper left sternal border. This murmur is more prominent in older patients, presumable due to development of a more extensive collateral circulation. The murmur of mitral regurgitation may be heard at the apex, radiating to the axilla; however, in young infants with heart failure there can be a surprising degree of regurgitation without a distinctive murmur.

The chest roentgenogram typically shows marked enlargement of the heart with posterior displacement of the esophagus by a large left atrium. There is pulmonary edema, and there may be atelectasis of the left lower lobe due to bronchial compression.

The electrocardiogram demonstrates the pattern of anterolateral infarction with deep Q wave in leads I and aV_L and abnormal R-wave progression across the precordium. Arrhythmias are frequent. The horizontal loop of the vectorcardiogram is clockwise and posteriorly oriented. The echocardiogram shows marked enlargement of the left atrium and ventricle with little or no left ventricular wall motion. The origin of the coronary artery can occasionally be imaged. Myocardial perfusion imaging with ^{201}Tl can help distinguish this from congestive cardiomyopathy.[413]

At cardiac catheterization, there may be an increase in saturation in the pulmonary artery if there is enough retrograde flow. There is usually some pulmonary hyper-

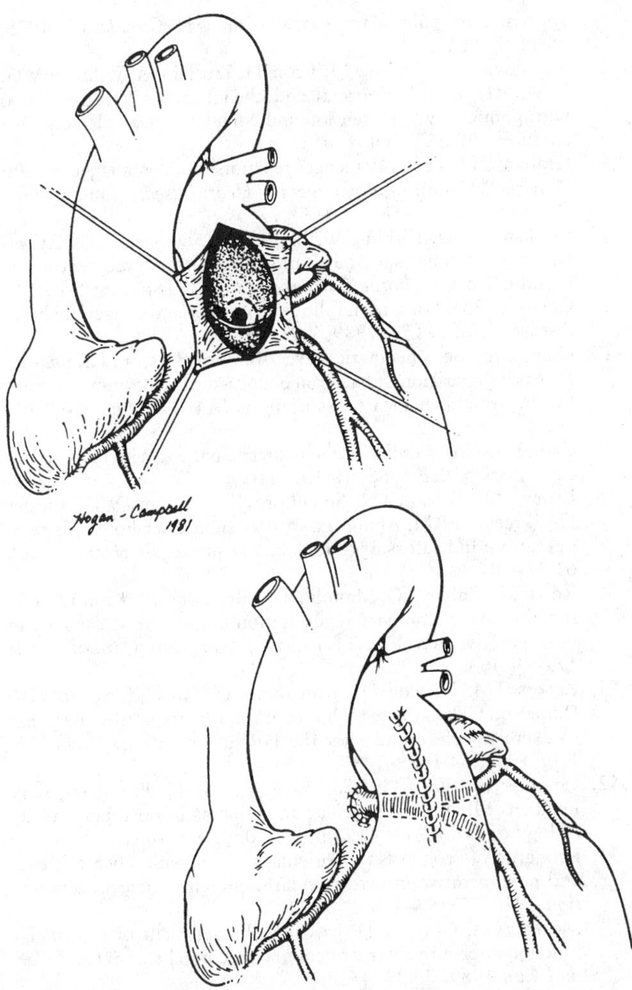

FIGURE 97-33 Transposition of anomalous left coronary artery from the pulmonary artery to the aorta. The orifice of the left coronary artery is excised from within the opened pulmonary artery (on cardiopulmonary bypass). The proximal segment of the left coronary artery and its branches, the circumflex and the left anterior descending branches, are mobilized to provide sufficient length for a tension-free anastomosis of the orifice, with a surrounding cuff of pulmonary arterial wall, to the left posterolateral wall of the aorta.

tension with very elevated pulmonary wedge pressure. Aortography or selective right coronary arteriography[288] demonstrates the collateral circulation filling the left coronary artery retrogradely with at least faint opacification of the main pulmonary artery.

Natural history and prognosis are indicated by the modes of presentation. Most patients die in infancy. Medical management is aimed at control of congestive heart failure and arrhythmias.

Surgical anastomosis to the aorta should be attempted to improve myocardial blood flow and prevent further myocardial damage.[414] The optimum age for operation has not been determined.[415] Clearly the risk is greater for infants, but this is also the group with the poorest natural prognosis.[416]

Antegrade left coronary arterial flow can be established in older children by interposition of autologous vein or synthetic grafts between the aorta and the anomalous left coronary artery, with subsequent ligation of the artery near its pulmonary arterial orifice.[417] Perfusion of the left coronary arterial system after ligation can also be accomplished by internal mammary or subclavian arterial anastomosis. Preferably, direct perfusion of the left coronary arterial orifice without ligation is accomplished in the infant by creation of a synthetic or autogenous tissue conduit from the aorta within the pulmonary artery[418] or excision of the orifice from the pulmonary artery with subsequent anastomosis to the ascending aorta[419] (Fig. 97-33).[417]

Assuming appropriate intraoperative myocardial protection, mortality is largely attributable to preexisting left ventricular infarction and failure, ventricular arrhythmias, and mitral regurgitation secondary to papillary muscle dysfunction and annular dilatation. These problems are most prevalent in critically ill infants requiring urgent surgery. Improvement in severely impaired left ventricular function following operation can be expected in operative survivors.[420] Low mortality and a good hemodynamic result should be anticipated in older patients having reasonable preoperative ventricular function.[421]

REFERENCES

1. Mitchell SC, Korones SB, Berendes HW: Congenital heart disease in 56,109 births. Incidence and natural history. *Circulation* 1971; 43:323–332.
2. Hoffman JIE, Christianson R: Congenital heart disease in a cohort of 19,502 births with long-term follow-up. *Am J Cardiol* 1978; 42:641–647.
3. Fyler DC: Report of the New England Regional Infant Cardiac Program. *Pediatrics* 1980; 65:II-375–II-461.
4. Nadas AS, Fyler DC: *Pediatric Cardiology,* 3d ed. Philadelphia, Saunders, 1972.
5. Hoffman JIE: Natural history of congenital heart disease: Problems in its assessment with special reference to ventricular septal defects. *Circulation* 1968; 37:97–125.
6. Keith JD, Rowe RD, Vlad P: *Heart Disease in Infancy and Childhood,* 3d ed. New York, Macmillan, 1978.
7. Adams FH, Emmanouilides GC, Riemenschneider TA (eds): *Moss' Heart Disease in Infants, Children, and Adolescents,* 4th ed. Baltimore, Williams & Wilkins, 1989.
8. Whittemore R: Maternal transmission of congenital heart disease. *Am J Cardiol* 1988; 61:499–500.
9. Nora JJ, Nora AH: The evolution of specific genetic and environmental counseling in congenital heart diseases. *Circulation* 1978; 57:205–213.
10. Kirby ML, Waldo KL: Role of neural crest in congenital heart disease. *Circulation* 1990; 82:332–340.
11. Ferencz C, Neill CA, Boughman JA, Rubin JD, Brenner JI, Perry LW: Congenital cardiovascular malformations associated with chromosome abnormalities: An epidemiologic study. *J Pediatr* 1989; 114:79–86.
12. Lipshultz SE, Frassica JJ, Orav EJ: Cardiovascular abnormalities in infants prenatally exposed to cocaine. *J Pediatr* 1991; 118:44–51.
13. Miao CY, Zuberbuhler JS, Zuberbuhler JR: Prevalence of congenital cardiac anomalies at high altitude. *J Am Coll Cardiol* 1988; 12:224–228.
14. Comline KS, Cross KW, Dawes GS (eds): *Fetal and Neonatal Physiology* (proceedings, Sir Joseph Barcroft Centenary Symposium). Cambridge, Cambridge University Press, 1973.
15. Rudolph AM: *Congenital Disease of the Heart: Clinical-Physiologic Considerations in Diagnosis and Management.* Chicago, Year Book, 1974.
16. Rudolph AM, Heymann MA: Neonatal circulation and pathophysiology of shunts. In: Levine HJ (ed): *Clinical Cardiovascular Physiology.* New York, Grune & Stratton, 1976: 597–619.
17. Dawes GS: *Foetal and Neonatal Physiology.* Chicago, Year Book, 1968.

18. Heymann MA, Rudolph AM: Effects of congenital heart disease on fetal and neonatal circulations. *Prog Cardiovasc Dis* 1972; 15:115–143.
19. Coceani F, Olley PM: Role of prostaglandins, prostacyclin, and thromboxanes in the control of prenatal patency and postnatal closure of the ductus arteriosus. In: Heymmann MA (ed): *Prostaglandins in the Perinatal Period.* New York, Grune & Stratton, 1980: 109.
20. Rudolph AM: Fetal and neonatal pulmonary circulation. *Annu Rev Physiol* 1979; 41:383–395.
21. Levin DL, Heymann MA, Kitterman JA, Gregory GA, Phibbs RH, Rudolph AM: Persistent pulmonary hypertension of the newborn infant. *J Pediatr* 1976; 89:626–630.
22. Fox WW, Duara S: Persistent pulmonary hypertension in the neonate: Diagnosis and management. *J Pediatr* 1983; 103:505–514.
23. Kirkpatrick BV, Krummel TM, Mueller DG, Ormazabal MA, Greenfield LJ, Salzberg AM: Use of extracorporeal membrane oxygenation for respiratory failure in term infants. *Pediatrics* 1983; 72:872–876.
24. Talner NS: Heart failure. In: Adams FH, Emmanouilides GC, Riemenschneider TA (eds): *Moss' Heart Disease in Infants, Children, and Adolescents,* 4th ed. Baltimore, Williams & Wilkins, 1989: 890–911.
25. Artman M, Graham TP Jr: Guidelines for vasodilator therapy of congestive heart failure in infants and children. *Am Heart J* 1987; 113:994–1005.
26. Menon G, Poskitt EM: Why does congenital heart disease cause failure to thrive? *Arch Dis Child* 1985; 60:1134–1139.
27. Levy RJ, Rosenthal A, Fyler DC, Nadas AS: Birthweight of infants with congenital heart disease. *Am J Dis Child* 1978; 132:249–254.
28. Rosenthal A, Castaneda A: Growth and development after cardiovascular surgery in infants and children. *Prog Cardiovasc Dis* 1975; 18:27–37.
29. Avery GB: *Neonatology: Pathophysiology and Management of the Newborn.* Philadelphia, Lippincott, 1975.
30. Somerville J: Gout in cyanotic congenital heart disease. *Br Heart J* 1961; 23:31–34.
31. Fischbein CA, Rosenthal A, Fischer EG, Nadas AS, Welch K: Risk factors of brain abscess in patients with congenital heart disease. *Am J Cardiol* 1974; 34:97–102.
32. Phornphutkul C, Rosenthal A, Nadas AS, Berenberg W: Cerebrovascular accidents in infants and children with cyanotic congenital heart disease. *Am J Cardiol* 1973; 32:329–334.
33. Beekman RH, Tuuri DT: Acute hemodynamic effects of increasing hemoglobin concentration in children with a right to left ventricular shunt and relative anemia. *J Am Coll Cardiol* 1985; 5:357–362.
34. Gidding SS, Stockman JA III: Effect of iron deficiency on tissue oxygen delivery in cyanotic congenital heart disease. *Am J Cardiol* 1988; 61:605–607.
35. Henriksson P, Varendh G, Lundstrom NR: Haemostatic defects in cyanotic congenital heart disease. *Br Heart J* 1979; 41:23–27.
36. Waldman JD, Czapek EE, Paul MH, Schwartz AD, Levin DL, Schindler S: Shortened platelet survival in cyanotic heart disease. *J Pediatr* 1975; 87:77–79.
37. Perloff JK, Rosove MH, Child JS, Wright GB: Adults with cyanotic congenital heart disease: Hematologic management. *Ann Intern Med* 1988; 109:406–413.
38. Aram DM, Ekelman BL, Ben Shachar G, Levinsohn MW: Intelligence and hypoxemia in children with congenital heart disease: Fact or artifact? *J Am Coll Cardiol* 1985; 6:889–893.
39. Rabinovitch M: Pulmonary hypertension. In: Adams FH, Emmanouilides GC, Riemenschneider TA (eds): *Moss' Heart Disease in Infants, Children, and Adolescents,* 4th ed. Baltimore, Williams & Wilkins, 1989: 856–886.
40. Blount SG Jr: Comparison of patients with ventricular septal defect at high altitude and sea level. *Circulation* 1977; 56:I-179–I-182.
41. Heath D, Edwards JE: The pathology of hypertensive pulmonary vascular disease: A description of six grades of structural changes in the pulmonary arteries with special reference to congenital cardiac septal defects. *Circulation* 1958; 18:533.
42. Rabinovitch M, Haworth SG, Castaneda AR, Nadas AS, Reid LM: Lung biopsy in congenital heart disease: A morphometric approach to pulmonary vascular disease. *Circulation* 1978; 58:1107–1122.
43. Rabinovitch M, Andrew M, Thom H, Trusler GA, Williams WG, Rowe RD, et al: Abnormal endothelial factor VIII associated with pulmonary hypertension and congenital heart defects. *Circulation* 1987; 76:1043–1052.
44. Graham TPJ: The Eisnemenger reaction and its management. In: Roberts WC (ed): *Adult Congenital Heart Disease.* Philadelphia, Davis, 1987: 567–581.
45. Blackstone EH, Kirklin JW, Bradley EL, DuShane JW, Appelbaum A: Optimal age and results in repair of large ventricular septal defects. *J Thorac Cardiovasc Surg* 1976; 72:661–679.
46. Gersony WM: Long-term follow-up of operated congenital heart disease. *Cardiol Clin* 1989; 7:915–923.
47. Committee on Rheumatic Fever, Endocarditis, and Kawasaki Disease: Prevention of bacterial endocarditis: Recommendations by the American Heart Association. *JAMA* 1990; 264:2919–2922.
48. Talner NS: Insurability of the pediatric patient with cardiac disease. *Pediatr Rev* 1988; 10:107–110.
49. Leung MP, Benson LN, Smallhorn JF, Williams WG, Trusler GA, Freedom RM: Abnormal cardiac signs after Fontan type of operation: Indicators of residua and sequelae. *Br Heart J* 1989; 61:52–58.
50. Rowe SA, Zahka KG, Manolio TA, Horneffer PJ, Kidd L: Lung function and pulmonary regurgitation limit exercise capacity in postoperative tetralogy of Fallot. *J Am Coll Cardiol* 1991; 17:461–466.
51. Zellers TM, Driscoll DJ, Mottram CD, Puga FJ, Schaff HV, Danielson GK: Exercise tolerance and cardiorespiratory response to exercise before and after the Fontan operation. *Mayo Clin Proc* 1989; 64:1489–1497.
52. Chandar JS, Wolff GS, Garson A Jr, Bell TJ, Beder SD, Bink Boelkens M, et al: Ventricular arrhythmias in postoperative tetralogy of Fallot. *Am J Cardiol* 1990; 65:655–661.
53. Krongrad E: Prognosis for patients with congenital heart disease and postoperative intraventricular conduction defects. *Circulation* 1978; 57:867–870.
54. Moreau GA, Graham TP Jr: Clinical assessment of ventricular function after surgical treatment of congenital heart defects. *Cardiol Clin* 1989; 7:439–452.
55. Turina MI, Siebenmann R, von Segesser L, Schonbeck M, Senning A: Late functional deterioration after atrial correction for transposition of the great arteries. *Circulation* 1989; 80:I-162–I-167.
56. Girod DA, Fontan F, Deville C, Ottenkamp J, Choussat A: Long-term results after the Fontan operation for tricuspid atresia. *Circulation* 1987; 75:605–610.
57. Graham TP, Bender HW, Spach MS: Ventricular septal defect. In: Adams FH, Emmanouilides GC, Riemenschneider TA (eds): *Moss' Heart Disease in Infants, Children, and Adolescents,* 4th ed. Baltimore, Williams & Wilkins, 1989: 189–209.
58. Moe DG, Guntheroth WG: Spontaneous closure of uncomplicated ventricular septal defect. *Am J Cardiol* 1987; 60:674–678.
59. Hoffman JI, Rudolph AM: The natural history of isolated ventricular septal defect with special reference to selection of patients for surgery. *Adv Pediatr* 1970; 17:57–79.
60. Engle MA, Kline SA, Borer JS: Ventricular septal defect. In: Roberts WC (ed): *Adult Congenital Heart Disease.* Philadelphia, Davis, 1987: 409–441.
61. Snider AR, Serwer GA: *Echocardiography in Pediatric Heart Disease.* Chicago, Year Book, 1990, 140–153.
62. Chin AJ, Alboliras ET, Barber G, Murphy JD, Helton JG, Pigott JD, et al: Prospective detection by Doppler color flow imaging of additional defects in infants with a large ventricular septal defect. *J Am Coll Cardiol* 1990; 15:1637–1642.
63. Murphy DJ Jr, Ludomirsky A, Huhta JC: Continuous-wave Doppler in children with ventricular septal defect: Noninvasive estimation of interventricular pressure gradient. *Am J Cardiol* 1986; 57:428–432.
64. Alpert BS, Cook DH, Varghese PJ, Rowe RD: Spontaneous closure of small ventricular septal defects: Ten-year follow-up. *Pediatrics* 1979; 63:204–206.
65. Trowitzsch E, Braun W, Stute M, Pielemeier W: Diagnosis, therapy, and outcome of ventricular septal defects in the 1st year of life: A two-dimensional colour-Doppler echocardiography study. *Eur J Pediatr* 1990; 149:758–761.

66. Weidman WH, Blount SG Jr, DuShane JW, Gersony WM, Hayes CJ, Nadas AS: Clinical course in ventricular septal defect. *Circulation* 1977; 56:I-156–I-169.
67. Rhodes L, Keane JF, Keane JP, Fellows KE, Jonas RA, Castaneda AR, et al: Long follow-up (to 43 years) of ventricular septal defect with audible aortic regurgitation. *Am J Cardiol* 1990; 66:340–345.
68. Gersony WM, Hayes CJ: Bacterial endocarditis in patients with pulmonary stenosis, aortic stenosis or ventricular septal defect. *Circulation* 1977; 56:I-84–I-87.
69. Anderson RC: Fetal and infant death, twinning and cardiac malformations in families of 2,000 children with and 500 without cardiac defects. *Am J Cardiol* 1976; 38:218–224.
70. Nolan SP: The origins of pulmonary artery banding. *Ann Thorac Surg* 1987; 44:427–429.
71. Albus RA, Trusler GA, Izukawa T, Williams WG: Pulmonary artery banding. *J Thorac Cardiovasc Surg* 1984; 88:645–653.
72. Warden HE, Cohen M, Read RC, Lillehei CW: Controlled cross circulation for open intracardiac surgery. *J Thorac Surg* 1954; 28:331.
73. DuShane JW, Kirklin JW, Patrick RT, Donald DE, Terry HR Jr, Burchell HB, et al: Ventricular septal defects with pulmonary hypertension: Surgical treatment by means of a mechanical pump-oxygenator. *JAMA* 1956; 160:950.
74. Kirklin JW, Barratt-Boyes BG: Ventricular septal defect. In: Kirklin JW, Barratt-Boyes BG (eds): *Cardiac Surgery*. New York, Wiley, 1986: 599–664.
75. Gumbiner CH, Takao A: Ventricular septal defect. In: Garson A Jr, Bricker JT, McNamara DG (eds): *The Science and Practice of Pediatric Cardiology*. Philadelphia, Lea & Febiger, 1990: 1002–1022.
76. Doty DB, McGoon DC: Closure of perimembranous ventricular septal defect. *J Thorac Cardiovasc Surg* 1983; 85:781–790.
77. Wells WJ, Lindesmith GG: Ventricular septal defect. In: Arciniegas E (ed): *Pediatric Cardiac Surgery*. Chicago, Year Book, 1985: 146–151.
78. Breckenridge IM, Stark J, Waterston DJ, Bonham Carter RE: Multiple ventricular septal defects. *Ann Thorac Surg* 1972; 13:128–136.
79. Aaron BL, Lower BR: Muscular ventricular septal defect repair made easy. *Ann Thorac Surg* 1975; 19:568–570.
80. Morris CD, Menashe VD: 25-year mortality after surgical repair of congenital heart defect in childhood. A population-based cohort study. *JAMA* 1991; 266:3447–3452.
81. Moller JH, Patton C, Varco RL, Lillehei CW: Late results (30 to 35 years) after operative closure of isolated ventricular septal defect from 1954 to 1960. *Am J Cardiol* 1991; 68:1491–1497.
82. Rizzoli G, Blackstone EH, Kirklin JW, Pacifico AD, Bargeron LM Jr: Incremental risk factors in hospital mortality rate after repair of ventricular septal defect. *J Thorac Cardiovasc Surg* 1980; 80:494–505.
83. Lynch JJ, Schuchard GH, Gross CM, Wann LS: Prevalence of right-to-left atrial shunting in a healthy population: Detection by Valsalva maneuver contrast echocardiography. *Am J Cardiol* 1984; 53:1478–1480.
84. Lewis FJ, Winchell P, Bashour FA: Open repair of atrial septal defects: Results in sixty-three patients. *JAMA* 1957; 165:922.
85. Bedford DE: The anatomical types of atrial septal defect: Their incidence and clinical diagnosis. *Am J Cardiol* 1960; 6:568.
86. Edwards JE: Classification of congenital heart disease in the adult. In: Roberts WC (ed): *Congenital Heart Disease in Adults*, Cardiovasc Clin Series 10/1. Philadelphia, Davis, 1979: 1–26.
87. Lucas RV Jr, Krabill KA: Anomalous venous connections, pulmonary and systemic. In: Adams FH, Emmanouilides GC, Riemenschneider TA (eds): *Moss' Heart Disease in Infants, Children, and Adolescents*, 4th ed. Baltimore, Williams & Wilkins, 1989: 582–617.
88. Ettedgui JA, Siewers RD, Anderson RH, Park SC, Pahl E, Zuberbuhler JR: Diagnostic echocardiographic features of the sinus venosus defect. *Br Heart J* 1990; 64:329–331.
89. Gumbiner CH, Hofschire PJ, Cheatham JP, Latson LA, Kugler JD, Fleming WH: Omphalocele associated with coronary sinus atrial septal defect: Report of two cases. *Pediatr Cardiol* 1990; 11:167–169.
90. Mahoney LT, Truesdell SC, Krzmarzick TR, Lauer RM: Atrial septal defects that present in infancy. *Am J Dis Child* 1986; 140:1115–1118.
91. Noonan JA: Syndromes associated with cardiac defects. In: Engle MA, Brest AN (eds): *Pediatric Cardiovascular Disease*. Philadelphia, Davis, 1981: 97–116.
92. Murphy JG, Gersh BJ, McGoon MD, Mair DD, Porter CJ, Ilstrup DM, et al: Long-term outcome after surgical repair of isolated atrial septal defect. Follow-up at 27 to 32 years. *N Engl J Med* 1990; 323:1645–1650.
93. Ludomursky A, Huhta JC: *Color Doppler of Congenital Heart Disease in the Child and Adult*. Mount Kisco, NY, Futura, 1987: 51–66.
94. Mehta RH, Helmcke F, Nanda NC, Pinheiro L, Samdarshi TE, Shah VK: Uses and limitations of transthoracic echocardiography in the assessment of atrial septal defect in the adult. *Am J Cardiol* 1991; 67:288–294.
95. Morimoto K, Matsuzaki M, Tohma Y, Ono S, Tanaka N, Michishige H, et al: Diagnosis and quantitative evaluation of secundum-type atrial septal defect by transesophageal Doppler echocardiography. *Am J Cardiol* 1990; 66:85–91.
96. Hamilton WT, Haffajee CE, Dalen JE, Dexter L, Nadas AS: Atrial septal defect secundum: Clinical profile with physiologic correlates. In: Roberts WC (ed): *Adult Congenital Heart Disease*. Philadelphia, Davis, 1987: 395–407.
97. Steele PM, Fuster V, Cohen M, Ritter DG, McGoon DC: Isolated atrial septal defect with pulmonary vascular obstructive disease—long-term follow-up and prediction of outcome after surgical correction. *Circulation* 1987; 76:1037–1042.
98. Rome JJ, Keane JF, Perry SB, Spevak PJ, Lock JE: Double-umbrella closure of atrial defects. Initial clinical applications. *Circulation* 1990; 82:751–758.
99. Hallman GL, Cooley DA, Gutgesell HP: *Surgical Treatment of Congenital Heart Disease*. Philadelphia, Lea & Febiger, 1987.
100. Trusler GA, Kazenelson G, Freedom RM, Williams WG, Rowe RD: Late results following repair of partial anomalous pulmonary venous connection with sinus venosus atrial septal defect. *J Thorac Cardiovasc Surg* 1980; 79:776–781.
101. Williams WH, Zorn-Chelton S, Raviele AA, Michalik RE, Guyton RA, Dooley KJ, et al: Extracardiac atrial pedicle conduit repair of partial anomalous pulmonary venous connection to the superior vena cava in children. *Ann Thorac Surg* 1984; 38:345–355.
102. St. John-Sutton MG, Tajik AJ, McGoon DC: Atrial septal defect in patients ages 60 years or older: Operative results and long-term postoperative follow-up. *Circulation* 1981; 64:402–409.
103. Daicoff GR, Brandenburg RO, Kirklin JW: Results of operation for atrial septal defect in patients forty-five years of age and older. *Circulation* 1967; 35:I-14–I-17.
104. Meyer RA, Korfhagen JC, Covitz W, Kaplan S: Long-term follow-up study after closure of secundum atrial septal defect in children: An echocardiographic study. *Am J Cardiol* 1982; 50:143–148.
105. Saalouke MG, Shapiro SR, Perry LW, Scott LP III: Isolated partial anomalous pulmonary venous drainage associated with pulmonary vascular obstructive disease. *Am J Cardiol* 1977; 39:439–444.
106. Rogers HM, Edwards JE: Incomplete division of the atrioventricular canal with patent interatrial foramen primum (persistent common cardioventricular ostium): Report of five cases and review of the literature. *Am Heart J* 1948; 36:28.
107. Rastelli GC, Ongley PA, Kirklin JW, McGoon DC: Surgical repair of the complete form of persistent common atrioventricular canal. *J Thorac Cardiovasc Surg* 1968; 55:299–308.
108. Rose V, Izukawa T, Moes CA: Syndromes of asplenia and polysplenia. A review of cardiac and non-cardiac malformations in 60 cases with special reference to diagnosis and prognosis. *Br Heart J* 1975; 37:840–852.
109. Ebels T, Anderson RH, Devine WA, Debich DE, Penkoske PA, Zuberbuhler JR: Anomalies of the left atrioventricular valve and related ventricular septal morphology in atrioventricular septal defects. *J Thorac Cardiovasc Surg* 1990; 99:299–307.
110. Ilbawi M, Cua C, DeLeon S, Muster A, Paul M, Cutilletta A, et al: Repair of complete atrioventricular septal defect with tetralogy of Fallot. *Ann Thorac Surg* 1990; 50:407–412.
111. Feldt RH, Porter CJ, Edwards WD, Puga FJ, Seward JB: Defects of the atrial septum and the atrioventricular canal. In: Adams FH, Emmanouilides GC, Riemenschneider TA (eds): *Moss' Heart Disease in Infants, Children, and Adolescents*, 4th ed. Baltimore, Williams & Wilkins, 1989: 170–189.

112. Seward JB, Tajik AJ, Edwards WD, Hagler DJ: *Two-Dimensional Echocardiographic Atlas,* vol 1, *Congenital Heart Disease*. New York, Springer, 1987: 270–292.
113. Snider AR, Serwer GA: *Echocardiography in Pediatric Heart Disease*. Chicago, Year Book, 1990: 154–162.
114. Nora JJ, Nora AH: Maternal transmission of congenital heart diseases: New recurrence risk figures and the questions of cytoplasmic inheritance and vulnerability to teratogens. *Am J Cardiol* 1987; 59:459–463.
115. Pacifico AD, Sand ME: Advances in the surgical management of congenital heart disease in infants and children. *Cardiovasc Clin* 1987; 17:177–219.
116. McGrath LB, Gonzalez–Lavin L: Actuarial survival, freedom from reoperation, and other events after repair of atrioventricular septal defects. *J Thorac Cardiovasc Surg* 1987; 94:582–590.
117. Castaneda AR, Mayer JE Jr, Joneas RA: Repair of complete atrioventricular canal in infancy. *World J Surg* 1985; 9:590–597.
118. Williams WH, Guyton RA, Michalik RE, Plauth WH Jr, Zorn Chelton S, Jones EL, et al: Individualized surgical management of complete atrioventricular canal. *J Thorac Cardiovasc Surg* 1983; 86:838–844.
119. Bailey SC, Watson DC: Atrioventricular septal defect repair in infants. *Ann Thorac Surg* 1991; 52:33–35.
120. Kadoba K, Jonas RA, Mayer JE, Castaneda AR: Mitral valve replacement in the first year of life. *J Thorac Cardiovasc Surg* 1990; 100:762–768.
121. Frid C, Thoren C, Book K, Bjork VO: Repair of complete atrioventricular canal. 15 years' experience. *Scand J Thorac Cardiovasc Surg* 1991; 25:101–105.
122. Merrill WH, Hammon JW Jr, Graham TP Jr, Bender HW Jr: Complete repair of atrioventricular septal defect. *Ann Thorac Surg* 1991; 52:29–32.
123. Studer M, Blackstone EH, Kirklin JW, Pacifico AD, Soto B, Chung GK, et al: Determinants of early and late results of repair of atrioventricular septal (canal) defects. *J Thorac Cardiovasc Surg* 1982; 84:523–542.
124. Berger TJ, Blackstone EH, Kirklin JW, Bargeron LM Jr, Hazelrig JB, Turner ME Jr: Survival and probability of cure without and with operation in complete atrioventricular canal. *Ann Thorac Surg* 1979; 27:104–111.
125. Danielson GK, Giuliani ER, Ritter DG: Successful repair of common ventricle associated with complete atrioventricular canal. *J Thorac Cardiovasc Surg* 1974; 67:152–158.
126. Vargas FJ, Coto EO, Mayer JE Jr, Jonas RA, Castaneda AR: Complete atrioventricular canal and tetralogy of Fallot: Surgical considerations. *Ann Thorac Surg* 1986; 42:258–263.
127. Vouhe PR, Neveux JY: Surgical repair of tetralogy of Fallot with complete atrioventricular canal. *Ann Thorac Surg* 1986; 41:342–344.
128. Danielson GK, Tabry IF, Ritter DG, Maloney JD: Successful repair of double-outlet right ventricle, complete atrioventricular canal, and atrioventricular discordance associated with dextrocardia and pulmonary stenosis. *J Thorac Cardiovasc Surg* 1978; 76:710–717.
129. Danielson GK, McMullan MH, Kinsley RH, DuShane JW: Successful repair of complete atrioventricular canal associated with dextroversion, common atrium, and total anomalous systemic venous return. *J Thorac Cardiovasc Surg* 1973; 66:817–822.
130. Alfieri O, Plokker M: Repair of common atrioventricular canal associated with transposition of the great arteries and left ventricular outflow obstruction. *J Thorac Cardiovasc Surg* 1982; 84:872–875.
131. McMullan MH, McGoon DC, Wallace RB, Danielson GK, Weidman WH: Surgical treatment of partial atrioventricular canal. *Arch Surg* 1973; 107:705–710.
132. Daliento L, Rizzoli G, Marchiori MC, Buja G, Milanesi O, Valente S, et al: Electrical instability in patients undergoing surgery for atrioventricular septal defect. *Int J Cardiol* 1991; 30:15–21.
133. Christie A: Normal closing time of the foramen ovale and the ductus arteriosus. *Am J Dis Child* 1930; 40:323.
134. Campbell M: Natural history of persistent ductus arteriosus. *Br Heart J* 1968; 30:4–13.
135. Kitterman JA, Edmunds LH Jr, Gregory GA, Heymann MA, Tooley WH, Rudolph AM: Patent ducts arteriosus in premature infants: Incidence, relation to pulmonary disease and management. *N Engl J Med* 1972; 287:473–477.
136. Thibeault DW, Emmanouilides GC, Nelson RJ, Lachman RS, Rosengart RM, Oh W: Patent ductus arteriosus complicating the respiratory distress syndrome in preterm infants. *J Pediatr* 1975; 86:120–126.
137. Siassi B, Blanco C, Cabal LA, Coran AG: Incidence and clinical features of patent ductus arteriosus in low-birthweight infants: A prospective analysis of 150 consecutively born infants. *Pediatrics* 1976; 57:347–351.
138. Krovetz LJ, Warden HE: Patent ductus arteriosus: An analysis of 515 surgically proven cases. *Dis Chest* 1962; 42:46–56.
139. Sahn DJ, Vaucher Y, Williams DE, Allen HD, Goldberg SJ, Friedman WF: Echocardiographic detection of large left to right shunts and cardiomyopathies in infants and children. *Am J Cardiol* 1976; 38:73–79.
140. Liao P, Su W, Hung J: Doppler echocardiographic flow characteristics of isolated patent ductus arteriosus: Better delineation by Doppler color flow mapping. *J Am Coll Cardiol* 1988; 12:1285–1291.
141. Stevenson JG: Fluid administration in the association of patent ductus arteriosus complicating respiratory distress syndrome. *J Pediatr* 1977; 90:257–261.
142. Krovetz LJ, Rowe RD: Patent ductus, prematurity and pulmonary disease. *N Engl J Med* 1972; 287:513–514.
143. Rashkind WJ, Mullins CE, Hellenbrand WE, Tait MA: Nonsurgical closure of patent ductus arteriosus: Clinical application of the Rashkind PDA Occluder System. *Circulation* 1987; 75:583–592.
144. Wessel DL, Keane JF, Parness I, Lock JE: Outpatient closure of the patent ductus arteriosus. *Circulation* 1988; 77:1068–1071.
145. Friedman WF, Hirschklau MJ, Printz MP, Pitlick PT, Kirkpatrick SE: Pharmacologic closure of patent ductus arteriosus in the premature infant. *N Engl J Med* 1976; 295:526–529.
146. Heymann MA, Rudolph AM, Silverman NH: Closure of the ductus arteriosus in premature infants by inhibition of prostaglandin synthesis. *N Engl J Med* 1976; 295:530–533.
147. Gersony WM, Peckham GJ, Ellison RC, Miettinen OS, Nadas AS: Effects of indomethacin in premature infants with patent ductus arteriosus: Results of a national collaborative study. *J Pediatr* 1983; 102:895–906.
148. Gay JH, Daily WJ, Meyer BH, Trump DS, Cloud DT, Molthan ME: Ligation of the patent ductus arteriosus in premature infants: Report of 45 cases. *J Pediatr Surg* 1973; 8:677–683.
149. Lewis CE Jr, Coen RW, Talbot W, Edwards WS: Early surgical intervention in premature infants with respiratory distress and patent ductus arteriosus. *Am J Surg* 1974; 128:829–834.
150. Adzick NS, Harrison MR, deLorimier AA: Surgical clip ligation of patent ductus arteriosus in premature infants. *J Pediatr Surg* 1986; 21:158.
151. Satur CR, Walker DR, Dickinson DF: Day case ligation of patent ductus arteriosus in preterm infants: A 10-year review. *Arch Dis Child* 1991; 66:477–480.
152. Hubbard C, Rucker RW, Realyvasquez F, Sperling DR, Hicks DA, Worcester CC, et al: Ligation of the patent ductus arteriosus in newborn respiratory failure. *J Pediatr Surg* 1986; 21:3–5.
153. Bell Thomson J, Jewell E, Ellis FH Jr, Schwaber JR: Surgical technique in the management of patent ductus arteriosus in the elderly patient. *Ann Thorac Surg* 1980; 30:80–83.
154. Ellis FHJ, Kirklin JW, Callahan JA, Wood EH: Patent ductus arteriosus and pulmonary hypertension: Analysis of patients treated surgically. *J Thorac Cardiovasc Surg* 1956; 31:268.
155. Frescura C, Thiene G, Giulia-Gagliardi M, Mazzucco A, Pellegrino PA, Daliento L, et al: Is lung biopsy useful for surgical decision making in congenital heart disease? *Eur J Cardiothorac Surg* 1991; 5:118–122.
156. Fremes SE, Patterson GA, Williams WG, Goldman BS, Todd TR, Maurer J: Single lung transplantation and closure of patent ductus arteriosus for Eisenmenger's syndrome. Toronto Lung Transplant Group. *J Thorac Cardiovasc Surg* 1990; 100:1–5.
157. Bridges ND, Perry SB, Parness I, Keane JF, Lock JE: Transcatheter closure of a large patent ductus arteriosus with clamshell septal umbrella. *J Am Coll Cardiol* 1991; 18:1297–1302.
158. Hosking MC, Benson LN, Musewe N, Dyck JD, Freedom RM: Transcatheter occlusion of the persistently patent ductus arteriosus: Forty-month follow-up and prevalence of residual shunting. *Circulation* 1991; 84:2313–2317.

159. Edwards JE, Burchell HB: Pathologic anatomy of deficiencies between the aortic root and the heart including aortic sinus aneurysms. *Thorax* 1957; 12:125–139.
160. Sakakibara S, Konno S: Congenital aneurysm of the sinus of Valsalva: Anatomy and classification. *Am Heart J* 1962; 63:405–424.
161. Burakovsky VI, Podsolkov VP, Sabirow BN, Nasedkina MA, Alekian BG, Dvinyaninova NB: Ruptured congenital aneurysm of the sinus of Valsalva: Clinical manifestations, diagnosis, and results of surgical corrections. *J Thorac Cardiovasc Surg* 1988; 95:836–841.
162. Shumaker HB Jr: Aneurysms of the aortic sinuses of Valsalva due to bacterial endocarditis with special reference to their operative management. *J Thorac Cardiovasc Surg* 1972; 63:896–902.
163. Shaffer EM, Snider AR, Beekman RH, Behrendt DM, Peschiera AW: Sinus of Valsalva aneurysm complicating bacterial endocarditis in an infant: Diagnosis with two-dimensional and Doppler echocardiography. *J Am Coll Cardiol* 1987; 9:588–591.
164. Kakos GS, Kilman JW, Williams TE, Hosier DM: Diagnosis and management of sinus of Valsalva aneurysms in children. *Ann Thorac Surg* 1974; 17:474–478.
165. Meyer J, Wukasch DC, Hallman GL, Cooley DA: Aneurysm and fistula of the sinus of Valsalva: Clinical considerations and surgical treatment in 45 patients. *Ann Thorac Surg* 1975; 19:170–179.
166. Doty DB: *Cardiac Surgery: A Looseleaf Notebook and Update Service*. Chicago, Year Book, 1985: Sinus V 1–4.
167. Nowicki ER, Aberdeen E, Friedman S, Rashkind WJ: Congenital left aortic sinus–left ventricle fistula and review of aortocardiac fistulas. *Ann Thorac Surg* 1977; 23:378–388.
168. Pan-Chih O, Ching-Heng T, Chen-Chun O, Chieh-Fu L: Surgical treatment of ruptured aneurysm of the aortic sinuses. *Ann Thorac Surg* 1981; 32:162–166.
169. Bonfils-Roberts EA, DuShane JW, McGoon DC, Danielson GK: Aortic sinus fistula—surgical considerations and results of operation. *Ann Thorac Surg* 1971; 12:492–502.
170. Clagett OT, Kirklin JW, Edwards JE: Anatomic variations and pathologic changes in 124 cases of coarctation of the aorta. *Surg Gynecol Obstet* 1954; 98:103.
171. Becker AE, Becker MJ, Edwards JE: Anomalies associated with coarctation of aorta: Particular reference to infancy. *Circulation* 1970; 41:1067–1075.
172. Rees AH, Elbl F, Villafane J, Solinger R, Mavroudis C, Harrison H: Surgical repair of atypical coarctation of the abdominal aorta in an infant. *Kentucky Med Assoc J* 1990; 88:62–65.
173. Moene RJ, Oppenheimer Dekker A, Wenink AC: Relation between aortic arch hypoplasia of variable severity and central muscular ventricular septal defects: Emphasis on associated left ventricular abnormalities. *Am J Cardiol* 1981; 48:111–116.
174. Ziemer G, Jonas RA, Perry SB, Freed MD, Castaneda AR: Surgery for coarctation of the aorta in the neonate. *Circulation* 1986; 74:I-25–I-31.
175. Parker FB Jr, Streeten DH, Farrell B, Blackman MS, Sondheimer HM, Anderson GH Jr: Preoperative and postoperative renin levels in coarctation of the aorta. *Circulation* 1982; 66:513–514.
176. Beekman RH, Robinow M: Coarctation of the aorta inherited as an autosomal dominant trait. *Am J Cardiol* 1985; 56:818–819.
177. Snider AR, Serwer GA: *Echocardiography in Pediatric Heart Disease*. Chicago, Year Book, 1990: 289–292.
178. Heymann MA, Berman W Jr, Rudolph AM, Whitman V: Dilatation of the ductus arteriosus by prostaglandin E_1 in aortic arch abnormalities. *Circulation* 1979; 59:169–173.
179. Lock JE, Keane JF, Fellows KE: *Diagnostic and Interventional Catheterization in Congenital Heart Disease*. Boston, Martinus Nijhoff, 1987: 99–102.
180. Beekman RH, Rocchini AP, Behrendt DM, Bove EL, Dick M, Crowley DC, et al: Long-term outcome after repair of coarctation in infancy: Subclavian angioplasty does not reduce the need for reoperation. *J Am Coll Cardiol* 1986; 8:1406–1411.
181. Maron BJ: Aortic isthmus coarctation. In: Roberts WC (ed): *Adult Congenital Heart Disease*. Philadelphia, Davis, 1987: 443–453.
182. Beekman RH, Rocchini AP, Behrendt DM, Rosenthal A: Reoperation for coarctation of the aorta. *Am J Cardiol* 1981; 48:1108–1114.
183. Barash PG, Hobbins JC, Hook R, Stansel HC Jr, Whittemore R, Hehre FW: Management of coarctation of the aorta during pregnancy. *J Thorac Cardiovasc Surg* 1975; 69:781–784.
184. Nora JJ, Nora AH: *Genetics and Counseling in Cardiovascular Diseases*. Springfield, IL, Charles C Thomas, 1978.
185. Sehested J: Evaluation of optimum time for surgical repair of coarctation of the aorta. *Surg Gynecol Obstet* 1978; 146:593–595.
186. Kirklin JW, Nadas AS: Editorial comments. In: Harvey WP, Kirkendall MM, Kirklin JW, et al (eds): *The Year Book of Cardiology—1979*. Chicago, Year Book, 1979: 286.
187. Kirklin JW, Barratt-Boyes BG: Coarctation of the aorta and aortic arch interruptions. In: Kirklin JW, Barratt-Boyes BG (eds): *Cardiac Surgery*. New York, Wiley, 1986: 1035–1080.
188. Trinquet F, Vouhe PR, Vernant F, Touati G, Roux PM, Pome G, et al: Coarctation of the aorta in infants: Which operation? *Ann Thorac Surg* 1988; 45:186–191.
189. Morris GC, Cooley DA, DeBakey ME, Crawford ES: Coarctation of the aorta with particular emphasis upon improved techniques of surgical repair. *J Thorac Cardiovasc Surg* 1960; 40:705.
190. Ravelo HR, Stephenson LW, Friedman S, Chatten J, Rashkind WJ, Vidas M, et al: Coarctation resection in children with Turner's syndrome: A note of caution. *J Thorac Cardiovasc Surg* 1980; 80:427–430.
191. Myers JL, Waldhausen JA: Management of complications following repair of coarctation of the aorta, patent ductus arteriosus, interrupted aortic arch, and vascular rings. In: Waldhausen JA, Orringer MB (eds): *Complications in Cardiothoracic Surgery*. St. Louis, Mosby Year Book, 1991: 135–148.
192. Reul GJ Jr, Kabbani SS, Sandiford FM, Wukasch DC, Cooley DA: Repair of coarctation of the thoracic aorta by patch graft aortoplasty. *J Thorac Cardiovasc Surg* 1974; 68:696–704.
193. Myers JL, Waldhausen JA, Pae WE Jr, Abt AB, Prophet GA, Pierce WS: Vascular anastomoses in growing vessels: The use of absorbable sutures. *Ann Thorac Surg* 1982; 34:529–537.
194. Cooper RS, Ritter SB, Rothe WB, Chen CK, Griepp R, Golinko RJ: Angioplasty for coarctation of the aorta: Long-term results. *Circulation* 1987; 75:600–604.
195. Brandt B III, Marvin WJ Jr, Rose EF, Mahoney LT: Surgical treatment of coarctation of the aorta after balloon angioplasty. *J Thorac Cardiovasc Surg* 1987; 94:715–719.
196. Allen HD, Marx GR, Ovitt TW, Goldberg SJ: Balloon dilation angioplasty for coarctation of the aorta. *Am J Cardiol* 1986; 57:828–832.
197. Goldman S, Hernandez J, Pappas G: Results of surgical treatment of coarctation of the aorta in the critically ill neonate. Including the influence of pulmonary artery banding. *J Thorac Cardiovasc Surg* 1986; 91:732–737.
198. Hammon JW Jr, Graham TP Jr, Boucek RJ Jr, Bender HW Jr: Operative repair of coarctation of the aorta in infancy: Results with and without ventricular septal defect. *Am J Cardiol* 1985; 55:1555–1559.
199. Tiraboschi R, Alfieri O, Carpentier A, Parenzan L: One stage correction of coarctation of the aorta associated with intracardiac defects in infancy. *J Cardiovasc Surg* 1978; 19:11–16.
200. Moreno NN, deCampo T, Kaiser GA, Pallares VS: Technical and pharmacologic management of distal hypotension during repair of coarctation of the aorta. *J Thorac Cardiovasc Surg* 1980; 80:182–186.
201. Pennington DG, Dennis HM, Swartz MT, Nouri S, Chen SC, Azzam F, et al: Repair of aortic coarctation in infants: Experience with an intraluminal shunt. *Ann Thorac Surg* 1985; 40:35–40.
202. Pollock JC, Jamieson MP, McWilliam R: Somatosensory evoked potentials in the detection of spinal cord ischemia in aortic coarctation repair. *Ann Thorac Surg* 1986; 41:251–254.
203. Gidding SS, Rocchini AP, Beekman R, Szpunar CA, Moorehead C, Behrendt D, et al: Therapeutic effect of propranolol on paradoxical hypertension after repair of coarctation of the aorta. *N Engl J Med* 1985; 312:1224–1228.
204. Williams WG, Shindo G, Trusler GA, Dische MR, Olley PM: Results of repair of coarctation of the aorta during infancy. *J Thorac Cardiovasc Surg* 1980; 79:603–608.
205. Bergdahl LA, Blackstone EH, Kirklin JW, Pacifico AD, Bargeron LM Jr: Determinants of early success in repair of aortic coarctation in infants. *J Thorac Cardiovasc Surg* 1982; 83:736–742.

206. Wagner HR, Ellison RC, Keane JF, Humphries OJ, Nadas AS: Clinical course in aortic stenosis. *Circulation* 1977; 56:I-147–I-156.
207. Whitmer JT, James FW, Kaplan S, Schwartz DC, Knight MJ: Exercise testing in children before and after surgical treatment of aortic stenosis. *Circulation* 1981; 63:254–263.
208. Snider AR, Serwer GA: *Echocardiography in Pediatric Heart Disease*. Chicago, Year Book, 1990, 242–250.
209. Bengur AR, Snider AR, Serwer GA, Peters J, Rosenthal A: Usefulness of the Doppler mean gradient in evaluation of children with aortic valve stenosis and comparison to gradient at catheterization. *Am J Cardiol* 1989; 64:756–761.
210. Sholler GF, Keane JF, Perry SB, Sanders SP, Lock JE: Balloon dilation of congenital aortic valve stenosis: Results and influence of technical and morphological features on outcome. *Circulation* 1988; 78:351–360.
211. Latson LA: Aortic stenosis: Valvular, supravalvular, and fibromuscular subvalvular. In: Garson A Jr, Bricker JT, McNamara DG (eds): *The Science and Practice of Pediatric Cardiology*. Philadelphia, Lea & Febiger, 1990: 1334–1352.
212. Sink JD, Smallhorn JF, Macartney FJ, Taylor JF, Stark J, de Leval MR: Management of critical aortic stenosis in infancy. *J Thorac Cardiovasc Surg* 1984; 87:82–86.
213. Keane JF, Bernhard WF, Nadas AS: Aortic stenosis surgery in infancy. *Circulation* 1975; 52:1138–1143.
214. Sandor GG, Olley PM, Trusler GA, Williams WG, Rowe RD, Morch JE: Long-term follow-up of patients after valvotomy for congenital valvular aortic stenosis in children: A clinical and actuarial follow-up. *J Thorac Cardiovasc Surg* 1980; 80:171–176.
215. Ankeney JL, Tzeng TS, Liebman J: Surgical therapy for congenital aortic valvular stenosis. A 23-year experience. *J Thorac Cardiovasc Surg* 1983; 85:41–48.
216. Ellis FHJ, Kirklin JW: Congenital valvular aortic stenosis: Anatomic findings and surgical technique. *J Thorac Surg* 1962; 43:199.
217. Fulton DR, Hougen TJ, Keane JF, Rosenthal AR, Norwood WI, Bernhard WF: Repeat aortic valvotomy in children. *Am Heart J* 1983; 106:60–63.
218. Lawson RM, Bonchek LI, Menashe V, Starr A: Late results of surgery for left ventricular outflow tract obstruction in children. *J Thorac Cardiovasc Surg* 1976; 71:334–341.
219. Williams WH: Heart valve replacement: Special problems in infants and children. In: Starek PJK (ed): *Heart Valve Replacement and Reconstruction*. Chicago, Year Book, 1987: 247–272.
220. Pelech AN, Dyck JD, Trusler GA, Williams WG, Olley PM, Rowe RD, et al: Critical aortic stenosis. Survival and management. *J Thorac Cardiovasc Surg* 1987; 94:510–517.
221. Gundry SR, Behrendt DM: Prognostic factors in valvotomy for critical aortic stenosis in infancy. *J Thorac Cardiovasc Surg* 1986; 92:747–754.
222. Duncan K, Sullivan I, Robinson P, Horvath P, de Leval M, Stark J: Transventricular aortic valvotomy for critical aortic stenosis in infants *J Thorac Cardiovasc Surg* 1987; 93:546–550.
223. Fleming WH, Sarafian LB: Aortic valve replacement with concomitant aortoventriculoplasty in children and young adults: Long-term follow-up. *Ann Thorac Surg* 1987; 43:575–578.
224. McKowen RL, Campbell DN, Woelfel GF, Wiggins JW Jr, Clarke DR: Extended aortic root replacement with aortic allografts. *J Thorac Cardiovasc Surg* 1987; 93:366–374.
225. Johnson RG, Williams GR, Razook JD, Thompson WM, Lane MM, Elkins RC: Reoperation in congenital aortic stenosis. *Ann Thorac Surg* 1985; 40:156–162.
226. Tveter KJ, Foker JE, Moller JH, Ring WS, Lillehei CW, Varco RL: Long-term evaluation of aortic valvotomy for congenital aortic stenosis. *Ann Surg* 1987; 206:496–503.
227. Hsieh KS, Keane JF, Nadas AS, Bernhard WF, Castaneda AR: Long-term follow-up of valvotomy before 1968 for congenital aortic stenosis. *Am J Cardiol* 1986; 58:338–341.
228. Feigl A, Feigl D, Lucas RV Jr, Edwards JE: Involvement of the aortic valve cusps in discrete subaortic stenosis. *Pediatr Cardiol* 1984; 5:185–189.
229. Wright GB, Keane JF, Nadas AS, Bernhard WF, Castaneda AR: Fixed subaortic stenosis in the young: Medical and surgical course in 83 patients. *Am J Cardiol* 1983; 52:830–835.
230. Choi JY, Sullivan ID: Fixed subaortic stenosis: Anatomic spectrum and nature of progression. *Br Heart J* 1991; 65:280–286.
231. Freedom RM, Culham JAG, Moes CAF: *Angiocardiography of Congenital Heart Disease*. New York, Macmillan, 1989.
232. Suarez de Tezo J, Pan M, Medina A, Romero M, Melian F, Segura J, et al: Immediate and follow-up results of transluminal balloon dilatation for discrete subaortic stenosis. *J Am Coll Cardiol* 1991; 18:1309–1315.
233. Kirklin JW, Ellis FHJ: Surgical relief of diffuse subvalvular aortic stenosis. *Circulation* 1961; 24:739.
234. Bjork VO, Holtquist G, Lodin H: Subaortic stenosis produced by abnormally placed anterior mitral leaflet. *J Thorac Cardiovasc Surg* 1961; 41:659.
235. McKay R, Ross DN: Technique for the relief of discrete subaortic stenosis. *J Thorac Cardiovasc Surg* 1982; 84:917–920.
236. Vogel M, Freedom RM, Brand A, Trusler GA, Williams WG, Rowe RD: Ventricular septal defect and subaortic stenosis: An analysis of 41 patients. *Am J Cardiol* 1983; 52:1258–1263.
237. Moses RD, Barnhart GR, Jones M: The late prognosis after localized resection for fixed (discrete and tunnel) left ventricular outflow tract obstruction. *J Thorac Cardiovasc Surg* 1984; 87:410–420.
238. Cooley Da, Garrett JR: Septoplasty for left ventricular outflow obstruction without aortic valve replacement: A new technique. *Ann Thorac Surg* 1986; 42:445–448.
239. Vouhe PR, Poulain H, Bloch G, Loisance DY, Gamain J, Lombaert M, et al: Aortoseptal approach for optimal resection of diffuse subvalvular aortic stenosis. *J Thorac Cardiovasc Surg* 1984; 87:887–893.
240. Ensing GJ, Schmidt MA, Hagler DJ, Michels VVR, Carter GA, Feldt RH: Spectrum of findings in a family with nonsyndromic autosomal dominant supravalvular aortic stenosis: A Doppler echocardiographic study. *J Am Coll Cardiol* 1989; 13:413–419.
241. Zalzstein E, Moes CAF, Musewe NN, Freedom RM: Spectrum off cardiovascular anomalies in Williams-Geuren syndrome. *Pediatr Cardiol* 1991; 12:219–223.
242. McGoon DC, Mankin HT, Vlad P, et al: The surgical treatment of supravalvular aortic stenosis. *J Thorac Cardiovasc Surg* 1961; 41:125.
243. Rastelli GC, McGoon DC, Ongley PA, Mankin HT, Kirklin JW: Surgical treatment of supravalvular aortic stenosis. Report of 16 cases and review of literature. *J Thorac Cardiovasc Surg* 1966; 51:873–882.
244. Doty DB, Polansky DB, Jenson CB: Supravalvular aortic stenosis. Repair by extended aortoplasty. *J Thorac Cardiovasc Surg* 1977; 74:362–371.
245. Keane JF, Fellows KE, LaFarge CG, Nadas AS, Bernhard WF: The surgical management of discrete and diffuse supravalvar aortic stenosis. *Circulation* 1976; 54:112–117.
246. Landes RG, Zavoral JH, Emery RW, Moller JH, Lindsay WG, Nicoloff DM: The surgical management of vascular abnormalities associated with supravalvular aortic stenosis. *J Thorac Cardiovasc Surg* 1978; 75:80–86.
247. Norman JC, Cooley DA, Hallman GL, Nihill MR: Left ventricular apical-abdominal aortic conduits for left ventricular outflow tract obstructions. Clinical results in eleven patients with a special composite prosthesis. *Circulation* 1977; 56:II-62–II-65.
248. Thevent A: Symmetric enlargement of the ascending aorta in supravalvular aortic stenosis of the diffuse type (an alternative to apico-aortic conduit). *J Cardiovasc Surg* 1981; 22:1–8.
249. Roberts WC: Anomalies usually silent until adulthood. In: Roberts WC (ed): *Adult Congenital Heart Disease*. Philadelphia, Davis, 1987: 646–656.
250. Leech G, Mills P, Leatham A: The diagnosis of a non-stenotic bicuspid aortic valve. *Br Heart J* 1978; 40:941–950.
251. Brandenburg RO Jr, Tajik AJ, Edwards WD, Reeder GS, Shub C, Seward JB: Accuracy of 2-dimensional echocardiographic diagnosis of congenitally bicuspid aortic valve: Echocardiographic-anatomic correlation in 115 patients. *Am J Cardiol* 1983; 51:1469–1473.
252. Hardy WE, Gnoj J, Ayres SM, Giannelli S Jr, Christianson LC: Pulmonic stenosis and associated atrial septal defects in older patients: Report of three cases, including one with calcific pulmonic stenosis. *Am J Cardiol* 1969; 24:130–134.
253. Koretzky ED, Moller JH, Korns ME, Schwartz CJ, Edwards JE: Congenital pulmonary stenosis resulting from dysplasia of valve. *Circulation* 1969; 40:43–53.
254. Li MD, Coles JC, McDonald AC: Anomalous muscle bundle of

the right ventricle: Its recognition and surgical treatment. *Br Heart J* 1978; 40:1040–1045.

255. D'Cruz IA, Agustsson MH, Bicoff JP, et al: Stenotic lesions of the pulmonary arteries: Clinical and hemodynamic findings in 84 cases. *Am J Cardiol* 1964; 13:441.
256. Rowe RD: Cardiovascular disease in the rubella syndrome. *Cardiovasc Clin* 1972; 5:62.
257. Stone FM, Bessinger FB Jr, Lucas RV Jr, Moller JH: Pre- and postoperative rest and exercise hemodynamics in children with pulmonary stenosis. *Circulation* 1974; 49:1102–1106.
258. Danilowicz D, Hoffman JI, Rudolph AM: Serial studies of pulmonary stenosis in infancy and childhood. *Br Heart J* 1975; 37:808–818.
259. Mody MR: The natural history of uncomplicated valvular pulmonic stenosis. *Am Heart J* 1975; 90:317–321.
260. Roberts WC, Shemin RJ, Kent KM: Frequency and direction of interatrial shunting in valvular pulmonic stenosis with intact ventricular septum and without left ventricular inflow or outflow obstruction: An analysis of 127 patients treated by valvulotomy. *Am Heart J* 1980; 99:142–148.
261. Noonan JA: Hypertelorism with Turner phenotype. A new syndrome with associated congenital heart disease. *Am J Dis Child* 1968; 116:373–380.
262. Cayler CG, Ongley P, Nadas AS: Relation of systolic pressure in the right ventricle to the electrocardiogram. *N Engl J Med* 1958; 258:979.
263. Lima CO, Sahn DJ, Valdes Cruz LM, Goldberg SJ, Barron JV, Allen HD, et al: Noninvasive prediction of transvalvular pressure gradient in patients with pulmonary stenosis by quantitative two-dimensional echocardiographic Doppler studies. *Circulation* 1983; 67:866–871.
264. Nakazawa M, Marka RA, Isabel Jones J, Jarmakani JM: Right and left ventricular volume characteristics in children with pulmonary stenosis and intact ventricular septum. *Circulation* 1976; 53:884–890.
265. Nadas AS (ed): Pulmonary stenosis, aortic stenosis, ventricular septal defect: Clinical course and indirect assessment (Report from the Joint Study on the Natural History of Congenital Heart Defects). *Circulation* 1977; 56:I-1–I-87.
266. Stanger P, Cassidy SC, Girod DA, Kan JS, Lababidi Z, Shapiro SR: Balloon pulmonary valvuloplasty: Results of the Valvuloplasty and Angioplasty of Congenital Anomalies Registry. *Am J Cardiol* 1990; 65:775–783.
267. Kan JS, Marvin WJ Jr, Bass JL, Muster AJ, Murphy J: Balloon angioplasty—branch pulmonary artery stenosis: Results from the Valvuloplasty and Angioplasty of Congenital Anomalies Registry. *Am J Cardiol* 1990; 65:798–801.
268. Marantz PM, Huhta JC, Mullins CE, Murphy DJ Jr, Nihill MR, Ludomirsky A, et al: Results of balloon valvuloplasty in typical and dysplastic pulmonary valve stenosis: Doppler echocardiographic follow-up. *J Am Coll Cardiol* 1988; 12:476–479.
269. Vancini M, Roberts KD, Silove ED, Singh SP: Surgical treatment of congenital pulmonary stenosis due to dysplastic leaflets and small valve annulus. *J Thorac Cardiovasc Surg* 1980; 79:464–468.
270. Litwin SB, Williams WH, Freed MD, Bernhard WF: Critical pulmonary stenosis in infants: A surgical emergency. *Surgery* 1973; 74:880–886.
271. Mistrot J, Neal W, Lyons G, Moller J, Lucas R, Castaneda A, et al: Pulmonary valvulotomy under inflow stasis for isolated pulmonary stenosis. *Ann Thorac Surg* 1976; 21:30–37.
272. Srinivasan V, Konyer A, Broda JJ, Subramanian S: Critical pulmonary stenosis in infants less than three months of age: A reappraisal of closed transventricular pulmonary valvotomy. *Ann Thorac Surg* 1982; 34:46–50.
273. McGoon MD, Fulton RE, Davis GD, Ritter DG, Neill CA, White RI Jr: Systemic collateral and pulmonary artery stenosis in patients with congenital pulmonary valve atresia and ventricular septal defect. *Circulation* 1977; 56:473–479.
274. Barbero-Marcial M, Atik E, Baucia JA, Pradel HO, Macruz R, Jatene AD: Reconstruction of stenotic or nonconfluent pulmonary arteries simultaneously with a Blalock-Taussig shunt. *J Thorac Cardiovasc Surg* 1988; 95:82–89.
275. Ring JC, Bass JL, Marvin W, Fuhrman BP, Kulik TJ, Foker JE, et al: Management of congenital stenosis of a branch pulmonary artery with balloon dilation angioplasty. Report of 52 procedures. *J Thorac Cardiovasc Surg* 1985; 90:35–44.
276. Cheatham JP: Pulmonary stenosis. In: Garson A Jr, Bricker JT, McNamara DG (eds): *The Science and Practice of Pediatric Cardiology*. Philadelphia, Lea & Febiger, 1990: 1382–1420.
277. Becker AE, Connor M, Anderson RH: Tetralogy of Fallot: A morphometric and geometric study. *Am J Cardiol* 1975; 35:402–412.
278. Rao BN, Anderson RC, Edwards JE: Anatomic variations in the tetralogy of Fallot. *Am Heart J* 1971; 81:361–371.
279. Higgins CB, Muldler DG: Tetralogy of Fallot in the adult. *Am J Cardiol* 1972; 29:837–846.
280. Bonchek LI, Starr A, Sunderland CO, Menashe VD: Natural history of tetralogy of Fallot in infancy: Clinical classification and therapeutic implications. *Circulation* 1973; 48:392–397.
281. Ruzyllo W, Nihill MR, Mullins CE, McNamara DG: Hemodynamic evaluation of 221 patients after intracardiac repair of tetralogy of Fallot. *Am J Cardiol* 1974; 34:565–576.
282. Taussig HB, Kallman CH, Nagel D, Baumgardner R, Momberger N, Kirk H: Long-time observations on the Blalock-Taussig operation: VIII. 20 to 28 year follow-up on patients with a tetralogy of Fallot. *Johns Hopkins Med J* 1975; 137:13–19.
283. Roberts WC, Friesinger GC, Cohen LS, Mason DT, Ross RS: Acquired pulmonic atresia: Total obstruction to right ventricular outflow after systemic to pulmonary arterial anastomoses for cyanotic congenital cardiac disease. *Am J Cardiol* 1969; 24:335–345.
284. Morgan BC, Guntheroth WG, Bloom RS, Fyler DC: A clinical profile of paroxysmal hyperpnea in cyanotic congenital heart disease. *Circulation* 1965; 31:66–69.
285. Guntheroth WG, Morgan BC, Mullins GL: Physiologic studies of paroxysmal hyperpnea in cyanotic congenital heart disease. *Circulation* 1965; 31:70–76.
286. Danilowicz DA: Delay in bone age in children with cyanotic congenital heart disease. *Radiology* 1973; 108:655–658.
287. Hagler DJ, Tajik AJ, Seward JB, Mair DD, Ritter DG: Wide-angle two-dimensional echocardiographic profiles of conotruncal abnormalities. *Mayo Clin Proc* 1980; 55:73–82.
288. Formanek A, Nath PH, Zollikofer C, Moller JH: Selective coronary arteriography in children. *Circulation* 1980; 61:84–95.
289. Dabizzi RP, Caprioli G, Aiazzi L, Castelli C, Baldrighi G, Parenzan L, et al: Distribution and anomalies of coronary arteries in tetralogy of Fallot. *Circulation* 1980; 61:95–102.
290. Bertranou EG, Blackstone EH, Hazelrig JB, Turner ME, Kirklin JW: Life expectancy without surgery in tetralogy of Fallot. *Am J Cardiol* 1978; 42:458–466.
291. Ponce FE, Williams LC, Webb HM, Riopel DA, Hohn AR: Propranolol palliation of tetralogy of Fallot: Experience with long-term drug treatment in pediatric patients. *Pediatrics* 1973; 52:100–108.
292. Heymann MA, Rudolph AM: Ductus arteriosus dilatation by prostaglandin E_1 in infants with pulmonary atresia. *Pediatrics* 1977; 59:325–329.
293. Garson A Jr, Gorry Ga, McNamara DG, Cooley DA: The surgical decision in tetralogy of Fallot: Weighing risks and benefits with decision analysis. *Am J Cardiol* 1980; 45:108–116.
294. Walsh EP, Rockenmacher S, Keane JF, Hougen TJ, Lock JE, Castaneda AR: Late results in patients with tetralogy of Fallot repaired during infancy. *Circulation* 1988; 77:1062–1067.
295. Neches WH, Park SC, Ettedgui JA: Tetralogy of Fallot and tetralogy of Fallot with pulmonary atresia. In: Garson A Jr, Bricker JT, McNamara DG (eds): *The Science and Practice of Pediatric Cardiology*. Philadelphia, Lea & Febiger, 1990: 1073–1100.
296. Kirklin JW, Blackstone EH: Editorial on papers by Naito, Wessel, and their colleagues. *J Thorac Cardiovasc Surg* 1980; 80:594–599.
297. Kirklin JW, Blackstone EH, Colvin EV, McConnell ME: Early primary correction of tetralogy of Fallot. *Ann Thorac Surg* 1988; 45:231–233.
298. Amato JJ, Marbey ML, Bush C, Galdieri RJ, Cotroneo JV, Bushong J: Systemic-pulmonary polytetrafluoroethylene shunts in palliative operations for congenital heart disease. Revival of the central shunt. *J Thorac Cardiovasc Surg* 1988; 95:62–69.
299. Arciniegas E, Farooki ZQ, Hakimi M, Green EW: Results of two-stage surgical treatment of tetralogy of Fallot. *J Thorac Cardiovasc Surg* 1980; 79:876–883.
300. Puga FJ, DuShane JW, McGoon DC: Treatment of tetralogy of Fallot in children less than 4 years of age. *J Thorac Cardiovasc Surg* 1972; 64:247–253.
301. Naito Y, Fujita T, Manabe H, Kawashima Y: The criteria for

reconstruction of right ventricular outflow tract in total correction of tetralogy of Fallot. *J Thorac Cardiovasc Surg* 1980; 80:574–581.
302. Coles JG, Kirklin JW, Pacifico AD, Kirklin JK, Blackstone EH: The relief of pulmonary stenosis by a transatrial versus a transventricular approach to the repair of tetralogy of Fallot. *Ann Thorac Surg* 1988; 45:7–10.
303. Fuster V, McGoon DC, Kennedy MA, Ritter DG, Kirklin JW: Long-term evaluation (12 to 22 years) of open heart surgery for tetralogy of Fallot. *Am J Cardiol* 1980; 46:635–642.
304. Wessel HU, Cunningham WJ, Paul MH, Bastanier CK, Muster AJ, Idriss FS: Exercise performance in tetralogy of Fallot after intracaradiac repair. *J Thorac Cardiovasc Surg* 1980; 80:582–593.
305. Gustafson RA, Murray GF, Warden HE, Hill RC, Rozar GE Jr: Early primary repair of tetralogy of Fallot. *Ann Thorac Surg* 1988; 45:235–241.
306. Borow KM, Green LH, Castaneda AR, Keane JF: Left ventricular function after repair of tetralogy of Fallot and its relationship to age at surgery. *Circulation* 1980; 61:1150–1158.
307. Ilbawi MN, Idriss FS, DeLeon SY, Muster AJ, Gidding SS, Berry TE, et al: Factors that exaggerate the deleterious effects of pulmonary insufficiency on the right ventricle after tetralogy repair. Surgical implications. *J Thorac Cardiovasc Surg* 1987; 93:36–44.
308. Backer CL, Idriss FS: Reoperation after initial repair of tetralogy of Fallot: Correction of residual or recurrent defects. In: Jacobs ML, Norwood WI (eds): *Pediatric Cardiac Surgery*. Boston, Butterworth-Heinemann, 1992: 91–104.
309. Leve M, Liberthson RR, Joseph RH, Seten CE, Eckner FA, Kunske RD, et al: The pathologic anatomy of Ebstein's disease. *Arch Pathol* 1970; 90:334–343.
310. Becker AE, Becker MJ, Edwards JE: Pathologic spectrum of dysplasia of the tricuspid valve. Features in common with Ebstein's malformation. *Arch Pathol* 1971; 91:167–178.
311. Kumar AE, Fyler DC, Miettinen OS, Nadas AS: Ebstein's anomaly: Clinical profile and natural history. *Am J Cardiol* 1971; 28:84–95.
312. Watson H: Natural history of Ebstein's anomaly of tricuspid valve in childhood and adolescence: An international co-operative study of 505 cases. *Br Heart J* 1974; 36:417–427.
313. Driscoll DJ, Mottram CD, Danielson GK: Spectrum of exercise intolerance in 45 patients with Ebstein's anomaly and observations on exercise tolerance in 11 patients after surgical repair. *J Am Coll Cardiol* 1988; 11:831–836.
314. Kastor JA, Goldreyer BN, Josephson ME, Perloff JK, Scharf DL, Manchester JH, et al: Electrophysiologic characteristics of Ebstein's anomaly of the tricuspid valve. *Circulation* 1975; 52:987–995.
315. Roberson DA, Silverman NH: Ebstein's anomaly: Echocardiographic and clinical features in the fetus and neonate. *J Am Coll Cardiol* 1989; 14:1300–1307.
316. Hernandez FA, Rochkind R, Cooper HR: The intracavitary electrocardiogram in the diagnosis of Ebstein's anomaly. *Am J Cardiol* 1958; 1:181–190.
317. Giuliani ER, Fuster V, Brandenburg RO, Mair DD: Ebstein's anomaly: The clinical features and natural history of Ebstein's anomaly of the tricuspid valve. *Mayo Clin Proc* 1979; 54:163–173.
318. Plowden JS, Kimball TR, Bensky A, Savani R, Flake AW, Warner BW, et al: The use of extracorporeal membrane oxygenation in critically ill neonates with Ebstein's anomaly. *Am Heart J* 1991; 121:619–622.
319. Westaby S, Karp RB, Kirklin JW, Waldo AL, Blackstone EH: Surgical treatment in Ebstein's malformation. *Ann Thorac Surg* 2981; 34:388–395.
320. Mair DD, Seward JB, Driscoll DJ, Danielson GK: Surgical repair of Ebstein's anomaly: Selection of patients and early and late operative results. *Circulation* 1985; 72:II-70–II-76.
321. Danielson GK: Ebstein's anomaly: Editorial comments and personal observations. *Ann Thorac Surg* 1982; 34:396–400.
322. Quaegebeur JM, Sreeram N, Fraser AG, Bogers AJ, Stumper OF, Hess J, et al: Surgery for Ebstein's anomaly: The clinical and echocardiographic evaluation of a new technique. *J Am Coll Cardiol* 1991; 17:722–728.
323. Oh JK, Holmes DR Jr, Hayes DL, Porter CB, Danielson GK: Cardiac arrhythmias in patients with surgical repair of Ebstein's anomaly. *J Am Coll Cardiol* 1985; 6:1351–1357.
324. Blake HAR, Hall J, Manion WC: Anomalous pulmonary venous return. *Circulation* 1965; 32:406–414.
325. Lucas RV Jr, Lock JE, Tandon R, Edwards JE: Gross and histologic anatomy of total anomalous pulmonary venous connections. *Am J Cardiol* 1988; 62:292–300.
326. Lucas RV Jr, Adams P Jr, Anderson RC, Varco RL, Edwards JE, Lester RG: Total anomalous pulmonary venous connection to the portal venous system: A cause of pulmonary venous obstruction. *Am J Roentgenol* 1961; 86:561.
327. Gathman GE, Nadas AS: Total anomalous pulmonary venous connection: Clinical and physiologic observations of 75 pediatric patients. *Circulation* 1970; 42:143–154.
328. Chin AJ, Sanders SP, Sherman F, Lang P, Norwood WI, Castaneda AR: Accuracy of subcostal two-dimensional echocardiography in prospective diagnosis of total anomalous pulmonary venous connection. *Am Heart J* 1987; 113:1153–1159.
329. Galioto FJ Jr, Fyler DC, Chameides L: Total anomalous pulmonary venous drainage (TAPVD): A 5 year review in New England. *Am J Cardiol* 1975; 35 (abstract):138.
330. Newfeld EA, Wilson A, Paul MH, Reisch JS: Pulmonary vascular disease in total anomalous pulmonary venous drainage. *Circulation* 1980; 61:103–109.
331. Harlan BJ, Starr A, Harwin FM: Total anomalous pulmonary venous connection. In: Harlan BJ, Harwin FM (eds): *Manual of Cardiac Surgery,* vol 2. New York, Springer, 1981: 333.
332. Kirklin JW: Surgical treatment for total anomalous pulmonary venous connection in infancy. In: Barratt-Boyes BG (ed): *Heart Disease in Infancy: Diagnosis and Surgical Treatment.* Edinburgh, Churchill Livingstone, 1973: 89–100.
333. Katz NM, Kirklin JW, Pacifico AD: Concepts and practices in surgery for total anomalous pulmonary venous connection. *Ann Thorac Surg* 1978; 25:479–487.
334. Turley K, Tucker WY, Ullyot DJ, Ebert PA: Total anomalous pulmonary venous connection in infancy: Influence of age and type of lesion. *Am J Cardiol* 1980; 45:92–97.
335. Yee ES, Turley K, Hsieh WR, Ebert PA: Infant total anomalous pulmonary venous connection: Factors influencing timing of presentation and operative outcome. *Circulation* 1987; 76:III-83–III-87.
336. Ward KE, Mullins CE: Anomalous pulmonary venous connections; pulmonary vein stenosis; atresia of the common pulmonary vein. In: Garson A Jr, Bricker JT, McNamara DG (eds): *The Science and Practice of Pediatric Cardiology.* Philadelphia, Lea & Febiger, 1992: 1145–1172.
337. Van Praagh R, Weinberg PM, Smith SD, Foran RB, Van Praagh S: Malpositions of the heart. In: Adams FH, Emmanouilides GC, Riemenschneider TA (eds): *Moss' Heart Disease in Infants, Children, and Adolescents,* 4th ed. Baltimore, Williams & Wilkins, 1989: 530–580.
338. VanPraagh R: Segmental approach to diagnosis. In: Fyler DC (ed): *Nadas' Pediatric Cardiology.* Philadelphia, Hanley & Belfus, 1992: 27–35.
339. VanPraagh S, Santini F, Sanders SP: Cardiac malpositions with special emphasis on visceral heterotaxy (asplenia and polysplenia syndromes). In: Fyler DC (ed): *Nadas' Pediatric Cardiology.* Philadelphia, Hanley & Belfus, 1992: 589–608.
340. Rooklin AR, McGeady SJ, Mikaelian DO, Soriano RZ, Mansmann HC Jr: The immotile cilia syndrome: A cause of recurrent pulmonary diseases in children. *Pediatrics* 1980; 66:526–531.
341. Fyler DC: D-transposition of the great arteries. In: Fyler DC (ed): *Nadas' Pediatric Cardiology.* Philadelphia, Hanley & Belfus, 1992: 557–575.
342. Paul MH: Complete transposition of the great arteries. In: Adams FH, Emmanoulides GC, Riemenschneider TA (eds): *Moss' Heart Disease in Infants, Children, and Adolescents,* 4th ed. Baltimore, Williams & Wilkins, 1989: 371–423.
343. Pasquini L, Sanders SP, Parness IA, Colan SD: Diagnosis of coronary artery anatomy by two-dimensional echocardiography in patients with transposition of the great arteries. *Circulation* 1987; 75:557–564.
344. Mandell VS, Lock JE, Mayer JE, Parness IA, Kulik TJ: The "laid back" aortogram: An improved angiographic view for demonstration of coronary arteries in transposition of the great arteries. *Am J Cardiol* 1990; 65:1379–1383.

345. Jonas RA, Giglia TM, Sanders SP, Wernovsky G, Nadal Ginard B, Mayer JE Jr, et al: Rapid, two-stage arterial switch for transposition of the great arteries and intact ventricular septum beyond the neonatal period. *Circulation* 1989; 80:I-203–I-208.
346. Rubay JE, de Halleux C, Jaumin P, Moulin D, Kestens Servaye Y, Lintermans J, et al: Long-term follow-up of the Senning operation for transposition of the great arteries in children under 3 months of age. *J Thorac Cardiovasc Surg* 1987; 94:75–81.
347. Hammon JW, Bender HW: Current status of atrial switch operations for transposition of the great arteries. In: Jacobs ML, Norwood WI (eds): *Pediatric Cardiac Surgery*. Boston, Butterworth-Heinemann, 1992: 35–47.
348. Williams WG, Trusler GA, Kriklin JW, Blackstone EH, Coles JG, Izukawa T, et al: Early and late results of a protocol for simple transposition leading to an atrial switch (Mustard) repair. *J Thorac Cardiovasc Surg* 1988; 95:717–726.
349. Cobanoglu A, Abbruzzese PA, Freimanis I, Garcia CE, Grunkemeier G, Starr A: Pericardial baffle complications following the Mustard operation. Age-related incidence and ease of management. *J Thorac Cardiovasc Surg* 1984; 87:371–378.
350. Jatene AD, Fontes VF, Souza LC, Paulista PP, Neto CA, Sousa JE: Anatomic correction of transposition of the great arteries. *J Thorac Cardiovasc Surg* 1982; 83:20–26.
351. Khanolkar UB, Kinare SG: Taussig-Bing complex—a pathologic study of eight cases. *Indian Heart J* 1990; 42:157–160.
352. Bauer EP, Bino MC, von Segesser LK, Laske A, Turina MI: Internal mammary artery anomalies. *Thorac Cardiovasc Surg* 1990; 312–315.
353. Litwin SB, Plauth WH Jr, Jones JE, Bernhard WF: Appraisal of surgical atrial septectomy for transposition of the great arteries. *Circulation* 1971; 43:I-7–I-10.
354. Gibbs JL, Qureshi SA, Wilson N, Smith RR, Yacoub MH: Doppler echocardiographic comparison of haemodynamic results of one- and two-stage anatomic correction of complete transposition. *Int J Cardiol* 1988; 18:85–92.
355. Lange PE, Pulss W, Sievers HH, Wessel A, Onnasch DG, Bernhard A, et al: Cardiac rhythm and conduction after two-stage anatomic correction of simple transposition of the great arteries. *Thorac Cardiovasc Surg* 1986; 34:22–24.
356. Castaneda AR: Simple transposition of the great arteries: The arterial switch operation in neonates. In: Jacobs ML, Norwood WI (eds): *Pediatric Cardiac Surgery*. Boston, Butterworth-Heinemann, 1992: 1–12.
357. Sievers HH, Lange PE, Wessel A, Onnasch DG, Berger F, Yacoub MH, et al: Up to 9 years of follow-up after anatomic correction of simple transposition of the great arteries. *Eur J Cardiothorac Surg* 1988; 2:318–323.
358. Quaegebeur JM, Rohmer J, Ottenkamp J, Buis T, Kirklin JW, Blackstone EH, et al: The arterial switch operation. An eight-year experience. *J Thorac Cardiovasc Surg* 1986; 92:361–384.
359. Penkoske PA, Westerman GR, Marx GR, Rabinovitch M, Freed MD, Norwood WI, et al: Transposition of the great arteries and ventricular septal defect: Results with the Senning operation and closure of the ventricular septal defect in infants. *Ann Thorac Surg* 1983; 36:281–288.
360. Wilcox BR, Henry GW, Anderson RH: The transmitral approach to left ventricular outflow tract obstruction. *Ann Thorac Surg* 1983; 35:288–293.
361. Abe T, Sugiki K, Izumiyama O, Komatsu S: A successful procedure for correction of the Taussig-Bing malformation. *J Thorac Cardiovasc Surg* 1984; 87:403–409.
362. Cohen DM, Williams WG: Arterial switch operations in infants and children with complex forms of transposition of the great arteries. In: Jacobs ML, Norwood WI (eds): *Pediatric Cardiac Surgery*. Boston, Butterworth-Heinemann, 1992: 13–34.
363. Hagler DJ, Ritter DG, Puga FJ: Double-outlet right ventricle. In: Adams FH, Emmanouilides GC, Riemenschneider TA (eds): *Moss' Heart Disease in Infants, Children, and Adolescents,* 4th ed. Baltimore, Williams & Wilkins, 1989:442–460.
364. Snider AR, Serwer GA: *Echocardiography in Pediatric Heart Disease*. Chicago, Year Book, 1990, 190–194.
365. Piccoli G, Pacifico AD, Kirklin JW, Blackstone EH, Kirklin JK, Bargeron LM Jr: Changing results and concepts in the surgical treatment of double-outlet right ventricle: Analysis of 137 operations in 126 patients. *Am J Cardiol* 1983; 52:549–554.
366. Anderson RH, Becker AE, Wilcox BR, Macartney FJ, Wilkinson JL: Surgical anatomy of double-outlet right ventricle—a reappraisal. *Am J Cardiol* 1983; 52:555–559.
367. Stewart S: Double-outlet right ventricle. A collective review with a surgical viewpoint. *J Thorac Cardiovasc Surg* 1976; 71:355–365.
368. Wilcox BR, Anderson RH: Lesions in abnormally connected hearts. In: Wilcox BR, Anderson RH (eds): *Surgical Anatomy of the Heart,* 2d ed. London, Gower Medical, 1992: 8.1–8.34.
369. Kirklin JW, Karp RA, McGoon DC: Surgical treatment of origin of both vessels from right ventricle, including cases with pulmonary stenosis. *J Thorac Cardiovasc Surg* 1964; 48:1026.
370. Gomes MM, Weidman WH, McGoon DC, Danielson GK: Double-outlet right ventricle with pulmonic stenosis. Surgical considerations and results of operation. *Circulation* 1971; 43:889–894.
371. Judson JP, Danielson GK, Puga FJ, Mair DD, McGoon DC: Double-outlet right ventricle. Surgical results, 1970–1980. *J Thorac Cardiovasc Surg* 1983; 85:32–40.
372. Silka MJ: Double-outlet ventricles. In: Garson A Jr, Bricker JT, McNamara DG (eds): *The Science and Practice of Pediatric Cardiology*. Philadelphia, Lea & Febiger, 1990: 1213–1232.
373. Freedom RM, Smallhorn JF: Double-outlet right ventricle. In: Freedom RM, Benson LN, Smallhorn JF (eds): *Neonatal Heart Disease*. London, Springer, 1992: 453–470.
374. Kirklin JW, Pacifico AD, Blackstone EH, Kirklin JK, Bargeron LM Jr: Current risks and protocols for operations for double-outlet right ventricle. Derivation from an 18 year experience. *J Thorac Cardiovasc Surg* 1986; 92:913–930.
375. Ruttenberg HD: Corrected transposition of the great arteries and splenic syndromes. In: Adams FH, Emmanouilides GC, Riemenschneider TA (eds): *Moss' Heart Disease in Infants, Children, and Adolescents,* 4th ed. Baltimore, Williams & Wilkins, 1989: 424–433.
376. Fyler DC: "Corrected" transposition of the great arteries. In: Fyler DC (ed): *Nadas' Pediatric Cardiology*. Philadelphia, Hanley & Belfus, 1992: 701–706.
377. Snider AR, Serwer GA: *Echocardiography in Pediatric Heart Disease*. Chicago, Year Book, 1990, 186–190.
378. Lundstrom U, Bull C, Wyse RK, Somerville J: The natural and "unnatural" history of congenitally corrected transposition. *Am J Cardiol* 1990; 65:1222–1229.
379. Hwang B, Bowman F, Malm J, Krongrad E: Surgical repair of congenitally corrected transposition of the great arteries: Results and follow-up. *Am J Cardiol* 1982; 50:781–785.
380. Fox LS, Kirklin JW, Pacifico AD, Waldo AL, Bargeron LM Jr: Intracardiac repair of cardiac malformations with atrioventricular discordance. *Circulation* 1976; 54:123–127.
381. Watson DC, Shapiro SR, Midgley FM, Scott LP: Surgical approach to corrected transposition of the great vessels and situs inversus with ventricular septal defect and systemic atrioventricular valve regurgitation. *Ann Thorac Surg* 1984; 38:520–521.
382. Nagai I, Kawashima Y, Fujita T, Mori T, Manabe H: Successful closure of ventricular septal defect through a left-sided ventriculotomy in corrected transposition of the great vessels. *Ann Thorac Surg* 1976; 21:492–498.
383. Russo P, Danielson GK, Driscoll DJ: Transaortic closure of ventricular septal defect in patients with corrected transposition with pulmonary stenosis or atresia. *Circulation* 1987; 76:III-88–III-92.
384. Kitamura S, Oyama C, Kawachi K, Miyagi Y, Morita R, Yamada Y, et al: A new method of closing the ventricular septal defect in corrected transposition of the great arteries. *Ann Thorac Surg* 1984; 38:640–643.
385. Mullins CE: Ventricular inversion. In: Garson A Jr, Bricker JT, McNamara DG (eds): *The Science and Practice of Pediatric Cardiology*. Philadelphia, Lea & Febiger, 1990: 1233–1245.
386. Kirklin JW, Barratt-Boyes BG: Congenitally corrected transposition of the great arteries. In: Kirklin JW, Barratt-Boyes BG (eds): *Cardiac Surgery: Morphology, Diagnostic Criteria, Natural History, Techniques, Results, and Indications*. New York, Wiley, 1986: 1263–1280.
387. Van Praagh R, David I, Van Praagh S: What is a ventricle? The single-ventricle trap. *Pediatr Cardiol* 1982; 2:79–84.
388. Elliott LP, Anderson RH, Bargeron LM Jr, Kirklin JK, White RD: Single ventricle or univentricular heart. In: Adams FH, Emmanouilides GC, Riemenschneider TA (eds): *Moss' Heart Disease in Infants, Children, and Adolescents,* 4th ed. Baltimore, Williams & Wilkins, 1989:485–503

389. Sahn DJ, Harder JR, Freedom RM, Duncan WJ, Rowe RD, Allen HD, et al: Cross-sectional echocardiographic diagnosis and subclassification of univentricular hearts: Imaging studies of atrioventricular valves, septal structures and rudimentary outflow chambers. *Circulation* 982; 66:1070–1077.
390. Shinebourne EA, Lau KC, Calcaterra G, Anderson RH: Univentricular heart of right ventricular type: Clinical, angiographic and electrocardiographic features. *Am J Cardiol* 1980; 46:439–445.
391. Freedom RM, Sondheimer H, Sische R, Rowe RD: Development of "subaortic stenosis" after pulmonary arterial banding for common ventricle. *Am J Cardiol* 1977; 39:78–83.
392. Shiraishi H, Silverman NH: Echocardiographic spectrum of double inlet ventricle: Evaluation of the interventricular communication. *J Am Coll Cardiol* 1990; 15:1401–1408.
393. Moak JP, Gersony WM: Progressive atrioventricular valvular regurgitation in single ventricle. *Am J Cardiol* 1987; 59:656–658.
394. Franklin RCG, Spiegelhatter DJ, Filho RIR, Macartney FJ, Anderson RH, Rigby ML, et al: Double inlet ventricle presenting in infancy: III. Outcome and potential for definitive repair. *J Thorac Cardiovasc Surg* 1991; 101:924–934.
395. Matsuda H, Kawashima Y, Kishimoto H, Hirose H, Nakano S, Kato H, et al: Problems in the modified Fontan operation for univentricular heart of the right ventricular type. *Circulation* 1987; 76:III-45–III-52.
396. Rothman A, Lang P, Lock JE, Jonas RA, Mayer JE, Castaneda AR: Surgical management of subaortic obstruction in single left ventricle and tricuspid atresia. *J Am Coll Cardiol* 1987; 10:421–426.
397. Freedom RM, Smallhorn JF: Hearts with a univentricular atrioventricular connection. In: Freedom RM, Benson LN, Smallhorn JF (eds): *Neonatal Heart Disease.* London, Springer, 1992: 498–521.
398. Sade RM: Surgical options in univentricular atrioventricular connection. In: Jacobs ML, Norwood WI (eds): *Pediatric Cardiac Surgery.* Boston, Butterworth-Heinemann, 1992: 48–69.
399. Colvin EV: Single ventricle. In: Garson A Jr, Bricker JT, McNamara DG (eds): *The Science and Practice of Pediatric Cardiology.* Philadelphia, Lea & Febiger, 1990: 1246–1279.
400. McKay R, Pacifico AD, Blackstone EH, Kirklin JW, Bargeron LM Jr: Septation of the univentricular heart with left anterior subaortic outlet chamber. *J Thorac Cardiovasc Surg* 1982; 84:77–87.
401. Feldt RH, Mair DD, Danielson GK, Wallace RB, McGoon DC: Current status of the septation procedure for univentricular heart. *J Thorac Cardiovasc Surg* 1981; 82:93–97.
402. Gale AW, Danielson GK, McGoon DC, Mair DD: Modified Fontan operation for univentricular heart and complicated congenital lesions. *J Thorac Cardiovasc Surg* 1979; 78:831–838.
403. McGoon DC, Danielson GK, Puga FJ: Univentricular heart. In: Glenn WWL, Baue AE, Geha AE (eds): *Thoracic and Cardiovascular Surgery.* Norwalk, CN, Appleton-Century-Crofts, 1983: 770–784.
404. McNamara JJ, Gross RE: Congenital coronary artery fistula. *Surgery* 1969; 65:59–69.
405. Liberthson RR, Sagar K, Berkoben JP, Weintraub RM, Levine FH: Congenital coronary arteriovenous fistula: Report of 13 patients, review of the literature and delineation of management. *Circulation* 1979; 59:849–854.
406. Jaffee RB, Glancy DS, Epstein SE, et al: Coronary arterial–right heart fistula: Long-term observations in seven patients. *Circulation* 1973; 47:133–143.
407. Oldham HN Jr, Ebert PA, Young WG, Sabiston DC Jr: Surgical management of congenital coronary artery fistula. *Ann Thorac Surg* 1971; 12:503–513.
408. Urruita SCO, Falaschi G, Ott DA, Cooley DA: Surgical management of 56 patients with congenital coronary artery fistulas. *Ann Thorac Surg* 1983; 35:300–307.
409. Pezzella AT, Falaschi G, Ott DA, Cooley DA: Congenital coronary artery-left heart fistulas: Report of three cases. *Cardiovasc Dis Bull Texas Heart Inst* 1981; 8:355–363.
410. Noren GR, Raghib G, Moller JH, Amplatz K, Adams P Jr, Edwards JE: Anomalous origin of the left coronary artery from the pulmonary trunk with special reference to the occurrence of mitral insufficiency. *Circulation* 1964; 30:171–179.
411. Hurwitz RA, Caldwell RL, Girod DA, Brown J, King H: Clinical and hemodynamic course of infants and children with anomalous left coronary artery. *Am Heart J* 1989; 118:1176–1181.
412. Wesselhoeft H, Fawcett JS, Johnson AL: Anomalous origin of the left coronary artery from the pulmonary trunk: Its clinical spectrum, pathology, and pathophysiology, based on a review of 140 cases with seven further cases. *Circulation* 1968; 38:403–425.
413. Gutgesell HP, Pinsky WW, DePuey EG: Thallium-201 myocardial perfusion imaging in infants and children: Value in distinguishing anomalous left coronary artery from congestive cardiomyopathy. *Circulation* 1980; 61:596–599.
414. Wilson CL, Dlabal PW, McGuire SA: Surgical treatment of anomalous left coronary artery from pulmonary artery: Follow-up in teenagers and adults. *Am Heart J* 1979; 98:440–446.
415. Kakou Guikahue M, Sidi D, Kachaner J, Villain E, Cohen L, Piechaud JF, et al: Anomalous left coronary artery arising from the pulmonary artery in infancy: Is early operation better? *Br Heart J* 1988; 60:522–526.
416. Driscoll DJ, Nihill MR, Mullins CE, Cooley DA, McNamara DG: Management of symptomatic infants with anomalous origin of the left coronary artery from the pulmonary artery. *Am J Cardiol* 1981; 47:642–648.
417. Arciniegas E, Farooki ZQ, Hakimi M, Green EW: Management of anomalous left coronary artery from the pulmonary artery. *Circulation* 1980; 62:I-180–I-189.
418. Takeuchi S, Imamura H, Katsumoto J, Hayashi I, Katohgi T, Yozu R: New surgical method for repair of anomalous left coronary artery from the pulmonary artery. *J Thorac Cardiovasc Surg* 1979; 78:7–11.
419. Vouhe PR, Baillot Vernant F, Trinquet F, Sidi D, de Geeter B, Khoury W, et al: Anomalous left coronary artery from the pulmonary artery in infants. Which operation? When? *J Thorac Cardiovasc Surg* 1987; 94:192–199.
420. Levitsky S, van der Horst RL, Hastreiter AR, Fisher EA: Anomalous left coronary artery in the infant: Recovery of ventricular function following early direct aortic implantation. *J Thorac Cardiovasc Surg* 1980; 79:598–602.
421. Moodie DS, Fyfe D, Gill CC, Cook SA, Lytle BW, Taylor PC, et al: Anomalous origin of the left coronary artery from the pulmonary artery (Bland-White-Garland syndrome) in adult patients: Long-term follow-up after surgery. *Am Heart J* 1983; 106:381–388.

Chapter 98

Adult Congenital Heart Disease

John E. Deanfield, M.B., D.Phil. ■ *Bernard J. Gersh, M.D.* ■
Douglas D. Mair, M.D.

INTRODUCTION

Congenital heart disease occurs in 5 to 10 per 1000 live births.[1] Without early treatment, the majority of patients would die in infancy or childhood, with only 5 to 15 percent surviving until puberty.[2] The advent of surgical procedures, from ligation of a patent arterial duct[3] in 1939 to the innovations of the 1990s as well as advances in medical treatment, has transformed the outlook for children with even complex defects. The majority now survive into adolescence and adult life (Chap. 97). This success story has radically altered both the size and complexity of the population of young adults with congenital heart disease. In the United States alone, well over a half million patients with functionally important congenital cardiac malformations have reached adulthood in the past three decades.[4] Despite the fact that most patients now surviving to adult life will have undergone surgery during childhood, "total correction" is not the rule.[5] The majority (if not all) require long-term surveillance, and many need reoperation. Other adults may require their first operation for congenital heart lesions that were well tolerated during childhood.

Both the "natural" survivors and the postoperative patients require specialized medical care. Arrhythmia is common, as are residual or deteriorating hemodynamic problems and endocarditis. Although adult cardiologists may be expert in one or more of these areas, the critical relationship between rhythm and hemodynamic status in hearts with complex circulations (such as after a Fontan operation or after intraatrial repair for transposition) may result in treatment errors by those inexperienced with congenital heart defects. Patients with cyanosis require special care because of polycythemia, bleeding, renal problems, and arthropathy and specific counseling and management regarding pregnancy. In addition to the medical problems, psychosocial problems such as the search for employment, life and health insurance, participation in sports, sexual activity, and contraception are of great importance to adolescents and young adults with congenital heart disease. Many of the "normal" ordeals of growing up are more difficult for this group in whom chronic illness, embarrassing scars, and/or exercise limitation may inhibit normal social intercourse and maturation.

MEDICAL CONSIDERATIONS

Many young adults with congenital heart disease have mild lesions that have not required and may not ever require surgery. The commonest defects in this category are small ventricular septal defect, mild pulmonary valve stenosis, mild aortic valve stenosis, and mitral valve prolapse (Table 98-1). Such patients need infrequent follow-up (e.g., biannual) to assess any progression in severity of the lesion, to reinforce the need for antibiotic prophylaxis against infective endocarditis (Chap. 94), and to obtain psychosocial advice. Other patients reach adult life with more complex defects that are still uncorrected. Some may still be candidates for palliative or definitive surgery, whereas in others surgery may no longer be possible, often because of the presence of irreversible pulmonary vascular disease. More and more survivors of surgery in childhood are now reaching adult life, and they now form the largest group of patients (Table 98-2). The majority need continuing medical surveillance as

TABLE 98-1

Common Congenital Heart Defects Compatible with Survival to Adult Life without Surgery or Interventional Catheterization

Mild pulmonary valve stenosis
Peripheral pulmonary stenosis
Bicuspid aortic valve
Mild subaortic stenosis
Mild supravalvar aortic stenosis
Small atrial septal defect
Small ventricular septal defect
Small patent ductus arteriosus
Mitral valve prolapse
Ostium primum atrial septal defect (atrioventricular septal defect)
Marfan's syndrome
Ebstein's anomaly
Corrected transposition (atrioventricular-ventriculoatrial discordance)
Balanced complex lesions (e.g., double-inlet ventricle with pulmonary stenosis)
Defects with pulmonary vascular obstructive disease (Eisenmenger syndrome)

late cardiovascular problems may result from hemodynamic disturbances, arrhythmia, and endocarditis. Such patients can also develop noncardiac problems as a consequence of their heart disease (e.g., secondary to cyanosis) and are, of course, susceptible to all the potential acquired "medical problems" of adulthood.

Hemodynamics

Study of the hemodynamic consequences of repaired and unrepaired congenital heart disease is a crucial aspect of long-term follow-up. Progressive congestive cardiac failure secondary to myocardial deterioration is the most common cause of disability and death in patients whose ventricles may have been subjected to many years of volume and pressure loading, often with chronic hypoxia. A significant number of the adult postoperative congenital heart disease patients have been repaired at older ages than is the current practice. This may result in greater preoperative damage and pulmonary vascular disease that may persist postoperatively. In the early era of open heart surgery myocardial protection was sometimes less than optimal, resulting in myocardial damage.

It should also be appreciated that postoperative circulations created by the repair of many congenital heart defects result in an adequate physiological repair (e.g., deoxygenated blood to lungs and oxygenated blood to the body) but often have very far from normal anatomy. For example, after the Mustard and Senning operation for transposition of the great arteries, the right ventricle remains on the systemic side of the circulation. Some of these patients have evidence of deteriorating right ventricular function, and there is increasing concern that this will become a major life-threatening problem with longer follow-up.[6] Similar concerns have been expressed for systemic ventricular function after the Fontan operation.[7] The different morphology and loading conditions for these ventricles suggest that standard indices of ventricular function, derived from studies of structurally normal hearts, may be inappropriate for such patients.[8] (See also Chap. 23.) Prospective serial studies are beginning to define "normal ranges" for congenital heart defects and to examine their "natural" and "unnatural" history.[9,10]

Residual hemodynamic defects are often present in repaired patients and may cause problems even many years after surgery. These may be amenable to further surgery (see below) or require long-term medical treatment. Standard medical therapy for the failing ventricle includes digitalis, diuretics, and afterload reducing agents (Chap. 26).

Cyanosis

Adults with congenital heart disease may have central cyanosis from right-to-left shunting secondary to their uncorrected cardiac defect or to pulmonary vascular disease (Eisenmenger's syndrome). (See Chap. 97.) The latter complication should be seen less frequently in years ahead as a result of the trend to early recognition and repair of congenital heart disease in infancy. Currently, however, a significant number of patients reach adult life with pulmonary vascular disease as a result of lesions such as large ventricular septal defect, atrioventricular septal defect, truncus arteriosus, and double-outlet right ventricle. Their pulmonary vascular resistance may already have been too high for surgical repair, at the time of diagnosis, or in others pulmonary vascular disease may have progressed despite repair of the congenital heart defect.

Cyanotic patients are prone to specific medical problems, including erythropoiesis, that may lead to polycythemia and hyperviscosity.[11] Many patients with cyanotic congenital heart disease establish a stable high hematocrit but few symptoms of hyperviscosity.[12] They have a low risk of stroke and do not require venesection.[13] In others, the hemoglobin concentration may rise progressively. Once it exceeds 20 g/dL, they are at risk

TABLE 98-2

Common Congenital Heart Defects Surviving to Adult Life after Surgery/Interventional Catheterization

Aortic valve disease, valvotomy or replacement
Pulmonary stenosis, valvotomy
Tetralogy of Fallot
Atrial septal defect
Ventricular septal defect
Atrioventricular septal defect
Transposition of the great arteries, atrial redirection
Complex transposition of the great arteries
Total anomalous pulmonary venous connection
Pulmonary atresia/ventricular septal defect
Fontan for complex congenital heart disease
Ebstein, tricuspid valve repair or replacement
Coarctation of the aorta
Mitral valve disease

from thromboembolic complications and may suffer from headache, dizziness, and fatigue.[14] Symptoms may be improved by judicious venesection to hemoglobin levels of 17 to 18 g/dL. This can be performed by the removal of 500 mL of blood and volume replacement with normal saline.[13,15] Overzealous venesection, however, may result in both acute and chronic problems, including cardiovascular collapse in patients with Eisenmenger's syndrome, iron depletion, microcytosis, and hyperviscosity in its own right.[16] The paradoxical anemia of polycythemic patients with iron deficiency due to repeated phlebotomy may be missed.

Patients with chronic cyanosis also develop defective hemostasis from abnormalities in platelet function and in the coagulation and fibrinolytic systems,[17] especially in patients with marked polycythemia. The risk of hemorrhage, especially at surgery, is well recognized and may be fatal. Hyperuricemia is common because of increased red cell turnover and renal dysfunction.[18] Arthralgia is well recognized, but gouty arthritis is rare and may be misdiagnosed. Other important problems include acne and renal impairment, which can deteriorate to renal failure as a result of relatively minor interventions, such as contrast medium injection at angiography.[19] Patients with right-to-left shunts are at risk of paradoxical embolus, which may cause a cerebrovascular accident or renal infarction. A cerebral abscess is a well-known complication of a septic embolus and must always be considered in the cyanotic patient with sudden-onset headache, somnolence, other neurologic symptoms, or low-grade fever.

The prognosis for patients with Eisenmenger's syndrome depends to a great extent on their management. A number of vasodilator drugs, including calcium channel blockers, angiotensin converting enzyme inhibitors, hydralazine, and nitrates, have been used, but no treatment has been shown to produce regression or alter the progress of pulmonary vascular disease.[20-22] Death may result from right-sided heart failure,[23] pulmonary hemorrhage, or arrhythmia.[23,24] It can also occur prematurely due to potentially avoidable complications such as inappropriate drug therapy or injudicious general anesthesia.

Progressive kyphoscoliosis has been recognized for many years as a complication of congenital heart disease.[25] This is common in cyanotic patients and in those with previous thoracotomy. The degree of deformity, if left untreated, may become profound and compromise pulmonary function. Treatment with bracing or insertion of a Harrington rod may be indicated even if the patient has an uncorrectable cardiac lesion, since the kyphoscoliosis may significantly reduce both the quality and quantity of life.

Infective Endocarditis

Patients with both unoperated and operated congenital heart disease are at risk from infective endocarditis. The wide variety of portals of entry include dental work; skin sepsis; obstetric/gynecologic, genito-urinary, and gastrointestinal interventions; cardiac catheterization; transesophageal echocardiography; and surgery.[26-30] There is also a risk of bacteremia and infective endocarditis in young adults who have their ears pierced or have a tattoo. Patients must be educated and preferably should carry an information card with them. The symptoms of endocarditis may be subtle, and the diagnosis must be considered in any patient who experiences unexplained malaise or fever. Injudicious prescription of antibiotics without previous blood culture may mask the problem and make bacteriological diagnosis and appropriate treatment difficult.

Life-long antibiotic prophylaxis against endocarditis (Chap. 94) is recommended for both unoperated and operated patients, but the specific indications and optimal regimes are still debated.[31,32] The American Heart Association Special Report on Prevention of Infective Endocarditis has stratified risk groups for the various lesions.[31] Prophylaxis is advocated for all lesions except secundum atrial septal defect closed by direct suture or a divided patent ductus arteriosus. (See Table 94-9.)

Electrophysiological Problems

Arrhythmias and conduction defects have a major impact on the prognosis and management of both unoperated and operated patients and have been linked to sudden death in a number of conditions.[33-35] The principles of diagnosis and treatment are similar to those employed in patients with arrhythmia due to other causes. (See Chap. 36.) In unoperated patients, chamber dilatation, myocardial hypertrophy, and fibrosis may all contribute to the genesis of arrhythmia. In operated patients, additional sinus or atrioventricular node damage and atrial and/or ventricular scarring may cause electrophysiological problems. Not only is the etiology multifactorial, but the clinical significance of arrhythmia depends very much on the hemodynamic context in which it occurs. Rhythm disturbances that might be benign in a structurally normal heart may be life threatening in congenital heart disease.

Supraventricular arrhythmia and sinus node injury not surprisingly occur most often in conditions with "atrial defects" or those requiring atrial surgery.[34,36] Abnormalities of sinus node function are common in patients with atrial septal defect, particularly the sinus venosus type,[37] and are often seen after Mustard or Senning operation for transposition of the great arteries.[38] Sinus node dysfunction has also been reported after surgery for tetralogy of Fallot, Fontan, and many other congenital heart lesions.[39,40] Clinical manifestations include sinus bradycardia, sinoatrial block, sinus arrest, and occasionally the tachybradycardia syndrome with paroxysmal atrial flutter and fibrillation. Although bradycardia has been postulated as the cause of sudden death in some conditions, current evidence indicates that tachyarrhythmia is usually a more likely explanation[41] (see below).

In sinus node disease, insertion of a pacemaker is indicated for patients with symptoms resulting from slow heart rate such as tiredness, dizziness, and syncope or for an extremely low heart rate. (See Chap. 40.) Indications in asymptomatic individuals are still controversial since the arrhythmia is benign in many cases. It should be noted that pacing may be difficult because of the complex underlying anatomy and lack of a suitable site for endocardial lead fixation. The choice of pacemaker will depend on the precise indication. The simplest VVI pacemaker may be adequate prophylaxis against bradycardia-related sudden death. In general, however, rate-responsive pacemakers are preferable and dual-chamber pacing may provide the best hemodynamics.[42,43] (See also Chap. 40.)

Injury to the atrioventricular (AV) node and proximal conduction tissue may result from surgery for lesions such as ventricular septal defect, AV septal defect, or tetralogy of Fallot. High-grade AV block was seen more commonly in the early era of surgery.[44] Transient complete AV block in the postoperative period has been shown to have prognostic significance in some reports, particularly if the site of damage is below the bundle of His. In a recent 30-year follow-up of ventricular septal defect repair at the Mayo Clinic, the development of transient complete heart block for over 72 h followed by resumption of sinus rhythm was a strong independent predictor of late mortality.[45] Whether or not transient perioperative AV block warrants permanent pacing and whether or not an invasive electrophysiological study can help stratify risk are unresolved.[36] Postoperative right bundle branch block is frequent after ventriculotomy and may be due to injury related to closure of a ventricular septal defect or to interruption of distal Purkinje fibers by ventriculotomy or muscle resection.[34–36] Occasionally, the electrocardiographic pattern of right bundle branch block with left axis deviation occurs (bifascicular block), and there may also be PR interval prolongation (trifascicular block).[46,47] Early reports suggested that these findings were harbingers of sudden cardiac death due to complete heart block.[48] More recent studies, however, have not substantiated this adverse prognosis.[49]

Tachyarrhythmias can be life threatening. Late sudden death has been reported in several lesions, both before and after repair. In general, the worse the disease (i.e., more complex anatomy and/or more extensive surgery), the greater the incidence of sudden death.[36] The identification of patients at risk and their management are important but controversial issues. After the Mustard and Senning operation atrial flutter with a rapid ventricular response is dangerous, especially when it occurs in association with right ventricular dysfunction or venous pathway obstruction.[50] Medical or electrical cardioversion should be promptly used to restore sinus rhythm, and drug therapy may need to be accompanied by pacemaker insertion. Recently, ablation (surgical or catheter) has been advocated for certain cases of atrial flutter. (See Chap. 43.) Atrial tachyarrhythmias are also common after the Fontan operation; sinus node injury, atrial suturing, and a dilated hypertensive right atrium probably contribute.[36,40] Modification of the operation to exclude the right atrium from the Fontan circuit, the *total cavopulmonary connection,* may reduce the incidence of potentially serious early and late rhythm disturbances.[41]

Ventricular arrhythmias are known to occur after open heart surgery, particularly repair of tetralogy of Fallot.[47,51–53] Studies using ambulatory electrocardiographic monitoring in postoperative patients have documented asymptomatic complex ectopy and nonsustained ventricular tachycardia in up to 50 percent of patients,[52–54] and up to 30 percent have inducible ventricular tachycardia at electrophysiological study.[55] Experimental and clinical studies have shown that the electrical substrate for reentry arrhythmia is present in the right ventricle.[56] In several reports, older age at surgery is a predisposing factor,[54,57] an observation that suggests factors present at the time of repair may be involved in the genesis of postoperative arrhythmia, in addition to the myocardial damage occurring at the time of surgery or during postoperative follow-up.[58] This is consistent with morphologic studies that have documented increasing fibrosis of the right ventricle as part of the natural history of defects such as tetralogy of Fallot.[59,60] The current practice of early surgical repair for tetralogy of Fallot may reduce the incidence of postoperative ventricular arrhythmia, and encouraging preliminary data support this view.[58,61] Other postulated risk factors include elevated right ventricular systolic pressure, reduced right ventricular ejection fraction, pulmonary regurgitation, and a ventriculotomy scar.[55,62,63] The clinical significance of nonsustained ventricular tachycardia and especially the indications for prophylactic, antiarrhythmic therapy remain unclear.[49] There is a disparity between the high frequency of ventricular arrhythmia and the much lower incidence of sudden death.[51,64,65] In the 30-year follow-up series from the Mayo Clinic, the risk of sudden death was highest in the first few years after repair without any evidence of an increasing hazard with time. The predictive value of an abnormal ambulatory electrocardiogram (ECG) or of electrophysiological study has not been established. Furthermore, prophylactic antiarrhythmic therapy has not been shown to be of value in asymptomatic patients with congenital heart defects. Such therapy may have proarrhythmic potential, be negatively inotropic, or have serious extracardiac side effects. At present, there is insufficient evidence to advocate prophylactic treatment for asymptomatic individuals. On the other hand, the rare patients with sustained ventricular tachycardia and symptoms or survivors of out-of-hospital cardiac arrest must be treated actively.

Risk stratification of patients with congenital heart lesions will undoubtedly be more refined in the future and will likely involve hemodynamic and electrophysiological testing both at rest and after exercise and evaluation of ventricular late potentials (Chap. 47) and heart rate variability.

Pregnancy

An increasing number of women with complex and postoperative congenital heart defects are reaching childbearing age. Advice is sought on both maternal and fetal risk as well as on the incidence of congenital heart disease in the offspring. Firm recommendations for many conditions are difficult as most experience has been gathered for patients with relatively simple defects such as secundum atrial septal defect and patent ductus arteriosus.[66] It has been estimated that congenital heart disease accounts for approximately 10 percent of heart disease cases in pregnancy and up to 1 percent of maternal deaths.[67]

There are profound changes in the maternal cardiovascular system during pregnancy, including a large (30 to 40 percent) increase in blood volume, a fall in peripheral vascular resistance, and an increase in cardiac output (approximately 40 percent).[68] (See also Chap. 113.) In general, women with left-to-right shunts or valvular regurgitation tolerate pregnancy well, whereas those with right-to-left shunts or valvar stenosis do less well.

Asymptomatic young women with small or moderate left-to-right shunts and normal pulmonary artery pressures can expect an uncomplicated pregnancy and labor. In the presence of a large left-to-right shunt, however, heart failure may be provoked or aggravated by pregnancy. Patients with cyanosis have the most problems in carrying a fetus to term and have a high incidence of early spontaneous abortion. In a recent review of 416 patients with congenital heart disease who had 822 pregnancies, 45 cyanosed mothers aged 15 to 41 years had 96 pregnancies. There was a clear relationship between the degree of hypoxia (rather than hyperviscosity) and fetal loss.[69] Meticulous care during pregnancy and delivery lessened the maternal complication rate, but this was still considerable (10 patients, 22 percent). Such patients require rest and a short labor as well as avoidance of dehydration and sepsis. In such situations, the decision as to whether or not to continue with the pregnancy depends on an assessment of the risk to the mother and fetus compared to the patient's desire to have children. An elevated pulmonary vascular resistance, from either Eisenmenger's syndrome or primary pulmonary hypertension, is a clear contraindication to pregnancy.[68] Although successful outcome is possible, maternal and fetal risks are high and advice against pregnancy should be given. If such patients are seen late in pregnancy and termination is not feasible, management should concentrate on maintenance of adequate preload and avoidance of vasodilatation. Patients with Marfan's syndrome and aortic root dilatation and patients with severe aortic stenosis are also at increased risk. While early reports suggested a high risk of aortic rupture and cerebral hemorrhage in patients with aortic coarctation,[70] more recent data have been more encouraging.[71] Fetal risk is increased, however, presumably as a result of compromised placental blood supply.

The management of pregnant women with prosthetic cardiac valves is a special problem because of the risk to the mother of thromboembolism and the risk to the fetus of anticoagulants (warfarin crosses the placenta and is teratogenic).[72–75] Depending on the condition involved and the mother's motivation and compliance, the use of subcutaneous heparin in the first and third trimesters and warfarin in midtrimester is one treatment option, although fetal loss, if not teratogenecity, is increased even with heparin. (See also Chap. 68.) Before prescribing any cardiovascular drug during pregnancy, the effects on both mother and fetus must be considered. Management of labor should be specifically directed toward avoidance of rapid changes in circulatory volume, blood pressure, or cardiac output. In most cases vaginal delivery is recommended, with careful attention to maternal position and analgesic agents. The American Heart Association no longer recommends endocarditis prophylaxis for vaginal delivery.[35] This, however, is not based on controlled data, and most cardiologists recommend antibiotics under these circumstances for almost all congenital heart defects.

Genetic Counseling

Genetic counseling should be provided for all potential parents with congenital heart disease, both male and female. The etiology of congenital heart disease remains unclear. (See Chap. 96.) It has been estimated that the cause of congenital heart disease is genetic in approximately 8 percent of cases (e.g., the Holt-Oram syndrome with autosomal dominant transmission of an atrial septal defect) and environmental in 2 percent (e.g., congenital rubella syndrome).[76] In the remainder, genetic and environmental factors are thought to interact.[77] The greater the number of affected first-degree relatives within the family, the greater the recurrence risk. Recurrence risks in siblings of patients with congenital heart disease are well documented and range between 1 and 8 percent.[78] For the affected potential parents, however, the recurrence risk in offspring is the key information and fewer data exist. In general, recurrence risks are considerably higher than in sibling studies. In a series of 233 women with congenital heart disease followed through 482 pregnancies, the overall incidence in offspring was 16.1 percent.[79] Certain forms of congenital heart disease recur more frequently than others; the recurrence risk appears to be higher in pregnancies from couples with affected mothers rather than fathers.

PSYCHOSOCIAL ASPECTS

During adolescence, a crucial transition occurs for the patient with congenital heart disease. By the end of the teenage years, the young adult needs to understand the nature and implications of his or her heart problem. Sensible advice and guidance must be available regarding employment, insurance, socialization, contraception, exercise, and sports.

Employment

Most patients can work and should have access to employment appropriate to their physical and intellectual capabilities. The report of the Natural History Study of Congenital Heart Defects suggested that, in comparison with national normal standards, among patients with ventricular septal defect, pulmonary stenosis, and aortic stenosis, a greater percentage achieved higher levels of education (college and beyond).[80] No similar data are yet available for large groups of patients with more complex defects, although their situation will undoubtedly prove worse. Despite the excellent potential of many adults with congenital heart disease, job discrimination is frequently encountered, even when a patient is cleared by a cardiologist.

Restrictions for employment exist for jobs in which the safety of others is the direct responsibility of an individual, such as driving a bus or truck. Most armed services exclude applicants with a cardiac history. The regulations for commercial airline pilots are clearer and subject to regular review. In Europe, a risk of sudden cardiac death or acute disability below 1 percent per annum is the maximum considered acceptable for multicrew flights and 0.1 percent for solo flights.[81] The number of congenital heart defects in which such low risk rates are clearly defined remains small.[82]

Insurance

In the absence of adequate long-term survival data for many operated and unoperated congenital heart lesions, life insurance may be difficult to obtain for many young adults. In 1986 only patients with very simple lesions were insured at regular rates.[83] These included mild pulmonary valve stenosis, uncomplicated corrected atrial septal defect, and ventricular septal defect and patent ductus arteriosus.

Psychosocial Development

Large controlled longitudinal studies of the psychosocial consequences of congenital heart disease are rare and difficult to interpret.[84] Most patients with congenital heart disease appear well adjusted but have subtle feelings of "difference" from their peers. Lack of self-esteem and fear of isolation are common.[85] These feelings are often compounded by frequent reminders that they are different through limitation of their activities compared to others, the presence of scars, cardiac symptoms, hospital visits, and family anxiety. As a result, adolescents and adults with congenital heart disease should be encouraged to lead as normal a life as possible and to discuss their heart disease openly. Anxiety about sexual activity, marriage, and childbirth are common, but patients often find these aspects difficult to discuss, particularly with the doctor in a regular clinic.[86] Often, such issues are best handled by the team caring for the patient, which may include a nurse, social worker, and psychologist. As the child with congenital heart disease matures, one of the most potent effects on his or her life is parental overprotection. In adolescents and young adults, this may result in enormous resentment and rebellion against all adult authority figures, including the doctor. Compliance with medical treatment and advice can be affected.

The impact of congenital heart disease on intellectual development is controversial. Interpretation of testing must take into account the very abnormal childhood experienced by many patients, with absence from schooling for medical reasons as well as decreased social interaction. In addition, patients have often had an overprotected childhood, and their attitude to testing procedures may be different. All studies of intellect exclude patients with genetic syndromes and other dysmorphic, somatic, or neurologic defects, but subtle abnormalities are easily missed.[87] Certain aspects of development appear to be more specifically affected by congenital heart disease. For example, walking is delayed in cyanotic children, but speech is not. This will affect the relevance of early IQ testing on later performance. Currently, data suggest that cyanosis is associated with mild intellectual impairment.[88–90] This is reduced by early corrective surgery, even involving cardiopulmonary bypass.

Contraception

Sexually active adolescents and young adults should be given appropriate advice about contraception.[91] In general, the low-dose estrogen oral contraceptive pill is safe for young women with congenital heart disease.[92] Exceptions include those with hypertension (e.g., associated with coarctation of the aorta) and those with pulmonary vascular disease or cyanosis with associated polycythemia. In such cases, a progesterone preparation is an alternative, although with a lower contraceptive efficacy.[93] Barrier methods, either using condom or diaphragm are safe and effective, but intrauterine devices should probably not be used because of the risk of endocarditis.[94] In women with severe pulmonary vascular disease or with lesions in which pregnancy would result in high maternal risk, laparoscopic sterilization should be considered.

Exercise/Sports

Exercise is of both physical and psychological benefit. It leads to improved cardiovascular fitness and decreased likelihood of obesity, hypertension, and ischemic heart disease.[95–97] Furthermore, participation in exercise and sports is part of normal socialization in adolescent and adult life. In many adults with congenital heart disease exercise capacity is diminished, even after surgery. Reduced performance may also reflect lack of regular exercise in protected individuals with congenital heart defects. This is often reinforced by doctors who, if in doubt, tend to limit exercise.

The Sixteenth Bethesda Conference provided recommendations for competition in athletics by patients with cardiovascular abnormalities,[98] but it remains difficult to make dogmatic recommendations.[99] In some cases, exercise capacity is clearly normal and the risk is minimal, as after closure of a small patent ductus arteriosus. In others, exercise capacity is limited and the risk is high, as in severe left ventricular hypertrophy. Between these extremes is a grey area in which recommendations must take into account the individual, the underlying cardiac defect, hemodynamic status, and the type of sport and form of exercise contemplated (e.g., isotonic or isometric, social or competitive, contact or noncontact). Formal testing should be performed (preferably including measurement of oxygen uptake), both as a measure of the effects of submaximal and maximal exercise and also as a reassurance to the patient. A 12-min walking test gives a good guide to functional capacity, whereas a treadmill protocol with more strenuous effort is employed to assess risk by revealing occult arrhythmia, ischemia, or fall in blood pressure (Chap. 16). Subjective estimates of exercise capacity are often inaccurate.

In general, volume overload, valve regurgitation, and left-to-right shunts are associated with good exercise tolerance, whereas pressure overload, valve stenosis, and right-to-left shunt are not. Recommendations for individual lesions are given in Tables 98-3 to 98-5. These should be considered as guidelines only, as adequate information to assess capacity and associated risk is not yet available for many conditions. Patients with fixed, elevated pulmonary vascular resistance have limited exercise capacity and for them exercise has considerable risk. As a result, most forms of active exercise should be avoided. The most controversial recommendations are those for aortic stenosis and Marfan's syndrome. It could be argued that exercise has an adverse effect on sudden death or the progression of left ventricular hypertrophy in the former (see Chap. 79) and may increase the risk

TABLE 98-3

Congenital Conditions in which Exercise Ordinarily Should Not Be Limited Other than by the Patient's Own Desire

- Left-to-right shunts without ventricular dysfunction or pulmonary vascular disease
- Mild-to-moderate valvar regurgitation
- Mild valvar stenosis
- Marfan's syndrome with normal aorta
- Most arrhythmias in the structurally normal heart, including Wolff-Parkinson-White syndrome
- Postoperative patients with excellent hemodynamic repairs, such as closure of atrial septal defect or some cases of tetralogy of Fallot

of progressive aortic dilatation in the latter (see Chap. 123). In the absence of formal data, however, we currently allow such patients to take part in a noncompetitive sport. In patients with Marfan's syndrome we measure the aortic root dimensions at frequent intervals. Patients with Marfan's syndrome and normal dimensions of the aortic root for age and size appear to have normal exercise capacity and no additional cardiovascular risk.

Supervised training programs for adults with congenital heart disease can improve aerobic fitness and increase the safe level at which they can participate in sports. Such programs also improve psychological adjustment and self-esteem.

SURGICAL CONSIDERATIONS

Reoperations

Reoperations in adults with congenital heart disease provide a particular challenge.[100] The risks are often higher than for primary procedures. Careful preoperative planning should include complete understanding of the cardiac anatomy and its relations, and study of previous operative reports. In a multicenter study catastrophic hemorrhage occurred in 144 patients during sternal reentry, with a 37 percent mortality.[101] Sternal reentry is particularly risky when the ventricle immediately beneath the sternum is a high-pressure chamber or when an extracardiac conduit lies in this position. Reentry via a different surgical approach (e.g., thoracotomy after sternotomy) can avoid adhesions and thus minimize bleeding. The current use of Gore-Tex membranes under the sternum may reduce the difficulties of future repeat procedures. Postoperative hemodynamic and respiratory problems are particularly common after reoperation because of the increased duration of surgery, previously scarred myocardium and/or lung disease, and greater use of blood products. The need for reoperation may come as a shock to patients and relatives who may have believed that childhood surgery was curative. As a result, resentment is frequent and tact is required. Indications for reoperation are shown in Table 98-6.

TABLE 98-4

Congenital Conditions in which Strenuous Sports Should Be Restricted but in which Lesser Levels of Exercise May Usually Be Allowed

- Mild hypertrophic cardiomyopathy
- Mild left ventricular outflow tract obstruction
- Marfan's syndrome with aortic root dilatation less than 5 cm
- Ventricular dysfunction with ejection fraction less than 40%
- Postoperative atrial redirection for transposition of the great arteries
- Hearts with univentricular atrioventricular connection (preoperative and postoperative)
- Some arrhythmias
- Some treated hypertensive patients after coarctation repair

TABLE 98-5

Congenital Conditions in which All Moderate and Strenuous Exercise Should Be Restricted

- Moderate and severe hypertrophic cardiomyopathy
- Moderate and severe pulmonary vascular disease
- Severe valvular stenosis
- Marfan's syndrome with aortic root more than 5 cm in diameter
- Long QT syndrome with exercise-induced ventricular tachycardia
- Postoperative patients with exercise-induced ventricular tachycardia

Inevitable Reoperation

Early repair of congenital heart defects that have involved insertion of a prosthetic valve or extracardiac

TABLE 98-6

Indications for Reoperation in Adults with Congenital Heart Disease

1. Inevitable reoperation after definitive repair: prosthetic valves, extracardiac conduits placed at an early age, and body size that becomes of inadequate size because of body growth
2. Residual defects after definitive repair: ventricular septal defect after tetralogy of Fallot and left AV valve regurgitation after AV septal defect repair
3. New/recurrent defects after definitive repair: subaortic stenosis, restenosis of aortic valve, pulmonary regurgitation in tetralogy of Fallot
4. Staged repair of complex defects: pulmonary atresia with ventricular septal defect
5. Unexpected complications: infective endocarditis
6. Heart/heart-lung transplantation for uncorrectable congenital heart disease
7. Patient operated on for congenital heart disease with new acquired heart disease: coronary disease

conduit commonly results in a need for reoperation to replace prostheses that are either too small or have undergone degeneration. Extracardiac conduits are commonly used for repair of pulmonary atresia with ventricular septal defect, truncus arteriosus, transposition with left ventricular outflow tract obstruction and/or ventricular septal defect, congenitally corrected transposition with left ventricular outflow tract obstruction, and/or ventricular septal defect and were used in early Fontan operations. Development of obstruction is influenced by the type of conduit, technique of insertion, and timing of the original operation. Heterografts have shown a high incidence of early obstruction. In one series replacement of 55 of 86 (64 percent) of heterograft conduits used for repair of truncus arteriosus was necessary after a mean interval of 4 years.[102] In another series of 143 survivors of conduit insertion, all had to be replaced by 10 years.[103] A homograft aorta or pulmonary artery and valve has also been used for the repair of pulmonary atresia with ventricular septal defect.[104] Homografts, fresh or frozen, in childhood, have not performed as well as initially hoped. Calcification and obstruction remain significant complications. However, because of their favorable handling characteristics, homografts remain the conduits of choice for most reconstructions.[107,108] Besides the conduit itself, improved operative technique and the use of a large conduit have clear beneficial influence on the need for early replacement. Patients with right-sided conduits need careful follow-up, particularly toward the end of the expected life of the conduit. Although conduit obstruction may be suspected from clinical examination, the signs of severe obstruction may be subtle and may be missed. As a result, replacement may be performed too late. The consequent major deleterious effects on right ventricular function increase the risk of surgery and may not be fully reversible. Regular, noninvasive evaluation by transthoracic or transesophageal echocardiography or magnetic resonance imaging is indicated in selected patients and may provide the information usually obtained by cardiac catheterization/angiography. Reoperation is usually indicated if the right ventricular pressure is near systemic or if there is evidence of deteriorating ventricular function.[109]

Residual/Recurrent Defects

Residual or recurrent defects may be difficult to distinguish unless careful assessment after the original repair has been performed. They may have a major impact on morbidity and mortality, as when major left AV valve regurgitation persists after repair of AV septal defect.[110] Much more long-term follow-up data are needed before guidelines for reoperation for relatively minor residual abnormalities, such as mild left AV valve regurgitation, in this situation can be established.

The reported need for reoperation after the commonly performed "corrective" operation for tetralogy of Fallot varies between 1.8 and 13 percent over a follow-up of up to 31 years.[111,112] Ventricular septal defect and right ventricular outflow tract obstruction are the commonest residual abnormalities. Pulmonary regurgitation is extremely common and inevitable after transannular patching as part of the original repair. The hemodynamic consequences of pulmonary regurgitation on the right ventricle are greater in the presence of other defects such as residual obstruction and/or ventricular septal defect. Pulmonary valve replacement has not been frequently required in the first two decades after repair but may become increasingly performed because of the late deleterious effects of pulmonary regurgitation on the right ventricle.[113] Current indications include progressive right ventricular dilatation and a decrease in exercise tolerance.[114] When surgery is performed before the development of right ventricular failure (often with tricuspid regurgitation and atrial flutter/fibrillation), both clinical status and right ventricular function improve.[115] The optimal method for assessing pulmonary regurgitation in serial follow-up has not been determined and therefore appropriate guidelines for intervention, are still not yet established.

Several studies have emphasized the palliative nature of aortic valvotomy in childhood.[116-118] Isolated aortic stenosis most frequently results from a bicuspid aortic valve, although in neonates and infants the structural abnormality of the aortic valve is more severe and the results of surgery even worse. (See Chap. 97.) In a series of 59 patients who underwent open aortic valvotomy at over 1 year of age, actuarial survival was 94 percent at 5 years but only 77 percent at 22 years. Reoperation was carried out in 36 percent, and the actuarial probability of reoperation was 44 percent at 22 years.[119] When serious events comprising death, reoperation, and endocarditis were grouped together, 92 percent were free of events at 5 years but only 39 percent at 22 years. Others have reported a similar long-term outcome.[116] The causes of restenosis have not been studied in detail but appear to be related to the degree of residual obstruction. The management of patients with aortic stenosis is likely to be influenced by balloon valvotomy in the young adult, in contrast to the disappointing impact of this technique in elderly patients.[119] (See also Chaps. 79 and 86.)

Staged Repair

For complex congenital heart disease, definitive repair may not be possible until the anatomy and physiology of the circulation have been improved by one or more palliative procedures as part of a staged approach to "correction." This course is often necessary for patients with pulmonary atresia and ventricular septal defect, hypoplastic pulmonary arteries, and multifocal pulmonary blood supply. Palliative procedures to increase flow to the central pulmonary arteries and unifocalization of pulmonary flow by anastomosis (direct or indirect) of collateral vessels to the pulmonary arteries may eventually result in the ability to perform a repair (conduit insertion between the right ventricle and pulmonary artery and ventricular septal defect closure) with an acceptable postoperative right ventricular/left ventricular pressure ratio.[120,121] Excellent surgical results have been reported from such an approach, but the long-term outcome is not yet available.[122]

Other situations in which definitive repair may be indicated in the young adult include complex congenital heart defects with one functioning ventricle palliated by a systemic-pulmonary shunt or pulmonary artery banding in childhood. In selected patients who fulfill the stringent criteria for a Fontan operation, it is likely that long-term results will be better after a Fontan operation than when the ventricle is left with a chronically increased load secondary to a systemic pulmonary shunt.[10] Again, however, disconcerting late problems have begun to be apparent after the Fontan operation, and more long-term data for the type of Fontan operations currently being performed are needed[123,124] (see below).

Unexpected Reoperations

Indications for unexpected reoperation include thrombosis in a low-flow circulation such as the Fontan, prosthetic valve failure or thrombosis, and infective endocarditis. The latter may be particularly difficult to diagnose in complex congenital heart disease where the site of vegetations may not be easy to image (e.g., in a Blalock-Taussig shunt). Reoperation in the patient with uncontrolled endocarditis carries a particularly high risk.

Heart/Heart-Lung Transplantation

Despite the major successes of the last three decades, an increasing number of patients survive to adult life with deteriorating clinical status. Their only remaining prospect may be a heart or heart-and-lung transplant. (See Chap. 32.) These patients often present specific surgical problems of multiple previous chest incisions, complex venous anatomy, and borderline pulmonary vascular resistance. In addition, the young adult with end-stage heart disease may not have the ideal social milieu to cope with the demands of transplantation, and they require considerable psychological support. The shortage of donors and the ability to monitor rejection in a single organ have stimulated great interest in single-lung transplantation for patients with primary pulmonary hypertension and Eisenmenger's syndrome (in conjunction with closure of the shunt). Such patients accounted for 23 percent of the single-lung transplants performed in 1990, and the use of this approach is increasing.[125]

First Operations for Congenital Heart Disease in Adults

The first surgical repair of a congenital heart defect may be required in the teenager or adult. This may be because the lesion has been mild and of little hemodynamic significance in childhood but has progressed in severity with time. Examples include a bicuspid aortic valve with progressive stenosis (see Chap. 79), Marfan's syndrome with aortic root dilatation (see Chap. 123), and Ebstein's anomaly with worsening symptoms. Alternatively, lesions such as small-to-moderate atrial septal defects may have been missed or misdiagnosed until adult life. In certain complex congenital heart defects, the combination of lesions produces a balanced hemodynamic state compatible with prolonged survival without intervention. Patients with double-inlet ventricle and pulmonary stenosis, complex pulmonary atresia, and tetralogy of Fallot may remain well until the second and even third decades of life before deteriorating.[126] The contemplation of heart surgery in an adolescent or young adult is often terrifying, implying the acceptance of the presence of a serious heart problem by the patient and his or her immediate friends and family. The scar on the chest may cause embarrassment, and the patient may be discriminated against both socially and at work. All these issues need to be dealt with sympathetically by the physician.

Noncardiac Surgery

Noncardiac surgery in adults with congenital heart disease when performed without adequate preparation is a major cause of avoidable morbidity and mortality. All the anesthetic risks encountered for cardiac reoperation apply equally to noncardiac surgery, but in the latter the patient may be managed by medical staff who may be unfamiliar with the significance of the congenital heart disease. Many patients with congenital heart defects are at increased risk for arrhythmia and from agents that depress ventricular function. The surgeon must be aware of the presence of a pacemaker or pacing leads that may affect the safe use of diathermy. Prophylaxis against infective endocarditis is usually indicated, and the choice of antibiotic regimen is dictated by the surgical procedure/intervention being undertaken. (See Chap. 94.) In patients with pulmonary vascular disease general anesthesia may have disastrous consequences with a sudden fall in systemic vascular resistance. Similar hemodynamic changes may induce a severe hypercyanotic spell in a patient with uncorrected tetralogy of Fallot, and meticulous pre-, intra-, and postoperative hemodynamic monitoring is mandatory together with the avoidance of vasodilating anesthetic agents, hypoxia, hypoventilation, and blood or volume loss. Cyanotic patients also have impaired hemostasis, and some patients may be taking anticoagulants. Intravenous lines, drugs, and infusions must be managed carefully in patients with intracardiac shunts, as air or emboli may reach the systemic circulation. The safety of noncardiac surgery in adults with congenital heart disease is greatly increased when physicians, anesthesiologists, and surgeons familiarize themselves with these issues, seek specialized advice, and if necessary, refer the patient to a team with more experience.

SPECIFIC LESIONS

General Considerations

Some lesions that are commonly seen in adult congenital heart disease practice both as a result of natural and unnatural survival are listed in Tables 98-1 and 98-2.

Interpretation of the literature on long-term outcome of congenital heart defects is hampered by a number of difficulties. First, follow-up is still short and numbers of survivors are small for many defects. The era of open heart surgery for congenital heart defects only began in the 1950s, and "correction" has only been attempted much more recently for many categories of patients now beginning to reach adult life (e.g., Fontan operation). Second, surgical practice has undergone a process of evolution during this time, with new operations for some lesions (e.g., transposition of the great arteries) or major change in operative technique for others (e.g., the Fontan operation). Third, major advances in cardiopulmonary bypass and myocardial protection have accompanied improved preoperative diagnosis and recognition of intracardiac anatomy, particularly of the disposition of the conduction tissues. Finally, for almost all lesions, the management philosophy has changed with a trend to early primary correction as opposed to initial palliation. For many defects, therefore, long-term outcome data relevant to current practice are not available.

Correct application of survival analysis is essential for interpretation of follow-up data.[127] In particular, the use of hazard functions providing an estimate of *instantaneous risk* is particularly valuable. The following section deals with some specific defects seen in adults with congenital heart disease.

Atrial Septal Defect

Atrial septal defects are among the most common congenital anomalies in adolescents and adults, accounting for up to 30 percent of congenital heart disease in this age group.[128,129] Approximately 75 percent of defects are ostium secundum defects, 20 percent are ostium primum defects (discussed below), 5 percent sinus venosus defects, and defects at other sites are rare.[130,131] (See Chap. 97.) Associated lesions include pulmonary stenosis, mitral valve prolapse, and mitral regurgitation. Atrial septal defects may be associated with other syndromes, including the Holt-Oram syndrome[132] (Fig. 10-2), and may be familial.[133] In the latter, conduction disease manifesting as prolongation of the PR interval and rarely heart block has been described.[133] Lutembacher's syndrome (atrial septal defect coexisting with mitral stenosis) is now very uncommon.

Natural History

Survival into adulthood is the rule, and patients living into their eighties and nineties have been reported.[128] Life expectancy, however, is not normal. Death during the first 20 years of life is infrequent, but after the age of 40 years, the mortality increases to about 6 percent per year.[134–136] Defects may go unrecognized for many years because symptoms are rare until later life and physical signs may be subtle. Later, the natural history is characterized by progressive symptoms and cardiomegaly, the development of atrial arrhythmias, right ventricular hypertrophy, and pulmonary hypertension. The mechanisms for the development of symptoms are multifactorial[128] and include the following:

1. Change in left ventricular compliance from superimposed hypertension or coronary artery disease that increases the shunt with age. Longstanding right ventricular volume overload, although relatively well tolerated, ultimately leads to right ventricular failure, and a marked increase in right ventricular volume can further compromise the left ventricle.
2. Supraventricular arrhythmias, particularly atrial fibrillation and flutter, increase with time and may cause symptoms and cardiac failure.
3. Progressive pulmonary vascular disease after the third decade of life.
4. Rarer complications, including systemic and pulmonary emboli, recurrent chest infections, and infective endocarditis (in patients with coexisting mitral valve disease).

Management

Surgical closure either by direct suture or use of a patch has been performed for almost 40 years (Chap. 97). Surgery carries a low risk (<1 percent operative mortality) provided the pulmonary vascular resistance is not significantly elevated.[131] In older patients, the indication for closure may be less clear. For example, in adults with additional cardiovascular disease, the early morbidity and mortality are increased and long-term benefit is less easy to demonstrate. Pulmonary vascular disease, which may preclude surgery, occurs in approximately 10 percent of untreated adults.

Recently, closure of atrial septal defect has been achieved in selected patients by use of a "clamshell" umbrella device inserted at cardiac catheterization.[137,138] Despite the encouraging early results, the current generation of atrial septal defect occluders has required modification due to a high incidence of strut fracture and a low, but significant, incidence of embolization. The attractions of closing defects without open heart surgery are obvious. Eventually, the transcatheter technique may supplant surgery as the method of choice for closure of many atrial septal defects and for patients with a patent foramen ovale and paradoxical emboli.

Late Results

In a recent study of patients undergoing surgical repair of an atrial septal defect between 1956 and 1960, late survival of patients undergoing operation at below 24 years of age was not significantly different from an age- and sex-matched control population. Late survival in patients aged 25 to 41 years was good but less than that of the control population, whereas repair after age 41 years was associated with significantly poorer late survival (Fig. 98-1). The combination of older age at operation and pulmonary hypertension had an additive effect on late mortality.[139] In this and other series, the propensity for atrial fibrillation and flutter increased as a function of age both before and after operation (Fig. 98-2).[139,140] Twenty-two percent of late deaths were due to stroke, and all occurred in patients with postoperative atrial fibrillation or flutter. These data support the current policy of repair at a preschool age (Chap. 97). A separate study of 66 patients who underwent closure of atrial septal defect between 60 and 78 years of age implied a benefit in survival in patients discharged from the hospital compared to unoperated historical age- and sex-matched controls.[141]

The near normal survival and low morbidity in patients undergoing repair within the first two decades of life have important implications for employment and insurance recommendations. Such patients should be encouraged to lead a normal life, and competitive sports should not be restricted in the absence of hemodynamic or electrophysiological sequelae. The risk of endocarditis in the absence of mitral valve disease is minimal. Patients

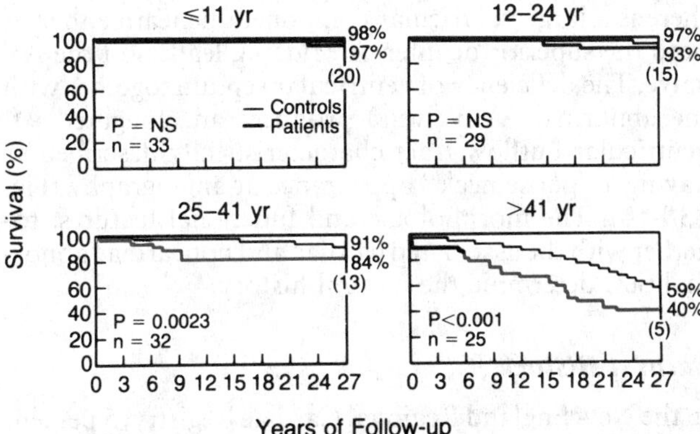

FIGURE 98-1 Long-term survival of perioperative survivors of atrial septal defect repair by age at time of operation. Controls are survival in an age- and sex-matched population. *(From Murphy JG, Gersh BJ, McGoon MD, et al: Long-term outcome after surgical repair of isolated atrial septal defects: Follow-up at 27–32 years. N Engl J Med 323:1645, 1990. Reproduced with permission from the publisher and authors.)*

who have undergone repair in the third decade of life or later require careful regular surveillance. Although late survival is good, the development of supraventricular arrhythmia and risk of cerebrovascular accident are of concern. Anticoagulation is indicated in patients with atrial fibrillation and should be considered in those with supraventricular tachycardia or atrial flutter in the absence of other contraindications. (See also Chaps. 36 and 68.)

Ventricular Septal Defect

Isolated ventricular septal defect, although one of the commonest congenital abnormalities in infants and children, is far less frequent in the adolescent and adult for several reasons.[128] First, most patients with a hemodynamically significant defect will have undergone repair in childhood; second, spontaneous decrease in size and closure is common for small or moderate perimembranous or muscular defects (this decreases in frequency with increasing age); and finally, patients with large unoperated defects may die earlier in life.[142] The spectrum of isolated ventricular septal defects in the adult is thus limited to the following four groups of patients: (1) those with small restrictive defects that were either small to begin with or have partially closed; (2) those with Eisenmenger's syndrome and a predominant right-to-left shunt with cyanosis[143] who need to be distinguished from those who develop secondary infundibular pulmonary stenosis, which can also decrease the left-to-right shunt and may result in cyanosis with shunt reversal[144] (see Chap. 97); (3) the occasional patient with a moderately restrictive defect in whom the diagnosis has been overlooked or who has not had closure in childhood; and (4) those who have had their defects closed in childhood.

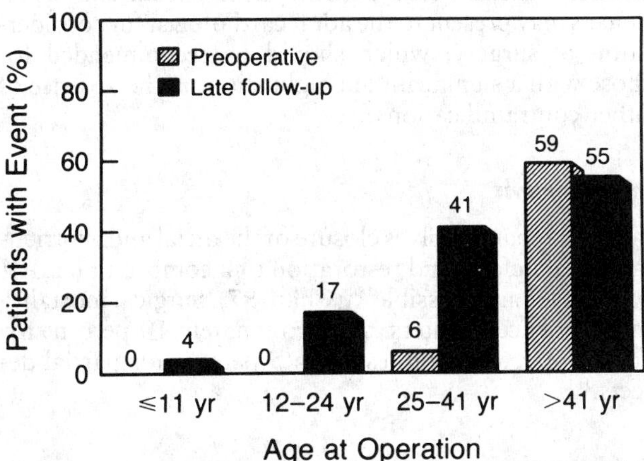

FIGURE 98-2 Incidence of atrial flutter or atrial fibrillation preoperatively and at late follow-up according to the age at operation after repair of atrial septal defect. *(From Murphy JG, Gersh BJ, McGoon MD, et al: Long-term outcome after surgical repair of isolated atrial septal defects: Follow-up at 27–32 years. N Engl J Med 323:1645, 1990. Reproduced with permission from the publisher and authors.)*

Natural History

The natural history of small restrictive ventricular septal defects is very favorable.[129] Nevertheless, the risk of infective endocarditis persists (developing in almost 4 percent of patients with ventricular septal defect) and lifelong prophylaxis is required. A subset of patients with perimembranous defects or defects in the outlet septum may develop aortic cusp prolapse and aortic regurgitation. This may be progressive and is often severe by the end of the second decade of life. As incompetence increases, the ventricular septal defect may become "closed" by the prolapsing cusp, but if left to develop, aortic valve replacement may be necessary.[145] Such defects are associated with a high risk of infective endocarditis. Severe and progressive pulmonary vascular disease is a feature of older patients with nonrestrictive large defects. Eisenmenger's syndrome is compatible with survival into young adult life, but the complications of right-sided heart failure, paradoxical emboli, and polycythemia usually result in death by the third decade. (See Chap. 97.) Occasionally, patients with moderate-sized ventricular septal defects and left-to-right shunts who did not develop pulmonary vascular disease present in adolescence and young adult life with symptoms of fatigue, effort intolerance, and respiratory infections.

Management

Patients with small ventricular septal defects are asymptomatic and should be managed conservatively. Continued medical follow-up is, however, helpful to remind patients about the need for infective endocarditis prophylaxis and to minimize inappropriate discrimination during the search for employment and insurance. Ventricular septal defects associated with aortic cusp prolapse and aortic regurgitation should be repaired even when the shunt is small in an effort to prevent progressive deterioration of the aortic valve. Surgical repair is indicated in the rare adult with a significant left-to-right shunt (pulmonary to systemic flow ratio exceeding 2 : 1) and a low pulmonary vascular resistance. The management of patients with large defects and infundibular narrowing causing right-to-left shunting and cyanosis is similar to that for tetralogy of Fallot (see below).

Unfortunately, adults are still seen with a large ventricular septal defect and pulmonary vascular disease. In those with borderline pulmonary vascular resistance (7 to 10 units/m^2) surgery may be attempted, but the benefits are unpredictable as the pulmonary vascular disease may progress despite closure of the defect.[146] (See Chap. 97.) Medical management and consideration for heart-lung or single-lung transplantation are the only realistic options for patients with established severe pulmonary vascular disease.

Late Results

Late results of surgery are good, but the life expectancy for the whole group is not normal. In a study of 145 operative survivors between 1956 and 1959, 30-year survival was 82 percent compared to 97 percent in age- and sex-matched controls.[44] Only 25 percent of patients in the series were over 10 years of age at surgery, and their 30-year survival of 70 percent was substantially lower than the 88 percent in patients under 2 years of age at operation. Thirty-year survival was 83 percent for patients aged 3 to 10 years at surgery. Older age at repair and preoperative pulmonary vascular disease are important predictors of late outcome. Postoperative conduction defects, especially right bundle branch block, are common, but complete heart block, which was seen in the early surgical experience, is now rare. Late ventricular arrhythmia has been reported, as after repair of tetralogy of Fallot.[147] The incidence of late sudden death, however, is extremely low, and prophylactic antiarrhythmic therapy in asymptomatic patients is not indicated.

The ability to close selected ventricular septal defects with transcatheter devices is exciting. A recent report described closure of 21 muscular ventricular septal defects in 12 patients, half of whom had complex heart defects.[148] All the defects were closed successfully, and subsequent cardiac surgery for associated lesions was performed in 11 of 12 patients.

In postoperative patients the risk of late infective endocarditis is very small providing the defect is isolated and is completely closed. Antibiotic prophylaxis, however, is often advised, particularly for 6 months postoperatively. Recommendations regarding physical activity and competitive sports require detailed evaluation, which may include exercise testing, cross-sectional echocardiography, and ambulatory electrocardiographic monitoring. The presence of abnormal left ventricular function, a more than trivial residual shunt, arrhythmia, or any degree of pulmonary hypertension mandates some restriction of physical activity.

Atrioventricular Septal Defect

The term *atrioventricular septal defect* describes the spectrum of lesions that have a defect at the site of the normal AV septum resulting in an abnormality involving the AV valves, ventricular architecture, and left ventricular outflow tract. A variety of different classifications have been used (Chap. 97), but the defects are usefully divided into "partial" and "complete" forms. In the former there is a large defect in the primum or inferior part of the atrial septum but no direct intraventricular communication (ostium primum defect). In the latter, there is a large ventricular component beneath either or both the superior or inferior bridging leaflets of the AV valve. The deficiency of ventricular septum together with the abnormal AV valve(s) produces an elongated left ventricular outflow tract characteristically described as having a "goose neck" appearance at angiography (Fig. 138-10). The morphologic and functional features, together with the associated cardiac and noncardiac abnormalities, determine the natural history.

Natural History

In the New England Regional Cardiac Registry, 5 percent of newborns with cardiac disease had AV septal defects with two-thirds being the "complete" form.[149] Down's syndrome is very frequently associated especially with complete defects. The noncardiac features, especially mental retardation, have a major influence on the management in adolescence and adult life.

The natural history of partial AV septal defects with little left AV valve regurgitation is similar to that of large secundum atrial septal defects (see above). A small number develop pulmonary vascular disease, and symptomatic deterioration in unoperated adults is often due to the onset of supraventricular arrhythmia. If the left AV valve is more than mildly regurgitant, the natural history is much worse, with a large left-to-right shunt, often with at least moderate pulmonary hypertension and early symptoms of cardiac failure. Patients with complete defects do even worse. Their course is characterized by the early development of pulmonary vascular disease (especially in patients with Down's syndrome who may have irreversible damage before their first birthday) with consequent right-to-left shunting and all the problems of patients with Eisenmenger's syndrome. As a result, surgery needs to be undertaken early if it is to be successful, and most uncorrected patients seen by the adolescent or adult cardiologist will have a pulmonary vascular resistance that is too high for repair (greater than 8 to 10 units/m^2). (See Chaps. 97 and 138.) Their outcome is poor, but survival into their thirties is possible. Uncorrected patients with partial AV septal defects may present to the adult cardiologist for consideration of surgery, which should be recommended for those with a significant left-right shunt in the absence of other contraindications.

Management

Surgical repair involves closure of the atrial and ventricular septal defects and restoration of a competent left AV valve as far as is possible[150] (Chap. 97). Surgical mortality in experienced centers is approximately 10 percent for complete defects and less than 5 percent for partial defects.[131]

Late Results

Patients with repair of both partial and complete forms of AV septal defect have now been followed for more than 20 years. Late results are good in the absence of pulmonary vascular disease and significant residual left AV valve regurgitation. Some patients with complete defects who were corrected later in childhood, before the need for correction in early infancy was appreciated, have developed progressive pulmonary vascular disease. This late complication should be greatly reduced in patients undergoing repair in the first 6 months of life, as is now technically feasible. (See Chap. 97.)

During long-term follow-up, careful attention must be paid to the status of the left AV valve. If the regurgitation increases in severity, reoperation and mitral valve replacement may be necessary.[110] Monitoring for arrhythmia at intervals is also currently recommended; in general, little intervention is usually required apart from lifelong infective endocarditis prophylaxis. Surgically repaired non-Down's patients without pulmonary vascular disease can often enjoy life without cardiovascular disability and should not be discouraged from competitive sports, pregnancy, or employment. Restrictions are clearly required for those with pulmonary vascular disease, left AV valve regurgitation, or mitral valve replacement on anticoagulants. Patients with Down's syndrome, both operated and unoperated, are demanding, and their families require considerable support from the physician as well as from the educational and social services. The recurrence risk of congenital heart disease in offspring of mothers with AV septal defect is higher than average, and potential parents should be counseled.

Tetralogy of Fallot

Tetralogy of Fallot is the most common form of cyanotic congenital heart disease seen in the adult. Nonetheless, in the developed world the unoperated patient with tetralogy of Fallot has fortunately become a rarity since the overwhelming majority of patients will have undergone palliation or more usually repair in childhood. From an anatomic and pathophysiological standpoint, the manifestations of tetralogy of Fallot are similar in all age groups, although hypercyanotic spells, which are often seen in infants and young children, are rare in adults. The development of systemic hypertension with age is a problem as this increases the afterload to both ventricles.[128,151] Although pulmonary blood flow may improve, this occurs at the expense of right ventricular failure. Acquired calcific aortic stenosis has similar effects. Aortic regurgitation may occur as a result of cusp prolapse in patients with aortic defect. If exacerbated by infective endocarditis, the volume overload is transmitted to both ventricles. The development of chronic obstructive lung disease is another manifestation of an acquired cardiopulmonary disease that may place the adult patient with tetralogy of Fallot at particular risk.

Natural History

Survival into the seventh decade is described,[152] but the natural history in the unoperated patient, which is determined by the severity of obstruction of the right ventricular outflow tract and pulmonary vasculature, is poor. Only 25 percent of patients reach the age of 10 years, 11 percent are alive at 20 years, 6 percent at age 30 years, but only 3 percent at age 40 years.[128,131,153] Complications of right-to-left shunting and polycythemia, which include stroke and cerebral abscess, are common and in many instances fatal. Patients are at continuing risk of infective endocarditis; the development of congestive heart failure in adolescence or early adult life is a major cause of death, as is arrhythmia. Myocardial fibrosis resulting from long-standing right ventricular pressure overload and hypoxemia are postulated mechanisms.[154] Prior palliative surgery with a Cooley or Waterston shunt (between the ascending aorta and right pulmonary artery) or a Potts shunt (between the descending aorta and the left pulmonary artery) can lead to the late development of pulmonary vascular disease.[155]

Management

The focus of medical treatment in unoperated patients is on the elevated hematocrit, bleeding disorders, and abnormal uric acid metabolism and the complications of pregnancy.

Repair is indicated in all suitable patients, and the principles and techniques are not significantly different in adults from those in children.[130] (See Chap. 97.) Most adults are suitable for repair, but the occasional patient with an underdeveloped pulmonary vascular bed may require a palliative shunt procedure. Intracardiac repair consists of closure of the ventricular septal defect and relief of right ventricular outflow tract obstruction. In some patients, this may require excision of the pulmonary valve and patch reconstruction of the annulus and outflow tract. In the occasional patient with an anomalous origin of the left coronary artery from the right coronary artery, a conduit between the right ventricle and pulmonary artery may be required.[131]

Late Results

Late survival is excellent, even in patients who underwent repair during the very early years of open heart surgery.[137] At the Mayo Clinic, the cumulative 30-year survival for patients undergoing successful surgery between 1956 and 1960 was 86 percent compared to 95 percent in age- and sex-matched controls (Fig. 98-3).[156] In a previous series of 396 hospital survivors of repair between 1955 and 1962 at the same institution 91 percent were alive at 20 years. At 30 years, 77 percent of the initial cohort of 106 patients undergoing surgery between 1954 and 1960 by Lillehei and associates were alive, including one patient who was 45 years of age at the time of operation.[157] Surgery cannot be considered "curative" as survival even in excellent series is slightly but significantly worse than for a matched control population. The risk factors for an adverse late outcome include older age at surgery, preoperative congestive heart failure, a previous Potts shunt, persistent right ventricular systolic hypertension, and a residual ventricular septal defect.[155,156] Late death may be sudden, due to tachyarrhythmia or, very rarely in the current era, due to conduction disease (see above). Left and right ventricular failure due to right ventricular pressure overload or left ventricular volume overload is another important cause of late mortality in older patients.[128]

The late functional outcome is excellent for the majority of patients. Most lead normal lives, but the results appear to be better in those undergoing surgery at a

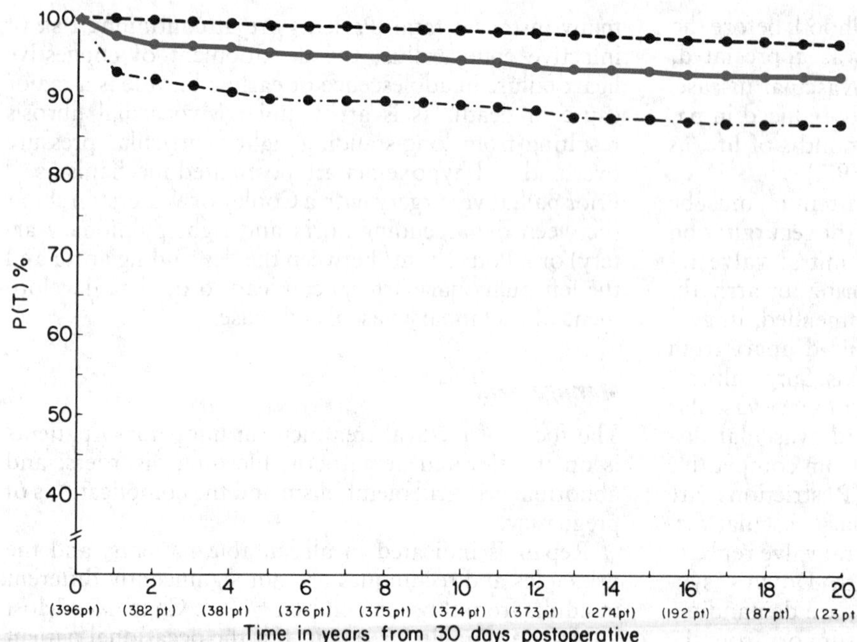

FIGURE 98-3 Probability of deterioration in operative survivors after repair of tetralogy of Fallot plotted against time in years. Time of deterioration is defined as the postoperative year in which late death (middle curve) or in which death, reoperation, or symptoms occurred (bottom curve). The top curve represents the controlled expected survival on the basis of an age- and sex-matched distribution. The number of patients at each follow-up interval is denoted in parentheses. *[From Fuster V, McGoon DC, Kennedy M, et al: Long-term evaluation (12–22 years) of open heart surgery for tetralogy of Fallot. Am J Cardiol 46:635, 1980. Reproduced with permission from the publisher and authors.]*

younger age.[158] Persistent or recurrent symptoms are usually the result of incomplete relief of right ventricular systolic hypertension or recurrent/residual ventricular septal defects. These problems are often manifest within the first few years after surgery and may require reoperation. Although pulmonary regurgitation does not appear to increase mortality, it may be associated with late impairment of exercise capacity and persistent cardiomegaly.[159] It may well become an increasing problem with very long follow-up, but the precise indications for pulmonary valve insertion are not yet clear.

Objective testing has emphasized the effects of older age at operation on subsequent exercise performance. Exercise performance is essentially normal in children repaired at below 5 years of age but is usually impaired when surgery is undertaken in adolescence or adulthood.[161] Ventricular arrhythmia is common during long-term follow up and again is related to the age at repair.[65] Few patients are symptomatic from arrhythmia, but a link with late sudden death has been postulated (see above).

Before unrestricted physical activity after repair of tetralogy of Fallot can be recommended, careful evaluation including cross-sectional echocardiography, electrocardiographic monitoring, and exercise testing should be undertaken. Normal activity including competitive sports seems reasonable if surgery has been performed at a young age, right and left ventricular function and size are normal, and there is no residual ventricular septal defect or significant right ventricular outflow tract obstruction and no worrisome arrhythmia. In those who do not fulfill these stringent criteria, the degree to which physical activity should be restricted must be individualized.

Pulmonary Stenosis

Isolated pulmonary valve stenosis is a common form of adult congenital heart disease and is characterized typically by a trileaflet valve with fused commissures. A dysplastic valve without commissural fusion occurs infrequently in otherwise normal children, but more commonly in patients with Noonan's syndrome[128] (Fig. 10-13). Subvalvar stenosis due to infundibular hypertrophy is usually a secondary phenomenon in response to obstruction to right ventricular outflow but may occur as a rare isolated entity. Supravalvar or peripheral pulmonary artery stenosis is also extremely uncommon as an isolated entity but is associated with tetralogy of Fallot and supravalvar aortic stenosis in William's syndrome (Fig. 10-25).

Natural History

Prolonged survival into adult life is common and depends upon the severity of obstruction. In patients with severe pulmonary stenosis, symptoms of right-sided failure increase with time due to progressive obstruction and alterations in right ventricular compliance.[161,162] In the Joint Study of the Natural History of Congenital Heart Disease, 19 percent of patients with severe stenosis aged 2 to 11 years and 37 percent aged 12 to 21 years were symptomatic. The natural history of moderate pulmonary stenosis in older patients is more favorable, with less tendency to progression. Patients with mild pulmonary stenosis (in contrast to those with mild aortic stenosis) at age exceeding 2 years rarely have symptoms and rarely develop progressive obstruction.[162] Associated right ventricular cavity hypoplasia, which is an important prognostic factor in neonates and infants, is much less relevant in those surviving to adulthood.

Management

Patients with mild stenosis are asymptomatic and require no intervention other than antibiotic prophylaxis against infective endocarditis. In patients with more severe stenosis (>40 mm gradient between the right ventricle and

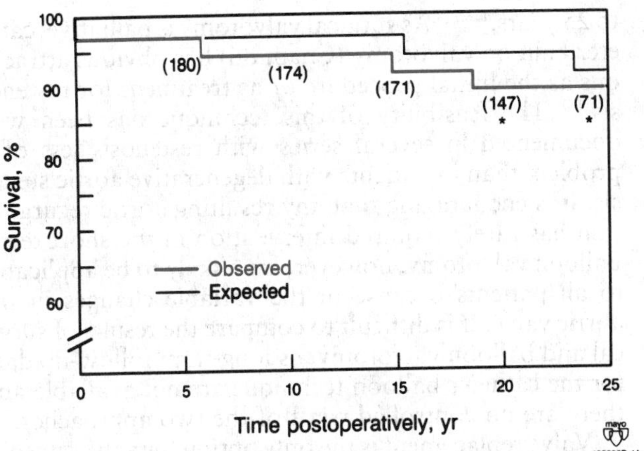

FIGURE 98-4 Long-term survival of perioperative survivors following surgical repair of isolated pulmonary stenosis and expected survival of age- and sex-matched control populations. Difference between expected and observed $P < 0.002$. *(From Kopecky SL, Gersh BJ, McGoon MD, et al: Long-term outcome of patients undergoing surgical repair of isolated pulmonary valve stenosis. Follow-up at 20–30 years. Circulation 78:1150, 1988. Reproduced with permission from the American Heart Association and authors.)*

pulmonary artery), intervention to reduce the severity should be considered even if asymptomatic.

Surgical valvotomy for isolated pulmonary stenosis has been successfully performed for more than 40 years. Perioperative morbidity and mortality are minimal beyond the neonatal period in patients without severe congestive cardiac failure or right ventricular dysplasia.[131] Late results are also excellent. In a study from the Mayo Clinic of patients undergoing surgery between 1956 and 1957, late survival for those undergoing valvotomy who are over 21 years of age was similar but not identical to an age- and sex-matched control population (Fig. 98-4). Among patients undergoing surgery at an older age, late survival, although still good, was less than that of the control population (Fig. 98-5).[163] This effect of age on late outcome, which was independent of the use of ventriculotomy and outflow patches and pulmonary regurgitation, is likely the result of long-standing pressure overload on the right ventricle. Late functional results are excellent, and pulmonary regurgitation is well tolerated in the short and medium term. More severe pulmonary regurgitation may result when a pulmonary valvectomy or transannular patch is required as may be the case for a small or dysplastic valve; the long-term consequences on the right ventricle and functional capacity are not yet well documented (see "Tetralogy of Fallot").

Surgical valvotomy is now rarely required after infancy because of the advent of catheter balloon pulmonary valvotomy.[164] In many institutions, balloon valvotomy is the initial procedure of choice at all ages even though most accumulated data apply to younger patients. In the series of 822 patients in the Valvuloplasty and Angioplasty of Congenital Heart Abnormalities (VACA) registry, gradient reduction was substantially worse in patients with dysplastic valves.[165] Interventional catheter procedures should be confined to centers with experienced operators.

Long-term follow-up data are not yet available. It appears that the excellent early results are maintained for at least 5 years, especially in older patients.[166] The late effects of pulmonary regurgitation resulting from the use of large balloons need to be determined. The risk of infective endocarditis in patients with mild pulmonary stenosis or in those with mild gradients after surgical or balloon valvotomy is low. Long-term follow-up is recommended to evaluate not only the right ventricular outflow tract gradient but also pulmonary regurgitation, right ventricular function, and exercise performance. In patients with good relief of pulmonary stenosis, no restriction of physical activities, including competitive sports, is required. In those with moderate residual obstruction or right ventricular dysfunction, exercise intensity should be reduced. (See also Chap. 86.)

Left Ventricular Outflow Tract Obstruction

Congenital left ventricular outflow tract obstruction may occur at valvar, subvalvar, and supravalvar levels. (See Chap. 97.) Aortic valve stenosis is a common abnormality in adults with congenital heart disease. It may either be an isolated defect or be associated with other lesions such as coarctation or ventricular septal defect. It is usually due to a bicuspid aortic valve, which may be present in 1 to 2 percent of the total adult population and is three to four times more common in males than in females.[167] Unicuspid and tricuspid stenotic valves are less common.[131] Subvalvar stenosis is due either to a discrete "membrane" below the aortic valve or less commonly to a fibromuscular tunnel.[168] Supravalvar stenosis is the least common variety of left ventricular outflow tract obstruction in adolescents and adults except in the context of William's syndrome.[169]

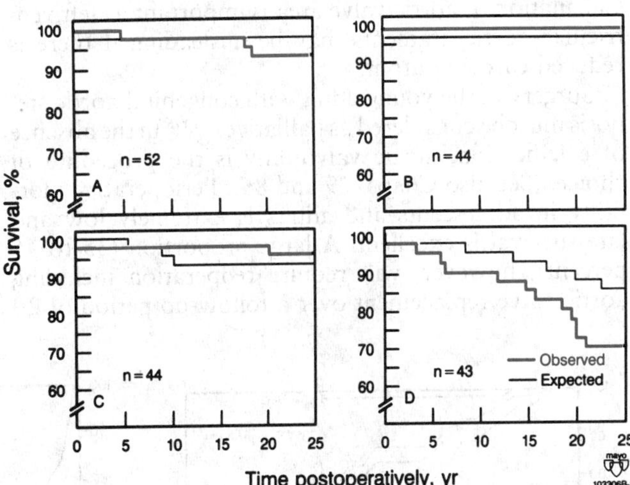

FIGURE 98-5 Long-term survival of perioperative survivors of surgical repair of pulmonary valve stenosis by age at time of operation. *A.* Ages 0 to 4 years. *B.* Ages 5 to 10 years. *C.* Ages 11 to 20 years. *D.* Ages 21 to 68 years. Expected is survival in an age- and sex-matched population. Values of *P* for comparison between the expected and observed survivals: 0.07, 0.34, 0.16, and <0.002 for panels *A, B, C,* and *D,* respectively. *(From Kopecky SL, Gersh BJ, McGoon MD, et al: Long-term outcome of patients undergoing surgical repair of isolated pulmonary valve stenosis. Follow-up at 20–30 years. Circulation 78:1150, 1988. Reproduced with permission from the publisher and authors.)*

Natural History

The natural history of congenital valvar aortic stenosis in adults is variable but is characterized by progressive stenosis with time (Fig. 98-6).[128] (See Chap. 79.) By the age of 45 years approximately half of all bicuspid aortic valves have some degree of narrowing. The severity of obstruction at the time of diagnosis correlates with the pattern of progression.[170] Bacterial endocarditis is relatively uncommon (1.8 to 2.7 cases per 100 patient years).[171] Slowly progressive aortic regurgitation is well recognized in young adulthood, but sudden deterioration is rare except as a sequel to infection.[172,173]

Discrete subaortic stenosis may cause rapidly progressive obstruction in childhood and young adult life. Progressive aortic regurgitation is common, and infective endocarditis is considered to be a particular hazard.[172,173] (See Chap. 97.) The natural history of supravalvar aortic stenosis is poor and survival to adulthood is exceptional.[128] The presence of associated congenital abnormalities and possibly premature coronary artery disease with systolic hypertension is likely a contributory factor to this adverse outcome.

Management

The development of symptoms (e.g., angina, exertional dyspnea, and syncope) mandates prompt intervention in aortic valve stenosis. (See Chap. 79.) In asymptomatic younger individuals, however, the documentation of severe aortic stenosis is, in itself, an indication for intervention.[174,175] Mild aortic stenosis in asymptomatic patients with gradients below 50 mm warrants careful surveillance. The management of patients in the intermediate group (gradients 50 to 75 mmHg) is more controversial, but evidence argues in favor of elective intervention. Calculation of aortic valve area is important as left ventricular–aortic gradients may be misleading if there is reduced cardiac output.

Surgery in the young adult with congenital aortic stenosis must be considered as palliative.[118,176] In the absence of calcification, aortic valvotomy is the procedure of choice. (See also Chaps. 79 and 86.) Perioperative mortality in adolescents and adults is extremely low and late survival is excellent. A large proportion (35 to 45 percent), however, will require reoperation including aortic valve replacement over a follow-up period of 20 to 25 years.[116,118] As surgical valvotomy is palliative, catheter balloon valvotomy (Chap. 86) has obvious attractions as the initial procedure or as treatment for restenosis.[177] The feasibility of this technique has been well documented in several series with restenosis less of a problem than in patients with degenerative aortic stenosis. It is encouraging that any resulting aortic regurgitation has rarely required intervention in the short term. Balloon valvotomy, however, is unlikely to be applicable to all patients because of the variable changes in the aortic valve. It is difficult to compare the results of surgical and balloon valvotomy, as long-term follow-up data for the catheter balloon technique are not available and there are no controlled trials of the two approaches.

Valve replacement is the only option for valves unsuitable for valvotomy, including those with significant calcification and regurgitation. The choice of prosthesis is discussed elsewhere (Chap. 79). The age and size of the patient are major considerations, as are individual characteristics that determine the safety of anticoagulation, such as the desire for future pregnancies.

Subaortic stenosis is usually amenable to more definitive surgical repair. This fact, in conjunction with the potential for progressive aortic regurgitation, justifies a more aggressive approach even in asymptomatic patients with lesser gradients.[178] Excision of the obstructive membrane together with a myectomy or myotomy is usually required. Subaortic stenosis occasionally recurs, and persistent or progressive aortic regurgitation may develop. Operative mortality is low, but the risks are greater in patients with "tunnel" forms of obstruction and in patients with obstruction at several levels. Some centers have reported promising results for catheter balloon dilatation of subaortic stenosis over short-term follow-up, but further evaluation of this technique is required.[179]

Hospital mortality for repair of supravalvar aortic stenosis is low, and late morbidity and mortality rates are also excellent. Nevertheless, residual abnormality such as aortic regurgitation or stenosis may persist after aortoplasty.

Medical follow-up of patients who have undergone surgical or balloon valvotomy should focus on the development of restenosis, the severity and progression of aortic regurgitation, and the constant hazard of infective endocarditis. Echocardiography has facilitated serial evaluation of gradients, valve areas, ventricular dimensions, function, and mass. The acceptable level of physi-

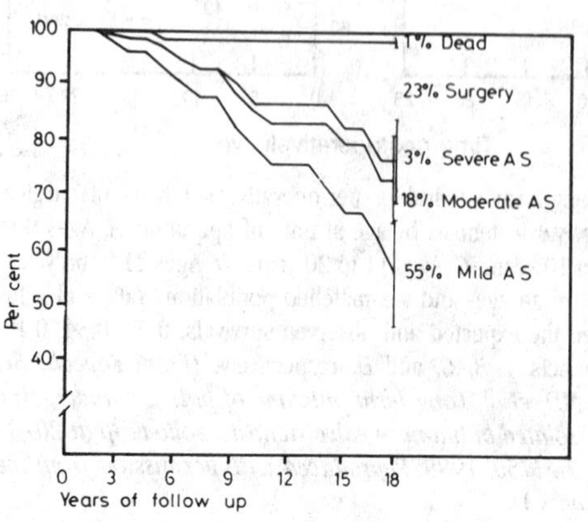

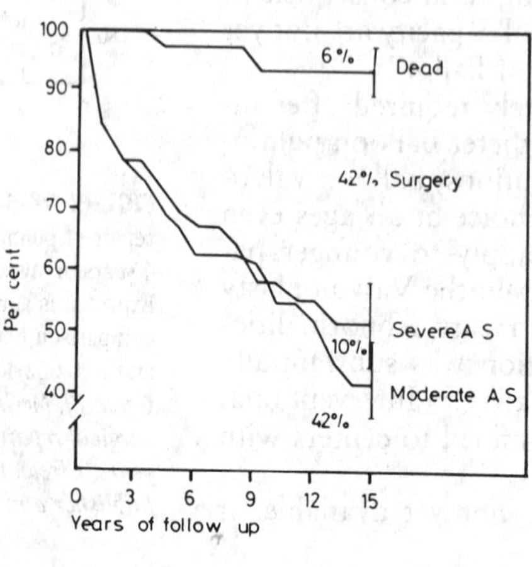

FIGURE 98-6 *Left:* Cumulative actuarial curves of 153 patients presenting with *mild* aortic stenosis. Bars show ±1 standard error in age at presentation 6.5 years (range 1 to 25 years); mean follow-up 8.8 years (range 1 to 26 years). *Right:* Cumulative actuarial curves of 54 patients presenting with *moderate* aortic stenosis. Conventions as in left-hand figure. Mean age at presentation 11.8 years (range 1 to 25 years). Mean follow-up 8.5 years (range 1 to 24 years). *(From Hossack KF, Neutze JM, Lowe JB, Barratt-Boyes BG: Congenital valvar aortic stenosis. Natural history and assessment for operation. Br Heart J 43:561, 1980. Reproduced with permission from the publisher and authors.)*

cal activity in patients with left ventricular outflow tract obstruction remains very controversial. It is debatable whether or not any patient who has had significant obstruction should be allowed to participate in competitive sports. We consider a residual gradient greater than 20 mmHg or persistent left ventricular hypertrophy to be contraindications to vigorous physical activity.[99] Before one approves strenuous activity in others, evaluation should include electrocardiographic monitoring and maximal exercise testing (Chap. 16).

Coarctation of the Aorta

Although coarctation of the aorta is a congenital malformation, nearly 20 percent of the cases presenting at the Mayo Clinic over a 20-year period were diagnosed initially in adolescence or adulthood. Most commonly, coarctation diagnosed at ages beyond childhood was discovered in asymptomatic patients in whom a routine physical examination for athletic participation or employment disclosed upper limb hypertension with diminished or absent femoral pulses. Coarctation of the aorta may occur anywhere along the descending aorta, even below the diaphragm, but more than 95 percent are located below the origin of the left subclavian artery and may involve the origin of this vessel. Usually, there is a discrete infolding of the aortic wall causing eccentric narrowing of the lumen. Frequently there is secondary aortic dilatation proximal and distal to the coarcted area (Fig. 14-1*B*).

Natural History

Isolated, severe aortic coarctation may cause congestive heart failure as early as the neonatal period. More frequently, however, coarctation producing symptoms during early infancy is associated with other congenital cardiovascular abnormalities such as ventricular septal defect, left ventricular outflow tract obstruction, or mitral valve abnormality. Many patients with undetected coarctation will remain symptom free until adolescence or early adulthood when symptoms such as headaches related to hypertension, leg fatigue, or leg cramps may develop. Occasionally, a major catastrophic event such as a cerebrovascular accident, infective endocarditis, or even rupture of the aorta is the first recognized symptom. A bicuspid aortic valve is found in approximately 25 to 50 percent of patients with coarctation, and these abnormal valves have a tendency to calcify in early or middle adult life, producing aortic stenosis. Calcific aortic stenosis may be the presenting condition, and subsequent investigation may disclose an additional coarctation of the aorta. In the era before surgical intervention, approximately 50 percent of patients with coarctation died within the first three decades, and 75 percent were dead by age 50.[180] Death was most frequently caused by a complication of hypertension such as stroke or aortic dissection, but other causes included endocarditis, endarteritis, and congestive heart failure.

Management

Infrequently, a mild degree of coarctation may be present and not justify intervention. In the great majority of cases, however, symptoms or the presence of significant upper body hypertension mandate surgical repair. On occasion, an asymptomatic adolescent or adult patient with a severe coarctation will be normotensive at rest because of well-developed collaterals around the coarctation site. Such patients have inappropriate hypertension with exercise, however, and should be repaired. There is evidence that residual hypertension and late complications are directly related to age at the time of repair.[181]

Surgery for coarctation has been available since 1945.[182] Various techniques have been used, including end-to-end anastomosis, patch grafting, and the use of the subclavian flap technique.[183] Aneurysmal or atherosclerotic changes in the aorta found in adolescents or adults may occasionally mandate the use of an interposition prosthetic graft. Surgery is performed without cardiopulmonary bypass, and the risk of death from operation is small. Serious morbidity is rare, but occasionally paraplegia secondary to spinal cord ischemia and bowel ischemia or infarction occur.[184] Some patients require antihypertensive medication because of transient postoperative hypertension for a short period, whereas in others hypertension may persist, requiring long-term treatment.

Balloon angioplasty of coarctation has been utilized, but the role of this technique remains controversial.[185] Immediate reduction of the degree of obstruction and gradient is usually possible but is achieved at the price of tearing both the aortic intima and media. Late aneurysm formation, presumably secondary to the disruption of the media, has been observed.[186] Currently, most centers do not perform catheter balloon angioplasty as the primary procedure for coarctation, reserving it for recoarctation, where it appears to have a much greater role.

Late Results

The Mayo Clinic has published late results in 646 patients with coarctation operated upon between 1946 and 1981.[181] The median age at operation was 16 years (range 1 week to 72 years) with 72 patients (11 percent) over age 35 years. Although survival was good (91 percent at 10 years, 72 percent at 30 years), the mean age of death was 38 years, confirming the previous finding that life expectancy is reduced for patients, even after repair. In this and other series reporting long-term follow-up, the most common cause of death was premature coronary artery disease with secondary myocardial infarction.[187,188] Other causes included congestive heart failure, stroke, and ruptured aortic aneurysm. Age at operation was a powerful prognostic factor. The older the patient, the greater the probability of premature death, making it highly likely that the duration of preoperative obstruction and hypertension is important in the etiology of arterial disease and subsequent cardiovascular events.

The incidence of recoarctation with all surgical techniques is low for repairs performed after infancy, but surgery in later years for associated abnormalities such as aortic and mitral valve disease may be required. The majority of survivors are asymptomatic, but there is a high incidence of late hypertension, despite satisfactory early fall in blood pressure after surgery and good relief of obstruction. In one series only 32 percent of patients were normotensive 30 years after repair and 25 percent were significantly hypertensive.[188] Long-term blood pressure surveillance is therefore mandatory as hypertension is directly related to many of the late vascular complications.[181,187,188] This incidence may decline significantly as more patients are diagnosed and repaired during infancy or early childhood.

Transposition of the Great Arteries

In complete transposition of the great arteries, the aorta arises from the right ventricle and the pulmonary artery from the left ventricle (discordant ventriculoarterial connection). As a result, the systemic and arterial circulations run "in parallel" rather than "in series" and predominantly desaturated blood enters the aorta. Oxygenation and survival depend on mixing between the systemic and pulmonary circulations at the atrial level in simple transposition (via a patent foramen ovale or atrial septal defect). (See Chap. 97.) In approximately half the cases there are associated anomalies: ventricular septal defect (30 percent), left ventricular outflow tract obstruction (5 to 10 percent), ventricular septal defect with left ventricular outflow tract obstruction (10 percent), patent ductus arteriosus, and more rarely coarctation of the aorta or AV valve anomalies.[189] These associated conditions affect both the natural history and surgical management.

Natural History

Transposition of the great arteries is relatively common, but the natural history is so poor that very few survive past childhood without intervention. For all varieties, actuarial survival at 1 month is 55 percent and at 1 year 10 percent.[190,191] The outlook is even worse for simple transposition with only 4 percent natural survival at 1 year.[192] Death is usually due to profound hypoxia and its hematological consequences. In transposition of the great arteries with large ventricular septal defect, severe hypoxia is rare, but patients do badly as a result of heart failure from excessive pulmonary flow and early pulmonary vascular disease.[92] Transposition with ventricular septal defect and left ventricular outflow tract obstruction presents with early hypoxia. Occasionally, prolonged survival into adult life may occur with a large atrial septal defect, ventricular septal defect, and/or patent ductus ateriosus with the development of pulmonary vascular disease (Eisenmenger's syndrome) or with associated ventricular septal defect and left ventricular outflow tract obstruction.

Management

The outlook has been transformed by the use of catheter balloon atrial septostomy.[193] In the late 1950s and early 1960s the Senning[194] and Mustard[195] operations involving atrial redirection of the systemic and pulmonary venous returns were introduced. These operations are usually performed between 3 and 12 months of age, with a trend over the years to earlier surgery. Both procedures have been undertaken with excellent early mortality (approximately 2 percent operative mortality and less than 10 percent for the whole early management protocols). Long-term follow-up for both procedures is now available with comparable late results apart from a lower incidence of baffle obstruction after the Senning operation.[196] Survival into adult life is common, and adult cardiologists are thus likely to see patients who have undergone these types of atrial redirection. Late problems, however, are now recognized, with sudden death, arrhythmia, tricuspid regurgitation, and right (systemic) ventricular dysfunction being the major concerns. These late complications have led to the increasing acceptance of the arterial switch operation as the operation of choice.[197] This procedure involves transection and reanastomosis of the great arteries (aorta to left ventricle, pulmonary artery to right ventricle) with coronary artery transfer. The mortality for this procedure has decreased, but the long-term results into adult life are not yet available. For transposition with ventricular septal defect, the mortality for atrial repair with ventricular septal defect closure has always been higher than for simple transposition, and arterial switch is the operation of choice. Transposition with ventricular septal defect and left ventricular outflow tract obstruction is usually palliated in infancy with a systemic to pulmonary shunt followed by repair by the Rastelli procedure in later childhood.[198] This involves closure of the ventricular septal defect to connect the left ventricle to the aorta and insertion of a valved conduit from the right ventricle to the pulmonary artery. Long-term results are good, but further surgery to replace the extracardiac conduit in adolescent and adult life is inevitable (see "Surgical Considerations").

Late Results

Two specific problems after atrial redirection have caused concern during long-term follow-up: arrhythmia and systemic ventricular dysfunction. Loss of sinus rhythm is progressive and has not been prevented by modification of surgical technique for either the Mustard or Senning operation.[38,199] In most cases, it is asymptomatic, but occasionally profound bradycardia may necessitate pacemaker insertion. There appears, however, to be no relation between loss of sinus rhythm and risk of sudden death. More worrisome is the development of atrial flutter. This arrhythmia has profound hemodynamic consequences after intraatrial repair and is a risk factor for sudden death, especially in the presence of right ventricular dysfunction. Deteriorating performance of the right ventricle supporting the systemic circulation has been reported in some patients, but the precise basis for this problem remains unclear.[200,201] Although a major concern, it is not yet known whether or not ventricular performance will inevitably deteriorate in the majority of patients and if so over what period.[202]

As most patients who have undergone intraatrial repair are well, clinical follow-up is directed largely at attempts to stratify risk for sudden death, which is currently difficult. Late death cannot be predicted merely from serial ECGs or ambulatory monitoring.[38] This difficulty underscores the need for a more sophisticated approach involving both electrophysiological and hemodynamic measurements. Assessment should include evaluation of cardiac performance at rest and exercise and evaluation of systemic and venous pathways. Transesophageal echocardiography appears useful in this situation. Heart transplantation should be considered in the patient who has severe right ventricular failure or disabling arrhythmias. An alternative approach is to perform pulmonary artery banding as preparation for conversion of the atrial repair to an arterial switch.[203] The rather limited information after arterial switch operation suggests that electrophysiological problems are much less prevalent.[204] The systemic left ventricle after the switch is at risk from the surgical procedure itself, potential myocardial ischemia from coronary distortion, as well as aortic regurgitation. Early results, however, are encouraging, but few patients have yet reached adult life.[205]

Congenitally Corrected Transposition (Atrioventricular and Ventriculoarterial Discordance)

In congenitally corrected transposition of the great arteries there is a discordant AV connection (right atrium to left ventricle and left ventricle to right atrium) and a discordant ventriculoarterial connection (left ventricle to pulmonary artery and right ventricle to aorta). As a result of the "double discordance," the systemic and pulmonary venous returns flow to the appropriate great arteries, hence the potentially confusing term "corrected transposition."

Natural History

In a small proportion of cases (approximately 10 percent in reported series, but this is probably an underestimate) there are no associated cardiac defects.[206,207] Such individuals are pink and asymptomatic and may survive undiagnosed until adult life. The only specific difference from normal hearts is the tendency to develop AV conduction problems and complete heart block. Complete heart block may be present from birth ($\approx$ 10 percent)[208] and is said to develop in about 2 percent of patients per year.[209] It is not clear whether or not the systemic right ventricle in patients with corrected transposition can maintain function over extended periods and whether or not this has an impact on outcome, since few studies have examined enough patients without associated defects over a long enough period. The majority of cases have a ventricular septal defect (90 percent) and/or pulmonary stenosis (80 percent).[206] Abnormalities of the tricuspid valve (systemic AV valve) are common and may be due to an intrinsic tricuspid valve abnormality such as Ebstein's malformation. These defects influence the natural history and surgical strategy required.

Management

Strategies and indications for surgery differ from those in patients in normal connections because of the potential for the operation to aggravate systemic ventricular dysfunction, systemic AV valve incompetence, or conduction problems. Palliative surgery in childhood is sometimes performed, as definitive repair may involve insertion of an extracardiac conduit. In a large retrospective study of 111 patients managed over a 20-year period, it was concluded that patients with symptomatic heart failure should be repaired before the systemic ventricle dilates and the tricuspid regurgitation becomes severe.[207] Patients with more than mild tricuspid regurgitation whose valves were not replaced did very poorly. In contrast, the patients with cyanosis did much better and the timing of intracardiac surgery can be delayed and be determined by the patient's symptoms.

Late Results

The long-term outcome of well-corrected patients is good, whereas those with severe symptomatic heart failure preoperatively do badly. Since repairs may involve insertion of an extracardiac conduit, prosthetic AV valve, and pacemaker, careful long-term follow-up is mandatory.

Complex Lesions

A number of complex congenital heart defects involve structural abnormalities that preclude the creation of a biventricular circulation. The changing nomenclature and classification that has been applied to these defects over the years is a major source of confusion. (See Chap. 97.) This group of patients includes those with double-inlet ventricle (single ventricle), absent right or left AV connection (tricuspid or mitral atresia), some cases of pulmonary atresia/intact ventricular septum and Ebstein's anomaly, and cases with straddling of an AV valve and hypoplastic left or right ventricles. The natural history of these defects is highly variable and depends to a large extent on the impact of the associated defects. In a recent report of 191 patients with double-inlet ventricle presenting in the first year of life, actuarial survival before definitive repair for the whole group was 57 percent at 1 year and 42 percent at 10 years.[126] On multivariate analysis, pulmonary stenosis, balanced pulmonary flow, and older age at presentation were factors favoring survival, whereas right atrial isomerism, common AV orifice, pulmonary atresia, obstruction to systemic output, and anomalous pulmonary venous return were detrimental. Despite the complex morphologic defects, prolonged natural survival is sometimes seen if the physiology is well balanced. The patients with double-inlet left ventricle with discordant ventriculoarterial connection and pulmonary stenosis with balanced pulmonary flow do best, with predicted actuarial survivals of 96 percent at 1 year and 91 percent at 10 years. Such patients may remain well past the third decade of life without intervention.[126]

Management

For most patients with complex congenital heart disease prolonged survival into adult life is only possible with one or more palliative operations (such as systemic to pulmonary shunt, Glenn shunt, pulmonary artery banding, and relief of systemic outflow obstruction) or after a Fontan-type procedure. With palliative surgery alone, clinical deterioration usually begins in the second decade of life and is often due to progressive ventricular dysfunction and/or AV valve regurgitation.[210–212]

The goals of management during childhood have been to maintain suitable anatomy and physiology for the Fontan circulation. A number of modifications of Fontan's original operation have been introduced.[124,213–215] The basic principle is to separate the systemic and pulmonary circuits by returning systemic venous blood to the pulmonary artery without incorporating a subpulmonary ventricle. This circulation is less "flexible" than one with two functioning ventricles; the operative risk and postoperative status are largely dependent on the patient's suitability. Most important are a low pulmonary vascular resistance and adequate ventricular function (both systolic and diastolic), allowing the circulation to operate with an acceptably low systemic venous pressure.[216] Careful preoperative hemodynamic assessment is vital to optimize patient selection. The operative risk varies considerably between institutions.

Long-Term Results

The early and medium-term results of the successful Fontan operation are excellent when compared to the preoperative status of the patients. Improvement in arterial saturation and exercise tolerance have been confirmed by objective testing.[215] The patients with the best hemodynamics can perform well at submaximal levels of exercise equivalent to most normal daily activities[216]; however, less encouraging long-term data are beginning to appear. Fontan's own analysis of 334 patients revealed a premature decline in survival and functional status and a late rise in hazard for which no risk factors could be identified other than the Fontan state per se.[124] Late problems include supraventricular arrhythmia, thrombus in the atria, and declining ventricular function.[123,124,217] Other concerns are the effects of nonpulsatile pulmonary flow favoring the development of pulmonary arteriovenous malformations as seen after the Glenn anastomosis.[218] Extrapolation of these data to current practice is difficult, but the Fontan procedure should be considered to be palliative, not curative.

Certain interesting surgical modifications have been introduced that may improve early and late hemodynamics and the functional results. Perforation of the patch at surgery (fenestrated Fontan) allows a hypertensive right atrium to decompress via a right to left shunt at the atrial level.[219] These holes may be closed later with an occlusion device at catheterization. Recent "Fontan" operations have excluded the right atrium from the circulation, creating a total cavopulmonary connection (superior vena cava to right pulmonary artery via a bidirectional Glenn anastomosis and inferior vena cava blood channeled to the pulmonary artery.[220] Data suggest improved flow and energy characteristics compared to the standard atriopulmonary connection and fewer early supraventricular arrhythmias.[44]

Ebstein's Anomaly of the Tricuspid Valve

Ebstein's anomaly is characterized by displacement of the proximal attachments of the tricuspid valve from the AV ring into the right ventricle. (See Chap. 97.) This structural abnormality divides the right ventricle into an "atrialized" portion and distal "ventricularized" portion. The severity is variable and accounts for the broad clinical spectrum, from severe disease causing fetal or neonatal death to mild disease compatible with natural survival as late as the eighth decade of life.[221] Ebstein's anomaly is an uncommon defect occurring in less than 1 percent of patients with congenital heart disease, but it is disproportionately represented in the adult congenital heart disease population because of its favorable natural history.

Natural History

The diagnosis of Ebstein's anomaly is now much easier with echocardiography, which has altered our understanding of the natural history. In a large collaborative study of Ebstein's anomaly reported in 1974 only 7 percent of patients were under 1 year of age.[221] Neonates presenting with Ebstein's anomaly comprise, not surprisingly, the worst end of the spectrum with a severe anatomic defect and a high incidence of associated abnormalities, particularly right ventricular outflow tract obstruction. Their poor outcome is predictable from their anatomy.[222] Those who survive this period with or without surgery may live into adult life, although there is continued morbidity and mortality throughout childhood. Many patients are minimally symptomatic in childhood and do not present until adolescence or adult life. Symptoms and signs, when they develop, include cyanosis due to right-to-left shunting at the atrial level, dyspnea secondary to hypoxia, and palpitation due to supraventricular arrhythmia. Ebstein's anomaly is often associated with ventricular preexcitation, which may involve one or more, usually right-sided, accessory pathways.[223] Approximately 25 to 30 percent of adults will have symptomatic arrhythmias that may be difficult to treat and can result in sudden death.[224] Progressive heart failure may develop with time and may be related not only to right-sided problems but also to left-sided abnormalities. Excessive fibrosis has been reported in the left ventricle, and left ventricular dysfunction may be induced on exercise.[222,225] Only 50 percent of adults with Ebstein's anomaly that were over 50 years old were cyanotic in one report,[226] and early cyanosis is an adverse risk factor for survival, as is congestive cardiac failure.[227]

Management

Outcome is poor in patients with increasing cyanosis, congestive cardiac failure, and uncontrolled arrhythmias and in those in New York Heart Association functional class III or IV. These features should therefore be taken as indications for surgery. In their absence, medical follow-up is appropriate as the risk is low. Objective assessment, however, of effort tolerance by periodic stress testing and monitoring of heart size is advisable.

Surgery may consist of repair or replacement of the tricuspid valve together with closure of the atrial septal defect to prevent cyanosis.[228] In the occasional patient, the atrial septal defect may be responsible for a left-to-right shunt and can be closed as the sole procedure. In others, the functional right ventricle is too small for a biventricular circulation, and a Fontan procedure may be the only option. The results of surgery are affected by the presence of arrhythmia. Uncontrolled preoperative supraventricular arrhythmia is a risk factor for early postoperative rhythm problems that may have serious hemodynamic consequences.[224] It is usually recommended that division of the accessory pathway be performed at the time of tricuspid valve surgery. The pathways are usually in the posteroseptal or right free wall position and may be multiple. A prolonged electrophysiological procedure on top of difficult tricuspid valve surgery may result in a very long operation. An alternative approach is to perform catheter radiofrequency ablation of the accessory pathway (Chap. 43) before surgery. Thus far, few such procedures have been done in patients with Ebstein's anomaly. In hearts with marked enlargement of the right atrium catheter ablation is challenging.

Marfan's Syndrome

Although this autosomal dominant syndrome is congenital in the sense that the patient was born with an abnormal gene (genes), the heart defect is usually acquired. The typical phenotypic features of tall, thin stature, pectus deformities, arachnodactyly, and high arched palate, by which the condition is currently diagnosed, may be obvious, subtle, or absent (Fig. 10-7). Cardiovascular complications occur in 30 to 60 percent of patients and are the cause of a decreased life expectancy.[229] Mitral valve prolapse is the commonest finding in the pediatric population,[230] but aortic root dilatation with a potential for aortic dissection or severe aortic valve regurgitation is the most serious later complication.[231] In a review of 257 patients seen between 1939 and 1972, the average age of death of the 72 patients who died was 32 years, with aortic root problems accounting for three-fourths of the deaths.[229]

Management

The risk of dissection is broadly related to the degree of dilatation of the aortic root. Dilatation can be followed serially by regular cross-sectional echocardiography, which should be performed at least annually. Particularly close monitoring is necessary during puberty and the rapid growth phase of adolescence. Treatment with beta blockade has been advocated for patients with evidence of aortic root enlargement, and elective aortic root surgery is recommended when the aorta exceeds 5 to 6 cm in diameter. The aortic valve may also need to be replaced. As regular long-term follow-up visits are required, patients with the Marfan syndrome are not uncommon in adult "congenital" heart clinics. In addition to their cardiac care, patients need expert help with skeletal and ocular problems, genetic counseling, advice on physical activity (see above), and general psychosocial support.

REFERENCES

1. Ferencz C, Rubin JD, McCarter RJ, Neill CA, Perry LW, Harper SI, et al: Congenital heart disease: Prevalence at live birth. *Am J Epidemiol* 1985; 121:31–36.
2. MacMahon B, McKeown T, Record RG: The incidence and life expectation of children with congenital heart disease. *Br Heart J* 1953; 15:121–129.
3. Gross RE, Hubbard JP: Surgical ligation of a persistent ductus arteriosus. *JAMA* 1939; 112:729–731.
4. Perloff JK: Congenital heart disease in adults. In: Kelly WN (ed): *Textbook of Internal Medicine*. Philadelphia, Lippincott, 1989: 223–235.
5. Stark J: Do we really correct congenital heart defects? *J Thorac Cardiovasc Surg* 1989; 97:109.
6. Graham TP, Atwood GF, Boucek RJ, Boerth RC, Bender HW: Abnormalities of right ventricular function following Mustard's operation for transposition of the great arteries. *Circulation* 1975; 52:678–684.
7. Penny DJ, Redington AN: Angiographic demonstration of incoordinate motion of the ventricular wall after the Fontan operation. *Br Heart J* 1991; 66:456–459.
8. Redington AN: Functional assessment of the heart after corrective surgery for complete transposition. *Cardiol Young* 1991; 1:84–90.
9. Graham TP, Franklin RCG, Wyse RKH, Gooch V, Deanfield JE: Left ventricular wall stress and contractile function in transposition of the great arteries after the Rastelli operation. *J Thorac Cardiovasc Surg* 1987; 93:775–784.
10. Gewillig MH, Lundstrom UR, Deanfield JE, Gooch VM, Franklin RCG, Graham TP, et al: Impact of the Fontan operation on left ventricular size and contractility. *Circulation* 1990; 81:118–127.
11. Rudolph AM, Nadas AS, Borges WH: Hematologic adjustment to cyanotic congenital heart disease. *Pediatrics* 1953; 11:454–464.
12. Territo MC, Rosove M, Perloff JK: Cyanotic congenital heart disease; haematologic management, renal function, and urate metabolism. In: Perloff JK, Child JS (eds): *Congenital Heart Disease in Adults*. Philadelphia, Saunders, 1991: 94–95.
13. Perloff JK, Rosove MH, Child JS, Wright GB: Adults with cyanotic congenital heart disease: Haematological management. *Ann Inter Med* 1988; 109:406–413.
14. Linderkamp O, Klose HJ, Betke K, Brodherr-Heberlein S, Buhlmeyer K, Kelson S, et al: Increased blood viscosity in patients with cyanotic congenital heart disease and iron deficiency. *J Pediatr* 1979; 59:567–569.
15. Oldershaw PJ, St John Sutton MS: Haemodynamic effects of haemocrit reduction in patients with polycythaemia secondary to cyanotic congenital heart disease. *Br Heart J* 1980; 44:584–588.
16. Rosove MH, Hocking WG, Canobbio MM, Perloff JK, Child JS, Skorton DJ: Chronic hypoxaemia and decompensated erythrocytosis in cyanotic congenital heart disease. *Lancet* 1986; 2:313–315.
17. Lusher JM: Diseases of coagulation: The fluid phase. In: Nathan DG, Oski FA (eds): *Haematology in Infancy and Childhood*, 3d ed. Philadelphia, Saunders, 1987: 1328–1329.
18. Young D: Hyperuricemia in cyanotic congenital heart disease. *Am J Dis Child* 1980; 134:902–903.
19. Ross EA, Perloff JK, Danovitch GM, Child JS, Canobbio MM: Renal function and urate metabolism in late survivors with cyanotic congenital heart disease. *Circulation* 1986; 73:396–400.
20. Packer M: Therapeutic application of calcium channel antagonists for pulmonary hypertension. *Am J Cardiol* 1985; 55:196–198.
21. Packer M: Vasodilation therapy for primary pulmonary hypertension. Limitations and hazards. *Ann Intern Med* 1985; 103:258–270.
22. Rich S, Kaufmann E, Levy PS: The effect of high doses of calcium-channel blockers in survival in primary pulmonary hypertension. *N Engl J Med* 1992; 327:76–81.
23. Morrison D, Sorenson S, Caldwell J, Ritchie J, Goldman S, Wright AL, et al: The effect of pulmonary hypertension on systolic function of the right ventricle. *Chest* 1983; 84:250–257.
24. Rounds S, Hill NS: Pulmonary hypertensive disease. *Chest*. 1984; 85:397–405.
25. Jordan CE, White RC Jr, Fischer KC, Neill C, Dorst JP: The scoliosis of congenital heart disease. *Am Heart J* 1972; 84:463–469.
26. Sullivan NM, Sutter VL, Mims MM, Marsh VH, Finegold SM: Clinical aspects of bacteremia after manipulation of the genitourinary tract. *J Infect Dis* 1973; 127:49–55.
27. DeSwiet M, Ramsey ID, Rees GM: Bacterial endocarditis after insertion of intrauterine contraceptive device. *Br Med J* 1975; 2:76–77.
28. Shull HJ Jr, Greene BM, Allen SD, Dunn GD, Schenker S: Bactere-

mia with upper gastrointestinal endoscopy. *Ann Intern Med* 1975; 83:212–214.

29. Görge G, Erbel R, Henrichs J, Wensschel H, Werner J, Meyer J: Positive blood cultures during transesophageal echocardiography (abstr). *J Am Coll Cardiol* 1990; 15:62A.
30. Sande MA, Levison ME, Lukas DA, Kaye D: Bacteremia associated with cardiac catheterisation. *N Engl J Med* 1969; 281:1104–1106.
31. Dajani AS, Bisno AL, Chung KJ, Durack DT, Freed M, Gerber MA, et al: Prevention of bacterial endocarditis. Recommendations by the American Heart Association. *JAMA* 1990; 264:2919–2922.
32. Working Party of the British Society for Antimicrobial Chemotherapy: The antibiotic prophylaxis of infective endocarditis. *Lancet* 1982; 2:1323–1326.
33. Godman MJ, Roberts NK, Izukawa T: Late postoperative conduction disturbances after repair of ventricular septal defect and tetralogy of Fallot. *Circulation* 1974; 49:214–221.
34. Stevenson WG, Klitzner T, Perloff JK: Electrophysiologic abnormalities. Natural occurrence and postoperative residua and sequelae. In: Child JS, Perloff JK (eds): *Congenital Heart Disease in Adults*. Philadelphia, Saunders, 1991: 259–295.
35. Vetter VL, Horowitz LN: Electrophysiologic residua and sequelae of surgery for congenital heart defects. *Am J Cardiol* 1982; 50:588–604.
36. Garson A Jr: Chronic postoperative arrhythmia. In: Gillette PC, Garson A Jr (eds): *Pediatric Arrhythmia: Electrophysiology and Pacing*. Philadelphia, Saunders, 1990: 667–678.
37. Boelens M, Friedli B: Sinus node function and conduction system before and after surgery for secundum atrial septal defect: An electrophysiologic study. *Am J Cardiol* 1984; 53:1415–1420.
38. Deanfield J, Camm J, Macartney F, Cartwright T, Douglas J, Drew J, et al: Arrhythmia and late mortality after Mustard and Senning operation for transposition of the great arteries: An eight year prospective study. *J Thorac Cardiovasc Surg* 1988; 96:569–576.
39. Weber HS, Hellenbrand WE, Kleinmann CS, Perlmutter RA, Rosenfeld LE: Predictors of rhythm disturbances and subsequent morbidity after the Fontan operation. *Am J Cardiol* 1989; 64:762–767.
40. Gewillig M, Wyse RK, de Leval MR, Deanfield JE: Early and late arrhythmia after the Fontan operation: Predisposing factors and clinical consequences. *Br Heart J* 1992; 67:72–79.
41. Balaji S, Gewillig M, Bull C, de Leval MR, Deanfield JE: Arrhythmias after the Fontan procedure: Comparison of total cavopulmonary connection and atriopulmonary connection. *Circulation* 1991; 84(suppl IV):162–167.
42. Ward DE, Clarke B, Schofield PM, Jones S, Dawkins K, Bennett D: Long term transvenous ventricular pacing in adults with congenital abnormalities of the heart and great arteries. *Br Heart J* 1983; 50:325–329.
43. Stewart WJ, DiCola VL, Hawthorne JW: Doppler ultrasound measurement of cardiac output in patients with physiologic pacemakers: Effects of left ventricular function and retrograde ventriculoatrial conduction. *Am J Cardiol* 1984; 54:308–312.
44. Fryda RJ, Kaplan S, Helmsworth JA: Postoperative complete heart block in children. *Br Heart J* 1971; 33:456–462.
45. Murphy JG, Gersh BJ, Warnes CA, McGoo MD, Mair DD, Porter CJ et al: The late survival after surgical repair of isolated ventricular septal defect (VSD). *Circulation* 1989; 80(suppl II):490.
46. Kulbertus HE, Coyne JJ, Hallidie-Smith KA: Conduction disturbances before and after surgical closure of ventricular septal defect. *Am Heart J* 1969; 77:123–131.
47. Deanfield JE, McKenna WJ, Hallidie-Smith KA: Detection of late arrhythmia and conduction disturbance after correction of tetralogy of Fallot. *Br Heart J* 1980; 44:577–583.
48. Wolff GS, Rowland TW, Ellison RC: Surgically induced right bundle branch block with left anterior hemiblock. *Circulation* 1972; 46:587–594.
49. Deanfield JE: Late ventricular arrhythmias occurring after tetralogy of Fallot: Do they matter? *Int J Cardiol* 1991; 30:143–150.
50. Gewillig M, Cullen S, Mertens B, Lesaffre E, Deanfield J: Risk factors for arrhythmia and death after Mustard operation for simple transposition of the great arteries. *Circulation* 1991; 84(suppl IV):187–192.
51. Quattlebaum TG, Varghese J, Neill CA, Donahoo JS: Sudden death among postoperative patients with tetralogy of Fallot: A follow-up study of 243 patients for an average of twelve years. *Circulation* 1976; 54:289–293.
52. Garson A, Nihill MR, McNamara DG, Cooley DA: Status of the adult and adolescent after repair of tetralogy of Fallot. *Circulation* 1979; 59:1232–1240.
53. Kavey RE, Blackman MS, Sondheimer HM: Incidence and severity of chronic ventricular dysrhythmia after repair of tetralogy of Fallot. *Am Heart J* 1982; 103:342–350.
54. Vaksmann G, Fournier A, Davignon A, Ducharme G, Houyel L, Fouron J-C: Frequency and prognosis of arrhythmias after operation "correction" or tetralogy of Fallot. *Am J Cardiol* 1990; 66:346–349.
55. Garson A Jr, Porter CB, Gillette PC, McNamara DG: Induction of ventricular tachycardia during electrophysiologic study after repair of tetralogy of Fallot. *J Am Coll Cardiol* 1983; 1:1493–1502.
56. Deanfield JE, McKenna W, Rowland E: Local abnormalities of right ventricular depolarization after repair of tetralogy of Fallot: A basis for ventricular arrhythmia. *Am J Cardiol* 1985; 55:522–526.
57. Deanfield JE, McKenna WJ, Presbitero P, England D, Graham GR, Hallidie-Smith K: Ventricular arrhythmia in unrepaired and repaired tetralogy of Fallot: Relation to age, timing of repair and haemodynamic status. *Br Heart J* 1984; 52:77–86.
58. Sullivan ID, Presbitero P, Gooch VM, Aruta E, Deanfield JE: Is ventricular arrhythmia in repaired tetralogy of Fallot an effect of operation or a consequence of the course of the disease? A prospective study. *Br Heart J* 1987; 58:40–44.
59. Jones M, Ferrans VJ: Myocardial degeneration in congenital heart disease: Comparison of morphologic findings in young and old patients with congenital heart disease associated with muscular obstruction to right ventricular outflow. *Am J Cardiol* 1977; 39:1051–1063.
60. Hegerty A, Anderson RH, Deanfield JE: Myocardial fibrosis in tetralogy of Fallot: Effect of surgery or part of the natural history? (abstr). *Br Heart J* 1988; 59:123.
61. Walsh ED, Rockenmacher S, Keane JF, Hougen TJ, Lock JE, Castaneda AR: Late results in patients with tetralogy of Fallot repaired during infancy. *Circulation* 1988; 77:1062–1067.
62. Kobayashi J, Hirose H, Nakano S, Matsuda H, Shirakura R, Kawashima Y: Ambulatory electrocardiographic study of the frequency and cause of ventricular arrhythmia after correction of tetralogy of Fallot. *Am J Cardiol* 1984; 54:1310–1313.
63. Horowitz LN, Vetter VL, Harken AH, Josephson ME: Electrophysiologic characteristics of sustained ventricular tachycardia after repair of tetralogy of Fallot. *Am J Cardiol* 1980; 46:446–452.
64. Dunnigam A, Pritzker MR, Benditt DG, Benson DW Jr: Life threatening ventricular tachycardias in later survivors of surgically corrected tetralogy of Fallot. *Br Heart J* 1984; 52:198–206.
65. Deal BJ, Scagliotti D, Miller SM, Gallastegni JL, Harriman RJ, Levitsky S: Electrophysiologic drug testing in symptomatic ventricular arrhythmias after repair of tetralogy of Fallot. *Am J Cardiol* 1987; 59:1380–1385.
66. de Swiet M: Management of congenital heart disease in pregnancy. In: Anderson RH, Macartney FJ, Shinebourne EA, Tynan M (eds): *Paediatric Cardiology*. Edinburgh, Churchill Livingstone, 1987: 1353–1361.
67. Naeye RL, Hagstrom JW, Talmadge BA: Postpartum death with maternal congenital heart disease. *Circulation* 1967; 36:304–312.
68. Perloff JK: Pregnancy in congenital heart disease. In: Perloff JK, Child JS (eds): *Congenital Heart Disease in Adults*. Philadelphia, Saunders, 1991: 124–140.
69. Presbitero P, Somerville J, Stone S, Aruta E, Spiegelhalter D: Pregnancy in cyanotic congenital heart disease: Maternal complications and factors influencing successful fetal outcome. *J Am Coll Cardiol* 1992; 19(suppl A):288A.
70. Mendelson CL: Pregnancy and coarctation of the aorta. *Am J Obstet Gynecol* 1940; 39:1014–1021.
71. Deal K, Colley CF: Coarctation of the aorta and pregnancy. *Ann Intern Med* 1973; 78:706–710.
72. Limet R, Grondin CM: Cardiac valve prosthesis, anticoagulation, and pregnancy. *Ann Thorac Surg* 1977; 23:337–341.
73. Lutz DJ, Noller KL, Spittell JA, Danielson GK, Fish CR: Preg-

nancy and its complications following cardiac valve prothesis. *Am J Obstet Gynecol* 1978; 131:460–468.

74. Hall JG, Pauli RM, Wilson KM: Maternal and fetal sequelae of anticoagulation during pregnancy. *Am J Med* 1980; 68:122–140.
75. Iturbe-Alessio I, Del Carmen Fonseca M, Mutchinik O, Santos MA, Zajarias A, Salazar E: Risks of anticoagulant therapy in pregnant women with artificial heart valves. *N Engl J Med* 1986; 315:1390–1393.
76. Nora JJ, Nora AH: The evolution of specific genetic and environmental counseling in congenital heart disease. *Circulation* 1978; 57:205–213.
77. Burn J: The aetiology of congenital heart disease. In: Anderson RH, Macartney FJ, Shinebourne EA, Tynan M (eds): *Paediatric Cardiology*. Edinburgh, Churchill Livingstone, 1987:15–63.
78. Allan LD, Crawford DC, Chita SK, Anderson RH, Tynan MJ: Familial recurrence of congenital heart disease in a prospective series of mothers referred for fetal echocardiography. *Am J Cardiol* 1986; 58:334–337.
79. Whittlemore R, Hobbins JC, Engle MA: Pregnancy and its outcome in women with and without surgical treatment of congenital heart disease. *Am J Cardiol* 1982; 50:641–651.
80. Weidman WH, Lenfant C, Hayes CJ, Kidd L, Keane JF, Gersony WM, et al: Symposium: The Report of the Natural History Study of Congenital Heart Defects: A 20-year follow-up. Presented at 61st Scientific Session of the American Heart Association, Washington DC, 1988.
81. Tunstall-Pedoe H: Acceptable risk in aircrew. *Eur Heart J* 1988; 9(suppl G):9–11.
82. Deanfield JE: Adult congenital heart disease with special reference to the data on long term follow-up of patients surviving to adulthood with or without surgical correction. *Eur Heart J*, 1992; 13(suppl H): 111–116.
83. Truesdell SC, Skorton DJ, Lauer RM: Life insurance for children with cardiovascular disease. *Pediatrics* 1986; 77:687.
84. Mahoney LT, Truesdell SC, Hamburgen M, Skorton DJ: Insurability, employability, and psychosocial considerations. Perloff JK, Child JS (eds): In: *Congenital Heart Disease in Adults*. Philadelphia, WB Saunders, 1991: 178–189.
85. Kellerman J, Zeltzer L, Ellenberg L, Dash J, Rigler D: Psychological effects of illness in adolescence. I. Anxiety, self-esteem, and perception of control. *J Pediatr* 1980; 97:126–131.
86. Zeltzer L, Kellerman J, Ellenberg L, Dash J, Rigler D: Psychologic effects of illness in adolescence. II. Impact of illness in adolescents—crucial issues and coping styles. *J Pediatr* 1980; 97:132–138.
87. Myers-Vando R, Steward MS, Folkins CH, Hines P: The effects of congenital heart disease on cognitive development, illness causality concepts, and vulnerability. *Am J Orthopsychiatr* 1979; 49:617–625.
88. Silbert A, Wolff P, Mayer B, Rosenthal A, Nadas A: Cyanotic heart disease and psychological development. *Pediatrics* 1969; 43:192–200.
89. Aram DM, Ekelman BL, Ben-Shachae G, Levinsohn MW: Intelligence and hypoxemia in children with congenital heart disease; fact or artifact? *J Am Coll Cardiol* 1985; 6:889–893.
90. Newburger JW, Silbert AR, Buckley LP, Fyler DC: Cognitive function and age at repair of transposition of the great arteries in children. *N Engl J Med* 1984; 310:1495–1499.
91. Huffman JW: Sex and the teenager. In: Huffman JW, Dewhurst JC, Capuaro VJ (eds): *The Gynecology of Childhood and Adolescence*, 2d ed. Philadelphia, Saunders, 1981: 527–542.
92. Bonnar J: Coagulation effects of oral contraception. *Am J Obstet Gyn* 1987; 157:1042–1048.
93. Fraser IS: Progestogens for contraception. *Austral Fam Phys* 1988; 17:882–885.
94. Whittemore R: Pregnancy and congenital heart disease. In: Adams FH, Emmanoulides GC, Riemenschneider TA (eds): *Heart Disease in Infants, Children and Adults*, 4th ed. Baltimore, Williams & Wilkins, 1989: 684–690.
95. Mayer JA, Bullen BA: Nutrition, weight control and exercise. In: Johnson WR, Buskurk ER (eds): *Science and Medicine of Exercise and Sport*. New York, Harper & Row, 1974: 259–275.
96. Rocchini AP, Katch V, Anderson J, Hinderliter J, Becque D, Martin M, et al: Blood pressure in obese adolescents: Effects of weight loss. *Paediatrics* 1988; 82:16–23.
97. Powell KE, Thompson PD, Casperen CJ, Kendrick KS: Physical activity and the incidence of coronary heart disease. *Ann Rev Public Health* 1987; 8:281–287.
98. Maron BJ, Epstein SE, Mitchell JH: Sixteenth Bethesda Conference. Cardiovascular abnormalities in the athlete: Recommendations regarding eligibility for competition. *J Am Coll Cardiol* 1985; 6:1185–1232.
99. Cullen S, Celermajer DS, Deanfield JE: Exercise in congenital heart disease. *Cardiol Young* 1991; 1:129–135.
100. Stark J, Pacifico AD (eds): *Reoperations in Cardiac Surgery*. Berlin, Springer-Verlag, 1989.
101. Dobell ARC, Jain AK: Catastrophic hemorrhage during redo sternotomy. *Ann Thorac Surg* 1984; 37:273–278.
102. Ebert PA, Turley K, Stanger P, Hoffman JIE, Hyemann MA, Rudolph AM: Surgical treatment of truncus arteriosus in the first 6 months of life. *Ann Surg* 1984; 200:451–456.
103. Jonas RA, Freed MD, Mayer JE Jr, Castaneda AR: Long-term follow-up of patients with synthetic right heart conduits. *Circulation* 1985; 72(suppl II):77–83.
104. Ross DN, Somerville J: Correction of pulmonary atresia with a homograft aortic valve. *Lancet* 1966; II:1446–1447.
105. Merin G, McGoon DC: Reoperation after insertion of aortic homograft as a right ventricular outflow tract. *Ann Thorac Surg* 1973; 16:122–126.
106. Park SC, Neches WH, Lenox CC, Zuberbuhler JR, Bahnson HT: Massive calcification and obstruction in a homograft after the Rastelli procedure for transposition of the great arteries. *Am J Cardiol* 1973; 32:860–864.
107. Shabbo FP, Wain WH, Ross DN: Right ventricular outflow reconstruction with aortic homograft conduit: Analysis of the long-term results. *Thorac Cardiovasc Surg* 1980; 28:21–25.
108. Di Carlo D, de Leval MR, Stark J: "Fresh" antibiotic sterilized aortic homografts in extracardiac valved conduits. Long-term results. *Thorac Cardiovasc Surg* 1984; 32:10–14.
109. Stark J: Reoperations in patients with extracardiac valved conduits. In: Stark J, Pacifico AD (eds): *Reoperations in Cardiac Surgery*. Berlin, Springer-Verlag, 1989: 271–290.
110. Studer M, Blackstone EH, Kirklin JW, Pacifico AD, Soto B, Chung GKT, et al: Determinants of early and late results of repair of atrioventricular septal (canal) defects. *J Thorac Cardiovasc Surg* 1982; 84:523–542.
111. Poirier RA, McGoon DC, Danielson GK, Wallace RB, Ritter DG, Moodie DS, et al: Late results after repair of tetralogy of Fallot. *J Thorac Cardiovasc Surg* 1977; 73:900–908.
112. Zhao H, Miller DC, Reitz BA, Shumway NE: Surgical repair of tetralogy of Fallot. Long-term follow-up with particular emphasis on late death and reoperation. *J Thorac Cardiovasc Surg* 1985; 89:204–220.
113. Ebert PA: Second operation for pulmonary stenosis or insufficiency after repair of tetralogy of Fallot. *Am J Cardiol* 1982; 50:637–640.
114. Wessel HU, Cunningham WJ, Paul MH, Nastanier CK, Muster AJ, Idriss FS: Exercise performance in tetralogy of Fallot after intracardiac repair. *J Thorac Cardiovasc Surg* 1980; 80:582–593.
115. Ilbawi MN, Idriss FS, Muster AJ, Wessel HU, Paul MH, De Leon SY: Tetralogy of Fallot with absent pulmonary valve. Should valve insertion be part of the intracardiac repair? *J Thorac Cardiovasc Surg* 1981; 81:906–915.
116. Presbitero P, Somerville J, Revel-Chion R, Ross D: Open aortic valvotomy for congenital aortic stenosis: Late results. *Br Heart J* 1982; 47:26–34.
117. Stewart JR, Paton BC, Blunt SG Jr, Swan H: Congenital aortic stenosis: Ten to twenty years after valvulotomy. *Arch Surg* 1978; 113:1248–1252.
118. Hsieh K, Keane JF, Nadas AS, Bernhard WF, Castaneda AR: Long term follow-up of valvulotomy before 1968 for congenital aortic stenosis. *Am J Cardiol* 1986; 58:338–341.
119. Rao PS, Thapar MK, Wilson AD, Levy JM, Chopra PS: Intermediate-term follow-up results of balloon aortic valvuloplasty in infants and children with special reference to causes of restenosis. *Am J Cardiol* 1989; 64:1356–1360.
120. Puga FJ, Leoni FR, Julsrud PR, Mair DD: Complete repair of pulmonary atresia, ventricular septal defect and severe peripheral arborization abnormalities of the central pulmonary arteries. Experience with preliminary unifocalization procedures in 38 patients. *J Thorac Cardiovasc Surg* 1989; 6:1018–1029.
121. Sullivan ID, Wren C, Stark J, de Leval M, Macartney FJ, Dean-

field JE: Surgical unifocalisation in pulmonary atresia and ventricular septal defect. A realistic goal? *Circulation* 1988; 78(suppl III):5–13.
122. Watterson KG, Wilkinson JL, Karl TR, Mee RBB: Very small pulmonary arteries: The central end-to-side shunt. *Ann Thorac Surg* 1991; 52:1132–1137.
123. Driscoll DJ, Offord KP, Felot RH, Schaff HV, Puga FJ, Danielson GK: Five to fifteen year follow-up after Fontan operation. *Circulation* 1992; 85:469–496.
124. Fontan F, Kirklin JW, Fernandez G, Costa F, Naftel DC, Tritto F, et al: Outcome after a "perfect" Fontan operation. *Circulation* 1990; 81:1520–1536.
125. Kaiett JM, Kaye MP: The Registry of the International Society for Heart and Lung Transplantation: Eight official report. *J Heart Transplant* 1991; 10:491–498.
126. Franklin RCG, Spiegelhalter DJ, Anderson RH, Macartney FJ, Filho RIR, Douglas JM, et al: Double inlet ventricle presenting in infancy: I. Survival without definitive repair. *J Thorac Cardiovasc Surg* 1991; 101:767–776.
127. Kaplan EL, Meier P: Nonparametric estimation from incomplete observations. *J Am Stat Assoc* 1958; 53:457–481.
128. Child JS, Perloff JK: Natural survival patterns: A narrowing base. In: Child JS, Perloff JK (eds): *Congenital Heart Disease in Adults*. Philadelphia, Saunders, 1991: 21–59.
129. Borow KM, Braunwald E: Congenital heart disease in the adult. In: Braunwald E (ed): *Heart Disease,* 3d ed. Philadelphia, Saunders, 1988: 976–1002.
130. Warnes CA, Fuster V, Driscoll DJ, McGoon DC: Atrial septal defect. In: Giuliani ER, Fuster V, Gersh BJ, McGoon MD, McGoon DC (eds): *Cardiology Fundamentals and Practise,* 2d ed, St Louis, Mosby Yearbook, 1991: 1622–1638.
131. Kirklin JW, Barratt-Boyes BG (eds): *Cardiac Surgery*. New York, Wiley, 1986: 463–497.
132. Massumi RA, Nutter DO: The syndrome of familial defects of the heart and upper extremities (Holt-Oram syndrome). *Circulation* 1966; 34:65–76.
133. Nora JJ, McNamara, Fraser FC: Hereditary factors in atrial septal defect. *Circulation* 1967; 35:448–456.
134. Perloff JD: Ostium secundum atrial septal defect—survival for 87–94 years. *Am J Cardiol* 1984; 53:388–389.
135. Craig RJ, Selzer A: Natural history and prognosis of atrial septal defects. *Circulation* 1968; 37:805–815.
136. Campbell M: Natural history of atrial septal defect. *Br Heart J* 1970; 32:820–826.
137. Lock JE: The adult with congenital heart disease. Cardiac catheterization as a therapeutic intervention. *J Am Coll Cardiol* 1991; 18:330–331.
138. Hellenbrand WE, Fahey JT, McGowan FX, Welton GG, Kleinman CS: Transesophageal echocardiographic guidance of transcatheter closure of atrial septal defect. *Am J Cardiol* 1990; 66:207–213.
139. Murphy JG, Gersh BJ, McGoon MD, Mair DD, Porter CJ, Ilstrup DM, et al: Long term outcome after surgical repair of isolated atrial septal defect. Follow up at 27 to 32 years. *N Engl J Med* 1990; 323:1645–1697.
140. Brandenburg RO Jr, Holmes DR Jr, Brandenburg RO, McGoon DC: Clinical follow-up study of paroxysmal supraventricular arrhythmias after operative repair of a secundum type atrial septal defect in adults. *Am J Cardiol* 1983; 51:273–276.
141. St John Sutton MG, Tajik AJ, McGoon DC: Atrial septal defect in patients aged 60 years or older: Operative results and long-term postoperative follow-up. *Circulation* 1981; 64:402–409.
142. Engle MA, Kline SA, Borer JS: Ventricular septal defect. In: Roberts WC (ed): *Adult Congenital Heart Disease*. Philadelphia, FA Davis, 1987: 409–441.
143. Wood P: The Eisenmenger syndrome or pulmonary hypertension with reversed central shunt. *Br Med J* 1958; 2:701–709.
144. Warnes CA, Fuster V, Driscoll DJ, McGoon DC: Ventricular septal defect. In: Giuliani ER, Fuster V, Gersh BJ, McGoon MD, McGoon DC (eds): *Cardiology: Fundamentals and Practice,* 2d ed. vol 2. St Louis, Mosby Year Book, 1991: 1639–1652.
145. Tatsuno K, Konno S, Sakakibara S: Ventricular septal defect with aortic insufficiency: Angiocardiographic aspects and a new classification. *Am Heart J* 1973; 85:13–21.
146. Cartmill TB, DuShane JW, McGoon DC, Kirklin JW: Results of repair of ventricular septal defect. *J Thorac Cardiovasc Surg* 1966; 52:486–499.
147. Blake RS, Chung EE, Wesley H, Hallidie-Smith KA: Conduction defects, ventricular arrhythmias and late death after surgical closure of ventricular septal defect. *Br Heart J* 1982; 47:305–315.
148. Bridges ND, Perry SB, Keane JF, Goldstein SAN, Mandell V, Mayer JE Jr, et al: Preoperative transcatheter closure of congenital muscular ventricular septal defects. *N Engl J Med* 1991; 324:1312–1317.
149. Report of the New England Regional Infant Cardiac Program. *Pediatrics* 1980; 65(suppl):441–444.
150. Rastelli GC, Ongley PA, Kirklin JW, McGoon DC: Surgical repair of the complete form of persistent common atrioventricular canal. *J Thorac Cardiovasc Surg* 1968; 55:299–308.
151. Abraham KA, Cherian G, Rao VD, Sukumar IP, Krishnaswami S, John S: Tetralogy of Fallot in adults: A report on 147 patients. *Am J Med* 1979; 66:811–816.
152. Phadke AR, Phadke SA, Handy M, Junnarkar RV: Acyanotic Fallot's tetralogy with survival to the age of 70 years: Case report. *Indian Heart J* 1977; 29:46–49.
153. Bertranou EG, Blackstone EH, Hazelrig JB, Turner ME, Kirklin JW: Life expectancy without surgery in tetralogy of Fallot. *Am J Cardiol* 1978; 42:458–466.
154. Deanfield JE, Ho S-Y, Anderson RH, McKenna WJ, Allwork SP, Hallidie-Smith KA: Late sudden death after repair of tetralogy of Fallot: A clinico-pathological study. *Circulation* 1983; 67:636–641.
155. Katz NM, Blackstone EH, Kirklin JW, Pacifico AD, Bargeron LM Jr: Late survival and symptoms after repair of tetralogy of Fallot. *Circulation* 1982; 65:403–410.
156. Murphy JG, Gersh BJ, McGoon MD, Mair DD, Ilstrup D, Porter CJ, et al: Long term (30 year) survival of patients undergoing complete repair of tetralogy of Fallot (abstr). *J Am Coll Cardiol* 1990; 15:205A.
157. Lillehei CW, Varco RL, Cohen M, Warden HE, Gott VL, DeWall RA, et al: The first open heart corrections of tetralogy of Fallot: A 26–31 year follow-up of 106 patients. *Ann Surg* 1986; 204:490–501.
158. Wennevold A, Rygg I, Lauridsen P, Efsen F, Jacobsen JR: Fourteen to nineteen-year follow-up after corrective repair for tetralogy of Fallot. *Scand J Thorac Cardiovasc Surg* 1982; 16:41–45.
159. Piccoli GP, Dickinson DF, Musumeci F, Hamilton DI: A changing policy for the surgical treatment of Fallot: Early and late results in 235 consecutive patients. *Ann Thorac Surg* 1982; 33:365–373.
160. Bjarke B: Oxygen uptake and cardiac output during submaximal and maximal exercise in adult subjects with totally corrected tetralogy of Fallot. *Acta Med Scand* 1975; 197:177–186.
161. Nugent EW, Freedom RM, Nora JJ, Ellison RC, Rowe RD, Nadas AS: Clinical course in pulmonary stenosis. *Circulation* 1977; 56(suppl I):I-38–I-47.
162. Mody MR: The natural history of uncomplicated valvular pulmonic stenosis. *Am Heart J* 1975; 90:317–321.
163. Kopecky SL, Gersh BJ, McGoon MD, Mair DD, Porter CH, Ilstrup DM, et al: Long-term outcome of patients undergoing surgical repair of isolated pulmonary valve stenosis. Follow-up at 20 to 30 years. *Circulation* 1988; 78:1150–1156.
164. Kan JS, White RI Jr, Mitchell SE, Gardner TJ: Percutaneous balloon valvuloplasty: A new method for treating congenital pulmonary valve stenosis. *N Engl J Med* 1982; 307:540–542.
165. Mullins CE, Latson LA, Neches WH, Colvin EV, Kan J: Balloon dilatation of miscellaneous lesions: Results of Valvuloplasty and Angioplasty of Congenital Anomalies Registry. *Am J Cardiol* 1990; 65:802–803.
166. Sullivan ID, Robinson PJ, Macartney FJ, Taylor JFN, Rees PG, Bull C, et al: Percutaneous balloon valvuloplasty for pulmonary valve stenosis in infants and children. *Br Heart J* 1985; 54:435–441.
167. Friedman WF, Johnson AD: Congenital aortic stenosis. In: Roberts WC (ed): *Adult Congenital Heart Disease*. Philadelphia, FA Davis, 1987: 357–374.
168. Kelly DT, Wulfsberg BA, Rowe RD: Discrete subaortic stenosis. *Circulation* 1972; 46:309–322.
169. Williams JCP, Barratt-Boyes BG, Lowe JB: Supravalvular aortic stenosis. *Circulation* 1961; 24:1311–1318.
170. Mills P, Leech G, Davies M, Leatham A: The natural history of a non-stenotic bicuspid aortic valve. *Br Heart J* 1978; 40:951–957.

171. Gersony WM, Hayes CJ: Bacterial endocarditis in patients with pulmonary stenosis, aortic stenosis or ventricular septal defect. *Circulation* 1977; 56(suppl I):I-84–I-87.
172. Fontana RS, Edwards JE: *Congenital Cardiac Disease: A Review of 357 Cases Studied Pathologically.* Philadelphia, Saunders, 1962.
173. Muna WFT, Ferrans VJ, Pierce JE, Roberts WC: Discrete subaortic stenosis in Newfoundland dogs: Association of infective endocarditis. *Am J Cardiol* 1978; 41:746–754.
174. Cohen LS, Friedman WF, Braunwald E: Natural history of mild congenital aortic stenosis elucidated by serial hemodynamic studies. *Am J Cardiol* 1972; 30:1–5.
175. Wagner HR, Ellison RC, Keane JF, Nadas AS, Bernhard WF, Castaneda AR: Long-term follow-up of valvotomy before 1968 for congenital aortic stenosis. *Am J Cardiol* 1986; 58:338–341.
176. Kugelmeier J, Egloff L, Real F, Rothlin M, Turina M, Senning A: Congenital aortic stenosis. Early and late results of aortic valvotomy. *Thorac Cardiovasc Surg* 1982; 30:91–95.
177. Bull C: Interventional catheterisation in infants and children (editorial). *Br Heart J* 1986; 56:197–200.
178. Somerville J, Stone S, Ross D: Fate of patients with fixed subaortic stenosis after surgical removal. *Br Heart J* 1980; 43:629–647.
179. Suarez de Lezo J, Pan M, Sancho M, Herrera N, Arizon J, Franco M, et al: Percutaneous transluminal balloon dilatation for discrete subaortic stenosis. *Am J Cardiol* 1986; 58:619–621.
180. Campbell M: Natural history of coarctation of the aorta. *Br Heart J* 1970; 32:633–640.
181. Cohen M, Fuster V, Steele PM, et al: Coarctation of the aorta: Long term follow-up and prediction of outcome after surgical correction. *Circulation* 1989; 80:840–845.
182. Gross RE, Hufnagel CA: Coarctation of the aorta. Experimental studies regarding its surgical correction. *N Engl J Med* 1945; 233:287–293.
183. Waldhausen JA, Whitman V, Werner JC, et al: Surgical intervention in infants with coarctation of the aorta. *J Thorac Cardiovasc Surg* 1981; 81:323–325.
184. Keen G: Spinal cord damage and operations for coarctation of the aorta. Aetiology, practice and prospects. *Thorax* 1987; 42:11–18.
185. Sperling DR, Dorsey TJ, Rowen M, Gazzaniga AB: Percutaneous transluminal angioplasty of congenital coarctation of the aorta. *Am J Cardiol* 1983; 51:562–564.
186. Ritter SB: Coarctation and balloons: Inflated or realistic? *J Am Coll Cardiol* 1989; 13:696–699.
187. Maron BJ, Humphries J, Rowe RD, et al: Prognosis of surgically corrected coarctation of the aorta. A 20 year postoperative appraisal. *Circulation* 1973; 47:119–126.
188. Presbitero P, Demarie D, Villani M, et al: Long-term results (15–30 years) of surgical repair of aortic coarctation. *Br Heart J* 1987; 57:462–467.
189. Fyler DC: Report of the New England regional cardiac infant program. *Pediatrics* 1980, 65:375–460.
190. Miller RA: Complete transposition of the great arteries. In: Morse DP (ed): *Congenital Heart Disease. Pathogenic Factors, Natural History, Diagnosis and Surgical Treatment.* Philadelphia, FA Davis, 1962: 74–75.
191. Keith JD, Neill CA, Vlad P, Rowe RD, Chute AL: Transposition of the great vessels. *Circulation* 1953; 7:830–838.
192. Leibman J, Cullum L, Belloc NB: Natural history of transposition of the great arteries. Anatomy and birth and death characteristics. *Circulation* 1969; 40:237–262.
193. Rashkind WJ, Miller WW: Creation of an atrial septal defect without thoracotomy: A palliative approach to complete transposition of the great arteries. *JAMA* 1966; 196:991–992.
194. Senning A: Surgical correction of transposition of the great vessels. *Surgery* 1959; 45:966–980.
195. Mustard WT: Successful two-stage correction of transposition of the great vessels. *Surgery* 1964; 55:469–472.
196. Turina MI, Seibenmann R, Segesser L, Schonbeck M, Senning A: Late functional deterioration after atrial correction for transposition of the great arteries. *Circulation* 1989; 80(suppl I):162–167.
197. Jatene AD, Fontes VF, Paulista PP, Souza LCB, Neger F, Galantier M, et al: Successful anatomic correction of transposition of the great vessels. A preliminary report. *Arg Braz Cardiol* 1975; 28:461–464.
198. Rastelli GG, Wallace RB, Ongley PA: Complete repair of transposition of the great arteries with pulmonary stenosis. A review and report of a case corrected by using a new surgical technique. *Circulation* 1969; 39:83–95.
199. Flinn CJ, Wolff GS, Dick M, Campbell RM, Borkal G, Casta A, et al: Cardiac rhythm after the Mustard operation for complete transposition of the great arteries. *N Engl J Med* 1984; 310:1635–1638.
200. Graham TP, Arwood GF, Boucek RJ, Boerth RF, Bender HW: Abnormalities of right ventricular function following Mustard's operation for transposition of the great arteries. *Circulation* 1975; 52:678–684.
201. Hagler DJ, Ritter DG, Mair DD, Tajik AJ, Seward JB, Fulton RE, et al: Right and left ventricular function after the Mustard procedure for transposition of the great arteries. *Am J Cardiol* 1979; 44:276–283.
202. Graham TP, Burger J, Bender HW, Hammon JW, Boucek RJ, Appleton S: Improved right ventricular function after intraatrial repair of transposition of the great arteries. *Circulation* 1985; 72:1145–1151.
203. Mee RBB: Severe right ventricular failure after Mustard or Senning operation. Two-stage repair: Pulmonary artery banding and switch. *J Thorac Cardiovasc Surg* 1986; 92:385–390.
204. Wernovsky G, Hougen TJ, Walsh Ep, Scholler GF, Colan SD, Sanders Sp, et al: Mid-term results after the arterial switch operation for transposition of the great arteries with intact ventricular septum: Clinical, hemodynamic, echocardiographic and electrophysiologic data. *Circulation* 1988; 77:1333–1344.
205. Colan SD, Trowitzsch E, Wernovsky G, Sholler GF, Sanders SP, Castaneda A: Myocardial performance after arterial switch operation for transposition of the great arteries with intact ventricular septum. *Circulation* 1988; 78:132–141.
206. Allwork SP, Bentall HH, Becker AD, Cameron H, Gerlis LM, Wilkinson JL, et al: Congenitally corrected transposition of the great arteries: Morphologic study of 32 cases. *Am J Cardiol* 1976; 38:910–923.
207. Lundstrom U, Bull C, Wyse RKH, Somerville J: The natural and "unnatural" history of congenitally corrected transposition. *Am J Cardiol* 1990; 65:1222–1229.
208. Friedberg DZ, Nadas AS: Clinical profile of patients with congenitally corrected transposition of the great arteries. A study of 60 cases. *N Engl J Med* 1970; 282:1053–1059.
209. Huhta JC, Maloney JE, Ritter DG, Ilstrup DM, Feldt RH: Complete atrioventricular block in patients with atrioventricular discordance. *Circulation* 1983; 67:1374–1377.
210. LaCorte MA, Dick M, Scheer G, LaFarge CG, Flyer DC: Left ventricular function in tricuspid atresia. Angiographic analysis in 28 patients. *Circulation* 1975; 52:996–1000.
211. Moodie DS, Ritter DG, Tajik AH, McGoon DC, Danielson GK, O'Fallon WM: Long-term follow-up after palliative operation for univentricular heart. *Am J Cardiol* 1984; 53:1648–1651.
212. Moodie DS, Ritter DG, Tajik AH, O'Fallon WM: Long-term follow-up in the unoperated univentricular heart. *Am J Cardiol* 1984; 53:1124–1128.
213. Fontan F, Baudet E: Surgical repair of tricuspid atresia. *Thorax* 1971; 26:240–248.
214. Choussat A, Fontan I, Besse P, Vallot F, Cahuve A, Bricand H: Selection criteria for Fontan's procedure. In Anderson RH, Shinebourne EA (eds): *Paediatric Cardiology.* Edinburgh, Churchill Livingstone, 1978: Chap 64
215. Fontan F, Deville C, Quagebeur J, Ottenkamp J, Sourdille N, Choussat A, et al: Repair of tricuspid atresia in 100 patients. *J Thorac Cardiovasc Surg* 1983; 85:647–660.
216. Gewillig MH, Lundstrom UR, Bull C, Wyse RKH, Deanfield JE: Exercise responses in patients after Fontan repair: Patterns and determinants of performance. *J Am Coll Cardiol* 1990; 15:1424–1432.
217. Matsuda H, Kawashima Y, Kishimoto H, Hirose H, Nakano S, Kato H, et al: Problems with the modified Fontan operation for univentricular heart of the right ventricular type. *Circulation* 1987; 76(suppl II):II-45–II-52.
218. Mathur M, Glenn WWL: Long term evaluation of cavopulmonary artery anastomosis. *Surgery* 1973; 74:889–916.
219. Bridges ND, Lock JE, Castaneda AR: Baffle fenestration with subsequent transcatheter closure. Modifications of the Fontan operation for patients at higher risk. *Circulation* 1990; 82:1681–1689.
220. de Leval MR, Kilner P, Gewillig M, Bull C: Total cavopulmonary connection: A logical alternative to atriopulmonary connection

for complex Fontan operations. *J Thorac Cardiovasc Surg* 1988; 96:682–695.

221. Watson H: Natural history of Ebstein's anomaly of the tricuspid valve in childhood and adolescence: An internation cooperative study of 505 cases. *Br Heart J* 1974; 36:417–427.
222. Celermajer DS, Dodd SM, Greenwald SE, Wyse RK, Deanfield JE: Morbid anatomy in neonates with Ebstein's anomaly of the tricuspid valve: Pathophysiologic and clinical implications. *J Am Coll Cardiol* 1992; 19:1049–1053.
223. Lev M, Gibson S, Millar RA: Ebstein's disease with Wolff-Parkinson-White syndrome: Report of a case with histopathologic study of possible conduction pathways. *Am Heart J* 1955; 49:724–741.
224. Till J, Celermajer D, Deanfield J: The natural history of arrhythmias in Ebstein's anomaly. *J Am Coll Cardiol* 1992; 19(suppl A):273A.
225. Saxena A, Fong LV, Tristram M, Ackery DM, Keeton BR: Late noninvasive evaluation of cardiac performance in mildly symptomatic older patients with Ebstein's anomaly of the tricuspid valve: Role of radionuclide imaging. *J Am Coll Cardiol* 1991; 17:182–186.
226. Genton E, Blount G: The spectrum of Ebstein's anomaly. *Am Heart J* 1967; 73:395–425.
227. Kumar AJ, Fyler DC, Miettinen OS, Nadas AS: Ebstein's anomaly. Clinical profile and natural history. *Am J Cardiol* 1981; 28:84–95.
228. Danielson GK, Fuster V: Surgical repair of Ebstein's anomaly. *Ann Surg* 1982; 196:499–504.
229. Murdoch JL, Walker BA, Halpern BI, Kuzma JW, McKusick VA: Life expectancy and causes of death in the Marfan syndrome. *N Engl J Med* 1972; 286:804–808.
230. Pyerlitz RE, Wappel MA: Mitral valve dysfunction in the Marfan syndrome. *Am J Med* 1983; 74:797–807.
231. Gott VL, Pyerlitz RE, Magovern GJ Jr, Cameron DE, McKusick VA: Surgical treatment of aneurysms of the ascending aorta in the Marfan syndrome. Results of composite graft repair in 50 patients. *N Engl J Med* 1986; 314:1070–1074.

PART XII

Pulmonary Hypertension and Pulmonary Heart Disease

Chapter 99

Pulmonary Hypertension

Alfred P. Fishman, M.D.

INTRODUCTION

The clinical manifestations, natural history, and reversibility of pulmonary (arterial) hypertension depend heavily on the etiology of this hemodynamic disorder and the segment of the pulmonary vascular bed that is primarily affected. For example, the effects of certain etiologies, such as hypoxia, are confined to the pulmonary precapillary bed (small muscular arteries and arterioles), leaving the more distal parts of the pulmonary vascular bed virtually unaffected.[1,2] In contrast, in primary pulmonary venous hypertension, the small veins and venules are primarily affected, the precapillary vessels undergo secondary changes, and the intervening capillary bed is virtually unaffected. In only rare circumstances, e.g., pulmonary hemangiomatosis,[3] is the pulmonary capillary bed directly involved.

Because of its large capacity, its great distensibility, its low resistance to blood flow, and the modest amounts of smooth muscle in the small arteries and arterioles, the pulmonary circulation is not predisposed to become hypertensive. Pulmonary arterial pressures increase when total cross-sectional area decreases, either through curtailment of the extent of the pulmonary arterial tree, by narrowing of the lumens of the resistance vessels, or by combinations of these two mechanisms. When pulmonary hypertension does occur, it is usually secondary to cardiac or pulmonary disease. Unexplained or "primary" pulmonary hypertension is rare. Nonetheless, although primary pulmonary hypertension is uncommon, it does provide an important clinical paradigm of obstructive pulmonary vascular disease that is free of clinical overlays arising from the diverse etiologies and pathogenetic mechanisms responsible for secondary pulmonary hypertension.

Mild or even moderate pulmonary (arterial) hypertension can exist for a lifetime without becoming evident clinically. For example, native residents at high altitude in whom mild to moderate pulmonary hypertension is a natural result of unremitting exposure to hypoxia can carry heavy loads and play a vigorous game of soccer without undue discomfort. When pulmonary hypertension does become manifest clinically, the symptoms are generally nonspecific (Table 99-1).

Definitions

Pulmonary *arterial* hypertension ("pulmonary hypertension") can occur acutely or, more often, chronically. The acute form is usually a result of either pulmonary embolism (Chap. 100) or the adult respiratory distress syndrome. This chapter deals with *chronic* pulmonary (arterial) hypertension.

Pulmonary *venous* hypertension is usually encountered clinically as a consequence of left ventricular failure or mitral valvular disease. Occasionally it may occur in the course of fibrosing mediastinitis. Only rarely is the entity known as primary pulmonary veno-occlusive disease encountered. Invariably, pulmonary venous hypertension elicits pulmonary *arterial* hypertension, which may obscure it clinically. The hallmarks of pulmonary venous hypertension are pulmonary congestion and edema. Pulmonary *venous* hypertension is said to exist when pulmonary venous (or left atrial) pressure exceeds 12 mmHg.

Cor pulmonale merely signifies enlargement of the

TABLE 99-1
Symptoms of Primary Pulmonary Hypertension

Dyspnea	Palpitations
Fatigue	Orthopnea
Dizziness	Cough
Syncope	Hoarseness
Chest pain	

right ventricle as a consequence of dilation, hypertrophy, or both.[4] Almost invariably, chronic cor pulmonale is secondary to chronic pulmonary hypertension, i.e., to a sustained increase in right ventricular work due to an increase in its afterload. If the load is inordinate, the right ventricle will fail, i.e., cor pulmonale will be accompanied by right ventricular failure.

NORMAL PULMONARY CIRCULATION

Structure

Immediately before birth, pulmonary arterial and aortic blood pressures are about equal and of the order of 70/40 with a mean of 50 mmHg. Immediately after birth, as the ductus arteriosus closes and the lungs begin breathing air, pulmonary arterial pressure falls rapidly to about one-half of systemic levels. Thereafter, pulmonary arterial pressures gradually decrease over weeks to reach adult levels.[5] (See also Chap. 97.)

In some neonates, the media of the small muscular arteries and arterioles fail to involute normally, the pulmonary circulation is hypoplastic, or pulmonary vascular tone is inordinately high. For any of these reasons, pulmonary hypertension persists and becomes life threatening. Currently, the treatment of choice is extracorporeal membrane oxygenation (ECMO), which is designed to bide time either for further development or for spontaneous regression of the pathological processes.[6]

In the normal adult at sea level, the small muscular arteries and arterioles in the lungs are thin walled and sparsely equipped with muscle; in the fetus and in the adult who has undergone prolonged exposure to chronic hypoxia, e.g., native residents at high altitude, the media of the arterioles are thickened and extend peripherally into precapillary vessels, i.e., the precapillary vessels undergo "remodeling."[7]

Endothelium and Endothelium–Smooth Muscle Interactions

In addition to its role as a semipermeable barrier between blood and interstitium, the endothelium serves a wide array of biologically important functions, the net effect of which is the processing of blood flowing through the lungs. Among these functions are the synthesis, uptake, storage, release, and metabolism of vasoactive substances; transduction of blood-borne signals; modulation of coagulation and thrombolysis; regulation of cell proliferation; engagement in the local inflammatory and proliferative reactions to injury; involvement in immune reactions; and angiogenesis.[8] (See also Chap. 2.) Some of the enzymes involved in these processes, such as the angiotensin converting enzyme, are found on the surface of endothelial cells; others, such as 5′-nucleotidase are found within the cell. All-in-all, it is appropriate to regard endothelium as an organ with diverse metabolic and endocrine functions, one that is unique because of its strategic disposition as the continuous monolayered lining of blood vessels throughout the body. It is also important to bear in mind that the lungs contain the largest expanse of endothelium in the body.

The cells that comprise the monolayered endothelial lining communicate not only with each other by anatomic junctions and bridges, but also with the underlying smooth muscle by way of biologically active substances.[9] This interaction participates in the setting of normal vasomotor tone as well as the change in vasomotor tone that follow the administration of vasoactive substances. It is not difficult to imagine that damage to the lining cells, proliferation of the intima, or hypertrophy of the smooth muscle will upset the normal interplay.

Endothelial injury disturbs normal endothelial function. Indeed, a variety of enzyme systems are currently being explored as possible tests for normal and abnormal pulmonary endothelium and, in patients with pulmonary vascular injury and/or occlusion, as a measure of the extent of the total endothelial surface area that is still being perfused. (See also Chaps. 2 and 56.)

Hemodynamics

For the adult pulmonary circulation, the definition of "normal" depends on the altitude. The normal pulmonary hemodynamics of adults residing at sea level and at altitude are compared in Table 99-2. At *sea level,* a cardiac output of 5 to 6 liters/min is associated with a pulmonary arterial pressure of about 20 mmHg systolic and 12 mmHg diastolic, with a mean of about 15 mmHg. At *altitude,* the same level of blood flow is associated with somewhat higher pressures (Table 99-2). Pulmonary arterial pressures tend to increase somewhat with age.

The large output ejected by the right ventricle is conveyed across the pulmonary circulation with only a mod-

TABLE 99-2
Values for Normal Pulmonary Circulation at Sea Level and Altitude

	Sea Level	Altitude (~15,000 ft)
Pulmonary arterial pressure (P_{PA}), mmHg	20/12, 15	38/14, 25
Cardiac output ($\dot{Q}$), L/min	6.0	6.0
Left atrial pressure (P_{LA}), mmHg	5.0	5.0
Pulmonary vascular resistance (PVR),* mmHg/L/ min (*R* units)	1.7	3.3

$$*\text{PVR} = \frac{P_{PA} - P_{LA}}{\dot{Q}} = \frac{15 - 5}{6} = 1.67\ R \text{ units.}$$ To convert *R* units to CGS units (dynes·s/cm[5]), multiply *R* units by 80.

est drop in pressure, e.g., a cardiac output of 5 to 6 liters/min is accompanied by a pressure drop of 5 to 10 mmHg between the pulmonary artery and left atrium (Table 99-2). Determination of pulmonary vascular resistance has proved to be a practical clinical tool for quantifying the hemodynamic state of the pulmonary circulation and for distinguishing between active and passive changes in the pulmonary resistance vessels, e.g., the effect of administering a vasodilator agent to a patient with pulmonary hypertension. It is calculated as the ratio of the difference in mean pressure at the two ends of the pulmonary vascular bed [pulmonary arterial minus left atrial pressures divided by the cardiac output (pulmonary blood flow)] (Table 99-2). In practice, since the left atrium may not be readily accessible, pulmonary wedge pressure is generally substituted for left atrial pressure.

Another approach to defining certain characteristics and the behavior of the pulmonary arterial tree, i.e., elastic properties and geometry, is the calculation of pulmonary arterial input impedance. This approach is of greater physiological than clinical value. It takes into account the pulsatile nature of pulmonary arterial pressures and flow. Like vascular resistance, it is defined as a ratio. But instead of a ratio involving *mean* pressures and blood flow, the ratio is of the amplitudes of pulsatile pressure to oscillatory flow near the beginning of the pulmonary artery at a particular frequency. Values for the ratio are obtained by resolving mathematically the pulsatile pressure and flow curves into their sinusoidal components.

Although calculated pulmonary vascular resistance has proved useful in assessing the state of the normal and abnormal pulmonary circulation, and even though a change in calculated resistance can often be helpful in deciding whether pulmonary vasoconstriction or vasodilation has occurred, translation of a calculated ratio into vasomotor activity has to be made with caution.[4] For example, changes in calculated pulmonary vascular resistance are not readily interpretable when a vasodilator agent evokes multiple hemodynamic changes simultaneously, e.g., simultaneous changes in pulmonary vascular pressures and blood flow. Also, clinical shortcuts, such as the use in the numerator of the pulmonary arterial pressure, per se, instead of the pressure *drop* between pulmonary artery and left atrium, deprives the calculation of any physiological meaning. Finally, the clinical implications of the calculated pulmonary vascular resistance depend on the effects that the hemodynamic changes exert on the work of the heart. For example, although two different vasodilators may elicit the same decrease in calculated pulmonary vascular resistance, the changes that they induce in cardiac output and pulmonary vascular pressures can result in different work loads on the heart: If one agent elicits a *decrease* in pulmonary arterial pressure along with an *increase* in cardiac output (an ideal response), it is more apt to be of long-term benefit than another agent that fails to decrease the pulmonary arterial pressure while increasing the cardiac output.

A considerable increase in cardiac output, i.e., three times that at rest, increases pulmonary arterial pressure in the normal lung by only a few millimeters of mercury. On the other hand, in pulmonary hypertensive states in which the distensibility and extent of the pulmonary vascular bed has been restricted by disease, lesser increments in pulmonary blood flow elicit more striking increases in pulmonary arterial pressure.

Changes in pulmonary blood volume are much more subtle than blood pressure or flow in their hemodynamic effects: they are also much more difficult to quantify. Clinical clues can be helpful in recognizing that the pulmonary blood volume has increased. Often a fullness of the pulmonary vascular pattern on the chest radiograph along with evidences of interstitial edema suggests that pulmonary blood volume has increased acutely. In chronic mitral stenosis or left ventricular failure, the pulmonary blood volume is not only increased but also redistributed toward the apices of the lungs, i.e., "cephalization."

Autonomic nerves to the pulmonary vascular tree play much less of a role in mediating vasoconstriction or vasodilation than do local stimuli, particularly hypoxia. Indeed, hypoxia can exert its pulmonary pressor effect in the isolated lung, i.e., that is devoid of external innervation. Acidosis reinforces the hypoxic pressor effect. The mechanism by which hypoxia exerts its local pressor effect is unknown.[2] Hypercapnia also exerts a pulmonary pressor effect, presumably by way of the local acidosis that it generates.

PULMONARY HYPERTENSION: GENERAL FEATURES

Clinical Manifestations

Pulmonary hypertension is a final common hemodynamic consequence of multiple etiologies and diverse mechanisms. As noted above, most cases of pulmonary hypertension are secondary (Table 99-3). Among the

TABLE 99-3

Etiologies of Chronic Pulmonary (Arterial) Hypertension

- I. **Secondary**
  - A. Cardiac diseases
    1. Acquired heart disease associated with pulmonary venous hypertension, e.g., left ventricular failure, mitral valve disease
    2. Congenital heart disease
  - B. Pulmonary diseases
    1. Chronic obstructive airways disease (chronic bronchitis and emphysema; chronic obstructive lung disease)
    2. Chronic interstitial lung disease
    3. Pulmonary vascular disease, e.g., thromboembolic disease; collagen vascular disease
  - C. Disorders leading to alveolar hypoventilation
    1. Abnormal chest bellows
    2. Disordered respiratory control
    3. Sleep apneas
- II. **Primary pulmonary hypertension**
- III. **Pulmonary Veno-occlusive disease**

underlying causes of pulmonary hypertension are mechanical compression and distortion of the resistance vessels of the lungs (e.g., by widespread pulmonary fibrosis), hypoxic vasoconstriction (e.g., in severe obstructive airways disease), intravascular obstruction (e.g., thromboemboli or tumor emboli), and combinations of mechanical and vasoconstrictive influences. However, the major importance of pulmonary hypertension is that it leads to cor pulmonale and right ventricular failure. Not uncommonly, attention is first drawn to the possibility of pulmonary hypertension by the unexpected discovery of right ventricular enlargement, generally a combination of hypertrophy and dilation. When pulmonary arterial pressures climb to systemic levels, right ventricular failure becomes inevitable.

Special Studies

The gold standard for the diagnosis of pulmonary hypertension is right-sided heart catheterization. This technique enables the direct determination of pulmonary arterial pressure, pulmonary wedge pressure (as an approximation of pulmonary venous pressure), pulmonary blood flow (cardiac output), and the responses of these parameters to interventions (vasodilators, oxygen, exercise). From the measurements and samples obtained during cardiac catheterization, pulmonary vascular resistance can be calculated (Table 99-2). As a rule, noninvasive methods are less reliable and less informative.

Chest Radiography

The findings on the chest radiograph depend on the duration of the pulmonary hypertension and the etiology. The characteristic findings of pulmonary hypertension are enlargement of the pulmonary trunk and hilar vessels in association with pruning of the peripheral pulmonary arterial tree (Fig. 99-1). Right-sided heart enlargement can be difficult to detect radiographically except when the right ventricle is greatly enlarged. In secondary pulmonary hypertension, changes in the lungs, e.g., hyperinflation, and in the position of the heart and diaphragm, often blur the radiologic changes of pulmonary hypertension and cor pulmonale.

Angiography, using contrast dyes, has little role in the work-up for pulmonary hypertension unless it is done "selectively" in the search for pulmonary emboli.[10]

The Electrocardiogram

This test can disclose enlargement of the right ventricle with respect to the left ventricle. It is much more reliable in respiratory disorders that do not involve the parenchyma of the lungs, e.g., alveolar hypoventilation and the sleep apneas, than in obstructive airways disease, parenchymal lung disease, or congenital or acquired heart disease.

Ultrasound

The amount of reliable information obtained by Doppler and two-dimensional echocardiography depends greatly on the commitment of individual clinics to standardizing and perfecting these indirect techniques. In general, Doppler techniques have proved useful in providing a measure of right ventricular thickness as an index of cor pulmonale. In some clinics, reliable estimates of the level of pulmonary hypertension have been obtained by determining regurgitant flows across the tricuspid and pulmonic valves using continuous-wave Doppler echocardiography.[11] In patients in whom the pulmonic valve has been visualized, its behavior during the cardiac cycle has also been used to estimate the level of pulmonary arterial pressure. Probably one of the more rewarding applications of echocardiography has been as an alternative to repeated cardiac catheterizations in tracing the course of the disease and in assessing the effects of therapeutic interventions, e.g., pulmonary vasodilators. (See also Chaps. 15 and 130.)

Lung Scans

Ventilation-perfusion scans are of most value in the diagnosis and exclusion of pulmonary thromboembolic disease (see below).

Radionuclide Studies

The response of the right ventricular ejection fraction to exercise is assessed in some clinics using radionuclide angiography. Scintigraphy using thallium 201 has also been useful in detecting hypertrophy of the right ventricle, i.e., cor pulmonale due to pulmonary hypertension. (See also Chap. 134.)

Lung Biopsy

The sampling of lung tissue by open thoracotomy is sometimes helpful in identifying the etiology of the pulmonary hypertension and, by excluding known etiologies, establishing the diagnosis of primary pulmonary hypertension. Attempts to predict responsiveness to vasodilators on the basis of lung biopsy have met with limited success.[12]

SECONDARY PULMONARY HYPERTENSION

Cardiac and/or respiratory diseases are the most common causes of secondary pulmonary hypertension. Pulmonary thromboembolic disease ranks third. Cardiac disease leads to pulmonary hypertension by increasing pulmonary blood flow, e.g., large left-to-right shunts, or by increasing pulmonary venous pressure, e.g., left ventricular failure. Almost invariably, secondary influences such as intimal proliferation in the pulmonary resistance vessels add a component of obstructive pulmonary vascular disease.[13] In respiratory disease, the predominant mechanism for the pulmonary hypertension is an increase in resistance to pulmonary blood flow arising from perivascular parenchymal changes coupled with pulmonary vasoconstriction due to hypoxia. In pulmonary thromboembolic disease, clots in various stages

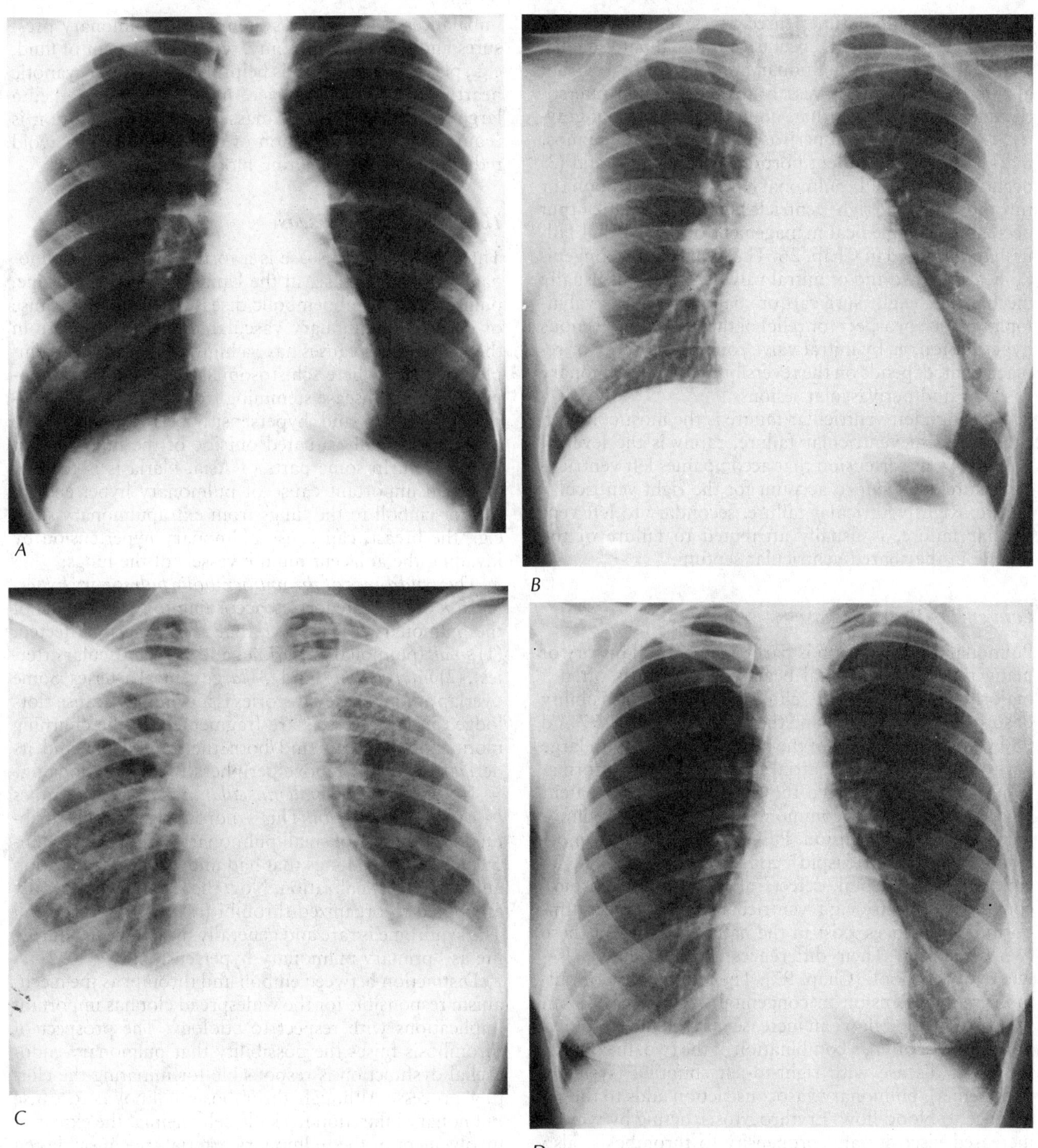

FIGURE 99-1 Cardiac silhouette in four patients with severe pulmonary hypertension on admission to the hospital: *A, B.* Primary pulmonary hypertension showing different stages in the evolution of cor pulmonale. *C.* Widespread pulmonary fibrosis. *D.* Systemic lupus erythematosus proven by lung biopsy. This radiograph is indistinguishable from that of primary pulmonary hypertension.

of organization and affecting pulmonary vessels of different size increase resistance to blood flow.[13]

Cardiac Disease

The mechanisms of pulmonary hypertension are usually quite different in acquired disorders of the left side of the heart from those of congenital heart disease.

Acquired Disorders of Left Side of Heart

Left ventricular failure is the most common cause of pulmonary hypertension. Among the various etiologies, myocardial disorders and lesions of the mitral and aortic valves predominate. Both types of lesions lead to an increase in pulmonary venous pressure that, in turn, evokes an increase in pulmonary arterial pressure. Presumably, the increase in pulmonary arterial pressure is reflex in origin. In time, three types of morphologic changes supervene: (1) occlusive intimal and medial changes not only in pulmonary venules and veins, but also in the precapillary vessels; (2) perivascular interstitial edema and fibrosis that, under the influence of gravity, cause vascular and perivascular changes to be most marked in the dependent portions of the lungs; and (3) occlusion of small pulmonary vessels by emboli or thrombi when the right ventricle fails and cardiac output decreases. The medical management of myocardial failure is considered in Chap. 26. The treatment of congenital heart disease and of mitral valvular disease is usually mechanical, e.g., surgical or balloon mitral valvuloplasty. The prospect for relief of the pulmonary venous hypertension, as by mitral valve commissurotomy or replacement, depends on the reversibility of the pulmonary vascular and perivascular lesions.[14]

Although left ventricular failure is the most common cause of right ventricular failure, rarely is the level of pulmonary hypertension that accompanies left ventricular failure sufficient to account for the right ventricular failure. Right ventricular failure, secondary to left ventricular failure, is usually attributed to failure of the muscle in the shared ventricular septum.

Congenital Heart Disease

Pulmonary hypertension is part of the natural history of many types of congenital heart disease and is often a major determinant of the clinical course, the feasibility of surgical intervention, and the outcome (Chaps. 97 and 98). Congenital defects of the heart associated with large left-to-right shunts, e.g., atrial septal defect, or abnormal communications between the great vessels, e.g., patent ductus arteriosus, are commonly associated with pulmonary arterial hypertension. Pulmonary hypertension occurs in both "pretricuspid" congenital defects, e.g., secundum atrial septal defect, and in "posttricuspid" congenital defects, e.g., ventricular septal defect. Important differences exist in the natural history of these two categories. Their differences are considered elsewhere in this book (Chap. 97). The major cause of pulmonary hypertension in congenital heart disease is an increase in blood flow, an increase in resistance to blood flow, or most often, a combination of the two. In congenital heart disease with right-to-left shunting (systemic hypoxemia), pulmonary vasoconstriction adds to the resistance to blood flow. Erythrocytosis, acting by way of increased viscosity and propensity to thrombosis, also contributes to the increase in resistance. Although the increase in pulmonary vascular tone elicited by hypoxia contributes to the increase in pulmonary vascular resistance, the predominant resistance is offered by anatomic changes in the walls of the small muscular arteries and arterioles. Patients with congenital heart disease and pulmonary hypertension who become pregnant are at increased risk of sudden death both in the course of delivery and immediately postpartum.

Depending on the nature of the congenital cardiac defect, vasodilators are sometimes helpful in diminishing heightened pulmonary vasomotor tone. Caution is required in administering such agents to patients with congenital heart disease because of the prospect of inducing imbalances between the systemic and pulmonary pressures and flows. Phlebotomy, with replacement of fluid, e.g., plasma or albumin, is helpful in congenital cyanotic heart disease in which severe hypoxemia has evoked a large increase in red cell mass. Once again, caution is required to avoid depletion of iron stores and to avoid reduction in the circulating blood volume.

Thromboembolic Disease

Thromboembolic disease is a form of occlusive pulmonary vascular disease. In the United States and Europe, pulmonary thromboembolic disease is a common cause of occlusive pulmonary vascular disease. Elsewhere in the world, other causes have a high incidence. For example, in Egypt, where schistosomiasis is endemic, pulmonary vascular disease stemming from ova lodged in pulmonary vessels and hypersensitivity reactions to the organism (usually situated outside of the lungs) is not uncommon. In some parts of Asia, filariasis is reputed to be an important cause of pulmonary hypertension. Tumor emboli to the lungs from extrapulmonary sites, e.g., the breast, can cause pulmonary hypertension by invading the adjacent minute vessels of the lungs.

The *syndromes of thromboembolic pulmonary hypertension* can be categorized according to the segments of the pulmonary arterial tree that are primarily affected: (1) *small* (pulmonary arterioles and small muscular arteries), (2) *intermediate,* and (3) *large* central arteries. Some overlap among these categories is inevitable because clots lodged in large vessels are fragmented by the churning motion of the heart and both the parent clot and its derivatives tend to move peripherally for final lodging.

1. *Occlusion of small muscular arteries and arterioles by organized thrombi.* This syndrome used to be attributed to a shower of small pulmonary emboli to the minute vessels of the lungs that had undergone organization and partial recanalization. Now the lesions are generally attributed to organized thrombi (rather than emboli).[15] The syndrome is rare and generally misdiagnosed during life as "primary pulmonary hypertension."

Distinction between emboli and thrombi as the mechanism responsible for the widespread clot has important implications with respect to etiology: The prospect of thrombosis raises the possibility that pulmonary endothelial dysfunction is responsible for initiating the clotting process. Although thrombosis is known to cause pulmonary infarction in sickle cell anemia, the extent of involvement of the pulmonary arterial tree in sickle cell disease is rarely sufficiently extensive to evoke pulmonary hypertension. Thrombi in the small muscular arteries and arterioles are common postmortem findings in pulmonary hypertensive patients who develop right-sided heart failure.

2. *Occlusion of intermediate pulmonary arteries by emboli.* This syndrome is by far the more common of the three.[15] It is caused by repeated clots, almost invariably released from vessels in the upper legs and thighs, that progressively amputate more and more of the pulmonary arterial tree. Ventilation-perfusion scans and selective angiography demonstrate the extent of the pulmonary vascular occlusion. (See Chap. 100.)

3. *Chronic proximal pulmonary thromboembolism.*

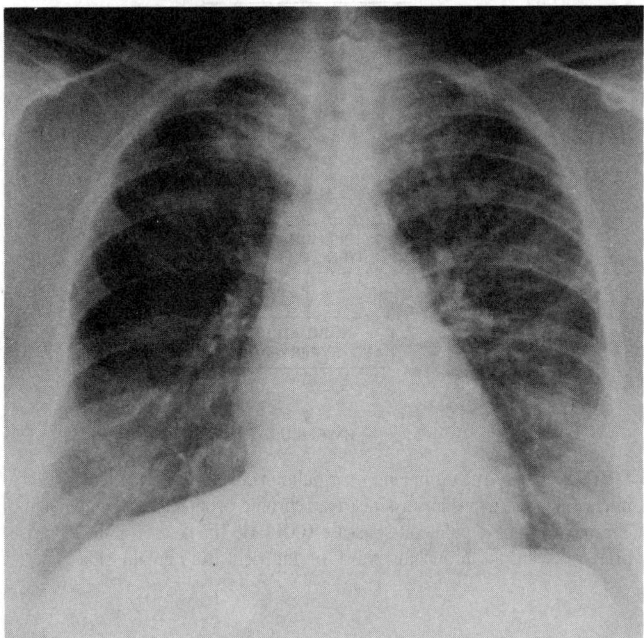

A

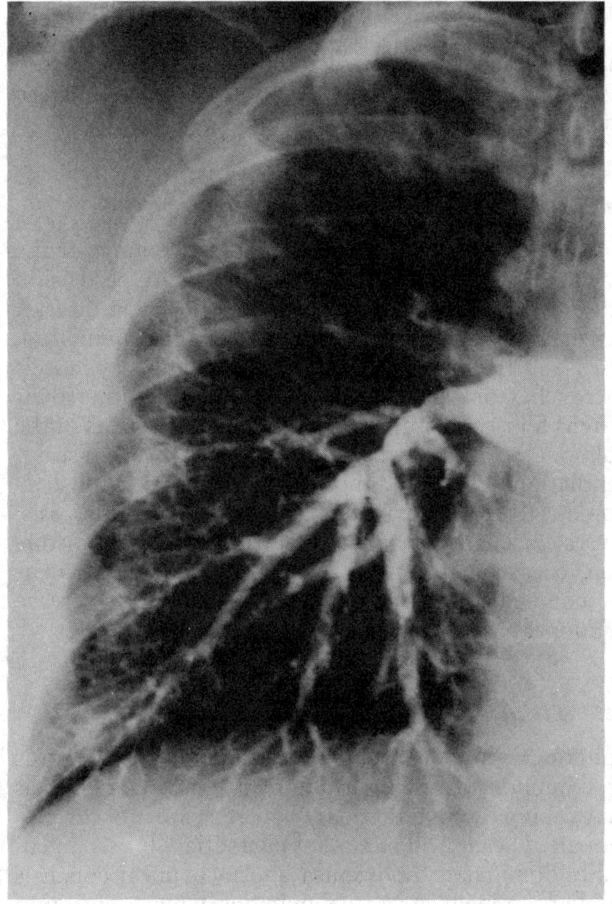

B

FIGURE 99-2 Pulmonary hypertension due to organized clot in central pulmonary arteries. Dramatic relief after pulmonary thromboendarterectomy. *A.* Chest radiograph. The right upper lobe is strikingly hypoperfused and the vasculature on the left is quite prominent, reflecting redirection of the pulmonary blood flow to open vessels. *B.* Angiogram. The flow to the right upper lung is interrupted by the large central clot.

In most survivors of acute massive pulmonary embolism, the hemodynamic, perfusion scan and angiographic abnormalities resolve. However, in a few, resolution fails to occur and organized large clots become incorporated into the walls of the major pulmonary arteries, leading to pulmonary hypertension (Fig. 99-2). Inadequacy of the local fibrinolytic mechanisms allows the clot to be incorporated into the pulmonary arterial wall, to propagate (antegradely and retrogradely), to obstruct large segments of the pulmonary vascular bed, and to decrease the compliance of the central pulmonary vessels. By the time the diagnosis is made, the obstructing lesions in the central pulmonary arteries have become part of the vessel walls by the processes of organization, fibrosis, endothelialization, and recanalization.[15]

The importance of recognizing *proximal* pulmonary thromboembolism as a cause of pulmonary hypertension is the possibility of relieving the pulmonary hypertension by surgical intervention, i.e., by pulmonary thromboendarterectomy. Ventilation-perfusion lung scanning is a cornerstone of diagnosis; it provides a measure of the distribution of pulmonary vascular resistances. As a rule, patients with proximal pulmonary thromboembolism will show two or more segmental-size perfusion defects. Perfusion defects that are segmental or larger call for cardiac catheterization both for hemodynamic assessment and for *selective* contrast pulmonary angiography. Segmental-sized defects are not seen in primary pulmonary hypertension. Selective angiography is essential for diagnosis since perfusion lung scans usually underestimate the severity of the central pulmonary arterial obstruction[16]; moreover, identification of the precise location and extent of the organized clot is necessary for surgical removal. The combination of clinical findings suggestive of pulmonary hypertension and segmental-sized perfusion defects calls for right-sided heart catheterization and selective pulmonary angiography. Fiberoptic angioscopy and magnetic resonance imaging are both under active investigation as modalities that may be helpful in defining the lesions of proximal thromboembolic pulmonary hypertension.[17] (See also Chap. 100.)

Surgery is advocated for patients with pulmonary hypertension who have persistent clot in lobar or more proximal pulmonary arteries after at least 6 months of anticoagulation. Thromboendarterectomy is done, generally via a median sternotomy, using deep hypothermic cardiopulmonary bypass with intermittent periods of circulatory arrest. Hemodynamic improvement is usually quite dramatic.

Respiratory Diseases and Disorders

Not only intrinsic pulmonary diseases but also respiratory disorders, i.e., disturbances in the respiratory muscle or in the control of breathing, can lead to pulmonary hypertension. Among the intrinsic lung diseases are those affecting the airways, e.g., chronic bronchitis, as well as those affecting the parenchyma. Among the respiratory disorders are the syndromes of alveolar hypoventilation and the sleep apneas.

Intrinsic Diseases of Lungs and/or Airways

Diseases that affect the parenchyma of the lungs or the tracheobronchial tree can elicit pulmonary hypertension in different ways depending on the underlying disease: In widespread interstitial fibrosis and/or inflammation, disease in the vicinity of the minute pulmonary vessels encroaches on vascular lumens, thereby limiting their distensibility and amputating peripheral segments of the pulmonary vascular tree; in obstructive airways disease, ventilation-perfusion abnormalities cause vasoconstriction due to arterial hypoxemia; in conglomerate fibrosis, several mechanisms act in concert: Mechanical distortion, encasement, and obstruction of vascular lumens are coupled with hypoxic vasoconstriction to increase pulmonary vascular resistance.

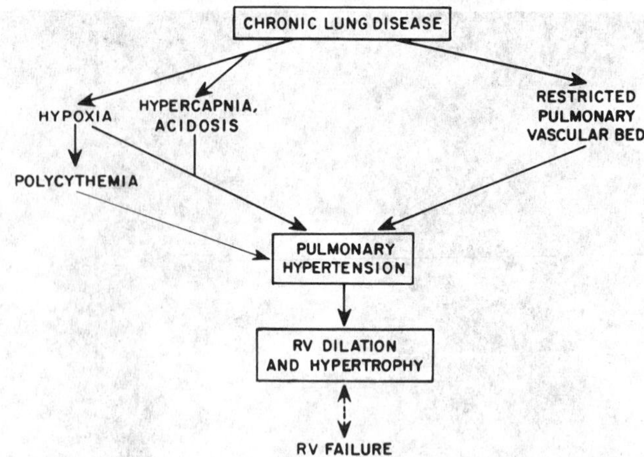

FIGURE 99-3 The evolution of cor pulmonale and right ventricular failure in chronic obstructive airways disease [chronic bronchitis and emphysema; chronic obstructive pulmonary disease (COPD)]. The factors on the left arise primarily from the bronchitis, those on the right from emphysema.

Interstitial Fibrosis

Pulmonary sarcoidosis, asbestosis, and radiation fibrosis are common causes of widespread pulmonary fibrosis that culminates in pulmonary hypertension and cor pulmonale. The clinical picture of interstitial fibrosis is generally dominated by dyspnea and tachypnea; cough is rarely prominent. As a rule, pulmonary hypertension of marked degree occurs toward the end of the illness when hypoxemia is present at rest and P_{CO_2} starts its climb toward hypercapnic levels (Fig. 99-1C). Cor pulmonale (right ventricular enlargement) and right ventricular failure are common sequelae.

Vasodilators have no proven place in dealing with the pulmonary hypertension associated with interstitial fibrosis. Oxygen therapy, particularly during daily activity or sleep, can be important in avoiding the hypoxic pulmonary pressor response. Corticosteroids often become the mainstay of therapy and often effect some symptomatic relief. The advent of single-lung transplantation has widened greatly the therapeutic horizons for dealing with widespread interstitial fibrosis.

Chronic Obstructive Airways Disease Chronic bronchitis and emphysema [chronic obstructive lung disease (COPD)] is the most common cause of pulmonary hypertension and cor pulmonale in patients with intrinsic pulmonary disease.[18,19] Even though chronic bronchitis and emphysema generally coexist, the predominant cause of the pulmonary hypertension is alveolar hypoxia resulting from chronic bronchitis; emphysema plays only a minor role, presumably by restricting the extent of the pulmonary vascular bed (Fig. 99-3). Cystic fibrosis illustrates the importance of chronic obstructive airways disease in evoking pulmonary hypertension since the disease in cystic fibrosis is virtually confined to the airways.

The indiscriminate use of COPD, without distinguishing between predominant bronchitis and predominant emphysema, tends to cloud the natural history of this spectrum of obstructive airway diseases. In essence, pulmonary hypertension (generally culminating in cor pulmonale) is encountered in two different settings: *episodically* in the "pink puffer," who only becomes hypoxemic during an acute respiratory infection, and *chronically* in the "blue bloater," within whom unremitting hypoxia is aggravated during an acute respiratory infection. In the blue bloater the course of the pulmonary hypertension is inexorably progressive. During a bout of respiratory failure, clinical distinction between a pink buffer and a blue bloater is often impossible. After recovery from the acute episode, however, distinction is usually quite simple.

The gold standard for diagnosing pulmonary hypertension in patients with chronic obstructive airways disease is right-sided heart catheterization. Less direct indices are used in some clinics.[20,21] One cardinal sign of pulmonary hypertension is right ventricular enlargement, i.e., dilation and hypertrophy; however, recognition of right ventricular enlargement can be difficult in obstructive airways disease because of hyperinflation and cardiac rotation.[22] Once suspicion is raised that the clinical picture of right ventricular failure stems from ventilation-perfusion abnormalities, an arterial blood sample will confirm that the P_{O_2} is low (P_{O_2} is from less than 40 to 50 mmHg), the P_{CO_2} is high ($P_{CO_2} > 50$ mmHg), and respiratory acidosis is present. Such arterial blood gas tensions are rare in left ventricular failure unless the patient is in frank pulmonary edema.

Electrocardiographic evidence of right ventricular enlargement is also often equivocal in patients with chronic obstructive airways disease (chronic bronchitis and emphysema; COPD) because of rotation and displacement of the heart, widened distances between electrodes and the cardiac surface, and the predominance of dilation over hypertrophy in the cardiac enlargement. Because of these limitations, it is not surprising that standard electrocardiographic criteria for right ventricular enlargement apply in about only one-third of patients with COPD who prove to have cor pulmonale at autopsy.

Consecutive changes in the electrocardiogram are often more useful than a single electrocardiogram in detecting right ventricular overload due to pulmonary hypertension. As the arterial P_{O_2} drops to distinctly subnormal levels, e.g., below 60 to 70 mmHg while awake, T waves tend to become inverted, biphasic, or flat in the right, precordial leads (V_1 to V_3); the mean electrical axis of the QRS shifts 30 degrees or more to the right of the patient's usual axis; ST segments become depressed in leads II, III, and aV_F; and right bundle branch block (incomplete or complete) often appears. These changes tend to reverse as arterial oxygenation improves. (See also Chap. 13.)

In the patient with chronic obstructive airways disease in whom pulmonary hypertension has been elicited or aggravated by a bout of bronchitis or pneumonia, the goal of therapy is to maintain tolerable levels of arterial oxygenation while waiting for the upper respiratory infection to subside. If the pulmonary hypertension is acute, modest enrichment of inspired air with oxygen, as by 28 percent oxygen delivered by a Venturi mask, generally suffices to relieve arterial hypoxemia and to restore pulmonary arterial pressures toward normal. Considerable improvement may also be accomplished even in the individual who has chronic pulmonary hypertension by sustained (virtually continuous) breathing of oxygen-enriched air that restores arterial P_{O_2} to nearly normal values.

Once the right ventricle has failed, cardiotonic agents can only be used cautiously because of the threat of arrhythmias posed by arterial hypoxemia and respiratory acidosis. Moreover, after adequate oxygenation has been achieved, the need for digitalis and diuretics often decreases since the hemodynamic burden on the right ventricle, i.e., the pulmonary arterial hypertension, decreases. Even though each episode of acute hypoxia and acidosis seems to elicit about the same increment in pulmonary arterial pressure, each bout of pulmonary hypertension appears to leave behind a slightly higher level of pulmonary hypertension after recovery.[18]

Arterial blood gas composition is the therapeutic compass to the control of pulmonary hypertension in chronic obstructive airways disease. The degree of hypoxia is usually underestimated by blood sampling since blood is drawn while the patient is awake and at rest, whereas hypoxemia is more marked during sleep and daily activity. In managing ambulatory patients, serial determinations of the hematocrit may serve as a practical clue to the occurrence of covert arterial hypoxemia, i.e., during sleep or activity. Once right ventricular failure has set in, however, there is no substitute for determining arterial P_{O_2} and P_{CO_2} as a guide to therapy. Ensuring the return of arterial oxygenation toward normal is much more vital than is the administration of cardiotonic measures. When respiratory infection has triggered the episode of pulmonary hypertension, a vital strategy for achieving a lasting improvement in arterial oxygenation is the administration of an appropriate antibiotic. While awaiting the salutary effects of antibiotic therapy, attention is paid to hydration, to postural drainage, and to adequate alveolar ventilation. The management of respiratory acidosis is described elsewhere in this volume.

Phlebotomy, once popular because of the prospect that increased blood viscosity contributes importantly to the pulmonary hypertension, has fallen into disuse. Polycythemia is rarely severe enough to be a serious problem in cor pulmonale that is associated with bronchitis and emphysema.

Vasodilators have recently been tried in various types of secondary pulmonary hypertension, including that due to chronic obstructive airways disease. The agents tried are the same as those outlined for *primary* pulmonary hypertension. They run the risk of aggravating arterial hypoxemia by exaggerating ventilation-perfusion abnormalities. Unfortunately, the efficacy of vasodilator agents in secondary pulmonary hypertension has proved to be far less impressive or predictable than in primary pulmonary hypertension. To date, the safest and most effective approach to pulmonary vasodilation in obstructive arterial hypoxemia is the use of oxygen-enriched inspired air.[22–24]

Conglomerate Fibrosis, Emphysema, and Chronic Bronchitis Pulmonary hypertension is uncommon in uncomplicated silicosis or tuberculosis. By contrast, in patients in whom smouldering, long-standing tuberculosis or conglomerate, massive fibrosis has shrunk and distorted the lungs, pulmonary hypertension is virtually the rule. The likelihood of pulmonary hypertension (and cor pulmonale) is enhanced by chronic pleurisy, fibrothorax, or excisional surgery, which exert their effects by a combination of all of these derangements. Although these combinations are generally complicated, the principles of management are those outlined above for obstructive airways disease. Unfortunately, therapeutic triumphs are uncommon because of the fixed anatomic changes.

Multiple System Diseases Pulmonary hypertension can be an important clinical complication of certain connective tissue diseases, notably scleroderma, lupus erythematosus, and dermatomyositis[25] (Fig. 99-1*D*). (See also Chap. 103.) Pulmonary hypertension has been reported to occur in about one-third of patients with scleroderma (systemic sclerosis), but in many of these the pulmonary hypertension is borderline. The cause of the pulmonary hypertension may be widespread interstitial pulmonary fibrosis, obliterative vascular disease, myocardial disease, or a combination of all three. Progressive systemic sclerosis (disseminated cutaneous systemic sclerosis) is almost invariably associated with rapidly progressive, diffuse interstitial fibrosis. In contrast, radiographic evidence of widespread pulmonary fibrosis may be less impressive in the CREST syndrome (calcinosis, long-standing Raynaud's phenomena, esophageal dysmotility, sclerodactyly, and telangiectasia) even though the pulmonary hypertension may be striking because of the obliterative vascular disease. Although Raynaud's phenomena occur in 95 percent of patients with progressive systemic sclerosis, particular attention has been paid to their occurrence in patients with the CREST syndrome because of its high incidence in this group and the possibility of "pulmonary Raynaud's phenomena."[26] It is unknown whether or not heightened pulmonary vasomotor reactivity is present in patients with systemic sclerosis. The contribution of pulmonary Raynaud's phenomena is of practical interest because of the prospect that patients with heightened pulmonary vascular tone might be better candidates for pulmonary vasodilator therapy than those in whom the pulmonary hypertension stems primarily from entrapment of the pulmonary resistance vessels by the fibrotic parenchymal process.[25]

Alveolar Hypoventilation in Patients with Normal Lungs

In patients with alveolar hypoventilation whose lungs are normal ("global" alveolar hypoventilation), the primary pathogenetic mechanism is alveolar hypoxia sometimes reinforced by respiratory acidosis.[19,27] In this respect, the ultimate cause(s) of pulmonary hypertension in *global* alveolar hypoventilation, as in *net* alveolar hypoventilation due to ventilation perfusion abnormalities, are the abnormal blood gases. The global alveolar hypoventilation in individuals with normal lungs generally originates either in an inadequate ventilatory drive (as after encephalitis), in covert obstruction of the upper airways (as in the sleep apnea syndromes), or in an ineffective chest bellows (as after paralytic poliomyelitis). Among the disorders associated with global alveolar hypoventilation are disorders of respiratory muscles, respiratory "centers" that are unresponsive to chemical stimuli, kyphoscoliosis, and extreme obesity. (See also Chaps. 101 and 104.)

Regardless of cause, the occurrence of pulmonary hypertension in patients with alveolar hypoventilation and normal lungs depends on the occurrence of sufficient alveolar and arterial hypoxia to elicit pulmonary hypertension. In some individuals, such as those with kyphoscoliosis, the stage for arterial hypoxemia and pulmonary hypertension is set by the mechanical limitations imposed by the deformed chest; the activities of daily life aggravate the situation by increasing metabolic demand, due to not only the increased activity, but also the heightened oxygen cost of breathing. In the sleep apnea syndromes, severe arterial hypoxemia and pulmonary hypertension that develops initially only during sleep may become self-perpetuating and carry over into wakefulness.[28] Cor pulmonale is a common result of the unrelieved pulmonary hypertension. Also, no matter how the alveolar hypoventilation has been initiated, an upper respiratory infection often topples this type of patient into respiratory failure, severe pulmonary hypertension, and right-sided heart failure.

For the patient in combined respiratory and cardiac (right ventricular) failure, the highest therapeutic priority is to improve oxygenation. Assisted ventilation, particularly during sleep, may be particularly helpful in those with sleep apnea, e.g., continuous positive airway pressure (CPAP) breathing. Success in avoiding alveolar and arterial hypoxia results in a decrease in pulmonary arterial pressures, thereby relieving the overburdened right ventricle. Recently, potent but short-acting pulmonary vasodilators, such as prostacyclin, have been advocated for urgent relief of right ventricular overload. In this category of patients, however, pharmacologic therapy is rarely needed because of the efficiency of the oxygen therapy and assisted ventilation in promoting pulmonary vasodilation.

PRIMARY (UNEXPLAINED) PULMONARY HYPERTENSION

Definition

Primary pulmonary hypertension is defined as pulmonary arterial hypertension of unknown cause. It is a diagnosis made by exclusion; all recognizable causes of pulmonary hypertension (Table 99-3) must be ruled out before the diagnosis of *primary* pulmonary hypertension can be made. The diagnosis presupposes that the seat of the disorder is in the pulmonary arterial tree. The occasional association of primary pulmonary hypertension and hepatic cirrhosis is a tantalizing aspect of the disease.[29] Pulmonary veno-occlusive disease (see below) is not included under the rubic of primary pulmonary hypertension even though its etiology is also unexplained: Although the pulmonary arterial tree does undergo secondary changes that cause pulmonary *arterial* hypertension along with the pulmonary *venous* hypertension, the pathologic features and pathogenetic mechanisms in pulmonary veno-occlusive disease are different and usually quite distinctive.

Primary pulmonary hypertension is a rare disease. Its prevalence is about 0.1 to 0.2 percent of all patients who come to autopsy. Based on the 194 patients entered into the National Registry for Primary Pulmonary Hypertension, the estimated incidence nationwide in the United States is about 400 new patients per year.[30] A total of about 1000 cases has been reported.

The clinical diagnosis of primary pulmonary hypertension rests on three different types of evidence: (1) clinical, radiographic, and electrocardiographic manifestations of pulmonary hypertension; (2) demonstration, by right-sided heart catheterization, of the typical hemodynamic constellation of abnormally high pulmonary arterial pressures and pulmonary vascular resistance in association with a normal pulmonary wedge pressure and a normal or low cardiac output; and (3) inability to attribute the pulmonary hypertension to a disorder of the heart, respiratory apparatus, or systemic circulation.

General Features

After puberty, females predominate, those between 10 and 40 years of age being most often affected. Before puberty, no sex difference is discernible. The textbook picture of a patient with primary pulmonary hypertension is that of a young woman in the prime of life who develops one or more of the symptoms in Table 99-1 without discernible cause. Sex and age are sometimes useful in distinguishing clinically between the likelihood of primary pulmonary hypertension and pulmonary thromboembolic disease. The latter generally favors men, particularly in their later years.

As a rule, median survival of patients can be predicted on the basis of the New York Heart Association functional classification: 6 months for class IV; $2\frac{1}{2}$ years for class III; 6 years for classes I and II. Unless interrupted by sudden death, the usual downhill course terminates in intractable right ventricular failure. Although this classification does provide a useful clinical guide, exceptions are not uncommon.[31]

Etiology

No matter what the etiology of primary pulmonary hypertension ultimately proves to be, the seat of the disease is the endothelium and its underlying smooth muscle, particularly of the small muscular arteries and arterioles. It seems reasonable that in response to some unknown stimulus, e.g., injury, the lining of these vessels proliferates to produce a state of widespread obstructive pulmonary vascular disease. Although this simple formulation may be reasonable from a global perspective, it glosses over many gaps in present understanding: Why is there localization to precapillary vessels? Does the restructured piled-up intimal lining behave the same as does normal endothelium? Does it process blood in the usual way? Does it elaborate enzymes normally and generate the usual biologically active substances? How do the piled-up cells of the intima communicate with each other and with the subintimal smooth muscle, which is generally hypertrophied? Are the thrombolytic mechanisms preserved or is the abnormal vascular lining predisposed to form clots? Unfortunately, few answers are available since, even though a great deal is now known about normal pulmonary endothelium, little is known about the endothelium and the endothelial–smooth muscle interplay of pulmonary hypertensive vessels.[8,9,32–34]

Uncertainty persists about whether or not the shared histologic pattern associated with primary pulmonary hypertension can be caused by diverse etiologies (Table 99-4).[35,36] This possibility of multiple etiologies complicates attempts to describe the natural history of the disorder. Moreover, the fact that etiology plays an important part in determining reversibility was exemplified by instances of recovery during the epidemic in some countries in Europe of "primary pulmonary hypertension" that followed the over-the-counter sale of Aminorex.[37] Thus, although the stereotypical young woman is apt to die within 2 to 3 years after the onset of symptoms, there are now many instances of longer life spans. Indeed, some patients are known to have lived 20 to 30 years or even longer after the clinical diagnosis was made.

Until recently, virtually all reports of primary pulmonary hypertension dealt with sporadic cases. An epidemic in Europe between 1967 and 1970 of primary pulmonary hypertension that was apparently linked to the over-the-counter sale of Aminorex, an anorectic agent, raised the prospect of hereditary predisposition since only one per thousand who took the drug developed pulmonary hypertension. Since then, about 25 families have been identified in which the disease seems to be hereditary.[38] The recent toxic oil epidemic in Spain reinforced the idea of individual susceptibility to toxic agents.[39] In familial primary pulmonary hypertension, the incidence is 7 percent (with a pattern of autosomal dominance and incomplete penetrance). One major insight provided by the families with primary pulmonary hypertension is that the pulmonary vascular lesions can be remarkably diverse in members of the same family. The familial incidence has raised questions about whether or not better family histories would reveal that some cases of primary pulmonary hypertension currently regarded as sporadic would, on searching inquiry, prove to be familial. (See also Chap. 96.)

TABLE 99-4

Suggested Mechanisms for Primary Pulmonary Hypertension

Sustained vasoconstriction	Most likely a contributing factor
Autoimmune mechanisms	Based on association with Raynaud's phenomenon and collagen vascular diseases, such as disseminated lupus erythematosus
Persistence of fetal pulmonary vascular bed	Questionably related to the adult syndrome
Dietary pulmonary hypertension	Suggested by outbreaks of pulmonary hypertension after ingestion of anoretic agent, Aminorex, and toxic oil; genetic predisposition seems to be involved
Combined portal and pulmonary hypertension	Pulmonary hypertension occurs in some patients with hepatic cirrhosis; possibly related to dietary pulmonary hypertension
Multiple pulmonary thrombi	Widespread occlusion of small muscular arteries and arterioles in the lungs, possibly due to unidentified endothelial injury
Familial pulmonary hypertension	A well-documented entity; possibility that some sporadic cases are really instances of the familial form of the disease

Pathology

The natural history of primary pulmonary hypertension depends on progressive attenuation of the pulmonary arterial tree, which gradually increases pulmonary vascular resistance to the point of eliciting right ventricular strain and failure. The seat of the disease is in the small pulmonary arteries (between 40 and 100 μm in diameter) and arterioles. The obliterative lesions affect one or more layers of these vessels. In some instances, medial hypertrophy predominates; in others, it is the intima that proliferates; in addition, evidence of inflammation is also present (Fig. 99-4).[12,40]

Clinicians have traditionally relied heavily on the pathologist for confirmation of the diagnosis of primary pulmonary hypertension. The pathologist can be helpful in three ways: (1) identifying a constellation of pulmonary precapillary lesions that are consistent with the clinical diagnosis of primary pulmonary hypertension, i.e., plexiform lesions, angiomatoid lesions, concentric intimal fibrosis and necrotizing arteritis; although the full-blown histologic picture is diagnostic, it is also uncommon to see all of these lesions in a single patient; (2) distinguishing between the obliterative vascular disease of primary pulmonary hypertension and those of pulmonary thromboembolic disease; the fibroelastosis that obliterates the vascular lumens of the small muscular arteries and arterioles in primary pulmonary hypertension is predominantly *concentric* whereas the organization of venous clots is generally *eccentric;* and (3) exclud-

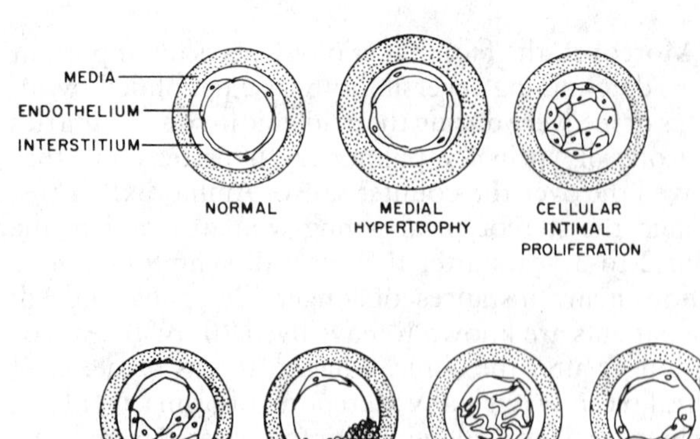

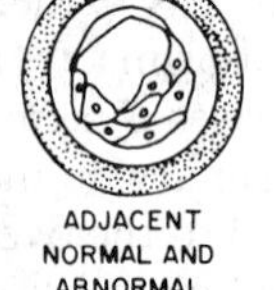

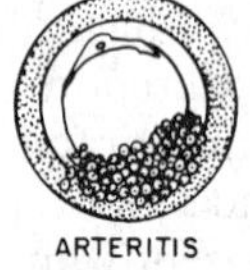

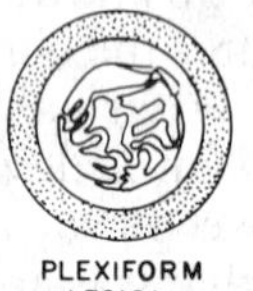

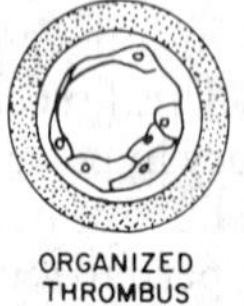

FIGURE 99-4 Vascular lesions in primary pulmonary hypertension. The plexiform lesion, once believed to be the histologic hallmark of primary pulmonary hypertension, has emerged as only one feature of a constellation of lesions.

ing known etiologies as the cause of the pulmonary hypertension, i.e., excluding secondary pulmonary hypertension. Thromboembolic disease is one entity that the pathologist can be helpful in excluding. Clots in small pulmonary arteries and arterioles are commonly found at autopsy in patients with primary pulmonary hypertension, particularly when right ventricular failure has set in. The pathologist is sometimes hard pressed to define the role of these clots—often relatively fresh in appearance—in the pathogenesis of the pulmonary hypertensive state. Although these clots may not have initiated the pulmonary hypertension process in primary pulmonary hypertension, it seems reasonable that they can aggravate and exaggerate pulmonary vascular obstruction.

Pathophysiology

The hemodynamic hallmarks of primary pulmonary hypertension in the resting patient have been indicated above: a combination of a high pulmonary arterial pressure, a normal or low cardiac output, and a normal left atrial (pulmonary wedge) pressure. As a result of this hemodynamic pattern, calculated pulmonary vascular resistance is high, generally leading to the logical conclusion that the resistance vessels, i.e., the small muscular arteries and arterioles, are the predominant sites of vascular obstruction. During exercise, as cardiac output increases, pulmonary arterial pressures increase further; the increments in pressure in the pulmonary hypertensive circuit are much more striking than in the normotensive pulmonary circulation.

Pulmonary vasodilators are currently administered acutely for testing the responsiveness of the pulmonary circulation.[41] Among these, prostacyclin has become the gold standard, but other vasodilators are often tried as well. Several clinical and hemodynamic changes are sought as desirable endpoints: (1) improvement in exercise tolerance; this increase in physical capacity is usually accompanied by an increase in cardiac output, which in turn improves oxygen delivery to peripheral organs and tissues; (2) a decrease in the level of pulmonary arterial hypertension, both at rest and during exercise; (3) a decrease in calculated pulmonary vascular resistance; optimally, this decrease should entail an increase in cardiac output (with minimal increase in heart rate) accompanied by a decrease in pulmonary arterial pressure; and (4) since pulmonary vasodilators are also systemic vasodilators, pulmonary vasodilation has to be effected without evoking undue systemic hypotension and tachycardia.

The combination of right-sided heart catheterization and vasodilator testing provides a comprehensive view of the hemodynamic state of the patient and a baseline for future noninvasive studies, such as serial echocardiograms.

Clinical Picture

In its early stages, the disease is difficult to recognize. In the sporadic case, the first clue is often an abnormal chest radiograph (Fig. 99-1) or electrocardiograph indicative of right ventricular hypertrophy (Fig. 99-5). Both are late manifestations. The existence of right ventricular enlargement is generally confirmed by echocardiography. By the time these changes appear, however, pulmonary hypertension is moderate to severe and generally long-standing. Initial complaints, particularly easy fatigability and chest discomfort, tend to be discounted, i.e., attributed to being "out of shape" except when the index of suspicion is high, e.g., as during an outbreak of "primary" pulmonary hypertension, such as that associated with the ingestion of Aminorex, or in patients with a history of familial pulmonary hypertension (Table 99-1).

When the disease is advanced, the activities of daily life are progressively circumscribed by increasing nonspecific discomfort. Dyspnea, particularly during exercise, becomes incapacitating. Some patients develop a nondescript type of chest pain along with breathlessness. Other common symptoms are weakness, fatigue, and syncope on effort (Table 99-1). Infrequently, an enlarged pulmonary artery causes hoarseness because of compression of the left recurrent laryngeal nerve. In time, right-sided heart failure develops.

Patients with severe pulmonary hypertension seem prone to sudden death. Death has occurred unexpectedly during normal activities, cardiac catheterization, and surgical procedures and after the administration of barbiturates or anesthetic agents. The mechanisms for sudden death are not clear. In a few instances, severe bradycardia and atrioventricular (AV) dissociation have preceded cardiac arrest.

It was noted above that as far as clinical manifestations and physical examination are concerned, primary pulmonary hypertension has an advantage over secondary pulmonary hypertension in that its manifestations are not complicated by those of underlying cardiac or respiratory disease. On physical examination, the jugular venous pulse usually shows a prominent *a* wave. Right ventricular hypertrophy causes a heave along the left sternal border, and a distinct systolic impulse is palpable over the region of the main pulmonary artery (Chap. 10). The pulmonic component of the second sound is markedly accentuated, the second heart sound is narrowly split, and an ejection click is heard in the pulmonic

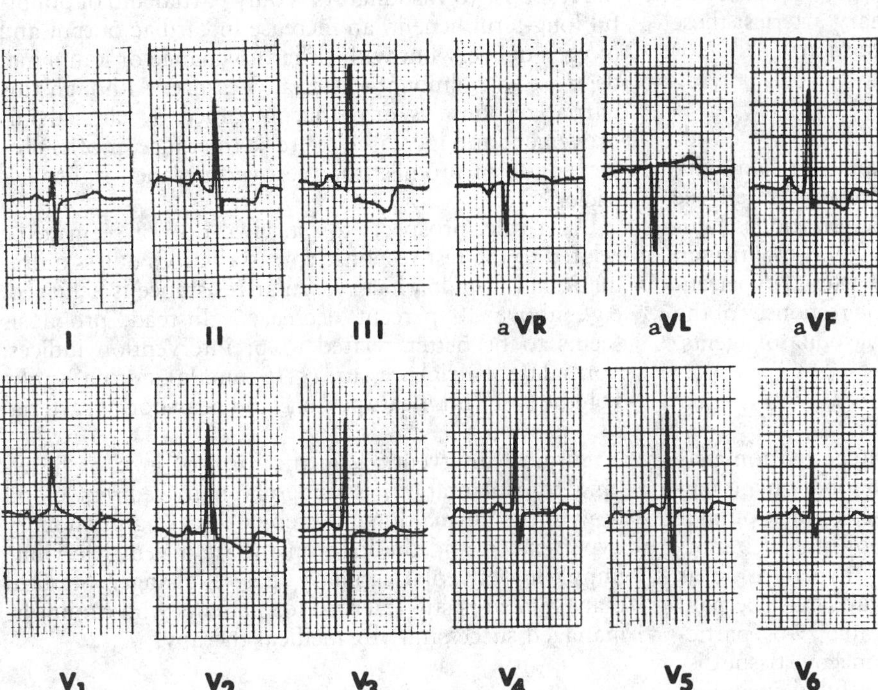

FIGURE 99-5 Electrocardiogram in patients with primary pulmonary hypertension and cor pulmonale.

area. Often a fourth heart sound emanating from the hypertrophied right ventricle is heard at the lower left sternal border. In some patients a midsystolic murmur is audible at the pulmonic area; as pulmonary arterial pressures approximate systemic arterial levels, the murmur of pulmonary valvular regurgitation often appears. (See also Chap. 11.)

The onset of right ventricular failure is accompanied by jugular venous distension and a gallop (S_3); inspiration intensifies the gallop. The liver becomes enlarged and tender and a hepatojugular reflux can be elicited; in time dilation of the failing right ventricle leads to tricuspid regurgitation manifested by a holosystolic murmur, best heard in the fourth interspace to the left of the sternum, that increases in intensity during inspiration. Tricuspid regurgitation is a feature of the echocardiographic findings. The liver develops expansile pulsations synchronous with the heart beat. Hydrothorax and ascites are uncommon even in the face of hepatomegaly and peripheral edema.

Special Studies

Direct determination of pulmonary circulatory pressures by right-sided heart catheterization is the only way to prove the diagnosis of pulmonary hypertension; however, other studies that are less direct can strongly suggest that it is present. Since the diagnosis of "primary" is one of exclusion, a variety of tests are undertaken, usually in the hope of identifying a more treatable disease than primary pulmonary hypertension.

Chest Radiography and Electrocardiography

In the early stages, the chest radiograph is generally normal. Later it shows cardiac enlargement in association with enlargement of the pulmonary trunk while the peripheral pulmonary arterial branches are attenuated; the lung fields appear oligemic (Fig. 99-1). Although fullness of the central pulmonary arterial trunks and peripheral "pruning" are distinctive, appearances vary somewhat from patient to patient in accord with the level and pace of the pulmonary hypertension and the age of the patient. (See also Chap. 14.) Radiographic evidence of right ventricular enlargement usually becomes overt only late in the course of the pulmonary hypertension. The electrocardiogram almost always shows right axis deviation, right ventricular enlargement, and usually, right atrial enlargement. (Chap. 13.)

The Echocardiogram

Two-dimensional echocardiography confirms the enlargement and hypertrophy of right atrium and ventricle, tricuspid regurgitation, and pulmonic valvular regurgitation.[42] At the same time, left ventricular structure and function are normal. The determination of right ventricular ejection fraction using radionuclide techniques can be helpful in evaluating the extent to which the excessive right ventricular afterload has compromised the right ventricle. This applies not only to primary pulmonary hypertension, but also to other disorders that lead to severe pulmonary hypertension, e.g., chronic obstructive airways disease and congenital heart disease. (See also Chap. 15.)

Lung Scans

The lung scan fails to disclose major perfusion defects. Angiography is done in selected cases to exclude pulmonary emboli. Lung scans can be particularly helpful, not only in excluding emboli in distal vessels, but also in calling attention to the possibility of large, long-standing organized clots in the major pulmonary arteries; these clots may be amenable to surgical resection.

Right-Sided Heart Catheterization

The results of cardiac catheterization are consistent with diffuse obliterative disease of the pulmonary arterial tree (see "Pathophysiology"). Cardiac catheterization is valuable in quantifying the hemodynamic abnormalities, in excluding cardiac causes of pulmonary arterial hypertension, and in assessing the hemodynamic responses of the heart and of pulmonary circulation to vasodilator agents.

Diagnosis

The diagnosis of primary pulmonary hypertension rests on two pillars: (1) the detection of pulmonary hypertension and (2) exclusion of known causes of high pulmonary arterial pressure. The history is of utmost importance. Before categorizing pulmonary hypertension as "primary" or "unexplained," due regard must be paid to the exclusion of known etiologies (Table 99-3), particularly thromboembolic disease and connective tissue disorders. Pulmonary function tests are useful in excluding diffuse pulmonary disorders, particularly interstitial fibrosis and granuloma. Serologic testing can point the way to covert connective tissue disorders. Abnormal liver function tests can signal the coexistence of portal and pulmonary hypertension. The value of cardiac catheterization in eliminating acquired or congenital heart disease has been indicated above. Unfortunately, by the time pulmonary hypertension complicating heart disease is recognized, the anatomic lesions are often far advanced so that the obliterative pulmonary vascular disease may be irreversible. One notable exception is the dramatic improvement that often follows surgical removal of organized clots from the walls of major pulmonary arteries.

Treatment

Until a few years ago, the prospects for treating primary pulmonary hypertension were entirely medical and empirical. Because of its rarity and high morbidity and mortality, a variety of approaches were used: vasodilators (nitrates, calcium channel blockers, diazoxide), anticoagulants (warfarin), cardiotonic agents (digoxin), diuretics (furosemide), and oxygen.[43] More recently, with the advent first of heart-lung transplantation and then of single-lung transplantation, the therapeutic options have increased considerably.

Goals and Prognosis

Medical management now centers around the use of pulmonary vasodilators in the hope of achieving a sustained decrease in pulmonary arterial pressure along with an increased or unchanged cardiac output, an increase in oxygen delivery to the tissues, and an unchanged systemic arterial blood pressure; calculated pulmonary vascular resistance would decrease concomitantly.[41,44] Unfortunately, this desirable hemodynamic constellation has proved difficult to achieve. Most often, the response to vasodilators is only partial and of doubtful long-term benefit: an increase in cardiac output and oxygen delivery but with either no change or a minimal decrease in pulmonary arterial pressure. Although this partial response is often accompanied by clinical improvement and increased exercise tolerance, it offers little long-term promise for the overburdened right ventricle.

As a rule, prospects for survival do not seem to be related to the test response to vasodilators unless a dramatic fall in pulmonary vascular resistance is achieved, e.g., above 30 percent decrease.[45] Instead, prognosis seems to be better related to preintervention indices: normal right atrial pressure (<10 mmHg), normal stroke volume (>17 mL/beats per m^2), and near-normal arterial oxygenation.

Surgical intervention, in the form of lung or heart-lung transplantation, is undertaken to redirect blood flow to the normal lung, thereby decreasing pulmonary hypertension and the load on the right ventricle while improving alveolar-capillary gas exchange. Surgical management is still reserved for patients who cannot be managed successfully by medical therapy.

Vasodilator Agents

Various agents have been tried over the years as pulmonary vasodilators. These include α-adrenergic antagonists, β-adrenergic agonists, diazoxide, hydralazine, nitrates, and angiotensin converting enzyme inhibitors. In general, these have not withstood the test of time. Experience has also taught that untoward reactions can occur with any pulmonary vasodilator even when low doses are used. However, two categories of agents continue to hold promise: calcium channel-blocking agents and arachidonic acid metabolites.[46]

Drugs That Block Calcium Transport

The designation *calcium channel blocker* refers to a heterogeneous group of agents of different structural, pharmacologic, and electrophysiological properties. (See also Chap. 67.) The agents in this category that are currently receiving the most clinical attention as potential pulmonary vasodilators are nifedipine and diltiazem. Of the two, nifedipine is the more popular. Verapamil, once used extensively, has fallen into disuse, largely because of its undesirable negative inotropic effect.

Nifedipine Nifedipine* is a synthetic agent that is unrelated to other vasoactive or cardiotonic drugs. It is a potent systemic vasodilator that is used for the treatment of coronary vasospasm. Although it has significant direct negative inotropic effects, these are usually not prominent clinically because of the reflex sympathetic stimulation of the heart; it does not possess antiarrhythmic properties. In an experimental model of pulmonary hypertension in the dog, it was thought to be more effective than either verapamil or diltiazem. It is now the agent of choice for empiric therapy. Both short- and long-acting preparations are available. The dosage is generally ti-

*This use is not listed in the manufacturer's directive.

trated to the maximal tolerable level based on avoiding untoward systemic effects, i.e., hypotension, headache, dizziness, and flushing.[47] Considerable caution is necessary in administering the higher dosages, however, because side effects can occur precipitously and be life threatening. In one study, 64 patients with primary pulmonary hypertension were treated with high doses of calcium channel blockers.[48] Seventeen patients responded to treatment with nifedipine (13 patients) or diltiazem (4 patients) and were alive after 5 years.

In some clinics, initial evaluation of pulmonary vasodilator capability using right-sided heart catheterization and test doses of Epoprostenol precedes the administration of nifedipine or diltiazem.[49] Acetylcholine can be useful as a substitute for Epoprostenol, which is still experimental. Almost invariably, those patients with favorable hemodynamic responses to Epoprostenol during this trial subsequently experience a favorable response to the maintenance use of a calcium channel blocker. Optimal dosage of the calcium channel blocker that is intended for oral maintenance therapy can also be estimated by administering escalating doses of the agent during the trial, either until the desired pulmonary hemodynamic effects are achieved or until systemic side effects preclude further increase in dosage. It should be emphasized that generalizations about the lasting value of vasodilator testing is difficult because of inconsistencies, especially with respect to increasing refractoriness as vasodilator therapy is continued, because of either progression of the disease or tachyphylaxis.[11]

Arachidonic Acid Metabolites

Epoprostenol (prostacyclin, PGI_2), a metabolite of arachidonic acid, continues to be a major focus of experimental attention as a pulmonary vasodilator. The lungs secrete prostacyclin into the blood stream where it has a short biological half-life, i.e., 2 to 3 min. In principle, it is attractive for the treatment of primary pulmonary hypertension on several accounts: (1) it is a pulmonary vasodilator; (2) it inhibits platelet aggregation; and (3) it inhibits proliferation of vascular smooth muscle. Unfortunately, it suffers the disadvantage of requiring continuous intravenous infusion, which is currently being done using portable pumps.[46] Analogues that can be given orally or by other noninvasive routes are being sought. Currently, its most effective use, aside from testing for pulmonary vascular responsivity, is to tide over responsive patients until the time of lung or heart-lung transplantation.

Most investigators continue to have high expectations for the exogenous prostaglandins, derivatives of arachidonic acid metabolism, as pulmonary vasodilators.[50,51] Among these are prostaglandin E_1 (PGE_1; Alprostadil) and Epoprostenol and its stable analogue, Lloprost. As yet, all share the disadvantage of requiring continuous intravenous infusion to be effective. (See also Chap. 30.)

Anticoagulant Therapy

Since 1984, when Fuster et al., in a nonrandomized clinical trial, showed that long-term survival was improved in patients with primary pulmonary hypertension by anticoagulant therapy (warfarin in low doses), some clinics routinely administer anticoagulants to patients with primary pulmonary hypertension.[52] Others delay until right-sided heart failure ensues. The high incidence of antemortem clots in the small pulmonary arteries and arterioles of patients with primary pulmonary hypertension support the practice of anticoagulation in primary pulmonary hypertension, at least when right ventricular failure is present. The usual regimens of anticoagulation are used. (See Chaps. 7 and 68.)

Heart-Lung and Lung Transplantation

Only one-third of patients with primary pulmonary hypertension are responsive to pulmonary vasodilator therapy, at least in the short term.[45] When pulmonary hypertensive disease has progressed, or threatens to progress, to the stage of right ventricular enlargement (cor pulmonale) and right ventricular failure, the physician and patient are left with few therapeutic options other than heart-lung or single-lung transplantation.[53,54] These procedures are currently being done at specialized centers, almost invariably handicapped by shortage of donor lungs. Not infrequently, a candidate for heart-lung or lung transplantation who has passed screening for transplantation can wait for 6 months to 1 year before a donor lung or heart-lung become available. In the interim, intensive rehabilitative measures, including nutritional support, is provided to tide the patient over the waiting period. In some institutions, prostacyclin, administered continuously by vein, is available as a pulmonary vasodilator to decrease the right ventricular overload.[53]

In the 1980s, heart-lung transplantation accounted for 40 percent of transplantation for end-stage, primary pulmonary hypertension. By the late 1980s, the percentage had fallen to 25 percent as the procedure became increasingly popular for treating Eisenmenger's syndrome, cystic fibrosis, and COPD. The anticipated survival rates now of combined heart-lung transplantation are 60 percent at 1 year and 56 percent at 2 years. The operative mortality is less than 20 percent. Although single-lung transplantation is gradually supplanting combined heart-lung transplantation, for many bilateral pulmonary disorders, combined heart-lung transplantation (or sequential single-lung transplantation) is still preferred for infectious diseases, such as cystic fibrosis or bronchiectasis.

In the last few years, single-lung transplantation, first used for idiopathic pulmonary fibrosis, has evolved as the operation of choice for end-stage primary pulmonary hypertension.[55] Originally, heart-lung transplantation was favored over single lung because of the fear that severe right ventricular failure was irremediable. Single-lung transplantation, however, by dropping pulmonary arterial pressures to near-normal levels, has proved to restore right ventricular function rapidly and dramatically even when the right ventricle is massively enlarged. As yet, relatively few single-lung transplants for primary pulmonary hypertension have been performed worldwide; however, the results have been impressive. At the end of 1990, 13 of 16 patients who had undergone single-lung transplantation had survived (67 percent survival).

Two aspects of transplantation merit emphasis: (1) intensive rehabilitation, before and after the surgery, are essential elements in influencing postoperative morbidity and mortality and (2) serious postoperative complications are common: rejection, infections, and disturbed healing of the airways. Chronic rejection, resulting in bronchiolitis obliterans, is particularly dreaded, but has a higher incidence after heart-lung than after single-lung transplantation.[56,57]

Prognosis

The diagnosis of primary pulmonary hypertension carries with it a poor prognosis for medical management unless pulmonary vasodilators succeed in decreasing pulmonary vascular resistance. Although death usually occurs within a few years after the onset of symptoms, instances of long-term survival do occur. As noted above, exceptions to the rule of a short and fatal course were highlighted by the Aminorex epidemic in patients in whom the drug was stopped. Experience with the toxic oil syndrome in Spain is in keeping with the Aminorex experience. At present, there is no specific medical treatment for primary pulmonary hypertension. Pulmonary vasodilators have, in about one-third of patients, improved exercise tolerance and the quality of life. The cause of death in patients managed medically is generally right ventricular failure. In some patients, sudden death terminates the illness.

Although surgical intervention is still in its infancy, many instances of dramatic improvement for at least 1 to 2 years after single-lung transplantation already exist. Although complications are generally manageable and optimism is high, longer term follow-up than 1 to 2 years is being awaited.

PULMONARY VENO-OCCLUSIVE DISEASE

This is the least common of all types of unexplained pulmonary hypertension. Not infrequently, the patient is thought to have primary arterial pulmonary hypertension until manifestations inconsistent with pulmonary precapillary disease, such as pulmonary congestion and edema, redirect attention to the pulmonary small veins and venules. Presumably the disorder begins as an inflammatory-thrombotic process in the small pulmonary veins and venules and ends in fibrous obliteration of the venous and venular lumens. Presumably as a secondary phenomenon, the distal pulmonary arterial tree also develops obstructive lesions that are generally proliferative ("reactive") rather than inflammatory in nature; the intervening capillary bed is remarkably normal. The pulmonary veno-occlusive lesions have been attributed to an inflammatory response to vascular injury followed by thrombosis and scarring. Among the postulated etiologies (based on exceedingly sparse evidence) are viral illness, chemotherapy, toxins, and mediastinal fibrosis.[58–60]

When the pulmonary hypertension is suspected of originating distal to the pulmonary capillary bed, mitral valve disease or myocardial dysfunction or even left atrial myxoma has a greater likelihood of being the cause than does primary pulmonary veno-occlusive disease. More esoteric etiologies for pulmonary venous hypertension to be excluded in arriving at the diagnosis are congenital atresia of pulmonary veins, fibrosing mediastinitis, and coexistent phlebitis of systemic and pulmonary veins.[59]

Clinical Picture

Predominantly children and young adults are affected, but the age has ranged from infancy to 48 years. There seems to be no sex difference. Although hints exist of possibly related familial cardiac disorders, the number of patients is too few to do more than raise suspicion of a familial or common environmental cause.

Clinical suspicion of this disorder generally arises when a patient with congested and edematous lungs proves to have a normal mitral valve and left ventricle. This stereotype is not always encountered, however, and some patients have carried the diagnosis of primary pulmonary arterial hypertension until autopsy disclosed the characteristic pulmonary venous lesions.

The cardinal signs are dyspnea and fatigue or exertion in conjunction with evidence of pulmonary hypertension; the pulmonary venous rather than pulmonary arterial etiology is suggested by radiologic evidence of postcapillary pulmonary hypertension without evidence of involvement of the left side of the heart (Fig. 99-6*A*). Pleural effusions are common. Cyanosis, syncope, hemoptysis, and finger clubbing have been inconsistent findings. Rarely, systemic embolization may occur.

Hemodynamics

Cardiac catheterization discloses a high pulmonary arterial pressure with a normal pulmonary wedge (and left ventricular end-diastolic) pressure. The low wedge pressure has been attributed to discontinuities and channels of high resistance between the pulmonary capillaries and the pulmonary and bronchial venous channels so that wedging interrupts all sources of flow distal to the area blocked by the catheter.

Pathology

Few lung biopsies have been done during life. At autopsy, both lungs are involved. The lungs are the seat of congestion, edema, and focal fibrosis, which may become extensive. The venous lesions may be more marked in one region than in another. Although the small pulmonary arteries as well as the small pulmonary veins are affected, the lesions are different (Fig. 99-6*B*). Most striking are the morphologic changes in the pulmonary veins and venules, which are narrowed or occluded by intimal proliferation and fibrosis; up to 95 percent of the veins and venules may be affected in this way, but complete occlusion is uncommon. Bronchial veins and bronchopulmonary anastomoses share in the occlusive process. Hypertrophy in the walls of the pulmonary arteries may be quite striking. In contrast to the pulmonary arterial and venous systems, the pulmonary capillary bed is generally unaffected. Thrombi in the pulmonary arteries are common.[58]

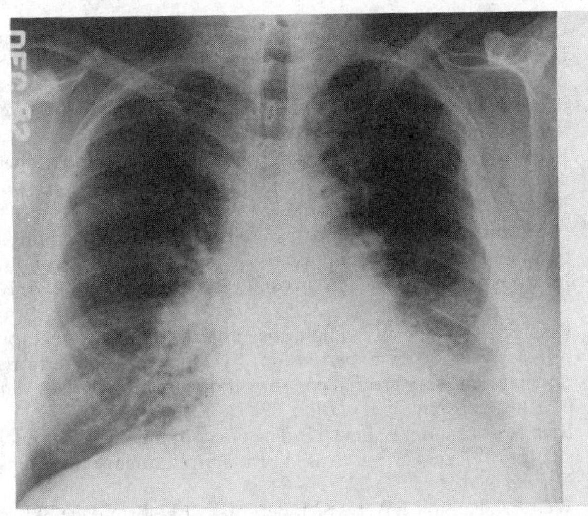

A

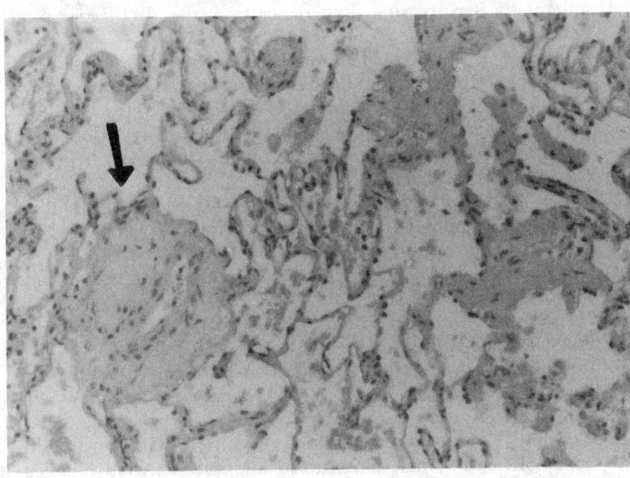

B

FIGURE 99-6 Pulmonary veno-occlusive disease proven by open lung biopsy. *A.* Chest radiograph. Pulmonary interstitial edema is marked at both bases. *B.* Lung biopsy. In addition to obliterative pulmonary venular disease, the pulmonary arterioles (arrow) showed intimal proliferation and medical hypertrophy. *(Courtesy of Dr. G.G. Pietra.)*

Treatment

Medical management has been disappointing, since the lesions are generally irreversible. An occasional patient has been reported to do well on pulmonary vasodilators.[59] The usual duration after recognition ranges from a few weeks in infants to several years in adults, with 7 being the maximum. These patients are also candidates for single-lung or heart-lung transplantation.

REFERENCES

1. Fishman AP: Hypoxia and its effects on the pulmonary circulation. How and where it acts. *Circ Res* 1976; 38:221–231.
2. Fishman AP: The enigma of hypoxic pulmonary vasoconstriction. In: Fishman AP (ed): *The Pulmonary Circulation: Normal and Abnormal.* Philadelphia, University of Pennsylvania Press, 1990: 109–130.
3. Faber CN, Yousem SA, Dauber JH, Griffith BP, Hardesty RL, Paradis IL: Pulmonary capillary hemangiomatosis. A report of three cases and a review of the literature. *Am Rev Respir Dis* 1989; 140:808–813.
4. Fishman AP: *The Pulmonary Circulation: Normal and Abnormal.* Philadelphia, University of Pennsylvania Press, 1990: 1–551.
5. Harris P, Heath D: The structure of the normal pulmonary blood vessels after infancy. In: Harris P, Heath D (eds): *The Human Circulation, Its Form and Function in Health and Disease.* Edinburgh, Churchill Livingstone, 1986: 30–47.
6. O'Rourke PP, Crone RK, Vacanti JP, Ware JH, Lillehei CW, Parad RB, et al: Extracorporeal membrane oxygenation and conventional medical therapy in neonates with persistent pulmonary hypertension of the newborn: A prospective randomized study. *Pediatrics* 1989; 84:967–973.
7. Reid LM: Vascular remodeling. In: Fishman AP (ed): *The Pulmonary Circulation: Normal and Abnormal.* Philadelphia, University of Pennsylvania Press, 1990: 259–282.
8. Ryan US: Endothelial processing of biologically active materials. In: Fishman AP (ed): *The Pulmonary Circulation: Normal and Abnormal.* Philadelphia, University of Pennsylvania Press, 1990: 69–84.
9. Evans JN, Coflesky JT: Endothelial and smooth muscle cell interaction. In: Fishman AP (ed): *The Pulmonary Circulation: Normal and Abnormal.* Philadelphia, University of Pennsylvania Press, 1990: 57–68.
10. Nicod P, Peterson K, Levine M, Dittrich H, Buchbinder M, Chappuis F, et al: Pulmonary angiography in severe chronic pulmonary hypertension. *Ann Intern Med* 1987; 107:565–568.
11. Beard JT II, Byrd BF III: Saline contrast enhancement of trivial Doppler tricuspid regurgitation signals for estimating pulmonary arterial pressure. *Am J Cardiol* 1988; 62:486–488.
12. Palevsky HI, Schloo BL, Pietra GG, Weber KT, Janicki JS, Rubin E, et al: Primary pulmonary hypertension. Vascular structure, morphometry, and responsiveness to vasodilator agents. *Circulation* 1989; 80:1207–1221.
13. Edwards WD: The pathology of secondary pulmonary hypertension. In: Fishman AP (ed): *The Pulmonary Circulation: Normal and Abnormal.* Philadelphia, University of Pennsylvania Press, 1990: 329–342.
14. Dev V, Shrivastava S: Time course of changes in pulmonary vascular resistance and the mechanism of regression of pulmonary arterial hypertension after balloon mitral valvuloplasty. *Am J Cardiol* 1991; 67:439–442.
15. Moser KM: Thromboembolic pulmonary hypertension. In: Fishman AP (ed): *The Pulmonary Circulation: Normal and Abnormal.* Philadelphia, University of Pennsylvania Press, 1990: 413–434.
16. Ryan KL, Fedullo PF, Davis GB, Vasquez TE, Moser KM: Perfusion scans underestimate the severity of angiographic and hemodynamic compromise in chronic thromboembolic pulmonary hypertension. *Chest* 1988; 93:1180–1185.
17. Ricou F, Nicod PH, Moser KM, Peterson KL: Catheter-based intravascular ultrasound imaging of chronic thromboembolic pulmonary disease. *Am J Cardiol* 1991; 67:749–752.
18. Weitzenblum E, Oswald M, Mirhom R, Kessler R, Apprill M: Evolution of pulmonary haemodynamics in COLD patients under long-term oxygen therapy. *Eur Respir J* 1989; 2(suppl 7):669S–673S.
19. Fishman AP: Cor pulmonale: General aspects. In: Fishman AP (ed): *Pulmonary Diseases and Disorders,* 2d ed. New York, McGraw-Hill, 1990: 999–1048.
20. Matthay RA, Shub C: Imaging techniques for assessing pulmonary artery hypertension and right ventricular performance with special reference to COPD. *J Thorac Imag* 1990; 5:47–67.
21. Tramarin R, Torbicki A, Marchandise B, Laaban JP, Morpurgo M: Doppler echocardiographic evaluation of pulmonary artery pressure in chronic obstructive pulmonary disease. A European multicentre study. *Eur Heart J* 1991; 12:103–111.
22. Maeda S, Katsura H, Chida K, Imai T, Kuboki K, Watanabe C, et al: Lack of correlation between P pulmonale and right atrial overload in chronic obstructive airways disease. *Br Heart J* 1991; 65:132–136.
23. Weitzenblum E, Sautegeau A, Ehrhart M, Mammoser M, Pelletier A: Long-term oxygen therapy can reverse the progression of pulmonary hypertension in patients with chronic obstructive pulmonary disease. *Am Rev Respir Dis* 1985; 131:493–498.
24. Brown G: Pharmacologic treatment of primary and secondary pulmonary hypertension. *Pharmacotherapy* 1991; 11:137–156.
25. Yousem SA: The pulmonary pathologic manifestations of the CREST syndrome. *Hum Pathol* 1990; 21:467–474.

26. Shuck JW, Oetgen WJ, Tesar JT: Pulmonary vascular response during Raynaud's phenomenon in progressive systemic sclerosis. *Am J Med* 1985; 78:221–227.
27. Fishman AP: Pulmonary hypertension and cor pulmonale. In: Fishman AP (ed): *Pulmonary Diseases and Disorders,* 2d ed. New York, McGraw-Hill, 1988: 999–1048.
28. Weitzenblum E, Apprill M, Krieger J, Ehrhart M, Kurtz D: Sleep disordered breathing and pulmonary hypertension. *Eur Respir J Suppl* 1990; 11:523S–526S.
29. Groves BM, Brundage BH, Elliott CG, Koerner SK, Fisher JD, Peter RH, et al: Pulmonary hypertension associated with hepatic cirrhosis. In: Fishman AP (ed): *The Pulmonary Circulation: Normal and Abnormal.* Philadelphia, University of Pennsylvania Press, 1990: 359–369.
30. Rich S: NIH Registry on Primary Pulmonary Hypertension: Baseline characteristics of the patients enrolled. In: Fishman AP (ed): *The Pulmonary Circulation: Normal and Abnormal.* Philadelphia, University of Pennsylvania Press, 1990: 451–458.
31. D'Alonzo GE, Barst RJ, Ayres SM, Bergofsky EH, Brundage BH, Detre KM, et al: Survival in patients with primary pulmonary hypertension. *Ann Intern Med.* 1991; 115:343–349.
32. Albelda SM: Role of growth factors in pulmonary hypertension. In: Fishman AP (ed): *The Pulmonary Circulation: Normal and Abnormal.* Philadelphia, University of Pennsylvania Press, 1990: 201–216.
33. Benitz WE: Inhibition of proliferation of vascular smooth muscle cells by heparin. In: Fishman AP (ed): *The Pulmonary Circulation: Normal and Abnormal.* Philadelphia, University of Pennsylvania Press, 1990: 187–200.
34. Hajjar KA, Nachman RL: Endothelial cell modulation of coagulation and fibrinolysis. In: Fishman AP (ed): *The Pulmonary Circulation: Normal and Abnormal.* Philadelphia, University of Pennsylvania Press, 1990: 231–244.
35. Voelkel NF, Weir EK: Etiologic mechanisms in primary pulmonary hypertension. In: Weir EK, Reeves JT (eds): *Pulmonary Vascular Physiology and Pathophysiology.* New York, Marcel Dekker, 1989: 513–539.
36. Koerner SK: Pulmonary hypertension: Etiology and clinical evaluation. *J Thorac Imag* 1988; 3:25–31.
37. Gurtner HP: Aminorex pulmonary hypertension. In: Fishman AP (ed): *The Pulmonary Circulation: Normal and Abnormal.* Philadelphia, University of Pennsylvania Press, 1990: 397–412.
38. Newman JH, Loyd JE: Familial pulmonary hypertension. In: Fishman AP (ed): *The Pulmonary Circulation: Normal and Abnormal.* Philadelphia, University of Pennsylvania Press, 1990: 301–313.
39. Lopez-Sendon J, Sanchez MAG, De Juan MJM, Coma-Canella I: Pulmonary hypertension in the toxic oil syndrome. In: Fishman AP (ed): *The Pulmonary Circulation: Normal and Abnormal.* Philadelphia, University of Pennsylvania Press, 1990: 385–396.
40. Pietra GG, Edwards WD, Kay JM, Rich S, Kernis J, Schloo B, et al: Histopathology of primary pulmonary hypertension. A qualitative and quantitative study of pulmonary blood vessels from 58 persons in The National Heart, Lung and Blood Institute, Primary Pulmonary Hypertension Registry. *Circulation* 1989; 80:1198–1206.
41. Weir EK: Acute vasodilator testing and pharmacological treatment of primary pulmonary hypertension. In: Fishman AP (ed): *The Pulmonary Circulation: Normal and Abnormal.* Philadelphia, University of Pennsylvania Press, 1990: 485–500.
42. Eysmann SB, Palevsky HI, Reichek N, Hackney K, Douglas PS: Echo/Doppler and hemodynamic correlates of vasodilator responsiveness in primary pulmonary hypertension. *Chest* 1991; 99:1066–1071.
43. Groves BM, Turkevich D, Donnellan K, Voelkel N, Robertson AD, Reeves JT: Current approach to treatment of primary pulmonary hypertension. *Chest* 1988; 93(suppl):175S–178S.
44. Palevsky HI, Fishman AP: The management of primary pulmonary hypertension. *JAMA* 1991; 265:1014–1020.
45. Reeves JT, Groves BM, Turkevich D: The case for treatment of selected patients with primary pulmonary hypertension. *Am Rev Respir Dis* 1986; 134:342–346.
46. Higenbottam T, Wheeldon D, Wells F, Wallwork J: Long-term treatment of primary pulmonary hypertension with continuous intravenous epoprostenol (prostacyclin). *Lancet* 1984; 1:1046–1047.
47. Rich S, Brundage BH: High-dose channel-blocking therapy for primary pulmonary hypertension: Evidence for long-term reduction in pulmonary arterial pressure and regression of right ventricular hypertrophy. *Circulation* 1987; 76:135–141.
48. Rich S, Kaufmann E, Levy PS: The effect of high doses of calcium-channel blockers on survival in primary pulmonary hypertension. *N Engl J Med* 1992; 327:76–81.
49. Weir EK, Rubin LJ, Ayres SM, Bergofsky EH, Brundage BH, Detre KM, et al: The acute administration of vasodilators in primary pulmonary hypertension. Experience from the NIH Registry on PPH. *Am Rev Respir Dis* 1989; 140:1623–1630.
50. Halpern SG, Shah PK, Lehrman S, Goldberg HS, Jasper AC, Koerner SK: Prostaglandin E_1 as a screening vasodilator in primary pulmonary hypertension. *Chest* 1987; 92:686–691.
51. Jones K, Higenbottam T, Wallwork J: Pulmonary vasodilation with prostacyclin in primary and secondary pulmonary hypertension. *Chest* 1989; 96:784–789.
52. Fuster V, Steele PM, Edwards WD, Gersh BJ, McGoon MD, Frye RL: Primary pulmonary hypertension: Natural history and the importance of thrombosis. *Circulation* 1984; 70:580–585.
53. Higenbottam TW: The criteria and preparation for heart-lung transplantation. In: Fishman AP (ed): *The Pulmonary Circulation: Normal and Abnormal.* Philadelphia, University of Pennsylvania Press, 1990: 511–521.
54. Reitz BA: Heart-lung transplantation. In: Fishman AP (ed): *Pulmonary Diseases and Disorders,* 2d ed. New York, McGraw-Hill, 1987; pt 18.
55. Calhoon JH, Grover FL, Gibbons WJ, Bryan CL, Levine SM, Bailey SR, et al: Single lung transplantation. Alternative indications and technique. *J Thorac Cardiovasc Surg* 1991; 101:816–824.
56. Estene M, Ketelbent P, Primo G, Yermault JC: Human heart-lung transplantation: Physiological aspects of the denervated lung and post transplant obliterative bronchiolitis. *Am Rev Respir Dis* 1987; 135:976–978.
57. Glanville AR, Baldwin JC, Burke CM, Theodore J, Robin ED: Obliterative bronchiolitis after heart-lung transplantation: Apparent arrest by augmented immunosuppression. *Ann Intern Med* 1987; 107:300–304.
58. Wagenvoort CA: Pulmonary veno-occlusive disease. In: Fishman AP (ed): *The Pulmonary Circulation: Normal and Abnormal.* Philadelphia, University of Pennsylvania Press, 1990: 343–352.
59. Liang MH, Stern S, Fortin PR, Louie DC, Marsh JD, Mudge GH Jr, et al: Fatal pulmonary venoocclusive disease secondary to a generalized venulopathy: A new syndrome presenting with facial swelling and pericardial tamponade. *Arthritis Rheum* 1991; 34:228–233.
60. Salzman GA, Rose UW: Prolonged survival in pulmonary veno-occlusive disease treated with nifedipine. *Chest* 1989; 95:1154–1156.

Chapter 100

Pulmonary Embolism

Joseph S. Alpert, M.D. ■ *James E. Dalen, M.D.*

Each year there are estimated to be approximately 100,000 deaths in the United States due primarily to pulmonary embolism and another 100,000, in patients who have other major diseases, in which it is a significant contributory cause. The majority of deaths occur in patients who are not treated because the diagnosis is not established.[1,2] The mortality of untreated pulmonary embolism is 20 to 30 percent. If the diagnosis is established and appropriate treatment instituted, mortality is less than 10 percent.[3]

In nearly all cases pulmonary embolism originates as deep venous thrombosis (DVT) in the proximal deep venous system in the lower legs.[4–6] Rudolf Virchow recognized deep venous thrombosis in 1858.[7] Some of the factors that predispose to DVT are shown in Table 100-1. The optimal strategy for preventing fatal pulmonary embolism is to recognize patients who are at increased risk of DVT and to institute appropriate prophylactic treatment. In order to reduce the incidence of pulmonary embolism, DVT must be prevented or, at the very least, recognized and treated.

DEEP VENOUS THROMBOSIS

Pathophysiology and Natural History

Virchow pointed out that three factors underlie the development of venous thrombosis: stasis, injury to the intima of the vein, and a hypercoagulable state. Experimental and clinical observations have subsequently confirmed the role of Virchow's triad in the genesis of DVT.[8–12] All three factors need not be present simultaneously for DVT to occur. It appears that stasis and intimal injury are the most important factors in the usual clinical course of events that leads to DVT.[13] The antiphospholipid syndrome and anticardiolipin antibodies are occasionally associated with venous thrombosis.[14,15]

Venous thrombosis appears to originate as a platelet nidus in the vicinity of the venous valves in the lower extremities. Disordered flow near these valves probably contributes to the formation of the platelet nidi.[16,17] Platelet aggregation and activation initiate the clotting cascade with subsequent formation of a red fibrin thrombus. The thrombus gradually grows in size as further platelets, fibrin, and red cells are incorporated. The intrinsic fibrinolytic system is also activated, attacking the fibrin framework of the thrombus. In some instances, the intrinsic fibrinolytic system is successful in dissolving the thrombus; in other situations, pieces of the thrombus break off and embolize to the pulmonary circulation. Residual venous thrombus becomes organized and incorporated into the venous wall.[8,9] (See also Chap. 7.)

It has long been recognized that patients with clinically evident malignancy are often at increased risk for venous thromboembolism and that an unusual form of venous thrombosis, thrombophlebitis migrans, may be a clue to the presence of occult cancer. Thrombophlebitis migrans involves superficial veins, often at atypical sites such as the arms. It may be migratory and resistant to anticoagulant therapy.

More than 90 percent of pulmonary emboli originate in the deep veins of the lower extremities.[4,5] Occasionally, DVT in pelvic veins or thrombi in the right heart give rise to pulmonary emboli. Thrombi localized to the deep venous system of the calf are of limited risk with respect to their tendency to embolize. Once such thrombi propagate into the popliteal vein and/or the veins of the thigh, however, the risk for pulmonary embolism increases

TABLE 100-1
Risk Factors for Deep Venous Thrombosis

Venous stasis, vascular injury, or secondary hypercoagulable states
Surgery (especially involving lower extremities or pelvis)
Trauma (especially fractured hip in the elderly and acute injury of the head and spinal cord)
Bed rest, immobility, stroke, or paralysis
Congestive heart failure, low cardiac output states
Malignancy
Pregnancy
Oral contraceptive agents, estrogen therapy
Obesity
Varicose veins
Inflammatory bowel disease
Advanced age
Prior thromboembolism
Nephrotic syndrome
Sepsis
Primary hypercoagulable state
Antithrombin III deficiency
Protein C deficiency
Protein S deficiency
Disorders of plasminogen and plasminogen activation
Paroxysmal nocturnal hemoglobinuria
Myeloproliferative disorders
Polycythemia vera
Heparin-induced thrombocytopenia
Lupus anticoagulant/anticardiolipin antibodies

TABLE 100-2
Techniques for the Prevention of Deep Venous Thrombosis

Graded compression stockings
Intermittent pneumatic compression
Anticoagulation
Intravenous heparin*
Adjusted dose subcutaneous heparin*
Low-dose subcutaneous heparin†
Low-molecular-weight heparin‡
Low-dose oral warfarin§
Minidose oral warfarin (1 mg/day)
Intravenous dextran
Dihydroergotamine‡
Hirudin‡

*Activated partial thromboplastin time 1.5–2.5 times control
†5000 units subcutaneously every 8–12 h
‡Currently not available in the United States
§Prothrombin time of 2.0 to 3.0 International Normalized Ratio

markedly.[18–22] The explanation may lie in the fact that calf thrombi are small and offer limited risk, even if they embolize. Thus, symptomatic pulmonary embolism usually stems from recurrent episodes of embolization that arise from thrombi in the proximal veins of the lower extremities. (See Table 125-2.)

Most episodes of calf DVT resolve without specific therapy. An occasional symptomatic individual will require anticoagulation. Above the knee, deep venous thrombosis gradually resolves during anticoagulant therapy. Two-thirds of patients will have complete resolution of DVT following 3 months of therapy. Ninety percent of patients will be normal 1 year after an episode of DVT that is treated with 3 months of anticoagulation. Individuals with DVT who receive no therapy frequently develop pulmonary embolism and/or chronic venous insufficiency of the lower extremities.

Prevention

There are multiple techniques to prevent DVT, as shown in Table 100-2.[23,24] Graduated compression stockings (GCS) are basic prophylaxis against deep venous thrombosis and are useful in most hospitalized patients with a single risk factor except those with severe peripheral arterial disease. Prophylactic regimens for specific patient groups are shown in Table 100-3. In medical patients with a factor for increased risk or surgical patients who are over 40 years of age and are undergoing major operations without contraindications, low-dose heparin, 5000 units subcutaneously every 8 to 12 h, is very effective in preventing DVT.[25,26] In patients at higher risk, e.g., in those undergoing hip replacement, in patients with hip fracture, and in men undergoing urologic procedures, low-dose subcutaneous heparin does not provide adequate protection. In these circumstances adjusted-dose heparin [activated partial thromboplastin time (APTT) 31 to 36 s 6 h after injection], low-dose warfarin [International Normalized Ratio (INR) 2.0 to 3.0],[27] intravenous dextran, or the combination of dihydroergotamine and low-dose heparin are more appropriate prophylaxis.[28,29] In patients at increased risk of bleeding, such as those undergoing neurosurgical procedures, intermittent pneumatic compression (IPC) boots have been shown to be effective.[30–32] In patients undergoing elective surgery, these prophylactic therapies should begin prior to the induction of anesthesia as DVT often begins while patients are anesthetized in the operating room. Aspirin and sulfinpyrazone have not been shown to be effective in preventing DVT. Hirudin[33,34] and low-molecular-weight heparin[35–40] appear very promising but are not currently available in the United States; neither is dihydroergotamine.

Diagnosis

If the prophylactic therapies listed above are instituted, the risk of DVT and its potentially lethal complication, pulmonary embolism, is greatly diminished. If prophylactic treatment is not used or if it fails, the clinician must recognize DVT as soon as possible in order to institute treatment to prevent pulmonary embolism. The classic signs of DVT, unilateral leg swelling and tenderness, occur in the minority of cases; most episodes of DVT are clinically silent. Venography or noninvasive tests of venous thrombosis should usually be performed when DVT is suspected.

The most sensitive and specific test for the recognition of DVT is venography[41,42]; but it is invasive and uncomfortable and is therefore seldom performed more than once on a given patient. (See also Chap. 128.)

TABLE 100-3

Prophylaxis against Deep Venous Thrombosis Pulmonary Embolism for Specific Patient Groups

Patient Group	Prophylaxis
Medical or surgical patients under 40 years of age with no clinical risk factors	Early ambulation
Medical patients with one or more risk factors (Table 100-1) or surgical patients over 40 years of age undergoing major operations but with no additional risk factors	GCS; LDH every 8–12 h or IPC
Surgical patients over 40 years of age undergoing major operations and with additional risk factors	GCS; adjusted dose subcutaneous heparin (dextran or IPC are alternatives in patients prone to hematomas or infection)
Very high risk general surgery patients with multiple risk factors	GCS; IPC and adjusted dose subcutaneous heparin (or dextran); in selected patients, perioperative warfarin (INR 2.0–3.0)
Total hip replacement	GCS; adjusted doses of warfarin (INR 2.0–3.0) or heparin (APTT 1.5–2.5 times control 6 h after injection); when available, LMWH (without laboratory control)
Hip fractures	GCS; warfarin (INR 2.0–3.0)
Knee surgery, neurosurgery	GCS; IPC
Acute spinal cord injury with paralysis	GCS; adjusted dose heparin (APTT 31–36 s 6 h after injection)
Multiple trauma	GCS; IPC; warfarin (INR 2.0–3.0) when feasible
Myocardial infarction	GCS; LDH (IVH if anterior infarct or increased risk factors)
Ischemic stroke with lower extremity paralysis	GCS; LDH (alternative: IPC, warfarin)
Long-term indwelling central vein catheter	GCS; warfarin, 1 mg/day
Hip or knee surgery in high risk patients with history of serious, previous pulmonary embolism	GCS; warfarin; consider prophylactic inferior vena cava filter

SOURCE: Modified from Dalen JE, Hirsh J (eds).[24]

NOTE: GCS = graded compression stockings; LDH = low-dose subcutaneous heparin; IPC = intermittent pneumatic compression; INR = International Normalized Ratio; APTT = activated partial thromboplastin time; LMWH = low-molecular-weight heparin; IVH = intravenous heparin.

Impedance plethysmography (IPG) (see Chap. 129) is extremely useful in evaluating patients with suspected DVT and can be performed in 15 to 20 min.[43–45] The correlation between unilaterally positive IPG and venography exceeds 90 percent. A bilaterally normal IPG nearly excludes proximal (above the knee) DVT. The test is less sensitive to DVT confined to the distal leg (below the knee). If the IPG is positive in both legs, venography should be performed (if available) because DVT may or may not be present.[46] The IPG is extremely useful in detecting DVT at the bedside.[18,43] (See also Chap. 129.)

Scanning the legs after the injection of fibrinogen labeled with ^{125}I is a very sensitive test for the diagnosis of DVT.[43] The disadvantage of this test is that the ^{125}I must be injected prior to the development of DVT. This test can be used preoperatively in patients who are at risk of intra- or postoperative DVT. (See also Chap. 134.)

The Doppler technique (Chap. 127) is another noninvasive test for the diagnosis of DVT, but its accuracy is highly dependent on the expertise of the operator. The sensitivity and specificity of this technique in detecting DVT vary widely in different medical centers. The same is true for other tests that have been suggested for the diagnosis of DVT, including the radionuclide venogram, duplex ultrasonography, and the radionuclide-labeled platelet scan. (See also Chap. 127.)

Treatment

If proximal DVT is detected, treatment includes intravenous heparin for 7 to 10 days, followed by oral warfarin therapy begun on day 2 to 3.[47,48] Heparin is given as an intravenous bolus of 5000 units, followed by an infusion of 1000 units per hour; the dosage is adjusted to produce an APTT between 1.5 and 2.5 times control. Warfarin anticoagulation should overlap heparin for 4 to 5 days. Without treatment, pulmonary embolism occurs in 50 percent of patients with proximal DVT. The probability of pulmonary embolism in patients with DVT limited to the distal lower extremity is less than 10 percent, and in this circumstance in an asymptomatic patient, many physicians would not institute heparin treatment. If DVT limited to the distal lower extremity is not treated with heparin, however, repeat IPG is usually indicated to make certain that there has not been extension to the proximal venous circulation.

Some advocate thrombolytic treatment with urokinase, streptokinase, or tissue plasminogen activator (TPA) in patients with symptomatic proximal DVT in order to prevent the postphlebitic syndrome. The incidence of the postphlebitic syndrome in patients treated with heparin is uncertain, however; at present, it is controversial whether or not fibrinolytic therapy prevents the postphlebitic syndrome in patients with DVT.

PULMONARY EMBOLISM

Pathophysiology and Natural History

Pulmonary embolism produces clinically important hemodynamic and respiratory pathophysiologic alterations. The major hemodynamic consequences of pulmonary embolism result from reduction in the cross-sectional area of the pulmonary vascular bed with associated increases in pulmonary vascular resistance and right ventricular afterload.[49–53] Because the reserve capacity of the pulmonary vascular bed is substantial, a single large embolic thrombus (or repeated smaller thrombi) must impact the pulmonary vascular bed before pulmonary vascular resistance and right ventricular afterload increase. In general, more than 50 percent of the pulmonary vascular tree must be occluded before pulmonary arterial pressure increases significantly.[49,50] Small increases in pulmonary arterial pressure resulting from hypoxic pulmonary vasoconstriction may be observed with more minor degrees of pulmonary embolism.[54] Patients with advanced cardiopulmonary disease, e.g., marked left ventricular failure, occasionally develop more severe hemodynamic abnormalities following modest episodes of pulmonary embolism.[52]

Increased right ventricular afterload leads to right ventricular dilatation and eventually failure, with decreased cardiac output and systemic arterial hypotension.[51,55] Dilatation of the right ventricle leads to a shift of the intraventricular septum into the left ventricular cavity. The result is a decrease in left ventricular capacitance and a modest reduction in left ventricular compliance.[56] Of course, left ventricular stroke volume decreases pari passu with falling right ventricular stroke volume. Individuals without prior heart or lung disease who have an acute pulmonary embolism that obstructs more than 50 percent of the pulmonary vascular bed rarely elevate pulmonary arterial or right ventricular systolic pressure above 60 mmHg. Higher values are often observed in patients with chronic, recurrent pulmonary embolism or in individuals with preexisting cardiopulmonary disease and acute pulmonary embolism.

The respiratory consequences of acute pulmonary embolism include the development of increased alveolar dead space, constriction of airway smooth muscle in lung zones with proximal embolism, hypoxemia, and hyperventilation.[54,55] Later in the course of the illness, regional loss of surfactant and pulmonary infarction may occur.

As soon as an embolus obstructs a pulmonary artery, blood flow ceases to the alveoli in that lung zone. Ventilation of these alveoli continues, thereby increasing alveolar dead space. Reduction of carbon dioxide tension in these alveoli results in proximal airway smooth-muscle constriction with a resultant decrease in alveolar ventilation. Teleologically, this is an attempt to correct the initial abnormal increase in alveolar dead space. Unfortunately, it is usually short-lived because carbon dioxide soon arrives in hypoperfused alveoli from adjacent perfused alveoli and from bronchial arterial collateral blood flow.

Arterial hypoxemia is quite common in patients with acute pulmonary embolism. Ventilation/perfusion mismatches and reduced cardiac output contribute to shunting of deoxygenated blood across the pulmonary vascular bed. In addition, patients with massive embolism and right ventricular failure may develop an intracardiac right-to-left shunt as right atrial dilatation stretches and opens a previously closed foramen ovale. Because right atrial pressure exceeds left atrial pressure in this setting, a right-to-left shunt of deoxygenated blood results. This opening of the foramen ovale can also allow a subsequent paradoxical embolus to enter the systemic circulation.

A minority of patients develop minimal or even no hypoxemia following acute pulmonary embolism, as the result of compensatory hyperventilation. Both the respiratory rate and the depth of respiration increase following acute pulmonary embolism. In general, the larger the embolism, the greater the depth of respiration but the slower the respiratory rate. Hyperventilation usually produces arterial hypocarbia and respiratory alkalosis. An occasional patient with massive embolism may develop hypercarbia despite marked hyperventilation.[56] Hyperventilation is probably the result of stimulation of stretch receptors in the pulmonary vascular bed, but this explanation remains controversial.[57] During the first 24 h following an episode of acute pulmonary embolism, alveolar surfactant is depleted, with resultant local atelectasis and edema.[58,59]

Pulmonary infarction or hemorrhage results when distal emboli totally occlude a small pulmonary artery.[60] Infarction following acute pulmonary embolism is often prevented since the pulmonary parenchyma has four sources of oxygen: the airways, the pulmonary arteries, bronchial arterial collateral circulation, and back-diffusion from the pulmonary veins. Some or all of these compensatory mechanisms may be compromised in patients with heart failure or intrinsic lung disease. Consequently, pulmonary infarction is more common under these circumstances.

Patients who survive an initial episode of pulmonary embolism usually do well if the diagnosis is made and appropriate therapy is instituted. The intrinsic fibrinolytic system of the pulmonary vascular bed initiates dissolution of thrombi. With heparin therapy alone, 36 percent of perfusion lung scan defects resolve within 5 days. At 2 weeks, 52 percent of defects have resolved; at 3 weeks, 73 percent; and at 1 year, 76 percent.[61] Arterial hypoxemia and chest roentgenographic abnormalities improve as the thromboemboli resolve.[62] Persistent pulmonary hypertension and chronic cor pulmonale from unresolved embolism are unusual.[63]

Diagnosis of Acute Pulmonary Embolus

One reason that the diagnosis of acute pulmonary embolism is frequently missed is that acute pulmonary embolism may present as one of three different clinical syndromes: pulmonary infarction (or hemorrhage), acute cor pulmonale, or acute "unexplained" dyspnea.[64] The pathophysiology, signs, and symptoms of these three syndromes are quite different. The differential diagnosis and the appropriate diagnostic workup are also different.

Pulmonary Infarction or Hemorrhage

This is the most common presentation of pulmonary embolism. More than 50 percent of all patients in whom pulmonary embolism is diagnosed have signs or symptoms of pulmonary infarction or hemorrhage. The classic symptom is the abrupt onset of pleuritic chest pain, with or without dyspnea. Hemoptysis occurs in a minority of patients. Pleuritic pain in patients with pulmonary infarction or hemorrhage may be caused by intraalveolar hemorrhage due to the influx of blood from the bronchial collateral circulation into obstructed portions of the distal pulmonary circulation.[60] Pulmonary angiography demonstrates submassive embolism with obstruction of distal branches of the pulmonary circulation.

Pulmonary hemorrhage due to bronchial arterial collateral flow usually causes a pulmonary infiltrate on the chest x-ray. Other chest film abnormalities include an elevated diaphragm due to splinting of respiration, or a small pleural effusion that is usually unilateral and may or may not be bloody. One or more of these three chest film abnormalities are present in more than two-thirds of patients with pulmonary infarction or hemorrhage.[65]

On physical examination, tachypnea with a respiratory rate greater than 20 per minute is nearly always present. Signs of right ventricular failure are absent. Examination of the lungs usually reveals rales, wheezes, or evidence of a pleural effusion. A pleural friction rub may be present. Evidence of deep venous thrombosis on physical examination is present in a minority of cases.

The principal differential diagnosis in patients with pulmonary infarction or hemorrhage includes viral or bacterial pneumonitis/pleuritis, which is suggested by a history of a viral prodrome, or of a shaking chill with fever or purulent sputum.

The most useful routine laboratory tests in patients with suspected pulmonary infarction or hemorrhage include the chest x-ray, white blood cell count (WBC) and differential, Grams's stain of sputum if available, and arterial blood gas analysis. The WBC, differential, and sputum examination help to diagnose bacterial pneumonia. Analysis of arterial blood gases in patients with pulmonary infarction or hemorrhage will nearly always demonstrate hypocapnia and respiratory alkalosis secondary to tachypnea. Since pulmonary infarction or hemorrhage usually occurs in patients with submassive pulmonary embolism, however, the arterial P_{O_2} may be in the normal range in patients without prior lung disease.

The most useful screening test for pulmonary embolism is the ventilation/perfusion (V/Q) lung scan.[64] (See Chap. 134.) The most specific finding for acute pulmonary embolism is the presence of large segmental perfusion defects that ventilate normally.[66,67] In the Prospective Investigation of Pulmonary Embolism Diagnosis (PIOPED) study, a normal perfusion scan excluded the diagnosis of pulmonary embolism with an accuracy of 98 percent.[68] A highly probable scan with multiple segmental or lobar perfusion defects that have normal ventilation patterns had a specificity of about 88 percent (Table 100-4). On the other hand, of the 931 patients in PIOPED who had a V/Q scan, only 13 percent were interpreted as high probability and 73 percent were either intermediate probability or low probability (Table 100-5). In addition, of the 251 patients who had pulmonary embolism documented by pulmonary angiography, only 40 percent had a high probability V/Q scan, 58 percent had scans interpreted as intermediate or low probability, and 2 percent had V/Q scans interpreted as near normal or normal (Table 100-6). Thus, patients suspected of having a pulmonary embolus who have an intermediate probability V/Q scan should be considered for either selective pulmonary angiography or additional tests to assess the lower extremities for DVT.

As noted earlier, IPG (Chap. 129) is useful in patients with suspected acute pulmonary embolism, in that it is positive in the majority of patients with acute pulmonary embolism.[20,45,69,70] If the diagnosis remains uncertain after evaluation of the clinical findings, IPG, and V/Q lung

TABLE 100-4
Results of Pulmonary Angiography in 731 Patients with V/Q Scan

V/Q Scan Interpretation	Percent with Angiographic Evidence of Pulmonary Embolism
High probability	88
Intermediate probability	33
Low probability	16
Near normal/normal	9

SOURCE: PIOPED Study.[68]

TABLE 100-5
Interpretations of V/Q Scans in 931 Patients Suspected of Having Pulmonary Embolism

High probability	13 percent
Intermediate probability	39 percent
Low probability	34 percent
Near normal/normal	14 percent

SOURCE: PIOPED Study.[68]

TABLE 100-6
Interpretations of V/Q Scans in 251 Patients with Pulmonary Embolism Documented by Pulmonary Angiography

High probability	40 percent
Intermediate probability	42 percent
Low probability	16 percent
Near normal/normal	2 percent

SOURCE: PIOPED Study.[68]

TABLE 100-7

Indications for Pulmonary Angiography

When examination of clinical findings, V/Q scan, and impedance plethysmography are inconclusive
When there are relative contraindications to anticoagulation
When thrombolytic therapy may be indicated
When inferior vena cava interruption or surgical therapy may be indicated
Recurrent pulmonary embolism, despite therapy
Young patient with uncertain predisposition to deep venous thrombosis

scan, selective pulmonary angiography may be indicated for a definitive diagnosis[69] (see Table 100-7). In some institutions, Doppler sonography (Chap. 127) or venography (Chap. 128) are also used (see below).

Acute Cor Pulmonale

Acute cor pulmonale, the most dramatic presentation of acute pulmonary embolism, occurs when pulmonary embolism obstructs more than 60 to 75 percent of the pulmonary circulation.

The normal response to acute pulmonary embolism is to increase cardiac output and right ventricular systolic pressure in order to overcome the increased resistance in the pulmonary circulation. Acutely, the normal right ventricle can increase its systolic pressure to about 50 to 60 mmHg. Acute increases in right ventricular systolic pressure above this level cause acute right ventricular dilatation and increased filling pressures. As the right ventricle dilates and fails, its stroke volume decreases, leading to decreased cardiac output, hypotension, and possible cardiac arrest.[70] Therefore, in addition to marked, acute dyspnea, patients with acute cor pulmonale may present with signs of decreased cardiac output: hypotension, syncope,[55] or cardiac arrest. On physical examination there are tachypnea and tachycardia and possibly hypotension. Signs of acute right ventricular failure—distended neck veins, right-sided S_3 gallop, and a parasternal heave—are usually present. The lungs may be clear, but signs of DVT may be present.

The most useful diagnostic tests in patients with suspected acute cor pulmonale are the electrocardiogram (ECG), measurement of central venous pressure, and arterial blood gas analysis. The ECG in patients with acute cor pulmonale will often show a new $S_1Q_3T_3$ pattern,[71] incomplete right bundle branch block, and/or signs of right ventricular ischemia.[72] The ECG helps to exclude acute myocardial infarction. Measurement of central venous pressure may be critical in diagnosing acute cor pulmonale in patients who present with systemic hypotension or cardiovascular collapse. If systemic arterial hypotension is due to acute cor pulmonale, right atrial and central venous pressure will be elevated.[70] Arterial blood gas analysis in patients with acute cor pulmonale usually, but not always, demonstrates hypoxemia as well as hypocapnia.[68,73,74] The chest x-ray is not helpful in the diagnosis of acute cor pulmonale and is often unremarkable.

Once the diagnosis of acute cor pulmonale is suspected, it should be confirmed by V/Q lung scan or pulmonary angiography. In unstable patients in whom surgical or thrombolytic therapy may be indicated, it is usually wise to proceed promptly to pulmonary angiography for definitive diagnosis (see Table 100-7).

Acute, Unexplained Dyspnea

The diagnosis of pulmonary embolism is most difficult in patients with submassive pulmonary embolism who do not sustain pulmonary infarction. The ECG remains normal, and there are no physical signs of right ventricular failure. If pulmonary infarction or hemorrhage does not occur, pleuritic pain is absent and there are no specific abnormalities on chest x-ray. In this circumstance, the primary symptom of acute pulmonary embolism is the sudden onset of dyspnea. The only abnormalities on physical examination are tachypnea, possibly tachycardia, and anxiety. The lungs are clear; there are no signs of acute right ventricular failure. Signs of DVT may be present or absent. Thus, many of the commonly obtained clinical variables are not abnormal.

The principal differential diagnoses in patients with acute dyspnea due to pulmonary embolism are left ventricular failure, pneumonia, and the hyperventilation syndrome. Left ventricular failure and pneumonia can usually be excluded by further history, physical examination, and chest x-ray. Patients presenting with dyspnea due to acute pulmonary embolism usually, but not always, have significant hypoxemia.[68,73] Measurement of arterial blood gases while the patient breathes room air may allow one to distinguish between potentially lethal pulmonary embolism and benign hyperventilation. On the other hand, some patients with pulmonary embolism have a normal arterial P_{O_2}.[68,73]

As with other syndromes of acute pulmonary embolism, IPG examination is very helpful, and the diagnosis should be confirmed by V/Q lung scan or pulmonary angiography.

Summary of Laboratory Tests in the Diagnosis of Pulmonary Embolism

Chest X-Ray

The chest x-ray is most useful in evaluating patients with pleuritic chest pain who are suspected of having pulmonary infarction or hemorrhage. Most patients with pulmonary infarction have an infiltrate, an elevated hemidiaphragm due to splinting, or a pleural effusion that is usually small and unilateral and may or may not be bloody.[65] In patients with acute cor pulmonale or acute unexplained dyspnea without pulmonary infarction or hemorrhage, the chest x-ray is usually normal or it may show subtle, nonspecific findings. The combination of unexplained dyspnea, arterial hypoxemia, and a normal chest x-ray should suggest the diagnosis of pulmonary embolism.[67]

Electrocardiogram

The ECG is most helpful in evaluating patients who have massive pulmonary embolism complicated by acute cor pulmonale. In these patients the ECG helps to exclude myocardial infarction and will often demonstrate the ECG correlates of acute cor pulmonale, i.e., a new $S_1Q_3T_3$ pattern, a new incomplete right bundle branch block, or signs of right ventricular ischemia.[65,71,72] These ECG findings are transient and resolve as right ventricular failure resolves. In patients with submassive pulmonary embolism, the ECG is not helpful. It may show nonspecific ST changes or sinus tachycardia. An occasional patient develops atrial fibrillation or flutter following an episode of pulmonary embolism.

Arterial Blood Gases

The vast majority of patients with acute pulmonary embolism have tachypnea; therefore, arterial blood gas analysis demonstrates hypocapnia and respiratory alkalosis.[65,68,73] The arterial P_{O_2} (breathing room air) is usually, but not always, decreased in patients with dyspnea due to pulmonary embolism.[65,68,73] In patients with pulmonary infarction or hemorrhage who have submassive pulmonary embolism, the arterial P_{O_2} may be normal or near normal, particularly if there is no prior pulmonary disease. The arterial blood gases should be measured while the patient is breathing room air. In patients receiving supplemental oxygen who do not have overt, significant, coexistent pulmonary disease, it is only necessary to discontinue supplemental oxygen for 5 to 10 min in order to assess baseline values.[74] It is important to emphasize that arterial blood gas changes are nonspecific and should not be used to make the diagnosis of pulmonary embolism. Similarly, a normal arterial P_{O_2} (780 mmHg) does not exclude the diagnosis.[68]

Ventilation/Perfusion Lung Scans (V/Q Scans)

Perfusion lung scans are extremely sensitive in detecting pulmonary embolism; a normal multiple-view perfusion scan essentially (98 percent) excludes acute pulmonary embolism.[64,65,66,68,75] Unfortunately, perfusion defects are not specific for pulmonary embolism; they may be the result of a wide variety of other pulmonary abnormalities. The specificity of perfusion lung scanning is increased by the use of a ventilation scan.

The scan abnormality most consistent with acute pulmonary embolism is the presence of multiple large segmental perfusion defects that ventilate normally.[64,66–68] The probability of pulmonary embolism with this set of findings exceeds 90 percent.

Unfortunately, as noted above, V/Q scan findings are very often nonspecific.[65,68,76,77] The perfusion scan may show defects that are nonsegmental, and the ventilation scan may show that these perfusion defects ventilate normally. In this circumstance, the diagnosis of acute pulmonary embolism is neither excluded nor confirmed. When this type of nonspecific lung scan is coupled with a strong clinical picture of pulmonary embolism and there is no other reasonable explanation for the patient's symptoms, it may be appropriate to proceed to selective pulmonary angiography and/or to treat for acute pulmonary embolism. The same nonspecific, lung-scan findings coupled with a weak clinical story for pulmonary embolism may be sufficient to make the diagnosis of pulmonary embolism unlikely. The IPG is especially helpful when the lung scan is nonspecific or of intermediate probability. If the IPG is negative, it is usually appropriate to conclude that the patient does not have pulmonary embolism. If the IPG is unilaterally positive, the diagnosis of pulmonary embolism should be pursued further by performing pulmonary angiography or peripheral venography.

The diagnosis of acute pulmonary embolism is not made by the results of the lung scan alone. The clinician must evaluate the clinical findings and the IPG (and arterial blood gas analysis, venography, and Doppler sonography, if performed) together with the results of the lung scan.

Echocardiography

Two-dimensional echocardiographic examination of patients with suspected and documented pulmonary embolism often yields clinically useful information.[78] (See Chap. 15.) Echocardiography may reveal thromboemboli trapped in the right heart chambers, right ventricular dilatation and/or dysfunction, shift of the interatrial septum, and shift of the interventricular septum into the left ventricular cavity with resultant diminution of left ventricular volumes. Coexisting valvular and/or myocardial abnormalities are also readily identified. Transesophageal echocardiography may demonstrate the presence of thrombi in the pulmonary arteries.

Pulmonary Angiography

Pulmonary angiography is the most accurate test for the diagnosis of acute pulmonary embolism.[79] Unfortunately, it is not available in all hospitals and has the disadvantage of being invasive. The mortality from pulmonary angiography is very low when performed by an experienced team[80]; however, the morbidity associated with this test is substantial. Therefore, we do not recommend that pulmonary angiography be performed in all patients in whom pulmonary embolism is suspected, but that the test be reserved for those patients with the specific indications noted in Table 100-7.

The primary contraindication to pulmonary angiography is a history of a severe systemic reaction to contrast media. Relative contraindications include the presence of high-grade ventricular ectopy, left bundle branch block, and coexisting life-threatening disease.[80] Pulmonary angiography should be performed with great caution in patients with suspected primary pulmonary hypertension. When angiography is performed in such patients, mainstream injections into the central pulmonary artery should be avoided. The use of stiff cardiac catheters is associated with an increased incidence of complications, including perforation of the heart.

Pulmonary angiography should be performed only by properly trained physicians. The complications of pulmonary angiography include those due to right-sided heart catheterization (arrhythmias, cardiac perforation) and reactions to contrast media. The ECG and systemic blood pressure should be monitored continuously. Right-sided heart pressures should be measured and recorded.

In patients with submassive pulmonary embolism, it is not necessary to perform main pulmonary arterial injections to visualize the entire pulmonary circulation. Rather, selective or subselective injections should be made into areas shown to have perfusion defects by lung scan. Injections of contrast medium by hand through a flexible, balloon-tipped catheter are often satisfactory.[81] The artery is occluded with the balloon, and the injection is made distal to the occlusion during cineangiography. The diagnostic finding of acute pulmonary embolism is the visualization of intraluminal clot.[79]

In patients with acute cor pulmonale due to massive pulmonary embolism, in whom pulmonary embolectomy may be indicated, mainstream injection into the main pulmonary artery with the use of cut film or cineangiography is appropriate. In this circumstance, the total pulmonary circulation, including the main and proximal right and left pulmonary arteries, must be visualized.

Venography

Venography, a test more widely available than pulmonary angiography, is useful in several circumstances.[41,42] In patients with nonspecific findings or intermediate probability by V/Q lung scan but a positive IPG, venography is appropriate. If the venogram demonstrates DVT, the treatment is the same as if acute pulmonary embolism had been documented. (See Chap. 128.)

D-Dimer

Preliminary studies indicate that the finding of a plasma concentration of D-dimer less than 500 mg/liter virtually rules out the diagnosis of pulmonary embolism.[82] Further studies are indicated.

Occult Malignancies and Pulmonary Embolism

Deep venous thrombosis and its complication, pulmonary embolism, may be clues to the presence of occult cancer, especially in young patients.[83] Malignancies may be present in a wide variety of locations, including the gastrointestinal tract, lung, breast, uterus, and prostate.

Given this association, the evaluation of the patient with venous thrombosis or pulmonary embolism should obviously include a complete history and physical examination, including breast and pelvic examination in women and examination of the prostate in men. Further diagnostic evaluation will be guided by the results of the history taking and physical examination. In the follow-up of patients with pulmonary embolism, the clinician should be alert to signs or symptoms of early cancer. This is particularly the case if no other factors predisposing to the development of DVT (Table 100-1) are present.

Paradoxical Embolism

Paradoxical embolism of the systemic circulation is a rare complication of DVT that may occur in patients who have an intracardiac defect (atrial septal defect, ventricular septal defect, patent ductus arteriosus, or pulmonary arteriovenous fistula) or a patent foramen ovale. Most reported cases of paradoxical embolism have occurred in patients with a patent foramen ovale,[84] which is present in about 27 percent of the adult population.[85] In order for a venous thrombus to cross a patent foramen ovale, the pressure in the right atrium must be greater than in the left atrium. The most common acute cause for right atrial pressure to exceed left atrial pressure is acute cor pulmonale secondary to acute massive pulmonary embolism.[84]

The usual clinical profile in a case of paradoxical embolism is that of massive pulmonary embolism causing acute cor pulmonale in a patient without prior heart disease but with a patent foramen ovale. The increased right atrial pressure causes a right-to-left shunt across the foramen ovale. If another venous thrombus is dislodged from the deep venous system, it may cross the foramen to enter and embolize the systemic circulation. The most common recognized site of systemic embolism is the brain.[86] Additional common recognized sites include the extremities and the coronary arteries.

Paradoxical embolism should be considered whenever systemic embolism occurs without the usual predisposing causes: atrial fibrillation, mitral valve disease, myocardial infarction, prosthetic heart valves, or cardiomyopathy. In this circumstance, evidence of pulmonary embolism should be sought. If there is evidence of acute pulmonary embolism in addition to unexplained systemic embolism, evidence of a right-to-left intracardiac shunt should be sought by means of indicator dilution curves,[87] angiography, transesophageal echocardiography, or contrast echocardiography.[88,89]

Paradoxical embolism tends to recur and is frequently fatal. If the diagnosis is confirmed during life, recurrence can be prevented by means of insertion of a filter in the inferior vena cava, interruption of the inferior vena cava, or closure of the intracardiac defect.

It should be noted that paradoxical embolism may occur without acute pulmonary embolism in patients with intracardiac defects complicated by right-to-left shunts and in patients with chronic cor pulmonale with right ventricular failure.[72]

Treatment of Acute Pulmonary Embolism

The therapeutic modalities available for patients with acute pulmonary embolism can be divided into two groups: prophylactic and definitive therapy. Prophylactic therapy is based on the concept that the body's intrinsic fibrinolytic system will dissolve thromboembolic material that finds its way into the pulmonary vascular bed. Such dissolution usually leads to resolution of the pathophysiologic changes associated with acute pulmonary embolism over a period of 7 to 14 days.[53] Thus, prophylactic therapy aims at preventing further embolic episodes. Examples of prophylactic therapy include anticoagulation with heparin or warfarin and inferior vena cava interruption (Table 100-3). Prophylactic therapy with anticoagulants is initiated as soon as the clinician has a high index of suspicion for an increased risk of DVT or pulmonary embolism.

Definitive therapy focuses on thromboemboli that have already arrived in the pulmonary vascular bed. Definitive therapy attempts to remove or dissolve such emboli in order to effect a more rapid resolution of the pathophysiologic sequelae of pulmonary embolism. Examples of definitive treatment for pulmonary embolism include thrombolytic agents and pulmonary embolectomy. Placement of an inferior vena cava filter is used to prevent further pulmonary emboli. Supportive measures, e.g., fluid and pressure administration, often precede or accompany definitive therapy and are terminated once the patient's hemodynamic status is stable.

Anticoagulation[3,24,90–95]

Intravenous heparin is the initial treatment of choice for most patients with acute pulmonary embolism. Heparin in a dosage higher than that required to block thrombin-fibrinogen interaction can relieve bronchoconstriction; heparin may also decrease the high pulmonary vascular resistance associated with acute pulmonary embolism. Several investigators have reported striking success with high-dose intravenous heparin in patients with massive pulmonary embolism, in whom the prognosis was guarded. Table 100-8 provides a dosage schedule for heparin tailored to the severity of the thromboembolic process.

The incidence of bleeding during heparin therapy is determined not by the dose of heparin but by defects in the walls of blood vessels. (See Chap. 68.) Therefore, contraindications to anticoagulants include conditions that predispose to bleeding, e.g., active peptic ulcer disease, esophageal varices, hemorrhagic diatheses, severe liver or kidney disease, severe hypertension, intracranial disease, and recent surgery on brain, spinal cord, joints, or genitourinary tract.

As noted in Table 100-8, heparin is continued for 7 to 10 days and should overlap oral warfarin therapy until a prothrombin time of INR = 2.0 to 3.0 (approximately 1.3 to 1.5 times control, using rabbit brain thromboplastin) is achieved. Warfarin is usually started at a dose of 5 to 10 mg/day for the first 3 days of therapy. Thereafter, warfarin dosage is adjusted according to the results of the prothrombin time. After the prothrombin time has been in the therapeutic range for 4 to 5 days, heparin is discontinued and fine regulation of the prothrombin time is achieved by altering the dosage of warfarin. Warfarin should be continued for as long as the patient has an underlying predisposition to thromboembolism, e.g., bed rest. In the patient with a fracture, this period of time should be for 2 months after the cast or traction is removed and the individual is ambulatory. If predisposition to thromboembolism is transitory, patients who have suffered an episode of acute pulmonary embolism should receive oral anticoagulation for 3 to 6 months. In the individual with permanent predisposition to thromboembolism, anticoagulation should be lifelong.

An alternative to daily oral warfarin is injection of subcutaneous heparin every 8 to 12 h for a minimum of 12 weeks. Subcutaneous heparin can be either fixed dose (i.e., 5000 units every 8 to 12 h) or adjusted dose to maintain the predose APTT at one-and-one-half times the control value.[24,96] (See Table 100-2 and Chap. 68.)

Some former anticoagulant regimens prolonged the prothrombin time to as much as two-and-one-half times control. Recent experience, however, favors more modest prolongation of the prothrombin time (INR of 2.0 to 3.0) without any resultant loss of therapeutic efficacy and with a decreased risk for hemorrhagic complications.[24,96] Heparin plasma activity is significantly shortened in some patients with acute pulmonary embolism, presumably as a result of active intravascular coagulation on the surface of pulmonary thromboemboli in the pulmonary vascular bed.[97] Administration of heparin as a continuous infusion results in fewer hemorrhagic complications than administration by the intermittent bolus tech-

TABLE 100-8

Heparin Regimens for the Treatment of Deep Venous Thrombosis and Pulmonary Embolism

Diagnosis	Heparin Dosage
Deep venous thrombosis without pulmonary embolism or with minor pulmonary embolism	5000 U IV loading dose followed by 1000–1500 U IV per hour; check activated partial thromboplastin time (APTT) 4–6 h after initiating infusion and adjust heparin dose to prolong APTT to 1.5–2.5 times control. Warfarin is started on day 2 to 3. Heparin is discontinued on day 7 to 10.
Major pulmonary embolism with or without right ventricular failure and hypotension	10,000 U IV loading dose followed by 1000–2000 U IV per hour; check APTT 4 h after initiating infusion and adjust heparin dose to prolong APTT to 1.5–2.5 times control (employ smaller loading and infusion dosage for smaller individuals or patients with hepatic and/or renal insufficiency). Warfarin is started on day 2 to 3 (if patient is stable) and heparin is discontinued on day 7 to 10.

nique.[98] Hemorrhagic complications of heparin are more common in elderly females than in any other patient group.[99]

Heparin can cause an immunologically mediated thrombocytopenia. (See Chap. 68.) Such decreases in platelet counts are usually asymptomatic but may occur in as many as 5 to 22 percent of patients receiving intravenous heparin. Because the onset of heparin-associated thrombocytopenia usually occurs 6 to 12 days after initiation of therapy, patients begun on heparin should have serial platelet counts. Occasionally, heparin-associated thrombocytopenia develops together with arterial thrombosis that may be life-threatening.[100,101]

Additional medical therapy is often required in patients with acute pulmonary embolism, regardless of whether prophylactic or definitive treatment is elected. For example, apprehension, pain, and respiratory distress usually respond to intravenous morphine sulfate as required. Oxygen is administered by nasal cannulae or mask. Hypotension or shock usually requires intravenous infusion of positive inotropic agents such as dobutamine, dopamine, or norepinephrine. (See also Chap. 30.)

Prophylactic Therapy: Venous Interruption[3,102–110]

Venous interruption is also a form of prophylactic therapy in that it is performed to prevent additional venous thromboemboli from reaching the pulmonary vascular bed. The first form of venous interruption to be performed was bilateral common femoral vein ligation. This type of venous interruption is simple to perform and entails minimal risk for the patient without heart disease as local anesthesia is employed. Further embolism occurs in 5 to 10 percent of cases, however, usually because clot is present above the tie at the time of surgery. Surgical interruption of the vena cava just below the renal veins carries a risk of 2 to 5 percent in patients without heart disease. If the patient has left-sided heart failure, the in-hospital mortality is approximately 20 percent; if left- and right-sided heart failure is present, the risk is 50 percent.[102] Essentially the same risk exists for femoral vein ligation in patients with heart failure because of the high mortality rate from recurrent thromboembolism in patients with prior cardiac decompensation. If a pelvic source of embolism exists, the left ovarian vein must also be ligated. In pregnant patients, this latter procedure does not result in interruption of pregnancy or prevent future pregnancies.

Interruption of the vena cava is highly effective in preventing further episodes of thromboembolism. Interruption of the inferior vena cava is indicated: (1) when embolism occurs in patients receiving appropriate anticoagulant therapy; (2) when anticoagulants are contraindicated; (3) when diseases predisposing to venous thrombosis and pulmonary embolism are prominent and persistent; (4) when septic embolism occurs; (5) when paradoxical embolism occurs; and (6) in some patients with massive embolism in whom a further episode of embolism would be fatal.

At present, the most common form of venous interruption is not surgery, but rather the insertion of a filter or umbrella into the inferior vena cava.[108] Schlosser reviewed the experience with more than 5000 patients who had undergone insertion of a Mobin-Uddin filter.[104] In these patients, nonfatal recurrent emboli occurred in 1.8 percent, and fatal recurrent embolism developed in 0.5 percent. When the 28-mm filter was employed in 2500 patients, nonfatal embolic recurrences occurred in only 0.5 percent of patients, and fatal recurrences were noted in 0.1 percent.[104] Filter migration is also said to be reduced with the 28-mm device.

Another popular inferior vena caval filter is the Kim-Ray Greenfield stainless-steel wire filter.[105] This device is inserted in a manner similar to that employed for the Mobin-Uddin filter, i.e., via a venous cutdown on the common femoral or internal jugular vein. Both of these approaches utilize local anesthesia, thereby avoiding the risks associated with the general anesthesia necessary for inferior vena caval clipping or ligation.

Morbidity following vena caval clipping or filter insertion is largely the result of subsequent total occlusion of the vena cava below the site of the clip or filter. In some series such occlusion was said to occur in 50 percent or more of patients who underwent these procedures. Occlusion of the inferior vena cava is much less frequent in patients with a Kim-Ray Greenfield filter than in those who have surgical inferior vena caval clipping or a Mobin-Uddin umbrella.[105] Morbid events secondary to total occlusion of the vena cava include postphlebitic limb syndrome, unilateral or bilateral leg swelling, and mild venous claudication.[106,107] It has been suggested that administration of anticoagulants following clip or umbrella insertion markedly reduces the incidence of vena caval occlusion and the attendant morbid events.[107] Inferior vena caval filters can also be inserted prophylactically in patients undergoing high-risk orthopedic surgical procedures.[109,110]

Prognosis of Patients Treated with Prophylactic Therapy

The excellent prognosis of patients with pulmonary embolism when the diagnosis is suspected and confirmed and prophylactic treatment is initiated has been documented.[3,63,111,112] Indeed, death secondary to pulmonary embolism is almost invariably the result of massive obstruction of the pulmonary vascular bed by thromboembolism.[3] Such patients usually die within minutes or hours following the acute episode, often before diagnosis and therapy are even considered. If the diagnosis is made and appropriate therapy is initiated, however, the outlook is often excellent, even in patients with massive embolism complicated by right ventricular failure without hypotension.[3] Patients with massive embolism, right ventricular failure, and systemic arterial hypotension are the subgroup who have the highest mortality.[3,63,112] As noted below, patients in this subgroup are often given for definitive therapy, since the prognosis is excellent for all other patient subgroups treated with less aggressive and invasive therapy, i.e., prophylactic therapy.

The overall hospital mortality for all patients treated for acute pulmonary embolism is 8 percent.[3] Individuals with massive pulmonary embolism obstructing 50 percent or more of the pulmonary vascular bed have an in-hospital mortality of 16 percent. As noted above, most of the deaths in these latter patients occur in individuals with right ventricular failure and systemic hypotension.[3] Preexisting heart disease also worsens the prognosis in patients with acute pulmonary embolism by predisposing them to the development of right ventricular failure and hypotension following the embolic event.

Resolution of pulmonary embolism occurs by two mechanisms: in vivo fibrinolysis and mechanical changes in the location of clots within the pulmonary vascular bed. The pressurized flow of blood near and around emboli shifts their position in the pulmonary vascular bed to more distal, and hence less compromising, locations. Embolic obstruction resolves by approximately 10 to 20 percent during the first 24 h after acute pulmonary embolism.[1,66] Complete resolution can occur as soon as 14 days after the acute event, but in most patients it remains incomplete for weeks.[66] The hemodynamic abnormalities associated with pulmonary embolism, i.e., pulmonary hypertension and right ventricular failure in patients with massive embolism, resolve as the pulmonary emboli resolve.[66,113]

Thus, the late prognosis of the patient with acute pulmonary embolism depends on two factors: (1) whether or not the diagnosis of pulmonary embolism is made and appropriate therapy is initiated, and (2) the presence of associated medical illness, e.g., heart disease. Further modest resolution of pulmonary embolism occurs for 3 to 4 months following discharge from the hospital. Thereafter, little, if any, further resolution occurs. Approximately two-thirds of patients with acute pulmonary embolism have complete resolution of their embolism. The remainder have partial resolution of much of the thromboembolic material. Very few patients with partial resolution of embolism develop chronic cor pulmonale. Only a rare patient with untreated or inadequately treated recurrent pulmonary embolism develops chronic cor pulmonale.[1,63] Recurrences of pulmonary embolism are uncommon in patients who are adequately treated and in whom appropriate prophylactic measures are undertaken.

Definitive Therapy: Rationale

As noted earlier, most patients with pulmonary embolism have an excellent prognosis if the diagnosis is suspected and confirmed and treatment is initiated. Individuals with massive embolism, right ventricular failure, and hypotension form a subgroup who have a high in-hospital mortality (32 percent).[2] One would expect these patients to benefit from a direct, definitive attack on the pulmonary vascular thromboemboli. This small minority of patients appear to benefit from thrombolytic dissolution of thromboemboli or even embolectomy. To date, however, unequivocal proof is still lacking that definitive therapy, in comparison with prophylactic therapy, leads to decreased mortality.

Definitive Therapy: Embolectomy[111,114–116]

Pulmonary embolectomy (Trendelenburg's operation) was introduced at the turn of the century but met with only occasional success. The introduction of cardiopulmonary bypass made successful performance of embolectomy more feasible. However, surgical mortality associated with embolectomy remains high, approximately 30 to 50 percent, because the operation is usually performed on patients who are in profound shock. Most individuals who require embolectomy die before it can be performed. Conversely, many patients who survive embolectomy might have survived with less vigorous therapy.[111]

The primary indications for embolectomy are the presence of right ventricular failure and systemic arterial hypotension requiring vasopressors in a patient with bilateral central pulmonary emboli documented by pulmonary angiography. In this setting, embolectomy can be lifesaving. In the absence of hypotension, pulmonary embolectomy is not indicated even if massive pulmonary embolism is documented by angiography. Such patients survive without embolectomy if further embolism is prevented by the administration of prophylactic therapy.[111]

Contraindications to pulmonary embolectomy include recurrent pulmonary embolism without angiographic evidence of occluded central pulmonary arteries, pulmonary arterial systolic pressure in excess of 70 mmHg, severe underlying heart disease complicated by heart failure, and marked pulmonary insufficiency secondary to severe pulmonary disease, i.e., chronic obstructive lung disease.

An alternative to operative pulmonary embolectomy, which requires a thoracotomy, is percutaneous pulmonary embolectomy employing a special catheter.[115,116] This technique involves percutaneous, transvenous introduction of a steerable suction catheter into the pulmonary artery under fluoroscopic guidance. Emboli are aspirated via the catheter, thereby removing them from the pulmonary vascular bed. Multiple retrievals of embolic material by the catheter are usually required before an improvement occurs in the abnormal pulmonary vascular hemodynamic pattern. A vena caval filter is usually inserted at the end of this procedure.[115] Experience with this technique is modest, and further work is required to define the applicability and success rate of catheter pulmonary embolectomy.

Definitive Therapy: Thrombolytic Therapy[117–133]

The search for an agent to dissolve thromboemboli in human beings has been long and complex. The agents that have been studied most extensively are streptokinase, urokinase, and TPA.

The efficacy of urokinase in the treatment of acute pulmonary embolism was assessed in a national cooperative trial sponsored by the National Heart, Lung and Blood Institute.[117] In this multicenter trial, half of the patients were treated with a 12-h infusion of urokinase, while the remainder received a 12-h infusion of heparin.[117] After completion of the 12-h infusions, therapy was the same in both groups: intravenous heparin followed by oral warfarin. Repeat pulmonary angiography demonstrated greater, albeit modest, resolution of embolism in the group treated with urokinase. Five days after the initial treatment, however, resolution of embolism as determined by lung scanning was the same in both groups. In-hospital mortality was the same for both groups.

Hemorrhagic complications were significant: moderate or severe bleeding occurred in 27 percent of the heparin-treated group and in 45 percent of the urokinase-treated patients.[117]

A second trial sponsored by the National Institutes of Health (NIH) compared a 24-h infusion of urokinase with an infusion of streptokinase in 167 patients with angiographically documented pulmonary embolism. Urokinase and streptokinase were equally effective.[118] There was no significant benefit derived from 24 h of thrombolytic infusion as compared with 12 h. Significant bleeding occurred in more than one-third of patients treated with urokinase or streptokinase; bleeding was sufficiently severe in 14 percent of patients to require transfusion.[118]

The 1980 NIH Consensus Conference on Thrombolytic Therapy and Thrombosis recommended that this form of treatment be widely applied to patients with documented pulmonary embolism with associated hemodynamic abnormalities.[118] Thrombolytic therapy, however, did not alter mortality secondary to pulmonary embolism in either of these two trials. Patients with massive embolism fared just as well with heparin (prophylactic) therapy as with thrombolytic (definitive) therapy. Another study demonstrated reduced morbidity with thrombolytic therapy as compared with routine anticoagulation.[119] In this study two indices of pulmonary function, pulmonary capillary blood volume and pulmonary diffusing capacity, were significantly better in pulmonary embolism patients treated with thrombolytic therapy than in individuals who received routine anticoagulation.[119]

Major concern persists about the incidence of bleeding complications in patients treated with thrombolytic therapy. Estimates of this incidence in early trials ranged from 5 to 45 percent.[120–123] Because estimates of bleeding complications with thrombolytic therapy varied, contraindications to this therapy were also variable depending on the investigator's perception of the risk of hemorrhage. On the basis of these early studies, it was difficult to determine firm indications for the use of thrombolytic agents in patients with acute pulmonary embolism. Genton concluded that thrombolytic therapy is potentially most useful in patients with documented massive pulmonary embolism and hemodynamic abnormalities, such as right ventricular failure and/or hypotension.[124] Recently, a multicenter randomized trial has documented improved right ventricular function and possibly a reduced number of adverse clinical events in patients with acute pulmonary embolism treated with TPA as compared with intravenous haparin.[125]

The dosage of urokinase for patients with acute pulmonary embolism is an initial intravenous infusion of 4400 IU per kilogram of body weight dissolved in 15 mL of sterile water given over 10 min. Maintenance therapy is then initiated: 4400 IU/kg per hour for a total of 12 h. Streptokinase is given as an initial loading dose of 250,000 IU dissolved in normal saline solution or 5% dextrose in water and administered over 30 min. Maintenance therapy consists of 100,000 IU/h for 24 h. Bell and Meek recommend determination of thrombin time, prothrombin time, partial thromboplastin time, and platelet count before initiating thrombolytic therapy in order to screen for preexisting coagulation disorders. During thrombolytic therapy, these investigators advise that thrombin times be measured every 4 to 8 h.[121] The thrombin time should be prolonged to between two and five times the normal control value in seconds to confirm that adequate fibrinolysis has been achieved.[121]

A number of studies have employed recombinant TPA (rTPA) in the thrombolytic therapy of acute pulmonary embolism.[23,125–133] In general, the studies have demonstrated that in selected patients thrombolytic therapy with rTPA can rapidly lyse pulmonary embolism and that it acts more rapidly and may cause less bleeding than urokinase. The usual dosage is 100 mg given intravenously over 2 h. It has also been administered at a rate of 0.6 mg/kg intravenously over 2 min.[134] (See also Chap. 69.)

At the present time, thrombolytic therapy is generally reserved for those patients who have hemodynamic embarrassment, right ventricular dysfunction, anatomically large pulmonary embolism, or extensive deep venous thrombosis. Additional data from ongoing clinical trials should document the full effect of thrombolytic therapy on morbidity and mortality. The contraindications to thrombolytic therapy are discussed in Chap. 69.

Pulmonary Embolism in Pregnancy[135–138]

Pulmonary embolism during pregnancy represents a difficult diagnostic and therapeutic problem. Lung scanning and pulmonary angiography involve ionizing radiation exposure for both mother and fetus. Consequently, the diagnosis often remains tentative. Therapy is also problematic since warfarin crosses the placenta and reaches the fetal circulation. It is usually wise to pursue the diagnostic evaluation of pulmonary embolism aggressively, even in pregnancy, because untreated pulmonary embolism carries a 30 percent mortality.[3]

The treatment of pulmonary embolism during pregnancy is hazardous.[135] Prophylactic therapy must continue throughout pregnancy and the puerperium. Heparin does not cross the placental barrier, but it is difficult to administer for more than 2 weeks and its use is associated with an increased rate of pregnancy complications as noted below. Warfarin derivatives cross the placenta and result in significant fetal teratogenesis and mortality. Interruption of the pregnancy to avert further embolism is usually not appropriate. Ligation of the femoral veins does not protect against emboli arising from pelvic and gluteal veins. Interruption of the inferior vena cava and left ovarian vein is a highly effective preventive procedure. This operation, however, entails a surgical risk of about 2 percent in experienced hands; there is little risk of miscarriage after the first trimester, and no interference with future pregnancies.[102] When pulmonary embolism occurs in the first trimester, the appropriate treatment is a 10-day course of heparin, followed by adjusted-dose subcutaneous heparin[108] administered by the patient at home. Heparin is used after delivery until the patient is fully ambulatory. In selected cases, inferior vena caval interruption is appropriate.

Hall et al. reviewed the complications associated with

anticoagulant therapy during pregnancy.[137] Heparin therapy was associated with hemorrhage (10 percent), spontaneous abortion (2 percent), stillbirths (13 percent), early infant mortality (7 percent), and chronic complications in 1 percent of surviving children. Warfarin therapy was complicated by fetal developmental abnormalities (nasal hypoplasia, mental retardation) in 7 percent of infants, spontaneous abortion (9 percent), and stillbirths (8 percent). Consequently, these authors recommend avoidance or termination of pregnancy in patients who require anticoagulant therapy.[137]

Chronic Pulmonary Embolism and Pulmonary Embolectomy[137–142]

Elective pulmonary embolectomy for chronic, unresolved pulmonary thromboembolism is considerably more successful than is the emergency operation. Daily et al. described four such patients, three of whom survived the operation and were markedly improved.[139] Moser et al. reported good results in 15 and 41 patients.[140,141] Benotti et al. identified 30 patients for whom extensive clinical and hemodynamic data were available.[142] The mean age was 45 years; most complained of dyspnea. Roentgenographic, arterial blood gas, and ECG findings were nonspecific; perfusion lung scans were invariably abnormal. Most patients had mild to moderate pulmonary hypertension at rest. Marked pulmonary hypertension developed during exercise. Operative mortality was 20 percent in the 20 patients who underwent elective pulmonary embolectomy, and operative results ranged from good to excellent.[142]

SPECIAL TYPES OF PULMONARY EMBOLISM

Robert C. Schlant, M.D. and Joseph S. Alpert, M.D.

Fat Embolism[145–172]

In 1861 Zenker[170] described the postmortem findings of fat emboli in the lungs, and in 1873 Bergmann[171] described the classic triad for the fat embolism syndrome (FES): dyspnea (respiratory insufficiency), confusion (neurologic dysfunction), and petechiae.

The entrance of free globules of fat into systemic veins most often occurs after fractures of long bones, especially fractures of the tibia and femur in automobile accidents. Fat may also enter the circulation following direct injury to subcutaneous fat tissue by contusion, concussion, burns, childbirth, poisoning, the use of a pump oxygenator, or high-altitude flights. Some less common causes include alcoholism, fatty metamorphosis of the liver, decompression sickness, sickle cell crisis, multiple blood transfusions, sternal-splitting incisions for cardiac surgery, and external cardiac massage.

The exact pathophysiology of FES is unknown and probably differs between patients.[166] At least some of the fatty emboli causing mechanical obstruction in the pulmonary circulation originate from traumatized bone, as myeloid tissue can occasionally be identified in the pulmonary vessels.[145,152,155] There is also evidence that physiobiochemical alterations in the natural emulsion of circulating fat can result in the production of macroglobules of fat that may act as emboli. Other physiobiochemical mechanisms suggested as contributing to the syndrome include the following: release of thromboplastin from traumatized tissues with resultant platelet aggregation; excess free fatty acidemia from the superimposition of fat on platelet aggregations; liberation of toxic free fatty acids in the lungs by enzymatic hydrolysis of embolic fat with subsequent pulmonary capillary leak and curtailment of lung surfactant activity[154]; release of vasoactive and bronchoactive substances such as bradykinin, histamine, or serotonin from pulmonary microthrombi; traumatic shock; and defects in the coagulation system.[150,151] The commonly observed sudden drop in hematocrit is usually related to blood loss in fractured extremities, extensive pulmonary hemorrhage, or, less frequently, associated disseminated intravascular coagulation (DIC). Thrombocytopenia frequently develops in individuals with fat embolism, probably as a result of platelet adhesion to fat droplets in the lung.[149]

The fat droplets vary in size and may obstruct small pulmonary arterial branches, including arterioles and capillaries. The fat globules may also traverse the pulmonary circulation and block arterioles and capillaries of the brain, skin, kidney, heart, and other organs.

Patients can develop the acute respiratory distress syndrome (ARDS) with extensive intrapulmonary hemorrhage and damage to pulmonary vascular endothelium and parenchyma. Clinically, it is frequently difficult to distinguish FES from ARDS.

Patients often have a lucid interval of 6 h to several days (typically, 24 to 40 h) following trauma before the first symptoms or signs of fat embolism are recognized. Most features of the syndrome result from fat emboli either to the lungs or to the brain.[159,164] Cardiorespiratory manifestations of pulmonary fat emboli include tachypnea, dyspnea, sinus tachycardia, hypoxemia, and pyrexia to 39.4°C (103°F). Individuals with severe respiratory distress may become cyanotic. Patients with fat embolism syndrome often have copious bronchial secretions, which may be hemorrhagic. The cerebral symptoms, which may occur simultaneously with or after the pulmonary symptoms, include headache, increasing irritability, disturbances of consciousness, disorientation, delirum, confusion, restlessness, convulsions, apathy, stupor, and coma. Focal cerebral syndromes may also occur.[168] As noted above, patients with fat embolism may present with, or develop, the full clinical picture of ARDS.[162] Oliguria and even anuria may develop.

Signs of systemic fat embolism include petechiae, especially on the anterior chest, axillary folds, neck, fundi, and conjunctivae. Rarely, fat emboli are seen in the retinal vessels. In some patients, the petechiae, whether spontaneous or induced, may be related to the associated thrombocytopenia, although small fat emboli may be found in biopsies of cutaneous capillaries adjacent to the petechiae.[172] The prothrombin time and partial thromboplastin time may be increased, and plasma fibrinogen may be reduced. The serum calcium level is often decreased, presumably because of the interaction between increased serum fatty acids and calcium; serum lipase and tributyrinase concentrations are usually elevated. A frozen section of clotted blood examined for fat may be of some diagnostic value early in the course of the fat embolism syndrome, particularly in patients with an arterial P_{O_2} less than 60 mmHg.[157,161] The findings of fat droplets in sputum or urine are also suggestive, but not diagnostic, of fat embolism.[148] Arterial hypoxemia is one of the earliest and most important laboratory findings. The chest roentgenogram usually shows extensive fluffy infiltrates; occasionally, only hazy, diffuse, fine stippling is seen throughout both lungs. The chest x-ray may also be compatible with pulmonary edema.[163]

There is no specific therapy for fat embolism; the most important principle is maintenance of pulmonary oxygenation and function. It is important to correct the arterial hypoxemia that is usually present and is occasionally quite marked. Supplemental inspiratory oxygen is usually required. Occasionally, assisted ventilation, with or without positive end-expiratory pressure (PEEP), is needed. Although 100% inspiratory oxygen may be necessary initially, this should later be reduced to 40% to avoid oxygen toxicity. Frequent determinations of arterial blood gas concentration are necessary. It has been suggested that massive doses of corticosteroids may decrease alveolar damage, although adequate clinical trials are lacking.[146,147,153,156,158–160,165,167] Doses usually employed are: hydrocortisone, 1 to 2 g/day, or methylprednisolone, 13 mg/kg per day, for 3 to 5 days. Schonfeld et al. demonstrated that prophylactic administration of methylprednisolone, 7.5 mg per kilogram of body weight, every 6 h for 12 doses to patients with long bone fractures reduced the development of signs and symptoms of the fat embolism syndrome.[167] Low-dose heparin was formerly recommended in order to decrease platelet adhesiveness. The stimulatory effect of heparin upon lipase activity in the lung is theoretically detrimental, however, since it might increase the amounts of toxic fatty acids in the lungs. Other former therapies that are no longer used include low-molecular-weight dextran,[150] intravenous ethyl alcohol, hypothermia, and various detergents.[149]

Air Embolism[173–182]

Air may enter the circulation during the course of intravenous infusions, pneumoperitoneum, knee-chest position in the puerperium, uterine douches, surgical procedures on the neck or brain, retroperitoneal air injection, irrigation of nasal sinuses, tubal or vaginal insufflation, urogenital sex,[179] rapid pressure decompensation, mechanical ventilation, or heart-lung bypass. The lethal dose varies with the age, condition, and position of the patient and the rapidity of air entry. Fatal air embolism can result from 5 to 15 mL of air per kilogram of body weight. Death results either from an "air lock" in the right ventricle or from air embolism to the lungs with resultant pulmonary vascular obstruction and secondary reflex pulmonary vasoconstriction.[173,174] It is likely that only very minute (if any) volumes of air traverse the pulmonary capillaries. Clinically, air embolism is associated with the sudden onset of dyspnea, shock, and cyanosis. Frequently, there is a loud, continuous churning or "mill-house" murmur or noise over the precordium produced by the mixing of air and blood in the right ventricle. Venous air embolism can also result in diffuse pulmonary injury with subsequent development of ARDS.[175] Marked ventilation-perfusion abnormalities can result from air in the pulmonary vascular bed.[177] Air bubbles in cardiac chambers can be detected by echocardiography.[180]

Treatment consists of turning the patient onto the left side with the head in a dependent position, in an effort to displace the air bolus from the right ventricular outflow tract to the right ventricular apex or right atrium and to trap the air in the superior portion of the right atrium. The air can then be aspirated through a needle or catheter inserted into the right ventricle. One should also administer 100% inspiratory oxygen.[178] Closed-chest cardiac massage has been used successfully, particularly when air embolism occurs during a neurosurgical or neck operation.[181]

Arterial air embolism can also occur and may produce embolic retinopathy, ventricular fibrillation, myocardial infarction, or cerebral symptoms including coma, confusion, hemiplegia, loss of memory, and seizures.[176,182] Air can enter the arterial system by many routes, including cardiac surgery, pneumothorax, paradoxical air embolism, artificial ventilation with high airway pressures, hemodialysis, and intraaortic balloon counterpulsation. Treatment is supportive, although hyperbaric oxygen has been employed with apparent benefit.

Amniotic Fluid Embolism[183–195]

Amniotic fluid embolism causing maternal mortality was first described in 1926 by Meyer[183] and was more firmly established as a clinical syndrome in 1941 by Steiner and Luschbaugh.[184] The incidence has been variably stated as being from 1 in 8000 to 1 in 80,000 live births. It remains one of the more common causes of maternal death during legal abortion, labor, delivery, and the immediate postpartum period. Predisposing factors are increased age and parity, premature placental separation, intrauterine fetal death, oversized baby, prolonged and vigorous labor with tumultuous uterine contractions, uterine rupture, large doses of oxytocin, meconium contamination of amniotic fluid, and abortion induced by intraamniotic injection of saline or glucose. It may also occur following amniocentesis.[193]

The amniotic fluid contains meconium, epithelial squamae, mucin, amorphous debris, lipids, bile pigments, lanugo, or any combination of these. It enters the maternal circulation either through the venous sinuses or the uteroplacental site or through the endocervical veins. The pulmonary embolic manifestations are primarily due to the solid contents of the amniotic fluid, since most experiments have indicated that filtered amniotic fluid produces minimal pulmonary vascular response. Occasionally, amniotic fluid material can be detected in the vessels of the lungs, heart, kidneys, and brain.[185] Recent evidence, however, suggests that cytologic techniques are not helpful in the diagnosis.[194,195]

Disseminated intravascular coagulation (DIC) develops in a significant number of patients who survive the initial pulmonary embolic event. It is produced by the entry into the circulation of large amounts of thromboplastic substances contained in the amniotic fluid. The coagulation cascade is initiated, leading to the consumption of factors V and VIII, prothrombin, and fibrinogen. If consumption proceeds more rapidly than repletion, deficiencies of these factors can develop. The fibrinolytic enzyme system is activated as a compensatory mechanism, resulting in the production of large amounts of fibrin degradation products; these act as inhibitors of thrombin, interfere with normal fibrin polymerization, and impair platelet function. This process can result in severe vaginal hemorrhage. Fibrin deposition throughout the microvasculature aggravates the pulmonary embolic manifestations and may produce systemic hypoperfusion with profound alteration in function of almost every organ in the body.

Clinically, most episodes of amniotic fluid embolism occur near the end of the first stage of labor and are manifested by the abrupt onset of severe dyspnea, hypotension or frank shock, tachypnea, tachycardia, cyanosis, evidence of acute cor pulmonale and pulmonary edema, and apprehension. The latter symptoms may progress rapidly to semicoma or coma. Generalized convulsions, cardiac arrest, and death may occur suddenly. Chest pain is relatively unusual. About 25 to 50 percent of patients die within the first hour, and the survivors are still at great risk of death from either irreversible shock or the subsequent development of profuse vaginal bleeding. There may be bleeding from venipuncture sites and all body orifices or into skin and mucosa. Acute renal failure may develop secondary to hypotension. The mortality in patients with the full-blown amniotic fluid embolism syndrome exceeds 80 percent.[189]

Laboratory findings usually reflect deficiencies of all coagulation factors, especially low fibrinogen levels and a low platelet count.

Treatment[184–190] consists of (1) general supportive measures for thromboembolism with hypotension and/or respiratory distress; (2) immediate evacuation of the uterus to remove the basic cause of the DIC process; (3) administration of fresh frozen plasma, platelets, and packed red blood cells as needed for anemia, hemorrhage, and/or hypotension; and (4) administration of cryoprecipitate (which contains fibrinogen and factor VIII) if bleeding persists and if fibrinogen and factor VIII are low.[189,190] Controversy exists regarding the use of fibrinogen, which promotes clotting and hemostasis, since theoretically it might produce more deposition of fibrin. The management of amniotic fluid embolism is greatly assisted by monitoring intraarterial blood pressure, central venous pressure, pulmonary artery pressure (with a balloon pulmonary artery catheter), and urinary output.[191,192]

Tumor Embolism[196–200]

In addition to pulmonary metastases from malignant tumors, acute and subacute cor pulmonale may result from emboli of malignant tissue cells to the pulmonary arteries and capillaries. These emboli may originate from the primary site of the tumor or from metastatic sites, such as the liver or inferior vena cava. Tumor emboli occur with virtually any type of malignancy but are more common in patients with renal carcinoma, primary hepatic carcinoma, gastric carcinoma, and trophoblastic tumors (chorioepithelioma). Rarely, pulmonary tumor embolism occurs in a patient without apparent malignancy, producing a syndrome of slowly progressive dyspnea and pulmonary hypertension.[200] (See also Chap. 111.)

Because trophoblastic tumors, even with extensive pulmonary metastases, may respond well to chemotherapy,[197,198] it is imperative to consider this diagnosis whenever a female patient has symptoms of acute dyspnea, pleurisy, cough, and/or hemoptysis or unexplained signs of pulmonary hypertension following a hydatidiform mole, abortion, or normal pregnancy. Occasionally, trophoblastic pulmonary emboli may not occur until several years after the initiating pregnancy, and the patient may have been asymptomatic in the interval. It is most common, however, for patients to describe amenorrhea, excessive menstrual bleeding or discharge, or other disturbance of menses. Since uterine curettage is often negative, the diagnosis is best established by measuring urinary gonadotropin excretion. Radiologic changes in the lungs resulting from metastasis of trophoblastic tumors may take one or more of the following forms: (1) discrete, usually well-defined, rounded opacities; (2) "snowstorm" patterns with multiple, small, less well defined opacities; and (3) changes resulting from embolic occlusion of the pulmonary arteries without invasion of the lung parenchyma. Of interest is one study of 50 asymptomatic puerperal patients, 13 of whom had pulmonary scan defects thought to be due to asymptomatic trophoblastic emboli.[199]

Cor pulmonale, i.e., right-sided heart failure, occasionally results from hematogenous or lymphatic spread of tumor. Cor pulmonale may be subacute, occurring over the course of a week or 10 days, or it may appear more slowly with a clinical picture of chronic right-sided heart failure.[196,200]

Rare Causes of Embolism

Among the many less common forms of pulmonary embolism are those due to cotton fiber, talc, hair, or other particulate matter in contaminated heroin or other illicit drugs; barium sulfate crystals after barium enema; vegetable material; bullets or shotgun shot; cardiac catheters or indwelling venous catheters; bone marrow, brain tissue, parasites, cardiac vegetations; form cells from rupture of atheromata in an enlarged pulmonary artery; liver cells; and bile thromboembolism.[201,202]

REFERENCES

1. Dalen JE, Alpert JS: Natural history of pulmonary embolism. *Prog Cardiovasc Dis* 1975; 17:259–269.
2. Anderson FA Jr, Wheeler B, Goldberg RJ, Hosmer DW, Patwardhan NA, Jovanovic B, et al: A population-based perspective of the hospital incidence and case-fatality rates of deep vein throm-

bosis and pulmonary embolism. *Arch Intern Med* 1991; 151:933–938.

3. Alpert JS, Smith R, Carlson J, Ockene IS, Dexter L, Dalen JE: Mortality in patients treated for pulmonary embolism. *JAMA* 1976; 236:1477–1480.
4. Sevitt S, Gallagher NG: Venous thrombosis and pulmonary embolism: A clinicopathologic study in injured and burned patients. *Br J Surg* 1961; 48:475–482.
5. Havig O: Source of pulmonary emboli. *Acta Chir Scand* 1977; 478:42–47.
6. Kakkar V, Howe CT, Flanc C, Clark WD: Natural history of post-operative deep venous thrombosis. *Lancet* 1969; 2:230–232.
7. Virchow RIK: *Cellular Pathology as Based upon Physiological and Pathohistology*, 7th Am. ed, Chance F, DeWitt RM (trans). New York, 1860, 236.
8. Wessler S, Reiner L, Freiman D, Reimer SM, Lertzman M: Serum-induced thrombosis. *Circulation* 1959; 20:864–876.
9. Freiman D, Wessler S, Lertzman W: Experimental pulmonary embolism with serum-induced thrombi aged in vivo. *Am J Pathol* 1962; 39:95–104.
10. Sevitt S: The structure and growth of valve-pocket thrombi in femoral veins. *J Clin Pathol* 1974; 27:517–521.
11. Wessler S: Studies in intravascular coagulation. III. The pathogenesis of serum-induced venous thrombosis. *J Clin Invest* 1955; 34:647–650.
12. Shattil SJ, Beunet J: Platelets in hemostasis. *Ann Intern Med* 1981; 94:108–113.
13. Moser KM: Venous thromboembolism. *Am Rev Respir Dis* 1990; 141:235–249.
14. Asherson RA, Khamashta MA, Ordi-Ros J, Derksen RHWM, Machin SJ, Barquinero J, et al: The "primary" antiphospholipid syndrome: Major clinical and serological features. *Medicine (Baltimore)* 1989; 68:366–371.
15. Ginsburg KS, Liang MH, Newcomer L, Goldhaber SZ, Schur PH, Hennekens CH, et al: Anticardiolipin antibodies and the risk for ischemic stroke and venous thrombosis. *Ann Intern Med* 1992; 117:997–1002.
16. Cotton LT, Clark C: Anatomic localization of venous thrombosis. *Ann R Coll Surg Engl* 1969; 36:214–222.
17. Kravis TC, Shibel EM, Brooks JD, Moser KM: Incorporation of radiolabeled fibrinogen into venous thrombi induced in dogs. *Circulation* 1974; 49:158–163.
18. Moser KM, LeMoine JR: Is embolic risk conditioned by location of deep venous thrombosis? *Ann Intern Med* 1981; 94:439–444.
19. Kakkar W, Howe CT, Nicolaides AW, Renney JT, Clarke MB: Deep vein thrombosis: Is there a high risk group? *Am J Surg* 1970; 120:527–530.
20. Huisman MV, Bulla HR, TenCate JW, Vreeden J: Serial impedance plethysmography for suspected deep venous thrombosis in outpatients. *N Engl J Med* 1986; 314:823–828.
21. Philbrick JT, Becker DM: Calf deep venous thrombosis: A wolf in sheep's clothing? *Arch Intern Med* 1988; 148:2131–2138.
22. Lagersted CL, Olsson CG, Fagher BO, Oquist BW, Albrechtsson U: Need for long-term anticoagulation treatment for symptomatic calf vein thrombosis. *Lancet* 1985; 2:515–518.
23. Goldhaber SZ, Morpurgo M: Diagnosis, treatment, and prevention of pulmonary embolism: Report of the WHO/International Society and Federation of Cardiology Task Force. *JAMA* 1991; 268:1727–1733.
24. Dalen JE, Hirsh J (eds): Third ACCP consensus conference on antithrombotic therapy. *Chest* 1992; 102 (suppl):303S–549S.
25. Kakkar VV: The logistic problems encountered in the multicenter trial of low-dose heparin prophylaxis. *Thromb Haemost* 1979; 41:105–113.
26. Halkin H, Goldberg J, Modan M, Modan B: Reduction of mortality in general medicine in-patients by low-dose heparin prophylaxis. *Ann Intern Med* 1982; 96:561–565.
27. Poller L, McKernon A, Thomson JM, Elstein M, Hirsch PJ, Jones JB: Fixed minidose warfarin: A new approach to prophylaxis against venous thrombosis after major surgery. *Br Med J* 1987; 295:1309–1312.
28. Kakkar VV, Stamatakis JD, Bentley PG, Lawrence D, de-Haas HA, Ward VP: Prophylaxis for postoperative deep-vein thrombosis, synergistic effect of heparin and dihydroergotamine. *JAMA* 1979; 241:39–42.
29. Pedersen B, Christiansen J: Thromboembolic prophylaxis with dihydroergotamine-heparin in abdominal surgery. *Am J Surg* 1983; 145:788–790.
30. Moser G, Krahenbuhl B, Barroussel R, Bene JJ, Donath A, Rohner A: Mechanical versus pharmacologic prevention of deep venous thrombosis. *Surg Gynecol Obstet* 1981; 152:448–450.
31. Coe NP, Collins REC, Klein LA, Bettmann MA, Skillman JJ, Shapiro RM, et al: Prevention of deep vein thrombosis in urological patients: A controlled, randomized trial of low-dose heparin and external pneumatic compression boots. *Surgery* 1978; 83:230–234.
32. Francis CW, Pellegrini VD, Marder VJ, Totterman S, Harris CM, Gabriel KR, et al: Comparison of warfarin and external pneumatic compression in prevention of venous thrombosis after total hip replacement. *JAMA* 1992; 267:2911–2915.
33. Markwardt F: Hirudin and derivatives as anticoagulant agents. *Thromb Haemost* 1991; 66:141–152.
34. Markwardt F (ed): Hirudin. *Semin Thromb Haemost* 1991; 17:79–159.
35. Levine MN, Hirsh J, Gent M, Turpie AG, Leclerc J, Powers PJ, et al: Prevention of deep vein thrombosis after elective hip surgery: A randomized trial comparing low molecular weight heparin with standard unfractionated heparin. *Ann Intern Med* 1991; 114:545–551.
36. Prandoni P, Lensing AWA, Büller HR, Carta M, Cogo A, Vigo M, et al: Comparison of subcutaneous low-molecular-weight heparin with intravenous standard heparin in proximal deep-vein thrombosis. *Lancet* 1992; 339:441–445.
37. Hull RD, Raskob GE, Pineo GF, Green D, Trowbridge AA, Elliott CG, et al: Subcutaneous low-molecular-weight heparin compared with continuous intravenous heparin in the treatment of proximal-vein thrombosis. *N Engl J Med* 1992; 326:975–982.
38. Hirsh J, Levine MN: Low molecular weight heparin. *Blood* 1992; 79:1–17.
39. Nurmohamed MT, Rosendaal FR, Büller HR, Dekker E, Hommes DW, Vandenbroucke JP, et al: Low-molecular-weight heparin versus standard heparin in general and orthopaedic surgery: A meta-analysis. *Lancet* 1992; 340:152–156.
40. Salzman EW: Low-molecular-weight heparin and other new antithrombotic drugs. *N Engl J Med* 1992; 326:1017–1019.
41. Rabinov K, Paulin S: Roentgen diagnosis of venous thrombosis in the leg. *Arch Surg* 1972; 104:134–139.
42. Hull R, Hirsh J, Sackett DL, Taylor DW, Carter C, Turpie AGG, et al: Clinical validity of a negative venogram in patients with clinically suspected venous thrombosis. *Circulation* 1981; 64:622–625.
43. Hull R, Hirsch J, Sackett DL, Stoddart G: Cost effectiveness of clinical diagnosis, venography, and noninvasive testing in patients with symptomatic deep-vein thrombosis. *N Engl J Med* 1981; 304:1561–1567.
44. Wheeler HB, O'Donnell JA, Anderson FA Jr, Benedict K Jr: Occlusive impedance phlebography: A diagnostic procedure for venous thrombosis and pulmonary embolism. *Prog Cardiovasc Dis* 1974; 17:199–205.
45. Hull R, Taylor DW, Hirsh J, Sackett DL, Powers P, Turpie AG, et al: Impedance plethysmography: The relationship between venous filling and sensitivity and specificity for proximal vein thrombosis. *Circulation* 1978; 58:898–902.
46. Curley FJ, Pratter MR, Irwin RS: The clinical implications of bilaterally abnormal impedance plethysmography. *Arch Intern Med* 1987; 147:125–129.
47. Hirsh J: Heparin. *N Engl J Med* 1991; 324:1565–1574.
48. Hull RD, Raskob GE, Hirsh J, Jay RM, Leclerc JR, Geerts WH, et al: Continuous intravenous heparin compared with intermittent subcutaneous heparin in the initial treatment of proximal vein thrombosis. *N Engl J Med* 1986; 315:1109–1114.
49. Dalen JE, Haynes FW, Hopper FG Jr, Evans GL, Bhardwaj P, Dexter L: Cardiovascular responses to experimental pulmonary embolism. *Am J Cardiol* 1967; 20:3–9.
50. Dexter L, Smith GT: Quantitative studies of pulmonary embolism. *Am J Med Sci* 1964; 247:641–650.
51. Vlahakes GJ, Turley K, Hoffman JIE: The pathophysiology of failure in acute right ventricular hypertension. Hemodynamic and biochemical correlations. *Circulation* 1981; 63:87–95.
52. McIntyre KM, Sasahara AA: Determinants of right ventricular function and hemodynamics after pulmonary embolism. *Chest* 1974; 65:534–543.

53. Sasahara AA, Cannilla JE, Morse RL, Sidd JJ, Tremblay GM: Clinical and physiologic studies in pulmonary thromboembolism. *Am J Cardiol* 1967; 20:10–20.
54. Alpert JS, Godtfredsen J, Ockene IS, Anas J, Dalen JE: Pulmonary hypertension secondary to minor pulmonary hypertension. *Chest* 1978; 73:795–797.
55. Thames MD, Alpert JS, Dalen JE: Syncope in patients with pulmonary embolism. *JAMA* 1969; 238:2509–2511.
56. Alpert JS: Effect of right ventricular dysfunction on left ventricular function. In: Kellerman JS (ed): *Advances in Cardiology*. Basel, Karger, 1986: 25–34.
57. Widdicombe JG: Reflex mechanisms in pulmonary thromboembolism. In: Moser KM, Stein M (eds): *Pulmonary Thromboembolism*. Chicago, Yearbook, 1973: 178–193.
58. Chernick V, Hodson WA, Greenfield LJ: Effect of chronic pulmonary artery ligation on pulmonary mechanisms and surfactant. *J Appl Physiol* 1966; 21:1315–1319.
59. Finley TN, Swensen EW, Clements JA, Gardner RE, Wright RR, Severinghaus JW: Changes in mechanical properties, appearance and surface activity of extracts of one lung following exclusion of its pulmonary artery in the dog. *Physiologist* 1960; 3:56.
60. Dalen JE, Haffajee CI, Alpert JS, Howe JP, Ockene IS, Paraskos JA: Pulmonary embolism, pulmonary hemorrhage and pulmonary infarction. *N Engl J Med* 1977; 296:1431–1435.
61. National Heart, Lung, and Blood Institute. Urokinase pulmonary embolism trial: Phase 1 results. *JAMA* 1970; 214:2163–2172.
62. Prediletto R, Paoletti P, Fornai E, Perissinotto A, Petruzzelli S, Formichi B, et al: Natural course of treated pulmonary embolism. Evaluation of perfusion lung scintigraphy, gas exchange and chest roentgenogram. *Chest* 1990; 97:554–561.
63. Parakos JA, Adelstein SJ, Smith RE, Rickman FD, Grossman W, Dexter L, et al: Late prognosis of acute pulmonary embolism. *N Engl J Med* 1973; 289:55–58.
64. Dalen JE, Dexter L: Pulmonary embolism. *JAMA* 1969; 207:1505–1507.
65. Szucs MM Jr, Brooks HL, Grossman W, Banas JS, Meister G, Dexter L, et al: Diagnostic sensitivity of laboratory findings in acute pulmonary embolism. *Ann Intern Med* 1971; 74:161–166.
66. Hull RD, Hirsh J, Carter CJ, Jay RM, Dodd PE, Ockelford PA, et al: Pulmonary angiography, ventilation lung scanning, and venography for clinically suspected pulmonary embolism with abnormal perfusion lung scan. *Ann Intern Med* 1983; 98:891–899.
67. Stein PD, Alavi A, Gottschalk A, Hales CA, Saltzman HA, Vreim CE, et al: Usefulness of noninvasive diagnostic tools for diagnosis of acute pulmonary embolism in patients with a normal chest radiograph. *Am J Cardiol* 1991; 67:1117–1120.
68. PIOPED Investigators: Value of the ventilation/perfusion scan in acute pulmonary embolism; results of the prospective investigation of pulmonary embolism diagnosis (PIOPED). *JAMA* 1990; 263:2753–2796.
69. Sasahara AA, Sharma GVRK, Parisi AF: New developments in the detection and prevention of venous thromboembolism. *Am J Cardiol* 1979; 43:1214–1224.
70. Dalen JE, Banas J Jr, Brooks H, Evans GL, Paraskos JA, Dexter L: Resolution rate of acute pulmonary embolism in man. *N Engl J Med* 1969; 280:1194–1197.
71. McGinn S, White PD: Acute cor pulmonale resulting from pulmonary embolism. *JAMA* 1935; 104:1473–1480.
72. Stein PD, Dalen JE, McIntyre KM, Sasahara AA, Wenger NK, Willis PW: The electrocardiogram in acute pulmonary embolism. *Prog Cardiovasc Dis* 1975; 17:247–257.
73. Huet Y, Lemaire F, Brun-Buisson C, Knaus WA, Teisseire B, Payen D, et al: Hypoxemia in acute pulmonary embolism. *Chest* 1985; 88:829–836.
74. Howe JP III, Alpert JS, Rickman FD, Spackman DG, Dexter L, Dalen JE: Return of arterial P_{O_2} values to baseline after supplemental oxygen in patients with cardiac disease. *Chest* 1975; 67:256–258.
75. Kipper MS, Moser KM, Kortman KE, Ashburn WL: Long term follow-up of patients with suspected pulmonary embolism and a normal lung scan. *Chest* 1982; 82:411–415.
76. Kelley MA, Carson JL, Palevsky HI, Schwartz JS: Diagnosing pulmonary embolism: New facts and strategies. *Ann Intern Med* 1991; 114:300–306.
77. Hull RD, Hirsh J, Carter CJ, Raskob GE, Gill GJ, Jay RM, et al: Diagnostic value of ventilation-perfusion lung scanning in patients with suspected pulmonary embolism. *Chest* 1985; 88:819–828.
78. Farfel Z, Shechter M, Vered Z, Rath S, Goor D, Gafni J: Review of echocardiographically diagnosed right heart entrapment of pulmonary emboli-in-transit with emphasis on management. *Am Heart J* 1987; 113:171–178.
79. Stein PD, O'Connor JF, Dalen JE, Pur-Shahriari AA, Hoppin FG, Hammond DT, et al: The angiographic diagnosis of acute pulmonary embolism: Evaluation of criteria. *Am Heart J* 1967; 73:730–741.
80. Dalen JE, Brooke HL, Johnson LW, Meister SG, Szucs MM, Dexter L: Pulmonary angiography in acute pulmonary embolism: Indications, techniques, and results in 367 patients. *Am Heart J* 1971; 81:175–185.
81. Benotti JR, Alpert JS, Dalen JE: Superiority of balloon-occlusion pulmonary cineangiography in the diagnosis of pulmonary embolism. (Abstract) *Chest* 1983; 84:341.
82. Bounameaux H, Cirafic P, de Moerloose P, Schneider P-A, Slosman D, Reber G, et al: Measurement of D-dimer in plasma as diagnostic aid in suspected pulmonary embolism. *Lancet* 1991; 337:196–200.
83. Gore JM, Appelbaum JS, Green HL, Dexter L, Dalen JE: Occult cancer in patients with acute pulmonary embolism. *Ann Intern Med* 1982; 96:556-560.
84. Meister SG, Grossman W, Dexter L, Dalen JE: Paradoxical embolism. Diagnosis during life. *Am J Med* 1972; 53:292–298.
85. Hagen PT, Scholz DG, Edwards WD: Incidence and size of patent foramen ovale during the first 10 decades of life: An autopsy study of 965 normal hearts. *Mayo Clin Proc* 1984; 59:17–20.
86. Dalen JE: Systemic embolism. In: Rippe JM, Irwin RS, Alpert JS, et al (eds): *Intensive Care Medicine*. Boston, Little, Brown, 1985: 209–217.
87. Banas J Jr, Meister SG, Gazzaniga AB, O'Connor NE, Haynes FW, Dalen JE: A simple technique for detecting small defects of the atrial septum. *Am J Cardiol* 1971; 28:467–471.
88. Higgins JR, Strunk BL, Schiller NB: Diagnosis of paradoxical embolism with contrast echocardiography. *Am Heart J* 1984; 107:375–377.
89. Lechat P, Mas JL, Lascault G, Loron P, Theard M, Klimczac M, et al: Prevalence of patent foramen ovale in patients with stroke. *N Engl J Med* 1988; 318:1148–1152.
90. Clagett GP, Saltzman EW: Prevention of venous thromboembolism. *Prog Cardiovasc Dis* 1975; 17:345–366.
91. Genton E, Hirsh J: Observations in anticoagulant and thrombolytic therapy in pulmonary embolism. *Prog Cardiovasc Dis* 1975; 17:335–343.
92. Barritt DW, Jordan SC: Anticoagulant drugs in the treatment of pulmonary embolism. A controlled trial. *Lancet* 1960; 1:1309–1312.
93. Kernohan RJ, Todd C: Heparin therapy in thromboembolic disease. *Lancet* 1966; 1:621–623.
94. Colman RW, Rubin RN: Prophylaxis and treatment of thromboembolism based on pathophysiology of clotting mechanisms. In: Fishman AP (ed): *Pulmonary Diseases and Disorders*, 2d ed. New York, McGraw-Hill, 1988: 1049–1057.
95. Hull R, Hirsh J, Jay R, Carter C, England C, Gent M, et al: Different intensities of oral anticoagulant therapy in the treatment of proximal vein thrombosis. *N Engl J Med* 1982; 307:1676–1681.
96. Hull R, Delmore T, Carter C, Hirsh J, Genton E, Gent M, et al: Adjusted subcutaneous heparin versus warfarin sodium in the long-term treatment of venous thrombosis. *N Engl J Med* 1982; 306:189–194.
97. Hirsh J, VanAken WG, Gallus AS, Dollery CT, Cade JF, Yung WL: Heparin kinetics in venous thrombosis and pulmonary embolism. *Circulation* 1976; 53:691–695.
98. Salzman EW, Deykin D, Shapiro RM, Rosenberg R: Management of heparin therapy—controlled prospective trial. *N Engl J Med* 1975; 292:1046–1050.
99. Jick H, Sloane D, Borda IT, Shapiro S: Efficacy and toxicity of heparin in relation to age and sex. *N Engl J Med* 1968; 279:284–286.
100. Bell WR, Tomasulo PA, Alving BM, Duffy TP: Thrombocytopenia occurring during the administration of heparin—a prospective study in 52 patients. *Ann Intern Med* 1976; 85:155–160.

101. King DJ, Kelton JG: Heparin-associated thrombocytopenia. *Ann Intern Med* 1984; 100:535–540.
102. Crane C: Venous interruption for pulmonary embolism: Present status. *Prog Cardiovasc Dis* 1975; 17:329–333.
103. Bomalaski JS, Martin GJ, Hughes RL, Yao JS: Inferior vena cava interruption in the management of pulmonary embolism. *Chest* 1982; 82:767–774.
104. Schlosser V: Umbrella filter implantation as prophylaxis against pulmonary embolism. *Eur Soc Cardiovasc Radiol* 1979; 23:329–331.
105. Greenfield LJ: Technical considerations for insertion of vena caval filters. *Surg Gynecol Obstet* 1979; 148:422–426.
106. Askew AR, Gardner AM: Long-term follow-up of partial caval occlusion by clip. *Am J Surg* 1980; 140:441–443.
107. Adelson J, Steer ML, Glotzer DJ, Skillman JJ, Simon M, Salzman EW: Thromboembolism after insertion of the Mobin-Uddin caval filter. *Surgery* 1980; 87:184–189.
108. Becker DM, Philbrick JT, Selby JB: Inferior vena cava filters: Indications, safety, effectiveness. *Arch Intern Med* 1992; 152:1985–1994.
109. Collins DN, Barnes LC, McCowan TC, Nelson CL, Carver DK, McAndrew MP, et al: Vena caval filter use in orthopaedic trauma patients with recognized preoperative venous thromboembolic disease. *J Orthop Trauma* 1992; 6:135–138.
110. Webb LX, Rush PT, Fuller SB, Meredith JW: Greenfield filter prophylaxis of pulmonary embolism in patients undergoing surgery for acetabular fracture. *J Orthop Trauma* 1992; 6:139–145.
111. Alpert JS, Smith RE, Ockene IS, Askenazi J, Dexter L, Dalen JE: Treatment of massive pulmonary embolism: The role of pulmonary embolectomy. *Am Heart J* 1975; 89:413–417.
112. Carson JL, Kelley MA, Duff A, Weg JG, Fulkerson WJ, Palevsky HI, et al: The clinical course of pulmonary embolism. *N Engl J Med* 1992; 326:1240–1245.
113. McIntyre KM, Sasahara AA: Hemodynamic and ventricular responses to pulmonary embolism. *Prog Cardiovasc Dis* 1974; 17:175–190.
114. Sautter RD, Myers WO, Ray JF III, Wenzel FJ: Pulmonary embolectomy: Review and current status. *Prog Cardiovasc Dis* 1975; 17:371–389.
114a. Meyer G, Tamisier D, Sors H, Stern M, Vouhé P, Makowski S, et al: Pulmonary embolectomy: A 20-year experience at one center. *Ann Thorac Surg* 1991; 51:232–236.
115. Greenfield LJ, Zocco JJ: Intraluminal management of acute massive pulmonary thromboembolism. *J Thorac Cardiovasc Surg* 1979; 77:402–410.
116. Timsit J-F, Reynaud P, Meyer G, Sors H: Pulmonary embolectomy by catheter device in massive pulmonary embolism. *Chest* 1991; 100:655–658.
117. Urokinase Pulmonary Embolism Study Group: The urokinase pulmonary embolism trial. *Circulation* 1973; 47(suppl 2):1–108.
118. Consensus Development Conference Report: Thrombolytic therapy in thrombosis: A National Institutes of Health consensus development conference. *Ann Intern Med* 1980; 93:141–144.
119. Sharma GVRK, Bueleston VA, Sasahara AA: Effect of thrombolytic therapy on pulmonary-capillary blood volume in patients with pulmonary embolism. *N Engl J Med* 1980; 303:842–845.
120. Marder VJ: Are we using fibrinolytic agents often enough? *Ann Intern Med* 1980; 93:136–137.
121. Bell WR, Meek AG: Guidelines for the use of thrombolytic agents. *N Engl J Med* 1979; 301:1266–1270.
122. Dalen JE: The case against fibrinolytic therapy. *J Cardiovasc Med* 1980; 5:798–804.
123. Sasahara AA: The case for fibrinolytic therapy. *J Cardiovasc Med* 1980; 5:794–797.
124. Genton E: Thrombolytic therapy of pulmonary thromboembolism. *Prog Cardiovasc Dis* 1979; 21:333–341.
125. Goldhaber SZ, Haire WD, Feldstein ML, Miller M, Toltzis R, Smith JL, et al: Alteplase versus heparin in acute pulmonary embolism: Randomized trial assessing right-ventricular function and pulmonary perfusion. *Lancet* 1993; 341:507–511.
126. Goldhaber SZ, Meyerovitz MF, Markis JE, Kim D, Kessler CM, Sharma GVRK, et al: Thrombolytic therapy of acute pulmonary embolism: Current status and future potential. *J Am Coll Cardiol* 1987; 10:96B–104B.
127. Verstraete M, Miller GAH, Bounameaux H, Charbonnier B, Colle JP, Lecorf G, et al: Intravenous and intrapulmonary recombinant tissue-type plasminogen activator in the treatment of acute massive pulmonary embolism. *Circulation* 1988; 77:353–360.
128. Goldhaber SZ, Kessler CM, Heit J, Markis J, Sharma GVRK, Dawley D, et al: Randomised controlled trial of recombinant tissue plasminogen activator versus urokinase in the treatment of acute pulmonary embolism. *Lancet* 1988;1:293–298.
129. PIOPED Investigators: Tissue plasminogen activator for the treatment of acute pulmonary embolism. *Chest* 1990; 97:528–533.
130. Goldhaber SZ: Thrombolysis for pulmonary embolism. *Prog Cardiovas Dis* 1991; 34:113–134.
131. Meyer G, Sors H, Charbonnier B, Kasper W, Bassand J-P, Kerr IH, et al: Effects of intravenous urokinase versus alteplase on total pulmonary resistance in acute massive pulmonary embolism: A European multicenter double-blind trial. *J Am Coll Cardiol* 1992; 19:239–245.
132. Dalla-Volta S, Palla A, Santolicandro A, Giuntini C, Pengo V, Visioli O, et al: PAIMS 2: Alteplase combined with heparin versus heparin in the treatment of acute pulmonary embolism. Plasminogen activator Italian Multicenter Study 2. *J Am Coll Cardiol* 1992; 20:520–526.
133. Diehl J-L, Meyer G, Igual J, Collignon MA, Giselbrecht M, Even P, et al: Effectiveness and safety of bolus administration of alteplase in massive pulmonary embolism. *Am J Cardiol* 1992; 70:1477–1480.
134. Levine M, Hirsh J, Weitz J, Cruickshank M, Neemeh J, Turpie AG, et al: A randomized trial of a single bolus dosage regimen of recombinant tissue plasminogen activator in patients with acute pulmonary embolism. *Chest* 1990; 98:1473–1479.
135. Evans G, Dalen JE, Dexter L: Pulmonary embolism during pregnancy. *JAMA* 1968; 206:320–326.
136. Hellgren M, Nygards EB: Long-term therapy with subcutaneous heparin during pregnancy. *Gynecol Obstet Invest* 1982; 13:76–89.
137. Hall JG, Pauli RM, Wilson KM: Maternal and fetal sequelae of anticoagulation during pregnancy. *Am J Med* 1980; 68:122–140.
138. Ginsberg JS, Hirsh J: Use of antithrombotic agents during pregnancy. *Chest* 1992; 102(suppl):385S–390S.
139. Daily PO, Johnston GG, Simmons CJ, Moser KM: Surgical management of chronic pulmonary embolism. *J Thorac Cardiovasc Surg* 1980; 79:523–531.
139a. DelCampo C: Pulmonary embolectomy: A review. *Can J Surg* 1985; 28:111–113.
140. Moser KM, Spragg RG, Utley J, Dailey PO: Chronic thrombotic obstruction of major pulmonary arteries: Results of thromboendarterectomy in 15 patients. *Ann Intern Med* 1983; 99:299–305.
141. Moser KM, Daily PO, Peterson KL, Dembitsky W, Vapnek JM, Shure D: Thromboendarterectomy for chronic major vessel thromboembolic pulmonary hypertension in 41 patients. Immediate and long-term results. *Ann Intern Med* 1987; 107:560–565.
141a. Moser KM, Anger WR, Fedulo PF: Chronic major-vessel thromboembolic pulmonary hypertension. *Circulation* 1990; 81:1735.
142. Benotti JR, Ockene IS, Alpert JS, Dalen JE: The clinical profile of unresolved pulmonary embolism. *Chest* 1983; 84:669–678.
143. Rich S, Levitsky S, Brundage BH: Pulmonary hypertension from chronic pulmonary thromboembolism. *Ann Intern Med* 1988; 108:425–434.
144. Lyerly HK, Sabiston DC: Surgical treatment of chronic pulmonary embolism. *Annu Rev Med* 1991; 42:507–517.
145. Gauss H: The pathology of fat embolism. *Arch Surg* 1924; 9:593–604.
146. Ashbaugh DG, Petty TL: The use of corticosteroids in the treatment of respiratory failure associated with massive fat embolism. *Surg Gynecol Obstet* 1966; 123:493–500.
147. Liljedahl S, Westermark L: Aetiology and treatment of fat embolism: Report of five cases. *Acta Anaesthesiol Scand* 1967; 11:177–194.
148. Tedeschi CG, Castelli W, Kropp G, Tedeschi LG: Fat macroglobulinemia and fat embolism. *Surg Gynecol Obstet* 1968; 126:83–90.
149. Warren S: Fat embolism. *Am J Pathol* 1946; 22:69–88.
150. Rokkanen P, Lahdensuu M, Kataja J, Julkunen H: The syndrome of fat embolism: Analysis of thirty consecutive cases compared

to trauma patients with similar injuries. *J Trauma* 1970; 10:299–306.

151. Bradford DS, Foster RR, Nossel HL: Coagulation alterations, hypoxemia, and fat embolism in fracture patients. *J Trauma* 1971; 10:307–321.
152. Peltier LF: The diagnosis and treatment of fat embolism. *J Trauma* 1971; 11:661–667.
153. Herndon JH, Riseborough EJ, Fischer JE: Fat embolism: A review of current concepts. *J Trauma* 1971; 11:673–680.
154. Fonte DA, Hausberger FX: Pulmonary free acids in experimental fat embolism. *J Trauma* 1971; 11:668–672.
155. Kerstell J: Pathogenesis of post-traumatic fat embolism. *Am J Surg* 1971; 121:712–715.
156. Fischer JE, Turner RH, Herndon JH, et al: Massive steroid therapy in severe fat embolism. *Surg Gynecol Obstet* 1971; 132:667–672.
157. Dines DE, Linscheid RL, Didier EP: Fat embolism syndrome. *Mayo Clin Proc* 1972; 47:237–240.
158. Rokkanen P, Alho A, Avikainen V, Karaharju E, Kataja J, Lahdensuu M, et al: The efficacy of corticosteroids in severe trauma. *Surg Gynecol Obstet* 1974; 138:69–73.
159. Moylan JA, Evenson MA: Diagnosis and treatment of fat embolism. *Annu Rev Med* 1977; 28:85–90.
160. Alho A, Saikku K, Eerola P, Koskinen M, Hamalainen M: Corticosteroids in patients with a high risk of fat embolism syndrome. *Surg Gynecol Obstet* 1978; 147:358–362.
161. Renne J, Wutheir R, House E, Cancro JC, Hoaglund FT: Fat macroglobulinemia caused by fractures or total hip replacement. *J Bone Joint Surg* 1978; 60A:613–618.
162. Oh WH, Mital MA: Fat embolism: Current concepts of pathogenesis, diagnosis and treatment. *Orthop Clin North Am* 1978; 9:769–779.
163. Curtis AM, Knowles GD, Putnam CE, McLoud TC, Ravin CE, Smith GJ: The three syndromes of fat embolism: Pulmonary manifestations. *Yale J Biol Med* 1979; 52:149–157.
164. Gossling HR, Donohue TA: The fat embolism syndrome. *JAMA* 1979; 241:2740–2742.
165. Guenter CA, Braun TE: Fat embolism syndrome. Changing prognosis. *Chest* 1981; 79:143–145.
166. Gossling HR, Pellegrini VD Jr: Fat embolism syndrome: A review of the pathophysiology and physiological basis of treatment. *Clin Orthop* 1982; 165:68–82.
167. Schonfeld SA, Ploysongsang Y, DiLisio R, Crissman JD, Miller E, Hammerschmidt DE, et al: Fat embolism prophylaxis with corticosteroids. A prospective study in high risk patients. *Ann Intern Med* 1983; 99:438–443.
168. Jacobson DM, Terrence CF, Reinmuth OM: The neurologic manifestations of fat embolism. *Neurology* 1986; 36:847–851.
169. Lindeque BG, Schoeman HS, Dommissee GF, Boeyens MC, Vlok AL: Fat embolism and the fat embolism syndrome. A double-blind therapeutic study. *J Bone Joint Surg (Br)* 1987; 69:128–131.
170. Zenker FA: *Beitrage zur Anatomie und Physiologie der Lunge.* Dresden, Braunsdorf, 1861.
171. Bergmann EB: Ein Fall tödlicher Fettembolie. *Klin Wochenschr* 1973; 10:385.
172. Whitaker AC: Traumatic fat embolism. Report of two cases with recovery. *Arch Surg* 1939; 38:182–189.
173. Berglund E, Josephson S: Pulmonary air embolization in the dog. I. Hemodynamic changes in repeated embolizations. *Scand J Clin Lab Invest* 1970; 26:97–103.
174. Josephson S: Pulmonary air embolization in the dog: II. Evidence and location of pulmonary vasoconstriction. *Scand J Clin Lab Invest* 1970; 26:113–123.
175. Ence TJ, Gong H Jr: Adult respiratory distress syndrome after venous air embolism. *Annu Rev Respir Dis* 1979; 119:1033–1037.
176. Marini JJ, Culver BH: Systemic gas embolism complicating mechanical ventilation in the adult respiratory distress syndrome. *Ann Intern Med* 1989; 110:699–703.
177. Hlastala MP, Robertson HT, Ross BK: Gas exchange abnormalities produced by venous gas emboli. *Respir Physiol* 1979; 36:1–17.
178. Yee ES, Verrier ED, Thomas AN: Management of air embolism in blunt and penetrating thoracic trauma. *J Thorac Cardiovasc Surg* 1983; 85:661–668.
179. Bray P, Myers RA, Cowley RA: Urogenital sex as a cause of nonfatal air embolism in pregnancy. *Obstet Gynecol* 1983; 61:653–657.
180. Rodigas PC, Meyer FJ, Haasler GB, Dubroff JM, Spotnitz HM: Intraoperative 2-dimensional echocardiography: Ejection of microbubbles from the left ventricle after cardiac surgery. *Am J Cardiol* 1982; 50:1130–1132.
181. Ericsson JA, Gottlieb JD, Sweet RB: Closed-chest cardiac massage in the treatment of venous air embolism. *N Engl J Med* 1964; 270:1353–1354.
182. Dedonis J, Schlant RC, Symbas PN: Arterial air embolism: An update. In: Hurst JW (ed): *Clinical Essays on the Heart*, vol. 3. New York, McGraw-Hill, 1984: 77–81.
183. Meyer JR: Emboli pulmonar amino-caseosa. Brasil Med 1926; 2:301–303.
184. Steiner PE, Luschbaugh CC: Maternal pulmonary embolism by amniotic fluid as a cause of obstetric shock and unexpected death in obstetrics. *JAMA* 1941; 117:1245.
185. Liban E, Raz S: A clinicopathologic study of fourteen cases of amniotic fluid embolism. *Am J Clin Pathol* 1969; 51:477–486.
186. Peterson EP, Taylor HB: Amniotic fluid embolism: An analysis of 40 cases. *Obstet Gynecol* 1970; 35:787–793.
187. Jewett JF: Amniotic-fluid infusion. *N Engl J Med* 1975; 292:973–974.
188. Morgan M: Amniotic fluid embolism. *Anaesthesia* 1979; 34:20–32.
189. Sterner S, Campbell B, Davies S: Amniotic fluid embolism. *Ann Emerg Med* 1984; 13:343–345.
190. Rodgers GP, Heymach GJ III: Cryoprecipitate therapy in amniotic fluid embolization. *Am J Med* 1984; 76:916–920.
191. Hogberg U, Joelsson I: Amniotic fluid embolism in Sweden, 1951–1980. *Gynecol Obstet Invest* 1985; 20:130–137.
192. Clark SL: Amniotic fluid embolism. *Clin Perinatol* 1986; 13:801–811.
193. Paterson WG, Grant KA, Grant JM, McLean N: The pathogenesis of amniotic fluid embolism with particular reference to transabdominal amniocentesis. *Eur J Obstet Gynecol Reprod Biol* 1977; 7:319–324.
194. Clark SL, Pavlova Z, Greenspoon J, Horenstein J, Phelan JP: Squamous cells in the maternal pulmonary circulation. *Am J Obstet Gynecol* 1986; 154:104–106.
195. Giampaola C, Schneider V, Kowalski BH, Bellaver LA: The cytologic diagnosis of amniotic fluid embolism: A critical reappraisal. *Diagn Cytopathol* 1987; 3:126–128.
196. Durhan JR, Ashley PF, Dorenclamp D: Cor pulmonale due to tumor emboli: Review of literature and report of a case. *JAMA* 1961; 175:757–760.
197. Bagshawe KD, Noble MIM: Cardiorespiratory aspects of trophoblastic tumors. *Q J Med* 1966; 35:39–54.
198. Li MC: Trophoblastic disease: Natural history, diagnosis and treatment. *Ann Intern Med* 1971; 74:102–112.
199. Ross M, Nowicki K, Rangarajan NS: Asymptomatic pulmonary embolism during pregnancy. *Obstet Gynecol* 1971; 37:131–133.
200. Margolis ML, Jarrell BE: Pulmonary tumor microembolism. *South Med J* 1985; 78:757–758.
201. Mehta S, Rubenstone AI: Pulmonary bile thromboemboli: A report of two cases. *Am J Clin Pathol* 1967; 47:490–496.
202. Dimmick JE, Bove KE, McAdams AJ, Benzing G: Fiber embolization—hazard of cardiac surgery and catheterization. *N Engl J Med* 1975; 292:685–687.

Chapter 101

Chronic Cor Pulmonale

John H. Newman, M.D. ■ *Joseph C. Ross, M.D.*

Cor pulmonale is a term that describes the pathological effects of lung dysfunction on the right side of the heart. The link between lung dysfunction and the right side of the heart in cor pulmonale is pulmonary hypertension. Because the pulmonary hypertension results from abnormal lung function, cor pulmonale is a form of secondary heart disease. Cor pulmonale occurs as a late manifestation of many diseases of the lung, but the common thread in each case is increased right ventricular afterload. Depending on severity and chronicity, the pulmonary hypertension leads to dilatation of the right ventricle with or without hypertrophy. The presence of overt right-sided heart failure is not essential to make the diagnosis of cor pulmonale, but right-sided heart failure is a common consequence. The clinical manifestations of cor pulmonale relate to alterations in cardiac output, salt and water homeostasis, and in most cases, gas exchange in the lung. Right-sided heart dysfunction secondary to left-sided heart failure, valvular dysfunction, or congenital heart disease is excluded in the definition of cor pulmonale.[1] Pulmonary venous obstruction may be considered as a cause of cor pulmonale. As a concept, cor pulmonale was introduced over 200 years ago, but the exact origin of the term is uncertain.[2] Osler[3] commented in the first edition of his textbook that "hypertrophy of the right ventricle . . . results from increased resistance in the pulmonary circulation, as in cirrhosis of the lung and emphysema." McGinn and White[4] apparently were the first to use the term *acute cor pulmonale* in the discussion of a case of massive thromboembolism in 1935. William Harvey's discussion of the relationship of the lung and right side of the heart in De Motu Cordis[5] showed remarkable insight into the limitations of that muscular structure.

INCIDENCE, ETIOLOGIES, AND PATHOLOGY

Emphysema and chronic bronchitis cause over 50 percent of cases of cor pulmonale in this country. The prevalence of cor pulmonale is difficult to determine because cor pulmonale does not occur in all cases of chronic lung disease and because routine physical examination and laboratory tests are relatively insensitive to the presence of pulmonary hypertension. The prevalence of chronic obstructive lung disease in the United States is about 15 million, directly resulting in approximately 70,000 deaths per year and contributing to about 160,000 other deaths.[6] It has been estimated that cor pulmonale accounts for 5 to 10 percent of organic heart disease. Cor pulmonale was present in 20 to 30 percent of admissions for heart failure in one study.[7] It is likely that cor pulmonale is a complication in a high percentage of cases. Gazes[8] found that 9.2 percent of cases of heart disease that came to autopsy had cor pulmonale.

Chronic cor pulmonale occurs most frequently in adult male smokers, although the incidence in women is increasing as heavy smoking in females becomes more prevalent. A list of all diseases that may lead to cor pulmonale would be extensive and is not included in this chapter, but the major types of disease processes are listed in Table 101-1. Two important causes of cor pulmonale, thromboembolism and primary pulmonary hypertension, are discussed in Chaps. 99 and 100.

Chronic Obstructive Pulmonary Disease

Chronic obstructive lung diseases (COPDs) cause cor pulmonale through several interrelated mechanisms, in-

TABLE 101-1

Etiologies of Chronic Cor Pulmonale by Mechanism of Pulmonary Hypertension

I. Hypoxic vasoconstriction
  A. Chronic bronchitis and emphysema, cystic fibrosis
  B. Chronic hypoventilation
    1. Obesity
    2. Sleep apnea
    3. Neuromuscular disease
    4. Chest wall dysfunction
  C. High-altitude dwelling and chronic mountain sickness (Monge's disease)
II. Occlusion of the pulmonary vascular bed
  A. Pulmonary thromboembolism, parasitic ova, tumor emboli
  B. Primary pulmonary hypertension
  C. Pulmonary venocclusive disease
  D. Fibrosing mediastinitis, mediastinal tumor
  E. Pulmonary angiitis from systemic disease
    1. Collagen vascular diseases
    2. Drug-induced lung disease
    3. Necrotizing and granulomatous arteritis
III. Parenchymal disease with loss of vascular surface area
  A. Bullous emphysema, α_1 antiproteinase deficiency
  B. Diffuse bronchiectasis, cystic fibrosis
  C. Diffuse interstitial disease
    1. Pneumoconiosis
    2. Sarcoid, idiopathic pulmonary fibrosis, histiocytosis X
    3. Tuberculosis, chronic fungal infection
    4. Adult respiratory distress syndrome
    5. Collagen vascular disease (autoimmune lung disease)
    6. Hypersensitivity pneumonitis

cluding hypoventilation, hypoxemia from ventilation/perfusion (V/Q) mismatch, and destruction of perfused surface area.[9] Patients with more prominent hypoxemia and alveolar hypoventilation develop erythrocytosis, edema, and early onset of cor pulmonale ("blue bloaters").[10] Patients in whom dyspnea on exertion is the most prominent symptom have less hypoventilation and less hypoxemia at rest and therefore develop cor pulmonale later ("pink puffers"). Some of the differences between blue bloaters and pink puffers may relate to ventilatory drives; patients with low drives may be more likely to fit the blue-bloater category, whereas pink puffers strive to maintain normal arterial pH and gas tensions.[11] Another hypothesis is that blue bloaters have more inflammatory bronchitis and that pink puffers suffer more from pure emphysema.[10] *Physical examination* in all forms of COPD shows an increase in the thoracic diameter, low diaphragms, hyperresonance to percussion, decreased breath sounds with expiratory wheezes, distant heart sounds, distended neck veins during expiration, and a palpable liver. Liver enlargement and leg edema are manifestations of right-sided heart failure and may or may not be present. The *chest roentgenogram* may show characteristic changes of emphysema such as hyperlucent lungs, bullae, increased anteroposterior (AP) diameter, and flattened diaphragm. In some cases, increased bronchovascular markings occur, suggestive of thickened or inflamed airways. On the other hand, the chest roentgenogram may not show characteristic findings or be indicative of the severity of the physiological impairment. *Pulmonary function tests* show an increased residual volume (RV) and total lung capacity (TLC), decreased forced vital capacity (FVC), and markedly decreased expiratory flow rates (FEV_1, FEF_{25-75}). *Arterial blood* studies at rest can be normal when disease is mild but in severe disease show decreased P_{O_2}, increased P_{CO_2}, and decreased pH. With cor pulmonale, P_{O_2} is likely to be below 55 torr. Desaturation increases with exercise and frequently during sleep. The V/Q inequality and hypoventilation both contribute to the hypoxemia. A P_{CO_2} above 45 torr at rest indicates general alveolar hypoventilation. (See also Chap. 17.) Asthma is a form of COPD that rarely, if ever, leads to chronic cor pulmonale.

Diffuse Interstitial Lung Disease

These patients have dyspnea, tachypnea, exercise intolerance, and occasionally, clubbing of the digits. Basilar rales are frequently heard on auscultation of the chest.[12] The *chest roentgenogram* shows diffuse reticular, reticulonodular, or fibrotic lesions, but the appearance does not always correlate well with physiological impairment. In some disease presentations such as desquamative interstitial pneumonitis, there may be an alveolar filling pattern. A lung biopsy is frequently required to identify the basic pathological process, and even then the exact etiology may not always be determined. Transbronchial biopsy can be diagnostic in some interstitial diseases such as sarcoidosis, and bronchoalveolar lavage may point to a diagnosis in many cases.[12] *Pulmonary function tests* show a restrictive process with reduced lung volumes, decreased compliance, and decreased diffusing capacity without airways obstruction. The forced expiratory volume in 1 (FEV_1) as a percentage of forced vital capacity (FVC) is usually at least 80 percent. At first, P_{O_2} decreases during exercise but is kept at normal levels at rest by hyperventilation. As the disease becomes more severe, P_{O_2} is low at rest. (See also Chap. 17.) The course and prognosis of interstitial lung disease depend on the specific etiology, and there is wide variation among and within diseases.[12,13] The presence of cor pulmonale in interstitial lung disease implies extensive severe lung dysfunction, and cor pulmonale may not occur even in end-stage disease.

Hypoventilation Syndromes

Some disorders (i.e., kyphoscoliosis) may impair or restrict mechanics of ventilation, causing *general* alveolar hypoventilation and alveolar hypoxia.[14] Extreme obesity may be associated with hypoventilation, cyanosis, polycythemia, and somnolence (without intrinsic lung disease), often called the Pickwickian syndrome.[15] Patients with daytime somnolence, morning headaches, and personality disturbances have been found to have periodic apnea during sleep associated with sleep deprivation, loud snoring, hypoxemia, and hypercapnia caused by upper airway obstruction (i.e., tongue, enlarged tonsils, or collapse of pharyngeal walls).[16] Brain stem abnormalities such as Arnold-Chiari malformation may also cause respiratory center depression and primary hypoventilation. The diagnosis of hypoventilation is confirmed by a depressed ventilatory response to inhaled CO_2, tests of pulmonary hyperventilation, or sleep studies. It has become apparent recently that disordered ventilation during sleep is a major component of many hypoventilation syndromes.[17] In all cases of hypoventilation, the main stimulus for pulmonary hypertension is hypoxic vasoconstriction, a response of the pulmonary arterioles to alveolar hypoxia. The respiratory acidosis that may accompany hypoventilation augments the vasoconstrictor response to hypoxia.

Chronic Mountain Sickness

Chronic pulmonary hypertension can develop during high-altitude dwelling in persons with normal lungs.[18] Pulmonary arterial pressure in normal humans increases as a function of the level of altitude, and the most important mechanism is the reduced partial pressure of alveolar O_2. The hypertensive response to high-altitude hypoxia is greater in men than in women and it is more prevalent in North Americans than in South Americans, suggesting racial differences. The chronic response is determined by the innate strength of hypoxic vasoconstriction and the degree of vascular remodeling in response to hypoxia. The ventilatory response to hypoxia also modifies the vascular changes. Persons with blunted ventilatory drives are more likely to become more hypoxic at high altitude and develop more hypertension. Hypercarbia augments the pressor response, and secondary erythrocytosis can worsen resistance to flow by an increase in blood viscosity. Nocturnal desaturation during sleep may exacerbate the process. Thus, the chronic pulmonary hypertension of high altitude is complex, and the chronic pulmonary vascular response is a result of many influences.[18]

Pulmonary Vascular Disease

Chronic cor pulmonale is a consequence of several diseases that involve the pulmonary vessels. Primary pulmonary hypertension and recurrent (or unresolved) pulmonary emboli are described in detail in Chaps. 99 and 100. Sickle cell disease, from SS or SC hemoglobinopathy, can cause cor pulmonale after multiple episodes of pulmonary infarction from focal pulmonary sickling or from thromboembolism.[19] Venocclusive disease is a rare disease of the veins that presents with pulmonary hypertension and pulmonary edema. There is at least one report of a beneficial response to immunosuppressive therapy in that disease.[20] Cirrhosis of the liver is usually associated with pulmonary vasodilation, but occasionally a disorder clinically and pathologically identical to primary pulmonary hypertension emerges.[21,22] Human immunodeficiency virus (HIV) positivity is a new cause of pulmonary vascular disease resembling primary pulmonary hypertension. (See also Chap. 107.) Collagen vascular diseases can cause cor pulmonale by primary vasculitis as well as by diffuse interstitial fibrosis. Systemic sclerosis, systemic lupus erythematosus (SLE), and rheumatoid arthritis (RA) are the collagen vascular diseases that most commonly cause pulmonary arteritis. Patients with SLE and RA frequently present with primary interstitial lung disease. Occasionally, the presentation is that of cor pulmonale without prominent interstitial disease but with primary pulmonary arteritis.[24] Cor pulmonale is not reported as a feature of Goodpasture's syndrome or idiopathic pulmonary hemosiderosis.

PATHOPHYSIOLOGY

Increased pulmonary vascular resistance (PVR) and pulmonary hypertension are central mechanisms in all cases of cor pulmonale. Physiological mechanisms of pulmonary arterial pressure are shown in Table 101-2. These variables can be described by Poiseuille's law. Fortunately, most pulmonary diseases and disorders do not produce enough pulmonary hypertension to cause cor pulmonale.

Normal Pulmonary Circulation

The primary function of this unique high-flow, low-pressure, low-resistance system is to provide blood for gas exchange, and it is ideally suited to optimize that function. It receives and transmits the entire cardiac output with a low pressure head primarily because of three characteristics: (1) pulmonary arteries are thin-walled with little resting muscular tone; (2) there is negligible vasomotor control by the autonomic nervous system at rest in the adult; and (3) many small arterioles and capillaries are nonperfused at rest and can be recruited when needed to expand the pulmonary vascular bed, resulting in a decreased PVR. Normal mean pulmonary artery

TABLE 101-2

Genesis of Pulmonary Hypertension: Poiseuille's Law

$$P_{PA} = CO\left(\frac{8}{\pi} n \frac{1}{N} \frac{1}{r^4}\right) + P_{LA}$$

where

CO	=	cardiac output (usually elevated in COPD; if PRV is fixed, increased CO will elevate PAP)
$\frac{8}{\pi}$	=	numerical constant related to tubular structure of vessels
n	=	blood viscosity (increased in polycythemia vera, secondary erythrocytosis and cryoglobulinemia)
N	=	number of perfused vessels of a particular radius (N is decreased in any occlusive or destructive disease; see Table 101-1)
$\frac{1}{r^4}$	=	radius of a vessel is a critical determinant of flow (r is decreased by vasoconstriction or luminal obstruction; change in r from 1 to 2 units increases resistance 16-fold)
P_{LA}	=	left atrial pressure; passive pulmonary hypertension can result from left atrial pressure elevation due either to LV or valve disease

pressure (PAP) is about 12 to 17 mmHg; PAP above 20 mmHg at rest suggests pulmonary hypertension. Flow of blood through pulmonary capillaries is accomplished by a pressure drop of only 5 to 9 mmHg (PA to LA), compared to an arterial to venous gradient of 90 mmHg in the systemic circuit. Thus, normal PVR is 10- to 20-fold less than systemic vascular resistance (See also Chaps. 5 and 99.)

Pulmonary Hypertension

The effective cross-sectional area of the pulmonary vascular bed must be reduced by more than 50 percent before any change in PAP can be detected at rest. Exercise causes increased PAP because of increased pulmonary blood flow in the normal bed, and exercise will dramatically raise PAP if the vascular bed is reduced. Obliterative vascular diseases increase PVR by vascular occlusion, while diffuse interstitial diseases act primarily by compression and obliteration of small vessels. It is now well established, however, that arteriolar constriction resulting from alveolar hypoxia is the predominant cause of pulmonary hypertension in chronic airway diseases.[1,25–27]

Pulmonary Arteriolar Constriction

The most important cause of pulmonary vasoconstriction is alveolar hypoxia. The mechanism of hypoxic pulmonary vasoconstriction is unknown. It is thought to be due either to mediator release from some unknown effector cell or a direct action of hypoxia on pulmonary vascular smooth muscle.[25] The degree of hypoxic vasoconstriction is dependent primarily on the alveolar P_{O_2}, and when alveolar P_{O_2} is about 55 torr, pulmonary artery pressure rises sharply (Fig. 101-1). When PAP is greater than 40 mmHg, arterial oxygen saturation is very likely

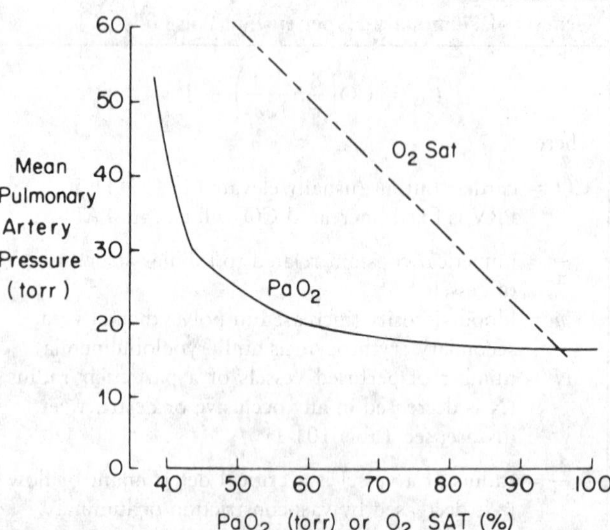

FIGURE 101-1 Pulmonary arterial pressure as a function of P_{O_2} or oxyhemoglobin saturation. Pulmonary arterial pressure rises sharply as P_{O_2} decreases below 55 torr. (*Redrawn from JT Reeves, RF Grover: High altitude pulmonary hypertension and pulmonary edema. Prog Cardiol 4:105, 1975, and from B Burrows, Am Rev Resp Dis 110:64, 1974.*)

TABLE 101-3
Pulmonary Vasomotor Tone

Dilator	Constrictor
Beta-adrenergic agonists	Alpha-adrenergic agonists
Histamine H_2	Histamine H_1
Prostacyclin (PGI_2), PGE_1	PGE_2, $PGF_{1\alpha}$, thromboxane A_2, PGD_2
Acetylcholine*	Serotonin
Oxygen	Hypoxia
Bradykinin	Angiotensin II
Vasoactive intestinal polypeptide	Platelet activating factor
Endothelial-derived relaxing factor	Leukotriene C_4/D_4
Atrial natriuretic peptide	Vasopressin

*The response of the pulmonary vascular bed is tone dependent. Acetylcholine is a vasodilator when the pulmonary circulation is preconstricted through the release of endothelial-derived relaxing factor.

less than 75 percent.[26] There is large individual variability in the hypoxic pressor response, and hypoxic vasoconstriction is enhanced by acidosis and blunted by alkalosis. Acidosis also has a mild direct pressor effect on the pulmonary circulation.[28] Extensive investigations into the mechanism of hypoxic vasoconstriction have shown that many local and circulating mediators of pulmonary vascular tone are capable of modulating the hypoxic pressor response but that no single mediator yet discovered is responsible (Table 101-3).

Hypoxic vasoconstriction in a region of lung where ventilation is diminished probably serves to maximize net arterial oxygenation by diverting blood from the hypoxic region to better ventilated areas. Because the pulmonary vascular bed is capable of large recruitment, localized hypoxic vasoconstriction does not cause pulmonary hypertension. Generalized hypoxia causes generalized hypoxic vasoconstriction and the development of pulmonary hypertension (Fig. 101-2). Obliteration of blood vessels was once thought to be the primary cause of hypertension in COPD, but it is clearly of secondary importance. In COPD, the first episodes of alveolar hypoxia may occur during sleep and gradually become more prevalent thereafter.[29] Any cause of alveolar hypoventilation (Table 101-1) can result in chronic cor pulmonale through the mechanism of hypoxic pulmonary vasoconstriction, even from entities as different as diffuse obstructive lung disease and kyphoscoliosis.[14] (See also Chap. 99.)

Other Factors That Increase Pulmonary Hypertension

After the cross-sectional area of the pulmonary vascular bed has become reduced, increases in cardiac output, heart rate, and blood volume or direct effects of acidosis and/or hypoxia on the myocardium may contribute to the pulmonary hypertension. Increased blood flow (i.e., exercise) requires the generation of a higher PAP, and in such a situation, the effects of hypoxia and acidosis will

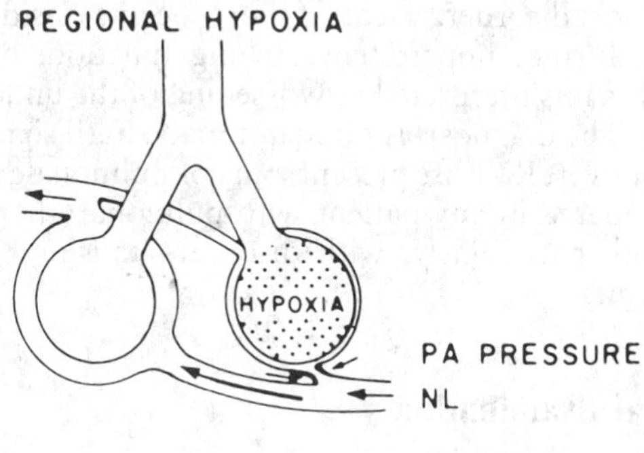

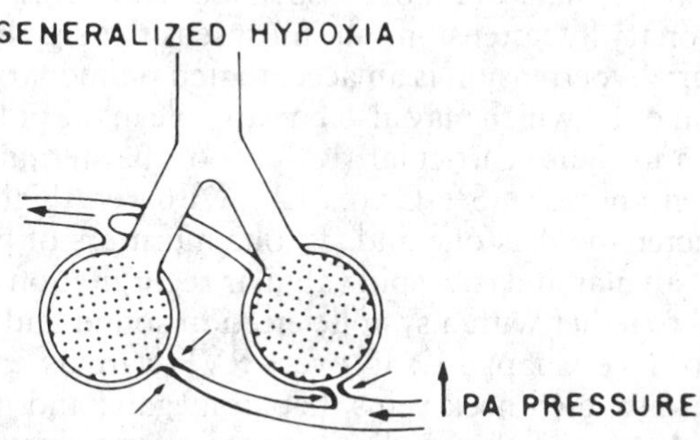

FIGURE 101-2 Hypoxic pulmonary vasoconstriction maximizes arterial oxygenation by diverting blood away from areas of regional hypoxia toward better ventilated zones. Generalized hypoxia causes generalized hypoxic vasoconstriction and results in pulmonary hypertension. (*From JH Newman: Pulmonary vascular reactivity in primary pulmonary edema. Semin Respir Med 4:299, 1983. Reproduced with permission of the publisher. Courtesy of JV Weil.*)

also be exaggerated.[26] Sustained hypoxemia causes secondary erythrocytosis. Blood viscosity increases rapidly after the hematocrit exceeds about 55 percent, raising PVR and also decreasing cerebral function. If left ventricular failure (LVF) is superimposed on an already reduced pulmonary vascular bed, a higher PAP will occur in response to a stimulus. Once established, pulmonary hypertension may be self-perpetuating. A sustained increase in PAP in patients with diffuse lung disease causes anatomic changes in the walls of small arteries, further increasing PVR and PAP.[30] Chronic hypoxia alone results in muscularization of pulmonary arterioles and exaggerated increases in PAP with stimuli.[31]

Right Ventricular Response to Pulmonary Hypertension

The right ventricle is thin walled and better able to handle an increase in volume load than to meet an increased pressure load. The primary cause of right ventricular failure (RVF), therefore, is a chronic pressure load (afterload). Small increases in PAP may result in large increases in right ventricular work. Pulmonary hypertension at rest indicates advanced disease, and at that stage small changes in blood flow will cause large increases in PAP.

Response of the right ventricle to pulmonary hypertension depends on the acuteness and severity of the pressure load. Acute cor pulmonale (see Chaps. 99 and 100) occurs after a sudden and severe stimulus (i.e., massive pulmonary emboli) with ventricular dilatation and failure but no hypertrophy. Chronic cor pulmonale, however, is associated with a more slowly evolving and slowly progressive hypertension,[32] and the response may include increased protein synthesis and right ventricular hypertrophy (RVH).[33] The severity of the hypertension, the rapidity with which it becomes severe, and the possible eventual onset of RVF are influenced by factors that intercede intermittently, such as (1) *alterations in ventilatory function*, causing alveolar pressure changes with effects on chamber function; (2) *alterations in gas exchange* with more or less severe hypoxemia, hypercapnia, and acidosis; and (3) *alterations in volume load* as influenced by exercise, heart rate, polycythemia, or renal retention of salt and water associated with cor pulmonale. At some stage, the myocardium is unable to function at the high pressure load, dilates, and fails. Right ventricular failure may occur relatively early in some patients with chronic bronchitis and emphysema because of sustained hypoxemia and hypercarbia but occurs later in patients with diffuse lung disease because the degree of RVH helps to maintain blood flow, even when PAP is high.[30] Significant pulmonary hypertension and RVH can occur in normal persons living at extreme altitude with no evidence for heart failure.[34] Thus the normal right ventricle can develop into an efficient high-pressure pump over time.

Left Ventricular Function in Cor Pulmonale

Dysfunction of the left ventricle occurs in some patients with cor pulmonale, but the evidence available indicates that cor pulmonale per se does not cause disease of the left heart. The likelihood, in most cases, is that left-sided heart dysfunction coexisting with cor pulmonale results from other known causes such as coronary ischemia or systemic hypertension. Left ventricular failure is a serious complication in cor pulmonale because the increase in lung water further impairs lung function, increases the work of breathing, increases pulmonary artery (PA) pressure, impairs gas exchange, and may induce respiratory failure. When underlying disease of the left ventricle is also present, the direct effects of hypoxia, hypercapnia, and acidosis arising from primary lung disease may precipitate left ventricular failure.[35,36]

Several lines of evidence point to direct effects of lung dysfunction and right ventricular hypertrophy on performance of the left ventricle.[36,37] Wide swings in transpulmonary pressure in obstructive lung disease can reduce left ventricular filling and increase left ventricular afterload.[38] Hypertrophy and elevated end diastolic pressure of the right ventricle in cor pulmonale can reduce left ventricular compliance and impair left ventricular filling through effects on the shared ventricular septum.[39] Despite these effects, most patients with chronic cor pulmonale demonstrate normal resting cardiac output, normal pulmonary artery wedge pressure, and normal resting left ventricular ejection fraction.[40] The majority of patients with abnormal left ventricular ejection fraction in either compensated or decompensated chronic lung disease probably have demonstrable coronary artery disease.

Edema Formation and Cor Pulmonale

Peripheral edema occurs in some cases of chronic cor pulmonale. The mechanism is poorly understood but is probably related to increased systemic venous pressure, hypercarbia, and hypoxemia.[41] The presence of pulmonary hypertension per se does not appear to be sufficient to cause fluid retention until right atrial pressure becomes elevated. Decreased clearance of aldosterone from the passively congested liver contributes to salt retention but is likely not an initiating event. Plasma volume is, however, increased in chronic cor pulmonale.[42]

Hypercarbia stimulates plasma renin activity, and hypercarbic, edematous patients with chronic obstructive lung disease have increased plasma levels of aldosterone and antidiuretic hormone.[43] This pattern occurs despite oxygen therapy in these patients. Thus, not only increased salt retention but also impaired water excretion contributes to edema in chronic hypercapnia. The role of atrial natriuretic peptide in water hemostasis in cor pulmonale remains to be evaluated. The renal effects of moderate hypoxia are less pronounced, unless the P_{O_2} is in the 30- to 45-torr range, where decrease in urine formation occurs. Other mechanisms of edema formation are increased systemic capillary hydrostatic pressure, related to increased venous pressure and blood volume, and perhaps a direct effect of hypoxia on peripheral tissue.

Many mechanisms appear to be operating to produce edema in chronic cor pulmonale, several of which are related to the primary pulmonary dysfunction. The exact pattern and sequence of events leading to edema is difficult to determine in any specific case. Pulmonary edema and pleural effusion are not seen as a consequence of chronic cor pulmonale.

COR PULMONALE: CLINICAL MANIFESTATIONS

Symptoms

Clinical manifestations of cor pulmonale are often obscured by the signs and symptoms of underlying disease and are, therefore, closely related to the pulmonary disease or disorder. It is necessary first to recognize the type and severity of lung disease and then to look for cor pulmonale.

There is no history that is specific for cor pulmonale. Episodes of leg edema, atypical chest pain, dyspnea on exertion, exercise-induced peripheral cyanosis, prior respiratory failure, and excessive daytime somnolence are all historical clues suggesting the presence of cor pulmonale. Chest pain may be due to strain or distortion of the chest wall (musculoskeletal) or may be related to right ventricular ischemia. Cough and complaints of easy fatigability are common. Some patients with nocturnal hypoventilation and sleep apnea may present with personality changes, mild systemic hypertension, and headache.

Left ventricular failure causes immediate effects on the pulmonary vascular bed and on lung function, producing rapid and dramatic respiratory symptoms. No such situation exists with cor pulmonale. The symptoms are mainly those related to progression of the underlying disease or disorder. Heart failure occurs insidiously, causing further impairment of lung function, but frequently is misinterpreted as worsening of the underlying disease. The diagnosis is often not made until significant RVH or overt RVF are present, but cor pulmonale should be considered in any patient with pulmonary hypertension and, particularly, with disorders causing chronic hypoxemia.

Physical Examination

The earliest signs are those associated with longstanding pulmonary hypertension. The most sensitive sign for pulmonary hypertension is an accentuated pulmonary component of S_2, which may also be palpable in the pulmonic area, and right ventricular (RV) lift of the sternum may be seen and felt. (See Chap. 10.) With very high PAP, characteristic diastolic and systolic murmurs of pulmonary valvular and tricuspid valvular regurgitation can be heard together with a systolic ejection sound and RV S_3 gallop. (See Chap. 11.) In overt RVF, cardiac enlargement, distended neck veins, hepatomegaly, and peripheral edema are present. Right ventricular failure is frequently accompanied by hypoxemia and cyanosis. Symptoms or signs suggestive of heart failure, such as dyspnea, orthopnea, peripheral edema, palpable liver, and distended neck veins, however, can be observed in patients with COPD without RVF. When neck veins are distended during inspiration as well as expiration, however, RVF is more likely present. Hyperinflated lungs alter the position of the heart and frequently make the examination difficult. The apical impulse and the RV lift are often not palpable and the RV S_3 gallop may be heard in the epigastrium. The heart sounds may be best heard in the subxiphoid area. Usually RVF is precipitated by an acute episode such as respiratory infection and is associated with significant hypoxemia, hypercapnia, and acidosis. Extremities may be warm due to peripheral vasodilation caused by hypercapnia.

Electrocardiogram

Electrocardiographic (ECG) patterns are influenced by many factors such as PAP, rotation, and displacement of the heart by hyperinflated lungs, arterial blood gases, myocardial ischemia, and metabolic disturbances. The value of the ECG in diagnosis of cor pulmonale, therefore, is dependent on the underlying disease and complicating conditions. Absence of changes indicating RV disease does not rule out cor pulmonale since the ECG may be normal in advanced cor pulmonale. The classic RVH pattern is seen more often when there is anatomic restriction of the pulmonary vascular bed. An example of RVH is shown in Fig. 101-3. The standard criteria for RV enlargement were absent in two-thirds of patients with COPD who had RVH on postmortem examination.[1] It has been suggested that when classical RVH changes are absent, diagnosis should be based on the combination of rS in V_5 to V_6, RAD, qR in a VR, and "P pulmonale."[44] Tall peaked P waves in leads II, III, AVF may reflect positional changes rather than right atrial enlargement. Right bundle branch block (RBBB) occurs in about 15

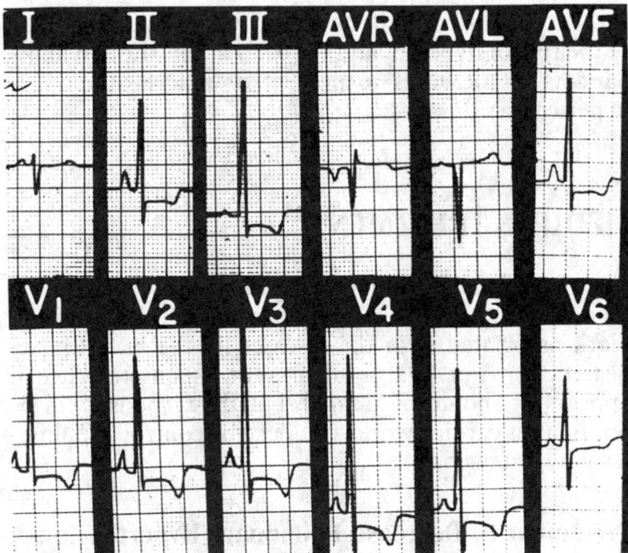

FIGURE 101-3 Electrocardiogram in a patient with cor pulmonale. The mean QRS axis was +120°. The tall, peaked P waves indicate right atrial enlargement. The tall R waves in leads V_1 to V_3 and deep S wave in V_6 and the associated T wave changes indicate right ventricular hypertrophy. (*From NF Voelkel, JT Reeves: Primary pulmonary hypertension. In Moser KM (ed): Pulmonary Vascular Diseases. New York, Marcel Dekker, 1979. Reproduced with permission of the publisher and the author. Courtesy of JR Pryor.*)

percent of patients.[44] A pattern of S_1, Q_3, and T_3 carries reasonable sensitivity and specificity for cor pulmonale in COPD.[45] Arrhythmias are infrequent in uncomplicated cor pulmonale but when present are mostly supraventricular and may reflect blood gas abnormalities, hypokalemia, or excess of drugs such as digitalis, theophylline, and beta agonists. Multifocal atrial tachycardia is associated with decompensated COPD and cor pulmonale, and is best treated by attention to the underlying disease rather than by antiarrhythmic drugs. Ventricular arrhythmias, when they occur, are associated with a high mortality.

Chest Roentgenogram

The radiographic findings of pulmonary hypertension in patients with normal lung parenchyma (such as early mitral stenosis) are well described.[46] Most diseases that cause cor pulmonale have grossly abnormal chest roentgenograms, and the radiologic diagnosis of pulmonary hypertension in these diseases is more difficult. Right ventricular enlargement may be difficult to detect in the vertical heart of emphysema, and comparison with previous films may be helpful. In the most obvious cases of cor pulmonale, there is RV and PA enlargement, but pulmonary hypertension precedes RV dilatation. One indicator of pulmonary hypertension is measurement of the dimensions of the right and left pulmonary arteries. Enlargement is considered to exist if the diameter of the right descending PA is greater than 16 mm[47] and the left descending PA is greater than 18 mm.[48] These findings occurred in 43 of 46 patients with known pulmonary hypertension, but the true sensitivity and specificity of these measurements are not known.

Echocardiogram

Advances in echocardiography make this a useful test in selected cases where cor pulmonale is suspected. The standard M mode is limited to detection of RV dilatation and is best able to display only the anteriormost RV wall near the interventricular septum. Two-dimensional echocardiography allows improved visualization of RV chamber size and wall thickness as well as changes in the interventricular septum resulting from RV hypertrophy.[49,50] Because the right ventricle is asymmetric, measurement of RV volume is difficult even with two-dimensional views. Right ventricular pressure overload is usually detected by hypertrophy of the anterior RV wall and by dilatation of the chamber. Hypertrophy of the septum can be found and septal encroachment into the left ventricular (LV) chamber can be seen. Right ventricular volume overload, as in atrial septal defect, causes dilatation as the predominant finding, often in association with abnormal ventricular septal motion.[51]

Doppler echocardiographic techniques have been developed to estimate pulmonary hypertension and to measure cardiac output. These techniques appear to be relatively accurate when PAP is above 30 mmHg but may not detect milder, but pathologically significant, pulmonary hypertension.[52,53] Doppler echocardiography may be useful for longitudinal follow-up of pharmacologic treatment of pulmonary hypertension cor pulmonale. (See also Chaps. 15 and 130.)

Nuclear Scan

Quantitative first-pass radionuclide angiocardiography is a useful technique for noninvasive assessment of RV function and shows an abnormal RV ejection fraction in patients with cor pulmonale.[54] Thallium 201 myocardial imaging can show RV free-wall thickening in patients with pulmonary hypertension, even when RVH is not detected by ECG.[55]

Right-Sided Heart Catheterization

Right-sided heart catheterization is the only technique available for the direct measurement of pulmonary artery pressure, pulmonary artery wedge pressure, and cardiac output. It is occasionally important in differentiating cor pulmonale from LV dysfunction when the clinical presentation is confusing. This is especially true in patients with primary pulmonary hypertension or unresolved pulmonary emboli, where airway function may appear normal, or with restrictive cardiomyopathy. (See Chaps. 91 and 99.) In cor pulmonale, PA diastolic pressure is significantly higher than wedge pressure, unlike LVF or mitral stenosis, where the diastolic-wedge pressure gradient is smaller in most patients (see Chap. 80). Mean PAP can be very high in obliterative vascular diseases but only moderately high in interstitial lung diseases.[56] In COPD, PAP is related to the level of hypoxemia and usually will be decreased by oxygen administration.[57] About 50 percent of patients with severe COPD will have pulmonary hypertension at rest; in those patients with normal resting values, PAP may rise with exercise.[58] Serial catheterization in patients with

COPD and pulmonary hypertension have revealed remarkable stability of pulmonary hemodynamics.[59]

USUAL STRATEGY OF WORKUP

Because of the diversity of diseases that cause cor pulmonale, no single strategy of workup exists. When lung parenchymal or airway disease is present, pulmonary function tests will frequently reveal the degree and nature of impairment. Spirometry, lung volumes (functional residual capacity), diffusing capacity for carbon monoxide, and an arterial blood sample for pH, P_{O_2}, and P_{CO_2} should be obtained. (See Chap. 17.) Transbronchial biopsy via a fiberoptic bronchoscope, bronchoalveolar lavage, and open lung biopsy are diagnostic options in patients with interstitial lung disease. The hematocrit, if elevated above 50 percent, gives a clue to the presence of chronic hypoxemia. Patients with cryptogenic pulmonary hypertension should receive a perfusion radionuclide lung scan to detect pulmonary emboli or other causes of obstruction of the pulmonary arteries. If pulmonary vasculitis is suspected, serum for antinuclear antibody, hepatitis B surface antigen, rheumatoid factor, and cryoglobulins can be screened.

Polysomnography should be performed in patients with cor pulmonale and any sign or symptoms of sleep apnea. Exercise tests will occasionally reveal desaturation or ventilatory limitations that denote significant lung dysfunction not appreciated on examination at rest. Doppler echocardiography is a reasonable addition to the noninvasive workup of a patient suspected to have pulmonary hypertension.

NATURAL HISTORY AND PROGNOSIS

Prognosis depends on control of the underlying lung disease and control of pulmonary hypertension, but the prognosis based on cor pulmonale alone may not be the same as for the underlying disease. Patients with COPD have hypoxic pulmonary hypertension that is to a great extent reversible, and RVF can be improved with appropriate therapy. Even with repeated episodes of RVF, some have long survivals.[10,54] The pink puffers tend to live longer than the blue bloaters.[10] Once RVF occurs, prognosis is poor; but even though RVF occurs most often in the terminal phase of illness, there are reports of 7- to 8-year survivals after the diagnosis of cor pulmonale.[60]

In patients with alveolar hypoventilation but no alteration in lung structure, the natural history is one of progressive worsening of pulmonary hypertension due to sustained hypoxemia, hypercapnia, and eventually, cor pulmonale and RVF. If alveolar ventilation is improved prior to the development of nonreversible changes in vessel walls, the prognosis is good.

Even with modern techniques for diagnosis and management, prognosis for the underlying disease has not been greatly improved. The prognosis for cor pulmonale, however, is much better because of newer techniques for early recognition of the problem, better understanding of the role of hypoxia, and the early application in many patients of measures to prevent or relieve pulmonary hypertension.

MEDICAL TREATMENT

Treatment of the primary lung disease is the focus of therapy and is the best way to reduce the RV pressure work associated with the disease. If RVF has not appeared, a major goal is to prevent its onset. When it appears, it should be treated, but the response will be poor unless cardiac work is reduced by control of pulmonary hypertension.

Treatment to Decrease Pulmonary Hypertension

Relief of hypoxia is of prime importance in reducing pulmonary hypertension, either to prevent or treat cor pulmonale. That may be done in two ways: (1) treatment of the underlying disease and (2) O_2 administration. Neither will lower PAP in all patients since hypertension is often intractable in those with an anatomic restriction of the pulmonary vascular bed. Most patients with chronic cor pulmonale have some hypoxic pulmonary vasoconstriction, and all should be treated with oxygen in amounts adequate to restore arterial O_2 tension to greater than 60 torr. Corticosteroids may be helpful in some patients with interstitial lung disease and patients with a bronchospastic component of COPD. Measures should be instituted to treat the systemic disease with which obliterative vascular disease is associated or to prevent further pulmonary emboli, if that is the problem.

In COPD, the primary focus is relief of hypoxemia by restoration of effective ventilation or by O_2 administration. Net alveolar ventilation may be improved by therapy, including bronchodilators for bronchospasm, antibiotics to prevent or treat acute exacerbations of bronchitis, bronchial toilet for removal of secretions, and avoidance of airway irritants such as tobacco smoke. Tranquilizers, sedatives, and narcotics must be avoided in unstable patients and patients with hypoventilation. Correction of hypoxia and acidosis may produce a striking reduction in PAP. In diseases that alter lung function but not structure, effective alveolar ventilation must be restored by treatment of the underlying disease or by use of mechanical ventilation. Ventilatory stimulants may be useful in some cases of decreased ventilatory drives.[61]

Adequate oxygenation may well prevent the onset of heart failure, both acutely and over a long period of time. Any patient with cor pulmonale and RVF should be given O_2 if it is required to restore P_{O_2} to levels above 60 torr, but it should be given cautiously when P_{CO_2} is high and the threat of respiratory acidosis is present. When low-flow nasal O_2 causes significant increases in P_{CO_2}, mechanical ventilation may be required to relieve hypoxia. Studies[27] have conclusively shown that home oxygen therapy, nocturnal or continuous, is beneficial in keeping patients with severe COPD functioning better for longer periods of time and may be effective both in treating cor pulmonale and in postponing its onset.

Treatment of Heart Failure

Cor pulmonale is heart disease, and while treatment of the lung disease and relief of hypoxia are necessary to reduce cardiac work, general principles also apply. Diuretics and phlebotomy can be appropriate measures for treatment of RVF. Pulmonary vasodilators are efficacious in some patients with primary pulmonary hypertension but are of uncertain value in cor pulmonale from COPD.[62] (See Chap. 99.)

Beneficial effects of digitalis are not as obvious as in LVF, and arrhythmias caused by digitalis may occur at relatively low serum levels in patients with hypoxia and acidosis. Susceptibility to digitalis intoxication is enhanced in pulmonary disease.[63] Its use in cor pulmonale, therefore, has been controversial. Nevertheless, studies[64] have shown that digitalis improves RV function in cor pulmonale, and it is an appropriate drug for treatment of RVF when given cautiously and in carefully controlled dosage levels. It should not be used during the acute phases of respiratory insufficiency when there are large fluctuations in levels of hypoxemia and acidosis but is reserved for the time when hypoxemia is stabilized. Heart rate cannot be used as a guide for the level of digitalization. It is also reasonable to question whether or not patients with cor pulmonale who continue to have overt RVF after relief of hypoxemia in intensive therapy for the underlying lung disease will benefit from the use of digitalis. Digitalis is appropriate if there is known or suspected concurrent LV systolic dysfunction.

Vasodilator therapy to reduce RV afterload has been recognized as a potential treatment strategy for years. Vasodilator therapy has the disadvantage of being secondary therapy, not aimed at the primary lung dysfunction. Vasodilator therapy has not become widespread because of uncertain benefit, small reductions in pulmonary hypertension, and occasional worsening of gas exchange.[62] (See also Chap. 99.)

Diuretics are effective in the treatment of RVF, and indications for their use are the same as in other forms of heart disease. Pulmonary function is improved by diuretics in patients with COPD who have hypervolemia.[65] The effects of diuretics should be carefully monitored by measurement of arterial P_{O_2}, P_{CO_2}, and pH, since acid-base abnormalities are often present in cor pulmonale. Contraction alkalosis can be a problem in hypercarbic patients with a large buffer base who have had vigorous diuresis.

Phlebotomy, when hematocrit is above 55 to 60 percent, may reduce PAP and PVR and, possibly, improve RV function.[66] The phlebotomy should be in small volumes (200 to 300 ml) and done cautiously.

SURGICAL TREATMENT

There is no surgical treatment for most diseases that cause chronic cor pulmonale. Pulmonary embolectomy is extremely efficacious for unresolved pulmonary emboli (Chap. 100). Adenoidectomy in children with chronic airway obstruction and uvulopalatopharyngeoplasty in some patients with sleep apnea can relieve cor pulmonale related to hypoventilation. Single-lung, double-lung, and heart-lung transplantations are all used for treatment of end-stage right-sided heart failure for several diseases complicated by cor pulmonale. The diseases most commonly treated by lung transplantation are primary pulmonary hypertension, emphysema, idiopathic pulmonary fibrosis, and cystic fibrosis.[61] The single- and double-lung transplant 2-year survival rate has risen to 60 percent, still lower than the approximately 80 percent for heart transplant alone. One interesting finding is that the RV can recover function after transplant even when severely stressed by chronic severe pulmonary hypertension. As of 1991, approximately 1600 single and double lung transplants were performed.[67]

REFERENCES

1. Fishman AP: State of the art: Chronic cor pulmonale. *Am Rev Resp Dis* 1976; 114:775–794.
2. Richards DW: The right heart and the lung with some observations on teleology. The J. Burns Amberson Lecture. *Am Rev Resp Dis* 1966; 94:691–702.
3. Osler W: *The Principles and Practice of Medicine*. New York, D. Appleton and Company, 1892: 628–640.
4. McGinn S, White PD: Acute cor pulmonale resulting from pulmonary embolism, its clinical recognition. *JAMA* 1935; 104:1473–1480.
5. Harvey W: *Exercitatio de Motu Cordis et Sanguinis in Animalibus*. Francofurti Guilielem Fitzeri, 1628, translated by CD Leake, Springfield, IL, Charles C Thomas, 1928.
6. Chronic Disease Reports: Chronic obstructive pulmonary disease, mortality. *MMWR* 1989; 38(32):549–552.
7. Chronic Obstructive Lung Disease: The health consequences of smoking. A report of the Surgeon General. Rockville, MD, U.S. Department of Health and Human Services, 1984: 189.
8. Gazes PC: *Clinical Cardiology: A Bedside Approach*. Chicago, IL, Yearbook Medical Publishers, 1975: 171.
9. Thurlbeck WM, Henderson JA, Fraser RG, Bates DV: Chronic obstructive lung disease. A comparison between clinical, roentgenologic, functional and morphological criteria in chronic bronchitis, emphysema, asthma and bronchiectasis. *Medicine* 1970; 49:81–145.
10. Filley GF, Beckwitt HJ, Reeves JT, Mitchell RS: Chronic obstructive bronchopulmonary disease. II. Oxygen transport in two clinical types. *Am J Med* 1968; 44:26–38.
11. Mountain R, Zwillich C, Weil J: Hypoventilation in obstructive lung disease. *N Engl J Med* 1978; 298:521–525.
12. Crystal RG, Bitterman PB, Rennard SI, Hance AJ, Keogh BA: Interstitial lung diseases of unknown cause (2 parts). *N Engl J Med* 1984; 310:154–166, 235–244.
13. Winterbauer RH, Hammer SP, Hallman KO, Hays JE, Pardee NE, Morgan EH, et al: Diffuse interstitial pneumonitis, clinicopathological correlations in 20 patients treated with Prednisone/Azathropine. *Am J Med* 1978; 65:661–672.
14. Bergofsky EH: Respiratory failure in disorders of the thoracic cage. *Am Rev Resp Dis* 1979; 119:643–669.
15. Burwell CS, Robin ED, Whaley RD, Bickelmann AG: Extreme obesity associated with alveolar hypoventilation—a Pickwickian syndrome. *Am J Med* 1956; 21:811–818.
16. Sackner MA, Landa J, Forrest T, Greeneltch D: Periodic sleep apnea: Chronic sleep deprivation related to intermittent upper airway obstruction and central nervous system disturbance. *Chest* 1975; 67:164–171.
17. Guilleminault C, Dement WC: *Sleep Apnea Syndromes*. New York, Allen R. Liss, 1978.
18. Grover RF: Chronic hypoxic pulmonary hypertension. In: Fishman AP (ed): *The Pulmonary Circulation: Normal and Abnormal*. Philadelphia, University of Philadelphia Press, 1990: 283–301.
19. Gerry JL, Buckley BH, Hutchins GM: Clinicopathologic analysis of cardiac dysfunction in 52 patients with sickle cell anemia. *Am J Cardiol* 1978; 42:211–216.

20. Wagenvoort CA: Pulmonary venocclusive disease, entity or syndrome? *Chest* 1976; 69:82–86.
21. Fritts HW: Systemic circulatory adjustments in hepatic disease. *Med Clin N Am* 1963; 47:563–578.
22. Segel N, Kay JM, Bayley TJ, Paton A: Pulmonary hypertension with hepatic cirrhosis. *Br Heart J* 1968; 30:575–578.
23. Coplan N, Shinony R, Ioachim H: Primary pulmonary hypertension associated with human immunodeficiency viral infection. *Am J Med* 1990; 89:96–99.
24. Perez D, Kramer N: Pulmonary hypertension in systemic lupus erythmatosus: Report of four cases and review of the literature. *Semin Arthritis Rheum* 1981; 11:177–181.
25. Bohr DF: The pulmonary hypoxic response. State of the field. *Chest* 1977; 71:244–246.
26. Burrows B: Arterial oxygenation and pulmonary hemodynamics in patients with chronic airways obstruction. *Am Rev Resp Dis* 1974; 110(suppl):64–70.
27. Nocturnal Oxygen Therapy Trial Group: Continuous or nocturnal oxygen therapy in hypoxemic chronic obstructive lung disease. A clinical trial. *Ann Intern Med* 1980; 93:391–398.
28. Enson Y, Guintini C, Lewis ML, Morris TQ, Ferrer MI, Harvey RM: The influence of hydrogen ion concentration and hypoxia on the pulmonary circulation. *J Clin Invest* 1964; 43:1146–1162.
29. Boysen PG, Block AJ, Wynne JW, Hunt LA, Flick MR: Nocturnal pulmonary hypertension in patients with chronic obstructive pulmonary disease. *Chest* 1979; 76:536–542.
30. Enson Y, Thomas HM, Bosken CH, Wood JA, Leroy EC, Blanc WA, et al: Pulmonary hypertension in interstitial lung disease: Relation of vascular resistance to abnormal lung structure. *Trans Assoc Am Phys* 1975; 88:248–255.
31. Fried R, Meyrick B, Rabinovitch M, Reid L: Polycythemia and the acute hypoxic response in awake rats following chronic hypoxia. *J Appl Physiol* 1983; 55:1167–1172.
32. Enson Y: Pulmonary heart disease: Relation of pulmonary hypertension to abnormal lung structure and function. *Bull NY Acad Med* 1977; 53:551–566.
33. Morkin E: Activation of synthetic processes in cardiac hypertrophy. *Circ Res* 1974; (suppl)35:37–48.
34. Grover RF: Pulmonary circulation in animals and man at high altitude. *Ann NY Acad Sci* 1965; 127:632–639.
35. Fishman AP: The left ventricle in chronic bronchitis and emphysema. *N Engl J Med* 1971; 285:402–404.
36. Murphy ML, Adamson J, Hutcheson F: Left ventricular hypertrophy in patients with chronic bronchitis and emphysema. *Ann Intern Med* 1974; 81:307–313.
37. Matthay RA, Berger HO: Cardiovascular function in cor pulmonale. In: *Clinics in Chest Medicine*. New York, Saunders, 1983; 4:269–295.
38. Buda AJ, Pinsky MR, Ingels NB, Daughters GT, Stinson EB, Alderman EL: Effect of intrathoracic pressure on left ventricular performance. *N Engl J Med* 1979; 301:453–459.
39. Bermis CE, Sehur JR, Borkenhagen D, Sonnenblick EH, Urschel CW: Influence of right ventricular filling pressure on left ventricular pressure and dimension. *Circ Res* 1974; 34:498–504.
40. Steele PS, Ellis JH, VanDyke D, Sutton F, Creagh E, Davies H: Left ventricular ejection fraction in severe chronic obstructive airways disease. *Am J Med* 1975; 59:21–28.
41. Berns AS, Schrier RS: The kidney in heart failure. In Suki WN, Eknoyan G (eds): *The Kidney in Systemic Disease*. New York, Wiley, 1981: 569.
42. Harvey RM, Ferrer MI, Richards DW, Cournand A: Influence of chronic pulmonary disease on the heart and circulation. *Am J Med* 1951; 10:719–738.
43. Farber MO, Roberts LR, Weinberger MH, Robertson GL, Fineberg NS, Manfredi F: Abnormalities of sodium and H_2O handling in chronic obstructive lung disease. *Arch Intern Med* 1982; 142:1326–1330.
44. Padmavati S, Raizada V: Electrocardiogram in chronic cor pulmonale. *Br Heart J* 1972; 34:658–667.
45. Murphy ML, Hutcheson F: The electrocardiographic diagnosis of right ventricular hypertrophy in chronic obstructive pulmonary disease. *Chest* 1974; 65:622–627.
46. Moore CB, Kraus WL, Dork DS: The relationship between pulmonary arterial pressure and roentgenographic appearance in mitral stenosis. *Am Heart J* 1959; 58:576–581.
47. Chang CH: The normal roentgenographic measurement of the right descending pulmonary artery in 1,085 cases. *Am J Roentgenol* 1962; 87:929–935.
48. Matthay RA, Schwarz MI, Ellis JH: Pulmonary artery hypertension in chronic obstructive pulmonary disease: Chest radiographic assessment. *Invest Radiol* 1981; 16:95–100.
49. Cacho A, Prokash R, Sarne R, Kaushik VS: Usefulness of two-dimensional echocardiography in diagnosing right ventricular hypertrophy. *Chest* 1983; 84:154–157.
50. Hagan A, DeMaria A: Diseases of the right heart. In: *Clinical Applications of Two-Dimensional Echocardiography*. Boston, Little Brown, 1985: 270.
51. Meyer RA, Schwartz DC, Benzing G, Kaplan S: Ventricular septum in right ventricular volume overload. An echocardiographic study. *Am J Cardiol* 1972; 30:349–353.
52. Schiller N: Pulmonary artery pressure estimation by Doppler and two-dimensional echocardiography. *Cardiol Clin* May 1990; 8(2):277–287.
53. Kitabatake A, Michitoshi I, Asao M, Masuyama T, Tanouchi J, Morita T, et al: Noninvasive evaluation of pulmonary hypertension by a pulsed Doppler technique. *Circulation* 1983; 68(2):302–309.
54. Berger HJ, Matthay RA, Loke J, Marshall RC, Gottschalk A, Zaret BL: Assessment of cardiac performance with quantitative radionuclide angiocardiography: Right ventricular ejection fraction with reference to findings in chronic obstructive pulmonary disease. *Am J Cardiol* 1978; 41:897–905.
55. Cohen HA, Baird MG, Rouleau JR: Thallium 201 myocardial imaging in patients with pulmonary hypertension. *Circulation* 1976; 54:790–795.
56. Bishop JM, Cross KW: Use of other physiological variables to predict pulmonary arterial pressure in patients with chronic respiratory disease: Multi-center study. *Eur Heart J* 1981; 2:509–517.
57. Stark RD, Finnegan P, Bishop JM: Long-term domiciliary oxygen in chronic bronchitis with pulmonary hypertension. *Br Med J* 1973; 3:467–470.
58. Schrijen F, Uffholtz H, Polu JM, Poincelot F: Pulmonary and systemic hemodynamic evolution in chronic bronchitis. *Am Rev Resp Dis* 1978; 117:25–31.
59. Weitzenblum E, Loiseau A, Hirth C, Mirhom R, Rasaholinjanahary J: Course of pulmonary hemodynamics in patients with chronic obstructive pulmonary disease. *Chest* 1979; 75:656–662.
60. Ferrer M: Cor pulmonale (pulmonary heart disease): Present-day status. *Am Heart J* 1975; 89:657–664.
61. Morgan EJ, Zwillich CW: The obesity-hypoventilation syndrome. *West J Med* 1978; 129:387–393.
62. Wiedemann H, Matthay R: Cor pulmonale in chronic obstructive pulmonary disease circulatory pathophysiology and management. *Clin Chest Med* 1990; 11:523–545.
63. Green LH, Smith TW: The use of digitalis in patients with pulmonary disease. *Ann Int Med* 1977; 87:459–465.
64. Smith DE, Bissett JK, Phillips JR, Doherty JE, Murphy ML: Improved right ventricular systolic time intervals after digitalis in patients with cor pulmonale and chronic obstructive pulmonary disease. *Am J Cardiol* 1978; 41:1299–1304.
65. Gertz I, Hedenstierna G, Wester PO: Improvement in pulmonary function with diuretic therapy in the hypervolemic and polycythemic patient with chronic obstructive pulmonary disease. *Chest* 1979; 75:146–151.
66. Weisse AB, Moschos CB, Frank MJ, Levinson GE, Cannilla JE, Regan TJ: Hemodynamic effects of staged hematocrit reduction in patients with stable cor pulmonale and severely elevated hematocrit levels. *Am J Med* 1975; 58:92–98.
67. Cooper JD: St. Louis International Lung Transplant Registry Report. St. Louis, MO, Aug. 1992.

PART XIII

The Heart and Systemic Disease or Conditions

Chapter 102

The Heart and Endocrine Disease

Joel Zonszein, M.D. ■ *Frederick S. Fein, M.D.* ■
Edmund H. Sonnenblick, M.D.

PITUITARY DISEASE

Pituitary Insufficiency

Pituitary tumors are the most common cause of hypopituitarism. Clinical features manifest deficiency of the individual hormones. In addition, headaches or visual field defects are caused by the space occupying lesion. Anterior pituitary function may also be impaired during severe illness. Pituitary necrosis, as in Sheehan's syndrome, has been reported in patients dying shortly after major cardiac surgery.[1] This may reflect the unfavorable outcome, since pathological studies of patients dying weeks after such surgical procedures do not have pituitary necrotic changes. Pituitary infarcts can also occur in 18 to 33 percent of patients maintained on mechanical respirators, particularly in those where circulatory function is compromised.[2] A milder and more transient form of hypopituitarism has been detected in as many as 15 percent of patients on ventilators.[3] Although this may have little or no clinical impact in the majority, its proper detection and treatment could be pivotal for appropriate care in some.

Acromegaly

The most common cause of acromegaly is a growth hormone– (GH-) producing pituitary adenoma. When excessive GH secretion takes place before epiphyseal closure, gigantism develops. Many of the GH effects are indirect and mediated through insulin-like growth factor I (IGF-I) or somatomedin C. The findings of elevated plasma GH levels, failure to suppress after a glucose challenge, and high plasma levels of IGF-I are utilized for the diagnosis and follow-up in the treatment of acromegaly.[4]

Cardiovascular Manifestations of Acromegaly

Growth hormone excess may lead to cardiovascular abnormalities; while some postulate that these are caused by hypertension alone,[5] others believe that the high morbidity is a direct result of prolonged and excessive GH exposure.[6] Correlation between elevation of GH and cardiac disease is unproven.[5,7]

Hypertension occurs in acromegaly three times more than in the general population.[5] It tends to be mild, responsive to conventional therapy, with regression occurring in some, after the successful treatment of GH excess. Hypertension in acromegaly may be secondary to GH-mediated sodium retention,[8] associated with low plasma renin.[9] The possibility of pheochromocytoma[10] or hyperaldosteronism[11] must be kept in mind, since they may represent a variant of the multiple endocrine neoplasia syndromes; thyrotoxicosis should be considered when tachyarrhythmias are present.[5]

In spite of the high incidence of hypertension and glucose intolerance, the occurrence of coronary artery disease or peripheral artery disease is surprisingly the same as a comparable ethnic, age- and sex-matched population.[5] The absence of elevated cholesterol and triglyceride levels may explain the lack of accelerated atherosclerosis in acromegaly.

Visceral enlargement is characteristic in acromegaly, and the heart is no exception. The extent of cardiomegaly may be disproportionately affected by concomitant hypertension, resulting in left ventricular hypertrophy[5] and/

or congestive heart failure.[12] Ventricular hypertrophy (either concentric or asymmetric septal hypertrophy) with preserved systolic function is common and readily demonstrated by echocardiography.[13] A characteristic form of acromegalic heart disease remains to be established.[5] Factors independent of diabetes, hypertension, or atherosclerotic disease may be responsible for this type of heart disease,[7] and indeed, congestive heart failure has been described in acromegaly without any of these factors.[14] Autopsy studies in acromegalic patients, however, have been unable to show a characteristic form of cardiac pathology.[12] Lowering excessive levels of GH can result in improvement in cardiac function.[7] The somatostatin analogue octreotide, in addition to its therapeutic value in acromegaly, is also beneficial in reversing some of the cardiovascular abnormalities.[15] Anesthesia and perioperative care is difficult in some due to increases in lung volume, tracheal thickness, and tongue size; these changes can also cause obstructive sleep apnea.[16] Since patients with acromegaly frequently have large pituitary tumors, anterior pituitary insufficiency may develop. The possibility of adrenal insufficiency should be considered, especially during surgery or other stressful events.

THYROID DISEASE

The heart is a major target organ for thyroid hormone action.[17] Thyroid hormone directly alters heart rate and velocity of myocardial contraction. Indirectly, it regulates tissue metabolism and extracellular fluid volume and distribution and may influence catecholamine effect. Both deficiency and excess of thyroid hormone can cause striking clinical cardiovascular derangements, particularly in the elderly and in those with underlying intrinsic heart disease.

Direct Effects of Thyroid Hormone on the Heart

Thyroid hormone–induced changes are mediated by the binding of triiodothyronine (T_3) to specific nuclear receptor proteins, resulting in increased transcription of T_3-responsive cardiac genes. The nuclear receptor for T_3 is the major molecule responsible for biological action. This receptor is a member of the ligand-activated transcription factor family and is encoded by cellular erythroblastosis A (c-*erb*-A) genes. Three T_3-binding isoforms of c-*erb* protein and two non-T_3-binding nuclear proteins have thus far been identified.[18] Thyroid hormone enhances cardiac protein synthesis and increases cardiac contractility.[19] Changes in myosin isoenzyme expression are the result of thyroid hormone effects on gene expression. The T_3 increases myocardial transcription of the myosin heavy chain– (MHC-) alpha gene and decreases the transcription of the MHC-beta gene, which leads to increased myosin adenosinetriphosphatase (ATPase) activity and an increased velocity of contraction.[19] Less chemical energy of ATP is used for contractile purposes and more of it goes to heat production,[20] resulting in decreased efficiency in the hyperthyroid heart. Thyroid hormone influences excitation-contraction coupling. The T_3-responsive messenger ribonucleic acids (mRNAs) have been identified, including those that increase sarcolemmal sodium pump sites by stimulating Na^+ and K^+-ATPase[21] and those responsible for the increase in the number of calcium channels.[22] It also causes a higher calcium influx across the sarcolemma[23] and stimulates plasma membrane Ca-ATPase activity. Thyroid hormone influences tissue content and plasma levels of atrial natriuretic factor.[24] Thyroid hormone added to chick embryonic heart increases the rate of spontaneous beating. In isolated segments of adult cardiac muscle, experimental hyperthyroidism is associated with increased rate of contraction and relaxation, with an abbreviation in contraction; hypothyroidism produces the converse effects.[25]

Indirect Effects of Thyroid Hormone on the Heart

One of the earliest responses to acute administration of thyroid hormone is a decline in systemic vascular resistance and a decrease in diastolic blood pressure, leading to a compensatory increase in cardiac contractility, heart rate, and cardiac output.[26] Conversely, in hypothyroidism, diastolic hypertension and increased vascular resistance are common.[27]

Catecholamine–Thyroid Hormone Interaction

Most manifestations of the hyperthyroid state such as tachycardia, palpitations, tremor, sweating, and central nervous system (CNS) hyperactivity mimic adrenergic hyperfunction; many of the symptoms of hypothyroidism resemble those of depressed sympathetic tone.[28] This correlation led to the assumption that thyrotoxicosis was a disease of excessive catecholamine secretion. The therapeutic utility of adrenergic receptor blockade in the symptomatic management of hyperthyroidism further supports this concept. In spite of these similarities, there is no evidence that thyroid hormone alters catecholamine plasma levels, nor is there an increased content of catecholamines in myocardium obtained from thyroid hormone–treated animals. Thyroid hormone increases cardiac sensitivity to beta-adrenergic agonists on the heart by an increased number, as well as affinity, of beta-adrenergic receptors. In humans, high doses of thyroid hormone do not increase metabolic and hemodynamic response to epinephrine,[29] in spite of the presence of increased density of beta-adrenergic receptors. It appears unlikely that increased catecholamine sensitivity is the explanation for the clinical and metabolic features of hyperthyroidism.[28]

Hyperthyroidism

Hyperthyroidism, or thyrotoxicosis, is the clinical state resulting from chronic exposure to elevated levels of thyroid hormone. The common types include autoimmune hyperthyroidism (Graves' disease), toxic multinodular goiter (Plummer's disease), and single or multiple hyperfunctioning adenomata of the thyroid.

The clinical manifestations of hyperthyroidism are quite protean and include weight loss with appetite preservation, diaphoresis, exertional dyspnea, heat intolerance, palpitations, easy fatigability, emotional lability, and weakness. These symptoms may be so mild or subtle that the patient is unaware of them. The most striking symptoms of hyperthyroidism are reflected by the cardiovascular system and may be the only manifestations of hyperthyroidism in the elderly. Physical examination frequently reveals a nervous and hyperkinetic individual with a hyperdynamic cardiovascular state. Fine hand tremor is common. The skin is warm and moist and palmar erythema may be present. The hair is fine and silky. Onycholysis (separation of distal nail from its bed) and acropachy ("drumstick" appearance of the fingers) can be found in severe and chronic cases. Proximal muscle weakness is common, with muscle wasting occasionally appearing. Lid retraction ("stare") and lid-lag are both manifestations of thyroid hormone excess. Asymmetric and soft goiter characteristic of autoimmune disease (Graves' disease) is usually present in the young; because of increased vascularity, a bruit can be audible. A nodular goiter with increased consistency is indicative of Plummer's disease, while a single palpable nodule suggests a "toxic adenoma" ("hot" nodule by nuclear scintiscan). Graves' disease is an autoimmune disorder in which, in addition to hyperthyroidism, "Graves' ophthalmopathy," pretibial myxedema, vitiligo, hepatosplenomegaly, and peripheral adenopathy may also be present.

Signs and symptoms of hyperthyroidism are variable and do not always correlate with the degree of elevation of circulating T_3 and T_4. In older individuals, manifestations of hyperthyroidism can be very subtle and virtually limited to the cardiovascular system. *Apathetic hyperthyroidism* is a term applied especially to the elderly who do not manifest the obvious signs and symptoms of thyrotoxicosis. The presence of a goiter is infrequent. Such patients may present with apathetic, placid facies and can be erroneously diagnosed as having malignancy or heart disease.

Cardiovascular Manifestations of Thyrotoxicosis

The most striking signs and symptoms are exhibited by the cardiovascular system.[30] Palpitations and exertional dyspnea are common; angina may be exacerbated in older individuals. The circulation is hyperdynamic, with a full bounding and rapid pulse even at rest. Atrial fibrillation is common, particularly in the elderly. Peripheral vasodilatation is accompanied with systolic hypertension and a low diastolic pressure. The precordial impulse is forceful and can often be visible. A short, high-pitched systolic murmur heard to the left of the sternal border, especially in the pulmonic valve area, is known as the "pulmonic scratch murmur." Functional mitral valve regurgitation can be present, and mitral valve prolapse is more frequent in hyperthyroid patients.[31] Dependent edema can be found in severe chronic cases and should not be confused with congestive heart failure or pretibial myxedema.

Congestive heart failure is uncommon in uncomplicated thyrotoxicosis. In patients with intrinsic heart disease, congestive heart failure may develop or worsen with hyperthyroidism. The prevalence of heart disease increases with age.[32] The paradox of left ventricular dysfunction, occurring in patients with hyperthyroidism, remains enigmatic.[33] Hyperthyroid individuals without overt congestive heart failure have increased cardiac index at rest, which further rises during exercise. In contrast, thyrotoxic patients in overt congestive heart failure have a high normal cardiac index that decreases during exercise. When these patients are rendered euthyroid, resting cardiac index nearly normalizes in both.

Beta-adrenergic blockade in hyperthyroidism results in a fall in cardiac index with increased pulmonary artery diastolic pressure in thyrotoxic patients with or without heart failure.[34] The changes are particularly profound in the former group. Therefore, beta-adrenergic blocking drugs should be avoided in hyperthyroid patients with overt heart failure unless this is rate related.

Atrial fibrillation (AF) is common in hyperthyroidism (10 to 25 percent),[35] is more frequent in men, and increases with age. In the elderly, atrial fibrillation can often be the major, or only, manifestation of thyrotoxicosis.[36] While AF is common in thyrotoxicosis, hyperthyroidism is not a common cause of AF,[37] and subclinical hyperthyroidism is a rare cause of AF.[38] Nonetheless, screening for hyperthyroidism in all patients with unexplained supraventricular tachycardia, irrespective of whether other typical clinical features are present, is recommended. In addition to an increased incidence of supraventricular tachyarrhythmias, hyperthyroidism may also cause or aggravate ischemia-related ventricular arrhythmias.

There is a high (8.5 percent) incidence of thromboembolic disease in hyperthyroidism, with cerebral emboli occurring in 53 percent.[39] In thyrotoxic patients with concomitant AF, arterial embolism is a more common event (10 to 40 percent).[39] Thromboembolic disease is particularly frequent in hyperthyroid patients with concomitant congestive heart failure, dilated left atrium, and mitral valve disease as well as during spontaneous or induced conversion of AF. The incidence of thromboembolic complications also increases with age.

Angina pectoris is rarely a manifestation of thyrotoxicosis in individuals without concomitant coronary artery disease (CAD). Ischemia is precipitated by an increased myocardial oxygen consumption in a setting of limited oxygen delivery.

Mitral valve prolapse syndrome occurs commonly in women with autoimmune thyroid disease.[40] This condition persists after correction of the hyperthyroid state and is seldom associated with significant mitral regurgitation, arrhythmias, or thromboembolism.[41] A distinct and reversible form of hemodynamically significant valvular regurgitation, associated with ventricular dilatation, has also been described in hyperthyroidism and is more prevalent in children.[42]

Diagnosis

In most patients with thyrotoxicosis, the diagnosis is suspected clinically and is confirmed by elevated serum levels of T_4 and T_3 and suppressed thyroid-stimulating hormone (TSH). With the advent of sensitive TSH assays,[43] it has become easier to differentiate between hyperthyroid and euthyroid states. Virtually all patients with primary hyperthyroidism have suppressed TSH levels, whereas TSH serum concentration is normal in euthyroid patients. A normal TSH serum concentration is the most cost-effective method of excluding hyperthyroidism, even when T_4 and/or T_3 levels are elevated. The TSH serum concentration alone, however, is not reliable in the management of patients with hypothalamic-pituitary thyroid disorders, in hospitalized patients with nonthyroidal illnesses, or in patients receiving medications (such as dopamine) that may affect serum TSH levels. In all these situations, determination of thyroid hormone levels is necessary. In complex cases, measurement of free thyroid hormone by dialysis methods may be required to establish the diagnosis.

Therapy

The main goal in the treatment of hyperthyroidism is the rapid achievement of the euthyroid state while avoiding therapeutic complications. Therapy remains empiric; whereas hyperthyroidism can be controlled, it can seldom be cured. Consequently, treatment results in changing one disease state, hyperthyroidism, for another, hypothyroidism. There is a diversity of opinion in the optimal management of thyrotoxic Graves' disease,[44] but since the cause of hyperthyroidism varies, treatment should be tailored individually.

The armamentarium available consists of drugs affecting production or release of thyroid hormone such as thionamides and iodide, medications that may improve symptomatology and decrease cardiovascular manifestations such as beta-adrenergic blockers, and definitive therapy resulting in thyroid ablation (either surgical subtotal thyroidectomy or radiation therapy with radioiodine). Thionamides such as methimazole and propylthiouracil (PTU) inhibit thyroid hormone synthesis. Propylthiouracil has the additional advantage of inhibiting the conversion of T_4 to T_3. Administered in high doses, it will totally block new hormone synthesis, but stored thyroid hormone will continue to be released. Metabolic improvement therefore takes an average of 6 weeks. Administration of iodide blocks the secretion of the stored hormone, blocks conversion of T_4 to T_3, and reduces the time it takes for thionamides to produce the euthyroid state. The most effective iodide preparation is sodium iodate, an organic iodide agent used for oral cholecystography. Since hyperthyroid glands avidly incorporate more iodine for new synthesis of thyroid hormone, thionamide therapy should be started several hours earlier to prevent iodide incorporation into thyroid hormones. The combination of inhibitors of synthesis, secretion, and conversion of T_4 and T_3 will result in progressive clinical improvement culminating in a laboratory and clinical remission within 3 to 4 weeks.

The addition of beta-adrenergic antagonists is critical for the rapid improvement of the cardiovascular manifestations; this effect is crucial in treating thyroid crisis. Beta-adrenergic blockers are rapidly metabolized in hyperthyroid patients; frequent and high doses are necessary. A pulse rate of 80 to 90 beats per minute indicates an adequate response. The use of longer acting beta-blocking adrenergic agents is also effective as they can be given with less frequency, achieving a similarly adequate response.[45] Beta-adrenergic blockers, including those that are more cardioselective, should be avoided in patients with asthma, obstructive pulmonary disease, heart block, and overt congestive heart failure unless the latter is rate related.

Aggressive therapy is indicated when there are significant cardiovascular symptoms such as in thyroid storm or when associated underlying medical conditions jeopardize the patient's well being. In these cases the use of beta-adrenergic blockers, which act immediately, is critical in addition to thionamides and iodide, which will reduce production and release of thyroid hormone in a slower fashion. Simultaneous treatment of the underlying medical conditions, normalization of fluid and electrolyte imbalance, and proper correction of other cardiopulmonary abnormalities are also crucial.

Radioactive iodine therapy, used for more than 50 years, has not been associated with an increased risk of cancer or reproductive mishaps; however, the calamities at Hiroshima and Chernobyl continue to deter people from receiving even low-dose organ-specific radiation. This modality is gaining popularity, becoming the treatment of choice for many patients over the age of 25.[46] Surgery is also effective and remains popular among some. It produces a rapid and permanent cure of hyperthyroidism in the great majority of patients. It is favored in toxic nodular goiters, particularly in those with large thyroid glands, and in patients with solitary toxic nodules. Thyroid surgery should be performed by an experienced surgeon but is inconvenient, expensive, and associated with short-lived discomfort as well as surgical complications in less experienced hands. Preoperative therapy with a beta-adrenergic antagonist alone is as effective as preoperative antithyroid drug and iodide therapy.[47]

Control of hyperthyroidism frequently reduces ischemia and angina and improves congestive heart failure. In addition to aggressive antithyroid therapy, management of patients with AF also includes slowing of the ventricular rate, anticoagulation, and cardioversion. The high ventricular rate in hyperthyroidism can be controlled with beta-adrenergic antagonists, calcium channel blockers, and/or digitalis glycosides. Myocardial sensitivity to digitalis glycosides is reduced in thyrotoxicosis, and large doses are required to control atrial arrhythmias. As hyperthyroidism lessens, serum levels of digoxin rise, increasing the chance of toxicity. Unless contraindicated, beta-adrenergic antagonists are more effective and a better choice than calcium channel blockers, which are less specific and less effective in reducing the pulse rate[48]; either of these approaches are preferred over the use of digitalis alone. (See also Chap. 36.)

Achievement of a euthyroid state often results in reversion of supraventricular arrhythmias to sinus rhythm.[49] Patients that spontaneously convert to regular sinus rhythm do so within 3 months after becoming euthyroid. When AF lasts longer than 3 to 4 months after achieving euthyroidism, intervention with medical or electrical cardioversion may be necessary.[49] Early cardioversion is generally avoided because of the high incidence of reappearance of supraventricular tachyarrhythmias.

Controversy over the use of anticoagulation in patients with thyrotoxicosis has partially been caused by lack of prospective studies. Recent clinical trials, however, have clearly demonstrated the benefits of oral anticoagulation agents in the primary prevention of systemic embolism.[50-53] In all three studies, warfarin-treated patients effectively and impressively decreased the rate of embolic phenomena in patients with atrial fibrillation.[51-53] Although prospective randomized control analyses are not available in hyperthyroidism, the significant reduction of thromboembolic complications in chronic AF in the nonhyperthyroid population can be extrapolated to the hyperthyroid patient population. (See also Chap. 68.) Low-dose aspirin appears to be less effective than oral anticoagulation,[51] but more research is needed to compare the effects of warfarin and aspirin.

Hypothyroidism

Hypothyroidism, or myxedema, is the clinical syndrome resulting from decreased production of T_4 and T_3. The vast majority of patients have primary hypothyroidism. Hypothyroidism may also result from pituitary (secondary) or hypothalamic (tertiary) disease. The etiology of adult primary hypothyroidism includes autoimmune hypothyroidism (Hashimoto's thyroiditis) and ablation of the thyroid after radioactive iodine therapy or thyroid surgery. Drugs such as amiodarone and lithium can also cause hypothyroidism, particularly in those with underlying autoimmune thyroid disease.

Manifestations of hypothyroidism are variable, proportionate to both the degree and duration of the thyroid hormone deficiency and the age of onset. The development of symptoms is insidious and includes weight gain without an increased appetite, dry skin, weakness, cold intolerance, memory impairment, deepening of the voice, constipation, lethargy, and menstrual abnormalities.[54] Physical examination reveals a dull expression, slow pulse, mild hypertension, dry yellowed skin, dry hair, periorbital puffiness, hair loss of the lateral aspects of the eyebrows, and delayed relaxation of the deep tendon reflexes. The presence of a goiter is common in younger patients (Hashimoto's) but is often absent in the elderly. Clinical features of hypothyroidism may be missed, particularly in the elderly.

Cardiovascular Manifestations of Hypothyroidism

Cardiac manifestations of hypothyroidism are the reverse of those seen in hyperthyroidism. There is decreased total body oxygen consumption, sinus bradycardia, reduced cardiac output, and elevated total peripheral vascular resistance. The pulse pressure tends to be narrow. Mild hypertension has been described, especially in older individuals.[55,56] Plasma renin, plasma aldosterone, and aldosterone production rates are all decreased in hypothyroid patients with hypertension.[57] Hypertension generally improves after thyroid hormone replacement.

Anatomic abnormalities of the heart in severe chronic myxedema include a dilated, pale, and flabby ventricle with myofibrillar swelling and fibrosis.[58] Cardiac output, stroke volume, heart rate, and plasma volumes are reduced in hypothyroidism.[59] Myocardial contraction and relaxation are slowed, with a prolonged duration of contraction.[60,61] Systolic time intervals and left ventricular isovolumic contraction times are also prolonged.[62] The reduced cardiac output coupled with an enlarged cardiac silhouette on chest x-ray and pleural and peritoneal effusions often lead to confusing hypothyroidism with congestive heart failure. In contrast to patients with reduced cardiac output from primary myocardial disease, cardiac output in hypothyroidism increases in response to exercise.[63] Although circulation times are prolonged, left- and right-sided intracardiac pressures are normal. Thus, uncomplicated hypothyroidism does not usually result in congestive heart failure. Thyroid replacement may lead to congestive heart failure, when underlying myocardial disease limits the ability of the heart to increase cardiac output. Typical electrocardiographic changes are sinus bradycardia, low-amplitude P waves and QRS complexes,[64] and atrioventricular or intraventricular conduction disturbances.[65] Nonspecific ST- and T-wave abnormalities and QT prolongation also occur.

Almost 95 percent of hypothyroid patients have hypercholesterolemia and hypertriglyceridemia.[66] Hypothyroidism increases all cholesterol subfractions: low-density lipoprotein (LDL), very low density lipoprotein (VLDL), and the protective high-density lipoprotein (HDL) cholesterol. Concentration of LDL receptors in fibroblasts, liver, and other tissues is decreased; thus LDL cholesterol accumulates in the blood because of a decreased clearance. Accumulation of VLDL may result from a decreased activity of lipoprotein lipase, without being sufficiently reduced as to cause fasting chylomicronemia. Reduced hepatic triglyceride lipase may explain the elevated HDL. Since the increased LDL cholesterol is not accompanied by proportional increment in total HDL cholesterol, it results in an unfavorable HDL-LDL cholesterol ratio. All these metabolic anomalies are reversed with treatment.

A direct association between thyroid status and coronary risk is controversial. Studies undertaken in the British Isles showed no association between cholesterol levels, coronary artery disease, and mild hypothyroidism.[67] Pathological studies, however, have shown a higher incidence of arteriosclerotic cardiovascular disease, especially in the presence of hypertension. Although coronary artery disease is common pathologically, angina pectoris is present in only 7 percent.[68] Further, the incidence of autopsy-proven myocardial infarction is not elevated in the hypothyroid population.[69] It is possible that lowered oxygen consumption in hypothyroidism protects against myocardial ischemia[70]; this can also explain the low prevalence of angina pectoris in these patients. In severe myxedema with increased blood pressure and elevated cholesterol, serious coronary atherosclerosis has been seen in individuals otherwise not at risk. This may be an important consideration when replacement therapy is undertaken.

Therapy of hypothyroidism may cause myocardial ischemia if the increased heart rate and augmented rate of myocardial contraction are not matched by a corresponding increase in coronary blood flow. This is an important consideration when therapy of hypothyroidism is undertaken. Evaluation of the hypothyroid patient with chest pain can be further complicated by the finding of elevated creatine kinase (CK).[71] While this elevation can imply myocardial injury, isoenzyme analysis often indicates that the source is skeletal muscle. Total CK levels are disproportionately elevated to cardiac isoenzymes, which are minimally increased, if at all. Further, the latter do not fluctuate rapidly, as is the case after myocardial damage.

Hypothyroidism causes effusions with a high protein content into serous cavities, probably caused by increased capillary permeability. Pericardial effusion is related to the severity and chronicity of hypothyroidism. It may be occasionally immense and asymptomatic, with the false diagnosis of heart failure being made by radiographic studies. In the past, such effusions were often the leading manifestations of hypothyroidism; however, the prevalence of pericardial effusion is now lower, most likely because of an earlier diagnosis and treatment.[72] There are generally no serious hemodynamic consequences, particularly since demands for cardiac output are low. These effusions can rarely result in cardiac tamponade.[73]

Diagnosis

The most important consideration in the diagnosis of hypothyroidism is to entertain the possibility. Elderly patients may present with noncharacteristic symptoms, and hypothyroidism can be overlooked.[74] In most cases the diagnosis is easily confirmed by a low T_4 concentration coupled with elevated plasma TSH concentration. The T_3 levels are not a good index of hypothyroidism as they may also be depressed in acutely or chronically ill patients without thyroidal disease.[75] There is a good correlation between the degree of hypothyroidism and both the depression in serum T_4 concentration and the elevation in plasma TSH. Hence, minimal elevation in TSH levels alone will not explain major clinical findings. While routine testing for hypothyroidism has a low yield in community screening programs, evaluation for thyroid dysfunction is useful and recommended in the elderly, particularly those admitted to geriatric units.[74] Only a minority of patients have secondary hypothyroidism (hypopituitarism), while T_4 concentrations are depressed, and TSH levels range from low to minimally elevated in this condition. In certain difficult clinical settings, measurement of free T_4 by equilibrium dialysis may be needed.[75]

Euthyroid Sick Syndrome

Significant alterations in thyroid hormone indices have been described in a variety of nonthyroidal illnesses (NTIs). It is now generally known that patients with acute NTI may have depressed thyroid hormone levels yet remain euthyroid—"euthyroid sick syndrome."[76] Seriously ill patients, such as those in a critical care unit, may have low T_4 levels but free T_4 levels are normal and hence they are euthyroid. With recovery from critical illness, T_4 and TSH levels may normalize. Repeat determinations of these hormone levels may indeed be a good diagnostic approach. In view of the rarity of secondary hypothyroidism and the high frequency of low T_4 levels in euthyroid critically ill patients, the finding of a normal TSH level is often sufficient to exclude the diagnosis of hypothyroidism.

Therapy

Therapy of hypothyroidism involves replacement with thyroid hormone. Since T_3 is primarily derived from extrathyroidal production from T_4, L-thyroxine is the preparation of choice. The full daily replacement dose of L-thyroxine will range from 1.5 to 2.0 μg/k per day. The most common administered dose is approximately 0.112 mg daily, although elderly patients usually need lower amounts. In hypothyroid patients receiving L-thyroxine replacement, TSH value alone provides a satisfactory and cost-effective assessment in nearly all cases. Reversal of the clinical manifestations of hypothyroidism may take months.

Therapy requires considerable prudence, particularly in the elderly or in those with underlying cardiovascular disease. In the latter, coronary blood flow may be limited during the period of increased cardiac demand and ischemia may result. In the presence of valvular heart disease, the high cardiac output can increase valvular gradients and potentially worsen symptoms. The development of angina, arrhythmias, and acute myocardial infarction are well-described complications of replacement therapy, especially when therapy is vigorous.[68] Therapy of patients with coronary artery disease consists of small initial doses of thyroxine (12.5 to 25 μg daily) with gradual, slow increments. This approach is recommended not only in patients with clinical signs and symptoms of coronary artery disease but also in overtly myxedematous patients without such features. Frequent cardiac monitoring is essential, and when evidence of myocardial ischemia occurs, the dose should be temporarily omitted. Concomitant therapy with antianginal drugs, such as nitrates, calcium channel blockers, and beta-adrenergic blockers, may be helpful. The latter two groups of drugs should be used with caution since symptomatic bradycardia and worsening of congestive heart failure can take place. In some cases, noninvasive or invasive evaluation of coronary blood flow should be considered prior to replacement therapy. Bypass surgery or angioplasty may be indicated.[70] During bypass surgery, special care is necessary. In the severely hypothyroid patient (myxedema coma), there is an increased sensitivity to many hypnotic and analgesic agents; an inability to excrete free water, with the propensity to develop hyponatremia; and an increased incidence of postoperative infections. With good anesthesia technique and careful monitoring in the perioperative period, surgery has been highly successful, without increased morbidity and/or prolonged hospital stay.[70]

Percutaneous transluminal coronary angioplasty (PTCA) can also be performed in mildly hypothyroid patients without increased mortality or major morbidity.[77]

AMIODARONE-INDUCED THYROID DYSFUNCTION

Amiodarone is an important source of exogenous iodine: It contains 37 percent iodine and provides 75 mg of iodine per 200-mg tablet. Iodine administration in these high doses may alter thyroid hormone production in patients with underlying thyroid disease. In some, iodide can provoke permanent hypothyroidism or thyrotoxicosis or generate a goiter.[78,79] Administration of milligram quantities of iodide typically results in a transient reduction of thyroid hormone secretion and a concomitant increase in TSH.[80] Amiodarone is also known to inhibit the various 5′-deiodinase isoenzymes,[81] decreasing the conversion of T_4 to T_3 in all tissues including the pituitary. The decrease in pituitary T_3 leads to an increase in plasma TSH, which increases T_4 production. A new equilibrium is reached in which T_4 levels are high, T_3 levels remain normal, and the patient is euthyroid. The compensatory increase in T_4 secretion during chronic therapy may be difficult to differentiate from "true hyperthyroidism," which amiodarone is also known to cause. Iodine-induced thyrotoxicosis, a well-known complication of amiodarone therapy, occurs in nearly 10 percent of patients who live in iodine-deficient regions.[82] Treatment with amiodarone can lead to thyroid dysfunction by uncovering an underlying thyroid disorder such as autoimmune thyroid disease[78] or nontoxic nodular goiter.[79] Recent reports also suggest a direct toxic effect of amiodarone, resulting in thyroid damage and leakage of thyroid hormone.[83] Sinus bradycardia, which almost invariably occurs with high doses of amiodarone, may suggest the presence of hypothyroidism.[84] Measurements of TSH, the most helpful test for primary hypothyroidism, may give misleading results in patients receiving amiodarone. In this particular situation, measurement of serum rT_3 concentration (biologically inactive thyroid hormone) may be helpful, as it is generally elevated in patients receiving amiodarone. Failure to show high serum levels of rT_3 in a patient receiving amiodarone may indicate hypothyroidism. When amiodarone-induced thyroid dysfunction occurs, discontinuation of the drug is indicated whenever possible. If amiodarone cannot be stopped, treatment of the associated thyroid dysfunction may be required. While hypothyroidism can easily be treated with thyroid replacement, amiodarone-induced thyrotoxicosis may be difficult to manage. It may require prolonged administration of thionamides as well as potassium perchlorate, a drug blocking iodide transport to the thyroid.[85] (See also Chap. 38 and 109.)

PARATHYROID DISEASE AND DISORDERS OF CALCIUM AND PHOSPHATE METABOLISM

Parathyroid Hormone Effects on the Cardiovascular System

Parathyroid hormone (PTH) has been shown experimentally to act directly on the heart by increasing the beating rate of cultured heart cells.[86] Prolonged exposure to high levels of PTH in animal studies increases myocardial calcium content, decreases energy production, and produces a transient decline in cardiac performance.[87] Vitamin D_3 affects cardiac function experimentally, and receptors for vitamin D_3 have been identified in the heart. In vitamin D_3–deficient rats, an increased cardiac contractility, hypertension, and elevated levels of CK have been demonstrated.[88]

Calcium has a positive inotropic effect on the myocardium in diverse clinical situations.[89] Left ventricular contractility varies directly with blood ionized calcium levels; however, the majority of patients who present with hypercalcemia or hypocalcemia have little evidence of myocardial dysfunction. Chronic hypercalcemia has been associated with calcium deposition in the heart, including coronary arteries, valves, and myocardial fibers.[90]

Chronic hypocalcemia can cause congestive heart failure,[91] which can be refractory to diuretic and digitalis therapy but responsive to calcium restoration.[92] Calcium infusion increases both cardiac output and blood pressure in hypoparathyroid patients without overt heart failure, suggesting that subclinical cardiac dysfunction may be present. Since calcium potentiates the action of digitalis, hypercalcemia can provoke digitalis toxicity. In hypercalcemia the plateau of the cardiac fiber action potential is abbreviated, which results in shortening of the ST segment and the QT interval. Hypocalcemia produces prolongation of the ST segment and QT interval. There have been rare reports of abnormal intraventricular conduction in patients with hypercalcemia.

The incidence of hypertension appears to be higher in hypercalcemic patients. Estimates of the prevalence of hypertension in patients with primary hyperparathyroidism vary; in a recent study an incidence of 48.3 percent was found in hyperparathyroidism compared to 34.8 percent in the control population.[93] Since the prevalence of hypertension in the general population is 20 to 30 percent, it remains uncertain whether or not there is a true association between hypertension and hyperparathyroidism. Surgical correction of hyperparathyroidism does not seem to have a beneficial effect on hypertension in the majority of patients,[94] but it may facilitate their management. Thiazide diuretics can cause transient hypercalcemia; when hypercalcemia persists, hyperparathyroidism is often unmasked.[95] Thiazides should be avoided in all patients with known hypercalcemia since they can further increase serum calcium. When diuretics are needed in such patients, loop diuretics should be used instead, as they are calciuric agents. (See Chap. 29.)

Hypophosphatemia and the Myocardium

Reversible left ventricular dysfunction can occur with both acute and chronic severe hypophosphatemia but is usually not significant in patients with serum phosphate levels greater than 1.5 mg/dL.[96]

ADRENAL DISEASE

Adrenal Insufficiency

A deficiency of cortisol occurs when adrenocorticotropic hormone (ACTH) secretion is impaired, as in hypopituitarism, or following withdrawal of long-term treatment with pharmacologic doses of glucocorticoids. Isolated aldosterone deficiency occurs commonly secondary to renin deficiency in certain patients with mild renal disease, especially diabetes mellitus (hyporeninemic hypoaldosteronism, or type IV renal tubular acidosis). In primary destructive adrenal disease (Addison's disease), both cortisol and aldosterone production are impaired.

Glucocorticoids have a major influence on the cardiovascular system. While the mechanisms are not clearly understood, there is evidence that glucocorticoids potentiate the vasoconstrictor response to catecholamines.[97] This effect is dramatic, and reversal of the hypotension of glucocorticoid deficiency can occur within minutes of glucocorticoid therapy. The rapidity of this effect precludes changes in plasma volume and is not related to any increase in myocardial catecholamine receptor number.[98] In Addison's disease, there is deficiency of both cortisol and aldosterone. Aldosterone deficiency causes impaired sodium reabsorption and potassium secretion in the renal distal tubule. This leads to the inability to conserve sodium and the propensity for volume depletion, especially when sodium intake is low, and during acute stressful events. Patients with Addison's disease have low blood pressure and cardiac output on the basis of both glucocorticoid and aldosterone deficiency; they are prone to vascular collapse when stressed.[98] Patients with Addison's disease also develop hyperkalemia with the associated cardiac and electrocardiographic changes (see Chap. 37). Cardiac size as judged by chest x-ray may appear somewhat small in these patients.

Cushing's Syndrome

Cushing's syndrome is the result of chronic exposure to elevated plasma levels of cortisol (hypercortisolism). The most common cause is therapy with glucocorticoids for nonendocrine disorders. Cushing's disease, which is characterized by a pituitary tumor and bilateral diffused adrenal hyperplasia, is the most frequent cause of endogenous hypercortisolism. Tumor hypercortisolism, caused by adrenal adenoma, adrenal carcinoma, and ectopic production of ACTH or corticotropin-releasing hormone (CRH) are less common.

Clinical features include obesity in 90 percent, hypertension in 85 percent, and glucose intolerance in 80 percent. Obesity in Cushing's syndrome tends to be central, with a rounded and full face ("moon face"), increased deposits in the periclavicular and cervical area ("buffalo hump"), and a large rounded abdomen. The extremities are thin, with muscle wasting and proximal muscle weakness—a reliable sign of Cushing's syndrome. Other catabolic effects include atrophy of the skin and underlying tissues, which manifests violaceous and wide striae, easy bruising, and a decreased skin barrier propensed to infections. Osteopenia and osteoporosis may result in pathological fractures. Excessive androgen production can be in part accountable for menstrual irregularities, hirsutism, and acne; clitoromegaly is a reliable sign of excessive androgen production often seen in adrenal carcinoma. Electrolyte abnormalities such as hypomagnesemia and hypercalcemia can be present; hypokalemic alkalosis can be indicative of ectopic ACTH production.

Hypertension is usually moderate, although malignant hypertension has been described. Very high cortisol production may cause a mineralocorticoid-like effect, volume expansion, and "low renin" hypertension. Since glucocorticoids may increase renin substrate, a subgroup of patients may have "high renin" hypertension. Glucocorticoid potentiation of vascular reactivity to catecholamines is an alternative explanation for hypertension.[97]

Patients with Cushing's syndrome often have concomitant glucose intolerance, hyperinsulinemia and/or overt diabetes, hypertension, obesity, and elevated plasma lipids. Thus, a high incidence of atherosclerosis might be expected in patients with prolonged disease. Cardiovascular complications of Cushing's syndrome, such as congestive heart failure and cerebrovascular accidents, may be the cause of death in 40 percent of untreated patients.[99]

A familial syndrome with inherited autosomal of X-linked dominant gene, in which affected members have "Carney's complex," consisting of primary pigmented nodular adrenocortical disease with hypercortisolism, cardiac myxomatous lesions, and cutaneous pigmentous lentigines has recently been described.[100]

Diagnosis and Treatment

In recent years, experience with simple tests for Cushing's syndrome has allowed physicians to effectively screen for this disease.[101] When normal subjects ingest 1 mg of dexamethasone at midnight, the next morning plasma cortisols are generally less than 5 μg/dL. A positive test (over 5 μg/dL) indicates the need for more extensive evaluation. Patients with Cushing's syndrome typically have elevated levels of urinary free cortisols (UFCs), a reflection of cortisol production by the adrenal gland. After a positive screening test and documentation of hypercortisolism, the different causes of increased cortisol production can be determined by manipulations of the hypothalamic-pituitary-adrenal axis. This is done by either suppression studies with dexamethasone or stimulation studies with CRH.[102] Anatomic localization of pituitary, adrenal, or ectopic sources resulting in hypercortisolism has greatly improved by means of better imaging techniques.[102] Measurement of ACTH levels in plasma from the inferior petrosal sinuses can distinguish ACTH-secreting pituitary adenomas from other causes of Cushing's syndrome.[103]

Transphenoidal pituitary adenomectomy has emerged as the treatment of choice for Cushing's disease.[104] When a pituitary lesion is not found by magnetic resonance imaging (MRI) or computerized tomography (CT) scan, petrosal sinus sampling may enable the neurosurgeon to do a partial hypophysectomy.

HYPERALDOSTERONISM, PHEOCHROMOCYTOMA

See Chapter 76.

SEX STEROIDS

The mechanism by which sex steroids affect CAD is closely linked to changes in lipid metabolism. Estrogen substantially decreases LDL cholesterol and raises HDL cholesterol, particularly HDL_2.[105] This beneficial effect is attenuated by progestins when combined with estrogen. Androgens have also a deleterious effect, by decreasing HDL, particularly HDL_2, and increasing LDL cholesterol.

Effects of Oral Contraceptives

An increased risk of hypertension, thromboembolic disease, and diabetes mellitus has been described in young women using oral contraceptives (OCs).[106] Hypertension takes place only in a few women on OCs, and it appears to be related to the overproduction of renin substrate by the liver.[107] The risk of deep-vein thrombophlebitis and thromboembolism can be three to four times higher in women receiving OCs,[108] but this is not the case in women receiving estrogen as replacement therapy.[109] The high incidence of vascular disease appears to be thrombotic, not atherosclerotic, and is not related to duration of OC use. Oral contraceptive administration to young women who smoke has been associated with an increased risk of myocardial infarction.[110] The high risk of developing CAD occurred in users over the age of 35 and/or with underlying risk factors such as hypertension, diabetes mellitus, and hyperlipidemia.[111] There is no reliable evidence that nonsmokers under age 45 or smokers under age 35 who use OCs have an increased likelihood of dying from myocardial infarction. Women under the age of 35 may still use OCs but should be advised to discontinue smoking. Women between the ages of 35 and 45 may use oral contraceptives if they do not smoke and do not have underlying risk factors for vascular disease. (See also Chap. 62.)

Oral contraceptives with high doses of progestin may cause glucose intolerance, which is related to the progestin dose as well as the user's age.[112] Caution is still recommended when these hormones are prescribed to patients with overt diabetes, glucose intolerance, or history of gestational diabetes. All progestins currently in use in the United States partly cancel the beneficial effects of estrogens in lipid metabolism and cause adverse lipid alterations.

Postmenopausal Estrogen Replacement

The average North American woman will be postmenopausal during one-third of her life span. The benefits of estrogen in postmenopausal women have been clearly established; they relieve menopausal symptoms, they reduce postmenopausal bone loss, with a 60 percent decline of hip fracture, and more important, they decrease the risk for CAD by 40 to 50 percent.[113] The Nurses Health Study showed a significant decrease in nonfatal myocardial infarction and fatal CAD among postmenopausal women taking estrogens.[113] These findings are supported by other studies. In the Leisure World retirement community in California study, mortality was reduced by 20 percent, mainly by lowering the rate of myocardial infarction among elderly women using estrogen replacement.[114] Three large cross-sectional angiographic studies have also shown a strong association of estrogen use with reduction of atherosclerosis.[115–117]

Estrogen replacement therapy is associated with a sixfold increase in endometrial cancer. The addition of progestin causes endometrial regression and reduces the incidence of cancer. Unfortunately, the combination of progestins with estrogens decreases the protective effect on CAD since progestins have an adverse effect on serum lipoproteins.

Epidemiologic studies suggest that estrogen replacement therapy also increases the incidence of breast cancer, with a relative risk of 1.3 in a metaanalysis.[118] This small change is important since breast cancer is a more common and a more lethal disease. Mammography before therapy and studies at intervals recommended by the American Cancer Society remain imperative for early detection. In contrast to endometrial cancer, progestins, when added to estrogens, do not appear to prevent the higher incidence of breast cancer.[119] Thus, the use of combination of estrogens and progestins is recommended in women with intact uterus, but the addition of progestin does not appear necessary in those who have undergone hysterectomy. When all benefits are carefully analyzed and compared against their risks, the potential advantage of estrogen replacement therapy is favored.[120]

HYPERINSULINEMIA

Insulin resistance, defined as higher than normal levels of insulin in the presence of normal or elevated levels of blood glucose, occurs in the majority of patients with impaired glucose tolerance, or non-insulin-dependent diabetes mellitus (NIDDM). It can also be found in about 25 percent of nonobese individuals with normal glucose tolerance.[121] Hyperinsulinemia has been identified as a risk factor for CAD, independent of hypertension, smoking, and elevated serum cholesterol.[121,122] The mechanism by which hyperinsulinemia causes atherosclerosis is not clear, but it may be by promoting proliferation and migration of arterial smooth-muscle cells as well as by stimulation of cholesterol synthesis in smooth-muscle and mononuclear cells.[123] Hyperinsulinemia may also promote atherosclerosis through its association with the other traditional risk factors.

Reaven[121] coined the term *syndrome X* to describe individuals with resistance to insulin-stimulated glucose uptake, glucose intolerance, hyperinsulinemia, increased levels of VLDL triglyceride, decreased levels of HDL cholesterol, and hypertension. This syndrome, now known as *hyperinsulinemia syndrome*, is distinguished from states of secondary insulin resistance such as obesity, diabetes, and a variety of uncommon autoimmune or endocrine disorders. Relative insulin deficiency may lead to high VLDL triglycerides and low HDL cholesterol.[124] Hyperinsulinemia may cause hypertension by promoting renal sodium retention, activating the sympathetic nervous system, and stimulating vascular smooth-muscle hypertrophy.[125] Insulin resistance is also closely related to obesity, particularly abdominal or lower body obesity, and other CAD risk factors.[125]

DIABETES MELLITUS

The prevalence of CAD is increased among patients with diabetes mellitus (DM).[126] It is the most frequent cause of death in non-insulin-dependent diabetes mellitus (NIDDM) and contributes significantly to mortality in insulin-dependent diabetes mellitus (IDDM).[127,128] The Framingham Study showed an increased incidence of myocardial infarction (MI), angina, and sudden death in patients with DM, particularly females.[129] The increased risk was independent of the usual risk factors for CAD,[130] and the influence of hyperglycemia on CAD mortality remains uncertain.[131]

Angiographic studies in patients with DM show a higher frequency of triple-vessel disease,[132,133] but it is less clear whether or not the changes are more diffuse. [128,132–134] The influence of glycemic control on CAD mortality is uncertain,[135] although normalization of blood glucose is advocated. Reduction of CAD risk in diabetics also depends on control of obesity, correction of hypertension, elimination of cigarette smoking, and improvement in the LDL-HDL cholesterol ratio.[130] The choice of certain antihypertensive agents (beta blockers and diuretics) in patients with DM may adversely influence glycemic control and hyperlipidemia. (See Chap. 77.) Caution is also needed when using beta blockers in patients with insulin-treated DM since hypoglycemia may be prolonged and unrecognized.

Myocardial infarction (MI) is the cause of death in about 20 percent of patients with DM.[136] This is the result of an increased incidence of CAD as well as increased mortality following MI, particularly in women.[137–139] This does not appear to be caused by larger infarctions.[140] Complications of MI such as congestive heart failure, cardiogenic shock, arrhythmias, and myocardial rupture are also more frequent.[137,141,142] Silent MI, a common feature of DM, is not limited to patients with autonomic neuropathy.[137,141,142] A correlation between glycemic control and increased mortality rate has been established.[143] Tight metabolic control during the immediate post-MI period has been associated with a decreased mortality rate.[144] The long-term mortality after MI is increased[138] and is associated with a higher incidence of reinfarction and chronic congestive heart failure.[138] Post-MI long-term treatment with timolol has been found to decrease mortality and nonfatal reinfarctions; a similar beneficial effect was found in nondiabetic individuals.[145] Silent ischemia commonly occurs in patients with DM and CAD, not necessarily in those with diabetic autonomic neuropathy.[146,147] Patients with concomitant peripheral vascular disease have a higher incidence of silent ischemia and infarction.[148]

Coronary artery bypass graft surgery (CABG) is frequently considered in the management of CAD in patients with DM. Short-term morbidity is increased, with a higher rate of sternotomy complications and renal failure.[134,149] Improvement in angina and late graft patency rates are similar in diabetics and nondiabetics.[150] Increased long-term mortality has also been reported following CABG.[134,150] Given the widespread use of angioplasty in the management of coronary artery disease, the influence of diabetes should be considered. Diabetes has not been associated with an increase in acute closure after single-vessel angioplasty in a large group of patients, primarily with single-vessel disease.[151] In patients with multivessel coronary disease undergoing multivessel angioplasty, the presence of diabetes predicted procedural failure and major ischemic procedural complications[152]; restenosis also occurs more frequently.[153]

Cardiac Autonomic Neuropathy

A patient can be considered to have cardiac autonomic neuropathy if two or more of the following tests are abnormal: (1) resting heart rate: Heart rate (HR) is determined after the patient is supine for 15 min; a resting HR of at least 100 beats per minute is abnormal; (2) beat to beat variability: The difference between the minimum and maximum heart rate is determined from electrocardiographic tracings obtained during periods of inspiration and expiration, with patients breathing six times per minute; a difference of at most 10 beats per minute is abnormal; (3) Valsalva maneuver: The ratio of the longest R-R interval after the maneuver to the shortest R-R interval during the maneuver is determined from electrocardiographic tracings, with patients blowing into a manometer and maintaining 40 mmHg for 15 s; an abnormal response is a ratio not exceeding 1.10; (4) heart rate response to standing: During electrocardiographic monitoring, the ratio of the R-R interval at the 30th beat after standing to the R-R interval at the 15th beat (30 : 15) is determined; a ratio of at most 1.00 is abnormal; (5) blood pressure response to standing: The fall in systolic blood pressure after 1 min of standing is determined by cuff sphygmomanometry; a fall of at least 30 mmHg is abnormal.[154]

Heart rate variability with respiration and standing is decreased in diabetics, especially in those with evidence of peripheral or autonomic neuropathy.[155–157] Defects in parasympathetic innervation, expressed as an increased resting HR and a decreased respiratory variation in HR, are more frequent and occur relatively early in DM.[158] Defects in sympathetic innervation, expressed as a decrease in the HR rise during standing, are less frequent and tend to occur later in the disease.[158] A prospective study of patients with DM with and without autonomic neuropathy revealed a markedly diminished survival in those with neuropathy with a substantial number of sudden deaths.[156]

An increased tendency to ventricular arrhythmias leading to sudden death may be associated with QT prolongation. A recent study showed a high incidence of QT prolongation at rest, especially after exercise, in diabetics with autonomic neuropathy, possibly reflecting autonomic imbalance.[159] The relationship of autonomic neuropathy to silent ischemia is uncertain at present. Postural hypotension commonly causes symptoms in diabetics with autonomic neuropathy, especially after bed rest, or when diuretics and/or other antihypertensive medications are used.

Cardiomyopathy

Clinical and pathological reports have documented the existence of a diabetic cardiomyopathy or heart muscle disease independent of coronary atherosclerosis.[160,161] An increased incidence of congestive heart failure even without clinical evidence of CAD or valvular heart disease can be found, especially in women.[162] Pathological studies have shown myocardial hypertrophy and interstitial fibrosis.[160,161] Controversy exists regarding the presence and significance of small-vessel disease, involving intramural coronary arteries, arterioles, and capillaries [128,160–162]; capillary microaneurysms have also been recently demonstrated.[163] Pathological studies have focused on the associated effects of hypertension on the development of diabetic cardiomyopathy. Postmortem studies revealed cellular hypertrophy and interstitial and myocytolytic necrosis with replacement fibrosis.[164] These changes are greater than what has been observed with either diabetes or hypertension alone. Diabetic cardiomyopathy may also occur in the setting of other atherosclerotic CAD; this may explain the increased frequency of congestive heart failure following MI.

Hemodynamic studies in patients with overt congestive heart failure show either dilated or restrictive cardiomyopathy.[161] (See Chaps. 89 and 91.) Systolic time intervals (STIs), especially preejection period and left ventricular ejection time are frequently abnormal, reflecting decreased contractility and/or a reduction in preload, possibly due to diminished left ventricular compliance.[165] Patients with microangiopathy are more likely to have abnormal STIs.[165] Treatment of hyperglycemia has been associated with partial normalization of STIs.[166] M-mode echocardiography has shown prolongation of isovolumic relaxation and slowing of ventricular filling.[167] Systolic function in patients with DM is frequently abnormal with concomitant hypertension but is less commonly affected in the normotensive.[167] Radionuclide studies have generally shown normal resting ejection fraction but a lower ejection fraction in response to dynamic exercise.[168] These abnormalities correlate with the presence of microangiopathy or autonomic neuropathy. Patients with diabetic autonomic neuropathy are more likely to have abnormal filling dynamics.[169] Young patients with DM have a high frequency of diastolic dysfunction demonstrated by pulsed Doppler echocardiography; the ratio of peak early to peak late (atrial) filling velocity is significantly lower in patients with DM.[170]

Experimental studies support the view that the diabetic state itself affects ventricular performance. Experimentally-induced diabetes in dogs is associated with reduced left ventricular compliance and increased interstitial connective tissue.[171] In diabetic rats, left ventricular papillary muscle shows marked slowing and prolongation of contraction with delayed relaxation.[172] With the development of diabetes, myosin ATPase decreases, with a shift in the isoenzyme form of myosin from the faster V_1 form to the slower V_3 form in some species;[173] this accounts for the decreased speed of muscle shortening. The delayed and slowed relaxation correlates with a reduction in the rate of Ca^{2+} binding of isolated sarcoplasmic reticulum.[174] All of these alterations are reversed by insulin treatment.[172] An important role for altered myocardial calcium metabolism in diabetes is suggested by the beneficial effects of verapamil on hemodynamic function and subcellular biochemistry in diabetic rats.[175]

The presence of hypertension combined with diabetes alters this relatively benign state in experimental animals as it does in humans. The importance of hypertension in accelerating complications should be emphasized, and careful blood pressure control is essential. The optimal mode of antihypertensive therapy remains to be established, but a drug that causes regression of ventricular hypertrophy and prevention of ongoing myocardial pathology would be ideal. Concomitant treatment of hyperglycemia is also recommended. (See also Chap. 77.)

REFERENCES

1. Kovacs K, Yeo J: Pituitary necrosis following major heart surgery. *Z Cardiol* 1975; 62:52–55.
2. Daniel PM, Spicer EJF, Treip CS: Pituitary necrosis in patients maintained on mechanical respirators. *J Pathol* 1973; 111:135–138.
3. Barber SG: Hypopituitarism and artificial ventilation. *Acta Endocrinol* 1979; 90:211–216.
4. Melmed S: Acromegaly. *N Engl J Med* 1990; 322:966–976.
5. McGuffin WL Jr, Sherman BM, Roth F, Gordon P, Kahn CR, Roberts WC, et al: Acromegaly and cardiovascular disorders: A prospective study. *Ann Intern Med* 1974; 81:11–18.
6. Csanady M, Gaspar L, Hogye M, Gruber N: The heart in acromegaly: An echocardiographic study. *Int J Cardiol* 1983; 2:349–357.
7. Hayward RP, Emanuel RW, Nabarro JD: Acromegalic heart disease: Influence of treatment of the acromegaly on the heart. *Q J Med* 1987; 62:41–58.
8. Snow MH, Piercy DA, Robson V, Wilkinson R: An investigation into the pathogenesis of hypertension in acromegaly. *Clin Sci Mol Med* 1977; 53:87–91.
9. Cain JP, Williams GH, Dluhy RG: Plasma renin activity and aldosterone secretion in patients with acromegaly. *J Clin Endocrinol* 1972; 34:73–81.
10. Anderson RJ, Lufkin EG, Sizemore GW, Carney JA, Sheps SG, Silliman YE: Acromegaly and pituitary adenoma with pheochromocytoma: A variant of multiple endocrine neoplasia. *Clin Endocrinol* 1981; 14:604–612.
11. Rioperez E, Botella JM, Valdivieso L, Ballesteros D, Diez L, Navas J: Conn's syndrome in a patient with acromegaly. *Horm Metab Res* 1981; 13:186–187.
12. Lie JT, Grossman SJ: Pathology of the heart in acromegaly: Anatomic findings in 27 autopsied patients. *Am Heart J* 1980; 100:41–52.
13. Savage DD, Henry WL, Eastman RC, Borer JS, Gorden P: Echocardiographic assessment of cardiac anatomy and function in acromegalic patients. *Am J Med* 1979; 67:823–829.
14. Jonas EA, Aloia JF, Lane FJ: Evidence of subclinical heart muscle dysfunction in acromegaly. *Chest* 1975; 67:190–194.
15. Chanson P, Timsit J, Masquest C, Warnet A, Guillausseau PJ, Berman P, et al: Cardiovascular effects of the somatostatin analog octreotide in acromegaly. *Ann Intern Med* 1990; 113:921–925.
16. Cadieux RJ, Kales A, Santen RJ, Bixler EO, Gordon R: Endoscopic findings in sleep apnea associated with acromegaly. *J Clin Endocrinol Metab* 1982; 55:18–22.
17. Levey GS: Thyroid and the heart. *Am J Med* 1990; 88:625.
18. Weinberger C, Thompson CC, Ong ES, Lebo R, Gruol DJ, Evans RM: The c-erb-A gene encodes a thyroid hormone receptor. *Nature (Lond)* 1986; 324:641–646.
19. Morkin E, Flink IL, Goldman S: Biochemical and physiological effects of thyroid hormone on cardiac performance. *Prog Cardiovasc Dis* 1983; 25:435–464.
20. Dillmann WH: Biochemical basis of the thyroid hormone action in the heart. *Am J Med* 1990; 88:626–630.
21. Gick GG, Ismail-Beigi F, Edelman IS: Thyroidal regulation of rat renal and hepatic Na, K-ATPase gene expression. *J Biol Chem* 1988; 263:16610–16618.
22. Kim D, Smith TW, Marsh JD: Effect of thyroid hormone on slow calcium channel function in cultured chick ventricular cells. *J Clin Invest* 1987; 80:88–94.
23. Rodgers RL, Black S, Katz S, McNeil JH: Thyroidectomy of SHR: effects on ventricular relaxation and on SR calcium uptake activity. *Am J Physiol* 1986; 250:H861–865.
24. Ladenson PW, Bloch KD, Seidman JG: Modulation of atrial natriuretic factor by thyroid hormone: Messenger ribonucleic acid and peptide levels in hypothyroid, euthyroid and hyperthyroid rat atria and ventricles. *Endocrinology* 1988; 123:652–657.

25. Buccino RA, Spann JF, Pool PE, Sonnenblick EH, Braunwald E: Influence of the thyroid state on the intrinsic contractile properties and energy stores of the myocardium. *J Clin Invest* 1967; 46:1669–1682.
26. Klein I: Thyroid hormone and the cardiovascular system. *Am J Med* 1990; 88:631–637.
27. Greattinger JS, Muenster JJ, Checchia CS, Grissom RL, Campbell JA: A correlation of clinical and hemodynamic studies in patients with hypothyroidism. *J Clin Invest* 1957; 37:502–510.
28. Levey GS, Klein I: Catecholamine–thyroid hormone interactions and the cardiovascular manifestations of hyperthyroidism. *Am J Med* 1990; 88:642–646.
29. Liggett SB, Shah SD, Cayer PE: Increased fat and skeletal muscle β-adrenergic receptors but unaltered metabolic and hemodynamic sensitivity to epinephrine in vivo in experimental human thyrotoxicosis. *J Clin Invest* 1989; 83:803–809.
30. Skelton CL: The heart and hyperthyroidism. *N Engl J Med* 1982; 307:1206–1208.
31. Brauman A, Algom M, Gilboa Y, Ramot Y, Golik A, Stryjer D: Mitral valve prolapse in hyperthyroidism of two different origins. *Br Heart J* 1985; 53:374–377.
32. Sandler G, Wilson GM: The nature and prognosis of heart disease in thyrotoxicosis. *Q J Med* 1959; 28:247–269.
33. Ladenson PW: Recognition and management of cardiovascular disease related to thyroid dysfunction. *Am J Med* 1990; 88:638–641.
34. Ikram H: The nature and prognosis of thyrotoxic heart disease. *Q J Med* 1985; 54:19–28.
35. Agner T, Abundal T, Thorsteinzson B, Agner E: A reevaluation of atrial fibrillation in thyrotoxicosis. *Dan Med Bull* 1984; 31:157–159.
36. Ciaccheri M, Cecchi F, Arcangeli C, Dolara A, Zuppiroli A, Pieroni C: Occult thyrotoxicosis in patients with chronic and paroxysmal isolated atrial fibrillation. *Clin Cardiol* 1984; 7:413–426.
37. Davidson E, Weinberger I, Rotenberg Z, Fuchs J, Agmon J: Atrial fibrillation. Cause and time of onset. *Arch Intern Med* 1989; 149:457–459.
38. Giladi M, Aderka D, Zeligman-Melatzki L, Finkelstein A, Ayalon D, Levo Y: Is idiopathic atrial fibrillation caused by occult thyrotoxicosis? A study of one hundred consecutive patients with atrial fibrillation. *Int J Cardiol* 1991; 30(3):309–313.
39. Bar-sela S, Ehrenfeld M, Eliakim M: Arterial embolism in thyrotoxicosis with atrial fibrillation. *Arch Intern Med* 1981; 141:1191–1192.
40. Marks AD, Channick BJ, Adlin EV, Kessler RK, Braitman LE, Denenberg BS: Chronic thyroiditis and mitral valve prolapse. *Ann Intern Med* 1985; 102:479–483.
41. Devereux RB, Kramer-Fox R, Kligfield P: Mitral valve prolapse: Causes, clinical manifestations, and management. *Ann Intern Med* 1989; 111:305–317.
42. Reynolds JL, Woody HB: Thyrotoxic mitral regurgitation. *Am J Dis Child* 1971; 122:544–548.
43. Ross DS, Daniels GH, Gouveia D: The use and limitations of a chemiluminescent thyrotropin assay as a single thyroid function test in an out patient endocrine clinic. *J Clin Endocrinol Metab* 1990; 71:764–769.
44. Wartofsky L, Glinoer D, Solomon B: Differences and similarities in the diagnosis and treatment of Graves' disease in Europe, Japan and the United States. *Thyroid* 1991; 1:129–135.
45. Gerst HP, Fildes J, Baylor P, Zonszein J: Long acting beta-adrenergic antagonists as preparation for surgery in thyrotoxicosis. *Arch Surg* 1986; 121:838–840.
46. Ingbar SH: The role of antiadrenergic agents in the management of thyrotoxicosis. *Cardiovasc-Rev Repts* 1981; 2:683.
47. Zonszein J, Santangelo RP, Mackin JF, Lee TC, Coffey RJ, Canary JJ: Propranolol therapy in thyrotoxicosis. A review of 84 patients undergoing surgery. *Am J Med* 1979; 66:411–416.
48. Clozel JP, Danchin N, Genton P, Thomas JL, Cherrier F: Effects of propranolol and of verapamil on heart rate and blood pressure in hyperthyroidism. *Clin Pharmacol Ther* 1984; 36:64–69.
49. Nakazawa HK, Sakurai K, Hamada N, Momotani N, Ito K: Management of atrial fibrillation in the postthyrotoxic state. *Am J Med* 1982; 72:903–906.
50. Hirsh J: Review article. Oral anticoagulant drugs. *N Engl J Med* 1991; 324:1865–1875.
51. Petersen P, Boyesen G, Godtfredsen J, Andersen ED, Andersen B: Placebo controlled, randomized trial of warfarin and aspirin for prevention of thromboembolic complications in chronic atrial fibrillation: The Copenhagen AFASAK study. *Lancet* 1989; 1:175–179.
52. Stroke prevention in Atrial Fibrillation Study Group Investigators: Preliminary report of the Stroke Prevention in Atrial Fibrillation Study. *N Engl J Med* 1990; 322:863–868.
53. The Boston Area Anticoagulation Trial for Atrial Fibrillation Investigators: The effect of low-dose warfarin on the risk of stroke in patients with non-rheumatic atrial fibrillation. *N Engl J Med* 1990; 323:1505–1511.
54. Bastenie PA, Bonnyns M, Vanhaelst L: Natural history of primary myxedema. *Am J Med* 1985; 79:91–100.
55. Saito I, Kunihiko I, Saruta T: Hypothyroidism as a cause of hypertension. *Hypertension* 1983; 5:112–115.
56. Klein I: Thyroid hormone and high blood pressure. In Laragh JH, Brenner BM, Kaplan NM (eds): *Endocrine Mechanisms in Hypertension,* vol 2. New York, Raven, 1989: 61–80.
57. Laragh JH, Sealey JE, Brunner HR: The control of aldosterone secretion in normal and hypertensive man. Abnormal renin-aldosterone patterns in low-renin hypertension. In: Laragh JH (ed): *Hypertension Manual.* New York, Yorke Medical Books, 1975: 197–225.
58. Hamolsky MW, Kurland GS, Freedberg AS: The heart in hypothyroidism. *J Chron Dis* 1961; 14:558–569.
59. Graettinger JS, Muenster JJ, Checchia CS, Grisson RL, Campbell JA: A correlation of clinical and hemodynamic studies in patients with hypothyroidism. *J Clin Invest* 1958; 37:502–510.
60. Vora J, O'Malley BP, Petersen S, McCullough A, Rosenthal FD, Barnett DB: Reversible abnormalities of myocardial relaxation in hypothyroidism. *J Clin Endocrinol Metab* 1985; 61:269–272.
61. Hillis WS, Bremner WF, Lawrie TDV, Thomson JA: Systolic time intervals in thyroid disease. *Clin Endocrinol* 1975; 4:617–624.
62. Farooki ZQ, Hoffman WH, Perry BL, Green EW: Myocardial dysfunction in hypothyroid children. *Am J Dis Child* 1983; 1:65–68.
63. Forfar JC, Muir AL, Toft AD: Left ventricular function in hypothyroidism. Responses to exercise and beta adrenoreceptor blockade. *Br Heart J* 1982; 48:278–284.
64. Jajiri J, Morita M, Higashi K, Fujii H, Fujii H, Nakamura N, et al: The cause of low voltage QRS complex in primary hypothyroidism. Pericardial effusion or thyroid hormone deficiency? *Jpn Heart J* 1985; 26:539–547.
65. Vanhaelst I, Neve P: Coronary artery disease in hypothyroidism. *Lancet* 1967; 2:800–802.
66. Elder J, McLelland A, O'Reilley DS, Packard CJ, Series JJ, Shepherd J: The relationship between serum cholesterol and serum thyrotropin, thyroxine and tri-iodothyronine concentrations in suspected hypothyroidism. *Ann Clin Biochem* 1990; 36:110–113.
67. Tunbridge WMG, Evered DC, Hall R, Appleton D, Bresis M, Clark F, et al: Lipid profiles and cardiovascular disease in the Whickham area with particular reference to thyroid failure. *Clin Endocrinol* 1977; 7:495–508.
68. Keating FR, Parkin TW, Selby JB, Dickinson LS: Treatment of heart disease associated with myxedema. *Prog Cardiovasc Dis* 1960; 3:364–381.
69. Steinberg AD: Myxedema and coronary artery disease. A comparative autopsy study. *Ann Intern Med* 1968; 68:338–344.
70. Becker C: Hypothyroid and atherosclerotic heart disease: Pathogenesis, medical management and the role of coronary artery bypass surgery. *Endocr Rev* 1985; 6:432–440.
71. Goldman J, Matz R, Mortimer R: High elevations of creatinine phosphokinase in hypothyroidism. *JAMA* 1977; 238:325–326.
72. Kabadi UM, Kumar SP: Pericardial effusion in primary hypothyroidism. *Am Heart J* 1990; 120(6):1393–1395.
73. Kelly JK, Butt JC: Fatal myxedema pericarditis in a Christian Scientist. *Am J Clin Pathol* 1986; 86(1):113–116.
74. Helfand M, Lawrence MC: Screening for thyroid disease. *Ann Intern Med* 1990; 112:840–849.
75. Gavin LA: The diagnostic dilemmas of hyperthyroxinemia and hypothyroxinemia. *Adv Intern Med* 1988; 33:185–203.
76. Wartofsky L, Burman KD: Alterations in thyroid function in patients with systemic illnesses: The "euthyroid sick syndrome." *Endocr Rev* 1982; 3:164–217.
77. Sherman SI, Ladenson PW: Percutaneous transluminal coronary angioplasty in hypothyroidism. *Am J Med* 1991; 90:367–370.
78. Rabinowe SL, Larsen PR, Antman EM, George KL, Friedman PL, Jackson RA, et al: Amiodarone therapy and autoimmune

thyroid disease: Elevation of a new monoclonal antibody defined T cell subset. *Am J Med* 1986; 81:53–57.
79. Kaplan J, Ish-Shalom S: Goiter and hypothyroidism during retreatment with amiodarone in a patient who previously experienced amiodarone-induced thyrotoxicosis. *Am J Med* 1991; 90:750–752.
80. Vagenakis AG, Rapoport B, Azizi F, Portnay GI, Braverman LE, Ingbar SH: Hyper-response to thyrotropin-releasing hormone by small quantities of thyroid hormones. *J Clin Invest* 1974; 54:913–918.
81. Burger A, Dinichert D, Nicod P, Jenny M, Lemarchard-Beraud T, Vallotton MB: Effect of amiodarone on serum triiodothyronine, reverse triiodothyronine, thyroxine and thyrotropin: A drug influencing peripheral metabolism in thyroid hormones. *J Clin Invest* 1976; 58:255–259.
82. Martino E, Safran M, Aghini-Lombardi F, Rajatanavin R, Lenziardi M, Fay M, et al: Environmental iodine intake and thyroid dysfunction during chronic amiodarone therapy. *Ann Intern Med* 1984; 101:28–34.
83. Lambert M, Unger J, De Nayer P, Brohet C, Gangji D: Evidence of thyroid damage in amiodarone-induced thyrotoxicosis suggestive of thyroid damage. *J Endocrinol Invest* 1990; 13:527–530.
84. Melmed S, Nademance R, Reed AW, Hendrickson JA, Singh BN, Hershman JM: Hyperthyroxinemia with bradycardia and normal thyrotropin secretion after chronic amiodarone administration. *J Clin Endocrinol Metab* 1981; 53:997–1001.
85. Martino E, Aghini-Lombardi F, Mariotti S, Lenziardi M, Baschieri L, Braverman LE, et al: Treatment of amiodarone associated thyrotoxicosis by simultaneous administration of potassium perchlorate and methimazole. *J Endocrinol Invest* 1986; 9:201–207.
86. Bogin E, Massry SG, Harary I: Effect of parathyroid hormone on rat heart cells. *J Clin Invest* 1981; 67:1215–1227.
87. Baczynski R, Massry SG, Kohan R, Masott M, Saglikes Y, Brautbar N: Effect of parathyroid hormone on myocardial energy metabolism in the rat. *Kid Intern* 1985; 27:718–725.
88. Weishaar RE, Simpson RU: Vitamin D_3 and cardiovascular function in rats. *J Clin Invest* 1987; 79:1706–1712.
89. Morgan JP: Abnormal intracellular modulation of calcium as a major cause of cardiac contractile dysfunction. *N Engl J Med* 1991; 325:625–632.
90. Roberts WC, Waller BF: Effect of chronic hypercalcemia on the heart: An analysis of 18 necropsy patients. *Am J Med* 1981; 71:371–384.
91. Connor TB, Rosen BL, Blaustein MP, Applefeld MM, Doyle LA: Hypocalcemia precipitating congestive heart failure. *N Engl J Med* 1982; 307:869–872.
92. Levine SN, Rheams CN: Hypocalcemic heart failure. *Am J Med* 1985; 78:1033–1035.
93. Heath H III, Hodgson SF, Kennedy MA: Primary hyperparathyroidism. *N Engl J Med* 1980; 302:189–193.
94. Lueg MC: Hypertension and primary hyperparathyroidism: A five-year case review. *South Med* 1982; 75:1371–1374.
95. Christensson T, Hellstrom K, Wengle B: Hypercalcemia and primary hyperparathyroidism: Prevalence in patients receiving thiazides as detected in a health screen. *Arch Intern Med* 1977; 137:1138–1142.
96. Vered Z, Battler A, Motro M: Left ventricular function in patients with chronic hypophosphatemia. *Am Heart J* 1984; 107:796–798.
97. Yard AC, Kadowitz PJ: Studies on the mechanism of hydrocortisone potentiation of vasoconstrictor responses to epinephrine in the anesthetized animal. *Eur J Pharmacol* 1972; 20:1–9.
98. Abrass IB, Scarpace PJ: Glucocorticoid regulation of myocardial beta-receptors. *Endocrinology* 1981; 108:977–980.
99. Plotz CM, Knowlton AI, Ragan C: The natural history of Cushing's syndrome. *Am J Med* 1952; 13:597–614.
100. Danoff A, Jormark S, Lorber D, Fleischer N: Adrenocortical micronodular dysplasia, cardiac myxomas, lentigines, and spindle cell tumors. *Arch Intern Med* 1987; 147:443–448.
101. Crapo L: Cushing's syndrome: A review of diagnostic tests. *Metabolism* 1979; 28:955–977.
102. Kaye TB, Crapo L: The Cushing's syndrome: An update on diagnostic tests. *Ann Intern Med* 1990; 112:434–444.
103. Oldfield EH, Doppman JL, Nieman LK, Chrousos GP, Miller DL, Katz DA, et al: Petrosal sinus sampling with and without corticotropin-releasing hormone for the differential diagnosis of Cushing's Syndrome. *N Engl J Med* 1991; 325:897–905.
104. Mampalalm TJ, Tyrell BJ, Wilson CB: Transsphenoidal microsurgery for Cushing disease. *Ann Intern Med* 1988; 109:487–493.
105. Walsh BW, Schiff I, Rosner B, Greenberg L, Ravnikar V, Sacks FM: Effects of postmenopausal estrogen replacement on the concentrations and metabolism of plasma proteins. *N Engl J Med* 1991; 325:1196–1204.
106. Webber LS, Hunter SM, Baugh JG, Srinivasan SR, Sklov MC, Berenson GS: The interaction of cigarette smoking, oral contraceptive use, and cardiovascular risk factor variables in children: The Bogalusa Heart Study. *Am J Publ Health* 1982; 72:266–274.
107. Boyd WN, Burden RP, Aber GM: Intrarenal vascular changes in patients receiving estrogen-containing compounds—A clinical, histological and angiographic study. *Q J Med* 1975; 44:415–431.
108. Royal College of General Practitioners: *Oral Contraceptive and Health: An Interim Report from the Oral Contraceptive Study of the Royal College of General Practitioners.* New York, Pitman Publishing, 1974.
109. Gambrell RD Jr: The menopause: Benefits and risk of estrogen-progestogen replacement therapy. *Fertil Steril* 1982; 37:457–474.
110. Mann JI, Vessey MP, Thorogood M, Doll SR: Myocardial infarction in young women with special reference to oral contraceptive practice. *Br Med J* 1975; 2:241–245.
111. Royal College of General Practitioners' Oral contraceptive study: Further analysis of mortality in oral contraceptive users. *Lancet* 1981; 1:541–546.
112. Godsland IF, Crook D, Simpson R: The effects of different formulations of oral contraceptive agents on lipid and carbohydrate metabolism. *N Engl J Med* 1990; 323:1375–1381.
113. Stampfer MJ, Colditz GA, Willett WC, Manson JE, Rosner B, Speizer FE, et al: Postmenopausal estrogen therapy and cardiovascular disease. Ten-year follow-up from the Nurses' Health Study. *N Engl J Med* 1991; 325:756–762.
114. Henderson BE, Ross RK, Paganini-Hill A, Mack TM: Estrogen use and cardiovascular disease. *Am J Obstet Gynecol* 1986; 154:1181–1186.
115. Sullivan JM, Vander Zwagg RV, Lemp GF, Hughes JP, Maddock V, Kroetz FW, et al: Postmenopausal estrogen use and coronary atherosclerosis. *Ann Intern Med* 1988; 108:358–363.
116. Gruchow HW, Anderson AJ, Barboriak JJ, Sobocinski KA: Postmenopausal use of estrogens and occlusion of coronary arteries. *Am Heart J* 1988; 115:954–963.
117. McFarland KF, Boniface ME, Hornung CA, Earnhardt W, Humphries JO: Risk factors and noncontraceptive estrogen use in women with and without coronary artery disease. *Am Heart J* 1989; 117:1209–1214.
118. Steinberg KK, Thacker SB, Smith SJ, Stroup DF, Zack MM, Flanders WD, et al: A meta-analysis of the effect of estrogen replacement therapy on the risk of breast cancer. *JAMA* 1991; 265:1985–1990.
119. Bergvist L, Adami HO, Persson I, Hoover R, Schairer C: The risk of breast cancer after estrogen and estrogen-progestin replacement. *N Engl J Med* 1989; 321:293–297.
120. Goldman L, Tosteson ANA: Uncertainty about postmenopausal estrogen (editorial). *N Engl J Med* 1991; 325:800–802.
121. Reaven GM: Role of insulin resistance in human disease. *Diabetes* 1988; 37:1595–1607.
122. Ducimetiere P, Eschwege E, Papoz L, Richard JL, Claude JR, Roseelin GE: Relationship of plasma insulin levels to the incidence of myocardial infarction and coronary heart disease mortality in a middle-age population. *Diabetologia* 1980; 19:205–210.
123. Stout RW: Insulin and atheroma—an update. *Lancet* 1987; 1:1077–1079.
124. Zavaroni I, Bonora E, Pagliara M, Dall'aglio E, Luchetti L, Buonanno G, et al: Risk factors for coronary artery disease in healthy persons with hyperinsulinemia and normal glucose tolerance. *N Engl J Med* 1989; 320:702–706.
125. Kaplan NM: The deadly quartet: Upper-body obesity, glucose intolerance, hypertriglyceridemia, and hypertension. *Arch Intern Med* 1989; 149:1514–1520.
126. Liebow IM, Hellerstein HK, Miller M: Arteriosclerotic heart disease in diabetes mellitus: A clinical study of 383 patients. *Am J Med* 1955; 18:438–447.
127. Knowles HD Jr: Long-term juvenile diabetes treated with unmeasured diet. *Trans Assoc Am Phys* 1971: 84:95–101.

128. Crall FV Jr, Roberts WC: The extramural and intramural coronary arteries in juvenile diabetes mellitus: Analysis of nine necropsy patients aged 19 to 38 years with onset of diabetes before age 15 years. *Am J Med* 1978; 64:221–230.
129. Kannel WB: Role of diabetics in cardiac disease: Conclusions from population studies. In: Zoneraich S (ed): *Diabetes and the Heart.* Springfield, IL, Charles C Thomas, 1978: 97–112.
130. Kannel WB: Lipids, diabetes, and coronary heart disease: Insights from the Framingham Study. *Am Heart J* 1985; 110:1100–1107.
131. Pan WH, Cedres LB, Liu K, Dyer A, Schoenberger JA, Shekelle RB, et al: Relationship of clinical diabetes and asymptomatic hyperglycemia to risk of coronary heart disease mortality in men and women. *Am J Epidemiol* 1986; 123:504–516.
132. Dortimer AC, Shenoy PN, Shiroff RA, Leaman DM, Babb JD, Liedtke AJ, et al: Diffuse coronary artery disease in diabetic patients: Fact or fiction? *Circulation* 1978; 57:133–136.
133. Abadie E, Masquet C, Guiomard A, Passa P: Coronary angiography in diabetic and non-diabetic patients with severe ischemic heart disease. *Diabet Metab* 1983; 9:53–57.
134. Salomon NW, Page US, Okies JE, Stephens J, Krause AH, Bigelow JC: Diabetes mellitus and coronary artery bypass. Short-term risk and long-term prognosis. *J Thorac Cardiovasc Surg* 1983; 85:264–271.
135. Keen H, Jarrett RJ, Ward JD, Fuller JH: Borderline diabetics and their response to tolbutamide. *Adv Metab Disord* 1973; 2(suppl):521–531.
136. Malins J: The prognosis and long-term course of diabetes. In: *Clinical Diabetes Mellitus.* London, Eyre and Spottiswoode, 1968: 462–474.
137. Partamian JO, Bradley RF: Acute myocardial infarction in 258 cases of diabetes. Immediate mortality and five-year survival. *N Engl J Med* 1965; 273:455–461.
138. Ulvenstam G, Aberg A, Bergstrand R, Johansson S, Pennert K, Vedin A, et al: Long-term prognosis after myocardial infarction in men with diabetes. *Diabetes* 1985; 34:787–792.
139. Abbott RD, Donahue RP, Kannel WB, Wilson PWF: The impact of diabetes on survival following myocardial infarction in men vs women. The Framingham Study. *JAMA* 1988; 260:3456–3460.
140. Jaffe AS, Spadaro JJ, Schechtman K, Roberts R, Geltman EM, Sobel BE: Increased congestive heart failure after myocardial infarction of modest extent in patients with diabetes mellitus. *Am Heart J* 1984; 108:31–37.
141. Bradley RF, Schonfeld A: Diminished pain in diabetic patients with acute myocardial infarction. *Geriatrics* 1962; 17:322–326.
142. Margolis JR, Kannel WS, Feinleib M, Dawber TR, McNamara PM: Clinical features of unrecognized myocardial infarction—silent and symptomatic. Eighteen year follow-up: The Framingham Study. *Am J Cardiol* 1973; 32:1–7.
143. Oswald GA, Corcoran S, Yudkin JS: Prevalence and risks of hyperglycemia and undiagnosed diabetes in patients with acute myocardial infarction. *Lancet* 1984; 1:1264–1267.
144. Clark RS, English M, McNeill GP, Newton RW: Effect of intravenous infusion of insulin in diabetics with acute myocardial infarction. *Br Med J* 1985; 291:303–305.
145. Gundersen T, Kjekshus J: Timolol treatment after myocardial infarction in diabetic patients. *Diabetes Care* 1983; 6:285–290.
146. Chipkin SR, Frid D, Alpert JS, Baker SP, Dalen JE, Aronin N: Frequency of painless myocardial ischemia during exercise tolerance testing in patients with and without diabetes mellitus. *Am J Cardiol* 1987; 59:61–65.
147. Nesto RW, Phillips RT, Ket KG, Hill T, Perper E, Young E, et al: Angina and exertional myocardial ischemia in diabetic and nondiabetic patients: Assessment by exercise thallium scintigraphy. *Ann Intern Med* 1988; 108:170–175.
148. Nesto RW, Watson FS, Kowalchuk GJ, Zarich SW, Hill T, Lewis SM, et al: Silent myocardial ischemia and infarction in diabetics with peripheral vascular disease: Assessment by dipyridamole thallium-201 scintigraphy. *Am Heart J* 1990; 120:1073–1077.
149. Verska JJ, Walker WJ: Aortocoronary bypass in the diabetic patients. *Am J Cardiol* 1975; 35:774–777.
150. Lawrie GM, Morris GC Jr, Glaeser DH: Influence of diabetes mellitus on the results of coronary bypass surgery. Follow-up of 212 diabetic patients ten to 15 years after surgery. *JAMA* 1986; 256:2967–2971.
151. Ellis SG, Roubin GS, King SB, Douglas JS, Weintraub WS, Thomas RG, et al: Angiographic and clinical predictors of acute closure after native vessel coronary angioplasty. *Circulation* 1988; 77:372–379.
152. Ellis SG, Vandormael MG, Cowley MJ, DiSciascio G, Deligonul V, Topol EJ, et al: Coronary morphologic and clinical determinants of procedural outcome with angioplasty for multivessel coronary disease. Implications for patient selection. *Circulation* 1990; 82:1193–1202.
153. Vandormael MG, Deligonul V, Kern MJ, Harper M, Presant S, Gibson P, et al: Multilesion coronary angioplasty: Clinical and angiographic followup. *J Am Coll Cardiol* 1987; 10:240–252.
154. Ewing DJ, Marty CN, Young RJ, Clarke BF: The value of cardiovascular autonomic function tests: 10 years experience in diabetes. *Diabetes Care* 1985; 8:491–498.
155. Lloyd-Mostyn RH, Watkins PJ: Defective innervation of heart in diabetic autonomic neuropathy. *Br Med J* 1975; 3:15–17.
156. Ewing DJ, Campbell IW, Clarke BF: The natural history of diabetic autonomic neuropathy. *Q J Med* 1980; 193:95–108.
157. Wheeler T, Watkins PJ: Cardiac denervation in diabetes. *Br Med J* 1973; 4:584–586.
158. Oikawa N, Umetsu M, Toyota T, Goto Y: Quantitative evaluation of diabetic autonomic neuropathy by using heart rate variations: Relationship between cardiac parasympathetic or sympathetic damage and clinical conditions. *Tohuku J Exp Med* 1986; 148:125–133.
159. Kahn JK, Sisson JC, Vinik AI: QT interval prolongation and sudden cardiac death in diabetic autonomic neuropathy. *J Clin Endocrinol Metab* 1987; 64:751–754.
160. Rubler S, Dlugash J, Yuceoglu YZ, Kumral T, Branwood AW, Grishman A: New type of cardiomyopathy associated with diabetic glomerulosclerosis. *Am J Cardiol* 1972; 30:595–602.
161. Regan TJ, Lyons MM, Ahmed SS, Levinson GE, Oldewurtel HA, Ahmad MR, et al: Evidence for cardiomyopathy in familial diabetes mellitus. *J Clin Invest* 1977; 60:885–899.
162. Kannel WB, Hjortland M, Castelli WP: Role of diabetes in congestive heart failure: The Framingham Study. *Am J Cardiol* 1974; 34:29–34.
163. Factor SM, Okun EM, Minase T: Capillary microaneurysms in the human diabetic heart. *N Engl J Med* 1980; 302:384–388.
164. Van Hoeven KH, Factor SM: A comparison of the pathological spectrum of hypertensive, diabetic and hypertensive-diabetic heart disease. *Circulation* 1990; 82:848–855.
165. Seneviratne BI: Diabetic cardiomyopathy: The preclinical phase. *Br Med J* 1977; 1:1444–1446.
166. Uusitopa M, Siitonen O, Aro A, Korhonen T, Pyorala K: Effects of correction of hyperglycemia on left ventricular function in non-insulin-dependent (type 2) diabetics. *Acta Med Scand* 1983; 213:363–368.
167. Shapiro LM, Howat AP, Calter MM: Left ventricular function in diabetes mellitus: I. Methodology and prevalence and spectrum of abnormalities. *Br Heart J* 1981; 45:122–128.
168. Vered A, Battler A, Segal P, Liberman D, Yerushalmi Y, Berezin M, et al: Exercise-induced left ventricular dysfunction in young men with asymptomatic diabetes mellitus (diabetic cardiomyopathy). *Am J Cardiol* 1984; 54:633–637.
169. Kahn JK, Zola B, Juni JE, Vinik AI: Radionuclide assessment of left ventricular diastolic filling in diabetes mellitus with and without cardiac autonomic neuropathy. *J Am Coll Cardiol* 1986; 7:1303–1309.
170. Zarich SW, Arbuckle BE, Cohen LR, Roberts M, Nesto RW: Diastolic abnormalities in young asymptomatic diabetic patients assessed by pulsed Doppler echocardiography. *J Am Coll Cardiol* 1988; 12:114–120.
171. Regan TJ, Ettinger PO, Kahn MI, Jesrani MV, Lyons MM, Oldewurtel HA, et al: Altered myocardial function and metabolism in chronic diabetes mellitus without ischemia in dogs. *Circ Res* 1974; 35:222–237.
172. Fein F, Strobeck JE, Malhotra A, Scheuer J, Sonnenblick EH: Reversibility of diabetic cardiomyopathy with insulin in rats. *Circ Res* 1981; 49:1251–1261.
173. Malhotra A, Penpargkul S, Fein FS, Sonnenblick EH, Scheuer J: The effect of streptozotocin-induced diabetes in rats on cardiac contractile proteins. *Circ Res* 1981; 49:1243–1250.
174. Penpargkul S, Fein F, Sonnenblick EH, Scheuer J: Depressed cardiac sarcoplasmic reticular function from diabetic rats. *J Mol Cell Cardiol* 1981; 13:303–309.
175. Afzal N, Pierce GN, Elimban V, Beamish RE, Dhalla NS: Influence of verapamil on some subcellular defects in diabetic cardiomyopathy. *Am J Physiol* 1989; 256:E453–E458.

Chapter 103

The Heart and Connective Tissue Disease

Bernadine P. Healy, M.D., ■ *Robert C. Schlant, M.D.* ■
Emilio B. Gonzalez, M.D.

The collagen vascular, or connective tissue, diseases represent a subset of the arthritides and rheumatic disorders. These disorders are systemic in nature, commonly linked by a diffuse abnormality of vasculature, and characterized by idiopathic, inflammatory lesions. Notably affected are joints, muscles, and connective tissue linings such as pleura and pericardium, and their inflammation accounts for the major symptoms. Serious morbidity and mortality, however, are most often linked to involvement of the kidneys, brain, and heart. Specific connective tissue diseases that may have major cardiac involvement include systemic lupus erythematosus, polyarteritis nodosa, giant-cell arteritis, rheumatoid arthritis, ankylosing spondylitis, polymyositis/dermatomyositis and progressive systemic sclerosis (Table 103-1). Their etiology remains uncertain. As their pathogenesis unveils, different causes become apparent, making their linkage under the common name of *collagen vascular* or *rheumatic disease* less appropriate.

SYSTEMIC LUPUS ERYTHEMATOSUS

Systemic lupus erythematosus (SLE) is one of the more common of the rheumatic diseases; it tends to affect women more than men and occurs most frequently in the second and third decades of life. A genetic predisposition to SLE has been suggested. Of unknown etiology, SLE is a form of hypersensitivity or autoimmune disorder. The sterile inflammatory process of SLE involves multiple organ systems and in particular, skin, joints, kidneys, brain, heart, and virtually all serous membranes. Systemic lupus erythematosus may present clinically in a variety of forms reflecting the target organ involved. Fevers, arthritis and arthralgias, skin rashes, and pleuritis are among the most common early signs of this condition. The immunologic abnormalities of SLE have been well characterized and enable it to be recognized despite the multiplicity and, frequently, the complexity of clinical presentations. Elevated serum gamma globulin concentrations and cryoproteins are common findings. The majority of patients have, at some point in the course of their illness, positive antinuclear antibodies (ANA). Less specific are anticytoplasmic antibodies, anticardiolipin (IgG-aCL) antibodies, antiphospholipid (aPL) antibodies, and rheumatoid factor, which are frequently identified. Serum complement is decreased in the majority of patients with SLE, and, insofar as serum complement is usually normal or elevated in other connective tissue disorders, such as rheumatoid arthritis, polyarteritis nodosa, scleroderma, and disseminated infections, this serologic test may be useful in diagnosis of SLE.[1,2] Certain patients with SLE are more likely to have elevated levels of antiphospholipid (aPL) antibodies, particularly those with recurrent venous thrombosis, thrombocytopenia, recurrent fetal loss, hemolytic anemia, livedo reticularis, leg ulcers, arterial occlusions, transverse myelitis, or pulmonary hypertension.[3] An increased prevalence of cardiac abnormalities has been reported in SLE patients with increased antiphospholipid or anticardiolipin antibody titers.[3–6]

TABLE 103-1
Primary Cardiac Manifestations of the Connective Tissue Diseases*

Disease	Pericardium	Myocardium	Endocardium (Valves)	Coronary Arteries
Systemic lupus erythematosus	++	+	++	+/−
Progressive systemic sclerosis	+	++	0	++
Polyarteritis nodosa	+/−	+	0	++
Ankylosing spondylitis	0	+/−	++	0
Rheumatoid arthritis	++	+	+	0
Polymyositis/dermatomyositis	++	++	+/−	+/−

*++ = major site of involvement; + = may be involved, but less frequently; +/− = rarely involved; 0 = not involved.

Lupus may run an acute, fulminating course, but most often is characterized by a chronic course marked with exacerbations and remissions, and the 10-year survival rate is reported in excess of 80 percent. When patients die of SLE, it is most often in the setting of acute renal failure, central nervous system disease, associated infection, or coronary artery disease (see below).

Primary Cardiac Involvement

Studies of patients with SLE have shown that a significant proportion have cardiac abnormalities.[1,2,4,7–27] In one prospective study of 74 patients with SLE, seven patients (9 percent) had typical Libman-Sacks verrucae and 6 (8 percent) had thickened, functionally impaired valves.[17] In addition to valvular thickening, or vegetations ("masses"), and mitral or aortic valvular regurgitation (or, occasionally, stenosis), there may be pericardial thickening or effusion, left ventricular regional or global systolic or diastolic dysfunction, or evidence of pulmonary hypertension.[28,29] Either valvular regurgitation or stenosis due to SLE can require valve replacement.[30] In most reports, cardiac abnormalities appear to be significantly more frequent in patients with elevated titers of anticardiolipin antibodies.[4,31–33] However, one study of valve disease in SLE did not find an increased frequency of valve disease in patients with aPL antibodies.[34]

Pericarditis

Systemic lupus erythematosus may cause a pancarditis with abnormalities of pericardium, endocardium, myocardium, and coronary arteries. Pericardial involvement is the most frequent of these, as observed clinically, by echocardiography, or at autopsy.[35,36] Clinical studies have described pericardial effusions at some point in the clinical course of over half of patients with active SLE, and an "idiopathic" benign pericarditis may antecede the other clinical signs of lupus in up to 4 percent of patients.[35] In the majority of SLE patients, the pericardial involvement is clinically silent and, if manifest, runs a benign course. On rare occasions lupus pericarditis may lead to pericardial constriction,[35,37] and acute cardiac tamponade.[38] Serological studies of pericardial fluid may be useful in diagnosis of lupus pericardial effusions, although in most instances the size of the pericardial effusion is not sufficiently large to allow aspiration.

A diffuse fibrofibrinous pericarditis is most typically associated with SLE. The pericardial fluid contains some mononuclear white cells, and occasionally LE cells. In patients with long-standing lupus who have been successfully treated with anti-inflammatory agents, pericarditis appears to occur with the same frequency, but at autopsy, the lesion is less extensive and more likely to be a healed fibrous, as opposed to a more active fibrinous, pericarditis.[36] Lupus erythematosus patients with pericarditis, particularly those who are debilitated by their systemic disease and renal failure and who additionally are immunosuppressed, are at increased risk for purulent pericarditis.[39] This is the most malignant and life-threatening consequence of the pericardial lesion.

Endocarditis and Valve Disease

The cardiovascular lesion of systemic lupus erythematosus that has received the most attention is the "atypical veruccous endocarditis" first described by Libman and Sacks in 1924,[40] long before lupus was recognized as a systemic disease. The lesions, as they were first described and subsequently attributed to systemic lupus erythematosus,[41] are fibrofibrinous, sterile vegetations which may develop on both surfaces of any of the four cardiac valves, but with a preponderance for the left-sided valves, particularly the undersurface of the mitral valve (Fig. 103-1). These *verrucae* are similar to those of nonbacterial thrombotic endocarditis (NBTE) or *marantic endocarditis,* the valve lesion that may occur in patients with debilitating illness or malignancies, particularly of the stomach or pancreas. The Libman-Sacks lesions may differ from marantic endocarditis in that focal necrosis of valve leaflets and mononuclear infiltrates may also be present. At times, hematoxylin bodies, which are believed to be a histological counterpart to the LE cells, may be identified within the lesions. While valvular vegetations in SLE (Libman-Sacks vegetations) are usually clinically silent, they can fragment and produce systemic emboli, and they can also become infected, producing infective endocarditis. Since the presence of vegetations are usually not apparent clinically except by echocardiography, it is prudent to recommend antibiotic prophylaxis against bacterial endocarditis (Chap. 94) when patients with SLE undergo procedures that may be associated with bacteremia. Echocardiographically, SLE has a characteristic appearance, with leaflet thickening

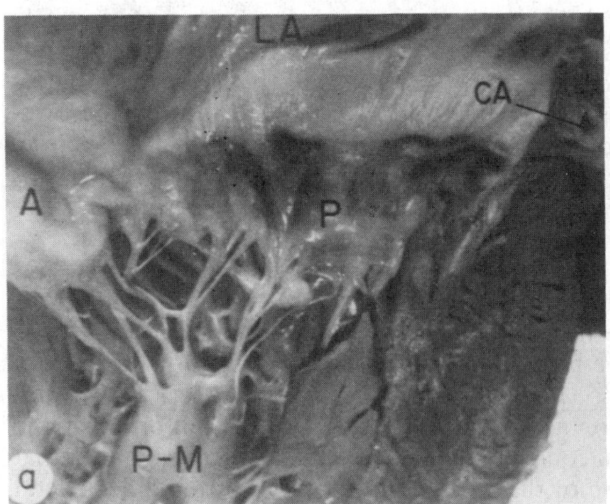

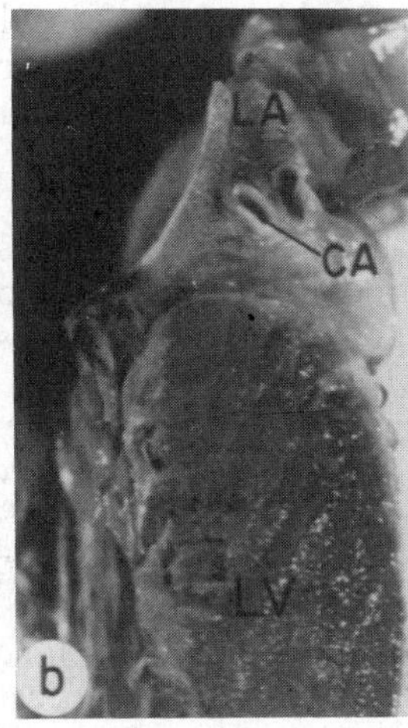

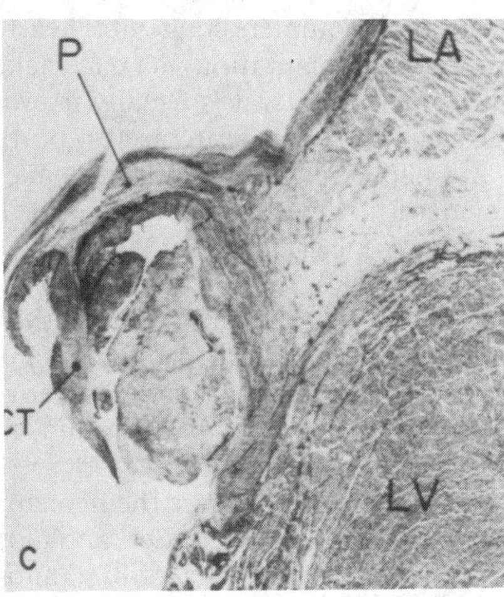

FIGURE 103-1 Shown is an example of Libman-Sacks endocarditis, which may occur in systemic lupus erythematosus. *A* and *B*. The left atrium (LA) and left ventricle (LV) are open. *B* and *C*. Fibrofibrinous "verrucae," present on the undersurface of the posterior leaflet (P) of the mitral valve, are often clinically silent. A, anterior leaflet of mitral valve; CA, left circumflex coronary artery; P-M, postero-medial papillary muscle; CT, chorda tendineae. H&E, ×8. *(From Bulkley BH, Roberts WC: The heart in systemic lupus erythematosus and the changes induced in it by corticosteroid therapy. Am J Med 1975; 58:243. Reproduced with permission from the publisher and author.)*

and valve masses.[34] The end-stage, or healed, form of the verrucous endocarditis of SLE is a fibrous plaque. In some instances, if the thrombotic lesions are extensive enough, their healing may be accompanied by focal scarring and deformity of the underlying valve tissue. It is probable that this healed, end-stage form of SLE endocarditis is most likely to lead to valvular dysfunction, and in particular to mitral or aortic regurgitation.[42–44] As with the pericardial disease, the verrucous endocardial lesions of SLE pose an increased risk of infective endocarditis, particularly in the immunosuppressed patient.

Myocarditis

Myocarditis is an uncommon cardiac manifestation of systemic lupus erythematosus with a prevalence of about 10 percent. Focal interstitial and perivascular mononuclear cell infiltrates associated with small areas of cell necrosis and replacement fibrosis may be observed at autopsy. Although a flagrant myocarditis with ventricular arrhythmias, heart block, and heart failure may occur, this is distinctly uncommon.

Several studies have suggested, however, that a subclincial cardiomyopathy may occur in association with SLE. Hemodynamic and echocardiographic studies have shown abnormalities in both systolic and diastolic function.[37] In many cases it is difficult to differentiate subtle abnormalities in cardiac function due primarily to an autoimmune attack on the myocardium from those due to the effect of systemic hypertension, coronary artery disease, or coexisting pericarditis.

Coronary Artery Disease

Acute myocardial infarction from coronary arteritis leading to death has been reported early in the course of SLE, particularly in young females. Studies of hearts in patients dying from SLE have demonstrated a high incidence of coronary atherosclerosis in patients who received treatment with corticosteroids for more than 2 to 3 years.[36,45,46] In one study of patients who had SLE for more than 2 to 3 years, death was more likely to be due to myocardial infarction than to SLE.[45] The exact mechanism(s) to explain this type of accelerated coronary atherosclerosis in lupus is unclear. It has been speculated that SLE may induce an underlying vasculopathy or arteritis that may facilitate premature atherogenesis from long-term corticosteroid treatment. In one study the presence of elevated antiphospholipid antibodies in patients with SLE correlated with left ventricular (global or segmental) dysfunction, verrucous valvular (aortic or mitral) thickening, global valvular (mitral or aortic) thickening and dysfunction, as well as mitral regurgitation and aortic regurgitation. Antiphospholipid antibodies are known to promote platelet aggregation[47] and to be associated with the presence of a clotting tendency, the so-called "lupus anticoagulant syndrome."[33] Abnormalities of the small intramural vessels of the heart include focal fibrinoid necrosis and thromboembolic occlusion, but are rarely associated with myocardial necrosis or fibrosis. Arteritis of the sinus node artery in association with scarring of both sinus and atrioventricular nodes has been reported[48] and may account for some of the rhythm and conduction disturbances seen in these patients.

Pregnancy and the Neonatal Lupus Syndrome

Neonatal lupus erythematosus is a rare syndrome that arises when the so-called anti-Ro (SSA) autoantibodies, mostly IgG, are formed and circulate in the pregnant patient, cross the placenta, and cause a lupus-like syndrome in the newborn with the appearance of a skin rash and transient cytopenias from passively acquired maternal autoantibodies. Since the half-life of IgG antibodies is approximately 21 to 25 days, the neonatal lupus syndrome in the baby is self-limiting and usually resolves in 3 to 6 months once all the IgG-containing anti-Ro maternal autoantibodies are gradually cleared by and from the neonate's circulation. An unfortunate exception is complete congenital heart block, which may require the implantation of a pacemaker. Once complete heart block occurs, it is usually irreversible. Second-degree heart block has been rarely reported as a component of the neonatal lupus syndrome, and one neonate has been described with first-degree heart block at birth that resolved 6 months later. Of interest, antibodies to the Ro (SSA) ribonucleoprotein complexes are present in over 85 percent of sera from mothers of infants with complete congenital heart block. In many patients, antibodies reactive to the La (SSB) antigen as well as the U1RNP protein particle are found in association with anti-Ro (SSA) antibodies.[49]

In the majority of cases the neonatal lupus syndrome is a relatively benign disorder, and most babies of mothers with anti-Ro (SSA)-La (SSB) or anti-U1RNP antibodies do not develop neonatal lupus. A pregnant woman with SLE with positive anti-Ro, anti-La, or anti-RNP antibodies has a risk of less than 3 percent of having a child with neonatal lupus and congenital heart block. On the other hand, the risk that this patient might have an infant with the neonatal lupus syndrome but without congenital heart block may be as high as 1 in 3. Interestingly, the neonatal lupus syndrome mediated by the presence of maternal anti-Ro antibodies can occur in children of mothers who do not have overt SLE; who may or may not meet criteria for a diagnosis of SLE; and who may or may not have a positive test for antinuclear antibodies.

The neonatal lupus syndrome with congenital heart block can be diagnosed by the appearance of fetal bradycardia around the 23d week of gestation. It is thought that the cardiac damage with conduction abnormalities in the neonate results from binding of the passively transferred pathogenic anti-Ro antibodies to Ro (SSA)/La (SSB) antigens present in the fetal heart. Whether or not these IgG anti-Ro antibodies represent "clinical markers" only and whether or not they are pathogenic is not known.[49] Of interest, all mothers of neonates with complete congenital heart block have been HLA-DR3 positive. If the mother is HLA-DR3 positive and has circulating IgG anti-Ro antibodies, the neonate is at risk regardless of its HLA-DR status.

Other cardiac abnormalities reported in the neonatal lupus syndrome include right bundle branch block, second-degree AV block, 2:1 AV block, patent ductus, arteriosus, patent foramen ovale, coarctation of the aorta, tetralogy of Fallot, atrial septal defect, hypoplastic right ventricle, ventricular septal defect, dysplastic pulmonic valve, mitral and tricuspid regurgitation, pericarditis, and myocarditis. In one study of idiopathic congenital complete heart block, accompanying heart disease occurred in one-third of patients and only two patients reached the age of 50 years without the need for a pacemaker.[50] In this study most pacemakers were inserted between the ages of 10 and 49 years.

Pregnant women with SLE should have a serum anti-Ro (SSA) antibody determination as early in pregnancy as possible. Prenatal treatment of established congenital heart block has consisted of the administration of prednisone or dexamethasone and plasmapheresis from week 23 on, although heart block has persisted in most cases. It is unclear whether or not aggressive anti-inflammatory therapy in an effort to diminish the generalized fetal insult and to lower the titers of circulating anti-Ro (SSA) antibodies makes a difference in fetal cardiac outcome. Fetal echocardiography is useful to follow the progression of the disease and also to help identify the presence of associated dysfunction in the fetal heart (decreased contractility, an increase in cardiac size, perhaps the presence of tricuspid regurgitation, pericardial effusions).

As noted, neither dexamethasone nor plasmapheresis have had much success in reversing intrauterine third-degree heart block. On the other hand, corticosteroids may be helpful to suppress an associated inflammatory response present in the form of pleuropericardial effusions or ascites in the fetus. Close monitoring of the clinical course in the prospective mother is also essential because of the risk of exacerbation of the SLE. If fetal bradycardia is present, an "intrauterine therapeutic approach" for as long as possible is recommended to allow for fetal maturation to occur. Ultrasound images may be useful to assess the degree of cardiac dysfunction if this is present. Following delivery, the neonatologist should be prepared to have a cardiac pacemaker implanted. Otherwise, all the other clinical and laboratory features of the neonatal lupus syndrome (with the exception of complete heart block and/or similar severe cardiac fetal disease, such as fibrosis from myocarditis) should slowly and gradually disappear over the first few months of the baby's life.

Women with lupus who are anti-Ro positive should be closely monitored during pregnancy as should mothers of babies previously born with congenital complete heart block. Pregnant patients who are Ro positive and whose babies have not had fetal bradycardia throughout most of the pregnancy should be reminded that congenital complete heart block is rare, and that the neonatal cutaneous lupus syndrome is benign and transient.

In adult patients with SLE, a significantly higher prevalence of myocarditis and conduction defects is found than in those who are anti-Ro negative or in healthy controls.[51] In general, myocarditis and conduction defects are reasonably common in adults with SLE and are associated with positive anti-Ro antibodies.

Secondary Effects of Systemic Lupus Erythematosus on the Heart

Many, if not most, of the clinically significant cardiac problems occurring in patients with SLE are secondary occurrences. Systemic hypertension, which is common in patients with SLE, particularly those with renal disease and long-standing steroid therapy, is the major cause of cardiac enlargement and heart failure. Severe pulmonary hypertension may occur in up to 14 percent of patients with SLE.[28,29] Uremic pericarditis may occur in patients with severe renal failure and be difficult to distinguish clinically from lupus erythematosus pericarditis.

Therapy

Therapy of cardiovascular lupus erythematosus is the therapy of the underlying disease and includes nonsteroidal anti-inflammatory drugs such as indocin, corticosteroids, and, in severe cases, cytotoxic agents such as azathioprine and cyclophosphamide. Systemic arterial hypertension, congestive heart failure, and arrhythmias should be treated with standard therapeutic measures. Lupus erythematosus valvulitis can require valve replacement[30,43,44]; and, rarely, pericardial effusions require pericardiocentesis.

POLYARTERITIS NODOSA

Polyarteritis nodosa is another disease entity of unknown cause that falls within the "collagen vascular" or connective tissue disorder spectrum. It is characterized by segmental necrotizing inflammation of the medium- to small-sized arteries throughout the body, resulting in disease and dysfunction of multiple organ systems. Commonly involved by polyarteritis are the skin, kidneys, gastrointestinal tract, spleen and lymph nodes, central nervous and musculoskeletal systems, and heart. Although the erythrocyte sedimentation rate and serum gamma globulins may be elevated in polyarteritis, and occasionally rheumatoid factor and antinuclear antibodies may be present, the final clinical diagnosis rests on the combination of multisystem disease and biopsy evidence of active arteritis.[52,53]

As inflammatory necrotizing arteritis may occur in a variety of disorders generally believed to fall outside the disease category of polyarteritis nodosa, other causes and types of arteritis are generally excluded before the diagnosis of polyarteritis nodosa is made. Specifically excluded and classed as separate entities are granulomatous or giant-cell arteritis, hypersensitivity angiitis, temporal arteritis, and arteritis involving the aorta and its major branches. Also, arteritis associated with other connective tissue disorders, when the latter are the major clinical disease form, is not recognized as representing polyarteritis nodosa.[53]

Cardiac Involvement in Polyarteritis Nodosa

The heart, and specifically the coronary arteries, is a frequent target of polyarteritis nodosa. Seen most commonly is a vasculitis of the distal extramural and subepicardial coronary arteries just as they penetrate the myocardium (Fig. 103-2). The lesions are characterized by inflammatory infiltration of media and adventitia. More advanced lesions show necrosis and inflammation of the full thickness of the vessel wall including the intima, with prominent involvement of the surrounding perivascular connective tissue (Fig. 103-2). More advanced lesions are frequently associated with thrombosis and focal aneurysmal dilatation due to the vascular necrosis. The latter is responsible for the nodular appearance of the arteries deemed characteristic of this disorder. A later stage of the vasculitic process is evident as the lesions heal, first showing the formation of granulation tissue and subsequently fibrous tissue replacement of the original components of the artery. In this healing phase, intimal proliferation leading to coronary artery luminal narrowing is evident.[54,55]

The coronary arterial disease of polyarteritis nodosa, not surprisingly, may lead to myocardial infarction. In keeping with the predominantly distal and intramural coronary involvement, the myocardial necrosis and subsequent replacement fibrosis tend to be focal and patchy throughout the left ventricle. This is in contrast to the large areas of grossly visible, regional, subendocardial, or transmural necrosis typically seen in the myocardial infarction caused by coronary atherosclerosis involving the extramural arteries.

Conduction system abnormalities have been identified in the hearts of patients with polyarteritis nodosa.[56,57] James and Birk[56] have pointed out that the size and location of the sinoatrial (SA) node and atrioventricular (AV) node arteries make them prime targets for polyarteritis. The perivascular inflammation of these vessels is more likely to lead to myocardial dysfunction, as the AV and SA node tissue closely surrounds these vessels and is included in the perivascular inflammatory reaction. Atrial and ventricular conduction disturbances may be a primary manifestation of polyarteritis, despite minimal involvement of vessels elsewhere in the heart.

Other cardiac abnormalities that may be seen in patients with polyarteritis nodosa are those that are likely secondary to the underlying systemic hypertension and renal disease. Cardiomegaly and left ventricular hypertrophy most often represent secondary cardiac manifestations of this disease. Similarly, pericarditis may develop in a patient with polyarteritis, but mostly in association with renal disease.

A new autoantibody identified in the serum of patients with systemic vasculitis, including Wegener's granulomatosis and polyarteritis nodosa, is the antineutrophil cytoplasmic antibody, or ANCA.[58] The ANCA test recognizes antibodies to azurophilic granules present in the cytoplasm of neutrophils. The antigen against which ANCA is directed is a 29 kDa serine proteinase. Approximately 90 percent of patients with Wegener's granulomatosis have positive so-called c-ANCA antibodies, the "c" describing the cytoplasmic staining observed under fluorescent microscopy. In contrast, most other vasculitides, including polyarteritis nodosa, tend to have a positive so-called p-ANCA antibody, the "p" describing the perinuclear staining observed in the immunofluorescent assay.

The antigen responsible for the p-ANCA antibody detection appears to be a myeloperoxidase. The detection of serum ANCA levels is a useful laboratory diagnostic marker in the evaluation of the systemic vasculitides. It is controversial whether or not the detection of a positive serum ANCA level obviates the need for a biopsy or angiogram. Serum ANCA levels may decline with appropriate steroid or cytotoxic therapy although this is not invariable. Rarely, positive ANCA antibodies, especially p-ANCA serum levels may be seen in inflammatory bowel diseases, such as Crohn's enteritis, Kawasaki's vasculitis, and tuberculosis.

Clinical Manifestations of Cardiac Disease in Polyarteritis

Despite the dramatic involvement of coronary arteries that may accompany polyarteritis nodosa, the most frequent cardiovascular abnormalities seen in patients with this disease are unrelated to the coronary arteries *per*

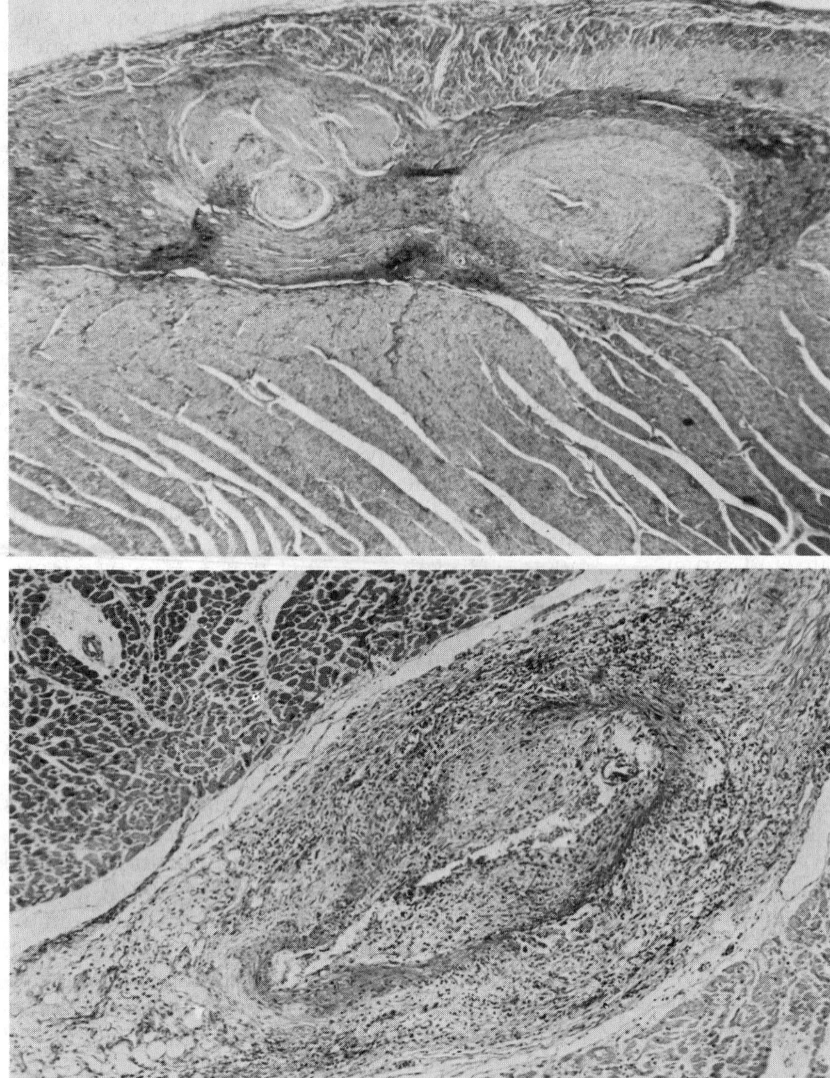

FIGURE 103-2 Polyarteritis nodosa. Examples of the necrotizing vasculitis affecting the extramural and intramural coronary arteries in polyarteritis. *Top.* Extramural coronary arteries. *Bottom.* Intramural coronary arteries. The intramural artery shows a necrotizing arteritis with inflammation involving the full thickness of the vessel. H&E, *top,* ×7; *bottom,* ×22.

se. Systemic hypertension occurs in approximately 90 percent of patients, and this in combination with chronic renal failure is the most likely cause of the congestive heart failure that may develop in up to 60 percent of patients with this disease.[52,53] Patients with polyarteritis nodosa may also develop acute myocardial infarction, which poses the diagnostic question of whether the myocardial injury is due to coronary arteritis with secondary thrombosis or to atherosclerosis, in a population which is typically middle-aged, male, steroid-treated, and susceptible to atherosclerotic coronary disease as well.

Therapy

Polyarteritis nodosa carries a generally poor prognosis, especially when hypertension and renal disease are present. Treatment of the heart disease in polyarteritis nodosa is directed at the specific cardiac dysfunction, and corticosteroid and other anti-inflammatory agents are administered for the underlying disease.[59] Corticosteroids are still the mainstay of therapy, although they may aggravate coexisting hypertension and even atherosclerosis. The use of anticoagulant therapy remains controversial.[52]

RHEUMATOID ARTHRITIS

Rheumatoid arthritis is characterized by its deforming erosion of the joints resulting from chronic synovial inflammation and proliferation. The most common of the connective tissue diseases, it tends to affect women twice as often as men and may run in families. Joint symptoms dominate its course, and symmetrical involvement of the hands and wrists is most common. Other joints of the upper and lower extremities and the temporomandibular and sternoclavicular joints may also be affected. More common systemic manifestations of rheumatoid arthritis include fevers, weight loss, anemia, subcutaneous rheumatoid nodules, and lymphadenopathy. Less frequently, pleuritis and a diffuse, necrotizing vasculitis may occur.

Pericardial Involvement in Rheumatoid Arthritis

Cardiac involvement is most uncommon in rheumatoid arthritis, but when it occurs, it may take a variety of forms. A diffuse, nonspecific fibrofibrinous pericarditis has been described in roughly 30 percent of patients with rheumatoid arthritis.[60] The pericarditis may be clinically silent in the majority of these patients, being overshadowed by pleuritis or joint pain. Its clinical course tends to be benign, but as in most instances of pericardial inflammation, sizable effusions may require pericardiocentesis, and pericardial constriction may necessitate pericardiectomy.[61] Chronic, symptomatic pericarditis in and of itself may require a course of corticosteroid therapy.

Myocardial and Endocardial Involvement in Rheumatoid Arthritis

Rarely rheumatoid nodules may focally infiltrate the heart, including the myocardium and the four cardiac valves (Fig. 103-3).[62,63] These nodules may lead to no symptoms, but if extensive enough, or strategically located, they may produce cardiac compromise. Rheumatoid nodules developing within the valve leaflets may result in mild valvular regurgitation; if the nodule becomes necrotic, perforation of the leaflet may occur and lead to severe valvular regurgitation.[63] The incidence of such valvular infiltration has been estimated at 1 to 2 percent from autopsy studies. Although distinctly uncommon, arrhythmias and conduction disturbances, including complete heart block,[62] and congestive heart failure may also result from rheumatoid myocarditis.

Therapy

As most of the cardiac lesions of rheumatoid arthritis are clinically silent, it not known whether or not the specific therapies used in rheumatoid arthritis, including salicylates, nonsteroidal anti-inflammatory agents, penicillamine, gold, and corticosteroids, are effective therapy for treating cardiac involvement. Conventional treatment of pericarditis, arrhythmias, and conduction disturbances that may occur in patients with rheumatic arthritis is utilized when these disorders produce clinical symptoms.

ANKYLOSING SPONDYLITIS

Ankylosing spondylitis, also called rheumatoid spondylitis, is now recognized as an entity related to, but distinct from, rheumatoid arthritis. Ankylosing spondylitis is

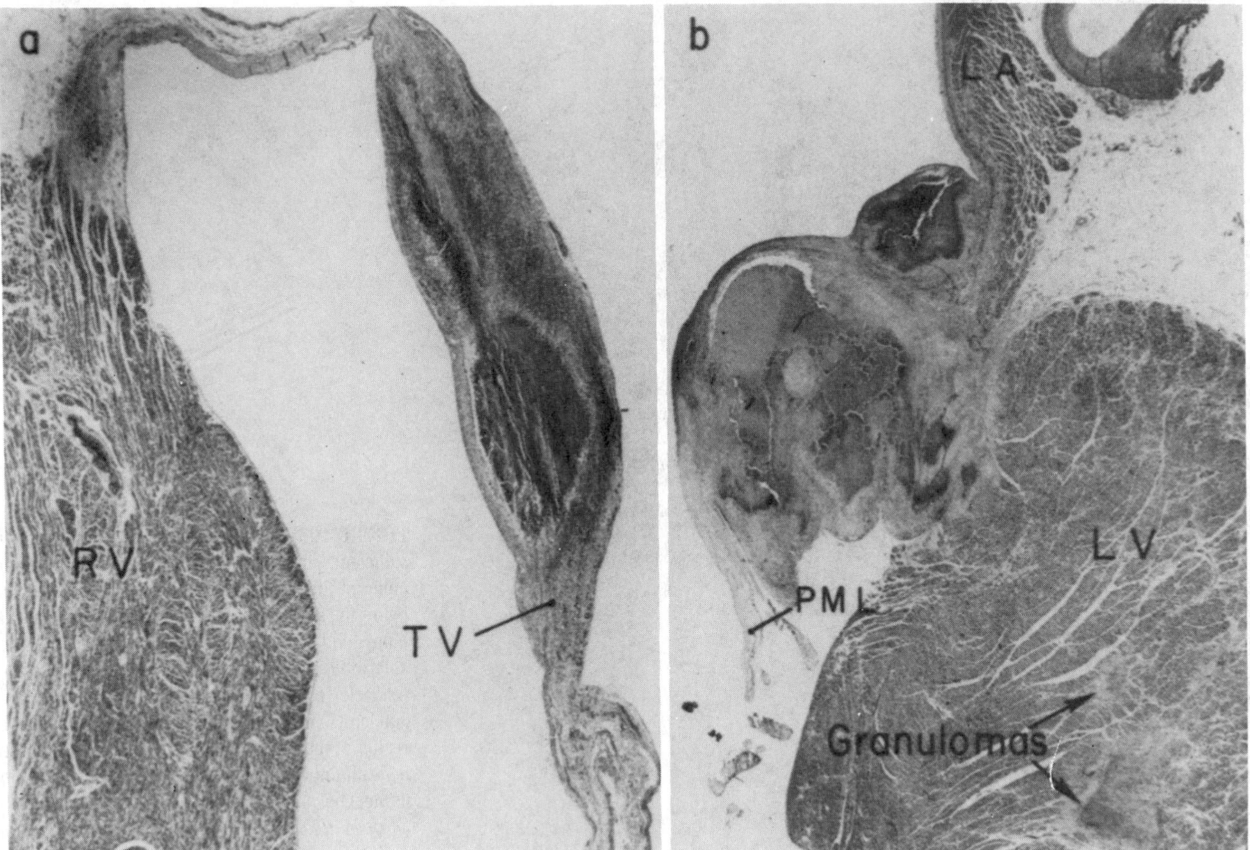

FIGURE 103-3 Rheumatoid arthritis. *A.* A tricuspid valve (TV) infiltrated by rheumatoid nodules. *B.* A mitral valve infiltrated by rheumatoid nodules. In addition, granulomas are present within the left ventricular (LV) wall. LA, left atrium; PML, posterior mitral leaflet; RV, right ventricle. *(A)* H&E, ×12; *(B)* H&E, ×6.5. *(From Roberts WC, Dangel JC, Bulkley BH: Nonrheumatic valvular cardiac disease: clinicopathologic survey of 27 different conditions causing valvular dysfunction. Cardiovasc Clin 1973; 5:333. Reproduced with permission from the publisher and author.)*

characterized by a progressive inflammatory lesion of the spine, leading to chronic back pain, deforming dorsal kyphosis, and, in its advanced stage, fusion of the costovertebral and sacroiliac joints with immobilization of the spine. This condition mainly affects men, generally first occurring early in life, but with a chronic progressive course of 20 to 30 years.[64] Identification of the HLA-B27 histocompatibility antigen in nearly all patients with ankylosing spondylitis has confirmed its genetic occurrence and also its relationship to other connective tissue states with a high prevalence of this antigen, such as Reiter's syndrome and juvenile arthritis.

The Heart in Ankylosing Spondylitis

Cardiovascular disease in ankylosing spondylitis takes the form of a sclerosing inflammatory lesion generally limited to the aortic root area. The inflammatory process, which extends immediately above and below the aortic valve, typically causes aortic regurgitation.[65,66] As the inflammatory process extends below the aortic valve, it may infiltrate the basal portion of the mitral valve (which is contiguous with the aortic valve) and cause mitral regurgitation.[67] Extension of the inflammatory lesion into the top of the ventricular septum, immediately below the aortic valve, accounts for the associated conduction disturbances (Fig. 103-4). Ventricular diastolic dysfunction may also occur.[68]

The major clinical manifestation of ankylosing spondylitis is aortic regurgitation, which may occur in up to 10 percent of patients with this condition, but mostly becomes manifest in the later years of the illness. For example, among patients with signs of spondylitis for 10 years, only 2 percent have clinical evidence of aortic regurgitation; by 30 years that number increases fivefold.[65]

Conditions that may be related to ankylosing spondylitis, including Reiter's syndrome and psoriatic arthropathy, can also develop an aortic root inflammatory lesion similar to ankylosing spondylitis.[69,70]

Therapy

Drug therapy for ankylosing spondylitis is primarily directed at relief of the pain and discomfort of back pain by salicylate or other anti-inflammatory agents, such as indomethacin and phenylbutazone. Corticosteroids are generally not used in this condition except when iritis occurs. The inflammatory lesion of the heart generally runs a clinically silent course until aortic regurgitation develops, and by that time an inflammatory component to the condition is not prominent. Accordingly, clinical evidence of cardiac involvement of ankylosing spondylitis is not an indication for corticosteroid therapy. Heart failure and conduction disturbances are managed conventionally. Not infrequently, however, the aortic regur-

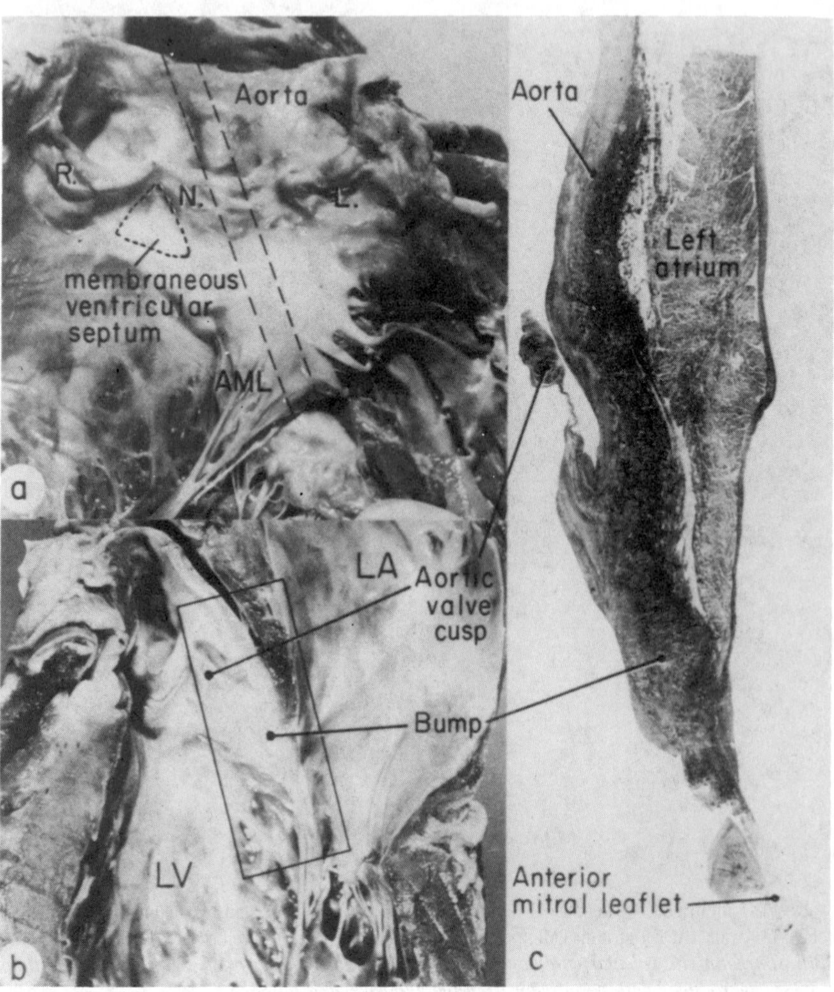

FIGURE 103-4 Ankylosing spondylitis. Aortic insufficiency, in this condition, results from the thickening of the aortic root. *A.* Immediately above and below the aortic valve. *B, C.* Leading to a subvalvular bump, and thickening of the base of aortic valve and anterior leaflet of mitral valve. *A.* The opened left ventricle (LV) with the right (R), noncoronary (N), and left (L) aortic valve cusps grossly thickened. The region of the membranous ventricular septum lying beneath the valve is the site of AV nodal conduction tissue. Phosphotungstic acid-hematoxylin stain, × 3. *(From Bulkley BH, Roberts WC: Ankylosing spondylitis and aortic regurgitation: description of the characteristic cardiovascular lesion from study of eight necropsy patients. Circulation 1973; 48:1014. Reproduced with permission from the American Heart Association, Inc. and the author.)*

gitation of ankylosing spondylitis may become severe enough to warrant aortic valve replacement,[65] and patients with aortic regurgitation should be monitored closely. (See also Chap. 79.)

PROGRESSIVE SYSTEMIC SCLEROSIS

Progressive systemic sclerosis (PSS) was first identified over two centuries ago and characterized by virtue of its striking skin manifestations; hence the name *scleroderma*. The systemic nature of this disease, and in particular its ability to affect the heart, became apparent much later. In 1943, Soma Weiss and coworkers[70] described a pattern in the cardiac dysfunction of nine patients with scleroderma and correlated these changes with abnormalities in the heart at autopsy in two patients. Moreover, they recognized that the cardiac disease was a manifestation of an underlying primary vascular disorder, or collagen vascular disease.

As we recognize scleroderma today, progressive systemic sclerosis is characterized by fibrous thickening of the skin and fibrous and degenerative alterations of the fingers, and of certain target organs, particularly the esophagus, small and large bowels, kidneys, lung, and heart. Central to this degenerative process are diffuse vascular lesions. Functionally, the vascular disorder is characterized by Raynaud's phenomenon, which is a prominent feature of scleroderma; Raynaud's disease of the digits is present in almost all patients with PSS and is the first clinical symptom in the majority. Structurally, the vascular lesions show intimal proliferation and adventitial scarring of small- and medium-sized vessels, including arterioles. The underlying pathophysiology of scleroderma that links structure and function is a Raynaud's phenomenon of visceral vasculature that leads to focal vascular lesions and parenchymal necrosis and fibrosis. This concept is supported by findings in the heart, as well as in the lungs and kidneys.[71-73] The underlying cause of the vascular disease PSS and the role of the immune system in the pathophysiology of scleroderma remain unclear. It has been suggested that PSS may be related to increased activity of endothelial cells, mast cells, and fibroblasts, perhaps under the influence of immigrant cells, such as the T cells, the macrophage, and the platelet.[74]

Like most connective tissue diseases, PSS may have variable clinical expression. Some patients may have predominantly skin involvement; others have minimal skin abnormalities but severe visceral disease which may therefore evade diagnosis.[75] The CREST (calcinosis, Raynaud's phenomenon, exophageal abnormality, sclerodactylia, telangiectasia) syndrome is one scleroderma variant that can manifest relatively mild skin changes limited to face and fingers, but severe lung disease with a primary pulmonary hypertension picture.[76] "Overlap syndromes" are seen when a patient with typical features of PSS also demonstrates features of systemic lupus erythematosus or rheumatoid arthritis. Although scleroderma may run a long and benign course, malignant renal, lung, or cardiac disease can occur with rapid deterioration and death at a young age.

The Cardiovascular System and PSS

Cardiovascular disease in patients with PSS is either due to a primary involvement of the heart by the sclerosing disease or secondary to disease of the kidney or lungs. In approaching PSS patients with cardiovascular disease, one must first make this distinction.

Primary PSS of the Heart

When the heart is involved directly by scleroderma, a myocardial fibrosis occurs. The fibrosis bears no direct relationship to large- or small-vessel occlusions or other anatomic abnormalities. The fibrosis tends to be patchy, involving all levels of the myocardium unpredictably, and the right ventricle as often as the left. Focal patchy myocardial cell necrosis may also be evident, and at autopsy over three-quarters of patients with myocardial PSS had foci of necrosis.[72,77] The myocardial necrosis associated with patent vasculature suggests strongly that the myocardial fibrosis of PSS does not occur *de novo*, but rather develops as most scars do, as the end-stage repair after tissue necrosis.[72,78] The type of necrosis evident in the heart of scleroderma patients is myofibrillar degeneration, or contraction band necrosis (Fig. 103-5). This lesion may develop if myocardium is subjected to transient occlusion with reperfusion—as would occur with vascular spasm. (It may also be induced experimentally by exposing myocardium to high doses of catecholamine.) Thus, the morphological characteristics of the myocardial lesion of primary cardiac PSS are consistent with a Raynaud's phenomenon of the heart. There is evidence that a Raynaud's phenomenon of the pulmonary arterioles may be responsible for the "primary" pulmonary hypertension-type lesion that may occur in PSS, and also that the kidneys in PSS can manifest Raynaud's-type phenomena. The concurrence of renal Raynaud's phenomenon when digital Raynaud's phenomenon was induced by cold water immersion in some patients with scleroderma was demonstrated by Cannon et al.[73] Thus, it is likely that the major visceral manifestations of PSS as seen in the heart, lungs, and kidney relate to the vascular spasm so evident and readily detectable in the digits; the necrosis and scarring of the fingertips that occur as a result of the reactivity also develop in the viscera similarly afflicted. Why the small vessels are hyperreactive and in spasm is not known, but a neurogenic component and defective endothelial-dependent vasodilatation are likely involved.

With regard to the heart *per se* the cause of the myocardial necrosis and fibrosis that develops in the setting of patent extramural and intramural vessels is not yet fully established. That the myocardial disease relates in part to immunologic abnormalities or to primary and unrestrained fibrous tissue proliferation remains a possibility. The growing body of evidence to date, however, suggests that the vascular system—and particularly the smaller arteries and arterioles—is the primary target organ of progressive systemic sclerosis, and that the cardiac sclerosis of scleroderma may be a consequence of focal intermittent and progressive ischemic injury.

As mentioned above, morphological study suggested a myocardial Raynaud's phenomenon because of the structural nature of the myocardial cell injury. Subse-

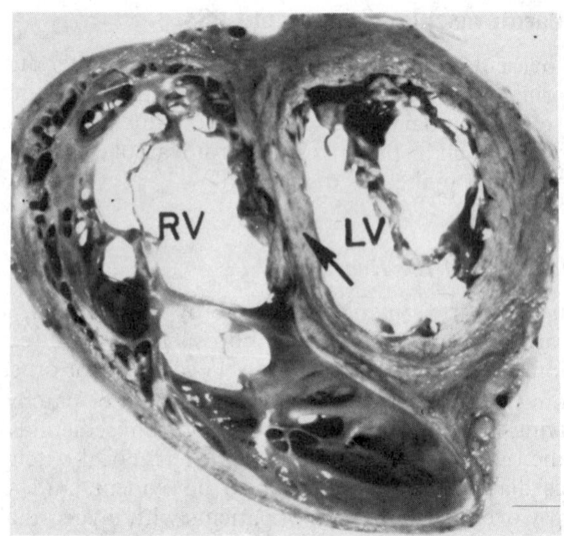

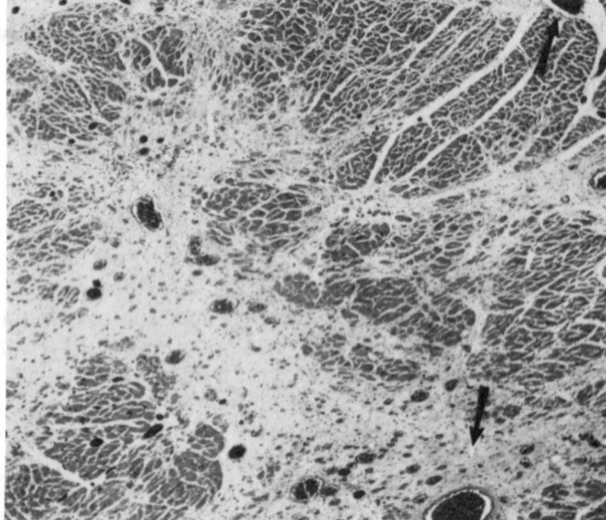

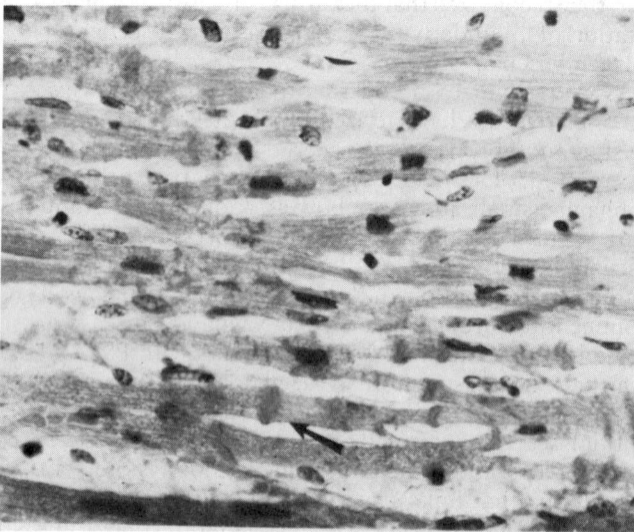

FIGURE 103-5 Progressive systemic sclerosis. *Top.* Cross section through the dilated right (RV) and left (LV) ventricle of a patient with cardiac PSS. Marked fibrous scarring of both ventricles is especially evident in the interventricular septum (arrow). *Bottom.* Photomicrograph of myocardium showing replacement fibrosis with patent intramural coronary arteries (arrows). *Bottom (right).* Higher-power magnification showing contraction-band necrosis of many fibers surrounding the areas of scar. H&E, ×45 and ×60. *(From Bulkley BH: Progressive systemic sclerosis: cardiac involvement. Clin Rheum Dis 1979; 5:131. Reproduced with permission from the publisher and author.)*

quently, several functional studies have suggested that microvascular spasm occurs in patients with cardiac scleroderma. Transient perfusion defects identified by ^{201}Tl-radionuclide imaging in the setting of patent coronary arteries have been indentified in patients with progressive systemic sclerosis and symptomatic cardiac disease, for example.[79] Other investigators have demonstrated reversible cold-induced myocardial perfusion defects, as well as cold-induced acute and reversible left ventricular dysfunction, in patients with scleroderma.[80,81] Decreased coronary reserve has also been reported in patients with widely patent coronary arteries.[82]

Clinical Manifestations of the PSS Myocardial Lesion

The clinical features of myocardial PSS include biventricular congestive heart failure, atrial and ventricular arrhythmias, myocardial infarction, angina pectoris, and sudden cardiac death.[78,83] These clinical manifestations reflect the underlying conditions of myocardial necrosis and fibrosis and may at times mimic ischemic heart disease due to coronary atherosclerosis. If the myocardial injury is extensive enough, leading to dilated hypodynamic ventricles, a syndrome resembling idiopathic dilated cardiomyopathy (Chap. 89) may be simulated.

The true incidence of the primary myocardial lesion of PSS is not known, and the extent to which clinical cardiac dysfunction reflects the typical myocardial lesion is not always apparent. Autopsy studies have suggested that up to 50 percent of patients with PSS have some evidence of increased scar tissue, and that up to 30 percent of patients have extensive lesions in their hearts.[78,84] Some clinical cardiac abnormality, including symptoms of heart failure or abnormal rhythm with conduction disturbances, may occur in 30 to 40 percent of patients with PSS, and in roughly one-half of them the cardiac disorder is due to primary myocardial scleroderma. Among those patients with severe morphologic myocardial involvement, clinically manifest cardiac disease is evident in close to 90 percent.[78]

Pericardial and Endocardial Disease

Pericarditis may occur in 20 percent or more of patients with PSS. Although in as many as two-thirds of patients with pericarditis the pericarditis is due to renal failure, there are some who develop a fibrofibrinous or fibrous pericarditis for which no other apparent cause is evident. Exudative pericardial effusions may accompany scleroderma pericarditis and have been reported to be as large as 1000 ml.[70] Rarely, constrictive pericarditis may result from the pericardial sclerosis.

Scleroderma is virtually unique among the connective tissue disorders in that it rarely, if ever, affects cardiac valves. Although mild, focal, nonspecific thickening of valve tissue has been described, no characteristic or consistent valve lesion has been recognized, either clinically or at autopsy.

Secondary Cardiovascular Disease in PSS

Since scleroderma most frequently manifests itself as renal and pulmonary parenchymal disease with pulmonary and systemic hypertension, cardiovascular disease secondary to these is common. Left vetricular hypertrophy and congestive heart failure may be associated with long-standing systemic hypertension and renal disease. Uremic pericarditis may occur. Cor pulmonale with marked right ventricular hypertrophy and right-sided heart failure may result from long-standing severe pulmonary scleroderma.

Pulmonary Hypertensive Disease of PSS

Although the pulmonary fibrosis of scleroderma had been known for years, the recognition of a "primary" pulmonary hypertensive lesion independent of parenchymal disease came later. Patients with this primary pulmonary vascular lesion tend to develop rapidly progressive dyspnea and right-sided congestive heart failure in the setting of clear lungs. Pulmonary pressures reach the systemic level and are refractory to treatment. Morphologically the pulmonary arterial lesions show the range of advanced alterations (medial and intimal hyperplasia, plexiform lesions, and necrotizing arteritis) seen in Eisenmenger syndromes and idiopathic primary pulmonary hypertension. Arterial vasospasm is believed to be a major component of "primary" pulmonary hypertension, and the association is supported by angiographic studies. On occasion vasodilators such as tolazoline may induce partial lowering of pressure, but the fixed pulmonary lesions and focal thrombotic occlusions that virtually always accompany the advanced stages of this condition make restoration of normal pressures unlikely. It is of interest that Raynaud's phenomenon of the digits accompanies idiopathic primary pulmonary hypertension in about one-third of patients,[85] suggesting that vascular hyperreactivity may be a common link between this idiopathic lung disease and scleroderma. (See Chap. 99.)

Although severe pulmonary hypertension is a less common manifestation of scleroderma, it is one that carries the gravest of prognoses. Sudden unexpected death is common in these patients, and hypotension and death may occur precipitously in the setting of what would appear to be relatively benign procedures such as pericardiocentesis or cardiac catheterization.

Treatment of PSS Cardiovascular Disease

There is no uniformly effective therapy for PSS cardiovascular disease.[44] Treatment consists of standard therapy for congestive heart failure and arrhythmias as they present. Nifedipine may improve myocardial perfusion abnormalities as well as systemic and pulmonary hemodynamics in patients with pulmonary hypertension due to PSS.[86,87] Nifedipine may also improve Raynaud's events involving the fingers. Captopril has also been shown to improve myocardial perfusion.[88,89] Other agents of potential therapeutic value for PSS cardiac disease include D-penicillamine and corticosteroids, but none has proved efficacy for either the systemic disease or its cardiac manifestations.

POLYMYOSITIS/DERMATOMYOSITIS

These idiopathic autoimmune inflammatory myopathies are rare in the United States with an estimated annual incidence of about 5 to 10 new patients per million. The clinical features include a typical heliotrope rash in dermatomyositis, with periorbital edema and the proximal muscle weakness present in both polymyositis (PM) and dermatomyositis (DM). Polymyositis is basically the same disease except for the absence of a skin rash.[90] Typical laboratory findings include an elevated serum creatine phosphokinase (CPK) level and elevation of other muscle enzymes such as a serum aldolase reflecting the presence of muscle breakdown from the inflammatory process. The so-called anti-Jo-1 antibody, which is detectable in the serum of some patients wth PM/DM, has been correlated with inflammatory arthritis, interstitial lung disease, and excess mortality, mostly due to respiratory failure. In PM/DM, typical changes in the electromyogram (EMG) include short-wave potentials, low-amplitude polyphasic units, and increased spontaneous activity with muscle fibrillation. A positive skeletal muscle biopsy of a proximal muscle such as the deltoid is often confirmatory.[91] In addition to skeletal muscle involvement, cardiac abnormalities may be present in up to 40 percent and include atrioventricular conduction defects, tachyarrhythmias, pericarditis with effusion, and a dilated, poorly contracting left ventricle. A type of myocarditis leading to congestive heart failure has been found in autopsy studies.[92] Rarely, coronary arteritis has been reported in polymyositis/dermatomyositis (PM/DM). Therefore, the evaluation of a middle-aged man with PM/DM who presents with chest pain, or even classic angina with an elevated serum CPK, may become a diagnostic challenge. In addition to coronary artery atherosclerosis, the differential diagnosis includes inflammatory myocarditis and coronary arteritis. Of significance, an increase in the MB-CPK may be "buried" in the marked elevation of CPK. If coronary angiography is suggestive of coronary vasculitis rather than typical atheromatous plaques, oral high-dose prednisone, 40 to 60 mg daily, is appropriate. This is also the usual initial therapeutic approach to patients with PM/DM even when no cardiac involvement is apparent.

There are no adequate large-scale, prospective, controlled clinical studies available comparing the efficacy of corticosteroid treatment with other immunosuppressive agents such as azathioprine (Imuran) and cyclophosphamide (Cytoxan).[92] At present, most rheumatologists, following an adequate initial trial of corticosteroid therapy with PM/DM, and in the face of suboptimal to no therapeutic response, institute treatment with methotrexate, azathioprine (Imuran), and cyclophosphamide (Cytoxan) in that order. The response to steroids in PM/DM is unpredictable, at best: some patients do exceedingly well on oral prednisone therapy while others are intractable to all agents. A subset of patients with PM/DM who have the so-called inclusion body myositis (IBM) are particularly intractable to anti-inflammatory treatment. This is also true for those patients who have a rare autoantibody called the anti-signal-recognition-particle antibody, or anti-SRP. Because some patients with PM/DM significantly benefit from an initial trial of high-dose oral or intravenous corticosteroid therapy, this therapy is usually used first. Preliminary trials with intravenous immunoglobulin (IVIG) appear promising in the treatment of PM/DM.

GIANT-CELL (CRANIAL, TEMPORAL, GRANULOMATOUS) ARTERITIS

Temporal arteritis is a systemic inflammatory vasculitis of unknown etiology that primarily involves extracranial vessels, especially branches of the external carotid artery, but can involve almost any artery in the body as well as some veins. Giant-cell arteritis (GCA) occurs almost exclusively in patients over 55 years of age. Common presenting symptoms include headaches, scalp tenderness, jaw claudication, visual disturbances including blindness, diplopia, weight loss, anemia, and, in about 50 percent of patients, musculoskeletal symptoms attributable to polymyalgia rheumatica, or PMR. Uncommon presentation of GCA include fever of unknown origin, chest pain from aortitis or myocardial infarction, aortic aneurysm,[93] coma, peripheral gangrene, peripheral neuropathies and large vessel involvement with limb claudication, aortic regurgitation, or stroke. Typical physical findings include tenderness of the temporal or occipital arteries, nodulations of the artery, a pulseless artery, and a tender scalp.

Most GCA patients have a greatly elevated Westergren erythrocyte sedimentation rate; however, a normal sedimentation rate has been rarely documented. The only specific diagnostic test is a temporal artery biopsy that demonstrates granulomatous arterial inflammation with disruption of the internal elastica lamina. Giant cells need not be present. Unfortunately, the positive yield for GCA in unilateral temporal artery biopsies is no greater than 60 percent, and a contralateral biopsy may be necessary.

Since the occurrence of "skip" lesions in histologic samples is well-known in GCA, a 3- to 4-cm section of artery should be examined. Angiography is generally not helpful in diagnosis or in selecting a biopsy site. High-dose prednisone therapy, 40 to 60 mg daily, is indicated to prevent blindness or to suppress inflammation in the presence of systemic involvement.

CHURG-STRAUSS SYNDROME

The Churg-Strauss syndrome, or allergic granulomatosis and angiitis, may be associated with left ventricular dilatation and a reduced ejection fraction, as well as mitral regurgitation, which may require valve replacement.[94] Left ventricular systolic function may improve significantly with corticosteroid therapy.[95]

ANTIPHOSPHOLIPID ANTIBODY SYNDROME

The antiphospholipid antibody syndrome (APS) has been defined by the presence of antiphospholipid (aPL) antibody or lupus anticoagulant, usually in high titer, and any or all of the following clinical events: recurrent arterial or venous thromboses, recurrent fetal losses, and thrombocytopenia.[96–101] Livedo reticularis is also frequently present. Clinically, the terms "anticardiolipin syndrome," "antiphospholipid syndrome," and "lupus anticoagulant syndrome" may usually be considered to be equivalent, although some individuals may have one antibody but not the other.[101] SLE is frequently present. Therapies to prevent fetal loss include aspirin, heparin, or high doses of prednisone, alone or in combination.[102]

There is an increased incidence of aortic or mitral regurgitation with the "primary" antiphospholipid syndrome,[97,103–107] as well as in patients with SLE who have aPL antibodies.[4,17,32,97,107–110] APS is frequently manifest by spontaneous small- and large-vessel arterial thrombosis in the cerebral and ocular circulations.[101,112–116] (See also Chap. 122.) There are no controlled trials of therapy to prevent arterial occlusion. Therapy has often included aspirin, warfarin, heparin, or corticosteroids.[112,115] One recent study found that an anticardiolipin antibody level was a risk factor for deep venous thrombosis or pulmonary embolus but not for ischemic stroke in healthy men.[116]

REFERENCES

1. Harvey AM, Shulman LE, Tumulty PA, Conley CL, Schoenrich EH: Systemic lupus erythematosus: A review of the literature and clinical analysis of 138 cases. *Medicine* 1954; 33:291–437.
2. Dubois EL: *Lupus Erythematosus: A Review of the Current Status of Discoid and Systemic Lupus Erythematosus and Their Variants,* 2d ed. New York, McGraw-Hill, 1974.
3. Alarcon-Segovia D, Deleze M, Oria CV, Sanchez-Guerrero J, Gomez-Pacheco L, Cabiedes J, et al: Antiphospholipid antibodies and the antiphospholipid syndrome in systemic lupus erythematosus: A prospective analysis of 500 consecutive patients. *Medicine* 1989; 68:353–365.
4. Nihoyannopoulos P, Gomez PM, Joshi J, Loizou S, Walport MJ, Oakley CM: Cardiac abnormalities in systemic lupus erythematosus: Association with raised anticardiolipin antibodies. *Circulation* 1990; 82:369–375.
5. O'Rourke RA: Antiphospholipid antibodies. A marker of lupus carditis? *Circulation* 1990; 82:636–638.
6. Khamashta MA, Cervera R, Asherson RA, Font J, Gil A, Coltart DJ, et al: Association of antibodies against phospholipids with heart valve disease in systemic lupus erythematosus. *Lancet* 1990; 335:1541–1544.
7. Brigden W, Bywaters EGL, Lessof MH, Ross IP: The heart in systemic lupus erythematosus. *Br Heart J* 1960; 22:1–16.
8. Chang RW: Cardiac manifestations of systemic lupus erythematosus. *Clin Rheum Dis* 1981; 8:197–206.
9. Bulkley BH, Roberts WC: Systemic lupus erythematosus as a cause of severe mitral regurgitation. *Am J Cardiol* 1975; 35:305–308.
10. Ansari A, Larson PH, Bates HD: Cardiovascular manifestations

of systemic lupus erythematosus. *Prog Cardiovasc Dis* 1985; 27:421–434.

11. Elkayam U, Weiss S, Lainado S: Pericardial effusion and mitral valve involvement in systemic lupus erythematosus: Echocardiographic study. *Am Rheum Dis* 1977; 36:349–353.
12. Doherty NE, Siegel RJ: Cardiovascular manifestations of systemic lupus erythematosus. *Am Heart J* 1985; 110:1257–1265.
13. Martinez-Costa X, Ordi J, Barbera J, Selva A, Bosch J, Vilardell M: High grade atrioventricular heart block in 2 adults with systemic lupus erythematosus. *J Rheumatol* 1991; 18:1926–1928.
14. Klinkhoff AV, Thompson CR, Reid GD, Tomlinson CW: M-mode and two-dimensional echocardiographic abnormalities in systemic lupus erythematosus. *JAMA* 1985; 253:3273–3277.
15. Mandell BF: Cardiovascular involvement in systemic lupus erythematosus. *Semin Arthritis Rheum* 1987; 17:126–141.
16. Doherty NE, Feldman G, Maurer G, Siegel RJ: Echocardiographic findings in systemic lupus erythematosus. *Am J Cardiol* 1988; 61:1144.
17. Galve E, Candell-Riera J, Pigrau C, Permanyer-Miralda G, Garcia-del-Castillo H, Soler-Soler J: Prevalence, morphologic types, and evolution of cardiac valvular disease in systemic lupus erythematosus. *N Engl J Med* 1988; 319:817–823.
18. Straaton KV, Chatham WW, Reveille JD, Koopman WJ, Smith SH: Clinically significant valvular heart disease in systemic lupus erythematosus. *Am J Med* 1988; 85:645–650.
19. Leung WH, Wong KL, Lau C-P, Wong C-K, Cheng C-H, Tai Y-T: Doppler echocardiographic evaluation of left ventricular diastolic function in patients with systemic lupus erythematosus. *Am Heart J* 1990; 120:82–87.
20. Leung WH, Wong KL, Lau CP, Wong C-K, Cheng C-H: Cardiac abnormalities in systemic lupus erythematosus: A prospective M-mode, cross-sectional and Doppler echocardiographic study. *Int J Cardiol* 1990; 27:367–375.
21. Crozier IG, Li E, Milne MJ, Nicholls MG: Cardiac involvement in systemic lupus erythematosus detected by echocardiography. *Am J Cardiol* 1990; 65:1145–1148.
22. Cujec B, Sibley J, Haga M: Cardiac abnormalities in patients with systemic lupus erythematosus. *Can J Cardiol* 1991; 7:343–349.
23. Enomoto K, Kaji Y, Mayumi T, Tusda Y, Kanaya S, Nagasawa K, et al: Frequency of valvular regurgitation by color Doppler echocardiography in systemic lupus erythematosus. *Am J Cardiol* 1991; 67:209–211.
24. Cervera R, Font J, Pare C, Azqueta M, Perez-Villa F, Lopez-Soto A, et al: Cardiac disease in systemic lupus erythematosus: Prospective study of 70 patients. *Ann Rheum Dis* 1992; 51:156–159.
25. Sturfelt G, Eskilsson J, Nived O, Truedsson L, Valind S: Cardiovascular disease in systemic lupus erythematosus: A study of 75 patients from a defined population. *Medicine* 1992; 71:216–223.
26. Sasson Z, Rasooly Y, Chow CW, Marshall S, Urowitz MB: Impairment of left ventricular diastolic function in systemic lupus erythematosus. *Am J Cardiol* 1992; 69:1629–1634.
27. Ong ML, Veerapen K, Chambers JB, Lim MN, Manivasagar M, Wang F: Cardiac abnormalities in systemic lupus erythematosus: Prevalence and relationship to disease activity. *Int J Cardiol* 1992; 34:69–74.
28. Asherson RA, Oakley CM: Pulmonary hypertension in SLE. *J Rheumatol* 1986; 13:1–5.
29. Asherson RA, Hingbottam TW, Xuan ATD, Khamashta MA, Hughes GRV: Pulmonary hypertension in a lupus clinic; experience with twenty four patients. *J Rheumatol* 1990; 17:1292–1298.
30. Alameddine AK, Schoen FJ, Yanagi H, Couper GS, Collins JJ Jr, Cohn LH: Aortic or mitral valve replacement in systemic lupus erythematosus. *Am J Cardiol* 1992; 70:955–956.
31. Ford PM, Ford SE, Lillicrap DP: Association of lupus anticoagulant with severe valvular heart disease in systemic lupus erythematosus. *J Rheumatol* 1988; 1:597–600.
32. Chartash EK, Lans DM, Paget SA, Qamar T, Lockshin MD: Aortic insufficiency and mitral regurgitation in patients with systemic lupus erythematosus and the antiphospholipid syndrome. *Am J Med* 1989; 86:407–412.
33. Leung WH, Wong KL, Lau C-P, Wong C-K, Liu HW: Association between antiphospholipid antibodies and cardiac abnormalities in patients with systemic lupus erythematosus. *Am J Med* 1990; 89:411–419.
34. Roldan CA, Shively BK, Lau CC, Gurule FT, Smith EA, Crawford MH: Systemic lupus erythematosus valve disease by transesophageal echocardiography and the role of antiphospholipid antibodies. *J Am Coll Cardiol* 1992; 20:1127–1134.
35. Hejtmancik MR, Wright JC, Quint R, Jennings FL: The cardiovascular manifestations of systemic lupus erythematosus. *Am Heart J* 1964; 119:119–130.
36. Bulkley BH, Roberts WC: The heart in systemic lupus erythematosus and the changes induced in it by corticosteroid therapy. A study of 36 necropsy patients. *Am J Med* 1975; 58:243–264.
37. Doherty NE, Siegel RJ: Cardiovascular manifestations of systemic lupus erythematosus. *Am Heart J* 1985; 110:1257–1265.
38. Ansari A, Larson PH, Bates HD: Cardiovascular manifestations of systemic lupus erythematosus: Current perspective. *Prog Cardiovasc Dis* 1985; 27:421–434.
39. Klacsmann PG, Bulkley BH, Hutchins GM: The changed spectrum of purulent pericarditis: An 86 year autopsy experience in 200 patients. *Am J Med* 1977; 63:666–673.
40. Libman E, Sacks B: A hitherto undescribed form of valvular and mural endocarditis. *Arch Intern Med* 1924; 33:701–737.
41. Gross L: The cardiac lesion in Libman-Sacks disease with a consideration of its relationship to acute diffuse lupus erythematosus. *Am J Pathol* 1940; 16:375–407.
42. Bulkley BH, Roberts WC: Systemic lupus erythematosus as a cause of severe mitral regurgitation: A new problem in an old disease. *Am J Cardiol* 1975; 35:305–338.
43. Paget SA, Bulkley BH, Grauer LE, Seningen R: Mitral valve disease of systemic lupus erythematosus: A cause of severe congestive heart failure reversed by valve replacement. *Am J Med* 1975; 59:134–139.
44. Seningen RP, Borer JS, Redwood DR, Bulkley BH, Paget SA: Libman-Sacks endocardoma: Diagnosis during life with radiographic, fluoroscopic and angiocardiographic findings. *Radiology* 1974; 113:597–598.
45. Urowitz MB, Bookman AAM, Koehler BE, Gordon DA, Smythe HA, Ogryzlo MA: The bimodal mortality pattern of systemic lupus erythematosus. *Am J Med* 1976; 60:221–225.
46. Petri M, Spence D, Bone LR, Hochberg MC: Coronary artery disease risk factors in the Johns Hopkins lupus cohort: Prevalence, recognition by patients, and preventive practices. *Medicine* 1992; 71:291–302.
47. Escolar G, Font J, Reverter JC, Lopez-Soto A, Garrido M, Cervera R, et al: Plasma from systemic lupus erythematosus patients with antiphospholipid antibodies promotes platelet aggregation: Studies in a perfusion system. *Arterioscl Thromb* 1992; 12:196–200.
48. James TN, Rupe CE, Monto RW: Pathology of the cardiac conduction system in systemic lupus erythematosus. *Ann Intern Med* 1965; 63:402–410.
49. Buyon JP, Winchester R: Congenital complete heart block: A human model of passively acquired autoimmune injury. *Arthritis Rheum* 1990; 33:609–614.
50. Reid JM, Coleman EN, Doig W: Complete congenital heart block. Report of 35 cases. *Br Heart J* 1982; 48:236.
51. Logar D, Kveder T, Rozman B, Dobovisek J: Possible association between anti-Ro antibodies and myocarditis or cardiac conduction defects in adults with systemic lupus erythematosus. *Ann Rheum Dis* 1990; 49:627–629.
52. Przybojewski JZ: Polyarteritis nodosa in the adult: Report of a case with repeated myocardial infarction and a review of cardiac involvement. *S Afr Med J* 1981; 60:512–518.
53. Alarcon-Segovia D: The necrotizing vasculitides: A new pathogenetic classification. *Sym Rheum Dis* 1977; 61:241–260.
54. Holsinger DR, Osmundson PJ, Edwards JE: The heart in periarteritis nodosa. *Circulation* 1962; 25:610–618.
55. Schrader ML, Hochman JS, Bulkley BH: The heart in polyarteritis nodosa: A clinicopathologic study. *Am Heart J* 1985; 109:1353–1359.
56. James TN, Birk RE: Pathology of the cardiac conduction system in polyarteritis nodosa. *Arch Intern Med* 1966; 117:561–567.
57. Thiene G, Valente M, Rossi L: Involvement of the cardiac conducting system in panarteritis nodosa. *Am Heart J* 1978; 95:716–724.
58. Charles LA, Jennette JC, Falk RJ: The role of HL60 cells in the detection of antineutrophil cytoplasmic autoantibodies. *J Rheum* 1991; 18:491–494.
59. Fauci AS, Haynes BF, Katz P: The spectrum of vasculitis: Clinical, pathologic, immunologic and therapeutic considerations. *Ann Intern Med* 1978; 89:660–676.

60. Bacon PA, Gibson DG: Cardiac involvement in rheumatoid arthritis: An echocardiographic study. *Ann Rheum Dis* 1974; 33:20–24.
61. Liss JP, Bachmann WT: Rheumatoid constrictive pericarditis treated by pericardiectomy: Report of a case and review of the literature. *Arthritis Rheum* 1970; 13:869–876.
62. Ahern M, Lever JV, Cosh J: Complete heart block in rheumatoid arthritis. *Ann Rheum Dis* 1983; 42:389–397.
63. Roberts WC, Dangel JC, Bulkley BH: Nonrheumatic valvular cardiac disease: A clinicopathologic survey of 27 different conditions causing valvular dysfunction. *Cardiovasc Clin* 1973; 5:333–446.
64. Julkunen H: Rheumatoid spondylitis—clinical and laboratory study of 149 cases compared with 182 cases of rheumatoid arthritis. *Acta Rheum Scand* 1962; 172(suppl 4):1–116.
65. Bulkley BH, Roberts WC: Ankylosing spondylitis and aortic regurgitation: Description of the characteristic cardiovascular lesion from study of eight necropsy patients. *Circulation* 1973; 48:1014–1027.
66. Kawasuji M, Hetzer R, Oelert H, Stauch G, Borst HG: Aortic valve replacement and ascending aorta replacement in ankylosing spondylitis: Report of three surgical cases and review of the literature. *Thorac Cardiovasc Surg* 1982; 30:310–314.
67. Roberts WC, Hollingsworth JF, Bulkley BH, Jaffe RB, Epstein SE, Stinson EB: Combined mitral and aortic regurgitation in ankylosing spondylitis: Angiographic and anatomic features. *Am J Med* 1974; 56:237–243.
68. Paulus HE, Pearson CM, Pitts W: Aortic insufficiency in 5 patients with Reiter's syndrome. *Am J Med* 1972; 53:461.
69. Gould BA, Turner J, Keeling DH, Hickling P, Marshall AJ: Myocardial dysfunction in ankylosing spondylitis. *Ann Rheum Dis* 1992; 51:227–232.
70. Weiss S, Stead EA, Warren JV, Bailey OT: Scleroderma heart disease: With a consideration of certain other visceral manifestations of scleroderma. *Arch Inter Med* 1943; 71:749.
71. Sackner AM, Akgun N, Kimbel P, Lewis DH: The pathophysiology of scleroderma involving the heart and respiratory system. *Ann Intern Med* 1964; 60:611.
72. Bulkley BH, Ridolfi RL, Salyer WR, Hutchins GM: Myocardial lesions of progressive systemic sclerosis: A cause of cardiac dysfunction. *Circulation* 1976; 53:483–490.
73. Cannon PJ, Hassar M, Case DB, Casarella WJ, Sommers SC, LeRoy EC: The relationship of hypertension and renal failure in scleroderma (progressive systemic sclerosis) to structural and functional abnormalities of the renal cortical circulation. *Medicine* 1974; 53:1–46.
74. Claman HN: On scleroderma: Mast cells, endothelial cells, and fibroblasts. *JAMA* 1989; 262:1206–1209.
75. Bulkley BH, Klacsmann PG, Hutchins GM: Angina pectoris, myocardial infarction and sudden death with normal coronary arteries: A clinicopathologic study of 9 patients with progressive systemic sclerosis. *Am Heart J* 1978; 95:563–569.
76. Salerni R, Rodnan GP, Leon DF, Shaver JA: Pulmonary hypertension in the CREST syndrome variant of progressive systemic sclerosis (scleroderma). *Ann Intern Med* 1977; 86:394–399.
77. Leinwand I, Duryee AW, Richter MN: Scleroderma (based on a study of over 150 cases). *Ann Intern Med* 1954; 41:1003–1041.
78. Bulkley BH: Progressive systemic sclerosis: Cardiac involvement. *Clin Rheum Dis* 1979; 5:131–149.
79. Follansbee WP, Curtiss EI, Medsger TA Jr, Steen VD, Uretsky BF, Owens GR, et al: Physiologic abnormalities of cardiac function in progressive systemic sclerosis with diffuse scleroderma. *N Engl J Med* 1984; 310:142–148.
80. Ellis WW, Baer AN, Robertson RM, Pincus T, Kronenberg MW: Left ventricular dysfunction induced by cold exposure in patients with systemic sclerosis. *Am J Med* 1986; 80:385–392.
81. Alexander EL, Firestein GS, Weiss JL, Heuser RR, Leitl G, Wagner HN Jr, et al: Reversible cold-induced abnormalities in myocardial perfusion and function in systemic sclerosis. *Ann Intern Med* 1986; 105:661–668.
82. Kahan A, Nitenberg A, Foult JM, Amor B, Menkes CJ, Devaux JY, et al: Decreased coronary reserve in primary scleroderma myocardial disease. *Arthritis Rheum* 1985; 28:637–646.
83. Smiley, JD: The many faces of scleroderma. *Am J Med Sci* 1992; 304:319–333.
84. D'Angelo WA, Fries JF, Masi AT, Shulman LE: Pathologic observations in systemic sclerosis (scleroderma): A study of fifty-eight autopsy cases and fifty-eight matched controls. *Am J Med* 1969; 46:428–440.
85. Walcott G, Burchell HB, Brown AL: Primary pulmonary hypertension. *Am J Med* 1970; 71:70–79.
86. Kahan A, Devaux JY, Amor B, Menkes CJ, Weber S, Nitenberg A, et al: Nifedipine and thallium-201 myocardial perfusion in progressive systemic sclerosis. *N Engl J Med* 1986; 314:1397–1402.
87. Alpert MA, Pressly TA, Mukerji V, Lambert CR, Mukerji B, Panayiotou H, et al: Acute and long-term effects of nifedipine on pulmonary and systemic hemodynamics in patients with pulmonary hypertension associated with diffuse systemic sclerosis, the CREST syndrome and mixed connective tissue disease. *Am J Cardiol* 1991; 68:1687–1690.
88. Kahan A, Devaux JY, Amor B, Menkes CJ, Weber S, Venot A, et al: The effect of captopril on thallium 201 myocardial perfusion in systemic sclerosis. *Clin Pharmacol Ther* 1990; 47:483–489.
89. Kazzam E, Caidahl K, Hällgren R, Gustafsson R, Waldenström A: Non-invasive evaluation of long-term cardiac effects of captopril in systemic sclerosis. *J Intern Med* 1991; 230:203–212.
90. Schwarz MI: Pulmonary and cardiac manifestations of polymyositis-dermatomyositis. *J Thorac Imaging* 1992; 7:46–54.
91. Plotz PH, Dalakas M, Leff RL, Love LA, Muller FW, Cronin ME: Current concepts in idiopathic inflammatory myopathies: Polymyositis, dermatomyositis, and related disorders. *Ann Intern Med* 1989; 111:143–157.
92. Dalakas MC: Polymyositis, dermatomyositis, and inclusion-body myositis. *N Engl J Med* 1991; 325:1487–1498.
93. Gonzalez EB, Varner WT, Lisse JR, Daniels JC, Hokanson JA: Giant-cell arteritis in the southern United States: An 11-year retrospective study from the Texas Gulf coast. *Arch Intern Med* 1989; 149:1561–1565.
94. Morgan JM, Raposo L, Gibson DG: Cardiac involvement in Churg-Strauss syndrome shown by echocardiography. *Br Heart J* 1989; 62:462–466.
95. Hasley PB, Follansbee WP, Coulehan JL: Cardiac manifestations of Churg-Strauss syndrome: Report of a case and review of the literature. *Am Heart J* 1990; 120:996–999.
96. Hughes GR: The anticardiolipin syndrome. *Clin Exp Rheumatol* 1985; 3:285–286.
97. Asherson RA, Khamashta MA, Ordi-Ros J, Derksen RH, Machin SJ, Barquinero J, et al: The primary antiphospholipid syndrome: Major clinical and serological features. *Medicine* 1989; 68:366–374.
98. Sammaritano LR, Gharavi AE, Lockshin MD: Antiphospholipid antibody syndrome: Immunologic and clinical aspects. *Semin Arthritis Rheum* 1990; 20:81–96.
99. McNeil HP, Chesterman CN, Krilis SA: Immunology and clinical importance of antiphospholipid antibodies. *Adv Immunol* 1991; 49:193–280.
100. Alarcon-Segovia D, Perez-Vasquez ME, Villa AR, Drenkard C, Cabiedes J: Preliminary classification criteria for the antiphospholipid syndrome within systemic lupus erythematosus. *Semin Arthritis Rheum* 1992; 21:275–286.
101. Lockshin MD: Antiphospholipid antibody syndrome. *JAMA* 1992; 268:1451–1453.
102. Pope JM, Canny CL, Bell DA: Cerebral ischemic events associated with endocarditis, retinal vascular disease and lupus anticoagulant. *Am J Med* 1991; 90:299-309.
103. Harris EN: Syndrome of the black swan. *Br J Rheumatol* 1987; 26:324–326.
104. Ford SE, Charrette EJP, Knight J, Pym J, Ford P: A possible role for antiphospholipid antibodies in acquired cardiac valve deformity. *J Rheumatol* 1990; 17:1499–1503.
105. Brenner B, Blumenfeld Z, Markiewicz W, Reisner SA: Cardiac involvement in patients with primary antiphospholipid syndrome. *J Am Coll Cardiol* 1991; 18:931–936.
106. Beynon HLC, Walport MJ: Antiphospholipid antibodies and cardiovascular disease. *Br Heart J* 1992; 67:281–284.
107. Galve E, Josep O, Barquinero J, Evangelista A, Vilardell M, Soler-Soler J: Valvular heart disease in the primary antiphospholipid syndrome. *Ann Intern Med* 1992; 116:293–298.
108. Anderson D, Bell D, Lodge R, Grant E: Recurrent cerebral ischemia and mitral valve vegetation in a patient with lupus anticoagulant. *J Rheumatol* 1987; 14:839–841.

109. D'Alton JG, Preston DN, Bormanis J, Green MS, Kraag GR: Multiple transient ischemic attacks, lupus anticoagulant and verrucous endocarditis. *Stroke* 1985; 16:512–514.
110. Cronin ME, Biswas R, Van der Straeton C, Fleisher TA, Klippel JH: IgG and IgM anticardiolipin antibodies in patients with lupus with cardiolipin antibody associated clinical syndromes. *J Rheumatol* 1988; 15:795–798.
111. Cowchock FS, Reece EA, Balaban D, Branch DW, Plouffe L: Repeated fetal losses associated with antiphospholipid antibodies: A collaborative randomized trial comparing prednisone to low-dose heparin treatment. *Am J Obstet Gynecol* 1992; 166:1318–1323.
112. Brey RL: Antiphospholipid antibodies and ischemic stroke. *Heart Dis Stroke* 1992; 1:379–382.
113. Antiphospholipid antibodies in stroke study group: Clinical and laboratory findings in patients with antiphospholipid antibodies and cerebral ischemia. *Stroke* 1990; 21:1268–1273.
114. Levine SR, Brey RL, Joseph CLM, Havstad S: Risk of recurrent thromboembolic events in patients with focal cerebral ischemia and antiphospholipid antibodies. *Stroke* 1992; 23(suppl):I-29–I-32.
115. Rosove MH, Brewer PMC: Antiphospholipid thrombosis: Clinical course after the first thrombotic event in 70 patients. *Ann Intern Med* 1992; 117:303–308.
116. Ginsburg KS, Liang MH, Newcomer L, Goldhaber SZ, Schur PH, Hennekens CH, et al: Anticardiolipin antibodies and the risk for ischemic stroke and venous thrombosis. *Ann Intern Med* 1992; 117:997–1002.

Chapter 104

The Heart and Obesity

James K. Alexander, M.D.

An increasing awareness of the potential for reversibility of the circulatory effects of obesity through weight reduction has been reflected by greater attention to relationships among obesity and hypertension, coronary disease, cardiomyopathy, and hypoventilation syndromes in recent years. These relations are briefly reviewed in this chapter together with some therapeutic implications and a short introduction to adipose tissue circulation.

ADIPOSE TISSUE CIRCULATION

Although adipose tissue is an active metabolic organ, oxygen delivery under resting conditions in individuals necessitates a blood flow of only 2 to 3 mL/min per 100 g as indicated by inert-gas washout techniques, or less than one-twentieth that of the brain.[1] However, passage of free fatty acids between blood and adipocytes is facilitated by a high capillary filtration coefficient, almost twice that of skeletal muscle, presumably due to increased capillary permeability.[2]

Of considerable importance is the degree to which adipose tissue serves as a blood volume reservoir and to which lipocyte metabolism is flow dependent. With hemorrhage-induced hypotension in dogs, the decrement in adipose tissue blood volume and flow is much greater than that in other organs, and adipose tissue oxygen uptake falls concomitantly.[3] In addition to metabolic demands and circulating blood volume, a variety of factors may produce profound hemodynamic alterations in the adipose tissue vascular bed, including sympathetic nervous influences, humoral agents, blood and tissue oxygen tension, blood pH, temperature, exercise, and mechanical compression.[4]

Histological studies have demonstrated "block devices" in the walls of small arteries and arterioles, with the capacity to regulate capillary blood flow.[5] Since adipose tissue blood flow is a function of both cell number and size,[6] increments in adipose depot volume secondary to either cellular hyperplasia or hypertrophy are accompanied by augmented flow. In extremely obese subjects, for example, in whom both hyperplasia and hypertrophy exist, adipose tissue flow may approximate one-half the total cardiac output at rest.[7] Weight loss in obese subjects involves reduction in adipocyte cell size but not number. Thus cardiac output falls as regression of adipocyte hypertrophy lowers total adipose tissue weight and flow,[8] although flow per kilogram adipose tissue actually increases as a result of increased adipocyte number.[9]

OBESITY AND HYPERTENSION

Epidemiologic studies clearly implicate obesity as a health hazard for hypertension, but correlation of the overall incidence of hypertension with obesity is of a low order,[10] highest in young men and black women.[11] A predominantly abdominal distribution of body fat appears to correlate better with the presence of hypertension than does relative weight or body mass,[12] and is often associated with a triad of obesity, hypertension, and hyperinsulinemia.[13] (See also Chap. 62.)

Mechanisms of hypertension with obesity differ from those of essential or renovascular hypertension, as suggested by the observations that (1) measurements of blood volume and renin levels of obese subjects do not correlate with the presence or absence of hypertension[14] and (2) systemic vascular resistance is less although cardiac output and pulse wave velocity are greater in obese than in lean hypertensive individuals.[14,15] The pathophysiology of hypertension with obesity is not yet defined. For several hypotheses advanced, involving elevated aldosterone levels, altered response to pressor agents, mechanical capillary compression in adipose depots, or elevated blood insulin levels, there is no firm supporting evidence.[16] In addition, some explanation must be found for the fact that most obese people are not hypertensive, and even with extreme obesity one-third are normotensive.[17]

Direct intraarterial pressure measurements indicate that hypertension is not artifactual in obese subjects.[17] A reasonable approximation of blood pressure level may be obtained when the degree of obesity is not extreme by utilizing a cuff containing a bladder 42 cm in length.[18] In very obese individuals with unusual arm configuration, difficulty in wearing the cuff, or inconsistent readings, direct intraarterial measurement is recommended before prolonged antihypertensive therapy is initiated.

Weight reduction, an important therapeutic consideration in obesity hypertension, brings about a decrement in blood pressure in a large percentage of such patients.[19,20] This decrement is poorly correlated with the amount of weight loss, often occurring early with a later plateau,[21,22] but may be associated with several other potentially desirable effects such as increased glucose tolerance and lesser insulin resistance,[23] reduced circulating blood volume and cardiac output, regression of myocardial hypertrophy,[24,25] and diminution of sympathetic tone.[26] If pharmacologic therapy is required for satisfactory long-term blood pressure control, use of thiazide diuretics and β-adrenergic blocking agents should probably be minimized in view of their potential for lowering high-density lipoprotein (HDL) cholesterol, reducing thermogenesis, and worsening insulin sensitivity.[27-30] (See also Chap. 77.)

OBESITY AND CORONARY HEART DISEASE

Excess mortality, largely due to cardiovascular disease, is associated with overweight greater than 30 to 40 percent above the norm.[31,32]

In men, no effect of obesity (relative weight greater than 20 percent of "ideal") can be demonstrated in early or late mortality rates after myocardial infarction.[33,34] But obese women appear to be at greater risk for early recurrence[35] and, if they are diabetic, for higher mortality.[36] Obesity does not emerge as a risk factor for sudden death due to coronary disease.[37]

Overall analysis of multidisciplinary studies does not identify obesity itself as an independent risk factor for coronary disease,[38,39] with some epidemiologic data to the contrary.[40] Recent studies suggest that the distribution of fat deposits, i.e., increased abdominal adipose tissue with augmentation in the ratio of waist to hip circumference, is a better predictor of cardiovascular disease than the degree of obesity.[12,41,42] Although weight reduction in obese subjects to "acceptable" levels for insurance purposes over the long term is associated with a decrement in cardiovascular mortality,[43,44] the effect of weight loss alone has not been delineated because alterations of established risk factors have usually taken place also. (See also Chap. 62.)

Despite extensive investigation, well-defined identification of mechanisms specific for obesity linking it to coronary disease through body somatotype, energy intake, blood lipids, serum uric acid, glucose tolerance, or hyperinsulinemia has proved elusive.[38]

Weight reduction in obese subjects commonly results in decrements of total serum cholesterol and triglycerides, but increments in HDL cholesterol are inconsistent,[45] often transient,[46] and poorly correlated with the amount of weight loss.[47,48]

Decrements in body weight greater than 20 percent may be required for symptomatic improvement in obese subjects with stable angina pectoris.[49] In obese persons with coronary disease subject to sleep apnea, serious arrhythmias may occur, disappearing on reversal of the apneic syndrome with weight loss.[50,51]

THE CARDIOMYOPATHY OF OBESITY

It is now well established that in morbidly obese individuals (i.e., body weight approximately 135 kg or more) there may develop a syndrome of chronic circulatory congestion associated with diastolic and sometimes systolic left ventricular dysfunction. Its pathological, physiological, and clinical features appear sufficiently distinctive to warrant characterization as obesity heart muscle disease or cardiomyopathy.[52]

In 1933, a roughly linear increment in heart weight with increasing body weight was demonstrated at necropsy,[53] and subsequent echocardiographic studies have established a similar relation for left ventricular mass with thickening of left ventricular septum and free wall in very obese subjects.[54] These findings are due to left ventricular hypertrophy in such persons, sometimes with accompanying right ventricular hypertrophy, and occasionally with fatty infiltration of the myocardium.[55,56]

Regional blood flow with marked obesity is characterized by a significant increase to adipose tissue, a modest increase to the splanchnic vascular bed, and little change in flow to other organs as compared to the setting of "ideal" or "average" weight.[7] This results in a high cardiac output at rest in absolute terms, directly related to the increment in body oxygen consumption,[57] but with a quasi-normal cardiac index. Circulating blood volume increases in direct proportion to cardiac output, leading to development of a central congestive circulatory state.[7,58] Thus, both left ventricular diastolic dysfunction associated with myocardial hypertrophy and increased pulmonary blood volume contribute to the evolution of pulmonary congestion. Elevated left ventricular diastolic pressure brings about pulmonary hypertension at rest or during exercise,[58-60] and in some cases a transpulmonary diastolic (pulmonary artery diastolic to wedge) pressure gradient is present, secondary to medial hypertrophy of small pulmonary arteries,[61,62] or hypoxic pulmonary vasoconstriction. (See also Chap. 99.)

Indexes of left ventricular systolic performance such as ejection fraction and velocity of circumferential fiber shortening may be normal or depressed.[63,64] The ratio of diastolic cavity radius to wall thickness is increased in patients with compromised ventricular systolic function, indicating an elevated ventricular wall tension, thought to be secondary to "inadequate" hypertrophy.[63]

Thus, two mechanisms appear to operate in the pathogenesis of recurrent bouts of circulatory congestion in patients with chronic severe exogenous obesity. In one group of patients, pulmonary and systemic vascular congestion develops as a consequence of chronic volume overload superimposed upon the effect of diminished diastolic ventricular compliance caused by ventricular hypertrophy. Left ventricular systolic performance is preserved in this group, and the symptoms and signs of pulmonary and systemic congestion are secondary to diastolic dysfunction alone. It is not unusual for patients with preserved left ventricular systolic performance to present with recurrent bouts of pulmonary and systemic congestion for many years (Fig. 104-1). In the other group, chronic volume overload and high cardiac output with or without accompanying hypertension result in a lesser degree of myocardial hypertrophy, such that the wall thickness–cavity radius ratio is reduced, ventricular wall stress is elevated, and left ventricular systolic dysfunction in superimposed. Since the clinical presentation in these two groups may be essentially the same, differentiation will usually require appraisal of left ventricular systolic function by echocardiographic, radionuclide, or angiographic techniques.

Although left ventricular function is preserved with moderate obesity,[64] limited observations suggest that the prevalence of a congestive circulatory state in extremely obese subjects is about 10 percent.[17] Body weight is usually twice the predicted norm or more, and rapid weight gain may precipitate or exacerbate congestive symptoms. Progressively increasing dyspnea and orthopnea are characteristic, whereas acute pulmonary edema is uncommon. The terminal phase is sometimes characterized by rapid weight gain due to fluid retention, with increasing somnolence, mental confusion, and coma.[61] Sudden death is common and is well documented by case reports.[65] Hypertension may or may not be present. Presystolic gallop (S_4) rhythm may be heard, but cardiac murmurs are usually absent. Frequent electrocardiographic findings include left deviation of the QRS axis in the frontal plane[66] or low-voltage right axis deviation and P pulmonale.[67] Despite gross anatomic involvement, electrocardiographic evidence of left ventricular hypertrophy is often absent.[52] Recurrent bouts of congestion predispose to the development of atrial fibrillation or flutter, in association with left atrial enlargement[52] (Fig. 104-1). Conduction defects secondary to fatty infiltration of the conduction system may be implicated in the predisposition to sudden death.[62,68]

Diuretic therapy is the most urgently indicated measure in the management of the obesity congestive state, together with judicious use of oxygen. Though cardioversion may be considered in an emergency setting, rapid ventricular rate in the presence of atrial fibrillation or flutter is usually controlled satisfactorily with digitalis administration. Early appraisal of left ventricular function by echocardiogram or radionuclide study may be helpful with regard to determining the need for an inotropic agent, as well as the potential for use of beta blockade

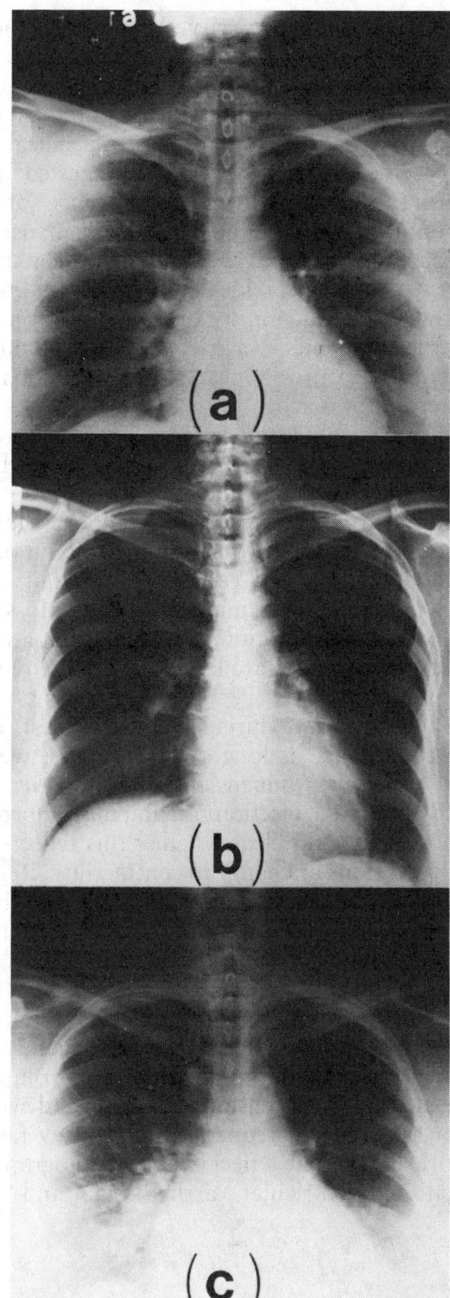

FIGURE 104-1 Chest films of a woman first presenting with severe pulmonary and systemic congestion. *A.* At age 29, weight 184 kg. *B.* At age 31, weight reduction to 157 kg was associated with decrements in heart size and pulmonary congestion. *C.* Recurrence of cardiomegaly and pulmonary congestion attended regain of weight at age 37. At age 43, weight 195 kg, echocardiogram demonstrated normal left ventricular systolic performance, with ejection fraction 64 percent, mean velocity of circumferential fiber shortening 1.36 cir/s. Left ventricular septal and posterior wall thicknesses were increased to 1.7 and 2.0 cm, respectively, and E–F slope was reduced to 30 mm/s, suggesting reduced left ventricular compliance. Left atrial dimension was enlarged to 5.2 cm. By age 48, atrial fibrillation had developed. *(From JK Alexander: The cardiomyopathy of obesity. Prog Cardiovasc Dis 27:325–334, 1985. Reproduced with permission from Grune & Stratton, Inc., and the author.)*

or calcium antagonists to control arrhythmia. Since there is no evidence of altered sodium–potassium–adenosine triphosphatase (Na-K-ATPase) activity with obesity,[69] and serum levels relate to lean body mass rather than total body weight,[70] higher digoxin dosage based on body weight may result in toxicity. Vasodilator therapy is indicated for control of severe hypertension and may be useful in the setting of left ventricular systolic dysfunction with elevated blood pressure or pulmonary hypertension. Although there are no studies specifically examining its efficacy in very obese congested subjects, considering the relatively high incidence of venous thrombophlebitis and pulmonary embolism, use of low-dose heparin prophylaxis would seem reasonable.

Achievement of near ideal weight or long-term significant weight reduction by dietary means seldom occurs in these patients. Gastric surgery in combination with dietary measures appears to be a reasonably safe and effective approach.[71–73]

Significant weight loss in subjects with marked obesity results in lowered blood pressure, reduced cardiac size, and favorable hemodynamic alterations.[8,25,59,74] Decrements in body oxygen consumption, blood volume, and cardiac output are proportional to the amount of weight loss. Blood volume and cardiac output fall approximately 30 mL and 30 mL/min per kg weight loss, respectively. Oxygen consumption, cardiac output, and stroke volume during exercise are less for the same work load after weight reduction.[69] Persistent elevation of left ventricular filling pressure during exercise suggests a decrement in compliance as long as 3 years after weight reduction.[74] Chamber dimensions fall, however, and if previously impaired, ejection fraction may improve with weight loss.[75] It is not clear whether this reflects altered loading conditions or change in contractility. Regression of hypertrophy as reflected by diminished wall thickness and left ventricular mass has been observed after weight reduction in some very obese individuals.[76]

Experimental and clinical studies indicate that marked dietary caloric restriction or fasting leads to diminished sympathetic nervous system activity, which, together with natriuresis and contraction of plasma volume, may provoke postural hypotension, dizziness, and syncope.[77] Rapid massive weight reduction induced by fasting or low-calorie diets may effect electrocardiographic QT prolongation, ventricular arrhythmia, and sudden death.[78]

SLEEP APNEA AND OBESITY HYPOVENTILATION SYNDROME

Although sleep apnea occurs in a variety of clinical settings, somewhat more than 50 percent of patients so afflicted are obese.[79] They are usually men, 40 to 60 years of age, with degrees of obesity varying from moderate to extreme. Daytime hypersomnia is frequent. Significant increases in systemic and pulmonary artery pressures occur cyclically during apnea, and with a rapid succession of apneic spells there may be a progressive rise in both.[80] Apnea may be accompanied by decrements in arterial O_2 tension to 50 mmHg or less, with moderate increases in CO_2 tension. Cardiac arrhythmias are frequent during apnea, involving sinus arrest, asystole up to 6 s, heart block, and ventricular tachycardia.[81] All of the hemodynamic and arrhythmic effects induced by sleep apnea may be reversed in some cases by tracheostomy, and when hypertension coexists, blood pressure may fall to or toward normal.[80,81]

A syndrome of hypoventilation, cyanosis, and somnolence, with resultant chronic hypoxemia, hypercapnia, respiratory acidosis, and polycythemia, occurs in about 5 percent of extremely obese persons.[17] The sequence of physiological events leading to the obesity hypoventilation syndrome may be initiated by the development of sleep apnea.[82] Transient bouts of hypoxia with apnea eventually cause blunting of the hypoxic ventilatory drive and, in conjunction with diminished chest wall compliance and increased respiratory work, a reduced ventilatory response to CO_2 as well. Chronic hypoxemia and hypercapnia stimulate pulmonary vasoconstriction, so that the effects of augmented pulmonary vascular resistance are superimposed upon the underlying hemodynamic derangements of severe obesity, namely, increased pulmonary blood volume and flow, with left atrial hypertension. Hypoventilation is reversible with weight reduction, and the attendant improvement in arterial blood gases is associated with a fall in pulmonary artery pressure and a reduction or elimination of the transpulmonary diastolic pressure gradient.[58] Several case reports document the disappearance of P pulmonale, T-wave inversion in leads V_1 to V_3 and right axis deviation after weight reduction in the electrocardiograms of obese subjects with hypoventilation syndrome.[67,83]

REFERENCES

1. Nielsen SL: Measurement of blood flow in adipose tissue from the washout of xenon-133 after atraumatic labeling. *Acta Physiol Scand* 1972; 84:187–196.
2. Oberg B, Rosell S: Sympathetic control of consecutive vascular sections in canine subcutaneous adipose tissue. *Acta Physiol Scand* 1967; 71:47–56.
3. Kovach AG, Rosell S, Sandar P, Koltay E, Kovach E, Tomka N: Blood flow, oxygen consumption and free fatty acid release in subcutaneous adipose tissue during hemorrhagic shock in control and phoenoxybenzamine-treated dogs. *Circ Res* 1970; 26:733–741.
4. Roddie IC: Circulation to skin and adipose tissue. In: *Handbook of Physiology*, sec 2, vol 3, *Peripheral Circulation*. Bethesda, MD, American Physiological Society, 1983; 306–309.
5. Curri SB, Merlen JF: Microvascular disorders of adipose tissue. *J Mal Vasc* 1986; 11:303–309.
6. DiGirolamo M, Eposito J: Adipose tissue blood flow and cellularity in the growing rabbit. *Am J Physiol* 1975; 299:107.
7. Alexander JK, Dennis EW, Smith WG, Amad KH, Duncan WC, Austin RC: Blood volume, cardiac output and distribution of systemic blood flow in extreme obesity. *Cardiovasc Res Cent Bull* 1962; 1:39–44.
8. Alexander JK, Peterson KL: Cardiovascular effects of weight reduction. *Circulation* 1972; 45:310–318.
9. Nielsen SL, Larsen O: Relationship of subcutaneous adipose tissue blood flow to thickness of subcutaneous tissue and total body fat mass. *Scan J Clin Lab Invest* 1973; 31:383–388.
10. Haynes RB: Is weight loss an effective treatment for hypertension? The evidence against. *Can J Physiol Pharmacol* 1986; 64:825–830.
11. MacMahon S, Cutlar J, Brittain E, Higgins M: Obesity and hypertension: Epidemiological and clinical issues. *Eur Heart J* 1987; (suppl B):57–70.
12. Bjorntorp P: Obesity and adipose tissue distribution as risk factors for the development of disease. A review. *Infusionstherapie* 1990; 17:24-27.
13. Black HR: The coronary artery disease paradox: The role of hyper-

insulinemia and insulin resistance and implications for therapy. *J Cardiovasc Pharmacol* 1990; 15:S26–S39.

14. Messerli FH, Christie B, DeCarvalho J, Aristimuno GC, Suarez DH, Dreslinski GR, et al: Obesity and essential hypertension: Hemodynamics, intravascular volume, sodium excretion, and plasma renin activity. *Arch Intern Med* 1981; 141:81–85.
15. Toto MJJ, Achimastos A, Asmar RG, Hughes CJ, Safar ME: Pulse wave velocity in patients with obesity and hypertension. *Am Heart J* 1986; 112:136–140.
16. Alexander JK: Blood pressure and obesity. In: Matarazzo JD, Weiss JM, Herd JA, Miller NE (eds): *Behavioral Health*. New York, Wiley, 1984: 877–886.
17. Alexander J, Amad K, Cole VW: Observations on some clinical features of extreme obesity with particular reference to cardiorespiratory effects. *Am J Med* 1962; 32:512–524.
18. Nielsen PE, Larsen B, Holstein P, Poulsen HL: Accuracy of auscultatory blood pressure measurements in hypertensive and obese subjects. *Hypertension* 1983; 5(1):122–127.
19. Rissanen A, Pietinen P, Siljamaki-Ojansuu U, Piirainen H, Reissel P: Treatment of hypertension in obese patients: Efficacy and feasibility of weight and salt reduction programs. *Acta Med Scand* 1985; 218:149–156.
20. Reisin E: Weight reduction in the management of hypertension: Epidemiologic and mechanistic evidence. *Can J Physiol Pharmacol* 1986; 64:818–824.
21. Cohen N, Flamenbaum W: Obesity and hypertension. Demonstration of a "floor effect." *Am J Med* 1986; 80:177–181.
22. Novi RF, Porta M, Lamberto M, Molinatti GM: Reductions of body weight and blood pressure in obese hypertensive patients treated by diet. A retrospective study. *Panminerva Med* 1989; 31:13–15.
23. Nobels F, vanGall L, deLeeuw I: Weight reduction with a high protein, low carbohydrate, calorie-restricted diet: Effects on blood pressure, glucose and insulin levels. *Neth J Med* 1989; 35:295–302.
24. Lavie CJ, Messerli FH: Cardiovascular adaptation to obesity and hypertension. *Chest* 1986; 90:275–279.
25. Alexander JK: Cardiac effects of weight reduction in obesity hypertension. In: F Messerli H (ed): *The Heart and Hypertension*. New York, Yorke Medical Books, 1987: 427–433.
26. Krieger DR, Landsberg L: Mechanisms in obesity-related hypertension: Role of insulin and catecholamines. *Am J Hypertens* 1988; 1:84–90.
27. Glueck CJ: Nonpharmacologic and pharmacologic alteration of high-density lipoprotein cholesterol: Therapeutic approaches to prevention of atherosclerosis. *Am Heart J* 1985; 110:1107–1115.
28. World Health Organization: Weight control in the management of hypertension. World Hypertension League. *Bull World Health Organ* 1989; 67:245–252.
29. Feher M: Antihypertensive drugs and the hypertensive diabetic patient. *J Hum Hypertens* 1990; 4:7–9.
30. Astrup AV: Obesity and diabetes as side-effects of beta-blockers. *Ugeskr-Laeger* 1990; 152:2905–2908.
31. Keys A: Overweight, obesity, coronary heart disease and mortality. *Nutr Rev* 1980; 38:297–307.
32. Sorlie P, Gordon T, Kannel WB: Body build and mortality: The Framingham Study. *JAMA* 1980; 243:1828–1831.
33. Pell S, D'Alonso C: A three-year study of myocardial infarction in a large employed population. *JAMA* 1961; 175:463–470.
34. Frank CW, Weinblatt E, Shapiro S, Sager RV: Physical inactivity as a lethal factor in myocardial infarction among men. *Circulation* 1966; 34:1022–1033.
35. Marmor A, Sobel BE, Roberts R: Factors presaging early recurrent myocardial infarction "extension." *Am J Cardiol* 1981; 48:603–610.
36. Tansey MJ, Opie LH, Kennally BM: High mortality in obese women diabetics with acute myocardial infarction. *Br Med J* 1977; 1:1624–1626.
37. Romo M, Ruosteeuoja R: Sudden coronary death: Incidence and common risk factors. *Adv Cardiol* 1978; 25:1–8.
38. Alexander JK: Obesity and coronary heart disease. In: Conner WE, Bristow JD (eds): *Coronary Heart Disease*. Philadelphia, Lippincott, 1985: 111–123.
39. Barrett-Connor EL: Obesity, atherosclerosis, and coronary artery disease. *Ann Intern Med* 1985; 103:1010.
40. Hubert AB, Feinleib M, McNamara PM, Castelli WP: Obesity as an independent risk factor for cardiovascular disease, a 26-year follow-up of participants in the Framingham Heart Study. *Circulation* 1983; 67:968–977.
41. vanGaal L: Body fat mass distribution. Influence on metabolic and atherosclerotic parameters in non–insulin dependent diabetics and obese subjects with and without impaired glucose tolerance. Influence of weight reduction. *Verh K Acad Geneeskd Bleg* 1989; 51:47–80.
42. Beykirch H, Reuter W, Hunecke I: Waist-hip and waist-thigh index in obesity especially in relation to weight reduction. *Z Gesamte Inn Med* 1989; 44:644–646.
43. Dublin LI: Relation of obesity to longevity. *N Engl J Med* 1953; 248:971–974.
44. Shephard WP, Marks HH: Life insurance looks at arteriosclerosis problem. *Minn Med* 1955; 38:736–741.
45. Marniemi J, Seppanen A, Hakala P: Long-term effects on lipid metabolism on weight reduction on lactovegetarian and mixed diet. *Int J Obes* 1990; 14:113–125.
46. Leighton RF: Management of the patient with a low HDL cholesterol. *Clin Cardiol* 1990; 13:521–532.
47. Ellis RW, Darga LL, Lucas CP: The short and long-term effects of a low-fat cholesterol-free, hypocaloric diet on serum triglyceride and cholesterol distribution in severely obese humans. *Int J Obes* 1987; 11:29–40.
48. Vermeulen A: Effects of a short-term (4 weeks) protein-sparing modified fast on plasma lipids and lipoproteins in obese women. *Ann Nutr Metab* 1990; 34:133–142.
49. Sharma B, Thadami U, Taylor SH: Cardiovascular effects of weight reduction in obese patients with angina pectoris. *Br Heart* 1974; 36:854–858.
50. Kryger M, Quesney LP, Holder D, Gloor P, MacLeod P: The sleep deprivation syndrome of the obese patient. *Am J Med* 1974; 56:531–539.
51. Shaw TRD, Carroll RJM, Craib IA: Cardiac and respiratory standstill during sleep. *Br Heart J* 1978; 40:1055–1058.
52. Alexander JK: The cardiomyopathy of obesity. *Prog Cardiovasc Dis* 1985; 27:325–334.
53. Smith HL, Willius FA: Adiposity of the heart. *Arch Intern Med* 1933; 52:911–931.
54. Lauer MS, Anderson KM, Kannel WB, Levy D: The impact of obesity on left ventricular mass and geometry. *JAMA* 1991; 266:231–236.
55. Amad KH, Brennan JC, Alexander JK: The cardiac pathology of obesity. *Circulation* 1965; 32:740–745.
56. Warnes CA, Roberts WC: The heart in massive (more than 300 pounds or 136 kilograms) obesity: Analysis of 12 patients studied at necropsy. *Am J Cardiol* 1984; 54:1087–1091.
57. White RI, Alexander JK: Body oxygen consumption and pulmonary ventilation in obese subjects. *J Appl Physiol* 1965; 20:197–201.
58. Kaltman AJ, Goldring RM: Role of circulatory congestion in the cardiorespiratory failure of obesity. *Am J Med* 1976; 60:645–653.
59. Bachman L, Freyschuss U, Hallberg D, Melcher A: Cardiovascular function in extreme obesity. *Acta Med Scand* 1973; 193:437–446.
60. Alandin-din A, Meterissian S, Lisbona R, MacLean LD, Forse RA: Assessment of cardiac function in patients who are morbidly obese. *Surgery* 1990; 108:809–818.
61. Alexander JK, Pettigrove JR: Obesity and congestive heart failure. *Geriatrics* 1967; 22:101–108.
62. James TN, Frame B, Coates EO: De subitaneis mortibus: III. Pickwickian Syndrome. *Circulation* 1973; 48:1311–1320.
63. Alexander JK, Woodard CB, Quinones MA, Gaasch WH: Heart failure from obesity. In: Mancini M, Lewis B, Cantaldo F. (eds): *Medical Complications of Obesity*. London, Academic Press, 1978.
64. Carabello BA, Gittens L: Cardiac mechanisms and function in obese normotensive persons with normal coronary arteries. *Am J Cardiol* 1987; 59:469–473.
65. MacGregor MI, Block AJ, Ball WC Jr: Serious complications and sudden death in the Pickwickian Syndrome. *Johns Hopkins Med J* 1970; 126:279–295.
66. Axelrad MA, Alexander JK: The electrocardiogram and cardiac anatomy in obesity. *Clin Res* 1965; 13:25.
67. Lillington GA, Anderson MA, Brandenburg RO: The cardiorespiratory syndrome of obesity. *Dis Chest* 1957; 32:1–20.
68. Balsaver AM, Morales AR, Whitehouse FW: Fat infiltration of myocardium as a cause of cardiac conduction defect. *Am J Cardiol* 1967; 19:261–265.

69. Beutler E, Kuhl W, Sacks P: Sodium-potassium-ATPase activity is influenced by ethnic origin and not by obesity. *N Engl J Med* 1983; 309:756–760.
70. Ewy GA, Groves BM, Ball MF, Nimmo L, Jackson B, Marcus F: Digoxin metabolism in obesity. *Circulation* 1971; 33:810–814.
71. Sugarman HJ, Baron PL, Fairman RP: Hemodynamic dysfunction in obesity hypoventilation syndrome and the effects of treatment with surgically induced weight loss. *Ann Surg* 1988; 207:604–613.
72. Benotti PN, Hollingshead J, Mascioli EA: Gastric restrictive operations for morbid obesity. *Am J Surg* 1989; 157:150–155.
73. Kral JG: Surgical treatment of obesity. *Med Clin North Am* 1989; 73:251–264.
74. Backman L, Freyschuss U, Hallberg D, Melcher A: Reversibility of cardiovascular changes in extreme obesity. *Acta Med Scand* 1979; 205:367–373.
75. Alpert MA, Terry BE, Kelly DL: Effect of weight loss on cardiac chamber size, wall thickness and left ventricular function in morbid obesity. *Am J Cardiol* 1985; 55:783–786.
76. Alpert MA, Terry BE, Kelly DL, Mukerji V: Effect of weight loss on left ventricular mass. *Circulation* 1990; 82(suppl III):750.
77. DeHaven J, Sherwin R, Hendler R, Felig P: Nitrogen and sodium balance and sympathetic-nervous system activity in obese subjects treated with a low calorie protein or mixed diet. *N Engl J Med* 1980; 302:477–482.
78. Van Itallie TB, Yang MU: Cardiac dysfunction in obese dieters: A potentially lethal complication of rapid, massive weight loss. *Am J Clin Nutr* 1984; 39:695–702.
79. Weitzman ED: The syndrome of hypersomnia and sleep-induced apnea. *Chest* 1979; 75:414–415.
80. Schroeder JS, Motta J, Guilleminault C: Hemodynamic studies in sleep apnea, In: Guilleminault C, Dement WC (eds): *Sleep Syndromes*. New York, Alan R Liss, 1978.
81. Tilkian A, Motta J, Guilleminault C: *Cardiac Arrhythmias in Sleep Apnea Syndromes*. New York, Alan R Liss, 1978.
82. Sharp JT, Barrocas M, Chokroverty S: The cardiorespiratory effects of obesity. *Clin Chest Med* 1980; 1:103–118.
83. Estes EH Jr, Sieker HO, McIntosh HD, Kelser GA: Reversible cardiopulmonary syndrome with extreme obesity. *Circulation* 1957; 16:179–187.

Chapter 105

Alcohol and Nutritional Disease

Timothy J. Regan, M.D.

HEART DISEASE IN ALCOHOLISM

Cardiomyopathy related to long-term alcohol abuse has gained renewed recognition in recent years. Alcoholism has been reported to be the most common identifiable etiologic factor, accounting for up to one-third of cases of congestive cardiomyopathy clinically[1] and 45 percent at autopsy.[2] Since the cardiovascular system may be affected by chronic alcohol abuse in a variety of ways, careful history taking is essential for patients with unexplained abnormalities related to any degree of cardiac decompensation, transient hypertension, arrhythmias, or chest pain.[3]

Clinical reports of cardiomyopathy have emphasized the problem of denial in eliciting a history of alcoholism. There is male predominance, and suggestive diagnostic aspects include a family history of chronic alcoholism, social disruption, and accident proneness. The major positive diagnostic feature is the history of ethanol ingestion in intoxicating amounts for many years, frequently marked by periods of "spree drinking." Often this information can be obtained only through persistent questioning of the patient or by communication with relatives.

That cardiac abnormalities can be present in the absence of other causes of heart disease has been suggested in multiple clinical studies. With the advent of technology enabling noninvasive as well as invasive evaluation of heart function, it has also become possible to evaluate cardiac involvement in subjects who abuse alcohol but have not yet developed clinical abnormalities.

Impaired diastolic relaxation of the left ventricle by echo Doppler appears to be an early manifestation of the subclinical abnormality[4]; diminished compliance has also been described.[5] A further stage includes left ventricular hypertrophy with increased wall thickness and normal internal diameter, which may progress to a modest degree of dilatation.[6] In the asymptomatic patient contractility may be diminished when evaluated directly[5] or noninvasively.[7] The type of beverage used does not appear to be a determinant, since these abnormalities have been observed in individuals using predominantly wine, beer, or spirits.

As with other causes of primary myocardial disease, a diffuse abnormality of the myocardium is present, unrelated to coronary atherosclerosis, arterial hypertension, or valvular or congenital heart disease. Although symptoms of congestive heart failure may be the most common presentation in primary myocardial disease of multiple etiologies, congestive heart failure may appear in fewer than half of the patients when they are first seen.[3] In a significant proportion, arrhythmias without congestive heart failure may be the first abnormality to arise. Chest pain is not uncommon, and classic angina pectoris may be the only symptom despite normal coronary arteriograms.

Heart Failure

As cardiac dysfunction in an alcoholic progresses to low-output failure, pulmonary congestion may lead to dyspnea on exertion or during sleep. Cardiomegaly may be moderate during an initial episode of decompensation in the absence of the mitral regurgitation related to papillary muscle insufficiency. After correction of heart failure, heart size may return to near normal. Occasionally a peripheral arterial or pulmonary embolism is the initial manifestation.

No consistent pattern of alcohol abuse is associated with the onset of heart failure. A period of intensified drinking may be reported, but in some patients recurrent illness can apparently occur after a period of abstinence. Since the addicted person may commonly delay seeking medical assistance for weeks or months, evidence of right-sided heart failure is not uncommon. Signs include distended jugular veins; enlarged, tender liver; and edema of the dependent portions of the body. Clinical evidence of peripheral neuropathy or hepatic cirrhosis is not usually associated with alcoholic cardiomyopathy.

The electrocardiogram (ECG) at this stage may be normal or may show nonspecific changes. Poor progression of the R wave across the precordium is fairly common, particularly as the disease advances; presumably this is the result of progression of ventricular disease and conduction delay. Evidence of left ventricular and atrial enlargement is common, and left anterior fascicular block occurs in a minority of patients, while left or right bundle branch block appears in approximately 10 percent.

The diagnosis of alcoholic heart muscle disease is often obscured when the patient presents with elevated arterial blood pressure. When seen in association with other causes of heart failure, hypertension is usually considered to be secondary to compensatory peripheral vasoconstriction during cardiac decompensation. In the alcoholic, hypertensive episodes may be frequent, particularly if measurements are made close to a period of ethanol intake. This response has also been reported during the late intoxication–early withdrawal period in up to one-half of noncardiac alcoholics observed in an out-patient setting, usually without the development of a classic withdrawal illness.[8] Other evidence of hypertension, such as retinopathy, usually is absent.

Arterial pressure may be moderately elevated for several days, with spontaneous decline thereafter to a normal level. Substantial elevations may require up to a week for spontaneous normalization and are usually associated with moderate sinus tachycardia. After a short period of abstinence, arterial pressures are normalized in all but 10 percent of noncardiac alcoholics; this represents the incidence of hypertension in a control group.[8] In a 1-year follow-up, the normotensive state was found to persist in patients who remained abstinent. In general, alcoholism is a risk factor for the development of systemic arterial hypertension. (See Chap. 75.)

Precipitating factors other than ethanol usually are not present; however, small isolated outbreaks appear to occur from time to time in association with the combination of ethanol abuse and the trace metals lead, cobalt, or arsenic. Several other factors have to be considered potentially important.

Clinically evident malnutrition usually is not present in the cardiac patient, although it is commonly associated with liver disease. In females, alcoholism-related heart failure is rare before menopause. Cigarette smoking is very common among persons addicted to alcohol. Since myopathic responses to chronic cigarette smoking have been seen experimentally, this factor may be more important than is generally recognized.

The course of alcoholic cardiomyopathy is variable, depending to a large degree on the extent of cardiac involvement. The outlook is relatively poor for patients who continue to ingest ethanol in substantial amounts. In one study, 64 alcoholic patients were followed over a 4-year period.[9] Fully one-third remained abstinent, and the mortality rate in this group was 9 percent, although only a minority exhibited clinical improvement paralleling the response to abstinence in persons with hepatic cirrhosis. Of those who remained actively alcoholic, more than one-half succumbed. Presumably, at certain stages of the disease the pathogenic mechanisms may continue unabated despite traditional pharmacologic management and abstinence from alcohol. The encouraging results of abstinence may well have been exaggerated, since this group of individuals seemed to have relatively mild cardiac disease on entrance into the study. Nevertheless the response to abstinence supports the view that the major etiologic element in this disease process is ethyl alcohol.

The choice of pharmacologic therapy for cardiac decompensation depends on the state of cardiac disease when the patient is first encountered. During the first episode of heart failure, if the patient has only modest cardiomegaly and pulmonary congestion, the patient may be managed initially by diuretics to diminish volume overload. As the disease progresses, there is a role for preload- and afterload-reducing agents and for digitalis, which is also useful in the control of atrial fibrillation. (See also Chap. 26.)

The role of cardiac transplantation in the treatment of alcoholic cardiomyopathy must be judged case by case. Obviously the patient should have discontinued the use of alcohol, and there should be no organic disease except the heart disease.

Arrhythmias

The patient may present initially with an arrhythmia. Cardiac arrhythmias developing in these circumstances are often considered idiopathic in origin, since little or no clinical evidence of heart disease may remain after resolution of the arrhythmias and the extent of alcohol use may not be known.

In one study, subjects without overt cardiomyopathy or cardiomegaly were selected on the basis of alcoholism, acute intoxication, and the presence of arrhythmias.[10] Supraventricular arrhythmias predominated, and atrial fibrillation was the most common arrhythmia. Cardioversion or pharmacologic intervention was frequently required, but sinus rhythm was restored spontaneously in some subjects. Plasma electrolyte levels on admission were mostly normal. During subsequent recurrences the same arrhythmias were present as during the original episodes. Several days after restoration of sinus rhythm, these patients were assessed by high-speed ECG. The observed moderate delays in conduction were considered the background for the genesis of the acute arrhythmias.[8] This phenomenon has been termed the "holiday heart" syndrome because of frequent presentation over holidays or weekends. The acute cardiac arrhythmia may occur in association with heavy ethanol consumption in a person who has chronically abused ethanol without other clinical evidence of heart disease. Under unusual circumstances, such as a prolonged period of sleeplessness, the arrhythmia may be induced acutely without chronic abuse.

In a prospective 5-year study of subjects, the risk ratio for supraventricular arrhythmia was 2.6 in those who usually consumed six or more drinks per day, compared to subjects with a monthly intake that averaged less than one per day.[11] This association was independent of age, sex, race, and smoking.

An evaluation of serial hospital admissions with ambulatory electrocardiographic recording during the intoxication and early withdrawal stages has revealed several points of interest.[12] Subjects were excluded if arrhythmias or evidence of cardiac ischemia were present on the admission ECG. Of the 60 patients monitored during the initial 12 or 24 h, 12 had high composite arrhythmia scores. This was due to the presence of ventricular premature contractions. On biochemical assays of the blood, high concentrations of plasma catecholamines were found. After baseline observations, therapy with propranolol reduced the incidence of arrhythmia. This response supports the view that the sympathetic nervous system has an important role in the genesis of these arrhythmias.

Magnesium deficiency is fairly common with chronic alcohol abuse, particularly in patients with severe withdrawal reactions. There is no clear evidence that isolated deficits of this cation give rise to arrhythmias. Another variable that is pertinent to arrhythmogenesis is sleep apnea and the attendant oxygen desaturation. This phenomenon has been described in asymptomatic individuals, but there are no data on the syndrome as associated with alcohol abuse. (See also Chap. 35.)

Sudden unexpected death in alcoholics has been reported from several countries. The phenomenon has been attributed to cardiac arrest; this attribution is supported by the observation of a reduced ventricular fibrillation threshold in an animal model of chronic alcoholism.[13] Young and middle-aged persons without coronary artery disease comprise 8 percent of all sudden deaths in one series.[14] A subsequent investigation in the Soviet Union revealed an incidence of 17 percent in the apparent absence of other toxins.[15] In many cases there was no evidence of cardiac hypertrophy, and liver involvement was often in the form of fatty liver rather than hepatic cirrhosis. Moderate alcoholemia was thought to reflect higher earlier blood alcohol levels, implying that the apparent cardiac arrest was related to declining blood levels of ethanol in the late intoxication periods. The sudden-death group has foci of fibrosis and necrosis with mononuclear cell infiltration. (See also Chap. 51.)

Determinants of Alcoholic Heart Disease

The evidence that ethanol and/or its metabolites are the etiologic basis for alcoholic cardiomyopathy is circumstantial. The major positive feature supporting this idea is the history of ethanol ingestion in intoxicating amounts over many years, frequently marked by periods of spree drinking.

Animal models have been shown to develop functional, biochemical, and morphologic abnormalities, but congestive heart failure and significant arrhythmias have not been reported. This may be related to an insufficient duration of ethanol exposure. Clinically, the reduced mortality rate in patients who become abstinent supports the view that ethanol is the major factor in development of the disease.[9]

It is noteworthy that development of the subclinical state is consistent with living in a family setting[7] and stable employment. In this study 60 percent of subjects were skilled laborers or office workers. The others were unskilled, but none were considered indigent. The duration of excessive intake averaged 16 years while the quantity of alcohol consumed appeared to approximate the over-six-drinks-per-day reported for the occurrence of atrial arrhythmias.[11] In addition to ethanol abuse several other factors that may affect the development of cardiomyopathy have been considered to be potentially important. Cigarette use is common in persons addicted to alcohol and may be contributory.[16] Clinically evident malnutrition, though often seen in association with alcoholic cirrhosis, particularly at the subclinical stage of the disease,[7] usually is not present in the cardiac patient. In females, alcoholic heart disease is rare prior to menopause.

Pathophysiology

With regard to mechanism, there is probably some direct effect of ethanol or its metabolites on cardiac function as well as a long-term neurohumoral influence on the heart that may interact with adaptive processes that tend to reduce pathological effects. While the pathogenesis of collagen accumulation—its synthesis and degradation—has not been defined, the early decrease of diastolic compliance of the left ventricle seen experimentally is most likely related to this alteration of interstitium.[17] After several years, left ventricular contractility may be impaired.[17,18] There is an associated accumulation of water and Na^+ in cardiac cells without a reduction of K^+, perhaps related to the altered membrane phospholipid composition. In view of the dilatation of sarcoplasmic reticulum observed by electron microscopy,[17] it has been postulated that dysfunction of the tubular membranes may limit the rate of Ca^{2+} availability to contractile protein, and thus diminish contractile performance, without a change in total Ca^{2+}.[18] Although high-energy phosphate levels are not altered, an inhibitory effect of long-term ethanol use on myosin adenosinetriphosphatase (ATPase) and Ca^{2+}-activated myofibrillar ATPase has been demonstrated.[16] (See also Chap. 25.)

One might expect protein synthesis in the cardiac cell to be adversely affected by chronic ethanol exposure. In experiments to determine the ability of chronic ethanol feeding to affect the process of myocardial hypertrophy during chronic aortic pressure overload,[19] however, the hypertrophic response was unimpaired. Moreover, ribonucleic acid, a determinant of protein synthesis, was not found to be diminished in alcoholic animals over a period of 14 weeks.[19]

When the disease is clinically evident, there appears to be some degree of impaired synthesis, or accelerated degradation, of contractile protein, since lysis of myofibrils is frequently observed on morphologic study of advanced alcoholic cardiomyopathy. This may precede the appearance of rapid clinical deterioration.

In examination of biopsy specimens from patients and of autopsy tissue preparations, no distinctive features have been revealed in patients with alcoholic heart disease as compared with idiopathic dilated cardiomyopathy or dilated cardiomyopathy from other causes.[20] Quite early in the prefailure stage there appears to be dilatation of the sarcoplasmic reticulum and the undifferentiated portion of the intercalated disk, but these changes are apparently obscured at later stages of disease, when considerable myocytolysis may be seen. An increase of fibrous tissue is a usual finding and may take the form of an increase in the interstitial collagen component or replacement of myocardial fibers. Small vessels are usually normal, but in the areas of fibrous tissue accumulation vessels may occasionally show wall thickening. It has been thought that these vascular abnormalities are secondary.[20]

VITAMIN DEFICIENCIES[21]

Thiamine

The key features of beriberi, or thiamine deficiency, though not readily reproducible in animals, include a high cardiac output associated with arteriolar vasodilatation. Although it has been the classic view that right ventricular failure is dominant when symptoms develop, several studies have documented a significant elevation of left ventricular end-diastolic and pulmonary capillary wedge pressures. The hemodynamic abnormalities are reversible with thiamine therapy. (See also Chap. 24.)

Other Vitamins

Unequivocal direct effects of vitamin A and niacin deficiencies on heart muscle in humans have not been established. Scurvy, however, can be associated with sudden death. Human volunteers on a vitamin C-deficient diet have reported dyspnea and chest pain associated with PR interval prolongation and ST-segment abnormalities. Electrocardiographic alterations can be reversed rapidly with parenteral vitamin C. In experimental vitamin B_6 deficiency in rats, cardiomyopathic changes were found postmortem, but the human counterpart has yet to be described. Excess doses of vitamin D in humans have been associated with deposits of calcium as well as with the shortened QT interval of hypercalcemia. Mild excesses of vitamin D_3 have been shown to intensify atherosclerosis in nonhuman primates.

Vitamin E and Selenium

In recent years a cardiomyopathy (Keshan's disease) affecting infants and children has been described in China. The disease is characterized by local myocardial necrosis, fibrosis, and hypercontraction bands. The disease has a regional distribution in agricultural areas where the selenium content of the staple grains and soil is reduced. Supplementation of the diet with selenium has been found effective as a preventive. In view of a seasonal variation, other factors may also be important. Although isolated selenium deficiency that produces cardiomyopathy has not been described in experimental animal models, a combination of selenium and vitamin E deprivations has been shown to produce diffuse patchy necrosis of the myocardium in young swine. An abnormality of cell lipid peroxidation has been thought to affect membrane lipids, with resultant disturbance of intracellular electrolyte and water composition as well as energy production. (See also Chap. 88.)

CACHEXIA

Severe weight loss in individuals of relatively normal initial body weight may have important cardiovascular consequences, particularly in infants and children. In an analysis of 93 malnourished children studied at autopsy in Costa Rica, there were 14 cases considered to have primary congestive heart failure resulting from either marasmus or kwashiorkor.[22] On histologic examination, interstitial edema was frequently observed. Substantial degrees of vacuolization within myocardial fibers with apparent disorganization of myofibrillar structure were observed.

The nutritional deficiency that characterizes protein-calorie undernutrition in more mature individuals has been studied by a number of investigators.[23] In human adult volunteers on a semistarvation regimen, significant reductions of heart rate, stroke volume, cardiac output, and heart size were observed during the development of cachexia. Cardiac output, however, did not appear to fall out of proportion to the diminished metabolic requirements. In addition, an echocardiographic study of patients with undernutrition secondary to a variety of chronic disease states found that the reduced cardiac output was associated with a diminished left ventricular end-diastolic diameter and mass. When adjusted for body weight, however, the cardiac index was higher than that of normal control subjects.

Anorexia nervosa influences the cardiovascular system in several respects. Observations of a group of individuals with anorexia nervosa showed that the systolic ejection phase indexes of left ventricular function were normal and responded normally to exercise. The patients in this study were considered to have an adult marasmus-type syndrome that did not significantly affect cardiac function; however, on two-dimensional echocardiography the left ventricular mass was found to be reduced to between one-half and two-thirds that of age- and sex-matched control subjects. This reduction was even greater when left ventricular mass was considered in relation to total body weight. Left ventricular afterload was reduced, while resting left ventricular function was normal. With the change in skeletal muscle mass the response to exercise was limited, with a lower peak oxygen consumption. In addition, there were reduced increments in heart rate and systolic blood pressure.

Analysis of substrates in systemic blood showed normal glucose responses to exercise; however, free fatty acid concentrations, which doubled in control patients during exercise, showed no change in the anorexic group. The ECG in anorexia nervosa is generally unremarkable, but some patients exhibit nonspecific ST- and T-wave changes. Although the QT interval is usually normal, prolongation has been described in association with sudden death, despite normal plasma electrolyte levels, as an apparently unusual event.

In primary protein-calorie undernutrition, the weight of the evidence indicates that the adult heart, though atrophied, will usually function normally prior to refeeding. Patients who recover from anorexia show improvement in heart rate, posterior wall dimension, systolic wall stress, and left ventricular internal dimension. Studies of young children, supported by some experimental data, suggest that substantial histologic abnormalities of the myocardium may occur. In some of the children studied, heart failure may be attributable to the undernutrition. A potential for arrhythmias and sudden death resulting from undernutrition has been postulated, but this has not been well established.

HYPERALIMENTATION

Therapeutic feeding by the enteric or parenteral route has assumed increasing importance in the treatment of a variety of acute illnesses. Although the initial hemodynamic changes during such therapy have not been delineated, the acute responses to oral feeding in normally nourished persons—particularly the cardiovascular changes—are of interest.

During oral feeding in human beings, a diet of mixed caloric composition induces an increase of cardiac output associated with a decline in systemic vascular resistance within 20 min after completion of a meal.[24] The rise in cardiac output is essentially due to an increase of stroke volume without a change in left ventricular filling pressure, implying an increase in contractility. In patients who have postprandial angina pectoris at rest, stroke volume is diminished while pulmonary wedge pressure is elevated.[24] (See Chap. 58.)

Patients with chronic cardiac disease may suffer forms of malnutrition similar to those described for the general hospital population.[25] An extreme form, the syndrome of *cardiac cachexia,* is attributable to anorexia, decreased intestinal absorption of food, and perhaps a change in the distribution of substrates absorbed into the circulatory system. Patients with cardiac cachexia appear to have increased morbidity and mortality rates in comparison to noncachectic patients similar in age, sex, and severity of heart disease. In a prospective study of cardiac patients undergoing surgery, the effects of short-term forced feeding of up to 1500 calories were evaluated.[26] The lack of effect on morbidity and mortality rates was perhaps related to the fact that feeding was begun just prior to operation and continued for approximately 5 days. The effects of longer term preparation of patients before surgery require investigation.

Adults with chronic undernutrition without underlying heart disease may develop heart failure during hyperalimentation.[23] Under the conditions of rapid repletion, a state resembling congestive heart failure may develop that is characterized by hypermetabolism and ventricular gallop but augmented cardiac output and normal left ventricular ejection fraction. Rapid resolution follows administration of diuretic therapy, slowing of the rate of hyperalimentation, and reduction of the daily intake of sodium.

During hyperalimentation some patients may develop hypophosphatemia. As in other circumstances producing this anion deficit, significant cardiac effects may ensue. In a study of patients with hypophosphatemia whose echocardiogram showed no mechanical defects, a significant increase in the incidence of arrhythmias was observed, without reduction in the plasma concentrations of other electrolytes.[27] Patients who exhibited nonsustained ventricular tachycardia were improved by normalization of plasma phosphate levels by oral supplements.

REFERENCES

1. Schwarz, F, Mall G, Zebe H, Schmitzer E, Mauthey J, Scheusten H: Determinants of survival in patients with congestive cardiomyopathy: Quantitative morphologic findings and left ventricular hemodynamics. *Circulation* 1984; 70:923–928.
2. Roberts WC, Siegel RJ, McManus BM: Idiopathic dilated cardiomyopathy: Analysis of 152 necropsy patients. *Am J Cardiol* 1987; 60:1340–1355.
3. Shirey EK, Proudfit WL, Hawk WA: Primary myocardial disease: Correlation with clinical findings, angiographic and biopsy diagnosis. *Am Heart J* 1980; 99:198–207.
4. Kupari M, Koskinen P, Suokas A, Ventila M: Left ventricular filling impairment in asymptomatic chronic alcoholics. *Am J Cardiol* 1990; 66:1473–1477.
5. Regan TJ, Levinson GE, Oldewurtel HA, Frank MJ, Weisse AB, Moschos CB: Ventricular function in noncardiacs with alcoholic fatty liver: Role of ethanol in the production of cardiomyopathy. *J Clin Invest* 1969; 48:397–407.
6. Mathews EC Jr, Gardin JM, Henry WL, Del Negro A, Fletcher R, Snow J: Echocardiographic abnormalities in chronic alcoholics with and without overt congestive heart failure. *Am J Cardiol* 1981; 47:570–578.
7. Urbano-Marquez A, Estruch R, Navarro-Lopez F, Grau JM, Mont L, Rubin E: The effects of alcoholism on skeletal and cardiac muscle. *N Engl J Med:* 1989; 320:409–415.
8. Regan TJ, Pathan A, Weisse AB, Eaddy C, Torres R: The contribution of arterial pressure to the cardiac dysfunction of chronic alcoholism, *Acta Med Scand* 1986; 703(suppl):273–280.
9. Demakis JG, Proskey A, Rahimtoola SH, Jamil M, Sutton GC, Rosen KM, et al: The natural course of alcoholic cardiomyopathy. *Ann Intern Med* 1974; 80:293–297.
10. Ettinger PO, Wu CF, DeLa Cruz CL Jr, Weisse AB, Ahmed SS, Regan TJ: Arrhythmias and the "holiday heart"; Alcohol-associated cardiac rhythm disorders. *Am Heart J* 1978; 95:555–562.
11. Cohen EJ, Klatsky AL, Armstrong MA: Alcohol use and supraventricular arrhythmia. *Am J Cardiol* 1988; 62:971–973.
12. Zim DH, Jacob MS, MacLeod SM, Sellers EM, T: TY: Propranolol and chlordiazepoxide effects on cardiac arrhythmias during alcohol withdrawal. *Alcoholism* 1980; 4:400–405.
13. Patel R, McArdle JJ, Regan TJ: Increased ventricular vulnerability in a chronic ethanol model despite reduced electrophysiologic responses to catecholamines. *Alcohol: Clin Exp Res.* 1991; 15:785–789.
14. Sarkioja T, Hirvonen J: Causes of sudden unexpected deaths in young and middle-aged persons. *Forensic Sci Intl* 1984; 24:247–261.
15. Vikhert AM, Tsiplenkova VG, Cherpachenka NM: Alcoholic cardiomyopathy and sudden cardiac death. *J Am Coll Cardiol* 1986; 8:3A–11A.
16. Rosengren A, Wilhelmsen L, Wedel H: Separate and combined effects of smoking and alcohol abuse in middle aged men. *Acta Med Scand* 1988; 223:111–118.
17. Thomas G, Haider B, Oldewurtel HA, Lyons MM, Yeh CK, Regan TJ: Progression of myocardial abnormalities in experimental alcoholism. *Am J Cardiol* 1980; 46:233–241.

18. Sarma JSM, Shigeaki I, Fischer R, Maruyama Y, Weishaar R, Bing BJ: Biochemical and contractile properties of heart muscle after prolonged alcohol administration. *J Mol Cell Cardiol* 1976; 8:951–972.
19. Whitman V, Schuler HG, Musselman J: Effects of chronic ethanol consumption on the myocardial hypertrophic response to a pressure overload in the rat. *J Mol Cell Cardiol* 1980; 12:519–572.
20. Olsen EGJ: The pathology of cardiomyopathies: A critical analysis. *Am Heart J* 1979; 98:385–392.
21. Watson R (ed): *Nutrition and Heart Disease,* vol 2. Boca Raton, FL, CRC Press, 1987: 19–71.
22. Piza J, Troper L, Cespedes R, Miller JH, Berenson GS: Myocardial lesions and heart failure in infantile malnutrition. *Am J Prop Med Hyg* 1971; 20:343–355.
23. Moodie DS: Anorexia and the heart: Results of studies to assess effects. *Postgrad Med* 1987; 81:46–55.
24. Figueras J, Singh GN, Ganz W, Swan HJC: Hemodynamic and electrocardiographic accompaniments of resting postprandial angina. *Br Heart J* 1979; 42:402–409.
25. Bistrian BR, Blackburn GL, Vitale J, Cochran D, Naylor J: Prevalence of malnutrition in general medical patients. *JAMA* 1976; 235:1567–1570.
26. Abel RM, Fischer JE, Buckley MJ, Barnett GO, Austen WG: Malnutrition in cardiac surgical patients: Results of a prospective randomized evaluation of early postoperative parenteral nutrition. *Arch Surg* 1976; 111:45–50.
27. Venditti F, Panezai F, Marotta C, Oldewurtel H, Regan TJ: Hypophosphatemia and cardiac arrhythmias. *J Min Elect Metab* 1987; 13:19–25.

Chapter 106

Syphilis and the Cardiovascular System

John Stone, M.D.

DEFINITION, ETIOLOGY, AND PATHOLOGY

The word *syphilis* derives from the title of a Latin poem of 1530 by Girolamo Fracastoro, a physician and poet from Verona.[1] Its literal etymology, in light of the human misery caused by the disease, is heavy with irony: *syn*, meaning "together," and *philein*, "to love." The euphemism for syphilis is *lues*, from the Latin root for *plague*, an implied verdict with which medical history strongly concurs.

Treponema pallidum, the spirochete that causes syphilis, results in human disease that is easily protean enough to qualify for its designation by earlier clinicians as "the great imitator." Luetic cardiovascular disease, like that in other organs, has its inception with the *primary* lesion, or chancre. The chancre is a painless shallow ulcer that may be genital or extragenital in location and is almost always transmitted venereally. The *secondary* stage of syphilis follows the chancre by 4 to 8 weeks; this stage is heralded by skin rash, malaise, fever, mucocutaneous ulcers, etc., and is triggered by wide vascular dissemination of the spirochete. The resultant arteritis sets the stage for *tertiary* lues, which involves the cardiovascular, neurological, and other systems and makes its appearance a few years to decades after the chancre.

Pathologically, the prime manifestation of cardiovascular syphilis is an *aortitis* that leads to *aortic aneurysms*, *aortic regurgitation*, and *coronary ostial disease*. Less common are distal aortic involvement, myocarditis, pulmonary arteritis, and myocardial gummata. In contrast to the more usual atheromatous involvement, the *proximal* aorta is most heavily involved in syphilis; the intima takes on a wrinkled "tree-bark" appearance, with plaque formation and thickening of the aortic wall. Microscopically, the *vasa vasorum* of the aorta are involved in an "endarteritis obliterans," with marked intimal proliferation and perivascular accumulation of lymphocytes and plasma cells. Patchy destruction of musculoelastic tissue is characteristic. The aortic valve leaflets in cardiovascular syphilis appear thickened, with rolled margins and separation of the cusps at the commissures. The myocardium often shows diffuse fibrosis, but large areas of infarction are uncommon.[2] Heggtveit's[3] necropsy study of luetic aortitis consisted of 100 cases ranging in age from 30 to 92 years. Aortic aneurysm was the most common complication (40 patients) followed by aortic regurgitation (29 cases) and coronary ostial stenosis (26 cases).

PATHOPHYSIOLOGY

Aortic aneurysms, either saccular or fusiform, may cause symptoms by putting pressure on adjacent structures: on the recurrent laryngeal nerve (causing hoarseness), on the bronchi (cough), on the superior vena cava (Fig. 106-1), or on the esophagus (causing dysphagia). Erosion of the sternum (Fig. 106-2) or vertebral bodies has been described. Rupture of the aneurysm into adjacent

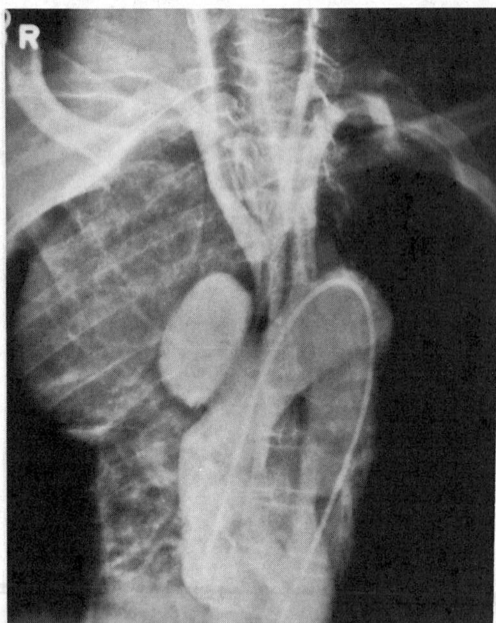

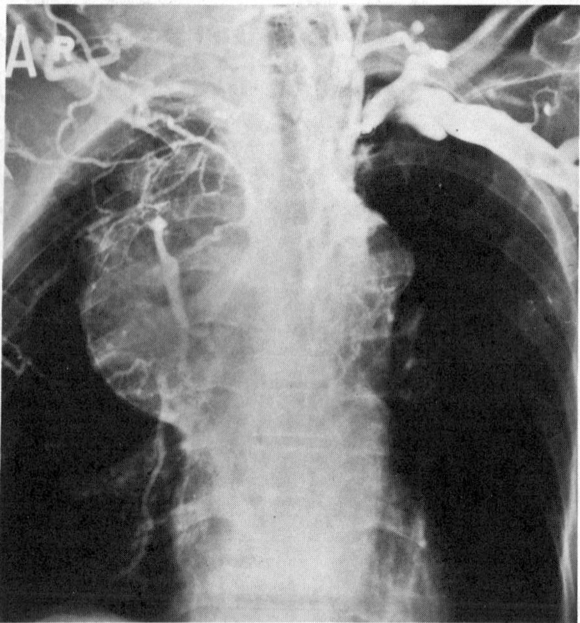

FIGURE 106-1 Superior vena caval obstruction in a patient with luetic aneurysm: *A. Aortogram* showing large two-chambered sacular aneurysm arising from the ascending aorta. *B Venogram* from the same patient showing impaired venous flow typical of the superior vena caval syndrome. *(X-rays courtesy of Dr. Wade H. Shuford, Department of Radiology, Emory University School of Medicine, and Grady Memorial Hospital, Atlanta, Georgia.)*

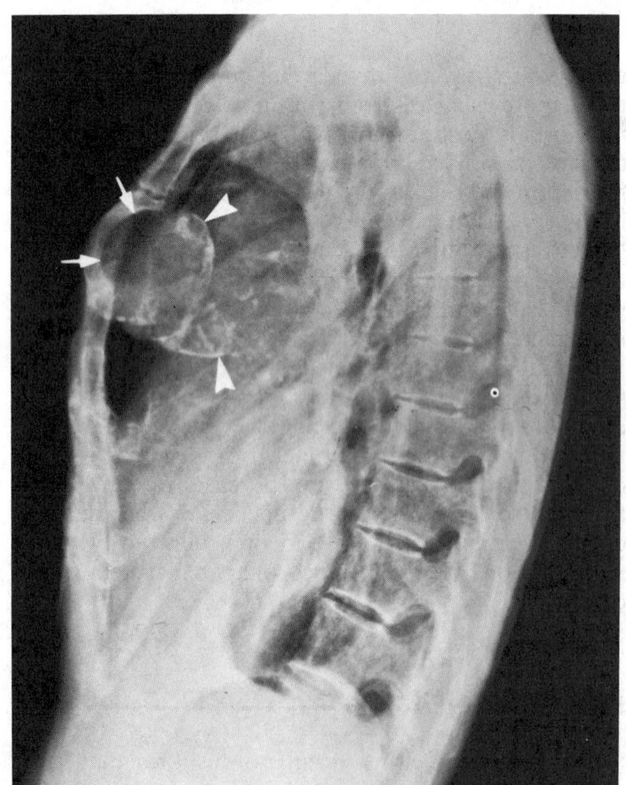

FIGURE 106-2 Lateral chest x-ray showing erosion of sternum (smaller arrows) and extensive "eggshell" calcification (larger arrows) in the wall of a luetic aneurysm. *(X-ray courtesy of Dr. Wade H. Shuford, Department of Radiology, Emory University School of Medicine, and Grady Memorial Hospital, Atlanta, Georgia.)*

structures (pulmonary artery, right side of the heart, thoracic cavity, etc.) may lead to rapid demise of the patient. Aortic dissection, however, is uncommon. Luetic aortic regurgitation ranges from mild to severe in degree. Coronary ostial stenosis caused by exuberant fibrosis may result in angina pectoris that seems clinically out of proportion to the aortic regurgitation present; rarely, a picture of congestive cardiomyopathy may result.[4]

CLINICAL MANIFESTATIONS

Clinical manifestations of cardiovascular syphilis may be divided conveniently into three categories: those secondary to aortic regurgitation, those secondary to aneurysm formation, and those secondary to coronary ostial disease; combinations do arise. All three forms of the disease require a high index of suspicion.

Symptoms

Patients with luetic aortic regurgitation may be free of symptoms early in the course of the disease. But gradually, if aortic regurgitation is more than trivial, left ventricular dilatation occurs, with the appearance of heart failure. Palpitations and a general awareness of the heartbeat often accompany the widened pulse pressure. Pain in various locations may result from expansion of the aneurysm (Fig. 106-3). Angina pectoris may occur because of aortic regurgitation, coronary ostial disease, or associated coronary atherosclerosis.

Physical Examination

Findings of the physical examination of patients with aortic regurgitation are most often similar to those for

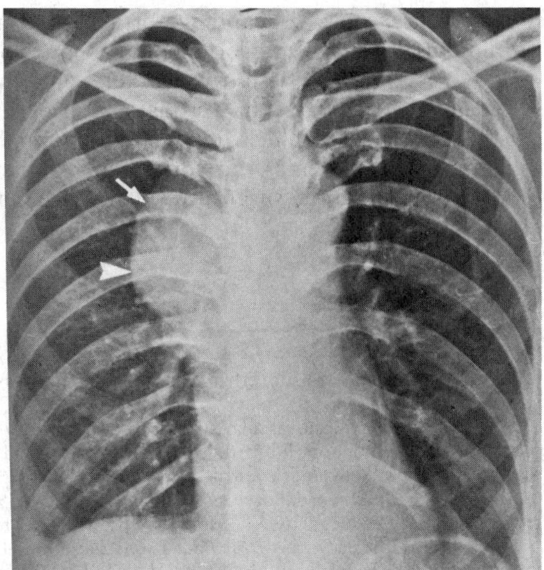

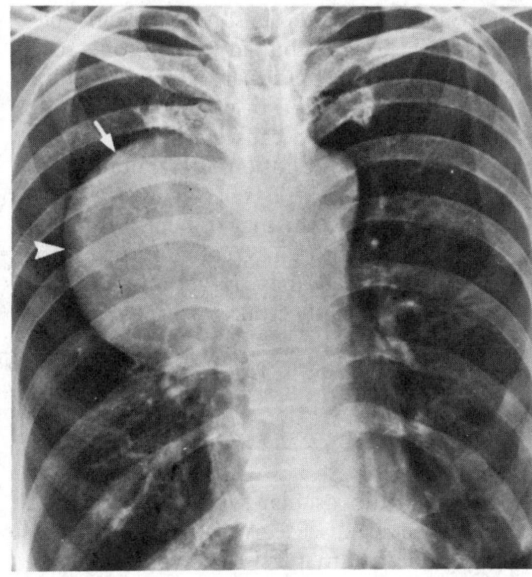

FIGURE 106-3 Posteroanterior chest films showing enlarging syphilitic aortic aneurysm: *A.* Earlier. *B.* Seven years later. *(X-rays courtesy of Dr. Wade H. Shuford, Department of Radiology, Emory University School of Medicine, and Grady Memorial Hospital, Atlanta, Georgia.)*

any patient with a significant aortic leak: a decrescendo diastolic murmur along the left sternal border; an Austin Flint diastolic rumble; and the peripheral findings for aortic regurgitation—the "collapsing" pulse, pistol-shot sounds and to-and-fro murmurs over peripheral arteries, pulsation in the capillary beds of the nails, and head bobbing synchronous with the pulse (de Musset's sign). Aortic closure may cause a "tambour" second sound, a musical-note-like ping that is slightly sustained to the ear. Harvey et al.[5] have emphasized that although most aortic diastolic murmurs, including those due to syphilis, are best heard along the *left* sternal border in the third and fourth intercostal spaces, when the murmur is louder to the *right* of the sternum, conditions associated with aortic root dilatation (e.g., syphilis, Marfan's syndrome, aortic sinusal aneurysm) may be present. An aortic valve cusp may become retroverted and produce a "cooing" diastolic murmur. The presence of aortic aneurysm may also cause a "tracheal tug" and pulsation of the sternoclavicular joint. (See also Chaps. 10, 11, and 79.)

Ancillary Data

Serological testing for syphilis ranges from the relatively less specific Venereal Disease Research Laboratory (VDRL) test to the highly sensitive and specific fluorescent treponemal antibody absorption test (FTA-ABS). The FTA-ABS test usually remains positive even when the VDRL has become negative as a result either of passage of time or of treatment. Interpretation of these tests may not be straightforward—biological false positives do occur—but a complete analysis of this problem is beyond the scope of this discussion.[6] Changes in the *electrocardiogram* are primarily those of left ventricular hypertrophy or myocardial ischemia. The *chest x-ray* may show prominence of the ascending aorta and enlargement of the cardiac chambers, especially the left ventricle. Linear "eggshell" calcification of the ascending aorta, though not specific for luetic aortitis, should point the clinician toward appropriate serological testing.[7] The *echocardiogram* may be helpful in detection and follow-up of the aortic aneurysm, estimation of the degree of aortic regurgitation, and assessment of left ventricular function. The diastolic mitral valve flutter that attends the Austin Flint rumble is also easily identified on the echocardiogram. *Angiography* and *coronary arteriography* will demonstrate and localize aortic aneurysm formation and help to define the anatomic basis for angina pectoris. Less invasive procedures, such as computed tomography and magnetic resonance imaging, are likely to play increasingly important roles in the future.

NATURAL HISTORY

The natural history of untreated syphilis has been reported in two large studies, the Oslo Study and the Tuskegee Study. In the Oslo Study,[8] cardiovascular syphilis was diagnosed in 10 percent of the patients; in the autopsy portion of the study, however, cardiovascular syphilis (usually aortitis) was found in 26 percent of those studied. In the Tuskegee Study,[9] among autopsied patients, aortitis was present in 50 percent of those who had a positive serological test. The interval between the appearance of the chancre and the onset of clinical cardiovascular syphilis varies greatly, from as few as 3 to 5 years to as many as 25 years or more. Coronary ostial stenosis requiring bypass grafts has been reported in a 25-year-old man.[10]

After the introduction of penicillin (PCN) therapy in the 1940s, the incidence of syphilis in the United States began to decline. In 1987, however, a significant increase in incidence was reported, especially in Florida, New York City, and California. The reported increases were largely in the heterosexual population. The figures are believed to reflect the known epidemiologic associations between sexually transmitted disease, acquired immunodeficiency syndrome (AIDS), and in some areas, intravenous drug abuse. One major public health concern is that this upsurge may presage an increase in congenital syphilis and other forms of the disease.[11] The human immunodeficiency virus, which causes AIDS, is known to modify the clinical manifestations of a number of diseases, notably tuberculosis. It has been suggested that AIDS may modify the natural history of neurosyphilis,[12] resulting in accelerated or more aggressive forms of the disease; whether or not AIDS may trigger an alteration in other forms of syphilis is uncertain.[13] (See also Chap. 107.)

TREATMENT

Medical therapy of cardiovascular syphilis must be tailored to the severity of the disease. A course of antibiotic therapy must be given for any persistent syphilitic infection. Penicillin (PCN) is still the most effective drug (benzathine PCN, 2.4 million units intramuscular once a week for 3 weeks, for a total of 7.2 million units) is the standard regimen. Doxycycline or ceftriaxone may be substituted in the penicillin-sensitive patient. Although evidence is lacking that antimicrobial agents benefit patients with cardiovascular syphilis, treatment as outlined above is recommended in part because about 15 percent of patients with cardiovascular syphilis have associated neurosyphilis.[14] If there is suspicion of neurosyphilis or if the patient is HIV-positive, consultation with an expert in sexually transmitted diseases should be obtained, since longer and higher dose therapy using the intravenous route may be necessary.[15] A lumbar puncture is recommended in patients who have unexplained neurological symptoms, evidence of treatment failure, very high nontreponemal antibody titer (VDRL or RPR), or other evidence of active syphilis (e.g., gumma), and in all patients who are HIV-positive.[16]

Antibiotic prophylaxis against endocarditis is indicated in patients with aortic regurgitation or luetic aneurysm at times of bacteremic risk. (See Chap. 94.) The usual medical strategies for congestive heart failure, such as digitalis, diuretics, and vasodilators, are useful. (See Chap. 26.) Surgery for patients with cardiovascular syphilis may include prosthetic aortic valve replacement, resection and grafting for aneurysmal disease, and endarterectomy or bypass grafting for coronary ostial disease. As in any case of long-standing aortic regurgitation, the timing of aortic valve replacement is a matter of controversy.[17] Preoperative assessment of left ventricular function, by ventriculography, coronary arteriography, and serial echocardiographic studies, should not only help to identify those patients who could benefit from surgery but also improve the surgical results.[18] (See Chap. 79.)

REFERENCES

1. Garrison FH: *History of Medicine.* Philadelphia, WB Saunders, 1929: 232–233.
2. Hudson REB: Cardiovascular syphilis. In: *Cardiovascular Pathology,* Vol 1. London, Edward Arnold, 1965: 1168–1190.
3. Heggtveit HA: Syphilitic aortitis. *Circulation* 1964; 29:346–355.
4. Holt S: Syphilitic ostial occlusion. *Br Heart J* 1977; 39:469–470.
5. Harvey WP, Corrado MA, Perloff JK: "Right-sided" murmurs of aortic insufficiency. *Am J Med Sci* 1963; 245:533–543.
6. Kampmeier RH: Syphilis. In: Evans AS, Feldman HA (eds): *Bacterial Infections of Humans.* New York and London, Plenum Medical Book Company, 1982: 553–577.
7. Higgins CB, Reinke RT: Nonsyphilitic etiology of linear calcification of the ascending aorta. *Radiology* 1974; 113:609–613.
8. Gjestland T: The Oslo study of untreated syphilis. *Acta Derm Venereol* 1955; 35(suppl 34):1–368.
9. Sparling PF: Syphilis. In: Wyngaarden JB, Smith LH (eds): *Cecil Textbook of Medicine.* Philadelphia, WB Saunders, 1985: 1650–1661.
10. Brown AP, Dawkins KD, Parker DJ: "Late" manifestations of cardiovascular syphilis occurring in a young man. *Br Heart J* 1987; 58:405–408.
11. *MMWR* 36: No. 25, pp 393–397, July 3, 1987. Increases in primary and secondary syphilis—United States.
12. Johns DR, Tierney M, Felsenstein D: Alteration in the natural history of neurosyphilis by concurrent infection with the human immunodeficiency virus. *N Engl J Med* 1987; 316:1569–1572.
13. *MMWR* 36: No. 29, pp 488–491. July 31, 1987. Tertiary syphilis deaths—South Florida.
14. Sparling PF: Sexually transmitted diseases. In: Wyngaarden JB, Smith LH, Bennett, JC (eds): *Cecil Textbook of Medicine.* Philadelphia, Saunders, 1992: 1751–1755.
15. Musher DM: Syphilis. In: Gorbach SL, Bartlett JG, Blacklow IVR (eds): *Infectious Diseases.* Philadelphia, Saunders, 1992:822–828.
16. Sanford JP: *Guide to Microbial Therapy.* Dallas, Antimicrobial Therapy, Inc., 1992.
17. Carabello BA, Usher BW, Hendrix GH, Assey ME, Crawford FA, Leman RB: Predictors of outcome for aortic valve replacement in patients with aortic regurgitation and left ventricular dysfunction: A change in the measuring stick. *J Am Coll Cardiol* 1987; 10:991–997.
18. Grabau W, Emanuel R, Ross D, Parker J, Hegde M: Syphilitic aortic regurgitation, an appraisal of surgical treatment. *Br J Vener Dis* 1976; 52:366–373.

Chapter 107

AIDS and the Cardiovascular System

Melvin D. Cheitlin, M.D.

Acquired immunodeficiency syndrome (AIDS) is caused by infection with a virus of the family Retroviridae. This group of retroviruses is comprised of enveloped ribonucleic acid (RNA) viruses possessing an RNA-dependent deoxyribonucleic acid (DNA) polymerase (reverse transcriptase). There are two classes of AIDS viruses known as human immunodeficiency virus 1 and 2 (HIV-1, HIV-2).

The most specific definition of infection by the HIV is by identification of the HIV organism in the tissues of the host. Since isolation of the virus is not easily done and therefore lacks sensitivity, a patient with repeated positive screening tests for antibodies to the HIV such as an enzyme-labeled immunoabsorbant assay (ELISA) confirmed by a supplemental test such as the Western blot immunofluorescence assay should be considered as being infected by the HIV.

A classification system for the different stages of HIV infection as proposed by the Centers for Disease Control (CDC) is helpful[1]:

Group I: Acute infection
Group II: Asymptomatic infection
Group III: Persistent generalized lymphadenopathy (PGL)
Group IV: Chronic disease—AIDS with constitutional disease (such as unexplained diarrhea, weight loss, or fever over 1 month), neurologic disease, secondary infectious diseases, secondary cancers (Kaposi's sarcoma, non-Hodgkin's lymphoma, primary lymphoma of the brain)

The recognition of human infection by HIV in 1981 represented the startling development of a modern epidemic with many of the aspects of epidemics of the past such as caused by poliomyelitis and Black Plague. This infection is due to a retrovirus that invades the nucleus of certain cells containing a specific receptor on their cell membranes and incorporates the DNA copy of the HIV in the host genetic material or genome. After an apparent incubation (dormant) period of a mean of 8 to 10 years, the virus can eventually express itself by releasing into the cytoplasm double-stranded DNA copies of the virus, killing the cell and invading other immune cells, usually T-helper lymphocytes, to the point that immune-defense mechanisms of the host are compromised.[2]

A long-term prospective study showed the actuarial rate of progression from time of infection to AIDS of 54 percent at 10 years after infection and an increasing progression after 5 years of infection.[3] About 30 percent of patients with PGL will progress to AIDS in 5 years.[4] At this point there is a breakdown of the body's defense against certain neoplastic changes, resulting in the development of non-Hodgkin's lymphoma and Kaposi's sarcoma. These complications lead inevitably, at least in a very high percentage of cases, to death.

At the beginning of the epidemic this organism in the United States struck mainly at the male homosexual population. Later it was found to be transmitted not only through sexual intercourse but also through blood-borne contamination, soon affecting the intravenous drug-user population and other populations receiving blood products and blood transfusions such as hemophiliacs.

From work with HIV-1, the usual way in which the

virus attacks cells is through interaction with a receptor on the surface membrane of the cell, the so-called CD4 receptor. This is present in T-helper lymphocytes. Macrophages, microglia, and Langerhan's cells may have other specific receptors for HIV other than CD4. Other cells seem to lack an HIV receptor and, therefore, are much less often found to be sites of infection; the myocardial cell is one such cell.

From the beginning of the epidemic it was recognized that the heart could be involved but that significant clinical involvement of the heart was unusual. Originally it was believed through autopsy studies that the heart was mainly involved because of pericarditis or because of metastatic Kaposi's sarcoma.[5,6] There were a few patients with nonbacterial thrombotic endocarditis (NBTE) reported, but this could be nonspecific since many of these patients have a wasting disease in which NBTE is not unusual.[7] On further review of autopsy series and clinical series and especially with the study of patients with AIDS who had echocardiography, it was apparent that abnormalities of the heart were seen frequently, even though clinical manifestations of heart disease still remained unusual.

AUTOPSY FINDINGS

The incidence of cardiac involvement at autopsy varies, depending on the definition of cardiac disease. In 15 autopsy series the incidence of cardiac involvement varies from none to 70 percent of the hearts, depending on whether or not lymphocytic infiltration with or without myocardial necrosis is included.[5-13] The presence of autopsy-proven cardiac involvement in patients who during life had clinically significant cardiac involvement is less impressive, especially if one includes the patients with localized, isolated collections of myocardial lymphocytes.

In evaluating autopsy reports, one often has difficulty in discerning how many patients had clinically significant abnormalities during life. In the large series of consecutive autopsies of AIDS patients, between 5 and 20 percent appear to have had cardiac lesions of potential clinical importance. These include patients with myocarditis with clinical manifestations, mainly with known pathogens, such as toxoplasmosis, clinically evident pericarditis, or nonbacterial endocarditis, which can cause systemic emboli.[14]

More important are the relatively few patients in whom the cause of death was listed as due to cardiac abnormality. The most common cause of death is respiratory failure and infection.[11,13,15] Neoplasm, lymphoma, and encephalopathy are also frequent causes of death.[16] Of 858 autopsied patients with AIDS from 15 series in the literature, only 9 (1 percent) had the cause of death listed as cardiac. If the cases with recognized etiology for heart disease are removed, only 0.5 percent of deaths were possibly due to HIV "myocarditis."

Right ventricular hypertrophy and/or dilatation was reported in 12 of 71 patients (16.9 percent)[12] and in 18 of 115 patients (15.7 percent).[11] Pericarditis varied in frequency from 3 of 41 (7.3 percent)[7] to 3 of 101 (3 percent).[9]

ECHOCARDIOGRAPHIC FINDINGS

Echocardiography in patients with either AIDS or PGL has been reported in a number of studies.[17-33] The prevalence of echocardiographic abnormalities varies from 15 to 60 percent and is higher if we include the finding of mitral valve prolapse, an echocardiographic abnormality that may be related to cachexia. The prevalence of left ventricular hypokinesis also varies from 12.5 to 41 percent in the three largest series.[19,20,22] In one series[19] four of the eight patients had congestive heart failure; one died and at autopsy had a dilated cardiomyopathy without evidence of inflammatory myocarditis or cardiac opportunistic infections. Only in this study[19] was clinical congestive heart failure mentioned. Dilated cardiomyopathy was seen only in the hospitalized patients.

The finding of pericardial effusion was common, varying from 20 to 40 percent.[20,22,23] The incidence of tamponade varies: In one series[20] of 18 patients with pericardial effusion, 5 (28 percent) had tamponade. In this report of 300 patients with AIDS, 16 (5 percent) had clinically apparent heart disease, due in most cases to opportunistic infection or tumor.[20] Over a period of 3 years at San Francisco General Hospital, Rapaport found that of 1171 patients hospitalized with AIDS, 88 (7.5 percent) had an echocardiogram ordered because of suspicion of cardiac disease (personal communication). Fifty-two (59 percent) of the echocardiograms had at least one abnormality. Sixteen of the 88 (18 percent) had either left ventricular dilatation and/or left ventricular hypokinesis, and 26 of the 88 (30 percent) had pericardial effusion. There were no control subjects.

A recent study[24] reported the results of echocardiography in 151 HIV-seropositive patients collected prospectively, 92 percent of whom were men with a median age of 37 years. Seventy-three percent were homosexual men. Thirteen percent were intravenous drug users, 74 percent of whom were in Walter Reed stages IV to VI, a classification using T_4 helper cell counts and clinical data.[5,25] One hundred seven patients (71 percent) had normal echocardiograms. Echocardiographic abnormalities attributed to HIV infection were present in 31 patients (20 percent). There was an association of abnormal echocardiographic findings with advanced clinical stages of the disease. The mortality during follow-up was the same for those with normal echocardiograms (35 of 102) as for those with abnormal echocardiograms (12 of 29) (p = .48). Even in those with the most advanced clinical disease, there was no independent prognostic significance of the echocardiographic cardiac involvement, with 44 percent of both echo-normal and echo-abnormal patients dying. This study shows a remarkably low incidence of HIV-associated echocardiographic abnormalities, most often asymptomatic pericardial effusion.

These studies suggest that the prevalence of echocardiographic abnormalities in HIV-positive patients depends on the stage of their clinical illness, with the sickest patients having the most abnormalities.

PERICARDIAL INVOLVEMENT

In general, pericardial effusion and pericarditis is the most commonly recognized cardiac involvement in

AIDS. At autopsy, Kaposi's sarcoma involvement and lymphoma may be clinically silent, accompanied by asymptomatic pericardial effusion, or may be clinically important because of pericardial tamponade.[26] Pericarditis due to specific organisms has been frequently reported. These organisms are most commonly *Mycobacterium tuberculosis*[20,27] or *M. avium-intracellulare*.[21] One study[20] reported pericardial tamponade in five patients and large pericardial effusions in six. Of the patients with clinical heart disease in this study, 22 percent had echocardiographic evidence of tamponade, and another 33 percent had large pericardial effusions.

At San Francisco General Hospital (SFGH), there has been a similar experience. In a consecutive series of 88 in-hospital AIDS patients who had echocardiograms, 36 (41 percent) had normal echocardiograms, and the most common abnormality, seen in 26 (30 percent), was pericardial effusion. We have recognized a total of 25 patients with AIDS or PGL who have pericardial disease. Ten of these patients had pericardiocentesis, of whom 8 (32 percent) presented with tamponade, 2 had pericardial windows, and 1 died and was autopsied. Another 2 patients, who had neither pericardiocentesis nor pericardial windows died and were autopsied. No etiology was found on examination of either fluid or tissue in all 12 patients.

The etiology of pericardial effusion or pericarditis is not obvious; it may be HIV infection or other opportunistic viral infections with Coxsackie virus or cytomegalovirus. In one recent report of 14 AIDS patients with pericardial effusion, 10 (71 percent) had tamponade.[29] Of the 14 patients, 8 (57 percent) had suggestive evidence of mycobacterial disease. Occasionally pericarditis has been reported to be caused by common organisms such as *Staphylococcus*,[30] *Cryptococcus neoformans*,[31] or *Herpes simplex* virus.[32]

MYOCARDIAL INVOLVEMENT

For a number of years involvement of the pericardium and myocardium with both common and unusual opportunistic infections and neoplasms, such as Kaposi's sarcoma and lymphoma, has been recognized. At times this involvement appears to be incidental and associated with the presence of organisms in many tissues including the heart. Often this involvement is not accompanied by signs of cell necrosis or even inflammation. At other times the infection is accompanied by an intense myocarditis. Opportunistic infection has included viruses (*H. simplex*, cytomegalovirus, and Coxsackie virus), bacteria, protozoa (*Toxoplasma gondii*), and fungi (*Candida albicans*, *C. neoformans*, and *Aspergillus fumigatus*).[33,34] Diagnoses of these specific infections have been made at autopsy but also have been made during life with myocardial biopsy. The importance of identifying a specific organism as the cause of the myocarditis rests in the potential for treatment,[35] for instance, amphotericin B and flucytosine for cryptococcosis. Grange and colleagues[36] reported a case of *T. gondii* myocarditis in a 58-year-old man with AIDS that was treated successfully with pyrimethamine and clindamycin.

The most common neoplasms are Kaposi's sarcoma and lymphoma of the non-Hodgkin's type.[5,6,11] With Kaposi's sarcoma the tumor involvement of the myocardium or pericardium is most frequently an incidental finding. On occasion a diagnosis of myocardial involvement by lymphoma is made on needle biopsy of the myocardium.

One study reported a collection of 21 cases of lymphoma in AIDS patients, 3 Hodgkin's and 18 non-Hodgkin's lymphoma of various histologic types, almost all of which were in the high-grade categories.[37] Unfortunately, they tend to be histologically aggressive tumors involving many organs and responding poorly to treatment. At times the patient presents with pericardial tamponade or even superior vena cava syndrome.[38–40] Echocardiography revealing infiltration into the myocardium and/or myocardial or pericardial masses is most helpful in establishing a diagnosis.

CARDIOMYOPATHY

In 1986 Cohen and colleagues[41] reported three patients with AIDS who had clinical, echocardiographic, and morphologic findings of dilated cardiomyopathy. All patients had a decreased ejection fraction, and two had congestive heart failure. All three patients died, and two had findings at autopsy compatible with myocarditis resulting in cardiomyopathy. Microscopic examination in both showed focal collections of inflammatory cells together with myofibrilar atrophy and myocardial necrosis. A subsequent report described 58 consecutively autopsied patients.[42] Seven (12 percent) had major clinical cardiovascular abnormalities, including four with congestive heart failure and others with ventricular tachycardia. All were late in the course of their disease. All patients with these major clinical cardiac abnormalities had focal myocarditis at autopsy. The etiology in these cases was not obvious but was believed to be viral myocarditis.

In another study of 71 patients with AIDS, 8 had left ventricular dilatation and decreased contractility and 4 had congestive heart failure.[19] In a similar echocardiographic study none of 102 AIDS patients had congestive heart failure, although 41 percent had left ventricular hypokinesia.[22]

In autopsy studies reported in the literature, cardiac causes of death have been rare, and clinically the incidence of congestive heart failure has been extremely small, although microscopic focal myocarditis is frequently described. In 14 studies reported in the literature, 1009 patients with AIDS were reported. A total of 8 died of cardiac involvement. One had *Cryptococcus* myocarditis, one had toxoplasmosis myocarditis, and five came from one institution.[12]

Symptomatic cardiomyopathy in association with HIV-1 infection is apparently unusual; however, echocardiographic evidence of left ventricular dysfunction is more common, especially in patients who are the furthest along in the course of the HIV disease. Individual reports of one to five cases of patients with either dilated left ventricle, hypokinetic left ventricle, or both have been reported frequently enough to require explanation.[41,43,44] Furthermore, the occurrence of cardiomyopathy in children, in whom a disease unrelated to HIV infection would be rare, further suggests a relationship between HIV disease and cardiomyopathy.[45]

Possible Reasons for Cardiomyopathy

There are many theories of the etiology of the occasional patient with congestive heart failure with a dilated, poorly contracting left ventricle. These explanations may well be related also to the more frequently observed echocardiographic reduction in left ventricular function with or without left ventricular dilatation. The most frequently mentioned etiology is that of myocarditis or postmyocarditis cardiomyopathy. There are occasional reports of virus being grown from cardiac muscle. In 1987 Calabrese and colleagues[46] were the first to report the culturing of HIV from a right ventricular myocardial biopsy from a patient with a hypokinetic right ventricle and a normal left ventricle.

There is little evidence that HIV itself invades the myocardial cell. The myocyte has no CD4 receptors, which are the major way by which the virus enters the cell. Although there are other ways and possibly other receptors by which the virus could invade the cell, no one has convincingly shown the virus or a portion of the viral DNA or RNA within the genome of the myocardial cell. One recent study reported detecting HIV nucleic acid sequences by in situ hybridization in cardiac tissue sections from 6 of 22 patients examined who died of AIDS.[43] The hybridization target was thought to be myocytes, but this could not be proven by this technique. Furthermore, the myocardial cells showing the positive hybridization signal were sparse, comprising only one or a few cells per section; the myocardium was normal by light microscopy; and none of the patients had clinical evidence of cardiac disease.

Other Theories for the Development of Cardiomyopathy

Opportunistic Infections

Patients with AIDS are exposed to and susceptible to multiple bacterial, viral, mycotic, and protozoal infections. Epstein-Barr virus and cytomegalovirus are both known to cause myocarditis in AIDS patients.[48,49] *Cryptococcus neoformans* and *T. gondii* myocarditis have been well described.[35,36,50] Myocarditis due to *M. avium-intracellulare* has been reported.[7] *Aspergillus* endocarditis and myocarditis have been reported.[51]

Dilated Cardiomyopathy as a Postviral Disorder

The study of patients with myocarditis without AIDS has shown that the myocarditis can be precipitated by viral infection and that the inflammatory reaction can progress when the virus is no longer recoverable from either the heart or even the patient. The viral infection precipitates an immune reaction either to viral antigen that cross reacts with a myocardial protein or to altered myocardial protein, which acts as a foreign antigen, thus precipitating the immune reactions that continue the myocardial necrosis and inflammatory cell infiltration.[52]

The evidence that congestive cardiomyopathy is precipitated by a previous viral myocarditis includes the biopsy finding of inflammatory infiltrate in some patients with dilated cardiomyopathy[53,54] and detection of increased elevated viral antibody titers and viral-specific RNA sequences in myocardial biopsies.[55] Thus, the cardiomyopathy can result from a previous infection with a number of organisms that are no longer recoverable from the myocardium.

Impairment of the Immune Mechanism Leading to Cardiomyopathy

Humorally mediated autoimmune reactions involving antimyosin antibodies may also be implicated in the development of cardiomyopathy.[56] Circulating cardiac autoantibodies have been identified in four of six AIDS patients with cardiomyopathy and in none of the HIV-positive patients without cardiomyopathy. In situ hybridization with genomic probes failed to show evidence of HIV or any other viruses within the heart muscle. Results of ELISA showed a high titer of immunoglobulin G antibody to myosin and to cardiac mitochondrial adenine nucleotide. In this study it was concluded that the cardiomyopathy may be related not to HIV infection of the heart but rather to autoimmunity.

Role of Cytokines in Myocarditis

Ho and colleagues[57] proposed a primary role for neuroglial cell damage from the cytolytic effect of release of substances termed cytokines from HIV-infected monocytes, the so-called innocent bystander destruction mechanism. Cytokines are biologically active mediators and are soluble proteins released by immune cells. Reversible myocardial depression is well documented in human and canine septic shock.[58,59] This was subsequently demonstrated to be due to a "myocardial depressant factor."[60] The exact nature of this myocardial depressant factor is not agreed upon but could be related to a variety of mediators of sepsis: endotoxin, cytokines, tumor necrosis factor (TNF), and interleukin 2.[61]

Other studies showed that the administration of endotoxin-released TNF caused depression of left ventricular function independent of left ventricular volume or loading conditions,[62] and elevated circulating levels of TNF have been noted in patients with severe chronic heart failure.[63] Increased circulating levels of TNF have been noted in patients with advanced HIV-1 infection.[64] This finding is consistent with a finding of increased production of the cytokine TNF by peripheral myocytes of patients with AIDS.[65]

Cachexia

Many patients with AIDS have marked weight loss and cachexia. In patients with anorexia nervosa wall motion as assessed by 2-D echo Doppler was found to be abnormal in 8 of 14 patients but not in control subjects; also, lower stroke volume was found in patients compared to controls, possibly because of decreased heart size.[66] Starvation and refeeding studies in animals have demonstrated myofibrillar atrophy and cardiac interstitial edema, which is accompanied by a decrease in left ventricular compliance and decreased peak systolic force.[67] These changes are thought to be due to protein-calorie malnutrition. Congestive heart failure may occur, especially during refeeding and recovery.[68,69]

after 12.8 months of therapy has been reported.[79] This myopathy is characterized by abnormal mitochondria with paracrystalloid inclusions. Whether or not this can occur in cardiac muscle in some patients is not clear.

Vitamin and Selenium Deficiency States

Cachectic people can have vitamin deficiency states; it is doubtful if many patients with cardiomyopathy have this as a prime etiology. However, selenium deficiency has been described together with reduced cardiac selenium levels in AIDS, similar to Keshan's disease seen in Chinese with selenium deficiency. In one study 10 patients with AIDS who had decreased left ventricular fractional shortening on echocardiography received sodium selenite for 23 days.[70,71] Six of eight showed a return toward normal of left ventricular fractional shortening within 21 days. Selenium deficiency has been reported to be common in malnourished pediatric patients with AIDS.[72]

Drug-induced Cardiomyopathy

The effect of drugs, both recreational and therapeutic, on myocardial function is not well delineated in patients with AIDS. In most patients with AIDS and cardiomyopathy, however, drugs do not seem to be the cause;[43,73] nevertheless, in patients with AIDS, drugs such as doxorubicin, alpha$_2$ interferon, and interleuken 2 have been shown to produce cardiomyopathy that is sometimes reversible. Recombinant alpha$_2$ interferon–related cardiomyopathy in patients treated for primary renal cancer has been reported.[74] One report described three cases of reversible cardiac dysfunction associated with alpha interferon therapy in AIDS patients with Kaposi's sarcoma.[75]

Cocaine use has been associated with myocarditis and dilated cardiomyopathy, which occasionally has been reported to be reversible.[76] Pentamidine has been reported to cause ventricular tachycardia.[77]

The most common currently used drug in AIDS, zidovudine (AZT), a nucleoside analogue, is a drug that inhibits replication of HIV in vitro, probably by inhibiting the reverse transcriptase enzyme, which is essential to the replication of the retrovirus. No adverse cardiac effects have been reported in phase 1 clinical trials, and one study failed to show cardiotoxicity;[78] however, a toxic mitochondrial myopathy caused by long-term AZT

Conclusions

It is thus apparent that clinical heart muscle disease and heart failure in AIDS is unusual. When it occurs, there may be explanations other than direct infection with HIV. The exact incidence of heart muscle disease in AIDS is as yet unknown but must be small, and the mechanisms that can cause failure are probably multiple.

CARDIOVASCULAR SURGERY IN AIDS PATIENTS

There has been an increased interest in the danger to the AIDS health care worker of becoming infected or of infecting patients and in the possibility of accelerating the disease through surgery. The problem is illustrated by the following questions:

1. Are we doing an expensive procedure that will cause prolonged hospitalization and probably not affect the outcome in AIDS patients?
2. What is the risk of accelerating the disease by surgery?
3. What is the risk of HIV infection to health care workers?
4. What is the risk of getting HIV infection during open heart surgery?

In general it is not wise to do expensive procedures with some degree of morbidity and mortality that result in prolonged hospitalization in patients with a limited lifespan due to their underlying disease. For this reason patients with AIDS should not be subjected to surgery that will most probably not significantly affect their survival. It is probable that 70 percent of patients found to have AIDS will die within 3 to 4 years of the diagnosis.[80] On the other hand, if patients with AIDS have medically uncontrollable symptoms, invasive procedures that can ameliorate these symptoms may be indicated.

The most frequent problem in which the question of cardiovascular surgery arises in a relatively young age subgroup is in the intravenous drug user with infective endocarditis and congestive heart failure. The presence of HIV disease in these patients, who overall have poor results from surgery, would mitigate for the patient's being treated medically for as long as possible.

HIV-positive patients and patients with PGL who have not had an opportunistic infection or cancer can have a prolonged course over many years and, in general, should be treated like patients without HIV disease. In this subgroup cardiovascular surgery should be considered for the usual indications.

The possibility that the progression of the HIV disease is accelerated by the immunologic challenge that occurs from cardiopulmonary bypass is largely unanswered. Instances of HIV-positive patients who developed AIDS shortly after open heart surgery have been reported. It is known that cardiopulmonary bypass produces temporary depression of phagocytic function and immune globulin production.[81] Cardiopulmonary bypass per se in HIV-negative patients causes prolonged abnormalities in the T_4/T_8 ratio up to 6 days postoperatively.[82] There is, therefore, a basis for concern that cardiopulmonary bypass surgery could accelerate the progression of HIV disease, and this must be taken into consideration.

Whether or not all patients undergoing cardiovascular surgery or other invasive procedures should have HIV testing is a matter of heated debate. Although the risk to health care personnel is small, HIV infection is usually tantamount to fatal infection; fear is great among both health care workers and the public. On the other hand, AIDS is an emotional subject, and patients who are known to be HIV positive may be subject to prejudice and discrimination. At present, HIV testing of both health care workers and patients is voluntary; however, there are proposed recommendations requiring disclosure to patients that a health care worker is HIV positive and informed consent from the patient before any invasive procedure is done. At present, there is only one instance of an HIV-positive dentist infecting five patients, probably from reuse of inadequately sterilized instruments. This matter is still under considerable debate.

Because of this risk, some cardiovascular surgeons and cardiologists are refusing to operate on or catheterize an HIV-positive person or a patient who will not allow an HIV test to be done. A survey was done of the attitudes of cardiac surgeons in the United States concerning operating on HIV-positive patients.[83] More than half responded, and two-thirds of these would perform open heart surgery on HIV-positive patients no matter how they had acquired their HIV infection. A quarter of the surgeons would not operate no matter how the HIV infection was acquired, and the rest were uncertain. Once the patient has gone from the HIV carrier state to AIDS, two-thirds of the cardiac surgeons would not operate. Ninety percent of those responding want to be able to test all their patients for HIV status.

The physician's fear of becoming infected with HIV is understandable, but like other professions that have personal dangers, the profession of the physician requires performance. Both the American College of Physicians and the American Medical Association currently have standards that state that a physician may not ethically refuse to treat a patient solely because he or she is HIV positive.

As of 1990, the literature has reported 18 health care workers who had no other risk factors and were known to be HIV negative at exposure who have seroconverted after exposure. The danger to health care personnel is greatest when exposure to blood and the chance of accidental needle or knife perforation or blood splash into the eyes or mouth are greatest. In one prospective study of 1307 consecutive procedures, accumulated exposure, parenteral or cutaneous, occurred in only 84 procedures (6.4 percent).[84] Parenteral exposure occurred in 1.7 percent. Knowledge of the patient's HIV status or awareness of the patient's high-risk status for such infection did not appear to influence the rate of exposure, suggesting that preoperative testing for HIV infection would not decrease the frequency of accidental exposure to blood.

In combined data from 14 prospective studies of the risk of HIV-1 transmission to health care workers, there were 2042 parenteral exposures in 1948 subjects. The chance of seroconversion was 0.29 percent per exposure (95 percent confidence interval, 0.13 to 0.7 percent), and in 668 people with 1051 total mucous membrane exposures there were no seroconversions (95 percent confidence limits, upper bound is 0.28 percent per exposure). The risk of a health care worker developing HIV seroconversion from work-related activities was very low, approximately one infection in 300 documented exposures to HIV-positive blood.[85]

REFERENCES

1. Centers for Disease Control: Classification system for human T-lymphotropic virus type III/lymphadenopathy-associated virus infections. *MMWR* 1986; 35:334–339.
2. Bacchetti P, Moss AR: Incubation period of AIDS in San Francisco (letter). *Nature* 1989; 338:251–253.
3. Lifson A, Hessol N, Rutherford GW, Buchbinder S, O'Malley P, Cannon L, et al: The natural history of HIV infection in a cohort of homosexual and bisexual men: Clinical manifestations, 1978–1989 (abstr). *Int Conf AIDS, Montreal* 1989; 5:60(T.A.O. 32).
4. Osmond D: Progression to AIDS in persons testing seropositive for antibody to HIV. In: Cohen PT, Sande MA, Volberding PA, (eds): *The AIDS Knowledge Base.* Waltham, MA, Medical Publishing Group, 1990: 1.1.6.
5. Silver MA, Macher AM, Reichert CM, Levens DL, Parrillo JE, Longo DL, et al: Cardiac involvement by Kaposi's sarcoma in acquired immune deficiency syndrome (AIDS). *Am J Cardiol* 1984; 53:983–985.
6. Welch K, Finkbeiner W, Alpers CE, Blumenfeld W, Davis RL, Smuckler EA, et al: Autopsy findings in the acquired immune deficiency syndrome. *J Am Med Assoc* 1984; 252:1152–1159.
7. Cammarosano C, Lewis W: Cardiac lesions in acquired immune deficiency syndrome (AIDS). *J Am Coll Cardiol* 1985; 5:703–706.
8. Roldan EO, Moskowitz L, Hensly GT: Pathology of the heart in acquired immunodeficiency syndrome. *Arch Pathol Lab Med* 1987; 111:943–946.
9. Wilkes MS, Fortin AH, Felix JC, Godwin TA, Thompson WG: Value of necropsy in acquired immunodeficiency syndrome. *Lancet* 1988; 2(8602):85–88.
10. Baroldi G, Corallo S, Moroni M, Repossini A, Mutinelli MR, Lazzarin A, et al: Focal lymphocytic myocarditis in acquired immunodeficiency syndrome (AIDS): A correlative morphologic and clinical study in 26 consecutive fatal cases. *J Am Coll Cardiol* 1988; 12:463–469.
11. Lewis W: AIDS: Cardiac findings from 115 autopsies. *Prog Cardiovasc Dis* 1989; 32:207–215.
12. Anderson DW, Virmani R, Reilly JM, O'Leary T, Cunnion RE, Robinowitz M, et al: Prevalent myocarditis at necropsy in the acquired immunodeficiency syndrome. *J Am Coll Cardiol* 1988; 11:792–799.
13. Magno J, Margaretten W, Cheitlin M: Myocardial involvement in acquired immunodeficiency syndrome: Incidence in a large autopsy study (abstr), *Circulation* 1988; 78(Suppl II):II–459.
14. Garcia I, Fainstein V, Rios A, Luna M, Mansell P, Reuben J, et al: Nonbacterial thrombotic endocarditis in a male homosexual with Kaposi's sarcoma. *Arch Intern Med* 1983; 143:1243–1244.
15. Moskowitz L, Hensley GT, Chan JC, Adams K: Immediate causes of death in acquired immunodeficiency syndrome. *Arch Pathol Lab Med* 1985; 109:735–738.
16. Murray JF, Garay SM, Hopewell PC, Mills J, Snider GL, Stover DE: Pulmonary complications of the acquired immunodeficiency syndrome: An update: Report of the second National Heart, Lung and Blood Institute workshop. *Am Rev Resp Dis* 1987; 135:504–509.
17. Fink L, Reichek N, St. John Sutton MG: Cardiac abnormalities in acquired immune deficiency syndrome. *Am J Cardiol* 1984; 54:1161–1163.
18. Kinney EL, Brafman D, Wright RJ II: Echocardiographic findings in patients with acquired immunodeficiency syndrome (AIDS) and AIDS-related complex (ARC). *Cathet Cardiovasc Diag* 1989; 16:182–185.
19. Himelman RB, Chung WS, Chernoff DN, Schiller NB, Hollander H: Cardiac manifestations of human immunodeficiency virus infection: A two-dimensional echocardiographic study. *J Am Coll Cardiol* 1989; 13:1030–1036.
20. Monsuez JJ, Kinney EL, Vittecoq D, Kitzis M, Rozenbaum W, d'Agay MF, et al: Comparison among acquired immune deficiency syndrome patients with and without clinical evidence of cardiac disease. *Am J Cardiol* 1988; 62:1311–1313.
21. Levy WS, Simon GL, Rios JC, Ross AM: Prevalence of cardiac abnormalities in human immunodeficiency virus infection. *Am J Cardiol* 1989; 63:86–89.
22. Corallo S, Mutinelli MR, Moroni M, Lazzarin A, Celano V, Repossini A, et al: Echocardiography detects myocardial damage in AIDS: Prospective study in 102 patients. *Eur Heart J* 1988; 9:887–892.
23. Hecht SR, Berger M, Van Tosh A, Croxson S: Unsuspected cardiac abnormalities in the acquired immune deficiency syndrome: An echocardiographic study. *Chest* 1989; 96:805–808.
24. Steffen HM, Müller R, Schrappe-Bächer M, Salzberger B, Fätkenheuer G, Wagner-Klein S, et al: Prevalence of echocardiographic abnormalities in human immunodeficiency virus 1 infection. *Am J Noninvas Cardiol* 1991; 5:280–284.
25. Redfield RR, Wright DC, Tramont EC: The Walter Reed staging

classification for HTLV-III/LAV infection: Special report. *N Engl J Med* 1986; 314:131–132.

26. Steigman CK, Anderson DW, Macher AM, Sennesh JD, Virmani R: Fatal cardiac tamponade in acquired immunodeficiency syndrome with epicardial Kaposi's sarcoma. *Am Heart J* 1988; 116:1105–1107.
27. D'Cruz IA, Sengupta EE, Abrahams C, Reddy HK, Turlapati RV: Cardiac involvement, including tuberculous pericardial effusion, complicating acquired immune deficiency syndrome. *Am Heart J* 1986; 112:1100–1102.
28. Woods GL, Goldsmith JC: Fatal pericarditis due to *Mycobacterium avium-intracellulare* in acquired immunodeficiency syndrome. *Chest* 1989; 95:1355–1357.
29. Reynolds M, Berger M, Hecht S, Kolokathis A, Horowitz SF: Large pericardial effusions associated with the acquired immune deficiency syndrome (AIDS) (abstr). *J Am Coll Cardiol* 1991; 17:221A.
30. Stechel RP, Cooper DJ, Greenspan J, Pizzarello RA, Tenenbaum MJ: Staphylococcal pericarditis in a homosexual patient with AIDS-related complex. *NY State J Med* 1986; 86:592–593.
31. Brivet F, Livartowski J, Herve P, Rain B, Dormont J: Pericardial cryptococcal disease in acquired immune deficiency syndrome (letter). *Am J Med* 1987; 82:1273.
32. Freedberg RS, Gindea AJ, Dieterich DT, Greene JB: Herpes simplex pericarditis in AIDS. *NY State J Med* 1987; 87:304–306.
33. Francis CK: Cardiac involvement in AIDS. *Curr Probl Cardiol* 1990; 15:571–639.
34. Zuger A, Louie E, Holzman RS, Simberkoff MS, Rahal JJ: Cryptococcal disease in patients with the acquired immunodeficiency syndrome: Diagnostic features and outcome of treatment: Clinical review. *Ann Intern Med* 1986; 104:234–240.
35. Kinney EL, Monsuez JJ, Kitzis M, Vittecoq D: Treatment of AIDS-associated heart disease. *Angiology* 1989; 40:970–976.
36. Grange F, Kinney EL, Monsuez JJ, Rybojad M, Derouin F, Khuong MA, et al: Successful therapy for *Toxoplasma gondii* myocarditis in acquired immunodeficiency syndrome. *Am Heart J* 1990; 120:443–444.
37. Ioachim HL, Cooper MC, Hellman GC: Lymphomas in men at high risk for acquired immune deficiency syndrome (AIDS): A study of 21 cases. *Cancer* 1985: 56:2831–2842.
38. Lloyd EA, Curcio CA: Lymphoma of the heart as an unusual cause of pericardial effusion: A case report. *S Afr Med J* 1980; 58:937–939.
39. Levitt LJ, Ault KA, Pinkus GS, Sloss LJ, McManus BM: Pericarditis and early cardiac tamponade as a primary manifestation of lymphosarcoma cell leukemia. *Am J Med* 1979; 67:719–723.
40. Goldfarb A, King CL, Rosenzweig BP, Feit F, Kamat BR, Rumancik WM, et al: Cardiac lymphoma in the acquired immunodeficiency syndrome. *Am Heart J* 1989; 118:1340–1344.
41. Cohen IS, Anderson DW, Virmani R, Reen BM, Macher AM, Sennesh J, et al: Congestive cardiomyopathy in association with the acquired immunodeficiency syndrome. *N Engl J Med* 1986; 315:628–630.
42. Reilly JM, Cunnion RE, Anderson DW, O'Leary TJ, Simmons JT, Lane HC, et al: Frequency of myocarditis, left ventricular dysfunction and ventricular tachycardia in the acquired immune deficiency syndrome. *Am J Cardiol* 1988; 62:789–793.
43. Kaminski HJ, Katzman M, Wiest PM, Enler JJ, Gifford DR, Rackley R, et al: Cardiomyopathy associated with the acquired immune deficiency syndrome. *J Acq Immune Defic Synd* 1988; 1:105–110.
44. Corboy JR, Fink L, Miller WT: Congestive cardiomyopathy in association with AIDS. *Radiology* 1987; 165:139–141.
45. Lipshultz SE, Chanock S, Sanders SP, Colan SD, Perez-Atayde A, McIntosh K: Cardiovascular manifestations of human immunodeficiency virus infection in infants and children. *Am J Cardiol* 1989; 63:1489–1497.
46. Calabrese LH, Proffitt MR, Yen-Lieberman B, Hobbs RE, Ratliff NB: Congestive cardiomyopathy and illness related to the acquired immunodeficiency syndrome (AIDS) associated with isolation of retrovirus from myocardium. *Ann Intern Med* 1987; 107:691–692.
47. Grody WW, Cheng L, Lewis W: Infection of the heart by the human immunodeficiency virus. *Am J Cardiol* 1990; 66:203–206.
48. Lafont A, Marche C, Wolff M, Perronne C, Witchitz S, Régnier B, et al: Myocarditis in acquired immunodeficiency syndrome (AIDS): Etiology and progress (abstr). *J Am Coll Cardiol* 1988; 11:196A.
49. Stewart JM, Kaul A, Gromisch DS, Reyes E, Woolf PK, Gowitz MH: Symptomatic cardiac dysfunction in children with human immunodeficiency virus infection. *Am Heart J* 1989; 117:140–144.
50. Acierno LJ: Cardiac complications in acquired immunodeficiency syndrome (AIDS): A review. *J Am Coll Cardiol* 1989; 13:1144–1154.
51. Cox JN, di Dió F, Pizzolato GP, Lerch R, Pochon N: *Aspergillus* endocarditis and myocarditis in a patient with the acquired immunodeficiency syndrome (AIDS): A review of the literature: Case report. *Virchows Archiv A (Pathological Anatomy and Histopathology)* 1990; 417:255–259.
52. Lowry PJ, Thompson RA, Littler WA: Cellular immunity in congestive cardiomyopathy: The normal cellular immune response. *Br Heart J* 1985; 53:394–399.
53. Zee-Cheng CS, Tsai CC, Palmer DC, Codd JE, Pennington DG, Williams GA: High incidence of myocarditis by endomyocardial biopsy in patients with idiopathic congestive cardiomyopathy. *J Am Coll Cardiol* 1984; 3:63–70.
54. Parrillo JE, Aretz HT, Palacios I, Fallon JT, Block PC: The results of transvenous endomyocardial biopsy can frequently be used to diagnose myocardial diseases in patients with idiopathic heart failure: Endomyocardial biopsy in 100 consecutive patients revealed a substantial incidence of myocarditis. *Circulation* 1984; 69:93–101.
55. Bowles NE, Richardson PJ, Olsen EGJ, Archard LC: Detection of Coxsackie-B-virus-specific RNA sequences in myocardial biopsy samples from patients with myocarditis and dilated cardiomyopathy. *Lancet* 1984; 1(8490):1120–1123.
56. Herskowitz A, Ansari AA, Neumann DA, Beschorner WE, Oliveira M, Chaisson RE, et al: Cardiomyopathy in acquired immunodeficiency syndrome: Evidence for autoimmunity (abstr). *Circulation* 1989; 80(Suppl II):II-322.
57. Ho DD, Pomerantz RJ, Kaplan JC: Pathogenesis of infection with human immunodeficiency virus. *N Engl J Med* 1987; 317:278–286.
58. Parker MM, Shelhamer JH, Bacharach SL, Green MV, Natanson C, Frederick TM, et al: Profound but reversible myocardial depression in patients with septic shock. *Ann Intern Med* 1984; 100:483–490.
59. Natanson C, Fink MP, Ballantyne HK, MacVittie TJ, Conklin JJ, Parrillo JE: Gram-negative bacteremia produces both severe systolic and diastolic cardiac dysfunction in a canine model that simulates human septic shock. *J Clin Invest* 1986; 78:259–270.
60. Parrillo JE, Burch C, Shelhamer JH, Parker MM, Natanson C, Schuette W: A circulating myocardial depressant substance in humans with septic shock: Septic shock patients with a reduced ejection fraction have a circulating factor that depresses *in vitro* myocardial cell performance. *J Clin Invest* 1985; 76:1539–1553.
61. Cunnion RE, Parrillo JE: Myocardial dysfunction in sepsis: Recent insights (editorial). *Chest* 1989; 95:941–945.
62. Suffredini AF, Fromm RE, Parker MM, Brenner M, Kovacs JA, Wesley RA, et al: The cardiovascular response of normal humans to the administration of endotoxin. *N Engl J Med* 1989; 321:280–287.
63. Levine B, Kalman J, Mayer L, Fillit HM, Packer M: Elevated circulating levels of tumor necrosis factor in severe chronic heart failure. *N Engl J Med* 1990; 323:236–241.
64. Lähdevirta J, Maury CPJ, Teppo AM, Repo H: Elevated levels of circulating cachectin/tumor necrosis factor in patients with acquired immunodeficiency syndrome. *Am J Med* 1988; 85:289–291.
65. Wright SC, Jewett A, Mitsuyasu R, Bonavida B: Spontaneous cytotoxicity and tumor necrosis factor production by peripheral blood monocytes from AIDS patients. *J Immunol* 1988; 141:99–104.
66. Goldberg SJ, Comerci GD, Feldman L: Cardiac output and regional myocardial contraction in anorexia nervosa. *J Adolesc Health Care* 1988; 9:15–21.
67. Abel RM, Grimes JB, Alonso D, Alonso M, Gay WA Jr: Adverse hemodynamic and ultrastructural changes in dog hearts subjected to protein-calorie malnutrition. *Am Heart J* 1979; 97:733–744.
68. Heymsfield SB, Bethel RA, Ansley JD, Gibbs DM, Felner JM, Nutter DO: Cardiac abnormalities in cachectic patients before and during nutritional repletion. *Am Heart J* 1978; 95:584–594.
69. Schocken DD, Holloway JD, Powers PS: Weight loss and the heart:

Effects of anorexia nervosa and starvation. *Arch Intern Med* 1989; 149:877–881.
70. Dworkin BM, Antonecchia PP, Smith F, Weiss L, Davidian M, Rubin D, et al: Reduced cardiac selenium content in the acquired immunodeficiency syndrome. *J Parenter Enter Nutr* 1989; 13:644–647.
71. Zazzo JF, Chalas J, Lafont A, Camus F, Chappuis P: Is nonobstructive cardiomyopathy in AIDS a selenium deficiency–related disease? (letter). *J Parenter Enter Nutr* 1988; 12:537–538.
72. Kavanaugh-McHugh A, Rowe S, Benjamin Y, Hutton N, Modin J, Ruff A, et al: Selenium deficiency and cardiomyopathy in malnourished pediatric AIDS patients (abstr). *Int Conf AIDS, Montreal* 1989; 5:329(T.B.P.256).
73. Kaul S, Fishbein MC, Siegel RJ: Cardiac manifestations of acquired immune deficiency syndrome: A 1991 update. *Am Heart J* 1991; 122:535–544.
74. Cohen MC, Huberman MS, Nesto RW: Recombinant alpha$_2$ interferon–related cardiomyopathy. *Am J Med* 1988; 85:549–551.
75. Deyton LR, Walker RE, Kovacs JA, Herpin B, Parker M, Masur H, et al: Reversible cardiac dysfunction associated with interferon alfa therapy in AIDS patients with Kaposi's sarcoma. *N Engl J Med* 1989; 321:1246–1249.
76. Chokshi SK, Moore R, Pandian NG, Isner JM: Reversible cardiomyopathy associated with cocaine intoxication. *Ann Intern Med* 1989; 111:1039–1040.
77. Wharton JM, Demopulos PA, Goldschlager N: Torsade de pointes during administration of pentamidine isethionate. *Am J Med* 1987; 83:571–576.
78. Richman DD, Fischl MA, Grieco MH, Gottlieb MS, Volberding PA, Laskin OL, et al: The toxicity of azidothymidine (AZT) in the treatment of patients with AIDS and AIDS-related complex: A double-blind, placebo-controlled trial. *N Engl J Med* 1987; 317:192–197.
79. Dalakas MC, Illa I, Pezeshkpour GH, Laukaitis JP, Cohen B, Griffin JL: Mitochondrial myopathy caused by long-term zidovudine therapy. *N Engl J Med* 1990; 322:1098–1105.
80. Centers for Disease Control: Acquired immunodeficiency syndrome—United States: update. *MMWR* 1986; 35:17–21.
81. Utley JR: The immune response. In: *Pathophysiology and Techniques of Cardiopulmonary Bypass,* vol 1. Baltimore, Williams & Wilkins, 1982: 132–144.
82. Pollock R, Ames F, Rubio P, Jones J, Reuben J, Wong W, et al: Protracted severe immune dysregulation induced by cardiopulmonary bypass: A predisposing etiologic factor in blood transfusion–related AIDS? *J Clin Lab Immunol* 1987; 22:1–5.
83. Condit D, Frater RWM: Human immunodeficiency virus and the cardiac surgeon: A survey of attitudes. *Ann Thorac Surg* 1989; 47:182–186.
84. Gerberding JL, Littell C, Tarkington A, Brown A, Schecter WP: Risk of exposure of surgical personnel to patients' blood during surgery at San Francisco General Hospital. *N Engl J Med* 1990; 322:1788–1793.
85. Henderson DK, Fahey BJ, Willy M, Schmitt JM, Carey K, Koziol DE, et al: Risk for occupational transmission of human immunodeficiency virus type 1 (HIV-1) associated with clinical exposures: A prospective evaluation. *Ann Intern Med* 1990; 113:740–746.

Chapter 108

The Heart and Kidney Disease

Deepak Kikeri, M.D. ■ *William E. Mitch, M.D.*

Cardiovascular disease is a major cause of morbidity and death in chronic dialysis patients.[1] Over 50 percent of deaths in patients in the European Dialysis and Transplant Registry were caused by cardiovascular disease; cardiac events accounted for 41.5 percent of deaths.[2] The cardiovascular mortality rate in end-stage renal disease (ESRD) patients is approximately three times higher than in nonuremic, age-matched subjects without kidney disease.[3]

Specific risk factors for cardiovascular morbidity in dialysis patients include the high prevalence of hypertension and diabetes mellitus, hyperlipidemia, hypotension during hemodialysis, and abnormalities in calcium and phosphate metabolism leading to hyperparathyroidism and vascular calcification. In addition, pericardial disease, infective endocarditis, and fluid and electrolyte disturbances can contribute significantly to cardiac dysfunction in ESRD.

CARDIOVASCULAR RISK FACTORS IN UREMIC PATIENTS

Systemic Arterial Hypertension

The majority of patients (80 to 90 percent) with ESRD develop systemic hypertension before beginning dialysis therapy. An expanded extracellular fluid volume (ECV)[4,5] and vasoconstriction mediated by the renin-angiotensin axis[5–9] likely play major roles in the pathogenesis of hypertension in patients with ESRD.

Hypertension due to sodium retention and ECV expansion in ESRD is associated with an increased cardiac output and/or increased total peripheral vascular resistance.[10] This is a different pattern from that of hypertensive subjects with normal renal function who usually have a normal cardiac output and a high peripheral resistance (see Chap. 75). The difference may be related to the anemia of ESRD, which causes a secondary increase in cardiac output.

Direct evidence that ECV expansion plays a critical role in the pathogenesis of hypertension of chronic renal failure (CRF) is found in studies demonstrating rapid resolution of hypertension in most patients after ECV is reduced substantially by vigorous dialysis.[5,6,11,12] Still, there is a small group (10 to 20 percent) of dialysis patients who exhibit dialysis-resistant hypertension. These patients have higher levels of plasma renin activity and the control of their hypertension may require bilateral nephrectomy. Even in this group, drugs inhibiting the renin-angiotensin axis can control hypertension, implicating the renin system in the pathogenesis of dialysis-resistant hypertension.[5,11–13] Interestingly, blood pressure in patients with dialysis-resistant hypertension may become sensitive to changes in ECV after bilateral nephrectomy[5,6,12] (see below).

The mechanisms for arterial vasoconstriction may be more complicated than activation of the renin system alone. For example, it has been proposed that a circulating inhibitor of Na:K-ATPase is important in mediating increased peripheral vascular resistance. In this scheme, inhibitors of the sodium pump cause an increase in intracellular sodium, which leads to an increase in intracellular calcium in vascular smooth muscle cells.[14,15] The increase in calcium stimulates vascular contraction.

Plasma levels of atrial natriuretic peptide (ANP), a vasodilator released in response to ECV expansion,[16,17] are increased in dialysis patients. The high level is rapidly reduced by decreasing ECV with dialysis.[15,18,19] Consequently, an inappropriately low ANP release in dialysis patients cannot be the cause of hypertension in ESRD.

The cornerstone of managing hypertension in dialysis patients is reducing the ECV effectively. This will require vigorous ultrafiltration during hemodialysis to obtain a true dry weight. The most common reason for *dialysis-resistant* hypertension is ECV expansion from inadequate ultrafiltration.

In patients who have persistent hypertension despite achieving dry weight, antihypertensive medications that inhibit the renin-angiotensin axis [beta blockers or angiotensin converting enzyme (ACE) inhibitors] would appear to be the logical choice because of the involvement of the renin system in the pathogenesis of hypertension. Other antihypertensive medications, including calcium channel blockers and minoxidil, can be effective in dialysis patients provided the ECV is reduced. The dosage of antihypertensive drugs should be adjusted for the degree of renal failure; generally, the drugs are withheld on the day of hemodialysis to prevent hypotension from occurring as ECV is reduced.

Bilateral nephrectomy is rarely necessary to treat dialysis-resistant hypertension. In fact, bilateral nephrectomy should be avoided because of the loss of residual renal function, a worsening of anemia, and potentially, more severe renal osteodystrophy. The most common reason for persistent hypertension is inadequate fluid removal and/or poor compliance in taking antihypertensive medications.

Diabetes Mellitus

Approximately 30 percent of all CRF patients who begin maintenance dialysis therapy are diabetic and have a significantly higher mortality rate than age-matched, nondiabetic patients. The most significant factor contributing to the high death rate in diabetic dialysis patients is coronary artery disease.[20,21] (See also Chap. 102.)

Hyperlipidemia

To document the status of plasma lipids, samples should be obtained after a 12-h fast and before the patient is given heparin during dialysis. Approximately 50 percent of patients with ESRD have high serum levels of triglycerides and low levels of high-density lipoprotein cholesterol.[22,23] Impaired degradation of very low density lipoprotein by lipoprotein lipase appears to be a major mechanism for the development of hypertriglyceridemia.[24–26] In patients treated by peritoneal dialysis, the high concentrations of glucose in the dialysate complicate the interpretation of serum triglycerides because glucose is converted to triglycerides.

Other factors that may contribute to hyperlipidemia in ESRD include the use of diuretics and beta blockers,[27–29] the use of acetate-buffered dialysis solutions[30] or a high glucose concentration in the dialysate,[31] and possibly, carnitine deficiency.[32] Heparin given to prevent clotting in the dialyzer will cause a transient fall in serum triglycerides by increasing the activity of lipoprotein lipase.[33–35] The change is transient, however, and during nondialysis periods serum triglycerides are high.

At present, there is no definite evidence that lowering plasma triglycerides improves survival.[36] Strategies for lowering triglycerides and low-density lipoprotein (LDL) cholesterol include restricting dietary fat, fish oil supplements, exercise, and avoiding alcohol or treatment with beta blockers or diuretics[37–42] (see Chap. 53). Clofibrate or gemfibrozil, among other drugs, may be effective but have been associated with the development of myositis and hepatotoxicity in dialysis patients (see Chap. 65). This makes it especially important to adjust the dosage for the degree of renal failure. Definitive evidence that treatment with antihyperlipidemic drugs prevents atherosclerosis in dialysis patients is lacking.

Hemodialysis-Associated Hypotension

Clinically significant hypotension occurs in approximately 25 percent of hemodialysis sessions.[43] In most cases, the consequences are minor, but acute myocardial and cerebral ischemia has been reported.

A common cause of hypotension during dialysis is excessive ultrafiltration leading to ECV depletion, decreased venous return, and cardiac output.[44] Moreover, rapid lowering of plasma osmolality as urea and other molecules are removed causes a shift of ECV to the intracellular compartment because these molecules do not move out of cells as rapidly as dialysis removes them from blood.[45,46] Finally, diffusion of solutes can also result in vasodilatation, which can interfere with the hemodynamic adaptation to reduced ECV.[47]

An important factor governing changes in plasma osmolality is the concentration of sodium in the dialysate. In the past, dialysates with a low sodium concentration was used to control hypertension. More efficient dialyzers now achieve higher rates of fluid removal (ultrafiltration) so higher concentrations of sodium in the dialysate can be used. This practice has reduced the number of hypotensive episodes.[48]

Until recently, acetate was used almost exclusively as the buffer in dialysate solutions. Unfortunately, acetate can impair blood pressure regulation because it is a powerful arterial vasodilator[49]; acetate can also cause hypoventilation and hypoxemia.[50] Currently, bicarbonate-based dialysate solutions are widely used and the ill-effects of acetate are infrequent.

Bioincompatibility of dialyzer membranes can activate the complement cascade and cause pulmonary shunting and hypoxemia. This is most often observed with cuprophane membranes and may be an important cause of hypotension during dialysis.[51] Newer dialysis membranes without cuprophane appear to cause less activation of the complement cascade.[52] Another cause of hypotension and, rarely, anaphylaxis is hypersensitivity to ethylene oxide, which is used to sterilize dialyzers.[53,54]

Other factors can increase the tendency toward hemodialysis hypotension: (1) cardiac dysfunction from longstanding hypertension, ischemic or valvular heart disease, other causes of cardiomyopathy, or pericardial tamponade; (2) changes in serum potassium and calcium causing decreased contractile force; (3) autonomic neuropathy (particularly in diabetic patients); (4) sepsis; (5) occult hemorrhage (e.g., retroperitoneal hemorrhage after femoral vein catheterization); and (6) use of antihypertensive medications on the day of dialysis.

To reduce the incidence of hypotension, a high-sodium, bicarbonate-buffered dialysate should be tried and the rate and extent of ultrafiltration monitored carefully. Antihypertensive medications should be avoided on hemodialysis days. Occasionally, switching from cuprophane to noncuprophane dialyzers or from dialyzers sterilized with gamma irradiation instead of ethylene oxide may be necessary, especially when complement activation or ethylene oxide allergy is believed to cause the hypotension. Management of hypotension usually includes reducing the ultrafiltration rate, placing the patient in the Trendelenburg position, and administering saline through the arteriovenous access. Oxygen administration may be useful in patients with ischemic heart disease.

Hyperparathyroidism

Secondary hyperparathyroidism is almost universal in dialysis patients. Hyperphosphatemia caused by failure to excrete dietary phosphates plays a major role in the pathogenesis of secondary hyperparathyroidism.[55] The mechanism for the effects of hyperphosphatemia includes a reduction in plasma-ionized calcium from direct complexing of calcium with phosphates. There also is reduced intestinal calcium absorption from binding of dietary calcium by phosphates in intestinal fluid plus decreased activity of 1α hydroxylase in proximal tubule cells leading to limited production of 1,25-dihydroxyvitamin D_3.[56] All of these factors reduce the level of ionized calcium and stimulate parathyroid hormone (PTH) secretion. There also is evidence that the ability of ionized calcium to regulate PTH secretion is abnormal in ESRD patients. This effect is most likely related to 1,25-dihydroxyvitamin D_3 deficiency.[57,58]

Unfortunately, many dialysis patients have an increased serum calcium X phosphate product (i.e., above 60 mg^2/dL^2). Morbidity in these patients includes vascular and soft-tissue calcification.[59–62] Calcification can occur in coronary and peripheral arteries[63] and in the myocardium.[64,65] Finally, it has been proposed that PTH can directly impair myocardial function,[66] but not all investigators agree.[67]

Prevention or treatment of secondary hyperparathyroidism is based on correcting hyperphosphatemia. This can be accomplished only if patients adhere to a diet containing less than 800 mg phosphorus per day. Generally, patients also need to take phosphate binders with meals. Calcium carbonate or acetate are the preferred agents, because they avoid the risk of aluminum toxicity (including osteomalacia, anemia, and encephalopathy). Although magnesium hydroxide is also effective, it is not used because of the risk of developing hypermagnesemia. Once hyperphosphatemia is corrected, a supplement of calcium is given to raise the total daily calcium intake above 1500 mg. At this level, neutral or positive calcium balance can be achieved.[68] If hypocalcemia persists and especially if there is evidence of secondary hyperparathyroidism, intravenous administration of 1,25-dihydroxyvitamin D_3 (calcitriol) can be used therapeutically. Vitamin D can also be given orally, but the risk of hypercalcemia is greater.

Just as it is rarely necessary to perform bilateral nephrectomy, subtotal parathyroidectomy also is rarely needed because severe hyperparathyroidism can be avoided. Prevention is emphasized not only to avoid surgery but also because hypocalcemia after parathyroidectomy is a serious problem. The patients usually must take so many calcium and vitamin D tablets that compliance is rare.

ISCHEMIC HEART DISEASE

Many studies have shown that coronary artery disease is a major cause of death in dialysis patients. It accounts for approximately 10 percent of the total mortality.[2,69,70] Risk factors for coronary artery disease include smoking, hypertension, type I or II diabetes mellitus, hyperlipidemia, and hyperparathyroidism.[71–74] (See also Chap. 62.) In addition, factors such as hypertension, ECV overload, anemia, hypotension and hypoxia during hemodialysis, and the arteriovenous fistula can adversely affect the balance between myocardial oxygen supply and demand. In one study, electrocardiographic changes of ischemia occurred during exercise in approximately 25 percent of dialysis patients.[75] In another study, myocardial uptake of thallium^{201} during exercise was abnormal in more than 50 percent of patients, many of whom were asymptomatic when the study was performed.[76] Myocardial ischemia and angina pectoris occur in some dialysis patients who have no evidence of significant narrowing of coronary arteries on angiography.[77]

The management of angina pectoris in uremic patients is similar to that used in patients without kidney disease except that drug dosages may have to be reduced (see Chap. 58). Nitrates, beta blockers, and calcium channel blockers are well tolerated but may need to be withheld before dialysis to avoid hypotension during dialysis. The hematocrit should be maintained above 30 percent, preferably by administering erythropoietin (if available) and iron (as needed) or by transfusion of packed red cells. Hypertension, ECV overload, and hyperparathyroidism should be controlled.

Treatment of angina pectoris that develops during hemodialysis includes (1) stopping ultrafiltration to avoid ECV depletion, (2) reducing blood flow through the dialyzer, and (3) administering oxygen. If there is associated hypotension, the patient should be placed in the Trendelenburg position and saline infused through the venous line before administering sublingual nitroglycerin. If there is no hypotension, nitroglycerin can be administered immediately with the blood pressure monitored closely. Finally, it should be emphasized that changes in serum potassium and ionized calcium during dialysis and between periods of dialysis may complicate interpretation of the electrocardiogram. Electrocardiograms obtained during angina while on dialysis will often differ from prior tracings taken off dialysis sessions with or without the presence of ischemia.

Acute and long-term management of myocardial infarction in ESRD patients is similar to that in nonuremic patients except that changes in ECV are more critical and usually require restricting salt and fluid intake plus judicious ultrafiltration. Rapid and/or excessive ultrafiltration should be avoided to prevent hemodynamic instability. Hypertension and anemia should be managed as noted above. Digoxin should be used cautiously in a reduced dosage with the plasma levels of digoxin and potassium frequently monitored. The concentration of potassium in the dialysate is commonly 2 meq/liter, but it is usually raised to 3 meq/liter to prevent drug-toxic arrhythmias in patients receiving digoxin. In such cases, dietary potassium must be restricted to prevent hyperkalemia between treatments. The use of antiarrhythmic drugs should be carefully monitored with serum levels.

The decision to perform cardiac angiography, with or without percutaneous transluminal coronary angioplasty or coronary artery bypass grafting, should be based upon the same criteria as for patients without kidney disease (see Chaps. 58 to 60). The dose of contrast dye should be minimized to prevent loss of residual renal function and fluid intake, including the dose of contrast, should be minimized to prevent fluid overload. It is not necessary to dialyze patients immediately after angiography unless there is concern about excess fluid or heart failure.

Dialysis should be performed just before cardiac surgery to optimize ECV status and avoid hyperkalemia. Although morbidity after coronary artery bypass grafting is higher in patients with renal failure, the mortality rate of coronary revascularization is not significantly higher than in patients with normal renal function.[78,79]

CONGESTIVE HEART FAILURE

Congestive heart failure accounts for 20 to 30 percent of the mortality in ESRD patients.[3,80] Echocardiograms reveal a high prevalence of "hypertrophic cardiomyopathy" characterized by left ventricular hypertrophy, asymmetric septal hypertrophy, and/or impaired contractility[81–87] ("uremic cardiomyopathy") as well as dilated cardiomyopathy.[88] Concentric left ventricular hypertrophy occurs in patients with current or previous systemic hypertension. Risk factors for myocardial dysfunction in dialysis patients include hypertension, persistent ECV expansion, anemia, the arteriovenous fistula, ischemic heart disease, metabolic acidosis, electrolyte disturbances (hyperkalemia, hypocalcemia), hyperparathyroidism, and possibly the uremic state itself. Hemodialysis can improve cardiac function dramatically,[81,89–98] presumably by controlling hypertension, correcting volume overload, removing uremic toxins, and normalizing blood pH and electrolyte levels (particularly ionized calcium[99] and potassium[100]).

In uremic patients who develop pulmonary edema, the pulmonary capillary pressure is lower than in nonuremic patients and is less than the plasma oncotic pressure. Thus, pulmonary capillary permeability is increased in uremic patients.[101,102]

The prevention of heart failure in dialysis patients requires strict control of ECV and hypertension. Salt and fluid restriction must be combined with adequate fluid removal to maintain the patient's weight as close as possible to the estimated dry weight. Since dialysis occurs only three times a week, dietary salt restriction is absolutely necessary. As noted, an inappropriately high "dry weight" is a common reason for persistent volume overload and hypertension in dialysis patients. Reasons for the error in assessing dry weight include an unsuspected loss of muscle mass (e.g., secondary to a catabolic illness) that is unrecognized because body weight does not change due to retained fluid. Finally, the influence of the arteriovenous fistula can be tested by occluding it and determining if the heart rate slows (Branham's sign). When this occurs, revision of the fistula may be required to decrease blood flow.

Management of heart failure includes bed rest and oxygen therapy plus removal of excess fluid by ultrafiltration while excluding other causes of heart failure such as myocardial infarction, arrhythmias, or infective endocarditis. If digitalis is used, appropriate adjustment of dosage and frequent monitoring of plasma levels are necessary.

PERICARDIAL DISEASE

Before dialysis was widely available, pericarditis was regarded as a preterminal event for uremic patients. The clinical incidence of pericarditis has since decreased from 50 percent to 5 to 20 percent.[103–105] Although pericarditis has become less common, it is still a problem.[105] Pericarditis in dialysis patients may be related to inadequate removal of uremic toxins; coincident diseases such as viral infections,[106] tuberculosis, or systemic lupus erythematosus; or drugs such as minoxidil[107] (see also Chap. 92). Pericarditis appears to occur less frequently in peritoneal dialysis patients compared to hemodialysis patients. It has been speculated that this difference is due to a higher clearance of "middle molecules" by peritoneal dialysis.[108]

The primary treatment for dialysis-associated pericarditis is intensive dialysis (e.g., daily hemodialysis for 1 to 2 weeks); heparin should be eliminated to avoid pericardial hemorrhage and tamponade. Unfortunately, intensive dialysis can cause hypokalemia, hypophosphatemia, and volume depletion. An important clue to the development of cardiac tamponade is severe hypotension during dialysis, especially in the absence of volume depletion. Besides dialysis, oral[109,110] or intrapericardial administration of corticosteroids[111] and indomethacin[112] have been used. The efficacy of indomethacin is questionable. Results from a prospective, double-blind study led to the conclusion that the predominant effect of indomethacin is to reduce fever.[113]

Pericardial effusion frequently complicates pericarditis, but cardiac tamponade is rare; the exact frequency is unknown. Small pericardial effusions are found in 15 to 20 percent of stable, asymptomatic dialysis patients.[114] It is unclear whether or not daily dialysis therapy is beneficial in these patients, but frequent evaluation of the size and hemodynamic importance of the effusion is prudent. Treatment of a large pericardial effusion by intensification of dialysis may result in improvement,[105,114] but if there is no improvement or if hemodynamic compromise occurs, surgical drainage of the pericardial effusion with or without pericardiectomy is indicated[105,115–121] (see Chap. 92).

Constrictive pericarditis is rare in dialysis patients even in patients with pericarditis.[122,123] It should be suspected when intractable right-sided heart failure in patients with a normal-sized or small heart is present. Cardiac catheterization can verify the diagnosis, and pericardiectomy is the definitive treatment (see Chap. 92).

INFECTIVE ENDOCARDITIS

Several factors predispose dialysis patients to infective endocarditis, the incidence of which may be as high as 3 to 5 percent.[124–126] These include uremia-associated immunocompromised state,[127,128] repeated puncture of the arteriovenous fistula, and infection of the arteriovenous access. In addition, calcific aortic or mitral valvular abnormalities, perhaps related to hyperparathyroidism, are present in approximately 10 percent of patients[90,129,130] and may serve as a nidus for infection. Bacteremia occurs in approximately 10 to 20 percent of dialysis patients.[131,132] *Staphylococcus aureus* is the most frequent organism,[126] although other microbes including *Staphylococcus epidermidis, Streptococcus viridans,* enterococci, and gram-negative organisms are also reported. The diagnosis of infective endocarditis may be difficult in uremic patients because of the frequency of bacteremia and because systolic and diastolic murmurs are common[133] (see also Chap. 94). Repeated blood cultures, physical examination, and 2-D and Doppler echocardiographic assessment are mandatory when infective endocarditis is suspected. Treatment of infective endocarditis consists of 4 to 6 weeks of parenteral antibiotics. (See Chap. 94.)

CARDIAC ARRHYTHMIAS

Risk factors for cardiac arrhythmias in dialysis patients include ischemic heart disease and calcification of the conduction system from secondary hyperparathyroidism plus pericarditis, hemodialysis-associated hypotension, acid-base and electrolyte disturbances (hyper- and hypokalemia, hyper- and hypocalcemia, hypermagnesemia), and hypoxemia during dialysis. Fortunately, serious arrhythmias are uncommon except in patients with underlying heart disease, those receiving digitalis, or those with severe hypokalemia.[134–138] Dialysis patients receiving digitalis have an excessive risk for atrial and ventricular arrhythmias during dialysis because of rapid shifts of potassium. Therefore, digitalis should be used only when necessary and at the lowest dosage necessary. As noted above, the potassium concentration in the dialysate can be raised to 3 meq/liter to decrease the risk of digitalis-toxic arrhythmias. This necessitates strict restriction of potassium intake to prevent hyperkalemia between dialyses to prevent hyperkalemia. Hyperkalemia is believed to be responsible for a significant fraction of the 10 percent death rate in dialysis patients due to cardiac arrest.[70]

RENAL FUNCTION IN HEART FAILURE

In heart failure, enhanced sympathetic activity and activation of the renin-angiotensin-aldosterone axis enhance salt reabsorption while vasopressin augments water reabsorption.[139–141] This causes ECV and plasma volume expansion leading to increased end-diastolic volume and edema. Circulating ANP levels are increased in heart failure despite the marked antinatriuresis.[21,142] Possibly, ANP modulates the antinatriuretic effects caused by sympathetic and renin system activation. Excessive vasopressin-induced water reabsorption can cause hyponatremia, which is a poor prognostic indicator.[143] (See also Chap. 25.)

Renal vasoconstriction in heart failure can be sufficiently severe to cause renal failure (prerenal azotemia), which is characterized by a blood urea nitrogen (BUN)–creatinine ratio that is greater than 10 : 1. It results from a selective decrease in urea clearance resulting from enhanced sodium reabsorption and a secondary increase in urea reabsorption. Additional features are oliguria, a low urinary sodium excretion, a high urine specific gravity and osmolality, and a normal urinalysis. Diuretic therapy may mask these characteristics by increasing urine flow and sodium excretion and reducing the urine specific gravity and osmolality. Factors that can precipitate or exacerbate renal failure include excessive diuresis, use of ACE inhibitors or nonsteroidal anti-inflammatory drugs (NSAIDs), and worsening cardiac function. When renal perfusion is reduced, glomerular filtration rate (GFR) becomes dependent on angiotensin II–induced efferent glomerular arteriolar constriction and vasodilator prostaglandins. Consequently, ACE inhibitors or NSAIDs can markedly decrease the GFR.[144,145] The ACE inhibitors and other antihypertensives (e.g., hydralazine) can also reduce glomerular filtration by causing systemic hypotension and reducing renal perfusion pressure.

The management of renal failure in heart failure patients is aimed primarily at improving cardiac function (see Chap. 26). The NSAIDs should be avoided, and diuretics should be used judiciously because excessive diuresis can cause renal failure directly and can predispose to ACE inhibitor–induced renal failure. Careful attention to urine flow, the BUN and serum creatinine, and potassium is mandatory.

RENAL FAILURE FOLLOWING CARDIAC CATHETERIZATION

Contrast Nephropathy

Risk factors for contrast-induced renal failure include diabetes mellitus, multiple myeloma, preexisting renal failure, volume depletion, heart failure, and the amount of contrast dye administered.[146–148] The renal failure is typically brief (approximately 5 to 7 days) and is associated with reduced urinary sodium excretion.[149] In high-risk patients, contrast dye studies should be avoided and noninvasive studies used to assess ventricular function and anatomy or the amount of contrast dye should be minimized. Volume expansion with saline prior to the studies may attenuate contrast nephropathy. There is some evidence that mannitol may be protective.[150]

Atheroembolic Nephropathy

This complication usually occurs in elderly patients with erosive aortic atherosclerosis who have embolization of cholesterol plaques to the kidneys during arterial catheterization. Serum creatinine rises sharply and usually does not return to normal levels. At times, renal failure may worsen, slowly leading to ESRD. Hypertension due to activation of the renin-angiotensin system may be present.[151] The urinalysis is typically normal. Atheroembolization to other locations such as the eyes (cholesterol plaques on fundoscopy), pancreas (pancreatitis), and skin (livedo reticularis or gangrene) may be present, suggesting the diagnosis.[152] Occasionally, immunologic activation may be suggested by an "active" urinary sediment with hematuria and cellular casts, hypocomplementemia, eosinophilia, and a high sedimentation rate.[153–155] Biopsy of an affected organ (e.g., skin, kidney) may help establish the diagnosis, but the absence of atheroemboli in a kidney biopsy does not exclude the diagnosis since affected vessels may be missed. There is no specific treatment.

THROMBOEMBOLIC RENAL ARTERIAL DISEASE

In contrast to atheroembolic renal disease, thromboembolic renal arterial disease (e.g., in patients with atrial fibrillation or after myocardial infarction) often causes renal infarction. Such patients may present with flank pain, proteinuria, and hematuria; the serum lactate dehydrogenase (LDH) levels are increased and renal failure may be evidenced by an increased serum creatinine, particularly if both kidneys are affected.[156–158] A radioisotope scan or renal arteriography will confirm the diagnosis. Therapy includes anticoagulation and possibly thrombolysis or surgical intervention.

CARDIAC DRUGS IN RENAL FAILURE

Digoxin

The volume of distribution of digoxin is reduced 30 to 50 percent in ESRD patients so the loading dose of digoxin should be reduced.[133] The maintenance dosage should be decreased because the primary route of elimination is by glomerular filtration of unmetabolized digoxin. Because of abnormal pharmacokinetics, only general guidelines for maintenance dosages are available: 0.0625 to 0.125 mg every other day can result in a therapeutic plasma level but regular monitoring is required. If a loading dose is not administered or if adjustments are made in the maintenance dose, the time required to attain a new steady state may be prolonged to approximately 3 weeks because of the longer half-life of digoxin in renal failure (4.4 days vs. 1.6 days in normal subjects[159]). Concomitant administration of quinidine or verapamil can increase plasma digoxin levels and clinical toxicity. (see Chaps. 27 and 109.)

Procainamide

As renal function decreases, so does the ability to eliminate unmetabolized procainamide; the half-life increases from approximately 3.5 to 16 h in renal failure.[160,161] In addition, the half-life of *N*-acetylprocainamide (NAPA), an active metabolite of procainamide primarily excreted by the kidneys, is markedly prolonged in renal failure.[161] Consequently, maintenance doses should be reduced or the intervals between dosages should be prolonged; close monitoring of plasma levels of both procainamide and NAPA is necessary (see also Chaps. 38 and 109). Since both compounds are removed by dialysis, a dose of procainamide should be administered after hemodialysis.

Phenytoin

Phenytoin is bound to plasma proteins, but with uremia, protein binding becomes abnormal, resulting in a higher concentration of free phenytoin.[162,163] Since most clinical laboratories measure the total phenytoin concentration or bound plus free drug, attempts to maintain a "therapeutic" level of phenytoin in CRF patients can cause toxicity. Fortunately, standard doses (e.g., 300 mg/day) often yield therapeutic levels of free phenytoin so no alteration in phenytoin dosage is recommended even though the plasma level may appear to be subtherapeutic. Toxicity is usually diagnosed from clinical signs (see Chap. 38).

Beta Blockers

Atenolol (Tenormin) and nadolol (Corgard) are eliminated primarily by the kidneys, so a dose reduction of 50 to 70 percent is necessary for CRF patients.[164] These drugs should be withheld the morning of a hemodialysis treatment because a significant fraction is removed by the dialysis procedure. The usual dose is given after dialysis (see also Chap. 66).

Nitroprusside

In dialysis or predialysis patients, thiocyanate will accumulate when nitroprusside is infused.[165] Thiocyanate can cause neurologic toxicity such as confusion, hyperreflexia, and seizures. Consequently, the dose of nitroprusside should be minimized and the drug given for as short a period as possible. Both cyanide and thiocyanate levels in plasma should be monitored to avoid toxicity (see also Chap. 30).

Angiotensin Converting Enzyme Inhibitors

The dose of these drugs should be reduced by approximately 50 percent in dialysis patients because they and their metabolites are excreted by the kidney. Accumulation of converting enzyme inhibitors can cause hematologic toxicity (see also Chap. 30). These drugs have two other types of toxic effects in predialysis patients. First, they can cause hyperkalemia by inhibiting angiotensin-stimulated aldosterone release, resulting in decreased potassium excretion and hyperkalemia. Second, they can cause rapid loss of renal function in patients with renal artery stenosis or with other conditions associated with activation of the renin-angiotensin system, including congestive heart failure.[144,166] The mechanism for the decrease in GFR is inhibition of angiotensin-induced constriction of the efferent glomerular arteriole, which dilates and leads to a decrease in the hydrostatic pressure across the glomerular capillary wall. These drugs should be withheld on the morning of a hemodialysis treatment to avoid hypotension.

Cyclosporine

The use of cyclosporine in heart transplant recipients is often associated with loss of renal function, and some patients progress to CRF (see also Chap. 32). Cyclosporine constricts both afferent and efferent glomerular arterioles, resulting in reduced GFR.[167] Proximal tubular injury with vacuolar changes, inclusion bodies, and giant mitochondria has been noted.[168] Cyclosporine usage may also lead to hyperkalemia and renal tubular acidosis.[169] These effects are usually reversible if the dose is reduced or the drug is discontinued. Renal failure resembling the hemolytic uremic syndrome has been associated with cyclosporine (possibly due to endothelial damage).[168] Finally, obliterative arteriopathy with interstitial fibrosis and glomerular sclerosis can occur.[168,170]

REFERENCES

1. Rostand SG, Brunzell JD, Cannon RO, Victor RG: Cardiovascular complications in renal failure. *J Am Soc Nephrol* 1991; 2:1053–1062.
2. Brynger H, Brunner FP, Chantler C, Donckerwoleke RA, Jacobs C, Kramer P, et al: Combined report on regular dialysis and transplantation in Europe, X, 1979. *Proc Eur Dial Transplant Assoc* 1980; 17:2–87.
3. Lazarus JM, Lowrie EG, Hampers CL, Merrill JP: Cardiovascular disease in uremic patients on hemodialysis *Kidney Int* (1975) (Suppl. 2): S167–S175.
4. Blumberg A, Nelp WB, Hegstrom RM, Scribner BH: Extracellular volume in patients with chronic renal disease treated for hypertension by sodium restriction. *Lancet* 1967; 2:69–73.
5. Vertes V, Cangiano JL, Berman LB, Gould A: Hypertension in end-stage renal disease. *N Engl J Med* 1991; 280:978–981.
6. Weidmann P, Maxwell MH, Lupu AN, Lewin AJ, Massry SG: Plasma renin activity and blood pressure in terminal renal failure. *N Engl J Med* 1991; 285:757–762.
7. Wilkinson R, Scott DF, Uldall PR, Kerr DNS, Swinney J: Plasma renin and exchangeable sodium in the hypertension of chronic renal failure—the effect of bilateral nephrectomy. *Q J Med* 1970; 39:377–394.
8. Kim KE, Onesti G, Schwartz AB, Chinitz JL, Swartz C: Hemodynamics of hypertension in chronic end-stage renal disease. *Circulation* 1972; 46:452–464.
9. Acosta JH: Hypertension in chronic renal disease. *Kidney Int* 1982; 22:702–712.
10. Kim KE, Onesti G, DelGuercio ET, Greco J, Fernandes M, Eidelson B, et al: Sequential hemodynamic changes in end-stage renal disease and the anephric state during volume expansion. *Hypertension* 1991; 2:102–110.
11. Lazarus JM, Hampers CL, Merrill JP: Hypertension in chronic renal failure. *Arch Intern Med* 1974; 133:1059–1066.
12. Stokes GS, Mani MK, Stewart JH: Relevance of salt, water, and renin to hypertension in chronic renal failure. *Br Med J* 1970; 3:126–129.
13. Vaughan ED, Carey RM, Ayers CR, Peach MJ: Hemodialysis-resistant hypertension: Control with an orally active inhibitor of angiotensin-converting enzyme. *J Clin Endocrinol Metab* 1991; 48:869–871.
14. Kelly RA, O'Hara DS, Mitch WE, Steinman TI, Goldszer RC, Solomon HS, et al: Endogenous digitalis-like factors in hypertension and chronic renal insufficiency. *Kidney Int* 1986; 30:723–729.
15. Deray G, Pernollet M-G, Devynck M-A, Zingraff J, Touan A, Rosenfeld J, et al: Plasma digitalislike activity in essential hypertension or end-stage renal disease. *Hypertension* 1986; 8:632–638.
16. Needleman P, Greenwald JE: Atriopeptin: A cardiac hormone intimately involved in fluid, electrolyte, and blood-pressure homeostasis. *N Engl J Med* 1986; 314:828–834.
17. Blaine EH: Role of atriopeptin in blood pressure regulation. *Am J Med Sci* 1988; 295(4):293–298.
18. Walker RG, Swainson CP, Yandle TG, Nicholls MG, Espiner EA: Exaggerated responsiveness of immunoreactive atrial natriuretic peptide to saline infusion in chronic renal failure. *Clin Sci* 1987; 72:19–24.
19. Saxenhofer H, Gnadinger MP, Weidmann P, Shaw S, Schohn D, Hess C, et al: Plasma levels and dialysance of atrial natriuretic peptide in terminal renal failure. *Kidney Int* 1987; 32:554–561.
20. Kjellstrand CM, Whitley K, Comty CM, Shapiro FL: Dialysis in patients with diabetes mellitus. *Diabet Nephrop* 1983; 2:5.
21. Shapiro FL, Comty CM: *Hemodialysis in Diabetics—1981 Update*, 2d ed. New York, Grune & Stratton, 1983: 333–343.
22. Goldberg AP, Herschel RH, Patsch W, Schechtman KB, Provilnce M, Weerts C, et al: Racial differences in plasma high-density lipoproteins in patients receiving hemodialysis. *N Engl J Med* 1983; 308:1245–1252.
23. Cramp DG, Tickner TR, Varghese DJ, Beale DJ, Moorhead JF, Wills MR: Plasma lipoprotein patterns in patients receiving dialysis therapy for chronic renal failure. *Clin Chim Acta* 1977; 76:233–236.
24. Goldberg AP, Applebaum-Bowden DM, Bierman EL, Hazzard WR, Haas LB, Sherrard DJ, et al: Increase in lipoprotein lipase during clofibrate treatment of hypertriglyceridemia in patients on hemodialysis. *N Engl J Med* 1979; 301:1073–1076.
25. Chan MK, Persaud J, Varghese Z, Moorhead JF: Pathogenic roles of post-heparin lipases in lipid abnormalities in hemodialysis patients. *Kidney Int* 1991; 25:812–818.
26. Murase T, Cattran DC, Rubenstein B, Steiner G: Inhibition of lipoprotein lipase by uremic plasma, a possible cause of hypertriglyceridemia. *Metabolism* 1975; 24:1279–1286.
27. Ames RP, Hill P: Elevation of serum lipid levels during diuretic therapy of hypertension. *Am J Med* 1976; 61:748–757.
28. Tanaka N, Sakaguchi S, Oshige K, Niimura T, Kanehisa T: Effect of chronic administration of propranolol on lipoprotein composition. *Metabolism* 1976; 25:1071–1075.
29. Harter HR, Meltzer VN, Tindira CA, Naumovich AD, Goldberg AP: Comparison of the effects of prazosin versus propranolol on plasma lipoprotein lipids in patients receiving hemodialysis. *Am J Med* 1986; 80:82–89.
30. Rorke SJ, Shippey W, Davidson WD: Acetate delivery to hemodialysis patients (abstr). *Kidney Int* 1975; 8:433.
31. Lindholm B, Norbeck HE: Serum lipids and lipoproteins during continuous ambulatory peritoneal dialysis. *Acta Med Scand* 1986; 220:143–151.
32. Lacour B, Chanard J, Haguet M, Basile C, Assan R, Di Giulio S, et al: Carnitine improves lipid anomalies in haemodialysis patients. *Lancet* 1980; 2:763–764.
33. Ibels LS, Reardon MF, Nestel PJ: Plasma post-heparin lipolytic activity and triglyceride activity in uremic and hemodialysis patients and renal allograft recipients. *J Lab Clin Med* 1976; 87:648–658.
34. Teraoka J, Matsui N, Nakagawa S, Takeuchi J: The role of heparin in the changes of lipid patterns during a single hemodialysis. *Clin Nephrol* 1982; 17:96–99.
35. Wessel-Aas T, Blomhoff JP, Wideroe T-E, Wirum E, Nilsen T: The effect of systemic heparinization on plasma lipoproteins and

toxicity in patients on hemodialysis and continuous ambulatory peritoneal dialysis. *Acta Med Scand* 1984; 216:85–92.
36. Ritz E, Augustin J, Bommer J, Gnasso A, Haberbosch W: Should hyperlipemia of renal failure be treated? *Kidney Int* 1985; 28:S-84–S-87.
37. Dornan TL, Gokal R, Pearce JS, Oliver DO, Ledingham JGG, Mann JI: Long-term dietary treatment of hyperlipidaemia in patients treated with chronic haemodialysis. *Br Med J* 1980; 281:1044.
38. Cattran DC, Steiner G, Fenton SSA, Ampil M: Dialysis hyperlipemia: Response to dietary manipulations. *Clin Nephrol* 1980; 13:177–182.
39. Golper TA: Therapy for uremic hyperlipidemia. *Nephron* 1991; 38:217–225.
40. Goldberg AP, Hagberg JM, Delez JA, Haynes ME, Harter HR: Metabolic effects of exercise training in hemodialysis patients. *Kidney Int* 1980; 18:754–761.
41. Hamazaki T, Nakazawa R, Tateno S, Shishido H, Isoda K, Hattori Y, et al: Effects of fish oil rich in eicosapentaenoic acid on serum lipid in hyperlipidemic hemodialysis patients. *Kidney Int* 1984; 26:81–84.
42. Rylance PB, Gordge MP, Saynor R, Parsons V, Weston MJ: Fish oil modifies lipids and reduces platelet aggregability in haemodialysis patients. *Nephron* 1986; 43:196–202.
43. Degoulet P, Reach I, Di Giulio S, Devries C, Rouby JJ, Aime F, et al: Epidemiology of dialysis induced hypotension. *Proc Eur Dial Transplant Assoc* 1981; 18:133–138.
44. Kinet J-P, Soyeur D, Balland N, Saint-Remy M, Collignon P, Godon J-P: Hemodynamic study of hypotension during hemodialysis. *Kidney Int* 1982; 21:868–876.
45. Rosa AA, Shideman J, McHugh R, Duncan D, Kjellstrand CM: The importance of osmolality fall and ultrafiltration rate on hemodialysis side effects. *Nephron* 1981; 27:134–141.
46. Keshaviah P, Shapiro F: A critical examination of dialysis-induced hypotension. *Am J Kid Dis* 1982; 2:290–301.
47. Rouby JJ, Rottembourg J, Durande J-P, Basset J-Y, Degoulet P, Glaser P, et al: Hemodynamic changes induced by regular hemodialysis and sequential ultrafiltration hemodialysis: A comparative study. *Kidney Int* 1980; 17:801–810.
48. Ogden DA: A double blind crossover comparison of high and low sodium dialysis. *Proc Clin Dial Transplant Forum* 1978; 8:157–164.
49. Aizawa Y, Ohmori T, Imai K, Nara Y, Matsuoka M: Depressant action of acetate upon the human cardiovascular system. *Clin Nephrol* 1977; 8:477–480.
50. Kraut J, Gafter U, Brautbar J, Miller J, Shinaberger J: Prevention of hypoxemia during dialysis by the use of sequential isolated ultrafiltration-diffusion dialysis with bicarbonate dialyzate. *Clin Nephrol* 1981; 15:181–184.
51. Hakim RM, Breillatt J, Lazarus JM, Port F: Complement activation and hypersensitivity reactions to dialysis membranes. *N Engl J Med* 1984; 311:878–882.
52. Amadori A, Candi P, Sasdelli M, Massai G, Favilla S, Passaleva A, et al: Hemodialysis leukopenia and complement function with different dialyzers. *Kidney Int* 1983; 24:775–781.
53. Dolovich J, Marshall CP, Smith EKM, Shimizu A, Pearson FC, Sugona MA, et al: Allergy to ethylene oxide in chronic hemodialysis patients. *Artif Organs* 1984; 8(3):334–337.
54. Grammer LC, Roberts M, Nicholls AJ, Platts MM, Patterson R: IgE against ethylene oxide–altered human serum albumin in patients who have had acute dialysis reactions. *Clin Immunol* 1984; 74:544–546.
55. Slatopolsky E, Caglar S, Pennell JP, Taggart DD, Canterbury JM, Reiss E, et al: On the pathogenesis of hyperparathyroidism in chronic experimental renal insufficiency in the dog. *J Clin Invest* 1971; 50:492–499.
56. Portale AA, Halloran BP, Murphy MM, Morris RC Jr: Oral intake of phosphorus can determine the serum concentration of 1,25-dihydroxyvitamin D by determining its production rate in humans. *J Clin Invest* 1986; 77:7–12.
57. Delmez JA, Tindira C, Grooms P, Dusso A, Windus DW, Slatopolsky E: Parathyroid hormone suppression by intravenous 1,25-dihydroxyvitamin D. *J Clin Invest* 1991; 83:1349–1355.
58. Dunlay R, Rodriguez M, Felsenfeld AJ, Llach F: Direct inhibitory effect of calcitriol on parathyroid function (sigmoidal curve) in dialysis. *Kidney Int* 1989; 36:1093–1098.
59. Mallick NP, Berlyne GM: Arterial calcification after vitamin-D therapy in hyperphosphataemic renal failure. *Lancet* 1968; 2:1316–1319.
60. Friedman SA, Novack S, Thomson GE: Arterial calcification and gangrene in uremia. *N Engl J Med* 1969; 280:1392–1394.
61. Rosen H, Friedman SA, Raizner AE, Gerstmann K: Azotemic arteriopathy. *Am Heart J* 1972; 84:250–255.
62. Ibels LS, Alfrey AC, Huffer WE, Craswell PW, Anderson JT, Weill R: Arterial calcification and pathology in uremic patients undergoing dialysis. *Am J Med* 1979; 66:790–796.
63. Lewin K, Trautman L: Ischaemic myocardial damage in chronic renal failure. *Br Med J* 1971; 4:151–152.
64. Terman DS, Alfrey AC, Hammond WS, Donndelinger T, Ogden DA, Holmes JH: Cardiac calcification in uremia. *Am J Med* 1971; 50:744–755.
65. Arora KK, Lacy JP, Schacht RA, Martin DG, Gutch CF: Calcific cardiomyopathy in advanced renal failure. *Arch Intern Med* 1975; 135:603–605.
66. McGonigle RJS, Fowler MB, Timmis AB, Weston MJ, Parsons V: Uremic cardiomyopathy: Potential role of vitamin D and parathyroid hormone. *Nephron* 1984; 36:94–100.
67. Gafter U, Battler A, Eldar M, Zevin D, Neufeld HN, Levi J: Effect of hyperparathyroidism on cardiac function in patients with end-stage renal disease. *Nephron* 1985; 41:30–33.
68. Hruska KA: Requirements for calcium, phosphorus and vitamin D. In: Mitch WE, Klahr S (eds.): *Nutrition and the Kidney.* Boston, Little, Brown, 1988: 104–130.
69. Lindner A, Charra B, Sherrard DJ, Scribner BH: Accelerated atherosclerosis in prolonged maintenance hemodialysis. *N Engl J Med* 1974; 290:697–701.
70. Wing AJ, Brunner FP, Brynger H, Jacobs C, Kramer P, Selwood NH, et al: Cardiovascular-related causes of death and the fate of patients with renovascular disease. *Contrib Nephrol* 1984; 41:306–311.
71. Bagdade JD: Accelerated atherosclerosis in patients on maintenance dialysis. *Adv Nephrol* 1980; 9:7.
72. Hahn R, Oette K, Mondorf H, Finke K, Sieberth HG: Analysis of cardiovascular risk factors in chronic hemodialysis patients with special attention to the hyperlipoproteinemias. *Atherosclerosis* 1983; 48:279–288.
73. Rostand SG, Gretes JC, Kirk KA, Rutsky EA, Andreoli TE: Ischemic heart disease in patients with uremia undergoing maintenance hemodialysis. *Kidney Int* 1979; 16:600–611.
74. Degoulet P, Legrain M, Reach I, Aime F, Devries C, Rojas P, et al: Mortality risk factors in patients treated by chronic hemodialysis. *Nephron* 1982; 31:103–110.
75. Bullock RE, Amer HA, Simpson I, Ward MK, Hall RJC: Cardiac abnormalities and exercise tolerance in patients receiving renal replacement therapy. *Br Med J* 1984; 289:1479–1484.
76. Dudczak R, Fridrich L, Derfler K, Kletter K, Frischauf H, Marosi L, et al: Myocardial studies in haemodialysis patients. *Proc Eur Dial Transplant Assoc* 1984; 21:251–261.
77. Roig E, Betriu A, Castaner A, Magrina J, Sanz G, Navarro-Lopez F: Disabling angina pectoris with normal coronary arteries in patients undergoing long-term hemodialysis. *Am J Med* 1981; 71:431–434.
78. Rottenbourg J, Mussat T, Gandjbaklch I, Barthelemy A, Toledano D, Gahl GM, et al: Open heart surgery in patients with end-stage renal disease. *Proc Eur Dial Transplant Assoc* 1983; 20:169.
79. Francis GS, Sharma B, Collins AJ, Helseth HK, Comty CM: Coronary-artery surgery in patients with end-stage renal disease. *Ann Intern Med* 1980; 92:499–503.
80. Jacobs C, Brunner FP, Chantler C, Donckerwolcke RA, Gurland HJ, Hathaway RA, et al: Combined report on regular dialysis and transplantation in Europe, VII, 1976. *Proc Eur Dial Transplant Assoc* 1977; 14:3–69.
81. Klein J, McLeish, K, Hodsden J, Lordon R: Hypertrophic cardiomyopathy: An acquired disorder of end-stage renal disease. *Trans Am Soc Artif Intern Organ* 1983; 29:120–127.
82. Lai KN, Ng J, Whitford J, Buttfield I, Fassett RG, Mathew TH: Left ventricular function in uremia: Echocardiographic and radionuclide assessment in patients on maintenance hemodialysis. *Clin Nephrol* 1984; 23:125–133.
83. Renger A, Muller M, Jutzler GA, Bette L: Echocardiographic evaluation of left ventricular dimensions and function in chronic hemodialysis patients with cardiomegaly. *Clin Nephrol* 1984; 21:164–168.

84. Bernardi D, Bernini L, Cini G, Ghione S, Bonechi I: Asymmetric septal hypertrophy and sympathetic overactivity in normotensive hemodialyzed patients. *Am Heart J* 1985; 109:539–545.
85. Bernardi D, Bernini L, Cini G, Geri AB, Urti DA, Bonechi I: Asymmetric septal hypertrophy in uremic-normotensive patients on regular hemodialysis. *Nephron* 1985; 39:30–35.
86. Miach PJ, Dawborn JK, Louis WJ, McDonald IG: Left ventricular function in uremia: Echocardiographic assessment in patients on maintenance dialysis. *Clin Nephrol* 1981; 15:259–263.
87. London GM, Faviani F, Marchais SJ, deVernejoul M-C, Guerin AP, Safar ME, et al: Uremic cardiomyopathy: An inadequate left ventricular hypertrophy. *Kidney Int* 1987; 31:973–980.
88. Parfrey PS, Harnett JD, Barre PE: The natural history of myocardial disease in dialysis patients. *J Am Soc Nephrol* 1991; 2:2–12.
89. Bornstein A, Zambrano SS, Morrison RS, Spodick DH: Cardiac effects of hemodialysis: Noninvasive monitoring by systolic time intervals. *Am J Med Sci* 1975; 269:189–192.
90. Scharf S, Wexler J, Longnecker RE, Blaufox MD: Cardiovascular disease in patients on chronic hemodialytic therapy. *Prog Cardiovasc Dis* 1980; 22:343–356.
91. Pedersen T, Rasmussen K, Cleemann-Rasmussen K: Effect of hemodialysis on cardiac performance and transmural myocardial perfusion. *Clin Nephrol* 1983; 19:31–36.
92. Nixon JV, Mitchell JH, McPhaul JJ Jr, Henrich WL: Effect of hemodialysis on left ventricular function. *J Clin Invest* 1983; 71:377–384.
93. Bornstein A, Gaasch WH, Harrington J: Assessment of the cardiac effects of hemodialysis with systolic time intervals and echocardiography. *Am J Cardiol* 1983; 51:332–335.
94. Gilmartin JJ, Duffy BS, Finnegan P, McCready N: Non-invasive study of left ventricular function in chronic renal failure before and after hemodialysis. *Clin Nephrol* 1983; 20:55–60.
95. Kramer W, Wizemann V, Kindler M, Thormann J, Grebe SF, Schutterle G, et al: Influence of fluid removal rate during hemodialysis on left ventricular performance and exercise tolerance in patients with coronary artery disease. *Clin Nephrol* 1984; 21:280–286.
96. Hung J, Harris PJ, Uren RF, Tiller DJ, Kelly DT: Uremic cardiomyopathy—effect of hemodialysis on left ventricular function in end-stage renal failure. *N Engl J Med* 1980; 230:547–551.
97. Ireland MA, Mehta BR, Shiu MF: Acute effects of haemodialysis on left heart dimensions and left ventricular function: An echocardiographic study. *Nephron* 1981; 29:73–79.
98. Madsen BR, Alpert MA, Whiting RB, Stone JV, Ahmad M, Kelly DL: Effect of hemodialysis on left ventricular performance. *Am J Nephrol* 1984; 4:86–91.
99. Henrich WL, Hunt JM, Nixon JV: Increased ionized calcium and left ventricular contractility during hemodialysis. *N Engl J Med* 1984; 310:19–23.
100. Chaignon M, Chen W-T, Tarazi RC, Nakamoto S, Salcedo E: Acute effects of hemodialysis on echographic-determined cardiac performance: Improved contractility resulting from serum increased calcium with reduced potassium despite hypovolemic-reduced cardiac output. *Am Heart J* 1982; 103:374–378.
101. Gibson DG: Haemodynamic factors in the development of acute pulmonary oedema in renal failure. *Lancet* 1966; 2:1217–1220.
102. Rackow EC, Fein IA, Sprung C, Grodman RS: Uremic pulmonary edema. *Am J Med* 1978; 64:1084–1088.
103. Wacker J, Merrill JP: Uremic pericarditis in acute and chronic renal failure. *JAMA* 1954; 156:764.
104. Ziegler TR, Lazarus JM, Young LS, Hakim R, Wilmore DW: Effects of recombinant human growth hormone in adults receiving maintenance hemodialysis. *J Am Soc Nephrol* 1991; 2:1130–1135.
105. Rutsky EA, Rostand SG: Treatment of uremic pericarditis and pericardial effusion. *Am J Kidney Dis* 1987; 10:2–8.
106. Osanloo E, Shalhoub RJ, Cioffi RF, Parker RH: Viral pericarditis in patients receiving hemodialysis. *Arch Intern Med* 1979; 139:301–303.
107. Houston MC, McChesney JA, Chatterjee K: Pericardial effusion associated with minoxidil therapy. *Arch Intern Med* 1981; 141:69–71.
108. Silverberg S, Oreopoulos DG, Wise DJ, Uden DE, Meindok H, Jones M, et al: Pericarditis in patients undergoing long-term hemodialysis and peritoneal dialysis. *Am J Med* 1977; 63:874–880.
109. Comty CM, Cohen SL, Shapiro FL: Pericarditis in chronic uremia and its sequels. *Ann Intern Med* 1971; 75:173–183.
110. Eliasson G, Murphy JF: Steroid therapy in uremic pericarditis. *JAMA* 1974; 229:1634–1635.
111. Buselmeier TJ, Simmons RL, Najarian JS, Mauer SM, Matas AJ, Kjellstrand CM: Uremic pericardial effusion. *Nephron* 1976; 16:371–380.
112. Minuth NW, Nottebohm GA, Eknoyan G, Suki WN: Endomethacin treatment of pericarditis in chronic hemodialysis patients. *Arch Intern Med* 1975; 135:807–810.
113. Spector D, Alfred H, Siedlecki M, Briefel G: A controlled study of the effect of indomethacin in uremic pericarditis. *Kidney Int* 1983; 24:663–669.
114. Goldberg M, Lazarus JM, Gottlieb MN, Lowrie EG, Merrill JP: Treatment of uremic pericardial effusion. *Proc Clin Dial Transplant Forum* 1975; 5:20.
115. Singh S, Newark K, Ishikawa I, Mitra S, Berman LB: Pericardiectomy in uremia. *JAMA* 1974; 228:1132–1135.
116. Ali-Regiaba S, Gay WA, Sullivan JF, Tapia L, David DS, White RP, et al: Treatment of uraemic pericarditis by anterior pericardiectomy. *Lancet* 1974; 2:12–14.
117. Luft FC, Kleit SA, Smith RN, Glover JL, Carr JB, de Quesada AM: Management of uremic pericarditis with tamponade. *Arch Intern Med* 1974; 134:488–490.
118. Morin JE, Hollomby D, Gonda A, Long R, Dobell ARC: Management of uremic pericarditis: A report of 11 patients with cardiac tamponade and a review of the literature. *Ann Thorac Surg* 1976; 22:588–592.
119. Leehey DJ, Daugirdas JT, Ing TS: Early drainage of pericardial effusion in patients with dialysis pericarditis. *Arch Intern Med* 1983; 143:1673–1675.
120. Daugirdas JT, Leehey DJ, Popli S, McCray GM, Gandhi VS, Pifarre R, et al: Subxiphoid pericardiostomy for hemodialysis-associated pericardial effusion. *Arch Intern Med* 1986; 146: 1113–1115.
121. Peraino RA: Pericardial effusion in patients treated with maintenance dialysis. *Am J Nephrol* 1983; 3:319–322.
122. Moraski RE, Bousvaros G: Constrictive pericarditis due to chronic uremia. *N Engl J Med* 1969; 281:542–543.
123. Wolfe SA, Bailey GF, Collins JJ Jr: Constrictive pericarditis following uremic effusion. *J Thorac Cardiovasc Surg* 1972; 63:540–544.
124. Dobkin JF, Miller MH, Steigbigel NH: Septicemia in patients on chronic hemodialysis. *Ann Intern Med* 1978; 88:28–33.
125. Leonard A, Raij L, Shapiro FL: Bacterial endocarditis in regularly dialyzed patients. *Kidney Int* 1973; 4:407–422.
126. Cross AS, Steigbigel RT: Infective endocarditis and access site infections in patients on hemodialysis. *Medicine* 1976; 55:453–466.
127. Goldblum SE, Reed WP: Host defenses and immunologic alterations associated with chronic hemodialysis. *Ann Intern Med* 1980; 93:597–613.
128. Ruiz P, Gomez F, Schrieber AD: Impaired function of macrophage Fc gamma receptors in end-stage renal disease. *N Engl J Med* 1990; 322:717–722.
129. Forman MB, Virmani R, Robertson RM, Stone WJ: Mitral annular calcification in chronic renal failure. *Chest* 1984; 85:367–371.
130. Maher ER, Curtis JR: Calcific aortic stenosis in chronic renal failure. *Lancet* 1985; 2:1007.
131. Keane WF, Shapiro FL, Raij L: Incidence and type of infections occurring in 445 chronic hemodialysis patients. *Trans Am Soc Artif Int Organ* 1977; 23:41–46.
132. Nsouli KA, Lazarus JM, Schoenbaum SC, Gottlieb MN, Lowrie EG, Shocair M: Bacteremic infection in hemodialysis. *Arch Intern Med* 1979; 139:1255–1258.
133. Orino E, Tanaka K, Tamura T, Sone S, Ogura T, Ichihara A: ATP-dependent reversible association of proteasomes with multiple protein components to form 26S complexes that degrade ubiquitinated proteins in human HL-60 cells. *FEBS Lett* 1991; 284:206–210.
134. Kyriakidis M, Voudiclaris S, Kremastinos D, Robinson-Kyriakidas C, Vyssoulis G, Zervakis D, et al: Cardiac arrhythmias in chronic renal failure. *Nephron* 1984; 38:26–29.
135. Weber H, Schwarzer C, Stummvoll HK, Joskowicz G, Wolf A, Steinbach K, et al: Chronic hemodialysis: High risk patients for arrhythmias? *Nephron* 1984; 37:180–185.

136. Forsstrom J, Heinonen E, Valimaki I, Antila K: Effects of haemodialysis on heart rate variability in chronic renal failure. *Scand J Clin Lab Invest* 1986; 46:665–670.
137. Blumberg A, Hausermann M, Strub B, Jenzer HR: Cardiac arrhythmias in patients on maintenance hemodialysis. *Nephron* 1983; 33:91–95.
138. Wizeman V, Kramer W, Funke T, Schutterle G: Dialysis-induced cardiac arrhythmias: Fact or fiction? *Nephron* 1985; 39:356–360.
139. Dzau VJ: Renal and circulatory mechanisms in congestive heart failure. *Kidney Int* 1987; 31:1402–1415.
140. Moss NG: Renal function and renal afferent and efferent nerve activity. *Am J Physiol* 1982; 12:F425–F433.
141. Mettauer B, Rouleau J-L, Bichet D, Juneau C, Kortas C, Barjon J-N, et al: Sodium and water excretion abnormalities in congestive heart failure. *Ann Intern Med* 1986; 105:161–167.
142. Sugawara A, Nakao K, Morii N, Yamada T, Itoh H, Shiono S, et al: Synthesis of atrial natriuretic polypeptide in human failing hearts. *J Clin Invest* 1992; 81:1962–1970.
143. Lee WH, Packer M: Prognostic importance of serum sodium concentration and its modification by converting-enzyme inhibition in patients with severe chronic heart failure. *Circulation* 1986; 73:257–267.
144. Packer M, Lee WH, Medina N, Yushak M, Kessler P: Functional renal insufficiency during long-term therapy with captopril and enalapril in severe chronic heart failure. *Ann Intern Med* 1987; 106:346–354.
145. Dzau VJ, Packer M, Lilly LS, Swartz SL, Hollenberg NK, Williams GH: Prostaglandins in severe congestive heart failure. *N Engl J Med* 1984; 310:347–352.
146. VanZee BE, Hoy WE, Talley TE, Jaenike JR: Renal injury associated with intravenous pyelography in nondiabetic and diabetic patients. *Ann Intern Med* 1978; 89:51–54.
147. Taliercio CP, Vlietstra RE, Fisher LD, Burnett JC: Risks for renal dysfunction with cardiac angiography. *Ann Intern Med* 1986; 104:501–504.
148. Holland MD, Galla JH, Sanders PW, Luke RG: Effect of urinary pH and diatrizoate on Bence Jones protein nephrotoxicity in the rat. *Kidney Int* 1985; 27:46–50.
149. Fang LST, Sirota RA, Ebert TH, Lichtenstein NS: Low fractional excretion of sodium with contrast media–induced acute renal failure. *Arch Intern Med* 1980; 140:531–533.
150. Anto HR, Chou S-Y, Porush JG, Shapiro WB: Infusion intravenous pyelography and renal function. *Arch Intern Med* 1981; 141:1652–1656.
151. Dalakos TG, Streeten DHP, Jones D, Obeid A: "Malignant" hypertension resulting from atheromatous embolization predominantly of one kidney. *Am J Med* 1974; 57:135–138.
152. McGowan JA, Greenberg A: Cholesterol atheroembolic renal disease. *Am J Nephrol* 1986; 6:135–139.
153. Richards AM, Eliot RS, Kanjuh VI, Bloemendaal RD, Edwards JE: Cholesterol embolism: A multiple-system disease masquerading as polyarteritis nodosa. *Am J Cardiol* 1965; 15:696–707.
154. Scully RE, Mark EJ, McNeely BU: Case records of the Massachusetts General Hospital. *N Engl J Med* 1986; 315:308–315.
155. Cosio FG, Zager RA, Sharma HM: Atheroembolic renal disease causes hypocomplementaemia. *Lancet* 1985; 2:118–121.
156. Lessman RK, Johnson SF, Coburn JW: Renal artery embolism. *Ann Intern Med* 1978; 89:477–482.
157. Winzelberg GG, Hull JD, Agar JWM, Rose BD, Pietka PG: Elevation of serum lactate dehydrogenase levels in renal infarction. *JAMA* 1979; 242:268–269.
158. London IL, Hoffstein P, Perkoff GT, Pennington TG: Renal infarction. *Arch Int Med* 1968; 121:87–90.
159. Jelliffe RW: An improved method of digoxin therapy. *Ann Intern Med* 1968; 69:703–717.
160. Gibson TP, Matusik EJ, Briggs WA: *N*-acetylprocainamide levels in patients with end-stage renal failure. *Clin Pharm Therap* 1976; 19:206–212.
161. Bennett WM, Muther RS, Parker RA, Feig P, Morrison G, Golper TA, et al: Drug therapy in renal failure: Dosing guidelines for adults. *Ann Intern Med* 1980; 93:286–325.
162. Reidenberg MM: The binding of drugs to plasma proteins and the interpretation of measurements of plasma concentrations of drugs in patients with poor renal function. *Am J Med* 1977; 62:466–470.
163. Letteri JM, Mellk H, Louis S, Kutt H, Durante P, Glazko A: Diphenylhydantoin metabolism in uremia. *N Engl J Med* 1971; 285:648–652.
164. Kirch W, Gorg ER: Clinical pharmacokinetics of atenolol—a review. *Eur J Drug Metab Pharmacokinet* 1982; 7:81.
165. Cohn JN, Burke LP: Nitroprusside. *Ann Intern Med* 1979; 91:752–757.
166. Hricik DE, Browning PJ, Kopelman R, Goorno WE, Madias NE, Dzau VJ: Captopril-induced functional renal insufficiency in patients with bilateral renal-artery stenoses or renal-artery stenosis in a solitary kidney. *Med Intell* 1983; 308:373–376.
167. Barros EJG, Boim MA, Ajzen H, Ramos OL, Schor N: Glomerular hemodynamics and hormonal participation on cyclosporine nephrotoxicity. *Kidney Int* 1987; 32:19–25.
168. Myers BD: Cyclosporine nephrotoxicity. *Kidney Int* 1986; 30:964–974.
169. Bantle JP, Nath KA, Sutherland DER, Najarian JS, Ferris TF: Effects of cyclosporine on the renin-angiotensin-aldosterone system and potassium excretion in renal transplant recipients. *Arch Intern Med* 1985; 145:505–508.
170. Myers BD, Sibley R, Newton L, Tomlanovich SJ, Bashkos C, Stinson E, et al: The long-term course of cyclosporine-associated chronic nephropathy. *Kidney Int* 1988; 33:590–600.

Chapter 109

Adverse Cardiovascular Drug Interactions

Lionel H. Opie, M.D., Ph.D.

The best known cardiovascular drug interaction is that between quinidine and digitalis, whereby quinidine elevates digoxin levels. This interaction "caught the eye" of cardiologists because it involved two classic drugs, which had been used in combination for many years. The knowledge of such an interaction alerted clinicians to the fact that apparently established properties of drugs could perhaps be explained more simply by drug interactions. For example, some arrhythmias thought to be caused by quinidine were probably evoked by the increased blood digoxin level.

Today a knowledge of cardiovascular drug interactions is regarded as basic to our understanding of cardiovascular drug pharmacologic properties. Such interactions can be either *pharmacokinetic*, whereby one agent interferes with the metabolism of another, or *pharmacodynamic*, whereby the hemodynamic properties of one agent are additive or subtractive to those of another. An example of the pharmacokinetic interaction is the decreased rate of hepatic metabolism of lidocaine during cimetidine therapy, with possible risk of lidocaine toxicity. An example of a pharmacodynamic interaction is when nifedipine is added to β-adrenergic blockade in the therapy of severe angina, sometimes with excess hypotension as a side effect.

This chapter will include discussions of the drug interactions of the major classes of cardiovascular drugs, following an established sequence of these drugs (Tables 109-1 to 109-7).[1]

β-ADRENERGIC BLOCKING DRUGS

β-Adrenergic blockers are subject to relatively few serious drug interactions (Table 109-1). An example of a pharmacokinetic interaction is that with cimetidine,[2] which reduces hepatic blood flow and therefore increases blood levels of propranolol and metoprolol, which are both metabolized in the liver. However, there is no interaction of cimetidine with β blockers such as atenolol, sotatol, and nadolol, which are not metabolized in the liver. Another pharmacokinetic interaction is when verapamil raises blood levels of metoprolol through a hepatic interaction[3]; presumably other β blockers metabolized by the liver may be subject to a similar interaction.

Now used with increasing frequency in the acute phase of myocardial infarction, β blockers may depress hepatic blood flow, thereby decreasing hepatic inactivation of lidocaine.[4] Thus β blockade increases lidocaine blood levels with enhanced risk of toxicity. An example of a pharmacodynamic interaction is that with nonsteroidal antiinflammatory drugs (NSAIDs), including indomethacin, which attenuate the antihypertensive effects of β blockers[5]; probably the mode of action is decreased formation of vasodilatory prostaglandins. (For the interaction of β blockers with disopyramide, see "Antiarrhythmic Agents," "Verapamil and β Blockers," and "Diltiazem." See also Chap. 66.)

TABLE 109-1
Drug Interactions of β-Adrenergic Blocking Agents

Cardiac Drug	Interacting Drugs	Mechanism	Consequence	Prophylaxis	Reference
		Hemodynamic Interactions			
All β Blockers	Calcium antagonists, especially nifedipine	Added hypotension	Risk of myocardial ischemia	Blood pressure control, adjust doses	27
	Verapamil or diltiazem	Added negative inotropic effect	Risk of myocardial failure	Check for CHF, adjust doses	13
	Flecainide	Added negative inotropic effect	Hypotension	Check LV function, flecainide levels	
		Electrophysiological Interactions			
All β Blockers	Verapamil	Added inhibition of SA, AV nodes	Bradycardia, asystole, complete heart block	Exclude "sick-sinus" syndrome, AV nodal disease,	11
	Diltiazem	Added negative inotropic effect	Excess hypotension	adjust dose, exclude predrug LV failure	30
		Hepatic Interactions			
Propranolol (P)	Cimetidine (C)	C decreases P metabolism	Excess propranolol effects	Reduce both drug doses	2
	Lidocaine (L)	Low hepatic blood flow	Excess lidocaine effects	Reduce lidocaine dose	4
Metoprolol (M)	Verapamil (V)	V decreases M metabolism	Excess M effects	Reduce M dose	3
	Cimetidine (C)	C decreases M metabolism	Excess M effects	Reduce both drug doses	90
Labetalol (L)	Cimetidine (C)	C decreases L metabolism	Excess L effects	Reduce both drug doses	91
		Antihypertensive Interactions			
β Blockers	Indomethacin (I), NSAIDs	I inhibits vasodilatory prostaglandins	Decreased antihypertensive effect	Omit indomethacin; use alternative drugs	5
		Immune Interacting Drugs			
Acebutolol	Other drugs altering immune status: procainamide, hydralazine, captopril	Theoretical risk of additive immune effects	Theoretical risk of lupus or neutropenia	Check antinuclear factors and neutrophils; low doses during cotherapy	(—)

CHF, congestive heart failure; LV, left ventricular; AV, atrioventricular. (—), Expected interaction, no reference.

NITRATES

The chief drug interactions of nitrates are pharmacodynamic (Table 109-2). For example, during triple therapy of angina pectoris (nitrates, β blockers, calcium antagonists), the efficacy of the combination may be lessened, probably because each drug can predispose to excess hypotension.[6] Even two components of triple therapy, such as diltiazem and nitrates, may interact adversely to cause excess hypotension.[7] Nonetheless high doses of diltiazem can improve persistent effort angina when added to maximum doses of propranolol and isosorbide dinitrate[8] without any report of significant hypotension. Therefore individual patients vary greatly in their susceptibility to the hypotension of triple therapy. (See also Chap. 30.)

CALCIUM ANTAGONISTS

Many of the interactions of calcium antagonists are pharmacodynamic (Table 109-2),[9] such as added effects on the atrioventricular (AV) or sinus nodes (verapamil or diltiazem plus β blockers or excess digitalis or amiodar-

TABLE 109-2

Drug Interactions of Nitrates and Calcium Antagonists

Cardiac Drug	Interacting Drugs	Mechanism	Consequence	Prophylaxis	Reference
		Nitrates			
All nitrates	Calcium antagonists	Excess vasodilation	Syncope, dizziness	Monitor BP	92
	Prazosin (PZ)	Excess vasodilation	Syncope, dizziness	Monitor BP and start with low PZ dose	
		Calcium Antagonist Drugs			
Verapamil (V)	β Blockers	SA and AV nodal inhibition Myocardial failure	Added nodal and negative inotropic effects	Care during cotherapy Check ECG, BP, heart size	11
	Cimetidine	Hepatic metabolic interaction	Blood V rises	Adjust dose	64
	Digitalis poisoning	Added SA and AV nodal inhibition	Asystole; complete heart block after IV verapamil	Avoid IV verapamil in digitalis poisoning	1
	Digoxin (D)	Decreased digoxin clearance	Risk of D toxicity	Halve D dose; blood D level	20
	Disopyramide	Pharmacodynamic	Hypotension, constipation	Check BP, LV, and gut	(—)
	Flecainide (F)	Added negative intropic effect	Hypotension	Check LV; F levels	
	Prazosin	Hepatic interaction	Excess hypotension	Check BP during cotherapy	23
	Quinidine (Q)	Added α-receptor inhibition; V decreases Q clearance	Hypotension; increased Q levels	Check Q levels and BP	24
	Theophylline (T)	Inhibition of hepatic metabolism	Increased blood T levels	Reduce T, check levels	26
Nifedipine (N)	β Blockers	Added negative inotropism	Excess hypotension	Check BP, use test dose of N	27
	Cimetidine	Hepatic metabolic interaction	Increased blood N levels	Decreased N dosage by 40%	93 64
	Digoxin (D)	Minor/modest changes in digoxin	Increased digoxin levels	Check D levels	94
	Prazosin (PZ)	PZ blocks α reflex to N	Postural hypotension	Test dose of N or PZ	29
	Propranolol (P)	N and P have opposite effects on blood liver flow	N decreases P levels; P increases N levels	Readjust P and N doses if needed	28
	Quinidine (Q)	N improves poor LV function; Q clearance faster	Decreased Q effect	Check Q levels	39
Diltiazem (D)	β Blockers	Added SA nodal inhibition; negative inotropism	Bradycardia, hypotension	Check ECG and LV function	30
	Cimetidine	Hepatic metabolic interaction	Increased D levels	Reduce D dose by one-third	64
	Cyclosporin (C)	Hepatic metabolism of C inhibited	Increased blood C levels	Decrease C dose	31
	Digoxin (D)	Some fall in D clearance	Only in renal failure	Check D levels	64
	Flecainide (F)	Added negative inotropic effect	Hypotension	Check LV; F levels	(—)
Nicardipine (see also nifedipine)	Cyclosporin (C)	Hepatic metabolism of C inhibited	Increased blood C levels	Decrease C dose	95
	Digoxin (D)	Decreased D clearance	Blood D doubles	Decrease D, D levels	68

SA, sinoatrial node; AV, atrioventricular node; LV, left ventricle; BP, blood pressure; ECG, electrocardiogram. (—), Expected interaction, no reference.

one), or on the systemic vascular resistance (for example, nifedipine plus β-blockers causing excess hypotension). However, it is now increasingly recognized that verapamil and diltiazem (but probably not nifedipine) especially inhibit the hepatic oxidation of some drugs the blood levels of which consequently increase. Such agents include cyclosporin (diltiazem), the antiepileptic carbamazepine (verapamil), prazosin (verapamil), theophylline (verapamil), and quinidine (verapamil). In addition, nifedipine especially and also verapamil tend to increase hepatic blood flow, potentially leading to enhanced first-pass metabolism of agents such as propranolol so that the blood levels fall. (See also Chap. 67.)

Verapamil (Calan, Isoptin) and β Blockers

Intravenous verapamil added to β-adrenergic blockade has the risk of added hypotension or added nodal inhibition.[10,11] In patients with angina pectoris already receiving β blockers, verapamil given intravenously[12] or orally[13] can reduce contractility,[13] increase heart size,[14] and cause sinus bradycardia.[15] By a hepatic pharmacokinetic interaction,[16] verapamil may raise blood levels of β blockers metabolized by the liver. Despite such hepatic interactions (e.g., verapamil with propranolol) in normal subjects, pharmacodynamic changes are more important.[17] Contraindications to the combination of verapamil and β blockade in the therapy of angina pectoris are preexisting depression of the sinoatrial (SA) or AV nodes and clinically detectable myocardial failure. The combination of verapamil plus β blockers improves myocardial function during exercise more than does either agent alone.[18] Verapamil plus a β blocker may have an added therapeutic effect in hypertension, but with a small risk of excess inhibition of heart rate, AV conduction, or left ventricular function.[19] (See Chap. 77.)

Other Drug Interactions with Verapamil

Digoxin

Verapamil can increase blood digoxin levels by over 50 percent.[20] The dose of digoxin must be cut to about half and blood levels of digoxin must then be rechecked. In digitalis toxicity, rapid intravenous verapamil is *absolutely contraindicated* because the sum of the inhibitory effects on the AV node of these two agents can be fatal. Experimentally, verapamil can inhibit the calcium-dependent delayed afterdepolarizations (DADs), which cause the ventricular automaticity found in digitalis toxicity. Yet intravenous verapamil should only be used in digitalis poisoning if the situation is desperate. Oral verapamil and digitalis can, however, be combined in the absence of digitalis toxicity or AV block, because their pharmacologic sites of action differ; however, the digoxin level needs monitoring. (See also Chap. 27.)

Verapamil-Prazosin

Verapamil may be combined with prazosin for hypertension with added and synergistic effects[21]; a hepatic pharmacokinetic interaction with enhanced bioavailability of prazosin may explain the synergistic effects.[22,23]

Verapamil-Quinidine

Verapamil and quinidine may interact to cause excess hypotension[24] either by combined inhibition of peripheral α receptors or by increase of quinidine levels[25]; the latter may be a hepatic interaction. (See Chap. 67.)

Verapamil-Disopyramide

Both verapamil and disopyramide are powerful negative inotropes, so that the combination can only be given when left ventricular function is carefully monitored.

Verapamil-Theophylline

Verapamil may inhibit the hepatic metabolism of theophylline to increase blood theophylline levels.[26]

Nifedipine (Procardia, Adalat)

The combination of nifedipine with β blockade is generally well tolerated except for the risk of hypotension.[27] Nifedipine and propranolol may have a pharmacokinetic interaction whereby blood levels of propranolol become increased; it is thought that nifedipine increases the hepatic blood flow so that propranolol breakdown in the liver is lessened.[28] Although nifedipine is an afterload reducer, it also has a direct negative inotropic effect. Hence combination with any other negative inotropic agent, not only β blockade but also disopyramide and others, should be undertaken with caution. Nifedipine combined with prazosin hydrochloride may cause excess hypotension[29] so that low initial additive doses are recommended. [See "Prazosin Hydrochloride (Minipress)."]

Diltiazem (Cardizem, Tildiem, Herbesser, Tilazem)

Like verapamil, diltiazem may increase blood digoxin levels. However, the rise is likely to be much less, and some studies report no increase at all. Diltiazem plus long-acting nitrates occasionally cause excess hypotension.[7] The combination of high-dose diltiazem with β blockade may cause bradycardia or hypotension.[30] Relatively few life-threatening interactions have been described for diltiazem, probably because intravenous diltiazem is relatively new. However, as the application of intravenous diltiazem increases, it can be expected to have a similar spectrum of drug interactions to that of intravenous verapamil. Diltiazem, metabolized by the liver, interacts with cyclosporin[31] so that the cyclosporin blood levels increase.

ANTIARRHYTHMIC AGENTS

During antiarrhythmic therapy numerous drug interactions are possible (Table 109-3).[32,33] Patients with serious ventricular arrhythmias frequently have associated angina (potentially necessitating calcium antagonists or β blockers) or heart failure (requiring digitalis and diuretics). Nausea, a common symptom of chronic cardiac patients, may require cimetidine. The most frequent drug interactions are with digoxin (quinidine and verapamil increasing levels), with diuretics (risk of QT prolongation with antiarrhythmics that prolong the action potential duration such as quinidine, disopyramide, amiodarone, and sotalol), and at the level of hepatic enzyme induction (cimetidine decreases hepatic metabolism of quinidine[34]; phenytoin and barbiturates have an opposite effect). There is also the risk of antiarrhythmic drug-drug interactions. Thus amiodarone when added to quinidine enhances the risk of QT prolongation while quinidine levels increase so that quinidine toxicity is also more likely.[33] (See also Chap. 38.)

Quinidine

Because quinidine increases blood digoxin levels, the dose of quinidine must be decreased and blood digoxin levels checked.[35] Quinidine may enhance the effects of other hypotensive agents, including verapamil,[24] or of agents inhibiting the sinus node (β blockers, verapamil, diltiazem, and methyldopa). Quinidine increases the effects of coumarin anticoagulants by a hepatic interaction.[36] When hepatic enzymes are induced by drugs such as phenytoin, phenobarbital, and rifampin (rifampicin), the hepatic metabolism of quinidine may markedly increase with decreased steady-state concentrations of quinidine.[37,38] Conversely, cimetidine can inhibit hepatic enzymes to decrease the metabolism of quinidine with opposite effects.[39] It appears that ranitidine has no such effects. Verapamil may increase quinidine levels.[25] Conversely, nifedipine may lower plasma quinidine levels, perhaps by causing left ventricular systolic function to improve.[40–42]

Hypokalemia decreases the antiarrhythmic effect of quinidine and predisposes to QT prolongation by quinidine. When quinidine is combined with other drugs that also prolong the QT interval, such as amiodarone or sotalol or thiazide diuretics, careful monitoring is required.[43]

Quinidine is a vagolytic drug and reduces the effects of procedures that enhance vagal activity such as carotid sinus massage. Quinidine also inhibits muscarinic receptors to reduce the effects of anticholinesterases in myasthenia gravis. (See also Chap. 36.)

Procainamide (Pronestyl)

Cimetidine inhibits the renal clearance of procainamide. The elimination half-life lengthens so that the dose of procainamide needs reduction.[44]

Disopyramide (Norpace)

Disopyramide is negatively inotropic, so that there is a potential danger of reduction of the cardiac output in patients already receiving other negative inotropes, such as the calcium antagonists (especially verapamil),[45] β blockers, or flecainide, or in patients with preexisting myocardial failure. It is also potentially dangerous to combine disopyramide with other drugs likely to depress nodal or conduction tissues, such as quinidine, digoxin, β blockade, and methyldopa. Disopyramide is ineffective in digitalis toxicity and should be avoided. There is no interaction between disopyramide and lidocaine. The concomitant use of disopyramide with other type I antiarrhythmic agents or β blockers should be reserved for life-threatening arrhythmias. The risk of QT prolongation requires that disopyramide not be combined with other drugs prolonging the QT interval, such as the tricyclics, and certain other antiarrhythmic agents, such as amiodarone or sotalol. Phenytoin[46] and other inducers of hepatic enzymes (barbiturates, rifampin) may lower disopyramide plasma levels. Pyridostigmine bromide may beneficially interact with disopyramide by inhibition of cholinesterase activity so that anticholinergic side effects of disopyramide are reduced.[47]

Lidocaine (Xylocaine; lignocaine)

In patients receiving cimetidine,[48] propranolol,[4] or halothane,[49] the hepatic clearance of lidocaine is reduced so that toxicity may occur more readily. Lidocaine may cause sinoatrial arrest, especially during coadministration of other agents potentially depressing nodal function,[50] including β blockers.

Tocainide (Tonocard)

There are presently no known adverse drug interactions involving tocainide.

Mexiletine (Mexitil)

Narcotics delay the gastrointestinal absorption of mexiletine. Rifampin (rifampicin), barbiturates and phenytoin all induce hepatic enzymes so that the plasma levels of mexiletine are reduced. Cimetidine should, but does not, increase plasma levels of mexiletine.[51] Rather cimetidine has a beneficial side effect of decreasing the gastrointestinal symptoms associated with mexiletine. Disopyramide and mexiletine when given together may predispose to a negative inotropic effect.[52] Mexiletine may, however, be combined with quinidine,[53,54] β-adrenergic blockade,[55] and amiodarone[56] provided that the appropriate contraindications for each drug are observed.

Encainide (Enkaid)

No known drug interactions are associated with encainide.

Flecainide (Tambocor)

Flecainide inhibits the sinus and AV nodal function so that combination with β blockers, verapamil, diltiazem, and digitalis requires care. Flecainide also has additive negative inotropic effects that may exaggerate those of β blockers,[57] verapamil, or disopyramide. Combined inhibitory effects on His-Purkinje conduction may arise during cotherapy with quinidine or procainamide and to a lesser extent with disopyramide. Flecainide blood levels are increased by amiodarone; the flecainide dose should be decreased by about one-third.[58] Studies of healthy volunteers suggest that (1) cimetidine delays the clearance of flecainide[59] and (2) flecainide increases blood digoxin levels.[57]

TABLE 109-3
Drug Interactions of Antiarrhythmic Drugs

Cardiac Drug	Interacting Drugs	Mechanism	Consequence	Prophylaxis	Reference
		Class IA			
Quinidine (Q)	Amiodarone	Added QT effects; blood Q rises	Torsades de pointes	Check QT, potassium	43 33
	Antibiotics (some)	Quinidine inhibits muscarinic receptors	Increased antibiotic-induced muscular weakness	Clinical care, drug levels	96
	Anticholinesterases	Quinidine inhibits muscarinic receptors	Decreased ACh efficacy in myasthenia gravis	Avoid Q if possible blood	96
	Antihypertensive agents β Blockers	Added hypotensive and added SA nodal effects	Hypotension, excess bradycardia	Regulate BP Check BP, ECG	(—) 97
	Cimetidine (C)	C inhibits oxidative metabolism of Q	Increased Q levels, risk of toxicity	Q levels, consider ranitidine	34 39
	Coumarin anticoagulants	Hepatic interaction with Q	Bleeding	Check prothrombin time	36
	Digoxin (D)	Decreased D clearance	Risk of D toxicity	Check D dose levels	35
	Diltiazem	Added inhibition of SA node	Excess bradycardia	Check ECG, heart rate	30
	Disopyramide	Added QT prolongation	Torsades de pointes	Check QT, potassium	43
	Diuretic, potassium losing	Hypokalemia and QT prolongation	Torsades de pointes	Check QT, potassium	98
	Hepatic enzyme inducers (phenytoin, barbiturates, rifampin)	Increased Q hepatic metabolism	Decreased Q levels	Q levels, doses	37
	Nifedipine	Increased Q clearance	Decreased Q levels	Q levels, doses	41 42
	Sotalol	Added QT prolongation	Torsades de pointes	Check QT, potassium	76
	Verapamil	Decreased Q clearance	Excess bradycardia	Check ECG, Q levels	24
	Warfarin	Hepatic interaction with Q	Bleeding	Check prothrombin time	36
Procainamide (P)	Captopril	Combined immune effects	Theoretical risk of neutropenia	Cotherapy with care	(—)
	Cimetidine	Decreased renal P clearance	Prolonged P half-life, excess P effect	Reduce P dose; consider ranitidine	44
Disopyramide (D)	Agents prolonging APD (quinidine, amiodarone, sotalol)	Added QT prolongation especially if hypokalemia	Torsades de pointes	Check QT, potassium	1
	β Blockers	Combined negative inotropism	Hypotension	Low doses	(—)
	Cimetidine	Hepatic D metabolism falls	Increased blood D levels		(—)
	Digitalis toxicity	Added SA, AV nodal depression	SA, AV block	Avoid D in digitalis toxicity	(—)
	Hepatic enzyme inducers (phenytoin, rifampin, barbiturates)	Enhanced D hepatic metabolism	Blood D levels fall; readjust D dose	Readjust D dose	46

TABLE 109-3
Drug Interactions of Antiarrhythmic Drugs *(continued)*

Cardiac Drug	Interacting Drugs	Mechanism	Consequence	Prophylaxis	Reference
	Drugs inhibiting SA or AV nodes/ conduction system (quinidine, β blockers, methyldopa, digoxin)	Pharmacodynamic additive effects	SA, AV block; conduction block	Check ECG; decrease doses	(—)
	Pyridostigmine	Inhibition of cholinesterase activity	Beneficial effect of P on D; harmful effect of D on P	In myasthenia gravis, avoid D	47
			Class IB		
Lidocaine (lignocaine)	Verapamil	Combined negative inotropism	Hypotension	Avoid IV D or V cotherapy	45
	Cimetidine	Decreased hepatic metabolism	Increased L levels	Decrease L infusion rate	48
	Halothane	Decreased hepatic blood flow	Increased L levels	Decrease L infusion rate	49
	Propranolol	Decreased hepatic blood flow	Increased L levels	Decrease L infusion rate	4
	Other β blockers	Decreased hepatic blood flow	Increased L levels	Decrease L infusion rate	99
Mexiletine	Hepatic enzyme inducers (phenytoin, barbiturates, rifampin)	Increased hepatic metabolism	Decreased plasma M levels	Increase M dose	(—)
			Class IC		
Flecainide (F)	Amiodarone	Unknown	Blood F rises; added effects on nodes, myocardium	Decrease F dose	58
	Digoxin (D)	Decreased D clearance	Blood D rises slightly	Check D level	57
	Drugs inhibiting SA or AV nodes, IV conduction or myocardial function	Pharmacodynamic, additive	SA, AV block; conduction block; negative inotropism	Decrease D dose	100
	Cimetidine	Decreased hepatic F loss	Blood F rises	Check F dose	59
Propafenone	Digoxin	Pharmacokinetic	Increased D level	Decrease D dose	60
			Class III		
Amiodarone (A)	Drugs prolonging QT interval (quinidine, disopyramide, phenothiazines, tricyclic antidepressants, thiazide diuretics, sotalol)	Pharmacodynamic additive effects	Torsades de pointes	Avoid low K+; avoid combinations	43
	Quinidine (Q)	Pharmacokinetic	Blood Q rises	Check Q levels	33
	Procainamide (P)	Pharmacokinetic	Blood P rises	Check P dose	33
Sotalol	(P) as above	Hypokalemia plus class III action	Torsades de pointes	Exclude low K+; use K+-retaining diuretic	76

APD, action potential duration; IV, intravenous; ACh, acetylcholine. (—), Expected interaction, no reference.

Propafenone (Rythmol, Arytmol, Rytmonorm)

Propafenone is a class IC antiarrhythmic drug; therefore it may interact adversely with other drugs, depressing nodal function or intraventricular conduction or the inotropic state. Nonetheless, propafenone can be combined with quinidine or procainamide at reduced doses of both drugs.[51] Propafenone substantially increases serum digoxin levels.[60]

Amiodarone (Cordarone)

The most serious interaction of amiodarone[43] is the potential for an additive proarrhythmic effect with other drugs prolonging the QT interval such as class IA antiarrhythmic agents, sotalol, phenothiazines, tricyclic antidepressants, and thiazide diuretics. Amiodarone does not normally depress the sinus node, yet may do so when combined with calcium antagonists such as verapamil or diltiazem.[9] In patients receiving warfarin, amiodarone prolongs the prothrombin time.[61]

Sotalol (Sotacor)

Cotherapy with any other agents that may cause hypokalemia (such as diuretics) or prolong the action potential duration (such as quinidine, disopyramide, amiodarone, or tricyclic antidepressants or probucol) may precipitate torsades de pointes.

Bretylium (Bretylol)

Experimentally, bretylium may worsen digitalis-induced ventricular tachycardia.[62] Nonetheless the drug may be lifesaving for patients with ventricular fibrillation thought to be induced by digitalis.[63]

POSITIVE INOTROPIC AGENTS (TABLE 109-4)

Digoxin

The *quinidine-digoxin* interaction is best known. Quinidine approximately doubles the blood digoxin levels, decreasing both renal and extrarenal clearance.[20,35,64] The previous dose of digoxin should be halved and the plasma digoxin rechecked. Quinine given for muscle cramps acts likewise.

The *verapamil-digoxin* interaction is equally significant; digoxin levels increase by 60 to 90 percent.[20,65] The *other calcium antagonists*, nifedipine and diltiazem, increase digoxin levels much less than verapamil.[64,66,67] Adjustment of the digoxin dose with these agents is usually not necessary except in the presence of renal failure (which decreases digoxin excretion). *Nicardipine* causes only a modest rise of digoxin levels.[65] *Nitrendipine*, however, resembles verapamil in approximately doubling the digoxin levels.[68] Thus there are no simple rules to explain which class of calcium antagonists or which specific agent is likely to increase digoxin levels significantly.

Among other vasodilators, *prazosin* increases digoxin levels in dogs by reduction of plasma and tissue binding.[69] Among antiarrhythmics other than quinidine or verapamil, *amiodarone* and *propafenone*[60] also elevate serum digoxin levels. The other antiarrhythmics, including procainamide and mexiletine, have no interaction with digoxin, except for a relatively small rise of digoxin levels with flecainide.[57]

When cotherapy elevates digoxin levels, the features of digitalis toxicity may depend on the agent added. With quinidine, tachyarrhythmias become more likely; amiodarone and verapamil seem to repress the ventricular arrhythmias of digitalis toxicity, so that bradycardia and AV block are more likely.[70]

Diuretics may indirectly precipitate digitalis toxicity by causing hypokalemia, which when really severe (plasma potassium below 2 to 3 meq/liter) may stop the tubular secretion of digoxin. Potassium-sparing diuretics (amiloride, triamterene, and spironolactone)[71] as well as captopril decrease digoxin clearance by about 20 to 30 percent. When these combinations with digoxin are used in the therapy of congestive heart failure, the blood digoxin level must be watched. Unexpectedly, spironolactone and its metabolite, canrenone, may decrease features of digitalis toxicity.[72] Nonetheless the combination digoxin-quinidine-spironolactone markedly elevates digoxin levels.[73]

The *gastrointestinal absorption* of digoxin may be decreased by cholestyramine, probably because of the binding of digoxin to the resin; digoxin should therefore be given several hours before the resin or else digoxin capsules may be used (Lanoxicaps; 0.2 mg = 0.25 mg of digoxin). Digoxin capsules also lessen interaction with kaolin-pectate, which reduces digoxin absorption, and with erythromycin and tetracycline, which inhibit gastrointestinal flora that inactivate digoxin and thereby increase digoxin blood levels. Cancer chemotherapeutic agents may damage intestinal mucosa to depress digoxin absorption. (See Chap. 27.)

SYMPATHOMIMETIC AGENTS

Dopamine (Intropin)

Dopamine is contraindicated during the use of cyclopropane or halogenated hydrocarbon anesthetics (enhanced risk of arrhythmias). Monoamine-oxidase inhibitors decrease the rate of dopamine metabolism by the tissues, and the dose of dopamine should be cut to one-tenth of usual.

Dobutamine (Dobutrex)

Dobutamine decreases plasma potassium and should be given with care together with diuretics, especially intravenous furosemide.

Amrinone (Inocor) and Milrinone (Primacor)

Amrinone and milrinone are phosphodiesterase inhibitors that may also provoke arrhythmias. During diuretic therapy, plasma K needs monitoring. When combined with digitalis, the digoxin level should not change, but digoxin toxicity should be guarded against because of multiple mechanisms for arrhythmia development. (See also Chap. 28.)

TABLE 109-4
Drug Interactions of Digitalis and Other Positive Inotropic Agents

Cardiac Drug	Interacting Drugs	Mechanism	Consequence	Prophylaxis	Reference
		Positive Inotropic Agents			
Digitoxin	Verapamil	Nonrenal clearance of digitoxin falls	Digitoxin levels up by one-third	Check digitoxin levels	101
	Other drugs interacting with digoxin	? Altered digitoxin clearance	? Digitoxin levels increase	Check digitoxin levels	
Digoxin (D)	Amiodarone	Reduced renal clearance of D	D level may double	Check D level; halve dose	70
	Captopril	Reduced D clearance	Blood D increases	Check D dose	102
	Diltiazem	Variable decrease of D clearance	Variable blood D increases	Check D level	66
	Diuretics; potassium-sparing amiloride/triamterene, spironolactone (S)	Reduced extrarenal D clearance	D levels up by 20%	Check D level	72
		S reduces renal D clearance	D levels increase	Complex effects; check D levels	72
	Nifedipine	Variable fall of D clearance	Variable blood D rises	Check D levels	64
	Nitrendipine	Reduced D clearance	Blood D doubles	Check D levels; halve dose	68
	Prazosin (PZ)	PZ displaces D from binding sites	Blood D rises	(Needs confirmation in humans)	69
	Propafenone	Not defined	D level increases	Check D level	60
	Quinidine, quinine	Reduced D clearance	Blood D doubles	Check D levels; halve dose	35
	Verapamil	Reduced D clearance	Blood D doubles or more	Check D levels; halve dose	20
		Sympathomimetic Inotropes			
Dobutamine Amrinone Milrinone	Thiazide diuretics	Additive hypokalemic effects	Arrhythmias	Check blood potassium	(—)*

* Expected interaction, no reference.

DIURETICS (TABLE 109-5)

Loop Diuretics

Loop diuretics, when given acutely and intravenously, may cause hypokalemia, precipitating digitalis toxicity.[74] Furosemide decreases renal clearance of lithium. Certain NSAIDs may antagonize the action of furosemide (and other diuretics). In normal subjects, concurrent captopril therapy lessens the diuretic effect of furosemide. (See also Chap. 29.)

Thiazide Diuretics

Steroids, estrogens, and indomethacin and other NSAIDs lessen the antihypertensive effect of thiazide diuretics[5] and may worsen congestive heart failure.[75] *Captopril* (Capoten) tends to be potassium retaining and may cause hyperkalemia if combined with other potassium retainers. Diuretic-induced hypokalemia may predispose to ventricular arrhythmias including torsades de pointes; usually there is additional therapy with antiarrhythmic agents such as sotalol,[76] quinidine, or amiodarone (all of which may prolong the QT interval). *Probenecid* interferes with the urinary excretion of thiazide and loop diuretics[74] so that diuretic efficacy is reduced. Diuretics may impair the renal clearance of *lithium* so that the blood level rises with risk of lithium toxicity.[77]

VASODILATORS (TABLE 109-6)

Nitroprusside (Nipride) and Hydralazine (Apresoline)

Nitroprusside and hydralazine may decrease digoxin levels, possibly as a result of increased tubular excretion.[78] On first principles, however, unloading agents may be expected to improve congestive heart failure, renal plasma flow, and renal excretion of digoxin. (See also Chap. 30.)

TABLE 109-5
Drug Interactions of Diuretics

Cardiac Drug	Interacting Drugs	Mechanism	Consequence	Prophylaxis	Reference
Diuretic					
Loop and thiazide	Indomethacin and other NSAIDs	Pharmacodynamic	Decreased antihypertensive effect	Adjust diuretic dose or add another agent	5
	Probenecid	Decreased intratubular secretion of diuretic	Decreased diuretic effect	Increase diuretic dose	74
	ACE inhibitors	Excess diuretics, high renins	Excess hypotension; prerenal uremia	Lower diuretic dose; test dose ACE inhibitor	103
Loop	Captopril	Possible interference with tubular secretion	Loss of diuretic efficacy of furosemide	Change to another ACE inhibitor	104

ACE, angiotensin converting enzyme.

Prazosin (Minipress)

There is an interaction with the calcium antagonists verapamil and nifedipine, so that excess or added hypotension results.[23,29] In the case of verapamil, part of the effect may be explained by a pharmacokinetic hepatic interaction.[23] Both nitrates and prazosin may cause syncope and these agents should be combined with care. Experimentally, prazosin may increase the plasma digoxin level.[69]

TABLE 109-6
Drug Interactions of Vasodilators and Angiotensin Converting Enzyme Inhibitors

Cardiac Drug	Interacting Drugs	Mechanism	Consequence	Prophylaxis	Reference
		Vasodilators			
Hydralazine/ nitroprusside	Digoxin (D)	Increased renal D excretion	Decreased D levels	Check D levels	78
Prazosin (P)	Nifedipine	Pharmacodynamic	Excess hypotension	Test dose of nifedipine	29
	Nitrates	Pharmacodynamic	Syncope, hypotension	Decrease P dose	23
	Verapamil	Hepatic metabolism	Synergistic antihypertensive effect	Adjust doses	23
		Angiotensin Converting Enzyme (ACE) Inhibitors			
	Diuretics	High renin levels in overdiuresed patients	"First" dose hypotension; risk of renal failure	Low test dose	103
	Potassium-sparing diuretics	Added potassium retention	Hyperkalemia	Avoid combination	105
Captopril	Loop diuretic	Possible interference with tubular secretion	Lessened diuretic effect of furosemide	Consider alternate ACE inhibitor therapy	104
Captopril (C)	Immunosuppressive drugs, procainamide, hydralazine, possibly acebutolol	Added immune effects	Increased risk of neutropenia	Avoid combination; check neutrophils	106
	Probenecid (P)	P inhibits tubular secretion of C	Small risk in C levels	Decrease dose of C	80

ANGIOTENSIN CONVERTING ENZYME INHIBITORS

In general, angiotensin converting enzyme (ACE) inhibitors have few drug interactions.[79] The most common one is with diuretics, with risk of excess hypotension in overdiuresed patients. The K^+-retaining diuretics or K^+ supplements together with captopril can cause hyperkalemia. Indomethacin and NSAIDs may decrease the antihypertensive effects of ACE inhibitors (and almost all antihypertensives). (See also Chaps. 30 and 77.)

Captopril (Capoten, Calan, Lopirin, Lopril)

Cotherapy of high-dose captopril with other drugs thought to alter or impair the immune status (such as hydralazine and procainamide) may predispose to neutropenia. Probenecid inhibits the renal tubular excretion of captopril, thereby increasing blood captopril levels[80]; doses of captopril may need downward adjustment. Captopril may decrease digoxin clearance by 20 to 30 percent.[71]

Enalapril (Vasotec, Xanef, Innovace, Renitec, Renivace)

Drug interactions are similar to those of captopril, except that the risk of neutropenia is less. It needs to be considered that the action of enalapril is longer lasting, and adverse hypotensive interactions with diuretics are therefore potentially more serious.

ANTITHROMBOTIC AGENTS (TABLE 109-7)

Aspirin

Blood levels of uric acid may be increased by both aspirin and thiazide diuretics, so that special care is required in patients with a history of gout.[81] Conversely, aspirin may decrease the uricosuric effects of sulfinpyrazone and probenecid. Aspirin also reduces the natriuretic effect of spironolactone. Aspirin-induced gastrointestinal bleeding may be a greater hazard in patients receiving corticosteroid therapy or NSAIDs. Antacids, by altering the pH

TABLE 109-7
Drug Interactions of Antithrombotic Agents

Cardiac Drug	Interacting Drugs	Mechanism	Consequence	Prophylaxis	Reference
Aspirin (A)	Hepatic enzyme inducers (barbiturates, phenytoin, rifampin)	Increased A metabolism	Decreased A effect	Adjust A dose; check A side effects	(—)*
	Sulfinpyrazone (S), probenecid (P)	A decreases urate excretion	Decreased uricosuric effect of S or P	Increase dose of S or P	81
	Thiazide diuretics	A decreases urate excretion	Hyperuricemia	Check blood urate	81
	Warfarin (W)	A is antithrombotic	Excess bleeding	Check prothrombin time	85
Sulfinpyrazone (S)	Warfarin	S displaces W from plasma proteins	Excess bleeding	Check prothrombin time	86
Warfarin (W)	Potentiating drugs				
	Allopurinol	Mechanism unknown	Excess bleeding	Check prothrombin time	84
	Amiodarone	Mechanism unknown	Sensitizes to W for 1–2 months	Avoid combination	61
	Aspirin	Added bleeding tendency	Excess bleeding	Check prothrombin time	85
	Cimetidine	Decreased W degradation	Increased blood W	Check prothrombin time	
	Quinidine	Hepatic interaction	Excess bleeding	Check prothrombin time	36
	Sulfinpyrazone	Displaces W from plasma proteins	Excess bleeding	Check prothrombin time	86
	Inhibitory drugs				
	Cholestyramine, Colestipol	Decrease absorption of W	Decreased W effect	Check prothrombin time	84

* Expected interaction, no reference.

of the stomach, may decrease the efficacy of enteric-coated preparations. Hepatic enzyme inducers (barbiturates, phenytoin, rifampicin) increase aspirin breakdown. Aspirin tends to cause hypoglycemia in patients receiving oral hypoglycemics or insulin. Aspirin, especially in high doses, may exaggerate a bleeding tendency and anticoagulant-induced bleeding.[82] Dipyridamole-warfarin causes less bleeding than aspirin plus warfarin in patients who have undergone bypass surgery.[83] All these drug interactions should be less intense if the aspirin doses are kept low, as is the current trend. (See also Chap. 68.)

Sulfinpyrazone (Anturane)

Sulfinpyrazone is highly bound to plasma proteins (98 to 99 percent) and may displace warfarin to precipitate bleeding. Like aspirin, sulfinpyrazone may sensitize patients given sulfonylureas and insulin to hypoglycemia.

Dipyridamole (Persantine)

Dipyridamole is a potent vasodilator, so that care is required when it is used in combination with other vasodilators.

Warfarin (Coumadin)

Warfarin may be subject to many (up to 80) drug interactions.[84] A good rule is to suspect interactions unless one can be sure. The safest rule is to tell patients having oral anticoagulation not to use any new or over-the-counter drugs without consultation and for the physician to carefully check out any added compounds. More frequent measurements of the prothrombin time are required when potentially interfering drugs are added.

Interfering Drugs

Interfering drugs include those that reduce absorption of vitamin K, warfarin (cholestyramine), or sulfinpyrazone and those that induce hepatic enzymes (barbiturates, phenytoin, rifampicin). The latter drugs increase the rate of warfarin metabolism in the liver. (See also Chap. 68.)

Potentiating Drugs

Other drugs decrease warfarin degradation to increase the anticoagulant effect, including a variety of antibiotics such as metronidazole (Flagyl) and co-trimoxazole (Bactrim). Cimetidine likewise inhibits hepatic degradation; ranitidine should not. Other potentiating drugs include the cardiovascular agents allopurinol, clofibrate, quinidine,[36] and amiodarone.[61] Amiodarone is especially dangerous because of its very long half-life. Drugs such as heparin also potentiate the risk of bleeding; there are large interindividual variations.[85] Very high doses of aspirin (six to eight tablets per day) may act differently by impairing synthesis of clotting factors. It must be restressed that sulfinpyrazone powerfully displaces warfarin from blood proteins, so that the dose of warfarin required may be reduced to only 1 mg in some patients.[86] (See also Chap. 68.)

Heparin

Physically, heparin is incompatible in a water solution with certain substances, including antibiotics, antihistamines, phenothiazides, and hydrocortisone. However, direct pharmacokinetic or pharmacodynamic drug interactions have not been described.

LIPID-LOWERING AGENTS (TABLE 109-8)

There are not many serious interactions. A number of lipid-lowering agents may interact with warfarin, either by decreased absorption (cholestyramine) or by hepatic interference (clofibrate, bezafibrate, gemfibrozil). Clofibrate and gemfibrozil increase warfarin effects. Probu-

TABLE 109-8
Drug Interactions of Lipid Lowering Agents

Cardiac Drug	Interacting Drugs	Mechanism	Consequence	Prophylaxis	Reference
Probucol	Thiazides, groups IA and III antiarrhythmics	Probucol-induced diarrhea with potassium loss?	QT prolongation	Check potassium; avoid combinations	107
Fibric acids (gemfibrozil, clofibrate, bezafibrate, fenobrate)	Warfarin	Hepatic interference	Risk of bleeding	Check prothrombin time	84
Bile acid sequestrants (cholestyramine, colestipol)	Warfarin (W)	Decreased absorption	Decreased W effect	Check prothrombin time	84
HMG CoA reductase inhibitors (lovastatin, pravastatin)	Fibrates, cyclosporine, erythromycin, nicotinic acid	Added risk of myositis	Rhabdomyolysis and risk of renal failure	Check creatine phosphokinase levels	108

col, in the presence of additional agents such as thiazide diuretics or group IA or III antiarrhythmics, may prolong QT interval and theoretically precipitate torsades de pointes. The HMG CoA reductase inhibitors such as lovastatin (Mevacor), simvastatin, and pravastatin should not be combined under ordinary circumstances with the fibric acid derivatives or cyclosporine because of the higher risk of myositis with rhabdomyolysis and possible renal failure. Concurrent therapy with nicotinic acid or erythromycin may also have an increased risk of rhabdomyolysis. Serum creatine kinase levels should be checked periodically, especially after increasing doses. (See also Chap. 65.)

ANTIHYPERTENSIVE DRUGS

Interactions for diuretics, β-adrenergic blockers, calcium antagonists, ACE inhibitors, and alpha$_1$-adrenergic blockers have already been considered. In general, NSAIDs interfere severely with antihypertensive efficacy of all antihypertensives.[87] An exception is nifedipine (and, presumably, other dihydropyridines).[88] Unlike other NSAIDs, aspirin[5] and sulindac may give relative protection from the negative interaction.[87] When calcium antagonists are used as antihypertensives, part of their effect is by natriuresis, so that adding a diuretic is often relatively ineffective.[89] (See also Chaps. 30 and 77.)

REFERENCES

1. Opie LH (ed): *Drugs for the Heart*, 2d ed. Orlando, FL, Grune & Stratton, 1987; 1–302.
2. Kirch W, Spahn H, Kohler H, Mutschler E: Influence of β-receptor antagonists on pharmacokinetics of cimetidine. *Drugs* 1983; 25(suppl 2):127–130.
3. McLean AJ, Knight R, Harrison PM, Harper RW: Clearance-based oral drug interaction between verapamil and metoprolol and comparison with atenolol. *Am J Cardiol* 1985; 55:1628–1629.
4. Ochs HR, Carstens G, Greenblatt DJ: Reduction in lidocaine clearance during continuous infusion and by coadministration of propranolol. *N Engl J Med* 1980; 303:373–377.
5. Webster J: Interactions of NSAIDs with diuretics and β-blockers: Mechanism and clinical implications. *Drugs* 1985; 30:32–41.
6. Tolins M, Weir K, Chesler E, Pierpont GL: "Maximal" drug therapy is not necessarily optimal in chronic angina pectoris. *J Am Coll Cardiol* 1984; 3:1051–1057.
7. Bruce RA, Hossack KF, Kusumi F, Day B, Kannagi T: Excessive reduction in peripheral resistance during exercise and risk of orthostatic symptoms with sustained-release nitroglycerin and diltiazem treatment of angina. *Am Heart J* 1985; 109:1020–1026.
8. Boden WE, Bough EW, Reichman MJ, Rich VB, Young PM, Korr KS, et al: Beneficial effects of high-dose diltiazem in patients with persistent effort angina on β-blockers and nitrates: A randomized, double-blind, placebo-controlled, cross-over study. *Circulation* 1985; 71:1197–1205.
9. Reicher-Reiss H, Neufeld HN, Ebner FX: Calcium antagonists—Adverse drug interactions. *Cardiovasc Drug Ther* 1987; 1:403–409.
10. Yeh R, Gulamhusein SS, Klein GJ: Combined verapamil and propranolol for supraventricular tachycardia. *Am J Cardiol* 1984; 53:757–763.
11. Ellrodt AG, Ault MJ, Riedinger MS, Murati GH: Efficacy and safety of sublingual nifedipine in hypertensive emergencies. *Am J Med* 1985; 79(suppl 4A):19–25.
12. Kieval J, Kirsten EB, Kessler KM, Mallon SM, Myerburg RJ: The effects of intravenous verapamil on hemodynamic status of patients with coronary artery disease receiving propranolol. *Circulation* 1982; 65:653–659.
13. Packer M, Meller J, Medina N, Yushak M, Smith H, Holt J, et al: Hemodynamic consequences of combined beta-adrenergic and slow calcium channel blockade in man. *Circulation* 1982; 65:660–668.
14. Johnston DL, Lesoway R, Humen DP, Kostuk WJ: Clinical and hemodynamic evaluation of propranolol in combination with verapamil, nifedipine and diltiazem in exertional angina pectoris: A placebo-controlled, double-blind, randomized, cross-over study. *Am J Cardiol* 1985; 55:680–687.
15. Winniford MD, Fulton KL, Corbett JR, Croft CH, Hillis LD: Propranolol-verapamil versus propranolol-nifedipine in severe angina pectoris of effort: A randomized, double-blind, cross-over study. *Am J Cardiol* 1985; 55:281–285.
16. Hamann SR, Kaltenborn KE, Vore M, Tan TG, McAllister RG Jr: Cardiovascular pharmacokinetic consequences of combined administration of verapamil and propranolol in dogs. *Am J Cardiol* 1985; 56:147–156.
17. Murdoch DL, Thomson GD, Thompson GG, Murray GD, Brodic MJ, McInnes GT: Evaluation of potential pharmacodynamic and pharmacokinetic interactions between verapamil and propranolol in normal subjects. *Br J Clin Pharmacol* 1991; 31:323–332.
18. Johnston DL, Gebhardt VA, Donald A, Kostuk WJ: Comparative effects of propranolol and verapamil alone and in combination on left ventricular function in patients with chronic exertional angina: A double-blind, placebo-controlled, randomized, cross-over study with radionuclide ventriculography. *Circulation* 1983; 68:1280–1289.
19. McInnes GT, Findlay IN, Murray G, Cleland JGF, Dargie HJ: Cardiovascular responses to verapamil and propranolol in hypertensive patients. *J Hypertens* 1985; 3(suppl 3):S219–S221.
20. Pedersen KE: Digoxin interactions: The influence of quinidine and verapamil on the pharmacokinetics and receptor binding of digitalis glycosides. *Acta Med Scand* 1985; (suppl 697):12–40.
21. Elliott HL, Pasanisi F, Meredith PA, Reid JL: Acute hypotensive response to nifedipine added to prazosin. *Br Med J* 1984; 288:238.
22. Pasanisi F, Elliott HL, Meredith PA, McSharry DR, Reid JL: Combined alpha-adrenoceptor antagonism and calcium channel blockade in normal subjects. *Clin Pharmacol Ther* 1984; 36:716–723.
23. Reid JL, Meredith PA, Pasanisi F: Clinical pharmacological aspects of calcium antagonists and their therapeutic role in hypertension. *J Cardiovasc Pharmacol* 1985; 7(suppl 4):S18–S20.
24. Maisel AS, Motulsky HJ, Insel PA: Hypotension after quinidine plus verapamil: Possible additive competition at alpha-adrenergic receptors. *N Engl J Med* 1985; 312:167–171.
25. Trohman RG, Estes DM, Castellanos A, Palomo AR, Myerburg RJ, Kessler KM: Increased quinidine plasma concentrations during administration of verapamil: A new quinidine-verapamil interaction. *Am J Cardiol* 1986; 57:706–707.
26. Hansten PD, Horn JR: Calcium channel blocker–induced drug interactions: Evidence for metabolic inhibition. *Drug Interact Newsl* 1986; 6:35–40.
27. Opie LH, White DA: Adverse interaction between nifedipine and beta-blockade. *Br Med J* 1980; 281:1462–1464.
28. Kleinbloesem CH, van Brummelen P, Sandberg THW, Danhof M, Breimer DD: Kinetic and haemodynamic interactions between nifedipine and propranolol in healthy subjects utilizing controlled rates of drug input. In: Kleinbloesem CH (ed): *Nifedipine: Clinical Pharmacokinetics and Haemodynamic Effects.* 's-Gravenhage, Drukkerij JH Pasmans BV, 1985: 151–165.
29. Kiss I, Farsang C: Nifedipine-prazosin interaction in patients with essential hypertension. *Cardiovasc Drugs Ther* 1989; 3:413–415.
30. Hung J, Lamb IH, Connolly SJ, Jutzky KR, Goris ML, Schroeder JS: The effect of diltiazem and propranolol, alone and in combination, on exercise performance and left ventricular function in patients with stable effort angina: A double-blind, randomized, and placebo-controlled study. *Circulation* 1983; 68:560–567.
31. Grino JM, Sabate I, Castelao AM, Alsina J: Influence of diltiazem on cyclosporin clearance. *Lancet* 1986; 2:1387.
32. Bigger JT, Giardina EG: Drug interactions in antiarrhythmic therapy. *Ann NY Acad Sci* 1984; 427:140–161.

33. Jaillon P: Antiarrhythmic drug interactions: Are they important? *Eur Heart J* 1987; 8(suppl A):127–132.
34. Hardy BG, Zador IT, Golden L, Lalka D, Schentag JJ: Effect of cimetidine on the pharmacokinetics and pharmacodynamics of quinidine. *Am J Cardiol* 1983; 52:172–175.
35. Hager WD, Fenster P, Mayersohn M, Perrier D, Graves P, Marcus FI, et al: Digoxin-quinidine interaction: Pharmacokinetic evaluation. *N Engl J Med* 1979; 300:1238–1241.
36. Koch-Weser J: Quinidine-induced hypoprothrombinemic hemorrhage in patients on chronic warfarin therapy. *Ann Intern Med* 1968; 68:511–517.
37. Dada JL, Wilkinson GR, Nies AJ: Interaction of quinidine with anticonvulsant drugs. *N Engl J Med* 1976; 294:699–702.
38. Twum-Barima Y, Carruthers SG: Quinidine-rifampicin. *N Engl J Med* 1981; 304:1466–1469.
39. Farringer JA, McWay-Hess K, Clementi WA: Cimetidine-quinidine interaction. *Clin Pharmacol* 1984; 3:81–83.
40. Green JA, Clementi WA, Porter C, Stigelman W: Nifedipine-quinidine interaction. *Clin Pharm* 1983; 2:461–465.
41. Farringer JA, Green JA, O'Rourke RA, Linn WA, Clementi WA: Nifedipine-induced alterations in serum quinidine concentrations. *Am Heart J* 1984; 108:1570–1572.
42. Van Lith RM, Appleby DH: Quinidine-nifedipine interaction. *Drug Intell Clin Pharm* 1985; 19:829–830.
43. Marcus FI: Drug interactions with amiodarone. *Am Heart J* 1983; 106:924–930.
44. Christian CO Jr, Meredith CG, Speeg KV Jr: Cimetidine inhibits procainamide clearance. *Clin Pharmacol Ther* 1984; 36:221–227.
45. Lee JT, Davy J-M, Kates RE: Evaluation of combined administration of verapamil and disopyramide in dogs. *J Cardiovasc Pharmacol* 1985; 7:501–507.
46. Kapil RP, Axelson JE, Mansfield IL, Edwards DJ, McErlane B, Mason MA, et al: Disopyramide pharmacokinetics and metabolism: Effect of inducers. *Br J Clin Pharmacol* 1987; 24:781–791.
47. Teichman SL, Fisher JD, Matos JA, Kim SG: Disopyramide-pyridostigmine: Report of a beneficial drug interaction. *J Cardiovasc Pharmacol* 1985; 7:108–113.
48. Feely J, Wilkinson GR, McAllister CB, Wood AJ: Increased toxicity and reduced clearance of lidocaine by cimetidine. *Ann Intern Med* 1982; 96:592–594.
49. Boyce JR, Cervenko FW, Wright FJ: Effects of halothane on the pharmacokinetics of lidocaine in digitalis-toxic dogs. *Can Anaesth Soc J* 1978; 25:323–328.
50. Jeresaty RM, Kahn AH, Landry AB Jr: Sinoatrial arrest due to lidocaine in a patient receiving quinidine. *Chest* 1972; 61:683–685.
51. Klein R, Huang SK, Southwest Cardiology Research Group: Combination therapy of propafenone with quinidine or procainamide: Enhanced efficacy and reduced side-effects (abstr). *J Am Coll Cardiol* 1985; 5:423.
52. Breithardt G, Selpel L, Abendroth RR: Comparative cross-over study of the effects of disopyramide and mexiletine on stimulus-induced ventricular tachycardia (abstr). *Circulation* 1980; 62(suppl 3):153.
53. Duff HJ, Roden D, Primm RK, Oates JA, Woosley RL: Mexiletine in the treatment of resistant ventricular arrhythmias: Enhancement of efficacy and reduction of dose-related side-effects by combination with quinidine. *Circulation* 1983; 67:1124–1128.
54. Greenspan AM, Spielman SR, Webb CR, Sokoff NM, Rae AP, Horowitz LN: Efficacy of combination therapy with mexiletine and a Type IA agent for inducible ventricular tachyarrhythmias secondary to coronary artery disease. *Am J Cardiol* 1985; 56:277–284.
55. Leahey EB, Heissenbuttel RH, Giardina EGV, Bigger JT Jr: Combined mexiletine and propranolol treatment of refractory ventricular tachycardia. *Br Med J* 1980; 2:357–358.
56. Waleffe A, Mary-Rabine L, Legrand V, Demoulin JC, Kulbertus HE: Combined mexiletine and amiodarone treatment of refractory recurrent ventricular tachycardia. *Am Heart J* 1980; 100:788–793.
57. Lewis GP, Holtzman JL: Interaction of flecainide with digoxin and propranolol. *Am J Cardiol* 1984; 53:52B–57B.
58. Shea P, Lal R, Kim SS, Schechtman K, Ruffy R: Flecainide and amiodarone interaction. *J Am Coll Cardiol* 1986; 7:1127–1130.
59. Maga TBT, Verbesselt R, Van Hecken A, Van Melle P, De Schepper PJ: Oral flecainide elimination kinetics: Effects of cimetidine (abstr). *Circulation* 1983; 68(suppl 3):416.
60. Hodges M, Salerno D, Granrud G: Double-blind placebo-controlled evaluation of propafenone in suppressing ventricular ectopic activity. *Am J Cardiol* 1984; 54:45D–50D.
61. Martinowitz U, Rabinovich J, Goldfarb D, Many A, Bank H: Interaction between warfarin sodium and amiodarone. *N Engl J Med* 1981; 304:671–672.
62. Gillis RA, Clancy MM, Anderson RJ: Deleterious effects of bretylium in cats with digitalis-induced ventricular tachycardia. *Circulation* 1973; 47:974–983.
63. Vincent JL, Dufaye P, Berre J, Kahn RJ: Bretylium in severe ventricular arrhythmias associated with digitalis intoxication. *Am J Emerg Med* 1984; 2:504–506.
64. Peipho RW, Culbertson VL, Rhodes RS: Drug interactions with the calcium-entry blockers. *Circulation* 1987; 75(suppl 5):181–194.
65. Lessem J, Bellinetto A: Interaction between digoxin and the calcium antagonists nicardipine and tiapamil. *Clin Ther* 1983; 5:595–602.
66. Kirch W, Hutt HJ, Dylewicz P, Qhnhaus EE: Dose-dependence of the nifedipine-digoxin interaction. *Clin Pharmacol Ther* 1986; 39:35–39.
67. Lessem JN: Interaction between Ca^{2+} antagonists and digitalis. *Cardiovasc Drugs Ther* 1988; 1:441–446.
68. Kirch W, Hutt HJ, Heidemann H, Ramsch K, Janisch HD, Ohnhaus EE: Drug interactions with nitrendipine. *J Cardiovasc Pharmacol* 1984; 6:S982–S985.
69. Plunkett LM, Gokhale RD, Vallner JJ, Tackett RL: Prazosin alters free and total plasma digoxin levels in dogs. *Am Heart J* 1985; 109:847–851.
70. Marcus FI: Pharmacokinetic interactions between digoxin and other drugs. *J Am Coll Cardiol* 1985; 5:82A–90A.
71. Waldorff S, Andersen JD, Heeboil-Nielsen N, Nielson OG, Moltre E, Sorensen V, et al: Spironolactone-induced changes in digoxin kinetics. *Clin Pharmacol Ther* 1978; 24:162–167.
72. Waldorff S, Hansen PB, Egeblad H, Berning J, Buch J, Kjaergard H, et al: Interactions between digoxin and potassium-sparing diuretics. *Clin Pharmacol Ther* 1983; 33:418–423.
73. Fenster PE, Hager WD, Goodman MM: Digoxin-quinidine-spironolactone interaction. *Clin Pharmacol Ther* 1984; 36:70–73.
74. Mudge GH: Diuretics and other agents employed in the mobilization of edema fluid. In: Gilman AG, Goodman LS, Gilman AG (eds): *The Pharmacological Basis of Therapeutics*, 6th ed. Macmillan, New York, 1980: 892–915.
75. Dzau VJ, Packer M, Lilly LS, Swartz SL, Hollenberg NK, Williams GH: Prostaglandins in severe congestive heart failure: Relation to activation of the renin-angiotensin system and hyponatremia. *N Engl J Med* 1984; 310:347–352.
76. McKibbin JK, Pocock WA, Barlow JB, Millar RN, Obel IW: Sotalol, hypokalaemia, syncope, and torsade de pointes. *Br Heart J* 1984; 51:157–162.
77. Jefferson JW, Kalin NH: Serum lithium levels and long-term diuretic use. *JAMA* 1979; 241:1134–1136.
78. Cogan JJ, Humphreys MH, Carlson CJ, Benowitz NL, Rapaport E: Acute vasodilator therapy increases renal clearance of digoxin in patients with congestive heart failure. *Circulation* 1981; 64:973–976.
79. Hodsman GP, Johnston CI: Angiotensin converting enzyme inhibitors: Drug interactions. *J Hypertens* 1987; 5:1–6.
80. Singhvi SM, Duchin KL, Willard DA, McKinstry DN, Migdalof BH: Renal handling of captopril: Effect of probenicid. *Clin Pharmacol Ther* 1982; 32:182–189.
81. Grayzel AI, Liddle L, Seegmiller JE: Diagnostic significance of hyperuricemia in arthritis. *N Engl J Med* 1961; 265:763–768.
82. Moroz L: Increased blood fibrinolytic activity after aspirin ingestion. *N Engl J Med* 1977; 296:525–529.
83. Chesebro JH, Fuster V, Elveback LR, McGoon DC, Pluth JR, Puga FJ, et al: Trial of combined warfarin plus dipyridamole or aspirin therapy in prosthetic heart valve replacement: danger of aspirin compared with dipyridamole. *Am J Cardiol* 1983; 51:1537–1541.
84. Stratton F, Chalmers DG, Flute PT, Lewis SM, MacIver J, Nelson MG: Drug interaction with coumarin derivative anticoagulants. *Br Med J* 1982; 285:274–275.

85. O'Reilly RA, Sahud MA, Aggeler PM: Impact of aspirin and chlorthalidone on the pharmacodynamics of oral anticoagulant drugs in man. *Ann NY Acad Sci* 1971; 179:173–186.
86. Bailey RR, Reddy J: Potentiation of warfarin action by sulphinpyrazone (letter). *Lancet* 1980; 1:254.
87. Houston MC: Nonsteroidal anti-inflammatory drugs and antihypertensives. *Am J Med* 1991; 90(suppl 5A):42S–47S.
88. Salvetti A, Magagna A, Abdel-Haq B, Lenzi M, Giovannetti R: Nifedipine interactions in hypertensive patients. *Cardiovasc Drugs Ther* 1990; 4:963–968.
89. Weinberger MH: The relationship of sodium balance and concomitant diuretic therapy to blood pressure response with calcium channel entry blockers. *Am J Med* 1991; 90(suppl 5A):15S–20S.
90. Kendall MJ, Laugher SJ, Wilkins MR: Ranitidine, cimetidine and metoprolol—a pharmacokinetic interaction study (abstr). *Gastroenterology* 1986; 90:1490.
91. Daneshmend TK, Roberts CJC: Reduction in labetalol first-pass metabolism following cimetidine (abstr). *Br J Clin Pharmacol* 1983; 15:153P.
92. Kubo SH, Fox SC, Prida XE, Cody RJ: Combined hemodynamic effects of nifedipine and nitroglycerin in congestive heart failure. *Am Heart J* 1985; 110:1032–1034.
93. Smith SR, Kendall MJ, Lobo J, Beerahee A, Jack DB, Wilkins MR: Ranitidine and cimetidine: Drug interactions with single dose and steady-state nifedipine administration. *Br J Clin Pharmacol* 1987; 23:311–315.
94. Kleinbloesem CH, van Brummelen P, Hilliers J, Moolenaar AJ, Breimer DD: Interaction between digoxin and nifedipine at steady-state in patients with atrial fibrillation. In: Kleinbloesem CH (ed): *Nifedipine: Clinical Pharmacokinetics and Haemodynamic Effects.* 's-Gravenhage, Drukkerij JH Pasmans BV, 1985; 167-173.
95. Bourbigot B, Guiserix J, Airiau J, Bressollette L, Morin JF, Cledes J: Nicardipine increases cyclosporin blood levels. *Lancet* 1986; 1:1447.
96. Aviado DM, Salem H: Drug action, reaction and interaction: I. Quinidine for cardiac arrhythmias. *J Clin Pharmacol* 1975; 15:477–485.
97. Loon NR, Wilcox CS, Folger W: Orthostatic hypotension due to quinidine and propranolol. *Am J Med* 1986; 81:1101–1104.
98. Roden DM, Woosley RL, Primm RK: Incidence and clinical features of the quinidine-associated long QT syndrome: Implications for patient care. *Am Heart J* 1986; 111:1088–1093.
99. Nattel S, Gagne G, Pineau M: The pharmacokinetics of lignocaine and β-adrenoceptor antagonists in patients with acute myocardial infarction. *Clin Pharmacokinet* 1987; 13:293–316.
100. Josephson MA, Kaul S, Hopkins J, Kvam D, Singh BN: Hemodynamic effects of intravenous flecainide relative to the level of ventricular function in patients with coronary artery disease. *Am Heart J* 1985; 109:41–45.
101. Kuhlmann J, Marcin S: Effects of verapamil on pharmacokinetics and pharmacodynamics of digoxin in patients. *Am Heart J* 1985; 110:1245–1250.
102. Cleland JGF, Dargie HJ, Pettigrew A, Gillen G, Robertson JI: The effects of captopril on serum digoxin and urinary urea and digoxin clearances in patients with congestive heart failure. *Am Heart J* 1986; 112:130–135.
103. Hodsman GP, Isles CG, Murray GD, Usherwood TP, Webb DJ, Robertson JI: Factors related to the first dose hypotensive effect of captopril: Prediction and treatment. *Br Med J* 1983; 286:832–834.
104. Toussaint C, Masselink A, Gentges A, Wambach G, Bonner G: Interference of different ACE inhibitors with the diuretic action of furosemide and hydrochlorothiazide. *Klin Wochenschr* 1989; 67:1138–1146.
105. Textor SC, Bravo EL, Fouad FM, Tarazi RC: Hyperkalaemia in azotemic patients during angiotensin-converting enzyme inhibition and aldosterone reduction with captopril. *Am J Med* 1982; 73:719–725.
106. Cooper RA: Captopril associated neutropenia: Who is at risk? *Arch Intern Med* 1983; 143:659–660.
107. Browne KF, Prystowsky EN, Heger JJ, Cerimele BJ, Finebera N, Zipes DP: Prolongation of the QT-interval induced by probucol: Demonstration of a method for determining QT-interval change induced by a drug. *Am Heart J* 1984; 107:680–684.
108. Tobert JA: Rhabdomyolysis in patients receiving lovastatin after cardiac transplantation. *N Engl J Med* 1988; 318:47–48.

PART XIV

Miscellaneous Causes of Heart Disease

Chapter 110

Effect of Noncardiac Drugs, Electricity, Poisons, and Radiation on the Heart

I. Sylvia Crawley, M.D. ■ *Robert C. Schlant, M.D.*

This chapter deals with a number of deleterious side effects of treatments[1] and environmental agents on the heart. Illnesses of human origin are not uncommonly the result of manufactured inventions and treatments, possibly cures, for other illnesses. Environmental factors are not necessarily under the control of human beings, but when they are, we must take the responsibility of their potential effects on our health.

NONCARDIAC DRUGS

Psychotropic Agents

The major cardiac effects of psychotropic agents are discussed. The reader is referred to reviews for more detailed discussion, including potential drug interactions, and literature citations.[2-4]

Tricyclic Antidepressants

Tricyclic antidepressants, including the tertiary (amitriptyline, doxepin, imipramine, trimipramine, clomipramine) and secondary (desipramine, nortriptyline, protriptyline) agents, have potentially serious cardiovascular effects. These dangers have been overemphasized, and with appropriate patient selection and monitoring, they can be used safely even in patients with cardiovascular disease.[2-5] The major effects include an increase in heart rate, orthostatic hypotension, electrocardiographic changes, and depression of ventricular function.

A slight increase in heart rate is common and may persist for days to months after discontinuing therapy.[6] The rate rarely exceeds 100 beats per minute. This effect is more common with the tertiary amines, especially amitriptyline.[4] Orthostatic hypotension occurs in up to 24 percent of patients and is more troublesome in patients with some degree of orthostasis prior to treatment.[2,3] This side effect is less common with nortriptyline and possibly with doxepin.[2]

The most common electrocardiographic changes include nonspecific ST- and T-wave changes and slight prolongation of QT interval, PR interval, and QRS duration.[2] PR prolongation is the result of prolonged HV conduction.[2,7] This effect on prolongation of conduction is minor and of no consequence in most patients; however, in patients with preexisting conduction system disease, especially bundle branch block, they should be used more cautiously.[8] The tricyclics have a quinidine-like property and may exert both antiarrhythmic and arrhythmogenic effects. The effectiveness of imipramine and nortriptyline as antiarrhythmic agents has been demonstrated in patients with and without depression.[9-11] Nortriptyline has also been shown to significantly suppress ventricular ectopy in patients without depression.[11] For both drugs these patients also had other evidence of heart disease. The antiarrhythmic efficacy of these drugs has not been established, and none of the patients studied had recognized sustained ventricular tachycardia. These studies do suggest that certain forms of ventricular ectopy are not a contraindication to the prudent use of tricyclic antidepressants. On the other hand, they should be avoided in the setting of ectopy possibly due to electrolyte abnormalities, type I antiarrhythmic drugs, or QT prolongation due to any cause.

Depression of left ventricular function is usually minimal with therapeutic doses. Severe preexisting left ventricular dysfunction is an important consideration, although patients with moderate dysfunction may be treated safely.[3,12] In some but not all reports, symptomatic orthostatic hypotension is more frequent in these patients, especially with imipramine.[12,13]

There are limited studies of the cardiovascular effects of clomipramine. The available data suggest that its electrocardiographic changes are similar to other tricyclics. Orthostatic hypotension and an increase in heart rate may occur.[14] At least one fatality due to clomipramine overdose is reported.[15]

Although the tricyclic antidepressants have potentially serious cardiac effects, they may be used safely in many patients with cardiovascular disease with appropriate considerations of their effects and drug interactions.

Tricyclic overdose frequently presents a special cardiac management problem. These patients should always receive prompt attention at the time of presentation with continuous electrocardiographic monitoring. Gastric lavage, catharsis, and repeated doses of charcoal are generally recommended. Prolonged gastric lavage may not be effective and can delay the use of activated charcoal.[16] Ipecac is not recommended because of the danger of aspiration. Gastric lavage may also be hazardous in the sedated or comatose patient, especially if seizures occur. Tracheal intubation may be indicated prior to gastric lavage.[17,18] A report of death related to aspiration of activated charcoal questions the efficacy of repeated dosing.[19] Because of potentially serious cardiovascular side effects, the use of physostigmine is not recommended.[17,20] Electrocardiographic abnormalities frequently include sinus tachycardia; prolongation of PR, QRS, and QT; ST- and T-wave changes; and bundle branch block. Rightward deviation of the frontal plane QRS axis with a terminal QRS axis of 130 to 270 is a frequent finding, and may be a better predictor of toxicity than QRS prolongation.[21] Sodium bicarbonate to maintain the pH over 7.45 may decrease unbound blood levels and transiently reduce conduction system defects. Since seizures may worsen metabolic acidosis, bicarbonate therapy is most important. Type I antiarrhythmics (quinidine, procainamide, disopyramide) should not be used. Beta-adrenergic blockers are not generally useful, and bretylium tosylate is questionably effective. Isoproterenol may be useful in suppressing ventricular ectopy and torsades de pointes ventricular tachycardia, but the latter usually requires temporary pacing.

The duration of cardiac monitoring after tricyclic overdose is controversial. Neither the initial drug level nor the degree of sinus tachycardia is predictive of major cardiac or central nervous system complications.[10,17] The majority of serious cardiac events occur in the first 6 h. Sinus tachycardia, QT and QRS prolongation, and right-axis deviation of the frontal terminal 40-ms QRS are important predictors of tricyclic toxicity, but these findings may be absent in some patients.[23] Intensive care unit admission may be unnecessary for selected patients whose management has included appropriate gastric lavage, catharsis, and repeated doses of activated charcoal and who are alert with active bowel sounds and have a normal electrocardiogram after 6 h of observation.[17,18,23] Underlying heart disease, polydrug ingestion, or other medical problems may dictate a longer observation. Differences in the tricyclics and some of the newer antidepressants must also be considered. Amoxapine may cause seizures with little effect on the electrocardiogram and is also recognized to cause acute renal failure.[20] It seems prudent to provide a minimum of 24 h of observation with continuous cardiac monitoring for most patients. When electrocardiographic effects are present, cardiac monitoring should be continued for at least 24 h after all signs of toxicity have resolved.[17,23] Hemodynamic monitoring may be necessary to provide appropriate therapy for hypotension. Profound peripheral vasodilation may require large volumes of intravascular fluids and vasopressors. Phenylephrine or norepinephrine is preferred to dopamine. Dobutamine is useful if a positive inotropic agent is needed.[17]

Other Antidepressants

Newer generation antidepressants may have fewer cardiovascular effects. Maprotiline does have the potential for effects similar to those of the tertiary and secondary tricyclic agents, especially with overdose.[24] Maprotiline was initially thought to have fewer cardiac effects, but subsequent experience has shown it to have a potential cardiac toxicity equal to that of the tricyclics.[25] Atrial flutter and torsades de pointes ventricular tachycardia have been reported with therapeutic doses.[26,27] There are few reported cases of severe cardiotoxicity to amoxapine even in overdose.[20,28] One series reported that 3 of 49 patients treated for amoxapine overdose had cardiac arrhythmias.[28] Ventricular premature beats, sinus tachycardia, and right bundle branch block have been reported.[28,29] Amoxapine overdose is more frequently associated with seizures and renal failure.[20,28] Trazodone has almost no anticholinergic effects and is less likely to cause tachycardia. Orthostatic hypotension is less frequent, and on the basis of animal studies, it is unlikely to cause problems with intracardiac conduction.[3] Overdose would be expected to be less complicated by cardiac effects.[3] In a number of reported cases of trazodone overdose no cardiac effects occurred.[28,30] There have been a few isolated case reports of adverse cardiac effects attributed to trazodone. Single cases of atrial and ventricular arrhythmias, sinoatrial node arrest, and complete heart block have been reported with "therapeutic" dose.[20,28,31] Some of these cases have occurred in elderly patients,[31] or with institution of a large initial dose in patients with significant preexisting heart disease.[32,33]

Fluoxetine, a serotonin uptake inhibitor, has little affinity for cholinergic receptors and causes few cardiovascular effects.[34,35] Minimal slowing of heart rate can occur. Sinus bradycardia and atrial tachyarrhythmias have been reported. Orthostatic hypotension may occur, especially with higher doses. It should be used with caution in the elderly and in patients with preexisting atrial arrhythmias or signs of sinus node dysfunction.[34] Significant effects on the conduction system have not been recognized.[35] Limited numbers of cases of overdose, some with blood levels 10 times therapeutic, have not demonstrated cardiac toxicity.[35]

Few cardiovascular effects have been demonstrated with bupropion. Limited studies in patients with left ventricular impairment, ventricular arrhythmias, or conduction system disease have shown few adverse effects.[2,13,36] Orthostatic hypotension is uncommon even in the presence of left ventricular impairment. Significant blood pressure elevation may occur, especially in patients with preexisting hypertension.[36] Despite the favorable cardiovascular profile, bupropion may be associated with significant risk of seizures.[36]

Monoamine Oxidase Inhibitors

Monoamine oxidase (MAO) inhibitors do not produce tachycardia and have little effect on cardiac conduction or myocardial contractility.[37] There have been few reports of cardiac arrhythmias.[2–4] They do frequently produce orthostatic hypotension, and for this reason they are usually avoided in certain patients with cardiac and cerebrovascular disease.

The potential interaction of MAO inhibitors with other drugs and tyramine-containing substances resulting in a hypertensive crisis limits the use of MAO inhibitors in many patients. Sublingual nifedipine, phentolamine, chlorpromazine, and captopril have been used in the treatment of hypertensive crisis.[2,3] Spontaneous hypertensive episodes not related to such interactions have also been reported with MAO inhibitors.[38] This interaction may persist for at least 2 weeks after discontinuing the drug.

Lithium

Lithium, as the citrate or carbonate salt, has infrequent cardiac effects in therapeutic doses, even in patients with heart disease.[39] Suppression of automaticity, especially of the sinus node, is the most common significant effect. Sinus node suppression with a slow escape rhythm may occur even with therapeutic doses and is probably more common in patients with preexisting sinus node disease or in patients taking other medications having a similar effect.[39] Permanent pacing has been used to allow continuation of lithium therapy.

Electrocardiographic changes are common and simulate hypokalemia. A decrease in amplitude or inversion of the T waves and U waves is common.[4,39] QT prolongation may occur. Although rare, PR prolongation, bundle branch block, and complete heart block are reported. Despite isolated reports of ventricular arrhythmias, lithium may have antiarrhythmic properties.[39]

There are no data to confirm the concern that lithium suppresses left ventricular function, although the long-term effects, especially in patients with pretreatment myocardial dysfunction, have not been studied.

Bradyarrhythmias are the most frequent cardiac effect of overdose and may require temporary transvenous pacing.[39] A reduced or absent anion gap may be a clue to the presence of lithium toxicity.[40]

Phenothiazine Antipsychotic Agents

Phenothiazine antipsychotic agents, particularly those of low potency, chlorpromazine and thioridazine, have significant cardiac effects.[41] An increase in heart rate occurs frequently, even to 100 beats per minute. Orthostatic hypotension is more frequent with parenteral than oral administration. T-wave changes in the electrocardiogram are common, occur variably in any patient, and are influenced by drugs and the fasting state. They may persist for 2 weeks after discontinuing therapy. QT prolongation may occur. Bundle branch block, complete heart block, and atrial and ventricular arrhythmias have been reported but are not common with therapeutic doses.[41]

Sudden death has occurred in patients receiving phenothiazines, but no risk factor can be identified. The mechanism of death is thought to be cardiac arrhythmia, either ventricular tachycardia or complete heart block.[41]

Overdose with the phenothiazines produce serious cardiovascular effects similar to those of the tricyclic agents, including electrocardiographic changes, hypotension, and arrhythmias. Torsades de pointes ventricular tachycardia also occurs.[41]

Chemotherapeutic Agents

Doxorubicin

Electrocardiographic changes during the course of therapy are common. They are not usually clinically important, regress in weeks to months, and generally do not predict subsequent cardiomyopathy. The most common are ST-T wave changes, but QRS changes may also occur and, less frequently, atrial or ventricular arrhythmias.[42,43] A reduction in QRS voltage has been used as a predictor of cardiomyopathy but is unreliable.[44,45]

Cardiomyopathy is the most serious cardiotoxic effect. The overall incidence of clinically apparent heart failure is reported in up to 9 percent of patients.[42] Subclinical left ventricular dysfunction is probably more frequent. In one series, 14 percent of 101 patients receiving at least 430 mg/m^2 developed clinical congestive heart failure while 21 percent of the asymptomatic patients also had abnormal resting left ventricular ejection fractions.[46]

A total dose of over 550 mg/m^2 is associated with a much higher incidence of cardiomyopathy of up to 30 percent.[42] Other factors that may increase the chance of cardiomyopathy even with doses below 550 mg/m^2 include prior radiation therapy,[44,47] the schedule of administration,[48] preexisting heart disease, uncontrolled hypertension,[44] and possibly the associated use of other chemotherapeutic agents.[42,44,49] A higher incidence is also reported in young children and older adults.[42,47] Serial assessment of left ventricular function may aid in the safe administration to selected patients with prior left ventricular dysfunction.[50] A study utilizing endomyocardial biopsy as a measure of myocardial damage failed to demonstrate an association with use of other chemotherapeutic agents, hypertension, age, or history of cardiac disease.[48] Continuous infusion over 48 to 96 h may also decrease cardiotoxicity.[51]

The clinical presentation of doxorubicin heart muscle disease is similar to that of idiopathic dilated cardiomyopathy. (See Chap. 89.) It usually occurs within days to a few months and mostly within the first year after therapy, but occasionally much later.[52] The hemodynamic and morphologic findings suggest a restrictive endomyocardial disease (Chap. 91) in some patients.[53] The clinical course is variable from an acute, fulminating heart failure and cardiogenic shock to a gradually progressive deterioration.[54] A few patients improve and appear to regress with medical therapy, but the overall mortality rate is reported to be as high as 61 percent.[42,55] The older patient, over age 45 years, is more likely to progress than the younger patient.[46]

A number of noninvasive methods have been utilized in an attempt to detect early evidence of left ventricular dysfunction in order to terminate therapy at a safer dosage or to provide greater antineoplastic effectiveness with higher doses without added risk to the myocardium. Systolic time intervals and echocardiography have not proved to produce adequate sensitivity or specificity.[56] Noninvasive assessment of end-systolic left ventricular function may provide better sensitivity and specificity, but further studies are needed.[57] The value of radionuclide determination of left ventricular ejection fraction, both at rest and with exercise, has been reported.[50] Serial determination of left ventricular ejection fraction during doxorubicin therapy may allow for higher doses without additional risk of congestive heart failure in certain patients.[58,59]

Endomyocardial biopsy (Chap. 33) and histopathological assessment of the degree of myocardial damage are thought to provide the most reliable measure of myocardial toxicity.[56,60] Its clinical usefulness is limited since it is invasive and requires special expertise. The validity of the histopathology in determining a safe dose is challenged. The histopathology is not specific for doxorubicin toxicity, and the myocellular damage seen on endomyocardial biopsy may not accurately reflect the extent of changes throughout the myocardium.[47,53] Coupled, however, with right-sided heart catheterization with resting and exercise hemodynamics it remains the most definitive method of evaluating dosage safety.[56,61]

Daunorubicin

The cardiac toxicity of daunorubicin is similar to that of doxorubicin. The electrocardiographic changes are similar. They are not related to dosage, are usually transient, and do not predict subsequent cardiomyopathy.[42,62] The overall incidence of cardiomyopathy seems to be slightly less than with doxorubicin. There are limited studies assessing relative risk. Total dosage less than 600 mg/m^2 is associated with an incidence of 1.5 percent; the incidence increases to 12 percent with a dosage over 1000 mg/m^2. Children seem to be at greater risk.[63] The onset of symptoms may be a little later than with doxorubicin, but there are some instances of development of myocarditis-pericarditis during treatment.[54,64] The literature also suggests that daunorubicin cardiomyopathy is less likely to respond to therapy. Available noninvasive studies for early detection are limited.[42]

Other Chemotherapeutic Agents

5-Fluorouracil may rarely cause myocardial ischemia or myocardial infarction.[42] Arrhythmias, congestive heart failure, cardiogenic shock, and sudden death have been reported.[42,65] This may represent coronary artery spasm or abnormalities of coagulation.[65,66] In one report the episodes of chest pain associated with ST-segment elevation and ventricular ectopy were prevented by the concomitant use of nifedipine or diltiazem hydrochloride during 5-fluorouracil administration.[66]

Vincristine and vindesine, both vinca alkaloids, have been reported to cause myocardial infarction.[42,67] Vindesine has also been reported to cause angina pectoris.[68] Orthostatic hypotension occurs in approximately 8 percent of patients receiving vincristine.[69]

Cyclophosphamide may cause myocardial necrosis when used in large doses, especially when combined with other agents.[42]

Mitoxantrone has been reported to cause congestive heart failure, impairment of left ventricular function, and histological changes in some patients.[70,71] The potential risk of cardiotoxicity remains to be determined.

Amsacrine (AMSA) may cause ventricular arrhythmias, especially in the presence of hypokalemia.[72] Prolongation of the QT interval, atrial arrhythmias, congestive heart failure, and sudden death are reported.[73,74] Mitomycin, busulfan, cisplatinum, and methotrexate rarely cause cardiac toxicity.[42]

Oral Contraceptive Agents

Soon after the introduction of oral contraceptive agents in the early 1960s, the potential risks for cardiovascular disease became apparent.[75] A number of studies demonstrated an increased incidence of hypertension, myocardial infarction, cerebrovascular accidents, and thromboembolic disease in users of oral contraceptives.[75–77] In the late 1970s and early 1980s low-dose formulations, less than 50 μg ethinyl estradiol, were introduced, and with the increasing frequency of their use the cardiovascular risks are thought to be considerably reduced.[78]

In contrast, menopausal estrogen replacement therapy is demonstrated to reduce the incidence and mortality of cardiovascular disease by many epidemiologic studies when estrogen replacement only is utilized.[79–81] More recent recommendations for the use of cyclic estrogen and progestin therapy to reduce the incidence of endometrial cancer cause uncertainty as to the potential deleterious effect on cardiovascular risk with the concomitant use of progestin.[80,82] (See also Chap. 62.)

Myocardial Infarction

The incidence of myocardial infarction in premenopausal women is rare, but this risk was reported to be three to four times greater in high-dose oral contraceptive users in general.[79] However, in certain subsets, the risk is even more striking. Users who also smoke have a 20.8-fold increased risk of myocardial infarction than those who neither smoke nor use the pill.[81] The greatest risk with this combination is in the older age group who also smoke cigarettes.[81] The risk of myocardial infarction is also significantly increased with other risk factors for coronary atherosclerotic heart disease. Most studies suggest that there is little residual cardiovascular risk in past users of oral contraceptives.[81,83] (See Chap. 62.)

The mechanism of myocardial infarction is unclear. A significant percentage of women under age 50 who have a myocardial infarction are oral contraceptive users, and many of these will not have angiographic evidence of atherosclerotic disease. Most often findings indicate a single-vessel discrete lesion or normal vessel.[82–84] Conversely, the occurrence of atherosclerotic coronary heart disease or myocardial infarction with normal coronary arteries in nonusers under age 50 is also recognized. The oral contraceptives are known to affect lipid metabolism, decrease glucose tolerance, cause hypertension, and adversely affect hemostasis (hypercoagulability), and these factors may contribute to coronary artery disease and/or thrombosis.[76,81,85] In addition, coronary spasm has also been implicated.[86] (See Chap. 62.)

Hypertension

A mild elevation of blood pressure occurs in 1 to 5 percent of patients. In some cases more significant elevation occurs but is usually reversible after discontinuing use.[87] A few instances of malignant hypertension have been reported.[87] Hypertension is more likely in users who are older or who have a past history or family history of hypertension.[77] The duration of use and the amount of estrogen in the preparation may also contribute.

The effects of these agents on the renin-angiotensin system and sodium metabolism have been investigated as possible mechanisms of the hypertension.[87] (See also Chap. 75.)

Thromboembolism

The relative risk of superficial or deep lag vein thrombosis or pulmonary embolism in oral contraceptive users is 4 to 10 times that of nonusers, representing a significant morbidity rate but rare death.[75,77] Factors that predispose to this complication are past history of thromboembolic disease, medical or surgical trauma, and the amount of estrogen in the agent.[77] This risk may be significantly reduced with preparations containing 50 to 80 μg or estrogen.[78,88] This risk is resolved within 1 month after nonuse. Smoking has not been implicated as an additional risk factor for this complication.[75,77] This effect is thought to result from a decrease in venous tone and an increase in coagulability caused by these agents.[75,77] (See also Chap. 100.)

Cerebrovascular Accidents

In early studies the risk of cerebrovascular events in oral contraceptive users was considered significant.[77] Other studies have found the risk to be small.[87] Factors that increase the chances of this complication include hypertension, smoking, migraine headaches, hypercholesterolemia, and possibly mitral valve prolapse.[89] Residual risk, especially for subarachnoid hemorrhage, after discontinuing use has been reported.[77]

As with myocardial infarction, cerebrovascular accidents seem to be related to more than atherosclerosis. Intimal hyperplasia and the hypercoagulable state may contribute to the pathogenesis.[77] (See Chap. 122.)

Use of Oral Contraceptive Agents

Prescribing practices for oral contraceptive agents have undergone considerable change since their introduction. Low-dose formulations and improved patient selection criteria have had a considerable positive impact on the risk-benefit ratio of their use.

Oral contraceptive agents should be avoided in patients with other risk factors for cardiovascular disease. Smoking appears to be the greatest risk for coronary heart disease and especially in the older individual.[87] The use of low-dose formulations in patients without hypertension, diabetes mellitus, thromboembolism, coronary artery heart disease, cerebrovascular accidents, recent surgery, or trauma provides a low-risk form of oral contraception while providing other protective effects.[78,85]

Blood pressure, lipid levels, and glucose tolerance should be monitored. Oral contraceptive therapy should be temporarily discontinued for at least 2 weeks prior to and after elective surgery, after trauma, or during any period of immobilization.[85]

Miscellaneous Agents

Cocaine

Cocaine is a water-soluble crystalline alkaloid that is derived from the *Erythroxylon* coca plant. It is often used as a topical anesthetic in rhinolaryngologic and ophthalmic surgery. In Europe and the United States, prior to World War I, it was thought to be nonaddicting and relatively safe. Since the 1970s there has been a second epidemic in its illicit use, and it has been estimated that 5 million people now use it regularly in the United States. It is usually taken by intranasal inhalation or snuffing, by smoking the "crack" variety, or by intravenous injection. The plasma half-life is approximately 50 to 90 min. The euphoriant effects last approximately 20 to 30 min when smoked or 60 to 90 min when used intranasally. Cocaine is metabolized by liver and plasma pseudocholinesterase to compounds that are water soluble and excreted in urine. Most, but not all, of the metabolites are pharmacologically inactive. Metabolites of cocaine can be detected in the urine for 1 to 2 days after administration and, occasionally, can be found for several more days.

The cardiovascular effects of cocaine are complex.[90–92] Its local anesthetic properties are due to its ability to block the initiation and conduction of electrical impulses within nerve cells. In the myocardium it blocks the fast sodium channel, producing a depression of depolarization and a slowing of conduction velocity. The refractoriness of atrial and ventricular muscle is also prolonged; in the electrocardiogram, the PR, QRS, and QT intervals may be prolonged.

A second major action of cocaine is to block the reuptake of catecholamines, including norepinephrine and dopamine, at the presynaptic level in both the central and the peripheral nervous systems and to increase the release of catecholamines from both central and peripheral stores.[90–92] These catecholamine-potentiating effects can lead to tachycardia, hypertension, mydriasis, and hyperthermia.

A third effect of cocaine is coronary vasoconstriction, which can result from two different mechanisms. The first is a direct vasoconstrictor effect upon vascular smooth muscle, an effect that is not endothelium dependent, but that is inhibited by nitroglycerin or calcium-blocking drugs but not by phentolamine, an alpha-adrenergic antagonist.[90–92] The second mechanism is coronary vasoconstriction that is mediated by alpha-adrenergic mechanisms and inhibited by phentolamine, an alpha-adrenergic antagonist.[93] Cocaine causes vasoconstriction of both nondiseased and diseased coronary artery segments, but its effect is especially marked in the latter.[94] It also produces significant constriction of smaller coronary arterioles.

Other effects of cocaine include a direct "toxic" effect on the myocardium; a direct negative inotropic effect presumably due to its inhibitory effect on sodium channels; an increase in intracellular calcium; possible increased platelet aggregation and thromboxane production and, in one case, protein C and antithrombin III deficiency; possible acceleration of atherosclerosis; and possible intimal hyperplasia of coronary vessels.[90–92]

The use of illicit cocaine has been associated with a wide variety of cardiovascular syndromes (Table 110-1). Acute pulmonary edema can result from acute, reversible myocarditis, which has sometimes been characterized by lymphocytic or eosinophilic infiltration and/or contraction band necrosis or from severe hypertension.[90–92] Some patients have electrocardiographic evidence or asymptomatic ("silent") myocardial ischemia during the first week or so of withdrawal.[95] Cocaine has also been reported to produce rhabdomyolysis; malignant hyperthermia; pneumothorax; diffuse alveolar hemorrhage; intestinal ischemia or gangrene; abruptio placentae; and perforation of the nasal septum. Central nervous system complications result from vasospasm or thrombosis and include infarction at all levels from the retina to the spinal cord, in addition to intracerebral, intraventricular, or subarachnoid hemorrhage.[90–92] Intravenous cocaine use is associated with an increased risk of endocarditis.

TABLE 110-1

Cardiovascular Complications of Cocaine

Sudden death
Acute myocardial infarction
Chest pain without myocardial infarction
Acute, reversible myocarditis
Irreversible heart muscle disease
Acute, severe hypertension
Acute aortic dissection, rupture
Electrocardiographic changes: sinus tachycardia, premature ventricular complexes, Wolff-Parkinson-White arrhythmias, ventricular tachycardia, torsades de pointes, ventricular fibrillation, prolongation of QTc, and early repolarization (ST-segment) changes
Pneumopericardium
Stroke
Subarachnoid hemorrhage
Accelerated coronary atherosclerosis
Intimal hyperplasia of coronary vessels

Myocardial ischemia or infarction can result from several mechanisms including an increase in myocardial oxygen requirements due to tachycardia and hypertension; vasoconstriction of epicardial or intramyocardial vessels either from the direct vasoconstrictor effect of cocaine or from alpha-adrenergic stimulation; platelet aggregation and coronary thrombosis; and underlying coronary atherosclerosis.[90–92] Of interest, myocardial infarction from cocaine does not appear to be related to the frequency or duration of usage or to the route of administration. The pain of infarction sometimes begins a number of hours after the use of cocaine. (See also Chap. 64.)

The evaluation of chest pain in individuals who have used cocaine can be very difficult.[96,97] The majority of patients do not develop enzymatic evidence of infarction, but their chest pain may not be different from those who do. In addition, many of the patients have ST-segment elevation, which is often most marked in precordial leads V_1 to V_3 due to normal variant, early repolarization changes (Chap. 13). These ST changes can mimic the changes of acute myocardial infarction. Total serum creatine kinase (CK) concentrations may be elevated, often from rhabdomyolysis.

There are no large adequate trials of the acute pharmacologic management of patients with chest pain following cocaine. A reasonable regimen includes therapy for acute cocaine intoxication, withdrawal, and addiction; aspirin (325 mg orally); and intravenous nitroglycerin. Calcium-blocking drugs such as nifedipine, diltiazem, verapamil, or nitrendipine may also be useful in the control of some cardiac arrhythmias, hypertension, and possibly coronary vasoconstriction. Beta-adrenergic blocking drugs such as propranolol can potentiate coronary vasoconstriction and, in general, should be avoided.[90–92] Occasionally, labetalol, which has both beta- and alpha-adrenergic blocking effects, is useful for control of blood pressure and tachycardia.

Patients should be carefully monitored for arrhythmias, and for serial changes in the 12-lead electrocardiogram and CK-MB levels. Echocardiography is useful to evaluate regional wall motion. Emergent coronary arteriography can sometimes be of great clinical value in determining whether or not the patient is sustaining an acute infarction. Thrombolytic therapy (see Chaps. 60 and 69) has been successfully employed in some patients but may be associated with a higher complication for subarachnoid hemorrhage and aortic dissection.

Several of the electrophysiological effects of cocaine are similar to those of class I antiarrhythmics (Chap. 38), and QT prolongation and ventricular arrhythmias, including torsades de pointes, may occur. Occasionally, transient second- or third-degree atrioventricular heart block may also occur. Correction of acidosis and correction of hypokalemia and hypomagnesemia appear to be useful.

It is possible that many patients with chest pain following cocaine use have sustained multiple, microfocal infarctions throughout the heart that are not in critical areas, do not produce regional wall abnormalities or fatal arrhythmias, and do not produce infarction of sufficient size to be detected by currently employed enzymatic techniques. If this is true, many of these patients may ultimately develop severe, irreversible ventricular scarring with dilatation and marked dysfunction.

Caffeine

Caffeine has a sympathomimetic amine effect on the cardiovascular system. Hemodynamic responses of acute administration include an increase in blood pressure and heart rate.[98] These effects can be blunted with chronic use depending on individual variations in plasma caffeine half-life[99] but are greater in the older individuals.[100] Blood pressure elevation is even greater during exercise.[101] The influence of caffeine consumption on therapy of hypertension has been emphasized.[101]

Caffeine is thought to have an arrhythmogenic effect on the heart.[100,101] Electrophysiological studies are limited. One study has demonstrated no change in conduction times; a shortened refractory period of the right atrium, atrioventricular node, and right ventricle; and an increased frequency of sustained tachycardia induced by the extrastimulus technique. This latter effect was especially frequent in patients with a prior history of arrhythmias.[102] One study has shown no arrhythmogenic effect with modest caffeine consumption.[103]

The mechanism of action of caffeine on the heart is not known.[100,102] Although elevations of catecholamines may occur with acute administration, this effect is less frequent with chronic use.[98,104] The role of caffeine as a risk factor for coronary artery disease is not well established.[100] Although one prospective study demonstrated a correlation between coffee consumption and risk of heart disease,[105] most studies have not, and the effects of coffee consumption, with or without caffeine, on cardiovascular disease remain controversial.[106,107]

Caffeine toxicity causes marked catecholamine release and may be associated with tachyarrhythmias, hypotension, metabolic acidosis, hyperglycemia, and hypokalemia.[108]

Theophylline

Theophylline has both chronotropic and ionotropic effects on the heart.[109] The most common cardiac effect with therapeutic doses is a slight increase in heart rate with minimal effects on blood pressure. Patients with severe obstructive lung disease or heart disease are subject to atrial and ventricular arrhythmias.[109] A significant positive inotropic effect by both oral and intravenous (aminophylline) administration has been demonstrated in human beings. This effect may be due to its direct effect on the heart, the release of catecholamines, or a reduction in peripheral resistance.[110] This inotropic effect may be attenuated in the presence of beta-adrenergic blockade.[111]

Toxicity is associated with sinus tachycardia, atrial and ventricular arrhythmias, and hypotension. Esmolol may be useful in the management of refractory ventricular arrhythmias.[111,112] Hypokalemia, hypercalcemia, hyperglycemia, hypophosphatemia, and metabolic acidosis may occur.[113–115] Dialysis may be helpful in patients with refractory arrhythmias or hypotension.[116] Dialysis is more likely to be indicated with acute overdose than with toxicity due to chronic use.[117] Toxicity due to sustained-release preparations may be prolonged.[118] Mexiletine interferes with theophylline clearance and may have an added arrhythmogenic effect.[119] Mexiletine should not be used in the treatment of ventricular arrhythmias associated with theophylline toxicity.

Terbutaline

Terbutaline is a selective beta$_2$-adrenergic agonist. It causes a slight increase in heart rate and pulse pressure without an increase in mean arterial pressure. Nonspecific T-wave changes (decreased amplitude) and J-point ST depression have been observed.[120–122] As with theophylline, atrial and ventricular arrhythmias may occur, especially in patients with preexisting heart disease or other precipitating factors. Occasionally, angina pectoris is worsened. Hypokalemia may occur.[123,124]

Terbutaline has been demonstrated to have a beneficial hemodynamic effect in patients with congestive heart failure and cardiogenic shock.[123,125–128]

The use of terbutaline in the treatment of premature labor may have significant cardiac complications.[129]

Albuterol

Albuterol (marketed as Salbutamol in Europe) is a highly selective beta$_2$-adrenergic agonist used as a bronchodilator and in the treatment of premature labor. It appears to have few cardiovascular effects, similar to terbutaline.[130] Similarly, hypokalemia may occur.[131] Potassium-losing diuretics may potentiate the hypokalemia, and high doses of potassium-sparing diuretics may be protective.[131] Aerosol therapy, since it produces effective bronchodilation with little systemic effects, has few cardiac effects.[132]

Overdose has fewer serious cardiac effects compared to theophylline.[133] Hypokalemia and sinus tachycardia occur, but serious cardiac arrhythmias are uncommon.[133]

Ergotamine

Ergotamine causes constriction of smooth muscles. There is constriction of peripheral vessels and an increase in blood pressure and peripheral vascular resistance.[134] Cardiac output may increase in patients with orthostatic hypotension.[134] The lower extremities are most commonly involved by peripheral vasoconstriction.[135] An aortic arch syndrome has been reported.[135] Intravenous sodium nitroprusside is useful in the therapy of prolonged vasoconstriction.[136]

The user of ergonovine maleate in the diagnosis of coronary artery spasm is recognized. (See also Chap. 58.) Ergotamine is frequently used in the treatment of migraine headaches. Myocardial infarction is a known complication of this therapy.[137]

An association of ergotamine and valvular heart disease has been reported. Aortic regurgitation and mitral regurgitation have been described.[138] Ergotamine and methysergide are chemically related. Either may cause pulmonary fibrosis, retroperitoneal fibrosis, and multivalvular heart disease (see later discussion, "Methysergide"). The occurrence of these side effects is less frequent with ergotamine.[138]

L-Dopa

L-Dopa has few cardiac effects in patients without heart disease. It does cause an increase in the amount of circulating dopamine, which may beneficially increase cardiac output in patients with heart failure.[139] Orthostatic hypotension is common, especially early in therapy, and is usually transient but may persist.[140] Because of the cardiac-stimulating effects of dopamine, arrhythmias, including sinus tachycardia and atrial and ventricular arrhythmias, may occur.[141] Levodopa may increase atrioventricular conduction.[141] These effects are more likely early in therapy or in patients with ischemic heart disease.[142] They are less likely with concomitant beta-adrenergic blockade.[141,142] Symptomatic postural hypotension may be treated with fludrocortisone acetate.[140]

Methysergide

Methysergide can cause retroperitoneal, pulmonary, and cardiac fibrosis. Cardiac involvement may affect the endocardium, myocardium, valves, and rarely the aorta.[143–145] The mitral and aortic valves are most commonly involved, but effects on the tricuspid and pulmonary valves have been reported.[143] Lesions are more frequently regurgitant than stenotic.[144] The mechanism is unknown, but the pathological conditions are similar to those seen in carcinoid heart disease. Periodic interruption of therapy with methysergide is recommended and thought to significantly reduce the incidence of cardiac involvement.[144] Patients should be monitored frequently for the development of murmurs during therapy. Methysergide should be discontinued when new murmurs are detected. Regression of the valvular lesion may occur, although valve replacement is required in some cases.[144] Patients with known valvular disease should not be given this drug.[143]

Low-Calorie Diets

Very low calorie diets have potentially serious cardiovascular effects including electrocardiographic changes, arrhythmias, and sudden death.[146,147] Atrial and ventricular arrhythmias may occur. In extreme cases QT prolongation and torsades de pointes ventricular tachycardia are reported. Potassium and magnesium deficiency, poor quality protein, and changes in the autonomic nervous system are possible mechanisms of this complication.[146,147] Some studies have shown no increase in cardiac arrhythmias during ambulatory monitoring or during stress testing with high-quality protein diets that include adequate vitamin and mineral supplements.[147,148]

Histamine H_2-Receptor Antagonist

Cimetidine infrequently causes any cardiac effects.[149,150] Although electrophysiological studies have not demonstrated any effect on sinus node function,[151,152] instances of severe bradycardia have been reported with oral and intravenous administration.[149,150] Hypotension, asystole, and atrial and ventricular arrhythmias have also been reported with intravenous use.[153] These complications appear more likely with larger doses, when given rapidly through a central venous line, or in patients with cardiac or renal disease.[149,150] The antagonist effect on histamine H_2 receptors in the heart has been postulated as the mechanism of these effects.[154] (See also Chap. 109.)

Ranitidine, another H_2-receptor antagonist, has also been reported to cause bradycardia.[155] Famotidine appears to have fewer hemodynamic effects with less frequent decrease in blood pressure compared to cimetidine.[156]

Ipecac

Patients with eating disorders may have significant cardiovascular changes. Dehydration and electrolyte abnormalities resulting from self-induced vomiting, laxative abuse, and use of diet pills and diuretics may cause significant electrocardiographic changes.[157] Ipecac may be used chronically and in large doses by these patients to induce vomiting. The principal alkaloids of ipecac are emetine and cephaeline. Emetine can have serious cardiovascular effects.[158,159] Electrocardiographic changes are frequent and include ST- and T-wave changes and prolongation of conduction.[158,159] Atrial and ventricular arrhythmias may occur and death has been reported.[160,161]

Chloroquine

Chloroquine and hydroxychloroquine are known to cause skeletal myopathy and rarely heart muscle disease. They may cause problems with myocardial function or the conduction system. Myocardial biopsy with electron microscopy is diagnostic, and the findings are like those found in skeletal myopathy.[162] Acute chloroquine poisoning causes hypotension, tachycardia, and prolongation of QRS and is usually fatal. A recent report suggests that mortality can be significantly decreased with aggressive use of mechanical ventilation, diazepam, and epinephrine.[163]

ELECTRICITY

This section deals with the cardiovascular effects of electrical injuries related to live wires and the electricity of nature—lightning. Iatrogenic problems related to electroconvulsive therapy (ECT) are also reviewed. Exposure to electrical fields has been implicated as a cause of adverse cardiac effects, but recent reviews have not revealed any clear-cut cause and effect.[164]

Environmental Accidents

Accidental contact with electricity may occur in the home, where children are particularly vulnerable,[165] or on the job, especially to electrical workers but also on any job in which electrical equipment is used. The hospital environment has become increasingly hazardous. There are approximately 1200 deaths related to electrical accidents per year.[166] Lightning injury also causes death to at least 100 people per year, representing a 30 percent mortality rate in reported cases.[167–169] People who are involved in outdoor activities, i.e., golfers, hikers, and farmers, are especially vulnerable. The Tazer, an electrical self-defense weapon, has also caused serious electrical injuries and death.[170]

Electrophysiology

The degree of total-body injury from electricity is determined by many factors: the amount of electrical energy delivered, the duration of the current, the resistance of the skin, the path of the current through the body, and the tissue damage along the way.[171] Alternating current, even of relatively low voltage, is of greater hazard than direct current since tetanic muscle contractions prevent the "let-go" phenomenon. Exposure to a current over the "let-go," but less than the ventricular fibrillation, threshold can cause respiratory arrest and death without direct cardiac effects.[168,172,173] Although burn injury is considered to be a common complication of electrical accidents, only about one-half of deaths due to contact with low voltage (less than 1000 V) are associated with burns.[173] High-tension wires (1000 V or greater) produce greater internal burn injuries, more like crush injuries, in addition to cardiovascular and central nervous system effects.[174] Lightning is of extremely high voltage but brief in duration and is a direct current.[167] Although deep burns do occur, they are less frequent, and a characteristic superficial burn is common.[175,176] A lightning strike may be direct, a side flash, or a stride potential (see below), and to some extent, this determines the extent and severity of injury.[177]

The path of the electrical current through the body, entry-to-exit sites, also determines the cardiac and central nervous system effects. A current path from arm to arm or arm to leg is more likely to cause direct cardiac effects. A vertical pathway of injury and extensive body surface burns are predictors of myocardial damage.[178] A stride potential, leg-to-leg, entry-to-exit sites, is infrequently associated with direct cardiac effects. A current path involving the head or a large current path from arm to arm may cause direct respiratory depression by its effect on the respiratory center.[168]

Cardiovascular Effects

A person struck by lightning may be comatose and without pulses or respirations. The immediate cardiac effect may be a direct result of the electrical current on the heart, causing asystole or ventricular fibrillation, or an indirect result of apnea and hypoxia, causing cardiac arrest.[176,179] Pulseless extremities may persist after normal cardiac activity resumes as a result of severe peripheral vasoconstriction.

During the hours following injury, other cardiac effects may be observed.[180–183] Sinus tachycardia and nonspecific ST- and T-wave changes are probably the most common. Arrhythmias, including ventricular ectopic beats, ventricular tachycardia, atrial ectopic beats, atrial tachycardia, and sinus bradycardia, may also occur. Conduction abnormalities including bundle branch block and, rarely, complete heart block are also reported. Acute myocardial infarction is rare but can occur and not become manifest for several hours after the injury.[177] This effect may be complicated by significant left ventricular dysfunction including pulmonary edema.[180,182,184] The ST- and T-wave changes, including prolongation of the QT interval, may be due to direct effects on the myocardium or may be secondary to electrical injury to the central nervous system. Intense catecholamine release may occur after injury and cause severe hypertension and tachycardia. One case of cardiac rupture has been reported.[185] These late cardiac effects may occur without initial cardiopulmonary arrest.

Victims of electrical accidents are subject to similar cardiac effects. Up to 36 percent of victims of electrical injury who seek medical care are found to have electrocardiographic changes, including cardiac arrhythmias or evidence of myocardial damage.[174,186] In fatal cases extensive focal necrosis of the myocardium and conduction system and contraction band necrosis in the smooth muscles of coronary arteries have been described. In addition, preexisting cardiac abnormalities may be more likely in patients with cardiac arrest related to electrical injury.[187] When electrical injury causes extensive burns and tissue necrosis, there may be additional secondary cardiac effects due to hypovolemia, electrolyte abnormalities, and infection.

Management and Prognosis

Immediate cardiopulmonary resuscitation should be instituted and continued for a prolonged period.[171,176,188] Spontaneous respirations may not occur for 30 min or more. Nonreactive pupils may be the result of transient central nervous system effects and are no contraindication to resuscitation attempts.[189] On the basis of reports of successful recovery after prolonged unconsciousness, it has been suggested that basal metabolism is significantly reduced after a lightning strike. In a lightning accident involving a number of victims, attention should be immediately directed to victims who are "apparently dead."[167,190] In such instances, death is rare when cardiopulmonary arrest does not occur.[167] In any electrical injury the victim may have complete cardiopulmonary arrest, respiratory arrest only, or only transient paralysis of extremities or muscles of respiration.

Since cardiac effects may not be immediately apparent, victims should be observed for development of arrhythmias or myocardial infarction.[182] Hypertension and tachycardia secondary to the catecholamine release may be managed with an intravenous beta-adrenergic blocking agent.[189]

Recovery from the cardiac effects of electrical injury

is usually good with electrocardiographic abnormalities resolving within a few weeks.[177,180] A number of patients who developed significant left ventricular dysfunction have been observed to return to near-normal myocardial function.[180,181,183] Some patients may have persistent left ventricular dysfunction.[191]

Electroconvulsive Therapy

Electroconvulsive therapy has been utilized in the treatment of various psychiatric illnesses since the late 1930s.[192] Morbidity during its early use was related to musculoskeletal injury as well as cardiopulmonary complications.[193] Present-day use is modified with pharmacologic agents that provide greater safety, although the major complications continue to be cardiovascular.[192,193]

The cardiac effects relate to the electroshock as well as to medications used to modify the response.[192] After the administration of atropine or scopolamine, general anesthesia is accomplished with a short-acting agent; muscle paralysis is achieved with succinylcholine chloride. The grand mal seizure is most commonly produced with an alternating current of 70 to 170 V for 0.1 to 1.0 s, applied either bilaterally or unilaterally to the head.[192] The onset of the seizure is associated with immediate vagal stimulation, which would produce a profound bradycardia without prior anticholinergic blockade. This is followed by a sympathetic stimulus with tachycardia and hypertension.[194] During the first few minutes after the seizure, cardiac arrhythmias may develop, including ventricular and atrial ectopic rhythms and brady- or tachyarrhythmias.[193,195] Additional electrocardiographic changes during this time may include ST- and T-wave changes, QRS changes, and QT prolongation.[195,196] The T-wave changes may simulate acute subendocardial infarction or hyperkalemia.[197,198] Although some electrocardiographic change is common, the changes are usually of short duration and of no clinical importance.[195,196] Acute pulmonary edema after ECT is reported, but it is unclear whether it is neurogenic or cardiac in origin.[199] Sudden death after ECT has been reported rarely.

Pathogenesis of Cardiovascular Effects

The stimulus of the electric shock to the central nervous system including the autonomic nervous system is responsible for many of the changes in heart rate and blood pressure, which are independent of any motor activity related to the seizure.[194] A significant transient elevation of catecholamines has been demonstrated and may contribute to the tachycardia and hypertension.[193,200] Increases in cardiac contractility and myocardial oxygen consumption may also result from catecholamine release.[201] In addition, the repolarization changes in the electrocardiogram are similar to those described with other problems of the central nervous system. (See Chaps. 13 and 122.)

The anesthetic agent may also contribute to the electrocardiographic changes. Whether methohexital causes fewer cardiovascular problems than thiopental sodium is controversial.[193,200] Hypoxia and/or respiratory acidosis may develop during the period of apnea immediately following the induction of general anesthesia and increase the chances of arrhythmias.[195] An increase in serum potassium due to both the effects of succinylcholine chloride and ECT may be seen. This increase, however, is small and rarely of clinical significance.[202] Preexisting heart disease or medications, especially cardiac or psychotropic agents, may also increase the risk of cardiovascular complications.

Recognition and Management

Preanesthetic assessment should be directed at identifying those patients with the greatest potential risk of major complications from ECT.[193,195] Uncontrolled hypertension, recent myocardial infarction, unstable angina pectoris, congestive heart failure, and arrhythmias may increase the risk of cardiovascular complications. Electrolyte abnormalities should be corrected prior to therapy, and the appropriateness of medications, especially cardiac and psychotropic agents, should be assessed. Preexisting pulmonary disease may also increase the chances of hypoxia and respiratory acidosis.

Attention to the anesthesia procedure regarding agents chosen, amount given, and ancillary respiratory support is also critical to the cardiopulmonary safety of the procedure. Cardiac monitoring should be done in all patients during and following the procedure until their full recovery from anesthesia.

Additional drug modification has been employed in selected patients. The use of small doses of a beta-adrenergic blocking agent given intravenously may blunt the tachycardia and hypertension and reduce the frequency of ventricular ectopic beats.[192,200] This can be especially useful in patients who are at risk of cardiac complications due to these effects. Pretreatment with lidocaine is reported to raise the seizure threshold to the shock stimulus, necessitating higher energy levels to effect a seizure.[203] A similar effect has been reported with clonidine.[204] Nitroprusside, begun intravenously just prior to the procedure, has also been used to blunt the hypertensive response.[205] There is one report of asystole associated with the administration of 1 mg of propranolol intravenously prior to ECT. This patient had electrocardiographic evidence of old myocardial infarction and was not given an anticholinergic agent prior to ECT.[206]

Patients who are on chronic anticoagulation with warfarin may be managed during ECT by the temporary use of intravenous heparin, which can be discontinued 6 to 8 h prior to and resumed shortly after the procedure.[207] Patients with permanent pacemakers also require special consideration. Currently used pacemakers are probably not affected by the ECT current.[208] Conversion to the fixed-rate mode with an external magnet over the generator may afford additional safety.[209]

Determinations of serum creatine phosphokinase (CK) activity have demonstrated a mild elevation of total levels in a few patients following ECT as the result of an increase in skeletal muscle fraction without elevations of the MB fraction.[210]

Although ECT frequently does cause transient electrocardiographic and hemodynamic changes, it continues to be a safe model of therapy for selected psychiatric illnesses. Attention to patient selection and the details of the procedure is an important determinant of its safety.[193]

Shock Wave Lithotripsy

Shock wave lithotripsy for the treatment of renal stones[211] and gall stones[212] has potential cardiac effects. The high-energy shock waves must be appropriately synchronized with the QRS of the electrocardiogram to avoid ventricular arrhythmias. The patient is immersed in a water bath, and proper electrical grounding is essential. Waterbath temperatures must be monitored to avoid hypo- or hyperthermia.[213] Hemodynamic alterations are usually minimal.[214] Supraventricular and ventricular arrhythmias may occur.[211,215] Second-generation lithotriptors do not require water immersion and deliver a smaller focus shock wave. These units may be safer but still can produce arrhythmias especially when not triggered by electrocardiography.[216] Endocarditis prophylaxis is recommended for patients with valvular heart disease.[217] Special precautions are necessary for patients with pacemakers.[218] These patients should have electrocardiography triggered treatment, and DDD modes should be reprogrammed to the VVI mode. Piezoelectric activity sensing rate responsive pacemakers implanted in the chest should have this mode deactivated. If implanted in the abdomen the piezoelectric crystal may be destroyed by the shockwave.[219] There is some concern that lithotripsy may contribute to the development of hypertension. Slight elevation of the diastolic blood pressure has been observed but without an increased incidence of hypertension (diastolic blood pressure of 90 mmHg or greater).[220]

POISONS

This section deals with a number of environmental contacts that demonstrate the ubiquitous nature of agents that can cause cardiac toxicity. The possible cardiac effects of these agents are reviewed. The reader is referred to other sources for their detailed toxicology.

Plants

Cardiac Glycoside-Like Effects

The oleander plant (*Nerium oleander*) contains oleandroside, oleandrin, and nerioside.[221,222] The lily of the valley plant (*Convallaria majalis*) contains convallarin, convallamarin, and convallatoxin.[221] The Jerusalem cherry contains solanocapsine (leaves) and solanine (berry), and the unripe berries of the jessamine (*Cestrum diurnum* and *C. nocturnum*) contain solanine.[221,222] Both the potato (*Solanum tuberosum*) plant and the green tubers also contain solanine.[223] Other plants known to contain substances with cardiac glycoside-like effects include milkweed (*Asclepias* species), *Hollarrhena* species of Asia, pheasant's eye (*Adonis vernalis*), green hellebore (*Helleborus viridis*), Christmas rose (*Helleborus niger*), and the wallflower (*Cheirina cheiri*).[222,224]

The cardiac effects of poisoning with these plants are similar to those of digitalis toxicity.[221,224,225]

Other Cardiotoxic Effects

The larkspur *(Delphinium)*, both the plant and the seed, contains delphinine, a substance similar to aconitine, which causes myocardial depression, cardiac arrhythmias, and hypotension.[221] The jimsonweed *(Datura stramonium)* contains a belladonna alkaloid, and the mature berries of the day-blooming or night-blooming jessamine contain a tropane-related alkaloid. Both have anticholinergic effects. The castor bean *(Ricinus communis)* contains ricin, a toxalbumin, which in severe cases causes hypotension and circulatory collapse.[224] Mistletoe *(Phorandendron serotinum)* (both the plant and berries) contains beta-phenethylamine and tyramine and can cause severe hypertension.[221] The Carolina jessamine *(Gelsemium sempervirens)* has mostly central nervous system effects, but the alkaloids gelsemine and gelsemicine have cardiac depressant effects.[221,225]

The ingestion of Chinese herbs containing aconite alkaloids can produce ventricular tachycardia or even fibrillation and death. No antidote is available, and clinical experience is very limited. Flecainide and amiodarone may be useful.[226]

Snakes and Scorpions

There are approximately 250 species of venomous snakes.[227] In the United States there are 19. Rattlesnakes, copperheads, and cottonmouths, all of the Crotalidae family, are responsible for the majority of bites. The coral snake, of the Elapidae family, is less frequently the cause.[229] Snake venom, in general, contains substances that affect the coagulation system; cellular components of the blood; endothelium of vessels; the nervous system, including the cardiorespiratory centers and myoneural junction; and the heart.[228] A specific snake venom, however, may have more effects on one system than another.[227] The cardiotoxins also are variable in any snake venom and are throught to have variable mechanisms of action and cardiac effects.[230] Animal studies have demonstrated that these cardiotoxins may augment myocardial contraction to systolic arrest or may have a negative inotropic effect. They may also cause cardiac arrhythmias.[230]

Animal studies demonstrate that certain *Crotalus* venoms cause a severe decrease in systemic arterial pressure and an increase in pulmonary artery pressure. The exact mechanism of these effects is unclear. A decrease in circulating blood volume due to venous pooling, especially in the lungs, and thromboembolism in the pulmonary vascular bed have been observed.[230] Clinically, there may be severe hypotension, which can be due to the negative inotropic effect of the venom on the myocardium, but may also be due to loss of intravascular volume due to increased permeability of blood vessels with plasma and blood loss in the tissues. Multiple pulmonary emboli are also seen in patients who survive 12 h or longer.[227]

Scorpion (order Scorpionida) venom can cause hypertension and electrocardiographic changes of myocardial infarction. Pulmonary edema may occur.[231] Arrhythmias, conduction disturbances, and myocarditis have been described.[232] Animal studies suggest that the scorpion toxin acts indirectly on the heart via the release of acetylcholine and catecholamines.[230]

Arthropods

Direct cardiac effects of the venom of bees, yellow jackets, hornets, and wasps (Hymenoptera order) are difficult to establish. Electrocardiographic changes of myocardial ischemia or infarction, chest pain, and pulmonary edema are reported.[231] These problems are usually associated with anaphylaxis and its treatment. Cardiac arrhythmias also occur in association with anaphylaxis or systemic symptoms. One case has been described in which arrhythmias occurred in the absence of systemic symptoms.[234]

Animal studies of bee venom have demonstrated major electrocardiographic changes, suggesting a direct cardiotoxic effect.[230]

Halogenated Hydrocarbons

Halogenated hydrocarbon exposure may occur in the home or in industrial environments. These substances are used in fire extinguishers as propellants, solvents, and refrigerants.[235] They are used in the manufacture of pesticides and plastics.[236] Cardiac effects include arrhythmias and sudden death.[237] These compounds depress myocardial contractility and sensitize the heart to the arrhythmogenic effects of epinephrine.[235] Cardiac effects may also result indirectly from hypoxia or the effects of these compounds on the central nervous system. Sudden death, presumably due to arrhythmias, may occur, or cardiopulmonary effects including pulmonary edema may occur hours after exposure.[236,237]

Carbon Monoxide

For many people, exposure to carbon monoxide is a potential environmental hazard of daily life. The industrial environment provides an even greater potential for poisoning.

Carbon monoxide has an affinity for hemoglobin that is much greater than that of oxygen. The cardiac effects are the result of hypoxia. These effects are determined by the degree of carbon monoxide exposure, the hemoglobin concentration, and the presence or absence of coronary or myocardial disease. A decrease in exercise performance occurs even in normal individuals with low-level exposure. Patients with angina pectoris have a greater reduction in exercise tolerance.[238]

Carbon monoxide poisoning causes myocardial ischemia most commonly manifest as ST- and T-wave changes on the electrocardiogram and atrial and ventricular arrhythmias.[239] Severe exposure can cause extensive myocardial necrosis and cardiomyopathy. Myocardial infarction may occur as a result of myocardial necrosis without coronary occlusion.[240]

RADIATION

The sensitivity of the heart to radiation is recognized as a potential cause of morbidity and mortality from radiation therapy to the mediastinum.[241] Pericardial disease is the most frequent complication with variable but frequent clinically significant manifestations. Myocardial effects are frequent but usually subclinical or mildly symptomatic. Infrequent but clinically important valvular problems can occur. Conduction defects, rarely progressing to complete heart block, have been reported.

The incidence of radiation heart disease is influenced by a number of variables. Radiation technology has evolved during the past 40 years.[242] Current techniques are designed to limit radiation exposure to the heart, and cardiac sequelae are considerably reduced.[241] Successful prolongation of life by radiation therapy for malignancies has allowed longer periods of observation for detection of radiation-induced heart disease. Noninvasive testing with echocardiography, stress testing, and nuclear imaging has allowed more sensitive methods of early detection.[243]

An understanding of the pathogenesis of radiation heart disease is based on animal studies that demonstrate the early and acute effects.[244,245] The pericardium, myocardium, endocardium, valves, conduction system, and coronary arteries may be affected by radiation. An acute exudative phase involving the pericardium, myocardium, endocardium, valves, and capillaries is followed by capillary endothelial damage. Progressive platelet and fibrin deposition and capillary destruction cause ischemia and fibrosis of the myocardium and conduction system.[242]

The exudative process, especially in the pericardium, is followed by progressive fibrosis and effusion. Pericardial thickening of either or both visceral and parietal layers is mild to severe and is associated with fibrinous to grossly bloody pericardial effusion. Valvular lesions and endocardial thickening result from cellular damage and fibrosis. Endothelial damage to the coronary arteries, loss of smooth-muscle cells, adventitial fibrosis and development of endothelial plaques are more likely in the proximal segments of the vessels, especially those located more anterior and adjacent to the radiation field.[242]

Pericardial Disease

Anatomic changes in the pericardium occur in the majority of patients, many without clinical findings. Clinically apparent pericardial involvement is most frequent 4 to 6 months after therapy.[241] Acute pericarditis, asymptomatic pericardial effusion, or both may occur. Cardiac and subcarinal shielding, equally weighted anterior and posterior ports, and a total dose of no more than 3000 rads given over a longer period have significantly reduced the incidence of radiation-induced heart disease, especially pericarditis. With such techniques the incidence of pericarditis is reported to be 2.5 percent.[241] Other etiologies for pericarditis must be considered in these patients. The pericardium may be involved by the malignancy. Such immunosuppressed patients are at risk of purulent pericarditis. Hypothyroidism, also a complication of radiation therapy, may also cause pericardial effusion.[241] Acute pericarditis, asymptomatic pericardial effusion, or both may not appear until 1 to 2 years after radiation therapy and rarely much later. In some cases it may be chronic and recurrent. Pericardial tamponade, constrictive pericarditis, and effusive constrictive pericarditis are also recognized to occur months to many years following radiation injury.[241–245]

The surgical management of post irradiation constrictive pericarditis may be especially difficult.[246] Surgical morbidity and mortality are significant, and long-term survival is less than 50 percent.[246] The extensive mediastinal and pericardial fibrosis makes complete pericardiectomy technically difficult to impossible. When large radiation doses have been used, there is a high incidence of associated heart disease, including coronary artery disease, myocardial dysfunction, conduction abnormalities, and valvular disease. Patient selection should consider any such concomitant cardiac involvement as well as the general nutritional status of the chronically ill patient. Significant underlying myocardial fibrosis and dysfunction contribute to the poor long-term improvement.[246]

Myocardial Disease

The extent and severity of myocardial fibrosis are variable. The anterior right ventricle is more susceptible than the more posterior left ventricle. The areas of fibrosis may be patchy or diffuse. With current radiation therapy techniques myocardial dysfunction is infrequent and usually mild.[243] Echocardiography and radionuclide ventriculography at rest and during exercise may show mild impairment of systolic function in some asymptomatic patients.[243] Due to the pathological process that results in myocardial fibrosis, there may be more significant impairment of diastolic function and rarely a severe restrictive cardiomyopathy.[241]

Valvular Disease

Radiation-induced valvular heart disease is infrequent.[241] Clinically apparent valvular dysfunction is appreciated years after radiation therapy. It is a gradually progressive process, and prolonged survival allows symptomatic valvular disease to manifest.[247] One review of 35 reported cases found that the mean time from radiation to clinically recognized valvular disease was 11.5 years and that symptoms developed at a mean of 5 years later.[247]

The most commonly involved valves are the aortic and mitral, with regurgitation more frequent than stenosis of either valve.[247] Lesions of the pulmonic and tricuspid valves are less frequent,[248] and subvalvular pulmonic stenosis has been described.[248,249]

Valve replacement has been undertaken but with limited success. Concomitant pericardial constriction is frequent, and coronary artery disease may also require surgical intervention.[241] Successful combined aortic and mitral valve replacement has been reported.[247]

Coronary Artery Disease

Premature coronary heart disease has been described in patients after radiation therapy.[249] Myocardial infarction has been reported in very young patients.[249] Long-term studies are inconclusive in documenting an increased cardiovascular morbidity.[241,242,248] The development of coronary artery disease is usually noted 10 years or more after radiation therapy.[250] A high incidence of left main and right ostial coronary disease has been noted.[250] Associated valvular disease is not uncommon.[250] Current radiation techniques make coronary artery disease a less likely complication.[242] The presence of hypercholesterolemia may be an additional risk factor for the development of radiation-induced coronary artery disease.[251]

Percutaneous transluminal coronary angioplasty and coronary artery bypass surgery have been successful in selected patients. The presence of extensive mediastinal and pericardial fibrosis, however, makes surgery technically difficult and sometimes precludes surgery.[247,250]

Conduction System Disease

Impairment of the conduction system including nodal and infranodal pathways may occur as a result of radiation.[241] Complete atrioventricular block may result from extensive fibrosis of the nodal tissues or the bundle branches.[249,252] Right bundle branch block is especially common, most likely related to the more anterior location of the right bundle.[241] Although up to 50 percent of patients may have some electrocardiographic abnormality, the incidence of complete heart block is rare.[240]

REFERENCES

1. Davies DM (ed): *Textbook of Adverse Drug Reactions*, 3d ed. New York, Oxford University Press, 1985.
2. Jefferson JW: Cardiovascular effects and toxicity of anxiolytics and antidepressants. *J Clin Psychiatry* 1989; 50:368–378.
3. Cole JO, Bodkin JA: Antidepressant drug side effects. *J Clin Psychiatry* 1990; 51(1, suppl):21–26.
4. Chutka DS: Cardiovascular effects of the antidepressants: Recognition and control. *Geriatrics* 1990; 45:55–67.
5. Raskind M, Veith R, Barnes R, Gumbrecht G: Cardiovascular and antidepressant effects of imipramine in the treatment of secondary depression in patients with ischemic heart disease. *Am J Psychiatry* 1982; 139:1114–1117.
6. Taylor DJE, Braithwaite RA: Cardiac effects of tricyclic antidepressant medication: A preliminary study of nortriptyline. *Br Heart J* 1978; 40:1005–1009.
7. Vohra J, Burrows G, Hunt D, Sloman G: The effect of toxic and therapeutic doses of tricyclic antidepressant drugs on intracardiac conduction. *Eur J Cardiol* 1975; 3:219–227.
8. Roose SP, Glassman AH, Giardina EGV, Walsh BT, Woodring S, Bigger JT: Tricyclic antidepressants in depressed patients with cardiac conduction disease. *Arch Gen Psychiatry* 1987; 44:273–275.
9. Connolly SJ, Mitchell B, Swerdlow CD, Mason JW, Winkle RA: Clinical efficacy and electrophysiology of imipramine for ventricular tachycardia. *Am J Cardiol* 1984; 53:516–521.
10. Giardina EGV, Barnard T, Johnson L, Saroff AL, Bigger JT Jr, Louie M: The antiarrhythmic effect of nortriptyline in cardiac patients with ventricular premature depolarizations. *J Am Coll Cardiol* 1986; 7:1363–1369.
11. Giardina EGV, Johnson LL, Vita J, Bigger JT Jr, Brem RF: Effect of imipramine and nortriptyline on left ventricular function and

blood pressure in patients treated for arrhythmias. *Am Heart J* 1985; 109:992–998.
12. Veith RC, Raskind MA, Caldwell JH, Barnes RF, Gumbrecht G, Ritchie JL al: Cardiovascular effects of tricyclic antidepressants in depressed patients with chronic heart disease. *N Engl J Med* 1982; 306:954–959.
13. Roose SP, Glassman AH, Giardina EGV, Johnson LL, Walsh BT, Bigger JT: Cardiovascular effects of imipramine and bupropion in depressed patients with congestive heart failure. *Clin Psychopharmacol* 1987; 7:247–251.
14. Faravelli C, Brat A, Marchetti G, Franchi F, Padeletti L, Michelucci A, et al: Cardiac effects of clomipramine treatment. *Neuropsychobiology* 1983; 9:113–118.
15. Swanson-Biearman B, Goetz CM, Dean BS, Krenzelok EP: Anafronil-overdose: A fatal outcome. *Vet Hum Toxicol* 1989; 31:378.
16. Watson WA, Leighton J, Guy J, Bergman R, Garriott JC: Recovery of cyclic antidepressants with gastric lavage. *J Emerg Med* 1989; 7:373–377.
17. Frommer DA, Kulig KW, Marx JA, Rumack B: Tricyclic antidepressant overdose: A review. *JAMA* 1987; 257:521–526.
18. Callaham M: Epidemiology of fatal tricyclic antidepressant ingestion: Implications for management. *Ann Emerg Med* 1985; 14:1–9.
19. Harsch HH: Aspiration of activated charcoal. *N Engl J Med* 1986; 314:318.
20. Kulig K: Management of poisoning associated with "newer" antidepressant agents. *Ann Emerg Med* 1986; 15:1039–1045.
21. Wolfe TR, Caravati EM, Rollins DE: Terminal 40-ms frontal plane QRS axis as a marker for tricyclic antidepressant overdose. *Ann Emerg Med* 1989; 18:348–351.
22. Bramble MG, Lishman AH, Purdon J, Diffey BL, Hall RJ: An analysis of plasma levels and 24-hour ECG recordings in tricyclic antidepressant poisoning: Implications for management. *Q J Med* 1985; 219:357–366.
23. Lavoie FW, Gansert GG, Weiss RE: Use of initial ECG findings and plasma drug levels in cyclic antidepressant overdose. *Ann Emerg Med* 1990; 19:696–700.
24. Parker J, Lahmeyer H: Maprotiline poisoning: A case of cardiotoxicity and myoclonic seizures. *J Clin Psychiatry* 1984; 45:312–314.
25. Knudsen K, Heath A: Effects of self poisoning with maprotiline. *Br Med J* 1984; 288:601–603.
26. Tollefson G, Lesar T, Herzog C: Atrial flutter and maprotiline: Case report. *J Clin Psychiatry* 1984; 45:31–33.
27. Herrmann HC, Kaplan LM, Bierer BE: Q-T prolongation and torsades de pointes ventricular tachycardia produced by the tetracyclic antidepressant agent maprotiline. *Am J Cardiol* 1983; 51:904–906.
28. Wedin GP, Oderda GM, Klein-Schwartz W, Gorman RL: Relative toxicity of cyclic antidepressants. *Ann Emerg Med* 1986; 15:797–804.
29. Bock JL, Cummings KC, Jatlow PI: Amoxapine overdose: A case report. *Am J Psychiatry* 1982; 139:1619–1620.
30. Lesar T, Kingston R, Dahms R, Saxena K: Trazodone overdose. *Ann Emerg Med* 1983; 12:221–223.
31. White WB, Wong SHY: Rapid atrial fibrillation associated with trazodone hydrochloride. *Arch Gen Psychiatry* 1985; 42:424.
32. Lippmann S, Bedford P, Manshadi M, Mather S: Trazodone cardiotoxicity. *Am J Psychiatry* 1983; 140:1383.
33. Aronson MD, Hafez H: A case of trazodone-induced ventricular tachycardia. *J Clin Psychiatry* 1986; 47:388–389.
34. Buff DD, Brenner R, Kirtane SS, Gilboa R: Dysrhythmia associated with fluoxetine treatment in an elderly patient with cardiac disease. *J Clin Psychiatry* 1991; 52:174–176.
35. Cooper GL: The safety of fluoxetine—an update. *Br J Psychiatry* 1988; 153(suppl 3):77–86.
36. Roose SP, Dalack GW, Glassman AH, Woodring S, Walsh BT, Giardina EGV: Cardiovascular effects of bupropion in depressed patients with heart disease. *Am J Psychiatry* 1991; 148:512–516.
37. Goldman LS, Alexander RC, Luchins DJ: Monoamine oxidase inhibitors and tricyclic antidepressants: Comparison of their cardiovascular effects. *J Clin Psychiatry* 1986; 47:225–229.
38. Keck PE, Carter WP, Nierenberg AA, Cooper TB, Potter WZ, Rothschild AJ: Acute cardiovascular effects of tranylcypromine: Correlation with plasma drug, metabolite, norepinephrine, and MHPG leves. *J Clin Psychiatry* 1991; 56:250–254.
39. Guttmacher LB, Goldstein MG: Treatment of the cardiac-impaired depressed patient. Part II: Lithium, carbamazine, and electroconvulsive therapy. *Psychiatr Med* 1988; 6:34–51.
40. Simard M, Gumbiner B, Lee A, Lewis H, Norman D: Lithium carbonate intoxication. A case report and review of the literature. *Arch Intern Med* 1989; 149:36–46.
41. Risch SC, Groom GP, Janowsky DS: Interfaces of psychopharmacology and cardiology, part 2. *J Clin Psychiatry* 1981; 42:47–59.
42. Von Hoff DD, Rozencweig M, Piccart M: The cardiotoxicity of anticancer agents. *Semin Oncol* 1982; 9:23–33.
43. Porembka DT, Lowder JN, Orlowski JP, Bastulli J, Lockrem J: Etiology and management of doxorubicin cardiotoxicity. *Crit Care Med* 1989; 17:569–572.
44. Minow RA, Benjamin RS, Lee ET, Gottlieb JA: Adriamycin cardiomyopathy—risk factors. *Cancer* 1977; 39:1397–1402.
45. Ali MK, Soto A, Maroongroge D, Bekheit-Saad S, Buzdar AV, Blumenschein GR, et al: Electrocardiographic changes after adriamycin chemotherapy. *Cancer* 1979; 43:465–471.
46. Dresdale A, Bonow RO, Wesley R, Palmeri ST, Barr L, Mathison D, et al: Prospective evaluation of doxorubicin-induced cardiomyopathy resulting from postsurgical adjuvant treatment of patients with soft tissue sarcomas. *Cancer* 1983; 52:51–60.
47. Isner JM, Ferrans VJ, Cohen SR, Witkind BG, Virmani R, Gottdiener JS, et al: Clinical and morphologic cardiac findings after anthracycline chemotherapy: Analysis of 64 patients studied at necropsy. *Am J Cardiol* 1983; 51:1167–1174.
48. Torti FM, Bristow MR, Howes AE, Aston D, Stockdale FE, Carter SK, et al: Reduced cardiotoxicity of doxorubicin delivered on a weekly schedule. *Ann Intern Med* 1983; 99:745–749.
49. Villani F, Comazzi R, Lacaita G, et al: Possible enhancement of the cardiotoxicity of doxorubicin when combined with Mitomycin C. *Med Oncol Tumor Pharmacother* 1985; 2:93–97.
50. Choi BW, Berger HJ, Schwartz BE, Alexander J, Wackers FJ, Gottschalk A, et al: Serial radionuclide assessment of doxorubicin cardiotoxicity in cancer patients with abnormal baseline resting left ventricular performance. *Am Heart J* 1983; 106:638–643.
51. Hortobagyi GN, Frye D, Buzdar AU, Ewer MS, Fraschini G, Hug V, et al: Decreased cardiac toxicity of doxorubicin administered by continuous intravenous infusion in combination chemotherapy for metastatic breast carcinoma. *Cancer* 1989; 63:37–45.
52. Goorin AM, Chauvenet AR, Perez-Atayde AR, Cruz J, McKone R, Libshultz SE: Initial congestive heart failure, six to ten years after doxorubicin chemotherapy for childhood cancer. *J Pediatr* 1990; 116:144–147.
53. Mortensen SA, Olsen HA, Baandrup U: Chronic anthracycline cardiotoxicity: Haemodynamic and histopathological manifestations suggesting a restrictive endomyocardial disease. *Br Heart J* 1986; 55:274–282.
54. Moreg JS, Oglon DJ: Outcomes of clinical congestive heart failure induced by anthracycline chemotherapy. *Cancer* 1992; 70:2637–2641.
55. Cohen M, Kronzon I, Lebowitz A: Reversible doxorubicin-induced congestive heart failure. *Arch Intern Med* 1982; 142:1570–1571.
56. McKillop JH, Bristow MR, Goris ML, Billingham ME, Bockemuehl K: Sensitivity and specificity of radionuclide ejection fractions in doxorubicin cardiotoxicity. *Am Heart J* 1983; 106:1048–1056.
57. Borow KM, Henderson IC, Neuman A, Colan S, Grady S, Papish S, et al: Assessment of left ventricular contractility in patients receiving doxorubicin. *Ann Inter Med* 1983; 99:750–756.
58. Schwartz RG, McKenzie WB, Alexander J, Sager P, Dsouza A, Manatunga A, et al: Congestive heart failure and left ventricular dysfunction complicating doxorubicin therapy, seven-year experience using serial radionuclide angiocardiography. *Am J Med* 1987; 82:1109–1118.
59. Palmeri ST, Bonow RO, Myers CE, Seipp C, Jenkins J, Green MV, et al: Prospective evaluation of doxorubicin cardiotoxicity by rest and exercise radionuclide angiography. *Am J Cardiol* 1986; 58:607–613.
60. Mason JW, Bristow MR, Billingham ME, Daniels JR: Invasive and noninvasive methods of assessing adriamycin cardiotoxic effects in man: Superiority of histopathologic assessment using endomyocardial biopsy. *Cancer Treat Rep* 1978; 62:857–864.
61. Kantrowitz NE, Bristow MR: Cardiotoxicity of antitumor agents. *Prog Cardiovasc Dis* 1984; 27:195–200.

62. Von Hoff DD, Rozencweig M, Layard M, Slavik M, Muggia FM: Daunomycin-induced cardiotoxicity in children and adults: A review of 110 cases. *Am J Med* 1977; 62:200–208.
63. Von Hoff DD, Layard M: Risk factors for development of daunorubicin cardiotoxicity. *Cancer Treat Rep* 1981; 65(suppl 4): 19–23.
64. Harrison DT, Sanders LA: Pericarditis in a case of early daunorubicin cardiomyopathy. *Ann Intern Med* 1976; 85:339–341.
65. Gradishar WJ, Vokes EE: 5-Fluorouracil cardiotoxicity: A critical review. *Ann Oncol* 1990; 1:409–414.
66. Kleiman NS, Lehane DE, Geyer CE Jr, Pratt CM, Young JB: Prinzmetal's angina during 5-fluorouracil chemotherapy. *Am J Med* 1987; 82:566–568.
67. Somers G, Abramow M, Wittek M, Naets JP: Myocardial infarction: A complication of vincristine treatment? *Lancet* 1976; 2:690.
68. Yancey RS, Talpaz M: Vindesine-associated angina and ECG changes. *Cancer Treat Rep* 1982; 66:587–588.
69. DiBella NJ: Vincristine-induced orthostatic hypotension: A prospective clinical study. *Cancer Treat Rep* 1980; 64:359–360.
70. Unverferth DV, Unverferth BJ, Balcerzak SP, Bashore TA, Neidhart JA: Cardiac evaluation of mitoxantrone. *Cancer Treat Rep* 1983; 67:343–350.
71. Schell FC, Yap H-Y, Blumenschein G, Valvdivieso M, Bodey G: Potential cardiotoxicity with mitoxantrone. *Cancer Treat Rep* 1982; 66:1641–1643.
72. McLaughlin P, Salvador PG, Cabanillas F, Legha SS: Ventricular fibrillation following AMSA. *Cancer* 1983; 52:557–558.
73. Vorobiof DA, Iturralde M, Falkson G: Amsacrine cardiotoxicity: Assessment of ventricular function by radionuclide angiography. *Cancer Treat Rep* 1983; 67:1115–1117.
74. Weiss RB, Grillo-Lopez AJ, Marsoni S, Posada JG Jr, Hess F, Ross BJ: Amsacrine-associated cardiotoxicity: An analysis of 82 cases. *J Clin Oncol* 1986; 4:918–928.
75. Stadel BV: Oral contraceptives and cardiovascular disease (first of two parts). *N Engl J Med* 1981; 305:612–618.
76. Stadel BV: Oral contraceptives and cardiovascular disease (second of two parts). *N Engl J Med* 1981; 305:672–677.
77. Dalen JE, Hickler RB: Oral contraceptives and cardiovascular disease. *Am Heart J* 1981; 101:626–639.
78. Derman RJ: Oral contraceptives and cardiovascular risk. *J Reprod Med* 1990; 34:747–765.
79. Stampfer MJ, Colditz GA, Willett WC, Manson JE, Rosner B, Speizer FE, et al: Postmenopausal estrogen therapy and cardiovascular disease. *N Engl J Med* 1991; 325:756–762.
80. Lobo RA: Estrogen and cardiovascular disease. *Ann NY Acad Sci* 1990; 592:286–294.
81. Barrett-Connor E, Bush TL: Estrogen and coronary heart disease in women. *JAMA* 1991; 265:1861–1867.
82. Goldman L, Tosteson ANA: Uncertainty about postmenopausal estrogen. *N Engl J Med* 1991; 325:800–802.
83. Stampfer MJ, Willett WC, Colditz GA, Speizer FE, Hennekens CH: A prospective study of past use of oral contraceptive agents and risk of cardiovascular disease. *N Engl J Med* 1988; 319:1313–1317.
84. Engle H-J, Lichtlen PR: Coronary atherosclerosis and myocardial infarction in young women—role of oral contraceptives. *Eur Heart J* 1983; 4:1–8.
85. Brown KH, Hammond CB: The risks and benefits of oral contraceptives. *Adv Intern Med* 1989; 34:285–306.
86. Jugdutt BI, Stevens GF, Zacks DJ, Lee SJ, Taylor RF: Myocardial infarction, oral contraception, cigarette smoking, and coronary artery spasm in young women. *Am Heart J* 1983; 106:757–761.
87. Hodsman GP, Robertson JIS, Semple PF, Mackay A: Malignant hypertension and oral contraceptives: Four cases with two due to the 30 μg oestrogen pill. *Eur Heart J* 1982; 3:255–259.
88. Gerstman BB, Piper JM, Friedman JP, Tomita DK, Kennedy AL, Ferguson WJ, et al: Oral contraceptive oestrogen and progestin potencies and the incidence of deep venous thromboembolism. *Int J Epidemiol* 1990; 19:931–936.
89. Elam MB, Viar MJ, Ratts TE, Chesney CM: Mitral valve prolapse in women with oral contraceptive-related cerebrovascular insufficiency: Associated persistent hypercoagulable state. *Arch Intern Med* 1986; 146:73–77.
90. Billman GE: Mechanisms responsible for the cardiotoxic effects of cocaine. *FASEB J* 1990; 4:2469–2475.
91. Isner JM, Chokshi SK: Cardiovascular complications of cocaine. *Curr Probl Cardiol* 1991; 16:95–123.
92. Kloner RA, Hale S, Alker K, Rezkalla S: The effects of acute and chronic cocaine use on the heart. *Circulation* 1992; 85:407–419.
93. Lange RA, Cigarroa RG, Yancy CW, Willard JE, Popma JJ, Sills MN, et al: Cocaine-induced coronary-artery vasoconstriction. *N Engl J Med* 1989; 321:1557–1562.
94. Flores ED, Lange RA, Cigarroa RG, Hillis LD: Effect of cocaine on coronary artery dimensions in atherosclerotic coronary artery disease: Enhanced vasoconstriction at sites of significant stenoses. *J Am Coll Cardiol* 1990; 16:74–79.
95. Nademanee K, Gorelick DA, Josephson MA, Ryan MA, Wilkins JN, Robertson HA, et al: Myocardial ischemia during cocaine withdrawal. *Ann Intern Med* 1989; 111:876–880.
96. Amin M, Gabelman G, Karpel J, Buttrick P: Acute myocardial infarction and chest pain syndromes after cocaine use. *Am J Cardiol* 1990; 66:1434–1437.
97. Gitter MJ, Goldsmith SR, Dunbar DN, Sharkey SW: Cocaine and chest pain: Clinical features and outcome of patients hospitalized to rule out myocardial infarction. *Ann Intern Med* 1991; 115:277–282.
98. Curatolo PW, Robertson D: The health consequences of caffeine. *Ann Intern Med* 1983; 98:641–653.
99. Smits P, Thien T, van't Laar A: Circulatory effects of coffee in relation to the pharmacokinetics of caffeine. *Am J Cardiol* 1985; 56:958–963.
100. Izzo JL Jr, Chosal A, Kwong T, Freeman RB, Jaenike JR. Age and prior caffeine use alter the cardiovascular and adrenomedullary response to oral caffeine. *Am J Cardiol* 1983; 52:769–773.
101. Lane JD: Caffeine and cardiovascular responses to stress. *Psychosom Med* 1983; 45:447–451.
102. Dobmeyer DJ, Stine RA, Leier CV, Greenberg R, Schaal SF: The arrhythmogenic effects of caffeine in human beings. *N Engl J Med* 1983; 308:814–816.
103. Graboys TB, Blatt CM, Lown B: The effect of caffeine on ventricular ectopic activity in patients with malignant ventricular arrhythmia. *Arch Intern Med* 1989; 149:637–639.
104. Robertson D, Hollister AS, Kincaid D, Workman R, Goldberg MR, Tung CS, et al: Caffeine and hypertension. *Am J Med* 1984; 77:54–60.
105. LaCroix AZ, Mead LA, Liang K-Y, Thomas CB, Pearson TA: Coffee consumption and the incidence of coronary heart disease. *N Engl J Med* 1986; 315:977–982.
106. Rosmarin PC, Applegate WB, Somes GW: Coffee consumption and serum lipids: A randomized, crossover clinical trial. *Am J Med* 1990; 88:349–356.
107. Grobbee DE, Rimm EB, Giovannucci E, Colditz G, Stampfer M, Willett W: Coffee, caffeine and cardiovascular disease in men. *N Engl J Med* 1990; 323:1026–1032.
108. Benowitz NL, Osterloh J, Goldschlager N, Kaysen G, Pond S, Forhan S: Massive catecholamine release from caffeine poisoning. *JAMA* 1982; 248:1097–1099.
109. Van Dellen RG: Theophylline: Practical application of new knowledge. *Mayo Clin Proc* 1979; 54:733–745.
110. Matthay RA, Berger HJ, Davies R, Loke J, Gottschalk A, Zaret BL: Improvement in cardiac performance by oral long-acting theophylline in chronic obstructive pulmonary disease. *Am Heart J* 1982; 104:1022–1026.
111. Seneff M, Scott J, Friedman B, Smith M: Acute theophylline toxicity and the use of esmolol to reverse cardiovascular instability. *Ann Emerg Med* 1990; 19:671–673.
112. Sessler CN, Cohen MD: Cardiac arrhythmias during theophylline toxicity. A prospective continuous electrocardiographic study. *Chest* 1990; 98:672–678.
113. Sawyer WT, Caravati EM, Ellison MJ, Krueger KA: Hypokalemia, hyperglycemia, and acidosis after intentional theophylline overdose. *Am J Emerg Med* 1985; 3:408–411.
114. McPherson ML, Prince SR, Atamer ER, Maxwell DB, Ross-Clunis H, Estep HL: Theophylline-induced hypercalcemia. *Ann Intern Med* 1986; 105:52–54.
115. Kearney TE, Manoguerra AS, Curtis GP, Ziegler MG: Theophylline toxicity and the beta-adrenergic system. *Ann Intern Med* 1985; 102:766–769.
116. Greenberg A, Piraino BH, Kroboth PD, Weiss J: Severe theophylline toxicity: Role of conservative measures, antiarrhythmic agents, and charcoal hemoperfusion. *Am J Med* 1984; 76:854–860.

117. Olson KR, Benowitz NL, Woo OF, Pond SM: Theophylline overdose: Acute single ingestion versus chronic repeated overmedication. *Am J Emerg Med* 1985; 3:386–394.
118. Corser BC, Youngs C, Baughman RP: Prolonged toxicity following massive ingestion of sustained-release theophylline preparation. *Chest* 1985; 88:749–750.
119. Kessler KM, Cox M, De Marchena EJ, Myerburg RJ: Proarrhythmia related to a kinetic and dynamic interaction of mexiletine and theophylline. *Am Heart J* 1989; 117:964–966.
120. Greefhorst APM, van Herwaarden CLA: Ventilatory and haemodynamic effects of terbutaline infusion during beta$_1$-selective blockade with metoprolol and acebutolol in asthmatic patients. *Eur J Clin Pharmacol* 1982; 23:203–208.
121. Whitsett TL, Manion CV, Wilson MF: Cardiac, pulmonary and neuromuscular effects of clenbuterol and terbutaline compared with placebo. *Br J Clin Pharmacol* 1981; 12:195–200.
122. Greefhorst APM, van Herwaarden CLA: Ventilatory and haemodynamic effects of prenalterol and terbutaline in asthmatic patients. *Eur J Clin Pharmacol* 1983; 24:173–178.
123. Wang RYC, Lee PK, Yu DYC, Tse TF, Chow MS: Terbutaline infusion in cardiogenic shock: Acute hemodynamic effects and clinical responses. *J Clin Pharmacol* 1983; 23:355–361.
124. Gross TL, Sokol RJ: Severe hypokalemia and acidosis: A potential complication of beta-adrenergic treatment. *Am J Obstet Gynecol* 1980; 138:1225–1226.
125. Wang RYC, Lee PK, Yu DYC, Tse TF, Chow MS: Myocardial metabolic effects of intravenous terbutaline in patients with severe heart failure due to coronary artery disease. *J Clin Pharmacol* 1983; 23:362–368.
126. Slutsky R: Hemodynamic effects of inhaled terbutaline in congestive heart failure patients without lung disease: Beneficial cardiotonic and vasodilator beta-agonist properties evaluated by ventricular catheterization and radionuclide angiography. *Am Heart J* 1981; 101:556–560.
127. Wang RYC, Tse TF, Yu DYC, Lee PK, Sum MS, Chow MS: Beneficial hemodynamic effects of intravenous terbutaline in patients with severe heart failure. *Am Heart J* 1982; 104:1016–1021.
128. Hooper WW, Slutsky RA, Kocienski DE, Witztum KF, Spragg RG, Ashburn WL, et al: Right and left ventricular response in subcutaneous terbutaline in patients with chronic obstructive pulmonary disease: Radionuclide angiographic assessment of cardiac size and function. *Am Heart J* 1982; 104:1027–1032.
129. Katz M, Robertson PA, Creasy RK: Cardiovascular complications associated with terbutaline treatment for preterm labor. *Am J Obstet Gynecol* 1981; 139:605–608.
130. Legge JS, Gaddie J, Palmer KNV: Comparison of two oral selective beta$_2$-adrenergic stimulant drugs in bronchial asthma. *Br Med J* 1971; 1:637–639.
131. Lipworth BJ, McDevitt DG, Struthers AD: Hypokalemic and ECG sequelae of combined beta-agonist/diuretic therapy. *Chest* 1990; 98:811–815.
132. Lee H, Izquierdo R, Evans HE: Cardiac response to oral and aerosol administration of beta agonists. *J Pediatr* 1983; 103:655–658.
133. Prior JG, Cochrane GM: Self-poisoning with oral salbutamol. *Br Med J* 1981; 282:1932.
134. Tfelt-Hansen P, Kanstrup I-L, Christensen NJ, Winkler K: General and regional haemodynamic effects of intravenous ergotamine in man. *Clin Sci* 1983; 65:599–604.
135. Feneley MP, Morgan JJ, McGrath MA, Egan JD: Transient aortic arch syndrome with dysphagia due to ergotism. *Stroke* 1983; 14:811–814.
136. Carr P: Self-induced myocardial infarction. *Postgrad Med J* 1981: 57:654–655.
137. Klein LS, Simpson RJ Jr, Stern R, Hayward JC, Foster JR: Myocardial infarction following administration of sublingual ergotamine. *Chest* 1982; 82:375–378.
138. Redfield MM, Nicholson WJ, Edwards WD, Tajik AJ: Valve disease associated with ergot alkaloid: Echocardiographic and pathologic correlations. *Ann Intern Med* 1992; 117:50–52.
139. Rajfer SI, Anton AH, Rossen JD, Goldberg LI: Beneficial hemodynamics effects of oral levodopa in heart failure. *N Engl J Med* 1984; 310:1357–1362.
140. Hoehn MM: Levodopa-induced postural hypotension: Treatment with fludrocortisone. *Arch Neurol* 1975; 32:50–51.
141. Goldberg LI, Whitsett TL: Cardiovascular effects of levodopa. *Clin Pharmacol Ther* 1971; 12:376–382.
142. Koch-Weser J: Drug Therapy of Parkinsonism. *N Engl J Med* 1976; 295:814–818.
143. Mason JW, Billingham ME, Friedman JP: Methysergide-induced heart disease: A case of multivalvular and myocardial fibrosis. *Circulation* 1977; 56:889–890.
144. Bana DS, MacNeal PS, LeCompte PM, Shah Y, Graham JR: Cardiac murmurs and endocardial fibrosis associated with methysergide therapy. *Am Heart J* 1974; 88:640–655.
145. Salner AL, Mullany LD, Cole SR: Methysergide induced mitral valvular insufficiency. *Conn Med* 1980; 44:6–8.
146. Pringle TH, Scorbie IN, Murray RG, Kesson CM, Maccuish AC: Prolongation of the QT interval during therapeutic starvation: A substrate for malignant arrhythmias. *Int J Obes* 1983; 7:253–261.
147. Atkinson RL: Low and very low calorie diets. *Med Clin N Am* 1989; 73:203–215.
148. Moyer CL, Holly RG, Amsterdam EA, Atkinson RL: Effects of cardiac stress during very-low-calorie diet and exercise program in obese women. *Am J Clin Nutr* 1989; 50:1324–1327.
149. Boyce MJ: Cimetidine and the cardiovascular system. In: Baron JH (ed): *Cimetidine in the 80's*. Edinburgh, Churchill Livingstone, 1981: 227–237.
150. Freston JW: Cimetidine: II. Adverse reactions and patterns of use. *Ann Intern Med* 1982; 97:728–734.
151. Gould L, Reddy CVR, Singh BK, Zen B: Electrophysiologic properties of cimetidine in man. *PACE* 1981; 4:3–7.
152. Engel TR, Luck JC: Histamine$_2$ receptor antagonism by cimetidine and sinus-node function. *N Engl J Med* 1979; 301:591–592.
153. MacMahon B, Bakshi M, Walsh MJ: Cardiac arrhythmias after intravenous cimetidine. *N Engl J Med* 1981; 305:832–833.
154. Cardiovascular histamine H_2 receptors (editorial). *Lancet* 1982; 2:421–422.
155. Koch-Weser J: Ranitidine: A new H_2-receptor antagonist. *N Engl J Med* 1983; 309:1368–1373.
156. Omote K, Namiki A, Nishikawa T, Hagiwara T, Iwasaki H, Tsuchida H: Haemodynamic effects of famotidine and cimetidine in critically ill patients. *Acta Anaesthesiol Scand* 1990; 34:576–578.
157. Mitchell JE, Seim HC, Colon E, Pomeroy C: Medical complications and medical management of bulimia. *Ann Intern Med* 1987; 107:71–77.
158. Palmar EP, Guay AT: Reversible myopathy secondary to abuse of Ipecac in patients with major eating disorders. *N Engl J Med* 1985; 313:1457–1459.
159. Manno BR, Manno JE: Toxicology of Ipecac: A review. *Clin Toxicol* 1977; 10:221–242.
160. Adler AG, Walinsky P, Krall RA, Cho SY: Death resulting from Ipecac syrup poisoning. *JAMA* 1980; 243:1927–1928.
161. Friedman EJ: Death from Ipecac intoxication in a patient with anorexia nervosa. *Am J Psychiatry* 1984; 141:702–703.
162. Ratliff NB, Estes ML, Myles JL, Shirey EK, McMahon JT: Diagnosis of chloroquine cardiomyopathy by endomyocardial biopsy. *N Engl J Med* 1987; 316:191–193.
163. Riou KB, Barriot P, Rimailho A, Baud FJ: Treatment of severe chloroquine poisoning. *N Engl J Med* 1988; 318:1–6.
164. Jauchem JR: Electromagnetic fields: Is there a danger? *Lancet* 1990; 336:884.
165. Thompson JC, Ashwal S: Electrical injuries in children. *Am J Dis Child* 1983; 137:231–235.
166. Hughes JH: Electrical injury. *Ariz Med* 1980; 37:760–762.
167. Cooper MA: Lightning injuries: Prognostic signs for death. *Ann Emerg Med* 1980; 9:134–138.
168. Bernstein T: Effects of electricity and lightning on man and animals. *J Forensic Sci* 1973; 18:3–11.
169. Duclos PJ, Sanderson LM, Klontz KC: Lightening-related mortality and morbidity in Florida. *Public Health Rep* 1990; 105:276–282.
170. Koscove EM: The Taser weapon: A new emergency medicine problem. *Ann Emerg Med* 1985; 14:1205–1208.
171. Dixon GF: The evaluation and management of electrical injuries. *Crit Care Med* 1983; 11:384–387.
172. Sances A Jr, Larson SJ, Myklebust J, Cusik JF: Electrical injuries. *Surg Gynecol Obstet* 1979; 149:97–108.
173. Wright RK, Davis JH: The investigation of electrical deaths: A report of 220 fatalities. *J Forensic Sci* 1980; 25:514–521.
174. Butler ED, Gant TD: Electrical injuries, with special reference to the upper extremities: A review of 182 cases. *Am J Surg* 1977; 134:95–101.

175. Kleinot S, Klachko DM, Keeley KJ: The cardiac effects of lightning injury. *S Afr Med J* 1966; 40:1141–1143.
176. Ghezzi KT: Lightning injuries. A unique treatment challenge. *Postgrad Med* 1989; 85:197–208.
177. Myers GJ, Colgan MT, Van Dyke DH: Lightning-strike disaster among children. *JAMA* 1977; 238:1045–1046.
178. Chandra NC, Siu CO, Munster AM: Clinical predictors of myocardial damage after high voltage electrical injury. *Crit Care Med* 1990; 18:293–297.
179. Strasser EJ, Davis RM, Menchey MJ: Lightning injuries. *J Trauma* 1977; 17:315–319.
180. Lewin RF, Arditti A, Sclarovsky S: Non-invasive evaluation of electrical cardiac injury. *Br Heart J* 1983; 49:190–192.
181. Jackson SHD, Parry DJ: Lightning and the heart. *Br Heart J* 1980; 43:454–457.
182. Kleiner JP, Wilkin JH: Cardiac effects of lightning stroke. *JAMA* 1978; 240:2757–2758.
183. Burda CD: Electrocardiographic changes in lightning stroke. *Am Heart J* 1966; 72:521–524.
184. Chia BL: Electrocardiographic abnormalities and congestive cardiac failure due to lightning stroke. *Cardiology* 1981; 68:49–53.
185. Kirchmer JT, Larson DL, Tyson KRT: Cardiac rupture following electrical injury. *J Trauma* 1977; 17:389–391.
186. Solem L, Fischer RP, Strate RG: The natural history of electrical injury. *J Trauma* 1977; 17:487–492.
187. James TN, Riddick L, Embry JH: Cardiac abnormalities demonstrated postmortem in four cases of accidental electrocution and their potential significance relative to nonfatal electrical injuries of the heart. *Am Heart J* 1990; 120:143–157.
188. Kobernick M: Electrical injuries: Pathophysiology and emergency management. *Ann Emerg Med* 1982; 11:633–638.
189. Hanson GC, McIlwraith GR: Lightning injury: Two case histories and a review of management. *Br Med J* 1973; 4:271–274.
190. Taussig HB: "Death" from lightning—and the possibility of living again. *Ann Intern Med* 1968; 68:1345–1353.
191. Homma S, Gillam LD, Weyman AE: Echocardiographic observations in survivors of acute electrical injury. *Chest* 1990; 97:103–105.
192. Weiner RD: The psychiatric use of electrically induced seizures. *Am J Psychiatry* 1979; 136:1507–1517.
193. Selvin BL: Electroconvulsive therapy—1987. *Anesthesiology* 1987; 67:367–385.
194. Brown ML, Huston PE, Hines HM, et al: Cardiovascular changes associated with electroconvulsive therapy in man. *AMA Arch Neurol Psychiatry* 1953; 69:601–608.
195. Gerring JP, and Shields HM: The identification and management of patients with a high risk for cardiac arrhythmias during modified ECT. *J Clin Psychiatry* 1982; 43:140–143.
196. Woodruff RA, Pitts FN, and McClure JN: The drug modification of ECT: I. Methohexital, Thiopental, and Preoxygenation. *Arch Gen Psychiatry* 1968; 18:605–611.
197. Gould L, Gopalaswamy C, Chandy F, Kim B: Electroconvulsive therapy-induced ECG changes simulating a myocardial infarction. *Arch Intern Med* 1983; 143:1786–1787.
198. Graybar G, Goethe J, Levy T, Phillips J, Youngberg J, Smith G: Transient large upright T-wave on the electrocardiogram during multiple monitored electroconvulsive therapy. *Anesthesiology* 1983; 59:467–469.
199. Buisseret D: Acute pulmonary edema following Grand Mal Epilepsy and as a complication of electric shock therapy. *Br J Dis Chest* 1982; 76:194–198.
200. Stoudemire A, Knos G, Gladson M, Markwalter H, Sung Y-F, Morris R, et al: Labetalol in the control of cardiovascular responses to electroconvulsive therapy in high-risk depressed medical patients. *J Clin Psychiatry* 1990; 51:508–512.
201. Mulgaokar GD, Dauchot PJ, Duffy JP, Anton AH: Noninvasive assessment of electroconvulsive induced changes in cardiac function. *J Clin Psychiatry* 1985; 46:479–482.
202. Bali IM: The effect of modified electroconvulsive therapy on plasma potassium concentration. *Br J Anaesth* 1975; 47:398–401.
203. Hood DD, Mecca RS: Failure to initiate electroconvulsive seizures in a patient pretreated with Lidocaine. *Anesthesiology* 1983; 58:379–381.
204. Elliott RL: Case report of a potential interaction between Clonidine and electroconvulsive therapy. *Am J Psychiatry* 1983; 140:1237–1238.
205. Giraulo D, Lind L, Salzman C, Pilon R, Elkins R: Sodium nitroprusside treatment of ECT-induced blood pressure elevations. *Am J Psychiatry* 1978; 135:1105–1106.
206. Decina P, Malitz S, Sackeim HA, Holzer J, Yudofsky S: Cardiac arrest during ECT modified by beta-adrenergic blockade. *Am J Psychiatry* 1984; 141:298–300.
207. Alexopoulos GS, Nasr H, Young RC, Wikstrom TR, Holzman SR: Electroconvulsive therapy in patients on anticoagulants. *Can J Psychiatry* 1982; 27:46–47.
208. Blitt CD: Electroconvulsive therapy with a cardiac pacemaker. *Anesthesiology* 1976; 45:580.
209. Abiuso P, Dunkelman R, Proper M: Electroconvulsive therapy in patients with pacemakers. *JAMA* 1978; 240:2459–2462.
210. Taylor PJ, Von Witt RJ, Fry AH: Serum creatinine phosphokinase activity in psychiatric patients receiving electroconvulsive therapy. *J Clin Psychiatry* 1981; 42:103–105.
211. Das G, Dick J, Fletcher MS, Webb DR, Bailey MJ, Kellett MJ: Extracorporeal shockwave lithotripsy: First 1000 cases at the London Stone Clinic. *Br Med J* 1987; 295:891–893.
212. Sackman M, Delius M, Sauerbruch T, Holl J, Weber W, Ippisch E, et al: Shock-wave lithotripsy of gallbladder stones. *N Engl J Med* 1988; 318:393–397.
213. Malhotra V: Hyperthermia and hypothermia as complications of extracorporeal shock wave lithotripsy. *Anesthesiology* 1987; 67:448.
214. Behnia R, Shanks CA, Ovassapian A, Wilson LA: Hemodynamic responses associated with lithotripsy. *Anest Analg* 1987; 66:354–356.
215. Walts LF, Atlee, JL III: Supraventricular tachycardia associated with extracorporeal shock wave lithotripsy. *Anesthesiology* 1986; 65:521–523.
216. Ector H, Janssens L, Baert L, DeGeest H: Extracorporeal shock wave lithotripsy and cardiac arrhythmias. *PACE* 1989; 12: 1910–1917.
217. Kroneman OC III, Brodsky MS, MacKenzie J, Hauser A: Endocarditis after lithotripsy (letter to ed). *Ann Intern Med* 1987; 106:777.
218. Landberg J, Abber J, Thuroff JW, Griffin JC: The effects of extracorporeal shock wave lithotripsy on pacemaker function. *PACE* 1987; 10:1142–1146.
219. Cooper D, Wilkoff B, Masterson M, Castle L, Belco K, Simmons T, et al: Effects of extracorporeal shock wave lithotripsy on cardiac pacemakers and its safety in patients with implanted cardiac pacemakers. *PACE* 1988; 11:1607–1616.
220. Lingeman JE, Woods JR, Toth PD: Blood pressure changes following extracorporeal shock wave lithotripsy and other forms of treatment for nephrolithiasis. *JAMA* 1990; 263:1789–1794.
221. Ellis MD: Poisonous plants. In: Ellis MD (ed): *Dangerous Plants, Snakes, Arthropods, and Marine Life,* Hamilton, IL, Hamilton Press, 1975: 3–81.
222. Van Stee EW: Cardiovascular toxicology: Foundations and scope. In: Van Stee EW (ed): *Cardiovascular Toxicology,* New York, Raven, 1982: 1–34.
223. Polson CJ, Green MA, Lee MR: *Clinical Toxicology,* 3d ed. Philadelphia, JB Lippincott, 1983: 401–402.
224. Moeschlin S: *Poisoning, Diagnosis, and Treatment,* New York Grune & Stratton, 1965: 543–544.
225. Akera T, Brown BS: Cardiovascular toxicology of cardiotonic drugs and chemicals. In: Van Stee EW (ed): *Cardiovascular Toxicology.* New York, Raven, 1982: 109–134.
226. Tai Y-T, But PP-H, Young K, Lau C-P: Cardiotoxicity after accidental herb-induced aconite poisoning. *Lancet* 1992; 340:1254–1256.
227. Russell FE: Pharmacology of animal venoms. *Clin Pharmacol Ther* 1967; 8:849–873.
228. Arena JM: *Poisoning, Toxicology, Symptoms, Treatment,* 4th ed. Springfield, IL, Charles C Thomas, 1979: 558–570.
229. Huang TT, Lewis SR, Lucas BS III: Venomous snakes. In: Ellis MD (ed): *Dangerous Plants, Snakes, Arthropods, and Marine Life.* Hamilton, IL, Hamilton Press, 1975: 123–142.
230. Lefer AM, Curtis MT: Cardiotoxicity of naturally occurring animal peptides. In: Stee EW (ed): *Cardiovascular Toxicology.* New York, Raven, 1982: 221–258.
231. Horen WP: Insect and scorpion sting. *JAMA* 1972; 221:894–898.
232. Alagesan R, Srinivasaraghavan J, Balambal R, Haranath K, Subramanyan N, Thiruvengadam KV: Transient complete right bundle branch block following scorpion sting. *J Indian Med Assoc* 1977; 69:113–114.

233. Levine HD: Acute myocardial infarction following wasp sting: Report of two cases and critical survey of the literature. *Am Heart J* 1976; 91:365–374.
234. Rowe SF, Greer KE, Hodge RH Jr: Electrocardiographic changes associated with multiple yellow jacket stings. *South Med J* 1979; 72:483–485.
235. Zakhari S, Aviado DM: Cardiovascular toxicology of aerosol propellants, refrigerants, and related solvents. In: Van Stee EW (ed): *Cardiovascular Toxicology*. New York, Raven, 1982: 281–314.
236. Polson CJ, Green MA, Lee MR: *Clinical Toxicology*, 3d ed. Philadelphia, JB Lippincott, 1983: 138–161.
237. Weill H: Cardiorespiratory effects of inhalant occupational exposures. *Circulation* 1981; 63:250A–252A.
238. Allred EN, Bleecker ER, Chaitman BR, Dahms TE, Gottlieb SO, Hackney JD, et al: Short-term effects of carbon monoxide exposure on the exercise performance of subjects with coronary artery disease. *N Engl J Med* 1989; 321:1426–1432.
239. Ilano AL, Raffin TA: Management of carbon monoxide poisoning. *Chest* 1990; 97:165–169.
240. Marius-Nunez AL: Myocardial infarction with normal coronary arteries after acute exposure to carbon monoxide. *Chest* 1990; 97:491–494.
241. Arsenian MA: Cardiovascular sequelae of therapeutic thoracic radiation. *Prog Cardiovasc Dis* 1991; 33:299–311.
242. Corn BW, Trock BJ, Goodman RL: Irradiation-related ischemic heart disease. *J Clin Oncol* 1990; 8:740–750.
243. Applefeld MM, Wiernik PH: Cardiac disease after radiation therapy for Hodgkin's disease: Analysis of 48 patients. *Am J Cardiol* 1983; 51:1679–1681.
244. Stewart JR, Fajardo LF: Radiation-induced heart disease. Clinical and experimental aspects. *Radiol Clin North Am* 1971; 9:511–513.
245. Fajardo LF, Stewart RJ: Pathogenesis of radiation-induced myocardial fibrosis. *Lab Invest* 1973; 29:244–257.
246. Ni Y, von Segesser LK, Turina M: Futility of pericardiectomy for postirradiation constrictive pericarditis. *Ann Thorac Surg* 1990; 49:445–448.
247. Carlson RG, Mayfield WR, Normann S, Alexander JA: Radiation-associated valvular disease. *Chest* 1991; 99:538–545.
248. Gustavsson A, Eskilsson J, Landberg, T, Svahn-Tapper G, White T, Wollmer P, et al: Late cardiac effects after mantle radiotherapy in patients with Hodgkin's disease. *Ann Oncol* 1990; 1:355–363.
249. Pohjola-Sintonen S, Totterman K-J, Salmo M, Siltanen P: Late cardiac effects of mediastinal radiotherapy in patients with Hodgkin's disease. *Cancer* 1987; 60:31–37.
250. McEniery PT, Dorosti K, Schiavone WA, Pedrick TJ, Sheldon WC: Clinical and angiographic features of coronary artery disease after chest irradiation. *Am J Cardiol* 1987; 60:1020–1024.
251. McReynolds RA, Gold GL, Roberts WC: Coronary heart disease after mediastinal irradiation for Hodgkin's disease. *Am J Med* 1976; 60:39–45.
252. Cohen SI, Bharati S, Glass J, Lev M: Radiotherapy as a cause of complete atrioventricular block in Hodgkin's disease. *Arch Intern Med* 1981; 141:676–679.

Chapter 111

Neoplastic Heart Disease

Robert J. Hall, M.D. ■ *Denton A. Cooley, M.D.*
Hugh A. McAllister, Jr., M.D. ■ *O. H. Frazier, M.D.*

Tumors of the heart, while uncommon, present in protean ways and have challenged the acumen of physicians since the seventeenth century. Antemortem diagnosis, however, was rare before 1950. Intracardiac myxoma was first diagnosed, with the aid of angiography, in 1952, with a subsequent attempt to remove the tumor surgically. The first successful removal with the use of cardiopulmonary bypass was performed in 1955.[1] Subsequently, increased clinical awareness, coupled with angiographic and noninvasive diagnostic techniques, has led to more frequently correct diagnoses.[2–5]

The heart may be the site of a primary tumor or may be invaded secondarily by malignancies that arise in adjacent or remote organs. Whether involved by primary or secondary tumors, neoplastic heart disease can be expressed in only limited ways (Table 111-1). In the presence of neoplastic disease, pericardial pain, effusion, tamponade, constriction, rapid increase in heart size, new heart murmurs, electrocardiographic changes, atrial or ventricular arrhythmias, atrioventricular (AV) block, and unexplained heart failure are suggestive of secondary invasion of the heart. The triad of obstruction, embolization, and constitutional manifestations characterizes intracavitary tumors, especially myxomas.

PRIMARY TUMORS OF THE HEART

Although they are less common than other tumors of the heart, primary tumors of the heart are far more challenging to both the physician and the surgeon. They usually present as intracavitary lesions, and more than 75 percent are benign.[6] Current surgical techniques permit removal and potential "cure" in a considerable number of patients with primary tumors, necessitating an awareness of the clinical and hemodynamic presentation of these tumors.

Primary tumors of the heart and pericardium are rare, occurring with a frequency of 0.001 to 0.28 percent in reported or collected postmortem series.[6] Myxomas are the most common of the primary tumors and constitute nearly 50 percent of all histologically benign tumors of the heart. The frequency and classification of 533 primary tumors and cysts of the heart and pericardium

TABLE 111-1
General Manifestations of Neoplastic Heart Disease

Pericardial involvement
- Pericarditis, pain
- Pericardial effusion
- Radiographic enlargement
- Arrhythmia, predominantly atrial
- Tamponade
- Constriction

Myocardial involvement
- Arrhythmias, ventricular and atrial
- Electrocardiographic changes
- Radiographic enlargement: generalized, localized
- Conduction disturbances and heart block
- Congestive heart failure
- Coronary involvement: angina, infarction

Intracavitary tumor
- Cavity obliteration
- Valve obstruction and valve damage
- Embolic phenomena: systemic, neurologic, coronary
- Constitutional manifestations

TABLE 111-2

Tumors and Cysts of the Heart and Pericardium

Type	Number	Percentage
Benign		
Myxoma	130	24.4
Lipoma	45	8.4
Papillary fibroelastoma	42	7.9
Rhabdomyoma	36	6.8
Fibroma	17	3.2
Hemangioma	15	2.8
Teratoma	14	2.6
Mesothelioma of the AV node	12	2.3
Granular cell tumor	3	
Neurofibroma	3	
Lymphangioma	2	
Subtotal	319	59.8
Pericardial cyst	82	15.4
Bronchogenic cyst	7	1.3
Subtotal	89	16.7
Malignant		
Angiosarcoma	39	7.3
Rhabdomyosarcoma	26	4.9
Mesothelioma	19	3.6
Fibrosarcoma	14	2.6
Malignant lymphoma	7	1.3
Extraskeletal osteosarcoma	5	
Neurogenic sarcoma	4	
Malignant teratoma	4	
Thymoma	1	
Leiomyosarcoma	1	
Liposarcoma	1	
Synovial sarcoma	1	
Subtotal	125	23.5
Total	533	100.0

SOURCE: HA McAllister, Jr, JJ Fenoglio, Jr: *Tumors of the Cardiovascular System.* Washington, DC, Armed Forces Institute of Pathology, 1978.

collected by the Armed Forces Institute of Pathology can be seen in Table 111-2.[7]

Cardiac Myxomas

Intracardiac myxoma is the most frequent benign tumor of the heart. While most (75 percent) are located in the left atrium, myxomas are also found in the right atrium (18 percent), right ventricle (4 percent), and left ventricle (4 percent).[7] Cardiac myxomas usually originate from the region of the fossa ovalis but may arise from a variety of locations within the atria.[7] Although myxomas have been reported as originating from the mitral annulus,[3] the mitral valve itself,[8] the aortic valve,[9] and the inferior vena cava,[10] it is likely that true myxomas only arise from the mural endocardium.[7]

Pathology

Attached to the endocardium by a broad base, myxomas are usually pedunculated, polypoid, and friable, although some may have a smooth surface and be rounded (Fig. 111-1). Sessile myxomas are uncommon.[3] A myxoma appears as a soft, gelatinous, mucoid, usually gray-white mass, often with areas of hemorrhage or thrombosis. They vary from 1 to 15 cm in diameter, with most measuring 5 to 6 cm (Fig. 111-1*A* and *B*).[7]

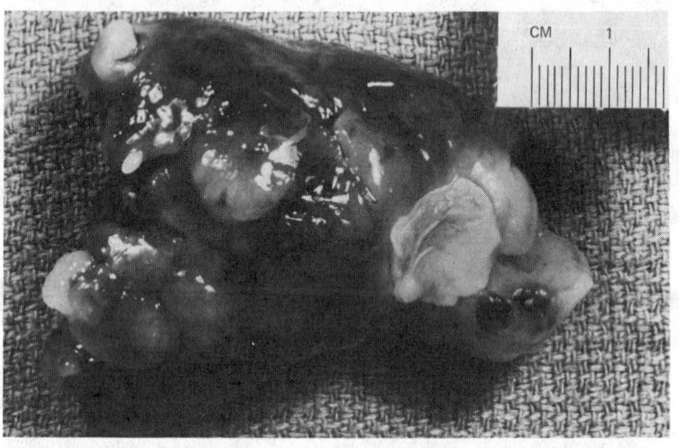

A

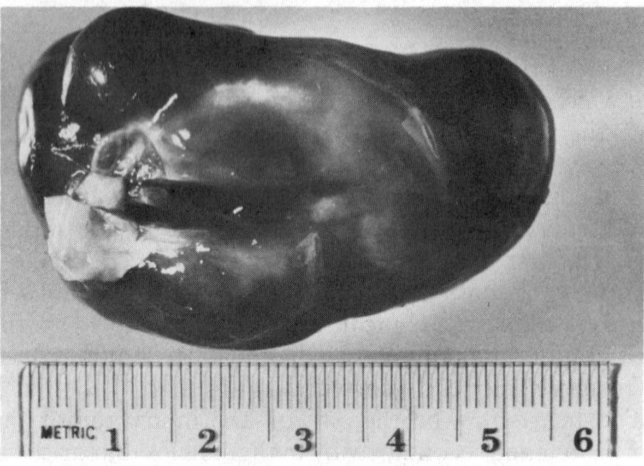

B

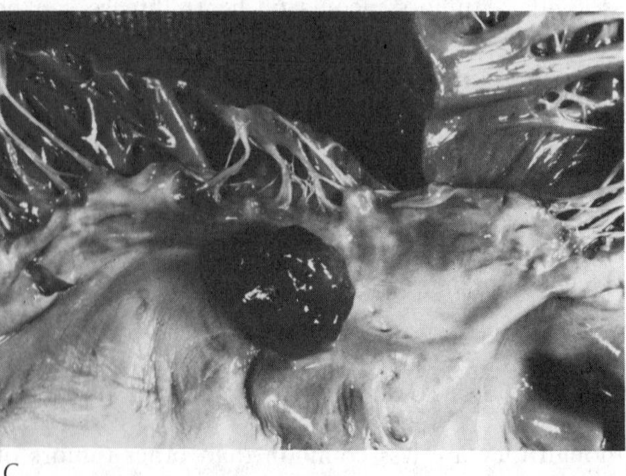

C

FIGURE 111-1 Left atrial myxomas. *A.* More polypoid and irregular. *B.* Smooth surfaced and rounded. Attachment to and portion of the atrial septum is seen on each tumor. *C.* An asymptomatic sessile myxoma attached above the posterior leaflet of the mitral valve was found coincidentally at necropsy.

On microscopic examination, the myxoma is composed of an acid mucopolysaccharide myxoid matrix in which polygonal cells (lepidic cells) and occasional blood vessels are embedded. Channels, often filled with red blood cells, communicate from the surface to deep within the tumor and are lined by endothelial-like cells resembling multipurpose mesenchymal cells, from which the tumor is purported to arise. Similar endothelial cells line the surface of the tumor; however, fibrin, erythrocytes, and organized thrombi also may be present on the surface. Cystic areas, focal or gross hemorrhage, calcification, glandular elements,[11] rarely bone formation, and even hematopoietic tissue constitute the multiple although uncommon variations that may be present.[7]

A neoplastic rather than a thrombotic origin of myxomas is supported by the ultrastructural characteristics of the tumor,[12–14] the results of biochemical analyses,[15] the cultural properties of the tumor cell,[7,16,17] and DNA analysis of the tumor.[18,19] Although myxomas can recur because of their incomplete removal[20,21] and distant growth of embolic myxomatous material has been observed,[20,22,23] the existence of a true malignant cardiac myxoma remains doubtful.[6] The occurrence of multiple tumors within the left atrium, bilaterally in each atrium,[24,25] or simultaneously in the atrium and ventricle,[26] raises the possibility of multicentric origin rather than metastasis of the tumor.

Age, Sex, and Familial Occurrence

Most patients with myxomas are from 30 to 60 years of age,[2] although myxomas have been discovered in children[27] and infants, neonates,[28] and the elderly.[29] Children have a higher incidence of ventricular myxomas than do adults.[27,30] A higher incidence in females has characterized most series.[2,3] Familial occurrence has been reported.[31,32] In these examples, males predominate, tumors are divided equally on both sides of the heart, and opposite atria are usually involved in afflicted members. In one report, three of four involved members had multiple myxomas.[32]

General or Constitutional Manifestations

Whereas asymptomatic patients with myxoma (Fig. 111-1C) have been reported,[26] most present with one or more effects of a triad of constitutional, embolic, and obstructive manifestations.[2,3] Cardiac myxomas provoke systemic illness in 90 percent of the patients, characterized by weight loss, fatigue, fever, anemia (often hemolytic), elevated sedimentation rate, and elevated serum immunoglobulin concentration formed in response to tumor embolization, degenerative changes within the tumor itself, or changes in the normal cardiac muscle. The globulin fraction most frequently elevated is immunoglobulin G (IgG), and immunoglobulin A (IgA) is involved only rarely.[2,16,33] A patient with coexisting cardiac myxoma and IgG multiple myeloma has been reported.[34] Less common findings are leukocytosis, thrombocytopenia, clubbing, Raynaud's phenomenon, and breast fibroadenomas.[2] Polycythemia may result from tumor production or erythropoietin.[35]

Patients with hemolytic anemia have features of intravascular mechanical destruction, which may be accompanied by pancytopenia. Hemolytic anemia is more likely to occur in patients with calcified myxomas, occurring more commonly in the right atrium. "Syndrome myxoma" characterizes a subset of patients with cardiac myxoma, associated with pigmented skin lesions and peripheral and endocrine neoplasms.[36,37] These patients, in contrast to those with "sporadic" myxoma, are usually younger, have a high frequency of familial myxoma, and more frequently have multiple and recurrent tumors. The protracted multisystemic symptoms produced by myxomas may mimic connective tissue disease and polyarteritis nodosa.[25,38,39]

Infected Myxoma

An intracavitary myxoma rarely becomes infected, and blood cultures have demonstrated a variety of organisms.[5,40–42] Most patients with infected myxomas experience major neurologic embolic events. Surgical resection should be carried out promptly before catastrophic embolic complications occur.[31,43]

Embolization

Systemic tumor embolization occurs in 40 to 50 percent of patients with left atrial myxoma,[2] with tumor fragments or surface clots most commonly embolizing to arteries in the brain, kidneys, and extremities. Rarely does a complete left atrial myxoma become detached and lodge in the aortic bifurcation.[42,44] The size and consistency of such an embolus may defy the usual technique of removal (using a Fogarty catheter from below) and require direct exploration of the aortic bifurcation.[45] Histological examination of emboli recovered at operation from a peripheral artery can aid in diagnosing an otherwise unsuspected intracardiac myxoma.[6,42,46,47] Systemic embolization, especially in a young patient with normal sinus rhythm, should arouse suspicion of a myxoma once bacterial endocarditis has been ruled out.

Tumor embolization of the *central nervous system* constitutes about one-half of all embolic events caused by left atrial myxomas,[47] may represent the first symptomatic manifestation,[16,22,47,48] and is more common in the left hemisphere.[49] Embolization may be to the extracranial or intracranial cerebral vessels, with the former being amenable to surgical removal.[22,48] Onset of the neurologic deficit may be gradual or sudden. Episodes of syncope can be mistaken for seizure activity and thus may delay recognition of the true cardiac cause.[47]

Intracranial arterial aneurysms secondary to myxomatous emboli have been demonstrated angiographically. Late rupture with intracranial hemorrhage has been reported.[22] Care must be taken to avoid embolization during surgical removal of an intracardiac myxoma, not only because of the immediate consequences of an embolic phenomenon, but also because viable metastatic foci may cause symptoms years later.[22] As a consequence, the patient who has sustained cerebral emboli is not necessarily "cured" even after the primary tumor is surgically removed.[49]

Retinal artery embolism can occur with transient[47] or permanent[50] visual impairment, confirmed by ophthalmoscopic[47] and histopathologic[50] evidence of particulate embolic matter in the retinal artery. Only rarely has occlusion of the retinal artery occurred in the absence of multifocal neurologic manifestations, usually in the distribution of the ipsilateral middle cerebral artery.

Coronary artery embolism associated with myxoma has been documented by both angiography in living patients and histology at postmortem study.[6,51] Myocardial infarction occasionally is the first manifestation of a myxoma.[51,52]

Left Atrial Myxoma

General Features Constitutional manifestations and embolic potential are common to varying degrees in patients with myxoma in any intracavitary location. The cardiac manifestations, symptoms, and physical findings are the consequence of the intracavitary mass and are unique to the particular location of the tumor. Myxomas of the left atrium may obstruct either the mitral or pulmonary venous orifices[53] and produce symptoms and manifestations of pulmonary venous hypertension, secondary pulmonary hypertension, and right-sided heart failure. The clinical symptoms include dyspnea on exertion, orthopnea, paroxysmal nocturnal dyspnea, acute pulmonary edema, cough, and hemoptysis, along with palpitations, chest pain, fatigue, and peripheral edema. Episodes of syncope or dizziness are frequent, and sudden death may occur. A marked effect of the severity of any symptom caused by a change in position of the patient, especially if recumbency relieves dyspnea,[2,54] is suggestive of myxoma, but this occurs infrequently.

Physical Examination On physical examination the first heart sound is loud and frequently split, with the second component corresponding to the tumor expulsion from the mitral orifice. The pulmonary component of the second sound is accentuated, and an early diastolic sound, the "tumor plop," is usually heard 80 to 120 ms after the aortic closure sound,[2,55] resembling, but not as sharp and of lower frequency than, an opening snap. The tumor plop may be confused with either an opening snap of the mitral valve or a third heart sound and follows the aortic closure sound at an interval that is intermediate between these events. Suspicion of a left atrial myxoma should be raised when one hears what is considered to be an inordinately early "third heart sound" associated with auscultatory features suggestive of mitral regurgitation or an unusually late low-pitched "opening snap" accompanying features that are consistent with severe mitral stenosis (Fig. 111-2).

An apical diastolic or systolic murmur or both are present in many patients. The auscultatory findings may vary from time to time or with a change in position of the patient.[2,54-56] Features of pulmonary hypertension are frequent and may result in a murmur of tricuspid regurgitation.[57] A shorter clinical history and the persistence of sinus rhythm are in contrast to features of rheumatic mitral valvular disease.

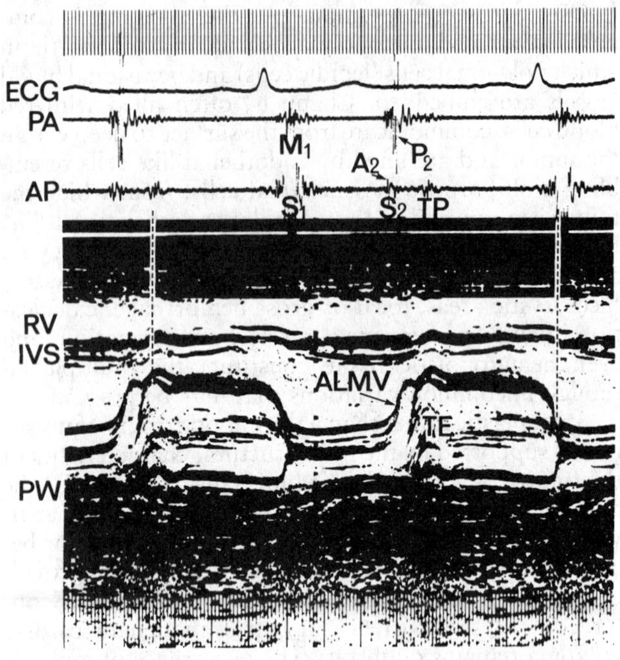

FIGURE 111-2 Recordings of a patient with a cystic left atrial myxoma including (*top*) the electrocardiogram, (*middle*) phonocardiograms from the pulmonary area (PA) at high frequency and from the apex (AP) at medium frequency, and (*bottom*) the echocardiogram at the level of the mitral valve. Time lines equal 0.01-s intervals. The right ventricle (RV), septum (IVS), and posterior wall (PW) of the left ventricle are identified. The loud component of the first sound (M_1) is delayed (Q to M_1 = 0.09 s). The pulmonic second sound (P_2) is accentuated. Multiple linear tumor echoes (TE) are seen behind the anterior leaflet to the mitral valve (ALMV), first appearing at the mitral level 0.04 s after onset of mitral opening and completing the forward movement 0.09 s after onset of mitral opening, at which point the "tumor plop" (TP) is recorded. The A_2–TP interval measures 0.10 s.

Electrocardiogram and Chest X-Ray Results of electrocardiography are nonspecific, reflecting hemodynamic alterations similar to those of mitral valvular disease; however, sinus rhythm is generally the rule. The chest roentgenogram reveals left atrial enlargement and the characteristic changes of pulmonary venous congestion and pulmonary hypertension. The absence of mitral valve calcification and the presence of a left atrium smaller than might be expected in a patient with presumed severe rheumatic mitral disease are helpful differentiating clues. Calcification may be evident in the tumor even on routine chest film,[58] but this is better visualized and motion is better appreciated on fluoroscopic examination.

The "wrecking-ball" effect of a calcified mobile myxoma may cause destruction of the mitral valve or rupture of the chordae tendineae and may produce severe mitral regurgitation.[54,59]

Echocardiography The value of ultrasound in the noninvasive diagnosis of intracavitary tumors has been well documented.[2,3,16,33] M-mode echocardiographic studies in patients with a prolapsing left atrial myxoma typically demonstrate a diminished EF slope of the anterior leaflet of the mitral valve, behind which a dense array of wavy tumor echoes is seen. These tumor echoes typically appear a short interval following the opening movement of the mitral leaflets, caused by the inertial lag in movement of the tumor after onset of diastole and opening of the mitral leaflets. The tumor plop coincides with the completion of this anterior movement of tumor echoes (Fig. 111-2). A similar array of tumor echoes may be seen in the left atrial chamber during ventricular systole. Precordial two-dimensional echocardiography [transthoracic echocardiography (TTE)] provides tomographic images of all four cardiac chambers and identifies the size, shape, point of attachment, and motion characteristics of left atrial myxomas.[4,33] Transesophageal echocardiography (TEE) permits superior imaging of the more posterior cardiac structures,[60] providing high-resolution views of especially their point of attachment, are better imaged by TEE (Figs. 111-3 and 131-6). (See Chap. 131.) Visualization of all four chambers permits recognition of multiple tumors[63] or tumors in less common locations.[64,65] Doppler assessment of mitral flow provides further information regarding the hemodynamic consequences of left atrial myxomas.[66]

Gated Radionuclide Cardiac Imaging Gated radionuclide imaging of the isotopically tagged blood pool also has resulted in detection of left atrial myxomas.[67] This technique has also defined intracavitary tumors in other chambers[67,68] and biatrial tumors.[24]

Other Imaging Techniques Cine-computed tomography provides precise spatial localization of intracardiac masses.[69,70] High resolution is similarly achieved by magnetic resonance imaging (MRI), which is demonstrating increased usefulness in the detection and characterization of intracardiac masses. The technique has been used to achieve excellent visualization of intracavitary atrial myxomas, providing information about the size, shape, attachment, and mobility of these tumors.[71-73]

Catheterization Cardiac catheterization invariably demonstrates significant pulmonary capillary wedge and pulmonary arterial hypertension.[2] A notch on the ascending limb of the left ventricular pressure curve results from expulsion of the myxoma from the left ventricle, which suddenly decreases left ventricular volume. When a large left atrial tumor or a left atrial ball thrombus obstructs the mitral orifice but does not prolapse into the left ventricular cavity, this notch is absent.[74] Similarly, a rapid y descent of the pulmonary wedge or left atrial pressure curve is the consequence of a sudden decrease of left atrial volume when the tumor prolapses into the left ventricle.[74] The notch, or "hold," on the rapid y descent appears to be caused by the slightly delayed tumor prolapse through the mitral orifice.[75] The large v wave, at times as high as 75 mmHg, even in the absence of significant mitral regurgitation, reflects the space-occupying effect of the tumor within the left atrium. When the clinical picture is that of mitral stenosis, these findings are highly suggestive of a space-filling defect in the atrium. Large left atrial myxomas that obstruct the mitral orifice without prolapsing into the left ventricle demonstrate a slow y descent.[74] Rarely, a left atrial myxoma is associated with a congenital atrial septal defect with an accompanying left-to-right shunt.[76]

Angiography Although angiography characterizes the size, location, and mobility of the tumor,[2] the efficacy of echocardiography and other imaging techniques has largely supplanted contrast angiography and usually permits immediate operative intervention without additional invasive studies.[4,33,35] Catheter passage or contrast injection into the chamber containing the myxoma risks embolization of tumor fragments.[77] Injection of contrast medium into the pulmonary artery, with attention paid

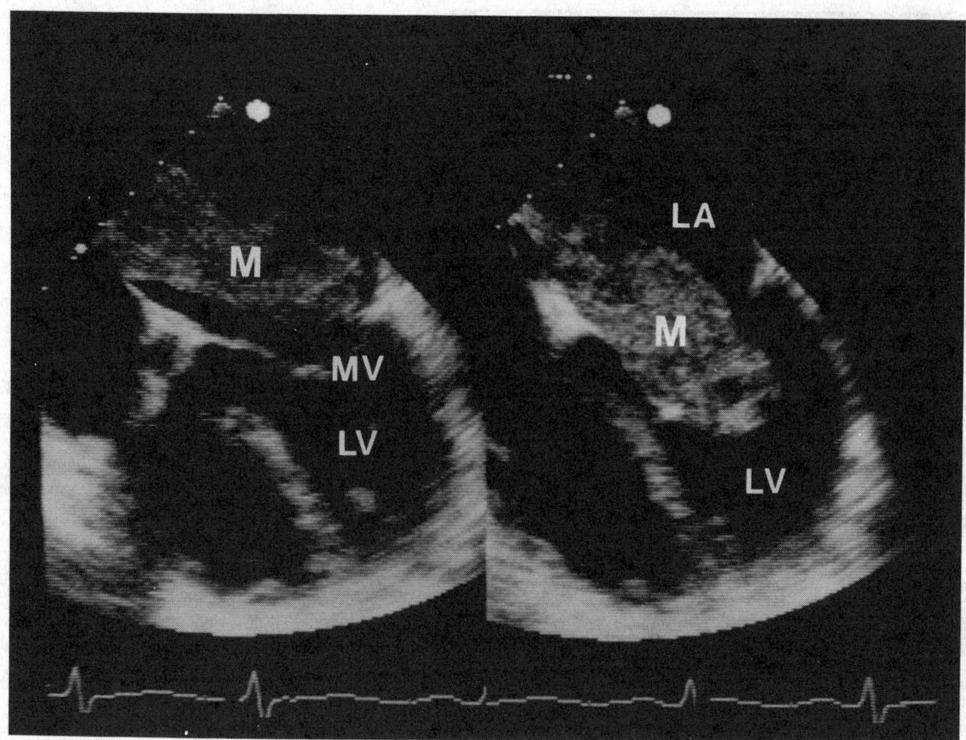

FIGURE 111-3 Transesophageal echocardiogram in the four-chamber view from a 50-year-old man who presented with exertional dyspnea and syncope. A large left atrial (LA) myxoma (M) attached to the interatrial septum is seen prolapsing across the mitral valve (MV) into the left ventricle (LV) in diastole (right panel). *(Courtesy of Susan Wilansky, M.D., Associate Director, Echocardiography Laboratory, St. Luke's Episcopal Hospital, Houston, Texas, and Bernardo Triestman, M.D.)*

to the levo phase of the angiogram, is diagnostic in all patients except those with small tumors.

Coronary Angiography Coronary angiography may demonstrate a vascular blush in the tumor from branches of both the right and left coronary arteries; and both left and right atrial myxomas and a right ventricular myxoma have been demonstrated in this manner.[78,79] Occasionally, an atrial myxoma in a patient with false-negative echocardiographic findings will be discovered in this fashion.[80] Neovascularization of a left atrial thrombus accompanying mitral stenosis may produce an appearance similar to a tumor blush.[81] Aneurysms and occlusion of the coronary artery caused by tumor emboli have also been demonstrated by coronary angiography.[80] The results of noninvasive imaging have proved sufficiently reliable and accurate in the diagnosis of left atrial myxoma that cardiac catheterization appears to be indicated primarily for patients with additional heart disease and for those over 40 years of age to rule out concomitant coronary artery disease.[79]

Differential Diagnosis Left atrial myxomas most often present as, and must be differentiated from, mitral valvular disease. At our institution, intracavitary myxomas were discovered in a ratio of approximately 1 per 100 patients presenting for mitral valve surgery.[2] Characteristically, the clinical course is relatively recent in origin, distinguishing myxoma from rheumatic mitral valvular disease; however, the course may occasionally span many years. Rarely, both conditions may coexist.[78] Fever, constitutional symptoms, and embolic phenomena mimic infective endocarditis; on rare occasions the myxoma itself may be infected. Muscle pain, skin rash, and Raynaud's phenomenon may simulate peripheral vasculitis,[82] and myxomatous emboli may be found on muscle biopsy.[30] Multiple systemic arterial aneurysms secondary to myxomatous embolization to the cerebral, pulmonary, renal, and muscular arteries have mimicked polyarteritis nodosa.[25,39] Similarly, coronary artery aneurysmal dilatation and myocardial infarction have been attributed to coronary myxoma embolization.[51,80] The clinical picture at times has been suggestive of acute rheumatic fever[83] and acute myocarditis.[84] The correct diagnosis will be suspected if the physician maintains a high index of clinical suspicion in patients with diverse and protean features, especially when cardiac, embolic, and constitutional manifestations coexist. Echocardiographic imaging of the heart has greatly facilitated the recognition of intracavitary tumors and results in detection in some patients who are asymptomatic.[5] Intracavitary thrombi may at times mimic intracardiac tumor masses (Fig. 111-4).[85]

Right Atrial Myxoma

Myxomas in the right atrial cavity constitute about one-fifth of all myxomas and tend to be more solid, have a wider attachment, and involve a greater amount of the atrial wall or septum than those in the left atrium. They originate from a variety of locations within the right atrium, including the inferior margin of the foramen ovale,[3,86] and characteristically produce tricuspid valve obstruction. A myxoma arising from the inferior vena cava has been reported.[10]

Clinical Manifestations Clinically, symptoms of low cardiac output and manifestations of systemic venous hypertension are present with a prominent jugular ve-

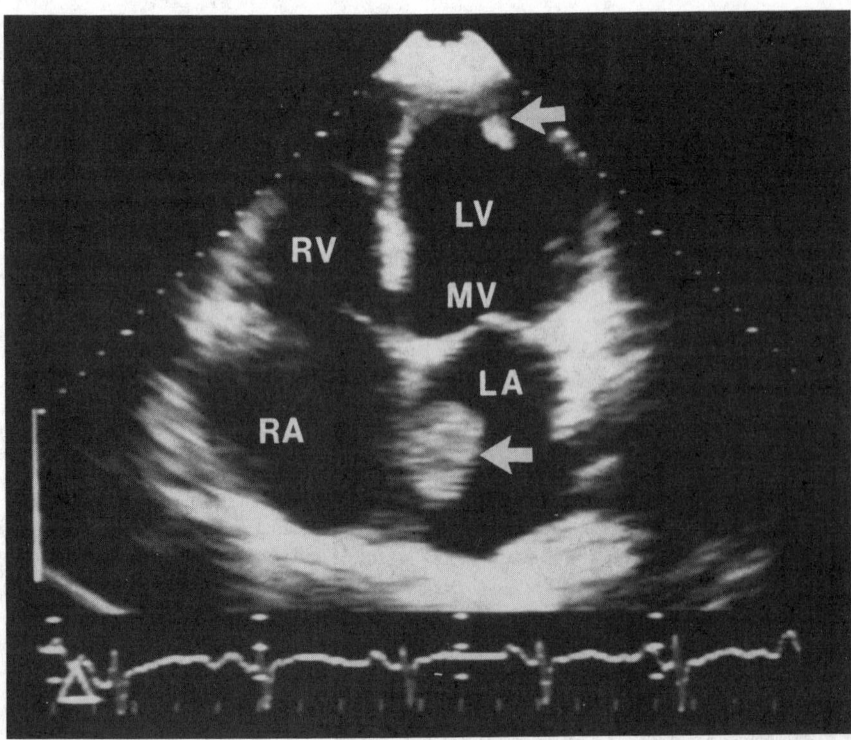

FIGURE 111-4 Two-dimensional echocardiogram, apical four-chamber view, of a patient with advanced congestive cardiomyopathy. Intracavitary masses (arrows), proved at autopsy to be thrombi, are present in the left atrium (LA) attached to the atrial septum (AS) and in the apex of the left ventricle (LV). The latter masses are both sessile and pedunculated. RA, right atrium; RV, right ventricle; MV, mitral valve. *(Courtesy of Carlos de Castro, M.D., Director, Noninvasive Laboratory, Department of Cardiology, St. Luke's Episcopal Hospital, Houston, Texas.)*

nous *a* wave, hepatomegaly, ascites, edema, and cyanosis,[68] which may be episodic and vary with the position of the patient. Persistence of normal sinus rhythm is common; however, sinus rhythm is also frequent in patients with rheumatic tricuspid stenosis. Intermittent episodes of syncope and abrupt onset of dyspnea, features never seen with rheumatic tricuspid stenosis,[54] are reported in one-third of these patients.[67] The pendular action of a prolapsing right atrial myxoma (wrecking-ball effect),[87] especially when it is calcified, may damage or destroy the tricuspid valve and produce severe tricuspid regurgitation.[54]

Pulmonary Emboli Whereas embolic tumor phenomena are reputed to occur less frequently with right than left atrial myxomas, pulmonary emboli have been reported,[86] at times are extensive,[87,88] and may produce irreversible pulmonary hypertension.[89] Wide dissemination of myxomatous embolization to the pulmonary arteries has been reported with active infiltration of the media[20] and formation of aneurysms.[25] Paradoxical embolization may occur if an interatrial communication exists.[31]

Systemic Manifestations Constitutional symptoms are less frequent in patients with a right atrial myxoma.[65] Anemia, polycythemia,[88,90] and cyanosis have been reported. Polycythemia and cyanosis may be caused by either right-to-left shunting through a patent foramen ovale or atrial septal defect,[31,91] low cardiac output and hypoxemic stimulation of the bone marrow, intravascular hemoconcentration,[90] or erythropoietin production by the tumor.[35] Mesenteric vasculitis of a nonembolic, probably autoimmune, origin has been reported.[92]

Auscultation On auscultation a loud early systolic sound may be heard. This sound occurs as late as 80 ms after the mitral component of the first sound and results from expulsion of the tumor from the right ventricle. A palpable tumor shock may coincide with this loud sound.[93] A crescendo murmur with inspiratory augmentation preceding this loud tumor expulsion sound is probably caused by early systolic tricuspid regurgitation while the valve is still held open by the tumor.[93] There may be a long diastolic murmur or, more commonly, only a late diastolic rumble, augmented by inspiration, accompanying atrial systole. If major injury to the tricuspid valve occurs, the murmur of tricuspid regurgitation will be present and large *v* waves will be seen in the jugular venous column. An early diastolic sound may be heard but is less constant than the tumor plop that accompanies a left atrial myxoma. The changing quality of the sound and murmurs, their closeness to the ear, and their frictionlike quality may mimic a pericardial rub.[65] Such sounds have been said to be an endocardial friction rub (see also Chap. 11).

Electrocardiogram and Chest X-Ray The results of electrocardiography are often normal, although right atrial enlargement frequently is suggested.[86] Low-voltage, right-axis deviation and varying degrees of right bundle branch block have been reported.[67] The chest roentgenogram may reveal some prominence or enlargement of the right atrial shadow and, occasionally, of the right ventricle. An important radiologic feature is the mild or moderate degree of cardiomegaly, considering the severe clinical state of the patients.[91] Calcification in the tumor may be recognized on plane film or at fluoroscopy and is more common in patients with myxomas in the right atrium.[2]

Echocardiography Whereas M-mode imaging poorly defines right atrial mass lesions, TTE and TEE provide excellent images of this region.[30,60,94,95] The latter provides more detail of the tumor and defines the site of attachment with greater clarity.[61–63] (See Chap. 131.)

Catheterization and Angiography Cardiac catheterization demonstrates elevated right atrial pressure, prominence of the *a* wave, and a diastolic gradient between the right atrium and right ventricle. Notching of the upstroke of the right ventricular pressure curve has been noted[86] and is similar to that seen in the left ventricle in patients with prolapsing left atrial myxomas. Similarly, a collapsing *y* descent has been described in the right atrium with marked inspiratory augmentation.[86] With current noninvasive imaging techniques, catheterization and angiography of the right-sided heart chambers are rarely necessary and risk embolization of tumor fragments to the pulmonary arteries.

Differential Diagnosis The clinical features of right atrial myxoma resemble those of rheumatic tricuspid valvular disease, although the latter is always accompanied by significant mitral and, frequently, aortic valve disease. There are many similarities to the manifestations of constrictive pericarditis and Ebstein's anomaly of the tricuspid valve. Episodic dyspnea, sudden syncope, and variability of symptoms and findings with position of the patient may serve as helpful clues. Changing murmurs, along with fever and anemia, can be suggestive of infective endocarditis. Tricuspid stenosis and regurgitation are prominent in patients with carcinoid syndrome, but involvement of the pulmonary valve and other features of a carcinoid tumor will usually serve to distinguish it from a right atrial myxoma. Obstruction of the right ventricular outflow tract may be the dominant finding in some examples of familial obstructive myopathy and may resemble a right atrial tumor. Pulmonary embolization of other diverse etiologies, with secondary thromboembolic pulmonary hypertension and right-sided heart failure, may be mimicked by right atrial myxoma. An awareness of the protean manifestations, along with evidence from echocardiographic imaging, usually facilitates a correct diagnosis.

Bilateral Atrial Myxoma

An atrial myxoma may pass through the foramen ovale and be present in both atria. The tumor is usually shaped like a dumbbell with the common stalk attached to the margin of the fossa ovalis. Among the cases reported, surgery was successful most often when the correct diagnosis was made preoperatively, emphasizing the importance of echographic exploration of all chambers.[24] Similar echocardiographic findings have been reported in patients with discrete tumors in each atrium.[63] Multichambered cardiac myxomas occasionally involve chambers other than the usual biatrial combination and are more frequent in familial occurrences.[31]

Left Ventricular Myxoma

A myxoma originates from the left ventricle in 2.5 to 4 percent of reported myxomas.[6,65] Recorded cases are found in the younger age groups, with most patients being under 30 years of age. Women are affected three times more often than are men, and a short duration of symptoms is also characteristic. Systemic emboli, mostly cerebral, occur in two-thirds of the patients, and constitutional symptoms are almost conspicuously absent. Emboli from left ventricular tumors may mimic multiple sclerosis.[96] Attacks of syncope occur in nearly half of the reviewed cases. Symptoms and physical findings are suggestive of aortic or subaortic obstruction. The location and movement of the tumor mass are demonstrated particularly well by TTE and by TEE.[97] (See Chaps. 15 and 131.) Echoes from an intracavitary left ventricular myxoma must be differentiated from left ventricular thrombi, which are usually apical but occasionally are pedunculated, and from ventricular septal rhabdomyomas. Left and right ventricular myxomas have been identified by MRI, which complements two-dimensional echographic findings and is of higher resolution than cardiac angiography.[98] (See Chap. 136.) Planning for surgical excision can be based upon noninvasive imaging without resorting to cardiac catheterization unless coexistent cardiac disease is suspected.[97,98]

Right Ventricular Myxoma

Myxomas of the right ventricle are as infrequent as those occurring in the left ventricle. The patient will have symptoms and manifestations of right-sided heart failure, syncope, unexplained fever, and a murmur consistent with pulmonary stenosis. An "ejection sound" has been reported, as well as delayed closure of the pulmonary valve. A right-sided tumor plop may be heard in diastole.[99] Calcium in the tumor may be recognized on the roentgenogram. A gradient across the right ventricular outlet is characteristic,[99] and the tumor can be visualized angiographically. Pulmonary emboli may occur.[100] Echocardiographic imaging, both TTE and TEE, will detect most right ventricular myxomas.[63,101] Transvenous intracardiac biopsy may be helpful in the differential diagnosis.[102] A right ventricular myxoma has been diagnosed in a neonate and has been successfully removed surgically.[28] Other tumors, producing similar outflow tract obstruction, rarely occur within the right ventricle.[103]

Surgery for Intracavitary Myxoma

Surgical resection of a myxoma is the only acceptable therapy and, in view of the dangers of embolization and sudden death, should be performed promptly. For complete removal of left atrial myxoma, we use a biatrial approach, excising a full thickness of interatrial septum if the tumor is attached to the region of the fossa ovalis (Fig. 111-5).[104,105] Right atrial myxomas are commonly attached to the fossa ovalis, and with right-sided tumors, a full thickness of atrial septum also should be resected. If a large portion of the septum is removed, a patch of knitted Dacron cloth should be used for repair to avoid distortion, dysrhythmia, or possible atrial septal defect. Since fragmentation and embolization of the tumor is an ever-present threat, vigorous palpation and other manipulations of the heart should be avoided until cardiopulmonary bypass is initiated.[22] We usually induce ventricular standstill with cardioplegia solution before manipulating the heart to reduce the possibility of fragmentation of the gelatinous tumor. Left atrial myxomas have been removed successfully during pregnancy, utilizing cardiopulmonary bypass, with subsequent uncomplicated completion of a full-term pregnancy.[106,107] Surgical removal of a right ventricular myxoma in a neonate has been reported.[28]

By its movement within the heart, the tumor may traumatize either AV valve, which may require replacement or repair by annuloplasty.[2] Arrhythmias and conduction disturbances may follow surgical removal of left atrial myxomas.[108] Recurrences of atrial myxomas are rare and usually occur within a 48-month period.[21]

Other Benign Primary Cardiac Tumors

Rhabdomyoma

The most frequent cardiac tumor in infants and children[6,109] is a rhabdomyoma, which is probably a hamartoma rather than a true neoplasm.[110] These tumors are usually multiple, most often involve the ventricular myocardium, and project into the cavity or move freely as a pedunculated mass.[109,111,112] Associated tuberous sclerosis is present in one-third of the patients.[113] Presenting symptoms may be caused by cardiac obstructive phenomena, arrhythmias, AV block, pericardial effusion, or even sudden death.[111,114,115] These tumors can mimic pulmonary stenosis and produce hypoxic spells like those seen with tetralogy of Fallot.[109] Ventricular outlet gradients,[116] angiographic abnormalities, echocardiography,[109,112,117–119] and MRI[120] can lead to demonstration of the tumor and successful surgical resection. Prenatal detection of an intracardiac rhabdomyoma by intrauterine echocardiography at 30 weeks gestation has been reported with ultimate surgical removal at 20 months of age.[121] Multiplicity of tumors does not contraindicate surgery, as these tumors appear to have little capacity for further growth. Pedunculated rhabdomyomas that arise from the left atrium and cause mitral stenosis have been reported.[114] Discrete and multiple myocardial hamartomas and rhabdomyomas have caused incessant ventricular tachycardia in infants and have been successfully removed surgically.[104,105,122–125]

Fibroma

Fibromas are usually ventricular and intramural. Although reported cases have occurred in the age range from newborn to 65 years, most occur in infants and children.[6,126] Calcification is common. Sudden death has been reported in nearly one-third of the patients, presumably due to involvement of the conduction system, pro-

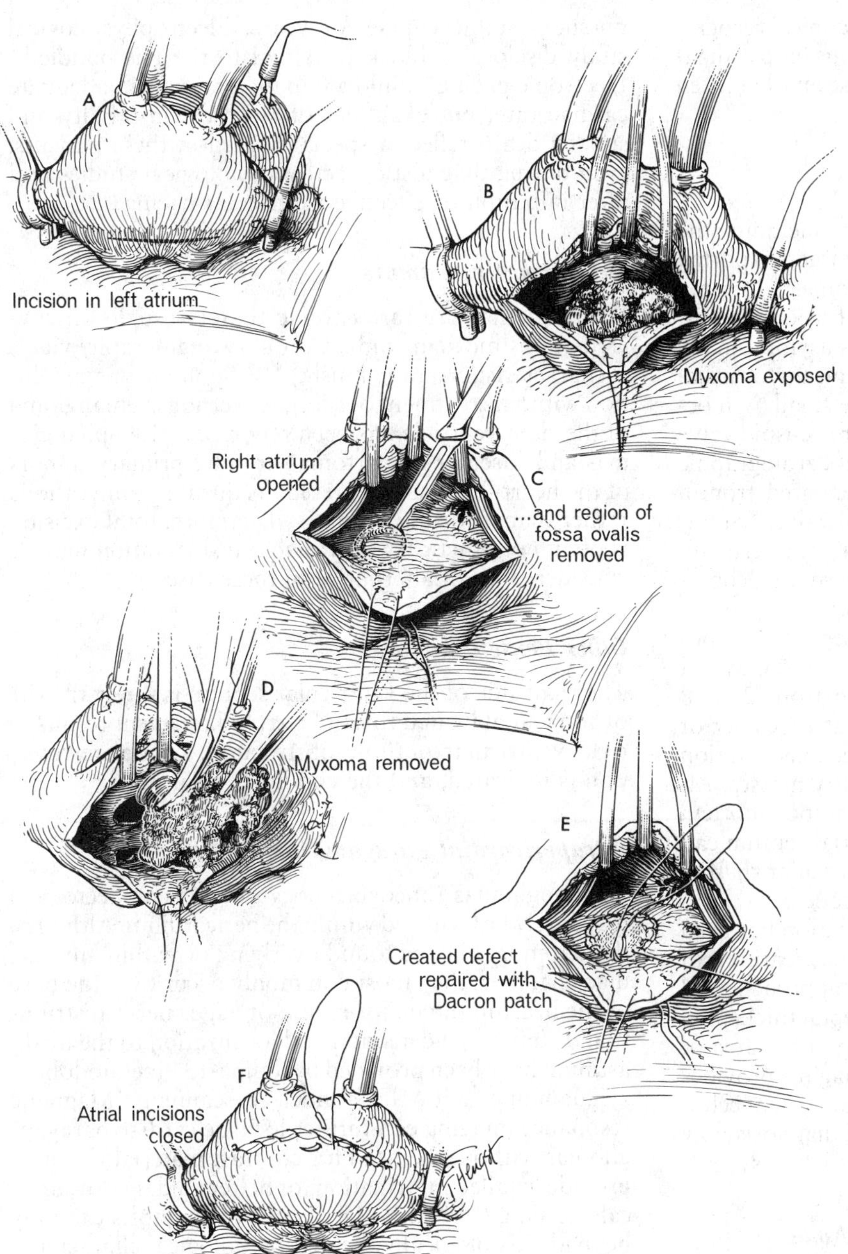

FIGURE 111-5 Drawing illustrating resection of a typical left atrial myxoma with a broad attachment to the interatrial septum near the fossa ovalis. The ascending aorta is cross-clamped and the left atrium is opened near the interatrial groove (*A*). After the pedicle of the tumor is located (*B*), a separate incision is made in the right atrium (*C*). The interatrial septum is opened near the fossa ovalis, and a portion of the interatrial septum is excised. The tumor is removed through the left atriotomy (*D*). The resultant atrial defect is closed with a knitted Dacron patch (*E*). The atrial chambers and atrioventricular valve areas should be thoroughly inspected for additional tumor implants or fragments before the atriotomy incisions are closed (*F*). *(From DA Cooley, Techniques in Cardiac Surgery, 2d ed. Philadelphia, WB Saunders, 1984: 324. Reproduced with permission from the publisher and author.)*

duction of arrhythmias, or obstruction of the outflow tract of the left ventricle.[126,127] Two-dimensional echocardiography accurately delineates intramural ventricular tumors.[128] Left axis deviation may occur as an interesting electrocardiographic feature. Total or partial resection of the tumor to relieve obstruction has been reported, with excellent probability of long-term survival.[104,125,127] Cardiac transplantation has been used in the management of a young adult with a nonresectable (1030-g) left ventricular fibroma.[129]

Papillary Fibroelastoma

Also referred to as papillomas or papillary fibromas, papillary fibroelastomas arise from the cardiac valves or occasionally from the ventricular endocardium, are most commonly seen in patients over 50 years of age, and have been traditionally seen as a coincidental finding at surgery or postmortem examination.[130] Grossly, these tumors resemble a sea anemone, with multiple papillary fronds attached to the endothelium by a short pedicle. There is a predilection for involvement of the aortic valve,[13] where angina and sudden death may result from coronary ostial occlusion caused by the fronds of the villous tumor.[6,13,131] Obstruction of the right ventricular outflow tract has been reported in a patient with a papillary tumor of the tricuspid valve.[132] Cerebral emboli from these lesions have also been reported.[133] The tumor is histologically different from Lambl's excrescences, which are degenerative in origin and usually situated on the ventricular aspect of the semilunar valve along the line of closure.[6,134,135] Papillary fibroelastomas are being discovered with increasing frequency by echocardiographic (TTE and TEE) imaging of the heart,[130,136-138] and successful surgical excision has followed clinical recognition.[130,133,134,136,138] Percutaneous transvenous biopsy diagnosis of a right atrial papillary fibroelastoma has been reported.[137]

Lipoma

Lipomas may occur throughout the heart, including the pericardium. They may be massive; the largest reported cardiac tumor was an intrapericardial lipoma.[139] Intrapericardial lipomas may cause pericardial effusion, be mistaken for a pericardial cyst, or present as asymptomatic cardiac or mediastinal enlargement.[140] Intramyocardial lipomas are encapsulated and usually are small.[6] An occasional lipoma arising from the mitral or tricuspid valve may resemble an atrial myxoma on echocardiographic examination[141] and must also be differentiated from a cyst[12,90,142] or lymphangioma of the mitral valve.[88] Surgical excision of lipomas yields excellent long-term results.[104] Tissue characterization by MRI permits preoperative identification of these fatty tumors.[143]

Lipomatous hypertrophy of the atrial septum is a nonencapsulated hyperplasia of adipose tissue and may not represent a true tumor. Varying in size from 2 to 8 cm, the tumescence may bulge into the atrial cavity or superior vena cava orifice[144] and become a consideration in the differential diagnosis of intracavitary masses. Although at times found coincidentally at postmortem study, lipomatous hypertrophy of the atrial septum can be associated with unexplained supraventricular rhythm and conduction disturbances, recurrent pericardial effusion,[145] and sudden death.[6,7,146] This association has been considered fortuitous by some observers. Features of both TTE, especially from the subcostal approach, and TEE[147] are distinctive and include atrial septal thickening with a bilobed appearance due to sparing of the area of the fossa ovalis. Magnetic resonance imaging provides noninvasive tissue characterization of lipomas that echocardiography does not provide.[148–150] The diagnosis may be confirmed by percutaneous transvenous biopsy.[151]

Mesothelioma of the Atrioventricular Node

The smallest tumor capable of producing sudden death by causing complete heart block or ventricular fibrillation is mesothelioma of the AV node.[6,152] Reported ages in patients have ranged from the newborn period to the ninth decade of life, with a strong female preponderance. Although the exact origin of these cystic tumors has been disputed, most researchers believe they arise from arrests in development[152,153]; also, other terms have been applied to them, such as lymphangioepithelioma[152] and congenital polycystic tumor of the AV node.[154,155] In vivo recognition has not been reported, although the cystic structure may exceed 3 cm in size. The tumor is usually large enough to be recognized grossly at postmortem examination and, despite its rare occurrence, should be suspected in all cases of sudden death without apparent cause, especially in children and young adults.[6,156,157] Most patients with mesothelioma of the AV node have demonstrated complete heart block and have recurrent attacks of Stokes-Adams syndrome. Even with complete heart block a narrow QRS is common, and these patients may pursue a stable course for years. Electrophysiological study discloses a block proximal to the His bundle.[156] Electronic pacing should aid in maintaining an adequate cardiac rate, but examples of electrical instability and sudden death reflect a special hazard in these patients, even during diagnostic electrophysiological studies and after initiation of effective ventricular pacing.[6,155]

Vasoformative Tumors

Hemangiomas are rare cardiac tumors usually discovered at postmortem study. Coronary angiography yields a characteristic tumor blush.[158,159] Spontaneous resolution without treatment of a large cavernous hemangioma of the right ventricle has been reported.[160] Lymphangiomas and vascular hamartomas are rare primary tumors of the heart that usually present as diffuse proliferations rather than as distinct tumors. Therefore, total excision is often not practical.[161] Cardiac transplantation may be considered as an alternative in these cases.

Other Benign Tumors

The right side of the ventricular septum is rarely the site of congenital benign thyroid rest. Enlargement results in right ventricular outflow obstruction. Complete resection is indicated, and the condition is curable.[162]

Intrapericardial Paraganglioma

Paragangliomas (pheochromocytoma, chemodectomas) may rarely be localized within the pericardium. Although these tumors may be found overlying or within any cardiac chamber, they most commonly occur over the base of the heart in the major region of vagus nerve distribution.[163] Improved detection and localization to the mediastinum have been provided by iodine-131 metaiodobenzylguanidine (^{131}I-MIBG) nuclear scanning. Magnetic resonance imaging can further localize cardiac paragangliomas without the need for contrast material and may provide detailed information for better guidance of surgical excision.[164–166] Although definitive diagnosis can only be made histologically, benign pathological characteristics do not necessarily predict a favorable outcome, as these tumors are highly vascular, adherent, and difficult to resect. Human cardiac explantation and autotransplantation have been applied to a patient with a large cardiac pheochromocytoma.[167]

Malignant Primary Tumors of the Heart

Angiosarcoma (Hemangiosarcoma)

Almost all primary malignant cardiac tumors are sarcomas, most frequently angiosarcomas,[168] and usually originate in the right atrium or pericardium.[102] Intense vascularity may produce a continuous murmur.[169] One-fourth of all angiosarcomas will, in part, be intracavitary with valvular obstruction and characteristically will manifest right-sided heart failure and pericardial tamponade with hemorrhagic fluid. Atrial angiosarcomas exhibit highly variable histological patterns, which may overlap those of Kaposi's sarcoma.[170] Echocardiography (Fig. 111-6*A*) and angiography are helpful in the diagno-

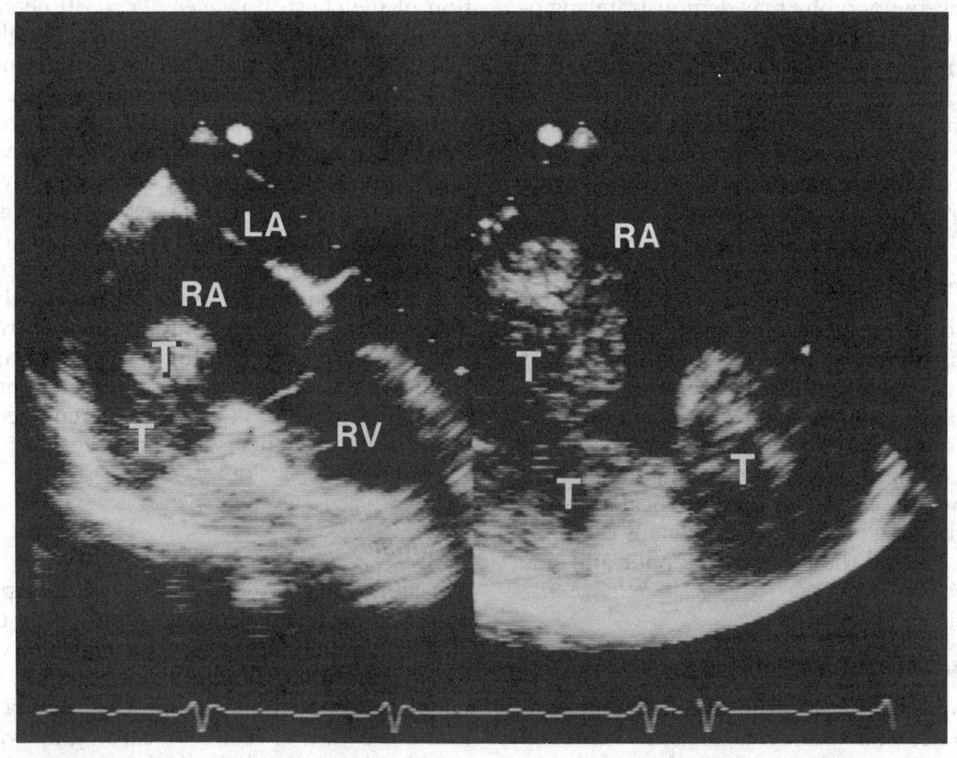

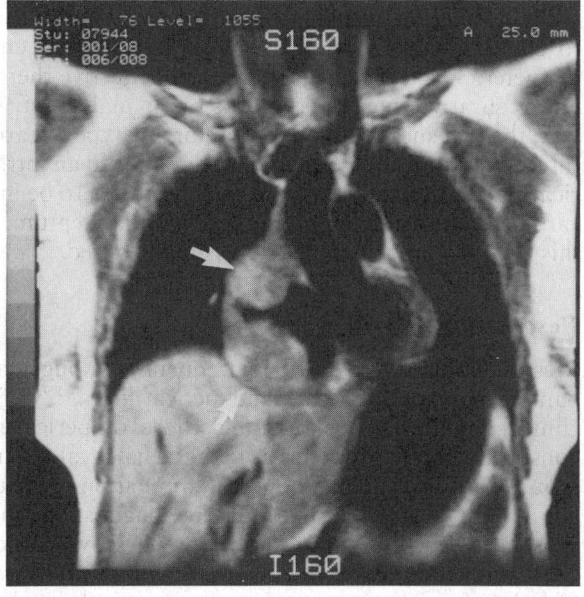

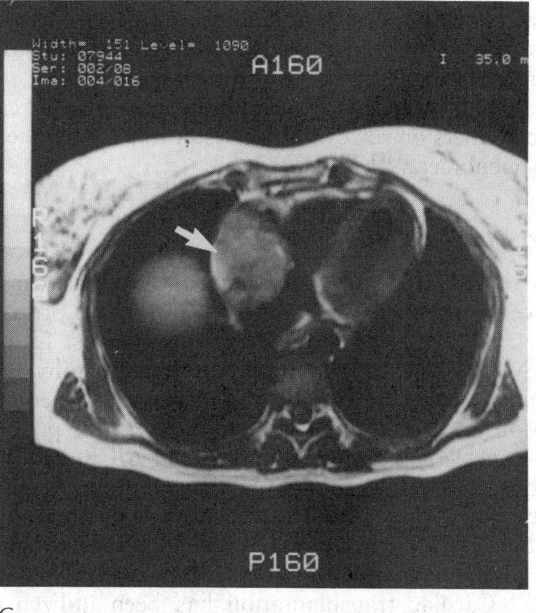

FIGURE 111-6 *A.* Biplane transesophageal echocardiogram from a 35-year-old woman who presented with shock of unknown cause. The horizontal plane seen on the left shows a tumor (T) in the right atrium (RA). The vertical plane on the right panel shows a large, bilobular tumor (T) adherent to the right atrial wall. Histology proved this to be an angiosarcoma. LA, left atrium; RV, right ventricle. *(Courtesy of Susan Wilansky, M.D., Associate Director, Echocardiography Laboratory, St. Luke's Episcopal Hospital, Houston, Texas.) B,C.* Arrowheads denote a dumbbell-shaped, intermediate signal intensity right atrial tumor, which is shown to abut the aorta in the coronal T1-weighted view and the tricuspid valve in the axial T1-weighted view. Note the loss of the usual high-signal intensity margin (fat) along the right lateral aspect of the aorta in the coronal plane. This raises concern for malignant invasion of the aortic wall. *(Courtesy of Clark L. Carrol, M.D., St. Luke's Episcopal Hospital, Texas Children's Hospital, and Texas Heart Institute, Houston, Texas.)*

sis.[171,172] Coronary angiography may demonstrate angiomatous vessels over the tumor area. The course is rapid, and widespread metastases make surgery impractical,[171] although tumor excision, radiation, and chemotherapy may offer some relief of symptoms and palliation.[6,104,105,125,169,170,172,173] An iatrogenic hemangiopericytoma of the right ventricle has been reported following intense radiotherapy to the cardiac area.[174]

Rhabdomyosarcoma

Rhabdomyosarcoma is the second most frequent primary sarcoma of the heart and, like angiosarcoma, is prevalent in males. There is no single chamber predilection; multiple sites are common, and significant obstruction of at least one valve is present in half of the patients.[175] Excision of the main tumor mass combined with radiation and chemotherapy has been advocated as the treatment for patients with primary malignant tumor of the heart, but in general the prognosis is poor and survival is short.[6,176–178]

Other Malignant Primary Tumors

Fibrosarcoma, liposarcoma,[179] primary malignant lymphoma,[180,181] and occasional sarcomas of other basic cell types constitute the remaining but infrequent primary malignant cardiac tumors.[6] The fibrous histiocytoma (Fig. 111-6) has a predilection for the left atrium[182,183] and has infrequently occurred adjacent to Dacron vascular grafts and to a mitral prosthetic valve, suggesting a possible mild carcinogenic effect of these materials.[184]

Malignant primary cardiac tumors may obstruct cardiac chambers or valves[185–188] or result in peripheral embolic phenomena.[182,189]

Surgery for Cardiac Tumors

Effective palliation and local control of the disease can be achieved with extensive resection of malignant primary tumors.[105,125,182,189–191] Echocardiography (Chaps. 15 and 131), MRI (Chap. 136), and computed tomography (CT) scanning (Chap. 135) are helpful in planning operative resection of cardiac tumors because these tests provide three-dimensional information (Fig. 111-6*B* and C).[73,192] Intraoperative echocardiography may be useful to guide surgical resection.[193] Adjuvant chemotherapy and radiation therapy are necessary to improve long-term prognosis, and the response to therapy can be assessed by MRI.[194] Cardiac transplantation has been utilized to completely resect an "inoperable" benign tumor[190] and an unresectable malignant primary cardiac neoplasm.[195] Cardiac explantation and autotransplantation may facilitate resection of some cardiac tumors.[167] (See also Chap. 32.)

Tumors of the Pericardium

Pericardial Cysts

Pericardial, or mesothelial, cysts are the most frequent benign "tumors" of the pericardium. They are usually found coincidentally on routine radiographic examination of the chest; however, 25 to 30 percent of the patients will have chest pain, dyspnea, cough, or paroxysmal tachycardia. Pericardial cysts occur most frequently in the third or fourth decade of life and are found equally among men and women.[196] The right costophrenic location is the most common, although they may present in the upper mediastinum.[197] Only rarely will the cyst connect with the pericardial cavity. Clinically and radiographically, they resemble other tumors of the pericardium such as hemangioma, lymphangioma, or lipoma as well as retrosternal hernia, a pericardial fat pad, and eventration of the diaphragm. Echocardiography[60,198] and CT[197] are most helpful in the differential diagnosis. Surgical excision completely relieves symptoms and confirms the diagnosis[6,13]; however, percutaneous aspiration of the cystic contents is an attractive alternative to surgical resection.[197]

Teratoma

Most teratomas are extracardiac yet intrapericardial and arise and receive their blood supply from the root of the aorta or pulmonary artery through the vasa vasorum. Most are found in infants and children, with a strong female preponderance.[6] One case has been diagnosed in utero by aid of fetal echocardiography.[199] Recurrent, nonbloody pericardial effusion is common in children with this tumor, and intrapericardial teratoma is the most likely diagnosis in this setting.[200] Embarrassment of cardiac function results from expansion of the tumor to considerable proportions, at times up to 15 cm in diameter. Surgical excision is the only effective therapy[6] and is curative since the tumor is rarely malignant.[201] In fact, the first successful operation for any type of cardiac tumor was done in 1938 when Beck removed an intrapericardial teratoma.[200] It is rare for a teratoma to be intracardiac and arise from the interventricular septum, but this type of tumor can be successfully excised.[202,203]

Mesothelioma

Mesothelioma ranks third in frequency among malignant tumors of the heart and pericardium.[7,204,205] The clinical manifestations resemble those of pericarditis, constrictive pericardial disease, and vena caval obstruction. Aspiration and histological examination of the usually bloody pericardial fluid may be diagnostic. Among those affected, males outnumber females by a ratio of 2 : 1, with the peak incidence occurring in the third to fifth decades. The prognosis is poor, surgical excision is usually impossible, and treatment with radiation and chemotherapy generally produces only temporary improvement.

Primary Tumors of the Aorta

Primary tumors of the aorta are rare. Occasionally, they are benign, but most frequently they are malignant sarcomas. Presentation may mimic aortic dissection, coarctation, atherosclerotic occlusive disease, and malignancies in other organs. All portions of the aorta may be involved, and distal metastases are common. Surgical extirpation will relieve the obstructive phenomena, but distant metastases usually lead to disease progression.[206,207]

SECONDARY TUMORS OF THE HEART

General Considerations

Metastatic tumors involve the heart, pericardium, or both, from a primary origin in some other organ 20 to 40 times more frequently than primary tumors of the heart.[208,209] These secondary tumors are more frequently carcinomas than sarcomas. Cardiac metastases occur most often in people older than 50 years of age; the incidence is equal in both sexes. The development of otherwise unexplained cardiac symptoms or manifestations, cardiac enlargement, tachycardia, arrhythmias, or heart failure in the presence of neoplastic disease is suggestive of cardiac metastases.

Frequency and Origin of Secondary Tumors

In a report by the Harvard Cancer Commission of 4375 autopsies of patients who died of cancer, myocardial metastases were present in 146 patients (3.4 percent).[208] In a series of 2547 consecutive autopsies performed at Walter Reed General Hospital, 980 cases of malignant disease were observed. The heart was the site of metastatic tumor in 5.7 percent of the cases and the heart, including the pericardium, in 13.9 percent.[209] In other series, cardiac metastases have been present in patients with malignant tumors in a range as wide as 1.5 to 21 percent.[210] An increased prevalence of secondary cardiac neoplasms in recent years may be related to more vigorous surgical and radiation treatment of patients with primary neoplasms.[211] The relative infrequency of cardiac metastases has been attributed to the strong kneading action of the heart, the metabolic peculiarities of striated muscle, rapid coronary blood flow, and lymphatic connections that drain afferently from the heart.[208]

Cardiac metastases occur with all types of primary tumors: carcinomas, sarcomas, leukemia, lymphomas,[212] Kaposi's sarcoma, etc. No malignant tumor tends particularly to metastasize to the heart, with the possible exception of malignant melanoma, which involves the myocardium in more than 50 percent of cases.[213] Cardiac metastases are most frequent, with bronchogenic carcinoma[214] and carcinoma of the breast occurring in one-third of the cases. Cardiac infiltration, often macroscopic, is seen in one-half of cases of leukemia and in one-sixth of cases of lymphoma.

Cardiac metastases are encountered with widespread systemic tumor dissemination; only rarely is metastatic tumor limited to the heart or pericardium. Carcinomatous metastases are generally grossly visible, multiple, discrete, small, white, firm nodules; microscopically, they resemble the primary tumor and the metastases in other organs. Diffuse infiltration is characteristic of sarcomatous metastases.

Metastatic tumors are classically thought to reach the heart by embolic hematogenous spread, lymphatic spread, or direct invasion, in descending order of frequency. Cardiac lymphatics are considered to be an important pathway of tumor metastases to the heart; lymphatic obstruction by tumor results in myocardial interstitial edema, and the secondary pressure on the myofibers may contribute to the eventual cardiac decompensation,[215] particularly in a patient with underlying atherosclerotic coronary heart disease. Lymphatic spread of tumors is particularly frequent with carcinoma of the bronchus and the breast; the proximity of the heart to major mediastinal lymphatic channels seems to explain the high incidence of cardiac metastases from mediastinal tumors.[210]

Manifestations

Secondary tumor involvement of the heart may be recognized as a pathological finding without clinical manifestations. More often, however, such involvement is symptomatic, and on rare occasions it may be the first or only expression of a remote primary tumor. Recognition of neoplastic heart disease is dependent on the physician's awareness of the probability of occurrence and diverse manners of presentation. At times, as with rapidly developing tamponade, recognition and appropriate therapy must be undertaken promptly. Secondary tumors of the heart may involve the pericardium, myocardium, endocardium, valves, and coronary arteries. Direct invasion of the heart through the venae cavae[216] or pulmonary veins[217] or through an expanding myocardial implant can produce an intracavitary tumor mass and result in obstruction to flow or cause valvular obstruction. Depending on the character and location of the cardiac lesion, a variety of manifestations may serve to identify cardiac involvement, especially in a patient with a known malignancy.

Pericardial Involvement

Pericardial involvement is often first manifested by chest pain, aggravated by inspiration, and a pericardial friction rub. Accumulation of fluid within the pericardium, often but not always bloody, may result in progressive cardiac enlargement on roentgenogram, with symptoms and signs of cardiac tamponade, and may be the first manifestation of a cardiac malignancy.[218] Clinically, the jugular venous pressure is increased, the arterial pressure is reduced, and "pulsus paradoxus" may be present. Reduced electrocardiographic QRS voltage can be expected. Electrical alternation, which is generally seen in patients with large effusions and serious tamponade,[219] may indicate the need for prompt pericardiocentesis. The echocardiogram demonstrates pericardial fluid and may demonstrate features of hemodynamic tamponade; diastolic collapse of the right atrium and ventricle[220,221]; inferior vena cava plethora with a blunted inspiratory response[222]; and altered inspiratory intracardiac Doppler flow velocities.[223–225] Pericardial effusion and tamponade may be the first manifestation of cardiac involvement by a malignancy.[218] The association of large quantities of pericardial fluid with tumor encasing the heart frequently results in persistent cardiac constriction, even after the fluid is withdrawn by pericardiocentesis.[210] Echocardiography and CT are both useful for detecting pericardial metastases (Fig. 111-7).[210,226,227]

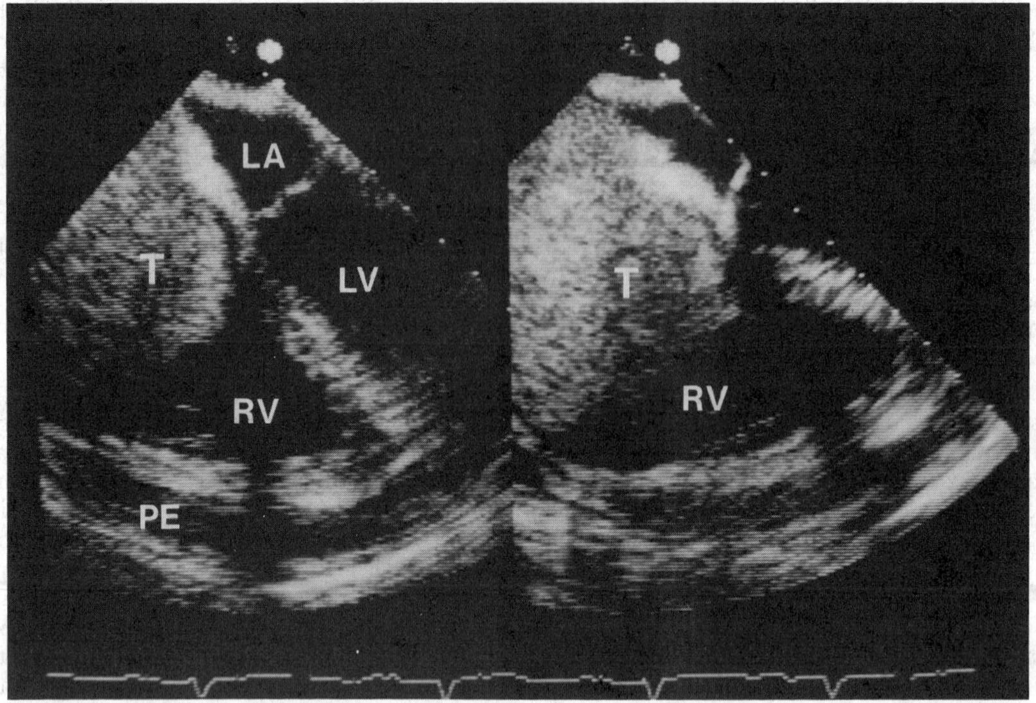

FIGURE 111-7 Transesophageal echocardiogram in a 55-year-old woman who presented with adenocarcinoma of the lung and obstructed superior vena cava syndrome. A large tumor (T) is seen in the right ventricle (RV) in systole *(left panel)* and diastole *(right panel)*. Subsequent images revealed that it originated from an obstructed superior vena cava. The echo-free space anterior to the right ventricle represented pericardial effusion (PE). LA, left atrium; LV, left ventricle. *(Courtesy of Susan Wilansky, M.D., Associate Director, Echocardiography Laboratory, St. Luke's Episcopal Hospital, Houston, Texas.)*

Myocardial Involvement

Atrial arrhythmias are common, probably because the atrium has less mobility and hence is invaded more often. Atrial flutter and fibrillation are frequent, and a patient with either one may be unusually resistant to conventional therapy. Ventricular extrasystoles and even serious ventricular arrhythmias[228] may accompany invasion of a tumor into the myocardium. Conduction disturbances and complete heart block have been reported.[229,230] Widespread muscle involvement by tumor invasion or obstruction of the cardiac lymphatic drainage system may cause congestive failure. Rarely, a pedunculated secondary tumor mass may produce a loud murmur and palpable thrill.[231] Myocardial damage and heart failure also may result from some of the chemotherapeutic agents used in the treatment of patients with neoplastic diseases, and combined radiotherapy and chemotherapy may synergistically increase cardiac damage.[232] (See Chap. 110.) The most frequent electrocardiographic abnormalities seen in patients with neoplastic heart disease are nonspecific changes of the ST segment and the T wave due to myocardial or pericardial involvement by the tumor. Pronounced and prolonged ST-segment elevation in the absence of myocardial infarction may occur with tumor invasion of the heart.[233]

Coronary Artery Involvement

In patients with malignant tumor, angina or myocardial infarction may result from concomitant atherosclerosis,[232] coronary occlusion by tumor embolization,[234] or external coronary compression by the tumor as well as from coronary fibrosis or accelerated atherogenesis in patients who have received radiation to the mediastinum.[232] The electrocardiographic pattern of myocardial infarction also can result from massive invasion of the myocardium by a tumor[232,235] or from a large pericardial effusion.[209,236]

Intracavitary Tumor

Extensions of tumors such as renal cell carcinoma,[216,237–239] hepatocellular carcinoma,[240,241] and uterine leiomyomatosis,[242–244] along the inferior vena cava and into the right atrium can present as an intracavitary obstructive mass. Leiomyosarcoma may be primary in the vena cava, most often the inferior, and extend directly into the heart.[245,246] Intracavitary metastases or an expanding myocardial tumor may progressively obliterate a cardiac chamber or result in a valvular obstruction[247–250] and, rarely, produce fever of unknown origin. Successful surgical resection has been reported.[105,239,241,245,252] Right atrial and tricuspid obstruction by an intracavitary mass can mimic pericardial constriction[251,252] from tumor invasion or from previous intensive radiotherapy to the mediastinum. Systemic or pulmonary emboli, so common with primary tumors of the heart, are uncommon with secondary tumors. Right-sided intracavitary thrombi may mimic primary or secondary tumors on echographic imaging of the heart.[253,254]

Diagnostic Studies

Echocardiography, TTE and TEE,[60,210,226,255] and CT scanning facilitate identification of pericardial effusion and intracavitary and pericardial masses (Fig. 111-7).[226,256–258] Magnetic resonance imaging provides a global view of cardiac anatomy and plays an important role in the diagnosis and evaluation of both primary and secondary tumors of the heart, providing information about the location, extent, and attachment of the tumor.[150,213,259] Pericardiocentesis may afford prompt symptomatic relief from pericardial tamponade and often provides a definitive cytologic diagnosis.[227] Ultrasound and fluoroscopic guidance aid in safe pericardial catheter placement. (See Chap. 93.) The results of endomyocardial biopsy may contribute to the diagnosis in some cases.[261,262] Bone formation in metastatic osteogenic sarcoma occasionally may be visible radiographically.[263]

Treatment

Malignant pericardial effusion usually recurs rapidly after pericardiocentesis. Depending on the cytological type and radiosensitivity of the tumor, radiation to the cardiac area, with or without systemic chemotherapy, is the treatment of choice.[227,264] The heart can tolerate 20 to 40 Gy, beyond which the risk of radiation-induced pericardial, myocardial, and valvular[265,266] damage is increased. Patients with malignant pericardial effusions have responded to systemic chemotherapy[267] and to intrapericardial administration of fluorouracil, radioactive gold (nitrogen mustard), and tetracycline.[227,268] Persistent reaccumulation of fluid may require surgical creation of a pericardial "window."[218,269–272] A pericardial-pleural "window" has also been produced with a percutaneous balloon catheter, without surgery.[273] Patients with myocardial administration of fluorouracil, radioactive gold (nitrogen mustard), and tetracycline.[227,268] Persistent reaccumulation of fluid may require surgical creation of a pericardial "window."[218,269–272] A pericardial-pleural "window" has also been produced with a percutaneous and prolong survival,[248,256,274–277] as may chemotherapy in the occasional patient. Documentation of tumor regression is possible with two-dimensional echo imaging.[278,279] Magnetic resonance imaging plays an important role in characterizing the three-dimensional extent and attachment of cardiac tumors. This information is of particular importance in planning a surgical approach aimed at either complete removal or palliative debulking of a tumor mass.[213] (See Chap. 136.)

Special Considerations

Leukemia

Leukemic infiltration of the heart is usually found at postmortem study and generally is not suspected before death.[210,280] Cardiac infiltrates are found in a majority of the postmortem studies of patients with acute leukemia, with most having pericardial involvement. Cardiac symptoms are unusual. Chronic lymphocytic leukemia reportedly has caused myocardial infiltration in some patients,[281] as well as mitral valve dysfunction[282] and congestive heart failure.[283] Myocardial rupture has been reported as an early manifestation of acute myeloblastic leukemia.[284] Massive pericardial effusion, often hemorrhagic,[285] and pericardial tamponade[286] have been reported, although overt pericardial effusion is not common. Management consists of pericardiocentesis and chemotherapy; occasionally, surgical decompression of the pericardium is necessitated by recurrent tamponade.[286] Infective endocarditis, commonly fungal, may complicate acute leukemia. Because of advances in treatment and improved long-term remission in patients with acute lymphoblastic leukemia, complicating infective endocarditis has been managed by valve replacement.[287]

Malignant Lymphoma

Involvement of the heart in patients with malignant lymphoma is common, although it is infrequently detected before death. Cardiac or pericardial metastases occur with both Hodgkin's and non-Hodgkin's lymphoma and result from lymphatic and hematogenous spread as well as direct extension from other intrathoracic masses, resulting in predominantly epicardial and pericardial involvement.[6] Cardiac involvement may occasionally be the direct cause of death, but antemortem detection is infrequent.[288]

Acquired Immunodeficiency Syndrome and Heart Neoplasms

Two varieties of malignancies involving the heart have been described in patients with acquired immunodeficiency syndrome (AIDS): Kaposi's sarcoma and, less commonly, malignant lymphoma.[289,290] Involvement of the heart by Kaposi's sarcoma may be primary or part of a widely disseminated process. The epicardium is a common location with involvement of the underlying myocardium. Clinical cardiac dysfunction is minimal, although fatal pericardial tamponade has been reported.[291] (See also Chap. 107.)

Lymphomas, usually of high-grade malignant characteristics, occur with increased frequency in patients with AIDS and other immunosuppressed states.[292] Both primary and, more commonly, secondary lymphomas involve the heart either as a diffuse infiltrative process or as focal nodules in any layer of the heart. Clinical features may be absent in approximately 50 percent of patients. When present, they include cardiomegaly, pericardial effusion, congestive failure, and progressive heart block.[289] Echocardiography is useful and demonstrates pericardial effusion, mass lesions, and wall motion abnormalities. Transvenous biopsy can be useful in making the diagnosis.[293]

CARCINOID HEART DISEASE

While carcinoid tumors are never primary in the heart and only rarely metastasize to the heart and pericardium,[294] products of the tumor produce a distinctive endocardial and valvular pathological pattern.[295] Carcinoid tumors originally were described by Oberdorfer in 1907.[295] Tumors producing the carcinoid syndrome most commonly arise in the gastrointestinal tract, but they may also arise in the bronchus, biliary tract, pancreas, testis,[295] and ovary.[296] Appendiceal carcinoids, although common, rarely metastasize or produce the carcinoid syndrome. Ileal carcinoids, containing cytoplasmic granules that take up and reduce silver salts (argentaffinity), frequently metastasize to the liver and produce the carcinoid syndrome. These carcinoids contain a high concentration of 5-hydroxytryptamine (5-HT), which is excreted mainly as 5-hydroxyindoleacetic acid (5-HIAA) in the urine. Bronchial, pancreatic, and gastric carcinoid tumors differ morphologically and histochemically, have a worse prognosis, and metastasize more widely than do ileal tumors. They also produce 5-HT and excrete 5-HIAA in the urine; however, the clinical picture may be atypical. Carcinoid tumors of the rectum have a negative argentaffin reaction and are not associated with abnormalities of 5-HT synthesis or the carcinoid syndrome. Whereas they bear no morphologic or histochemical relation to the more typical carcinoid tumor, carcinomas of the bronchus, pancreas, or thyroid may occasionally secrete humoral substances that produce the carcinoid syndrome. In gastrointestinal carcinoid disease, the syndrome is produced by secretion of tumor products into the systemic circulation, which unfortunately delays its recognition until after liver metastases are present. The carcinoid syndrome, which results from the systemic effect of circulating vasoactive amines, consists of cutaneous flushing,[297] intestinal hypermobility, bronchial constriction, edema, and cardiac lesions.[298] Coronary artery spasm has been reported.[299]

Cardiac Lesions

Cardiac lesions are more commonly found in the right side of the heart than in the left. Left-sided involvement occurs with bronchial tumors, in the presence of an intraatrial communication,[300] or in the absence of such a communication when there is extensive right-sided heart involvement. Glistening grossly, white-yellow deposits are found on the pulmonary and tricuspid valves and, to varying degrees, on the right atrial and ventricular endocardium. Contraction of these deposits leads predominantly to pulmonary stenosis and tricuspid regurgitation and, occasionally, may produce a restrictive type of myopathy.[295] Mitral valve involvement may result in both stenosis and regurgitation. On microscopic examination (Fig. 111-8) the endocardial lesions consist of superficial deposits of fibrous tissue beneath a normal endothelium.[301,302] Metastatic lesions may be found in the myocardium. Both 5-HT and bradykinin have been implicated in the pathogenesis of the cardiac lesions.[295]

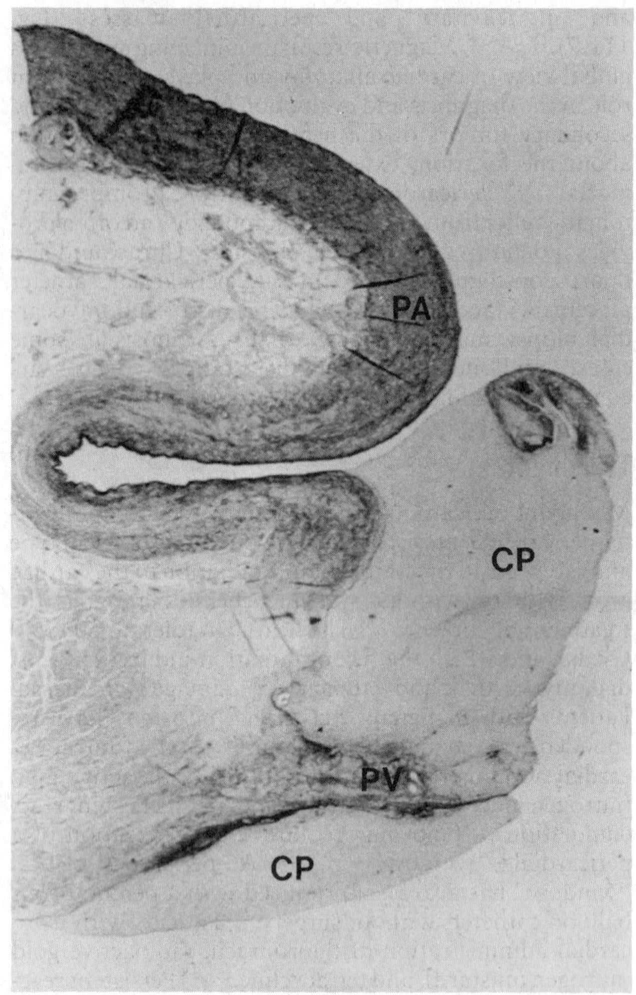

FIGURE 111-8 In carcinoid heart disease, there is either focal or diffuse plaquelike thickening of valvular and mural endocardium. When the pulmonary valve is involved, as in this patient, deposition of the fibrous tissue is almost exclusively on the arterial aspect of the valve cusps. PA, pulmonary artery; CP, carcinoid plaque; PV, pulmonary valve. (Movat Pentachrome × 10.)

Clinical Manifestations

Carcinoid heart disease[295] cannot be recognized clinically until cardiac murmurs and signs of right-sided heart failure develop, especially elevated jugular venous pressure with inspiratory augmentation of the *v* wave, which is characteristic of tricuspid regurgitation. A harsh, holosystolic, lower sternal border murmur with inspiratory accentuation is common, frequently followed by an early diastolic filling sound and diastolic rumble. A left upper sternal midsystolic murmur of pulmonary stenosis may or may not be identified separately. Murmurs of concomitant left-sided heart valvular involvement are rarely identified. There may be a parasternal heave and systolic pulsation of the liver, although enlargement and multinodular irregularity of the liver, ascites, and edema may be features of hepatic metastases without cardiac involvement.

Roentgenography of the chest will show the lung fields to be clear and the pulmonary trunk to be normal in size; the heart may be normal in size or show evidence of right ventricular and atrial enlargement. The electrocardiogram (ECG) may show evidence of right atrial enlargement, but right ventricular hypertrophy is rare. Echo imaging reveals right ventricular volume overload and abnormal right-sided valves. The tricuspid valve is typically thickened, retracted, and fixed in a semiopen position. Doming of the tricuspid valve may be present when the valve is predominantly stenotic.[303] Color-flow Doppler imaging will identify tricuspid valve regurgitation. The echographic changes are distinctive of carcinoid heart disease, are useful in following its progression, and may aid in detecting subclinical involvement.[295,303,304]

Transesophageal echocardiography enhances the diagnostic accuracy and, additionally, reveals thickening of the right atrial wall.[305]

Cardiac catheterization usually reveals predominant tricuspid regurgitation with a large, right atrial systolic wave as well as some degree of tricuspid diastolic gradient. Angiography demonstrates thickening and doming of both the pulmonary and tricuspid valves. Injection of contrast medium into the pulmonary artery provides evidence of pulmonary regurgitation, which is rarely appreciated clinically from auscultation of a separate diastolic murmur. A large transpulmonary valve gradient and marked elevation of right ventricular pressure are unusual. Low cardiac output with a wide arteriovenous oxygen difference usually dominates the picture by the time cardiac catheterization is performed.

Diagnosis of carcinoid heart disease depends on clinical recognition of the characteristic right-sided heart findings in the setting of systemic features of the carcinoid syndrome. The diagnosis is sometimes made only after the tricuspid valve has been replaced.[295] In cases of ileal carcinoid disease, clinical recognition of multinodular deformity, along with radionuclide or CT imaging of the enlarged liver, serves to identify the prerequisite metastases to this organ.[295] Carcinoid tumors that originate in the location that can release metabolic products outside the portal circulation do not share the latter characteristics. Urinary excretion of 5-HIAA is markedly elevated, and heavy diversion of tryptophan to this metabolic pathway may result in profound hypoproteinemia and nicotinamide deficiency (pellagra).

Treatment

Current chemotherapeutic programs are at least partially effective in some patients with extensive liver metastases. When hepatic metastases are present, removing the primary ileal lesion is indicated only if it is large and is producing mechanical obstruction. Occasionally, large hepatic metastases are few in number and resection may afford symptomatic relief. Catheter embolization may permit segmental hepatic ablation in selected patients. In contrast, removal of an extraportal primary tumor can result in rapid resolution of cardiac failure. Some of the manifestations of the carcinoid syndrome may be blocked by alpha-adrenergic blockers, serotonin antagonists,[295,306] and somatostatin analogues.[307,308]

Valve Replacement

Because heart failure is a frequent cause of disability and death when carcinoid heart disease complicates the carcinoid syndrome, tricuspid valve replacement and pulmonary valvotomy, with outflow tract enlargement if necessary, have been recommended when hemodynamically indicated.[295,296] Since the mechanism of valvular fibrosis in this entity is unknown, implantation of a bioprosthetic valve is generally not recommended, although use of tissue valves has been reported by several groups.[295,309] Carcinoid plaque extending onto bioprosthetic valves as early as 8 months after surgery has been reported.[295] Balloon valvuloplasty for tricuspid and pulmonary stenoses caused by carcinoid heart disease has been reported.[310]

Only a small number of patients have had valve surgery; however, selected patients have experienced clinical improvement even in the presence of extensive hepatic metastases, reflecting the slow progression and potential for long-term survival with this tumor.[295,311-313] Anesthetic considerations require an understanding of the effects of release of humoral substances. With proper care and planning, general anesthesia can be conducted with minimal risk.[295,307,314]

REFERENCES

1. Newman HA, Cardell AR, Pritchard RW: Intracardiac myxomas: Literature review and report of six cases, one successfully treated. *Am Surg* 1966; 33:219–230.
2. Peters MN, Hall RJ, Cooley DA, Leachman RD, Garcia E: The clinical syndrome of atrial myxoma. *JAMA* 1974; 230:695–701.
3. St John Sutton MG, Mercier LA, Giuliani ER, Lie JT: Atrial myxomas: A review of clinical experience in 40 patients. *Mayo Clin Proc* 1980; 55:371–376.
4. Pechacek LW, Gonzalez-Camid F, Hall RJ, Garcia E, de Castro CM, Leachman RD, et al: The echocardiographic spectrum of atrial myxoma: A ten-year experience. *Texas Heart Inst J* 1986; 13:179–195.
5. Markel ML, Waller BF, Armstrong WF: Cardiac myxoma. A review. *Medicine (Baltimore)* 1987; 66:114–125.
6. McAllister HA Jr: Primary tumors and cysts of the heart and pericardium. In: Harvey WP (ed): *Current Problems in Cardiology*. Chicago, Year Book Medical, 1979.
7. McAllister HA Jr, Fenoglio JJ Jr: *Tumors of the Cardiovascular System*. Washington, DC, Armed Forces Institute of Pathology, 1978.
8. Sandrasagra FA, Oliver WA, English TAH: Myxoma of the mitral valve. *Br Heart J* 1979; 42:221–223.
9. Gorlach, G, Hagel KJ, Mulch J, Scheld HH, Moosdorf R, Fitz H, et al: Myxoma of the aortic valve in a child. *J Cardiovasc Surg (Torino)* 1986; 27:679–680.
10. Devig PM, Clark TA, Aaron BL: Cardiac myxoma arising from the inferior vena cava. *Chest* 1980; 78:784–786.
11. Goldman BI, Frydman C, Harpaz N, Ryan SF, Loiterman D: Glandular cardiac myxomas. Histologic, immunohistochemical, and ultrastructural evidence of epithelial differentiation. *Cancer* 1987; 59:1767–1775.
12. Feldman PS, Horvath E, Kovacs K: An ultrastructural study of seven cardiac myxomas. *Cancer* 1977; 40:2216–2232.
13. Fine G: Primary tumors of the pericardium and heart. *Cardiovasc Clin* 1973; 5:207–238.
14. Wold LE, Lie JT: Scanning electron microscopy of intracardiac myxoma. *Mayo Clin Proc* 1981; 56:198–200.
15. Bashey RI, Nochumson S: Cardiac myxoma: Biochemical analyses and evidence for its neoplastic nature. *NY State J Med* 1979; 79:29–32.
16. Glasser SP, Bedynek JL, Hall RJ, Hopeman AR, Treasure RL, McAllister HA Jr, et al: Left atrial myxoma: Report of a case including hemodynamic, surgical, histologic and histochemical characteristics. *Am J Med* 1971; 50:113–122.
17. Dewald GW, Dahl R, Spurbeck JL, Carney JA, Gordon H: Chromosomally abnormal clones and nonrandom telomeric translocations in cardiac myxomas. *Mayo Clin Proc* 1987; 62:558–567.
18. Seidman JD, Berman JJ, Hitchcock CL, Becker RL, Mergner W, Moore W, et al: DNA analysis of cardiac myxomas: Flow cytometry and image analysis. *Hum Pathol* 1991; 22:494–500.
19. Kotylo PK, Kennedy JE, Waller BF, Sample RB: DNA analysis of atrial myxomas. *Chest* 1991; 99:1203–1207.
20. Read RC, White HJ, Murphy ML, Williams D, Sun CN, Flanagan WH: The malignant potentiality of left atrial myxoma. *J Thorac Cardiovasc Surg* 1974; 68:857–868.
21. Cleveland DC, Westaby S, Karp RB: Treatment of intra-atrial cardiac tumors. *JAMA* 1983; 249:2799–2802.
22. Desousa AL, Muller J, Campbell R, Batnitzky S, Rankin L: Atrial

myxoma: A review of the neurological complications, metastases, and recurrences. *J Neurol Neurosurg Psychiat* 1978; 41:1119–1124.
23. Pastakia B: Malignant atrial myxoma presenting as intercranial mass (letter). *Chest* 1979; 75:531–532.
24. Dashkoff N, Boersma RB, Nanda NC, Gramiak R, Andersen MN, Subramanian S: Bilateral atrial myxomas: Echocardiographic considerations. *Am J Med* 1978; 65:361–366.
25. Leonhardt ET, Kullenberg KP: Bilateral atrial myxomas with multiple arterial aneurysms—A syndrome mimicking polyarteritis nodosa. *Am J Med* 1977; 62:792–794.
26. Morgan DL, Palazola J, Reed W, Bell HH, Kindred LH, Beauchamp GD: Left heart myxomas. *Am J Cardiol* 1977; 40:611–614.
27. Steinke WE, Perry LW, Gold HR, McClanathan JE, Scott LP: Left atrial myxoma in a child. *Pediatrics* 1972; 49:580–589.
28. Balsara RK, Pelias AJ: Myxoma of right ventricle presenting as pulmonic stenosis in a neonate. *Chest* 1983; 83:145–146.
29. Davison ET, Mumford D, Zamah Q, Horowitz R: Left atrial myxoma in the elderly. Report of four patients over the age of 70 and review of the literature. *J Am Geriatr Soc* 1986; 34:229–233.
30. Burech DL, Teska DW, Haynes RE: Right atrial myxoma in a child. *Am J Dis Child* 1977; 131:750–752.
31. Powers JC, Falkoff M, Heinle RA, Nanda NC, Ong LS, Weiner RS, et al: Familial cardiac myxoma: Emphasis on unusual clinical manifestations. *J Thorac Cardiovasc Surg* 1979; 77:782–788.
32. Crawford FA Jr, Selby JH Jr, Watson D, Joransen J: Unusual aspects of atrial myxoma. *Ann Surg* 1978; 188:240–244.
33. Fyke FE III, Seward JB, Edwards WD, Miller FA, Reeder GS, Schattenberg TT, et al: Primary cardiac tumors: Experience with 30 consecutive patients since the introduction of two-dimensional echocardiography. *J Am Coll Cardiol* 1985; 5:1465–1473.
34. Graham SL, Sellers AL: Atrial myxoma with multiple myeloma. *Arch Intern Med* 1979; 139:116–117.
35. Burns ER, Schulman IC, Murphy MJ Jr: Hematologic manifestations and etiology of atrial myxoma. *Am J Med Sci* 1982; 284:17–22.
36. Vidaillet HJ Jr, Seward JB, Fyke FE III, Su WPD, Tajik AJ: "Syndrome myxoma": A subset of patients with cardiac myxoma associated with pigmented skin lesions and peripheral and endocrine neoplasms. *Br Heart J* 1987; 57:247–255.
37. Danoff A, Jormark S, Lorber D, Fleischer N: Adrenocortical micronodular dysplasia, cardiac myxomas, lentigines, and spindle cell tumors. Report of a kindred. *Arch Intern Med* 1987; 147:443–448.
38. Kaminsky ME, Ehlers K, Engle ME, Klein AA, Levin AR, Subramanian VA: Atrial myxoma mimicking a collagen disorder. *Chest* 1979; 75:93–95.
39. Boussen K, Moalla M, Blondeau P, Ayed HB, Lie JT: Embolization of cardiac myxomas masquerading as polyarteritis nodosa. *J Rheumatol* 1991; 18:283–285.
40. Rajpal RS, Leibsohn JA, Leikweg WG, Gross CM, Olinger GN, Rose HD, et al: Infected left atrial myxoma with bacteremia simulating infective endocarditis. *Arch Intern Med* 1979; 139:1176–1178.
41. Joseph P, Himmelstein DU, Mahowald JM, Stullman WS: Atrial myxoma infected with candida: First survival. *Chest* 1980; 78:340–343.
42. Schweiger MJ, Hafer JG Jr, Brown R, Gianelly RE: Spontaneous cure of infected left atrial myxoma following embolization. *Am Heart J* 1980; 99:630–634.
43. Flynn W, Garcia-Rinaldi R, Roehm JO Jr, Crawford ES: Surgical treatment of infected right atrial myxoma. *Ann Thorac Surg* 1979; 27:242–245.
44. Bradham RR, Gregorie HB Jr, Howell JS Jr, Rivers CF, Barnwell WH: Aortic obstruction from embolizing cardiac myxoma. *J S C Med Assoc* 1979; 75:7–10.
45. Yeoh NTL, Clegg JF: Massive embolism from cardiac myxoma. *Angiology* 1981; 32:819–821.
46. Chadda KD, Pochaczevsky R, Gupta PK, Lichstein E, Schwartz IS: Nonprolapsing atrial myxoma; Clinical, echocardiographic, and angiographic correlations. *Angiology* 1978; 29:179–186.
47. Tipton BK, Robertson JT, Robertson JH: Embolism to the central nervous system from cardiac myxoma: Report of two cases. *J Neurosurg* 1977; 47:937–940.
48. Thompson JR, Simmons CR: Arterial embolus: Manifestation of unsuspected myxoma. *JAMA* 1974; 228:864–865.
49. Roeltgen DP, Weimer GR, Patterson LF: Delayed neurologic complications of left atrial myxoma. *Neurology (NY)* 1981; 31:8–13.
50. Cogan DG, Wray SH: Vascular occlusions in the eye from cardiac myxomas. *Am J Ophthalmol* 1975; 80:396–403.
51. Tanabe J, Williams RL, Deithrich EB: Left atrial myxoma: Association with acute coronary embolization in an 11-year-old boy. *Pediatrics* 1979; 63:778–781.
52. Cheitlin MD, McAllister HA Jr, de Castro CM: Myocardial infarction without atherosclerosis. *JAMA* 1975; 231:951–959.
53. Stevens LH, Hormuth DA, Schmidt PE, Atkins S, Fehrenbacher JW: Left atrial myxoma: Pulmonary infarction caused by pulmonary venous occlusion. *Ann Thorac Surg* 1987; 43:215–217.
54. Harvey WP: Clinical aspects of cardiac tumors. *Am J Cardiol* 1968; 21:328–343.
55. Martinez-Lopez JI: Sounds of the heart in diastole. *Am J Cardiol* 1974; 34:594–601.
56. Goodwin JF: The spectrum of cardiac tumors. *Am J Cardiol* 1968; 21:307–314.
57. Cecil MP, Silverman ME: Tricuspid valve honk due to pulmonary hypertension secondary to left atrial myxoma. *Am J Cardiol* 1991; 67:321.
58. Sharratt GP, Grover ML, Monro JL: Calcified left atrial myxoma with floppy mitral valve. *Br Heart J* 1979; 42:608–610.
59. Case Records of the Massachusetts General Hospital, Weekly Clinicopathological Exercises: Case 42-1973. *N Eng J Med* 1973; 289:853–859.
60. Reeder GS, Khandheria BK, Seward JB, Tajik AJ: Transesophageal echocardiography and cardiac masses. *Mayo Clin Proc* 1991; 66:1101–1109.
61. Obeid AI, Marvasti M, Parker F, Rosenberg J: Comparison of transthoracic and transesophageal echocardiography in diagnosis of left atrial myxoma. *Am J Cardiol* 1989; 63:1006–1008.
62. Mugge A, Daniel WG, Haverich A, Lichtlen PR: Diagnosis of noninfective cardiac mass lesions by two-dimensional echocardiography: Comparison of the transthoracic and transesophageal approaches. *Circulation* 1991; 83:70–78.
63. Vargas-Barron J, Romero-Cardenas A, Villegas M, Keirns C, Gomez-Jaume A, Delong R, et al: Transthoracic and transesophageal echocardiographic diagnosis of myxomas in the four cardiac cavities. *Am Heart J* 1991; 121:931–933.
64. O'Neil MB Jr, Grehl TM, Hurley EJ: Cardial myxomas: A clinical diagnostic challenge. *Am J Surg* 1979; 138:68–76.
65. Meller J, Teichholz LE, Pichard AD, Matta R, Litwak R, Herman MV: Left ventricular myxoma: Echocardiographic diagnosis and review of the literature. *Am J Med* 1977; 63:816–823.
66. Panidis IP, Mintz GS, McAllister M: Hemodynamic consequences of left atrial myxomas as assessed by Doppler ultrasound. *Am Heart J* 1986; 111:927–931.
67. Case Records of the Massachusetts General Hospital, Weekly Clinicopathological Exercises: Case 14-1978. *N Engl J Med* 1978; 298:834.
68. Meyers SN, Shapiro SE, Barresi V, DeBoer AA, Pavel DI, Gracey DR, et al: Right atrial myxoma with right to left shunting and mitral valve prolapse. *Am J Med* 1977; 62:308–314.
69. Bateman TM, Sethna DH, Whiting JS, Chaux A, Berman DS, Forrester JS: Comprehensive noninvasive evaluation of left atrial myxomas using cardiac cine-computed tomography. *J Am Coll Cardiol* 1987; 9:1180–1183.
70. Seifert P, Chomka EV, Stagl R, Swarner D, Brundage BH, Levitsky S: Application of the cine computed tomographic scan for precise localization of the origin of an atrial myxoma: Surgical implications. *Ann Thorac Surg* 1986; 42:469–470.
71. Pflugfelder PW, Wisenberg G, Boughner DR: Detection of atrial myxoma by magnetic resonance imaging. *Am J Cardiol* 1985; 55:242–243.
72. Go RT, O'Donnell JK, Underwood DA, Feiglin DH, Salcedo EE, Pantaja M, et al: Comparison of gated cardiac MRI and 2D echocardiography of intracardiac neoplasms. *Am J Roentgenol* 1985; 145:21–25.
73. Freedberg RS, Kronzon I, Rumancik WM, Liebeskind D: The contribution of magnetic resonance imaging to the evaluation of intracardiac tumors diagnosed by echocardiography. *Circulation* 1988; 77:96–103.
74. Sung RJ, Ghahramani AR, Mallon SM, Richter SE, Sommer LS, Gottlieb S, et al: Hemodynamic features of prolapsing and nonprolapsing left atrial myxoma. *Circulation* 1975; 51:342–349.

75. Ognibene AJ, Nelson WP: Atrial myxoma: Comments on hemodynamic alterations—Report of a case. *Dis Chest* 1967; 52:699–701.
76. Hamer JPM, Nieveen J, Bergstra A, Blickman JR, Homan Van der Heide JN: Left atrial myxoma moving from right atrium to left ventricle. *Acta Med Scand* 1979; 205:527–534.
77. Pindyck F, Peirce EC II, Baron MG, Lukban SB: Embolization of left atrial myxoma after transseptal cardiac catheterization. *Am J Cardiol* 1972; 30:569–571.
78. Shapiro MR, Cohen MV, Grose R, Spindola-Franco H: Diagnosis of left atrial myxoma by coronary angiography eight years following open mitral commissurotomy. *Am Heart J* 1983; 105:325–327.
79. Chow W-H, Chow T-C, Tai Y-T, Yip ASB, Cheung K-L: Angiographic visualization of "tumour vascularity" in atrial myxoma. *Eur Heart J* 1991; 12:79–82.
80. Stewart JA, Warnica JW, Kirk ME, Winsberg F: Left atrial myxoma: False negative echocardiographic findings in a tumor demonstrated by coronary arteriography. *Am Heart J* 1979; 98:228–232.
81. Bochna AJ, Falicov RE: Diagnosis of intracardiac thrombi in mitral stenosis and left ventricular dysfunction: Use of selective coronary arteriography. *Arch Intern Med* 1980; 140:759–762.
82. Huston KA, Combs JJ Jr, Lie JT, Giuliani ER: Left atrial myxoma simulating peripheral vasculitis. *Mayo Clin Proc* 1978; 53:752–756.
83. Lortscher RH, Toews WH, Nora JJ, Wolfe RR, Spangler RD: Left atrial myxoma presenting as rheumatic fever. *Chest* 1974; 66:302–303.
84. Neches WH, Park SC, Lenox CC, Zuberbuhler JR, Siewers RD: Left atrial myxoma: Clinical presentation suggesting acute myocarditis. *JAMA* 1974; 229:1906–1907.
85. Warda M, Garcia J, Pechacek LW, Massumkhani A, Hall RJ: Auscultatory and echocardiographic features of mobile left atrial thrombus. *J Am Coll Cardiol* 1985; 5:379–382.
86. Roguin N, Amikam S, Riss E: Prolapsing right atrial myxoma: Clinical and haemodynamic considerations. *Br Heart J* 1977; 39:577–580.
87. Hickie JB, Gibson H, Windsor HM: "The wrecking ball": Right atrial myxoma. *Med J Aust* 1970; 2:82–86.
88. Vidne B, Atsmon A, Aygen M, Levy MJ: Right atrial myxoma: Case report and review of the literature. *Isr J Med Sci* 1971; 7:1196–2000.
89. Muroff LR, Johnson PM: Right atrial myxoma presenting as nonresolving pulmonary emboli: Case report. *J Nucl Med* 1976; 17:8920–8922.
90. Siggillino JJ, Crawley CJ, Clauss RH, Reed GE, Tice DA: Myxoma of the right atrium with polycythemia. *Arch Intern Med* 1963; 111:178–183.
91. Natarajan P, Vijayanagar RR, Eckstein PF, Bognolo DA: Right atrial myxoma with atrial septal defect: A case report and review of the literature. *Cathet Cardiovasc Diagn* 1982; 8:267–272.
92. Park JM, Garcia RR, Patrick JK, Waagner D, Anuras S: Right atrial myxoma with a nonembolic intestinal manifestation. *Pediatr Cardiol* 1990; 11:164–166.
93. Massumi R: Bedside diagnosis of right heart myxomas through detection of palpable tumor shocks and audible plops. *Am Heart J* 1983; 105:303–310.
94. Lyons SV, McCord J, Smith S: Asymptomatic giant right atrial myxoma: Role of transesophageal echocardiography in management. *Am Heart J* 1991; 121:1555–1558.
95. Smith ST, Hautamaki K, Lewis JW Jr, Serwin J, Alam M: Transthoracic and transesophageal echocardiography in the diagnosis and surgical management of right atrial myxoma. *Chest* 1991; 100:575–576.
96. Albers GW, Avalos SM, Weinrich M: Left ventricular tumor masquerading as multiple sclerosis. *Arch Neurol* 1987; 44:779–780.
97. Wrisley D, Rosenberg J, Giambartolomei A, Levy I, Turiello C, Antonini T: Left ventricular myxoma discovered incidentally by echocardiography. *Am Heart J* 1991; 121:1554–1555.
98. Camesas AM, Lichtstein E, Kramer J, Liebeskind D, Kronzon I, Tyras D, et al: Complementary use of two-dimensional echocardiography and magnetic resonance imaging in the diagnosis of ventricular myxoma. *Am Heart J* 1987; 114:440–442.
99. Hada Y, Wolfe C, Murray GF, Craige E: Right ventricular myxoma. Case report and review of phonocardiographic and auscultatory manifestations. *Am Heart J* 1980; 100:871–877.
100. Gonzalez A, Altieri PI, Marquez E, Cox RA, Castillo M: Massive pulmonary embolism associated with a right ventricular myxoma. *Am J Med* 1980; 69:795–798.
101. Nass PC, Neimeyer MG, Brutel-de-la-Riviere A, Brune DF, Plokker HW: Left atrial and right ventricular cardiac myxoma. A case report. *Eur J Cardiothorac Surg* 1989; 3:468–470.
102. Adachi K, Tanaka H, Toshima H, Morimatsu M: Right atrial angiosarcoma diagnosed by cardiac biopsy. *Am Heart J* 1988; 115:482–485.
103. Betancourt B, Defendini EA, Johnson C, De Jesus M, Pavia-Villamil A, Cruz AD: Severe right ventricular outflow tract obstruction caused by an intracavitary cardiac neurilemoma: Successful surgical removal and postoperative diagnosis. *Chest* 1979; 75:522–524.
104. Cooley DA: Surgical management of cardiac tumors. In: Kapoor AS, Reynolds RD (eds): *Cancer and the Heart*. New York, Springer-Verlag, 1986: 126–134.
105. Murphy MC, Sweeney MS, Putnam JB Jr, Walker WE, Frazier OH, Ott DA, et al: Surgical treatment of cardiac tumors: A 25-year experience. *Ann Thorac Surg* 1990; 49:612–618.
106. Casarotto D, Bortolotti U, Russo R, et al: Surgical removal of a left atrial myxoma during pregnancy. *Chest* 1979; 75: 390–392.
107. Trimakas AP, Maxwell KD, Berkay S: Fetal monitoring during cardiopulmonary bypass for removal of a left atrial myxoma during pregnancy. *Johns Hopkins Med J* 1979; 144:156–160.
108. Bateman TM, Gray RJ, Raymond MJ, Chaux A, Czer LS, Matloff JM: Arrhythmias and conduction disturbances following cardiac operation for the removal of left atrial myxomas. *J Thorac Cardiovasc Surg* 1983; 86:601–607.
109. Mahoney L, Schieken RM, Doty D: Cardiac rhabdomyomas simulating pulmonic stenosis. *Cathet Cardiovasc Diagn* 1979; 5:385–388.
110. Fenoglio JJ Jr, McAllister HA Jr, Ferrans VJ: Cardiac rhabdomyoma: A clinicopathologic and electron microscopic study. *Am J Cardiol* 1976; 38:241–251.
111. Howanitz EP, Teske DW, Qualman SJ, Finck S, Kilman JW: Pedunculated left ventricular rhabdomyoma. *Ann Thorac Surg* 1986; 41:443–445.
112. Spooner EW, Farina MA, Shaher RM, Foster ED: Left ventricular rhabdomyoma causing subaortic stenosis—The two-dimensional echocardiographic appearance. *Pediatr Cardiol* 1982; 2:67–71.
113. Guereta LG, Burgueros M, Elorza MD, Alix AG, Benito F, Gamallo C: Cardiac rhabdomyoma presenting as fetal hydrops. *Pediatr Cardiol* 1986; 7:171–174.
114. Kuehl KS, Perry LW, Chandra R, Scott LP III: Left ventricular rhabdomyoma: A rare cause of subaortic stenosis in the newborn infant. *Pediatrics* 1970; 46:464–468.
115. Violette EJ, Hardin NJ, McQuillen EN: Sudden unexpected death due to asymptomatic cardiac rhabdomyoma. *J Forensic Sci* 1981; 26:599–604.
116. Pillai R, Kharma N, Brom AG, Becker AE: Mitral valve origin of pedunculated rhabdomyomas causing subaortic stenosis. *Am J Cardiol* 1991; 67:663–664.
117. Milner S, Abramowitz JA, Levin SE: Rhabdomyoma of the heart in a newborn infant: Diagnosis by echocardiography. *Br Heart J* 1980; 44:224–227.
118. Duncan WJ, Rowe RD, Freedom RM, Izukawa T, Olley PM: Space-occupying lesions of the myocardium: Role of two-dimensional echocardiography in detection of cardiac tumors in children. *Am Heart J* 1982; 104:780–785.
119. Marx GR, Bierman FZ, Matthews E, Williams R: Two-dimensional echocardiographic diagnosis of intracardiac masses in infancy. *J Am Coll Cardiol* 1984; 3:827–832.
120. Boxer RA, LaCorte MA, Singh S, Shapiro J, Schiller M, Goldman M, et al: Diagnosis of cardiac tumors in infants by magnetic resonance imaging. *Am J Cardiol* 1985; 56:831–832.
121. Boxer RA, Seidman S, Singh S, LaCorte MA, Pek H, Goldman M, et al: Congenital intracardiac rhabdomyoma: Prenatal detection by echocardiography, perinatal management, and surgical treatment. *Am J Perinatol* 1986; 3:303–305.
122. Ott DA, Garson A, Cooley DA, McNamara D: Definitive operation for refractory cardiac tachyarrhythmia in children. *J Thorac Cardiovasc Surg* 1985; 90:681–689.
123. Garson A Jr, Smith RT Jr, Moak JP, Kearney DL, Hawkins EP, Titus JL, et al: Incessant ventricular tachycardia in infants: Myocardial hamartomas and surgical cure. *J Am Coll Cardiol* 1987; 10:619–626.

124. Kearney DL, Titus JL, Hawkins EP, Ott DA, Garson A Jr: Pathologic features of myocardial hamartomas causing childhood tachyarrhythmias. *Circulation* 1987; 75:705–710.
125. Reece IJ, Cooley DA, Frazier OH, Hallman GL, Powers PL, Montero CG: Cardiac tumors: Clinical spectrum and prognosis of lesions other than classical benign myxoma in 20 patients. *J Thorac Cardiovasc Surg* 1984; 88:439–446.
126. Reul GJ Jr, Howell JF, Rubio PA, Petersen PK: Successful partial excision of an intramural fibroma of the left ventricle. *Am J Cardiol* 1975; 36:262–265.
127. Williams DB, Danielson GK, McGoon DC, Feldt RH, Edwards WD: Cardiac fibroma. Long-term survival after excision. *J Thorac Cardiovasc Surg* 1982; 84:230–236.
128. Biancaniello TM, Meyer RA, Gaum WE, Kaplan S: Primary benign intramural ventricular tumors in children: Pre- and postoperative electrocardiographic, echocardiographic, and angiocardiographic evaluation. *Am Heart J* 1982; 103:852–857.
129. Jamieson SW, Gaudiani VA, Reitz BA, Oyer PE, Stinson EB, Shumway NE: Operative treatment of an unresectable tumor of the left ventricle. *J Thorac Cardiovasc Surg* 1981; 81:797–799.
130. Gorton ME, Soltanzadeh H: Mitral valve fibroelastoma. *Ann Thorac Surg* 1989; 47:605–607.
131. Israel DH, Sherman W, Ambrose JA, Sharma S, Harpaz N, Robbins M: Dynamic coronary ostial obstruction due to papillary fibroelastoma leading to myocardial ischemia and infarction. *Am J Cardiol* 1991; 67:104–105.
132. Anderson KR, Fiddler GI, Lie JT: Congenital papillary tumor of the tricuspid valve: An unusual cause of right ventricular outflow obstruction in a neonate with trisomy E. *Mayo Clin Proc* 1977; 52:665–669.
133. Kasarskis EJ, O'Connor W, Earle G: Embolic stroke from cardiac papillary fibroelastomas. *Stroke* 1988; 19:1171–1173.
134. Cha SD, Incarvito J, Chang KS, Maranhao V, Gooch AS: Giant Lambl's excrescences of papillary muscle and aortic valve: Echocardiographic, angiographic, and pathologic findings. *Clin Cardiol* 1981; 4:51–54.
135. Fitzgerald D, Gaffney P, Dervan P, Doyle CT, Horgan J, Nelligan M: Giant Lambl's excrescence presenting as a peripheral embolus. *Chest* 1982; 81:516–517.
136. de Virgilio C, Dubrow TJ, Robertson JM, Siegel S, Ginzton L, Nussmeier M, et al: Detection of multiple cardiac papillary fibroelastomas using transesophageal echocardiography. *Ann Thorac Surg* 1989; 48:119–121.
137. Schwinger ME, Katz E, Rotterdam H, Slater J, Weiss EC, Kronzon I: Right atrial papillary fibroelastoma: Diagnosis by transthoracic and transesophageal echocardiography and percutaneous transvenous biopsy. *Am Heart J* 1989; 118:1047–1050.
138. Wolfe JT III, Finck SJ, Safford RE, Persellin ST: Tricuspid valve papillary fibroelastoma: Echocardiographic characterization. *Ann Thorac Surg* 1991; 51:116–118.
139. Moulton AL, Jaretzki A III, Bowman FO Jr, Silverstein EF, Bregman D: Massive lipoma of heart. *NY State J Med* 1976; 76:1820–1825.
140. Shumacker HB Jr, Leshnower AC: Extracavitary lipoma of the heart: Operative resection. *Ann Thorac Surg* 1974; 18: 411–414.
141. Barberger-Gateau P, Paquet M, Desaulniers D, Chenard J: Fibrolipoma of the mitral valve in a child: Clinical and echocardiographic features. *Circulation* 1978; 58:955–958.
142. Leatherman L, Leachman RD, Hallman GL, Cooley DA: Cyst of the mitral valve. *Am J Cardiol* 1968; 21:428–430.
143. Tuna IC, Julsrud PR, Click RL, Tazelaar HD, Bresnahan DR, Danielson GK: Tissue characterization of an unusual right atrial mass by magnetic resonance imaging. *Mayo Clin Proc* 1991; 66:498–501.
144. McNamara RF, Taylor AE, Panner BJ: Superior vena caval obstruction by lipomatous hypertrophy of the right atrium. *Clin Cardiol* 1987; 10:609–610.
145. Tschirkov A, Stegaru B: Lipomatous hypertrophy of interatrial septum presenting as recurring pericardial effusion and mistaken for constrictive pericarditis. *Thorac Cardiovasc Surg* 1979; 27:400–403.
146. Voigt J, Agdal N: Lipomatous infiltration of the heart. An uncommon cause of sudden, unexpected death in a young man. *Arch Pathol Lab Med* 1982; 106:497–498.
147. Kindman LA, Wright A, Tye T, Seale W, Appleton C: Lipomatous hypertrophy of the interatrial septum: Characterization by transesophageal and transthoracic echocardiography, magnetic resonance imaging, and computed tomography. *J Am Soc Echocardiogr* 1988; 1:450–454.
148. Applegate PM, Tajik AJ, Ehman RL, Julsrud PR, Miller FA Jr: Two-dimensional echocardiographic and magnetic resonance imaging observations in massive lipomatous hypertrophy of the atrial septum. *Am J Cardiol* 1987; 59:489–491.
149. Fisher MS, Edmonds PR: Lipomatous hypertrophy of the interatrial septum. Diagnosis by magnetic resonance imaging. *J Comput Tomogr* 1988; 12:267–269.
150. Lund JT, Ehman RL, Julsrud PR, Sinak LJ, Tajik AJ: Cardiac masses: Assessment by MR imaging. *AJR* 1989; 152:469–473.
151. Stone GW, O'Kell RT, Good TH, Hartzler GO: Lipomatous hypertrophy of the interatrial septum: Diagnosis by percutaneous transvenous biopsy. *Am Heart J* 1990; 119:406–408.
152. Manion WC, Nelson WP, Hall RJ, Brierty PE: Benign tumor of the heart causing complete heart block. *Am Heart J* 1972; 83:535–542.
153. Fenoglio JJ, Jacobs DW, McAllister HA Jr: Mesothelioma of the atrioventricular node. *Cancer* 1977; 40:721–727.
154. Paulson SM, Kristensen IB: So-called mesothelioma of the atrioventricular node. *J Submicrosc Cytol* 1981; 13:667–674.
155. James TN, Galakhov I: De subitaneis mortibus. XXVI. Fatal electrical instability of the heart associated with benign congenital polycystic tumor of the atrioventricular node. *Circulation* 1977; 6:667–678.
156. Hellemans IM, van Hemel NM, Kooyman CA: Atrioventricular block in childhood caused by mesothelioma. *PACE* 1981; 4:216–220.
157. Evans DW, Stovin PG: Fatal heart block due to mesothelioma of the atrioventricular node. *Br Heart J* 1986; 56:572–574.
158. Raabe DS, Fischer JC, Brandt RL: Cavernous hemangioma of the right atrium: Presumptive diagnosis by coronary angiography. *Cathet Cardiovasc Diagn* 1976; 2:389–395.
159. Boden WE, Funk EJ, Carleton RA, Benham I, Khan AH, Lasser A, et al: Left ventricular hemangioma masquerading as *Mycoplasma* pericarditis. *Am Heart J* 1983; 106:771–774.
160. Palmer TE, Tresch DD, Bonchek LI: Spontaneous resolution of a large cavernous hemangioma of the heart. *Am J Cardiol* 1986; 58:184–185.
161. Trout HH, McAllister HA Jr, Giordano JM, Rich NM: Vascular malformations. *Surgery* 1985; 97:36–41.
162. Grigg LE, Downey W, Tatoulis J, Hunt D: Benign congenital intracardiac thyroid and polycystic tumor causing right ventricular outflow tract obstruction and conduction disturbance. *J Am Coll Cardiol* 1987; 9:225–227.
163. Hui G, McAllister HA Jr, Angelini P: Left atrial paraganglioma: Report of a case and review of the literature. *Am Heart J* 1987; 113:1230–1234.
164. Saad MF, Frazier OH, Hickey RC, Samaan NA: Intrapericardial pheochromocytoma. *Am J Med* 1983; 75:371–376.
165. Conti VR, Saydjari R, Amparo EG: Paraganglioma of the heart. The value of magnetic resonance imaging in the preoperative evaluation. *Chest* 1986; 90:604–606.
166. Fisher MR, Higgins CB, Andereck W: Magnetic resonance imaging of an intrapericardial pheochromocytoma. *J Comput Assist Tomogr* 1985; 9:1103–1105.
167. Cooley DA, Reardon MJ, Frazier OH, Angelini P: Human cardiac explantation and autotransplantation: Application in a patient with a large cardiac pheochromocytoma. *Texas Heart Inst J* 1985; 12:171–176.
168. Panella JS, Paige ML, Victor TA, Semerdjian RA, Hueter DC: Angiosarcoma of the heart. Diagnosis by echocardiography. *Chest* 1979; 76:221–223.
169. Bjerregaard P, Baandrup U: Haemangioendotheliosarcoma of the heart. Diagnosis and treatment. *Br Heart J* 1979; 42:734–737.
170. Janigan DT, Husain A, Robinson NA: Cardiac angiosarcomas. A review and a case report. *Cancer* 1986; 57:852–859.
171. Marni E, Pedroni E, Magrini U, Mariani P, Richichi I, Vigano M: Angiosarcoma of the heart: Report of a case in a 9-year-old boy. *Med Pediatr Oncol* 1983; 11:336–338.
172. Miller HI, Keren G, Shapira I, Ghosh P, Vidne B: Primary angiosarcoma of the heart detected by two-dimensional echocardiography. *Isr J Med Sci* 1986; 22:900–902.
173. Wakely PE Jr: Angiosarcoma of the heart in an adolescent. *Arch Pathol Lab Med* 1987; 11:472–475.
174. Schmid KW, Thurner J Jr, Gruenewald K: Hemangiopericytoma of the heart following treatment of Hodgkin's disease. A case report. *Virchows Arch [A]* 1987; 411:485–488.

175. Schmaltz AA, Apitz J: Primary rhabdomyosarcoma of the heart. *Pediatr Cardiol* 1982; 2:73–75.
176. Nagata K, Irie K, Morimatsu M, Nakashima T, Eriguchi N, Koga M: Rhabdomyosarcoma of the right ventricle. *Acta Pathol Jpn* 1982; 32:843–849.
177. Sholler GF, Hawker RE, Nunn GR, Bale P, Bergin M: Primary left ventricular rhabdomyosarcoma in a child: Noninvasive assessment and successful resection of a rare tumor. *J Thorac Cardiovasc Surg* 1987; 93:465–468.
178. Schwartz JE, Schwartz GP, Judson PL, Siebel JE Jr, Trumbull HR: Complete resection of a primary cardiac rhabdomyosarcoma: Case report, review of the literature, and management recommendations. *Cardiovasc Dis Bull Texas Heart Inst* 1979; 6:413–424.
179. Cafferty LL, Epstein JI: Primary liposarcoma of the right atrium. *Hum Pathol* 1987; 18:408–410.
180. Cairns P, Butany J, Fulop J, Rakowski H, Hassaram S: Cardiac presentation of non-Hodgkin's lymphoma. *Arch Pathol Lab* 1987; 111:80–83.
181. Scully RE, Mark EJ, McNeely WF, McNeely BU: Case records of the Massachusetts General Hospital: Case 22-1987. *N Engl J Med* 1987; 316:1394–1404.
182. Minamiji K, Yamasaki T, Nakao M, Furomoto M, Yoshida Y: 201 Tl and 67 Ga uptake in malignant fibrous histiocytoma of the heart. *Chest* 1986; 89:303–306.
183. Laya MF, Mailliard JA, Bewtra C, Levin HS: Malignant fibrous histiocytoma of the heart. A case report and review of the literature. *Cancer* 1987; 59:1026–1031.
184. Holtzman E, Schiby G, Segal P, Priel I: Malignant fibrous histiocytoma complicating mitral valve replacement. *J Am Coll Cardiol* 1986; 7:956–960.
185. Frandsen NE, Andersen G, Nielsen JR: Malignant mesenchymoma of the heart presenting as mitral stenosis. *Acta Med Scand* 1981; 209:235–237.
186. Donovan VM, Summer W, Hutchins GM: Left atrial leiomyosarcoma: Manifestation as unexplained pulmonary vascular disease. *Arch Intern Med* 1982; 142:1923–1925.
187. Terashima K, Aoyama K, Nihei K, Nito T, Imai Y, Takahashi K, et al: Malignant fibrous histiocytoma of the heart. *Cancer* 1983; 52:1919–1926.
188. Ceretto WJ, Miller ML, Shea PM, Gregory CW, Vieweg WV: Malignant mesenchymoma obstructing the right ventricular outflow tract. *Am Heart J* 1981; 101:114–115.
189. Mori K, Itoh H, Kanaya H, Onoe T, Ohka T, Lin S, et al: Malignant fibrous histiocytoma of the heart. *Jpn Circ J* 1983; 47:188–193.
190. Dein JR, Frist WH, Stinson EB, Miller DC, Baldwin JC, Oyer PE, et al: Primary cardiac neoplasms. Early and late results of surgical treatment in 42 patients. *J Thorac Cardiovasc Surg* 1987; 93: 502–511.
191. Putman JB Jr, Sweeney MS, Colon R, Lanza LA, Frazier OH, Cooley DA: Primary cardiac sarcomas. *Ann Thorac Surg* 1991; 51:906–910.
192. Rienmüller R, Tiling R: MR and CT for detection of cardiac tumors. *Thorac Cardiovasc Surg* 1990; 38:168–172.
193. Mora F, Mindich BP, Guarino T, Goldman ME: Improved surgical approach to cardiac tumors with intraoperative two-dimensional echocardiography. *Chest* 1987; 91:142–144.
194. Szucs RA, Rehr RB, Yanovich S, Tatum JL: Magnetic resonance imaging of cardiac rhabdomyosarcoma: Quantifying the response to chemotherapy. *Cancer* 1991; 67:2066–2070.
195. Horn M, Phebus C, Blatt J: Cancer chemotherapy after solid organ transplantation. *Cancer* 1990; 66:1468–1471.
196. Feigin DS, Fenoglio JJ, McAllister HA, Madewell JR: Pericardial cysts: A radiologic-pathologic correlation and review. *Radiology* 1977; 125:15–20.
197. Stoller JK, Shaw C, Matthay RA: Enlarging, atypically located pericardial cyst. Recent experience and literature review. *Chest* 1986; 89:402–406.
198. Pezzano A, Belloni A, Faletra F, Binaghi G, Colli A, Rovelli F: Value of two-dimensional echocardiography in the diagnosis of pericardial cysts. *Eur Heart J* 1983; 4:238–246.
199. De Geeter B, Kretz JG, Nisand I, Eisenmann B, Kieny MT, Kieny R: Intrapericardial teratoma in a newborn infant: Use of fetal echocardiography. *Ann Thorac Surg* 1983; 35:664–666.
200. Reynolds JL, Donahue JK, Pearce CW: Intrapericardial teratoma: A cause of acute pericardial effusion in infancy. *Pediatrics* 1969; 43:71–78.
201. MacDonald S, Fay JE, Lynn RM: Intrapericardial teratoma: A continuing challenge. *Can J Surg* 1983; 26:81–82.
202. Maeta H, Hiyama T, Okamura K, Iriyama T, Yamaguchi T, Tamura T, et al: Successful excision of intracardiac teratoma. *J Thorac Cardiovasc Surg* 1982; 83:909–913.
203. Costas C, Williams RL, Fortune RL: Intracardiac teratoma in an infant. *Pediatr Cardiol* 1986; 7:179–181.
204. Sytman AL, MacAlpin RN: Primary pericardial mesothelioma: Report of two cases and review of the literature. *Am Heart J* 1971; 81:760–769.
205. Yilling FP, Schlant RC, Hertzler GL, Krzyaniak R: Pericardial mesothelioma. *Chest* 1982; 81:520–523.
206. Mason MS, Wheeler JR, Gregory RT, Gayle RG: Primary tumors of the aorta: Report of a case and review of the literature. *Oncology* 1982; 39:167–172.
207. Borislow DS, Floyd WL, Sane DC: Primary aortic sarcoma mimicking aortic dissection. *Am J Cardiol* 1989; 64:549–551.
208. Prichard RW: Tumors of the heart: Review of the subject and report of one hundred and fifty cases. *Arch Pathol* 1951; 51:98–128.
209. DeLoach JF, Haynes JW: Secondary tumors of heart and pericardium: Review of the subject and report of one hundred thirty-seven cases. *Arch Intern Med* 1953; 91:224–249.
210. Kutalek SP, Panidis IP, Kotler MN, Mintz GS, Carver J, Ross JJ: Metastatic tumors of the heart detected by two-dimensional echocardiography. *Am Heart J* 1985; 109:343–349.
211. Lockwood WB, Broghamer WL Jr: The changing prevalence of secondary cardiac neoplasms as related to cancer therapy. *Cancer* 1980; 45:2659–2662.
212. McDonnell PJ, Mann RB, Bulkley BH: Involvement of the heart by malignant lymphoma: A clinicopathologic study. *Cancer* 1982; 4:944–951.
213. Emmot WW, Vacek JL, Agee K, Moran J, Dunn MI: Metastatic malignant melanoma presenting clinically as obstruction of the right ventricular inflow and outflow tracts. Characterization by magnetic resonance imaging. *Chest* 1987; 92:362–364.
214. Weg IL, Mehra S, Azueta V, Rosner F: Cardiac metastasis from adenocarcinoma of the lung. Echocardiographic-pathologic correlation. *Am J Med* 1986; 80:108–112.
215. Kline IK: Cardiac lymphatic involvement by metastatic tumor. *Cancer* 1972; 29:799–808.
216. Kadir S, Coulam CM: Intracaval extension of renal cell carcinoma. *Cardiovasc Intervent Radiol* 1980; 3:180–183.
217. Onuigbo WI: Direct extension of cancer between pulmonary veins and the left atrium. *Chest* 1972; 62:444–446.
218. el Allaf D, Burette R, Pierard L, Limet R: Cardiac tamponade as the first manifestation of cardiothoracic malignancy: A study of 10 cases. *Eur Heart J* 1986; 7:247–253.
219. Hernandez-Lopez E, Chahine RA: Simultaneous electrical and mechanical alternans in pericardial effusion: Echocardiographic documentation. *Arch Intern Med* 1980; 140:840–842.
220. Conrad SA, Byrnes TJ: Diastolic collapse of the left and right ventricles in cardiac tamponade. *Am Heart J* 1988; 115:475–478.
221. Levine MJ, Lorell BH, Diver DJ, Come PC: Implications of echocardiographically assisted diagnosis of pericardial tamponade in contemporary medical patients: Detection before hemodynamic embarrassment. *J Am Coll Cardiol* 1991; 17:59–65.
222. Himelman RB, Kircher B, Rockey DC, Schiller NB: Inferior vena cava plethora with blunted respiratory response: A sensitive echocardiographic sign of cardiac tamponade. *J Am Coll Cardiol* 1988; 12:1470–1477.
223. Picard MH, Sanfilippo AJ, Newell JB, Rodriguez L, Guerrero JL, Weyman AE: Quantitative relation between increased intrapericardial pressure and Doppler flow velocities during experimental cardiac tamponade. *J Am Coll Cardiol* 1991; 18:234–242.
224. Hatle LK, Appleton CP, Popp RL: Differentiation of constrictive pericarditis and restrictive cardiomyopathy by Doppler echocardiography. *Circulation* 1989; 79:357–370.
225. Burstow DJ, Oh JK, Bailey KR, Seward JB, Tajik AJ: Cardiac tamponade: Characteristic Doppler observations. *Mayo Clin Proc* 1989; 65:312–324.
226. Moncada R, Baker M, Salinas M, Demos TC, Churchill R, Love L, et al: Diagnostic role of computed tomography in pericardial heart disease: Congenital defects, thickening, neoplasms, and effusions. *Am Heart J* 1982; 103:263–282.
227. Kralstein J, Frishman W: Malignant pericardial diseases: Diagnosis and treatment. *Am Heart J* 1987; 113:785–790.

228. Sheldon R, Isaac D: Metastatic melanoma to the heart presenting with ventricular tachycardia. *Chest* 1991; 99:1296–1298.
229. Redwine DB: Complete heart block caused by secondary tumors of the heart: Case report and review of literature. *Tex Med* 1974; 70:59–64.
230. Kubac G, Doris I, Ondro M, Davey PW: Malignant granular cell myoblastoma with metastatic cardiac involvement: Case report and echocardiogram. *Am Heart J* 1980; 100:227–229.
231. Esper RJ, Machado RA, Schapira L, de la Fuente LM, Favolaro RG: Loud systolic and diastolic murmurs originating on a right atrial metastatic tumor. *Chest* 1987; 91:926–927.
232. Kopelson G, Herwig KJU: The etiologies of coronary artery disease in cancer patients. *Int J Radiat Oncol Biol Phys* 1978; 4:895–896.
233. Hartman RB, Clarke PI, Schulman P: Pronounced and prolonged ST segment elevation. Pathognomonic sign of tumor invasion of the heart. *Arch Intern Med* 1982; 142:1917–1919.
234. Virmani R, Khedekar R, Robinowitz M, McAllister HA Jr: Tumor embolization in coronary artery causing myocardial infarction. *Arch Pathol Lab Med* 1983; 107:243–245.
235. Lubell DL, Goldfarb CR: Metastatic cardiac tumor demonstrated by ^{201}Thallium scan. *Chest* 1980; 78:98–99.
236. Salem BI, Schnee M, Leatherman LL, de Castro CM, Benrey J: Electrocardiographic pseudo-infarction pattern: Appearance with a large posterior pericardial effusion after cardiac surgery. *Am J Cardiol* 1978; 42:681–685.
237. Nakayama DK, Norkool P, deLorimier AA, O'Neill JA Jr, D'Angio GJ: Intracardiac extension of Wilms' tumor. A report of the National Wilms' Tumor Study. *Ann Surg* 1986; 204:693–697.
238. Rothenberg DM, Brandt TD, D'Cruz I: Computed tomography of renal angiomyolipoma presenting as right atrial mass. *J Comput Assist Tomogr* 1986; 10:1054–1056.
239. Shahian DM, Libertino JA, Zinman LN, Leonardi HK, Eyre RC: Resection of cavoatrial renal cell carcinoma employing total circulatory arrest. *Arch Surg* 1990; 125:727–731.
240. Chua SO, Chiang CW, Lee YS, Lin SH, Liaw YF: Moving right atrial mass associated with hepatoma: Two cases detected by echocardiography. *Chest* 1986; 89:148–150.
241. Fujisaki M, Kurihara E, Kikuchi K, Nishikawa K, Uematsu Y: Hepatocellular carcinoma with tumor thrombus extending into the right atrium: Report of a successful resection with the use of cardiopulmonary bypass. *Surgery* 1991; 109:214–219.
242. Maurer G, Nanda NC: Two-dimensional echocardiographic identification of intracardiac leiomyomatosis. *Am Heart J* 1982; 103:915–917.
243. Garcia FA, Villaneuva RA, Narciso FV, Aventura AP: Intravenous leiomyomatosis of the uterus and pelvis presenting as a cardiac tumor. *Ann Thorac Surg* 1986; 42(suppl 6):41–43.
244. Schlosser V, Siebers JW, Kasper W, Bohm N: Vascular tumor in the heart. *J Cardiovasc Surg (Torino)* 1987; 28:132–134.
245. Griffin AS, Sterchi JM: Primary leiomyosarcoma of the inferior vena cava: A case report and review of the literature. *J Surg Oncol* 1987; 34:53–60.
246. Lupetin AR, Dash N, Beckman I: Leiomyosarcoma of the superior vena cava: Diagnosis by cardiac gated MR. *Cardiovasc Intervent Radiol* 1986; 9:103–105.
247. Birmingham CL, Peretz DI: Metastatic carcinoma presenting as obstruction to the right ventricular outflow tract: Report of a case and review of the literature. *Am Heart J* 1979; 97:229–232.
248. Stark RM, Perloff JH, Glick HJ, Hirshfeld JW, Devereux RB: Clinical recognition and management of cardiac metastatic disease: Observations in a unique case of alveolar soft-part sarcoma. *Am J Med* 1977; 63:653–659.
249. Steffens TG, Mayer HS, Das SK: Echocardiographic diagnosis of a right ventricular metastatic tumor. *Arch Intern Med* 1980; 140:122–123.
250. Bartels P, O'Callaghan WG, Peyton R, Sethi G, Maley T: Metastatic liposarcoma of the right ventricle with outflow tract obstruction: Restrictive pathophysiology predicts poor surgical outcome. *Am Heart J* 1988; 115:696–698.
251. Kaku K, Kawashima Y, Kitamura S, Morgan E, Labotka R: Resection of leiomyosarcoma originating in internal iliac vein and extending into heart via inferior vena cava. *Surgery* 1981; 89:604–611.
252. Luck SR, DeLeon S, Shkolnik A, Morgan E, Labotka R: Intracardiac Wilms' tumor: Diagnosis and management. *J Pediatr Surg* 1982; 17:551–554.
253. Van Osdol KD, Hall RJ, Warda M, Massumi A, Klima T: Right ventricular thrombus: Clinical and diagnostic features. *Tex Heart Inst J* 1983; 10:359–364.
254. Heitzman M, Gibson TC, Tabakin BS: A right-sided cardiac mass. *Arch Intern Med* 1984; 144:1813–1815.
255. Schrem SS, Colvin SB, Weinreb JC, Glassman E, Kronzon I: Metastatic cardiac liposarcoma: Diagnosis by transesophageal echocardiography and magnetic resonance imaging. *J Am Soc Echocardiogr* 1990; 3:149–153.
256. Watts FB Jr, Zingas AP, Das L, Cushing BA: Computed tomographic diagnosis of an intracardiac metastasis from osteosarcoma. *J Comput Tomogr* 1983; 7:271–272.
257. Wolverson MK, Grider RD, Sundaram M, Heiberg E, Johnson F: Demonstration of unsuspected malignant disease of the pericardium by computed tomography. *J Comput Tomogr* 1980; 4:330–333.
258. Gross BH, Glazer GM, Francis IR: CT of intracardiac and intrapericardial masses. *AJR* 1983; 140:903–907.
259. Salcedo EE, Cohen GI, White RD, Davison MB: Cardiac tumors: Diagnosis and management. *Curr Probl Cardiol* 1992; 17:73–137.
260. Gatenby RA, Hartz WH, Kessler HB: Percutaneous catheter drainage for malignant pericardial effusion. *J Vasc Interv Radiol* 1991; 2:151–155.
261. Hanley PC, Shub C, Seward JB, Wold LE: Intracavitary cardiac melanoma diagnosed by endomyocardial left ventricular biopsy. *Chest* 1983; 84:195–198.
262. Gosalakkal JA, Sugrue DD: Malignant melanoma of the right atrium: Antemortem diagnosis by transvenous biopsy. *Br Heart J* 1989; 62:159–160.
263. Seibert KA, Rettenmier CW, Waller BF, Battle WE, Levine AS, Roberts WC: Osteogenic sarcoma metastatic to the heart. *Am J Med* 1982; 73:136–141.
264. Quraishi MA, Costanzi JJ, Hokanson J: The natural history of lung cancer with pericardial metastases. *Cancer* 1983; 51:740–742.
265. Warda M, Khan A, Massumi A, Mathur V, Klima T, Hall RJ: Radiation-induced valvular dysfunction. *J Am Coll Cardiol* 1983; 2:180–185.
266. McAllister HA Jr, Hall RJ: Iatrogenic heart disease. In: Cheng TO (ed): *The International Textbook of Cardiology.* New York, Pergamon, 1986: 871–873.
267. Primrose WR, Clee MD, Johnston RN: Malignant pericardial effusion managed with vinblastine. *Clin Oncol* 1983; 9:67–70.
268. Sheppard FA, Morgan C, Evans WK, Ginsberg JF, Watt D, Murphy K: Medical management of malignant pericardial effusion by tetracycline sclerosis. *Am J Cardiol* 1987; 60:1161–1166.
269. Chan A, Rischin D, Clarke CP, Woodruff RK: Subxiphoid partial pericardiectomy with or without sclerosant instillation in the treatment of symptomatic pericardial effusions in patients with malignancy. *Cancer* 1991; 68:1021–1025.
270. Hankins JR, Satterfield JR, Aisner J, Wiernik PH, McLaughlin JS: Pericardial window for malignant pericardial effusion. *Ann Thorac Surg* 1980; 30:465–471.
271. Prager RL, Wilson CH, Bender HW Jr: The subxiphoid approach to pericardial disease. *Ann Thorac Surg* 1982; 34:6–9.
272. Alcan KE, Zabetakis PM, Marino ND, Franzone AJ, Michelis MF, Bruno MS: Management of acute cardiac tamponade by subxiphoid pericardiotomy. *JAMA* 1982; 247:1143–1148.
273. Palacios IF, Tuzcu EM, Ziskind AA, Younger J, Block PC: Percutaneous balloon pericardial window for patients with malignant pericardial effusion and tamponade. *Cathet Cardiovasc Diagn* 1991; 22:244–249.
274. Melvin KN, Howard RJ, Rakowski H, Goldman BS, El-Maraghi NRH: Embryonal carcinoma of the testis with metastases to the right atrium. *Can J Surg* 1983; 26:86–88.
275. Poole GV Jr, Meredith JW, Breyer RH, Mills SA: Surgical implications in malignant cardiac disease. *Ann Thorac Surg* 1983; 36:484–491.
276. Lagrange JL, Despins P, Spielman M, Le Chevalier T, de Lajartre AY, Fontaine F, et al: Cardiac metastases: Case report on an isolated cardiac metastasis of a myxoid liposarcoma. *Cancer* 1986; 58:2333–2337.
277. Pillai R, Blauth C, Peckham M, Hendry W, Barrett A, Goldstraw P: Intracardiac metastases from malignant teratoma of the testis. *J Thorac Cardiovasc Surg* 1986; 92:118–120.

278. Wiske PS, Gillam LD, Blyden G, Weyman AE: Intracardiac tumor regression documented by two-dimensional echocardiography. *Am J Cardiol* 1986; 58:186–187.
279. Atay AE, Alpert MA, Kleinsteuber WK, Freelon RL: Prolonged survival associated with spontaneous disappearance of untreated right atrial intracavitary metastasis. *Am Heart J* 1987; 114:437–440.
280. Terry LN, Kligerman MM: Pericardial and myocardial involvement by lymphomas and leukemias. *Cancer* 1970; 25:1003–1008.
281. Schwartz JB, Shamsuddin AM: The effects of leukemic infiltrates in various organs in chronic lymphocytic leukemia. *Hum Pathol* 1981; 12:432–440.
282. Meltzer V, Korompai FL, Mathur VS, Guinn GA: Surgical treatment of leukemic involvement of the mitral valve. *Chest* 1975; 67:119–121.
283. Applefeld MM, Milner SD, Vigorito RD, Shamsuddin AM: Congestive heart failure and endocardial fibroelastosis caused by chronic lymphocytic leukemia. *Cancer* 1980; 46:1479–1484.
284. Björkholm M, Ost A, Biberfeld P: Myocardial rupture with cardiac tamponade as a lethal early manifestation of acute myeloblastic leukemia. *Cancer* 1982; 50:1867–1869.
285. Cassis N Jr, Porterfield J, Rogers JS: Massive hemopericardium as the initial manifestation of chronic myelogenous leukemia. *Arch Intern Med* 1982; 142:2193–2194.
286. Liepman MK, Goodlerner S: Surgical management of pericardial tamponade as a presenting manifestation of acute leukemia. *J Surg Oncol* 1981; 17:183–188.
287. Crofts MA, Morgan-Capner P, Sharp JC, Mcleod AA, Keates JR, Jackson G, et al: Fungal endocarditis in a patient with acute leukaemia treated by valve replacement. *Br Med J* 1982; 284:574–575.
288. Wong DWH, Guthaner DF, Gordon EP, Mitchell RS: Lymphoma of the heart. *Cathet Cardiovasc Diagn* 1984; 10:377–384.
289. Acierno L: Cardiac complications in acquired immunodeficiency syndrome (AIDS): A review. *J Am Coll Cardiol* 1989; 13:1144–1154.
290. Lewis W: AIDS: Cardiac findings from 115 autopsies. *Prog Cardiovasc Dis* 1989; 32:207–215.
291. Steigman CK, Anderson DW, Macher AM, Sennesh JD, Virmani R: Fatal cardiac tamponade in acquired immunodeficiency syndrome with epicardial Kaposi's sarcoma. *Am Heart J* 1988; 116:1105–1107.
292. Goldfarb A, King CL, Rosenzweig BP, Feit F, Kamat BR, Rumancik WM, et al: Cardiac lymphoma in the acquired immunodeficiency syndrome. *Am Heart J* 1989; 118:1340–1344.
293. Andress JD, Polish LB, Clark DM, Hossack KF: Transvenous biopsy diagnosis of cardiac lymphoma in an AIDS patient. *Am Heart J* 1989; 118:421–423.
294. Schiller VL, Fishbein MC, Siegel RJ: Unusual cardiac involvement in carcinoid syndrome. *Am Heart J* 1986; 112:1322–1323.
295. Strickman NE, Hall RJ: Carcinoid heart disease. In: Kapoor AS, Reynolds RD (eds): *Cancer and the Heart.* New York, Springer-Verlag, 1986: 135–156.
296. Artaza A, Beiner JA, Gonzalez M, Aranda I, de Teresa EG, Pulpon LA: Carcinoid heart disease: Report of a case secondary to a pure carcinoid tumour of the ovary. *Eur Heart J* 1985; 6:800–805.
297. Sane DC, Feldman JM: A blush from the heart. *Chest* 1987; 92:360–361.
298. Mattingly TW: The functioning carcinoid tumor: A serendipity in diagnosis. *Trans Am Clin Climatol Assoc* 1965; 77:190–204.
299. Topol EJ, Fortuin NJ: Coronary artery spasm and cardiac arrest in carcinoid heart disease. *Am J Med* 1984; 77:950–952.
300. Millward MJ, Blake MP, Byrne MJ, Hung J, Gibson P: Left heart involvement with cardiac shunt complicating carcinoid heart disease. *Aust NZ J Med* 1989; 19:716–717.
301. McAllister HA Jr: Endocrine diseases and the cardiovascular system. In: Silver MD (ed): *Cardiovascular Pathology,* 2d ed. New York, Churchill Livingstone, 1991: 1181–1204.
302. Lundin L, Funa K, Hansson HE, Wilander E, Oberg K: Histochemical and immunohistochemical morphology of carcinoid heart disease. *Pathol Res Pract* 1991: 187:73–77.
303. Forman MB, Byrd BF, Oates JA, Robertson RM: Two-dimensional echocardiography in the diagnosis of carcinoid heart disease. *Am Heart J* 1984; 107:492–496.
304. Davies MK, Lowry PJ, Littler WA: Cross-sectional echocardiographic feature in carcinoid heart disease. A mechanism for tricuspid regurgitation in this syndrome. *Br Heart J* 1984; 51:355–357.
305. Lundin L, Landelius J, Andren B, Oberg K: Transesophageal echocardiography improves the diagnostic value of cardiac ultrasound in patients with carcinoid heart disease. *Br Heart J* 1990; 64:190–194.
306. Grahame-Smith DG: The carcinoid syndrome. In: Bondy PK, Rosenberg LE (eds): *Metabolic Control and Disease,* 8th ed. Philadelphia, Saunders, 1980: 1695–1707.
307. Kvols LK, Moertel CG, O'Connell MJ, Schutt AJ, Rubin J, Hahn RG: Treatment of the malignant carcinoid syndrome. Evaluation of a long-acting somatostatin analogue. *N Engl J Med* 1986; 315:663–666.
308. Oates JA: The carcinoid syndrome. *N Engl J Med* 1986; 315:702–704.
309. Ridker PM, Chertow GM, Karlson EW, Neish AS, Schoen FJ: Bioprosthetic tricuspid valve stenosis associated with extensive plaque deposition in carcinoid heart disease. *Am Heart J* 1991; 121:1835–1838.
310. Mullins PA, Hall JA, Shapiro LM: Balloon dilatation of tricuspid stenosis caused by carcinoid heart disease. *Br Heart J* 1990; 63:249–250.
311. Kay JH: Eleven-year follow-up after tricuspid valve replacement and pulmonic valvulotomy in the carcinoid syndrome (letter). *Am J Cardiol* 1984; 53:651.
312. Codd JE, Drozda J, Merjavy J: Palliation of carcinoid heart disease. *Arch Surg* 1987; 122:1076–1077.
313. Lundin L, Hansson HE, Landelius J, Oberg K: Surgical treatment of carcinoid heart disease. *J Thorac Cardiovasc Surg* 1990; 100:552–561.
314. Nielsen MS, Manners JM: Valve replacement in carcinoid syndrome. Anaesthetic management for tricuspid and pulmonary valve surgery. *Anaesthesia* 1979; 34:494–499.

Chapter 112

Traumatic Heart Disease

Panagiotis N. Symbas, M.D.

Accidental or intentional trauma is the leading cause of death, hospitalization, and loss of working days in our society, particularly among young people.[1-3] Cardiac and/or great-vessel injuries are a major contributor to this mortality and morbidity.[4] The heart or great vessels may be injured from penetrating and nonpenetrating trauma. Also, as the diagnostic and therapeutic modalities for the management of heart diseases have become more complex and more invasive, mechanical injuries to the heart due to iatrogenic trauma have become increasingly important. These result from the complications of various diagnostic, therapeutic, and resuscitative procedures, including cardiac catheterization, percutaneous coronary angioplasty,[5,6] percutaneous aortic or mitral valvuloplasty,[7,8] insertion of pacemaker leads[9] or Swan-Ganz catheters,[10] closed and open chest cardiac massage, and electric defibrillation.[11,12] The increasing use of invasive catheters has also led to the more frequent migration of these catheters to the heart or pulmonary vascular beds[13-15] and of nonbacterial thrombotic endocarditis and bacterial endocarditis.

Two other types of cardiac trauma not due to mechanical injury warrant separate classification. The first type includes injury to the heart from ionizing radiation, which predominantly causes pericarditis but may also result in myocardial injury.[16-18] The second includes the group of cardiac injuries due to electric current,[19,20] which may cause asystole, ventricular fibrillation, other arrhythmias, and myocardial injury. (See also Chap. 110.)

Many nonpenetrating injuries and an occasional penetrating injury of the heart are well tolerated. Thus, the majority of these lesions are diagnosed infrequently, since their initial clinical manifestation may be none or relatively mild, and the lesion may be overlooked unless a high index of suspicion is maintained and specific studies are obtained.[21,22] Frequently, these cardiac injuries are overshadowed by the more overt manifestations of cerebral, abdominal, or musculoskeletal trauma. For these reasons and because only the more severe injuries are reflected in autopsy studies, the actual incidence of traumatic heart disease remains obscure.

PENETRATING INJURIES

Penetrating injuries usually are observed with wounds of the precordium but may also be associated with wounds elsewhere in the chest, neck, or upper abdomen. They usually are due to missile or knife wounds but occasionally are caused by a missile embolus reaching the heart through the venous system or by a needle migrating through the esophagus.

Penetrating Cardiac Trauma

Although penetrating cardiac trauma frequently involves only the free cardiac wall, injury to cardiac valves, chordae tendineae, papillary muscles, atrial or ventricular septum, coronary arteries, and conduction system may occur. The multiplicity of heart and great vessel lesions that may be produced by penetrating wounds is indicated in Table 112-1.

The relative frequency of a single, free cardiac wall penetrating wound is due to its area of exposure on the anterior chest wall. In decreasing order of frequency the structures affected are the right ventricle, left ventricle, right atrium, and left atrium.[23] The cardiac wounds may

TABLE 112-1

Penetrating Wounds of the Heart

1. Pericardial damage
    a. Laceration or perforation
    b. Hemopericardium with or without cardiac tamponade
    c. Serofibrinous or suppurative pericarditis
    d. Pneumopericardium
    e. Constrictive pericarditis
2. Myocardial damage
    a. Laceration
    b. Penetration or perforation
    c. Retained foreign body
    d. Structural defects
        (1) Aneurysm formation
        (2) Septal defects
        (3) Aorticocardiac fistula
3. Valvular injury
    a. Leaflet or cusp injury
    b. Papillary muscle or chordae tendineae laceration
4. Coronary artery injury
    a. Laceration or thrombosis with or without myocardial infarction
    b. Arteriovenous fistula
    c. Aneurysm
5. Embolism
    a. Foreign body
    b. Thrombus (septic or sterile)
6. Infective endocarditis
7. Rhythm or conduction disturbances

be single or multiple; the latter are more commonly caused by missiles.[23,24] Over 50 percent of victims with penetrating cardiac trauma succumb shortly after injury.[25] The remaining survive for varying periods of time; many can recover completely if treated immediately.

The pathophysiological consequences and clinical manifestations of penetrating injuries to the heart depend upon the size and site of the wound, the mode of injury, and especially the state of the pericardial wound.[1,26] When the pericardial wound remains open and bleeding occurs freely into the pleural space, there are signs and symptoms of hemothorax and loss of circulating blood volume. When there is intrapericardial hemorrhage with a sealed pericardial wound, cardiac tamponade (Chaps. 92 and 93) is the presenting clinical picture. The diagnosis of cardiac injury should be suspected in a patient with chest, lower neck, epigastric, or especially precordial penetrating wounds and with symptoms and signs of cardiac tamponade and/or hemothorax and loss of circulating blood volume. The management of penetrating wounds of the heart consist of immediate thoracotomy and cardiorrhaphy.[23,25,27–34] When this cannot be done or while appropriate arrangements are being made for thoracotomy, the patient's blood volume should be expanded; pericardiocentesis is done only to provide time for a safe operation.[23,35]

Residual or Delayed Sequelae or Penetrating Cardiac Trauma

Patients with penetrating cardiac wound should be closely observed immediately postoperatively and after discharge for clinical manifestation of residual or delayed sequelae from the penetrating cardiac wounds. Such sequelae may include the following: (1) ventricular or atrial septal defect; (2) injury of valve cups, leaflets, or chordae tendineae; (3) aortocardiac, aortic pulmonary, or coronary artery to coronary vein or to cardiac chamber communication; (4) ventricular aneurysms; (5) posttraumatic or postoperative pericarditis; and (6) electrocardiographic abnormalities.[36,37] When symptoms and signs of structural defect are detected, echocardiography and/or cardiac catheterization should be performed to define the lesion and its hemodynamic significance and determine the proper mode of therapy.[36,38]

Recurrent posttraumatic pericarditis, which is similar to the postcardiotomy syndrome seen after cardiac surgery, occurs in approximately 20 percent of all cases of penetrating heart wounds. Symptomatic management is the treatment of choice for this syndrome unless cardiac tamponade or other sequelae, such as purulent or constrictive pericarditis, require surgical intervention.

Missile wounds may also result in the presence of a projectile within the heart following either a direct injury to the heart or an injury to a systemic vein with subsequent migration of the missile to the heart. The missile or the thrombus associated with it may embolize into the systemic or pulmonary arteries.[39–41] Bacterial endocarditis may also occur if the projectile is not completely embedded in the myocardium.[42,43] Also, several patients with projectiles in the heart have developed cardiac neurosis with an almost maniac desire for removal of the foreign body.[44] In many patients, however, the retained missile in the heart has resulted in no ill effects over a long period of observation.[45,46] Therefore, the treatment of missiles in the heart should be individualized according to the patient's clinical course and the location, size, composition, and shape of the missile.[45,46] Symptomatic missiles should be removed. Similarly, missiles free or partially protruding in a left cardiac chamber should be removed, because their embolization to the systemic arterial system may have serious consequences.[45,46] Missiles in the right side of the heart may either be removed or be left to embolize in the pulmonary vascular bed, from which they can be easily retrieved.[40] Intramyocardial or intrapericardial bullets or pellets are generally tolerated well and may be left in place.

A missile that has embolized to the systemic circulation should be surgically removed without delay unless it has resulted in a significant neurologic deficit.[41] Projectiles adjacent to or embedded within the wall of one of the great or coronary arteries should be extracted to prevent subsequent erosion and bleeding.

Coronary Artery Penetrating Trauma

Coronary artery injuries can result in cardiac tamponade and varying degrees of myocardial ischemia or myocardial infarction. The management of these wounds is dependent on the amount of myocardium at risk. Wounds of major branches of the coronary arterial system are repaired or bypassed, whereas small terminal vessels are ligated.[47] Coronary artery aneurysms and arteriovenous fistulas are rare sequelae of injury, and their treatment should be individualized.[48]

Aortic and Great-Vessel Penetrating Trauma

The pathophysiology of penetrating wounds to the great vessels is quite similar to that of penetrating wounds to the heart and is dependent upon whether the site of the wound is intra- or extrapericardial.[49,50] In addition to the obvious results of either immediate or delayed hemorrhage, a penetrating wound of a great vessel may result in the formation of a false aneurysm, with possible subsequent rupture, or of an arteriovenous fistula, producing either immediate or latent signs and symptoms of congestive heart failure.[51] Traumatic arteriovenous fistulas occasionally are complicated by the development of bacterial endarteritis and endocarditis.[52] These traumatic vascular lesions should be detected and repaired as soon as possible.

NONPENETRATING INJURIES

The vast majority of the blunt injuries to the heart are due to automobile accidents, although other forms of trauma from contact sports, altercations, falls, etc., may also result in such an injury. The cardiac injury usually is caused by direct compressing or decelerating forces delivered to the chest or rarely by an indirect force delivered to the abdomen or even to the extremities that results in a marked increase of the intravascular pressures. A wide variety of injuries are produced by nonpenetrating trauma (Table 112-2).

TABLE 112-2

Nonpenetrating Trauma of the Heart

1. Pericardial injury
   a. Hemopericardium
   b. Rupture or laceration
   c. Serofibrinous pericarditis
   d. Constrictive pericarditis
2. Myocardial injury
   a. Contusion
   b. Rupture of free cardiac wall, early or delayed
   c. Rupture of septum
   d. Aneurysm
   e. Laceration
3. Disturbances of rhythm or conduction
4. Valve injury
   a. Rupture of valve leaflets, cusp, or chordae tendineae
   b. Contusion of papillary muscle
5. Coronary artery injury
   a. Thrombosis with or without myocardial infarction
   b. Arteriovenous fistula
   c. Laceration with or without myocardial infarction
6. Great-vessel injury
   a. Rupture
   b. Aneurysm formation
   c. Aorta–cardiac chamber fistula
   d. Thrombotic occlusion

Cardiac Contusion

Contusion of the heart usually refers to blunt injury to the heart causing identifiable histopathological changes within the myocardium. The pathological lesions of myocardial contusion vary considerably in extent and character, ranging from small areas of petechiae or ecchymosis, which may be either subepicardial or subendocardial, to contusion of the full thickness of the myocardial wall with or without rupture of the heart.[1] Histologically, various degrees of subepicardial or intramyocardial hemorrhage or disruption of the myocardial fibers and leukocyte infiltration and edema may be present.[1] The forces that produce nonpenetrating lesions of the heart and great vessels are such that external evidence of chest injury may be meager or nondetectable in almost one-third of the traumatized patients. This lack of evidence of chest wall injury and the frequent absence of symptoms from the cardiac or vascular injury along with the common presence of other more obvious injuries to the body may impede the early diagnosis of a cardiovascular injury.

Patients with contusion of the heart are frequently asymptomatic, but they may complain of pain that is identical in character, location, and radiation to the pain of myocardial ischemia and/or myocardial infarction.[53] In patients with severe contusion of the heart, all the clinical features of a well-developed myocardial infarction may be present. They may complain of typical chest pain starting immediately after or within several hours following the trauma.[54] An angina-like syndrome may also be caused by the contusion, which is usually transient unless there is concomitant coronary artery injury or occult atherosclerotic coronary heart disease.[55] Coronary thrombosis may result from nonpenetrating trauma, but this is rare and is usually associated with existing atherosclerotic coronary artery disease.[56] In 546 necropsy cases of nonpenetrating cardiac trauma, not one instance of coronary thrombosis was found. Dyspnea and hypotension may also be presenting symptoms. In mild or moderate myocardial contusion, these signs may be transient and are usually absent. Cardiac failure is relatively rare, and when present, the possibility of an associated cardiac injury, such as rupture of the ventricular septum or of one of the cardiac valves, is great. Hemopericardium, with or without signs and symptoms of cardiac tamponade, may be associated with myocardial contusion. Laceration of a coronary artery from nonpenetrating injury also may rarely occur, producing cardiac tamponade or a coronary artery fistula.[57]

The diagnosis of cardiac contusion should be suspected in all patients with significant blunt trauma, particularly to the precordium. Unfortunately, none of the currently available diagnostic tests for myocardial contusion can conclusively establish the diagnosis in all patients. The appropriate use and interpretation of the available tests, however, assist in the diagnosis of myocardial contusion with reasonable accuracy.

Electrocardiography has been the most widely used test for the diagnosis of contusion of the heart.[58–60] Various electrocardiographic abnormalities have been considered indicative of cardiac contusion, such as nonspecific ST-T or Q-wave changes, supraventricular tachyarrhythmias, and ventricular arrhythmias, including fibrillation, which is usually the cause of death at the time of the traumatic impact.[58] On the other hand, a variety of other clinical conditions,[61–65] which frequently are present in traumatized patients, i.e., pain, anxiety, hemorrhage, hypoxia, hypokalemia, head trauma, alcohol or cocaine, may cause many of these abnormalities. Therefore, the presence of these other causes must be excluded before the electrocardiographic abnormalities are attributed to contusion of the heart.

Elevation of the serum level of the MB fraction of creatinine kinase (CK) has been extrapolated from use in acute myocardial infarction as a diagnostic aid in patients with cardiac contusion. Other clinical conditions that cause elevation in this enzyme, i.e., tachyarrhythmias and skeletal muscle diseases, including major trauma (see Chap. 60), need to be excluded before an abnormal level is ascribed to contusion of the heart.[66–69]

Radioisotope imaging of the heart in dogs with experimentally produced cardiac contusion has identified the area of injury only in animals with full-thickness contusion.[70] Therefore, this is of diagnostic value only in a limited number of patients since the incidence of full-thickness contusion is rare in patients surviving the initial traumatic impact.

Two-dimensional transthoracic and transesophageal echocardiography are useful in the diagnosis of cardiac contusion and particularly of the structural lesions associated with cardiac contusion.[71–74] The sensitivity and specificity of these tests for diagnosing contusion of the heart, however, has not been clearly defined.

The treatment of myocardial contusion is symptomatic. Appropriate limitation of activity and prevention and early treatment of arrhythmias are the most important therapeutic measures. The possible increased sensitivity of the heart to medications must also be considered when one is deciding what drugs to use in the patient with recent trauma.

Anticoagulants should not be administered because they may cause bleeding within the myocardium or pericardial space. Digitalis should be used in the presence of congestive heart failure or atrial fibrillation, and antiarrhythmic agents should be used for control of ectopic rhythms. If the myocardial contusion is severe, support with inotropic drugs (Chap. 28) may be necessary. When all these measures fail, balloon counterpulsation may be utilized.[75,76]

Cardiac Rupture

Although minor, insignificant myocardial contusion of the right ventricle is the most frequent lesion, the most fatal lesion is rupture of the heart. Myocardial rupture is extremely difficult to treat because of the rapid demise of the patient. Very often, when traumatic cardiac rupture occurs, it is only one of many severe body injuries that could have resulted in death. Although rupture of the heart commonly is not amenable to therapy, there have been reports of successful surgical repair.[52] Rupture of the atrium or the interventricular septum may not be rapidly fatal, and successful surgical correction of the injury is often possible. In the case of interventricular septal rupture, surgical repair is accomplished optimally after medical therapy has allowed for the hemodynamic stabilization of the patient.

Residual or Delayed Sequelae of Blunt Injury to the Heart

Contusion of the heart usually heals with little or no obvious scar or impairment of cardiac function. Large contusions, however, may cause a decrease in cardiac output, and extensive necrosis may lead to either rupture or, rarely, to congestive heart failure and formation of a true or false aneurysm.[77,78] Cardiac aneurysms may cause arrhythmias, congestive heart failure, rupture, and mural thrombosis with embolism. Because of these complications, surgical repair of traumatic aneurysm is usually advisable. Localized areas of necrosis and hemorrhage involving the cardiac conduction system may produce varying degrees of atrioventricular block or any of the different types of intraventricular conduction defects.[26]

The most commonly injured valve in the surviving patients is the aortic valve, with aortic regurgitation characteristically causing the rapid development of congestive heart failure.[79] Injury of the atrioventricular valves is an infrequent result of nonpenetrating cardiac injury and usually occurs in the presence of severe cardiac trauma resulting in death. Rupture of the mitral valve leaflet may have somewhat similar hemodynamic consequences to aortic valve injury but is rarely encountered clinically. In contrast, tricuspid valve injury may be tolerated for years before surgical correction is required.[80]

Papillary muscle or chordae tendineae rupture occurs more frequently than rupture of valve leaflets. Cardiac contusion may also cause papillary muscle dysfunction with secondary mitral or tricuspid regurgitation.[81] The clinical outcome depends on whether the structures involved are on the right side of the heart, where the lesion may be well tolerated, or on the left side, where the high-pressure system can lead to more serious hemodynamic sequelae. The murmurs produced by these lesions are generally typical of valvular regurgitation, but unusual high-pitched systolic and diastolic murmurs of variable loudness may also result. (See Chap. 11.) Traumatic tricuspid regurgitation may be present despite the absence of any detectable murmur.[82] Prompt and correct diagnosis by echocardiographic, hemodynamic, and angiographic studies is important. Hemodynamically significant valvular injury should undergo valvuloplasty or replacement.

Pericardial lesions are often overlooked and heal without incident. Hemopericardium may occur but usually is due to the coexisting myocardial injury. When the hemorrhage is severe, cardiac tamponade will rapidly occur. When the oozing of blood or serum into the peri-

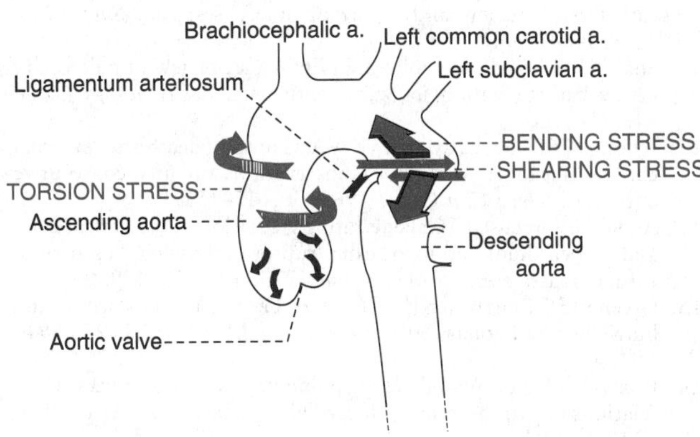

FIGURE 112-1 Diagrammatic illustration of the forces acting upon the aortic wall during rupture of the aorta from blunt trauma *(From PN Symbas: Traumatic Injuries of the Heart and Great Vessels. Springfield IL, Charles C Thomas, Springfield IL, 1971: 153. Reproduced with permission from the publisher and author.)*

cardium is slow, however, dilatation of the pericardial sac can develop over an extended period of time.

Posttraumatic pericarditis, which is similar to the post–myocardial infarction syndrome, develops less frequently with blunt than with penetrating cardiac injuries. The symptoms and signs of posttraumatic pericarditis are similar to those of pericarditis produced by a wide variety of causes. When hemopericardium or hydropericardium is suspected, echocardiography can confirm the diagnosis. Pericardial laceration is usually well tolerated, but herniation of the heart may occur, leading to more serious consequences and death.[83,84]

Aortic Rupture

Rupture of the aorta is the most common blunt injury of the great vessels. Rupture or avulsion of the innominate, carotid, or left subclavian arteries or the venae cavae have also been observed. Because of the variety of mechanical forces produced by blunt trauma (Fig. 112-1) combined with anatomic factors,[86] the most common sites of rupture of the aorta from blunt injury are the descending aorta just distal to the origin of the left subclavian artery (aortic isthmus) and the ascending aorta just proximal to the origin of the brachiocephalic artery.[85,86] Because of the high incidence of severe cardiac injury in patients with rupture of the ascending aorta, most patients who survive aortic rupture for a sufficient period of time to receive definitive surgical correction are those who have sustained rupture of the aortic isthmus.[85] Occasionally, rupture at other sites of the descending and even the abdominal aorta may occur. About 20 percent of the patients with aortic rupture survive the original injury. A false aneurysm is formed in these patients at the site of rupture, the wall of which consists of adventitia and/or parietal pleura and other mediastinal structures. The intactness of these structures maintains continuity of the circulation.

The common manifestations of traumatic rupture of the aorta are chest and/or midscapular pain; a new murmur; increased pulse amplitude; and hypertension of the upper extremities.[87] Some patients, however, are surprisingly free of any major symptoms or signs from the aortic rupture. Hoarseness, evidence of a superior vena cava syndrome, paraplegia, and anuria are rare manifestations. Although there are occasionally no obvious signs of external injury, patients with rupture of the aorta usually have associated injuries of the skeleton, abdomi-

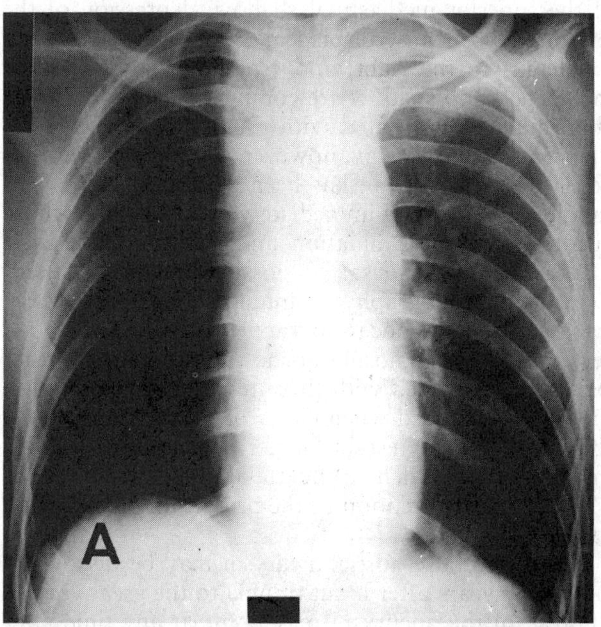

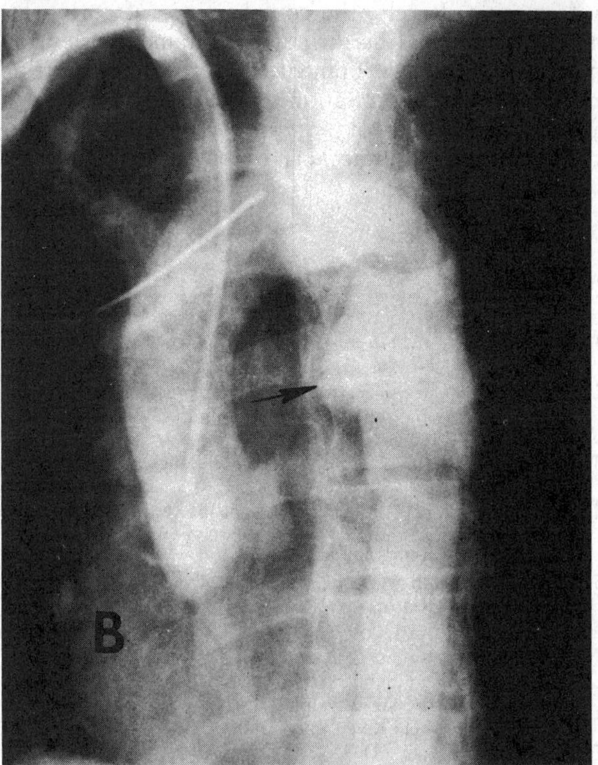

FIGURE 112-2 *A.* Chest roentgenogram of a young male who shortly before admission was involved in an automobile accident. Note the mediastinal widening. *B.* Aortogram the same day showing a false aneurysm distal to the origin of the left subclavian artery and two filling defects, one proximal and one distal to the aneurysm.

nal viscera, or central nervous system. These coexisting injuries may mask the signs of aortic rupture. For this reason, any patient who has sustained severe blunt trauma or who has been exposed to major deceleration forces should be suspected of having aortic rupture if there is an increased pulse pressure, upper extremity hypertension, and especially widening of the upper mediastinal silhouette. Chest roentgenography is of great diagnostic value in patients with aortic rupture. Widening of the superior mediastinal shadow, depression of the left main bronchus, displacement of the trachea and esophagus to the right, and especially obliteration of the aortic knob shadow are common roentgenographic abnormalities associated with this injury (Fig. 112-2). The most definitive way, however, to establish the diagnosis of aortic rupture has been by aortography. This should be performed immediately in all patients whose history, physical examination, and particularly the chest roentgenogram suggest the possibility of this injury. Computed tomography scanning[88] and particularly transesophageal echocardiography[74] (see Chap. 131) are very useful in diagnosing aortic rupture. Until further experience is gained with these tests, however, caution should be exercised when either of them is used as the sole technique for establishing the diagnosis. Surgical treatment should then be undertaken as soon as possible, with particular attention to the protection of the spinal cord.

A chronic false aortic aneurysm may be discovered months or years after blunt trauma to the great vessels. Rupture of the aneurysm may occur at any time after its formation. Rarely, the complications of peripheral embolization from the thrombus contained within the aneurysm or the development of bacterial endoaortitis or chronic pseudocoarctation may occur.[89,90] Because of the relative instability of these aneurysms and the potential complications, surgical correction is the treatment of choice.

REFERENCES

1. Symbas PN: *Cardiothoracic Trauma*. Philadelphia, Saunders, 1989.
2. Environmental Health Services Division, Centers for Disease Control: Unintentional and intentional injuries. *MMWR* 1982; 31:240, 245–248.
3. Cost of injury—United States: A report to Congress. *JAMA* 1989; 262:2803–2804.
4. Kemmerer WT, Eckert WG, Gathwright JB, Reemtsma K, Creech O Jr: Patterns of thoracic injuries in fatal traffic accidents. *J Trauma* 1961; 1:595–599.
5. Bredlau CE, Roubin GS, Leimgruber PP, Douglas JS Jr, King SB 3d, Gruentzig AR: In-hospital morbidity and mortality in patients undergoing elective coronary angioplasty. *Circulation* 1985; 72:1044–1052.
6. Gaul G, Hollman J, Simpendorfer C, Franco I: Acute occlusion in multiple lesion coronary angioplasty: Frequency and management. *J Am Coll Cardiol* 1989; 13:283–288.
7. Safian RD, Berman AD, Diver DJ, McKay LL, Come PC, Riley MF, et al: Balloon aortic valvuloplasty in 170 consecutive patients. *N Engl J Med* 1988; 319:125–130.
8. Nobuyoshi M, Hamasaki N, Kimura T, Nosaka H, Yokoi H, Yasumoto H, et al: Indications, complications and short-term clinical outcome of percutaneous transvenous mitral commissurotomy. *Circulation* 1989; 80:782–792.
9. Meyer JA, Millar K: Perforation of the right ventricle by electrode catheters: A review and report of nine cases. *Ann Surg* 1968; 168:1048–1060.
10. Shah KB, Rao TL, Laughlin S, El Etr AA: A review of pulmonary artery catheterization in 6,245 patients. *Anesthesiology* 1984; 61:271–275.
11. Bynum WR, Conell RM, Hawk WA: Causes of death after external cardiac massage: Analysis of observations on fifty consecutive autopsies. *Cleve Clin Quart* 1963; 30:147–151.
12. Agdal N, Jorgensen TG: Penetrating laceration of the pericardium and myocardium and myocardial rupture following closed chest cardiac massage. *Acta Med Scand* 1973; 194:477–479.
13. Greene JF Jr, Fitzwater JE, Clemmer TP: Septic endocarditis and indwelling pulmonary artery catheters. *JAMA* 1975; 233:891–892.
14. Pace NL, Horton W: Indwelling pulmonary artery catheters. Their relationship to aseptic endocardial vegetation. *JAMA* 1975; 233:893–894.
15. Bloomfield DA: Techniques of nonsurgical retrieval of iatrogenic foreign bodies of the heart. *Am J Cardiol* 1971; 27:538–545.
16. Cohn KE, Stewart JR, Fajardo LF, Hancock EW: Heart disease following radiation. *Medicine* 1967; 46:281–298.
17. Morton DL, Glancy DL, Joseph WL, Adkins PC: Management of patients with radiation-induced pericarditis with effusions: A note on the development of aortic regurgitation in two of them. *Chest* 1973; 64:291–297.
18. De Silva RA, Graboys TB, Podrid PJ, Lown B: Cardioversion and defibrillation. *Am Heart J* 1980; 100:881–895.
19. Bernstein T: Effects of electricity and lightning on man and animals. *J Forensic Sci* 1973; 18:3–11.
20. Jackson SH, Parry DJ: Lightning and the heart. *Br Heart J* 1980; 43:454–527.
21. Moritz AR, Atkins JP: Cardiac contusions: An experimental and pathologic study. *Arch Pathol* 1938; 25:445–462.
22. Samson PC: Battle wounds and injuries of the heart and pericardium: Experiences in forward hospitals. *Ann Surg* 1948; 127:1127–1149.
23. Symbas PN, Harlaftis N, Waldo WJ: Penetrating cardiac wounds: A comparison of different therapeutic methods. *Ann Surg* 1976; 183:377–381.
24. Symbas PN: *Cardiothoracic Trauma: Current Problems in Surgery*. St. Louis, MO, Mosby Year Book, 1991: 742–797.
25. Sugg WL, Rea WJ, Ecker RR, Rose EF, Shaw RR: Penetrating wounds of the heart. An analysis of 459 cases. *J Thorac Cardiovasc Surg* 1968; 56:531–545.
26. Parmley LF, Mattingly WT, Manion WC: Penetrating wounds of the heart and aorta. *Circulation* 1958; 17:953.
27. Borja AR, Lansing AM, Ransdell HT Jr: Immediate operative treatment for stab wounds of the heart: Experience with fifty-four consecutive cases. *J Thorac Cardiovasc Surg* 1970; 59:622–667.
28. Beall AC Jr, Patrick TA, Okies JE, Bricker DL, DeBakey ME: Penetrating wounds of the heart. Changing patterns of surgical management. *J Trauma* 1972; 12:468–473.
29. Trinkle JK, Marcos J, Grover FL, Cuello LM: Management of the wounded heart. *Ann Thorac Surg* 1974; 17:230–236.
30. Mattox KL, Limacher MC, Feliciano DV, Colosimo L, OMeara ME, Beall AC Jr, et al: Cardiac evaluation following heart injury. *J Trauma* 1985; 25:758–765.
31. Demetriades D: Cardiac penetrating injuries: Personal experience of 45 cases. *Br J Surg* 1984; 71:95–97.
32. Marshall WG Jr, Bell JL, Kouchoukos NT: Penetrating cardiac trauma. *J Trauma* 1984; 24:147–149.
33. Ivatury RR, Rohman M, Steichen FM, Gunduz Y, Nallathambi M, Stahl WM: Penetrating cardiac injuries: Twenty-year experience. *Am Surg* 1987; 53:310–317.
34. Trinkle JK, Toon RS, Franz JL, Arom KV, Grover FL: Affairs of the wounded heart: Penetrating cardiac wounds. *J Trauma* 1979; 19:467–472.
35. Cooper FW Jr, Stead EA Jr, Warren JV: The beneficial effect of intravenous infusions in acute cardiac tamponade. *Ann Surg* 1944; 120:822–825.
36. Symbas PN, DiOrio DA, Tyras DH, Ware RE, Hatcher CR Jr: Penetrating cardiac wounds: Significant residual and delayed sequelae. *J Thorac Cardiovasc Surg* 1973; 66:526–532.
37. Symbas PN: *Traumatic Heart Disease: Current Problems in Cardiology*. St. Louis, MO, Mosby Year Book, 1991: 539–582.
38. Whisennand HH, Van Pelt SA, Beall AC Jr, Mattox KL, Espada

R: Surgical management of traumatic intracardiac injuries. *Ann Thorac Surg* 1979; 28:530–536.
39. Bland EF, Beebe GW: Missiles in the heart: A 20 year follow up report of world war cases. *N Engl J Med* 1966; 274:1039–1046.
40. Symbas PN, Hatcher CR Jr, Mansour KA: Projectile embolus of the lung. *J Thorac Cardiovasc Surg* 1968; 56:97–103.
41. Symbas PN, Harlaftis N: Bullet emboli in the pulmonary and systemic arteries. *Ann Surg* 1977; 185:318–320.
42. Decker HR: Foreign bodies in the heart and pericardium: Should they be removed? *J Thorac Surg* 1939; 9:62.
43. Harken DE: Experiments in intracardiac surgery. I. Bacterial endocarditis. *J Thorac Surg* 1942; 11:656–670.
44. Turner GG: Bullets in the heart for 23 years. *Surgery* 1942; 9:832–852.
45. Symbas PN, Picone AL, Hatcher CR Jr, Vlasis SE: Cardiac missiles: A review of the literature and personal experience. *Ann Surg* 1990; 211:639–648.
46. Symbas PN, Vlasis SE, Picone AL, Hatcher CR Jr: Missiles in the heart. *Ann Thorac Surg* 1989; 48:192–194.
47. Heitzman EJ, Heitzman GC: Myocardial infarction following penetrating wounds of the heart. *Am J Cardiol* 1961; 7:283–287.
48. Konecke LL, Spitzer S, Mason D, Kasparian H, James PM Jr: Traumatic aneurysm of the left coronary artery. *Am J Cardiol* 1971; 27:221–223.
49. Symbas PN, Sehdava JS: Penetrating wounds of the thoracic aorta. *Ann Surg* 1970; 171:441–450.
50. Symbas PN, Kourias E, Tyras DH, Hatcher CR Jr: Penetrating wounds of the great vessels. *Ann Surg* 1974; 179:757–762.
51. Symbas PN, Schlant RC, Logan WD Jr, Lindsay J, Mac Connell K, Zakaryia M: Traumatic aorticopulmonary fistula complicated by postoperative low cardiac output treated with dopamine. *Ann Surg* 1967; 165:614–619.
52. Parmley LF Jr, Orbison JA, Hughes CW, Mattingly TW: Acquired arteriovenous fistulas complicated by endarteritis and endocarditis lenta due to *Streptococcus faecalis*. *N Engl J Med* 1954; 250:305–309.
53. Kissane RW: Traumatic heart diseases, especially myocardial contusion. *Postgrad Med* 1954; 15:114–119.
54. Kissane RW: Traumatic heart disease: Nonpenetrating injuries. *Circulation* 1952; 6:421–425.
55. Stern T, Wolf RY, Reichart B, Harrington OB, Crosby VG: Coronary artery occlusion resulting from blunt trauma. *JAMA* 1974; 230:1308–1309.
56. Levy H: Traumatic coronary thrombosis with myocardial infarction; postmortem study. *Arch Intern Med* 1949; 84:261–276.
57. Forker AD, Morgan JR: Acquired coronary artery fistula from nonpenetrating chest injury. *JAMA* 1971; 215:289–291.
58. Louhimo I: Heart injury after blunt thoracic trauma: An experimental study on rabbits. *Acta Chir Scand Suppl* 1968; 380:1–60.
59. Dolara A, Morando P, Pampaloni M: Electrocardiographic findings in 98 consecutive nonpenetrating chest injuries. *Dis Chest* 1967; 52:50–56.
60. Jones FL Jr: Transmural myocardial necrosis after nonpenetrating cardiac trauma. *Am J Cardiol* 1970; 26:419–422.
61. Potkin RT, Werner JA, Trobaugh GB, Chestnut CH III, Carrico CJ, Hallstrom A, et al: Evaluation of noninvasive tests of cardiac damage in suspected cardiac contusion. *Circulation* 1982; 66:627–631.
62. Bayer MJ, Burdick D: Diagnosis of myocardial contusion in blunt chest trauma. *JACEP* 1977; 6:238–242.
63. Hoffman B: The genesis of cardiac arrhythmias. *Prog Cardiovasc Dis* 1966; 8:319–329.
64. Marriott HT, Nizet PM: Physiologic stimuli simulating ischemic heart disease. *JAMA* 1967; 200:715.
65. Tindall GT, Iwata K, McGraw CP, Vanderveer RW: Cardiorespiratory changes associated with intracranial pressure waves: Evaluation of these changes in 27 patients with head injuries. *South Med J* 1975; 68:407–412.
66. Guzy PM: Creatine phosphokinase–MB (CPK-MB) and the diagnosis of myocardial infarction. *West J Med* 1977; 127:455–460.
67. Rapaport E: Serum enzymes and isoenzymes in the diagnosis of acute myocardial infarction. *Mod Concepts Cardiovasc Dis* 1977; 46:43–46.
68. Marmor A, Alpan G: Specificity of creatine kinase MB isoenzyme for myocardial injury. *Clin Chem* 1978; 24:2206.
69. Snow N, Richardson JD, Flynt LM Jr: Myocardial contusion implication for patients with multiple traumatic injuries. *Surgery* 1982; 92:744–750.
70. Gonzalez AC, Harlaftis N, Gravanis M, Symbas PN: Imaging of experimental myocardial contusion: Observations and pathologic correlations. *Am J Roentgenol* 1977; 128:1039–1040.
71. Miller FA Jr, Seward JB, Gersh BJ, Tajik AJ, Mucha P Jr: Two-dimensional echocardiographic findings in cardiac trauma. *Am J Cardiol* 1982; 50:1022–1027.
72. King RM, Mucha P Jr, Seward JB, Gersh BJ, Farnell MB: Cardiac contusion: A new diagnostic approach utilizing two-dimension echocardiography. *J Trauma* 1983; 23:610–614.
73. Skorton DJ, Collins SM, Nichols T, Pandian NG, Bean JA, Kerber RE: Quantitative texture analysis in two-dimensional echocardiography: Application to the diagnosis of experimental myocardial contusion. *Circulation* 1983; 68:217–223.
74. Shapiro NG, Yanofsky SD, Trapp I, Purham RM, Labovitz A, Sear JE, et al: Cardiovascular evaluation in thoracic blunt trauma using transesophageal echocardiography (TEE). *J Trauma* 1991; 131:835–839.
75. Saunders CR, Doty DB: Myocardial contusion: Effect of intra-aortic balloon counterpulsation on cardiac output. *J Trauma* 1978; 18:706–708.
76. Snow N, Luca AE, Richardson JD: Intra-aortic balloon counterpulsation for cardiogenic shock from cardiac contusion. *J Trauma* 1982; 22:426–429.
77. Killen DA, Gobbel WG Jr, France R, Vix VA: Post-traumatic aneurysm of the left ventricle. *Circulation* 1969; 39:101–108.
78. Singh R, Nolan SP, Schrank JP: Traumatic left ventricular aneurysm: Two cases with normal coronary angiograms. *JAMA* 1975; 234:412–414.
79. Payne DD, DeWeese JA, Mahoney EB, Murphy GW: Surgical treatment of traumatic rupture of the normal aortic valve. *Ann Thorac Surg* 1974; 17:223–229.
80. Liu S, Sako Y, Alexander CS: Traumatic tricuspid insufficiency. *Am J Cardiol* 1970; 26:200–204.
81. Schroeder JS, Stinson EB, Bieber CP, Wexler L, Shumway NE, Harrison DC: Papillary muscle dysfunction due to nonpenetrating chest trauma, recognition in a potential cardiac donor. *Br Heart J* 1972; 34:645–647.
82. Marvin RF, Schrank JP, Nolan SP: Traumatic tricuspid insufficiency. *Am J Cardiol* 1973; 32:723–726.
83. Munchow OBG, Carter R, Vannix RS, Anderson FS: Cardiac arrest due to ventricular herniation. Report of a case of two successful cardiac resuscitations. *JAMA* 1960; 173:1350–1351.
84. Anderson M, Fredens M, Olesson KH: Traumatic rupture of the pericardium. *Am J Cardiol* 1971; 27:566–569.
85. Parmley LF, Mattingly TW, Manion WC, Jahnke EJ Jr: Nonpenetrating traumatic injury of the aorta. *Circulation* 1958; 17:1086–1101.
86. Symbas PN, Tyras DH, Ware RE, DiOrio DA: Traumatic rupture of the aorta. *Ann Surg* 1973; 178:6–12.
87. Symbas PN, Tyras DH, Ware RE, Hatcher CR Jr: Rupture of the aorta: A diagnostic triad. *Ann Thorac Surg* 1973; 15:405–410.
88. Fenner MN, Fisher KS, Sergel NL, Porter DB, Metzmoker CO: Evaluation of possible traumatic thoracic aortic injury using aortography and CT. *Am Surg* 1990; 56:497–499.
89. Stryker WA: Traumatic saccular aneurysms of the thoracic aorta. *Am J Clin Pathol* 1948; 18:152–161.
90. Kinley CE, Chandler BM: Traumatic aneurysm of thoracic aorta: A case presenting as a coarctation. *Can Med Assoc J* 1967; 96:279–281.

PART XV

Special Physiological Conditions and the Cardiovascular System

Chapter 113

Heart Disease and Pregnancy

John H. McAnulty, M.D. ■ *James Metcalfe, M.D.* ■ *Kent Ueland, M.D.*

Throughout the world, maternal heart disease is still most often due to rheumatic fever.[1,2] In the United States and other western societies, congenital heart disease is now predominant.[3,4,5] Whatever the cause, heart disease in a pregnant woman may affect the well-being of both the mother and the fetus.[6] Potential dangers to the mother fall into several categories. First, by imposing a hemodynamic burden, pregnancy may result in her disability or death. On the basis of recorded experience, pregnancy is particularly dangerous to women with some specific cardiac abnormalities; these include Eisenmenger's syndrome,[7] primary pulmonary hypertension,[8] Marfan's syndrome,[9] and significant mitral stenosis.[10] Concern for maternal and fetal safety is sufficient to consider prevention or interruption of pregnancy in women with these and other abnormalities[11] (Table 113-1). At a minimum, counseling and close clinical attention is required.

Second, pregnancy may aggravate preexisting maternal heart disease. Ventricular dysfunction may worsen, bacterial endocarditis can occur, and in women with rheumatic heart disease, pregnancy may increase the chance of a recurrence of rheumatic fever.[10,12,13]

Third, in rare instances, pregnancy may cause heart disease. A peripartum cardiomyopathy may develop in individuals with previously normal hearts.[14–16]

In women with heart disease, fetal health may be jeopardized for a number of reasons. The fetus depends on an adequate and continuous supply of well-oxygenated maternal blood to the uterus and is at risk of abnormal organogenesis or death should this supply be compromised. When maternal heart disease is severe, this risk is significant; fetal wastage exceeds 50 percent in women with severe congenital heart disease.[6,17,18]

In addition, if the mother or father[19] has congenital heart disease, the fetus has an increased likelihood of being born with heart disease. Congenital heart disease is recognized in 0.8 percent of all live births in the United States.[17–19] If one of the parents has congenital heart disease, the offspring has up to a 15 percent chance of having a similar abnormality[20–26] (Table 113-2). This increases to 50 percent when the abnormality is an autosomal dominant trait, as is the case with hypertrophic cardiomyopathy or with Marfan's syndrome (see also Chaps. 96 and 97). Finally, even if the mother and fetus survive pregnancy, the child has an increased chance of

TABLE 113-1

Cardiovascular Abnormalities Placing a Mother and Infant at Extremely High Risk

Advise *Avoidance* or *Interruption* of Pregnancy:
- Pulmonary hypertension
- Dilated cardiomyopathy with congestive failure
- Marfan Syndrome with dilated aortic root
- Cyanotic congenital heart disease
- Symptomatic obstructive lesions

Pregnancy Counseling and Close Clinical Follow-up Required:
- Prosthetic valve
- Coarctation of the aorta
- Marfan Syndrome
- Dilated cardiomyopathy in asymptomatic women
- Obstructive lesions

SOURCE: From McAnulty JH, et al.[11] Reproduced with permission from the publisher and authors.

TABLE 113-2

Congenital Heart Disease in the Offspring of a Parent with Congenital Heart Disease

Congenital Heart Defect in a Parent	Risk of Congenital Heart Disease in Offspring If One Parent Is Affected,*† Percentage
Intracardiac shunts	
ASD	3–11
VSD	4–22
PDA	4–11
Obstruction to flow	
Left-sided obstruction‡	3–26
Right-sided obstruction	3–22
Complex abnormalities	
Tetralogy of Fallot	4–15
Ebstein's anomaly	Uncertain
Transposition of the great arteries	Uncertain

* The higher number in each range comes from one large series.[20] The incidence of congenital heart disease in the offspring tends to be closer to the lower numbers for most other reported series.[23, 25, 26]
† The risk in obstructive lesions is decreased by corrective surgery prior to pregnancy.[20]
‡ Includes coarctation, aortic stenosis, discrete subaortic stenosis, supravalvular stenosis. It does not include IHSS: with this, the child has a 50 percent chance of having IHSS.
SOURCE: McAnulty JH, Metcalfe J, Ueland K: Cardiovascular disease. In: Burrow GN, Ferris TF (eds): *Medical Complications during Pregnancy*. Philadelphia, Saunders, 1988. Reproduced with permission from the publisher and authors.

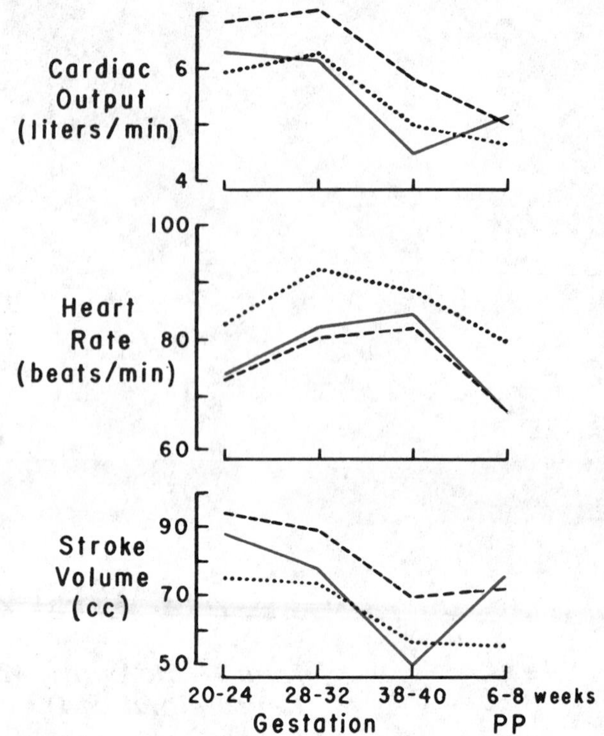

FIGURE 113-1 The effects of time in gestation and of maternal position on the cardiovascular system of the mother. Data were obtained at three periods during gestation and once postpartum. Solid line = supine; broken line = side; dotted line = sitting.

losing its mother because of the mortality rate associated with heart disease.

CARDIOVASCULAR ADJUSTMENTS AT VARIOUS STAGES OF PREGNANCY

Changes in the cardiovascular system during a normal pregnancy are remarkable, so it is not surprising that certain maternal cardiac abnormalities are not well tolerated (Fig. 113-1). Even in the woman without heart disease, the hemodynamic adjustments can result in symptoms and signs that are sometimes difficult to distinguish from those associated with cardiac abnormalities.

Sodium and water retention occur. Total body water increases steadily throughout pregnancy by 6 to 8 liters; most is extracellular.[27] Sodium retention results in an excess accumulation of 500 to 900 meq by the time of delivery. Plasma volume begins to increase as early as 6 weeks after conception, approaches its maximum in the second trimester[28] (Fig. 113-2), and approximates $1\frac{1}{2}$ times normal by the time of delivery.[29] Complex interactions of the renin-angiotensin-aldosterone system, reproductive hormones, prostaglandins, and atrial natriuretic factor contribute to these volume changes.[30,31,32] There is also an increase in red blood cell mass, but proportionally it is not as great as the increase in plasma volume, and thus the hematocrit falls. Peak hemodilution occurs at 24 to 26 weeks with a gradual increase in hematocrit in the third trimester (see Fig. 113-2). The hematocrit resulting from pregnancy is rarely less than 30 percent. Although these changes contribute to the hemodynamic alterations of pregnancy, they do not adequately explain all of them.

The most significant hemodynamic change occurring in the maternal circulation during pregnancy is an increase in resting cardiac output (Fig. 113-1). This begins early in the first trimester and reaches levels of 30 to 50 percent above values in nonpregnant individuals by the middle trimester.[29,33–40] The cardiac output may remain elevated to this degree throughout the rest of the pregnancy, but it is sensitive to changes in position, which affect venous return to the heart.[29,38,39] Early in pregnancy the increase in resting cardiac output is due mainly to an increase in stroke volume, a variable which falls later in pregnancy coincident with the progressive elevation in heart rate.[29,37–39] Initially the increased cardiac output is associated with a decreased arteriovenous oxygen difference, but this gradually widens as resting oxygen consumption increases progressively and at term reaches a level 20 percent above that of the nonpregnant state.[29]

As shown in Fig. 113-1, when measurements are made in the supine position, the resting cardiac output of the woman near term in pregnancy is, on the average, lower than that of the postpartum woman. This decrement is attributed to compression of the inferior vena cava by the enlarged uterus, which results in a decreased venous return and an average fall in cardiac output of 0.6 liter/

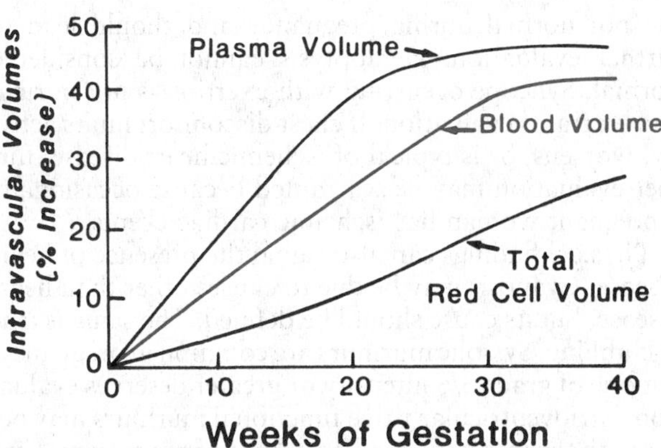

FIGURE 113-2 Schematic representations of the percent increases in the intravascular volumes that occur during pregnancy. Plasma volume increases by approximately 50 percent and total red cell volume by approximately 25 percent, causing a 40 percent increase in total blood volume.

min, when compared to that measured in the left lateral position,[39] even in women with adequate venous collaterals. In a few women, presumably those whose collaterals are not well developed, maintenance of the supine position may result in alarming hypotension and bradycardia, a vasovagal syndrome which has been called the "supine hypotensive syndrome of pregnancy."[41] With standing, there is a 1.2 liters/min fall in cardiac output.[39] During labor, cardiac output increases with each uterine contraction (compared with the time between contractions), but the magnitude of the increase varies, depending on the anesthesia used and on body position.[42]

Immediately after vaginal delivery, cardiac output may increase by as much as 60 to 80 percent. With a cesarean section there may be a transient fall in output and blood pressure.[42] In the postpartum period relative bradycardia is common, and resting cardiac output falls progressively to normal levels. The majority of the hemodynamic changes of pregnancy approach normal within a few weeks. Some may persist for as long as seven months postpartum.[43] Lactation may partially explain this, as the threefold increase in mammary blood flow may persist until weaning.[44]

The increase in cardiac output is associated with a fall in systemic vascular resistance. This occurs early in pregnancy and is associated with a slight fall in mean arterial blood pressure, which returns to the level of the nonpregnant state before delivery.[29,37–39] The changes in cardiac output and total systemic vascular resistance do not accurately reflect changes in the resistance of specific vascular beds that regulate the distribution of the increased maternal cardiac output. A schematic summary of the distribution of cardiac output in a resting woman at several stages of pregnancy is shown in Fig. 113-3. This is a composite, using data from a variety of studies, but the general outlines are probably correct. By the end of the first trimester, uterine flow has increased by only 50 to 100 mL/min over that of the nonpregnant state; it increases to 200 mL/min above the baseline at term.[44–47] In twin pregnancies uterine flow is even higher. This progressive expansion of uterine blood flow is out of phase with the total rise in resting maternal cardiac output, which reaches its peak in the middle trimester.

When redistribution of flow is required in order to

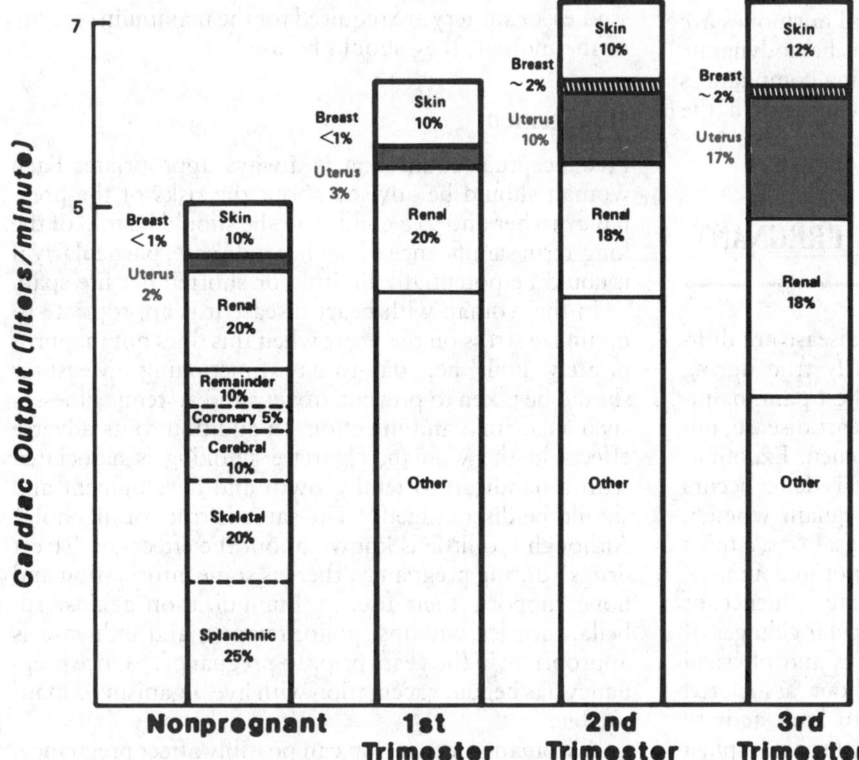

FIGURE 113-3 The distribution of increased cardiac output in association with human pregnancy. The data are fragmentary, especially early in pregnancy, and nonexistent in the postpartum period. The change in flow to each region is labeled.

serve the mother, uterine blood flow falls.[48,49] Excitement, heat, exercise, and decrease in venous return have all been shown to result in decreased uterine blood flow. Though exercise may temporarily divert blood flow from the pregnant uterus and affect the fetus as assessed by a fall in fetal heart rate, it is not apparent that this transient diversion has any permanent detrimental effect on the baby.[50,51] This question has become more important with the increasing enthusiasm for exercise in this country. The type of exercise affects maternal hemodynamics and perfusion of the uterus. As an example, maximal exercise by swimming causes less fetal bradycardia than the same level of cycling.[50] Regular endurance aerobic exercise has been associated with a reduction in birth weight. Since most of the reduction is due to a decrease in neonatal fat mass, it is not clear if this is detrimental.[52] There is not enough evidence available to suggest that the healthy pregnant woman should avoid recreational exercise.

The hemodynamic responses of a pregnant woman to exercise are different from those of a nonpregnant woman. For a given level of exercise in the sitting position, there is a greater increase in oxygen consumption compared to that of the nonpregnant state.[36–40,43,53–55] This is associated with a relatively smaller rise in arteriovenous oxygen difference than that produced by the same exercise in nonpregnant women.

The mechanisms evoking the hemodynamic changes of pregnancy are not clear. Recognizing the similarity between the hemodynamic changes of human pregnancy and those found in patients with an arteriovenous fistula, Burwell et al. suggested that the low-resistance shunt created by the placental vascular bed might be the basis for the hemodynamic change.[56] It is now recognized that maternal cardiac output increases long before there is any significant change in uterine blood flow, so Burwell's explanation is not adequate for the observed changes in resting cardiac output. At the present time it seems most likely that changes in the levels of steroid hormones are the most significant contributors to the hemodynamic changes of pregnancy, possibly by altering compliances throughout the maternal vascular system and in the heart.[57–58]

CLINICAL EVALUATION OF THE PREGNANT WOMAN

The recognition and definition of heart disease are difficult at any time, and this is particularly true during pregnancy. Easy fatigability, dyspnea, chest pain, palpitations, and syncope are symptoms of heart disease, but all are common in normal pregnant women. Examination may be equally misleading. Peripheral edema occurs in as many as 80 percent of normal pregnant women, and pulmonary rales, visible neck vein pulsations, a third heart sound, and systolic murmurs are not uncommon.

Although it is difficult to differentiate evidence of heart disease from the normal cardiovascular changes of pregnancy, there are symptom complexes and physical findings that should cause concern about associated heart disease. Dyspnea severe enough to limit activity and true orthopnea or paroxysmal nocturnal dyspnea are not normal during pregnancy and should lead to further evaluation. Hemoptysis cannot be considered normal. Syncope occurring with exertion is not normal and warrants evaluation. If chest discomfort limits activity, worsens, or is typical of ischemic heart disease, further evaluation may be warranted because occasionally a pregnant woman has ischemic cardiac events.[57–63]

Physical findings can also signal the presence of heart disease. Cyanosis may be due to causes other than heart disease, but its cause should be defined. The same is true of clubbing. Systolic murmurs are common in pregnancy, but one of grade 3/6 intensity or greater deserves evaluation. Atrioventricular valve functional murmurs may occur with the increased cardiac output of pregnancy,[64] but a diastolic murmur is so unusual that it warrants the diagnosis of heart disease if care is taken to exclude internal mammary flow sounds (the mammary soufflé) and a venous hum which has a diastolic component; both are common in normal pregnancy.

GENERAL CONSIDERATIONS

Each patient and each cardiac lesion must be considered individually, but some aspects of the diagnosis and management of heart disease during pregnancy apply in all cases.

Health Priorities

Fetal well-being should be considered as part of each diagnostic and management consideration, but the highest priority should be given to maternal health. If there are alternatives to drug intervention, such as appropriate manipulation of the environment or maternal activity, these measures are preferable. But if drugs, diagnostic studies, or surgery are required for the maximum security of the mother, they should be used.

Management

Preconceptual counseling is always appropriate. Each woman should be advised about the risks of the pregnancy to her and to a child, and she should be told of the long-term significance of her heart disease, particularly if it could be potentially limiting or shorten her life span.

In the woman with heart disease it is appropriate to minimize stress on the heart when this does not inappropriately limit her day-to-day functioning. Measures should be taken to prevent anxiety and systemic illnesses such as anemia and infection. In addition to its adverse effects in the woman, cigarette smoking is associated with a handicap to fetal growth and development and should be discouraged.[65] The same is true for alcohol.[66] Although too little is known about the effects of "street drugs" during pregnancy, there is some information and none supports their use.[67,68] Immunization against rubella, measles, mumps, polio, tetanus, and influenza is appropriate in the years prior to pregnancy.[69] Once pregnancy has begun, vaccination with live organisms is inadvisable.

A woman's occupation can possibly affect pregnancy.

As noted earlier, there is a fall in cardiac output with standing.[39] This observation is worthy of consideration when combined with evidence that women who work in the standing position at an occupation continued throughout pregnancy tend to have smaller than expected children.[70] The "stress" of standing, or of exercise, in a healthy mother, and the effect on blood flow to the fetus is not sufficient to advise avoidance of either. In the woman with heart disease, which may already adversely affect uterine blood flow, activity should, at least, be kept at a level below that which causes symptoms.

Each lesion is unique and must be considered separately, but certain issues must be considered with every cardiac lesion. The hemodynamic status must be assessed with each visit and a decision made about the need for diagnostic studies or intervention. Antibiotic prophylaxis against endocarditis using the recommendations of the American Heart Association is as applicable to pregnancy as to the nonpregnant state.[71] In addition, antibiotic prophylaxis against bacterial endocarditis is recommended during labor and delivery in individuals with valve abnormalities and some congenital lesions. It is recognized that the benefit of this approach has not been documented, but the low risk and expense associated with antibiotic prophylaxis make its use appropriate.

In individuals with a history of rheumatic fever and particularly in those with rheumatic heart disease, antibiotic prophylaxis is indicated to prevent recurrences.[72]

Thromboembolic events occur often enough in individuals with heart disease to address the need for anticoagulation therapy. If it is required, warfarin should be avoided. It crosses the placental barrier and puts the fetus at risk of abnormal development and hemorrhage. (See "Anticoagulants.") Alternatives to warfarin, including the self-administration of subcutaneous heparin, should be used for the woman who is pregnant.

CARDIOVASCULAR DISEASE IN PREGNANCY

Each of the abnormalities discussed in the remainder of this chapter is covered in detail in other sections of this book. We will relate them to pregnancy and will consider (1) the potential problems during pregnancy, emphasizing the effects of the normal hemodynamic changes on each lesion (Table 113-3); (2) the demonstrated risk to the mother and fetus; and (3) the management of mother and fetus during pregnancy.

Rheumatic Fever

Clinically recognized rheumatic fever is uncommon in the United States,[1,73] and when it does occur, it is associated with less severe heart disease.[74] However, there are regions in the United States where the incidence is increasing,[75] and it remains a problem throughout much of the world.[1,73] In addition, it has been suggested that rheumatic fever is more likely to occur during pregnancy,[10,11] a reason for the more aggressive use of antibiotic prophylaxis in pregnant women and in women capable of pregnancy. Myocarditis occurring during pregnancy may be due to other causes, but its occurrence should raise the consideration of rheumatic fever, particularly in women with a previous episode. When congestive heart failure develops, it should be treated with standard therapy. (See also Chap. 78.)

Valve Disease

Mitral Valve Disease

Significant heart disease in women usually involves the mitral valve and is rheumatic in origin.

Mitral Stenosis The increased cardiac output, tachycardia, and fluid retention of pregnancy may double the resting pressure gradient across a stenotic mitral valve[76,77] resulting in hemodynamic deterioration in the patient with mitral stenosis. Symptoms attributable to an increase in left atrial pressure with associated pulmonary vascular congestion and bronchial vein distension occur in up to 25 percent of patients with mitral stenosis during pregnancy.[8,10] They usually become apparent by the 20th week and may be aggravated still further at the time of labor and delivery with the associated increases in heart rate and cardiac output. Maternal death from pulmonary edema may occur but is rare when there is careful attention to the management of congestive heart failure.[8,10,78] Although potentially at risk from the elevated left atrial pressure, the patient with significant mitral stenosis also depends on this pressure to fill the left ventricle adequately and thus to maintain cardiac output. The pregnant woman is liable to sudden shifts in the distribution of blood volume and is, therefore, at increased risk of a sudden decline in left atrial pressure and a consequent dramatic fall in cardiac output. This may also increase maternal and fetal morbidity and may be the explanation for the death of women with mitral stenosis who had no previous congestive heart failure.[10]

Management of the patient with mitral stenosis should include prophylaxis against rheumatic fever[72] and endocarditis.[71] When severe mitral stenosis is identified prior to pregnancy, mitral commissurotomy or balloon valvotomy (Chap. 86) should be undertaken before conception (see Chap. 80). When a woman with mitral stenosis becomes pregnant, no definitive treatment is needed unless symptoms develop, but restriction of activity to minimize symptoms is appropriate. If symptoms of pulmonary congestion develop, attempts should be made to control them with further restriction of activity and sodium intake. If an arrhythmia develops or pulmonary congestion persists, standard medical therapy is required. Should these symptoms be unremitting despite medical therapy, mitral commissurotomy or valve replacement can be performed, but fetal loss may be as high as 33 percent.[79,80] Balloon valvotomy is preferable for most women, particularly late in pregnancy when the effects of radiation from the catheterization are less likely to affect fetal development.[81,82] If thromboembolic complications develop, anticoagulation therapy is required, but again, warfarin derivatives should be avoided if possible because of the danger to the fetus.[83–87]

TABLE 113-3

Effects of Pregnancy on Heart Disease

Cardiac Lesion	Relevant Hemodynamic Change in Pregnancy	Result	Time of Greatest Risk	Demonstrated Risks	Management
Myocardial Disease					
Rheumatic fever; myocarditis; cardiomyopathy	↑ Blood volume ↑ Cardiac output	↑ Pulmonary capillary pressure ↓ Cardiac output	> 12 weeks	Uncommon: ↑ Maternal morbidity	Treat pulmonary congestion Avoid pregnancy if left ventricular failure is present
Valve Deformities					
Mitral stenosis	↑ Cardiac output ↑ Heart rate ↑ Blood volume ↓ Pulmonary vascular resistance	↑ Pulmonary capillary pressure	> 12 weeks (when hemodynamic changes become significant)	↑ Maternal morbidity and mortality from pulmonary congestion and pulmonary edema ↓ Fetal growth and ↑ fetal loss	Limit demands for cardiac output, based on symptoms Avoid tachycardia Treat tachyarrhythmia
	Obstruction of inferior vena cava by uterus Blood loss at delivery	↓ Venous return ↓ LA filling ↓ LV filling ↓ Cardiac output	Late in pregnancy when supine (labor, delivery, surgery) and post partum	Possible explanation of some maternal deaths	Maintain venous return, especially if symptoms of ↓ cardiac output occur
Mitral regurgitation (includes mitral prolapse when complicated by important mitral regurgitation)	↑ Blood volume	↑ Pulmonary capillary pressure	> 12 weeks	Uncommon: pregnancy is usually uneventful	Rx of pulmonary congestion if it occurs (restrict sodium intake, diuretics)
Aortic stenosis	Obstruction of inferior vena cava by uterus Blood loss at delivery	↓ Venous return ↓ LV filling ↓ Cardiac output	Late in pregnancy when supine (labor, delivery, surgery) and post partum	↑ Maternal mortality uncommon because aortic stenosis is rare in pregnancy	Maintain venous return Strict limitation of activity, and if symptoms persist, proceed to valve surgery or interruption of pregnancy
Aortic regurgitation	↑ Blood volume	↑ Pulmonary capillary pressure	> 12 weeks	Uncommon: pregnancy is usually uneventful	Rx of pulmonary congestion if it occurs (restrict sodium intake, diuretics)
Pulmonary stenosis	Obstruction of inferior vena cava by uterus Blood loss at delivery	↓ Venous return ↓ LV filling ↓ Cardiac output	Late in pregnancy when supine (labor, delivery, surgery) and post partum	Uncommon: pregnancy is usually uneventful	Maintain venous return

TABLE 113-3

Effects of Pregnancy on Heart Disease* (*Continued*)

Cardiac Lesion	Relevant Hemodynamic Change in Pregnancy	Result	Time of Greatest Risk	Demonstrated Risks	Management
Congenital Lesions					
Shunts: Left-to-right (septal defect, patent ductus)	↑ Cardiac output ↑ Blood volume ↑ Pulmonary vascular resistance	↑ Pulmonary capillary pressure	>12 weeks	Uncommon: pregnancy is usually uneventful	Rx of pulmonary congestion if it occurs (restrict sodium intake, diuretics)
Right-to-left (Eisenmenger's syndrome, tetralogy of Fallot)	↓ Peripheral vascular resistance Obstruction of inferior vena cava by uterus Blood loss at delivery	↑ Shunting and ↓ venous return ↓ Pulmonary blood flow	Late in pregnancy when supine (labor, delivery, surgery) and post partum	↑ Maternal mortality due to sudden death ↓ Fetal growth and ↑ fetal loss	Avoid pregnancy Maintain venous return
Coarctation of the aorta	Obstruction of inferior vena cava by uterus	↓ Venous return ↓ LV filling ↓ Cardiac output	Late in pregnancy when supine (labor, delivery, surgery) and post partum	Uncommon: pregnancy is usually uneventful	Maintain venous return
	↑ Blood volume ↑ Pulse pressure ↑ Steroid hormones ? Tendency to ↑ hypertension	Distension of aortic root	>12 weeks	Aortic rupture Dissection of aorta Rupture of intracranial aneurysm	Delay pregnancy until Rx optimal Treat hypertension and minimize ↑ pulse pressure
Pulmonary Hypertension					
Any cause	Obstruction of inferior vena cava by uterus Blood loss at delivery	↓ Venous return ↓ LV filling ↓ Cardiac output	Late in pregnancy when supine (labor, delivery, surgery) and post partum	↑ Maternal mortality due to sudden death	Avoid pregnancy Maintain venous return Try to lower pulmonary vascular resistance
Developmental Abnormalities					
Hypertrophic cardiomyopathy (Idiopathic hypertrophic subaortic stenosis)	Obstruction of inferior vena cava by uterus ↑ Heart rate Blood loss at delivery	↓ Venous return ↓ LV filling ↓ LV obstruction ↓ Cardiac output	>12 weeks	↑ Maternal morbidity during pregnancy	Maintain venous return β-adrenergic blockade to ↓ LV outflow obstruction
	↑ Blood volume	↑ Pulmonary capillary pressure		↑ Maternal morbidity during pregnancy	Rx of pulmonary congestion, especially diuretics
Marfan's syndrome	↑ Blood volume ↑ Pulse pressure ↑ Steroid hormones	Distension of aortic root	> 12 weeks	↑ Maternal mortality from aortic dissection or rupture	Avoid pregnancy Minimize ↑ pulse pressure

* This table summarizes the theoretical basis for concern about specific heart lesions in relation to the cardiovascular changes which normally occur during pregnancy. Under "Management" we list specific recommendations for each lesion, omitting consideration of general recommendations for prophylaxis against rheumatic fever and bacterial endocarditis, maintenance of general health, and precautions against anemia, infections, anxiety, and fatigue. The statement *Avoid pregnancy* means that the lesion has a documented high risk during pregnancy. Accordingly, in our opinion, pregnancy is inadvisable, and if it occurs, an early interruption is advised.

Mitral Regurgitation Mitral regurgitation from any cause is generally well tolerated during pregnancy. Unlike mitral stenosis, it may be due to a variety of causes, and it is of value to understand its etiology in considering the management during pregnancy. When it is caused by rheumatic fever, antibiotic prophylaxis against streptococcal infection is indicated. The presence of mitral regurgitation necessitates prophylaxis against endocarditis at the time of labor and delivery (see also Chap. 94). Occasionally, the hemodynamic alterations of a normal pregnancy can overwhelm the capabilities of the heart with a regurgitant mitral lesion and result in symptoms of congestive heart failure. These should be treated in the routine manner. In our experience surgery for mitral regurgitation has not been necessary during pregnancy.

Mitral Valve Prolapse The mitral valve prolapse syndrome warrants discussion not because it is dangerous but because it is common, occurring in 5 to 10 percent of young adults.[88,89] There is some familial tendency toward the development of the syndrome, but there is no clear genetic pattern of inheritance. Pregnancy, with its changes in vascular resistance and blood volume, may alter the physical findings in the syndrome, either enhancing or diminishing them. It is not clear that the occasional problems associated with the syndrome (endocarditis, arrhythmia, cerebral emboli, or mitral regurgitation) are more likely to occur during pregnancy,[90–92] and no treatment is recommended except the use of prophylactic antibiotics at the time of labor and delivery in those with a heart murmur (see also Chap. 80).

Aortic Valve Disease

Aortic Stenosis Usually a congenital abnormality,[93] aortic stenosis is more common in males than in females and so is infrequently encountered during pregnancy. It is so rare that we may have underestimated its danger in the past. A woman with aortic stenosis may very rarely have difficulty during pregnancy with volume overload and associated congestive heart failure, but it is hypovolemia that puts these patients at greatest potential risk. Any significant fall in venous return can result in a dramatic fall in cardiac output with resulting cerebral or cardiac ischemia. In addition, with this fall in cardiac output, uterine blood flow may be compromised. With aortic stenosis maternal mortality rates up to 17 percent have been reported during pregnancy.[94] Mortality seems to be most likely to occur when the patient is predisposed to hypovolemia, for example, at the time of interruption of pregnancy, at which time the mortality rate approaches 40 percent.[94,95] A fetal mortality rate of 32 percent has also been noted in these women.

If a woman is found to have severe aortic stenosis prior to pregnancy, surgical correction before conception is advisable. This not only offers protection to the mother and fetus but also decreases the incidence of congenital heart disease in the infant.[20] In most women of this age, a commissurotomy suffices. If a valve must be inserted prior to pregnancy, the issue of long-term anticoagulation therapy should be considered a relative indication for use of a bioprosthesis rather than a mechanical prosthesis. In the patient with aortic stenosis who is already pregnant, measures to prevent hypovolemia and to restrict activity are appropriate. If symptoms develop, activity should be limited still further. If symptoms are progressive and cannot be controlled, aortic valve surgery, or possibly balloon valvotomy,[96] should be performed (see also Chap. 79).

Aortic Regurgitation Like aortic stenosis, aortic regurgitation is not common in young women, and like the other major regurgitant lesion, mitral regurgitation, it is usually well tolerated during pregnancy. Should heart failure develop, standard treatment is appropriate. Antibiotic prophylaxis at the time of labor and delivery is indicated. If aortic regurgitation develops in a patient with endocarditis and if the infection is not rapidly controlled or if hemodynamic deterioration occurs, early surgery should be considered despite the pregnancy. The mortality rate associated with medical therapy alone is high in such patients[97] (see also Chap. 79).

Pulmonary and Tricuspid Valve Disease

Pulmonary valve lesions are uncommon in pregnancy. Significant stenosis should be corrected prior to pregnancy. If it is recognized after conception, treatment is unnecessary unless the mother is symptomatic despite restriction of activity. If mechanical correction is necessary during pregnancy, balloon valvotomy (Chap. 94) would seem optimal.

Doppler echocardiographic evidence of tricuspid regurgitation is common[98] but severe disease is not. With an increase in intravenous drug use, this may change. When present, tricuspid regurgitation is well tolerated during pregnancy, and no special considerations are in order other than prophylaxis against bacterial endocarditis (see also Chap. 81).

Congenital Heart Disease

An increasing number of women with congenital heart disease are reaching childbearing age and many are capable of conception. Each abnormality has its unique relation to pregnancy.[4,78] Some considerations applicable in all cases were discussed in the beginning of the chapter.

Pulmonary Hypertension

It is recognized that pulmonary hypertension may not be simply the result of congenital heart disease and that it is frequently related to some of the abnormalities discussed below, but its danger warrants emphasis here. *Pulmonary hypertension is a contraindication to pregnancy.* Whether hypertension is primary (with no recognizable cause) or secondary (due to prolonged left-to-right shunting, drug abuse, or recurrent pulmonary emboli), the risks to the lives of the mother and the child are significant. The maternal mortality rate approaches 50 percent in those with primary pulmonary hypertension,[18] and when the hypertension is due to Eisenmenger's syndrome, the maternal mortality rate ranges from 30 to 70 percent.[17,78] Death may occur during gestation or the postdelivery period. The fetal mortality rate exceeds 40 percent even when the mother survives. If pregnancy occurs in a woman with pulmonary hypertension, interruption should be recommended. If this recommendation is not accepted, aggressive attempts to prevent hypovolemia are essential, especially during and after delivery. A sudden fall of venous return limits the ability of the right ventricle to pump blood through the fixed pulmonary vascular resistance, often resulting in a cascading hemodynamic and metabolic deterioration with subsequent death (see also Chap. 97).

Congenital Heart Disease without Associated Cyanosis

Left-to-Right Shunts Some women with left-to-right shunts reach adulthood and become pregnant, occasionally with no previous recognition of the cardiac abnormality. Others undergo surgical correction prior to pregnancy, but residual defects may remain. Although left-to-right shunting increases the chance of pulmonary hypertension, right ventricular failure, arrhythmias, emboli, and congestive heart failure, it is not clear that these complications are made more likely by pregnancy. The degree of shunting is affected by the relative resistances in the systemic and pulmonary vascular circuits; both fall during pregnancy and the changes are normally similar, so there is no significant alteration in the degree of shunting during pregnancy.[29] Those with shunts also have right ventricular volume overload. Like other volume overload conditions, pregnancy is reasonably well tolerated.

Patients with uncomplicated atrial septal defects tolerate pregnancy well unless there are associated complex cardiac or congenital abnormalities. Women with a ventricular septal defect or patent ductus arteriosus are more likely to have had their cardiac abnormality recognized and corrected prior to pregnancy, but if they have not, they, too, tolerate a pregnancy well. The offspring of these women have a 4 to 10 percent[20–26] incidence of congenital cardiac defects (Table 113-2), an incidence which is not affected by surgical correction prior to pregnancy[26] (see also Chaps. 96 and 97).

With any left-to-right shunting there is a risk of thrombosis and emboli, but routine anticoagulation therapy is not appropriate. Should congestive heart failure develop from a left-to-right shunt, standard therapy is indicated.

Obstructive Lesions Obstructive lesions of the left side of the heart include the previously discussed aortic valve stenosis, and also supra- as well as subaortic valve stenosis. In general, surgical correction prior to pregnancy for any of these lesions may protect the mother during pregnancy and, of interest, may significantly reduce the incidence of congenital heart disease in the offspring.[20] This suggests that the hemodynamic effects of left ventricular obstructive lesions influence fetal development, presumably by affecting uterine perfusion.

Although there are a variety of left ventricular obstructive disease processes, two syndromes warrant some discussion: coarctation of the aorta and hypertrophic obstructive cardiomyopathy.

Although *coarctation of the aorta* usually affects males, it may occur in women and may be associated with a bicuspid aortic valve. Coarctation and its associated lesions shorten life span, but affected individuals often reach childbearing age and may conceive. These individuals are at risk of aortic root dissection and of cerebral hemorrhage due to rupture of associated intracranial aneurysms and complications of prolonged hypertension. The risk of these events is even higher during pregnancy, with an overall maternal mortality rate in these patients of approximately 3 percent.[8,99] Cardiovascular complications, particularly aortic rupture or dissection, are common in those who survive.[99–101] Should pregnancy occur in a patient with a coarctation, treatment of hypertension is indicated. Care should be taken to prevent major swings in blood pressure, and prophylactic antibiotics against endocarditis are appropriate (see also Chap. 97).

Hypertrophic obstructive cardiomyopathy is recognized with increasing frequency and is usually inherited as an autosomal dominant condition (see also Chap. 90). Because its dynamic characteristics are affected by changes in ventricular volume and vascular resistance, it might be expected that pregnancy would not be well tolerated. The normal fall in peripheral vascular resistance during pregnancy and the tendency to hypotension due to obstructed venous return or to blood loss at the time of delivery both tend to increase the outflow tract obstruction, an undesirable consequence. In addition, the emotional variations and the intermittent discomfort of pregnancy, labor, and delivery are likely to be associated with increased catecholamine levels, which may also increase outflow obstruction. An increase in both the number and the severity of symptoms has been noted in women with obstructive cardiomyopathy during pregnancy,[102–104] and a death due to ventricular tachycardia has been reported.[105]

Management of patients with hypertrophic obstructive cardiomyopathy should include avoidance of hypovolemia. Beta-adrenergic blocking agents have been used at the time of labor and delivery,[102] but it is not clear that their use is necessary on a prophylactic basis.[104] If the patient develops angina or tachyarrhythmia, these drugs may be instituted during pregnancy, though the potential effects of beta-adrenergic blockade on the fetus should be considered. Prophylactic antibiotics are needed at the time of labor and delivery as these women are at risk of developing endocarditis on their mitral valve.

Obstructions to right ventricular outflow are also preferably corrected prior to pregnancy. This not only will decrease maternal morbidity but, as with correction of left-sided obstructive lesions, may decrease the incidence of congenital heart disease in the offspring.[20] If pregnancy occurs prior to correction, however, a safe pregnancy results in most cases. Treatment should be directed toward preventing intravascular volume depletion. The dangers of right ventricular obstruction due to increased pulmonary vascular resistance have been emphasized in the discussion of pulmonary hypertension.

Cyanotic Congenital Heart Disease

Congenital cardiac lesions resulting in cyanosis are frequently complex and deserve individual consideration. An increasing number of women with cyanotic congenital heart disease are living three to four decades and are becoming pregnant.[4,106]

Women with *tetralogy of Fallot* may accomplish a full-term pregnancy, but they and their fetuses are at increased risk of morbidity and mortality.[4,106] In addition, as with any form of cyanotic heart disease, the children are likely to be small at birth and fetal wastage is high. Alterations in pulmonary or peripheral vascular resistance and in venous return may cause sudden changes in pulmonary or peripheral blood flow, which may result in symptoms or death. Surgical correction of the cardiac lesion prior to pregnancy reduces maternal risk, almost to that of normal women.[20,26,107] The fetal risk is also reduced, but the baby continues to have an increased chance of having congenital heart disease[20,21,108] (Chap. 97).

Even women with *transposition of the great arteries* (some with single ventricles) may become pregnant. Maternal risk is difficult to evaluate because "therapeutic interruption" is carried out in many series, but a woman can survive pregnancy.[20] Fetal loss, however, approaches 50 percent. Partial or complete surgical correction of the lesion prior to pregnancy decreases the spontaneous abortion rate.

Marfan's Syndrome

It may be difficult to make the diagnosis of Marfan's syndrome (it has been recommended that ocular lens subluxation and aortic root disease be documented before the diagnosis is definite)[9] but it is important to do so because pregnancy is particularly dangerous for affected women. First, half the offspring inherit the problem. Second, the life span of a parent with Marfan's syndrome is reduced to half of normal; this must be considered when contemplating the future of the child. Third, and perhaps most important, the risk of death from aortic rupture or dissection is high during pregnancy,[101,109] particularly if the aortic root is enlarged (>40 mm by echocardiogram has been used as one criteria).[110,111] For all these reasons, women with Marfan's syndrome should be advised to avoid pregnancy. If the diagnosis of Marfan's syndrome is definite, the risks of pregnancy are so high that interruption should be recommended. Should the parents elect to continue with the pregnancy, the mother's activity should be restricted and hypertension should be prevented. Beta blockade has not yet been clearly proved to be of value when used on a prophylactic basis, but its use in pregnant patients with Marfan's syndrome seems reasonable. Prophylactic antibiotics against endocarditis should be used with labor and delivery because of the high incidence of associated mitral valve prolapse and bicuspid aortic valves.

Congestive (Dilated) Cardiomyopathies

Pregnancy should be avoided by women with idiopathic dilated cardiomyopathy (Chap. 89). This strong recommendation does not result from studying a large number of patients with idiopathic dilated cardiomyopathy or secondary cardiomyopathy (Chap. 88). Rather, it comes from the observation that myocardial dysfunction is the feature associated with increased maternal and fetal mortality in many forms of heart disease.

A concern for maternal safety in women with a dilated cardiomyopathy also comes from observations of those who develop this problem as a result of pregnancy. This *peripartum cardiomyopathy* occurs almost exclusively in the third trimester or in the first six postpartum weeks. It is this timing that suggests pregnancy is the cause. In women whose ventricular function does not return to normal, subsequent pregnancies are associated with exacerbation of the disease and with a maternal mortality approaching 50 percent.[14,112,113] When ventricular function returns to normal after pregnancy, a subsequent safe pregnancy is possible,[114] but maternal mortality still approaches 10 percent.[113] With this *peripartum cardiomyopathy*, pathological changes are similar to those of other types of dilated cardiomyopathies.[112] Small studies suggest that an endomyocardial biopsy is likely to reveal an inflammatory process and that azathioprine and prednisone may favorably affect outcome.[16,115] In the United States, peripartum cardiomyopathy occurs most commonly in black women, especially in those who are multiparous, older, or pregnant (or postpartum) with twins, and those whose pregnancy is complicated by hypertension.[14,15] If pregnancy occurs, treatment should include limitation of activity. If heart failure occurs and persists despite standard treatment, interruption of pregnancy must be considered.

Coronary Artery Disease

Myocardial infarction and angina pectoris during pregnancy have been reported.[59–62,116] The causes of the coronary obstruction have been thromboemboli, dissection, and presumed spasm, as well as atherosclerosis. Kawasaki's disease is being recognized with increased frequency[117] and has already been implicated as a cause of myocardial infarction in pregnancy[118] (see also Chap. 64). If a coronary disease syndrome is recognized, standard medical therapy is most appropriate, but coronary bypass surgery[63] and angioplasty[119] have also been utilized.

Cardiac Arrhythmias

Pregnant women frequently experience dizziness, palpitations, and syncope, but arrhythmias are also not uncommon during pregnancy[2,120] and should be considered a possible cause. As in the nonpregnant state, if a tachyarrhythmia is demonstrated, management should be undertaken with deliberate effort to avoid drug treatment. Attempts to manipulate the environment in terms of eliminating stimulants (especially caffeine), fatigue, and anxiety are always appropriate. When medical treatment is required, standard medications should be used. If cardioversion is necessary, it appears to be tolerated without problems to the mother and child.[121] As in the nonpregnant state, drug treatment of asymptomatic atrial or ventricular premature beats, or runs of premature beats,[122] is not justified.

Bradyarrhythmias may also occur during pregnancy.[2,120] They generally do not require treatment unless they result in symptoms or in clear compromise of maternal hemodynamics. Even complete heart block, which in this age group is most likely to be congenital in origin, is consistent with successful pregnancy.[123] The indications for insertion of a permanent pacemaker are not changed by a pregnancy[124] (see Chap. 40).

Pregnancy and Cardiac Surgery

Valve Surgery

Individuals who have undergone commissurotomy or surgical repair of a valve almost always have a residual deformity. They should be managed in the same way as other patients with valve disease. The use of antibiotics at the time of labor and delivery is advised (Chap. 94), and those with rheumatic valve disease should take antibiotics chronically to prevent recurrences of rheumatic fever (Chap. 78). Patients who are symptomatic from the valve disease despite surgery require careful evaluation and consideration of further surgery before pregnancy is undertaken. Some do not attain sufficient relief from surgery to permit a safe pregnancy.

Prosthetic Valves

A prosthetic heart valve is a relative contraindication for pregnancy. This recommendation is influenced by the maternal mortality rate of 1 to 5 percent, the 20 to 40 percent incidence of congestive heart failure, emboli bleeding, infections, or severe arrhythmias during pregnancy,[11,86,125–128] and the greater than 5 percent/year chance of severe complications or death that the mother faces indefinitely.[129] If a couple elects to accept those risks and the woman becomes pregnant, the type of prosthesis she has influences management.

All patients with *mechanical* prosthetic heart valves require full anticoagulation therapy. Because of the risks to the fetus from the warfarin derivatives, women with mechanical prostheses should be instructed in the use of heparin therapy when contemplating pregnancy or when pregnant.[83,84,130–133] Low-dose ("minidose") heparin does not adequately prevent embolic events,[131] so full-dose subcutaneous heparin is required (see also Chap. 68).

The single advantage of bioprosthetic heart valves over mechanical prostheses is their lower susceptibility to thrombosis and thromboembolic events. This lower susceptibility allows freedom from anticoagulant therapy. For this reason, it is an advantage for a young woman planning pregnancy to have a tissue valve. A disadvantage to the tissue prosthesis is the high likelihood of the eventual need for valve replacement.[128] If an individual with a heterograft valve has an embolic event, anticoagulants (heparin during pregnancy) should be instituted (see also Chap. 80).

Prophylactic antibiotics must be used at the time of dental and surgical procedures and at the time of labor and delivery by women with a mechanical or a tissue prosthesis. If endocarditis develops in a pregnant woman with a prosthetic valve, aggressive antibiotic therapy must be instituted (Chap. 94). If the infection is not immediately controlled, replacement of the prosthesis is required.

Pregnancy after Surgery for Congenital Lesions

The risks of pregnancy in patients with cardiovascular disease depend on the residual lesions and the type of surgery. Surgical correction, even if not complete, increases maternal safety and fetal viability and decreases the chance of congenital heart disease in the infant.[20] Patients with persistent pulmonary hypertension are at high risk of maternal and fetal mortality. If residual defects are present, or if a patch, conduit, or artificial valve has been inserted, antibiotics should be used in dental and surgical procedures and with labor and delivery (see Chap. 94).

Pregnancy after Cardiac Transplantation

Many cardiac transplant recipients are women of childbearing age. While successful pregnancies after transplantation have been reported,[134] the potential hazards to the mother and the fetus include maternal heart failure, immunosuppressive therapy, maternal infections, and serial diagnostic studies. The potential for a shortened maternal life span should also be remembered when a patient is counseled about the advisability of pregnancy (see Chap. 32).

THE USE OF CARDIOVASCULAR DRUGS IN PREGNANCY

It is best to avoid medications during pregnancy when possible. However, if the cardiovascular function of the mother indicates the need for a drug, it should not be withheld.[132,135–137]

Diuretics

Diuretics should be reserved for women with congestive heart failure uncontrolled by sodium restriction and those with hypertension.[137,138] Although it was once advised that they be used in an uncomplicated pregnancy to prevent preeclampsia, this is now discouraged. There are some potential risks to the fetus from using thiazide diuretics in pregnancy.

Inotropic Agents

Indications for the use of digitalis are not changed by pregnancy. Both digoxin and digitoxin cross the placental barrier, and fetal serum levels approximate those in the mother.[139] The same dose of digoxin, in general, yields lower maternal serum levels during pregnancy than in the nonpregnant state, so measurement of blood levels may be required if the desired clinical effect is not achieved. Digitalis may shorten the duration of gestation and labor, possibly because of an effect on the myometrium similar to the inotropic effect of digitalis on the myocardium.[140]

When intravenous inotropic or vasopressor agents are required, the standard agents (dopamine, norepinephrine, dobutamine) may be used, but the fetus is jeopardized because all the available preparations result in decreased uterine blood flow and may stimulate uterine contractions.

Adrenergic Receptor Blockade

Studies suggesting that beta blockers may decrease umbilical blood flow,[141] initiate premature labor,[142] and result in a small and infarcted placenta with a potential for low birth weight infants[143] have led to concerns about their use. However, they have been employed for such a large number of pregnant women without adverse effects[143,144] that their use for the usual indication seems appropriate. The β_1 selective drugs in particular have been associated with successful, uncomplicated pregnancies.[144,145] All the available beta-blocking agents cross the placenta, are present in human breast milk, and can reach significant clinical levels in the fetus or the newborn. If these agents are used during pregnancy it is appropriate to monitor fetal heart rate, as well as the newborn infant's heart rate, blood sugar, and respiratory status after delivery, carefully.[135,136]

Antiarrhythmic Agents

All of the antiarrhythmic drugs cross the placenta and are excreted in breast milk. Fetal serum levels can approach those of the mother. While this feature has been used on occasion to treat fetal arrhythmias,[145,146] there is insufficient accumulated information to know whether or not these drugs put the fetus, or child, at risk.[136,137]

Lidocaine is the preferred drug for a dangerous ventricular rhythm requiring urgent treatment. Intravenous procainamide or quinidine are alternatives if lidocaine fails. Bretylium tosylate is a third choice, because it may adversely affect uterine perfusion.

If chronic oral antiarrhythmic drug is essential, quinidine has been used most frequently without clear adverse effects unique to pregnancy.[147] It is, of course, a drug that should be used with concern in any population.[148] There is some information available about procainamide, disopyramide,[149-151] adenosine,[152] mexiletine,[153] flecainide,[153,154] and amiodarone.[155,156] Each of these should be avoided unless absolutely required for maternal protection.

Calcium Channel Blocking Agents and Adenosine

Nifedipine, verapamil, and diltiazem have not been demonstrated to adversely affect pregnancy.[107,108] Each, however, is a peripheral vasodilator and may lower blood pressure sufficiently to decrease uterine blood flow. Each crosses the placenta and is found in breast milk, but adverse effects on the fetus or infant have not been reported. Verapamil is as effective in managing supraventricular arrhythmias during pregnancy as at other times.[151] Adenosine has been successfully used in pregnancy to treat paroxysmal supraventricular tachycardia without recognized adverse effects.[152]

Vasodilator Agents

Although none of the vasodilators is contraindicated, the preload and afterload reducers have the potential for adversely affecting uterine perfusion.[136] Many also cross the placenta and fetal effects have not been well defined. Hydralazine and the nitrate preparations have been most frequently used with good fetal tolerance. There is little information available on the effects of captopril,[157] enalopril, or lisinopril on the fetus, but perinatal renal dysfunction associated with maternal use of angiotensin-converting enzyme (ACE) inhibitors is a reason to use alternative drugs when possible.[158] Nitroprusside use may result in fetal accumulation of thiocyanate and cyanide, but its use is justified in life-threatening situations.[159]

Anticoagulants

Concerns about the use of anticoagulants in pregnancy have already been expressed. The warfarin derivatives pose the usual significant risks to the mother: a 1 to 5 percent chance per year of a significant bleeding episode and up to a 10 percent chance per year of a minor hemorrhage. The fetus is at an even higher risk because warfarin derivatives cross the placenta. Fetal exposure during the first 2 months results in a 15 to 25 percent incidence of malformations from the so-called warfarin embryopathy syndrome (facial abnormalities, optic atrophy, digital abnormalities, epithelial changes, and mental impairment).[85,86,160,161] Although organogenesis is reasonably complete by the end of the first trimester, fetal risk continues: warfarin increases the chance of fetal bleeding or maternal intrauterine bleeding and may cause mental or visual impairment of the fetus. Safety from this drug is not granted in the third trimester either, as the risk of hemorrhage persists, particularly at the time of labor and delivery. Although pregnancy has been well tolerated and successfully accomplished in patients on long-term anticoagulant therapy,[125] it is best to avoid warfarin derivatives whenever possible. One alternative is to use no anticoagulants, but in some patients, particularly those with prosthetic heart valves or recurrent embolic episodes, this is not acceptable. The preferred alternative is the use of heparin, which does not cross the placental barrier. Although the mother continues to be at risk of bleeding, fetal development is not endangered. Women can be instructed in the outpatient use of heparin, and its use is preferable to that of warfarin,[130-132] particularly at the time of conception and in the first trimester.[86]

Antiplatelet agents increase the chance of maternal bleeding and cross the placenta. The most commonly used of them, aspirin, is associated with an increased incidence of abortion and fetal growth retardation.[162] It does not increase the incidence of cardiac malformation in the newborn,[163] but its inhibition of prostaglandin synthesis may result in closure of the ductus arteriosus during fetal life.[164] (See also Chap. 68.)

OBSTETRIC DRUGS AND THEIR CARDIAC EFFECTS

Drugs Used to Stimulate the Uterus

Significant hemodynamic changes may be associated with attempts to induce or suppress labor. The injection of hypertonic solutions into the uterus to produce abortion may result in hypervolemia and, if saline is used, hypernatremia. Prostaglandins E_2 and F_{2a} are employed as agents for inducing labor, both at term and in therapeutic abortion. Hemodynamic alterations are not observed in the low doses generally recommended.

Drugs Used to Quiet the Uterus

Ethyl alcohol administered intravenously in hypertonic concentrations is frequently used to avert premature labor. Its use is no longer recommended. Ritodrine, isoxsuprine, hydrochloride, terbutaline, and other beta-sympathomimetic amines are sometimes used to stop premature labor. All cause an increase in heart rate and contractility and should not be used when diabetes, hypertension, or heart disease complicates pregnancy. The use of ritodrine and terbutaline at term has been associated with pulmonary edema.[165,166] Evidence to date indicates that the pulmonary edema is not due to left ventricular failure. It responds promptly to cessation of the beta-sympathomimetic amine and administration of diuretics.

Drugs Used at Delivery

Adequate analgesia for pain minimizes the hemodynamic burden of labor and reduces the danger of pulmonary edema precipitated by tachycardia. The anesthetic technique employed for delivery should depend on the training and competence of the anesthesiologist. Subarachnoid block, epidural block using an anesthetic solution containing epinephrine, and balanced general anesthesia (thiopental sodium, nitrous oxide, oxygen, and succinylcholine) are all associated with major, although transient, hemodynamic changes.[42,167–169] Epidural anesthesia without epinephrine in the anesthetic solution is the most effective of the techniques explored so far in maintaining hemodynamic stability.[42] Scopolamine is contraindicated because of the restlessness and tachycardia it evokes, and atropine should be used in minimal doses and with caution. A term delivery in a well-managed patient offers the best hope of a successful outcome for both mother and child. Although term cesarean section has historically been associated with a high maternal mortality rate in patients with mitral stenosis, with modern techniques and in skilled hands, surgical delivery may be preferable to labor for the rare patient in or on the verge of pulmonary edema at term.[170]

DIAGNOSTIC PROCEDURES FOR HEART DISEASE DURING PREGNANCY

The use of diagnostic procedures should be considered especially carefully during pregnancy because of potential risks to the mother and the child. Unless the normal changes of pregnancy are recognized, the findings may be misinterpreted. An electrocardiogram, though safe, should be obtained only when indicated to help deal with specific clinical problems. Nonspecific ST-T abnormalities have been reported during pregnancy, but their significance is not clear. There has also been a suggestion that a shift in the electrical axis on the electrocardiogram occurs during pregnancy, but these findings have not been universally accepted.[171]

All x-ray procedures should be avoided, particularly in early pregnancy. There is the risk of abnormal fetal organogenesis or of increased incidence of malignancy, particularly leukemia.[172] If x-ray procedures are required for maternal safety, risks to the fetus can be minimized by use of abdominal shielding, but attempts should be made to focus the radiation away from the fetus and to delay the study to as late in pregnancy as possible.[172]

Radionuclide studies should be avoided during pregnancy. Although many radionuclides should attach to albumin and thus not reach the fetus, separation can occur and fetal exposure is possible.

Cardiac catheterization should be avoided because of the dangers of fluoroscopic exposure and because of the potentially adverse effects of introducing foreign material into the cardiovascular system of a pregnant woman. However, if the woman is at particular risk from her heart disease, the procedure should be performed. It is important to emphasize that any woman who is about to undergo x-ray examination or cardiac catheterization should be questioned about the possibility of being pregnant.

A cardiac ultrasound evaluation is of no known risk to the mother or to the fetus, but it should be performed only when clinically indicated.

REFERENCES

1. Padmavati S: Rheumatic fever and rheumatic heart disease in developing countries. *Bull WHO* 1978; 56:543–550.
2. McFaul PB, Dornan JC, Lamki H, Boyle D: Pregnancy complicated by maternal heart disease. A review of 519 women. *Br J Obstet Gynecol* 1988; 95:861–867.
3. Bitsch M, Johansen C, Wennevold A, Osler M: Maternal heart disease. A survey of a decade in a Danish university hospital. *Acta Obstet Gynecol Scand* 1989; 68:119–124.
4. Pitkin RM, Perloff JK, Koos BJ, Beall MH: Pregnancy and congenital heart disease. *Ann Intern Med* 1990; 112:445–454.
5. Oakley CM: Pregnancy in heart disease: Pre-existing heart disease. *Cardiovasc Clin* 1989; 19:57–80.
6. Burwell CS, Metcalfe J: *Heart Disease and Pregnancy: Physiology and Management.* Boston, Little, Brown, 1958.
7. Jones AM, Howitt G: Eisenmenger syndrome in pregnancy. *Br Med J* 1956; 1:1627–1630.
8. Szekely P, Snaith L: *Heart Disease and Pregnancy.* Edinburgh, London, Churchill Livingstone, 1974: 171.
9. Pyeritz RE, McKusick VA: The Marfan's syndrome: Diagnosis and management. *N Engl J Med* 1979; 300:772–778.
10. Szekely P, Turner R, Snaith L: Pregnancy and the changing pattern of rheumatic heart disease. *Br Heart J* 1973; 35:1293–1303.
11. McAnulty JH, Morton MJ, Ueland K: The heart and pregnancy. *Curr Probl Cardiol* 1988; 13:589–665.
12. Lewis BV, Parsons M: Chorea gravidarum. *Lancet* 1966; 1: 284–286.
13. Ueland K, Metcalfe J: Acute rheumatic fever in pregnancy. *Am J Obstet Gynecol* 1966; 95:586–587.
14. Damakis JG, Rahimtoola SH, Sutton GC, Meadows WR, Szanto PB, Tobin JR, et al: Natural course of peripartum cardiomyopathy. *Circulation* 1971; 44:1053–1061.
15. Homans DC: Peripartum cardiomyopathy. *N Engl J Med* 1985; 312:1432–1437.
16. Midei MG, DeMent SH, Feldman AM, Hutchings GM, Baughman KL: Peripartum myocarditis and cardiomyopathy. *Circulation* 1990; 81:922–928.

17. Neilson G, Galca EG, Blunt A: Eisenmenger's syndrome and pregnancy. *Med J Aust* 1971; 1:431–434.
18. Dawkins K, Burke CM, Billingham M, Jamieson SW: Primary pulmonary hypertension and pregnancy. *Chest* 1986; 89:383–388.
19. Whittemore R, Wells JA, Castellsague-Pique X, Holabird N: Congenital heart defects in the second generation—A comparative study. (Abstr.) *Am J Cardiol* 1991; 66:524A.
20. Whittemore R, Hobbins JC, Engle MA: Pregnancy and its outcome in women with and without surgical treatment of congenital heart disease. *Am J Cardiol* 1982; 50:641–651.
21. Whittemore R: Congenital heart disease: Its impact on pregnancy. *Hosp Pract* 1983; 18:65–74.
22. Mitchell SC, Korones SB, Berendes HW: Congenital heart disease in 56,109 births: Incidence and natural history. *Circulation* 1971; 43:323–332.
23. Nora JJ, Nora AH: The evolution of specific genetic and environmental counseling in congenital heart diseases. *Circulation* 1978; 57:205–213.
24. Roberts N: A predictive study of congenital heart disease and need for care. *West J Med* 1978; 120:19–25.
25. Rose V, Gold RJM, Lindsay G, Allen M: A possible increase in the incidence of congenital heart defects among the offspring of affected parents. *J Am Coll Cardiol* 1985; 6:376–382.
26. Morris CD, Menashe VD: Recurrence of congenital heart disease in offspring of parents with surgical correction. (Abstr.) *Clin Res* 1985; 33:68A.
27. Lindheimer MC, Katz AL: Sodium and diuretics in pregnancy. *N Engl J Med* 1973; 299:891–894.
28. Chesley LC: Plasma and red cell volumes during pregnancy. *Am J Obstet Gynecol* 1972; 112:440–450.
29. Metcalfe J, Ueland K: Maternal cardiovascular adjustments to pregnancy. *Prog Cardiovasc Dis* 1974; 16:363–374.
30. Schrier RW: Pathogenesis of sodium and water retention in high-output and low-output cardiac failure, nephrotic syndrome, cirrhosis and pregnancy. *N Engl J Med* 1988; 319:1065–1072.
31. Milsom I, Hedner J, Hedner T: Plasma atrial natriuretic peptide (ANP) and maternal hemodynamic changes during normal pregnancy. *Acta Obstet Gynecol Scand* 1988; 67:717–722.
32. Adesanya CO, Anjorin FI, Sada IA, Parry EH, Sagnella GA, MacGregor GA: Atrial natriuretic peptide, aldosterone, and plasma renin activity in peripartum heart failure. *Br Heart J* 1991; 65:152–154.
33. Lees MM, Taylor SH, Scott DB, Kerr MG: A study of cardiac output at rest throughout pregnancy. *J Obstet Gynaecol Br Commonw* 1967; 74:319–328.
34. Rubler S, Damani PM, Pinto ER: Cardiac size and performance during pregnancy estimated with echocardiography. *Am J Cardiol* 1977; 40:534–540.
35. Katz R, Karliner JS, Resnick R: Effects of natural volume overload state (pregnancy) on left ventricular performance in normal human subjects. *Circulation* 1978; 58:434–441.
36. Capeless EL, Clapp JF: Cardiovascular changes in early phase of pregnancy. *Am J Obstet Gynecol* 1989; 161:1449–1453.
37. Easterling TR, Benedetti TJ, Schmucker BC, Millard SP: Maternal hemodynamics in normal and preeclamptic pregnancies: A longitudinal study. *Obstet Gynecol* 1990; 76:1061–1069.
38. Robson SC, Hunter S, Boys RJ, Dunlop W: Serial study of factors influencing changes in cardiac output during human pregnancy. *Am J Physiol* 1989; 256:H1060–H1065.
39. Clark SL, Cotton DB, Pivarnik JM, Lee W, Hankins GDV, Benedetti TJ, et al: Position change and central hemodynamic profile during normal third-trimester pregnancy and post partum. *Am J Obstet Gynecol* 1991; 164:883–887.
40. Vered Z, Poler SM, Gibson P, Wlody D, Perez JE: Noninvasive detection of the morphologic hemodynamic changes during normal pregnancy. *Clin Cardiol* 1991; 14:327–334.
41. Kerr MG: The mechanical effects of the gravid uterus in late pregnancy. *J Obstet Gynaecol Br Commonw* 1965; 72:513–529.
42. Ueland K, Akamatsu TJ, Eng M, Bonica JJ, Hansen JM: Maternal cardiovascular dynamics: VI. Cesarean section under epidural anesthesia without epinephrine. *Am Obstet* 1972; 114:775–780.
43. Sady MA, Haydon BB, Sady SP, Carpenter MW, Thompson PD, Coustan DR: Cardiovascular response to maximal cycle exercise during pregnancy and at two and seven months post partum. *Am J Obstet Gynecol* 1990; 162:1181–1185.
44. Thoresen M, Wesche J: Doppler measurements of changes in human mammary and uterine blood flow during pregnancy and lactation. *Acta Obstet Gynecol* 1988; 67:741–745.
45. Assali NS, Rauramo L, Peltonen T: Measurement of uterine blood flow and uterine metabolism: VII. Uterine and fetal blood flow and oxygen consumption in early human pregnancy. *Am J Obstet Gynecol* 1960; 79:86–98.
46. Metcalfe J, Romney SAL, Ramsey LH, Reid DE, Burwell CS: Estimation of uterine blood flow in normal human pregnancy at term. *J Clin Invest* 1955; 34:1632–1638.
47. Thaler I, Manor D, Itskovitz J, Rottem S, Levit N, Timor-Tritsch I, et al: Changes in uterine blood flow during human pregnancy. *Am J Obstet Gynecol* 1990; 162:121–125.
48. Roman-Ponce H, Thatcher WW, Caton D, Barron DH, Wilcox CJ: Effects of thermal stress and epinephrine on uterine blood flow in ewes. *J Anim Sci* 1978; 46:167–174.
49. Clapp JF: The effects of maternal exercise during pregnancy on uterine blood flow and pregnancy outcome. In: Moawad AH, Lindheimer MD (eds): *Uterine and Placental Blood Flow*. New York, Marson, 1982.
50. Watson WJ, Katz VL, Hackney AC, Gall MM, McMurray RG: Fetal responses to maximal swimming and cycling exercise during pregnancy. *Obstet Gynecol* 1991; 77:382–386.
51. Rauramo I, Forss M: Effect of exercise on maternal hemodynamics and placental blood flow in healthy women. *Acta Obstet Gynecol Scand* 1988; 67:21–25.
52. Clapp JF III, Capeless EL: Neonatal morphometrics after endurance exercise during pregnancy. *Am J Obstet Gynecol* 1990; 163:1805–1811.
53. Guzman CA, Caplan R: Cardiorespiratory response to exercise during pregnancy. *Am J Obstet Gynecol* 1970; 108:600–605.
54. Ueland K, Novy MJ, Metcalfe J: Cardiorespiratory responses to pregnancy and exercise in normal women and patients with heart disease. *Am J Obstet Gynecol* 1973; 115:4–10.
55. Sady SP, Carpenter MW, Thompson PD, Sady MA, Haydon B, Coustan DR: Cardiovascular response to cycle exercise during and after pregnancy. *J Appl Physiol* 1989; 66:336–341.
56. Burwell CS, Strayhorn WD, Flickinger D, Corlette MB: Circulation during pregnancy. *Arch Intern Med* 1938; 62:979–1003.
57. Hart MV, Hosenpud JD, Hohimer AR, Morton MJ: Hemodynamics during pregnancy and sex steroid administration in guinea pigs. *Am J Physiol* 1985; 249:R-179–185.
58. Hoversland AS, Parer JT, Metcalfe J: Hemodynamic adjustments in the pygmy goat during pregnancy and early postpartum. *Biol Reprod* 1974; 10:578–588.
59. Ciraulo DA, Markovitz A: Myocardial infarction in pregnancy associated with a coronary artery thrombus. *Arch Intern Med* 1979; 139:1046–1047.
60. Beary JF, Summer WR, Bulkley BH: Postpartum acute myocardial infarction: A rare occurrence of uncertain etiology. *Am J Cardiol* 1979; 43:158–161.
61. Ahronheim JH: Isolated coronary periarteritis: Report of a case of unexpected death in a young pregnant woman. *Am J Cardiol* 1977; 40:287–290.
62. Jewett J: Two dissecting coronary-artery aneurysms post partum. *N Engl J Med* 1978; 298:1255–1256.
63. Majden JF, Walinsky P, Cowchock SF, Wagner RJ, Plzak L Jr: Coronary artery bypass surgery during pregnancy. *Am J Cardiol* 1983; 52:1145–1151.
64. Cutforth R, MacDonald CB: Heart sounds and murmurs in pregnancy. *Am Heart J* 1966; 71:741–747.
65. Meyer MB, Tonascia JA: Maternal smoking, pregnancy complications, and perinatal mortality. *Am J Obstet Gynecol* 1987; 128:494–502.
66. Rosett HL, Weiner L: Alcohol and the fetus: a clinical perspective In: *Fetus Clinical Perspective*. New York, Oxford University Press, 1984.
67. Rodgers BD, Lee RV: Drug abuse. In: Burrow GN, Ferris TF (eds): *Medical Complications During Pregnancy*, 3d ed. Philadelphia, Saunders, 1988: 570–581.
68. Casnoff IJ, Burns WJ, Schnoll SH, Burns KA: Cocaine use in pregnancy. *N Engl J Med* 1985; 313:666–669.
69. Rimland D, McGowan JE, Shulman JA: Immunization for the internist. *Ann Intern Med* 1976; 85:622–629.
70. Naeye RL, Peters EC: Working during pregnancy: Effects on the fetus. *Pediatrics* 1982; 69:724–727.
71. Dajani AS, Bisno AL, Chung KJ, Durack DT, Freed M, Gerber MA, et al: Prevention of bacterial endocarditis—Recommenda-

tions by the American Heart Association. *JAMA* 1990; 264:2919–2922.
72. Dajani AS, Bisno AL, Chung KJ, Durack DT, Gerber MA, Kaplan EL, et al: Prevention of rheumatic fever. *Circulation* 1988; 78:1082–1086.
73. Krause RM: The influence of infection on the geography of heart disease. *Circulation* 1979; 60:972–976.
74. Massell BF, Chute CG, Walker AM, Kurland GS: Penicillin and the marked decrease in morbidity and mortality from rheumatic fever in the United States. *N Engl J Med* 1988; 318:280–286.
75. Veasy LG, Widemeier SE, Orsmond GS, Ruttenberg HD, Boucek MM, Roth SJ, et al: Resurgence of acute rheumatic fever in the intermountain area of the United States. *N Engl J Med* 1987; 316:421–427.
76. McAnulty JH: Rheumatic heart disease. In: Gleicher N (ed): *Principles and Practice of Medical Therapy in Pregnancy,* 2d ed. Norwalk, CT, Appleton and Lange, 1992.
77. Bryg RJ, Gordon PR, Kudesia VS, Bhatia RK: Effect of pregnancy on pressure gradient in mitral stenosis. *Am J Cardiol* 1989; 63:384–386.
78. Metcalfe J, McAnulty JH, Ueland K: *Pregnancy and Heart Disease.* Boston, Little, Brown, 1986.
79. Commerford PJ, Hastie T, Beck W: Closed mitral valvotomy: Actuarial analysis of results in 654 patients over 12 years and analysis of preoperative predictors of long-term survival. *Ann Thorac Surg* 1982; 33:473–479.
80. Bernal JM, Miralles PJ: Cardiac surgery with cardiopulmonary bypass during pregnancy. *Obstet Gynecol Surv* 1986; 41:1–6.
81. Mangione JA, Zuliani MF, Del Castillo JM, Nogueira EA, Arie S: Percutaneous double balloon mitral valvuloplasty in pregnant women. *Am J Cardiol* 1989; 64:99–102.
82. Esteves CA, Auristela IOR, Braga SLN, Harrison JK, Sonsa JEMR: Effectiveness of percutaneous balloon mitral valvotomy during pregnancy. *Am J Cardiol* 1991; 68:930–934.
83. Hall JG, Pauli RM, Wilson KM: Maternal and fetal sequelae of anticoagulation during pregnancy. *Am J Med* 1980; 68:122–140.
84. Merrill LK, VerBurg DJ: The choice of long-term anticoagulants for the pregnant patient. *Obstet Gynecol* 1976; 47:711–714.
85. Stevenson RE, Burton M, Frelauto GH, Taylor HA: Hazards of oral anticoagulants during pregnancy. *JAMA* 1985; 243:1549–1551.
86. Iturbe-Alessio I, Fonseca MC, Mutchnik O, Santos MA, Zajarias A, Salazar E: Risks of anticoagulant therapy in pregnant women with artificial heart valves. *N Engl J Med* 1986; 315:1390–1393.
87. Sareli P, England MJ, Berk MR, Marcus RH, Epstein M, Driscoll J, et al: Maternal and fetal sequelae of anticoagulation during pregnancy in patients with mechanical heart valve prostheses. *Am J Cardiol* 1989; 63:1462–1465.
88. Devereux RB, Perloff JK, Reichek N, Josephson ME: Mitral valve prolapse. *Circulation* 1976; 54:3–14.
89. Procacci PM, Savran SV, Schreiter SL, Bryson AL: Prevalence of clinical mitral-valve prolapse in 1,169 young women. *N Engl J Med* 1976; 294:1086–1088.
90. Shapiro EP, Trible EL, Robinson JC, Estruch MT, Gottlieb SH: Safety of labor and delivery in women with mitral valve prolapse. *Am J Cardiol* 1985; 56:806–807.
91. Cowles T, Gonik B: Mitral valve prolapse in pregnancy. *Semin Perinatol* 1990; 14:34–41.
92. Degani S, Abinader EG, Scharf M: Mitral valve prolapse and pregnancy: A review. *Obstet Gynecol Surv* 1989; 44:642–649.
93. Roberts WC: The congenitally bicuspid aortic valve: A study of 85 autopsy cases. *Am J Cardiol* 1970; 26:72–83.
94. Arias F, Pineda J: Aortic stenosis in pregnancy. *J Reprod Med* 1978; 20:229–232.
95. Easterling TR, Chadwick HS, Otto CM, Benedetti TJ: Aortic stenosis in pregnancy. *Obstet Gynecol* 1988; 72:113–118.
96. Angel JL, Chapman C, Knuppel RA, Moraless WJ, Sims CJ: Percutaneous balloon aortic valvuloplasty in pregnancy. *Obstet Gynecol* 1988; 72:438–440.
97. McAnulty JH, Rahmitoola SH: Surgery for infective endocarditis. *JAMA* 1979; 242:77–79.
98. Limacher MC, Ware JA, O'Meara ME, Fernandez GC, Young JB: Tricuspid regurgitation during pregnancy: Two dimensional and pulsed Doppler echocardiographic observations. *Am J Cardiol* 1985; 55:1059–1062.
99. Deal K, Wooley CF: Coarctation of the aorta and pregnancy. *Ann Intern Med* 1973; 78:706–710.
100. Barash PG, Hobbins JC, Hook R, Stansel HC Jr, Whittemore R, Hehre FW: Management of coarctation of the aorta during pregnancy. *J Thorac Cardiovasc Surg* 1975; 69:781–784.
101. Barrett JM, VanHooydonk JD, Bochm FH: Pregnancy related rupture of arterial aneurysms. *Obstet Gynecol Surv* 1982; 37:557–566.
102. Kolibash AJ, Ruis DE, Lewis RP: Idiopathic hypertrophic subaortic stenosis in pregnancy. *Ann Intern Med* 1975; 82:791–794.
103. Turner GM, Oakley CM, Dixon HG: Management of pregnancy complicated by hypertrophic obstructive cardiomyopathy. *Br Med J* 1968; 4:281–284.
104. Oakley GD, McGarry K, Limb DG, Oakley CM: Management of pregnancy in patients with hypertrophic cardiomyopathy. *Br Med J* 1979; 1:1749–1750.
105. Shah DM, Sunderji SG: Hypertrophic cardiomyopathy and pregnancy: Report of a maternal mortality and review of literature. *Obstet Gynecol Surv* 1985; 40:444–448.
106. Patton DE, Lee W, Cotton DB, Miller J, Carpenter RJ Jr, Huhta J, et al: Cyanotic maternal heart disease in pregnancy. *Obstet Gynecol Surv* 1990; 45:594–600.
107. Singh H, Bolton PJ, Oakley CM: Pregnancy after surgical correction of tetralogy of Fallot. *Br Med J* 285, 1982.
108. Zellers TM, Driscoll DJ, Michels VV: Prevalence of significant congenital heart defects in children of parents with Fallot's Tetralogy. *Am J Cardiol* 1990; 65:523–526.
109. Murdoch JL, Walker BA, Helpern BL, Kuzma JW, McKusick VA: Life expectancy and causes of death in the Marfan syndrome. *N Engl J Med* 1972; 2986:804–808.
110. Pyeritz RE: Maternal and fetal complications of pregnancy in the Marfan syndrome. *Am J Med* 1981; 71:784–790.
111. Mor-Yosef S, Younis J, Granat M, Kedari A, Milgalter A, Schenker JG: Marfan's syndrome in pregnancy. *Obstet Gynecol Surv* 1988; 43:382–385.
112. O'Connell JB, Costanzo-Mordin MR, Surbranian R, Robinson JA, Wallis DE, Scanlon PJ: Peripartum cardiomyopathy: Clinical, hemodynamic, histologic and prognostic characteristics. *J Am Coll Cardiol* 1986; 8:52–56.
113. Elkayam U, Ostrzega EL, Shotan A: Peripartum cardiomyopathy. In: Gleicher N (ed): *Principles and Practice of Medical Therapy in Pregnancy,* 2d ed. Norwalk, CT, Appleton and Lange, 1992.
114. Sutton MS, Cole P, Plappert M, Saltzman D, Goldhaber S: Effects of subsequent pregnancy on left ventricular function in peripartum cardiomyopathy. *Am Heart J* 1991; 121:1776–1778.
115. Melvin KR, Richardson PJ, Olsen EG, Daly K, Jackson G: Peripartum cardiomyopathy due to myocarditis. *N Engl J Med* 1982; 308:731–734.
116. Frenkel Y, Barkai G, Reisin L, Rath S, Mashiach S, Battler A: Pregnancy after myocardial infarction: Are we playing safe? *Obstet Gynecol* 1991; 77:822–825.
117. Gersony WM: Diagnosis and management of Kawasaki disease. *JAMA* 1991; 265:2699–2703.
118. Nolan TE, Savage RW: Peripartum myocardial infarction from presumed Kawasaki's disease. *South Med J* 1990; 83:360–361.
119. Cowan NC, de Belder MA, Rothman MT: Coronary angioplasty in pregnancy. *Br Heart J* 1988; 59:588–592.
120. Mendelson CL: Disorders of the heartbeat during pregnancy. *Am J Obstet Gynecol* 1956; 72:1268–1301.
121. Schroeder JS, Harrison DC: Repeated cardioversion during paroxysmal atrial tachycardia during 3 successive pregnancies. *Am J Cardiol* 1971; 27:445–446.
122. Chandra NC, Gates EA, Thamer M: Conservative treatment of paroxysmal ventricular tachycardia during pregnancy. *Clin Cardiol* 1991; 14:347–350.
123. Abramovici H, Faktor JH, Gonen Y, Brandes JM, Amikam S: Maternal permanent bradycardia: Pregnancy and delivery. *Obstet Gynecol* 1984; 63:381–383.
124. Jaffe R, Gruber A, Fejgin M, Altaras M, Ben-Aderet N: Pregnancy with an artificial pacemaker. *Obstet Gynecol Surv* 1987; 42: 137–139.
125. Casanegra P, Aviles G, Maturana G, Dubernet J: Cardiovascular management of pregnant women with a heart valve prosthesis. *Am J Cardiol* 1975; 36:802–806.
126. Deviri E, Levinsky L, Yuchezkel M, Levy MJ: Pregnancy after valve replacement with porcine xenograft prosthesis. *Surg Gynecol Obstet* 1985; 160:437–443.
127. Vitali E, Donatelli F, Quaini E, Groppelli G, Pellegrini A: Pregnancy in patients with mechanical prosthetic heart valves. Our

experience regarding 98 pregnancies in 57 patients. *J Cardiovasc Surg* 1986; 27:221–227.
128. McAnulty JH, Blair N, Walance C, Ueland K: Prosthetic heart valves and pregnancy: Maternal and infant outcome. (Abstr.) *J Am Coll Cardiol* 1986; 7:117A.
129. Bloomfield P, Wheatley DJ, Prescott RJ, Miller HC: Twelve-year comparison of a Bjork-Shiley mechanical heart valve with porcine bioprostheses. *N Engl J Med* 1991; 324:573–579.
130. Hellgren M, Mygards E-B: Long-term therapy with subcutaneous heparin during pregnancy. *Gynecol Obstet Invest* 1982; 13: 76–89.
131. Brabeck MC: Ambulatory management of thromboembolic diseases during pregnancy with continuous infusion of heparin. *JAMA* 1987; 257:1790–1791.
132. Ginsbert JS, Kowalchuk G, Hirsh J, Brill-Edwards P, Burrows R: Heparin therapy during pregnancy. *Arch Intern Med* 1989; 149:2233–2236.
133. Wang RY, Lee PK, Chow JS, Chen WW: Efficacy of low-dose, subcutaneously administered heparin in treatment of pregnant women with artificial heart valves. *Med J Aust* 1983; 2:126–128.
134. Kirk EP: Organ transplantation and pregnancy. *Am J Obstet Gynecol* 1991; 164:1629–1634.
135. Brinkman CR III, Woods JR Jr: Effects of cardiovascular drugs during pregnancy. *Cardiovasc Med* 1976; 1:231–251.
136. Tamari I, Eldar M, Rabinowitz M, Nuefeld HN: Medical treatment of cardiovascular disorders during pregnancy. *Am Heart J* 1982; 104:1357–1363.
137. Ueland K, McAnulty JH, Ueland FR, Metcalfe J: Special considerations in the use of cardiovascular drugs. *Clin Obstet Gynecol* 1981; 24:809–823.
138. Collins R, Yusuf S, Peto R: Overview of randomized trials of diuretics in pregnancy. *Br Med J* 1985; 290:17–23.
139. Rogers MC, Willerson JT, Goldblatt A, Smith TW: Serum digoxin concentrations in human fetus, neonate and infant. *N Engl J Med* 1972; 298:1010–1013.
140. Weaver JB, Person JF: Influence of digitalis on time of onset and duration of labor in women with cardiac disease. *Br Med J* 1973; 3:519–520.
141. Chez RA, Ehrenkrantz RA, Oakes GK, et al: Effects of adrenergic agents on ovine umbilical and uterine blood flows. In: Longo LD, Reneau DD (eds): *Fetal and Newborn Cardiovascular Physiology,* vol 2. *Fetal and Newborn Circulation.* New York and London, Garland STPM Press, 1978: 1.
142. Barden TP, Stander RW: Myometrial and cardiovascular effects of an adrenergic blocking drug in human pregnancy. *Am J Obstet Gynecol* 1968; 101:91–99.
143. Rubin PC: Beta-blockers in pregnancy. *N Engl J Med* 1982; 305:1323–1326.
144. Rubin PC, Butters L, Clark D, Sumner D, Beifield A, Pledger D, et al: Obstetric aspects of the use in pregnancy-associated hypertension of the beta-adrenoreceptor antagonist atenolol. *Am J Obstet Gynecol* 1984; 150:389–392.
145. Frishman WH, Chesner M: Beta-adrenergic blockers in pregnancy. *Am Heart J* 1988; 115:147–152.
146. Perry JC, Ayres NA, Carpenter RJ Jr: Fetal supraventricular tachycardia treated with flecainide acetate. *J Pediatr* 1991; 118:303–305.
147. Hill LM, Malkasian GD Jr: The use of quinidine sulfate throughout pregnancy. *Obstet Gynecol* 1979; 54:366–368.
148. Salerno DM: Quinidine, worse than adverse? *Circulation* 1991; 84:2196–2198.
149. Leonard RF, Braun TE, Levy AM: Initiation of uterine contractions by disopyramide during pregnancy. *N Engl J Med* 1978; 299:84–85.
150. Tadmor OP, Keren A, Rosenak D, Gal M, Shaia M, Hornstein E, et al: The effect of disopyramide on uterine contractions during pregnancy. *Am J Obstet Gynecol* 1990; 162:482–486.
151. Rotmensch HH, Elkayam U, Frishman W: Antiarrhythmic drug therapy during pregnancy. *Ann Intern Med* 1983; 98:487–497.
152. Podolsky SM, Varon J: Adenosine use during pregnancy. *Ann Emerg Med* 1991; 20:1027–1028.
153. Lownes HE, Ives TJ: Mexiletine use in pregnancy and lactation. *Am J Obstet Gynecol* 1987; 157:446–447.
154. Wagner X, Jouglard J, Moulin M, Miller AM, Petitjean J, Pisapia A: Coadministration of flecainide acetate and sotalol during pregnancy: Lack of teratogenic effects, passage across the placenta, and excretion in human breast milk. *Am Heart J* 1990; 119: 700–702.
155. McKenna WJ, Harris L, Rowlan E, Whitelaw A, Storey G, Holt D: Amiodarone therapy during pregnancy. *Am J Cardiol* 1983; 51:1231–1233.
156. Foster CJ, Love HG: Amiodarone in pregnancy. Case report and review of the literature. *Int J Cardiol* 1988; 20:307–316.
157. Fiocci R, Lijnen P, Fagard R, Staessen J, Amery A, Van Assche F, et al: Captopril during pregnancy. *Lancet* 1984; 2:1153.
158. Hanssens M, Keirse MJ, Vankelecom F, Van Assche FA: Fetal and neonatal effects of treatment with angiotensin converting enzyme inhibitors in pregnancy. *Obstet Gynecol* 1991; 78: 128–135.
159. Stempel JE, O'Grady JP, Morton MJ, Johnson KA: Use of sodium nitroprusside in complications of gestational hypertension. *Obstet Gynecol* 1982; 60:533–538.
160. Pauli RM, Madden JD, Kranzler KJ, Culpepper W, Port R: Warfarin therapy initiated during pregnancy and phenotypic chondrodysplasia punctata. *J Pediatr* 1976; 88:506–508.
161. Fillmore SJ, McDevitt E: Effects of coumarin compounds on the fetus. *Ann Intern Med* 1970; 73:731–735.
162. Corby DG: Aspirin in pregnancy and fetal effects. *Pediatrics* 1978; 62:930–937.
163. Werler MM, Mitchell AA, Shapiro S: The relation of aspirin use during the first trimester of pregnancy to congenital cardiac defects. *N Engl J Med* 1989; 321:1639–1642.
164. Rudolph AM: Effects of aspirin and acetaminophen in pregnancy and in the newborn. *Arch Intern Med* 1981; 141:358–363.
165. Elliot HR, Abdulla U, Haves PJ: Pulmonary oedema associated with ritodrine infusion and betamethasone administration in premature labour. *Br Med J* 1978; 2:799–800.
166. Hosenpud JD, Morton MJ, O'Grady JP: Cardiac stimulation during ritodrine hydrochloride tocolytic therapy. *Obstet Gynecol* 1983; 62:52–58.
167. Roberts SL, Chestnut DH: Anesthesia for the obstetric patient with heart disease. *Clin Obstet Gynecol* 1987; 30:601–610.
168. Ramanathen J, Sibai BM: Obstetric anesthesia for complicated pregnancy. In: Gleicher N (ed): *Principles and Practice of Medical Therapy in Pregnancy,* 2d ed. Norwalk, CT, Appleton and Lange, 1992.
169. Patton DE, Lee W, Miller J, Jones M: Maternal, uteroplacental, and fetoplacental hemodynamic and Doppler velocimetric changes during epidural anesthesia in normal labor. *Obstet Gynecol* 1991; 77:17–19.
170. Ferraris G, Gambotto C: Cesarean section as the method of choice for patients with cardiac decompensation. *Minerva Ginecol* 1972; 14:198–205.
171. Schwartz DB, Schamroth L: The effect of pregnancy on the frontal plane QRS axis. *J Electrocardiol* 1979; 12:279–281.
172. Mitchell MS, Capizzi RL: Neoplastic diseases. In: Burrow GN, Ferris TF (eds): *Medical Complications During Pregnancy.* Philadelphia, Saunders, 1988.

Chapter 114

Exercise and the Heart: Acute Hemodynamics, Conditioning Training, the Athlete's Heart, and Sudden Death

Peter M. Buttrick, M.D. ■ James Scheuer, M.D.

In recent years considerable interest has been focused on the effects of exercise conditioning on the cardiovascular system. This is due to clinical studies that suggest that exercise increases longevity and decreases the risk and symptoms of cardiovascular disease and to animal studies that show a reduced vulnerability to ischemic insult and lethal arrhythmias in the isolated hearts of conditioned animals. Also, hypertrophy of the heart secondary to dynamic physical conditioning has intrigued cardiac physiologists because it represents a unique form of cardiac hypertrophy associated with normal or enhanced cardiac function and coronary reserve. This contrasts with hypertrophy associated with chronic systolic overload, as observed in patients with long-standing hypertension or aortic stenosis, in which impaired cardiac function and depressed coronary reserve can be seen.

The current concept that exercise contributes to cardiovascular health must be contrasted with the historical view that prolonged exercise causes severe heart disease as evidenced by cardiac enlargement, significant arrhythmias, and electrocardiographic abnormalities. While this historical misconception has largely been corrected, the modern-day explosion of interest in exercise and physical fitness threatens to create a new myth of "biological arrogance" that implies that exercise can prevent or cure cardiac illness. In reality, exercise and conditioning may have broad-based, though modest, salutary effects on the heart. Exercise training, however, is not universally beneficial or even safe.

This chapter will provide physicians with an understanding of the physiological responses that accompany acute exercise and the chronic cardiovascular adaptations that occur as a result of physical conditioning. Several excellent recent reviews of various aspects of exercise conditioning have been published.[1-3]

ACUTE HEMODYNAMICS

The chronic cardiac adaptations that develop as a result of conditioning reflect acute hemodynamic responses to repeated imposed loads. In this context, it is important to distinguish the acute load posed by isotonic (dynamic) exercise, which produces large increases in both cardiac output and oxygen consumption (V_{O_2}) and a fall in systemic vascular resistance, from isometric (static) exercise, which acutely increases systemic vascular resistance while producing only minimal changes in cardiac output and V_{O_2}[4]. Cardiovascular data illustrating these distinc-

TABLE 114-1

Cardiovascular Data from Eight Normal Subjects at Rest and While Performing Either Isometric* or Isotonic† Exercise

	Rest	Isometric	Isotonic
Cardiac output (liters/min)	5.7 ± 0.3	6.8 ± 0.7	21.9 ± 1.0
Heart rate (beats/min)	70 ± 7	110 ± 6	164 ± 4
Stroke volume (mL)	85 ± 7	62 ± 5	131 ± 5
Mean atrial pressure (mmHg)	94 ± 3	118 ± 6	124 ± 4
Systemic vascular resistance (dyn · s/cm^5)	1352 ± 103	1466 ± 131	461 ± 56
V_{O_2} (mL/min)	324 ± 33	556 ± 42	2758 ± 472

SOURCE: Adapted from Bezucha et al.[4] Reproduced with permission from the publisher and author.
*Sustained contraction of the extensor muscles of the lower extremities at 30% of maximal effect.
†Two-legged cycling at 82% of V_{O_2} max.

tions from eight normal subjects performing either isometric (in this case sustained contraction of the knee extensor muscles against a fixed load) or isotonic (two-legged exercise on a cycling ergometer) exercise are shown in Table 114-1. It should be emphasized, however, that most competitive athletes perform a combination of isotonic and isometric conditioning, and the resultant cardiac adaptations probably reflect the combined effects of these hemodynamic loads.

Isotonic, or Dynamic, Exercise

The acute cardiovascular response to isotonic, or dynamic, exercise involves complex and integrated hemodynamic and neurohumoral functions that culminate in increased oxygen delivery to and extraction by the exercising muscles. In normal sedentary individuals there is a 10-fold increase in oxygen consumption from rest to maximal exertion.[5] In well-trained athletes the increase in maximal oxygen consumption can be as great as 20 to 30 times resting values, and indeed maximal oxygen consumption (V_{O_2max}) is widely regarded as a measure of the training effect or the degree of fitness.[6]

The various factors that contribute to oxygen consumption can be illustrated by rearranging the Fick equation:

$$V_{O_2} = \text{HR} \times \text{SV} \times [A - V_{O_2}]$$

where V_{O_2} is oxygen consumption, HR is heart rate, SV is stroke volume, and $[A - V_{O_2}]$ is the difference between arterial and mixed venous oxygen content.

With acute dynamic exercise, heart rate, stroke volume, and $[A - V_{O_2}]$ all increase, and the net result is a marked increase in V_{O_2}.

The earliest hemodynamic response to acute dynamic exercise is probably a fall in systemic vascular resistance that reflects a marked vasodilatation of the resistance vessels in the exercising muscle. This is most marked at mild levels of exercise, with only minimal further decreases in vascular resistance occurring at nearly maximal work loads. The hemodynamic effects of this reflex are twofold: afterload falls and the cardiac output is redistributed. During maximal effort in human beings, more than 80 percent of cardiac output may be directed to working muscle compared with only 18 percent at rest.[7] In experimental animals a 5- to 15-fold increase in blood flow to peripheral muscle has been reported.[8] Many factors contribute, including local autoregulation that may be mediated by a fall in tissue P_{O_2} or by the release of locally acting vasodilators such as adenosine and lactic acid, and the effects of circulating catecholamines and stimulation of sympathetic vasodilatory nerve fibers. In addition, vasoconstriction of the splanchnic and renal circulation also likely occurs during acute exercise so that blood flow to these organs may actually fall, further redistributing cardiac output. A schematic representation of the distribution of blood flow at rest and during peak exercise is shown in Fig. 114-1. Note the marked increase in flow both to the coronary arteries and to active skeletal muscles and the decrease in flow to other organs.

During sustained dynamic exercise, skeletal muscle metabolism is primarily aerobic. Therefore, it is appropriate that the increased demand for adenosine triphosphate (ATP) generation and utilization is met by a correspondingly large increase in oxygen supply. The aerobic capacity of exercising muscle is considerable and is far greater than that of the splanchnic and renal circulations, which are disproportionally perfused at rest. For this reason, oxygen extraction increases and mixed venous oxygen content decreases during acute exercise. In addition, during sustained dynamic exercise the local oxygen requirements of the *exercising* muscle are only partially met by the large increases in local flow. Therefore, at maximal exercise loads local oxygen extraction may also increase. With chronic conditioning, the aerobic capacity of skeletal muscle increases further, as evidenced by a marked increase in the activity of the enzymes of oxidative metabolism in tissue homogenates and by an increase in the size and number of mitochondria per unit of muscle.[2]

With acute dynamic exercise, the most striking cardiovascular alteration is an increase in heart rate, which is much greater in human beings than in smaller animals. Changes in heart rate correlate with both cardiac output and V_{O_2}.[9] The main cause of the rise in heart rate with exercise is sympathetic stimulation. This is demonstrated by the attenuating effects of beta-adrenergic blockade. Parasympathetic withdrawal also plays a definite but lesser role. During maximal effort, changes in heart rate alone cannot completely account for the improved cardiac output; in fact, clear increases in stroke volume have been shown to occur in human beings and also in

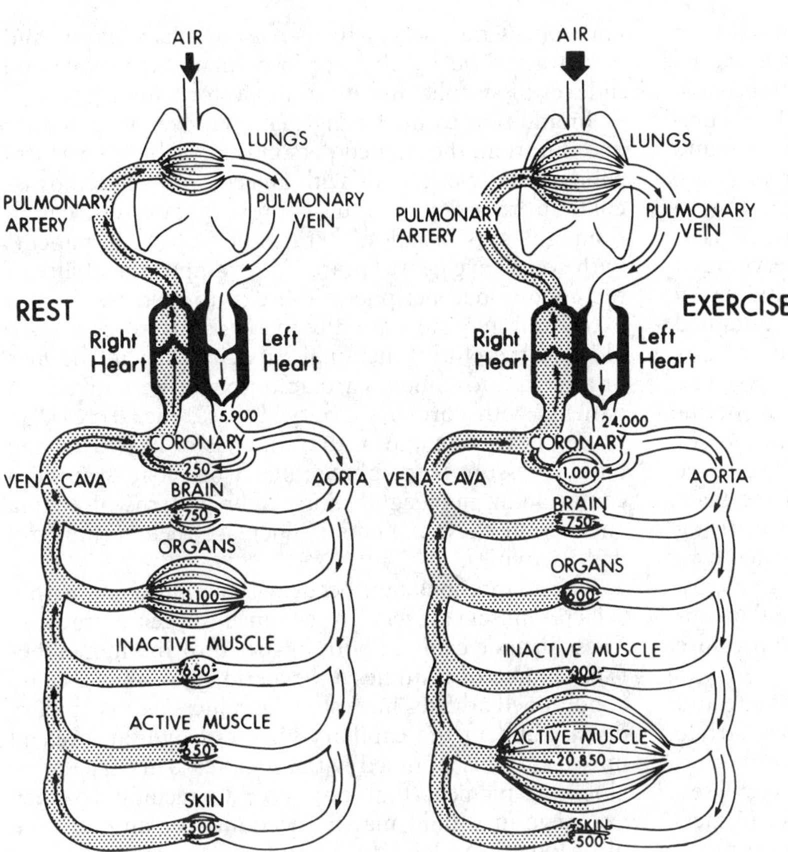

FIGURE 114-1 Schematic representation of the cardiopulmonary system at rest (*left*) and during peak isotonic upright exercise (*right*). During exercise, there are significant increases in blood flow to the exercising muscles and the coronary circulation, and flow to the organ falls. (*Adapted from JH Mitchell, G Blomqvist: N Engl Med 284:1018, 1971. Reproduced with permission from the publisher and author.*)

experimental animals in studies in which heart rate and afterload were precisely controlled.[10] The increase in stroke volume results from a variety of factors, foremost among which are Frank-Starling effects. With acute exercise, in addition to the decrease in systemic vascular resistance mentioned above, there is an increase in venous return. This is probably mediated by sympathetic vasoconstriction of the large-capacitance veins as well as by the pumping effects of muscular contraction. It is more prominent with supine than with upright exercise. The hemodynamic effect of these volume shifts is an increase in end-diastolic volume, and the concept of diastolic or volume loading has been proposed as a feature of dynamic exercise conditioning. Studies in both dogs and human beings have shown that the increase in end-diastolic volume is most marked at maximal work loads, suggesting that both exercise type and intensity are important factors in determining the diastolic volume load to which exercised hearts are exposed. This point is quite pertinent when evaluating the prevalence and degree of cardiac hypertrophy in physically conditioned subjects. In addition, with acute exercise most researchers have reported an independent increase in inotrophy manifested by a decrease in end-systolic volume, an increase in maximum *dP/dt,* and an increase in fractional shortening, although given the changes in preload and afterload associated with acute exercise, this is hard to establish with certainty. The increased inotrophy probably also is related to acute catecholamine effects as well as to intrinsic cardiac adaptations. The increases in cardiac output and stroke volume are paralleled by a marked increase in systolic blood pressure. Diastolic blood pressure remains unchanged and may even fall slightly, reflecting the significant decrease in peripheral vascular resistance. Therefore, mean arterial pressure increases only moderately.

Thus, the acute hemodynamic response to dynamic exercise is well adapted to provide large amounts of oxygen to exercising muscle for oxidative metabolism. This is accomplished by both central and peripheral adaptations. Heart rate, stroke volume, and $[A - V_{O_2}]$ difference increase significantly. In addition, there is a marked decrease in systemic vascular resistance and an increase in venous return. The increase in cardiac output is preferentially directed toward working muscle. (See also Chap. 5.)

Isometric, or Static, Exercise

The acute cardiovascular responses to isometric exercise differ importantly from those to isotonic exercise. With isometric exercise a discrete muscle group is called upon to sustain a muscular contraction without performing external work. Since the muscle group involved tends to be small, the absolute oxygen requirements necessary to sustain the effort are proportionally modest. In the example shown in Table 114-1, V_{O_2} increases from 324 to only 556 mL/min with isometric exercise, compared with 2758 mL/min with an isotonic effort; however, the oxygen costs of isometric and isotonic work for a given muscular effort are similar. The increase in cardiac output required to maintain this level of oxygen consumption is also proportionally lower.

The oxygen requirements of the isometrically contracting muscle are not easily met by an increase in regional blood flow. Local vasodilatation is limited by a mechanical compression of the resistance vessels caused by sustained muscular contraction.[11] In fact, blood flow to the contracting muscle may actually fall. The combination of limited flow and increased metabolic demand appears to evoke a locally mediated pressor response that probably represents an important adaptation to maintain regional perfusion. This pressor response is at least in part mediated locally by an afferent nerve track originating in muscle, as demonstrated by studies in which an isometrically exercised muscle was maintained in an ischemic state with an occluding cuff after exercise.[12] As long as the cuff remained inflated, systemic arterial pressure was elevated; with release of the occlusion, pressure promptly normalized. The magnitude of the pressure response is proportional both to the relative tension sustained in the working muscle and the mass of the muscle groups involved, although a surprising increase in mean arterial pressure can be generated by a sustained contraction of relatively small muscle groups. For example, hand grip at 40 percent of maximal voluntary effort for 3 min can increase mean arterial pressure by 25 to 30 mmHg.

In the presence of this increase in arterial pressure and in the absence of an increase in venous return, stroke volume usually falls. Thus, the most significant mechanism available to the heart to maintain an increased cardiac output is an increase in the heart rate. In fact, the response of the heart rate to isometric exercise, given the modest metabolic needs of the exercising muscle groups, is quite exaggerated.

Thus, the acute hemodynamic loads placed on the heart during these two exercise modes are quite distinct. With dynamic exercise, there is a decrease in systemic vascular resistance and an increase in venous return leading to an increase in end-diastolic volume and stroke volume. With static loads, mean arterial pressure and systemic vascular resistance increase, venous return may decrease, and stroke volume actually falls. In its most pure state, dynamic exercise has been described as a volume (or diastolic) load whereas static exercise represents a pressure (or systolic) load. Importantly, dynamic (in contrast to static) exercise, by virtue of the large associated increases in cardiac output and V_{O_2}, stresses the entire cardiovascular system, and thus, repetitive bouts of exercise may induce a spectrum of physiological cardiovascular adaptations (see below).

CHRONIC ADAPTATIONS

With conditioning induced by chronic repetitive bouts of dynamic exercise, a number of cardiovascular adaptations develop, the effect of which is to enhance the ability of the organism to respond to exercise loads of varying type, intensity, and duration. The best single indicator of the functional capacity of the cardiovascular system is maximal oxygen consumption ($\dot{V}_{O_2max}$), and with conditioning this may increase as much as two- to threefold. About half of this increase is a reflection of adaptations that occur within the periphery to enhance oxygen extraction, and about half is due to a central cardiovascular component that serves to increase cardiac output and is characterized by changes in cardiac dimensions and indexes of systolic and diastolic performance.[13]

In addition to increasing maximal exercise intensity and duration, the trained person is also able to perform submaximal work loads with an economy of cardiovascular effort, and it is in this context that exercise conditioning has its broadest therapeutic impact. In patients with congestive heart failure, for example, the ability of the conditioned peripheral muscles to increase oxygen extraction may substantially increase anaerobic threshold and therefore functional capacity even in the face of a fixed and limited cardiac output. Alternatively, in patients with coronary artery disease, the decrease in resting heart rate and in the response of heart rate and blood pressure to a submaximal work load seen with conditioning may significantly alter patterns of angina and permit these patients to increase their meaningful daily activities.

The adaptations that occur with conditioning within skeletal muscle all serve to enhance oxygen extraction. These include changes both in structure and in metabolism. Numerous studies in experimental animals and conditioned athletes have shown an increase in capillary density and in the capillary-fiber ratio within skeletal muscle.[2,14] This, coupled with an increase in tissue myoglobin, a pigment that can serve to facilitate oxygen exchange in a fluid matrix, accounts for an increased diffusion of oxygen to the oxidative machinery of the muscle cells. In addition, the muscle cells themselves have enhanced respiratory capacity. This is a reflection of the absolute increase in the size and number of mitochondria per cell and an increase in the level of respiratory enzyme capacity per mitochondrion. The myriad biochemical changes that occur within muscle cells and fibers of different types have been well reviewed.[2,13]

As mentioned above, the ability of the periphery to increase oxygen extraction accounts for approximately 50 percent of the increased V_{O_2max} observed during exercise with training. In situations where cardiac output increases only minimally, however, the rise in oxygen extraction predominates. In fact, oxygen extraction may increase to such an extent within skeletal muscle that the increment in limb blood flow may be lower for any submaximal level of work in conditioned versus sedentary individuals. This is of practical benefit for patients with a limited cardiac reserve.

Cardiac adaptations that occur with conditioning have been more difficult to define precisely in human beings, in whom duration, mode, and intensity of conditioning protocols vary and among whom longitudinal studies are relatively rare. Therefore, much information has been derived from studies in inbred strains of animals subjected to carefully defined exercise protocols. These data can then be extrapolated to fit the available information for human beings. It is clear, however, that with conditioning in both human beings and experimental animals significant alterations in cardiac structure and function occur that allow the heart to increase its stroke volume markedly. In athletes, during submaximal exercise a normal cardiac output is seen at a reduced heart rate compared with unconditioned controls, and at peak exercise intensity athletes have a marked increase in cardiac output at an equivalent heart rate. The mechanisms underlying this augmentation in cardiac performance reflect Frank-Starling effects (an increase in end-diastolic volume) and probably also augmented mechanisms of both myocardial contraction and relaxation.

The primary cardiac adaptation that occurs with training is an increase in heart size. In trained human beings, both longitudinal and cross-sectional echocardiographic studies have been done in trained athletes.[15] The left ventricular mass is increased approximately 50 percent in elite athletes compared with age-matched sedentary controls. This is predominantly due to an increase in resting end-diastolic dimension, although both posterior and septal wall thickness may slightly increase (rarely to more than 14 mm). In trained swimmers and runners, this translates into an increase in ventricular diastolic volume up to 60 to 80 percent. In longitudinal studies of swimmers and army recruits before and after intense conditioning programs of 8 to 9 weeks, similar although less marked findings have been observed.[16,17] Interestingly, these changes largely regress within 3 weeks of the cessation of training. Representative echocardiograms (ECGs) from endurance-trained athletes and from isometrically trained athletes are shown in Fig. 114-2. In animal studies, where it is possible to control populations and the nature and degree of conditioning precisely, identical patterns of cardiac enlargement have been seen. In general, the increase in heart weight is 20 to 30 percent versus age-matched controls, and there are clear increases in diastolic dimension with preserved (or even reduced) systolic dimension. In general, the magnitude of the change in cardiac mass and dimension reflects the intensity of the training program, and protocols that do not increase V_{O_2} to greater than 70 percent of maxi-

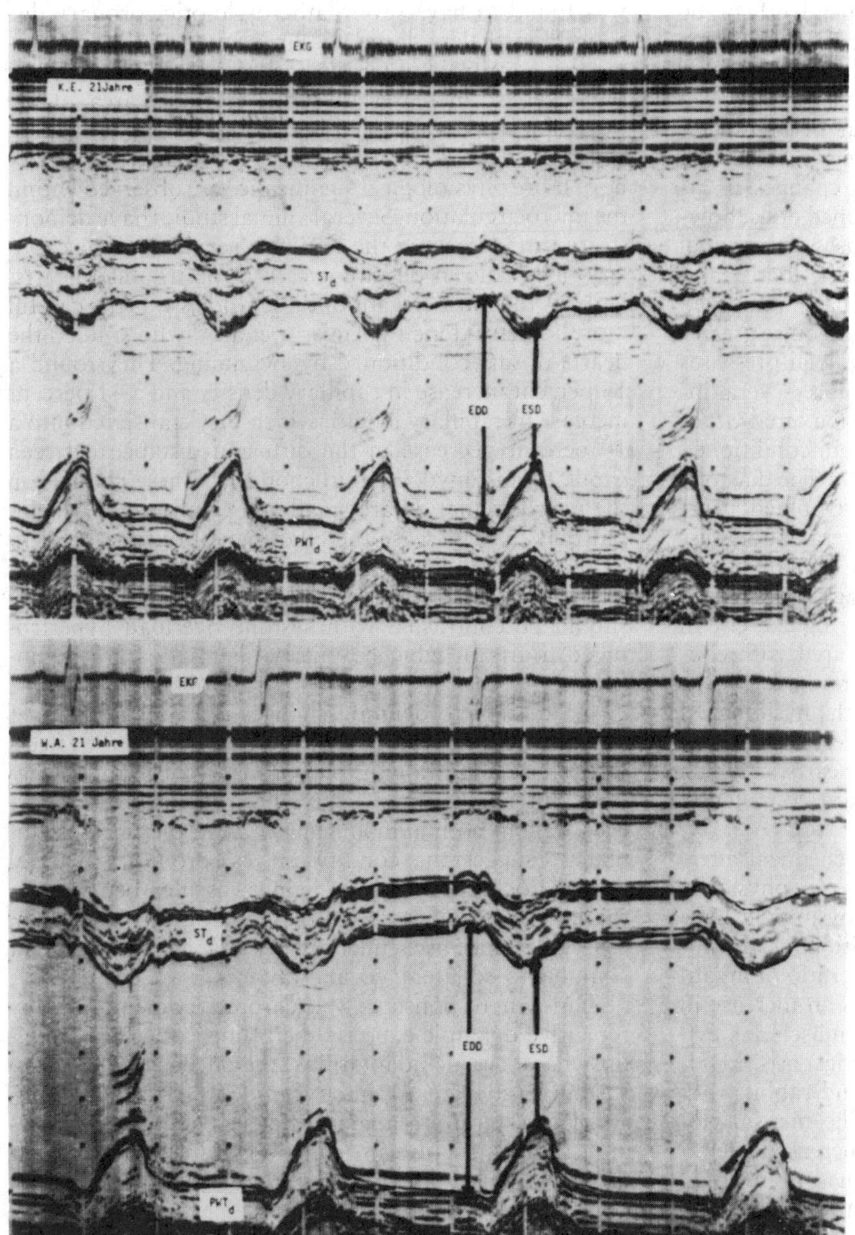

FIGURE 114-2 Representative echocardiograms from athletes trained for isometric and isotonic exercise. The left ventricle of a weight lifter (*top panel*) has an increased septal and posterior wall thickness, and that of a long-distance runner (*bottom panel*) has an increased left ventricular end-diastolic dimension. (*From J Keul, H-H Dickhuth, M Lehmann: Circ Res 48:I-162, 1981. Reproduced with permission from the American Heart Association and author.*)

mum tend not to evoke this adaptation. The cardiac hypertrophy seen in response to the physiological stress of dynamic exercise conditioning should be contrasted with the hypertrophy secondary to pathological overload states such as hypertension and aortic stenosis, in which the increase in cardiac mass primarily reflects an increase in wall thickness with relatively preserved (at least until the late stages of illness) cavitary dimension.

The reasons cardiac dimension and mass increase with conditioning are not completely understood, but a number of factors have been identified that probably contribute. First, in a trained individual there is an increase in parasympathetic tone and a resultant bradycardia. Diastolic filling time is increased, and ventricular dilatation occurs. Also, during dynamic exercise the ventricles are exposed to an additional volume load, which in itself can lead to cardiac hypertrophy characterized by an increase in the number of mitochrondia in series and a pattern of eccentric cardiac hypertrophy.

That the mechanical properties of the physiologically hypertrophied muscle are enhanced independently of the Frank-Starling effects of increased end-diastolic volume has been suggested in studies of human beings and demonstrated in animal studies. In human beings, enhanced systolic performance during exercise has been difficult to demonstrate both because of the insensitivity of the methods employed and because of the changes in afterload that occur during exercise. In trained dogs, however, Barnard et al.[18] have shown increases in maximal *dP/dt* at submaximal and maximal work loads, and Stone[19] has shown that trained dogs have improved pumping ability at similar heart rates and require greater volume infusions to achieve similar left atrial pressures compared with controls. In smaller animals, several investigators have shown an increase in maximal *dP/dt* and in fractional shortening in hearts from conditioned rats under extreme loading conditions.[1,10,20] The diastolic properties of the physiologically hypertrophied heart have not been studied as extensively. Several studies using noninvasive imaging techniques in human beings have shown enhanced early diastolic filling and increased rates of peak myocardial lengthening during exercise in the hearts of conditioned athletes compared with controls,[21,22] and studies in isolated rat hearts have shown an increase in maximal negative *dP/dt* with physiological hypertrophy.[20] All these studies are in clear contrast to work in systolic overload hypertrophied hearts, in which peak shortening and relaxation rates are consistently reduced.

A number of ultrastructural and biochemical alterations have been identified in the hearts of physically conditioned animals that underlie the physiological adaptations outlined above.[2,13] With conditioning, the absolute myocyte size increases, as does the ratio of myofibrils and mitochondria per cell. There is an increase in the respiratory capacity of the cardiac muscle, as evidenced by an increase in lactic dehydrogenase (LDH) and pyruvate kinase activities. In rats and rabbits (but not in human beings) an increase in the myosin isoenzyme of the V_1 ($\alpha\alpha$) type, which has increased adenosine triphosphatase (ATPase) activity, has been noted and correlated with the improved contractile performance seen in these hearts. In addition, alterations in sarcoplasmic reticulum and sarcolemmal function have been identified in conditioned hearts from a variety of species, suggesting alterations in calcium uptake and release that may account for the enhanced diastolic capabilities of these hearts.[23]

Adaptations also occur within the coronary circulation both at the level of the large epicardial vessels and within the microcirculation.[3,24] These adaptations probably help accommodate the large increases in coronary flow that occur during acute exercise. An early anecdotal report worth mentioning is the autopsy study of Clarence DeMar, who at the time of his death at age 70 had run more than 1000 long-distance races. At postmortem evaluation, his epicardial vessels were without atherosclerosis and were two to three times as large as those usually observed in septuagenarians.[25] Of course, this uncontrolled observation must be juxtaposed against examples such as that of Jim Fixx, the exercise enthusiast, who suffered a myocardial infarction while jogging and was found to have severe atherosclerotic coronary disease. Nonetheless, large necropsy studies in human beings and control studies in both dogs and rats suggest that exercise increases the cross-sectional area of the large epicardial vessels, although the functional significance of these changes is unknown. Changes that may be of more physiological significance are observed within the microcirculation. Several animal studies have demonstrated an increase in the capillary density and the capillary-fiber ratio in physiologically hypertrophied hearts. Perhaps the most elegant of these studies was the careful morphometry done by Anversa et al.,[26] who studied the hearts of rats conditioned by swimming. They found a 16 percent increase in capillary density and a 41 percent increase in capillary length, which they translated into a 10 percent decrease in the diffusion distance between capillary and myocyte mitochondria. These changes in the microcirculation are small and of uncertain benefit, but they may increase the efficiency of oxygen delivery to the physiologically stressed myocardium. Also, this adaptation in physiologically hypertrophied hearts should be contrasted with systolic overload hypertrophied hearts in which capillary-fiber ratios are diminished.

In addition to defining changes in capillary number and density, several investigators have studied the effects of exercise conditioning on coronary collateral formation. The results to date have been inconclusive; however, data in both human beings[27] and experimental animals[28–30] suggest that conditioning can promote collateral growth to a potentially ischemic vascular bed. Again, the clinical significance of these changes is uncertain, especially since ischemia per se is a far more potent stimulus to collateral formation.

Thus, in response to the chronic load imposed by repetitive dynamic exercise the trained organism develops characteristic adaptations, the effect of which is to sustain large increases in oxygen delivery to the periphery. The respiratory capacity of skeletal muscles increases and cardiac structure and function is altered to maintain an increased stroke volume without adverse metabolic cost.

GENDER DIFFERENCES IN CARDIOVASCULAR RESPONSE TO EXERCISE

The relative incidence of cardiovascular disease in women is increasing. Nevertheless, there is a remarkable paucity of literature describing the unique physiological responses of women to acute and chronic exercise. Even large population-based epidemiologic studies describing the cardiovascular benefits of physical fitness have mainly been limited to men. Some conclusions can be drawn, however, from the literature published to date.

In general, the physiological responses and adaptations of women to exercise are qualitatively similar to those seen in men. That is, acute dynamic exercise results in a decrease in peripheral vascular resistance and increases in venous return, stroke volume, and peripheral oxygen extraction. Acute static exercise increases peripheral vascular resistance with relatively modest changes both in stroke volume and in $[A - V_{O_2}]$. There are gender-specific differences that help identify and explain the significantly (50 percent) reduced maximal aerobic capacity seen in women relative to men when V_{O_2max} is expressed as liters per minute.[31] First, if V_{O_2max} is adjusted to lean body mass (women have a higher percentage of body fat), the difference is reduced to about 10 to 15 percent. This probably reflects a true gender-specific difference in oxygen transport and delivery since women have a lower hemoglobin concentration and a smaller blood volume than men, although differences in fitness cannot be ruled out.

Women have a smaller cross-sectional muscle mass than men (70 to 85 percent, depending on conditioning status), although both the absolute number of muscle fibers and the fiber-type distribution in an individual muscle group appear to be similar.[32] The mechanism(s) underlying skeletal muscle hypertrophy in men relative to women is unknown. Both estrogen and androgen receptors exist in muscle, and the well-described effects of anabolic steroids on muscle mass suggests that this phenomenon may be hormonally mediated. The greater absolute (isometric) strength in men is a reflection of the increased muscle mass, since strength normalized to cross-sectional muscle area is similar.[33] Interestingly, however, the capacity to perform isotonic exercise as measured by time to muscle fatigue is probably greater in women than in men. The women's world record for the marathon is approximately 90 percent of that for men, and women generally do better than men in endurance swimming competitions despite their reduced muscle mass. This might reflect estrogen effects on muscle metabolism. Several lines of evidence both in experimental animals and humans suggest that estrogen results in preferential utilization of fatty acids as substrate during exercise with a relative sparing of glycogen stores.[34]

The cardiac (central) response to acute dynamic exercise differs somewhat in unconditioned men and women, which may have significant clinical implications. Both genders increase stroke volume during acute isotonic exercise, although careful radionucleotide studies in humans as well as animal studies suggest that they do so through slightly different mechanisms. In general, men tend to increase their ejection fraction during moderate to marked exercise with little or no increase in end-diastolic volume whereas women tend to increase end-diastolic volume without a significant increase in ejection fraction.[35] This may be due to differences in cardiac structure (male hearts are larger, although when adjusted for lean body mass, they are equivalent in size), differences in afterload, or real differences in inotropy (chronic testosterone administration in experimental animals has been shown to have a potent inotropic effect[36]). Regardless, the lack of a rise in ejection fraction during treadmill exercise stress testing in a woman should not be presumed to reflect cardiac pathology and may in fact be a manifestation of her normal physiology.

THE ATHLETE'S HEART

The most important distinctions that a cardiologist is called upon to make in the assessment of an athlete are (1) recognition of the distinctive physical and laboratory features that characterize the athlete's heart that themselves are manifestations of the physiological adaptation to conditioning and (2) recognition of cardiac pathological conditions in patients who happen to be athletic.

The general physical examination of the athlete includes some characteristic but unusual features.[37,38] Notable is a resting bradycardia, generally between 40 and 60 beats per minute. In addition, the normal respiratory variation in heart rate may be exaggerated. Blood pressure and jugular venous pulsations are normal. The left ventricular enlargement discussed above may be apparent on palpation of the precordium but is usually subtle, and a widely displaced apex impulse should alert the physician to concurrent cardiac disease. The first and second heart sounds are normal; however, both S_3 and S_4 are heard in up to 50 percent of athletes. These sounds are maximal in the supine position and are without clinical significance. Short, midsystolic murmurs are quite common, presumably reflecting the large stroke volume. The presence of a thrill or a diastolic murmur warrants further investigation.

Electrocardiographic alterations are often seen.[39] Sinus bradycardia and sinus arrhythmia are extremely common and may be quite dramatic, with sinus pauses of up to 2.5 s. Therefore, it is not surprising that junctional escape beats are also frequently observed. First-degree atrioventricular (AV) block may be found in approximately 20 percent of athletes, and periods of Möbitz I second-degree AV block may also be observed.[40] These abnormalities are presumably vagally mediated, as they disappear with exercise or atropine administration.

The clinical significance of bradycardia in athletes poses an intriguing problem for the consulting physician. This is illustrated by a recent study that contrasted 16 patients who undertook heavy exercise and developed postural syncope or Stokes-Adams attacks (group 1) with 37 elite asymptomatic athletes (group 2).[41] Ambulatory ECG recordings showed heart rates between 30 and 40 in both groups; however, electrophysiological study revealed significant conduction abnormalities in approximately half the group 1 patients. Eight group 1 patients became asymptomatic with deconditioning, and the remainder required permanent pacemaker insertion. Group 2 patients required no specific intervention. This study highlights the distinction between the physiological adaptations seen in the elite athletes in group 2 and the true abnormal findings in the group 1 patients that were perhaps worsened by the increased vagal tone associated with exercise conditioning.

Supraventricular and ventricular premature contractions occur in athletes, but probably no more frequently than in the general population. Certainly the development of a malignant supraventricular or ventricular tachycardia should not be ascribed to the athlete's heart syndrome and warrants further investigation.

Changes in P-wave and QRS morphology are commonly observed in trained athletes. Increases in P-wave voltage suggesting left or right atrial enlargement are commonly seen. An increase in QRS voltage suggesting left or right ventricular hypertrophy is seen in approximately 50 percent of athletes and is often associated with T-wave inversion in the inferior leads. Axis deviation and QRS prolongation are not commonly seen and should alert the physician to the presence of intrinsic cardiac disease. An elevated early takeoff of the T wave is common, as is T-wave inversion in the anterior leads (juvenile T-wave pattern). Downsloping ST-T changes indicating abnormal repolarization (so-called strain) are unusual, although they may occur, particularly in subjects who perform predominantly isometric exercises, such as weight lifting.

The chest x-ray in a conditioned athlete often reveals cardiomegaly. This has been recognized since the 1920s, when it was incorrectly thought to reflect significant underlying heart disease. The heart is generally globular in shape, and the cardiothoracic ratio is between 0.5 and 0.6. A disproportionate increase in the size of any one cardiac chamber is not observed.

A large number of echocardiographic studies have described the nature of the athlete's heart.[15] They are alluded to above and are illustrated in Fig. 114-2. In general, isotonically trained athletes have a slight (less than 20 percent) increase in wall thickness, a slight increase in diastolic dimension, and a normal or even slight decrease in systolic dimension reflecting preserved or augmented systolic function. In contrast, isometrically conditioned athletes may show a concentric pattern of left ventricular hypertrophy. A recent ECG of nearly 1000 elite athletes defined the limits of cardiac hypertrophy associated with exercise conditioning.[42] This study found that left ventricular wall thickness of greater than 13 mm was very uncommon in athletes and virtually limited to athletes training in rowing sports; wall thicknesses exceeding 16 mm were not seen. The presence of asymmetrical septal hypertrophy is distinctly unusual, although it can occur. In such cases it may be difficult to distinguish between physiological hypertrophy and hypertrophic obstructive cardiomyopathy, which may pose a risk of sudden death during exercise (Chap. 90). It may therefore be necessary in these rare cases to screen first-degree relatives and/or advise a period of deconditioning during which regression of hypertrophy should be noted in athletes but not in patients with a hypertrophic myopathy.

The athlete's heart presents the clinician with a spectrum of abnormalities that reflect physiological adaptations to the conditioned state, not intrinsic pathological conditions. It is important for the clinician to recognize these adaptations and distinguish them from real cardiac disease, such as "sick-sinus" syndrome or hypertrophic obstructive cardiomyopathy, which are as likely to occur in athletes as in any other segment of the population.

EXERCISE AND SUDDEN DEATH

Cardiovascular death during exercise is extremely rare.[43,44] The annual incidence of sudden death in individuals under age 30 is between 2 and 7 per 100,000, of which approximately 8 percent are exercise related. In individuals over age 30 the incidence of sudden death is between 50 and 60 per 100,000, with approximately 2 to 3 percent of these deaths occurring during exercise. Estimated mortality rates during various modes of exercise range from 1 death per 396,000 person-hours of jogging to 1 per 13,000 to 26,000 person-hours of cross-country skiing.

Several autopsy studies of victims who died during vigorous activities indicate that most of these individuals had either recognized or occult cardiac disease.[43] As might be suspected, the epidemiologic pattern of deaths was quite different in young (below age 35) and older (above age 35) populations. The largest studies of young patients are those of Maron et al.[45] and Waller.[46] Structural cardiac disease was identified in 85 to 97 percent. The most common entity identified was congenital anomalies of the coronary arteries in 30 patients (35 percent). Hypertrophic obstructive cardiomyopathy was second in frequency and was found in 19 cases (22 percent). Other diagnoses included coronary artery disease (5 percent), mitral valve prolapse (4 percent), rupture or dissection of the aorta (3 percent), and dilated myopathy and myocarditis (1 percent). Another large European study[47] found a high incidence of arrhythmogenic right ventricular dysplasia. In studies of older populations,[46,48] up to two-thirds of patients who died during exercise had an overt history of coronary artery disease, and the majority of the remainder had recognizable coronary risk factors. Other, far less prevalent abnormalities that were reported to contribute to death during exercise in this older population included cardiomyopathies, valvular heart disease, aortic disease, abnormalities of conduction, and primary arrhythmogenic disorders.

These pathological findings have important implications for the identification of patients at risk. In the low-risk, younger age group the search for an individual with significant cardiac disease presents significant problems of both accuracy and expense. While it is not feasible to perform noninvasive diagnostic studies on all active young individuals prior to participation in a vigorous exercise program, the American Medical Association Committee on Medical Aspects of Sports recommends that students taking part in vigorous athletics undergo a physical examination before competing. Certainly individuals with a history or ECG consistent with a tachyarrhythmia, a conduction abnormality, or an AV bypass tract ought to be evaluated further, and some should be excluded completely from athletics. Similarly, the appreciation of a murmur consistent with a coronary anomaly, hypertrophic obstructive cardiomyopathy, mitral valve prolapse, or aortic root disease would mandate further evaluation. Among older patients, in whom the major risk factor for sudden death is coronary artery disease, it is prudent to perform an exercise stress test in all patients with known coronary artery disease and all others with risk factors or symptoms suggesting occult coronary artery disease prior to enrollment in a program of vigorous physical activity.

A final question is whether or not exercise conditioning may actually protect against cardiovascular death, especially in patients with either overt or covert coronary artery disease who are at high risk. With conditioning, the resting heart rate is decreased and the major determinant of myocardial oxygen demand, the product of heart rate and blood pressure, is lower for any submaximal work load.[49] Coronary capillarity and capacitance may increase, and myocardial oxygen demands and coronary flow per gram of myocardium at any submaximal work load are decreased. All these factors would tend to increase the intensity level necessary to provoke coronary ischemia. In addition, blood rheology may be altered so as to diminish platelet aggregability,[50,51] and the increase in circulating high-density lipoprotein (HDL) cholesterol may actually retard the development of atherosclerotic heart disease.[52] In isolated rat hearts, physical training increases the ventricular fibrillation threshold during hypoxia and ischemia.[53] It is therefore attractive to postulate that conditioning may delay the onset of clinical coronary artery disease and actually prolong life in populations at risk.

The epidemiologic evidence necessary to support this conclusion is compelling and includes a number of large longitudinal studies compiled over the past decade. The first is a mortality study of over 6000 San Francisco stevedores.[54] Careful records of their physical activities were kept as part of their employment record, and an analysis indicated that heavy work (greater than 5.2 kcal/min) significantly decreased the relative risk of fatal myocardial infarction over the 21 years of follow-up. Morris et al.[55] surveyed nearly 18,000 British civil servants with sedentary jobs about their leisure time activities and subdivided them into two groups depending on whether they exercised vigorously (greater than 7.5 kcal/min) outside of work or were sedentary. After 8 years of follow-up, the relative risk for the development of symptomatic coronary artery disease was decreased by 50 percent in the physically active group and was independent of age, smoking history, or body habitus. More recently, Paffenbarger et al.[56] surveyed habitual energy output and correlated it with death and the onset of symptomatic coronary artery disease in nearly 17,000 male Harvard alumni who were followed over 16 years. Rates of first coronary attack were 25 to 30 percent lower among alumni who expended 2000 kcal or more per week during exercise compared with the less active males. Mortality rates were lower among the physically active subjects and were independent of coronary risk factors. Especially noteworthy was the observation that energy expenditure at a later age was the primary determinant of risk (or benefit) and was independent of activity at a younger age. Similar data have been reported in large studies from Puerto Rico and Finland and from a retrospective analysis of the Framingham patient registry. (See also Chap. 62 and 63.)

A second approach has been to evaluate the role of exercise in the secondary prevention of myocardial infarction and cardiovascular death in patients who have sustained a prior infarction. This has been attempted by several groups.[57–59] Inadequate patient numbers, inadequate control groups, and incomplete compliance with the exercise programs make these studies difficult to interpret. Nonetheless, vigorous supervised physical activity after myocardial infarction was not associated with an adverse outcome, and in fact, a trend toward increased survival was identified in patients who complied with a long-term exercise program in several of these studies.

Thus, it is reasonable to conclude not only that carefully prescribed physical conditioning is safe but also that for the majority of the population, including selected patients with coronary artery disease, it may be of benefit in preventing or at least postponing the onset of symptomatic coronary artery disease.

REFERENCES

1. Schaible TF, Scheuer J: Cardiac adaptations to chronic exercise. *Prog Cardiovasc Dis* 1985; 27:297–324.
2. Holloszy JO, Booth FW: Biochemical adaptations to endurance exercise in muscle. *Ann Rev Physiol* 1976; 28:273–291.
3. Cohen MV: Coronary and collateral blood flows during exercise and myocardial vascular adaptations to training. *Exer Sport Sci Rev* 1983; 11:55–98.
4. Bezucha GR, Lenser MC, Hanson PG, Nagle FJ: Comparison of hemodynamic responses to static and dynamic exercise. *J Appl Physiol* 1982; 53:1589–1593.
5. Bruce RA, Kusumi F, Hosmer D: Maximal oxygen intake and normographic assessment of functional aerobic impairment in cardiovascular disease. *Am Heart J* 1973; 85:546–562.
6. Saltin B, Astrand PO: Maximal oxygen uptake in athletes. *J Appl Physiol* 1967; 23:353–358.
7. Zelis R, Flaim S: Alterations in vasomotor tone in congestive heart failure. *Prog Cardiovasc Dis* 1982; 24:437–459.
8. Vatner SF, Franklin D, Higgins CB, Patrick T, Brunwald E: Left ventricular response to severe exertion in untethered dogs. *J Clin Invest* 1972; 51:3052–3060.
9. Hellerstein HK, Ader R: Relationship between per cent maximal oxygen (% max VO2) uptake and per cent maximal heart rate (% MHR) in normals and cardiac (ASHD) (abstract). *Circulation* 1971; 43(suppl 2):76.
10. Saltin B, Blomqvist G, Michell JH: Response to exercise after bedrest and after training. *Circulation* 1968; 38(suppl V):V-1–V-78.
11. Asmussen E: Similarities and dissimilarities between static and dynamic exercise. *Circ Res* 1981; 48:(suppl 2):I3–10.
12. Hanson P, Nagle F: Isometric exercise: Cardiovascular responses in normal and cardiac populations. In: Hanson P (ed): *Exercise and the Heart, Cardiology Clinics*. Philadelphia, WB Saunders, 1987: 157–170.
13. Rowell LB: Human cardiovascular adjustments to exercise and thermal stress. *Physiol Rev* 1974; 54:75–159.
14. Hermansen L, Wachtlova M: Capillary density of skeletal muscle in well trained and untrained men. *J Appl Physiol* 1971; 30:860–863.

15. Maron BJ: Structural features of the athlete's heart as defined by echocardiography. *J Am Coll Cardiol* 1986; 7:190–203.
16. Ehsani AA, Hagberg JM, Hickson RC: Rapid changes in ventricular dimensions and mass in response to physical conditioning and deconditioning. *Am J Cardiol* 1972; 42:52–56.
17. Frick MH, Sjogran A-L, Perasalo J, Pajunen S: Cardiovascular dimension and moderate physical training in young men. *J Appl Physiol* 1970; 29:452–455.
18. Barnard RJ, Duncan HW, Baldwin KM, Grimditch G, Buckberg GD: Effects of intensive exercise training on myocardial performance and coronary blood flow. *J Appl Physiol* 1980; 49:444–449.
19. Stone HL: Cardiac function and exercise training in conscious dogs. *J Appl Physiol* 1977; 42:824–832.
20. Schaible TF, Scheuer J: Cardiac function in hypertrophied hearts from chronically exercised female rats. *J Appl Physiol* 1981; 50:1140–1145.
21. Matsuda M, Sugishita Y, Koseki S, Ito I, Akatsuka T, Takámatsu K: Effect of exercise on left ventricular diastolic filling in athletes and nonathletes. *J Appl Physiol* 1983; 52:323–328.
22. Granger CB, Karimeddini MK, Smith V-E, Shapiro HR, Katz AM, Riba AL: Rapid ventricular filling in left ventricular hypertrophy: Physiologic hypertrophy. *J Am Coll Cardiol* 1985; 5:862–868.
23. Scheuer J, Buttrick PM: The cardiac hypertrophic response to physiologic and pathologic overload. *Circulation* 1987; 75:I-63–69.
24. Scheuer J: Effects of physical training on myocardial vascularity and perfusion. *Circulation* 1982; 66:491–495.
25. Currens JH, White PD: Half a century of running: Clinical physiologic and autopsy findings in the case of Clarence DeMar (Mr. Marathon). *N Engl J Med* 1961; 265:988–993.
26. Anversa P, Levicky V, Beghi C, McDonald SL, Kikkawa Y: Morphometry of exercise-induced right ventricular hypertrophy in the rat. *Circ Res* 1983; 52:57–64.
27. Froelicher V, Jensen D, Atwood JE, McKirnan MD, Gerber K, Slutsky R, et al: Cardiac rehabilitation: Evidence for improvement in myocardial perfusion and function. *Arch Phys Med Rehabil* 1980; 61:517–522.
28. Eckstein RW: Effect of exercise and coronary artery narrowing on coronary collateral circulation. *Circ Res* 1957; 5:230–235.
29. Cohen MV, Yipintsoi T, Malhotra A, Penpargkal S, Scheur J: Coronary collateral stimulation by exercise in dogs with stenotic coronary arteries. *J Appl Physiol* 1978; 45:797–805.
30. Roth DM, White FC, Nichols ML, Doggs SL, Longhurst JC, Bloor CM: Effect of long-term exercise on regional myocardial function and coronary collateral development after gradual coronary artery occlusion in pigs. *Circulation* 1990; 82:1778–1789.
31. Drinkwater BL: Women and exercise: Physiological aspects. *Exer Sport Sci Rev* 1984; 12:21–51.
32. Costill D, Daniels J, Evans W, Fink W, Krahenbuhl G, Saltin B: Skeletal muscle enzyme and fiber type composition in male and female track athletes. *J Appl Physiol* 1976; 40:149–154.
33. Astrand PO, Rodahl K: *Textbook of Work Physiology, Physiologic Basis of Exercise.* New York, McGraw-Hill, 1986: 343–344.
34. Kendrick ZV, Steffan CA, Rumsey WL, Goldberg DI: Effect of estradiol on tissue glycogen metabolism in exercised oophorectomized rats. *J Appl Physiol* 1987; 63:492–496.
35. Higgenbotham MB, Morris KG, Coleman RD, Cobb FR: Sex-related differences in the normal cardiac responses to upright exercise. *Circulation* 1984; 70:357–366.
36. Scheuer J, Malhotra A, Schaible TF, Capasso J: Effects of gonadectomy and hormonal replacement on rat hearts. *Circ Res* 1987; 61:12–19.
37. Huston TP, Puffer JC, Rodney WM: The athletic heart syndrome. *N Engl J Med* 1985; 313:24–32.
38. Crawford MH, O'Rourke RA: The athlete's heart. *Adv Intern Med* 1979; 24:311–329.
39. Zehender P, Meinertz T, Keul J, Just H: ECG variants and cardiac arrhythmias in athletes: Clinical relevance and prognostic importance. *Am Heart J* 1990; 119:1378–1391.
40. Meytes I, Kaplinsky E, Yahini JH, Hanne-Paparo N, Neufeld HN: Wenckebach AV block: A frequent feature following heavy physical training. *Am Heart J* 1975; 90:426–430.
41. Ector H, Verlinden M, Vanden Eynde E, Bourgois J, Herman L, Fagard R, et al: Bradycardia syncope and sports. *Lancet* 1984; 2:591–594.
42. Pelliccia A, Maron BJ, Spataro A, Proschan MA, Spirito O: The upper limit of physiologic cardiac hypertrophy in highly trained elite athletes. *N Engl J Med* 1991; 324:295–301.
43. Thompson PD, Mitchell JH: Exercise and sudden cardiac death: Protection or provocation. *N Engl J Med* 1984; 311:914–915.
44. McCaffrey FM, Braden DS, Strong WB: Sudden cardiac death in young athletes. A review. *Am J Dis Child* 1991; 145:177–183.
45. Maron BJ, Epstein SE, Roberts WE: Causes of sudden death in competitive athletes. *J Am Coll Cardiol* 1986; 7:204–214.
46. Waller BF: Exercise-related sudden death in young (age ≤ 30) and old (age > 30) conditioned subjects. In: Wenger NC (ed): *Exercise and the Heart,* 2d ed. Philadelphia, FA Davis, 1985.
47. Corrado D, Thiene G, Nava A, Rossi L, Pennelli N: Sudden death in young competitive athletes. Clinical pathologic correlations in 22 cases. *Am J Med* 1990; 89:588–596.
48. Waller BF, Roberts WC: Sudden death while running in conditioned runners age 40 or over. *Am J Cardiol* 1980; 45:1292–1300.
49. Amsterdam EA, Dressendorfer R, Mason DT, et al: Exercise training in coronary heart disease: Physiological rationale, clinical indications and practical application. In: Mason DT (ed): *Advances in Heart Disease*, vol 2. New York, Grune & Stratton, 1978: 345–362.
50. Dix CJ, Hassall DG, Bruckdorfer KR: The increased sensitivity of platelets to prostacyclin in marathon runners. *Thromb Haemost* 1984; 51:385–387.
51. Williams RS, Logue EE, Lewis JL, Barton T, Stead NW, Wallace AG, et al: Physical conditioning augments the fibrinolytic response to venous occlusion in healthy adults. *N Engl J Med* 1980; 302:987–991.
52. Wood PD, Williams PT, Haskell WL: Physical activity and high density lipoproteins. In: Mill NE, Miller GJ (eds): *Clinical and Metabolic Aspects of High Density Lipoproteins.* New York, Elsevier, 1984.
53. Noakes TD, Higginson L, Opie LH: Physical training increases ventricular fibrillation thresholds of isolated rat hearts during normoxic, hypoxic and regional ischemia. *Circulation* 1983; 67:24–30.
54. Paffenbarger RS, Hale WE: Work activity and coronary heart mortality. *N Engl J Med* 1975; 292:545–550.
55. Morris JN, Everitt MG, Pollard R, Chave SP, Semmence AM: Vigorous exercise in leisure time: Protection against coronary heart disease. *Lancet* 1980; ii:1207–1210.
56. Paffenbarger RS, Hyde RT, Wing AL, Hsieh CC: Physical activity, all-cause mortality and longevity in college alumni. *N Engl J Med* 1986; 314:605–613.
57. Shaw LW: Effects of prescribed exercise program on mortality and cardiovascular morbidity in patients after a myocardial infarction. *Am J Cardiol* 1981; 48:39–46.
58. Shephard RJ, Corey P, Kavanagh T: Exercise compliance and the prevention of a recurrence of myocardial infarction. *Med Sci Sports Exer* 1981; 13:1–5.
59. Naughton J: Role of physical activity as a secondary intervention for healed myocardial infarction. *Am J Cardiol* 1985; 55:21D–26D.

Chapter 115

Cardiovascular Aging and Adaptation to Disease

Steven P. Schulman, M.D. ■ *Myron L. Weisfeldt, M.D.*

DIFFICULTIES IN THE STUDY OF AGING

Many have a preconception that cardiovascular function and other functions decrease substantially during later life. This bias is certainly related to the fact that cardiovascular disease is so widely prevalent in our population. Since its prevalence and severity increase with age, the perception is that nearly every older American has "heart trouble."[1-3] Also, when cardiovascular function is objectively decreased in an older individual and there is no apparent etiology, the changes are ascribed to aging. As discussed in this chapter, this bias is for the most part unfounded and, in fact, is not substantiated if one examines a *disease-free* older population.

In order to understand the magnitude and mechanisms of age-related changes in cardiovascular function, we must be clear about definitions and limitations of available information. First, it is important to note the use, in this context, of the term *aging*. Although aging occurs during all phases of life, the early changes, i.e., those occurring during the phase of growth and development, are not the subject of this discussion. The cardiovascular changes that are discussed are those that occur during *adulthood*.

Second, it is often extremely difficult to dissociate aging from disease. For example, for many years it had been controversial what level of systolic blood pressure represents a normal age-associated increase and what level indicates the presence of a disease, i.e., systemic hypertension. Many thought an elevated systolic blood pressure was part of "normal" aging. It is now recognized that although systolic blood pressure does gradually increase with age, an elevated systolic blood pressure is a strong risk factor for the development of future cardiovascular disease and lowering elevated systolic blood pressure with medications reduces the risk.[4,5] In attempting to distinguish truly age-related changes from those of disease, one should note several important factors. In Western man, the autopsy prevalence of ischemic disease in those over 60 years of age is approximately 50 percent.[1-3] Thus, only studies in which significant efforts are made to eliminate subjects with ischemic heart disease can appropriately be viewed as an examination of aging separate from disease. It is reassuring that many of the recent observations of cardiovascular function that change with aging are predictable from studies in experimental animals. In nonhuman species ischemic heart disease is not common. Similar aging changes in the cardiovascular system in many species would support the notion of universal aging changes rather than unrecognized disease as the cause.

Third, there are many factors that affect cardiovascular function over the life span of the animal that may or may not be referred to as aging-induced changes. These include environmental factors such as temperature and toxins and life-style, including the quality of nutrition and the degree of cardiovascular fitness or conditioning. There may also be age-associated alterations in the function of other organ systems, such as the thyroid gland, which secondarily affect the heart. Although the broad outline of age-associated changes in cardiovascular function can now be formulated from available data in human beings and experimental animals, many issues of secondary determination of age-associated alterations in cardiovascular function remain to be settled.

Finally, it should be recognized not only that there is difficulty in dissociating disease from aging but also the manifestations of cardiovascular disease in any given individual may, in part, be age-determined. Thus, aging may increase or decrease the rate of disease progression. In addition, the severity of the disease-induced functional decline likely depends on the aging substrate upon which the disease is superimposed. The response to treatment in the individual with cardiovascular disease may also be determined in part by aging. For example, there is some evidence of a decrease, with aging, in the potency of the inotropic response to digitalis glycosides and catecholamines.[6–11] (See also Chap. 27.) Such an age-associated decrease in response to pharmacologic agents may well affect the response to treatment in any given older individual with severe heart disease.

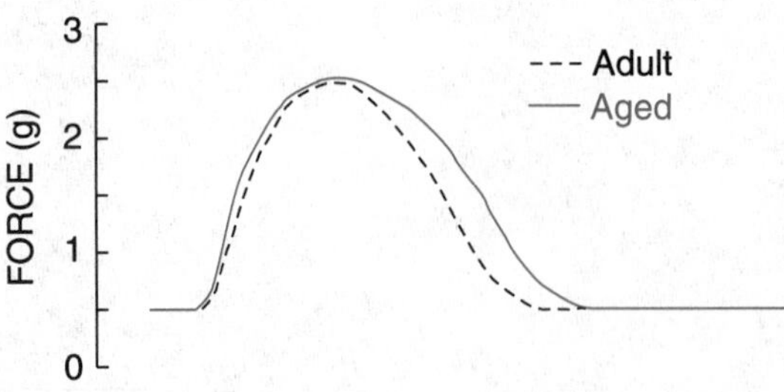

FIGURE 115-1 Typical isometric twitch in a young adult (- - - - -) and in aged (——) isolated cardiac muscle. Note that the rate of rise in tension and maximum tension achieved do not differ with age but that the duration of contraction is prolonged, primarily due to slowed and delayed relaxation.

NORMAL AGING

Cardiovascular Aging as a Selective Process

Age-related cardiovascular changes appear in a selective, rather than nonspecific, fashion.[12] Again, the common belief is that all aspects of bodily function decrease similarly with aging. For the cardiovascular system this does not appear to be the case. The ability of the cardiac muscle to develop tension is well maintained with aging[13] as is the inotropic response of the cardiac muscle to direct stimulation of the myofibrils with calcium.[7] Such observations predict the relatively normal global left ventricular function at rest.[14,15] In contrast, there is a striking decrease in the response to stimulation of beta-sympathetic receptors of cardiovascular tissues.[6,9,12] This decrease in beta-sympathetic response manifests itself in decreased inotropic response of cardiac muscle, decreased arterial vasodilating response, and decreased heart rate, or chronotropic response. With left ventricular loading induced by exercise and other causes, there is enhanced use of the Frank-Starling mechanism to compensate for the increased work load and lower inotropic state due to the decreased response to catecholamines.[14,16]

Function of the Cardiac Muscle

Isolated cardiac muscle from rats, guinea pigs, and other species shows, with aging, a remarkable maintenance of ability to develop tension when studied in vitro. As shown in Fig. 115-1, the rate of rise in tension and the maximum tension achieved under isometric conditions are unchanged with age. The lack of change in tension development, or the rate of tension rise, holds over the entire working range of muscle length.[13]

There appears to be a small decrease in the velocity of shortening in cardiac muscle from senescent animals. This may be related to a decrease in adenosine triphosphatase (ATPase) activity of the myofibrils, as studies show a progressive decrease in calcium-activated myosin ATPase activity with age.[17,18] It should also be noted that stiffness increases with age, which tends to increase shortening velocity.[9]

The most striking and consistent change in mechanical performance of isolated cardiac muscle from senescent animals is prolonged duration of contraction and relaxation (Fig. 115-1).[19] The durations of contraction and relaxation are thought to be determined in part by the sarcoplasmic reticulum as well as by the duration of calcium entry during depolarization. The age-associated prolongation of relaxation can be attributed to both a decrease in the velocity of myocardial sarcoplasmic calcium uptake with increased age[20] and a prolongation of the action potential duration.[21] In younger animals a similar prolongation of relaxation and decreased velocity of calcium uptake by sarcoplasmic reticulum is seen following hypertrophy due to pressure overload. There is some degree of hypertrophy present in animals with aging. This hypertrophy may be secondary to the increased impedance to left ventricular ejection as a result of stiffer arteries and dropout or death of a few myocardial cells.[22] In experimental animals the age-associated prolongation of relaxation and the decreased velocity of calcium uptake by the sarcoplasmic reticulum can be decreased by intense exercise.[23] Thus, it is possible that the age-associated prolongation of duration of contraction is a reflection of both the age-associated mild hypertrophy of cardiac muscle and deconditioning due to a lower overall level of physical activity.

The conclusion from studies on the function of isolated cardiac muscle function with age is that the ability to develop tension and the rate of tension development are normal but that there is some prolongation of the duration of contraction due to a delayed and decreased rate of relaxation. The velocity of shortening, particularly at low loads, is also decreased.

Left Ventricular Function in Human Beings at Rest

Paralleling these features of the function of isolated cardiac muscle in experimental animals are studies of left ventricular function in human beings.[12,14–16] Studies utilizing both echocardiographic and radionuclide scintigraphy for assessment of left ventricular volumes have shown that resting left ventricular function is well maintained with age in healthy subjects.[14–16] Similar to animal models, left ventricular mass and wall thickness also increase with age in healthy individuals, likely due to the age-related increase in afterload (see below).

In contrast to normal systolic function and similar to the prolongation in contraction duration noted in animal models, there is a slowed and delayed early diastolic left ventricular relaxation under resting conditions in man.[24] As a result, a number of studies utilizing noninvasive techniques have shown a decrease in indices reflecting the velocity of left ventricular filling during the rapid early diastolic filling phase of the cardiac cycle.[15,25] This decrease in rapid filling may be consequent to several age-related changes including a prolongation of the time constant of relaxation,[26] mild left ventricular hypertrophy,[15] an increase in afterload,[27] an increase in left ventricular chamber stiffness,[28] and an increase in regional heterogeneity in filling among left ventricular segments.[29] Unlike previously mentioned animal studies, it appears the more sedentary life-style associated with aging does not influence the age-related decrease in early filling as senior endurance athletes have a similar decrease in left ventricular peak filling as age-matched sedentary subjects.[29a] The end-diastolic volume is maintained in healthy elderly subjects because of an increase in the atrial contribution to late left ventricular filling.[30]

In summary, in a normal person at rest there is no major age-associated change in left ventricular systolic function; however, evidence of the prolonged relaxation that characterizes aging cardiac muscle can be easily identified in human beings at rest. Signs include a prolonged isovolumic phase of diastole and slowed early diastolic left ventricular filling.

CARDIOVASCULAR AGING AND ADAPTATION TO DISEASE

Although the changes in relaxation are not of sufficient magnitude to have a major impact on resting cardiac function or on the cardiovascular response to exercise when disease is not present, prolonged relaxation may influence overall cardiac function of the older individual in the presence of disease. This is particularly important in coronary and hypertensive heart disease, two common diseases in the elderly that further decrease early diastolic filling.[31,32] In the setting of ischemic heart disease, for example, one would predict that delayed and prolonged relaxation would tend to compromise subendocardial blood flow. This may be particularly true with tachycardia, since prolonged relaxation would accentuate the detrimental effect of an abbreviated diastole. If relaxation is prolonged, left ventricular diastolic pressure is, on average, higher potentially compromising subendocardial blood flow during tachycardia. Similarly, in elderly patients with hypertension and left ventricular hypertrophy, dyspnea and/or fatigue may occur with the tachycardia associated with exercise because of an increase in left ventricular end-diastolic pressure and an inability to increase end-diastolic volume because of impaired filling of the ventricle.[33] Prolonged relaxation in the aged may contribute to the well-recognized fact that symptoms of cardiac arrhythmias, including dyspnea and syncope, occur at a slower heart rate in older than in younger individuals. The depressed response to catecholamines and an increase in vascular load may also impair the cardiovascular adaptation to disease.

Depressed Response to Catecholamines

Studies of isolated cardiac muscle show a striking decrease in the response of tissue from older animals to certain inotropic factors, particularly catecholamines and digitalis glycosides.[7–11] In terms of both the response of cardiac muscle to calcium and the response of myofibrils upon direct exposure to calcium following chemical removal of the cell membrane, the inotropic response to calcium is well sustained. This fact and the maintained intrinsic cardiac muscle function with increasing age indicate that myofibrillar contractile function is selectively well maintained with aging. In contrast, the striking decrease in the inotropic response to catecholamines suggests a defect in signal recognition/transduction that normally leads to increased myofibrillar contractile activity.

The age-associated decrease in the inotropic response to catecholamines is *not* principally receptor mediated.[11] Beta-adrenergic receptor number and affinity in cardiac muscle from rats appear unchanged. The mechanism of the decrease in inotropic response is probably decreased calcium mobilization by the intracellular signals resulting from catecholamine stimulation. The ability of catecholamines to enhance relaxation, in contrast to the inotropic response, is not impaired.[12]

Thus, in senescent myocardium, the duration of contraction is shortened by catecholamines in the face of a markedly diminished inotropic effect. This results in a significantly lower peak tension developed by isolated cardiac muscle of senescent, as opposed to young adult, animals in the presence of beta-sympathetic stimulation (Fig. 115-2).

The inotropic response to postextrasystolic potentiation in cardiac muscle from senescent animals is well maintained and similar to the calcium response.[7] The response to digitalis glycosides in cardiac muscle of both rats and dogs, however, is markedly decreased with age. In the dog the toxic effect of digitalis, in terms of producing ventricular tachycardia, is unchanged with age, so that the therapeutic-to-toxic ratio is much less favorable in the senescent than in the young adult dog.[8] It is unclear, however, whether or not these observations in experimental animals are applicable in human beings.

Peripheral Vasculature

Several age-associated changes in arterial mechanical properties demonstrated in animal models and in man[28,34,35] increase the load that the central vasculature presents to the left ventricle during ejection. These consist of alterations in the composition and distribution of elastin and collagen in central arteries that cause a stiffening of the vasculature and changes in the distal arterioles. These age-related changes lead to increases in both mean systemic vascular resistance, which is the nonpulsatile component of afterload, and characteristic impedance and pulse wave velocity, the pulsatile components of afterload, which have been demonstrated during cardiac catheterization in patients without hypertension

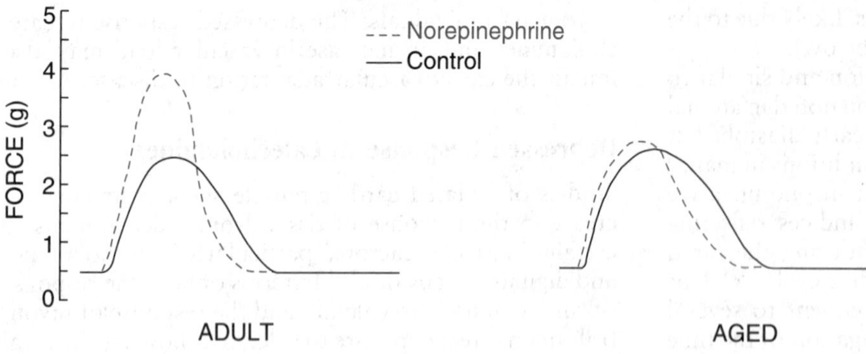

FIGURE 115-2 Typical isometric twitch in a young adult and in aged isolated cardiac muscle before (——) and after (- - - - -) exposure to norepinephrine. There is no significant increase in maximum tension or rate of tension development in aged muscle although the enhanced relaxation effect due to the catecholamines is relatively unaffected by age.

or coronary artery disease.[36,37] Additionally, noninvasive measurements performed on a population of rural Chinese, who have a very low prevalence of hypertension and atherosclerosis, demonstrate a direct relationship between age and arterial pulse wave velocity.[27]

The increase in arterial stiffness that occurs with age almost certainly is the major factor contributing to the increase in echocardiographically determined left ventricular mass and is probably an important contributor to the age-associated increase in systolic blood pressure, which is observed even in healthy individuals.[9,12,15] The most striking age change in the arterial vasculature parallels directly the age change in cardiac muscle, that is, a decrease in the response to beta-sympathetic stimulation.[6,38] There is a distinct age-associated decrease in the vasodilating response of rat aorta to beta-sympathetic stimulation. That this is a specific decrease in the response to beta-sympathetic stimulation is shown by the fact that the response to other vasodilating agents, such as nitroglycerin, is relatively well maintained with age. Similarly, in man, an age-related decrease in forearm vasodilation to an isoproterenol infusion has been demonstrated.[39]

With exercise, cardiac output rises markedly. Systolic blood pressure reflects the net effect of the increased filling of all arterial structures as a result of augmented cardiac output and arterial vasodilatation through beta-sympathetic stimulation. From the observations in isolated aorta, one can speculate that during exercise a major factor in augmenting the load on the left ventricle during ejection in older individuals is decreased arterial vasodilation. Thus, left ventricular systolic load rises to a higher level in older than in younger adult humans. Strong support for this notion has been obtained during exercise studies in beagle dogs. These studies show that dynamic impedance to left ventricular ejection is greater during exercise, but not at rest, in 10- to 14-year-old dogs than in 1- to 4-year-old dogs.[22] The lower impedance during exercise in the young dogs can be entirely eliminated by beta-sympathetic blockade. Thus, the load on the left ventricle during ejection is the same in adult and senescent animals following beta blockade, whereas before beta blockade the load is much greater in the older dogs. These observations, therefore, support the concept that in the young adult, sympathetic arterial vasodilation acts to decrease left ventricular load. In the aged dog this response to beta stimulation is lost, and systolic pressure and ventricular load are much greater. Beta blockade eliminates the capacity for vasodilation in the young adult animal and renders the hemodynamic response of the young dog very similar to that of the aged dog. One of the major unanswered questions about the peripheral vascular response of the older individual is the influence of age on the ability of exercising skeletal muscle to effect vasodilatation and augment blood flow. Reduced diversion of blood from the splanchnic and renal beds to exercising skeletal muscle may also be an important factor in the age-associated decline in exercise capacity.

Other Aspects of the Intrinsic Cardiovascular Response

In addition to the altered inotropic and vasodilator response to beta-sympathetic stimulation, there is a clear age-associated decrease in the chronotropic response to catecholamines in both animal models and man.[10,39] The maximum heart rate response to beta-sympathetic stimulation has been shown to be diminished in the senescent beagle dog both before and after vagal blockade. Older healthy subjects have a smaller increase in heart rate following an isoproterenol infusion than younger subjects.

Although the studies to date are not extensive, there appears to be no major age-associated alteration in coronary vascular structure. There are some anatomic data suggesting an age-associated decrease in the capillary density, but this decrease is accounted for partly by the mild hypertrophy discussed above. The few studies that have been performed to assess vasodilating ability of the coronary vasculature show no major age-associated alterations except for decreased beta-sympathetic coronary arterial vasodilation. For many years it was thought that there was a marked age-associated decrease in overall left ventricular function ascribable to altered coronary flow due to diminished capillary density or to altered oxygen delivery on the basis of increased resistance to oxygen diffusion. Studies have not supported these conclusions, however, and this particular theory of cardiovascular aging has fallen from favor. Such a mechanism of cardiovascular aging would, of course, conflict directly with the evidence in senescent animals of maintained intrinsic cardiac muscle function and normal inotropic response of cardiac muscle and the left ventricle to certain types of inotropic stimulation, such as calcium and postextrasystolic potentiation.

Cardiovascular Response to Exercise in Human Beings

The age-associated decrease in exercise capacity and the decrease in maximum rate of oxygen consumption during exercise have long been of interest.[12,28,40,31] (See also Chap. 114.) On the basis of early studies that claimed to demonstrate a marked decrease in resting cardiac function in normal aging people, it used to be held that the major factor in the decrease in exercise ability with age was a diminished ability to augment cardiac output.

Although no study to date has clearly identified the factors that limit exercise ability in normal human beings, the age-associated reduction is not due to a straightforward limitation of the ability to increase cardiac output due to a marked reduction of overall cardiac function. Among the possible mechanisms of the decrease are any or all of the following:

- Increased work of breathing or overall decrease in pulmonary function
- Decreased blood flow to skeletal muscle
- Alterations in metabolism in skeletal muscle and/or sensation of fatigue
- Psychologic factors
- Indirect mechanisms whereby the physiological alterations that occur in cardiac function with age lead to an increased sense of fatigue or increased respiratory demands.

Although the question of what factor or factors limit exercise ability with age cannot be answered definitively now, the age-associated alterations in cardiovascular response to exercise that occur at each level of work performance up to the maximal level for an individual can be examined in a descriptive manner.

Figure 115-3 lists four factors that determine maximal cardiac output during exercise or any other form of stress. They are maximal heart rate, the maximal cardiac inotropic state, minimal impedance to left ventricular ejection, and the maximal use of the Frank-Starling mechanism. (See also Chap. 114.) If there is a change in any one of the factors in the direction indicated, and if the other three factors are held constant, there would be an augmentation of cardiac output. In contrast, a change in any of these factors in the opposite direction reduces maximal cardiac output. This assumes that there is no limitation in venous return. If heart rate or contractility does not increase to the same degree or if impedance to left ventricular ejection does not decrease as much in the elderly compared to the young adult subjects, maximum cardiac output capacity is lower. Finally, limitations in the use of the Frank-Starling mechanism may also limit maximum cardiac output capacity. On the other hand, if

CONTRIBUTE TO EXERCISE CARDIAC OUTPUT	AGED	AGED AT SAME WORKLOAD
HEART RATE INCREASE	LESS	LOWER HEART RATE
AFTERLOAD DECREASE INOTROPY INCREASE	LESS LESS	LARGER END-SYSTOLIC VOLUME
FRANK-STARLING USE	MORE	LARGER END-DIASTOLIC AND STROKE VOLUMES

FIGURE 115-3 Factors that contribute to increased cardiac output during stress and the influence of age on the response of these factors to exercise stress.

the Frank-Starling mechanism and increased fiber length could be utilized, this reserve mechanism may compensate for alterations in the other three variables that might otherwise limit exercise capacity. It is, in fact, this pattern of exercise response that has been shown to be present in normal aging human beings. There is a clear decrease in the maximum heart rate response to exercise in the elderly. There is also evidence of a decrease in cardiac inotropic response and an increase in impedance to ejection during exercise. These three age-associated alterations in cardiovascular function serve to diminish maximum cardiac output capacity. There appears to be, though, a readily available and effective use of the Frank-Starling mechanism that compensates significantly in normal elderly individuals, thus maintaining cardiac output at high work load levels.

These conclusions are based on an extensive study of 61 normal individuals from the Baltimore Longitudinal Study on Aging.[14] The Baltimore Longitudinal Study population is a group of individuals who have been volunteer research subjects for up to 30 years. These individuals have appeared for general medical evaluation, including detailed description of cardiovascular status, on a biennial basis. Thus, within this population, subjects can be screened to eliminate, with some confidence, those with manifest cardiovascular disease. All subjects who participated had no evidence of cardiovascular disease based on a detailed history, physical examination, and electrocardiographic stress testing. Those subjects over the age of 40 had no evidence of ischemic heart disease on exercise thallium testing. These individuals performed bicycle exercise while gated cardiac blood pool scans (see Chap. 114) were obtained at each level of exercise up to the maximum. Absolute left ventricular volumes and cardiac output were measured.

In these subjects at rest there was a slightly higher systolic blood pressure with increasing age, but no change in left ventricular end-diastolic volume, left ventricular end-systolic volume, or ejection fraction. With exercise, there were three major age-associated alterations in the measured cardiovascular variables. First, as expected, there was a lower heart rate response to exercise at each work load level that is likely related to the decreased chronotropic sympathetic response associated with aging noted above. Second, in the younger individuals, the end-systolic volume diminished with exercise, reflecting enhanced inotropic state and effective vasodilation of the arterial vasculature related to the normal beta-sympathetic response to exercise. In the elderly individuals end-systolic volume did not decrease with exercise. This almost certainly reflects both the decreased cardiac inotropic response and a decreased aortic vasodilator response or increased impedance to ejection, as suggested by the animal studies discussed above. Third, there was a striking increase in the end-diastolic volume with exercise in the elderly individuals. In the normal younger individuals there was a minimal increase in end-diastolic volume at any level of exercise. Thus, the younger individuals did not utilize the Frank-Starling mechanism to augment stroke volume and cardiac output; they relied completely and successfully on an augmented heart rate, the inotropic state of the ventricle, and a decrease in impedance to ejection. In the elderly individuals, with each stepwise increase in exercise there was a stepwise increase in end-diastolic volume that was greater than the increase in end-systolic volume, thus augmenting stroke volume and indicating a reliance on and effective utilization of the Frank-Starling mechanism. Thus, there was an age-associated increase in stroke volume, at any level of exercise, ascribable to enhanced use of the Frank-Starling mechanism. This greater increase in stroke volume in the elderly compensated for the lower heart rate response to exercise and resulted in maintenance of the cardiac output at all levels of exercise, so that cardiac output was the same in elderly and younger individuals at any specific exercise work load. (See also Chap. 114.)

In summary, the cardiac output response to exercise is unchanged at any given level of work load in normal human beings from age 20 to 80 years. There is a marked difference, though, in the mechanisms used to increase exercise cardiac output in younger and older subjects. The adrenergically mediated responses, an increase in heart rate, a decrease in end-systolic volume, and the reduction of impedance to left ventricular ejection were all less in the elderly. This is compensated for, however, by an increased use of the Frank-Starling mechanism, reflected by a progressive step-by-step increase in end-diastolic volume as exercise work load increases. Further support for an age-related decrease in beta-adrenergic responsiveness as a key determinant of the differences in the mechanism to increase exercise cardiac output comes from studies of participants who received intravenous propranolol prior to exercise testing. Young beta-blocked subjects have a large increase in their end-diastolic volume at peak exercise, similar to elderly, non-beta-blocked subjects.[29a]

There is clinical utility in use of the ejection fraction at rest and at exercise in the identification of heart disease and in assessing severity and prognosis. Ejection fraction is the fraction of the end-diastolic volume ejected during systole, or the stroke volume divided by end-diastolic volume. Age changes in ejection fraction must be understood to avoid error in assessing the health of elderly subjects—such as ascribing to aging what is normal to disease or to disease what is normal to aging. As noted above, resting ejection fraction is unchanged with age. During exercise the ejection fraction tends to increase less in elderly individuals than in young individuals. The increase in ejection fraction in younger individuals reflects the decrease in end-systolic volume with maintenance of end-diastolic volume and thus both inotropic stimulation of the left ventricle and the vasodilating response of the central vasculature during exercise. In the elderly individual, the ejection fraction increases less with exercise, than in younger individuals, probably due to decreased beta-adrenergic responsiveness reflected in failure to decrease end-systolic volume, and to decreased arterial vasodilatation.[41a]

Importantly, these age-related changes are not immutable. A recent study demonstrates that healthy elderly subjects who undergo 1 year of conditioning have a significant increase in maximal oxygen consumption.[42] Cardiac function evaluated during bicycle exercise by gated blood pool scanning was significantly different following exercise training. Exercise ejection fraction at peak exercise and the increase in ejection from rest to peak exercise were greater following exercise training. End-systolic volume, which did not change from rest to exercise at baseline, decreased significantly during exercise following training. Exercise stroke volume and cardiac output were also significantly greater following training. Potential mechanisms for this improvement following exercise training include an increase in beta-adrenergic sensitivity and/or a decrease in arterial stiffness or afterload.

Importantly, ejection fraction increases from rest to exercise in both healthy sedentary and athletic elderly subjects. Thus, a decrease in ejection fraction from rest to exercise would likely reflect the presence of disease and not be due only to aging. (See also Chap. 114.) Furthermore, left ventricular function during exercise is likely to be affected more severely by disease in the elderly than in young individuals. With reduced sympathetic responsiveness and increased load, the Frank-Starling reserve is used even in the absence of disease. There may be less reserve available for use in the presence of additional stresses superimposed by disease.

CARDIOVASCULAR DISEASE IN AGING

Hypertension

There is a modest increase in diastolic pressure during the early portion of adulthood, which levels off around age 55. The prevalence of diastolic hypertension also levels off in midlife.[43] In contrast, systolic blood pressure increases progressively with increasing age, as does the prevalence of isolated systolic hypertension.[44] Although systolic and diastolic blood pressures are both independent risk factors for the development of cardiovascular disease, systolic blood pressure is the stronger predictor of risk in the elderly.[4] The prevalence of left ventricular hypertrophy, identified by electrocardiography and echocardiography, also increases with age and is an independent risk factor for the development of cardiovascular disease.[45,46] This high prevalence of isolated systolic hypertension and left ventricular hypertrophy, as well as an age-specific response to different classes of antihypertensive agents, arises from age-associated hemodynamic changes. These include the previously mentioned increase in aortic stiffness that is also manifest in the hypertensive population.[27] Furthermore, peripheral vascular resistance increases and cardiac output declines with increasing age in persons with hypertension.[47] This hemodynamic profile of an increase in aortic stiffness and peripheral vascular resistance, in addition to the decrease in beta-sympathetic responsiveness in the elderly, suggests that older hypertensive subjects might respond better to arteriolar vasodilators than to beta-blockers.[31]

Several large randomized trials evaluating medical therapy for diastolic hypertension have clearly demonstrated a benefit of therapy in the elderly.[44] Elderly subjects randomized to treatment have a reduction in cardiovascular mortality and stroke compared to those on placebo.[48] A recent randomized trial in elderly subjects with isolated systolic hypertension has demonstrated that treatment reduces stroke in long-term follow-up compared to placebo.[5] Although left ventricular mass is also a significant risk factor for the development of cardiovascular disease, whether or not antihypertensive therapy that causes regression of cardiac mass further reduces cardiovascular risk has not yet been determined.[49]

Ischemic Heart Disease

Although age is the most important risk factor for manifest ischemic heart disease, the potency of other specific risk factors is so significant that a severe form of the disease can occur at any age. Since, in general, age is associated with more severe, diffuse atherosclerosis and more damage to the left ventricle, almost all clinical manifestations of ischemic heart disease have a higher mortality rate and a worse outcome in the older population. Thus, mortality rates in acute myocardial infarction, unstable angina, heart failure, and arrhythmias are all increased in the elderly. It is not surprising that evidence of functioning collateral vessels is greater in older individuals, who likely have had a longer duration of disease, than in younger individuals. The presence of these collaterals likely indicates not only some protection against acute occlusive episodes (and thus the association of age and non-Q-wave myocardial infarction[50]) but also increased overall severity of disease with each of the vessels having more severe atherosclerosis.

The clinical assessment of the elderly patient with coronary artery disease is often limited by the coexistence of diseases that make interpretation of symptoms difficult.[51] Thus, in the elderly objective parameters such as stress test results are important in assessing and diagnosing ischemic heart disease. Treadmill testing is also useful to detect silent ischemia, which occurs with increasing frequency in the elderly and is a strong risk factor for the developent of future symptomatic cardiac disease.[52] Additionally, elderly subjects often present with atypical symptoms of acute myocardial ischemia and infarction or the acute myocardial infarction is often completely unrecognized.[53]

In general, therapy of ischemic heart disease is not age specific. The high mortality associated with acute ischemic syndromes in the elderly, however, often dictates an aggressive approach to management. Thrombolytic therapy in acute myocardial infarction has been demonstrated to reduce mortality.[54] Several large, placebo-controlled trials of thrombolytic therapy have included elderly patients and demonstrated significant reductions in short-term mortality, averaging about 17 percent.[54–56] In absolute terms, the net benefit of thrombolytic therapy is greatest in the elderly because of the high mortality in this age group. Although the elderly have an increased risk of intracerebral hemorrhage compared to younger patients,[57] other comorbid conditions, such as hypertension, cerebrovascular disease, and diabetes, must be taken into account, and age alone is not necessarily a criterion to exclude a patient from receiving thrombolytic therapy. (See also Chap. 60.)

The use of percutaneous transluminal angioplasty or coronary artery bypass surgery as therapy for ischemic heart disease in the elderly is somewhat controversial. The high prevalence of comorbid conditions and more advanced atherosclerosis places the elderly patient at increased risk of morbidity and mortality from mechanical revascularization; yet, where appropriate, the results of surgical therapy of ischemic heart disease in older individuals are rewarding. Angioplasty or bypass surgery can result in marked symptomatic improvement in the elderly, particularly in those patients with unstable angina, postinfarction angina, or ischemic pulmonary edema.[58–61] (See also Chaps. 70 and 73.)

Congestive Heart Failure

Recent demographic studies suggest that the prevalence of congestive heart failure is increasing in men and women of all races, with an approximate doubling in the number of hospital discharges for congestive heart failure between 1973 and 1986.[62] While age-specific rates of hospital discharges for heart failure have been stationary for younger patients, the increase in the prevalence of heart failure is entirely accounted for by the steep rise in the number of elderly heart failure patients. This age-associated increase in the prevalence of heart failure is consequent to at least two interacting factors. First, there is a marked age-associated increase in the prevalence of coronary artery disease and systemic arterial hypertension,[2,44] which are the two most common cardiovascular diseases that cause myocardial damage.[63] Second, there are age-related cardiovascular changes that ordinarily do not limit cardiac function; however, in the setting of myocardial damage these may cause symptomatic heart failure to become manifest.

The age-associated factors that may affect the severity of heart failure include an increase in both the pulsatile (arterial stiffness and wave reflections) and nonpulsatile (systemic vascular resistance) components of afterload.[35] The previously mentioned increase in arterial stiffness with age also holds true in a heart failure population.[64] This increase in impedance to left ventricular ejection would tend to aggravate congestive symptoms, particularly with exercise or stress. In addition, the age-associated decrease in sympathetic responsiveness limits the ability of the older person to augment heart rate and cardiac function in the presence of superimposed heart disease, particularly in the setting of acute depression of left ventricular function. Finally, the decrease in early left ventricular filling and the presumptive increase in left ventricular filling pressures during exercise alluded to above may worsen heart failure symptoms, especially in association with diseases that also impair left ventricular filling, such as coronary artery disease and systemic arterial hypertension.

The treatment of congestive heart failure in the elderly is complicated by an age-associated decrease in renal function and an increase in cerebral vascular disease, both of which would increase the risks of drug side effects. (See also Chap. 116.) As discussed above, animal studies suggest that the toxicity of digitalis in terms of inducing arrhythmias in the elderly individual is similar to that in the young or middle-aged adult, but the increase in inotropy associated with the administration of digitalis glycosides seems to be diminished in both isolated heart muscle and the intact left ventricle of the aged animal. The applicability of these data to human beings is uncertain, but they do indicate some possibility that digitalis glycosides may be less beneficial and potentially more toxic in this age group. (See Chap. 27.) Vasodilator therapy of mild heart failure is often more appropriate in an elderly individual. This therapy for the elderly patient with heart failure is especially attractive in the setting of increased impedance to ejection and likely decreased inotropic responsiveness to other agents. The decrease in mortality with vasodilator therapy added to therapy with digoxin and diuretics that has been demonstrated in patients with symptomatic heart failure holds for the subgroup of heart failure patients over the age of 70 years.[65] In patients who have normal left ventricular systolic function but symptomatic diastolic heart failure from impaired left ventricular filling, beta blockers or calcium channel blockers may be beneficial.[66,66a] (See also Chap. 26.)

Electrophysiology

Loss of pacemaker and conducting cells in otherwise normal hearts has been identified in the elderly.[67] Thus, there appears to be some age-associated predisposition in the elderly to sinus node dysfunction as well as to abnormalities of conduction in the atrioventricular (AV) node and the His-Purkinje system, including the bundle branches.

Supraventricular and ventricular arrhythmias also increase in frequency with aging[68] but have not been associated with specific evidence of cardiovascular disease. It would appear that arrhythmias in the elderly are to be approached in the same fashion as in younger individuals, i.e., those that are asymptomatic or unassociated with evidence of distinct cardiac disease can be viewed as less serious than ventricular arrhythmias associated with evidence of left ventricular dysfunction and/or ischemia. (See also Chap. 36.) In the post–myocardial infarction patient, both older and younger subjects benefit from beta-blocker therapy with a reduction in sudden death.[69] Furthermore, life-threatening ventricular arrhythmias are common in the elderly patient with severe coronary disease and left ventricular dysfunction. As in younger subjects, aggressive management of survivors of cardiac arrest or elderly patients with hypotensive ventricular tachycardia seems justified.[70] Antiarrhythmic therapy selected from electrophysiological testing and/or placement of the automatic implantable cardioverter defibrillator is well tolerated in the elderly and leads to improved mortality when compared to theoretical survival curves.[71]

Valvular Heart Disease

The most frequent valvular heart disease in the elderly is calcific aortic stenosis. (See Chap. 79.) In the sixth or seventh decade this condition is most often due to congenitally bicuspid valve whereas in the more elderly patients calcific aortic stenosis is more likely due to primary aortic degenerative changes.[72] The development of clinically significant aortic stenosis may be very rapid in this age group, as calcification and severe scarring occur rather abruptly. In some patients the disease may progress from mild aortic stenosis to very severe obstruction within 6 to 18 months. Also, animal studies show that there may be a lessened hypertrophic response to increased impedance to left ventricular ejection in the elderly. Isoyama et al.[73] have shown less hypertrophy of the left ventricle in older rats subject to the same increase in left ventricular pressure as young rats (following aortic banding). Failure to hypertrophy and normalized wall stress in the elderly could also contribute to the appearance of heart failure following valve regurgitation[74] or myocardial infarction.

Clinical recognition of valvular aortic stenosis may be difficult in the elderly. Systolic murmurs are common from a number of etiologies, and the murmur of significant aortic stenosis may be difficult to distinguish from the others. The association of left ventricular hypertrophy helps to identify the severity of the condition. By far the most helpful study one can perform in screening an elderly subject for significant aortic stenosis is a Doppler echocardiogram looking for severe aortic valve calcification with decreased mobility and a significant Doppler gradient. (See Chap. 130.) Nonetheless, it appears that asymptomatic elderly patients with significant aortic stenosis by echocardiography can be carefully followed without surgical intervention until the first sign of symptoms appears.[75] Surgical therapy with aortic valve replacement often results in marked improvement in the elderly subject with symptomatic aortic stenosis.[76] Aortic regurgitation may result from degenerative changes within the proximal aorta and valve although symptomatic aortic regurgitation is unlikely. (See also Chap. 79.) It should be remembered that there is some increase in susceptibility to bacterial endocarditis in patients with degenerative aortic valve disease. Instructions regarding antibiotic prophylaxis should be imparted as vigorously in the elderly as they are in young individuals with evidence of valvular disease. (See Chap. 94.)

With regard to the mitral valve, symptomatic mitral regurgitation in the elderly is most often related to ischemic heart disease and papillary muscle dysfunction. Myxomatous degeneration of the mitral valve rather than rheumatic heart disease is probably the next leading cause of mitral regurgitation. The most common cause of mitral stenosis in the elderly is rheumatic disease, which at times may not result in symptoms until the patient reaches old age. The diagnosis may be more difficult in this age group because calcification of the valve may decrease the intensity of the first heart sound and the opening sound, and diminished cardiac output may decrease the intensity of the diastolic rumble. Doppler echocardiography is very useful in diagnosing the presence of significant disease. (See Chap. 130.) Balloon valvuloplasty should be considered for elderly patients who are not surgical candidates with mitral stenosis.[77] (See Chap. 86.)

REFERENCES

1. White NK, Edwards JE, Dry TJ: The relationship of the degree of coronary atherosclerosis with age in men. *Circulation* 1950; 1:645–654.
2. Elveback L, Lie JT: Continued high incidence of coronary artery disease at autopsy in Olmsted County, Minnesota, 1950 to 1979. *Circulation* 1984; 70:345–349.

3. Tejada C, Strong JP, Montenegro MR, et al: Distribution of coronary and aortic atherosclerosis by geographic location, race, and sex. *Lab Invest* 1968; 18:509–526.
4. Kannel WB: Blood pressure and the development of cardiovascular disease in the aged. In: Caird FI, Dall JLC, Kennedy RD (eds): *Cardiology in Old Age.* New York and London, Plenum, 1976: 143–175.
5. SHEP Cooperative Research Group: Prevention of stroke by antihypertensive drug treatment in older persons with isolated systolic hypertension. Final results of the Systolic Hypertension in the Elderly Program (SHEP). *JAMA* 1991; 265:3255–3264.
6. Fleish JH: Further studies of the effect of aging on beta-adrenoreceptor activity of rat aorta. *Br J Pharmacol* 1971; 42:311–313.
7. Gerstenblith G, Spurgeon HA, Froehlich JP, et al: Diminished inotropic responsiveness to ouabain in aged rat myocardium. *Circ Res* 1979; 44:517–523.
8. Guarnieri T, Spurgeon HA, Froehlich JP, et al: Diminished inotropic response but unaltered toxicity to acetylstrophanthidin in the senescent beagle. *Circulation* 1979; 60:1548–1554.
9. Lakatta EG, Yin FCP: Myocardial aging: Functional alterations and related cellular mechanisms. *Am J Physiol* 1982; 242(*Heart Circ Physiol* 11):H927–H941.
10. Yin FCP, Spurgeon HA, Greene HL, et al: Age-associated decrease in heart rate response to isoproterenol in dogs. *Mech Aging Dev* 1979; 10:17–25.
11. Guarnieri T, Filburn CR, Zitnik G, et al: Contractile and biochemical correlates of beta-adrenergic stimulation of the aged heart. *Am J Physiol* 1980; 239(*Heart Circ Physiol* 8):H501–H508.
12. Weisfeldt ML (ed): *The Aging Heart: Its Function and Response to Stress.* New York, Raven, 1980.
13. Weisfeldt ML, Loeven WA, Shock NW: Resting and active mechanical properties of carneae from aged male rats. *Am J Physiol* 1977; 220:1921–1927.
14. Rodeheffer RJ, Gerstenblith G, Becker LC, et al: Exercise cardiac output is maintained with advancing age in healthy human subjects: Cardiac dilation and increased stroke volume compensate for a diminished heart rate. *Circulation* 1984; 69:203–213.
15. Gerstenblith G, Frederiksen J, Yin FCP, et al: Echocardiographic assessment of a normal adult aging population. *Circulation* 1977; 56:273–278.
16. Yin FCP, Raizes GS, Guarnieri T, et al: Age-associated decrease in ventricular response to hemodynamic stress during beta-adrenergic blockade. *Br Heart J* 1978; 40:1349–1355.
17. Alpert NR, Gale HH, Taylor N: The effect of age on contractile protein ATPase activity and the velocity of shortening. In: Tanz RD, Kalaler F, Kobentz J (eds): *Factors Influencing Myocardial Contractility.* New York, Academic, 1967: 127–144.
18. Bhatnager GM, Walford GD, Beard E, et al: Dissociation of time to peak force (TPF) and myofibrillar ATPase activity (MF-ATPase) with aging of the myocardium. *J Mol Cell Cardiol* 1984; 16:203–218.
19. Lakatta EG, Gerstenblith G, Angell CS, et al: Prolonged contraction duration in aged myocardium. *J Clin Invest* 1975; 55:61–68.
20. Froehlich JP, Lakatta EG, Beard E, et al: Studies of sarcoplasmic reticulum function and contraction duration in young adult and aged rat myocardium. *J Mol Cell Cardiol* 1978; 10:427–438.
21. Wei JY, Spurgeon HA, Lakatta EG: Excitation-contraction coupling in rat myocardium: Alterations with adult aging. *Am J Physiol* 1984; 246:H784–H791.
22. Yin FCP, Weisfeldt ML, Milnor WR: The role of aortic input impedance in the decreased cardiovascular response to exercise with aging in the dog. *J Clin Invest* 1981; 68:28–38.
23. Spurgeon HA, Steinback MF, Lakatta EG: Prolonged contraction duration in senescent myocardium is prevented by exercise. *Physiologist* 1980; 23:56–67.
24. Harrison TR, et al: The relation of age to the duration of contraction, ejection, and relaxation of the normal human heart. *Am Heart J* 1964; 67:189–199.
25. Miller TR, Grossman SJ, Schectman KB, et al: Left ventricular diastolic filling in the healthy elderly. *Am J Cardiol* 1986; 58:531–535.
26. Hirota Y: A clinical study of left ventricular relaxation. *Circulation* 1980; 62:756–763.
27. Avolio AP, Fa-Quan L, Wei-Qiang L, et al: Effects of aging on arterial distensibility in populations with high and low prevalence of hypertension: Comparison between urban and rural communities in China. *Circulation* 1985; 71:202–210.
28. Gerstenblith G, Lakatta EG, Weisfeldt ML: Age changes in myocardial function and exercise response. *Prog Cardiovasc Dis* 1976; 19:1–21.
29. Bonow RO, Vitale DR, Bacharach SL, et al: Effects of aging on asynchronous left ventricular regional function and global ventricular filling in normal human subjects. *J Am Coll Cardiol* 1988; 11:50–58.

29a. Schulman SP, Lakatta EG, Fleg JL, Laketta L, Becker LC, Gerstenblith G: Age-related decline in left ventricular filling at rest and exercise. *Am J Physiol* 1992; 263 *(Heart Circ Physiol):* H1932–H1938.

30. Arora RR, Machac J, Goldman ME, et al: Atrial kinetics and left ventricular diastolic filling in the healthy elderly. *J Am Coll Cardiol* 1987; 9:1255–1260.
31. Schulman SP, Weiss JL, Becker LC, et al: The effects of antihypertensive therapy on left ventricular mass in elderly patients. *N Engl J Med* 1990; 322:1350–1356.
32. Bonow RO, Bacharach SL, Green MV, et al: Impaired left ventricular diastolic filling in patients with coronary artery disease: Assessment with radionuclide angiography. *Circulation* 1981; 64:315–323.
33. Kitzman DW, Higginbotham MB, Cobb FR, et al: Exercise intolerance in patients with heart failure and preserved left ventricular systolic function: Failure of the Frank-Starling mechanism. *J Am Coll Cardiol* 1991; 17:1065–1072.
34. Hallock P, Benson IC: Studies of the elastic properties of human isolated aorta. *J Clin Invest* 1937; 16:595–602.
35. Yin FCP: The aging vasculature and its effect on the heart. In: Weisfeldt ML (ed): *The Aging Heart,* New York, Raven, 1980: 137–213.
36. Nichols WW, O'Rourke MF, Avolio AP, et al: Effects of age on ventricular-vascular coupling. *Am J Cardiol* 1985; 55:1179–1184.
37. Merrillon JP, Motte G, Masquet C, et al: Relationship between physical properties of the arterial system and left ventricular performance in the course of aging and arterial hypertension. *Eur Heart J* 1982; 3(suppl A):95–102.
38. Fleisch JH, Hooker CS: The relationship between age and relaxation of vascular smooth muscle in the rabbit and rat. *Circ Res* 1976; 38:243–249.
39. Van Brummelen P, Buhler FR, Kiowski W, at al: Age-related decrease in cardiac and peripheral vascular responsiveness to isoprenaline: Studies in normal subjects. *Clin Sci* 1981; 60:571–577.
40. Strandell T: Circulatory studies on healthy old men. *Acta Med Scand* 1964; (suppl 414):1–44.
41. Dehn MM, Bruce RA: Longitudinal variations in maximal oxygen uptake with age and activity. *J Appl Physiol* 1972; 33:805–807.

41a. Lakatta EG: Cardiovascular regulatory mechanisms in advanced age. *Physiol Rev* 1993; 73:413–467.

42. Ehsani AA, Ogawa T, Miller TR, et al: Exercise training improves left ventricular systolic function in older men. *Circulation* 1991; 83:96–103.
43. Hypertension Detection Follow-up Group: Blood pressure studies in 14 communities: A two-stage screen for hypertension. *JAMA* 1977; 237:2385–2391.
44. Applegate WB: Hypertension in elderly patients. *Ann Intern Med* 1989; 110:901–915.
45. Kannel WB, Gordon T, Castelli WB, et al: Electrocardiographic left ventricular hypertrophy and risk of coronary heart disease. The Framingham Study. *Ann Intern Med* 1970; 72:813–822.
46. Levy D, Garrison RJ, Savage DD, et al: Left ventricular mass and incidence of coronary heart disease in an elderly cohort. *Ann Intern Med* 1989; 110:101–107.
47. Lund-Johansen P: Hemodynamics in essential hypertension at rest and during exercise—a 20-year follow-up study. *Ann Clin Res* 1988; 20(suppl 48):31–38.
48. European Working Party on High Blood Pressure in the Elderly: Mortality and morbidity results from the European Working Party on High Blood Pressure in the Elderly Trial. *Lancet* 1985; 1:1349–1354.
49. Pfeffer MA, Pfeffer JM: Reversing cardiac hypertrophy in hypertension. *N Engl J Med* 1990; 322:1388–1390.
50. Nicod P, Gilpin E, Dittrich H, et al: Short-and long-term clinical outcome after Q wave and non-Q wave myocardial infarction in a large population. *Circulation* 1989; 79:528–536.
51. Frishman WH, DeMaria AN, Ewy GA: Clinical assessment. *J Am Coll Cardiol* 1987; 10:48A–51A.

52. Fleg JL, Gerstenblith G, Zonderman AB, et al: Prevalence and prognostic significance of exercise-induced silent myocardial ischemia detected by thallium scintigraphy and electrocardiography in asymptomatic volunteers. *Circulation* 1990; 81:428–436.
53. Nadelmann J, Frishman WH, Ooi WL, et al: Prevalence, incidence and prognosis of recognized and unrecognized myocardial infarction in persons aged 75 years or older: The Bronx Aging Study. *Am J Cardiol* 1990; 66:533–537.
54. ISIS-2 (Second International Study of Infarct Survival) Collaborative Group: Randomized trial of intravenous streptokinase, oral aspirin, both or neither among 17,187 cases of suspected acute myocardial infarction: ISIS-2. *Lancet* 1988; 2:349–360.
55. Wilcox RG, Olsson CG, Skene AM, et al: Trial of tissue plasminogen activator for mortality reduction in acute myocardial infarction: Anglo-Scandinavian study of early thrombolysis (ASSET). *Lancet* 1988; 2:525–530.
56. AIMS Trial Study Group: Effect of intravenous APSAC on mortality after acute myocardial infarction: Preliminary report of a placebo-controlled clinical trial. *Lancet* 1988; 1:545–549.
57. International Study Group: In-hospital mortality and clinical course of 20,891 patients with suspected acute myocardial infarction randomized between alteplase and streptokinase with or without heparin. *Lancet* 1990; 336:71–75.
58. Gersh BJ, Kronmal RA, Frye RL, et al: Coronary arteriography and coronary artery bypass surgery: Morbidity and mortality in patients aged 65 years or older: A report from the coronary artery surgery study. *Circulation* 1983; 67:483–491.
59. Horneffer PJ, Gardner TJ, Manolio TA, et al: The effects of age on outcome after coronary bypass surgery. *Circulation* 1987; 76(suppl V):V-6–V-12.
60. Kunis R, Greenberg H, Yeoh CB, et al: Coronary revascularization for recurrent pulmonary edema in elderly patients with ischemic heart disease and preserved ventricular function. *N Engl J Med* 1985; 313:1207–1210.
61. Raizner AE, Hust RG, Lewis JM, et al: Transluminal coronary angioplasty in the elderly. *Am J Cardiol* 1986; 57:29–32.
62. Ghali RK, Cooper R, Ford E: Trends in hospitalization rates for heart failure in the United States, 1973–1986. Evidence for increasing population prevalence. *Arch Intern Med* 1990; 150:769–773.
63. Pomerance A: Pathology of the heart with and without cardiac failure in the aged. *Br Heart J* 1965; 27:697–710.
64. Carroll JD, Shroff S, Wirth P, et al: Arterial mechanical properties in dilated cardiomyopathy. Aging and the response to nitroprusside. *J Clin Invest* 1991; 87:1002–1009.
65. CONSENSUS Trial Study Group: Effects of enalapril on mortality in severe congestive heart failure. Results of the Cooperative North Scandinavian Enalapril Survival Study (CONSENSUS). *N Engl J Med* 1987; 316:1429–1435.
66. Topol EJ, Traill TA, Fortuin NJ: Hypertensive hypertrophic cardiomyopathy in the elderly. *N Engl J Med* 1985; 312:277–283.
66a. Wei JY: Age and the cardiovascular system. *N Engl J Med* 1992; 327:1735–1739.
67. Lev M: The pathology of complete atrioventricular block. *Prog Cardiovasc Dis* 1964; 6:317–326.
68. Gleg JL, Kennedy HL: Cardiac arrhythmias in a healthy elderly population: Detection by 24-hour ambulatory electrocardiography. *Chest* 1982; 81:301–307.
69. Norwegian Multicenter Study Group: Timolol-induced reduction in mortality and reinfarction in patients surviving acute myocardial infarction. *N Engl J Med* 1981; 304:801–807.
70. Tresh DD, Platia EV, Guarnieri T, et al: Refractory symptomatic ventricular tachycardia and ventricular fibrillation in elderly patients. *Am J Med* 1987; 83:399–404.
71. Tresh DD, Troup PH, Thakur RK, et al: Comparison of efficacy of automatic implantable cardioverter defibrillator in patients older and younger than 65 years of age. *Am J Med* 1991; 90:717–724.
72. Seltzer A: Changing aspects of the natural history of valvular aortic stenosis. *N Engl J Med* 1987; 317:91–98.
73. Isoyama S, Wei JY, Izumo S, et al: The effect of age on the development of cardiac hypertrophy produced by aortic constriction in the rat. *Circ Res* 1987; 61:337–342.
74. Isoyama S, Grossman W, Wei JY: Effect of age on myocardial adaptation to volume overload in the rat. *J Clin Invest* 1988; 81:1850–1857.
75. Pellikka PA, Nushimura RA, Bailey KR, et al: The natural history of adults with asymptomatic hemodynamically significant aortic stenosis. *J Am Coll Cardiol* 1990; 15:1012–1017.
76. Edmunds LH, Stephenson LW, Edie RN, et al: Open-heart surgery in octonogenarians. *N Engl J Med* 1988; 319:131–136.
77. Tuzcu EM, Block PC, Griffin BP, Newell JB, Palacias IF: Immediate and long-term outcome of percutaneous mitral valvotomy in patients 65 years and older. *Circulation* 1992; 85:963–971.

Chapter 116

Geriatric Considerations in Cardiovascular Therapy

Paul E. Nolan, Jr., Pharm.D. ■ *Frank I. Marcus, M.D.*

Mortality rates for cardiovascular disease have declined in most countries over the past decade.[1] The decline in cardiovascular mortality can be attributed in part to specific medical and surgical interventions.[2] Cardiovascular disease remains the major cause of mortality in the aged population worldwide, however, particularly in industrialized nations.[1] When one considers projections that, well into the next century, an increasing proportion of the population will be 65 years of age and older,[3] it becomes evident that clinicians will be treating an increasing number of elderly patients with cardiovascular disease. Therefore, it is important that clinicians understand the effects of age that potentially influence cardiovascular therapy in elderly patients.

OVERVIEW OF GERIATRIC CLINICAL PHARMACOLOGY

Although there is considerable interindividual variability, many physiological functions decline with age.[4] These physiological changes potentially result in alterations in the clinical pharmacokinetics and pharmacodynamics of cardiovascular drugs.[5] In addition, the elderly are susceptible to a variety of chronic illnesses,[6] some of which may further modify the disposition and response to cardiovascular drugs.

Table 116-1 provides a summary of geriatric clinical pharmacology.

Absorption

Several physiological alterations occur within the gastrointestinal tract in the elderly.[7] These include prolonged gastric emptying time, elevated gastric pH, decreased splanchnic blood flow, reduced gastrointestinal motility, and decreased absorptive surface area. In general, however, specific measurements of absorptive and digestive functions appear to be well maintained throughout the normal aging process.[8] In addition, the absorption of most drugs is generally unaltered in the elderly[7]; however, age-related decreases in hepatic blood flow may result in enhanced oral bioavailability of highly extracted drugs (e.g., propranolol, verapamil) that undergo extensive first-pass hepatic metabolism.[7]

Distribution

Body Composition

In the elderly total body weight and lean body mass often decrease, but the percentage of fat weight increases.[9,10] Furthermore, lean body mass is lower and percentage of fat is greater in elderly females as compared to elderly males.[10] Consequently drugs that are relatively lipophilic (e.g., lidocaine) may demonstrate an increased volume of distribution in the elderly. The increased distribution of lipophilic drugs (e.g., lidocaine) may demonstrate an increased volume of distribution in the elderly. The increased distribution of lipophilic drugs may prolong their

TABLE 116-1
Summary of Geriatric Clinical Pharmacology

Pharmacokinetic/ Physiological Process	Observed Physiological Changes	Potential Clinical Consequences
Absorption	Prolonged gastric emptying time Elevated gastric pH Decreased splanchnic blood flow Reduced gastrointestinal motility Decreased absorptive surface area	Absorption of drugs may be altered Increased absorption of drugs that undergo extensive first-pass metabolism
Distribution		
Body composition	Decreased body weight and lean body mass; increased percentage of fat weight	Increased volume of distribution and half-life of lipophilic drugs Reduced volume of distribution and elevated plasma concentrations of hydrophilic drugs
Protein binding	Decreased serum albumin Increased serum α-acid glycoprotein	Decreased protein binding of acidic drugs Increased protein binding of basic drugs
Hepatic metabolism	Decreased hepatic blood flow and hepatic size	Decreased excretion of drugs that are highly dependent on either hepatic blood flow or on intrinsic activity of hepatic microsomal enzymes for elimination
Renal function	Decreased renal blood flow, glomerular filtration, and renal tubular secretion	Decreased excretion of drugs that are highly dependent upon the kidney for elimination

elimination. On the other hand, a hydrophilic drug such as digoxin may have a reduced volume of distribution that could result in higher plasma concentrations.

Protein Binding

In healthy elderly, plasma concentrations of albumin tend to decrease and those of α_1-acid glycoprotein (AAG) may slightly increase.[11] In addition, concentrations of albumin may be further depleted and those of AAG further increased in the elderly because of the existence of disease states that modify these proteins. An acidic compound (e.g., phenytoin) has a greater affinity for albumin whereas basic drugs (e.g., lidocaine, disopyramide) demonstrate a greater affinity for AAG. Theoretically, basic drugs should therefore have a decreased unbound or free plasma concentration and acidic drugs an increased free concentration in the aged. Many cardiovascular drugs do not show significant changes in protein binding in disease-free elderly.[11]

Hepatic Metabolism

In addition to protein binding, the metabolism of drugs by the liver is determined by the intrinsic activity of hepatic microsomal enzymes, hepatic blood flow, and hepatic volume or size[12] Recent evidence demonstrates that the in vitro activity of many microsomal enzymes responsible for phase I hepatic metabolism (i.e., oxidation, reduction, and hydrolysis) is unchanged in elderly humans.[13,14] In addition, substrate affinity of hepatic microsomal monooxygenases is unaffected by age.[15] Phase II reactions (e.g., glucuronidation) also are generally unaltered in the elderly.[7]

Hepatic blood flow and hepatic size decline with age.[16,17] These decreases are most notable in elderly females.[17] The reduction in hepatic blood flow may result in a decrease in clearance of drugs that are highly dependent upon hepatic blood flow for elimination (e.g., lidocaine, verapamil). For drugs with clearance principally dependent on the intrinsic activity of phase I hepatic microsomal enzymes (e.g., quinidine), the observed age-related reductions in elimination may result from the decreases in hepatic volume and size, which probably diminishes the absolute content and therefore overall functional activity of hepatic monooxygenases.

Polymorphic Hepatic Metabolism

Several cardiovascular drugs are metabolized by hepatic enzymes that have a genetically founded polymorphic distribution. Data for *N*-acetyltransferase, a nonmicrosomal enzyme with a trimodal distribution (i.e., homozygous rapid, heterozygous rapid, and homozygous slow acetylators), suggest that an age-related reduction in activity occurs.[18] This should result in a higher proportion of slow acetylators in the elderly. *N*-acetyltransferase is implicated in the metabolism of procainamide and hydralazine. On the other hand, limited evidence suggests that debrisoquine hydroxylase, an enzyme that metabolizes propafenone, encainide, flecainide, and some β-adrenergic blockers in extensive metabolizers of these compounds, demonstrates no change in phenotypic distribution with age.[19]

Renal Function

The elimination of drugs that undergo renal excretion may diminish in the elderly because various aspects of renal physiological function generally deteriorate with age.[20] Renal blood flow, glomerular filtration, and renal tubular secretion often decrease in the elderly. Creatinine clearance, an estimate of glomerular filtration, also frequently declines; however, there is no reduction in creatinine clearance in about one-third of the elderly.[21] Serum creatinine, an indicator of the equilibrium between the production and excretion of creatinine, should not be assumed to reflect reliably renal function in the elderly because the production of creatinine diminishes secondary to a decrease in muscle mass. Therefore, creatinine clearance should either be measured or estimated by any one of several predictive equations.[22] These equations, however, may be inaccurate in the debilitated elderly nursing home patient.[23]

Miscellaneous

Environmental Influences

Several other factors may modify the clinical pharmacology of cardiovascular drugs in the elderly. For example, environmental influences, such as cigarette smoking and alcohol ingestion, can induce hepatic microsomal enzymes, thereby enhancing the elimination of many drugs.[24] Interestingly, selected hepatic enzyme systems may respond differently to the inducing effect of smoking in the elderly relative to younger individuals.[24]

Nutritional Factors

The human diet can potentially alter the disposition of drugs.[24] High-protein diets increase the rates of hepatic drug oxidation. Cruciferous vegetables such as cabbage and brussel sprouts can also enhance hepatic oxidative metabolism. Although there is a lack of investigation of the interaction between advanced age and diet on drug metabolism, nutritional factors may play a role in altering hepatic drug metabolism in the elderly.

Ethnic Differences

There is some evidence for interethnic variability in drug metabolism and responsiveness.[25] There is a greater prevalence of slow acetylators among Caucasians and blacks as compared to either Chinese or Japanese individuals.[25] Therefore, more individuals in the former groups may be at greater risk for developing drug-induced systemic lupus erythematosus during the chronic administration of procainamide or hydralazine. With respect to drug responsiveness, Chinese individuals are more sensitive to the β-blocking and hypotensive actions of propranolol despite a higher clearance of propranolol.[25]

Gender Differences

Gender differences may play an important role in the disposition of some cardiovascular drugs. For lidocaine, the half-life is longer and the volume of distribution is larger in females than in males.[26] In addition, there may be greater age-related reduction in the total body clearance of lidocaine in elderly males as compared to elderly females.[27] The total body clearance of propranolol is greater in males than females because of sex-related differences in selected metabolic pathways.[28]

Stereospecific Considerations

Many cardiovascular drugs are clinically available as 50:50 racemic mixtures of two enantiomers that frequently differ in their pharmacokinetic and pharmacologic properties.[7] Examples encompass the antiarrhythmic drugs disopyramide, mexiletine, tocainide, propafenone, sotalol, and flecainide; virtually all β-adrenergic antagonists including propranolol, metoprolol, and atenolol; and the calcium channel antagonist, verapamil. It remains to be determined whether or not the disposition and activity of the enantiomers of many of these compounds are altered as a consequence of aging.

Drug Interactions

The elderly are at increased risk for having drug interactions because of concurrent illnesses and the resultant polypharmacy.[7] In addition, specific drug interactions can be magnified in the elderly secondary to age and disease-related changes in physiological functions.[7] Drug interactions may result from alterations in either pharmacokinetics or pharmacodynamics.[29] An overview of cardiovascular drug interactions is beyond the scope of this chapter. The reader is referred to Chap. 109 and to a recent review of clinically important drug interactions.[29]

Cardiovascular, Adrenergic, and Neuroendocrine Changes

A number of cardiovascular, adrenergic, and neuroendocrine changes occur during the normal aging process, and these may modify the response to cardiovascular drugs.[5,30]

Cardiovascular Changes

Resting heart rate and left ventricular systolic shortening are diminished in the healthy elderly.[31] Ventricular performance, however, is preserved, in part by an increase in ventricular wall thickness.[31] (See Chap. 115.) Exercise heart rate is also reduced, but cardiac output is maintained by enhanced cardiac dilation and increased stroke volume.[32] The compliance in large arteries consistently decreases with age, but there are inconclusive data for age-related changes in resistance vessels.[5]

In addition to those age-related changes, which normally occur within the cardiovascular system, the prevalence of congestive heart failure (CHF) rises progressively with increasing age for both males and females.[33] Congestive heart failure may alter drug metabolism and elimination as a result of hypoperfusion to the liver and kidney.[34] It may also modify the pharmacodynamics of antiarrhythmic drugs such as encainide and flecainide, which are more likely to cause proarrhythmia in patients with poor left ventricular function.[35]

Adrenergic Changes

Although concentrations of plasma norepinephrine are increased in the elderly, baroreflex sensitivity to both hypertensive and hypotensive stimuli is blunted during normal human aging.[30] Cardiac β_1-adrenergic receptor responsiveness also declines with age.[5] Consequently, the inotropic and chronotropic effects of β_1 agonists are diminished in the elderly. Vascular β_2-receptor sensitivity appears to be maintained as evidenced by a normal response to intravenous isoproterenol in older individuals.[36] This observation, however, could possibly result from age-related alterations in isoproterenol pharmacokinetics. This finding contrasts with those reported for isolated arterioles from aged experimental animals and following localized intraarterial administration of isoproterenol to humans.[36] There is no apparent effect of age on α_1-adrenoceptor sensitivity.[37]

Neuroendocrine Changes

Activity of the renin-angiotensin-aldosterone system (RAAS) declines with age.[30] Circulating levels of renin, angiotensin II, and aldosterone are subsequently decreased and may contribute to a diminished ability to conserve sodium. Plasma concentrations of atrial natriuretic factor (ANS) increase with age and may contribute to the reduction in RAAS activity.[30] In the elderly patient with essential hypertension, however, there is an increase in total body exchangeable sodium despite elevated ANF plasma levels. Finally, the elderly may manifest disturbances in water balance secondary to a reduction in intravascular volume, diminished thirst following water deprivation, altered vasopressin secretion, and declining glomerular filtration.[30]

Pharmacodynamic Changes in the Elderly

Many reports suggest that there is an increased response or enhanced sensitivity (i.e., altered pharmacodynamics) to numerous cardiovascular and noncardiovascular drugs in the elderly.[38] Often, these exaggerated pharmacologic responses can be explained by age-dependent changes in pharmacokinetics.[38] Some changes in pharmacodynamics in the elderly may be an indirect effect either of the normal aging process (e.g., decreased baroreflex sensitivity) or of underlying and perhaps previously undetected disease processes. Nonetheless, clinicians should be aware of the potential for altered response to cardiovascular drugs in elderly patients.

SELECTED CARDIOVASCULAR DRUGS

Antiarrhythmics

Quinidine

In the elderly the total body clearance, renal clearance, and nonrenal clearance of quinidine are decreased and the half-life is increased.[39,40] There is no change in the protein binding and volume of distribution of quinidine in the healthy elderly.[39] In addition, elderly patients may be at a potentially greater risk for accumulating the active metabolite, 3-hydroxyquinidine.[41] Elevated concentrations of this metabolite may contribute to the occurrence of quinidine-induced cardiotoxicity such as ventricular tachycardia or excessive prolongation of the QRS interval.[42]

Procainamide

Two reports indicate that the elimination of procainamide is diminished in elderly patients.[43,44] Reductions in the renal clearance and possibly the nonrenal clearance of procainamide are the probable mechanisms. These reductions in clearance probably explain the longer half-life of procainamide in the aged. Furthermore, the clearance of *N*-acetylprocainamide (NAPA) is decreased,[43] the half-life is extended,[45] and the steady-state NAPA-to-procainamide serum concentration ratios are increased[44] in the elderly.

Disopyramide

The pharmacokinetics of both total (protein-bound plus unbound) and unbound disopyramide are altered in the elderly.[46,47] For total disopyramide the total body clearance is reduced, the volume of distribution is increased, and the half-life is prolonged in the elderly.[46] Although there is no change in the protein binding of disopyramide in the elderly, steady-state serum concentrations of unbound disopyramide are greater due to the reduced clearance of unbound disopyramide.[46] The serum concentrations of mono-*N*-dealkyldisopyramide, the major metabolite of disopyramide, also tend to be higher in the elderly.[46,47] Interestingly, cigarette smoking may induce the metabolism of disopyramide to a greater extent in aged individuals.[46] The elderly also appear more likely to experience the anticholinergic adverse effects of disopyramide.[47]

Lidocaine

There is disagreement regarding age-related changes in the pharmacokinetics of lidocaine,[27,48–50] particularly among single-dose investigations.[27,48,49] Some single-dose studies report an increase in the half-life of lidocaine but no change in the clearance of lidocaine in elderly subjects.[48,49] On the other hand, another single-dose study describes a decrease in clearance in elderly males but not in elderly females relative to sex-matched young control groups.[27] Nevertheless, following continuous infusion of lidocaine in elderly patients with acute myocardial infarction, the total body clearance of lidocaine decreases and the serum concentration of lidocaine rises with or without concomitant heart failure.[50] The protein binding of lidocaine is apparently increased in the elderly.[49]

Mexiletine

The rate, but not the extent, of absorption of oral mexiletine is decreased in the elderly.[51] The elderly also tend to have a prolonged half-life and a reduction in the oral clearance of mexiletine.

Flecainide

The oral clearance and half-life of flecainide in elderly subjects are similar to young volunteers following single oral doses of flecainide.[52] With chronic oral dosing in elderly subjects, however, there is a decrease in oral clearance and an increase in half-life of flecainide, perhaps due to time-dependent changes in the hepatic metabolism of flecainide.[52]

Amiodarone

An ongoing clinical investigation should reveal whether or not there are significant pharmacokinetic differences for amiodarone in the elderly. During chronic treatment for either recurrent sustained ventricular tachycardia or fibrillation, however, advanced age was associated with an increased likelihood for developing amiodarone-induced adverse effects.[53] It is not known whether this is a direct pharmacodynamic effect of amiodarone in the aged or is a secondary phenomenon due to altered pharmacokinetics.

Propafenone

The metabolism and elimination of propafenone is polymorphic and stereoselective.[54] Extensive metabolizers of propafenone (i.e., generally 90 percent or greater for most populations[19]), but not poor metabolizers, form the active metabolite 5-hydroxypropafenone. Thus, for propafenone the total body clearance is greater and the half-life is shorter in extensive as compared to poor metabolizers. In addition, plasma concentrations of the S-(+)-enantiomer are almost twice as great as that of the R-(−)-enantiomer. This stereoselective elimination is independent of metabolic phenotype. Presently, there is a lack of information directly comparing the pharmacokinetics of propafenone between young and healthy subjects or patients.

Moricizine

Following single doses of moricizine to both young and elderly healthy volunteers, the total body clearance is approximately 50 percent less and the half-life is almost twice as long in the elderly group.[55] In addition, plasma concentrations of two of the major metabolities of moricizine are elevated in the elderly volunteers. Plasma protein binding is similar in both healthy young and elderly subjects. A steady-state pharmacokinetic comparison between young and elderly subjects should be performed because moricizine induces its own metabolism during chronic dosing.[56]

Sotalol

In otherwise healthy elderly hypertensive patients, the total body clearance and renal clearance of racemic sotalol (i.e., DL-sotalol) are reduced 40 to 50 percent and the half-life is increased about 60 percent relative to healthy young subjects.[57] The alterations in the elimination of racemic sotalol in the elderly are predominantly secondary to age-related decreases in creatinine clearance. Elderly patients may also manifest greater reductions in blood pressure than younger hypertensives following racemic sotalol.[57]

Digoxin

Several pharmacokinetic parameters of digoxin are altered in the elderly.[58] These include a reduction in the volume of distribution and total body clearance and an increase in half-life.[58] In addition, the rate of absorption of digoxin from tablets is slowed in the elderly, but the extent of absorption is unchanged[58]; however, there also may be a reduction in the extent of absorption of digoxin from digoxin capsules in the elderly.[59]

The pharmacodynamics of digoxin may be modified in the elderly. In several species there is an apparent age-related increased sensitivity to digitalis glycosides.[60,61] In elderly humans with congestive heart failure, an increase in resting left ventricular ejection fraction may occur at relatively low (0.4 to 1.0 ng/mL) serum digoxin concentrations.[62] In addition, the elderly appear to remain at risk for digoxin toxicity as a result of altered digoxin pharmacokinetics and/or pharmacodynamics despite a recently reported diminished incidence of digoxin toxicity.[63] (See also Chap. 27.)

Vasodilators

Angiotensin Converting Enzyme Inhibitors

Despite lower circulating concentrations of renin, angiotensin converting enzyme inhibitors (ACEIs) are frequently effective in the management of hypertension in the aged.[64] The hypertensive elderly, however, may have exaggerated pharmacodynamic responses to those ACEIs that are principally renally eliminated (e.g., enalapril, lisinopril, quinapril, ramipril, and others) secondary to an age-related decrease in glomerular filtration.[65,66]

The benefit of ACEIs in elderly patients with New York Heart Association (NYHA) class IV congestive heart failure (CHF) is clearly established by the results of the Cooperative North Scandinavian Enalapril Survival Study (CONSENSUS), in which the mean age for the treatment group was 71 years.[67] Other studies, in which the mean age of the patients treated with ACEIs is at least 60 years, also demonstrate favorable effects in less severe CHF.[68,69] In general, both short- and long-acting ACEIs are well tolerated by older patients with CHF.[70] Another study, however, suggests that the very elderly with CHF (mean age 83 years) may be relatively intolerant of ACEIs, and that beginning doses of ACEIs should be low (e.g., 1.25 mg of enalapril) to minimize the occurrence of adverse effects.[71]

Nitrates

Although formal pharmacokinetic studies of nitrates are lacking in elderly human beings, older animals have a longer half-life and a larger volume of distribution but no change in total body clearance of nitrates.[72] With respect to pharmacodynamics, elderly patients generally exhibit greater reductions in clinical estimates of ventricular preload, suggesting that venous smooth muscle in the aged is more sensitive to the relaxant effects of organic nitrates.[72] Hypotension and bradycardia may occur more commonly in elderly patients with acute myocardial infarction who are administered nitroglycerin. A dampened baroreceptor response to the hypotensive effects of nitroglycerin may be the underlying mechanism. Therefore, smaller doses of nitrates should be used in elderly patients. There is currently no information regarding any age-related differences in the rate or extent of development of tolerance to organic nitrates.

Hydralazine

Hydralazine undergoes phenotype-dependent, extensive first-pass metabolism that results in greater bioavailability in slow acetylators.[73] Furthermore, the first-pass metabolism is apparently saturable.[73] The total body clearance and volume of distribution of hydralazine appear to be decreased in older hypertensive patients versus young, healthy volunteers.[73] In addition, the half-life is apparently longer in the older group. These dissimilarities may reflect differences in methodologies[73] or actual changes in rates of acetylation in the aged.[18] Although a four-times-daily hydralazine regimen was used in the Vasodilator Heart Failure Trial (VHeFT),[69] less frequent administration (e.g., every 8 h) may provide satisfactory dosing in the elderly.

Calcium Channel Blockers

Although many calcium channel-blocking drugs are now clinically available and used in the management of hypertension, chronic stable angina, and other cardiovascular disorders, this section will be limited to a discussion of verapamil, diltiazem, and nifedipine. The reader is referred to a recent review for information about the newer calcium channel antagonists.[74] For verapamil, diltiazem, and nifedipine, both the normotensive and hypertensive elderly have a reduced clearance and prolonged half-life relative to younger controls, perhaps due to decreased first-pass extraction.[5] In addition, the elderly hypertensive patient may have an increased antihypertensive effect that is generally unaccompanied by a reflex tachycardia. The latter effect may indicate impaired baroreflex activity. Interestingly atrioventricular conduction delay is relatively less frequent in elderly patients without underlying conduction disturbances as compared to younger patients for both verapamil and diltiazem.[5]

β-Adrenergic Antagonists

β-adrenergic antagonists are extensively prescribed for the treatment of hypertension, arrhythmias and chronic stable angina and to decrease mortality after myocardial infarction. The pharmacodynamic response to β_1-receptor antagonists generally declines with advanced age.[5] Although this observation suggests a diminished pharmacotherapeutic role for β_1-selective and β_1-nonselective antagonists in the elderly, particularly in the treatment of hypertension,[64] the results of the Systolic Hypertension in the Elderly Program (SHEP) demonstrate the value of β-adrenergic blockade as step 2 therapy in the treatment of isolated systolic hypertension in the elderly.[75]

Various investigators have reported a decreased clearance and corresponding increased steady-state concentrations for several β blockers in the elderly.[5] Another group, however, recently showed an age-related increase in half-life for each of the enantiomers of propranolol but no changes in the unbound oral clearance for either enantiomer at steady state.[76]

REFERENCES

1. Uemura K: International trends in cardiovascular diseases in the elderly. *Eur Heart J* 1988; 9(suppl D):1–8.
2. Goldman L, Cook EF: The decline in ischemic heart disease mortality rates. An analysis of the comparative effects of medical interventions and changes in lifestyle. *Ann Intern Med* 1984; 101:825–846.
3. Frye RL, Higgins MW, Beller GA, Benson JA, Sorer JS, Curry CL, et al: Task force III: Major demographic and epidemiologic trends affecting adult cardiology. *J Am Coll Cardiol* 1988; 12:840–846.
4. Abernethy DR, Azarnoff DL: Pharmacokinetic investigations in elderly patients. Clinical and ethical considerations. *Clin Pharmacokinet* 1990; 19:89–93.
5. Abernethy DR: Altered pharmacodynamics of cardiovascular drugs and their relation to altered pharmacokinetics in elderly patients. *Clin Geriatr Med* 1990; 6:285–292.
6. Valkenburg HA: Epidemiologic considerations of the geriatric population. *Gerontology* 1988; 34(suppl 1):2–10.
7. Dawling S, Crome P: Clinical pharmacokinetic considerations in the elderly. An update. *Clin Pharmacokinet* 1989; 4:236–263.
8. Arora S, Kassarjian Z, Krasinski SD, Croffey B, Kaplan MM, Russell RM: Effect of age on tests of intestinal and hepatic function in healthy humans. *Gastroenterology* 1989; 96:1560–1565.
9. Forbes GB, Reina JC: Adult mean body mass declines with age: Some longitudinal observations. *Metabolism* 1970; 19:653–663.
10. Fulop T, Worum I, Csongor J, Foris G, Leovey A: Body composition in elderly people. *Gerontology* 1985; 31:6–14.
11. Wallace SM, Verbeeck RK: Plasma protein binding of drugs in the elderly. *Clin Pharmacokinet* 1987; 12:41–72.
12. Vestal RE: Aging and determinants of hepatic drug clearance. *Hepatology* 1989; 9:331–334.
13. Schmucker DL, Woodhouse KW, Wang RK, Wynne H, James OF, McManus M, et al: Effects of age and gender on in vitro properties of human liver microsomal monooxygenases. *Clin Pharmacol Ther* 1990; 48:365–374.
14. Garcia-Agundez J, Luengo A, Benitez J: Aminopyrine *N*-demethylase activity in human liver microsomes. *Clin Pharmacol Ther* 1990; 48:490–495.
15. Wynne HA, Mutch E, James OFW, Wright P, Ralins MD, Woodhouse KW: The effect of age upon the affinity of microsomal monooxygenase enzymes for substrate in human liver. *Age Ageing* 1988; 17:401–405.
16. Marchesini G, Bua V, Brunori A, Bianchi G, Pisi P, Fabbri A, et al: Galactose elimination capacity and liver volume in aging man. *Hepatology* 1988; 8:1079–1083.
17. Wynne HA, Cope LH, Mutch E, Rawlins MD, Woodhouse KW, James OF: The effect of age upon liver volume and apparent liver blood flow in healthy man. *Hepatology* 1989; 9:297–301.
18. Iselius L, Evans DAP: Formal genetics of isoniazid metabolism in man. *Clin Pharmacokinet* 1983; 8:541–544.
19. Steiner E, Bertilsson L, Sawe J, Bertling I, Sjoqvist F: Polymorphic debrisoquin hydroxylation in 757 Swedish subjects. *Clin Pharmacol Ther* 1988; 44:431–435.
20. Meyer BR, Bellucci A: Renal function in the elderly. *Cardiol Clin* 1986; 4:227–234.
21. Lindeman RD, Tobin J, Shock N: Longitudinal studies on rate of decline in renal function with age. *J Am Geriatr Soc* 1985; 33:278–285.
22. Luke DR, Halstenson CE, Opsahl JA, Matzke GR: Validity of creatinine clearance estimates in the assessment of renal function. *Clin Pharmacol Ther* 1990; 48:503–508.
23. Drusano GL, Muncie HL, Hoopes JM, Damron DJ, Warren JW: Commonly used methods of estimating creatinine clearance are inadequate for elderly debilitated nursing home patients. *J Am Geriatr Soc* 1988; 36:437–441.
24. Anderson KE: Influences of diet and nutrition on clinical pharmacokinetics. *Clin Pharmacokinet* 1988; 14:325–346.
25. Wood AJJ, Zhou HH: Ethnic differences in drug disposition and responsiveness. *Clin Pharmacokinet* 1991; 20:350–373.
26. Wing LMH, Miners JO, Birkett J, Foenander T, Lillywhite K, Wanwimolrok S: Lidocaine disposition—sex differences and effects of cimetidine. *Clin Pharmacol Ther* 1984; 35:695–701.
27. Abernethy DR, Greenblatt DJ: Impairment of lidocaine clearance in elderly male subjects. *J Cardiovasc Pharmacol* 1983; 5:1093–1096.

28. Walle T, Walle K, Cowart D, Conradi EC: Pathway-selective sex differences in the metabolic clearance of propranolol in human subjects. *Clin Pharmacol Ther* 1989; 46:257–263.
29. McInnes GT, Brodie MJ: Drug interactions that matter. A critical reappraisal. *Drugs* 1988; 36:83–110.
30. Phillips PA, Hodsman GP, Johnston CI: Neuroendocrine mechanisms and cardiovascular homeostasis in the elderly. *Cardiovasc Drug Ther* 1990; 4:1209–1214.
31. Merino A, Alegria E, Castello R, Martinez-Caro D: Influence of age on left ventricular contractility. *Am J Cardiol* 1988; 62:1103–1108.
32. Rodeheffer RJ, Gerstenblith G, Becher LC, Fleg JL, Weisfeldt ML, Lakatta EG: Exercise cardiac output is maintained with advancing age in healthy human subjects; cardiac dilatation and increased stroke volume compensate for a diminished heart rate. *Circulation* 1984; 69:201–213.
33. Kannel WB, Belanger AJ: Epidemiology of heart failure. *Am Heart J* 1991; 121:951–957.
34. Shammas FV, Dickstein K: Clinical pharmacokinetics in heart failure. *Clin Pharmacokinet* 1988; 15:94–113.
35. Herre JM, Titus C, Oeff M, Eldar M, Franz MR, Griffin JC, et al: Inefficacy and proarrhythmic effects of flecainide and encainide for sustained ventricular tachycardia and ventricular fibrillation. *Ann Intern Med* 1990; 113:671–676.
36. Klein C, Hiatt WR, Gerber JG, Nies AS: Age does not alter human vascular and nonvascular β_2-adrenergic responses to isoproterenol. *Clin Pharmacol Ther* 1988; 44:573–578.
37. Klein C, Gerber JG, Payne NA, Nies AS: The effect of age on the sensitivity of the α_1 adrenoceptor to phenylephrine and prazocin. *Clin Pharmacol Ther* 1990; 47:535–539.
38. Feely J, Coakley D: Altered pharmacodynamics in the elderly. *Clin Geriatr Med* 1990; 6:269–283.
39. Ochs HR, Greenblatt DJ, Woo E, Smith TW: Reduced quinidine clearance in elderly persons. *Am J Cardiol* 1978; 42:481–485.
40. Drayer DE, Hughes M, Lorenzo B, Reidenberg MM: Prevalence of high (3S)-3-hydroxyquinidine/quinidine ratios in serum, and clearance of quinidine in cardiac patients with age. *Clin Pharmacol Ther* 1980; 27:72–75.
41. Ackerman BH, Olsen KM: Accumulation of 3-hydroxyquinidine following chronic quinidine therapy. *DICP Ann Pharmacother* 1991; 25:867–869.
42. Bowers LD, Nelson KM, Connor R, Lais CJ, Krauss E: Evidence supporting (3S)-3-hydroxyquinidine-associated cardiotoxicity. *Ther Drug Monitor* 1985; 7:308–312.
43. Reidenberg MM, Camacho M, Kluger J, Drayer DE: Aging and renal clearance of procainamide and acetylprocainamide. *Clin Pharmacol Ther* 1980; 28:732–735.
44. Bauer LA, Black D, Gensler A, Spinkle J: Influence of age, renal function and heart failure on procainamide clearance and *N*-acetylprocainamide serum concentrations. *Int J Clin Pharmacol Ther Toxicol* 1989; 27:213–216.
45. Galeazzi RL, Omar-Amberg C, Karlaganis G: *N*-acetyl-procainamide kinetics in the elderly. *Clin Pharmacol Ther* 1981; 29:440–446.
46. Bonde J, Pedersen LE, Bodtker S, Angelo HR, Svendsen TL, Kampmann JP: The influence of age and smoking on the elimination of disopyramide. *Br J Clin Pharmacol* 1985; 20:453–458.
47. Roberto P, Vitaliano B, Donatella P, Raffaella M, Sergio B, Gabriella C: Disopyramide pharmacokinetics in the elderly after single oral administration. *Pharmacol Res Comm* 1988; 20:1025–1034.
48. Nation RL, Triggs EJ: Lignocaine kinetics in cardiac patients and aged subjects. *Br J Clin Pharmacol* 1977; 4:439–448.
49. Cusack B, O'Malley K, Lavan J, Noel J, Kelly JG: Protein binding and disposition of lignocaine in the elderly. *Eur J Clin Pharmacol* 1985; 29:323–329.
50. Cusson J, Nattel S, Matthews C, Talajic M, Lawand S: Age-dependent lidocaine disposition in patients with acute myocardial infarction. *Clin Pharmacol Ther* 1985; 37:381–386.
51. Grech-Belanger O, Barbeau G, Kishka P, Fiset C, LeBoeuf E, Blouin M: Pharmacokinetics of mexiletine in the elderly. *J Clin Pharmacol* 1989; 29:311–315.
52. McQuinn RL, Weeks CE, Kvam DC, Fredell PA, Carlson GL, Miller AM, et al: Pharmacokinetics of flecainide in elderly subjects (abstr). *Clin Pharmacol Ther* 1986; 39:210.
53. Herre JM, Sauve MJ, Malone P, Griffin JC, Helmy I, Langberg JJ, et al: Long-term results of amiodarone therapy in patients with recurrent sustained ventricular tachycardia or ventricular fibrillation. *J Am Coll Cardiol* 1989; 13:442–449.
54. Hii JTY, Duff HG, Burgess ED: Clinical pharmacokinetics of propafenone. *Clin Pharmacokinet* 1991; 21:1–10.
55. Pieniaszek HJ, Young SM, Davidson AF, Benedek IH: Moricizine pharmacokinetics in young and elderly volunteers (abstr). *J Clin Pharmacol*1992; 32:755.
56. Siddoway LA, Schwartz SL, Barbey JT, Woosley RL: Clinical pharmacokinetics of moricizine. *Am J Cardiol* 1990; 65:21D–25D.
57. Ishizaki T, Hirayama H, Tawara K, Nakaya H, Sato M, Sato K: Pharmacokinetics and pharmacodynamics in young normal and elderly hypertensive subjects: A study using sotalol as a model drug. *J Pharmacol Exp Ther* 1980; 212:173–181.
58. Cusack B, Kelly J, O'Malley K, Noel J, Lavan J, Horgan J: Digoxin in the elderly: Pharmacokinetic consequences of old age. *Clin Pharmacol Ther* 1979; 25:772–776.
59. Pouwels M-JM, Hooymans PM, Van der Aa GC, Gribnau FW: Comparison of steady-state serum concentrations of digoxin in tablets (Lanoxin) and capsules (Lanoxicaps) in the elderly. *DICP Ann Pharmacother* 1991; 25:1043–1046.
60. Marsh AJ, Lloyd BL, Taylor RR: Age dependence of myocardial Na^+-K^+-ATPase activity and digitalis intoxication in the dog and guinea pig. *Circ Res* 1981; 48:329–333.
61. Katano Y, Kennedy RH, Stemmer PM, Temma K, Akera T: Aging and digitalis sensitivity of cardiac muscle in rats. *Eur J Pharmacol* 1985; 113:167–178.
62. Ware JA, Snow E, Luchi JM, Luchi RJ: Effect of digoxin on ejection fraction in elderly patients with congestive heart failure. *J Am Geriatr Soc* 1984; 32:631–635.
63. Mahdyoon H, Battilana G, Rosman H, Goldstein S, Gheorghiade M: The evolving pattern of digoxin intoxication: Observations at a large urban hospital from 1980 to 1988. *Am Heart J* 1990; 120:1189–1194.
64. Lopez LM: Hypertension in the elderly: Conventional wisdom revisited. *Pharmacotherapy* 1991; 11:225–236.
65. Hockings N, Ajayi AA, Reid JL: Age and the pharmacokinetics of angiotensin converting enzyme inhibitors enalapril and enalaprilat. *Br J Clin Pharmacol* 1986; 21:341–348.
66. Kelly JG, O'Malley K: Clinical pharmacokinetics of the newer ACE inhibitors. *Clin Pharmacokinet* 1990; 19:177–196.
67. The CONSENSUS Trial Study Group: Effects of enalapril on mortality in severe congestive heart failure. Results of the Cooperative North Scandinavian Enalapril Survival Study (CONSENSUS). *N Engl J Med* 1987; 316:1429–1435.
68. The SOLVD Investigators: Effect of enalapril on survival in patients with reduced left ventricular ejection fractions and congestive heart failure. *N Engl J Med* 1991; 325:293–302.
69. Cohn JN, Johnson G, Ziesche S, Cob F, Francis G, Tristani F, et al: A comparison of enalapril with hydralazine-isosorbide dinitrate in the treatment of chronic congestive heart failure. *N Engl J Med* 1991; 325:303–310.
70. Giles TD, Fisher MB, Rush JE: Lisinopril and captopril in the treatment of heart failure in older patients. *Am J Med* 1988; 85(suppl 3B):44–47.
71. O'Neill CJA, Bowes SG, Sullens CM, Royston JP, Hunt WB, Denham MJ, et al: Evaluation of the safety of enalapril in the treatment of heart failure in the very old. *Eur J Clin Pharmacol* 1988; 35:143–150.
72. Alpert JS: Nitrate therapy in the elderly. *Am J Cardiol* 1990; 65:23J–27J.
73. Ludden TM, McNay JL, Shepherd AMM, Lin MS: Clinical pharmacokinetics of hydralazine. *Clin Pharmacokinet* 1982; 7:185–205.
74. Abernethy DR, Schwartz JB: Pharmacokinetics of calcium antagonists under development. *Clin Pharmacokinet* 1988; 15:1–14.
75. SHEP Cooperative Research Group: Prevention of stroke by antihypertensive drug treatment in older persons with isolated systole hypertension. *JAMA* 1991; 265:3255–3264.
76. Lalonde RL, Tenero DM, Burlew BS, Herring VL, Bottorff MB: Effects of age on the protein binding and disposition of propranolol stereoisomers. *Clin Pharmacol Ther* 1990; 47:447–455.

PART XVI

Emotions and the Cardiovascular System

Chapter 117

The Heart, Emotional Stress, and Psychiatric Disorders

Robert S. Eliot, M.D. ■ *Hugo M. Morales-Ballejo, M.D.*

Numerous instances of persons' dying suddenly after an emotional upset have been recorded. There is now evidence documenting many of the profound interrelationships of the brain and stress on human and animal physiology and confirming the link between emotions and some illnesses or death.

Stress remains to be well defined. In the context of this discussion, *stress* is considered to be the body's response to real or imagined events perceived as requiring some adaptive response and/or producing strain. This allows us then to differentiate between *stress*—the internally mediated adaptive response—and *stressors*—the stimuli.

Obviously stresses cover a range—from mild annoyances to death threats, from momentary scares to never-ending tension—with a corresponding spectrum of responses.

PHYSIOLOGY

The central nervous system controls cardiovascular functions through the baroreceptors and numerous afferent and efferent neuroendocrine connections of the autonomic nervous system. In reviews of animal experiments and clinical studies,[1-3] it was concluded that stress effects are mediated largely by increases in cortisol and catecholamines. The effects are further modulated by various neuropeptides, vagal stimulation, circadian influences, adaptive mechanisms, genetic susceptibilities, and the presence of defects or disease.

In the conscious pig stressful stimuli can increase its vulnerability to ventricular fibrillation.[4] This effect is blocked by adaptation, by intracerebral injection of a beta blocker, or by blockade of frontocortical projections to the brainstem cardiovascular nuclei. It is postulated that the pathway goes from the frontal lobes to the frontocortical brainstem, which stimulates autonomic outflow (norepinephrine), increases cyclic adenosine monophosphate (cAMP), and decreases extracellular potassium ions.

Stress responses are often divided into several patterns: those involving active coping ("fight or flight"), those associated with an aversive situation or long-term monitoring (vigilance), and those characterized by subordination, in which active coping is attempted but not successful. In the fight-or-flight reaction, the release of catecholamines raises the blood pressure and heart rate, with increased cardiac output and decreased total peripheral resistance. The vigilance response, which seems to be mediated by the pituitary-adrenocortical system, results in elevated blood presssure with increased total peripheral resistance but decreases in both heart rate and cardiac output.

In studies of psychosocial effects on mice, plasma cortisol levels were highest in submissive animals, lower in subordinate animals, and lowest in dominant animals.[5] Catecholamine levels showed the opposite pattern, being highest in dominant animals. Similar patterns have been observed in other animal groups and in human beings as well. Three categories of human reactions have been described: effort without distress, effort with distress, and distress without effort.[6] In experiments with healthy subjects performing a choice-reaction task with a high degree of control or a vigilance task with no control, subjects reported they were pleasantly challenged by the high-control task and felt some distress from the low-control task. Epinephrine increased in both, but cortisol decreased in the former and increased in the latter.

The stress of public speaking can increase platelet activation as well as serum levels of the catecholamines epinephrine and norepinephrine.[7] Propranolol treatment moderates the heart rate and systolic blood pressure during the stress period but does not block the catecholamine or platelet responses.

It has been postulated that acute (coping) response to stress is designed to provide the necessary energy for fight or flight and to protect against loss of blood and metabolites.[8] The subordinate and submissive types of responses also are appropriate animal behavior, generally minimizing injury while promoting survival of species. In the normal course of events these responses are called into play for short periods and are not harmful. On the other hand, it is important to consider whether or not these reactions lead to harmful disease processes, and if so, how?

PATHOPHYSIOLOGY

Hypertension (See also Chap. 75)

A review of animal and human studies concluded that stress alone can elevate blood pressure but that it has not been proved to lead to sustained hypertension.[9] In the presence of other potentiators such as genetic susceptibility or salt loading, however, stress might act as a trigger. Supporting the latter finding were studies with salt-sensitive rats, spontaneously hypertensive rats, children of hypertensive parents, and rats with one kidney. Structural adaptations to the increased pressure might then reinforce or stabilize the pressure condition.[10]

Atherosclerosis

One theory of the pathogenesis of atherosclerosis[11] involves several phases: (1) injury to the vascular intima; (2) adherence of platelets to the injured area, with release of growth factor and other substances that stimulate platelet adhesion, smooth-muscle growth, and attraction of macrophages; (3) ingestion of lipids by macrophages and thickening of vascular tissue by smooth-muscle proliferation and macrophage invasion; and (4) plaque enlargement by the secretion of fibrin and continuation of the previous process. (See Chap. 54.) The physiological and metabolic stress effects can aggravate the process at any phase: Raised blood pressure may increase the possibility of intimal damage; and lipid mobilization and increased platelet adherence may accelerate the growth of the atherosclerotic plaque.

Increased neurohormonal activity (adrenocortical, sympathetic, renin angiotensin systems) due to stress contributes to endothelial cell dysfunction. An abnormal endothelium may become an ineffective barrier unable to retard platelets and monocytes from adhering to the blood vessel wall. In this circumstance, excessive release of growth-promoting factors and increased infiltration of lipids into the vessel wall may lead to rapid progression of the atherosclerotic lesion.[12] (See Chap. 2.)

In studies of the extent of atherosclerosis in stressed and unstressed male macaque monkeys, stress was induced by frequent disruptions of social groupings.[13] In unstressed animals little disease was seen in monkeys on low-fat diets. On an atherogenic diet, dominant animals showed minimal lesions, and subordinate animals had moderate amounts of disease. Conversely, among the stressed monkeys, lesions were more prominent in the dominant than in the subordinate animals regardless of the diet; however, the extent of atherosclerosis was magnified 30-fold on the high-fat diet. In studies of female macaques,[14] dominant females seemed to be protected from atherosclerosis; subordinate females and ovariectomized females were as affected as the males in the same groups, and unstable groupings did not increase the involvement. Apparently disruption of social groupings that was very stressful to competitive males was not as stressful to the females because they do not fight as aggressively for status as the males do.

In human studies, serum cholesterol levels have been observed to rise during periods of stress such as medical students' examination period, soldiers' training with demolition weaponry, and anticipation of surgery.[15] Lipid levels are even more labile. In the course of a stress interview blood lipids may rise as much as 159 percent.[15]

Increased activity of the sympathetic nervous system influences lipid metabolism. Activation of alpha$_1$ receptors and possibly angiotensin may inhibit lipoprotein lipase activity, leading to elevated very low density lipoprotein (VLDL) triglyceride and decreased high-density lipoprotein (HDL) cholesterol levels. Sympathetic activation may also increase cholesterol by impairing LDL clearance. [12] In one study cholesterol levels correlated positively with measures of depression, hostility, and emotional instability; they correlated negatively with motivation and happiness.[16]

Ischemia

Many mechanisms, either alone or in combination, can lower the oxygen supply to the heart or increase its demands, resulting in myocardial ischemia. (See Chap. 5.) Atherosclerotic lesions, thrombi, and vasospasm (all of which may be related to stress reactions) can decrease the blood supply to an area of the heart. Increased heart rate and increased total systemic resistance, possibly stress related, add to the oxygen demand. (See Chap. 57.)

Ambulatory monitoring of persons with known coronary artery disease has shown that asymptomatic ("silent") ischemia occurs quite often, particularly in association with a stressful activity such as public speaking. (See also Chaps. 45 and 58.) Patients awaiting the results of coronary angiography had more episodes of silent ischemia than they experienced during a later, less anxious period. Those with higher levels of urinary cortisol and urinary norepinephrine had a greater number of episodes of ischemia.[17] Even normal persons may respond to stressors with increases in heart rate and changes in electrical irritability of the heart.[18]

Activation of the sympathetic nervous system as measured by increases in catecholamine levels correlates with the circadian pattern of blood pressure elevation and the increased incidence of silent myocardial ischemia and cardiovascular events during the early to midmorning hours. (See Chaps. 58 to 60.)

Sudden Death

Ventricular fibrillation, the principal mechanism of sudden death, may be triggered by injury to the brain, by ischemia from coronary vasospasm or thrombi, or by exacerbation of a preexisting conduction defect.

In experiments with dogs, it was noted that the vulnerability to ventricular fibrillation increased when the animals were put into cages where they had previously received shocks as compared with their vulnerability in a cage where they were always left undisturbed.[19] The dogs' vulnerability also increased when they were angry (the anger being induced by moving a dish of food from the subject to a second dog).

Sympathetic activation is also implicated by the finding that dogs given infusions of catecholamines such as norepinephrine or isoproterenol may have "contraction band" myocardial lesions that are similar to the lesions of skeletal muscle ruptured by overcontraction. Such lesions were noted in 86 percent of sudden cardiac death victims[20] including those with no evidence of atherosclerosis. In addition, they have been observed in crime victims who died despite the absence of physical assault,[21] in test pilots who lost control of their aircraft, in patients with pheochromocytoma,[22] and in cocaine-induced sudden death[23]; that is, in situations where there may be large endogenous releases of catecholamines. The mechanism may be a change in cell permeability that permits calcium overloading of the myocardial cells. In studies with dogs, pretreatment with beta blockers[24] or calcium channel blockers[25] decreased the damage produced by infusion of norepinephrine or isoproterenol.

THE ROLE OF ENVIRONMENT

Although physicians recognize the impact of behavior on disease, we tend to overlook the importance of the environment in which that behavior takes place. The interaction between the individual and the environment is important, as stress is largely a product of the environmental context.

Social status, interactions with other people, and changes in such social elements impact on health. When people change jobs, move their place of residence, or make other major life alterations, the risk of heart disease may increase two to three times, independent of such factors as age, sex, race, cigarette smoking, cholesterol, blood pressure history, physical activity, and obesity.

One study found that hypertension was less prevalent among blacks living in areas of Detroit with low ecologic stress than among their counterparts living in high-stress areas.[26]

There are also data suggesting that in black children there seems to be an interaction between stress and sodium sensitivity, such that the combination of being black, being on a high-salt diet, and being exposed to stress produces higher than expected increases in blood pressure.[27]

A study of Japanese migrants to the Bay area of California found a marked increase in coronary artery disease (CAD)—up to fivefold—compared with Japanese who remained in Japan.[28] Among the Japanese migrants in California, however, there was a group who had almost the same low incidence of coronary disease as those who remained in Japan. The major CAD risk factors did not appear to account for the difference. This suggested that mobility per se was not a major risk factor for the migrants. The main difference between the groups appeared to be the degree of social support.[29] The group with the higher rate had become acculturated and had adopted "Western ways." Those with low incidence of heart disease had closer ties with other members of the Japanese ethnic group and more closely maintained the language, diet, and customs.

A study in a more general population verified the importance of social support networks.[30] Connections were evaluated on the basis of criteria such as marital status, membership in clubs, and church or synagogue attendance. Follow-up over the next 9 years revealed that those with fewer connections at the beginning of the study had a mortality rate two to three times higher than those with the greatest number of associations, even when taking into account such factors as age, race, cigarette smoking, serum cholesterol, blood pressure, family history, physical activity, obesity, socioeconomic status, and self-reported health status. Curiously, the data were for all forms of death, not just heart disease.

The protective effects of social support help to explain two questions raised by morbidity data: (1) why certain risk factors are related not just to one disease but to a variety of diseases, (2) why the recognized risk factors such as cigarette smoking, high blood pressure, and elevated serum cholesterol often relate imperfectly to disease incidence and outcome. It may be that some people are partially protected from the adverse effects of these factors by the positive effects of social support.

In Syme's view, life changes are important primarily when they disrupt relationships, as they do with job changes, residential moves, divorce, or the loss of loved ones.[28] Even the difference between male and female risks in CAD may be partially related to social support, as men seem to have fewer intimate ties.

The effect of social contact can also be seen in animal studies. Rabbits that were fondled and petted while on a high-cholesterol diet had a markedly lower rate of atherogenesis than a matched group that was not fondled.[31] In nonhuman primates, it was noted that affiliative behaviors such as grooming lower the heart rate and may have a protective effect, since increased heart rates have been correlated with increased atherosclerosis.[14]

Social Class

Socioeconomic factors can also influence health. The lower the socieconomic status, the higher the rates of many diseases. The reasons for this difference are not clearly understood. Hypotheses include poor nutrition, poor medical care, and heavy infectious burden, but these variables do not entirely account for the differences.

In one study[30] a poor area was compared with a more affluent area. The incidence of hypertension was 50 percent higher in the poor area regardless of considerations of social interaction, medical care, smoking, and other accepted risk factors. Among a group of more affluent people living in the area, however, the pattern of hypertension reflected that of the poor area as a whole rather than that of the similar income group in the affluent area. Interviews with the individuals revealed fears of robbery and violence, and there was evidence that the distribution of hypertension correlated with the number of police and fire department calls, suggesting that the increased mortality among lower socioeconomic classes might be related to greater environmental stress levels.

Work

In the work environment, architectural layout, danger, and excessive noise (unwanted sound) can all impact on stress and health. Other stressors such as time pressures like those of assembly-line workers, responsibility for others' safety as with air-traffic controllers, nonsupportive superiors, and work overload have been reported to be associated with increased incidences of hypertension, myocardial infarction, or other illnesses.[32]

Much occupational stress seems to derive from feelings of lack of control. Among San Francisco bus drivers, hypertension was noted to be more prevalent among drivers than applicants and the local population.[28] An analysis of 2000 drivers and the conditions under which they worked indicated that the bus schedules were unrealistic and rigid and that the drivers were harassed and penalized for not maintaining them.

It has been suggested that it is not only job demand but also latitude of control in the job that strongly influence maintenance of health and well-being.[6] In laboratory tests of normal individuals given a timed task, persons reported less distress when allowed to select their own pace than when they had no control, and physiologically they demonstrated lower cortisol levels when in control. In the Framingham Study, a higher incidence of coronary heart disease was noted among women having high job demands but poor supervision.[33]

The control hypothesis is the underlying explanation for how one reacts to stress. Certainly not all stress is bad, and in fact, some types—those events that are perceived as new, interesting, and challenging, for example—are often beneficial. At the other end of the spectrum is deleterious stress associated with fear, uncertainty, and doubt that may lead to loss of control over the situation and its outcome. Lost control or lack of it can lead to a period of perceived struggle with increased neurohormonal activity (cortisol, catecholamines, angiotensin) (Fig. 117-1). The so-called hot reactor responds to these situations with marked swings in blood pressure during the day, especially during working hours (circadian pattern).[34]

Awareness of the patient's environment—cultural background, socioeconomic condition, work status, family situation—can provide the insight for effective counseling, intervention, and prevention. By identifying detrimental factors in the environment, the physician can help the patient to find areas where change is possible or to cope with unchangeable aspects. This might prevent continuing stress and adverse health consequences.

HISTORY

It has been said that "50% of visits to doctors are for complaints without an ascertainable biological base."[35] It is important for the physician to know what the patient perceives as the reason for the visit even if it is a repeat visit by an individual under treatment.

PSYCHOLOGIC EFFECTS

Several syndromes combine anxiety and cardiovascular symptoms, including functional cardiac disorders, mitral valve prolapse, and panic disorder. The presence of any of these obviously does not rule out CAD, since this can be present in addition to one of the other syndromes. There is also overlap among the anxiety disorders, and their relationship is unclear. (See Chap. 118.)

Patients with atypical chest pain and normal resting electrocardiograms often have some type of esophageal disease, but they may have coronary disease or even both. Panic disorder is also common in such cases. In one study[36] 43 to 61 percent of patients with chest pain and negative coronary arteriography findings had panic disorder, compared to only 5 to 23 percent of patients with pain and positive arteriography findings. (See Chap. 118.)

In the authors' experience, patients with high pain thresholds or denial are more apt to have or develop hypertensive and ischemic heart disease than those with high levels of anxiety.

Therapy is important for patients with chest pain even when CAD has been ruled out, since the pain can be disabling. In one study,[37] at 17-month follow-up, a large percentage of patients still believed their problem was heart disease and more than half were unable to work because of the pain.

PANIC DISORDER, SOLDIER'S HEART, ANXIETY NEUROSIS, MITRAL VALVE PROLAPSE, AND OTHER CONDITIONS

Panic Disorder (See Chap. 118)

One study estimated that 15 percent of a cardiologist's patients have panic disorder, which can be of two types: that relating to external danger (exogenous) and that seeming to occur spontaneously (endogenous).[38] There was less of a preponderance of females in the exogenous type, and it did not seem to be genetically determined as did the endogenous type. The endogenous type was noted to respond better to pharmacologic treatment (monoamine oxidase inhibitors and tricyclic antidepressants), and the exogenous type was noted to be amenable to behavioral therapy.

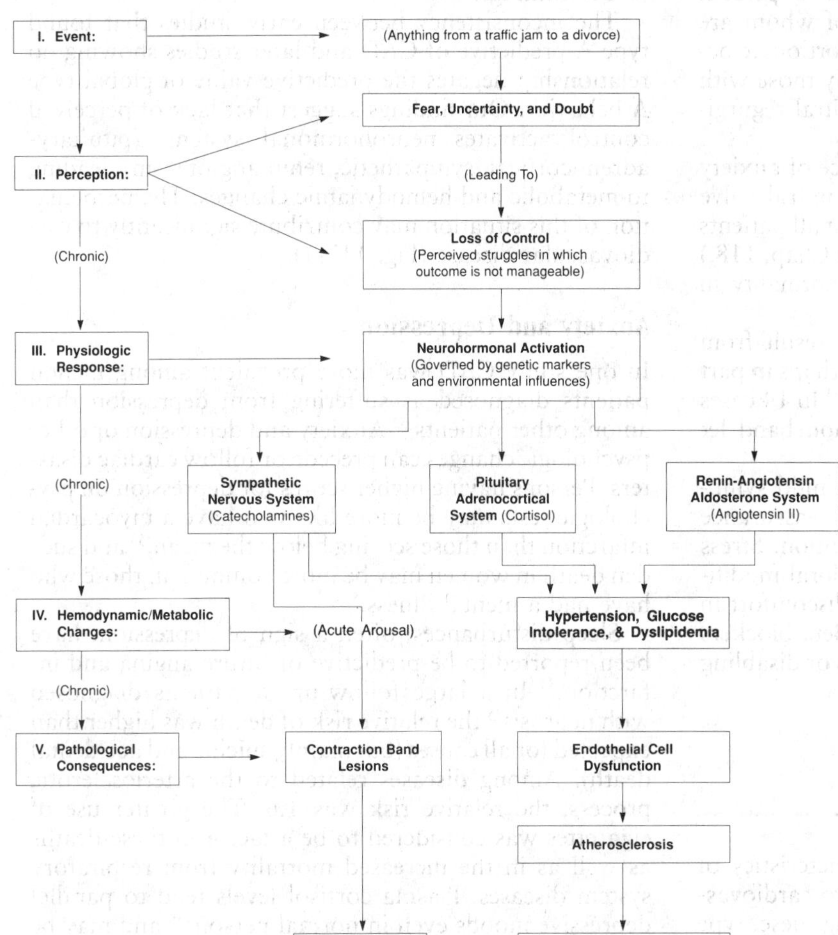

FIGURE 117-1 Conceptual diagram of how a perceived loss of control over outcome may provoke acute and chronic neurohormonal responses. When loss of control becomes chronic, pathophysiological consequences may ensue as diagrammed.

Our studies revealed that alprazolam not only has a strong anxiolytic effect but also it decreases adrenergic drive similarly to beta blockade.[39] Its short duration of action combined with these effects makes alprazolam an effective agent for controlling anxiety and panic in patients with cardiovascular disease.

Soldier's Heart

Perhaps the most dramatic associations of stress with the heart are those seen in soldiers during war, although, rather surprisingly, these are rarely associated with typical CAD. Wooley[40] has traced the history of this nervous condition through its various aliases from DaCosta's description of the "irritable heart" among soldiers in the Civil War to neurocirculatory asthenia, soldier's heart, anxiety neurosis, mitral valve prolapse (MVP) syndrome, and autonomic dysfunction states. Whether or not these are really all one and the same is not clear; there are undoubtedly many overlaps in the diagnoses. Nevertheless, all can be associated with periods of cardiac-type symptoms, usually without evidence of recognizable disease. In some cases the symptoms are related to emotional stress or exercise effort, and many patients also suffer from anxiety. (See Chaps. 80 and 118.)

Anxiety Neurosis

Patients with anxiety neurosis have complaints of a moderate to severe degree of dyspnea, palpitations, chest pain, nervousness, anxiety, or fatigue. Among the most commonly reported aggravating factors are emotion-provoking situations, illness, hard physical labor, pregnancy, and military service. Dyspnea is one of the more common and characteristic symptoms, and cases with marked respiratory complaints have been termed "respiratory neurosis."[41] Generally the patient feels respiratory distress both at rest and with exertion, but the degree of effort necessary to produce dyspnea varies extraordinarily according to emotional state. Sighing respirations are characteristic and are a helpful diagnostic sign. Most of these patients have precordial, nonanginal pain that is characterized either as fleeting sticks and stabs and/or as dull and aching left thoracic pain of prolonged duration.

Mitral Valve Prolapse (See Chap. 80)

In one study of symptomatic patients evaluated for mitral valve prolapse syndrome, both symptoms and outcome were similar in those with and without echocardiographic evidence of prolapse.[42] There may be two separate conditions sharing a similar pathway of expression.

Mitral valve prolapse is found in about 5 percent of the general population, the majority of whom are asymptomatic. One report found a disproportionate occurrence of complications in men, especially those with a previously identified heart murmur of mitral regurgitation.[43]

Although there may be a higher incidence of anxiety and panic disorders among patients with mitral valve prolapse, this is not well established and not all patients with panic disorder have the condition. (See Chap. 118.) The common denominator may be an abnormality in adrenergic control mechanisms.

Sudden death, which is very rare, may result from repolarization changes and arrhythmias, perhaps in part the result of traction on a papillary muscle.[44] In 14 cases coming to autopsy examination, contraction band lesions were not found in any.[45]

In asymptomatic patients or those with mild symptoms, no treatment is indicated other than reassurance of the generally benign nature of the condition. Stress management, relaxation techniques, behavioral modification, and other measures can minimize discomfort in those whose symptoms are stress related. Beta blockers may be indicated for some with palpitations or disabling chest pain. (See Chap. 118.)

CORONARY-PRONE BEHAVIOR

Attempts have been made to relate characteristics of behavior and personality to susceptibility to cardiovascular illnesses, with varying success. Among these, type A behavior is most often cited.[46] Individuals of type A are characterized by a sense of time urgency, explosive speech patterns, hostility, and competitiveness among other features. In the Western Collaborative Group Study (WCGS)[47] and other studies of middle-class American men, individuals with extreme type A patterns demonstrated two to four times the risk of developing CAD as individuals of type B (those lacking the type A characteristics). Later studies of different populations, however, failed to show significant differences in risk of death.

Subsequent attention addressed individual aspects of the type A concept and focused on anger and hostility. It was postulated that type A persons feel a greater need to be in control and become upset when, as often happens, things do not go according to plan and are beyond their control. In several large studies, measures of hostility, anger-in, and anger-out have correlated with CAD incidence, at least among younger men.[48] Unexpressed anger was also noted in high-renin hypertensive patients.[49] The Western Electric Study found a correlation between hostility scores from the Minnesota Multiphasic Personality Index (MMPI) and coronary atherosclerosis.[50] Even individuals of type B with high hostility were more likely to have significant occlusion than low-hostility type A individuals. Hostility indexes were positively associated with the 20-year risk of death from CAD and all causes combined. Suppressed anger, particularly with regard to one's spouse, correlated with mortality in the 12-year Tecumseh follow-up.[51] The effect was strongest in combination with elevated systolic blood pressure (>140 mmHg).

The inconsistency between early studies that found type A predictive of CAD and later studies showing no relationship negates the predictive value of global type A behavior. Our findings suggest that lack of perceived control activates neurohormonal systems (pituitary-adrenocortical, sympathetic, renin angiotensin), leading to metabolic and hemodynamic changes. The perpetuation of this situation may contribute significantly to cardiovascular disease (Fig. 117-1).

Anxiety and Depression

In one study CAD was more prevalent among mental patients diagnosed as suffering from depression than among other patients.[52] Anxiety and depression or other psychologic changes can precede or follow cardiac disasters. Persons having higher scores for depression on psychologic tests may be more likely to have a myocardial infarction than those scoring below the mean,[53] and sudden death in women may be more common in those who have had a mental illness.[54]

Sleep disturbances, often a sign of depression, have been reported to be predictive of future angina and infarction.[53] In a large follow-up of patients diagnosed with neurosis[55] the relative risk of death was higher than expected for all causes (but mainly suicide and accidental death). Among diseases related to the arteriosclerotic process, the relative risk was 1.6. The greater use of cigarettes was considered to be a factor in these deaths as well as in the increased mortality from respiratory system diseases. Plasma cortisol levels tend to parallel depressive moods even in normal persons[56] and may be significantly elevated in persons diagnosed as depressed.

PHYSIOLOGICAL OVERREACTIVITY (HOT REACTING)

The physiological reactions that mediate the effects of personality and behavior on disease have been studied. Laboratory-induced mental stress reactivity, however, does not necessarily follow type A-B patterns: Exaggerated cardiovascular response ("hot reacting") is often observed in individuals of type B and can be absent in type A patients. Our study found the correlation between overreactivity and type A behavior to be only about 0.1 to 0.3.[57]

Reactivity patterns reportedly differ between adolescents with and without family history of hypertension. Those with a positive family history demonstrated greater elevations of both heart rate and diastolic blood pressure readings after such stressors as mental arithmetic, Stroop color test, and shock avoidance.[58]

Hypertensive patients and, perhaps, those destined to develop hypertension have a greater than expected increase in blood pressure when challenged with a simple video game or math problem.[59] The clinical value of blood pressure reactivity testing is its correlation with the working time blood pressure, which has been found to be better than casual blood pressure measurements in

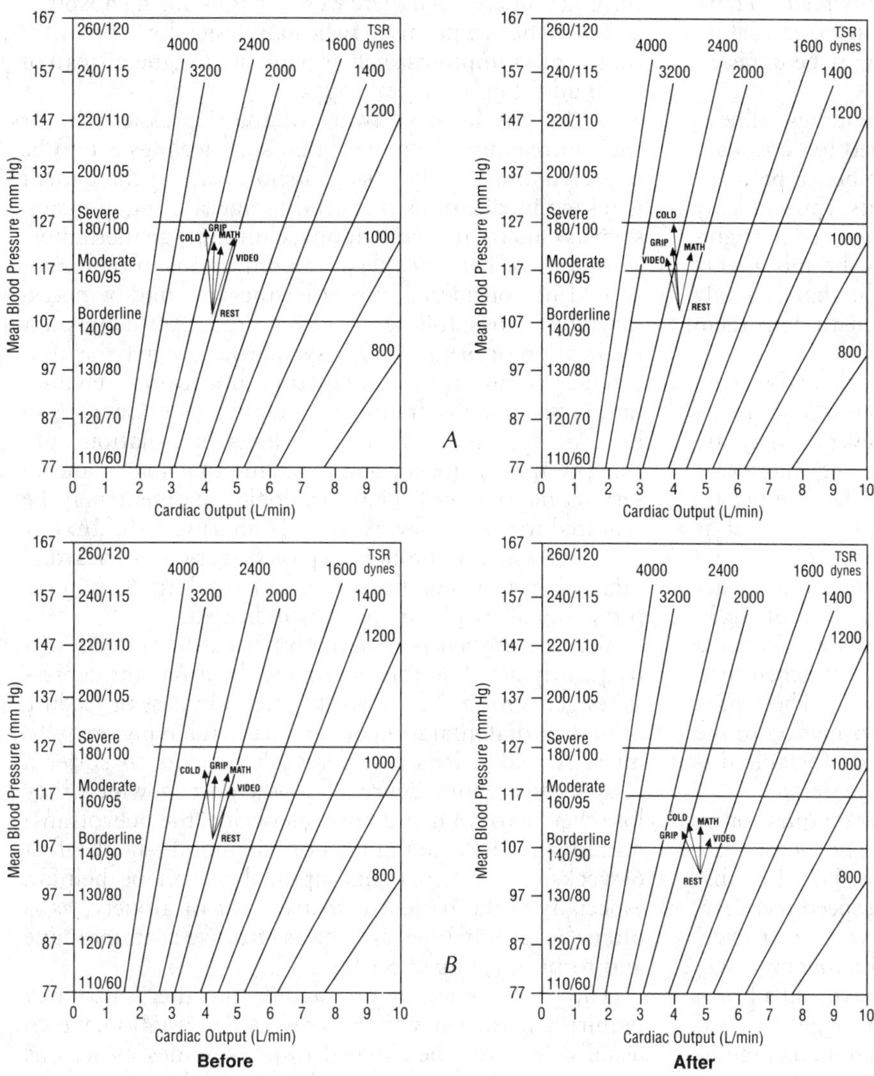

FIGURE 117-2 Cardiovascular reactivity graphs displaying levels of mean blood pressure in millimiters of mercury (vertical axis), cardiac output in liters per minute (horizontal axis), and total systemic resistance (TSR) in dynes·s·cm^{-5} (radiated lines). Blood pressure was obtained using oscillometric apparatus. Cardiac output was measured by ensemble averages of signals obtained from an impedance cardiograph. Measurements were taken during a standardized protocol at baseline (rest) and during different challenges. The arrows indicate the changes from baseline during hand grip (grip), cold pressor (cold), computerized video game (video), and mental arithmetic (math) tests. The average hemodynamics were obtained during a double-blind placebo-controlled study of 20 labile and mild hypertensives.[65] *A.* Ten patients before and 2 h after oral ingestion of placebo. No significant changes were noted. *B.* Ten patients before and 2 h after oral ingestion of diltiazem, 120 mg. Significant decrease in blood pressure was obtained due to reduction in total systemic resistance.

predicting future target organ damage or complications of hypertension.[60–62] Increased activity of the sympathetic nervous system may be an important component of the circadian pattern of blood pressure elevation and the increased incidence of cardiovascular events in the morning hours between 7 A.M. and noon, after awakening, and assuming the upright position.

Using our standardized alpha- and beta-adrenergic low-challenge stress test with impedance cardiography monitoring, we can determine not only the elevated levels of blood pressure during stress but also the hemodynamics involved.[63,64] Using this technique during pharmacologic intervention, we can determine whether the blood pressure changes are mediated by cardiac output, total systemic resistance, or both.[65] The results before and after pharmacologic intervention can be graphically displayed in a way that clearly identifies the levels of reactivity and the hemodynamics (Fig. 117-2).

Coronary Care Unit Anxiety and Psychosis

Obviously the effects of stress can be most detrimental when the heart is already injured. Reducing anxiety and stress in patients facing open heart surgery and those suffering infarction is crucial.

In the hospital, nurses play a major role in determining the mental state of their patients and thus the rate of their recovery. The mechanistic aspects of the intensive care unit or coronary care unit (CCU) and the impersonal concern with technical equipment and numbers tend to make the patient feel dehumanized, helpless, and hopeless. The touch of a hand or a few words of reassurance addressed directly to him or her is calming and restores hope. Patients may be anxious and somewhat confused and disoriented. Anxiolytic agents are required by many patients, especially those who show heightened reactions to stresses such as physicians on rounds and alarm bells.[66] We agree with those physicians who favor giving every myocardial infarction patient a short-acting tranquilizer to prevent or relieve anxiety. A good choice is alprazolam, a benzodiazepine that may decrease epinephrine and norepinephrine[39,67] and does not exacerbate an underlying depression as some other tranquilizers may. (See also Chap. 60)

Some patients use denial to cope with their fear. Those who reject the reality of their illness may balk at the necessity of treatment. Those who accept the reality of the illness but deny its seriousness actually seem to have a better prognosis,[68] at least in the acute phase. Thus, total elimination of denial at this stage may be unnecessary and unwise.

The combination of strange surroundings, illness, medications, and disturbed sleep can lead to "coronary care unit psychosis" in a significant number of patients. This is especially likely for elderly patients who suddenly find themselves out of control and immobilized in frightening surroundings. Such patients may be mistakenly treated as psychotic or senile, when all that is really needed is some familiar place or person to help them touch base and become reoriented.

Patients are less likely to become disoriented if there are windows and clocks to indicate time of day and if they are talked *to* rather than *about* even if they are unable to reply. In some instances, we strongly advocate a role for the family physician in the CCU. The person who has just had a myocardial infarction may feel as though he or she has been cut off from everything. It can be reassuring to see a physician who knows him or her well. Some of today's cardiologists tend to be more technically oriented and may seem to be more concerned with the machines to which the patient is attached than with the human being they are monitoring. The family physician may be more able to relay information to the family members, who may feel more comfortable discussing their concerns with a familiar physician.

For the heart attack patient, an important question to be discussed in the CCU is, Why now? The factors that led to or were associated with the event should be discussed in order to tailor management to speed recovery, return the patient to gainful life, and prevent recurrence. This is also the "golden moment" for initiating improvements in life-style. Those who feel they have had a brush with death are particularly amenable to suggestions for behavioral change such as smoking cessation, diet modification, and relaxation therapy. (See Chap. 62.)

Convalescent Depression

At some period during recovery, depression frequently sets in. This may occur as early as 3 to 5 days after the myocardial infarction or surgery or appear later after the patient has left the hospital. It has been likened to the mourning for a loss: in this case a sense of lost potential or lost physical ability.[68] Generally the depression is transient, and talking about the individual's concerns may be the best treatment. A patient's stress level can be markedly reduced through reassurance as to the normalcy and transience of such conditions as physical weakness and memory lapses and by an open discussion of financial and domestic problems that are worrisome. Authoritative information can dispel concerns caused by harmful "myths" about cardiac conditions and aid in adaptive coping by both patients and family. It has been pointed out that appropriate information contributes to adaptive coping by correcting unrealistic appraisals of threat, by reducing uncertainty and thus increasing the sense of control, and by suggesting new (more appropriate) coping strategies.[69]

At times, the patient may become depressed after returning home, even if there were no signs during hospitalization. The symptoms may be manifested by "somatization" with symptoms such as pain and fatigue instead of or in addition to mental signs.

If the physician is aware of the depression, he or she can reassure the patient that such feelings are to be expected and usually pass in a short time. If the patient is taking medications that tend to aggravate depression such as cimetidine, methyldopa, clonidine, guanethidine, reserpine, or beta blockers,[70] modifications in treatment should be considered. No other therapy may be necessary, but close follow-up is required. Antidepressant medication or professional psychiatric care may be indicated in some cases. Participation in a formal rehabilitation program is frequently helpful. (See Chap. 63.) Loss of appetite, insomnia, feelings of isolation, and general apathy are among the signs that may indicate serious depression.[68] Pharmacologic treatment may be required for only a few weeks. Ordinarily, if the anxiety and depression that follow bypass surgery or myocardial infarction have not been resolved by 3 to 6 months, professional psychiatric care is indicated.

Because of their potential adverse cardiac effects, it is frequently not desirable to employ the usual antidepressant agents for at least 6 weeks after a bypass procedure or myocardial infarction or for a patient having arrhythmias. Actually, it is rare for such patients to suffer a severe endogenous depression—the sort in which they lose their serotonin and norepinephrine, the neurotransmitters that help maintain normal mood—in the first 6 weeks. In such patients alprazolam can be helpful, especially if the patient displays a lot of anxiety, as is often the case. It appears to be as effective as imipramine and to produce its effect faster.[71]

The patient's family or "significant other" also may require help to deal with the stress of the situation, which usually involves heightened responsibilities as well as care of an agitated patient. The crisis situation of the heart attack or the cardiac surgery and the resulting role changes and stresses can unleash emotional problems up to 2 years later and may have an adverse effect on relationships.[72]

Although physicians and surgeons find sexual matters difficult to discuss with their patients, this area is a major concern for most cardiac patients. Physicians should try to overcome their reticence and offer information in an objective, nonthreatening fashion that will allay fears and anxiety. Resumption of sexual activity may be very important in the marital relationship during the stressful readjustment period. Most patients are capable of the physical exertion required (5 METS at orgasm),[73] which is about the equivalent of climbing a flight of stairs briskly. On the other hand, angina during intercourse is a possibility and can be devastating to a patient. Therefore, it may be advisable for some patients to use nitroglycerin prior to sexual activity, particularly before the first attempt after hospitalization.

Although cardiac rehabilitation programs are usually thought of as primarily exercise programs, they also offer psychologic benefits that tend to help resolve transient depression. As with many special medical conditions, other patients who have been through the experience can provide meaningful psychosocial support. There is empathy among the members, and they encourage each other. Patients who have participated in a comprehensive rehabilitation program are more likely to return to work and to report a more satisfactory quality of life.[74] (See Chap. 63.) Patients who are deemed ineligible for an exercise program may be the ones needing more psychologic counseling.

PHARMACOLOGY

Among the most important considerations in choosing a pharmacologic agent are the interaction of the drug with other treatment modalities, its effect on the patient's other disease conditions, and its overall effect on the patient's quality of life. Beta blockers and other agents prescribed because of their cardiovascular effects also can alter mood and mental acuity. (See Chap. 66.) Agents prescribed to combat depression or other mental conditions can affect the heart and/or interact with cardiovascular agents to alter their effectiveness or to induce side effects. The physician should be very familiar with the state of the person's cardiovascular system as well as the person's psychologic makeup.

Anxiety

For treating anxiety without depression, all the minor tranquilizers (benzodiazepines) are about equally effective. The choice depends on the half-life desired. Those with short half-lives are preferred for the elderly, who are very susceptible to toxic buildup leading to oversedation. On the other hand, if treatment with a short half-life is stopped too suddenly, the patient may experience seizures.[75] This can be avoided with proper tapering. If the patient cannot be trusted to take the medication as ordered, it is best to use one with a long half-life as it has a built-in tapering effect. Titrating from very low dose levels is the rule of thumb for pharmacologic management of the elderly. The minor tranquilizers do not affect blood pressure, cause cardiovascular problems, or interact with the medications commonly prescribed for hypertension or diabetes.

In the hospital, the short-acting tranquilizers are preferred in most cases; but for home use, the patient's compliance behavior determines which drug is preferable. Alprazolam has some antidepressant side effects when compared to the other minor tranquilizers.[71] It has a short half-life that also makes it suitable for outpatient management. It is safe for use in the presence of serious cardiovascular problems, including arrhythmias, postbypass state, infarction, angina, and silent ischemia.[67]

Depression

For a significantly depressed patient with severe cardiovascular disease, electroconvulsive shock treatments (ECT) may be the safest antidepressant,[76] but the risks associated with the anesthesia and shock must be considered.

Tricyclic antidepressants are often used for depression. In general, however, these agents should not be used within 6 weeks of an infarction or in the presence of congestive heart failure, decompensation, or rhythm and conduction disturbances. Slow titration and electrocardiographic monitoring are recommended. Certain tricyclics, such as amitriptyline and imipramine, can produce postural hypotension. The hypotensive effect can be minimized by using divided doses instead of the one-a-day form.

Some tricyclics may interact with other medications. For instance, when imipramine is used together with cimetidine, the cimetidine potentiates the imipramine and the dosage must be carefully monitored to avoid toxicity.

If a very depressed patient cannot use tricyclics because of cardiac problems and does not allow ECT, one can employ a monoamine oxidase (MAO) inhibitor. This is possible only if the patient is cooperative and willing to maintain the necessary restrictions. As their name implies, these agents interfere with the enzyme that degrades serotonin and norepinephrine. To prevent precipitating a hypertensive crisis, patients must avoid foods containing tyramine (cheese, wine, pickled herring, etc.) as well as all decongestants. In other respects these drugs are very safe.

The Elderly

The elderly have the most cardiovascular disease but also have the most sensitivity to medications. When the forward blood flow slows, the kidneys, which have already lost nephrons, are not as well perfused, and renal insufficiencies progress further. (See also Chap. 116.) Thus, the elderly are in danger of toxic buildup, and with tricyclics this can lead to arrhythmias, ventricular fibrillation, and sudden death.

Hypertensive Patients

Many antihypertensive agents can cause depression, particularly methyldopa and reserpine. With clonidine, guanethidine, and propranolol, the incidence is about 1 percent, provided doses are moderate. The patient who becomes depressed from taking an antihypertensive and who, for various reasons, cannot use the alternative antihypertensives, can be given an antidepressant, but the patient must be cooperative, educated in the problems and limitations, and carefully monitored.

If there is depression that precludes the use of tricyclics, it is possible to treat both the depression and the hypertension with MAO inhibitors, as long as the patient is careful to avoid the tyramine foods, particularly cheese, beer, and wine. (See also Chap. 77.)

Psychosis

Major tranquilizers, the neuroleptics, are not often employed, mainly because of the risk of tardive dyskinesia. They are also likely to cause disturbances in ventricular repolarization with large doses, and it is suspected that ventricular arrhythmias related to their use may be the cause of the occasional sudden death during long-term treatment.[77]

If the patient does develop a psychosis such as the intensive care unit psychosis, a low dosage of haloperidol may be prescribed. It is the least detrimental to the cardiovascular system but can cause extrapyramidal effects such as stiffness, nervousness, anxiety, and restlessness, which necessitate additional treatment. Fortunately the intensive care unit problems usually clear up in a few days.

Cooperation between the cardiologist and the psychiatrist is necessary when severe mental conditions develop in patients with cardiovascular disorders or vice versa.

REFERENCES

1. Schneiderman N: Behavior, autonomic function, and animal models of cardiovascular pathology. In: Dembroski TM, Schmidt TH, Blumchen G (eds): *Biobehavioral Bases of Coronary Heart Disease.* Basel, Karger, 1983: 304–364.
2. Herd JA: Cardiovascular disease and hypertension. In: Gentry WD (ed): *Handbook of Behavioral Medicine.* New York, The Guilford Press, 1984: 222–281.
3. Corr PB, Pitt B, Natelson BH, Reis DJ, Shine KI, Skinner JE: Task Force 3: Sudden cardiac death: Neural-chemical interactions. *Circulation* 1987; 76 (suppl 1): 208–214.
4. Skinner JE: Psychosocial stress and sudden cardiac death: Brain mechanisms. In: Beamish RE, Singal PK, Dhalla NS (eds): *Stress and Heart Disease.* Boston, Martinus Nijhoff Publishing, 1983: 44–59.
5. Henry JP: Coronary heart disease and arousal of the adrenal cortical axis. In: Dembroski TM, Schmidt TH, Blumchen G (eds): *Biobehavioral Bases of Coronary Heart Disease.* Basel, Karger, 1983: 365–381.
6. Frankenhaeuser M: The sympathetic-adrenal and pituitary-adrenal response to challenge: Comparison between the sexes. In: Dembroski TM, Schmidt TH, Blumchen G (eds): *Biobehavioral Bases of Coronary Heart Disease.* Basel, Karger, 1983: 91–105.
7. Levine SP, Towell BL, Suarez AM, Knierem LK, Harris MM, George JN: Platelet activation and secretion associated with emotional stress. *Circulation* 1985; 71:1129–1134.
8. Theorell T: Physiological issues in establishing links between psychosocial factors and cardiovascular illness. In: *Breakdown in Human Adaptation to "Stress."* Boston, Martinus Nijhoff Publishers, 1984: 241–250.
9. Brody MJ, Natelson BH, Anderson EA, Folkow B, Levy MN, Obrist PA, et al: Task Force 3: Behavioral mechanisms in hypertension. *Circulation* 1987; 76(suppl 1):95–100.
10. Folkow B: Psychosocial and central nervous influences in primary hypertension. *Circulation* 1987; 76(suppl 1):10–19.
11. Ross R, Faggiotto A, Bowen-Pope D, Raines E: The role of endothelial injury and platelet and macrophage interactions in atherosclerosis. *Circulation* 1984; 70(suppl 3):77–82.
12. Dzau VJ: Atherosclerosis and hypertension: Mechanisms and interrelationships. *J Cardiovasc Pharmacol* 1990; 15(suppl 5):S59–S64.
13. Clarkson TB, Weingand KW, Kaplan JR, Adams MR: Mechanisms of atherogenesis. *Circulation* 1987; 76(suppl 1): 20–28.
14. Clarkson TB, Kaplan JR, Adams MR, Manuck SB: Psychosocial influences on the pathogenesis of atherosclerosis among nonhuman primates. *Circulation* 1987; 76(suppl 1):29–40.
15. Dimsdale JE, Herd JA: Variability of plasma lipids in response to emotional arousal. *Psychosom Med* 1982; 44:413–430.
16. van Doornen LJP, Orlebeke KF: Stress, personality and serum-cholesterol level. *J Human Stress* 1982; 8:24–29.
17. Freeman LJ, Nixon PGF, Sallabank P, Reaveley D: Psychological stress and silent myocardial ischemia. *Am Heart J* 1987; 114:477–482.
18. Lown B, DeSilva RA, Reich P, Murawski BJ: Psychophysiologic factors in sudden cardiac death. *Am J Psychiatry* 1980; 137:1325–1335.
19. Verrier RL, Lown B: Behavioral stress and cardiac arrhythmias. *Ann Rev Physiol* 1984; 46:155–176.
20. Baroldi G, Falzi G, Mariani F: Sudden coronary death: A postmortem study in 208 selected cases compared to 97 "control" subjects. *Am Heart J* 1979; 98:20–31.
21. Cebelin MS, Hirsch CS: Human stress cardiomyopathy: Myocardial lesions in victims of homicidal assaults without internal injuries. *Hum Pathol* 1980; 11:123.
22. Szakacs JE, Cannon A: L-norepinephrine myocarditis. *Am J Clin Pathol* 1958; 30:425–434.
23. Tazalaar HD, Karch SB, Stephens BG, Billingham ME: Cocaine and the heart. *Hum Pathol* 1987; 18:195–199.
24. Pieper GM, Clayton FC, Todd GL, Eliot RS: Temporal changes in endocardial energy metabolism following propranolol and the metabolic basis for protection against isoprenaline cardiotoxicity. *Cardiovasc Res* 1979; 13:207–214.
25. Todd GL, Sterns DA, Plambeck MS, Joekel CS, Eliot RS: Protective effects of slow channel calcium antagonists on noradrenaline-induced myocardial necrosis. *Cardiovasc Res* 1986; 20:645–651.
26. Harburg E, Schull WJ, Erfurt JC, Schork MA, Rice R: A family set method for estimating heredity and stress: I. A pilot survey of blood pressure among Negroes in high and low stress areas, Detroit, 1966–1967. *J Chronic Dis* 1970; 23:83–92.
27. Faulkner B, Kushner H, Khalsa DK, Canessa M, Katz S: Sodium sensitivity, growth and family history of hypertension in young blacks. *J Hypertens* 1986; 4(suppl 5):S-381–S-383.
28. Syme SL: Socioenvironmental factors in heart disease. In: Beamish RE, Singal PK, Dhalla NS (eds): *Stress and Heart Disease,* Boston, Martinus Nijhoff Publishing, 1985: 60–70.
29. Marmot MG, Syme SL: Acculturation and coronary heart disease in Japanese Americans. *Am J Epidemiol* 1976; 104:225–247.
30. Berkman LF, Syme SL: Social networks, host resistance, and mortality: A nine-year follow-up study of Alameda county residents. *Am J Epidemiol* 1979; 109:186–204.
31. Nerem RM, Levesque MJ, Cornhill JF: Social environment as a factor in diet-induced aortic atherosclerosis in rabbits. *Science* 1980; 208:1475–1476.
32. McLean AA: *Work Stress.* Reading, MA, Addison-Wesley Publishing Company, 1979.
33. Haynes SG, Feinleib M: Women, work and coronary heart disease: Prospective findings from the Framingham Heart Study. *Am J Public Health* 1980; 70:133–141.
34. Eliot RS: Stress and the heart. *Postgrad Med* 1992; 92:237–248.
35. Kleinman A, Eisenberg L, Good B: Culture, illness, and care. *Ann Intern Med* 1978; 88:251–258.
36. Katon W: Panic disorder: Epidemiology, diagnosis, and treatment in primary care. *J Clin Psychiatry* 1986; 47(suppl 10):21–27.
37. Ockene IS, Shay MY, Alpert JS, Weiner BH, Dalen JE: Unexplained chest pains in patients with normal coronary arteriograms. *N Engl J Med* 1980; 303:1249–1252.
38. Claycomb JB: 15% of cardiology patients at risk for panic disorder (Wright State University School of Medicine Dayton, Ohio Symposium on Personality and Emotional Factors in Heart Disease). *Intern Med News* 1987; 20:35–37, March 1–14.
39. Morales-Ballejo HM, Eliot RS, Boone JL: Influence of alprazolam-placebo on the hemodynamic changes caused by stress (abstr). *Am J Hypertens* 1990; 3(5):2:99A.
40. Wooley CF: From irritable heart to mitral valve prolapse: British army medical reports, 1860 to 1870. *Am J Cardiol* 1985; 55:1107–1109.
41. Christie RV: Some types of respiration in the neuroses. *Q J Med* 1935; 4:427.
42. Retchin SM, Fletcher RH, Earp JA, Lamson N, Waugh RA: Mitral valve prolapse: Disease or illness. *Arch Intern Med* 1986; 146:1081–1084.
43. Devereux RB, Hawkins I, Kramer-Fox R, Lutas EM, Hammond IW, Spitzer MC et al: Complications of mitral valve prolapse: Disproportionate occurrence in men and older patients. *Am J Med* 1986; 81:751–758.
44. Jeresaty RM: Sudden death in the mitral valve prolapse—click syndrome. *Am J Cardiol* 1976; 37:317–318.
45. Chesler E, King RA, Edwards JE: The myxomatous mitral valve and sudden death. *Circulation* 1983; 67:632–639.
46. Friedman M, Rosenman RH: Association of specific overt behavior pattern with increases in blood cholesterol, blood clotting time, incidence of arcus senilis and clinical coronary heart disease. *JAMA* 1959; 169:1286–1296.

47. Rosenman RH, Brand RJ, Jenkins CD, Friedman M, Strauss R, Wurm M: Coronary heart disease in the Western Collaborative Group Study: Final follow-up experience of $8\frac{1}{2}$ years. *JAMA* 1975; 233:872–877.
48. Dembroski TM, MacDougall JM: Beyond global type A: Relationships of paralinguistic attributes, hostility, and anger-in to coronary heart disease. In: Field T, McAbe P, Schneiderman N (eds): *Stress and Coping*. Hillsdale, NJ, Lawrence Erlbaum, 1985: 223–242.
49. Esler M, Julius S, Zweifler A, Randall O, Harburg E, Gardiner H, et al: Mild high-renin essential hypertension: Neurogenic human hypertension? *N Engl J Med* 1977; 296:405–411.
50. Williams RB Jr, Barefoot JC, Shekelle RB: The health consequences of hostility. In: Chesney MA, Rosenman RH (eds): *Anger and Hostility in Cardiovascular and Behavioral Disorders*. Washington, DC, Hemisphere Publishing, 1985: 173–185.
51. Julius M, Harburg E, Cottingham EM, Johnson EH: Anger-coping types, blood pressure, and all-cause mortality: A follow-up in Tecumseh, Michigan (1971–1983). *Am J Epidemiol* 1986; 124:220–233.
52. Jefferson JW: Biologic treatment of depression in cardiac patients. *Psychosomatics* 1987; 26(suppl 11):31–36.
53. Appels A: The year before myocardial infarction. In: Dembroski TM, Schmidt TH, Blumchen G (eds): *Biobehavioral Bases of Coronary Heart Disease*. Basel, Karger, 1983: 18–37.
54. Talbott E, Kuller LH, Perper J, Murphy PA: Sudden unexpected death in women: Biologic and psychosocial origins. *Am J Epidemiol* 1981; 114:671–682.
55. Sims A: Neurosis and mortality: Investigating an association. *J Psychosom Res* 1984; 28:353–362.
56. Chodzko-Zajko WJ, O'Connon PJ: Plasma cortisol, the dexamethasone suppression test and depression in normal adult males. *J Psychosom Res* 1986; 30:313–320.
57. Ruddel H, Langewitz W, McKinney ME, Todd GL, Buell JC, Eliot RS: Hemodynamic responses during the type A interview: A comparison with mental challenge and a clinical interview. *J Autonom Nerv Syst* 1986; (suppl):685–688.
58. Jorgensen RS, Houston BK: Family history of hypertension, gender, and cardiovascular reactivity and stereotypy during stress. *J Behav Med* 1981; 4:175–189.
59. Horan MJ, Lenfant C: Epidemiology of blood pressure and predictors of hypertension. *Hypertension* 1990; 15(suppl I):I-120–I-124.
60. Perloff D, Sokolow M, Cowan R: The prognostic value of ambulatory blood pressures. *JAMA* 1983; 249:2792–2798.
61. Devereux RB, Pickering TB, Harshfield GA, Kleinert HD, Denby L, Clark L, et al: Left ventricular hypertrophy in patients with hypertension: Importance of blood pressure responses to regularly recurring stress. *Circulation* 1983; 68:470–476.
62. Morales-Ballejo HM, Eliot RS, Boone JL, Hughes JS: Psychophysiologic stress testing as a predictor of mean daily blood pressure. *Am Heart J* 1988; 116:673–681.
63. McKinney ME, Miner MH, Ruddel H, McIlvain HE, Witle H, Buell JC, et al: The standardized mental stress test protocol: Test-retest reliability and comparison with ambulatory blood pressure monitoring. *Psychophysiology* 1985; 22:453–563.
64. Eliot RS: The dynamics of hypertension—An overview: Present practices, new possibilities, and new approaches. *Am Heart J* 1988; 116:583–589.
65. Morales-Ballejo HM, Boone JL, Eliot RS: Influence of diltiazem-placebo on the hemodynamic changes caused by stress in mild hypertensives. *Clin Res* 1991; 39(2):433A.
66. Tesar GE, Hackett TP: Psychiatric management of the hospitalized cardiac patient. *J Cardiopul Rehabil* 1985; 5:219–225.
67. Stratton JR, Halter JB: Effect of a benzodiazepine (alprazolam) on plasma epinephrine and norepinephrine levels during exercise stress. *Am J Cardiol* 1985; 56:136–139.
68. Knapp D, Blackwell B: Emotional and behavioral problems in cardiac rehabilitation patients. *J Cardiac Rehabil* 1985; 5:112–123.
69. Anderson MP: Psychological aspects of cardiovascular disorders and rehabilitation. In: Peterson LH (ed): *Cardiovascular Rehabilitation*. New York, Macmillan, 1983: 94–117.
70. Ouslander JG, Small GW: Management of depression in the elderly patient with physical illness. *Geriatr Med Today* 1984; 3:90–96.
71. Feighner JP, Aden GC, Fabre LF, Rickels K, Smith WT: Comparison of alprazolam, imipramine, and placebo in the treatment of depression. *JAMA* 1983; 249:3057–3064.
72. Dracup K, Meleis A, Baker K, Edlefsen P: Family-focused cardiac rehabilitation: A role supplementation program for cardiac patients and spouses. *Nurs Clin North Am* 1984; 19:113–124.
73. Nemec ED, Mansfield L, Kennedy JW: Heart rate and blood pressure responses during sexual activity in normal males. *Am Heart J* 1976; 92:274–277.
74. Ben-Ari E, Kellerman JJ, Fisman E, Pines A, Peled B, Drury Y: Benefits of long-term physical training in patients after coronary artery bypass grafting—a 58-month follow-up and comparison with a nontrained group. *J Cardiopul Rehabil* 1986; 6:165–170.
75. Gold M, Lydiard RB, Carman J: *Advances in Psychopharmacology: Predicting and Improving Treatment Response*. Boca Raton, FL, CRC Press, 1984.
76. Neshkes RE, Jarvik LF: Depression in the elderly: Current management concepts. *Geriatrics* 1986; 41:51–58.
77. AMA Drug Evaluations, 5th ed. 1983: 225–226.

Chapter 118

Panic Attacks and the Cardiovascular System

David V. Sheehan, M.D. ■ *B. Ashok Raj, M.D.*

HISTORICAL REVIEW

Panic disorder, with its mixture of psychological and severe paroxysmal autonomic symptoms, mimics disease in varied organ systems in the body. It is chameleon-like in its presentations and has challenged the diagnostic skills of clinicians from the eighteenth century to the present time. Well-documented descriptions of this disorder are found in the literature of the mid-nineteenth century. The descriptions tend to focus on the somatic symptoms of anxiety, particularly palpitations, chest pain, shortness of breath, and choking or smothering sensations.

War stimulated many studies of this disorder in the military. In 1867, Maclean,[1] a professor of military medicine, described 252 cases of valvular disease without murmurs. He blamed the heavy knapsacks, chest straps, and tunics that the soldiers wore for their "irritable-heart" symptoms. They abolished these accouterments, but the symptoms persisted. According to Skerritt,[2] in 1870 Myers, a surgeon in the Coldstream Guards, observed that functional heart disorder was more common in the army than in the navy or Metropolitan Police. Meanwhile, Coote[3] in 1858 described a syndrome of inframammary discomfort in women that included various pains, globus, variability of temperatures, irregular pulse, palpitations, vomiting, and constipation. He felt that it was due to a local vascular problem while others attributed its etiology to muscular disorder, uterine dysfunction, or spinal curvature. In 1871 Da Costa,[4] a Philadelphia physician, produced his classic work on the irritable heart based on his experience treating American Civil War veterans.

By 1880, Beard and others popularized the term *neurasthenia* to cluster a number of common symptoms like headache, pain, noise in the head, fears, and sweating, rather than just the cardiovascular symptoms or weakness. In 1894 Freud[5] separated from neurasthenia a syndrome with a smaller group of symptoms and called it *anxiety neurosis*. This disorder included free-floating anxiety and anxiety attacks, with cardiac and other symptoms, that led to the development of phobias.

The medical literature during the World War I has many papers pertaining to "soldier's heart." In 1917 Sir Thomas Lewis[6] introduced the term *effort syndrome* as a substitute for the prevailing British Army terminology *disordered action of the heart*. In 1918 Oppenheimer et al.[7] introduced the term *neurocirculatory asthenia* as a convenient term to describe a syndrome characterized by nervous and circulatory symptoms and associated with an increased predisposition to fatigue. In 1920 MacKenzie[8] suggested that the heart abnormalities were only part of a larger general condition, a "war neurosis," with patients resembling psychoneurotic casualties. Concurrently, Culpin[9] noted the association between effort syndrome, anxiety symptoms, and phobias and suggested that treatment should be focused on the underlying nervous disorder and not on the heart.

In the post-World War I years, the term *cardiac neurosis* was used increasingly to describe a syndrome of excessive worry about heart disease, even when organic heart disease was present (Schnur, 1939).[10] At this time, hyperventilation was identified either as a part of the effort syndrome or as an independent disorder.

During World War II, the focus shifted back to the effort syndrome. In 1941 Wood[11] concluded that Da Costa's syndrome and effort syndrome were the same. He advocated support and reassurance rather than physical rehabilitation as the desirable treatment. Maxwell Jones and Sir Aubrey Lewis[12] found that about 30 percent of the patients also had a psychiatric diagnosis of anxiety state. Jones[13] later noted in 1948 that these patients would stop exercise at lower blood lactate levels than controls due to their fear of damage to their hearts—an "effort phobia."

The irritable-heart concept continued to resurface in the descriptions of "hyperkinetic heart syndrome" by Gorlin[14] in 1962 and the "hyperdynamic beta-adrenegic circulatory state" by Frohlich et al.[15] in 1966. The cardinal feature of this latter condition was the presence of a hyperkinetic circulation with cardiac awareness, exercise intolerance, labile episodic hypertension, and high resting pulse rate. Infusion of isoproterenol induced hysterical outburst in these individuals and propranolol blocked the symptoms. This led Frohlich to speculate that these individuals had increased reactivity of beta-adrenergic receptors.

In 1968 Barlow et al.[16] confirmed with phonocardiography and angiography that nonejection, midsystolic clicks, and late systolic murmurs heard on auscultation originated from the mitral valve. In 1976 Wooley[17] suggested that Da Costa's syndrome, the effort syndrome, and neurocirculatory asthenia were all probably just earlier descriptions of the mitral valve prolapse (MVP) syndrome. (See also Chap. 80.)

EPIDEMIOLOGY

In the epidemiologic catchment area study, anxiety and phobic disorders were the most common disabling psychiatric disorders in the United States. Lifetime prevalence rates were estimated as 8.3 percent of the general adult population.[18] In this study, panic disorder had a lifetime prevalence of 1.5 percent of the general population (2.1 percent for females and 0.6 percent for males).[18] The criteria used to identify panic disorder were the Research Diagnostic Criteria (RDC). These criteria are more restrictive than the criteria of the *Diagnostic and Statistical Manual of Mental Disorders*, third edition, revised (DSM-III-R), which accommodates some cases that would have previously been diagnosed as generalized anxiety disorder and most cases of agoraphobia.[19] Based on DSM-III-R criteria, lifetime prevalence rates of panic disorder are estimated to be 3 or 4 percent of the general population. It is estimated, based on the conservative Epidemiologic Catchment Area Study findings, that 2.6 million people in the United States have panic disorder; based on the broader definition of panic disorder in the DSM-III-R, 6 million people are affected.

AGE OF ONSET

The age-of-onset distribution of panic disorder is uniform and unimodal with a peak in the twenties.[21] The mean age of onset is 23 years.[31] Panic disorder rarely starts before the age of 15 or after the age of 40. It is twice as common in the 25-to-44 age group as in the 45-to-64 age group. After the age of 65, prevalence drops to approximately one-twelfth that of the 18-to-45 age group.

Although the unimodal age-of-onset distribution is difficult to explain in psychological terms, it is consistent with a biologic illness model of panic disorder, in which the disorder appears to afflict women preferentially in their child-bearing years.

GENDER DISTRIBUTION

Seventy-five to 80 percent of the victims of panic disorder are women.[21–24] There is no evidence that this gender difference is related to educational status, ethnic background, or social status. The higher risk of women for panic disorder contrasts with the equal gender distribution in some other anxiety disorders, such as obsessive-compulsive disorder.

GENETICS

Increasing data suggest that panic disorder is a genetically inherited disease. There is evidence of an increased concordance in monozygotic as compared to dyzygotic twins,[25,26] and the lifetime morbidity risk among first-degree relatives has been found to be 15 to 25 percent.[27,28] There is also evidence from the Yale Family Genetics Study that patients who are comorbid for panic disorder and major depression have "increased rates of major depression, anxiety disorders (phobia, panic disorder, and generalized anxiety disorder), and alcoholism compared with the first degree relatives of normal controls and depressed probands without an anxiety disorder."[29] Within families, the transmission pattern for panic disorder is consistent with inheritance for an autosomal dominant gene or with single-locus genetics.[28,30] Preliminary findings from a recent genetic linkage study suggest that panic disorder may be coded by a gene on chromosome 16, position Q22.[28]

CLINICAL DESCRIPTION

The Symptom Cluster

Although panic disorder as a diagnostic label was first used in 1980 in the DSM-III (the American Psychiatric Association's official classification of psychiatric disorders), a similar cluster of symptoms was known in medicine for centuries under a variety of aliases. The unique clinical feature of panic disorder is the occurrence of unexpected unprovoked panic attacks at some point in the patient's history. In making a diagnosis, it is preferable to focus attention on the unexpected, unprovoked paroxysmal nature of these symptom attacks rather than on the word *panic*. A panic attack is defined as any attack with at least 4 of the possible 13 symptoms listed in Table 118-1. It is not defined by any judgment of the

TABLE 118-1
Symptoms of Panic Attack

1. Shortness of breath (dyspnea) or smothering sensations
2. Dizziness, unsteady feelings, or faintness
3. Palpitations or accelerated heart rate (tachycardia)
4. Trembling or shaking
5. Sweating
6. Choking
7. Nausea or abdominal distress
8. Depersonalization or derealization
9. Numbness or tingling sensations (paresthesias)
10. Flushes (hot flashes) or chills
11. Chest pain or discomfort
12. Fear of dying
13. Fear of going crazy or of doing something uncontrolled

intensity of the attack. The patient does not need to have an intense, cognitive feeling of panic or show signs of overt anxiety to the clinician. For example, the patient may experience skipping or racing of the heart, dizziness, a choking sensation, or pain in the left side of the chest. These symptoms may be accompanied by some cognitive anxiety, although this may not be intense. Such an attack is labeled a panic attack because the four symptoms occur suddenly and unexpectedly within a 10-min period. The important point in making an accurate diagnosis is to focus on whether or not any of the attacks are unexpected and on counting the number of symptoms in each of the patient's attacks rather than focusing on the intensity of each attack.

The majority of patients have two to four unexpected, unprovoked anxiety attacks per week. Typically, they last about 15 to 20 min with some lasting only 1 or 2 min and others lasting more than 1 h. There is considerable variability in the number of symptoms that occur during each attack, many attacks having only one or two symptoms while others may have as many as 10 or 12 symptoms. The typical attack usually has four to eight symptoms, with the attack accompanied by considerable cognitive anxiety.

It has been widely assumed that a feeling of being mentally anxious is always present during the attacks. Approximately 20 percent of the attacks in panic disorder occur in the absence of any subjective, cognitive sense of anxiety. Certain symptoms—notably left-sided mammary chest pain, pressure, or discomfort, lightheadedness, and paresthesias—frequently occur in the absence of mental anxiety, especially when they occur as isolated somatic symptoms.

Symptom Progression over Time

The symptoms of panic disorder appear to follow an orderly progression over time and do not appear to occur in the random haphazard fashion that was previously believed. A common sequence of stages is given in Table 118-2.

The disorder first begins in about 50 percent of cases with a full unexpected panic attack, while in the rest it first begins with attacks limited to only one or two symptoms (limited-symptom attacks) that may occur in the absence of feeling mentally anxious. For example, the patient may experience an episode of tachycardia or paresthesias or feel acutely short of breath for no apparent reason, and several days later other symptoms from the cluster may occur, again in isolation or in pairs. Later, an attack may occur with four or more symptoms during the same attack. The patient may experience great alarm or a fear of dying or losing control or running away.

Because the attacks often occur in an unexpected, unprovoked manner, patients may be unable to find any psychosocial reason to explain their symptoms. They interpret the events as an expression of a medical illness. Usually they first seek evaluation from an internist or a family physician rather than a psychiatrist. If one symptom dominates in their symptom cluster, they may seek the specialist who is expert in that area. For example, if they are troubled by skipping or racing of their heart, they may first consult a cardiologist. The clinician then reassures them that "there is nothing seriously wrong" and that their disorder is "just stress and nerves." They are encouraged to minimize the stress and conflict in their lives and to rest, and are reassured that the symptoms will then remit. Use of a stress and conflict model to conceptualize this disorder and the physician's reassurance that there is "nothing wrong" rarely helps, although much was made of the value of this management strategy in the past. It can no longer be recommended as a useful strategy for managing this disorder. Clinicians can no longer rely on the stress/conflict model of conceptualizing panic disorder to treat panic disorder.

Within weeks the patient usually has another unexpected panic attack and is again at a loss to explain why the attack occurred in the absence of stress or conflict. Because the physician used a stress/conflict model to identify it as an anxiety disorder and the attack occurred in the absence of stress or conflict, the patient interprets this to mean that he or she does not have an anxiety disorder. The patient often assumes that he or she has an exotic medical illness and begins to search for a specialist who has the diagnostic sophistication or the appropriate technology to make an accurate diagnosis. The patient engages in excessive health worries and goes doctor shopping in search of a solution. Reassurances that there is nothing medically wrong quickly vanish with the next attack. Panic attacks are so terrifying that they counteract all reassurances and convince the patient that indeed there is something physically wrong and that the last

TABLE 118-2
Common Stages of Panic Disorder

Stage 1: Limited-symptom attacks
Stage 2: Panic attacks
Stage 3: Health worries
Stage 4: Limited phobias
Stage 5: Extensive phobias
Stage 6: Demoralization, depression

physician obviously misunderstood the illness. These patients are often labeled hypochondriacs and feel embarrassed because they recurrently call their physicians with somatic complaints in spite of no evidence of medical illness.

The majority of patients have attacks unexpectedly in a variety of situations and often begin to fear and avoid situations that they associate with their bad attacks. If the unexpected attacks continue, the phobias begin to generalize further, and patients often progress to a stage of extensive phobic avoidance behavior and some become housebound.

Approximately 50 to 60 percent of patients eventually develop a secondary demoralization depression and lose hope. Twenty percent of patients with panic disorder report suicide attempts, and 12 percent of patients with panic attacks report suicide attempts.[31] In 1872 Darwin[32] put it succinctly, "If we expect to suffer, we are anxious. If we have no hope of relief, we despair."

If the unexpected attacks are very frequent and intense, the patient usually progresses through these stages (Table 118-2) very rapidly. If the unexpected attacks lessen in intensity, the disorder may temporarily stop at one of the stages and not progress further until the frequency and the intensity of the attacks increase. If the unexpected attacks stop completely, as they do in about 15 percent of all cases, the disorder moves through the stages in reverse until there is a spontaneous remission of all symptoms. In the majority of cases; however, there is a progression from unexpected attacks to progressive phobic avoidance behavior and increasing depression over time.

Life Course

Panic disorder has a chronic, fluctuating course during the middle years of life. As many as 50 percent of the victims are disabled to some degree, and 73 to 92 percent are symptomatic when reevaluated up to 20 years after initial diagnosis.[2,33,34]

Patients with panic disorder also have an excess mortality from suicide and, among males, from cardiovascular disease when compared with controls matched for age and sex.[35]

ATYPICAL/MASKED PRESENTATIONS OF PANIC IN CARDIOLOGY

In cardiology panic disorder is most likely to be found in patients presenting with atypical chest pain and MVP.

Atypical Chest Pain and Panic Disorder

Anxiety is the most common cause of chest pain and is usually experienced as a sharp stabbing sensation in the left inframammary region[36] (Chap. 19). Traditionally, this diagnosis is made by exclusion of all cardiac and other physical causes. The typical patient presenting in primary care will get a physical examination, enzyme studies, and an electrocardiogram (ECG). Depending on the findings, there may be further testing and cardiology consultation. The range of tests include ECGs, 24-h ambulatory ECG, stress ECG, and myocardial perfusion scintigraphy. Findings inconclusive of cardiac disease, in the presence of persistent complaints of chest pain, may lead to a referral for a coronary angiogram.

In cases with minimal disease or normal coronary arteries (NCAs), patients are reassured that their chest pains are not due to coronary artery disease but are left with no other explanation for their symptoms. They may be told to lose weight, stop smoking, or reduce stress. They may be referred to a gastroenterologist to rule out esophageal spasm syndrome, since this disorder is reported in 17 to 100 percent of patients with chest pain and NCAs.[37,38] In one study of 25 patients with esophageal manometric abnormalities consistent with diffuse spasm syndrome, 84 percent met criteria for a psychiatric diagnosis, most frequently anxiety and depression.[39] Follow-up studies of patients with chest pain and NCAs have shown that mortality rates for these patients are no higher than those expected for the general population.[40–42] When they are evaluated from the standpoint of function, however, a different picture emerges. Despite being told they have normal coronary arteries on angiogram, in one study[43] a majority continued to complain of chest pain, 44 percent still believed they had heart disease, 51 percent were unable to work because of the chest pain, and 25 percent continued to use cardiac medications. In another study,[44] 90 percent visited the emergency room during the follow-up period complaining of chest pain, and 9 percent had a second normal coronary arteriogram.

This syndrome of chest pain with NCAs has been studied psychiatrically. In these studies, 33 to 48 percent of subjects meet criteria for panic disorder.[45–48] This is much higher than the 2 to 5 percent rate in the community or in controls with chest pain and coronary artery disease. The studies suggest a chest pain syndrome secondary to an anxiety disorder such as panic. The pain is usually atypical, is more likely to occur in a younger female, and is accompanied by palpitations, multiple somatic complaints, multiple phobias, and depression. It is less likely to be associated with a positive stress test. Of interest, panic disorder patients cannot be distinguished on the basis of risk factors for coronary artery disease (CAD) such as presence of diabetes, hypertension, hyperlipidemia, smoking, obesity, or a family history of CAD. This observation that chest pain secondary to panic disorder is more likely to be atypical or nonanginal in character is supported by a study of outpatients attending a cardiology clinic,[49] which evaluated patients with atypical or nonanginal chest pain with or without CAD for the presence of panic disorder. Of 74 patients with atypical or nonanginal chest pain without CAD, 59 percent had panic disorder. Fifty percent of 30 subjects with atypical or nonanginal chest pain and CAD met criteria for panic disorder. Overall, the literature supports an association between atypical or nonanginal chest pain and panic disorder.

Mitral Valve Prolapse

In 1963 Barlow[16] established MVP as a separate and distinct disorder. To this day, however, there is debate about whether or not MVP and panic disorder are identical, separate and distinct, or overlap to a certain degree[50] (Chap. 80). Clinically, both conditions are most common in women of child-bearing years and run in families. Symptoms common to both include palpitations, tachycardia, lightheadedness, dizziness, actual or near syncope, fatigue, dyspnea, and chest pain atypical of angina pectoris. The reported incidence of MVP in panic disorder ranges from 0 percent[51] to 40 to 50 percent.[52–55] Two studies[56,57] found rates of 8 and 15 percent, and this was not considered significantly higher than the rates expected for the general population. The variability in results may be due to study size, diagnostic methods, and criteria for MVP. A recent study[58] of 131 consecutive patients with panic disorder presenting to a psychiatric clinic rather than to cardiology used strict criteria for diagnosing MVP. The diagnosis of definite MVP was made in 34 percent of these subjects and probable MVP in another 5 percent.[58]

The prevalence of panic disorder in patients with MVP has been less extensively investigated. In a comparison of subjects with MVP, cardiac controls, and normal controls,[59] the rates of panic disorder were 12, 6, and 4.5 percent, respectively. Although the results were in the expected direction, the differences were not statistically significant. The rate of panic attacks, however, was significantly higher in patients with MVP (25 percent) than in controls (4.5 percent). The diagnosis of panic disorder was much more likely in the female subjects. In other studies, rates of 16 percent[60] and 0 percent[61] have been reported.

Overall, the literature supports an association between the two disorders, even if it does not explain it. For the cardiologist in practice, MVP should serve as a marker for the possible existence of an associated panic disorder in patients who are persistently somatic and excessively disabled from their cardiovascular symptoms.

Electrocardiogram

Electrocardiographic abnormalities, often labile, limited to T-wave inversion, mostly involving leads II, III, and aV_F but occasionally involving leads I, aV_L and V_4, V_5, and V_6, have been reported in anxiety neurosis/panic disorder.[62–64] On the other hand, two studies found no difference in the frequency of T-wave abnormalities in anxiety neurosis and healthy controls.[65,66] No other characteristic ECG abnormaltiy is found in anxiety neurosis/panic disorder.

CONSEQUENCES OF PANIC DISORDER

There are serious and widespread medical and psychiatric consequences to missing the diagnosis or inadequately treating the disorder.

Medical Consequences

Significantly higher rates of hypertension and peptic ulcer have been reported in patients with panic disorder as compared to controls.[67,68] Increased mortality from cardiovascular disease and suicide has been reported for males with panic disorder in some studies[69,70] but not in others.[4,71–74] Examination of the New Haven portion of the Epidemiologic Catchment Area Program suggests that the risk of stroke in persons with a lifetime diagnosis of panic disorder is twice that in persons with or without other psychiatric disorder.[75] A study[76] of patients awaiting cardiac transplant for idiopathic dilated cardiomyopathy found a high rate of panic disorder among these patients compared to controls who had heart failure from CAD, rheumatic, or congenital heart disease. In the majority of cases, the panic disorder preceded the onset of heart failure. It has been suggested that panic disorder patients may exhibit mild left ventricular hypertrophy or dilatation.[77]

Another consequence of panic disorder is overutilization of medical services. Patients with panic disorder are two to three times more likely to use the services of an emergency room for an emotional problem than are patients with depression.[78] These patients have numerous somatic complaints, and the vast majority believe they have a physical disorder. In one study,[79] 70 percent had 12 or more symptoms each, and 70 percent of another sample had seen 10 or more physicians for somatic complaints.[80]

Some of the testing may not be inexpensive or benign. For example, subjects presenting with chest pain may end up having unnecessary coronary angiograms. Of those with normal coronary arteries and chest pain, about 33 percent will meet criteria for panic disorder.[47]

Psychiatric Consequences

In a review of suicide in anxiety disorders, 6 to 60 percent of deaths during follow-up are attributed to suicide.[81] The variation in rates depends on the sample studied, with higher rates being observed in studies of panic disorder patients who had been hospitalized. In that population, 20 percent of deaths during follow-up are due to suicide.[69,70,82] Data from a community-based study of psychiatric disorders[83] showed that 7 percent of people with uncomplicated panic disorder reported a suicide attempt at some time in their lives, and the rate goes up to 20 percent if comorbid conditions coexist. These rates are similar to that observed for depression.

Criteria for diagnosis of lifetime alcohol abuse is seen in 13 percent of Americans, in 18 percent of those with depression, and in 27 percent of patients with panic disorder. Panic disorder patients are also more likely to be given symptomatic treatment and to take medications for insomnia, dizziness, and nausea. As a group they are at high risk for unnecessary polypharmacy.

TREATMENT

Panic disorder is now usually treated with a sequence of distinct approaches. The first and most critical of these is the use of antipanic medication to control the unexpected attacks. Because antipanic medications alone rarely lead to complete timely resolution of phobic avoidance, in vivo exposure behavior therapy is usually necessary to reduce phobic avoidance and anticipatory anxiety. If there are psychosocial problems complicating recovery, psychotherapy is indicated, but it is not routinely imposed on all patients with panic disorder. Finally, to protect the patient against future relapse, to equip them if they do relapse, and to insure good compliance to the other treatment steps, it is important to educate the patients about their illness and the rationale for the treatments used. Relaxation treatment and exercise programs are ineffective in the treatment of panic disorder. Indeed, marked exercise exacerbates the symptoms of panic disorder by increasing blood levels of lactic acid, to which they are hypersensitive.

MEDICATION CHOICES

Although only one medication (alprazolam) has to date been formally approved by the U.S. Food and Drug Administration for the treatment of panic disorder, there is good evidence suggesting that several classes of medications may be effective. Several studies suggest that benzodiazepines,[84–86] tricyclic antidepressants,[80,87–89] and monoamine oxidase (MAO) inhibitors[80,89–91] are effective.

Although not all benzodiazepines, tricyclics, or MAO inhibitors have been systematically studied for panic disorder, clinical experience and case reports suggest that most, if not all, the drugs within these classes are usually effective when appropriately dosed. There is conflicting evidence on the value of trazodone in panic disorder; Charney et al.[92] found it ineffective (albeit using low doses), while in our experience it is frequently effective if given in adequate doses. The newest class of "antidepressants," the selective serotonin uptake inhibitors (SSUIs)[93] (e.g., fluoxetine,[94] fluvoxamine,[95] sertraline, paroxetine, and citalopram), are also frequently effective for panic disorder. The antidepressants are effective in panic disorder even in the absence of any depressive symptoms.[80] Not all antidepressants are effective in panic disorder, bupropion hydrochloride[96] and amoxapine hydrochloride being the exceptions. Buspirone is a nonbenzodiazepine anxiolytic that has been found effective in the treatment of generalized anxiety disorder.[97–100] Although it causes no sedation or ataxia, does not have a withdrawal syndrome, and is a well-tolerated anxiolytic, it is not better than placebo in the treatment of panic disorder,[101] even when given in high doses.[102]

MEDICATION COMPARISONS

Although alprazolam is the most thoroughly studied and most widely prescribed medication for panic disorder, the preliminary evidence suggests that it may not be unique among benzodiazepines in this regard. Noyes et al.[103] have found diazepam was effective, while Tesar et al.[104] reported that clonazepam was as effective as alprazolam. In our experience almost every available (nonhypnotic) benzodiazepine appears to have some antipanic effects if correctly dosed.

Although imipramine is the most extensively studied tricyclic antidepressant for panic disorder, there is currently no evidence that it is superior (or inferior) to any other tricyclic for panic disorder. Phenelzine is the most thoroughly studied MAO inhibitor for panic disorder, although both tranylcypromine and isocarboxazid also appear effective. Tranylcypromine appears to be both subjectively better tolerated and slightly less potent overall in severe panic disorder than phenelzine.

The different classes of antipanic drugs have not all been systematically compared with each other. A study comparing phenelzine, imipramine, and placebo found evidence that phenelzine was superior to imipramine on a few but not all outcome measures.[80] A later study replicated this difference and found alprazolam overall not statistically different from either phenelzine or imipramine, although it was less effective in controlling the depressive dimensions of the disorder.[89] Phenelzine had a greater effect on disability measures and appeared to be a more potent rehabilitator with its energizing, mood-elevating, confidence-enhancing effects.[89] Phenelzine appears to have a margin of superiority over other antipanic drugs especially in severe and chronic cases.

To date there are no adequate studies comparing the SSUIs with the other classes of antipanic drugs. Preliminary case series suggest they are similar in potency to the tricyclics but perhaps a little less potent than the hydrazine MAO inhibitors.

MEDICATION USE

The majority of failures on antipanic drugs occur because the doses used are too low and the duration of treatment is too short. Attention to these two issues is critical to good medication management. Practical guidelines for the use of MAO inhibitor[105–107] and benzodiazepine[108,109] therapy in panic disorder are available.[110]

TREATMENT OF RESIDUAL PHOBIC AVOIDANCE

After the medication dosage has been adjusted correctly, some patients continue to have residual phobias that are a learned complication of having panic attacks. In vivo exposure behavior therapy is the most effective type of behavior therapy for these phobias. The cardiologist should seek consultation from a behavior therapist (either a psychiatrist or psychologist) to implement this behavioral treatment.

LONG-TERM TREATMENT

If psychosocial problems complicate recovery, psychotherapy is indicated. The relapse rate is in excess of 70 percent, and many patients will require long-term medication management. It is useful to give patients an opportunity every 12 months to see if they need to continue with their antipanic drug. If they suffer a recurrence, it is wise quickly to restart the antipanic drug and maintain them on it for at least another year.

REFERENCES

1. Maclean WC: Diseases of the heart in the British Army: The cause and the remedy. *Br Med J* 1867; i:161–164.
2. Skerritt PW: Anxiety and the heart—A historical review. *Psychol Med* 1983; 13:17–25.
3. Coote C: Inframammary pain. *Br Med J* 1858; i:502–503.
4. Da Costa JM: On irritable heart: A clinical study of a functional cardiac disorder and its consequences. *Am J Med Sci* 1871; 61:17–52.
5. Freud S: *On the Grounds for Detaching a Particular Syndrome from Neurasthenia under the Description 'Anxiety Neurosis.' The Standard Edition of the Complete Psychological Works of Sigmund Freud,* vol 3 (1893–1899). London, Hogarth, 1894.
6. Lewis T: *Report upon Soldiers Returned as Cases of 'Disordered Action of the Heart' (DAH) or 'Valvular Disease of the Heart' (VDH).* Medical Research Committee, Special Report Series, No. 8. London, 1917.
7. Oppenheimer BS, Rothschild MA: The psychoneurotic factor in the 'Irritable heart of soldiers.' *Br Med J* 1918; ii:29–31.
8. MacKenzie J: The soldiers heart and war neurosis: A study in symptomatology. *Br Med J* 1920; i:491–494, 530–534.
9. Culpin M: The psychological aspect of the effort syndrome. *Lancet* 1920; ii:184–186.
10. Schnur S: Cardiac neurosis associated with organic heart disease. *Am Heart J* 1939; 18:153–165.
11. Wood PW: Da Costa's syndrome (or effort syndrome). *Br Med J* 1941; i:767–772, 805–811, 845–851.
12. Jones M, Lewis A: Effort syndrome. *Lancet* 1941; i:813–818.
13. Jones M: Physiological and psychological responses to stress in neurotic patients. *J Ment Sci* 1948; 94:392–427.
14. Gorlin R: The hyperkinetic heart syndrome. *JAMA* 1962; 182:823–829.
15. Frohlich ED, Dustan HP, Page IH: Hyperdynamic beta-adrenergic circulatory state. *Arch Intern Med* 1966; 117:614–619.
16. Barlow JB, Bosman CK, Pocock WA, Marchand P: Late systolic murmurs and non ejection ("mid-late") systolic clicks: An analysis of 90 patients. *Br Heart J* 1968; 30:203–218.
17. Wooley CF: Where are the diseases of yesteryear? Da Costa's syndrome, soldiers heart, the effort syndrome, neurocirculatory asthenia and the mitral valve prolapse syndrome. *Circulation* 1976; 53:749–751.
18. Robins LN, Helzer JE, Weissman MM, Oruaschel H, Gruenberg E, Burke JD Jr, et al: Lifetime prevalence of psychiatric disorders at three sites. *Arch Gen Psychiatry* 1984; 41:949–959.
19. American Psychiatric Association: *Diagnostic and Statistical Manual of Mental Disorders*, 3d revised ed. Washington, DC, American Psychiatric Association, 1987.
20. McGlynn TJ, Metcalf HL: *Diagnosis and Treatment of Anxiety Disorders: A Physician's Handbook.* Washington, DC, American Psychiatric Press, 1989.
21. Sheehan DV, Sheehan KE, Minichello WE: Age of onset of phobic disorders: A re-evaluation. *Compr Psychiatry* 1981; 22(6):544–553.
22. Marks IM, Lader M: Anxiety states (anxiety neurosis): A review. *J Nerv Ment Dis* 1973; 156:3–18.
23. Weissman MM, Leaf PJ, Holzer CE III, Merikangas KR: Epidemiology of anxiety disorders. *Psychopharmacol Bull* 1985; 21:538–541.
24. Ballenger JC, Burrows GR, DuPont RL Jr, Lesser IM, Noyes R Jr, Pecknold JC, et al: Alprazolam in panic disorder and agoraphobia: Results from a multicenter trial. Efficacy in short term treatment. *Arch Gen Psychiatry* 1988; 45:413–422.
25. Torgersen S: Genetic factors in anxiety disorders. *Arch Gen Psychiatry* 1983; 40:1085–1089.
26. Hopper JL, Judd FK, Derrick PL, Macaskill GT, Burrows GD: A family study of panic disorder: Reanalysis using a regressive logistic model that incorporates a sibship environment. *Gen Epidemiol* 1990; 7:151–161.
27. Crowe RR, Noyes R, Pauls DL, Slymen D: A family study of panic disorder. *Arch Gen Psychiatry* 1983; 40:1065–1069.
28. Crowe RR, Noyes R, Wilson AF, Elston RC, Ward LJ: A linkage study of panic disorder. *Arch Gen Psychiatry* 1987; 44:933–937.
29. Ballenger JC, Burrows GD, DuPont RL Jr., Lesser IM, Noyes R Jr, Pecknold JC: Alprazolam in panic disorder and agoraphobia: Results from a multicenter trial. Efficacy in short term treatment. *Arch Gen Psychiatry* 1988; 45:413–422.
30. Pauls DL, Bucher KD, Crowe RR, Noyes R Jr: A genetic study of panic disorder pedigrees. *Am J Hum Genet* 1980; 32:639–644.
31. Weissman MM, Klerman GL, Markowitz JS, Ouellette R: Suicidal ideation and suicide attempts in panic disorder and panic attacks. *New Engl J Med* 1989; 321:1209–1214.
32. Darwin C: *The Expressions of the Emotions in Man and Animals.* London, Murray, 1872.
33. Greer S: The prognosis of anxiety states. In: Lader MH (ed): *Studies of Anxiety.* London, Royal Med. Psychological Assoc., 1969: 151–157.
34. Wheeler EO, White PD, Reed EW, Cohen ME: Neurocirculatory asthenia (anxiety neurosis, effort syndrome, neurasthenia). A twenty-year follow-up study of one hundred and seventy-three patients. *J Am Med Assoc* 1950; 142:878–889.
35. Coryell W, Noyes R, Clancy J: Excess mortality in panic disorder: A comparison with primary unipolar depression. *Arch Gen Psychiatry* 1982; 39:701–703.
36. Kitt TM: Recurrent atypical chest pain. *Hosp Phys* 1986; 11:57–64.
37. Dart AM, Davies AH, Dalal J, Ruttley M, Henderson AH: "Angina" and normal coronary arteriograms: A follow-up study. *Eur Heart J* 1980; 1:97–100.
38. Brand DL, Martin D, Pope CE: II. Esophageal manometrics in patients with angina like chest pain. *Digest Disord Sci* 1977; 22:300–304.
39. Clouse RE, Lustman PJ: Psychiatric illness and contraction abnormalities of the esophagus. *N Eng J Med* 1983; 309:1377–1342.
40. Bruschke AV, Proudfit WB, Sones FM: Clinical course of patients with normal and slightly or moderately abnormal coronary arteriograms. A follow-up study of 500 patients. *Circulation* 1973; 47:936–945.
41. Isner JM, Salem DN, Banas JS, Levine HJ: Long term clinical course of patients with normal coronary arteriography: Follow-up study of 121 patients with normal or nearly normal coronary arteriograms. *Am Heart J* 1981; 102:645–653.
42. Kemp HG, Vokonoas PS, Cohn PF, Gorlin R: The anginal syndrome associated with normal coronary arteriograms. Report of a six-year experience. *Am J Med* 1973; 54:735–742.
43. Ockene IS, Shay MJ, Alpert JS, Weiner BH, Dalen JE: Unexplained chest pain in patients with normal coronary arteriograms: A follow-up study of functional status. *N Eng J Med* 1980; 303:1249–1252.
44. Lavey EB, Winkle RA: Continuing disability of patients with chest pain and normal coronary arteriograms. *J Chronic Dis* 1979; 32:191–196.
45. Bass C, Wade C: Chest pain with normal coronary arteries: A comparative study of psychiatric and social morbidity. *Psychol Med* 1984; 14:51–61.
46. Katon W, Hall ML, Russo J, Cormier L, Hollifield M, Vitaliano PP: Chest pain: Relationship of psychiatric illness to coronary arteriographic results. *Am J Med* 1988; 84:1–9.
47. Beitman BD, Lamberti JW, Mukerji V, DeRosear L, Basha I, Schmid L: Panic disorder in patients with angiographically normal coronary arteries. A pilot study. *Psychosomatics* 1987; 28:480–484.
48. Mukerji V, Beitman BD, Alpert MA, Lamberti JW, DeRosear L, Basha IM: Panic attack symptoms in patients with chest pain and angiographically normal coronary arteries. *J Anxiety Disord* 1987; 1:41–46.
49. Beitman BD, Basha I, Flaker G, DeRosear L, Mukerji V, Trombka L, et al: Atypical or nonanginal chest pain. Panic disorder or coronary artery disease? *Arch Intern Med* 1987; 147:1548–1552.
50. Gottlieb SH: Mitral valve prolapse: From syndrome to disease. *Am J Cardiol* 1987; 60:53J–58J.
51. Hickey AJ, Andrew G, Wilchen DE: Independence of mitral valve prolapse and neurosis. *Br Heart J* 1983; 50:333–336.
52. Kantor JS, Zitrin CM, Zeldis SM: Mitral valve prolapse syndrome in agoraphobic patients. *Am J Psychiatry* 1980; 137:467–470.
53. Venkatesh A, Pauls DL, Browe R, Noyes R Jr, Van Valkenburg C, Martins JB, et al: Mitral valve prolapse in anxiety neurosis (panic disorder). *Am Heart J* 1980; 100:302–305.
54. Pariser SF, Jones BA, Pinta ER, Young ER, Fontana ME: Panic attacks: Diagnostic evaluation of 17 patients. *Am J Psychiatry* 1979; 136:105–106.
55. Gorman JM, Fyer AF, Glicklich J, King DL, Klein DF: Mitral

valve prolapse and panic disorders: Effect of imipramine. In: Klein DF, Rabkin JG (eds): *Anxiety: New Research and Changing Concepts.* New York, Raven, 1981: 317–326.

56. Mavissakalian M, Salerni R, Thompson ME, Michelson L: Mitral valve prolapse and agoraphobia. *Am J Psychiatry* 1983; 140:1612–1614.
57. Shear MK, Devereux RB, Kramer-Fox R, Mann JJ, Frances A: Low prevalence of mitral valve prolapse in patients with panic disorder. *Am J Psychiatry* 1984; 141:302–303.
58. Liberthson R, Sheehan DV, King ME, Weyman AE: The prevalence of mitral valve prolapse in patients with panic disorders. *Am J Psychiatry* 1986; 143:511–515.
59. Kane JM, Woerner M, Zeldis S, Kramer R, Saravay S: Panic and phobic disorders in patients with mitral valve prolapse. In: Klein DF, Rabkin JG (eds): *Anxiety: New Research and Changing Concepts.* New York, Raven, 1981: 327–340.
60. Hartman N, Kramer R, Brown WT, Devereux RB: Panic disorder in patients with mitral valve prolapse. *Am J Psychiatry*, 1982; 139:669–670.
61. Mazza DL, Martin D, Spacavento L, Jacobsen J, Gibbs H: Prevalence of anxiety disorders in patients with mitral valve prolapse. *Am J Psychiatry* 1986; 143:349–352.
62. Graybiel A, White PD: Inversion of the T waves in lead I or II of the electrocardiogram in young individuals with neurocirculatory asthenia, with thyrotoxicosis, in relation to certain infections and following paroxysmal ventricular tachycardia. *Am Heart J* 1935; 10:345.
63. Wendkos MH, Logue RB: Unstable T waves in leads II and III in persons with neurocirculatory asthenia. *Am Heart J* 1946; 31:711.
64. Levander-Lindgren M: Studies in neurocirculatory asthenia (DA Costa's syndrome): I. Variations with regard to symptoms and some pathophysiological signs. *Acta Med Scand* 1962; 172:665.
65. Kannel WB, Dawber TR, Cohen ME: The ECG neurocirculatory asthenia (anxiety neurosis or neurasthenia): A study of 203 neurocirculatory patients and 757 healthy controls in the Framingham study. *Ann Intern Med* 1958; 49:1351.
66. Cohen ME, White PD, Johnson RE: Neurocirculatory asthenia, anxiety neurosis, or the effort syndrome. *Arch Intern Med* 1948; 81:260.
67. Noyes R, Clancy J, Hoenk PR, Slymen DJ: The prognosis of anxiety neurosis. *Arch Gen Psychiatry* 1980; 37:173–178.
68. Katon W: Panic disorder and somatisation: A review of 55 cases. *Am J Med* 1984; 77:101–106.
69. Coryell W, Noyes R, Clancy J: Excess mortality in panic disorder. *Arch Gen Psychiatry* 1982; 39:701–703.
70. Coryell W, Noyes R, House JD: Mortality among outpatients with panic disorder. *Am J Psychiatry* 1986; 143:508–510.
71. Wheeler EO, White PD, Reed EW, Cohen ME: Neurocirculatory asthenia (anxiety neurosis, effort syndrome, neurasthenia): A twenty year follow-up study of 173 patients. *JAMA* 1950; 142:878.
72. Martin RL, Cloninger R, Guze SB, Clayton PJ: Mortality in follow up of 500 psychiatric outpatients. *Arch Gen Psychiatry* 1985; 42:47–66.
73. Black DW, Warrack G, Winokur G: The Iowa record-linkage study. III. Excess mortality among patients with "functional disorders." *Arch Gen Psychiatry* 1985; 42:82–88.
74. Winokur G, Black DW: Psychiatric and medical diagnosis as risk factors for mortality in psychiatric patients. A case controlled study. *Am J Psychiatry* 1987; 144:208–211.
75. Weissman MM, Markowitz JS, Ouellete R, Greenwald S, Kahn JP: Panic disorder and cardiovascular/cerebrovascular problems: Results from a community survey. *Am J Psychiatry* 1990; 147:1504–1508.
76. Kahn JP, Drusin RE, Klein DF: Idiopathic cardiomyopathy and panic disorder: Clinical association in cardiac transplant candidates. *Am J Psychiatry* 1987; 144:1327–1330.
77. Kahn JP, Gorman JM, King DL, Fyer AJ, Liebowitz MR, Klein DF: Cardiac left ventricular hypertrophy and chamber dilatation in panic disorder patients: Implications for idiopathic dilated cardiomyopathy. *Psychiatry Res* 1990; 32:55–61.
78. Markowitz JS, Weissman MM, Ouellette R, Lish JD, Klerman GL: Quality of life in panic disorder. *Arch Gen Psychiatry* 1989; 46:984–992.
79. Sheehan DV, Sheehan KH: The classification of anxiety and hysterical states. I. Historical review and empirical delineation. *J Clin Psychopharmacol* 1982; 1:235–244.
80. Sheehan DV, Ballenger JC, Jacobson G: Treatment of endogenous anxiety with phobic, hysterical and hypochondriacal symptoms. *Arch Gen Psychiatry* 1980; 37:51–59.
81. Noyes R: Suicide and panic disorder: A review. *J Affect Disord* 1991; 22:1–11.
82. Allgulander C, Lavori PN: Excess mortality among 3,302 patients with pure anxiety neurosis. *Arch Gen Psychiatry* 1991; 48:599–602.
83. Weissman M, Klerman G, Markowitz J, Ouellette R: Suicidal ideation and suicide attempts in panic disorder and attacks. *N Eng J Med* 1989; 321:1209–1213.
84. Sheehan DV, Coleman JH, Greenblatt DJ, Jones KJ, Levine PH, Orsulak PJ, et al: Some biochemical correlates of panic attacks with agoraphobia and their response to a new treatment. *J Clin Psychopharmacol* 1984; 4:66–75.
85. Chouinard G, Annable L, Fontaine R, Solyom L: Alprazolam in the treatment of generalized anxiety and panic disorders: A double blind placebo controlled study. *Psychopharmacology* 1982; 77:229–233.
86. Sheehan DV, Uzogara E, Coleman JH, Greenblatt DJ, Jones KJ, Levine P, et al: The treatment of panic attacks with agoraphobia with alprazolam and ibuprofen: A controlled study (abst). *Am Psychiatr Assoc Annu Meeting,* Toronto, Canada, 1982.
87. Klein DF: Delineation of two drug-responsive anxiety syndromes. *Psychopharmacologia* 1964; 5:397–408.
88. Klein DF: Importance of psychiatric diagnosis in prediction of clinical drug effects. *Arch Gen Psychiatry* 1967; 16:118–126.
89. Sheehan DV, Claycomb JB, Surman OS, Gelles L, Gallo J, LeGros J: The relative efficacy of alprazolam, phenelzine and imipramine in treating panic attacks and phobias (abstr). *Scientif Proc 137th Annu Meeting Am Psychiatr Assoc, Los Angeles* 1984: 83.
90. Solyom L, Heseltine GFD, McClure DJ, Solyom C, Ledwidge B, Steinberg G: Behaviour therapy versus drug therapy in the treatment of phobic neurosis. *Can Psychiatr Assoc J* 1973; 18:25–32.
91. Tyrer P, Candy J, Kelly DA: A study of the clinical effects of phenelzine and placebo in the treatment of phobic anxiety. *Psychopharmacologia* 1973; 32:237–254.
92. Charney DS, Woods SW, Goodman WK, Rifkin B, Kinch M, Aiken B, et al: Drug treatment of panic disorder: The comparative efficacy of imipramine, alprazolam, and trazodone. *J Clin Psychiatry* 1986; 47:580–586.
93. Sheehan DV, Zak JP, Miller JA, Fanous BSL: Panic disorder: The potential role of serotonin reuptake inhibitors. *J Clin Psychiatry* 1988; 49(Suppl 8):30–36.
94. Gorman JM, Liebowitz MR, Fryer AJ: An open trial of fluoxetine in the treatment of panic attacks. *J Clin Psychopharmacol* 1987; 7:329–332.
95. den Boer JA, Westenberg HG, Klamerbeek WD, Verhoeven WMA, Kahn RS: Effect of serotonin uptake inhibitors in anxiety disorders: A double-blind comparison of clomipramine and fluvoxamine. *Int Clin Psychopharmacol* 1987; 2:21–32.
96. Sheehan DV, Davidson J, Manschreck TC, Van Wyck-Fleet J: Lack of efficacy of a new antidepressant (bupropion) in the treatment of panic disorder with phobias. *J Clin Psychopharmacol* 1983; 31:28–31.
97. Goldberg HL, Finnerty R: Comparison of buspirone in two separate studies. *J Clin Psychiatry* 1982; 43(12, sec 2):87–91.
98. Richels K, Weisman K, Norstad N, Singer M, Stoltz D, Brown A, et al: buspirone and diazepam in anxiety: A controlled study. *J Clin Psychiatry* 1982; 43(12, sec 2):81–86.
99. Feighner JP: A double blind comparison of buspirone and diazepam in outpatients with generalized anxiety disorder. *J Clin Psychiatry* 1982; 43(12, sec 2):103–107.
100. Wheatley D: Buspirone: Multicenter efficacy study. *J Clin Psychiatry* 1982; 43(12, sec 2):92–94.
101. Sheehan DV, Raj BA, Sheehan KH, Soto S: Is buspirone effective for panic disorder? *J Clin Psychopharmacol* 1990; 10(1):3–11.
102. Sheehan DV, Raj BA, Harnett-Sheehan K, Soto S, Knapp E: The relative efficacy of high dose buspirone and alprazolam in the treatment of panic disorder: A double blind placebo controlled study. *Acta Psychiatr Scand.* Accepted for publication, 1993.
103. Noyes R Jr, Anderson DJ, Clancy J, Crowe RR, Slymen DJ, Ghoneim MM, et al: Diazepam and propranolol in panic disorder and agoraphobia. *Arch Gen Psychiatry* 1984; 41:287–292.
104. Tesar GE, Rosenbaum JF, Pollack MH, Otto MW, Sachs GS,

Herman JB: Double-blind placebo-controlled comparison of clonazepam and alprazolam for panic disorder. *J Clin Psychiatry* 1991; 52(2):69–76.
105. Sheehan DV, Claycomb JB: The use of MAO inhibitors in clinical practice. In: Manschreck TC (ed): *Psychiatric Medicine Update.* Massachusetts General Hospital Review for Physicians. New York, Elsevier, 1983: 143–162.
106. Sheehan DV, Claycomb JB, Kouretas N: Monoamine oxidase inhibitors: Prescription and patient management. *Int J Psychiatry Med* 1980; 10(2):99–121.
107. Sheehan DV: Traitement des troubles anxieuc par les antidepresseurs. *Actualities Med Int Psychiatrie* 1986; 1(1), suppl:104–123.
108. Sheehan DV, Raj BA: Benzodiazepine treatment of panic disorder. In: Noyes R Jr, Roth M, Burrows GD (eds.): *Handbook of Anxiety*, vol 4: *The Treatment of Anxiety.* Amsterdam, Elsevier Science, 1990: 169–206.
109. Sheehan DV: Benzodiazepines in panic disorder and agoraphobia. *J Affect Disord* 1987; 13:169–181.
110. Sheehan DV, Raj A: Monoamine oxidase inhibitors. In: Last CG, Hersen M (eds): *Handbook of Anxiety Disorders.* Elmsford, NY, Pergamon, 1988: 478–503.

Chapter 119

Iatrogenic Heart Disease and Related Problems

J. Willis Hurst, M.D. ■ *W. Proctor Harvey, M.D.*

Iatrogenic heart disease[1–6] is usually defined as *physician-induced heart disease*. The word *iatrogenic* is derived from two Greek words, *iatros* (physician) and *gignesthai* (to be born, from which is derived the word *genesis*). This simple definition is not adequate because problems other than those caused by physicians are often labeled as iatrogenic disease. Accordingly, it is time to refine and expand the definition or to create a new word that encompasses sources of error other than those caused by physicians.

A REFINED AND EXPANDED DEFINITION

The following discussion supports the concept that the definition of iatrogenic should be refined and expanded. Whereas physicians are involved in all of the problems discussed, their involvement is remote in many of them.

- Nonmedical reporters commonly interpret and report on articles that appear in recent medical journals. Many times, their reports are misleading and the reporters, of course, never realize that they disturb some of their readers and listeners who may assume they have heart disease from the information they receive. These problems can be labeled iatrogenic because the original articles were written by physicians. This seems unfair, because the reporters made the error and improperly influenced the readers or listeners.
- The level of cholesterol and blood pressure can be measured at the grocery store. This often leads the abnormally health conscious person to abuse the opportunity by frequent measurements of his or her blood lipids or blood pressure. When the information is misused or is inaccurate, no one blames the grocery store. Although a physician may have encouraged the development of self-examination, it seems unfair to blame physicians for such errors that result from patient behavior.
- In years past physicians usually functioned alone. Today, physicians often head a team, and although the physicians are ultimately responsible for a patient's care, it is impossible for them to perform or supervise every task and to control the conversation of others who may not appreciate the sensitivity of patients. To blame only the physician without recognizing the problems caused by other personnel seems unfair.
- Certain patients are abnormally susceptible to comments they hear, whereas the same comments may have no effect on other patients.[4] Emotionally stable patients, when told they have heart disease, respond with initial disbelief and may seek another medical opinion in an effort to disprove the initial diagnosis. On the other hand, emotionally unstable patients will accept the physician's statement that there is an unimportant heart murmur as if it were a death sentence. They conclude that the physician is not telling them how seriously damaged their heart really is; they seek other medical opinions, not to clarify the problem, but to obtain and accept the worst assessment of the lot. At times, it is impossible for a physician to say anything that is not misconstrued by the patient. In this situation, it is not proper to

blame only the physician for the problems that emerge.

- Iatrogenic heart disease can be said to be present when a physician diagnoses heart disease in a patient whose heart is normal or when a physician interprets a patient's heart disease as being more serious than it actually is. The word iatrogenic is properly used when either of these events occur.
- In this day of high-technology and therapeutic options there is an increased chance of diagnostic or therapeutic misadventure. Obviously, the use of some diagnostic and therapeutic procedures, including the use of drugs, is associated with a small number of complications even when they are used with great skill. Accordingly, it is necessary to separate the complications that occur despite the use of great professional skill from the complications that occur as a result of professional skill that is less than desirable. The word iatrogenic is properly used when the complications of a diagnostic or therapeutic procedure (including the use of drugs) occur as a result of less desirable professional skill. On the other hand, it is unfair to blame *every* undesired complication on the physician.

If all of the preceding problems are to be labeled as iatrogenic, we must forget the Greek origin of the word; the word must not imply that the physician is solely responsible for the problem. A new understanding of the word must take into account nonphysician sources of information, the large number of individuals who talk to patients, the emotionally disturbed patient who receives all information as "bad news," patients who have been led to believe their heart disease is worse than it is (not simply patients who have no heart disease but have been misdiagnosed as having heart disease), and diagnostic and therapeutic misadventures.

THE CREATION OF A NEW WORD

A wordsmith might create a word like *erraregenic* heart disease to imply that the original source of the trouble was some sort of an error (the word *error* is derived from the Latin word *errare*). Such a word highlights the fact that the fault is not *always* due to a physician. Should such a word be accepted, the circumstances would be analyzed to determine where the specific fault lay.

Recognizing that the new word is not likely to be accepted and used, we have based the following discussion on the refined and expanded definition of the word iatrogenic.

IATROGENIC HEART DISEASE PRODUCED BY DRUGS, PROCEDURES, AND OPERATIONS

Drugs

All drugs can produce undesirable side effects. The physician must discuss the likelihood of their occurrence with the patient whenever drugs are prescribed. When treating a patient, the physician must weigh the value of a drug with its complications against the danger of the disease when the drug is not used. When should the undesired side effects of drug treatment be labeled iatrogenic? The side effects can be labeled as being iatrogenic when the physician is not aware that the the undesired side effects of a drug outweigh the value of the drug in treating a disease that is self-limited or when another less toxic drug could be used. The word iatrogenic can also be used when a physician fails to recognize the undesirable effect of a drug but persists in continuing the drug.

All drugs used to control cardiac arrhythmias may produce cardiac arrhythmias. The proarrhythmic effect of antiarrhythmic drugs can, in fact, be lethal. (See also Chap. 38.)

Drugs used to control systemic hypertension can produce postural hypotension, syncope, and cardiac arrhythmias (mostly bradyarrhythmias). (See also Chap. 77.)

Nitrates given for angina pectoris may cause postural hypotension and syncope. (See also Chap. 30.)

Beta-blocking drugs used for angina or hypertension may precipitate the "sick-sinus syndrome," atrioventricular block, heart failure, and postural hypotension. (See also Chap. 66.)

Calcium channel-blocking drugs given for angina pectoris or hypertension may produce cardiovascular problems. Verapamil may contribute to the development of sick-sinus syndrome and atrioventricular block and decreased myocardial contractility. Nifedipine may aggravate angina pectoris in a small percentage of patients and, under certain circumstances, may decrease myocardial contractility. Diltiazem may also produce a decrease in contractility and bradyarrhythmia secondary to marked sinus node slowing. Caution should be exercised when combining beta blockers and diltiazem or verapamil since underlying conduction system disease such as sick-sinus syndrome may be made manifest. (See also Chap. 67.)

Diuretics such as furosemide, ethacrynic acid, chlorothiazide, and hydrochlorothiazide, which produce potassium and magnesium loss by the kidneys, may precipitate cardiac arrhythmias. Patients who take diuretics that spare the loss of potassium may develop hyperkalemia and its serious cardiac complications, especially if they continue to take potassium chloride or if renal function deteriorates. (See also Chaps. 29 and 36.)

Acetylsalicylic acid (aspirin) given to decrease the incidence of transient ischemic attacks or to prevent coronary thrombosis may produce serious gastrointestinal bleeding. (See also Chap. 68.)

Thrombolytic agents such as streptokinase or tissue plasminogen activator (tPA) may produce cerebral hemorrhage. (See also Chap. 69.)

Digitalis may produce ventricular arrhythmias and atrioventricular block. When a diuretic that produces potassium loss is given to a patient receiving digitalis, the stage is set for many arrhythmias, including atrial tachycardia with atrioventricular block and ventricular tachycardia. (See also Chap. 27.)

Tricyclic drugs given to patients with psychiatric

problems may produce bundle branch block. Doxorubicin and daunorubicin given for neoplastic disease may produce cardiomyopathy. (See also Chaps. 88 and 110.)

Procedures and Operations

The *misinterpretation of the electrocardiogram* continues to be a major cause of iatrogenic heart disease. Some patients seem compelled to ask technicians, "What does it show?" Some technicians are virtually obsessed with giving an answer, which may, in a susceptible patient, lead to iatrogenic heart disease.

A physician may not realize that serious coronary disease can be present and the electrocardiogram can remain normal. On the other hand, certain abnormalities in the electrocardiogram may mislead the inexperienced physician to state that the patient has had a myocardial infarction when in reality the tracing shows the configuration of the Wolff-Parkinson-White abnormality or some other pseudoinfarct pattern.

Exercise electrocardiography may yield results that stimulate a physician to state that coronary disease is present. Every physician must remember that false-positive responses for ischemia occur in 10 percent of middle-aged males who have positive responses and that false-positive responses occur in about 50 percent of young women who have positive responses.

The *computer interpretation* and "read-out" of electrocardiograms have created enormous problems. The patient or an inexperienced physician may read the computer interpretation and fail to realize that the computer interpretation is often incorrect. At the time of this writing elected public officials have decreed that the computer can interpret electrocardiograms. Let it be stated—loud and clear—that computers cannot read electrocardiograms.

New *technology* always brings a new array of misinterpretations that may lead to iatrogenic heart disease. A decrease in ejection fraction with exercise determined by *technetium ventriculography* in a 70-year-old inactive male may be due to aging rather than coronary artery disease. An anterior septal reperfusion abnormality determined by a *thallium stress test* may be due to isolated left bundle block rather than coronary atherosclerosis. (See also Chap. 134.) Unimportant catheter-induced coronary spasm may be misinterpreted as being due to obstructive coronary disease. The misuse of the results of *echocardiography* is a common cause of iatrogenic heart disease. The echo-Doppler identification of minor amounts of valve regurgitation may lead the physician to diagnose aortic, mitral, pulmonic, and tricuspid regurgitation when none is present. (This phenomenon may occur in normal persons.) (See also Chap. 130.) Topping the list of misadventures is the physician's improper explanation of the presence of minor degrees of mitral valve prolapse. (See also Chap. 80.)

The insertion of a *Swan-Ganz catheter* may cause thrombophlebitis, pulmonary embolism, and cardiac arrhythmias.

Radiation of the chest for neoplastic disease may be followed by constrictive pericarditis, accelerated coronary atherosclerosis, and myocardial disease.

The expected complications of *cardiac surgical procedures* are discussed in the chapters dealing with the specific operations.

IATROGENIC HEART DISEASE PRODUCED BY THE MISINTERPRETATION OF CLINICAL INFORMATION

Much could be written about the misinterpretation of symptoms. Perhaps the most common problem in this regard is assuming a patient has or does not have coronary disease from the interpretation of the history of chest pain. Skilled cardiologists have learned that their error rate is considerable.

The results of the physician's examination may be misinterpreted or overemphasized. Suppose a systolic click is heard at the apex. This may lead reflexly to ordering an echocardiogram and to an excessively long or weighty discussion about the problems of mitral valve prolapse. Whereas most patients have no symptoms from the benign variety of mitral valve prolapse, an improper explanation of the condition may cause iatrogenic heart disease. Seasoned consultants cannot always erase the fear that has been engendered by the initial discussion of the condition. The emotionally disturbed patient may even thank the physician for finding such a terrible condition while commenting that all the previous physicians simply missed the diagnosis and were uninformed because they attributed the symptoms to anxiety. The following case report by W. P. H. makes still another point. In this patient an imagined systolic click led to iatrogenic heart disease.

A 31-year-old single woman, who was a respected and successful businesswoman, was referred for cardiovascular evaluation because of symptoms of weakness, a feeling of faintness, palpitation, and periods of chest discomfort. She also had discomfort (numbness) in her left upper extremity that also involved her left hand and fingers.

When first evaluated by her physician over 1 year earlier, she was told she had mitral valve prolapse. An echocardiogram was reported to her as showing mitral valve prolapse. She also related that she was informed that she had systolic click(s) of the mitral valve, and on follow-up visits to her physician she was told that this auscultatory evidence was detected each time.

Other studies including routine laboratory work, electrocardiograms, and x-rays of her heart and lungs were normal. Her symptoms continued and became more frequent and bothersome.

Subsequently, she was seen for evaluation in our hospital as an outpatient. The physical examination indicated normal findings. Her blood pressure was also normal and without postural hypotension. The examination of her heart was normal. No click(s), murmurs, or gallop sounds were present despite the examiner's looking specifically for them in various positions, including sitting, standing, squatting supine, and the left lateral position. Her previous echocardiogram(s) performed at the other hospital were not available. Repeat echocardiograms at our institution (two dimensional and M mode) were obtained and carefully and specifically searched for evidence of mitral valve prolapse; none was found. Thus, the clinical diagnosis of no heart disease was supported.

Her true diagnosis was obtained as follows. During the physical examination she was asked to hyperventilate. Shortly after starting to hyperventilate, she became anxious and weak and had chest discomfort and dizziness. She also experienced numbness in her upper extremities, particularly in the left arm and hand. Bilateral carpopedal spasm developed, and she was told to stop hyperventilating. She stated these symptoms reproduced those she thought were due to her mitral valve prolapse.

The diagnosis of hyperventilation syndrome, which explained her symptoms, was thereby made. She was reassured that mitral valve prolapse was not present and that she had no heart disease. This was welcome news to her, since she had believed that she had a serious heart condition. The mechanism of her hyperventilation was explained to her, as well as measures of prevention of future attacks.

IATROGENIC PROBLEMS AND DISABILITY PRODUCED BY PREVENTIVE AND REHABILITATIVE EFFORTS

Paul Dudley White did much to dispel the notion that hard work caused coronary artery disease. In fact, he believed the opposite. As time passed, scientific studies supported his view. Four decades ago a patient with myocardial infarction was placed on strict bed rest for several weeks and was not permitted to return to work for several months. Unnecessary retirement was commonplace. This type of iatrogenic disability is less common today but it still occurs.

There are patients who are *cholesterol level fanatics.* Their serum cholesterol may be 180 mg/dL or less, yet they have their blood cholesterol level determined several times each year. They remain on a strict low-cholesterol, low-fat diet, and most of their conversation with others relates to the subject. To eat a meal with them becomes a lecture on their will power. Such people are, in fact, emotionally disabled. The physician is usually unable to diminish the patients' obsession with the subject even when their coronary arteriograms are normal at the age of 70.

There are patients who are *exercise fanatics.* They exercise excessively in an effort to prevent heart disease, and should they have a myocardial infarction, they spend most of their time in a rehabilitation program. Rehabilitation programs are superb for many patients, but a few patients overuse them and spend most of their time in rehabilitation routines. When this occurs, they become rehabilitation cripples. Their rehabilitation process rehabilitates them to spend more time in the rehabilitation process. When this occurs, rehabilitation has failed because a successful program should encourage the patient to participate in many activities—mental and physical. Such behavior by a patient is not solely the physician's fault, but the physician involved should make every effort to lead the patient to a more realistic type of rehabilitation. The following brief case report by J. W. H. makes the point:

Mr. Smith, a man in his late sixties, had mitral valve replacement for severe mitral regurgitation due to myxomatous degeneration of the mitral valve. Prior to cardiac surgery he had heart failure and atrial fibrillation. His blood pressure was 120/80 mmHg, his serum cholesterol was 190 mg/dL, and his coronary arteriogram was normal. After uneventful mitral valve replacement, he entered a rehabilitation program.

When he visits the office, he brings many records showing his blood cholesterol level, his exercise progress, and many sophisticated measurements that show he is doing well. Any effort on my part (J. W. H.) to suggest that maybe he is overdoing it is met with an extended discussion of the exercise program and the details of his diet. He is disabled because his every thought centers on his rehabilitation program. He smiles and waits for me to congratulate him on his will power. I sit bewildered as to why he had an exercise stress test performed when he is on digitalis for atrial fibrillation.

THE PREVENTION OF IATROGENIC HEART DISEASE

Our goal should be to eliminate the following: the undersired effects of cardiac drugs and the complications of diagnostic and therapeutic procedures; the misinterpretation of symptoms, physical signs, and results of diagnostic testing; and the improper use of preventive measures. It is unrealistic to believe that such a worthy goal can be reached, but we must try.

We must be aware of the words that cause anxiety in patients and the words that comfort patients. The following essay, entitled "Words: Good and Bad," by J. W. H., illustrates the distinction. It is reproduced here with permission from the publisher.[7]

Words can produce comfort to patients or they can frighten patients. Words can lead patients to be happy or push them to a state of despair and depression. Words used by physicians and other health personnel may be more destructive to the peace of mind of patients than the much-discussed machines that belong to this era of high technology.

Words are designed to convey the thoughts of one person to another person. We must realize their impact on patients and should check to be certain the words that have been used have not been misinterpreted. The list of words below illustrates the point:

WORDS THAT ARE HARMFUL

"You have a 'dead zone' in your heart." This sentence may be uttered after the physician has inspected the electrocardiogram, viewed the results of radionuclide scan or studied the left ventriculogram of a patient who has had a myocardial infarction.

Many patients react unfavorably to the word "dead." Obviously, no one likes to believe any part of the body is dead.

"Your echocardiogram shows what I thought. You remember I said you had a systolic click and late systolic murmur. Your echo shows marked prolapse of the mitral valve." This statement can frighten patients. The word "prolapse" is often interpreted as having an ominous meaning.

"You have heart failure." This sentence is commonly used after the physician finds evidence of pump dysfunction. The patients may interpret such words as meaning the heart will soon stop beating. Many patients live in great fear after hearing such words.

"You have digitalis intoxication." Many patients wonder about the seriousness of this problem. It is, at times, serious but patients may interpret the word "intoxication" to be far more serious than the physician means it to be.

"You must be admitted to the coronary care unit because you may have a serious rhythm disturbance." These words, followed by a hasty action, may lead patients to believe that they are surely dying.

"This aortic graft may last you 5 years." The patient may interpret this as meaning the graft will burst in 5 years.

"The survival curve for patients like you shows that 80% of the patients are alive at 5 years." The patient may interpret this sentence as meaning that he or she will live only 5 years.

"The equipment broke down again." This sentence makes the patient feel insecure and anxious.

"Mr. Brown, please move over." "Mr. Smith, do you feel well?" "Mr. Jones, hold your breath." "Don't move, Mr. Johnson." When these sentences are said to the *same* patient by the physician or technician the patient feels dehumanized.

WORDS THAT ARE HELPFUL

"You have an area of tough scar tissue in your heart. The heart attack you had has healed with some scar tissue. We have made some progress in our attempts to prevent heart attacks and we will apply this knowledge to you." Something like this can be said to a patient after a heart attack. The words *dead tissue* need not be used.

"You have a common condition of the heart valve. As a rule, it is of little importance. I am happy to state that it is not serious in your case." An echocardiogram need not be done in all patients with a midsystolic click and late apical systolic murmur.

"You have some congestion in your lungs and we will add some medication to assist the pumping action of your heart." This statement is less frightening than using the term heart failure.

"You are experiencing some of the side effects of digitalis, indicating that we must adjust the dosage for you." All drugs produce undesired effects and the words "digitalis intoxication" or "digitalis poisoning" seem inappropriate and unduly frightening.

"We will place you in the safe environment of the coronary care unit. The nurses are especially trained to make observations. It is a very safe place, you should be there about two days and your rehabilitation will begin there. You see, I expect you to return to work." Three points are made in this "conversation." The word "safe" is used. Patients react favorably to this word. The expected amount of time in the coronary care unit is stated indicating the patient should not be there a large number of days. Finally, rehabilitation and return to work are emphasized.

"We have made a lot of progress in the field and most aortic grafts last a long time." The duration of graft patency should be discussed very carefully or the patient will live in unwarranted fear.

"Recent studies show that the operation places you in a much better position as far as your future is concerned." This statement gives the patient an open-ended and optimistic view of the future, whereas the mention of survival curves and the percentage of survivors at a specific point in time are frightening to the patient.

"I will have the equipment checked. These days, specially trained people keep our equipment running properly." To say, "Our equipment has broken down again" is not necessary. The patient should not share in previous unrelated experiences that are described by a frustrated person.

"Mr. Brown, please hold your breath a moment. Thank you. Mr. Brown, move a little to the side now. Thank you. You are good at following instructions. Are you comfortable?" This conversation indicates the patient's proper name is used consistently and, in addition, a note of concern is shown by the person who is performing the test on Mr. Brown.

The following suggestions by W. P. H. will bring comfort to patients and their families.

Some cardiovascular disease terms, or conversations, should be avoided in the presence of patients. "Decomp." can be used instead of "heart failure." Many patients associate the term "gallop" with a dire event because they remember it was used for "galloping consumption," "gallop" denoting severe and rapid progression. We should say: "S_3, S_4, VDG, ADG."

I have also learned to explain to my patients that when the ECG term *block* is used, it is an electrical description, and does not connote blockage of blood in the heart or circulation. An experienced registered nurse instructor was referred for evaluation because she had developed left bundle branch block on her electrocardiogram. Upon examination she appeared unusually concerned and nervous. I said, "I'll bet you might be thinking that 'bundle branch block' means a 'blockage of blood.'" She said "Yes." I assured her that this was not so. She said, "Thank God, I thought this meant I was likely to have sudden death in the near future." This was 12 years ago and she is still doing well.

With patients having valve prolapse, I stress the good aspects and prognosis of this common cardiac lesion. Avoid bringing up the rare dire complication of sudden death (unless the patient has been aware of this or, of course, if the patient is unnecessarily frightened by this possibility). Make a point to explain that about 90 percent of patients need no treatment except an explanation and reassurance.

Because the patient is in contact with personnel other than the physician, it is useful to discuss periodically the problem of iatrogenic heart disease with the staff.

Finally, physicians should ask their patients to relate their perceptions of their problems to them after the physicians have discussed the conditions with them. By this act physicians can at least clear up any misperception patients have regarding their cardiovascular problems.

REFERENCES

1. Auerback A, Gliebe PA: Iatrogenic heart disease; common cardiac neurosis. *JAMA* 1945; 129:338–341.
2. Weinberg HB: Iatrogenic heart disease. *Ann Intern Med* 1953; 38:9–22.
3. Hart AD: Iatrogenics and cardiac neurosis—Critique. *JAMA* 1954; 156:1133–1138.
4. Wheeler EO, Williamson CR, Cohen ME: Heart scare, heart surveys, and iatrogenic heart disease; emotional and symptomatological effects of suggesting to one hundred sixty-two adults that they might have heart disease. *JAMA* 1958; 167:1096–1102.
5. Harrison TR, Reeves TJ: The psychologic management of patients with cardiac disease. *Am Heart J* 1965; 70:136–138.
6. Sevin BH: Mitral valve prolapse, panic states, and anxiety. *Psychiatr Clin North Am* 1987; 10:141–150.
7. Hurst JW: Words—good and bad. *Am J Cardiol* 1984; 54:444–445.

PART XVII

Environmental Factors and the Cardiovascular System

Chapter 120

The Influence of Environmental Factors on the Cardiovascular System

Robert F. Grover, M.D., Ph.D. ■ John T. Reeves, M.D.
Loring B. Rowell, Ph.D. ■ Claude A. Piantadosi, M.D.
Herbert A. Saltzman, M.D.

Cardiovascular function is regulated to preserve two vital functions, tissue oxygenation and normal body temperature. For example, during muscular exercise, the oxygen supply to the working muscles must be increased, and concurrently the increased heat generated must be dissipated. Humans are often subjected to environmental factors that stress cardiovascular regulation severely. Exposure to the atmospheric hypoxia of high altitude reduces muscular working capacity in spite of major adaptations to preserve tissue oxygenation. In hot environments, temperature regulation must compete with increased demands for oxygen during exercise, and here again, working capacity is reduced. Regrettably, our environment is now frequently contaminated with noxious substances, one of the most lethal of which is carbon monoxide. Here, artificial manipulation of the patient's environment by means of hyperbaric oxygen may assist in preserving tissue oxygenation and thereby be lifesaving. To the patient with cardiovascular disease, adaptation to such environmental stresses as heat, cold, or the hypoxia of high altitude becomes an even greater challenge. We shall examine how the body meets these challenges.

HIGH ALTITUDE

Each year millions of people visit the mountainous regions of the western United States for recreation. With modern transportation, rapid ascent to resort areas at 8000 to 9500 ft in altitude is a common occurrence. Major highways cross mountain passes above 11,000 ft, and during the summer season, half a million people drive to the summits of Pike's Peak and Mt. Evans, both exceeding 14,000 ft (4267 m). Just how severe is the stress of such altitudes?

To begin with, ascent to high altitude means exposure to a decrease in total atmospheric pressure and a parallel decrease in the partial pressure of oxygen (P_{O_2}) we breathe. At sea level, the inspired P_{O_2} is 150 mmHg; it is 125 mmHg at 5000 ft (1524 m), 100 mmHg at 10,000 ft (3048 m), and about 80 mmHg at 14,000 ft (4267 m). This is the atmospheric hypoxia to which people are exposed in the Rocky Mountains.

Circulatory Oxygen Transport

Arterial Oxygenation

Within the lung, the inspired P_{O_2} is lowered by the presence of carbon dioxide and water vapor. Furthermore, there is imperfect matching of blood flow to regional ventilation. Consequently, the arterial P_{O_2} perfusing the body, which ranges from about 80 to 90 mmHg at sea level, is reduced to 45 to 50 mmHg at 14,000 ft (4267 m).

Although the arterial P_{O_2} on the summit of Pike's Peak

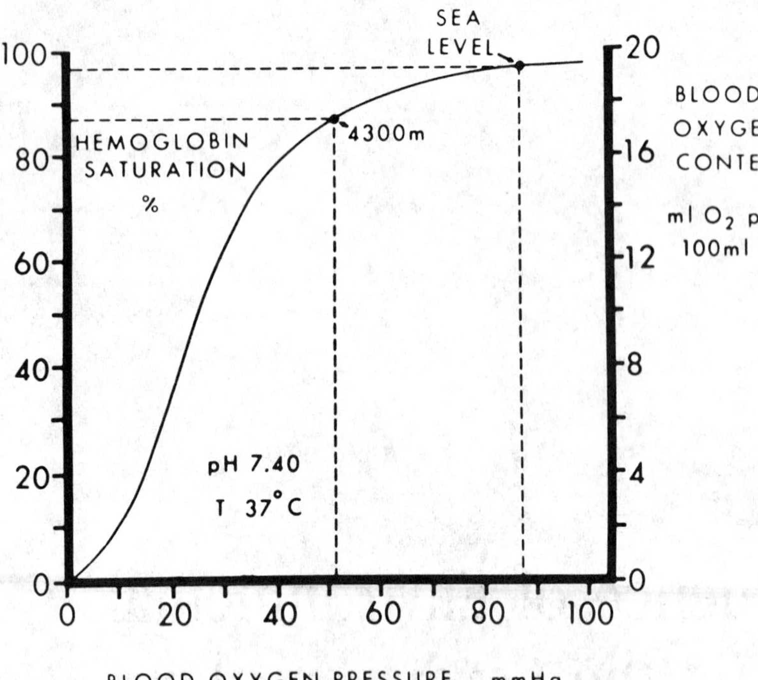

FIGURE 120-1 As a consequence of the sigmoid shape of the hemoglobin-oxygen dissociation curve, the large decrease in arterial oxygen pressure (tension) on ascent from sea level to 14,000 ft (4300 m) in altitude results in only a small decrease in hemoglobin saturation and blood oxygen content. [*From RF Grover: Man living at high altitudes. In: JD Ives, RG Barry (eds): Arctic and Alpine Environments, London, Methuen, 1974: 822. Reproduced with permission of the publisher and author.*]

is only half as great as at sea level, this does not mean that the quantity of oxygen in the blood has been reduced to one-half. That is because of the nonlinear oxygen-binding characteristics of hemoglobin. The relation between oxygen tension and oxygen saturation is defined by the hemoglobin-oxygen dissociation curve (Fig. 120-1). From this it can be seen that following adaptation to 14,000 ft (4267 m), the arterial oxygen saturation is still 85 percent compared with 95 percent at sea level. Thus, a 50 percent decrease in arterial P_{O_2} causes only a 10 percent reduction in saturation. At the more modest altitudes at which the tourist and ski resorts are situated, the fall in saturation is even less. The moderate nature of this hypoxemia should be emphasized, since many of our concepts regarding high altitude are based on much more severe hypoxic tests.

The effect of a decrease in saturation on the actual amount of oxygen in the blood (arterial O_2 content) depends on the hemoglobin concentration. With a normal hemoglobin of 15 g/dL, when saturation falls to 85 percent, the arterial O_2 content is reduced from 19 to 17 mL/dL (Fig. 120-1). Within the first few hours or days at high altitude, however, plasma volume decreases while total red blood cell mass initially remains unchanged.[1] Consequently, hematocrit rises, and with it hemoglobin concentration, which increases the O_2-carrying capacity of the blood. This offsets the fall in saturation and restores the arterial O_2 content to preascent values (Fig. 120-2). In other words, after a week at high altitude, even though the saturation is 85 percent, the quantity of oxygen in 100 mL of blood (milliliters of oxygen per deciliter) has been restored to normal. Even during heavy

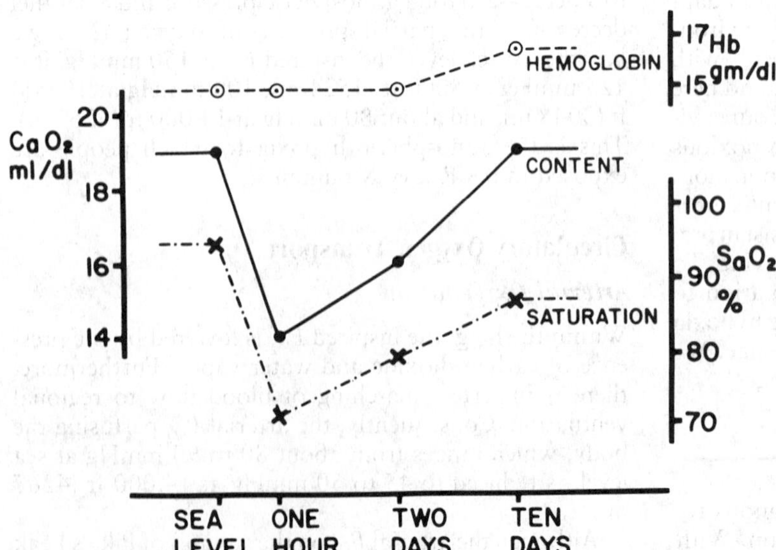

FIGURE 120-2 Arterial blood oxygenation during adaptation to high altitude. Following the initial fall, arterial saturation (S_aO_2) improves with increasing ventilation. Concurrently, hemoconcentration increases hemoglobin (Hb) concentration and hence the O_2-carrying capacity of the blood. The net result is restoration of arterial O_2 content (C_aO_2) to preascent values.

exercise at altitude, arterial O_2 content is well maintained because there is further hemoconcentration, which tends to offset the added decrease in saturation.[2] True polycythemia, reflecting an increase in total red blood cell mass resulting from bone marrow stimulation, begins to appear after about 10 days but requires many weeks of residence at altitudes high enough to cause a sustained reduction in arterial saturation before a new plateau in red cell mass is established.[3]

Cardiac Output

Since the transport of oxygen by the circulation depends not only on the quantity of oxygen in each unit of blood (arterial O_2 content) but also on the number of these units of blood pumped by the heart per minute, i.e., cardiac output, let us examine the latter, including its components, heart rate (HR) and stroke volume. With ascent to high altitude, HR increases[4] as a result of hypoxic stimulation of the sympathetic nervous system but with no change in parasympathetic activity.[4] This tachycardia increases cardiac output, which offsets initial hypoxemia and preserves oxygen transport; however, this early tachycardia may not be sustained. Within a day or two, resting HR returns to preascent values, and even the tachycardia of exercise may diminish[4] (Fig. 120-3). Surprisingly, cardiac stroke volume also decreases by as much as 25 percent during the first week at high altitude.[1] As a result of these circulatory adjustments, cardiac output, both at rest and during exercise, plateaus at levels about 20 percent below the corresponding values at sea level[1] (Fig. 120-3). Consequently, even though the quantity of O_2 in the arterial blood has been restored to normal by hemoconcentration, the amount of O_2 transported to the body is now reduced by the low cardiac output (Fig. 120-4). For the body to remain normally oxygenated, extraction of O_2 from arterial blood must be increased. Direct measurements in normal humans, both at rest and during exercise, confirm this increase in extraction (widening of the arteriovenous difference in blood O_2 content).[1]

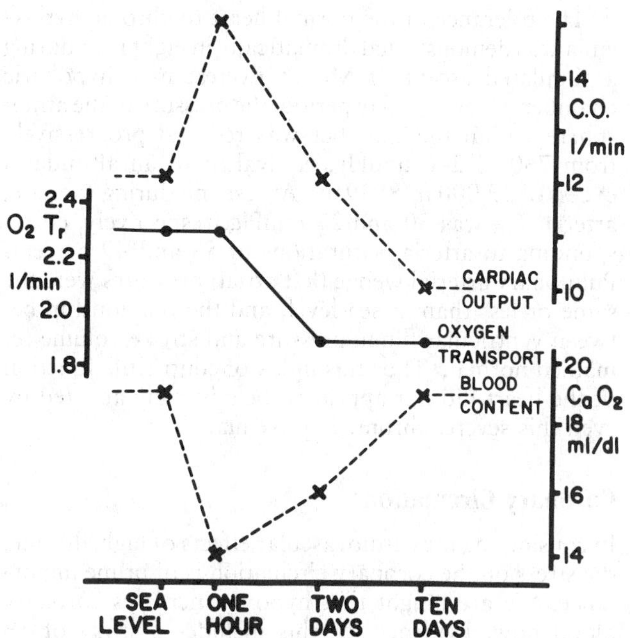

FIGURE 120-4 Oxygen transport (O_2Tr) by the systemic circulation during submaximal exercise. Upon ascent to high altitude, the fall in arterial blood O_2 content (C_aO_2) is offset by an increase in cardiac output (CO). Although C_aO_2 is restored within 10 days, the fall in CO to subnormal levels results in a net reduction in O_2Tr, which then requires a greater O_2 extraction from the blood to preserve O_2 delivery.

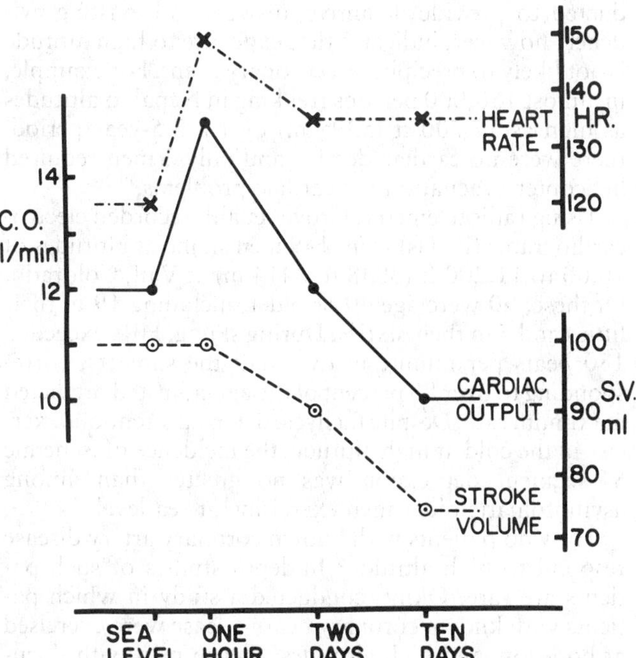

FIGURE 120-3 Time course of alterations in exercise heart rate (HR), stroke volume (SV), and cardiac output (CO) during adaptation to high altitude. After 10 days, CO is subnormal because of a significant decrease in SV.

Myocardial Function

By what mechanism does stroke volume decrease? Observations made with M-mode echocardiography in normal individuals demonstrated a progressive decrease in both end-diastolic and end-systolic diameters of the left ventricular chamber over the first week at high altitude.[5] Volumes calculated from these diameters indicated a progressive decrease in stroke volume that was highly correlated with the decrease in end-diastolic volume while ejection fraction remained normal.

Initially, the decline in diastolic volume appears to reflect the reduction in blood volume from hemoconcentration. Stroke volume, however, remains decreased even after several weeks when true polycythemia has restored blood volume to preascent values. During this period of adaptation, circulating norepinephrine and systemic vascular resistance rise, suggesting that ventricular afterload may now be suppressing stroke volume. All indices of contractility remain normal,[5] indicating that myocardial function is not compromised at moderate or even very high altitude. Hence, the decrease in stroke volume reflects the operation of normal physiogenic mechanisms rather than any impairment of myocardial function.

The tolerance of the normal heart to chronic hypoxemia was demonstrated dramatically in eight men during a simulated ascent of Mount Everest in a hypobaric chamber. Over a 40-day period, the pressure of the atmosphere within the chamber was reduced progressively from 760 to 240 mmHg, equivalent to an altitude in excess of 29,000 ft (8839 m). At rest and during exercise, arterial P_{O_2} was 30 and 27 mmHg, respectively, corresponding to arterial saturations of 58 and 49 percent. Pulmonary arterial wedge (left atrial) pressures were the same or less than at sea level, and the relationship between ventricular filling pressure and stroke volume remained normal.[6] Thus this index of contractile function of the heart did not appear to be adversely affected by even this severe, chronic hypoxemia.

Coronary Circulation

In considering the cardiovascular effects of high altitude, the stress on the coronary circulation is of prime importance. We are taught that hypoxia increases coronary blood flow. Evidence for this includes a study of 19 young men in whom breathing 10 percent O_2 nearly doubled coronary blood flow.[7] However, breathing 10 percent O_2 at sea level yields inspired O_2 tensions equivalent to sudden exposure to 18,000 ft (5486 m), so such evidence does not apply directly to tourists ascending to 10,000 ft (3048 m) over several days. Here, again, the situation becomes clear when one thinks in terms of oxygen transport.

Oxygenation of the myocardium requires a balance between demand and supply. The primary determinants of demand are HR, systolic pressure (the so-called double product), and myocardial contractility. (See also Chap. 5.) Ascent to high altitude increases myocardial O_2 demand, primarily through increased HR. Such increased demand must be met by an increase in O_2 supply. In general, this is accomplished by increasing coronary blood flow, since O_2 extraction from the coronary arterial blood (coronary arteriovenous O_2 difference) is always nearly maximal. If the altitude is sufficiently high to lower saturation and arterial O_2 content as well, less O_2 will be available for extraction, and compensation requires even greater flow. Hence, with initial ascent to high altitude, coronary blood flow will be increased in proportion to the increase in HR and the decrease in arterial saturation.

Increase in Oxygen Extraction

Within a few days at high altitude, HR will decrease and arterial O_2 content will be restored by hemoconcentration (Figs. 120-2 and 120-3). Both adjustments will tend to return coronary flow to preascent levels. In addition, a third important but subtle factor that permits coronary flow to decrease even further operates. This is a decrease in the affinity of hemoglobin for O_2, which is another aspect of adaptation to high altitude. Within the red blood cell, the concentration of 2,3-diphosphoglycerate (2,3-DPG) increases, producing a "right shift" in the hemoglobin dissociation curve,[8] lowering the saturation at any given tension. Because of the sigmoid shape of the dissociation curve, this right shift has little effect on arterial O_2 loading; however, it facilitates O_2 unloading from peripheral capillary blood.

Normal Decrease in Coronary Blood Flow

The coronary circulation is regulated to maintain the coronary sinus P_{O_2} constant at 18 mmHg. The corresponding saturation will be lowered from 34 percent at sea level to 22 percent at 10,200 ft (3109 m) as a consequence of the right shift in the dissociation curve.[9] Consequently, O_2 extraction from the coronary blood will increase significantly (wider coronary arteriovenous O_2 difference),[9] and less coronary blood flow will be needed to supply the myocardial O_2 requirements (Fig. 120-5). Literally, the right shift in the dissociation curve *permits* coronary flow to decrease. Direct measurements in normal humans studied first at sea level and again after adaptation to high altitude show a consistent decrease in coronary flow, both at rest and during exercise.[9] A decrease in coronary flow at high altitude is surprising but entirely consistent with the operation of normal physiological mechanisms designed to preserve the constancy of myocardial tissue P_{O_2} (coronary sinus P_{O_2}). The decrease in coronary flow is required to prevent a rise in coronary sinus P_{O_2}. There is no evidence of myocardial ischemia or hypoxia. Neither is there any impairment to increasing coronary flow when required to meet increased O_2 demands, as during exercise.

Coronary Artery Disease

Does visiting high altitude pose a special risk for the patient with coronary artery disease? How do you advise the 55-year-old man from Atlanta who is contemplating a skiing vacation to Colorado? These are very practical questions, but well-controlled studies have not been conducted to provide definitive answers. All existing evidence, however, indicates that exposure to high altitude is not likely to precipitate a coronary event. For example, in almost 150,000 persons trekking in Nepal to altitudes as high as 17,700 ft (5395 m) over a 3.5-year period, there were no cardiac deaths, and only 3 men required helicopter evacuation for cardiac problems.[10]

Using radiotelemetry, Grover et al.[11] recorded electrocardiograms (ECGs) from 149 men skiing at altitudes of 10,00 to 11,200 ft (3048 to 3414 m) at Vail, Colorado. Of these, 90 were age 40 or older, including 19 in their fifties and 5 in their sixties. During skiing, HRs exceeded 150 beats per minute in over half the subjects, corresponding to over 80 percent of the age-adjusted predicted maximum rate. Despite tachycardia from strenuous exercise in the cold at high altitude, the incidence of ischemic ST-segment depression was no greater than among asymptomatic older men exercising at sea level.

How do patients with known coronary artery disease respond to high altitude? In-depth studies of such patients are rare. Okin[12] conducted a study in which patients with known coronary heart disease were exercised at both low and high altitudes. Eleven men with documented previous myocardial infarction and/or angina performed a standardized step test, first at their resident altitude of 5200 ft (1585 m), and again after driving into the mountains to 8000 ft (2438 m) and then to 10,400

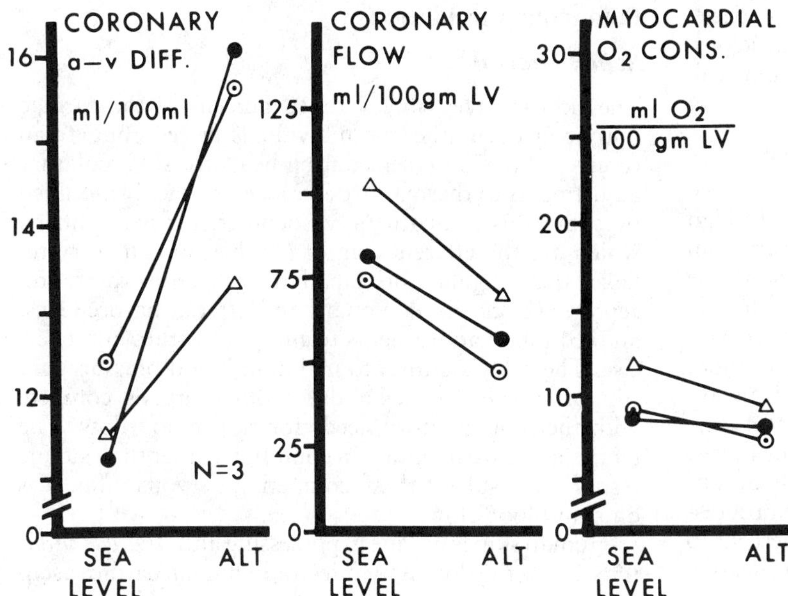

FIGURE 120-5 Alterations in the coronary circulation of the normal human heart following adaptation to 10,200 ft in altitude. Oxygen extraction from coronary blood increases, i.e., there is a significant widening of the coronary arteriovenous difference in O_2 content. This permits coronary flow (Q_{cor}) to decrease while maintaining myocardial O_2 consumption unaltered. [*From RF Grover: Mechanisms augmenting coronary arterial oxygen extraction. In: JHK Vogel (ed): Myocardial infarction—A New Look at an Old Subject. (Advances in Cardiology, vol 9.) Basel/New York, S. Karger, 1973; 97. Reproduced with permission of the publisher and author.*]

ft. Although HR during exercise was greater at the higher altitudes (70 percent of predicted maximum based on age), no patient who had a normal Master's test at 5200 ft (1585 m) had a positive Master's test at higher altitude, and no patient developed symptoms at higher altitude they did not have at 5200 ft (1585 m). Hence ischemic changes could not be produced in these patients with known coronary heart disease despite ascent from 5200 ft (1585 m) to 8000 (2438 m) and 10,400 ft (3170 m).

In another study,[13] a hypobaric chamber was employed to simulate ascent to high altitude. Thirty men with proven stabilized ischemic heart disease performed a double Master's two-step exercise test at sea level. Within a week they entered a decompression chamber and over 10 min were taken to a simulated altitude of 15,000 ft (4572 m). After 40 min of rest, they repeated the exercise test; they were then returned to ground level. None of the subjects manifested any symptoms or arrhythmias during exercise testing at ground level or in the decompression chamber. The response to the Master's test was positive in 17 of the subjects at sea level and increased slightly to 20 at simulated altitude.

Considering the available evidence, given a patient with stable coronary artery disease and a reasonably good exercise tolerance at sea level, there is no justification for advising such a patient to avoid travel to high altitude.

Paradoxically, prolonged residence at high altitude may actually reduce mortality from coronary heart disease. Mortimer et al.[14] analyzed age-adjusted mortality rates for atherosclerotic heart disease in populations living at different altitudes in New Mexico. For males, although not for females, mortality rates declined progressively from low to high altitude; the rate above 6500 ft (1981 m) was only 72 percent of the rate below 3700 ft (1128 m). This decline in rate was not explained by ethnic or socioeconomic factors and was concluded to be a true consequence of the higher altitude. The increased vascularity of the myocardium[15] in high-altitude residents may be a protective factor. In addition, left ventricular work may actually be less in high-altitude residents because of lower systemic arterial blood pressure[16] and lower heart rate.

Pulmonary Circulation

Pulmonary Hypertension

Airway hypoxia stimulates pulmonary vasoconstriction, but when hypoxia is induced acutely, alveolar P_{O_2} must be reduced below 70 mmHg before a significant rise in pulmonary arterial pressure is seen.[17] This means that with ascent to high altitude, little or no pulmonary hypertension would be observed in the visitor to altitudes below 10,000 ft (3048 m). When the airway hypoxia is sustained for months, however, as during residence at high altitude, impressive pulmonary hypertension does develop.[17] Among residents of Leadville, Colorado, living at 10,200 ft (3109 m), resting pulmonary arterial pressures on the average are twice as high as those of individuals living at sea level. Mean pressures range from 11 to 45 mmHg at rest and frequently exceed 60 mmHg during exercise.[17] This increased work load on the right ventricle is reflected in the ECG as a rightward shift in the mean QRS axis and right ventricular enlargement.[18] Although these findings differ from those usually encountered in normal sea level residents, the pulmonary hypertension of high altitude is generally benign, nonprogressive, and reversible with descent to lower altitude. Hence, it should not be considered cardiovascular disease, and the term *cor pulmonale,* if used, is misleading.

In special circumstances, the hypoxic pulmonary hypertension of high altitude may not be entirely benign. It may delay the usual postnatal resolution of the normally high pulmonary arterial pressure in the fetus[19] and result in "persistent fetal circulation" of the newborn that may be fatal.[20] Although high-altitude pulmonary hypertension appears well tolerated by the human right ventricle, it becomes so severe in cattle that heart failure develops, and the resulting edema produces what cattle raisers call *brisket disease.*[21]

High-Altitude Pulmonary Edema

Although the vast majority of people ascending to high altitude experience no pulmonary problems (apart from an awareness of the normal increase in ventilation), the occasional individual will develop acute high-altitude pulmonary edema (HAPE). The incidence is between 1 and 10 per 10,000 persons ascending rapidly to altitudes above 8000 ft (2438 m).[22,23] Symptoms almost always appear during the first 2 to 7 days at such altitudes. The patient has undue shortness of breath, cyanosis, tachycardia, moist rales, fatigue, and frequently a nonproductive cough. Untreated, HAPE tends to be progressive and fatal, whereas recovery is prompt on descent to lower altitude. During the episode of HAPE, the heart is not enlarged and heart failure is absent. This is a form of noncardiac pulmonary edema that occurs in otherwise healthy and comparatively young individuals[22,23] with no underlying cardiovascular or pulmonary disease.[24] Despite intensive research, the pathogenesis of HAPE remains uncertain. Either the lung vessel permeability has increased such that a water and protein leak overwhelm the capacity of the lymphatic drainage or high pressure within the vessels forces fluid into the lungs, perhaps even rupturing pulmonary capillaries. Probably both mechanisms operate, since they would be mutually reinforcing.[25] The consensus is that HAPE is part of the spectrum of acute mountain sickness with relative hypoventilation and abnormal fluid retention as underlying factors.[26] Consequently, respiratory stimulation, as by administration of acetazolamide, is both a rational and an effective mode of prophylaxis for HAPE.

Although acute severe pulmonary hypertension is usually present during an episode of HAPE, the relation between these two conditions is not clear. Probably pulmonary hypertension per se does not precipitate the pulmonary edema. On the other hand, the presence of elevated intravascular pressure would tend to augment fluid leakage. This may explain why nifedipine, which prevents hypoxic pulmonary vasoconstriction,[27] has proved effective in both preventing and treating HAPE.[28] Furthermore, the increased pulmonary vascular reactivity in chronically hypoxic children living at high altitude may contribute to their predisposition to reentry HAPE.[29] (See also Chaps. 25 and 99.)

HEAT STRESS

Humans adjust to heat stress mainly by altering the vasomotor state of the skin to regulate heat exchange with the environment. Thermal balance is further modified by sweating and shivering. This section deals with adjustments of the systemic cutaneous and other regional circulations to regulate blood pressure and blood volume distribution along with body temperature. Reviews of this topic can be consulted for further details.[30,31]

Cutaneous Circulation

Reflex Control[32–34]

The skin receives only 5 to 10 percent of the cardiac output in normothermic individuals at rest, but it can receive 50 to 70 percent during heat stress. Circulatory adjustments to thermal stress can be drastically modified by cutaneous sympathetic vasoconstrictor nerve fibers, which are the efferent arm of (1) thermoregulatory reflexes that originate principally in cutaneous thermoreceptors, (2) cardiopulmonary and arterial baroreflexes, and (3) reflex adjustments to upright posture and exercise. The body's efforts to maintain blood pressure and support metabolic demands of other organs compete with thermoregulatory needs for skin blood flow. The temperature we maintain in conditions other than supine rest is the result of these competing nervous influences on skin blood flow.

Human skin is unique in possessing an *active vasodilator* system, the dominant effector in human cardiovascular response to rising core temperature (not skin temperature), accounting for almost all the increase in skin blood flow. The mechanism of active cutaneous vasodilation is still unknown. It requires intact sympathetic innervation and is somehow functionally linked to sweat gland function, inasmuch as patients with congenital absence of sweat glands (and intact sympathetic nerves) cannot vasodilate the skin or adequately regulate body temperature.[35] A rise in skin blood flow markedly increases the volume of blood within the compliant venous plexuses where it passes at reduced linear velocity just below the skin surface, increasing transcutaneous heat transfer. Cutaneous veins have a rich sympathetic nerve supply that reflexively controls the volume near the body surface in response to heat and cold. They are not responsive to baroreflexes, but they do constrict during exercise. As will be discussed, the shift in blood volume into cutaneous veins is the major regulatory problem in human cardiovascular adjustment to heat stress.

Circulatory Adjustments to Heat Stress

Supine Rest

In normal resting individuals,[30,31] heat stress can greatly increase cardiac output and total skin blood flow; however, responses vary widely because of differences in thermal conditions, duration of exposure, posture, internal temperature, and methodology. During supine rest, the cardiovascular system's capacity to increase cardiac output and skin blood flow is great during direct, whole-body heating designed to generate a maximum response by raising body skin temperature, as shown in Fig. 120-6. Cardiac output increases by 6 to 7 liters/min, a rise of 2.8 liters/min per degree Celsius (°C) increase in right atrial blood temperature. As blood flow to other major vascular beds decreases, the increase in cardiac output goes to skin, as reflected by the increase in forearm skin blood flow in Fig. 120-6. Arterial blood pressure is well maintained. Similar changes in blood flow are seen in patients with erythroderma; their chronically high skin blood flow leads to high-output failure with edema, venous congestion, hepatomegaly, and cardiac

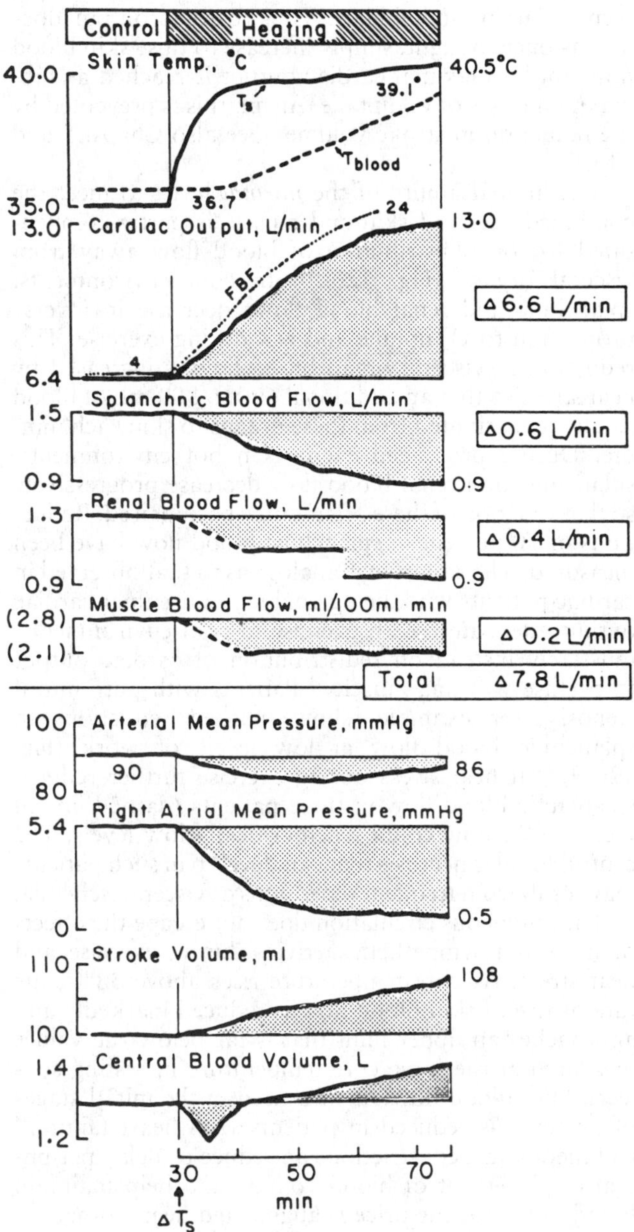

FIGURE 120-6 Average maximal circulatory responses to direct whole-body heating. The initial and final values and time course are shown for skin temperature (T_s), rectal temperature (T_r), and T_{blood} (right atrium) and each cardiovascular variable. Contributions of increased cardiac output (in 12 men) and reduced regional blood flows to total skin blood flow (7.8 liters/min) are shown in boxes on the right. Note that arterial pressure is well maintained, but right atrial pressure fell markedly while stroke volume increased. (*From LB Rowell: Human cardiovascular adjustments to exercise and thermal stress. Physiol Rev, 54:75, 1974. Reproduced with permission of the publisher and the author.*)

enlargement along with renal and gastrointestinal abnormalities.[36] Paraplegic patients show blunted responses to increased core temperature.[37] The cause is unknown; loss of thermal sensors in the spinal cord may contribute.[31] The rise in skin blood flow is also subnormal in patients with diabetic neuropathy,[38] undoubtedly because of defective neural control of skin blood vessels.

Hyperthermia per se increases sympathetic nervous activity, which causes regional vasoconstriction that, in turn, increases the fraction of cardiac output available for skin and alters the distribution of blood volume. Plasma norepinephrine concentration and plasma renin activity increase in proportion to core temperature; however, the renin-angiotensin system adds little to the neurogenic vasoconstriction elicited from thermoreceptors in the hypothalamus and spinal cord.[39]

Because high rates of skin blood flow increase the volume of blood in compliant cutaneous veins, translocation of blood volume from other regions is required to minimize the reduction in central blood volume (CBV) and cardiac filling pressure. The distribution of blood volume is altered most by splanchnic vasoconstriction, which reduces the pressure within a capacious venous bed that contains approximately 20 percent of total blood volume. Since splanchnic veins are normally at their maximum compliance, large decrements in intravenous volume will accompany small pressure changes. Central mobilization of blood volume is enhanced by the fall in right atrial pressure (Fig. 120-6) caused by the large pressure gradient that develops between central and cutaneous veins at high rates of skin blood flow. We cannot say whether or not blood volume is actively expressed from visceral organs by venoconstriction, but the fall in right atrial pressure along with splanchnic vasoconstriction favors a *passive* mobilization. The *increase* in stroke volume under these conditions (Fig. 120-6) suggests an increase in myocardial contractile force. Since much of the energy needed to force blood back to the heart is provided by the left ventricle (venous return to the heart is also aided by compression of peripheral veins by exercising skeletal muscles, by the abdominothoracic pump, and by ventricular suction of the right ventricle; see Chap. 5), an increase in myocardial contractile force would be highly advantageous during heat stress. It follows that patients in mild congestive heart failure may develop acute left ventricular failure during heat stress.[40] Also, the reduction in filling pressure caused by cutaneous vasodilation creates severe problems for patients with stenotic valvular lesions and reduced ventricular compliance.

Standing at Rest

When humans stand up, hydrostatic forces displace blood volume into dependent veins with approximately 600 mL moving into the legs.[41] In association with increases in skin blood flow and cutaneous venous compliance, blood volume in the legs increases an additional 200 mL.[41] This effect decreases further the return of blood to the heart and creates more severe orthostatic problems. Central blood volume and filling pressure decrease as illustrated in Fig. 120-7. Right and left ventricular outputs can only be transiently maintained by depletion of preventricular sumps, i.e., thoracic and splanchnic veins and the pulmonary vasculature. Cardiac output falls as a result of the marked decrease in stroke volume. Without vasoconstriction in skin to supplement that occurring in other organs, syncope would occur rapidly. In short, we defend ourselves against heat syncope by cutaneous vasoconstriction, not venoconstriction; but vasoconstriction merely reduces the rate at which dependent cutaneous veins fill and thus delays

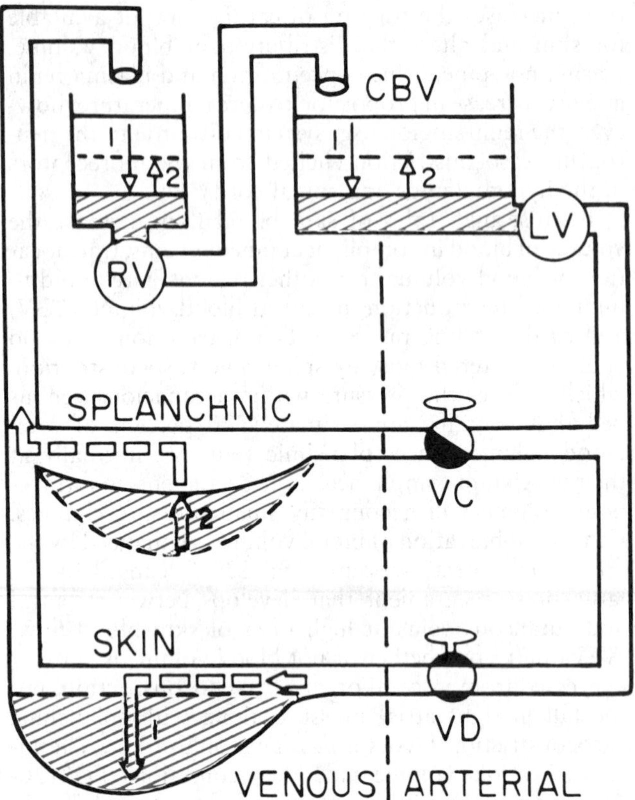

FIGURE 120-7 Schematic illustration of effects of skin vasodilation (VD) on preventricular volume sumps for right (RV) and left (LV) ventricles. As skin veins fill, venous return is transiently reduced so that preventricular sumps are depleted. CBV represents central or thoracic blood volume. Reduction in CBV is partially compensated by passive [caused by arteriolar vasoconstriction (VC)] expulsion of blood volume from splanchnic organs.

rather than prevents syncope. In addition, vasoconstriction of the splanchnic region serves to minimize reduction of CBV.

Exercise

As during rest, cutaneous venous volume increases when heat stress and exercise are combined despite the pumping action of muscle contraction.[42] In cool environments, the cutaneous veins of the legs refill so slowly after each compression by contracting muscle that their average pressure and volume remain low. In contrast, during heat stress these veins refill so rapidly after each contraction that average venous volume is increased markedly.[41] Venous volume is further increased by the loss of venoconstriction and the increase in compliance. Reductions in CBV, ventricular filling pressure, and stroke volume ensue, so that during moderate to heavy exercise, cardiac output is maintained by increased HR but is *not* increased to meet the additional demands for skin blood flow (Fig. 120-8). Because of the decrease in stroke volume, HR approaches maximal values at submaximal levels of O_2 uptake so that eventually cardiac output is reduced below normal and demands for skin and muscle blood flow cannot be met. Even the most severe hyperthermia does not increase total skin blood flow to levels seen in supine individuals. Thus, cardiac output does not, as once thought, simply increase to raise skin blood flow until a maximal cardiac output is reached at submaximal levels of O_2 uptake. Again, this is prevented by the reduction in stroke volume. (See also Chaps. 5 and 114.)

The limited ability of the *normal* heart to meet the combined needs of skin and muscle is partly compensated for by redistribution of blood flow away from visceral organs (Fig. 120-9). In cool environments, splanchnic and renal blood flows decrease in inverse proportion to O_2 uptake and HR during exercise. This reduction in visceral organ blood flow is increased by heat stress so that an additional 600 to 800 mL of blood can be redistributed from these organs to skin each minute. During prolonged exercise in hot environments, splanchnic and renal blood flow decrease progressively so that function of these organs may be impaired. Reductions of 70 percent in splanchnic blood flow have been measured. The situation is analogous to that observed in cardiac patients who, being unable to raise their cardiac output adequately with exercise in cool environments, must rely instead on redistribution of cardiac output to perfuse working muscle.[43] Patients with pure mitral stenosis, for example, show marked reductions in splanchnic blood flow at low levels of work (Fig. 120-9).[44] If heat stress during exercise further reduces splanchnic blood flow in these patients (dashed line in Fig. 120-9), flow could reach critically low levels. The central lobular necrosis that can develop in such patients may result from frequent repetitions of visceral ischemia.

The cutaneous circulation does not escape the effects of increased sympathetic activity during exercise and heat stress. As core temperature rises above 38°C, the rate of rise of skin blood flow is reduced markedly and approaches an upper limit that is far below the values measured at the same core temperature in resting subjects. Skin blood flow, as measured in the initial stages of exercise, is reduced in patients with heart failure.[45] Cutaneous vasoconstriction can reduce or delay peripheral displacement of blood volume and help maintain blood flow, but the price is augmented heat storage.

In the overall regulatory scheme, regulation of blood pressure during heat stress appears to have precedence unless core temperature rises beyond tolerable limits, at which point regulation fails. Such failure is most likely in patients with stenotic valvular lesions and reduced ventricular compliance because of the large reductions in cardiac filling pressure associated with heat stress. In addition, critical hepatic and renal functions are likely to be disrupted by increased diversion of their blood flow. This would be most likely in patients with low output whose perfusion of visceral organs was chronically reduced at rest.

COLD STRESS

Exercise in a cold environment, as in shoveling snow, is considered particularly stressful to patients with effort angina; however, the mechanism by which cold produces angina remains obscure. In the familiar cold pressor test, intense discomfort is produced by immersion of the hand

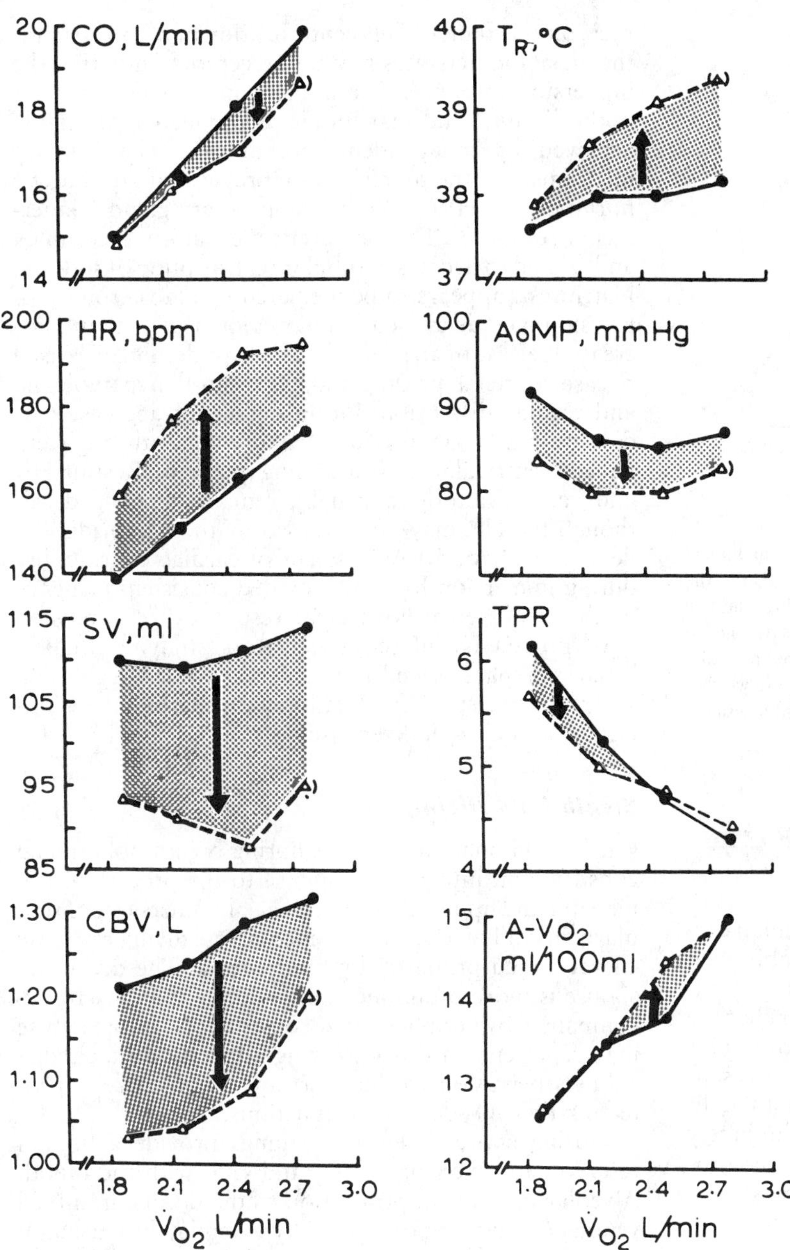

FIGURE 120-8 Summary of cardiovascular responses to graded exercise in hot (43.3° △---△) and neutral (25.6°C, ● — ●) environments. Arrows show the direction of change in each variable with heating (variables coded as in Fig. 120-6). Average data from six men.

in ice water or application of ice to the forehead. Reflex sympathetic stimulation is produced, resulting in a rise in systolic blood pressure (± 12 mmHg) accompanied by a modest increase in HR that is, however, less in older men (+4 beats per minute) than in younger men (+10 beats per minute).[46] This elevation of the rate-pressure product increases cardiac work, i.e., myocardial O_2 demand, which is met by an increase in coronary blood flow.[47] In patients with coronary disease, however, there is a paradoxical decrease in coronary blood flow.[48] A discrepancy between myocardial O_2 demand and supply appears to be the basis for angina in this circumstance.

A less severe stimulus than the cold pressor test can also provoke angina. When coronary disease patients inhaled very cold air (−20°C), some experienced typical angina chest pain even though there was only minimal change in blood pressure or HR, no increase in myocardial O_2 consumption, no change in coronary blood flow, and no angiographic evidence of coronary artery constriction. This suggests that cold air constricts minute coronary collaterals or other blood vessels specifically affecting blood flow to potentially ischemic regions of the myocardium.[49] This is at rest. (See also Chap. 58.)

Exercise performance in cold environment has also been examined in men with effort angina and a history of cold intolerance.[50] During submaximal exercise on a bicycle ergometer, systolic blood pressure, HR, and the rate-pressure product were significantly higher, and angina developed at a lower work load, when the room temperature was −10°C rather than +20°C. Similar results could also be obtained by having the subjects inhale very cold air (−35°C) during exercise in an otherwise warm room (+20°C). Skin cooling, however, was considered far more important than the inhalation of only moderately cold air (−10°C) in stressing the heart, presumably due to greater sympathetic stimulation.

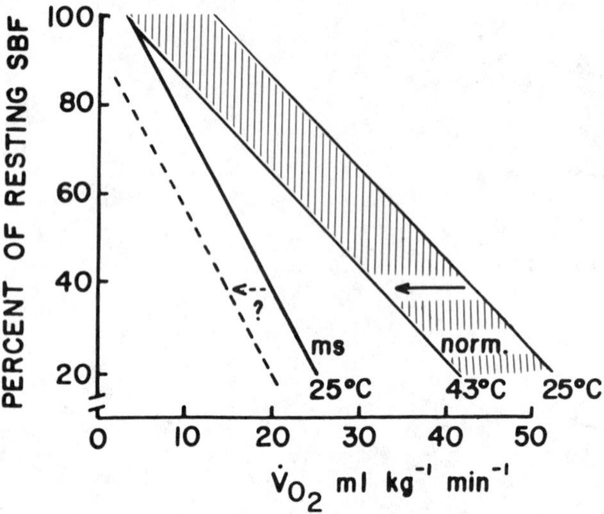

FIGURE 120-9 Summary of splanchnic vascular responses to upright exercise in normal subjects at 25 and 43°C environmental temperature. The shaded region marks the highly significant 20 percent reduction in splanchnic blood flow (SBF) at any given $\dot{V}_{O_2}$ in the heat in normal subjects. On the left is the regression line from seven patients with pure mitral stenosis (ms), who show much greater reduction in flow at any given $\dot{V}_{O_2}$. It is not known whether these patients show further reduction in flow in the heat. (Dashed line shows result of predicted 20 percent reduction.)[30,31]

DIVING AND HYPERBARIC MEDICINE

Diving Medicine

Underwater diving induces responses by the human cardiovascular system that have become reasonably well understood in recent years. In addition to these physiological responses, emergencies sometimes occur that are associated with profound alterations in cardiovascular function. Divers are also subject to the same cardiovascular illnesses that occur in conventional settings. In addition, the risk of an ensuing fatal consequence is infinitely greater should an acute myocardial infarction or cerebrovascular accident occur during diving.

Diving and Immersion

Alterations in the physical environment encountered by the diver breathing air include increases in barometric pressure, density of the breathing gas, inspired P_{O_2}, inspired pressure of nitrogen, and loss of body heat to the surrounding water.[51–54] The most characteristic cardiovascular response to these physical forces, both individually and collectively, has been bradycardia. Alterations in circulatory pressures, resistances, and cardiac output occur primarily in association with immersion and hypothermia.

Simple immersion in thermoneutral water produces remarkable adjustments in cardiopulmonary and renal function. These physiological responses, attributable to the effects of increased hydrostatic pressure outside the body, include dehydration, ventilatory restriction, and increased cardiac output. Hydrostatic pressure from immersion increases the pressure gradient across the diaphragm and decreases venous compliance in the lower extremities. These combined effects increase intrathoracic blood volume. This centralization of blood distends the atria and activates mechanoreceptors, initiating the immersion response. The immersion response includes both diuretic and natriuretic components, probably achieved by independent mechanisms. The primary mechanism of the diuresis is suppression of antidiuretic hormone (ADH) release by the pituitary gland (Gauer-Henry response). The natriuretic mechanism is complex and related to decreased tubular reabsorption of sodium. Natriuresis appears to be mediated by aldosterone suppression via decreased renin-angiotensin activity, increased release of atrial natriuretic peptide, and increased release of renal prostaglandins. Central hypervolemia and cardiac distension during immersion increase cardiac output by improving stroke volume through enhanced ventricular-diastolic filling (preload). Resting HR and cardiac afterload usually remain unchanged, although the HR may be increased by the Bainbridge reflex. (See Chap. 5.) Assessment of cardiac contractility during immersion has not provided consistent evidence of change. The cardiovascular responses to immersion have proved useful to investigators studying weightlessness in space as well as disorders of volume regulation such as congestive heart failure, chronic renal insufficiency, and chronic liver disease.

Breath-Hold Diving

Cardiopulmonary alterations during breath-hold diving constitute an integrated response to the process of immersion and apnea. Apnea and facial immersion, particularly in cold water, elicit an incomplete diving response characterized primarily by bradycardia. The diving response is more pronounced in children and may be accompanied by peripheral vasoconstriction. This response may represent an O_2-conserving adaptation that redistributes perfusion to the heart and brain thereby protecting their O_2-dependent functions.

During a breath hold, the lungs provide a limited reservoir for exchange of O_2 and CO_2 with the blood. Alveolar P_{O_2} falls in proportion to the decline in mixed venous P_{O_2}, leading to arterial hypoxemia, decreased O_2 transport, and anaerobic metabolism. Arterial hypoxemia also elicits chemoreceptor activity, which produces peripheral vasoconstriction and helps direct a limited O_2 supply to the heart and brain. With a breath hold, the alveolar P_{CO_2} rises in proportion to both pulmonary blood flow and the diffusion gradient for CO_2 between mixed venous blood and the air spaces. As CO_2 production increases, the mixed venous P_{CO_2} rises and leads to further increases in the alveolar P_{CO_2}. The point at which the high P_{CO_2} causes breathing to resume is called the break point. The time to the break point can be extended by maneuvers that lower the P_{CO_2}, e.g., hyperventilation. Importantly, hyperventilation does not increase the O_2 store of the body significantly because the increase in alveolar P_{O_2} produced by lowering alveolar P_{CO_2} has little effect on the O_2 content of arterial blood. Therefore, hyperventilation extends the time to the break point but may lead to severe hypoxemia before the CO_2 break point is reached. These gas exchange processes during a breath hold are affected by underwater descent when thoracic compression decreases the volume of the lungs and raises the partial pressures of the gases in the alveoli. During ascent from the breath-hold dive, the lung reexpands and alveolar P_{O_2} and P_{CO_2} decline. If the dive has been unusually long, e.g., after a period of hyperventilation, the diver may experience profound hypoxemia and loss of consciousness while approaching the surface. This phenomenon, known as shallow-water blackout, is responsible for a significant number of drownings every year.

Near Drowning

The physical environment of underwater divers and swimmers is deceptively dangerous, and relatively minor injuries or accidents may produce catastrophic results. Such catastrophes are usually the result of inhalation of water into the airways (near drowning) and subsequent asphyxia. Effective pulmonary gas exchange ceases and the victim suffers hypoxic injuries to the brain, heart, and kidneys. Pulmonary injury is also very prominent, and the adult respiratory distress syndrome complicates near drowning in nearly half of the cases. Prolonged hypoxia leads to diffuse neuronal damage, compromise of the blood-brain barrier, and cerebral edema. As in other cases of severe cerebral hypoxia, the neurologic outcome is uncertain.

The effects of near drowning on the heart are complex. Atrial and ventricular arrhythmias, particularly ventricular fibrillation, often complicate near drowning in both fresh and salt water. These arrhythmias have been associated in animal studies with large and rapid shifts in electrolyte concentrations. Human cases generally do not provide strong evidence for such a pathophysiological mechanism; however, pathological studies of the human heart after either fresh water or salt water drowning demonstrate changes consistent with catecholamine excess. This suggests that intense adrenergic stimulation precipitates the rhythm disturbances. Myocardial infarction also may occur in patients with coronary artery disease as either a cause or an effect of an episode of near drowning.

Decompression Sickness

A major physical consequence of diving with compressed gases is the uptake of inert gas, e.g., nitrogen, by the tissues of the body.[55–58] The elimination of nitrogen or other inert gas from the body after a pressure decrease during ascent from depth or to altitude is known as decompression. Decompression sickness (DCS) occurs primarily during rapid decompression when nitrogen, dissolved in body tissues and no longer in equilibrium with a falling barometric pressure, undergoes a change in physical state. Bubbles form within tissues and venous blood, producing diverse clinical manifestations. Evolution of gas in body tissues may occur during decompression after hyperbaric exposures to more than 2 atmospheres (atm) absolute or greater, or during rapid ascent from sea level to less than 0.5 atm absolute (18,000 ft, or 5486 m). Explosive decompression of a pressurized aircraft cabin is a familiar example of the latter circumstance. Decompression sickness is more likely to occur in association with severe exercise, after prolonged hyperbaric exposures, and with excessive body fat. These associations are related to increased uptake of inert gas by body tissues. Other aggravating factors include increasing age, fatigue, and preexisting vascular disease, presumably related to impaired gas transport from tissues to the external environment. Decompression sickness also occurs less frequently with regular hyperbaric exposures. This acclimatization phenomenon has led to much speculation concerning mechanisms. A favored explanation is a decrease in the number of gas nuclei that act as loci for bubble formation during decompression. The mechanical effects of bubbles alone do not entirely explain the pathophysiology of decompression sickness. Gas bubbles in blood and tissues may produce a variety of secondary manifestations related to the effects of surface activity at the gas-to-blood interface. In serious decompression sickness, there may be loss of intravascular fluid and hemoconcentration, activation of complement, platelet aggregation, procoagulant activity, and release of vasoactive compounds such as serotonin, histamine, and bradykinin.

The clinical manifestations of decompression sickness are diverse. Overt clinical signs and symptoms are more likely to occur when bubbles lodge in regions wherein ischemia evolves with associated pain and/or perturbed function. For convenience the clinical manifestations are classified as being either mild (type 1) or severe (type 2). Both mild and severe manifestations of decompression sickness may be present in up to one-third of these patients. Accordingly, a careful search for subtle type 2 manifestations is mandatory in every instance. The common manifestations of both mild and severe decompression sickness are listed in Table 120-1.

The most characteristic manifestation of mild decompression sickness is characterized most often by pain that is ordinarily localized within or near limb joints. After excursion dives in which compressed air is breathed, the pain is far more likely to occur in the *upper* rather than the lower limbs. After prolonged exposure to compressed air, as in the case of caisson workers, or after deep helium-oxygen saturation diving, pain typically occurs in the *lower* rather than the upper limbs. The initial symptom may be numbness. Characteristically, the discomfort becomes progressively more severe, and debili-

TABLE 120-1

Signs and Symptoms of Decompression Sickness

1. Type 1 (mild)
   a. Extremities: pain (bends), paresthesia, numbness, edema
   b. Skin: pruritis, mottling, rash, pallor, urticaria
2. Type 2 (severe)
   a. Central nervous system: loss of consciousness, scintillating scotomas, Ménière's syndrome, vertigo, staggering gait, aphasia, paresis or paralysis, sensory loss, bladder and bowel paralysis
   b. Cardiorespiratory: substernal distress, paroxysmal coughing, shock, tachypnea, asphyxia (chokes), hemoconcentration, platelet–red cell aggregates
   c. Systemic: extreme fatigue

tating pain may evolve, requiring potent analgesic management. At times, local edema and mottling may occur over the site of the pain. Typically the pain subsides completely or lessens substantially during prompt recompression with oxygen breathing. Trials of recompression and oxygen breathing, singly or in combination, may be employed diagnostically as well as therapeutically. Untreated, limb pain will subside gradually; however, complete resolution of the pain is likely to require several days. The cutaneous manifestations of mild decompression sickness include pruritis and patchy vasodilation, consistent with vascular stasis. Urticaria and edema may occur as well. Many patients also complain of malaise; the etiology is obscure.

Severe (type 2) decompression sickness is characterized by neurologic or cardiorespiratory involvement. Manifestations are diverse, multiple, and unpredictable. The natural history is variable in the absence of recompression therapy. In fulminant cases, cardiorespiratory arrest and death may occur. Permanent serious neurologic sequelae including paraplegia also may occur. In other instances, severe neurologic deficits resolve gradually over intervals of weeks and months despite the absence of appropriate treatment. Severe decompression sickness involving the cardiorespiratory system is characterized by retrosternal discomfort, dyspnea, cough, tachypnea, and extreme fatigue. A sharp "catch" sensation during inspiration is characteristic. Divers refer to this symptom as "chokes." Postural hypotension, oliguria, hemoconcentration, and hypovolemic shock also may occur.

Neurologic decompression sickness involves the spinal cord relatively often. The latter manifestation reflects the consequences of ischemic injury, produced by bubble-induced stasis in the epidural venous plexus. The onset is often insidious with initial mild symptoms of limb paresthesia and weakness. Minutes to hours later, paralysis often occurs, commonly with impairment of bladder and bowel function. Girdle pain is a noteworthy early symptom. Visual disturbances, headaches, abnormal behavior, vertigo, nystagmus, nausea, and vomiting may develop as manifestations of upper central nervous system (CNS) and labyrinthine involvement. Migraine-like symptoms may occur, particularly in patients with histories of true migraine headaches. A significant number of serious cases of DCS arise from venous gas emboli crossing a patent foramen ovale during or shortly after ascent. This cardiac anomaly, normally present in about 20 to 35 percent of the general population, is thought to be a risk factor for development of serious DCS. The associated risk is probably a function of the extent of bubble formation in the venous system during and after decompression.

Management of decompression sickness is straightforward and very successful. Prompt recompression in a hyperbaric chamber and breathing of 100 percent oxygen with short air breaks lead to relief of symptoms within a few minutes in most cases. With appropriate treatment, the recovery rate approximates 95 percent. The rationale for treatment is based on the twin principles that (1) reexposure to hyperbaric pressures facilitates the return of gas bubbles to the physically dissolved state and (2) breathing pure oxygen lowers the concentration of inert gas in venous blood, thereby increasing the gradient for removal of nitrogen from tissue and hence from the bubbles within the tissue. Clearly the best responses to treatment are achieved when recompression is prompt. In more severe cases of decompression sickness, other forms of ancillary therapy may be beneficial, including volume repletion and possibly administration of corticosteroids. Details of treatment schedules are outlined fully in the U.S. Navy Diving Manual.[56] These tables represent treatment standards. Fortunately for the patient, even serious neurologic disability may respond to recompression therapy after a delay of several days. Furthermore, the prognosis for full recovery is good even when the initial response is incomplete. Complete recovery has been observed to require as much as 2 years in some cases.

Intraarterial Gas Embolism

In compressed-air diving, arterial air (or gas) embolism may occur during ascent to the surface, particularly when the diver fails to exhale normally.[55-59] Under these circumstances, as ambient hydrostatic pressure decreases during the ascent, gas within the lungs expands reciprocally according to Boyle's law. One important consequence of this reciprocal action may not be apparent. At greater depths, a partial ascent equivalent to a barometric change of 1 atm will be associated with only a small increase in gas volume; i.e., a change from 10 to 9 atm causes only a 10 percent increase in gas volume. At shallow depths, the consequences are much greater; i.e., a change from 2 to 1 atm will result in a 100 percent increase in gas volume. Failure to exhale under these circumstances may create pressure gradient exceeding the compliance of lung tissue. If this positive pressure gradient between alveolar gas and the pulmonary interstitium leads to alveolar disruption and pulmonary interstitial emphysema, soft tissue or mediastinal emphysema, pneumothorax, or pneumopericardium may follow. Free gas may also enter pulmonary venous blood and travel through the left side of the heart to the arterial circulation. Air may then disburse throughout the arterial system including the coronary and renal arteries. The most common clinical manifestations occur within the distribution of the carotid arteries, however, leading to acute profound cerebral dysfunction characterized by loss of consciousness, seizures, and paralysis. In contrast to DCS, the gas bubbles of arterial gas embolization do not arise from a physical change of the state of dissolved gas in tissues; and depending on the degree of pulmonary overdistension, the amount of gas disseminated into the arterial system may be very large. This severe complication of ascent can occur rapidly after only brief exposures or at very shallow depths in circumstances under which decompression sickness is not a diagnostic consideration. In the absence of adequate treatment, a severe CNS deficit from air embolism is more likely to be permanently disabling or lethal than is DCS. Recompression therapy should commence within minutes if a satisfactory clinical outcome is to be achieved. The principles of management are similar to those elaborated for DCS, but the magnitude, length, and number of recompression treatments are generally greater. A number of case reports describe incremental benefit from longer hyperbaric exposures configured in days rather than hours. Some observers report resolution of neurologic deficits, in some cases even after delays of treatment of more than 24 h.

Serious intraarterial gas embolism also occurs in other circumstances, for example, as a result of explosive decompression of pressurized aircraft, after accidental trauma to the great vessels, during blast injury to the thorax, and in the hospitalized patient. Arterial gas embolism in the hospital setting is not infrequent but is often unrecognized as a complication of various diagnostic and therapeutic procedures (Table 120-2). Air may enter the arterial system directly, as during cardiovascular surgery and radiodiagnostic procedures, or after venous air embolism, when acute pulmonary hypertension permits air to cross a patent foramen ovale. In the patient with serious underlying illness, the presence of a major arterial gas embolism may impose very difficult therapeutic choices for the physician. Oxygen therapy alone is not likely to produce a good functional recovery, but even when hyperbaric oxygen therapy is practical, the prognosis is relatively guarded. Whenever possible, the same principles of treatment should be employed for air embolism in the hospitalized patient as in the diver.

Hyperbaric Oxygen Therapy[60–66]

General Principles

Hyperbaric oxygen therapy is defined as breathing 100 percent oxygen at greater than normal atmospheric pressures. This is achieved in special environmental chambers containing pressurized gas and at the same time providing adequate technological support for patient care. The important advantage of hyperbaric pressures is in overcoming the barrier to increased O_2 transport imposed by limited solubility of O_2 in plasma. Whereas 100 mL of blood equilibrated at P_{O_2} of 110 mmHg contains only 0.3 mL of physically dissolved O_2, the latter amount can be increased to almost 6 mL at 3 atm absolute by the breathing of 100 percent oxygen. Under these circumstances, the P_{O_2} in arterial blood will approach 2000 mmHg. The clinical rationale for the use of hyperbaric oxygen has been based on the following three principles: (1) the function of hypoxic vital organs can be maintained or restored even in the setting of decreased perfusion; (2) specific beneficial pharmacologic effects can be achieved with high oxygen pressures; and (3) removal of bubbles within tissues can be expedited greatly by the combined effects of increased hydrostatic pressure to reduce bubble size and high pressures of oxygen to accelerate washout of dissolved inert gas by providing a much greater diffusive outward gradient for elimination of inert gas molecules from the bubble. The latter principle is fully exploited in the treatment of decompression sickness and arterial gas embolism, as outlined above. The second principle provides the rationale for use of hyperbaric oxygen in gas gangrene and other anaerobic infections. Application of the first principle, maintaining or restoring the function of hypoxic or ischemic tissues, is relevant in many cardiovascular diseases and in the management of injured tissues with microcirculatory compromise.

The potential applicability of hyperbaric oxygen as therapy for ischemic tissues has been constrained greatly by two major biological problems: (1) profound ischemia is likely to prevent delivery of O_2 to the hypoxic target, and (2) the potential toxicity of oxygen to the lungs and CNS rules out high and continuous levels of exposure. As a practical matter, CNS and pulmonary oxygen toxicities are avoided by limiting exposures to generally less than 3 atm absolute for intervals of time shorter than 90 to 120 min. In practice, these intermittent limited exposures are well tolerated, and judgments of therapeutic efficacy are based on the success of single or repetitive treatment profiles conforming to these criteria. There are only a limited number of standard indications for hyperbaric oxygen therapy in clinical practice (Table 120-3), and most observations concerning therapy of cardiovascular diseases with hyperbaric oxygen are anecdotal. Several of these applications are discussed in greater detail below, although the reader is referred to other sources for discussion of the role of adjunctive hyperbaric oxygen in the management of infectious diseases.

Carbon Monoxide Intoxication

Acute carbon monoxide (CO) intoxication is the leading cause of accidental poisoning in the United States.[64,65] Uptake of CO by the body impairs O_2 transport to tissues by two mechanisms. First, arterial O_2 content is decreased in a manner analogous to anemia because hemo-

TABLE 120-2

Hospital Procedures Sometimes Associated with Intraarterial Air Embolism

1. Deep venous catheter insertion, use, and removal
2. Radiodiagnostic injections of contrast dye into arterial system
3. Cardiovascular surgery
4. Neuroradiographic and neurosurgical procedures including myelography
5. Hemodialysis
6. Positive pressure ventilation
7. Transbronchial biopsy

TABLE 120-3

Indications for Hyperbaric Oxygen Therapy

1. Hyperbaric oxygen as a primary modality
   a. Decompression sickness
   b. Intraarterial air or gas embolism
   c. Carbon monoxide intoxication
   d. Exceptional blood loss (anemia)
2. Hyperbaric oxygen as an adjunctive modality
   a. Gas gangrene
   b. Necrotizing soft tissue infections involving anaerobic organisms
   c. Poorly healing ulcers, wounds, and compromised skin grafts in selected patients
   d. Refractory osteomyelitis
   e. Osteoradionecrosis

globin binds CO with a 200-fold greater affinity than O_2. Second, carboxyhemoglobin shifts the oxyhemoglobin dissociation curve to the left, adversely affecting the release of O_2 from the remaining binding sites on the hemoglobin molecule. The net result of high carboxyhemoglobin levels is tissue hypoxia. Despite compensatory increases in blood flow, there may be serious functional consequences for hypoxia-sensitive organs such as the heart and the brain. At high carboxyhemoglobin levels, severe tissue hypoxia may set the stage for secondary mechanisms of CO toxicity related to intracellular binding of CO. When tissue P_{O_2} is low, CO may compete successfully for O_2 binding sites on intracellular hemoproteins such as myoglobin and mitochondrial oxidase, cytochrome aa_3. This effect has potentially serious consequences for myocardial performance when myocardial O_2 demands are high, particularly in the presence of coronary artery disease.

Clinical manifestations of acute CO intoxication include headache, confusion, visual disturbance, unconsciousness, seizures, and pulmonary edema. In untreated patients, the consequences of severe intoxication may lead to death. Metabolic acidosis and rhabdomyolysis may accompany serious intoxication. Patients with mild CO poisoning are likely to recover without specific treatment other than removal from the noxious gaseous environment. With more severe forms of intoxication, the outlook is uncertain. The severity of the clinical illness often does not correlate with the measured carboxyhemoglobin level but corresponds more closely to the extent and the duration of the exposure. Patients with any form of CNS impairment, evidence of myocardial ischemia, or carboxyhemoglobin levels above 25 percent merit aggressive therapeutic intervention. The rationale for treatment with hyperbaric oxygen is based primarily on more rapid removal of the CO from hemoglobin and tissue sites. Because O_2 and CO compete for hemoglobin and many tissue binding sites, hyperbaric oxygenation greatly accelerates CO elimination. Furthermore, O_2 dissolved in plasma under hyperbaric conditions effectively bypasses any impediment to oxygen transport imposed by carboxyhemoglobin. Potentially lethal cerebral hypoxia may be averted as a consequence. Twenty minutes of exposure to 100 percent oxygen at 2.4 atm absolute will be accompanied by release of CO from the blood equivalent to that obtained after 5 h of breathing uncontaminated air. Sixty to 90 min of hyperbaric oxygen therapy at this pressure is sufficient to reduce carboxyhemoglobin saturation to well below 10 percent. Prompt recovery is the rule if treatment can be initiated before extensive irreversible brain injury has occurred.

Although the rational for the use of hyperbaric oxygen to treat acute CO poisoning is strong and anecdotal clinical experience positive, it has been difficult to prove the efficacy of hyperbaric oxygen in clinical trials. Part of this problem relates to the inability to identify and gather significant numbers of high-risk patients with CO poisoning, administer the therapy promptly and effectively, and obtain adequate long-term follow-up of the patients.

The use of hyperbaric oxygen also has been suggested to reverse the toxic effects of other poisonous gases, such as hydrogen cyanide and hydrogen sulfide, which, like CO, interfere with cellular respiration by binding to cytochrome aa_3. Unlike that for CO, however, this binding process for these gases is not competitive with O_2. Consequently, reports of successful treatment of cyanide and hydrogen sulfide poisoning with hyperbaric oxygen go unexplained at present. Nevertheless, prompt oxygen administration may protect tissue viability and provide a useful adjunct to the standard antidotes.

Ischemic Heart Disease

The early enthusiasm for therapeutic hyperbaric oxygen generated hope for benefit in ischemic heart disease in the 1960s. One important observation obtained largely from experimental animals was that hyperbaric oxygen exerted a predictable antiarrhythmic effect. Human observations have been sparse because available pharmacologic agents are generally successful and much easier to employ in the setting of ischemia. The implications of this antiarrhythmic effect, however, have continued to be of interest to investigators.

The concept of minimizing myocardial damage from myocardial infarction by the employment of hyperbaric oxygen has been tested experimentally, with variable results. Aside from scattered anecdotal observations, only one controlled trial has been performed in human beings. In this series, overall mortality of patients treated with hyperbaric oxygen at 2 atm absolute was lower than that of control patients. The diversity among patients and comparable excellent results from other centers using conventional management precluded definitive interpretation, however. At this time, hyperbaric oxygen is viewed as being of unproven value in the treatment of ischemic heart disease. The advent of fibrinolytic therapy and newer invasive techniques that appear to improve the clinical outcome of patients with serious myocardial infarction makes it unlikely that hyperbaric oxygen will be employed widely in the management of these patients. The therapy also has limited investigational interest, particularly in view of experimental concerns that reperfusion after acute coronary occlusion may lead to tissue injury from reactive oxygen species formed as a result of metabolic responses provoked by the ischemia.

Cerebrovascular Insufficiency

The improvement of techniques for reestablishing cerebral blood flow has led to renewed interest in surgical management of chronic cerebrovascular insufficiency.[66] Surgeons have been reluctant to undertake risky interventions, however, in the absence of knowledge as to whether or not the neurologic deficit could be reversed if arterial blood flow were restored. One approach to this difficult problem has been the diagnostic use of hyperbaric oxygen. Very limited observations to date suggest that reversal of neurologic impairment associated with brief exposures to hyperbaric oxygen identifies a population of patients likely to respond well to cerebral revascularization.

In a small fraction of patients suffering from acute cerebrovascular accidents, the neurologic deficit has been reversed dramatically by exposure to hyperbaric oxygen. More often than not, however, the reversal has proved to be temporary. Thereafter, in the absence of means for providing long-term benefit, widespread therapeutic employment has not seemed justifiable. In the future, however, prompt administration of hyperbaric oxygen, combined with a therapy that restores blood flow, may allow long-term salvage of neurologic function in selected patients.

Peripheral Vascular Insufficiency

Medical management of chronic atherosclerotic peripheral vascular disease is associated with relatively limited benefit. (See Chap. 124.) Accordingly, there has been considerable interest in alternative therapy. Hyperbaric oxygen has yielded limited results, however, as might be expected when the fundamental problem of vascular compromise is not altered by the treatment modality. Therapeutic intervention with hyperbaric oxygen may be beneficial when superimposed acute problems such as infection or compromised skin grafts occur.

Vasculitis, involving the skin and extremities, is more reversible than atherosclerotic vascular insufficiency. Benefit from intermittent treatment with hyperbaric oxygen has been described for forms of vasculitis causing ischemic injury associated with ulceration.

Problem Wounds

The application of hyperbaric oxygen to manage pain and ulceration caused by chronic wounds is based upon observations that tissue P_{O_2} is low and wound healing impaired in regions within the distribution of a compromised peripheral circulation. Furthermore, tissue hypoxia is a common feature of both acute and chronic wounds. Tissue P_{O_2} measurements have indicated that wound hypoxia is often sufficient to impair leukocyte function and collagen synthesis in the tissues. In selected chronic wounds, the oxygen tension can be increased with hyperbaric oxygen treatment and wound healing enhanced. Clinical treatment profiles vary, and optimal treatment schedules have not been determined for most wounds.

Another special circumstance associated with poor microcirculatory function and low tissue P_{O_2} is chronic radiation injury. In this setting, chronic pain, ulceration, and tissue necrosis are common and difficult to manage. There is experimental evidence that repetitive treatments with hyperbaric oxygen increase collagen synthesis and capillary proliferation within the injured tissues. The results are better oxygenation and more rapid wound healing, so that supplemental therapy with oxygen is no longer necessary.

REFERENCES

1. Alexander JK, Hartley LH, Modelski M, Grover RF: Reduction of stroke volume during exercise in man following ascent to 3100 m altitude. *J Appl Physiol* 1967; 23:849–858.
2. Dempsey JA, Reddan WG, Birnbaum ML, Forster HV, Thoden JS, et al: Effects of acute though lifelong hypoxic exposure on exercise pulmonary gas exchange. *Respir Physiol* 1971; 13:62–89.
3. Weil JV, Jamieson G, Brown DW, Grover RF, et al: The red cell mass–arterial oxygen relationship in normal man. *J Clin Invest* 1968; 47:1627–1639.
4. Grover RF, Weil JV, Reeves JT: Cardiovascular adaptation to high altitude. In: Pandolf KB (ed): *Exercise and Sport Sciences Reviews,* vol 14. New York, Macmillan, 1986: 269–302.
5. Alexander JK, Grover RF: Mechanism of reduced stroke volume at high altitude. *Clin Cardiol* 1983; 6:301–303.
6. Reeves JT, Groves BM, Sutton JR, Wagner PD, Cymerman A, et al: Operation Everest II: Preservation of cardiac function at great altitude. *J Appl Physiol* 1987; 63:531–539.
7. Hellems HK, Ord JW, Talmers FN, Christensen RC: Effects of hypoxia on coronary blood flow and myocardial metabolism in normal human subjects (abstr). *Circulation* 1957; 16:893.
8. Eaton JW, Brewer GJ, Grover RF: Role of red cell 2,3-diphosphoglycerate in adaptation of man to altitude. *J Lab Clin Med* 1969; 73:603–609.
9. Grover RF, Lufschanowski R, Alexander JK: Alterations in the coronary circulation of man following ascent to 3,100 m altitude. *J Appl Physiol* 1976; 41:832–838.
10. Shlim DR, Houston R: Helicopter rescues and deaths among trekkers in Nepal. *JAMA* 1989; 261:1017–1019.
11. Grover RF, Tucker CE, McGroarty SR, Travis RR: The coronary stress of skiing at high altitude. *Arch Intern Med* 1990; 150:1205–1208.
12. Okin JT: Response of patients with coronary heart disease to exercise at varying altitudes. *Adv Cardiol* 1970; 5:92–96.
13. Khanna PK, Dham SK, Hoon RS: Exercise in an hypoxic environment as a screening test for ischaemic heart disease. *Aviat Space Environ Med* 1976; 47:1114–1117.
14. Mortimer EA Jr, Monson RR, MacMahon B: Reduction in mortality from coronary heart disease in men residing at high altitude. *N Engl J Med* 1977; 296:581–585.
15. Kayar SR, Banchero N: Myocardial capillarity in acclimation to hypoxia. *Pfluegers Arch* 1985; 404:319–325.
16. Marticorena E, Ruiz L, Severino J, Galvez J, Penaloza D: Systemic blood pressure in white men born at sea level: Changes after long residence at high altitudes. *Am J Cardiol* 1969; 23:364–368.
17. Grover RF: Chronic hypoxic pulmonary hypertension. In: Fishman AP (ed): *The Pulmonary Circulation—Normal and Abnormal.* Philadelphia, University of Pennsylvania Press, 1990: 283–299.
18. Pryor R, Weaver WF, Blount SG Jr: Electrocardiographic observations of 493 residents living at high altitude (10,150 ft). *Am J Cardiol* 1965; 16:494–499.
19. Reeves JT, Grover RF: High-altitude pulmonary hypertension and pulmonary edema. In: Yu PN, Goodwin JF (eds): *Progress in Cardiology,* vol 4. Philadelphia, Lea & Febiger, 1975: 99–118.
20. Sui GJ, Lui YH, Cheng XS, Anand IS, Harris E, Harris P, et al: Subacute infantile mountain sickness. *J Pathol* 1988; 155:161–170.
21. Reeves JT, Wagner WW Jr, McMurtry IF, Grover RF: Physiological effects of high altitude on the pulmonary circulation. In: Robertshaw D (ed): *Environmental Physiology III: International Review of Physiology,* vol 20. Baltimore, University Park Press, 1979: 289–310.
22. Sophocles AM, Bachman J: High-altitude pulmonary edema among visitors to Summit County, Colorado. *J Fam Pract* 1983; 17:1015–1017.
23. Sophocles AM Jr: High-altitude pulmonary edema in Vail, Colorado, 1975–1982. *West J Med* 1986; 144:569–573.
24. Grover RF, Hyers TM, McMurtry IF, Reeves JT: High-altitude pulmonary edema. In: Fishman AP, Renkin EM (eds): *Pulmonary Edema.* Bethesda, MD, American Physiological Society, 1979: 229–240.
25. Reeves JT, Schoene B: When lungs on mountains leak: Studying pulmonary edema at high altitudes (editorial). *N Engl J Med* 1991; 325:1306–1307.
26. Hackett PH, Rennie D, Hofmeister SE, Grover RF, Grover EB, Reeves JT: Fluid retention and relative hypoventilation in acute mountain sickness. *Respiration* 1982; 43:321–329.
27. McMurtry IF, Davidson AB, Reeves JT, Grover RF: Inhibition of hypoxic pulmonary vasoconstriction by calcium antagonists in isolated rat lungs. *Circ Res* 1976; 38:99–104.
28. Bärtsch P, Maggiorini M, Ritter M, Noti C, Vock P, Oelz O: Prevention of high altitude pulmonary edema by nifedipine. *N Engl J Med* 1991; 325:1284–1289.
29. Scoggin CH, Hyers TM, Reeves JT, Grover RF: High altitude

pulmonary edema in the children and young adults of Leadville, Colorado. *N Engl J Med* 1977; 297:1269–1272.

30. Rowell LB: Cardiovascular aspects of human thermoregulation. *Circ Res* 1983; 52:367–379.
31. Rowell LB: Cardiovascular adjustments to thermal stress. In: Shepherd JT, Abboud FM (eds): *Handbook of Physiology,* sec 2, *The Cardiovascular System,* vol III, *Peripheral Circulation and Organ Blood Flow.* Bethesda, MD, American Physiological Society, 1983: 967–1023.
32. Greenfield ADM: The circulation through the skin. In: Hamilton WF, Dow P (eds): *Handbook of Physiology,* vol 2. Bethesda, MD, American Physiological Society, 1963: 1325–1351.
33. Shepherd JT: *Physiology of the Circulation in Human Limbs in Health and Disease.* Philadelphia, WB Saunders, 1963.
34. Rowell LB: Reflex control of the cutaneous vasculature. *J Invest Dermatol* 1977; 69:154–166.
35. Brengelmann GL, Freund PR, Rowell LB, Olerud JE, Kraning KK: Absence of active cutaneous vasodilation associated with congenital absence of sweat glands in man. *Am J Physiol* 1981; 240:H571–H575.
36. Shuster S: Systemic effects of skin disease. *Lancet* 1967; 2:907–912.
37. Freund PR, Brengelmann GL, Rowell LB, Halar E: Attenuated skin blood flow response in hyperthermia in paraplegic man. *J Appl Physiol* 1984; 56:1104–1109.
38. Greeson TP, Freedman RI, Levan NE, Wong, WH: Cutaneous vascular responses in diabetics. *Microvas Res* 1975; 10:8–16.
39. Escourrou P, Freund PR, Rowell LB, Johnson DG: Splanchnic vasoconstriction in heat-stressed man—role of the renin-angiotensin system. *J Appl Physiol* 1982; 52:1438–1443.
40. Ansari A, Burch GE: Influence of hot environments on the cardiovascular system. *Arch Intern Med* 1969; 123:371–378.
41. Gauer OH, Thron HL: Postural changes in the circulation. In: Hamilton WF, Dow P (eds): *Handbook of Physiology,* vol 3. Bethesda, MD, American Physiological Society, 1965: 2409–2439.
42. Rowell LB: *Human Circulation—Regulation During Physical Stress,* New York, Oxford University Press, 1986.
43. Wade OL, Bishop JM: *Cardiac Output and Regional Blood Flow.* Oxford, Blackwell Scientific, 1962.
44. Blackmon JR, Rowell LB, Kennedy JW, Twiss RD, Conn RD: Physiological significance of maximal oxygen intake in pure mitral stenosis. *Circulation* 1967; 36:497–510.
45. Zelis R, Mason DT, Braunwald E: Partition of blood flow to the cutaneous and muscular beds of the forearm at rest and during leg exercise in normal subjects and in patients with heart failure. *Circ Res* 1969; 24:799–806.
46. LeBlanc J, Côté J, Dulac S, Dulong-Turcot F: Effects of age, sex, physical fitness on responses to local cooling. *J Appl Physiol* 1978; 44:813–817.
47. Neill WA, Duncan DA, Kloster F, Mahler DJ: Response of the coronary circulation to cutaneous cold. *Am J Med* 1974; 56:471–476.
48. Mudge GH Jr, Grossman W, Mills RM, Lesch M, Braunwald E: Reflex increase in coronary vascular resistance in patients with ischemic heart disease. *N Engl J Med* 1976; 295:1333–1337.
49. Hattenhauer M, Neill WA: The effect of cold air inhalation on angina pectoris and myocardial supply. *Circulation* 1975; 51:1053–1058.
50. Lassvik CT, Areskog N-H: Angina pectoris during inhalation of cold air. Reactions to exercise. *Br Heart J* 1980; 43:661–667.
51. Bert P: *La Pression Barométrique* (trans Hitchcock MA). Columbus, OH, College Book Co, 1943.
52. Bennett PB, Elliott DH (eds): *The Physiology and Medicine of Diving,* 3d ed. San Pedro, CA, Best Publishing Co, 1982.
53. Salzano JV, Stolp B, Moon RE, Camporesi EM: Exercise at 47 and 66 ATA. In: Bachrach AJ, Matzen MM (eds): *Underwater Physiology VII,* proceedings of Seventh Symposium on Underwater Physiology. Bethesda, MD, Undersea Medicine Society, 1981: 181.
54. Lin YC: Circulatory functions during immersion and breath-hold dives in humans. *Undersea Biomed Res* 1984; 11:123–138.
55. Boycott FE, Damant GCC, Haldade JS: Prevention of compressed air illness. *J Hyg* 1908; 8:342–443.
56. *U.S. Navy Diving Manual,* NAVSEA, 0994–LP–001–9020. Department of the Navy, Washington, DC, 1981.
57. Bühlmann AA: *Decompression–Decompression Sickness.* New York, Springer-Verlag, 1984.
58. Miller JN, Fagraeus L, Elliott DH, Shields TG, Grimstad J, Bennett PB: Nitrogen-oxygen saturation therapy in serious cases of compressed air decompression sickness. *Lancet* 1978; 2:169–171.
59. Moon RE, Camporesi EM, Kisslo JA: Patent foramen ovale and decompression sickness in divers. *Lancet* 1989; 1:513–514.
60. *Hyperbaric Oxygen Therapy: A Committee Report.* Undersea and Hyperbaric Medical Society, Bethesda, MD, 1989.
61. Holback KH, Wassman H, Banatelli AT: A method to identify and treat reversible alterations of brain tissue. In: Schmiedek T (ed): *Microsurgery for Stroke.* New York, Springer-Verlag, 1977: 169–176.
62. Heyman A, Saltzman HA, Whalen RE: The use of hyperbaric oxygenation in the treatment of cerebral ischemia and infarction. *Circulation* 1966; 33(suppl 2):20–27.
63. Tsuru M, Nakagawa Y, Kitaoka K, Kwahigashi H: Treatment of cerebral ischemia by hyperbaric oxygenation. In: Shiraki K, Matsuoka S (eds): *Hyperbaric Medicine and Underwater Physiology.* Kitakyushu, Japan, Fukuoka Printing Co, 1983: 315–327.
64. Piantadosi CA: The role of hyperbaric oxygen in carbon monoxide, cyanide and sulfide intoxication. *Respir Care* 1991; 4:215–231.
65. Davis JC, Hunt TK: *Problem Wounds. The Role of Oxygen.* New York, Elsevier, 1988.
66. Camporesi EM, Barker AC (eds): *Hyperbaric Oxygen Therapy. A Critical Review.* Bethesda, MD, Undersea and Hyperbaric Medical Society, 1991.

Chapter 121

Occupation and Cardiovascular Disease

Nanette Kass Wenger, M.D.

OCCUPATIONAL TOXIC EXPOSURES AND CARDIOVASCULAR RISK

General Considerations

Associations of occupations with cardiovascular diseases primarily involve potential occupational toxic exposures.[1] Improved industrial hygiene and increased automation have decreased toxic occupational exposures; hazards result predominantly from leaks, blowouts, equipment breakdown, and the like. Occupational toxic exposures can be classified as physical, biological, or chemical. Physical exposures include extremes of oxygen pressure, barometric pressure, gravity, acceleration, noise, temperature, and humidity (Chap. 120). Biological agents are involved in laboratory-acquired infections or in work in endemic areas; allergy or hypersensitivity to medications or vaccines may be considered an iatrogenic toxic exposure. Many chemical agents enter the body by inhalation, skin absorption, or ingestion; these agents may produce cardiovascular toxicity (Chap. 110) by a direct effect on the myocardium, by impairment of the oxygen-carrying capacity of the blood, or (as with organic phosphorous insecticides) by cholinesterase inhibition, clinically evident as intense parasympathetic stimulation.

Occupational toxic exposures may also mimic cardiovascular disease.[2] Toxic gases or fumes can induce pulmonary edema with retrosternal pain or discomfort, mimicking myocardial infarction. Differentiation is important, as morphine is contraindicated because concomitant central nervous system toxicity and respiratory depression result from some chemical toxicities. Digitalis is generally ineffective, and immediate therapy includes administration of oxygen, bronchodilator and corticosteroid drugs, antibiotics for secondary infection, and tracheostomy if needed.[3]

South American miners working at high altitudes in the Andes who develop "high-altitude heart disease" (see Chaps. 99 and 101) may be considered to have occupational heart disease.

Firefighters' chronic occupational exposure to carbon monoxide results in increased blood concentrations of carboxyhemoglobin, even in nonsmoking firefighters; changes in cardiac serum enzyme levels in one study suggested myocardial damage.[4] Carbon monoxide exposure with increased blood carboxyhemoglobin levels such as occurs in steel and foundry workers has not been documented to accelerate atherogenesis; nevertheless, increased symptoms in patients known to have coronary disease occur with exposure to carbon monoxide.[5]

Exposure to halogenated hydrocarbon, fluorocarbon solvents, and propellants has been associated with cardiac arrhythmias[6] and sudden death.

Nitrate Exposure and Withdrawal

Employees with coronary heart disease involved in the manufacture of explosives using glyceric nitrol esters such as nitroglycol experience an occupational hazard: nitroglycol is 180 times more volatile than nitroglycerin and is easily absorbed via the lungs and skin. Such workers developed angina during the weekend that disappeared on their returning to work; sudden death also occurred during the weekend, with deprivation of the nitroglycol vasodilation that was present during the workweek.[2] These workers also frequently had severe headaches on Monday and Tuesday, but not during the remainder of the week.

Chest pain and sudden death have occurred as "withdrawal symptoms" in workers without apparent coronary heart disease after prolonged nitroglycerin and other nitrate exposures; the time of increased risk is 1 or 2 days after cessation of exposure, suggesting that rebound vasospasm may be the etiology. Exertional and emotional stimuli did not precipitate the pain; but coronary spasm, reversed by nitroglycerin, has been documented by angiography during nitrate withdrawal.[7] Another possibility is that chronic exposure to vasodilators may provoke compensatory homeostatic vasoconstriction; its persistence during nitroglycerin withdrawal may result in myocardial ischemia.

Carbon Disulfide

Epidemiologic data show an increased risk of coronary death[5] in workers involved in the manufacture of viscose rayon and of carbon tetrachloride due to chronic exposure to carbon disulfide fumes. The risk appears related to the carbon disulfide exposure, although risk is accentuated when concomitant hypertension and older age are present.[8] The mechanism of the toxic effect has not been elucidated.

Occupational and Vascular Hand Trauma

Repeated, prolonged occupational hand trauma, as encountered among machinists, welders, plumbers, iron and steel workers, and miners who use hand-held vibrating tools such as high-frequency pneumatic hammers and chain saws, may result in severe ischemia of the digits. (See also Chap. 124.) This traumatic vasospastic disease occurred almost predictably in 40 percent of lumberjacks (tree fellers) after 3 to 5 years of occupational exposure and in 70 percent at 11 to 15 years. Preventive measures such as use of antivibration saw handles have markedly decreased the prevalence of this problem in Finnish forest workers.[9]

Cardiovascular changes similar to those encountered in endurance athletes have been described with vibration disease[10]; they include an increased left ventricular ejection fraction, due mainly to an increase in left ventricular end diastolic dimension, and a decreased resting heart rate.

Atherosclerotic Coronary Artery Disease and Occupation

A number of studies relate the incidence and severity of clinical coronary artery disease to differences in occupational physical activity.[11] The relation of emotional stress associated with occupational responsibilities to coronary atherosclerosis, as well as to hypertension, remains controversial (Chaps. 62 and 117). A 1985 conference on Behavioral Medicine and Cardiovascular Disease concluded that a growing body of evidence on occupational stress implicated high work demand and responsibility with few opportunities to control the job situation might be associated with increased coronary artery disease. Further research and intervention were recommended.[12]

Conflicting associations are described between occupation and coronary artery disease. White collar workers are reported to have a lower risk of fatal coronary artery disease than blue collar workers, even when conventional coronary risk factors are comparable. Whether occupation per se or other uncontrolled variables are the determinants requires elucidation.[13] In a Swedish study,[14] low social class, as defined by occupation, was related to the incidence of coronary artery disease and nonfatal myocardial infarction, even in multivariate analysis. In Finland, however,[15] high occupational physical workload was described to engender coronary risk; however, the high-energy demand, with heavy dynamic and static work components, has not been separated from socioeconomic status. Meta-analyses of physical activity,[16] including occupational physical activity, have shown an increased relative risk of coronary death in sedentary occupations (particularly evident in well-designed studies). An increased risk for myocardial infarction mortality was described among U.S. working police officers (but not firefighters)[17] and for coronary artery disease among Swedish bus and tram drivers (but not taxi drivers).[18] Socioeconomic status, job psychologic stress, and exposure to air pollutants are among the variables requiring examination, as the differences just cited are not explicable by standard coronary risk attributes.

EMPLOYMENT OF THE CARDIAC PATIENT

General Considerations

Ramifications of employment or reemployment of cardiac patients relate to early rehabilitation; to selective placement depending on the type of heart disease and functional capacity; to effects of work and the work environment on the heart disease; to education of the patient, employer, labor union, and physician; to insurance, law, and worker's compensation decisions; and to industry experience with cardiac patients as employees.[19]

The proceedings of the Bethesda Conference of the American College of Cardiology on insurability and employability of the patient with ischemic heart disease[20] highlighted the lack of uniformity both of assessment of medical impairment by physicians and of administrative guidelines for disability determination by governmental agencies and organizations; comparable problems are present in the public and private sectors.

The Council on Occupational Health of the American Medical Association has addressed the problem of employable patients with heart disease in an article entitled "Employability of Workers Handicapped by Certain Diseases: A Guide for Employers and Physicians"[121]:

> **Patients with cardiac disease can work. Most patients with cardiac disease should work, usually in gainful employment. Many patients with cardiac disease achieve satisfactory rehabilitation on their own. Many, however,**

achieve it only by painstaking attention to the varied factors of professionally guided rehabilitation. The extent of the pathologic symptoms and the apparent limitation of cardiac reserve are often not as important as the emotional factors and the resiliency with which the patient adjusts to his disease.

The physician's alertness, ingenuity, flexibility, and maturity are needed to cope successfully with the variety of factors involved in any individual case. Many forms of assistance are available in the medical profession, in the industrial community, and among the social agencies. The great number of persons involved makes their successful rehabilitation important to industry, and community and to the nation.*

The physical work demands of most occupations have been reduced by automation and mechanization, and only about 5 percent of occupations in the United States currently entail heavy work. Exercise-based risk stratification procedures, used to guide clinical care, can also evaluate a patient's capability to fulfill specific job requirements.[20] Energy expenditure at work is commonly less than at exercise testing, owing to the intermittent activity of work.[22]

Although so-called heart laws[20] in a number of states define that myocardial infarction in police officers and firefighters is job related, without regard to medical evidence (postulated to reflect cumulative lifelong job stress), recent evidence suggests that even age-mandated retirement of these professionals is not warranted. At older age, high physical activity on the job is rarely required and public safety is unlikely to be adversely affected.[23]

Legislative Considerations

Social Security Disability

Policies and current regulations for the determination of cardiovascular disability under titles II and XVI of the Social Security Act (P.L. 96-265, P.L. 96-473), published by the Social Security Administration, define *severe cardiac impairment* as resulting from one or more of three consequences of heart disease: congestive heart failure, ischemia (with or without necrosis) of heart muscle, and conduction disturbances and/or arrhythmias resulting in cardiac syncope. Criteria are provided for evaluating impairment; the documentation needed to support the evaluation is also described.[24] Revisions of these criteria, as suggested by an expert cardiovascular panel, were published in the *Federal Register* in 1991[25]; these revisions, designed to assess functional rather than structural impairments as the basis for entitlement for disability payments, are currently being evaluated for implementation. Social Security law defines *disability* as "the inability to engage in *any* substantial gainful activity by reason of any medically determinable physical or mental impairment. . ." Current legislation mandates review of all cases of nonpermanent disability at least every 3 years and of all other cases as appropriate. Review determinations are based on contemporary definitions of disability for the initial claims, rather than on the policies prevailing at the time disability benefits were awarded. Although the law does not mandate medical recovery for cessation of disability status and payments, some federal courts have required demonstration of medical improvement before disability benefits can be terminated.

Federal Motor Carrier Safety Regulations[26,27]

The Federal Highway Administration of the U.S. Department of Transportation requires a waiver to permit driving (Section 391.41) by individuals with a clinical diagnosis of myocardial infarction, angina pectoris, coronary insufficiency, thrombosis, or cardiovascular disease known to be accompanied by or likely to cause syncope, dyspnea, collapse, or congestive cardiac failure. Suggestions for certification include a normal resting and exercise electrocardiogram, no residual complications or physical limitations, and no use of medications likely to interfere with safe driving. Coronary bypass surgery and pacemaker implantation are considered remedial procedures and not cardiovascular conditions; they do not automatically disqualify drivers, but the final determination is based on the underlying cardiac condition. Specific blood pressure levels are provided to determine eligibility to drive of patients with hypertension; and antihypertensive medications must be unlikely to interfere with alertness, judgment, coordination, or other prerequisites of driving.

In general, sudden cardiac death rarely results in catastrophic motor vehicle accidents; drivers usually can bring their vehicle to a safe roadside position. Similar safety data have been described among Canadian public safety officers, London Transport bus drivers, and truck and private vehicle drivers in Dade County, Florida.[23] Nevertheless, a number of states in the United States prohibit driving after a syncopal episode; and several have specific regulations for syncope due to cardiac arrhythmia.[28] No distinction is made between arrhythmias managed medically or with implantable cardioverter defibrillators.

Robinson and Mulcahy[29] emphasize the safety of returning public service vehicle drivers to work following myocardial infarction; they suggest that risk stratification of coronary patients may enable further relaxation of licensing regulations for low-risk coronary patients.

Federal Aviation Administration

The flying status of pilots following successful coronary bypass surgery has generated considerable controversy and concern.[30] As of May 1982, no pilot with coronary disease significant enough to have required treatment is eligible for unrestricted medical certification by the U.S. National Transportation Safety Board (NTSB).

The NTSB, a nonmedical group, had previously ordered the Federal Aviation Administration (FAA) to medically certify pilots with surgically treated coronary disease, returning them to active private and commercial flight status without restriction.[31] These pilots were individuals with complete myocardial revascularization who had not had myocardial infarction and were asymptom-

*Reprinted with permission of the Helen Dwight Reid Educational Foundation. Published by Heldref Publication, Washington, DC. Copyright 1968.

atic after surgery; all their major risk factors had been reversed and their exercise electrocardiograms were normal. Under the new regulations, the FAA medical evaluation, as performed by the federal air surgeon, may impose operational limitations on pilots after successful coronary bypass surgery and may specify requirements for subsequent medical evaluation. This latter approach is in accord with the recommendations of an American College of Cardiology Bethesda Conference on cardiovascular problems associated with aviation safety.[30] Data from the Coronary Artery Surgery Study (CASS) Registry[32] suggest that nonsmoking, nonhypertensive persons (considered comparable to airline pilots) without prior myocardial infarction and with well-preserved left ventricular function who have a normal maximal exercise test following coronary bypass surgery are at low risk for cardiac events in the initial 7 years; their risk is comparable to that of a similarly aged U.S. male population. This information is relevant for the licensing both of airline pilots and of others in transportation industry occupations where there is concern for public safety.

The issue of aircrew licensing after coronary bypass surgery requires review. Conventional coronary risk factors appear to affect adversely the complication-free time after coronary bypass surgery.[33] Parker[34] suggests a plan for follow-up evaluations.

Patients with prosthetic heart valves are generally considered unfit to pilot airplanes because of their unacceptable risks of thromboembolism and anticoagulation complications.[35] Interim suggestions are also offered for licensing of flying personnel with congenital heart lesions with a low risk of complications either before or after surgical correction[36] as well as those with arrhythmias and conduction abnormalities.[37–39]

Worker's Compensation Considerations

Causal relation between occupation and heart disease from the viewpoint of worker's compensation decisions and awards requires only that the employee has been subjected to unusual or excessive physical or emotional strain in the course of work prior to development of angina pectoris or acute myocardial infarction. The administration of these "heart cases," however, varies widely among the states.[40] Compensation has also been awarded both on the basis of ordinary work activity as causally related to heart disease and on the basis that the cumulative physical and mental strain of a lifetime of work may culminate in an acute coronary episode.[41] Medical committees[19] properly emphasize that these attitudes often negate efforts to rehabilitate cardiac patients and hamper their employment or reemployment. (See also Chaps. 142 and 143.)

REFERENCES

1. Goldhaber SZ: Cardiovascular effects of potential occupational hazards. *J Am Coll Cardiol* 1983; 2:1210–1215.
2. Weill H: Cardiorespiratory effects of inhalant occupational exposures. *Circulation* 1981; 63:250A–252A.
3. Kleinfeld M: Acute pulmonary edema of chemical origin. *Arch Environ Health* 1965; 10:942–946.
4. Sammons JH, Coleman RL: Firefighters' occupational exposure to carbon monoxide. *J Occup Med* 1974; 16:543–546.
5. Rosenman KD: Cardiovascular disease and environmental exposure. *Br J Ind Med* 1979; 36:85–97.
6. Speizer FE, Wegman DH, Ramirez A: Palpitation rates associated with fluorocarbon exposure in a hospital setting. *N Engl J Med* 1975; 292:624–626.
7. Klock JC: Nonocclusive coronary disease after chronic exposure to nitrates: Evidence for physiologic nitrate dependence. *Am Heart J* 1975; 89:510–513.
8. Nurminen M, Mutanen P, Tolonen M, Hernberg S: Quantitated effects of carbon disulfide exposure, elevated blood pressure and aging on coronary mortality. *Am J Epidemiol* 1982; 115:107–118.
9. Pyykko I, Korhonen O, Farkkila M, Starck J, Aatola S, Jantti V: Vibration syndrome among Finnish forest workers, a follow-up from 1972 to 1983. *Scand J Work Environ Health* 1986; 12:307–312.
10. Matoba T, Itaya M, Toyomasu K, Tsuiki T, Toshima H, Kuwahara H: Increased left ventricular function as an adaptive response in vibration disease. *Am J Cardiol* 1983; 51:1223–1226.
11. Kannel WB, Belanger A, D'Agostino R, Israel I: Physical activity and physical demand on the job and risk of cardiovascular disease and death: The Framingham Study. *Am Heart J* 1986; 112:820–825.
12. Tyroler HA, Haynes SG, Cobb LA, Irvin CW Jr, James SH, Kuller LH, et al: Conference on Behavioral Medicine and Cardiovascular Disease, February 3–7, 1985, Sea Island, GA, Task Force 1: Environmental Risk Factors in Coronary Artery Disease. *Circulation* 1987; 76(suppl I):I-139–I-144.
13. Buring JE, Evans DA, Fiore M, Rosner B, Hennekens CH: Occupation and risk of death from coronary heart disease. *JAMA* 1987; 258:791–792.
14. Rosengren A, Wedel H, Wilhelmsen L: Coronary heart disease and mortality in middle aged men from different occupational classes in Sweden. *Br Med J* 1988; 297:1497–1500.
15. Ilmarinen J: Work and cardiovascular health: Viewpoint of occupational physiology. *Ann Med* 1989; 21:209–214.
16. Berlin JA, Colditz GA: A meta-analysis of physical activity in the prevention of coronary heart disease. *Am J Epidemiol* 1990; 132:612–628.
17. Dubrow R, Burnett CA, Guite DM, Brockert JE: Ischemic heart disease and acute myocardial infarction mortality among police officers. *J Occup Med* 1988; 30:650–654.
18. Rosengren A, Anderson K, Wilhelmsen L: Risk of coronary heart disease in middle-aged male bus and tram drivers compared to men in other occupations: A prospective study. *Int J Epidemiol* 1991; 20:82–87.
19. American Heart Association: Report of the Committee on Stress, Strain, and Heart Disease. *Circulation* 1977; 55:825A–835A.
20. Insurability and Employability of the Patient with Ischemic Heart Disease. 20th Bethesda Conference of the American College of Cardiology, October 3–4, 1988, Washington, DC. *J Am Coll Cardiol* 1989; 14:1003–1044.
21. American Medical Association Council on Occupational Health: Employability of Workers Handicapped by Certain Diseases: A Guide for Employers and Physicians. *Arch Environ Health* 1968; 17:389–397.
22. Hellerstein HK: Vocational aspects of rehabilitation: Work evaluation. In: Wenger NK, Hellerstein HK (eds): *Rehabilitation of the Coronary Patient,* 3d ed. New York, Churchill Livingstone, 1992: 523–542.
23. Shephard RJ: Public safety officers and cardiac disease. *J Cardiopulmon Rehabil* 1992; 12:51–55.
24. U.S. Department of Health and Human Services, Social Security Administration: *Disability Evaluation Under Social Security.* Washington, DC, U.S. Department of Health Services, SSA Publication No. 05-10089, February 1986.
25. U.S. Department of Health and Human Services, Social Security Administration: Revised medical criteria for determination of disability cardiovascular system. Social Security Administration, 20 CFR Part 404, RIN 0960-AA99. *Federal Register* 1991; 56:31266–31276.
26. U.S. Department of Transportation, Federal Highway Administration: The regulatory criteria for evaluation under Section 391.41(b)(4)(b)(6), *Federal Register,* Washington, DC, U.S. Gov-

ernment Printing Office, November 23, 1977, rev. October 1983 (nonsubstantive).

27. U.S. Department of Transportation, Federal Highway Administration: *Conference on Cardiac Disorders and Commercial Drivers.* Washington, DC Office of Motor Carriers. Pub. No. FHWA-MC-88-040, December 1987.
28. Strickberger SA, Cantillon CO, Friedman PL: When should patients with lethal ventricular arrhythmias resume driving? An analysis of state regulations and physician practices. *Ann Intern Med* 1991; 115:560–563.
29. Robinson K, Mulcahy R: Return to employment of professional drivers following myocardial infarction. *Irish Med J* 1986; 79:31–34.
30. Task Force III: Recommendations for postoperative patients with ischemic heart disease. Cardiovascular Problems Associated with Aviation Safety. Eighth Bethesda Conference of the American College of Cardiology, April 25–26, 1975, Washington, DC. *Am J Cardiol* 1975; 36:610.
31. Sands MJ Jr: Sounding board: Aviator medical certification after coronary-artery surgery. *N Engl J Med* 1982; 307:52–54.
32. Chaitman BR, Davis KB, Dodge HT, Fisher LD, Pettinger M, Holmes DR, et al: Should airline pilots be eligible to resume active flight status after coronary bypass surgery? A CASS Registry Study. *J Am Coll Cardiol* 1986; 8:1318–1324.
33. Hammond IW, Lee ET, Davis AW, Booze CF Jr: Prognostic factors related to survival and complication-free times in airmen medically certified after coronary surgery. *Aviat Space Environ Med* 1984; 55:321–331.
34. Parker DJ: The airline pilot after coronary artery bypass grafting. *Eur Heart J* 1984; 5(suppl A):77–79.
35. Parker DJ: The patient after cardiac valve surgery—risks and complications. *Eur Heart J* 1984; 5(suppl A):141–145.
36. Macartney FJ: Flying and congenital heart disease. *Eur Heart J* 1984; 5(suppl A):147–154.
37. Campbell RWF: Ventricular ectopic activity and its relevance to aircrew licensing. *Eur Heart J* 1984; 5(suppl A):95–98.
38. Bennett D: Atrial fibrillation. *Eur Heart J* 1984; 5(suppl A):89–93.
39. Canaveris G, Nau GJ: Intraventricular conduction disturbances in flying personnel: Development and prognosis of bifascicular blocks. *Aviat Space Environ Med* 1984; 58:683–689.
40. Barth PS, Hunt HA: Occupational disease in the law: The handling of heart cases and the by-accident provision. In Barth PS, Hunt HA (eds): *Workers' Compensation and Work-Related Illnesses and Disease.* Cambridge, MA, MIT Press, 1980: 105–114.
41. Warshaw LJ: Heart cases under workmen's compensation laws. *J Occup Med* 1967; 9:349–352.

PART XVIII

Diseases of the Great Vessels and Peripheral Vessels

SECTION A

Diagnosis and Treatment of Diseases of the Great Vessels and Peripheral Vessels

Chapter 122

Cerebrovascular Disease and Neurologic Manifestations of Heart Disease

Louis R. Caplan, M.D.

Most vascular diseases have a tendency to affect both the heart and the brain. In addition, cardiac diseases often lead to secondary lesions and dysfunction within the brain, and central nervous system (CNS) diseases can affect the heart and its function.

BRAIN AND CEREBROVASCULAR COMPLICATIONS OF HEART DISEASE

Cerebral complications occur when: (1) the heart pumps unwanted materials into the circulation that reach the brain (embolism); (2) pump function fails and the brain is hypoperfused; or (3) drugs given to treat cardiac disease have neurologic side effects.

Cardiogenic Brain Embolism

Etiology

Until recently, the diagnostic criteria of cardiogenic embolism were very restrictive. It was diagnosed when sudden focal neurologic signs, maximal at onset, developed in a patient with a peripheral systemic embolism and a cardiogenic source of embolism such as recent myocardial infarction or rheumatic mitral stenosis. By these criteria, cardiogenic embolism was diagnosed in only 3 to 8 percent of stroke patients.[1–3] None of these criteria are secure. In various stroke registries,[4–7] about 10 to 20 percent of patients did not have maximal symptoms at outset. Many other cardiac lesions are now well-accepted sources of emboli, e.g., atrial fibrillation. Only about 2 percent of patients with cardiogenic brain embolism[4] have clinically recognized peripheral emboli. In necropsy studies of patients with brain embolism, however, infarcts are commonly found in the spleen and kidneys and other organs. The symptoms of peripheral embolism are often so minor and nonspecific (transient abdominal discomfort, leg cramp, etc.) that they are seldom diagnosed correctly.

Before the advent of echocardiography, fully 30 percent of patients with stroke were believed to have cardiogenic embolism.[4] Later studies that used stricter criteria attributed 17 percent,[5] 22 percent,[8] and 14 percent[6] of strokes to cardiogenic embolism. With more advanced diagnostic techniques more cardiac abnormalities are recognized, and in the Lausanne Stroke Registry 305 (23 percent) of 1311 patients with a first stroke had a potential cardiac source of embolism.[7,9] Because many patients have coexisting cardiac and extracranial vascular disease,[9–11] the exact criteria for the diagnosis of cardiac embolism remain controversial.

Cardiac sources can be divided into three groups[9]: (1) *cardiac wall abnormalities*, e.g., cardiomyopathies, hypokinetic and akinetic ventricular regions after myocardial infarction, atrial septal aneurysms, ventricular aneurysms, atrial myxomas and other tumors, septal defects, and patent foramen ovale; (2) *valve disorders*, e.g., rheumatic mitral and aortic disease, prosthetic valves, bacterial endocarditis, nonbacterial thrombotic endocarditis, mitral valve prolapse, and mitral annulus calcification; and (3) *arrhythmias*, especially atrial fibrillation and "sick-sinus" syndrome.

Some sources have much higher rates of initial and recurrent embolism. The Stroke Data Bank[12] divided potential sources into *strong* (valve surgery, atrial fibrillation, sick-sinus syndrome, ventricular aneurysm, akinetic segments, mural thrombi, cardiomyopathy, diffuse ventricular hypokinesia) and *weak* (myocardial infarct over 6 months old, aortic and mitral stenosis and regurgitation, congestive failure, mitral valve prolapse, mitral annulus calcification, hypokinetic ventricular segments).

Even within individual cardiac sources, e.g., atrial fibrillation, there are differences in risk depending on many factors. For example, in atrial fibrillation, associated heart disease, patient age, duration, chronic versus intermittent, and atrial size may influence embolic risk. A potential cardiac source of embolism does not mean that a stroke was actually caused by an embolus from the heart. Coexistent occlusive cerebrovascular disease is common. In the Lausanne registry, among patients with potential cardiac embolic sources, 11 percent of patients had severe cerebral occlusive disease (>75 percent stenosis) and 40 percent had mild to moderate stenosis proximal to brain infarcts.[9]

Mitral valve prolapse (MVP) continues to be a controversial issue. (See Chap. 80.) Several clinical series indicate that MVP is associated with stroke.[13–16] Morphologic lesions, such as thrombi and fibrous lesions, clearly suggest embolism[17–19]; fibrin-platelet depositions on the surfaces of the mitral leaflets have been noted,[16–18] as well as thrombi in the angle between the posterior mitral valve leaflet and the left atrial wall.[16,19,20] Patients with MVP also have other disorders such as atrial fibrillation, syncope, and migraine. The rate of recurrence of stroke in patients with MVP as the only known cause is very low.[15,16] Given the very high incidence of MVP, the frequency of MVP-related stroke is extremely low.[16–21] Most neurologists feel that warfarin anticoagulants are ordinarily not indicated in prophylaxis of patients with MVP, even after an initial stroke. Aspirin prophylaxis (160 to 325 mg/day) would, however, be advisable. Demonstration of an intracardiac thrombus by echocardiography would change that recommendation to warfarin in individual high-risk patients. (See also Chap. 80.)

Mitral annulus calcification (MAC) is an important but frequently unrecognized cause of embolism. Ulceration and extrusion of calcium through overlapping cusps has been seen at necropsy,[22] thrombi have been found on valves attached to the ulcerative process, and calcific emboli have been seen in surgical embolectomies.[16,22,23] Several series show a convincing relationship between MAC and brain emboli or stroke.[5,22,24–26] Bacterial endocarditis can also develop on the MAC.

More patients have cardiogenic embolism than are presently diagnosed. Clinical features and brain investigations such as computed tomography (CT) or cerebral angiography may suggest emboli, but often a source cannot be identified. These cases, which are termed *infarcts of unknown causes* (IUC) in the Stroke Data Bank,[6,27,28] may involve 40 percent of patients.

Nonbacterial thrombotic endocarditis and Libman-Sachs endocarditis[29] are also important sources of brain embolism. In infective endocarditis, embolic complications are common.[30] Mycotic aneurysms can cause fatal subarachnoid bleeding. Bleeding can also result from vascular necrosis as a result of an infected embolus.[30] Embolization usually stops when the infection is controlled.[30] Warfarin does not prevent embolization and is probably contraindicated unless there are other important lesions such as a prosthetic valve or life-threatening pulmonary embolism. (See also Chap. 94.) In children and young adults with congenital heart defects, especially those with right-to-left shunts and polycythemia, brain abscess is an important complication. (See also Chap. 97.)

Emboli can arise from sources other than the heart, such as proximal arteries (intraarterial or local embolism), leg veins (paradoxical emboli), fat in the liver or bones (fat embolism), and materials introduced by the patient or physician (drug particles or air).[11] The types of embolic material can also vary (Table 122-1).[11]

Clinical Findings

Anterior Circulation Recipient Sites Balloons placed into the circulation always follow the same flow patterns,[31] and anterior circulation material reaches the middle cerebral arteries (MCA) and their branches.[31] The commonest sites are the mainstem MCA, the upper or lower divisions of the MCA, or their branches. The upper division of the MCA supplies the frontal and parietal lobes above the sylvian fissure, and the inferior division supplies the convexal temporal and inferior parietal lobes.[32,33] Resultant neurologic deficits include the following:

TABLE 122-1
Embolic Materials

Cardiac	Intraarterial
1. Red fibrin-dependent thrombi	1. Red fibrin-dependent thrombi
2. White platelet-fibrin nidi	2. White platelet-fibrin nidi
3. Material from marantic endocarditis	3. Combined fibrin-platelet and fibrin-dependent clots
4. Bacteria from vegetations	4. Cholesterol crystals
5. Calcium from valves and mitral annulus calcification	5. Atheromatous plaque debris
6. Myxoma cells and debris	6. Calcium from vascular calcifications
	7. Air
	8. Mucin from tumors
	9. Talc or microcrystalline cellulose from injected drugs

MCA Upper Division Contralateral hemiparesis, hemisensory loss; aphasia (left hemisphere); lack of awareness of deficit, neglect of the left space, motor impersistence (right hemisphere)[34]

MCA Inferior Division Wernicke-type fluent aphasia, agitation, right upper quadrant anopia (left hemisphere); agitation and hyperactivity, left neglect, poor drawing and copying (right hemisphere)[33]

MCA Mainstem Infarcts—usually features of both upper and inferior division infarcts.

Posterior Circulation Recipient Sites Vertebrobasilar territory symptoms are commonly attributed to local disease within that circulation without consideration of possible cardiogenic embolism. In the major registries,[4–6,9] however, about 20 percent of emboli of cardiac origin go to the posterior circulation. Twenty percent is expected, as about one-fifth of cerebral blood flow goes to this circulation. In the posterior circulation, certain recipient sites are favored:

Posterior Cerebral Artery (PCA)[33,35] Particles and clots go to the most distal part of the system; the PCA is the terminal vessel in the vertebrobasilar circuit. The hallmark of PCA lesions is hemianopia and/or hemisensory loss contralateral to the infarct. Patients with left PCA infarcts also commonly cannot read or name colors but retain the ability to write and spell.[33] Amnesia is sometimes prominent and may last for up to 6 months. Right PCA infarction is often associated with left visual neglect.

Top of the Basilar Artery[36,37] The major clinical features are apathy and sleepiness; abnormal vertical gaze; and hallucinations, unusual reports, and other behavioral abnormalities.[36] Bilateral PCA infarction is present, and the clinical findings include bilateral visual field loss, amnesia, and severe agitation and delirium.[36]

Vertebral Artery (VA) Intracranially and Its Posterior Inferior Cerebellar Artery (PICA) Branch[38] Somewhat larger emboli may occlude an intracranial VA and cause cerebellar infarction involving mostly the posterior inferior surface.[38,39] Ataxia, vomiting, and occipital headache are the commonest signs.

Onset and Course

Many embolic strokes have their onset during rest or sleep. Sudden coughing or sneezing or arising at night to urinate can precipitate embolism. Although the deficit is most often maximal at outset, 11 percent of embolic stroke patients in the Harvard Stroke Registry had a stuttering or stepwise course, whereas 10 percent had fluctuations or progressive deficits. Later progression, if it occurs, is usually within the first 48 h. Progression is usually due to distal passage of emboli. "Nonsudden embolus" is explained by the embolus moving from its initial location, as demonstrated by angiography to a more distal branch.[40] Early angiography has a very high rate of showing intracranial emboli, but angiography after 48 h demonstrates a much lower rate of blockage.[4,41] More recently, transcranial Doppler (TCD) sonography shows a high incidence of MCA blockage acutely in patients with sudden onset hemispheric strokes but later, thrombolysis and normalization of the intracranial blood velocities occur.[42] As in all large infarcts, brain edema and swelling may develop during the 24 to 72 h after the stroke, with headache, decreased alertness, and worsening of the neurologic signs. The edema is often cytotoxic (inside cells) and may not respond to corticosteroid treatment.

Diagnostic Testing

Emboli usually cause occlusion of distal branches and produce surface infarcts that are roughly triangular with the apex of the triangle pointing inward. CT and magnetic resonance imaging (MRI) can suggest the presence of embolism by the location and shape of the lesion, the presence of multiple superficial wedge-shaped infarcts in multiple different vascular territories, hemorrhagic infarction, and visualization of a thrombus within arteries. In a series of 60 patients with cardiogenic sources of embolism studied by CT in whom occlusive atherosclerotic cerebrovascular disease had been excluded, 56 had superficial large or small cortical or subcortical infarcts, and only 4 had deep infarcts.[43] Emboli can block the MCA and cause solely deep infarcts because the superficial territory has good collateral flow; these infarcts are called *striatocapsular* because they involve the internal capsule and the adjacent basal ganglia, which are supplied by lenticulostriate branches of the MCA.[44] Occasionally, tiny emboli may cause small deep or superficial infarcts.

MRI is probably more sensitive for the detection of brain infarcts than CT, and it is also superior in detecting hemorrhagic infarction by imaging hemosiderin. Hemorrhagic infarction has long been considered characteristic of embolism, especially when the vessel leading to the infarct is patent.[45] The mechanism of hemorrhagic infarction is related to reperfusion of an ischemic zone, which occurs with spontaneous passage of the embolus after iatrogenic opening of an occluded artery (e.g., endarterectomy, fibrinolytic treatment) or after restoration of the circulation after a period of systemic hypoperfusion. Hemorrhage occurs into proximal reperfused regions of brain infarcts.[46] At times, it is also possible to image the acute embolus on CT.[11,47,48] In unselected series of stroke patients, transthoracic echocardiography (TTE) (Chap. 15) has been variably useful in defining a source.[49–51] TTE is useful in patients with known cardiac disease to clarify potential embolic sources and heart function,[5] in young patients without stroke risk factors, and in stroke patients who do not have lacunar infarction or ultrasound evidence of intrinsic atherostenosis of a major extracranial and intracranial artery. Transesophageal echocardiography (TEE) (Chap. 131) provides much better visualization of the aorta, atria, cardiac valves, and septal regions. Reports of TEE suggest that the diagnostic yield is 2 to 10 times that of TTE.[52–55] Ulcerative aortic plaques, atrial septal aneurysms, and atrial septal defects are also much better seen with TEE. The use of an echo-enhancing agent like agitated saline helps detect intracardiac shunts.

Echocardiography has definite limitations. Particles

the size of 2 mm can block major brain arteries but are probably beyond the imaging resolution of current echocardiographic technology.[11] Also, thromboembolism is a dynamic process. When a clot forms in the heart and embolizes, there may be no residual evidence until a clot reforms.[11] Cardiac thrombi may be imaged differently or sequential echocardiograms[56]; even large intracardiac thrombi seen on one echocardiogram can disappear later.[57] Platelet scintigraphy using platelets labeled with radionuclides may be helpful in localizing cardiac and intraarterial sources, but its sensitivity and specificity are undefined.[58]

Prevention and Treatment

Early studies showed that warfarin was effective in preventing brain embolism in patients with rheumatic mitral stenosis and atrial fibrillation (AF). Previously, the intensity of anticoagulation was higher than currently employed, and brain hemorrhages and other bleeding complications were more common. Excellent trials have shown that low-dose warfarin [International Normalized Ratio (INR) 2.0 to 3.0] is also effective in preventing brain emboli in patients with nonrheumatic AF.[59–69]

In the Copenhagen Atrial Fibrillation, Aspirin, Anticoagulation (AFASAK) study, 1007 patients (median age 74.2 years) with chronic, nonrheumatic AF were assigned to warfarin (INR 2.8 to 4.2), aspirin (75 mg/day), or placebo.[59] The study was halted prematurely when an analysis of efficiency reached a predetermined level of significance in favor of treatment with warfarin. The principal outcome was the composite of ischemic or hemorrhagic stroke, transient ischemic attack (TIA), and systemic embolism. The observed reduction for warfarin compared to placebo was 64 percent, an absolute risk reduction of 3.5 percent per year. A subsequent report of an analysis by intention to treat, which excluded TIA and minor stroke, indicated a risk reduction of about 50 percent ($p < .05$) and an absolute reduction of about 1.5 percent per year.

The Stroke Prevention in Atrial Fibrillation (SPAF) study evaluated both warfarin and aspirin in patients with nonrheumatic AF.[60,64] The study evaluated two groups of patients on the basis of their eligibility for warfarin. In group 1, 627 patients who were judged to be eligible for warfarin were randomized to open-label warfarin (INR of 2.8 to 4.5; prothrombin time, 1.3 to 1.8 × control) or double-blind to either aspirin (325 mg daily, enteric coated) or matching placebo. In group 2, 703 patients who were considered ineligible for warfarin were randomized in double-blind fashion to aspirin (325 mg daily, enteric coated) or matching placebo. The principal outcome, which was a composite of ischemic stroke and system embolism, was significantly decreased during a mean follow-up of 1.3 years. The outcome of disabling ischemic stroke or vascular death was reduced by warfarin by 54 percent ($p = .11$), an absolute reduction of 2.6 percent per year. Aspirin also decreased the principal outcome in both study groups. The risk reduction was 42 percent ($p = .02$), and the absolute reduction was 2.7 percent per year. The outcome of disabling stroke or death was reduced 22 percent by aspirin ($p = .33$), or an absolute reduction of about 1 percent per year.

In the Boston Area Anticoagulation Trial for Atrial Fibrillation (BAATAF), 420 patients with nonrheumatic AF and with a mean age of 68 years were randomized unblinded to a warfarin group (target prothrombin time ratio, 1.2 to 1.5 × control; INR of 1.5 to 2.7) or to a control group who were allowed to take aspirin.[62] The principal outcome was ischemic stroke or systemic embolism, and the mean follow-up was 2.2 years. The incidence of stroke was reduced by 86 percent in the warfarin group compared to control ($p = .002$), equivalent to an absolute risk reduction of 2.6 percent per year. There was no demonstrable benefit of aspirin; however, the study was not designed to test the efficiency of aspirin.

In the Canadian Atrial Fibrillation Anticoagulation (CAFA) study, 187 patients were randomized to warfarin (INR target range 2.0 to 3.0) and 191 to placebo.[65] The principal outcome was the composite of nonlacunar stroke, noncentral nervous system embolism, and fatal or intracranial hemorrhage. The relative risk reduction produced by warfarin was 37 percent ($p = .17$). The study was prematurely terminated when the preliminary results of the Copenhagen AFASAK and SPAF studies became known.

The Veterans Affairs Stroke Prevention in Nonrheumatic Atrial Fibrillation study was a randomized, double-blind, placebo-controlled study to evaluate low-intensity anticoagulation with warfarin (prothrombin time ratio of 1.2 to 1.5, corresponding to an INR of 1.4 to 2.8) in male veterans.[69] The placebo group ($n = 265$) and the warfarin group ($n = 260$) were followed for an average of 1.7 and 1.6 years, respectively. Subjects receiving warfarin had a 79 percent reduction in the risk of cerebral infarction. None of the 18 patients in this study or the 52 patients in the SPAF study who had lone AF had a cerebral infarction.

A follow-up analysis of the SPAF study identified three risk factors for thromboembolism: recent congestive heart failure, history of hypertension, and previous thromboembolism. It was concluded that anticoagulation with warfarin was not indicated in patients who had none of the three risk factors and were therefore at a low risk for thromboembolism (2.5 percent per year). In such patients the dangers of anticoagulant therapy may outweigh its benefits.[66,67] The potential benefit of aspirin versus warfarin is being assessed in the SPAF II study. In the meantime, aspirin (325 mg daily) would appear to be reasonable and safe therapy for patients with lone, nonrheumatic AF who are under 60 years of age and who have none of the three identified risk factors.[66–69] In other patients with AF, long-term oral warfarin therapy (INR of 2.0 to 3.0) should be used unless there is a contraindication.[68,69]

The effects of anticoagulation on embolism from other cardiac conditions have not been well studied.The rate of recurrence of stroke in patients with MVP is so low that warfarin is not routinely recommended for prophylaxis except when a thrombus is seen on echocardiography. (See also Chap. 80.) Warfarin may not be effective in preventing calcific, myxomatous, bacterial, and fibrin-platelet emboli; and some researchers have suggested that warfarin may worsen cholesterol crystal embolization.[70]

The timing of the initiation of warfarin anticoagulation after embolic stroke remains controversial. Embolic brain infarcts often become hemorrhagic, and serious brain hemorrhage has occurred after anticoagulation.[71–74] Large infarcts, hypertension, bolus of large heparin doses, and excessive anticoagulation have been associated with hemorrhage. Because most hemorrhagic transformations occur within 48 h, the recommendations of the Cerebral Embolism Task Force were to avoid early anticoagulation in patients with large infarcts or hemorrhagic transformation on repeat CT.[75,76] Later studies, however, support the view that anticoagulation can be undertaken without hemorrhagic transformation.[74,77] The risk of reembolism must be balanced against the small but definite risk of important bleeding. If the patient has a large brain infarct, heparin should be delayed and bolus heparin infusions should be avoided. On the other hand, if the risk for reembolism is high, immediate heparinization is advisable, whereas if the risk seems low, it is prudent to delay anticoagulants for at least 48 h and possibly even for a period of 2 to 3 weeks.[75,76]

Brain Hypoperfusion Due to Cardiac Pump Failure

In patients undergoing cardiopulmonary resuscitation (CPR), the heart is often able to recover in individuals whose brain has been irreversibly damaged by ischemic-anoxic damage. Cardiologists should be familiar with the pathology, signs, and prognosis of brain dysfunction after periods of circulatory failure.

Different brain regions have selective vulnerability to hypoxic-ischemic damage. Those regions that are most remote and at the edges of major vascular supply are more liable to injury. These zones have usually been referred to as "border zones" or "watersheds."

The cerebral cortex is most vulnerable to injury. The damage may be diffuse or "laminar," involving layers of the cortex. The hippocampus is one of the most vulnerable areas.[78–81] In the brain, the border zone regions are between the ACA and MCA and the MCA and PCA. The damage is usually most severe in the posterior parieto-temporo-occipital region and in frontal areas most remote from the heart and thus called *distal fields*. A similar border zone exists in the cerebellum between the cerebellar arteries, and in the brainstem between medial and lateral arteries. The basal ganglia and thalamus are most involved if hypoxia is severe but some circulation is preserved. This situation applies most to hanging, strangulation, drowning, and carbon monoxide exposure.[82] Cerebellar neurons, especially Purkinje cells, may also be selectively injured.[83]

When circulatory arrest is complete and abrupt, brainstem nuclei are especially vulnerable to necrosis, especially in young humans and experimental animals.[84] When hypoxia and ischemia are especially severe, the spinal cord may also be damaged.[85,86] When cortical damage is very severe and protracted, cytotoxic edema causes massive brain swelling, with cessation of blood flow and brain death.

Clinical Findings

Very severe damage leads to severe injury to the cortex and brainstem and irreversible coma and brain death. When initially examined, the patient has no brainstem reflexes (pupillary, corneal, and oculovestibular and oculocephalic reflexes) and no response to stimuli except perhaps decerebration. These findings do not improve, and respiratory control is absent or lost.

When cerebral cortical damage is very severe but brainstem ischemic changes are reversible, brainstem reflexes are preserved but there is no meaningful response to the environment. Automatic facial movements such as blinking, tongue protrusion, and yawning usually persist. The eyes may rest slightly up and move from side to side. When this state does not improve, it is referred to as the *persistent vegetative state*,[80,86a,87] or "wakefulness without awareness."[80] Laminar necrosis also often causes seizures. These are often multifocal myoclonic twitches or jerks of the facial and limb muscles, which are very difficult to control with anticonvulsants; oversedation should be avoided.

With severe border-zone injury, there is weakness of the arms and proximal lower extremities with preservation of face and leg and foot movement (the so-called man in a barrel syndrome). With less severe ischemia, the symptoms and signs are predominantly visual. Patients speak of difficulty in seeing and cannot integrate the features of large objects or scenes despite retained ability to see small objects in some parts of their visual fields. Reading is impossible. There are features of Balint's syndrome[88,89] including: asimultagnosia, i.e., seeing things piecemeal or sequentially; optic ataxia, i.e., poor eye-hand coordination; and optic apraxia, i.e., difficulty in directing gaze. Apathy and inertia are also common and are due to frontal lobe border-zone damage. Amnesia is also very common. Patients cannot make new memories and have patchy, retrograde amnesia for events during and before the hospitalization. This Korsakoff-type of syndrome is due to hippocampal damage and sometimes is not reversible. Amnesia may be accompanied by visual abnormalities, apathy, and confusion or may be an isolated cognitive deficit.

Action myoclonus (the Lance-Adams syndrome)[83] is thought to be due to cerebellar damage. This disorder is characterized by arrhythmic fine or coarse jerking, especially on attempted movement. Reaching for an object may be accompanied by gross oscillation and tremorlike movements. Gait ataxia is also common. The findings are worsened by stress and emotion and suppressed somewhat by barbiturates and diazepam.[90]

Prognosis

Shortly after resuscitation or arrest, patients with less severe cerebral injuries show some signs of reactivity to the environment. Eye opening and restless limb movements develop. The eyes may fixate on objects. Noise, a flashlight, or a gentle pinch arouses the patient to avoid or react to the stimulus. Soon the patient awakens fully and may begin to speak. Cognitive and behavioral abnormalities may be detected after awakening, depending on the degree of injury.

Prognostic signs and variables have been extensively studied.[89,91] The initial neurologic findings and their course are helpful in predicting outcome.[91] Among all patients who responded with meaningful responses to pain at 1 h, all survivors had preserved intellectual function.[91] Patients who do not respond to pain by 24 h either die or remain in a vegetative state. Being comatose predicts a poor prognosis.[93,94] Thus, two simple observations, the presence or absence of coma and the response to pain, predict neurologic outcome very early.[94] After hypoxic-ischemic insults, the outcome can be analyzed progressively at 3, 7, and 14 days after the event.[94]

In a study in Seattle of out-of-hospital cardiac arrests, patients who did not awaken died on average 3.5 days after arrest.[95,96] Of 459 patients, 183 never awakened (39 percent). Among those who did awaken, 91 (32 percent) had persistent neurologic deficits.[95] Prognosis could be made by analysis of pupillary light reflexes, eye movements, and motor responses.[96] Bystander initiation of CPR was not significantly related to awakening,[96] in contrast to another study that found that outcome was better if CPR was started by bystanders before the emergency team arrived.[97] Patients awake on admission were included in one study[97] but excluded in the other.[96] After in-hospital CPR, pneumonia, hypotension, renal failure, cancer, and a housebound state before hospitalization were significantly related to death in the hospital.[98] (See also Chaps. 51 and 52.)

Diagnostic Testing

Neurologic imaging and other tests have proved to be relatively unhelpful, in contrast to the neurologic examination. CT is used to exclude other causes of coma such as brain hemorrhage. Electroencephalography (EEG) is helpful in studying cortical activity in unresponsive patients and in assessment of brain death. Similarly, the absence of responses to visual and somatosensory stimuli is a poor prognostic sign. TCD may be helpful in the evaluation of brain death.[99–101]

Treatment

Other than maintaining adequate circulation and oxygenation, treatment has not been very helpful in improving outcome. Increased blood sugar correlates with poor outcome,[102] and experimental animals subjected to circulatory arrest do worse if they have been fed glucose before the arrest.[103–104] Blood calcium and the presence of free radicals and excitatory neurotoxins have all been postulated to effect neuronal cell death.[104–106] A multifaceted approach to therapy has been most successful to date.[107] The treatment of hypoxic-ischemic patients clearly needs more study and trials.

Neurologic Effects of Cardiac Drugs

The neurologic side effects of several cardiovascular agents can mimic or cause stroke. (See also Chap. 109.)

Digitalis can cause visual hallucinations, yellow vision, and general confusion.[108,109] Digitalis levels need not be elevated, and the symptoms disappear with cessation of the drug.

Quinidine can cause confusion with delirium, seizures and coma, vertigo, tinnitus, and visual blurring.[110] Chronic cognitive and behavioral changes and "quinidine dementia" are less well known. Alzheimer's dementia may be diagnosed and may disappear on cessation. Similar experience has been seen with lithium.

Patients may become acutely comatose while being treated with intravenous lidocaine. This has been associated with the accidental administration of very large doses; more common CNS effects of less extreme toxicity include sedation, irritability, and twitching. The latter may progress to seizures accompanied by respiratory depression.

NEUROLOGIC AND CEREBROVASCULAR COMPLICATIONS OF CARDIAC SURGERY

The incidence of some change in intellectual function and behavior after cardiac surgery is quite high. Fortunately, most changes are reversible with time. The reported incidence of neurologic complications after cardiac surgery varies widely from 7 to 61 percent for transient complications and from 1.6 to 23 percent for permanent complications.[111,112] Prospectively, transient complications have been noted in fully 61 percent of patients.[113] Similarly, in another series, 16.8 percent of patients had stroke or encephalopathy after coronary artery bypass surgery (CABS); the encephalopathies usually cleared, and only 2 percent of patients had severe strokes.[114]

Atherothrombotic, Hemodynamically Mediated Brain Infarcts

A major concern has been that the hemodynamics and circulatory stress of heart surgery will lead to underperfusion of areas supplied by already stenosed or occluded arteries, leading to brain infarcts. This concern underlies neck auscultation for bruits, ultrasound carotid artery testing, and even cerebral angiography prior to CABS. Hemodynamically induced infarction, however, is a very rare complication of heart surgery. Embolism is much more common and a much greater concern. Patients with carotid bruits have a very low rate of stroke after elective surgery.[114,115] In a retrospective study of CABS patients with known carotid disease, ipsilateral strokes occurred in 1.1 percent of arteries with 50 to 90 percent stenosis, in 6.2 percent of arteries with >90 percent stenosis, and in only 2 percent of vessels with carotid occlusion.[116,117] Stroke rates tend to be lower in those undergoing a combined as opposed to a staged procedure,[118] but definitive conclusions as to the proper management of combined cerebral and coronary artery disease await the outcome of clinical trials. Intracranial flow and velocity do not show significant changes in patients with high-grade carotid stenosis during CABS.[119]

Most studies have relied on clinical localization of focal deficits and inference about their mechanisms. A neuroradiology study reviewed neuroimaging results from 30 patients with acute strokes in relation to CABS.[120] Only one had strong evidence of a hemodynamic atherostenotic mechanism. Thrombotic infarction may occur in the days following surgery when the cessation of anticoagulation and the activation of coagulation factors may promote hypercoagulability.

Brain Embolism

A strong point against a hemodynamic cause of many strokes is their timing. Strokes occur more frequently *after* recovery from the anesthetic. If the mechanism of stroke were hemodynamic, the major circulatory stress would be intraoperative and patients would awaken with the deficit. In only one of the studies cited did the authors record the timing of the CABS-related strokes.[120] In that study only 17 percent of patients had the deficit noted immediately postoperatively. The distribution of infarcts and their multiplicity in the neuroradiologic study were most consistent with embolism.[120] It was concluded that cerebral infarction associated with CABS is more frequently caused by cerebral embolization than by cerebral hypoperfusion. Embolic infarcts may involve either the anterior or the posterior circulation.[114,120] In our series of postoperative, posterior circulation strokes, the majority were embolic and followed cardiac surgery.[121]

Emboli may arise from preexisting cerebrovascular lesions or postoperative arrhythmias. Mounting evidence links operative and postoperative embolism to aortic ulcerative atherosclerotic lesions. Cross-clamping of the ascending aorta or aortotomy may liberate cholesterol or calcific plaque debris.[114]

After cardiac surgery, severe bilateral, predominantly border-zone infarcts have been reported, and the small arteries of the brain and other viscera (heart, kidney, spleen, pancreas) may be packed with birefringent cholesterol crystal emboli.[122] TEE makes it possible to detect protruding ulcerative plaques in the aorta preoperatively and intraoperatively.[123–125] In one patient with repeated peripheral emboli, the protruding atherosclerotic plaque was removed surgically.[123] Intraaortic atherosclerotic debris identified by TEE has been found to be associated with embolic events.[124] Intraoperative B-mode ultrasonography with the probe placed on the aorta has also been used to detect severe aortic atherosclerotic plaques.[125] Ultrasonic imaging showed aortic atheromas in 58 percent of patients, whereas visual examination and palpation detected plaques in only 24 percent.[125] Atherosclerosis of the ascending aorta is an important risk factor for post-CABS stroke.[126]

In some patients, hypercoagulability related to surgery can precipitate occlusive thrombosis in atherostenotic arteries, and the newly formed thrombus can lead to intraarterial embolism. It is apparent that cardiac, aortic, and intraarterial embolisms account for the vast majority of cardiac surgery–related focal neurologic deficits.

Encephalopathy

Gilman described a diffuse CNS disorder following open heart surgery; it is characterized by altered levels of consciousness and activity and confusion[127] and is now termed an *encephalopathy*. Clinical and imaging studies do not show important focal neurologic signs or large focal infarcts. The incidence of this encephalopathic process varies.[112] In one series, 57 of 1669 (34 percent) CABS patients had postoperative mental state changes including delirium and encephalopathy.[128] In the Cleveland Clinic prospective series, 11.6 percent were "encephalopathic" on the fourth postoperative day.[114] The encephalopathy likely has multiple causes. Embolization of particulate matters has been considered to be the leading cause and this has led to technical improvements, including the introduction of membrane rather than bubble oxygenators and on-line filtration.[117] These technical advances have led to a decrease in the risk of macroemboli (>25 mm) as a cause, but they cannot protect against microemboli of air, fat, or particles.[117]

A necropsy study of patients who died after cardiopulmonary bypass or angiography has awakened interest in this subject.[110,127] Focal, small capillary and arteriolar dilatations (SCADs) were commonly found in the brain.[129] About one-half of the SCADs show birefringent crystalline material within the dilated capillaries. SCADs could, at least in part, explain the decreased cerebral blood flow found during cardiopulmonary bypass.[31] SCADs are iatrogenically generated microemboli, but as yet their origin is unknown. Their morphology is most consistent with air or fat.[125]

Other causes of encephalopathy are common. Hypoxic-ischemic insults due to hypotension and hypoperfusion do occur. A very common cause of encephalopathy in the postoperative period, however, is the use of drugs. Particularly important are haloperidol, narcotics, and sedatives. Morphine is sometimes used heavily intraoperatively, and opiate withdrawal with restlessness and hyperactivity can result. Agitation and restlessness are often early signs of organic encephalopathy and may lead to the administration of haloperidol, barbiturates, phenothiazines, or benzodiazepines for calming and sedation. When these drugs wear off and the patient begins to awaken, agitation may occur and more sedatives may be given. Haloperidol may produce rigidity, restlessness, agitation, hallucinations, and confusion. In experimental animals, haloperidol delays recovery from strokes by months and its use is not advised.[130,131] Phenothiazines and sedatives are also problematic; in general, use of sedatives and narcotics should be minimized and tapered as soon as feasible.

Intracranial Hemorrhage after Cardiac Surgery

Occasionally, intracerebral or subarachnoid hemorrhages have been reported after cardiac surgery, most commonly in children who have had repair of congenital heart disease[132] or after cardiac transplantation.[133] The postulated mechanism involves an abrupt increase in brain blood flow with rupture of small intracranial arteries unprepared for the new load. Generally, there is a prolonged period of low cardiac output that is suddenly increased by the operation. Abrupt increases in brain blood flow or pressure in other situations have also been associated with intracerebral hemorrhage.[134]

Peripheral Nerve Complications

Brachial plexus and peripheral nerve lesions frequently develop after cardiac surgery and can be confused with CNS complications.[135] In one series new peripheral nervous system deficits occurred in 13 percent of patients.[135] The commonest deficit is a unilateral brachial plexopathy characterized by shoulder pain and usually weakness and numbness of one hand. It is probably caused by positioning of the arm during surgery with traction on the lower trunk of the brachial plexus. Ulnar, peroneal, and saphenous nerve injuries are also common and are also related to positioning. Diaphragmatic and vocal cord paralysis are likely related to local effects of the cardiac surgery on the recurrent laryngeal and phrenic nerves.

CARDIAC EFFECTS OF BRAIN LESIONS

The field of neurocardiology is relatively new.[136] Information is beginning to emerge on cardiac muscle changes (myocytolysis), arrhythmias, pulmonary edema, electrocardiographic (ECG) changes, and sudden death due to brain disease and sudden emotional stresses.

Cardiac Lesions

The two most common lesions found in the heart in patients dying with acute CNS lesions are patchy regions of myocardial necrosis and subendocardial hemorrhages. The changes can range from eosinophilic staining of cells with preserved striations to transformation of myocardial cells into dense eosinophilic bands. These changes have been referred to as *myocytolysis.*[137] Subendocardial petechiae and frank hemorrhages are also noted. These lesions were described in the 1950s[136-139] but were thought initially to be rare.[138,140] One study found a very high incidence of myocardial changes in patients dying of brain lesions that increase intracranial pressure rapidly.[141] Stress-related release of catecholamines and possibly corticosteroids may be responsible, at least in part, for the cardiac lesions found in patients with CNS lesions.[142-146]

Electrocardiographic and Enzyme Changes

In stroke patients, especially those with subarachnoid hemorrhage, an ECG syndrome occurs that is characterized by prolonged QT interval; giant, wide, roller-coaster, inverted T waves; and U waves.[147] These changes were termed *cerebral T waves.*[142] Subsequent studies showed that patients with stroke who had continuous electrocardiographic monitoring had a high incidence of T-wave and ST-segment changes, various arrhythmias, and cardiac enzyme abnormalities. ECG changes may include prolonged QT interval, depressed ST segments, flat or inverted T waves, and U waves.[148-150] Less often, tall peaked T waves and elevated ST segments are noted. (See also Chap. 13.)

Cardiac and skeletal muscle enzymes, including CK-MG, are often abnormal in stroke patients.[151-154] During the 4 to 7 days after stroke, there is usually a slow rise and later fall in serum CK-MB levels, a pattern quite different from that found in acute myocardial infarction (Chap. 60); the temporal pattern of cardiac isoenzyme release is more compatible with a smoldering low-grade necrosis such as patchy, focal myocytolysis.[138,151] The ST-segment and T-wave abnormalities and cardiac arrhythmias correlate significantly with raised levels of CK-MB in stroke patients.[138]

Arrhythmias

All types of cardiac arrhythmias have been found in stroke patients, most frequently sinus bradycardia and tachycardia and premature ventricular contractions.[148-150] Some arrhythmias are manifestations of primary cardiac problems, but others are undoubtedly secondary to the brain lesions. Sinus tachycardia and bradycardia are maximal on the first day after intracerebral hemorrhage.[155] Ventricular bigeminy, atrioventricular dissociation and block, ventricular tachycardia, atrial fibrillation, and bundle branch blocks are found less often.[155] All arrhythmias are more common with brainstem compression.

Pulmonary Edema

Acute pulmonary edema may complicate strokes, especially subarachnoid hemorrhage (SAH) and posterior circulation ischemia and hemorrhage.[138,156] Pulmonary edema has been observed in 70 percent of cases of fatal SAH and correlates with the severity and suddenness of development of raised intracranial pressure.[157]

Centrally mediated sympathetic discharges such as those caused by increased intracranial pressure produce intense systemic vasoconstriction.[138] Blood shifts from the high-resistance systemic circulation to the lower-resistance pulmonary circulation. Increased pulmonary capillary pressure leads to pulmonary hypertension and rupture of pulmonary vessels with lung hemorrhage. The pulmonary edema fluid has a high protein content and can develop despite normal cardiac function.[138,158]

Sudden Death

Sudden death associated with stressful situations, including so-called voodoo death, must involve central nervous system mechanisms.[159-162] The presumed mechanism of sudden death, ventricular fibrillation, can be reliably elicited by stimulation of cardiac sympathetic nerves both in the normal and ischemic heart.[163] Ischemia reduces the threshold for ventricular fibrillation.[138,161,164] Stress must cause CNS stimulation that triggers autonomic activation. Sudden vagotonic stimulation can cause sudden bradycardia and cardiac standstill. The effects of vagal stimulation on the development of ventricular arrhythmias is uncertain.[163] Patients with lateral medullary and lateral pontine infarcts affecting reticular formation structures die unexpectedly; these patients have a high incidence of various types of autonomic dysregulation, such as labile blood pressure, syncope, tachycardia, and flushing.[21,38,165]

COEXISTENT VASCULAR DISEASES AFFECTING BOTH HEART AND BRAIN

Atherosclerosis

The most common and most important vascular disease that affects both the brain and the heart is atherosclerosis. The most frequent cause of death in stroke patients is coronary artery disease,[166] and extracranial and intracranial arterial atherosclerosis[167] is common in patients with coronary artery disease.

Pathology and Predominant Sites of Disease

In white men the predominant atherosclerotic lesions involve the origins of the internal carotid artery (ICA) and the vertebral artery (VA) origins in the neck.[168] Fatty streaks and flat plaques first affect the posterior wall of the common carotid artery (CCA) opposite the flow divider between the ICA and the external carotid artery (ECA), a region of low sheer stress.[169,170] Atherosclerotic plaques at this site do not differ from plaques in the aorta or coronary arteries. (See Chap. 55.) Plaques at first probably expand gradually and encroach on the lumen of the ICA and sometimes the CCA (Fig. 122-1). Atheromatous plaques often develop concurrently at the VA origin or spread from the parent subclavian artery to involve the VA origin.[171] When plaques reach a critical size, they affect turbulence, flow, and motion of the arteries causing complications to develop within the plaques. Cracking, ulcerations, and mural thrombi develop, and the overlying endothelium is badly damaged with the development of occlusive thrombi.[172] Fresh thrombi that are loosely adherent to the vascular wall rapidly propagate and embolize. Because the ICA has no nuchal branches, clot often propagates cranially, usually extending as far as the first branch of the ophthalmic artery, which arises from the intracranial siphon portion of the ICA. In the VA, collateral channels from the ECA and thyrocervical trunk usually provide collateral channels that reconstitute the VA in the neck and limit the propagation of the thrombus. During the 2 to 3 weeks after the development of an occlusive thrombus, the clot gradually organizes and is much less likely to propagate or embolize. The reduction in cranial blood flow caused by severe stenosis or occlusion of the ICA or VA leads to the development of collateral circulation that is usually adequate.

Figure 122-2 shows diagrammatically the sites of predilection for development of atherosclerosis in the cerebral circulation. Note the concentration of these sites at branch points and flow dividers.

There are important race and sex differences in the distribution of cerebral atherosclerosis.[173–175] White men are especially prone to develop lesions of the ICA and VA origins. Patients with ICA-origin disease have a high incidence of hypercholesterolemia, coronary artery disease, and peripheral vascular occlusive disease. Perhaps with the exception of the basilar artery (BA) and the ICA siphon, intracranial occlusive disease develops only after extracranial disease is well established in this group. In contrast, blacks and individuals of Chinese, Japanese, and Thai ancestry have a much higher incidence of intracranial occlusive disease and a rather low frequency of extracranial disease.[173,176–178] Intracranial disease is more prevalent in women and is also found in diabetics. Of interest, patients with intracranial occlusive disease may not have a high incidence of coronary or peripheral vascular occlusive disease.

Mechanisms of Ischemia

Ischemia in patients with occlusive lesions is caused by two different mechanisms—hypoperfusion and embolism. Hypoperfusion develops only when there is a critical reduction in luminal diameter or perfusion pressure sufficient to reduce distal flow. When flow is reduced slowly, the brain vasculature has a remarkable capacity to develop collateral circulation. Patients with severe ICA-origin occlusive disease remain asymptomatic despite marked decrease in blood flow.[173,179,180] Even when vascular occlusion is abrupt, e.g., tying neck arteries to treat brain aneurysms, surprisingly few patients develop symptoms of brain ischemia. In most patients, within a few days or at most 2 weeks following an arterial occlusion, collateral circulation develops maximally and stabilizes.

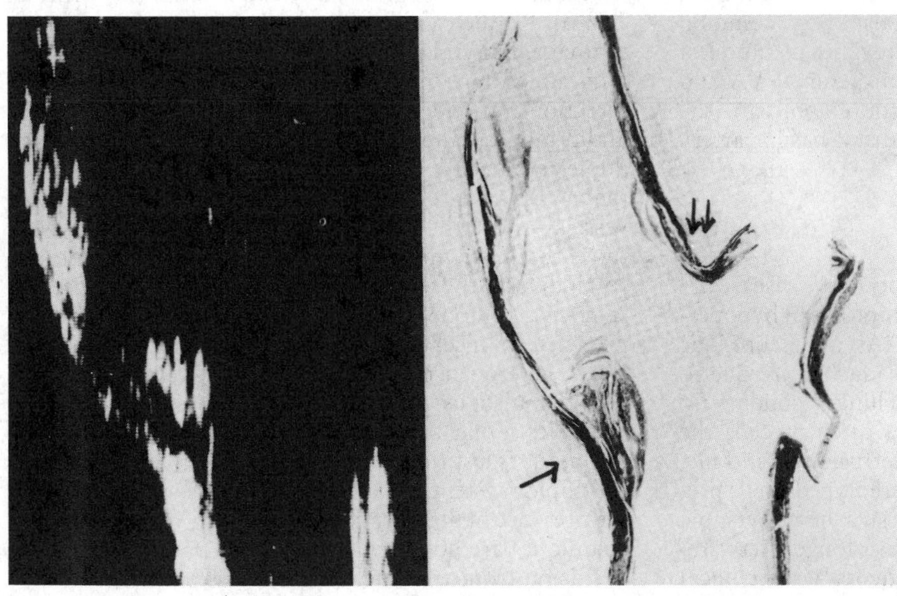

FIGURE 122-1 *A.* B-mode ultrasonic image showing plaque at internal carotid artery origin. *B.* A carotid specimen. The plaque (single arrow) is opposite the flow divider between the internal and external carotid arteries (two arrows). (*From M Hennerici, W Steinke: Abbildende Ultraschallverfahren (B-scan) in Duplex system. In: Durchbluntungsstorungen des Gehirns—neue diagnostiche Möglichkeiten. Gutersloh, Bertelsmann, 1987, with permission.*)

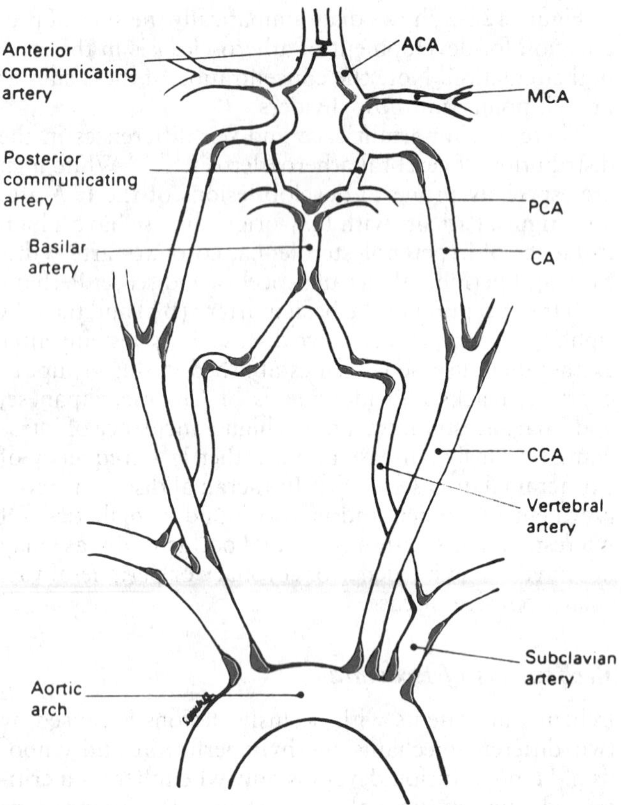

FIGURE 122-2 Sites of predilection for atherosclerotic narrowing: black areas represent plaques. (*From LR Caplan, RW Stein: Stroke: A Clinical Approach. Boston, Butterworth, 1986, with permission.*)

Intraarterial embolism is probably a much more frequent and important cause of brain infarction than hypoperfusion. In patients with anterior circulation infarcts, angiography shows a very high incidence of intraarterial intracranial emboli distal to an ICA thrombosis.[24,41,177,181] These emboli most often involve the MCA and its branches. If angiography is repeated or performed later than 48 h after the stroke, the MCA occlusion is not present.[4] Intraarterial emboli often fragment and move distally. Intraarterial embolism is also very common in the posterior circulation, where the commonest donor sites are the VA origin and intracranial VA and the most frequent recipient sites for emboli are the intracranial VA, the PCA, and the distal basilar artery bifurcation.[36,182]

Clinical Findings

Many patients with atherosclerotic occlusive disease are asymptomatic. The most frequent symptoms of hypoperfusions or embolism are headache, TIAs, and neurologic signs related to brain infarction. Headaches are due to vascular distension or to brain swelling secondary to infarction. Unaccustomed headaches often precede the stroke.[183] TIAs are caused by hypoperfusion or intraarterial emboli. Frequent, very brief stereotyped spells precipitated by postural changes suggest a hemodynamic mechanism. In contrast, emboli cause longer, less frequent attacks.[173,178,184] In many patients with clinical TIAs, i.e., with no lasting symptoms or signs, neuroimaging tests show brain infarcts.[185] Strokes may have various temporal features such as being maximal at outset, fluctuating, stepwise, or gradually progressive. The pattern is related to the adequacy of collateral circulation and the propagation and embolization of occlusive thrombi.

The neurologic signs depend on the region of brain that is ischemic. Table 122-2 outlines the most frequent clinical patterns found in the territories of the major extracranial and intracranial arteries.[38,168,186]

Diagnostic Testing

In the majority of patients the nature and severity of the brain and vascular lesions causing the stroke can be defined. CT and MRI should be able to localize the brain lesion, distinguish between infarct and hemorrhage, and determine the location, extent, and size of the process. CT or MRI is usually the first test in patients with suspected stroke because the information allows the clinician to exclude nonvascular disease such as tumor or abscess; to differentiate hemorrhage from ischemia from subdural hematoma; to identify the vascular territory involved; and to define the extent of brain tissue already damaged.

The vascular territory involved should be inferred by the nature of the neurologic symptoms and signs and the location of the brain lesion on CT or MRI. Echocardiography, especially TEE, has dramatically improved the ability to detect potential cardiac sources of emboli. (See also Chaps. 15 and 131.)

Ultrasound techniques can be used to screen for obstructive lesions in the major extracranial and intracranial arteries in both the anterior (carotid) circulation and the posterior (vertebrobasilar) arteries. For extracranial use the two most important are *B-mode scans* and *Doppler spectra,* both pulsed and continuous wave (CW) Doppler. The anatomy of the carotid bifurcation (the CCA, proximal ICA, and ECA) and the proximal VAs can be imaged by high-frequency, 5 to 10 MHz, B-mode ultrasound systems, which provide images of the vessels in real time both longitudinally and in cross-section (Fig. 122-3). Plaque calcifications and clot are often difficult to image. Pulsed Doppler registers frequency shifts from moving columns of blood. Doppler analysis can show the direction and velocity of blood flow. Multigated Doppler and B-mode scanning are now used together in so-called duplex systems.[187,188] The duplex system is probably more than 90 percent effective in separating three groups of vessels—those that are normal or minimally narrowed, those that have moderate disease (30 to 70 percent narrowing), and those with severe narrowing (>70 percent stenosis). B-mode scanning can sometimes suggest the presence of ulceration or hemorrhage in plaques that show heterogeneous, unusual shaped images.[189] CW Doppler also uses a movable probe to measure flow velocities along the carotid and vertebral arteries; the technique is less time consuming and less expensive than the duplex system and in expert hands is very accurate in the presence of high-grade stenosis.[187,188,190,191] Ultrasound techniques are not very accurate in separating complete occlusion from very high degrees of stenosis.

TCD ultrasound can be used to analyze the presence

TABLE 122-2

Common Signs in Cerebrovascular Occlusive Disease at Various Sites

ICA origin	Ipsilateral transient monocular blindness; MCA and ACA signs
ICA siphon (proximal to ophthalmic artery)	Same as ICA origin
ICA siphon (distal to ophthalmic artery)	MCA and ACA signs
ACA	Contralateral weakness of the lower limb and shoulder shrug
MCA	Contralateral motor, sensory, and visual loss Left Aphasia Right Neglect of left space, lack of awareness of deficit, apathy, impersistence
AChA	Contralateral motor, sensory, and visual loss, usually without cognitive changes
Subclavian artery (proximal to VA)	Lack of arm stamina, cool hand, transient dizziness, veering, diplopia
VA origin	Same as subclavian, but no ipsilateral arm or hand findings
VA intracranially	Lateral medullary syndrome; staggering and veering (cerebellar infarction)
BA	Bilateral motor weakness; ophthalmoplegia and diplopia
PCA	Contralateral hemianopia and hemisensory loss Left Alexia with agraphia Right Neglect of left visual space

NOTE: ICA = internal carotid artery; ACA = anterior cerebral artery; MCA = middle cerebral artery; AChA = anterior choroidal artery; VA = vertebral artery; BA = basilar artery; PCA = posterior cerebral artery.

of intracranial arterial stenoses and to provide information about the intracranial effects of extracranial lesions. The technique takes advantage of the soft spots in the temporal bones and natural foramina (the orbit and foramen magnum) that provide windows for ultrasound recording. The depth and angle of the probe recording can be varied, allowing recording of velocities and sound spectra from all the major intracranial arteries.[42,99,192] Major obstructive lesions should be detectable by the use of both extracranial ultrasound and TCD. Continuous recording of intracranial arteries with TCD is a very sensitive and accurate method for detecting emboli passing under the probes.[185,193]

Magnetic resonance angiography (MRA) provides an additional method of imaging both the extracranial and intracranial arteries for areas of stenosis and occlusion.[177,194] Standard catheter angiography is warranted when ultrasound and MRA have not sufficiently defined

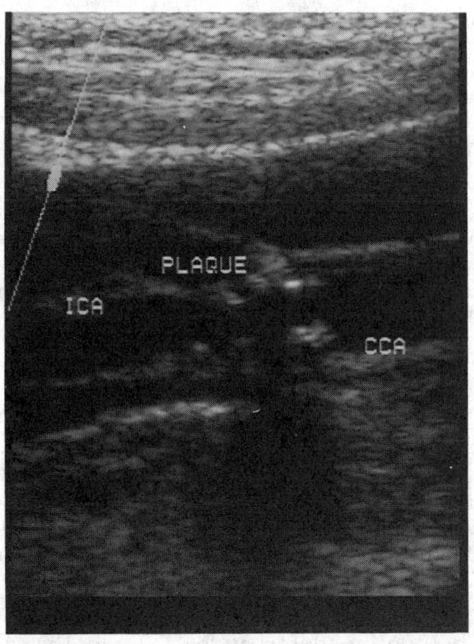

A

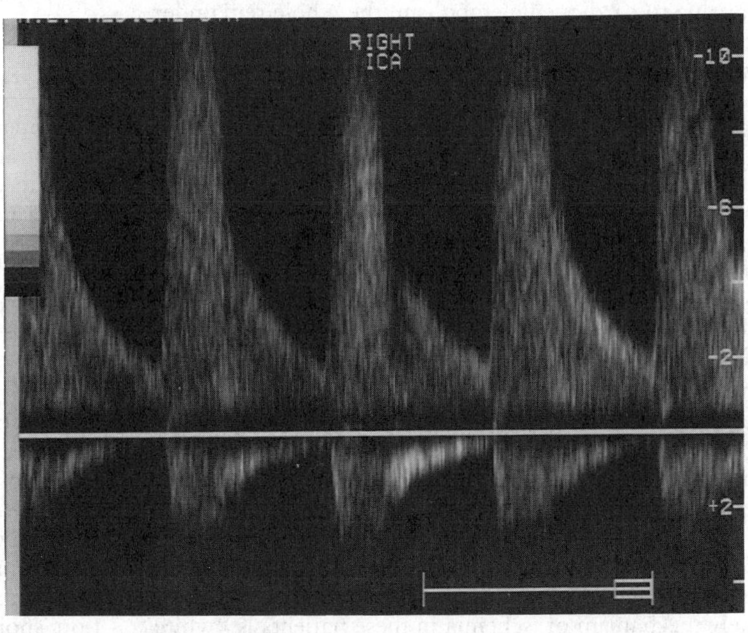

B

FIGURE 122-3 Duplex scan of carotid artery plaque. *A*. B-mode ultrasonic image showing plaque protruding into internal carotid artery (ICA) lumen. *B*. Doppler spectra at level of plaque showing high voltage related to stenosis.

the vascular lesion and treatment is clincially feasible.[177,186]

Treatment

For rational treatment, the following should be known: the location, nature, and severity of the occlusive lesion; the location, extent, and reversibility of the brain lesion; and the blood constituents and coagulability.[186,195] Treatment should *not* be guided solely by the temporal pattern of the symptoms such as TIA, progressing stroke, or so-called completed stroke.[188,196] These time courses do not predict the cause and mechanism of ischemia, do not tell if an infarct is present, and do not identify patients who will have further or recurrent ischemia.[196]

The physician should first decide whether or not any specific therapy is indicated. Very severe neurologic deficits, serious intercurrent illnesses (dementia, cancer, etc.), and psycho-socioeconomic considerations may make patients not suitable for specific treatments. If treatment is feasible, the next questions are what brain tissue is at risk for further ischemia and what is the benefit/risk ratio of specific treatments? To determine the tissue at risk, the clinician considers the cause and the deficit. For example, a man with a slight hemiplegia due to a small lacunar infarct in the anterior limb of the internal capsule may have infarcted the entire tissue supplied by an occluded small artery. In that case, treatment would consist of controlling hypertension, the cause of his microvasculopathy. If, however, that same patient has a small cortical infarct in the precentral gyrus due to ICA disease, the rest of the ICA territory is at risk for further ischemia and aggressive treatment would be warranted. Suppose a patient has a moderate-sized MCA infarct. If the patients were a Chinese woman with intrinsic atherosclerotic disease of that MCA, she might have little tissue at risk for further ischemia. No aggressive treatment should be given. If that same woman's infarct was due to cardiogenic embolism, the whole remainder of the brain is at risk for further damage from another embolus.

Patients who have little tissue at risk are not candidates for specific therapy. If there is considerable residual at-risk tissue, the guidelines in Table 122-3 are used to guide treatment, which depends upon the location and severity of the causative vascular lesion. Carotid endarterectomy (CEN) has been shown to be effective in symptomatic patients with severe ICA stenosis (>70 percent).[191,197,198] Studies now in progress should determine if CEN will prove superior to medical therapy for asymptomatic patients. To be effective, the operative mortality and morbidity of CEN must not be greater than 2 to 4 percent.[191,197-199] Surgery is also feasible on the extracranial vertebral artery in selected patients with intraarterial embolism from this site or with intractable posterior hemodynamic ischemia, a rare occurrence.[200]

For minor and moderate degrees of stenosis in extracranial and intracranial arteries, agents that alter platelet aggregation and adhesion are recommended. The most likely mechanism of ischemia in these patients is "white clot"—platelet fibrin emboli. Aspirin,[201,202] ticlopidine,[203,204] and many of the nonsteroidal anti-inflammatory drugs have antiplatelet effects, as do the omega-3 fish oils containing eicosopentanoic acid. Aspirin is usually selected first because of the potentially serious side effects of ticlopidine. (See Chap. 68.)

For patients with severe stenosis of large intracranial arteries, warfarin is recommended if there are no contraindications. The prothrombin time should be kept at an INR of 2.0 to 3.0 (about 1.5 times control). Anticoagulation should be continued for at least 2 months. The presence of occlusion should be detectable by duplex system, TCD, and/or MRI. The same regimen is used for patients with severe extracranial stenosis who are not

TABLE 122-3
Suggested Use of Anticoagulants and Platelet Antiaggregants

Heparin (Standard Dose)
Short term, 2–4 weeks. Usually given by intravenous infusion keeping APTT between 60 and 100 s (1.5–2 × control APTT). 1. Immediate therapy of definite-origin cerebral embolism (large cerebral infarct, hypertension, bacterial endocarditis, or sepsis would delay or contraindicate this use). 2. Patients with severe stenosis or occlusion of the ICA origin, ICA siphon, MCA, vertebral artery, or basilar artery with less than a clinical deficit. Subsequent treatment could be warfarin or surgery.
Heparin (Subcutaneous Minidose)
For prophylaxis of deep vein occlusion in patients immobilized by stroke (unless contraindicated). (See Chap. 100.)
Warfarin
Usually overlapped with heparin; keeping prothrombin time around INR of 2.0–3.0 (approximately 1.3–1.5 × control). 1. Long term (>3 months) a. Patients with cardiogenic cerebral embolization and rheumatic heart disease, atrial fibrillation with large atria or prior cerebral embolism, prosthetic valves, and some hypercoagulable states. b. Patients with severe stenosis of the ICA origin, ICA siphon, MCA stem, vertebral artery, and basilar artery. Used until studies show artery has been occluded for at least 3 weeks. 2. Short term (3–6 weeks) a. Patients with recent occlusion of the ICA, MCA, vertebral, or basilar arteries.
Platelet Antiaggregants (Aspirin, Ticlopidine)
1. Patients with plaque disease of the extracranial and intracranial arteries without severe stenosis. 2. Patients with polycythemia or thrombocytosis and related ischemic attacks.

NOTE: APTT = activated partial thromboplastin time; ICA = internal carotid artery; MCA = middle cerebral artery; INR = International Normalized Ratio.

operative candidates or who refuse surgery. For patients with complete occlusions when first seen, heparin and then warfarin are prescribed for 2 to 3 months.

At present, thrombolytic treatment with streptokinase or recombinant tissue plasminogen activator (rTPA) is experimental and is used only in investigational protocols.[205,206] Reperfusion can lead to breakage of ischemic capillaries and hemorrhagic infarction and frank hemorrhage.

Because all patients with atherosclerosis are at risk of developing more lesions, control of risk factors is very important and should be begun in the hospital. Risk factors include smoking, hyperlipidemia, obesity, inactivity, and hypertension. (See also Chap. 62.) Blood pressure should not be excessively lowered during the acute ischemic period as this may decrease flow in collateral arteries.[207,208] Blood pressure therapy and control can be instituted 3 to 4 weeks after the stroke. Rehabilitation must also begin early.[186,209]

Management of Coexistent Coronary and Cerebrovascular Disease

Many patients have both coronary and cerebrovascular occlusive disease, and risk factor control is especially important. In candidates for both CABS and CEN there is controversy regarding which surgery should be done first or whether or not both procedures should be done together under the same anesthetic. In general, the most symptomatic system should be operated on first. Thus, if the patient has severe coronary disease with active cardiac ischemia but asymptomatic severe extracranial occlusive disease, he or she should have a CABS procedure and no CEN. On the other hand, if the patient has active cerebrovascular symptoms (recent TIAs or nondisabling stroke within 3 months) and minor or stable coronary symptoms, a CEN would be in order without a CABS. If the patient has both active coronary and cerebrovascular symptoms, the CEN and CABS should be performed together.[210-212] The reasons for this view are as follows: (1) The morbidity and mortality of the two procedures done together are considerably higher than either alone. The stroke risk is especially high.[211] (2) Patients with asymptomatic bruits[115] or even severe stenosis have a very low rate of stroke due to hemodynamic changes during CABS or other surgery. Most operative and postoperative strokes are embolic. (3) With good medical care, the risk of myocardial infarction during CEN in patients with stable coronary disease is relatively low. (See also Chap. 125.)

It is important to define the extent of cerebrovascular disease preoperatively by noninvasive means (ultrasound and/or MRA) as well as to define cardiac and coronary artery anatomy and function when indicated. Staged surgical procedures are sometimes warranted. In some patients with excessive surgical risks, anticoagulation represents an alternative treatment. Clearly, optimum medical therapy should be instituted preoperatively unless symptoms are emergent.

Systemic Arterial Hypertension

High blood pressure, both acute and chronic, damages deep, penetrating, small intracranial arteries; accelerates the development of atherosclerosis in the extracranial and large intracranial arteries; and results in ischemic syndromes of lacunar infarction,[207,208] diffuse ischemic changes to white matter and basal gray structures (Binswanger's disease), or intracerebral hemorrhage. Hypertension is also frequent in patients with aneurysmal SAH and may contribute to enlargement and rupture of congenital and acquired aneurysms.

Hypertension especially damages the deep arteries that penetrate perpendicularly from the major intracranial arteries (Fig. 122-4). Serial sections of these arteries in patients with hypertension show characteristic abnormalities consisting of focal microaneurysmal enlargements and small hemorrhagic extravasations through the arterial walls. Subintimal foam cells may obliterate the lumen, and pink-staining amorphous fibrinoid material is found within the walls of the small arteries. The media is often considerably thickened. In places the vessels are often replaced by whorls, tangles, and wisps of connective tissue that completely obliterate the usual vascular layers, causing segmental arterial disorganization as a consequence of *lipohyalinosis* and *fibrinoid degeneration*.[213,214] Microaneurysms are particularly common in patients with hypertensive intracerebral hemorrhages and in hypertensive older patients.[134,215-218]

The two major patterns of brain ischemia in patients with hypertension are *discrete lacunar infarcts* and a more *diffuse patchy white and gray matter degeneration with gliosis*. Both are thought to be most often caused by lipohyalinosis. The term *lacune* (hole) refers to small, deep infarcts caused by lipohyalinosis of the penetrating artery feeding the ischemic brain.[213] Other vascular pathological processes such as microdissections and tiny emboli also cause lacunes.[213,214] Some patients are normotensive and have miniature atherosclerotic lesions (so-called microatheromas) at the orifices of the branches or

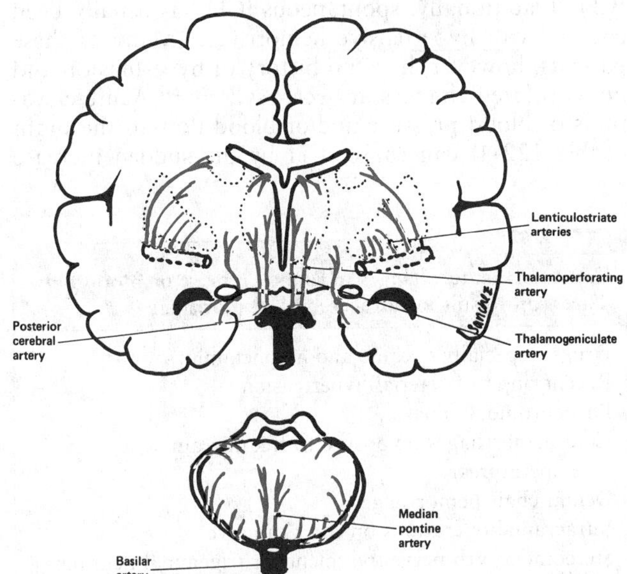

FIGURE 122-4 Deep penetrating arteries prone to the development of lipohyalinosis and microaneurysms. Occlusion of these arteries cause lacunar infarcts, and rupture of these arteries causes intracerebral hemorrhage. (*From LR Caplan, RW Stein: Stroke: A Clinical Approach. Boston, Butterworth, 1986, with permission.*)

within the parent arteries blocking or extending into the branches.[207,208,213,214,218–221] Amyloid angiopathy can cause small, deep infarcts in normotensive and hypertensive patients. Single lacunes cause discrete clinical syndromes.[208,222,223] The most common are pure motor hemiparesis,[224] pure sensory stroke,[225] ataxic hemiparesis,[226] and the dysarthria–clumsy hand syndrome.[227]

Since the advent of CT and MRI, it has become widely appreciated that hypertensive patients with lacunes often have more diffuse changes in the white matter of the brain, referred to as *leukoariosis*.[228] The clinical picture consists of acute strokes; subacute progression of neurologic signs; dementia, especially the frontal lobe apathetic type; gait disorder; and Parkinsonian, pyramidal, and pseudobulbar signs.[229–232] The clinical signs and gross pathology are identical to those partially described by Otto Binswanger in 1894 and 1895[233] and by his students Alzheimer and Nissl.[229,233,234] The deep arteries are thickened and hyalinized and show lipohyalinosis and sometimes amyloid angiopathy in regions of white matter atrophy and gliosis. Invariably, lacunar infarcts are also found. The pathogenesis most likely is related to diffuse vascular narrowing in deep arteries and altered microvascular flow and perfusion. Some studies suggest altered hemorheology and increased blood viscosity,[232] and some patients have had polycythemia vera.[229] The diagnosis is made from the clinical picture, the CT and MRI findings, and the absence of cortical infarcts, larger artery occlusive disease, or cardioembolic sources.

Hypertensive Intracranial Hemorrhage

Intracerebral hemorrhage (ICH) accounts for about 10 percent of all strokes.[4,6] Head trauma, vascular malformations, bleeding diatheses, drugs (especially amphetamines and cocaine), amyloid angiopathy, and intracranial aneurysms account for some cases.[235] The majority of patients without these conditions have a spontaneous ICH. Traditionally, spontaneous ICH has usually been equated wth hypertensive hemorrhage. Many of these patients, however, have no history of hypertension and no associated changes at necropsy.[134,236,237] Acute elevations of blood pressure and/or blood flow to the brain (Table 122-4) can cause ICH by the sudden increase in blood pressure causing breakage of capillaries and arterioles.[134]

TABLE 122-4

Causes of Acute Changes in Blood Pressure or Blood Flow That Can Result in Intracerebral Hemorrhage

Drugs, especially cocaine and amphetamines
Recent onset of arterial hypertension
Pheochromocytoma
Cold hemorrhages (exposure to freezing ambient temperatures)
Dental chair hemorrhages
Intracranial operations on the Vth nerve
Stereotactic Vth nerve treatment for trigeminal neuralgia
Carotid endarterectomy (reflex hypertension and reperfusion)
Cardiac transplantation, especially in children
Surgical repair of congenital heart disease in children
Migraine

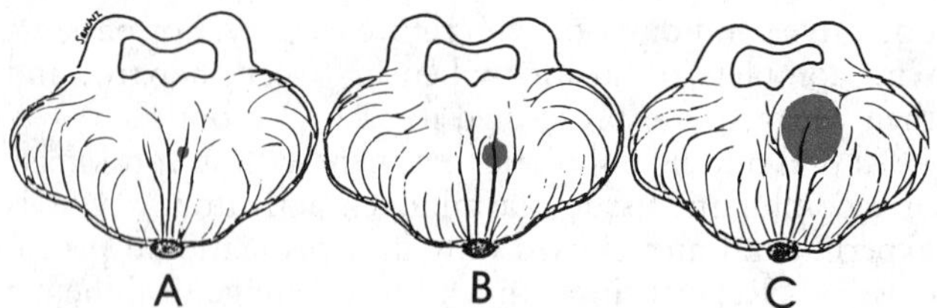

FIGURE 122-5 Gradual evolution of a hypertensive pontine intracerebral hematoma. *A.* The earliest leakage of blood from a paramedian penetrating artery. *B.* and *C.* The hematoma has grown. (*From LR Caplan, RW Stein: Stroke: A Clinical Approach. Boston, Butterworth, 1986, with permission.*)

Hypertensive ICH issues from the deep penetrating arteries, so the location parallels the distribution of these arteries. Hematomas develop in the same sites as lacunes, the most frequent being the putamen/internal capsule (30 to 40 percent), caudate nucleus (8 percent), lobar white matter (20 percent), thalamus (15 percent), pons (10 percent), and cerebellum (10 percent).[186,238] In fatal hematomas, microaneurysms and lipohyalinosis are prevalent in penetrating arteries, but the hematomas obscure findings in the middle of the lesions.[239] Along the outside, circumferentially, fibrin globules represent rupture sites.[239] Arterioles or capillaries rupture in the center of the lesion, suddenly increasing local tissue pressure and leading to pressure on adjacent capillaries and their rupture. As the hematoma gradually grows on its periphery (Fig. 122-5), local tissue pressure and finally intracranial pressure increase until the hematoma is contained. Alternatively, the pressure is decompressed by the lesion emptying into the ventricular system or into the subarachnoid space at the brain surface.

Clinical Findings Contrary to popular belief, patients with ICH have a gradual evolution of neurologic signs; symptoms do not begin abruptly as in SAH.[238,240] The first neurologic signs are related to the bleeding site, e.g., left putaminal hematoma patients might first notice right arm weakness or numbness, whereas cerebellar hematoma patients stagger and feel off balance. As the hematoma grows, focal signs worsen. When and if the hematoma increases sufficiently in size to increase intracranial pressure, headache, vomiting, and decreased levels of alertness develop.[185,238,240] In the presence of small restricted hemorrhages, headache is absent and the patient remains alert. The course and findings mimic so-called progressing ischemic stroke. Headache is absent or not a very prominent symptom in more than half of the patients with ICH. Loss of consciousness is also not invariable but is a bad prognostic sign when present. Clinical localization of the hematoma rests on an analysis of pupillary responses, eye movements, and the presence and distribution of motor signs.

Diagnosis CT accurately shows the location, size, shape, and extent of hematomas. Also shown is the presence of ventricular and surface drainage, surrounding edema, and pressure shifts in surrounding tissues. MRI in the patient with an acute hematoma is more difficult to interpret, but old hematomas are more readily shown by imaging hemosiderin-containing cavities. MRI is also superior in suggesting arteriovenous malformations and cavernous angiomas. Lumbar puncture is seldom warranted. Atypical location, absence of hypertension, and abnormal vascular echoes on MRI are indications for angiography.

Prognosis and Treatment[186,238,241] Coma, increased intracranial pressure, and large hematoma size (>3 cm in one dimension on CT) all indicate a poor prognosis.[241] Ordinarily, severe systemic hypertension should be reduced but not excessively. The hematoma causes increased intracranial pressure, and the spinal fluid pressure and pressure in the dural sinuses increase pari passu. Patients with ICH can die from raised pressure. In order to perfuse the brain and to maintain the arterial-venous pressure gradient, the systemic arterial pressure must rise. Overzealous reduction of systemic blood pressure may make the patient worse. The patient's state of alertness and neurologic signs are carefully monitored, together with the blood pressure.

Recent hematomas in the brain lobes, cerebellum, and right putamen are sometimes drained surgically without leaving a major deficit, at times using stereotactic equipment with CT guidance. The indications for drainage are increased pressure and the presence of lesions that require removal (tumor, arteriovenous malformations, aneurysm). When hematomas resolve, they leave a hole disconnecting but not destroying the overlying cortex.

In general, small hematomas resolve well without specific therapy except blood pressure control, whereas massive hematomas usually kill or maim patients before they can be treated. Medium-sized hematomas (2 to 4 cm), which increase pressure and cause worsening signs or decreased consciousness while the patient is under observation, are indications for drainage if the hematoma is favorably located.

Subarachnoid Hemorrhage

SAH is not directly caused by hypertension in most cases, although an abrupt increase in blood pressure (e.g., due to cocaine or amphetamines) can sometimes lead to SAH, as can a bleeding diathesis, trauma, or amyloid angiopathy. The most frequent lesions causing SAH are abnormal vessels such as aneurysms and vascular malformations on or near the surface of the brain. SAH describes bleeding directly into the subarachnoid space with rapid dissemination into the cerebrospinal fluid (CSF) pathways. Usually the blood is suddenly released under systemic arterial pressure, causing an abrupt rise in intracranial pressure and producing headache, vomiting, and interruption of conscious behavior and memory, at least temporarily.[242] In some patients, the jet and spread of blood cause neckache, backache, or sciatica instead of headache. Patients are usually agitated and restless or sleepy and have a stiff neck.

The most frequent cause of SAH is leakage from a berry aneurysm. Often there has been a past history of a "warning leak," that is, a sudden-onset headache unusual for the patient that lasts days and usually prevents normal daily activities.[242,243] Aneurysms are most often located at bifurcations of major intracranial arteries. The commonest sites are the ICA–posterior communicating artery junction, the ACA–anterior communicating artery junction, and the MCA bifurcation. CT can often suggest the site of rupture if blood is pooled locally near a typical site.[244,245] Large aneurysms are occasionally visible on contrast-enhanced CT or MRI. Lumbar puncture is very important in the diagnosis of SAH.[246] The absence of blood in the CSF effectively excludes the diagnosis of SAH if the fluid is examined within 24 h of the onset of the headache, although bleeds that are very small in volume or older than 72 h can be missed. The CSF pressure, presence of xanthochromia, and quantification of the hemoglobin and bilirubin content of the CSF by spectrophotometry can help quantitate and date the bleeding and document increased intracranial pressure.[246]

The two most important complications of aneurysmal SAH are rebleeding and brain ischemia due to vasoconstriction (so-called vasospasm). Once an aneurysm has ruptured, either a tiny cap of platelets and fibrin seals the point of rupture or continued bleeding is fatal. Lysis of the fibrin cap initiates rebleeding. Surgical clipping of the aneurysmal sac or obliteration of the aneurysm by endovascular use of balloons or other devices should be attempted before rebleeding occurs.

Vasoconstriction of arteries is thought to be due to blood or blood products that bathe the adventitia of arteries.[247–250] In the presence of a large accumulation of blood, there is a much higher incidence of arterial vasoconstriction and resultant brain ischemia and infarction.[251] Delayed ischemia can also develop postoperatively as manipulation of vessels can precipitate or potentiate vasoconstriction. The clinical findings in patients with vasoconstriction confirmed by angiography are often those of diffuse brain swelling such as headache, decreased alertness, and confusion. When vasoconstriction is focal or multifocal, the clinical findings are those of focal ischemia such as hemiparesis, aphasia, hemianopia, etc. Vasoconstriction usually has its onset 3 to 5 days after hemorrhage, and the peak time for constriction is days 5 to 9; vasoconstriction usually improves after the second week unless there is rebleeding.[252]

Vasoconstriction has been detected by angiography in 30 to 70 percent of patients with SAH, depending on the timing of the study.[247,253] Severe vasoconstriction is manifested by a lumen size of <0.5 mm, delayed anterograde flow, and evidence of collateral filling distal to the vasoconstricted vessel. TCD is effective in monitoring for the presence of vasoconstriction, which increases blood flow velocity.[99,254,255] Single-photon emission computed tomography (SPECT) can also show regions of poor perfusion and document the presence of delayed ischemia.[256]

Many treatments have been tried to prevent or treat vasoconstriction after SAH.[257] These include removal of blood by lumbar puncture or at the time of early surgery,[258] pharmacologic agents such as calcium channel blockers to minimize contraction of the arterial wall, and hypervolemia to prevent ischemia by maintaining perfusion. At present, the most popular approaches are early surgery, nimodipine (a calcium channel blocker), and hypervolemic therapy, especially after aneurysmal clipping. Hypovolemia is common after SAH, as is hyponatremia. Hypervolemia does not reverse the vasoconstriction but helps maintain brain perfusion.

Coagulopathies

Hypercoagulability and bleeding due to decreased coagulability affect most body organs, including the brain and heart. An increased tendency for clotting can be caused by abnormalities of the formed blood elements or serologic factors.[258–260] Increased numbers of red blood cells and platelets and qualitative abnormalities such as sickle-cell disease can cause excess intravascular clotting, especially in the presence of dehydration and reduced plasma volume. Excessive platelet activation, or so-called sticky platelets, can also explain increased coagulability but has proved hard to measure reliably in vitro.[261,262] The level of β thromboglobulin is a good marker for platelet activation. (See also Chap. 7.) Serologic abnormalities may be congenital or acquired. Decreased amounts of natural anticoagulants (antithrombin III, protein C, and protein S) can cause hypercoagulability.[258–260] These proteins may be decreased in patients with hypoproteinemia, especially that due to the nephrotic syndrome and urinary protein loss.[261] Fibrinogen levels and the levels of the various coagulation factors such as factors VIII and XI may also be high in patients with excess clotting. (See also Chap. 7.) In many patients with excess clotting, e.g., those on high-dose estrogen birth control pills, pregnant women, and patients with cancer, serologic and standard coagulation tests (in vitro) cannot clarify the mechanism of the excessive clotting in vivo. Stroke patients may have serologic evidence of platelet activation and increased fibrin formation but decreased natural fibrinolytic and anticoagulant activity.[260]

Recently, measurement of various serum antiphospholipid antibodies has elicited considerable interest. The usually measured substances are the so-called lupus anticoagulant[263–265] and anticardiolipin antibodies. Increased activity of antiphospholipid antibodies (APLA) is found in patients with systemic lupus erythematosus, AIDS, giant-cell arteritis, and Sneddon's syndrome[266–268] (livedo reticularis and strokes) and in association with the use of many drugs (e.g., phenytoin, phenothiazines, procainamide, hydralazine, and quinidine).[263–265,269] When the APLAs are not associated with other conditions and the patient has clinical evidence of excess clotting, the disorder is considered to be primary and is referred to as the *primary APLA syndrome*.[270–272] Patients with APLAs have an increased incidence of spontaneous abortions, venous occlusive disease of the legs and pulmonary embolism, brain infarcts (often multiple), thrombocytopenia, and false-positive syphilis serologic tests. Some older patients with APLAs also have important risk factors for stroke.[269–272]

Patients with systemic illnesses often have elevated erythrocyte sedimentation rates, and strokes and pulmonary emboli often follow and complicate myocardial infarction. (See Chap. 60.) Customarily, such brain infarcts have been attributed to cardiogenic embolism, but some undoubtedly are secondary thromboses precipitated by increased levels of acute-phase reactant coagulation proteins. Cancer, especially mucinous adenocarcinoma, has been associated with multiple vascular occlusions, large and tiny brain infarcts, and venous and arterial occlusions.[273]

Deficient coagulability can lead to serious intracranial bleeding. The hemorrhage can be into the brain (ICH), cerebrospinal fluid (SAH), or the subdural and epidural compartments. Thrombocytopenia, hemophilia, and leukemia are common conditions leading to intracranial hemorrhage. The most common iatrogenic cause of bleeding is anticoagulation with heparin or warfarin.[274,275] Brain hemorrhage has also been described after fibrinolytic treatment of patients with coronary artery disease[276,277] and after rTPA infusion to treat cerebrovascular occlusive disease.[205,206] (See also Chaps. 60 and 69.)

Anticoagulant-related ICH, which is often a catastrophic complication with high morbidity and mortality, is relatively rare considering the frequency of anticoagulant usage. Anticoagulant-related hemorrhages develop more insidiously and evolve more slowly more often than do other causes of ICH.[238,274] Many are erroneously attributed to brain ischemia, especially if anticoagulants had been prescribed to treat TIAs. Any patient taking anticoagulants who develops CNS symptoms should be considered to have anticoagulant-related ICH until CT or MRI excludes the diagnosis. The hematoma grows slowly and insidiously increases intracranial pressure. Many patients require surgical drainage of their hematomas to ensure survival. Anticoagulants should be stopped immediately, and their effect reversed by fresh frozen plasma or vitamin K. It is probably safe to resume anticoagulation 10 days to 2 weeks after the ICH if indicated, e.g., for prophylaxis in patients with artificial heart valves.[278] In patients treated with fibrinolytic agents, hemorrhages are most often lobar or cerebellar and may be multiple. ICH may be more common when there is a past stroke, when heparin or other agents that affect coagulation are given with or after fibrinolytic agents, and when there is a hemostatic defect secondary to treatment.[276,277]

Arterial Dissections

Aortic dissections involving the innominate or carotid arteries (Chap. 123) are a well-known cause of stroke or other manifestations of cerebral ischemia. Less well known are the syndromes produced by dissections of the extracranial and intracranial arteries, which are especially likely to occur in young, active individuals without risk factors for atherosclerosis or stroke but after trauma or chiropractic or other neck manipulations. They are also associated with fibromuscular dysplasia, Marfan's syndrome, pseudoxanthoma elasticum, and migraine.

The dissection starts with a tear in the media and spreads longitudinally (Fig. 122-6). It can disrupt adventitial fibers or even rupture through the adventitia to produce an extravascular hematoma and a false or pseudoaneurysm within muscle and connective tissue. Intracranially, such a rupture can produce SAH. Other dissections may produce arterial obstruction and secondary thrombosis of the narrowed vascular lumen. Most recognized cerebral vascular dissections occur in the extracranial vessels, particularly the pharyngeal portion

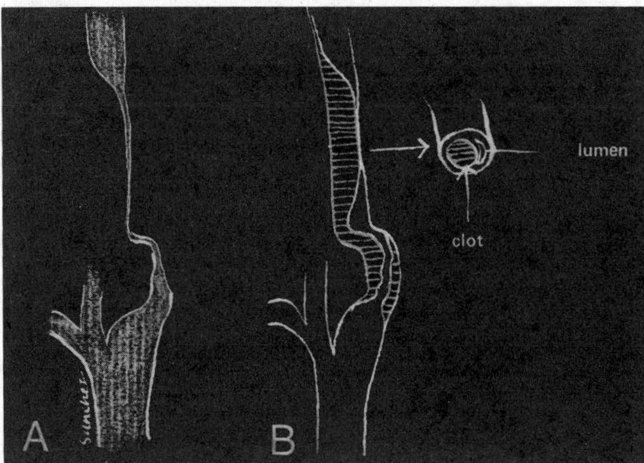

FIGURE 122-6 Diagrams of a carotid artery dissection. *A.* Shows the lumen encroached upon by the intramural clot. *B.* The dissection is cross-hatched. (*From LR Caplan, RW Stein: Stroke: A Clinical Approach. Boston, Butterworth, 1986, with permission.*)

of the internal carotid artery or the nuchal vertebrae arteries.[279–283]

Extracranial dissections produce sharp pain and throbbing headache; brain and retinal ischemic episodes, which may occur in rapid-fire attacks, or "carotid allegro"[284]; and pressure on adjacent structures. Strokes, usually from embolization of clots, are common but often have a benign course. Intracranial dissections have a poorer prognosis, often with vascular rupture and SAH.

The diagnosis is confirmed by angiography, CT, or MRI. Ultrasound studies can be helpful in suggesting the diagnosis of dissection in the neck.[285]

Treatment consists of the use of heparin acutely, followed by warfarin for 6 to 12 weeks to prevent intraarterial thrombus and peripheral embolus. Intracranial dissections with SAH have been treated surgically.[281,286,287] Surgery on extracranial dissections has also been performed,[280] but the results are not clearly superior to medical management.

REFERENCES

1. Aring C, Merritt H: Differential diagnosis between cerebral hemorrhage and cerebral thrombosis. *Arch Intern Med* 1935;56: 435–456.
2. Whisnant J, Fitzgibbons J, Kurland L, Sayre GP: Natural history of stroke in Rochester, Minnesota 1945–1954. *Stroke* 1971;2:11–22.
3. Matsumoto N, Whisnant J, Kurland L, Okazaki H: Natural history of stroke in Rochester, Minnesota 1955–1969. *Stroke* 1973;4:2–29.
4. Mohr J, Capland LR, Melski J, Duncan G, Goldstein R, Kistler JP, et al: The Harvard Cooperative Stroke registry: A prospective study. *Neurology* 1978;28:754–762.
5. Caplan LR, Hier D, D'Cruz I: Cerebral embolism in the Michael Reese Stroke Registry. *Stroke* 1983;14:530–536.
6. Foulkes MA, Wolf PA, Price TR, Mohr JP, Hier DB: The Stroke Data Bank: Design, methods, and baseline characteristics. *Stroke* 1988;19:547–554.
7. Bogousslavsky J, Van Melle G, Regli F: The Lausanne Stroke Registry: Analysis of 1000 consecutive patients with first strokes. *Stroke* 1988;19:1083–1092.
8. Kunitz S, Gross C, Heyman A, Kase C, Mohr JP, Price TP, et al: The pilot stroke data bank: Definition, design and data. *Stroke* 1984;15:740–746.
9. Bogousslavsky J, Cachin C, Regli F, Despland PA, Van Melle G, Kappenberger L: Cardiac sources of embolism and cerebral infarction—clinical consequences and vascular concomitants: The Lausanne Stroke Registry. *Neurology* 1991;41:855–859.
10. Halperin J, Hart RG: Atrial fibrillation and strokes: New ideas, persisting dilemmas. *Stroke* 1988;19:937–941.
11. Caplan LR: Of birds and nests and brain emboli. *Rev Neurol (Paris)* 1991;147:265–273.
12. Kittner SJ, Sharkness CM, Sloan M, Price TR, Dambrosia JM, Tuhrim S, et al: Infarcts with a cardiac source of embolism in the NINDS Stroke Data Bank: Neurological examination. *Neurology* 1991;41:(in press)
13. Barnett HJM, Jones MW, Boughner DR, Kostuk WJ: Cerebral ischemic events associated with prolapsing mitral valve. *Arch Neurol* 1976;33:777–782.
14. Barnett HJM, Bougher DR, Taylor DW, Cooper PE, Kostuk WJ, Nichol PM: Further evidence relating mitral valve prolapse to cerebral ischemic events. *N Engl J Med* 1980;302:139–144.
15. Sandok BA, Giuliani ER: Cerebral ischemic events in patients with mitral valve prolapse. *Stroke* 1982;13:448–450.
16. Lauzier S, Barnett HJM: Cerebral ischemia with mitral valve prolapse and mitral annulus calcification. In: Furlan AJ (ed): *The Heart and Stroke.* London, Springer, 1987:63–100.
17. Pomerance A: Ballooning deformity (mucoid degeneration) of atrioventricular valves. *Br Heart J* 1969;31:343–351.
18. Pomerance A, Davies MJ: Strokes: A complication of mitral leaflet prolapse. *Lancet* 1977;2:1186.
19. Kostuk WJ, Boughner DR, Barnett HJM, Silver MD: Strokes: A complication of mitral-leaflet prolapse. *Lancet* 1977;2:313–316.
20. Hanson MR, Conomy JP, Hodgman JR: Brain events associated with mitral valve prolapse. *Stroke* 1980;11:499–506.
21. Jones HR, Naggar CZ, Selyan MP, Downing ZZ: Mitral valve prolapse and cerebral ischemic events. A comparison between a neurology population with stroke and a cardiology population with mitral valve prolapse observed for 5 years. *Stroke* 1982;13:451–453.
22. Pomerance A: Pathological and clinical study of calcification in the mitral valve ring. *J Clin Pathol* 1970;23:354–361.
23. Fulkerson PK, Beaver BM, Auseon JC, Graven HL: Calcification of the mitral annulus—etiology, clinical associations, complications and therapy. *Am J Med* 1979;66:967–977.
24. DeBono DP, Warlow CP: Mitral annulus calcification and cerebral or retinal ischemia. *Lancet* 1979;2:383.
25. Korn D, DeSanctis RW, Sell S: Massive calcification of the mitral annulus. A clinicopathological study of fourteen cases. *N Engl J Med* 1962;267:900–909.
26. Benjamin EJ, Plehn JF, D'Agostino RB, Belanger AJ, Comai K, Fuller DL, et al: Mitral annular calcification and the risk of stroke in an elderly cohort. *N Engl J Med* 1992;327:374–379.
27. Sacco RL, Ellenberg JH, Mohr JP, Tatemichi T, Hier DB, Price TR, et al: Infarcts of undetermined cause: The NINCDS Stroke Data Bank. *Ann Neurol* 1989;25:382–390.
28. Mohr JP: Infarct of unclear cause. In: Furlan AJ (ed): *The Heart and Stroke.* London, Springer, 1987:101–116.
29. Galve E, Candell-Riera J, Pigrau C, Permanyu-Miralda G, Garcia del Castillo H, Soler-Soler J: Prevalence, morphology, types and evaluation of cardiac valvular disease in systemic lupus erythematosus. *N Engl J Med* 1988;319:817–823.
30. Kanter MC, Hart RG: Neurologic complications of infective endocarditis. *Neurology* 1991;41:1015–1020.
31. Gacs G, Merel MD, Bodosi M: Balloon catheter as a model of cerebral emboli in humans. *Stroke* 1982;13:39–42.
32. Caplan LR, Kelly M, Kase CS, Hier DB, White JL, Tatemichi T, et al: Infarcts of the inferior division of the right middle cerebral artery; mirror image of Wernicke's aphasia. *Neurology* 1986;36:1015–1020.
33. Caplan LR: Posterior cerebral artery syndromes. In: Vinken P, Bruyn G, Klawans H, Toole J (eds): *Cerebrovascular Disease,* vol I. New York, North Amsterdam, 1989:409–415.
34. Fisher CM: Left hemiplegia and motor impersistence. *J Nerv Ment Dis* 1956;123:201–218.
35. Pessin MS, Lathi E, Cohen MB, Kwan E, Hedges TR, Caplan LR: Clinical features and mechanisms of occipital infarction in

the posterior cerebral artery territory. *Ann Neurol* 1987;21:290–299.
36. Caplan LR: Top of the basilar syndrome: Selected clinical aspects. *Neurology* 1980;30:72–79.
37. Mehler MF: The rostral basilar artery syndrome: Diagnosis, etiology, prognosis. *Neurology* 1989;39:9–16.
38. Caplan LR: Vertebrobasilar occlusive disease. In: Barnett HJM, Mohr JP, Stein B, Yatsu F (eds): *Stroke: Pathophysiology, Diagnosis, and Management.* New York, Churchill Livingstone, 1985:549–620.
39. Amarenco P: The spectrum of cerebellar infarctions. *Neurology* 1991;41:973–979.
40. Fisher CM, Perlman A: The nonsudden onset of a cerebral embolism. *Neurology* 1967;17:1025–1032.
41. Fieschi C, Argentino C, Lenzi GL, Sacchetti ML, Toni D, Bozzao L: Clinical and instrumental evaluation of patients with ischemic stroke within the first six hours. *J Neurol Sci* 1989;91:311–322.
42. Kushner MJ, Zanotte EM, Bastianiello S, Mancini G, Sachetti M, Carolei A, et al: Transcranial doppler in acute hemispheric brain infarction. *Neurology* 1991;41:109–113.
43. Ringlestein EB, Koschorke S, Holling A, Thron A, Lambertz H, Minale C: Computed tomographic patterns of proven embolic brain infarcts. *Ann Neurol* 1989; 26:759–765.
44. Bladin PF, Berkovic SF: Striatocapsular infarction. *Neurology* 1984;34:1423–1430.
45. Fisher CM, Adams RD: Observations on brain embolism. *J Neuropathol Exp Neurol* 1951;10:92–94.
46. Fisher CM, Adams RD: Observations on brain embolism with special reference to hemorrhagic infarction. In: Furlan AJ (ed): *The Heart and Stroke.* London, Springer, 1987:17–36.
47. Gacs G, Fox AJ, Barnett HJ, Vinuela F: CT visualization of intracranial arterial thromboembolism. *Stroke* 1983;14:756–763.
48. Tomsick T, Brott T, Barsan W, Broderick J, Haley C, Levy D, et al: Thrombus localization with emergency cerebral computed tomography. *Stroke* 1990;21:180.
49. Bergerson G, Shah P: Echocardiography unwarranted in patients with cerebral ischemic events. *N Engl J Med* 1981;304:489.
50. Greenland P, Knopman D, Mikell F, Asinger R, Anderson D, Good D: Echocardiography in diagnostic assessment of stroke. *Ann Intern Med* 1981;95:51–54.
51. Donaldson R, Emmanuel R, Earl C: The role of two-dimensional echocardiography in the detection of potentially embolic intracardiac masses in patients with cerebral ischemia. *J Neurol Neurosurg Psychiatry* 1981;44:803–809.
52. Tegeler CH, Downes TR: Cardiac imaging in stroke. *Stroke* 1991;22:1206–1211.
53. Pop G, Sutherland GR, Koudstaal PJ, Sit TW, de Jong G, Roelandt JR: Transesophageal echocardiography in the detection of intracardiac embolic sources in patients with transient ischemic attacks. *Stroke* 1990;21:560–565.
54. Zenker G, Ecbel R, Kramer G, Mohr-Kahaly S, Drexler M, Harnoncourt K, et al: Transesophageal echocardiography in young patients with cerebral ischemic events. *Stroke* 1988;19:345–348.
55. Tunick PA, Perez JL, Kronzon I: Protruding atheromas in the thoracic aorta and systemic embolization. *Ann Intern Med* 1991;115:423–427.
56. Yasaka M, Yamaguchi T, Miyashita T, Park YO, Sawada T, Omae T: Predisposing factors of recurrent embolization in cardiogenic cerebral embolism. *Stroke* 1990;21:1000–1007.
57. DeWitt LD, Pessin MS, Pandian NG, Pauker SG, Sonnenberg FA, Caplan LR: Benign disappearance of ventricular thrombus after embolic stroke, a case report. *Stroke* 1988;19:393–396.
58. Ezekowitz MD, Wilson DA, Smith EO, Burow RD, Harrison L, Parker D, et al: Comparison of Indium-III platelet scintigraphy and two-dimensional echocardiography in the diagnosis of left ventricular thrombi. *N Engl J Med* 1982;306:1509–1513.
59. Petersen P, Boysen G, Godtfredsen J, Andersen ED, Andersen B: Placebo-controlled, randomized trial of warfarin and aspirin for prevention of thromboembolic complications in chronic atrial fibrillation: The Copenhagen AFASAK Study. *Lancet* 1989;1:175–179.
60. Stroke Prevention in Atrial Fibrillation Study Group Investigators: Preliminary report of the Stroke Prevention in Atrial Fibrillation Study. *N Engl J Med* 1990;322:863–868.
61. Chesebro JH, Fuster V, Halperin J: Atrial fibrillation—risk marker for stroke. *N Engl J Med* 1990;323:1556–1558.
62. The Boston Area Anticoagulation Trial for Atrial Fibrillation Investigators: The effect of low-dose warfarin on the risk of stroke in patients with nonrheumatic atrial fibrillation. *N Engl J Med* 1990;323:1505–1511.
63. Cairns JA, Connolly SJ: Nonrheumatic atrial fibrillation. Risk of stroke and role of antithrombotic therapy. *Circulation* 1991;84:469–481.
64. Stroke Prevention in Atrial Fibrillation Investigators: The stroke prevention in atrial fibrillation trial: Final results. *Circulation* 1991;84:527–539.
65. Connolly SJ, Laupacis A, Gent M, Roberts RS, Cairns JA, Joyner C: Canadian Atrial Fibrillation Anticoagulation (CAFA) study. *J Am Coll Cardiol* 1991;18:349–355.
66. The Stroke Prevention in Atrial Fibrillation Investigators: Predictors of thromboembolism in atrial fibrillation: I. Clinical features of patients at risk. *Ann Intern Med* 1992;116:1–5.
67. The Stroke Prevention in Atrial Fibrillation Investigators: Predictors of thromboembolism in atrial fibrillation: II. Echocardiographic features of patients at risk. *Ann Intern Med* 1992;116:6–12.
68. Pritchett ELC: Management of atrial fibrillation. *N Engl J Med* 1992;326:1264–1271.
69. Ezekowitz MD, Bridgers SL, James KE, Carliner NH, Colling CL, Gornick CC, et al: Randomized trials of warfarin for atrial fibrillation. *N Engl J Med* 1992;327:1451–1453.
70. Moldveen-Geronimus M, Merriam JC: Cholesterol embolization: From pathologic curiosity to clinical entity. *Circulation* 1967;35:946–953.
71. Shields RW, Laureno R, Lachman T, Victor M: Anticoagulant-induced hemorrhage in acute cerebral embolism. *Ann Neurol* 1982;12:75.
72. Lieberman A, Hass WK, Pinto R, Isom W, Kupersmith M, Bear G, et al: Intracranial hemorrhage and infarction in anticoagulated patients with prosthetic heart valves. *Stroke* 1978;9:18–24.
73. Drake ME, Shin C: Conversion of ischemic to hemorrhagic infarction by anticoagulant administration. Report of two cases with evidence from serial computed tomographic brain scans. *Arch Neurol* 1983;40:44–46.
74. Cerebral Embolism Study Group: Immediate anticoagulation of embolic stroke: A randomized trial. *Stroke* 1983;13:668–676.
75. Cerebral Embolism Task Force: Cardiogenic brain embolism. *Arch Neurol* 1986;43:71–84.
76. Cerebral Embolism Task Force: Cardiogenic brain embolism: The second report of the Cerebral Embolism Task Force. *Arch Neurol* 1989;46:727–743.
77. Pessin MS, Estol CJ, Lafranchise EF, Caplan LR: Safety of anticoagulation in hemorrhagic infarction. *Neurology* 1991;41:263.
78. Brierley J, Meldrum B, Brown A: The threshold and neuropathology of cerebral "anoxic-ischemic" cell change. *Arch Neurol* 1973;29:367–373.
79. Brierley JB, Adams JH, Graham DI, Simpson JA: Neurocortical death after cardiac arrest: A clinical, neurophysiological report of two cases. *Lancet* 1971;2:560–565.
80. Dougherty JH, Rawlinson DG, Levy DE, Plum F: Hypoxic-ischemic brain injury and the vegetative state: Clinical and neuropathologic correlation. *Neurology* 1981;31:991–997.
81. Cummings JL, Tomiyasu U, Read S, Benson DF: Amnesia with hippocampal lesions after cardiopulmonary arrest. *Neurology* 1984;34:679–681.
82. Dooling E, Richardson EP: Delayed encephalopathy after strangling. *Arch Neurol* 1976;33:196–199.
83. Lance J, Adams RD: The syndrome of intention and action myoclonus as a sequel to hypoxic encephalopathy. *Brain* 1963;86:111–133.
84. Gilles F: Hypotensive brainstem necrosis. *Arch Pathol* 1969;88:32–41.
85. Silver JR, Buxton PH: Spinal stroke. *Brain* 1974;97:539–550.
86. Caronna JJ, Finkelstein S: Neurological syndromes after cardiac arrest. *Stroke* 1978;9:517–520.
86a. Jennett B, Plum F: Persistent vegetative state after brain damage: A syndrome in search of a name. *Lancet* 1972;1:734–737.
87. Levy DE, Knill-Jones RP, Plum F: The vegetative state and its prognosis following non-traumatic coma. *Ann NY Acad Sci* 1978;315:293–306.
88. Hacaen H, Ajuriaguerra J: Balint's syndrome and its minor forms. *Brain* 1954;77:373–400.
89. Caplan LR: Neurology of the acute cardiac. In: Donoso E, Cohen

S (eds): *Critical Cardiac Care*. New York, Stratton International Medical Books, 1979:183–197.

90. Sherwin I, Redman W: Successful treatment in action myoclonus. *Neurology* 1969;19:846–850.
91. Willoughby J, Leach B: Relation of neurological findings after cardiac arrest to outcome. *Br Med J* 1974;3:437–439.
92. Plum F, Caronna J: Can one predict outcome of medical coma? In: *Outcome of Severe Damage to the Central Nervous System. A CIBA Foundation Symposium*. New York, Elsevier, 1975: 121–139.
93. Bell JA, Hodgson HJ: Coma after cardiac arrest. *Brain* 97;97:361–372.
94. Levy D, Carrona JJ, Singer BH, Lapinski RH, Frydman H, Plum F: Predicting outcome from hypoxic-ischemic coma. *JAMA* 1985;253:1420–1426.
95. Longstreth WT, Inui TS, Cobb LA, Copass MK: Neurologic recovery after out-of-hospital cardiac arrest. *Ann Intern Med* 1983;38:588–592.
96. Longstreth WT, Diehr P, Inui TS: Prediction of awakening after out-of-hospital cardiac arrest. *N Engl J Med* 1983;308: 1378–1382.
97. Thompson RG, Hallstrom AP, Cobb LA: Bystander-initiated cardiopulmonary resuscitation in the management of ventricular fibrillation. *Ann Intern Med* 1979;90:737–740.
98. Bedell SE, Delbanco TG, Cook EF, Epstein FH: Survival after cardiopulmonary resuscitation in the hospital. *N Engl J Med* 1983;309:569–576.
99. Caplan LR, Brass LM, DeWitt LD, Adams RJ, Gomez C, Otis S, et al: Transcranial doppler ultrasound: Present status. *Neurology* 1990;40:696–700.
100. Kirkham F, Levin S, Padayachee T, Kyme M, Neville B, Gosling R: Transcranial pulsed doppler ultrasound findings in brainstem death. *J Neurol Neurosurg Psychiatry* 1987;50:1504–1513.
101. Ropper A, Kehne S, Wechsler L: Transcranial doppler in brain death. *Neurology* 1987;37:1733–1735.
102. Longstreth WT, Inui TS: High blood glucose level on hospital admission and poor neurological recovery after cardiac arrest. *Ann Neurol* 1984;15:59–63.
103. Myers C, Yamaguchi S: Nervous system effects of cardiac arrest in monkeys. *Arch Neurol* 1977;34:65–74.
104. Plum F: What causes infarction in ischemic brain. *Neurology* 1983;33:222–233.
105. Collins RC, Dobkin BH, Choi DW: Selective vulnerability of the brain: New insights into the pathophysiology of stroke. *Ann Intern Med* 1989;110:992–1000.
106. Albers G, Goldberg M, Choi D: *N*-methyl-D-aspartate antagonists: Ready for clinical trial in brain ischemia? *Ann Neurol* 1989;25:398–403.
107. Giswold S, Safar P, Rao G, Moosy J, Kelsey S, Alexander H: Multifaceted therapy after global brain ischemia in monkeys. *Stroke* 1984;15:803–812.
108. Volpe BT, Soave R: Formal visual hallucinations as digitalis toxicity. *Ann Intern Med* 1979;91:868–869.
109. Closson RG: Visual hallucinations as the earliest symptoms of digoxin intoxication. *Arch Neurol* 1983;40:386.
110. Gilbert GJ: Quinidine dementia. *JAMA* 1977;237:2093–2094.
111. Slogoff S, Girgis KZ, Keats AS: Etiologic factors in neuropsychiatric complications associated with cardiopulmonary bypass. *Anesth Analg* 1982;61:903–911.
112. Gilman S: Neurological complications of open heart surgery. *Ann Neurol* 1990;28:475–476.
113. Shaw PJ, Bates D, Cartlidge NEF, Heaviside D, Julian DG, Shaw DA: Early neurological complications of coronary artery bypass surgery. *Br Med J* 1985;291:1384–1387.
114. Breuer AC, Furlan AJ, Hanson MR, Lederman RJ, Loop FD, Cosgrove DM: Central nervous system complications of coronary artery bypass graft surgery: Prospective analysis of 421 patients. *Stroke* 1983;14:682–687.
115. Ropper AH, Wechsler LR, Wilson LS: Carotid bruit and the risk of stroke in elective surgery. *N Engl J Med* 1982;307:1388–1390.
116. Furlan AJ, Craciun AR: Risk of stroke during coronary artery bypass graft surgery in patients with internal carotid artery disease documented by angiography. *Stroke* 1985;16:797–799.
117. Sila C: Neuroimaging of cerebral infarction associated with coronary revascularization. *AJNR* 1991;12:817–818.
118. Hertzer NR, Loop FD, Beven EG, O'Hara PJ, Krajewski LP: Surgical staging for simultaneous coronary and carotid disease: A study including prospective randomization. *J Vasc Surg* 1989;9:455–463.
119. VonReutern G-M, Hetzel A, Birnbaum D, Schlosser V: Transcranial doppler ultrasound during cardiopulmonary bypass in patients with internal carotid artery disease documented by angiography. *Stroke* 1988;19:674–680.
120. Hise JH, Nippu ML, Schnitker JC: Stroke associated with coronary artery bypass surgery. *AJNR* 1991;12:811–814.
121. Tettenborn B, Sloan M, Haley EC, Price TR, Estol C, Pessin MS, et al: Post-operative brainstem cerebellar strokes. *Neurology* 1990;40(suppl):325.
122. Price DL, Harris J: Cholesterol emboli in cerebral arteries are a complication of retrograde aortic profusion during cardiac surgery. *Neurology* 1970;20:1207–1214.
123. Tunick PA, Culliford AT, Lamparello PJ, Kronzon I: Atheromatosis of the aortic arch as an occult source of multiple systemic emboli. *Ann Intern Med* 1991;114:391–392.
124. Karalis DG, Chandrasekaran K, Victor MF, Ross JJ, Mintz GS: Recognition and embolic potential of intraaortic atherosclerotic debris. *J Am Coll Cardiol* 1991;17:73–78.
125. Marshall JNG, Barzilai B, Kouchoukos N, Saffitz J: Intraoperative ultrasonic imaging of the ascending aorta. *Ann Thorac Surg* 1989;48:339–344.
126. Gardner TJ, Horneffer PJ, Manolio TA, Pearson TA, Gott VL, Baumgartner WA, et al: Stroke following coronary artery bypass grafting: A ten-year study. *Ann Thorac Surg* 1985; 40:574–581.
127. Gilman S: Cerebral disorders after open-heart operations. *N Engl J Med* 1965;272:489–498.
128. Coffey CE, Massey EW, Roberts KB, Curtis S, Jones RH, Pryor DB: Natural history of cerebral complications of coronary artery bypass graft surgery. *Neurology* 1983;33:1416–1421.
129. Moody DM, Bell MA, Challa VR, Johnston WE, Prough DS: Brain microemboli during cardiac surgery or aortography. *Ann Neurol* 1990;28:477–486.
130. Feeney DM, Gonzalez A, Law WA: Amphetamine, haloperidol and experience interact to affect the rate of recovery after motor cortex injury. *Science* 1982;217:855–857.
131. Houda DA, Feeney DM: Haloperidol blocks amphetamine induced recovery of binocular depth perception after bilateral visual cortex lesions in the cat. *Proc West Pharmacol Soc* 1985;28:209–211.
132. Humphreys RP, Hoffman JH, Mustard WT, Trusler GA: Cerebral hemorrhage following heart surgery. *J Neurosurg* 1975;43:671–675.
133. Sila CA: Spectrum of neurologic events following cardiac transplantation. *Stroke* 1989;20:1586–1589.
134. Caplan LR: Intracerebral hemorrhage revisited. *Neurology* 1988;38:624–627.
135. Lederman RJ, Breuer AC, Hanson MR, Furlan AJ, Loop FD, Cosgrove D, et al: Peripheral nervous system complications of coronary artery bypass graft surgery. *Ann Neurol* 1982;12:297–301.
136. Natelson BH: Neurocardiology: An interdisciplinary area for the 80's. *Arch Neurol* 1985;42:178–184.
137. Schlesinger MJ, Reiner L: Focal myocytolysis of heart. *Am J Pathol* 1955;31:443–459.
138. Norris JW, Hachinski V: Cardiac dysfunction following stroke. In: Furlan AJ (ed): *The Heart and Stroke*. London, Springer, Verlag, 1987:171–183.
139. Smith RP, Tomlinson BE: Subendocardial hemorrhages associated with intracranial lesions. *J Pathol Bacteriol* 1954;68: 327–334.
140. Cropp GJ, Manning GW: Electrocardiographic changes simulating myocardial ischemia and infarction associated with spontaneous intracranial hemorrhage. *Circulation* 1960;22:25–38.
141. Kolin A, Norris JW: Myocardial damage from acute cerebral lesions. *Stroke* 1984;15:990–993.
142. Samuels MA: Electrocardiographic manifestations of neurologic disease. *Semin Neurol* 1984;4:453–459.
143. Myers MG, Norris JW, Hachinski V, Sole MJ: Plasma norepinephrine in stroke. *Stroke* 1981;12:200–204.
144. Marion DW, Segal R, Thompson ME: Subarachnoid hemorrhage and the heart. *Rev Neurosurg* 1986;18:101–106.
145. Haggendal J, Johansson G, Jonsson L, Thoren-Tolling K: Effect of propranolol on myocardial cell necrosis and blood levels of catecholamines in pigs subjected to stress. *Acta Pharmacol Toxicol* 1982;50:58–66.

146. Hunt D, Gore J: Myocardial lesions following experimental intracranial hemorrhage. *Am Heart J* 1972;83:232–236.
147. Burch GE, Myers R, Abildskov JA: A new electrocardiographic pattern observed in cerebrovascular accidents. *Circulation* 1954;9:719–723.
148. Dimant J, Grob D: Electrocardiographic changes and myocardial damage in patients with acute cerebrovascular accidents. *Stroke* 1977;8:448–455.
149. Rolak LA, Rokey R: Electrocardiographic features. In: Rolak LA, Rokey R (eds): *Coronary and Cerebral Vascular Disease.* Mt. Kisco, NY, Futura, 1990:139–197.
150. Goldstein DS: The electrocardiogram in stroke: Relationship to pathophysiological type and comparison with prior tracings. *Stroke* 1979;10:253–259.
151. Puleo P: Cardiac enzyme assessment. In: Rolak L, Rokey R (eds): *Coronary and Cerebral Vascular Disease.* Mt. Kisco, NY, Futura, 1990;199–216.
152. Fabinyi G, Hunt D, McKinley L: Myocardial creatine kinase isoenzyme in serum after subarachnoid hemorrhage. *J Neurol Neurosurg Psychiatry* 1977;40:818–820.
153. Neil-Dwyer G, Cruickshank J, Stratton C: Beta-blockers, plasma total creatine kinase and creatine kinase myocardial isoenzyme, and the prognosis of subarachnoid hemorrhage. *Surg Neurol* 1986;25:163–168.
154. Myers MG, Norris JW, Hachinsky VC, Weingert ME, Sole MJ: Cardiac sequelae of acute strokes. *Stroke* 1982;13:838–842.
155. Stober T, Sen S, Anstatt T, Bette L: Correlation of cardiac arrythmias with brainstem compression in patients with intracerebral hemorrhage. *Stroke* 1988;19:688–692.
156. Hoff JT, Nishimura M: Experimental neurogenic pulmonary edema in cats. *J Neurosurg* 1978;18:383–389.
157. Wier BK: Pulmonary edema following fatal aneurysmal rupture. *J Neurosurg* 1978;49:502–507.
158. Theodore J, Robin ED: Pathogenesis of neurogenic pulmonary edema. *Lancet* 1975;2:749–751.
159. Engel GL: Psychologic factors in instantaneous cardiac death. *N Engl J Med* 1976;294:664–665.
160. Engel GL: Psychologic stress, vasodepressor (vasovagal) syncope and sudden death. *Ann Intern Med* 1978;89:403–412.
161. Lown B: Sudden cardiac death: The major challenge confronting contemporary cardiology. *Am J Cardiol* 1979;43:313–328.
162. Lown B, Temte JV, Reich P, Gaughan C, Registeen Q, Hai H: Basis for recurring ventricular fibrillation in the absence of coronary heart disease and its management. *N Engl J Med* 1976;294:623–629.
163. Talman WT: Cardiovascular regulation and lesions of the central nervous system. *Ann Neurol* 1985;18:1–12.
164. Schwartz PJ, Stone HL, Brown AM: Effects of unilateral stellate ganglion blockage on the arrhythmias associated with coronary occlusion. *Am Heart J* 1976;92:589–599.
165. Haws CW, Burgess MJ: Effects of bilateral and unilateral stellate stimulation on canine refractory periods at sites of overlapping innervation. *Circ Res* 1978;42:195–198.
166. Adams H, Kassell N, Mazuz H: The patients with transient ischemic attacks. Is this the time for a new therapeutic approach? *Stroke* 1984;15:371–375.
167. Hennerici M, Aulich A, Sandmann W, Freund HJ: Incidence of asymptomatic extracranial arterial disease. *Stroke* 1981;12: 750–758.
168. Caplan LR: Cerebrovascular disease: Large artery occlusive disease. In: Appel S (ed): *Current Neurology,* vol 87. Chicago, Year Book, 1988:179–226.
169. McMillan DE: Blood flow and the localization of atherosclerotic plaques. *Stroke* 1985;16:582–587.
170. Zarins CK, Giddins DP, Bharadvaj BK, Sottivrai VS, Mabon R: Carotid bifurcation atherosclerosis. *Circ Res* 1983;53:502–514.
171. Hutchinson EC, Yates DO: The cervical portion of the vertebral artery, a clinicopathologic study. *Brain* 1956;79:319–331.
172. Fisher CM, Ojemann RG: A clinico-pathologic study of carotid endarterectomy plaques. *Rev Neurol (Paris)* 1986;142:573–589.
173. Caplan LR, Gorelick PB, Hier DB: Race, sex, and occlusive vascular disease: A review. *Stroke* 1986;17:648–655.
174. Gorelick PB, Caplan LR, Hier DB, Patel D, Langenberg P, Pessin MS, et al: Racial differences in the distribution of posterior circulation occlusive disease. *Stroke* 1985;16:785–790.
175. Gorelick PB, Caplan LR, Hier DB, Patel D, Parker S: Racial differences in the distribution of anterior circulation occlusive cerebrovascular disease. *Neurology* 1984;34:54–59.
176. Feldmann E, Daneault N, Kwan E, Ho K, Pessin MS, Langenberg P, et al: Chinese-white differences in the distribution of occlusive cerebrovascular disease. *Neurology* 1990;40:1541–1545.
177. Caplan LR, Wolpert SM: Angiography in patients with occlusive cerebrovascular disease: A stroke neurologist and neuroradiologist's views. *AJNR* 1991;12:593–601.
178. Pessin MS, Duncan GW, Mohr JP, Poskanzer DC: Clinical and angiographic features of carotid transient ischemic attacks. *N Engl J Med* 1977;296:358–362.
179. Chambers BR, Norris JW: Outcome in patients with asymptomatic neck bruits. *N Engl J Med* 1986;315:860–865.
180. Hennerici M, Hulsbomer HB, Rautenberg W, Hefter H: Spontaneous history of asymptomatic internal carotid occlusion. *Stroke* 1986;17:718–722.
181. Ringelstein EB, Zeumer H, Angelou D: The pathogenesis of strokes from internal carotid artery occlusion: Diagnostic and therapeutical implications. *Stroke* 1983;14:867–875.
182. Caplan LR, Tettenborn B: Embolism in the posterior circulation. In: Berguer R, Caplan L (eds): *Vertebrobasilar Arterial Disease.* St Louis, Quality Med Publ, 1991;52–65.
183. Gorelick PB, Hier DB, Caplan LR, Langenberg P: Headache in acute cerebrovascular disease. *Neurology* 1986;36:1445–1450.
184. Pessin MS, Hinton RC, Davis KR, Duncan G, Roberson G, Ackerman R, et al: Mechanism of acute carotid stroke. *Ann Neurol* 1979;6:245–252.
185. Russell D, Madden KP, Clark WM, Sandset PM, Zivin JA: Detection of arterial emboli using doppler ultrasound in rabbits. *Stroke* 1991;22:253–258.
186. Caplan LR: *Stroke: A Clinical Approach,* 2d ed. Boston, Butterworths, 1992:195–271.
187. Hennerici M, Freund H: Efficacy of C-W Doppler and duplex system examinations for the evaluation of extracranial carotid disease. *J Clin Ultrasound* 1984;12:155–161.
188. Caplan LR: TIAs—we need to return to the question, what is wrong with Mr. Jones? *Neurology* 1988;791–793.
189. O'Donnell TF, Erdoes L, Mackey WC, McCullough J, Shepard A, Heggerick P: Correlation of B-mode ultrasound imaging and arteriography with pathologic findings at carotid endarterectomy. *Arch Surg* 1985;120:443–449.
190. Zwiebel WJ, Zagzebski JA, Crummy AB, Hirscher M: Correlation of peak doppler frequency with lumen narrowing in carotid stenosis. *Stroke* 1982;13:386–391.
191. Caplan LR, Pessin MS: Symptomatic carotid artery disease and carotid endarterectomy. *Annu Rev Med* 1988;39:273–299.
192. Hennerici M, Rautenberg W, Sitzer G, Schwartz A: Transcranial doppler ultrasound for the assessment of intracranial arterial flow velocity. I. Examination technique and normal values. *Surg Neurol* 1986;315:860–856.
193. Spencer MP, Thomas GI, Nicholls SC, Sauvage LR: Detection of middle cerebral artery emboli during carotid endarterectomy using transcranial doppler ultrasonography. *Stroke* 1990; 21:415–423.
194. Edelman RR, Mattle HP, Atkinson DJ, Hoogewoud HM: MR angiography. *AJR* 1990;154:937–946.
195. Caplan LR: Treatment of cerebral ischemia: Where are we headed? *Stroke* 1984;15:571–574.
196. Caplan LR: Are terms such as completed stroke or RIND of continued usefulness? *Stroke* 1983;14:431–433.
197. North American Symptomatic Carotid Endarterectomy Trial (NASCET) Collaborators: Beneficial effect of carotid endarterectomy in symptomatic patients with high-grade carotid stenosis. *N Engl J Med* 1991;325:445–453.
198. European Carotid Surgery Trialist's Collaborative Group: MRC European Carotid Surgery Trial: Interim results for symptomatic patients with severe (70–99 percent) or with mild (0–29 percent) carotid stenosis. *Lancet* 1991;1:1235–1243.
199. Caplan LR: Carotid artery disease (editorial). *N Engl J Med* 1986;315:886–888.
200. Berguer R, Caplan LR (eds): *Vertebrobasilar Arterial Disease.* St. Louis, Quality Med Publ, 1991:201–261.
201. Fields WS, Lemak NA, Frankowski RF, Hardy RJ: Controlled trial of aspirin in cerebral ischemia. *Stroke* 1977;8:301–314.
202. Canadian Cooperative Study Group: A randomized trial of aspirin and sulfinpyrazone in threatened stroke. *N Engl J Med* 1978;299:53–59.
203. Hass WK, Easton JD, Adams HP, Pryse-Phillips W, Molony BA, Anderson S, et al: A randomized trial comparing ticlopidine

hydrochloride with aspirin for the prevention of stroke in high risk patients. *N Engl J Med* 1989;321:501–507.

204. Warlow CP: Ticlopidine, a new antithrombotic drug: But is it better than aspirin for long term use? *J Neurol Neurosurg Psychiatry* 1990:53:185–187.
205. DelZoppo G, and the rtPA Acute Stroke Study Group: An open, multicenter trial of recombinant tissue plasminogen activator in acute stroke. A progress report. *Stroke* 1990;20(suppl 10): 174–175.
206. DelZoppo G: Fibrinolytic therapy in thromboembolic vertebrobasilar insufficiency. In: Berguer R, Caplan LR (eds): *Vertebrobasilar Arterial Disease.* St. Louis, Quality Med Publ, 1991: 179–192.
207. Caplan LR: Intracranial branch atheromatous disease. *Neurology* 1989;39:1246–1250.
208. Caplan LR: Lacunar infarction: A neglected concept. *Geriatrics* 1976;31:71–75.
209. Caplan LR: A general therapeutic perspective on stroke treatment. In: Dunkel R, Schmidley J (eds): *Stroke in the Elderly: New Issues Is Diagnosis, Treatment and Rehabilitation.* New York, Springer, 1987:60–69.
210. Pettigrew LC: Surgical considerations. In: Rolak L, Rokey R (eds): *Coronary and Cerebral Vascular Disease.* Mt Kisco, NY, Futura, 1990:349–377.
211. Hertzer NR, Loop FD, Beven EG: Management of coexistent carotid and coronary artery disease: A surgical viewpoint. In: Furlan A (ed): *The Heart and Stroke.* London, Springer, 1987:305–318.
212. Easton JD, Hart RG: Asymptomatic carotid artery disease in patients undergoing open heart surgery: A neurologic viewpoint. In: Furlan A (ed): *The Heart and Stroke.* London, Springer, 1987:319–327.
213. Fisher CM: The arterial lesions underlying lacunes. *Acta Neuropathol* 1969;12:1–15.
214. Fisher CM: Lacunes, small deep cerebral infarcts. *Neurology* 1965;15:774–784.
215. Rosenblum WI: Miliary aneurysms and "fibrinoid" degeneration of cerebral blood vessels. *Hum Pathol* 1977;8:133–139.
216. Cole F, Yates P: Intracerebral microaneurysms and small cerebrovascular lesions. *Brain* 1966;90:759–767.
217. Fisher CM: Pathological observations in hypertensive cerebral hemorrhage. *J Neuropathol Exp Neurol* 1971;30:536–550.
218. Fisher CM: Cerebral miliary aneurysms in hypertension. *Am J Pathol* 1972;66:314–324.
219. Fisher CM, Caplan LR: Basilar artery branch occlusion: A cause of pontine infarction. *Neurology* 1971;21:900–905.
220. Fisher CM: Bilateral occlusion of basilar artery branches. *J Neurol Neurosurg Psychiatry* 1977;40:1182–1189.
221. Mohr JP: Lacunes. *Stroke* 1982;13:3–11.
222. Miller V: Lacunar stroke, a reassessment. *Arch Neurol* 1983;40:129–134.
223. Fisher CM: Lacunar strokes and infarcts: A review. *Neurology* 1982;32:871–876.
224. Fisher CM: Pure motor hemiplegia of vascular origin. *Arch Neurol* 1965;13:30–44.
225. Fisher CM: Pure sensory stroke and allied conditions. *Stroke* 1982;13:434–447.
226. Fisher CW: Ataxic hemiparesis. *Arch Neurol* 1978;35:126–128.
227. Fisher CM: A lacunar stroke, the dysarthric-clumsy hand syndrome. *Neurology* 1967;17:614–617.
228. Hachinski VC, Potter P, Merskey H: Leukoaraiosis. *Arch Neurol* 1987;44:21–23.
229. Caplan LR, Schoene W: Subcortical arteriosclerotic encephalopathy (Binswanger disease): Clinical features. *Neurology* 1978;28:1206–1219.
230. Babikian V, Ropper AH: Binswanger's disease: A review. *Stroke* 1987;18:2–12.
231. Caplan LR: Binswanger's disease. In: Vinken P, Bruyn G, Klawans H (eds): *Handbook of Clinical Neurology. Neurobehavioral Disorders,* vol 2(46), Fredericks JAM (ed). Amsterdam, Elsevier, 1985:317–321.
232. Caplan LR: Binswanger's disease. *Curr Opin Neurol Neurosurg* 1988;1:57–62.
233. Blass JP, Hoyer S, Nitsch R: A translation of Otto Binswanger's article, "The delineation of the generalized progressive paralysis?" *Arch Neurol* 1991;48:961–972.
234. Olszewski J: Subcortical arteriosclerotic encephalopathy. *World Neurology* 1962;3:359–373.
235. Kase CS: Intracerebral hemorrhage: Non-hypertensive causes. *Stroke* 1986;17:590–594.
236. Bahemuka M: Primary intracerebral hemorrhage and heart weight: A clinicopathological case-control review of 218 patients. *Stroke* 1987;18:531–536.
237. Brott T, Thalinger K, Hertzberg V: Hypertension as a risk factor for spontaneous intracerebral hemorrhage. *Stroke* 1986;17: 1078–1083.
238. Caplan LR: Intracerebral hemorrhage. In: Tyler HR, Dawson D (eds): *Current Neurology,* vol 2. Boston, Houghton Mifflin, 1979:185–205.
239. Fisher CM: Pathological observations in hypertensive cerebral hemorrhages. *J Neuropathol Exp Neurol* 1971;30:536–550.
240. Caplan LR, Mohr JP: Intracerebral hemorrhage: An update. *Geriatrics* 1978;33:42–52.
241. Tuhrim S, Dambrosia JM, Price TR, Mohr JP, Wolf PA, Heyman A, et al: Prediction of intracerebral hemorrhage survival. *Ann Neurol* 1988;24:258–263.
242. Adams HP, Jergenson DD, Kassell NF, Sahs AL: Pitfalls in the recognition of subarachnoid hemorrhage. *JAMA* 1980; 244:794–796.
243. Ostergaard JR: Warning leaks in subarachnoid hemorrhage. *Br Med J* 1990;301:190-191.
244. Caplan LR: Computed tomography and stroke. In: McDowell F, Caplan LR (eds): *Cerebrovascular Survey Report for the National Institute of Neurological and Communicative Disorders and Stroke (NINCDS),* revised. Washington, DC, NINCDS, 1985:61–74.
245. Weisberg L: Computed tomography in aneurysmal subarachnoid hemorrhage. *Neurology* 1979;29:802–808.
246. Caplan LR, Flamm ES, Mohr JP, Toole J, Plum F, Fisher CM, et al: Lumbar puncture and stroke. *Stroke* 1987;18:540A–544A.
247. Heros R, Zervas NT, Varsos V: Cerebral vasospasm after subarachnoid hemorrhage: An update. *Ann Neurol* 1983;14:599–608.
248. Kassell N, Sasaki T, Colohan A, Nazar G: Cerebral vasospasm following aneurysmal subarachnoid hemorrhage. *Stroke* 1985;16:562–572.
249. MacDonald RL, Wier BK: A review of hemoglobin and the pathogenesis of cerebral vasospasm. *Stroke* 1991;22:991–982.
250. Wilkins RH: Attempts at prevention or treatment of intracranial arterial spasm: An update. *Neurosurgery* 1986;18:808–825.
251. Fisher CM, Kistler JP, Davis JM: Relation of cerebral vasospasm to subarachnoid hemorrhage visualized by computerized tomographic scanning. *Neurosurgery* 1980;6:1–9.
252. Weir B, Grace M, Hansen J, Rothberg C: Time course of vasospasm in man. *J Neurosurg* 1978;48:173–178.
253. Kwak R, Niizuma H, Ohi T, Suzuki J: Angiographic study of cerebral vasospasm following rupture of intracranial aneurysms. I. Time of the appearance. *Surg Neurol* 1979;11:257–262.
254. Harders A, Gilsbach J: Time course of blood velocity changes related to vasospasm in the circle of Willis measured by transcranial doppler ultrasound. *J Neurosurg* 1987;66:718–728.
255. Sloan MA, Haley EC, Kassell NF, Henry ML, Stewart SR, Beskin RR, et al: Sensitivity and specificity of transcranial Doppler ultrasonography in the diagnosis of vasospasm following subarachnoid hemorrhage. *Neurology* 1989;39:1514–1518.
256. Davis S, Andrews J, Lichtenstein M, Kagi A, Tress B, Rossiter S, et al: A single-photon emission computed tomography study of hypoperfusion after subarachnoid hemorrhage. *Stroke* 1990;21:252–259.
257. Wilkins RH: Attempted prevention or treatment of intracranial arterial spasm: A survey. *Neurosurgery* 1980;6:198–210.
258. Hart RG, Kanter MC: Hematologic disorders and ischemic stroke: A selective review. *Stroke* 1990;20:1111–1121.
259. Coull BM, Goodnight SH: Current concepts of cerebrovascular disease and stroke: Antiphospholipid antibodies, prothrombotic states and stroke. *Stroke* 1990;21:1370–1374.
260. Feinberg WM, Bruck DC, Ring ME: Hemostatic markers in acute stroke. *Stroke* 1989;20:592–597.
261. Holliday P, Mammen E, Buday J, Gilroy J, Barnhart M: "Sticky platelet" syndrome and cerebral infarction. *Neurology* 1983; 33:(suppl 2):145.
262. Wu K, Hoak J: Increased platelet aggregation in patients with transient ischemic attacks. *Stroke* 1975;6:521–524.
263. Hart R, Miller V, Coull B, Bril V: Cerebral infarction associated with lupus anticoagulants: Preliminary report. *Stroke* 1984; 15:114–118.

264. Levine SR, Welch KMA: The spectrum of neurologic disease associated with antiphospholipid antibodies, lupus anticoagulants, and anticardiolipin antibodies. *Arch Neurol* 1987;44: 876–883.
265. Kushner M, Simonian N: Lupus anticoagulant, anticardiolipin antibodies and cerebral ischemia. *Stroke* 1989;20:225–229.
266. Levine SR, Langer SL, Albers JW, Welch KMA: Sneddon's syndrome: An antiphospholipid antibody syndrome. *Neurology* 1988;38:798–800.
267. Rebollo M, Vol JF, Garijil F, Quintana F, Bercinao J: Livedo reticularis and cerebrovascular lesions (Sneddon's syndrome): Clinical, radiologic, and pathologic features in eight cases. *Brain* 1983;106:965–979.
268. Bruyn RP, VanderVeen JP, Donker AJ, Valk J, Wolters EC: Sneddon's syndrome: Case report and literature review. *J Neurol Sci* 1987;79:243–253.
269. Antiphospholipid Antibodies in Stroke Study Group (APASS): Clinical and laboratory findings in patients with antiphospholipid antibodies and cerebral ischemia. *Stroke* 1990;21: 1268–1273.
270. DeWitt LD, Caplan LR: Antiphospholipid antibodies and stroke. *AJNR* 1991;12:454–456.
271. Askerson RA: A "primary antiphospholipid syndrome"? (editorial). *J Rheumatol* 1988;15:1742–1746.
272. Coull BM, Boudette DN, Goodnight SH, Briley DP, Hart R: Multiple cerebral infarction and dementia associated with anticardiolipin antibodies. *Stroke* 1987;18:1107–1112.
273. Amico L, Caplan LR, Thomas C: Cerebrovascular complications of mucinous cancers. *Neurology* 1989;39:522–526.
274. Kase C, Robinson R, Stein R, DeWitt LD, Hier D, Harp D, et al: Anticoagulant-related intracerebral hemorrhage. *Neurology* 1985;35:943–948.
275. Caplan LR: Anticoagulation for cerebral ischemia. *Clin Neuropharmacol* 1986;9:399–414.
276. Bovill EG, Terrin ML, Stump DC, Berke AD, Frederick M, Collen D, et al: Hemorrhagic events during therapy with recombinant tissue-type plasminogen activator, heparin, and aspirin for acute myocardial infarction. *Ann Intern Med* 1991;115:256–265.
277. Kase CS, Pessin MS, Zivin JA, Del Zoppo GJ, Furlan AJ, Buckley JW, et al: Intracranial hemorrhages following coronary thrombolysis with tissue plasminogen activator. *Am J Med* 1992;92:384–390.
278. Babikian V, Kase C, Pessin M, Caplan L, Gorelick P: Resumption of anticoagulation after intracranial bleeding in patients with prosthetic valves. *Stroke* 1988;19:407–408.
279. Hart RG, Easton JD: Dissections of cervical and cerebral arteries. *Neurol Clin North Am* 1983;1:255–282.
280. Anson J, Crowell RM: Cervicocranial arterial dissection. *Neurosurgery* 1991;29:89–96.
281. Caplan LR, Zarins CK, Hemmati M: Spontaneous dissection of the extracranial vertebral arteries. *Stroke* 1985;16:1030–1036.
282. Mas JL, Bousser MG, Hasboun D, Laplane D: Extracranial vertebral artery dissections. *Stroke* 1987;18:1037–1047.
283. Mokri B, Houser W, Sandok B, Piepgras D: Spontaneous dissections of the vertebral arteries. *Neurology* 1988;38:880–885.
284. Ojemann RG, Fisher CM, Rich JC: Spontaneous dissecting aneurysms of the internal carotid artery. *Stroke* 1972;3:434–440.
285. Hennerici M, Steinke W, Rautenberg W: High-resistance doppler flow pattern in extracranial carotid dissection. *Arch Neurol* 1989;46:670–672.
286. Berger MS, Wilson CB: Intracranial dissecting aneurysms of the posterior circulation. *J Neurosurg* 1984;61:882–894.
287. Friedman AH, Drake CG: Subarachnoid hemorrhage from intracranial dissecting aneurysm. *J Neurosurg* 1984;60:325–334.

Chapter 123

Diagnosis and Treatment of Diseases of the Aorta

Joseph Lindsay, Jr., M.D. ■ *Michael E. DeBakey, M.D.* ■
Arthur C. Beall, M.D.

The aorta, structurally and functionally uncomplicated, manifests disease in a limited number of ways. Weakness of its wall may result in aneurysm, dissection, or rupture. Narrowing of the main trunk may occur but does so less frequently than does obstruction of the origin of a main branch. In contrast to this limited variety of clinical manifestations stands an array of disease processes capable of involving the aorta.

ETIOLOGIC AND PATHOGENETIC CONSIDERATIONS IN AORTIC DISEASE

Medial Changes of Aging

With advancing age the aortic media undergoes characteristic histological changes. These include fragmentation of elastic fibers and loss of smooth-muscle cell nuclei, so-called medionecrosis.[1] Moreover, collagenous tissue and basophilic ground substance replace the lost medial structures. Although the degree to which these changes are present in any one individual may vary, they appear to be an almost universal consequence of aging. Tortuosity and ectasia of the aorta commonly develop, and the loss of the normal "Windkessel" function of the aorta may contribute an increase in systolic blood pressure in some older individuals.

Atherosclerosis[2,3]

Aortic atherosclerosis is so prevalent in the Western world that its absence in middle life and beyond is noteworthy. Its first manifestation, "fatty streaks," are recognized in childhood. These focal collections of intracellular lipid appear as yellow, circumscribed, flat, or slightly raised intimal lesions. Of interest, they are common even in societies in which serum cholesterol measurements are low. By young adulthood some, but not all, of these fatty streaks have evolved into "fibrous plaques," firm, pale, gray, elevated lesions. They are comprised of lipid-laden smooth-muscle cells surrounded by proteoglycans and by a matrix of lipid, collagen, and elastic fibers. Their central core of amorphous, yellow material consists of extracellular lipid and cell debris. With the passage of time many of these plaques become ulcerated and calcified. Overlying thrombus is common. Initially an intimal process, the larger and more complex lesions penetrate the underlying media producing scarring and atrophy. (See Chaps. 54 and 55.)

Aortic atherosclerosis varies in severity from individual to individual. Diabetes, hypercholesterolemia, smoking, and hypertension are among the major identified risk factors.

Atherosclerosis, characteristically most severe in the abdominal aorta, tends to spare the ascending segment. Involvement is severe in the latter only in a few special situations. In patients with diabetes mellitus, atherosclerosis is frequently of great severity throughout the aorta. Individuals with type II hyperlipoproteinemia are a second exception to the rule that the ascending aorta is spared.[4] Finally, atherosclerosis can be of great severity overlying areas of syphilitic aortitis involving the ascending segment. (See Chap. 106.) At least two explanations have been advanced for the predilection of atherosclerosis for the infrarenal aorta.[5] First, the velocity and pulsatile characteristics of blood flow in that segment differ from those found in the proximal aortic segments. Such differences may influence the interface of blood with the aortic wall so as to favor plaque development in the infrarenal segment. Second, the wall of the abdominal aorta is thinner, has fewer elastic lamellae, and has more smooth-muscle fibers. Moreover, it lacks the rich network of vasa vasorum found in the proximal aorta.

Aortic atherosclerosis is manifest clinically in three major ways: aneurysm, obstruction of the infrarenal aorta, and embolization from atheromatous plaques to distal arterial beds.[6]

Medial Degeneration

Aortic aneurysm and medial dissection provide clinical evidence of a defective aortic media in a variety of acquired disorders. Atherosclerosis, syphilis, and other forms of aortitis may underlie these manifestations, and systemic hypertension often participates in their genesis.

There is, however, a characteristic lesion that testifies to the presence of a predominantly medial defect (or more likely, defects). In such cases, aneurysmal dilatation of the ascending aorta extends proximally into the aortic sinuses and ends distally just short of the innominate artery. The descriptive term *anuloaortic ectasia* has been applied.[7] A histological lesion, *cystic medial necrosis,* was for many years considered to be the hallmark of medial degeneration. More recent observations suggest that this light microscopic lesion is neither specific nor accurately named.[1,8–10] The defect or defects almost certainly lie at a biochemical and subcellular level.[11]

Anuloaortic ectasia is the characteristic aortic lesion of *Marfan's syndrome.*[7,12] The prototypical "Florence flask" or "onion bulb" appearance reflects the severity of the medial degeneration in the aortic root. Rupture of such aneurysms or aortic regurgitation secondary to aortic root dilatation is responsible for most of the premature deaths. Aortic dissection is somewhat less common if one excludes the intimal tears and associated limited medial disruptions commonly encountered within the aneurysm.

In the most complete presentation of Marfan's syndrome, skeletal, ocular, and cardiovascular anomalies are present and a family history of similar abnormalities exists.[7,12] Long extremities, particularly long, thin, hands and feet ("arachnodactyly"), and sparse muscle mass are outstanding musculoskeletal aberrations. Subluxed or frankly dislocated lenses attributable to lax supporting ligaments are characteristic. In addition to aortic aneurysm, myxomatous transformation of the aortic and mitral valves may produce valvular incompetence. Despite its close association with Marfan's syndrome, anuloaortic ectasia occurs most often in individuals with no other detectable congenital or hereditable anomaly.

Aortic aneurysm and dissection closely mimicking the characteristic aortic lesion of Marfan's syndrome are found in a variety of other congenital or hereditable disorders. For example, similar lesions have been reported in patients with congenital anomalies of the aortic valve,[13] aortic coarctation,[13] Turner's syndrome,[14] polycystic kidneys,[15] Ehlers-Danlos syndrome,[16] and osteogenesis imperfecta.[17]

Exceptionally, medial degeneration severe enough to result in aneurysm, rupture, or dissection is found in the main pulmonary arteries or in the aorta distal to the ascending segment.

Aortitis

Infective Aortitis[18,19]

Bacteria may spread to the aortic wall directly from contiguous tissue, but more frequently invading organisms are blood borne, entering the aortic wall from the lumen or from the vasa vasorum. Since the intact endothelium is quite resistant to bacterial invasion, a previously damaged area almost always provides the site for infection. For this reason secondarily infected aneurysms are more common than are aneurysms resulting solely from bacterial infection.

Osler introduced the term *mycotic aneurysm* to describe aneurysms resulting from septic emboli originating in *subacute* infective endocarditis.[18] An infected embolus lodging in a branch point of a distal artery forms the nidus for such a process, but because the large bore of the aorta offers few opportunities for the lodgment of small bits of infected material, embolization to the vasa vasorum has been hypothesized to explain the rare aortic aneurysm complicating endocarditis. In the antibiotic era it is far more common to encounter bacterial aortitis attributable to contiguous spread of infection from the aortic valve to the adjacent aortic wall and adjacent tissue.[20] The resulting perivalvular abscesses may disrupt the junction between the aorta and the fibrous cardiac skeleton producing aortocameral fistulas or damage to the conduction system.[21]

Blood-borne organisms not related to endocarditis may also invade the aortic wall, particularly at sites of aneurysm or in nonaneurysmal areas severely involved with atherosclerosis. A variety of organisms may be responsible, but *Staphylococcus aureus* and, especially, *Salmonella* species have been most frequently encountered.[18,19,22] In fact, *Salmonella* may be responsible for a third to a half of such infections.[18,22] An unusual ability of this organism to invade endothelium has been demonstrated, and it has been suggested that this genus may produce aortic infection in areas of relatively normal endothelium.[23]

The bacteremia responsible for an aortic infection need not be clinically apparent. Thus, an unexplained persistent febrile illness, particularly in an older man in whom aortic atherosclerosis may be anticipated, may reflect an infected aortic segment.

Rupture of a secondarily infected aneurysm or of a "mycotic" aneurysm created by the aortitis is inevitable unless resection of the infected segment under cover of effective antibiotic therapy can be accomplished. Antibiotics alone are not sufficient to prevent rupture.

An increased susceptibility to *Salmonella* infections exists among patients with acquired immunodeficiency syndrome. As yet only a few cases of aortic infection in this condition have been recorded, but more may be anticipated. A variety of therapeutic and ethical issues result.[24]

Direct extension from a pyogenic or tuberculous pulmonary or mediastinal infection to the aorta may also occur. Aneurysm, rupture, or fistula may ensue. Syphilitic aortitis is reviewed in Chap. 106.

Nonspecific Aortitis—Takayasu's Disease[25–28]

Narrowing of an aortic segment or of one of its branches, aneurysm formation, or aortic regurgitation may be produced by an arteritis for which no specific etiology can be found. It may occur as an isolated abnormality or be associated with noninfectious inflammatory involvement of other organs as in, for example, lupus erythematosus or rheumatoid arthritis.

Takayasu's arteritis, named for the Japanese ophthalmologist who first called attention to the fundoscopic findings of the disease, is the prototype. Because of its predilection for the brachiocephalic vessels, this arteritis has been labeled *"pulseless" disease* and *aortic arch syndrome.* The classic form occurs with the greatest frequency in the Orient. However, patients with nonspecific aortitis presenting in a manner quite similar to this prototype are encountered worldwide. Whether they represent similar or identical disease processes is uncertain.

The description to follow will focus on the prototypical illness described in the Orient. The reader may infer that variations on the theme will be encountered elsewhere.

Etiology The etiology of Takayasu's arteritis is unknown. No infectious agent has been identified. Clinical and serologic data suggest an *autoimmune* process. Recently, a genetic predisposition has been suggested because of clustering of the disorder in certain families and because of the frequency of similar histocompatibility antigens in these kindred.[29]

Pathology Histological examination discloses a granulomatous arteritis during active stages of the disease. The microscopic appearance is remarkably similar to that in giant-cell arteritis and in the aortitis associated with seronegative spondylitis. In later stages medial degeneration, fibrous scarring, intimal proliferation, and thrombosis result in narrowing of the affected vessel. Aneurysm formation is observed rather less commonly than are stenosis and aortic rupture or dissection.

Detailed angiographic examination has provided a great deal of information about the distribution of the stenotic lesions.[27] The left subclavian artery, particularly in its midportion, is narrowed in about 90 percent of instances. The right subclavian, the left carotid, and the brachiocephalic trunk follow closely with regard to frequency of stenosis. Ishikawa[27] detected lesions in the thoracic aorta by angiography in two-thirds of his series. Involvement of the abdominal aorta was identified in half, but in only about 12 percent was there aortoiliac involvement. He found angiographic evidence of pulmonary arteritis in about half. Pulmonary hypertension may be found at catheterization. In patients studied at the Mayo Clinic[25] involvement of the abdominal aorta and renal and superior mesenteric arteries was even more frequent than in the Japanese series.

Clinical Features Manifestations of the illness appear during the second or third decade in 70 to 80 percent of instances, but it has been reported in childhood and in middle life. Women are eight or nine times more often affected than are men.

During the early, or "prepulseless," period of the illness, constitutional manifestations—such as fever, night sweats, malaise, nausea and vomiting, weight loss, arthralgia, and skin rash—are frequently encountered. The patient may experience Raynaud's phenomenon, and splenomegaly may be present. Laboratory study may disclose an elevated erythrocyte sedimentation rate, anemia, and serum protein abnormalities.

Claudication or numbness of an upper extremity due to subclavian artery narrowing and evidence of ischemia of the central nervous system occur with great frequency. Postural dizziness or frank syncope usually reflects cerebral ischemia due to narrowing of the brachiocephalic arteries.

Narrowing of the aorta proximal to the renal arteries or of the renal arteries accounts for some, if not all, of the hypertension observed in more than half of aortitis patients. It must be remembered that difficulty may be encountered in accurately measuring arterial pressure because of arch vessel stenosis.

Cardiac manifestations may result from aortic regurgitation, coronary artery narrowing, or severe hypertension. Dilatation of the aortic root commonly accompanies the aortic valve incompetence. Angina pectoris, heart failure, and myocardial infarction are reported. Biopsy evidence has been presented for the presence of myocarditis in some patients.[30] Pericarditis has been observed clinically, but more commonly healed pericarditis is noted at necropsy.

The retinopathy to which Takayasu first directed attention is believed to result from ischemia of the retina. Ocular ischemia may also be manifested by transient loss of vision, cataracts, corneal opacity, and iridial atrophy. Blindness is a common complication.

Involvement of the visceral arteries occasionally results in splanchnic ischemia, and intermittent claudication due to aortoiliac obstruction may occur.

Recently attention has been directed toward the special problems that may arise during pregnancy in patients with this disorder.[31,32] Hypertension is a frequent and troublesome problem, but the outcome for mother and child is acceptable when meticulous obstetrical care is provided.

Prognosis[33,34] Disability and death occur with severe aortitis. One-third to one-quarter of patients will have a significant event or will die within 5 years. Those with few or no ischemic complications at the time of diagnosis fare better and have a good 5- and 10-year prognosis. In addition to the presence of complications at diagnosis, the presence of severe hypertension or of cardiac involvement predicts a shortened life expectancy.

Cerebrovascular accidents and blindness are the most common major events. Congestive heart failure and aortic rupture or dissection are less frequent.

Management The benefits of any specific therapy have been difficult to assess since the disease typically runs a chronic course. Adrenocorticoids appear to be effective in suppressing the inflammation of the active phase. Immunosuppressive therapy has also been utilized.[26,30] Operative treatment may relieve symptoms from arterial obstruction, and percutaneous angioplasty has been utilized with favorable initial results.[35,36]

Giant-Cell Arteritis[37,38]

Giant-cell arteritis (temporal arteritis, polymyalgia rheumatica) involves extracranial arteries, including the aorta in 10 to 13 percent of cases. Its peak incidence in late life seems to set it apart from other varieties of nonspecific arteritis. It may also produce narrowing of the brachiocephalic arteries, aneurysm of the ascending aorta, aortic regurgitation, and aortic dissection. Unlike Takayasu's arteritis, giant-cell arteritis rarely involves the descending thoracic or abdominal aorta.

Aortitis in HLA-B27-Associated Spondyloarthropathies

Although the etiology of neither ankylosing spondylitis nor Reiter's syndrome is known, more than 90 percent of individuals afflicted with one of these disorders have the histocompatibility antigen HLA-B27, an antigen quite infrequent in the general population. This observation may provide a clue to a common pathogenetic mechanism.[39]

Aortitis has been demonstrated to accompany a sizeable minority of patients with these disorders.[40] Moreover, it may be present in some patients with the HLA-B27 antigen who are not afflicted with spondyloarthropathy. Patients with the antigen can be identified with considerable frequency among subjects with lone aortic regurgitation or conduction abnormalities.[39]

On histological examination the inflammatory aortic lesion found in association with these disorders resembles that of syphilis. Focal destruction of the medial elastic tissue is seen, but that layer is not thickened as are the intima and adventitia. An obliterative arteritis of the vasa vasorum may be present.[40]

Unlike syphilis, the process is largely limited to the aortic wall behind and immediately above the sinuses of Valsalva. The thickening of the adventitia and the intimal proliferation extend below the aortic valve to involve the membranous ventricular septum and the base of the anterior leaflet of the mitral valve.[40] The aortic valve cusps are thickened and retracted and their edges rolled.

Such aortitis is more frequent in patients with spondylitis of long duration, in those with peripheral joint complaints in addition to spondylitis, and in patients with associated iritis.

As is the case with syphilis, aortic regurgitation is the most frequent clinical manifestation of these forms of aortitis. Extension of the aortitis onto the interventricular ventricular septum occasionally results in atrioventricular conduction abnormalities. Either of these clinical manifestations may be severe and life threatening. (See also Chap. 79.)

Congenital Anomalies of the Aorta

Patent ductus arteriosus, coarctation of the aortic isthmus, aortopulmonary window, aneurysm of the aortic sinuses, and anomalies of the aortic arch are considered in the section of this text dealing with congenital heart disease. (See Chaps. 97 and 98.)

Pseudocoarctation of the Aorta

Congenital kinking, so-called pseudocoarctation of the aorta, may be detected during the investigation of a mediastinal mass or of a systolic murmur. An abnormally elongated thoracic aorta tethered to the ligamentum arteriosum produces a silhouette shaped like an S or a 3 on radiographic examination. Thus, it may resemble true coarctation. However, rib notching is not present. Exclusion of hemodynamically significant coarctation may require sophisticated imaging or the demonstration that no pressure difference exists between the upper and the lower aortic segments. True coarctation may coexist, and congenital cardiovascular anomalies similar to those found in true coarctation may be associated.

Some authorities believe the abnormality to be a sharp downward angulation of the aorta at the attachment of the ligamentum arteriosum as a result of elongation of the fourth aortic arch.[41] Others consider the embryologic defect to be the same as for typical isthmic coarctation. However, in these cases the narrowing is not severe enough to result in significant obstruction.[42]

Abdominal Coarctation of the Aorta

Although rare, hemodynamically significant narrowing of the descending thoracic or abdominal aorta deserves attention because it affects young people and because it often produces life-threatening hypertension that is surgically correctable.[43,44] Although it most often appears to be a congenital lesion, at least some examples appear to result from healed aortitis.[45] For this reason, some writers prefer the term *middle aortic syndrome.*

The narrowed aortic segment may be quite focal, but diffuse hypoplasia of the abdominal aorta and iliac arteries may be encountered.

Commonly involved in this process, the renal arteries may be stenosed, hypoplastic, or thrombosed. As a consequence, severe hypertension is the most common presenting complaint. Involvement of the visceral arteries may result in ischemia in their distribution. Intermittent claudication from involvement of the iliac arteries is more frequent than in patients with coarctation at the aortic isthmus.

On examination, similarities to the more common postductal coarctation will be noted. Upper extremity hypertension will be present together with feeble pulses and hypotension in the legs. Attention may be directed to the unusual location of the stenosis by a bruit in the lumbar or umbilical area.

Operative treatment is usually required since severe hypertension significantly shortens the life expectancy of patients with this disorder.

CLINICAL MANIFESTATIONS OF AORTIC DISEASE

Aneurysm[46,47]

Aneurysms, areas of focal or diffuse dilatation of the aorta, develop at sites of congenital or acquired medial weakness. Hypertension, frequently present in patients with aneurysm, exposes weakness that might otherwise not be manifest and, in addition, probably accelerates degeneration of the aortic wall. Once begun, aneurysm formation is promoted by physical laws, particularly that of LaPlace. (See Chap. 5.) Expansion and rupture often result unless the patient succumbs to intercurrent disease before this can occur.

Fusiform and *saccular* aneurysms are described. In the former, circumferential dilatation, the result of a diffuse area of weakness, produces a spindle-shaped deformity. In the latter, balloon-like dilatation occurs, beginning at a relatively narrow neck. Many aneurysms are not pure examples of either. In either variety, by the time the aortic wall has been stretched to aneurysmal size, little or no recognizable aortic tissue remains; the wall of the aneurysmal sack is composed of fibrous tissue.

Whether fusiform or saccular, the lumen of the aneurysm virtually always contains laminated thrombus. Such clots may be extensive enough to fill a saccular aneurysm or to cover the circumference of a fusiform aneurysm. For this reason angiographic opacification of the aortic lumen often does not clearly delineate the size or extent of the aneurysm.

Aneurysms may result from a variety of causes. Congenital medial weakness producing aortic dilatation has been discussed in the previous section. With the declining incidence of syphilitic aortitis, damage to the aortic wall by an inflammatory process, either infectious or nonspecific, is uncommon. Saccular aneurysms are often encountered in regions of the aorta weakened by aortic dissection.

Despite this variety of possibilities, atherosclerosis appears to be responsible for the great majority of aortic aneurysms. Furthermore, because of the predilection of atherosclerosis for the infrarenal aorta, the majority are located in that segment. It may, however, be simplistic to attribute all such lesions to atherosclerosis. Recently, data have been put forward that suggest the possibility that an underlying biochemical or ultrastructural defect of the media contributes to the development of an aneurysm in many patients.[48,49]

Thoracic Aneurysm

Etiology and Pathologic Anatomy As noted above, anuloaortic ectasia, the typical aortic lesion of medial degeneration, has been described as a Florence flask or onion bulb aorta. These are apt descriptors since the dilatation is greatest in the proximal ascending aorta, including the aortic sinuses. The diameter quickly tapers so that it approaches a normal dimension before the takeoff of the innominate artery. The most frequent aortic manifestation of Marfan's syndrome, anuloaortic ectasia is more often encountered in individuals with no musculoskeletal or ocular manifestations of that disorder. Limited or extensive medial dissection may complicate this lesion.[7,50]

Saccular aneurysms of the aorta frequently follow aortic dissection when operative repair is not carried out. Moreover, they may develop in the descending thoracic aorta even after successful operative repair of a dissection involving the ascending aorta.[51] Such aneurysms may gradually expand over time and require operative treatment months or years after the acute event.

Syphilitic aneurysms are still occasionally encountered. The ascending aorta and arch are the segments most often affected, but the aortic dilatation often extends into the aortic sinuses and the descending aortic segment. Syphilitic aneurysms are more often saccular than fusiform. (See also Chap. 106.)

The most common thoracic aneurysms, those attributable to atherosclerosis, typically are located in the descending thoracic segment and may extend into the arch. They tend to be fusiform, but this is not invariable. They often extend over a considerable length and some extend into the abdomen. An associated abdominal aneurysm is quite frequent and should be sought whenever an atherosclerotic thoracic aneurysm is encountered.[46]

Clinical Manifestations[52,53] Aneurysms limited to the ascending aorta rarely produce symptoms directly unless they are undergoing active expansion or rupture. Findings of aortic regurgitation often draw the attention of an examiner and lead to detection of the aneurysm by one of the imaging techniques. Since the aortic root is located within the cardiac silhouette and the entire ascending aorta within the pericardial space, dilatation may not be readily appreciated on a chest radiograph. Echocardiography, especially transesophageal, is more often valuable. (See Chaps. 15 and 131.)

Although often asymptomatic and detected fortuitously in the course of an incidental chest radiograph, aneurysms involving the arch or descending thoracic segments are more likely to produce symptoms than are those confined to the ascending aorta. These segments are fixed by the brachiocephalic arteries and lie in a position to compress a variety of mediastinal structures as well as the thoracic spine. Compression of the tracheobronchial tree may be attended by cough or dyspnea. Tracheal deviation or "tug" may be detected on physical examination. Pressure on the esophagus may result in dysphagia, rarely quite severe. Hoarseness may result from the compression of the recurrent laryngeal nerve. Adjacent vascular structures may be compressed, resulting in pulmonary arterial stenosis or superior vena caval obstruction.

Chest pain, described as deep and aching or throbbing, has been the most frequent symptom reported in patients with thoracic aneurysm. Pain may be associated with erosion of the rib cage or vertebrae. The appearance of pain clearly related to an aneurysm must be regarded as a signal of expansion and threatened rupture.

Rupture can be the initial manifestation of a thoracic aneurysm. Massive, usually fatal hemorrhage into the mediastinum, pleural space, esophagus, or tracheobronchial tree ensues. Rupture of an aneurysm of the ascending aorta, because of the intrapericardial location of that structure, results in acute hemopericardium and cardiac tamponade. Hemoptysis may precede by days or weeks fatal hemorrhage in descending thoracic aneurysms that have become adherent to adjacent lung. Rarely, aneurysms may rupture into adjacent vascular structures, producing aortovenous or aortopulmonary fistulas.

Diagnostic Studies The aorta may now be imaged by a variety of modalities. Of these, the chest radiograph (Chap. 14) and transthoracic echocardiography (Chap.

15) are the most readily available and are especially useful for screening purposes. Aortography, computerized tomography (Chap. 135), magnetic resonance imaging (Chap. 136), and transesophageal echocardiography (Chap. 131) all provide detailed information regarding the aorta's anatomy.

Natural History and Prognosis Most of the data concerning the natural history of thoracic aortic aneurysms come from retrospective analyses of hospital experience,[52,53] but some are available from epidemiologic studies.[54] If anuloaortic ectasia and aortic dissection are excluded, the vast majority of cases studied have been examples of atherosclerotic aneurysms involving the descending aortic segment. Joyce et al.'s[52] classic review suggests a 50 percent 5-year and a 70 percent 10-year mortality. More recent studies have suggested that the 5-year mortality may approach 75 percent.[53,54] One-third to one-half of deaths result from rupture of the aneurysm; most of the remainder are a consequence of other vascular diseases. The location of the aneurysm did not influence the mortality rate, but advanced age, an aneurysm more than 6 cm in size, the presence of hypertension, and the association of other cardiovascular disease all increased the risk of death. The presence of symptoms, a reflection of a large aneurysm or one threatening to rupture, was associated with a reduced rate of survival.

The natural history of patients with anuloaortic ectasia may be even more grim. In one series, 52 of 56 patients with Marfan's syndrome died as a consequence of aortic disease.[55] The average age at death was 32 years.

Treatment Surgical repair constitutes the only known effective treatment for thoracic aneurysms. It is urgently indicated in patients with a large aneurysm (6 cm or larger), especially if symptoms suggest expansion or compression of an adjacent structure. Cardiac failure from aortic regurgitation or aortocameral fistula may also necessitate early operative treatment. Resection is less urgent in small, asymptomatic aneurysms.

Consideration of the severity of associated diseases is also important in selection of patients for surgery. Compared with the patient who has no other disease, the individual with associated coronary or cerebrovascular disease has a greater operative risk and a smaller risk of dying from rupture of the aneurysm before succumbing to the associated vascular disease.

Surgical treatment consists in replacing the resected aneurysmal segment with a Dacron graft attached to relatively normal aorta proximally and distally. Specific surgical procedures vary with the site of the aneurysm and the need for maintaining circulation to distal parts of the body during the necessary period of aortic occlusion (Fig. 123-1). Accordingly, thoracic aneurysms are divided into those affecting the ascending aorta,[56] those affecting the transverse arch of the aorta containing origins of the brachiocephalic vessels, and those affecting the descending thoracic aorta distal to the left subclavian artery.

For aneurysms of the ascending aorta, total cardiopulmonary bypass is required.[57] The myocardium is protected by cold cardioplegia during the period that the coronary ostia are exposed. The aneurysm is opened,

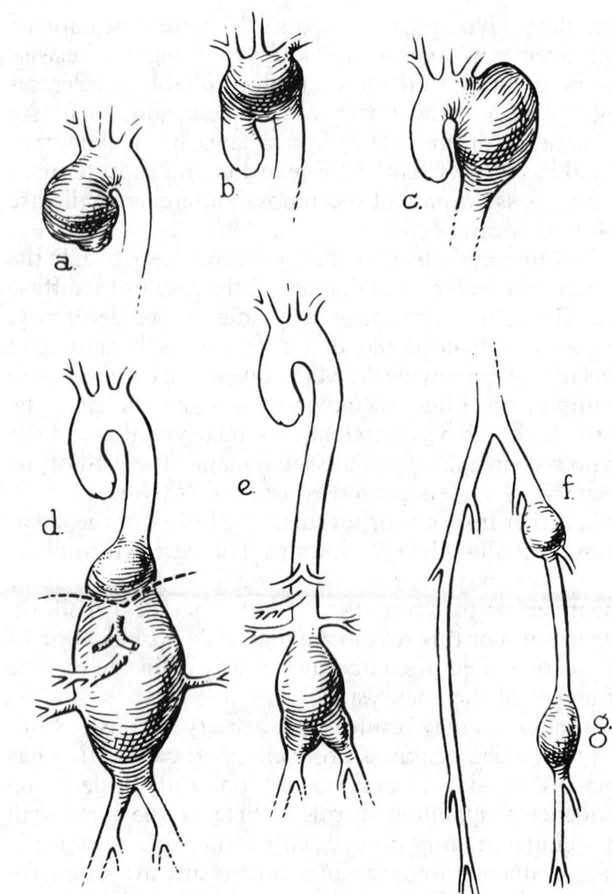

FIGURE 123-1 Most frequent sites of aneurysms of the aorta and major arteries. *A.* Fusiform aneurysm of the ascending aorta. *B.* Fusiform aneurysm of the aortic arch involving the brachiocephalic, carotid, and subclavian arteries. *C.* Fusiform aneurysm of the descending portion of the aortic arch. *D.* Large fusiform thoracoabdominal aneurysm involving the celiac, superior mesenteric, and renal arteries. *E.* Fusiform aneurysm of the abdominal aorta and iliac arteries. *F.* Fusiform aneurysm of the femoral artery. *G.* Fusiform aneurysm of the popliteal artery.

and a woven albumin-coated Dacron graft is sutured in place from within the aneurysm with continuous sutures. Finally, the aneurysmal sac is trimmed and sutured around the graft. If the aneurysm is associated with aortic valve incompetency, the leaflets are excised and a composite albumin-coated Dacron graft and prosthetic valve is sutured in place to the aortic annulus with interrupted sutures, after which the coronary ostia are sutured to an appropriate opening made in the Dacron graft. The distal anastomosis of the graft is performed as previously described.

For aneurysms of the transverse arch of the aorta, total cardiopulmonary bypass is also required. Additionally, profound hypothermia is used to protect the brain during temporary absence of circulation to the brachiocephalic vessels. A woven albumin-coated Dacron graft is sutured to relatively normal aorta proximally and distally from within the aneurysm, and the brachiocephalic, left common carotid, and left subclavian arteries are attached individually to appropriate openings in the graft. It is often possible to preserve the relatively normal aortic wall segment from which these vessels arise and simply anastomose this segment to an appropriate opening made in the graft for this purpose. The walls of the aneurysm are trimmed and sutured together around the grafts.

Aneurysms arising distal to the left common carotid artery do not require extracorporeal circulation.[58,59] Although we previously recommended left atrial–to–femoral artery bypass, femoral-femoral partial cardiopulmonary bypass, hypothermia, or temporary shunts around the aneurysm during the period of aortic occlusion, in recent years we have not used these adjuncts because they did not prevent certain complications, particularly spinal cord ischemia, which occurs in about 3 to 4 percent of the patients, and they were associated with a number of complications. The aorta is clamped proximally and distally to the aneurysm while the blood pressure is controlled proximally by the intravenous administration of nitroprusside, and the aneurysm is opened. Bleeding from the orifices of the intercostal arteries is controlled within the aneurysm by figure-of-eight sutures, and a woven albumin-coated Dacron graft is sutured to relatively normal aorta proximal and distal to the aneurysm. If one or two large intercostal arteries are present, they are attached to openings made in the graft. Finally, the walls of the aneurysm are trimmed and sutured around the graft.

Results of these methods of surgical treatment have been most encouraging. The surgical mortality rate for all aneurysms of the ascending or descending thoracic aorta is about 15 percent, although it is somewhat higher for those affecting the transverse arch and origins of the brachiocephalic vessels. Follow-up studies on these patients for almost 40 years provide evidence of maintenance of good results with long-term survival.[59] Deaths during this period have usually been due to associated diseases or other causes, although aneurysms occasionally develop in later years in other parts of the aorta and require surgical treatment.

Abdominal Aneurysm

Etiology Traditionally, virtually all abdominal aneurysms have been attributed to atherosclerosis. Recent recognition of familial clustering of these lesions and identification of biochemical and molecular defects in the media of individuals with aneurysm have led to the realization that it may be too simplistic to consider atherosclerosis as the sole pathogenetic mechanism.[48,49]

Rarely, a traumatic, congenital, or mycotic abdominal aneurysm is encountered, and occasionally it may occur as a residual of aortic dissection or in patients with Marfan's syndrome.

Pathological Anatomy Abdominal aneurysms are, as a rule, fusiform but may be saccular. They are located, in almost all instances, distal to the renal arteries, extend to the aortic bifurcation, and often involve the iliac arteries (Fig. 123-1). Exceptionally, they extend above the renal arteries. In that case, the origins of not only the renal arteries but also the major visceral arteries may be involved. Such involvement complicates operative management.

Five to 10 percent of abdominal aneurysms are accompanied by an intense inflammatory and fibrotic reaction in the anterior and lateral periaortic tissue,[60,61] a process histologically similar to retroperitoneal fibrosis. It has been suggested that these "inflammatory aneurysms" result from hypersensitivity to an antigen or antigens in the atherosclerotic plaque.

The clinical presentation of inflammatory aneurysms may suggest the threat of rupture since abdominal pain may be associated and the aneurysm may be tender. Systemic manifestations such as weight loss and an elevated erythrocyte sedimentation rate are reported. The difficulty of operative repair is increased.

Clinical Manifestations[62–64] Men are three or four times more likely to have an atherosclerotic abdominal aneurysm than women. The typical patient is in the seventh or eighth decade. Most are symptomatic and are detected in the course of an examination directed at unrelated symptoms.

Pain that can definitely be attributed to the aneurysm, especially when it is of recent onset, likely heralds rupture. Characteristically constant and located in the midabdomen, lumbar region, or pelvis, the pain may be severe and may be described as having a boring quality. Detection of an aneurysm that is tender to palpation carries much the same threat of rupture.

Unless the patient is obese, physical examination almost always discloses an abdominal mass in the epigastrium, slightly to the left of the midline. If definite expansile movement can be detected, the diagnosis of abdominal aneurysm is reasonably secure. Bruits may be audible, and femoral pulses are reduced in some patients.

Rupture may be the initial manifestation. Rapid exsanguination may result from free rupture into the peritoneal cavity. Fortunately, more often the rupture is directed into the retroperitoneal space, where hemorrhage may be retarded. Abdominal pain and evidence of occult blood loss may persist for hours or days, allowing time for diagnosis and operative treatment. Rarely, the rupture is confined for several days to a few weeks. In such instances, the patient may present a puzzling diagnostic picture consisting of abdominal pain, fever, and slight to moderate blood loss.[65] Recognition of the nature of the illness can be lifesaving since secondary rupture always ensues.

Rarely, rupture occurs into an adjacent retroperitoneal structure. When a communication develops with the venae cavae or other large vein, a loud continuous murmur in the abdomen and high-output congestive heart failure may ensue.[65] Rupture into the duodenum results in gastrointestinal bleeding,[65] but aortoduodenal fistulas are more common after graft replacement of the infrarenal aorta.

An unruptured aneurysm may also produce serious complications. Acute thrombosis may mimic saddle embolism. Furthermore, embolization of thrombus or atherosclerotic debris from aneurysms (and indeed from severely atherosclerotic, but nonaneurysmal, segments) to the lower extremities is far more frequent than is generally appreciated.[65] Secondary bacterial infection of an aortic aneurysm gives rise to fever, leukocytosis, and abdominal pain. Such infections lead to rupture of the aneurysm. Antibiotics, as a rule, neither eradicate the infection nor prevent the rupture.[18,65]

Diagnostic Studies[66] Anteroposterior or cross-table lateral radiographs of the abdomen often confirm the presence of aneurysm by demonstrating the characteristic "egg-shell" calcification of its wall. Imaging with ultrasound provides reproducible measurements of the dimensions of the aneurysm, and computed radiographic tomography and magnetic resonance imaging provide a more definitive confirmation of the diagnosis. Aortography can be reserved for instances in which additional information regarding the extent of the aneurysm or the degree of involvement of branch arteries is required. The aortogram, a depiction of the luminal contour, may be misleading since the aneurysm is characteristically filled or lined with thrombus.

Natural History[66–69] Rupture of an abdominal aneurysm is a frequent cause of death. The risk of rupture appears greatest for larger aneurysms (those greater than 5 cm in diameter). There is, therefore, general agreement that individuals with aneurysms of this size and an acceptable anesthetic risk should undergo operative treatment. Aneurysms smaller than 4 cm appear rarely to rupture and do not ordinarily require surgery unless they become larger. Those whose diameter is more than 4 cm but less than 5 cm fall into a gray zone in which there is disagreement regarding the desirability of operation.

Commonly associated with abdominal aneurysms are coronary and cerebrovascular disease.[70] Two characteristics of these patients are noteworthy. They are both less likely to die of rupture because of the lethality of their "organ-fixed" atherosclerosis and they incur a greater operative risk for aneurysmectomy. It is important to recognize that given appropriate preoperative screening for coronary disease with dipyridamole-thallium scintigraphy or coronary arteriography and appropriate treatment of the coronary disease, the risk of aneurysmectomy is acceptable in such patients.[71]

Treatment Since operative repair of abdominal aneurysms can now be accomplished with a mortality rate well under 5 percent,[72] surgery can be recommended for all patients except those with advanced associated disease.

Symptomatic aneurysms require urgent surgical treatment since early rupture can be confidently predicted. A ruptured abdominal aneurysm is a surgical emergency. Prompt surgical treatment can save most of these patients. Death is otherwise inevitable.

Surgery for an abdominal aortic aneurysm does not require maintenance of the distal circulation.[72,73] The aorta is clamped proximally between the aneurysm and the renal arteries, the iliac arteries are clamped distally, and the aneurysm is opened. Bleeding from the orifices of the lumbar arteries is controlled from within the aneurysm by figure-of-eight sutures. If the aortic bifurcation is not affected by the aneurysm, an albumin-coated Dacron tube graft may be used to restore circulation. If the bifurcation and the proximal iliac arteries are affected, an albumin-coated Dacron bifurcation graft is required. From within the aneurysm the graft is sutured proximally to normal aorta and distally to the aortic bifurcation or individually to the iliac arteries. Finally, the aneurysmal walls are trimmed and sutured over the graft.

We have used this method of treatment in more than 10,000 patients for almost 40 years. The surgical risk depends primarily on the presence or absence of rupture, associated heart disease or hypertension, and patient's age. Our experience has shown that the 5- to 10-year survival rate for patients operated on for aneurysms of the abdominal aorta closely parallels that for comparable age groups in the normal population. Surgical treatment is therefore recommended for all patients with aneurysms of the abdominal aorta unless a surgical contraindication exists.

Aortic Dissection

Pathological Anatomy[74–76]

Longitudinal cleavage of the aortic media by a dissecting column of blood characterizes aortic dissection. The split in the media, not usually circumferential, often occupies about half of the circumference of the aorta and may extend through the entire length of the vessel. The plane of dissection typically follows the greater curvature of the ascending aorta and the arch. Most often located lateral to the true lumen in the descending aorta, it may be medial and may spiral "barber pole" fashion about the long axis of the aorta.

The *false channel* created by this splitting of the medial elastic lamina communicates almost invariably with the *true lumen* through an intimal tear located near its proximal end (Fig. 123-2). Such tears are often single and transverse in orientation, but exceptions are frequent. *Secondary* or *reentry* tears, located more distally along the false channel, are also quite common.

The ascending aorta is involved in about two-thirds of all instances of aortic dissection. The intimal (*entry*) tear in this most common variety is located a few centimeters above the aortic valve. The medial cleavage may not extend beyond the ascending aorta, but far more frequently it extends beyond the arch, often to the aortoiliac bifurcation.

Dissections that do not include the ascending aorta, the second most common anatomic variety, account for about a quarter of all cases. In typical examples, the proximal limit of the medial hematoma lies just beyond the origin of the left subclavian artery. The medial split extends distally for varying distances, often to the aortoiliac bifurcation.

A small number of cases do not follow these two patterns. In some, the medial cleavage is short and limited to the arch or to the descending thoracic or abdominal segments. A few seem to lack an intimal tear. In one rather frequently encountered variation, an entry tear is located just beyond the left subclavian artery, but the dissection extends proximally into the ascending aorta.

The most widely applied nomenclature is that of DeBakey[68] (Fig. 123-3). In this classification, proximal dissection falls into type I and those originating beyond the arch into type III. Type II includes those involving the ascending aorta only, a small heterogenous group. Apart from length, many are indistinguishable from type I.

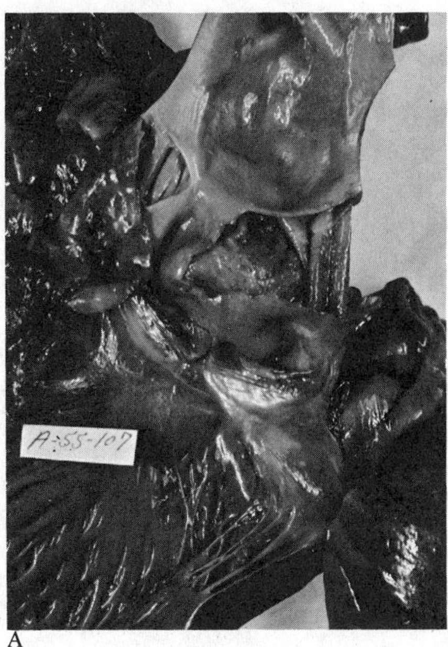

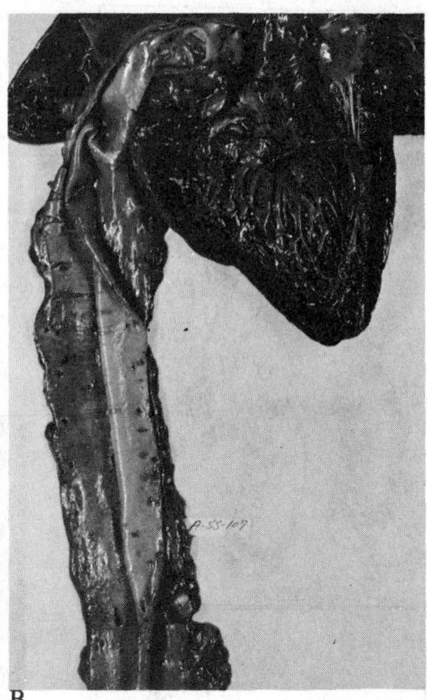

FIGURE 123-2 Dissecting aortic aneurysm. *A.* The large intimal rent may be seen a few centimeters above the aortic cusps. *B.* The false channel created by the dissecting hematoma is shown. Notice the clearly sheared layers of aortic media.

Others originate within chronic fusiform dilatation of the ascending aorta. In such instances, multiple intimal tears and limited medial splitting are characteristic.

Death from aortic dissection most often occurs from disruption of the outer wall of the false channel opposite the entrance tear. Rupture of proximal dissection therefore produces hemopericardium and cardiac tamponade. Hemorrhage into the mediastinum or either pleural space may occur. Typically, external rupture of distal dissection results in a bloody left pleural effusion. Death from external rupture, while often abrupt, may be delayed by temporary cessation of hemorrhage attributable to falling arterial pressure and increasing tension in the periaortic tissue. Dramatic clinical syndromes result in those rare instances in which the false channel ruptures into the right-sided heart chambers producing a large left-to-right shunt.

In approximately half of patients with proximal dissection, medial hematoma undermines the aortic valve, rendering it incompetent. Fortunately, very serious hemodynamic consequences of aortic regurgitation appear infrequently during the acute phase.

Obstruction of a branch vessel of the aorta accompanies type I dissection in about half of patients. This complication is less frequent in those with type III. The results may be catastrophic, particularly in patients with type I, since in them the coronary and cerebral circulations are jeopardized. Obstruction of renal or splanchnic arteries may produce life-threatening complications in either type. Severe hypertension and acute renal failure may attend renal artery involvement. The iliac arteries are the branch arteries most frequently compromised. Potentially disabling but usually not immediately life threatening, narrowing of these arteries may produce dramatic, painful ischemia of the lower extremities.

The aortic wall that has been weakened by aortic dissection but that does not rupture during the acute phase is often the site of subsequent aneurysm formation. Such rupture constitutes a major threat to the survivor of the initial illness.

Pathogenesis[1,8–10,77,78]

Arterial hypertension seems clearly to be a factor in the genesis of aortic dissection. An elevated blood pressure, or evidence of its existence, can be found in 80 percent of patients. In most, no conclusive evidence of a medial defect can be identified, and no heritable or congenital basis for suspecting such a defect is apparent. The mechanism by which hypertension promotes the process remains unclear. Increased arterial pressure must certainly expose any existing weakness of the aortic wall and may, in addition, accentuate the degenerative processes of aging that promote such weakness.

The frequency with which dissecting hematoma is noted in Marfan's syndrome, in certain other congenital and heritable conditions, and in experimental lathyrism provides a strong argument for the importance of an underlying medial defect in at least some individuals with this disorder. Indeed, histological evidence of degeneration of elastin or of smooth-muscle cells in the aortic media of such patients has long been noted. Recent studies, however, have thrown considerable doubt on the specificity of the classic histological findings. These newer studies indicate that such findings are frequently absent in patients with dissection and that remarkably similar changes may be found in older patients without dissection. It seems likely that the fundamental medial defect or defects may be unrecognizable by light microscopy. Studies of the ultrastructure, biochemistry, and molecular biology of aortic dissection are promising.

The role of the intimal (entry) tear in the genesis of medial dissection is debated. Many investigators feel that it exposes the media to blood under luminal pressure and that the resulting shear forces initiate and propagate the medial cleavage. Others propose that medial weakness leads to hemorrhage from the vasa vasorum. The resulting intramural hematoma cleaves the medial layers. In this hypothesis the intimal tears are secondary. The infrequent cases in which no intimal tear can be identified are cited as evidence for this scenario.

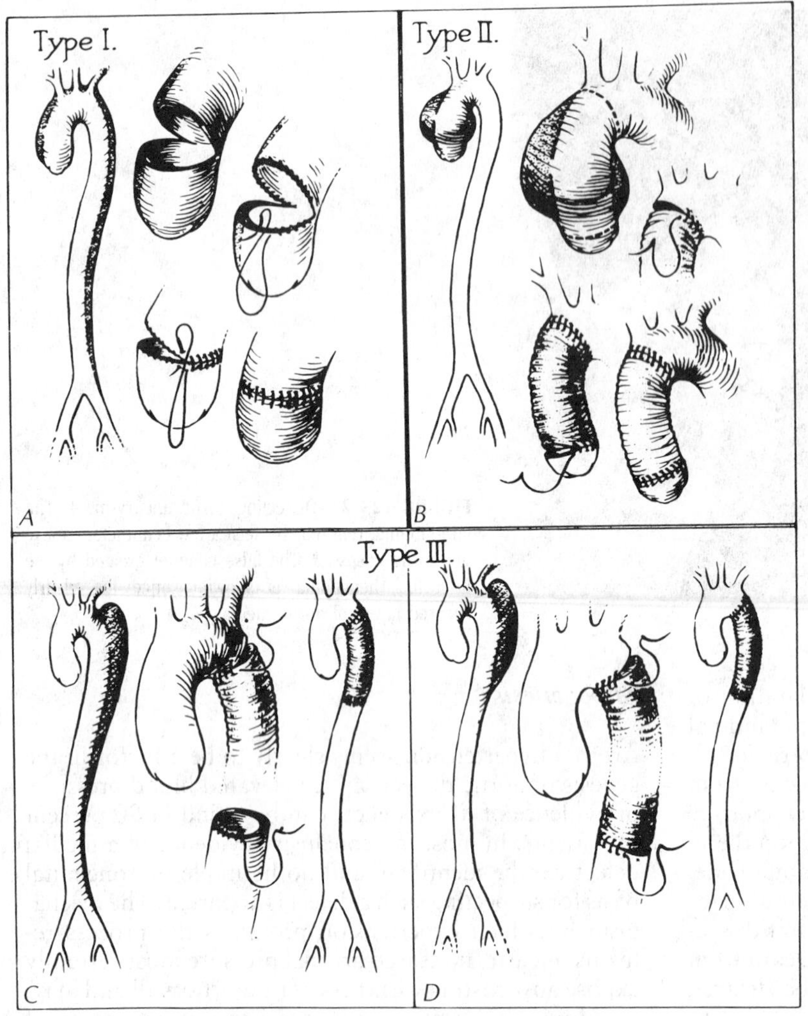

FIGURE 123-3 Surgical classification of dissecting aneurysms of the aorta based on anatomic and pathological patterns of the lesions and their respective methods of surgical treatment.

Clinical Manifestations[74,75,79–81]

Most common in the fifth through the seventh decades of life, aortic dissection has been reported in children as well as the very old. Men are affected at least twice as commonly as women.

Certain congenital lesions of the aorta (e.g., coarctation and bicuspid aortic valve) are associated with increased frequency of dissection.[13] A greater-than-expected incidence is encountered in patients with aortic stenosis, often originating at the site where a jet of blood strikes the aortic intima. It also occurs in patients with certain heritable disorders such as Marfan's and Turner's syndromes.

Iatrogenic vascular trauma, a complication of cardiac catheterization, coronary bypass surgery, cardiopulmonary bypass, or intraaortic balloon counterpulsation, may produce extensive aortic dissection.

Many writers have concluded that pregnancy, either because of its effects on the aortic wall or because of attendant hemodynamic stress, predisposes to medial dissection.[82] Such a conclusion is not unreasonable since half or more of the reports of aortic dissection in women younger than 40 years have occurred during pregnancy. Since the total number reported is relatively small (certainly in relation to the frequency of pregnancy) and since most reports concern one or a few cases, it is possible that selective reporting accounts for this association. (See Chap. 113.)

History Sudden, excruciating pain, presumably attributable to the progress of the medial cleavage, announces the onset of dissection in 90 percent of instances. Patients may describe the pain as "cutting," "ripping," or "tearing," but such vivid descriptors cannot always be elicited.

Those afflicted most commonly locate the discomfort in the anterior chest, somewhat less frequently in the interscapular area, and less often in the epigastrium or the lumbar region. Since these locations often are the site of pain from more common processes (e.g., myocardial infarction or cholecystitis), the examiner must be alert to the possibility of aortic dissection in any patient with pain in these sites in whom the more common diagnoses are not immediately obvious.

Two features of the pain of dissection help to separate it from that of other conditions. The discomfort of dissection may not build in intensity, as in the case of other disorders producing severe pain in the trunk. Rather, it is at its most intense from its inception. Moreover, it often is located either simultaneously or sequentially in more than one of the four sites mentioned above. Suspicion should be aroused particularly by pain occurring both above and below the diaphragm.

A sudden neurologic episode accompanies the onset of most instances of "painless" aortic dissection. Syncope is the most frequent neurologic event and a particularly ominous sign. It seems always to reflect external rupture, almost always of the ascending aorta into the pericardial space. Less frequently, focal neurologic signs reflect arterial occlusion of the cerebral or spinal circulation.

When pain is not prominent, occlusion by the dissection of the femoral or the subclavian artery may be the predominant clinical feature. Arterial embolism may be simulated.

Rarely, the acute episode goes entirely unrecognized by the patient. In such instances, diagnostic study of patients who have an abnormal chest film, aortic regurgitation, or obstruction of an arterial branch of the aorta uncovers chronic dissection.

Physical Examination Although none are diagnostic of dissection, physical findings that greatly increase the probability of its presence can often be detected on examination. The murmur of aortic regurgitation can be heard in about half of all patients with acute type I dissection. Loss or diminution of an arterial pulse may also be detected in half. One or the other of these cardinal findings is present in all but a small minority of that subgroup. In contrast, patients with dissection limited to the descending aorta less frequently have pulse deficits and uncommonly have a murmur of aortic regurgitation. Thus, these patients often have none of these confirmatory findings.

The frequency with which hypertension underlies aortic dissection has been mentioned, and a majority of patients presenting with dissection will have high arterial pressure. Many others will be able to provide a history of high blood pressure. Even in those with neither a history of hypertension nor a measurable blood pressure elevation, physical examination will often reveal left ventricular hypertrophy or vascular changes in the optic fundi. Blood pressure elevations during the acute process may be modest during the acute process, but particularly in those with type III dissection, extraordinarily high readings can be encountered. The arm blood pressure may be higher in one arm than in the other if the dissection involves the vascular supply of one. Renal ischemia, a consequence of renal artery involvement, has been invoked to explain diastolic blood pressures that may reach 140 to 160 mmHg or more.

Twenty percent of patients with dissection involving the ascending aorta present with hypotension. Such a presentation requires immediate consideration of operative treatment since external rupture almost always is responsible.

Laboratory Studies Of the routine diagnostic studies, only the chest x-ray provides diagnostic information of much value. The aortic shadow is abnormal in 80 to 90 percent of cases,[80] but may also be abnormal in many instances in patients who do not have dissection.[83] Dilatation of the ascending aorta, reflected by protrusion of its shadow from the right side of the mediastinum, is a characteristic finding in proximal dissection. Dilatation of the aortic knob and descending thoracic aorta is typical of distal disease (Fig. 123-4). Certain other findings—for example, progressive widening of the aortic silhouette on serial films, a lobulated or serrated margin of the aortic shadow, or a *double-lumen* effect created by a less radiopaque false channel—are less frequent but more specific. The same may be said for detection of intimal calcification more than 6 mm inside the margin of the aorta.

For confirmation of the diagnosis, either computed tomography after intravenous administration of contrast material or transesophageal echocardiography (Chap. 131) may be employed with confidence. Both have high sensitivity and specificity. Magnetic resonance imaging (Chap. 136) can also provide detailed images of the aorta. Its value is limited in acutely ill patients because of the time required to obtain the images and the relative inaccessibility of the patient during the process.[84,85]

An aortogram, accomplished by means of contrast injection through a catheter placed in the aorta, may be required to provide an understanding of the extent of the dissection and details regarding the involvement of branch vessels. Two aortic channels can usually be identified because of the variation in intensity and timing of their opacification. Moreover, the aortogram may identify a linear lucency representing the aortic intima and media separating the two channels (Figs. 123-5 and 123-6). At times the false channel is not opacified because of thrombosis. In such cases, the true lumen appears to be compressed and to lie at a distance from the margins of the aortic shadow. The resulting appearance of a thickened aortic wall can also be produced by thrombosis within an aneurysm, aortitis, or mediastinal hema-

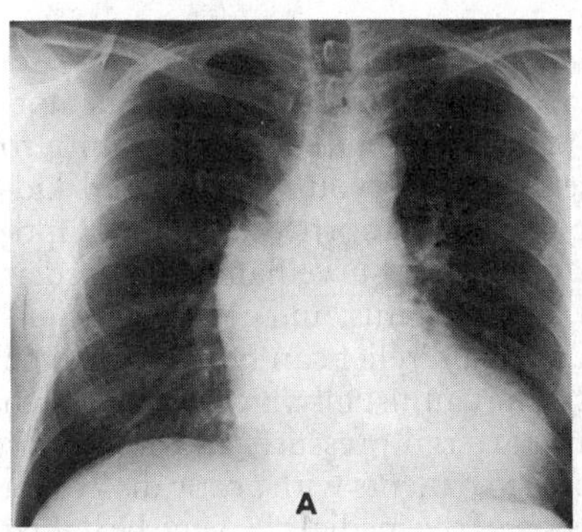

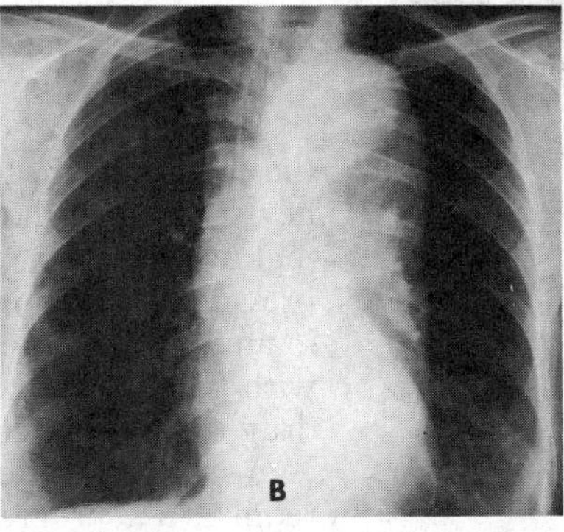

FIGURE 123-4 *A.* Type I aortic dissection. Characteristic appearance on chest roentgenogram. Note the marked dilatation of the ascending aorta. The aorta may appear normal on the roentgenogram early in the course of aortic dissection. *B.* Type III aortic dissection. In contrast to type I, marked distortion of the aortic arch and dilation of the descending portions are typical, as seen in this radiograph of a patient with dissection beginning distal to the arch vessels.

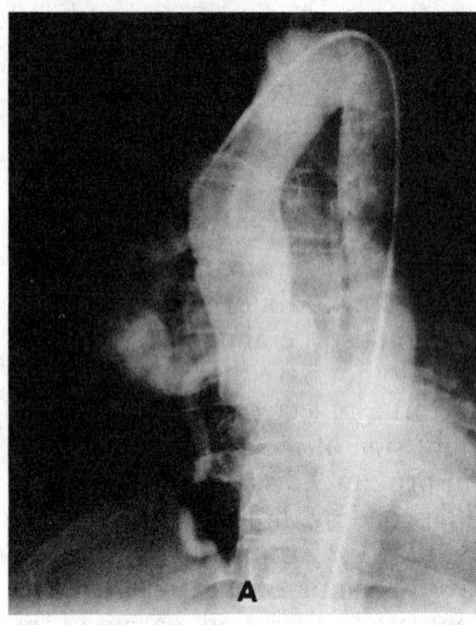

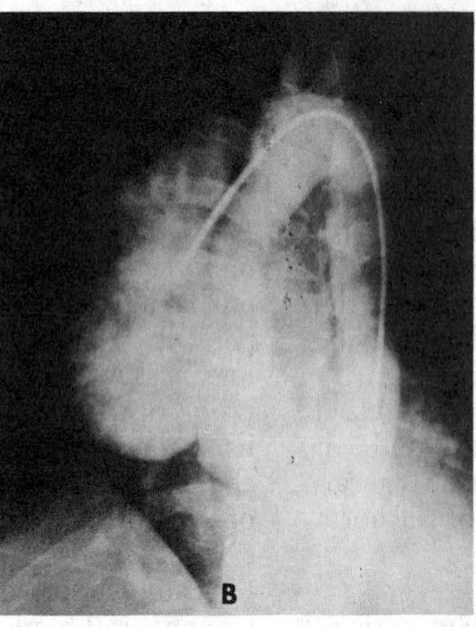

FIGURE 123-5 Serial frames from an aortogram of a patient with type I aortic dissection. Contrast material is seen to fill a tremendously dilated false channel. This accounts for the dilatation of the ascending aorta noted in Fig. 123-4.

toma or tumor. These can usually be distinguished from dissection because in these the aortic lumen is not significantly compressed.

Natural History and Prognosis[74,75,79,80,86,87]

We must look to older reports of aortic dissection for information about the natural history of the process. Since the mid-1960s virtually all patients have received either operative intervention or aggressive pharmacologic treatment. From the classic work of Hirst and his associates[86] and others[79,80] it can be estimated that 35 percent of patients succumb within the initial 24 h and that the mortality rate continues to be high during the first and second weeks. Fifty percent die within 48 h, 70 percent by 1 week, and 80 percent by 2 weeks.

Certain subgroups are identifiable. Hypotension (blood pressure less than 100 mmHg) usually indicates aortic rupture and nearly certain early death. Almost all such patients have involvement of the ascending aorta; one-quarter of those with such involvement present in this way. In contrast, the prognosis for survival during the first 2 weeks is relatively good for those with type III dissection. Older reports indicate that about half survive without aggressive treatment. Without modern therapeutic intervention, the mortality rate of patients with type I or II dissection who are hypertensive or normotensive is intermediate between these extremes.

Patients who survive the first 2 weeks continue to experience a high mortality rate in the first year. About half of the survivors die within 3 months and an additional 10 percent within 1 year of the onset of their illness. The lucky few who pass the first anniversary apparently may expect reasonable longevity. Late deaths may be due to cerebrovascular complications of hypertension, heart failure from severe aortic regurgitation, or rupture of a saccular aneurysm of the residual false channel.

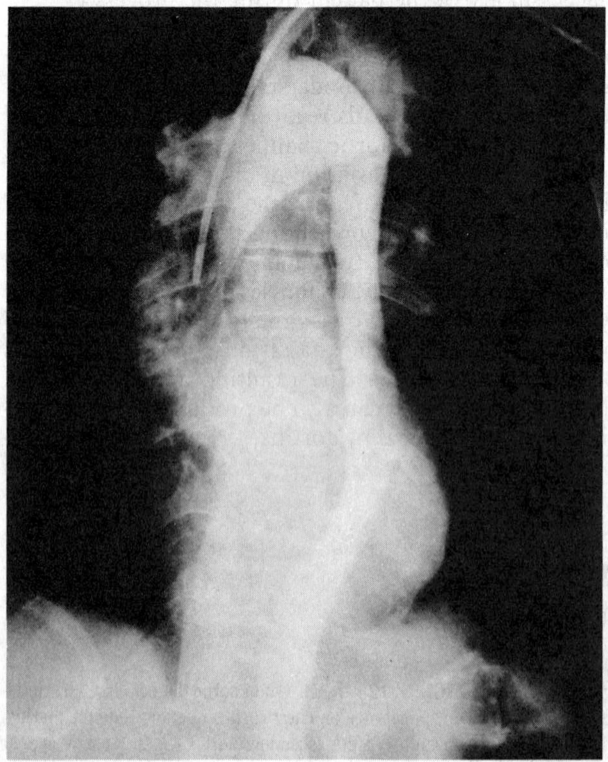

FIGURE 123-6 Aortic dissection, type III. A typical aortogram of a patient with aortic dissection beginning distal to the arch vessels. The narrowed true lumen is filled with contrast material and does not occupy the entire aortic shadow. Contrast material can be seen entering the false channel just beyond the left subclavian artery.

Treatment[74,75,87,88]

Sudden life-threatening complications—such as very severe hypertension, cardiac tamponade, massive hemorrhage, severe aortic regurgitation, or ischemic injury to the myocardium, the central nervous system, and kidneys—threaten the patient with aortic dissection. Optimal management requires close surveillance of vascular pressures, urine flow, mental status, and neurologic signs in an intensive care unit. Pain relief can be difficult even with potent narcotics but can usually be obtained with drug therapy to reduce arterial pressure.

A successful outcome in patients with aortic dissection requires that progression of the medial cleavage be halted and that external rupture of the weakened aortic wall be prevented. Inasmuch as the aortic defect is structural, operative treatment represents the most effective long-term remedy. There is, in addition, evidence to suggest that aggressive antihypertensive treatment lessens the stress on the aortic wall and thus the likelihood on progression of the dissection and of rupture of the weakened wall.[88] Such therapy is widely employed prior to and, in selected instances, as an alternative to surgical management.

When hypotension is not present and the diagnosis of acute dissection has been confirmed, intravenous antihypertensive medication should be initiated as quickly as possible. Sodium nitroprusside (Chap. 3 and 77) combined with a beta-adrenergic blocking agent such as propranolol is currently most frequently employed. The therapeutic goal is a systolic pressure of 100 to 120 mmHg. The target blood pressure level may require upward adjustment upon detection of evidence of hypoperfusion of vital organs. Furthermore, downward adjustment may be necessary if the pain of dissection persists and adequate cerebral function and urine flow are maintained.

Intravenous labetalol may prove to be a useful alternative to the combination of nitroprusside and a beta-adrenergic blocking agent. Hydralazine, minoxidil, and diazoxide cannot be recommended since they produce reflex stimulation of the left ventricle and consequently an increase in the rate of rise of aortic pressure.

Not all patients with acute aortic dissection have elevated blood pressure. Hypotension, it has been noted, reflects aortic rupture and dictates emergency operation. Some individuals have pressures only slightly higher than the 100 to 120 mmHg target level for antihypertensive treatment. Pharmacologic treatment is of dubious value in such patients, although beta-adrenergic blockade may be tried as a means of reducing the rate of rise of aortic pressure.

As noted, operative treatment must be considered in all patients, but certain subgroups can be recognized whose clinical presentation dictates the timing of the surgery. At one extreme are those who are hypotensive on admission and whose need for emergency operation has already been noted. On the other hand, operative treatment may never be an option in those of advanced years or associated cardiac, renal, or pulmonary disease. Further, it may not be justified in patients with severe neurologic injury from the dissection. In these inoperable individuals, antihypertensive therapy is continued indefinitely by converting the drug regimen to an oral one that avoids vasodilators.

For patients whose dissection involves the ascending aorta, operative repair should be undertaken as soon as the patient can be stabilized and appropriate diagnostic information compiled. Such patients are in grave danger of a fatal complication despite effective antihypertensive therapy. By contrast, for those with uncomplicated type III dissection, it is now believed that operation during the acute phase does not improve survival beyond that achieved with drug treatment.[89] Younger patients and those who are relatively good operative risks may benefit from operation in the subacute phase to protect them from eventual rupture of a residual saccular aneurysm.

The surgical technique for aortic dissection varies with the origin of the dissecting process and its extent (Fig. 123-3).[90-92] For type I aneurysms (Figs. 123-4 and 123-5), the procedure consists in transection of the ascending aorta with use of cardiopulmonary bypass, obliteration of the false lumen by approximation of the inner and outer walls of the dissecting process with a continuous suture proximally and distally, and end-to-end anastomosis of the transected aorta. In patients for whom this method of direct repair is not applicable, it may be necessary to resect the proximal segment and restore vascular continuity by means of an albumin-coated Dacron patch or tube graft. Many patients have aortic valve incompetence secondary to loss of commissural support of the valve leaflets. This condition may be corrected in some by suture approximation of the inner and outer layers of the dissecting process with resultant resuspension of the valve, although other patients may require prosthetic valve replacement.

Surgical treatment for type II aneurysms consists essentially in resection and graft replacement of the entire ascending aorta with use of cardiopulmonary bypass. Aortic valve incompetence is more common in this type than in type I and is less often amenable to reparative techniques because of the usually more chronic nature of the dissecting process. Under such circumstances prosthetic replacement of the aortic valve usually is performed concomitantly with graft replacement of the ascending aorta.

Surgical treatment for type III aneurysms (Fig. 123-6) consists of resection of the descending thoracic aorta above the level of the origin of the dissecting process (usually at, or just below, the origin of the left subclavian artery), obliteration of the distal false passage by suture closure of the inner and outer layers, and replacement of the excised segment with an aortic graft. In some patients in whom the dissecting process is extensive distally, a thoracoabdominal approach may be necessary.

Analysis of experience with more than 1000 patients treated by these surgical methods at Baylor College of Medicine indicates gratifying results. The surgical mortality rate has been steadily reduced with some variation depending on the type and stage of the disease, being about 15 percent in type I, 5 percent in type II, and 12 percent in type III. Long-term results extending over 35 years are also gratifying, with an overall 10-year survival rate of about 35 percent. In type II this survival rate is over 50 percent.[92,93]

Acquired Occlusive Disease of the Aorta and Its Major Branches

Chronic Occlusive Disease of the Arch Vessels

Etiology and Pathology Atherosclerosis accounts for more than 90 percent of instances of occlusion of the brachiocephalic, carotid, and subclavian arteries. Takayasu's arteritis, luetic aortitis, neoplastic obstruction, and trauma account for almost all the remainder. Lesions tend to be located at arterial bifurcations and are therefore characteristically found at the origin of the arch vessels and at the bifurcation of the common carotid arteries. The proximal left subclavian artery is the most common site of an obstructing lesion.

Clinical Manifestations Occlusion at the origin of one of the arch vessels often does not produce symptoms because of the many possibilities for collateral connections. Upper extremity ischemia is particularly unusual. The occurrence of symptoms of cerebral ischemia suggests that more than one lesion is present, that there are lesions in more distal arteries, that collateral circulation is compromised, or that a *steal syndrome* is present. Details of the clinical manifestations of cerebrovascular disease are discussed in Chap. 122.

The steal syndromes are of particular interest. In its classic presentation, *subclavian steal* is triggered by vigorous motion of the arm on the side of severe proximal subclavian arterial occlusion. Symptoms of cerebral ischemia result. Because of the subclavian occlusion, blood flow to the arm cannot be increased sufficiently to maintain arterial pressure in the face of exercise-induced vasodilation and blood is "stolen" from the cerebral circulation. That is, blood delivered to the brain through the carotid arteries is diverted via the circle of Willis and proceeds in a direction opposite from that of normal flow through the ipsilateral vertebral artery to the exercising arm. In *brachiocephalic artery steal,* a much more unusual problem, retrograde flow through the ipsilateral carotid artery may be an additional hazard.

Meticulous assessment of the carotid, temporal, and upper extremity pulses; measurement of the blood pressure in both arms; and careful auscultation for bruits in the neck and supraclavicular areas detect brachiocephalic occlusive disease.

Laboratory Studies Noninvasive techniques have been developed to aid in the assessment of the severity of arterial obstruction in this area. These techniques are particularly pertinent to the evaluation of a patient with a carotid bruit. The pressure within the arterial system distal to the carotid obstruction may be assessed by ocular pneumoplethysmography, a technique by which the pressure in the ophthalmic artery is estimated. Ultrasound techniques employing the Doppler principle may provide useful information regarding blood flow in the obstructed artery and may demonstrate reversal of flow in steal syndromes. Duplex scans often are helpful in identifying ulcerative plaques in carotid artery. (See Chap. 127.) Definitive identification of the severity and location of the occlusion depends on arteriography. This may be accomplished via the transfemoral catheter approach, but intravenous arteriography employing digital subtraction imaging may obviate the need for this examination.

Treatment

Occlusive diseases of the vessels arising from the aortic arch are amenable to surgical treatment when segments distally in the neck are patent. This condition is best considered as proximal or distal occlusion, although both may occur in the same patient. Distal occlusion usually affects the carotid bifurcations or origins of the vertebral arteries.

Proximal occlusion usually occurs in the vessels at or near their origins from the aortic arch and is best corrected by the bypass procedure. The proximal end of a graft is attached to the side of the ascending aorta, and the distal end or ends of the graft are attached to patent arterial segments in the neck or supraclavicular region distal to the occlusion. The ascending aorta is exposed through a second or third right anterior intercostal incision. Using a partial occlusion clamp, the surgeon anastomoses the proximal end of the graft to the ascending aorta end to side. The patent distal arterial segments are exposed through separate incisions in the neck and supraclavicular regions. The distal end of the graft is drawn retrosternally through a tunnel made by blunt dissection and is attached to the side of the patent distal segment. In patients with multiple occlusive segments, the appropriate limbs are attached to the sides of the other patent arterial segments. Knitted Dacron velour tubes 6 to 8 mm in diameter are used for this purpose.

Results of this form of treatment have been very gratifying. In virtually all patients with only proximal occlusion of vessels arising from the aortic arch, normal circulation has been restored. In patients with combined proximal and distal occlusion, the success rate varies with the ability to correct the distal occlusion.

Abdominal Angina

Patients with abdominal angina may be treated by endarterectomy, excision and graft replacement, or bypass graft, the last procedure being preferable for most patients.[94] The abdominal aorta is exposed between the renal and common iliac arteries. The proximal end of the graft is attached to the side of the abdominal aorta in this region, and the other end of the graft is carried behind the transverse mesocolon and stomach and sutured to the side of the normal hepatic or splenic artery. Since the occlusive process usually does not affect the trifurcation of the celiac artery, attachment of the graft to the hepatic or splenic arteries provides complete revascularization of the celiac distribution. One end of a second tube is sutured to the side of the graft, and the other end is carried through a tunnel in the small-intestinal mesentery under the duodenum and attached to the side of the superior mesenteric artery distal to the site of occlusion. Knitted Dacron velour tubes 8 mm in diameter are used in most patients.

Renovascular Hypertension

In Chaps. 75 and 76, renal arterial occlusive disease is discussed as a cause of hypertension. Surgical treatment for renovascular hypertension is directed toward correction of renal ischemia.[95,96] Patients with well-localized disease may be treated by endarterectomy and patch-graft angioplasty. For more extensive segmental occlusion, the end-to-side bypass principle is preferred. The proximal end of an 8-mm Dacron velour graft is attached to the abdominal aorta below the origin of the renal arteries, and the distal end of the graft is attached to the side of the renal artery distal to the obstruction. Bifurcation grafts are, of course, required in the treatment of bilateral disease when this method is used. The bypass graft method has been particularly effective in restoring normal circulation to both the kidneys and the lower limbs in patients with combined occlusive disease of the aorta, iliac arteries, and renal arteries.[97,98] The proximal end of the renal arterial graft is attached to the side of the aortic segment of the aortoiliac bypass graft in these patients. In a small number of patients, reconstructive surgery is impossible because of the site and extent of the disease. In these, total or partial nephrectomy may be required.

The use of renal artery angioplasty is discussed in Chap. 126.

Chronic Obstruction of the Infrarenal Aorta[99,100]

Etiology and Pathogenesis Atherosclerosis underlies all but a few instances of chronic obstruction of the infrarenal aorta. Rarely, infrarenal coarctation, aortitis, or clinically silent embolism or in situ thrombosis produce this situation.

Rupture of atherosclerotic plaques sets the stage for mural thrombus and gradual progression of luminal narrowing and, in many instances, complete occlusion of the terminal aorta. Collateral vessels connecting the lumbar and inferior mesenteric arteries with branches of the internal iliac and common femoral arteries ameliorate the effects of the aortic narrowing. Thus, the symptoms of lower extremity ischemia typically progress over months or years. This indolent course may, however, be punctuated by abrupt acceleration of symptoms, the result of a sudden increase in the size of the obstructing thrombus or its extension to a significant collateral. On the other hand, progression to complete occlusion may be entirely asymptomatic.

Data have been offered to suggest that the pathogenesis of aortoiliac atherosclerosis may differ from that of atherosclerosis in more distal segments of the arterial tree.[101] Those with aortoiliac narrowing are younger and present with a shorter duration of symptoms than do patients with femoropopliteal obstruction. It has been reasoned that in the normal course of events the narrowing in the more distal femoropopliteal arteries appears first. Only when other factors intrude, the reasoning continues, does "premature" atherosclerotic narrowing in the infrarenal aorta appear—thus the younger age.

Anatomic characteristics of the aortoiliac bifurcation that produce an aortic impedance mismatch may be responsible.[101] An iliac bifurcation angle more acute than normal has been observed in some patients,[102] and in others, the aorta and iliac arteries are smaller than average.[103]

Clinical Manifestations Men are affected far more often than women. The mean age of patients in most series falls in the sixth decade, but some are much younger. The usual "risk factors" for atherosclerosis are found with great frequency.

Seventy years after the original description by Rene Leriche[104] of the syndrome associated with this process, its cardinal features still apply. Pain or tiredness in the lower back, buttocks, or thighs produced by exertion and relieved by brief periods of rest are hallmarks of aortoiliac obstruction. Claudication may occur in the calf or foot in association with the more proximal distress and can be the sole complaint. Men often complain of inability to maintain a penile erection.

Absence of or reduction in the femoral pulse is typical. More distal pulses in the legs are reduced or absent, and bruits are commonly audible over femoral arteries and in the midline of the abdomen near the umbilicus. Low skin temperature, diminished hair growth, atrophy of the skin and subcutaneous tissue, and diminished muscle bulk in the lower limbs are common but not universal signs. Frank gangrene is not common, and amputation for ischemia is therefore seldom required.

The findings in patients with aortoiliac obstruction overlap those in patients with femoropopliteal narrowing. A firm identification of involvement of the aortoiliac segment may be difficult on clinical grounds. To further complicate matters, in many patients obstructing lesions are present at both levels. Fortunately, modern imaging techniques have made diagnosticians less dependent on clinical findings for the localization of the level of arterial obstruction.

Natural History and Prognosis The survival rate for patients with the Leriche syndrome appears to be lower than for those in a control population matched for age and sex, but death rarely results for the aortoiliac disease. Coronary and cerebrovascular diseases are largely responsible for the higher death rate. Significant morbidity or death occasionally follows occlusion of the renal arteries by proximal extension of the thrombotic process.

Treatment Chronic aortoiliac occlusion may be partial or complete and may occur alone or may be associated with femoropopliteal occlusive disease as discussed in Chap. 124. For aortoiliac occlusion, the end-to-side bypass with a flexible, knitted, albumin-coated Dacron bifurcation graft is the preferable method of treatment.[91] One end of the graft is attached to the side of the uninvolved abdominal aorta above the obstruction, and the other ends are drawn through tunnels made behind the peritoneum and attached to the sides of distal patent segments, either in the external iliac arteries or in the common femoral arteries opposite the origins of the deep femoral arteries in the groins. (See also Chap. 125.)

In the absence of femoropopliteal occlusive disease, this method has been successful in restoring normal distal circulation in about 98 percent of patients. Even in patients with combined aortoiliac and femoropopliteal disease, bypass of the aortoiliac occlusion alone with revascularization of the deep femoral arterial system may be adequate to relieve symptoms. If symptoms are not relieved, extension of the bypass to the popliteal region can be considered. Follow-up observations in these patients for almost 40 years have provided evidence of maintenance of good long-term results with a relatively low recurrence rate of about 5 percent if only the aortoiliac region is occluded.[105]

Percutaneous transluminal angioplasty devised by Gruntzig[106,107] has been used in several centers in the treatment of iliac and femoropopliteal obstructive atherosclerotic disease. The early success rate appears to be satisfactory, but the long-term patency rate remains to be determined. This technique is applicable in highly selected cases of a relatively short segment of well-localized stenotic occlusion. (See Chap. 126.)

Acute Aortoiliac Obstruction[108–110]

Etiology A rare event, sudden occlusion of the terminal aorta may result from a large ("saddle") embolus, from in situ thrombosis of a severely atherosclerotic aorta or of an aneurysm, from trauma, or as a result of aortic dissection.

When either dissection or trauma is responsible, the clinical picture usually leaves little doubt as to the reason for the aortic occlusion. Most emboli large enough to occlude the terminal aorta are thrown off from the heart. Thus, embolus must be considered when acute aortoiliac occlusion occurs in patients with mitral stenosis, atrial fibrillation, or recent myocardial infarction. Rarely embolization of a vegetation from fungal endocarditis may be large enough to occlude the aortic bifurcation.

In situ thrombosis of an aneurysm or of a severely atherosclerotic aorta may develop when blood flow through these vessels is considerably reduced, as may be the case in shock or congestive heart failure.

Clinical Manifestations Unlike gradually progressive obstruction, abrupt total or near total interruption of flow through the terminal aorta or common iliac arteries produces acute, limb-threatening ischemia. Although the clinical picture will vary depending on the presence of preexisting collaterals, the full-blown syndrome is characterized by the abrupt onset of pain, typically severe and located in the lumbar area, the buttocks, the perineum, the abdomen, and the legs. Numbness, paresthesia, dysesthesia, and finally paralysis of the affected limb dominate the picture. Pulses are absent in the legs, although at times faint femoral pulsations may be detected. The legs are cold and pale. Unless circulation is restored, massive muscle necrosis may produce myoglobinuria, renal failure, acidosis, and hyperkalemia. (See also Chap. 124.)

Treatment In contrast to chronic aortoiliac occlusion, acute obstruction to blood flow does not allow for the formation of collateral circulation. Immediate operation is necessary for survival. The procedure used depends on the cause of the occlusion.

Treatment for aortic dissection has been discussed above. Acute aortoiliac occlusion due to trauma with an intimal tear producing dissection may be corrected by the bypass graft technique described for chronic aortoiliac occlusion. In patients with acute aortoiliac occlusion due to a saddle embolus, consideration also must be given to treatment of the underlying disease, such as concomitant open mitral commissurotomy at the time of embolectomy, in order to prevent recurrent embolization to such vital organs as the brain.

Although aortoiliac embolectomy may be performed directly through an incision in the distal aorta or proximal iliac arteries, this approach requires laparotomy in a severely ill patient, and it does not provide the means for removing the more distally lodged embolic material often present in these patients. The preferable approach is to expose both common femoral arteries in the groins and, through transverse arteriotomies, to remove, with balloon-tipped Fogarty catheters, the embolic material lodged proximally and distally.[111] Care must be taken to prevent further embolization in the opposite leg while these catheters are passed proximally. Even large amounts of embolic material in the distal aorta itself can be safely removed in this manner, with use of a local anesthetic when the general condition of the patient contraindicates general anesthesia.

Restoration of circulation usually is good after such procedures. Subsequent mortality rates, however, remain high because of the underlying disease that caused the saddle embolus in many of these patients, particularly those with myocardial infarction and a mural thrombus. Nevertheless, by the use of a local anesthetic and Fogarty catheters, surgery is possible in virtually all patients. (See also Chap. 125.)

REFERENCES

1. Schlatmann TJM, Becker AE: Histologic changes in the normal aging aorta: Implications for dissecting aortic aneurysm. *Am J Cardiol* 1977; 39:13–20.
2. Ross R, Glomset JA: The pathogenesis of atherosclerosis. *N Engl J Med* 1976; 295:369–377,420–425.
3. Ross R: The pathogenesis of atherosclerosis—An update. *N Engl J Med* 1986; 314:488–500.
4. Roberts WC, Ferrans VJ, Levy RI, Fredrickson DS: Cardiovascular pathology in hyperlipoproteinemia. *Am J Cardiol* 1973; 31:557–570.
5. Zarins CK, Glagov S, Giddens DP, Ku DN: Hemodynamic factors and atherosclerotic change in the aorta. In: Bergan JJ, Yao JST (eds): *Aortic Surgery*. Philadelphia, Saunders, 1989: 17–25.
6. Tunick PA, Perez JL, Kronzon I: Protruding atheromas in the thoracic aorta and systemic embolization. *Ann Intern Med* 1991; 115:423–427.
7. Savunen T: Annulo-aortic ectasia—A clinical, structural and biochemical study. *Scand J Thorac Cardiovasc Surg* 1986; (suppl 37):1–45.
8. Wilson SK, Hutchins GM: Aortic dissecting aneurysms—Causative factors in 204 patients. *Arch Pathol Lab Med* 1982; 106:175–180.
9. Schlatmann TJM, Becker AE: Pathogenesis of dissecting aneurysm of the aorta—Comparative histopathologic study of significance of medial changes. *Am J Cardiol* 1977; 39:21–26.
10. Nakashima Y, Kurozumi T, Sueishi K, Tanaka K: Dissecting aneurysm: A clinicopathologic and histopathologic study of 111 autopsied cases. *Hum Pathol* 1990; 21:291–296.
11. Hollister DW, Godfrey M, Sakai LY, Pyeritz RE: Immunohistologic abnormalities of the microfibrillar-fiber system in the Marfan Syndrome. *N Engl J Med* 1990; 323:152–159.
12. Pyeritz RE, McKusick VA: The Marfan Syndrome: Diagnosis and management. *N Engl J Med* 1979; 300:772–777.
13. Roberts CS, Roberts WC: Dissection of the aorta associated with congenital malformation of the aortic valve. *J Am Coll Cardiol* 1991; 17:712–716.
14. Subramaniam PN: Case report: Turner's syndrome and cardiovascular abnormalities: A case report and review of the literature. *Am J Med Sci* 1989; 297:260–262.
15. Nunez L, O'Connor LF, Pinto AG, Gil-Aguado M, Gutierrez M: Annuloaortic ectasia and adult polycystic kidney—A frequent association. *Chest* 1986; 90:299–300.
16. Leier CV, Call TD, Fulkerson PK, Wooley CF: The spectrum of defects in the Ehlers-Danlos Syndrome, types I and III. *Ann Intern Med* 1980; 92:171–178.
17. Hortop J, Tsipouras P, Hanley JA, Maron BJ, Shapiro JR: Cardiovascular involvement in osteogenesis imperfecta. *Circulation* 1986; 73:54–61.
18. Ewart JM, Burke ML, Bunt TJ: Spontaneous abdominal aortic infections: Essentials of diagnosis and management. *Am Surg* 1983; 49:37–50.

19. Atnip RG: Mycotic aneurysms of the suprarenal abdominal aorta: Prolonged survival after in situ aortic and visceral reconstruction. *J Vasc Surg* 1989; 10:635–641.
20. Saner HE, Asinger RW, Homans DC, Helseth HK, Elsperger KJ: Two-dimensional echocardiographic identification of complicated aortic root endocarditis: Implications for surgery. *J Am Coll Cardiol* 1987; 10:859–868.
21. David TE, Komeda M, Brofman PR: Surgical treatment of aortic root abscess. *Circulation* 1989; 80:I-269–I-274.
22. Oz MC, McNicholas KW, Serra AJS, Spagna PM, Lemole GM: Review of *Salmonella* mycotic aneurysms of the thoracic aorta. *J Cardiovasc Surg* 1989; 30:99–103.
23. Cohen PS, O'Brien TF, Schoenbaum SC, Medeiros AA: The risk of endothelial infection in adults with *Salmonella* bacteremia. *Ann Intern Med* 1978; 89:931–932.
24. Dupont J-R, Bonavita JA, DiGiovanni RJ, Spector HB, Nelson SC: Acquired immunodeficiency syndrome and mycotic abdominal aortic aneurysms: A new challenge? Report of a case. *J Vasc Surg* 1989; 10:254–257.
25. Hall S, Barr W, Lie JT, Stanson AW, Kazmier FJ, Hunder GG: Takayasu's arteritis: A study of 32 North American patients. *Medicine* 1985; 64:89–99.
26. Shelhamer JH, Volkman DJ, Parillo JE, Lawley TJ, Johnston MR, Fauci AS: Takayasu's arteritis and its therapy. *Ann Intern Med* 1985; 103:121–126.
27. Ishikawa K: Diagnostic approach and proposed criteria for the clinical diagnosis of Takayasu's arteriopathy. *J Am Coll Cardiol* 1988; 12:964–972.
28. Hall S, Buchbinder R: Takayasu's arteritis. *Rheum Dis Clin North Am* 1990; 16:411–422.
29. Takeuchi Y, Matsuki K, Saito Y, Sugimoto T, Juji T:HLA-D region genomic polymorphism associated with Takayasu's arteritis. *Angiology* 1990; 41:421–426.
30. Talwar KK, Chopra P, Narula J, Shrivastava S, Singh SK, Sharma S, et al: Myocardial involvement and its response to immunosuppressive therapy in nonspecific aortoarteritis (Takayasu's disease)—A study by endomyocardial biopsy. *Int J Cardiol* 1988; 23:323–334.
31. Ishikawa K, Matsuura S: Occlusive thromboaortopathy (Takayasu's disease) and pregnancy: Clinical course and management of 33 pregnancies and deliveries. *Am J Cardiol* 1982; 50:1293–1300.
32. Wong VCW, Wang RYC, Tse TF: Pregnancy and Takayasu's arteritis. *Am J Med* 1983; 75:597–601.
33. Ishikawa K: Survival and morbidity after diagnosis of occlusive thromboaortopathy (Takayasu's Disease). *Am J Cardiol* 1981; 47:1026–1032.
34. Subramanyan R, Joy J, Balakrishnan KG: Natural history of aortoarteritis (Takayasu's disease). *Circulation* 1989; 80:429–437.
35. Park JH, Han MC, Kim SH, Oh BH, Park YB, Seo JD: Takayasu arteritis: Angiographic findings and results of angioplasty. *Am J Roentgenol* 1989; 153:1069–1074.
36. Sharma S, Rajani M, Kaul U, Talwar KK, Vishwa D, Shrivastava S: Initial experience with percutaneous transluminal angioplasty in the management of Takayasu's arteritis. *Br J Radiol* 1990; 63:517–522.
37. Klein RG, Hunder GG, Stanson AW, Sheps SG: Large artery involvement in giant cell (temporal) arteritis. *Ann Intern Med* 1975; 83:806–812.
38. Mitnick HJ, Tunick PA, Rotterdam H, Esposito R: Antemortem diagnosis of giant cell aortitis. *J Rheumatol* 1990; 17:708–711.
39. Bergfeldt L, Insulander P, Lindblom D, Moller E, Edhag O: HLA-B27: An important genetic risk factor for lone aortic regurgitation and severe conduction system abnormalities. *Am J Med* 1988; 85:12–18.
40. Bulkley BH, Roberts WC: Ankylosing spondylitis and aortic regurgitation: Description of the characteristic cardiovascular lesion from study of eight necropsy patients. *Circulation* 1973; 48:1014–1027.
41. Hoeffel JC, Henry M, Mentre B, Louis JP, Pernot C: Pseudocoarctation or congenital kinking of the aorta: Radiologic considerations. *Am Heart J* 1975; 89:428–436.
42. Smyth PT, Edwards JE: Pseudocoarctation, kinking or buckling of the aorta. *Circulation* 1972; 46:1027–1032.
43. Graham LM, Zelenock GB, Erlandson EE, Coran AG, Lindenauer SM, Stanley JC: Abdominal aortic coarctation and segmental hypoplasia. *Surgery* 1979; 86:519–529.
44. Cohen JR, Birnbaum E: Coarctation of the abdominal aorta. *J Vasc Surg* 1988; 8:160–164.
45. Lande A: Takayasu's arteritis and congenital coarctation of the descending thoracic and abdominal aorta: A critical review. *Am J Roentgenol* 1976; 127:227–233.
46. Roberts WC: Pathology of arterial aneurysms. In: Bergan JJ, Yao JS (eds): *Aneurysms. Diagnosis and Treatment*. New York, Grune & Stratton, 1982: 17–43.
47. Dobrin PB: Pathophysiology and pathogenesis of aortic aneurysms: Current concepts. *Surg Clin North Am* 1989; 69:687–703.
48. Powell J, Greenhalgh RM: Cellular, enzymatic, and genetic factors in the pathogenesis of abdominal aortic aneurysms. *J Vasc Surg* 1989; 9:297–304.
49. Reilly JM, Tilson MD: Incidence and etiology of abdominal aortic aneurysms. *Surg Clin North Am* 1989; 69:705–711.
50. Svensson LG, Crawford ES, Coselli JS, Safi HJ, Hess KR: Impact of cardiovascular operation on survival in the Marfan patient. *Circulation* 1989; 80(suppl I):I-233–I-242.
51. Heinemann M, Laas J, Karck M, Borst HG: Thoracic aortic aneurysm after acute type A aortic dissection: Necessity for follow-up. *Ann Thorac Surg* 1990; 49:580–584.
52. Joyce JW, Fairbairn JF II, Kincaid OW, Juergens JL: Aneurysms of the thoracic aorta. A clinical study with special reference to prognosis. *Circulation* 1964; 29:176–181.
53. Pressler V, McNamara JJ: Thoracic aortic aneurysm. Natural history and treatment. *J Thorac Cardiovasc Surg* 1980; 79:489–498.
54. Bickerstaff LK, Pairolero PC, Hollier LH, Melton LJ, Van Peenen HJ, Cherry KJ, et al: Thoracic aortic aneurysms: A population-based study. *Surgery* 1982; 92:1103–1108.
55. Murdoch JL, Walker BA, Halpern BL, Kuzma JW, McKusick VA: Life expectancy and causes of death in the Marfan syndrome. *N Engl J Med* 1972; 286:804–808.
56. DeBakey ME, Noon GP: Aneurysms of the thoracic aorta. *Med Concepts Cardiovasc Dis* 1975; 44:53–58.
57. DeBakey ME, Noon GP: Aneurysms of the sinuses of valsalva. In: Sabiston DC, Spencer FC (eds): *Gibbon's Surgery of the Chest*, 3d ed. Philadelphia, Saunders, 1976:903–913.
58. Crawford ES, Rubio PA: Reappraisal of adjuncts to avoid ischemia in the treatment of aneurysms of the descending thoracic aorta. *J Thorac Cardiovasc Surg* 1973; 66:693–704.
59. DeBakey ME, McCollum CH, Graham JM: Surgical treatment of aneurysms of the descending thoracic aorta: Long-term results in 500 patients. *J Cardiovasc Surg* 1978; 19:571–576.
60. Sterpetti AV, Hunter WJ, Feldhaus RJ, Chasan P, McNamara M, Cisternino S, et al: Inflammatory aneurysms of the abdominal aorta: Incidence, pathologic, and etiologic considerations. *J Vasc Surg* 1989; 9:643–650.
61. Gaylis H, Isaacson C: Abdominal inflammatory aortic aneurysms. In: Bergan JJ, Yao JT (eds): *Aortic Surgery*. Philadelphia, Saunders, 1989: 267–292.
62. Johnston KW, Scobie TK: Multicenter prospective study of nonruptured abdominal aortic aneurysms. I. Population and operative management. *J Vasc Surg* 1988; 7:69–81.
63. Rutherford RB, McCroskey BL: Ruptured abdominal aortic aneurysms: Special considerations. *Surg Clin North Am* 1989; 69:859–868.
64. Sullivan CA, Rohrer MJ, Cutler BS: Clinical management of the symptomatic but unruptured abdominal aortic aneurysm. *J Vasc Surg* 1990; 11:799–803.
65. Bower TC, Cherry KJ Jr, Pairolero PC: Unusual manifestations of abdominal aortic aneurysms. *Surg Clin North Am* 1989; 69:745–754.
66. Bandyk DF: Preoperative imaging of aortic aneurysms: Conventional and digital subtraction angiography, computed tomography scanning, and magnetic resonance imaging. *Surg Clin North Am* 1989; 69:721–735.
67. Cronenwett JL, Murphy TF, Zelenock GB, Whitehouse WM Jr, Lindenauer SM, Graham LM, et al: Actuarial analysis of variables associated with rupture of small abdominal aneurysms. *Surgery* 1985; 98:472–483.
68. Nevitt MP, Ballard DJ, Hallett JW Jr: Prognosis of abdominal aortic aneurysm: A population-based study. *N Engl J Med* 1989; 321:1009–1014.
69. Lederle FA: Management of small abdominal aortic aneurysms. *Ann Intern Med* 1990; 113:731–732.
70. Roger VL, Ballard DJ, Hallett JW Jr, Osmundson PJ, Puetz PA,

Gersh BJ: Influence of coronary artery disease on morbidity and mortality after abdominal aortic aneurysmectomy: A population-based study, 1971–1987. *J Am Coll Cardiol* 1989; 14:1245–1252.

71. Graor RA: Preoperative evaluation and management of coronary and carotid artery occlusive disease in patients with abdominal aortic aneurysms. *Surg Clin North Am* 1989; 69:737–743.
72. DeBakey ME, Crawford ES, Cooley DA, et al: Aneurysms of the abdominal aorta: Analysis of graft replacement therapy one to eleven years after operation. *Ann Surg* 1964; 160:622–639.
73. DeBakey ME: Aneurysmectomy of the abdominal aorta. *Surg Tech Illus* 1976; 1:5–20.
74. Crawford ES: The diagnosis and management of aortic dissection. *JAMA* 1990; 264:2537–2541.
75. DeSanctis RW, Doroghazi RM, Austen WG, Buckley MJ: Aortic dissection. *N Engl J Med* 1987; 317:1060–1067.
76. Roberts WC: Aortic dissection: Anatomy, consequences, and causes. *Am Heart J* 1981; 101:195–214.
77. Larson EW, Edwards WD: Risk factors for aortic dissection: A necropsy study of 161 cases. *Am J Cardiol* 1984; 53:849–855.
78. Carson MW, Roach MR: The strength of the aortic media and its role in the propagation of aortic dissection. *J Biomechanics* 1990; 23:579–588.
79. Lindsay J Jr, Hurst JW: Clinical features and prognosis in dissecting aneurysm of the aorta: A reappraisal. *Circulation* 1967; 35:880–888.
80. Slater EE, DeSanctis RW: The clinical recognition of dissecting aortic aneurysm. *Am J Med* 1976; 60:625–633.
81. Eagle KA, Quertermous T, Kritzer GA, Newell JB, Dinsmore R, Feldman L, et al: Spectrum of conditions initially suggesting acute aortic dissection but with negative aortograms. *Am J Cardiol* 1986; 57:322–326.
82. Williams GM, Gott VL, Brawley RK, Schauble JF, Labs JD: Aortic disease associated with pregnancy. *J Vasc Surg* 1988; 8:470–475.
83. Jagannath AS, Sos TA, Lockhart SH, Saddekni S, Sniderman KW: Aortic dissection: Analysis of the usefulness of plain chest radiographic findings. *Am J Radiol* 1986; 147:1123–1126.
84. Anderson MW, Higgins CB: Should the patient with suspected acute dissection of the aorta have MRI, CAT scan, or aortography as the definitive study? *Cardiovasc Clin* 1990; 21/1:293–304.
85. Adachi H, Kyo S, Takamoto S, Kimura S, Yokote Y, Omoto R: Early diagnosis and surgical intervention of acute aortic dissection by transesophageal color flow mapping. *Circulation* 1990; 82(suppl IV):IV-19–IV-23.
86. Hirst AE Jr, Johns VJ Jr, Kime SW Jr: Dissecting aneurysms of the aorta: A review of 505 cases. *Medicine* 1958; 37:217–279.
87. Doroghazi RM, Slater EE, DeSanctis RW, Buckley MJ, Austen WG, Rosenthal S: Long-term survival of patients with treated aortic dissection. *J Am Coll Cardiol* 1984; 3:1026–1034.
88. Asfoura JY, Vidt DG: Acute aortic dissection. *Chest* 1991; 99:724–729.
89. Glower DD, Fann JI, Speier RH, Morrison L, White WD, Smith LR, et al: Comparison of medical and surgical therapy of uncomplicated descending aortic dissection. *Circulation* 1990; 82(suppl IV):IV-39–IV-46.
90. DeBakey ME, Beall AC Jr, Cooley DA, Crawford ES, Morris GC Jr, Garrett HE, et al: Dissecting aneurysms of the aorta. *Surg Clin North Am* 1966; 46:1045–1055.
91. DeBakey ME: The development of vascular surgery. *Am J Surg* 1979; 137:697–738.
92. DeBakey ME, McCollum DH, Crawford ES, Morris GC Jr, Howell J, Noon GP, et al: Dissection and dissecting aneurysms of the aorta: Twenty-year follow-up of five hundred twenty-seven patients treated surgically. *Surgery* 1982; 92:1118–1134.
93. DeBakey ME: Surgical treatment for acute and chronic dissection of the aorta. In: Ernst CB, Stanley JC (eds): *Current Therapy in Vascular Surgery*. Toronto, BC Decker, 1987: 93–96.
94. McCollum CH, Graham JM, DeBakey ME: Chronic mesenteric arterial insufficiency: Results of revascularization in 33 cases. *South Med J* 1976; 69:1266–1268.
95. DeBakey ME, Morris GC Jr, Morgen RO, et al: Lesions of the renal artery: Surgical technic and results. *Am J Surg* 1964; 107:84–96.
96. DeBakey ME, McCollum CH III: Atherosclerotic occlusive disease, section V in surgical management of atherosclerotic vascular disease. In: Gross HL (ed): *Atherosclerosis*. Kalamazoo, The Upjohn Company, 1977: 81–96.
97. Lawrie GM, Morris GC Jr, Soussou ID, Starr DS, Silvers A, Glaeser DH, et al: Late results of reconstructive surgery for renovascular disease. *Ann Surg* 1980; 191:528–533.
98. Lawrie GM, Morris GC Jr, DeBakey ME: Long-term results of treatment of the totally occluded renal artery in 40 patients with renovascular hypertension. *Surgery* 1980; 88:753–759.
99. Brewster DC: Clinical and anatomical considerations for surgery in aortoiliac disease and results of surgical treatment. *Circulation* 1991; 83(suppl I):I-42–I-52.
100. Bergan JJ: Variations of the Leriche syndrome. In: Bergan JJ, Yao JST (eds): *Aortic Surgery*. Philadelphia, Saunders, 1989: 149–159.
101. Stubbs DH, Kasulke RJ, Kapsch DN, Nichols WK, Silver D: Populations with the Leriche syndrome. *Surgery* 1981; 89:612–616.
102. Sharp WV, Donovan DL, Teague PC, Mosteller RD: Arterial occlusive disease: A function of vessel bifurcation angle. *Surgery* 1982; 91:680–685.
103. Palmaz JC, Carson SN, Hunter G, Weinshelbaum A: Male hypoplastic infrarenal aorta and premature atherosclerosis. *Surgery* 1983; 94:91–94.
104. Leriche R, Morel A: The syndrome of thrombotic obliteration of the aortic bifurcation. *Ann Surg* 1948; 127:193–204.
105. DeBakey ME: Patterns of atherosclerosis and rates of progression. In: Paoletti R, Gotto AM Jr (eds): *Atherosclerosis Reviews*, vol 3. New York, Raven, 1978: 1–56.
106. Gruntzig A, Hopff H: Perkutane Rekanalisation Chronischer Arterieller Verschlusse Mit Einem Neuen Dilatationskatheter. *Dtsch Med Wochenschr* 1974; 99:2502–2510.
107. Gruntzig A: Perkutane Dilatation von Kronarstenosen: Beschreibung eines neuen Kathetersystems. *Klin Wochenschr* 1976; 54:543–545.
108. Schatz IJ, Stanley JC: Saddle embolus of the aorta. *JAMA* 1976; 235:1262–1263.
109. Busuttil RW, Keehn G, Milliken J, Paredero VM, Baker JD, Machleder HI, et al: Aortic saddle embolus: A twenty-year experience. *Ann Surg* 1983; 197:698–706.
110. Webb KH, Jacocks MA: Acute aortic occlusion. *Am J Surg* 1988; 155:405–407.
111. DeBakey ME, Lawrie GM: Acquired diseases of the aorta. In: Edlich RF, Spyker DA (eds): *Current Emergency Therapy '85*. Rockville, MD, Aspen Systems Corporation, 1985:417–421.

Chapter 124

The Diagnosis and Management of Diseases of the Peripheral Arteries and Veins

John W. Joyce, M.D.

Diseases of the arteries and veins are common, recurrent events in active medical practice. The vascular system parallels the heart in that its many structural and hydraulic disorders cause major symptoms and findings that are so often accessible to the eye, ear, and hand. Clinical syndromes are clearly defined, and diagnosis is usually established through knowledge of the natural history of each entity and by a competent historical and physical examination. Both invasive and indirect testing modalities are well developed and can provide confirmation, quantitation, and in some instances, clarification of the diagnosis.

Assessment of the vascular system is an intrinsic component of a general examination and an essential extension for evaluation of many cardiac problems. The vascular bed can reflect primary cardiac disease in micro- and macroembolic events, endocarditis, congestive failure, tricuspid and aortic incompetence, and complicating venous thromboembolism. In turn, cardinal cardiac manifestations such as dyspnea, syncope, edema, congestive failure, hypertension, aortic valve disease, chest pain, and angina pectoris can be caused by arterial and venous disorders (Fig. 124-1). Several congenital heart problems have both valvular and aortic components. Of fundamental importance is appreciation of the comorbidity of atherosclerosis in the aorta, carotid, renal, visceral, and peripheral arteries in the examination and treatment of coronary artery disease. This chapter presents a synopsis of information essential for the diagnosis and treatment choices of the major arterial and venous diseases.

CLINICAL ASSESSMENT OF ARTERIAL DISEASE: HISTORICAL FEATURES

Certain general information is always pertinent in the assessment of arterial disease. This includes the patient's age, sex, and associated problems; the presence of risk factors for atherosclerosis; and knowledge of prior trauma, procedures, and drug use. Specific symptoms are evaluated for tempo, progression, factors that aggravate or alleviate, and their relationship to other medical events. Interrogation of others and prior records are often essential when the patient is impaired. Claudication and ischemic distress are the major symptoms of occlusive arterial disease.

Claudication

Claudication is a stereotyped, reproducible distress in muscle groups brought on by sustained exercise and relieved by 3 to 6 min of rest. The distress may be described as numbness, weakness, giving away, aching, cramping, or pain. It may change character and location with progression of the causative lesion. Claudication

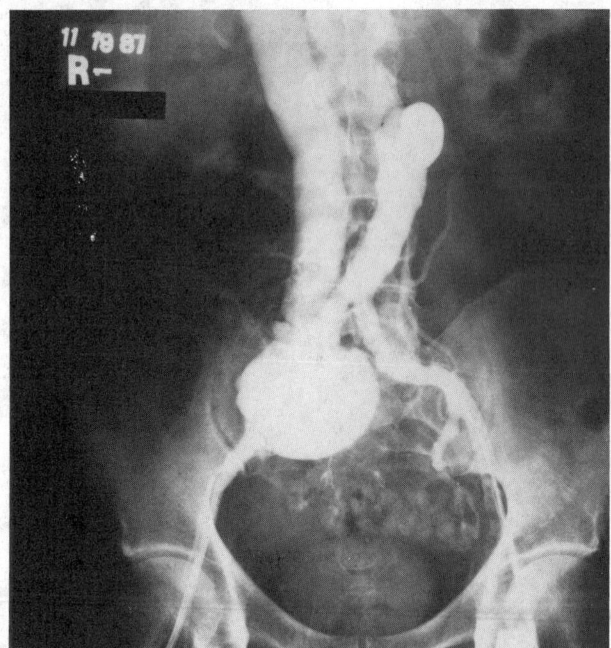

FIGURE 124-1 This 72-year-old man led a vigorous life until hospitalized twice in 1 month for progressive fatigue, dyspnea, orthopnea, and paroxysmal nocturnal dyspnea. A continuous bruit in the right lower quadrant, noted during his second hospital stay, defined the cause of his high-output cardiac failure. Rupture of an iliac artery aneurysm into the adjacent iliac vein, shown in this aortogram, was repaired and he regained his prior vitality.

occurs at shorter distances when the work load is increased by a rapid pace, carrying a burden, and walking uphill or over rough terrain. Abrupt decreases in claudication distance signal thrombosis in situ of occlusive or aneurysmal disease or, on occasion, embolization from these sources or the heart and proximal vessels. Claudication limits often decrease after a period of inactivity but improve to prior levels with reconditioning.

It is essential to establish that the distress occurs in muscle groups, that relief is timely, and that it does not occur at rest. When these criterion are not met, musculoskeletal or neurologic disorders should be suspected. Claudication as defined is a most reliable symptom. Quantitation by history alone, however, is quite variable because of differences in pace, work load, and estimates of distance. Standardized treadmill testing utilizing ankle/brachial indices at rest and after duplication of symptoms provides confirmation of the diagnosis and quantitation of claudication distance for follow-up and can identify various pain syndromes not of arterial origin.

The site of claudication localizes the occlusive process when this is a single, focal lesion. Foot claudication results from pedal and low calf occlusive disease, calf and pedal distress from tibioperoneal trunk lesions, and low calf discomfort from popliteal disease. Superficial femoral disease causes claudication of the entire calf, and both thigh and calf symptoms occur with common femoral and external iliac lesions. Dependent on the distribution of the process, aortoiliac occlusive disease may produce unilateral or bilateral claudication of the calf, thigh, buttocks, and occasionally the low back. The symptoms usually progress from distal to cephalad but may be limited to the calf or buttocks and thighs. This may reflect that individual patient's particular gait or associated involvement of the internal iliac arteries. When the occlusive process is at multiple levels, the initial site of claudication usually reflects the most distal significant lesion, or the area with the least collateral flow. Many patients with bilateral disease on examination will report unilateral symptoms. This occurs because the symptomatic leg has a more critical lesion that reaches the threshold of claudication before a lesser lesion in the contralateral limb.

Variants of Claudication

Two causes of leg distress induced by exercise can be perplexing. In the first, a classic claudication history is obtained, yet on examination pulses are normal and proximal bruits may not be noted. This is clarified by having the patient ascend the examining table steps repetitively until the symptoms are reproduced, then promptly repeating the exam. Pedal pulses will now be absent, the feet will appear pale, and bruits will occur at the aortoiliac, femoral, or popliteal areas. Both symptoms and findings will clear with a few minutes of rest. Treadmill testing can further define the syndrome; ankle/brachial indices will be normal at rest, drop with exercise, and then recover. Vasospasm was thought to explain this quandary.[1] However, arteriography will demonstrate early occlusive disease of the aortoiliac, femoral, or popliteal arteries, usually of atherosclerotic origin[2]; entrapment or adventitial cystic disease of the popliteal artery can also cause the syndrome[3]; and popliteal entrapment is suspected when pedal pulses disappear with passive dorsiflexion or active plantar flexion of the foot. The phenomenon of "vasospastic claudication" is explained by a stenosis, subcritical at rest, that diverts flow into dilated muscular beds just distal to it with exercise, depriving downstream arteries of pressure and flow.[2] Of note, arterial spasm induced by ergot toxicity causes a fixed lesion and abnormal examination findings.

A second variant is pseudoclaudication. It may be of neurogenic or muscular origin. The patient with neurogenic claudication will describe exercise-induced distress. This often has a dysthetic quality; however, it clears slowly or may require a specific posture for relief, and clumsiness may develop as walking progresses. Of importance, the distress also occurs with prolonged standing or in given fixed positions. The arterial examination is normal at rest and after exercise. A history of current or prior back distress should be sought. Compression of the distal spinal cord by hypertrophic bone, disc protrusion, or tumor causes the syndrome.[4] When arterial and neurogenic diseases coexist, the dominant lesion can usually be identified by observing the symptoms during exercise and measuring the arterial indices.[5] Muscular distress induced by exercise is common in amyotrophic lateral sclerosis, muscular dystrophy, and the McArdle syndrome. The muscular deficits are apparent to history and examination, and exercise testing will clarify the status of the arterial system.

Ischemic Distress

With severe perfusion deficits, the patient can experience persistent distress of two types: rest pain and ischemic neuropathy. Rest pain is constant, agonizing, and confined to the digits, foot, or hand. It may localize to focal sites of infarction, ulceration, or infection. Such small lesions can occur with vasculitis, microembolization, or thrombosis but more often represent trauma to an area of poor perfusion from chronic occlusive disease. The patient may be unaware of injury, but it is important to inquire of new shoes, ingrown nails, or recent trimming of callus or nails. Rest pain is first noted at night, interrupting sleep, and may be partially relieved by hanging the limb dependent, sleeping in a chair, or walking about. Large doses of anodynes are required, the pain can suppress appetite and weight, and the patient may become depressed. The area is tender and sensitive to touch, clothing, and bedding. Muscular atrophy and contractures of ankle, knee, and hip joints can ensue when the limb is protected by fixed postures and immobility.

Ischemic neuropathy is constant distress described as aching, throbbing, burning, pulling, or tearing. It is diffuse, often affecting the entire lower leg or forearm, and may shift its focus of intensity. Momentary jabs or lancinating pain are often experienced. Paroxysms of exacerbation lasting hours may occur, and these may be accompanied by a diffuse cyanosis and coolness of the skin.

THE ARTERIAL EXAMINATION

The presence or absence of pulses, aneurysms, and bruits and their quantitation are the essence of the arterial examination. Specific problems, to be discussed later, can require these extensions: the Allen test, evaluation of perfusion, exercise testing, and the thoracic outlet maneuvers. It is also fundamental that the skin and body habitus be noted and the ocular fundus viewed when indicated. When repetitive examinations are confirmed by the subsequent course or objective tests, confidence in these skills grows quickly.

Pulses

Arteries routinely palpated are the radial, ulnar, subclavian, carotid, aortic, femoral, popliteal, posterior tibial, and dorsalis pedis. When a pulse is abnormal or absent, its course should be traced as far as muscle or bony anatomy allows. Collateral arteries are sought under several circumstances: scapular and rib with thoracic coarctation, superficial epigastric and hypogastric with abdominal coarctation, and geniculates with chronic popliteal occlusion. The temporal and occipital arteries are palpated when temporal arteritis is suspected.

The following techniques will serve the examiner well:

1. Both patient and examiner should be in a relaxed position.
2. Use the surface area of three or more fingers when possible.
3. Control and relax any nearby joint with the other hand.
4. Begin with light pressure, increasing and varying it for difficult examinations.
5. Avoid use of the thumb, as the examiner's pulse can be transmitted.

The most challenging pulse is the pulse not found. The history and ancillary findings may support that it should be absent. When in doubt, Doppler signals and pressures can establish whether the pulse is absent or just obscured.

Individual arteries are palpated sequentially as the arm, neck, trunk, and legs are examined. Paired vessels are compared. Blood pressure is taken bilaterally, and a difference of 10 mmHg or more is significant if duplicated after several readings. The following pulses are easily identified. The radial pulse is quite accessible, particularly when the examiner uses a second hand to relax the wrist tendons into flexion. The posterior tibial is identified by controlling the ankle with one hand and cupping three to four fingers of the other hand about the posterioinferior surface of the medial malleolus. The subclavian pulse is best felt with the patient sitting and by curling two to three fingers into the supraclavicular space and slowly increasing pressure. The common femoral artery is easily felt just below the inguinal ligament. The limb should be uncrossed and rotated laterally to relieve muscle tension. Firm pressure may be required for the obese patient. Examination of the carotid is done with gentle pressure of two to three fingers, palpating the artery from the clavicle to the mandibular angle. It is prudent to examine each carotid individually and with the patient semirecumbent. Of note, what seems to be a normal internal carotid may actually be the external carotid, which is prominent because the internal carotid is highly diseased.

Certain pulses can be difficult. The dorsalis pedis is commonly felt between the tendons of toes 1 and 2, two to three inches below the joint crevice. It may, however, be more lateral and is sometimes congenitally absent. The abdominal aorta is examined with the patient supine on a firm surface, knees flexed, and arms at the side. Examination is initiated with the gentle pressure of eight fingers spread across the epigastrium to appreciate any diffuse pulsation. Then two or three fingers of each hand are gradually brought deeper on either side of the aorta until its pulsation and dimensions are defined. With a difficult exam, it is helpful to coach the patient to breath and relax, warning that modest discomfort may be felt and penetrating deeper with each expiration. The popliteal can be challenging when musculoskeletal structures are prominent or relaxation is poor. It is best approached with the patient supine, the knee relaxed into the cradle of eight examining fingers, and varying the pressure according to the resistance felt. When a pulse is not found, it may sometimes be located by palpating lower between the heads of the gastrocnemius muscle. Popliteal examination should routinely include both of these sites and is not completed until the adductor muscle mass distal to the adductor hiatus is compressed between both hands. Aneurysms can occur at any of these three locations (Fig. 124-2).

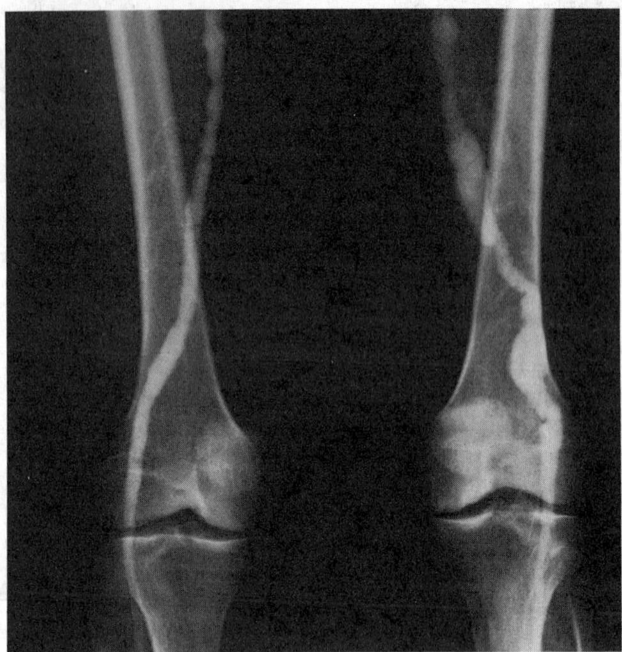

FIGURE 124-2 Popliteal artery aneurysmal disease located at the adductor hiatus. This is a common site for aneurysms and is easily overlooked unless the area is routinely examined. The popliteal arteries are normal at the joint crevice. Typical arteriomegaly is seen in both superficial femoral arteries.

The ulnar, a particularly important parallel vessel because of the impact of wrist punctures, is subject to variation and not infrequently is obscured by tendons. The *Allen test* can ascertain its patency. The test depends upon the integrity of the radial, ulnar, and palmar arch arteries. It is performed by occluding the radial or ulnar artery with firm digital pressure, having the patient exsanguinate the hand by making a fist and then relaxing both the hand and wrist. When the noncompressed artery is patent, flushing will occur within 3 s. Delayed refilling is diagnostic of occlusive disease in the noncompressed vessel and may also define digital or microcirculatory deficits when focal refilling is slow in the digits.[6] It is imperative that the wrist be relaxed to avoid false-positive results caused by ligamentous compression.[7] Thus, the Allen test is valuable in assessing occlusive disease of the radial, ulnar, palmar, and digital arteries.

Aneurysms

Arterial aneurysms are a major cause of death and disability. Early detection allows definitive repair. The three most common aneurysms are accessible to examination; 40 to 60 percent of abdominal aortic and almost all popliteal and femoral aneurysms are detected by examination.[8–11]

The size and pulsatility of paired arteries are of similar magnitude, and ectasia is suspected when a pulse is larger or more forceful than others in a given patient. *Aneurysm* is defined as a focal enlargement of one and a half or more times larger than the usual diameter of that artery. The diagnosis of aneurysm is established when a palpable, often visible pulsation is transmitted to the fingers on each side of an enlarged vessel. A mass pulsating on only part of its surface represents a mass with a transmitted pulse. Lesions adjacent to the abdominal aorta producing this phenomenon include mesenteric and pancreatic cysts, horseshoe kidney, and retroperitoneal tumors. Tortuosity of the right carotid, abdominal aorta, or wrist arteries can mimic an aneurysm. Ultrasound or angiographic studies may be needed to clarify this question when examination is uncertain.

Abdominal aortic aneurysms are detected by the technique described. The mass may be found below the ziphoid, above the umbilicus, but more often fills the epigastrium. Most aneurysms center left of the midline, but tortuosity may swing the mass more to the right on occasion. Slight patient discomfort is usual, but significant tenderness suggests an inflammatory aneurysm, recent expansion, or a contained rupture. When the mass extends below the umbilicus, it may represent either extension into the iliac arteries or a large, overlapping aortic aneurysm. Isolated iliac aneurysms are usually hidden in the pelvis, and less than a fifth are detected by abdominal or digital examination of the rectum or pelvis. Most are found incidental to imaging or symptoms.[12] Femoral aneurysms are often first noted by the patient, but popliteal lesions are easily overlooked unless the popliteal space is routinely examined at all three sites described (Fig. 124-2). Femoral and popliteal aneurysms are often first detected when the patient presents with acute thrombosis, distal micro- or macroembolization, or edema from venous compression or thrombosis.[10,11]

Most thoracic and thoracoabdominal aneurysms are diagnosed incidental to imaging procedures. Both are also found during investigation of pain and thoracic aneurysms, during the pursuit of aortic valve incompetence, cough, dysphagia, hemoptysis, or dysphonia. Physical signs are late manifestations of thoracic aneurysms and include those of aortic valve incompetence, unilateral or bilateral jugular venous distension, and pulsatility in the upper intercostal spaces or of the precordium. Carotid and axillosubclavian aneurysms are easily diagnosed by palpation, and some present with local pain, thrombosis, or distal embolic complications.[13,14] Visceral aneurysms are rarely large enough to be palpated, 3 to 5 percent present as rupture, and the majority are found incidental to surgery or imaging.[15,16]

Bruits

Bruits represent turbulent flow in arteries or veins and can be induced by stenosis, extrinsic compression, aneurysm, and hyperdynamic flow. In superficial arteries the turbulence may be of enough magnitude to be palpable as a thrill. The proximal limit of a bruit defines the site of the lesion. Bruits usually transmit an additional 4 to 6 cm, or further downstream in vessels with high-velocity flow. Both the pitch and duration of a bruit are informative. Coarse, low-pitched bruits are generated in larger vessels such as the proximal limb arteries, carotid, or aorta, while bruits of a higher pitch occur in smaller arteries or mark a high-grade stenosis in any vessel. Duration and pitch increase as a stenosis progresses, but a bruit may disappear when a certain critical narrowing is reached. In turn, an early stenosis may be silent until flow increased by exercise, emotion, or drugs generates a bruit.

A continuous bruit is heard throughout systole and diastole and is repeated without pause in the next cardiac cycle. It is nearly pathognomonic of arteriovenous fistula at the site of its greatest intensity. Continuous bruits occur at acquired fistula of named arteries and veins (Fig. 124-1); over multiple congenital fistulae of the liver, lung, soft tissue, or skull; and over areas of tumor necrosis or prior biopsies. There are three innocent bruits, the first being the classic jugular venous hum of the youthful. It is heard with the patient upright and clears with the Valsalva maneuver, with head rotation, or when the patient reclines. Bruits are sometimes heard in the supraclavicular space or epigastrium of young patients. The supraclavicular bruit disappears with shoulder hyperabduction.[17] The epigastric bruit may represent coeliac compression or organic visceral or renal artery stenosis. In the absence of hypertension, azotemia, or intestinal symptoms, it can be observed.[18]

Extensions of the Arterial Examination

The value of the Allen test in establishing patency of the radial, ulnar, and digital arteries has been discussed. The exercise test was described for the patient having a positive claudication history but negative exam ("vasospastic" claudication). It is just as useful for the patient with a positive examination but negative history. The work load imposed exceeds the patient's usual activity level, and claudication is experienced, confirming the examination. In a third application, observation and interrogation during exercise may clarify an unclear history or separate claudication from other symptoms.

Pedal perfusion has been traditionally tested by timing elevation pallor and venous refilling. With the patient supine, both feet are elevated to 60 degrees for 1 min. If no pallor is seen, perfusion is judged normal, the appearance of pallor before 15 s suggests poor healing capacity, and pallor without elevation is indicative of severe ischemia. The patient then sits upright and refilling of the pedal veins is timed. Normal filling occurs in less than 15 s, filling between 30 and 45 s suggests slow healing, and values beyond 60 s confirm severe ischemia. Venous incompetence invalidates venous filling times, and the test is not practical with significant edema or obesity. Grossly abnormal tests correlate well with the presence of rest pain or ulceration.

The several thoracic outlet maneuvers screen arterial, venous, and neurologic compression syndromes of the shoulder girdle. They are best understood with a full discussion of these complex entities.[19]

The Skin

Occlusive arterial disease can alter skin temperature, color, and nutrition. Skin temperature is reduced in the zone of reduced perfusion caused by acute or chronic occlusive disease. Differences are best felt with the dorsum of the fingers, and comparisons to the contralateral or proximal limb should be made. Profound coolness indicates severe ischemia. Generalized coolness may denote shock, hemorrhage, or poor cardiac output. Chronically cool hands and feet reflect the basic vasomotor tone of some patients. Limbs with neurologic damage, immobility, and reflex sympathetic dystrophy are often cool. Edema can accompany these states, obscuring pulses. Doppler systolic indices will differentiate occlusive disease from these vasomotor changes.

Skin color varies with blood flow and therefore with temperature, activity, and emotional stimuli. A red or purplish color of the forefoot is common with chronic ischemia and increases with dependency. It represents chronic arteriolar dilation in response to inadequate flow. Pallor can be seen with acute ischemia or on elevation with chronic ischemia. Skin chronically deprived of blood can become thin, translucent, and shiny. Thick calluses and nails may develop. Age and various dermatologic disorders can also cause these findings, and a circulatory deficit should be established before a causal role is presumed.

Additional skin lesions and color changes will be described in subsequent sections discussing vasomotor and microcirculatory syndromes.

CLINICAL SYNDROMES

Chronic Occlusive Arterial Disease

Atherosclerosis obliterans is the usual cause of chronic occlusive disease of the extremities. This includes patients under age 35.[20] Coexistent coronary disease is clinically apparent in 40 percent or more, and additional occult disease is found by screening patients whose exercise is limited by claudication.[21,22] It is the major cause of operative death and subsequent shortened life span.[21,23] In addition there is at least a 15 percent prevalence of carotid occlusive disease and abdominal aortic aneurysms in males beyond 65 years of age.[21,24,25] Sound management requires a careful analysis of the entire cardiovascular system. The limb lesion often serves as the initial marker of these comorbid conditions and of the risk factors of smoking, hypertension, and hyperlipidemia that accelerate the atherosclerotic process.

Natural History

Occlusive disease can manifest as asymptomatic pulse reductions or bruits, claudication, ischemic syndromes, and microcirculatory embolic events. Common sites of focal lesions are the aortoiliac, superficial femoral (often at the adductor hiatus), and popliteal arteries. These present as claudication when collateral vessels are patent. This can be stable or progress slowly over several years when risk factors are controlled. Over 80 percent of such patients avoid ischemic complications or amputation for 5 or more years.[26,27] Up to 15 percent of those who continue smoking undergo amputation within 5 years, however, and diabetics have an amputation rate of 25 percent within 9 years.[26,28] Ischemic complications are more frequent when two or three levels (aortoiliac, femoropopliteal, tibioperoneal) are diseased, or significant collaterals are impaired. Such diffuse disease usually reflects significant risk factors. Superimposed thrombosis in situ or chronic lesions can abruptly shorten claudica-

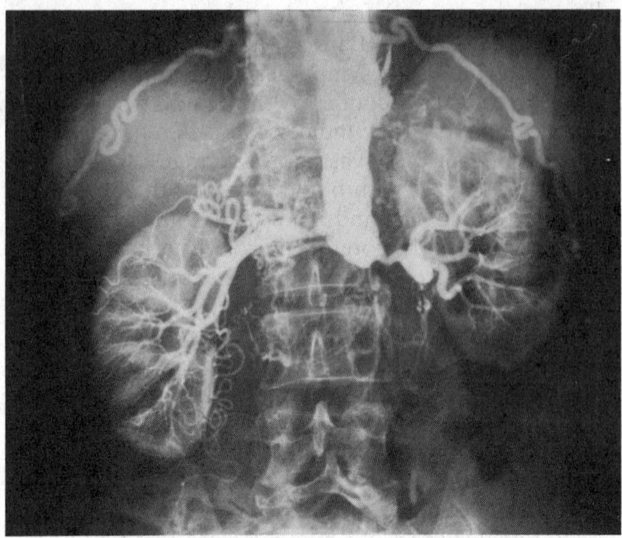

FIGURE 124-3 Classic juxtarenal aortic occlusion. These lesions start as significant plaque at the aortic bifurcation, and thrombus propagates proximally until the high flow into the renal arteries limits its progression. Subsequent renal artery occlusion leads to premature death unless repair is accomplished. This 42-year-old male smoker presented with uncontrolled hypertension and claudication. Note the hypertrophied intercostal arteries serving as collaterals to the legs.

tion distance or cause distal ischemia. As noted before, many ulcers and infarcts are caused by trauma to a limb with borderline perfusion.

Clinical Strategy

Ideally, all patients would be returned to normal by a procedure. The majority, however, are not limited enough to warrant repair, with its morbidity and mortality, and in some repair is precluded by coexistent disease or by technical limitations. The usual logic is establishment of a diagnosis clinically and quantification by the vascular laboratory, reserving angiography for those patients needing repair. Surgical indications are limiting claudication, ischemic complications, and removal of proximal sites causing microembolization. This logic should be extended to include angiography to establish specific etiology in young patients; when an unusual, treatable lesion is suspected; and when juxtarenal occlusion of the aorta with azotemia or hypertension is detected (Fig. 124-3). If the renal arteries are stenotic in this latter syndrome, surgery can prevent premature death from renal failure.[29] The efficacy of percutaneous balloon angioplasty also extends this strategy: 80 to 90 percent of isolated stenosis or short occlusions of the aortoiliac and femoropopliteal systems can be successfully treated with low mortality and morbidity and reasonable 5-year durability.[30] Arteriography or ultrasound imaging are justified when such lesions are suspected.

Medical Therapy

Vasodilating drugs do not improve claudication.[31] These agents improve only cutaneous flow and may accelerate healing of minor wounds when ischemia is mild. Anticoagulants do not alter the natural course of atherosclerosis. They are utilized when a clotting disorder or a cardiac source of embolism is identified. Pentoxifylline, 400 mg orally three times daily, can improve claudication distance 30 to 60 percent in some patients.[32,33] More significant help for most patients is a walking program of 30 to 45 min (with interruptions for claudication) performed four or more days weekly. This frequently increases walking distance by 200 percent or more.[34] Patients with occlusive disease should receive careful instruction in good foot care. Regular follow-up is required to monitor disease progression, to detect other atherosclerotic manifestations, and to control risk factors.

Other Causes

Leg claudication and ischemia can result from numerous causes, most of which are given in Table 124-1. Many are suggested by the history or clinical constellation (acute arterial occlusion, aortic dissection, temporal and Takayasu arteritis, radiation therapy, ergot use, and competitive cycling), some by physical findings (coarctation, pseudoxanthoma elasticum, occluded aneurysms), and others only through imaging. The distinctive features of several of these causes warrant a brief profile.

After an isolated case report by von Winiwarter, Buerger described a progressive, distal arteriopathy of all four extremities affecting young Jewish male smokers that he speculated was of infectious origin. The disease he named as thromboangiitis obliterans is now known to affect women in growing numbers, is seen from age 15 to 50 years in all races, and is a vasculitis of small and medium-sized arteries and veins most likely generated as an autoimmune reaction to any form of tobacco use. The acute pathology is panvasculitis accompanied by an inflammatory intraluminal thrombus that starts in digital vessels and progresses cephalad in a few short years. It may skip from low calf vessels to the popliteal artery. Involvement of the profunda femoris, iliac, coronary, cerebral, or upper arm vessels is occasional. Patients present with digital sensitivity or ischemia, pedal or low calf claudication, or Raynaud's phenomenon. Both legs and often both arms are involved at the time of presentation. Linear or nodular distal superficial thrombophlebitis is common. Biopsy of acute lesions, particularly accessible veins, is diagnostic, and angiographic features are characteristic. Progressive tissue loss is inevitable until

TABLE 124-1
Causes of Leg Claudication

Atherosclerosis obliterans	Temporal arteritis
Acute arterial occlusion	Takayasu arteritis
Occluded aneurysms	Popliteal entrapment
Thromboangiitis obliterans	Adventitial cystic disease
Fibromuscular dysplasia	Aortic coarctation (thoracic, abdominal)
Aortic dissection	Pseudoxanthoma elasticum
Radiation fibrosis	Primary arterial tumor
Retroperitoneal fibrosis	Cyclist's lesion
Ergot toxicity	

tobacco is stopped and then stability or improvement will be seen. Surgical sympathectomy and intravenous prostacyclin analogues can accelerate healing of ischemic lesions, but amputation of damaged digits and limbs is often needed.[35–37]

Two congenital lesions peculiar to youthful claudicants are noteworthy. The popliteal artery can be entrapped by the medial gastrocnemius or various muscular and ligamentous bands, causing claudication and later occlusion. Second, adventitial cystic disease is a slowly enlarging growth in the popliteal, or occasionally common femoral artery, analogous in structure and content to a ganglion. It also causes claudication and subsequently occludes. Both warrant surgical repair upon diagnosis, but often are discovered only after occlusion or distal embolization.[38,39]

Takayasu arteritis involves the iliofemoral system, and temporal arteritis involves the profunda femoral, superficial femoral, and distal vessels in 5 to 10 percent of cases. This is usually bilateral and results in claudication that progresses briskly over a few months. Ischemia is rare. Both have characteristic clinical and laboratory findings. Arteriographic features are typical. These arteritides are unique among all arteriopathies in that stenotic lesions are significantly improved in their acute phase by steroid therapy. Adjunctive cytotoxic drugs are also useful.[40–42]

Ergot toxicity can induce Raynaud's phenomenon, claudication, acute ischemia, or tissue infarction depending on the dose taken. It is usually seen with overuse of rectal suppositories for migraine. Symptoms recede over several days when the drug is stopped. Intravenous nitroprusside can effectively lyse the arterial spasm in a few hours.[43]

Acute Arterial Occlusion

The mechanisms causing acute arterial occlusion may place both life and limb in jeopardy. Significant acute or chronic cardiac disease coexists with most thrombotic or embolic occlusions. It is the major determinant of immediate and long-term survival, and death exceeds limb loss in all major reports. Acute arterial occlusion is an event of high priority that requires prompt evaluation of the limb, heart, and other problems common to these patients.[44–46]

Etiology

The classic logic of approach to acute arterial occlusions defines etiology in three generic groups—trauma, thrombosis in situ, and embolism—each with a subset of specific mechanisms. Attention to arterial integrity is of prime importance in all penetrating (including medical interventions), crushing, and deceleration injuries and fractures. In situ thrombosis occurs with both occlusive and aneurysmal disease. Any of the lesions listed in Table 124-1—aneurysms, clotting disorders, but predominantly atherosclerosis with its multiple manifestations and risk factors—can be the substrate of thrombosis.

A small percentage of acute emboli come from proximal occlusive or aneurysmal arterial lesions, but the majority originate in the heart. Both the left ventricle and atrium may harbor thrombus, and ischemic heart disease now exceeds valvular problems as a source of emboli.[47] Atrial fibrillation is common to both. Emboli tend to be multiple, be recurrent, and distribute randomly, most to the legs but with a significant incidence of cerebral, renal, visceral, and arm events.[48] Venous thrombi from the right heart or limbs can pass across septal defects and cause arterial events, often cerebral. Such paradoxical embolism can be both a diagnostic and a therapeutic challenge.[49]

There are two exceptions to the diagnostic triad. First are the branch vessel deficits of aortic dissection that may be subtle on exam, attributed to other causes, or confusing because no history of chest pain is given. The second is ergot toxicity, usually diagnosed only when the question of drug use is asked.[43]

Manifestations

The site and spectrum of manifestations are dependent on the location of the occlusion and the status of collateral and distal arteries. The presentation may be the silent loss of a pulse, a sudden reduction in walking distance, or a major clinical event. Acute occlusion is abrupt, evolving over moments or a few hours: The tempo of onset does not differentiate embolic from thrombotic events.[50] Examination defines absent pulses and distal ischemia of varying degrees manifest by skin pallor and coolness, muscle tenderness or hardness, and reduced motor and sensory power. Coolness begins several inches distal to the occlusion and helps localize its site, similar to claudication in chronic disease. When collateral is also obstructed, the coolness approximates the obstructed site. Clot fragmentation can abruptly reduce the findings, while proximal progression reflects clot propagation.

Management

Immediate measures are directed to urgent care of all associated problems (usually cardiac) and protection of the limb from trauma by a bulky dressing. Heparin is given to prevent clot propagation and venous thromboembolism and to control embolic sources when present.[44,51] It can be reversed quickly if surgery follows. Etiology is established at the original assessment. Angiography is required to plan repair when there is preexisting occlusive or aneurysmal disease or the etiology is uncertain. Many surgeons will perform balloon embolectomy without angiography when an embolic source is certain and the vessel is previously normal.

Ideally all acute occlusions warrant repair, and its urgency is governed by the degree of ischemia. Severe ischemia is manifest by pallor at rest, profound coolness, tender or hard muscles, and loss of motor and sensory power; repair must be within hours of onset to salvage the limb. Not infrequently acute or unstable cardiac disease makes risks prohibitive for either repair or an inevitable early amputation required to prevent toxicity. The Fogarty embolectomy catheter defuses this dilemma. Time is taken to stabilize the patient, and the procedure is then accomplished through local incisions under infiltrative anesthesia, with minimal risk.[52,53] Lysis of acute emboli and prosthetic graft thrombi has evolved as a viable alternative when not contraindicated.[54]

Prevention

Acute arterial occlusion is often preventable. The need for meticulous technique during interventional procedures is apparent. Conditions known to cause occlusion warrant definitive treatment. Surgical lesions include aneurysms, thoracic outlet arteriopathy, adventitial cystic disease and popliteal entrapment syndromes, and atrial myxoma. Treatable medical disorders include vasculitis, hematologic problems, and in particular, cardiac disease prone to atrial or ventricular thrombi; atrial fibrillation, acute myocardial infarction, profound congestive failure, cardiomyopathy, and prosthetic valves all warrant chronic antithrombotic therapy with warfarin. (See Chap. 68.)

Microcirculatory Disorders

Digital and microcirculatory ischemia may present as focal digital cyanosis, skin petechiae, infarction, or gangrene and may be accompanied by livedo reticularis and Raynaud's phenomenon. Lesions may be single but are usually multiple and can be acute or chronic findings. Most initial lesions heal spontaneously with little or no tissue loss, but recurrences are common, compound the ischemia, and can result in loss of phalanges, digits, or large areas of skin (Fig. 124-4).

Etiologic mechanisms can be grouped in three categories: (1) trauma in an area of preexistent occlusive disease, (2) atherothrombotic emboli, and (3) humoral and systemic disease (Table 124-2). The source of microemboli is almost always proximal ulcerative plaque or aneurysm and only rarely the heart, in contrast to macroembolic events. Solitary lesions showering atheroemboli are readily treated surgically.[55] When lesions are found at several levels, surgical choices are more difficult. Suprarenal and thoracoabdominal ulcerative or aneurysmal disease can cause progressive azotemia or intestinal ischemia and require a formidable repair.[56] Thromboulcerative disease of the entire aorta can shower randomly to the brain, viscera, kidneys, skin, and muscle. Anemia, leukocytosis, elevated sedimentation rate, azotemia, and abnormal urinary sediment are usually noted, and the syndrome is differentiated from vasculitis by biopsy.[57] Microembolic events are usually spontaneous but may be precipitated by surgery, instrumentation, and anticoagulant therapy.[56]

The hematologic syndromes listed can cause blue digits, but several can also thrombose large arteries and veins. Most have specific treatment. The vasculitides present with multiple cyanotic or infarcting digits, Raynaud's phenomenon, splinter hemorrhages, and livoid skin lesions that often infarct. Systemic lupus erythematosus can be accompanied by a circulating anticoagulant causing large-artery and vein thrombosis. This can be suppressed by anticoagulation[58] (Chap. 103). Digital ischemia with advanced malignancy is rare and may be explained by a coagulopathy, cold agglutinins, cryoglobulins, thrombocytosis, or marantic endocarditis.

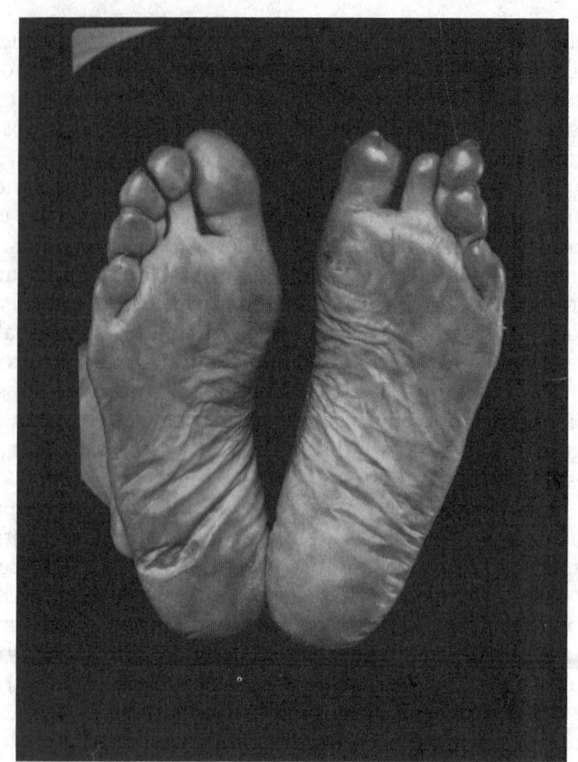

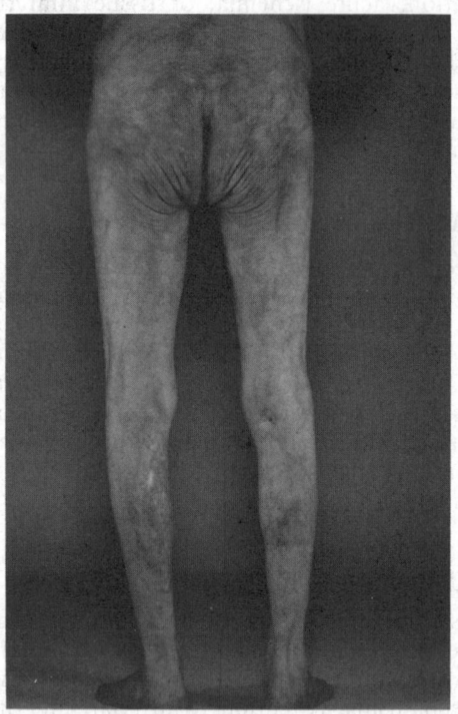

FIGURE 124-4 *A.* Cyanotic toe pads, livoid plantar skin, and prior tissue loss typical of recurrent showers of atherothrombotic microemboli. This 73-year-old man presented because of ischemic rest pain of the left great toe. *B.* In the patient described in *A,* extensive secondary livedo reticularis was seen only from the waist down. These microcirculatory phenomena led to the diagnosis and successful repair of a 7-cm abdominal aortic aneurysm.

TABLE 124-2
Etiologic Mechanisms: Categories

I. Occlusive disease:
  Trauma
II. Microembolism:
  Spontaneous
  Instrumentation
  Surgery
  Anticoagulation
III. Specific diseases:
  Vasculitis
  Hematologic disease
  Ergot toxicity
  Cold injury
  Malignancy
  Hepatitis-B antigenemia
  Hematologic disorders
    Polycythemia vera
    Thrombocytosis
    Intravascular coagulopathy
    Cryoglobulins
    Cold agglutinins
    Circulating anticoagulant
    Thrombotic thrombocytopenia purpura
    Heparin-induced thrombocytopenia

Vasospastic Disorders

The color and warmth of the acral parts vary considerably from person to person in a normal population, reflecting individual vasomotor tone. Livedo reticularis, acrocyanosis, and Raynaud's phenomenon are distinctive clinical syndromes manifest by abnormal color and temperature changes of the skin. These are induced or intensified as a result of stimuli from cold, emotion, or drugs and cause spasm in digital arteries, arterioles, and perhaps venules. The syndromes are usually a benign, life-long, primary process, and features of each may combine in a given patient. All three syndromes have important secondary causes. Careful clinical examination and selective testing will usually confirm the specific etiology and define prognosis and the direction of therapy.

Livedo Reticularis

Livedo reticularis is characterized by a persistent, symmetrical, bluish meshlike pattern on the extremities and sometimes the trunk that is variable in its extent and intensity. It is most apparent after stimulation by cold or emotion and fades with warmth and exercise. It is often first seen in childhood or at puberty and is more common in women and fair-skinned individuals. It is so frequent in its milder form that it is overlooked or considered a variant of normal skin, which it is. The skin overall is often somewhat cool. It is postulated that spasm of cutaneous arterioles with secondary dilation of the capillaries and venules causes slow flow, increased oxygen uptake, and more reduced oxyhemoglobin, producing the color changes. Primary livedo reticularis is not uncommonly seen with acrocyanosis and primary Raynaud's disease. Treatment is rarely needed.

Secondary livedo reticularis is patchy, focal, or asymmetric in distribution, of late onset, and may be complicated by local infarction or ulceration. The lesions are sometimes elevated or tender. Causes of the secondary syndrome include atherothrombotic emboli (Fig. 124-4), systemic and cutaneous vasculitis, amantadine and beta blocker therapy, and limbs with neurogenic disuse, including reflex sympathetic dystrophy. Therapy is directed at the underlying cause, and vasodilators may be of some help.

Hemosiderin deposition can occur in secondary and on occasion with primary livedo reticularis. *Erythema ab igne* can be confused with livedo reticularis. This is a focal, well-defined livoid pattern with broader branches and is reddish. It is frequently stained with hemosiderin and is caused by chronic exposure to local heat from devices or a fireplace.

Acrocyanosis

This is a benign persistent cyanotic discoloration and coolness of the hands and fingers, sometimes the feet, seen predominantly in women. Mild local edema is not uncommon, and on occasion as associated hyperhidrosis can be most bothersome and require treatment. It is painless and does not ulcerate. Cold and emotion will intensify and warmth and exercise will ameliorate the findings. It is a bothersome cosmetic defect for some. Nifedipine, 10 to 20 mg, or prazosin, 1 to 5 mg, each given three times daily often reduces the symptoms. A modest degree of acrocyanosis is sometimes seen in limbs immobilized by neurogenic deficits. Rarely, beta blockade will induce the syndrome.

Raynaud's Phenomenon

The diagnosis of Raynaud's phenomenon is made from a reliable history alone. It is difficult to demonstrate, even with ice immersion, as generalized cooling is usually needed to bring out the findings. The syndrome is defined as episodes of blue or white color changes of the digits, often followed by reactive hyperemia during recovery, and induced by cold or emotional stimuli. Most patients describe the white phase, some blue to white, a few blue only, and most note the subsequent hyperemia. A dead, numb feeling, but rarely pain, accompanies the ischemic phase, and dysthetic, throbbing, or painful sensations are common in recovery. Fingers are involved more often than toes, initially distal phalanges and later all, but rarely the palm. Thumbs are often spared. Recovery time is 3 to 10 min but can exceed 1 h in advanced cases, usually of secondary origin.

The prime question is whether the patient has a primary, benign vasospastic phenomenon or a secondary disease. Allen and Brown[59] defined primary Raynaud's phenomenon as episodes of color changes that were bilateral and symmetrical, were induced by cold or emotion, and were not accompanied by gangrene, ulceration, or evidence of other disease for a period of 2 years. It has since been shown that secondary forms may evolve years later in some patients.[60–62]

Secondary forms of Raynaud's phenomenon are numerous. They include almost any form of acute or chronic occlusive arterial disease, occupational lesions such as hypothenar hammer and vibratory tool syndromes, connective tissue disorders, neurogenic stimuli from reflex dystrophy, carpal tunnel and thoracic outlet syndromes, hematologic disorders, and various drugs and random causes. Trophic skin changes, ulceration, and infarction are common to obstructive forms of Raynaud's disease. Unilateral involvement indicates a secondary process.[63]

Most patients with primary Raynaud's phenomenon require no therapy and quickly learn to keep not only hands but the whole body warm. Treatment of secondary forms is directed to their cause when feasible. Nifedipine, prazosine, guanethidine, and phenoxybenzamine, alone or in combination, can suppress the vasospasm in some patients. Sympathectomy rarely produces lasting benefit to either form.

Aneurysmal Disease

Effective repair of aneurysms has been defined for several decades. The indications and risks of surgery are discussed in Chap. 125. For this large group of patients to benefit from repair, it is essential that the lesion be identified and that the ancillary disease so often present be assessed.

Examination techniques and the role of imaging have been presented earlier. Appreciation of three general characteristics of aneurysms adds to the logic of approach. First, most aneurysms progressively enlarge; the tempo for degenerative etiologies extends over years, while infectious or traumatic lesions progress in days or months. Second, aneurysms tend to be multiple. Five to 10 percent of patients with an aortic aneurysm and 50 percent or more with peripheral aneurysms will have additional lesions.[64–65] A final generalization reviews aneurysm behavior. Rupture is the dominant threat of thoracic and abdominal aortic, iliac, and visceral artery aneurysms, while thrombosis, microembolism, and macroembolism are rare. In contrast, the latter complications are typical of carotid and limb aneurysms and rupture is rare. Any aneurysm can cause dysfunction of adjacent structures by compression or can form fistula with contiguous viscera or veins (Fig. 124-1). Ascending thoracic aorta aneurysms may cause aortic valve incompetence or dissect, particularly when caused by cystic medial disease or congenital defects of the arterial wall.

Patients should be screened for aneurysmal disease by examination or various imaging techniques in two sets of circumstances: certain clinical problems and in specific settings. Aneurysms should be considered with discovery of an aneurysm elsewhere, unexplained occlusion of a distal artery, microembolic syndromes, limb edema possibly caused by aneurysm compression or fistula, and any continuous bruit. Aneurysms should be sought with given diseases known to cause them, including syphilis, the heritable disorders of connective tissue, several of the vasculitides, and atherosclerosis. Hypertension, smoking, and age predispose to aneurysm formation; the lesion was found in 15 percent of males over age 65 screened by ultrasound,[66] and a familial tendency for aneurysms in both males and females has been identified.[67]

The current mortality and morbidity of aneurysm repair come from chronic medical problems rather than from surgical complications. The remarkable success of contemporary surgery is dependent on the recognition and perioperative care of the multiple problems common to these patients. The patient should be free of infection to minimize the chance of graft infection. A simple hematologic screen will exclude bleeding disorders, intravascular coagulopathy, and platelet deficits. A history of prior venous thromboembolic disease warrants postoperative prophylaxis. The kidneys should be screened for renal artery stenosis, obstructive uropathy, and horseshoe kidney. Surgery can be performed with serum creatinine values below 4 mg/dL. Values above this level do not preclude surgery, but the need for dialysis increases.[68,69] Spirometry and blood gas values predict the need for pulmonary preparation and later ventilatory support. Death from respiratory failure is rare, even in patients with a P_{O_2} of less than 50 torr, forced expiratory flow (FMEF) less than 26 percent of predicted normal, and those on oxygen.[70] (See also Chap. 17.)

Carotid surgery screening by Duplex ultrasound is logical for those patients with bruits or a prior history of stroke or transient ischemic attacks. Angiography and possible prophylactic repair is warranted with significant bilateral stenosis found on scanning and those with recent ischemic events.[71] (See also Chap. 122.) Significant hypertension, congestive failure, and hazardous rhythm problems should be identified and treated before repair. Critical aortic stenosis should not be overlooked. Coronary artery disease is the major determinant of both operative and long-term survival of the patient with atherosclerotic aneurysmal disease. A logical screening protocol is essential for all patients. (See Chap. 139.)

Upper Extremity Arterial Disease

The diagnosis of these lesions can be demanding for three reasons: Experiences are less common, the etiology is more varied, and the combinations of associated vasospastic and microcirculatory disorders are more frequent. The principles of diagnosis and treatment learned from the leg provide a reliable background logic, and upper extremity lesions are also categorized as acute and chronic occlusive disease, microcirculatory and vasospastic disorders, and aneurysmal disease. Most problems are seen in one or more of three anatomic zones: at or near the origins of the brachiocephalic arteries in the chest, the axillosubclavian area, or the hand. Lesions in the muscular portion of the arm are less frequent, often the result of embolic occlusion, direct or iatrogenic trauma, and on occasion vasculitis, fibromuscular dysplagia, or embolic infections. When required, noninvasive testing should survey the entire limb, and angiography should include the aortic arch and extend through the hand, with vasodilation adequate for the delineation of the digital arteries.

Chronic atherosclerotic occlusive disease is seen almost only at the origin of the innominate or, most often, left subclavian arteries. Claudication is infrequent or modest because of the intermittent use of the arm and its excellent collateral. Radiologic or ultrasound evidence of "steal" from the vertebrae is not uncommon, but any neurologic symptoms are most often explained by associated carotid disease rather than the primary lesion.[72] Acute macroemboli come predominantly from the heart and only occasionally from proximal aneurysmal or occlusive lesions. Most acute in situ occlusions reflect direct or iatrogenic trauma, aneurysm thrombosis, and the occasional clotting disorder. Acute or chronic microcirculatory disease of the hands may be generated by any of the numerous mechanisms listed in Table 124-2. Most are caused by connective tissue or hematologic disorders, emboli from proximal occlusive and aneurysmal disease, or occupational trauma. Raynaud's phenomenon may accompany any acute or chronic occlusive process. It may also reflect neural irritation at the thoracic outlet. Aneurysms are rare, usually located in the proximal brachiocephalic or axillosubclavian arteries and atherosclerosis, trauma, or the outlet syndrome are the usual etiologies. Thrombosis, distal micro- and macroemboli, and a painful mass are common presentations. Rupture is rare except with infected lesions.[73]

Several specific entities should be remembered. Thromboangiitis obliterans may present initially with Raynaud's phenomenon or hand ischemia. It is bilateral, leg involvement is usual, and its clinical features, selective testing, and angiography separate it from other causes of hand ischemia.[74] The arteriopathic variant of the *thoracic outlet syndrome* almost always harbors an osseous lesion (most commonly cervical rib) that causes a poststenotic aneurysm, or less frequently, a stenosis. As noted, these complicate by thrombosis, distal micro- or macroembolization, and Raynaud's phenomenon, alone or in combination (Fig. 124-5). Treatment is surgical.[75] Many patients with Takayasu's syndrome and a tenth of those with temporal arteritis have lesions of the proximal arm arteries. Limiting arm claudication develops over just a few months, but the process can be halted or improved by steroid therapy.[40,41] Repetitive trauma to the hypothenar area from using the hand as a hammer on wrenches, levers, or other devices causes occlusion or aneurysm formation of the ulnar artery at the hammate bone. Digital ischemia and Raynaud's phenomenon of one or more digits can result from distal emboli. Improvement follows if the trauma is stopped, but continued manifestations require surgical treatment.[76] Vibratory tools such as chainsaws, grinders, and jackhammers can induce hand dysthesias and Raynaud's phenomenon after several years. Symptoms initially occur during use, later becoming chronic, but ischemia is a rare and late occurence.[77]

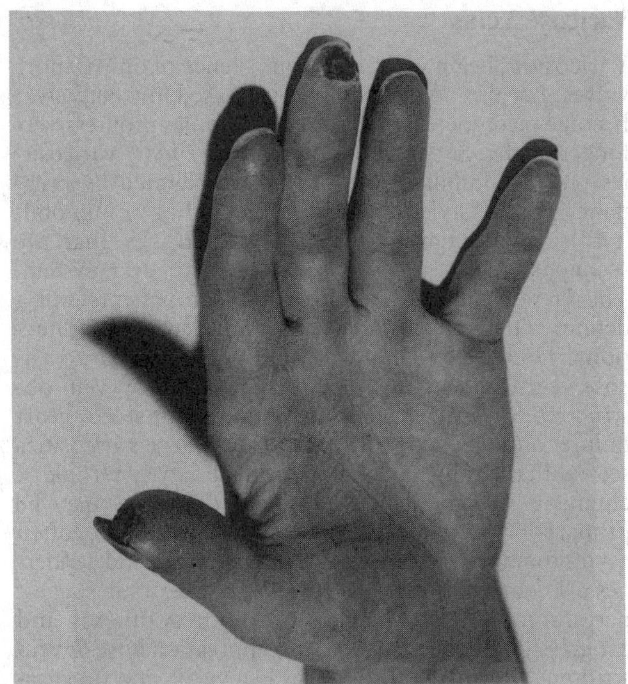

A

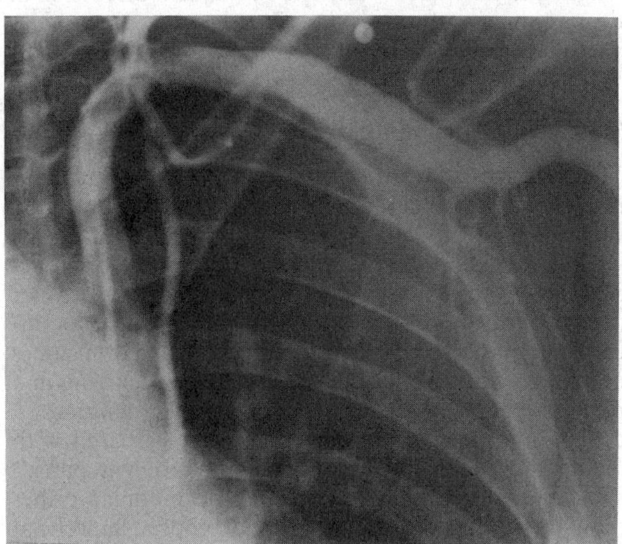

B

FIGURE 124-5 *A.* This 24-year-old house painter presented with rest pain and ischemic ulcers of digits 1 and 3. He had experienced bilateral arm claudication for 2 years and Raynaud's phenomenon for 9 months before admission. Steroids had been given for a diagnosis of vasculitis. *B.* For the patient described in *A,* radial and ulnar pulses were normal. Hyperabduction and costoclavicular maneuvers were abnormal bilaterally. Cervical ribs were noted on cervical spine roentgenograms. Note the subtle shadow suggesting thrombus in the mid-upper portion of the poststenotic aneurysm. The digital lesions healed slowly following resection of the cervical and first rib, aneurysmorraphy, and cervical sympathectomy. A similar, asymptomatic lesion on the right was subsequently repaired.

VENOUS DISEASE

Diseases of the venous system are always challenging. Superficial lesions that are so common and apparent may disarm the clinician, preventing a search for underlying mechanisms that can alter diagnosis and treatment. Deep disease of the limb and central veins can be subtle and easily overlooked, exposing the patient to the risk of thromboembolism. In contrast, what appears as obvious deep vein thrombosis is often explained by venous compression or several other diseases causing edema and distress. Objective testing that defines the diagnosis is required regularly in contrast to the arterial system. Medical treatment is undergoing constant refinement; surgical management of certain syndromes is evolving, and the literature of venous disease is growing rapidly.[78–79]

Varicose Veins

Varicosities begin with the incompetence of one or more valves. Local venous pressure is increased, further valves become incompetent, and the vein becomes progressively longer, wider, and tortuous over time. Primary varicosities reflect a familial trait and are accelerated by pregnancy and life-styles requiring long standing or immobility. It is essential to recognize varicosities that are secondary to disease of the perforator or deep system. The Trendelenburg test is useful in lean patients, but a definitive deferential is best accomplished with bidirectional Doppler or Duplex ultrasound. Secondary varicose veins are caused by perforator and deep vein obstruction or incompetence, chronic right-sided heart failure, and arteriovenous fistula. The large varicosities seen with the congenital Klippel-Trenaunay syndrome of cutaneous hemangioma and hemihypertrophy may be primary or secondary. Primary varicosities are often asymptomatic but can cause local distress and tenderness. Edema and stasis changes are rare and suggest perforator or deep vein disease. Both symptoms and progression can be managed by compression hose or vein stripping. Recurrent thrombosis in a varix, and subcutaneous or external hemorrhage warrant stripping. Sclerotherapy is effective for varicosities a few centimeters in length and for spider veins. The subsequent discussion of deep venous insufficiency describes the care of secondary varicosities.

Superficial Thrombophlebitis

The presence of a warm, tender, erythematous, and indurated linear lesion in the anatomic course of a superficial vein is diagnostic. Ultrasound can clarify the diagnosis when features are atypical. The process most often occurs in a varix or at sites of indwelling catheters or needles. Phlebitis following illicit drug use may be infected. It may also be seen after direct trauma or in zones of severe acute arterial ischemia. Lesions occurring in a previously normal vein, whether single or migratory, can be idiopathic but more often are associated with malignancy, thromboangiitis obliterans, or vasculitis.[80] The lesions of the latter two may be modular rather than linear and require diagnostic biopsy. Superficial thrombophlebitis is usually self-limited, but healing can be accelerated by rest, intermittent warmth, and anti-inflammatory agents. Septic lesions are treated with culture-specific antibiotics and may require drainage. Systemic anticoagulation is appropriate for lesions that progress despite conservative care and those located where the lesser or greater saphenous veins enter the deep system.[81]

Deep Venous Thrombosis

The diagnosis of deep venous thrombosis should be objectively documented when feasible for three reasons. First, this establishes the need for treatment to accelerate healing, to prevent clot propagation, and to prevent the sequelae of chronic venous insufficiency and pulmonary embolism. A firm diagnosis facilitates treatment choices when anticoagulation is contraindicated. Second, if the diagnosis is disproved, the cost of treatment and the risks of hemorrhage, heparin-induced thrombocytopenia, and warfarin necrosis are avoided.[82,83] Third, other diagnoses are sought when thrombosis is not found. The cardinal manifestations of deep vein thrombosis are increased venous pattern, edema, and muscle turgidity and discomfort. These findings, however, may be absent or subtle. Edema has many systemic causes, and a broad spectrum of mechanisms can mimic phlebitis (Table 124-3).

Less than half of patients presenting with venous thrombosis have the diagnosis confirmed when tested objectively.[84,85] Each test must also be selected carefully. The various forms of plethysmography, isotope venography, and bidirectional Doppler may be 95 percent sensitive to thigh obstructions, but less so below and above this level, and do not differentiate thrombosis from external compression. Fibrinogen scanning is most sensitive to calf thrombosis, but any tissue irritation can cause false positives. Ultrasound imaging, particularly with color, is highly sensitive below the groin and has excellent accuracy when positive below the knee. All of these tests are adequate when they correlate with the clinical findings. Venography remains the most definitive test, but care must be paid to inadequate filling or defects caused by dilution from collaterals without contrast.[86]

Anticoagulation with heparin and subsequently warfarin for 12 to 16 weeks is highly effective in preventing clot propagation and pulmonary embolism. (See Chaps. 68 and 100.) Heparin-induced thrombocytopenia is avoided by monitoring platelets at 2- to 3-day intervals, and warfarin necrosis is avoided by overlapping heparin with warfarin for 4 to 5 days.[82,83] The risk of major hemorrhage from anticoagulation is 1 to 2 percent when laboratory control is precise and attention is paid to drugs enhancing warfarin.[87] Thrombus isolated to the calf is less threatening, but upward of 20 percent extend proximally and 10 percent embolize. Laboratory surveillance of the lesion is required if anticoagulants are not used.[88] Caval occlusive procedures, particularly filters causing minimal obstruction, are used when anticoagulants are contraindicated or have failed. It has become clear that thrombolytic agents (Chap. 69), when given early and not contraindicated, can reduce the postphle-

TABLE 124-3
The Swollen Leg: Differential of Local Causes

Deep venous thrombosis	Acute arthritis with edema
Congestive episodes	Neurogenic pain with orthostatic tissue edema
Acute cellulitis	Tendonitis with orthostatic edema
Lipedema	Achilles
Lymphedema	Adductor
Muscle hemorrhage	Anserine
Trauma	Venous compression
Blood dyscrasia	Baker's cyst
Anticoagulants	Aneurysm
Muscle tear	Bone muscle tumor
Ruptured Baker's cyst	Femoral bursitis
Sustained cramp	May-Thurner syndrome
Factitial	
Ortho, vascular surgery	

bitic syndrome.[87] Prophylactic anticoagulation, in various protocols, protects those at bedrest who are predisposed to thrombosis. This includes patients with prior thromboembolism, congestive failure, major skeletal trauma or surgery, debility, obesity, and age.[78,79,89] (See Chap. 100.)

When thromboembolic events occur without the usual stimuli of stasis or venous injury, a search for acquired or congenital clotting defects, malignancy, and immune disorders is appropriate. Such screening is valuable even when negative in planning the duration of treatment and establishing prognosis.

Central Venous Thrombosis

Occlusion of the superior (SVC) or inferior vena cava (IVC) may be an acute thrombotic event or occur gradually, reflecting slow obstruction with subsequent thrombosis. The acute syndromes produce massive regional swelling and discomfort. Venous collaterals are prominent in chronic occlusion, and those of the IVC syndrome are best appreciated with the patient upright. Malignancy is the cause of over 80 percent of SVC and about half of IVC obstruction. Benign causes of the SVC syndrome include a growing incidence caused by indwelling catheters and fibrosing mediastinitis.[90] Inferior vena caval obstruction is often an extension from leg thrombosis, and both syndromes may be the initial manifestation of a clotting problem. Lytic therapy may clear thrombosis if given early. Bypass surgery is effective and durable in select instances of both syndromes.[91] Acute and chronic hepatic vein thrombosis presents with varying degrees of hepatic failure and ascites. Clotting disorders, tumors, and congenital venous anomalies are the usual causes.[92] Acute axillosubclavian thrombosis is often attributed to unusual effort, and many of these have an associated outlet lesion. Compression by tumor or aneurysm, indwelling catheters, and clotting defects are other causes. Lytic therapy can be effective when given early and should be followed by anticoagulation. Those with local outlet lesions can be further improved by subsequent balloon dilation or surgery.[93]

Chronic Venous Insufficiency

Chronic deep venous incompetence or obstruction causing venous hypertension in the upright position produces this common syndrome. It is characterized by leg edema, venous dilation, and intradermal deposition of proteins and hemosiderin. Later, cutaneous findings of fibrosis, lichenification, cellulitis, and ulceration follow. Edema of the foot and toes distinguishes lymphedema from the edema of chronic venous insufficiency (Fig. 124-6). Symptoms include heavy congested limbs, venous claudication, pruritis, and skin ulceration that is often painful. Prior deep venous thrombosis, chronic right-sided heart failure, or arteriovenous fistula produces the syndrome. Increased ambulatory pressure can be confirmed by direct measurement or plethysmography. Both incompetence and obstruction can be documented by bidirectional Doppler, ultrasound, or colored Duplex scanning and venography.[94] Successful management has two stages: the initial healing of the skin including ulcer grafting when required and then lifelong control of venous hypertension utilizing elastic hose generating 30 to 40 mmHg of compression. Repair or replacement of incompetent proximal valves and bypass of iliocaval obstruction are promising in a select subset of patients. The initial durability of these operations is encouraging.[95,96]

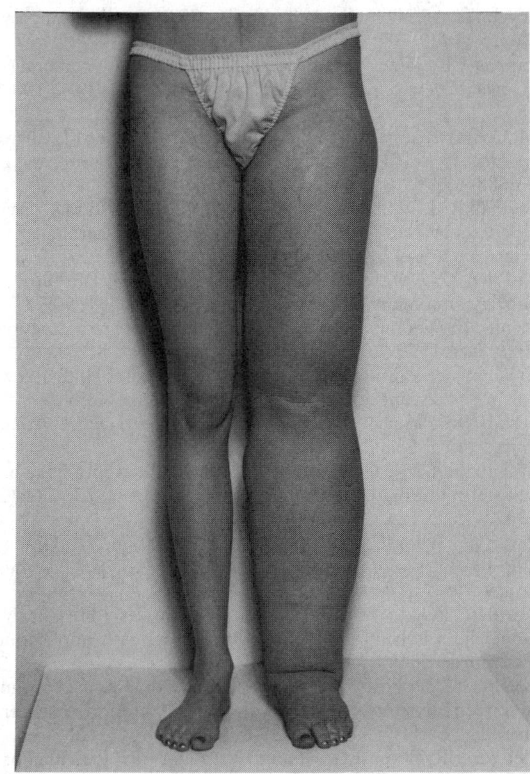

FIGURE 124-6 Massive painless edema and skin thickening in a 19-year-old woman that had evolved in less than 2 years. This constellation of historical and physical events is diagnostic of lymphedema praecox.

REFERENCES

1. Leary WV, Allen EV: Intermittent claudication as a result of arterial spasm induced by walking. *Am Heart J* 1941; 22:719–725.
2. DeWeese JA: Pedal pulses disappearing with exercise. *N Engl J Med* 1960; 262:1214–1217.
3. Barnett AJ, Dugdale L, Ferguson I: Disappearing pulse syndrome due to myxomatous degeneration of the popliteal artery. *Med J Austral* 1966; 2:355–358.
4. Kavanaugh GJ, Svein HJ, Holman CB, Johnson RM: "Pseudoclaudication" syndrome produced by compression of the cauda equina. *JAMA* 1968; 206:2477–2481.
5. Goodreau JJ, Creasy JK, Flanigan DP, Burnham SJ, Kudrna JC, Schafter MF, et al: Rational approach to the differentiation of vascular and neurogenic claudication. *Surgery* 1978; 84:749–757.
6. Allen EV: Thromboangiitis obliterans: Methods of diagnosis of chronic occlusive arterial lesions distal to the wrist with illustrative cases. *Am J Med Sci* 1929; 178:237–244.
7. Kamienski RW, Barnes RW: Critique of the Allen test for continuity of the palmar arch assessment by Doppler ultrasound. *Surg Gynec Obstet* 1976; 142:861–864.
8. Lederle FA, Walker JM, Reinke DB: Selective screening for abdominal aortic aneurysms with physical examination and ultrasound. *Arch Intern Med* 1988; 148:1753–1756.
9. Littooy FN, Steffan G, Greisler HP, White TL, Barker WH: Use of sequential B-mode ultrasonography to manage abdominal aortic aneurysms. *Arch Surg* 1989; 124:419–421.

10. Wychulis AR, Spittell JA Jr, Wallace RB: Popliteal aneurysms. *Surgery* 1970; 68:942–951.
11. Pappas CK, James JM, Bernatz PE, Schirger A: Femoral aneurysms: Review of surgical management. *JAMA* 1964; 190:489–493.
12. McCready RA, Pairolero PC, Gilmore JC, Kazmier FJ, Cherry KJ Jr, Hollier LH: Isolated iliac artery aneurysms. *Surgery* 1983; 93:688–693.
13. Zwolak RM, Whitehouse WM, Knake JE, Bernfeld BD, Zelenock GB, Cronenwett JL, et al: Atherosclerotic extracranial carotid artery aneurysms. *J Vasc Surg* 1984; 1:415–422.
14. Pairolero PC, Walls JT, Payne WS, Hollier LH, Fairbairn JF II: Subclavian-axillary artery aneurysms. *Surgery* 1981; 90:757–763.
15. Stanley JC, Thompson NW, Fry WJ: Splanchnic artery aneurysms. *Arch Surg* 1970; 101:689–697.
16. Trastek VF, Pairolero PC, Joyce JW, Hollier LH, Bernatz PE: Splenic artery aneurysms. *Surgery* 1982; 91:694–699.
17. Perloff JK: *Physical Examination of the Heart and Circulation.* Philadelphia, Saunders, 1982: 215.
18. McLaughlin MJ, Colapinto RF, Hobbs BB: Abdominal bruits: Clinical and angiographic correlation. *JAMA* 1975; 232:1238–1242.
19. Beven EG: Thoracic outlet syndromes. In: Young JR, Graor RA, Olin JW, Bartholomew JR (eds): *Peripheral Vascular Diseases.* St. Louis, Mosby Year Book, 1991: 497–509.
20. Pairolero PC, Joyce JW, Skinner CR, Hollier LH, Cherry KJ: Lower limb ischemia in young adults: Prognostic implications. *J Vasc Surg* 1984; 1:459–464.
21. Szilagyi ED, Elliott JP Jr, Smith RF, Reddy DJ, McPharlin M: A thirty-year survey of the reconstructive surgical treatment of aortoiliac occlusive disease. *J Vasc Surg* 1986; 3:421–436.
22. Hertzer NR, Beven EG, Young JR, O'Hara PJ, Ruschhaupt WF III, Graor RA, et al: Coronary artery disease in peripheral vascular patients: A classification of 1000 coronary angiograms and results of surgical management. *Ann Surg* 1984; 199:223–233.
23. Criqui MH, Langer RD, Fronek A, Feigelson HS, Klauber MR, McCann TJ, et al: Mortality over a period of 10 years in patients with peripheral arterial disease. *N Engl J Med* 1992; 326:381–386.
24. Turnipseed WD, Berkoff MA, Belzer FO: Postoperative stroke in cardiac and peripheral vascular disease. *Ann Surg* 1980; 192:365–368.
25. Collin J, Araujo L, Walton J, Lindsell D: Oxford screening programme for abdominal aortic aneurysm in men ages 65 to 74 years. *Lancet* 1988; ii:613–615.
26. Juergens JL, Barker NW, Hines EA Jr: Arteriosclerosis obliterans: Review of 520 cases with special reference to pathogenic and prognostic factors. *Circulation* 1960; 21:188–195.
27. Imperato AM, Kim GE, Davidson T, Crowley JG: Intermittent claudication: Its natural course. *Surgery* 1975; 78:795–799.
28. Schadt DC, Hines EA Jr, Juergens JL, Barker NW: Chronic atherosclerotic occlusion of the femoral artery. *JAMA* 1961; 175:937–940.
29. Starrett RW, Stoney RJ: Juxtarenal aortic occlusion. *Surgery* 1974; 76:890–897.
30. Johnston KW, Colapinto RF: Peripheral arterial transluminal dilation: Early results. *Can J Surg* 1982; 25:532–534.
31. Coffman JD: Principles of conservative treatment of occlusive arterial disease. In: Spittel JA Jr (ed): *Clinical Vascular Disease.* Philadelphia, FA Davis, 1983: 1–13.
32. Porter JM, Cutler BS, Lee BY, Reich T, Reichle FA, Scogin JT, et al: Pentoxifylline efficacy in the treatment of intermittent claudication: Multicenter controlled double-blind trial with objective assessment of chronic occlusive arterial disease patients. *Am Heart J* 1982; 104:66–72.
33. Porter JM, Baur GM: Pharmacologic treatment of intermittent claudication. *Surgery* 1982; 92:966–971.
34. Ekroth R, Dahllof AG, Gundevall B, Holm J, Scherstein T: Physical training of patients with intermittent claudication: Indications, methods, and results. *Surgery* 1978; 84:640–643.
35. Lie JT: The rise and fall and resurgence of thromboangiitis obliterans (Buerger's disease). *Acta Pathol Jpn* 1989; 39:153–158.
36. Mills JL, Taylor LM Jr, Porter JM: Buerger's disease in the modern era. *Am J Surg* 1987; 154:123–129.
37. Fiessinger JN, Schafter M: Trial of iloprost versus aspirin treatment for critical limb ischaemia of thromboangiitis obliterans. *Lancet* 1990; 335:555–557.
38. Collins PS, McDonald PT, Lim RC: Popliteal artery entrapment: An evolving syndrome. J Vasc Surg 1989; 10:484–490.
39. Ishikawa K: Cystic adventitial disease of the popliteal artery and of other stem vessels in the extremities. *Jpn J Surg* 1987; 17:221–229.
40. Klein RG, Hunder GG, Stanson AW, Sheps SG: Large artery involvement in giant cell (temporal) arteritis. *Ann Intern Med* 1975; 83:806–812.
41. Hall S, Barr W, Lie JT, Stanson AW, Kazmier FJ, Hunder GG: Takayasu arteritis: A study of 32 North American patients. *Medicine* 1985; 64:89–99.
42. Shelhamer JH, Volkman DJ, Parrillo JE, Lawley TJ, Johnston MR, Fauci AS: Takayasu's arteritis and its therapy. *Ann Intern Med* 1985; 103:121–126.
43. Wells KE, Steed DL, Zajko AB, Webster MW: Recognition and treatment of arterial insufficiency from cafergot. *J Vasc Surg* 1986; 4:8–15.
44. Green RM, DeWeese JA, Rob CG: Arterial embolectomy before and after the Fogarty catheter. *Surgery* 1975; 77:24–33.
45. Blaisdell FW, Steele M, Allen RE: Management of acute lower extremity arterial ischemia due to embolism and thrombosis. *Surgery* 1978; 84:822–834.
46. Abbott WM, Maloney RD, McCabe CC, Lee CE, Wirthlin LS: Arterial embolism: A 44 year perspective. *Am J Surg* 1982; 143:460–464.
47. Hight DW, Tilney NL, Couch NP: Changing clinical trends in patients with peripheral arterial emboli. *Surgery* 1976; 79:171–176.
48. Darling RC, Austen WG, Linton RR: Arterial embolism. *Surg Gynecol Obstet* 1967; 124:106–114.
49. Meister SG, Grossman W, Dexter L, Dalen JE: Paradoxical embolism: Diagnosis during life. *Am J Med* 1972; 53:292–298.
50. McKechnie RE, Allen V: Sudden occlusion of the arteries of the extremities: A study of 100 cases of embolism and thrombosis. *Surg Gynecol Obstet* 1936; 63:231–240.
51. Holm J, Schersten T: Anticoagulant treatment during and after embolectomy. *Acta Chir Scand* 1972; 138:683–687.
52. Fogarty TJ, Cranley JJ, Krause RJ, Strasser ES, Hafner CD: A method for extraction of arterial emboli and thrombi. *Surg Gynec Obstet* 1963; 116:241–244.
53. Thompson JE, Weston AS, Sigler L, Raut PS, Austin DJ, Patman RD: Arterial embolectomy after acute myocardial infarction: A study of 31 patients. *Ann Surg* 1970; 171:979–986.
54. McNamara TO, Fischer JR: Thrombolysis of peripheral arterial and graft occlusions: Improved results using high-dose urokinase. *Am J Roentgenol* 1985; 144:769–775.
55. Karmody AM, Powers SR, Monaco VJ, Leather RP: "Blue toe" syndrome: An indication for limb salvage surgery. *Arch Surg* 1976; 111:1263–1268.
56. Hollier LH, Kazmier FJ, Ochsner J, Bowen JC, Procter CD: "Shaggy" aorta syndrome with atheromatous embolization to visceral vessels. *Ann Vasc Surg* 1991; 5:439–444.
57. Richards AM, Eliot RS, Kanjuh VI, Bloemendaal RD, Edwards JE: Cholesterol embolism: A multiple-system disease masquerading as polyarteritis nodosa. *Am J Cardiol* 1965; 15:696–707.
58. Gastineau DA, Kazmier FJ, Nichols WL, Bowie EJW: Lupus anticoagulant: An analysis of the clinical and laboratory features of 219 cases. *Am J Hematol* 1985; 19:265–275.
59. Allen EV, Brown GE: Raynaud's disease: A critical review of minimal requisites for diagnosis. *Am J Med Sci* 1932; 183:187–200.
60. DeTakats G, Fowler EF: Raynaud's phenomenon. *JAMA* 1962; 179:99–106.
61. Priollet P, Vayssairat M, Housset E: How to classify Raynaud's phenomenon: Long-term follow-up study of 73 cases. *Am J Med* 1987; 87:494–498.
62. Gifford RW Jr, Hines EA Jr: Raynaud's disease among women and girls. *Circulation* 1957; 16:1012–1021.
63. Coffman JD: *Raynaud's Phenomenon.* New York, Oxford, 1989.
64. Dent TL, Lindenauer M, Ernst CB, Fry WJ: Multiple arteriosclerotic aneurysms. *Arch Surg* 1972; 105:338–344.
65. Joyce JW, Fairbairn JR II, Kincaid OW, Juergens JL: Aneurysms of the thoracic aorta: A clinical study with special reference to prognosis. *Circulation* 1964; 29:176–181.
66. Bergqvist D, Bengtsson J, Sternby NH: Associated atherosclerotic manifestations. In: Greenhalgh RM, Mannick JA (eds): *The Cause and Management of Aneurysms.* London, Saunders, 1990: 47.

67. Johansen K, Koepsell T: Familial tendency for abdominal aortic aneurysms. *JAMA* 1986; 256:1934–1936.
68. Johnson KW, Scobie TK: Multicenter prospective study of nonruptured abdominal aortic aneurysms. Population and operative management. *J Vasc Surg* 1988; 7:69–81.
69. Cohen JR, Mannick JA, Couch NP, Whittemore AD: Abdominal aortic aneurysm repair in patients with preoperative renal failure. *J Vasc Surg* 1986; 3:867–870.
70. Hollier LJ, Reigel MM, Kazmier FJ, Pairlero PC, Cherry KJ, Hallett JW Jr: Conventional repair of abdominal aortic aneurysm in the high risk patient: A plea for abandonment of nonresective therapy. *J Vasc Surg* 1986; 3:712–717.
71. Hart RG, Easton JD: Management of cervical bruits and carotid stenosis in preoperative patients. *Stroke* 1983; 14:290–297.
72. Walker PM, Paley D, Harris KA: What determines the symptoms associated with subclavian artery occlusive disease. *J Vasc Surg* 1985; 2:154–157.
73. Bower TC, Pairolero PC, Hallett JW Jr, Cherry KJ: Brachiocephalic aneurysms: The case for early recognition and repair. *Ann Vasc Surg* 1991; 5:125–132.
74. Hirai M, Shionaya S: Arterial obstruction of the upper limb in Buerger's disease; its incidence and primary lesion. *Br J Surg* 1979; 66:124–128.
75. Kieffer E: Arterial complications or thoracic outlet syndrome. In: Bergan JJ, Yao JST (eds): *Evaluation and Treatment of Upper and Lower Extremity Circulatory Disorders.* New York, Grune & Stratton, 1984.
76. Conn J Jr, Bergan JJ, Bell JL: Hypothenar hammer syndrome: Posttraumatic digital ischemia. *Surgery* 1970; 68:1122–1127.
77. Vibration Syndrome: Current Intelligence Bulletin 38. Washington DC, National Institute of Occupational Safety and Health, 1982.
78. Hirsh J, Hull RD: *Venous Thromboembolism: Natural History, Diagnosis and Management.* Boca Raton, CRC Press, 1987.
79. LeClerc JR: *Venous Thromboembolic Disorders.* Philadelphia, Lea and Febiger, 1991.
80. Zimran A, Shilo S, Dallberg L, Herskro C: Chronic cutaneous polyarteritis nodosa simulating recurrent thrombophlebitis. *Isr J Med Sci* 1985; 21:154–156.
81. Plate G, Eklof B, Jensen R, Oblin P: Drop vein thrombosis, pulmonary embolism, and acute surgery in thrombophlebitis of the long saphenous vein. *Acta Chir Scan* 1985; 151:242–246.
82. Ansell J, Deykin D: Heparin-induced thrombocytopenia and recurrent thromboembolism. *Am J Hematol* 1980; 8:325–333.
83. Colp MS, Minifee PK, Wolma FS: Coumadin necrosis: A review of the literature. *Surgery* 1988; 103:271–277.
84. Haeger K: Problems of acute deep vein thrombosis: The interpretation of signs and symptoms. *Angiology* 1969; 20:219–223.
85. Barnes RW, Wu KK, Hoak JC: Fallibility of the clinical diagnosis of venous thrombosis. *JAMA* 1975; 234:605–607.
86. LeClerc JR, Illegcas F, Jarzem P: Diagnosis of deep vein thrombosis. In: LeClerc J (ed): *Venous Thromboembolic Disorders.* Philadelphia, Lea and Febiger, 1991: 176–228.
87. Robitaille P, LeClerc JR, Brave G: Treatment of venous thromboembolism. In: LeClerc J (ed): *Venous Thromboembolic Disorders.* Philadelphia, Lea and Febiger, 1991: 267–302.
88. Kakkar VV, Howe CT, Nicholdes AN, Rennen JG, Clark MB: Deep vein thrombosis of the legs: Is there a higher risk group? *Am J Surg* 1970; 120:527–530.
89. Hyers TM, Hull RD, Weg JG: Antithrombosis therapy for venous thromboembolic disease. *Chest* 1989; 95(suppl):375–515.
90. Parish BM, Marschke RF Jr, Dines DE, Lee RE: Etiologic considerations in superior vena cava syndromes. *Mayo Clin Proc* 1981; 56:407–413.
91. Lochridge SK, Kibbe WP, Doty DB: Obstruction of the superior vena cava. *Surgery* 1979; 85:14–19.
92. Lillimoe KD, Cameron JL: The Budd-Chiari syndrome. In: Rutherford RB (ed): *Vascular Surgery.* Philadelphia, Saunders, 1989: 1195–1202.
93. Kunkel JM, Machleder HI: Treatment of Paget-Schroetter syndrome: A staged, multidisciplinary approach. *Arch Surg* 1989; 124:1153–1158.
94. Nicholaides A, Christopoulos D, Vasdekis S: Progress in the investigation of chronic venous insufficiency. *Ann Vasc Surg* 1989; 3:278–292.
95. Kistner RL, Ferris EB: Technique of surgical reconstruction of femoral vein valve. In: Bergan JJ, Yao JST (eds): *Operative Techniques of Vascular Surgery.* New York, Grune & Stratton, 1980.
96. Gruss JD: Various bypass for chronic venous insufficiency. In: Bergan JJ, Yao JST (eds): *Venous Disorders.* Philadelphia, Saunders, 1991.

Chapter 125

The Surgical Treatment of Peripheral Vascular Disease

Thomas F. Dodson, M.D. ■ *Robert B. Smith, III, M.D.*

Arterial surgery, as practiced within the scope of general vascular surgery, is in the vast majority of cases directed toward palliative management of atherosclerotic occlusive disease. The first part of this chapter addresses the most commonly performed reconstructions for chronic arterial insufficiency, with the exception of aortic procedures, which are considered in Chap. 123. The remainder of the current chapter is devoted to a description of the surgical management of the most common venous disorders: varicose veins, venous thromboembolism, and the postthrombotic limb.

CAROTID ENDARTERECTOMY

The majority of transient ischemic attacks (TIAs) and fixed neurologic deficits are thought to result from embolization of material from ulcerated plaques, but reduced regional blood flow related to a severely stenotic or totally occluded internal carotid artery also accounts for some ischemic deficits.[1-3] Over the past 30 years carotid endarterectomy has become a widely debated, but generally effective, and relatively safe operation for direct intervention in the stroke-prone patient. It is now one of the most frequently performed surgical procedures in general vascular surgery.

Carotid endarterectomy is a relatively low stress operative procedure[4] for which blood transfusions are seldom required. Most carotid surgery is performed with the patient under general endotracheal anesthesia, but some surgeons prefer local or cervical block anesthesia. Studies in the past decade have confirmed reductions in both hospital stay and hospital costs in patients selected for regional anesthesia.[5-8]

After operation, carotid endarterectomy patients should ideally be observed in an intensive care unit setting overnight. In both the recovery room and the intensive care unit, careful attention must be given to fluctuations in blood pressure. Appropriate pharmacologic therapy is begun promptly if any trend toward significant hypotension or hypertension is observed, since either can be associated with an increase in postoperative neurologic deficits. Most patients require little in the way of analgesia and are able to be out of bed and return to a regular diet the morning after operation. The majority are discharged from the hospital on the third or fourth day; usually sutures are removed on the day of release from the hospital. Both aspirin and dipyridamole are prescribed for their antiplatelet effect during the first 4 weeks following operation.[9,10] Because of its cost and questionable efficacy, however, dipyridamole is discontinued after 1 month, but aspirin (81 mg) is continued indefinitely.[11] Both the timing and the choice of medications for antithrombotic therapy are subjects of much debate at present.[12-14] (See Chap. 68.)

Among practitioners of carotid endarterectomy, the technical feature that produces the most controversy is whether or not to insert an indwelling shunt intraoperatively (Fig. 125-1). It is generally felt that as many as 80

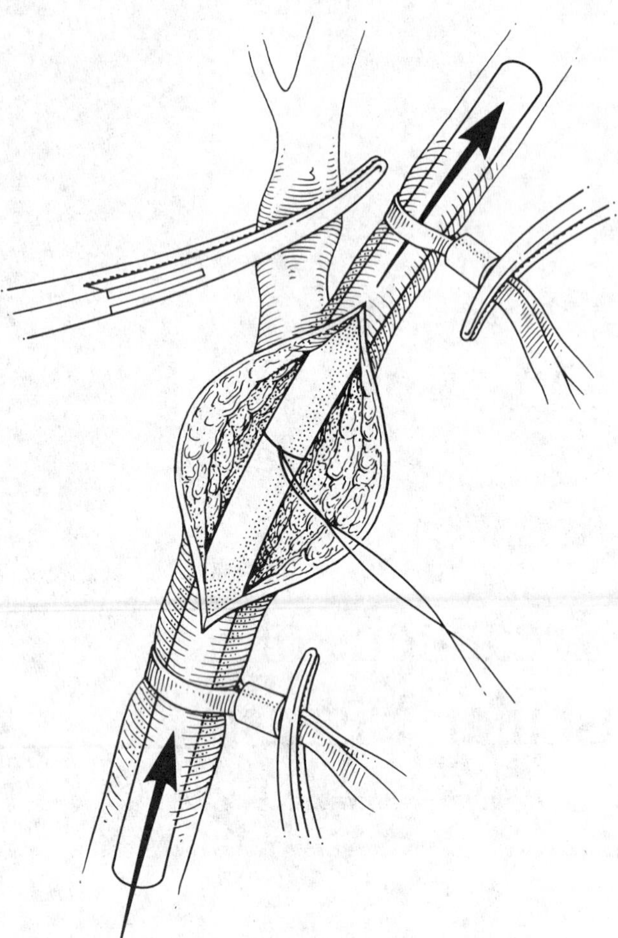

FIGURE 125-1 Indwelling shunt in place to preserve internal carotid flow during the endarterectomy.

percent of patients can undergo operation safely without the use of a shunt; the remaining 20 percent constitute the potentially threatened group. Among surgeons who are not inclined to shunt routinely, it is acknowledged that a shunt should be used for patients with total occlusion of the opposite internal carotid artery and for those with history of a previous cerebrovascular accident. (See also Chap. 122.)

Carotid endarterectomy for properly selected candidates provides dependable prophylaxis against a cerebrovascular accident. Although the appropriate indications for carotid endarterectomy have been a source of much debate, new data are allowing clinical decisions to be made on firmer ground. Both the North American Symptomatic Carotid Endarterectomy Trial (NASCET) and the European Carotid Surgery Trialists' Collaborative Group (ECST) have recently published data showing that symptomatic patients who have stenoses of 70 to 99 percent (characterized as "severe" stenoses) benefit from undergoing surgery.[15,16] Those patients with high-grade stenoses who were symptomatic and underwent operation had an absolute reduction of 17 percent in the risk of ipsilateral stroke at 2 years.[17] In fact, this information prompted NASCET investigators to issue a "Clinical Alert" to physicians in the United States and Canada.[18] Symptomatic patients with moderate degrees of stenosis (30 to 69 percent) are still currently under investigation.

Asymptomatic patients with varying degrees of carotid stenosis pose the greatest problems with respect to indications for operative intervention. It has been clearly demonstrated that a carotid bruit is a better indicator of a cardiac ischemic event than of a stroke.[19] In trying to justify the indications for operation in these patients, the authors have chosen to depend on the data provided by investigators from Seattle. In patients with 80 percent or greater carotid stenosis, 35 percent of such patients had a stroke, TIA, or carotid occlusion within 6 months of the discovery of the lesion, and 45 percent had similar events within 1 year.[20,21] Therefore, we currently recommend operation to patients who are asymptomatic but have carotid stenoses of 75 to 80 percent. (See also Chap. 122.)

Early postoperative morbidity related to carotid endarterectomy can be divided into central nervous system complications and all other problems. The incidence of perioperative stroke is quite low in the hands of experienced surgeons, but even the most senior surgeon has an occasional unexpected neurologic complication.[22] Fortunately, the majority of these are focal and transient; they are due presumably to microscopic embolization during the operative procedure or immediately thereafter. All that is necessary in these situations is supportive treatment, since the majority of small deficits clear completely within a few days. Approximately 1 to 2 percent of patients, however, have evidence of a more severe hemispheric defect at the time of recovery from anesthesia or as a new event hours or days after the procedure. Those that occur immediately postoperatively can often be attributed to thrombosis of the arteriotomy site, perhaps due to technical difficulty in the closure or to an unrecognized intimal flap. Such patients can be helped by immediate return to the operating room for reexploration of the arteriotomy.[23] If the vessel is found to be occluded, it should be reopened and a thrombectomy accomplished with the addition of a vein patch angioplasty. If at reoperation the artery is pulsating normally throughout its course, however, an operative angiogram should be performed to search for a correctable defect. Hemispheric neurologic deficits that occur later in the hospital stay are more ominous in nature and usually less responsive to reoperation. If the patient is stable, a repeat angiogram should be performed promptly to exclude an active lesion, such as a vessel partially occluded by intraluminal thrombus.

Local complications related to the cervical wound are variable in frequency and severity. Postoperative cervical hematomas are rather common but are generally of little consequence and rarely require surgical evacuation. Wound infections are extremely unusual. Cranial nerve injuries due to the transection of such major nerves as the vagus or hypoglossal are rare complications of primary endarterectomy procedures[24,25]; they occur with greater frequency among carotid reoperations. Most peripheral nerve complications are the result of contusion rather than transection and typically resolve over weeks or months. Death in the hospital following endarterectomy is most often attributable to myocardial infarction or to complications of a perioperative stroke. A mortality rate of 1 to 2 percent is considered acceptable, as is a serious neurologic morbidity rate of 1 to 2 percent. Even these low rates must be scrutinized carefully, however, in centers where carotid endarterectomy is undertaken with asymptomatic patients. In order to justify preventive surgery of this type, the team must be satisfied that prophylactic endarterectomy in their hands carries an extremely low risk of undesirable consequences.

UPPER EXTREMITY REVASCULARIZATION

Chronic arterial insufficiency of the upper extremity is most often due to occlusive disease of the aortic arch branches near their origin, either the subclavian artery or the brachiocephalic trunk. Symptoms may be limited to ischemic manifestations of the arm and hand or may include posterior circulation insufficiency of the brain due to subclavian steal syndrome. Patient selection for surgical intervention is extremely important in this group of disorders, as many patients have few or no symptoms and should not be subjected to an operative procedure simply for correction of an anatomic or radiologic finding.[26,27] Individuals who are significantly limited by arm claudication or those who have symptomatic subclavian steal syndrome should be thoroughly evaluated by vascular examination and complete angiography. Since the patterns of occlusive lesions are quite variable, any surgical procedure must be carefully planned. Generally, extrathoracic bypass procedures are preferred if a normal donor artery is available; otherwise, a transthoracic procedure may be required to originate a prosthetic bypass from the aortic arch itself. If an extra-anatomic bypass is feasible, the operation imposes a low degree of surgical stress, and there is little likelihood of the need for blood transfusions. General anesthesia is preferred, but selected operations for poor-risk patients can be performed with local anesthesia if necessary. (See also Chap. 124.)

Atheromatous occlusive disease of the subclavian artery is the most common lesion involving the proximal aortic arch branches. Extraanatomic revascularization of this vessel can be achieved by one of several techniques, depending on the pattern of obstruction and the relationship of the artery in question to a patent donor vessel. In general, shorter Dacron or Gore-Tex bypasses are preferred, and the ipsilateral common carotid artery is used to originate the graft, assuming the carotid system on that side is fully patent both proximally and distally. Otherwise, the subclavian graft can be originated from the opposite common carotid or the configuration of subclavian-subclavian or axillary-axillary bypass can be used. In the infrequent patient with symptomatic occlusion of the axillary or brachial artery, saphenous vein bypass is the procedure of choice.[28,29]

Late patency rates following proximal aortic arch revascularization procedures are excellent (80 to 90 percent), and the great majority of patients have long-term relief of symptoms. The operative mortality rate is about 2 percent, and the risk of serious postoperative complications is correspondingly low.

INFRAINGUINAL LOWER EXTREMITY BYPASSES

Although the busy vascular surgeon sees a wide variety of vascular problems, patients with intermittent claudication are frequent visitors to the vascular office.[30,31] The authors feel that mere limitation in desired walking distance is not a strong indication for operative intervention, but that severely limited ambulation, inability to work, or inability to carry out the daily functions of living are sufficient reasons for careful evaluation. Since smoking is so common in the patients, the first step is usually directed toward cessation of all tobacco use. A structured exercise program is the next part of a "conservative" approach to patients with claudication.[32] Because of its cost and its failure to affect the majority of claudicants, pentoxifylline is rarely recommended.[33] Since the natural history of claudication is "relatively benign," a nonoperative approach seems indicated for the majority of patients.[31,34] In those patients who have truly disabling claudication, operative intervention is associated with a low mortality (0.8 percent) and a primary 5-year patency rate approaching 80 percent when autogenous veins are used as the bypass graft.[35] (See also Chap. 124.)

For occlusive disease distal to the inguinal ligament and with the indications for operation being present or impending tissue loss, revascularization by means of a femoropopliteal bypass graft is the preferred surgical approach, and autogenous saphenous vein is the conduit of choice.[36–42] These procedures produce a moderate degree of surgical stress and can be performed with either regional or general anesthesia.

When the subject's own saphenous vein or arm veins are not suitable or when it is necessary to minimize the operating time because of the patient's general condition, alternative graft materials such as polytetrafluoroethylene (PTFE),[43–45] human umbilical vein,[46–48] or, rarely, knitted Dacron may be used. Inability to utilize autogenous tissue for vascular reconstruction—the patient's own long or short saphenous vein or arm veins—has ranged from as high as one-third of patients[49] to as low as 4 percent of patients subjected to operation.[50] After the conduit has been selected, the next important decision is the location of the distal anastomosis: Whether it should be connected to the proximal portion of the popliteal artery above the knee or to the distal segment below the knee. Findings on the preoperative angiogram and the surgeon's personal preference both influence this choice. The next point in the decision tree is whether to reverse the vein or use it "in situ." This is currently a controversial issue in vascular surgery, and strong proponents exist on both sides of the issue.[51,52] Recent data have suggested that there is "no significant difference" in overall patency rates between the two types of vein grafts at 3 years and that vascular surgeons should be adept at both procedures.[53–55] Table 125-1 presents the current results with various types of bypass grafts.

In some situations it is necessary to accomplish the distal anastomosis to one of the tibial branches rather than to the popliteal artery itself. An additional incision may be necessary to permit access to the anterior tibial artery, posterior tibial artery, or distal peroneal artery.

TABLE 125-1
Current Results of Femoropopliteal/Femorodistal Bypass Grafts

Bypass Graft	Above the Knee	Below the Knee	Infrapopliteal	Reference
Reversed saphenous vein for claudication and limb salvage	5 yr primary: 77% 5 yr cum: 76%	5 yr primary: 80% 5 yr cum: 86%	5 yr primary: 69% 5 yr cum: 77%	51
In situ saphenous vein for claudication and limb salvage	—	5 yr cum: 79%	5 yr cum: 74% (proximal tibial) 5 yr cum: 71% (distal tibial)	52
In situ saphenous vein for limb salvage	—	—	5 yr cum: 80%	57
Arm veins for limb salvage	—	—	5 yr primary: 51% (all levels) 5 yr cum: 57% (all levels)	56
Gore-Tex for claudication	5 yr primary: 57%	—	—	45
Gore-Tex for claudication and limb salvage	5 yr cum: 42%	5 yr cum: 28%	5 yr cum: 12%	44
Umbilical vein for claudication and limb salvage	—	5 yr cum: 57% (above and below knee)	25 yr cum: 32%	47

Primary: initial procedure only; cum: initial plus other procedures.

A number of institutions are now reporting successful series of grafts to the pedal arteries.[58–60] Lower extremity tissue loss, once thought to preclude successful revascularization, can now also be dealt with by a combination of free tissue transfer combined with distal revascularization.[61] This aggressive approach to revascularization of the threatened extremity has led to an overall diminution in the number of primary amputations performed for lower limb ischemia. Veith and colleagues[62] noted a drop in the primary amputation rate from 41 percent (1974) to 5 percent (1989). This was accomplished with a procedural mortality rate of 3 percent in over 2800 patients. Interestingly, recent data from Johns Hopkins noted *no* decline in lower extremity amputations over the period 1979 to 1989—data that go against Veith's report and conventional assumption.[63] Autogenous veins should be used for tibial or pedal bypass, if at all possible, since other conduits are associated with higher failure rates over the succeeding years.

Postoperatively, the patient is encouraged to begin early ambulation but is cautioned to avoid extremes of knee joint flexion; frequent elevation of the limb minimizes postoperative lymphedema. Aspirin and dipyridamole are prescribed postoperatively for their antiplatelet effect. Just as in patients undergoing operation for carotid disease, the dipyridamole is discontinued after 1 month, and aspirin (81 mg) is continued indefinitely. Patients who have poor runoff, who require nonautologous vascular reconstruction, or who have thrombosis in the postoperative period are considered for prolonged warfarin therapy. The data, however, are not convincing with respect to anticoagulation in this subset of patients.[43,64,65]

The vascular surgeon is obligated to follow all patients with lower extremity revascularizations periodically on a permanent basis. The authors see each patient 4 to 6 weeks after the surgical procedure, every 6 months for 2 years, and yearly thereafter. While current reports of peripheral arterial surgery document mortality rates of 1 to 4 percent,[42,44] in general, the higher mortality rates are found in patients operated upon with severe ischemia. It should be remembered that in this subgroup of high-risk patients, over one-half will be dead within 5 years. Howell and colleagues added emphasis to this fact with their finding that in patients with an ankle/brachial index less than or equal to 0.30, 64 percent expired within 6 years. They concluded that this degree of peripheral vascular ischemia carried a "malignant prognosis."[66]

Revascularization by means of a bypass graft may fail early as a result of arterial thrombosis due to technical difficulties, hypercoagulability, or poor choice of procedure relative to impaired inflow or outflow. Late graft thrombosis is usually attributable to progression of atheromatous disease or obstruction from intimal hyperplasia. In either early or late graft occlusions, patency generally can be restored and maintained by prompt intervention. More serious graft-related complications include perigraft sepsis and false aneurysm formation at the host graft suture line.[67,68] When these problems are promptly and correctly diagnosed, they too can be treated effectively; otherwise, life and limb may be in jeopardy.

MESENTERIC VASCULAR INSUFFICIENCY

Postprandial abdominal pain and weight loss are the hallmark symptoms of chronic mesenteric arterial insufficiency. *Abdominal angina* usually occurs in a setting of generalized arterial occlusive disease and is characterized by significant occlusions of one or more of the major visceral arterial trunks—celiac, superior mesenteric, and inferior mesenteric.[69] Timely diagnosis requires a high level of suspicion *and* performance of an abdominal aortogram with the patient positioned in both the anteroposterior and lateral views in order to demonstrate the origins of the visceral arteries in profile. The patient with mesenteric insufficiency symptoms and angiographic demonstration of significant occlusion or stenosis should be considered for prompt revascularization, since untreated abdominal angina frequently culminates in transmural infarction of the intestine, with a high associated mortality rate. The magnitude of the surgical procedure necessary to revascularize one or more of the visceral arteries constitutes a severe surgical stress, especially to the elderly patient with associated cardiopulmonary problems.[70] General anesthesia is necessary, and blood transfusions may be required perioperatively. Severely malnourished individuals may benefit from a preoperative buildup period of central hyperalimentation.[71,72]

Correction of a tight stenosis or occlusion of the celiac and superior mesenteric arteries is usually achieved by means of a vascular bypass from the abdominal aorta, but local endarterectomy is preferred in some centers.[73] Repair of the inferior mesenteric artery can be accomplished either by performing patch angioplasty or by reimplanting that vessel onto an aortic prosthesis interposed as a part of the same procedure. Visceral bypass grafts can be performed with autogenous saphenous vein or one of the prosthetic tubes, either PTFE or knitted Dacron. The level of the abdominal aorta chosen to originate the vascular graft depends on the vessel to be revascularized, the body habitus of the patient, and the degree of atherosclerotic involvement of the aorta as evident on the preoperative angiogram. In general, the authors prefer to originate the bypass from the supraceliac abdominal aorta at the diaphragm, since that segment of the vessel seldom contains calcified atherosclerotic plaques.[74] Hollier and colleagues[75] and Hallett and coworkers[76] at the Mayo Clinic have shown that revascularization of as many stenotic or occluded vessels as possible helps to protect against later recurrence of mesenteric symptomatology.

Postoperatively, the patient should be observed in the intensive care unit setting for a day or two, with particular attention to proper volume replacement. Most patients are eating well and ready to be discharged from the hospital 7 to 9 days after operation. Operative mortality for elective mesenteric or celiac bypass should not exceed 5 to 9 percent, but the incidence of serious postoperative morbidity is substantial, including thrombosis of the graft, sometimes with resultant acute bowel ischemia; intraabdominal bleeding; and the usual array of problems seen after major abdominal vascular surgery, such as myocardial ischemia, pulmonary insufficiency, urinary tract sepsis, and wound complications. In the Emory series reported by Rheudasil et al.,[74] postoperative complications occurred in 54 percent of patients. Although survivors of visceral revascularization procedures usually have good long-term patency of the graft, the patients must be followed closely as there is a small incidence of late graft failure with development of recurrent symptoms. Follow-up surveillance of the mesenteric revascularization can be accomplished by ultrasonography[77] or by digital subtraction angiography. If graft thrombosis occurs, prompt reoperation should be entertained, provided the patient is an acceptable surgical candidate; otherwise, intestinal gangrene may ensue.

TREATMENT OF VARICOSE VEINS OF THE LOWER EXTREMITY

The term *varicose veins* refers to the dilated, tortuous, incompetent veins of the lower extremity, usually involving tributaries of the main vessel of the greater or lesser saphenous systems. It has been estimated that 10 to 20 percent of the adult population in the United States has varicose veins. The diagnosis is easily established by physical examination, but the important differential between primary and secondary varicosities may not be readily evident. Moreover, the mere existence of venous varicosities in the leg does not require therapeutic intervention; the patient must have sufficient symptoms to justify surgical care. Patient complaints regarding varicose veins can usually be divided into two categories: cosmetic and organic. The latter includes local aching, burning, heaviness, or fatigue of the limb associated with periods of limb dependency. Many of the complaints of discomfort can be controlled by the faithful use of properly fitted, knee-length elastic surgical hose, thus precluding the need for a surgical procedure.[78] Cosmetic concerns, however, cannot be solved by simply prescribing compression stockings. (See also Chap. 124.)

If surgical care of the varicosities is selected, it is important to identify any secondary varicose veins related to disease of the deep venous system since this problem may require an altogether different therapeutic approach. The differential diagnosis can usually be made by a combination of careful history, physical examination, and studies in the noninvasive vascular laboratory[79]; if not, ascending and descending phlebography may be performed to clarify the functional status of the deep veins. (See Chap. 128.) Interventional management of primary varicose veins should be tailored to the needs of the individual patient and may include one or more of a combination of several options: sclerotherapy, local excision-ligation, and an extensive stripping procedure. In earlier years the greater saphenous vein was frequently stripped from the saphenofemoral junction to the ankle. Currently, however, there is much less enthusiasm for total removal of the greater saphenous trunk, as it has been realized that such extensive surgery often is not required to achieve the desired result and the intact remnant of saphenous vein may be useful at some later date as a conduit for coronary or peripheral vascular reconstructions. Recent data, derived from duplex ultrasonography, has also demonstrated that varicose vein valvular incompetence is a complex and heterogeneous process and that surgical therapy should be directed to the patient's specific pattern of incompetence.[80] (See also Chap. 127.)

Sclerotherapy of varicose veins is performed in the physician's office.[81] It is best reserved for small nests of primary or recurrent superficial varicosities and is not as useful for the primary treatment of sizable tortuous systems. The candidate for surgical removal of varicosities can be treated on an ambulatory surgery basis if the process is relatively limited.[82] Inpatient care, including administration of a regional or general anesthetic, is required for more extensive multiple ligations or stripping procedures, especially if both legs are to be treated. Once considered the cornerstone of varicose vein operations, ligation and stripping of saphenous and varicose veins is infrequently performed today.

A well-performed, complete excision of varicose veins should provide durable protection from local recurrence for a number of years. If small varicosities are missed or recur within the first few months, they can be managed readily by transcutaneous sclerotherapy or by simple ligation and excision under local anesthesia in the office. Patient education and careful follow-up should serve to maintain control of varicose veins over an extended period of time, but the patient must understand that the condition tends to reappear with time and that more than one surgical procedure may be required.[83] Surgical mortality for varicose vein removal should approach zero, and the risk of serious complications is quite small. Minor problems such as impaired wound healing, hematoma formation, or infection do occur but should be readily responsive to appropriate local measures.

TABLE 125-2

Risk Factors for Pulmonary Embolism

Past history of venous thromboembolism
Advancing age
Obesity (greater than 20% over ideal weight)
Acute paralysis or other conditions resulting in lack of mobility
Heart disease, especially cardiac arrhythmias and congestive heart failure
Cancer of lung, gastrointestinal and genitourinary tracts
Major operations, particularly those resulting in extended periods of immobility
Postpartum patients
Women receiving oral contraceptives who are hospitalized
Trauma patients, particularly with trauma to the lower extremities, spine, and pelvis
Patients with inflammatory bowel disease (probably)
Patients with gram-negative infections (possibly)

SOURCES: Coon and coworkers.[87–90]

SURGICAL TREATMENT OF VENOUS THROMBOEMBOLISM

Approximately 630,000 individuals have a pulmonary embolus in the United States each year, and of this number approximately 11 percent (67,000) die within 1 h of the event.[84–86] Because the incidence of this potentially lethal problem is so high, it is important to have some idea of the potential risk factors that might contribute to the onset of a pulmonary embolus. Investigators at the University of Michigan have delineated many of these factors (Table 125–2).[87–90] Consideration should be given to anticoagulant prophylaxis in such patients. Although as many as 20 percent of all hospitalized patients may be candidates for thromboembolism prophylaxis, a recent review indicated that only one-third of patients at risk actually received prophylactic treatment.[91]

Since the great majority of thromboembolic events start in the veins of the lower extremity, proper treatment of deep venous thrombosis in the leg is a subject of great importance. Standard treatment for acute lower extremity venous thrombosis, however, does not usually involve surgical intervention. Most of the patients with acute thrombophlebitis can be managed successfully by inpatient medical therapy. The drug of choice, heparin, is administered to prevent additional thrombus formation or propagation of existing thrombus.[92] Continuous intravenous infusion of heparin to maintain activated partial thromboplastic time at approximately twice the control level is most effective, but careful regulation of the heparin infusion is necessary to prevent excessive anticoagulant effect and to diminish hemorrhagic complications.[93] In past years we have continued the heparin for approximately 10 days, with warfarin (Coumadin) being added on days 5 to 10. Recent data have suggested, however, that the overall hospital course may be shortened to approximately 5 days by beginning the warfarin on the first day of in-hospital therapy.[94] In that series the frequency of documented recurrent venous thromboembolism was low and essentially the same in both treatment groups. Patients with iliofemoral thrombosis and those with major pulmonary emboli represented only a small fraction of patients in the study cited and probably should be excluded from such "short course" therapy. Strict laboratory control of warfarin dosage is required to maintain effective anticoagulation since excessive variations in drug effect increase the risk of serious complications, such as bleeding. Oral anticoagulation with warfarin (Coumadin) is usually continued for a total duration of 3 months.[65] Although it has previously been taught that a therapeutic range of 1.5 to 2.0 times the control for prothrombin time (PT) is the "ideal," we now know that a less intense therapeutic range is associated with equally effective protection against pulmonary embolus but with a much lower incidence of bleeding secondary to the anticoagulation.[95,96] The thrombolytic drugs streptokinase and urokinase have been advocated by some for treatment of acute thrombophlebitis in the effort to achieve prompt lysis of intraluminal clot and thereby preserve venous valvular function.[97–99] If these drugs are to be effective, they should be administered within a few days after the onset of venous thrombosis. The value of lytic agents in enhancing natural clot dissolution is limited by side effects and by the fact that old thrombi become increasingly resistant to lysis. We await current, prospective, randomized studies to delineate the appropriate role of thrombolytic agents versus traditional anticoagulation. (See also Chaps. 68, 69, and 100.)

Surgical thrombectomy of the iliofemoral venous system is rarely performed in the current era because of concern about the previously documented high rate of recurrent thrombosis and little, if any, reduction in long-term sequelae.[100] Earlier operation and utilization of a temporary arteriovenous fistula may improve the dismal results of years past.[101–104] Thrombectomy may be useful in instances of *phlegmasia cerulean dolens* or impending venous gangrene that is unresponsive to standard anticoagulant therapy.[105] Thrombolytic therapy might also be considered in such cases, but the experience in the literature reports small numbers of patients, and it is difficult to base new therapy on such minimal data.[106]

Interruption of the inferior vena cava (IVC) is generally reserved for instances of recurrent pulmonary embolism occurring in spite of adequate medical treatment and for patients in whom heparin therapy is contraindicated. Caval interruption has undergone a major metamorphosis in the past half century: from initial IVC ligation to placement of a partially occluding external device and then to the transvenous placement of an "umbrella" to trap clot within its spokes. The initial transvenous filter had an unacceptably high caval thrombosis rate (approximately 60 percent), and the Greenfield filter was introduced in 1973 to overcome this disadvantage.[107] A retrospective review of Greenfield filters from 1977 to 1981 indicated a patency rate of 97 percent in 33 patients.[108] Although this was initially a bulky device and often difficult to place, its superior patency rate made it the standard of surgical therapy. Investigators are now, however, broadening the indications for the use of an advanced device because of its ease of placement, reliability, and low morbidity and mortality.[109]

Since the Greenfield filter has recently been modified to permit percutaneous introduction, it is rarely necessary for patients to go to the operating room for caval interruption.[110,111] In an analysis of the transition from surgical to percutaneous Greenfield filters, Hye and colleagues[112] noted that the cost of percutaneous placement was approximately 60 percent that of surgical placement. Given the already expanded indications for caval interruption, the increased ease of placement has the potential for overutilization.[113]

Interestingly, the search for even better filter devices has not stopped, and new designs are currently being evaluated.[114] It is important to note that partial interruption by any method may be converted to complete obstruction by thrombosis in situ or by migration of distal thrombi that impinge on the obstructing device. Secondary obstruction of the vena cava adds to the consequences of deep venous thrombosis by aggravating any chronic venous hypertension, thus increasing the risk of chronic edema and venous ulceration.

THE POSTTHROMBOTIC LIMB

Although the pathophysiology of the postphlebitic syndrome, with its edema, hyperpigmentation, and ulceration, is a subject of much debate, the consequences are well known and common. In a prospective study conducted by Strandness and colleagues,[115] pigmentation developed in 15 of 61 limbs (23 percent) affected by acute deep vein thrombosis. Nearly 90 percent of limbs with pigmentation had either occluded or incompetent veins. Ulceration later developed in three of the patients in their study.

The nonoperative approach to chronic venous insufficiency involves three major components: education, elevation, and compression.[116] If the edema or ulcerations are resistant to prolonged elevation and the wearing of elastic stockings, the addition of a leg compression pump to be used either periodically during the day or for prolonged periods at night may aid in their resolution.[117] Wound care for postphlebitic ulcerations is currently undergoing an explosion of new developments.[118] In our institution, the enterostomal therapy nurses have become essential to the ongoing management of venous stasis ulcers and other chronic wounds. Operative procedures other than skin grafting have been unusual in our experience, although other investigators have accumulated a large experience with venous valve reconstruction and crossover grafts to relieve chronic venous hypertension in selected patients.[119,120] (See also Chap. 124.)

REFERENCES

1. Whisnant JP, Fitzgibbons JP, Kurland LT, Sayre GP: Natural history of stroke in Rochester, Minnesota, 1945 through 1954. *Stroke* 1971; 2:11–22.
2. Mohr JP, Caplan LR, Melski JW, Goldstein RJ, Duncan GW, Kistler JP, et al: The Harvard Cooperative Stroke Registry: A prospective registry. *Neurology* 1978; 28:754–762.
3. Mohr JP: Natural history and pathophysiology of brain infarction. *Circulation* 1991; 83(suppl I):I-172–I-175.
4. Mackey WC, O'Donnell TF, Callow AD: Cardiac risk in patients undergoing carotid endarterectomy: Impact on perioperative and long-term morbidity. *J Vasc Surg* 1990; 11:226–234.
5. Muskett A, McGreevy J, Miller M: Detailed comparison of regional and general anesthesia for carotid endarterectomy. *Am J Surg* 1986; 152:691–694.
6. Corson JD, Chang BB, Shah DM, Leather RP, DeLeo BM, Karmody AM: The influence of anesthetic choice on carotid endarterectomy outcome. *Arch Surg* 1987; 122:807–812.
7. Hafner CD, Evans WE: Carotid endarterectomy with local anesthesia: Results and advantages. *J Vasc Surg* 1988; 7:232–239.
8. Godin MS, Bell WH III, Schwedler M, Kerstein MD: Cost effectiveness of regional anesthesia in carotid endarterectomy. *Am Surg* 1989; 55:656–659.
9. Chesebro JH, Fuster V, Elveback LR, Clements IP, Smith HC, Holmes DR, et al: Effect of dipyridamole and aspirin on late vein-graft patency after coronary bypass operations. *N Engl J Med* 1984; 310:209–214.
10. Edwards WH, Edwards WH Jr, Mulherin JL Jr, Jenkins JM: The role of antiplatelet drugs in carotid reconstructive surgery. *Ann Surg* 1985; 201:765–770.
11. Fitzgerald GA: Medical intelligence: Dipyridamole. *N Engl J Med* 1987; 316:1247–1256.
12. Pfisterer M, Burkart F, Jockers G, Meyer B, Regenass S, Burckhardt D, et al: Trial of low-dose aspirin plus dipyridamole versus anticoagulants for prevention of aortocoronary vein graft occlusion. *Lancet* 1989; 2:1–6.
13. Gavaghan TP, Gebski V, Baron DW: Immediate postoperative aspirin improves vein graft patency early and late after coronary artery bypass graft surgery. *Circulation* 1991; 83:1526–1533.
14. Goldman S, Copeland J, Moritz T, Henderson W, Zadina K, Ovitt T, et al: Starting aspirin therapy after operation: Effects on early graft patency. *Circulation* 1991; 84:520–526.
15. European Carotid Surgery Trialists' Collaborative Group: MRC European Carotid Surgery Trial: Interim results for symptomatic

patients with severe (70–99%) or with mild (0–29%) carotid stenosis. *Lancet* 1991; 337:1235–1243.
16. North American Symptomatic Carotid Endarterectomy (NASCET) Steering Committee: North American Symptomatic Carotid Endarterectomy Trial: Methods, patient characteristics, and progress. *Stroke* 1991; 22:711–720.
17. North American Symptomatic Carotid Endarterectomy Trial Collaborators: Beneficial effect of carotid endarterectomy in symptomatic patients with high-grade stenosis. *N Engl J Med* 1991; 325:445–453.
18. North American Symptomatic Carotid Endarterectomy Trial Investigators: Clinical Alert: Benefit of carotid endarterectomy for patients with high-grade stenosis of the internal carotid artery. *Stroke* 1991; 22:816–817.
19. Chambers BR, Norris JW: Outcome in patients with asymptomatic neck bruits. *N Engl J Med* 1986; 315:860–865.
20. Roederer GO, Langlois YE, Jager KA, Primozich JF, Beach KW, Phillips DJ, et al: The natural history of carotid arterial disease in asymptomatic patients with cervical bruits. *Stroke* 1984; 15:605–613.
21. Lees RS: The natural history of carotid artery disease. *Stroke* 1984; 15:603–604.
22. Thompson JE: Complications of carotid endarterectomy and their prevention. *World J Surg* 1979; 3:155–165.
23. Perdue GD: Management of postendarterectomy neurologic deficits. *Arch Surg* 1982; 117:1079–1081.
24. Hertzer NR, Feldman BJ, Beven EG, Tucker HM: A prospective study of the incidence of injury to the cranial nerves during carotid endarterectomy. *Surg Gynecol Obstet* 1980; 151:781–784.
25. Sannella NA, Tober RL, Cipro RP, Pedicino JF, Donovan E, Gabriel N: Vocal cord paralysis following carotid endarterectomy: The paradox of return of function. *Ann Vasc Surg* 1990; 4:42–45.
26. Fields WS, Lemak NA: Joint study of extracranial arterial occlusion. *JAMA* 1972; 222:1139–1143.
27. Hafner CD: Subclavian steal syndrome. *Arch Surg* 1976; 111:1074–1080.
28. Garrett HE, Morris GC, Howell JF, DeBakey ME: Revascularization of upper extremity with autogenous vein bypass graft. *Arch Surg* 1965; 91:751–757.
29. McCarthy WJ, Flinn WR, Yao JST, Williams LR, Bergan JJ: Result of bypass grafting for upper limb ischemia. *J Vasc Surg* 1986; 3:741–746.
30. Criado E, Ramadan F, Keagy BA, Johnson G Jr: Intermittent claudication. *Surg Gynecol Obstet* 1991; 173:163–170.
31. Coffman JD: Intermittent claudication—Be conservative. *N Engl J Med* 1991; 325:577–578.
32. Radack K, Wyderski RJ: Conservative management of intermittent claudication. *Ann Intern Med* 1990; 113:135–146.
33. Green RM, McNamara J: The effects of pentoxifylline on patients with intermittent claudication. *J Vasc Surg* 1988; 7:356–362.
34. Imparato AM, Kim GE, Davidson T, Crowley JG: Intermittent claudication: Its natural course. *Surgery* 1975; 78:795–799.
35. Kent KC, Donaldson MC, Attinger CE, Couch NP, Mannick JA, Whittemore AD: Femoropopliteal reconstruction for claudication: The risk to life and limb. *Arch Surg* 1988; 123:1196–1198.
36. Bergan JJ, Veith FJ, Bernhard VM, Yao JST, Flinn WR, Gupta SK, et al: Randomization of autogenous vein and polytetrafluoroethylene grafts in femoral-distal reconstruction. *Surgery* 1982; 92:921–930.
37. Hall RG, Couplant GAE, Lane R, Delbridge L, Appleberg M: Vein, Gore-Tex or a composite graft for femoropopliteal bypass. *Surg Gynecol Obstet* 1985; 161:308–312.
38. Tilanus HW, Obertop H, Van Urk H: Saphenous vein or PTFE for femoropopliteal bypass. *Ann Surg* 1985; 202:780–782.
39. Veith FJ, Gupta SK, Ascer E, White-Flores S, Samson RH, Scher LA, et al: Six-year prospective multicenter randomized comparison of autologous saphenous vein and expanded polytetrafluoroethylene grafts in infrainguinal arterial reconstructions. *J Vasc Surg* 1986; 3:104–114.
40. Veterans Administration Cooperative Study Group 141: Comparative evaluation of prosthetic, reversed, and in situ vein bypass grafts in distal popliteal and tibial-peroneal revascularization. *Arch Surg* 1988; 123:434–438.
41. Taylor LM Jr, Porter JM: Clinical and anatomic considerations for surgery in femoropopliteal disease and the results of surgery. *Circulation* 1991; 83(suppl I):I-63–I-69.
42. Londrey GL, Ramsey DE, Hodgson KJ, Barkmeier LD, Sumner DS: Infrapopliteal bypass for severe ischemia: Comparison of autogenous vein, composite, and prosthetic grafts. *J Vasc Surg* 1991; 13:631–636.
43. Flinn WR, Rohrer MJ, Yao JST, McCarthy WJ III, Fahey VA, Bergan JJ: Improved long-term patency of infragenicular polytetrafluoroethylene grafts. *J Vasc Surg* 1988; 7:685–690.
44. Whittemore AD, Kent KC, Donaldson MC, Couch NP, Mannick JA: What is the proper role of polytetrafluoroethylene grafts in infrainguinal reconstruction? *J Vasc Surg* 1989; 10:299–305.
45. Prendiville EJ, Yeager A, O'Donnell TF Jr, Coleman JC, Jaworek A, Callow AD, et al: Long-term results with the above-knee popliteal expanded polytetrafluoroethylene graft. *J Vasc Surg* 1990; 11:517–524.
46. Harris JP, Farey L, Stephen MS, Sheil AGR, May J: Limitations of human umbilical vein grafts. *Surgery* 1984; 96:23–28.
47. Dardik H, Miller N, Dardik A, Ibrahim IM, Sussman B, Berry SM, et al: A decade of experience with the glutaraldehyde-tanned human umbilical cord vein graft for revascularization of the lower limb. *J Vasc Surg* 1988; 7:336–346.
48. Jarrett F, Hirsch SA: Reoperation for complications of stabilized human umbilical vein grafts. *Am J Surg* 1989; 158:438–442.
49. Killewich LA, Bartlett ST: The "all-autogenous" tissue policy for infrainguinal reconstruction questioned. *Am J Surg* 1990; 160:552–555.
50. Kent KC, Whittemore AD, Mannick JA: Short-term and midterm results of an all-autogenous tissue policy for infrainguinal reconstruction. *J Vasc Surg* 1989; 9:107–114.
51. Taylor LM Jr, Edwards JM, Porter JM: Presenter status of reversed vein bypass grafting: Five-year results of a modern series. *J Vasc Surg* 1990; 11:193–206.
52. Leather RP, Shah DM, Chang BB, Kaufman JL: Resurrection of *in situ* saphenous vein bypass: 1000 cases later. *Ann Surg* 1988; 208:435–442.
53. Watelet J, Cheysson E, Poels D, Menard JF, Papion H, Saour N, et al: In situ versus reversed saphenous vein for femoropopliteal bypass: A prospective randomized study of 100 cases. *Ann Vasc Surg* 1986; 1:441–452.
54. Harris PL, How TV, Jones DR: Prospectively randomized clinical trial to compare in situ and reversed saphenous vein grafts for femoropopliteal bypass. *Br J Surg* 1987; 74:252–255.
55. Wengerter KR, Veith FJ, Gupta SK, Goldsmith J, Farrell E, Harris PL, et al: Prospective randomized multicenter comparison of in situ and reversed vein infrapopliteal bypasses. *J Vasc Surg* 1991; 13:189–199.
56. Andros G, Harris RW, Salles-Cunha SX, Dulawa LB, Oblath RW, Apyan RL: Arm veins for arterial revascularization of the leg: Arteriographic and clinical observations. *J Vasc Surg* 1986; 4:416–427.
57. Mannick JA, Whittemore AD, Donaldson MC: Clinical and anatomic considerations for surgery in tibial disease and the results of surgery. *Circulation* 1991; 83(suppl I):I-81–I-85.
58. Harris HW, Rapp JH, Reilly LM, Orlando PA, Krupski WC, Goldstone J: Saphenous vein bypass to pedal arteries: An aggressive strategy for foot salvage. *Arch Surg* 1989; 124:1232–1236.
59. Andros G, Harris RW, Salles-Cunha SX, Dulawa LB, Oblath RW: Lateral plantar artery bypass grafting: Defining the limits of foot revascularization. *J Vasc Surg* 1989; 10:511–521.
60. Gloviczki P, Morris SM, Bower TC, Toomey BJ, Naessens JM, Stanson AW: Microvascular pedal bypass for salvage of the severely ischemic limb. *Mayo Clin Proc* 1991; 66:243–253.
61. Cronenwett JL, McDaniel MD, Zwolak RM, Walsh DB, Schneider JR, Reus WF, et al: Limb salvage despite extensive tissue loss. *Arch Surg* 1989; 124:609–615.
62. Veith FJ, Gupta SK, Wengerter KR, Goldsmith J, Rivers SP, Bakal CW, et al: Changing arteriosclerotic disease patterns and management strategies in lower-limb-threatening ischemia. *Ann Surg* 1990; 212:402–414.
63. Tunis SR, Bass EB, Steinberg EP: The use of angioplasty, bypass surgery, and amputation in the management of peripheral vascular disease. *N Engl J Med* 1991; 325:556–562.
64. Arfvidsson B, Lundgren F, Drott C, Scherstén T, Lundholm K:

Influence of coumarin treatment on patency and limb salvage after peripheral arterial reconstructive surgery. *Am J Surg* 1990; 159:556–560.
65. Hirsh J: Oral anticoagulant drugs. *N Engl J Med* 1991; 324:1865–1875.
66. Howell MA, Colgan MP, Seeger RW, Ramsey DE, Sumner DS: Relationship of severity of lower limb peripheral vascular disease to mortality and morbidity: A six-year follow-up study. *J Vasc Surg* 1989; 9:691–697.
67. Freischlag JA, Moore WS: Infection in prosthetic vascular grafts. In: Rutherford RB (ed): *Vascular Surgery,* 3d ed. Philadelphia, Saunders, 1989: 510–521.
68. Freischlag JA, Moore WS: Anastomotic aneurysms. In: Rutherford RB (ed): *Vascular Surgery,* 3d ed. Philadelphia, Saunders, 1989: 522–528.
69. Mikkelsen WP: Intestinal angina: Its surgical significance. *Am J Surg* 1957; 94:262–269.
70. Rogers DM, Thompson JE, Garrett WV, Talkington CM, Patman RD: Mesenteric vascular problems: A 26-year experience. *Ann Surg* 1982; 195:554–565.
71. Veterans Affairs Total Parenteral Nutrition Cooperative Study Group: Perioperative total parenteral nutrition in surgical patients. *N Engl J Med* 1991; 325:525–532.
72. Detsky AS: Parenteral nutrition—Is it helpful? *N Engl J Med* 1991; 325:573–575.
73. Stoney RJ, Reilly LM, Ehrenfeld WK: Chronic mesenteric ischemia and surgery for chronic visceral ischemia. In: Wilson SE, Veith FJ, Hobson RW II, Williams RA (eds): *Vascular Surgery, Principles and Practice.* New York, McGraw-Hill, 1987: 672–684.
74. Rheudasil JM, Stewart MT, Schellack JV, Smith RB III, Salam AA, Perdue GD: Surgical treatment of chronic mesenteric arterial insufficiency. *J Vasc Surg* 1988; 9:495–500.
75. Hollier LH, Bernatz PE, Pairolero PC, Payne WS, Osmundson PJ: Surgical management of chronic intestinal ischemia: A reappraisal. *Surgery* 1981; 90:940–946.
76. Hallett JW Jr, James ME, Ahlquist DA, Larson MV, McAfee MK, Cherry KJ Jr: Recent trends in the diagnosis and management of chronic intestinal ischemia. *Ann Vasc Surg* 1990; 4:126–132.
77. Eidt JF, Harward T, Cook JM, Kahn MB, Troilett R: Current status of duplex Doppler ultrasound in the examination of the abdominal vasculature. *Am J Surg* 1990; 160:604–609.
78. Chant ADB, Magnussen P, Kershaw C: Support hose and varicose veins. *Br Med J* 1985; 290:204.
79. Nicolaides AN, Vasdekis SN, Christopoulos D: Detection and quantification of venous reflux. In: Bernstein EF (ed): *Recent Advances in Noninvasive Diagnostic Techniques in Vascular Disease.* St. Louis, Mosby, 1990: 219–243.
80. Hanrahan LM, Kechejian GJ, Cordts PR, Rodriguez AA, Araki CA, LaMorte WW, et al: Patterns of venous insufficiency in patients with varicose veins. *Arch Surg* 1991; 126:687–691.
81. Goldman MP: Clinical methods for sclerotherapy of varicose veins. In: Goldman MP (ed): *Sclerotherapy, Treatment of Varicose Veins and Telangiectatic Leg Veins.* St. Louis, Mosby Year Book, 1991: 266–290.
82. Goren G, Yellin AE: Ambulatory stab evulsion phlebectomy for truncal varicose veins. *Am J Surg* 1991; 162:166–174.
83. Lofgren EP, Lofgren KA: Recurrence of varicose veins after the stripping operation. *Arch Surg* 1971; 102:111–114.
84. Dalen JE, Alpert JS: Natural history of pulmonary embolism. *Prog Cardiovasc Dis* 1975; 17:259–270.
85. Alpert JS, Smith R, Carlson CJ, Ockene IS, Dexter L, Dalen JE: Mortality in patients treated for pulmonary embolism. *JAMA* 1976; 236:1477–1480.
86. Dalen JE, Paraskos JA, Ockene IS, Alpert JS, Hirsh J: Venous thromboembolism: Scope of the problem. *Chest* 1986; 89 (suppl):370S–373S.
87. Coon WW, Coller FA: Clinicopathologic correlations in thromboembolism. *Surg Gynecol Obstet* 1959; 109:259–269.
88. Coon WW, Coller FA: Some epidemiologic considerations of thromboembolism. *Surg Gynecol Obstet* 1959; 109:487–501.
89. Coon WW: Epidemiology of venous thromboembolism. *Ann Surg* 1977; 186:149–164.
90. Coon WW: Risk factors in pulmonary embolism. *Surg Gynecol Obstet* 1976; 143:385–390.
91. Wheeler HB, Anderson FA Jr: Prophylaxis against venous thromboembolism in surgical patients. *Am J Surg* 1991; 161:507–511.
92. Hirsh J: Heparin. *N Engl J Med* 1991; 324:1565–1574.
93. Salzman EW, Deykin D, Shapiro RM, Rosenberg R: Management of heparin therapy: Controlled prospective trial. *N Engl J Med* 1975; 292:1046–1050.
94. Hull RD, Raskob GE, Rosenbloom D, Panju AA, Brill-Edwards P, Ginsberg JS, et al: Heparin for 5 days as compared with 10 days in the initial treatment of proximal venous thrombosis. *N Engl J Med* 1990; 322:1260–1264.
95. Hull R, Hirsh J, Jay R, Carter C, England C, Gent M, et al: Different intensities of oral anticoagulant therapy in the treatment of proximal-vein thrombosis. *N Engl J Med* 1982; 307:1676–1681.
96. Hirsh J, Levin MN: The optimal intensity of oral anticoagulant therapy. *JAMA* 1987; 258:2723–2726.
97. Graor RA, Young JR, Risius B, Ruschhaupt WF: Comparison of cost effectiveness of streptokinase and urokinase in the treatment of deep vein thrombosis. *Ann Vasc Surg* 1987; 1:524–528.
98. Graor R: Thrombolytic therapy for deep vein thromboses and pulmonary emboli. In: Bergan JJ, Yao JST (eds): *Venous Disorders.* Philadelphia, Saunders, 1991: 170–181.
99. Criado E, Johnson G Jr: Venous disease. In: Wells SA Jr (ed): *Current Problems in Surgery.* St. Louis, Mosby Year Book, 1991: 339–400.
100. Lansing AM, Davis WM: Five-year follow-up study of iliofemoral venous thrombectomy. *Ann Surg* 1966; 168:620–628.
101. Plate G, Einarsson E, Ohlin P, Jensen R, Qvarfordt P, Eklöf B: Thrombectomy with temporary arteriovenous fistula: The treatment of choice in acute iliofemoral venous thrombosis. *J Vasc Surg* 1984; 1:867–876.
102. Rutherford RB: Role of surgery in iliofemoral thrombosis. *Chest* 1986; 89(suppl):434S–437S.
103. Swedenborg J, Hägglöf R, Jacobsson H, Johansson J, Johnsson H, Larsson S, et al: Results of surgical treatment for iliofemoral venous thrombosis. *Br J Surg* 1986; 73:871–874.
104. Juhan C, Cornillon B, Tobiana F, Schlama S, Barthelemy P, Denjean-Massia JP: Patency after iliofemoral and iliocaval venous thrombectomy. *Ann Vasc Surg* 1987; 1:529–533.
105. Nachbur BH, Ris HB: Thrombectomy in acute deep vein thrombosis: Long-term follow-up. In: Bergen JJ, Yao JST (eds): *Venous Disorders.* Philadelphia, Saunders, 1991: 182–197.
106. Elliot MS, Immelman EJ, Jeffery P, Benatar SR, Funston MR, Smith JA, et al: The role of thrombolytic therapy in the management of phlegmasia caerulea dolens. *Br J Surg* 1979; 66:422–424.
107. Greenfield LJ, McCurdy JR, Brown PP, Elkins RC: A new intracaval filter permitting continued flow and resolution of emboli. *Surgery* 1973; 73:599–606.
108. Gomez GA, Cutler BS, Wheeler HB: Transvenous interruption of the inferior vena cava. *Surgery* 1983; 93:612–619.
109. Rohrer MJ, Scheidler MG, Wheeler HB, Cutler BS: Extended indications for placement of an inferior vena cava filter. *J Vasc Surg* 1989; 10:44–50.
110. Denny DF Jr, Dorfman GS, Cronan JJ, Greenwood LH, Morse SS, Yoselevitz M: Greenfield filter: Percutaneous placement in 50 patients. *Am J Radiol* 1988; 150:427–429.
111. Pais SO, Tobin KD: Percutaneous insertion of the Greenfield filter. *Am J Radiol* 1989; 152:933–938.
112. Hye RJ, Mitchell AT, Dory CE, Freischlag JA, Roberts AC: Analysis of the transition to percutaneous placement of Greenfield filters. *Arch Surg* 1990; 125:1550–1553.
113. Todd GJ, Sanderson J, Nowygrod R, Benvenisty A, Reemtsma K: Recent clinical experience with the vena cava filter. *Am J Surg* 1988; 156:353–358.
114. Grassi CJ: Inferior vena caval filters: Analysis of five currently available devices. *Am J Radiol* 1991; 156:813–821.
115. Strandness DE Jr, Langlois Y, Cramer M, Randlett A, Thiele BL: Long-term sequelae of acute venous thrombosis. *JAMA* 1983; 250:1289–1292.
116. Johnson G Jr, Ramadan FM: Nonoperative management of chronic venous insufficiency. In: Ernst CB, Stanley JC (eds): *Current Therapy in Vascular Surgery,* 2d ed. Philadelphia, BC Decker, 1991: 974–977.
117. Smith PC, Sarin S, Hasty J, Scurr JH: Sequential gradient pneu-

matic compression enhances venous ulcer healing: A randomized trial. *Surgery* 1990; 108:871–875.
118. Alvarez O, Rozint J, Meehan M: Principles of moist wound healing: Indications for chronic wounds. In: Krasner D (ed): *Chronic Wound Care: A Clinical Source Book for Health Care Professionals.* King of Prussia, PA, Health Management Publications, 1990: 266–281.
119. Raju S, Fredericks R: Valve reconstruction procedures for nonobstructive venous insufficiency: Rationale, techniques, and results in 107 procedures with two- to eight-year follow-up. *J Vasc Surg* 1988; 7:301–310.
120. Wilson NM, Rutt DL, Browse NL: Repair and replacement of deep vein valves in the treatment of venous insufficiency. *Br J Surg* 1991; 78:388–394.

Chapter 126

Angioplasty of Peripheral Blood Vessels

Benjamin Signer, M.D. ■ *Michael D. Dake, M.D.* ■
Lewis Wexler, M.D.

In 1964, Dotter and Judkins[1] first described percutaneous enlargement of a stenotic arterial lumen utilizing coaxial catheter dilatation. Further refinements by Van-Andel[2] and Porstmann[3] led to the development by Grüntzig and Hopff[4] of a wire-guided balloon catheter that could be inflated to a predicted diameter, relieving vascular stenosis and improving blood flow. This chapter will review these developments as well as discuss the indications, results, complications, and current research aimed at improving percutaneous transluminal angioplasty (PTA).

PATHOPHYSIOLOGY

The understanding of how PTA works has evolved considerably since Dotter and Judkins first postulated that the success of the procedure was due to mechanical compaction of compressible atheromatous plaque. Although plaque redistribution may play a role in the Dotter method, current work shows that the mechanism of PTA is multifactorial and results from a combination of events affecting all three layers of the vascular wall. Balloon dilatation causes a fracture of the atheromatous plaque with concurrent dehiscence of the intima from the media.[5-14] The resulting clefts between the media and the intima correspond to the luminal defects visualized on post-PTA arteriograms.[14] Endothelial damage with exposure of the media to the blood stream apparently stimulates a poorly controlled intimal hyperplasia that may result in restenosis. (See also Chaps. 70 and 71.)

Angioplasty can cause a spectrum of injury to the media, ranging from stretching and incomplete tears to disruption and rupture.[5-15] The sequelae of medial trauma may play a pivotal role in both atheromatous and disease-free portions of the arterial wall. Several studies have shown that overstretching of the media correlates histologically with disruption of smooth-muscle intracellular junctions and necrosis of medial myocytes. Since dilatation to the point of adventitial deformation can lead to undesired complications such as aneurysm formation and arterial rupture, less aggressive stretching of the media results in the "controlled" injury required for the success of PTA.[16]

BALLOON AND GUIDE WIRE TECHNOLOGY

A brief review of some of the characteristics of balloon catheters and guide wires will aid in understanding how advancements in design have led to improved outcomes following PTA.

Compliance describes the degree of balloon stretching in response to increases in inflation pressure. Balloons having low compliance will increase their diameter in a linear fashion as pressure increases. Early PTA balloons, such as those made from latex and polyvinyl chloride, were highly compliant and would readily stretch beyond their nominal maximal diameter. This not only would result in a decrease in dilating force on the vessel but also would increase susceptibility to balloon rupture at a lower pressure.[17] More importantly, balloon overdilation may yield to vessel rupture during a procedure.[18] Additionally, permanent balloon deformations can lead to vessel trauma upon attempted removal, due to roughening of the surface and irregularities in balloon profile. Utilization of low-compliance material such as polyethylene and polyurethane has helped to decrease these problems.

Trackability refers to the ability of a catheter to slide over a guide wire with minimal resistance and without incurring a change in wire position. While the skills of the operator and the uniqueness of the anatomic situation are important factors in advancing the catheter and wire to the stenotic site, intrinsic properties of the guide wire and catheter are also important in achieving this goal. Catheters must maintain longitudinal integrity so axial forces applied at the proximal end are received at the catheter tip. Other important properties include minimal friction between the catheter lumen and guide wire and sufficient lateral flexibility of the catheter to traverse vascular tortuosity and irregularities.

The wire must have sufficient firmness to provide the catheter support as it negotiates tortuous anatomic pathways. Concurrently, guide wires must be adequately flexible to neither traumatize the vessel nor impede advancement through diseased vasculature. A wide variety of guide wires encompassing a spectrum of stiffness, cross-sectional diameter, and tip flexibility have been designed. In addition, wires with angled tips and attachable steering devices are available to aid in navigating through challenging lesions.[16]

Profile refers to the longitudinal cross-sectional diameter of a balloon catheter. Integration and fixation of the balloon to the distal catheter as well as the degree of taper at the catheter tip are important elements in determining catheter profile. Low-profile devices with smooth, almost imperceptible transitions from the tip to the shaft facilitate catheter passage through stenotic vessels. Fewer complications at the vascular entry site are incurred due to decrease in catheter diameter.[16]

PHARMACOLOGIC ADJUNCTS

Percutaneous transluminal angioplasty is a "controlled" injury to the arterial wall causing both platelet aggregation and fibrin deposition at the site of endothelial damage. These factors likely contribute to myointimal hyperplasia at the angioplasty site. In order to reduce thrombus formation and limit possible restenosis, these processes must be addressed.

Pharmacologic adjuncts to PTA are used to prevent thrombus formation, remove thrombus incurred during a procedure, or eradicate preexisting thromboses. Vasospasm produced before or during angioplasty may be lessened with pharmacotherapy. The following is a brief discussion of several agents frequently used in PTA.

Aspirin

Aspirin is a nonspecific inhibitor of cyclooxygenase[19] (Chap. 68). It blocks the production of thromboxane A_2 while allowing the synthesis of prostacyclin to continue within the endothelium. Percutaneous transluminal angioplasty initiates the evolution of myocytes that migrate to the region of traumatized intima where they form fibromuscular elastic deposits. Platelet-derived growth factor is one of several agents that can initiate this smooth-muscle proliferation. This process may be inhibited, in part, by aspirin. Thus, aspirin acts by multiple processes to decrease thrombosis by altering platelet function and deposition.

Although aspirin has been shown to inhibit cyclooxygenase in vitro, results of in vivo tests remain controversial. This may be due to individual patient differences in volume of distribution and gastrointestinal absorption. In addition, other metabolic pathways for platelet activation have been identified that are not deactivated by aspirin. The ideal dosage of aspirin has not been determined.[20–24] Most physicians give 81 to 325 mg/day at the time of PTA and continue this regimen for an indefinite period. (See also Chap. 68.)

Heparin

Fibrin deposition can be controlled by heparin, which accelerates the ability of antithrombin III to neutralize several clotting factors within the intrinsic and common coagulation pathways (Chap. 68). This decreases the conversion of fibrinogen to fibrin. By decreasing fibrin accumulation, thrombosis is prevented and platelet accumulation minimized. Heparin may also indirectly decrease vasoconstriction by decreasing platelet aggregation and the resultant generation of thromboxane A_2.

Heparin (2 to 4 units/mL) may be incorporated into flush solutions utilized in diagnostic angiography and is commonly given as an intraarterial bolus (50 to 100 units/kg of body weight) after crossing a lesion just prior to PTA. Administration earlier in an angioplasty procedure may increase the risk of bleeding at the puncture site, especially if multiple catheter exchanges are needed during attempts to negotiate a tight lesion.

Full anticoagulation is not usually prescribed following PTA. Exceptions include small-vessel angioplasty, poor distal runoff, marked intimal irregularity secondary to PTA, and procedure-induced vasospasm or embolus. The half-life of heparin is dose dependent and is prolonged in patients with hepatic and renal dysfunction. Although the effects of heparin can be reversed by protamine, many prefer to use this agent only in special circumstances, such as an inability to maintain groin hemostasis by conventional methods. Protamine should not be given to patients taking NPH insulin as it can cause fatal anaphylactic reactions. (See also Chap. 71.)

Nitroglycerin

Arterial vasospasm may be induced following irritation of a stenosed vessel by balloon catheters and guide wires. Small vessels such as the renal arteries and infrapopliteal vessels are most susceptible. Stasis induced by vasospasm must be treated immediately in order to avert platelet aggregation and subsequent thrombosis. Vasodilators may prevent or treat this problem and also assist in traversing eccentrically diseased atherosclerotic lesions. Pharmacologic dilation of the disease-free segment of the stenosis may facilitate guide wire passage, making PTA feasible. Adjuncts commonly used to relieve vasospasm are nitrates, tolazoline, papaverin, and calcium channel-blocking agents.

Nitroglycerin may be used in PTA as a rapid acting direct dilator of both arterial and venous smooth muscle (Chap. 30). It is administered intraarterially (100 to 200 μg bolus) to avoid inactivation by the liver on first pass. It has also been given transdermally following PTA to prevent postprocedure vasospasm. Hemodynamic monitoring when administering intraarterial nitroglycerin is important. Nitroglycerin can not only cause hypotension but also reflex tachycardia, leading to increased cardiac work and possible angina pectoris.

Calcium Blockers

Calcium channel-blocking agents prevent coupling of free cytoplasmic calcium with a calmodulin substrate inhibiting increased actin/myosin interaction and subsequent vasoconstriction (Chap. 67). Calcium channel blockers produce arterial, but not venous, smooth-muscle relaxation. Nifedipine (10 mg) is administered sublingually, prior to PTA. A needle is inserted into the capsule and its liquid contents squirted under the patient's tongue. If the patient is already receiving a calcium channel blocker, there is no need to administer nifedipine prior to PTA. Like nitroglycerin, nifedipine may induce hypotension and reflex tachycardia. (See also Chaps. 70 and 71.)

INDICATIONS

The key determinant for success of PTA is proper patient selection. Anatomically, short focal lesions no longer than 3 to 4 cm are considered ideal for PTA. Treatment of stenoses longer than 7 cm are generally associated with poorer outcomes. Examples of favorable anatomic lesions include focal stenoses of the abdominal aorta, aortic bifurcation, common and external iliac arteries, and superficial femoral and popliteal arteries. Short iliac, superficial femoral, and popliteal artery occlusions may also be prime candidates for PTA.

Additional lesions amenable to treatment with somewhat less success include long segment stenoses of the iliac and superficial femoral arteries and short stenoses within infrapopliteal arteries. Unfavorable results from PTA are more frequently found in the lesions longer than 15 cm within the aforementioned arteries; stenotic segments bordering aneurysmal defects, especially in the iliac vesssesl; and acute thrombotic occlusions. Lesions previously deemed "contraindicated" to angioplastic therapy may be attempted, however, if the patient is a poor surgical risk, has a short life expectancy, or is a compromised operative candidate due to previous saphenous vein harvesting. In such instances, PTA may be performed on lesions harboring undesirable anatomic characteristics in an effort to preserve an imperiled extremity.[25]

Complementary technologies have expanded the realm of lesions previously considered untreatable. Experience with thrombolytic therapy has shown that certain occlusions may be transformed into stenotic lesions amenable to PTA. Therefore, a trial of regional thrombolysis, e.g., transcatheter urokinase infused at the site of the occlusion, may be given in selected patients prior to angioplasty.

Percutaneous transluminal angioplasty may also serve as a useful adjunct to surgical procedures, such as the treatment of anastamotic stenoses, ameliorating stenoses in native vessels where compromised inflow or runoff threaten graft patency, and alleviating stenoses to provide additional distal limb flow that facilitates conversion of a proximal amputation into a more distal level of amputation.[16]

The spectrum of problems that may benefit from PTA includes blue toe syndrome,[26,27] stenoses associated with dialysis access,[28,29] subclavian artery steal syndrome[30,31] and other supraaortic stenoses,[32,33] chronic mesenteric ischemia,[34] Budd-Chiari syndrome,[35,36] and portal-systemic shunt complications.[37]

LOWER EXTREMITY ISCHEMIA

The initial workup of patients with lower extremity ischemia consists of a careful history, physical examination, and noninvasive vascular studies (ankle/arm indices, Doppler waveform analysis, and pulse-volume recordings)[38] (Chaps. 127 to 129). Suggested standards for reports dealing with lower extremity ischemia have been published.[39] Other causes of lower extremity pain, such as lumbar disk disease, primary and metastatic neoplasm, and osteoarthroses should be ruled out.

In general, lifestyle-limiting claudication, rest pain, nonhealing foot ulcers, and impending gangrene are typical indications for angioplasty.

Abdominal Aorta

Angioplasty of the abdominal aorta may be divided into two groups: a rare group with exclusive involvement of the lower abdominal aorta[40–42] and a more common group with lesions extending into the common iliac arteries.[40,43–45] Most patients are young women with a long history of cigarette smoking. Initial technical success has been high, with few complications. Angioplasty at the bifurcation requires bilateral retrograde advancement of balloon catheters from the femoral arteries into the distal aorta and proximal iliac arteries with simultaneous inflation. Long-term results from this "kissing-balloon" technique[43] have been very good (Table 126-1) and compare favorably with surgical interventions (Table 126-2).

Iliac Artery

Atherosclerotic stenosis involving the iliac arteries represents the set of lesions in which peripheral PTA is most

TABLE 126-1

Results of PTA for Lower Extremity Ischemia

Location	Patency (%) 0–12 months	13–24 months	25–36 months	37–48 months	49–60 months
Aorta*	80–100	80–89	70–86	70	—
Iliac†					
Stenosis	81–100	98	70–93	92	60–86
Occlusion	72–86	—	56	—	48
Femoropopliteal‡					
Stenosis	81–100	75–81	68–73	61–72	61–70
Occlusion	82–92	—	62–69	61–69	60–69
Infrapopliteal¶	75–97	89	—	—	—

*From refs. 40, 43–46.
† From refs. 46–49.
‡ From refs. 52–54.
¶ From refs. 56, 57.

frequently performed. Fewer technical demands are associated with iliac artery PTA compared with angioplasty of more distal lesions; this may add to its success and acceptance. Other conditions amenable to PTA include prior surgery, radiation therapy, fibromuscular dysplasia, retroperitoneal fibrosis, and Takayasu's arteritis. Long-term patency has been very successful[46–49] (Table 126-1).

Stenoses of the iliac arteries play a major role in producing claudication of the lower extremities. Although rest pain and tissue loss are frequently caused by more distal lesions, PTA of iliac artery lesions may improve inflow to patients with additional disease of the femoropopliteal or tibioperoneal systems, thereby increasing the success of subsequent bypass graft surgery. In patients with severe disease and coexistent iliac artery stenoses, PTA may improve inflow mitigating against or minimizing the extent of amputation.

Treatment of iliac artery *occlusions* by PTA has a lower success rate than treatment of *stenoses*.[48] More recently, angioplasty of total occlusions has been preceded by localized thrombolytic therapy consisting of direct infusion of urokinase into the thrombus in an effort to improve patency and reduce distal embolization. Although initial reports are encouraging, long-term data are not available. Patency rates following treatment of isolated external iliac artery stenosis are less than achieved following PTA of common iliac artery lesions. A combined life-table analysis following PTA in patients with common and/or external iliac artery stenosis and/or occlusion showed a cumulative patency rate at 1, 2, and 5 years to be 78, 74, and 62 percent, respectively.[50] In the future the results of PTA may more closely approach the results of surgery since many of the older studies were performed prior to the use of high-pressure balloon catheters. These devices can yield improved results in highly calcified vessels. The results combining thrombolytic treatment with angioplasty and the use of vascular stents to treat dissections caused by balloon angioplasty may also improve long-term success rates.

There are other potential advantages to PTA of iliac lesions. The cost may be less than surgery and general anesthesia is not utilized. Male sexual function is not compromised, as may occur in patients undergoing bypass graft surgery due to dissection of the parasympathetic nerve fibers located at the aortic bifurcation. In addition, angioplasty does not preclude future surgical bypass procedures. In one series, mortality from elective aortoiliac and aortofemoral reconstruction was 3 to 4 percent and was much higher in patients above the age of 75,[51] compared to essentially no mortality from PTA. (See also Chap. 125.)

Femoropopliteal Arteries

The technical approach for PTA of the femoral and popliteal arteries is the same, and the results and complica-

TABLE 126-2

Results of Surgical Vascular Reconstuction for Lower Extremity Ischemia

Procedure	Patency (%) 0–12 months	13–24 months	25–36 months	37–48 months	49–60 months	120 months
Aortobifemoral bypass graft	—	—	—	—	85	70–75
Femoropopliteal bypass graft	98	80	78	75	67	—
Femorodistal bypass graft	89	83	78	78	73	—

SOURCE: Becker et al.[16]

tions are similar. Short stenotic or occlusive lesions are ideal candidates for femoral or popliteal angioplasty. Lesions greater than 7 cm in length have less favorable results. Angioplasty performed in patients with claudication has a higher degree of success than in cases where limb salvage is the primary indication for the procedure. Similarly, heavily calcified lesions are more difficult to dilate and more susceptible to restenoses and/or reocclusion.

While the success of femoropopliteal PTA may be defined as achieving a technically satisfactory angiographic result, the resolution of clinical symptoms and improvement in noninvasive vascular studies are equally important indicators. Improvement in skin color and temperature, augmentation of previously absent or diminished pulses, and resolution of rest pain and claudication are clinical signs of success. Improvement in ankle-arm indices of at least 0.15 is a positive laboratory finding. (See also Chap. 127.)

Pharmacologic adjuncts are more frequently used in treating femoropopliteal and infrapopliteal lesions than in the aorta and iliac arteries. Diseased peripheral arteries are more susceptible to decreased blood flow from stenoses due to their naturally progressive diminution in caliber. Since the rate of platelet aggregation and subsequent thrombus formation are inversely proportional to regional blood flow, antiplatelet agents such as aspirin and heparin should be used aggressively. Similarly, calcium channel-blocking agents and nitrates should be employed both during and following PTA to prevent vasospasm.

Femoropopliteal angioplasty is an acceptable initial procedure in appropriate anatomic candidates. In addition to the advantages noted previously, femoropopliteal PTA permits the preservation of the saphenous veins, reserving their use for future coronary or peripheral vascular reconstruction. Although the patency rates from femoropopliteal angioplasty are somewhat lower[52–55] (Table 126-1), they compare favorably with surgical results (Table 126-2).

In a prospective, randomized comparison of PTA with vascular reconstruction, a life-table analysis of 49 patients treated by PTA for femoropopliteal stenosis and occlusion showed cumulative patency rates of 69, 59, and 59 percent at 1, 2, and 4 years, respectively. This compared with 77, 70, and 69 percent cumulative patency in a similar number of patients at the same time intervals treated with surgical intervention.[50]

Consideration must be given to the perioperative mortality reported for infrainguinal reconstructions, which range from 2.2 percent in patients under 75 to 6.7 percent in the over-75-year age group.[51] In addition, the 5-year survival following infrainguinal surgical reconstruction was only 48 percent, largely due to fatal coronary events. The operative mortality and disappointing long-term patient survival make PTA an attractive alternative to surgery in selected patients. (See also Chap. 125.)

Infrapopliteal Arteries

Although published experience is limited, the development of low-profile balloons and steerable guide wires, coupled with the utilization of agents to lessen vasospasm, has led to improved results in treating stenoses and occlusions of the tibial arteries. Indications for the procedure include rest pain, ischemic ulceration, and gangrene. Initial results[56,57] have compared favorably with both PTA performed at more proximal locations and with surgical care (Tables 126-1 and 126-2). Infrapopliteal PTA may also be considered preoperatively to provide a more proximal level for distal anastomoses. In such instances, proximal lesions should be adequately treated prior to performance of infrapopliteal PTA.

RENAL VASCULAR INSUFFICIENCY

An estimated one million individuals have renovascular hypertension (RVH) in the United States.[58] In most patients RVH may be controlled with available drugs. (See Chaps. 76 and 77.) Some patients, however, have poor compliance to multiple-drug therapies or are unable to tolerate the side effects of the medications. In addition, a decrease in blood pressure caused by therapy may further decrease blood flow through a stenotic renal artery, further accelerating the loss of renal function.

Although the surgical correction of RVH improves long-term survival, many patients with RVH have coexistent renal failure and coronary artery disease and are poor candidates for general anesthesia. The incidence of major morbidity with renal surgical bypass is 20 percent,[59] with the operative mortality reported ranging from 1.1 to 5.4 percent.[60] Approximately 15 percent of patients undergo nephrectomy in the course of the procedure.[59] In selected patients percutaneous transluminal renal angioplasty (PTRA) may be a suitable treatment alternative, relieving renal artery stenosis (RAS) and lowering blood pressure.

Atherosclerotic disease is the cause of RVH in approximately 50 to 70 percent of patients, with fibromuscular dysplasia (FMD) accounting for the overwhelming majority of the remainder. (See also Chap. 76.)

It is uncertain who will benefit from PTRA. The diagnosis of RVH is enhanced by the presence of increased renin activity in blood from the renal vein of the ischemic kidney. Unilateral increases in renal vein renin can also positively predict a favorable outcome following surgical revascularization.[61] The absence of this finding, however, is not a contraindication to PTRA. Approximately 40 percent of patients with RAS but no unilateral increase in renal vein renin will still benefit following PTRA.[62] The measurements of renal vein renin may be less meaningful in patients receiving chronic beta blockade or angiotensin converting enzyme (ACE) inhibitor therapy. (See Chap. 76.)

In limited studies, patients with atherosclerotic disease are more likely to have progression in arterial luminal narrowing than individuals with FMD. Patients with FMD who have undergone PTRA have had significantly better results from the procedure compared to patients with RVH secondary to atherosclerotic disease.

A review of several studies[58,59,62–65] with an average follow-up of 6 to 24 months shows that a larger number of patients with FMD (Table 126-3) are cured of RAS utilizing PTRA compared to those with atherosclerotic disease (Table 126-4). Of 187 patients followed, 61 per-

TABLE 126-3

Percutaneous Transluminal Renal Angioplasty: Fibromuscular Dysplasia

Number of patients	Average Follow-up (months)	Overall (%) % Total	Overall (%) C	Overall (%) I	Overall (%) F	Unilateral (%) % Total	Unilateral (%) C	Unilateral (%) I	Unilateral (%) F	Bilateral (%) % Total	Bilateral (%) C	Bilateral (%) I	Bilateral (%) F	Reference
187	6	25	38	55	6	—	—	—	—	—	—	—	—	65
60	22	42	50	32	18	—	—	—	—	—	—	—	—	64
88	16	23	25	60	15	65	31	12	17	35	15	70	15	62
47	6	24	85	15	0	—	—	—	—	—	—	—	—	59
89	16	35	93		7	90	46	32	21	10	100	0	0	63
98	24	28	37	63	0	—	—	—	—	—	—	—	—	58

Abbreviations: C = cured—patient no longer needs medication to treat hypertension, diagnostic blood pressure (DBP) ≤ 90 mmHg with ≥10 mmHg decrease following PTRA; I = improved—DBP decreases 15% from pre-PTRA levels, medication still required, DBP between 90 and 110 mmHg; F = failed—DBP > 110 mmHg; DBP falls less than 15% from pre-PTRA levels.

cent had RAS secondary to atherosclerotic disease; at 6 months, 89 percent of this group demonstrated benefit from PTRA.[65] In the same study, 25 percent of patients had RAS secondary to FMD and benefit was demonstrated in 93 percent. With life-table analysis, the 5-year cumulative patency rate in the group with atherosclerotic disease was 80 percent, and it was 89 percent in the group with FMD.[65] Several factors contribute to these findings. Patients with atherosclerotic disease are older and more frequently have bilateral disease than do those with FMD. In FMD the stenosis lies either within the main renal artery or its branch vessels, whereas atherosclerotic lesions tend to be more proximal and to involve the ostium of the artery. In such cases, angioplasty may displace but not fracture the plaque, yielding poorer results.[66] Given the older age and more diffuse nature of the disease in patients having RAS due to atherosclerosis, essential hypertension may be an additional factor contributing to their hypertension.

Percutaneous transluminal renal angioplasty may also be utilized to dilate renal transplant arterial stenoses.[67–69] The incidence of RAS in renal transplant patients ranges from 1 to 25 percent.[68] Etiologies include atherosclerotic disease involving the transplant and/or donor segment of the renal artery, FMD, and stenosis at the surgical anastomosis. Initial technical success was 84 percent in one small series.[69] Patients with an end-to-end anastomosis to the internal iliac artery have a decreased success

TABLE 126-4

Percutaneous Transluminal Renal Angioplasty: Atherosclerotic Disease (conducted in 6 studies)

Number of patients	Average Follow-up (months)	Overall (%) % Total	Overall (%) C	Overall (%) I	Overall (%) F	Ostial (%) % Total	Ostial (%) C	Ostial (%) I	Ostial (%) F	Nonostial (%) % Total	Nonostial (%) C	Nonostial (%) I	Nonostial (%) F
187	6	61	11	78	10	33	6	72	22	67	15	82	3
60	22	58	29	48	23	—	—	—	—	—	—	—	—
88	16	68	15	50	35	33	0	25	75	—	—	—	—
47	6	73	15	44	41	65	9	36	55	35	25	58	17
89	16	57	84		16	10	0	0	100	39	20	45	35
98	24	66	23	71	6	—	—	—	—	—	—	—	—

Number of patients	Average Follow-up (months)	Unilateral (%) % Total	Unilateral (%) C	Unilateral (%) I	Unilateral (%) F	Bilateral (%) % Total	Bilateral (%) C	Bilateral (%) I	Bilateral (%) F	Reference
187	6	—	—	—	—	—	—	—	—	65
60	22	—	—	—	—	—	—	—	—	64
88	16	63	25	47	28	37	5	41	54	62
47	6	—	—	—	—	—	—	—	—	59
89	16	59	17	30	53	41	10	5	85	63
98	24	—	—	—	—	—	—	—	—	58

Abbreviations: C = cured—patient no longer needs medication to treat hypertension, diagnostic blood pressure (DBP) ≤ 90 mmHg with ≥10 mmHg decrease following PTRA; I = improved—DBP decreases 15% from pre-PTRA levels, medication still required, DBP between 90 and 110 mmHg; F = failed—DBP > 110 mmHg, DBP falls less than 15% from pre-PTRA levels.

rate of PTRA compared with patients having an end-to-side anastomosis with the external iliac artery. Restenosis occurs in approximately 20 percent of patients and is successfully treated with redilatation in 86 percent.

COMPLICATIONS

The risks of PTA may be classified into major and minor complications. In a comprehensive review of 4662 PTAs of peripheral and renal arteries, major complications occurred in 5.7 percent.[16] The most common complications were thrombus and embolism (4.8 percent), followed by arterial rupture and perforation (0.26 percent), death (0.23 percent), limb and kidney loss (0.21 percent), and arteriovenous fistula (0.09 percent). Minor complications occurred in approximately 4.6 percent of cases. Hematoma, pseudoaneurysm, and minor entry site injury combined to represent 3.7 percent of the total. Transient acute tubular necrosis occurred in less than 0.88 percent of patients. The incidence of patients requiring surgery or other forms of treatment for complications was 2.5 percent.

REFERENCES

1. Dotter CT, Judkins MP: Transluminal treatment of arteriosclerotic obstructions: Descriptions of a new technique and a preliminary report of its application. *Circulation* 1964; 30:654–670.
2. VanAndel GJ (ed): *Percutaneous Transluminal Angioplasty: The Dotter Procedure: A Manual for the Radiologist.* Amsterdam, Excerpta Medica, 1976.
3. Porstmann W: Ein neuer Korsett-ballonkatheter zur transluminale rekanalisation nach Dotter unter besonderer Berucksichtigung von obliterationen an der beckenarterien. *Radiol Diagn (Berl)* 1973; 14:239–244.
4. Grüntzig A, Hopff M: Perkutane Rekanalisation chronischer arterieller verschlusse mit ein em neuer Dilatations Katheter: Modifikation der Dotter-Tecknik. *Dtsch Med Wochenschr* 1974; 99:2502–2510.
5. Block PC, Baughman KL, Pasternak RC, Fallon JT: Transluminal angioplasty: Correlation of morphologic and angiographic findings in an experimental model. *Circulation* 1980; 61:778–785.
6. Block PC, Myler RK, Stertzer S, Fallon JT: Morphology after transluminal angioplasty in human beings. *N Engl J Med* 1981; 305:382–385.
7. Saffitz JE, Totty WG, McClennan BL, Gilula LA: Percutaneous transluminal angioplasty: Radiological pathological correlation. *Radiology* 1981; 141:651–654.
8. Faxon DP, Weber VJ, Haudenschild C, Gottsman SB, McGovern WA, Ryan TJ: Acute effects of transluminal angioplasty in three experimental models of atherosclerosis. *Arteriosclerosis* 1982; 2:125–133.
9. Block PC: Mechanism of transluminal angioplasty. *Am J Cardiol* 1984; 53:69C–71C.
10. Wolf GL, LeVeen RF, Ring EJ: Potential mechanisms of angioplasty. *Cardiovasc Intervent Radiol* 1984; 7:11–17.
11. Lyon RT, Zarins CK, Lu C-T, Yang C-F, Glasgov S: Vessel, plaque and lumen morphology after transluminal balloon angioplasty: Quantitative study in distended human arteries. *Arteriosclerosis* 1987; 7:306–314.
12. Waller BF: Pathology of transluminal balloon angioplasty used in the treatment of coronary heart disease. *Hum Pathol* 1987; 18:476–484.
13. Zollikofer CL, Redha FH, Bruhlmann WF, Uhlschmid GK, Vlodaver Z, Castaneda-Zuniga WR, et al: Acute and long-term effects of massive balloon dilation on the aortic wall and vasa vasorum. *Radiology* 1987; 164:145–149.
14. Castaneda-Zuniga WR, Formanek A, Tadavarthy M, Vlodaver Z, Edwards JE, Zollikofer CL, et al: The mechanism of balloon angioplasty. *Radiology* 1980; 135:565–571.
15. Kinney TB, Chin AK, Rurik GW, Finn JC, Shoor PM, Hayden WG, et al: Transluminal angioplasty: A mechanical pathophysiological correlation of its physical mechanisms. *Radiology* 1984; 153:85–89.
16. Becker GJ, Katzen BT, Dake MD: Noncoronary angioplasty. *Radiology* 1989; 170:921–940.
17. Abele J: Balloon catheters and transluminal dilation: Technical considerations. *Am J Roentgenol* 1980; 135:901–906.
18. Zollikofer CL, Salomonowitz E, Castaneda-Zuniga WR, Brühlman WF, Amplatz K: The relation between arterial and balloon rupture in experimental angioplasty. *Am J Roentgenol* 1985; 144:777–779.
19. Hamberg M, Svensson J, Samuelsson B: Thromboxanes: A new group of biologically active compounds derived from prostaglandin endoperoxides. *Proc Natl Acad Sci USA* 1975; 2:2994–2998.
20. Harter HR, Burch JW, Majerus PN, Stanford N, Delmez JA, Anderson CB, et al: Prevention of thrombosis in patients on hemodialysis by low-dose aspirin. *N Engl J Med* 1979; 301:577–579.
21. Preston FE, Whipps S, Jackson CA, French AJ, Wyld PJ, Stoddard CJ: Inhibition of prostacyclin and platelet thromboxane A_2 after low dose aspirin. *N Engl J Med* 1981; 304:76–79.
22. Weksler BB, Pett SB, Alonso D, Richter RC, Stelzer P, Subramanian V, et al: Differential inhibition by aspirin of vascular and platelet prostaglandin synthesis in atherosclerotic patients. *N Engl J Med* 1983; 308:800–805.
23. Fuster V, Badimon L, Badimon JJ, Chesebro JH: The pathogenesis of coronary artery disease and the acute coronary syndromes (first of two parts). *N Engl J Med* 1992; 326:242–250.
24. Fuster V, Badimon L, Badimon JJ, Chesebro JH: The pathogenesis of coronary artery disease and the acute coronary syndromes (second of two parts). *N Engl J Med* 1992; 326:310–318.
25. Dake MD: Peripheral angiography, angioplasty, atherectomy, laser techniques, thrombolysis, and stents. *Curr Op Radiol* 1990; 2:239–249.
26. Brewer ML, Kinnison ML, Perler BA, White RI: Blue toe syndrome: Treatment with anticoagulants and delayed percutaneous transluminal angioplasty. *Radiology* 1988; 166:31–36.
27. Kumpe DA, Zwerdinger S, Griffin DJ: Blue digit syndrome: Treatment with percutaneous angioplasty. *Radiology* 1988; 16:37–44.
28. Glanz S, Gordon DH, Butt KMH, Hong J, Lipkowitz GS: The role of percutaneous angioplasty in the management of chronic hemodialysis fistulas. *Ann Surg* 1987; 206:777–781.
29. Ingram TL, Reid SH, Tisnado J, Cho SR, Posner MP: Percutaneous transluminal angioplasty of brachiocephalic vein stenoses in patients with dialysis shunts. *Radiology* 1988; 166:45–47.
30. Burke DR, Gordon RL, Mishkin JD, McLean GK, Meranze SG: Percutaneous transluminal angioplasty of subclavian arteries. *Radiology* 1987; 164:699–704.
31. Erbstein RA, Wholey MH, Smoot S: Subclavian artery steal syndrome: Treatment by percutaneous transluminal angioplasty. *Am J Roentgenol* 1988; 151:291–294.
32. Kachel R, Endert G, Basche S, Grossmann K, Glaser FH: Percutaneous transluminal angioplasty (dilatation) of carotid, vertebral, and innominate artery stenosis. *Cardiovasc Intervent Radiol* 1987; 10:142–146.
33. Vitek JJ, Keller S, Duvall ER, Gupta KL, Chandra-Sekar B: Brachiocephalic artery dilatation by percutaneous transluminal angioplasty. *Radiology* 1986; 158:779–785.
34. Odurny A, Sniderman KW, Colapinto RF: Intestinal angina: Percutaneous transluminal angioplasty of the celiac and superior mesenteric arteries. *Radiology* 1988; 167:59–62.
35. Yamada R, Sato M, Kawabata M, Nakatsuka H, Nakamura K, Kabayashi N: Segmental obstruction of the hepatic inferior vena cava treated by transluminal angioplasty. *Radiology* 1983; 149:91–96.
36. Furui S, Yamauchi T, Ohtomo K, Tsuchiya K, Makita K, Takenaka E: Hepatic inferior vena cava obstructions: Clinical results of treatment with percutaneous transluminal laser-assisted angioplasty. *Radiology* 1988; 166:673–677.
37. Ruff RJ, Chaung VP, Alspaugh JP, Casarella WJ, Tuten TU, Gaylord GM: Percutaneous vascular intervention after surgical shunting for portal hypertension. *Radiology* 1987; 164:469–474.
38. Barnes RW: Noninvasive diagnostic assessment of peripheral vascular disease. *Circulation* 1991; 83:120–127.

39. Rutherford RB, Flanigan DP, Gupta SK, Johnston KW, Karmody A, Whittemore AD: Suggested standards for reports dealing with lower extremity ischemia. *J Vasc Surg* 1986; 4:80–94.
40. Odurny A, Colapinto RF, Sniderman KW, Johnston KW: Percutaneous transluminal angioplasty of abdominal aortic stenosis. *Cardiovasc Intervent Radiol* 1989; 12:1–6.
41. Charlebois N, Saint-Georges G, Hudon G: Percutaneous transluminal angioplasty of the lower abdominal aorta. *Am J Roentgenol* 1986; 146:369–371.
42. Heeney D, Bookstein J, Daniels E, Warmath M, Horn J, Rowley W: Transluminal angioplasty of the aorta. Report of 6 cases in women. *Radiology* 1983; 148:81–83.
43. Tegtmeyer CJ, Kellum CD, Kron IL, Mentzer RM Jr: Percutaneous transluminal angioplasty in the region of the aortic bifurcation. The two-balloon technique with results and long-term follow-up study. *Radiology* 1985; 157:661–665.
44. Morag B, Rubinstein Z, Kessler A, Schneiderman J, Levinkopf M, Bass A: Percutaneous transluminal angioplasty of the distal abdominal aorta and its bifurcation. *Cardiovasc Intervent Radiol* 1987; 10:129–133.
45. Yakes WF, Kumpe DA, Brown SB, Parker SH, Lattes RG, Cook PS: Percutaneous transluminal aortic angioplasty: Techniques and results. *Radiology* 1989; 172:965–970.
46. Johnston KW, Rae M, Hogg-Johnston SA, Colapinto RF, Walker PM, Baird RJ: 5-year results of a prospective study of percutaneous transluminal angioplasty. *Ann Surg* 1987; 206:403–413.
47. vanAndel GJ, vanErp WFM, Krepel VM, Breslau PJ: Percutaneous transluminal dilatation of the iliac artery: Long-term results. *Radiology* 1985; 156:321–323.
48. Colapinto RF, Stronell RD, Johnston WK: Transluminal angioplasty of complete iliac obstructions. *Radiology* 1986; 146:859–862.
49. Katzen BT, VanBreda A: Transluminal angioplasty of the iliac arteries. *Semin Intervent Radiol* 1985; 2:196–205.
50. Wilson SE, Wolf GL, Cross AP: Percutaneous transluminal angioplasty versus operation for peripheral arteriosclerosis. Report of a prospective randomized trial in a selected group of patients. *J Vasc Surg* 1989; 9:1–9.
51. Plecha FR, Bertin VJ, Plecha EJ, Avellone JC, Farrell CJ, Hertzer NR, et al: The early results of vascular surgery in patients 75 years of age and older: An analysis of 3259 cases. *J Vasc Surg* 1985; 2:769–774.
52. Gardiner GA Jr, Meyerovitz MF, Harrington DP, Boxt LM, Taus RH, Marx M, et al: Dissection complicating angioplasty. *Am J Roentgenol* 1985; 145:627–631.
53. Hewes RC, White RI Jr, Kaufman SL, Chang R, Kadir S, Kinnison ML, et al: Long-term results of superficial femoral artery angioplasty. *Am J Roentgenol* 1986; 146:1025–1029.
54. Krepel VM, vanAndel GJ, van Erp WFM, Breslau PJ: Percutaneous transluminal angioplasty of the femoropopliteal artery: Initial and long-term results. *Radiology* 1985; 156:325–328.
55. Morgenstern BR, Getrajdman GI, Laffey KJ, Bixon R, Martin EC: Total occlusions of the femoropopliteal artery: High technical success rate of conventional balloon angioplasty. *Radiology* 1989; 172:937–940.
56. Schwarten DE, Cutcliff WB: Arterial occlusive disease below the knee: Treatment with percutaneous transluminal angioplasty performed with low-profile catheters and steerable guide wires. *Radiology* 1988; 169:71–74.
57. Brown KT, Schoenberg NY, Moore ED, Saddekni S: Percutaneous transluminal angioplasty of infrapopliteal vessels: Preliminary results and technical considerations. *Radiology* 1988; 169:75–78.
58. Tegtmeyer CJ, Kellum CD, Ayers C: Percutaneous transluminal angioplasty of the renal artery. Results and long-term follow-up. *Radiology* 1984; 153:77–84.
59. Miller GA, Ford KK, Braun SD, Newman GE, Moore AV Jr, Malone R: Percutaneous transluminal angioplasty vs. surgery for renovascular hypertension. *Am J Roentgenol* 1985; 144:447–450.
60. Stanley JC: Renovascular hypertension: Surgical treatment. *Urol Radiol* 1981; 3:205–208.
61. Pickering TG, Sos TA, Vaughn ED Jr, Case DB, Sealey JE, Harshfield GA, et al: Predictive value and changes of renin secretion in hypertensive patients with unilateral renovascular disease undergoing successful renal angioplasty. *Am J Med* 1984; 76:398–404.
62. Martin LG, Price RB, Casarella WJ, Sones PJ, Wells JO Jr, Zellmer RA, et al: Percutaneous angioplasty in clinical management of renovascular hypertension: Initial and long-term results. *Radiology* 1985; 155:629–633.
63. Sos TA, Pickering TG, Sniderman K, Saddekni S, Case DB, Silane MF, et al: Percutaneous transluminal renal angioplasty in renovascular hypertension due to atheroma or fibromuscular dysplasia. *N Engl J Med* 1983; 309:274–279.
64. Kuhlmann U, Greminger P, Grüntzig A, Schneider E, Pouliadis G, Lüscher T, et al: Long-term experience in percutaneous transluminal dilatation of renal artery stenosis. *Am J Med* 1985; 79:692–698.
65. Klinge J, Mali WPTM, Puijlaert CBAJ, Geyskes GG, Becking WB, Feldberg MAM: Percutaneous transluminal angioplasty: Initial and long-term results. *Radiology* 1989; 171:501–506.
66. Cicuto KP, McLean GK, Oleaga JA, Freiman DB, Grossman RA, Ring EJ: Renal artery stenosis: Anatomic classification for percutaneous transluminal angioplasty. *Am J Roentgenol* 1981; 137:599–601.
67. Raynaud A, Bedrossian J, Remy P, Brisset J-M, Angel C-Y, Gaux J-C: Percutaneous transluminal angioplasty of renal transplant arterial stenoses. *Am J Roentgenol* 1986; 146:853–857.
68. Gerlock AJ Jr, MacDonell RC Jr, Smith CW, Muhletaler CA, Parris WCV, Johnson HK: Renal transplant arterial stenosis: Percutaneous transluminal angioplasty. *Am J Roentgenol* 1983; 140:325–331.
69. Lohr JW, MacDougall ML, Chonko AM, Diederich DA, Grantham JJ, Savin VJ: Percutaneous transluminal angioplasty in transplant renal artery stenosis: Experience and review of the literature. *Am J Kid Dis* 1986; 7:363–367.

SECTION B

Special Diagnostic Techniques for the Evaluation of the Great Vessels and Peripheral Vessels

Chapter 127

Doppler Methods for Analysis of Arterial and Venous Disorders

D. E. Strandness, Jr., M.D.

The introduction of ultrasonic methods in clinical medicine has permitted the characterization of both normal and abnormal flow states associated with a variety of cardiovascular diseases.[1] The most useful method of evaluating arterial and venous disorders has been with Doppler ultrasound.[2,3] The use of this method has been possible because of the ease of access of ultrasound to large- and medium-sized vessels and to the small arteries of the digits as well.

Since the initial human studies in the 1960s, considerable improvements have been made in the Doppler systems themselves. There is also greater understanding of the pathophysiology of the effects of disease on arterial and venous pressure-flow relations.

INSTRUMENTATION

The types of devices available and currently in use vary from simple pocket-sized units to complex systems that combine B mode with pulsed Doppler systems; these are currently in the forefront of the entire field.[4,5] Furthermore, it is clear that progress in the analysis of the velocity data will become extremely important in the detection of the early lesions of atherosclerosis and in the study of their progression over time.

Continuous Wave System

Continuous mode transmission of sound waves is widely used for the bedside evaluation of arterial and venous disorders. The transmitting frequencies employed range from 5 to 10 MHz. These provide the necessary tissue penetration to reach the large- and medium-sized arteries and veins of the limbs.[4] The Doppler frequency shifts are satisfactory for analogue recordings or audible interpretation. These systems permit both an estimation of the velocity of flow and its direction as well.

Ultrasonic Duplex Scanning

An important development in ultrasonic vascular diagnosis has been the combining of pulsed Doppler with imaging methods. This combination not only provides an image of the underlying blood vessels, but also permits selective sampling of the velocities across areas of interest. The imaging will permit the detection of atherosclerotic lesions and venous thrombi[5-7] while also permitting an estimate to be made of the extent of narrowing that might be present. More recently, color Doppler has been added to the systems, making it possible to immediately depict the flow within the visualized segments.[8] This facilitates the examination and in some circumstances provides a precise diagnosis.

ARTERIAL SYSTEM

Normal Physiology, Peripheral Arteries

Arterial pressure measurements show a slight decrease in the mean pressure but an amplification of the systolic pressure between the level of the central aorta and the pedal arteries. Thus, the systolic pressure recorded at the ankle is normally greater than that recorded in the arm. This ankle/arm index is therefore normally 1.0 or greater.[9]

The velocity patterns show three basic directional changes with each pulse cycle: (1) forward flow during systole, (2) transient flow reversal in early diastole, and (3) a small, forward flow component in middiastole to late diastole.[10] This pattern is normally found from the level of the common femoral artery down to, and including, the pedal arteries.

Following exercise, the systolic pressure at the ankle normally either shows no change or increases in the poststress period.[11] At very high work loads (near maximum) there may be a transient fall in systolic pressure at the ankle, but there is a rapid return to normal after cessation of walking (within 1 to 2 min).

Effects of Arterial Narrowing and Occlusion, Peripheral Arteries

With the development of atherosclerosis, progressive narrowing and sometimes occlusion of the arteries occurs, which forces the blood through high-resistance collateral channels. This results in a fall in the pulse and the mean blood pressure distal to the occlusion, with a fall in the ankle/arm index.[9] The magnitude of the decrease is a reflection of the extent of the disease. Values between 0.5 and 1.0 are seen with occlusion of a single segment; values below 0.5 are observed with multilevel disease. After treadmill exercise, the ankle pressure falls and requires an abnormally long recovery time; this is a reflection of the degree of ischemia and the extent of the functional disability.[11]

The velocity patterns distal to sites of disease are also altered, with a loss of the reverse-flow component, a reduction in peak velocity, and a monophasic signal that is above zero flow levels.[6] The standard sites from which these recordings are made include the common femoral, superficial femoral, popliteal, and pedal arteries (Chap. 124). The Doppler frequency shift is most commonly processed by fast Fourier transform spectrum analysis.

It is possible to use the duplex scanner to examine the arterial system from the abdominal aorta to the arteries below the knee. Hemodynamically significant stenoses (greater than 50 percent reduction in diameter) are noted by a greater than 100 percent increase in peak systolic velocity within the narrowed segment.[6] Occlusions are noted by the presence of a plaque within the artery and the lack of flow in the visualized vessel. Color flow is particularly useful below the groin, where over 50 percent stenoses can be detected by the presence of turbulent flow and a bruit. Turbulent flow is recognized by the random admixture of colors beyond the stenosis. The arterial wall vibration that produces the bruit is seen by the appearance of a Doppler shift due to tissue movement adjacent to the narrowed segment.

Normal Physiology, Extracranial Arterial System

Flow in the extracranial arteries has characteristics that are entirely different from those observed in the peripheral arteries.[12] The common carotid artery supplies blood to the external carotid artery; this is a relatively high resistance circuit as compared with the internal carotid artery, which is in a low-resistance bed. Thus, flow to the brain is quasi-steady and is normally above zero. On the other hand, the flow pattern in the external carotid artery often goes to, or approaches, zero in late systole and diastole. It has been noted, using pulsed Doppler studies, that flow through the normal carotid bulb is complex, with the development of boundary layer separation in the posterolateral aspect of the sinus. This is a region of low shear and is the site where the atheromatous plaque first develops. These flow phenomena can now be examined by duplex scanning to study the effects of early disease on velocity patterns.

Effects of Arterial Narrowing and Occlusion, Extracranial Arteries

The most common site at which atherosclerosis develops is the carotid bifurcation. This leads to progressive changes that range from stenosis of varying degrees to total occlusion of the internal carotid artery. The velocity patterns in the common carotid artery retain their quasi-steady flow until the stenosis in the internal carotid approaches total occlusion. Under these circumstances, flow in the common carotid artery commonly goes to zero or may even reverse in early diastole.

The flow velocity through the stenosis increases by an amount related to the degree of narrowing. The backscattered frequency from the area of stenosis shows a greater Doppler shift because of the greater flow velocity. The amount of shift also depends on the transmitted frequency and the cosine of the angle of incidence of the sound beam. A further observation is that as flow becomes disturbed or turbulent because of changes in lumen diameter, the usual narrow band of frequencies normally associated with systole becomes widened, producing spectral broadening. Knowledge of these relations and of the operating characteristics of the Doppler system used permits estimates of the degree of stenosis to be made with an acceptable degree of accuracy.[12]

The diagnosis of the degree of narrowing depends on the accurate detection of the velocity through suspected areas of narrowing. For stenoses in the range of 50 to 79 percent diameter reductions, the peak systolic velocity exceeds 125 cm/s. For the very tight stenosis (>80 percent), the peak systolic velocity will exceed 145 cm/s.

Considerable experience with the application of duplex scanning to the carotid arteries is available. When used to study the carotid bifurcation, the test has a sensitivity of 98 percent and a specificity of 92 percent. Stenoses can be easily detected and distinguished from total occlusion—a fact of considerable clinical importance.

The technique can be used in the following applications: (1) screening of asymptomatic patients with cervical bruits, (2) evaluation of the carotid bifurcation in patients undergoing major arterial procedures and aortocoronary bypass grafting, (3) assessment of patients with symptoms suggestive of transient cerebral ischemia, and (4) long-term follow-up.[10,12,13]

The progression of the atherosclerotic plaque can be

monitored by repeat duplex scanning. There is evidence that the very tight stenoses exceeding 80 percent are frequently associated with the development of transient ischemic attacks, strokes, and total occlusion of the internal carotid artery.[13] This fact is of importance given the recent results of the randomized clinical trials that have shown carotid endarterectomy to be of great benefit in symptomatic patients with greater than 70 percent stenoses.[14,15] The availability of duplex scanning makes it possible to identify these patients without having to resort to arteriography as the screening procedure.

In addition, it is possible to monitor the outcome after carotid endarterectomy. In approximately 10 to 20 percent of patients, a high-grade restenosis may develop secondary to myointimal hyperplasia. These lesions are smooth, in contrast to the atherosclerotic plaque, and in most circumstances do not appear to be associated with the development of transient ischemic attacks. Duplex scanning has been useful for monitoring these changes in order to relate the degree of progression of disease to the clinical outcome.

VENOUS SYSTEM

Normal Physiology

Under resting conditions, venous return is largely determined by the intrathoracic and intraabdominal pressure changes that accompany respiration.[16] Normally, flow in the major leg veins decreases or goes to zero with inspiration, because the intraabdominal pressure exceeds venous pressures. With expiration, venous pressures exceed intraabdominal pressures and flow increases. In the presence of competent valves, coughing, deep breathing, or a Valsalva maneuver does not result in flow reversal in the major veins of the limbs.

Effects of Venous Occlusion and Valvular Incompetence

Acute venous thrombosis, which is a common in-hospital problem, alters the flow pattern in a predictable manner.[16] Since the obstructed segment offers added resistance, flow is diverted via collateral channels in proportion to the extent of the resistance change, depending also on the location of the occlusion. The detection of deep vein thrombi is best done by the use of duplex scanning. Thrombi are detected by the visualization of the thrombus and lack of compressibility of the involved segment. In cases where the thrombus is not echogenic enough to be seen, the lack of detectable flow is also a useful diagnostic parameter.[7] Duplex scanning is considered to be the test of choice with an accuracy that appears to be equal to venography.

When the valves are destroyed and rendered incompetent secondary to venous thrombosis, there is reversal of flow with coughing, a Valsalva maneuver, or limb compression proximal to the site being examined. In establishing the site and extent of involvement, it is important not only to assess the deep veins in the usual location, but also to assess the superficial veins. In practice, the greater and lesser saphenous veins are examined as well as the perforating veins, which empty into the posterior arch vein in the lower one-third of the leg.

It appears that most of the sequelae of venous thrombosis can be explained by the loss of competence of the valves in the deep venous system.[17] With loss of valve competence, ambulatory venous hypertension and edema lead to hyperpigmentation and ulceration along the inner aspect of the lower leg.

Chronic venous obstruction in the ileofemoral venous segment often leads to the development of venous claudication.[18] This entity consists of a bursting pain in the thigh during exercise that is relieved by elevation. It can be suspected by a reduction in venous outflow measured by strain gauge plethysmography.

With the availability of duplex scanning to document venous occlusion and plethysmographic methods to assess venous function, it is now possible to completely assess both the superficial and deep veins. New information is now available to help promote our understanding of venous function and those diseases that affect the venous system.

REFERENCES

1. Satomura S: Study of flow patterns in peripheral arteries by ultrasonics. *J Acoust Soc Jpn* 1959; 15:151–153.
2. Strandness DE Jr, McCutcheon EP, Rushmer RF: Application of transcutaneous Doppler flowmeter in evaluation of occlusive arterial disease. *Surg Gynecol Obstet* 1966; 122:1039–1045.
3. Strandness DE Jr: *Duplex Scanning in Vascular Disorders*. New York, Raven, 1990.
4. Strandness DE Jr, Schultz RD, Sumner DS, Rushmer RF: Ultrasonic flow detection: A useful technic in the evaluation of peripheral vascular disease. *Am J Surg* 1967; 113:311–320.
5. Phillips DJ, Powers JE, Eyer MK, Blackshear WM Jr, Bodily KC, Strandess DE Jr, et al: Detection of vascular disease using the duplex scanner III. *Ultrasound Med Biol* 1980; 6:205–218.
6. Kohler TR, Nance DR, Cramer MM, Vandenberghe N, Strandness DE Jr: Duplex scanning for diagnosis of aortoiliac and femoropopliteal disease. *Circulation* 1987; 76:1074–1080.
7. Killewich LA, Bedford GR, Beach KW, Strandness DE Jr: Diagnosis of deep venous thrombosis: A prospective study comparing duplex scanning to contrast venography. *Circulation* 1989; 79:810–814.
8. Merritt CR: Doppler color flow imaging. *J Clin Ultrasound* 1987; 15:591–597.
9. Carter SA: Role of pressure measurements in vascular disease. In: Bernstein EF (ed): *Noninvasive Diagnostic Techniques in Vascular Disease*, 2d ed. St. Louis, Mosby, 1982: 317–343.
10. Strandness DE Jr: Duplex scanning and the vascular surgeon. *J Cardiovasc Surg* 1987; 28:235–252.
11. Strandness DE Jr: Exercise testing in the evaluation of patients undergoing direct arterial surgery. *J Cardiovasc Surg* 1970; 11:192–204.
12. Taylor DC, Strandness DE Jr: Carotid artery duplex scanning. *J Clin Ultrasound* 1987; 15:635–644.
13. Moneta GL, Taylor DC, Nicholls SC, Bergelin RO, Zierler RE, Kazmers A, et al: Operative versus nonoperative management of asymptomatic high-grade internal carotid artery stenosis: Improved results with carotid endarterectomy. *Stroke* 1987; 18:1005–1010.
14. MRC European Carotid Surgery Trial: Interim results for symptomatic patients with severe (70–99%) or mild (0–29%) carotid stenosis. European Trialists Collaborative Group. *Lancet* 1991; 337:1235–1242.
15. North American Symptomatic Carotid Endarterectomy Trial Col-

laborators: Beneficial effect of carotid endarterectomy in symptomatic patients with high-grade carotid stenosis. *New Engl J Med* 1991; 325:445–463.

16. Barnes RW: Doppler ultrasonic diagnosis of venous disease. In: Bernstein EF (ed): *Noninvasive Diagnostic Techniques in Vascular Disease*, 2d ed. St. Louis, Mosby, 1982; 452–458.
17. Strandness DE Jr, Langlois YE, Cramer MM, Randlett A, Thiele BL: Long-term sequelae of acute venous thrombosis. *JAMA* 1983; 250:1289–1292.
18. Killewich L, Martin R, Cramer MM, Beach KW, Strandness DE Jr: The pathophysiology of venous claudication. *J Vasc Surg* 1984; 4:507–511.

Chapter 128

Phlebography

Renate L. Soulen, M.D. ■ **Michael C. Soulen, M.D.**

INDICATIONS

Radiographic visualization of the venous system is useful as a road map for central venous catheter placement, balloon dilatation, or for venous sampling; for delineation of tumors or vascular malformations; for assessment of trauma, venous insufficiency, and suitability of veins for bypass grafting or shunts; and, above all, for the diagnosis of venous thrombosis. This chapter will consider only the latter.

Deep vein thrombosis remains a common cause of serious morbidity and mortality, yet eludes reliable diagnosis on the basis of history and physical examination alone.[1] Although radionuclide and noninvasive techniques have contributed greatly to the diagnosis, phlebography remains the "gold standard" and, when properly performed, has an accuracy approaching 100 percent.[2,3]

TECHNIQUE

Upper Extremity and Mediastinal Phlebography

Thirty milliliters of a 60 percent aqueous contrast medium are injected relatively slowly (e.g., 5 mL/s) through a needle in the dorsum of the hand or, when the problem is clearly intrathoracic, in the basilic or brachial vein, while serial films of the extremity and chest are obtained with the patient supine. At the completion of injection, during filming of the axilla and chest, the arm is elevated 90°, thereby creating a good bolus and promoting emptying of the arm. If the mediastinum is of interest, both upper extremities are injected simultaneously and both are elevated in order to prevent spurious filling defects from unopacified blood. We prefer hand injection so that the injection site is kept in view and injection can be stopped immediately should extravasation be seen. An adequate study can be obtained even when hand injected through a 23-gauge needle. A leaded shield and the distance permitted by extra connecting tubing protect the operator. The veins are further cleared of contrast medium by infusion of saline solution or 5% glucose in water through the same needle while the films are processed.

Lower Extremity Phlebography

Though unanimity is lacking as to the optimal method, variations of the technique of Rabinov and Paulin[4] are the most widely accepted. The key features of the technique are that the patient is semierect, the leg of interest is non-weight-bearing, and the injection of contrast medium is made with no tourniquet on. This requires a tilt table as well as hand grips and axillary support for patients unable to bear weight on the contralateral leg. Contrast medium is injected into as distal and medial a vein as possible. Retrograde insertion of the needle facilitates filling of the foot veins and thereby the deep calf veins into which they drain. We inject 100 mL by hand, taking a lateral film of the foot after 25 mL; anteroposterior, lateral, and internal oblique views of the calf and knee after 75 mL; anteroposterior and lateral views of the thigh after completion of injection; and an anteroposterior film of the abdomen and pelvis immediately after elevation of the leg and calf massage during infusion of saline solution or 5% glucose in water. The table is then immediately lowered to the horizontal, and infusion of the flush solution is continued while the films are processed. Operator protection is as previously de-

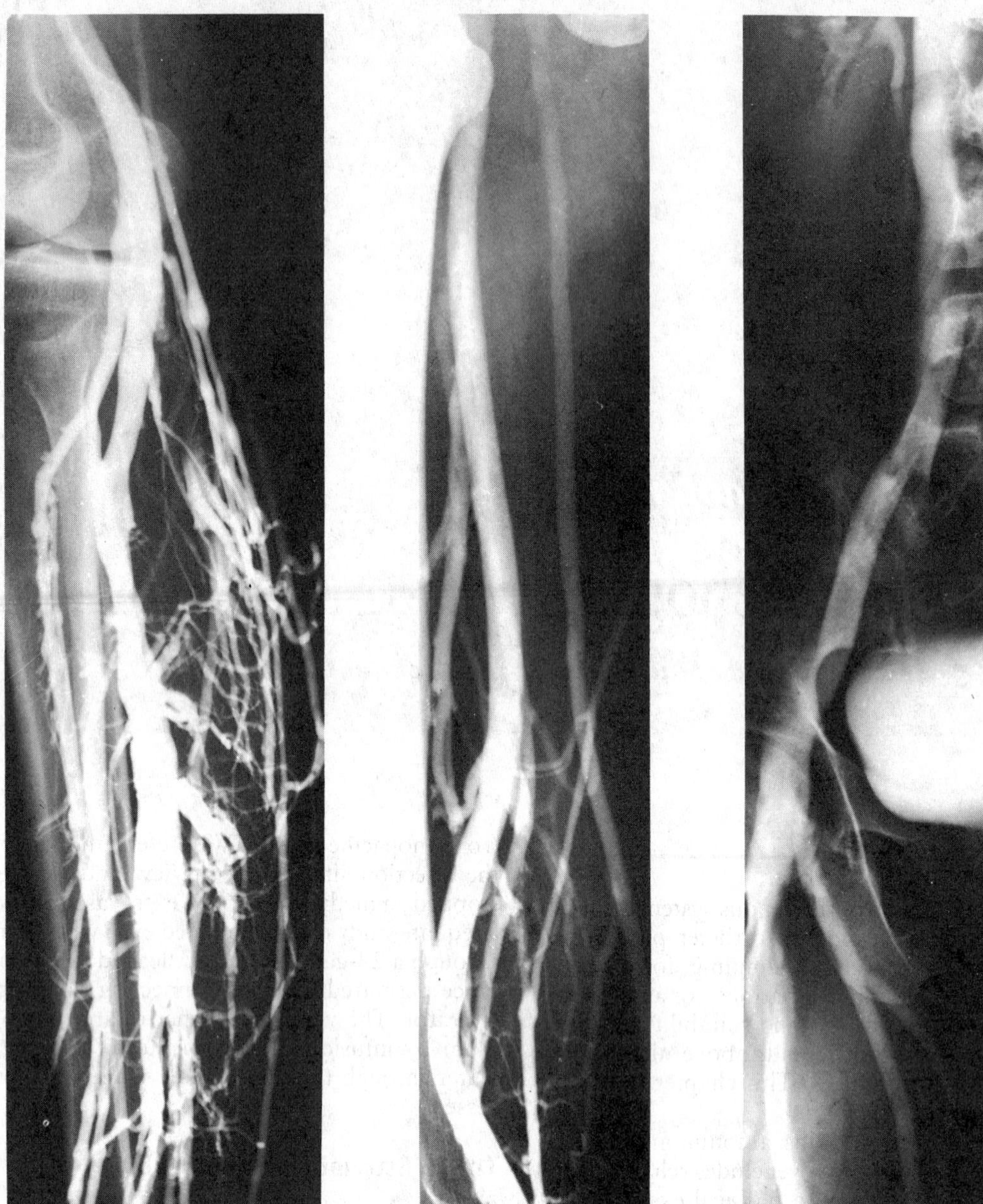

FIGURE 128-1 Normal phlebogram. Note excellent opacification of the entire deep venous system. *A*. Lateral film of the lower leg. *B*. The thigh. *C*. Abdomen and pelvis. Film of the foot and additional views of the calf and thigh, included in all examinations, are not shown.

scribed. Excellent opacification of the entire deep venous system is obtained without fluoroscopy (Fig. 128-1). In the presence of many superficial varicosities, stereoscopic views of the calf may be helpful, or an ankle tourniquet may be used to reduce opacification of the superficial veins. Retrograde injection into a superficial vein of the lower leg, with a tourniquet just below the knee, may provide an alternative to venous cutdown in patients with no available foot veins. We give 30 to 50 mg lidocaine through the same venipuncture site immediately before the contrast medium in order to reduce discomfort and to protect the venous endothelium.[5]

The Rabinov-Paulin technique prevents artifacts due to layering of the contrast medium and to extrinsic compression of intrinsically normal veins by tourniquet or muscle contraction. Consequently, failure to opacify a major deep vein can confidently be attributed to obstruction, *providing* the feeding foot veins have been adequately filled. The foot film serves three important purposes: (1) it permits determination of this filling, (2) it documents presence or absence of injection site extravasation, and (3) it demonstrates disease if present. Deep vein thrombosis limited to pedal veins has been reported in 10 percent of patients whose phlebograms include the foot and has been associated with pulmonary embolism.[6]

Though a large calf hematoma or other mass could lead to obstruction, in the great majority of patients, failure to opacify a deep vein in whole or in part equates with thrombotic occlusion of indeterminate age. Presence of collaterals lends further support to this diagnosis. Demonstration of a broad intraluminal filling defect, characteristically with tapered antegrade tail (Fig.

128-2), permits diagnosis of acute deep vein thrombosis. Destruction of valves and irregular filling defects reflect the postphlebitic state and deep vein incompetence.

RELATION TO OTHER TECHNIQUES

Doppler ultrasound (Chap. 127), impedence plethysmography (Chap. 129), and phleborheography share the advantages of having bedside capability and minimal risk, but the disadvantages of being nonspecific and dependent on alterations in flow for diagnosis. Consequently, the false-negative rate for clots limited to the lower leg is high, extrinsic disease cannot be distinguished from intrinsic venous disease, and nonthrombotic diseases that alter venous flow, such as severe arterial insufficiency or heart failure, may render studies uninterpretable. Color flow duplex ultrasound imaging, which permits determination of the presence or absence of filling defects within the lumen of visualized veins, provides specificity but does not reliably visualize the deep veins of the calf or pelvis.[7] Nonetheless, its high positive predictive value (99 percent) and reasonable sensitivity (93 percent) for femoropopliteal thrombus have made color flow duplex imaging (Chap. 127) a popular initial test for patients with suspected deep vein thrombosis. Phlebography is then reserved for patients with equivocal ultrasound results, negative results in a high-risk setting, or when detection of infrapopliteal or iliac thrombus would alter management. Outcome analysis supports withholding treatment on the basis of a negative compression ultrasound exam.[8] The fibrinogen uptake test (Chap. 134) is also a bedside test with virtually no risk and with a high degree of sensitivity for clots forming below the knee. However, reliable interpretation requires at least a 24-h delay from the time of radionuclide injection; clot outside a vein cannot be distinguished from clot inside a vein (limiting its use in the high-risk orthopedic surgery group); and edema, cellulitis, and arthritis also produce high counts. Magnetic resonance imaging (Chap. 136) is a noninvasive nonbedside examination that demonstrates both intrinsic and extrinsic venous disease as well as unrelated disease (such as calf hematoma) that can mimic venous thrombosis. It has replaced phlebography for evaluation of venous abnormalities in the chest and is the most accurate noninvasive technique for evaluating the inferior vena cava and major pelvic veins.[9,10] Recent studies suggest magnetic resonance may replace diagnostic limb phlebography as scanner access and costs improve.[11] In comparison, phlebography is not a bedside test and carries small, though potentially serious, risks; to date, however, it remains the only widely available technique that is specific and highly accurate and provides an immediate definitive answer. Thus, in the setting of possible deep vein thrombosis today, phlebography is recommended only for cases in which the clinical picture and noninvasive results are discordant, and when such studies are negative in a high-risk setting.

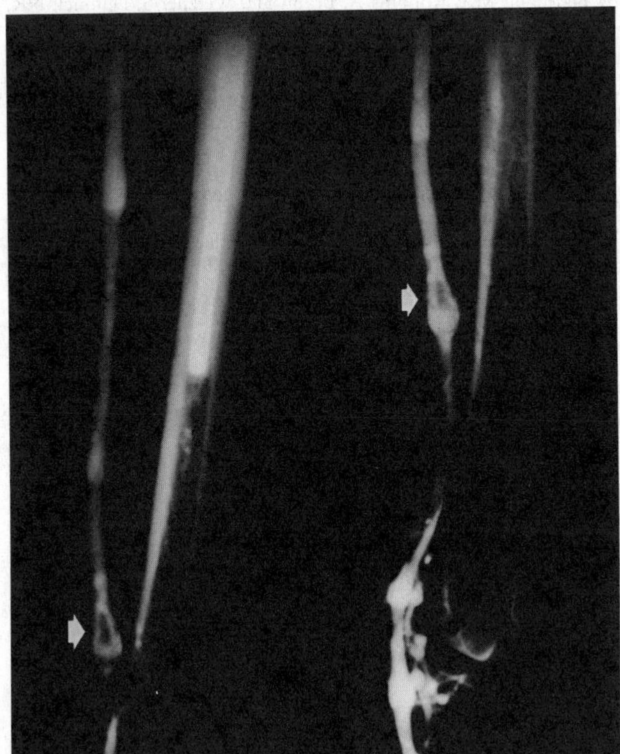

FIGURE 128-2 Acute nonoccluding thrombus in the superficial femoral vein of an asymptomatic patient post ipsilateral hip replacement. Frontal and lateral views of the thigh show a flame-shaped filling defect (arrow) originating in a valve cusp. The sharp border and the typical antegrade taper in two right-angled views distinguish the clot from a defect secondary to inflow of unopacified blood. Impedence plethysmography was normal in this limb.

COMPLICATIONS

In a large prospective study of patients receiving intravenous contrast media, adverse reactions varying from nausea to cardiovascular collapse occurred in 12.7 percent of those receiving ionic agents and 3.1 percent in those receiving nonionics. The incidence of severe reactions was 0.22 percent and 0.04 percent respectively with no contrast-related fatalities.[12] Current data are insufficient to determine a difference in mortality. Though patients with a positive allergy history have twice the incidence of untoward reactions as those without, these reactions are unpredictable and may occur on first exposure to contrast medium or after prior uneventful exposure. Though nonionics cost an order of magnitude more than ionic contrast agents, their use is recommended in medically unstable patients and in those with a history of asthma, allergy, or prior reaction to contrast media.

The hyperosmolality of conventional ionic intravascular agents produces an increase in plasma volume, endothelial injury, and variable degrees of discomfort during injection. The large volume of contrast medium needed for lower limb phlebography can thus cause pulmonary edema in patients in borderline or frank cardiac failure. If phlebography is deemed urgent in such a high-risk patient, pretreatment with intravenous furosemide and use of nonionic contrast medium are recommended. The endothelial injury leads to a mural inflammatory response which, in turn, promotes thrombosis. The variation in the reported incidence of postphlebography thrombosis, from negligible to 48 percent,[13,14] is the result of widely disparate phlebography techniques and criteria for the postphlebographic diagnosis. There is general agreement, however, that (1) damage is lessened by keeping endothelial exposure time minimal; (2) a newly positive fibrinogen uptake test postphlebography reflects mural inflammation, not necessarily with clot; and (3) correlation between the postphlebography syndrome of pain and swelling and evidence of deep vein thrombosis on objective reexamination is poor. The incidence of postphlebography syndrome and of newly positive fibrinogen uptake test, and the magnitude of discomfort during injection, have all been reduced by dilution of standard contrast agents and, most dramatically, by nonionic agents whose osmolality approaches that of blood.[14,15] There is, however, no reduction in objective evidence of postphlebographic thrombosis.[15,16] Administration of heparin has been advocated as a preventive measure,[17] but has not proved protective in our hands.[18] Transient renal failure induced by contrast medium may follow phlebography in patients with preexisting impaired renal function. Good hydration minimizes this risk.

Extravasation of contrast medium at the puncture site causes a chemical cellulitis which may progress to ulceration, necrosis, and, very rarely, gangrene requiring amputation. The likelihood of necrosis is greater in the presence of arterial or venous insufficiency and when extravasation provokes regional vascular spasm. The importance of constant puncture site monitoring cannot be overemphasized. Immediate cessation of injection, elevation, and warm soaks minimize injury.

REFERENCES

1. Kakkar VV: Deep vein thrombosis: Detection and prevention. *Circulation* 1975; 51:8–19.
2. Hull R, Hirsh J, Sackett DL, Taylor DW, Carter C, Turpie AGG, et al: Clinical validity of a negative venogram in patients with clinically suspected venous thrombosis. *Circulation* 1981; 64:622–625.
3. Lea Thomas M: *Phlebography of the Lower Limb.* Edinburgh, Churchill Livingstone, 1982: 85.
4. Rabinov K, Paulin S: Roentgen diagnosis of venous thrombosis in the leg. *Arch Surg* 1972; 104:134–144.
5. Ritchie WGM: The effect of contrast media on normal and inflamed canine veins. *Invest Radiol* 1974; 9:444–455.
6. Lea Thomas M, O'Dwyer JA: A phlebographic study of the incidence and significance of venous thrombosis in the foot. *Am J Roentgenol* 1978; 130:751–754.
7. Rose SC, Zwiebel WJ, Nelson BD, Priest DL, Knighton RA, Brown JW, et al: Symptomatic lower extremity deep vein thrombosis: accuracy, limitations, and role of color flow Doppler imaging in diagnosis. *Radiology* 1990; 175:639–644.
8. Vaccaro JP, Cronan JJ, Dorfman GS: Outcome analysis of patients with normal compression ultrasound examinations. *Radiology* 1990; 175:645–649.
9. Brammer WM: Diagnosing deep venous thrombosis in the 1990s. *J Okla State Med Assoc* 1991; 84:101–106.
10. Kabala JE, Gillatt DA, Persad RA, Penry JB, Gingell JC, Chadwick D: Magnetic resonance imaging in the staging of renal cell carcinoma. *Br J Radiol* 1991; 64:683–689.
11. Vukov LF, Berquist TH, King BF: Magnetic resonance imaging for calf deep venous thrombophlebitis. *Ann Emerg Med* 1991; 20:497–499.
12. Katayama H, Yamaguchi K, Kozuka T, Takashima T, Seez P, Matsuura K: Adverse reactions to ionic and nonionic contrast media. *Radiology* 1990; 175:621–628.
13. Lea Thomas M: *Phlebography of the Lower Limb.* Edinburgh, Churchill Livingstone, 1982: 54.
14. Albrechtsson U, Fagher B, Lagerstedt C, Larusdottir H, Olsson CG, Westling H, et al: Double-blind comparison between Iohexol and Metrizoate in phlebography of the lower limb. *Acta Rad* 1983; 366(suppl):58–64.
15. Bettmann MA, Robbins A, Braun SD, Wetzner S, Dunnick NR, Finkelstein J: Contrast venography of the leg: Diagnostic efficacy, tolerance, and complication rates with ionic and nonionic contrast media. *Radiology* 1987; 165:113–116.
16. Hagen B: Systemic and local reactions during phlebography of the legs with special regard to delayed complications. *Radiology* 1985; 23:260–264.
17. Minar E, Ehringer H, Sommer G, Marosi L, Czembirek H: Prevention of postvenographic thrombosis by heparin flush: Fibrinogen uptake measurement. *Am J Roentgenol* 1984; 143:629–632.
18. Ritchie WGM, Soulen RL, Rogers PW: Effect of phlebography on the ^{125}I uptake test. *Am J Roentgenol* 1979; 133:855–858.

Chapter 129

Impedance Plethysmography

Thom W. Rooke, M.D.

Over the past 30 years impedance plethysmography (IPG) has become the best studied and most widely employed of the so-called functional diagnostic tests for deep venous thrombosis.[1-3] Unlike "anatomic" tests such as venography or echo Doppler (duplex) ultrasound scanning (i.e., tests that directly image the thrombi), functional tests like IPG identify the presence of venous thrombi by detecting the hemodynamic abnormalities they produce. Because IPG relies on indirect evidence of venous obstruction, it is subject to more false positives and negatives than are imaging tests; nevertheless, the ease of performance, low cost, and reasonable overall accuracy continue to make IPG a useful screening and/or diagnostic tool in appropriate settings.

PRINCIPLES

The basic principles that underlie IPG are relatively simple.[4] A high-frequency, low-intensity electrical current (too weak to be felt by the subject) is passed between two electrodes that encircle the lower limb (Fig. 129-1). Encircling the limb within these electrodes are two other electrodes between which voltage measurements are made. The magnitude of the voltage difference between these "measuring" electrodes is dependent upon the electrical impedance of the underlying limb as predicted by Ohm's law; in turn, the electrical impedance is dependent upon the volume of blood (or other fluid) within the limb. Changes in limb blood volume thus change the electrical impedance and voltage.

To test for the presence of deep venous thrombosis, the patient lies supine with the legs slightly flexed and elevated. A pneumatic compression cuff is placed around the thigh and inflated to a pressure above that of venous pressure but below arterial pressure (typically 40 to 60 mmHg); this produces venous occlusion (i.e., during cuff inflation blood can flow into the leg but not out). As blood becomes trapped distal to the cuff, the volume of the leg increases and the electrical impedance and voltage change (Fig. 129-2*A*). After a certain inflation period (typically 1 to 2 min), the cuff is rapidly deflated and

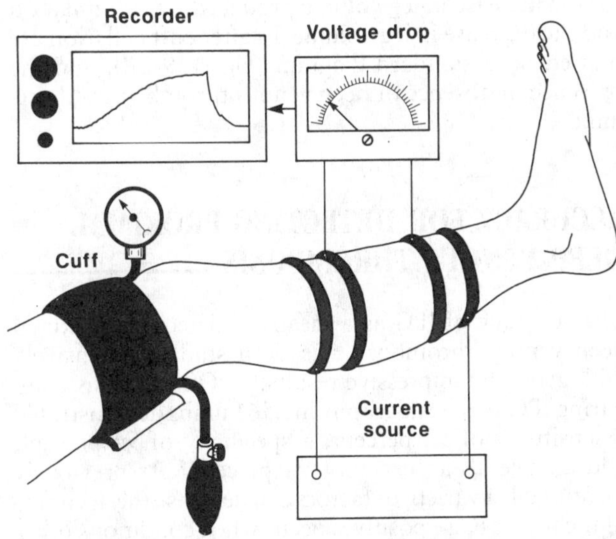

FIGURE 129-1 Schematic representation of IPG. A high-frequency, low-intensity electrical current is passed between the two outer electrodes, and the voltage change is measured between the two inner electrodes. An inflatable thigh cuff is used to produce venous occlusion.

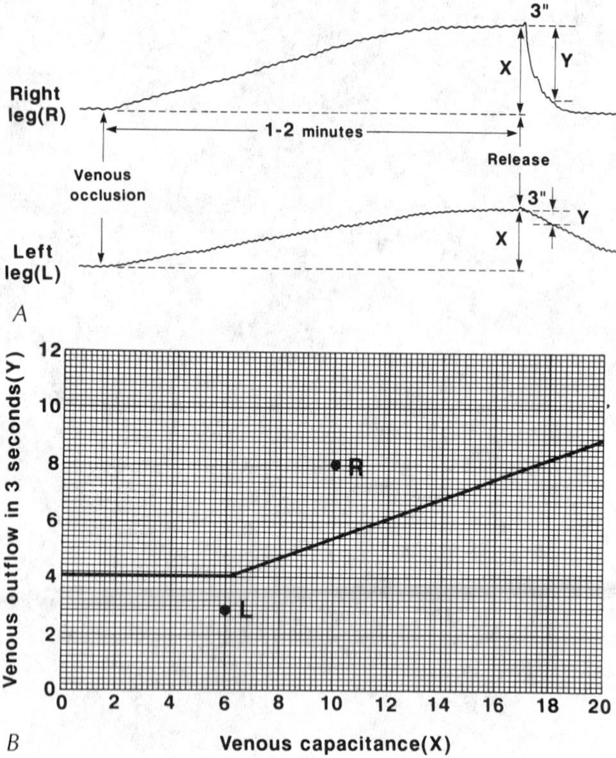

FIGURE 129-2 *A.* An IPG tracing from a normal right limb (above) and an obstructed left limb (below). When venous obstruction is present, IPG is typically affected in two ways. (1) The rise in leg volume occurring during venous occlusion is decreased (because the deep venous thrombosis has already occluded venous outflow and thus causes limb distension and a reduction in limb compliance). (2) The decrease in leg volume occurring during the first 3 s following cuff deflation is reduced (i.e., the rate of venous outflow is reduced). *B.* The changes in volume produced by cuff inflation and deflation can be plotted on a standard diagram. The line separating normal (above) from abnormal (below) has been empirically derived by comparing IPG results from limbs with and without deep venous thrombosis, as determined using a "gold standard" such as venography for the diagnosis.

venous flow is allowed to resume. As blood drains from the limb, the volume and voltage rapidly change. Values for the increase in leg volume produced by cuff inflation and the decrease in leg volume 3 s after cuff deflation are plotted on a standard diagram (Fig. 129-2*B*), and the presence or absence of deep venous thrombosis is determined.

ACCURACY FOR DETECTING PROXIMAL DEEP VENOUS THROMBOSIS

The accuracy of IPG as a means of detecting proximal deep venous thrombosis has been studied extensively with generally impressive results.[1,5-7] One analysis comparing IPG with venography in 2561 limbs demonstrated a sensitivity of 93 percent, a specificity of 94 percent, and an overall accuracy of 94 percent.[1] As previously mentioned, a variety of factors can decrease the accuracy of the test.[8,9] False positives occur when conditions other than acute deep venous thrombosis cause or mimic venous obstruction; the most common examples of these include elevated pressure from congestive heart failure or any other cause (this usually gives a bilaterally positive result), extrinsic vein compression, or "old" nonrecanalized venous thrombi. In contrast, false-negative tests are usually due to below-the-knee (distal) thrombi or nonoccluding proximal thrombi. As one would predict, the accuracy of IPG is variable and depends upon the subgroup of patients being studied.[10,11] For example, although there is ample documentation that the test is useful when applied to symptomatic patients,[1] concern has been raised about its reliability as a tool for screening high-risk asymptomatic patients.[12] Other pitfalls to testing include unsuitable body habitus (such as morbid obesity or severe limb edema) and inability on the part of the patient to cooperate during the examination (as occurs with patients who are comatose or in those with severely reduced limb mobility due to recent limb fracture, joint replacement, or other cause).

PROGNOSTIC VALUE FOR PREDICTING PULMONARY EMBOLISM

Despite potential pitfalls with its sensitivity and specificity, IPG appears to offer considerable prognostic information about the likelihood of a subsequent pulmonary embolism in patients suspected of having deep venous thrombosis. (See also Chap. 100.) In one report involving

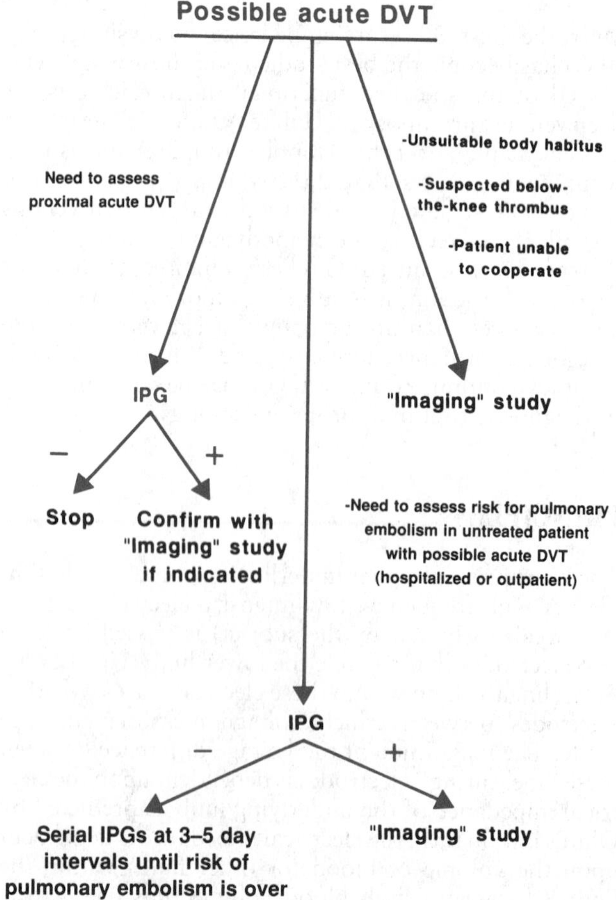

FIGURE 129-3 Algorithm for the use of IPG in the diagnosis of acute deep venous thrombosis (DVT). (See also Chap. 100.)

short-term follow-up on 1074 patients with bilaterally negative IPG there were no fatal pulmonary emboli and only a 1 percent incidence of clinical suspicion for nonfatal pulmonary emboli. Other plethysmographic (i.e., functional) techniques, such as strain gauge plethysmography or phleborheography, have demonstrated similar good results.[1]

CONCLUSIONS

In summary, the IPG remains best suited for use with cooperative, anatomically suitable patients in whom there is either a clinical suspicion of acute proximal deep venous thrombosis or a need to demonstrate that the patient is not at high risk for pulmonary embolism if anticoagulation therapy is withheld.[13,14] The algorithm in Fig. 129-3 has proven to be a useful guideline for the clinical application of the test. Note that IPG is not recommended for making the diagnosis of calf deep venous thrombosis or in situations where body habitus or poor cooperation makes testing difficult. In addition, abnormal IPG should usually be verified with ultrasound duplex scanning or venography, especially in situations where congestive heart failure, bilaterally positive IPG,[15] extrinsic compression, or other causes of false-positive findings are possible. (See also Chap. 100.)

REFERENCES

1. Wheeler HB, Anderson FA Jr: Can noninvasive tests be used as the basis for treatment of deep vein thrombosis? In: Bernstein EF (ed): *Noninvasive Diagnostic Techniques in Vascular Disease,* 3d ed. St. Louis, CV Mosby, 1985: 805–818.
2. Rosner NH, Doris PE: Diagnosis of femoropopliteal venous thrombosis: Comparison of duplex sonography and plethysmography. *Am J Roentgenol* 1988; 150:623–627.
3. Hirsh J: Diagnosis of venous thrombosis and pulmonary embolism. *Am J Cardiol* 1990; 65:45C–49C.
4. Wheeler HB, Penny BC: Impedance plethysmography: Theoretic, experimental, and clinical considerations. In: Bernstein EF (ed): *Noninvasive Diagnostic Techniques in Vascular Disease,* 3d ed. St. Louis, CV Mosby, 1985: 119–132.
5. Huss RD, Raskob GE, LeClerc JR, Jay RM, Hirsh J: The diagnosis of clinically suspected venous thrombosis. *Clin Chest Med* 1984; 5:439–456.
6. Izzo KL, Aquino E: Deep venous thrombosis in high-risk hemiplegic patients: Detection by impedance plethysmography. *Arch Phys Med Rehab* 1986; 67:799–802.
7. Brown JG, Ward PE, Wilkinson AJ, Mollan RAB: Impedance plethysmography. *J Bone Joint Surg (Br)* 1987; 69:264–267.
8. Patterson RB, Fowl RJ, Keller JD, Schomaker W, Kempczinski RF: The limitations of impedance plethysmography in the diagnosis of acute deep venous thrombosis. *J Vasc Surg* 1989; 9:725–730.
9. Vaccaro P, Van Aman M, Miller S, Fachman J, Smead WL: Shortcomings of physical examination and impedance plethysmography in the diagnosis of lower extremity deep venous thrombosis. *Angiology* 1987; 38:232–235.
10. Comerota AJ, Katz ML, Greenwald LL, Leefmans E, Czeredarczuk M, White JV: Venous duplex imaging: Should it replace hemodynamic tests for deep venous thrombosis? *J Vasc Surg* 1990; 11:53–61.
11. Comeroto AJ, Knight LC, Maurer AH: The diagnosis of acute deep venous thrombosis: Noninvasive and radioisotopic techniques. *Ann Vasc Surg* 1988; 2:406–424.
12. Comerota AJ, Katz ML, Grossi RJ, White JV, Czeredarczuk M, Bowman G, et al: The comparative value of noninvasive testing for diagnosis and surveillance of deep vein thrombosis. *J Vasc Surg* 1988; 7:40–49.
13. Hull RD, Raskob GE, Carter CJ: Serial impedance plethysmography in pregnant patients with clinically suspected deep vein thrombosis. *Ann Intern Med* 1990; 112:663–667.
14. Huisman MV, Buller HR, Ten Cate JW, Vreeken J: Serial impedance plethysmography for suspected deep venous thrombosis in outpatients. *N Engl J Med* 1986: 314:823–828.
15. Curley FJ, Pratter MR, Irwin RS, Anderson FA Jr, Phillips DA, Doherty PW, et al: The clinical implications of bilaterally abnormal impedance plethysmography. *Arch Intern Med* 1987; 147:125–129.

PART XIX

Special Diagnostic Ultrasound Techniques Used in the Evaluation of the Cardiovascular System

Chapter 130

Technique of Doppler and Color Flow Doppler in the Evaluation of Cardiac Disorders and Function

Alan S. Pearlman, M.D.

The use of ultrasonic techniques for cardiovascular diagnosis is termed *echocardiography*. This term actually refers to two broad families of techniques: echocardiographic *imaging* of cardiovascular structure and dynamics (Chap. 15), and *Doppler* echocardiographic assessment of cardiovascular blood flow direction and velocity. These diagnostic methods are complementary rather than competitive and are best used in an integrated fashion.

TECHNIQUE

This chapter emphasizes the clinical applications of Doppler echocardiography, but a brief review of certain technical features is appropriate. Doppler physics and instrumentation are discussed more fully elsewhere.[1]

Doppler Principles

The cardiac chambers and great vessels appear sonolucent in echocardiographic images because blood cells are too small to reflect ultrasonic waves of the frequencies used in clinical practice. Blood cells do cause *scattering* of ultrasonic energy, however, much as fog droplets cause scattering of light. Although only small amounts of the incident energy are scattered back to the ultrasound transducer, this does provide a means to record the direction and velocity of blood cell motion.

Johann Christian Doppler, an Austrian physicist, studied the motion of the stars by analyzing the color of the light they emitted. He hypothesized that the motion of a star away from an observer on Earth would increase the wavelength (and thus reduce the frequency) of the light it emitted. Conversely, motion of a star toward Earth would shorten the wavelength (and increase the frequency) of its emitted light. Thus, an observer on Earth would perceive that stars had different colors, depending on their direction of motion.

Adaptation of Doppler's theory to acoustics forms the basis for Doppler echocardiography. When an ultrasound beam encounters moving blood cells, the frequency of the ultrasonic energy scattered back to the transducer differs from that of the originally broadcast ultrasound. The difference in frequencies is termed the *Doppler shift*; its magnitude is determined by the direction and velocity of blood flow, according to the Doppler equation:

$$V = \frac{C(F_r - F_t)}{2F_t(\cos\theta)}$$

where V is the blood velocity, C is the speed of sound in soft tissue (approximately 1540 m/s), F_r is the frequency of return signal, F_t is the frequency of transmitted signal, and θ is the intercept angle between the direction of blood flow and the ultrasound beam.

The quantity $F_r - F_t$ is the Doppler shift, or ΔF. Note that F_t is a constant frequency determined by the ultrasonic transducer, while C is essentially uniform in soft tissue (including blood). When these constants are combined and expressed as k, the Doppler equation can be rewritten as $\triangle F = kV \cos \theta$. Angle θ must therefore be determined in order to calculate blood flow velocity from the measured Doppler shift. The cosine function is maximum (1.0) when angle $\theta = 0$; as θ increases, its cosine decreases in a nonlinear fashion. Therefore, the Doppler shift measured by the ultrasonic instrument is maximum when angle θ is as near as possible to 0 (or 180°). As θ increases from 0, its cosine decreases and so does the measured Doppler shift. At an intercept angle of 90° ($\cos 90° = 0$), no Doppler shift is recorded, regardless of blood flow velocity. In practice, the ultrasound instrument measures the Doppler shift, assumes that $\cos \theta = 1.0$, and calculates flow velocity from the Doppler equation.

Most echocardiographic devices integrate Doppler echocardiography with two-dimensional imaging. Even when blood flow direction is demonstrated using Doppler color flow imaging, tomographic views demonstrate cardiac structures only in two dimensions. The intercept angle between the ultrasound beam and the blood flow direction is a three-dimensional angle, however, and the true spatial intercept angle cannot be measured directly with current echocardiographic techniques. If blood flow velocity is determined from the measured Doppler frequency shift, the *calculated* velocity can never be larger than *actual* velocity so long as $\cos \theta$ is assumed to be 1.0 (i.e., angle $\theta = 0$). If angle correction is attempted by visually estimating angle θ and substituting its cosine in the Doppler equation, then it is possible for the *calculated* velocity to be equal to, smaller than, or larger than the *actual* velocity, depending on the accuracy of the angle estimate. Most investigators do not use angle correction, but rather try to align the Doppler beam with the direction of blood flow and adjust angulation so as to record the maximum Doppler shifts. When no higher flow velocity can be detected despite diligent searching from multiple orientations, the operator assumes that a near-zero intercept angle has been achieved.

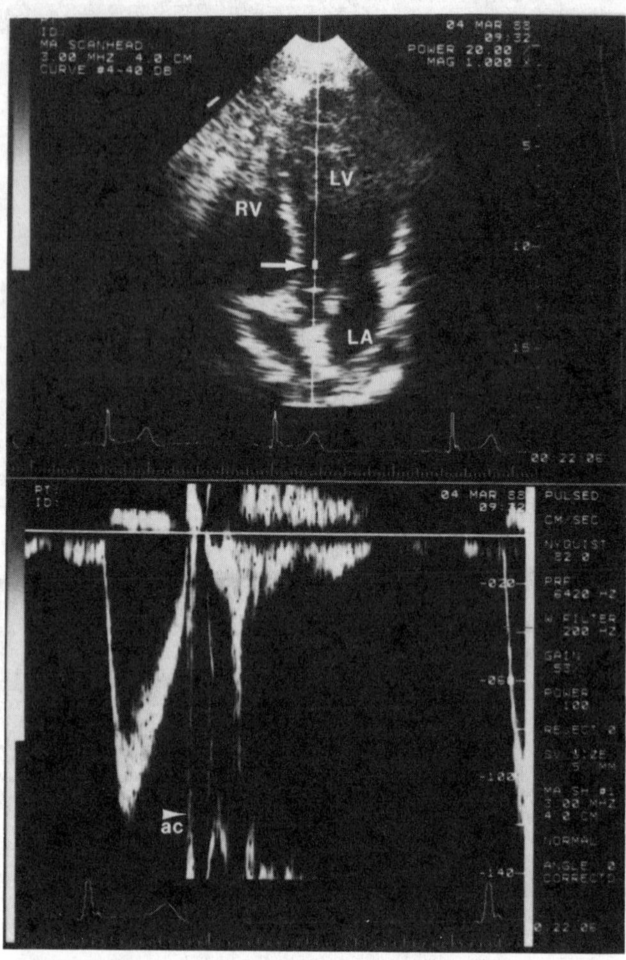

FIGURE 130-1 Normal left ventricular outflow, pulsed wave Doppler recording. *Top*: Apical five-chamber image, showing orientation of the Doppler cursor. Doppler shifts are recorded from the region of the sample volume (arrow) in the outflow tract of the left ventricle. LV, left ventricle; LA, left atrium; RV, right ventricle. *Bottom*: Spectral Doppler recording of velocity in centimeters per second (vertical axis) as a function of time (horizontal axis). During systole, flow away from the transducer is shown as a deflection below the baseline. The spectrum is narrow during the acceleration phase of ejection and shows minimal broadening during deceleration. The timing of aortic closure (ac) (arrowhead) coincides with the end of anterograde systolic flow.

Doppler Outputs

Clinical instruments detect Doppler shifts not from individual blood cells but rather from groups of blood cells passing through the ultrasound beam. When adjacent blood cells move with velocities and directions similar to those of their neighbors, a situation termed *organized* (or *laminar*) *flow*, the moving blood cells all cause similar Doppler shifts. As blood flow accelerates and decelerates during the cardiac cycle (Fig. 130-1), the corresponding Doppler shifts (and flow velocities) are relatively uniform at any instant. When adjacent blood cells move with varying velocities or in differing directions, a situation termed *disturbed* (or *turbulent*) *flow*, they cause a broad spectrum of simultaneous Doppler shift frequencies (Fig. 130-2). Accordingly, Doppler echocardiography can be used to determine not only the direction and velocity but also the pattern (organized vs. disturbed) of blood flow.

Doppler echocardiography typically employs transducers that emit ultrasound frequencies in the range of 2 to 5 million cycles per second. The magnitude of the Doppler shifts induced by flowing blood is within the audible range (0 to 20,000 cycles per second). Organized flow causes tonal (musical) signals, while disorganized flow causes a broad spectrum of noisy (dissonant) signals. An appreciation of the pitch, quality, and timing of the Doppler shifts helps the examiner to recognize, optimize, and record the Doppler signals. More precise measurement of the velocity and timing of blood flow requires a graphic output. Such a graphic display is generated by means of frequency spectrum analysis techniques, which provide a record of blood velocity as a function of time (Fig. 130-1). By convention, blood flow toward the transducer is plotted above the zero-velocity baseline, while flow away from the transducer is plotted below the baseline. Doppler signal intensity is depicted in gray scales. A simultaneous electrocardiographic tracing is recorded to aid in timing.

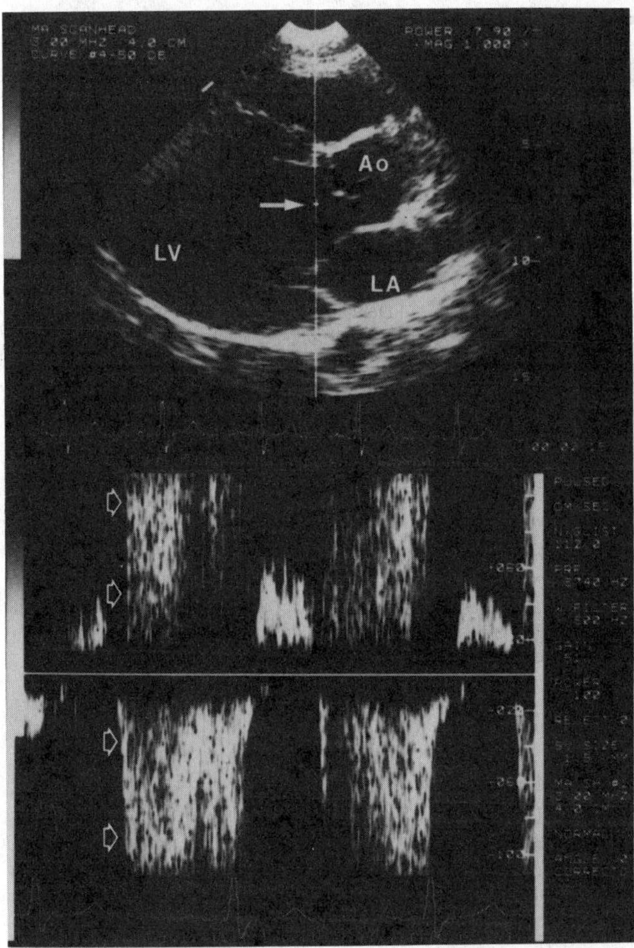

FIGURE 130-2 Aortic regurgitation, pulsed wave Doppler recording. *Top:* Parasternal long-axis image, showing orientation of the Doppler cursor and location of the sample volume (arrow) in the center of the outflow tract, on the left ventricular side of the aortic leaflets. LV, left ventricle; Ao, aorta; LA, left atrium. *Bottom:* Spectral Doppler recording. Diastolic regurgitant flow is disturbed, and thus multidirectional, causing a broad spectrum of Doppler shifts (open arrows) that last through diastole.

It is possible to record Doppler signals from multiple locations, almost simultaneously. Tomographic Doppler echocardiographic "images" of blood flow velocity and direction are displayed in color. Color Doppler can also be used to examine flow at multiple sites along a given scan line, with the resultant signals displayed in a color time-motion (Q/M) format.

Doppler Instrumentation

Most ultrasound instruments can be used for both echocardiographic imaging and Doppler blood flow evaluation. Four basic Doppler modalities are available. The user can select among these modes and use them as needed to answer the clinical question(s). It may be necessary to use special transducers in order to optimize certain Doppler modes.

Pulsed Wave Doppler

Pulsed wave Doppler (PWD) uses a single piezoelectric element alternately as transmitter and receiver. A brief burst of ultrasound is emitted by the transducer, which then switches automatically to function as a receiver until signals from the depth of interest have returned to the transducer. The cycle then repeats. Since the speed of sound in soft tissue and blood is essentially constant, the time required for an ultrasonic burst to travel to a given depth, interact with moving blood cells, and return to the transducer defines the distance between the transducer and the region of Doppler sampling. The sampling rate is related inversely to the transit time from the transducer to the depth of interest and back. The return signal is analyzed for Doppler shifts only during a brief time period, whose onset can be adjusted in relation to the time of burst emission. Accordingly, Doppler shifts can be measured at specific points along the axis of the ultrasound beam. The region of Doppler sampling is termed the *sample volume*; its position is indicated along a cursor line superimposed on a two-dimensional image of the heart (Fig. 130-1). The major advantage of PWD is its ability to record flow velocity and direction at specific locations within the cardiac chambers or great vessels. Pulsed wave Doppler has a relatively slow sampling rate, however, limiting its utility for quantitating high flow velocities.

Continuous Wave Doppler

Continuous wave Doppler (CWD) employs a transducer that includes two piezoelectric crystals (or groups of crystals): One functions constantly as a transmitter, while the other acts constantly as a receiver. The instrument continuously compares the frequencies of backscattered ultrasound signals to that of the broadcast sound energy and calculates the corresponding blood flow velocities. Because CWD detects Doppler shifts from all blood cells that move through the ultrasound beam, regardless of their distance from the transducer, a CWD velocity curve displays a variety of simultaneous velocities (Fig. 130-3). Continuous wave Doppler is ideal for recording high flow velocities because of its high sampling rate. Unfortunately, CWD provides no range information; the examiner cannot determine with certainty where along the ultrasound beam the recorded signals originated. Continuous wave Doppler and PWD are quite complementary, since the limitations of one technique are the strengths of the other.

High Pulse Repetition Frequency Doppler

High pulse repetition frequency (HPRF) Doppler is a modified PWD technique developed to record high flow velocities while retaining some range specificity.[2] In conventional PWD, the rate at which successive ultrasound bursts can be emitted—the *pulse repetition frequency (PRF)*— is determined by the depth of the sample volume; the deeper the region of interest, the lower the PRF. High pulse repetition frequency Doppler utilizes the fact that blood cells moving through the sample volume do not scatter all of the ultrasonic energy back to the transducer. Some of the energy continues along the original line of transmission, and this can be used to interrogate flowing blood at a greater depth. For example, consider recording flow just below the aortic valve leaflets, 12 cm

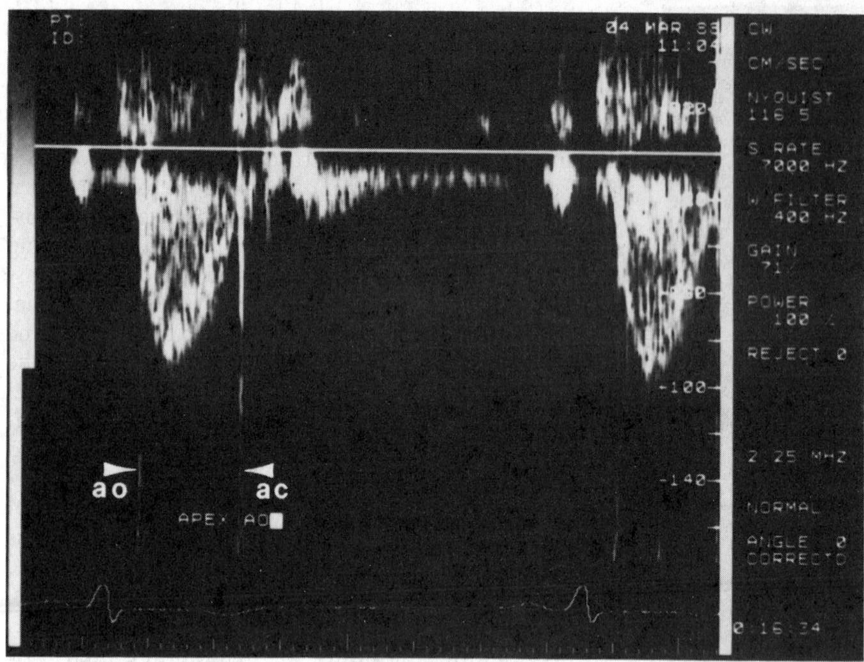

FIGURE 130-3 Normal left ventricular outflow, continuous wave Doppler, recorded from the same subject as in Fig. 130-1, using a nonimaging Doppler transducer to orient the ultrasound beam across the left ventricular outflow tract and aortic valve. Systolic ejection flow velocities appear below the baseline and are enveloped by clicks representing aortic opening and aortic closure. ao, aortic opening; ac, aortic closure. Since Doppler shifts are recorded along the entire ultrasound beam, a broad spectrum of velocities is recorded with the highest velocities arising in the narrowest area. Signals from flow across the mitral valve, adjacent to the left ventricular outflow tract, can be seen above the baseline in diastole.

from the transducer, from the cardiac apex (Fig. 130-4*A*). If flow velocity at this site were too high to be recorded accurately by standard PWD, the examiner could place the primary sample volume at 6 cm depth (Fig. 130-4*B*). Ultrasound energy from a given pulse would arrive at this depth approximately 40 μs after it left the transducer, and backscattered signals would return to the transducer 80 μs after pulse emission. At the same time, some of the ultrasound energy from the original emission would arrive at the level of the left ventricular outflow tract, 12 cm from the transducer. Backscattered energy from this site would arrive back at the transducer at exactly the same time as energy from the second burst returned to the transducer from the 6-cm depth. In this way, the sampling rate determined by a 6-cm sample volume depth (double that usually available at 12 cm) can be used to examine at both 6 and 12 cm. Similarly, by placing the primary sample volume at 4 cm, the examiner can sample simultaneously at depths of 4, 8, and 12 cm, thereby tripling the PRF usually available at 12 cm (Fig. 130-4C). Usually HPRF Doppler is implemented so that signal strength declines as PRF is increased, a characteristic that sometimes limits its utility. However, HPRF Doppler allows measurement of high velocities selectively from two serial stenoses, such as subaortic and valvular aortic stenosis. Moreover, its relatively narrow beam pattern occasionally makes HPRF Doppler useful in distinguishing between two high-velocity jets that lie adjacent to each other, such as medially directed mitral regurgitation and forward ejection across a stenotic aortic valve.

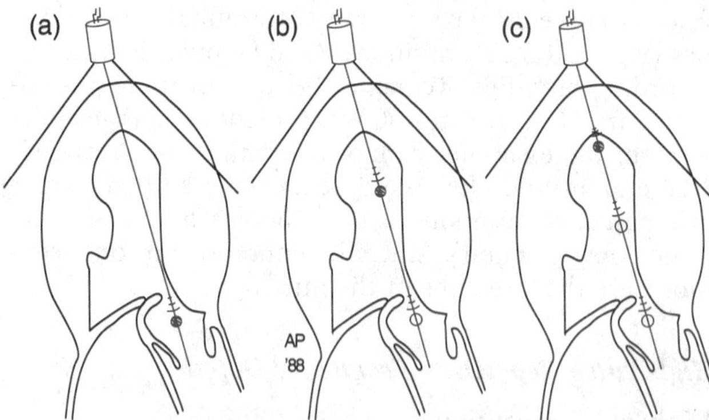

FIGURE 130-4 Schematic illustrating examination of left ventricular ejection flow in obstructive hypertrophic cardiomyopathy using high pulse repetition frequency pulsed Doppler. *A.* Apical long-axis schematic showing the sample volume (shaded circle) positioned in the left ventricular outflow chamber, 12 cm from the transducer. *B.* The primary sample volume has been repositioned at the level of the papillary muscle base, 6 cm from the transducer, thereby doubling the pulse repetition frequency compared to that of *A*. At this higher sampling rate, left ventricular outflow can be interrogated by a secondary sample volume (open circle). *C.* The primary sample volume is positioned in the left ventricular apex, 4 cm from the transducer, thereby tripling the sampling rate of *A* and creating two secondary sample volumes (open circles) at 8- and 12-cm depth. This approach can allow interrogation of high-velocity flow, with a sampling frequency high enough to prevent aliasing, while retaining some range specificity.

Doppler Color Flow Imaging

Another modified pulsed Doppler technique, color flow imaging (CFI), provides real-time, two-dimensional images of flowing blood. Other synonyms include *color flow Doppler, color flow mapping*, and *two-dimensional Doppler*. In essence, CFI uses pulsed Doppler to record blood flow direction and velocity at a series of several hundred sequential sampling depths along a given ultrasound beam. Beam direction is scanned rapidly across an examining sector. In this fashion, blood flow can be interrogated in real time at a large number of depths across a wedge-shaped, variable-sized (typically 30° to 60°) sector of view. Because frequency spectrum analysis is computationally complex and time consuming, Doppler CFI instead employs an instantaneous frequency estimator to determine the dominant frequency at each of the sample sites along each individual scan line. Usually, the Doppler shift between successive samples at each sampling depth is estimated using an autocorrelation technique. For display purposes, velocity components directed toward the transducer are assigned one primary color, while flow velocities directed away from the transducer are assigned a different color. Since each site is sampled four to eight times in rapid succession, variance in the Doppler shifts (which may indicate flow disorganization, as occurs secondary to valvular obstruction, regurgitation, or intracardiac shunting) can be encoded by admixing a third primary color with those denoting flow direction. In one popular display format (Plate X, 130-1) flow toward the transducer is encoded in red and flow away from the transducer is encoded in blue. Brighter shades are assigned to higher velocities. Disturbed flow is denoted by admixture of green-yellow shades, causing a mosaic of turquoise-blue and red-orange colors. These colors are then mapped onto a two-dimensional echocardiographic sector image. Although it is a tomographic technique, Doppler CFI bears a superficial resemblance to angiographic imaging.

Doppler examinations are best performed in conjunction with two-dimensional echocardiography (Chap. 15), which provides an anatomic orientation. Proper positioning of the transducer depends on the information sought. To measure flow velocity, one must use examining windows that align the ultrasound beam coaxial with the direction of blood flow. To detect regions of flow disturbance in which blood cells move in multiple directions, a variety of examining windows should be used.

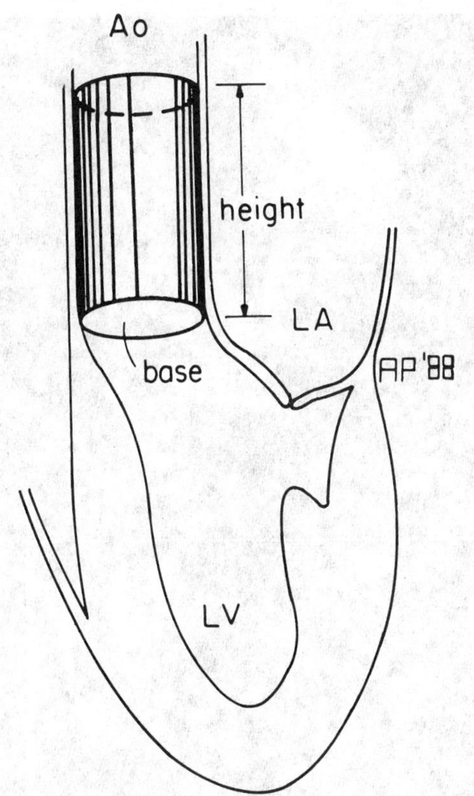

FIGURE 130-5 Diagram illustrating the concept of ultrasonic stroke volume measurement. Blood ejected from the left ventricle during a single systole would fill a segment of aorta whose shape is cylindrical. Thus, stroke volume could be determined by measuring the base and height of this cylinder. LV, ventricle; Ao, aorta; LA, left atrium.

HEMODYNAMIC MEASURES AVAILABLE FROM DOPPLER DATA

A number of important hemodynamic measures can be made by using Doppler echocardiographic data. Most of these measures are derived from spectral (pulsed or continuous wave) Doppler velocity curves. Useful information also can be obtained by analyzing regions of normal and disturbed flow.

Stroke Volume Determination

Doppler echocardiographic measurement of stroke volume is conceptually straightforward.[3] Consider ejection of blood into the ascending aorta, for example. If the aorta were a straight tube of uniform diameter, then the blood propelled out of the left ventricle during a single systole would fill a cylindrical volume (Fig. 130-5). This volume could be calculated as the product of base times height. The base would represent the area (A) of a cross section of the aortic root, determined from aortic diameter (D) according to the formula $A = \pi (D/2)^2$. The height of the cylinder can be determined from the Doppler flow velocity curve; since velocity measures distance per unit time, the integral of velocity is a measure of distance. Thus, the area under the systolic velocity-time curve represents the *stroke distance*, the distance that an average blood cell travels during systole.

The technical requirements for accurate ultrasonic measurement of stroke volume deserve emphasis. Cross-sectional area and flow velocity-time integral should be measured at the same intracardiac site. For example, if PWD is used to record systolic flow velocity in the ascending aorta, then aortic diameter should be measured at the level of the sample volume (Fig. 130-6). If CWD is used to record aortic flow velocity, however, aortic diameter should be measured at the narrowest part of the aorta since the highest flow velocity, which determines the outer edge of the CWD tracing, occurs in the narrowest portion of the vessel. Diameter is squared in calculating cross-sectional area, so the examiner must record and measure diameters with great care, ideally employing those imaging windows that allow measurement of dimensions using axial rather than lateral ultrasound resolution. Unfortunately, accurate determination of flow velocity requires that the ultrasound beam be parallel to the direction of flow. Accordingly, dimension measures and flow velocities often are recorded from different examining windows, nonsimultaneously. Beat-to-beat changes in stroke volume due to varying filling periods or altered loading conditions can influence the accuracy of measurement.

Doppler determination of stroke volume is based on several important assumptions. Since the ultrasound

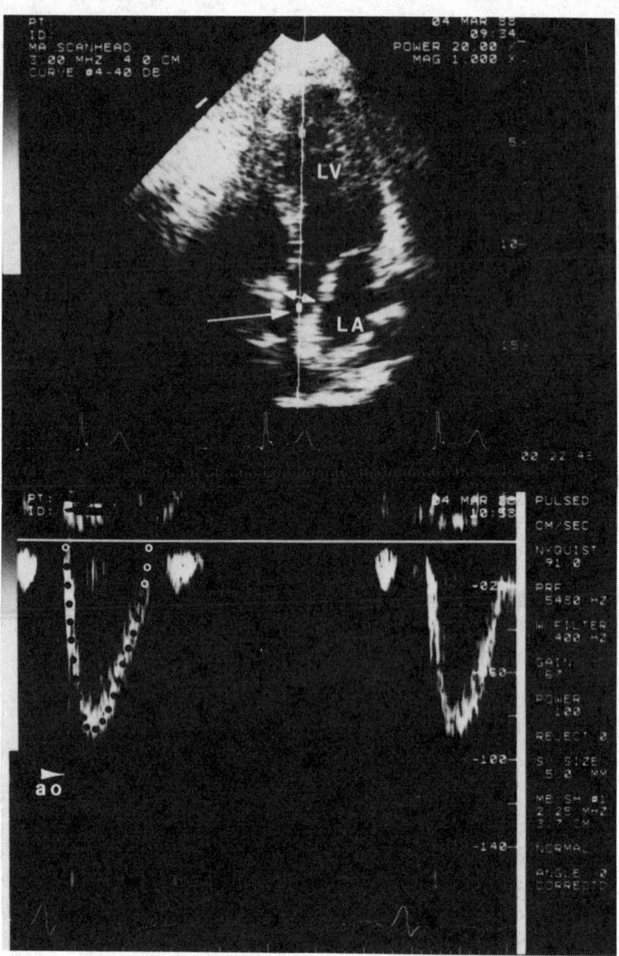

FIGURE 130-6 Normal ascending aortic flow, pulsed wave Doppler recording. *Top*: Apical four-chamber image, showing orientation of the Doppler cursor. The sample volume (long arrow) is positioned in the ascending aorta. Aortic diameter (double-headed arrow) could be measured from this view if needed for stroke volume determination, but a high parasternal long-axis view would be preferable. *Bottom*: Systolic flow shows brisk acceleration with a narrow spectrum and minimal spectral broadening during deceleration. The velocity-time integral, determined by tracing the area enclosed by the curve (dots added for emphasis), represents the stroke distance. Note the aortic opening (arrowhead) click that coincides with rapid flow acceleration and denotes the location of the sample volume just beyond the aortic valve plane. ao, aortic opening; LV, left ventricle; LA, left atrium.

beam must be aligned coaxially with the direction of blood flow, the examiner assumes that blood flow parallels the walls of the cardiac chambers and great vessels. Moreover, it is assumed that the recorded velocity-time integral accurately represents the average spatial velocity across the region interrogated. This assumes that flow in the area of recording is laminar and blunt in profile. Thus, volumetric flow cannot be measured from regions of flow disorganization. Determination of cross-sectional area usually assumes that the area has a simple shape, such as a circle or an ellipse. The area measured is assumed to represent the average area during the period of flow (even though instantaneous area may change during the cardiac cycle), and the anatomic cross section is assumed to be filled by flowing blood. While these assumptions are reasonable, none is strictly true.

Keeping the preceding cautions in mind, experienced investigators have demonstrated that Doppler echocardiographic stroke volume measures appear to be accurate when compared to available reference standards.[3–5] It is notable that when indicator dilution, Fick, and angiographic stroke volumes are compared,[6,7] although agreement is linear, it is by no means perfect. The lack of complete agreement among the "gold standard" methods for stroke volume determination suggests that they may be flawed as standards of reference.

Several intracardiac locations can be used for ultrasonic determination of stroke volume. Stroke volume can be determined from measures of vessel cross-sectional area and Doppler velocity-time integral recorded from the ascending aorta.[4] Left ventricular (LV) stroke volume also can be determined from systolic diameter and velocity-time integral data recorded in the LV outflow tract.[5] Pulmonary artery flow and diameter both can be recorded from the high parasternal position, thereby providing a measure of right ventricular (RV) output[8,9]; however, it is often difficult to measure pulmonary artery diameter accurately in adults.

Stroke volume also can be measured in diastole at the mitral valve level using an apical approach to record the flow velocity waveform. Transmitral flow volume can be measured at the level of the mitral leaflet tips using pulsed Doppler to record flow velocity. The diastolic velocity-time integral then is multiplied by the average diastolic mitral orifice. The average diastolic mitral orifice area is calculated by first measuring the maximum early diastolic mitral area from a parasternal short-axis image of the mitral leaflet tips. Next, the ratio of the mean to the maximum diastolic mitral leaflet separation is determined from the mitral M-mode tracing. This ratio is then multiplied by the maximum mitral orifice area to determine the average mitral diastolic opening. This somewhat cumbersome approach has been used successfully in animal[10] and clinical[8] studies.

The mitral annulus level provides a computationally simpler approach to determining transmitral stroke volume. Pulsed Doppler sampling is used from the apical examining window to measure the diastolic velocity-time integral at the annulus level. Annular diameter can be measured from apical four-chamber, apical long-axis, or parasternal long-axis views. Cross-sectional area can be computed either by assuming that the annulus is elliptical in shape[11] and using two orthogonal annular diameters or by assuming a circular annular shape and using a single diameter to calculate its area.[5] Investigators do not agree as to which method is more accurate.

Finally, stroke volume can be determined from systolic diameter and velocity-time integral measures made in the RV outflow tract[12] or from diastolic diameter and velocity-time integral recorded at the tricuspid annular level.[13]

Careful Doppler stroke volume measures from two different intracardiac sites show good agreement when the same volume of flow actually passes through both sites. In patients with normal aortic and mitral valves, Lewis et al.[5] demonstrated excellent agreement between stroke volumes measured during systole in the LV outflow tract and during diastole at the mitral annular level. Although measurement of stroke volumes at numerous sites in an individual subject is time consuming and impractical, the possibility of measuring echo Doppler stroke volumes at different locations within the heart and great vessels can be useful. When a value from one site is suspect, data from other sites may provide an internal check. Moreover, when one site cannot be used for volume flow determination, another appropriate location usually is available. For example, stroke volume cannot be measured in the ascending aorta in the presence of valvular aortic stenosis because the profile of flow velocities is not blunt and because the high-velocity aortic flow jet does not fill the aortic root. However, systolic volumetric flow can be measured accurately from the LV outflow tract.[14]

Differences in flow volumes measured at different intracardiac sites, expected in patients with regurgitant valves or intracardiac shunts,[5,8,9,12] can be used to determine the severity of the lesion, as discussed below.

Measurement of Time Intervals

A variety of time intervals have been used to evaluate systolic and diastolic ventricular function. Although classically measured from invasive pressure recordings or external pulse wave and phonocardiographic tracings, the timing and duration of isovolumic contraction, ventricular ejection, isovolumic relaxation, and ventricular filling can also be determined from Doppler velocity curves (Fig. 130-7).

For example, analysis of the systolic Doppler velocity curve recorded in the ascending aorta allows determination of LV ejection duration, acceleration time (onset of flow to peak ejection velocity), and deceleration time.[15] Average and instantaneous measures of acceleration, as well as instantaneous and maximum velocities, also can be determined. From the diastolic mitral flow velocity curve, one can measure total and fractional diastolic duration and the phases of rapid filling, diastasis, and atrial contraction.[16] The interval from cessation of mitral flow to onset of aortic flow defines the period of isovolumic LV contraction; the interval between the end of aortic flow and the beginning of mitral flow describes the period of isovolumic LV relaxation. Comparable right-sided intervals can be measured from pulmonary and tricuspid valve velocity curves.

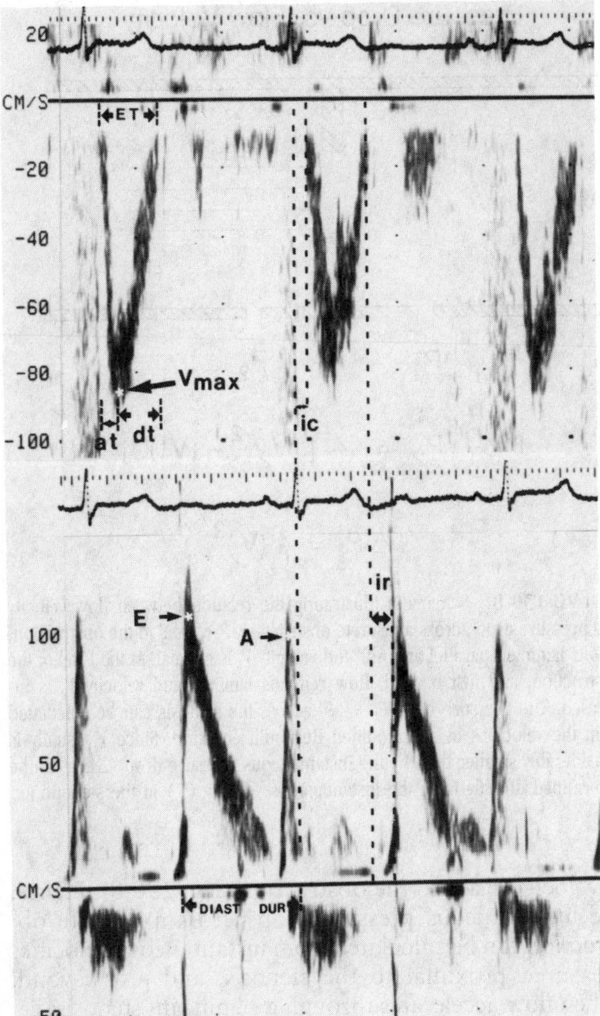

FIGURE 130-7 Measurement of time intervals from Doppler velocity curves. *Top*: Left ventricular ejection velocity recorded from the left ventricular outflow tract of a normal subject by using pulsed wave Doppler. Ejection velocity is plotted on the vertical axis in centimeters per second, and time on the horizontal axis; the distance between pairs of large marks represents 200 ms. Ejection time is measured from the onset to end of ejection flow. Acceleration time is measured from the onset of ejection to the time of maximum velocity. Deceleration time is measured from the time of maximum velocity to the end of ejection. ET, ejection time; AT, acceleration time; V_{max}, maximum velocity; DT, deceleration time. *Bottom*: Left ventricular inflow velocity recorded at the mitral leaflet tips in the same subject using pulsed wave Doppler. The time scale and heart rate are identical to those for ejection recordings. The duration of diastole is measured from onset to end of mitral inflow. Peak flow velocities during early diastole and atrial systole are labeled. By aligning the ejection and filling curves so that the QRS complexes coincide, the duration of isovolumic contraction and relaxation can be measured. DIAST DUR, duration of diastole; E, early diastolic peak velocity; A, atrial systolic peak velocity; IC, isovolumic contraction; IR, isovolumic relaxation.

Determination of Pressure Gradients

One of the most valuable uses of Doppler velocities is for calculating pressure gradients noninvasively. Gradients across discrete narrowings in the heart or great vessels can be determined by using a modification of Bernoulli's theorem, according to which the pressure drop across a discrete stenosis can be related to energy lost for three purposes: to accelerate flowing blood through the narrowed area (*convective acceleration*), to overcome inertial forces during valve opening and closure (*inertial component*), and to overcome resistance (*viscous friction*) as flowing blood cells come into contact with the edges of the obstructive orifice.[17] Typically, valvular stenoses are not so severe that viscous friction is important. Moreover, once a stenotic valve is open, inertial losses are minimal. Accordingly, energy is expended primarily in order to accelerate blood flow through the discrete narrowing and thereby to maintain the rate of volumetric flow.

The modified Bernoulli equation, which neglects viscous friction and inertial components, states that $P_1 - P_2 = 4(V_2^2 - V_1^2)$, where P_1 is pressure proximal to the discrete obstruction, P_2 is pressure distal to the obstruction, V_1 is velocity proximal to the obstruction, and V_2

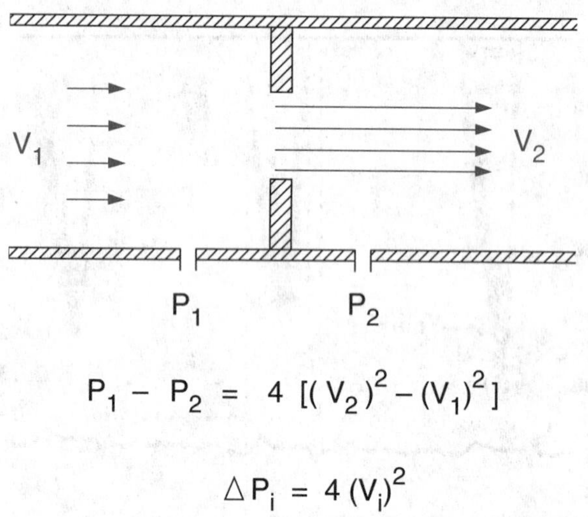

FIGURE 130-8 Schematic illustrating the relation between flow velocity and pressure drop across a discrete obstruction. Proximal to the obstruction, flow is laminar (parallel arrows) and velocity V_1 is normal. At the level of the obstruction, and just beyond, flow remains laminar and velocity V_2 is increased. The pressure drop $P_1 - P_2$ across the stenosis can be calculated from the velocities by the modified Bernoulli equation. Since V_1 usually is considerably smaller than V_2, the instantaneous pressure drop $(\Delta P)_i$ can be determined directly from the instantaneous velocity (V_i) in the stenotic jet.

is velocity distal to the obstruction (Fig. 130-8). Hence, the instantaneous pressure drop across a discrete obstruction can be calculated from instantaneous velocities measured proximal to the stenosis, and just beyond. When flow accelerates through a significant stenosis, velocity in the stenotic jet is substantially higher than that proximal to the obstruction. Since these velocities are then squared in calculating the pressure drop (ΔP), the proximal velocity usually can be neglected. In this case, the Bernoulli equation can be simplified to $\Delta P_i = 4(V_i)^2$, where ΔP_i represents the instantaneous gradient at the time of stenotic jet velocity V_i. Note that when distal velocity does not exceed proximal velocity by a substantial amount, *both* velocity terms should be used to calculate pressure drops; otherwise, the simplified Bernoulli equation overestimates the instantaneous pressure drop.

Experimental and clinical investigations have used Doppler velocity measures to calculate instantaneous, maximum, and mean pressure gradients across a variety of discrete stenoses and compared these to direct manometric gradients. Excellent agreement has been evident when Doppler and manometric gradients have been measured simultaneously and with proper technique.[18,19] The use of Doppler pressure gradients to assess specific cardiac defects is discussed in more detail below. (See also Chaps. 79 to 83.)

Evaluation of Flow Disturbances

Doppler measurements of flow velocities, volumes, and gradients all assume that blood flow is organized and laminar. Many cardiovascular lesions, however, cause flow disorganization (*turbulence*). The multiple directions and velocities of blood cells in a region of disturbed flow make it difficult to use Doppler techniques to measure flow velocity or volume, but the presence and spatial distribution of a flow disturbance can provide useful information.

Conventional PWD is ideal for detecting flow disturbances[20] and has been proved a reliable means to confirm the presence or absence of valvular regurgitation. The spatial extent of a flow disturbance can be assessed with standard PWD, which allows the examiner to determine whether the disturbance is localized, generalized, or intermediate in distribution.[21] This approach is time consuming and tedious, however, since the examiner must move the Doppler sample volume sequentially across a given chamber (using the two-dimensional echo image as a guide) to map both the depth and breadth of the region of disturbed flow. Most investigators now use Doppler CFI to delineate regions of disturbed flow in a tomographic format.[22] The use of flow disturbance assessment to evaluate valvular regurgitant severity is discussed below.

CLINICAL APPLICATIONS

First used to study cardiac function more than 30 years ago,[23,24] Doppler echocardiography now is employed for a number of applications. The clinical uses of Doppler echocardiography can be considered in terms of several broad categories: measurement of ventricular performance, assessment of valvular function, and evaluation of shunt lesions. Each is discussed in more detail.

Measurement of Ventricular Performance

Ventricular Systolic Function

Stroke volume and cardiac output determined from echo Doppler measures of cross-sectional area and velocity-time integral are useful in describing the systolic function of both left and right ventricles. Echo Doppler stroke volumes agree well with invasive standards of reference,[4,5,8–14] and they are atraumatic, inexpensive, and well suited for repeated use. Thus, they have been used for serial evaluation of changes in stroke volume during exercise in patients with coronary artery disease[25] and during vasodilator treatment in patients with heart failure.[26] By providing a *global* assessment that is independent of *regional* abnormalities, Doppler measures complement echocardiographic imaging for evaluating ventricular systolic performance.

It should be emphasized that stroke volumes show a wide range of normal, and they are altered by changes in ventricular loading conditions. Therefore, a single stroke volume or cardiac output determination can be misleading, and these measures need to be interpreted in the context of clinical and other laboratory data. This proviso applies not only to echo Doppler measures but also to other techniques for volume flow measurement.

Doppler measures of ejection velocity and flow acceleration also can be used to describe ventricular systolic performance. Rushmer[27] described the ventricle as an impulse generator and noted that the peak velocity of ventricular ejection and its rate of acceleration both increased with exercise and decreased with ischemic dysfunction. More recently, clinical investigators have used both pulsed and continuous wave Doppler to quantitate changes in aortic peak flow velocity and acceleration in patients during exercise testing.[25,28–30] Blunted increases in peak velocity and acceleration were noted in patients with significant coronary artery disease.[30] Linear relations between Doppler measures (aortic peak velocity, average acceleration, and maximum acceleration) and LV systolic function (ejection fraction, *dP/dt*) also have been described.[30,31] In patients with detectable mitral regurgitation, it is also possible to determine average left ventricular *dP/dt* from the time course of mitral regurgitant velocity during early systole (recorded using CWD) as an independent means to quantitate global ventricular systolic performance.[32]

Similar approaches can be applied to evaluating RV systolic function. For example, systolic flow in the RV outflow tract accelerates more rapidly than normal in patients with pulmonary hypertension,[33] suggesting an increase in right ventricular *dP/dt*. The rate of pressure rise in the right ventricle is reduced when this chamber fails, and Doppler tricuspid regurgitant velocity curves can reflect this functional impairment.[34] Since the complexities of RV geometry make it difficult to evaluate global systolic function, Doppler methods for quantitating RV output, ejection velocity, and acceleration rate seem particularly appealing.

Ventricular Diastolic Function

Doppler recordings of diastolic flow through the atrioventricular valves provide a means to characterize the magnitude and time course of ventricular filling and thereby offer some insights about global ventricular diastolic function. Many different LV diastolic indexes have been described.[35,36] Doppler curves can be used to define a variety of *time intervals*, such as the periods of isovolumic relaxation (aortic closure to mitral opening), rapid filling, early diastole, and atrial contraction. The *peak velocities* that occur during early filling (E) and after atrial contraction (A) can be measured. Rates of flow *acceleration* and *deceleration* during early diastole can be calculated. Peak and mean *filling rates* and *filling fractions* can be computed from the diastolic transmitral velocity curve (recorded at the level of the mitral annulus using PWD) and the annular cross-sectional area. Finally, Doppler *area fractions* can be measured by integrating areas under different portions of the mitral flow velocity curve. Various abnormalities have been reported in different clinical settings; for example, patients with abnormal LV relaxation may demonstrate prolonged Doppler isovolumic relaxation times,[16] patients with hypertension or hypertrophic cardiomyopathy may have reduced transmitral E velocities and E/A ratios,[16] and patients with myocardial ischemia may show decreased Doppler area fractions during rapid filling.[37]

While the ability to record the time course of ventricular filling atraumatically is exciting, diastolic ventricular filling and diastolic ventricular function are not synonymous.[38] A number of technical and physiological pitfalls deserve emphasis. Mitral diastolic flow velocity must be recorded by orienting the Doppler beam coaxial with the direction of flow; hence, good apical examining windows are important. Peak early and late diastolic velocities do not occur at the same level of the LV inflow tract.[39,40] While there is not general agreement as to whether transmitral diastolic velocities should be recorded at the mitral leaflet tips or annulus, it is clear that range-gated pulsed Doppler must be used and sample volume position must be specified. Transmitral velocities only reflect ventricular filling *rates* when multiplied by mitral orifice area measurements.[35] Mitral orifice area changes more dramatically at the leaflet tips than at the annulus; the latter sampling site may be easier for determining instantaneous filling rate.

It is also noteworthy that transmitral velocity curves are affected by a number of variables in addition to ventricular relaxation and diastolic compliance. An increase in heart rate shortens the diastolic intervals, lowers E velocity, and lowers the E/A ratio. The E velocity and E/A ratio decline with increasing age,[41] and these measures also are affected by the atrioventricular sequence (PR interval). Finally, preload[42,43] exerts an important influence on ventricular filling. Increases in left atrial pressure at the time of mitral valve opening, which may result from mitral regurgitation, LV failure, or atrial contraction during ventricular systole, cause an increase in mitral E velocity, E/A ratio, and early filling fractions even in those patients with disorders (e.g., hypertrophic cardiomyopathy, aortic stenosis) that would be expected to cause abnormal diastolic function. Ventricular diastole is complex,[38] includes both active and passive phases, and is subject to the influence of ventricular systolic function, mitral valve competence, atrial contractile performance and timing, and loading conditions. The examiner who uses transmitral flow velocities as a means to understand ventricular diastolic function must keep these complexities in mind. (See also Chaps. 23 and 25.)

Restricted cardiac filling may result from pericardial constriction or tamponade, and not from myocardial dysfunction. In tamponade, recent studies suggest that cardiac volume is fixed, causing right and left ventricular filling to compete. (See also Chap. 92.) This situation can be demonstrated by Doppler evaluation of right- and left-sided flow velocities during the respiratory cycle.[44] In constriction, ventricular filling terminates abruptly in early diastole,[45] and pulmonary (or hepatic) venous flow recordings may show prominent reversals with atrial systole[46] despite the absence of further ventricular filling.

Intracardiac Pressure Estimation

Certain intracardiac pressures can be estimated using Doppler flow velocity recordings. In patients with tricuspid regurgitation, peak tricuspid regurgitant velocity provides a valuable means to calculate peak systolic pulmonary artery pressure.[47] According to the simplified Bernoulli equation, the peak velocity of tricuspid regurgitation indicates the maximum systolic pressure difference between the right ventricle and atrium, which should occur at the time of peak RV systolic pressure. Maximum RV–right atrial pressure differences calculated from Doppler tricuspid regurgitant velocities agree closely with those measured simultaneously by catheter.[34,47] Peak RV pressure can be determined by adding right atrial pressure to the calculated pressure difference. Peak RV pressure is the same as peak systolic pulmonary artery pressure, unless there is RV outflow obstruction.

Right atrial pressure can be estimated by inspecting the neck veins, but this is not always accurate.[47] Right atrial pressure can be approximated by considering the clinical setting; right atrial pressure varies from approximately 0 to 20 mmHg, being low when tricuspid function is normal or intravascular volume is low and high when tricuspid regurgitation is severe or RV failure is present. Some workers have suggested using an arbitrary value (such as 10 mmHg) for right atrial pressure. Imaging of the inferior vena cava (using subcostal two-dimensional echocardiography) can help estimate mean right atrial pressure.[48] If the vena cava is normal in size and its caliber decreases by 50 percent or more during inspiration, mean right atrial pressure is low (approximately 5 mmHg). If the vena cava is engorged and its caliber is relatively constant during inspiration, this denotes that mean right atrial pressure is high (approximately 15 mmHg). Intermediate findings are noted with intermediate degrees of right atrial hypertension.

While difficulties in estimating right atrial pressure precisely do limit the accuracy and repeatability of Doppler peak RV systolic pressure measures, peak tricuspid regurgitant velocity alone may indicate whether or not a patient has significant pulmonary hypertension. For example, if tricuspid regurgitant velocity is 4.0 m/s, RV pressure exceeds right atrial pressure by 64 mmHg. Such a patient has significant pulmonary hypertension regardless of the level of right atrial pressure.

Estimation of peak systolic pulmonary artery pressure from tricuspid regurgitant velocity is especially useful because tricuspid regurgitation is prevalent in subjects without clinical evidence of heart disease and in patients with various cardiac disorders. In patients with minimal amounts of tricuspid regurgitation, it may be difficult to measure peak regurgitant velocity from CWD curves. In this case, it is possible to increase the intensity of the regurgitant Doppler signal using intravenous injection of contrast microbubbles.[49]

Pulmonary artery systolic pressures also can be determined from the pulmonary closure–tricuspid opening interval measured from Doppler recordings of pulmonary and tricuspid valve flow.[50] This approach recognizes that if right atrial pressure remains relatively normal, the isovolumic relaxation period lengthens as pulmonary artery pressures rise. Using phonocardiography to measure the duration of RV isovolumic relaxation, one can estimate pulmonary artery systolic pressure from a nomogram utilizing the heart rate and pulmonary closure–tricuspid opening interval.[51] Good agreement between estimates of pulmonary systolic pressure determined by using Doppler measures of RV isovolumic relaxation and the nomogram, and catheter pressure measurements, also has been noted.[50] This approach, however, tends to underestimate actual pulmonary systolic pressures in patients with elevated right atrial pressures.

The time from onset to peak velocity (also referred to as *acceleration time*) of RV ejection flow provides a third Doppler approach to determining pulmonary artery pressures. Several groups have noted that pulmonary acceleration time shortens as pulmonary artery pressures increase, and empiric regression equations relating Doppler acceleration times to measured pulmonary artery pressure have been reported.[33,52,53] Although all have used pulsed Doppler techniques to measure pulmonary acceleration time, some authors have sampled in the RV outflow tract just proximal to the pulmonic valve,[33,53] while others have recorded just distal to the valve in the main pulmonary artery.[52] In the latter site, care must be taken to avoid positioning the sample volume near the medial wall, where acceleration times may be shorter than in the center of the vessel. Some authors have found the best agreement between acceleration times and pulmonary artery pressures[52]; others have reported better correlations by using time interval ratios such as acceleration time/RV ejection duration[33] or preejection period/acceleration time.[53] A short acceleration can result from tachycardia alone; some writers suggest correcting for heart rate and others do not, but most agree that acceleration times are less reliable predictors of right-sided pressure when heart rate exceeds 100 beats per minute. The studies cited, and others, describe empiric relations between Doppler acceleration time measures and directly (although not always simultaneously) determined pulmonary artery pressures, but different authors report different mathematical relations. Doppler pulmonary acceleration time can be measured in nearly all patients. This interval, however, appears to give an approximate range of pulmonary artery pressure rather than a precise numerical value.

Pulmonic regurgitant velocities provide a final Doppler approach to pulmonary pressures. Pulmonic regurgitation is prevalent in clinically normal individuals as well as patients with a variety of cardiac disorders. Masuyama et al.[54] reasoned that initial diastolic pulmonic regurgitant velocity would reflect the pressure difference between the pulmonary artery and the right ventricle at the time of minimum RV diastolic pressure and that this velocity should increase when pulmonary artery pressure becomes elevated. They described close agreement between initial diastolic pulmonic regurgitant velocity and catheter measures of the initial diastolic gradient between the pulmonary artery and the right ventricle. They also noted agreement between end-diastolic pulmonary arterial–RV gradients measured by catheter and by Doppler. This led to the suggestion that pulmonary end-diastolic pressure could be calculated from end-diastolic pulmonic regurgitant velocity if one could determine right atrial pressure.

The multiple Doppler methods for estimating right-sided pressures provide internal checks, and at least one is feasible for nearly all patients.[55] On the other hand, none of these methods works for every patient, some appear to have relatively broad confidence limits, and they are not ideal for monitoring small changes in right-sided pressures.

It is also possible to determine LV end-diastolic pressure from Doppler recordings in patients with aortic regurgitation by calculating the end-diastolic pressure difference between the aorta and the left ventricle from end-diastolic aortic regurgitant velocity using the simplified Bernoulli equation. This noninvasive pressure difference then is subtracted from diastolic cuff pressure to yield LV end-diastolic pressure. For example, if the systemic arterial diastolic pressure were 80 mmHg and end-diastolic aortic regurgitant velocity were 4 m/s (indicating a gradient of 64 mmHg), then LV end-diastolic pressure would be 16 mmHg. Good agreement between Doppler estimates and direct measures of LV end-diastolic pressure has been reported in patients with substantial aortic regurgitation.[56] This approach depends on accurate measurement of end-diastolic regurgitant velocity, which in turn requires sufficient regurgitation to demonstrate clearly the high-velocity components and proper alignment of the Doppler beam and the regurgitant jet. Diastolic arterial cuff pressure may not be identical to central aortic diastolic pressure, and small errors in either diastolic aortic pressure or end-diastolic gradient determination may lead to large errors in the calculated end-diastolic pressure. In practice, this approach often overestimates LV end-diastolic pressure, especially when aortic regurgitation is mild.

Assessment of Valvular Function

Echocardiographic images demonstrate the *anatomy* and *etiology* of valvular lesions (Chap. 15), while Doppler techniques provide functional information about the *hemodynamic significance* of the lesions. Thus, valvular disorders are best evaluated by using the combination of imaging and Doppler techniques.

Valvular Stenosis

Blood passing through a stenotic valve demonstrates characteristic flow dynamics (Fig. 130-8). Proximal to the stenosis, flow is laminar. Blood passing through the stenotic orifice remains laminar, but its velocity must increase in order to maintain the volumetric rate of flow. Beyond the valve orifice, the kinetic energy in the high-velocity stenotic jet is dissipated as vortices of flow move radially away from the flow centerline, and velocities decline as flow moves downstream. Important quantitative hemodynamic information can be derived from the stenotic jet velocity.

Stenosis severity can be determined by calculating the pressure gradient across the stenotic valve from the recorded Doppler flow velocity using the equation $\Delta P = 4(V)^2$. Many investigators have used Doppler velocities to calculate pressure gradients in patients with valvular aortic stenosis,[57–62] mitral stenosis,[58,63,64] pulmonic stenosis,[59,65,66] or pulmonary artery bands.[59] The same approach has been used to determine the intracavitary subaortic gradient in hypertrophic cardiomyopathy.[67] In general, these studies all have demonstrated excellent agreement between Doppler and manometric pressure gradients. Since Doppler flow velocities are angle-dependent, the examiner must search systematically from a number of transducer positions and orientations in order to record maximum jet velocity. Valvular stenoses often cause oblique jets (especially in acquired aortic stenosis), and the direction of the stenotic jet cannot be inferred from the orientation of the valve leaflets. Doppler CFI can be helpful for visualizing stenotic jet orientation. While certainly feasible for mitral stenosis, CFI of aortic stenosis jets has proved to be difficult. Often, all that is seen is a spray of disturbed systolic flow filling the ascending aorta, with no clearly recognizable jet direction. Therefore, the examiner must search thoroughly from a variety of examining windows, assuming that the highest recorded jet velocity represents a position at which the Doppler beam and flow jet are nearly coaxial. Since pressure gradients vary with changes in volumetric flow, nonsimultaneous comparisons between Doppler and catheter measures may be difficult to interpret. Additionally, proper catheter technique requires that pressure be measured simultaneously on each side of the discrete obstruction in order to avoid downstream pressure augmentation.

Certain Doppler measures are particularly useful for specific lesions.

Aortic Stenosis Careful in vitro and in vivo studies have documented that transaortic gradients can be determined accurately from Doppler velocities.[18,60,68] Nonetheless, the relation between Doppler and invasive gradients can be confusing. Doppler velocities correspond to instantaneous pressure gradients; the pressure gradient calculated from the highest systolic Doppler velocity represents the maximum instantaneous pressure gradient across the stenotic valve. This is not the same as the "peak-to-peak" pressure gradient across the stenotic aortic valve that frequently is reported at cardiac catheterization. In fact, LV pressure reaches its maximum value earlier in systole than does aortic root pressure (Fig. 130-9). Although the peak-to-peak pressure gradient is readily measured and convenient, it is not a gradient that actually exists in time, and it cannot be measured directly by Doppler. Note that the peak-to-peak gradient typically is smaller than the maximum instantaneous pressure gradient.[60]

Mean pressure gradients by both Doppler and manometric techniques show excellent agreement.[60,61,68] Moreover, the mean gradient reflects the average obstruction to LV ejection created by the stenotic aortic valve. Therefore, many echocardiographers use mean systolic gradients to express aortic stenosis severity. Determination of Doppler mean gradient requires measurement of instantaneous velocity at multiple points through systole (Fig. 130-9), computation of the corresponding instantaneous gradients, and calculation of the average systolic gradient from these multiple instantaneous gradients. This is done by digitizing the aortic jet velocity curve (typically recorded by using CWD), with the calculations performed by a computer in the Doppler instrument or in an off-line analysis system. Excellent linear agreement between Doppler maximum and mean transaortic gradients in aortic stenosis patients has been demonstrated.[69,70] Thus, it is possible to calculate the mean gradient directly from the measured maximum transaortic gradient.

Regardless of how they are measured, gradients reflect not only the degree of stenosis but also the transvalvular volumetric flow rate. Classically, the orifice area of a stenotic cardiac valve is determined by using the hydraulic formula derived by Gorlin and Gorlin,[71] which states that the valve orifice area is directly proportional to the volume of transvalvular flow and inversely proportional to the square root of the transvalvular pressure gradient. (See also Chap. 79.) The authors recognized that valve

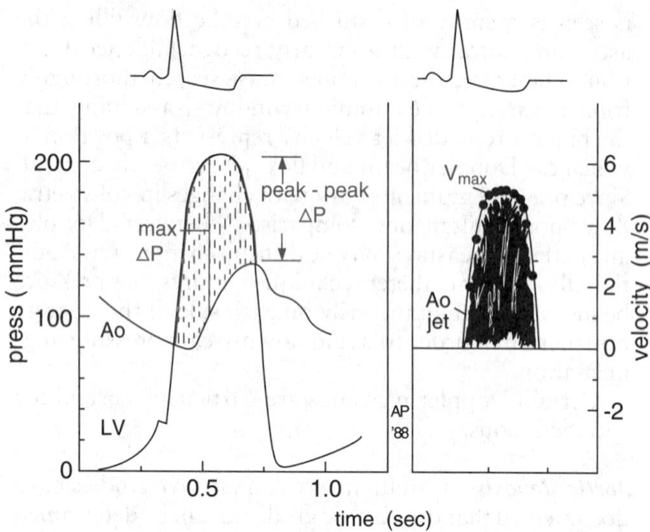

FIGURE 130-9 Diagram illustrating the relation between systolic pressure gradient and aortic velocity in valvular aortic stenosis. *Left:* A dynamic systolic gradient between left ventricular and aortic pressures is evident. Assuming proper alignment of the pressure tracings, a series of instantaneous pressure differences (dashed lines) can be measured, and the mean systolic gradient can be calculated. The gradient between peak systolic left ventricular pressure and peak systolic aortic pressure can also be determined, even though these two peaks are nonsimultaneous. Note that the maximum instantaneous gradient is always larger than the peak-to-peak gradient. LV, left ventricular, Ao, aortic; max $\triangle P$, maximum instantaneous gradient; peak-peak $\triangle P$, peak left ventricular to peak aortic gradient. *Right*: Schematic continuous wave Doppler recording of aortic jet velocity from above the valve (i.e., from the suprasternal or right parasternal window). Using the simplified Bernoulli equation, instantaneous pressure gradients can be determined from the instantaneous velocities and mean gradient can be calculated. Maximum $\triangle P$ can be determined as $4(V_{max})^2$. Ao jet, aortic jet velocity.

area would be inversely proportional to the velocity of blood flow across the valve; since techniques for measuring flow velocity were not then available, they substituted pressure gradient (which is related to the square of velocity) in their formula. Since Doppler techniques measure both transvalvular volume flow and pressure gradient, Doppler data could be used in the Gorlin formula to calculate aortic valve orifice area.

Most investigators, however, prefer a more direct approach (the *continuity equation*), which is based on the concept that during systolic ejection, the same volume of flow passes through both the LV outflow tract and the stenotic aortic valve orifice. As discussed earlier, stroke volume can be calculated as the product of flow cross-sectional area (CSA) and flow velocity-time integral (VTI). Hence, when systolic stroke volume is measured in the left ventricular outflow tract (LVOT) and in the stenotic aortic valve orifice (AoV),

$$CSA_{LVOT} \times VTI_{LVOT} = CSA_{AoV} \times VTI_{AoV}$$

If one measures the cross-sectional area of the LV outflow tract, the velocity-time integral of the systolic velocity curve recorded in the LV outflow tract, and the velocity-time integral of the aortic stenosis jet, one can compute CSA_{AoV}, the functional aortic valve orifice area.[61,62,69,72] A number of investigators have used this approach to determine aortic valve orifice area in patients with valvular aortic stenosis. As with the Gorlin equation, one must measure the volume of anterograde flow through the stenotic aortic valve. The majority of adults with acquired aortic stenosis have some coexisting aortic regurgitation.[70] Therefore, volumetric flow measured at another site is not necessarily the same as systolic transaortic flow volume. In order to determine aortic valve area by the continuity equation, LV outflow tract diameter is measured high in the outflow tract, just proximal to the plane of the aortic annulus. We assume that the outflow tract is circular in cross section, relatively constant in area during systole, and effectively filled by flow. We measure the velocity-time integral in the LV outflow tract by using pulsed Doppler from an apical examining window and positioning a relatively large sample volume (to optimize recording of spatial average velocity) just proximal to the stenotic aortic valve. The jet of high-velocity flow through the stenotic aortic valve is recorded from whichever transducer window yields the highest flow velocity, usually by using CWD. Aortic valve area then can be calculated from these data (Fig. 130-10). In patients with aortic stenosis, agreement between aortic orifice areas determined from echocardiographic measures using the continuity equation and orifice areas determined from catheterization data using the Gorlin formula has been quite good.[61,69,72–74] Since the ratio of peak velocities in the LV outflow tract and stenotic aortic jet is nearly identical to the ratio of velocity-time integrals,[75] peak flow velocities can be substituted in the continuity equation.[72,75] In aortic stenosis, valve orifice areas carefully measured by echo Doppler techniques provide relatively equivalent information to that available from catheterization data,[69,76] with the potential for considerable cost savings and a reduction in morbidity.[69,77] It should be emphasized that these measures do require a methodical approach, careful attention to technique, and substantial experience before they can be substituted for catheterization data.

Mitral Stenosis Transmitral peak and mean diastolic gradients can be determined from measured Doppler velocities by using the simplified Bernoulli equation.[63,64] Color flow imaging can be used to identify the direction of the diastolic mitral jet and to help in aligning the Doppler beam, necessary for accurate gradient determination. Since these jets are almost always oriented toward the cardiac apex, it usually is sufficient to search thoroughly from the apical window for the highest spectral jet velocity. Doppler and manometric measurements demonstrate excellent agreement for mitral stenosis patients[58,63,64] for both maximum and mean diastolic gradients. Since mitral gradients vary with volume flow, even changing on a beat-to-beat basis when atrial fibrillation causes varying cycle lengths, gradients alone are of limited value for expressing stenosis severity.

One can calculate functional mitral valve area in mitral stenosis by using the continuity equation. Mitral valve area is determined by dividing the stroke volume by the stenotic jet velocity-time integral. Stroke volume can be measured in the LV outflow tract or main pulmonary artery, and the mitral stenotic jet is recorded from the apical window by using CWD. This method compares well to valve areas calculated from catheterization

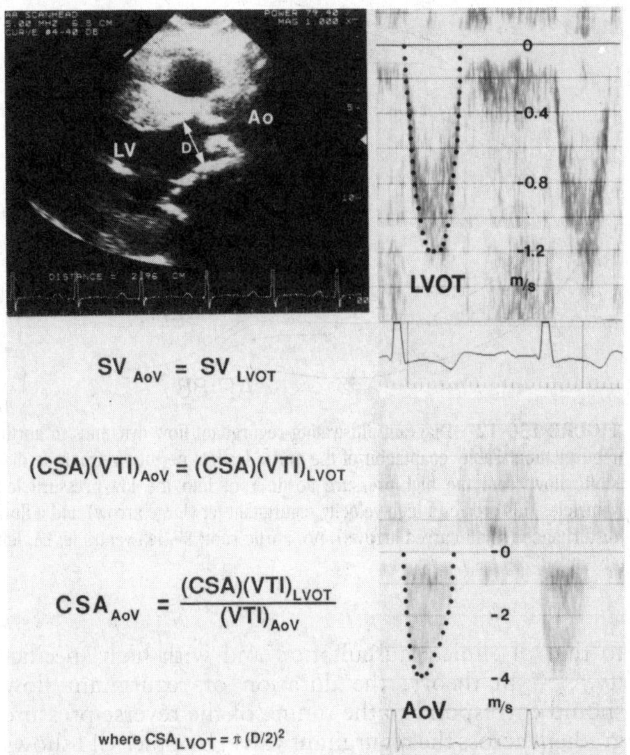

FIGURE 130-10 Determination of aortic valve area using the continuity equation. *Top left:* Midsystolic parasternal long-axis image from a young man with mixed aortic stenosis and insufficiency. Left ventricular outflow tract diameter is indicated (double-headed arrow). LV, left ventricular, D, diameter, Ao, aorta. *Top right:* Left ventricular outflow tract velocity, recorded from the cardiac apex by pulsed wave Doppler. The velocity-time integral is determined by tracing the edge of the velocity-time curve (dots added for emphasis). LVOT, left ventricular outflow tract. *Bottom right:* The jet of high-velocity flow through the stenotic aortic valve is recorded from the cardiac apex by continuous wave Doppler. The velocity-time integral is denoted by the dots. AoV, aortic valve. *Bottom left*: The continuity equation states that the volume of flow (stroke volume) through the left ventricular outflow tract is equal to that through the stenotic aortic valve. Stroke volume is equal to the product of cross-sectional area and flow velocity-time integral. The equation can be solved for stenotic aortic valve area. SV, stroke volume; LVOT, left ventricular outflow tract; AoV, aortic valve; CSA, cross-sectional area; VTI, flow velocity-time integral; CSA_{AoV}, stenotic aortic valve area.

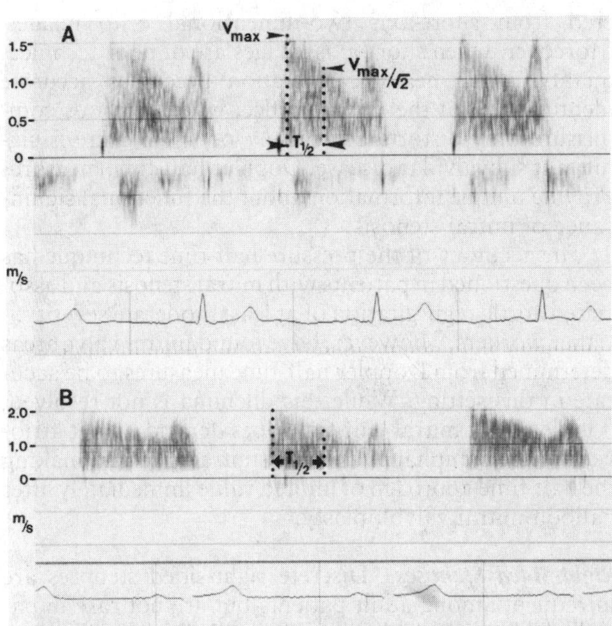

FIGURE 130-11 Evaluation of mitral stenosis severity by the pressure half-time technique. *A.* Continuous wave Doppler recording from the cardiac apex in a patient with moderate mitral stenosis. Pressure half-time ($T_{1/2}$) is measured in milliseconds from the time of maximum diastolic velocity V_{max} to the time at which velocity drops to $V_{max}\sqrt{2}$. In this patient, $T_{1/2}$ is 226 ms, indicating a mitral valve area of 1 cm^2. *B.* Severe mitral stenosis, with a slower rate of velocity decline. In this patient, $T_{1/2}$ = 319 ms; mitral valve area = 0.7 cm^2.

data in patients with pure mitral stenosis and in those with mitral stenosis and associated aortic regurgitation.[78] In the majority of patients with mitral stenosis, who also have some degree of mitral regurgitation, however, the volume of diastolic flow across the mitral valve cannot be determined by measuring left or right ventricular outflow. In this situation, the continuity equation valve area would underestimate the true functional mitral orifice area.

Many echocardiographers use a simpler Doppler technique to determine mitral orifice area from the rate of decline of the transmitral pressure gradient (Fig. 130-11). Using catheter measures, Libanoff and Rodbard[79] observed that the diastolic transmitral pressure gradient is maximum at the point of mitral valve opening, thereafter falling in a linear fashion. In order to determine the rate of pressure decay, they measured the time required for the maximum initial pressure gradient to decline by 50 percent, referring to this interval as the *pressure half-time*. The pressure half-time was prolonged from normal in patients with mitral stenosis, and the degree of prolongation was inversely related to the valve orifice area. The half-time was found to be relatively independent of the diastolic filling period, the presence and degree of mitral regurgitation, and the transvalvular flow volume during exercise. The pressure half-time can be determined directly from the transmitral diastolic flow velocity curve, since the instantaneous transmitral diastolic flow velocity is directly proportional to the square root of the corresponding instantaneous pressure gradient. Since gradient is proportional to the square of velocity, the *Doppler pressure half-time* is the time required for the initial maximum velocity to decline to a level 70 percent of the maximum initial velocity (i.e., initial velocity divided by the square root of 2). Doppler measures by Hatle et al.[80] confirmed that the Doppler pressure half-time increases as the mitral valve area decreases. Hatle observed empirically that patients with catheterization mitral valve areas of approximately 1.0 cm^2 had Doppler half-times of approximately 220 ms,[80] a value that has been more recently confirmed.[81] Thus, the mitral orifice area can be calculated by dividing 220 ms/cm^2 by the Doppler half-time, measured in milliseconds. Mitral valve areas derived by the Doppler half-time technique generally are in good agreement with catheterization data,[58,81,82] and these measures are relatively unaffected by mitral volumetric flow, heart rate, and presence or absence of coexisting mitral regurgitation.[83] The Doppler half-time method provides an excellent "check" on diastolic mitral orifice areas planimetered from short-axis two-dimensional echo images. Moreover, when short-axis images are of poor technical quality, when heavy calcification precludes accurate identification of the mitral orifice, when previous commissurotomy distorts the valve,[82] or when there is significant subvalvular disease, Doppler half-time measures provide unique information about the functional significance of mitral stenosis.

The accuracy of the pressure half-time technique has been questioned in patients with mitral stenosis and associated aortic regurgitation of at least moderate severity.[78] Other workers,[84] however, have found mitral valve areas determined from Doppler half-time measures to be accurate in this setting. While this dilemma is not resolved, it is clear that mitral half-time does depend on net atrioventricular compliance and transmitral gradient, making the half-time approach of limited value immediately after balloon mitral valvuloplasty.[85]

Right-Sided Stenoses Discrete right-sided stenoses are infrequent among adult patients but are not rare in patients with congenital heart disease. Valvular, subvalvular, and pulmonary arterial stenoses may occur in isolation or in association with ventricular septal defects. Pulmonary artery bands, used to restrict pulmonary blood flow in certain shunt lesions, may become functionally stenotic. (See also Chaps. 97 and 98.) Patients with rheumatic valvular disease may develop tricuspid stenosis (Chap. 81).

Doppler techniques for pressure gradient and valve area determination can be used to evaluate discrete right-sided stenoses. Pressure gradients across stenotic pulmonic valves and pulmonary artery bands have been measured accurately[59,65,66] by using the simplified Bernoulli equation. Serial stenoses in the RV outflow tract can be detected and gradients quantitated by using HPRF Doppler, and semilunar valve areas can be determined.[86] Mean pressure gradients and valve areas can be calculated in patients with rheumatic tricuspid stenosis. In this circumstance, however, relatively small gradients may be significant, and there are no good reference standard measures for valve orifice area.

Valvular Regurgitation

The flow dynamics of blood traveling retrograde through an incompetent valve are similar to those of valvular stenosis, except that flow direction is reversed. A regurgitant valve provides a regurgitant orifice (usually small) through which blood can flow from the chamber distal to the valve (whose pressure is high) into the chamber proximal to the valve (whose pressure is low). Accordingly, valvular regurgitation involves a pressure drop across a small flow orifice, thereby causing a high-velocity retrograde flow jet within and just beyond the regurgitant orifice and a flow disturbance that fills a portion of the "receiving" chamber (Fig. 130-12).

A variety of investigators have documented that disturbed flow detected proximal to a closed valve (using range-gated Doppler) accurately reflects the presence of valvular regurgitation, compared to selective cineangiographic results.[20,21,87,88] In several studies, pulsed Doppler detected valvular regurgitation with a sensitivity superior

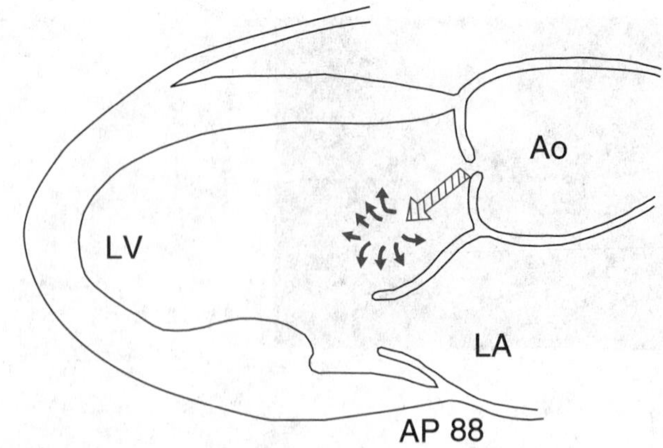

FIGURE 130-12 Diagram illustrating regurgitant flow dynamics in aortic regurgitation. Faulty coaptation of the aortic leaflets permits retrograde diastolic flow from the high-pressure aortic root into the low-pressure left ventricle. This creates a high-velocity regurgitant jet (large arrow) and a flow disturbance (small curved arrows). Ao, aortic root; LV, left ventricle; LA, left atrium.

to that of clinical auscultation and with high specificity.[20,87,88] In theory, the duration of regurgitant flow should correspond to the timing of the reverse pressure gradient across the regurgitant valve. Doppler CFI shows that some regurgitant jets are narrow and that they move (with the regurgitant valve plane) during the cardiac cycle. When a localized flow disturbance that moves during the cardiac cycle is interrogated by a narrow ultrasound beam that cannot track flow motion, the region of Doppler sampling may intersect the flow disturbance during only a portion of the cardiac cycle. The same phenomenon can be observed using Doppler CFI, since a narrow regurgitant jet may move in the elevational plane and thus "disappear" from the tomographic plane being imaged. Accordingly, for example, mild mitral regurgitation sometimes may seem not to be holosystolic when recorded by pulsed Doppler. With the broader beam of CWD, however, one often can demonstrate that regurgitation really is holosystolic.

Another reliable marker of valvular regurgitation is retrograde high-velocity flow, usually best demonstrated by CWD. When a patient has multivalvular disease, one must be particularly careful to distinguish the origin of high-velocity jets. For example, if a patient has calcific aortic stenosis and mitral annular calcification, one would need to distinguish the high-velocity systolic jet of aortic stenosis from that of mitral regurgitation. Both of these flow jets would be directed away from the cardiac apex. The timing of the spectral Doppler velocity curves is crucial; since mitral regurgitation begins and ends at the points of LV and left atrial pressure crossover, this lesion always begins earlier and lasts longer than aortic stenosis.[89] Similarly, aortic regurgitation begins earlier and ends later than forward flow across a stenotic mitral valve. Careful attention to the timing of onset and the duration of high-velocity jets usually allows accurate identification.

A number of methods for determining the severity of valvular regurgitation have been described. Some of these are semiquantitative; others provide numerical measures of regurgitant volume and regurgitant fraction.

Certain methods can be applied to any regurgitant valve, while others are particularly well suited to specific lesions. In judging the accuracy of these techniques, it is important to recognize that so-called gold standards have important physiological and methodologic limitations. The severity of valvular regurgitation changes as impedance to forward ejection is altered; thus, nonsimultaneous comparisons between Doppler results and alternate methods must be interpreted cautiously, especially if similar loading conditions were not known to be present at the time of the different investigations. While angiographic data often are used as a reference standard, qualitative and quantitative angiographic methods do not show good agreement.[7] The former techniques are widely available, but the results are influenced by contrast load, chamber size, and interobserver variability. The latter methods are not used widely and are technically demanding. Moreover, disagreement between angiographic and indicator dilution (including Fick) measures of stroke volume in patients with normal valves[7] suggests that quantitative angiographic regurgitant volumes may not be free of error.

Aortic Regurgitation A number of Doppler techniques are useful in judging the severity of aortic regurgitation. Probably the most popular qualitative approach is known as *flow mapping*. Originally developed using nonimaging pulsed Doppler,[21] flow mapping assumes that the spatial distribution of the regurgitant flow disturbance reflects the severity of regurgitation. Now, most workers use Doppler CFI (Plate X, 130-2) to determine whether the flow disturbance is localized, intermediate in distribution, or widespread (corresponding in general to mild, moderate, and severe regurgitation). Some investigators have recommended measuring jet length,[21] while others have emphasized measuring the width of the regurgitant jet as a percentage of the LV outflow tract diameter, or the cross-sectional area of the regurgitant jet,[90] In these studies, regurgitant mapping results generally have been concordant with semiquantitative angiographic findings (although Doppler and invasive measures were not made simultaneously). When used in conjunction with clinical and other echocardiographic data, flow mapping usually does indicate whether regurgitation is hemodynamically unimportant, significant, or somewhere in between.

Nonetheless, a number of technical cautions must be kept in mind. Regurgitant flow disturbances have a three-dimensional spatial distribution, and their orientation may not be coaxial to a given tomographic imaging plane. Therefore, a variety of transducer positions and orientations and multiple examining windows should be used to prevent underestimating regurgitant jet distribution.[90] Because Doppler CFI demonstrates the regurgitant disturbance in a real-time tomographic format, this method would seem preferable to standard, single range-gate Doppler for depicting the distribution of a regurgitant lesion. The latter technique, however, may offer slightly better sensitivity. The area of a regurgitant disturbance varies during the cardiac cycle, and beat-to-beat changes can be seen when changes in regurgitant volume result from variations in cycle length or loading conditions. For a given volume of regurgitation, the size of a regurgitant jet also depends to an important degree on whether it is a "free" jet directed into the center of the receiving chamber or a "constrained" jet that runs along (and is deformed by) one of the walls of the receiving chamber. Finally, the distribution of aortic regurgitation is determined not only by aortic regurgitant volume but also by diastolic driving pressure, regurgitant orifice size and shape, and the size and distensibility of the left ventricle. Thus, flow mapping provides only a semiquantitative assessment of regurgitant severity.

A simple qualitative method for determining aortic regurgitant severity involves analyzing the relative intensity of the CWD regurgitant flow velocity curve (Fig. 130-13). This technique assumes that the strength of the aortic regurgitant jet signal is proportional to the number of blood cells passing retrograde through the regurgitant orifice. Although the number of blood cells flowing retrograde through the valve in diastole never equals the volume of forward transaortic systolic flow, the percentage of blood cells that leak backward during diastole increases as regurgitation becomes progressively more se-

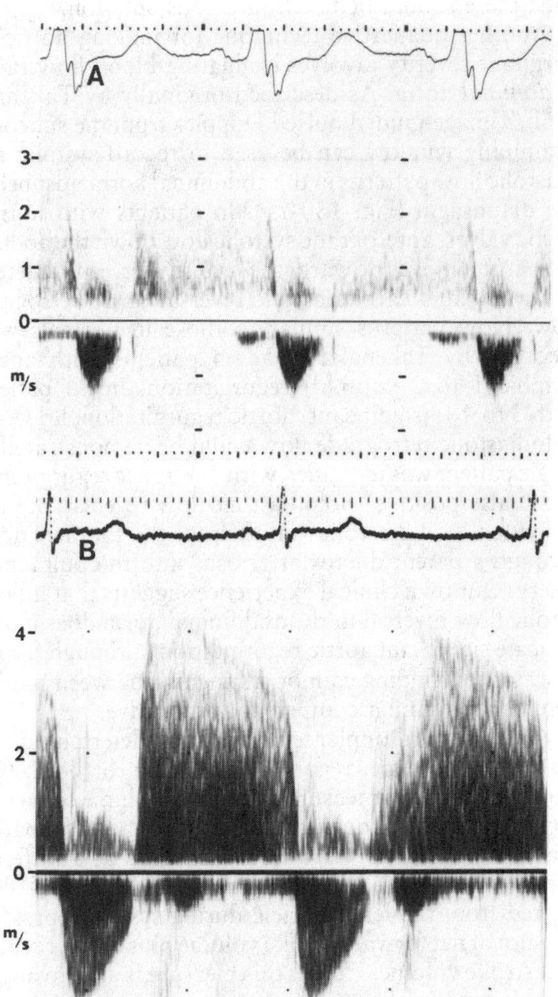

FIGURE 130-13 Assessment of aortic regurgitant severity from continuous wave Doppler regurgitant signal intensity. *A*. Mild regurgitation causes a faint diastolic regurgitant waveform (compare to anterograde systolic signal intensity), in which high-velocity components are recorded poorly. *B*. Severe regurgitation causes an intense regurgitant waveform.

vere. The intensity of the spectral Doppler signal depends on ultrasound signal strength, examination depth, and instrument gain settings in addition to the number of blood cells in the regurgitant flow stream. Thus, regurgitant signal strength must be compared to the intensity of the anterograde flow signal. When aortic regurgitation is mild, the waveform is typically faint, and it cannot always be recorded throughout diastole. As a narrow jet of mild aortic regurgitation moves during the cardiac cycle, the Doppler waveform may differ in timing from beat to beat. When aortic regurgitation is severe, the regurgitant spectral waveform is well defined and near equal in intensity to that of anterograde flow through the aortic valve. Such a waveform appears consistent from cycle to cycle and is easily recorded. Intermediate degrees of regurgitation are manifest by intermediate waveform patterns and intensities. It should be emphasized that for this analysis, both retrograde and anterograde flow velocity curves must be optimized. Slight transducer angulations may be needed to optimize the two curves, because forward and retrograde flow are not always coaxial. If changes in instrument gain are needed to record optimal anterograde and retrograde flow signals, these should be taken into consideration.

Another qualitative technique for judging aortic regurgitant severity involves evaluating blood flow in the *abdominal* aorta. As described originally by Takenaka et al.,[91] image-guided pulsed Doppler from the subcostal examining window can be used to record systolic and diastolic flow patterns in the abdominal aorta, just below the diaphragm (Fig. 130-14). In patients with normal aortic valves, anterograde systolic flow down the abdominal aorta moves toward the transducer, and there is either minimal early diastolic reversal or no retrograde flow. Flow patterns similar to those in normals were recorded by Takenaka et al. in patients with angiographic 1 to 2+ (mild) regurgitation. In all patients with 3 to 4+ (significant) aortic regurgitation, however, holodiastolic retrograde flow could be demonstrated. A single patient was identified with 1+ aortic regurgitation and "false-positive" holodiastolic flow reversal, but this individual had diastolic runoff from the thoracic aorta through a patent ductus arteriosus into the pulmonary artery. Our own clinical experience suggests that holodiastolic flow reversal in the abdominal aorta does indeed indicate significant aortic regurgitation, although the absence of this finding cannot distinguish between modest regurgitation and a competent aortic valve.

A number of Doppler techniques can determine aortic regurgitant volume, regurgitant fraction, or both. One approach involves measuring the total volume of systolic flow that passes through the aortic valve and comparing this value to net forward flow measured at a different site.[92–94] In aortic regurgitation, the volume of flow ejected from the left ventricle during systole represents the sum of net forward stroke volume plus aortic regurgitant stroke volume. Hence, this measure is akin to angiographic stroke volume in a patient with pure aortic regurgitation. Net forward stroke volume can be measured at the level of the mitral annulus[93,94] or pulmonary artery,[92] so long as there is no mitral or pulmonic regurgitation. The difference between transaortic stroke volume and forward stroke volume represents aortic regurgitant vol-

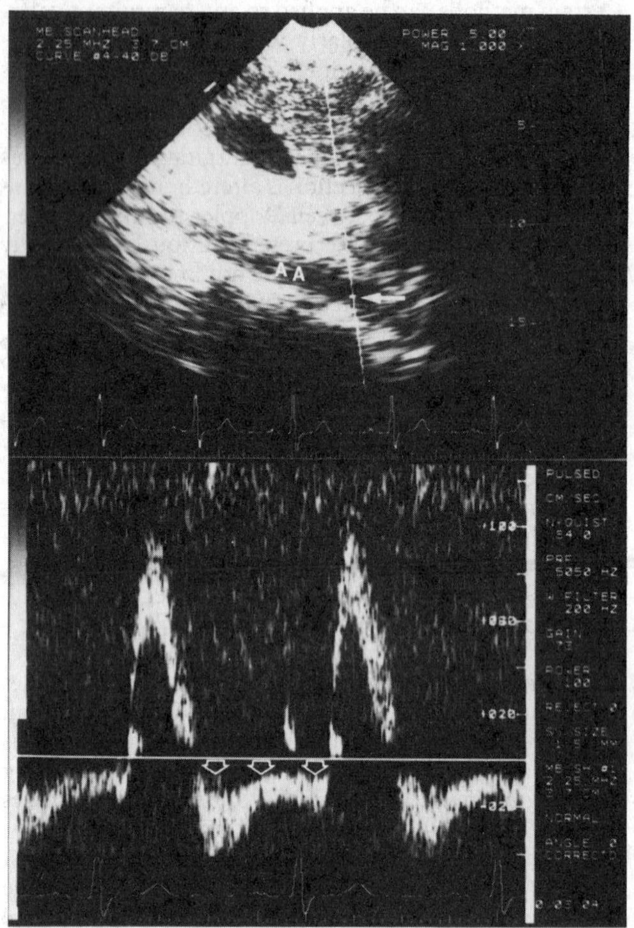

FIGURE 130-14 Assessment of aortic regurgitant severity from pulsed Doppler recording of abdominal aortic flow. *Top*: Subcostal image showing the Doppler sample volume (arrow) positioned in the abdominal aorta. Systolic flow is oriented toward the transducer. AA, abdominal aorta. *Bottom*: Pulsed Doppler velocity curve shows anterograde systolic flow above the baseline and retrograde flow that lasts throughout diastole (open arrows). This indicates severe regurgitation.

ume; the quotient aortic regurgitant volume/total stroke volume represents aortic regurgitant fraction. Good agreement between ultrasonic and invasive aortic regurgitant fractions generally has been reported,[92–94] although some authors question the accuracy of this approach.[95] The ultrasonic approach can still be employed when a patient has both aortic and mitral regurgitation, since it still allows selective measurement of aortic regurgitant volume. In such a patient, aortic regurgitant volume could be calculated as the difference between total systolic transaortic stroke flow (measured in the LV outflow tract or ascending aorta) and net forward stroke volume (measured in the pulmonary artery, assuming the absence of pulmonic regurgitation). Mitral regurgitant volume also could be measured as the difference between total diastolic transmitral stroke volume and net forward stroke volume in the pulmonary artery. Thus, in a patient with both aortic and mitral regurgitation, Doppler echocardiographic measures could define the actual volume of regurgitation through each of the two leaky valves. In contrast, the difference between angiographic LV stroke volume and net forward (Fick or thermodilution) stroke volume would represent the sum of aortic plus mitral regurgitant volume. As data from Kitabatake et al.[92] indicate, aortic regurgitant fractions are smaller by Doppler than by angiography in patients with both aortic and mitral regurgitation, as would be expected. In this situation, the Doppler aortic regurgitant fraction more accurately reflects the degree of aortic regurgitation.

A variation on this technique involves comparing diastolic and systolic flow velocity integrals recorded in the *thoracic* aorta. This technique uses pulsed Doppler to record flow velocity curves in the descending thoracic aorta from the suprasternal window.[96] The systolic velocity-time integral is proportional to total LV stroke volume; the diastolic velocity-time integral is proportional to the volume of aortic regurgitation. If the cross-sectional area of the aorta was constant during the cardiac cycle, the diastolic/systolic velocity-time integral ratio would represent the aortic regurgitant fraction. The aorta pulsates, however, and its cross-sectional area may be considerably larger during systole than during diastole. Thus, the ratio of diastolic to systolic velocity integrals tends to overestimate regurgitant fraction. This can be corrected by multiplying by the ratio of diastolic to systolic aortic cross-sectional areas, which is determined by calculating the ratio of the squares of the average aortic diastolic and systolic diameters. This approach yielded regurgitant fractions that compared closely to simultaneous angiographic aortic regurgitant fractions in 30 patients with varying degrees of aortic regurgitation.[96] Moreover, this technique was able to track directional changes in regurgitant fraction resulting from changes in heart rate and afterload.

A final means to quantitating aortic regurgitant severity stems from the fact that the aortic regurgitant velocity curve reflects the time course of the diastolic aortic–LV pressure gradient. The pressure gradient is highest at the onset of diastole and falls thereafter. As regurgitation becomes more severe, LV pressure rises more rapidly during diastole, and aortic diastolic pressure falls faster.[19] Thus, the more severe the regurgitation, the faster should be the rate of decline in aortic regurgitant velocity. Several investigators have recorded aortic regurgitant velocity curves by CWD and measured deceleration slopes and velocity half-times.[56,97–99] In these studies, the time course of aortic regurgitant velocity generally did reflect the severity of the lesion. Doppler and angiographic measures were nonsimultaneous, however, and there was overlap between deceleration slopes (or Doppler half-times) in adjacent angiographic grades of aortic regurgitation. It is important to remember that the time course of the aortic regurgitant velocity curve simply reflects the time course of the corresponding gradient, which is influenced by other factors besides regurgitant severity. When the left ventricle is poorly compliant (as in a patient with mixed aortic stenosis and regurgitation, or associated ischemic ventricular damage) or when aortic systolic pressure is very high, the aortic regurgitant velocity decay may be steep even when regurgitation is not severe. When analyzing the meaning of a given velocity profile, one must consider the hemodynamic milieu.

Mitral Regurgitation Many of the same methods just described also can be applied to mitral regurgitation. Flow mapping using CFI (Plate XI, 130-3) or image-guided pulsed Doppler can identify whether the mitral regurgitant flow disturbance is localized, widespread, or intermediate in degree.[100–102] Some investigators have suggested that the length of the regurgitant jet[100] can define the severity of mitral regurgitation. Other workers recommend measuring the maximal regurgitant jet area,[101] while still others prefer the percentage of the left atrial cross section filled by the regurgitant flow disturbance.[102] We believe that a number of factors must be considered when measuring color Doppler regurgitant disturbances to define the severity of mitral regurgitation. For a given quantity of valvular regurgitation, the size of the color Doppler regurgitant disturbance will depend on transducer frequency, pulse repetition frequency, high-pass filtering, instrument gain, driving pressure, and receiving chamber size.[103] In addition, the direction of the regurgitant jet exerts an important influence on jet size depicted by color Doppler imaging.[104] In particular, jets that pass obliquely along the atrial surface of a mitral leaflet and then along the atrial wall (a frequent observation with mitral prolapse or leaflet flail) are unable to entrain blood circumferentially. Thus, oblique "wall jets" typically are considerably smaller than unconstrained "free jets" when regurgitant volumes and driving pressures are comparable. Considering these provisos, we prefer to use Doppler flow mapping to develop a qualitative sense of whether mitral regurgitation is mild, moderate, or severe, recognizing the important influence of jet direction.

It is also noteworthy that when mitral regurgitation is mapped from the cardiac apex, ultrasound signal strength decreases as depth from the transducer increases. When signal strength is low, it may not be possible to detect mitral regurgitation deep in the left atrium even though the regurgitant disturbance actually is widespread. This is a particular problem for patients with large left ventricles and atria (in whom the superior portion of the atrium is very far from the transducer) and for those with highly reflective mitral valves (leaflet or annular calcification, or prostheses) that attenuate signal strength. For this reason, the regurgitant disturbance should be imaged from multiple views, including parasternal as well as apical windows. Examination from the precordium, as compared to the apex, usually permits Doppler sampling closer to the transducer, which may lead to improved signal strength.

Mitral regurgitant signal strength can be assessed by CWD and judged by comparison to the intensity of forward flow across the mitral valve.[105] This approach indicates qualitatively whether regurgitation is mild, severe, or intermediate in degree. The technical cautions discussed for aortic regurgitation again apply. The mitral regurgitant velocity curve also reflects the time course of the systolic pressure difference between the left ventricle and left atrium.[18] A "shoulder" or "cutoff" on the downslope of the mitral regurgitant velocity curve denotes early dissipation of the ventricular-atrial pressure difference in late systole, indicating a left atrial v wave[105] and suggesting that regurgitation is hemodynamically significant.

As noted earlier, mitral regurgitant volume and regurgitant fraction can be measured by comparing the volume of diastolic flow through the mitral valve with systolic flow into the aorta or pulmonary artery (assuming the absence of aortic or pulmonic regurgitation, respectively). In patients with isolated mitral regurgitation, Rokey et al.[93] measured diastolic transmitral stroke volume (from annular diameter and velocity-time integral) and net forward stroke volume (from LV outflow tract diameter and systolic velocity-time integral). The difference between these two measures was used to calculate regurgitant volumes and fractions, which showed good agreement with invasive measures. Blumlein and colleagues[106] traced end-diastolic and end-systolic endocardial borders in apical two-dimensional echo images to compute total LV stroke volume and Doppler measures to determine forward flow through the aortic valve. These workers also noted good agreement between non-invasive and invasive regurgitant volumes.

Recently, several groups have recommended using color Doppler techniques to image the area of flow acceleration proximal to the regurgitant orifice as a means to calculating regurgitant flow rates and volumes. This approach entails measuring the area (in square centimeters) of a hemispheric-shaped isovelocity surface, and the flow velocity (in centimeters per second) at that surface, to determine the flow rate (in milliliters per second) proximal to the regurgitant orifice. Regurgitant orifice area then can be determined by dividing by regurgitant velocity. In vitro studies[107–109] support the accuracy of this approach, which has promise for future use in clinical investigations.

Finally, Doppler techniques for estimating right-sided pressures (discussed earlier) are of great value in judging the hemodynamic significance of mitral regurgitation. When these methods suggest low pulmonary pressures, severe mitral regurgitation is unlikely. If pulmonary pressures are elevated substantially, particularly in the absence of other causes, then the possibility of severe mitral regurgitation warrants serious consideration.

Tricuspid and Pulmonic Regurgitation These lesions frequently are evident by Doppler investigation in asymptomatic subjects who have no auscultatory, radiographic, electrocardiographic, or echocardiographic evidence of heart disease.[110] The velocity and time course of the regurgitant spectral Doppler signals usually correspond well to those expected from pressure differences between the right-sided chambers. Therefore, we believe these signals truly indicate small amounts of *physiological regurgitation* across the right-sided valves. The Doppler signals of physiological regurgitation typically are faint, and they may vary from beat to beat as the heart moves during the respiratory cycle. Color flow images typically demonstrate a localized flow disturbance with a narrow origin. The right-sided heart chambers are normal in size. Similar findings suggest that "physiological" mitral regurgitation occurs in a significant number of patients without clinical mitral valve disease. Doppler evidence of aortic regurgitation is unusual in patients who do not have abnormal aortic leaflets or aortic root disease.[110]

Pathological right-sided regurgitation can be suspected when Doppler regurgitant signals are intense, easily recorded, consistent from cycle to cycle, and relatively widespread by flow mapping evaluation. The right-sided heart chambers usually are enlarged. It should be possible to calculate regurgitant volumes from differences between anterograde flow through the regurgitant valve and net forward flow measured at a different site; however, good reference standards are not available to document the accuracy of this approach. A useful index of tricuspid regurgitant severity involves analyzing the direction and timing of flow velocity in the middle hepatic vein, recorded by image-guided spectral or color Doppler from the subcostal window.[111] Normally, the hepatic vein drains into the right atrium as the latter expands during ventricular systole. With increasing tricuspid regurgitation, the systolic component of the hepatic vein flow curve (corresponding to the *x* descent of the jugular venous tracing) is blunted. With severe tricuspid regurgitation, systolic flow reversal (corresponding to a large *c-v* wave) occurs.

Prosthetic Valve Function

Doppler echocardiographic methods frequently are used to study prosthetic valve function and to document the nature and severity of prosthetic malfunction. The general alterations in flow dynamics that characterize stenosis and regurgitation of native valves also pertain to prosthetic valves. Thus, anterograde flow velocity is increased when prosthetic stenosis is present, while a retrograde high-velocity jet and a flow disturbance in the chamber receiving the regurgitant flow characterize prosthetic valve regurgitation.

Quantitative assessment of these abnormalities generally follows the approaches outlined for native valve disorders. Instantaneous and mean gradients can be determined by using the simplified Bernoulli equation.[112–116] Aortic valve functional orifice area can be calculated by using the continuity equation.[117] Mitral valve functional orifice area can be determined from pressure half-time measures (using the formula Valve area = 220/half-time) for bioprosthetic and tilting disc mechanical valves.[114,116] Regurgitant severity can be estimated[114–116] by spectral or color Doppler flow mapping, retrograde signal strength, or differential volume flow techniques. In general, these Doppler techniques have been able to identify significant prosthetic stenosis and/or regurgitation in small numbers of patients.[113–117]

The design and construction of valvular prostheses make it difficult to use Doppler techniques to assess prosthesis function quantitatively. Echogenic stents and sewing rings in nearly all valves and reflective occluders in mechanical valves cause significant attenuation of ultrasound signal strength in all Doppler modes,[118] limiting the sensitivity for detecting flow abnormalities on the side of the prosthesis away from the transducer. This is an important problem when examining for suspected prosthetic mitral regurgitation, since acoustic "masking" of the left atrium by the prosthetic valve may conceal Doppler evidence of regurgitation. For this reason, color Doppler investigation via the transesophageal window is of particular value for detecting the presence, mechanism, and degree of prosthetic mitral regurgitation.[119]

Moreover, there are many different prosthesis types and designs, each with its own functional and hemodynamic characteristics. Ranges of forward flow velocities have been reported[113–116] for different kinds of prosthetic valves thought *clinically* to be functioning normally; however, only small numbers of individual valves of a particular size and type have been included in these series. Furthermore, the velocity of anterograde flow across a prosthesis does vary with cardiac output and, at least for aortic valve prostheses, also with prosthesis size.[120] Calculation of valve orifice area from the continuity equation or consideration of the ratio of flow velocities just distal and proximal to the valve may help in distinguishing high gradients due to obstruction from those due to increased flow volumes.[117] The spatial profile of forward flow velocities may be quite complex in certain kinds of prostheses,[121] however, and forward flow jets may be oblique. Obtaining accurate velocity and gradient measures may be difficult in these cases.

Many bioprostheses as well as mechanical prostheses normally do permit some leakage.[122,123] Pulse duplicator studies have demonstrated that the amount of this "physiological" backflow, while usually small, does vary with loading conditions and heart rate.[122] Most patients with clinically normal prostheses have Doppler features suggesting that regurgitation, when present, is mild. Many patients with clinically significant regurgitation have Doppler evidence of widely distributed, intense regurgitation.[113–115,119] Nonetheless, given the problems with ultrasound signal strength, acoustic masking, and regurgitant severity estimation just noted, it is not always possible to distinguish between "physiological' and "pathological" prosthetic regurgitation using transthoracic Doppler techniques.

Evaluation of Shunt Lesions

Intracardiac shunts can be documented by demonstrating flow through the abnormal communication. By definition, shunt flow is abnormal in direction and often high in velocity. Both spectral and color flow Doppler techniques are useful in detecting intracardiac shunts. In general, shunt severity can be determined by measuring volumetric flows at different locations within the heart and great vessels.[8,9,12,124]

Ventricular Septal Defect

In patients with ventricular septal defect, flow through the ventricular septum can be demonstrated by pulsed, continuous, or flow imaging Doppler techniques. Many defects are perimembranous, with left-to-right shunt flow; in these patients, precordial long- and short-axis views are especially good for demonstrating flow in systole toward the transducer. Defects may be variable in location, however, and so it is important to use apical and subcostal windows as well. Multiple defects are most easily demonstrated by using Doppler CFI. In general, the velocity of flow through a small ventricular septal defect is high, since there is a large pressure drop from the left to the right ventricle. Large ventricular septal defects may allow equalization of pressure, in which case shunt flow velocity will not be high. A postjet flow disturbance within the RV body can be demonstrated by using pulsed Doppler or CFI. Compared with angiographic findings, Doppler can detect ventricular septal defect with a sensitivity of 95 to 100 percent and a high specificity.[125] Doppler findings clearly complement two-dimensional echocardiographic images and are of particular value in patients with defects that are too small to detect confidently by two-dimensional imaging. (See also Chap. 97.)

Since the defect diameter is difficult to measure reliably, the volume of shunt flow through a ventricular septal defect cannot be measured at the site of the actual defect but rather must be determined at a downstream site. Immediately distal to the septal defect, flow often is nonlaminar. Hence, it may not be possible to measure volume flow in the RV outflow tract or even in the main pulmonary artery. In this case, volumetric flow through the pulmonary circulation can be measured at the level of the mitral valve. Systemic volume flow is measured in the ascending aorta. The ratio between pulmonary and systemic flow volumes has correlated well to catheterization measures of the Q_p/Q_s ratio in both experimental and clinical studies.[8,125] These results support the role of Doppler in estimating the magnitude of shunting through a ventricular septal defect.

Atrial Septal Defect

Flow through an atrial septal defect can be demonstrated by color (Plate XI, 130-4) or spectral Doppler techniques.[126–128] While precordial and apical windows often can demonstrate left-to-right shunt flow, the subcostal window usually offers best alignment of the ultrasound beam with the shunt flow.[126] Shunting often can be detected in both late systole and diastole. In most patients with atrial septal defect, shunt flow velocities are low (in the range of 1 m/s), because of the small pressure drop between the two atria. Therefore, flow through the atrial septum can be demonstrated by using standard pulsed Doppler. Most secundum defects are relatively large and can be imaged directly by two-dimensional echocardiography. The thin septum primum portion covering the fossa ovalis often "drops out" in apical and parasternal views even when the atrial septum is functionally intact, however, and Doppler findings can be of great help in deciding if a septal defect is present. Care should be taken not to mistake normal systemic venous inflow (which often tracks along the right side of the atrial septum) for interatrial shunt. Attention to the timing of flow is important, but when there is a question about the Doppler findings, contrast or transesophageal echocardiography may be necessary.

Shunt magnitude can be quantitated by measuring pulmonary volume flow in the pulmonary artery and systemic volume flow in the aorta. The ratio between these two measures corresponds well to the Q_p/Q_s ratio determined at catheterization.[8,9,12] Color Doppler measures of the diameter of the flowstream through the atrial septal defect also have correlated with shunt magnitude at catheterization, with a defect measuring 1.5 cm or larger, indicating a Q_p/Q_s of at least 2:1.[127]

Patent Ductus Arteriosus

Persistent patency of the ductus arteriosus, infrequent in adults, is common in newborns and an important cause of neonatal respiratory distress. Left-to-right shunting through a ductus arteriosus must be diagnosed correctly before proper medical or surgical management can be carried out. Unfortunately, clinical findings are not always diagnostic. (See also Chaps. 97 and 98.)

Left-to-right flow through a patent ductus arteriosus can be demonstrated by imaging the main pulmonary artery, usually from a high parasternal approach. By color Doppler imaging, systolic flow is seen to pass from the right ventricle into the pulmonary artery, directed away from the transducer. Normally, no appreciable backflow is recorded. When a patent ductus arteriosus is present, retrograde flow from the aorta into the pulmonary artery is readily demonstrated. Spectral Doppler interrogation shows that ductal flow persists throughout diastole in patients without significant elevation of pulmonary artery pressure, while diastolic ductal flow is abbreviated in those with significant pulmonary hypertension.[128]

In patent ductus arteriosus, the profile of flow in the pulmonary artery is nonblunt, so that volume flow cannot be measured at that site. In order to quantitate the Q_p/Q_s ratio, systemic flow is measured in the RV outflow tract (which is relatively cylindrical in shape). Pulmonary flow can be measured in either the mitral orifice or the ascending aorta, since the total volume of shunt flow passes through both of these sites. Good agreement between pulmonary/systemic flow ratios measured by Doppler and by catheterization in children with patent ductus arteriosus has been reported.[8]

LIMITATIONS

Several technical limitations deserve reemphasis. First, compared to echocardiographic imaging, Doppler echocardiography typically depends upon low-amplitude signals, since the amount of ultrasonic energy backscattered from blood cells is substantially smaller than that reflected from interfaces between the myocardium and the blood pool. Distinguishing Doppler signals from background noise sometimes is difficult, particularly when ultrasound penetration is poor or when flow is examined at a great distance from the transducer. Second, accurate measurement of blood flow velocity using Doppler echocardiography requires orientation of the ultrasound beam parallel to the direction of blood flow in three-dimensional space, so the possibility of velocity underestimation must always be kept in mind. Unless angle correction is attempted or jet identity is incorrect, however, velocity overestimation ought not to occur. Third, Doppler CFI demonstrates flow vectors tomographically, whereas intracardiac blood flow has three-dimensional components that may be spatially complex. While comprehensive flow assessment can be carried out using multiple examining windows and transducer orientations, this can be tedious and may be of limited use when flow volume varies from beat to beat, as during an arrhythmia. Finally, Doppler is a demanding technique that requires of the examiner a good ear for Doppler frequencies, understanding of hemodynamics, and considerable patience.

GENERAL RECOMMENDATIONS

Doppler techniques give hemodynamic information, while two-dimensional echocardiography and M-mode echocardiography (Chap. 15) provide a structural assessment. Hence, these techniques supplement each other and offer intrinsic checks. For example, Doppler can be used to determine whether or not apparent echo dropout in the ventricular or atrial septum actually represents a septal defect, and echocardiographic images provide anatomic landmarks for Doppler interrogation. Similarly, measurement of the mitral orifice area by two-dimensional echocardiography can be checked against pressure half-time results determined by Doppler. Hence, Doppler techniques should be used together with two-dimensional and M-mode echocardiography as part of the comprehensive ultrasonic evaluation of the patient with known or suspected heart disease. In our laboratory, we use Doppler routinely, making those flow measures that appear important in the context of the clinical presentation and other examination findings. We first survey for structural abnormalities and then use imaging and Doppler in an interactive manner. At the present time, we find Doppler echocardiography clinically useful in (1) evaluating ventricular systolic and diastolic performance and estimating right-sided heart hemodynamics; (2) measuring pressure gradients and valve orifice areas in stenotic valves or other discrete narrowings; (3) detecting valvular regurgitation and estimating its hemodynamic significance; (4) evaluating valvular prosthesis function; and (5) establishing the presence and determining the significance of intracardiac shunts. Doppler echocardiography is an established and important part of the comprehensive cardiac ultrasound examination.

REFERENCES

1. Nanda NC: Doppler Echocardiography, 2d ed. Philadelphia, Lea & Febiger, 1993: 3–56.
2. Otto CM, Pearlman AS: Measurement of high flow velocities using pulsed Doppler echocardiography. *Echocardiography* 1985; 2:141–152.
3. Williams GA, Labovitz AJ: Doppler estimation of cardiac output: Principles and pitfalls. *Echocardiography* 1987; 4:355–374.
4. Huntsman LL, Stewart DK, Barnes SR, Franklin SB, Colocousis JS, Hessel EA: Noninvasive Doppler determination of cardiac output in man—clinical validation. *Circulation* 1983; 67:593–602.
5. Lewis JF, Kuo KC, Nelson JG, Limacher MC, Quinones MA: Pulsed Doppler echocardiographic determination of stroke volume and cardiac output: Clinical validation of two new methods using the apical window. *Circulation* 1984; 70:425–431.
6. Hillis LD, Firth BG, Winniford MD: Analysis of factors affecting the variability of Fick versus indicator dilution measurements of cardiac output. *Am J Cardiol* 1985; 56:764–768.
7. Croft CH, Lipscomb K, Mathis K, Firth BG, Nicod P, Tilton G, et al: Limitations of qualitative angiographic grading in aortic or mitral regurgitation. *Am J Cardiol* 1984; 53:1593–1598.
8. Barron JV, Sahn DJ, Valdes-Cruz LM, Lima CO, Goldberg SJ, Grenadier E, et al: Clinical utility of two-dimensional Doppler echocardiographic techniques for estimating pulmonary to systemic blood flow ratios in children with left to right shunting atrial septal defect, ventricular septal defect or patent doctus arteriosus. *J Am Coll Cardiol* 1984; 3:169–178.
9. Dittman H, Jacksh R, Voelker W, Karsch K-R, Seipel L: Accuracy of Doppler echocardiography in quantification of left to right

shunts in adult patients with atrial septal defect. *J Am Coll Cardiol* 1988; 11:338–342.

10. Fisher DC, Sahn DJ, Friedman MJ, Larson D, Valdes-Cruz LM, Horowitz S, et al: The mitral valve orifice method for noninvasive two-dimensional echo Doppler determinations of cardiac output. *Circulation* 1983; 67:872–877.
11. de Zuttere D, Touche T, Saumon G, Nitenberg A, Prasquier R: Doppler echocardiographic measurement of mitral flow volume: Validation of a new method in adult patients. *J Am Coll Cardiol* 1988; 11:343–350.
12. Kitabatake A, Inoue M, Asao M, Ito H, Masuyama T, Tanouchi J, et al: Noninvasive evaluation of the ratio of pulmonary to systemic blood flow in atrial septal defect by duplex Doppler echocardiography. *Circulation* 1984; 69:73–79.
13. Meijboom EJ, Horowitz S, Valdes-Cruz LM, Sahn DJ, Larson DF, Lima CO: A Doppler echocardiographic method for calculating volume flow across the tricuspid valve. *Circulation* 1985; 71:551–556.
14. Otto CM, Pearlman AS, Gardner CL, Enomoto D, Togo T, Tsuboi H, et al: Experimental validation of Doppler echocardiographic measurement of volume flow through the stenotic aortic valve. *Circulation* 1988; 78:435–441.
15. Gardin JM, Iseri LT, Elkayam U, Tobis J, Childs W, Burn CS, et al: Evaluation of dilated cardiomyopathy by pulsed Doppler echocardiography. *Am Heart J* 1983; 106:1057–1065.
16. Spirito P, Maron BJ, Bonow RO: Noninvasive assessment of left ventricular diastolic function: Comparative analysis of Doppler echocardiographic and radionuclide angiographic techniques. *J Am Coll Cardiol* 1986; 7:518–526.
17. Richards KL: Doppler echocardiographic quantification of stenotic valvular lesions. *Echocardiography* 1987; 4:289–303.
18. Currie PJ, Hagler DJ, Seward JB, Reeder GS, Fyfe DA, Bove AA, et al: Instantaneous pressure gradient: A simultaneous Doppler and dual catheter correlative study. *J Am Coll Cardiol* 1986; 7:800–806.
19. Nishimura RA, Tajik AJ: Determination of left-sided pressure gradients by utilizing Doppler aortic and mitral regurgitant signals: Validation by simultaneous dual catheter and Doppler studies. *J Am Coll Cardiol* 1988; 11:317–321.
20. Grayburn PA, Smith MD, Handshoe R, Friedman BJ, DeMaria AN: Detection of aortic insufficiency by standard echocardiography, pulsed Doppler echocardiography, and auscultation. *Ann Intern Med* 1986; 104:599–605.
21. Ciobanu M, Abbasi AS, Allen M, Hermer A, Spellberg R: Pulsed Doppler echocardiography in the diagnosis and estimation of severity of aortic insufficiency. *Am J Cardiol* 1982; 49:339–343.
22. Miyatake K, Okamoto M, Kinoshita N, Izumi S, Owa M, Takao S, et al: Clinical applications of a new type of real-time two-dimensional flow imaging system. *Am J Cardiol* 1984; 54:857–868.
23. Satumora S: Ultrasonic Doppler method for the inspection of cardiac functions. *J Acoust Soc Am* 1957; 29:1181–1185.
24. Franklin DL, Schlegel W, Rushmer RF: Blood flow measured by Doppler frequency shift of back-scattered ultrasound. *Science* 1961; 134:564–565.
25. Maeda M, Yokota M, Iwase M, Miyahara T, Hayashi H, Sotobata I: Accuracy of cardiac output measured by continuous wave Doppler echocardiography during dynamic exercise testing in the supine position in patients with coronary artery disease. *J Am Coll Cardiol* 1989; 13:76–83.
26. Elkayam U, Gardin JM, Berkley R, Hughes CA, Henry WL: The use of Doppler flow velocity measurement to assess the hemodynamic response to vasodilators in patients with heart failure. *Circulation* 1983; 67:377–383.
27. Rushmer RF: Initial ventricular impulse—a potential key to cardiac evaluation. *Circulation* 1964; 29:268–283.
28. Daley PJ, Sagar KB, Wann LS: Supine versus upright exercise: Doppler echocardiographic measurement of ascending aortic flow velocity. *Br Heart J* 1985; 54:562–567.
29. Mehta N, Bennett DE: Impaired left ventricular function in acute myocardial infarction assessed by Doppler measurement of ascending aortic blood velocity and maximum acceleration. *Am J Cardiol* 1986; 57:1052–1058.
30. Mehdirad AA, Williams GA, Labovitz AJ, Bryg RJ, Chaitman BR: Evaluation of left ventricular function during upright exercise: Correlation of exercise Doppler with post-exercise two-dimensional echocardiographic results. *Circulation* 1987; 75:413–419.
31. Sabbah HN, Khaja F, Brymer JF, McFarland TM, Albert DE, Snyder JE, et al: Noninvasive evaluation of left ventricular performance based on peak aortic blood acceleration measured with a continuous-wave Doppler velocity meter. *Circulation* 1986; 74:323–329.
32. Bargiggia GS, Bertucci C, Recusani F, Raisaro A, de Servi S, Valdes-Cruz LM, et al: A new method for estimating left ventricular *dP/dt* by continuous wave Doppler-echocardiography. *Circulation* 1989; 80:1287–1292.
33. Kitabatake A, Inoue M, Asao M, Masuyama T, Tanouchi J, Morita T, et al: Non-invasive evaluation of pulmonary hypertension by a pulsed Doppler technique. *Circulation* 1983; 68:302–309.
34. Hatle L, Angelsen B: *Doppler Ultrasound in Cardiology,* 2d ed. Philadelphia, Lea & Febiger, 1985: 172–173.
35. Rokey R, Kuo LC, Zoghbi WA, Limacher MC, Quinones MA: Determination of parameters of left ventricular diastolic filling with pulsed Doppler echocardiography: Comparison with cineangiography. *Circulation* 1985; 71:543–550.
36. Nishimura RA, Abel MD, Hatle LK, Tajik AJ: Assessment of diastolic function of the heart: Background and current applications of Doppler echocardiography. Part II. Clinical studies. *Mayo Clin Proc* 1989; 64:181–204.
37. Labovitz AJ, Lewen MK, Kern M, Vandormael M, Deligonal U, Kennedy HL, et al: Evaluation of left ventricular systolic and diastolic dysfunction during transient myocardial ischemia produced by angioplasty. *J Am Coll Cardiol* 1987; 10:748–755.
38. Thomas JD, Weyman AE: Echocardiographic Doppler evaluation of left ventricular diastolic function. Physics and physiology. *Circulation* 1991; 84:977–990.
39. Dittrich HC, Blanchard DG, Wheeler HA, McCann HA, Donaghey LB: Influence of Doppler sample volume location on the assessment of changes in mitral inflow velocity profiles. *J Am Soc Echo* 1990; 3:303–309.
40. Jaffe WM, Dewhurst TA, Otto CM, Pearlman AS: Influence of Doppler sample volume location on ventricular filling velocities. *Am J Cardiol* 1991; 68:550–552.
41. Bryg RJ, Williams GA, Labovitz AJ: Effect of aging on left ventricular diastolic filling in normal subjects. *Am J Cardiol* 1987; 59:971–974.
42. Stoddard MF, Pearson AC, Kern MJ, Ratcliff J, Mrosek DG, Labovitz AJ: Influence of alteration in preload on the pattern of left ventricular diastolic filling as assessed by Doppler echocardiography in humans. *Circulation* 1989; 79:1226–1236.
43. Thomas JD, Choong CYP, Flachskampf FA, Weyman AE: Analysis of the early transmitral Doppler velocity curve: Effect of primary physiologic changes and compensatory preload adjustment. *J Am Coll Cardiol* 1990; 16:644–655.
44. Gonzalez MS, Basnight MA, Appleton CP, Carucci M, Henry C, Olajos M: Experimental cardiac tamponade: A hemodynamic and Doppler echocardiographic reexamination of the relation of right and left heart ejection dynamics to the phase of respiration. *J Am Coll Cardiol* 1991; 18:243–252
45. Hatle LK, Appleton CP, Popp RL: Differentiation of constrictive pericarditis and restrictive cardiomyopathy by Doppler echocardiography. *Circulation* 1989; 79:357–370.
46. Klein AL, Tajik AJ: Doppler assessment of pulmonary venous flow in healthy subjects and in patients with heart disease. *J Am Soc Echo* 1991; 4:379–392.
47. Yock PG, Popp RL: Noninvasive estimation of right ventricular systolic pressure by Doppler ultrasound in patients with tricuspid regurgitation. *Circulation* 1984; 70:657–662.
48. Kircher BJ, Himelman RB, Schiller NB: Noninvasive estimation of right atrial pressure from the inspiratory collapse of the inferior vena cava. *Am J Cardiol* 1990; 66:493–496.
49. Himelman RB, Stulbarg M, Kircher B, Lee E, Kee L, Dean NC, et al: Noninvasive evaluation of pulmonary artery pressure during exercise by saline-enhanced Doppler echocardiography in chronic pulmonary disease. *Circulation* 1989; 79:863–871.
50. Hatle L, Angelsen BAJ, Tromsdal A: Non-invasive estimation of pulmonary artery systolic pressure with Doppler ultrasound. *Br Heart J* 1981; 45:157–165.
51. Burstin L: Determination of pressure in the pulmonary artery by external graphic recordings. *Br Heart J* 1967; 29:396–404.

52. Kosturakis D, Goldberg SJ, Allen HD, Loeber C: Doppler echocardiographic prediction of pulmonary arterial hypertension in congenital heart disease. *Am J Cardiol* 1984; 53:1110–1115.
53. Isobe M, Yazaki Y, Takaku F, Koizumi K, Hara K, Tsuneyoshi H, et al: Prediction of pulmonary arterial pressure in adults by pulsed Doppler echocardiography. *Am J Cardiol* 1986; 57:316–321.
54. Masuyama T, Kodama K, Kitabatake A, Sato H, Nanto S, Inoue M: Continuous-wave Doppler echocardiographic detection of pulmonary regurgitation and its application to noninvasive estimation of pulmonary artery pressure. *Circulation* 1986; 74:484–492.
55. Chan K-L, Currie PJ, Seward JB, Hagler DJ, Mair DD, Tajik AJ: Comparison of three Doppler ultrasound methods in the prediction of pulmonary artery pressure. *J Am Coll Cardiol* 1987; 9:549–554.
56. Grayburn PA, Handshoe R, Smith MD, Harrison MR, DeMaria AN: Quantitative assessment of the hemodynamic consequences of aortic regurgitation by means of continuous wave Doppler recordings. *J Am Coll Cardiol* 1987; 10:135–141.
57. Hatle L, Angelsen B, Tromsdal A: Non-invasive assessment of aortic stenosis by Doppler ultrasound. *Br Heart J* 1980; 43:284–292.
58. Stamm RB, Martin RP: Quantification of pressure gradients across stenotic valves by Doppler ultrasound. *J Am Coll Cardiol* 1983; 2:707–718.
59. Stevenson JG, Kawabori I: Non-invasive determination of pressure gradients in children: Two methods employing pulsed Doppler echocardiography. *J Am Coll Cardiol* 1984; 3:179–192.
60. Currie PJ, Seward JB, Reeder GS, Vlietstra RE, Bresnahan DR, Bresnahan JF, et al: Continuous-wave Doppler echocardiographic assessment of severity of calcific aortic stenosis: A simultaneous Doppler-catheter correlative study in 100 adult patients. *Circulation* 1985; 71:1162–1169.
61. Skjaerpe T, Hegrenaes L, Hatle L: Non-invasive estimation of valve area in patients with aortic stenosis by Doppler ultrasound and two-dimensional echocardiography. *Circulation* 1985; 72:810–818.
62. Otto CM, Pearlman AS, Comess KA, Reamer RP, Janko CL, Huntsman LL: Determination of the stenotic aortic valve area in adults using Doppler echocardiography. *J Am Coll Cardiol* 1986; 7:509–517.
63. Holen J, Aaslid R, Landmark K, Simonsen S: Determination of pressure gradient in mitral stenosis with a non-invasive ultrasound Doppler technique. *Acta Med Scand* 1976; 199:455–460.
64. Hatle L, Brubakk A, Tromsdal A, Angelsen B: Non-invasive assessment of pressure drop in mitral stenosis by Doppler ultrasound. *Br Heart J* 1978; 40:131–140.
65. Lima CO, Sahn DJ, Valdes-Cruz LM, Goldberg SJ, Barron JB, Allen HD, et al: Noninvasive prediction of transvalvular pressure gradient in patients with pulmonary stenosis by quantitative two-dimensional echocardiographic Doppler studies. *Circulation* 1983; 67:866–871.
66. Johnson GL, Kwan OL, Handshoe S, Noonan JA, DeMaria AN: Accuracy of combined two-dimensional echocardiography and continuous wave Doppler recordings in the estimation of pressure gradient in right ventricular outlet obstruction. *J Am Coll Cardiol* 1984; 3:1013–1018.
67. Sasson Z, Yock PG, Hatle LK, Alderman EL, Popp RL: Doppler echocardiographic determination of the pressure gradient in hypertrophic cardiomyopathy. *J Am Coll Cardiol* 1988; 11:752–756.
68. Smith MD, Dawson PL, Elion JL, Booth DC, Handshoe R, Kwan OL, et al: Correlation of continuous wave Doppler velocities with cardiac catheterization gradients: An experimental model of aortic stenosis. *J Am Coll Cardiol* 1985; 6:1306–1314.
69. Otto CM, Pearlman AS: Doppler echocardiography in adults with symptomatic aortic stenosis: Diagnostic utility and cost-effectiveness. *Arch Intern Med* 1988; 148:2553–2560.
70. Otto CM, Nishimura RA, Davis KB, Kisslo KB, Bashore TM: Doppler echocardiographic findings in adults with severe symptomatic valvular aortic stenosis. *Am J Cardiol* 1991; 68:1477–1484.
71. Gorlin R, Gorlin SG: Hydraulic formula for calculation of the area of the stenotic mitral valve, other cardiac valves, and central circulatory shunts. *Am Heart J* 1951; 41:1–29.
72. Zoghbi WA, Farmer KL, Soto JG, Nelson JG, Quinones MA: Accurate noninvasive quantification of stenotic aortic valve area by Doppler echocardiography. *Circulation* 1986; 73:452–459.
73. Richards KL, Cannon SR, Miller JF, Crawford MH: Calculation of aortic valve area by Doppler echocardiography: A direct application of the continuity equation. *Circulation* 1986; 73:964–969.
74. Teirstein P, Yeager M, Yock PG, Popp RL: Doppler echocardiographic measurement of aortic valve area in aortic stenosis: A noninvasive application of the Gorlin formula. *J Am Coll Cardiol* 1986; 8:1059–1065.
75. Otto CM, Pearlman AS, Gardner CL, Kraft CD, Fujioka MC: Simplification of the Doppler continuity equation for calculating stenotic aortic valve area. *J Am Soc Echo* 1988; 1:155–157.
76. Galan A, Zoghbi WA, Quinones MA: Determination of severity of valvular aortic stenosis by Doppler echocardiography and relation of findings to clinical outcome and agreement with hemodynamic measurements determined at cardiac catheterization. *Am J Cardiol* 1991; 67:1007–1012.
77. Shah PM, Graham BM: Management of aortic stenosis: Is cardiac catheterization necessary? *Am J Cardiol* 1991; 67:1031–1032.
78. Nakatani S, Masuyama T, Kodama K, Kitabatake A, Fujii K, Kamada T: Value and limitations of Doppler echocardiography in the quantification of stenotic mitral valve area: Comparison of the pressure half-time and the continuity equation methods. *Circulation* 1988; 77:78–85.
79. Libanoff AJ, Rodbard S: Atrioventricular pressure half-time. Measure of mitral valve orifice area. *Circulation* 1968; 38:144–150.
80. Hatle L, Angelsen B, Tromsdal A: Noninvasive assessment of atrioventricular pressure half-time by Doppler ultrasound. *Circulation* 1979; 60:1096–1104.
81. Gonzalez MA, Child JS, Krivokapich J: Comparison of two-dimensional and Doppler echocardiography and intracardiac hemodynamics for quantification of mitral stenosis. *Am J Cardiol* 1987; 60:327–332.
82. Smith MD, Handshoe R, Handshoe S, Kwan OL, DeMaria AN: Comparative accuracy of two-dimensional echocardiography and Doppler pressure half-time methods in assessing severity of mitral stenosis in patients with and without prior commissurotomy. *Circulation* 1986; 73:100–107.
83. Bryg RJ, Williams GA, Labovitz AJ, Aker U, Kennedy HL: Effect of atrial fibrillation and mitral regurgitation on calculated mitral valve area in mitral stenosis. *Am J Cardiol* 1986; 57:634–638.
84. Grayburn PA, Smith MD, Gurley JC, Booth DC, DeMaria AN: Effect of aortic regurgitation on the assessment of mitral valve orifice area by Doppler pressure half-time in mitral stenosis. *Am J Cardiol* 1987; 60:322–326.
85. Thomas JD, Wilkins GT, Choong CYP, Abascal VM, Palacios IF, Block PC, et al: Inaccuracy of mitral pressure half-time immediately after percutaneous mitral valvotomy: Dependence on transmitral gradient and left atrial and ventricular compliance. *Circulation* 1988; 78:980–993.
86. Kosturakis D, Allen HD, Goldberg SJ, Sahn DJ, Valdes-Cruz LM: Noninvasive quantification of stenotic semilunar valve areas by Doppler echocardiography. *J Am Coll Cardiol* 1984; 3:1256–1262.
87. Esper RJ: Detection of mild aortic regurgitation by range-gated pulsed Doppler echocardiography. *Am J Cardiol* 1982; 50:1037–1043.
88. Saal AK, Gross BW, Franklin DW, Pearlman AS: Noninvasive detection of aortic insufficiency in patients with mitral stenosis by pulsed Doppler echocardiography. *J Am Coll Cardiol* 1985; 5:176–181.
89. Hatle L, Angelsen B: *Doppler Ultrasound in Cardiology*, 2d ed. Philadelphia, Lea & Febiger, 1985: 142.
90. Perry GJ, Helmcke F, Nanda NC, Byard C, Soto B: Evaluation of aortic insufficiency by Doppler color flow mapping. *J Am Coll Cardiol* 1987; 9:952–959.
91. Takenaka K, Dabestani A, Gardin JM, Russell D, Clark S, Allfie A, et al: A simple Doppler echocardiographic method for estimating severity of aortic regurgitation. *Am J Cardiol* 1986; 57:1340–1343.
92. Kitabatake A, Ito H, Inoue M, Tanouchi J, Ishihara K, Morita T, et al: A new approach to noninvasive evaluation of aortic regurgitant fraction by two-dimensional Doppler echocardiography. *Circulation* 1985; 72:523–529.
93. Rokey R, Sterling LL, Zoghbi WA, Sartori MP, Limacher MC,

Kuo LC, et al: Determination of regurgitant fraction in isolated mitral or aortic regurgitation by pulsed Doppler two-dimensional echocardiography. *J Am Coll Cardiol* 1986; 7:1273–1278.

94. Zhang Y, Nitter-Hauge S, Ihlen H, Rootwelt K, Myhre E: Measurement of aortic regurgitation by Doppler echocardiography. *Br Heart J* 1986; 55:32–38.
95. Iliceto S, D'Ambrosio G, Amico A, Tota F, Piccini G, Marangelli V, et al: Errors in measurement of stroke volume for invasive and echo-Doppler evaluations of valvular regurgitant fractions: Clinical evaluation and computer simulation. *Eur Heart J* 1990; 11:355–360.
96. Touche T, Prasquier R, Nitenberg A, de Zuttere D, Gourgon R: Assessment and follow-up of patients with aortic regurgitation by an updated Doppler echocardiographic measurement of the regurgitant fraction in the aortic arch. *Circulation* 1985; 72:819–824.
97. Masuyama T, Kodama K, Kitabatake A, Nanto S, Sato H, Uematsu M: Noninvasive evaluation of aortic regurgitation by continuous-wave Doppler echocardiography. *Circulation* 1986; 73:460–466.
98. Teague SM, Heinsimer JA, Anderson JL, Sublett K, Olson EG, Voyles WF, et al: Quantification of aortic regurgitation utilizing continuous wave Doppler ultrasound. *J Am Coll Cardiol* 1986; 8:592–599.
99. Labovitz AJ, Ferrara RP, Kern MJ, Bryg RJ, Mrosek DG, Williams GA: Quantitative evaluation of aortic insufficiency by continuous wave Doppler echocardiography. *J Am Coll Cardiol* 1986; 8:1341–1347.
100. Miyatake K, Izumi S, Okamoto M, Kinoshita N, Asonuma H, Nakagawa H, et al: Semi-quantitative grading of severity of mitral regurgitation by real-time two-dimensional Doppler flow imaging technique. *J Am Coll Cardiol* 1986; 7:82–88.
101. Spain MG, Smith MD, Grayburn PA, Harlamert EA, DeMaria AN, O'Brien M, et al: Quantitative assessment of mitral regurgitation by Doppler color flow imaging: Angiographic and hemodynamic correlations. *J Am Coll Cardiol* 1989; 13:585–590.
102. Helmcke F, Nanda NC, Hsiung MC, Soto B, Adey CK, Goyal RD, et al: Color Doppler assessment of mitral regurgitation with orthogonal planes. *Circulation* 1987; 75:175–183.
103. Stevenson JG: Two-dimensional color Doppler estimation of the severity of atrioventricular valve regurgitation: Important effects of instrument gain setting, pulse repetition frequency, and carrier frequency. *J Am Soc Echo* 1989; 2:1–10.
104. Chen C, Thomas JD, Anconina J, Harrigan P, Mueller L, Picard MH, et al: Impact of impinging wall jet on color Doppler quantification of mitral regurgitation. *Circulation* 1991; 84:712–720.
105. Hatle L, Angelsen B: *Doppler Ultrasound in Cardiology,* 2d ed. Philadelphia, Lea & Febiger, 1985: 177–188.
106. Blumlein S, Bouchard A, Schiller NB, Dae M, Byrd BF III, Ports T, et al: Quantitation of mitral regurgitation by Doppler echocardiography. *Circulation* 1986; 74:306–314.
107. Recusani F, Bargiggia GS, Yoganathan AP, Raisaro A, Valdes-Cruz LM, Sung H-W, et al: A new method for quantification of regurgitant flow rate using color Doppler flow imaging of the flow convergence region proximal to a discrete orifice: An *in vitro* study. *Circulation* 1991; 83:594–604.
108. Utsunomiya T, Ogawa T, Doshi R, Patel D, Quan M, Henry WL, et al: Doppler color flow "proximal isovelocity surface area" method for estimating volume flow rate: Effects of orifice shape and machine factors. *J Am Coll Cardiol* 1991; 17:1103–1111.
109. Bargiggia GS, Tronconi L, Sahn DJ, Recusani F, Raisaro A, De Servi S, et al: A new method for quantitation of mitral regurgitation based on color flow Doppler imaging of flow convergence proximal to regurgitant orifice. *Circulation* 1991; 84:1481–1489.
110. Kostucki W, Vandenbossche J-L, Friart A, Englert M: Pulsed Doppler regurgitant flow patterns of normal valves. *Am J Cardiol* 1986; 58:309–313.
111. Pennestri F, Loperfido F, Salvatori MD, Mongiardo R, Ferrazza A, Guccione P, et al: Assessment of tricuspid regurgitation by pulsed Doppler ultrasonography of the hepatic veins. *Am J Cardiol* 1984; 54:363–368.
112. Holen J, Simonsen S, Froysaker T: An ultrasound Doppler technique for the non-invasive determination of the pressure gradient in the Bjork-Shiley mitral valve. *Circulation* 1979; 59:436–442.
113. Williams GA, Labovitz AJ: Doppler hemodynamic evaluation of prosthetic (Starr-Edwards and Bjork-Shiley) and bioprosthetic (Hancock and Carpentier-Edwards) cardiac valves. *Am J Cardiol* 1985; 56:325–332.
114. Sagar KB, Wann LS, Paulsen WHJ, Romhilt DW: Doppler echocardiographic evaluation of Hancock and Bjork-Shiley prosthetic valves. *J Am Coll Cardiol* 1986; 7:681–687.
115. Panidis IP, Ross J, Mintz GS: Normal and abnormal prosthetic valve function as assessed by Doppler echocardiography. *J Am Coll Cardiol* 1986; 8:317–326.
116. Wilkins GT, Gillam LD, Kritzer GL, Levine RA, Palacios IF, Weyman AE: Validation of continuous-wave Doppler echocardiographic measurements of mitral and tricuspid prosthetic valve gradients: A simultaneous Doppler-catheter study. *Circulation* 1986; 74:786–795.
117. Rothbart RM, Castriz JL, Harding LV, Russo CD, Teague SM: Determination of aortic valve area by two-dimensional and Doppler echocardiography in patients with normal and stenotic bioprosthetic valves. *J Am Coll Cardiol* 1990; 15:817–824.
118. Sprecher DL, Adamick R, Adams D, Kisslo J: In vitro color flow, pulsed and continuous wave Doppler ultrasound masking of flow by prosthetic valves. *J Am Coll Cardiol* 1987; 9:1306–1310.
119. Khandheria BK, Seward JB, Oh JK, Freeman WK, Nichols BA, Sinak LJ, et al: Value and limitations of transesophageal echocardiography in assessment of mitral valve prostheses. *Circulation* 1991; 83:1956–1968.
120. Teoh KH, Fulop JC, Weisel RD, Ivanov J, Tong CP, Slattery SA, et al: Aortic valve replacement with a small prosthesis. *Circulation* 1987; 76(suppl III):123–131.
121. Baumgartner H, Khan S, DeRobertis M, Czer L, Maurer G: Effect of prosthetic aortic valve design on the Doppler-catheter gradient correlation: An *in vitro* study of normal St. Jude, Medtronic-Hall, Starr-Edwards and Hancock valves. *J Am Coll Cardiol* 1992; 19:324–332.
122. Dellsperger KC, Wieting DW, Baehr DA, Bard RJ, Brugger J-P, Harrison EC: Regurgitation of prosthetic heart valves: Dependence on heart rate and cardiac output. *Am J Cardiol* 1983; 51:321–328.
123. Flachskampf FA, O'Shea JP, Griffin BP, Guerrero L, Weyman AE, Thomas JD: Patterns of normal transvalvular regurgitation in mechanical valve prostheses. *J Am Coll Cardiol* 1991; 18:1493–1498.
124. Valdes-Cruz LM, Horowtiz S, Mesel E, Sahn DJ, Fisher DC, Larson D, et al: A pulsed Doppler echocardiographic method for calculation of pulmonary and systemic flow: Accuracy in a canine model with ventricular septal defect. *Circulation* 1983; 68:597–602.
125. Stevenson JG, Kawabori I, Dooley T, Guntheroth WG: Diagnosis of ventricular septal defect by pulsed Doppler echocardiography. *Circulation* 1978; 58:322–326.
126. Shub C, Tajik AJ, Seward JB: Clinically "silent" atrial septal defect: Diagnosis by two-dimensional and Doppler echocardiography. *Am Heart J* 1985; 110:665–667.
127. Pollick C, Sullivan H, Cujec B, Wilansky S: Doppler color-flow imaging assessment of shunt size in atrial septal defect. *Circulation* 1988; 78:522–528.
128. Stevenson JG: The use of Doppler echocardiography for detection and estimation of severity of patent ductus arteriosus, ventricularseptal defect, and atrial septal defect. *Echocardiography* 1987; 4:321–346.

Chapter 131

Transesophageal Echocardiography

Alan Appelbe, M.B.B.S. ■ *Randolph P. Martin, M.D.*

Transesophageal echocardiography (TEE) has emerged as an important new technique for the assessment of cardiac structure and function. The use of TEE is rapidly increasing among cardiologists, cardiac anesthesiologists, and cardiac surgeons. Simultaneously, TEE probe technology and applications of the procedure continue to develop.

While TEE has distinct advantages when compared to transthoracic echocardiography (TTE) (Table 131-1), TEE echocardiography is not a substitute for the skilled use of TTE. Transesophageal echocardiography has proved to be of extreme value and offers additional diagnostic information among patients with presumed or known prosthetic/native mitral valve dysfunction for infective endocarditis lesions and their complications, in the assessment of intracardiac masses, in the diagnosis of thoracic aortic disease, in the detection of cardiac sources of embolus, and as an intraoperative/postoperative monitoring technique among cardiac and noncardiac surgical patients.

TABLE 131-1
Comparison of TTE and TEE

	TTE	TEE
Transducer frequency	2.5–3.5 mHz	5 mHz
Resolution	Lower	Higher
Posterior structures (left atrium/descending aorta)	Far field	Near field
Chest wall and lung interference	Limitation	Nil
Invasiveness	Noninvasive	Semi-invasive
Risk	Nil	Small/finite

HISTORY

In 1976, Frazin and Associates[1] first reported the acquisition of M-mode echocardiograms from a transesophageal approach using an ultrasound transducer mounted on a coaxial cable. The first two-dimensional TEE images were obtained in 1977.[2] These early TEE probes were cumbersome and found limited application. In 1980, Hanrath et al.[3] widened the application of TEE by developing an innovative TEE probe that used phased array technology and miniaturization. Subsequent developments include the evolution of smaller higher-resolution transducers, incorporation of pulse wave and color flow Doppler, incorporation of continuous wave Doppler, and development of biplane and multiplane TEE.

INSTRUMENTATION

Commercially available adult TEE probes consist of a phased array ultrasound transducer mounted on the tip of a modified gastroscope (Fig. 131-1). The handle of the probe has two control knobs that enable right and

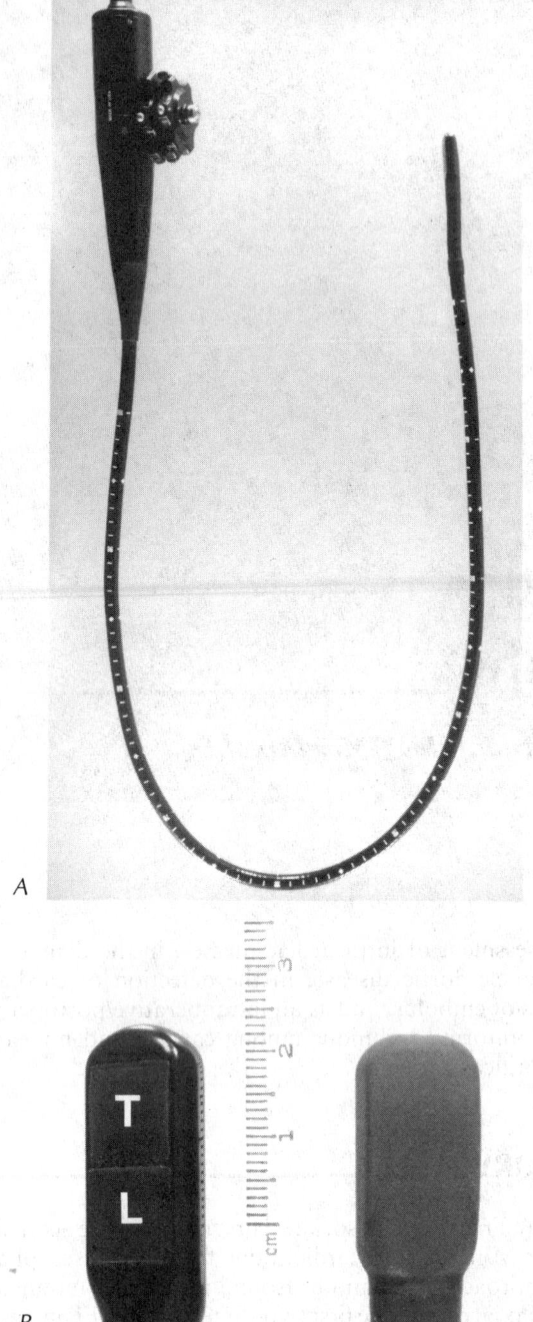

FIGURE 131-1 *A.* Transesophageal echocardiography probe. The probe is a 100-cm modified gastroscope. There are two control knobs present on the handle of the probe. The larger inner knob controls anterior and posterior flexion and the smaller outer knob controls leftward and rightward angulation. *B.* Close-up views of the transducer of a biplane (on the left) and single-plane TEE probe (on the right). Note the centers of the biplane transducers are separated by a distance of 12 mm. *T = transverse, L = longitudinal.*

left lateral flexion and anterior and posterior flexion. Single-plane TEE probes generally incorporate a 64-element phased array transducer that images in the transverse plane. The current generation of biplane TEE probes has two 48- or 64-element transducers (Fig. 131-1*B*). Importantly, only one imaging plane is active at any one time, and the centers of the two transducers are separated by 10 to 15 mm. This separation of the transducers means that when switching between planes, one does not obtain an orthogonal view at the same level. The adult TEE probe has a shaft diameter of 9 mm and a tip diameter of 14 mm. This size limits the use of TEE in pediatric patients, a limitation that has been overcome by the introduction of probes with shaft diameters of 7 mm and less.

The present generation of TEE probes allows two-dimensional and M-mode echocardiography as well as pulse wave, continuous wave, and color flow Doppler. Safety aspects and care of the probe includes careful maintenance with regular electrical safety checks and cleaning and sterilization of the probe between patients. Since ultrasound transducers produce heat while in use, TEE probes include a temperature sensor at the tip and an automatic cutoff mechanism to avoid thermal injury to the esophagus.

EXAMINATION TECHNIQUE

In the awake patient, preparation for the performance of TEE includes obtaining a history of any gastrointestinal symptoms or known esophageal disorder (Table 131-2). Informed consent should be obtained. Above and beyond informed consent, establishing rapport with the patient (verbal sedation) is very important. Except in emergency situations such as aortic dissection, TEE should be performed after at least a 4-h fast. The procedure room must be equipped with an oxygen supply, suction equipment,

TABLE 131-2
Summary of Contraindications for Performance of TEE

Summary of Contraindications for Performance of TEE
Absolute Contraindications
Large esophageal varices or recent bleed
Carcinoma of esophagus or tumor invading esophagus
Esophageal diverticulum (Zenker's)
Ruptured esophagus, tracheoesophageal fistula
Esophageal stricture
Mallory-Weiss tear; esophageal ulcer, severe esophagitis
Dysphagia of unknown etiology
Cervical spine instability
Relative Contraindications
Grade 1 varices
Meal < 4 h
Esophageal stricture successfully dilated
Mild esophagitis
Oropharyngeal deformity or surgery
Gastric ulcer
Not Contraindications
Nasogastric tube
Hiatus hernia
Duodenal ulcer
Tracheostomy
Critically ill
Elderly

blood pressure monitor, and resuscitation supplies. In most centers, oxygen saturation is monitored using a pulse oximeter. In the awake patient, TEE is generally performed in the left lateral decubitus position to facilitate removal of secretions and lower the risk of aspiration.

Ten percent lidocaine aerosol spray is used to achieve local anesthesia of the hypopharynx and to suppress the gag reflex. In selected patients, intravenous sedation (commonly midazolam) is used while the patient's vital signs are carefully monitored. In some centers, the majority of ambulatory patients are performed unsedated. This practice may reduce the incidence of complications such as aspiration and respiratory depression. An anticholinergic agent such as glycopyrrolate may be used to reduce salivation, but as with intravenous sedation, its use should be tailored to the individual patient.

ANATOMY AND IMAGING PLANES

The tomographic images obtained using TEE are confusing and disorientating when first seen. The relationship between the esophagus and the heart dictates the rather "unnatural" perspective from which TEE images are obtained. The cognitive problems of dealing with this new imaging perspective are compounded by the lack of uniformity in image orientation by different users, the "keyhole" nature of all ultrasound images, and the clarity of the images, which allows minute normal structural details to be seen. Since the heart's orientation in the chest is variable, nonstandard views are commonly obtained, and when manipulating the TEE probe, one cannot follow a simple recipe of maneuvers to obtain the standard views. In order to perform TEE competently, one must understand the three-dimensional anatomy of the heart from the perspective of the esophagus. This is best achieved by the supervised performance and/or observation of at least 50 TEEs. A systematic approach to image acquisition is mandatory to minimize the risk of overlooking abnormalities.

Although a selection of standard views is presented in this chapter, multiple other views are available. Following introduction of the TEE probe, one advances the tip of the probe to approximately 30 cm from the incisors in order to position the TEE probe behind the mid left atrium at the level of the base of the heart (Figs. 131-2

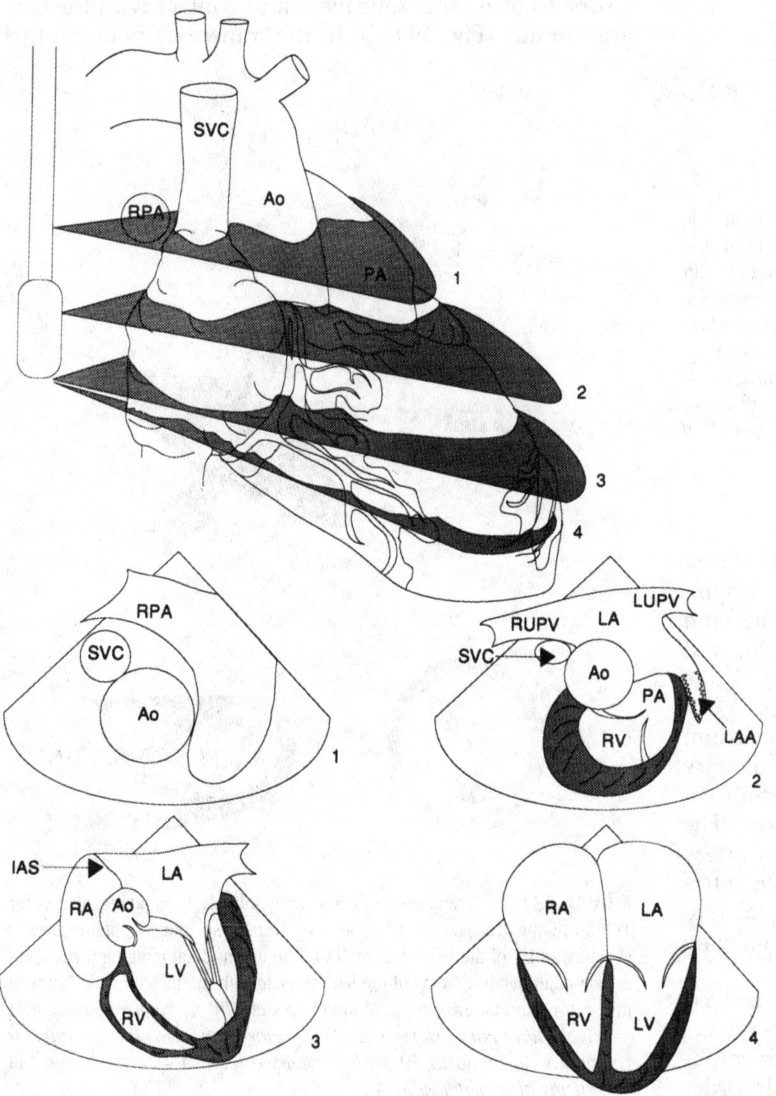

FIGURE 131-2 Selection of transverse imaging planes for TEE. Plane 1 is at the level of the right pulmonary artery (RPA). Plane 2 is at the level of the left atrial appendage (LAA) and the right and left upper pulmonary veins (RUPV, LUPV). Plane 3 is at the level of the aortic valve and left ventricular outflow tract (LVOT). To obtain a four-chamber view (plane 4), posterior flexion of the tip of the probe is required to bring the imaging plane into line with the axis of the left ventricle (LV). *SVC = superior vena cava, Ao = aorta, PA = pulmonary artery, LA = left atrium, RV = right ventricle, IAS = interatrial septum.*

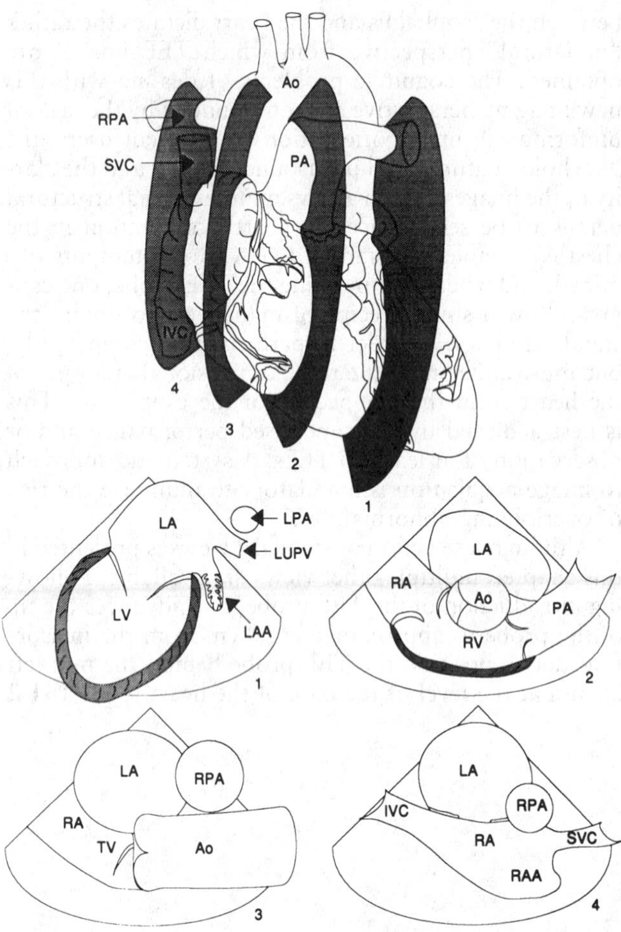

FIGURE 131-3 Standard longitudinal imaging planes for TEE. Plane 4 is in line with the superior vena cava (SVC) and right atrium (RA). Plane 3 is in line with the ascending aorta (Ao). However, further angulation of the tip of the probe would be required to align the plane with the left ventricular outflow tract and ascending aorta. Plane 2 is aligned with the right ventricular (RV) outflow tract. Plane 1 is the left ventricular inflow view. *PA = pulmonary artery, RPA = right pulmonary artery, IVC = inferior vena cava, LA = left atrium, LUPV = left upper pulmonary vein, LAA = left atrial appendage, LV = left ventricle, TV = tricuspid valve, RAA = right atrial appendage.*

and 131-3). In the transverse imaging plane at this level, examination of the aortic valve, aortic root, left atrium, left atrial appendage, right atrium, pulmonary veins, and proximal coronary arteries is carried out. In this and other positions, repeated minor remanipulation of the tip of the probe is required to optimize the images. Withdrawal of the probe above the level of the left atrium allows the main pulmonary artery, the right pulmonary artery, superior vena cava, ascending aorta, and a variable portion of the left pulmonary artery to be seen. The ascending aorta above the level of the pulmonary artery is obscured in the transverse imaging plane by the interposed trachea and main airways. This "blind zone" represents an important limitation of the transverse imaging plane.

Advancing the TEE probe below the level of the base of the heart in the transverse imaging plane gives images of the mitral valve, left atrium, left ventricle, interventricular septum, right ventricle, and right atrium. In order to obtain a four-chamber view of the left ventricle, the tip of the TEE probe is flexed posteriorly to bring the transverse imaging plane into line with the long axis of the left ventricle.

In the longitudinal (also called sagittal) imaging plane at the level of the mid left atrium, four standard views are obtained (Fig. 131-3). With the imaging plane rotated to the left, the left ventricular inflow view is obtained showing the left atrium, left atrial appendage, mitral valve, and anterior and inferior walls of the left ventricle. Clockwise rotation around the long axis of the probe moves the imaging plane toward the right and brings the right ventricular outflow tract, pulmonary valve, and main pulmonary artery into view. Further clockwise rotation brings the ascending aorta into view, and further rotation toward the right brings the right atrium and superior vena cava into view.

The ascending aorta and aortic valve are "cut" obliquely in the standard transverse and longitudinal imaging planes (Fig. 131-3). Right and left angulation of the tip of the TEE probe is required to produce orthogonal views of the aortic valve and ascending aorta.

An additional standard position for TEE imaging is the transgastric position, which is reached by advancing the probe into the stomach and flexing the tip of the probe to bring the transducer into contact with the gastric fundus (Fig. 131-4). In the transverse plane in this

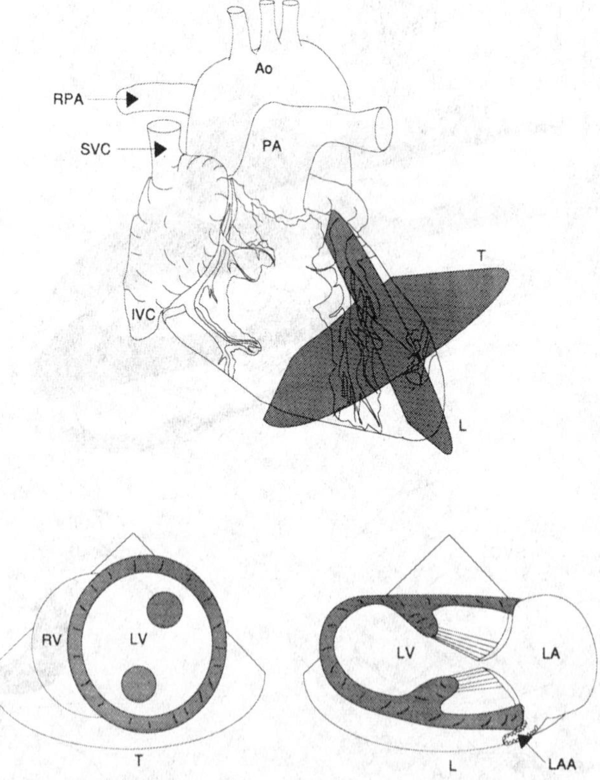

FIGURE 131-4 Transverse (T) and longitudinal (L) imaging planes for TEE from the transgastric position. The transverse imaging plane gives a short-axis view of the left ventricle (LV). The longitudinal imaging plane gives a "two-chamber-like" view of the left ventricle with the inferior wall (apex of the sector) and anterior walls of the LV in view. *RV = right ventricle, RPA = right pulmonary artery, SVC = superior vena cava, IVC = inferior vena cava, Ao = aorta, PA = pulmonary artery, LA = left atrium, LAA = left atrial appendage.*

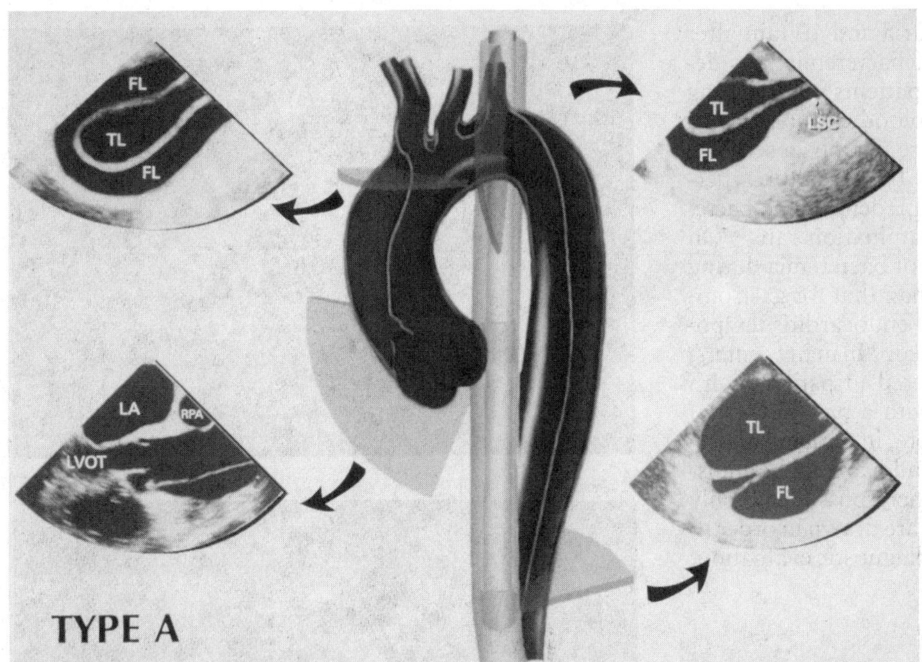

FIGURE 131-5 Transverse and longitudinal transesophageal imaging planes for the aorta in a patient with a type A aortic dissection. *TL = true lumen, FL = false lumen, LSC = left subclavian artery, LA = left atrium, RPA = right pulmonary artery, LVOT = left ventricular outflow tract.*

position, a short-axis-like view of the left ventricle is obtained. The left ventricular wall motion at the midventricular level can be observed from this position. In the longitudinal view at this level the inferoposterior and anterior walls of the left ventricle are seen as well as the papillary muscles and subvalvular apparatus of the mitral valve. The fact that the true apex of the left ventricle is usually not seen has important limitations for the detection of apical left ventricular thrombi and the measurement of left ventricular volumes and ejection fractions using TEE.

The thoracic aorta should be examined as part of the routine TEE examination. In the midesophagus, rotation of the probe to face posteriorly and toward the left brings the descending aorta into view (Fig. 131-5). Advancing and withdrawing the TEE probe using the transverse imaging plane allow the intimal surface of the aorta to be examined. Withdrawal of the probe to 20 to 25 cm reveals the transverse aortic arch and distal portions of the ascending aorta. In the longitudinal plane, the origins of the great vessels can be seen. Examination of the transverse aortic arch is generally performed last since the tip of the probe is close to the upper esophageal sphincter, which is uncomfortable for the patient and may result in probe displacement.

SAFETY AND COMPLICATIONS

Despite the semi-invasive nature of TEE, it has an excellent safety record. A series[4] of 10,419 TEE examinations performed at 15 European centers documented complications necessitating interruption of the TEE in only 0.18 percent of cases. These complications included bronchospasm, hypoxia, nonsustained ventricular tachycardia, third-degree atrioventricular (AV) block, angina pectoris, and minor pharyngeal bleeding. In this series, there was one death related to perforation of the esophagus in a patient with an unsuspected carcinoma of the lung.

In a series of 1110 consecutive TEE examinations performed at the Mayo Clinic,[5] complications included nonsustained ventricular arrhythmias (0.3 percent), nonsustained atrial arrhythmias (0.3 percent), congestive heart failure (0.2 percent), laryngospasm (0.2 percent), and parotid swelling. One death occurred in this series in a patient who suffered an acute episode of respiratory distress 5 to 10 min after completion of an uncomplicated TEE. Resuscitation was unsuccessful, and at autopsy the esophagus was normal, but there was microscopic evidence of myocarditis.

Because manipulation of the TEE probe is performed "blindly," perforation of the esophagus is of great concern. The incidence of perforation in esophagogastroscopies performed by gastroenterologists ranges from 0.02 to 0.03 percent. Only one reported case of perforation of the esophagus due to TEE has been reported.[4] To avoid this complication, the operator should never exert force to perform a TEE and should exclude patients with significant esophageal disease (Table 131-2). When esophageal disease is present and the safety of TEE is uncertain, a gastroenterologist should be consulted. Particular care is warranted in the elderly and unconscious patients.

Uncommon complications reported with TEE include a Mallory-Weiss tear,[6] endotracheal placement of the probe,[7] and unilateral vocal cord paralysis during prolonged TEE in neurosurgical patients in the upright position.[8] An intramural hematoma of the esophagus with subsequent rupture into the thorax has been reported[4] in one patient treated with thrombolytic therapy immediately after TEE.

The risk of patients developing endocarditis following TEE and the need for prophylactic antibiotics remain controversial. Transesophageal echocardiography is often performed on patients at increased risk of infective endocarditis. Bacteremia during upper gastrointestinal endoscopy with biopsy or esophageal dilation occurs in 4 to 8 percent of patients.[9,10] In a series of 100 consecutive

TEEs, with blood cultures drawn at 5 and 10 min after the procedure, a 7 percent rate of bacteremia was detected.[11] By contrast, a series of 85 patients[12] undergoing TEE revealed no bacteremia with blood cultures drawn at 15 and 30 min after the procedure. Finally, a series of 47 patients undergoing TEE with blood cultures performed both before and after the TEE detected no bacteremia above the background contamination rate.[13] On the basis of available data, the risk of bacteremia during TEE appears to be similar or less than that for gastrointestinal endoscopy. A single case of endocarditis temporally related to TEE has been reported.[14] In many centers, antibiotic prophylaxis is administered in patients with prosthetic valves and in patients with a past history of endocarditis. (See Chap. 94.) Of note, in patients undergoing TEE for suspected infective endocarditis, administration of antibiotics is avoided where possible or only given after sufficient blood cultures are drawn in order to minimize the interference with the diagnostic evaluation.

INDICATIONS FOR TEE

Intracardiac Masses

Transesophageal echocardiography offers significant advantages over TTE for the detection and assessment of intracardiac tumors[15,16] and intracardiac thrombi.[15,17,18]

A study of 93 consecutive patients[15] with intracardiac thrombi or tumors underscores the value of TEE compared to TTE. In this series 32 patients had paracardiac or cardiac tumors other than myxoma. Transesophageal echocardiography detected 100 percent of these tumors, whereas TTE detected 83 percent. Transesophageal echocardiography was superior in locating tumors involving the superior vena cavae, pulmonary artery or descending thoracic aorta, and masses anterior to the heart. Transesophageal echocardiography provided only limited information regarding the extracardiac extent of tumors, and tissue characterization of the tumor was not possible. In this same series, 15 patients had myxomas. Transesophageal echocardiography provided enhanced morphologic details such as cysts within the myxoma and provided more accurate anatomic details, in particular, the exact site of attachment of the tumor (Fig. 131-6). The use of TEE in selected patients may help to differentiate myxomas from thrombi.

In this same series of 93 patients,[15] 43 patients had intracardiac thrombi. For the 26 patients with thrombi in the body of the left atrium, TTE had a sensitivity of 69 percent versus 100 percent for TEE. Twelve patients had left atrial appendage thrombi, all of which were detected by TEE (Fig. 131-10) but none by TTE. The high sensitivity of TEE for left atrial thrombi, especially left atrial appendage thrombi, compared to TTE has been confirmed in other series.[17,18] Visualization of thrombi at the apex of the left ventricle is difficult.[15] With further experience with biplane and multiplane TEE, this limitation may be overcome.

Transesophageal echocardiography is indicated in a patient in whom a cardiac or paracardiac mass is suspected and in whom transthoracic echocardiographic findings are inconclusive or in whom further definition of the morphology and site of attachment of an intracardiac tumor is required.

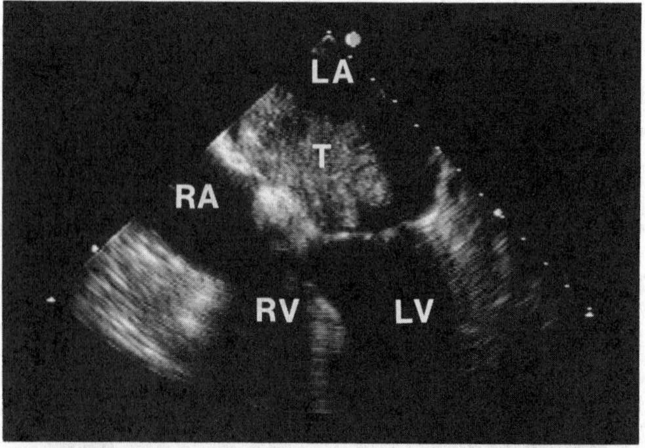

A

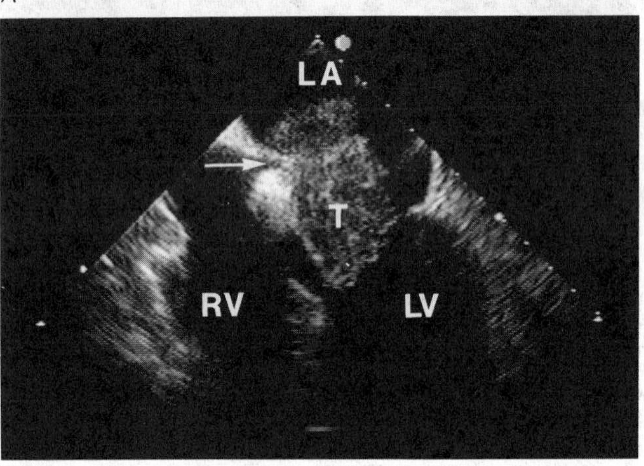

B

FIGURE 131-6 *A.* Systolic frame in the transverse imaging plane showing a left atrial myxoma (T). *B.* During diastole the left atrial myxoma (T) prolapses through the mitral valve (MV). The site of attachment to the fossa ovalis (arrow) can be seen. *LA = left atrium, RA = right atrium, LV = left ventricle, RV = right ventricle.*

INFECTIVE ENDOCARDITIS

The use of TTE for infective endocarditis has been hampered by its low diagnostic sensitivity. Transesophageal echocardiography has a far greater potential for the detection of vegetations because of its superior image quality.

A prospective study of 96 patients[19] with suspected endocarditis revealed a sensitivity of 100 percent for the detection of vegetations by TEE versus a sensitivity of 63 percent by TTE. The specificity was high for both techniques at 98 percent. Transesophageal echocardiography was sensitive for the detection of vegetations of all sizes, whereas the detection of vegetations by TTE was inversely related to their size (100 percent if greater than 10 mm, 69 percent if 5 to 10 mm, 25 percent if below 5 mm). With its ability to detect small vegetations, TEE may facilitate the diagnosis of infective endocarditis at an earlier stage.

A second large series[20] comparing TTE to TEE involved 62 consecutive patients with suspected endo-

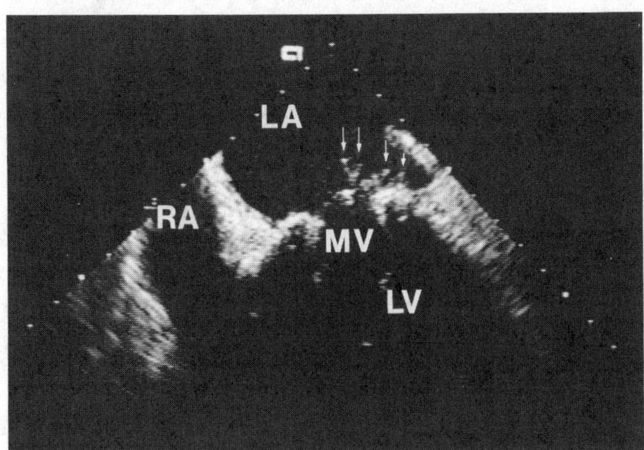

FIGURE 131-7 Transesophageal four-chamber view showing a prosthetic mitral valve with multiple vegetations present (arrows) attached to the sewing ring at the valve. These vegetations measuring up to 1 cm in length were not visible on transthoracic echo. *RA = right atrium, LV = left ventricle, LA = left atrium, MV = mitral valve orifice.*

carditis and 16 healthy controls. Using the presence of a vegetation, abscess, or leaflet perforation as echocardiographic criteria for the diagnosis of endocarditis, TEE had a sensitivity of 94 percent versus 44 percent for TTE. The specificity was high for both techniques. Importantly in this second study, TEE findings had a definite impact on many patients' management in whom the TTE was inconclusive.

Transesophageal echocardiography is a proven value for prosthetic valve endocarditis (Fig. 131-7), particularly for detection of vegetations on the atrial surface of mitral prosthetic valves.[21] It can also detect other nonvalvular sources of sepsis such as pacemaker lead infections.[22,23]

Transesophageal echocardiography also enhances the detection of complications of infected endocarditis including mitral valve chordal rupture, mycotic aneurysms,[21] fistulous connections,[24] secondary mitral valve involvement in aortic valve endocarditis[25] (Fig. 131-8),

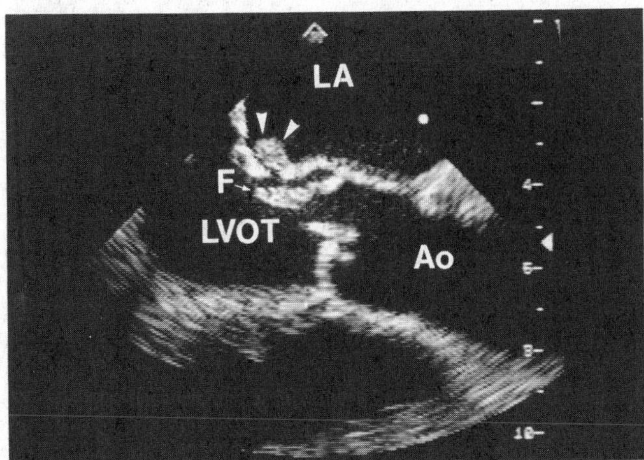

FIGURE 131-8 Longitudinal TEE view of the left ventricular outflow tract (LVOT) and ascending aorta (Ao). The noncoronary cusp of the aortic valve is flail (F), and there is secondary involvement of the anterior leaflet of the mitral valve (arrow heads). *LA = left atrium.*

and abscess cavities. In a series of 118 patients[26] with infected endocarditis documented by surgery or autopsy, 46 regions of abscess formation were present. Transesophageal echocardiography had a much higher sensitivity than TTE (87 percent versus 28 percent) for the detection of abscesses. Furthermore, the mortality rate was higher in those with abscesses, suggesting that TEE facilitates the identification of patients with a worse prognosis who warrant early intervention.

Transesophageal echocardiography complements the traditional methods of investigation of infective endocarditis. Because of its high sensitivity and enhanced ability to detect complications, TEE should be considered in all patients with suspected or proven endocarditis, especially those with mitral prosthetic valves.

AORTIC DISEASE

Due to the intimate relationship between the thoracic aorta and the esophagus, TEE provides high-resolution images of aortic anatomy and blood flow. This is particularly true for the descending thoracic aorta, which is poorly visualized by TTE.

Transesophageal echocardiography is of great value in the diagnosis of aortic dissection (Fig. 131-5). It allows visualization of the intimal flap and entry site, differentiation of the true and false lumens, detection of pericardial and left pleural effusions, and assessment of myocardial and aortic valve function.

The diagnostic accuracy of TEE for aortic dissection is very high. The reported sensitivity of TEE for diagnosis of aortic dissection ranges from 97 to 100 percent and specificity from 98 to 100 percent.[27-31] In the largest reported series[27] 164 patients with suspected aortic dissection were studied using a combination of TTE and TEE. The sensitivity of TEE was 99 percent and specificity was 98 percent. Transesophageal echocardiography proved superior to aortography and computed tomography (CT) scan. Importantly the three diagnostic errors that occurred in this series using TEE all involved the ascending aorta. Two false-positive diagnoses were made due to reverberation artifacts in the ascending aorta that mimicked intimal flaps. One false negative occurred because using single-plane TEE, the ascending aorta is partially obscured by the interposed airways. Biplane TEE may largely circumvent these problems.[31]

Patients with acute aortic dissection often are critically ill and have a high early mortality. In this setting TEE has advantages over aortography, computerized axial tomography, and magnetic resonance imaging. Transesophageal echocardiography can be applied rapidly at the patient's bedside and allows a more aggressive surgical approach to be applied. The use of TEE for the diagnosis of aortic disease other than aortic dissection has been less adequately explored. For thoracic aortic aneurysms, TEE allows aortic diameter and wall thickness to be measured; color flow Doppler allows angiographic-like visualization of aortic blood flow velocities and allows distinction between thrombus within an aneurysm and a thrombosed false lumen of a dissection. In the only systematic study of thoracic aortic aneurysms using TEE, 15 of 15 thoracic aneurysms were completely and correctly diagnosed.[32]

Limitations of TEE for the assessment of the thoracic aorta included its limited ability to assess branch vessel involvement and the risk of overestimation of aortic diameter and wall thickness due to oblique tomography images of a tortuous aorta.

CONGENITAL HEART DISEASE INCLUDING ATRIAL SEPTAL DEFECTS

Transesophageal echocardiography is superior to TTE for the detection of atrial septal defects (ASD).[33–35] From the esophageal position, high-resolution images of the interatrial septum are obtained due to the proximity of the interatrial septum to the posterior aspect of the heart. Furthermore, the ultrasound beam can be directed almost perpendicular to the interatrial septum. Not only does TEE offer the ability to detect abnormalities of the interatrial septum, but identification of the proper insertion of the pulmonary veins can be readily obtained in most patients. Currently, TEE may offer hope in sending selected patients with an ASD to surgery without the need for an invasive procedure.

In a series of 41 patients[35] with the clinical diagnosis of ASD, the sensitivity of TTE for the detection of the defects was 80 percent versus 100 percent for TEE. It was notable that of the eight patients with sinus venosus ASDs, TTE only detected two, whereas TEE detected all eight. In all cases TEE allowed clear visualization of partial anomalous pulmonary venous return associated with sinus venosus ASD.

The high-quality images obtained allow the size of the ASD to be measured directly. These measurements correlate well with surgical estimates of the defect size.[36,37] Preliminary work suggests that the size of the defect correlates well with the shunt flow ratio (QP/QS) measured by cardiac catheterization.[36,37] In addition, quantitative assessment of ASD shunt volume flow is possible by the use of pulse wave Doppler and measurement of the defect size.[36,37]

Transesophageal echocardiography may become the procedure of choice for assessment of ASDs because it gives the anatomy of the atrial septum, determination of the number, and the insertion of the pulmonary veins as well as provides useful hemodynamic information.

Transesophageal echocardiography has also been used to assess other congenital anomalies in both pediatric and adult populations. Transesophageal echocardiography can provide substantial additional information over TTE and cardiac catheterization, most notably for abnormalities of systemic pulmonary venous drainage, descending aorta disease, AV valve malformation, subaortic stenosis, and atrial baffle function[38] and following a Fontan procedure.[39] The valve of TEE is the setting of congenital heart disease is attained where TEE is performed by an experienced echocardiographer fully conversant with the morphology and hemodynamic features of complex congenital heart disease.

PROSTHETIC VALVES

Echocardiography and Doppler examination of prosthetic valves from the transthoracic approach are hindered by the acoustic shadowing produced by the metallic portions of the valve and sewing ring. Transesophageal echocardiography circumvents many of these imaging difficulties.

Transesophageal echocardiography is far more sensitive than TTE in the detection and quantitation of pathological regurgitation[40] of prosthetic mitral valves. Furthermore, valvular and paravalvular leaks can be differentiated and the exact site of the regurgitant orifice localized. Transesophageal echocardiography is so sensitive that the minor degree of "physiological" regurgitation present in normal prosthetic valves is readily detected. Each particular prosthetic valve has its own particular pattern of regurgitation.[41,42] An abnormal morphology of prosthetic valves is more clearly visualized by TEE, which is also more sensitive for the detection of vegetations (Fig. 131-7), thrombi, abscesses, and flail bioprosthetic leaflets.[40]

The advantages of TEE for the examination of aortic prosthetic valves are less clear. Quantitation of regurgitation and examination of the anterior portion of the sewing ring present particular difficulties. On the other hand, the detection of vegetations and abscess cavities on aortic prostheses is superior by TEE.[26,43] The examination of prosthetic aortic valves is particularly difficult when a mitral prosthesis is also present due to the acoustic shadowing that the mitral valve produces. Some of these limitations of TEE for prosthetic aortic valves may be overcome by the use of biplane and multiplane TEE from a transgastric position.

NATIVE MITRAL VALVE DISEASE

Transesophageal echocardiography provides consistently superior images of the mitral valve, which allows the accurate identification of abnormalities. The availability of detailed anatomic information regarding the mitral valve apparatus has become increasingly important in the era of mitral valve repair. The use of TEE aids in the identification of potentially repairable valves and the planning of the surgical procedure.

The detection of ruptured chordae and flail mitral valve leaflets is greatly enhanced by the use of TEE[44–47] (Fig. 131-9). In the two largest studies comparing TEE and TTE[45,47] containing a total of 55 patients undergoing mitral valve surgery, the sensitivity of TEE was 100 percent for the detection of ruptured chordae and flail leaflet. The sensitivity of TTE was 65 to 70 percent for the detection of a flail leaflet and only 35 percent for the detection of ruptured chordae. The specificity of TEE findings was high with only one false positive for ruptured chordae due to a healed vegetation.

The high-resolution two-dimensional images of the mitral valve provide an estimate of the likely severity of mitral regurgitation. However, the two principal means of assessing the severity of mitral regurgitation from a

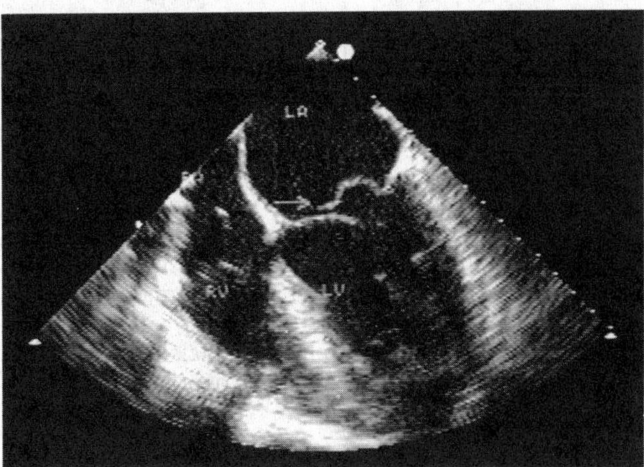

FIGURE 131-9 Transesophageal four-chamber view. The posterior leaflet of the mitral valve overrides the anterior leaflet due to ruptured chordae tendinea (arrow). *LA = left atrium, RA = right atrium, LV = left ventricle, RV = right ventricle.*

transesophageal approach are color flow mapping and pulmonary venous flow patterns. The ability to accurately grade the severity of mitral regurgitation by TEE is critically important, particularly during mitral valve repair surgery, where this judgment must be made both accurately and rapidly.

Color flow mapping has proven to be a clinically useful means of estimating the severity of mitral regurgitation by a transthoracic approach despite numerous technical limitations.[48] Firm guidelines for semiquantitation of mitral regurgitation severity by TEE using color flow mapping have not been established. It is, however, apparent that the criteria used in TEE cannot be used for TTE.[49] First, there are numerous technical differences between the two techniques including the higher-frequency transducer and proximity of the transducer to the mitral regurgitation. Transesophageal echocardiography also allows visualization of low-velocity swirling flow in the left atrium from the pulmonary venous inflow, which can merge with the mitral regurgitation jet, leading to overestimation of its size. Furthermore, from a transthoracic approach, the best correlation between angiographic grading of mitral regurgitation and color flow mapping is achieved by using the ratio of the jet area to left atrial area.[48] This approach cannot be used in TEE because the left atrial area cannot be measured since the whole left atrium cannot be included in any one view. In studies comparing TTE and TEE, TEE is more sensitive for the detection of mitral regurgitation,[49] but more importantly, mitral regurgitant jet areas are systematically larger by TEE.[49,50] This can lead inexperienced observers to overestimate the severity of mitral regurgitation by TEE.

In a group of 51 patients[50] studied by biplane TEE, a maximal jet area more than 7 cm^2 correlated with severe mitral regurgitation (MR). A maximal jet area between 4 and 7 cm^2 correlated with moderate MR; a jet area between 1.5 and 4 cm^2 correlated with angiographically mild MR; and a jet area less than 1.5 cm^2 was not detected on angiography. In this biplane TEE study, the best correlation between angiographic grades and color flow grades was achieved by using the maximal jet area seen in either plane. Biplane TEE allows a more accurate appreciation of the three-dimensional shape of the mitral regurgitation jet and gives a more accurate estimation of its severity.

A major limitation of color flow mapping and measurement of jet areas is that the shape and area of the regurgitant jet is substantially modified by interaction with adjacent solid boundaries.[51] Eccentric jets that strike the left atrial wall entrain less fluid and will be smaller than central jets of mitral regurgitation.[52] The pattern of flow in the pulmonary veins provides a second independent method of estimation of severity of mitral regurgitation by TEE and is particularly helpful with eccentric jets.

Transesophageal echocardiography with pulse wave Doppler provides a highly detailed and reproducible measurement of pulmonary venous flow patterns. The pattern of flow has been shown to reflect changes in left atrial pressure.[53] Increasing degrees of mitral regurgitation result in a decrease in the forward flow in the pulmonary veins during ventricular systole with a compensatory increase in the pulmonary venous diastolic flow. Considerable overlap in flow patterns is seen with mild to moderate degrees of mitral regurgitation; however, reversed flow in the pulmonary veins is observed with severe mitral regurgitation. Reversed systolic flow in the pulmonary veins is both a sensitive (greater than 90 percent) and specific (greater than 90 percent) sign of severe mitral regurgitation.[54,55] Both the right and the left upper pulmonary veins should be sampled since flow patterns can be discordant between the different pulmonary veins, particularly where mitral regurgitant jets are eccentric.[55]

DETECTION OF INTRACARDIAC SOURCES OF EMBOLI

The heart and thoracic aorta are increasingly recognized as a source of cerebrovascular and peripheral ischemic events. The use of TTE to detect cardiac sources of embolism has typically been unrewarding.[56] By comparison, TEE identifies potential cardiac sources of emboli in the majority of patients presenting with unexplained stroke. In a series of 79 patients[57] with cryptogenic stroke, TEE identified a potential cardiac source of embolism in 57 percent of patients compared with 15 percent by TTE. Even in patients with no clinical cardiac disease, potential sources of embolism were detected in 39 percent of patients by TEE.

Transesophageal echocardiography is sensitive for the detection of a wide range of cardiac abnormalities associated with systemic embolism, including left atrial thrombi, atrial septal defects, patent foramen ovale, atrial septal aneurysm, intracardiac tumors, left atrial spontaneous contrast, and aortic atherosclerotic debris.

The sensitivity of TTE for the detection of thrombi within the body of the left atrium is 60 percent.[57] Transthoracic echocardiography, however, has a much lower sensitivity (15 percent) for detection of thrombi within the left atrial appendage. This so-called blind spot represents a critical limitation of TTE since 50 percent[58] of left atrial thrombi occur within the left atrial appendage. On the other hand, TEE offers detailed images of the left atrium, including the left atrial appendage. The sensitivity and specificity of TEE for the detection of left atrial and left atrial appendage thrombi is close to 100 percent[15,17,18,57,59] (Fig. 131-10).

From a transesophageal approach, the interatrial septum is in the near field and high-resolution images are obtained. Not surprisingly, abnormalities of the interatrial septum are clearly visualized, including atrial septal aneurysms and patent foramen ovale. Both of these lesions have been associated with an increased incidence of unexplained stroke.[60–62] Transesophageal echocardiography is more sensitive than TTE for the detection of atrial septal aneurysms and patent foramen ovale.[57,59] With the use of TEE, thrombotic material has been visualized within atrial septal aneurysms,[60] and emboli from the venous system have been seen straddling the foramen ovale.[63]

Spontaneous echo contrast or "smoke" has been detected more frequently since the introduction of TEE.[64,65] Left atrial spontaneous contrast is noted in conditions that favor stasis of blood including atrial fibrillation, mitral stenosis, and left atrial enlargement.[65,66] By comparison, the presence of mitral regurgitation lessens the frequency of spontaneous contrast.[66] Left atrial spontaneous contrast shows a very strong association with the presence of left atrial thrombi, with 80 to 100 percent of patients with left atrial thrombi having spontaneous contrast.[65–68] Of particular clinical importance, left atrial spontaneous contrast is an independent predictor of thromboembolic risks in patients with mitral valve disease[66,67] and nonvalvular atrial fibrillation.[66]

Transesophageal echocardiography allows the visualization of the aortic intima with great resolution. Intimal irregularity, thickening, and mobile atheromatous material can all be readily detected. With the advent of this sensitive method to examine the aortic intima, it has become apparent that the aorta is an important source of emboli in patients with unexplained stroke and arterial emboli. In a series of 556 patients undergoing TEE, intraaortic atherosclerosis was detected in 7 percent of cases.[69] Intraaortic atherosclerotic debris was associated with embolic events. Moreover, the incidence of embolism was higher when the debris was pedunculated and highly mobile (8 of 11) than when it was immobile (3 of 25). In addition, the incidence of embolism was 27 percent in those patients with mobile atheroma undergoing invasive procedures. In a separate study[70] of 72 patients with a history of transient ischemic attack or stroke, TEE revealed widespread atherosclerotic debris in 44 percent of patients.

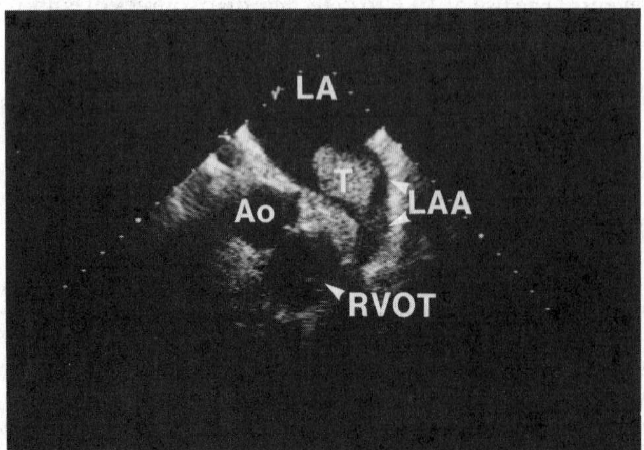

FIGURE 131-10 Transesophageal echocardiography image of the left atrial appendage (LAA) in the transverse plane. A thrombus (T) is present in the orifice of the left atrial appendage. *LA = left atrium, Ao = aorta, RVOT = right ventricular outflow tract.*

INTRAOPERATIVE TEE

Intraoperative TEE has emerged as a new technique by which cardiac surgeons and anesthesiologists can more precisely define the operative anatomy, immediately assess the outcome of surgery, and more accurately monitor left ventricular function without interfering with the operating field.

Intraoperative TEE has had its greatest impact in the assessment of valve repair and replacement.[71,72] Transesophageal echocardiography performed before the patient is placed on bypass precisely defines the anatomy, and aids in the selection of the appropriate operative procedure. Transesophageal echocardiography with color flow Doppler after cardiopulmonary bypass, gives instant feedback to the surgeon regarding the adequacy of repair and guides further intervention.[73,74] In patients undergoing mitral valve repair, intraoperative TEE is now performed routinely in many centers.

Transesophageal echocardiography also allows continuous intraoperative monitoring of left ventricular global and regional function. Left ventricular function is monitored in the transgastric short-axis view at the mid papillary muscle level. By the detection of regional wall motion abnormalities, TEE is a sensitive and early indicator of myocardial ischemia.[75] New regional wall motion abnormalities following coronary artery bypass graft surgery are predictive of an adverse clinical outcome.[76]

With the advent of TEE probes with a smaller diameter, TEE is emerging as a useful new tool in surgical decision making during repair of congenital defects.[77] In a series of 224 patients undergoing surgery for congenital defects, TEE detected new unsuspected findings in 21 percent of patients and had some effect on the operative procedure in 47 percent of patients.

TEE IN THE CRITICALLY ILL

Transthoracic echocardiography is often unsatisfactory in critically ill patients due to limited image quality. Transesophageal echocardiography may be helpful in this setting since high-quality images can consistently be obtained. The procedure can be performed at the patient's bedside, and even in hemodynamically unstable patients, TEE can be performed safely.[78,79]

TEE DURING BALLOON CATHETER MITRAL COMMISSUROTOMY

Transesophageal echocardiography has proved useful during invasive procedures for better visualization of the three-dimensional anatomy and detection of complications during balloon mitral commissurotomy.[80,81] It allows the detection of left atrial thrombi,[18] better localization of the atrial septal puncture site, immediate assessment of a newly created atrial septal defect,[82] mitral valve gradient or regurgitation, and the detection of complications such as tamponade.

FUTURE DIRECTIONS

Transesophageal echocardiography has also been applied in the setting of transcatheter closure of atrial septal defects.[83] Preliminary data suggest that the addition of TEE to fluoroscopy may make this intervention safer, easier, and more effective. The high-resolution images available by TEE allow visualization of the proximal portions of the coronary arteries in a high percentage of patients.[84] Pulse Doppler and color flow Doppler can be used to measure proximal coronary artery blood flow.[85] Preliminary reports suggest that using biplane TEE, luminal narrowing, particularly of the left main coronary artery, can be accurately detected.[86]

REFERENCES

1. Frazin L, Talano JV, Stephanides L, Loeb HS, Kopel L, Gunnar RM: Esophageal echocardiography. *Circulation* 1976; 54:102–108.
2. Hisanaga K, Hisanaga A, Nagata K, Yoshida S: A new transesophageal real-time two-dimensional echocardiographic system using a flexible tube and its clinical application. *Proc Jpn Soc Ultrason Med* 1977; 32:43–44.
3. Hanrath P, Kremer P, Langenstein BA, Matsumoto M, Bleifield W: Transösophageale echokardiographie: ein neues verfahrn zur dynamischen ventrikelfunktionsanalyse. *Dtsch Med Wochenschr* 1981; 106:523–552.
4. Daniel WG, Erbel R, Kasper W, Visser CA, Engberding R, Sutherland GR, et al: Safety of transesophageal echocardiography: A multicenter survey of 10,419 examinations. *Circulation* 1991; 83:817–821.
5. Khandheria BK, Seward JB, Tajik AJ: Transesophageal echocardiography. In: Braunwald E (ed): *Heart Disease: A Textbook of Cardiovascular Medicine*, 3d ed. Philadelphia, WB Saunders, 1992:290.
6. Dewhirst WE, Stragand JJ, Fleming BM: Mallory-Weiss tear complicating intraoperative transesophageal echocardiography in a patient undergoing aortic valve replacement. *Anesthesiology* 1990; 73:777–778.
7. Fagan LF Jr, Weiss R, Castello R, Labowitz AJ: Transtracheal placement and imaging with a transesophageal echocardiographic probe. *Am J Cardiol* 1991; 67:909–910.
8. Cucchiari RF, Nugent M, Seward JB, Messick JM: Air embolism in upright two dimensional transesophageal echocardiography. *Anesthesiology* 1984; 60:353–355.
9. Baltch AL, Bunac I, Agrawal A, O'Connor P, Bram M, Malarino E: Bacteremia after upper gastrointestinal endoscopy. *Arch Intern Med* 1971; 137:594–597.
10. Shorvan PJ, Eykyn PJ, Cotton PB: Gastrointestinal instrumentation, bacteremia, and endocarditis. *Gut* 1983; 24:1078–1093.
11. Dennig K, Sedlmayr V, Selig B, Rudolph W: Bacteremia with transesophageal echocardiography (abstr). *Circulation* 1989; 80:II473.
12. Chandrasekaran K, Bansal RC, Minz GS, Ross JJ, Shah PM: Impact of transesophageal color flow Doppler echocardiography in current cardiology practice. *Echocardiography* 1990; 7:115–145.
13. Steckelberg JM, Khandheria BK, Anhalt JP, Ballard DJ, Seward JB, Click RL, et al: Prospective evaluation of the risk of bacteremia associated with transesophageal echocardiography. *Circulation* 1991; 84:177–180.
14. Foster E, Kusumoto FM, Sobol SM, Schiller NB: Streptococcal endocarditis temporally related to transesophageal echocardiography. *J Am Soc Echocardiogr* 1990; 3:424–427.
15. Mügge A, Daniel WG, Haverich A, Lichtlen PR: Diagnosis of noninfective cardiac mass lesions by two-dimensional echocardiography. *Circulation* 1991; 83:70–78.
16. Obeid AI, Marvasti M, Parker F, Rosenberg J: Comparison of transthoracic and transesophageal echocardiography in diagnosis of left atrial myxoma. *Am J Cardiol* 1989; 63:1006–1008.
17. Aschenberg W, Schlüter M, Kremer P, Schröder E, Siglow V, Bleifeld W: Transesophageal two-dimensional echocardiography for the detection of left atrial appendage thrombus. *J Am Coll Cardiol* 1986; 7:163–166.
18. Kronzon I, Tunick PA, Glassman E, Slater J, Schwinger M, Freedberg RS: Transesophageal echocardiography to detect atrial clots in candidates for percutaneous transseptal mitral balloon valvuloplasty. *J Am Coll Cardiol* 1990; 16:1320–1322.
19. Erbel R, Rohmann S, Drexler M, Mohr-Kahaly S, Gerharz CD, Iversen S, et al: Improved diagnostic value of echocardiography in patients with infective endocarditis by transesophageal approach. A prospective study. *Eur Heart J* 1988; 9:43–53.
20. Shively BK, Gurule FT, Roldan CA, Leggett JH, Schiller NB: Diagnostic value of transesophageal compared with transthoracic echocardiography in infective endocarditis. *J Am Coll Cardiol* 1991; 18:391–397.
21. Taams MA, Gussenhoven EJ, Bos E, De Jaegere P, Roelandt J, Sutherland G, et al: Enhanced morphological diagnosis in infective endocarditis by transesophageal echocardiography. *Br Heart J* 1990; 63:109–113.
22. Porkolab FL, Weinbaum DL, Lerberg DB, Phillips JC: The source of recurrent bacteremia identified by trans-esophageal echocardiography. *Ann Intern Med* 1990; 112:628–629.
23. Zehender M, Büchner C, Geibel A, Kasper W, Meinertz T, Just H: Diagnosis of hidden pacemaker lead sepsis by transesophageal echocardiography and a new technique for lead extraction. *Am Heart J* 1989; 118:1050–1053.
24. Bansal RC, Graham BM, Jutzy KR, Shakudo M, Shah PM: Left ventricular outflow tract to left atrial communication secondary to rupture of mitral-aortic intervalvular fibrosa in infective endocarditis: Diagnosis by transesophageal echocardiography and color flow imaging. *J Am Coll Cardiol* 1990; 15:499–504.
25. Karalis DG, Bansal RC, Hauck AJ, Ross JR, Applegat PM, Jurtzy KR, et al: Transesophageal recognition of subaortic complications in aortic valve endocarditis. Clinical and surgical implications. *Circulation* 1992; 86:353–362.
26. Daniel WG, Mügge A, Martin RP, Lindert O, Hausmann D, Nonnast-Daniel B, et al: Improvement in the diagnosis of abscesses associated with endocarditis by transesophageal echocardiography. *N Engl J Med* 1991; 324:795–800.
27. Erbel R, Mohr-Kahaly S, Rennollet H, Brunier J, Drexler M, Wittlich N, et al: Diagnosis of aortic dissection: The value of transesophageal echocardiography. *Thorac Cardiovasc Surgeon* 1987; 35:126–133.
28. Erbel R, Engberding R, Daniel W, Roelandt J, Visser C, Rennollet H: Echocardiography in diagnosis of aortic dissection. *Lancet* 1989; 1:457–461.
29. Sasaki S, Yoshida H, Matsui Y, Sakuma M, Yashuda K, Tanade T: The value of recent noninvasive medical imagings in diagnosis of dissecting aortic aneurysm: Further investigation on transesophageal echocardiography and MRI. *Kyobu Geka* 1989; 42:297–302.
30. Kasper W, Hofmann T, Meinertz T, Billmann P, Byrtus M, Lang K, et al: Diagnosis of thoracic aortic aneurysms and dissections using transesophageal echocardiography. *Z Kardiol* 1986; 75:609–615.
31. Hashimoto S, Kumada T, Osakada G, Kubo S, Tokunaga S, Tamaki S, et al: Assessment of transesophageal Doppler echography in dissecting aortic aneurysm. *J Am Coll Cardiol* 1989; 14:1253–1262.

32. Taams MA, Gussenhowen WJ, Schippers LA, Roelandt J, Van Herwerden LA, Bos E, et al: The value of transesophageal echocardiography for diagnosis of thoracic aorta pathology. *Eur Heart J* 1988; 9:1308–1316.
33. Hanrath P, Schlutter M, Langenstein BA, Polster J, Engel S, Kremer P, et al: Detection of ostium secundum atrial septal defects by transesophageal cross sectional echocardiography. *Br Heart J* 1983; 49:350–358.
34. Weigel JT, Seward JB, Hagler DJ, Khanderia BK, Tajik JA: Transesophageal echocardiography in 21 atrial septal defects with incomplete precordial echocardiography (abstr). *Circulation* 1989; 80(suppl II):II-474.
35. Kronzon I, Tunick PA, Freedberg RS, Trehan N, Rosenzweig BP, Schwinger ME: Transesophageal echocardiography is superior to transthoracic echocardiography in the diagnosis of sinus venosus atrial septal defect. *J Am Coll Cardiol* 1991; 17:537–542.
36. Mehta RH, Helmcke F, Nanda NC, Hsiung M, Pacifico AD, Hsu TL: Transesophageal Doppler color flow mapping assessment of atrial septal defect. *J Am Coll Cardiol* 1990; 16:1010–1016.
37. Morimoto K, Matsuzaki M, Tohma Y, Ono S, Tanaka N, Michishige H, et al: Diagnosis and quantitative evaluation of secundum-type atrial septal defect by transesophageal Doppler echocardiography. *Am J Cardiol* 1990; 66:85–91.
38. Kaulitz R, Stümper OFW, Geuskens R, Sreeram N, Elzenga NJ, Chan CK, et al: Comparative values of the precordial and transesophageal approaches in the echocardiographic evaluation of atrial baffle function after an atrial correction procedure. *J Am Coll Cardiol* 1990; 16:686–694.
39. Stümper O, Sutherland GR, Geuskens R, Roelandt JR, Bos E, Hess J: Transesophageal echocardiography in evaluation and management after a Fontan procedure. *J Am Coll Cardiol* 1991; 17:1152–1160.
40. Nellessen U, Schnittger I, Appleton CP, Masuyama T, Bolger A, Fischell TA, et al: Transesophageal two-dimensional echocardiography and color Doppler flow velocity mapping in the evaluation of cardiac valve prostheses. *Circulation* 1988; 78:848–855.
41. Mohr-Kahaly S, Kupferwasser I, Erbel R, Oelert H, Meyer J: Regurgitant flow in apparently normal valve prostheses: Improved detection and semiquantitative analysis by transesophageal two-dimensional color-coded Doppler echocardiography. *J Am Soc Echocardiogr* 1990; 3:187–195.
42. Van den Brink RBA, Visser CA, Basart DCG, Düren DR, De Jong AP, Dunning AJ: Comparison of transthoracic and transesophageal color Doppler flow imaging in patients with mechanical prostheses in the mitral valve position. *Am J Cardiol* 1989; 63:1471–1474.
43. Dittrich HC, McCann HA, Walsh TP, Blanchard DG, Oppenheim GE, Waack TC, et al: Transesophageal echocardiography in the evaluation of prosthetic and native aortic valves. *Am J Cardiol* 1990; 66:758–760.
44. Alam M, Sun I: Superiority of transesophageal echocardiography in detecting ruptured mitral chordae tendineae. *Am Heart J* 1991; 121:1819–1821.
45. Hozumi T, Yoshikawa J, Yoshida K, Yamaura Y, Akasaka T, Shakudo M: Direct visualization of ruptured chordae tendineae by transesophageal two-dimensional echocardiography. *J Am Coll Cardiol* 1990; 16:1315–1319.
46. Himelman RB, Kusumoto F, Oken K, Lee E, Cahalan MK, Shah PM, et al: The flail mitral valve: Echocardiographic findings by precordial and transesophageal imaging and Doppler color flow mapping. *J Am Coll Cardiol* 1991; 17:272–279.
47. Sochowski RA, Chan KL, Ascah KJ, Bedard P: Comparison of accuracy of transesophageal versus transthoracic echocardiography for the detection of mitral valve prolapse with ruptured chordae tendineae (flail mitral leaflet). *Am J Cardiol* 1991; 67:1251–1255.
48. Utsunomiya T, Ogawa T, King SW, Sunada E, Lobodzinski SM, Henry WL, et al: Pitfalls in the display of color Doppler jet areas: Combined variability due to Doppler angle, frame rate, and scanning direction. *Echocardiography* 1990; 7:739–745.
49. Smith MD, Harrison MR, Pinton R, Kandil H, Kwan OL, DeMaria AN: Regurgitant jet size by transesophageal compared with transthoracic Doppler color flow imaging. *Circulation* 1991; 83:79–86.
50. Yoshida K, Yoshikawa J, Yamaura Y, Hozumi T, Akasaka T, Fukaya T: Assessment of mitral regurgitation by biplane transesophageal color Doppler flow mapping. *Circulation* 1990; 82:1121–1126.
51. Cape EG, Yoganathan AP, Weyman AE, Levine RA: Adjacent solid boundaries alter the size of regurgitant jets on Doppler color flow maps. *J Am Coll Cardiol* 1991; 17:1094–1102.
52. Chen C, Thomas JD, Anconina J, Harrigan P, Mueller L, Picard MH, et al: Impact of impinging wall jet on color Doppler quantification of mitral regurgitation. *Circulation* 1991; 84:712–720.
53. Rajagoplan B, Bertram CD, Stallard T, Lee GJ: Blood flow in pulmonary veins: III. Simultaneous measurements of their dimensions, intravascular pressure and flow. *Cardiovasc Res* 1979; 13:684–692.
54. Castello R, Pearson AC, Lenzen P, Labowitz AJ: Effect of mitral regurgitation on pulmonary venous velocities derived from transesophageal echocardiography color-guided pulsed Doppler imaging. *J Am Coll Cardiol* 1991; 17:1499–1605.
55. Klein AL, Obarski TP, Stewart WJ, Casale PN, Pearce GL, Husbands K, et al: Transesophageal Doppler echocardiography of pulmonary venous flow: A new marker of mitral regurgitation severity. *J Am Coll Cardiol* 1991; 18:518–526.
56. Pearson AC: Transthoracic echocardiography vs. transesophageal echocardiography in detecting cardiac source of embolism. *Echocardiography* 1993; 10:397–403.
57. Shresta NK, Moreno FL, Narcisco FV, Torres L, Calleja HB: Two-dimensional echocardiography diagnosis of left atrial thrombus in rheumatic heart disease: A clinicopathologic study. *Circulation* 1983; 67:341–347.
58. Jordan NA, Schiefly CH, Edwards JE: Mural thrombus and arterial embolism in mitral stenosis. *Circulation* 1951; 3:363–367.
59. Hofmann T, Kasper W, Meinertz T, Geibel A, Just H: Echocardiographic evaluation of patients with clinically suspected arterial emboli. *Lancet* 1990; 336:1421–1424.
60. Schneider B, Hanrath P, Vogel P, Meinertz T: Improved morphologic characterization of atrial septal aneurysm by transesophageal echocardiography: Relation to cerebrovascular events. *J Am Coll Cardiol* 1990; 16:1000–1009.
61. Webster MWI, Smith HJ, Sharpe DN, Chancellor AM, Swift DL, Bass NM, et al: Patent foramen ovale in young stroke patients. *Lancet* 1988; ii:11–12.
62. Lechat P, Mas JL, Lascault G, Loron P, Theard M, Klimczac M, et al: Prevalence of patent foramen ovale in patients with stroke. *N Engl J Med* 1988; 318:1148–1152.
63. Nagelhout DA, Pearson AC, Labovitz AJ: Diagnosis of paradoxic embolism by transesophageal echocardiography. *Am Heart J* 1991; 121:1552–1554.
64. Erbel R, Stern H, Ehrenthal W, Schreiner G, Treese N, Kramer G, et al: Detection of spontaneous echocardiography: Spontaneous echocardiographic contrast. *Clin Cardiol* 1986; 9:245–252.
65. Castello R, Pearson AC, Labovitz AJ: Prevalence and clinical implications of atrial spontaneous contrast in patients undergoing transesophageal echocardiography. *Am J Cardiol* 1990; 65:1149–1153.
66. Black IW, Hopkins AP, Lee LCL, Walsh WF, Jacobson BM: Left atrial spontaneous echo contrast: A clinical and echocardiographic analysis. *J Am Coll Cardiol* 1991; 18:398–404.
67. Daniel WG, Nellesen U, Schröder E, Nonnast-Daniel B, Bednarski P, Nikutta P, et al: Left atrial spontaneous echo contrast in mitral valve disease: An indicator for an increased thromboembolic risk. *J Am Coll Cardiol* 1988; 11:1204–1211.
68. Chen YT, Kan MN, Chen JS, Lin WW, Hwang DS, Chang M, et al: Contributing factors to formation of left atrial spontaneous echo contrast in mitral valvular disease. *J Ultrasound Med* 1990; 9:151–155.
69. Karalis DG, Chandrasekaran K, Victor MF, Ross JJ Jr, Mintz GS: Recognition and embolic potential of intraaortic atherosclerotic debris. *J Am Coll Cardiol* 1991; 17:73–78.
70. Pop G, Sutherland GR, Koudstaal PJ, Sit TW, De Jong G, Roelandt JRTC: Transesophageal echocardiography in the detection of intracardiac embolic sources in patients with transient ischemic attacks. *Stroke* 1990; 21:560–565.
71. Sheikh KH, De Bruijn NP, Rankin JS, Clements FM, Stanley T, Wolfe WG, et al: The utility of transesophageal echocardiography and Doppler color flow imaging in patients undergoing cardiac valve surgery. *J Am Coll Cardiol* 1990; 15:363–373.
72. Dahm M, Iversen S, Schmid FX, Drexler M, Erbel R, Oelert H: Intraoperative evaluation of reconstruction of the atrioventricular

valves by transesophageal echocardiography. *Thorac Cardiovasc Surgeon* 1987; 35:140–142.

73. Reichert SLA, Visser CA, Moulijn AC, Suttorp MJ, v.d. Brink RBA, Koolen JJ, et al: Intraoperative transesophageal color-coded Doppler echocardiography for evaluation of residual regurgitation after mitral valve repair. *J Thorac Cardiovasc Surg* 1990; 100:756–761.
74. Marwick TH, Stewart WJ, Currie PJ, Cosgrove DM: Mechanisms of failure of mitral valve repair: An echocardiographic study. *Am Heart J* 1991; 122:149–153.
75. Wohlgelernter D, Jaffee CC, Cabiu HS, Yeatman LA, Cleman M: Silent ischemia during coronary occlusion produced by balloon inflation: Relation to regional myocardial dysfunction. *J Am Coll Cardiol* 1987; 10:491–498.
76. Leung JM, O'Kelly B, Browner WS, Tubau J, Hollenberg M, Mangano DT, et al: Prognostic importance of postbypass regional wall-motion abnormalities in patients undergoing coronary artery bypass graft surgery. *Anesthesiology* 1989; 71:16–25.
77. Dan M, Bonato R, Mazzucco A, Bortolotti U, Faggian G, Giron G, et al: Value of transesophageal echocardiography during repair of congenital heart defects. *Ann Thorac Surg* 1990; 50:637–643.
78. Oh JK, Seward JB, Khandheria BK, Gersh BJ, McGregor CGA, Freeman WK, et al: Transesophageal echocardiography in critically ill patients. *Am J Cardiol* 1990; 61:1492–1495.
79. Chan KL: Transesophageal echocardiography for assessing cause of hypotension after cardiac surgery. *Am J Cardiol* 1988; 15:1142–1143.
80. Jaarsma W, Visser CA, Suttorp MJ, Haagen FDH, Ernest SMPG: Transesophageal echocardiography during percutaneous balloon mitral valvuloplasty. *J Am Soc Echocardiogr* 1990; 3:384–391.
81. Ballal RS, Mahan EF III, Nanda NC, Dean LS: Utility of transesophageal echocardiography in interatrial septal puncture during percutaneous mitral balloon commissurotomy. *Am J Cardiol* 1990; 66:230–232.
82. Kronzon I, Tunick PA, Goldfarb A, Freedberg RS, Chinitz L, Slater J, et al: Echocardiographic and hemodynamic characteristics of atrial septal defects created by percutaneous valvuloplasty. *J Am Soc Echocardiogr* 1990; 3:64–71.
83. Hellenbrand WE, Fahey JT, McGowan FX, Weltin GG, Kleinman CS: Transesophageal echocardiographic guidance of transcatheter closure of atrial septal defect. *Am J Cardiol* 1990; 66:207–213.
84. Taams MA, Gussenhoven EJ, Cornel JH, The SHK, Roelandt JRTC, Lancée CT, et al: Detection of left coronary artery stenosis by transesophageal echocardiography. *Eur Heart J* 1988; 9:1162–1166.
85. Iliceto S, Marangelli V, Memmola C, Rizzon P: Transesophageal Doppler echocardiography evaluation of coronary blood flow velocity in baseline conditions and during dipyridamole-induced coronary vasodilation. *Circulation* 1991; 83:61–69.
86. Yoshida K, Yoshikawa J, Hozumi T, Yamaura Y, Akasaka T, Fukaya T, et al: Detection of left main coronary artery stenosis by transesophageal color Doppler and two-dimensional echocardiography. *Circulation* 1990; 81:1271–1276.

Chapter 132

Exercise and Stress Echocardiographic Testing

Michael H. Crawford, M.D. ■ *Charles F. Presti, M.D.*

DESCRIPTION

Exercise is believed to be the best stress for testing myocardial performance. The addition of cardiac imaging to the standard electrocardiographic exercise test adds information of value concerning myocardial function and perfusion. Perfusion is best assessed by radionuclide techniques, but inferences can be made about the adequacy of myocardial blood flow by evaluating ventricular function. Exercise echocardiography appears to be ideally suited for the assessment of myocardial function. It is completely noninvasive, requires no radiation exposure, and is readily applicable to most exercise-testing situations. The information obtained from the exercise echocardiogram relates primarily to regional wall motion and left ventricular function, but as with any echocardiographic study, important information is also provided about valvular structure and function, chamber size, wall thickness, and pericardial abnormalities.

Although developed more than a decade ago, exercise two-dimensional echocardiography languished in research laboratories until digital image acquisition and processing were commercially available. This technology overcame the biggest barrier to the application of echocardiography to exercise testing—respiratory interference.[1] Digital acquisition permits the capture of high-quality images obtained at end expiration that are then displayed in cine-loop format. Digital display also permits the side-by-side display of rest and exercise echocardiograms, which may enhance the ability to detect subtle abnormalities in regional wall motion. This technological advance combined with higher quality images in general from the newer generation echocardiographs has increased imaging success rates to 95 percent or better.

Two-Dimensional Echocardiographic Imaging Technique

Exercise echocardiographic imaging can be obtained during supine or upright bicycle exercise or treadmill exercise. Images can be monitored continuously during bicycle exercise but are assessed consistently only before and immediately after treadmill exercise because of the difficulty of recording adequate images at peak treadmill exercise. All the common chest wall transducer locations have been used for exercise echocardiography. The apical two- and four-chamber views are the most commonly used views during either bicycle or treadmill exercise. These images provide a biplane evaluation of left ventricular function, and data from both images can be acquired without moving the transducer location. Also, the apical views are essential for visualization of the left ventricular apex, an area commonly affected by coronary artery disease.[2] Subcostal views provide a biplane assessment of left ventricular function and have been successfully applied during upright bicycle exercise in normal individuals and patients undergoing rehabilitation after a myocardial infarction.[3] Parasternal views can be difficult to obtain during exercise because of exaggerated chest wall movement. Application of echocardiography to the recovery phase of exercise, for example, after treadmill exercise, allows for enhanced utilization of the parasternal long- and short-axis views, which may provide important information not seen in other views.[4]

The selection of bicycle or treadmill exercise echocardiography has generated some controversy. Bicycle exercise was frequently used by early researchers because work load is more readily quantitated and the competing radionuclide angiographic techniques used bicycle exercise. Clinicians began using immediate posttreadmill exercise imaging because treadmills were more readily available in the clinical setting and this approach was believed to be technically easier. Although there is little comparative data available, the results of both techniques in the clinical arena are comparable for the following reasons. Since imaging can be obtained at peak exercise during bicycle exercise, it should be more sensitive for detecting small, quickly reversible areas of myocardial ischemia. This advantage, however, is mitigated by the fact that most patients do not achieve high work loads with bicycle exercise and echo imaging is more challenging, especially during upright bicycle. Treadmill exercise requires immediate postexercise imaging, but since higher work loads can be achieved on the treadmill and image quality is better postexercise in the supine position, clinical results are equivalent to bicycle stress.

RESULTS

Detection of Coronary Artery Disease

The normal response to exercise is for all myocardial segments to develop hyperdynamic motion during and immediately after the exercise. An abnormal exercise response consists of the development of segmental hypokinesis, akinesis, or dyskinesis during or immediately after exercise[2] (Fig. 132-1). Several studies have compared the results of exercise echocardiography with those of coronary angiography.[3,5–10] Three criteria have been formulated for diagnosing coronary artery disease by two-dimensional echocardiography: (1) resting wall motion abnormality, (2) exercise-induced wall motion abnormality, and (3) abnormal response of ejection fraction to exercise.

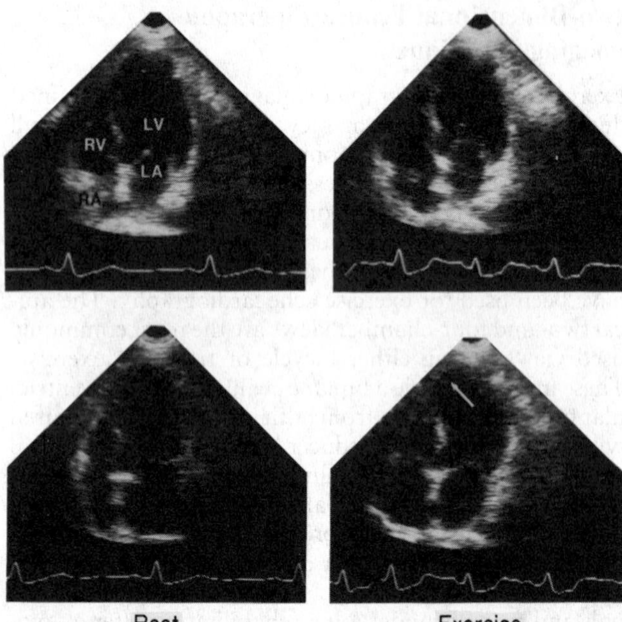

FIGURE 132-1 Apical four-chamber view in end-diastole (top) and end-systole (bottom) at rest and at peak exercise. Note normal apical-systolic contraction at rest and dyskinesis (arrow) at peak exercise in this patient with a high grade left anterior descending coronary artery lesion. RV = right ventricle, RA = right atrium, LV = left ventricle, LA = left atrium.

It appears from these studies that if a wall motion abnormality is seen at rest or develops during exercise, the sensitivity for detecting coronary artery disease ranges from 69 to 100 percent. When only new wall motion abnormalities or worsening of existing wall motion abnormalities are used as a criterion for diagnosing coronary artery disease, the sensitivity decrease slightly, ranging from 61 to 86 percent. The specificity of using either resting wall motion abnormality or new or worsening wall motion abnormality ranges in these studies from 75 to 100 percent and increases when only new or worsening wall motion abnormalities seen during exercise are considered.

The range in sensitivities seen in these studies reflects the influence of a variety of factors, including both the extent of coronary artery disease and the degree of ischemia elicited. Patients with multivessel coronary artery disease are more easily identified by two-dimensional echocardiography than are patients with less extensive or single-vessel disease (Table 132-1). If multivessel coronary artery disease is more prevalent in one study population than in another, the sensitivity of detecting coronary artery disease in all likelihood will be higher in that report. Likewise, for any given extent of coronary artery disease, the more profound the ischemia induced during exercise, the greater the likelihood of detecting a wall motion abnormality. Differences in the exercise work load achieved will be determined by the age, sex, and functional status of the population studied as well as the exercise protocol itself, and so the degree of ischemia elicited may vary from study to study.

It should also be noted that calculation of the sensitivity and specificity of exercise echocardiography based on coronary arteriography has significant shortcomings, as coronary arteriography, which describes anatomy, cannot truly validate the exercise echocardiographic test, which assesses myocardial function and depends on the induction of myocardial ischemia. Nevertheless, these studies indicate that the detection of a new or worsening wall motion abnormality is highly specific for identifying the presence of coronary artery disease. The absence of this finding does not necessarily exclude the possibility of coronary artery disease but does make its presence unlikely.

TABLE 132-1

Results of Exercise Two-Dimensional Echocardiography for the Detection of Coronary Artery Disease

Sensitivity	
Single-vessel disease	75 %
Multivessel disease	95 %
All coronary artery disease	85 %
Specificity	90 %

Risk Stratification after Myocardial Infarction

Early postmyocardial infarction patients with reduced global left ventricular function or persistent myocardial ischemia have a higher risk of subsequent events. The former is a potent predictor of subsequent death, and the latter is highly predictive of subsequent unstable angina, infarction, and the need for coronary artery bypass surgery or angioplasty. Both of these poor prognostic features can be detected by means of cardiac imaging performed at rest and during exercise. Two-dimensional exercise echocardiography has been used to risk-stratify patients after uncomplicated acute myocardial infarction.[11,12] The addition of echocardiographic imaging to postmyocardial infarction treadmill exercise testing provides additional information to that obtained from the exercise electrocardiogram (ECG) alone. Thus, patients who develop new exercise-induced wall motion abnormalities appear to have a higher incidence of multivessel coronary artery disease as well as a worse short-term prognosis in terms of recurrent infarction, need for coronary artery bypass grafting, and cardiac death. The risk for subsequent cardiac events appears to be especially increased in patients who develop exercise-induced wall motion abnormalities in areas remote from the infarct, indicating additional myocardium at risk.

Exercise Doppler Echocardiography

Doppler echocardiography provides an additional noninvasive means of assessing ventricular performance during exercise. Aortic Doppler velocity recordings can be obtained reproducibly in almost all patients during exercise. Using the product of Doppler mean aortic flow velocity and proximal ascending aortic area derived from two-dimensional echocardiographic imaging, it is possible to calculate stroke volume and cardiac output. Also, peak velocity achieved during exercise and the time to peak velocity are additional measures of exercise ventricular systolic function. Exercise-induced changes in Doppler measurements of aortic flow velocity and derived cardiac outputs correlate well with changes in cardiac output determinations by the traditional methods of Fick oximetry and thermodilution in normal subjects.[13]

Because Doppler measurements of aortic blood flow velocity are indicative of global left ventricular function, this technique is not sensitive or specific for the detection of coronary artery disease. Studies have demonstrated that normal patients could be distinguished from those with severe coronary artery disease, but those with milder disease could not be discriminated from normal patients.[14,15] Since left ventricular performance is a powerful predictor of post–myocardial infarction, Doppler aortic velocity recordings during exercise have been applied to the risk stratification of patients early after myocardial infarction.[16] Comparative studies have shown that exercise-induced wall motion abnormalities on two-dimensional echo imaging have greater predictive value than Doppler measurements performed simultaneously in uncomplicated early postinfarction patients.[17]

Experimental studies in humans have shown that transient myocardial ischemia induced by percutaneous coronary balloon angioplasty,[18] rapid atrial pacing,[19] or dipyridamole infusion[20] resulted in abnormalities of the Doppler transmitral flow velocity profile suggestive of diastolic dysfunction. Consequently, there was enthusiasm that if similar abnormalities could be induced during exercise, this would represent a simple stress echo Doppler technique for detecting coronary artery disease. Unfortunately, studies in patients with known coronary artery disease and demonstrable exercise-induced wall motion abnormalities on echocardiographic imaging did not show consistent Doppler transmitral flow velocity abnormalities.[21] The Doppler velocity profile was related to changes in systolic performance, which suggests that exercise-induced ischemic left ventricular dysfunction affects transmitral velocity differently than the ischemia induced by other means. Thus, Doppler echocardiographic assessment of systolic or diastolic left ventricular performance during exercise is less useful than evaluating segmented wall motion abnormalities for the detection of myocardial ischemia.

COMPARISON WITH OTHER TECHNIQUES

Comparison with Exercise Electrocardiography

Abnormal resting ECGs due to prior infarctions, left ventricular hypertrophy, conduction abnormalities, or drug effects contribute to a relative lack of sensitivity of exercise electrocardiography for diagnosing coronary artery disease. In comparison with the exercise ECG, exercise echocardiography appears to have similar to slightly better sensitivity in identifying single-vessel coronary artery disease.[3,5–9] Exercise echocardiography is significantly better than the exercise ECG in identifying patients with multivessel disease. The specificity of exercise two-dimensional echocardiography is comparable to that of the exercise ECG. Thus, the addition of two-dimensional echocardiography to the exercise ECG significantly improves sensitivity in diagnosing coronary artery disease without reducing specificity, especially in patients with a nondiagnostic exercise ECG. (See Chap. 16.)

Comparison with Radionuclide Techniques

In comparison with thallium-201 single-photon computed tomography (SPECT), wall motion abnormalities identified by two-dimensional echocardiography correlate very well with the area of the defect demonstrated on SPECT. Additionally, there is excellent concordance between demonstration of irreversible thallium-201 scintigraphy defects and resting wall motion abnormalities on two-dimensional echocardiography and between reversible thallium-201 scintigraphy defects and exercise-induced wall motion abnormalities as seen on two-dimensional echocardiography. These data help substantiate the ischemic basis of the exercise-induced wall motion abnormalities seen on two-dimensional echocardiography and confirm the ability of echocardiography to localize areas of regional ischemia. Sensitivity for the detection of angiographically demonstrated coronary artery disease was similar by both techniques ranging from 60 percent for one-vessel disease to 94 percent for three-vessel disease. Specificity was 88 percent for echo and 81 percent for SPECT in a study of 112 patients.[22]

Both two-dimensional echocardiography and radionuclide angiography rely on segmental and global assessment of left ventricular function. Both can be applied to exercise testing, although two-dimensional echocardiography is less cumbersome and can be used during both bicycle and treadmill exercise while radionuclide angiography is limited to use during bicycle exercise. Either first transit or equilibrium radionuclide angiography techniques can be used. The former offers beat-by-beat analysis of left ventricular function similar to two-dimensional echocardiography, but if multiple analyses are to be made, significant time must be allowed for washout and additional radiation exposure is necessary. Sequential assessment of left ventricular function can be achieved by means of equilibrium radionuclide angiography, but beat-by-beat analysis cannot be done and multiple projections cannot be used during exercise.

The sensitivity for diagnosing coronary artery disease based on either wall motion or ejection fraction analysis is slightly higher for two-dimensional echocardiography than for radionuclide angiography with similar degrees of specificity.[3,6,8,9] This difference most likely reflects the advantage of using multiple imaging planes and beat-by-beat analysis of wall motion, as can be done using two-dimensional echocardiography. (See also Chap. 134.)

NONEXERCISE STRESS TESTING

The noninvasive evaluation of the patient who cannot exercise adequately is a common clinical problem. The use of intravenous dipyridamole to produce differences in regional myocardial perfusion in patients wirh coronary artery disease has become popular with thallium-201 scintigraphy or positron emission tomography to detect regional perfusion defects. The use of dipyridamole echocardiography has been championed by Italian investigators.[23] Studies have shown very high specificity for the detection of coronary artery disease, but sensitivity has been only 60 to 74 percent. Also, high doses are required for these results, and adverse effects are experienced by two-thirds of patients studied.[24] In the United States dobutamine stress echocardiography has been more popular because experimental studies have suggested that dobutamine is superior to vasodilators for inducing wall motion abnormalities.[25] Clinical studies have shown the sensitivity of dobutamine-induced wall motion abnormalities detected by echocardiography for identifying patients with angiographically documented coronary artery disease to be 89 percent with a specificity of a negative study of 85 percent. Side effects are relatively infrequent (18 percent) with few being severe enough to stop the infusion.[26] Thus, in patients who cannot exercise, dobutamine stress echocardiography seems to be an excellent alternative.

Transesophageal Stress Echocardiography

Transesophageal echocardiography combined with stress produced either by atrial pacing utilizing electrodes on the probe[27–29] or by the infusion of dipyridamole,[30] has been found to have satisfactory specificity and sensitivity in selected patients with no substantial complications. Some patients studied with atrial pacing have had chest discomfort from esophageal stimulation. The procedure primarily evaluates changes in regional wall motion. This semi-invasive procedure appears useful in highly selected patients who are unable to perform dynamic exercise. The diagnostic accuracy of the procedure remains to be determined in larger series performed in other laboratories, particularly since the evaluation of wall motion is often difficult.

SUMMARY AND RECOMMENDATIONS

As echocardiography has advanced from M-mode to two-dimensional imaging and higher resolution imaging units and as digital computer analysis systems have been introduced, most patients referred for assessment of left ventricular function at rest and during exercise can be evaluated with echocardiography. The technique is readily adapted to most exercise facilities, is noninvasive, requires no radiation exposure, and provides beat-by-beat analysis of left ventricular function. Clinical studies comparing two-dimensional echocardiography during exercise in patients with coronary artery disease have demonstrated sensitivity and specificity for identifying the presence of coronary artery disease comparable to those of radionuclide angiography and thallium-201 scintigraphy and superior to those of exercise electrocardiography. Exercise echocardiography is clinically useful in (1) diagnosing coronary artery disease in patients who are likely to have a nondiagnostic electrocardiographic response to exercise, (2) diagnosing patients in whom a simultaneous assessment of left ventricular function and evidence of inducible myocardial ischemia is desirable, (3) evaluating the functional significance of angiographically "subcritical" coronary stenosis, and (4) risk stratifying patients after uncomplicated myocardial infarction.

REFERENCES

1. Feigenbaum H: Exercise echocardiography. *J Am Soc Echocardiogr* 1988; 1:161–166.
2. Crawford MH, Amon KW, Vance WS: Exercise 2-dimensional echocardiography: Quantification of left ventricular performance in patients with severe angina pectoris. *Am J Cardiol* 1983; 51:1–6.
3. Gintzon LE, Conant R, Brizendine M, Lee F, Mena I, Laks MM: Exercise two-dimensional echocardiography: A new method of segmental wall motion analysis. *Am J Cardiol* 1984; 53:805–811.
4. Presti CF, Armstrong WF, Feigenbaum H: Comparison of echocardiography at peak exercise and after bicycle exercise in evaluation of patients with known or suspected coronary artery disease. *J Am Soc Echocardiogr* 1988; 1:119–126.
5. Armstrong WF, O'Donnell J, Dillion JC, McHenry PL, Morris SN, Feigenbaum H: Complementary value of two-dimensional exercise echocardiography to routine treadmill exercise testing. *Ann Intern Med* 1986; 105:829–835.
6. Limacher MC, Quinones MA, Poliner LR, Nelson JG, Winters WL, Waggoner AD: Detection of coronary artery disease with exercise two-dimensional echocardiography. *Circulation* 1983; 67:1211–1218.

7. Robertson WS, Feigenbaum H, Armstrong WF, Dillon JC, O'Donnell J, McHenry PW, et al: Exercise echocardiography: A clinically practical addition in the evaluation of coronary artery disease. *J Am Coll Cardiol* 1983; 2:1085–1091.
8. Visser VA, vanderWieken RL, Kan G, Lie KI, Busemann-Sokele E, Meltzer RS, et al: Comparison of two-dimensional echocardiography with radionuclide angiography during dynamic exercise for the detection of coronary artery disease. *Am Heart J* 1983; 106:528–535.
9. Crawford MH, Petru MA, Amon KW, Sorensen SG, Vance WS: Comparative value of 2-dimensional echocardiography and radionuclide angiography for quantitating changes in left ventricular performance during exercise limited by angina pectoris. *Am J Cardiol* 1984; 53:42–46.
10. Armstrong WF, O'Donnell J, Ryan T, Feigenbaum H: Effect of prior myocardial infarction and extent and location of coronary artery disease or accuracy of exercise echocardiography. *J Am Coll Cardiol* 1987; 10:531–538.
11. Applegate RJ, Dell'Italia LJ, Crawford MH: Usefulness of two-dimensional echocardiography during low-level exercise testing early after uncomplicated acute myocardial infarction. *Am J Cardiol* 1987; 60:10–14.
12. Jaarsma W, Visser CA, Funke Kupper AJ, Res JCJ, Van Eenige MJ, Roos JP: Usefulness of two-dimensional exercise echocardiography shortly after myocardial infarction. *Am J Cardiol* 1986; 57:86–90.
13. Christie J, Sheldahl LM, Tristani FE, Sagar KB, Ptacin MJ, Wann S: Determination of stroke volume and cardiac output during exercise: Comparison of two-dimensional and Doppler echocardiography, Fick oximetry, and thermodilution. *Circulation* 1987; 76:539–547.
14. Bryg RJ, Labovitz AJ, Mehdirad AA, Williams GA, Chaitman BR: Effect of coronary artery disease on Doppler-derived parameters of aortic flow during upright exercise. *Am J Cardiol* 1986; 58:14–19.
15. Harrison MR, SMith MD, Friedman BJ, DeMaria AN: Uses and limitations of exercise Doppler echocardiography in the diagnosis of ischemic heart disease. *J Am Coll Cardiol* 1987; 10:809–817.
16. Mehta N, Bennett D, Mannering D, Dawkins K, Ward DE: Usefulness of noninvasive Doppler measurement of ascending aortic blood velocity and acceleration in detecting impairment of the left ventricular functional response to exercise three weeks after acute myocardial infarction. *Am J Cardiol* 1986; 58:879–884.
17. Riesmeyer JS, Crawford MH: Superiority of exercise two-dimensional echocardiography versus ascending aorta Doppler for the identification of jeopardized myocardium post–myocardial infarction. *Coronary Artery Dis* 1990; 1:591–595.
18. Labovitz AJ, Lewen MK, Kern M, Vandormael M, Deligonal U, Kennedy HL: Evaluation of left ventricular systolic and diastolic dysfunction during transient myocardial ischemia produced by angioplasty. *J Am Coll Cardiol* 1987; 10:748–755.
19. Iliceto S, Amico A, Marangelli V, D'Ambrosio G, Rizzon R: Doppler echocardiographic evaluation of the effect of atrial pacing-induced ischemia on left ventricular filling in patients with coronary artery disease. *J Am Coll Cardiol* 1988; 11:953–961.
20. Lattanzi F, Picano E, Masini M, De Prisco F, Distante A, L'Abbate A: Transmitral flow changes during dipyridamole-induced ischemia. *Chest* 1989; 95:1037–1042.
21. Presti CF, Walling AD, Montemayor I, Campbell JM, Crawford MH: Influence of exercise-induced myocardial ischemia on the pattern of left ventricular diastolic filling: A Doppler echocardiographic study. *J Am Coll Cardiol* 1991; 18:75–82.
22. Quinones MA, Verani MS, Haichin RM, Mahmarian JJ, Suarez J, Zoghbi WA: Exercise echocardiography versus thallium-201 single photon emission computed tomography in the evaluation of coronary artery disease: Analysis of 292 patients. *Circulation* 1992; 85:1026–1031.
23. Picano E, Distante A, Masini M, Morales MA, Lattanzi F, L'Abbate A: Dipyridamole-echocardiography test in effort angina pectoris. *Am J Cardiol* 1985; 56:452–456.
24. Picano E, Lattanzi F, Mansini M, Distante A, L'Abbate A: High-dose dipyridamole echocardiography test in effort angina pectoris. *J Am Coll Cardiol* 1986; 8:848–854.
25. Fung AY, Gallagher RP, Buda AJ: The physiologic basis of dobutamine as compared with dipyridamole stress interventions in the assessment of critical coronary stenosis. *Circulation* 1987; 76:943–951.
26. Sawada SG, Segar DS, Ryan T, Brown SE, Dohan AM, Williams R, et al: Echocardiographic detection of coronary artery disease during dobutamine infusion. *Circulation* 1991; 83:1605–1614.
27. Lambertz H, Kreis A, Trumper H, Hanrath P: Simultaneous transesophageal atrial pacing and transesophageal two-dimensional echocardiography: A new method of stress echocardiography. *J Am Coll Cardiol* 1990; 16:1143–1153.
28. Zabalgoitia M, Gandhi DK, Abi-Mansour P, Rosenblum J: Transesophageal stress echocardiography: Detection of coronary artery disease in patients with normal resting left ventricular contractility. *Am Heart J* 1991; 122:1456–1463.
29. Flachskampf FA, Hoffmann R, Hanrath P: Transesophageal stress echocardiography. *Coronary Artery Dis* 1992; 3:364–368.
30. Agati L, Renzi M, Sciomer S, Vizza DC, Voci P, Penco M: Transesophageal dipyridamole echocardiography for diagnosis of coronary artery disease. *J Am Coll Cardiol* 1992; 19:765–770.

Chapter 133

Intravascular Ultrasound

Steven E. Nissen, M.D.

Recent advances in microelectronic and piezoelectric technology have permitted development of miniaturized ultrasound devices capable of real-time tomographic intravascular and intracardiac imaging.[1–7] Initial coronary and peripheral vascular studies have provided unique, detailed cross-sectional images of the vessel lumen and arterial wall not previously obtainable in vivo by any other technique.[8–12] Pilot studies have also demonstrated the feasibilty of intracavitary imaging of both right- and left-sided cardiac chambers.[13] The success of initial investigations has resulted in the emergence of new applications for intravascular imaging in diagnostic and therapeutic catheterization.[10–17]

RATIONALE FOR INTRALUMINAL IMAGING

Limitations of Angiography

Although angiography has endured for several decades as the predominant method for determining the severity of coronary artery disease (CAD), multiple investigators have questioned the accuracy and reproducibility of coronary arteriography.[18–26] These studies have described discrepancies between angiography and postmortem anatomy, and report significant intra- and interobserver variability in the interpretation of angiograms. Recent investigations have documented significant disparities between the angiographic severity of lesions and the physiological consequences of stenoses.[26]

Angiography depicts three-dimensional coronary anatomy from a two-dimensional silhouette of the vessel lumen, (Chap. 138). Necropsy studies however, demonstrate that coronary obstructions are frequently complex and eccentric, a phenomenon exaggerated by complex alterations in luminal shape produced by interventions such as balloon angioplasty.[27] Although angiographic methods usually describe lesion severity by the percentage of luminal area reduction, necropsy studies demonstrate that atherosclerotic CAD is usually diffuse and contains no truly normal segment from which to calculate percentage of stenosis.[22] In the setting of diffuse narrowing, percentage of luminal reduction will always underestimate lesion severity.

Potential Advantages of Ultrasound

Intravascular ultrasound has several unique properties that are theoretically valuable in the detection and quantitation of CAD. The cross-sectional perspective of intravascular ultrasound permits visualization of the full 360° circumference of the vessel wall, not just two surfaces. Thus, measurement of the lumen area is not dependent on radiographic projection and can be determined by planimetry directly from a tomographic image.[6,10,11] The ability of ultrasound to penetrate tissue enables characterization of the intramural anatomy of the vessel wall in normal and atherosclerotic segments. Because plaque morphology is an important determinant of the prognosis and natural history of CAD, intravascular ultrasound may provide important incremental diagnostic information valuable in management of CAD. The tomographic perspective of ultrasound enables characterization of CAD in vessels that are difficult to assess by conventional angiographic techniques, including diffusely diseased segments and eccentric plaques.

INTRAVASCULAR IMAGING TECHNOLOGY

Intraoperative studies using epicardial high-frequency transducers verified the feasibility of ultrasound assessment of CAD, but the technique was impractical for routine examinations.[28] Initial efforts to develop miniaturized transducers for intraluminal examination began nearly 20 years ago, but only recently have such efforts yielded success.[2-9] Since the transducer is placed in close proximity to the vessel wall, high frequencies (20 to 50 MHz) can be employed to provide excellent theoretical resolution (axial below 100 μm and lateral below 250 μm). Two dissimilar technical approaches to intraluminal transducer design have emerged: mechanically rotated devices and multielement electronic arrays. (Fig. 133-1) Multielement designs generally result in catheters with greater mechanical flexibility, while mechanical probes offer greater acoustic power. Each design has yielded small intravascular devices suitable for coronary imaging (1.1 to 1.8 mm in diameter), typically generating images at 10 to 30 frames per second for storage on videotape.

Visualization of small coronary arteries necessitates imaging close to the surface of the catheter, which requires addressing the troublesome problem of transducer *ring-down artifact.* The ring-down phenomenon is characterized by high-amplitude oscillations of the piezoelectric transducer material that obscures imaging of structures located close to the catheter surface. The initial mechanical probe designs utilized a small ultrasound element directly rotated by a drive shaft that traversed the length of the catheter (Fig. 133-1, top panel). Several recent approaches employ a rotating acoustic mirror to permit a longer signal path from the transducer to the vessel lumen (Fig. 133-1, middle panel). This modification confines the ring-down signal within the catheter and permits imaging close to the surface of the device. In an electronic array design, the transducer is surface mounted, but the ring-down may be reduced or eliminated by digital subtraction[6,9,11] (Fig. 133-1, bottom panel). For both mechanical and electronic designs, a movable guide wire is usually employed to facilitate subselective coronary cannulation.

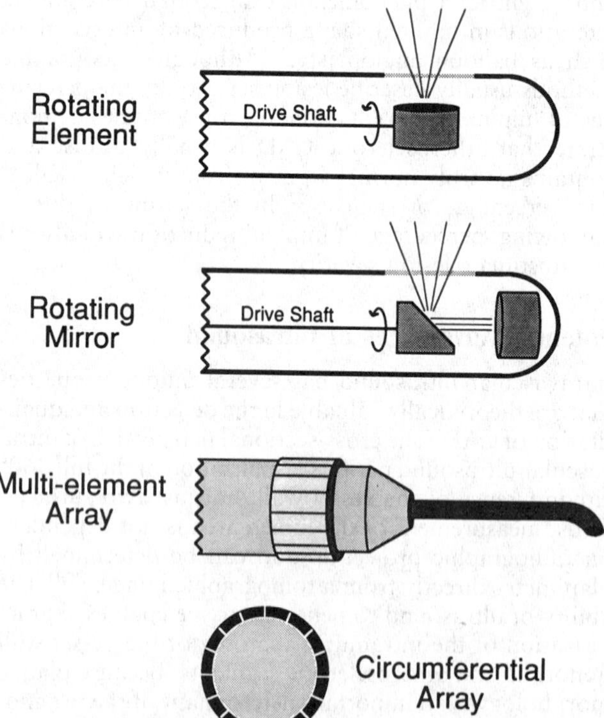

FIGURE 133-1 Schematic illustration of the design of intravascular ultrasound devices. One approach generates a 360° image by directly rotating a single transducer element (top panel), while other designs reflect the ultrasound beam using a rotating mirror (middle panel). The rotating mirror design reduces the impact of transducer *ring-down artifact* (see text). An alternate design utilizes a multielement electronic array (bottom panel).

Limitations of Current Devices

For safe coronary imaging, the transducer-tipped catheter must be small and flexible to enable safe passage into the tortuous vessels frequently encountered in humans. Current technology has permitted reduction of mechanical probe sizes to 3.9 F (1.30 mm) and electronic designs to 3.5 F (1.17 mm). Normal first-order epicardial coronaries typically range from 1.0 to 5.0 mm, while atherosclerotic lumina can reach 0.1 mm. Accordingly, no probe is currently capable of imaging moderately severe stenoses prior to balloon angioplasty. Further reductions in transducer size may be difficult because transducer miniaturization limits available acoustic power and thus signal-to-noise ratio.

All tomographic imaging techniques, including intravascular ultrasound, are vulnerable to distortion produced by oblique imaging planes. Thus, a vessel with a circular cross-sectional profile will appear elliptical whenever the transducer is not orthogonal to the long axis of the vessel. This phenomenon can represent a confounding variable in quantitative measurements. Non-orthogonal orientation is more prevalent in the larger vessels encountered during peripheral vascular imaging, and the small size of the coronaries limits the extent of possible angulation. For mechanical probes, rotation speed may increase or decrease because of mechanical drag, particularly when the drive shaft is bent by a tortuous coronary, producing geometric distortion of the image, a phenomenon known as *nonuniform rotational distortion.*

HUMAN CORONARY IMAGING

Safety

Although intracoronary instrumentation is required, initial studies of intravascular ultrasound during diagnostic catheterization have demonstrated few serious untoward effects.[6,9,11] Transient coronary spasm has been noted, but no deaths or vessel dissections were reported in initial studies. The imaging device can be occlusive when advanced into stenoses or small distal vessels, but patients generally do not experience chest pain if the catheter is promptly withdrawn. Coronary ultrasound has also been employed as an adjunct to interventional procedures such as balloon angioplasty with few untoward effects.[10] Patients with acute coronary syndromes have been studied, including patients examined immediately following myocardial infarction.[29] Most protocols avoid instrumentation of patients in whom estimated coronary diameter is too small to safely accommodate the device (3.5 to 5.5 F, 1.17 to 1.83 mm). Intravenous heparin (5000 to 10,000 units) has been routinely employed prior to imaging, although there are no controlled studies of the necessity for anticoagulation.

Normal Coronary Anatomy

Several investigators have characterized anatomy by intravascular ultrasound based on in vitro comparisons of ultrasound appearance and tissue histology.[30–32] There are, however, significant differences between ultrasound anatomy visualized in vitro and in vivo. Necropsy specimens not distended by physiological pressure collapse to a lumen cross-sectional area less than one-third in vivo size. The contraction of vessels in vitro results in a bunching or corrugation of vessel wall structures that alters the acoustic properties of the tissue.[33] Other investigations have abnormalities in patients with atherosclerotic CAD[11,34] (Fig. 133-2).

A distinctly laminar appearance to the normal vessel wall is reported in many, but not all, normal individuals, although the genesis of these ultrasound layers remains controversial. In some normal subjects, a discrete linear ultrasonic reflectance is observed at the acoustic interface between the lumen and intima (Fig. 133-2). Other normal subjects may exhibit an intimal leading edge that poorly reflects ultrasound, a phenomenon that leads to *dropout* of ultrasound signals. Thus, distinct laminations of the vessel wall are absent at 30 to 50 percent of the coronary sites in normal patients.[11,34]

When an intimal leading edge is observed, the maximal thickness averages less than 0.20 mm, and most investigators consider a normal value to be less than 0.20 to 0.30 mm.[10,11,34] These values are greater than the histologic thickness of the intima and reflect the intrinsic axial resolution of the ultrasound device, not precise anatomic boundaries. When a distinct subintimal sonolucent layer is evident (50 to 70 percent of normal segments), the maximal thickness averages less than 0.20 mm (Fig. 133-2). One hypothesis proposes that the characteristic sonolucent zone represents normal media. However, differences in the ultrasound anatomy of muscular (usually laminar) and elastic (usually monolayered) arteries have been reported. Some of the disparate findings in normal individuals may also reflect dissimilarities in instrumentation (electronic vs. mechanical probes) or selection of normal subjects (young vs. old).

Morphology of Coronary Atherosclerosis

Although ultrasound dropout is frequently observed in normal segments, it is less prevalent in diseased vessels.[11] A variety of intravascular ultrasound features are identified in patients with atherosclerotic CAD. The thickness of the intimal leading-edge or sonolucent zone is abnormally increased in many patients with CAD, although the ultrasound appearance differs significantly among available imaging devices. Mechanical ultrasound probes visualize coronary plaques as variable echogenic intraluminal encroachments, usually with a thin sonolucent subintimal band thought by some investigators to represent normal media (Fig. 133-3). Necropsy studies, however, demonstrate that the media is often attenuated or completely absent in atherosclerotic segments, thus complicating the identification of structural landmarks. Studies using electronic probes report a variably increased intimal leading edge, often with a distinctly thickened sonolucent subintimal band thought to represent atherosclerotic plaque of low acoustic reflectance

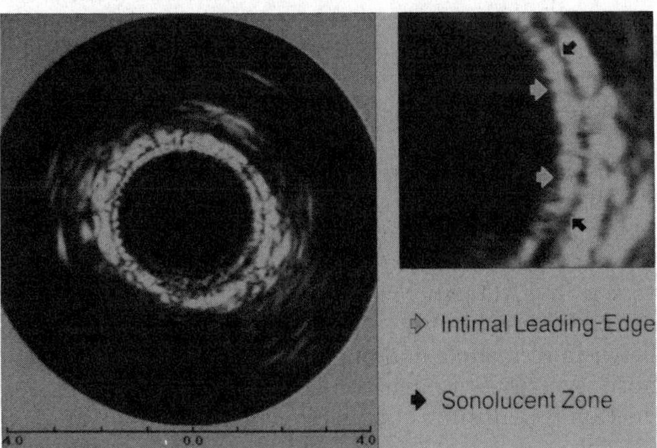

FIGURE 133-2 Intravascular ultrasound image of the coronary in a normal subject with a scale in millimeters (left panel). These images were obtained with a multielement imaging probe. A 250 percent magnification of a portion of the vessel wall is shown in the right panel. The light gray arrows indicate a thin linear ultrasound reflectance at the border between the lumen and intima. The black arrows identify a subadjacent sonolucent zone. The ultrasound catheter appears as a central dark circular structure. (*Reproduced with permission of Circulation and the American Heart Association.*)

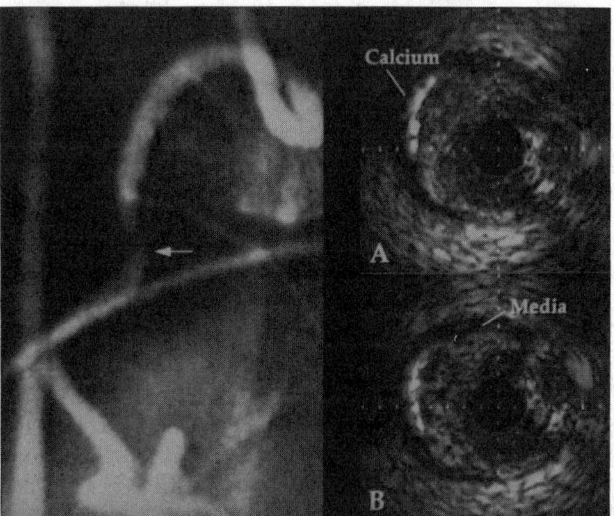

FIGURE 133-3 Angiogram and intravascular ultrasound image of the right coronary before (*A*) and after (*B*) mechanical atherectomy. The arrow in the left panel illustrates the lesion and imaging site prior to treatment. Plaque removal is evident at 4 to 5 o'clock in the image in *B*. For mechanical probes, the sonolucent zone is thought to represent normal media. Also identified is an area of plaque calcification. (*Courtesy of Paul Yock, M.D., and CVIS Corporation.*)

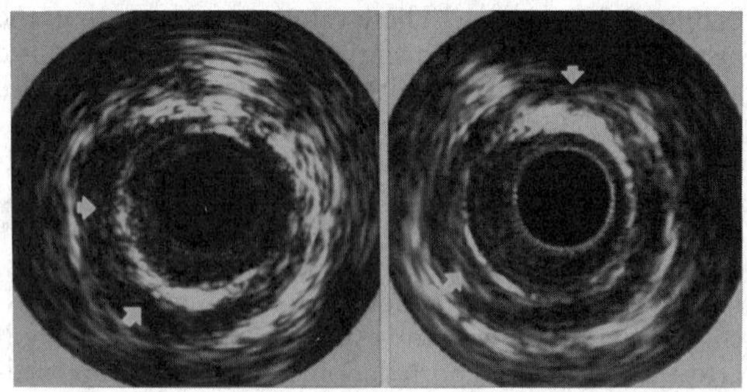

FIGURE 133-4 Atherosclerotic coronary wall morphology imaged with a multielement electronic ultrasound device. In the left panel, the arrows identify a crescentic sonolucent plaque that appears to bulge the vessel wall outward (compensatory remodeling). In the right panel, a concentric sonolucent plaque is illustrated, the thickest portion identified by the arrow at 7 o'clock. At 12 o'clock, an arrow identifies a fibrocalcific plaque that shadows underlying structures. (*Left panel image reproduced with permission of Circulation and the American Heart Association.*)

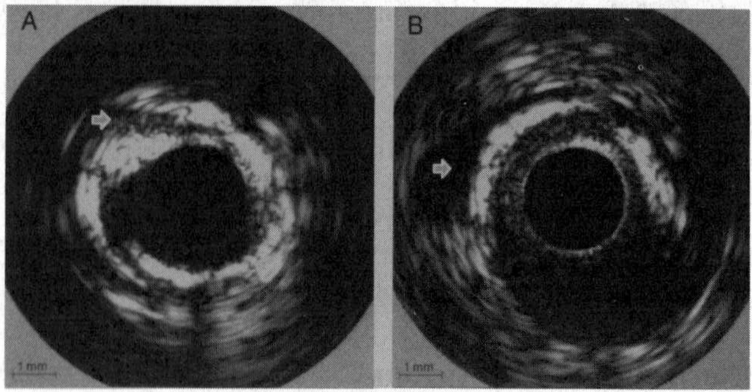

FIGURE 133-5 Ultrasound appearance at two angioplasty sites. *A.* Arrow indicates a discontinuity in the plaque, presumably representing a large fracture or dissection. *B.* A false lumen is evident at the site of the arrow. (*Reproduced with permission of Circulation and the American Heart Association.*)

(Fig. 133-4). It must be emphasized that ultrasound provides images based on the acoustic reflectance of tissue, not actual histology.

With either mechanical or electronic devices, atherosclerotic vessels often exhibit both abnormal thickening and increased echogenicity of the intimal leading edge (Fig. 133-4). Presumably, these more echogenic "hard plaques" represent areas of greater intimal fibrosis with more specular ultrasound reflections. In the most extreme examples, dense plaques impede ultrasound transmission, thus "shadowing" underlying structures (Fig.133-4, right panel). These heavily fibrotic or calcified intimal atherosclerotic lesions reduce transmission of the low-energy, high-frequency ultrasound signals, thus obscuring the underlying structure of the arterial wall. Accordingly, the presence of extensive "shadowing" plaques may preclude measurement of total atheroma area becasue the full thickness of the vessel wall is not visualized.

Intravascular ultrasound with electronic probes at segments containing an angiographic luminal irregularity frequently reveals a crescentic sonolucent band encroaching upon the lumen (Fig. 133-4, left panel). In many patients, both lesions, thickening of the intimal leading edge and broad sonolucent plaques, coexist at a single site or at different locations (Fig. 133-4, right panel). At some sites, the sonolucent band is thickened but symmetrical, lending a distinctive triple-layer appearance to the vessel.

Plaque morphology is somewhat different with current mechanical probes, exhibiting a more echogenic plaque, often with a subadjacent sonolucent zone thought to represent normal media (Fig.133-3). For both types of devices, the adventitia appears as a third, deeper layer of the arterial wall and varies widely in appearance (Figs. 133-2 to 133-5). A distinct interface at the trailing edge of this adventitial layer is not apparent except within bypass grafts. Since this layer likely represents the tissues encasing the vessel, the ambiguity of the trailing edge often precludes measurement of total vessel wall thickness.

Wall Morphology: Angiographically Normal Sites

Atherosclerotic abnormalities in coronary wall morphology are commonly detected at sites in which no lesion is present by angiography.[11,34,35] In the presence of any luminal irregularity by angiography, intravascular ultrasound often demonstrates CAD at all other examined coronary sites.[35] More than 75 percent of angiographically normal sites in CAD patients demonstrate one or more abnormalities by intravascular ultrasound.[35] The extent of disease in angiographically normal vessels confirms the finding, previously reported from necropsy studies, that coronary disease is frequently more diffuse than apparent by angiography. In some cases, it is evident that preservation of angiographic lumen size was a consequence of compensatory remodeling of the vessel wall (Fig. 133-4, left panel).

Quantitative Luminal Measurements

Precise quantitation of vascular dimensions from a tomographic perspective represent an important potential application of intravascular ultrasound. In normal subjects, the correlation between angiographic and ultrasound coronary diameter is close, r = 0.87 to r = 0.92.[11,34] In patients with eccentrically diseased coronary lumina, the correlation between ultrasound and angiographic diameters is only moderate, r = 0.78.[11] This reduced correlation is probably explained by the irregular, noncircular cross-sectional profile of atherosclerotic vessels in CAD patients that cannot be adequately portrayed by angiography. There are also major differences between ultrasonic and angiographic assessment of stenosis severity—comparison of cross-sectional area reduction reveals only a moderate correlation, r = 0.63.[11]

Assessment of Angioplasty Results

A poor correlation has been reported for comparisons of ultrasound and angiographic assessment of residual stenosis following balloon angioplasty.[10,16] Measurements of luminal cross-sectional area following angioplasty are generally smaller by ultrasound than by angiography.[10,16] These differences may represent enhancement of the apparent angiographic diameter of the vessel produced by extraluminal contrast within cracks or splits in the intima and/or media of the vessel. Because balloon dilation distorts the vessel lumen and wall, the reported differences between angiographic and ultrasonic measurements probably reflect the differences between silhouette and tomographic imaging of complex, eccentric lumina following angioplasty.

After balloon angioplasty, a spectrum of ultrasound morphologic findings has been found, including complex cracks, splits, and dissections in the vessel wall[10,16] (Fig. 133-5). Some investigators have speculated that intravascular ultrasound would be particularly valuable in detecting angioplasty-related complications such as dissection or intraluminal thrombus.[10] It is difficult, however, to distinguish therapeutic from pathologic dissection by intravascular ultrasound.[16] Thrombus has acoustic properties similar to blood and may also be difficult to clearly differentiate. In addition to assessment of the angioplasty site, ultrasound permits evaluation of the luminal dimensions and the extent of atherosclerotic disease in "normal" segments, which is reported to be useful for balloon sizing.

EMERGING CORONARY APPLICATIONS

Published studies support several emerging applications for intravascular ultrasound. Precision measurement of coronary luminal diameter and cross-sectional area may have incremental value in assessment of eccentrically diseased vessels. The tomographic perspective of intravascular ultrasound is likely superior to planar methods such as angiography for cross-sectional area measurement.[11] The advantages of tomographic imaging are particularly evident in the assessment of the results of these catheter-based revascularization procedures because it is difficult for angiography to characterize the complex alterations in the vessel wall produced by balloon, laser, or atherectomy procedures. Residual stenosis measurements by ultrasound and angiography are often disparate following "successful" angioplasty. The ability of intravascular imaging to independently assess residual lesions is an important evolving application.

Unlike angiography, which depicts only the effects of atherosclerosis on the lumen, intravascular ultrasound permits evaluation of the actual pathological site of the disease. The ability to image atherosclerotic wall abnormalities in vivo has considerable research potential and is currently contributing to scientific understanding of the anatomy and pathology of CAD. Measurements of the size and morphologic characteristics of plaques may provide the most precise means yet developed to assess disease progression or regression. Intravascular ultrasound has demonstrated greater sensitivity than angiography in the detection of CAD and commonly detects atherosclerosis in angiographically normal segments.[10,11,35] Intravascular ultrasound has also been applied to evaluation of angiographically normal coronaries following cardiac transplantation, often revealing occult intimal thickening.[34]

The indications for intravascular ultrasound during coronary angioplasty continue to evolve. Ultrasound imaging provides precise measurements of the cross-sectional area of the residual lumen and atheroma.[10] The morphology of the vessel wall following revascularization may hold important clues to phenomena such as restenosis and abrupt occlusion. However, the value of ultrasound anatomy in predicting the short- and long-term complications of angioplasty is not yet defined. Technical developments are expanding the practicality of intravascular ultrasound during angioplasty. Current advances include smaller probes and combination devices incorporating both intravascular ultrasound and an angioplasty balloon.[15,37] Combination devices enable imaging before, during, and after angioplasty without catheter exchange. Long-term studies comparing ultrasound anatomy to clinical outcome are in progress and likely will establish the ultimate value of intravascular ultrasound following angioplasty.

Noncoronary Applications

Studies have demonstrated the feasibility of intravascular imaging of peripheral vessels.[12] Imaging of the pulmonary arteries has been successfully performed and the technique appears promising as a means to detect chronic thrombi causing pulmonary hypertension.[36] Other investigators have demonstrated the feasibility of intracardiac ultrasound, although clinical applications for this imaging approach have not yet emerged. Three-dimensional reconstruction of coronary and peripheral vessels has been demonstrated, although the incremental value of this method of image display has not yet been defined.[37]

Future Research and Development

The technology and clinical role for intravascular ultrasound examination of the coronaries is rapidly evolving. Important technical advances include further reductions in the size of imaging catheters and development of improved combination devices with diagnostic and therapeutic capability. In addition to the combination of imaging transducers with an angioplasty balloon, current investigational devices include transducers mounted on atherectomy devices and laser systems. If such devices provide practical assistance to revascularization procedures, combination imaging and therapy devices have the potential to become the future standard for angioplasty techniques. Imaging catheters are also under development that incorporate a tip-mounted Doppler flow probe to allow simultaneous cross-sectional area and flow velocity measurements. Such a device may provide continuous beat-to-beat assessment of coronary blood flow in vivo. Forward looking probes have been proposed as means to evaluate coronaries with diameters smaller than existing transducers.

These technical developments will likely expand the applicability of intravascular ultrasound in diagnostic and therapeutic cardiac catheterization. The precise role of this new imaging modality will be determined by current research examining the value of plaque morphology in defining the extent, natural history, and optimal treatment of CAD.

REFERENCES

1. Bom N, Lancee CT, Van Egmond FC: An ultrasonic intracardiac scanner. *Ultrasonics* 1972; 10:72–76.
2. Yock PG, Johnson EL, Linker DT: Intravascular ultrasound: Development and clinical potential. *Am J Cardiac Imaging* 1988; 2:185–193.
3. Pandian NG, Kreis A, Brockway B, Isner JM, Sacharoff A, Boleza E, et al: Ultrasound angioscopy: Real-time, two dimensional, intraluminal ultrasound imaging of blood vessels. *Am J Cardiol* 1988; 62:113–116.
4. Roelandt JR, Bom NY, Serruys PW: Intravascular high-resolution real-time, two-dimensional echocardiography. *Int J Cardiac Imaging* 1989; 4:63–67.
5. Hodgson JM, Graham SP, Savakus AD, Dame SG, Stephens DN, Dhillon PS, et al: Clinical percutaneous imaging of coronary anatomy using an over-the-wire ultrasound catheter system. *Int J Cardiac Imaging* 1989; 4:187–193.
6. Nissen SE, Grines CL, Gurley JC, Sublett K, Haynie D, Diaz C, et al: Application of a new phased-array ultrasound imaging catheter in the assessment of vascular dimensions: In vivo comparison to cineangiography. *Circulation* 1990; 81:660–666.
7. Bessen M, Moriushi M, McLeay L, McRae M, Henry WL: Intravascular ultrasound cross-sectional arterial imaging before and after balloon angioplasty in vitro. *Circulation* 1989; 80:873–882.
8. Yock P, Linker D, Angelsen B: Two-dimensional, intravascular ultrasound: Technical development and initial clinical experience. *J Am Soc Echocardiogr* 1989; 4:296–304.
9. Hodgson JM, Graham SP, Sheehan H, Savakus AD: Percutaneous intracoronary ultrasound imaging: Initial applications in patients. *Echocardiography* 1990; 7:403–413.
10. Tobis JM, Mallery J, Mahon D, Lehmann K, Zalesky P, Griffith J, et al: Intravascular ultrasound imaging of human coronary arteries in vivo. *Circulation* 1991; 83:913–926.
11. Nissen SE, Gurley JC, Grines CL, Booth DC, McClure R, Martin Berk MD, et al: Intravascular ultrasound assessment of lumen size and wall morphology in normal subjects and coronary artery disease patients. *Circulation* 1991; 84:1087–1099.
12. Isner JM, Rosenfield K, Kelly S, Losordo DW, DeJesus ST, Palefsky P, et al: Percutaneous intravascular ultrasound examination as an adjunct to catheter-based interventions: Preliminary experience in patients with peripheral vascular disease. *Radiology* 1990; 175:61–70.
13. Pandian NG, Weintraub A, Schwartz SL, Kumar R, Kosay BS, Katz SE, et al: Intravascular and intracardiac ultrasound imaging: Current research and future directions. *Echocardiography* 1990; 7:377–387.
14. Kimura BJ, Fitzgerald PJ, Sudhir K, Amidon TM, Strunk BL, Yock PG: Guidance of directed coronary atherectomy by intracoronary ultrasound imaging. *Am Heart J* 1992; 124:1365–1369.
15. Cacchione JG, Reddy K, Richards E, Sheehan H, Hodgson JM: Combined intravascular ultrasound/angioplasty balloon catheter: Initial use during PTCA. *Cathet Cardiovasc Diagn* 1991; 24:99–101.
16. Gurley JC, Nissen SE, Grines CL, Booth DC, Fischer C, DeMaria AN: Comparison of intravascular ultrasound and angiography following percutaneous transluminal angioplasty (abstr). *Circulation* 1990; 82(suppl III): III-72.
17. Isner JM, Rosenfield K, Losordo DW, Rose L, Langevin RE, Razvi S, et al: Combination balloon-ultrasound imaging catheter for percutaneous transluminal angioplasy. *Circulation* 1991; 84:739–754.
18. Arnett EN, Isner JM, Redwood CR, Kent KM, Baker WP, Ackerstein H, et al: Coronary artery narrowing in coronary heart disease: Comparison of cineangiographic and necropsy findings. *Ann Intern Med* 1979; 91:350–356.
19. Grodin CM, Dydra I, Pastgernac A, Campeau L, Bourassa MG: Discrepancies between cineangiographic and post-mortem findings in patients with coronary artery disease and recent myocardial revascularization. *Circulation* 1974; 49:703–709.
20. Blackenhorn DH, Curry PJ: The accuracy of arteriography and ultrasound imaging for atherosclerosis measurement: A review. *Arch Pathol Lab Med* 1982; 106:483–490.
21. Isner JM, Kishel J, Kent KM: Accuracy of angiographic determination of left main coronary arterial narrowing. *Circulation* 1981; 63:1056–1061.
22. Roberts WC, Jones AA: Quantitation of coronary arterial narrowing at necropsy in sudden coronary death. *Am J Cardiol* 1979; 44:39–44.
23. Vlodaver Z, Frech R, van Tassel RA, Edwards JE: Correlation of the antemortem coronary angiogram and the postmortem specimen. *Circulation* 1973; 47:162–168.
24. Zir LM, Miller SW, Dinsmore RE, Gilber JP, Harthorne JW: Interobserver variability in coronary angiography. *Circulation* 1976; 53:627–632.
25. Galbraith JE, Murphy ML, Desoyza N: Coronary angiogram interpretation: Interobserver variability. *JAMA* 1981; 240:2053–2059.
26. White CW, Wright CB, Doty DB, Hirtza LF, Eastham CL, Harrison DG, et al: Does visual interpretation of the coronary arteriogram predict the physiologic importance of a coronary stenosis? *N Engl J Med* 1984; 310:819–824.
27. Waller BF: "Crackers, breakers, stretchers, drillers, scrapers, shavers, burners, welders, and melters": The future treatment of atherosclerotic coronary artery disease? A clinical-morphologic assessment. *J Am Coll Cardiol* 1989; 13:969–987.
28. McPherson DD, Hiratzka LF, Lamberth WC, Brandt B, Hunt M, Kieso RA, et al: Delineation of the extent of coronary atherosclerosis by high frequency epicardial echocardiography. *N Engl J Med* 1987; 316:304–309.
29. Nissen SE, Gurley JC, Booth DC, Berk MR, Yamagishi M, Fischer C, et al: Differences in intravascular ultrasound plaque morphology in stable and unstable patients (abstr). *Circulation* 1991; 84(suppl II):II-436.
30. Gussenhoven EJ, Essed CE, Lancee CT, Mastik F, Frietman P, Van Egmond FC, et al: Arterial wall characteristics determined by intravascular ultrasound imaging: An in vitro study. *J Am Coll Cardiol* 1989; 4:947–952.
31. Potkin BN, Bartorelli AL, Gessert JM, Necille, RF, Almagor Y, Robert WC, et al: Coronary artery imaging with intravascular high-frequency ultrasound. *Circulation* 1990; 81:1575–1585.
32. Nishimura RA, Edwards WD, Warnes CA, Reeder GS, Holmes DR, Tajik AJ, et al: Intravascular ultrasound imaging: In vitro validation and pathologic correlation. *J Am Coll Cardiol* 1990; 16:145–154.
33. Gurley JC, Nissen SE, Fischer DC, O'Connor WN, DeMaria AN: Is the tri-layer arterial appearance an artifact? Differences between *in vivo* and *in vitro* intravascular ultrasound (abstr). *J Am Coll Cardiol* 1991; 17(suppl A):112A.
34. St Goar FG, Pinto FJ, Alderman EL, Fitzgerald PJ, Stadius ML, Popp RL: Intravascular ultrasound imaging of angiographically normal coronary arteries: An in vivo comparison with quantitative angiography. *J Am Coll Cardiol* 1991; 18:952–958.
35. Nissen SE, Gurley JC, Grines CL, Booth DC, Fischer C, DeMaria AN: Coronary atherosclerosis is frequently present at angiographically normal sites: Evidence from intravascular ultrasound in man (abstr). *Circulation* 1990; 82(suppl III):III-459.
36. Pandian NG, Weintraub A, Kreis A, Schwarz SL, Konstam MA, Salem DN: Intracardiac, intravascular, two dimensional high-frequency imaging of the pulmonary artery and its branches in humans and animals *Circulation* 1990; 81:2007–2012.
37. Isner JM, Rosenfield K, Losordo DW, Rose L, Langevin RE, Razvi S, et al: Combination balloon-ultrasound imaging catheter for percutaneous transluminal angioplasty. *Circulation* 1991; 84:739–754.

PART XX

Diagnostic Radionuclide and Nuclear Techniques Used in the Evaluation of the Cardiovascular System

Chapter 134

Nuclear Cardiology

Lynne L. Johnson, M.D. ■ *Gerald M. Pohost, M.D.*

The application of radionuclide tracers for detection and risk assessment of heart disease has evolved into an important clinical discipline over the past two decades. The present chapter will critically describe the important radionuclide procedures, both their strengths and their weaknesses. The first section of this chapter explains the basic principles and components for radionuclide imaging of the heart, including instrumentation, methods of acquiring images, methods of displaying images, image processing, and both qualitative and quantitative approaches to image analysis. Then each of the major areas of nuclear cardiology will be described in detail, including methods to assess myocardial perfusion, viability, and metabolism; methods to assess heart function; approaches for detection and sizing of acutely infarcted myocardium; and approaches for the evaluation of inflammation and thrombosis.

Nuclear cardiology is a discipline based on the use of radioactive tracer pharmaceuticals to derive images that help assess normal and abnormal physiological, biochemical, metabolic, or even immunologic processes in vivo. Since only a minute quantity of material need be administered, there is no alteration of the physiologic or pathologic process being evaluated. The number of molecules of a given compound that are injected are so few that there is no detectable biological effect. The only potential risk of a nuclear cardiology procedure is the low-dose radiation exposure. The exposure is typically less than 1 rad of total body radiation and less than 5 rads of exposure to a single organ. To understand this better, the total body radiation exposure associated with a radionuclide tracer study is approximately equivalent to the radiation exposure of a person living at an elevation of one mile above sea level (e.g., Denver) over a 5-year period. Such studies also roughly approximate the radiation dose of a standard upper gastrointestinal series and are substantially less than that associated with a coronary angiographic study. In the latter case, the radiation exposure to the sternum is in the range of 25 rad. In view of the extremely low risk from these studies, nuclear cardiology methods are generally considered to be noninvasive techniques.

The weakness of the nuclear cardiology methods is that they have limited spatial and temporal resolution. Spatial resolution varies between 0.5 mm for state-of-the-art positron emission tomography (PET) systems to 1.5 cm for single-photon emission computed tomography (SPECT) methods. Most single-photon planar imaging procedures have a spatial resolution of about 1 cm. Also, since only a limited dose of radionuclide is administered, acquisition times vary considerably. A planar thallium myocardial imaging study, or a gated ventricular function study, requires around 5 to 10 min per view, or 20 to 30 min for the two- or three-view imaging sequence. A SPECT thallium study requires 20 to 30 min to acquire.

BASIC PRINCIPLES OF NUCLEAR CARDIOLOGY

Instrumentation

Nuclear cardiology utilizes radionuclides which emit electromagnetic radiation by virtue of a change in the energy state of their atomic nucleus. The radiation that is detected is in the form of gamma rays or x-rays. The quantum particle of such radiation is known as a photon.

The interactions that make such electromagnetic radiation or photons visible are photoelectric absorption and Compton scatter. The light flashes that result are known as scintillations. The gamma or x-ray photons deposited in tissue account for the small radiation dose described in units called rads (radiation absorbed dose). Many of the emitted photons are detectable by the gamma (scintillation) camera.

Gamma Camera

The gamma or scintillation camera allows imaging of the distribution of the gamma or x-ray photons emitted by a radionuclide in the body. There are three basic types of gamma cameras: (1) the Anger camera (or the single crystal gamma camera); (2) the multicrystal camera; and (3) the positron camera.

Anger Camera

In 1958, Hal Anger described the most important imaging device for radionuclide studies, the single-crystal gamma camera, frequently referred to as the Anger Camera.[1] This device has withstood the test of time and continues to be the most commonly employed instrument for clinical radionuclide imaging. The Anger camera uses a relatively thin (0.25- to 0.50-in. thick), flat, large (approximately 10 to 15 in. in diameter) sodium iodide crystal. Between the crystal and the patient is a piece of flat lead machined with numerous holes, called a collimator. The holes are generally arranged in a parallel fashion. The collimator allows gamma or x-ray photons that emanate from the patient to strike the crystal. Scattered photons and those originating from regions outside of the field of view of the gamma camera will be absorbed by the lead collimator. The gamma photons that traverse the holes of the collimator interact with the crystal to produce scintillations which are detected by the photomultiplier tubes (Fig. 134-1). The photomultiplier tube converts scintillations into an electrical signal. The greater the observed intensity, the greater the electrical signal. The photomultiplier tubes closest to the scintillation will observe more light than those farther away. The electronic outputs from all of the photomultiplier tubes are fed into an electronic processor which determines the position of the scintillation from the outputs of the photomultiplier tubes.[2]

Before scintillations are displayed to the observer, they are filtered through an electronic device known as a pulse height analyzer.[3] This device allows only electrical signals that emanate from a pre-set range of energies to pass through. In this way, a window is made to accept only those photons with energies around the photopeak(s) of a radionuclide. For nuclear cardiology procedures, the two most commonly employed radionuclides—^{99m}Tc and ^{201}Tl—have totally different settings for the pulse height analyzer due to the differences in the energies of the photons emitted. Technetium-99m has a single photopeak of 140 keV. It is customary to set the window at 20 percent of the photopeak energy, or 28 keV centered around the 140 keV photopeak. Thallium-201 has multiple photopeaks; the lower energy x-ray photons are located at 68 to 84 keV and are customarily included within the pulse height analyzer's window. Many laboratories select a second window to encompass the 170 keV photopeak.

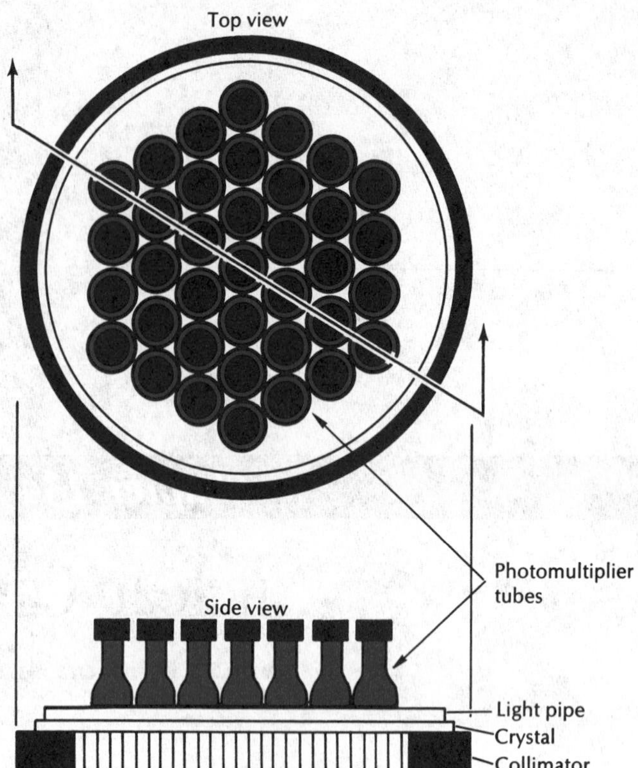

FIGURE 134-1 Illustration of the location of the collimator, the sodium iodide crystal, and the photomultiplier (PM) tubes in an Anger type gamma camera. The top view shows the hexagonal array of the 37 PM tubes. The PM tubes can also be arranged in a circular array. Gamma photons emanating from the heart can transverse the open holes of the lead collimator to strike the crystal and produce a scintillation. The light pipe conducts the scintillation to the photomultiplier tubes. The PM tubes amplify the signal to generate an image. [*From FD Roll (ed): Nuclear Medicine: Physics, Instrumentation, and Agents. St. Louis, Mosby, 1977:234. Reproduced with permission from the publisher and the editor.*]

Since the time of Anger's initial description, the single-crystal gamma camera has been improved substantially. The photomultiplier tube has become more efficient and smaller, allowing a greater number of tubes to be included in the camera. The crystal has become thinner and the electronics less noisy. Certain cameras are now digital, allowing direct connection between the photomultiplier tubes and an imaging computer.[4] The use of an imaging computer, whether with an analog or a digital Anger camera, has become standard. The computer allows acquisition and display of multiple-frame gated blood pool imaging studies to assess ventricular function, computation of ejection fraction, optimal display of myocardial images with the ability to manipulate both contrast and intensity, quantitation of the distribution and redistribution of radionuclides in myocardial perfusion imaging studies, and tomographic acquisition and display (known as single-photon emission computed tomography, or SPECT).

Single-Photon Emission Computed Tomography

Single-photon emission computed tomography (SPECT) is most commonly performed with one Anger camera head mounted on a gantry. The gantry rotates the gamma camera(s) around the patient.[5] SPECT cameras are also available with two or even three heads to increase acquisition speed. In the case of SPECT using one Anger camera head, the camera generally rotates in a circular orbit 180° around the patient from the right anterior oblique to the left posterior oblique orientation. The camera head stops at predetermined positions (e.g., every 6°, with 32 stops) and acquires imaging data for a preselected time (40 s at each stop for ^{201}Tl). After the acquisition time period is complete for one position, the camera rotates to the next stop where another acquisition is made, and so on. To increase imaging speed, certain newer SPECT systems can acquire counts continuously not only while the detector is stopped but also while it is moving. Such systems are useful for the new myocardial perfusion agent, ^{99m}Tc teboroxime, which remains in the myocardium for a relatively short time. After all of the images are acquired, the computer, using an approach similar to that of x-ray computed tomography—i.e., filtered backprojection—reconstructs the images into a series of parallel tomographic slices.[6] There are more potential technical pitfalls to performing SPECT imaging than planar imaging and careful attention must be paid to center of rotation correction and patient motion during acquisition.

SPECT generates images of slices through the heart (e.g., from apex to base, from septum to posterolateral wall, or from superior to inferior wall). SPECT should be differentiated from conventional planar imaging. With the planar method, images are generated from photons originating in all portions of the heart (two-dimensional projection of a three-dimensional object). With SPECT, images represent tomographic slices through the heart. SPECT has improved contrast over planar imaging, improved anatomical localization of defects, and increased ability to detect small defects over planar imaging. In nuclear cardiology, SPECT is most commonly employed in conjunction with myocardial perfusion imaging with ^{201}Tl or one of the ^{99m}Tc-based myocardial perfusion agents.

Multicrystal Gamma Camera

Instead of using a single sodium iodide crystal, as in the Anger camera, the multicrystal camera uses a rectangular array of crystals. Each crystal is coupled to a photomultiplier tube by means of a fiberoptics conduit.[7] Cameras constructed in this way can record substantially more counts than the conventional Anger camera, due to a lower dead time (the time during which the camera electronics processes the electrical pulse associated with each scintillation and is unable to respond to another scintillation pulse). For example, a conventional Anger camera can respond to a count rate (or pulse rate) of up to 200,000 counts per second, while a multicrystal camera can detect over 600,000 counts per second. The digital Anger camera has the ability to measure count rates of up to 400,000 counts per second. Continued improvements in each type of camera will lead to even better performance.

The main use of the multicrystal camera is for first-pass ventricular function studies. These studies are performed using the injection of a bolus of technetium pertechnetate or technetium-99m labeled radiopharmaceutical. Since the multicrystal camera has a high count rate, it is better able to cope with the great number of counts contained in a radionuclide bolus injection as it passes through the central circulation, allowing reasonable estimates of right and left ventricular ejection fractions. The first-pass approach can be applied following serial injections of technetium pertechnetate over a fairly short time interval before background activity from the previous dose(s) interferes with measurement accuracy. With the advent of the new ^{99m}Tc-labeled myocardial perfusion agents, it is possible to inject a single tracer dose as a bolus and obtain a first-pass ejection fraction measurement at peak exercise in addition to images depicting myocardial perfusion.

Positron Camera

Positron emission (computed) tomography (PET) utilizes a gamma camera that detects photons resulting from positron annihilation. When a positron interacts with an electron, the two particles annihilate one another and produce two high-energy gamma photons of 511 keV oriented in opposite directions. The PET camera generally consists of several concentric rings of crystals forming a cylinder into which the patient is placed.[8] Crystals are oriented in pairs on opposite sides of the ring 180° apart. If the two gamma photons generated by the positron annihilation strike opposite crystals nearly simultaneously, a scintillation is recorded in the resultant image. If one gamma photon strikes a crystal without another gamma photon striking the opposite crystal, no signal is registered. Thus, PET cameras have a built-in mechanism to exclude background scatter and photons originating from planes outside the field of interest. While positron emission tomography is an excellent cardiologic research tool, to date its only clinical advantage over single photon methods is in the assessment of myocardial viability in patients with ischemic heart disease and wall motion abnormalities who are being considered for revascularization.[9] Positron radionuclides generally have a short half-life. Most are produced by a small on-site cyclotron. Recently, less expensive small linear accelerators have provided an alternative to the cyclotron. One PET radionuclide of potential value for myocardial perfusion imaging, rubidium-82, is generator-produced, obviating the need for an on-site particle accelerator. Rubidium, which is similar to thallium, behaves like potassium in the myocardium. The particle accelerator generated radionuclides that have been used in cardiology include ^{11}C, ^{13}N, ^{15}O, and ^{18}F. These radionuclides are incorporated into radiopharmaceuticals such as ^{11}C-palmitic acid, ^{13}N-ammonia, and ^{18}F-fluorodeoxyglucose.

The Computer

Computers are now routinely used for acquisition, display, and analysis of radionuclide images and are considered an essential component of a nuclear cardiology laboratory. A computer system is now used for virtually every nuclear cardiology procedure. The computer system allows display of gated radionuclide angiocardiograms and first-pass studies as movies at 20 to 32 frames per second. Myocardial perfusion images are acquired using a computer for display and quantitative analysis.

RADIONUCLIDE METHODS TO ASSESS MYOCARDIAL PERFUSION AND VIABILITY

The most unique aspect of nuclear cardiology is its ability to assess myocardial perfusion and viability. At the present time there are no other methods that provide this information in a cost-effective way. Nevertheless, high-speed magnetic resonance imaging of a bolus of paramagnetic material as it traverses the myocardium, or even of specific paramagnetic agents to depict myocardial perfusion, are under development and could ultimately provide an alternative (see Chap. 136).

^{201}Tl remains the radionuclide of choice for assessment of both myocardial perfusion and viability. Newer technetium-based agents have somewhat more desirable imaging characteristics but at present do not afford the same opportunity to assess viability as does thallium. These agents include the technetium isonitrile known as sestamibi and technetium BATO complex known as teboroxime. The PET agents, ^{82}Rb and $^{13}NH_3$, are also used for myocardial perfusion imaging.

Thallium-201

Thallium-201 is a cyclotron-produced radionuclide with a half life of 73 h. It emits a cluster of x-rays between 68 to 82 keV; however, it also has photopeaks at 135 and 165 keV. The rationale for its use as a myocardial-imaging agent stems from its similarity to potassium (K^+) in biological systems and to its primarily intracellular distribution. Both ionic potassium (K^+) and thallium (Tl^+) have similar hydrate ionic radii, and both are thought to be transported across the cell membrane by the sodium-potassium ATPase pump.[10]

Thallium Kinetics

To understand the clinical utility of thallium, it is important to understand its kinetics. Thallium kinetics are best described by considering its behavior both in the blood pool as well as in the myocardium. This is most easily done by considering the two phases of thallium distribution: initial distribution and delayed distribution, commonly referred to as redistribution.

Initial Distribution of ^{201}Tl After injection of a bolus of thallous-201 chloride (TlCl), cardiac blood pool activity rises rapidly to a peak and falls more gradually as the thallium is extracted very efficiently by the tissues of the body. Afterwards, blood pool activity declines slowly as the thallium is excreted. After injection of an intravenous bolus of thallium, approximately 5 percent of the injected dose, representing the percentage of the cardiac output delivered to the coronary circulation, distributes to the myocardium. The myocardium extracts approximately 80 to 90 percent of the thallium passing through the coronary circulation.[11,12] Skeletal muscle, kidney, liver, and gonadal tissue also efficiently extract thallium. The time interval from injection to peak myocardial thallium activity depends on myocardial perfusion.[13] If thallium is administered at rest, the time to peak myocardial thallium activity is delayed. If thallium is administered at maximal exercise or with vasodilators, the time to peak myocardial thallium activity is early. Peak myocardial thallium activity distal to a coronary stenosis will be delayed relative to myocardium supplied by a nonstenotic coronary artery. Regions supplied by normal and stenotic arteries are responsible for the defect(s) observed on myocardial images.

Due to its very efficient extraction, the initial distribution of thallium in the myocardium is very closely related to myocardial perfusion.[14,15] Myocardial extraction of thallium from the blood is related to blood flow, however, and thus to exposure of the myocardium to the blood: The more prolonged the exposure, the more effective the extraction, and conversely. For example, at very high flow rates, such as that induced by the coronary vasodilators dipyridamole and adenosine, myocardial extraction may decrease.[16,17] Extraction of thallium by the myocardium may also be affected by severe hypoxia, insulin, ß-adrenergic blocking agents, and digitalis, although the effect does not appear to be clinically important.[12]

Like potassium, initial thallium extraction is affected by myocardial viability. In a perfusion-independent model using cultured fetal rat hearts, myocardial thallium extraction was not affected until the hearts showed evidence of death, as determined by the presence of lactic dehydrogenase (LDH) in the culture medium.[18] Even under conditions that simulated severe ischemia, such as addition of lactic acid, anoxia, and deprivation of glucose and other oxidizable substrates, myocardial thallium extraction in this model was relatively normal. These data suggest that thallium extraction by the myocardium occurs only in the presence of viability, and myocardial extraction occurs at a relatively normal rate even in the presence of severe ischemia. In summary, the initial distribution of thallium is related to perfusion and myocardial viability.

Redistribution After the initial distribution of thallium, myocardial and blood pool activity continue to change (Fig. 134-2*A*). There is an increase in myocardial thallium activity to peak and then slow clearance, which ultimately parallels the decrease in blood pool thallium. In myocardial zones jeopardized by significant stenoses, peak activity is delayed and thallium concentration is lower relative to the nonjeopardized myocardium.[19] Because the clearance from all viable myocardium will parallel blood pool activity, clearance is more rapid from higher flow regions than from lower flow regions. Thallium activity in the normal and underperfused myocardium approach one another over time.[14] Complete thallium redistribution can occur only in the absence of myocardial scar.

The persistent thallium defect, however, is not specific for nonviable myocardium. Up to 50 percent of viable myocardial segments will demonstrate persistent defects within the conventional 3- to 4-h follow-up imaging interval.[20] Generally, the basis for this appears to be more rapid clearance of thallium from the blood pool with less

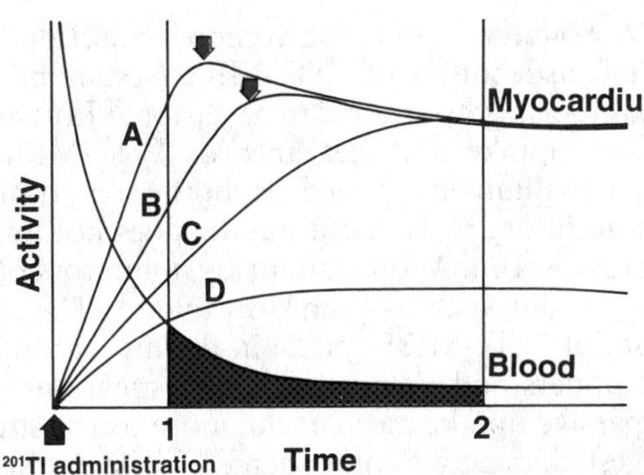

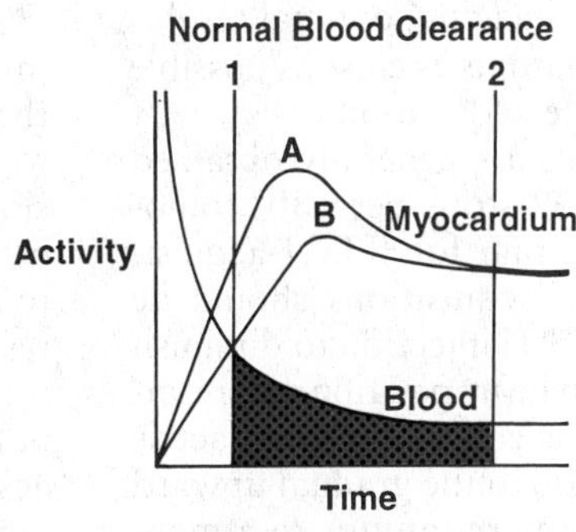

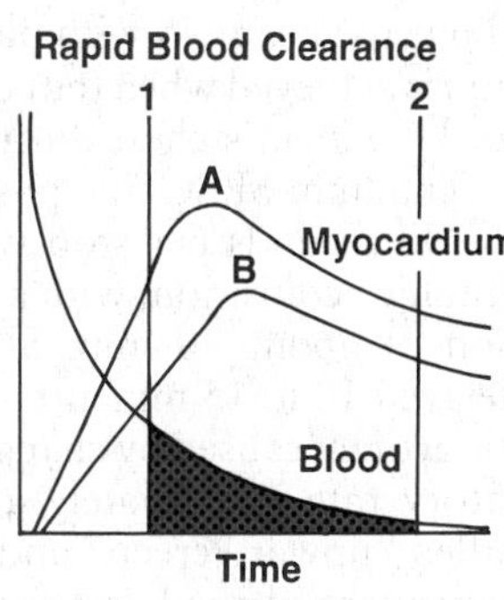

FIGURE 134-2. *A.* Time activity curves after intravenous administration of ^{201}Tl. Immediately after intravenous administration of ^{201}Tl, blood activity rises rapidly and then falls exponentially as the tracer is distributed throughout the body. Myocardium efficiently extracts the ^{201}Tl and rises to peak (blue arrows) as a function of the rate at which the tracer circulates through the myocardium (a function of flow and blood concentration). The time to peak is earliest and the peak highest when perfusion is maximal in the distribution of a normal coronary artery, i.e., at peak exercise or with dipyridamole or adenosine infusion. When myocardial exposure to ^{201}Tl (termed "the input function") is reduced, the time activity curve for myocardial thallium reaches a later and lesser peak. After peak, myocardial thallium activity begins to clear, at first, rapidly and then more slowly. Ultimately, it will clear at a rate that is parallel to the rate of clearance of ^{201}Tl activity from the blood. If curve A represents territory supplied by a normal coronary artery, curve B represents territory supplied by a coronary artery with significant disease, and curve C a territory supplied by a coronary artery with even more advanced disease. Images acquired at time 1 will show a defect in the territory represented by curves B and C. (Note that time 1 intercepts curves B and C at a substantially lower level of activity than the intersection of time 1 with curve A.) By time 2, the defect has resolved, i.e., it has demonstrated redistribution. Curve D represents myocardial ^{201}Tl activity in a territory with myocardial scar. Under these circumstances, ^{201}Tl activity increases minimally related to surrounding viable myocardium. Images acquired at times 1 and 2 will demonstrate a persistent defect. If blood pool activity clears rapidly, the opportunity for redistribution to occur is lessened and fixed defects can be observed in viable myocardial segments. *B.* Myocardial time activity curves in normal (A) and ischemic (B) territories are plotted for a patient with a normal blood clearance (left) and for a patient with rapid blood clearance. When blood activity is normal, thallium redistribution occurs. In contrast, when blood pool activity clears rapidly, thallium input is reduced, and redistribution is not evident within the usual 3 to 4 h time frame. Thus, redistribution is evident between 1 and 2 under the conditions illustrated on the left but will not occur under the circumstances illustrated on the right. Viability usually can be documented either by administering a second dose of ^{201}Tl or by repeating the imaging study at a later time (12 to 48 h). The "input function" for blood ^{201}Tl is stippled and can be seen to be substantially greater with normal blood clearance than with rapid blood clearance.

residual thallium available for re-uptake (Fig. 134-2*B*). There are two methods to get thallium into these persistent defects in viable myocardial territory. The first is to obtain follow-up images 24 to 48 h after the initial injection.[21] This will lead to resolution of the defects in over 75 percent of viable myocardial territory. Another method is to give a second injection of thallium to boost the blood pool activity 3 to 4 h after the initial injection.[22] This technique also appears to lead to fill-in of over 75 percent of viable myocardial defects.

Under certain circumstances, in patients with reduced regional resting blood flow, myocardial activity will gradually increase in the affected region and demonstrate redistribution. These findings have been reported in patients with unstable angina pectoris, refractory angina, or patients with down regulation of wall motion in the underperfused territory, known as "hibernating myocardium."[23-26] When thallium is administered to such patients, even in the resting state, an initial defect can be observed to show, at least, partial redistribution by 3 to 4 h. The redistribution of thallium in the asynergic segment documents viability.

Planar Imaging with ^{201}Tl

There are two basic approaches to myocardial perfusion imaging: conventional planar imaging and single photon emission computed tomography, or SPECT. Generally, three views are obtained for planar imaging: the anterior, an intermediate (45°) left anterior oblique (LAO), and a steep (70°) LAO, or left lateral view. For the anterior and intermediate LAO projections, the patient lies supine on the imaging table, while for the steep LAO, or left lateral projection, the patient is placed in the right lateral decubitus position with his/her left side against the collimator to reduce the possibility of attenuation of inferior wall activity by the diaphragm.

Planar images are acquired for a preset time of 8 to 10 min per view, using a low-energy, medium-resolution collimator. Imaging should be initiated 5 min after administration of ^{201}Tl. Usually, the imaging sequence begins in the anterior projection, followed by the 45° LAO projection, and then the steep LAO projection. The anterior view is obtained first to allow assessment of pulmonary thallium activity immediately post exercise. Delayed imaging to detect "redistribution" is generally obtained at 3 to 4 h after ^{201}Tl injection. To further assess viability in patients with persistent defects at 3 to 4 h, a second injection of 1 mCi ^{201}Tl is administered and imaging repeated 5 to 10 min later.[22] Alternatively, if it is convenient for the patient, a repeat late imaging sequence is performed. Since myocardial thallium activity is relatively low at the time of the very late sequence, images are acquired for a longer period (e.g., 15 min per view).

SPECT Thallium Imaging

The patient is placed in the supine position on the imaging pallet for SPECT acquisitions. The camera rotates through a 180° circular orbit from 45° right anterior oblique (RAO) to 45° left posterior oblique position in a step-and-shoot mode. The patient's arms are placed above the head. As with planar imaging, optimal resolution is achieved when the collimator is as close as possible to the patient's chest during the acquisition.

Thallium SPECT acquisitions are generally obtained for 40 seconds per stop with 32 stops per 180° tomographic acquisition, with a total time for SPECT acquisition of about 30 min. SPECT acquisitions should be delayed 10 to 15 min after the ^{201}Tl injection to diminish the artifact caused by changes in heart position and respiratory rate immediately after exercise. This artifact is called "upward creep" and refers to the gradual upward movement of the heart from a more inferior to a more superior position within the chest.[27] During the 10 to 15 min period prior to initiation of SPECT imaging, a planar image is acquired in the anterior projection to assess thallium lung activity. SPECT imaging is again performed 3 to 4 h after thallium administration to assess redistribution, following reinjection, or on repeat late imaging as needed. The raw tomographic image data are then reconstructed into a three-dimensional object, which is sliced in three planes for display. First, a transaxial tomogram oriented to the body planes is reconstructed from the multiple projection images using a process known as filtered backprojection. Then, this initial tomogram is reoriented to the intrinsic cardiac axes and displayed as short axis, vertical, and horizontal long axis slices.

Technetium-Based Perfusion Agents

Two new ^{99m}Tc-based perfusion agents are now available for clinical use: ^{99m}Tc-sestamibi and ^{99m}Tc-teboroxime. The physical characteristics and biologic behavior of thallium and the two ^{99m}Tc-based agents are compared in Table 134-1.

^{99m}Tc-Methoxy Isobutyl Isomitrile

Technetium-99m methoxy isobutyl isonitrile (^{99m}Tc-MIBI) is a relatively new myocardial perfusion imaging agent with the advantages associated with ^{99m}Tc: (1) a single photopeak of 140 keV in an optimal range for imaging with an Anger camera; (2) a relatively short half life of 6 h, allowing safe administration of up to eight times the dose of ^{201}Tl; and (3) on-site preparation using a commercially available kit and a technetium generator.

^{99m}Tc-MIBI Kinetics After intravenous injection, the myocardial distribution of ^{99m}Tc-MIBI (sestamibi) like that of thallium is proportional to perfusion.[28] In contrast to thallium, uptake and clearance of ^{99m}Tc-MIBI are slower than thallium in cultured newborn rat myocardial cells.[29] In addition, ^{99m}Tc-MIBI uptake does not appear to be altered by 10 m*M* ouabain or by inhibitors of the respiratory chain such as 5 m*M* cyanide.[30] The exact mechanism of ^{99m}Tc-MIBI uptake in the myocardium is not well understood. While early investigations suggested a passive uptake mechanism, more recent studies have suggested an active component.[31-33] The extraction fraction of ^{99m}Tc-MIBI is lower than that of ^{201}Tl.[34]

Sestamibi has relatively stable myocardial concentrations with little washout over a 3 to 4 h period with very low blood levels (Fig. 134-3).[35] Accordingly, it does not demonstrate the redistribution phenomenon and cannot be used to fully assess myocardial viability after a single dose of the radiopharmaceutical. Thus, due to its clinically insignificant redistribution, two injections of sestamibi must be made, one at rest and a second at peak stress, or with dipyridamole infusion. The uptake of ^{99m}Tc-MIBI is similar to that of ^{201}Tl in animal models of myocardial ischemic insult.[36] In this model of ischemic insult, ^{99m}Tc-MIBI uptake appears to require viability in the same way that thallium does. It has also been shown that ^{99m}Tc-MIBI demonstrates comparable uptake to ^{201}Tl in stunned myocardium.[37]

Immediately following reperfusion, perfusion tracer distribution reflects myocardial blood flow and not viability; that is, the defect size may be smaller in extent than the infarct size.[38] The clinically insignificant redistribution of sestamibi up to 1 to 2 h following injection, however, makes it a good agent for assessing the extent of myocardial salvage following reperfusion.[39-41] One dose of the tracer is injected prior to the administration of thrombolytic therapy and imaging performed several hours later. The initial defect size represents both necrotic and "salvaged" but hypoperfused myocardium ("region at risk"). The patient is reinjected and reimaged 24 h later. The later defect delineates the final infarct size. The difference between the two defects represents the salvaged myocardium.

^{99m}Tc-MIBI Imaging In contrast to thallium imaging in which initial and delayed acquisitions can be made following a single tracer injection, ^{99m}Tc-MIBI images can

TABLE 134-1
Single Photon Perfusion Agents

	Thallium-201	Sestamibi (^{99m}Tc)	Teboroxime (^{99m}Tc)
Chemical form	Element	Isonitrile	BATO complex
Charge	Cation	Cation	Neutral
Effective dose equivalent	1.05 rem/3 mCi	1.06 rem/30 mCi	1.78 rem/30 mCi
Target organ	Kidney	Upper GI	Upper GI
Peak extraction fraction	0.75–0.85	0.40–0.60	0.80–0.90
Myocardial clearance $T_{1/2}$ at rest	3–4 h	> 6 h	10–15 min
Reuptake from blood levels	Yes	No	No
Redistribution	Yes	No	Yes

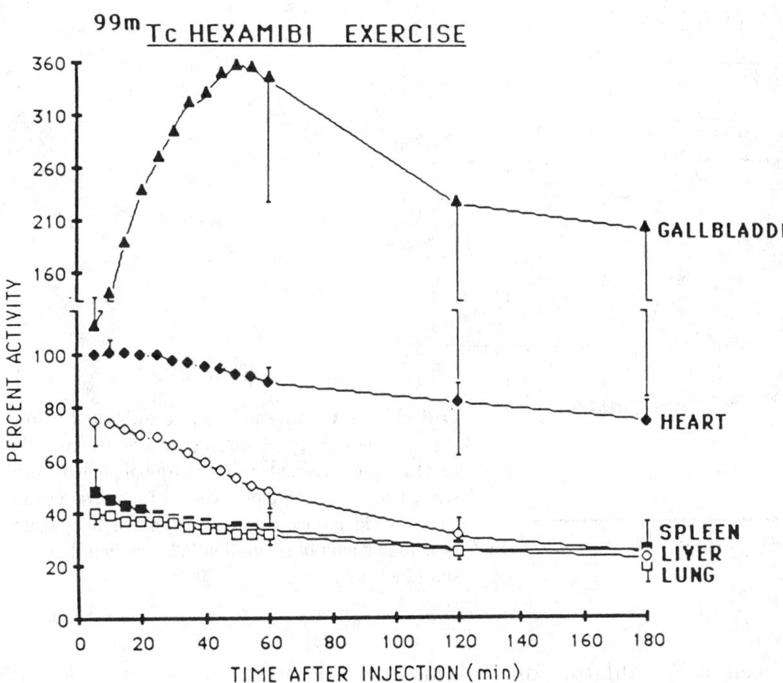

FIGURE 134-3 Time activity plots for the organs identified in five normal volunteers following an injection of ^{99m}Tc-sestamibi during exercise. Myocardial activity shows little clearance over time. Gallbladder activity peaks soon after injection and then decreases. Clearance of tracer from the hepatobiliary tree is hastened by giving the patient whole milk after the completion of exercise. Optimal imaging time is 30 to 60 min following exercise to allow intestinal activity to fall while myocardial activity remains relatively constant. (*From Wackers et al: J Nucl Med 30:305, 1989. Reproduced with permission from the publisher and authors.*)

be acquired only after two separate injections of tracer. One injection of the agent is made at the time of peak exercise and the other in the resting state. There are two potential protocols: (1) a same-day protocol in which the study at rest is performed first with administration of a low dose (7 to 10 mCi) of ^{99m}Tc-MIBI, followed in 2 to 3 h by a second injection of a higher dose (20 to 30 mCi) of the agent at peak exercise[42]; or (2) a separate day approach in which the rest and exercise studies are performed 24 h apart.

After administraton of ^{99m}Tc-MIBI, imaging by either planar or SPECT approaches is performed 1 h after the rest injection and 30 min following the stress injection to allow clearance of the agent from liver and gallbladder. Clinically significant redistribution of myocardial activitiy is not observed in the first 1 to 2 h following injection. Because the count rate is higher than that for thallium imaging due to the substantially higher injected dose, twice the number of projection images are acquired and a high-resolution collimator is used for ^{99m}Tc-MIBI imaging, and the image quality is somewhat better than that for thallium. The time per projection is shorter than that for thallium so that the total acquisition can be kept under 25 min. The time per projection is 25 to 30 s for the low dose of ^{99m}Tc-MIBI and 20 s for the high dose.

The high myocardial count rate from the relatively large administered dose makes it possible to obtain electrocardiographic (ECG) gated SPECT images in a clinically acceptable time. Such gated tomograms displayed in a movie format depict left ventricular wall thickening (at rest). Using this technique, exercise perfusion and resting function can be obtained using a single tracer dose.

^{99m}Tc-Teboroxime Kinetics

^{99m}Tc-Teboroxime is a member of a class of neutral lipophilic technetium-containing complexes. It is chemically different from the cationic complexes which include ^{99m}Tc-MIBI (sestamibi).[43] Like thallium, ^{99m}Tc-teboroxime exhibits high myocardial extraction and distributes in proportion to regional myocardial perfusion.[44–46] The high extraction of teboroxime is maintained at higher levels of myocardial blood flow than is observed with either thallium or sestamibi.[47] For this reason, teboroxime is suited for use with pharmacologic vasodilators, such as dipyridamole or adenosine, which increase myocardial blood flow by greater increments over resting flow than occurs during exercise. In contrast to the other agents, teboroxime clears rapidly from the myocardium even at rest, with a half-life for myocardial clearance of 6 to 10 min.[48] This clearance rate is faster at higher flows associated with exercise or pharmacologic vasodilation (Fig. 134-4). Regional washout rates of teboroxime are related to regional myocardial blood flow.[47] Ischemic defects in some patients can demonstrate rapid redistribution and may obviate the need for a second rest injection.[49] The standard imaging protocols with this agent however, include two injections of tracer, one at stress and one at rest.

^{99m}Tc-Teboroxime Imaging In view of the rapid myocardial washout of this agent, images must be acquired rapidly. For planar imaging, subjects usually are imaged upright (either seated or standing) in front of the gamma camera to minimize scatter from the substantial hepatic uptake of this tracer.[49] Acquisition should begin 1 to 2 min after stress. Each of the three views is completed in about 60 s and one total acquisition completed in under 4 min. Two separate injections of ^{99m}Tc-teboroxime are made at rest and at peak exercise. For each study, 12 to 20 mCi of the agent are administered. Stress studies are generally performed first, followed within 1 to 1.5 h by resting studies.

It is also necessary to complete a SPECT acquisition as rapidly as possible, e.g., within 6 min or even 3 min

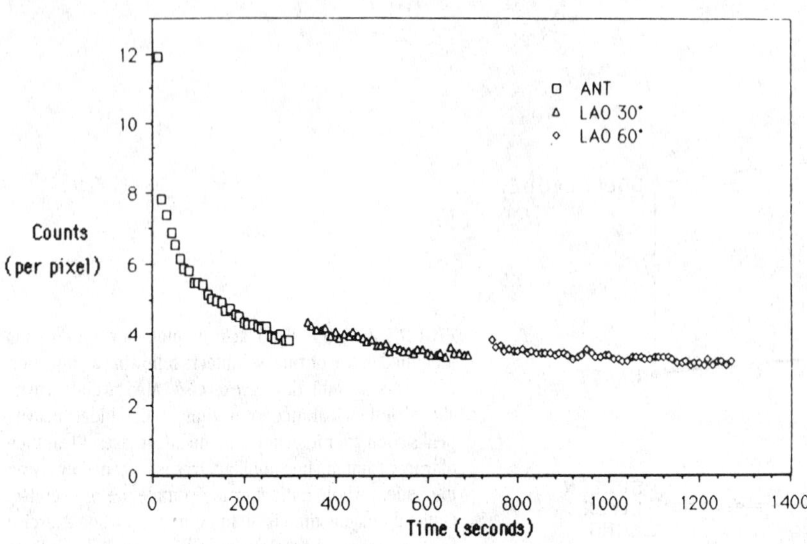

FIGURE 134-4 Myocardial time activity curve following injection of ^{99m}Tc teboroxime at peak exercise. The breaks in the curve and change in symbol plotted represent change in imaging projections. The curve demonstrates rapid myocardial wash-out which necessitates prompt initiation of acquisition following injection and short imaging times.

of injection. High-quality SPECT images have been obtained on cameras capable of continuous step and shoot acquisition or multihead cameras. Interference from hepatic activity can be reduced by volume masking and by using computerized interpolative background subtraction.

PET Perfusion

Although there are three positron radionuclides which can be used for myocardial perfusion imaging, two are cyclotron-produced and short-lived, ^{15}O water and ^{13}N ammonia, and, therefore, are not widely available. The third, rubidium-82 (^{82}Rb), is generator-produced and, although it has a very short half-life (75 s), it can be administered intravenously during infusion of dipyridamole to diagnose and assess the severity of coronary artery disease. In contrast to single-photon methods, a positron emitter can be used to quantitate regional myocardial blood flow in milliliters per minute per gram with the use of mathematical modeling.

The major theoretical advantages of PET assessment of regional distribution of myocardial blood flow over single-photon tomographic imaging include the superior resolution associated with the intrinsic collimation of positron emitters and the ability to correct for tissue attenuation of photons routinely. Tissue attenuation varies widely among patients and accounts for some "false positive" defects on single-photon studies. Few investigators have compared directly the diagnostic accuracy of SPECT and PET myocardial perfusion in the same group of subjects. Available data show comparable sensitivities of the two techniques for diagnosis of CAD and for determination of the distribution of diseased coronary arteries.[50,51]

CLINICAL APPROACHES TO MYOCARDIAL PERFUSION IMAGING

Both thallium and the technetium-based agents can be administered during exercise stress, infusion of the vasodilators dipyridamole or adenosine, or in unstable patients at rest.

Graded Exercise Testing

In stable patients who are able to exercise, either treadmill or bicycle exercise can be used to stress the myocardium with resultant increases in regional myocardial perfusion under normal circumstances. In the presence of significant coronary artery stenoses, stress- or vasodilator-induced increments in perfusion will be reduced or absent. For optimal perfusion imaging, patients should be advised to fast for approximately 12 h prior to the study. Since it is important to achieve a high level of cardiac work for optimal results, β-adrenergic and calcium channel blockers should be discontinued for 24 to 48 h prior to the exercise test. It is possible to perform the test while the patient is on these agents, but sensitivity and specificity are reduced. Also, long-acting nitrates should be discontinued 6 h before the exercise stress test. The safety of discontinuation of the anti-ischemic medications must be determined for each patient.

A maximal symptom-limited stress test should be performed with the patient exercising to the point of fatigue, dyspnea, or chest discomfort that prevents further exercise. In addition, exercise should be stopped if serious arrhythmias or hypotension occur, even if the patient is asymptomatic. The exercise is considered adequate if the patient's heart rate reaches at least 85 percent or more of peak age-predicted heart rate. Submaximal exercise protocols are performed in patients assessed prior to hospital discharge after myocardial infarction. In such cases, exercise is begun at a lower level and is increased more gradually and stopped after 9 min, or at 75 percent of peak predicted heart rate.

When the patient has achieved his/her highest level of exercise, 2.0 to 4.0 mCi of ^{201}Tl, 20 to 30 mCi of ^{99m}Tc-MIBI, or 15 to 20 mCi of ^{99m}Tc-teboroxime is administered intravenously. Following injection of the perfusion imaging agent, the patient is encouraged to continue to exercise for an additional 60 to 90 s.

Pharmacologic Stress

Dipyridamole

Dipyridamole is a coronary vasodilator that can be administered intravenously in stable patients who are unable to exercise adequately.[52] Similar to exercise stress, dipyridamole infusion leads to an increase in myocardial blood flow, which is attenuated in the distribution of significantly diseased coronary arteries. Myocardial perfusion images will demonstrate defects in the distribution of such vessels. As with exercise, patients should fast for 12 h prior to the study, but must also abstain from drinking caffeine-containing beverages, such as coffee, tea, and certain cola drinks, which antagonize the effects of adenosine. Also, all medications containing xanthines, such as theophylline, must be held for at least 36 h prior to the study.

At the time of the study, an intravenous line is started and dipyridamole is given by slow IV push at a rate of 0.14 mg/kg over 4 min (total dose = 0.56 mg/kg). Four min after completing the infusion, ^{201}Tl (2.0 to 4.0 mCi) is administered intravenously. In patients who can tolerate it, low level treadmill exercise may be performed following termination of dipyridamole infusion to further enhance the dipyridamole effect. Tracer is administered after 1 min of treadmill exercise.

Side effects are fairly common during or after dipyridamole infusion, and include headache, nausea, and/or chest pain.[53] If any of these symptoms becomes severe, a bolus of aminophylline (100 mg), a direct antagonist of adenosine, can be administered intravenously to quickly reverse them. If possible, the administration of aminophylline should be delayed for at least 1 min after administration of the perfusion agent.

While dipyridamole testing is quite safe, it is associated with a small but definite risk. In a series of 3911 patients who were evaluated using dipyridamole in conjunction with thallium testing, nonfatal myocardial infarction occurred in 4 and death in 2.[54] The risk of dipyridamole testing is generally felt to be similar to that of exercise stress testing.

Dipyridamole myocardial imaging is reserved for stable patients who are unable to exercise because of peripheral vascular, musculoskeletal, or neurologic disease. In addition, dipyridamole can be substituted for exercise in patients who are unlikely to achieve an adequate heart rate response during exercise stress. These include patients on β-adrenergic blocking agents and patients who are poorly motivated. Dipyridamole should not be used in patients who have unstable myocardial ischemic syndromes, such as unstable angina pectoris or acute myocardial infarction, or in patients with critical aortic stenosis and hypertrophic cardiomyopathy. Also, it should not be administered to patients with asthma, since it may exacerbate bronchospasm.

Adenosine

Dipyridamole works by blocking cellular reuptake of adenosine, a potent coronary vasodilator, and raising adenosine levels at the site of vascular smooth muscle cells.[55] Adenosine infusion may be used instead of dipyridamole for inducing hyperemia with resultant perfusion defects in the distribution of coronary arteries with significant stenoses, and has been shown to be as effective as dipyridamole for detecting coronary artery disease.[55] The side effects of the adenosine infusion are similar to but more frequent than those observed with dipyridamole. The plasma half-life of adenosine is very short. Thus, untoward effects generally are relieved immediately when the infusion is stopped.

Dobutamine

Dobutamine is a beta agonist, increases demand on the heart by its inotropic and chronotropic actions, and can induce angina and regional ischemia with concomitant wall motion abnormalities or reversible perfusion defects on thallium scintigraphy.[56] Incremental infusion of dobutamine can be used to assess patients unable to exercise and potentially unable to tolerate dipyridamole, such as those with asthma and/or those on xanthines (see also Chap. 28).

Image Interpretation

Qualitative Analysis of Planar Images

Myocardial perfusion images are always evaluated qualitatively, and most laboratories utilize additional strategies for quantitative and computer-assisted interpretations. A normal myocardial perfusion imaging study is depicted in Fig. 134-5. Almost all of the radiopharmaceutical in the heart is distributed to the left ventricular myocardium. The right ventricular myocardium is usually seen as a much less intense and thinner structure and is better visualized after dipyridamole infusion than exercise stress, and with ^{99m}Tc-MIBI than with ^{201}Tl (Fig. 134-6). Splanchnic activity is more prominent in resting studies, exercise studies achieving a low level of exercise, dipyridamole studies, and adenosine studies. In the ante-

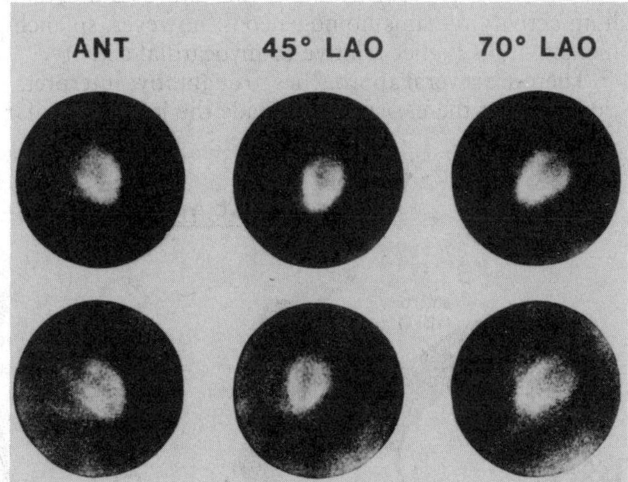

FIGURE 134-5 Normal ^{201}Tl study showing homogenous distribution of the radiotracer in the anterior (ANT), 45° LAO and 70° LAO projections. Images acquired early are depicted in the top row, while images acquired 3 to 4 h later are illustrated in the bottom row. It should be noted that reduced activity in the region of the apex on the ANT view is consistent with normal apical thinning. Also, activity seems to decrease from apex to base related to the increase distance from the gamma camera crystal between apex and base. [*From G Pohost, R O'Rourke (eds): Principles and Practice of Cardiac Imaging. Boston, Little Brown, 1991: 196. Reproduced with permission of the publisher and editors.*]

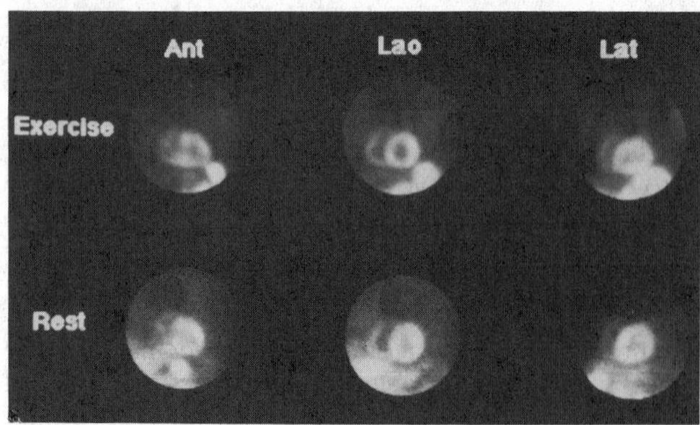

FIGURE 134-6 Three view (ungated) planar ^{99m}Tc-sestamibi scans performed following injection at peak exercise. Note the clear visualization of the right ventricular free wall. There are septal and apical defects on the LAO and ANT views, respectively, which demonstrate fill-in on the "Rest" injected images (bottom row).

rior view, the normal perfusion study demonstrates homogeneous distribution of the radiopharmaceutical in a U-shaped configuration, with the base of the U corresponding to the mitral valve plane. In the 45° left anterior oblique view, left ventricular myocardial activity appears as a donut pattern, or in a U-shaped configuration with the base of the U facing upward. In the 70° left anterior oblique view, tracer uptake appears as a U with its base facing upward and to the right. The normal perfusion pattern demonstrates homogeneous myocardial activity throughout the U or donut pattern. A possible exception to this pattern is the left ventricular apex which appears to have less activity due to the fact that the apex is frequently thinner than the remainder of the left ventricular myocardium. For this reason, the apex in any projection is the most difficult segment to evaluate. Interobserver variability for the apex is highest.[57] Under normal conditions in the "redistribution" or resting studies, thallium activity remains homogeneous; however, splanchnic activity is higher relative to myocardial activity.

There are several approaches to qualitative interpretation. One of the easiest is to divide the left ventricular activity into three segments in each of the three projections (Fig. 134-7). In the anterior projections, the segments are the anterolateral, apical, and inferior. In the 45° LAO projection, the segments are the lateral, apical inferior, and septal. And in the 70° LAO projection, the segments are the posteroinferior or posterolateral, inferioapical, anteroapical, and anteroseptal. Segments are graded on a scale of 0 to 2, with 2 representing normal activity, 1 representing definitely decreased activity, and 0 representing no activity. Half scores are also used as follows: 1.5 represents slight decrease in activity, and 0.5 represents severe decrease in activity. Images are best interpreted with two or more observers.[57] Disagreements between observers are settled by consensus. An increase in grade by one or more between the stress and the delayed or resting imaging sequence is considered to represent "redistribution," or ischemic but viable myocardium (Fig. 134-8). No change or a change by less than one grade is considered to be a persistent defect and may represent either ischemia or scar. Patients who have thallium defects that are present 3 to 4 h later should undergo reinjection or 24-h follow-up study. Both the reinjection and the 24-h studies are graded as described above.

An advantage of thallium imaging is that an unusual increase in pulmonary activity in the absence of chronic obstructive pulmonary disease is diagnostic of left heart failure.[58–60] Abnormally increased pulmonary thallium activity is readily detected when there is substantial contrast between the lungs and the mediastinum, which contains very little thallium activity. Qualitatively, lung thallium activity can be graded on a scale of 0 to 2+ (Fig. 134-9). When lung activity approximates the most intense left ventricular myocardial segment, it is graded as 2+. If the lungs are readily observed but the activity is substantially less than the most intense myocardial segment, lung activity is considered to be 1+. If the lungs are difficult to observe, the activity is considered to be zero. To quantitate lung thallium activity, computer-generated regions of interest are drawn over the heart and over a segment of the left lung to obtain average counts per pixel in the two regions. A lung/myocardial

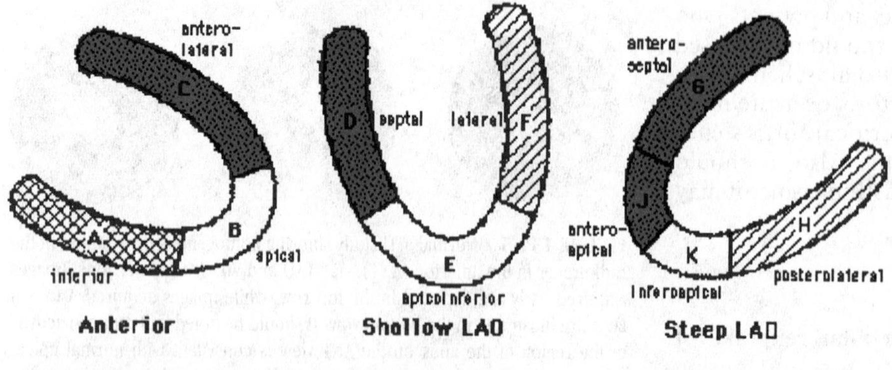

FIGURE 134-7 Schematic diagram of the 10 left ventricular segments commonly used in myocardial perfusion imaging. Also, the most likely vascular supply is indicated for each segment. LAD = left anterior descending, LCF = left circumflex, RCA = right coronary artery.

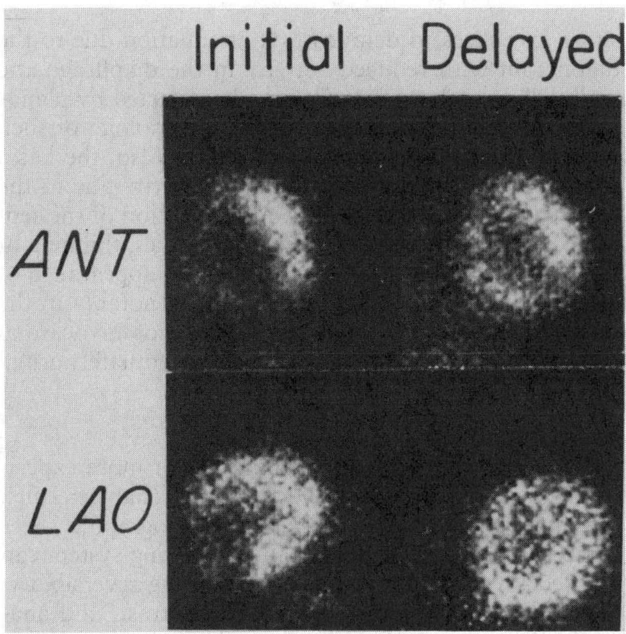

FIGURE 134-8 Example complete ^{201}Tl redistribution. Thallium-201 imaging study in the anterior (ANT) and 45° left anterior oblique (LAO) projections. Both the early (initial) and 3-h delayed (delayed) images are displayed. The initial images show defects in the inferior, inferioapical, and septal segments. The delayed images demonstrate complete redistribution.

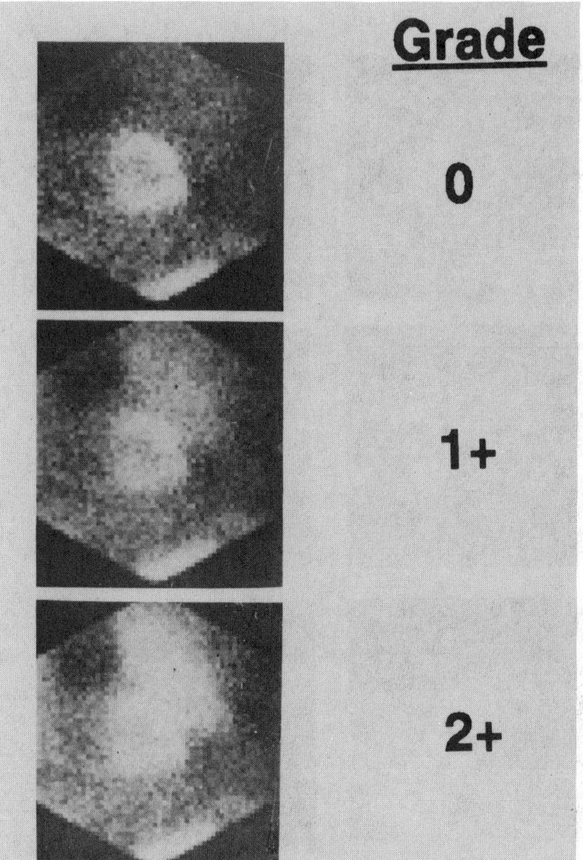

FIGURE 134-9 Qualitative scoring of lung ^{201}Tl activity. Anterior ^{201}Tl images depict myocardial and lung activity. Lung activity can be qualitatively evaluated by comparing it to peak myocardial activity. If the left lung borders are not clearly defined it is grade 0. If the borders of the lung are well defined, but the activity is substantially less than that of peak myocardial activity, it is graded at 1+. If lung activity is equivalent to peak myocardial activity, it is grade 2+. Abnormally increased lung activity can be seen in either left-sided heart failure or chronic obstructive lung disease. In congestive left-sided heart failure, lung activity decreases substantially on the delayed image, while in chronic lung disease it usually persists.

activity ratio greater than 0.5 is abnormal.[61] Patients with lower levels of exercise or beta-blockade, however, occasionally can exhibit abnormal ratios.

With both thallium and teboroxime studies, a decrease in the size of the left ventricular cavity between initial and delayed or rest imaging studies suggests left ventricular failure. Normally, the exercise-injected left ventricle is either smaller or equal in size to that at rest. Both increased lung thallium activity and transient left ventricular dilation are considered to be signs of left ventricular failure, consistent with severe coronary artery disease.[62] Of course, patients with any condition leading to left-sided heart failure, such as valvular disease or cardiomyopathy can demonstrate increased lung thallium activity. Also, patients with a cardiomyopathy or left ventricular volume overload can demonstrate transient left ventricular dilation. The additional presence of reversible perfusion defects is highly suggestive of a coronary etiology.

Artifacts

A major problem interfering with accurate interpretation of myocardial perfusion images, somewhat more so with the lower energy thallium-201, is the artifacts produced by soft tissue attenuation. Among the most common artifacts is that due to breast attenuation in women. On planar images, overlaying breast tissue can produce apparent defects in the anterolateral wall (anterior view), upper septum (45° LAO view), and anteroseptal wall (70° LAO view) (Fig. 134-10). A clue to breast attentuation is the appearance of a border of attenuation continuing from myocardium into the surrounding background region. The borders of the breasts can be best observed in an image that has not been subjected to background subtraction or to contrast enhancement. Other structures may also attenuate thallium activity, including the diaphragm (attenuation of inferior wall activity in the 70° LAO projection, or in more dramatic cases, in the anterior projection). A dilated right ventricle can attenuate inferior wall activity, and pacemakers can produce discrete defects occasionally observed in the anterolateral segment (anterior projection). It is important to note that changes in the position of attenuating soft tissue, particularly the breasts, can lead to the misdiagnosis of redistribution with a defect on the initial imaging study and partial or total resolution on a subsequent study. Despite the higher energy of ^{99m}Tc and use of high resolution collimators for imaging the technetium perfusion tracers, attenuation artifacts are not eliminated.

Computer Analysis of Planar Studies

There are several strategies for computer-assisted quantitative analysis of myocardial perfusion images.[63–65] Generally, the approaches involve interpolative background

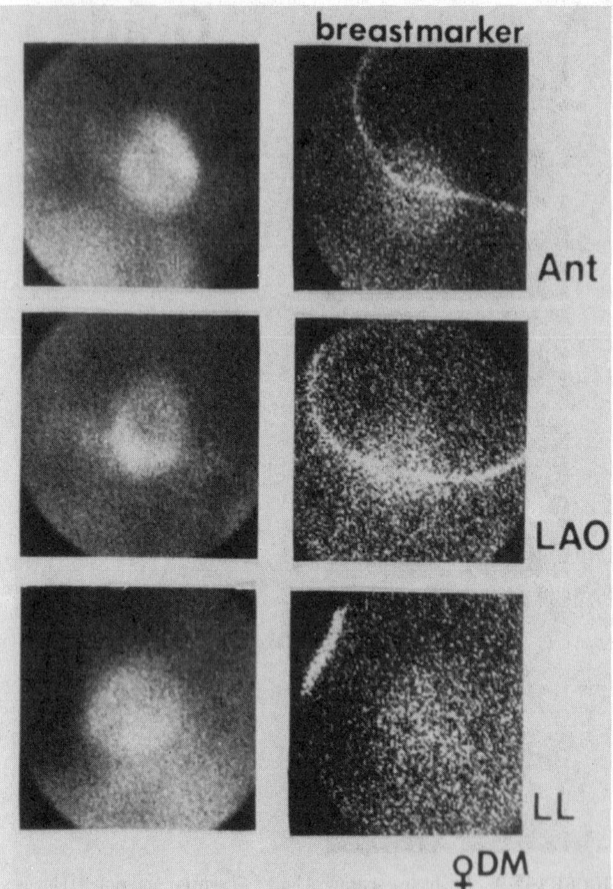

FIGURE 134-10 Three planar thallium images on a female patient are displayed on the left panel. Reduced counts due to breast attenuation are best seen in the anterolateral wall in the LAO view. The three images displayed in the right panel are planar images of plastic tubing filled with small concentration of technetium, placed under the breast fold, and imaged in the three standard views ("breastmarker"). The markers outline the left breast and help localize the attenuating tissue on the planar thallium images. (*From FJT Wackers, JA Mattera: Optimizing planar Tl-201 imaging: Computer quantification. Cardiology 20:107, 1990. Reproduced with permission from the publisher and the authors.*)

subtraction and circumferential plots of tracer activity to depict regional change in activity between the initial and delayed "redistribution" (thallium) or rest (sestamibi) images (Fig. 134-11). The computerized approaches lead to more reproducible results but should only be used to assist with qualitative interpretation. In this way, the computerized data provide a "second opinion" to coordinate subjective interpretations.

Qualitative Interpretation of SPECT Studies

Normal Appearance A SPECT imaging study is generally displayed in several orientations. In the recommended format for display, the short axis tomographic slices are displayed from apex to base, while the long axis slices are displayed in two orthogonal orientations, horizontal from superior to inferior and vertical from septum to lateral wall (Fig. 134-12). The short axis tomographs generally show homogeneous thallium activity with a donut pattern. It is common, however, for the basal short axis slices to demonstrate attenuation due to the diaphragm with reduced activity in the diaphragmatic wall. While such attenuation can be detected by planar imaging, SPECT imaging obscures the etiology of such attenuation, a disadvantage of SPECT. Also, the basal septum can appear to have reduced activity due to the reduced myocardial thickness in this portion of the septum. Finally, as with planar imaging studies, thinning of the left ventricular apex can lead to the appearance of less activity in the apical segment, most notably in the long axis slices. The higher resolution of myocardial imaging with sestamibi can further accentuate normal apical thinning.

Qualitative Interpretation Again, two or more experienced observers are desirable for most reliable results. As with planar interpretations the tomographic slices can be divided into segments and a scoring system can be used for localizing defects and scoring reversibility. The tomographic nature, improved contrast, and anatomical detail of SPECT compared to planar imaging offers more accurate localization of defects to particular vascular territories and improves the sensitivity to detect small defects (Fig. 134-13). (See also Fig. 134-1, Plate XII.) SPECT imaging is superior to planar imaging for depicting defects in the left circumflex artery territory (Fig. 134-14).

Quantitative Interpretation Techniques have been developed to perform quantitative analysis of tomographic scans.[66,67] In the method most widely available, circumferential profiles are generated on short axis slices. Normal profiles are generated and the patient's count profiles compared to the normal data file. Like planar quantitation, computerized data provide a "second opinion" for the qualitative interpretation.

In addition to detection of ischemia and infarction, SPECT can be used to evaluate chamber size and morphology in nonischemic disease. For example, in patients with dilated cardiomyopathy, short axis slices demonstrate increased LV volumes and decreased wall thickness (Fig. 134-15). Since these images are acquired without gating, the apparent thickness of the myocardium is not only related to its actual thickness but also to its motion; i.e., the less the motion, the thinner it appears. In hypertrophic cardiomyopathy, both marked upper septal hypertrophy and cavity obliteration are suggested by the SPECT ^{201}Tl study.

"Bull's Eye" Display

An approach that complements the interpretation of the tomographic slices is a computer generated display that resembles a target called a "bull's eye." This "bull's eye" display method uses the short axis slices that are telescoped together into a circular array in which the apex is represented by the center of the array and the base is represented by the perimeter of the array. The polar display map is divided into the territories of the three major coronary arteries. The color scale displayed is related to the count density or to the degree of reduc-

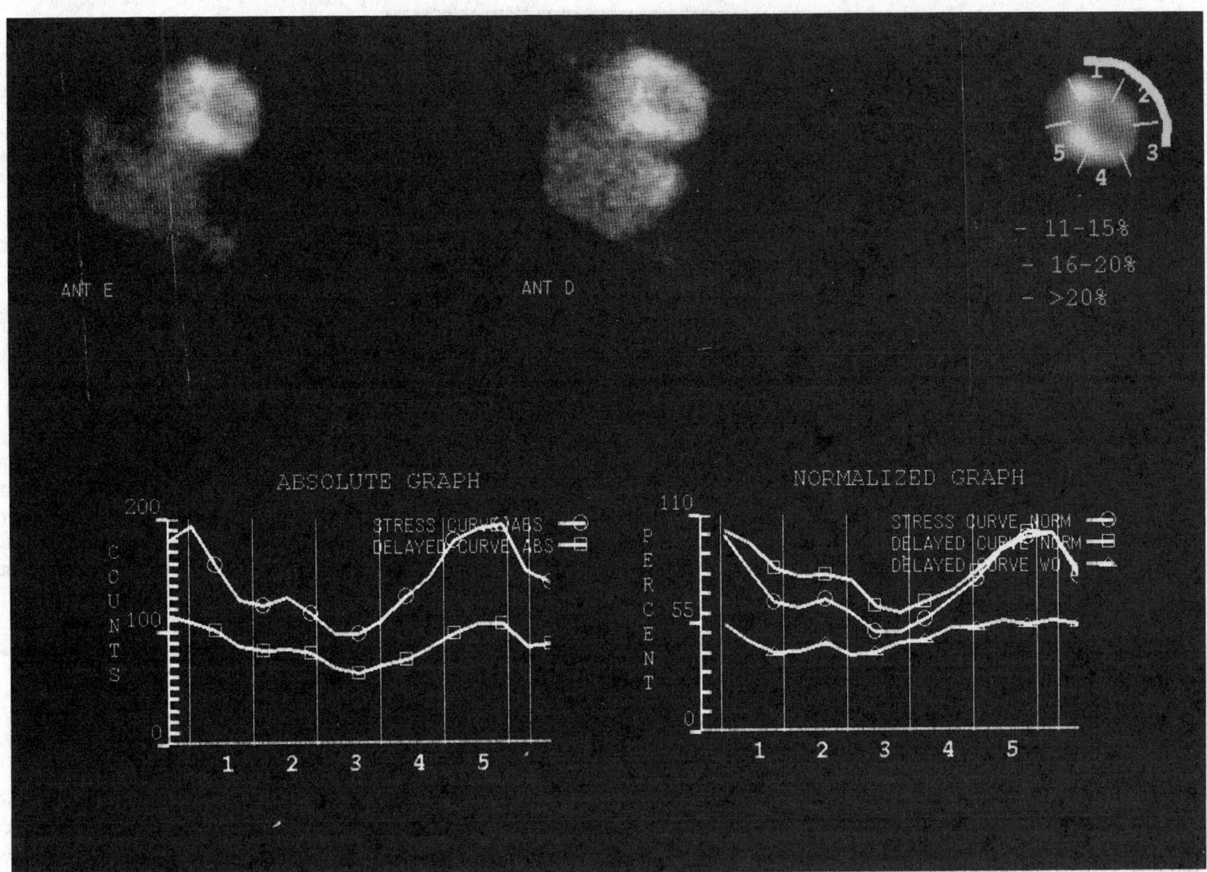

FIGURE 134-11 Computer-assisted analysis of planar ^{201}Tl images. The anterior view was selected for this illustration although the 45° or 70° LAO projections were also analyzed. It is evident by inspection that there is a defect in the anteroapical walls on the early (E) image which fills in the delayed (D) image. The program rotates the D image until it optimally matches the E image, performs interpolative background subtraction, divides the heart into five sectors, which results in the image shown in the upper right part of the figure, and then computes the normalized count differences. The count differences are then color coded with different colors selected to represent an 11 to 15 percent difference, a 16 to 20 percent difference, and a difference greater than 20 percent. A graphic display of the data is depicted on the bottom. The counts are plotted for transmural activity for segments 1–5 (from anterobase to posterior base). The graphs show counts (per pixel) on the y axis and segment number on the x axis. The graph on the left shows the absolute counts over the sectors for the stress and delayed images. If tracer uptake were perfectly homogeneous, two superimposed horizontal lines would be observed. Since tracer distribution is never perfectly homogeneous due to normal apical thinning and variable attenuation, plots are never linear. The difference between these two plots represents the amount of radiotracer clearance. In the graph on the right the delayed curve is normalized to the hottest pixel in the stress curve. In this program, counts that remain 80 percent of peak or higher are considered to be normal. If the two curves were superimposable, there would be no redistribution. In this example, the stress curve is below the delayed curve for sectors 1–3 (anterior wall). The degree of difference between the two curves can be expressed as percentage defect severity.

tion below two standard deviations of the normal mean for each vascular territory. (See Fig. 134-2, Plate XII.)

Artifacts

The computer process of reconstruction can produce artifactual defects on the reconstructed slices if the center of rotation is incorrect or if the patient moves during the acquisition. The same soft tissue attenuation artifacts seen on planar images also produce artifacts in SPECT images (Table 134-2). Because SPECT images are highly processed, these artifacts are more difficult to detect. Breast tissue in females is a common source of artifact, and the distribution is similar to that for planar images (anterolateral, upper septal, anteroseptal, and posterolateral). Persistent defects in these territories in women may or may not be related to breast attenuation. Again, if the breast changes position relative to the heart be-

TABLE 134-2
Common Artifacts on Planar Thallium Scans

Segment with Defect	Cause
AL, PL, AB, US (fixed)	Breast (same positions between serial images)
AL, PL, AB, US (transient)	Breast change (change in position on serial images)
IN, D, PB	Overlying diaphragm, enlarged RV
AL (discrete circle)	Pacemaker pulse generator
Diffuse with small papillary muscle "hot spot"	LV hypertrophy

Legend: AL = anterolateral; PL = posterolateral; AB = anterobasal; US = upper septum; IN = inferior; D = diaphragmatic; PB = posterobasal.

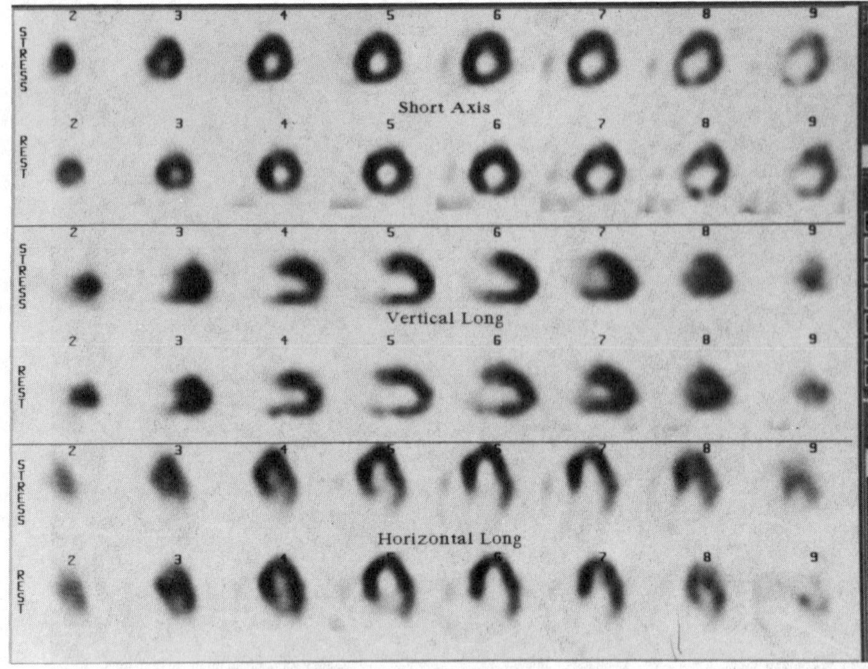

FIGURE 134-12 Tomographic slices two pixels in thickness from a ^{99m}Tc sestamibi study in a standard display. The top two rows show short axis tomographs from apex to base with stress above, rest below. Note the "donut" pattern of tracer uptake in this patient without perfusion defects. The middle two rows show the vertical long axis slices displayed from lateral wall to septum. The apex is pointed toward the right. The lower two rows depict the horizontal long axis slices with the apex pointed upward. The septal wall is always shorter than the lateral wall in this projection.

tween the initial and delayed acquisitions, defects may appear artifactually to fill in, thereby suggesting ischemia. Diaphragmatic attenuation can lead to the appearance of fixed defects in the inferior or posterior segments. Finally, a focal area of increased activity, or "hot spot," can be seen in the anterolateral wall on either planar or SPECT images and may represent unusual accumulation of activity in the anterolateral or the inferior papillary muscle. This type of hot spot is most commonly seen in patients with LVH and can lead to the misinterpretation that activity in the remainder of the myocardium is abnormally reduced. More rapid clearance of thallium from such hot spots can lead to the appearance of extensive redistribution in a patient with normal coronary arteries. The rapid myocardial washout and early hepatic uptake of ^{99m}Tc-teboroxime make these tomographic scans more subject to reconstruction artifacts than the other two tracers; however, high-quality tomograms can be acquired in 3 to 4 min (Fig. 134-16).

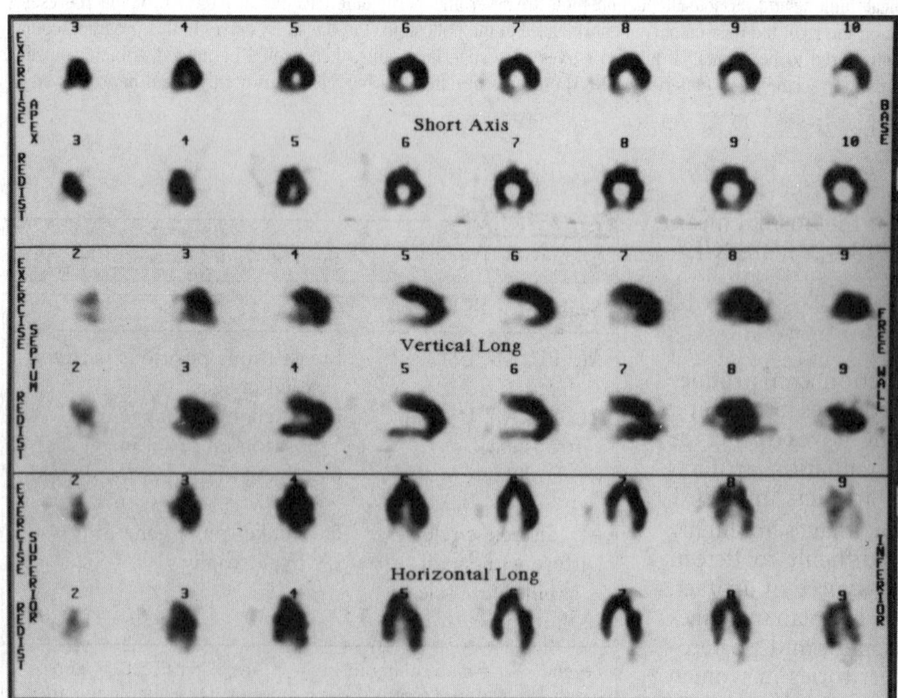

FIGURE 134-13 Tomographic slices two pixels in thickness from a thallium stress and 4-h redistribution study in standard display. There is an inferoposterior defect on the initial tomographic slices that shows almost complete redistribution at 4 h. This scan was read as showing ischemia in the distribution of the RCA.

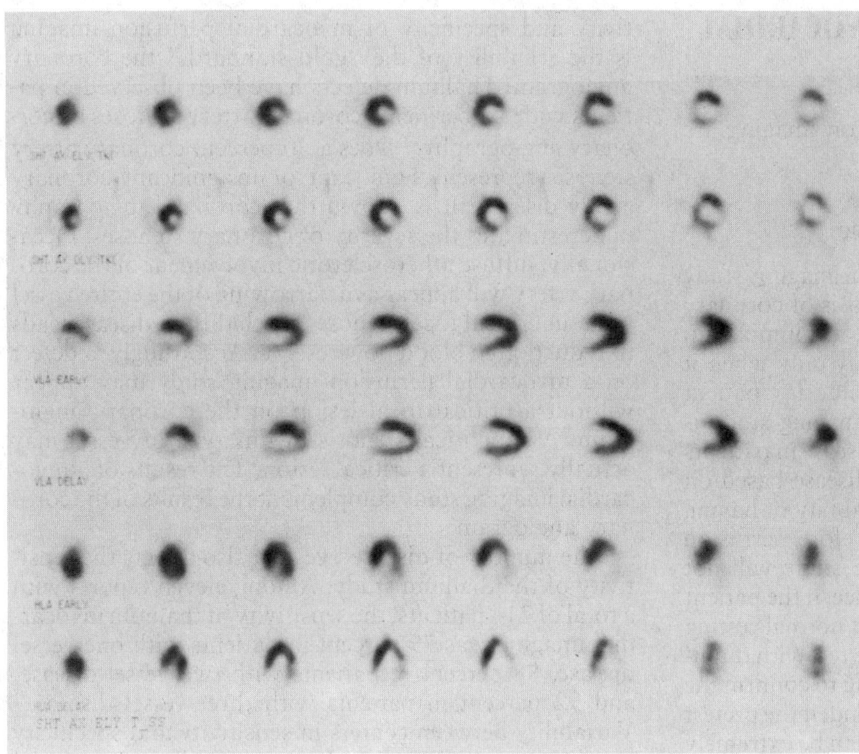

FIGURE 134-14 Tomographic slices one pixel thick from a thallium stress and 4-h redistribution study. The vertical long axis slices are displayed from lateral wall to septum and the horizontal long axis slices are displayed from superior to inferior walls. There is an inferolateral defect on the initial tomographic slices that shows minimal redistribution at 4 h and no further change following thallium reinjection (not shown). This scan was read as showing infarction in the distribution of the LCF artery.

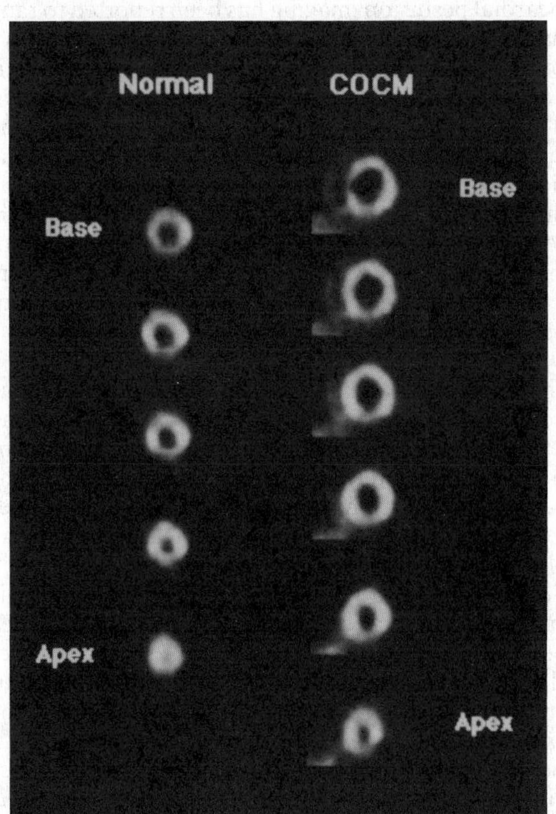

FIGURE 134-15 ^{201}Tl tomographic short axis slices displayed from base to apex from a normal subject (left column) and from a patient with dilated cardiomyopathy (right column). The dilation of the left ventricular cavity in the cardiomyopathy patient is apparent.

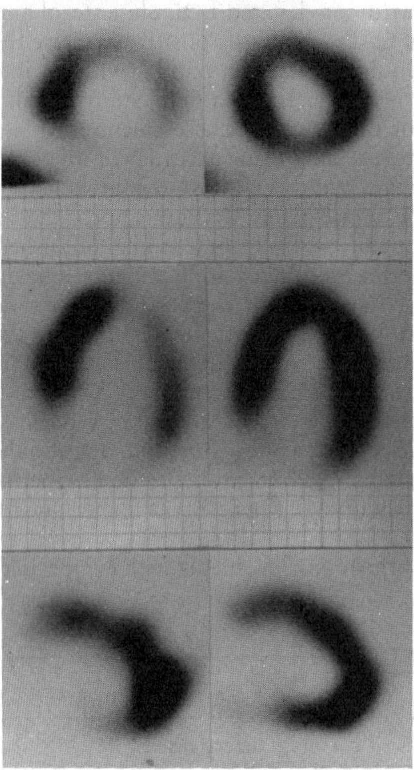

FIGURE 134-16 Representative slices from tomographic scans obtained immediately following an exercise injection (left) and immediately following a rest injection (right) of ^{99m}Tc teboroxime. Short axis slices are on the top, horizontal long axis slices in the middle, and vertical long axis slices on the bottom. There are extensive defects involving the anterolateral and inferopost-erolateral walls on the exercise study, which fill in almost completely on the rest study consistent with extensive ischemia in the territory of the left circumflex and right coronary arteries. (*Courtesy of Squibb Diagnostics.*)

CLINICAL APPLICATIONS OF MYOCARDIAL PERFUSION IMAGING

The applications of myocardial perfusion imaging are listed in Table 134-3.

Diagnosis of Coronary Artery Disease

The addition of a myocardial perfusion imaging study can improve the accuracy for the diagnosis of coronary artery disease over an ECG exercise test. It is important, however, to order the radionuclide study only when it will add information of incremental value for patient management. A myocardial perfusion imaging study is not indicated to detect coronary artery disease in patients in whom there is a high likelihood of disease based on other available information. If the probability of having coronary artery disease is 90 percent before perfusion imaging, the results of the radionuclide study will not change the odds substantively. For instance, if the patient has a history of typical angina pectoris, a normal resting ECG and a positive ECG-graded exercise test with duplication of anginal pain, additional imaging to confirm the diagnosis is unnecessary. On the other hand, if the pretest probability is 50–50, the imaging study can be extremely helpful in substantially raising or lowering the likelihood for disease.[68] For example, an asymptomatic 50-year-old man with an elevated LDL cholesterol and a family history of CAD who had a positive exercise ECG but no angina would represent a patient with an intermediate risk. In this case, the thallium study would be quite helpful for the diagnostic assessment.

To date, the diagnostic accuracy of myocardial perfusion imaging has been most comprehensively studied using the exercise planar thallium approach with qualitative interpretation. Forty-nine studies published in 1977–1985 described a total of 4678 patients. The mean sensitivity and specificity in these studies were 82 and 88 percent, respectively.[69] Patients with prior myocardial infarction are more readily detectable and studies in such patients exhibit a higher sensitivity than studies in patients without myocardial infarction. When assessing the diagnostic accuracy of any method, one should consider patient referral bias. In studies with a higher percentage of patients with MI, sensitivity is higher due to selection bias alone.

One of the major problems with evaluating the sensitivity and specificity of myocardial perfusion imaging is the reliability of the "gold standard," the coronary angiogram. Thallium defects have been observed in patients with "subcritical" coronary artery stenoses by coronary angiography.[70] Does a 30 percent coronary artery stenosis represent significant or insignificant coronary artery disease? It is known that coronary angiography underestimates the severity of coronary stenoses. Occasionally, diffuse atherosclerotic involvement of the coronary artery will appear as a narrowing of the entire vessel without critical focal stenoses. Such diffuse disease leads to reduction in blood flow reserve. Accordingly, a defect on a myocardial perfusion imaging study may appear without a critical focal lesion on the coronary angiogram. A subcritical stenosis in this type of vessel may actually represent a critical lesion. The results of a myocardial imaging study complement the results of the coronary angiogram.

The number of diseased vessels also affects the sensitivity of the thallium study. Among eleven reports with a total of 714 patients, the sensitivity of thallium myocardial imaging was 79 percent in patients with one-vessel disease, 88 percent in patients with two-vessel disease, and 92 percent in patients with three-vessel disease.[71] Variability between centers in sensitivity and specificity is related to patient population as well as inter- and intraobserver variability for interpretation of both the myocardial imaging study and the coronary angiographic study. Inter- and intraobserver variability for myocardial perfusion imaging has been reported to range from 3 to 16 percent and 4 to 11 percent, respectively.[72] Another factor contributing to differences in sensitivity and specificity at different institutions is related to physician acceptance of the thallium study. In institutions with good confidence in the results of the test, coronary angiography is usually not performed in patients with normal thallium scans and is performed in those with abnormal scans. This practice leads to a reduction in the number of patients with normal coronary angiograms and and an apparent increase in sensitivity with a decrease in specificity.[73]

Dipyridamole or adenosine can be administered in lieu of exercise in patients who cannot perform adequate exercise, such as patients with peripheral vascular disease and claudication, or orthopedic problems, or patients who cannot adequately increase myocardial demand due to β-adrenergic blocking agents. The sensitivity and specificity results for these pharmacologic approaches are similar to results reported for exercise.[53,55]

To date, the sensitivity and specificity of myocardial perfusion imaging for disease detection does not appear to be significantly affected by the radiopharmaceutical used (^{201}Tl, ^{99m}Tc-sestamibi, or ^{99m}Tc-teboroxime). Furthermore, while SPECT imaging may provide other information, it has not improved the accuracy of the myocardial perfusion study over the planar approach. It increases sensitivity but decreases specificity (Table 134-4).

Several factors can lead to reduced sensitivity and specificity in myocardial perfusion imaging (Table 134-5). For exercise studies, submaximal exercise may not increase myocardial demand enough to provoke ischemia. Both β-adrenergic and calcium channel blocking

TABLE 134-3
Clinical Applications of Myocardial Imaging

Diagnosis of coronary artery disease
Localization of coronary arteries with significant disease
Evaluation of myocardial viability
Assessment of functional significance of a known coronary artery lesion
Risk stratification
- In patients with stable coronary artery disease
- Post-myocardial infarction
- Prior to major noncoronary surgery

Assess efficacy of revascularization or medical therapy

TABLE 134-4

Exercise Thallium Imaging to Detect Coronary Artery Disease

	No. of Patients	Sensitivity	No. of Patients	Specificity
Planar				
Qualitative	3115	0.82	1563	0.88
Quantitative	579	0.89	139	0.68
SPECT				
Qualitative	357	0.94	53	0.77
Quantitative	660	0.95	135	0.61

SOURCE: Modified from Maddahi J, Rodrigues E, Berman DS.[69]

agents can reduce myocardial stress level with a similar outcome. Drugs that interfere with the action of dipyridamole or adenosine, such as aminophylline and, to a lesser extent, β-adrenergic and calcium channel blocking agents will reduce myocardial activity and lead to reduced sensitivity. Anything that reduces the amount of radiopharmaceutical delivered to the heart will reduce sensitivity and specificity, including subcutaneous infiltraton of the radiopharmaceutical dose, or arm vein uptake of the agent (most notably with ^{201}Tl). As already discussed, soft tissue attenuation can adversely affect specificity by producing artifacts that are interpreted as significant defects. Left bundle branch block (LBBB) has been reported to reduce tracer activity in the absence of coronary artery disease. This may be related to dysynchronous motion of the interventricular septum, which impinges on diastole filling time at high heart rates. Reconstruction artifacts on SPECT images contribute to the lower specificity of this imaging modality.

Evaluation of Myocardial Viability

A defect on a myocardial perfusion imaging study performed soon after the injection of the radiopharmaceutical may be related to the inability of the myocardium to extract the agent (myocardial scar or infarction) or to relatively lower perfusion to that segment. There are three strategies for assessing the viability of an initial defect on a stress perfusion image: (1) delayed imaging several hours later, (2) delayed imaging 12 or more hours after injection, and (3) imaging after a second injection at rest. The first two approaches are only useful with thallium; the third approach can be used with either the thallium or technetium-based methods. A major problem with the two-injection technique is that defects may persist with the injection at rest in the presence of a severe coronary stenosis associated with diminished baseline flow (such as that observed with "hibernating myocardium").[74] Therefore, if a coronary stenosis is severe, the rest injection will demonstrate a defect similar to that of the exercise injection, that would be interpreted as consistent with nonviable myocardium.

The kinetics of thallium provide a means for assessing viability after a single injection of the agent by obtaining an initial imaging sequence and then, after 3 or 4 h, a follow-up imaging sequence. Defects that fill in are viable, while up to 50 percent of those that do not fill in may still be viable. The reason for persistence of a defect in a viable myocardial segment is most likely related to thallium content in the blood. If the blood level of thallium is relatively high, the redistribution phenomenon will occur more readily, but if the blood level of thallium is relatively low, the defect is likely to persist.[75] Accordingly, if the follow-up imaging study demonstrates persistent defects only, a second injection of thallium can be made in the resting state to boost the blood thallium levels. This approach will lead to partial or total resolution in approximately 50 percent of persistent thallium defects[22] (Fig. 134-17). Alternatively, a repeat imaging sequence can be performed 24 h or more after the initial study to allow the low thallium in the blood more time to gain access to the hypoperfused but viable myocardial segment. Over 50 percent of thallium defects that persist by the 3 to 4 h study will resolve 24 h or later.[21]

It is important to note that if a defect shows convincing evidence of resolution, even if it is only partial, viability has been established. Conversely, partial defect fill in occurring over 4 h of redistribution may be hidden by thallium reinjection in the presence of severely diminished resting blood flow (Fig. 134-18). We recommend, therefore, that when using thallium, a "redistribution" imaging study should be performed 3 to 4 h after the initial dose is administered. If no redistribution is found, a second injection of 1.0 mCi of ^{201}Tl should be given and the imaging study repeated. If all defects persist and the issue of viability is a major question, a 24-h imaging study should be performed.

While ^{99m}Tc-sestamibi appears to behave like thallium with regard to its myocardial extraction by viable versus nonviable myocardial tissue,[37] the very low blood levels

TABLE 134-5

Factors Reducing Sensitivity and Specificity of Myocardial Perfusion Imaging

Submaximal exercise
Beta blockers or calcium channel blockers
Reduction in dose to myocardium
  Radionuclide infiltration during injection
  Uptake of the agent in the arm vein
Soft tissue attenuation
Inadequate response to dipyridamole or adenosine
Intraventricular conduction delay, especially left bundle branch block
SPECT reconstruction artifacts

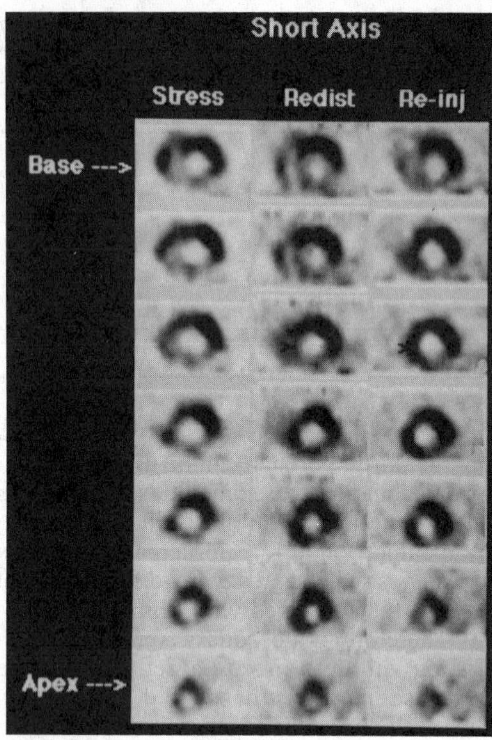

FIGURE 134-17 Short axis slices of the ^{201}Tl tomograms obtained after exercise stress (left), 4 h later (Redist) (center), and following thallium reinjection (Re-inj) (right). There are both anteroseptal, apical, and infero-posterolateral defects on the stress images with some redistribution into the anteroseptal defect at 4 h and further redistribution following reinjection (arrows).

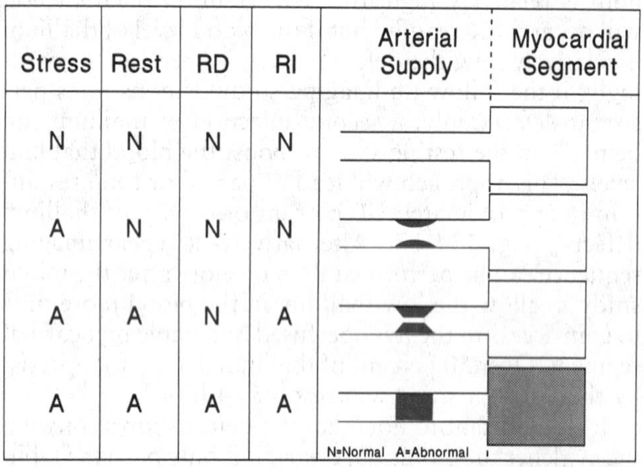

Stress	Rest	RD	RI	Arterial Supply	Myocardial Segment
N	N	N	N		
A	N	N	N		
A	A	N	A		
A	A	A	A		

N=Normal A=Abnormal

FIGURE 134-18 Anticipated results of ^{201}Tl images after stress (Stress), at rest (Rest), with redistribution (RD), and after reinjection (RI) for four clinical situations. These clinical situations are schematically depicted from top to bottom on the right-hand side of the illustration (myocardial segments are coded as white for viable and gray for nonviable). Included are: normal arterial supply; coronary stenosis compromising stress but not rest myocardial perfusion; severe coronary stenosis compromising resting blood flow ("hibernating myocardium"); total coronary occlusion nonviable myocardial segment. In the four vertical columns to the left, the results of the thallium image are indicated as normal (N) or abnormal (A). It is of interest to note that in the situation of "hibernating myocardium," thallium distribution with either stress or at rest will be abnormal, as will thallium distribution with reinjection. The only means to distinguish between viable and nonviable myocardium in this particular case is to use thallium redistribution imaging at 3 to 4 h, or if necesssary, later.

of the agent following the initial first-pass extraction do not allow clinically relevant redistribution. Defects on stress studies are further evaluated by imaging after a rest injection. It should be noted that this two-injection approach is better than 4 h thallium redistribution to detect defect reversibility.[76] A study comparing two injections of sestamibi with thallium reinjection, however, has not been reported. If viability is the question, ^{201}Tl is the agent of choice.

Clinical Rationale for Assessment of Viability

Markedly reduced, or absent, segmental ventricular wall motion does not necessarily indicate absence of viability, even in patients with historic or ECG evidence of myocardial infarction. Such wall motion abnormalities can occur in patients with severe coronary artery disease and reduced resting blood flow ("hibernating" myocardium); in patients with acute myocardial infarction after reperfusion therapy, ("stunned" myocardium); and in patients with acute infarcted or scarred myocardium. In patients with reduced or absent wall motion, the reversibility of the wall motion abnormality following interventional therapy can be predicted by thallium imaging.[77] Occasionally, patients with extensive coronary artery disease have severe heart failure due to ischemic depression of ventricular function. Coronary artery bypass graft surgery in such patients can lead to substantial improvement in ventricular function with reduction in heart failure.[78] Such patients may appear to be candidates for cardiac transplantation, yet coronary artery bypass surgery may lead to substantial improvement, obviating the need for transplantation. Occasionally, thallium defects will persist on delayed and reinjected images, but the myocardium may still be viable. In cases where all defects persist, PET imaging of both perfusion with ^{13}N-ammonia and metabolic activity with ^{18}F-fluorodeoxyglucose can demonstrate viability. Segments with perfusion defects and a shift from fatty acid to glucose metabolism are viable and will improve function after revascularization.[79]

Risk Stratification

Perhaps the most important application of myocardial perfusion imaging is the assessment of risk for subsequent infarction or death. Myocardial perfusion imaging for risk assessment has been evaluated in three major categories of patients: (1) stable coronary artery disease; (2) post myocardial infarction; and (3) prior to major noncoronary surgery.

Risk Assessment in Stable Patients

One of the first studies to demonstrate the utility of ^{201}Tl to assess risk evaluated 139 stable patients.[80] Thirty-nine patients had previous myocardial infarctions, while 100 did not. Several clinical parameters were examined to determine their ability to predict subsequent myocardial infarction and/or death. All patients underwent both thallium exercise testing and coronary angiography. Computer-displayed planar thallium studies were interpreted qualitatively by two observers. Many clinical parameters were assessed in this study including age, gender, dosage of ß-adrenergic blocking agents, angina pectoris functional class, result of exercise ECG, ejection fraction, number of vessels with significant coronary disease, and several thallium parameters. The thallium imaging parameters included number of transient defects, number of persistent defects, total number of defects, and lung activity score. By logistic regression analysis, the chi square values for those 39 patients with previous myocardial infarction indicated that the ejection fraction was the best predictor of mortality. For the 100 patients without previous myocardial infarction, the number of transient thallium defects was the best predictor of ensuing myocardial infarction or death during the 3 to 5 year follow-up period. Several subsequent studies further corroborated both the low risk of patients with normal thallium studies and the higher risk of patients with positive thallium studies.[81–86]

Investigators have demonstrated the prognostic significance of increased ^{201}Tl lung activity.[87] Generally, however, in patients without previous myocardial infarction, it is the extent of myocardium that demonstrates thallium redistribution that is the best predictor of subsequent myocardial infarction.[88]

Risk Assessment After Myocardial Infarction

The resting ejection fraction is an excellent predictor of subsequent events in patients after myocardial infarction. Nevertheless, extensive thallium defects, the presence of residual ischemia (reversible defect), and the presence of increased lung activity are useful criteria after myocardial infarction for predicting subsequent cardiac events. Combined perfusion and infarct-avid imaging also have been reported to be of value for risk assessment soon after acute myocardial infarction.[89]

Risk Assessment Before Major Noncardiac Surgery

Several studies have established the utility of dipyridamole-thallium imaging prior to major noncardiac peripheral vascular surgery for predicting coronary events postoperatively. In one of the first studies, 48 patients were evaluated prior to peripheral vascular surgery.[90] Eight patients sustained a postoperative cardiac ischemic event, including myocardial infarction or unstable angina pectoris. All eight of these patients demonstrated redistribution on their preoperative dipyridamole thallium studies. Conversely, in the 40 patients who had no cardiac ischemic event postoperatively, there was a significantly lower incidence of patients (8 patients or 20 percent) with thallium redistribution on their preoperative dipyridamole thallium study. In four subsequent studies, including a total of 575 patients, 54 patients had myocardial infarction, or death associated with noncardiac vascular surgery. Eighty-seven percent of patients with a postoperative event demonstrated thallium redistribution on their preoperative dipyridamole study. In patients without a postoperative event, 64 percent demonstrated no evidence of thallium redistribution on their preoperative thallium-dipyridamole study. The results of this and other studies indicate that dipyridamole-thallium myocardial imaging is an excellent approach to preoperative risk assessment in patients with a medium to high probability of coronary artery disease and in need of major noncardiac surgery[91–93] (see also Chap. 139).

MYOCARDIAL INFARCT IMAGING

There are two radiopharmaceuticals in clinical use to detect and size acute myocardial infarction and help to determine prognosis after infarction based on their localization in necrotic myocardium ("hot spot" imaging agents). The first agent, ^{99m}Tc stannous pyrophosphate (^{99m}Tc-PPi), is a bone-imaging agent that was incidentally observed to localize in acutely infarcted myocardium in a patient undergoing bone scanning for detection of metastatic disease in 1974.[94] The second agent, indium-111 (^{111}In) labeled specific antibody (antimyosin) to cardiac myosin, is a Fab fragment of a murine monoclonal antibody directed against human heavy-chain cardiac myosin. Perfusion-imaging agents such as ^{201}Tl and ^{99m}Tc-sestamibi have been used to localize and size myocardial infarction based on the size and location of the perfusion defects.[95–100] Perfusion defects in the setting of acute myocardial infarction, however, may represent either necrosis or reduced blood flow at rest due to ongoing ischemia. Occasionally, nontransmural infarction may not be detected by perfusion imaging.

Pharmacokinetics and Biodistribution of Technetium Pyrophosphate

^{99m}Tc pyrophosphate was initially developed as a bone-imaging agent. The radiolabel, ^{99m}Tc, is generator-produced and widely available. Pyrophosphate is readily prepared by adding ^{99m}Tc to a sterile vial containing stannous pyrophosphate. The radionuclide is rapidly cleared from the blood pool with a clearance half $T_{1/2}$ of about 15 min. Imaging is commonly performed 2 to 4 h after tracer injection.[101] The mechanism of uptake into the necrotic myocardium is presumed to be pyrophosphate binding to intracellular Ca^{2+}.[102,103] During severe cell ischemia, there are shifts of electrolyte concentrations between the intracellular and extracellular spaces. The intracellular concentration of calcium increases, leading to mitochondrial calcium deposition as the cell is irreversibly damaged. The radiotracer traverses the disrupted sarcolemma to bind with intracellular calcium. Studies in laboratory animals suggest that pyrophosphate binds to severely (but reversibly) ischemic, as well as irreversibly damaged myocardial cells; this limits the specificity of the agent.[104] Another drawback of this radiotracer is uptake of pyrophosphate into the ribs, which can interfere with visualization of small areas of myocardial tracer uptake, especially with planar imaging. Pyrophosphate localization can be demonstrated as early as 10 to 12 h postinfarction and is most likely to be clinically observable between 24 and 72 h. Images usually remain positive until days 6 to 14 postinfarction but can remain positive for weeks or months, especially in patients with large anterior infarctions. This finding implies chronic ongoing ischemia or ventricular aneurysm formation.[105]

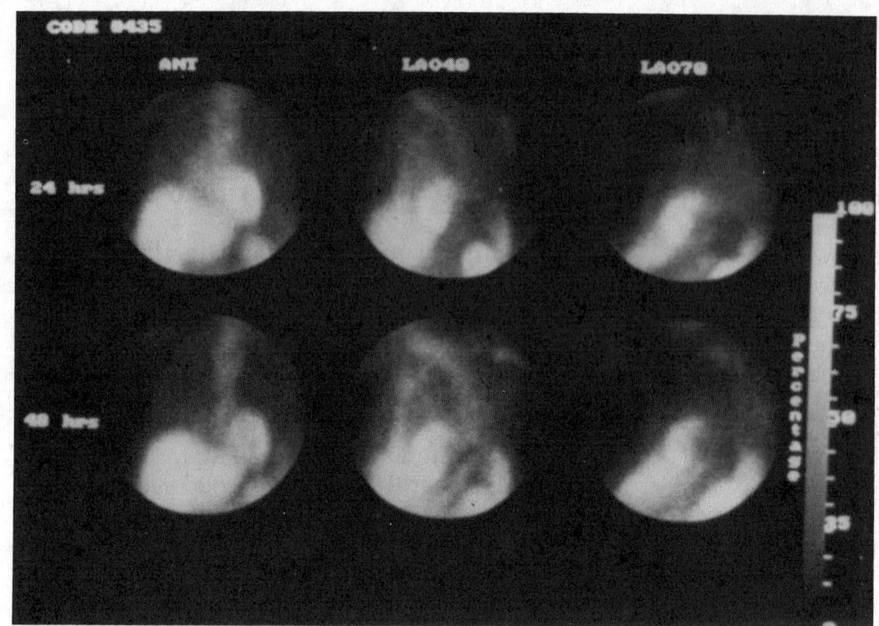

FIGURE 134-19 Planar images of ^{111}In antimyosin uptake acquired 24 h postinjection (top row) and 48 h postinjection (bottom row). In the anterior projection there appears to be diffuse myocardial uptake because the septum is viewed enface in this projection. In the oblique views the radiolabeled antibody is seen to be localized to the anteroseptal, apical, and anterior walls (left anterior descending artery territory). Uptake is also seen in the liver and left kidney.

Pharmacokinetics and Biodistribution of Antimyosin Antibody

The antimyosin antibody used in clinical practice is a monoclonal Fab fragment of a murine antibody directed specifically against human heavy-chain cardiac myosin. In a series of experiments in laboratory animals, antimyosin uptake was found specifically to indicate myocardial necrosis.[106–108] The antibody fragment can only gain access to and bind with the antigen (heavy-chain myosin) when the myocardial cell membrane is disrupted, a process that indicates irreversible cell damage. The antibody fragment can be bound via a chelating agent to ^{111}In. Indium-111 has a reasonable energy spectrum for clinical imaging but a relatively long half-life of 72 h (limiting dosage) and is cyclotron-produced (limiting availability). A technetium-labeled antibody fragment has been developed but is not clinically available.[109] Since antimyosin is a large molecule, its clearance from the blood pool is relatively slow. The $T_{1/2}$ for blood pool clearance is 6 to 12 h.[110] By 24 h after injection, the blood pool has cleared sufficiently in the majority of patients to yield reasonable infarct imaging (Fig. 134-19). In 12 to 20 percent of patients, however, the blood pool activity precludes obtaining a diagnostic scan at 24 h and imaging must be repeated at 48 h.[111] In addition to necrotic myocardium, antimyosin also localizes in liver and kidneys. Liver activity can obscure uptake in myocardial inferior wall. Antimyosin images can remain positive for up to 9 months postinfarction.[112] These late positive scans presumably represent antibody binding to heavy-chain myosin fragments imbedded in scar. Alternatively, it may represent ongoing subclinical ischemic damage. Table 134-6 compares the properties of the two infarct-avid radiopharmaceuticals.

Sensitivity and Specificity for Detection of Myocardial Infarction

One of the most definitive studies of pyrophosphate was carried out in 52 patients who underwent planar imaging studies at the time of acute myocardial infarction, subsequently died, and underwent necropsy. The predictive indices for the recognition of microscopic or gross myocardial infarction by the radionuclide imaging technique were evaluated.[113] The sensitivity was 89 percent, the specificity 100 percent; the predictive value for a positive scan was 100 percent and for a negative scan 72 percent. For antimyosin, a multicenter clinical trial was conducted to evaluate the sensitivity and specificity of planar imaging using the ECG and serum creatine kinase (CK-MB) fraction as the standards against which the imaging results were compared. In 340 patients, the clinical parameters were considered to give a definitive diagnosis of acute myocardial infarction. The sensitivity of antimyosin was 94 percent for Q-wave infarctions and 82

TABLE 134-6
"Hot Spot" Infarct Imaging Agents

Agent	Binding Site	Window for Positivity	Time from Injection to Imaging, h	Noncardiac Uptake
^{99m}Tc-pyrophosphate	Intracellular Ca^{2+}	2–14 days	4	Bone
^{111}In-antimyosin	Heavy chain cardiac myosin	Immediate up to 9 mo	24–48	Liver, kidney

percent for non-Q infarctions. The specificity was 95 percent.[114] Most of the false negative scans occurred in patients with infarction involving the inferoposterior segments. Both pyrophosphate and antimyosin scans have been reported to be positive in some patients with unstable angina pectoris. In the multicenter antimyosin trial, 37 percent of patients with a clinical diagnosis of unstable angina had positive scans. Such uptake is thought to represent myocardial necrosis indicating that there is a continuum of degree of necrosis from unstable angina to transmural infarction.

The use of "hot spot" imaging to confirm the diagnosis of acute myocardial infarction in a patient in whom the ECG and enzymes are already diagnostic is not necessary. For diagnosis, the imaging study should be reserved for patients in whom the routine clinical tests are not diagnostic, such as small enzyme rises with equivocal ECG changes, an uninterpretable ECG due to intraventricular conduction delay (IVCD), left bundle branch block (LBBB) with equivocal enzymes, or an ECG showing an infarct pattern of indeterminate age and a recent history suggestive of myocardial infarction or after cardiac surgery when ECG and serum enzymes are difficult to interpret (Table 134-7).

Infarct Sizing

Both techniques for imaging of recently infarcted myocardium have been shown to be capable of assessing infarct size using SPECT in both laboratory animal models and in patients.[115–120] The laboratory studies have shown that these approaches are useful in both early reperfused and late nonreperfused infarcts.[120] The infarct-sizing technique involves applying a threshold value for activity to each tomographic slice. This threshold value represents a percentage of the highest counts in that slice as validated experimentally. All of the voxels (cubic volume elements in the image) demonstrating tracer uptake above the threshold level are defined as infarct and summed. The volume is determined using an externally placed radioactive standard of known length and multiplied by the specific gravity of heart muscle to yield grams of myocardium infarcted. Infarct size can also be expressed as percentage of the total left ventricular (LV) mass using dual isotope tomographic imaging of thallium in addition to the infarct-avid radiopharmaceutical.[119–121] Infarct size as percentage of total myocardium has been correlated with predischarge left ventricular ejection fraction (LVEF) in patients with their first myocardial infarction. From the resultant regression equation, ejection fraction falls below normal (0.50) when 23 percent or more of left ventricular myocardium is infarcted. This corresponds to an infarct size of about 40 g.[119–121] When simultaneous tomographic imaging of ^{111}In antimyosin antibody and ^{201}Tl is performed in patients with non-Q-wave infarctions, localization of both tracers in the area of the infarction is frequently observed, suggesting an admixture of viable and necrotic myocardium. In a nongated tomogram, transmural distribution in tracer localization cannot be resolved. Therefore, nontransmural infarctions cannot be accurately measured using a threshold technique.

TABLE 134-7

Diagnostic Indications for "Hot Spot" Acute Myocardial Imaging

Small enzyme rise with equivocal ECG changes
Uninterpretable ECG due to LBBB with equivocal enzymes
ECG showing infarct pattern of indeterminate age and a history consistent with MI 2–7 days earlier
After cardiac surgery when serum enzymes and ECG are difficult to interpret

Determination of Prognosis: Dual Isotope Imaging

Infarct size assessed visually from planar images, or quantitated by SPECT imaging using either pyrophosphate or antimyosin has been shown to be predictive of postinfarction cardiac events, including heart failure and death.[105,119,121] This is not surprising since the extent of infarct tracer localization relates inversely to the LVEF and a low predischarge LVEF is known to be an excellent predictor of death after infarction.[122,123]

Another approach to assessing prognosis from a "hot spot" imaging approach is to combine it with perfusion imaging obtained simultaneously. For technical reasons, ^{201}Tl and ^{111}In can be simultaneously imaged with less interference between tracers than occurs between technetium and thallium. The thallium distribution soon after injection is related to perfusion of viable myocardium, and antimyosin localization denotes necrosis. Regions of myocardium in which neither tracer is found represent either scar or viable, but hypoperfused, myocardium at further ischemic risk. Three patterns of thallium and antimyosin localization have been reported in patients imaged to 72 to 96 h after onset of chest pain: matches, mismatches, and overlap.[89] In the matching pattern, the location and extent of antimyosin uptake corresponds to that of the thallium defect. In a mismatch, the thallium defect is either more extensive than the region of antimyosin uptake, or there is an additional unmatched thallium defect in a different vascular territory (Fig. 134-20). In an overlapping pattern, there is both antimyosin and thallium uptake in the same myocardial segments. The latter pattern has been observed in nontransmural infarction and is often seen after reperfusion therapy. In a study correlating patterns of uptake of the two tracers on simultaneously acquired SPECT scans performed 72 to 96 h after the onset of chest pain, patients with either mismatching patterns and/or overlapping patterns had a higher incidence of further ischemic events in the 6 weeks following hospital discharge, including infarct extension, recurrent angina, or ischemia on exercise stress test.[89]

RADIONUCLIDE ANGIOCARDIOGRAPHY (RNA)

Two techniques exist for assessment of ventricular performance using radionuclides: the first-pass technique

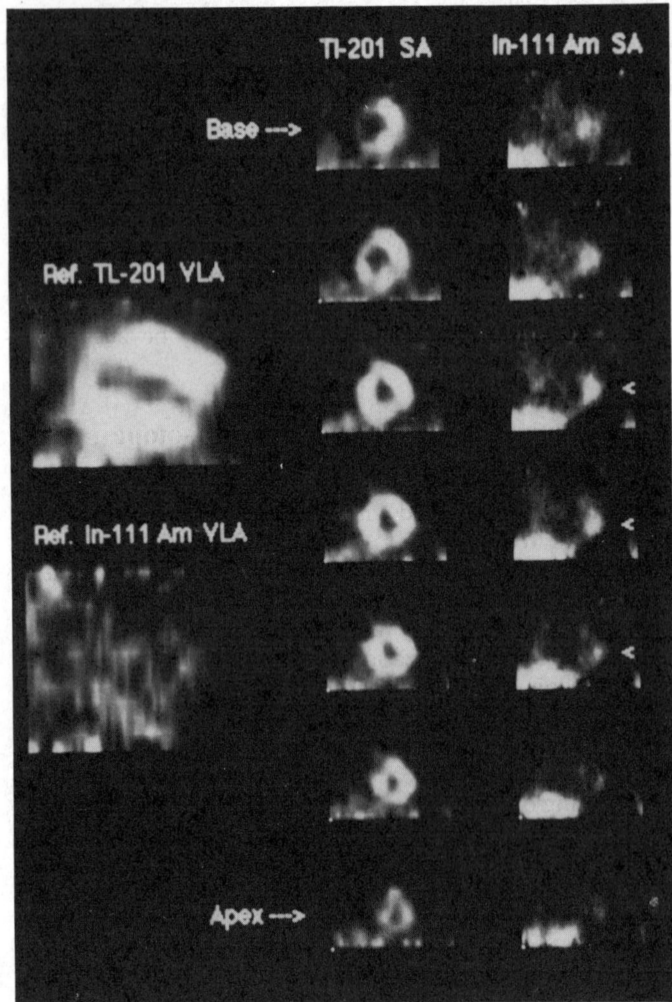

FIGURE 134-20 Example of simultaneously acquired tomograms of a perfusion tracer, ^{201}Tl, and a necrosis avid tracer, ^{111}In antimyosin, in a patient in the early postinfarction period. Reference vertical long axis slices are displayed on the left with thallium on the top and ^{111}In antimyosin on the bottom, and corresponding short axis slices are displayed on the right from base to apex with thallium to the left and antimyosin to the right. There is a mild thallium defect in the lateral wall of the left ventricle and uptake of antimyosin in the lateral wall of the corresponding short axis slices (arrows). This pattern of overlap of the two tracers is seen in nontransmural infarctions. There is in addition an apical thallium defect without apical antimyosin uptake, seen on the vertical long axis slice. This unmatched thallium defect outside the territory of the acute infarction was due to ischemia in the distribution of the distal LAD.

and gated blood pool imaging. Information that can be derived from these studies include assessment of left or right ventricular ejection fraction, regional wall motion, left ventricular volumes, and diastolic function (see Table 134-8 for gated blood pool imaging and Table 134-9 for the first-pass technique). These two techniques differ in optimal instrumentation, choice of radiotracer, optimal patient positions for acquisition, data analysis, presentation, and interpretation. Both techniques, however, have in common a quantitative count-based and geometry-independent method for calculating the left ventricular ejection fraction in contrast to echocardiography, which uses either a qualitative assessment of left ventricular global function or a model-dependent measurement. Ejection fraction calculated using either of the radionuclide techniques is accurate and reproducible.[124–126] Although the ejection fraction is not strictly an index of contractility since it is affected by preload, afterload, and heart rate, it is, nevertheless, a very useful clinical parameter to assess left ventricular performance at rest, or to assess changes associated with therapy or an intervention (see also Chaps. 23 and 25). The relative advantages and limitations of each of the two radionuclide methods to assess ventricular function must be understood to apply them optimally.

TABLE 134-8

Data Available From a Resting Multigated Blood Pool Study
Detailed analysis of wall motion in three views
LVEF
RVEF
LVEDV
Diastolic indices
Phase mapping
Stroke volume ratio for regurgitant fraction

TABLE 134-9

Data Available From a Resting First-Pass Study
Wall motion in one view
LVEF
RVEF
LVEDV, SV, CO
Diastolic indices
Transit times
Shunt detection and quantitation

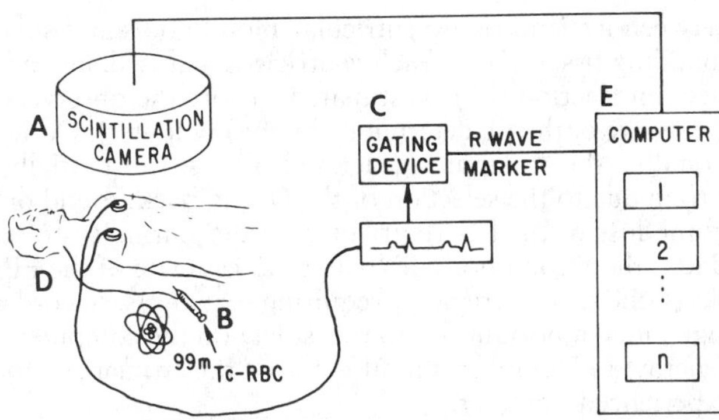

FIGURE 134-21 Schematic diagram of the method for acquiring a multigated blood pool imaging study. The gamma camera head (A) is positioned directly over the patient's chest for anterior view acquisition. Electrodes are previously placed on the patient's shoulders (and lower abdomen) so that they do not interfere with cardiac blood pool activity (D). The ECG is recorded, and a gating device generates signals with each R wave. These signals indicate to the imaging computer (E) to initiate a new acquisition cycle. The heart cycle is divided into a number of consecutive components. Each of these components is stored in sequence by the computer (E), e.g., 1,2,. . . *N*. Finally, ^{99m}Tc-labeled red blood cells are administered intravenously (B). [*From DS Berman, DJ Mason (eds): Clinical Nuclear Cardiology. New York, Grune & Stratton, 1981. Reproduced with permission from the publisher and the editors.*]

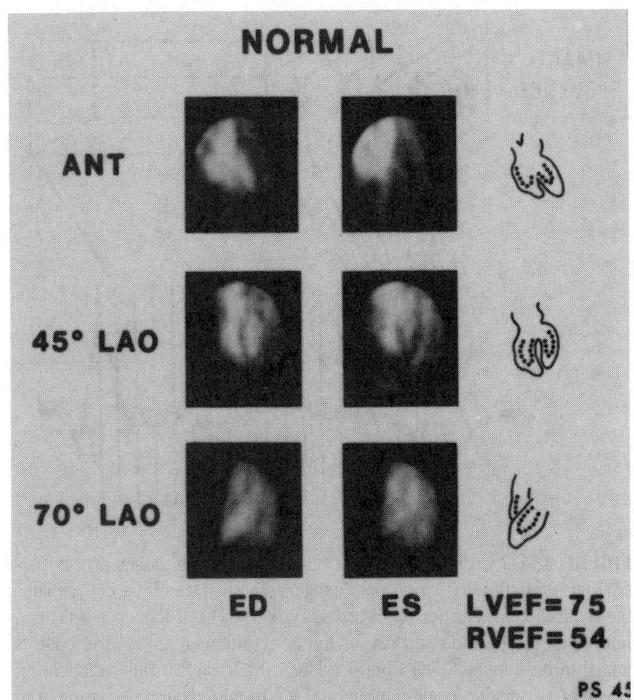

FIGURE 134-22 End-diastolic (ED) and end-systolic (ES) frames from a normal equilibrium multigated blood pool imaging study acquired in the anterior (ANT), 45°, and 70° LAO projections. Outlines, drawn by hand, from the end-diastolic (solid lines) and end-systolic (dashed lines) images are illustrated in the right column. The computer-measured counts from the left ventricular and right ventricular blood pools provided an ejection fraction estimate of 0.75 and 0.54, respectively. The RV ejection fraction measurement is substantially less reliable than the LVEF due to the overlapping and adjacent right atrial. [*From DS Berman, DT Mason (eds): Clinical Nuclear Cardiology. New York, Grune & Stratton, 1981. Reproduced with permission.*]

Gated Blood Pool Imaging

The gated blood pool imaging method (multigated acquisition, or MUGA) uses ^{99m}Tc-pertechnetate labeled to the patient's red blood cells to retain it within the blood pool (Fig. 134-21). The labeling process involves the intravenous injection of stannous pyrophosphate, which binds to red blood cell membranes. Then, ^{99m}Tc-pertechnetate is administered and binds to the red-cell-bound stannous pyrophosphate. Technetium remains within the blood pool and, because the heart has the largest blood pool within the chest, the chambers can then be imaged with an Anger camera (Fig. 134-22).

Red Blood Cell Labeling

The most efficient labeling technique involves the intravenous injection of stannous pyrophosphate followed in 15 to 20 min by removal of 2 to 3 cc of the patient's blood into a heparinized syringe containing 20 to 30 mCi of ^{99m}Tc.[127,128] The blood is incubated outside of the patient for 10 min allowing highly efficient radionuclide labeling of the small aliquot of blood, which is then reinjected and distributed throughout the blood volume.

ECG Gating and Acquisition

Imaging is performed by synchronizing acquisition to the R wave of the ECG (Fig. 134-23). Each R-R interval is subdivided into a preselected number of windows of equal duration. For a resting study, 28 to 32 frames are selected with an acquisition time of 6 to 10 min. This will yield a reasonable temporal resolution for accurate identification of frames representing end-diastole and end-systole in the time activity curve. For an exercise study with more rapid heart rates, half of the number of frames are selected to optimize image quality. Counts are accumulated sequentially for each successive R-R interval and stored in the imaging computer. Counts from summation of several hundred successive cardiac cycles are displayed as a continuous loop movie. Gated blood pool imaging can be performed on patients with atrial or ventricular premature beats using specialized software. Windows can be set prior to beginning an acquisition, and all beats that fall outside the window are rejected in the formation of the imaging sequence. With this approach, a meaningful left ventricular ejection fraction value can be measured in almost any patient, even those with atrial fibrillation.

The Anger camera is positioned over the supine patient on the imaging table so that the cardiac blood pool is in the center of the field of view as can be determined using the persistence oscilloscope. The "best septal" (45° to 50°) LAO view is acquired first, in which the septum separating the left and right ventricles appears of homogeneous thickness from top to bottom. This view is used for calculation of left ventricular ejection fraction. Some degree of angulation of the Anger camera head toward the feet is also used to minimize atrial overlap. Accuracy of the left ventricular ejection fraction calculation depends on optimal isolation of the left ventricle from adjacent cardiac structures. From the best septal angle, the detector is rotated 45° toward the next view, which is an anterior study. In addition to the anterior and

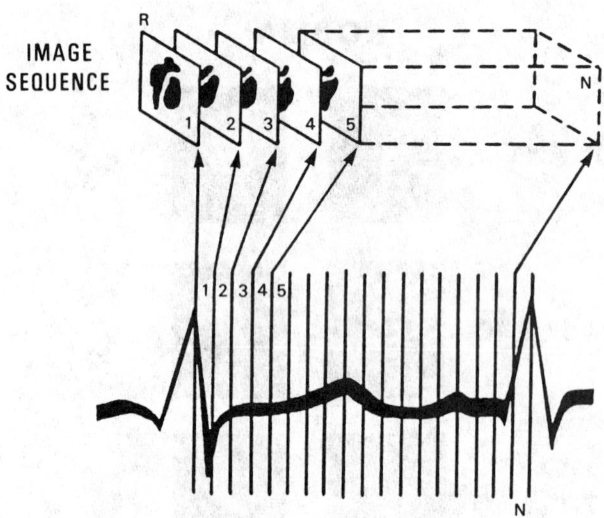

FIGURE 134-23 Schematic illustration showing the gating process for equilibrium multigated blood pool imaging. The R wave of the ECG initiates the acquisition process for each cardiac cycle. The ECG R-R interval is divided into 18 or more windows. Data for the first window of the cardiac cycle is added to the summed data from previous cardiac cycles. This results in an image of reasonable quality during a 5- to 10-min acquisition period. The same is true of each of the subsequent intervals. Since the R-R interval is never precisely the same from beat to beat, image quality may be lower in later frames. In atrial fibrillation, many of the last frames in the sequence show reduced activity since the shorter R-R intervals do not contribute data to the later frames. Once the acquisition is complete, the computer-stored images are displayed in sequence as a movie. [*From DS Berman, DT Mason (eds): Clinical Nuclear Cardiology. New York, Grune & Stratton, 1981. Reproduced with permission from the publisher and the editors.*]

"best septal" LAO view, one other projection is usually acquired for assessment of regional wall motion: either the left lateral or the 60° left posterior oblique (the inverse of the 30° right anterior oblique). Each resting acquisition is completed after acquisition of a predetermined number of counts in the range of 200,000 to 250,000 (6 to 10 min).

Qualitative Assessment of the Gated Blood Pool Study (MUGA)

Initial evaluation of the MUGA study consists of an overall qualitative assessment. The observer should have substantial experience with MUGA interpretations. First, the cardiac chambers and other landmarks are identified: left ventricle, overlying right ventricle, portions of left and right atria, superior and inferior vena cavae, aorta and pulmonary artery in the anterior view; left and right ventricles, left and right atria in the "best septal" LAO view; and left ventricle and left atrium in the steep LAO, or LPO, view. The size of the chambers and great vessels is assessed. The thickness of the left ventricular myocardium is judged to be normal, thinned, or hypertrophied. The configuration of the interventricular septum is assessed to determine if there is disproportionate thickening of the upper septum as can be seen in hypertrophic cardiomyopathy.[129] The anterior and "best septal" LAO views are studied to detect pericardial effusion, which is seen as a prominent photon-deficient space between left and right ventricular blood pools and surrounding tissue. Then, each ventricle is assessed, and an ejection fraction (EF) is estimated (before the observers are aware of the EF determined by the computer). Occasionally, the computer-generated EF is substantially wrong due to the selection of the wrong background or to the loss of the left ventricular border during systole. Under these conditions, a "ballpark" estimate of the EF alerts one to a discrepancy requiring reanalysis. Accordingly, it is important not to rely solely on the computer-generated EF number if it differs from the estimate of an experienced observer.

Finally, regional wall motion is assessed. The LV silhouette is evaluated for aneurysm, which is usually observed as an apical (or occasionally inferior or posterior wall) bulge in the end-systolic image with dyskinesis of the involved segment. For qualitative analysis of regional wall motion, the three views are divided into segments (Fig. 134-24). Wall motion for each segment can be graded on a semiquantitative scale. For example, 3 = normal, 2 = mild hypokinesis, 1 = moderate to severe hypokinesis, 0 = akinesis, and −1 = dyskinesis. Because the right ventricle overlies the inferior wall of the left ventricle in the anterior view, inferior wall motion should only be assessed in the lateral, or LPO, view. Quantitative computer algorithms have been developed and are commercially available, although it is not clear that these programs add substantially to the qualitative interpretation. In addition, qualitative assessment of right ventricular function is made in the "best septal" LAO view. Under certain circumstances, the interventricular septum moves paradoxically, i.e., into the RV in systole and back into the LV in diastole. Such paradoxical septal motion can be seen in a variety of conditions, including after septal MI when the interventricular septum is thin and such motion actually represents dyskinesis (Table 134-10).

Measurement of Left Ventricular Ejection Fraction (LVEF)

With the best septal LAO view, the computer detects the borders of the LV using a threshold or second derivative

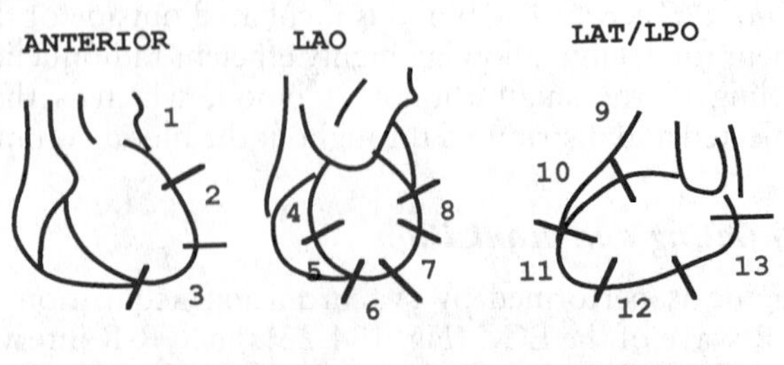

FIGURE 134-24 Schematic display of division of the left ventricle into 13 segments in the three-view gated blood pool images for semiquantitative assessment of region wall motion.

TABLE 134-10
Causes of Paradoxical Septal Motion

Causes of Paradoxical Septal Motion
Left bundle branch block
Right ventricular paced rhythm
After heart surgery using cardiopulmonary bypass
Congenital absence of the pericardium
Right ventricular volume overload (e.g., atrial septal defect or tricuspid regurgitation)
Septal infarction

technique. The image may be enhanced using spatial and temporal smoothing to aid in border definition, especially in studies with relatively lower counts or with high background activity. An initial end-diastolic region of interest is drawn by the observer around the computer-displayed left ventricle and a time versus activity curve is generated from either the fixed end-diastolic region or from multiple left ventricular regions adjusted frame by frame throughout the cardiac cycle. A background region is identified just outside the left ventricular region of interest and average background counts are subtracted from each LV pixel of each frame of the cycle. LVEF is calculated from the background corrected end-diastolic and end-systolic frames (Fig. 134-25).

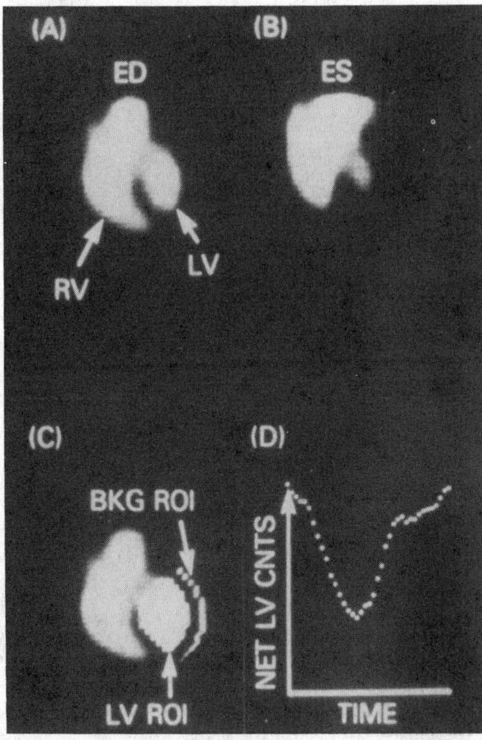

FIGURE 134-25 Panels *A* and *B* depict gated blood pool images at the end-diastolic and end-systolic frames. Panels *C* and *D* demonstrate the left ventricular region selected for measurement of left ventricular ejection fraction and the region of interest adjacent to the left ventricle selected as background. The average counts per pixel in the background region are assumed to represent the same background counts in the left ventricular region. The background corrected time activity curve is displayed in panel *D*.

Right Ventricular Ejection Fraction

No study has yet compared radionuclide studies of right ventricular ejection fraction (RVEF) with a reliable gold standard, such as magnetic resonance imaging. Nevertheless, RVEF values generated are clinically useful for assessing right ventricular function in patients with cor pulmonale and inferior wall infarction.[130–134]

There are two methods for quantitating RVEF using radionuclide gated blood pool imaging. In one method, the gated equilibrium approach is used.[135] Regions of interest are used to outline the right ventricular blood pool at end-diastole and end-systole. Average background counts are determined from a region adjacent to the right ventricle and subtracted from the end-diastolic and end-systolic images. The major problem with this technique is accurately determining the right ventricular borders at end-diastole and end-systole. In the second method, a "gated first pass" acquisition is performed. The patient is first injected with stannous pyrophosphate. Twenty to 30 min later, the gamma camera detector is positioned over the patient to obtain an anterior projection, and a bolus of ^{99m}Tc-pertechnetate is injected through a large right antecubital vein, while an ECG-gated acquisition is performed. Acquisition is terminated when the bolus is seen in the pulmonary artery. The standard gated software is used to compute the RVEF. During systole, the right atrial blood pool is pulled into the right ventricular region of interest and, therefore, separate regions of interest for end-diastole and end-systole are selected. Subsequently, a standard three-view equilibrium study is performed. The advantage of the "gated first pass" technique is the temporal separation of RA and RV activity. The drawback is that the studies have relatively fewer counts using a standard Anger camera.

Stroke Count Ratios

The difference between ventricular end-diastolic and end-systolic counts is proportional to ventricular stroke volume. In the absence of either interventricular shunting or valvular regurgitation, the stroke volume from the two ventricles is equivalent. The degree to which the ratio of the stroke counts is greater than or less than unity is a quantitative index of the degree of left or right ventricular volume overload. Using the imaging computer, regions of interest are drawn around the left ventricular and right ventricular blood pools. A stroke count ratio is derived by dividing the left ventricular stroke counts by the right ventricular stroke counts. A normal ratio is about 1.5 due to the greater overlap of the right atrium and ventricle in comparison to the overlap of the left atrium and ventricle. Ratios above 2.0 indicate left ventricular volume overload due to mitral or aortic regurgitation,[136–138] or ventricular septal defect, or patent ductus arteriosus. Ratios below 1.0 indicate right ventricular volume overload, tricuspid regurgitation, or atrial septal defect. Several studies have found a good correlation between angiographically quantitated regurgitation and stroke count ratios.[136,137] When the LV is dilated with an ejection fraction less than 30 percent, the ventricular stroke count ratio is inaccurate.

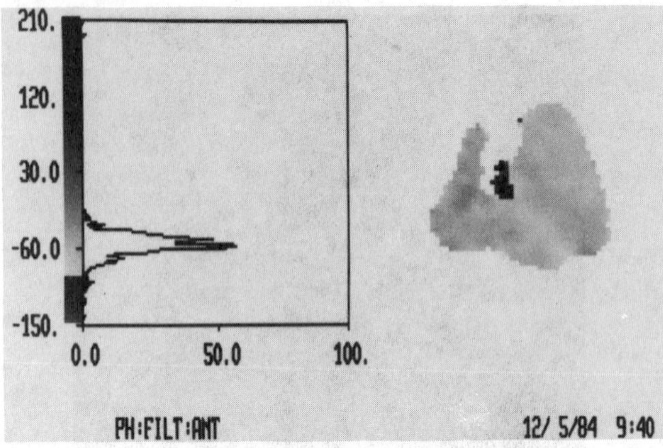

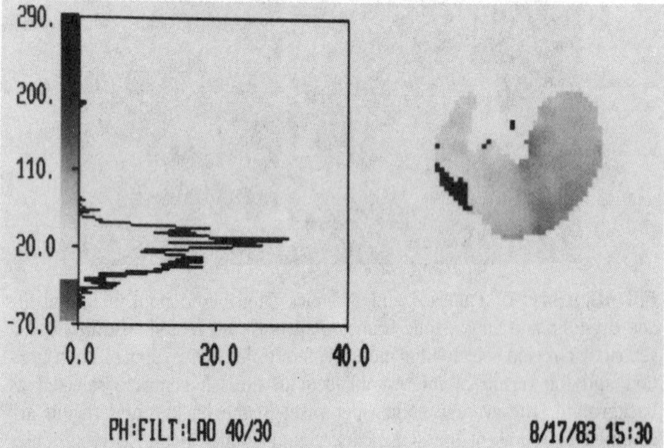

FIGURE 134-26 Panels *A* and *B* show phase images (right) and ventricular phase histograms (left). The phase histograms show the range of phase angles on the *y* axis and the number of pixels in the phase image with each phase angle on the *x* axis. The gray scale has been selected to highlight those pixels with earliest ventricular phase angles in black. Panel *A* in the anterior projection shows the earliest phase angles localized to the upper septum (normal), and panel *B* in the anterior projection shows the earliest phase angles localized to the right ventricular free wall in a patient with WPW and right anterior bypass tract.

Phase and Amplitude Images

Amplitude images depict the rate of change of counts from end-diastole to end-systole. Such images are useful for identifying the boundaries of the left and right ventricles. Accordingly, they are helpful for computing stroke count ratios.[139] Phase images display the pattern of contractile motion. Assuming that activation and contraction are coupled, a map of the spread of activation over the atria and ventricles can be generated.[140,141] This can be of value for localization of bypass tracts in patients with preexcitation syndromes, such as the Wolf-Parkinson-White syndrome (Fig. 134-26). The earliest point of left ventricular activation can be identified by a method of triangulation from phase images generated from the three standard views.[142] The technique can be used as an adjunct to electrophysiologic mapping for tract localization. The ability to localize the initial point of left ventricular activation can also aid in localizing the focus of a ventricular tachyrhythmia.

Diastolic Function

Dividing the cardiac cycle into 28 to 32 frames allows assessment of ventricular relaxation rates and, thus, diastolic function. In normal sinus rhythm, the three phases of diastole can be clearly defined using the time activity curve: rapid diastolic filling, diastasis, and atrial systole (Fig. 134-27). Changes in the configuration of the curve occur in diseases that affect left ventricular stiffness such as hypertrophy. As the ventricle becomes less compliant, the rate of early filling decreases.

Several diastolic indices have been described and investigated. Two of the most useful indices are peak filling rate (normalized to end-diastolic counts)[143,144] and time to peak filling.[144] Both indices are affected by heart rate. The normal value for peak filling rate at heart rates less than 100 is greater than 2.5 EDV/s, and time to peak is less than 180 ms. Assessment of diastolic function during exercise is unreliable due to high heart rate with encroachment of the atrial component of diastolic filling on peak filling at short cycle lengths.

The parameters of diastolic function become abnormal in pathologic processes that affect passive myocardial stiffness, such as hypertrophy, myocardial infiltration, and fibrosis.[145] In addition, diastolic function becomes abnormal in pathologic processes that affect myocardial energy production, such as ischemia. In the presence of even mild reduction in nutrient flow, which can occur at rest in coronary artery disease, abnormalities in diastolic indices can be observed on gated blood pool imaging.[146] Abnormalities in diastolic filling detected by gated blood pool imaging are among the earli-

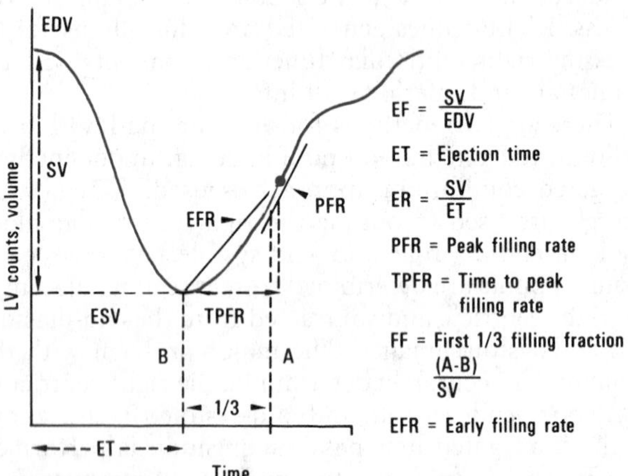

FIGURE 134-27 Time-activity curve derived from an equilibrium multigated blood pool study at rest. Left ventricular counts are indicated on the *y* axis and time on the *x* axis. The curve begins at end diastole, and its amplitude is proportional to the end-diastolic volume (EDV). The nadir of the curve represents end-systolic activity (ESV). Stroke volume counts (SV) are the difference between ED counts and ES counts. The systolic portion of the curve is to the left of the nadir and occurs during the ejection time (ET). The ejection rate (ER) is the stroke volume divided by the ET. The diastolic portion is to the right. Diastolic function is frequently measured with reference to the point at which the ventricular filling rate is at its peak. The slope of the line drawn between the radius and the point of peak filling is the early filling rate (EFR). The peak filling rate (PFR) is calculated by measuring the slope of a 100-ms segment of the filling portion of the curve centered on the point of peak filling. The first third of the filling fraction (FF) is another calculated index of diastolic function.

est and most sensitive changes that occur at rest in patients with coronary artery disease. These abnormalities, however, are not very specific. A major clinical application of the diastolic function analysis is to assess the effect of treatment for ischemic heart disease either using medication or revascularization.

Left Ventricular Volume Measurements

The most commonly reported approach for measuring left ventricular volumes from gated blood pool studies uses a count-based method. With this method, the counts are determined in the left ventricular region of interest. Left ventricular counts are corrected for attenuation. Finally, counts are converted to volume using the counts per cubic centimeter of a blood sample. While this approach has been validated against x-ray contrast cineangiography,[147–149] it is cumbersome to perform since it involves the counting of blood samples and acquisition of additional images with radioactive markers to calculate attenuation. Therefore, it is not recommended for routine clinical use.

A geometric area–length approach for measuring left ventricular end-diastolic volume from gated blood pool imaging studies has been validated against x-ray contrast cineangiography.[150] Such an approach depends on the ability to separate the left ventricle from adjacent structures in a view depicting its long axis. The "best septal" LAO view imaged using a 30° caudal tilt comes closest to fulfilling these conditions. A specialized collimator with its parallel holes slanted at a 30° angle can be used to acquire such images. End-systolic volume can be calculated by determining ejection fraction and substituting the area–length determined value for end-diastolic volume.

$$EF = \frac{EDV - ESV}{EDV} = 1 - \frac{ESV}{EDV}$$

Therefore,

$$ESV = EDV(1 - EF)$$

First-Pass Technique

The first-pass technique utilizes a high-count-rate gamma camera (ideally a multicrystal camera) to acquire data after the injection of a bolus of ^{99m}Tc-pertechnetate. Counts are recorded in a dynamic mode as the bolus passes through the central circulation. The gamma camera detector is positioned in front of the patient to obtain a straight anterior projection. Determination of LVEF with this technique relies on the fact that most of the activity is normally located in the right ventricle and left ventricle at different times (Fig. 134-28). Thus, each ventricle can be assessed without substantial interference from the background activity of the other ventricle. Anything that breaks up the bolus before it arrives in the left ventricle will decrease the reliability of the LVEF measurement. In addition to poor injection techniques, the physiologic conditions that reduce the accuracy of the first-pass LVEF determination include tricuspid regurgitation, pulmonary hypertension, atrial septal defect, and mitral regurgitation. While the gated equilibrium blood pool approach is the technique of choice to measure LVEF in patients with any of these conditions, the first-pass approach remains the optimal method for determination of RVEF.

Hemodynamic Data from First-Pass Studies

The left ventricular ejection fraction is measured from the time activity curve of the bolus of activity as it passes through the left ventricle.[151] The time activity curve has a sawtooth appearance with each high frequency oscillation representing an individual cardiac cycle. The peaks represent end-diastoles and the troughs end-systoles (Fig. 134-3, Plate XIII). The counts from the peaks or troughs are summed for the number of beats the isotope is in the left ventricle, which varies from about 3 to 20 depending on the transit time and cardiac output. The resultant end-diastolic and end-systolic images are corrected for background activity (although it is considerably less than

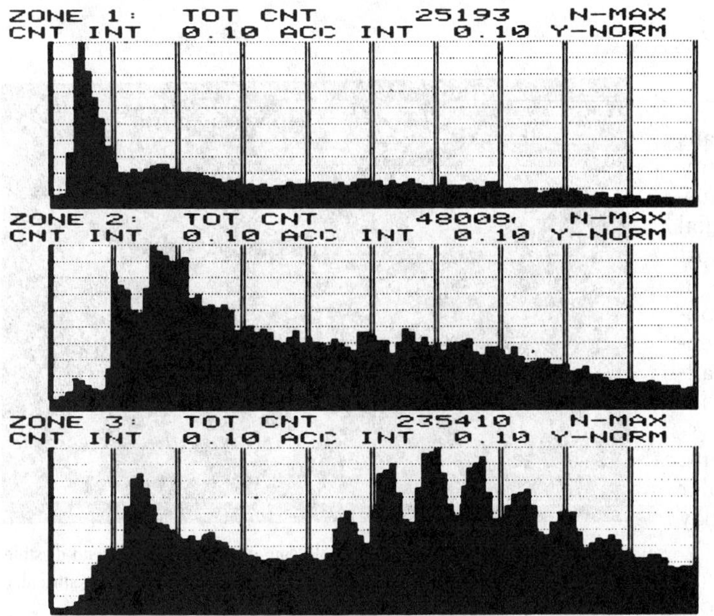

FIGURE 134-28 First-pass acquisition of a bolus injection of ^{99m}Tc using a multicrystal scintillation camera. Regions over the superior vena cava (top panel), right ventricle (middle panel), and left ventricle (bottom panel) were selected; counts are displayed on the *y* axes, time on the *x* axes. Temporal separation of the bolus in the different regions is demonstrated. The top panel shows a single narrow peak of counts representing a compact bolus of ^{99m}Tc in the superior vena cava. The sawtooth pattern of activity seen on the bottom panel represents the left ventricular phase of the bolus passage. Each high frequency oscillation represents an individual cardiac cycle; the peaks are end-diastoles, the troughs are end-systoles.

with the blood pool method), and the left ventricular ejection fraction is computed as

ED counts − ES counts/ED counts − background

A cardiac cycle is generated from component images of the time activity curve and can be viewed in movie format for wall motion analysis. In addition, a regional ejection fraction image can be derived. In this image, the magnitudes of regional ejection fractions are color coded (e.g., red for high and blue for low ejection fractions) and mapped for the entire left ventricle. Such an approach is particularly useful for assessing regional wall motion in nonborder-forming walls.

Left ventricular volumes can be determined by outlining the LV region and by using the area-length method analogous to x-ray cineangiography. From the end-diastolic volume and LVEF, end-systolic and stroke volumes and cardiac output can be calculated.

RVEF can be calculated using a gated first-pass approach with digital Anger camera, or an ungated first-pass approach with a multicrystal or digital Anger camera. Either first-pass approach is a better method for measuring RVEF than the gated equilibrium blood pool approach because the right ventricular activity is temporally separated from other cardiac chambers.

Diastolic function can also be assessed using the first-pass technique.[152,153] The theoretical disadvantage of the first-pass technique is that there is incomplete mixing of tracer with blood as the bolus washes into and out of the LV. The advantage of this technique over gated blood pool imaging is that it is derived from relatively few cardiac cycles which reduces the impact of variations in cardiac cycle length.

Finally, first-pass acquisition is useful for left-to-right shunt detection and quantitation.[154] In the absence of a left-to-right shunt, the time activity curve in a region of interest drawn over a segment of right lung demonstrates a single peak with an exponential decrease in activity. In the presence of a left-to-right shunt, the recirculating tracer may produce a second peak. Curves can be fitted to both the primary and secondary peaks to quantitate shunt size.[155]

Clinical Applications of Resting Radionuclide Angiography (Table 134-11)

The gated blood pool imaging study provides a means to assess ejection fraction, regional wall motion, chamber size, and approximate size of the great vessels. Thus, the test is useful for prognostication after myocardial infarction and in valvular heart disease. One of the most frequent applications of gated blood pool imaging is to elucidate the cause of dyspnea. A dilated, poorly contracting left ventricle or the presence of a large left ventricular aneurysm confirms systolic left ventricular failure, whereas a thick-walled elongated ventricle with abnormal diastolic parameters suggests diastolic dysfunction as a possible cause of the patient's symptoms. A normal left ventricular study with right ventricular dilation and dysfunction suggests a pulmonary etiology for the dyspnea.

Left ventricular aneurysm and pseudoaneurysm are readily detected by three-view multigated blood pool imaging. Aneurysm is suggested by an akinetic or dyskinetic segment (most commonly at the apex), which is associated with a bulging of the chamber at end-systole (Fig. 134-29). A pseudoaneurysm is suggested by a large aneurysmal dilation with a narrow neck connecting it to the main body of the ventricle.

Enlargement of the left ventricle with a normal or near normal ejection fraction suggests left ventricular volume overload. If the aorta appears dilated, aortic regurgitation is the likely etiology (Fig. 134-30), whereas if the left atrium is dilated, mitral regurgitation is suggested. Enlargement of the left ventricle with segmental contraction abnormalities suggests coronary artery disease with previous myocardial infarction(s). Dilation of all four chambers with global hypokinesis of the ventricles most likely represents idiopathic dilated cardiomyopathy (Fig. 134-31). (See also Chap. 89.) Isolated thickening of the intraventricular septum, particularly the upper septum and obliteration of the LV apex with contraction is seen in hypertrophic cardiomyopathy.[156] Elongation of the left ventricle, lack of base-to-apex shorten-

TABLE 134-11

Clinical Applications of Resting RNA
Document the diagnosis of LV systolic failure (low LVEF)
Distinguish systolic from diastolic dysfunction in patient with dyspnea thought to be cardiac in etiology
Quantitate degree of valvular regurgitation
Detect and quantitate intracardiac shunts
Follow cardiac function in patients on chemotherapy
Assess prognosis post-MI
Localize LV scar
Assess RV function in patients with cor pulmonale or acute inferior MI (RV infarction)
Distinguish congestive cardiomyopathy from ischemic LV dysfunction
Assess effects of interventions (surgical or medical) on LV function

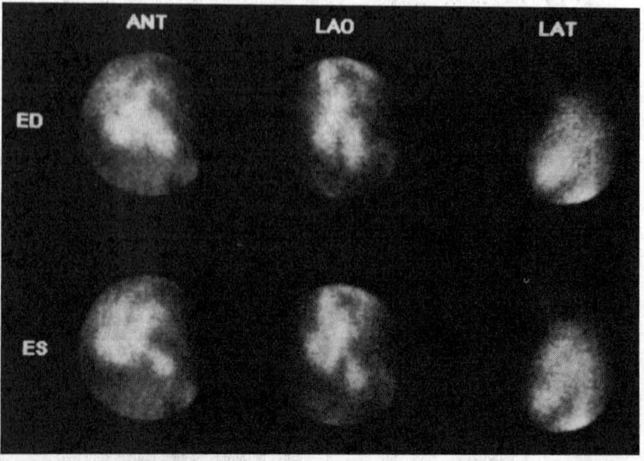

FIGURE 134-29 Gated blood pool scans in three views at end-diastole (top) and end-systole (bottom) showing a discrete apical left ventricular aneurysm.

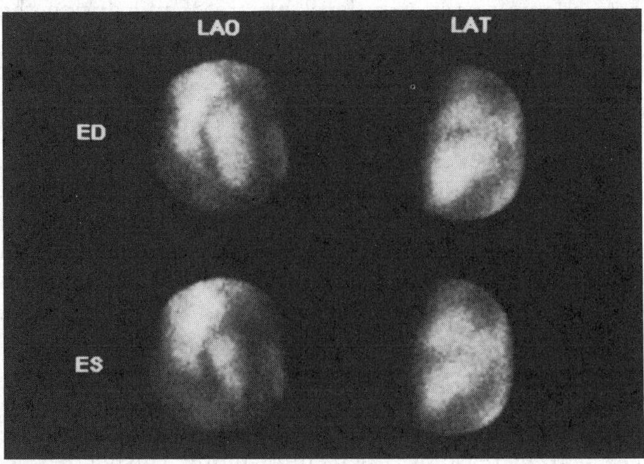

FIGURE 134-30 Gated blood pool scans in two views at end-diastole (top) and end-systole (bottom) showing marked dilation of the left ventricle with preserved systolic function compatible with left ventricular volume overload. The patient had severe aortic regurgitation.

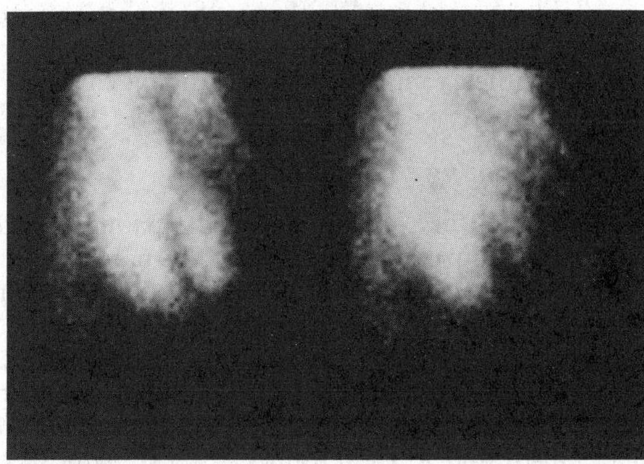

FIGURE 134-32 Gated blood pool imaging study in the left anterior oblique projection in a patient with a recent right ventricular (RV) myocardial infarction. Comparison of the end-diastole (left) image with the end-systolic (right) image demonstrates poor RV function but normal left ventricular function. Gated blood pool scanning is an excellent method for detecting RV involvement in patients with inferior wall myocardial infarction.

ing during contraction, thickening of the interventricular septum and free wall, and prominence of the papillary muscles is seen in left ventricular hypertrophy (LVH) secondary to hypertension or aortic stenosis. It is important to be careful not to misinterpret the lack of base-to-apex shortening of the LV as apical asynergy. Enlargement of the right ventricle and/or main pulmonary artery with reduced RVEF are observed in association with cor pulmonale or primary pulmonary hypertension. Dilation and poor right ventricular (RV) function in association with acute inferior wall infarction suggests the diagnosis of RV infarction (Fig. 134-32). Dilation of the right ventricle, paradoxical septal motion, and normal or near normal RV function are observed in association with RV volume overload. RV volume overload can be seen with tricuspid regurgitation or atrial septal defect. The blood pool image can also be helpful in detecting extracardiac abnormalities. Aneurysms of the thoracic aorta, and poststenotic dilation, and dilation of the main pulmonary artery can be seen. A

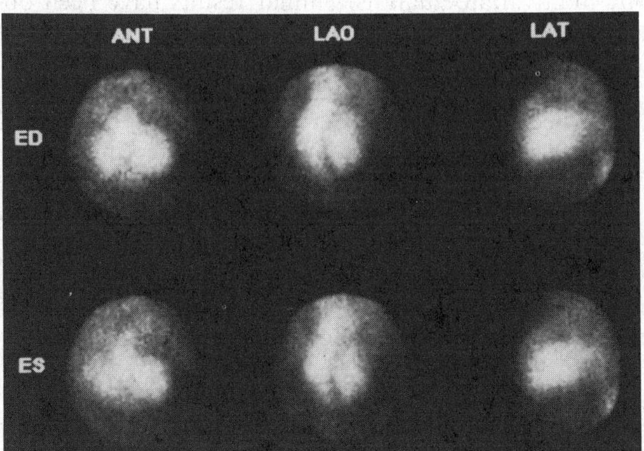

FIGURE 134-31 Gated blood pool imaging study in three views at end-diastole (top) and end-systole (bottom). There is dilatation and global hypokinesis of both ventricles.

photon-free "halo" around the left and right ventricular blood pools, when seen in several views, suggests pericardial effusion, but care must be taken not to be misled by breast attenuation in a female patient. The echocardiogram is the test of choice to diagnose pericardial effusion.

In addition to its qualitative diagnostic utility, radionuclide cineangiography can be used to assess prognosis in the post-myocardial-infarction patient. Several studies have demonstrated that the LVEF (at rest) is an independent variable predicting survival post infarction.[122,123] Serial evaluation of LVEF by radionuclide cineangiography has been reported to be useful for detection of doxorubicin cardiotoxicity.[157,158] Also, serial gated blood pool studies have been used to detect changes in LV systolic function after cardiac surgery. Radionuclide-cineangiographically determined ejection fraction was found to decrease substantially in the early hours after coronary artery bypass graft surgery. Serial studies demonstrated that ejection fraction returned toward normal by 12 h after discontinuation of the bypass pump.[159] Also, the response to drugs that affect LV systolic and/or diastolic function can be followed by serial gated blood pool studies.[160,161] Finally, the effects of revascularization on diastolic filling have been assessed.[162]

Exercise Radionuclide Cineangiography

Ejection fraction and wall motion can be assessed during exercise stress using either "first-pass" or gated equilibrium blood pool imaging. Both approaches can be applied using upright bicycle exercise. With the equilibrium approach, exercise can also be performed semi-supine or supine. Peak exercise studies are compared to studies at rest. Patients tend to be more limited by leg fatigue with supine exercise.

Methods

Exercise radionuclide cineangiography can be performed using either "first-pass" or gated equilibrium imaging. The approach used depends on the type of gamma camera available. As with studies at rest, "first-pass" imaging requires a camera capable of acquiring data at a high speed, i.e., either a multicrystal or a digital camera.

First-Pass Imaging

With traditional first-pass imaging, the patient is exercised using an upright bicycle with the patient's arms around the camera head and his/her chest flush against the collimator. Workload is increased every 3 min. At peak exercise, a bolus of 15 mCi ^{99m}Tc-pertechnetate is injected IV.[163] Motion artifacts are minimal due to the stable position of the chest and the very short acquisition time (25 ms/frame × 1000 frames = 25 s). After recovery, a second bolus of 15 mCi ^{99m}Tc-pertechnetate is given to obtain data at rest. First-pass radionuclide angiography can also be performed using either ^{99m}Tc-sestamibi or ^{99m}Tc-teboroxime. In this way, function is assessed using the first-pass approach and myocardial perfusion assessed by subsequent imaging of the distribution of the radiopharmaceutical (Fig. 134-33).[164]

Gated Equilibrium Imaging

Exercise gated blood pool imaging requires that the patient's chest remain in a relatively stationary position for the duration of exercise.[165] This can be accomplished by using a special table with the bicycle ergometer attached at the "foot" end and a series of straps to secure the patient's chest in a relatively fixed position. This table allows exercise to be performed either supine, semisupine (i.e., midway between sitting and supine), or upright. Electrodes are connected to the patient to allow continuous monitoring, periodic recording of the ECG, and synchronization of data acquisition with the R wave for gating. The head of the gamma camera is positioned to acquire imaging from the "best septal" orientation, i.e., the interventricular septum is similar in thickness from top to bottom. Exercise is performed in 3-min stages. During the first minute of each stage, the heart rate adapts to the new level of stress, and during the second and third minutes of each stage, imaging is performed. A stable ECG signal for gating is essential for technical success. In contrast to the "first-pass" approach, this method provides LVEF measurements at each stage of exercise.

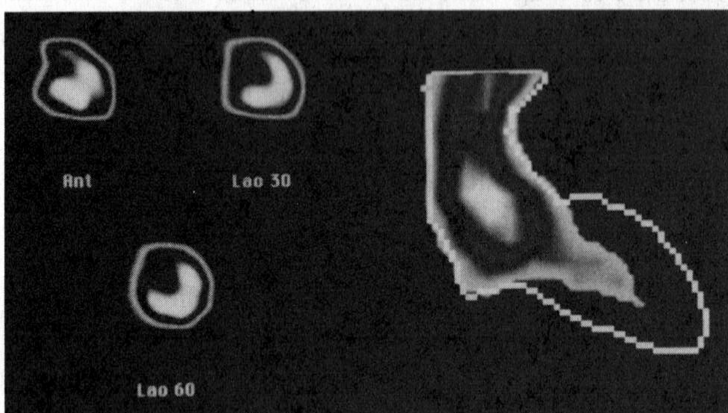

FIGURE 134-33 Perfusion and LVEF by the first-pass technique obtained with a single injection of a ^{99m}Tc-based myocardial perfusion tracer (Tc-99m teboroxime). The study was performed with the patient standing. The three planar images (Ant, 30° LAO, and 60° LAO) are displayed and show a normal perfusion pattern for a patient in the upright position. The ventricular function image displayed in the right panel with end-diastolic perimeter and end-systolic image superimposed shows normal wall motion. The computed ejection fraction was 0.74.

A study at rest as described previously is performed prior to the exercise study. Rest imaging is performed supine first to obtain three views to assess regional wall motion and then in the upright or semi-supine position to match the exercise study.

Clinical Applications of Exercise RNA

The widely accepted normal response of LVEF to exercise is to increase by 5 percent or more. This increase is due both to the Frank Starling mechanism with increased end-diastolic volume from increased venous return and to the positive inotropic effects of circulating catecholamines.[166] The response, however, is blunted normally in older subjects.[167] In younger patients, no change or a fall in LVEF during exercise indicates left ventricular dysfunction due either to ischemia or to intrinsic myocardial disease. An abnormal LVEF response to exercise is sensitive but not specific for coronary artery disease.[168] Accordingly, perfusion imaging is superior to exercise radionuclide cineangiography for diagnosis of coronary artery disease. A fall in LVEF combined with appearance of a new regional wall motion abnormality increases the specificity of this technique for detecting coronary artery disease; however, it is impractical to perform exercise RNA in multiple views. Using a single view, i.e., anterior view for the first-pass approach or the best septal LAO for the gated blood pool method, limits sensitivity in comparison to the multiple views or the SPECT acquisition used with myocardial perfusion imaging. Nevertheless, exercise radionuclide cineangiography can play a role in prognostication for patients with coronary artery disease.

In the largest series of patients undergoing exercise RNA for the assessment of coronary artery disease, the first-pass technique was used.[169] In this series, the LVEF at peak exercise was found to be the single most important predictor of reduced 5-year, event-free survival by multivariate analysis. Similar results have been obtained in a smaller sample size using the gated blood pool approach.[170] The ejection fraction response and the appearance of new regional contraction abnormalities have been reported to indicate the extent of residual jeopardized myocardium in patients after myocardial infarction.[171]

Normally, RVEF also increases with exercise. In the presence of proximal right coronary artery (RCA) disease, the RVEF has been observed to decrease. Thus, the ejection fraction response of the two ventricles to exercise can be discordant as a function of the distribution of the coronary artery disease.[172]

Exercise duration has been demonstrated to be of value for determining the time for aortic valve replacement in patients with asymptomatic aortic regurgitation.[173] However, the role of ejection fraction at peak exercise for timing of aortic valve replacement is unclear. One problem is that "peak exercise" depends on the fitness of the patient. Exercise ejection fraction measured at the time of the anaerobic threshold has been reported to be less dependent on fitness than peak exercise.[174] Two parameters to determine the optimal time for valve replacement in aortic regurgitation that are useful and easily obtained are resting LVEF and exercise duration.[175] This information can be acquired by resting radionuclide cineangiography for ejection fraction determination and treadmill exercise testing for assessment of exercise duration. These studies should be repeated annually in patients with severe aortic regurgitation (see also Chap. 79). The gated blood pool approach is the preferred RNA technique to follow these patients because it offers the additional information of stroke volume ratios which allows quantitation of the severity of regurgitation.

Finally, exercise radionuclide angiography is useful to differentiate cardiac from pulmonary etiologies in patients with exertional dyspnea.[134]

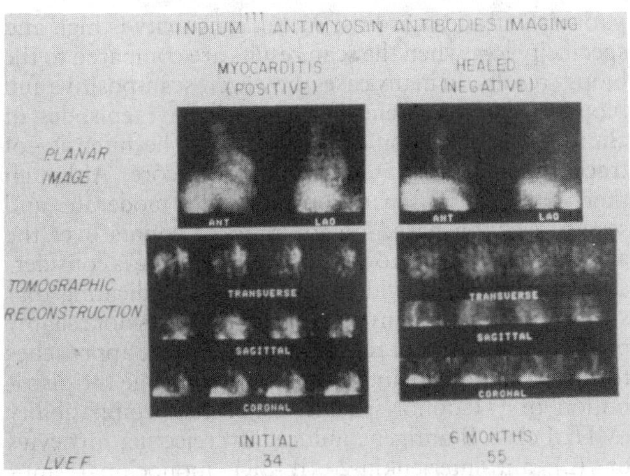

FIGURE 134-34 ^{111}In antimyosin antibody planar and tomographic images in a patient with myocarditis showing a diffuse pattern of uptake (left) which became negative 6 mo later (right) as the patient's ventricular function improved. This was documented by the rise in LVEF shown on the bottom. (*Courtesy of Dr. William Dec.*)

IMAGING OF MYOCARDIAL INFLAMMATION

Myocarditis and cardiac allograft rejection involve both inflammatory infiltrates and myocyte necrosis. Accordingly, the radionuclide-imaging strategies for detection of these two conditions utilize approaches to label inflammatory infiltrates or necrotic myocytes. Lymphocytes tagged with ^{111}In have been used as a means for labeling inflammatory cells. It is a technically difficult procedure and blood pool background activity makes imaging of the myocardial inflammation difficult.

Gallium-67

Gallium-67 (^{67}Ga) is a gamma-emitting radionuclide with multiple-energy photopeaks and relatively long half-life, which is taken up into sites of inflammation and sites of hematological and other malignancies. Because imaging of gallium is cumbersome, its clinical usefulness has declined as other agents, especially radiolabeled antibodies, have been developed. Myocardial uptake of ^{67}Ga is observed in patients with viral myocarditis and new onset cardiomyopathy.[176] Conversion of the scan from positive to negative has been observed to correspond to clinical improvement in patients with myocarditis.[177] Gallium uptake also can be observed in patients with sarcoidosis localized to sites throughout the body corresponding to involvement of organs including the heart with the granulomatous process.[178]

Indium-111 Antimyosin

^{111}In-labeled antimyosin has been used to identify both myocarditis and cardiac allograft rejection in patients with recent onset of heart failure, i.e., less than 6 months.[179] Using the endomyocardial biopsy as the gold standard, one group found that the sensitivity of antimyosin for detecting myocarditis was 83 percent but the specificity was only 53 percent. Low specificity was attributed, in part, to persistent blood pool activity and to false negative biopsies due to sampling error.[180] In support of the latter explanation was the spontaneous improvement in left ventricular function that occurred in biopsy-negative and scan-positive patients supporting the diagnosis of an inflammatory, partially reversible, myocardial process (Fig. 134-34).

Myocyte necrosis is a hallmark of cardiac allograft rejection. Antimyosin imaging has been performed in several series of patients after cardiac transplant in close proximity to the endomyocardial biopsy (Fig. 134-35).[181–184] The findings are similar to the results in

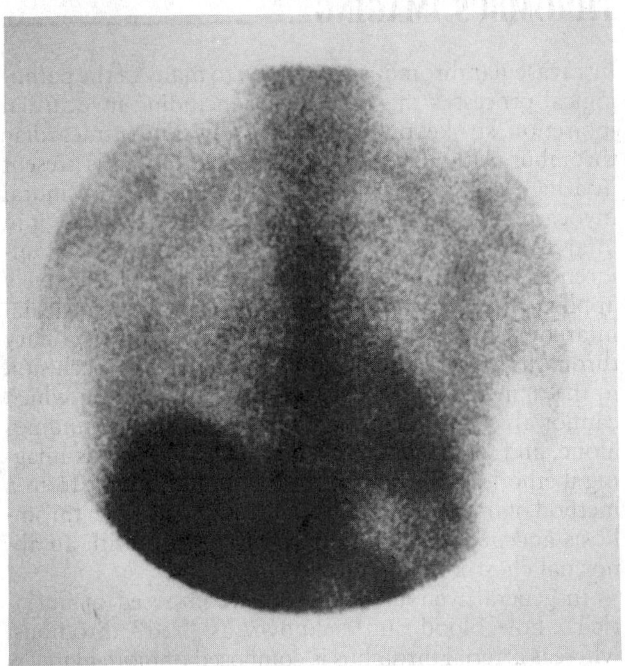

FIGURE 134-35 Planar scan acquired 48 h following injection of ^{111}In antimyosin antibody into a cardiac transplant patient. The scan shows diffuse myocardial uptake. The patient had moderately severe rejection by endomyocardial biopsy including histopathological evidence for myocyte necrosis. (*Courtesy of Ignasio Carria, M.D.*).

patients with myocarditis. Again, sensitivity is high and specificity low when the scan results are compared to the biopsy results. In many cases, however, scan-positive and biopsy-negative patients went on to have episodes of clinical rejection soon after the scan. The intensity of tracer uptake correlates with biopsy score. Although there is a general separation into mild, moderate, and severe rejection based on the ratio of counts over the allograft normalized to the lung counts, there is considerable overlap of individual data points, indicating that such quantitation of myocardial uptake does not reliably predict the severity of rejection. More recent approaches for detecting transplant rejection are to image the distribution of (1) donor-specific major histocompatibility (MHC) class II antigens induced on rejecting myocytes or (2) anti-interleukin-2 (IL-2R) monoclonal antibodies.[185,186]

A late complication in patients after cardiac transplantation, which has been evaluated using radionuclide-imaging methods, is vasculopathy. Coronary atherosclerosis occurs in 40 to 50 percent of patients surviving 5 years following transplant.[187] Since the transplanted heart is denervated, patients do not develop angina with ischemia and frequently present with sudden death.[188] As a result of the diffuse nature of the atherosclerotic process, even the coronary arteriogram may show no significant discrete stenosis.[189,190] Two studies examined perfusion imaging as a means to diagnose allograft vasculopathy and showed poor diagnostic accuracy.[191,192] However, a more recent study demonstrated fair sensitivity and specificity values using treadmill exercise and SPECT imaging with either ^{201}Tl or ^{99m}Tc sestamibi as the perfusion agent.[193]

THROMBUS IMAGING

Intravascular thrombus is common to many of the pathological processes that affect man including myocardial infarction, stroke, pulmonary embolus, and intracardiac thrombus. Although coronary artery thrombus is present in a high percentage of patients with acute transmural myocardial infarction, it is not as consistently present in infarct-related vessels in non-Q-wave myocardial infarction.[194,195] Thrombolytic therapy could be effectively applied in selected patients with non-Q-wave myocardial infarction if a means existed to image intracoronary thrombus noninvasively. Another problem is reocclusion in the immediate post-PTCA period, a condition which cannot always be determined from the clinical findings alone, and which would benefit from a thrombus-imaging method. Other diagnoses that would benefit from a method of imaging thrombi include deep leg-vein thrombosis and pulmonary embolism in patients with an abnormal chest x-ray.

In general, venous thrombus is composed of fibrin-rich whole blood and is known as "red" thrombus, whereas arterial thrombus is composed of more platelets and is therefore known as "white" thrombus. While there is a broad spectrum in composition of arterial and venous thrombi, imaging arterial thrombi has involved labeled platelets and imaging venous thrombi has used labeled fibrinogen, or fibrin. The radiotracer methods of imaging need to label the thrombus rapidly with minimal blood pool activity.

Platelet Imaging

For more than a decade, thrombus imaging has been performed using autologous platelets labeled with ^{111}In. Such labeled platelets have been used to image mural thrombi. Several studies have compared platelet imaging to 2-D echocardiography for detection of mural thrombus in patients with anterior infarctions or cardiomyopathy.[196,197] Indium-labeled platelet imaging was specific but less sensitive than echocardiography. Nevertheless, it appears that radiolabeled platelet imaging can detect thrombus activity and predict systemic embolization better than the echo.[198] The labeling technique is time consuming and laborious. Because the average life span of a platelet is approximately nine days, blood pool activity is a problem, and diagnostic images are not obtained until as late as 48 or 72 h after IV administration. Further, the dosimetry of ^{111}In is unfavorable due to its relatively long half life. To overcome such technical drawbacks, monoclonal antibodies to components of activated platelets have been developed using hybridoma technology. One platelet antibody under investigation is called S12, an Fab′ fragment of an antibody directed against glycoprotein membrane protein 140 (GMP-140), which is a component of alpha granules that upon platelet activation is translocated from the internal to the external platelet membrane. The Fab′ fragment is labeled with ^{99m}Tc and thus has favorable energy and dosimetry. In a rabbit model of atherosclerosis induced by arterial injury, uptake of ^{99m}Tc-labeled S12 antibody to platelet alpha granules at sites of arterial endothelial injury was observed.[199] Another antibody to platelet presently under development—50H.19—is against the glycoprotein IIb/IIIa complex present on the platelet membrane. Fab′ monoclonal antibody fragments of this antibody labeled with ^{99m}Tc have been used to image experimental thrombi in both peripheral veins and arteries.[200] Larger amounts of this antibody can decrease platelet aggregation in vitro, prolong the bleeding time in vivo, and prevent coronary artery reocclusion after reperfusion in an animal model.[201-204] Both of these platelet antibodies (S12 and 50H.19) have fairly rapid blood pool clearances allowing imaging at about 2 h after injection. Other approaches to intravascular thrombus imaging involving platelets include labeling and administering platelet components such as the protein, thrombospondin,[205] and annexin-V, a substance which becomes exposed on the platelet surface with activation.[206]

Fibrin Imaging

Early studies using ^{131}I and ^{125}I labeled fibrinogen demonstrated uptake in acute coronary artery thrombi, both in an experimental preparation and in patients.[207,208] Labeled fibrinogen leads to high blood pool activity and both iodine radiotracers have poor imaging properties. Hui et al. were the first to develop an antifibrin antibody without crossreactivity with fibrinogen.[209] This antibody, called 59D8, as well as another antibody against the same fibrin region, called T2G1s, have been demon-

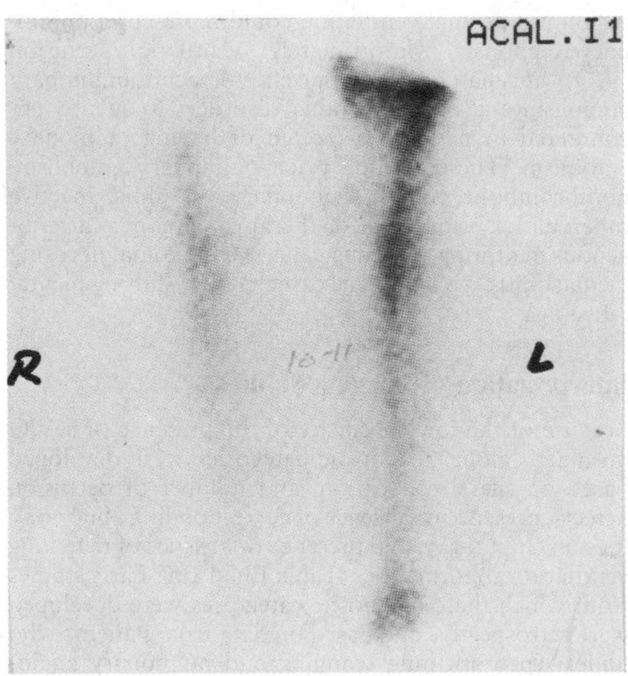

FIGURE 134-36 Image depicting the distribution of ^{99m}Tc-labeled antifibrin antibody in a 71-year-old woman 11 days after a total knee replacement. The image was acquired 6 h after IV administration of the monoclonal antibody. Antibody distribution on the left calf corresponded to a region with an acute deep vein thrombosis as documented by radiographic venography. *(From GM Pohost, R O'Rourke: Principles and Practice of Cardiovascular Imaging. Boston, Little, Brown, 1991: 286. Reproduced with permission.)*

strated to allow imaging of both arterial and venous thrombi.[210,211] Clinical trials using 59D8 to diagnose venous thrombotic disease have been reported[212–214] (Fig. 134-36). This approach was demonstrated to be reasonably accurate for diagnosing deep venous thrombosis without false positives but with a substantial incidence of false negative scans. Sequential imaging helps improve the sensitivity over a single imaging procedure. Concomitant heparin therapy does not appear to affect accuracy.[213]

Another antifibrin antibody, GC4, is targeted to partially digested fibrin. This epitope is exposed even later in the process of thrombus formation than the epitope to which T2G1s is targeted. Radiolabeled T2G1s and GC4 were compared in a dog model in which both antibodies were injected and the ratios of uptake of the two were compared in fresh and 3-day-old thrombus.[215] The GC4 antibody was found to bind more avidly to older thrombus than the T2G1s. Therefore, GC4 may be a better agent for use in diagnosis of deep vein thrombosis since patients usually present with formed clot.

One study evaluated an antifibrin antibody (64C5) for imaging pulmonary emboli in an animal model.[216] These investigators found that this antibody to fibrin could detect larger pulmonary emboli.

Other Approaches to Imaging Thrombus and Atherosclerotic Plaque

Another approach to imaging intravascular thrombi is to use radiolabeled t-PA. To be used successfully, the enzyme must be inactivated so that it will not lyse the clot and produce radiolabeled degradation products that increase background and decrease image quality. Ord et al. modified t-PA to reduce release of such radiolabeled degradation products from the liver.[217] These investigators attempted to image coronary and carotid thrombi in a canine model. They could not visualize a coronary thrombus using a modified t-PA labeled with ^{131}I and planar imaging. However, using ^{123}I labeling to optimize imaging properties of the tracer and SPECT imaging to improve image contrast, they were able to depict carotid thrombi.

Finally, the ability to image atherosclerotic plaque would provide a means to assess the activity and location of the disease. At the present time, radionuclide imaging of atherosclerotic plaque in man is suboptimal. The most promising approach involves the use of ^{99m}Tc-labeled low density lipoprotein (LDL). Sequestration of LDL was demonstrated by planar imaging in carotid, iliac, and femoral vessels in patients.[218] These investigators also found that the extent of LDL uptake correlated with plaque activity as assessed by histopathologic evaluation. The more active the plaque, the more abundant the foam cells and macrophages.

LUNG SCANNING

The incidence of pulmonary embolism is not well known but among hospitalized patients is probably substantial. Left untreated, the mortality from pulmonary embolism has been estimated to be about 30 percent. Anticoagulation significantly improves outcome in patients who have a high probability of pulmonary embolism, while the risks from hemorrhage secondary to anticoagulation are outweighed by the therapeutic benefits. In a patient unlikely to have pulmonary embolism, however, the risks of anticoagulation are not justified. The clinical suspicion for pulmonary embolism arises frequently in the care for hospitalized patients on the medical and surgical services (see also Chap. 100).

Establishing a diagnosis of pulmonary embolism from clinical information and routine laboratory data is usually not possible. The symptoms and signs of pulmonary embolism are nonspecific, and the highest incidence is among hospitalized patients with comorbid disease such as heart and lung disease, which further confounds interpretation. Dyspnea is the most common symptom but is difficult to distinguish from intrinsic lung disease or heart failure. Chest pain, when present, may be confused with pleurisy, pneumonia, or myocardial infarction. The classic triad of dyspnea, chest pain, and hemoptysis occurs in only about 20 percent of patients.

Abnormalities in several routine laboratory tests including arterial blood gases, ECG, and chest film may be helpful in supporting the diagnosis but are also nonspecific. The laboratory test that is considered the "gold standard" for pulmonary embolism is pulmonary angiography. This procedure, however, is invasive, costly, and not without risk, especially in patients with pulmonary hypertension. Practically, pulmonary angiography cannot be performed on all patients suspected of having pulmonary embolism because of the large number of hospitalized patients in whom this diagnosis is entertained. A more noninvasive screening test is necessary. Despite all of its shortcomings as outlined below, lung scanning remains a very frequently ordered test.

Method

Lung scanning combines the imaging of regional lung perfusion and the imaging of pulmonary ventilation.[219–221] To image regional perfusion, radiolabeled particles are injected slowly into an arm vein. Either ^{99m}Tc macroaggregated albumin or ^{99m}Tc serum albumin microspheres can be used (10–60 μm in size). These radioactive particles are trapped in the pulmonary capillaries and precapillary arterioles. Accordingly, the distribution of these macroaggregates or microspheres is closely related to regional pulmonary blood flow. In a healthy person, only 0.1 percent of the cross-sectional area of the pulmonary vascular bed is occluded by the microspheres and therefore may have no effect on cardiac output. In patients with chronic lung disease and in those with primary pulmonary hypertension, the pulmonary vascular bed is reduced and the number of particles administered must be reduced to maintain a safety margin for maintenance of flow through the pulmonary bed. An adequate perfusion lung scan consists of at least six views: anterior, posterior, left and right lateral views, and left and right posterior oblique views. Multiple views are necessary to visualize the pulmonary segments adequately.

Pathologically, a pulmonary embolism represents the occlusion of a pulmonary artery by embolic material leading to regional reduction in blood flow; this can be detected by perfusion-imaging defects, or "cold" areas. However, many other conditions can also produce regional reductions in blood flow. These include extrinsic compression of pulmonary vessels due to tumor or disease of the vessel walls, such as vasculitis; compressed lung; bronchial–pulmonary collaterals; arteriovenous communications; pulmonary venous hypertension; and alveolar hypoxia.

The addition of ventilation scanning improves the specificity of perfusion scanning alone to detect pulmonary embolism. Ventilation scanning is performed using inhalation of radioisotopes of noble gases or aerosols, including ^{133}Xe, ^{127}Xe, ^{81m}Kr, and ^{99m}Tc-monodispersed aerosol. Ventilation scanning protocols differ somewhat among laboratories. Generally, when using ^{133}Xe; ventilation imaging is performed in the posterior view and includes wash-in, equilibrium, and wash-out phases. The equilibrium phase image shows the aerated volume of lung. In most normals, xenon is cleared in approximately 1 to 3 min during the wash-out phase. This phase is the most sensitive for detection of air trapping due to the airway obstruction of chronic obstructive lung disease, which can appear as "cold" zones on a lung perfusion image. If ventilation imaging is performed using a ^{99m}Tc DTPA aerosol, the same six static images are obtained as in the perfusion scan; however, since the radionuclide is the same, the dynamics of wash-in and wash-out cannot be evaluated.

Ventilation imaging detects regional airway abnormalities producing defects that may not be apparent on the chest film.[219–221] A lung segment that has reduced perfusion but normal ventilation could represent a pulmonary embolism. Unfortunately, ventilation-perfusion (V/Q) "mismatch" is not specific for acute pulmonary embolism and occurs in other disorders frequently encountered in patients suspected of having pulmonary embolism. These include prior pulmonary embolism, nonthrombotic emboli, pulmonary vasculitis, inactive tuberculosis, prior radiation therapy, pulmonary arteriovenous malformation, lung cancer, lymphoma, fibrosing mediastinitis, a Swan-Ganz catheter, and shifting pleural effusions.

Interpretation of Imaging Studies

Because of the low specificity of the presence of a V/Q mismatch alone, diagnostic categories were developed based on the size, location, and number of perfusion defects, presence or absence of corresponding abnormalities on chest x-ray, and presence or absence of matching ventilation abnormalities (Table 134-12).[222] Early studies from which these diagnostic categories were developed were retrospective and based on data from patients who underwent both lung scanning and pulmonary angiography. More recently, the results of an NIH-sponsored multicenter prospective clinical trial were reported. The trial was called the PIOPED trial (Prospective Investigation of Pulmonary Embolism Diagnosis), and the purpose of the trial was to determine the true sensitivity and specificity of the lung scan.[223] It included 6 clinical centers that enrolled 1493 patients, 931 of whom completed V/Q scanning and 755 of whom underwent pulmonary angiography, which was considered to represent the "gold standard." Based on the results of those patients who underwent angiography, the prevalence of pulmonary embolism was 33 percent. Scans were classified into high, intermediate (indeterminant), and low probability categories on the basis of criteria similar to those described above (Table 134-12). From the sample of 931 scans, 13 percent were interpreted as high probability, 39 percent as medium probability, 34 percent as low probability, and 13 percent as normal. The sensitivity of a high probability scan was low (41 percent), but the specificity high (97 percent). If high and intermediate results were lumped together, the sensitivity increased to 82 percent, but the specificity fell to 52 percent. For all three categories together, the overall sensitivity was 98 percent, but the specificity was down to 10 percent. Taking into account the incidence of pulmonary embolism in the population, the positive predictive value for a high probability scan was 88 percent; lower in patients with prior pulmonary embolism. The negative predictive value for a low probability scan was 84 percent, and if all clinical data were added together to establish the presumptive diagnosis, the negative predictive value rose to 88 percent.

The criteria for determining when to perform pulmonary angiography in patients with suspected pulmonary embolism and abnormal V/Q scans are controversial, but the following is one approach. A normal lung scan study rules out a pulmonary embolism, and no further tests need to be performed. A high probability lung scan confirms the diagnosis and indicates anticoagulation and consideration of thrombolysis (Fig. 134-37). A low prob-

TABLE 134-12
Lung Scan Interpretation

Interpretation	Description	Percentage with PE
Normal/very low probability	No perfusion defects Nonsegmental perfusion defects (due to small effusion, cardiomegaly, or elevated diaphragm)	0
Low probability	Any perfusion defect with a larger radiographic abnormality Small segmental defect with normal CXR Small V/Q mismatch	<10
Intermediate	One moderate segmental V/Q mismatch without any radiographic abnormality Widespread severe COPD Perfusion defects not falling into other categories	20–40
High	Two or more large segmental perfusion defects without corresponding ventilation or radiographic defects Two or more moderate segmental perfusion defects (>25% and <75% of a segment) without matching ventilation or radiographic defects and one large mismatched segmental defect Four or more moderate unmatched perfusion defects	>85

ability scan in a patient with a low clinical likelihood for pulmonary embolism and without unexplained abnormal supportive laboratory data rules out significant pulmonary embolism and obviates the need for further work-up. Reports on follow-up of these patients show they do not develop subsequent episodes of pulmonary embolism.[224] In a patient with a high clinical suspicion for pulmonary embolism and a low probability scan, however, further diagnostic work-up, including evaluation of the leg veins by plethysmography, venography,

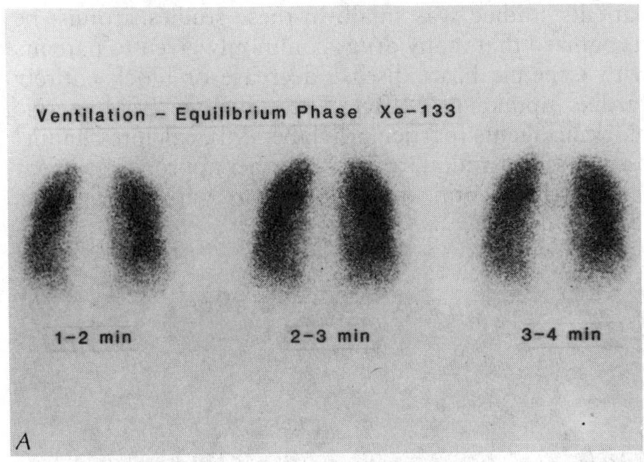

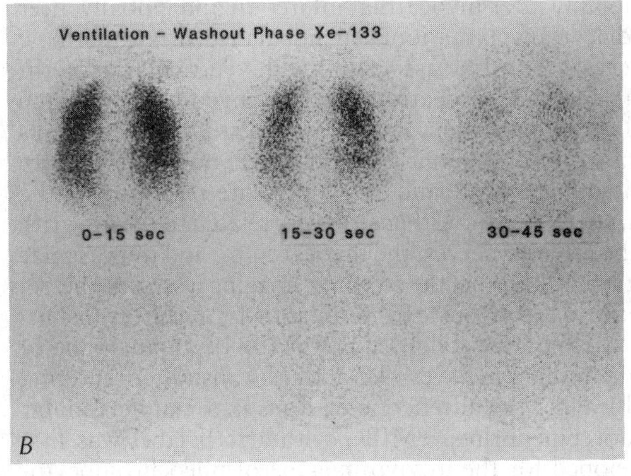

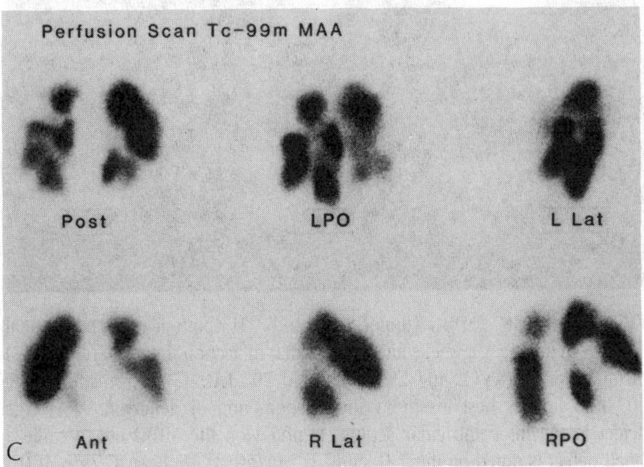

FIGURE 134–37 *A.* Homogenous distribution of xenon-133 during the equilibrium phase of the ventilation study reflects normal patency of the bronchial tree in both lungs. *B.* Rapid and symmetrical clearance of ^{133}Xe during the wash-out phase excludes obstructive lung disease. *C.* Multiple bilateral segmental and subsegmental defects on six standard views of the perfusion scintigram obtained with 4 mCi of ^{99m}Tc MAA in the same patient are typical for high-probability study for pulmonary embolus. (*Courtesy of Eva Dubovsky, M.D.*)

or antifibrin imaging, should be performed. If peripheral venous thrombosis is documented, the patient should be anticoagulated as if he/she had a pulmonary embolism. If the leg vein studies are negative, and the clinical suspicion is still high, then the patient should undergo pulmonary angiography. Decision-making paths for the intermediate probability scans are similar to those outlined for low probability scans (see also Chap. 100).

The results of the lung scan, clinical history, other supportive laboratory data, and evaluation of the peripheral veins can aid the physician in his/her decision concerning anticoagulation therapy in over half of the patients who present with clinical symptoms suggesting pulmonary embolism. In the remaining patients, pulmonary angiography will be necessary to confirm or exclude the diagnosis. Another radionuclide imaging approach that has the potential to improve sensitivity and specificity is intravascular thrombus imaging using radiolabeled antiplatelet or antifibrin antibodies. To date, however, data from animal studies suggest that only large, central emboli can be successfully imaged using these techniques.

CARDIAC SYMPATHETIC NEURONAL IMAGING

The sympathetic nerves of the autonomic nervous system are important for the regulation of cardiac function. The integrity of the sympathetic nerves is interrupted regionally after myocardial infarction and globally after cardiac transplantation. An imbalance in sympathetic innervation can be associated with ventricular arrhythmias and sudden death in the prolonged QT syndrome and in patients after myocardial infarction.[225] Methods to study the adrenergic nervous system noninvasively are limited. Heart rate and blood pressure responses of the heart to exercise or other stress are related to the integrity of the afferent nerves, the myocardium, and the vascular system. Radionuclide receptor imaging assesses the response of the myocyte to stimulation by a neurotransmitter. Metaiodobenzylguanidine (MIBG), an analogue of guanethidine, behaves like a neurotransmitter, entering and leaving the adrenergic neurons in a manner similar to norepinephrine.[226] MIBG with an ^{131}I label was first developed for the in vivo imaging of pheochromocytomas.[227,228] More recently the agent has been labeled with ^{123}I, which has much better imaging properties and dosimetry than ^{131}I, and applied to in vivo imaging of the cardiac adrenergic nervous system.[229]

Cardiac imaging with ^{123}I MIBG has been largely restricted to use as a research tool and has limited availability as a clinical test due to the limited production and resultant high cost of ^{123}I.[230] Purified ^{123}I has excellent imaging properties with a 13.3-h half-life and a 159 keV photopeak. It is cyclotron produced, however, and has three undesirable impurities (^{124}I, ^{125}I, ^{126}I) that increase the radiation dose. Thus, another factor contributing to its cost is the process of ^{123}I purification.

There are two pathways for cardiac uptake of MIBG: high affinity uptake by postganglionic sympathetic nerves, and nonspecific (extraneuronal) uptake probably representing simple diffusion.[231] Neuronally bound MIBG is retained, whereas the extraneuronally bound tracer is rapidly metabolized and not retained.[232] Images obtained 3 to 4 h after injection are thought to represent essentially neuronally bound MIBG. Another approach to minimizing contamination of activity from extraneuronal uptake is to administer clonidine, a drug that inhibits extraneuronal myocardial uptake of catecholamines prior to administration of MIBG.[223]

A number of experimental studies have demonstrated that MIBG uptake is an indicator of adrenergic integrity (or injury) and function.[234] Cardiac uptake of MIBG is blocked by imipramine, which blocks high affinity uptake of norepinephrine, and by reserpine, which blocks norepinephrine storage.[226] In addition, competitive uptake between MIBG and norepinephrine analogs (phenylpropanolamine) has been demonstrated.[226] Uptake of MIBG is decreased with injury to adrenergic neurons.[232]

MIBG imaging has been applied to the detection of myocardial sympathetic imbalance after myocardial infarction. The efferent sympathetic nerves travel over the epicardial surface of the heart from base to apex and are interrupted in the myocardial territory distal to regions of transmural myocardial infarction. In one study, both MIBG and thallium imaging were performed after myocardial infarction. Regions with decreased MIBG uptake and homogenous thallium uptake were observed[235] that could identify patients with sympathetic imbalance at risk for malignant ventricular arrhythmias (Fig. 134-38). The sensitivity and specificity of this imaging approach could not be assessed, however, since the number of patients studied was small. In these studies, it must be recognized that many drugs commonly given to patients with ischemic heart disease decrease or block entirely cardiac uptake of MIBG. These include β-adrenergic blocking agents (particularly labetalol), calcium channel blockers, and amiodarone.[236] Another approach to imaging for the identification of patients with sympathetic

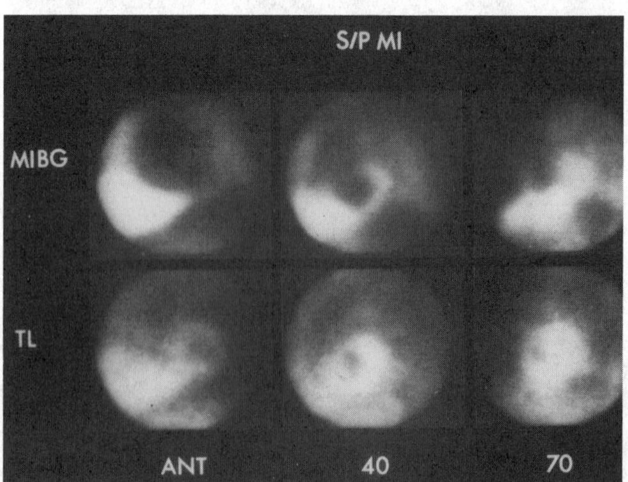

FIGURE 134-38 MIBG (upper row) and ^{201}Tl (bottom row) myocardial imaging in a patient 2 weeks after myocardial infarction. Images are depicted in the anterior (ANT), 40° LAO (40), and 70° LAO (70) projections. The 40° LAO images best exemplify the phenomenon of denervation. A large defect in the interventricular septum is noted on the MIBG image while a small defect is noted on the ^{201}Tl study. (*Courtesy of Michael W. Dae, M.D.*)

imbalance after infarction is to use the β-receptor antagonist iodocyanopindolol labeled with ^{123}I. This agent has been used experimentally to demonstrate intact adrenergic receptors in regions of ^{201}Tl uptake and absent MIBG uptake.[237]

Abnormal MIBG studies can be found in association with neuropathies presumably involving the cardiac sympathetic nerves. Sudden death has been reported in patients with the prolonged QT syndrome and MIBG/^{201}Tl mistmatches.[234] Diffusely decreased cardiac uptake of MIBG has been found in patients with generalized neuropathy due to diabetes mellitus or the Shy Drager syndrome.[234] Abnormal MIBG studies have been reported in patients with inherited and acquired neuropathies.

In addition to patients with coronary artery disease and neuropathy patients, abnormal MIBG studies have been reported in patients with idiopathic dilated cardiomyopathy and after cardiac transplantation documenting sympathetic denervation and reinnervation. In patients with idiopathic dilated cardiomyopathy, MIBG imaging demonstrates moderate to marked diffuse reduction compared to normals; myocardial wash-out measured over 16 h is also faster when compared to normals.[238,239] It was hypothesized that the diffuse decrease in myocardial uptake of the radiotracer reflects damage to sympathetic neurons, and faster wash-out reflects the increase in autonomic nervous system activity in this condition, i.e., higher than normal levels of circulating norepinephrine.[238] Also, it has been observed that cardiac uptake of MIBG correlated with ejection fraction and with myocardial norepinephrine concentrations measured from endomyocardial biopsy specimens.

In a small group of postcardiac transplant patients imaged within 6 months of surgery, graft uptake of MIBG was <10 percent of normal in the first 2 h and negligible by 16 h.[238] Serial PET imaging studies done after cardiac transplantation using the epinephrine analog, ^{11}C-HED, demonstrated absence of uptake soon after transplantation; this is consistent with total cardiac denervation. But there was focal uptake in the anterolateral left ventricular wall 1 year or more after transplantation, which is consistent with focal reinnervation.[240]

METABOLIC IMAGING

Although myocardial metabolism can be evaluated with single-photon-emitting radiotracers, PET imaging presently provides the best noninvasive approach for the clinical assessment of cardiac metabolism. The other modality that can evaluate myocardial metabolism in vivo is magnetic resonance spectroscopy. While this tool is presently in its research phase, it has great promise as a clinically relevant methodology for the future.

To study myocardial metabolism, several positron-emitting radiotracers have been used. Carbon-11 provides an important radionuclide that can be incorporated into several relevant molecular species such as fatty acids, glucose, lactate, pyruvate, ketone bodies, acetate, and amino acids.[241] Fluorine-18 with a half-life of approximately 2 h has been coupled to 2-deoxyglucose to form ^{18}F-fluoro-2-deoxyglucose as a means to assess glycolytic metabolism. ^{11}C has been incorporated into palmitic acid to form a fatty acid tracer to study oxidative metabolism. Finally, ^{11}C-labeled acetate has been used for evaluating the activity of the tricarboxylic cycle. These three radiopharmaceuticals (^{18}F-fluorodeoxyglucose, ^{11}C-palmitic acid, and ^{11}C-acetate) have been used to assess the metabolic consequences of an ischemic insult.[242]

For cardiologic purposes, the most clinically relevant PET agent is ^{18}F-fluorodeoxyglucose, which is used in conjunction with a myocardial perfusion tracer to assess myocardial viability in patients with ischemic heart disease.[243,244] Generally, ^{13}N-ammonia is administered to assess regional myocardial perfusion, however, ^{82}Rb can also be used to evaluate perfusion. Defects in the distribution of the perfusion tracer may represent ischemia or infarction. Ischemic zones are metabolically active and will extract fluorodeoxyglucose as evidence of anaerobic glycolysis. Glycolytic activity also can be observed in nonischemic portions of the myocardium. The PET approach, using a perfusion tracer and fluorodeoxyglucose, appears to be the best noninvasive method for assessing viability. In view of its cost, however, most clinicians will settle for a thallium study with redistribution and/or reinjection as the cost-effective means for assessing viability.

Positron emission tomography has also been used to evaluate metabolism in patients with cardiomyopathy. In idiopathic dilated cardiomyopathy, myocardial distribution of ^{11}C-palmitate has been observed to be heterogeneous.[245,246] This could merely represent interspersed fibrosis commonly observed in cardiomyopathies. In patients with hypertrophic cardiomyopathy, the pattern of uptake of the perfusion agents ^{13}N-ammonia and ^{18}F-fluorodeoxyglucose was normal, even in the subendocardial region.[247] In contrast, in Duchenne's muscular dystrophy, the pattern of uptake of these two tracers was similar to patterns seen in ischemia with abnormal zones corresponding to regions of hypokinesis generally in the posterolateral wall.[248]

REFERENCES

1. Anger HO: Scintillation camera. *Rev Sci Inst* 1958; 29:27–32.
2. Sorenson JA, Phelps ME: The Anger Camera: Performance characteristics. In: *Physics in Nuclear Medicine.* Philadelphia, Saunders, 1987:298–317.
3. Sorenson JA, Phelps ME: Pulse-height spectrometry. In: *Physics in Nuclear Medicine.* Philadelphia, Saunders, 1987:219–237.
4. Esser PD (ed): *Digital Imaging: Clinical Advances in Nuclear Medicine.* New York, Society of Nuclear Medicine, 1982.
5. Williams DL, Ritchie JL, Harp GD, Caldwell JH, Hamilton GW, Eisner RL, et al: Preliminary characterization of the properties of a transaxial whole-body single-photon tomograph: Emphasis on future application to cardiac imaging. In: Esser PD (ed): *Functional Mapping of Organ Systems.* New York, Society of Nuclear Medicine, 1981:149–160.
6. Brooks RA, DiChiro G: Theory of image reconstruction in computed tomography. *Radiology* 1975; 117:561–572.
7. Grenier RP, Bender MA, Jones RH: A computerized multicrystal scintillation gamma camera. In: Hine G, Thorenson JA (eds): *Instrumentation in Nuclear Medicine,* Vol. 2. New York, Academic, 1974:101–134.
8. Phelps ME, Hoffman EJ, Mullani NA, Higgins CS, Ter-Pogossian MM: Design considerations for a positron emission transaxial tomograph (PET III). *Trans Nucl Sci* 1976; NS-23:516–522.

9. Bonow RO, Berman DS, Gibbons RJ, Johnson LL, Rumberger JA, Schwaiger M, et al: Cardiac positron emission tomography. *Circulation* 1991; 84:447–454.
10. Zimmer L, McCall D, D'Addabbo L, Whitney K: Kinetics and characteristics of thallium exchange in cultured cells. (Abstr.) *Circulation* 1979; 60(II):138.
11. Leppo JA, Meerdink DJ: Comparative myocardial extraction of two technetium labeled BATO derivatives (SQ30217,S32014) and thallium. *J Nucl Med* 1990; 31:67–74.
12. Welsh HF, Strauss HW, Pitt HB: The extraction of thallium-201 by the myocardium. *Circulation* 1977; 56:188-191.
13. Okada RD, Jacobs ML, Daggett WM, Leppo J, Strauss HW, Newell JB, et al: Thallium-201 kinetics in nonischemic canine myocardium. *Circulation* 1982; 65:70–77.
14. Pohost GM, Zir LM, Moor RH, McKusick KA, Guiney TE, Beller GA: Differentiation of transiently ischemic from infarcted myocardium by serial imaging after single dose of thallium-201. *Circulation* 1977; 55:294–302.
15. Nielson AP, Morris KG, Murdock R, Bruno FP, Cobb FR: Linear relationship between the distribution of thallium-201 and blood flow in ischemic and nonischemic myocardium during exercise. *Circulation* 1980; 61:797–801.
16. Strauss HW, Pitt B: Noninvasive detection of subcritical coronary arterial narrowings with a coronary vasodilator and myocardial perfusion imaging. *Am J Cardiol* 1977; 39:403–406.
17. Gould KL: Noninvasive assessment of coronary stenoses by myocardial perfusion imaging during pharmacologic coronary vasodilation. *Am J Cardiol* 1978; 41:267–278.
18. McCall D, Zimmer L, D'Addabbo L, Whitney K: Modification of thallium-201 uptake in cultured myocardial cells. (Abstr.) *Circulation* 1979; 60:138.
19. Okada RD, Pohost GM: Effect of decreased blood flow and ischemia on myocardial thallium clearance. *J Am Coll Cardiol* 1984; 3:744–750.
20. Bonow RD, Dilsizian V, Cuocolo A, Bacharach SL: Identification of viable myocardium in patients with chronic coronary artery disease and left ventricular dysfunction: Comparison of thallium scintigraphy with reinjection and PET imaging with ^{18}F-fluorodeoxyglucose. *Circulation* 1991; 83:326–337.
21. Kiat H, Berman DS, Maddahi J, Yang LD, Van Train K, Rozanski A, et al: Late reversibility of tomographic myocardial thallium-201 defects: An accurate marker of myocardial viability. *J Am Coll Cardiol* 1988; 12:1456–1463.
22. Dilsizian V, Rocco T, Freedman NMT, Leon MB, Bonow RO: Enhanced detection of ischemic but viable myocardium by the reinjection of thallium after stress-redistribution imaging. *N Engl J Med* 1990; 323:141–146.
23. Berger BC, Watson DD, Burwell LR, Crosby IK, Wellons HA, Teates CD, et al: Redistribution of thallium at rest in patients with stable and unstable angina and the effect of coronary artery bypass surgery. *Circulation* 1979; 60:1114–1125.
24. Gerwitz H, Beller GA, Strauss HW, Dinsmore RE, Zir LM, McKusick KA, et al: Transient defects on resting thallium scans in patients with coronary artery disease. *Circulation* 1979; 59:707–713.
25. Wackers FJT, Lie KL, Liem KL, Sokole EB, Samson G, van der Shoot JB, et al: Thallium-201 scintigraphy in unstable angina pectoris. *Circulation* 1978; 57:738–742.
26. Brown KA, Okada RD, Boucher CA, Phillips HR, Strauss HW, Pohost GM: Serial thallium-201 imaging at rest in patients with unstable and stable angina pectoris: Relationship of myocardial perfusion at rest to presenting clinical syndrome. *Am Heart J* 1983; 106:70–77.
27. Friedman J, Van Train K, Maddahi J, Hasegawa B, Bietendorf J, Waxman A, et al: "Upward creep" of the heart: A frequent source of false positive reversible defects on ^{201}Tl stress redistribution SPECT. (Abstr.) *J Nucl Med* 1986; 27:899.
28. Okada RD, Glover D, Gaffney T, Williams S: Myocardial kinetics of technetium-99m-hexakis-2-methoxy-2-methylpropylisonitrile. *Circulation* 1988; 77:491–498.
29. Maublart JC, Gachon P, Moins N: Hexakis (2-methoxy isobutyl isonitrile) ^{99m}Tc + thallium-201 chloride uptake and release in cultured myocardial cells. *J Nucl Med* 1988; 29:48–54.
30. Meerdink DJ, Leppo JA: Comparison of hypoxia and ouabain effects on the myocardial uptake kinetics of technetium-99m hexakis 2-methoxyisobutyl isonitrile and thallium-201. *J Nucl Med* 1989; 30:1500–1506.
31. Piwnica-Worms D, Kronauge JF, Holman BL, Lister-James J, Davison A, Jones AG: Hexakis (carbomethoxyisopropylisonitrile) technetium (I), a new myocardial perfusion imaging agent: Binding characteristics in cultured chick heart cells. *J Nucl Med* 1988; 29:55–61.
32. Piwnica-Worms D, Kronauge JF, Delmon L, Holman BL, Marsh JD, Jones AG: Effect of metabolic inhibition on technetium-99m-MIBI kinetics in cultured chick myocardial cells. *J Nucl Med* 1990; 31:464–472.
33. Chiu ML, Kronauge JF, Piwnica-Worms D. Effect of mitochondrial and plasma-membrane potentials on accumulation of hexakis (2-methoxyisobutylisonitrile)-technetium(I) in cultured mouse fibroblasts. *J Nucl Med* 1990; 31:1646–1653.
34. Leppo JA, Meerdink DJ: Comparison of the myocardial uptake of a technetium-labeled isonitrile analogue and thallium. *Circ Res* 1989; 65:632–639.
35. Wackers FJT, Berman DS, Maddahi J, Watson DD, Beller GA, Strauss HW, et al: Technetium-99m-hexakis 2-methoxy-isobutyl isonitrile: Human biodistibution, dosimetry, safety, and preliminary comparison to thallium-201 for myocardial perfusion imaging. *J Nucl Med* 1989; 30:301–311.
36. Canby RC, Silber S, Pohost GM: Relations of myocardial imaging agents ^{99m}Tc-MIBI and ^{201}Th to myocardial blood flow in a canine model of myocardial ischemic insult. *Circulation* 1990; 81:289–296.
37. Sinusas AJ, Watson DD, Cannon JM, Beller GA: Effect of ischemia and post ischemic dysfunction on myocardial uptake of technetium-99m labeled methoxyisobutyl isonitrile and thallium-201. *J Am Coll Cardiol* 1989; 14:1785–1793.
38. Okada RD, Pohost GM: The use of preintervention and postintervention thallium imaging for assessing the early and late effects of experimental coronary arterial reperfusion in dogs. *Circulation* 1984; 69:1153–1160.
39. Wackers FJT: Thrombolytic therapy for myocardial infarction: Assessment of efficacy by myocardial perfusion imaging with technetium-99m-sestamibi. *Am J Cardiol* 1990; 66:36E–41E.
40. Wackers FJT, Gibbons RJ, Verani MS, Kayden DS, Pellika PA, Behrenbeck T, et al: Serial quantitative planar technetium-99m-isonitrile imaging in acute myocardial infarction: Efficacy for noninvasive assessment of thrombolytic therapy. *J Am Coll Cardiol* 1989; 14:861–873.
41. Gibbons RJ, Verani MS, Behrenbeck T, Pellika PA, O'Connor MK, Mahmarian JJ, et al: Feasibility of tomographic ^{99m}Tc-hexakis-2-methoxy-2-methylpropylisonitrile imaging for the assessment of myocardial area at risk and the effect of treatment in acute myocardial infarction. *Circulation* 1989; 80:1277–1286.
42. Taillefer R, Laflamme L, Dupras G, Picard M, Pheneuf DC, Leveille J: Myocardial perfusion imaging with ^{99m}Tc-methoxy-isobutyl-isonitrile (MIBI): Comparison of short- and long-time intervals between rest and stress injection: Preliminary results. *Eur J Nucl Med* 1987; 13:515–522.
43. Narra RK, Nunn AD, Kuczynski BL, Feld T, Wedeking P, Eckelman WC: A neutral technetium-99m complex for myocardial imaging. *J Nucl Med* 1989; 30:1830–1837.
44. Stewart RE, Hutchins GD, Brown D, McClanahan TB, Gallagher KP, Petry NS, et al: Myocardial retention and clearance of the flow tracer ^{99m}Tc SQ30217 in canine heart. (Abstr.) *J Nucl Med* 1989; 30:860.
45. Marshall RC, Leidholdt EM Jr, Barnett CA: Single pass myocardial extraction and retention of a ^{99m}Tc isonitrile vs. ^{201}Tl. (Abstr.) *Circulation* 1990; 76:218.
46. Leppo JA, Meerdink DJ: Comparative myocardial extraction of two technetium-labeled BATO derivatives (SQ30217, SQ32014) and thallium. *J Nucl Med* 1990; 31:67–74.
47. Stewart RE, Schwaiger M, Hutchins GD, Chiao PC, Gallagher KP, Nguyen N, et al: Myocardial clearance kinetics of technetium-99m SQ30217: A marker of regional myocardial blood flow. *J Nucl Med* 1990; 31:1183–1190.
48. Seldin DW, Johnson LL, Blood DK, Muschel M, Smith KF, Wall RM, et al: Myocardial perfusion imaging with technetium-99m SQ30217: Comparison with thallium-201 and coronary anatomy. *J Nucl Med* 1989; 30:312–319.
49. Hendel RC, McSherry B, Karimeddini M, Leppo JA: Diagnostic value of a new myocardial perfusion agent, teboroxime (SQ30217) utilizing a rapid planar imaging protocol: Preliminary results. *J Am Coll Cardiol* 1990; 16:855–861.
50. Tamaki N, Yonekura Y, Senda M, Yamashita K, Koide H, Saji

H, et al: Value and limitation of stress thallium-201 single photon emission computed tomography: Comparison with nitrogen-13 ammonia positron tomography. *J Nucl Med* 1988; 29:1181–1188.

51. Stewart R, Kalus M, Molina E, Gacioch G, Squicciarini S, Hutchins G, et al: Rubidium-82 versus thallium-201 SPEC for the diagnosis of regional coronary artery disease. (Abstr.) *Circulation* 1989; 80:209.
52. Fitzgerald GA: Dipyridamole. *N Engl J Med* 1987; 316:1247–1257.
53. Leppo J, Boucher CA, Okada RD, Newell JB, Strauss HW, Pohost GM: Serial thallium-201 myocardial imaging after dipyridamole infusion: Diagnostic utility in detecting coronary stenosis and relationship to regional wall motion. *Circulation* 1982; 66:649–657.
54. Rozanski A: Personal communication.
55. Verani MS, Mahmarian JJ, Hixson JB, Boyce TM, Staudacher RA: Diagnosis of coronary artery disease by controlled coronary vasodilation with adenosine and thallium-201 scintigraphy in patients unable to exercise. *Circulation* 1990; 82:80–87.
56. Pennell DJ, Underwood SR, Swanton RH, Walker JM, Ell PJ: Dobutamine thallium myocardial perfusion tomography. *J Am Coll Cardiol* 1991; 18:1471–1479.
57. Okada RD, Boucher CA, Kirshenbaum HK, Kushner FG, Strauss HW, Block PC, et al: Improved diagnostic accuracy of ^{201}Tl stress test using multiple observers and criteria derived from interobserver analysis of variance. *Am J Cardiol* 1980; 46:619–624.
58. Boucher CA, Zir LM, Beller GA, Okada RD, McKusick KA, Strauss HW, et al: Increased lung uptake of thallium-201 during exercise myocardial imaging: Clinical hemodynamic and angiographic implications in patients with coronary artery disease. *Am J Cardiol* 1980;46:189–196.
59. Bingham JB, McKusick K, Strauss HW, Boucher CA, Pohost GM: Influence of coronary artery disease on pulmonary uptake of thallium-201. *Am J Cardiol* 1980;46:821–826.
60. Kusher FG, Okada RD, Kirschenbaum HD, Boucher CA, Strauss HW, Pohost GM: Lung thallium-201 uptake after stress testing in patients with coronary artery disease. *Circulation* 1981;63: 341–347.
61. Levy R, Rozanski A, Berman DS, Garcia E, Van Train K, Maddahi J, et al: Analysis of the degree of pulmonary thallium-201 washout in patients with coronary artery disease. *J Am Coll Cardiol* 1983;2:719–728.
62. Weiss AT, Bateman DS, Lew AS, Nielsen J, Potkin B, Swan HJC, et al: Transient ischemic dilatation of the left ventricle on stress thallium-201 scintigraphy: A marker of severe and extensive coronary artery disease. *J Am Coll Cardiol* 1987;9:752–759.
63. Burow RD, Pond IM, Schafer AW, Becker L: Circumferential profiles: A new method for computer analysis of thallium-201 myocardial perfusion images. *J Nucl Med* 1979;20:771–777.
64. Watson DD, Campbell NP, Read ED, Gibson RS, Teates CD, Beller GA: Spatial and temporal quantitation of planar thallium myocardial images. *J Nucl Med* 1981;22:557–584.
65. Goris ML, Daspit SG, McLaughlin P, Kriss JP: Interpolative background subtraction. *J Nucl Med* 1976;17:744–747.
66. Garcia EV, Van Train K, Maddahi J, Prigent F, Friedman J, Areeda J, et al: Quantification of rotational thallium-201 myocardial tomography. *J Nucl Med* 1985;26:17–26.
67. Van Train K, Berman D, Garcia EV, Berger HJ, Sands M, Friedman J, et al: Quantitative analysis of stress thallium-201 myocardial scintigrams: A multicenter trial. *J Nucl Med* 1986;27:17–25.
68. Diamond GA, Forrester JS: Analysis of probability as an aid to the clinical diagnosis of coronary artery disease. *N Engl J Med* 1979;300:1350–1358.
69. Maddahi J, Rodrigues E, Berman DS: Assessment of myocardial perfusion by single-photon agents. In: Pohost GM, O'Rourke RA (eds): *Principles and Practice of Cardiovascular Imaging*. Boston, Little Brown, 1991:202–204.
70. Marcus ML, Skorton DJ, Johnson MR, Collins SM, Harrison DG, Herber RE: Visual estimates of percent diameter coronary stenosis: "A battered gold standard." *J Am Coll Cardiol* 1988; 11:882–885.
71. Maddahi J, Rodrigues E, Berman DS: Assessment of myocardial perfusion by single-photon agents. In: Pohost GM, O'Rourke RA (eds): *Principles and Practice of Cardiovascular Imaging*. Boston, Little Brown, 1991:203.
72. Massie BM, Botvinick EH, Brundage BH: Correlation of thallium-201 scintigraphs with coronary anatomy: Factors affecting region by region sensitivity. *Am J Cardiol* 1979;44:616–622.
73. Rozanski A, Diamond G, Berman D, Forrester J, Morris D, Swan HJC: The declining specificity of exercise radionuclide ventriculography. *N Engl J Med* 1983;309:518–522.
74. Dilsizian V, Smeltzer WR, Freedman NMT, Dextras R, Bonow RO: Thallium reinjection after stress-redistribution imaging: Does 24-hour delayed imaging after reinjection enhance detection of viable myocardium? *Circulation* 1991;83:1237–1255.
75. Budinger TF, Pohost GM, Bischoff P: Thallium-201 integral concentration over 2 hours explains persistent defects in patients with redistribution evidence of myocardial infarction on electrocardiogram. (Abstr.). *Circulation* 1987;76:64.
76. Antunes ML, Johnson LL, Rodney RA, Gibbons JF, Vaccarino RA, Bhatia K, et al: Is stress/rest sestamibi superior to stress/four hour redistribution thallium for assessing myocardial viability? (Abstr.). *Circulation* 1991;84:314.
77. Rozanski A, Berman DS, Gray R, Levy R, Raymond M, Maddahi J, et al: Use of thallium-201 redistribution scintigraphy in the preoperative differentiation of reversible myocardial dyssynergy. *Circulation* 1981;64:936–944.
78. Piggott JD, Kouchoukos NT, Oberman A, Cutler GR: Late results of surgical and medical therapy for patients with CAD and depressed LV function. *J Am Coll Cardiol* 1985;5:1036–1045.
79. Marshall RC, Tillisch JH, Phelps ME, Huang SC, Carson R, Henze E, et al: Identification and differentiation of resting myocardial ischemia in man with positron computed tomography, ^{18}F-labeled fluorodeoxyglucose and ^{13}N-ammonia. *Circulation* 1983;67:766–778.
80. Brown KA, Bricker CF, Okada RD, Guiney TE, Newell JD, Strauss HW, et al: The prognostic value of exercise thallium imaging in patients presenting for evaluation of chest pain. *J Am Coll Cardiol* 1983;1:944–1001.
81. Staniloff HM, Forrester JM, Berman DS, Swan HJC: Prediction of death, myocardial infarction, and worsening chest pain using thallium scintigraphy and exercise electrocardiography. *J Nucl Med* 1986;27:1842–1848.
82. Pamelia FX, Gibson RS, Watson DD, Craddock GB, Sirowatka J, Beller GA, et al: Prognosis with chest pain and normal thallium-201 exercise scintigrams. *Am J Cardiol* 1985;55:920–926.
83. Ladenheim ML, Pollock BH, Rozanski A, Berman DS, Staniloff HM, Forrester JS, et al: Extent and severity of myocardial hypoperfusion as predictors of prognosis in patients with suspected coronary artery disease. *J Am Coll Cardiol* 1986;7:464–471.
84. Kotler TS, Maddahi J, Berman DS, Diamond GA: Is thallium scintigraphy better than coronary angiography for prognosis? (Abstr.) *Circulation* 1986;74:512.
85. Kotler TS, Maddahi J, Kiat H, Berman D, Diamond G: Benefit from surgery in patients with triple vessel coronary artery disease may be predicted by evidence of ischemia on exercise-redistribution ^{201}Tl scintigraphy. *Clin Nucl Med* 1987;12:14.
86. Maddahi J, Kiat H, Resser K, Areeda J, VanTrain K, Cohen I, et al: Prediction of coronary events by ^{201}Tl quantitation of jeopardized myocardium and clinical and exercise test variables. (Abstr.) *J Nucl Med* 1988;29:770.
87. Gill JB, Ruddy TD, Newell JB, Finkelstein DM, Strauss HW, Boucher CA: Prognostic importance of thallium uptake by the lungs during exercise in coronary artery disease. *N Engl J Med* 1987;317:1485–1489.
88. Kaul S, Finkelstein DM, Homma S, Leavitt M, Okada RD, Boucher CA: Superiority of quantitative exercise thallium-201 variables in determining long-term prognosis in ambulatory patients with chest pain: A comparison with cardiac catheterization. *J Am Coll Cardiol* 1988;12:25–34.
89. Johnson LL, Seldin DW, Keller AM, Wall RM, Bhatia K, Bingham C, et al: Dual isotope thallium and indium antimyosin SPECT imaging to identify acute infarct patients at further ischemic risk. *Circulation* 1990;81:37–45.
90. Boucher CA, Brewster DC, Darling RC, Okada RD, Strauss HW, Pohost GM: Determination of cardiac risk by dipyridamole thallium imaging before peripheral vascular surgery. *N Engl J Med* 1985;312:389–394.
91. Eagle KA, Singer DE, Brewster DC, Darling AC, Mulley AG, Boucher CA: Dipyridamole thallium scanning in patients undergoing vascular surgery. *JAMA* 1987;257:2185–2189.
92. Gibson RS, Watson DD, Craddock GS, Crampton RS, Kaiser DL,

Denny MJ, et al: Prediction of cardiac events after uncomplicated myocardial infarction: A prospective study comparing predischarge exercise thallium-201 scintigraphy and coronary angiography. *Circulation* 1983;66:321–336.

93. Leppo JA, O'Brien J, Rotwendler JA, Getchell JD, Lee VW: Dipyridamole thallium-201 scintigraphy in the prediction of future cardiac events after acute myocardial infarction. *N Engl J Med* 1984;310:1014–1018.
94. Shen AC, Jennings RB: Myocardial calcium and magnesium in acute ischemic injury. *Am J Pathol* 1972;67:417–433.
95. Keyes JW Jr, Brady TJ, Leonard PF, Svetkoff DB, Winter SM, Rogers WL, et al: Calculation of viable and infarcted myocardial mass for thallium-201 tomograms. *J Nucl Med* 1981;22:339–343.
96. Pringent F, Maddahi J, Garcia EV, Satoh Y, Van Train K, Berman DS: Quantification of myocardial infarct size by thallium-201 single photon emission computed tomography: Experimental validation in dog. *Circulation* 1986;74:852–861.
97. Pringent F, Maddahi J, Garcia EV, Resser K, Lew AS, Berman DS: Comparative methods for quantifying myocardial infarct size by thallium–201 SPECT. *J Nucl Med* 1987;28:325–333.
98. Holman BS, Moore SC, Shulkin PM, Kirsch CM, English RJ, Hill TC: Quantitation of perfused myocardial mass using thallium-201 and emission computed tomography. *Invest Radiol* 1983;4:322–326.
99. Verani MS, Jeroudi MO, Mahmarian JJ, Boyce TM, Borges-Neto S, Patel B, et al: Quantification of myocardial infarction during coronary occlusion and myocardial salvage after reperfusion using cardiac imaging with technetium-99m hexakis 2-methoxyisobutyl isonitrile. *J Am Coll Cardiol* 1988;12:1573–1581.
100. Sinusas AJ, Trautman KA, Bergin JD, Watson DD, Ruiz M, Smith WH, et al: Quantification of "area of risk" during coronary occlusion and degree of myocardial salvage after reperfusion with technetium-99m methoxyisobutyl-isonitrile. *Circulation* 1990; 82:1424–1437.
101. Willerson JT, Parkey RW, Poliner LR, Buja LM, Bonte FY: Radionuclide imaging in acute myocardial infarction. *Cardiovasc Med* 1978;69–85.
102. Buja M, Parkey RW, Dees JH, Stokely EM, Harris RA, Bonte FJ, et al: Morphologic correlates of technetium-99m stannous pyrophosphate imaging of acute myocardial infarction in dogs. *Circulation* 1975;52:596–607.
103. Buja LM, Tofe A, Kulkarni PV, Mukherjee A, Parkey RW, Francis MD, et al: Sites and mechanisms of localization of technetium-99m phosphorus radiopharmaceuticals in acute myocardial infarcts and other issues. *J Clin Invest* 1977;60:724–740.
104. Beller GA, Khaw BA, Smith TW: Localization of radiolabeled cardiac myosin-specific antibody in myocardial infarcts. Comparision with technetium-99m stannous pyrophosphate. *Circulation* 1977;55:74–78.
105. Buja LM, Poliner LR, Parkey RW, Pulido JC, Hutcheson D, Platt MR, et al: Clinicopathological study of persistently positive technetium-99m stannous pyrophosphate myocardial scinitigrams and myocytolytic degeneration post myocardial infarction. *Circulation* 1977;56:1016–1023.
106. Khaw BA, Fallon JT, Beller GA, Haber E: Specificity of localization of myosin-specific antibody fragments in experimental myocardial infarction: Histologic, histochemical, autoradiographic and scintigraphic studies. *Circulation* 1979;60:1527–1531.
107. Khaw BA, Scott J, Fallon JT, Cahill SL, Haber E, Homcy C: Myocardial injury: Quantification by cell sorting initiated with antimyosin fluorescent spheres. *Science* 1982;217:1050–1053.
108. Framie LH, Lopez JA, Khaw BA, Fallon JT, Haber E, Powell WJ: Early membrane damage during coronary reperfusion. Detection by radiolabeled anti-cardiac myosin (Fab') 2. *J Clin Invest* 1983;72:535–544.
109. Weber RW, Boutin RH, Nedelmen MA, Lister-James J, Dean RT: Enhanced kidney clearance with an ester-linked ^{99m}Tc-radiolabeled antibody Fab'-chelator conjugate. *Bioconjugate Chemistry* 1990;2:431–437.
110. Khaw BA, Yasuda T, Gold HK, Leinbach RC, Johns JA, Kanke M, et al: Acute myocardial infarction imaging with ^{111}In-labeled monoclonal antimyosin Fab. *J Nucl Med* 1987;28:1671–1678.
111. Johnson LL, Seldin DW, Becker LC, LaFrance N, Liberman HA, James C, et al: Antimyosin imaging in acute transmural myocardial infarction: Results of a multicenter clinical trial. *J Am Coll Cardiol* 1989; 13:27–35.
112. Tamaki N, Yamada T, Matsumori A, Yoshida A, Fujita T, Ohtani H, et al: Indium-111 antimyosin antibody imaging for detecting different states of myocardial infarction: Comparison with ^{99m}Tc-pyrophosphate imaging. *J Nucl Med* 1990; 31:136–142.
113. Poliner LR, Buja LM, Parkey RW, Bonte FJ, Willerson JT: Clinicopathological findings in 52 patients studied by ^{99m}Tc-stannous pyrophosphate myocardial scintigraphy. *Circulation* 1979; 59: 257–267.
114. Berger H, Lahiri A, Leppo J, Makler T, Maddahi J, Mintz G, et al: Antimyosin imaging in patients with ischemic chest pain: Initial results of phase III multicenter trial. *J Nucl Med* 1988; 29:805–806.
115. Lewis SE, Devous MD, Corbett JR, Izquierdo C, Nicod P, Wolfe CL, et al: Measurement of infarct size in acute canine myocardial infarction by single photon emission computed tomography with technetium-99m pyrophosphate. *Am J Cardiol* 1984; 54: 193–199.
116. Corbett JR, Lewis SE, Wolfe CL, Jansen DE, Lewis M, Rellas JS, et al: Measurement of myocardial infarct size in patients by technetium pyrophosphate single photon tomography. *Am J Cardiol* 1984; 54:1231–1236.
117. Wolfe CL, Lewis SE, Corbett JR, Parkey RW, Buja M, Willerson JT: Measurement of myocardial infarction fraction using single photon emission computed tomography. *J Am Coll Cardiol* 1985; 6:145–151.
118. Jansen DE, Corbett J, Wolfe CL, Lewis SE, Gabliani G, Filipchuk N, et al: Quantification of myocardial infarction: A comparison of single photon-emission computed tomography with pyrophosphate to serial plasma MB-creatine kinase measurement. *Circulation* 1985; 72:327–333.
119. Antunes ML, Seldin DW, Wall RM, Johnson LL: Measurement of acute Q wave myocardial infarct size with single photon emission computed tomographic imaging of indium-111 antimyosin. *Am J Cardiol* 1989; 63:777–783.
120. Johnson LL, Lerrick KS, Coromilas J, Seldin DW, Esser PD, Zimmerman JM, et al: Measurement of infarct size and percentage myocardium infarcted in a dog preparation with single photon emission computed tomography, thallium-201, and indium-111 monoclonal antimyosin Fab. *Circulation* 1987; 76:181–190.
121. Antunes ML, Tresgallo ME, Seldin DW, Bhatia K, Johnson LL: Effect of infarct size measured from antimyosin SPECT scans on left ventricular remodeling. *J Am Coll Cardiol* 1991; 18:1263–1270.
122. Mukharji J, Rude RE, Poole K, Gustafson N, Thomas LJ, Strauss HW, et al: Risk factors for sudden death after acute myocardial infarction: 2 year follow-up. *Am J Cardiol* 1984;54:31–36.
123. Multicenter Postinfarction Research Group: Risk stratification and survival after myocardial infarction. *N Engl J Med* 1983; 309:331–336.
124. Kaul S, Boucher CA, Okada RD, Newell JB, Strauss H, Pohost GM: Sources of variability in radionuclide angiographic assessment of ejection fraction: A comparison of first pass and gated equilibrium techniques. *Am J Cardiol* 1983; 53:823–828.
125. Marshall RC, Berger HJ, Reduto LA, Gottschalk A, Zaret BL: Variability in sequential measures of left ventricular performance assessed with radionuclide angiocardiography. *Am J Cardiol* 1978; 41:531–536.
126. Upton MT, Rerych SK, Newman GE, Bounous EP, Jones RH: The reproducibility of radionuclide angiographic measurements of left ventricular function in normal subjects at rest and during exercise. *Circulation* 1980; 62:126–132.
127. Callahan RJ, Froelich JW, McKusick KA, Leppo J, Strauss HW: A modified method for the in-vivo labelling of red blood cells with ^{99m}Tc: Concise communication. *J Nucl Med* 1982; 23:315–318.
128. Srivastava SC, Straub R, Som P, Yamamoto K: Optimization and evaluation of the in-vitro method for labelling red blood cells in whole blood with ^{99m}Tc. (Abstr.) *J Nucl Med* 1984; 25:128.
129. Pohost GM, Vignola PA, McKusick KE, Block PC, Myers GS, Walker HJ, et al: Hypertrophic cardiomyopathy: Evaluation by gated cardiac blood pool scanning. *Circulation* 1977; 55:92–99.
130. Rigo P, Murray M, Taylor DR, Weisfeldt ML, Kelly DT, Strauss HW, et al: Right ventricular dysfunction detected by gated scintiphotography in patients with acute inferior myocardial infarction. *Circulation* 1975; 52:268–274.
131. Maddahi J, Shah PK, Berman DS, Pichler M, Matsuoka DT,

Forrester JS, et al: Assessment of right ventricular ejection fraction in evolving acute myocardial infarction by multiple gated equilibrium scintigraphy: Hemodynamic correlates and prognostic significance. (Abstr.) *Am J Cardiol* 1979; 43:37.

132. Shah PK, Maddahi J, Berman DS, Pichler M, Swan HJC: Scintigraphically detected predominant right ventricular dysfunction in acute myocardial infarction: Clinical and hemodynamic correlates and implications for therapy and prognosis. *J Am Coll Cardiol* 1985; 6:1264–1272.
133. Reduto LA, Berger HJ, Cohen LS, Gottschalk A, Zaret BL: Sequential radionuclide assessment of left and right ventricular performance following acute myocardial infarction. *Ann Intern Med* 1978; 78:441–447.
134. Berger HJ, Matthay RA, Loke J, Marshall RC, Gottschalk A, Zaret BL: Assessment of cardiac performance and quantitative radionuclide angiocardiography: Right ventricular ejection fraction with reference to findings in chronic obstructive and pulmonary disease. *J Am Coll Cardiol* 1978; 41:897–905.
135. Maddahi J, Berman DS, Matsouka DT, Waxman AD, Stankus KE, Forrester JS, et al: A new technique for assessing right ventricular ejection fraction using rapid multiple-gated equilibrium cardiac blood pool scintigraphy: Description validation and finding in chronic coronary artery disease. *Circulation* 1979; 60:581-589.
136. Rigo P, Alderson PO, Robertson RM, Becker LC, Wagner HN: Measurement of aortic and mitral regurgitation by gated cardiac blood pool scans. *Circulation* 1979; 60:306-312.
137. Lam W, Pavel D, Byrom E, Sheikh A, Best D, Rosen K: Radionuclide regurgitant index: Value and limitations. *Am J Cardiol* 1981; 47:292–298.
138. Urguhart J, Patterson RE, Packer M, Goldsmith SJ, Horowitz SF, Litwak R, et al: Quantification of valve regurgitation by radionuclide angiography before and after valve replacement surgery. *Am J Cardiol* 1981; 47:287–291.
139. Makler PT Jr, McCarthy DM, Velchik MG, Goldstein HA, Alavi A: Fourier amplitude ratio: A new way to assess regurgitation. *J Nucl Med* 1983; 24:204–207.
140. Botvinick EH, Frais MA, Shosa DW, O'Connell JW, Pacheo-Alvarez JA, Scheinman M, et al: An accurate means of detecting and characterizing abnormal patterns of ventricular activation by phase imaging analysis. *Am J Cardiol* 1982; 50:289–298.
141. Botvinick E, Dunn R, Frais M, O'Connell W, Shosa D, Herkens R, et al: The phase image: Its relationship to patterns of contraction and conduction. *Circulation* 1982; 65:551–560.
142. Johnson LL, Seldin DW, Yeh HL, Spotnitz HM, Reiffel JA: Phase analysis of gated blood pool scintigraphic images to localize bypass tracts in Wolff-Parkinson-White syndrome. *J Am Coll Cardiol* 1986; 8:67–75.
143. Bacharach SL, Green MV, Borer JS, Hyde JE, Farkas SP, Johnson GS: Left ventricular peak ejection rate, filling rate, and ejection fraction-frame rate requirements at rest and exercise: Concise communication. *J Nucl Med* 1979; 20:189-193.
144. Mancini GBJ, Slutsky RA, Norris SL, Bhargava V, Ashburn WL, Higgins CB: Radionuclide analysis of peak filling rate, filling fraction, and time to peak filling rate. *Am J Cardiol* 1983; 51:43–51.
145. Inouye S, Massie B, Loge D, Topic N, Silverstein D, Simpson P, et al: Abnormal left ventricular filling: An early finding in mild to moderate systemic hypertension. *Am J Cardiol* 1984; 53:120–126.
146. Bonow RO, Bacharach SL, Green MV, Kent KM, Rosing DR, Lipson LC, et al: Impaired left ventricular diastolic filling in patients with coronary artery disease: Assessment with radionuclide angiography. *Circulation* 1981; 64:315–323.
147. Links JM, Becker LC, Shindledecker JG, Guzman P, Burow RD, Nickeloff EL, et al: Measurement of absolute left ventricular volume from gated blood-pool studies. *Circulation* 1982; 65:82–91.
148. Verani MS, Gaeta J, LeBlanc AD, Paliner LR, Phillips L, Lacy JL, et al: Validation of left ventricular volume measurements by radionuclide angiography. *J Nucl Med* 1985; 26:1394–1401.
149. Burns RJ, Nitkin RS, Weisel RD, Houle S, Prieur TG, McLaughlin PR, et al: Optimized count-based scintigraphic left ventricular volume measurement. *Can J Cardiol* 1985; 1:42–46.
150. Seldin DW, Esser PD, Nichols AB, Ratner SJ, Alderson PO: Left ventricular volume determined from scintigraphy and digital angiography by a semi-automated geometric method. *Radiology* 1983; 149:809–813.
151. Marchall RC, Berger HJ, Costin JC, Freedman GS, Wolberg G, Cohen LS, et al: Assessment of cardiac performance with quantitative radionuclide angiocardiography: Sequential left ventricular ejection fraction normalized left ventricular ejection rate and regional wall motion. *Circulation* 1978; 57:320–329.
152. Anderson PAW, Rerych SK, Moore TE, Jones RH: Accuracy of left ventricular end-diastolic dimension determinations obtained by radionuclide angiocardiography. *J Nucl Med* 1981; 22:500–505.
153. Aroney CN, Ruddy TD, Dighero H, Fifer MA, Boucher CA, Palacios IF: Differentiation of restrictive cardiomyopathy from pericardial constriction: Assessment of diastolic function by radionuclide angiography. *J Am Coll Cardiol* 1989; 13:1007–1014.
154. Anderson P, Jones RH, Sabiston DC: Quantitation of left to right cardiac shunts by radionuclide angiography. *Circulation* 1974; 49:512–516.
155. Askenazi J, Ahnberg D, Korngold E, LaFarge CG, Maltz DL, Treves S, et al: Quantitative radionuclide angiography: Detection and quantitation of left to right shunts. *Am J Cardiol* 1976; 37: 382–387.
156. Pohost GM, Vignola PA, McKusich KE, Block PC, Myers GS, Walker HJ, et al: Hypertrophic cardiomyopathy. *Circulation* 1977; 55:92–99.
157. Alexander J, Dainiak N, Berger HJ, Goldman L, Johnstone D, Reduto L, et al: Serial assessment of doxorubicin cardiotoxicity in quantitative radionuclide angiocardiography. *N Engl J Med* 1979; 300:278–283.
158. Choi BW, Berger HJ, Schwartz PE, Alexander J, Wackers FJT, Gottschalk A: Serial radionuclide assessment of doxorubicin cardiotoxicity in cancer patients with abnormal baseline resting left ventricular performance. *Am Heart J* 1983; 106:638–643.
159. Phillips HR, Carter JE, Okada RD, Levine FH, Boucher CA, Osbakken M, et al: Serial changes in left ventricular ejection fraction in the early hours after aortocoronary bypass grafting, *Chest* 1983; 83:28–34.
160. Bonow RO, Leon MB, Rosing DR, Kent KM, Lipson LC, Bacharach SL, et al: Effect of verapamil and propranolol on left ventricular systolic and diastolic filling in patients with coronary artery disease: Radionuclide angiographic studies at rest and during exercise. *Circulation* 1987; 65:1337–1350.
161. Bonow RO, Rosing DR, Bacharach SL, Green MV, Kent RM, Lipson LC, et al: Effect of verapamil on left ventricular systolic function and diastolic filling in patients with hypertrophic obstructive cardiomyopathy. *Circulation* 1981; 64:787–796.
162. Bonow RO, Kent KM, Rosing DR, Lipson LC, Bacharach SL, Green MV, et al: Improved left ventricular diastolic filling in patients with coronary artery disease after percutaneous transluminal coronary angioplasty. *Circulation* 1982;66:1159–1167.
163. Rerych SK, Scholz PM, Newman GE, Sabiston DC, Jones RH: Cardiac function at rest and during exercise in normals and in patients with coronary artery disease: Evaluation by radionuclide angiography. *Ann Surg* 1978;187:449–464.
164. Potts JM, Borges-Neto S, Smith LR, Jones RH: Comparision of bicycle and treadmill radionuclide angiography. *J Nucl Med* 1991;32:1918–1922.
165. Borer JS, Bacharach SL, Green MV, Kent KM, Epstein SE, Johnston GE: Real-time radionuclide cineangiography in the noninvasive evaluation of global and regional left ventricular function at rest and during exercise in patients with coronary artery disease. *N Engl J Med* 1977;296:839–844.
166. Poliner LR, Dehmer GJ, Lewis SE, Parkey RW, Blomquist CG, Willerson JT: Left ventricular performance in normal subjects: A comparison of the responses to exercise in the upright and supine positions. *Circulation* 1980;62:528–634.
167. Port S, Cobb FR, Coleman E, Jones RH: Effect of age on the response of the left ventricular ejection fraction to exercise. *N Engl J Med* 1980;303:1133–1137.
168. Jones RH, McEwan P, Newman GE, Port S, Reryon SK, Scholz PM, et al: Accuracy of diagnosis of coronary artery disease by radionuclide measurement of left ventricular function during rest and exercise. *Circulation* 1981;64:586–600.
169. Lee KL, Pryor DB, Pieper KS, Harrell FE, Califf RM, Mark DM, et al: Prognostic value of radionuclide angiography in medically treated patients with coronary artery disease. *Circulation* 1990;82:1705–1717.
170. Bonow RO, Kent KM, Rosing DR, Lan KKG, Lakatos E, Borer JS, et al: Exercise-induced ischemia in mildly symptomatic pa-

tients with coronary artery disease and preserved left ventricular function. *N Engl J Med* 1985;311:1339–1345.

171. Morris DD, Rozanski A, Berman DS, Diamond GA, Swan HJC: Non-invasive prediction of the angiographic extent of coronary artery disease following myocardial infarction: Comparison of clinical exercise electrocardiographic and ventriculographic parameters. *Circulation* 1984;70:192–201.
172. Johnson LL, McCarthy DM, Sciacca RR, Cannon HJ: Right ventricular ejection fraction during exercise in patients with coronary artery disease. *Circulation* 1979;60:1284–1291.
173. Bonow RO, Borer JS, Rosing DR, Henry WL, Pearlman AS, McIntosh CL, et al: Preoperative exercise capacity in symptomatic patients with aortic regurgitation as a predictor of postoperative left ventricular function and long-term prognosis. *Circulation* 1980;62:1280–1290.
174. Boucher CA, Kanarek DJ, Okada RD, Hutter AM, Strauss HW, Pohost GM: Exercise testing in aortic regurgitation: Comparison of radionuclide left ventricular ejection fraction with exercise performance at the anaerobic threshold and peak exercise. *Am J Cardiol* 1983;1:801–808.
175. Bonow RO, Rosing DR, Kent KM, Epstein SE: Timing of operation for chronic aortic regurgitation. *Am J Cardiol* 1982;50:325–336.
176. O'Connell JB, Henkin RE, Robinson JA, Subramanian R, Scanlon PJ: Gallium-67 imaging in patients with dilated cardiomyopathy and biopsy proven myocarditis. *Circulation* 1984;70:58–62.
177. O'Connell JB, Robinson JA, Henkin RE, Gunnar RM: Immunosuppressive therapy in patients with cardiomyopathy and myocardial uptake of gallium-67. *Circulation* 1981;64:780–786.
178. Forman MB, Sandlwer MP, Sachs GA, Kronenberg MU, Powers TA: Radionuclide imaging in myocardial sarcoidosis-demonstration of myocardial uptake of technetium pyrophosphate and gallium. *Chest* 1983;83:578–580.
179. Dec GW, Palacios I, Yasuda T, Fallon JT, Khaw BA, Strauss HW, et al: Antimyosin antibody cardiac imaging: Its role in the diagnosis of myocarditis. *J Am Coll Cardiol* 1990;16:97–104.
180. Chow LH, Radio SJ, Sears TD, McManus BM: Insensitivity of right ventricular endomyocardial biopsy in the diagnosis of myocarditis. *J Am Coll Cardiol* 1989;14:915–920.
181. Frist W, Yasuda T, Segall G, Khaw BA, Strauss HW, Gold H, et al: Noninvasive detection of human cardiac transplant rejection with indium-111 antimyosin (Fab) imaging. *Circulation* 1987;76:81–85.
182. Ballester-Rodes M, Carrio-Gasset I, Abadal-Berini L, Obrador-Mayol D, Berna-Roqueta L, Caralps-Riesa JM: Patterns of evolution of myocyte damage after human heart transplantation detected by indium-111 monoclonal antimyosin. *Am J Cardiol* 1988;62:623–627.
183. Carrio I, Berna L, Ballester M, Estorch M, Obrador D, Cladellas M, et al: Indium-111 antimyosin scintigraphy to assess myocardial damage in patients with suspected myocarditis and cardiac rejection. *J Nucl Med* 1988;29:1893–1900.
184. Allen MD, Tsuboi H, Togo T, Eary JF, Gordon D, Thomas R, Reichenbach DD: Detection of cardiac allograft rejection and myocyte necrosis by monoclonal antibody to cardiac myosin. *Transplantation* 1989;48:923–928.
185. Isobe M, Strauss HW, Haber E: Noninvasive detection of cardiac rejection by I-123-labeled monoclonal antibody that binds to monomorphic determinants of MHC IA antigen. (Abstr.) *Circulation* 1991;84:644.
186. Eisen HJ, Belland SE, Perloff LJ: Scintigraphic detection of early cardiac transplant rejection using radiolabeled anti-interleukin-2 receptor monoclonal antibodies. (Abstr.) *Circulation* 1991; 84(II):643.
187. Eich DM, Johnson DE, Hastillo A, Thompson JA, Barnhart GR, Ko D, et al: Accelerated coronary atherosclerosis in cardiac transplantation. *Cardiovasc Clinics* 1990;20:199–211.
188. Schroeder JS, Hunt SA: Chest pain in heart transplant recipients. *N Engl J Med* 1991;324:1805–1807.
189. Gao SZ, Alderman EL, Schroeder JS, Silverman JF, Hunt SA: Accelerated coronary vascular disease in the heart transplant patient: Coronary arteriographic findings. *J Am Coll Cardiol* 1988;12:334–340.
190. Johnson DE, Alderman EL, Schroeder JS, Gao SZ, Hunt S, DeCampli WM, et al: Transplant coronary artery disease: Histopathologic correlations with angiographic morphology. *J Am Coll Cardiol* 1991;17:449–457.
191. McKillop JH, Goris ML: Thallium-201 myocardial imaging in patients with previous cardiac transplantation. *Clin Radiol* 1981;32:447–449.
192. Smart FW, Ballantyne CM, Cocanougher B, Farmer CA, Sekela ME, Noon GP, et al: Insensitivity of noninvasive tests to detect coronary artery vasculopathy after heart transplant. *Am J Cardiol* 1991;67:243–247.
193. Rodney RA, Johnson LL, Barr M, et al: Comparison of exercise SPECT thallium-20 and sestamibi for detection of cardiac allograft atherosclerosis. (Abstr.) *J Am Coll Cardiol* 1992;19:173A.
194. DeWood MA, Spores J, Notske R, Mouser LT, Burroughs R, Golden MS, et al: Prevalence of total coronary occlusion during the early hours of transmural myocardial infarction. *N Engl J Med* 1980;303:897–902.
195. DeWood MA, Stifter WF, Simpson WF, Spores J, Eugster GS, Judge TP, et al: Coronary arteriographic findings soon after non-Q wave myocardial infarction. *N Engl J Med* 1986;315:417–423.
196. Stratton JR, Ritchie JL, Hamilton GW, Hammermeister KE, Harker LA: Left ventricular thrombi: In vivo detection by indium-111 platelet imaging and two dimensional echocardiography. *Am J Cardiol* 1981;47:874–881.
197. Ezekowitz MD, Wilson DA, Smith EO, Burow RD, Harrison LH, Parker DE, et al: Comparison of indium-111 platelet scintigraphy and two-dimensional echocardiography in the diagnosis of left ventricular thrombi. *N Engl J Med* 1982;306:1509–1513.
198. Stratton JR, Ritchie JL: Indium-111 platelet imaging of left ventricular thrombi, predictive value for systemic emboli. *Circulation* 1990;81:1182–1189.
199. Miller DD, Boulet AJ, Tio FO, Garcia OJ, Guy DM, McEver RP, et al: In vivo technetium-99m S12 antibody imaging of platelet alpha granules in rabbit endothelial neointimal proliferation after angioplasty. *Circulation* 1991;83:224–236.
200. Som P, Oster ZH, Yamamoto K, Sacker DF, Brill AB, Newell RD, et al: Radioimmunoimaging of experimental thrombi in dogs using technetium-99m labeled monoclonal antibody fragments reactive with human platelets. *J Nucl Med* 1986;27:1315–1320.
201. Mickelson JK, Simpson PJ, Lucchesi BR: Antiplatelet monoclonal (Fab')2 antibody directed against platelet GPIIb/IIIa receptor complex prevents coronary artery thrombosis in the canine heart. *J Mol Cell Cardiol* 1989;21:393–405.
202. Coller BS, Scudder LE, Berger HJ, Juliucci JD: Inhibition of human platelet function in vivo with a monoclonal antibody. *Ann Intern Med* 1988;109:635–638.
203. Yasuda T, Gold HK, Fallon JT, Leinbach RC, Guerrero JL, Scudder LE, et al: Monoclonal antibody against the platelet glycoprotein (GP)IIb/IIIa receptor prevents coronary artery reocclusion after reperfusion with recombinant tissue-type plasminogen activator in dogs. *J Clin Invest* 1988;81:1284–1291.
204. Coller BS, Scudder LE: Inhibition of dog platelet function by in vivo infusion of (Fab')2 fragments of a monoclonal antibody to the platelet glycoprotein IIb/IIIa receptor. *Blood* 1985;66:1456–1459.
205. Perlman SB, Folts JD, Hammes RJ, Besozzi MC, Masher DF: The accumulation of a platelet protein, thrombospondin, at the site of arterial thrombus formation: Preliminary report. *Eur J Nucl Med* 1987;12:492–495.
206. Thiagarajan P, Tait JF: Binding of annexin V/placental anticoagulant protein I to platelets. *J Bio Chem* 1990;265:17420–17423.
207. Mochos CB, Oldewurtel HA, Lahiri K, Manskopf G, Regan TJ: Incorporation of ^{131}I-fibrinogen in a coronary artery thrombus, detected in vivo with a scintillation camera. *Cardiovasc Res* 1974;8:715–720.
208. Erhardt LR, Lundman T, Mellstedt H: Incorporation of I-125 labelled fibrinogen into coronary arterial thrombi in acute myocardial infarction in man. *Lancet* 1973;387–390.
209. Hui KY, Haber E, Matsueda GR: Monoclonal antibodies to synthetic fibrin-like peptide bind to human fibrin but not fibrinogen. *Science* 1983;222:1129–1131.
210. Cequeira MD, Stratton JR, Vracko R, Schaible TF, Ritchie JL: Noninvasive arterial thrombus imaging with ^{99m}Tc-monoclonal antifibrin antibody. *Circulation* 1992;85:298–304.
211. Knight LC, Maurer AH, Ammar IA, Shealy DJ, Mathis JA: Evaluation of indium-111 labeled antifibrin antibody for imaging vascular thrombi. *J Nucl Med* 1988;29:494–502.
212. DeFaucal P, Peltier P, Planchon B, Dupas B, Touze MD, Baron D, et al: Evaluation of indium-111 labeled antifibrin monoclonal

antibody for the diagnosis of venous thrombotic disease. *J Nucl Med* 1991;32:787–791.

213. Alavi A, Palevsky HI, Gupta N, Meranze S, Kelley MA, Jatlow AD, et al: Radiolabeled antifibrin antibody in the detection of venous thrombosis: Preliminary results. *Radiology* 1990;175: 79–85.
214. Jung M, Kletter K, Dudczak R, Koppensteiner R, Minar E, Kahle P, et al: Deep vein thrombosis: Scintigraphic diagnosis with indium-111 labeled monoclonal antifibrin antibodies. *Radiology* 1989;173:469–475.
215. Rosebrough SF, McAfee JG, Grossman ZD, Kudryk BJ, Ritter-Hrncirik CA, Witanowski LS, et al: Thrombus imaging: A comparison of radiolabeled GC4 and T2G1s fibrin-specific monoclonal antibodies. *J Nucl Med* 1990;31:1048–1057.
216. Kanke M, Matsueda GR, Strauss HW, Yasuda T, Liau CS, Khaw BA: Localization and visualization of pulmonary emboli with radiolabeled fibrin-specific monoclonal antibody. *J Nucl Med* 1991; 32:1254–1260.
217. Ord JM, Hasapes J, Daugherty A, Thorpe SR, Bergmann SR, Sobel BE: Imaging of thrombi with tissue-type plasminogen activator rendered enzymatically inactive and conjugated to a residualizing label. *Circulation* 1992; 85:288–297.
218. Lees AM, Lees RS, Schoen FJ, Isaacsohn JL, Fischman AJ, McKusick KA, et al: Imaging human atherosclerosis with Tc-99m labeled low density lipoproteins. *Atherosclerosis* 1988; 8:461–470.
219. Sostman HD, Gottschalk A: Detection of pulmonary emboli. In: Gottschalk A, Hoffer PB, Potchen EJ (eds): *Diagnostic Nuclear Medicine.* Baltimore, Williams & Wilkins, 1988:502–537.
220. Biello DR: Radiological (scintigraphic) evaluation of patients with suspected pulmonary thromboembolism. *JAMA* 1987; 257: 3257–3259.
221. Biello DR, Mattar AG, McKnight RC, Siegel BA: Ventilation-perfusion studies in suspected pulmonary embolism. *Am J Radiol* 1979; 133:1033–1037.
222. Mettler FA, Guiberteau MJ: *Essentials of Nuclear Medicine Imaging.* Philadelphia, Saunders, 1991:141–176.
223. The Pioped Investigators: Value of the ventilation/perfusion scan in acute pulmonary embolism—Results of the prospective investigation of pulmonary embolism diagnosis. *JAMA* 1990; 263: 2753–2759.
224. Lee ME, Biello DR, Kumar B, Siegel BA: Low probability ventilation-perfusion scintigrams: Clinical outcomes in 99 patients. *Radiology* 1985; 156:497–500.
225. Inoue H, Zipes PD: Results of sympathetic denervation in the canine heart: Supersensitivity that may be arrhythmogenic. *Circulation* 1987: 75:877–887.
226. Sisson JC, Wieland DM, Sherman D, Mangner TJ, Tobes MC, Jacques S: Metaiodobenzylguanidine as an index of the adrenergic nervous system integrity and function. *J Nucl Med* 1987; 28:1620–1624.
227. Wieland DM, Wu JL, Brown LE, Mangner TJ, Swanson DP, Bierwalters WH: Radiolabeled adrenergic neuron blocking agents: Adrenomedullary imaging with (^{131}I) iodobenzylguanidine. *J Nucl Med* 1980; 21:349–353.
228. Manger WM, Hoffmen BB: Heart imaging in the diagnosis of pheochromocytoma and assessment of catecholamine uptake. *J Nucl Med* 1983; 24:994.
229. Kline RC, Swanson DP, Wieland DM, Thrall JH, Gross MD, Pitt B, et al: Myocardial imaging in man with I-123 meta-iodobenzylguanidine. *J Nucl Med* 1981; 22:129–132.
230. Kulkarni PV, Corbett JR: Radioiodinated tracers for myocardial imaging. *Semin Nucl Med* 1990; 20:119–129.
231. Tobes MC, Jacques S, Wieland DM, Sisson JC: Effect of uptake-one inhibitors on the uptake of norepinephrine and metaiodobenzylguanidine. *J Nucl Med* 1985; 26:897–907.
232. Dae MW, O'Connell JW, Botvinick EH, Ahearn T, Yee E, Huberty JP, et al: Scintigraphic assessment of regional cardiac adrenergic innervation. *Circulation* 1989; 79:634–644.
233. Minando JD, Tuli MM, Wellman HN, Zipes DP: Scintigraphic evidence of canine myocardial sympathetic denervation. (Abstr.) *Circulation* 1986; 74:437.
234. Sisson JC, Shapiro B, Meyers L, Mallette S, Mangner TJ, Wieland DM, et al: Metaiodobenzylguanidine to map scintigraphically the adrenergic nervous system in man. *J Nucl Med* 1987; 28: 1625–1636.
235. Stanton MS, Tuli MM, Radtke NL, Heger JJ, Miles WM, Mock BH: Regional sympathetic denervation after myocardial infarction in humans detected noninvasively using ^{123}I-metaiodobenzylguanidine. *J Am Coll Cardiol* 1989; 14:1519–1520.
236. Fagret D, Wolf JE, Comet M: Myocardial uptake of meta-I-123-iodobenzylguanidine in patients with myocardial infarct. *Eur J Nucl Med* 1989; 15:624–628.
237. Sisson JC, Wieland DM, Johnson JW, Bolgos GL, Malak TA, VanDort ME, et al: Scintigraphy of adrenergic receptors and neurons in myocardial infarcts. (Abstr.) *J Nucl Med* 1989; 30:767.
238. Glowniak JV, Turner FE, Gray LL, Palac RT, Langunas-Solar MC, Woodward WR: Iodine-123 metaiodobenzylguanidine imaging of the heart in idiopathic congestive cardiomyopathy and cardiac transplants. *J Nucl Med* 1989; 30:1182–1191.
239. Schofe J, Spielmann R, Schuchert A, Weber K, Schiuter M: Iodine-123 meta-iodobenzylguanidine scintigraphy: A noninvasive method to demonstrate myocardial adrenergic nervous system disintegrity in patients with idiopathic dilated cardiomyopathy. *J Am Coll Cardiol* 1988; 12:1252–1258.
240. Schwaiger M, Hutchins GM, Kalff V, Rosenspine K, Hada MS, Mallette S, et al: Evidence for regional catecholamine uptake and storage sites in the transplanted human heart by positron emission tomography. *J Clin Invest* 1991; 87:1681–1690.
241. Schwaiger M, Hicks R: The clinical role of metabolic imaging of the heart by positron emission tomography. *J Nucl Med* 1991; 32:565–578.
242. Schwaiger M, Brunken R, Grover-McKay M, Krivokapich J, Child J, Tillisch JH, et al: Regional myocardial metabolism in patients with acute myocardial infarction assessed by positron emission tomography. *J Am Coll Cardiol* 1986; 8:800–808.
243. Marshall RC, Tillisch JH, Phelps ME, Huang SC, Cason R, Henze E, et al: Identification and differentiation of resting myocardial ischemia and infarction in man with positron computed tomography, ^{18}F-labeled fluorodeoxyglucose and ^{13}N ammonia. *Circulation* 1983; 67:766–768.
244. Tillisch J, Brunken R, Marshall R, Schwaiger M, Mandelkern M, Phelps M, et al: Reversibility of cardiac wall motion abnormalities predicted by positron emission tomography. *N Engl J Med* 1986; 314;884–888.
245. Geltman EM, Smith JL, Beecher D, Ludbrook PA, Ter-Pogossian MM, Sobel BE: Altered regional myocardial metabolism in congestive cardiomyopathy detected by positron tomography. *Am J Med* 1983; 74:773–785.
246. Schelbert HR, Henze E, Sochor H, Grossman RG, Huang S-C, Barrio JR, et al: Effects of substrate availability on myocardial ^{11}C-palmitate kinetics by positron emission tomography in normal subjects and patients with ventricular dysfunction. *Am Heart J* 1986; 111:1055–1064.
247. Grover-McKay M, Schwaiger M, Krivokapich J, Perloff JK, Phelps ME, Schelbert HR: Regional myocardial blood flow and metabolism at rest in mildly symptomatic patients with hypertrophic cardiomyopathy. *J Am Coll Cardiol* 1989; 13:317–324.
248. Perloff JK, Henze E, Schelbert HR: Alterations in regional myocardial metabolism, perfusion, and wall motion in Duchenne muscular dystrophy studied by radionuclide imaging. *Circulation* 1984; 69:33–42.

Chapter 135

Computed Tomography of the Heart

Bruce H. Brundage, M.D.

In 1983 the introduction of the ultrafast computed tomography (CT) scanner for clinical use opened a new area of cardiac imaging. Previous attempts to use conventional x-ray transmission CT to evaluate the heart had been severely limited because of motion artifact created by cardiac contraction and relaxation. Some modicum of success was achieved with conventional CT in the evaluation of aortic disease.[1] The relative lack of aortic motion permitted reasonable imaging of aortic dissection and aortic aneurysms.[2] There was also some success in the evaluation of patency of coronary artery bypass grafts using this technique.[3] However, the advent of ultrafast CT has relegated conventional CT to a relatively unimportant role in the diagnosis of cardiovascular disease.

TECHNOLOGY

Ultrafast CT is a unique technology that utilizes a powerful electron beam and has a scanner with no moving parts. Conventional CT is limited in its evaluation of the heart because an x-ray tube is mechanically rotated around the thorax, which requires 1 to 2 s. The ultrafast CT scanner projects an electron beam that passes through a magnetic coil that focuses and bends the electron beam to strike a series of fixed tungsten targets that encircle the thorax (Fig. 135-1). The beam is swept magnetically along the tungsten targets in an arc of 210°. The x radiation generated from the tungsten target passes through the thorax and is attenuated by the intervening structures before striking the twin fixed detector array opposite the targets. The electron beam can be swept along the tungsten target in 50 ms, and after an 8-ms interscan delay the procedure can be repeated. This sequence translates into a scanning frequency of 17 scans per second. The x-ray generated by each tungsten target is collimated to strike the twin adjacent detector arrays. Thus, for each beam sweep two adjacent 8-mm sections of anatomy are imaged. Since there are four tungsten targets, the electron beam can be cascaded across each target in sequence so that in a period of seven heart beats, eight adjacent slices are obtained. There is a 4-mm gap between targets so eight adjacent scan levels represent 8 cm of anatomy.

IMAGING PROTOCOLS

Three imaging protocols are employed for cardiac imaging with ultrafast CT. The most commonly employed protocol, known as the cine mode because the images obtained can be displayed on a television screen in a movie format, creates real-time cross-sectional views of the beating heart. This imaging mode is particularly useful for assessing ventricular function and valve motion (Fig. 135-2). The flow mode imaging protocol is used to evaluate blood flow. In this mode each scan is gated to the electrocardiogram, assuring that sequential images are obtained at the same point in the cardiac cycle. This assures that there will be excellent registration of the images when a scan series is obtained following the intra-

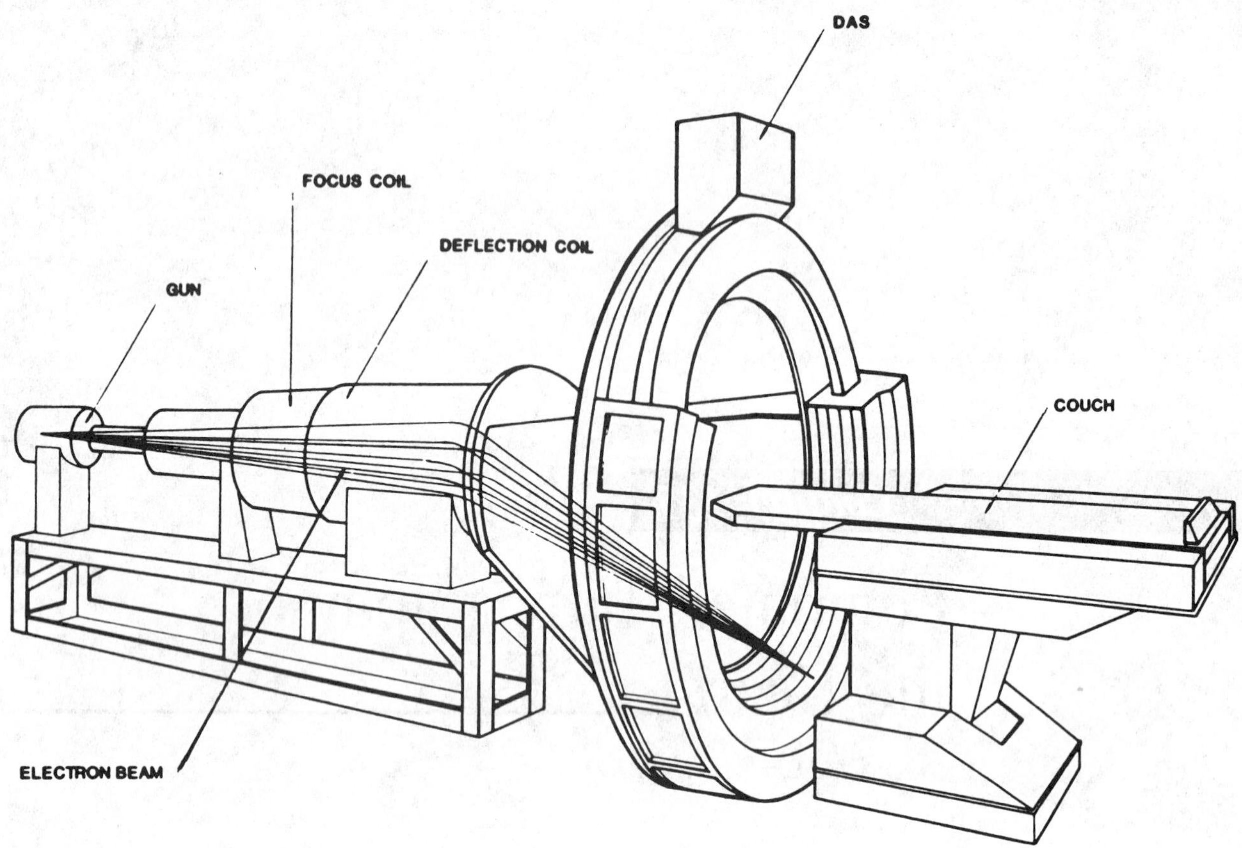

FIGURE 135-1 Cutaway diagram of the ultrafast CT scanner depicts the electron beam emitting from the electron gun and being focused on the tungsten target by the magnetic deflection coil. DAS = immediate memory.

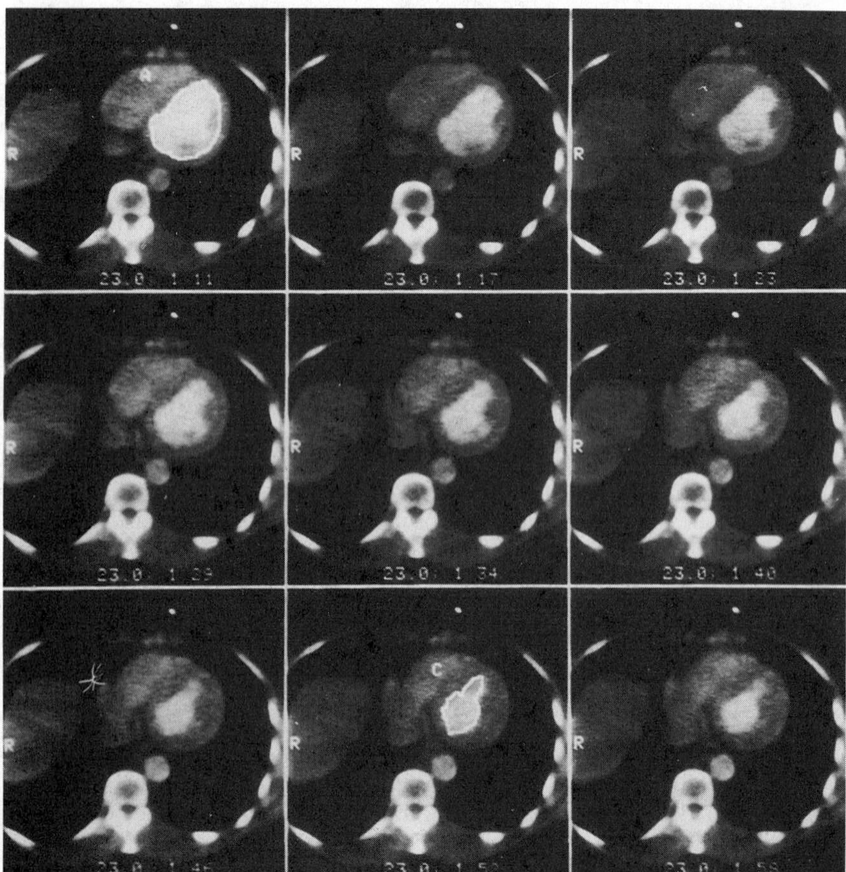

FIGURE 135-2 An 8-mm CT slice of the mid–left ventricle imaged for one complete cardiac cycle at 58-ms intervals. A = end diastole; C = end systole.

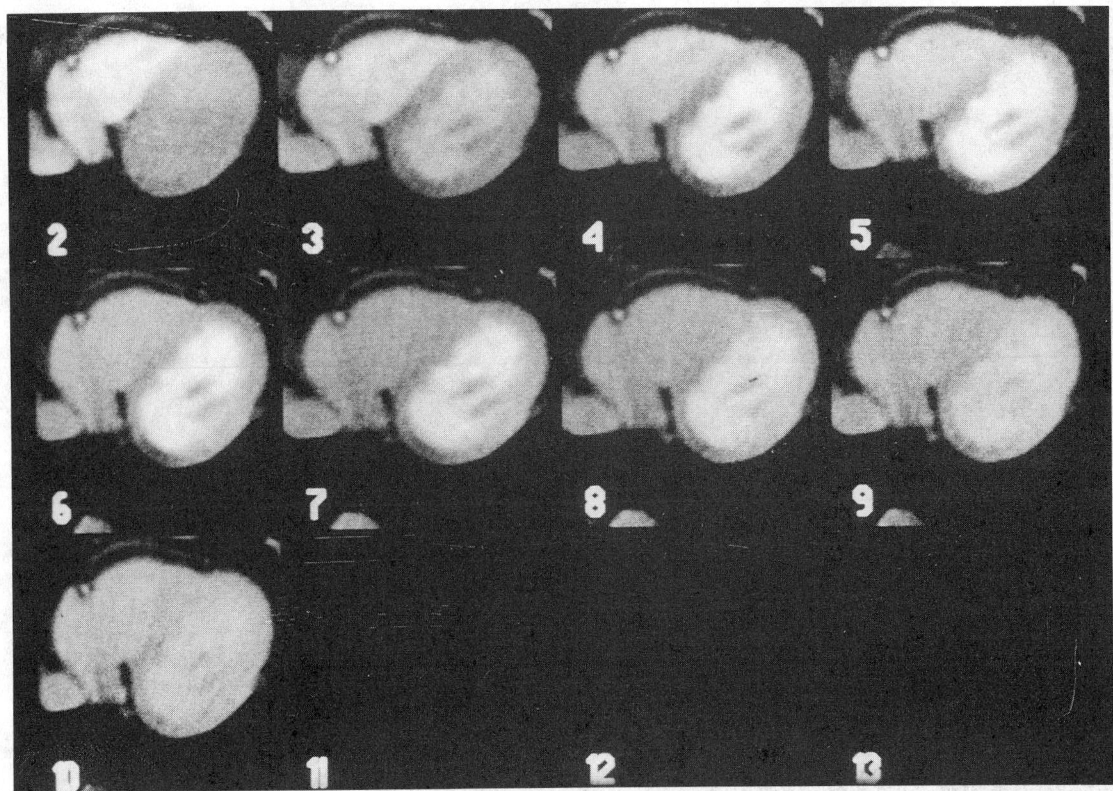

FIGURE 135-3 An 8-mm CT slice of the mid–right ventricle and mid–left ventricle scanned (50 ms) every other cardiac cycle at end diastole. *(From BH Brundage, MJ Lipton, L Cox: What is the role of CT scanning of the heart? In: SH Rahimtoola (ed): Controversies in Coronary Heart Disease, Cardiovascular Clinics. Philadelphia, F.A. Davis, 1983: 91–112. Reproduced with permission from the publisher and the author.)*

venous injection of an iodine contrast medium. The entrance, progressive enhancement, and egress of the iodine through the various cardiac chambers or within the myocardium itself can then be analyzed by time-density curves (Fig. 135-3). Each image is acquired in 50 ms and up to 20 images can be obtained during one imaging sequence. Interscan interval is a function of heart rate. The volume imaging protocol is very similar to traditional imaging protocols employed by conventional CT scanners. Single images, usually gated to the electrocardiogram, are acquired and then the patient couch is moved 3 or 8 mm (depending on slice thickness desired) and another single gated scan is obtained. This sequence can be repeated for up to 40 contiguous scans axially encompassing 12 to 32 cm of anatomy (see Figs. 135-7 and 135-14 as examples). The acquisition time for each scan is 50 ms or multiples of that interval if high image resolution is desired. The spatial resolution is 1.6 mm^3 in the 50-ms mode and 0.8 mm^3 in the 100-ms mode.

The cine mode imaging protocol is used to provide precise assessment of right and left ventricular global and regional systolic and diastolic function (Fig. 135-4).[4–6] Multiple images of the entire right and left ventricle are obtained during intravenous contrast enhancement of the cavities throughout one cardiac cycle. Measurements of ejection fraction and cardiac volumes are obtained by computing end-systolic and end-diastolic volumes from the summation of the individual volumes of each slice[5,7] (Fig. 135-2). Usually 8 slices (averaging 1 cm in thickness) will encompass the left and right ventricles. However, when cardiac enlargement is present, 12 slices may be required. This is accomplished by summating images from two and occasionally three scanning periods. As long as the heart rate is the same during each imaging sequence, accurate cardiac volumes and ejection fractions are obtainable.

A radial area technique has been developed for determining regional left ventricular function.[8] Each slice of the left ventricle is divided into 12 equal regions and the wall motion is displayed graphically or numerically. With the same analysis program it is also possible to quantify regional systolic wall thickening. Border definition of the endocardium and epicardium for this program can be determined visually by the operator or with a computer-assisted edge detection method. Assessment of global and regional ventricular function can be obtained at rest and during bicycle exercise.[8] The configuration of the scanner couch and gantry facilitates assessment of cardiac function during bicycle exercise (Fig. 135-1). Function can also be assessed by ultrafast CT during various pharmacologic stresses including intravenous inotropic drugs and dipyridamole.[9,10] Frame-by-frame analysis of cardiac volumes during diastole provides an accurate depiction of the ventricular volume curve. Maximum peak filling rate, time to maximum peak filling rate, and *dv*/*dt* can be computed.[6] The results are comparable to those obtained by radioisotope techniques. The cine mode imaging protocol can also be used to measure accurately myocardial volume.[11] Assuming a uniform specific gravity for myocardium of 1.005, myocardial

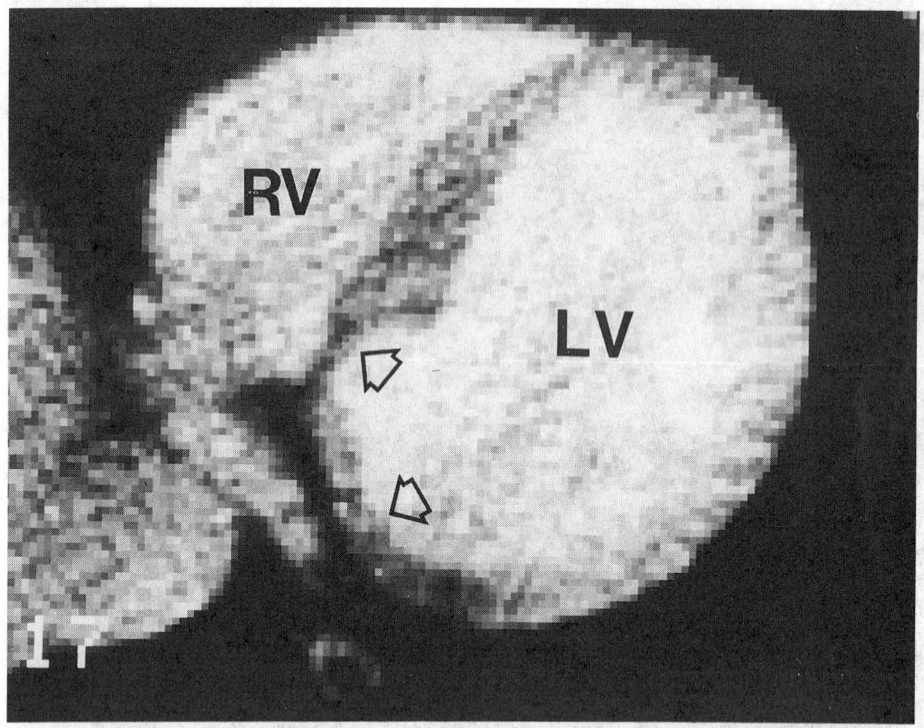

A

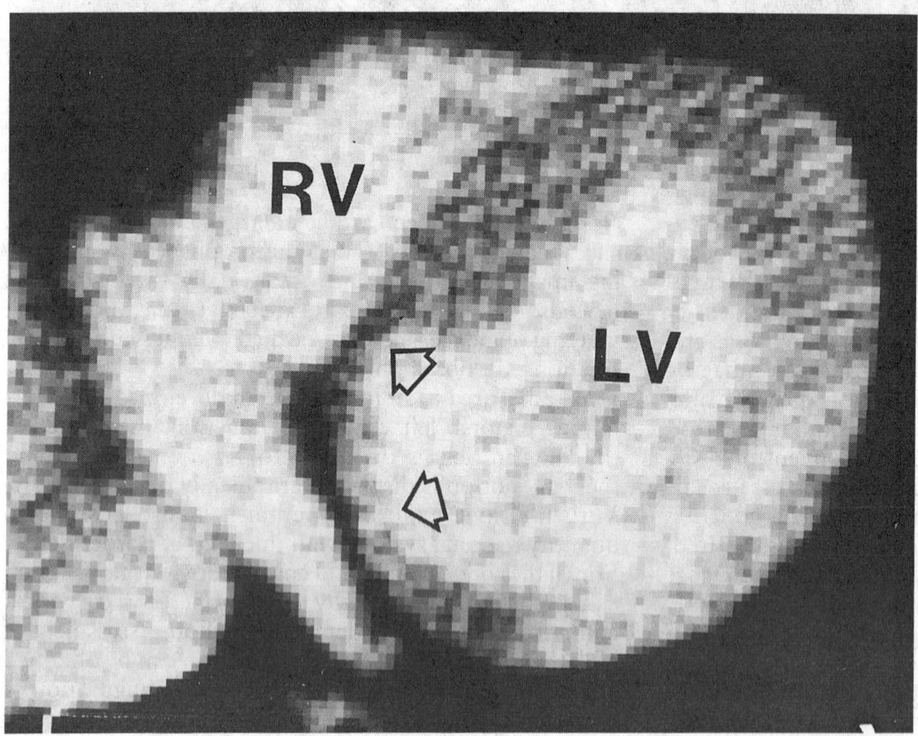

B

FIGURE 135-4 *A.* End-diastolic scan of the right (RV) and left (LV) ventricles. Arrows depict an area of posterior LV thinning due to an old myocardial infarction. *B.* End-systolic scan of the area in *A.* Note the lack of posterior wall thickening (arrows).

mass can be computed from myocardial volume. Several investigators have demonstrated remarkable precision for the measurement of both right and left ventricular mass with excellent intraobserver, interobserver, and interstudy reproducibility.[12,13] Ultrafast CT may well be the new gold standard for the measurement of myocardial mass.

The flow mode imaging protocol is employed to measure cardiac output and myocardial blood flow. Following the intravenous injection of a known amount of iodinated contrast material, analysis of the time-density curves in the pulmonary artery, left ventricle, or aorta will provide an accurate estimate of cardiac output provided the dead space between the injection site and the central circulation is known. Several investigators have verified accurate measurement of cardiac output using ultrafast CT.[14,15] The most important use of flow mode imaging protocol, however, is the assessment of tissue

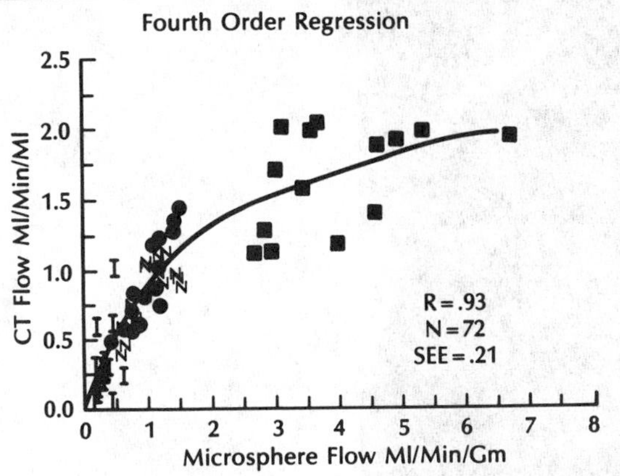

FIGURE 135-5 Ultrafast CT measurement of myocardial flows in dogs are correlated with radioisotope microsphere measurements: (○) Baseline state; (■) pharmacologic vasodilation. I = ischemic myocardium; N = nonischemic myocardium. *(From CJ Wolfkiel et al: Measurement of myocardial blood flow by ultrafast computed tomography. Circulation 76:1262–1273, 1987. Reproduced with permission from the publisher and the author.)*

perfusion, in particular, myocardial blood flow. Myocardial blood flow is quantified by analysis of the myocardial time-density curves. Wolfkiel et al.[16] demonstrated that intravenous injections of small amounts of contrast medium (0.35 mL/kg) could be employed to measure accurately regional myocardial blood flow in resting or basal states and during temporary regional ischemia (Fig. 135-5). However, during high blood flow states such as produced with pharmacologic vasodilation, compared to radioactive microspheres, ultrafast CT measurements of blood flow were inappropriately low. This underestimation at high flows appears to be due to the washout of the iodinated indicator from the myocardium before all indicator has reached the myocardium. Several methods have been proposed for analyzing the myocardial time-density curves. The simplest measures the change in myocardial density and relates that to the blood pool time-density curves [$F/V = C_m / \int_0^\infty C_i(t)\,dt$]. Several corrections or modifications have been suggested to overcome underestimation at high flows, but at present this problem remains unsolved.[17,18] In an attempt to circumvent the problem of early washout and beam hardening, several investigators have employed direct intraaortic injection of the contrast medium and have demonstrated excellent correlation between ultrafast CT and radioactive microsphere flow measurement over a wide range of flows including those following pharmacologic vasodilation.[18,19] Obviously the requirement of intraaortic injection of contrast medium seriously limits the clinical usefulness of this technique for measuring myocardial blood flow at the present time. However, research in progress suggests that myocardial blood flow may be measurable over a wide range of flows using intravenous contrast injections.[20]

Similar flow measurement techniques have been tested for the evaluation of pulmonary lung perfusion as well.[21] Much more work needs to be done in this area before the clinical value of ultrafast CT for assessing pulmonary tissue perfusion is known.

The volume imaging protocol is primarily employed when detailed evaluation of cardiovascular anatomy is required. High-resolution scanning (0.8 mm^3 spatial resolution) with thin, 3-mm slices is usually employed with this imaging protocol. Coronary artery calcification, aortic intimal dissection, and pulmonary artery embolization (see below) are examples of conditions for which this protocol can be used.

CORONARY ARTERY DISEASE

The greatest clinical experience with the use of ultrafast CT has been in the evaluation and study of coronary artery disease. Based on successes with conventional CT to assess coronary artery bypass graft patency, ultrafast CT was evaluated soon after its clinical availability for this use (Fig. 135-6). A multicenter prospective study evaluated the accuracy of ultrafast CT compared to graft angiography and demonstrated a sensitivity of 89 percent, a specificity of 96 percent, and a predictive accuracy exceeding 92 percent.[22] The technique appears to work equally well for saphenous vein grafts and internal mammary artery grafts. The major drawback of ultrafast CT in evaluating bypass grafts is the difficulty in differentiating fully patent grafts from those that are partially obstructed. Several approaches to this problem have been suggested, including measurement of graft flow velocity and comparison of graft time-density curves to aortic curves before and after pharmacologic vasodilation.[23,24] Further investigation is warranted as the clinical utility of assessment of graft patency would be greatly enhanced if the quality of flow could also be determined.

Ultrafast CT can identify acute myocardial infarction as a region of absent or markedly reduced resting myocardial blood flow (Fig. 135-7). Imaging the left ventricle using the flow mode protocol is the best technique. Relatively few data are available regarding the accuracy of this technique, but in one small study of 20 patients comparison of ultrafast CT, thallium perfusion scintigraphy, and technitium pyrophosphate scanning demonstrated ultrafast CT to be the most sensitive and specific.[25] Several investigators have reported the value of ultrafast CT for the evaluation of ventricular remodeling following acute myocardial infarction.[26,27] The combination of regional wall motion analysis using the cine mode protocol and assessment of myocardial blood flow by the flow mode protocol may prove useful in determining residual risk area after acute infarction.[28-30] Equivalent areas of hypokinesis/akinesis and resting hypoperfusion indicate completed infarction. Conversely, a large area of hypokinesis with only a small central area of hypoperfusion suggests substantial myocardium is at risk. Ultrafast CT is a relatively untapped imaging resource for the assessment of acute myocardial infarction and holds great promise in this regard.

The excellent spatial and temporal resolution of ultrafast CT make it an ideal method for evaluating left ventricular aneurysm and associated thrombus.[31,32] Regional wall motion abnormalities characteristic of ventricular aneurysms are easily detected as is the intracavitary filling defect of the often associated thrombus (Fig. 135-8). One study suggests that ultrafast CT may be

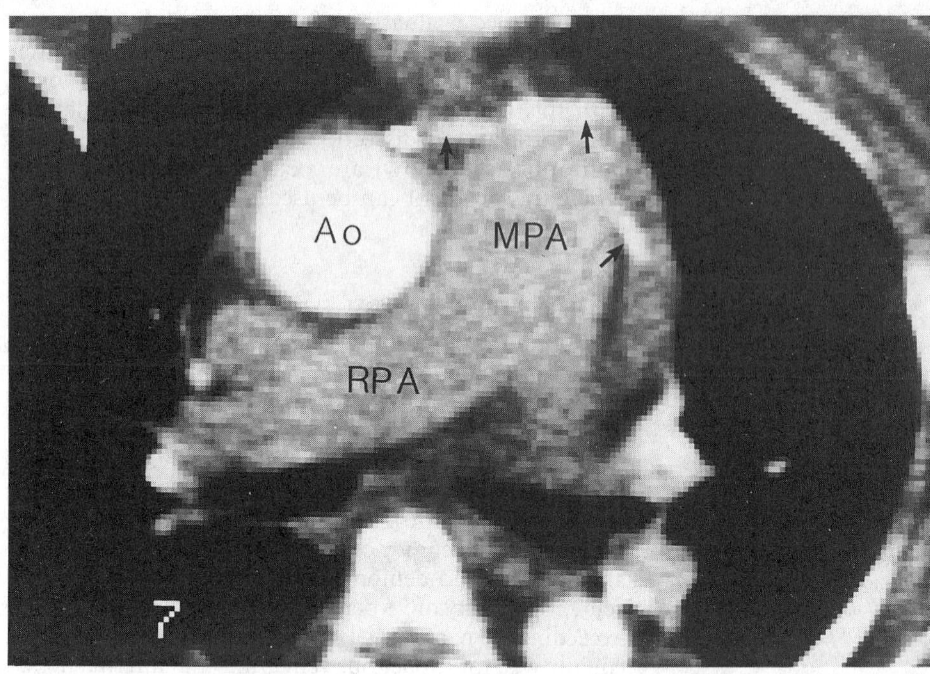

FIGURE 135-6 During maximal contrast enhancement of the ascending aorta (A), a patent branching saphenous vein coronary bypass graft (arrows) is clearly seen. MPA = main pulmonary.

superior to echocardiography in the detection of left ventricular thrombus.[31]

Ultrafast CT is useful in the evaluation of patients with chest pain and suspected coronary artery disease. In one study of patients presenting with chest pain and undergoing coronary arteriography, the ejection fraction response to exercise and the presence or absence of exercise-induced wall motion abnormalities were used successfully for differentiating patients with chest pain and coronary artery disease from those with chest pain and no coronary artery disease[8] (Fig. 135-9). The positive predictive accuracy was 92 percent for ultrafast CT compared to 63 percent for stress electrocardiography and 70 percent for thallium-201 myocardial scintigraphy. It

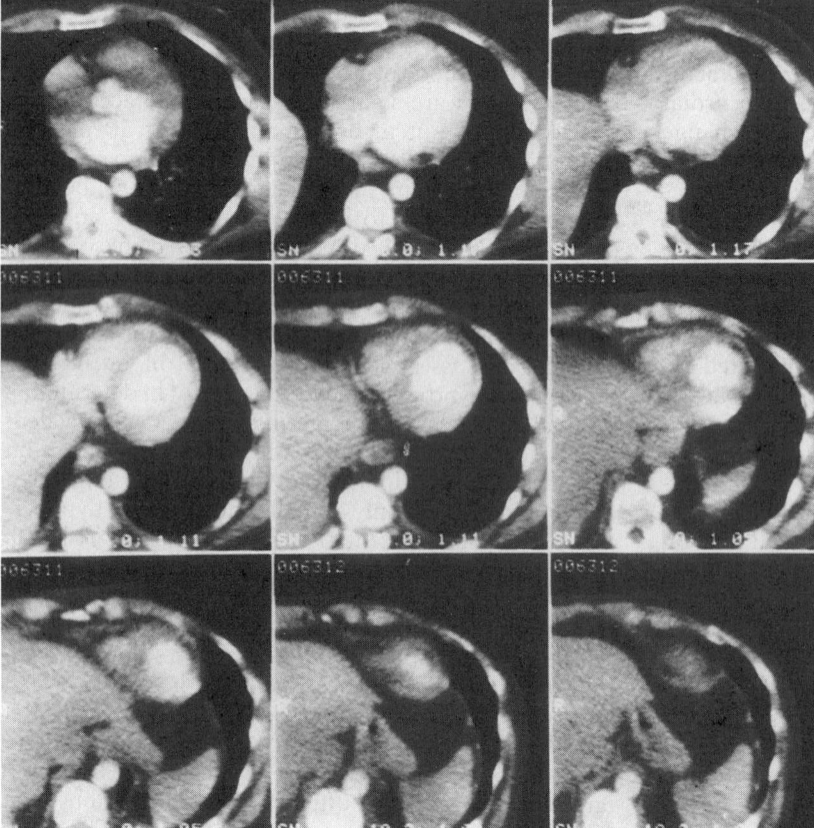

FIGURE 135-7 Fifty-millisecond contrast-enhanced ultrafast CT scans gated to end-diastole include the left ventricle from base (top left) to apex (bottom right). An acute myocardial infarction identified by the absence of myocardial enhancement is seen in panel 6 but is also apparent in several adjacent scans. *(From BH Brundage, E Chomka: Evaluation of acute myocardial infarction by computed tomography. In: BH Brundage (ed): Comparative Cardiac Imaging. Rockville, MD, Aspen, 1990:223–229. Reproduced with permission from the publisher and the author.)*

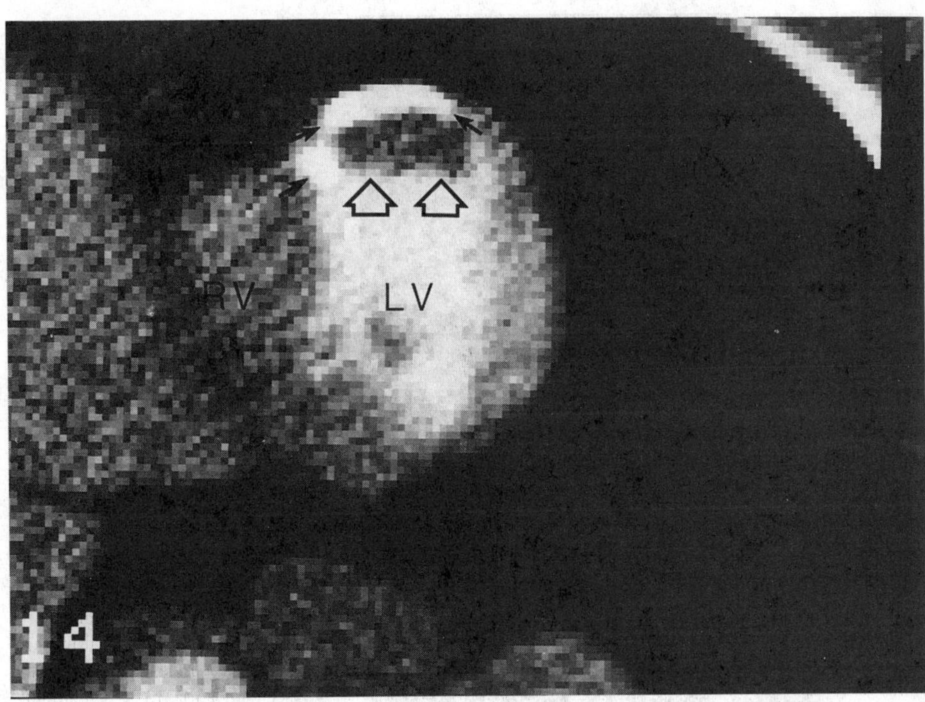

FIGURE 135-8 Calcified (small solid arrows) left ventricular (LV) aneurysm contains a large thrombus outlined by contrast enhancement. RV = right ventricle.

has also been shown that exercise ultrafast CT may be useful in the evaluation of the post–myocardial infarction patient prior to discharge from the hospital. When compared to low-level exercise thallium scintigraphy, ultrafast CT better differentiated multivessel and single-vessel disease.[30]

One of the more promising applications of ultrafast CT is the detection of coronary calcium (Fig. 135-10). Several investigators have demonstrated that the presence of coronary calcium detected by ultrafast CT is predictive of obstructive coronary artery disease; the sensitivity approaches 100 percent, and the specificity ranges from 60 to 90 percent.[33-35] In asymptomatic populations, ultrafast CT may be useful for identifying patients at risk for future coronary events so that clinicians can focus their risk factor reduction strategies on the most appropriate patients. One investigative group has shown that the progression of coronary artery calcification is more rapid in patients with symptomatic coronary artery disease than in those with coronary artery calcium but no symptoms.[36] Studies in progress are evaluating the value of serial quantification of coronary artery calcium to track the progression of coronary artery disease and to determine if risk factor prevention strategies are effective in slowing or reversing the progression of the disease as marked by the calcium content.

While current slice thickness and spatial resolution of ultrafast CT scanners are not sufficient to permit clinically diagnostic intravenous coronary angiography, the diagnosis of patients with Kawasaki's disease or anomalous origin of the coronary artery is possible with current ultrafast CT technology.[37] Future improvements in spatial resolution and slice thickness may soon make it feasible to perform diagnostic coronary angiography with ultrafast CT.[38]

VALVULAR HEART DISEASE

Echocardiography remains the standard for the evaluation of valvular heart disease; however, ultrafast CT offers several possible advantages in selected patients. Precise and accurate measurement of cardiac volumes has been demonstrated by several investigators. Reiter and coworkers[5] demonstrated in animals that ultrafast CT measurements of aortic regurgitant volume correlate well with measurements made by electromagnetic flow

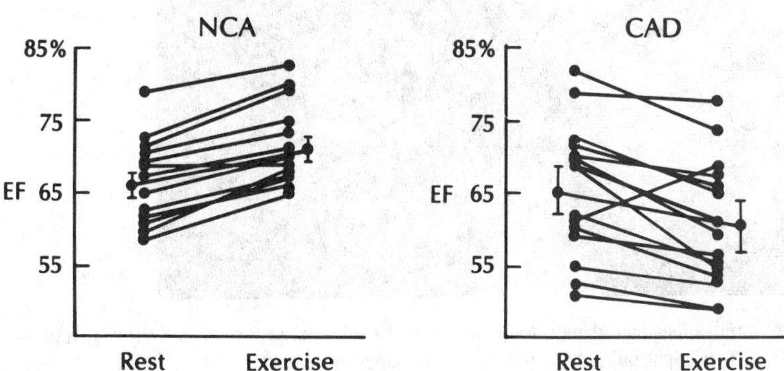

FIGURE 135-9 Ejection fraction (EF) response to bicycle exercise determined by ultrafast CT scanning is contrasted between chest pain patients with normal coronary arteries (NCAs) and those with coronary artery disease (CAD) as defined by coronary arteriography. *(From E Roig et al: Exercise ultrafast computed tomography for the detection of coronary artery disease. J Am Coll Cardiol 13:1073–1081, 1989. Reproduced with permission from the publisher and the author.)*

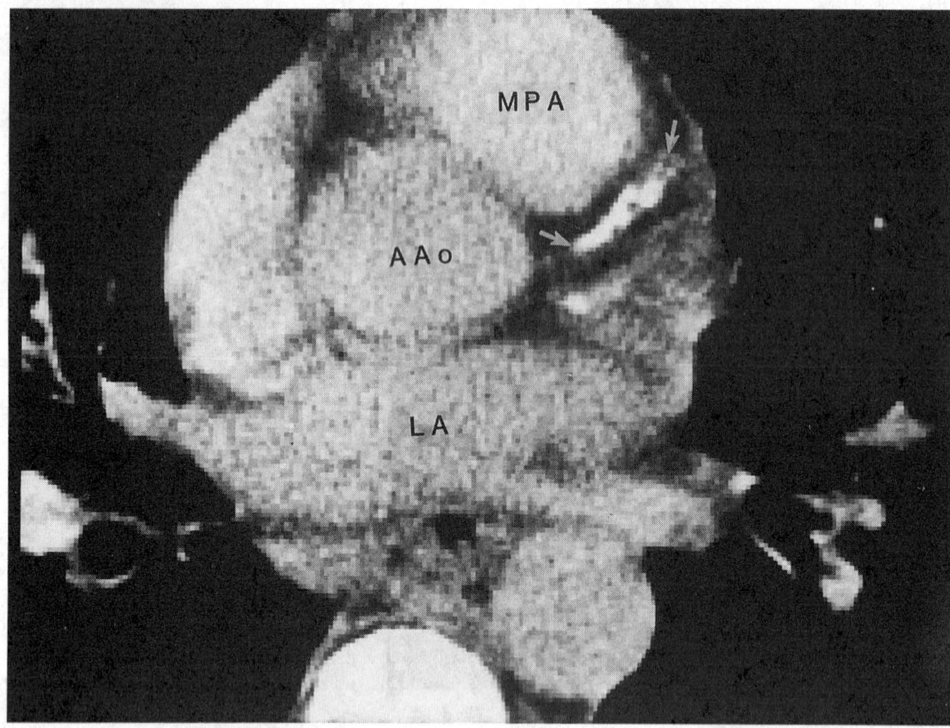

FIGURE 135-10 Densely calcified (arrows) left anterior descending coronary artery is easily detected on this nonenhanced ultrafast CT scan. AAo = ascending aorta; LA = left atrium; MPA = main pulmonary artery.

probes. In patients with isolated aortic or mitral regurgitation, determination of right ventricular and left ventricular volumes provides an accurate measurement of regurgitant volume. The degree of accuracy achieved has not been possible with other imaging techniques, including biplane ventriculography.

Several studies have demonstrated that CT can identify successfully left atrial thrombus[31,39] (Fig. 135-11). One study comparing ultrafast CT with echocardiography suggests that ultrafast CT may be more sensitive than transthoracic echocardiography.[31] To date there have been no comparisons of transesophageal echocardiography and ultrafast CT. However, ultrafast CT is significantly less invasive than transesophageal echocardiography.

Valve function and anatomy can be imaged by ul-

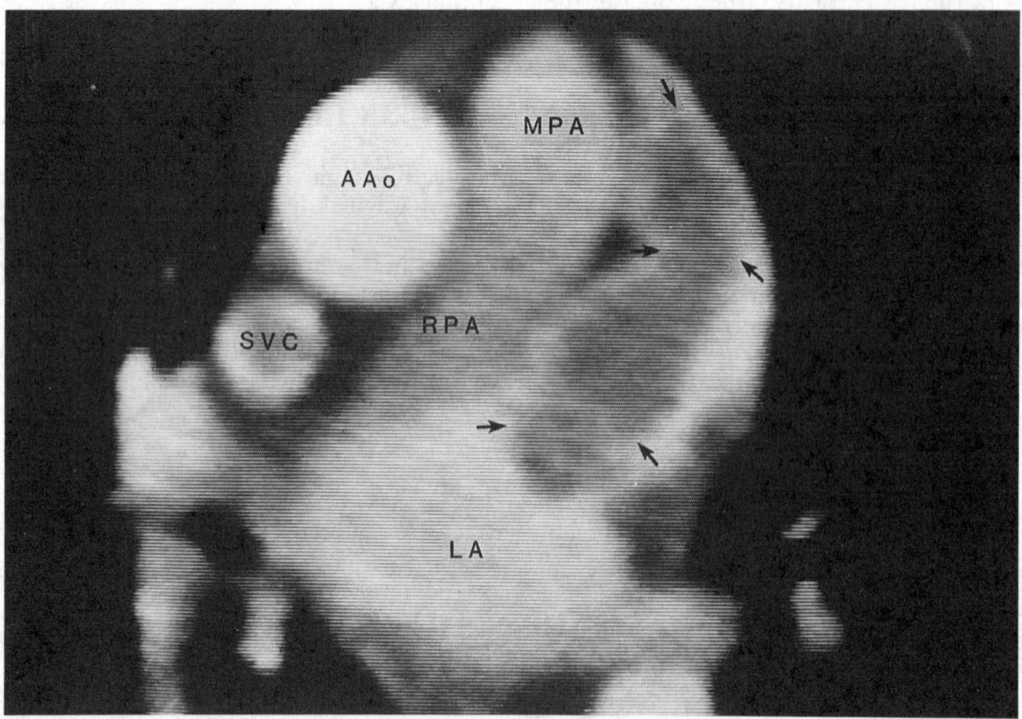

FIGURE 135-11 Contrast-enhanced ultrafast CT image of the left atrial appendage demonstrates the presence of a large thrombus (arrows). AAo = ascending aorta; LA = left atrium; MPA = main pulmonary artery; RPA = right pulmonary artery; SVC = superior vena cava.

trafast CT, but echocardiography remains the procedure of choice if an adequate acoustic window is available. In those patients where body habitus, obesity, or hyperinflation of the lungs prevents adequate images by echocardiography, ultrafast CT is a reasonable alternative. Prosthetic valve function can be assessed by ultrafast CT because the streak artifacts created by motion are minimized. Detection of valve ring abscess has also been reported.[40]

DISEASES OF THE GREAT VESSELS

Conventional CT has been widely employed for the assessment of aortic dissection. (See also Chap. 123.) Movement due to aortic pulsation and patient respiration, however, sometimes creates motion artifact that may conceal dissected intima. Ultrafast CT with its rapid image acquisition overcomes this drawback (Fig. 135-12). To date there are no comparative studies of ultrafast CT with conventional CT, nuclear magnetic resonance imaging, or echocardiography. Stanford[41] demonstrated excellent results when comparing ultrafast CT images with findings at surgery or autopsy. Ultrafast CT has advantages of speed and minimal invasiveness over conventional angiography, including tomographic image format. Comparative studies with transesophageal echocardiography and nuclear magnetic resonance are needed, but the speed with which ultrafast CT can be performed could well make it the procedure of choice for diagnosing dissection. Ultrafast CT also is useful in assessing thoracic and abdominal aortic aneurysms.[41] Excellent definition of the extent of the aneurysm and the amount of intraaneurysmal thrombus has been demonstrated (Fig. 135-12). Other abnormalities of the aorta such as sinus of Valsalva aneurysm, supervalvular aortic stenosis, and coarctation have been well demonstrated by this technique.[42–44]

Abnormalities of the pulmonary artery are also well visualized by ultrafast CT. Chronic pulmonary artery thromboembolism can be diagnosed, and the determination of the proximal extent of the thrombus, which is critical in planning surgical therapy, is well delineated (Fig. 135-13). Recent reports suggest that ultrafast CT also may prove to be a useful tool in the detection of acute pulmonary thromboembolism and that relatively small emboli are detectable.[45] Furthermore, tissue perfusion imaging techniques provide a type of "lung scan" that is a useful adjunct to the anatomic information provided.[21]

PERICARDIAL DISEASE

Ultrafast CT is well suited to the assessment of pericardial disease because of its tomographic representation of cardiac anatomy, high spatial resolution, and excellent density resolution.[46] Calcific constrictive pericarditis is easily diagnosed by ultrafast CT, and the distribution of the calcification, its thickness, and its extension into the visceral pericardium and myocardium are well defined (Fig. 135-14). Such geographic demonstration is helpful in planning the surgical treatment. The surgeon can focus on those areas of pericardium where the removal of the calcified pericardium is feasible. As with two-dimensional echocardiography, diastolic properties of the left ventricle can be evaluated using the cine mode.[6] Alterations in early and late diastolic filling are easily detected. Superior and inferior vena cava cross-sectional areas are good indicators of the degree of elevation of right ventricular diastolic and atrial filling pressures.

Pericardial effusion can also be evaluated by ultrafast

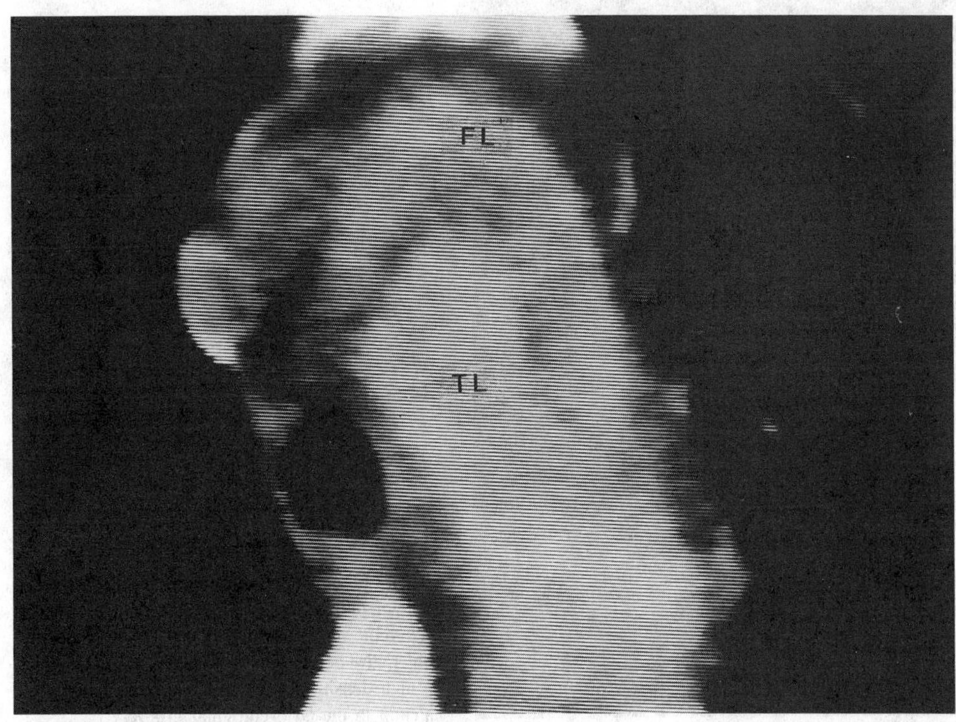

FIGURE 135-12 True (TL) and false (FL) lumens of an aortic isthmus dissection are defined during contrast enhancement.

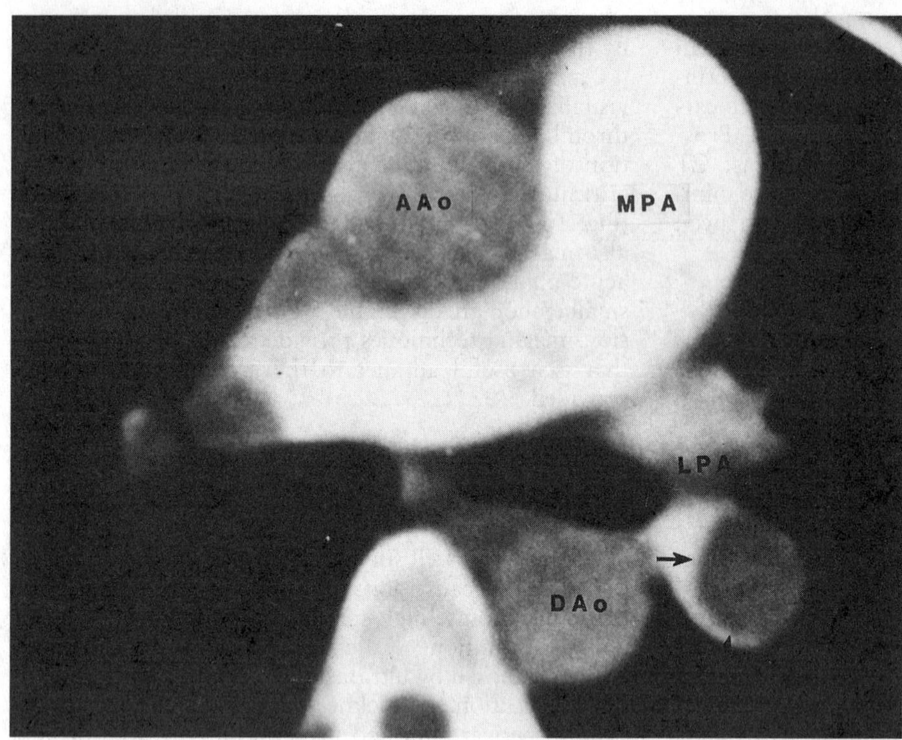

FIGURE 135-13 Large left pulmonary artery (LPA) chronic thrombus (arrows) is outlined by contrast medium on this high resolution ultrafast CT scan. AAo = ascending aorta; DAo = descending aorta; MPA = main pulmonary artery.

CT, although the density of the pericardial fluid is usually very similar to that of the myocardium so the exact amount cannot be determined unless intravenous contrast medium is used to enhance the myocardium. The cine mode is used to evaluate left and right ventricular function simultaneously. Tamponade can be detected by abnormalities in septal and right ventricular free-wall motion and right atrial filling characteristics similar to those described with echocardiography. (See also Chaps. 15 and 92.)

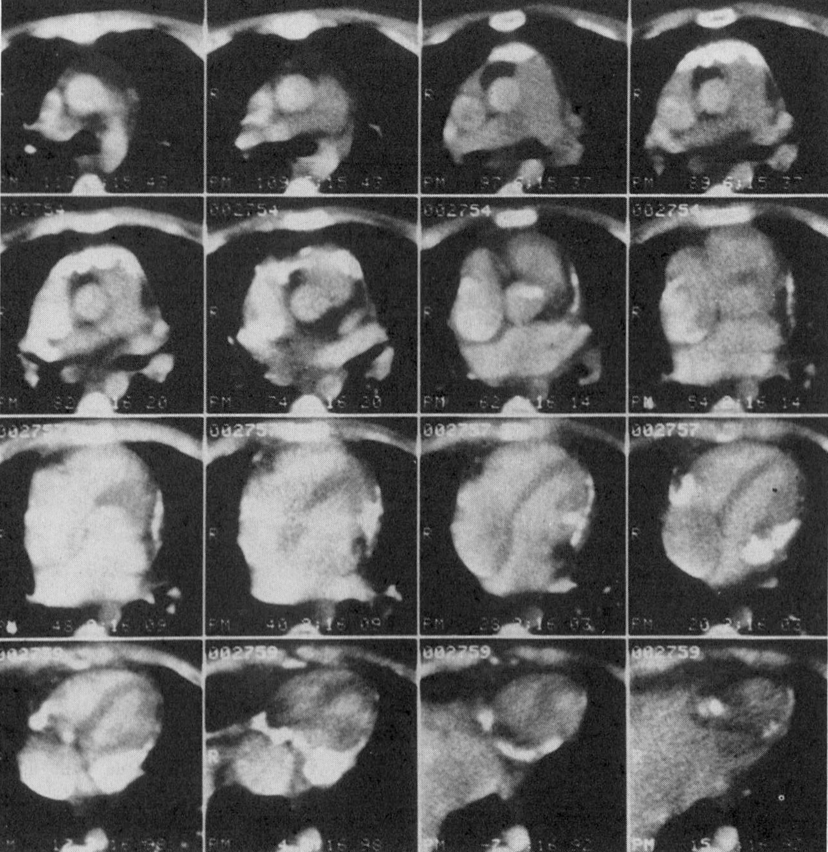

FIGURE 135-14 One-centimeter adjacent contrast-enhanced ultrafast CT scans from the aortic arch to the ventricular apex in a patient with calcific constrictive pericarditis. The calcium is identified by its high density (white). Note the large amount of calcium in the atrioventricular groove.

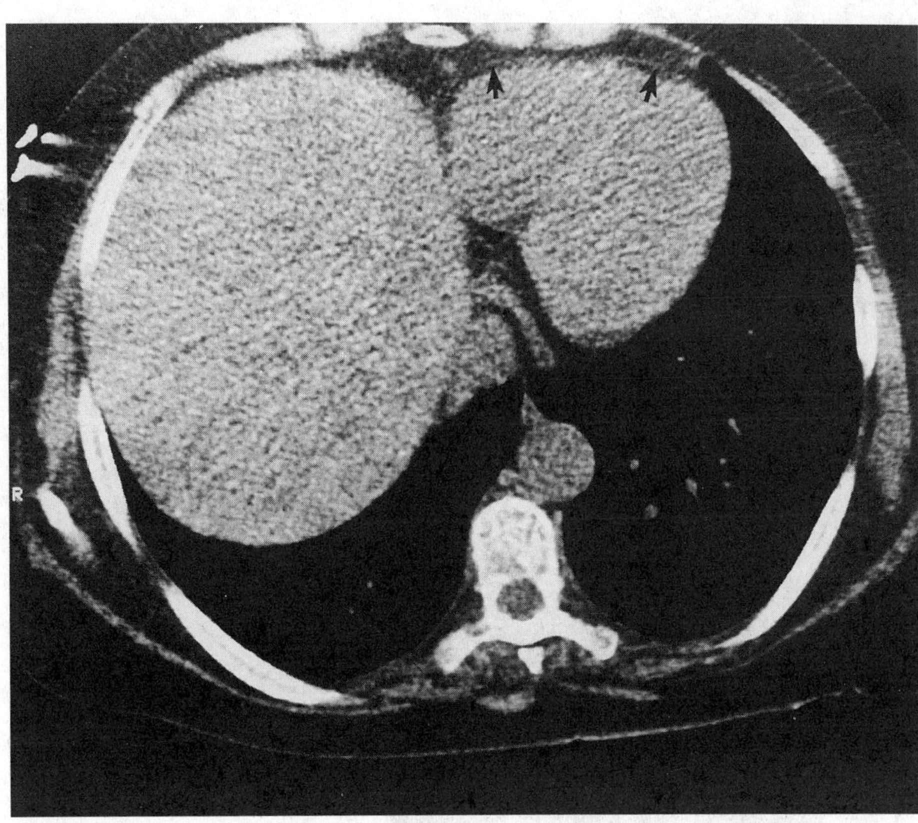

FIGURE 135-15 Ultrafast CT scan defines a normal thin anterior pericardium (arrows) in a patient thought to have constrictive pericarditis after echocardiography and cardiac catheterization.

Ultrafast CT is particularly well suited to assess pericardial involvement with metastatic tumors because it permits visualization of the mediastinum at the same time. The extent and location of pericardial involvement is therefore easily identified.

The high spatial resolution of ultrafast CT makes it possible to determine pericardial thickness, particularly over the anterior wall of the right ventricle (Fig. 135-15). The pericardium is silhouetted by the epicardial fat and the surrounding lung tissue. This allows an accurate measurement of pericardial thickness and is useful in cases in which it is difficult to determine whether there is pericardial constriction or myocardial restriction. A pericardial thickness in excess of 4 mm in patients with abnormal hemodynamics is strong evidence for pericardial constriction.

MYOCARDIAL DISEASE

The myocardium of both the right and left ventricle can be visualized in its entirety with ultrafast CT. Therefore, both precise measurement of myocardial mass and evaluation of right and left ventricular function are possible, and evaluation of diseases of the myocardium is optimized.[4,5,11–13] Ventricular hypertrophy of any cause can be quantified and serially evaluated, such as evaluation of regression of ventricular hypertrophy following the treatment of hypertensive heart disease or correction of aortic valve stenosis. Since both ventricular volumes and wall thickness can be determined accurately, when coupled with pressure analysis, global and regional wall stresses can be measured. In patients with hypertrophic cardiomyopathy the distribution and severity of the hypertrophic process can be quantified.[47] Also, systolic and diastolic ventricular function can be measured. Furthermore, assessment of mitral valve motion is also possible.

In idiopathic dilated cardiomyopathy quantitation of systolic and diastolic ventricular function and measurement of chamber volumes and wall stress before and after vasodilator treatment may be useful. (See also Chaps. 23 and 89.) Clues to the etiology of the dilated cardiomyopathy may also be acquired. Arrhythmogenic right ventricular dysplasia may be identified by careful analysis of right ventricular endocardial anatomy.[48] Furthermore, phase analysis of the left ventricular and right ventricular activation-contraction sequence can be used to identify the focus of ventricular tachycardia.[49] Ultrafast CT has also been used to identify unspecified cardiac abnormalities in patients with lone atrial fibrillation.[50]

CONGENITAL HEART DISEASE

The use of ultrafast CT to diagnose congenital heart disease is well described.[51] In addition to the obvious advantages of cross-sectional high-resolution imaging for defining cardiac structural abnormalities, ultrafast CT can also be used to quantify intracardiac shunts,[52] assess right and left ventricular function,[4,5] measure myocardial mass,[11–13] and evaluate valvular function (Fig. 135-16). With the indicator dilution technique, quantification of cardiac shunts by ultrafast CT has an accuracy equivalent to that of radioisotope methods.[52] Ultrafast CT has been used to diagnose atrial septal defect,[53] supravalvular aortic stenosis,[43] Ebstein's anomaly,[54] congenital

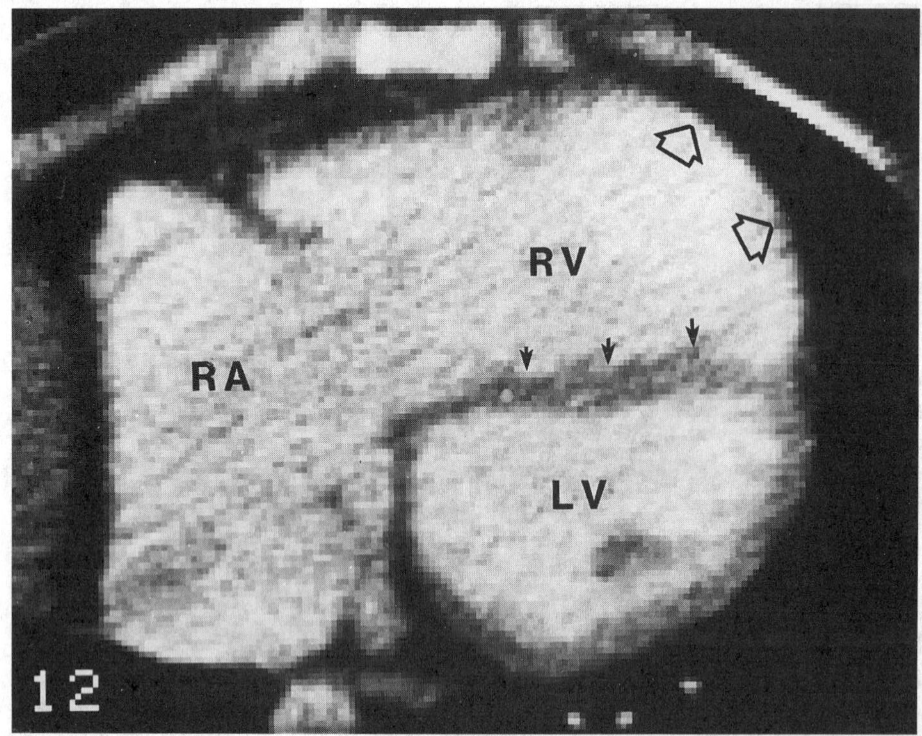

A

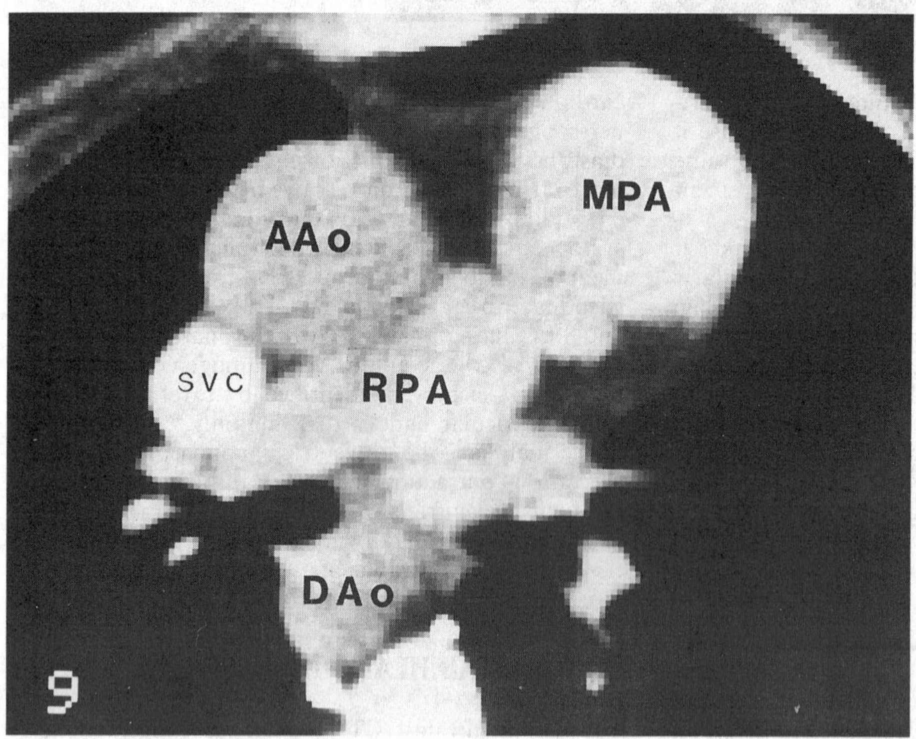

B

FIGURE 135-16 Postoperative ultrafast CT study of a patient operated for tetralogy of Fallot demonstrates (*A*) right ventricular dilation and aneurysm (open arrows) with paradoxical diastolic flattening of the interventricular septum due to severe tricuspid regurgitation. The same study (*B*) revealed residual stenosis of the right pulmonary artery (RPA). AAo = ascending aorta; DAo = descending aorta; LV = left ventricle; MPA = main pulmonary artery; RA = right atrium; SVC = superior vena cava.

arteriovenous fistulae,[42] conotruncal abnormalities,[55] cor triatriatum,[56] and ventricular septal defect.[57] The experience with ultrafast CT to diagnose congenital heart disease is small, but its ability to acquire images rapidly, its high spatial resolution, and its capacity to evaluate function, flow, and anatomy with a single diagnostic test offer great promise.

CARDIAC TUMORS

Intracardiac tumors are well visualized by ultrafast CT with intravenous contrast enhancement. Reports diagnosing both right[58] (Fig. 135-17) and left[59] atrial myxomas have been published. Ultrafast CT can also be useful for the evaluation of cardiac metastatic tumor. The excel-

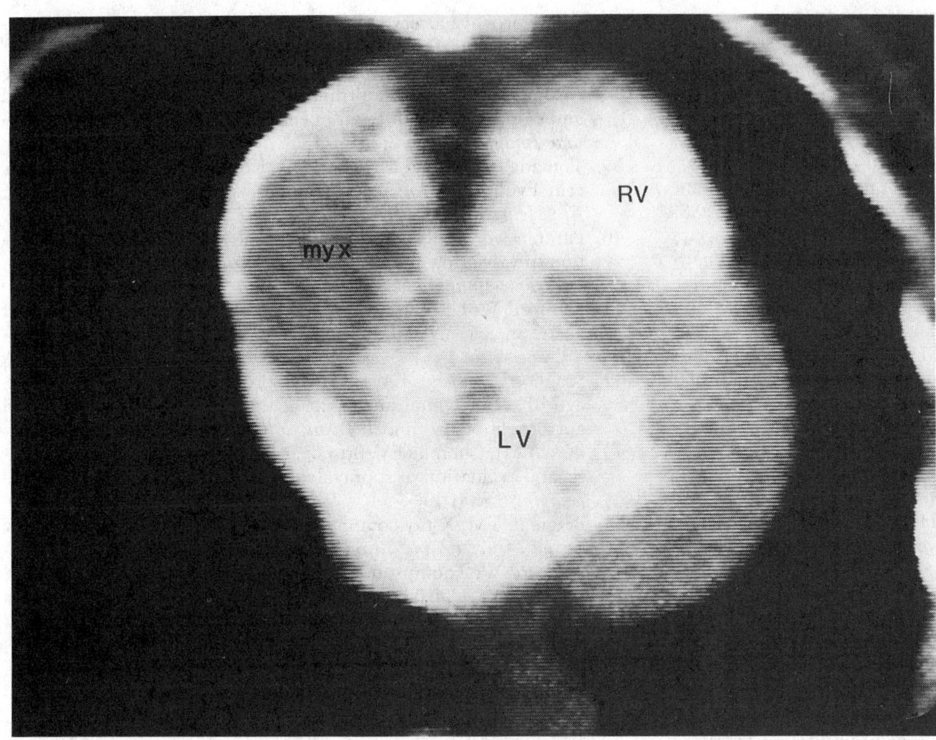

FIGURE 135-17 Large right atrial myxoma (myx) is depicted by contrast enhanced cine CT. LV = left ventricle; RV = right ventricle. *(From P Seifert et al: Application of the cine computed tomographic scan for precise localization of the origin of an atrial myxoma: Surgical implications. Ann Thorac Surg 42:467–470, 1986. Reproduced with permission from the publisher and the author.)*

lent visualization of adjacent mediastinal, pulmonary, and chest wall structures makes it useful in staging the tumor as well as suggesting its primary source. (See also Chap. 111.)

SUMMARY

Ultrafast CT is a new technology that has only been clinically available for a short time. In this interval it has been demonstrated to be useful in evaluating all forms of cardiac disease. In addition to providing excellent definition of normal and pathologic anatomy, its ability to evaluate both right and left ventricular global and regional function, provide precise measurements of cardiac volumes and myocardial mass, and assess myocardial tissue perfusion makes it a particularly unique and potentially powerful diagnostic tool. In the coming years ultrafast CT can be expected to receive much wider utilization.

REFERENCES

1. Gonda RL, Gutierrez OH, Azodo MVU: Mycotic aneurysms of the aorta: Radiologic features. *Radiology* 1988; 168:343–346.
2. Godwin JD, Herfkens RJ, Skioldebrand CG, Federle MP, Lipton MJ: Evolution of dissections and aneurysms of the thoracic aorta by conventional and dynamic CT scanning. *Radiology* 1980; 136:125–136.
3. Brundage BH, Lipton MJ, Herfkens RJ, Berninger WH, Redington RW, Chatterjee K, et al: Detection of patent coronary bypass grafts by computed tomography: A preliminary report. *Circulation* 1980; 61:826–831.
4. Feiring AJ, Rumberger JA, Rieter SJ, Collins SM, Skorton DJ, Rees M, et al: Sectional and segmental variability of left ventricular function: Experimental and clinical studies using ultrafast computed tomography. *J Am Coll Cardiol* 1988; 12:415–425.
5. Reiter SJ, Rumberger JA, Feiring AJ, Stanford W, Marcus ML: Precision of measurements of right and left ventricular volume by cine computed tomography. *Circulation* 1986; 74:890–900.
6. Rumberger JA, Weiss RM, Feiring AJ, Stanford W, Hajduczok ZD, Rezai K, et al: Patterns of regional diastolic function in the normal human left ventricle: An ultrafast computed tomographic study. *J Am Coll Cardiol* 1989; 14:119–126.
7. Rich S, Chomka EV, Stagl R, Shanes JG, Kondos GT, Brundage BH: Determination of left ventricular ejection fraction using ultrafast computed tomography. *Am Heart J* 1986; 112:392–396.
8. Roig E, Chomka EV, Castaner A, Campo A, Heras M, Rich S, et al: Exercise ultrafast computed tomography for the detection of coronary artery disease. *J Am Coll Cardiol* 1989; 13:1073–1081.
9. Lanzer P, Garrett J, Sievers R, O'Connell WO, Botvinick E, Higgens CB: Quantitation of regional myocardial function by cine computed tomography: Pharmacologic changes in wall thickness. *J Am Coll Cardiol* 1986; 8:682–692.
10. Bell MR, Rumberger JA, Stanson AW, Sheedy PF: Rapid and minimally invasive measurement of flow reserve with ultrafast CT (abstr). *Circulation* 1991; 84(II):678.
11. Feiring AJ, Rumberger JA, Reiter SJ, Skorton DJ, Collins SM, Lipton MJ, et al: Determination of left ventricular mass in dogs in rapid acquisition cardiac computer tomography. *Circulation* 1985; 72:1355–1364.
12. Roig E, Georgiou D, Chomka EV, Wolfkiel C, Logalbo-Zak C, Rich S, et al: Reproducibility of left ventricular myocardial volume and mass measurements by ultrafast computed tomography. *J Am Coll Cardiol* 1991; 18:990–996.
13. Hajduczok ZD, Weiss RM, Stanford W, Marcus ML: Determination of right ventricular mass in humans and dogs with ultrafast computed tomography. *Circulation* 1990; 82:202–212.
14. Wolfkiel CJ, Ferguson JL, Chomka EV, Law WR, Brundage BH: Determination of cardiac output by ultrafast computed tomography. *Am J Physiol Imaging* 1986; 1:117–123.
15. Garrett J, Lanzer P, Jaschke W, Botvinick E, Sievers R, Higgens CB, et al: Measurement of cardiac output by cine computed tomography. *Am J Cardiol* 1985; 56:657–661.
16. Wolfkiel CJ, Ferguson JL, Chomka EV, Law WR, Labin IN, Tenzer ML, et al: Measurement of myocardial blood flow by ultrafast computed tomography. *Circulation* 1987; 76:1262–1273.

17. Rumberger JA, Feiring AJ, Lipton MJ, Higgins CB, Ell SR, Marcus ML: Use of ultrafast computed tomography to quantitate regional myocardial perfusion: A preliminary report. *J Am Coll Cardiol* 1987; 9:59–69.
18. Wang T, Wu X, Cheng N, Ritman EL: Myocardial blood flow estimated by synchronous, multislice, high-speed computed tomography. *IEEE Med Imaging* 1989; 8:70–77.
19. Weiss RM, Hajduczok JD, Marcus ML: A new cine CT algorithm for quantitation of myocardial perfusion (abstr). *Circulation* 1988; 78(II):98A.
20. Canty JM, Srinivasan G: First-pass myocardial extraction of non-ionic contrast is dependent upon vasomotor tone; estimates at rest and following vasodilation using fast CT (abstr). *Circulation* 1991; 84(II):678.
21. Larsen RL, Bridges CR, Beck KC, Hoffman EA: Regional pulmonary blood flow via cine-xray computed tomography (abstr). *FASEB J* 1990; 4:A1074.
22. Stanford W, Brundage BH, Mac Millan R, Bateman TM, Chomka EV, Lipton MJ, et al: Sensitivity and specificity of assessing coronary bypass graft patency with ultrafast computed tomography: Results of a multicenter study. *J Am Coll Cardiol* 1988; 12:1–7.
23. Whiting JS, Bateman TM, Sethna DH: Quantitation of saphenous vein bypass graft flow using intravenous contrast ultrafast CT (abstr). *Circulation* 1986; 74(II):41.
24. Rumberger JA, Feiring AJ, Hiratzka LE, Reiter SJ, Stanford W, Marcus ML: Determination of changes in coronary bypass graft flow rate using cine-CT (abstr). *J Am Coll Cardiol* 1986; 7:155A.
25. Brundage BH, Hart K, Chomka E, Kieras K, Pietras RJ, Pavel D: Detection, location and sizing of acute myocardial infarction by fast, computed tomography (abstr). *Clin Res* 1985; 33:172A.
26. Rumberger JA, Reed JE, Behrenbeck T: Serial changes in regional infarct and noninfarct wall thickness after anterior wall myocardial infarction (abstr). *Circulation* 1991; 84(II):475.
27. Hajduczok ZD, Stanford W, Weiss RM: Serial assessment of ventricular remodeling after infarction in humans (abstr). *Circulation* 1991; 84(II):475.
28. Chomka EV, Wolfkiel CJ, Claudio J, Brundage BH: Combined perfusion and functional imaging of the left ventricle in patients with recent myocardial infarction by ultrafast computed tomography. *J Am Coll Cardiol* 1987; 9:151A.
29. Halmann M, Sideman S, Marcus M, Bayar R: Superimposition of the coronary tree on the three dimensional reconstructed left ventricle: Comparison of risk region to aneurysm mapping (abstr). *Circulation* 1991; 84(II):678.
30. Pietras RJ, Ashley WW, Bertsch MJ, De Graff JA, Wen TW, Quintana J, et al: Prediction of morbidity post myocardial infarction by treadmill thallium 201 and exercise ultrafast computed tomography (abstr). *Circulation* 1989; 80(II):309.
31. Helgason CM, Chomka E, Louie E, Rich S, Zajoc E, Roig E, et al: The potential role for ultrafast cardiac computed tomography in patients with stroke. *Stroke* 1989; 20:465–472.
32. Lessick J, Sideman S, Azhari H, Marcus M, Orenadir E, Beyer R: Regional three-dimensional geometric ventricle with fibrous aneurysms: A cine computed tomography study. *Circulation* 1991; 84:1172–1186.
33. Tannenbaum SR, Kondos GT, Veselick KE, Pendergast MR, Brundage BH, Chomka EV: Detection of calcific deposits in coronary arteries by ultrafast computed tomography and correlation with angiography. *Am J Cardiol* 1989; 63:870–871.
34. Agatston AS, Janowitz WR, Hildner FJ, Zusmer AR, Viamonte M, Detrano R: Quantification of coronary artery calcium using ultrafast computed tomography. *J Am Coll Cardiol* 1990; 15:827–832.
35. Simons DB, Schwartz RS, Sheedy PF, Breen JF, Rumberger JA: Non-invasive detection of anatomic coronary artery disease by ultrafast CT: A quantitative pathologic study (abstr). *J Am Coll Cardiol* 1991; 17:104A.
36. Janowitz WR, Agatston AS, Viamonte M: Comparison of serial quantitative evaluation of calcific coronary artery plaque by ultrafast computed tomography in persons with and without obstructive coronary artery disease. *Am J Cardiol* 1991; 68:1–6.
37. Frey EE, Matherne GP, Mahoney LT, Soto Y, Stanford W, Smith WL: Coronary artery aneurysms due to Kawasaki disease: Diagnosis with ultrafast CT. *Radiology* 1988; 167:725–726.
38. Napel S, Rutt B, Pflugfelder P: Three dimensional images of the coronary arteries from ultrafast computed tomography: Method and comparison with two-dimensional arteriography. *Am J Cardiac Imaging* 1989; 3:237–243.
39. Tomada H, Hoshiai M, Tagawa R, Koide S, Kawada S, Shotsu A, et al: Evolution of left atrial thrombus with computed tomography. *Am Heart J* 1980; 100:306–310.
40. Paramesworam R, Roman C, Eldredge WJ, Maranhao V: Detection of valve ring abscess by ultrafast computed tomography. *Am J Cardiac Imaging* 1988; 2:229–231.
41. Stanford W: Ultrafast computed tomography in the diagnosis of aortic aneurysms and dissections. *J Thorac Imaging* 1990; 5:32–39.
42. Scagliotti D, Fisher EA, Deal BJ, Gordon D, Chomka EV, Brundage BH: Congenital aneurysm of the left sinus of Valsalva and aorto-pulmonary tunnel. *J Am Coll Cardiol* 1986; 7:443–445.
43. Bertch MJ, Chomka EV, Brundage BH: Ultrafast CT in the diagnosis and evaluation of supravalvular aortic stenosis. *Am J Cardiac Imaging* 1988; 1:47–54.
44. Bateman TM: X-ray computed tomography of the cardiovascular system. *Curr Probl Cardiol* 1991; 16:771–829.
45. Stanford W, Thompson BH, Landas SK, Geraghty JJ, Reiner TJ, Jabro MN, et al: High resolution ultrafast CT in the diagnosis of experimental pulmonary embolisms (abstr). *Circulation* 1991; 84(II):156.
46. Rees M, Mac Millan R, Flicker S, Fender B, Clark D: Rapid-acquisition computed tomography demonstration of chronic calcified pericardial constriction. *J Comput Tomogr* 1986; 10:183–186.
47. Chomka EV, Wolfkiel CJ, Rich S, Shanes JG, Tamboli H, Brundage BH: Ultrafast computed tomography: A new method for the evaluation of hypertrophic cardiomyopathy. *Am J Noninvas Cardiol* 1987; 1:140–151.
48. Dery R, Lysbon MJ, Garrett JS, Abbott J, Higgins CB, Sheinman MM: Cine-computed tomography of arrhythmogenic right ventricular dysplasia. *J Comput Assist Tomogr* 1986; 10:120–123.
49. Martino JB, Fisher DJ, Collins SM, Stanford W: Phase analysis of cine computed tomography identifies sites of origin of ventricular tachycardia in patients (abstr). *J Am Coll Cardiol* 1991; 17:284A.
50. Hopson JR, Weiss RM, Stanford W, Kringle G: Cine computed tomographic abnormalities in "lone" atrial fibrillation (abstr). *Circulation* 1990; 82(III):58.
51. Eldredge WJ, Flicker S: Evaluation of congenital heart disease using cine-CT. *Am J Cardiac Imaging* 1987; 1:38–50.
52. Mac Millan RM, Rees MR, Eldredge WJ, Maranhao V, Clark D: Quantitation of shunting at the atrial level using rapid acquisition computed tomography with comparison to cardiac catheterization. *J Am Coll Cardiol* 1986; 7:946–948.
53. Skotvicki R, Maranhao V, Clark D, Flicker S, Eldredge J: Detection of atrial septal defect by cine CT scanning. *Cath Cardiovasc Diag* 1986; 12:103–106.
54. Garrett JS, Schiller NB, Botvinick EH, Higgins CB, Lipton MJ: Cine-computed tomography of Ebstein's anomaly. *J Comput Assist Tomogr* 1986; 10:664–666.
55. Bali C, Fisher EA, Chomka E, Brundage BH: Cine computed tomography in conotruncal abnormalities (abstr). *Clin Res* 1987; 35:260A.
56. Mac Millan RM, Rees MR, Maranhao V, Clark DL: Cine-computed tomography of cor triatriatum. *J Comput Assist Tomogr* 1986; 10:124–125.
57. Eldredge WJ, Rees M, Flicker S, Clark DL: Cine-CT scanning of the ventricular septum for the diagnosis of ventricular septal defect (abstr). *Circulation* 1985; 72(III):27.
58. Seifert P, Chomka EV, Stagl R, Swarner D, Brundage BH, Levitsky S: Application of the cine computed tomographic scan for precise localization of the origin of an atrial myxoma: Surgical implications. *Ann Thorac Surg* 1986; 42:467–470.
59. Bateman TM, Sethna DH, Whiting JS, Chaux A, Berman DS, Forrester JS: Comprehensive non-invasive evaluation of left atrial myxoma using cardiac cine-computed tomography. *J Am Coll Cardiol* 1987; 9:1180–1183.

Chapter 136

Magnetic Resonance Imaging of the Heart and Great Vessels

Roderic I. Pettigrew, Ph.D., M.D.

PHYSICAL FUNDAMENTALS

The physical phenomenon of nuclear magnetic resonance (NMR) was first described by Felix Block and Edward Purcell and colleagues in 1946.[1,2] In 1952 Block and Purcell jointly received the Nobel Prize in physics for this discovery, which became a major analytical tool of chemists over the subsequent 20 years. It was not until 1973, however, that Paul Lauterbur produced the first two-dimensional image, a very low resolution scan of two small glass tubes filled with water.[3] Not surprisingly, an additional 10 years was required to develop and refine the hardware and the computer software techniques needed to obtain clinically useful in vivo human cardiovascular images. Currently, NMR can be used to simultaneously evaluate cardiac and vascular structure, chamber and valve function, blood flow, and to some extent, myocardial tissue character while producing images with superb morphologic detail. When the phenomenon of NMR is used to produce images, this technique is now popularly referred to simply as *magnetic resonance imaging (MRI),* ostensibly to prevent the public concerns associated with any term that includes "nuclear."

Nuclear magnetic resonance can be observed only when the *nuclear* component of an atom contains an odd number of either neutrons or protons and is placed in a static *magnetic* field.[4] Because of the odd number of nucleons, the nucleus has intrinsic spin about its own axis and also precesses about the direction of the static magnetic field, much like a gyroscope or a spinning top that precesses, or sweeps out a cone-shaped path, about the direction of the earth's gravitational pull. This nucleus can then be stimulated from its "ground," or "resting," state to a higher energy level by exposure to a second magnetic field that oscillates. When the stimulating magnetic field is oscillating at a frequency that exactly matches the precessional frequency of the nucleus, the stimulating field and the target nucleus are said to be in *resonance,* a condition that results in maximal excitation of the target nucleus. When the stimulating field is turned off, the excited nucleus relaxes back to its resting state over a time characteristic of the chemical environment in which the nucleus resides. This time period, aptly called the *spin-lattice* or *T_1 relaxation* time, is simply the time needed for 63 percent of the excited nuclei to return to their initial resting state. A second type of relaxation process in which the initial coherent alignment of the newly excited nuclei dissipates over time also occurs. This loss of coherence is due to the destructive interference between the local tiny magnetic fields of each nucleus and those of its neighbors. The time that characterizes this process is referred to as the spin-spin or T_2 relaxation time and also reflects chemical structure, having a direct relationship with the extent of molecular motion (i.e., T_2 is longer for liquids than for solids). The T_2 is simply the time required for the maximally coherent spin alignment to be reduced by 63 percent.

Magnetic resonance imaging is based on the observation that there are significant differences in the fundamental NMR parameters of the hydrogen nucleus (a proton) in different tissues.[4,5] These parameters are (1) proton density, (2) T_1 relaxation time, (3) T_2 relaxation time, and (4) flow of protons. A fifth parameter, chemical shift, gives rise to NMR spectra but is not typically used in conventional cardiac imaging. When the hydrogen nucleus, a proton, is excited within the body, it can produce a detectable electric signal whose spatial location may be determined by causing the static magnetic field strength to vary with position. This in turn causes the frequency of the signal to indicate its spatial origin. Once the originating location of the signal is determined through mathematical signal data analysis, an image can be constructed in which the shade of gray on a scale from black to white is made to be proportional to the NMR signal strength. This signal strength depends on the composite effects of all the fundamental NMR parameters. However, the NMR process can be executed with a variety of techniques specifically chosen to emphasize the relative contribution of any of these parameters to the image intensity. This is referred to as "weighting" the image to a specific fundamental parameter. The image contrast, therefore, depends largely on the difference between the emphasized fundamental NMR parameter values for the tissues of interest. Of the various fundamental NMR parameters, the relaxation times exhibit the greatest differences for tissues, as opposed to proton density weighted images, which exhibit little contrast. When visualization of intracardiac, transvalvular, or intravascular flow patterns is sought, techniques that highlight flow effects are employed, as discussed below.

Because the relaxation times for myocardium, epicardial fat, and blood differ by at least 200 percent, the magnetic resonance image contrast is markedly superior to that obtained with conventional x-ray computed tomography, which reflects much smaller soft tissue x-ray attenuation differences of the order of 10 to 15 percent (Table 136-1, Fig. 136-1). This high degree of soft tissue contrast in MRI allows cardiac imaging to be accomplished without the necessity of administering a contrast medium, which is required in conventional or cine x-ray computed tomography, cardiac catheterization, and nuclear medicine procedures. In addition, the sensitivity of MRI to flowing protons further increases the contrast between moving blood and cardiac chamber or vascular walls. When desired, the sensitivity to flow can be used to directly visualize intracardiac shunts and regurgitant jets in valvular insufficiency. Since these high-contrast images can be obtained with electrocardiographic gating during small time windows of approximately 5 to 25 ms sequentially spaced throughout the cardiac cycle, dynamic or cine studies can be constructed. This makes the study of cardiac function possible.

TABLE 136-1

Representative NMR Relaxation Times and X-ray Attenuation Coefficients

	T_1 (ms)	T_2 (ms)	u (cm^{-1})
Fat	175	100	0.18*
Myocardium	550	45	0.20*
Blood (static)	900	360	~0.20†
Acute myocardial infarction	~630	~55	~0.20†

T_1 = spin-lattice or longitudinal relaxation time; T_2 = spin-spin or transverse relaxation time; u = x-ray attenuation coefficient at 70 keV.

*Data obtained from Johns HE, Cunningham JR: *Physics of Radiology*, 4th ed. Springfield, IL, Charles C Thomas, 1983.

†Approximate, estimated from *.

Thus, MRI is a versatile technique which can be used routinely to obtain several basic categories of clinically useful information: (1) excellent definition of normal and pathological detail in three dimensions (3D), allowing wall thickness, chamber volumes, valve areas, vessel cross sections, and lesion location and sizes to be accurately measured; (2) limited tissue characterization of paracardiac and intracardiac masses, pericardial effusions, infiltrative lesions, and myocardial infarction due to differences in relaxation times and resulting signal intensity; (3) evaluation of global and regional biventricular function, including measurements of absolute systolic wall thickening, severity of valvular insufficiency, radial shortening, ejection fraction, stroke volume, and cardiac output; and (4) blood flow quantification with both instantaneous and integrated blood velocity measurements within vessels over the cardiac cycle, permitting the measurements of forward and reverse cardiac output and pulmonic and systemic flow ratios. This per-

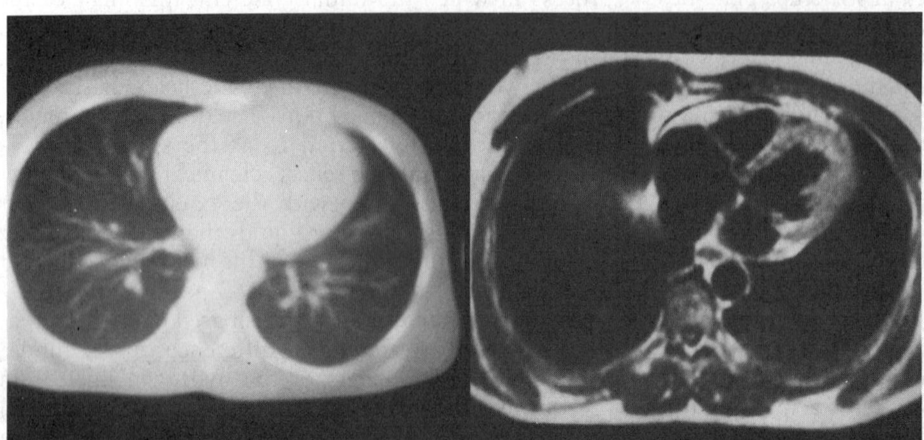

FIGURE 136-1 Transverse x-ray computed tomography (*A*) and MRI (*B*) sections through the heart. Superior MRI depiction of morphologic detail results from greater soft tissue and blood contrast, due to large MRI relaxation time differences versus small x-ray attenuation differences. (*From Casarella WJ, Ball TI, Bernardinio ME, et al: Magnetic resonance imaging: Current clinical applications (pt 2). Emory Univ J Med 1:197, 1987. Reproduced with permission from the publisher and authors.*)

mits MRI to be clinically useful in evaluating a wide variety of cardiovascular diseases as outlined in Table 136-2.

TECHNIQUES AND NORMAL ANATOMY

As already indicated, the appearance and signal intensity of tissues in an MR image depend heavily on the type of imaging technique used. Currently, two techniques that are complementary in the appearances of the images they generate and in the type of information that can be obtained with them are widely used. These are electrocardiographic gated spin echo and fast gradient echo imaging.[5–14] This second approach is referred to by a variety of acronyms that are different for each manufacturer of MRI systems. These include FAME (fast acquisition with multiphase excitation), FLASH (fast low-angle shot), and GRASS (gradient recalled acquisition in the steady state).[12–14] Variations of these basic conventional techniques have given rise to more recent ones (e.g., "turbo FLASH") which can generate images in less than 1 s, as opposed to the several minutes required for current conventional approaches.[15] Additional specialized techniques that have begun to have increasing utilization are spin phase-velocity mapping for flow quantification, myocardial tagging to assess regional and intramyocardial wall thickening, regional strain, and deformation dynamics.[16–18] These techniques are briefly described below.

Spin echo imaging is particularly useful for evaluating cardiac structure, paracardiac and intracardiac masses and thrombi, and acute and remote myocardial infarction.[10,11] The fast gradient echo technique is excellent for evaluating regurgitant lesions, intracardiac shunts, and flow within vessels.[14,19–22] Either technique can be used to measure right and left ventricular volumes and quantitative functional indexes, e.g., biventricular ejection fractions, biventricular stroke volumes, cardiac output, radial shortening, and systolic wall thickening.[14,19–29] (For a more detailed description of how these procedures are technically executed, see Refs. 7 and 11–13.)

With the spin echo technique, the NMR signal is retrieved at a time that is typically 20 to 30 ms after the proton is excited. This signal is referred to as an *echo,* and the time at which this echo is obtained is simply called the *echo time* (TE). The first signal to be received is called the *first echo.* This procedure can be executed in such a way that a *second echo* signal is obtained at a later time which is typically approximately twice that at which the first echo was retrieved, i.e., typically at a TE of 60 to 90 ms. Spin echo images generated with both echoes are useful. The images obtained with the shorter echo times have a better signal-to-noise ratio and excellent contrast between epicardial fat, myocardium, and rapidly flowing blood. Thus, images obtained with the first echo tend to be most useful for defining anatomic features. The first echo image, however, does not usually exhibit good lesion contrast for pathologic tissues which are characterized by increases in T_1 and T_2. This is so because the first echo image exhibits a signal intensity that reflects a mixture of T_1 and T_2 influences, and these have opposing effects on signal intensity. That is, an increase in T_1 causes a decrease in signal intensity; an increase in T_2 produces an increase in signal intensity. The second echo image with TE = 60 ms or longer is typically more T_2 weighted, having more time for T_2 decay (relaxation) to occur. Thus, the second echo image is more often useful in detecting lesions characterized by abnormally long or shortened T_2 times, e.g., acute myocardial infarction, myocardial scar, and cardiac masses.

A normal spin echo study (Fig. 136-2) is characterized by a relatively dark signal intensity for rapidly flowing intracardiac blood, particularly during systole and early diastole. During late to end diastole, the signal intensity for relatively slow flowing blood may be bright. In the normal cardiac image, the structures that are typically identified, in order of decreasing spin echo signal inten-

TABLE 136-2
Cardiovascular Applications of MRI

Disorder	MRI Information
Congenital heart disease	Three-dimensional structure Biventricular function, pre- and postoperative Shunt identification Valve areas Severity of valve regurgitation
Aortic aneurysm, dissection, coarctation	Cross-sectional area Site of dissection/intimal flap Thrombus identification Location of important branches
Ischemic heart disease	Site and extent of infarction and sequelae Viable myocardium versus scar Ventricular aneurysms, thrombi Segmental wall motion and systolic thickening Global function and indexes, e.g., RVEF, LVEF, CO
Cardiac masses	Lesions, site and extent Resectability Functional consequence Limited tissue characterization
Cardiomyopathies	Myocardial function/dysfunction Hypertrophic site and distribution Myopathic vs. reactive hypertrophy Ventricular mass
Valvular heart disease	Visualization of regurgitant jets Regurgitant fractions/volumes Valve area Chamber volumes
Pericardial disease	Thickened pericardium Intrapericardial adhesions Effusion volume Transudative vs. exudative Functional consequence

NOTE: RVEF, LVEF = right and left ventricular ejection fractions; CO = cardiac output.

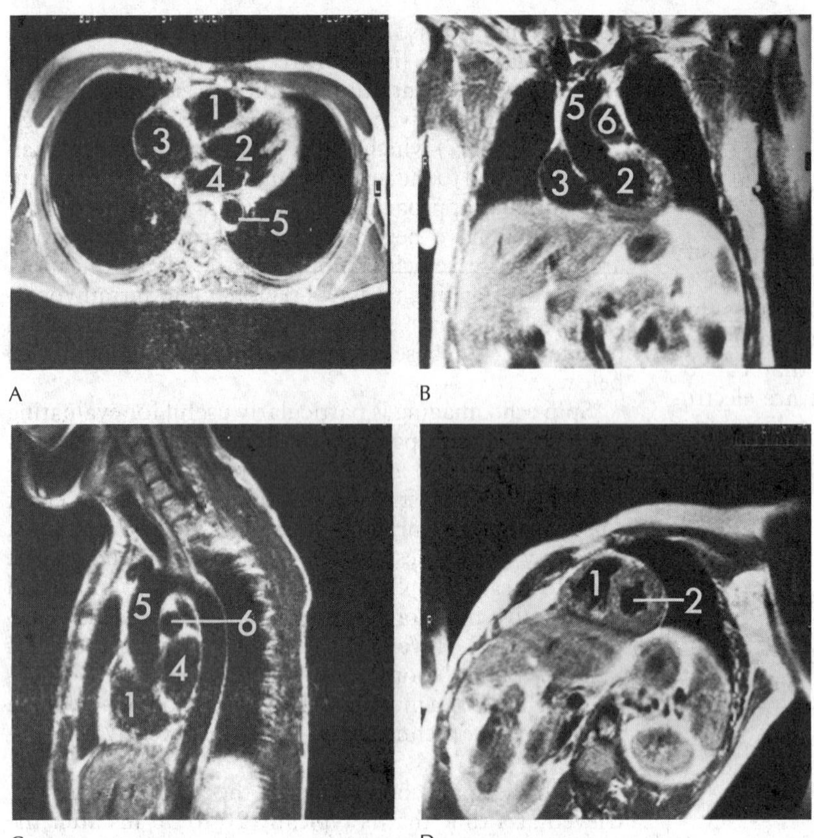

FIGURE 136-2 Normal sections: transverse (*A*), coronal (*B*), sagittal (*C*), and short axis (*D*). (1) Right ventricle; (2) left ventricle; (3) right atrium; (4) left atrium; (5) aorta; (6) pulmonary artery.

sity, are (1) pericardial and epicardial fat, (2) cardiac valves, (3) myocardium, (4) flowing intracardiac and intravascular blood, and (5) pericardial space/fluid.[8–10] Normally the pericardial and epicardial fat, as well as the subcutaneous fat, constitute the brightest tissue in an image. Both cardiac valves and the myocardium have a more medium gray-level intensity, although cardiac valves are typically only imaged with the spin echo technique when they are closed. (As discussed below, the valve leaflets may be visualized throughout the cardiac cycle with the fast gradient echo technique.) The dark signal intensity of rapidly flowing blood results in high contrast with the cardiac valves, atrial and ventricular septa, papillary muscles, myocardial wall, and walls of the great vessels and their branches.

In order to obtain a dynamic study with the spin echo technique (Fig. 136-3), one acquires a series of excitations of multiple slices encompassing the cardiac chambers, with each slice at a different phase of the cardiac cycle. This procedure is repeated with successive permutations of the phase at which a slice is excited, so that after a sufficient number of permutations, each slice is imaged at enough phases of the cardiac cycle to permit cine display.[7–11] In a 20-min acquisition time, one can typically obtain six to seven 1-cm-thick short-axis slices spanning both ventricular chambers, with each slice imaged at 12 to 14 phases over the first approximate 500 to 600 ms of the cardiac cycle. This results in images being obtained at intervals of approximately 40 ms, permitting adequate evaluation of systolic ventricular function.[11] Obviously, however, this approach does not permit diastolic function to be evaluated.

The fast gradient echo technique generates an echo in a time that is quite short compared to that of conventional spin echo imaging.[12–14] Typically, the gradient echoes are obtained at 4 to 12 ms and are obtained at rapid successive intervals of 25 to 40 ms throughout the cardiac cycle. This permits one or more slices to be rapidly imaged at a relatively large number of phases (typically 16 or more) of the cardiac cycle. Because of the significantly shorter echo times, this technique produces images characterized by bright signal intensity from rapidly flowing blood. In direct contrast to the spin echo images, the signal intensity from flowing blood in gradient echo images generally increases as the flow velocity increases. Flow disturbances such as those found with regurgitant jets or intracardiac shunts produce an absence of signal due to an immediate loss of the coherent alignment of the spinning protons within these flow patterns. A cine display of these gradient echo images yields high-temporal-resolution dynamic studies that permit both wall motion and wall thickening dynamics as well as regurgitant jets and shunts to be directly visualized.[20–22] This technique is also useful for the assessment of false lumen flow in aortic dissection and other vascular anomalies and the evaluation of flow patterns in congenital heart disease.[14]

A normal study obtained with this technique is shown in Fig. 136-4. Note that normally flowing blood is typically bright in the chambers and vessels; however, there is less contrast between the soft tissues than is obtained with spin echoes. As a result, infiltrative lesions, myocardial infarction, and even some small noncalcified masses may not be as readily seen with gradient echo imaging as with spin echoes. Thus, these techniques are complementary. The technique that is used is dictated by the

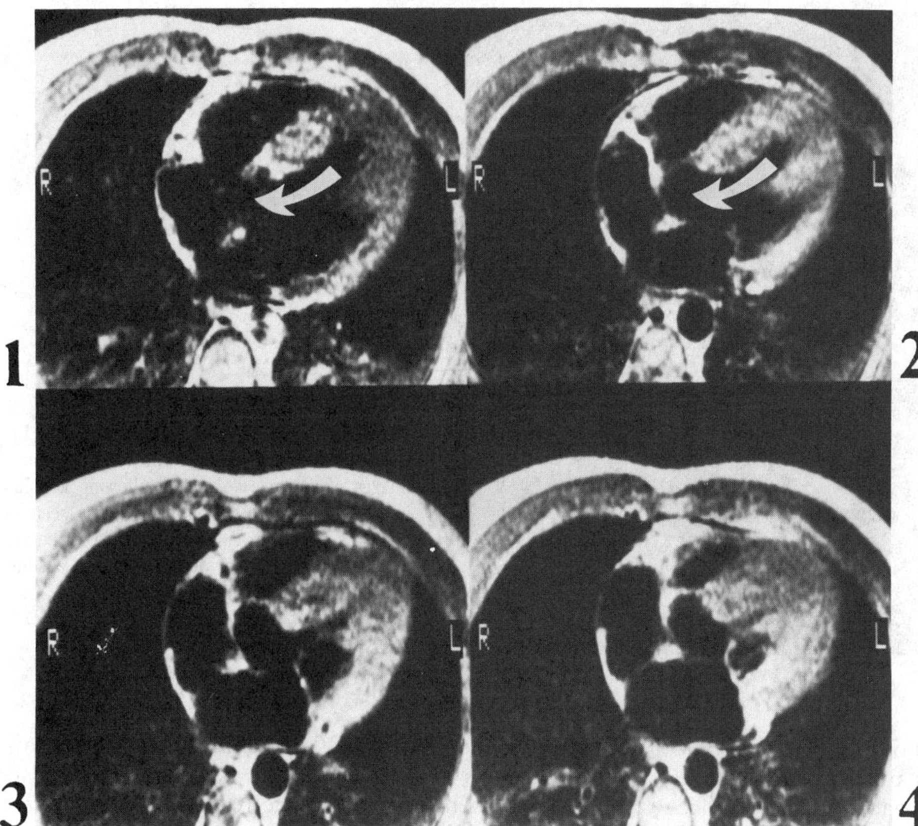

FIGURE 136-3 Spin echo images of same section obtained at four successive systolic phases of the cardiac cycle. Complete typical sequence generates similar images at 12 to 14 phases through cardiac cycle. These can be displayed in a cine mode to evaluate function. Note progressive systolic wall dynamics and partial obstruction of left ventricular outflow tract (arrow) in patient with hypertrophic cardiomyopathy.

clinical problem being investigated, although our routine approach involves a combination of both procedures to take advantage of the complementary contrast features.

Ultrafast Imaging

A recently developed dynamic technique that acquires images at 300 to 500 ms has been shown to have potential for assessing myocardial perfusion by contrast agent tracking.[15] This technique uses a very rapid, repeated acquisition of gradient echoes. Following a preparation pulse, the gradient echo sequence is implemented after a brief delay time that is chosen to optimize T_1 or T_2 contrast in the myocardium. The gradient echo sequence is then rapidly repeated with a TE of approximately 2 ms. With rapid repetitions of the excitation pulse every 4 ms

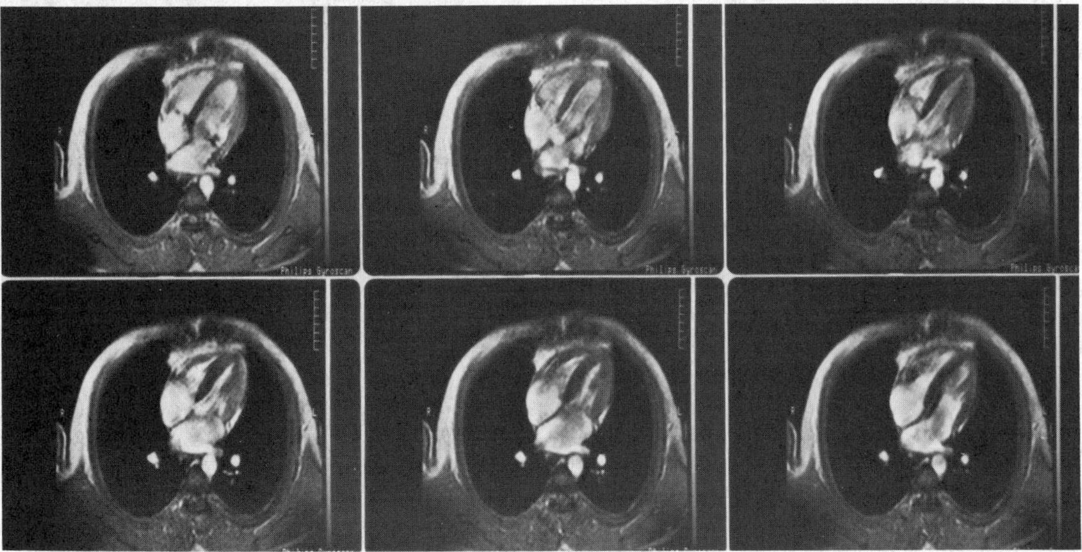

FIGURE 136-4 Normal fast gradient echo multiphase images of same transverse section through the ventricles and atria. Six successive phases are shown; images at 16 cardiac phases are usually obtained and displayed in a cine mode. Note contrast reversal versus spin echo images. Blood in chambers is normally bright; myocardium is gray.

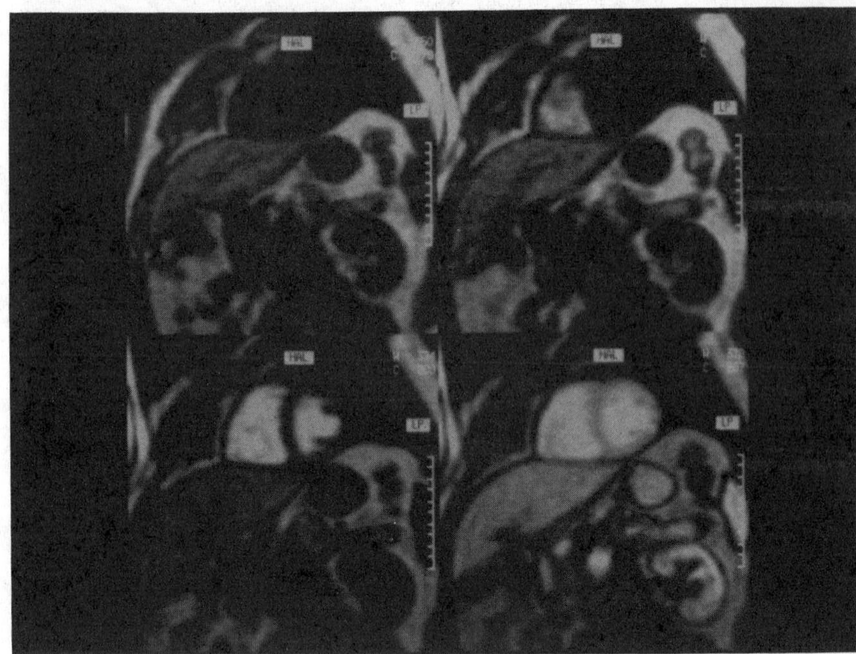

FIGURE 136-5 First-pass cardiac perfusion. Ultrafast (340 ms) sequential turboFLASH short-axis images of the heart obtained following a bolus injection of Gd-DTPA. Contrast agent is seen to enter the right ventricular (upper right), then the left ventricular (lower left), and myocardium (lower right). (*Courtesy of Daniel Finelli, University Hospitals of Cleveland, Ohio, and Siemens Medical Systems.*).

(TR = 4 ms), an image composed of 64 lines of resolution can be acquired in approximately 300 ms. While this temporal resolution is too broad and the cardiac detail is too coarse to supplant conventional functional imaging techniques, the rapid acquisition of complete images in this time frame is suitable for visualizing the transit of a contrast agent through the myocardium. This method may be suitable for assessing regional myocardial perfusion, as has been reported recently[15] (Fig. 136-5).

An even faster imaging technique is that of echo planar or instant imaging, in which single-snapshot images are acquired in 40 ms or less.[30-32] These images are acquired following the generation of either a conventional spin echo or gradient echo with subsequent rapid acquisition of all the data required to form a complete image within the subsequent 30 to 40 ms. This ultrafast technique is achieved by rapid switching or oscillation of the phase-encoding imaging gradient throughout the envelope of the single spin or gradient echo signal. In this case, all of the lines of data in the image matrix are acquired within the time of a single echo, resulting in the ultrafast imaging times. This data acquisition method results, of course, in a decreased signal-to-noise ratio, but with a favorable trade-off in the total study time. Since the echo planar innovation can be applied after the generation of either a spin or gradient echo, the contrast features are similar to those of dark blood T_2-weighted spin echo images or bright blood gradient echo sequences.[32]

When implemented in these modes, dynamic studies of a single section can be obtained at a rate of from seconds (typically 16 heartbeats) to real time (Fig. 136-6). Consequently, these techniques should be useful for imaging cardiac and ventricular function and also for assessing myocardial perfusion when used in conjunction with paramagnetic contrast agents.[15,33]

Coronary MRI angiograms have also been recently demonstrated using 15 to 20 s bright blood image acquisition schemes (Fig. 136-7). The basic approach also uses the gradient echo sequence repeated at very brief intervals of approximately 10 ms to acquire multiple lines of image resolution per heart beat. By acquiring eight image lines per heart beat, the entire 128 line image matrix can be filled in 16 total cardiac cycles. Respiratory motion artifacts and degradation of image quality can

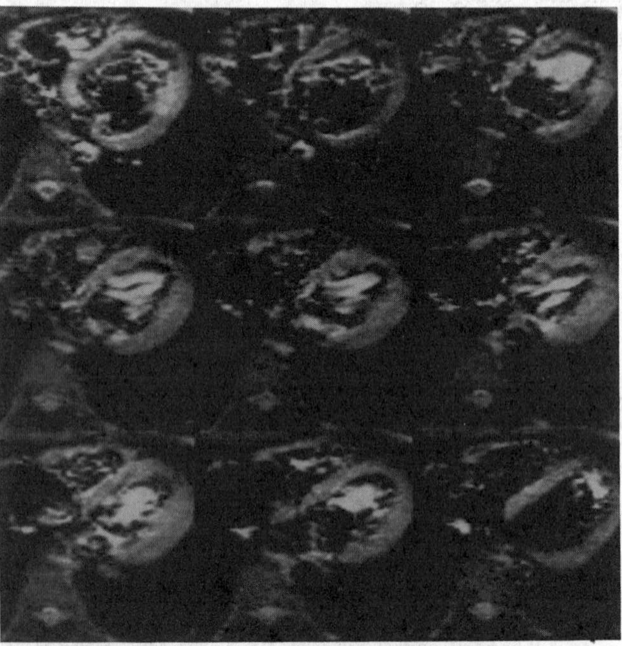

FIGURE 136-6 Ultrafast spin echo cine. By incrementing the delay from the R-wave trigger over 16 successive cycles, a series of instant 56-ms images are acquired at 16 points in the cardiac cycle. One image was acquired every other heartbeat. TE = 26 ms, matrix = 128 × 128. Images at nine of the points are shown. (*Courtesy of R. Rezedzian, Ph.D., Advanced NMR, Inc.*)

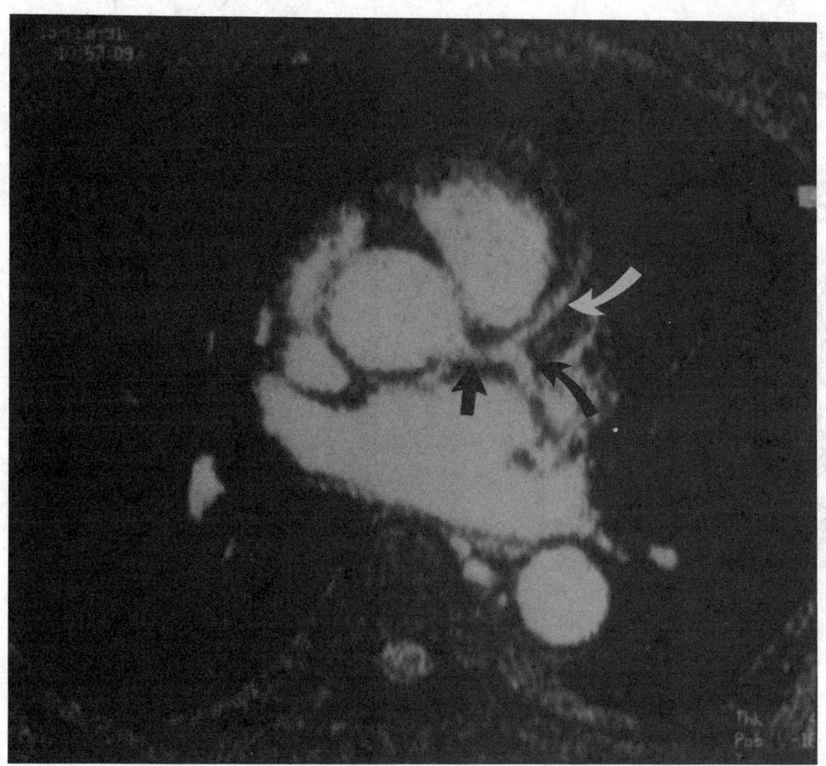

FIGURE 136-7 MR angiogram of the proximal left coronary artery. Transverse tomographic image shows the left main (straight arrow), left anterior descending (curved white arrow), and proximal left circumflex (curved black arrow) coronary arteries. Image was obtained in approximately 15 s during suspended respiration and illustrates early efforts towards MR coronary angiography. (*Courtesy of Robert Edelman, M.D., Beth Israel Hospital, Boston, Massachusetts.*)

be completely eliminated by simple breath holding for this brief period. This typically allows visualization of the coronary arteries. Active research is currently under way to refine this technology for potential routine application.[33a,33b] Thus, these ultrafast techniques indicate that future applications of cardiac MRI in acquired heart disease will not only include the assessment of cardiac structure, function, tissue character, and intravascular flow but also should allow the assessment of relative regional myocardial perfusion. Consequently, in the future, MRI may play an important role in the assessment and management of coronary artery disease and its manifestations.

Flow Quantification

One can also quantify the velocity of blood flow when imaged by either of the basic cardiac NMR techniques.[16,34–39] Because blood flow signal is obtained for such a wide range of velocities with the gradient echo sequence, this technique is the most suitable for flow velocity quantification. With this sequence implemented in a cine mode, flow velocities can be measured throughout the cardiac cycle.[16,39]

Phase-velocity quantification is based on the observation that as spins move with a velocity along an imaging magnetic field gradient, they acquire a shift in their angular position relative to stationary spins. This is called a spin phase shift, which is proportional to the velocity with which the spins move. This shift in the phase angle of the spins is a parameter contained within the detected NMR signal and can be readily measured.[16,34–39] Specifically, the composite NMR signal (1) gives rise to the conventional modulus image, where the image signal intensity is simply related to the magnitude of the MRI signal, and (2) can be used to generate a phase image where the signal intensity is proportional to the shift in spin phase relative to the stationary spins. This phase image, therefore, provides a pixel-by-pixel mapping of spin velocities, providing that both the strength of the imaging gradient and the time during which the spins are exposed to the gradient are known or are calibrated. Since these features of the sequence gradient waveforms can be explicitly prescribed, it is possible to define the gradient waveforms such that a desired amount of spin phase is acquired per unit velocity. This parameter is commonly referred to as the velocity sensitivity (expressed in cycles per centimeter per second).[16,34–39]

In order to display flow in two opposite directions, a gray scale for displaying the spin phases is chosen so that zero phase shift is medium gray. Spins that move into the scanner will typically acquire positive phase shifts of 0 to 180°. These are assigned a proportional intensity from midgray to white (Fig. 136-8). Spins that move in the opposite direction will acquire negative phase shifts of 0 to − 180°. These are assigned a proportional intensity from medium gray to black.

An additional and particularly useful extension of this type of adjustment of the phase shift acquired by moving spins is the use of gradient waveform modifications to completely eliminate any spin phase shift per unit velocity, i.e., flow velocity sensitivity equal to 0. When this is done, it is referred to as flow velocity compensation and is very useful in that it reduces or eliminates flow-related and motion artifact.[40,41] The general term used to describe gradient shaping to compensate and reverse motion-induced spin phases is *gradient moment nulling*. In general, gradient moment nulling can be applied to compensate for spin phase shifts induced not only by the velocities with which spins move but also by the higher order

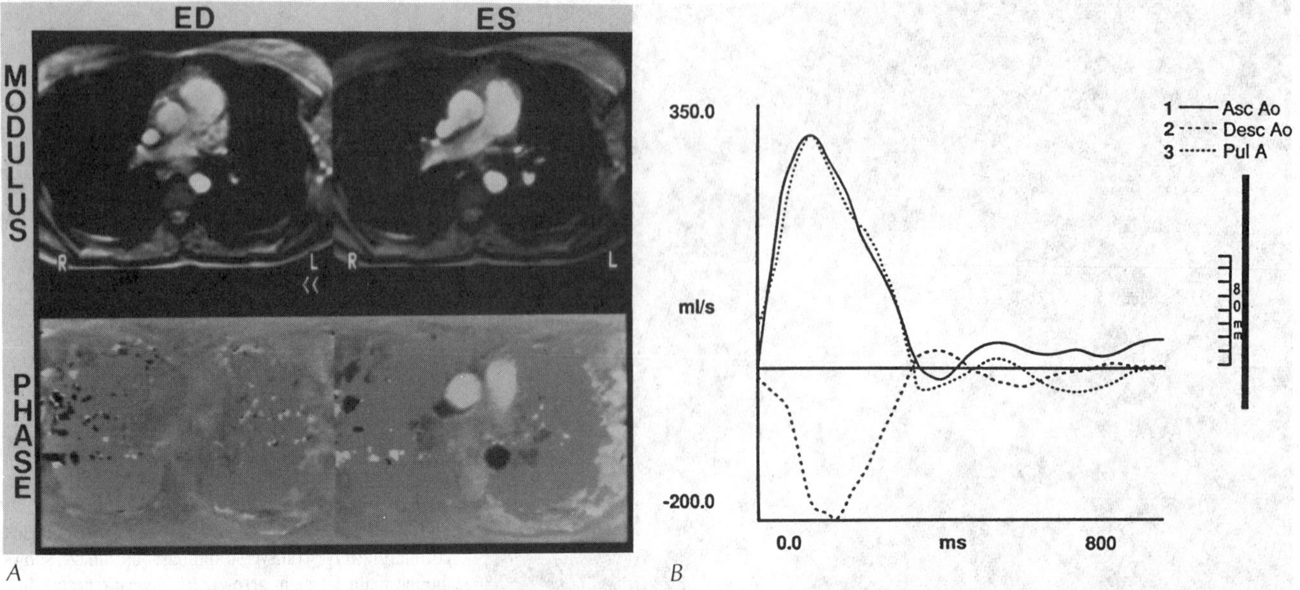

FIGURE 136-8 *A.* Modulus and phase images at end diastole (ED) and end systole (ES) of a normal transaxial section at the level of the main pulmonary artery. *B.* Flow-time curves obtained after quantification of the aortic and pulmonic flow velocities at 16 points through the cardiac cycle. Measurement of cross-sectional vascular areas was used to compute flow in milliliters per second from directly measured velocities in centimeters per second: (———) ascending aorta; (-------) descending aorta; (··········) pulmonary artery. (*From Pettigrew RI: Dynamic magnetic resonance imaging in acquired heart disease. Seminars in Ultrasound, CT, and MR 12:61–91, 1991. Reproduced with permission from the publisher and author.*)

components of motion including acceleration and jerk. For most routine applications, the compensation for velocity-induced spin phase shifts alone is used.

Myocardial Tagging

In 1988, Zerhouni et al.[17] introduced a technique that allowed the noninvasive marking or tagging of specific segments of the myocardium at a specified point in the cardiac cycle, so that the functional behavior of this specifically tagged segment could be observed throughout the remainder of the heart cycle. This technique offered a tool for studying detailed aspects of myocardial mechanics that previously had been possible only with invasive opaque or physical markers placed on the myocardium.

As originally described and implemented, the technique of myocardial tagging produced a series of radial stripes of signal void with equally distant angular spacing across the end-diastolic image of the myocardium. Shortly after this technique was developed, Axel and Dougherty[42] introduced a tagging method that imposed a two-dimensional grid of signal void on a spin echo or gradient echo image (Fig. 136-9). While the original radial tagging technique permitted the observation and study of mechanical features such as myocardial twist and strain,[18] the grid approach more easily permitted assessment of intrawall dynamics. Consequently,

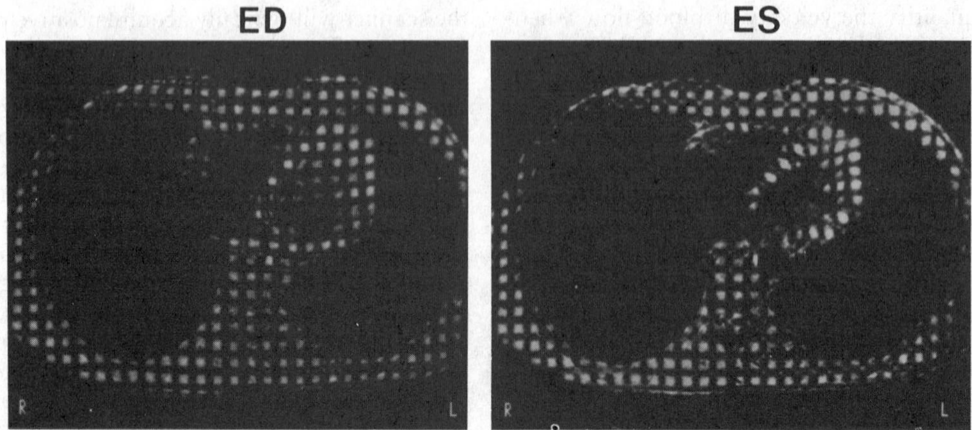

FIGURE 136-9 Myocardial tagging of a transaxial section using the spatial modulation of magnetization technique is shown at end diastole (ED) and end systole (ES). Note the regional and transmural differences in systolic deformation of the initially tagged squares or tiles. (*From Pettigrew RI: Dynamic magnetic resonance imaging in acquired heart disease. Seminars in Ultrasound, CT, and MR 12:61–91, 1991. Reproduced with permission from the publisher and author.*)

subendocardial versus subepicardial mechanics can be assessed.[43]

Early clinical applications of these unique techniques indicate potential utility in (1) objectively assessing wall motion abnormalities, (2) assessing regional myocardial mechanics, (3) distinguishing thrombus (no grid deformation) from slow flow (grid deformation at end systole), and (4) observing the effects of drug therapies on regional myocardial function by observing variances in the deformation of the tagged segments.[17,18]

TABLE 136-3

Functional Information Obtained with Dynamic MRI
1. Chamber volumes: biventricular ejection fractions, forward cardiac output, regurgitant volume/fraction
2. Myocardial wall dynamics: regional diastolic wall thickness and systolic wall thickening, radial shortening, strain, intramyocardial thickening
3. Valvular regurgitation: visualization of regurgitant jets, measurement of regurgitant fractions
4. Intracardiac and vascular flow: shunt visualization, vessel patency/obstruction assessment; flow quantification, Q_P/Q_S

RESULTS

Ventricular Function

When dynamic fast gradient echo imaging is employed, both chamber and valvular function can be evaluated. When this technique is combined with spin echo imaging, a rather comprehensive evaluation of cardiac structure and of chamber and valvular function with limited tissue characterization are accomplished (Table 136-2). Thus, a particularly attractive feature of MRI of the cardiovascular system is that these composite techniques allow a single MRI examination to determine all of the quantitative functional indexes (Table 136-3), which usually necessitate many other noninvasive studies. Moreover, since MRI allows direct planimetry of end-diastolic and end-systolic volumes, these measurements can be obtained in principle quite accurately (Fig. 136-10). This is so because with MRI there are no geometric assumptions such as those required for noninvasive volume determinations with contrast and conventional nuclear ventriculography, in which it is assumed that all ventricles have an ellipsoidal shape. From the measurements of biventricular volumes at end diastole and end systole, biventricular ejection fractions, stroke volumes, cardiac outputs, and regurgitant fractions in cases of isolated valvular dysfunction can be calculated (Fig. 136-11). The ability to directly visualize all regions of the myocardium with MRI also permits absolute wall thickness and systolic wall thickening to be assessed in three dimensions. This is a more accurate index of myocardial contractility than is wall motion alone. As indicated below, a number of centers have validated many of these measurements (Tables 136-4 and 136-5) and explored the clinical values of these parameters as derived by MRI.[19-29] The measurement of ventricular volumes of in vitro and in vivo canine hearts has correlated closely with the measurements at autopsy.[23-25] One study reported a correlation coefficient of 0.94 with a standard error of estimate (SEE) of 14 g when in vivo MRI cardiac mass measure-

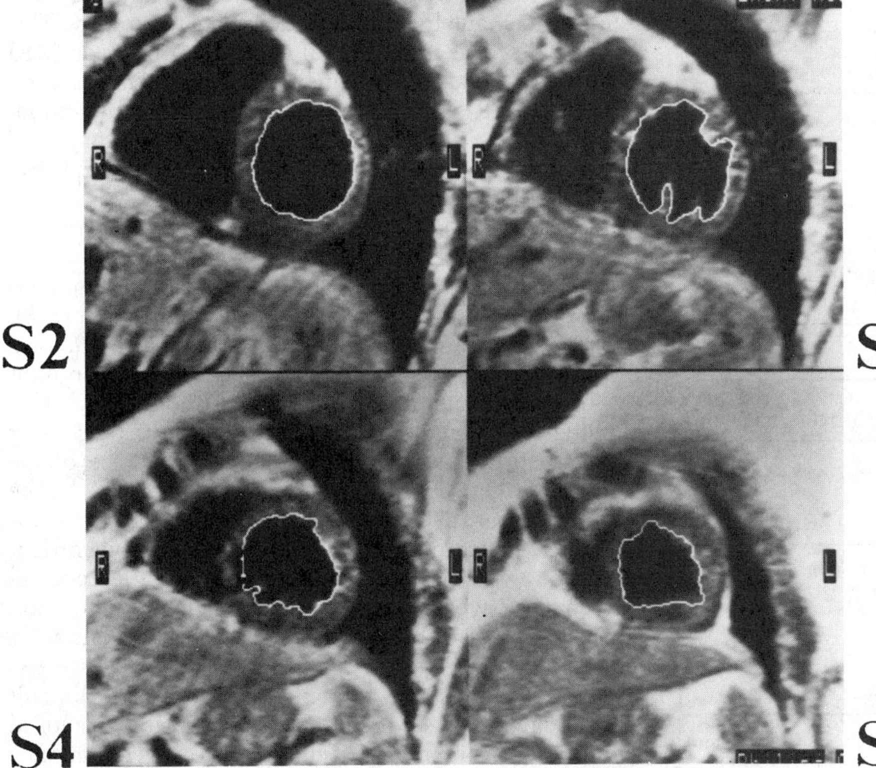

FIGURE 136-10 The central four of six successive short-axis sections that span the ventricles from base (S2) progressing toward apex (S5). Each section is at end diastole. Planimetry and summation of the ventricular volume of each section yield direct determination of end-diastolic volume. Process is repeated at end systole to determine end-systolic volume, stroke volume, ejection fraction, and cardiac output. Measurement for both ventricles can also yield regurgitant fraction. Note that no geometric assumptions about ventricular shape are made.

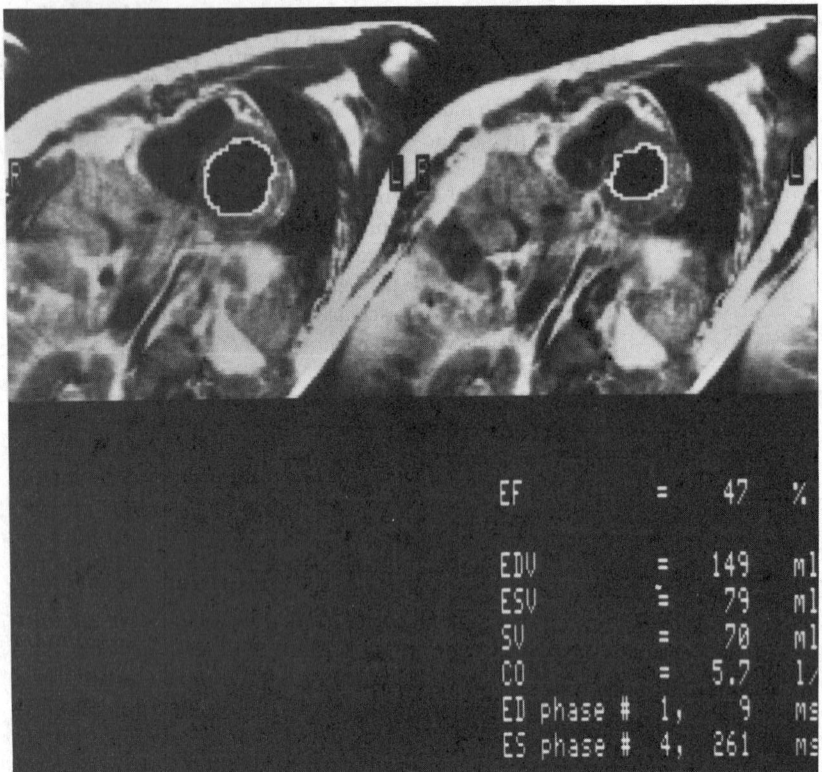

FIGURE 136-11 Quantitative indexes of cardiac function shown in bottom right quadrant were obtained by the process described in Fig. 136-10. One representative section from a complete set of seven short-axis sections spanning the ventricular chambers is shown. *Left:* End diastole. *Right:* End systole.

ments were compared to those made immediately following canine sacrifice.[25] Our own phantom and ex vivo porcine heart volume measurements obtained from MRI images have agreed within 3 percent with the actual volumes obtained by direct measurement. Interobserver agreement among multiple experienced observers who performed planimetry of the endocardial margins has been consistently well within 10 percent. Other researchers have similarly reported low interobserver variability for biventricular volumes measured from a series of successive tomographic images that encompass the ventricles at end diastole and end systole.[16]

The ejection fractions derived from direct MRI measurements have also been validated by several investigators[19,27,28] (Table 136-5). As shown, we have found an overall correlation coefficient of 0.92 between the MRI-derived left ventricular ejection fractions and the measurements made by radionuclide ventriculography. This is typical of the close level of correlation between MRI and the reference measurements in several studies. Consequently MRI is currently well established as a methodology that accurately measures ventricular volumes and all volume-derived functional indexes such as ejection fraction, stroke volume, and cardiac output. Typical normal functional indexes as measured by MRI are presented in Table 136-4.

When using the fast gradient echo technique to semiquantitatively evaluate the severity of a regurgitant lesion (Figs. 136-12 and 136-13), studies have also found a good correlation between the grading of the regurgitant lesion by MRI and by Doppler echocardiography.[20] This finding has been similarly reported by investigators at other institutions who have compared the size of the regurgitant jet relative to the receiving chamber, to the same comparative measurement as viewed by color Doppler echocardiography. Moreover, since biventricular stroke volumes can be measured, the difference between these two in the presence of a single valvular lesion permits one also to measure the regurgitant volume or regurgitant fraction.

Wall thickness measurements have been more difficult to validate because of the absence of a gold standard noninvasive comparative technique. However, comparisons with echocardiography in normal individuals and

TABLE 136-4

Normal MRI Left Ventricular Volumes

n	EDVI (mL/m²)	ESVI (mL/m²)	Mean EF (%)	Reference
10	57 ± 9	17 ± 4	70	24
13	63 ± 8	26 + 6	59	11

NOTE: EDVI = end-diastolic volume index; ESVI = end-systolic volume index; EF = ejection fraction.

TABLE 136-5

MRI Left Ventricular Ejection Fraction Correlations

Standard	Number of Patients	Correlation	Reference
Cath	20	r = .95, SEE = 3%	27
Cath	11	r = .88	28
RNV	50	r = .92, SEE = 6%	11

NOTE: Cath = contrast ventriculography; RNV = radionuclide ventriculography; SEE = standard error of estimate.

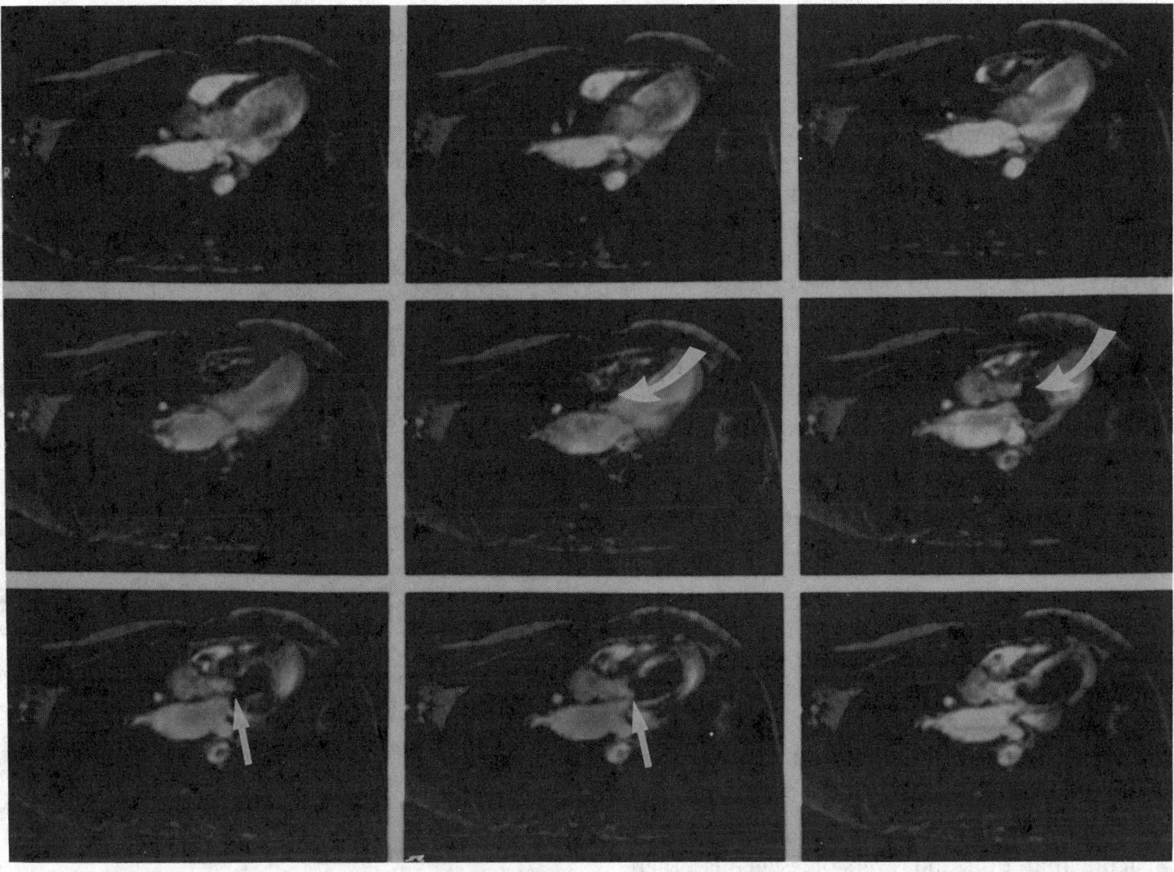

FIGURE 136-12 Aortic regurgitation and mitral stenosis. Mitral stenosis produces a dark, flame-shaped jet of signal void (arrows) across the mitral valve during diastole (phases 7 to 9). Moderate aortic regurgitation (curved arrows) is also present in phases 5 to 9. The two jets become confluent in the latter three phases. (*From Pettigrew RI: Dynamic magnetic resonance imaging in acquired heart disease. Seminars in Ultrasound, CT, and MR 12:61–91, 1991. Reproduced with permission from the publisher and author.*)

in patients with hypertrophic cardiomyopathy[44] have agreed within 1 or 2 mm, i.e., within the error of each technique. In addition, although not direct proof, the accuracy of the ejection fractions derived from planimetry of the endocardial end-systolic and end-diastolic margins as well as the documented accuracy of in vivo left ventricular (LV) mass measurements indicate that MRI is a superb methodology for evaluating systolic wall thickening over three dimensions. This can be measured circumferentially from the tomographic short axis slices (see next section). Care should be taken, however, not to take measurements on the basalmost slice because of

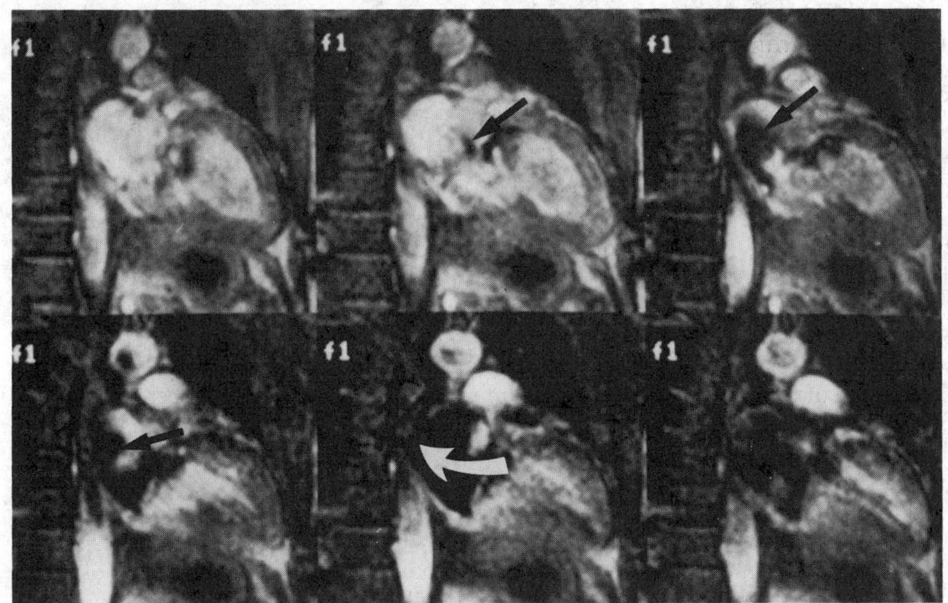

FIGURE 136-13 Severe mitral regurgitation with progressive regurgitant jet (arrows) shown in sequential systolic images of same long-axis section obtained with fast gradient echo technique. Note abnormal loss of signal in left atrium due to regurgitant flow disturbance. Signal in left atrium is completely lost (curved arrow) during late systole.

the normal basal descent of this section toward the apex during ventricular systole. The cine display of either dynamic spin echo images or fast gradient echo images permits one to assess qualitatively regional and global wall motion in a fashion analogous to contrast or radionuclide ventriculography. Our experience and the literature indicate that this is an excellent modality for assessing qualitative and quantitative biventricular function and that it not only provides all of the information indicated above but also permits evaluation of the pericardium, great vessels, and general cardiovascular morphology. In a direct comparison of 20 patients imaged by gated equilibrium radionuclide ventriculography we have found MRI to be slightly superior for evaluating segmental wall motion, apparently because of the tomographic images and direct visualization of wall thickening dynamics afforded by MRI. Thus, the comprehensive nature of MRI makes it particularly well suited to evaluating left ventricular function as well as right ventricular function, which has long been difficult to quantitatively assess by other techniques. This comprehensive feature and the inherent three-dimensionality make MRI the most complete noninvasive method for the assessment of cardiac function.

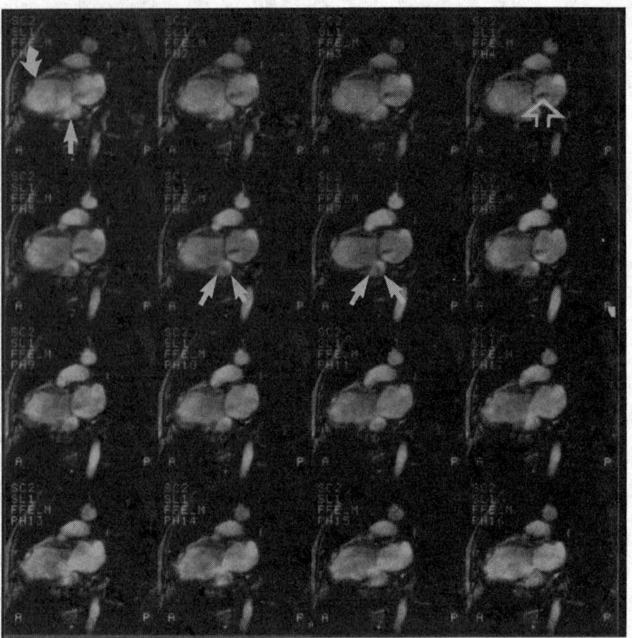

FIGURE 136-14 Sequential vertical long-axis images of a patient with poor global contraction, remote anterior infarction (curved arrow), and an inferobasal aneurysm (arrows). Also note mild mitral regurgitation (open arrowhead). (*From Pettigrew RI: Dynamic magnetic resonance imaging in acquired heart disease. Seminars in Ultrasound, CT, and MR 12:61–91, 1991. Reproduced with permission from the publisher and author.*)

Ischemic Heart Disease: Remote and Acute Myocardial Infarction

In the spectrum of ischemic heart disease (remote infarction, acute infarction, and reversible ischemia), there are four basic MRI findings: (1) regional thinning of the infarcted myocardial wall, (2) infarct age–dependent change in signal intensity, (3) decreased regional systolic wall thickening and motion, and on occasion (4) increased intracavitary signal adjacent to the infarcted myocardium. Of these, the first three are significant.

In remote infarction, segmental wall thinning (Fig. 136-14) and decreased regional systolic wall thickening (Fig. 136-15) appear to be the most frequent and reliable findings.[10,11,45] Normally the LV wall thickness at end diastole is approximately 10 ± 2 mm, and the thickness increases by 35 to 70 percent at end systole.[46,47] Segmental wall thinning is seen as a discrete area that is significantly thinner than the adjacent segments (Fig. 136-16). Since this thinning is due to a loss of myocardium, it should be evident at all phases of the cardiac cycle, including diastole. Decreased to absent thickening of such a segment in systole is consistent with remote infarction and scar (Fig. 136-14). Note, however, that some less common diseases, such as postinflammatory sarcoidosis, can produce similar findings.

The signal intensity of remotely infarcted regions may also be decreased on T_2-weighted spin echo images. This T_2 signal reduction is due to a decrease in the water content of scar tissue as compared with normal myocardium. Occasionally, one may also observe increased intracavitary blood signal adjacent to the site of infarction due to locally sluggish blood flow.[9,11,48] This finding, however, is less prevalent than wall thinning and subnormal systolic thickening.[11,45,46] When viewed dynamically, a small infarct zone may move as it is pulled along by adjacent areas that exhibit normal-to-increased systolic thickening. Direct measurement of the thickness at end diastole and end systole, however, reveals decreased systolic wall thickening. In subendocardial infarction one may see a mild degree of diastolic wall thinning but a relatively normal percentage of thickening of the remaining thickness of viable myocardium.

In acute myocardial infarction, classically the infarcted site may appear as a segmental area of increased signal intensity (Fig. 136-17) on an image obtained with the second echo or an echo time of at least 60 ms, although the sensitivity improves as the TE increases to about 90 ms. This finding has been reported in canines and in humans for infarcts of approximately 1 day to 2 to 3 weeks of age.[45,49–52] The prolonged T_2 which results in the bright signal intensity on the late echo image is apparently due to increased water content and local edema. In our experience, which has largely involved infarctions treated by thrombolytic therapy or balloon angioplasty, and as reported by others, this type of edematous change may not always be observed.[45] Perhaps the most reliable indicator of acute infarction is a segmental decrease in systolic wall thickening[11,45] (Fig. 136-18). Since fibrosis and scarring typically begin to develop after approximately 2 weeks or more postinfarction, the end-diastolic wall thickness for acute infarctions will usually appear normal. When imaged dynamically with the *gradient echo cine technique,* not only are the abnormal wall dynamics apparent, but one may also observe the acutely infarcted region as an area of decreased signal intensity.[53] One animal study has indicated that this signal alteration may be related to hemorrhage with subsequent iron deposition.[54]

Increased intracavitary signal adjacent to acutely infarcted regions may be seen on spin echo images and is due to sluggish blood flow adjacent to the hypokinetic wall segment. One should note, however, that this find-

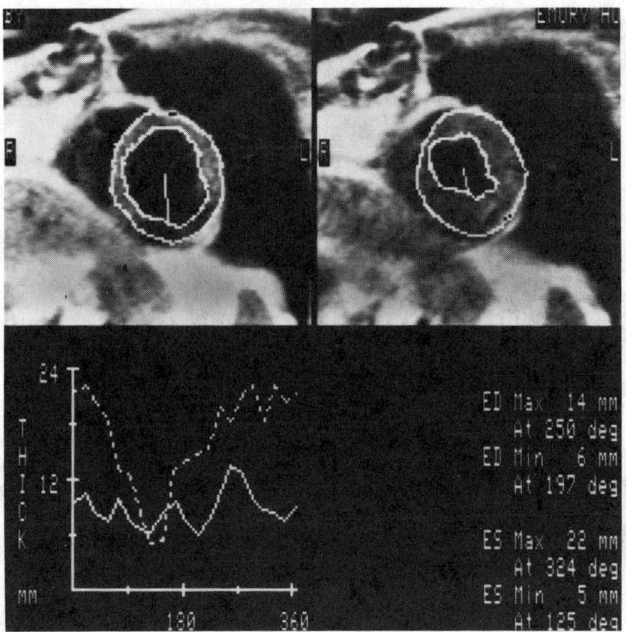

FIGURE 136-15 Radial wall thickening of one short-axis section with endocardial and epicardial edges outlined. *Left:* At end diastole. *Right:* At end systole. Graph at bottom left shows radial wall thickness at end diastole (solid line) and at end systole (broken line) clockwise from inferior wall (0°). Note absence of systolic thickening of infarcted anteroseptal segment (~140°) with compensatory hypercontractility of inferior lateral segments.

ing can also be observed in normal volunteers, particularly along the inferolateral segment between the papillary muscles, and thus is not a specific finding for myocardial infarction.[9,11] Its presence in normal individuals is most likely related to imaging during a slow phase of the cardiac cycle during which blood signal intensity on spin echo images is brightest.

Viable Myocardium versus Scar

Canine studies of brief reversibly ischemic insults indicate that there are no detectable changes from MR images in the relaxation times.[55-57] We have observed that the immediate loss of contractility associated with acute reversible ischemia can be detected by MRI as a decrease in normal systolic wall thickening.[56] Other studies have indicated that the administration of paramagnetic contrast agents may aid in the detection of ischemia by marking areas of relative hypoperfusion in a fashion analogous to that of perfusion imaging with radioactive thallium. Our current experience in comparing resting dynamic MRI studies with thallium studies indicates that *viable* myocardium may be detected with MRI by assessing systolic wall thickening, a parameter known to correlate with the level of myocardial perfusion. It appears that myocardial scar (i.e., *remote* infarction) can be distinguished from viable myocardium on the basis of the presence of diastolic wall thinning and concomitant absent systolic wall thickening. The presence of viable myocardium is established when active systolic thickening is observed. With "stunned" or "hibernating" myocardium the MRI findings are an approximately normal diastolic wall thickness with a diminished systolic thickening and no abnormal signal intensity (Fig. 136-18). Since in some cases of acute infarction there may not be increased T_2-weighted signal intensity, however, distinction between infarcted and stunned myocardium may be difficult in the acute setting.[11] Future use of paramagnetic perfusion agents, viability markers, or pharmacologic stress may be used to make this distinction.

Currently, only resting myocardial disease can be definitely assessed, and while this technique may be used to distinguish viable myocardium from scar, it cannot be used for screening disease of the coronary arteries. Multiple centers are pursuing the evaluation of paramagnetic perfusion markers that may be administered to the patient at peak stress and followed by subsequent MRI, as is similarly done with thallium myocardial perfusion imaging.[15,33] If this were accomplished, the advantage that MRI might offer would be the improved anatomic detail and resolution of MRI (~2 mm) versus that of thallium imaging (~18 mm) in conjunction with the direct measures of diastolic wall thickness and systolic wall thickening, ventricular volumes, ejection fractions, cardiac output, and regurgitant fractions.

Contrast Enhancement of Infarction and Perfusion

A number of recent reports have demonstrated the potential for infarct enhancement by using paramagnetic or

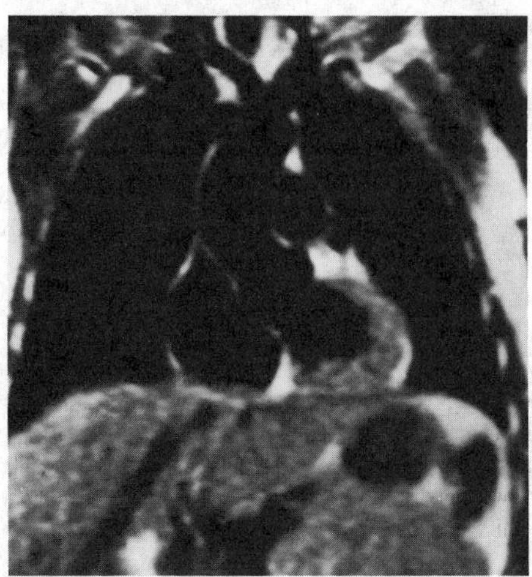

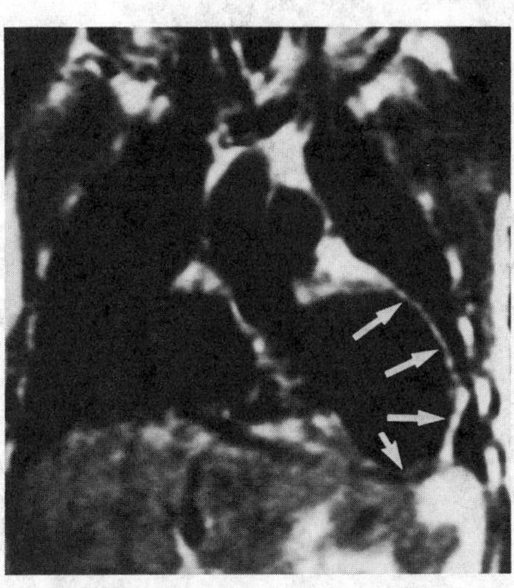

FIGURE 136-16 Coronal sections. *A.* Normal left ventricular wall thickness. *B.* Marked anteroapical thinning exemplifying a remote transmural infarction.

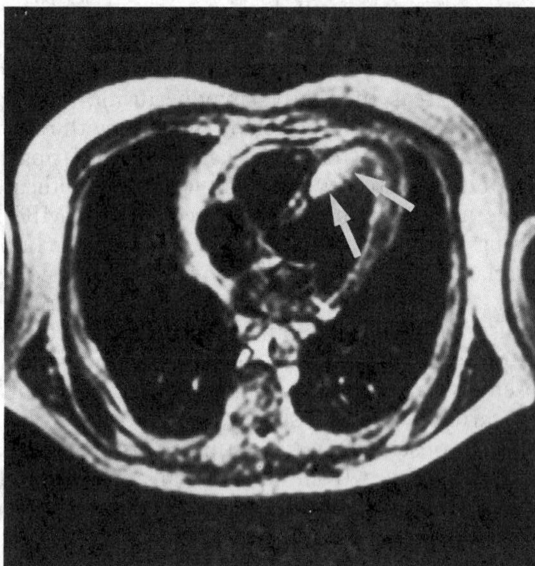

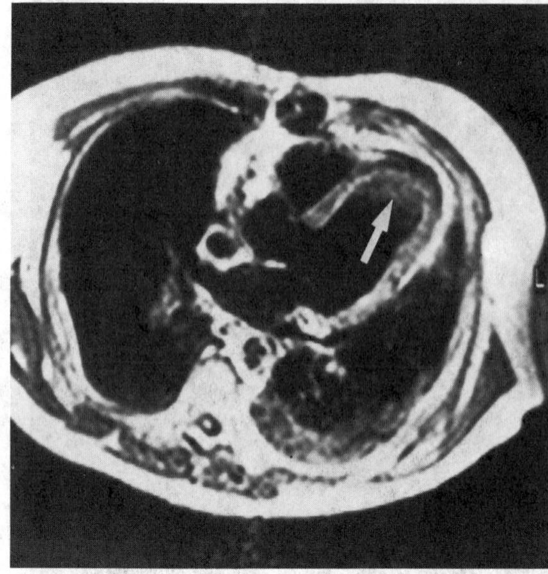

FIGURE 136-17 Tranverse sections. *A*. Acute infarction with distinctly increased signal intensity (arrows) on section echo image (TE = 60 ms). *B*. Same patient imaged 6 weeks later shows apical thrombus (arrow). [*From Casarella WJ, Ball TI, Bernardino ME, et al: Magnetic resonance imaging: Current clinical applications (pt 2). Emory Univ J Med 1(3):200, 1987. Reproduced with permission from the publisher and authors.*]

superparamagnetic agents. Early work in this area used gadolinium diethylenetriamine pentaacetic acid (Gd-DTPA), which has been shown to improve visualization and detection of acute infarction by generating a brighter region postcontrast (Fig. 136-19) in a significant percentage of cases.[58,59] A recent study in dogs with acute infarction indicates considerable promise for an iron oxide–based agent for clearly delineating acutely infarcted myocardium and distinguishing this from viable myocardium.[60] This agent appears to mark the intact, viable myocardium with a loss of signal intensity. This loss of signal is due to T_2 relaxation enhancement and magnetic susceptibility effects that destroy spin coherence. Infarcted regions are not perfused with this agent and, thus, appear as bright areas that sharply contrast the dark viable myocardium on spin echo images.[60] Additional studies with these and other agents are needed to define their eventual clinical role, although it appears quite likely that a perfusion, viability, and infarction enhancement agent ultimately will be found.

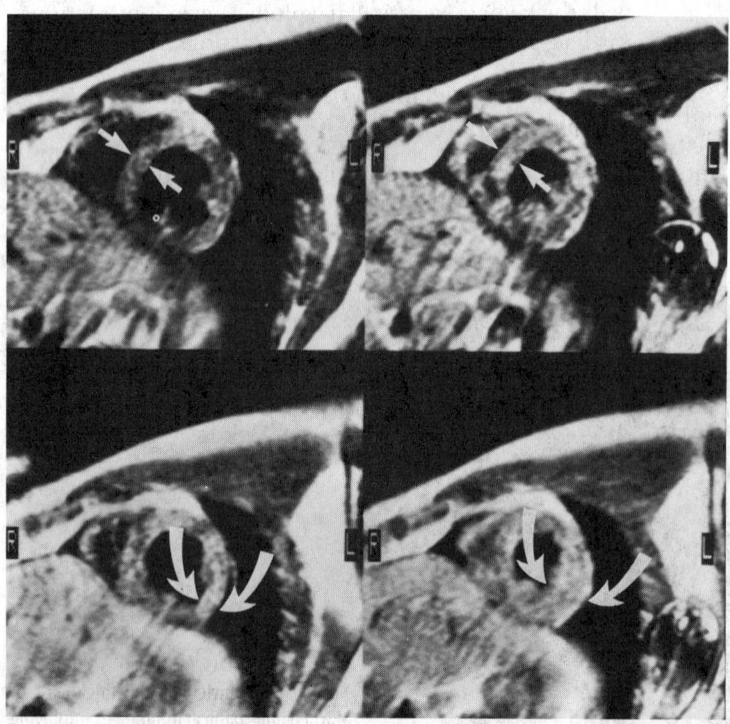

FIGURE 136-18 Stunned myocardium (arrows) versus subendocardial infarction. *A, B.* Two sections imaged at end diastole (ED) and end systole (ES). Note lack of thickening of anteroseptal segment (arrows) versus normal-to-increased thickening of inferior and lateral walls (curved arrows).

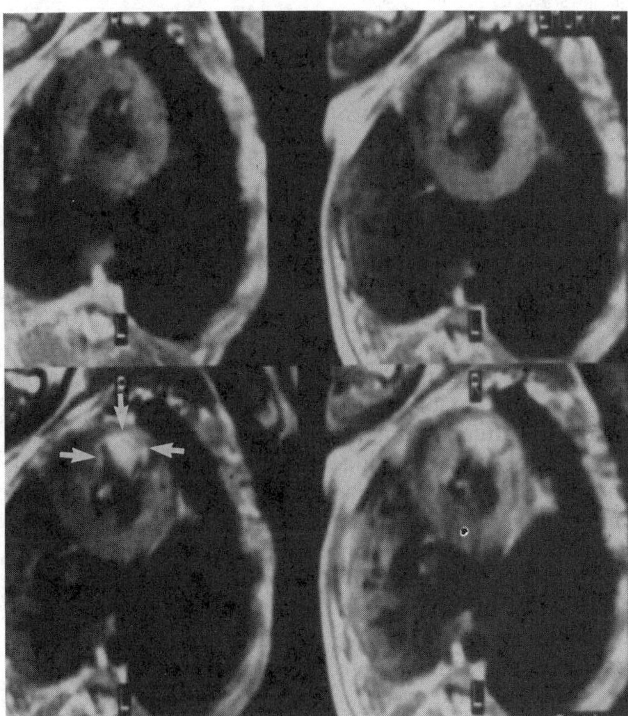

FIGURE 136-19 Contrast agent–enhanced acute infarction. Transverse spin echo (TE = 30 ms) section of a dog's heart before intervention (upper left). Following LAD ligation (upper right) there are equivocal apical intensity changes that enhance (arrows) after Gd-DTPA (bottom left). In the final image (bottom right), obtained 15 min after Gd-DTPA, clearance of the agent reduces previous enhancement.

Cardiomyopathies

In hypertrophic cardiomyopathy (Fig. 136-3), MRI has been shown to be superior to echocardiography and ventriculography in delineating the precise site and extent of the hypertrophic process.[44,61] Since MRI is not body habitus dependent and does not have any visualization blind spots, it serves as a good adjunctive modality to imaging this disease process when the echocardiographic examination is not definitive. Our experience has shown MRI to be a good alternative technique in the assessment of the spectrum of hypertrophic forms. Here, again, the ability to directly measure systolic wall thickening is useful and may assist in determining whether or not the hypertrophic process is myopathic, i.e., primary, or reactive. In cardiomyopathies, we have observed the percentage of systolic wall thickening to be decreased (typically less than 30 percent); the percentage of systolic wall thickening in reactive myocardial hypertrophy is typically normal to increased. (See also Chap. 90.)

In idiopathic dilated cardiomyopathy, ventricular dilatation and poor global systolic function can be evaluated both qualitatively and quantitatively. In particular, ventricular volumes, ejection fraction, and cardiac output can be quantified and followed as indices of responsiveness to medical therapy.

Restrictive cardiomyopathies may have normal systolic function but should have small end-diastolic volumes consequent to the restricted diastolic filling. In addition, diastolic relaxation (i.e., diastolic function) may be abnormal. Although there has been some early investigation of diastolic function, at present this parameter has not been fully explored or well characterized quantitatively by cardiac MRI and remains an area for additional investigation.[62] Nonetheless, restrictive cardiomyopathies should be readily distinguishable from constrictive pericarditis by demonstrating a normal appearing pericardium/pericardial space. (See also Chap. 91.)

Cardiac Masses and Thrombi

A number of reports have suggested that MRI is superior to other studies in the depiction of the site and extent of cardiac masses, such as atrial myxomas (Fig. 136-20), intracardiac neoplasms, and paracardiac cyst, all of which can be imaged with relative ease by MRI.[63–65] In addition to identifying these masses, usually one can distinguish between a lipomatous tumor (Fig. 136-21), lymphoma, myxomas, and paracardiac cyst on the basis of spin echo image signal intensity and mass structure. Of these masses, cysts are typically extremely bright (i.e., slightly brighter than fat), lipomas are similar to subcutaneous fat, lymphomas are mildly brighter than myocardium, and myxomas are isointense to slightly brighter than the myocardium. If Gd-DTPA is administered, vascular tumors become significantly brighter than the myocardium. Imaging of calcified masses may be difficult since little to no NMR signal is derived from heavily calcified structures.

Although ventricular or atrial thrombi can often be seen as abnormal areas of increased intracavitary signal adjacent to the myocardium (Fig. 136-17), occasionally slow-moving blood may appear with a similar signal intensity.[9,66] When dynamic studies are obtained, this differential diagnosis may be resolved by simply viewing

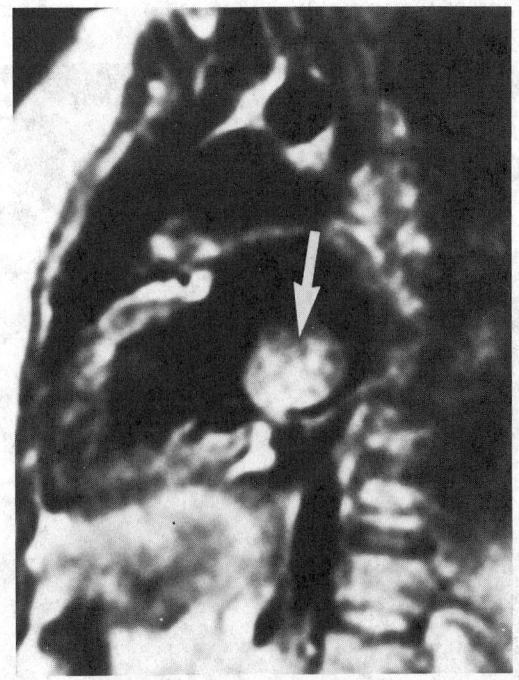

FIGURE 136-20 Vertical long-axis section showing a large myxoma (arrow) in the left atrium.

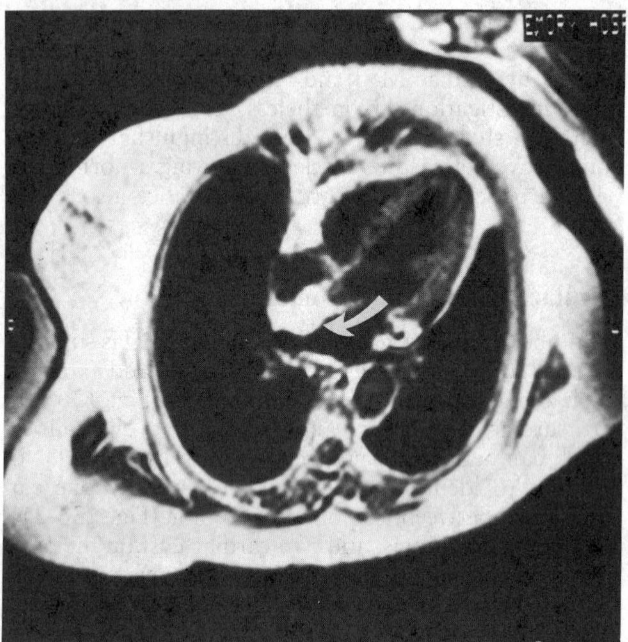

FIGURE 136-21 Lipomatous hypertrophy of the atrial septum (arrow) is evident as an intensely bright mass with signal intensity equivalent to that of subcutaneous fat.

the dynamic study during which slow-moving blood can be seen to fluctuate in signal intensity, whereas the signal intensity of the thrombus is generally constant. If only static images are available, the later or second echo image may be useful in helping to resolve this differential. On the second echo image, slow-moving blood may have an increased signal intensity in comparison to the first echo image due to a phenomenon known as *even echo spin rephasing*.[67] Thrombi, conversely, may show a decrease in signal intensity because of a short T_2 and consequent signal intensity decay.[10] When imaged with a cine gradient echo sequence, thrombus is typically seen as a constant filling defect throughout the heart cycle. If phase-velocity mapping is used, thrombus will have no velocity and thus no spin phase shift, but slow flow will cause some spin phase shift.

Pericardial Disease

The normal pericardial space is typically seen by MRI as a very thin (approximately 2-mm) dark line just between the bright epicardial and pericardial fat. Several investigators[68,69] have reported clear depiction of pericardial effusions (Fig. 136-22), pericardial cysts, and inflammatory pericardial processes, such as uremic pericarditis. With the latter, the inflamed pericardium and intrapericardial adhesions produce an abnormally bright signal intensity due to a prolonged T_2 or shortened T_1 of the inflamed pericardial fluid. This abnormal bright appearance of the pericardial fluid on spin echo images appears to be typical of exudative effusions. One report[70] has highlighted the ability of MRI to accurately identify exudative versus transudative pericardial effusions, simply based on the signal intensity of the effusion relative to that of myocardium. Transudative effusions were noted to have signal intensity less than that of myocardium, while exudative effusions all had signal intensity equivalent to or greater than that of myocardium. This difference is probably due to a short T_1 of the exudative fluid in which the protein content is high. The relatively increased signal of exudative effusions has been reported specifically in uremic pericarditis where the inflamed pericardium and intrapericardial adhesions may be visualized.[10,69,70] In constrictive pericarditis, the pericardium may appear as a thickened area of variable but likely increased signal intensity (relative to myocardium). In addition, the functional consequence of the pericardial abnormality may be assessed by both qualitative inspection and quantitative analysis of the cine images.

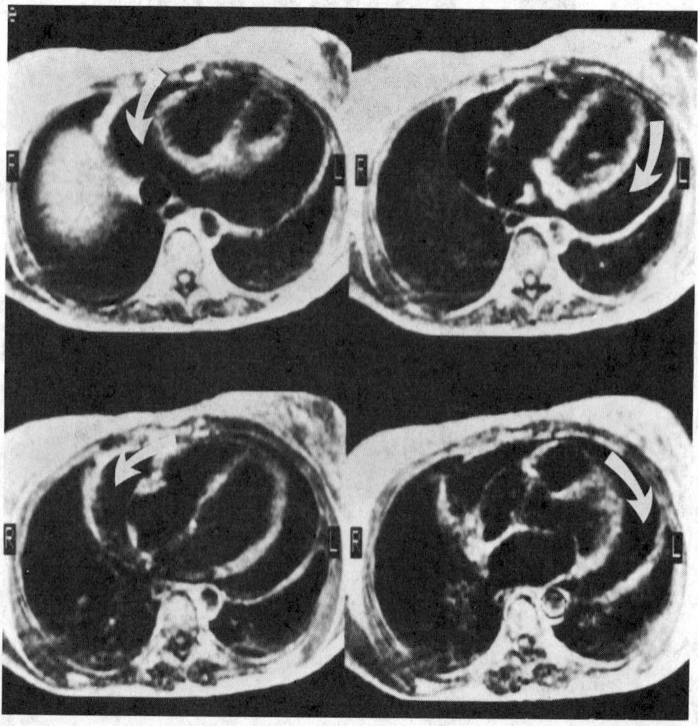

FIGURE 136-22 Massive pericardial effusion (arrows). *A–D.* Four successive transverse sections progressing caudally. Primary disease is scleroderma with transudative effusion that typically has a dark signal intensity, as shown, versus the bright signal intensity associated with exudative or loculated effusions.

Vascular Abnormalities

In contrast to conventional x-ray computed tomography, MRI allows vessels and vascular walls to be clearly identified and easily distinguished from surrounding mediastinal tissues. This capability results from the excellent contrast afforded by the relative absence of signal associated with rapidly flowing blood. Thus, direct visualization of aortic aneurysms, aneurysmal clots, and aortic dissection with depiction of the true and false lumina can be made (Fig. 136-23).[71,72] The location of important branches in aortic dissection and identification of flow in the false lumen can usually be established without the need for an intravascular contrast agent, particularly when dynamic studies are obtained. A cardiac cycle–dependent modulation of intraluminal signal intensity in cine images is convincing evidence of flow in the channel in question. This is readily apparent on visual inspection of the dynamic studies. The ability to image in any arbitrary plane allows sections to be obtained in the plane of the vascular abnormality and further facilitates accurate measurements of the dimensions of the various vascular segments. Recently, the ability to generate three-dimensional MRI angiograms of the great vessels has been realized (Fig. 136-24). This image can be rotated to allow viewing over 180° to clarify the three-dimensional vascular relationships (Plate XII, 136-1). In addition, with MRI flow velocity mapping, flow rates (in milliliters per minute) can be quantified in most vessels larger than approximately 6 mm in diameter.

In pulmonary hypertension, characteristic enlargement of a pulmonary artery can be detected. Moreover, increased spin echo signal intensity within the enlarged vessel during the systolic phases has been correlated with severe pulmonary artery hypertension and pressures greater than 90 mmHg.[10] This increased signal intensity during a phase of normally rapid blood flow is indicative of abnormally slow rates comparable to or less than those typically obtained at late diastole.

Blood flow in venous or arterial disease can be quantified. Although quantitative velocity measurements of venous blood flow are not routinely made, previous dog studies have demonstrated that they can be readily made and that they correlate closely with invasive direct measures.[73] As demonstrated above, a modified version of a fast gradient echo technique has been used to measure quantitatively velocities in the ascending aorta and pulmonary artery.[16] In the future, cross-sectional area measurements coupled with these types of quantitative flow determination may also allow routine calculations of pressure gradients across areas of vessel stenosis.

ADVANTAGES OVER OTHER TECHNIQUES

MRI versus Contrast and Radionuclide Ventriculography at Rest

Magnetic resonance imaging has several advantages when compared to both contrast and radionuclide ventriculographic techniques. First, MRI allows evaluation of both right and left ventricular global and segmental function in a tomographic mode. In addition, there is direct high-resolution visualization of the myocardium and systolic wall thickening, whereas with either ventriculographic technique one only infers the behavior of the myocardial wall from the motion of the blood-endocardium interface. Moreover, this is done from a series of dynamic planar (two-dimensional) images versus the three-dimensional tomographic slices obtained with MRI. Consequently, overlapping structures, which may conceal or diminish the appreciation of regional wall abnormalities with either of the other ventriculographic techniques, are not a problem with MRI.

Because MRI is a dynamic three-dimensional imaging technique, biventricular volumes can be directly mea-

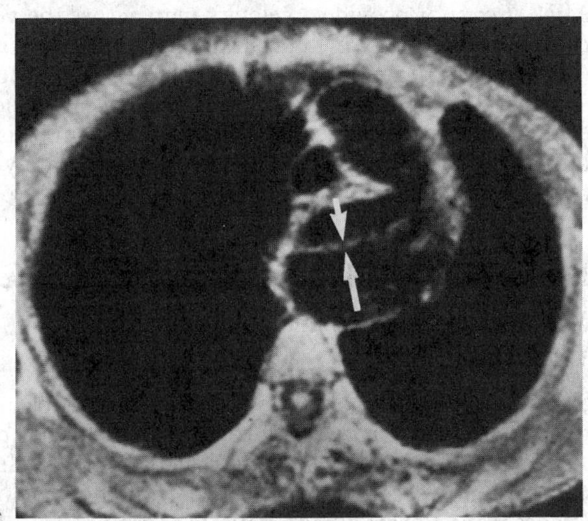

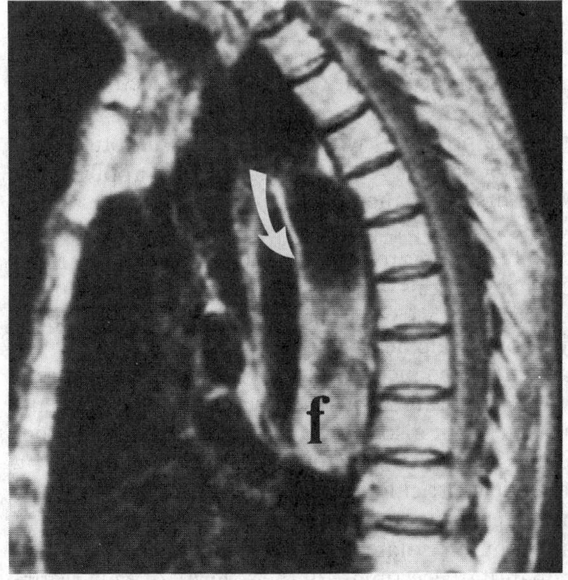

FIGURE 136-23 Dissecting aortic aneurysm shown in a transverse section at the level of the aortic arch (*A*) and in a sagittal section (*B*). Intimal flap is seen originating in proximal descending aorta (arrows in *A*) and is also clearly seen in *B* (curved arrow). Bright signal intensity in false lumen (F) is slow blood flow and not thrombus, since images obtained at other phases of the cardiac cycle showed significant intensity changes.

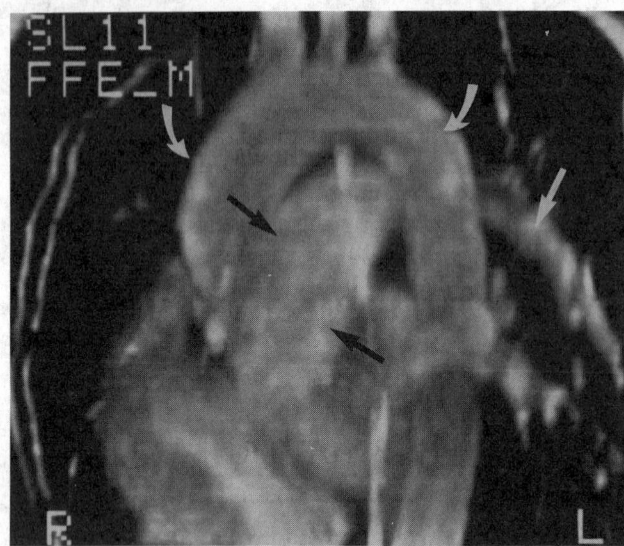

FIGURE 136-24 Magnetic resonance imaging angiogram of the great vessels. Left lateral view shows the aortic arch with upper extremity branches, proximal descending aorta (curved arrow), main pulmonary artery (black arrow) anterior to the ascending aorta, and the left pulmonary artery (white straight arrow). Similar images can be generated for any arbitrary view angle and displayed in a cine loop to create a rotating three-dimensional holographic type display for enhanced visualization of vascular structures.

sured without the significant geometric assumptions that are used in the Dodge methodology, which assumes that the left ventricle has a revolved ellipsoidal shape. In patients who have sustained a previous myocardial infarction with consequent regional deviations from this idealized ellipsoid of revolution and in those with dilated congestive myopathies, one would expect that the volume estimations would have varying degrees of accuracy. This variation in accuracy is related to the extent to which the assumed ellipsoidal geometry matches the actual ventricular configuration. With MRI, in which no such geometric assumptions are made, the accuracy of the measurements should vary minimally with the shape of the ventricle. Thus, these theoretical considerations and the clinical experience to date at a number of academic centers indicate that MRI is a more accurate technique for measurement of ventricular volumes.[23-25,28,29] Similarly, the problems with geometric assumptions described with contrast ventriculography also apply to radionuclide first-pass angiocardiography. With the radionuclide first-pass technique geometric assumptions appear to be even more problematic in that the ventricular chamber margins are less distinct and the apparent chamber size can vary significantly with the orientation and position of the heart within the thorax.

Magnetic resonance imaging not only offers theoretically more accurate ventricular volume measurements noninvasively but also allows the measurement of other functional indexes that cannot be easily obtained by radionuclide ventriculographic techniques. This includes the measurement of regurgitant volumes and forward cardiac output in isolated or compound valvular disease, a semiquantitative estimate of the severity of each regurgitant lesion when there are multiple valvular abnormalities, and pulmonic and aortic flow rates (e.g., Q_P/Q_S). Again, the ability to directly visualize diastolic wall thickness and systolic wall thickening allows wall abnormalities to be identified with greater specificity than do ventriculographic techniques. Additional MRI information includes visual three-dimensional contrast-free angiograms and measurements of the great vessels, quantification of vascular flow rates (in milliliters per minute), and assessment of the pericardium, including measurements of effusion volumes. With recent improvements in software techniques, a comprehensive cardiac MRI examination can be performed in a time that allows the cost to be competitive with radionuclide equilibrium blood pool imaging at our institution. Since the information provided by MRI both includes and exceeds that provided by gated blood pool imaging, we consider a dynamic MRI examination of this type to be more cost-effective. Table 136-6 gives a comparison of MRI and other resting noninvasive imaging modalities based on the current literature and the experience of the author and colleagues.

MRI versus Echocardiography

The major advantage of MRI versus echocardiography (transthoracic and transesophageal) is that MRI is tomographic and three dimensional, with each successive tomographic section being imaged equally well. Thus, in contrast to echocardiography, MRI views all the segments of the ventricles with equal clarity and resolution. In addition, MRI is not body habitus dependent, as is transthoracic echocardiography, and obese and/or barrel-chested patients do not pose a problem if their maximum thorax diameter does not exceed the diameter of the MRI patient tube (typically 50 to 60 cm, depending on the manufacturer). Moreover, MRI has the ability to image the great vessels in any plane and to generate three-dimensional angiograms without contrast media (Fig. 136-24). Although echocardiography provides excellent evaluation of cardiac valvular function, it is not suitable for accurate chamber volume, ejection fraction, cardiac output, and regurgitant volume or regurgitant fraction measurements, which can be obtained with MRI. In addition, while it can measure blood flow velocities, unlike MRI, it cannot provide a velocity map across the vessel cross section from which accurate integrated flow rates (in milliliters per minute) can be obtained (Fig. 136-8). Thus, MRI provides a more complete three-dimensional evaluation of cardiovascular structure with some quantitative functional indexes which are not accurately obtained by echocardiography (Table 136-6).

DISADVANTAGES

MRI versus Contrast and Radionuclide Ventriculography

The major limitation of MRI versus contrast ventriculography is the current inability to measure chamber pressures. Ongoing studies indicate that pressure gradients across stenoses can be established from flow velocity images using the modified Bernoulli equation, as is done with Doppler echocardiography. Measurements of intraventricular or atrial pressures, however, do not seem

TABLE 136-6
Comparison of Resting Noninvasive Imaging Modalities

Feature	Modality			
	ECHO	First Pass	GBP	MRI
Three-dimensional structure	+ +	0	+	+ + + +
Wall tissue character	+	0	0	+ +
Wall motion	+ + +	+	+ + +	+ + +
Wall thickening	+ + +	0	0	+ + + +
Functional indexes	+ +	+ +	+ +	+ + +
Valvular disease	+ + + +	0	0	+ + +
Blood flow/regurgitant	+ + +	0	0	+ + +
Body habitus independence	+ +	+ + + +	+ + + +	+ + + +
Lack of non-viz areas	+	0	+ + +	+ + +
Noninvasiveness	+ + + +	+ + +	+ + +	+ + + +

NOTE: ECHO = two-dimensional color echocardiography; First Pass = first-pass angiocardiography; GBP = gated equilibrium blood pool imaging: 0, of no utility; +, little utility; + +, fair utility; + + +, good utility; + + + +, excellent utility.

theoretically likely. The temporal resolution of contrast ventriculography is significantly better than that obtained with current dynamic MRI techniques, which in some instances image the late diastolic phases less completely. Thus, while diastolic function can be evaluated by the fast gradient echo cine technique, it may be currently evaluated better by contrast ventriculography.

The major disadvantage of MRI versus radionuclide ventriculography is the inability to evaluate ventricular function under physical stress, as can be done with either the gated blood pool or first-pass radionuclide ventriculographic technique. As a consequence, an evaluation for coronary artery disease is not currently routine with MRI. A number of recent studies indicate that paramagnetic contrast agents and/or new ultrafast imaging techniques used in conjunction with pharmacologic stress will permit routine coronary artery disease detection and myocardial characterization in the future. Dobutamine stress MRI has also been recently demonstrated to be effective in identifying partial coronary artery stenosis in animals and in a human study and thus may soon become a routine procedure.[74,75]

MRI versus Echocardiography

The major disadvantages of MRI versus echocardiography are the nonportability of the MRI study and, at some centers, the moderately higher cost. In addition, because echocardiography is in real time, it also generally images valve leaftlets and vegetations with greater clarity.

The cost difference, however, may have a significant regional variation. At our institution, the price of a comprehensive MRI examination exceeds that of color Doppler echocardiography by approximately $200. When the transesophageal approach is used, the price differential is about $100.

COMPLICATIONS

Among the early attractive features of MRI were its noninvasiveness and apparent saftey in that it required no exogenous contrast medium and had no demonstrable or theoretical side effects. The worldwide experience with MRI over the last 10 years has show that this complication-free expectation was indeed well founded, as there have been no reported side effects from the use of *conventional* MRI. Some precautions and contraindications to MRI do, however, exist.[76,77] These include the absolute contraindications of cardiac pacemakers, recent arterial aneurysmal clips, and cochlear implants. Placement of a cardiac pacemaker in a magnetic resonance imager may result in cessation of the pacemaker function or artificial rapid pacing, and aneurysmal and cochlear clips may be dislodged by the magnetic field of the imager.[78,79]

Multiple prosthetic cardiac valves have been tested to determine whether either significant dislodgement or heating may occur while in a magnetic resonance imager.[76] In one series of valves tested, only pre-6000 Starr-Edwards valves (manufactured prior to 1964) exhibited enough deflection and image distortion in field strengths exceeding 0.35 T to be of concern for imaging when there is a clinical question of valve dehiscence.[76] Hence, although it is unlikely that even pre-1964 valves that are well secured will be affected by a magnetic resonance imager, imaging of patients with these valves is not recommended.

Thus, in summary, dynamic cardiac MRI is a cost-effective study that offers a rather comprehensive evaluation of cardiac structure and function at rest. Its major current clinical limitation is its lack of routine use to screen for coronary artery disease. Few contraindications to MRI exist, and conventional MRI in noncontraindicated patients has no associated biological side effects.[80]

REFERENCES

1. Bloch R, Hansen WW, Packard ME: Nuclear induction. *Phys Rev* 1946; 69:127.
2. Purcell EM, Torrey HC, Pound RV: Resonance absorption by nuclear magnetic moments in a solid. *Phys Rev* 1946; 69:37–38.

3. Lauterbur PC: Image formation by induced local interactions: Examples employ nuclear magnetic resonance. *Nature* 1973; 242:190–191.
4. Pykett IL, Newhouse JH, Buonanno FS, Brady TJ, Goldman MR, Kistler JP, et al: Principles of nuclear magnetic resonance imaging. *Radiology* 1982; 143:157–168.
5. Fullerton GD: Basic concepts for nuclear magnetic resonance imaging. *Magn Reson Imaging* 1982; 1:39–55.
6. Lanzer P, Barta C, Botvinick EH, Wiesendanger HU, Modin G, Higgins CB: ECG-synchronized cardiac MR imaging: Method and evaluation. *Radiology* 1985; 155:681–686.
7. Crooks LE, Barker B, Chang H, Feinberg D, Hoenninger JC, Watts JC, et al: Magnetic resonance imaging strategies for heart studies. *Radiology* 1984; 153:459–465.
8. Herfkens RJ, Higgins CB, Hricak H, Lipton MJ, Crooks LE, Lanzer P, et al: Nuclear magnetic resonance imaging of the cardiovascular system: Normal and pathologic findings. *Radiology* 1983; 147:749–759.
9. von Schulthess GK, Fisher M, Crooks LE, Higgins CB: Gated MR imaging of the heart: Intracardiac signals in patients and healthy subjects. *Radiology* 1985; 156:125–132.
10. Higgins CB: Overview of MR of the heart. *Am J Roentgenol* 1986; 146:907–918.
11. Pettigrew RI: Dynamic cardiac MR imaging: Techniques and applications. *Radiol Clin North Am* 1989; 27:1183–1203.
12. van der Meulen P, Groen JP, Cuppen JJ: Very fast MR imaging by field echoes and small angle excitation. *Magn Reson Imaging* 1985; 3:297–299.
13. Frahm J, Haase A, Matthaei D: Rapid NMR imaging of dynamic processes using the FLASH technique. *Magn Reson Med* 1986; 3:321–327.
14. Pettigrew RI, Ziffer JA, Churchwell AL, Parks WJ, Baron M: Fast gradient echo imaging at 0.5T: Assessment of cardiac function and valvular dysfunction. *Dynam Cardiovasc Imag* 1987; 1:220–226.
15. Atkinson DJ, Burstein DD, Edelman RR: First-pass cardiac perfusion: Evaluation with ultrafast MR imaging. *Radiology* 1990; 174(3 pt 1):757–762.
16. Firmin DN, Nayler GL, Klipstein RH, Underwood SR, Rees RS, Longmore DB: In vivo validation of MR velocity imaging. *J Comput Assist Tomogr* 1987; 11:751–756.
17. Zerhouni EA, Parrish DM, Rogers WJ, Yang A, Shapiro EP: Human heart tagging with MR imaging—A method for non-invasive assessment of myocardial motion. *Radiology* 1988; 169:59–63.
18. McVeigh ER, Zerhouni EA: Noninvasive measurement of transmural gradients in myocardial strain with MR imaging. *Radiology* 1991; 180:677–683.
19. Semelka RC, Tomei E, Wagner S, Mayo J, Kondo C, Suzuki J, et al: Normal left ventricular dimensions and function: Interstudy reproducibility of measurements with cine MR imaging. *Radiology* 1990; 174:763–768.
20. Pflugfelder PW, Landzber GS, Cassidy MM, Cheitlin MD, Schiller NB, Auffermann W, et al: Comparison of cine MR imaging with Doppler echocardiography for the evaluation of aortic regurgitation. *Am J Roentgenol* 1989; 152:729–732.
21. Utz JA, Herfkens RJ, Heinsimer JA, Shimakawa A, Glover G, Pelc N: Valvular regurgitation: Dynamic MR imaging. *Radiology* 1988; 168:91–94.
22. Holmvang G, Edelman R, Pearlman JF, Marshall JE, Brady TJ, Kantor HL: Study of valvular regurgitation by CINE-NMR: Comparison to color Doppler flow MAPS (abstr). *Circulation* 1987; 76(suppl IV):IV-30.
23. Rehr RB, Malloy CR, Filipchuk NG, Peshock RM: Left ventricular volumes measured by MR imaging. *Radiology* 1985; 156:717–719.
24. Sechtem U, Pflugfelder PW, Gould RG, Cassidy MM, Higgins CB: Measurement of right and left ventricular volumes in healthy individuals with cine MR imaging. *Radiology* 1987; 163:697–702.
25. Caputo GR, Tscholakoff D, Sechtem U, Higgins CB: Measurement of canine left ventricular mass by using MR imaging. *Am J Roentgenol* 1987; 148:33–38.
26. Fisher MR, von Schulthess GK, Higgins CB: Multiphase cardiac magnetic resonance imaging: Normal regional left ventricular wall thickening. *Am J Roentgenol* 1985; 145:27–30.
27. Stratemeier EJ, Thompson R, Brady TJ, Miller SW, Saini S, Wismer GL, et al: Ejection fraction determination by MR imaging: Comparison with left ventricular angiography. *Radiology* 1986; 158:775–777.
28. Utz JA, Herfkens RJ, Heinsimer JA, Bashore T, Califf R, Glover G, et al: Cine MR determination of left ventricular ejection fraction. *Am J Roentgenol* 1987; 148:839–843.
29. Markiewicz W, Sechtem U, Higgins CB: Evaluation of the right ventricle by magnetic resonance imaging. *Am Heart J* 1987; 113:8–15.
30. Mansfield P: Real-time echo-planar imaging by NMR. *Br Med Bull* 1984; 40:187–189.
31. Chapman B, Turner R, Ordidge RJ, Doyle M, Cawley M, Coxon R, et al: Real-time movie imaging from a single cardiac cycle by NMR. *Magn Reson Med* 1987; 5:246–254.
32. Rzedzian R, Pykett I: Instant images of the human heart using a new, whole-body MR imaging system. *Am J Roentgenol,* 1987; 149:245–250.
33. Kantor HL, Rzedzian RR, Pykett I, Berliner E, Brady T, Buxton R: Transient effects of gadolinium-DTPA and dysprosium-DTPA intravenous infusion on myocardial NMR image intensity using high speed NMR imaging. Book of Abstracts. *Soc Magn Res Med* 1988; 1:256.
33a. Edelman RR, Manning WJ, Burstein D, Paulin S: Coronary arteries: Breath hold MR angiography. *Radiology* 1991; 181:641–643.
33b. Wang SJ, Hu BS, Macovski A, Nishimura DG: Improved coronary angiography using fast selective inversion recovery (abstr). Book of Abstracts. *Soc Magn Reson Med* 1991: 337.
34. Moran PR: A flow velocity zeugmatographic interface for NMR imaging in humans. *Magn Reson Imaging* 1982; 1:197–203.
35. van Dijk P: Direct cardiac NMR imaging of heart wall and blood flow velocity. *J Comput Assist Tomogr* 1984; 8:429–436.
36. Pettigrew RI, Dannels W: Use of standard gradients with compound oblique angulation for optimal quantitative, MR flow imaging in oblique vessels. *Am J Roentgenol* 1987; 148: 405–409.
37. Pettigrew RI, Dannels W, Galloway JR, Pearson T, Millikan W, Henderson JM, et al: Quantitative phase-flow MR imaging in dogs by using standard sequences: Comparison with in vivo flowmeter measurements. *Am J Roentgenol* 1987; 148:411–414.
38. Meier D, Maier S, Bosiger P: Quantitative flow measurements on phantoms and on blood vessels with MR. *Magn Reson Med* 1988; 8:25–34.
39. Nayler GL, Firmin DN, Longmore DB: Blood flow imaging by cine magnetic resonance. *J Comput Assist Tomogr* 1986; 10:715–722.
40. Firmin DN, Nayler GL, Kilner PJ, Longmore DB: The application of phase shifts in NMR for flow measurement. *Magn Reson Med* 1990; 14:230–241.
41. Puttany PM, Phillips JJ, Chiu LC, Lipcamon JD, Duerk JL, McNally JM: Motion artifact suppression technique (MAST) for MR imaging. *J Comput Assist Tomogr* 1987; 11:369–377.
42. Axel L, Dougherty L: Heart wall motion: Improved method of spatial modulation of magnetization for MR imaging 2. *Radiology* 1989; 172:349–350.
43. Palmon L, Reichek N, Yeon S, Bergy P, Axel L, Hoffman E, et al: Circumferential myocardial segment shortening in concentric left ventricular hypertrophy due to hypertension. Book of Abstracts. *Soc Magn Reson Med* 1990; 1:271.
44. Maron BJ, Dwyer AJ, Knop R, Bonow RO, Doppman JL: Efficacy of nuclear magnetic resonance in the diagnosis and the identification of distribution of left ventricular hypertrophy in hypertrophic cardiomyopathy (abstr). *J Am Coll Cardiol* 1985; 5:434.
45. Johnston DL, Mulvagh SL, Cashion RW, O'Neill PG, Roberts R, Rokey R, et al: Nuclear magnetic resonance imaging of acute myocardial infarction within 24 hours of chest pain onset. *Am J Cardiol* 1989; 64:172–179.
46. Pflugfelder PW, Sechtem UP, White RD, Higgins CB: Quantification of regional myocardial function by rapid cine MR imaging. *Am J Roentgenol* 1988; 150:523–529.
47. Fisher MR, von Schulthess GK, Higgins CB: Multiphase cardiac magnetic resonance imaging: Normal regional left ventricular wall thickening. *Am J Roentgenol* 1985; 145:27–30.
48. McNamara MT, Higgins CB: Magnetic resonance imaging of chronic myocardial infarcts in man. *Am J Roentgenol* 1986; 146:315–320.
49. Pflugfelder PW, Wisenberg G, Prato FS, Carroll SE, Turner KL: Early detection of canine myocardial infarction by magnetic resonance imaging in vivo. *Circulation* 1985; 71:587–594.
50. McNamara MT, Higgins CB, Schechtmann N, Botvinick E, Lipton MJ, Chatterjee K: Detection and characterization of acute myocar-

dial infarction in man with use of gated magnetic resonance. *Circulation* 1985; 71:717–724.

51. Tscholakoff D, Higgins CB, Sechtem U, Caputo G, Derugin N: MRI of reperfused myocardial infarct in dogs. *Am J Roentgenol* 1986; 146:925–930.
52. Rokey R, Verani MS, Bolli R, Kuo LC, Ford JJ, Wendt RE, et al: Myocardial infarct size qualification by MR imaging early after coronary artery occlusion in dogs. *Radiology* 1986; 158:771–774.
53. Meese RB, Herfkens RJ, Negro-Vilar R, Spritzer C, Bashore TM: Rapid dynamic magnetic resonance imaging of the heart in evaluation of acute myocardial infarction (abstr). *Circulation* 1987; 76(suppl IV):IV-31.
54. Lotan C, Miller SK, Reeves R, Cranny G, Pohost G: High-field MR imaging: Evidence of the presence of hemorrhagic regions in infarcted canine myocardium (abstr). *Radiology* 1988; 169:37.
55. Tscholakoff D, Higgins CB, McNamara MT, Derugin N: Early-phase myocardial infarction: Evaluation by MR imaging. *Radiology* 1986; 159:667–672.
56. Pettigrew RI, Patterson RE, Malveaux E, Dannels W, Eisner R, Casarella W: Early myocardial ischemia assessed by MRI *in vivo:* Cardiac dynamics (annual meeting, Society of Magnetic Resonance in Medicine, 5th Annual Meeting). Book of Abstracts. *Soc Magn Reson Med* 1986; 2:394.
57. McNamara MT, Tscholakoff D, Revel D, Soulen R, Schechtmann N, Botvinick E, et al: Differentiation of reversible and irreversible myocardial injury by MR imaging with and without gadolinium-DTPA. *Radiology* 1986; 158:765–769.
58. de Roos A, Doornbos J, van der Wall EE, van Voorthuisen AE: MR imaging of acute myocardial infarction: Value of Gd-DTPA. *Am J Roentgenol* 1988; 150:531–534.
59. Nishimura T, Kobayashi H, Ohara Y, Yamada N, Haze K, Takamiya M, et al: Serial assessment of myocardial infarction by using gated MR imaging and Gd-DTPA. *Am J Roentgenol* 1989; 153:715–720.
60. Pettigrew RI, Brownell AL, Holmvang G, Rozenman Y, Kantor H, Southern J, et al: Iron oxide MRI of myocardial tissue blood delivery post acute infarction: Comparison with quantitative PET (abstr). *Circulation* 1987; 76:44.
61. Higgins CB, Byrd BF III, Stark D: Magnetic resonance imaging of hypertrophic cardiomyopathy. *Am J Cardiol* 1985; 55:1121–1126.
62. Markiewicz W, Sechtem U, Higgins CB: Evaluation of the right ventricle by magnetic resonance imaging. *Am Heart J* 1987; 113:8–15.
63. Amparo EG, Higgins CB, Farmer D, Gamsu G, McNamara M: Gated MRI of cardiac and paracardiac masses: Initial experience. *Am J Roentgenol* 1984; 143:1151–1156.
64. Go RT, O'Donnell JK, Underwood DA, Feiglin DH, Salcedo EE, Pantoja M, et al: Comparison of gated cardiac MRI and 2D echocardiography of intracardiac neoplasms. *Am J Roentgenol* 1985; 145:21–25.
65. Conces DJ, Vox VA, Klatte EC: Gated MR imaging of left atrial myxomas. *Radiology* 1985; 156:445–447.
66. Zeitler E, Kaiser W, Schuierer G, Stetter E, Oppelt A, Rogalsky W: Magnetic resonance imaging of clots in the heart and vascular system. *Radiology* 1985; 28:105–108.
67. Waluch V, Bradley WG: NMR even echo rephasing in slow laminar flow. *J Comput Assist Tomogr* 1984; 8:594–598.
68. Stark DD, Higgins CB, Lanzer P, Lipton MJ, Schiller N, Crooks LE, et al: Magnetic resonance imaging of the pericardium: Normal and pathologic findings. *Radiology* 1984; 150:469–474.
69. Soulen RL, Stark DD, Higgins CB: Magnetic resonance imaging of constrictive pericardial disease. *Am J Cardiol* 1985; 55:480–484.
70. Mulvagh SL, Rokey R, Vick GW III, Johnston DL: Usefulness of nuclear magnetic resonance imaging for evaluation of pericardial effusions, and comparison with two-dimensional echocardiography. *Am J Cardiol* 1989; 64:1002–1009.
71. Dinsmore RE, Liberthson RR, Wismer GL, Miller SW, Liu P, Thompson R, et al: Magnetic resonance imaging of thoracic aortic aneurysms: Comparison with other imaging methods. *Am J Roentgenol* 1986; 146:309–314.
72. Amparo EG, Higgins CB, Hricak H, Sollitto R: Aortic dissection: Magnetic resonance imaging. *Radiology* 1985; 155:399–406.
73. Pettigrew RI, Dannels W, Galloway JR, Pearson T, Millikan W, Henderson JM, et al: Quantitative phaseflow MR imaging in dogs by using standard sequences: Comparison with in vivo flow-meter measurements. *Am J Roentgenol* 1987; 148:411–414.
74. Pennell DJ, Underwood SR, Manzara CC, Mohiaddin RH, Poole-Wilson PA, Ell PJ, et al: Magnetic resonance imaging of reversible myocardial ischemia during dobutamine stress. Book of Abstracts. *Magn Reson Med* 1990; 1:116.
75. Pettigrew RI, Martin S, Eisner RL, Oh D, Leyendecker J, Schmarkey S, et al: Catecholamine stress cine MRI to detect partial coronary artery stenosis. Book of Abstracts. *Magn Reson Med* 1991; 1:243.
76. Soulen RL, Budinger TF, Higgins CB: Magnetic resonance imaging of prosthetic heart valves. *Radiology* 1985; 154:705–707.
77. Pavlicek W, Geisinger M, Castle L, Borkowski GP, Meaney TF, Bream BL, et al: The effects of nuclear magnetic resonance on patients with cardiac pacemakers. *Radiology* 1983; 147:149–153.
78. Hayes DL, Holmes DR Jr, Gray JE: Effect of 1.5 tesla nuclear magnetic resonance imaging scanner on implanted permanent pacemakers. *J Am Coll Cardiol* 1987; 10:728–786.
79. Shellock FG: MR imaging of metallic implants and materials: A compilation of the literature. *Am J Roentgenol* 1988; 151:811–814.
80. Budinger TF: Nuclear magnetic resonance NMR in vivo studies: Known thresholds for health effects. *J Comput Assist Tomogr* 1981; 5:800–811.

Chapter 137

Positron Emission Tomography

Heinrich R. Schelbert, M.D.

The study of the human heart with conventional radionuclide techniques has remained confined to mostly ventricular function and relative distributions of regional myocardial blood flow. Positron emission tomography (PET) exceeds these capabilities and offers the opportunity to prove and quantify regional functional processes in the human heart spanning blood flow, biochemical reaction rates, substrate fluxes, and receptors. The large number of positron-emitting and biologically active tracers, the truly quantitative imaging capability, and the in vivo application of tracer kinetic principles are unique features of this technology. These advantages permit a more comprehensive evaluation and characterization of the human heart's physiology and pathophysiology.

TOOLS FOR PROBING MYOCARDIAL TISSUE FUNCTION

Fundamental to the uniqueness of PET are (1) the large number of available physiologically active radiotracers; (2) the quantitative imaging capability; and (3) the in vivo application of tracer kinetic principles. Positron-emitting isotopes of elements that constitute major parts of living matter like carbon 11 (^{11}C), nitrogen 13 (^{13}N), and oxygen 15 (^{15}O) can be inserted into biomolecules without disturbing their physiological properties. The high specific activity of these compounds (activity per mass) permits administration of minute quantities that do not exert a mass effect and thus do not perturb the very process to be studied (Table 137-1). As their physical half-life is only short, functional processes can be measured at short time intervals. The radioactivity concentrations of these tracers in tissues like arterial blood and myocardium and their changes over time can be measured noninvasively. The time-activity curves derived from serially acquired tomographic images are fitted with operational equations based on tracer kinetic models and yield quantitative estimates of regional functional processes. Tracer kinetic models describe the kinetics of a given tracer in tissue. As only the activity concentrations of a given tracer label is measured externally, these models relate the externally derived signal to the metabolic fate of the tracer label and its relationship to the functional process under study. A more detailed description of the technical features specific to PET is available in the literature.[1–4]

Several aspects of myocardial tissue function can now be evaluated or quantified (see also Table 137-1).

Myocardial Blood Flow

Several approaches for the quantitative evaluation and, in particular, quantification of regional myocardial blood flow exist. Tracers like ^{82}Rb, ^{13}N ammonia, and the more recently developed copper (II) pyruvaldehyde *bis*-(N^4-thiosemicarbazone) (^{62}Cu PTSM) are retained in myocardium in proportion to blood flow. After they are administered intravenously, images of their regional activity concentrations depict the relative distribution of myocardial blood flow at the time of tracer injection. Each tracer offers advantages and disadvantages. For example, because ^{82}Rb is available through generator based push-button operated infusion systems, its use in the clinical setting is logistically easy.[5] The short physical half-life of only 75 s permits serial studies at time intervals of only about 10 min and thus enables evaluation

TABLE 137-1

Positron-Emitting Tracers for Probing Myocardial Tissue Function

A. Myocardial Blood Flow	
^{15}O water	
^{13}N ammonia	
^{82}Rb	
^{62}Cu PTSM	
B. Myocardial Metabolism	
^{18}F 2-fluoro-2-deoxyglucose	Exogenous glucose utilization
^{11}C palmitate	Myocardial fatty acid metabolism
^{11}C acetate	Tricarboxylic acid cycle flux, oxygen consumption
^{15}O oxygen	Oxygen extraction
^{13}N or ^{11}C amino acids	Amino acid metabolism, protein synthesis
C. Neuronal Control	
^{11}C hydroxyephedrine	Uptake and storage of catecholamine by adrenergic nerve endings
^{11}C CGP 12177	β Adrenoreceptors
^{11}C MQNB	Muscarinic receptors
D. Others	
^{18}F mizonidazole	Hypoxic/ischemic myocardium

of changes in regional blood flow in response to physiological or pharmacologic interventions. At the same time, the short physical half-life may result in low count and, thus, statistically noisy images. The longer physical half-life of ^{13}N ammonia (10 min), by contrast, produces images of higher count rates and thus of higher diagnostic quality[6,7] but requires longer intervals for serial studies (40 to 60 min). Because it is cyclotron produced, its use must be coordinated with cyclotron runs, which may be cumbersome for stress intervention studies. The newly developed ^{62}Cu PTSM offers the advantages of a generator-produced tracer and of a longer physical half-life but has been reported to yield images of lesser contrast because it is less avidly extracted by myocardium. Its clinical utility remains to be established further.[8,9]

Common to these tracers of flow is their nonlinear response to blood flow as a result of a curvilinear decline of the first-pass extraction fractions with increasing flows (Fig. 137-1). However, tracer kinetic models developed and validated in animal experiments compensate for the nonlinear response so that the noninvasive estimates of blood flow linearly trace changes in blood flow. Because the capillary and sarcolemmal membranes exert only a negligible barrier effect on the exchange of ^{15}O water, this particular tracer is, in theory, most ideally suited for measurements of blood flow.[10] The tracer is also metabolically inert while the uptake and retention of ^{13}N ammonia or of ^{82}Rb is potentially susceptible to alterations in regional myocardial metabolism. Animal experiments have, however, failed to demonstrate significant effects of metabolism.[11,12]

Regardless of the tracer employed, each approach requires rapid acquisition of serial images and generation of regional time-activity curves that are then submitted to fitting with a tracer specific operational equation. Because ^{15}O water is present in both the myocardium and arterial blood (i.e., the left ventricular cavity), this approach requires correction for blood pool activity with ^{15}O-labeled carbon monoxide, which may reduce count densities and thus cause statistically noisy images.[13,14]

Each approach offers comparable estimates of blood flow at rest or during pharmacologic vasodilation in human myocardium (Table 137-2). Differences pertain to the error sensitivity of each method, which appears to be highest for the ^{15}O water method as evidenced by the relatively high coefficient of variation.[13–17]

Myocardial Glucose Utilization

As shown schematically in Fig. 137-2, the initial metabolic step of exogenous glucose metabolism can be evaluated and quantified with ^{18}F 2-fluoro-2-deoxyglucose. This radiolabeled glucose analogue exchanges across the capillary and sarcolemmal membranes in proportion to glucose, with which it then competes for hexokinase for phosphorylation to ^{18}F deoxyglucose-6-phosphate.[18–21] Unlike its natural counterpart, the phosphorylated glucose analogue is a poor substrate for glycogen formation, glycolysis, the fructose-pentose shunt. The rate of dephosphorylation is very low in myocardium. Lastly, the phosphorylated analogue is relatively impermeable to the cell membrane and becomes virtually trapped in the cell. Images of the myocardial ^{18}F activity concentrations acquired about 40 to 60 min after tracer injection (to allow time for phosphorylation) therefore reflect the relative distributions of exogenous glucose utilization rates. Because the compound traces only the initial steps of glucose utilization (up to the branch point between glycogen synthesis and glycolysis; Fig. 137-2), it offers no direct information on glycolytic rates, oxidative metabolism, or glycogen synthesis. One might argue, however, that in states of glycogen depletion, as for example, during ischemia, exogenous glucose serves as the major source of glycolytic flux, and thus, ^{18}F deoxyglucose may in fact offer some estimates of glycolytic rates.

The tissue kinetics of ^{18}F deoxyglucose have been described by a unidirectional transport model[18–21] that allows quantification of regional rates of myocardial glucose utilization through relatively simple, rapid, and computationally efficient analysis approaches.[22,23] Typi-

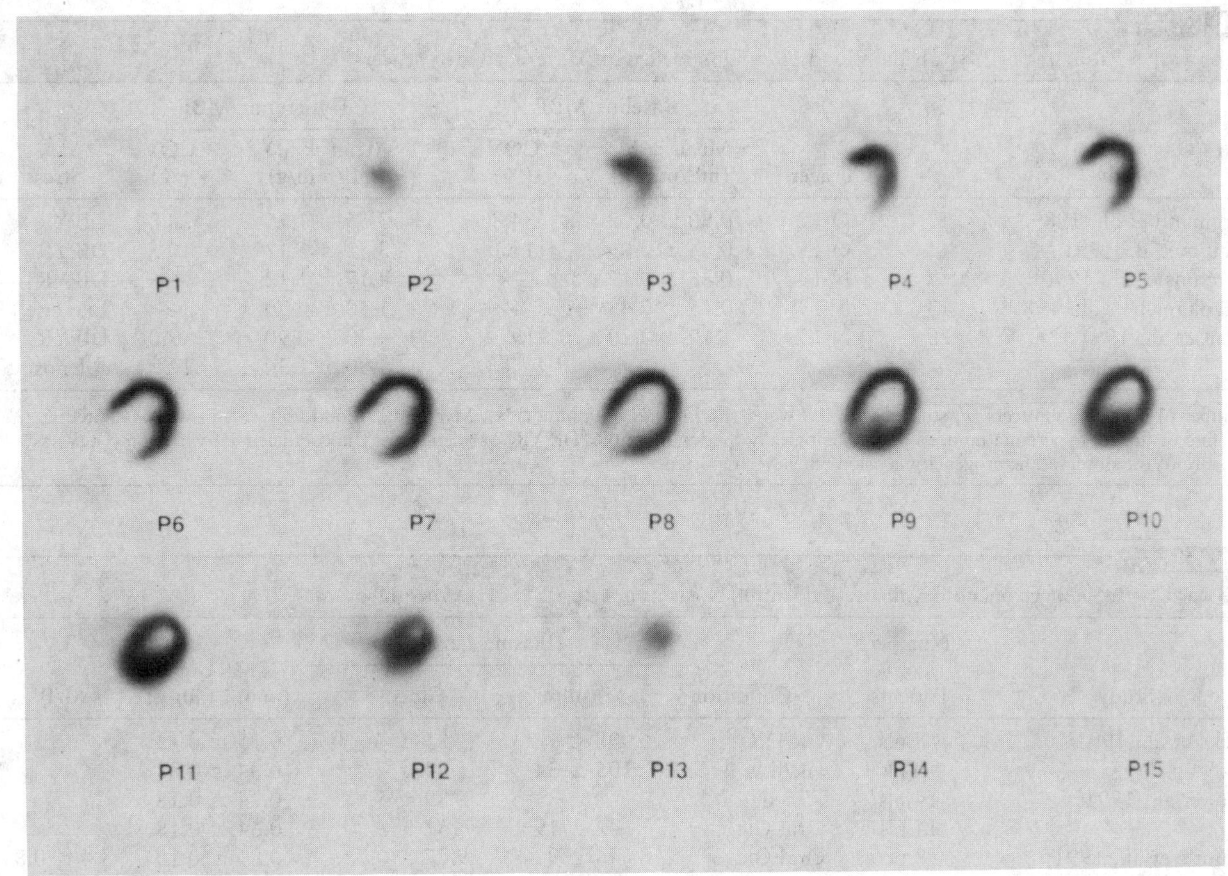

A

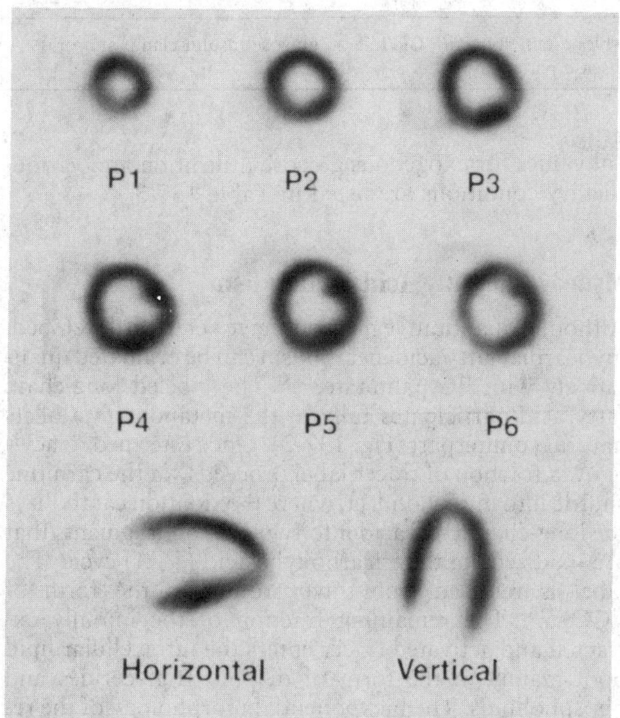

B

FIGURE 137-1 Tomographic images in a normal volunteer after intravenous injection of ^{18}F deoxyglucose. *A.* Contiguous transaxial images as routinely acquired with current PET. The images begin at the anterobasal wall of the left ventricle (P1) and proceed by 7-mm steps to the mid-left ventricle (P6 to P8) and to the inferior diaphragmatic portion of the left ventricle (P12 to P13). The images are viewed from the subject's feet (top anterior, bottom posterior, right = left and left = right). Note the homogeneous uptake of tracer throughout the left ventricular myocardium. The free right ventricular wall is visualized faintly. Also note the anterior and the posterior papillary muscles. *B.* Short, horizontal and vertical long axis cuts of the left ventricular myocardium as reconstructed from the set of transaxial images in the same normal volunteer.

TABLE 137-2
Noninvasive Estimates of Myocardial Blood Flow Obtained with Different Flow Tracers

Study	*n*	Tracer	Baseline MBF Mean ± SD (mL/min/g)	Baseline MBF COV (%)	Hyperemic MBF Mean ± SD (mL/min/g)	Hyperemic MBF COV (%)	Stress
Bergmann et al., 1989[13]	11	O-15	0.90 ± 0.22	34.8	3.55 ± 1.15	28.8	DIPYR
Araujo et al., 1991[14]	11	O-15	0.84 ± 0.09	15.1	3.52 ± 1.12	10.5	DIPYR
Hutchins et al., 1990[15]	7	N-13	0.88 ± 0.17	—	4.17 ± 1.12	—	DIPYR
Krivokapich et al., 1989[17]	13	N-13	0.75 ± 0.43	—	1.50 ± 0.70	—	Exercise
Chan et al., 1991[16]	20	N-13	1.10 ± 0.20	19	4.40 ± 0.90	9.0	DIPYR
					4.30 ± 1.30	12	Adenosine

Number of normal volunteers (*n*) studied with ^{15}O water (^{15}O) or ^{13}N ammonia (^{13}N). Myocardial blood flow (MBF) was evaluated at baseline or during hyperemia induced pharmacologically by dipyridamole (DIPYR) or adenosine. The coefficient of variation (COV) as a measure of the observed heterogeneity is listed whenever reported.

TABLE 137-3
Myocardial Rates of Exogenous Glucose Utilization Measured with PET ^{18}F Deoxyglucose

Study	Number of Patients	Condition	Plasma Levels Insulin	Plasma Levels Glucose	MRGlc (mmol/min/g)	M/B
Hicks et al., 1991[24]	8 nls	Glc/INC	98 ± 18	85 ± 7	0.35 ± 0.12	
	9 nls	Glc/INS + FFA	105 ± 34	84 ± 7	0.34 ± 0.08	
Choi et al., 1991[22]	14 nls	Fasted	8 ± 3	89 ± 5	0.24 ± 0.18	
	14 nls	Oral Glc	42 ± 19	152 ± 32	0.64 ± 0.18	
Knuutie et al., 1991[25]	8 pts	Oral Glc	46 ± 9	9.77 ± 0.78	0.80 ± 0.10	5.4 ± 0.8
	8 pts	Glc/INS	89 ± 1	5.1 ± 0.1	0.88 ± 0.10	18.1 ± 2.3
vom Dahl et al., 1991[26]	10 pts	Oral Glc	—	107 ± 28	0.40 ± 0.10	4.1 ± 1.5
	7 pts	Glc/INS	—	85 ± 4	0.50 ± 0.10	6.8 ± 2.5

MRGlc = rate of exogenous glucose utilization; M/B = myocardium-to-blood activity ratio; Glc/INS = glucose-insulin clamp and oral glucose loading; values are given for normals (nls) and coronary artery disease patients (pts).

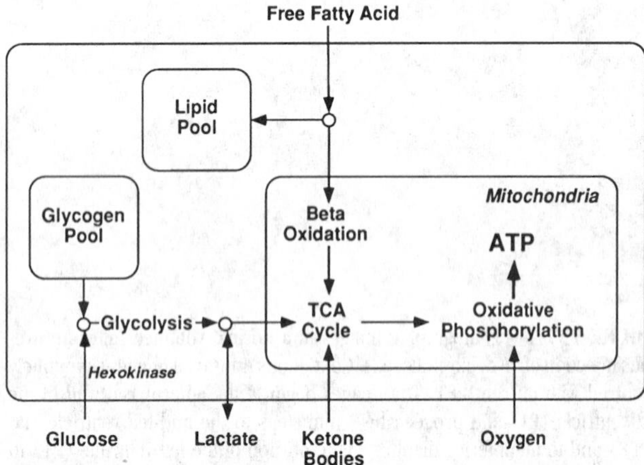

FIGURE 137-2 Highly simplified schematic representation of myocardial substrate metabolism. As described in the text, several of the major metabolic pathways can be evaluated with PET. For example, the initial transmembranous exchange and the hexokinase-mediated phosphorylation reaction from glucose to glucose-6-phosphate can be measured with ^{18}F deoxyglucose. The uptake of long-chain free fatty acid, the initial activation step, and the subsequent distribution of free fatty acid between the endogenous lipid pool and direct oxidation [via β oxidation and the tricarboxylic acid (TCA) cycle] can be evaluated with ^{11}C palmitate. Substrate flux through the TCA cycle and, by inference, oxidative metabolism and oxygen consumption can be measured with ^{11}C acetate.

cal values for exogenous glucose utilization and various dietary conditions are listed in Table 137-3.

Myocardial Fatty Acid Metabolism

Although quantitative methods have yet to be developed, myocardial fatty acid metabolism can be evaluated qualitatively with ^{11}C palmitate.[27–31] The labeled long-chain fatty acid participates fully in the metabolic fate of its natural counterpart (Fig. 137-2). Once esterified to acyl-CoA, a fraction of tracer label proceeds via the carnitine shuttle into mitochondria, where β oxidation catabolizes the long-chain fatty acid into two-carbon fragments that are oxidized via the tricarboxylic acid (TCA) cycle. The label is released from myocardium in the form of $^{11}CO_2$.[32,33] The remaining fraction of the initially extracted and activated tracer enters the intracellular lipid pool mainly in the form of di- and triglycerides and phospholipids. The biexponential morphology of the recorded tissue time-activity curve reflects the metabolic fate of the tracer (Fig. 137-3). The slow turnover rate of the intracellular lipid pool accounts for the slow clearance phase while the rapid clearance curve component corresponds to the fraction of tracer that has entered oxidative pathways directly and its rate of oxidation.

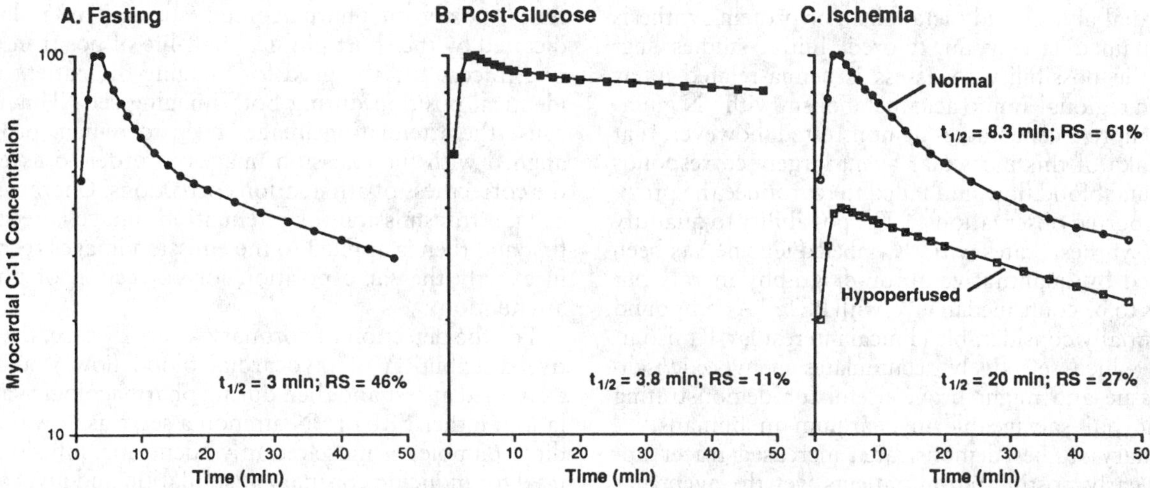

FIGURE 137-3 Evaluation of myocardial fatty acid metabolism with ^{11}C-labeled palmitate. The idealized time-activity curves were reconstructed from serially acquired images following tracer administration in a normal volunteer after an overnight fast (*A*), following glucose loading (100 g orally) (*B*), and in a patient with chronic coronary artery disease (*C*). The biexponential clearance curve morphology corresponds to the fractional tracer distribution between a small, rapid turnover pool (rapid clearance phase; corresponding to oxidation of tracer to ^{11}C CO_2 and its release) and a large, slow turnover pool (endogenous lipids). As demonstrated by biexponential least square curve fitting, the size (RS) and slope ($t_{1/2}$) of the rapid clearance phase decline from the fasted to the glucose-loaded state, reflecting a decrease in the fraction of tracer that becomes immediately oxidized and thus a decline in the rate of fatty acid oxidation in exchange for a proportionate increase in glucose oxidation. As seen in *C*, the initial uptake as well as the size and slope are markedly reduced in hypoperfused myocardium, indicating a disproportionate segmental decline in fatty acid oxidation in the hypoperfused myocardium.

Because ischemia reduces the rate of fatty acid oxidation and of TCA cycle activity, the relative size and rate of the rapid clearance curve component on the ^{11}C myocardial time-activity curve typically decline during acute myocardial ischemia.[31,34] A disproportionately greater fraction of tracer label then enters the slower turnover, endogenous lipid pool.[33] Estimates of fatty acid oxidation during ischemia, however, are complicated by enhanced back diffusion of nonmetabolized tracer.[34,35]

Preferential utilization of a given fuel substrate such as glucose, lactate, or free fatty acid depends on their concentrations in arterial blood, which in turn are affected by fasting, carbohydrate ingestion, or physical stress.[36] Changes in preferential substrate utilization can be demonstrated with both ^{11}C palmitate and ^{18}F deoxyglucose.[19,23,36] In the presence of high free fatty acid and low glucose and insulin levels, the preferential use of free fatty acid is reflected on the ^{11}C palmitate curve by the large relative size of the rapid clearance phase and its steep slope (both corresponding to increased fatty acid oxidation) and the low or even undetectable ^{18}F deoxyglucose uptake. Ingestion of carbohydrates raises plasma glucose levels, stimulates insulin secretion and depresses fatty acid levels (Table 137-3). The shift to myocardial glucose utilization is reflected by a decline in the size and slope of the rapid clearance phase of ^{11}C palmitate and by an increase in myocardial ^{18}F deoxyglucose uptake.

Myocardial Oxygen Consumption

Preliminary studies have demonstrated the possibility of measuring myocardial oxygen consumption from the product of oxygen extraction (by ^{15}O oxygen) and myocardial blood flow (by ^{15}O water).[37,38] While this approach awaits validation, the most widely applied method relies on ^{11}C acetate. The tracer rapidly accumulates in myocardium, rapidly clears from blood, and produces high signal-to-background images.[39–45] It directly traces the flux of substrate through the TCA cycle as the final oxidative pathway common to most substrates. The rate of clearance from myocardium derived from serially acquired images corresponds to the TCA cycle activity and, because of its close coupling to oxidative phosphorylation, to oxidative metabolism and myocardial oxygen consumption. It should be emphasized, however, that the tracer yields not mass fluxes but rather rate constants that can be converted into units of O_2 per minute per gram of myocardium. Unlike ^{11}C palmitate or ^{18}F deoxyglucose, the clearance rate of ^{11}C acetate from myocardium is relatively insensitive to changes in myocardial preferential substrate utilization.

Neuronal Control of Cardiac Function

Recent investigations have focused on the development, validation, and application of tracers of myocardial neuronal control. For example, initial studies with ^{11}C *meta*-hydroxyephedrine, a catecholamine analogue, has demonstrated the possibility to evaluate noninvasively uptake and storage of catecholamines by adrenergic nerve endings and, by implication, density and function of adrenergic neurons.[46] Other studies have employed β-adrenoreceptor ligands labeled with ^{11}C (for example, the experimental compound ^{11}C CGP-12177) for evaluating and quantifying β-receptor concentrations or ^{11}C-labeled methiodide salt of quinuclidinyl benzylate (MQNB) for the study and quantification of muscarinic receptors.[47,48]

Other Aspects of Myocardial Tissue Function

Despite a relatively large number of available ^{11}C- or ^{13}N-labeled amino acids, their potential utility for exploring myocardial amino acid metabolism or protein synthesis has remained largely unexplored. Initial studies suggested the possibility to assess ischemia-related alterations in regional amino acid metabolism with ^{13}N glutamate[49]; more recent studies demonstrated, however, that the uptake of this particular agent largely corresponds to regional blood flow and failed to reproduce the previously reported observations.[50] The possibility to quantify protein synthesis rates with ^{11}C-labeled leucine has been suggested by quantitative autoradiography in rats but remains to be confirmed in vivo with PET.[51] A compound of potentially considerable clinical interest is ^{18}F misonidazole, which selectively accumulates in hypoxic/ischemic tissue and might prove useful for demonstrating ischemic but salvageable myocardium in humans.[52–54] Preliminary studies demonstrated increased tracer uptake in early postinfarction patients, yet the agent has remained unsatisfactory because of low myocardium-to-blood-pool uptake ratios.

CLINICAL APPLICATIONS

The relatively high startup and operational cost of PET, including installation, operation, and maintenance of a scanner, cyclotron, and radiopharmaceutical synthesis laboratory, and related technical and operational complexities have delayed the rapid transfer and widespread dissemination of this new technology into the clinical environment. However, a more widespread clinical acceptance is currently gaining momentum as investigational studies have demonstrated the value of PET to contribute to diagnosis, characterization, treatment, and monitoring of disease. In the cardiovascular area, the diagnosis and characterization of coronary artery disease and the identification of viable myocardium have been foremost.

Diagnosis and Characterization of Coronary Artery Disease

Detection of Coronary Artery Disease

Unlike conventional radionuclide approaches, which employ flow tracers primarily during physical stress and at rest for the detection of coronary artery disease, PET relies mostly on pharmacologic stress. This is largely dictated by the short physical half-life of positron-emitting tracers and the need for imaging the patient in an identical position during both imaging sets. This is because the attenuation images need to remain properly aligned with the emission images in order to ascertain the correctness of attenuation corrections. Characteristically, a transmission (or attenuation) image is recorded first and then is applied to the emission images recorded in exactly the same position for correction of photon attenuation.

For the detection of coronary artery disease, the relative distribution of myocardial blood flow is initially examined at rest and then during pharmacologic vasodilation. Either ^{82}Rb or ^{13}N ammonia serve as flow tracers; dipyridamole, or more recently adenosine, infusions are used for inducing coronary vasodilation and myocardial hyperemia. As both tracers are retained in myocardium in proportion to blood flow, the resulting images depict the distribution of myocardial blood flow at baseline and during hyperemia. The approach identifies true resting flow defects as well as attenuated responses of regional blood flow to hyperemia as a consequence of coronary stenosis. The baseline and hyperemia flow images are analyzed by visual inspection, by circumferential activity profile techniques, or by polar map approaches based on circumferential activity profiles or reoriented short-axis cuts of the left ventricular myocardium. While most investigations have relied on visual analysis, studies are currently in progress to explore the utility and diagnostic accuracy of more quantitative approaches. One laboratory employs a "semiquantitative" approach where myocardial tracer activity concentrations are normalized to the total administered activity.[4] Although the approach accounts for the nonlinear response in tracer uptake and the systemic effects of vasodilatory drugs, it assumes these changes to be constant. Given the recently reported interpatient variability of myocardial blood flow responses to pharmacologic vasodilation as determined by truly quantitative studies (Table 137-2), the validity of these assumptions may be limited.

Several clinical investigations have confirmed the high diagnostic performance of PET for the detection of coronary artery disease (Table 137-4).[7,55–58] In a total of 556 patients with angiographically proven coronary artery disease, sensitivities ranged from 87 to 97 percent and specificities from 78 to 100 percent. Most of these studies

TABLE 137-4
Detection of Coronary Artery Disease by Positron Emission Tomography

Study	Number of Patients	Tracer	Stress	Sensitivity (%)	Specificity (%)
Schelbert et al., 1982[7]	32	N	DIP	97	100
Demer et al., 1989[56]	193	N, Rb	DIP	94	95
Tamaki et al., 1988[55]	48	N	EX	88	90
Go et al., 1990[57]	202	Rb	DIP	93	78
Stewart et al., 1991[58]	81	Rb	DIP	87	82

Tracer: Rb = ^{82}Ru and N = ^{13}N ammonia. DIP = intravenous dipyridamole; EX = supine bicycle exercise.

compared rest or stress-induced flow defects to arteriographic findings by visual analysis, and most defined a 50 to 70 percent diameter luminal narrowing as significant stenosis. Given the well-known limitation of visual analysis, Demer et al.[56] graded stenosis severity by estimates of coronary flow reserve, obtained by quantitative coronary arteriography. Coronary arteries were classified as moderately to severely stenosed if the predicted coronary flow reserve was less than 3, as intermediate if the coronary flow reserve ranged from 3 to 4, and as minimal for coronary flow reserve values greater than 4. According to this classification, 94 percent of vessels with moderate to severe, 49 percent of vessels with intermediate, and 5 percent of vessels with minimal stenosis flow reserves were accurately identified with PET and pharmacologic vasodilatory stress.

Comparison of PET to Conventional Techniques

While impressive, the diagnostic accuracy of PET must be compared to that of more conventional approaches. Demer et al.[56] indirectly compared their findings to those of another laboratory using thallium single-photon emission computed tomography (SPECT) but the same angiographic approach for defining stenosis severity. In this comparison, PET outperformed thallium tomographic imaging. Both studies defined stenosis severity by the angiographically predicted coronary flow reserve. Moderate to severe coronary stenoses were detected with a 95 percent sensitivity by PET and a 72 percent sensitivity by thallium SPECT, intermediate stenoses with a 49 percent sensitivity by PET while none was detected by SPECT. Goldstein et al.[59] subsequently demonstrated that the angiographically determined coronary flow reserve did in fact significantly correlate with the relative myocardial flow reserve by PET and pharmacologically induced hyperemia.

Other studies compared both techniques in the same patients (Table 137-5). An early study used supine bicycle stress and ^{13}N ammonia in 48 patients with coronary artery disease and failed to demonstrate significant differences in the diagnostic performance of PET and SPECT.[55] A more recent report examined the relative merits of PET and SPECT in 202 patients during the same pharmacologic stress.[57] Myocardial blood flow was evaluated with ^{82}Rb at baseline and again 4 min after dipyridamole infusion. About 8 to 9 min later, or a total of 12 to 13 min after the end of the dipyridamole infusion, ^{201}Tl was injected and SPECT imaging performed within 10 min. As shown in Table 137-5, PET and SPECT exhibited comparable specificities while PET demonstrated a significantly higher sensitivity than SPECT. The results were similar when only 132 of the 202 patients without prior cardiac events such as angioplasty or bypass grafting were analyzed. A second study[58] reported somewhat different findings in 81 patients. Again, all patients underwent rest and dipyridamole stress imaging with ^{82}Rb and PET; for the ^{201}Tl SPECT study, 38 (or 47 percent) of the patients underwent treadmill stress testing and the remaining 43 (or 53 percent) pharmacologic stress with dipyridamole. In that study, PET and SPECT exhibited comparable sensitivities; however, the specificity was higher for PET than for SPECT. The findings did not differ between patients submitted to treadmill stress testing and patients with pharmacologically induced hyperemia for thallium SPECT.

Thus, both studies demonstrated an improvement in the diagnostic accuracy for PET yet differed in terms of higher sensitivities and specificities. While it might be argued that in the study by Go et al.[57] the hyperemic effects of dipyridamole had dissipated at the time of the thallium injection and thus accounted for the lower sensitivity of thallium SPECT, continuous coronary sinus flow measurements have demonstrated an average decay half-time of 33 min for the hyperemic response. This would amount to an average decline in the hyperemic response over a period of 8 to 9 min of about 15 to 18 percent,[60] which is unlikely to explain fully the significantly lower sensitivity of SPECT thallium imaging. More plausible is the gain in specificity in the study by Stewart et al.[58] It most likely resulted from the adequate correction of photon attenuation and thus a reduction of falsely positive findings. Although the reasons for the observed differences between both studies remain unclear, image analysis at different points of the receiver operating curve (ROC) might be one possible explanation. It is also likely that the absence of a significant difference between PET and SPECT findings in the first study[55] might be attributed to the first-generation, less advanced imaging instrumentation used in this study and the use of supine bicycle exercise rather than of pharmacologic stress.

On balance, the reported studies demonstrate a statistically significant gain in diagnostic accuracy for the detection of coronary artery disease by PET. Although larger clinical trials will be needed for defining more clearly the diagnostic gain, current information nevertheless indicates an improved diagnostic accuracy that

TABLE 137-5

Comparison of PET and SPECT for Detection of Coronary Artery Disease

Study	Number of Patients	Sensitivity (%)		Specificity (%)	
		SPECT	PET	SPECT	PET
Tamaki et al., 1988[55]	48	81	88	94	90
Go et al., 1990[57]	203	78	93*	80	78
Stewart et al., 1991[58]	81	84	84	53	88†

$^{*}p < .001$
$^{\dagger}p < .05$

might eliminate additional diagnostic procedures like coronary arteriography and might be cost effective.

Quantitative Studies of Blood Flow

Particularly intriguing is the possibility to quantify regional myocardial blood flow and its response to physical or pharmacologic stress in myocardium supplied by normal and stenosed coronary arteries. In normal myocardium, moderate supine bicycle exercise has been shown to produce only a 2.2-fold increase that paralleled the increase in rate pressure product as an index of cardiac work and thus, by inference, oxygen consumption[17] (Table 137-2). More prominent increases, in the range of three to five times the baseline blood flow, have been demonstrated with intravenous dipyridamole or, more recently, with intravenous adenosine.[14–16,61] While these agents produced hyperemia independent of oxygen demand, intravenous dobutamine, recently advocated as a pharmacologic stress agent, increases myocardial oxygen consumption, which in normal myocardium is paralleled by an appropriate increase in myocardial blood flow.[62] Infusion rates of 40 μg dobutamine/min per kilogram of body weight raised myocardial blood flow 2.8 times from 0.82±0.22 to 2.21±0.37 mL/min per g. This increase was paralleled by a proportionate 2.8-fold increase in the rate pressure product as an index of cardiac work.

Responses to blood flow in myocardium subtended by stenosed coronary arteries have been observed to be attenuated relative to those in normal myocardium[14,61] but normalized after successful coronary angioplasty.[63] Of interest is that one study observed an increase rather than an anticipated decrease of blood flow with pharmacologic vasodilation in territories supplied by coronary collaterals.[64] In collateral dependent myocardium, blood flow increased with dipyridamole from 0.70±0.10 to 1.43±0.73 mL/min per g as compared to an increase from 0.88±0.21 to 3.0±1.3 mL/min per g in normal myocardium. While this observation argues against a coronary steal, it does not exclude it as the technique measures only transmural flows. A subendocardial decrease might have been offset by a subepicardial increase in blood flow.

Quantification rather than qualitative evaluation of blood flow at rest and in response to pharmacologic interventions offers several advantages. It might improve the accuracy with which the functional significance of coronary stenosis and the response to therapeutic interventions (both pharmacologic and interventional) can be assessed and might prove especially useful in patients with balanced lesions or left main coronary artery disease. It further might aid in the characterization of patients with anginalike symptoms but normal coronary arteries (syndrome X), although initial preliminary studies have remained inconclusive in this area.[65,66] For example, in about half of 15 such patients, myocardial blood flow reserve was markedly attenuated due to increased baseline blood flows. An extension of these studies with dobutamine stress and ^{11}C acetate revealed an attenuated increase in oxidative metabolism. Quantitative measurements of blood flow might also provide explanations for ischemic symptoms in patients with left ventricular hypertrophy but normal coronary arteries.[67] Important for such evaluations will be the establishment of normal values for baseline and maximum achievable blood flow with pharmacologic vasodilation as well as for myocardial flow reserves. The latter appears to be related to age.[68] Myocardial flow reserve as the ratio of hyperemic to baseline flows was found to be 27 percent lower in older than in younger, apparently healthy volunteers (mean ages 25±4 and 55±9 years). Similarly, baseline flows as the numerator of flow reserve are related to the rate pressure product and thus to cardiac work, thereby influencing the observed flow reserve values. Thus, use of absolute maximum achievable blood flows may be more useful.[17,69]

Assessment of Myocardial Viability

Myocardial viability pertains to a segmental impairment of contractile function that is potentially reversible. Distinction of a potentially reversible from an irreversible impairment of contractile function is frequently of considerable clinical importance but remains diagnostically challenging. This is because both types share a number of common features, such as similar degrees of abnormal systolic wall motion, reduced blood flow, and electrocardiographic abnormalities.[70] Persistence of metabolic activity for maintaining vital but energy-requiring processes such as cellular homeostasis and transmembrane ion concentration gradients is critical for cell survival and is a key feature of potentially reversible dysfunctional or viable myocardium. Some residual blood flow must persist for removal of inhibitory metabolites.

Diagnostic approaches to the identification of viable myocardium target one or two of these key features. Positron emission tomography evaluates regional myocardial blood flow and preserved metabolic activity.[71,72] It entails two procedural steps: First myocardial blood flow is evaluated with ^{82}Rb, ^{13}N ammonia, or in some laboratories, with ^{15}O water. This is followed by examining the relative distribution of exogenous glucose utilization with intravenous ^{18}F deoxyglucose (Fig. 137-4 to 137-7). Both image sets are then analyzed for regional abnormalities in blood flow and glucose utilization and their relationship by visual inspection, circumferential profile analysis approaches,[71,72] or more recently, polar mapping of the relative distribution of blood flow and glucose metabolism and regional tracer uptake differences.[73]

Several patterns of blood flow and glucose utilization may occur in dysfunctional myocardial segments.[72] In pattern A blood flow and ^{18}F deoxyglucose uptake are within normal limits. In pattern B blood flow is reduced but ^{18}F deoxyglucose is normal, increased relative to blood flow or relative to the tracer uptake in normal myocardium ("blood flow–metabolism mismatch"). In pattern C both blood flow and ^{18}F deoxyglucose uptake are reduced concordantly. How well each of these patterns identifies a reversible or irreversible impairment of contractile function has been examined against the functional outcome after revascularization in several studies.[72,74–76] As listed in Table 137-6, patterns A and B were 78 to 85 percent accurate in predicting an improve-

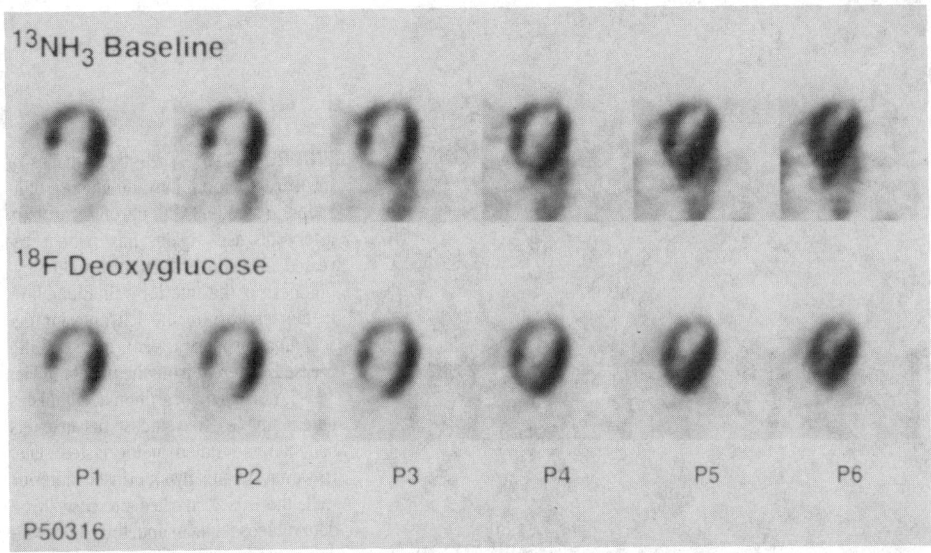

FIGURE 137-4 Transaxial images of myocardial blood flow and glucose utilization obtained in a patient with chronic coronary artery disease and akinesis of the anterior wall. Note the extensive perfusion defect in the anterior wall on the ^{13}N ammonia images associated with a concordant decrease in ^{18}F deoxyglucose uptake. The concordant decrease in tracer uptake is referred to as blood flow–metabolism match.

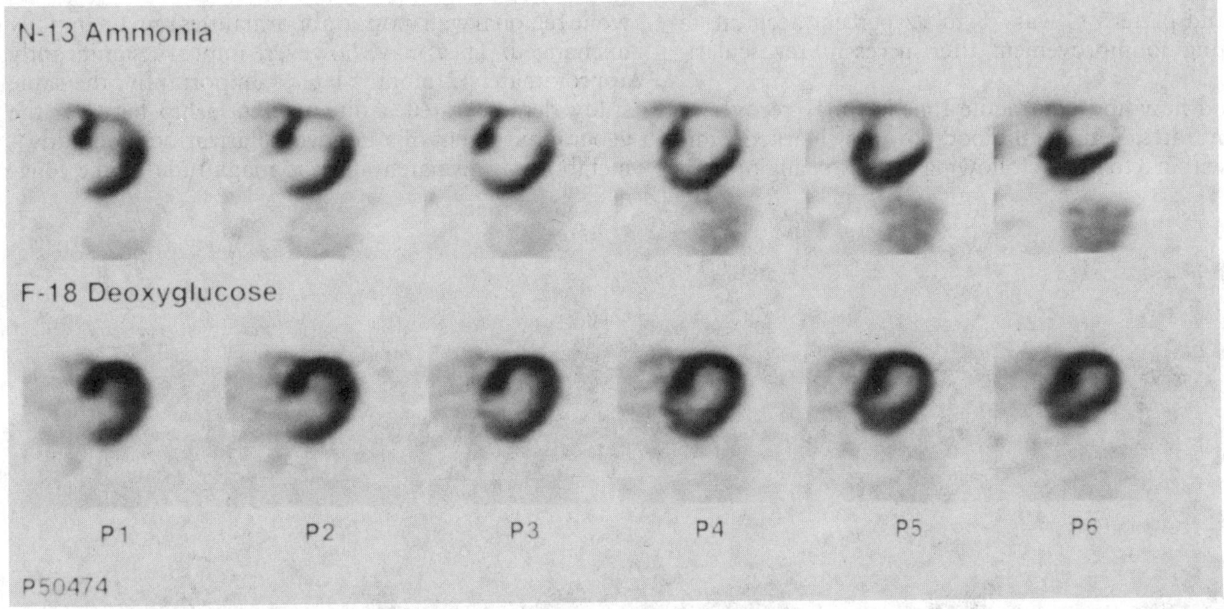

FIGURE 137-5 Transaxial images of myocardial blood flow and exogenous glucose utilization in a patient with chronic coronary artery disease and impaired wall motion of the anterior wall. Again, note the extensive flow defect in the territory of the left anterior descending involving the anterior wall and the anterior septum. However, different from the example shown in Fig. 137-4, ^{18}F deoxyglucose uptake is preserved or even enhanced in the hypoperfused myocardium. This discordant uptake of the metabolic and blood flow tracer is referred to as blood flow–metabolism mismatch.

TABLE 137-6

Predictive Value of Blood Flow Metabolism Patterns of PET for Functional Outcome after Interventional Revascularization

Study	Number of Patients	Number of Dysfunctional Segments	Predictive Accuracy (%)	
			Positive	Negative
Tillisch et al., 1986[72]	17	67	85	92
Tamaki et al., 1989[74]	22	46	78	78
Tamaki et al., 1991[75]	11	56	80	100

Positive predictive accuracy listed as a postinterventional improvement in regional wall motion with either normal blood flow or glucose metabolism or a mismatch. The negative predictive accuracy indicates a lack of postinterventional improvement in segments with blood flow–metabolism matches.

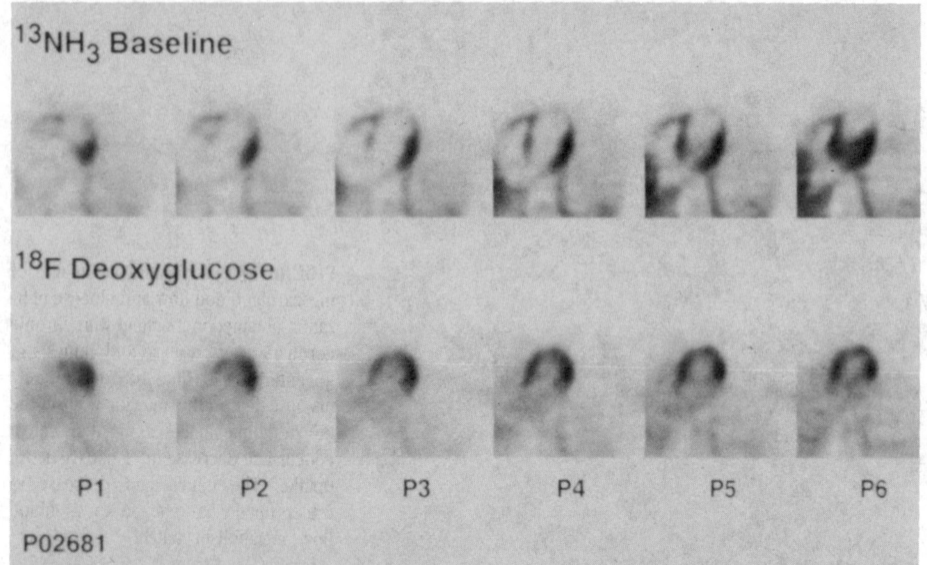

FIGURE 137-6 Transaxial images of myocardial blood flow and glucose utilization in a patient with chronic coronary artery disease. Again, this patient revealed on echocardiography severe hypokinesis of the anterior wall. Blood flow in the territory of the left anterior descending coronary artery is markedly decreased; different from the patient in Fig. 137-5, normal myocardium accumulates little if any ^{18}F deoxyglucose because this patient was studied in the fasted state. However, in the hypoperfused anterior wall, there is a marked increase in ^{18}F deoxyglucose uptake and, thus, in exogenous glucose utilization.

ment and pattern C was 78 to 92 percent accurate in predicting no improvement after successful revascularization.

Blood flow and contractile function may recover at different rates. Segmental blood flow may markedly improve within 3 to 4 days following successful angioplasty while regional wall motion abnormalities remain initially unchanged. They may, however, improve significantly approximately 2 months later.[76] Importantly, the same study demonstrated a direct relationship between the geographic extent of a prerevascularization blood flow–metabolism mismatch and the magnitude of the long-

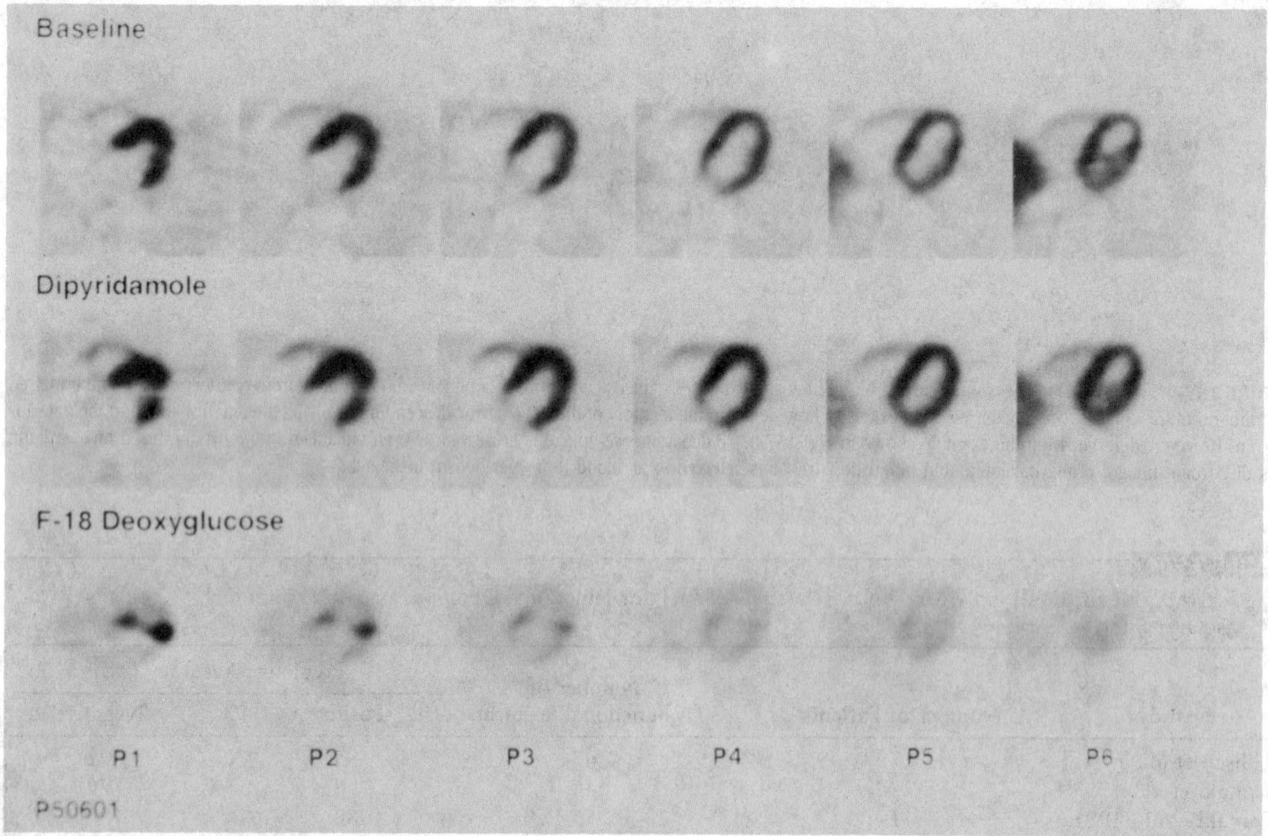

FIGURE 137-7 Transaxial images of blood flow at baseline and during dipyridamole-induced hyperemia as well as of glucose utilization in a patient with coronary artery disease. Note the small area of decreased ^{13}N ammonia uptake in the anterolateral wall on the baseline blood flow images. The hyperemia study confirms that this defect is not artifactual but rather related to coronary artery disease as it becomes more extensive during pharmacologic vasodilation. The glucose uptake images reveal in the same segment an enhancement of exogenous glucose utilization.

term wall motion improvement. Within the same context, earlier studies had demonstrated that extensive blood flow–metabolism mismatches or normal blood flow and metabolism in large dysfunctional segments were associated with an improvement in global left ventricular function, whereas left ventricular ejection fractions remained unchanged when blood flow–metabolism mismatches were absent or involved only a small fraction of the left ventricular myocardium.[72] Lastly, repeat coronary arteriography revealed that 95 percent of coronary artery bypass grafts to segments with blood flow–metabolism mismatches remained patent.[74] This was different for grafts to segments with blood flow–metabolism matches. At 5 to 7 weeks after revascularization, 70 percent of such grafts were found to be obstructed. Thus, these data provide considerable support for the notion that normal or relatively increased glucose metabolism accurately identified a reversible impairment of contractile function and that PET might predict the magnitude of a postrevascularization improvement in global left ventricular function.

Possible Mechanisms of Blood-Metabolism Patterns

Several mechanisms might account for reversible impairments of contractile function. While necrosis or scar tissue formation almost always accounts for the irreversible impairment or loss of contractile function, *myocardial hibernation, myocardial stunning,* or possibly, *repetitive stunning* might underlie the reversible impairment of contractile function.[77,78] (See also Chap. 57.) It is possible that pattern A, or normal blood flow and glucose metabolism in dysfunctional segments, might signify pure stunning, whereas pattern B, or segmentally reduced flow associated with sustained glucose utilization, is consistent with hibernation as a more chronic form of dysfunction or even represents a functional and metabolic adaptation to a chronic reduction in supply. It should be emphasized that the operational term *blood flow–metabolism match* does not infer complete absence of viable myocardium. Conversely, the term *mismatch* does not infer that all myocardium is in fact viable. Rather, more often than not, normal myocytes and compromised by salvageable myocytes coexist in the same myocardial segment together with fibrotic tissue. The assessment of their fractional distribution is important. For example, the presence of only normal myocardium and scar tissue might result in a concordant reduction of blood flow and metabolism. Conversely, substantial amounts of compromised but salvageable myocytes together with some normal myocytes and fibrotic tissue presumably cause a blood flow–metabolism mismatch and account for a functional improvement upon restoration of blood flow. These considerations would also explain why regional wall thickness failed to adequately discriminate between viable and nonviable myocardium.[79] Questions like whether the magnitude of an improvement of contractile function depends on the magnitude of residual glucose metabolic activity or the degree of reduced blood flow remain to be explored. Less clear is the reason for the augmented glucose utilization. While this is known to occur in acute myocardial ischemia, its mechanism remains largely undefined in more chronic conditions.[80–83] (See also Chap. 6A.) It is equally uncertain whether the enhanced glucose utilization is exclusively anaerobic or oxidative. In chronic dog studies, the fraction of glucose that was metabolized anaerobically was increased in reperfused relative to normal myocardium, despite adequate blood flow and oxygen delivery.[84] The sustained increase in anaerobic glycolysis might be consistent with the augmented lactate release in chronic coronary artery disease patients.[85] It is also possible that the preferential glucose utilization by "hibernating myocardium" might in fact represent an adaptative process as this particular substrate is more oxygen efficient than, for example, free fatty acid.

Dietary Standardization

As mentioned earlier, normal myocardium can freely change between various substrates, depending on their substrate concentrations and the endocrine milieu. This does not appear to be true for acutely ischemic, stunned, or otherwise compromised myocardium that fails to fully participate in normal shifts in preferential substrate usage. For example, changes in glucose utilization in compromised and dysfunctional myocardium in response to changes in plasma substrate levels are attenuated in animal experiments and in patients.[72,74,86] Therefore, when patients with chronic coronary artery disease are examined under fasting conditions with preferential use of fatty acid by normal myocardium, glucose utilization is increased in absolute terms in "viable myocardium." Conversely, if patients are studied after oral glucose loading, glucose utilization in viable myocardium may actually be reduced in absolute terms, though less than blood flow. Thus, evaluation of patients in the fasted state more accurately uncovers viable myocardium.

Unfortunately, there are several limitations to this approach. First, while it might be sensitive, the amount of viable myocardium identified might be small and inconsequential for an improvement in contractile function. Second, use of ^{18}F deoxyglucose in the fasted state frequently results in diagnostically suboptimal or even uninterpretable images.[87] Thus, most laboratories prefer an approach where glucose (100 g) is administered orally about 1 h prior to the ^{18}F deoxyglucse injection, which prompts a decline in free fatty acid levels and secretion of insulin, enhances the uptake of tracer in normal myocardium and its clearance from blood, and results in images of superior diagnostic quality.[88] Other approaches have included euglycemic hyperinsulinemic clamp. From the data in Table 137-3, it is unclear whether or not this more tedious approach produces more consistent glucose metabolic rates and results in greater standardization. More complex is the use of ^{18}F deoxyglucose in patients with diabetes mellitus in whom careful monitoring of plasma glucose levels and possible administration of insulin are needed.

Prediction of Long-Term Morbidity and Mortality

The observed patterns of blood flow and metabolism on PET are also predictive of longer-term morbidity and mortality. Several reports have reported significantly different long-term fates for patients with and without blood flow–metabolism mismatches. Over a 2.1-year follow-up period in 48 patients, the presence of a blood flow–metabolism mismatch was associated with a significantly higher morbidity and mortality than in patients without mismatches.[89] Patients included in this study had only modestly reduced left ventricular function (LVEF about 47 percent). Even more striking differences were reported for a 1-year follow-up period. In 82 patients with severe left ventricular dysfunction (mean LVEF 34 percent), a mismatch pattern was associated with a 1-year mortality of 30 percent as compared to 8.3 percent for patients with only matches. Similar data were recently obtained in our laboratory in more than 100 patients.[90] The 1-year mortality for patients with an average ejection fraction of only less than 35 percent was 30 percent for patients with and only 8.6 percent for patients without mismatches. Interventional revascularization appeared to significantly reduce the mortality in mismatch patients in both studies, to 3.9 percent in the study by Eitzman et al.[91] and to 9.1 percent in the study by Maddahi et al.[90] Revascularization resulted in both studies in an improvement of congestive heart failure symptoms in patients with but not in patients without mismatches.

Comparison to Other Diagnostic Approaches

Most widely applied for the identification of myocardial viability is the ^{201}Tl stress redistribution approach using single-photon emission computed tomography. While the standard 4-hr redistribution approach underestimates the incidence of viable myocardium by as much as 50 percent when defects failed to resolve,[92–95] modifications of the standard approach, as, for example, 24 h or more delayed imaging[96] and ^{201}Tl reinjection,[97,98] have markedly improved its diagnostic accuracy. Preliminary studies in our laboratory in patients with severely depressed left ventricular function and congestive heart failure have revealed persistent limitations of the delayed ^{201}Tl imaging approach. Again, nearly 50 percent of fixed segments on late redistribution continue to exhibit metabolic evidence of myocardial viability on PET.[99] Conversely, segments with partial defect resolution on late redistribution imaging failed to exhibit metabolic activity after ^{18}F deoxyglucose administration. Comparative studies of the ^{201}Tl reinjection and the PET approach have revealed somewhat discordant observations. In one study in 20 patients, 63 percent of all irreversible defects on ^{201}Tl reinjection revealed persistent metabolic activity.[79] On the other hand, in segments with severely reduced blood flow, ^{201}Tl reinjection and ^{18}F deoxyglucose were equally effective in identifying myocardial viability. In a second study,[75] about 25 percent of all irreversible defects on thallium reinjection were found to be viable on PET. The accuracy of the PET findings was confirmed in a subset of 11 patients after surgical revascularization, where blood flow metabolism patterns were more accurate than the ^{201}Tl approach in predicting the functional outcome after successful revascularization.

Viability in Acute Myocardial Infarction

Relative or absolute segmental increases in glucose utilization have also been observed in patients early after an acute myocardial infarction. Blood flow–metabolism mismatch patterns were present in about half of the myocardial segments subtended by the infarct vessels. Studies in relatively small patient populations suggest that the prevalence of this pattern is independent of acute coronary thrombolysis.[81,100] Rather, persistence of metabolic activity statistically correlates with vessel patency or the presence of residual or even normal antegrade blood flow through the infarct vessel. While collateral blood flow may potentially account for the sustained metabolic activity, no statistically significant correlations were found, presumably as a result of the relatively small patient population study.

At present, it remains uncertain whether or not the blood flow–metabolism pattern in acute infarct patients is similarly predictive of the long-term outcome of contractile function. In one study, none of the segments with blood flow–metabolism matches revealed a significant improvement in contractile function when reexamined on two-dimensional echocardiography at an average of 6 weeks after the acute event.[81] On the other hand, contractile function improved in half of the segments with an early postinfarction mismatch. It should be emphasized that this improvement occurred spontaneously as none of the patients underwent interventional revascularization. The observations seem to suggest that function does not improve in segments with blood flow–metabolism matches. The spontaneous improvement in contractile function in half of the mismatch segments suggests “stunning” early after the infarction, whereas the absence of an improvement in the remainder of the mismatched segments may have been due to progression of ischemia to necrosis (as no revascularization was attempted) or due to myocardial hibernation. More recent data suggest that if revascularized, segments with blood flow–metabolism mismatches do in fact improve contractile function.[101]

Other Approaches with PET for Assessment of Myocardial Viability

Given the large number of available positron-emitting tracers, other aspects of myocardial ischemia can readily be assessed and other criteria and methods be developed for identifying potentially reversible contractile dysfunction. One approach has employed ^{11}C acetate as a measure of oxidative metabolism in compromised myocardium.[102] Preliminary findings in acute myocardial infarct as well as chronic coronary artery disease patients have suggested that ^{11}C acetate offers comparable accuracies to ^{18}F deoxyglucose for predicting the long-term outcome in contractile function after interventional revascularization.[102] The available information precludes an evaluation of the criteria used in these studies for distinguishing between reversible and irreversible impairment of contractile function. As oxidative metabolism parallels blood flow, it also will be necessary to define better to what extent measurements of oxidative metabolism are superior to flow measurements for the identification of myocardial viability.

The recently advocated ^{82}Rb uptake and retention approach is particularly intriguing, especially in the clinical environment for it requires only a single tracer injection of the logistically easy-to-use generator-produced agent

^{82}Rb.[103] Data in animal experiments obtained with nonimaging devices had indicated that myocardium injured only reversibly retains the cation ^{82}Rb while it clears from irreversibly injured myocardium.[104] The approach entails acquisition of an early and a late phase image after ^{82}Rb administration. The initial image presumably depicts blood flow, whereas the late image depicts active and energy-requiring retention of tracer or cations in myocardium. Increases in defect sizes or new defects in tracer activity concentrations on the late relative to the early phase images identify myocardium as irreversibly injured, whereas retention of the rubidium cations identifies myocardium as viable. Compared to ^{18}F deoxyglucose uptake in patients with recent myocardial infarction and to the ^{18}F deoxyglucose uptake in patients with coronary artery disease, this new approach appeared to provide comparable, if not superior, information. Additional studies are required to examine the value and validity of this approach compared to postrevascularization changes in regional contractile function as the true test for "viability."

The water perfusable tissue index seems equally promising.[105] It determines the extravascular tissue density from the transmission and an ^{15}O carbon monoxide blood pool image and employs ^{15}O-labeled water to estimate the fraction of the extravascular tissue that is capable of exchanging water rapidly. Implicit in this approach is that the fraction of extravascular tissue that does not exchange water represents scar tissue or irreversibly injured myocardium. As discussed earlier, the fraction of nonreversibly injured myocardium in a given myocardial segment should be useful for predicting an improvement in contractile function. Preliminary studies in patients after an acute myocardial infarction and coronary thrombolysis as well as in patients with chronic coronary artery disease supports the validity of this concept.[106,107] In acute myocardial infarct patients, contractile function consistently improved if less than 30 percent of the extravascular tissue density had sustained an irreversible ischemic injury. Similarly encouraging were observations in chronic coronary artery disease patients in whom the water perfusable tissue index accurately predicted a postrevascularization improvement in contractile function. In the latter study, however, the index did not differ significantly from that in normal myocardium for those segments that improved function, implying that the ischemic injury had been relatively mild. Further studies are needed to apply the approach to more severe conditions of ischemic injury, to validate the approach in terms of delineating scar tissue and viable myocardium, and to define to what extent the approach will be able to distinguish between normal and ischemically compromised myocardium. It also will be important to reconcile findings by this approach with biopsy and histologic studies that indicated a considerable variability in the degree of scar tissue formation relative to the presence or absence of wall motion abnormalities or relative to a postinterventional recovery of wall motion.[108–110]

Clinical Role of PET for Assessing Myocardial Viability

While conventional approaches such as late thallium redistribution scintigraphy or ^{201}Tl reinjection perform diagnostically rather accurately in patients with mild or moderate depression of left ventricular function (Chap. 134), experience in our laboratory has found these approaches to be of limited accuracy in patients with severely depressed left ventricular function and congestive heart failure symptoms. At the same time, these patients frequently pose a considerable diagnostic and therapeutic dilemma. The dominant factor leading to the functional depression of left ventricular performance often remains unclear. Interventional revascularization is associated with a considerable morbidity and mortality while the therapeutic benefits remain unpredictable. Thus, these patients often face the critical choice between interventional revascularization, pharmacologic management, and if appropriate, cardiac transplantation.

These patients are, however, most likely to benefit diagnostically and therapeutically from viability studies with PET. First, blood flow–metabolism imaging has been found useful for identifying the leading cause of poor left ventricular function. Positron emission tomography is 85 percent accurate in distinguishing between idiopathic dilated cardiomyopathy and end-stage coronary artery disease.[111] Blood flow and glucose utilization are homogeneous in idiopathic dilated cardiomyopathies, whereas end-stage coronary artery disease is associated with large, discrete reductions in blood flow corresponding to vascular territories. Moreover, the metabolism part of the approach determines whether these flow defects are mostly due to scar tissue formation or are associated with stunning or hibernation. Obviously, if such regions of hibernation or stunning occupy a significant portion of the left ventricular myocardium, revascularization would be expected to result in an improvement in global left ventricular function and in relief or amelioration of congestive heart failure symptoms. Such patients therefore might be assigned to coronary artery bypass grafting or coronary angioplasty,[112] whereas patients with idiopathic dilated cardiomyopathy or end-stage coronary artery disease but only scar tissue are more likely candidates for pharmacologic management or cardiac transplantation. The indication or even need for revascularization procedures is supported further by the observed high first-year mortality in those patients with blood flow–metabolism mismatches or evidence of viable myocardium who did not undergo revascularization (see above).

Less certain at present is the role of PET in postinfarction patients. Initial experience suggests that patients with blood flow–metabolism mismatches might benefit from surgical revascularization or angioplasty.

SUMMARY AND CONCLUSIONS

Positron emission tomography offers the opportunity for probing and quantifying a wide range of functional processes in the human heart. While of considerable interest in the research environment, the utility and potential value of these probes in the diagnosis and characterization of human cardiovascular disease remains largely unexplored. Clinical investigations have demonstrated an impressive accuracy with which PET detects coronary artery disease, provides estimates of its severity, and permits characterization of its metabolic and functional consequences. Positron emission tomography offers numerous possibilities to explore other cardiac disorders, to contribute to a better understanding of their underlying pathophysiology, and to improve their characterization in the clinical environment and to monitor responses to therapy.

ACKNOWLEDGMENTS

The author acknowledges Eileen Rosenfeld's skillful secretarial assistance in preparing this manuscript and Wendy Wilson for preparing the illustrations.

REFERENCES

1. Phelps M, Mazziotta J, Schelbert H: *Positron Emission Tomography and Autoradiography*. New York, Raven, 1986.
2. Marcus M, Schelbert H, Skorton D, Wolf GL: *Cardiac Imaging*. Philadelphia; Saunders, 1991.
3. Reivich A: *Positron Emission Tomography*. New York, Alan R Liss, 1985.
4. Gould K: *Coronary Artery Stenosis*. New York, Elsevier, 1990.
5. Gould KL: Identifying and measuring severity of coronary artery stenosis. Quantitative coronary arteriography and positron emission tomography. *Circulation* 1988; 78:237–245.
6. Schelbert HR, Phelps ME, Hoffman EJ, Huang SC, Selin CE, Kuhl DE: Regional myocardial perfusion assessed with N-13 labeled ammonia and positron emission computerized axial tomography. *Am J Cardiol* 1979; 43:209–218.
7. Schelbert HR, Wisenberg G, Phelps ME, Gould KL, Henze E, Hoffman EJ, et al: Noninvasive assessment of coronary stenoses by myocardial imaging during pharmacologic coronary vasodilation. VI. Detection of coronary artery disease in man with intravenous N-13 ammonia and positron computed tomography. *Am J Cardiol* 1982; 49:1197–1207.
8. Shelton ME, Green MA, Mathias CJ, Welch MJ, Bergmann SR: Kinetics of copper-PTSM in isolated hearts: A novel tracer for measuring blood flow with positron emission tomography. *J Nucl Med* 1989; 30:1843–1847.
9. Shelton ME, Green MA, Mathias CJ, Welch MJ, Bergmann SR: Assessment of regional myocardial and renal blood flow with copper-PTSM and positron emission tomography. *Circulation* 1990; 82:990–997.
10. Bergmann SR, Fox KAA, Rand AL, McElvany KD, Welch MJ, Markham J, et al: Quantification of regional myocardial blood flow in vivo with H215O. *Circulation* 1984; 70:724–733.
11. Schelbert HR, Phelps ME, Huang SC, MacDonald NS, Hansen H, Selin C, et al: N-13 ammonia as an indicator of myocardial blood flow. *Circulation* 1981; 63:1259–1272.
12. Goldstein RA, Mullani NA, Marani SK, Fisher DJ, Gould KL, O'Brien HA Jr: Perfusion imaging with rubidium-82: II. Effects of pharmacologic interventions on flow and extraction. *J Nucl Med* 1983; 24:907–915.
13. Bergmann SR, Herrero P, Markham J. Weinheimer CJ, Walsh MN: Noninvasive quantitation of myocardial blood flow in human subjects with oxygen-15-labeled water and positron emission tomography. *J Am Coll Cardiol* 1989; 14:639–652.
14. Araujo L, Lammertsma A, Rhodes C, McFalls E, Iida H, Rechavia E, et al: Noninvasive quantification of regional myocardial blood flow in coronary artery disease with oxygen-15-labeled carbon dioxide inhalation and positron emission tomography. *Circulation* 1991; 83:875–885.
15. Hutchins G, Schwaiger M, Rosenspire K, Krivokapich J, Schelbert H, Kuhl D: Noninvasive quantification of regional blood flow in the human heart using N-13 ammonia and dynamic positron emission tomographic imaging. *J Am Coll Cardiol* 1990; 15:1032–1042.
16. Chan S, Brunken R, Phelps M, Schelbert H: Maximal myocardial blood flow during adenosine infusion is comparable to that of intravenous dipyridamole (abstr). *J Nucl Med* 1991; 32:969.
17. Krivokapich J, Smith GT, Huang SC, Hoffman EJ, Ratib O, Phelps ME, et al: 13N ammonia myocardial imaging at rest and with exercise in normal volunteers. Quantification of absolute myocardial perfusion with dynamic positron emission tomography. *Circulation* 1989; 80:1328–1337.
18. Sokoloff L, Reivich M, Kennedy C, Des Rosiers MH, Patlak CS, Pettigrew KD, et al: The [14C]-deoxyglucose method for the measurement of local cerebral glucose utilization: Theory, procedure and normal values in the conscious and anesthetized albino rat. *J Neurochem* 1977; 28:897–916.
19. Phelps ME, Hoffman EJ, Selin CE, Huang SC, Robinson G, MacDonald N, et al: Investigation of [18F] 2-fluoro-2-deoxyglucose for the measure of myocardial glucose metabolism. *J Nucl Med* 1978; 19:1311–1319.
20. Ratib O, Phelps ME, Huang SC, Henze E, Selin CE, Schelbert HR: Positron tomography with deoxyglucose for estimating local myocardial glucose metabolism. *J Nucl Med* 1982; 23:577–586.
21. Gambhir SS, Schwaiger M, Huang SC, Krivokapich J, Schelbert HR, Nienaber CA, et al: Simple noninvasive quantification method for measuring myocardial glucose utilization in humans employing positron emission tomography and fluorine-18 deoxyglucose. *J Nucl Med* 1989; 30:359–366.
22. Choi Y, Hawkins R, Huang S, Gambhir S, Brunken R, Phelps M, et al: Parametric images of myocardial metabolic rate of glucose generated from dynamic cardiac PET and 2-[^{18}F]fluoro-2-deoxy-*d*-glucose studies. *J Nucl Med* 1991; 32:733–738.
23. Choi Y, Hawkins R, Brunken R, Huang S, Kuhle W, Chen K, et al: Evaluation of regional heterogeneity of myocardial glucose metabolism in normal humans using dynamic FDG-PET. *J Nucl Med* 1991; 32:938.
24. Hicks R, Herman W, Kalff V, Molina E, Wolfe E, Hutchins G, et al: Quantitative evaluation of regional substrate metabolism in the human heart by positron emission tomography. *J Am Coll Cardiol.* 1991; 18:101–111.
25. Knuuti J, Nuutila P, Ruotsalainen U, Saraste M, Härkönen R, Ahonen A, et al: Euglycemic hyperinsulinemic clamp and oral glucose load in stimulating myocardial glucose utilization during positron emission tomography (abstr). *J Nucl Med* 1991; 32:988.
26. vom Dahl J, Hicks R, Hermann W, Lee K, Wolfe E, Hutchins G, et al: Insulin substitution significantly improves the quality of myocardial tissue viability studies with FDG-PET in patients with diabetes mellitus (abstr). *J Nucl Med* 1991; 32:988.
27. Hoffman EJ, Phelps ME, Weiss ES, Welch MJ, Coleman RE, Sobel BE, et al: Transaxial tomographic imaging of canine myocardium with 11C-palmitic acid. *J Nucl Med* 1977; 18:57–61.
28. Klein MS, Goldstein RA, Welch MJ, Sobel BE: External assessment of myocardial metabolism with 11C-palmitate in rabbit hearts. *Am J Physiol* 1979; 237:H51–H58.
29. Weiss ES, Hoffman EJ, Phelps ME, Welch MJ, Henry PD, Ter-Pogossian MM, et al: External detection and visualization of myocardial ischemia with 11C-substrates in vitro and in vivo. *Circ Res* 1976; 39:24–32.
30. Schön HR, Schelbert HR, Najafi A, Robinson G, Huang SC, Barrio J, et al: C-11 labeled palmitic acid for the noninvasive evaluation of regional myocardial fatty acid metabolism with positron computed tomography. I. Kinetics of C-11 palmitic acid in normal myocardium. *Am Heart J* 1982; 103:532–547.
31. Schelbert HR, Henze E, Schön HR, Najafi A, Hansen H, Huang SC, et al: C-11 palmitic acid for the noninvasive evaluation of regional myocardial fatty acid metabolism with positron computed tomography. IV. In vivo demonstration of impaired fatty acid oxidation in acute myocardial ischemia. *Am Heart J* 1983; 106:736–750.
32. Wyns W, Schwaiger M, Huang SC, Buxton DB, Hansen H, Selin C, et al: Effects of inhibition of fatty acid oxidation on myocardial kinetics of C-11 labeled palmitate. *Circ Res* 1991; 65:1787–1797.
33. Rosamond TL, Abendschein DR, Sobel BE, Bergmann SR, Fox KAA: Metabolic fate of radiolabeled palmitate in ischemic canine myocardium: Implications for positron emission tomography. *J Nucl Med* 1987; 28:1322–1329.
34. Schön HR, Schelbert HR, Najafi A, Hansen H, Robinson GR, Huang SC, et al: C-11 labeled palmitic acid for the noninvasive evaluation of regional myocardial fatty acid metabolism with positron computed tomography. II. Kinetics of C-11 palmitic acid in acutely ischemic myocardium. *Am Heart J* 1982; 103:548–561.

35. Fox KAA, Abendschein DR, Ambos HD, Sobel BE, Bergmann SR: Efflux of metabolized and nonmetabolized fatty acid from canine myocardium. Implications for quantifying myocardial metabolism tomographically. *Circ Res* 1985; 57:232–243.
36. Schelbert HR, Henze E, Schön HR, Keen R, Hansen HW, Selin C, et al: C-11 palmitate for the noninvasive evaluation of regional myocardial fatty acid metabolism with positron computed tomography. III. In vivo demonstration of the effects of substrate availability on myocardial metabolism. *Am Heart J* 1983; 105:492–504.
37. Merlet P, Mazoyer B, Dubois-Rande J, Raynaud L, Valette H, Crouzel C, et al: Assessment of coronary reserve in man using intravenous bolus 15O-water and positron emission tomography (PET): A comparison with intra coronary Doppler study (abstr). *J Nucl Med* 1991; 32:998.
38. Bol A, Iida H, Essamri B, Vanbutsele R, Labar D, Grandin C, et al: Assessment of myocardial oxidative reserve with PET: Comparison of C-11 acetate kinetics with quantitation of metabolic rate of oxygen (MRO2) using 0-15 02. *J Nucl Med* 1991; 32:988–989.
39. Brown M, Marshall DR, Burton BS, Sobel BE, Bergmann SR: Delineation of myocardial oxygen utilization with carbon-11-labeled acetate. *Circulation* 1987; 76:687–696.
40. Brown MA, Myears DW, Bergmann SR: Noninvasive assessment of canine myocardial oxidative metabolism with 11C-acetate and positron emission tomography. *J Am Coll Cardiol* 1988; 12:1054–1063.
41. Buxton DB, Schwaiger M, Nguyen A, Phelps ME, Schelbert HR: Radiolabeled acetate as a tracer of myocardial tricarboxylic acid cycle flux. *Circ Res* 1988; 63:628–634.
42. Buxton DB, Nienaber CA, Luxen A, Ratib O, Hansen H, Phelps ME, et al: Noninvasive quantitation of regional myocardial oxygen consumption in vivo with [1-11C] acetate and dynamic positron emission tomography. *Circulation* 1989; 79:134–142.
43. Armbrecht JJ, Buxton DB, Schelbert HR: Validation of [1-11C] acetate as a tracer for noninvasive assessment of oxidative metabolism with positron emission tomography in normal, ischemic, post-ischemic and hyperemic canine myocardium. *Circulation* 1991; 81:1594–1605.
44. Armbrecht JJ, Buxton DB, Brunken RC, Phelps ME, Schelbert HR: Regional myocardial oxygen consumption determined noninvasively in humans with [1-11C] acetate and dynamic positron tomography. *Circulation* 1989; 80:863–872.
45. Henes CG, Sergmann SR, Walsh MN, Sobel BE, Geltman EM: Assessment of myocardial oxidative metabolic reserve with positron emission tomography and carbon-11 acetate. *J Nucl Med* 1989; 30:1489–1499.
46. Schwaiger M, Kalff V, Rosenspire K, Haka M, Molina E, Hutchins G, et al: Noninvasive evaluation of sympathetic nervous system in human heart by positron emission tomography. *Circulation* 1990; 82:457–464.
47. Delforge J, Janier M, Syrota A, Crouzel C, Vallois JM, Cayla J, Lançon J, et al: Noninvasive quantification of muscarinic receptors in vivo with positron emission tomography in the dog heart. *Circulation* 1990; 82:1494–1504.
48. Delforge J, Syrota A, Lançon J, Nakajima K, Loc'h C, Janier M, et al: Cardiac beta-adrenergic receptor density measured in vivo using PET, CGP 12177, and a new graphical method. *J Nucl Med* 1991; 32:739–748.
49. Zimmerman R, Tillmanns H, Knapp WH, Helus F, Georgi P, Rauch B, et al: Regional myocardial nitrogen-13 glutamate uptake in patients with coronary artery disease: Inverse poststress relation to thallium-201 uptake in ischemia. *J Am Coll Cardiol* 1988; 11:549–556.
50. Krivokapich J, Barrio J, Huang S, Schelbert H: Dynamic positron tomographic imaging with nitrogen-13 glutamate in patients with coronary artery disease: Comparison with nitrogen-13 ammonia and fluorine-18 fluorodeoxyglucose imaging. *J Am Coll Cardiol* 1990; 16:1158–1167.
51. Hashimoto T, Buxton DB, Ackermann RF, Huang SC, Phelps ME, Schelbert HR: Regional rates of protein synthesis in rat myocardium by quantitative autoradiography and C-14 leucine. *Circulation* 1989; 80:II-637.
52. Shelton M, Dence C, Hwang D, Herrero P, Welch M, Bergmann S: In vivo delineation of myocardial hypoxia during coronary occlusion using fluorine-18 fluoromisonidazole and positron emission tomography: A potential approach for identification of jeopardized myocardium. *J Am Coll Cardiol* 1990; 16:477–485.
53. Revenaugh J, Caldwell J, Martin G, Rasey J, Krohn K: A Comparison of F-18 fluorodeoxyglucose (FDG) and H-3-fluoromisonidazole (FISMO) uptake during low-flow ischemia (abstr) *J Nucl Med* 1991; 32:1028.
54. Revenaugh J, Caldwell J, Martin G, Grierson J, Krohn K: Positron emission tomography (PET) imaging of myocardial hypoxia with 18F-fluoromisonidazole (FMISO) in post myocardial infarction patients (abstr). *Circulation* 1991; 84:II-424.
55. Tamaki N, Yonekura Y, Senda M, Yamashita K, Koide H, Saji H, et al: Value and limitation of stress thallium-201 single photon emission computed tomography: Comparison with nitrogen-13 ammonia positron tomography. *J Nucl Med* 1988; 29:1181–1188.
56. Demer LL, Gould KL, Goldstein RA, Kirkeeide RL, Mullani NA, Smalling RW, et al: Assessment of coronary artery disease severity by positron emission tomography. Comparison with quantitative arteriography in 193 patients. *Circulation* 1989; 79:825–835.
57. Go R, Marwick T, MacIntyre W, Saha G, Neumann D, Underwood D, et al: A prospective comparison of rubidium-82 PET and thallium-201 SPECT myocardial perfusion imaging utilizing a single dipyridamole stress in the diagnosis of coronary artery disease. *J Nucl Med* 1990; 31:1899–1905.
58. Stewart R, Schwaiger M, Molina E, Popma J, Gacioch G, Kalus M, et al: Comparison of rubidium-82 positron emission tomography and thallium-201 SPECT imaging for detection of coronary artery disease. *Am J Cardiol* 1991; 67:1303–1310.
59. Goldstein R, Kirkeeide R, Demer L, Merhige M, Nishikawa A, Smalling R: Relation between geometric dimensions of coronary artery stenoses and myocardial perfusion reserve in man. *J Clin Invest* 1987; 79:1473–1478.
60. Brown BG, Josephson MA, Peterson RB, Pierce CD, Wong M, Hecht HS, et al: Intravenous dipyridamole combined with isometric handgrip for near maximal acute increase in coronary flow in patients with coronary artery disease. *Am J Cardiol* 1981; 48:1077–1085.
61. Walsh MN, Geltman EM, Brown MA, Henes CG, Weinheimer CJ, Sobel BE, et al: Noninvasive estimation of regional myocardial oxygen consumption by positron emission tomography with carbon-11 acetate in patients with myocardial infarction. *J Nucl Med* 1989; 30:1798–1808.
62. Krivokapich J, Huang S, Schelbert H: Response of absolute myocardial blood flow to dobutamine assessed with nitrogen-13 ammonia and dynamic positron emission tomography. *J Am Coll Cardiol* 1991; 17:379A.
63. Walsh MN, Geltman EM, Steele RL, Kenzora JL, Ludbrook PA, Sobel BE, et al: Augmented myocardial perfusion reserve after coronary angioplasty quantified by positron emission tomography with H215O. *J Am Coll Cardiol* 1990; 15:119–127.
64. McFalls EO, Araujo LI, Lammertsma A, Pupita G, Jones T: The assessment of coronary flow and flow reserve in patients with collateral-dependent myocardium using positron emission tomography (PET) (abstr). *Circulation* 1989; 80:II-639.
65. Senneff M, Bergmann S, Henes C, Sobel B, Geltman E: Impaired myocardial oxidative metabolism assessed with positron emission tomography (PET) in patients with chest pain and normal coronary arteries (abstr). *J Nucl Med* 1990; 31:713.
66. Geltman E, Henes C, Senneff M, Sobel B, Bergmann S: Increased myocardial perfusion at rest and diminished perfusion reserve in patients with angina and angiographically normal coronary arteries. *J Am Coll Cardiol* 1990; 16:586–595.
67. Camici P, Chiriatti G, Oorenzoni R, Bellina R, Gistri R, Italiani G, et al: Coronary vasodilation is impaired in both hypertrophied and nonhypertrophied myocardium of patients with hypertrophic cardiomyopathy: A study with nitrogen-13 ammonia and positron emission tomography. *J Am Coll Cardiol* 1991; 17:879–886.
68. Senneff M, Geltman E, Bergmann S, Hartman J: Noninvasive delineation of the effects of moderate aging on myocardial perfusion. *J Nucl Med* 1991; 32:2037–2042.
69. Czernin J, Brunken R, Porenta G, Buxton D, Tillisch J, Phelps M, et al: Rate pressure product determines blood flow and oxygen consumption in remote myocardium of patients with acute infarction (abstr). *J Nucl Med* 1991; 32:989.
70. Brunken R, Tillisch J, Schwaiger M, Child JS, Marshall R, Man-

delkern M, et al: Regional perfusion, glucose metabolism and wall motion in chronic electrocardiographic Q-wave infarctions. Evidence for persistence of viable tissue in some infarct regions by positron emission tomography. *Circulation* 1986; 73:951–963.

71. Marshall RC, Tillisch JH, Phelps ME, Huang SC, Carson RC, Henze E, et al: Identification and differentiation of resting myocardial ischemia and infarction in man with positron computer tomography 18F-labeled fluorodeoxyglucose and N-13 ammonia. *Circulation* 1983; 67:766–778.
72. Tillisch J, Brunken R, Marshall R, Schwaiger M, Mandelkern M, Phelps M, et al: Reversibility of cardiac wall motion abnormalities predicted by positron tomography. *N Engl J Med* 1986; 314:884–888.
73. Porenta G, Kuhle W, Czernin J, Ratib O, Brunken R, Phelps M, et al: Semiquantitative assessment of myocardial viability and flow from cardiac PET polar maps (abstr). *J Nucl Med* 1991; 32:927.
74. Tamaki N, Yonekura Y, Yamashita K, Saji H, Magata Y, Senda M, et al: Positron emission tomography using fluorine-18 deoxyglucose in evaluation of coronary artery bypass grafting. *Am J Cardiol* 1989; 64:860–865.
75. Tamaki N, Ohtani H, Yamashita K, Magata Y, Yonekura Y, Nohara R, et al: Metabolic activity in the areas of new fill-in after thallium-201 reinjection: Comparison with positron emission tomography using fluorine-18-deoxyglucose. *J Nucl Med* 1991; 32:673–678.
76. Nienaber C, Brunken R, Sherman C, Yeatman L, Gambhir S, Krivokapich J, et al: Metabolic and functional recovery of ischemic human myocardium after coronary angioplasty. *J Am Coll Cardiol* 1991; 18:966–978.
77. Braunwald E, Kloner RA: The stunned myocardium: Prolonged, postischemic ventricular dysfunction. *Circulation* 1982; 66:1146–1149.
78. Rahimtoola SH: A perspective on the three large multicenter randomized clinical trials of coronary bypass surgery for chronic stable angina. *Circulation* 1985; 72:V-123–V-135.
79. Bonow R, Dilsizian V, Cuocolo A, Bacharach S: Identification of viable myocardium in patients with chronic coronary artery disease and left ventricular dysfunction: Comparison of thallium scintigraphy with reinjection and PET imaging with F-18-fluorodeoxyglucose. *Circulation* 1991; 83:26–37.
80. Camici P, Araujo LI, Spinks T, Lammertsma AA, Kaski JC, Shea MJ, et al: Increased uptake of 18F-fluorodeoxyglucose in postischemic myocardium of patients with exercise-induced angina. *Circulation* 1986; 74:81–88.
81. Schwaiger M, Brunken R, Grover-McKay M, Krivokapich J, Child J, Tillisch JH, et al: Regional myocardial metabolism in patients with acute myocardial infarction assessed by positron emission tomography. *J Am Coll Cardiol* 1986; 8:800–808.
82. Schwaiger M, Brunken R, Krivokapich J, Child J, Tillisch J, Phelps ME, et al: Beneficial effect of residual antegrade flow on tissue viability as assessed by positron emission tomography in patients with myocardial infarction. *Eur Heart J* 1987; 8:981–988.
83. Pierard L, De Landsheere C, Berthe C, Rigo P, Kulbertus H: Identification of viable myocardium by echocardiography during dobutamine infusion in patients with myocardial infarction after thrombolytic therapy: Comparison with positron emission tomography. *J Am Coll Cardiol* 1990; 15:1021–1031.
84. Schwaiger M, Schelbert HR, Ellison D, Hansen H, Yeatman L, Vinten-Johansen J, et al: Sustained regional abnormalities in cardiac metabolism after transient ischemia in the chronic dog model. *J Am Coll Cardiol* 1985; 6:336–347.
85. Wisneski JA, Gertz EW, Neese RA, Gruenke LD, Craig JC: Dual carbon-labeled isotope experiments using D-[6-14C] glucose and L-[1,2,3-13C3] lactate: A new approach for investigating human myocardial metabolism during ischemia. *J Am Coll Cardiol* 1985; 5:1138–1146.
86. Vaghaiwalla Mody F, Buxton DB, Krivokapich J, Hansen HA, Selin CE, Schelbert HR: Attenuated response of glucose metabolism in reperfused canine myocardium to changes in substrate levels (abstr). *J Am Coll Cardiol* 1990; 15:80A.
87. Berry J, Baker J, Pieper K, Hanson M, Hoffman J, Coleman R: The effect of metabolic milieu on cardiac PET imaging using fluorine-18-deoxyglucose and nitrogen-13-ammonia in normal volunteers (abstr). *J Nucl Med* 1991; 32:1518–1525.
88. Choi Y, Brunken R, Hawkins R, Huang S-C, Buxton D, Hoh C, et al: Determinants of myocardial glucose utilization assessed with dynamic FDG PET. *Circulation* 1991; 84:II-425.
89. Tamaki N, Yonekura Y, Kawamoto M, Magata Y, Sasayama S, Takahashi N, et al: Simple quantification of regional myocardial uptake of fluorine-18-deoxyglucose in the fasting condition. *J Nucl Med* 1991; 32:152–157.
90. Maddahi J, DiCarli M, Davidson M, Khanna S, Rokhsar S, Tillisch J, et al: Prognostic significance of PET assessment of myocardial viability in patients with left ventricular dysfunction (Abstr). *J Am Coll Cardiol* 1992; 19:142A.
91. Eitzman D, Al-Aouar Z, Kanter L, Hepner A, vom Dahl J, Kirsch M, et al: Clinical outcome in patients with advanced coronary artery disease following PET viability studies (abstr). *J Nucl Med* 1991; 32:1011.
92. Brunken R, Schwaiger M, Grover-McKay M, Phelps ME, Tillisch J, Schelbert HIR: Positron emission tomography detects tissue metabolic activity in myocardial segments with persistent thallium perfusion defects. *J Am Coll Cardiol* 1987; 10:557–567.
93. Brunken RC, Kottou S, Nienaber CA, Schwaiger M, Ratib OM, Phelps ME, et al: PET detection of viable tissue in myocardial segments with persistent defects at Tl-201 SPECT. *Radiology* 1989; 172:65–73.
94. Gibson RS, Watson DD, Taylor GJ, Crosby IK, Wellons HL, Holt ND, et al: Prospective assessment of regional myocardial perfusion before and after coronary revascularization surgery by quantitative thallium-201 scintigraphy. *J Am Coll Cardiol* 1983; 1:804–815.
95. Liu P, Kiess MC, Okada RD, Block PC, Strauss HW, Pohost GM, et al: The persistent defect on exercise thallium imaging and its fate after myocardial revascularization: Does it represent scar or ischemia? *Am Heart J* 1985; 110:996–1001.
96. Kiat H, Berman DS, Maddahi J, Yang LD, Van Train K, Rozanski A, et al: Late reversibility of tomographic myocardial thallium-201 defects: An accurate marker of myocardial viability. *J Am Coll Cardiol* 1988; 12:1456–1463.
97. Dilsizian V, Rocco T, Freedman N, Leon M, Bonow R: Enhanced detection of ischemic but viable myocardium by the reinjection of thallium after stress-redistribution imaging. *N Engl J Med* 1990; 323:141–146.
98. Ohtani H, Tamaki N, Yonekura Y, Mohiuddin I, Hirata K, Ban T, et al: Value of thallium-201 reinjection after delayed SPECT imaging for predicting reversible ischemia after coronary artery bypass grafting. *Am J Cardiol* 1990; 66:394–399.
99. Brunken RC, Vaghaiwalla Mody F, Hawkins RA, Phelps ME, Schelbert HR: Positron tomography detects glucose metabolism in segments with 24 hour tomographic thallium defects (abstr). *Circulation* 1988; 78:II-91.
100. Czernin J, Porenta G, Brunken R, Chan S, Kuhle W, Phelps M, et al: Oxidative and glycolytic metabolic tissue characterization in patients with acute infarction using dynamic PET (abstr). *J Nucl Med* 1990; 31:774.
101. Czernin J, Porenta G, Brunken R, Bennet R, Tillisch J, Phelps M, et al: Metabolic and functional fate of viable myocardium by PET early after acute infarction (abstr). *Am Coll Cardiol* 1991; 17:120A.
102. Gropler RJ, Siegel BA, Perez JE, Bergmann SR, Kopitsky RG, Sobel BE, et al: Recovery of contractile function in viable but dysfunctional myocardium is dependent upon maintenance of oxidative metabolism. *J Am Coll Cardiol* 1990; 15:203A.
103. Gould L, Yoshida K, Hess M, Haynie M, Mullani N, Smalling R: Myocardial metabolism of fluorodeoxyglucose compared to cell membrane integrity for the potassium analogue rubidium-82 for assessing infarct size in many by PET. *J Nucl Med* 1991; 32:1–9.
104. Goldstein RA: Kinetics of rubidium-82 after coronary occlusion and reperfusion. Assessment of patency and viability in open-chested dogs. *J Clin Invest* 1985; 75:1131–1137.
105. Iida H, Rhodes C, de Silva R, Yamamoto Y, Araujo L, Maseri A, et al: Myocardial tissue fraction—correction for partial volume effects and measure of tissue viability. *J Nucl Med* 1991; 32:2169–2175.
106. Yamamoto Y, De Silva R, Rhodes C, Araujo LI, Iida H, Rechavia E et al: A new strategy for the assessment of viable myocardium and regional myocardial blood flow using ^{15}O-Water and Dynamic Positron Emission Tomography. *Circulation* 1992;86:167–178.

107. DeSilva R, Yamamoto Y, Rhodes C, Iida H, Nihoyannopoulas P, Davies G et al: Detection of hibernating myocardium using H_2 ^{15}O and Positron Emission Tomography (PET) (abstr). *J Am Coll Cardiol* 1992;19:141A.
108. Flameng W, Suy R, Schwarz F, Borgers M, Piessens J, Thone F, et al: Ultrastructural correlates of left ventricular contraction abnormalities in patients with chronic ischemic heart disease: Determinants of reversible segmental asynergy post-revascularization surgery. *Am Heart J* 1981; 102:846–857.
109. Stinson E, Billingham M: Correlative study of regional left ventricular histology and contractile function. *Am J Cardiol.* 1977; 39:378–383.
110. Cabin HS, Soni Clubbs K, Vita N, Zaret BL: Regional dysfunction by equilibrium radionuclide angiography: A clinicopathologic study evaluating the relation of degree of dysfunction to the presence and extent of myocardial infarction. *J Am Coll Cardiol* 1987; 10:743–747.
111. Vaghaiwalla Mody F, Brunken R, Warner-Stevenson L, Nienaber C, Phelps M, Schelbert H: Differentiating cardiomyopathy of coronary artery disease from non-ischemic dilated cardiomyopathy utilizing positron tomography. *J Am Coll Cardiol* 1991; 17:373–383.
112. Louie H, Laks H, Milgalter E, Drinkwater D, Hamilton M, Brunken R, et al: Ischemic cardiomyopathy: Criteria for coronary revascularization and cardiac transplantation. *Circulation* 1991; 84:III-290–III-295.

PART XXI

Diagnostic Techniques of Cardiac Catheterization and Vascular Angiography

Chapter 138

Techniques of Cardiac Catheterization Including Coronary Arteriography

Robert H. Franch, M.D. ■ *Spencer B. King III, M.D.* ■
John S. Douglas, Jr., M.D.

In 1929, Werner Forssman, a resident surgeon at Eberswalde, catheterized his right atrium from a left antecubital vein cutdown, utilizing self-fluoroscopy with a mirror. The position of the catheter tip was verified by a roentgenogram.[1-3] The extensive use of the catheter by Cournand in the early 1940s in the study of human cardiovascular physiology led his group and those of Dexter, McMichael, and Bing to explore the use of this technique for the study of heart disease.[4] At Emory University in 1945 Brannon, Weens, and Warren described the hemodynamics of atrial septal defect in four patients.[5] From these beginnings steady advances in methods occurred.[6-12] Catheterization then spread from the laboratory to the bedside, to yield physiological data and to guide treatment. Now, palliative or even corrective interventions involving valves, arteries, and septal defects may accompany the catheterization study.[13,14]

PREPARATIONS FOR CARDIAC CATHETERIZATION

A relaxed meeting with the patient and the patient's family serves to lessen apprehension, correct any misunderstanding, and establish rapport. Since catheterization is frequently the first major step on the road to cardiac surgery, a tolerable experience fosters an optimistic attitude in the patient and family toward future events. The physician who is to perform the catheterization should obtain the history, examine the patient, and review the current chest x-ray, electrocardiogram (ECG), echocardiogram, and past catheterization and surgical records and angiocardiograms. It is mandatory to have the old operative note in hand if the patient has had complex palliation or repair. A clinical diagnosis is made, and a catheterization protocol is designed to answer pertinent specific questions. The catheterization protocol may be modified as data become available during the procedure.

The patient's education booklet about the procedure is usually read by the patient prior to securing informed consent. Anticoagulants are stopped, and the prothrombin time is brought to less than 16 s before a percutaneous arterial catheterization. Serum levels of creatinine, urea nitrogen, and potassium are noted. A patient with chronic renal disease is well hydrated; prophylaxis for past allergy to contrast media is given.[15] Breakfast is withheld for a morning procedure; for an afternoon procedure, coffee or juice is permitted and lunch is withheld. In our experience prophylactic antibiotics are not necessary. In children, a combination of 6.25 mg of promethazine (Phenergan), 6.25 mg of chlorpromazine (Thorazine), and 25 mg of meperidine hydrochloride (Demerol) per milliliter of mixture provides excellent sedation.[16] The intramuscular dose for a child is 0.5 to 2.0 mL, depending on the age and weight, and is given 1 h before the procedure. The mixture is not given intravenously, nor is it given again after the initial loading dose. If additional sedation is required, small doses of intravenous diazepam may be used. In selected adults, diazepam (Valium) or midazolam (Versed) may be given intravenously. Subcutaneous 0.5 to 2 percent lidocaine (Xylocaine) is given, depending on the age of the patient. Occasionally, particularly in adults, vagal slowing of the pulse, nausea, and perspiration are noted. Intravenous atropine is antidotal. Full systemic heparinization is not used routinely during a diagnostic study.

It is desirable that the laboratory be fully involved daily in diagnostic work. General efficiency is increased, costly equipment and space are utilized, and most important, all personnel become confident and knowledgeable with experience. Certainly the most important ingredient in the laboratory is the thoroughly experienced technical-professional team. The procedure must move briskly. The primary objective is to make an accurate diagnosis at one sitting, with the least possible risk and discomfort to the patient. After the procedure, a preliminary labeled single-page diagram in the patient's chart can accurately present the essence of complex catheterization findings.[17]

Outpatient left-sided heart and coronary artery studies require careful selection of patients and an experienced support team.[18–20] The American College of Cardiology and the American Heart Association have published the criteria in Table 138-1 with regard to patients who require inpatient cardiac catheterization.[21]

Most of the criteria in Table 138-1 would lead to hospitalization of the patient. Others have stated that if a patient is stable enough to be at home before cardiac catheterization, an outpatient catheterization can be considered and a decision following the procedure can be made based on the patient's tolerance of the procedure and the catheterization findings. This approach is most relevant when a catheterization laboratory is in or adjacent to a hospital. The cost savings per case with outpatient procedures remains significant. Although some physicians have performed cardiac catheterization of stable, low-risk patients in freestanding facilities, the lack of support in this environment is a potential liability and it is not recommended.

TABLE 138-1

The Clinical Characteristics of Patients Who Require Supervision after Catheterization and Would Not Be Candidates for Ambulatory Cardiac Catheterization

High risk for vascular complications
Morbid obesity
Severe peripheral vascular disease
Mechanical prosthetic valve
General debility or cachexia
Low ejection fraction (≤35%)
Anticoagulation or bleeding diathesis
Uncontrolled systemic hypertension
Patient's home a significant distance from catheterization laboratory
Diabetes mellitus that is difficult to control
Chronic corticosteroid use
History of radiographic contrast material allergy
Severe chronic obstructive lung disease
Less than 21 years of age or complex congenital heart disease, regardless of age
Recent stroke (within 1 month)
Severe ischemia during stress testing
Pulmonary hypertension
Arterial desaturation

TECHNIQUES

Catheterization of the Right Side of the Heart: Percutaneous Venous

Percutaneous femoral or median cubital vein catheterization usually permits reuse of the vein. The femoral vein is entered medial to the common femoral artery pulse. To extend the range of the percutaneous technique, a thin tubular sheath is advanced over a short introducer catheter into the lumen of the vein (Fig. 138-1). This temporary conduit may then be used to introduce a variety of closed-tip catheters. Two catheters can be inserted through a single femoral vein puncture site by initially placing two guide wires through the femoral vein sheath; the maneuver is repeated to insert an additional catheter.[22] If the hepatic portion of the inferior vena cava (IVC) is absent, the azygos vein channels the catheter tip into the right superior vena cava (SVC) and thence into the right atrium (Fig. 138-2). In order to cross the tricuspid valve from the IVC, bending the catheter tip against the right atrial wall may be required. If atrial ectopy occurs, the catheter tip can be looped in a hepatic vein and then advanced into the right atrium. The tip is then rotated from the lateral right atrial wall clockwise (cw) across the anterior atrial wall and through the tricuspid valve followed by a slight counterclockwise (ccw) turn to the anterolateral position in the right ventricle and then cw to place the tip via the outflow track into the main pulmonary artery and then into the left pulmonary artery, its direct continuation. The foramen ovale is entered with the tip pointed leftward and 45° posteriorly. The SVC lies posteriorly and is entered by making a 60° ccw turn from the lateral right atrial border with a straight catheter tip. The foramen ovale is probe patent in approximately 20 to 35 percent of adults.

The internal jugular vein or the subclavian vein may also be used to insert a balloon catheter percutaneously. The latter catheter produces little ectopy since the advancing force is distributed over the surface of the balloon. The tricuspid valve is easily crossed from this approach. If a right-to-left shunt is present, the balloon should be filled with CO_2, and the side arm of the sheath flushed regularly. (See also Chap. 18.)

Rarely if a venous cutdown is necessary, the right basilic or right median cubital (but not the cephalic) vein is preferred. Care should be taken not to mistake the superficial radial, ulnar, or accessory brachial arteries for veins. From the left arm, the catheter tip may enter a persistent left SVC, exiting via the coronary sinus into the right atrium in an awkward position for entering the right ventricle. A deep inspiration often enables the

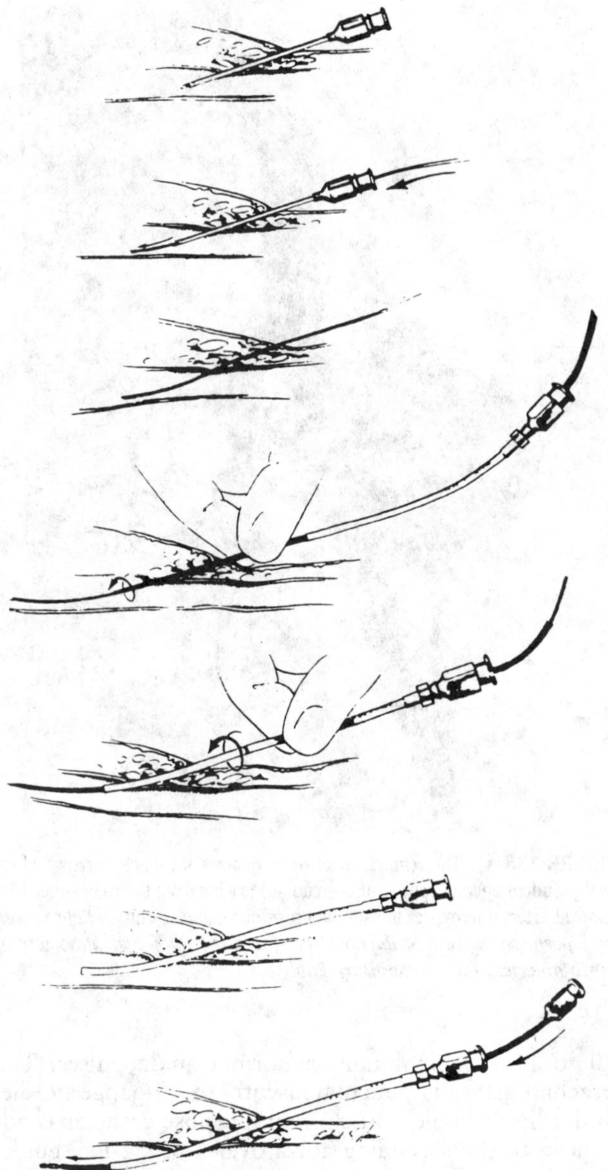

FIGURE 138-1 Percutaneous sheath catheterization of the femoral vein. Following venous puncture, a spring guide wire is introduced into the vein. The needle is withdrawn, leaving the guide in the vein. A Teflon dilator–venous sheath assembly is advanced in a rotary motion over the guide into the vein. The Teflon dilator and the guide wire are removed, leaving the flexible sheath in the vein. Various types of catheters, including closed-tip side-hole catheters, can now be inserted using the sheath as a conduit. (*Courtesy of Drs. W. H. Neches and C. E. Mullins.*)

catheter tip to pass the subclavian vein—brachiocephalic vein junction. The seating of a conventional catheter tip in the pulmonary artery wedge position may be difficult if severe pulmonary artery hypertension or extreme enlargement of the right side of the heart is present. A flow-directed balloon catheter may then be used. Clues to inadvertent coronary sinus catheterizations are (1) the acute angle that the catheter shaft makes as it enters the coronary sinus, especially in the right anterior oblique position; (2) the marked desaturation of coronary sinus blood; and (3) the posterior position of the catheter in the lateral view.

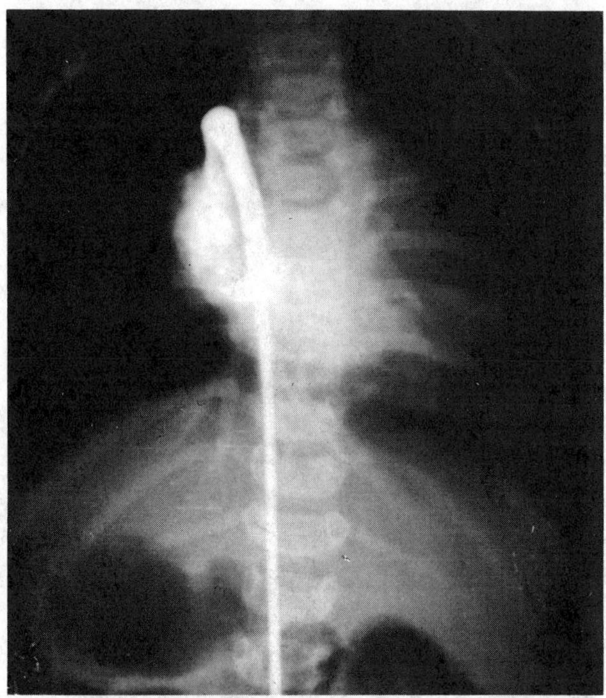

FIGURE 138-2 Selective opacification of the azygos vein. If the hepatic portion of the inferior vena cava is absent, the catheter tip enters the right atrium superiorly via the azygos vein.

In order to enter the pulmonary artery in patients with transposition of the great arteries and an intact ventricular septum, a balloon catheter is passed across the inevitably present interatrial communication to the left atrium and then superiorly looped in the left ventricular outflow tract, from which it enters the pulmonary artery readily. In postsurgical patients with pulmonary valve atresia the pulmonary artery may also be entered via a subclavian (Blalock) or aorticopulmonary (Waterston or Potts) shunt.[23] (See also Chap. 97.)

Catheterization of the Left Side of the Heart

Percutaneous Technique

In 1953, Seldinger described the use of a flexible metal leader to introduce a polyethylene tube into the artery. The Seldinger technique is used in the common femoral and less often in the axillary or brachial arteries in carrying out catheterization of the left side of the heart. The common femoral artery, 4 cm in length, begins at the inguinal ligament and ends at its bifurcation into the deep and superficial femoral arteries at the inferior cortical margin of the head of the femur (Fig. 138-3). The inguinal crease, especially in an obese patient, tends to be inferior to the ligament. In this case, a puncture at or below the crease may involve the superficial femoral artery, and lack of posterior bony support results in poor compression with the chance of bleeding and pseudoaneurysm formation[24] (Fig. 138-4). A skin puncture site chosen 3 cm below the inguinal ligament (not the crease) allows the common femoral artery to be entered at a point where it is compressible against the head of the femur. A needle containing a stylet with a Doppler crystal

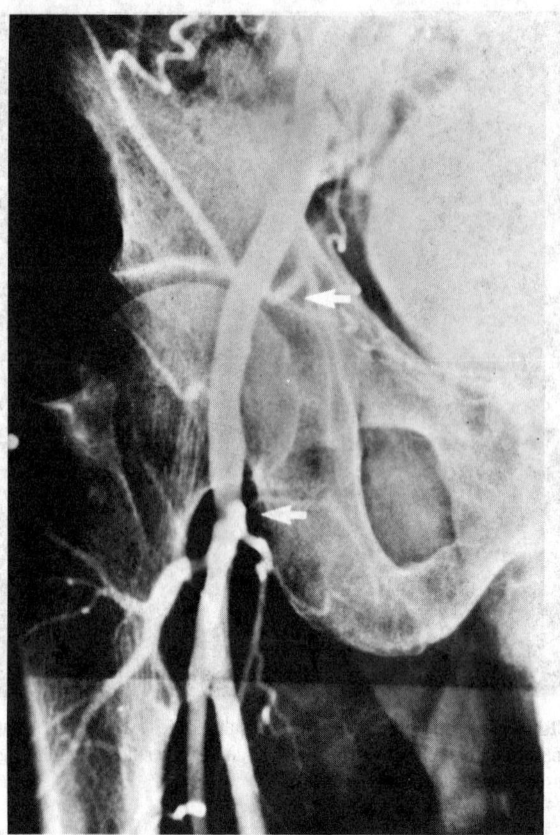

FIGURE 138-3 Right femoral arteriogram in the frontal view. The common femoral artery (CFA) extends from the inguinal ligament near the origin of the inferior epigastric and deep circumflex iliac artery (upper arrow) to its division into the deep and superficial femoral artery (lower arrow). The CFA courses over the medial femoral head, ending just beyond its inferior cortical margin. The inguinal crease should not be used as a landmark, since it bears no fixed relation to the CFA. Puncture the skin at a 40° angle 3 to 4 cm below the *inguinal ligament* to enter the CFA over the femoral head, allowing a firm compression site and avoiding the superficial femoral artery.

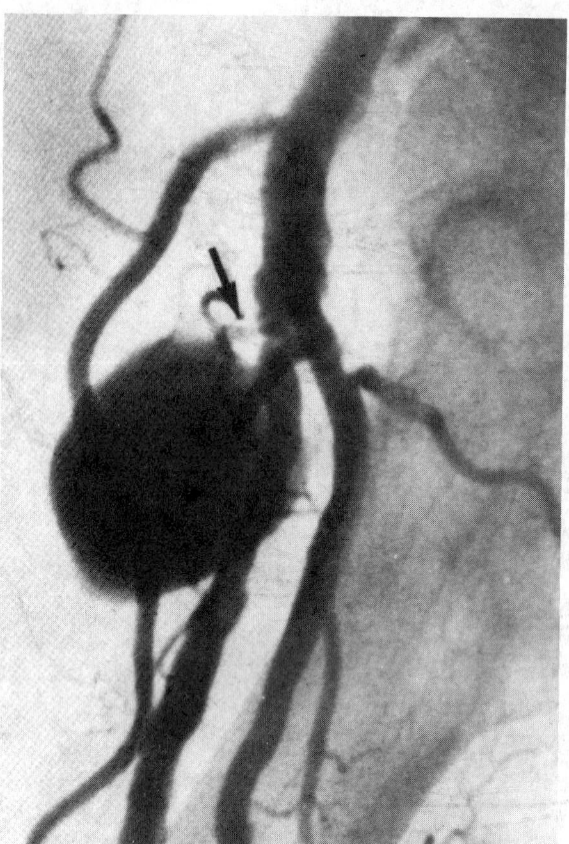

FIGURE 138-4 The femoral arteriogram shows the neck (arrow) of an oval pseudoaneurysm (pulsating hematoma) arising from the right superficial femoral artery (arrow) at the site of a previous catheter entry. (*Reproduced with permission from S. Rapoport et al and the Radiological Society of North America, Inc., Supervisory Publisher.*)

at its tip is useful in locating the poorly palpable artery or in finding a vein. External rotation of the leg and slight adduction help fixate the artery. The artery is punctured at a 45° angle transfixing the anterior and posterior wall. The guide wire is inserted only when the needle spurt is maximal. Resistance to insertion usually indicates an intramural or extravascular position of the needle or entry into a side branch artery by the guide. The catheter is inserted into the artery over the guide wire, or a sheath assembly may be used, facilitating catheter introduction in a very obese patient or if scar tissue is superficial to the artery (Fig. 138-5). The catheter sheath reduces bleeding during manipulation and reduces discomfort during catheter changes.[25] An arterial pressure may be monitored through a side port in the sheath. Guide wires with torsional control of a flexible distal tip aid passage through a tortuous iliac artery, as does a right Judkins catheter, alone or with a guide.[26,27] The guide tip is kept at the level of the diaphragm, and the catheter is advanced to this level. The catheter is aspirated and then flushed with heparinized saline solution. Occasionally, small particles of plaque material may be found in the aspirate. The femoral and foot pulses are palpated prior to withdrawal. The artery is compressed manually for 10 to 15 min, maintaining normal ankle pulses. The brachial artery is punctuated with an 18-gauge needle, and a no. 7 French 80-cm multipurpose catheter is advanced to the ascending aorta over a 0.032-in J-guide. Five thousand units of heparin is then given. A sheath is not routinely used, nor is protamine given. An arm board is applied for 6 h. Rarely, the right subclavian artery will rise aberrantly as the last root vessel of a left aortic arch, precluding easy access to the ascending aorta from the right brachial artery. Percutaneous left-sided heart catheterization via an aortofemoral or axillary-femoral synthetic bypass graft has been surprisingly free of complications. A potential hazard is disruption of the pseudointima with subsequent thrombosis.

The normal aortic valve is easily crossed retrogradely with the catheter tip. Even in aortic valve stenosis, the left ventricle is entered in nearly all cases. By slowly withdrawing the catheter tip from its looped position in the left aortic sinus, wall-to-wall exploration of the severely stenotic valve is possible. A straight-tip guide wire may enhance this maneuver.[28] Left and right Judkins, left Amplatz, and pigtail catheters have all been used to center the guide wire in the aortic root to achieve more effective probing of the stenotic orifice.[29–31]

In selected patients who have aortic and mitral valve disk or ball-valve prosthesis, a brief direct percutaneous puncture through the palpable apex of the left ventricle

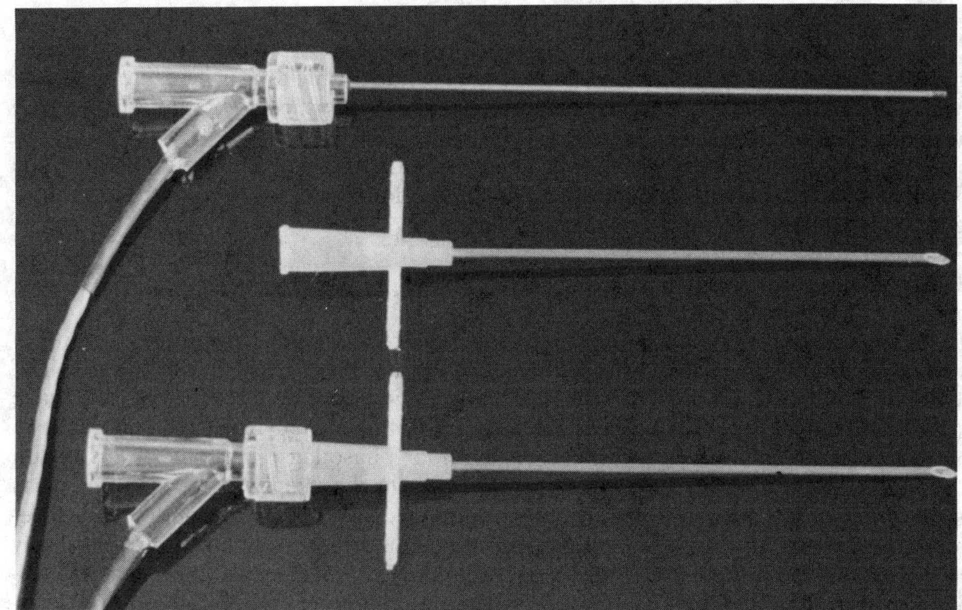

FIGURE 138-5 A Doppler probe with a coaxial cable arising from a side arm (*top*) slides inside a standard 18 gauge needle (*bottom*). The needle tip is directed to the front wall of the femoral artery (a high-pitched pulsatile signal) or to the front wall of the femoral vein (low-frequency rushing sound). Sounds intensify maximally in the midintraluminal position after puncture is made. (*Reproduced with permission from the Peripheral Systems Group, the ACS Company.*)

is surprisingly free of complications. Left ventricular angiography may be performed through the cannula. Retrograde catheterization of the left ventricle via a prosthetic aortic disc valve is not difficult but should be avoided if possible. Valvular incompetence is induced, and the catheter may become entrapped in the disk valve mechanism.[32,33] In contrast, tissue valves can be crossed without significant hazard.

In cases with both femoral and axillary artery disease, selective coronary arteriography has been performed via a translumbar approach utilizing a sheath.[34]

Arterial Cutdown

The cutdown technique for left-sided heart study usually utilizes the brachial artery. After the administration of 100 units/kg of heparin intravenously, the anterior wall of the exposed artery is punctured with the tip of an 18-gauge needle. The opening is enlarged slightly with a small forceps, permitting insertion of the tapered catheter. The arteriotomy is closed either by a previously placed, very small purse string loop or by one or two interrupted sutures. If brisk bleeding does not occur from both proximal and distal artery segments, thrombectomy is performed with a balloon catheter.

Transseptal Approach Transseptal catheterization may be used to enter the left atrium.[35] From the right femoral vein percutaneously, a 71-cm-long needle is advanced inside a dilator catheter-sheath system to a position beneath the ledge of the limbus fossae ovalis in the right atrium. The needle is then bared to puncture the atrial septum.[36–38] Entry into the left atrium is confirmed by a clear continuous pressure tracing. The dilator is then pushed across the septum. The needle tip is pulled back into the dilator, and when both are well in the left atrium, the sheath is slid over them to also enter the left atrium; needle and dilator are then withdrawn. The sheath permits various preformed open- or closed-tip catheters or large guide wires to be passed into the left atrium and left ventricle. A carbon-dioxide-filled balloon catheter may be passed from the left atrium to the left ventricle to the ascending aorta.[39–40] Biplane fluoroscopy, continuous pressure recording, a catheter in the aortic root, and knowledge of the size and position of the left atrium following pulmonary artery angiography are helpful in positioning the transseptal needle. The left atrium is difficult to enter if there is deformity of the thoracic or lumbar spine or if there is a very large right atrium. Other relative contraindications to transseptal catheterization include marked dilatation of the aortic root and other anatomic distortions of the inferior cava or atria. The procedure is not done if there is intraatrial thrombus or tumor.

Retrograde catheterization of the left atrium from the left ventricle in the right anterior oblique (RAO) projection utilizes a tapered flexible catheter that forms a clockwise loop in the left ventricle as it passes to the left atrium.[41] A pigtail catheter has been similarly used.[42]

EQUIPMENT

Catheters

Disposable single-use catheters in a wide range of sizes, shapes, and lengths with end and/or side holes are available for diagnostic use. The ideal nonpreformed catheter is soft enough to permit bending as required, has memory to hold its shape, and has enough strength or body to permit the curve of the tip to be advanced intact. Torque control is improved by incorporating a thin wire braid in the walls. Transmission of torque to the catheter tip in the ascending aorta is damped by a tortuous iliac artery. The torque is received instead by the proximal part of the catheter, resulting in coiling or potential knotting in the iliac artery. Preformed catheters are made to serve a specific function with a minimum of manipulation. Catheters should have smooth, regular surfaces to reduce thrombogenicity. Atrial septostomy with a fluid-filled balloon catheter or with a controlled folding surgical blade at the catheter tip[43] improves shunting and increases systemic arterial saturation in patients with transposition of the great arteries. A precompressed ivalon plug inserted by catheter has been used to close the patent ductus arteriosus. Loop-snare catheters are used for nonthoracotomy retrieval of intraluminal cardiovascular foreign bodies.[44] A ring-shaped ceramic crystal mounted at the distal tip of a 4F catheter gives an estimation of instantaneous arterial flow velocity using the Doppler technique.[45] A catheter-tip electromagnetic probe is also used to measure blood flow velocity.[46] Stroke volume is derived by utilizing the diameter of the aorta, determined angiographically or by ultrasound. A Doppler pulmonary artery catheter can provide continuous instantaneous cardiac output values, assuming a flat velocity profile.[47]

A 1.8-mm-diameter intravascular fiber-optic catheter inserted either directly in the operating room or via a no. 10 French guiding catheter is used to visualize the coronary arteries.[48] The coronary arteries may also be studied by intravascular, intracoronary echographic catheters. (See Chap. 133.) Hydrogen gas is detected within 4 s of inhalation with extreme sensitivity by a pacing catheter electrode positioned at the site of a left-to-right shunt or downstream from it.

Used in treating valvular pulmonic stenosis[49] and coarctation of the aorta,[14] pulmonary valvuloplasty and aortic angioplasty balloons up to 4 cm long with an inflation diameter up to 20 mm are made of high-tensile-strength polyethylene. Inflation to 3 to 4 atm with a 20-mL plastic syringe is usual. The lumen between the no. 8 or 9 French catheter and the balloon is large, permitting deflation in less than 7 s, decreasing the occlusion time.[50] A balloon catheter is used to size a secundum atrial septal defect, especially if umbrella closure is to be done.[51] Test balloon occlusion of aortopulmonary collaterals mimic the effects of planned surgical closure. In patients with pulmonary atresia and intact ventricular septum who have had surgical relief of the pulmonary atresia, the atrial septal defect can be temporarily closed with a balloon catheter in order to direct all the systemic venous return to the small right ventricle, testing its response.

Radiation Exposure

A qualified radiologic physicist should check the catheterization facilities, and secondary or scattered radiation should be minimized. Radiation intensity varies inversely with the square of the distance; i.e., if the distance to the source is doubled, the amount of radiation will be only one-quarter as much. One should select the smallest possible collimation and keep the image intensifier as close to the patient as possible. The U-arm position that places the x-ray tube to the examiner's side of the table causes the greatest exposure as a result of scattered radiation from the patient. Two film badges should be worn, one at the belt beneath the 0.5-mm equivalent lead apron and the other at the collar level outside the apron. The eyes, gonads, and red bone marrow have a whole-body limit of 5 rem (roentgen equivalent man) per year; any specific organ, such as the thyroid or skin, has a yearly limit of 15 rem. Lead glass spectacles and a thyroid collar reduce radiation to the eye by one-half and to the thyroid by 90 percent.[52] A floating or preferably a floor-length screen is needed for added shielding.[53] The maximal permissible dose, or "safe" exposure, for catheterization lab personnel is 100 mrem/week monitored by an unshielded left collar badge. If possible, women of childbearing age should have studies done within 10 days after the onset of menstruation.

Pressure-Recording System

If the heart rate is 60 to 120 beats per minute, the fundamental frequency of the basic wave is 1 to 2 per s. The first 10 to 20 harmonic components of the pressure wave occur up to a rate of 10 to 20 Hz; it is important to detect them without phase lag or amplitude distortion since they contribute to the steeply rising or falling parts of the pressure curve. A properly responding pressure-recording system should have a high natural frequency and optimal damping. A high natural frequency is obtained by using a bubble-free, saline solution–filled system of minimum length whose catheter and connector tubings have stiff walls and wide bores. Many catheter-tubing transducer systems are underdamped.[54] To achieve optimal damping, a damping needle or tube is placed between the catheter and the transducer. This extends the output-input ratio of the pressure wave in a nearly uniform manner (unity + 5 percent) to as close as possible to the natural frequency of the system. The values for both frequency response and damping coefficient are obtained by introducing a square-wave pressure input to the catheter system and by measuring the amplitude ratio of any two successive peak pressure amplitudes and the time interval between peaks (Fig. 138-6). For clinical cardiac catheterization, a manometer system with a uniform dynamic response greater than 20 Hz is desirable.

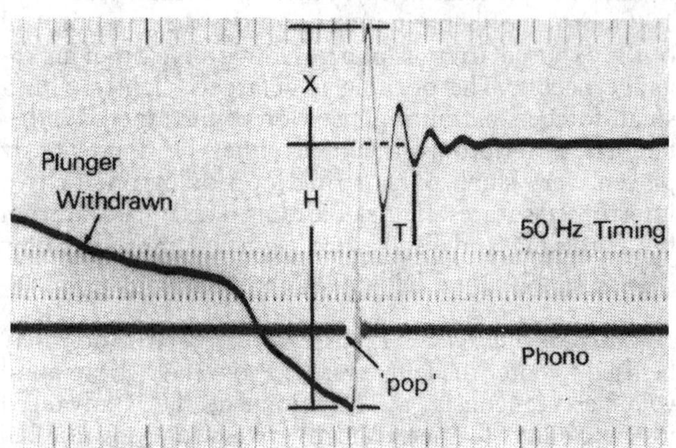

FIGURE 138-6 In order to measure the frequency response of a catheter transducer system, an abrupt transient input pressure is applied to the catheter tip (a plunger is pulled free of an air-filled syringe); the pressure oscillations are recorded at a fast paper speed and measured. X = height of the initial overshoot; H = end height of the recorded deflection; T = period of free oscillation, 0.08 s. The natural frequency is 13 Hz; the useful range is 4 Hz. The amplitude ratio of two successive peak amplitudes is 0.59, and the damping coefficient is 0.17. This underdamped system is optimally damped by the addition of a narrow-bore tube between catheter and transducer. (*Reproduced with permission of Irex Corporation.*)

An additional limiting factor in pressure recording is the superimposition of artifacts on the pressure pulse by the accelerating and decelerating movements imparted to the fluid-filled cardiac catheter by the beating heart. Distortion of the catheter-obtained phasic pressure waveform by motion artifact is avoided with the use of a catheter-tip, side-mounted, ultraminiature semiconductor gauge.

Oxygen Analysis

The total oxygen content of the blood may be determined by the classical Van Slyke manometric technique or, more rapidly, by gas chromatography or mass spectrometry. Small samples of blood from a syringe may be analyzed by direct photo-oximetry, by a membrane electrode, or after hemolysis, by a precision spectrophotometer. A fiber-optic reflection oximeter catheter permits intracardiac oxygen saturation measurements without withdrawal of blood.[55]

Analysis of expired air for oxygen and carbon dioxide may be made by gas analyzers or infrared or mass spectroscopy.[56] Oxygen consumption can also be measured throughout the procedure using a flow-through hood technique. The arteriovenous O_2 difference and thermal or dye dilution values for cardiac output can be substituted into the Fick equation and used to check the direct measurement of oxygen consumption against the calculated one.

DATA OBTAINED AT CATHETERIZATION

One must be familiar with the limitations of cardiac catheterization in order to avoid mistakes in diagnosis. There may be technical errors in obtaining the data, or properly recorded data may be misinterpreted or may not be specific.

Pressure Measurements

High-fidelity phasic pressure curves are usually not obtained from the ventricles or great arteries by conventional recording systems. The underdamped curve gives falsely high systolic and falsely low diastolic readings, and the overdamped curve has a smooth shape with disappearance of the incisura. The shape of the ventricular or great-artery pressure trace is occasionally of diagnostic aid. An abrupt fall in pressure in early diastole (early diastolic dip) followed by a sudden rise to a high end-diastolic pressure plateau occurs in abnormal compliance states such as constrictive pericarditis and restrictive cardiomyopathy. In isolated pulmonary stenosis the configuration of the right ventricular pressure curve is frequently peaked or triangular, but it is trapezoidal if a large ventricular septal defect is associated with the pulmonary stenosis.

In valvular pulmonary stenosis, the pulse pressure is frequently greater in the left pulmonary artery than in the right pulmonary artery because flow is preferentially directed into the left pulmonary artery and kinetic energy is translated into lateral pressure. In bilateral branch pulmonary artery stenosis, the proximal main pulmonary artery shows a wide pulse pressure with a low dicrotic notch (Fig. 138-7). In supravalvular aortic stenosis, the coanda effect makes the right branchial and right carotid artery peak pressures greater than those on the left. A giant A wave in the right atrium is characteristic of valvular pulmonary stenosis but not of tetralogy of Fallot. A large V wave on the pulmonary artery wedge pressure tracing may or may not mean that severe mitral regurgitation is present.[57]

Left ventricular end-diastolic pressure (LVEDP) is recorded on a high-sensitivity scale and is measured where the downslope of the A wave in the left ventricle coincides with the initial upstroke of the left ventricular pressure. The LVEDP may also be measured at the peak of the R wave of the ECG. An elevated LVEDP reflects an alteration in the ventricular pressure-volume relation or a decrease in diastolic compliance of the ventricle. An increased LVEDP occurs commonly with a dilated failing left ventricle but may also be noted in a small ventricular cavity with thick walls or in a normal-size left ventricular cavity during an acute ischemic attack. (See Chaps. 23 and 25.)

In order to measure the maximal rate of rise of left ventricular pressure, or peak *dP/dt*, a high-fidelity pressure record is needed, obtained ideally via a catheter-tip transducer. This value is influenced by preload and afterload in addition to the contractile state. The preejection phase index *dP/dt/P*, where *P* is the left ventricular pressure during isovolumic systole, reflects the velocity of shortening of contractile elements but also responds to changes in preload. (See also Chap. 23.) In daily practice,

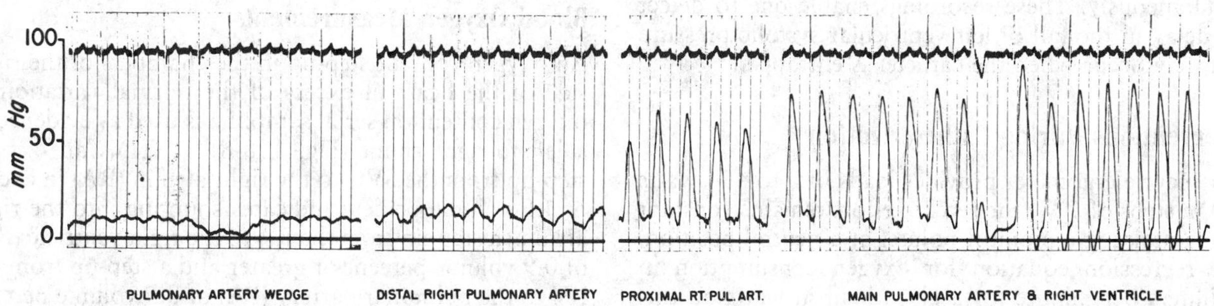

FIGURE 138-7 Pressure record in multiple congenital stenosis of the right and left pulmonary artery branches, illustrating a systolic pressure differential between the distal, proximal, and main pulmonary artery. There are systolic hypertension and a wide pulse pressure in the proximal right and main pulmonary arteries, related to a reduction in the capacity of the pulmonary artery compression chamber.

ejection phase indexes derived from the conventional left ventricular angiogram are used to assess left ventricular function.[58] The ejection fraction is commonly employed as an index of ventricular contractility but is sensitive to changes in preload and afterload as well.

A satisfactory pulmonary artery wedge pressure provides a good estimate of left atrial mean pressure.[59] Some change in waveform and phase shift (0.06-s time delay) occurs in the transmitted signal when compared with the direct left atrial pressure record. End-expiratory pulmonary artery diastolic pressure agrees within 2 to 4 mmHg with mean pulmonary artery wedge pressure in the absence of increased pulmonary arteriolar resistance. Pulmonary vein wedge pressure does not give an accurate estimate of the pulmonary artery pressure in the presence of pulmonary artery hypertension.

Pressure recording permits measurement of either the peak or the mean pressure differential across a stenotic semilunar or atrioventricular (AV) valve or a segmentally narrowed blood vessel. If possible, simultaneous pressure recordings across a valve should be obtained, especially if there is atrial fibrillation. If the pulmonary artery wedge is used as an estimate of left atrial mean pressure, the waveform and amplitude should be confirmed at a second site. The error in assessing the mitral valve area in mitral stenosis may be large when the measured pressure differential is small. Because of the slow fall of the *y* descent in the wedge position, the mitral valve gradient may be overestimated by 3 to 4 mmHg when compared with the gradient obtained with a direct left atrial pressure.[60] A pullback record across the semilunar valve performed with a catheter having multiple paired side holes may show a false zone of composite ventricular and great-artery pulses resulting from the simultaneous recorded pressures through proximal and distal side holes. Occasionally a gradient may be overlooked if the catheter tip cannot be advanced well into the ventricle so that it washes into the aorta in systole and falls into the left ventricle in diastole. In a case of proximal infundibular pulmonary stenosis, if the pullback is at the cranial aspect of the tricuspid valve, the catheter may fall back into the right atrium from the right ventricular outflow tract very quickly, missing the gradient.

Left ventricular cavity obliteration with catheter entrapment may result in spurious pressure gradient. To detect an intraventricular gradient, the left ventricular pressure should be checked in the inflow and outflow, i.e., submitral and subaortic, positions simultaneously and in the apical versus the inflow or outflow positions simultaneously. These recordings enable one to detect the delay in the fall of left ventricular systolic pressure that may occur when the catheter is entrapped.[61]

Interventions during Catheterization

Our bicycle ergometer provides loads of 0 to 450 watts (W) in steps of 5 W; the level of effort remains constant by maintaining a monitor pointer at a neutral position. The regression equation for oxygen consumption in milliliters per minute for a given load in watts on this ergometer is $V_{O_2} = 13.16\ W + 254\ mL$. An increase in cardiac output of 0.6 liter/min or greater for each 100 mL of oxygen consumed presumes a normal response. If the oxygen consumption is increased 200 to 250 mL/min by supine use of a bicycle ergometer, an increase or arteriovenous difference greater than 30 mL/liter is considered abnormal. When the pulmonary artery oxygen saturation falls to substantially less than 30 percent during exercise, the upper limit of circulatory stress is being approached. Normally, during exercise, LVEDP falls and stroke work increases; if left ventricular performance is impaired, LVEDP rises and stroke work rises; and in severe dysfunction, stroke work fails to increase despite an increase in LVEDP. Isometric hand-grip exercise increases heart rate, systemic mean pressure, and cardiac output. A fall in left ventricular stroke work and a sharp rise in LVEDP during the grip test indicate poor left ventricular reserve.

All patients with mitral stenosis who have normal or mildly increased pulmonary artery and wedge pressures at rest should have the mitral gradient and cardiac output rechecked during exercise. In normal patients pulmonary artery pressure with exercise rises minimally, usually no higher than 25 mmHg mean. In a patient with a repaired ventricular septal defect and residual pulmonary vascular disease, the pulmonary artery pressure may be at the upper limits of normal or slightly increased at rest but may double with low-level exercise.

Rapid atrial pacing may be used as a stress intervention. In normal individuals, LVEDP falls as the heart rate is increased. If a paced patient with coronary artery disease is unable to meet the increased myocardial oxygen demand, the LVEDP rises in the early postpacing period and excess lactate is noted in coronary sinus blood. In patients with tetralogy of Fallot, atrial pacing produces a drop in arterial oxygen saturation and an increase in right-to-left shunting by increasing dynamic right ventricular outflow tract obstruction.

In hypertrophic cardiomyopathy, isoproterenol, amyl nitrite, exercise, tilting, and the Valsalva maneuver intensify or provoke a systolic outflow tract pressure differential, whereas a purely vasopressor amine, phenylephrine, decreases the outflow tract pressure gradient. (See Chap. 90.)

The response of cardiac output to vasodilator drugs in the patient with cardiac failure can be assessed. In patients with primary pulmonary artery hypertension, a 30 percent decrease in pulmonary vascular resistance and a 10 percent decrease in mean pulmonary artery pressure is the usual criterion for a positive response to pulmonary vasodilator drugs.[62] (See Chap. 99.)

Blood Oxygen Measurements

An oxygen content step-up in the chambers of the right side of the heart in excess of the normal variation in oxygen content on serial sampling is used as evidence of a left-to-right shunt (Fig. 138-8).[63,64] Thus an oxygen step-up from the SVC to the right atrium (RA) in excess of 1.9 volume percent indicates shunting into the right atrium; a step-up from the RA to the right ventricle (RV) of 0.9 volume percent or greater and a step-up from the RV to the pulmonary artery (PA) of 0.5 volume percent or greater indicates a left-to-right shunt at the right ventricular and pulmonary artery levels, respectively. By these criteria, false-positive results are rare, but false-

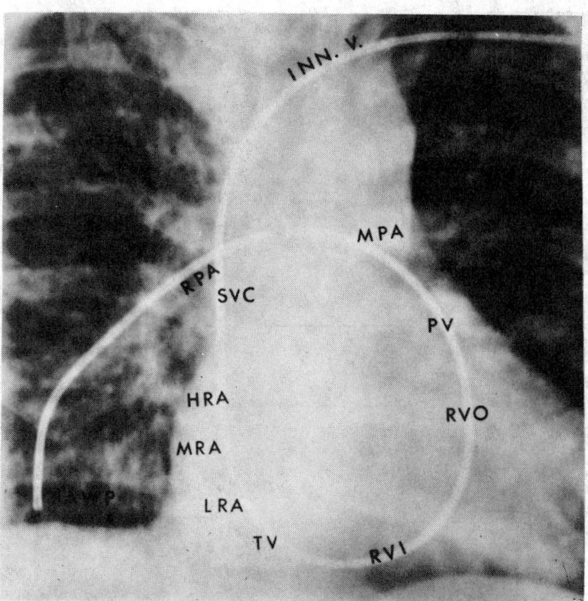

FIGURE 138-8 Sites of blood sampling during catheterization of the right side of the heart. Catheter introduced from the left basilic vein into the right pulmonary artery. INN.V = innominate vein (brachiocephalic vein); SVC = superior venae cavae; HRA, MRA, LRA = high, mid-, and low right atria; RVI, RVO = right ventricular inflow and outflow tracts; TV, PV = tricuspid and pulmonary valves; MPA, RPA = main and right pulmonary arteries; PAWP = pulmonary artery wedge position.

negative results occur in patients with small shunts. In an anemic or polycythemic patient, the detection of shunting is best reflected by the step-up in percentage oxygen saturation rather than the step-up in volume percent, since the latter is dependent on the hemoglobin concentration.[65,66]

Studies show that sensitivity in detecting left-to-right shunts is improved if numerous serial blood samples are withdrawn in rapid succession for oximetry. If two sets of interrupted samples are taken from the SVC, RA, RV, and PA, a 9 percent saturation increase between the SVC and the RA indicates an atrial shunt; a 5 percent saturation increase between the RA and the RV a ventricular shunt; and a 3 percent saturation increase between the RV and the PA a pulmonary artery shunt. Sensitivity can be improved if blood samples are obtained in multiple pairs in a rapid serial sweep without flushing with saline solution between samples. The rise in oxygen saturation step-up for a given left-to-right shunt is related to the saturation of mixed venous blood (MVB). For example, if the MVB is 85 percent, a 5 percent step-up represents a 2 : 1 shunt; if MVB is 75 percent, a 10 percent step-up is needed; if the MVB is 65 percent, a 15 percent step-up indicates a 2 : 1 shunt. The results of the blood oxygen analysis should be reviewed before the catheterization is completed. Left-to-right shunts less than 20 percent of pulmonary flow are not detectable by oximetry. Since no oximetric criteria exist for exclusion of a shunt, selective angiography and/or the use of a hydrogen (platinum) electrode provide maximal sensitivity and reliability in excluding small shunts. The presence of an increased oxygen step-up in the right side of the heart should be closely correlated with angiographic findings.

Catheter Position

The catheter position may be useful in identifying the anatomic location of an intracardiac defect (Fig. 138-9). In crossing a membranous ventricular septal defect in the anteroposterior view, the catheter inserted from the arm passes into the ascending aorta from the right ventricle in a hairpin loop and enters the pulmonary artery from the right ventricle in a wider U loop (Fig. 138-10). A patent ductus arteriosus is frequently entered as the tip of the catheter points to the "roof" of the junction of the main and left pulmonary arteries. Failing direct catheter passage, a flexible-spring guide wire, introduced while the venous catheter tip rests in the main pulmonary artery, readily passes through the ductus into the descending aorta; in aorticopulmonary septal defect, the tip passes directly up the ascending aorta from the main pulmonary artery. When the catheter tip enters a pulmonary vein within the heart shadow, angiography or a dye curve is necessary to ascertain whether the pulmonary vein drains into the left or the right atrium. A secundum atrial septal defect is more easily crossed from the leg approach, a sinus venosus defect from an arm approach, and an ostium primum defect from either approach. If the tricuspid valve is congenitally displaced into the right ventricle, the pressure transition from the right ventricle to the right atrium may occur while the catheter tip is far to the left of the spine. Simultaneous intracardiac electrocardiography is confirmatory (Fig. 138-11).

Flow and Shunt Calculations

Fick Method

Cardiac Output In 1870 Adolph Fick expounded a theory for the measurement of blood flow that he never used in the laboratory: "The total uptake or release of a substance by an organ is the product of the blood flow to the organ and of the arteriovenous concentration of the substance." The cardiac output may be calculated given the following three values: total oxygen consumption of 300 mL/min, arterial blood oxygen content of 19 mL per deciliter of blood, and mixed venous blood oxygen content of 14 mL per deciliter of blood. The cardiac output, in liters per minute, is equal to the oxygen consumption divided by the arteriovenous oxygen difference multiplied by 10 (to convert the latter to liters). In this case the cardiac output equals 6.0 liters/min. Cardiac output may be related to the body surface area (BSA) as the cardiac index. Assuming a BSA of 2.0 m^2, the cardiac index would be $\frac{6}{2}$, or 3 liters/min per m^2. Because of laminar flow from the coronary sinus and the cavae and in the right atrium, mixed venous blood is best obtained from the pulmonary artery. Under conditions of exercise, a minimum of 3 min is usually required to obtain a steady state preliminary to expired air and blood collection. In a given person, repeated measurements of the cardiac output at rest by the Fick technique may vary to a maximum of ±17 percent, presuming a continued steady state.

Shunt Calculations Shunt calculations utilizing the Fick principle tend to be approximations since complete mixing of venous and shunted blood may not occur. Also,

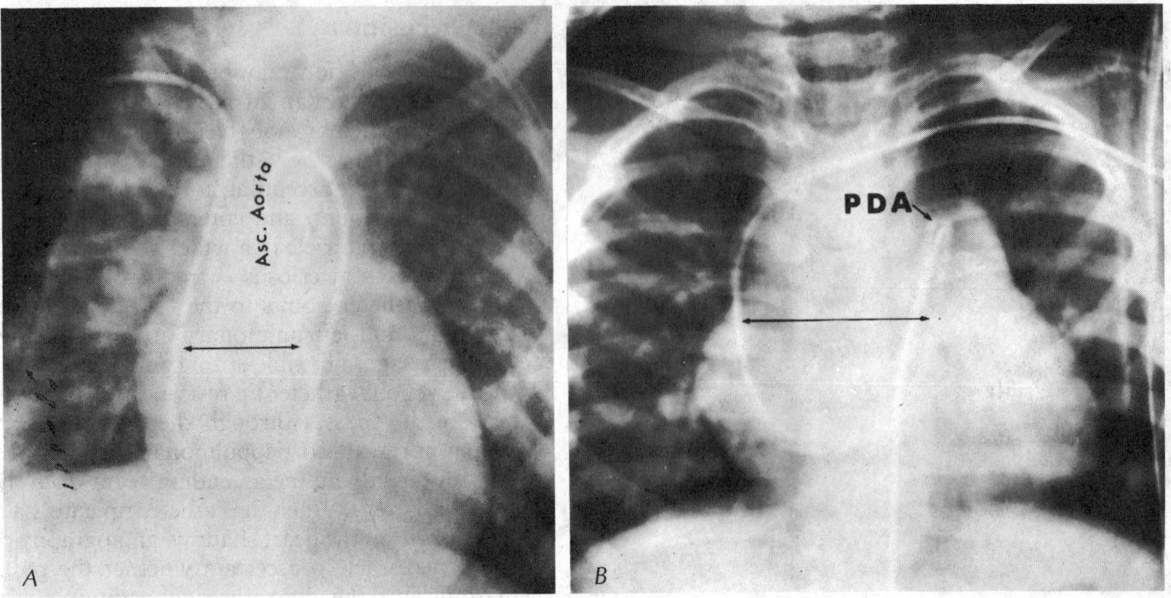

FIGURE 138-9 Anteroposterior roentgenograms that demonstrate the difference in width of the catheter loop when (*A*) the catheter tip passes in a hairpin loop (arrow) from the right ventricle to the ascending aorta via a ventricular septal defect and (*B*) the catheter tip passes in a wide U loop (arrow) from the right ventricle to the pulmonary artery, thence to the descending thoracic aorta via a patent ductus arteriosus (PDA).

as the arteriovenous oxygen narrows, small errors in the analysis or in the collection of blood samples make large variations in the calculated pulmonary blood flow possible. The calculation of shunt flow, however, is useful; it provides a quantitative index that is combined with clinical findings to determine whether or not surgery is advisable.

Numerous formulas have been developed, but those listed below are the ones used most often. The oxygen capacity is the maximal amount of oxygen that will combine with hemoglobin and that will be dissolved in plasma at a high P_{O_2}. One gram of hemoglobin can combine with 1.36 mL of oxygen. The amount of oxygen dissolved in plasma is dependent upon the solubility coefficient of oxygen, the temperature, and the partial pressure of oxygen. At 37°C, the solubility coefficient is

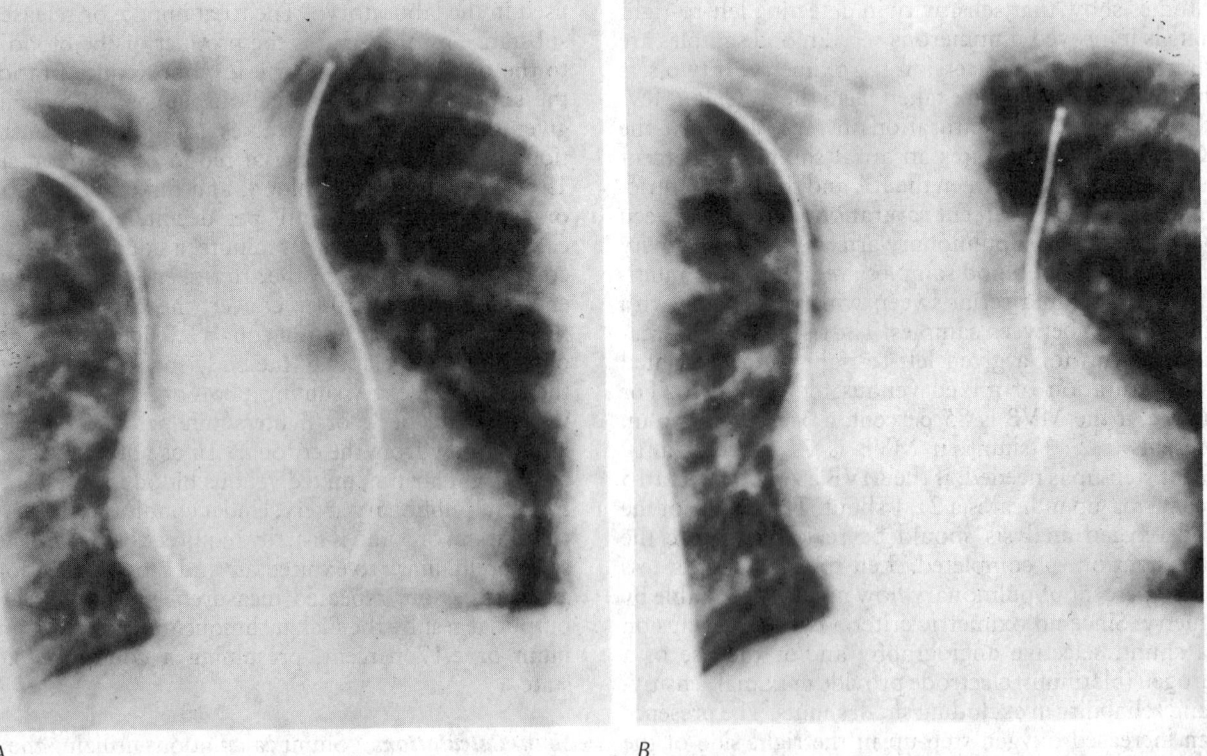

FIGURE 138-10 *A.* The catheter tip passes from the right superior vena cava to the right atrium, thence to the coronary sinus, thence to the left superior vena cava. *B.* The catheter tip passes from the left superior vena cava to an anomalous left upper lobe pulmonary vein.

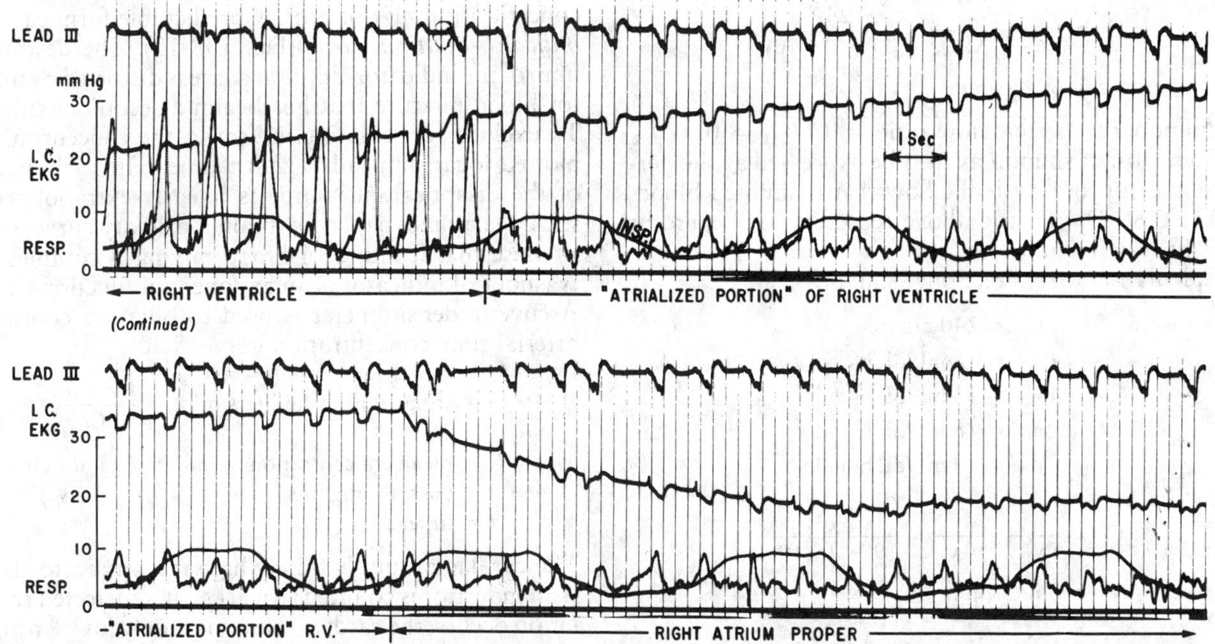

FIGURE 138-11 The use of the intracavitary electrocardiogram (I.C. EKG) and simultaneous pressure recording in a diagnosis of Ebstein's disease. Lead III of the standard electrocardiogram shows a short PQ interval and a prolonged QRS complex associated with Wolff-Parkinson-White syndrome. The I.C. EKG of the "atrialized portion" of the right ventricle resembles the I.C. EKG of the right ventricle, but the pressure pulse of the atrialized portion of the right ventricle is the same as that of the right atrium proper. This finding suggests displacement of the tricuspid valve into the right ventricle. The I.C. EKG in the right atrium proper shows characteristic peaked biphasic P waves and reduction in voltage of the QRS.

such that the amount of oxygen dissolved in plasma is 0.03 mL/mmHg per liter. With an oxygen tension of about 100 mmHg about 3 mL of oxygen is dissolved per liter of blood. This small amount is usually ignored, although when the patient is breathing 100 percent oxygen, a considerable amount of oxygen can be dissolved in plasma. Oxygen content is related to both the hemoglobin concentration and the oxygen saturation. The oxygen content equals 1.36 × Hb (g/dL) × O_2 sat (%)/100.

1. Calculation of left-to-right shunt:

Total oxygen consumption (V_{O_2})	240 mL/min
Pulmonary artery blood oxygen content (PA_{O_2})	17 mL/dL blood
Mixed venous blood oxygen content (MV_{O_2})	15 mL/dL blood
Arterial blood oxygen content (Sa_{O_2}) (assumed to equal pulmonary venous oxygen content)	19 mL/dL blood

$$\text{Pulmonary flow } (Q_p) = \frac{V_{O_2}}{Sa_{O_2} - PA_{O_2}} = \frac{240}{19 - 17(10)} = 12 \text{ liters/min}$$

$$\text{Systemic flow } (Q_s) = \frac{V_{O_2}}{Sa_{O_2} - MV_{O_2}} = \frac{240}{19 - 15(10)} = 6 \text{ liters/min}$$

a. Pulmonary flow/systemic flow ratio $= Q_p/Q_s = \frac{12}{6} = 2$.

b. If one substitutes for Q_s and Q_p in the above formula and reduces to a common denominator, the pulmonary flow–systemic flow ratio is obtained from a formula requiring only the oxygen saturation. Assuming an oxygen capacity of 20 volumes percent, the following blood oxygen saturations for the above samples are Sa = 95 percent, PA = 85 percent, and MV = 75 percent.

$$\frac{Q_p}{Q_s} = \frac{Sa_{O_2}\% - MV_{O_2}\%}{Sa_{O_2}\% - Pa_{O_2}\%} = \frac{95 - 75}{95 - 85} = 2$$

c. Left-to-right shunt may also be expressed as the percentage of total pulmonary flow that is shunted blood. The 2:1 Q_p/Q_s ratio above then represents a 50 percent left-to-right shunt.

2. Calculation of right-to-left shunt:

$$V_{O_2} = 240 \text{ mL/min}$$
$$MV_{O_2} = 13 \text{ mL/dL blood}$$
$$Sa_{O_2} = 17 \text{ mL/dL blood}$$

Pulmonary vein blood oxygen content is as follows:

$$PV_{O_2} = 19 \text{ mL/dL blood}$$

(assumed to be 98 percent of oxygen capacity + 0.3 mL of dissolved oxygen)

$$Q_p = \frac{V_{O_2}}{PV_{O_2} - MV_{O_2}} = \frac{240}{19 - 13(10)} = 4 \text{ liters/min}$$

$$Q_s = \frac{V_{O_2}}{Sa_{O_2} - MV_{O_2}} = \frac{240}{17 - 13(10)}$$

$$= 6 \text{ liters/min}$$

Pulmonary/systemic flow ratio = Q_p/Q_s = 0.7

Right-to-left shunt may also be expressed as the percentage of total systemic flow that is shunted blood. The 0.66 Q_p/Q_s ratio above represents a 33 percent right-to-left shunt.

3. Calculation of bidirectional shunt*:

$$V_{O_2} = 240 \text{ mL/min}$$
$$PA_{O_2} = 15 \text{ mL/dL blood}$$
$$MV_{O_2} = 13 \text{ mL/dL blood}$$
$$Sa_{O_2} = 18 \text{ mL/dL blood}$$
$$PV_{O_2} = 19 \text{ mL/dL blood}$$

$$Q_p = \frac{V_{O_2}}{PV_{O_2} - PA_{O_2}} = \frac{240}{19 - 15(10)}$$

$$= 6 \text{ liters/min}$$

$$Q_s = \frac{V_{O_2}}{Sa_{O_2} - MV_{O_2}} = \frac{240}{18 - 13(10)}$$

$$= 4.8 \text{ liters/min}$$

$$Q_{ep} = \frac{V_{O_2}}{PV_{O_2} - MV_{O_2}} = \frac{240}{19 - 13(10)}$$

$$= 4.0 \text{ liters/min}$$

Left-to-right shunt = $Q_p - Q_{ep} = 6 - 4$ = 2 liters/min

Right-to-left shunt = $Q_s - Q_{es} = 4.8 - 4.0$ = 0.8 liters/min

Indicator-Dilution Technique

Cardiac Output: Dye Method The cardiac output, or the mean volume rate of flow, may be determined by using a modification of the standard concentration equation used for the determination of a static fluid volume such as the blood volume:

$$V = \frac{I}{C}$$

where V = fluid volume, mL

I = indicator added to fluid, mg

C = concentration of indicator in each milliliter of fluid, mg/mL

For determination of a moving fluid volume,

$$\text{Cardiac output} = \frac{I}{Ct}$$

where t = time required for all indicator-fluid mixture to pass sampling site once

If the indicator particles are injected into the circulation as a bolus and measured in the initial passage at a downstream site, they distribute themselves in a time-concentration plot of grossly predictable form called an *indicator-dilution curve* (Fig. 138-12). The descending limb of the indicator-dilution curve is distorted by indicator-blood mixture that has begun a second circulation. To exclude recirculating indicator, the concentration is plotted logarithmically against time. The early portion of the disappearance slope is linearly extrapolated on semilogarithmic paper to obtain a primary curve, on the premise that if indicator-blood mixing is complete, the washout of indicator is an exponential function of time. A cuvette densitometer is used to obtain a continuous arterial time-concentration curve. Thus,

$$\text{Cardiac output (in liters/min)} = \frac{I \times 60 \text{ s}}{Ct}$$

where C = mean concentration of indicator in one circulator passage, mg/liter

t = time, s

The cardiac output is falsely high if an indicator is lost. If an indicator is counted twice, i.e., if undetected recirculation occurs, the cardiac output is falsely low. An analog computer provides rapid calculation of cardiac output from dye-dilution curves and detects whether or not logarithmic decay of indicator concentration has occurred. The Stewart-Hamilton formula assumes constant heart rate and stroke volume and a linear runoff in the pulmonary artery. Values for cardiac output obtained with the indicator-dilution technique compare closely with those obtained by the Fick method.[67]

In the absence of shunt, the indicator-dilution curve shows an uninterrupted buildup slope, a sharp concentration peak, a steep disappearance slope, and a prominent recirculation peak. Two major types of distortion are produced by central shunting. In a left-to-right shunt, there is decreased peak concentration of dye, a gentle disappearance slope (prolonged disappearance time), and absence of the recirculation peak. These alterations are produced by the recirculation of indicator particles through the lungs, resulting in a slow release of indicator to the peripheral circulation. The typical curve produced by a venoarterial, or right-to-left, shunt shows deformity of the buildup slope by an abnormal or early-appearing hump, or reflection, representing indicator that has been shunted from right to left. The distortion in contour of the indicator-dilution curve in valvular regurgitation is similar to that occurring with left-to-right shunts. Efforts have been made to predict all or part of the curve from certain other curve components. The cardiac output obtained by the forward-triangle method compares favorably with the classical Hamilton method. In this technique, the initial portion of the indicator-dilution curve is considered to be a triangle. The area of this triangle multiplied by a constant gives the area of the primary dilution curve. Intracardiac shunts can be detected and quantified by indicator dilution curves.[68]

Cardiac Output: Thermodilution Technique The thermodilution technique was introduced by Fegler in 1953 to measure volume flow rate.[69] A precalibrated bead thermistor-tipped catheter or a multiple-lumen, flow-directed thermistor catheter is placed in the pulmonary artery. Ten milliliters of iced (5°C) or room temperature

*Effective pulmonary flow Q_{ep} is that volume of systemic venous blood that, after returning to the right atrium, actually reaches the pulmonary capillaries. It is equal to effective systemic blood flow Q_{es}.

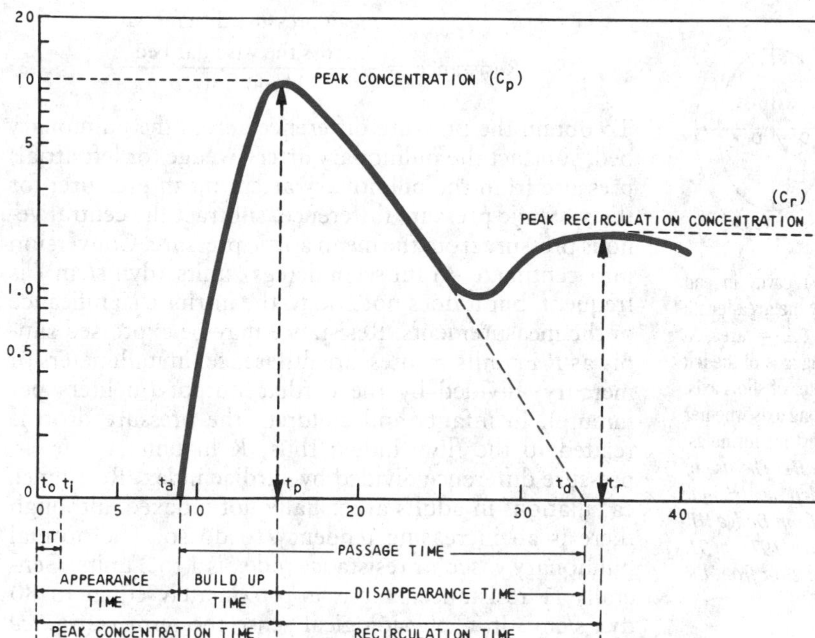

FIGURE 138-12 Time and concentration components of a normal indicator-dilution curve that has been replotted semilogarithmically, with extrapolation of the declining slope of concentration to eliminate the effect of recirculated indicator. The logarithm of the concentration on the ordinate is plotted against time on the abscissa. t_o = time of onset of injection of the indicator slug; t_i = time from t_o to the end of the injection; t_a = time from t to the first detectable appearance of indicator at the sampling site; t_p = time from t_o to the peak (maximal) concentration of the indicator; t_d = time when the declining concentration of indicator reaches a minimally detectable value; t_r = time from t_o to the time of the secondary concentration peak due to systemic recirculation of indicator; IT = the injection time. *(From Wood EH, Swan HJC: Definition of terms and symbols for description of circulatory dilution curves. J Appl Physiol 6:797, 1954. Modified and reproduced with permission from the publisher and authors.)*

(22°C) dextrose solution is injected rapidly (<4 s) through a second lumen into the right atrium. As the cold dextrose-blood mixture is initially ejected from the right ventricle, the pulmonary artery temperature drops maximally and then progressively rises in a beat-to-beat disappearance slope as the cold dextrose-blood mixture is washed out of the ventricle. The recirculation phase is negligible. Recording the curve allows assessment of the technical adequacy of the study. The area under the time-temperature curve is electronically integrated and the cardiac output is computed by the Stewart-Hamilton formula. The difference between successive determinations should be less than 10 percent. Since there is no gold standard for cardiac output, the results are compared with the dye dilution and Fick techniques and are noted to correlate well,[70] except in low cardiac output states where the Fick method is preferable. If severe tricuspid or pulmonary regurgitation or significant left-to-right shunting is present, the peak is attenuated and the downslope of the curve is prolonged and the thermal dilution cardiac output will likely be unreliable.[6,71] In general, in using thermal dilution, a true directional change in cardiac output is reflected by an observed change of ±10 percent.

Ventricular Volume Measurements

Left ventricular volume is estimated by selective injection of contrast medium into the left ventricle or left atrium. The image of the opacified left ventricular cavity is obtained either by a large film changer or by cineangiography. Biplane views used include frontal and lateral, right and left anterior oblique, or half-axial left anterior oblique and conventional right anterior oblique.[72–74] A single-plane mode using the frontal or the right anterior oblique projection is often adequate.[75–76] In the classic biplane technique each shadow of the left ventricular cavity is treated as an ellipse. The long axis of the ventricle (L_m) and the two mutually perpendicular short axes at its midpoint (D_a and D_1) are measured, and the volume (V) is calculated from the formula for volume of an ellipsoid:

$$V = \frac{4}{3}\pi \times \frac{D_a}{2} \times \frac{D_1}{2} \times \frac{L_m}{2}$$

or

$$V = \frac{\pi}{6} \times D_a \times D_1 \times L_m$$

In the single-plane method, the long axis and one short axis are measured; the second nonvisible short axis is assumed to equal the first; thus

$$V = \frac{\pi}{6} \times L_m \times D_1^2$$

More often, in either the biplane or single-plane method, the short-axis dimension is derived from the measured long axis and the area (A) of the left ventricular shadow, treated as an ellipse (area-length method of Dodge) (Fig. 138-13):

$$A = \pi L_m \frac{D}{4}$$

Corrections are made for magnification due to the divergence of the x-ray beam.[77] A calibrated grid or circular reference marker is filmed at the estimated level of the left ventricle. The true grid size equals the size measured on the projected film times a correction factor. More magnification may occur in the periphery than in the center of the field (pin cushion effect) due to spherical aberration in the lens system. Geometric and nongeometric count-based radionuclide techniques for calculation of ventricular volumes are well validated.

If the left ventricle of a postmortem heart specimen is filled with contrast material and filmed, the calculated estimate of the volume of the left ventricle is higher than the known volume of the left ventricle. An appropriate regression equation for both single-plane[75,76] and bi-

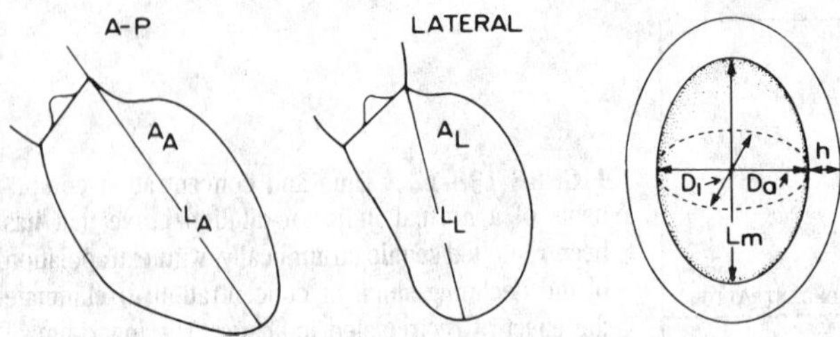

FIGURE 138-13 Dimensions of the left ventricular (LV) cavity in end diastole used for the calculation of the ventricular volume by the area-length method, biplane technique. A-P = anteroposterior plane; A_a, A_l = area, A-P and area lateral plane (planimetry); L_a, L_l = length or long axis of the left ventricle, A-P and lateral plane (measured); D_a, D_l = diameter of short axis, A-P and lateral plane (derived); L_m = maximum length or long axis whether from the A-P or lateral plane; h = wall thickness, LV. See text for formulas. (*Left and middle portion of figure from Sandler H, Dodge HT: The use of single plane angiocardiograms for the calculation of left ventricular volume. Am Heart J 75:325, 1968. Right portion of figure from Dodge HT: Hemodynamic aspects of cardiac failure. Hosp Pract January 1971, p. 91. Illustration by Tagawa B, Miller A. Reproduced with permission from the publishers and authors.*)

plane[72,74] techniques has been derived to adjust for this initial overestimate. The left ventricular end-diastolic volume is normally 70 ± 20 mL/m², and the end-systolic volume is 24 ± 10 mL/m². The forward stroke volume obtained by left ventriculography agrees well with indicator dilution and Fick determinations. The ejection fraction of the left ventricle is 0.67 ± 0.08; values below 0.55 are usually considered abnormal. Diastolic left ventricular wall thickness measured by angiography is 9 mm for women and 12 mm for men, and left ventricular wall mass is 76 g/m² for women and 99 g/m² for men.[78]

The total stroke volume obtained by left ventriculography is used to assess the severity of mitral and aortic valve regurgitation. Total stroke volume minus forward stroke volume equals regurgitant stroke volume. The regurgitant fraction equals regurgitant stroke volume divided by total stroke volume. Severe valvular regurgitation has a regurgitant fraction of 0.50 or greater (Fig. 138-14).

Right ventricular volume is estimated by applying Simpson's rule or the area-length method to the cavity silhouettes after biplane angiography.[79] The end-diastolic volume of the right ventricle in normal persons is 81 ± 12 mL/m².[80] The opacified left atrial shadow is represented as an ellipsoid so that left atrial volume can also be calculated in the biplane mode; the normal left atrial maximal volume is 63 ± 16 mL with a mean volume of 35 + 8.7 mL.[81]

Resistance

By Poiseuille's law, the flow varies directly with the fourth power of the radius of a tube; resistance varies inversely with the fourth power of the radius. Vascular resistance to blood flow in systemic, pulmonary, or regional vascular beds is estimated by analogy to Ohm's law:

$$\text{Resistance} = \frac{\text{pressure (in volts)}}{\text{flow (in amperes)}}$$

or

$$\text{Resistance} = \frac{\text{mean pressure differential across the vascular bed}}{\text{blood flow}}$$

To obtain the pressure difference across the pulmonary bed, subtract the pulmonary artery wedge (or left atrial) pressure from the pulmonary artery mean pressure; for the systemic pressure difference, subtract the central venous pressure from the mean aortic pressure. Conversion into centimeter-gram-second (cgs) units (dyn·s/cm⁵) is frequent, but it does not add to the intrinsic significance of the measurements. Resistance may be expressed simply as R in units = pressure difference (in millimeters of mercury) divided by the cardiac output (in liters per minute). In infants and children, the pressure drop is related to the flow index; thus, R in units × m² = pressure difference divided by cardiac index. Resistance calculations in adults are usually not indexed, although there is an increasing tendency to do so. The normal pulmonary vascular resistance index is 1 to 2 units. Generally, 1 resistance unit is approximately equal to 80 dyn·s/cm⁵. In a physiological sense the term *resistance* avoids specific definition. A change in resistance usually implies a change in a cross-sectional area of the vascular bed but does not indicate the mechanism behind the change. Passive widening of the vessels by increases in intravascular flow as well as the opening of previously closed channels may produce changes in resistance similar to those of active vasomotion. Subnormal calculated pulmonary vascular resistance is noted in the patient who has a large atrial septal defect with normal pulmonary artery pressure. Clinically, the resistance figure is useful in quantitating the extent of pulmonary vascular disease; thus a patient with a pulmonary vascular resistance of 10 units per m² probably would not benefit from closure of a septal defect. (See Chap. 97.)

Calculation of Valve Areas

The equation for calculation of valve area (Torricelli's orifice equation) uses a standard hydrokinetic formula

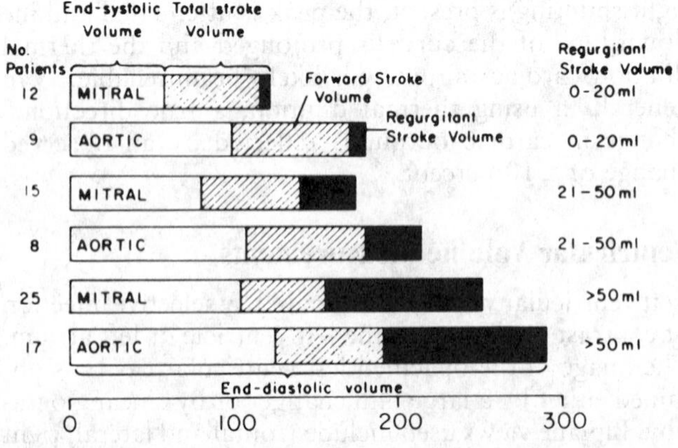

FIGURE 138-14 The mean values for left ventricular volumes obtained by ventriculography in patients with minimal, moderate, and marked aortic and mitral valve regurgitation. The entire bar represents the end-diastolic volume in milliliters. The total stroke volume equals the forward plus the regurgitant stroke volume. (*From Jones JW, Rackley CE, Bruce RA, et al: Left ventricular volumes in valvular heart disease. Circulation 29:887, 1964. Reproduced with permission from the American Heart Association, Inc., and the authors.*)

for a rounded-edge orifice or a short tube. When flow occurs across a narrow orifice, the pressure differential is related to the conversion of pressure energy into kinetic energy. The Gorlin formula for calculation of valve area is derived from two standard orifice formulas, describing flow and velocity.[82]

Formula I

$$F = AVC_c$$

where F = volume rate of flow during the time the valvular orifice is open, mL/s of diastole or systole
A = area of fixed orifice, cm^2
V = velocity flow, cm/s
C_c = coefficient of orifice contraction compensating for the physical phenomenon of reduction of the orifice stream to an area less than the area of the actual orifice.

Formula II

$$V^2 = C_v^2\, 2gh \quad \text{or} \quad V = C_v\sqrt{2gh}$$

where V = as above
C_v = coefficient of velocity (allowing for some loss in conversion of pressure energy to velocity)
g = gravity acceleration (980 cm/s per s)
h = pressure head or differential across the orifice, cmH_2O

Combining I and II

$$A = \frac{F}{C_c \times C_v\sqrt{2gh}} \qquad A = \frac{F}{C \times 44.3\sqrt{P_1 - P_2}}$$

where C = discharge coefficient (an orifice constant obtained by comparing calculated with measured valve areas at postmortem, which combines C_c, C_v, conversion factor, mmHg to cmH_2O, other unknown factors)
$44.3 = \sqrt{2g} = \sqrt{1960}$
$h = P_1 - P_2$
= pressure differential across the orifice, mmHg

The duration of ventricular filling or emptying is measured in seconds from pullback or simultaneous pressure records obtained immediately upstream and downstream from the valve. The systolic or diastolic time per beat multiplied by the heart rate gives the number of seconds in each minute during which either filling or emptying occurs across the atrioventricular or semilunar valve, respectively. Thus, the volume rate of flow in milliliters per second of systole or diastole is the mean volume rate of flow (cardiac output in milliliters per minute) divided by the filling or emptying time in seconds per minute.

A sample calculation of mitral valve area is as follows:

Cardiac output (CO) = 5000 mL/min
Diastolic filling period (DFP) beat = 0.38 s/beat
Pulse rate = 90 beats/min
DFP/min = 34 s/min
Left atrial mean diastolic pressure (LAP) = 30 mmHg
Left ventricular mean diastolic pressure (LVDP) = 5 mmHg
C = 0.85 (orifice constant for the mitral valve)[83]

$$\text{Mitral valve flow (MVF)} = \frac{\text{CO}}{\text{DFP/min}} = \frac{5000\ \text{mL/min}}{34\ \text{s/min}} = 147\ \text{mL/s of diastole}$$

$$\text{Mitral valve orifice area (MAV)} = \frac{\text{MVF}}{0.85 \times 44.5\sqrt{\text{LAP} - \text{LVDP}}} = \frac{147}{38\sqrt{25}} = 0.8\ \text{cm}^2$$

The calculation for the aortic valve area is as follows:

$$\text{AVA (in cm}^2) = \frac{F}{C \times 44.5\sqrt{P_1 - P_2}} = \frac{\text{aortic valve flow (mL/s of systole)}}{1 \times 44.5\sqrt{\text{LVS} - \text{ASP}}}$$

where LVS = left ventricular systolic mean pressure, mmHg
ASP = aortic systolic mean pressure, mmHg*
C = orifice constant coefficient (value of 1 for the aortic valve)

Similarly, orifice areas may be calculated for the tricuspid and pulmonary valves, using an orifice constant of 1.0. The approximations and systematic errors in the formula do not detract from their usefulness in providing objectivity in the classification of patients with valvular disease. Valve orifices may not be constant but may be flow and pressure dependent. Modifications of the widely used Gorlin formula have been made. To estimate aortic valve area, the Bache formula uses either the peak-to-peak or the maximum systolic gradient, thus avoiding planimetry.[85] Hakki omits the heart rate, the ejection or filling period, and the empiric constant. He uses the square root of either the mitral mean, aortic mean, or aortic peak pressure gradients divided into the cardiac output. In the absence of bradycardia or tachycardia, the Hakki mitral or aortic valve area generally agrees with the Gorlin areas.[86,87] The Cannon formula omits taking the square root of the mean transvalvar gradient (ΔP), stating that at any given valve area, flow is a linear function of ΔP.[88] If flow is normal, reducing a valve orifice diameter to less than half or the cross-sectional area to one-fourth is generally required to offer significant obstruction. A significantly reduced mitral valve area is 1 cm^2; aortic valve area is 0.7 cm^2. Calculation of the orifice area of a stenotic valve in the presence of associated valvular regurgitation must take into consideration the added regurgitant flow or the severity of the

*If the femoral artery is used, the aortic gradient from the simultaneous left ventricular–femoral artery pressure tracing should be averaged with the gradient obtained from the tracing that is realigned to correct for the central to peripheral time lag of the femoral pulse.[84]

stenosis will be overestimated. To obtain an estimate of mitral or aortic regurgitant volume, the forward stroke volume (Fick) should be subtracted from total angiographic left ventricular stroke volume. (See Chaps. 79 and 80.)

SELECTIVE ANGIOGRAPHY

Since 1947, when contrast medium was first injected through a rubber catheter placed in the right ventricle,[89] the technique of selective angiography has been continually refined. In the patient with valvar or congenital heart disease, the diagnosis is often initially made by noninvasive imaging. Catheterization and angiography are then done as directed studies in order to provide physiological data and additional anatomic detail. A catheter with a large lumen facilitates rapid low-pressure delivery of a single bolus of the contrast agent. A closed-end catheter with laterally directed openings reduces recoil. A balloon-tipped angiographic catheter with proximal side holes is easy to manipulate and induces less ectopy than do conventional catheters (Fig. 138-15). A power injector delivers the desired volume of contrast media at a preselected maximal flow rate. In adults with complex cyanotic congenital heart disease, a large NIH catheter (up to 12F) inserted via the femoral vein can deliver 70 to 80 mL of contrast media in 2 s without recoil.

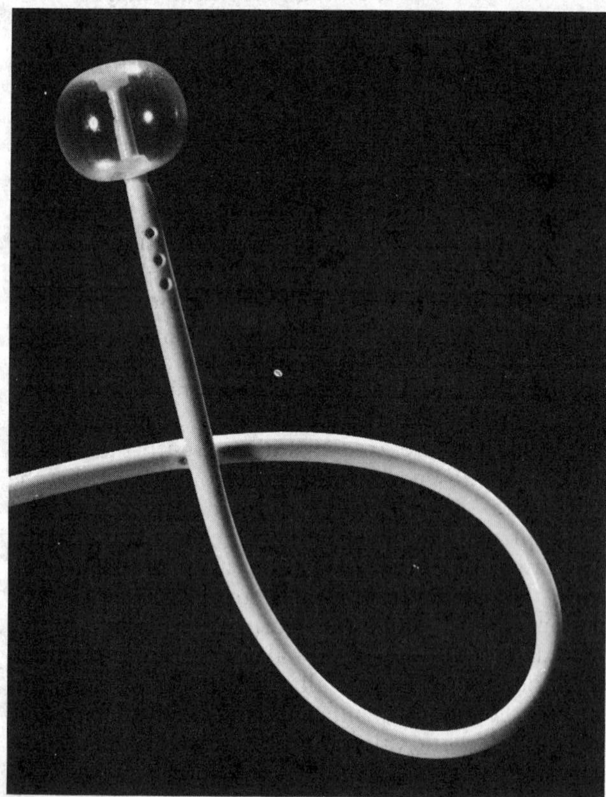

FIGURE 138-15 A Berman balloon angiographic catheter permits easy access to the right ventricle, the pulmonary artery, and if an atrial septal defect is crossed, the left ventricle and even the aorta. Maximum flow rates of contrast media are 5, 14, and 20 mL/s for nos. 5, 6, and 7 French catheters, respectively; myocardial staining and ventricular ectopy are reduced by this method. (*Courtesy of Critikon, a Johnson & Johnson Company.*)

Positioning the catheter in the apex of either ventricle or in the great arteries is done by using a tip deflector wire and by taking advantage of septal defects.

Contrast Media

In 1923, Osborn noted that the urinary bladder of luetic patients treated with oral and intravenous sodium iodide became opaque to x-rays because of the absorption of photons by iodine.

All contrast media contain three iodine molecules attached to a fully substituted benzene ring. The fourth position in the standard ionic agent is taken up by sodium or methylglucamine as cation; the remaining two positions of the benzene ring have side chains of diatrizoate or metatrizoate or iothalamate. All media are excreted predominantly by glomerular filtration. The normal half-time of excretion is 20 min; biliary excretion is 1 percent. A dose of 2 mL/kg of medium may be scaled up or down in relation to total body weight, size of the heart chambers, systemic blood flow, degree of left-to-right shunting, severity of pulmonary vascular disease, and clinical status of the patient. Since significant hemodynamic changes may rapidly follow the administration of contrast media, serial injections should ideally be spaced in time as the clinical status of the patient dictates. Marked systemic vasodilatation occurs within 30 s, accompanied by transient decrease in arterial pressure returning to control or slightly higher levels within 1 or 2 min.[90] A peak increase in cardiac output occurs at 2 min, and an increase in left ventricular ejection time index is noted within 1 min, reflecting the transient increase in stroke volume modified by the negative inotropic effect of the contrast medium. In 1 to 2 min, the plasma volume increases 2 to 14 percent and the plasma osmolality increases to 3 to 9 percent. Transient hypervolemia and depressed contractility are in part responsible for the elevation of left atrial and left ventricular end-diastolic pressure.

To reduce the osmotic effects of contrast medium, the number of dissolved particles must be decreased[91] or the molal concentration of iodine per particle must be increased (Fig. 138-16). New generation, nonionic, monomer, and ionic dimer contrast agents have approximately the same viscosity and iodine concentration but have only one-half or less the osmolality of the ionic agents, e.g., iopamidol and ioxaglic acid (ioxaglate), 796 and 560 mosmol/kg H_2O, respectively, versus 1689 mosmol/kg H_2O for diatriozate sodium.[92] The advantages of the new agents include less hemodynamic loading,[93–95] patient discomfort, binding of ionic calcium,[96] depression of myocardial function and blood pressure, and possibly less anaphylactoid reaction. A disadvantage is the high cost that leads to a policy of selected use.[97] Also, while standard contrast media have a moderate anticoagulant effect, nonionic media have only a slight anticoagulant effect, and the catheter and syringe containing them should thus be kept free of blood.[98,99] The principal use of the new agents may be in very ill patients, especially infants in heart failure[100]; in adults with extremely poor left ventricular function; in patients with renal disease, especially in diabetics; and in patients with a history of serious reaction to contrast media or with

CONTRAST MEDIA

	Standard Agents	New Generation Agents	
	High Osmolality	Low Osmolality	
Structure	Ionic Monoacid Monomer	Non-Ionic Monomer	Ionic Monoacid Dimer
Benzene Rings	One	One	Two
Cation	One	None	One
Moles of Iodine	Three	Three	Six
Particles in Solution	Two	One	Two
Molal Concentration Of Iodine Per Particle	1.5	3.0	3.0
Side Chains	Ditrizoate[1] Metrizoate[2] Iothalamate[3]	Metrizamide[4] Iopamidol[5] Iohexol[6]	Ioxaglate[7]
Proprietary Names	[1]Renografin 76 Angiovist Hypaque [2]Isopaque [3]Conray	[4]Amipaque [5]Isovue [6]Omnipaque	[7]Hexabrix

FIGURE 138-16 Comparison of structure, iodine per particle, and side chain between standard and new contrast media. The number next to the proprietary name identifies the side chain it contains.

multiple allergies. If standard high-osmolality agents are used, those that are non–calcium binding may produce less negative inotropic effect and less ventricular fibrillation.[101]

Filming Methods

Cineangiography uses intensification and amplification fluoroscopy and provides reliable filming by a 35-mm movie camera as well as television monitoring and tape or disc recording.[102] Though the detail of the individual cine frame lacks the spatial resolution of the cut-film screen angiogram, the motion itself increases visual perception by noise averaging and use of the integrating (5 frames per second) or persistence ability of the eye (0.2 s). The circular image of the phosphor is usually overframed on relatively slow 35-mm film with an 18 × 24-mm useful film area. Finally, meticulous attention to film processing and the film type is essential to obtaining the desired contrast and image detail. For coronary angiography high-contrast, sharp, white images on a dark background are desired; in the congenital heart patient a wide gray scale helps to define the anatomy by supplying varying opacification density. Biplane cineangiography with biplane video recording is highly desirable in the study of complex congenital heart defects, especially in infancy. The total amount of contrast medium is significantly reduced, and chamber and great-vessel relations are better defined.

To perform computer-enhanced digital angiography, the catheterization laboratory image intensifier and video camera are linked to an analog-to-digital converter, computer system, and digital storage device. The analog video signal is digitized into a series of discrete numerical values that represent continuous voltage fluctuation and can be stored on disks. The images are acquired in the standard cineradiographic mode and are simultaneously stored on film via the cine camera and digitized from the video image. The digital information is enhanced for display by a real-time image processor and is stored on a digital disk for further processing. In single-plane acquisition, exposure rates of 15, 30, and 60 frames per second in a 512 × 512 matrix are available. In simultaneous biplane acquisition, 15 and 30 frames per second are possible. Enhanced images can be recalled and reviewed to allow selection of a freeze frame. The selected image can be stored and displayed on a separate monitor. A real-time image processor enhances and smooths the fluoroscopic image. For difficult projections, pulsed fluoroscopy is available on demand at approximately half the cine dose level, the last 5 s of which can be stored on digital disk for instant review. Varying degrees of enhancement, frame rates, and exposure times can be selected from a preprogrammed push-button module. Analytical programs include subtraction capabilities, ventricular ejection fraction, edge enhancement, and regional and global wall motion. An image mask is made electronically by reversing the polarity of the background image of bone and tissue. The mask is then superimposed on the angiographic image. The positive and negative images of the competing tissue background cancel, leaving the digital subtraction angiogram. Arterial stenosis quantification and 2X zoom magnification can be performed in postprocessing. A hand-held infrared control device permits image review and freeze-frame storage during the study. It can be placed in a sterile bag and operated by the cardiologist at tableside. Postcase review and additional image processing are accomplished via the view panel. Hard-copy images of selected frames, which are particularly useful for interventional procedures, can be recorded via video paper, x-ray film, or laser copier. In practice, the resolution of the digital arteriogram from the hard disk approaches that of cine film. Thus, once a practical way of permanent image archiving is established and if a standard compatible system for exporting image data is developed, digital angiography is likely to replace film in the catheterization laboratory.

Positioning

Universal positioning capability of the x-ray and intensifier tubes by using stands of L-, U-, or C-arm configuration permits angled views of a supine patient. Two profile views of the curved ventricular septum (VS) are needed. They are made in degrees of axial obliquity and cranial angulation as follows: (1) The 40° left anterior oblique (LAO) and 30° cranial position (four-chamber view) outlines the posterior third of the ventricular septum, the valve plane in AV canal defects, and the four heart chambers without superimposition. (2) The 60° LAO and 30° cranial position (long axial view) outlines the anterior two-thirds of the ventricular septum, the membranous ventricular septal defect, and the left ventricular outflow tract. An elongated right anterior oblique (RAO) view, which is useful for seeing the right ventricular infundibulum and supracristal ventricular septal defect, is obtained by 30° axial right anterior oblique and 40° cranial angulation. The main pulmonary artery and its bifurcation are seen in the frontal position with 30° of cranial angulation; a steep LAO position with marked cranial angulation is also used.[107] Patient positioning for angulated views using a fixed horizontal tube and vertical biplane tubes has been elegantly outlined.[103,104]

A successful procedure results when a rapid injection of the proper volume of contrast medium is made through an adequate-sized catheter, properly positioned, with detailed attention to radiologic technique and to the position of the x-ray tube or tubes.

Uses of Angiography

Right atrial angiography is useful in defining (1) the tricuspid valve in Ebstein's anomaly and tricuspid atresia or stenosis, (2) myxoma or thrombus, (3) juxtaposition of right atrial appendage in cyanotic congenital heart disease, (4) the right atrial border in effusion or tumor, and (5) atrial septal defect with right-to-left shunting or occasionally an anomalous pulmonary vein by reflux. In the lateral position a right ventricular injection is used in order to study the caliber and the level of obstruction to right ventricular outflow and the relation of the great vessels to the right ventricle (Figs. 138-17 and 138-18). A pulmonary artery injection may be used to fill the left side of the heart in order to detect a left-to-right shunt and to detect the site of partial (Fig. 138-19) or total anomalous venous drainage of the pulmonary veins and to visualize the pulmonary artery and its branches. An atrial septal defect is best defined by selectively injecting the right upper-lobe pulmonary vein rather than the left atrium itself. In patients with an endocardial cushion defect and an ostium primum atrial defect, selective left ventricular (LV) angiography shows relative elongation (Swan's neck) of the LV outflow tract and shortening of the LV inflow tract due to deficiency of the upper part of the inlet ventricular septum (Fig. 138-20). To identify the pulmonary arteries in cases of pulmonary atresia with ventricular septal defect or to identify one pulmonary artery in cases where a shunt procedure has inadvertently produced discontinuity between right and left branches, a hand injection of contrast media into an end-hole balloon catheter occluding a pulmonary vein or into a conventional catheter in the pulmonary vein wedge position will frequently retrogradely opacify the ipsilateral pulmonary artery back to its main confluence.[105–107] The size and site of origin of multiple systemic-to-pulmonary-artery collaterals arising from the descending aorta should be defined.

Valve Regurgitation

Injections made above the aortic valve serve to detect aortic regurgitation. In milder degrees of aortic regurgitation, a regurgitant jet is noted; opacification is limited

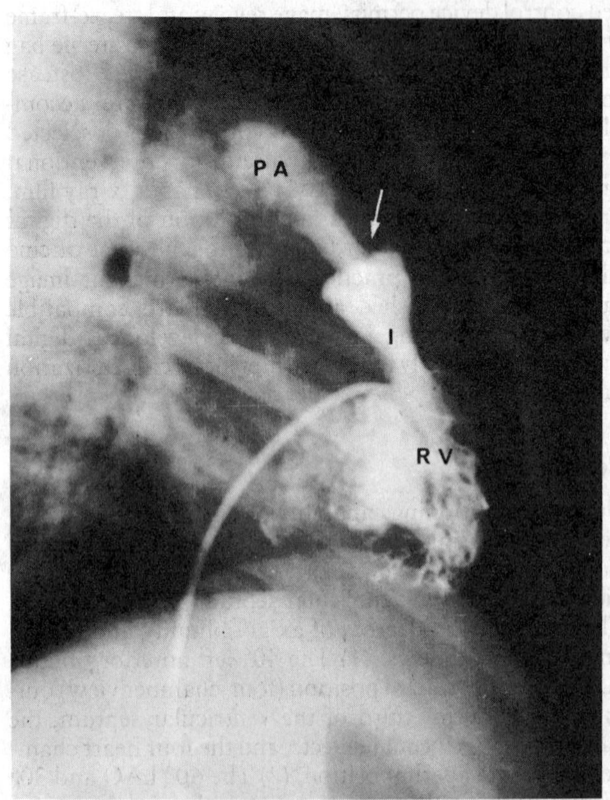

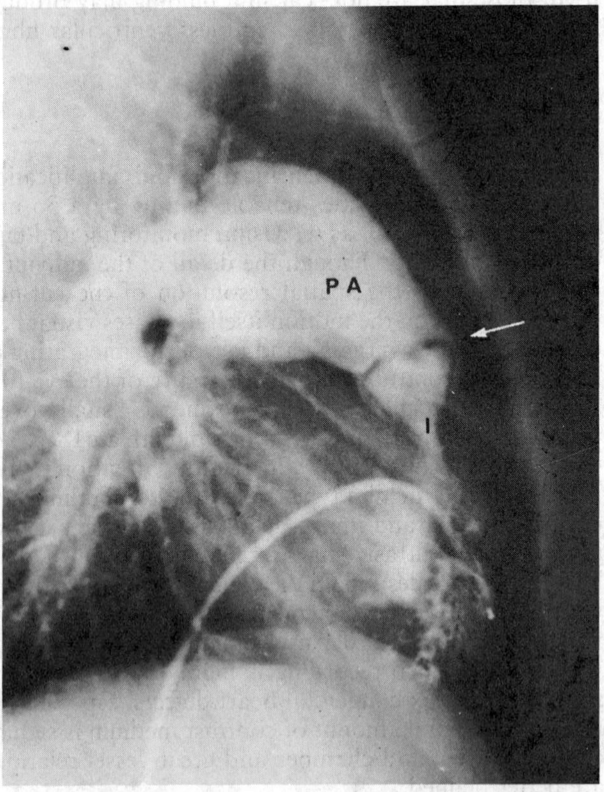

FIGURE 138-17 *A.* Valvular pulmonary stenosis (lateral view). Right ventricular injection of opaque medium. Contrast material exits through central orifice of pulmonary valve in form of a jet (arrow). RV = right ventricle; I = infundibulum of right ventricle; PA = pulmonary artery. *B.* Valvular pulmonary stenosis (lateral view). Right ventricular injection of opaque medium reveals bulging of fused cusps (arrow) into dilated pulmonary artery and narrowing of infundibulum of right ventricle.

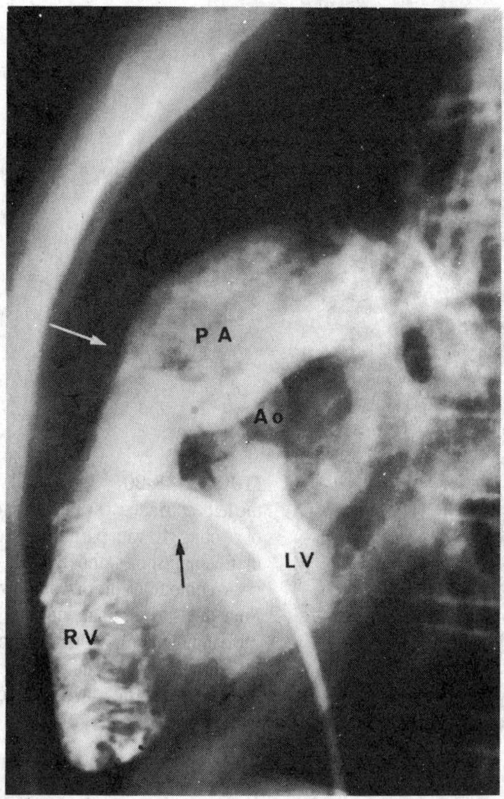

FIGURE 138-18 Ventricular septal defect and pulmonary hypertension (lateral view). Right ventricular injection reveals normal outflow and moderate-sized ventricular septal defect (bottom arrow) in membranous portion of ventricular septum. Contrast material passes into the aorta. Observe large size of main pulmonary artery and normal pulmonary valve (top arrow). PA = pulmonary artery; Ao = aorta; RV = right ventricle; LV = left ventricle.

to the left ventricular outflow tract, clearing with each systole (grade 1), or faint, persistent, incomplete opacification of the left ventricular cavity (grade 2) occurs. In grades 3 and 4, no distinct jet is seen, and dense complete opacification of the left ventricle occurs either progressively or in one or two diastolic cycles, and left ventricular density exceeds aortic density in the severe case. After an aortic injection, the size and mobility of a stenotic aortic valve may be visualized by negative-contrast washout of the opacified aorta with nonopaque ventricular blood. In the LAO view the mouthlike opening of a bicuspid aortic valve is seen. A left ventricular injection may display the level of obstruction to left ventricular outflow. In patients with endocardial cushion defect, the frontal view may show a radiolucent notch in the anterior mitral valve leaflet or between the superior and inferior bridging leaflets of the AV valve; the left ventricular outflow tract has an elongated or gooseneck appearance in early diastole while the inflow tract is shortened.

Left ventricular injection in the RAO view is used to detect and grossly quantitate mitral regurgitation. The angiographic criteria for grading mitral regurgitation are somewhat subjective, and so disagreement may arise between observers in assessing the degree of reflux. In grades 1 and 2 mitral regurgitation, a narrow- to moderate-width regurgitant jet of slight to moderate density is noted; minimum to moderate opacification of the left atrium clears quickly. In grades 3 and 4, a well-defined jet is absent and left atrial opacification is intense, immediate, and lingering, and so the left atrium appears denser than the left ventricle or aorta in grade 4 mitral regurgitation. In mitral valve prolapse, which is shown best in a lateral projection with slight cranial angulation, all or a

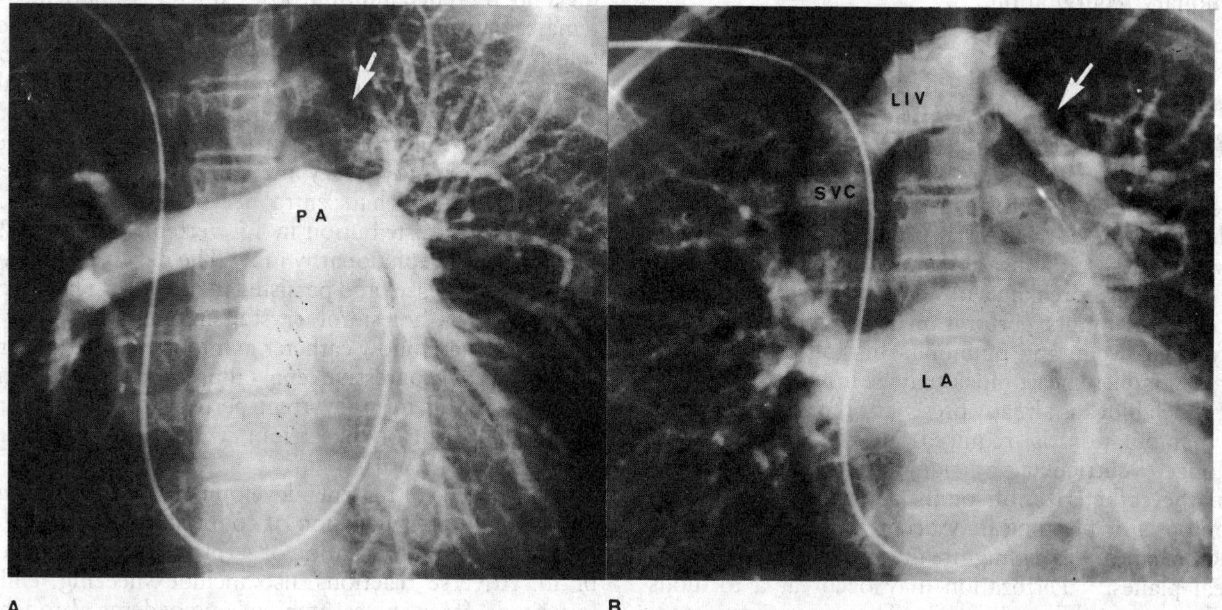

FIGURE 138-19 Partial anomalous drainage of pulmonary veins (frontal view). *A.* The catheter has been introduced into the right atrium and ventricle and positioned in the main pulmonary artery (PA), where selective injection is performed. *B.* Pulmonary venous phase. A large pulmonary vein (arrow) drains the upper lobe of the left lung, with anomalous venous return to the left brachiocephalic vein. SVC = superior vena cava; LA = left atrium.

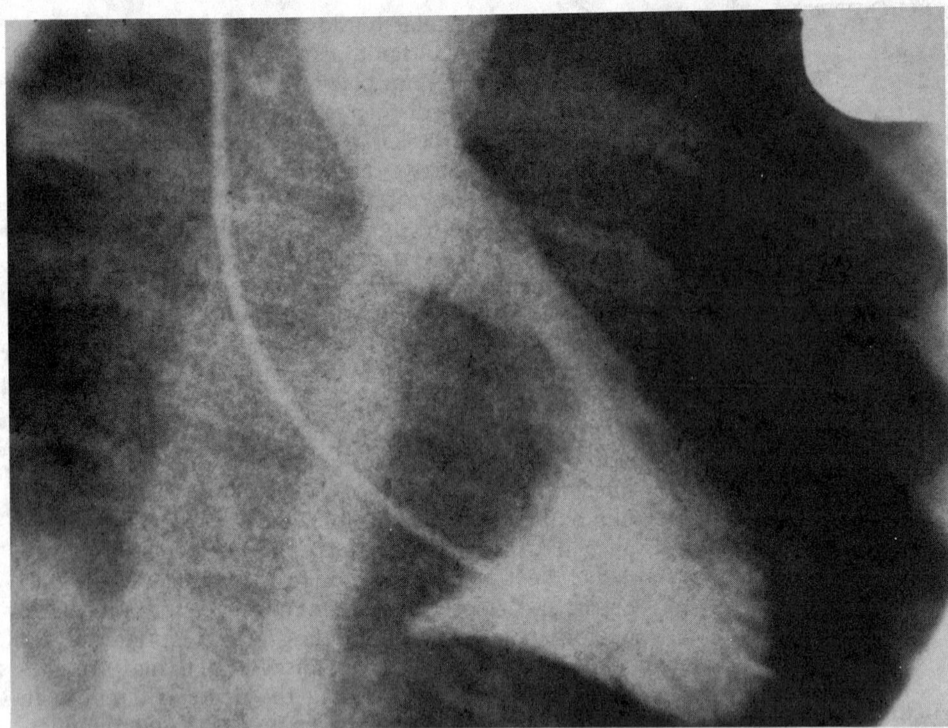

FIGURE 138-20 The frontal view of the left ventricular (LV) cineangiogram of a young girl with partial atrioventricular canal shows the typical swan's neck contour of the LV outflow tract. Note the shorter than normal mitral valve annulus to LV apex distance (the LV inflow tract) in comparison to the LV apex to aortic valve distance (LV outflow tract).

portion of one or both leaflets balloon above the mitral annulus in systole with or without associated mitral valve regurgitation. A normal mitral valve may leak if ectopic beating occurs. Unlike disc or ball valves, prosthetic tissue valves can be crossed with the catheter tip without interfering with valve function. Selective RV angiography in the RAO or lateral position via a pigtail catheter lying in the apex of the right ventricle gives adequate evaluation of tricuspid regurgitation.[108] Reflux into the superior vena cava and inferior vena cava is associated with severe tricuspid regurgitation. A properly placed main pulmonary artery catheter will detect significant pulmonary regurgitation.

COMPLICATIONS OF CARDIAC CATHETERIZATION AND ANGIOGRAPHY

An experienced operator can carry out catheterization of the right side of the heart without difficulty in practically all cases. Complications may include knotting of the catheter[109]; breakage of the guide wire; excessive blood loss in infants; perforation of the atrium, ventricle, or coronary vein; and pulmonary infarction or hemorrhage. Complete heart block may be induced if left bundle branch block is already present or if prolonged catheter manipulation is required in a cyanotic infant. Prolonged ventricular or atrial arrhythmia may occur.

In the catheterization of the left side of the heart, thrombosis or bleeding may occur at the percutaneous puncture site and may migrate into fascial and retroperitoneal planes.[110] Perforation may occur at a tortuous subclavian or pelvic arterial site. The commonest vascular complication is femoral arterial pseudoaneurysm or pulsating hematoma, in part due to the increased use of heparin postcatheterization (Fig. 138-4). Pseudoaneurysm following catheterization may be detected by color Doppler flow imaging. In systole a high-velocity flow signal moves into the sac of the pseudoaneurysm from the small puncture site in the superficial or common femoral artery; in diastole there is a low-flow velocity from the sac into the femoral artery retrogradely. In the presence of the femoral artery to femoral vein fistula there is a constant-flow signal from the artery to the vein.[111,112] Among 23,000 patients (72 percent males) at Emory University Hospital who had coronary artery angiography via the percutaneous femoral approach using a no. 8 French multipurpose catheter, 14 patients (12 females and 2 males) required femoral artery thrombectomy. The smaller femoral artery of the female is more prone to thrombotic occlusion than is that of the male. Arteriovenous fistula occurs uncommonly. Cerebral embolism may result from plaque dislodgment or fibrin clot. In 30,000 coronary artery and left ventricular catheterizations 35 patients had central nervous system complications (carotid distribution in 15, vertebrobasilar in 20, and diffuse encephalopathy in 2). The deficit resolved in one-half of all cases and persisted in one-half. There were two deaths. Cholesterol crystal embolization shower syndrome may follow catheter manipulation in the aorta and results in progressive renal failure. Transseptal puncture may result in inadvertent perforation of the aorta or the free wall of the atrium, with resultant cardiac tamponade.

Ten percent of patients develop nausea and vomiting immediately after injection of contrast media, probably related to direct stimulation of serotonin receptors in the brain. Adverse reactions also include sneezing, chills, low-grade fever, hives, itching, angioedema, bronchospasm, and shock.[113] Since no anticontrast media immunoglobulin E (IgE) is found, these reactions are anaphylactoid rather than being true anaphylaxis. The mechanism may be related to activation of kallikrein, classical or alternate complement, or intrinsic coagulation systems or to direct hyperosmolar or chemical cytoxocity.[114] Rare reactions include parotitis (iodide mumps), glossitis, and pancreatic edema. A two-dose oral corticosteroid regimen (methylprednisolone 32 mg) given 12 and 2 h before standard contrast media injection significantly reduces acute allergic reactions. Diphenhydramine hydrochloride, cimetidine hydrochloride, and ephedrine sulfate, singly or combined, have been added to prednisone.[115] Patients at high risk for contrast media nephropathy usually have preexisting renal failure or diabetes with renal disease. Good hydration before the procedure is essential, and mannitol and loop diuretics may be used to diminish the induced renal insufficiency. The mechanism of contrast nephrotoxicity is related in part to renal cortical vasoconstriction and to tubular cell toxicity.[116–118] The risk of renal insult is still present with low-osmolality media. There is no difference in the rise in serum creatinine postangiography in either low- or high-risk groups whether ionic or nonionic contrast media are used.[119,120] Pulmonary edema following angiography may be caused by volume overload and a negative inotropic effect.[121] (See also Chap. 29.)

In desperately ill cyanotic infants and in those with marked ventricular dysfunction or severe valvular obstruction, the desire for films that display the cardiac anatomy spectacularly should be tempered by the potential consequences of large doses of contrast medium in this setting.

CORONARY ARTERIOGRAPHY AND LEFT VENTRICULOGRAPHY

Coronary arteriography remains the standard by which all methods of diagnosing coronary artery disease are measured. It is the primary method of defining coronary anatomy in living patients. To accomplish this in a safe, reliable, and reproducible manner, adherence to certain principles of performance and interpretation is required.[122–124]

Coronary arteriography provides not only an anatomic map of the coronary arteries, including the site, severity, and shape of stenotic lesions, but also the characteristics of distal vessels in terms of size, presence of atherosclerotic disease, mass of myocardium served, a rough index of differential coronary flow, identification of collateral vessels, and an estimate of their functional importance.[125–134] Intracoronary thrombi can be recognized, although it is clear from angioscopic studies that coronary arteriography is relatively insensitive in the detection of thrombi. In addition, the presence of coronary spasm can be ascertained by using provocative maneuvers.[135–140] The functional significance of a coronary stenosis can be assessed by directly measuring coronary flow both at rest and during an intense coronary dilator stimulus. The difference between resting and maximal coronary flow is the coronary flow reserve capacity of the coronary bed. Coronary flow reserve can be measured in the coronary arteriography laboratory using a digital subtraction technique or by intracoronary Doppler techniques.[141]

Left ventricular catheterization makes possible measurements of left ventricular pressure at rest, with exercise, or after pharmacologic agents. Left ventriculography enables one to make a visual analysis of wall motion. Ventricular systolic and diastolic volume and ejection fraction can be calculated. Careful correlation of the coronary arteriogram and left ventriculogram permits identification of stenotic and potentially bypassable arteries serving viable myocardium. Left ventricular wall motion can be further evaluated by the addition of stress such as atrial pacing, pharmacologic agents, or exercise. Augmenting left ventricular contraction by the use of nitrates, catecholamines, or postextrasystolic beats may permit the identification of left ventricular wall segments that have a potential for improved function after revascularization surgery.[142–144] The presence of associated valvular heart disease may be determined. In patients who have undergone surgery previously, patency of grafts and status of the native coronary arteries can be ascertained. In certain children with congenital heart disease, the location of the coronary arteries can be determined as an aid to planning surgical correction.[145,146]

Techniques of Coronary Arteriography

Sones ushered in the modern era of coronary arteriography in 1958 when he developed a safe and reliable method of selective coronary arteriography.[125] The Sones technique utilizes an antecubital incision over the brachial artery. The artery is exposed, and a woven Dacron catheter (Sones USCI) is passed into the brachial artery and maneuvered through the axillary and subclavian arteries into the ascending aorta. Manipulation techniques depend on defecting the soft, tapered catheter tip off the aortic valve cusps up to the coronary orifices. The Sones technique has stood the test of time. The advantages are that it requires only one catheter, aortoiliac disease is avoided, and the operator is close to the aortic root and therefore gets the best feel of the catheter tip. The disadvantages are that an antecubital dissection, arteriotomy, and arterial closure are needed. Manipulation skills and precise knowledge of the aortic root anatomy are required. A detailed description of the Sones technique has been published.[147]

Percutaneous arterial catheterization, described in 1953 by Seldinger[148] (Fig. 138-1), was first used to study the coronary arteries as reported by Rickets and Abrams in 1962.[149] Modification of catheters was made by Amplatz et al.[150] and by Judkins[151] in 1967. The Judkins technique requires three preformed catheters: one for each coronary artery and a pigtail catheter for the left ventricular injection. The Judkins technique is much easier to learn; paradoxically, this may be its major drawback. The femoral artery is punctured below the inguinal ligament, and a left coronary artery catheter is passed over the guide wire into the aorta. After the catheter is flushed and good pressure tracings are obtained from the tip, the catheter is advanced until it engages the left coronary orifice. The preformed shape of the catheter holds it against the inside of the aortic curve, enabling the tip to spring into the left coronary orifice. The tip is made in four lengths for use with different-sized aortic roots. After the left catheter is removed, the appropriate-sized right coronary catheter is inserted over a guide wire and positioned above the right coronary orifice, where it is rotated clockwise. The tip will descend and will be held against the outside curve of the aorta, causing it to spring into the right coronary orifice. Left ventricular studies are performed by replacing the coronary catheters with the pigtail catheter. A detailed description of the Judkins technique has also been published.[152]

This technique has the advantages of a percutaneous approach; the disadvantages are the requirement for multiple catheter exchanges and a potential increased rick of emboli to the coronary or cerebral circulation. Complications may arise from the ease of entry of the catheter tip into the coronary arteries. Some poorly trained angiographers have applied this technique without proper appreciation of the devastating consequences of catheter obstruction of the left main coronary artery. Methods of avoiding serious complications of catheter emboli, including systemic heparinization and catheter debriding techniques, have reduced complications in active centers.

In an attempt to combine the advantages of the Sones and Judkins techniques, the single-catheter percutaneous femoral approach was first applied by Schoonmaker in 1968, and the use of this technique was reported by Schoonmaker and King.[153] This technique has been employed at Emory University Hospital in over 50,000 studies since 1972.

Performance of Coronary Arteriography

The description of our technique of coronary arteriography is brief; a more detailed description has been published.[154] It is the authors' belief that one cannot become expert in performing coronary arteriography by reading. Only through training in an active laboratory and performing hundreds of coronary arteriograms under close supervision can the physician gain a proper appreciation of the potential hazards of coronary arteriography so that they can be avoided.[155]

A close physician-patient relationship is essential to reduce fear of the examination. The patient is seen before the procedure, and a thorough history, physical examination, and description of the procedure are completed. Patients with mild or stable symptoms may undergo coronary arteriography as outpatients unless noninvasive studies indicate the likely presence of severe anatomic problems such as left main coronary artery stenosis. Exclusionary criteria for outpatient catheterization were discussed earlier in this section.[19–21] In most laboratories, outpatient catheterization studies are performed with smaller diameter catheters of a no. 5 to no. 7 French size. Propranolol and nitrates are usually continued up to and through the procedure. An intravenous line is routinely started for administration of 0.6 mg of atropine and 5 to 10 mg of diazepam when sedation is needed. The intravenous line is also essential as a port for the administration of additional drugs during the procedure as needed if pain or hypotension occurs or if congestive failure is aggravated. Electrocardiographic monitoring is performed throughout the procedure. Atropine, lidocaine, propranolol, furosemide, corticosteroids, an antihistamine, nitroglycerin, epinephrine and other vasopressors, and narcotics should be readily available for intravenous administration. Heparin and antibiotics are not routinely administered in our laboratory. Patients with a history of anaphylactoid reactions to contrast media are pretreated with antihistamines and corticosteroids.

A three-way stopcock manifold is connected to lines for pressure monitoring, contrast medium, and heparinized saline solution. A clear catheter is maintained by intermittent flushing with saline solution and contrast medium. The femoral artery is catheterized by the Seldinger technique, and a multipurpose polyurethane catheter is inserted into the descending aorta, where it is flushed before being advanced around the aortic arch without a guide wire. The catheter is advanced to the left ventricle, where, following pressure measurements and test injections to exclude catheter-tip entrapment, 32 to 40 mL of contrast medium is injected over 4 s. This slow injection allows adequate visualization without recoil of the end-hole and side-hole catheter. Filming is routinely done in the RAO view or in a biplane mode using right anterior and left anterior oblique views.

Essential to any coronary arteriographic technique is a thorough knowledge of aortic root anatomy (Fig. 138-21). Usually the left coronary orifice arises from the left sinus of Valsalva, which is posterior and to the left. The right coronary artery usually arises from the right sinus of Valsalva, which is anterior. Because of extensive variation in the position, size, and number of orifices, considerable experience is required to avoid failure to identify and study one of the arteries. Left coronary cannulation is performed in the following manner: The tip of the catheter is placed in the non-coronary cusp which lies posterior and to the left (toward the spine in the right anterior oblique view). As the catheter is advanced with a slight clockwise rotation, the tip flips up into the left coronary ostium or into the left cusp. From the left coronary cusp, the catheter tip can be rotated posteriorly and advanced superiorly into the left coronary ostium (Fig. 138-21). Right coronary artery catheterization is

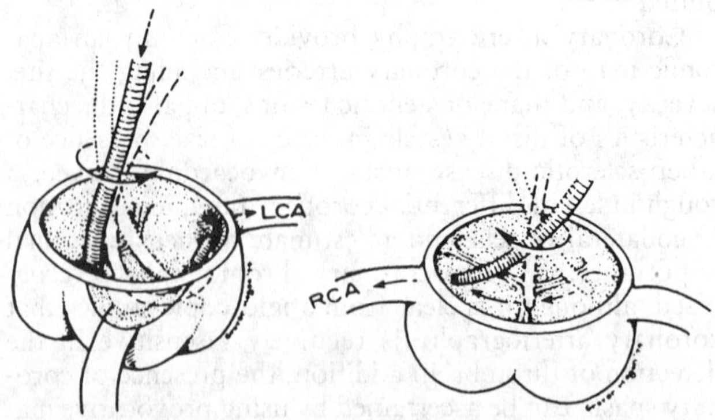

FIGURE 138-21 *Left.* A 30° right anterior oblique view of the aortic root demonstrating the left coronary orifice. *Right.* A 60° left anterior oblique view of the aortic root demonstrating location of the right coronary orifice. (*From Schoonmaker FW, King SB: Coronary arteriography by the single catheter percutaneous femoral technique. Circulation 50:737, 1974. Reproduced with permission from the American Heart Association, Inc., and the authors.*)

done by positioning the tip of the catheter above the left coronary cusp and rotating clockwise so that the tip sweeps along the anterior aortic root until it reaches the right coronary ostium (Fig. 138-21). An alternative method is to advance the catheter tip in the right cusp. It curls into the right orifice. When the operator is unsuccessful in reaching one or the other coronary orifices, the catheter is removed and replaced by an appropriate Judkins or other preformed catheter.

All injections into the coronary arteries are preceded by aspiration of a small amount of contrast medium into the hand-held syringe (to exclude the possibility of air embolism) and are monitored visually until the contrast medium clears. Pressure monitoring is done after these injections. Hypotension following coronary injection usually clears spontaneously or with coughing, which transiently increases aortic pressure and enhances clearing of contrast medium. If hypotension lasting more than a few seconds occurs, especially in a patient with severe proximal coronary artery disease, a pressor agent in an adequate dose to obtain a quick response is started promptly. Adequate coronary perfusion pressure is essential in these patients. If congestive heart failure is aggravated by the effect of contrast medium, the first drug used is sublingual nitroglycerin; furosemide may be needed, however. When chest pain occurs, nitrates are given sublingually or intravenously and the catheter is repositioned in the left ventricle to monitor left ventricular end-diastolic pressure. If pain continues or ST-segment elevation occurs, coronary injection may reveal coronary spasm. Intracoronary nitroglycerin or sublingual nifedipine usually provides prompt relief. If severe elevation of end-diastolic pressure occurs, the patient may be propped up and given additional nitrates and oxygen. When tachycardia accompanied by adequate or elevated blood pressure develops during angina, 1-mg increments of propranolol may be given intravenously, producing dramatic relief. Hypertension is treated with nifedipine, 10 mg sublingually. Narcotics are used for pain that is not promptly relieved by nitroglycerin, nifedipine, and propranolol. Ventricular fibrillation, a rare occurrence, is promptly corrected with the defibrillator. All laboratory personnel must be thoroughly trained in cardiopulmonary resuscitation, as unstable patients may develop life-threatening arrhythmias before, during, and after angiography. Minor anaphylactoid reactions are treated with antihistamines; more serious reactions are treated with the addition of epinephrine and corticosteroids.[155] Maximal safety is obtained when an expert angiographer performs a brief but complete study, obtaining all clinically pertinent information with a minimal number of injections. Because of the osmotic diuresis induced by the contrast media, intravenous and oral fluid supplements are required after catheterization, and postural hypotension must be checked for when the patient is allowed up.

Interpretation of the Coronary Arteriogram

Once of interest to angiographers and surgeons only, the viewing and interpretation of coronary angiograms should now be of vital interest to cardiologists if they are to make informed decisions about their patients.

The coronary arteriogram should be viewed in a systematic fashion. Because coronary anatomy can be quite variable, one needs to view the films with an eye toward making sure the entire left ventricular epicardial surface and septum are adequately supplied and that no gaps exist. If significant gaps are found, an occluded or anomalous artery is likely. The coronary arteries should be viewed one at a time, and some division of arterial segments such as the one suggested by the American Heart Association[156] should be made (Fig. 138-22). Areas of foreshortening and overlap should be examined in other views to convince the observer that there is not a hidden lesion. It is helpful for several observers to study the arteriogram. As each segment is viewed, a systematic scoring and recording system is mandatory if consistency is to be maintained and no segments are to be overlooked.

Angiographic Views

Filming is done in a number of projections such that all coronary arteries can be visualized throughout their lengths and significant disease can be detected and quantified. Multiple views in the transverse plane (Figs. 138-23 to 138-25) were utilized until 1973, when Bunnell reported the advantages of obtaining views incorporating sagittal angulation of the x-ray beam along the long axis of the body (Fig. 138-26). The use of these views (Figs. 138-27 and 138-28) greatly enhances the ability to visualize the proximal left coronary artery, unmasking lesions that would otherwise be missed in up to 20 percent of patients and significantly improving diagnosis in an additional 30 to 40 percent.[157-159] The evolution of a new generation of x-ray equipment to obtain these views has revolutionized coronary arteriography.[160] In most laboratories, standard views of the left coronary artery

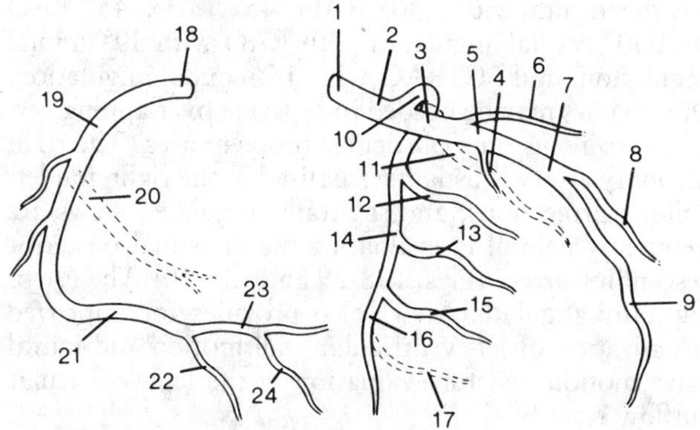

FIGURE 138-22 Diagram of the coronary circulation. Each arterial segment is evaluated carefully in all views and the degree of stenosis is determined. Left main coronary artery 1, 2: left anterior descending coronary artery 3, 5, 7, 9; diagonal branches 6, 8; major septal perforating branch 4; circumflex coronary artery in the atrioventricular groove 10, 14, 16; ramus intermedius 11; obtuse marginal branches 12, 13, 15; posterior descending branch of the circumflex coronary artery if present 17; right coronary artery in the atrioventricular groove 18, 19, 21, 23; large right ventricular branch of the right coronary artery 20; posterior descending branch of the right coronary artery 22; left ventricular branch of the right coronary artery 24. (*From King SB III, Douglas JS Jr: Coronary Arteriography and Angioplasty. New York, McGraw-Hill, 1985, p. 363. Reproduced with permission from the publisher and authors.*)

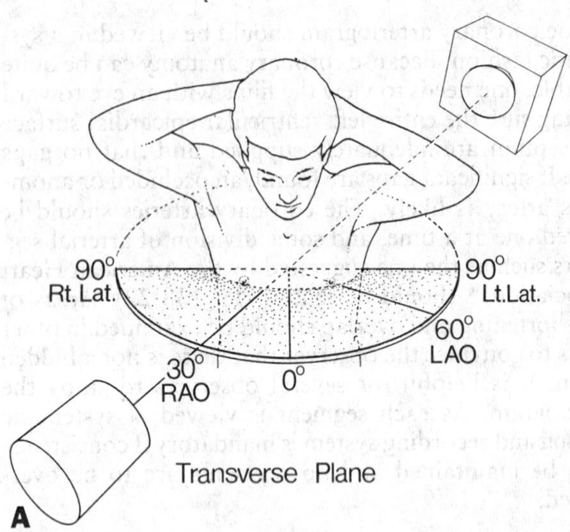

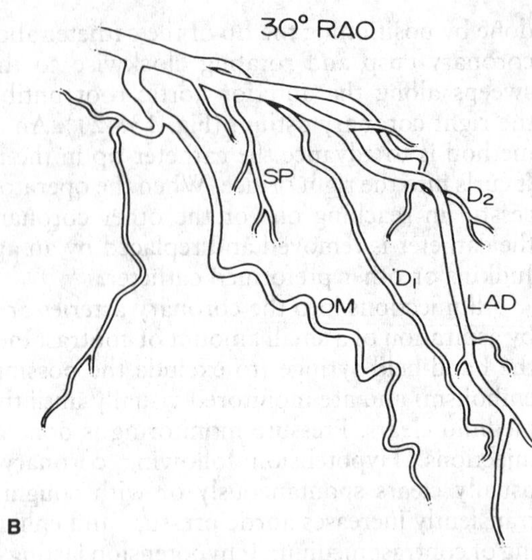

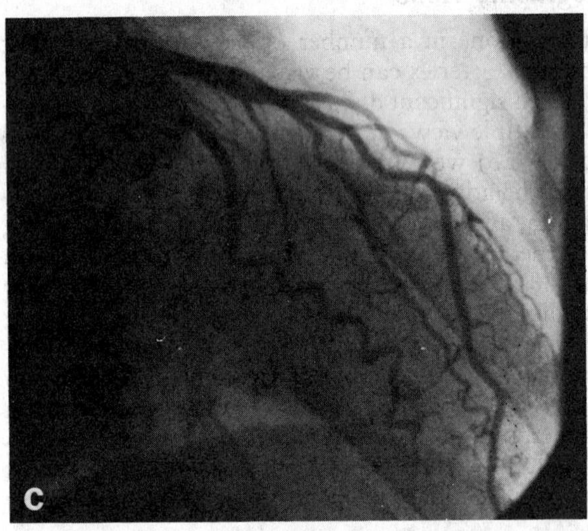

FIGURE 138-23 Diagrammatic representation of the standard right anterior oblique (RAO) view of the left coronary angiogram, the direction of the x-ray beam, and the position of the overhead image intensifier. Most of the left coronary artery is well visualized in this projection, although there is considerable overlap of the mid-left anterior descending artery and the diagonal branches. When the left main, circumflex, and diagonal branches have a leftward initial course, the long axis of these arterial segments is projected away from the image intensifier, preventing optimal visualization from the RAO view. The image intensifier is placed anteriorly in an RAO position relative to the patient. (*From King SB III, Douglas JS Jr, Morris DC: New angiographic views for coronary arteriography. In: Hurst JW (ed): Update IV: The Heart. New York, McGraw-Hill, 1981: 203. Reproduced with permission from the publisher, editor, and authors.*)

are the frontal view, 30° RAO, 45° LAO, 45° LAO with 30° cranial angulation, 30° RAO with 30° cranial angulation, and 30° RAO with 15° caudal angulation. Other views may be needed to separate overlapping vessels or to focus on a particular problem area. The right coronary artery is usually visualized in the right and left oblique projections, and sagittally angulated views are frequently helpful in evaluating the proximal posterior descending artery (Figs. 138-29 and 138-30). The use of sagittally angulated views also provides for improved visualization of left ventricular wall motion and mitral valve motion and for evaluation of the left ventricular outflow tract.[160]

The Left Coronary Artery

The ostium of the left coronary artery originates from the left sinus of Valsalva near the sinotubular ridge. The main left coronary usually courses to the left and slightly anterior. After a quite variable length, it gives rise at near right angles to the circumflex artery and continues in a straight line as the anterior descending artery (Figs. 138-31 and 138-32). The left orifice and the left main coronary artery are best seen in a direct frontal view or in a shallow LAO or RAO projection or a shallow LAO with 30° cranial angulation. The diagonal artery may arise between the circumflex and anterior descending arteries as a trifurcation of the left main coronary artery, or the diagonal branch may originate from the anterior descending artery and course over the anterolateral free wall of the left ventricle. The diagonal branches are seen on the side in the RAO view; however, the origin is obscured by overlap with the anterior descending artery (Figs. 138-31 and 138-32). The LAO view separates the anterior descending artery and diagonals somewhat; however, because of the frequent horizontal orientation of these arteries, there may be considerable foreshortening. Cranial angulation of the overhead intensifier with shallow LAO or RAO rotation is most helpful in separating the proximal anterior descending artery and its diagonal branches (Figs. 138-27 and 138-29). The anterior descending artery continues in the AV groove toward the apex, giving rise at nearly right angles to the septal perforating arteries that go deep into the muscular septum. The first septal perforator may arise before or after the first diagonal and is usually the largest septal artery. The septal vessels differ from the epicardial arteries in that they are straighter and move little with cardiac action, in contrast to the buckling of epicardial arteries that frequently occurs with systole. The left anterior de-

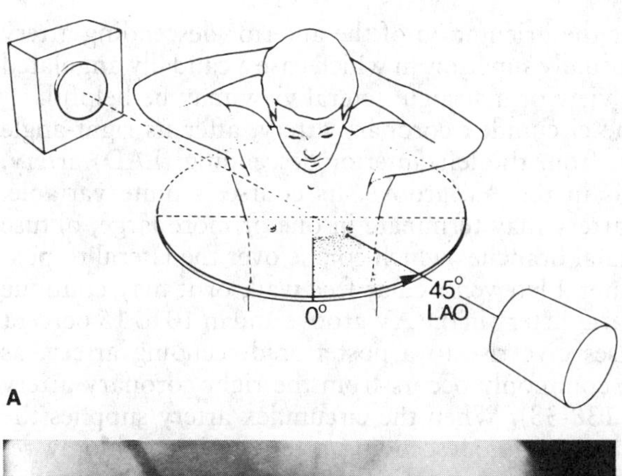

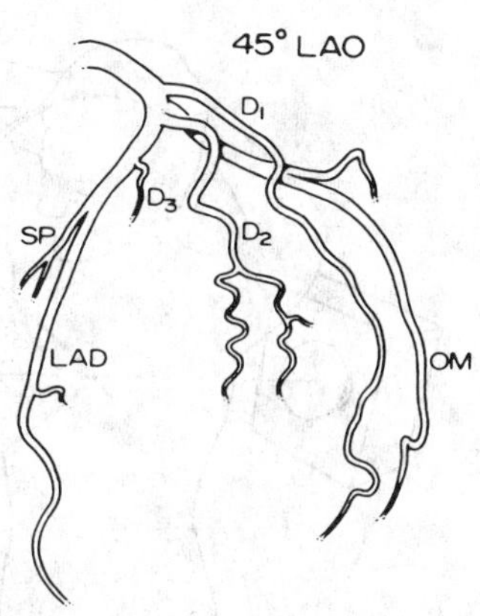

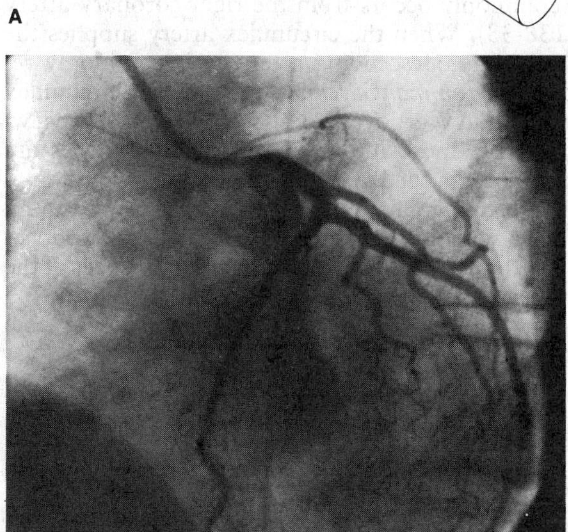

FIGURE 138-24 Diagrammatic representation of the left anterior oblique (LAO) left coronary angiogram and the direction of the x-ray beam in this view. The value of this view depends in large part on the orientation of the long axis of the heart. When the heart is relatively horizontal, the left anterior descending (LAD) coronary artery and diagonal branches are seen end-on throughout much of the course. In this illustration, the longitudinal axis is an intermediate position and there is moderate foreshortening of the anterior descending and diagonal branches in their proximal portions (compare with Fig. 138-27). The LAO projection is frequently inadequate to visualize the proximal LAD and its branches; the left main segment, which is directed toward the image tube and therefore foreshortened; and the proximal circumflex coronary artery, which may be obscured by overlapping vessels, as in this illustration. The LAO projection is frequently used to visualize the distal LAD and its branches, the mid-circumflex coronary artery in the atrioventricular (AV) groove, and the distal right coronary artery that is filling via collaterals from the left coronary artery. The image intensifier is above the patient in an LAO position. *(From King SB III, Douglas JS Jr, Morris DC: New angiographic views for coronary arteriography. In: Hurst JW (ed): The Heart, Update IV. New York, McGraw-Hill, 1981: 204. Reproduced with permission from the publisher, editor, and authors.)*

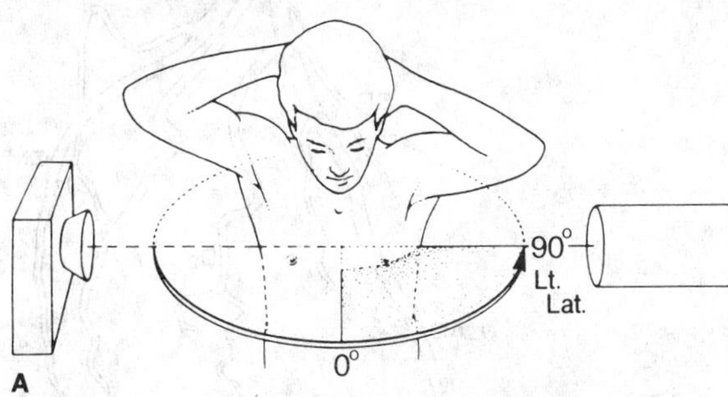

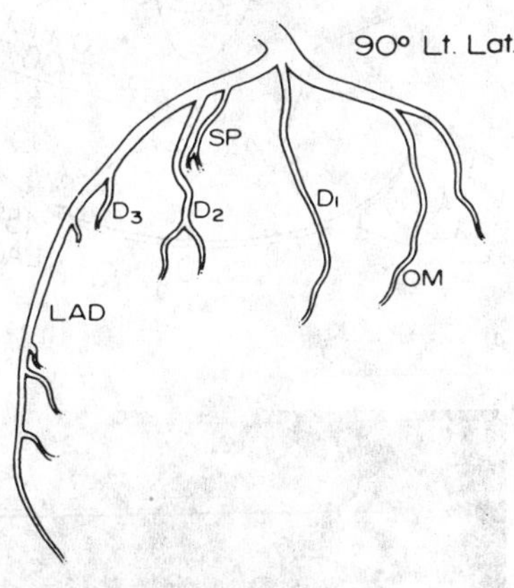

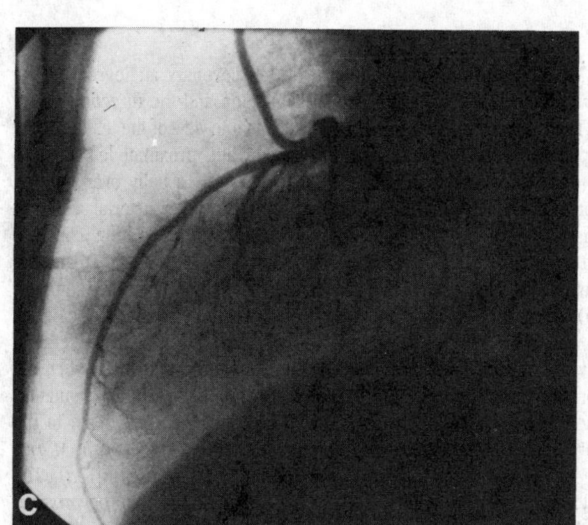

FIGURE 138-25 Diagrammatic illustrations of the left lateral or 90° LAO view of the left coronary arteriogram and direction of the x-ray beam. The left lateral view of the left coronary artery is most useful for analyzing the proximal and mid-LAD by avoiding overlap with the diagonal branches, which commonly take an inferior course from the LAD in this projection. The most proximal portion of the diagonal branches may not be well visualized since the long axis of these segments may be in the direction of the x-ray beam. The leftward-directed left main segment is foreshortened in this view (compare with Fig. 138-27). In this view, the image intensifier is placed on the patient's left, and the x-ray beam has a right-to-left direction in the horizontal plane. *(From King SB III, Douglas JS Jr, Morris DC: New angiographic views for coronary arteriography. In: Hurst JW (ed): The Heart, Update IV. New York, McGraw-Hill, 1981: 205. Reproduced with permission from the publisher, editor, and authors.)*

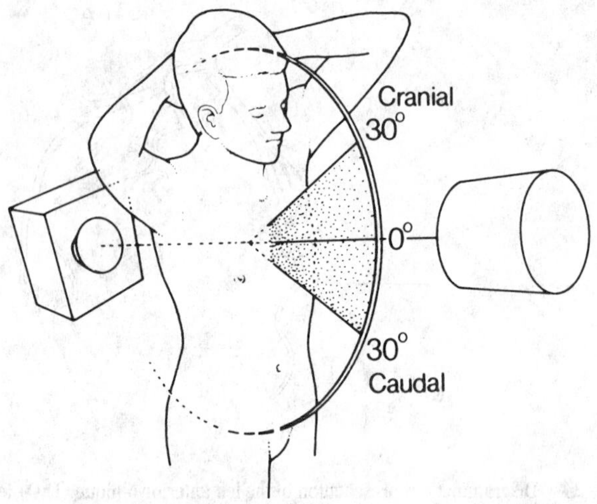

FIGURE 138-26 Illustration of sagittal angulation of x-ray beam in coronary arteriography. (*From King SB III, Douglas JS Jr, Morris DC: New angiographic views for coronary arteriography. In: Hurst JW (ed): The Heart, Update IV. New York, McGraw-Hill, 1981: 205. Reproduced with permission from the publisher, editor, and authors.*)

scending artery usually continues around the apex but may end short of the apex in association with an unusually long posterior descending artery. The anterior descending artery is usually best visualized in the RAO view and in a cranially angulated shallow oblique view unless the orientation of the anterior descending artery is unusually superior, in which case a caudally angulated LAO view or a straight lateral view may be helpful.

The circumflex coronary artery, after its right-angle origin from the left anterior descending (LAD) artery, travels in the AV groove. Its course is quite variable. The artery may terminate in one or more large, obtuse marginal branches which course over the lateral to posterolateral left ventricular free wall, or it may continue as a large artery in the AV groove and in 10 to 15 percent of cases give rise to a posterior descending artery, as more commonly occurs from the right coronary artery (Fig. 138-33). When the circumflex artery supplies the major posterior descending artery, it is commonly referred to as a *dominant circumflex artery*. The circumflex artery in the AV groove is best seen in the LAO view, but surgically more important marginal branches are visualized best in the RAO view. Occasionally proximal stenoses in the circumflex artery are best viewed in an RAO view with 15° caudal angulation, which produces a view as though looking from the superior aspect of the liver toward the left shoulder.

The Right Coronary Artery

The right coronary artery orifice is normally located in the right sinus of Valsalva. It may be high near the sinotubular ridge or above it, in the midsinus, or occasionally low near the aortic valve. The artery commonly courses

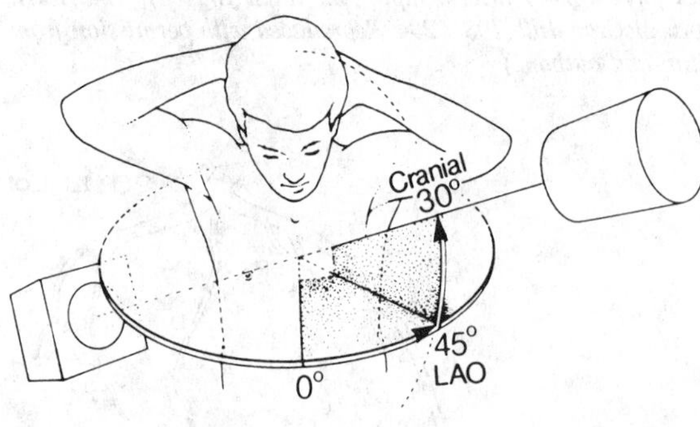

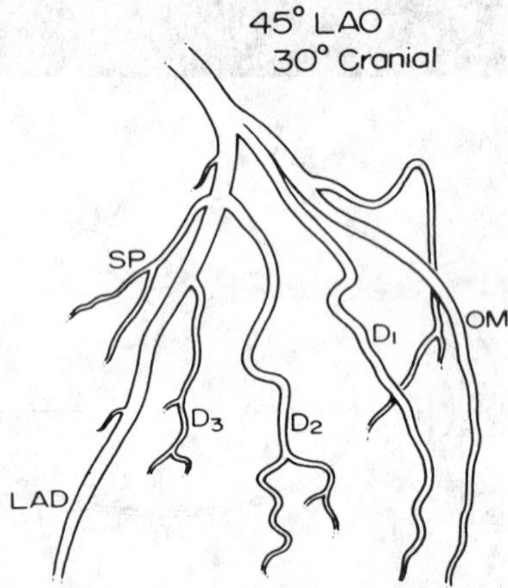

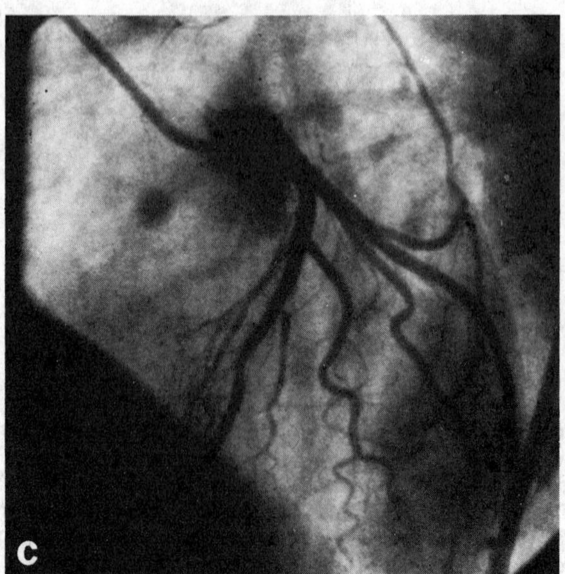

FIGURE 138-27 Diagrammatic illustration of the left coronary angiogram in the 45° left anterior oblique (LAO) with 30° cranial angulation and the direction of the x-ray beam used to produce this view. This is the most valuable view of the left coronary artery in most patients. Foreshortening of the left main and proximal left anterior descending and diagonal branches present in the LAO view is usually overcome by cranial angulation of the image intensifier. The proximal left coronary arterial segments are frequently visualized at an angle almost perpendicular from their long axis. The ostium of the left main coronary artery, the most proximal portion of the LAD, and the origin of the diagonal branches are usually well visualized without overlap (compare with Fig. 138-24). Some overlap may occur with branches of the proximal circumflex coronary artery, and this is frequently overcome by using a 60° LAO with 30° cranial angulation. The value of the LAO with cranial angulation is considerably less when the proximal left coronary artery is superiorly directed, in which case caudal angulation of the image intensifier is frequently helpful. The direction of the x-ray beam in the 45° LAO with 30° angulation is demonstrated. (*From King SB III, Douglas JS Jr, Morris DC: New angiographic views for coronary arteriography. In: Hurst JW (ed): The Heart, Update IV. New York, McGraw-Hill, 1981: 206. Reproduced with permission from the publisher, editor, and authors.*)

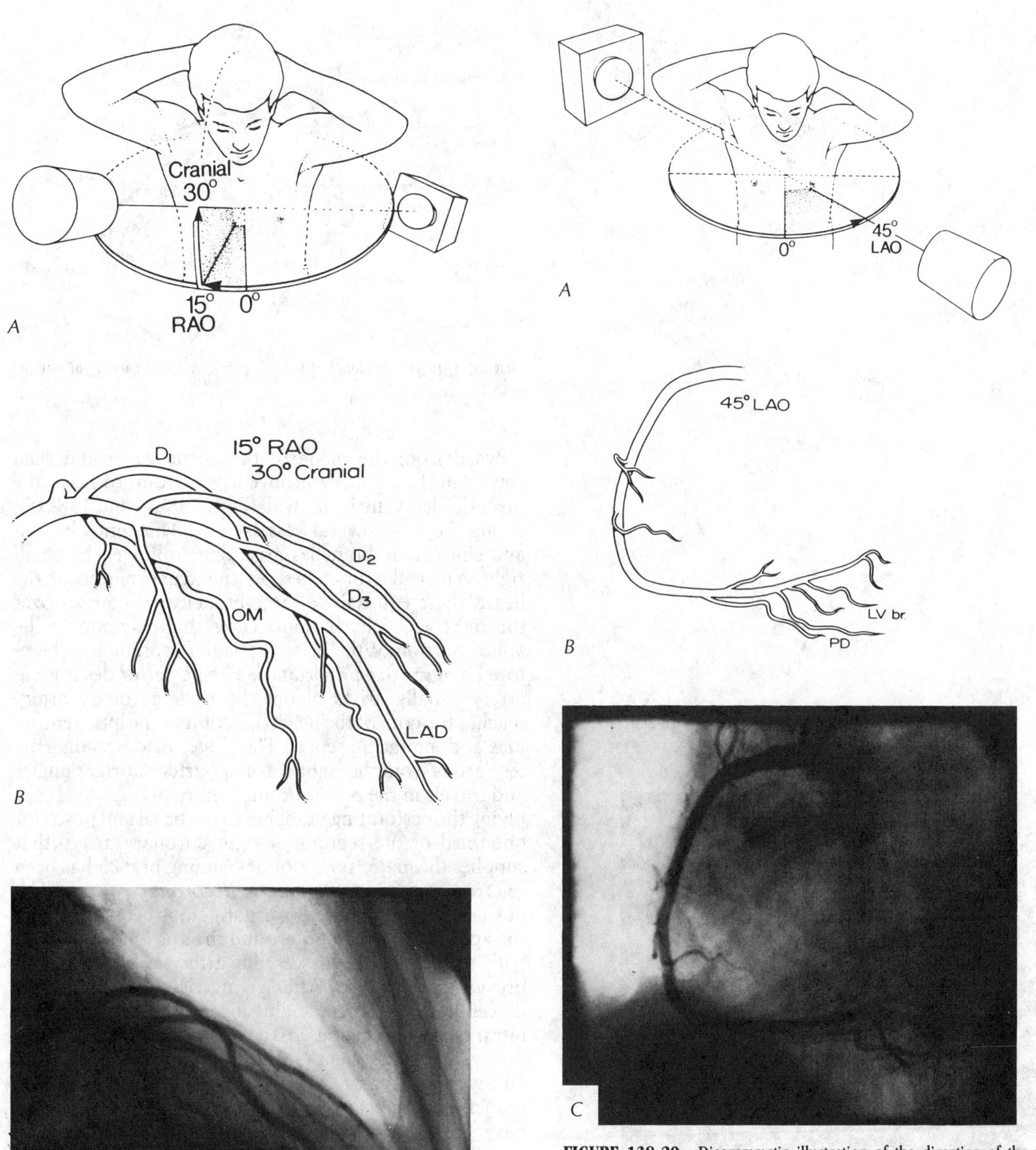

FIGURE 138-28 Diagrammatic illustration of the direction of the x-ray beam and the left coronary angiogram in the 15° RAO with 30° cranial angulation. This view is particularly helpful in analyzing the mid-left anterior descending artery and the diagonal branch points. Overlap with diagonal branches is usually avoided. The origin of the circumflex artery may be well seen, as in this illustration. (*From King SB III, Douglas JS Jr, Morris DC: New angiographic views for coronary arteriography. In: Hurst JW (ed): The Heart, Update IV. New York, McGraw-Hill, 1981: 208. Reproduced with permission from the publisher, editor, and authors.*)

FIGURE 138-29 Diagrammatic illustration of the direction of the x-ray beam and the right coronary artery in the 45° LAO projection. This view is excellent for visualizing the proximal mid and distal right coronary artery in the AV groove since the direction of the x-ray beam is perpendicular to these arterial segments. Ostial lesions of the right coronary artery are not well visualized if the proximal right coronary artery takes an anterior direction from the aorta and therefore originates in a direction parallel to the x-ray beam. This can usually be overcome by turning to a more severe left oblique projection. The posterior descending and left ventricular branches of the right coronary artery, which pass down the posterior aspect of the heart toward the apex, are severely foreshortened since the long axis of these vessels is in the same direction as the x-ray beam. The proximal posterior descending branches can be visualized by cranial angulation of the overhead intensifier (see Fig. 138-30) or from a right oblique view. The image intensifier is in the standard LAO position. (*From King SB III, Douglas JS Jr, Morris DC: New angiographic views for coronary arteriography. In: Hurst JW (ed): The Heart, Update IV. New York, McGraw-Hill, 1981: 208. Reproduced with permission from the publisher, editor, and authors.*)

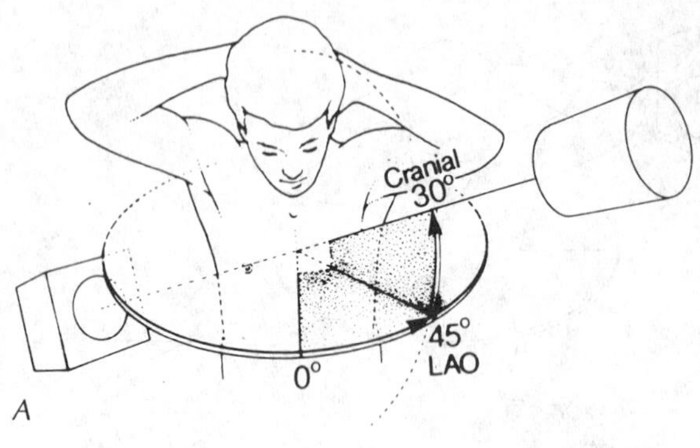

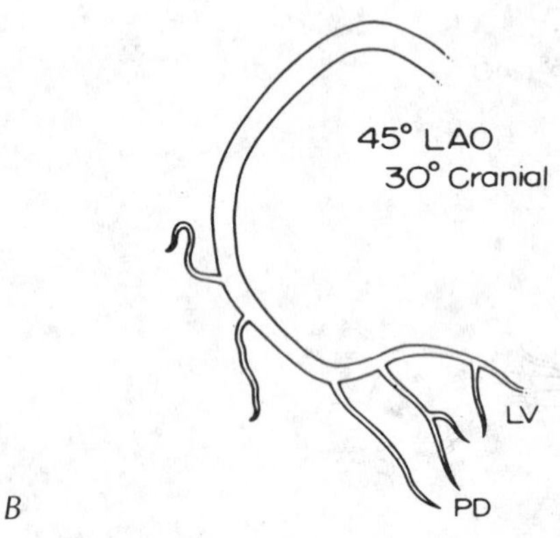

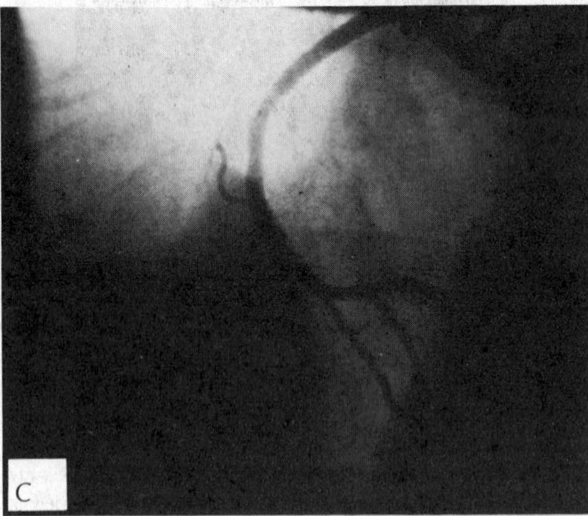

FIGURE 138-30 Diagrammatic illustration of the direction of the x-ray beam and the right coronary artery in 30° LAO with 30° cranial angulation. Cranial angulation of the image intensifier overcomes the problem of foreshortening of the posterior descending and left ventricular branches observed in Fig. 138-29. Lesions in the posterior descending or left ventricular branches can be well visualized. When the right coronary artery originates anteriorly from the aorta, the proximal portion of the vessel is frequently well seen in this projection. With anomalous origin of the left anterior descending artery from the right coronary artery, this view is helpful since the standard LAO view produces considerable foreshortening of the anomalous artery. The direction of the x-ray beam is the same as in Fig. 138-27. (*From King SB III, Douglas JS Jr, Morris DC: New angiographic views for coronary arteriography. In: Hurst JW (ed): The Heart, Update IV. New York, McGraw-Hill, 1981: 210. Reproduced with permission from the publisher, editor, and authors.*)

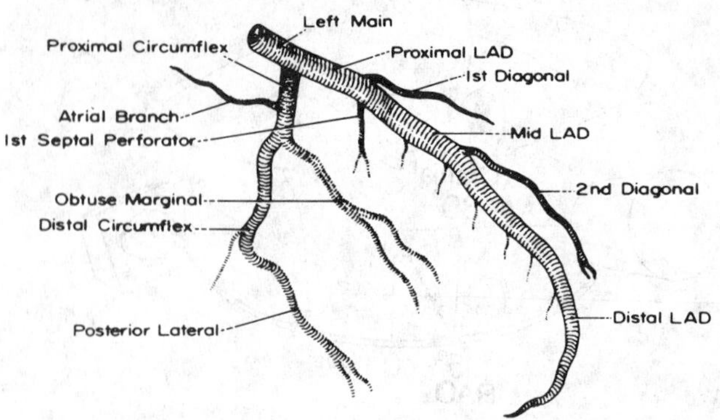

FIGURE 138-31 Anatomy of the left coronary tree in the right oblique view.

upward from the plane of the aortic valve and then travels in the right AV groove as a conduit to reach the posterior left ventricular wall (Figs. 138-34 and 138-35). Along the way, several vessels arise. The conus branch and sinus node branches arise first, followed by small right ventricular branches. At the acute margin of the heart, there is usually a large branch that courses over the right ventricle. In some cases this may supply the apical portion of the interventricular septum and therefore be of greater importance. The posterior descending artery usually arises before the right coronary artery reaches the crux of the heart (junction of the interventricular and interatrial septa). The posterior descending artery arises from the right coronary artery at right angles and travels in the posterior interventricular groove, supplying the perforating branches to the basal and posterior one-third of the septum. A right coronary artery that supplies the major posterior descending branch has been referred to as a *dominant right coronary artery.* The posterior descending artery usually stops before reaching the apex, but it may curl around the apex in association with a short anterior descending artery to form the loop previously described. After giving rise to the posterior descending artery, the right coronary artery becomes intramyocardial at the crux, gives rise to the AV node artery, and subsequently returns to the surface, making an inverted U curve (Fig. 138-35). The left ventricular branches of the right coronary artery are variable and cover the same area as the posterolateral branches of a large circumflex system. The proximal conduit portion of the right coronary artery is well seen in standard RAO and LAO views. However, because of its horizontal orientation, the origin of the posterior descending artery is well seen in the RAO view but foreshortened in the LAO view; to overcome this, cranial angulation of the intensifier is necessary. Pathological studies indicate that lesions at the takeoff of the posterior descending artery are frequently overlooked if standard oblique views in the transverse plane are used.

Grading Stenoses

Visual inspection of the coronary arteriogram has traditionally been used to assess the severity of coronary artery stenosis. In our laboratory, a system of analyzing

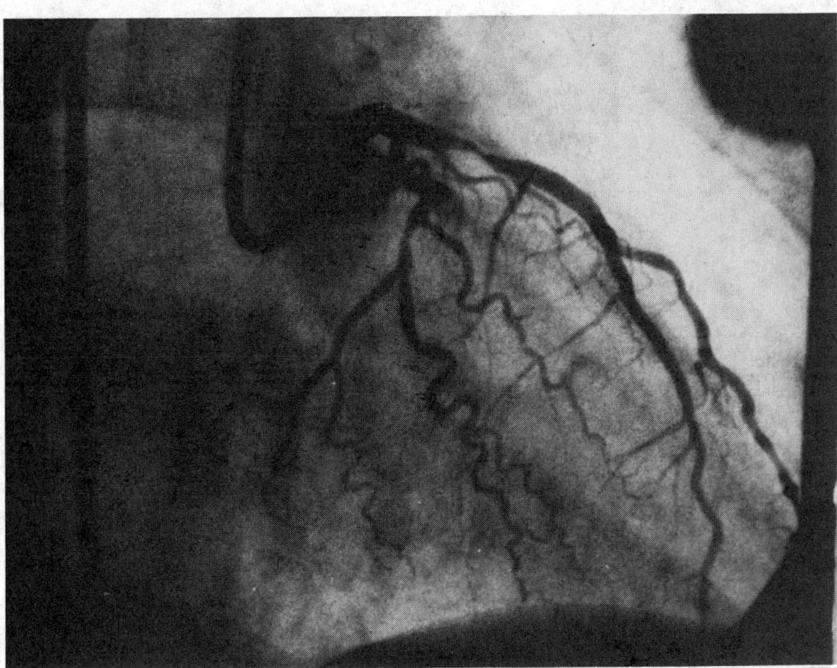

FIGURE 138-32 Right anterior oblique view of the left coronary artery showing high-grade stenosis of the left anterior descending proximal to the first septal perforating branch.

each arterial segment has been used, and the degree of stenosis is recorded as a reduction in lumen diameter expressed as a percentage, with total occlusion being 100 percent. Measurement of cineangiograms has been done with a programmable digital caliper system. In each available projection, the frame showing the most severe stenosis in end diastole is chosen for measurement. The percentage of diameter stenosis recorded is a mean value of the measurements from two or three available projections. This method has been shown to reduce observer variability. Although cross-sectional area reduction is the measurement of greatest physiological importance, use of diameter stenosis is in keeping with the American Heart Association recommendation that the diameter method be adopted for grading coronary artery stenoses.[156] A 50 percent reduction in diameter is equivalent to a 75 percent reduction in cross-sectional area, and a 75 percent reduction in diameter is equal to a 90 percent reduction in cross-sectional area. It is of great importance to identify which method of expressing stenosis is used. From the standpoint of surgically significant lesions, it has been our practice to consider stenoses with greater than 50 percent diameter reduction or 75 percent cross-sectional area reduction as lesions that may produce myocardial ischemia. Lesions in series and long stenoses are of added importance. Quantitative computerized methods for calculating coronary artery stenosis are used for clinical investigations and are also increasingly utilized for routine clinical coronary arteriography.[161] Techniques employing edge detection algorithms are often applied clinically.

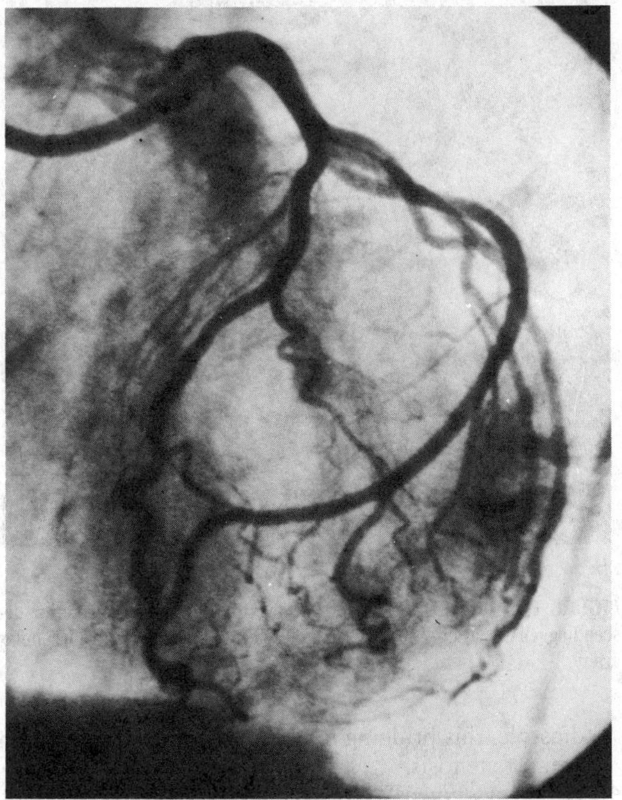

FIGURE 138-33 LAO view of the left coronary artery demonstrating dominant circumflex coronary artery giving rise to the posterior descending artery.

Pitfalls in Coronary Arteriography

There are a number of pitfalls in coronary arteriography that should be looked for and avoided.

1. *Short left main or double left coronary orifices.* When the left main orifice is very short or absent, selective injection of the anterior descending or circumflex arteries may be made (Fig. 138-36). If on viewing an arteriogram, no circumflex or anterior descending artery is seen filling either primarily or through collaterals from the right coronary artery, the possibility that the artery was missed by subselective injection must be entertained.

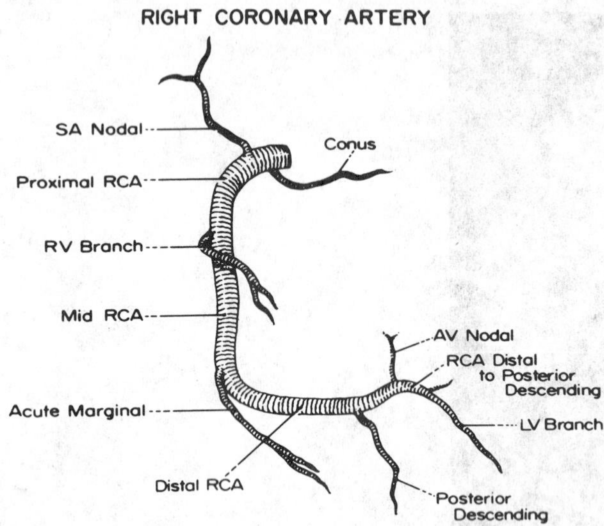

FIGURE 138-34 Anatomy of the right coronary tree.

2. *Orifice lesions.* The left and right coronary artery orifices need to be seen on a tangent with the aortic sinuses. Some backflow from the orifices is needed if the catheter is lying within the left main or proximal right coronary artery to avoid missing an orifice lesion.
3. *Myocardial bridges.* The anterior descending, diagonal, and marginal branches not uncommonly dip intramyocardially, and the overlying myocardium may act to compress the artery during systole (Fig. 138-37). If the coronary artery is not viewed carefully in diastole, this bridging may give the appearance of an area of stenosis.[162–165]
4. *Foreshortening.* When possible, avoid reading lesions in segments that are seen only coming toward or away from the image intensifier. Dense opacification of seg-

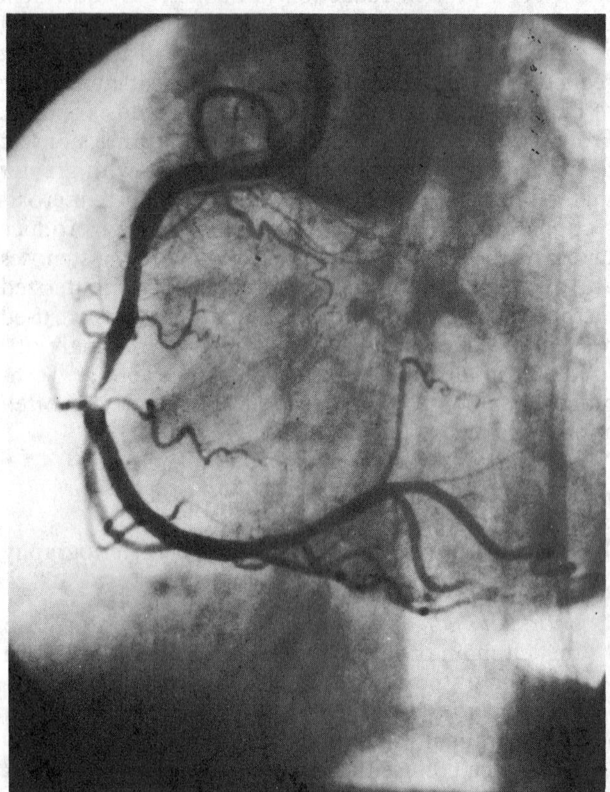

FIGURE 138-35 LAO view of the right coronary artery (RCA) with high-grade lesion in its midportion.

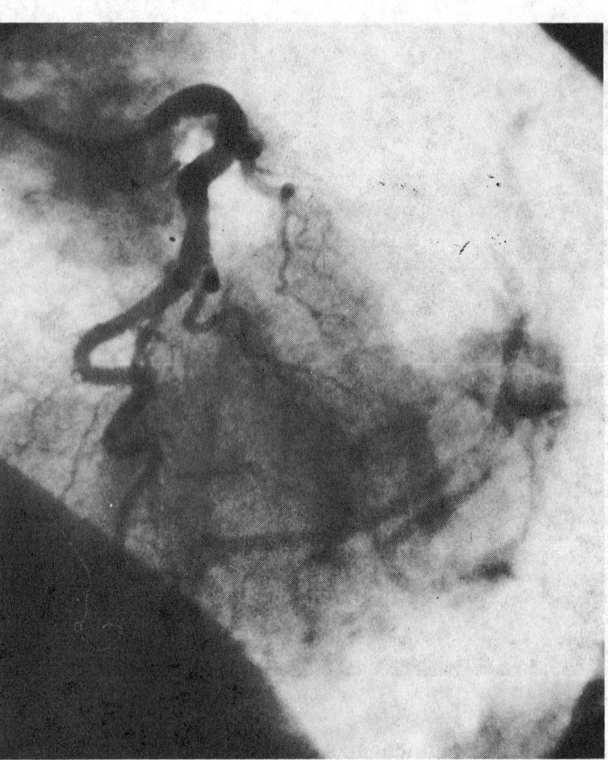

A

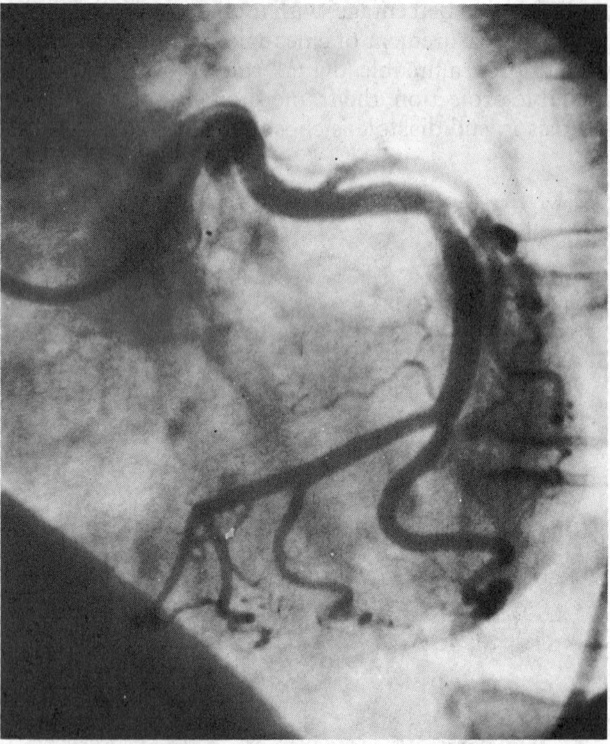

B

FIGURE 138-36 *A.* LAO view of selective injection into left anterior descending (LAD) artery. *B.* LAO view of selective injection into circumflex artery.

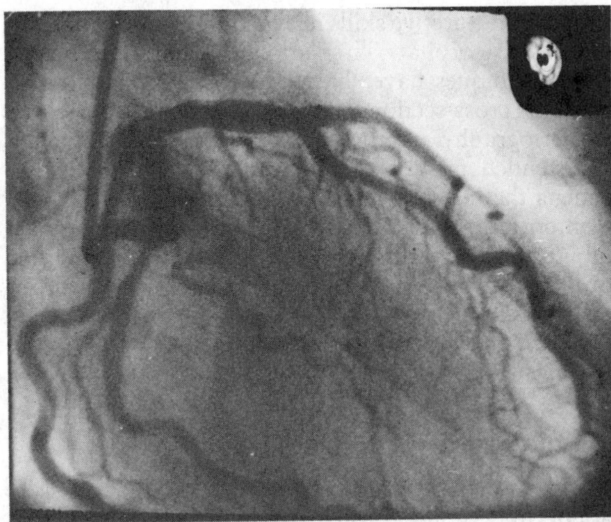

A

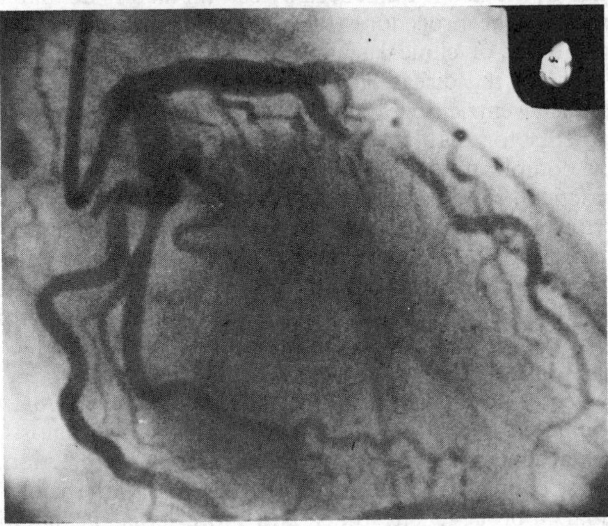

B

FIGURE 138-37 RAO view of left coronary artery system. *A.* Diastolic appearance of anterior descending artery showing smooth lumen. *B.* Systolic appearance showing obliteration of the lumen by an overriding muscular bridge.

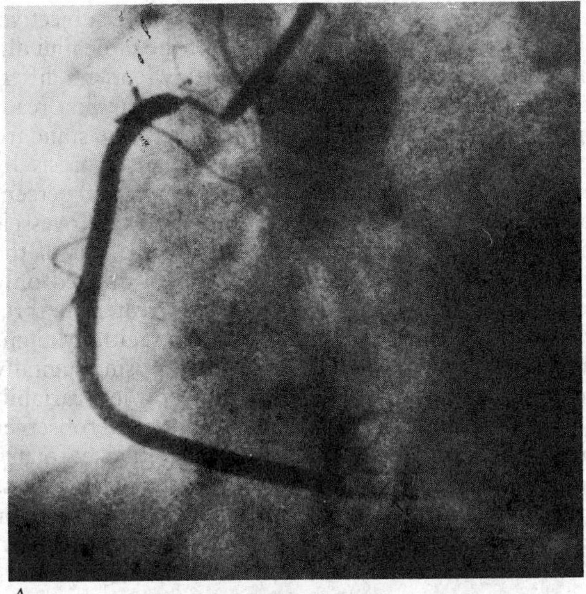

A

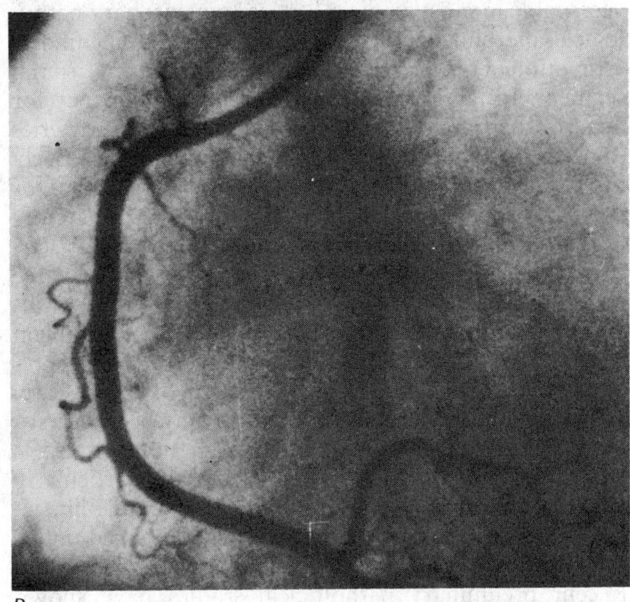

B

FIGURE 138-38 *A.* LAO view of right coronary injection showing pericatheter spasm. *B.* Same view following nitroglycerin, showing relief of spasm.

ments seen end-on may produce the appearance of a lesion in an intervening segment.

5. *Coronary spasm.* Catheter-induced spasm may give the appearance of a lesion (Fig. 138-38). When spasm is suspected (usually at the catheter tip in the right coronary artery), nitrates should be given and the injection should be repeated in 5 to 10 min. Spontaneous coronary artery spasm is a separate problem, and when this is suspected, nitrates and atropine are avoided since the atropine may play a role in blocking coronary artery spasm. Provocation with ergot derivatives will identify most patients with spontaneous coronary artery spasm.[135–139]
6. *Anomalous coronary arteries.* Coronary arteries may arise from ectopic locations, or a single coronary artery may be present.[166–185] Only by ensuring that the entire epicardial surface has an adequate arterial supply can one be confident that all branches have been visualized.
7. *Totally occluded arteries or vein grafts.* Absence of vascularity in a portion of the heart may indicate total occlusion of its arterial supply. Usually, however, collateral channels permit visualization of the distal occluded artery unless it is an acute occlusion.[186–190] Vessels filled solely by collaterals have very little pressure supporting their walls and may appear smaller than their actual lumen size, giving a false sense of pessimism about the possibilities for surgical anastomosis.

Limitations of Coronary Arteriography

In spite of significant improvements in the quality of coronary arteriographic studies as a result of improved x-ray imaging systems, there remain a number of limitations of the method. Film interpretation is subjective. Different angiographers may interpret the same film differently, and the same angiographer may render a different interpretation at a time remote from the first reading.[191,192] It has been reported that the average standard deviation of estimation of any segmental stenosis by experienced angiographers may be as high as 20 percent and that disagreement about the number of major vessels with 70 percent stenosis may occur 30 percent of the time.[192] These reported studies, however, utilized only views in the transverse plane, imposing greater interpretive burdens than are encountered when sagittally angulated views one obtained. Further studies using sagitally angulated views would be expected to show less variability in interpreting coronary arteriograms. Interobserver and intraobserver variability in interpreting coronary ateriograms is not unlike interpretive differences in chest x-rays or other diagnostic studies involving human error and judgment. Routine use of several readers has been shown to reduce interpretive error.[192] Although correlation of angiography with postmortem findings has been acceptable in most studies,[193–206] certain coronary pathological-anatomic factors may favor angiographic underestimation of the degree of stenosis present in any arterial segment. In large part, this is due to the tendency for diffuse atheromatous narrowing of the coronary arteries to occur. In attempting to grade stenosis of an obviously narrow segment, one may not have a normal segment for comparison or may choose for comparison an apparently normal segment which in fact has diffuse tabular narrowing.[196–198] This leads to underestimation of the degree of stenosis present. Pathological studies currently available probably overestimate the frequency of this problem since the pathological material available for study represents the severest end of the spectrum of the disease. Eccentric atherosclerotic plaques also may be underestimated unless the minor axis of the stenotic lumen is visualized. Sagittally angulated views are particularly valuable in this regard. Very discrete membrane-like lesions, which fortunately are rare, may be missed unless they are visualized directly in the plane of the lesion. Recent preliminary pathological studies have shown poor correlation between left main coronary stenosis at autopsy and that at angiography, especially in the presence of a short left main coronary artery, and point up the importance of sufficient angiographic views and excellent interpretive skills in evaluating this critical portion of the coronary circulation.[199] Quantitative computer techniques have shown excellent correlation between the cross-sectional luminal area of stenotic lesions at arteriography and direct planimetered measurements of distended postmortem specimens.[200] Dynamic phenomena that are not active at the time of the study may be important. "Hit and run" events such as coronary embolization or thrombosis with subsequent resolution, coronary artery spasm, and even primary coronary artery dissection may leave left ventricular scars but not result in coronary angiographic findings.

Risk of Coronary Arteriography

As with any invasive procedure, there is a finite risk to patients undergoing coronary arteriography. The magnitude of the risk is influenced by certain factors definable prior to the procedure (skill of the angiographer and instability of clinical symptoms) but primarily by the extent of the disease found at coronary arteriography and left ventriculography.[127,153,201,202] Physicians referring patients for coronary arteriograms must be aware of the complication rate in a given laboratory and, when practical, should achieve stability of clinical symptoms prior to study. That is not to say that unstable patients should not be studied, but the physician must balance the risk of the procedure and potential benefit against the risk of not doing the procedure. The frequency of major complications has decreased in active centers (Table 138-2).

Major complications are of two types. *Local arterial complications* consist of arterial occlusion or stenosis, hematoma formation, false aneurysm, and infection. These complications occur more frequently with the brachial approach. The other and more lethal group of complications relates to *thromboembolic events* or depression of myocardial function due to infarction or acute ischemia. Thromboemboli are more commonly due to multiple catheter and guide wire exchanges during which thrombus material is stripped from the catheter surface at the puncture site only to be deposited on a subsequent catheter, as suggested by Takaro and associates.[207] The addition of systemic heparinization was felt to have reduced thromboembolic complications in some

TABLE 138-2
Complications of Coronary Arteriography

	CASS*		SOC CARD Angiography[204]†	Abrams and Adams[201]			
				Femoral		Brachial	
	1979[202]	1983[205]	1990	H	NH	H	NH
Death	0.0020	0.0007	0.0011	0.0016	0.0015	0.0010	0.0030
Myocardial infarction	0.0025	0.0027	0.0005	0.0018	0.0023	0.0014	0.0023
Cerebral emboli	0.0003	0.0007	0.0007	0.0008	0.0010	0.0008	0.0009
Arterial complications	0.0080	0.0082	0.0038				
Ventricular fibrillation	0.0063	0.0038	0.0043				

* CASS = Coronary Artery Surgery Study.
† Society for Cardiac Angiography and interventions.
NOTE: H = systemic heparin; NH = no systemic heparin.

laboratories. The early CASS report[202] and that by Abrams and Adams,[201] however, found that the use of heparin did not influence complication rates. Of equal or greater importance may be the routine use of catheter debriding techniques with vigorous aspiration and flushing of the catheter in the abdominal aorta to dislodge any retained thrombus material. Minor allergic reactions to contrast media in the form of urticaria occur commonly, but anaphylactic and pyrogenic reactions are exceedingly rare.[208–210] Radiation exposure to the patient, estimated as 20 to 45 R, has little risk unless multiple restudies are needed.

Reported mortality rates related to coronary arteriography range from 0.05 to 4 percent, and virtually all deaths occur in patients with severe, multivessel coronary disease or left main coronary artery stenosis.[151,201,202–204,207] A widely quoted acceptable mortality rate for coronary arteriography is 0.1 percent. Case selection, however, may play an important role in deter-

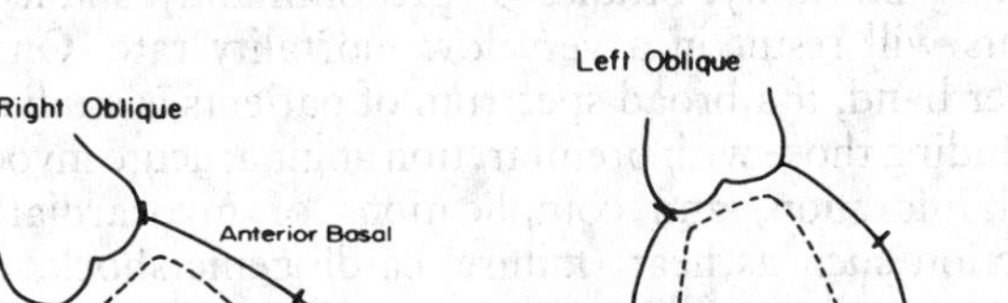
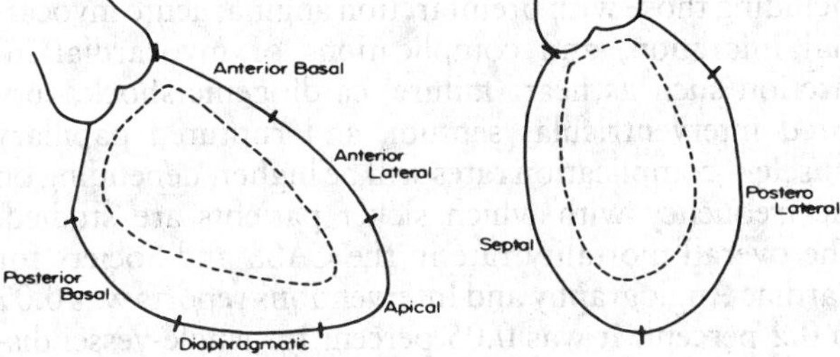

FIGURE 138-39 Left ventricular wall silhouette in RAO and LAO views.

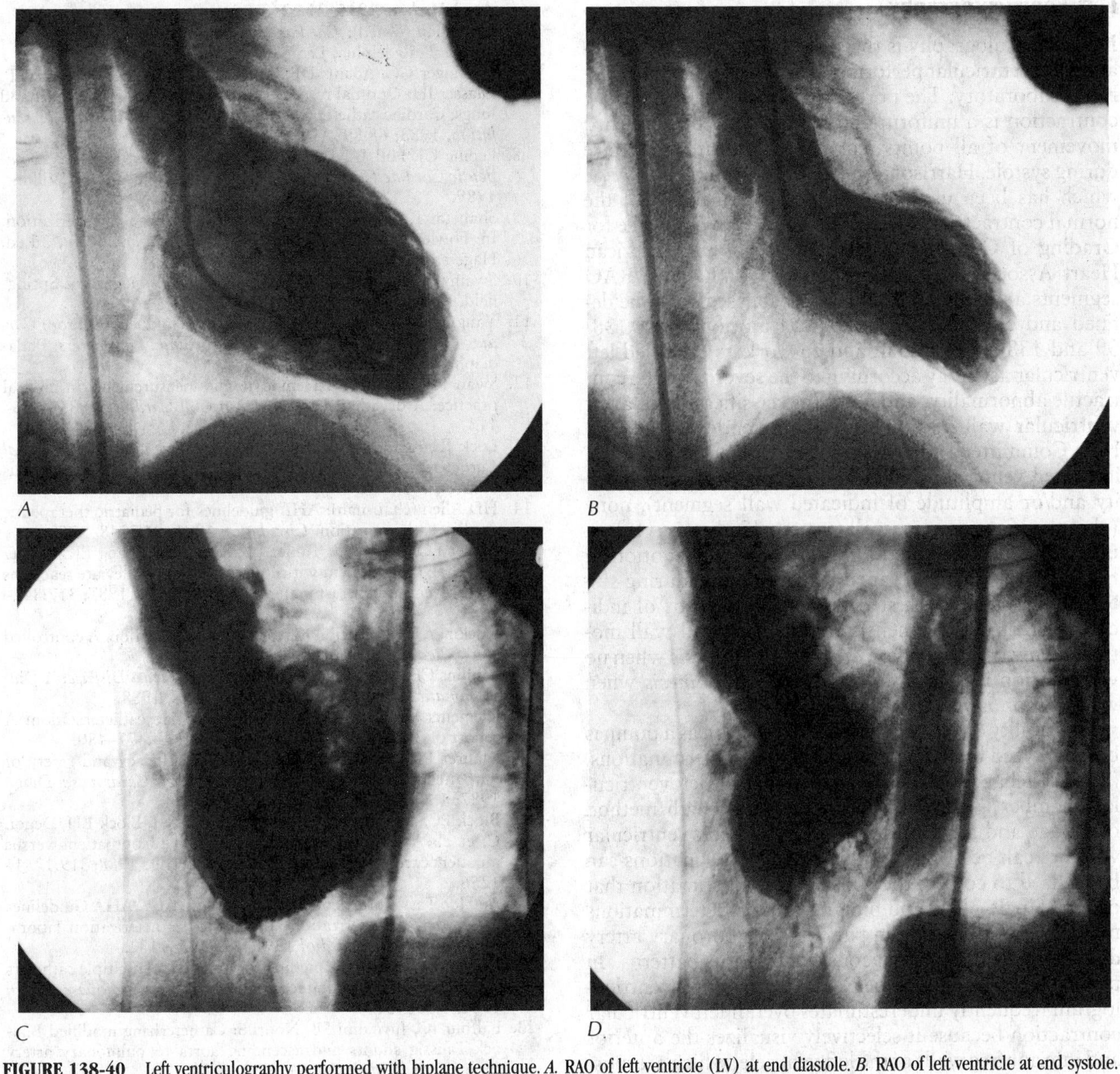

A

B

C

D

FIGURE 138-40 Left ventriculography performed with biplane technique. *A.* RAO of left ventricle (LV) at end diastole. *B.* RAO of left ventricle at end systole. (Notice contraction abnormality of anterior wall.) *C.* LAO at end diastole. *D.* LAO at end systole.

mining mortality. Studies in predominantly stable patients will result in a very low mortality rate. On the other hand, if a broad spectrum of patients is studied—including those with preinfarction angina, acute myocardial infarction, and complications of myocardial infarction such as heart failure, cardiogenic shock, ruptured interventricular septum, and ruptured papillary muscle—complication rates will be higher, depending on the frequency with which sicker patients are studied. The overall mortality rate in the CASS and Society for Cardiac Angiography and Interventions reports was 0.07 to 0.2 percent. It was 0.05 percent for single-vessel disease, 0.07 percent for double-vessel disease, 0.012 percent for triple-vessel disease, and 0.8 percent in patients with left main coronary artery stenosis.[202,205] The point to be made is that laboratory and surgical teams must be prepared to act in the best interest of severely ill patients and not be overly concerned with an arbitrary mortality figure.

Left Ventriculography

Left ventriculography is the standard method for evaluating left ventricular performance in the coronary angiography laboratory. The normal pattern of left ventricular contraction is a uniform and almost concentric inward movement of all points along the endocardial surface during systole. Harrison[211] introduced the term *asynergy*, which has been used to indicate a disturbance of the normal contraction pattern. The Ad Hoc Committee for Grading of Coronary Artery Disease of the American Heart Association[156] has recommended that five RAO segments and two LAO left ventricular segments be defined and characterized as to wall motion (Figs. 138-39 and 138-40). Herman and co-workers classified left ventricular asynergy according to the severity of the contractile abnormality, and a similar classification of a left ventricular wall motion was recommended by the Ad Hoc Committee; normal (normal wall motion of the indicated ventricular segment), reduced (reduced velocity and/or amplitude of indicated wall segment), none (absence of appropriate wall motion of indicated ventricular segment), dyskinetic (paradoxical wall motion of the indicated segment), aneurysmal (bulging during systole and diastole with sharply defined margins of indicated ventricular segment), and/or undefined wall motion. Many angiographers use the term *akinesis* when no wall motion is present and the term *hypokinesis* when wall motion is reduced.

The ability of the left ventricle to function as a pump is best analyzed by left ventricular volume determinations. (See also Chap. 23.) If it is assumed that the left ventricular chamber is ellipsoid and if the area-length method of Dodge and associates is employed,[213] left ventricular volumes can be calculated and regression equations can be utilized to correct the consistent overestimation that occurs. Single-plane and biplane volume determinations may differ significantly in patients with coronary artery disease and nonhomogeneous contraction patterns. In particular, the single-plane RAO or lateral left ventriculogram frequently underestimates overall left ventricular contraction because it selectively visualizes the anterior and inferior free walls of the left ventricle, which are most commonly involved in myocardial infarction. Vogel and associates[214] found that the single-plane RAO left ventriculogram underestimated ejection fraction in 70 percent of patients with coronary artery disease. For this reason, biplane left ventriculography is frequently desirable in evaluating patients with coronary artery disease.

REFERENCES

1. Liljestrand G: In "Le Prix Nobel en 1956," Nobel Foundation, Stockholm, 1957.
2. Steckelberg JM, Ulietstra RE, Ludwig J, Mann RJ: Werner Forssman (1904–1979) and his unusual success story, *Mayo Clin Proc* 1979; 54:746–748.
3. Forssman W: Die Sondierung des rechten Herzens, *Berl Klin Wochenschr* 1929; 8:2085–2087.
4. Cournand A: Cardiac catheterization: Development of the technique, its contribution to experimental medicine and its initial application to man. *Acta Med Scand* 1975; 579(suppl):7–32.
5. Brannon ES, Weens HS, Warren JV: Atrial septal defect: Study of hemodynamics by the technique of right heart catheterization. *Am J Med Sci* 1945; 214:248–251.
6. Grossman W (ed): *Cardiac Catheterization and Angiography,* 4th ed. Philadelphia, Lea & Febiger, 1991.
7. Friesinger GC, Adams DF, Bourassa MG, Carlson E, Elliot LP, Glasser IH: Optimal resources for examination of the heart and lungs: Cardiac catheterization and radiographic facilities. *Circulation,* 1983; 68:893A–930A.
8. Pepine CJ, Hill JA, Lambert CR (eds): *Diagnostic and Therapeutic Cardiac Catheterization.* Baltimore, Williams & Wilkins, 1989.
9. Shabetai R, Adolph RJ: Principles of cardiac catheterization. In: Fowler NO (ed): *Cardiac Diagnosis and Treatment,* 3d ed. Hagerstown, Harper & Row, 1980: 106.
10. Swamy S, Segal LI, Mouli S: *Percutaneous Angiography.* Springfield, IL, Charles C Thomas, 1977.
11. Yang SS, Bentivoglio LG, Maranhao V, Goldberg H: *From Cardiac Catheterization Data to Hemodynamic Parameters.* Philadelphia, FA Davis, 1980.
12. Swan HJC, Ganz W: Hemodynamic measurements in clinical practice: A decade in review. *J Am Coll Cardiol* 1983; 1:103–113.
13. Lock JE, Keane JF, Fellows KE: *Diagnostic and Interventional Catheterization in Congenital Heart Disease.* Boston, Martinus Nijhoff, 1987.
14. HD Allen (chairman): AHA guidelines for pediatric therapeutic cardiac catheterization. *Circulation* 1991; 84:2248–2258.
15. Lasser EC, Berry CC, Talner LB, Santini LC, Lang EK, Gerber FH, et al: Pretreatment with corticosteroids to alleviate reactions to intravenous contrast material. *N Engl J Med* 1987; 317:845–849.
16. Ruckman RN: Sedation for cardiac catheterization: A controlled study. *Pediatr Cardiol* 1980; 1:263–268.
17. Mullins CE, Mayer DC (eds): *Congenital Heart Disease: A Diagrammatic Atlas.* New York, Alan R Liss, 1988.
18. Clements SD, Gatlin S: Outpatient cardiac catheterization: A report of 3000 cases. *Clin Cardiol* 1991; 14:477–480.
19. Mahrer PR, Young C, Magnusson PT: Efficacy and safety of outpatient cardiac catheterization. *Cathet Cardiovasc Diagn* 1987; 13:304–308.
20. Block PC, Ockene I, Goldberg RJ, Butterly J, Block EH, Degon C, et al: A prospective randomized trial of outpatient versus inpatient cardiac catheterization. *N Engl J Med* 1988; 319:1251–1256.
21. Ad Hoc Task Fore, Pepine CJ (chairman): ACC/AHA Guidelines for cardiac catheterization and cardiac catheterization laboratories. *J Am Coll Cardiol* 1991; 18:1149–1182.
22. Cooper MW: A simple method for insertion of multiple catheters through a single venipuncture site. *Cathet Cardiovasc Diagn* 1982; 8:305–310.
23. Balfour IC, Juveidini SB, Nouri S: Catheterizing modified Blalock-Taussig shunts and ascending aorta to pulmonary artery shunts. *Am J Cardiol* 1991; 68:279–280.
24. Rapoport S, Sniderman KW, Morse SS, Proto MH, Ross GR:

Pseudoaneurysm: A complication of faulty technique in femoral artery puncture. *Radiology* 1985; 154:529–530.

25. Hillis LD: Percutaneous left heart catheterization and coronary arteriography using a femoral artery sheath. *Cathet Cardiovasc Diagn* 1979; 5:393–399.
26. Wholey MH: A newly designed directionally controlled guidewire. *Cathet Cardiovasc Diagn* 1986; 12:66–70.
27. Leimgruber PP, Talley JD, Gruentzig AR: Use of a steerable coronary guidewire facilitating catheterization of atherosclerotic and tortuous peripheral vessels. *Am J Cardiol* 1986; 58:187–189.
28. Nicholson WJ: Multipurpose A2 catheter approach to left heart catheterization in severe aortic stenosis. *Clin Cardiol.* 1988; 11:697–700.
29. Baur HR, Mruz GL, Erickson DL, Van Tassel RL: New technique for retrograde left heart catheterization in aortic stenosis. *Cathet Cardiovasc Diagn* 1982; 8:299–304.
30. Laskey WK: Percutaneous retrograde left ventricular catheterization in aortic valve stenosis. *Cathet Cardiovasc Diagn* 1986; 12:75–79.
31. MacDonald RG, Feldman RL, Pepine CJ: A modified catheter system for retrograde left ventricular catheterization in aortic valve stenoses. *Cathet Cardiovasc Diagn* 1985; 11:433–439.
32. Kober G, Hilgermann R: Catheter entrapment in a Bjork-Shiley prosthesis in aortic position. *Cathet Cardiovasc Diagn* 1987; 13:262–265.
33. Horstkotte D, Jehle J, Loogen F: Death due to transprosthetic catheterization of a Bjork-Shiley prosthesis in the aortic position. *Am J Cardiol* 1986; 58:566–567.
34. Nath PH, Soto B, Holt JH, Satler LF: Selective coronary angiography by translumbar aortic puncture. *Am J Cardiol* 1983; 52:425–426.
35. O'Keefe JH, Vlietstra RE, Hanley PC, Seward JB: Revival of the transseptal approach for catheterization of the left atrium and ventricle. *Mayo Clin Proc* 1985; 60:790–795.
36. Mullins CE: Transseptal left heart catheterization: Experience with a new technique in 520 pediatric and adult patients. *Pediatr Cardiol* 1983; 4:239–246.
37. Laskey WK, Kusiak V, Untereker WJ, Hirshfeld JW: Transseptal left heart catheterization: Utility of a sheath technique. *Catheter Cardiovasc Diagn* 1982; 8:535–542.
38. Croft CH, Lipscomb K: Modified technique of transseptal left heart catheterization. *J Am Coll Cardiol* 1985; 5:904–910.
39. Lam W, Juska J, Pietras R: Transseptal balloon catheterization of the left ventricle in adult valvular heart disease. *Am Heart J* 1984; 107:147–152.
40. Kotoda K, Hosegawa T, Mizumo A, Saigusa M: Transseptal left heart catheterization with Swan-Ganz flow directed catheter. *Am Heart J* 1983; 105:436–439.
41. Shirey EK, Sones MF: Retrograde transaortic and mitral valve catheterization. *Am J Cardiol* 1966; 18:745–753.
42. Iskandrian AS, Bemis CE, Kimbiris D, Owens J: Retrograde catheterization of left atrium. *Br Heart J* 1979; 42:715–718.
43. Ali Kahn MA, Bucher JT, Mullins CE, Yousef AL, Nihill MR, et al: Blade atrial septostomy: Experience with the first 50 procedures. *Cathet Cardiovasc Diagn* 1991; 23:257–262.
44. Fisher RG, Ferreyro R: Evaluation of current techniques for nonsurgical removal of intravascular iatrogenic foreign bodies. *Am J Radiol* 1978; 130:541–548.
45. Sibley DH, Millar HD, Hartley CJ, Whitlow PL: Subselective measurement of coronary blood flow velocity using a steerable Doppler catheter. *J Am Coll Cardiol* 1986; 8:1332–1340.
46. Nichols WW, Pepine CJ, Conti CR, Feldman RL, Christie LG: Evaluation of a new catheter mounted electromagnetic velocity sensor during cardiac catheterization. *Cathet Cardiovasc Diagn* 1980; 16:97–113.
47. Ehlers KC, Mylrea KC, Waterson CK, Adkins JM: Cardiac output measurements: A review of current techniques and research. *Ann Biomed Engin* 1986; 14:219–239.
48. Spears JR, Marais HJ, Serier J, Pomerantzeff O, Geyer RP, Sipzener RS: In vivo coronary angioscopy. *J Am Coll Cardiol* 1983; 1:1311–1314.
49. Rocchini AP, Kveselis DA, Crowley D, Dick M, Rosenthal A: Percutaneous balloon valvuloplasty for treatment of congenital pulmonary valvar stenosis in children. *J Am Coll Cardiol* 1984; 3:1005–1012.
50. Mitchell SE, White RI Jr, Kan J, Tolkoff J: Improved balloon catheters for large vessel and valvular angioplasty. *Am J Roentgenol* 1984; 142:571–572.
51. Rao PS, Langhough R: Relationship of echocardiography shunt flow and angiographic size to the stretched diameter of the atrial septal defect. *Am Heart J* 1991; 122:505–508.
52. Finci L, Meier B, Steppenino G, Roy P, Rutishauser W: Radiation exposure during diagnostic catheterization and single and double vessel percutaneous transluminal coronary angioplasty. *Am J Cardiol* 1987; 60:1401–1403.
53. Gertz EW, Wisneski JA, Gould RG, Akin JR: Improved radiation protection for physicians performing cardiac catheterization. *Am J Cardiol* 1982; 50:1283–1286.
54. Gardner RM, Hollingsworth KW: Optimizing the ECG and pressure monitoring. *Crit Care Med* 1986; 14:651–658.
55. Krovetz LJ, Brenner JI, Polanyi M: Application of an improved intracardiac fiber optic system. *Br Heart J* 1978; 40:1010–1013.
56. Dehmer GJ, Firth BG, Hillis LD: Oxygen consumption in adult patients during cardiac catheterization. *Clin Cardiol* 1982; 5:436–540.
57. Fuchs RM, Heuser RR, Yin FCP, Brinker JA: Limitations of pulmonary wedge V waves in diagnosing mitral regurgitation. *Am J .Cardiol* 1982; 49:849–854.
58. Dodge HT, Sheehan FH: Quantitative contrast angiography for assessment of ventricular performance in heart disease. *J Am Coll Cardiol* 1983; 1:73–81.
59. Lange RA, Moore DM Jr, Cigarroa RG, Hillis LD: Use of pulmonary capillary pressure to assess severity of mitral stenosis. Is true left atrial pressure needed in this condition. *J Am Coll Cardiol* 1989; 13:825–829.
60. Hosenpud JD, McAnulty JH, Morton MJ: Overestimation of mitral valve gradients obtained by phasic pulmonary artery wedge pressure. *Cathet Cardiovasc Diagn* 1983; 9:283–290.
61. Falicov RE, Resnekov L: Mid ventricular obstruction in hypertrophic cardiomyopathy. *Br Heart J* 1977; 39:701–705.
62. Palevsky HI, Long W, Crow J, Fishman AP: Prostacyclin and acetylcholine as screening agents for acute pulmonary vasodilator responsiveness in primary pulmonary hypertension. *Circulation* 1990; 82:2018–2026.
63. Hillis DL, Firth BG, Winniford MD: Variability of right sided cardiac oxygen saturations in adults with and without intracardiac left to right shunting. *Am J Cardiol* 1986; 58:129–132.
64. Glamann DB, Lange RA, Hillis LD: Incidence and significance of a "step-down" in oxygen saturation from SVC to PA. *Am J Cardiol* 1991; 68:695–697.
65. Freed MD, Miettinen OS, Nadas AS: Oximetric detection of intracardiac left-to-right shunts. *Br Heart J* 1979; 42:690–694.
66. Autman EM, Marsh JD, Green LH, Grossman W: Blood oxygen measurements in the assessment of intracardiac left to right shunts: A critical appraisal of methodology. *Am J Cardiol* 1980; 46:265–271.
67. Bloomfield DA: *Dye Curves: The Theory and Practice of Indicator Dilution.* Baltimore, University Park Press, 1974.
68. Hillis DL, Winniford MD, Jackson JA, Firth BG: Measurement of left to right intracardiac shunting in adults: Oximetric versus indicator dilution techniques. *Cathet Cardiovasc Diagn* 1985; 11:467–472.
69. Levett JM, Replogle RL: Thermodilution cardiac output: A critical analysis and review of the literature. *J Surg Res* 1979; 27:392–404.
70. Fischer AP, Benis AM, Jurado RA, Seely E, Teirstein P, Litwak RS: Analysis of errors in measurement of cardiac output by simultaneous dye and thermal dilution in cardiothoracic surgical patients. *Cardiovasc Res* 1978; 12:190–199.
71. Hamilton MA, Stevenson LW, Woo RN, Child JS, Tillisch JH: Effect of tricuspid regurgitation on the reliability of the thermodilution cardiac output technique in congestive heart failure. *Am J Cardiol* 1989; 64:945–948.
72. Dodge HT, Sandler H, Ballew DW, Lord JD Jr: The use of biplane angiocardiography for the measurement of left ventricular volume in man. *Am Heart J* 1960; 60:762–776.
73. Als AV, Paulin S, Aroesty JM: Biplane angiographic volumetry using the right anterior oblique and half-axial left anterior oblique technique. *Radiology* 1978; 126:511–514.
74. Wynne J, Green LH, Mann T, Levin D, Grossman W: Estimation of left ventricular volumes in man from biplane cineangiograms filmed in oblique projections. *Am J Cardiol* 1978; 41:726–732.
75. Sandler H, Dodge HT: The use of single plane angiocardiograms

for the calculation of left ventricular volume in man. *Am Heart J* 1968; 75:325–334.
76. Kennedy JW, Trenholme SE, Kasser IS: Left ventricular volume and mass from single plane cineangiocardiograms. *Am Heart J* 1970; 80:343–352.
77. Sheehan FH, Mitten-Lewis S: Factors influencing accuracy in left ventricular volume determination. *Am J Cardiol* 1989; 64:661.
78. Kennedy JW, Baxley WA, Figley MM, Dodge HT, Blackmon JR: Quantitative angiocardiography: I. The normal left ventricle in man. *Circulation* 1966; 34:272–278.
79. Shimazaki Y, Kawashima Y, Mori T, Beppu S, Yokota K: Angiographic volume estimation of right ventricle. *Chest* 1980; 77:390–395.
80. Gentzler RO II, Briselli MF, Gault JH: Angiographic estimation of right ventricular volume in man. *Circulation* 1974; 50:324–330.
81. Murray JA, Kennedy JW, Figley MM: Quantitative angiocardiography: II. The normal left atrial volume in man. *Circulation* 1968; 37:800–804.
82. Gorlin R, Gorlin G: Hydraulic formula for calculation of area of stenotic mitral valve, other cardiac valves and central circulatory shunts. *Am Heart J* 1951; 41:1–29.
83. Cohen MV, Gorlin R: Modified orifice equation for the calculation of mitral valve area. *Am Heart J* 1972; 84:839–840.
84. Folland ED, Parisi AF, Carbone C: Is peripheral arterial pressure a satisfactory substitute for ascending aortic pressure when measuring aortic valve gradients? *J Am Coll Cardiol* 1984; 4:1207–1212.
85. Bache RJ, Jorgensen CR, Wang Y: Simplified estimation of aortic valve area. *Br Heart J* 1972; 34:408–411.
86. Hakki AH: A simplified valve formula for the calculation of stenotic cardiac valve areas. *Circulation* 1981; 63:1050–1055.
87. Angel J, Soler-Soler J, Anivarro I, Domingo E: I. Hemodynamic evaluation of stenotic cardiac valves. II. Modification of the simplified formula for mitral and aortic valve area calculation. *Cathet Cardiovasc Diagn* 1985; 11:127–138.
88. Cannon SR, Richards KL, Crawford M: Hydraulic estimation of stenotic orifice area: A correction of the Gorlin formula. *Circulation* 1985; 71:1170–1178.
89. Chavez I, Dorbecker N, Celis A: Direct intracardiac angiocardiography: Its diagnostic value. *Am Heart J* 1947; 33:560.
90. Brown R, Rahimtoola SH, Davis GD, Swan HJC: The effects of angiocardiographic contrast medium on circulatory dynamics in man: Cardiac output during angiocardiography. *Circulation* 1965; 31:234–290.
91. Almen T: Experience from 10 years of development of water soluble nonionic contrast media. *Invest Radiol* 1980; 15:S283–288.
92. Bettmann MA: Angiographic contrast agents: Conventional and new media compared. *Am J Roentgenol* 1982; 139:787–794.
93. Kern MJ: Selection of radiocontrast media in cardiac catheterization. Comparative physiology and clinical effects of nonionic and ionic dimeric formulations. *Am Heart J* 1991; 122:195–201.
94. Gwilt DJ, Nagle RE: Contrast media for left ventricular angiography: A comparison between cardio-conray and iopamidol. *Br Heart J* 1984; 51:427–430.
95. Gertz EW, Wisneski JA, Chiu D, Akin JR, Hu C: Clinical superiority of a new nonionic contrast agent (iopamidol) for cardiac angiography. *J Am Coll Cardiol* 1985; 5:250–258.
96. Morris TW, Sahler LG, Violante M, Fischer HW: Reduction of calcium activity by radiopaque contrast media. *Radiology* 1983; 148:55–59.
97. McClennan BL: Ionic and nonionic iodinated contrast media: Evolution and strategies for use. *Am J Roentgenol* 1990; 155:225–233.
98. Brogan WC III, Hillis LD, Lange RA: Contrast agents for cardiac catheterization: Conceptions and misconceptions. *Am Heart J* 1991; 122:1129–1135.
99. Robertson HJF: Blood clot formation in angiographic syringes containing nonionic contrast media. *Radiology* 1987; 162:621–622.
100. Dissessa TG, Zednikova M, Hiraishi S, Jarmakani JM, Higgins CB, Friedman WF: The cardiovascular effects of metrizamide in infants. *Radiology* 1983; 148:687–691.
101. Hirshfield JW Jr: Cardiovascular effects of contrast agents. *Am J Cardiol* 1990; 66(suppl):9F–17P.
102. Levin DC, Dunham LR, Stueve R: Causes of cine image quality deterioration in cardiac catheterization laboratories. *Am J Cardiol* 1983; 52:881–886.
103. Soto B, Pacifico AD: *Angiocardiography in Congenital Heart Malformations.* Mount Kisco, NY, Futura Publishing, 1990.
104. Bargeron LM Jr, Elliott LP, Soto B, Bream PR, Curry GC: Axial cineangiography in congenital heart disease: I. Concept, technical and anatomic considerations. *Circulation* 1977; 56:1075–1093.
105. Nihill MR, Mullins CE, McNamara DG: Visualization of the pulmonary arteries in pseudotruncus by pulmonary vein wedge angiography. *Circulation* 1978; 58:140–147.
106. Keane JF, McFaul R, Fellows K, Lock J: Balloon occlusion angiography in infancy: Methods, uses and limitations. *Am J Cardiol* 1985; 56:495–497.
107. Garcia-Medina V, Bass J, Braunlin E, Krabell KA, Pylers L, Castanida-Zuniga WR, et al: A useful projection for demonstrating the bifurcation of the pulmonary artery. *Pediatr Cardiol* 1990; 11:147–149.
108. McGrath LB, Chen C, Bailey BN, Cha SD, Fernandez J, Lamb GW, et al: Determination of the need for tricuspid valve replacement value of pre-operative right ventricular angiography. *J Invas Cardiol* 1991; 3:35–40.
109. Thomas HA, Stevers RE: Nonsurgical reduction of arterial catheter knots. *Am J Roentgenol* 1979; 132:1018–1019.
110. Trerotola SO, Kuhlman JE, Fishman EK: Bleeding complications of femoral catheterization: CT evaluation. *Radiology* 1990; 174:37–40.
111. Cohen GI, Chan KL: Physical examination and echo Doppler study in the assessment of femoral artery complications following cardiac catheterization. *Cathet Cardiovasc Diag* 1990; 21:137–143.
112. Fellmeth BD, Roberts AC, Bookstein JJ, Freischlag JA, Forsythe JR, Buckner NK, et al: Postangiographic femoral artery injuries: nonsurgical repair with US-ultrasound guided compression. *Radiology* 1991; 178:671–675.
113. Lalle AF: Contrast media reactions: Data analysis and hypothesis. *Radiology* 1980; 134:1–12.
114. Cohan RH, Dunnick NR: Intravascular contrast media: Adverse reactions. *Am J Roentgenol* 1987; 149:665–670.
115. Greenberger PA, Patterson R, Tapio CM: Prophylaxis against repeated radiocontrast media reactions in 857 cases. *Arch Intern Med* 1985; 145:2197–2200.
116. Dawson P: Contrast agent nephrotoxicity: An appraisal. *Br J Radiol* 1985; 58:121–124.
117. Dawson P: Chemotoxicity of contrast media and clinical adverse effects: A review. *Invest Radiol* 1985; 20(suppl):84–91.
118. Katzberg RW, Morris TW, Schulman G: Reactions to intravenous contrast media. *Radiology* 1983; 147:327–334.
119. Parfrey PS, Griffiths SM, Barrett MB, Paul MD, Genge M, Withers J, et al: Contrast material-induced renal failure in patients with diabetes mellitus, renal insufficiency or both. *N Engl J Med* 1989; 320:143–149.
120. Schwab SJ, Hlatky MA, Pieper KS: Contrast nephrotoxicity: A randomized controlled trial of a nonionic and an ionic contrast agent. *N Engl J Med* 1989; 320:149–153.
121. Greganti MA, Flowers W Jr: Acute pulmonary edema after the intravenous administration of contrast media. *Radiology* 1979; 132:583–585.
122. Ross J Jr (Chairman): Guidelines for coronary angiography: A report of the American College of Cardiology/American Heart Association Task Force on assessment of diagnostic and therapeutic cardiovascular procedures (Subcommittee on Coronary Arteriography). *Circulation* 1987; 76(4):963A.
123. Pepine CJ, Allen HD, Bashore TM, Brinker JA, Cohn LH, Dillon JC, et al: ACC/AHA Guidelines for Cardiac Catheterization Laboratories. *Circulation* 1991; 84:2213–2247.
124. Bashore TM: State of the art of coronary angiography. *J Invas Cardiol* 1991; 3(suppl B):47B–59B.
125. Sones FM Jr, Shirey EK: Cine coronary arteriography. *Mod Concepts Cardiovasc Dis* 1962; 31:735.
126. Abrams HL, Adams DF: The coronary arteriogram: I and II. Structural and functional aspects. *N Engl J Med* 1969; 281:1276–1285, 1336–1342.
127. Conti ER: Coronary arteriography. *Circulation* 1977; 55:227–237.
128. Verani MS: The functional significance of coronary collateral vessels: Anecdote confronts science. *Cathet Cardiovasc Diagn* 1983; 9:333–337.

129. Schwarz F, Schuler G, Hoffmann M, Kubler W: Recruitment of collaterals following acute coronary occlusion reduces infarct size in man. *J Am Coll Cardiol* 1983; 1:591.
130. Hamby RI, Aintablian A, Schwartz A: Reappraisal of the functional significance of the coronary collateral circulation. *Am J Cardiol* 1976; 38:304–309.
131. Nohara R, Kambara H, Murakami T, Kadota K, Tamaki S, Kawai C: Collateral function in early acute myocardial infarction. *Am J Cardiol* 1983; 52:955–959.
132. Mehmel HC, Schwarz F, Schuler G, Maurer W, Tillmanns H, Senges J: The functional result of intracoronary streptokinase therapy after myocardial infarction may be determined by collaterals. *Circulation* 1981; 64(suppl IV):IV–194.
133. Rentrop P, Merx W, Mathey D, Blanke H, Rutsch W, Karsch KR: Functional results of streptokinase-reperfusion in relation to collaterals and duration of symptoms. *Circulation* 1981; 64(suppl IV):IV–194.
134. Helfant RH, Vokonas PS, Gorlin R: Functional importance of the human coronary collateral circulation. *N Engl J Med* 1971; 284:1277–1281.
135. Heupler FA Jr: Syndrome of symptomatic coronary arterial spasm with nearly normal coronary arteriograms. *Am J Cardiol* 1980; 45:873–881.
136. Curry RC, Pepine CJ, Sabom M, Feldman RL, Christie LG, Conti CR: Effects of ergonovine in patients with and without coronary artery disease. *Circulation* 1977; 56:803–809.
137. Conti CR, Curry RC, Christie LG, Pepine CJ: Clinical use of provocative pharmacoangiography in patients with chest pain. *Adv Cardiol* 1979; 26:44–54.
138. Oliva P, Potts D, Pluss R: Coronary arterial spasm in Prinzmetal angina: Documentation by coronary arteriography. *N Engl J Med* 1973; 288:746.
139. Waters DD, Szlachcic J, Bonan R: Comparative sensitivity of exercise, coldpressor and ergonovine testing in provoking attacks of variant angina in patients with active disease. *Circulation* 1983; 67:310–315.
140. Maseri A, Severi S, DeNes M, Marzilli M, Ballestra AM, Parodi O, et al: "Variant" angina: One aspect of a continuous spectrum of vasospastic myocardial ischemia: Pathogenic mechanisms, estimated incidence and clinical and arteriographic findings in 138 patients. *Am J Cardiol* 1978; 42:1019–1035.
141. O'Neill WW, Walton JA, Bates ER, Calfer HT, Aueron PM, LeFree MT, et al: Criteria for successful coronary angioplasty as assessed by alterations in coronary vasodilatory reserve. *J Am Coll Cardiol* 1984; 3:1382–1390.
142. Helfant RH, Pine R, Meister SG, Feldman MS, Trout RG, Banka VS: Nitroglycerin to unmask reversible asynergy: Correlation with post coronary bypass ventriculography. *Circulation* 1974; 50:108–113.
143. Horn HR, Teichholz LE, Cohn PF, Herman MV, Gorlin R: Augmentation of left ventricular contraction pattern in coronary artery disease by inotropic catecholamine: The epinephrine ventriculogram. *Circulation* 1974; 49:1063–1071.
144. Dyke SH, Cohn PF, Gorlin R, Sonnenblick EH: Detection of residual myocardial function in coronary artery disease using post extrasystolic potentiation. *Circulation* 1974; 50:694–699.
145. Formanek A, Nath PH, Zollikofer C, Moller JH: Selective coronary arteriography in children. *Circulation* 1980; 61:84–95.
146. Dabizzi RP, Caprioli G, Aiazzi L, Castelli C, Baldrighi G, Parenzan L, et al: Distribution and anomalies of coronary arteries in tetralogy of Fallot. *Circulation* 1980; 61:95–102.
147. Heupler FA Jr: Coronary arteriography and left ventriculography: Sones technique. In: King SB III, Douglas JS Jr (eds): *Coronary Arteriography*. New York, McGraw-Hill, 1984: 137–181.
148. Seldinger SI: Catheter replacement of the needle in percutaneous arteriography: A new technique. *Acta Radiol* 1953; 39:368.
149. Ricketts HJ, Abrams HL: Percutaneous selective coronary cine arteriography. *JAMA* 1962; 181:620.
150. Amplatz K, Formanek G, Stranger P, Wilson W: Mechanics of selective coronary artery catheterization via femoral approach. *Radiology* 1967; 89:1040–1047.
151. Judkins MP: Selective coronary arteriography: I. A percutaneous transfemoral technique. *Radiology* 1967; 89:815–824.
152. Judkins MP, Judkins EJ: The Judkins technique. In: King SB III, Douglas JS Jr (eds): *Coronary Arteriography*. New York, McGraw-Hill, 1984: 182–217.
153. Schoonmaker FW, King SB III: Coronary arteriography by the single catheter percutaneous femoral technique: Experience with 6,800 cases. *Circulation* 1974; 50:735–740.
154. King SB III, Douglas JS Jr: Catheterization techniques in coronary arteriography and left ventriculography: Multipurpose techniques. In: King SB III, Douglas JS Jr (eds): *Coronary Arteriography*. New York, McGraw-Hill, 1984: 239–274.
155. Douglas JS Jr, King SB III: Complications of coronary arteriography: Management during and following the procedure. In: King SB III, Douglas JS Jr (eds): *Coronary Arteriography*. New York, McGraw-Hill, 1984: 302–313.
156. Austin WG, Edwards JE, Frye RL, Gensini GC, Gott VL, Griffith LSC, et al: A reporting system on patients evaluated for coronary artery disease: Report of the ad hoc committee for grading coronary artery disease, Council on Cardiovascular Surgery, American Heart Association. *Circulation* 1975; 51(suppl 4):30.
157. Bunnell IL, Greene DG, Tandom RN, Arani DT: The halfaxial projection: A new look at the proximal left coronary artery. *Circulation* 1973; 48:1151–1156.
158. Aldridge HE, McLoughlin MJ, Taylor KW: Improved diagnosis in coronary cine arteriography with routine use of 110 oblique views and cranial and caudal angulations. *Am J Cardiol* 1975; 36:468–473.
159. Frederick PR, Fry WH, Russell JG, Marshall HW: Longitudinal angulation in coronary arteriography: Apparatus and evaluation. *Cathet Cardiovasc Diagn* 1977; 3:305–311.
160. King SB III, Douglas JS Jr, Morris DC: New angiographic views for coronary arteriography. In: Hurst JW (ed): *The Heart, Update IV*. New York, McGraw-Hill, 1980: 275.
161. McMahon MM, Brown BG, Cukingnan R, Rolett EL, Bolson E, Frimer M, et al: Quantitative coronary angiography: Measurement of the "critical" stenosis in patients with unstable angina and single vessel disease without collaterals. *Circulation* 1979; 60:106–113.
162. Kramer JR, Kitazume H, Proudfitt WL, Sones FM Jr: Clinical significance of isolated coronary bridges: Benign and frequent condition involving the left anterior descending artery. *Am Heart J* 1982; 103:283–288.
163. Ishimori T, Raizner AE, Chahine RA, Awdeh M, Luchi RJ: Myocardial bridges in man: Clinical correlations and angiographic accentuations with nitroglycerin. *Cathet Cardiovasc Diagn* 1977; 3:59–65.
164. Kitazume H, Kramer JR, Krauthamer D: Myocardial bridges in obstructive hypertrophic cardiomyopathy. *Am Heart J* 1983; 106:131–135.
165. Brugada P, Bar FW, DeZwaan C, Roy D, Green M, Wellens HJ: "Sawfish" systolic narrowing of the left anterior descending coronary artery: An angiographic sign of hypertrophic cardiomyopathy. *Circulation* 1982; 66:800–803.
166. Engel HJ, Torres C, Page HL: Major variations in anatomical origin of the coronary arteries. *Cathet Cardiovasc Diagn* 1975; 1:157–169.
167. Chaitman BR, Lesperance J, Saltiel J, Bourassa MG: Clinical, angiographic, and hemodynamic findings in patients with anomalous origin of the coronary arteries. *Circulation* 1976; 53:122–131.
168. Donaldson RM, Raphael M, Radley-Smith R, Yacoub MH, Ross DN: Angiographic identification of primary coronary anomalies causing impaired myocardial perfusion. *Cathet Cardiovasc Diagn* 1983; 9:237–249.
169. Ogden JA: Congenital anomalies of the coronary arteries. *Am J Cardiol* 1970; 25:474–479.
170. Benge W, Martins JB, Funk DC: Morbidity associated with anomalous origin of the right coronary artery from the left sinus of Valsalva. *Am Heart J* 1980; 99:96–100.
171. Antopol W, Kugel MA: Anomalous origin of the left circumflex coronary artery. *Am Heart J* 1933; 8:802.
172. Donaldson RM, Raphael MJ: Missing coronary artery: Review of technical problems in coronary arteriography resulting from anatomical variants. *Br Heart J* 1982; 47:62–72.
173. Kimbiris D, Iskandrian AS, Segal BL, Bemis CE: Anomalous aortic origin of the coronary arteries. *Circulation* 1978; 58:606–615.
174. Page HL Jr, Engel HJ, Campbell WB, Thomas CS Jr: Anomalous origin of the left circumflex coronary artery: Recognition, angiographic demonstration, and clinical significance. *Circulation* 1974; 50:768–773.
175. Levin DC, Fellows KE, Abrams HL: Hemodynamically signifi-

cant primary anomalies of the coronary arteries, angiographic aspects. *Circulation* 1978; 58:25–34.
176. Moodie DS, Gill GC, Loop FD, Sheldon WC: Anomalous left main coronary artery originating from the right sinus of Valsalva: Pathophysiology, angiographic definition, and surgical approaches. *J Thorac Cardiovasc Surg* 1980; 80:198–205.
177. Mustafa I, Gula G, Radley-Smith R, Durrer S, Yacoub MH: Anomalous origin of the left coronary artery from the anterior aortic sinus: A potential cause of sudden death: Anatomic characterization and surgical treatment. *J Thorac Cardiovasc Surg* 1981; 82:297–300.
178. Chaitman BR, Lesperance J, Saltiel J, Bourassa MG: Clinical, angiographic and hemodynamic findings in patients with anomalous origin of the coronary arteries. *Circulation* 1976; 53:122–131.
179. Liberthson RR, Dinsmore RE, Fallon JT: Aberrant coronary artery origin from the aorta: Report of 18 patients: Review of literature and delineation of natural history and management. *Circulation* 1979; 59:748–754.
180. Thompson SI, Vieweg WV, Alpert JS, Hagan AD: Anomalous origin of the right coronary artery from the left sinus of Valsalva with associated chest pain: Report of two cases. *Cathet Cardiovasc Diagn* 1976; 2:397–402.
181. Roberts WC, Siegel RJ, Zipes DP: Origin of the right coronary artery from the left sinus of Valsalva and its functional consequences: Analysis of 10 necropsy patients. *Am J Cardiol* 1982; 49:863–868.
182. Brandt B III, Martins JB, Marcus ML: Anomalous origin of the right coronary artery from the left sinus of Valsalva. *N Engl J Med* 1983; 309:596–598.
183. Ogden JA, Goodyer AVN: Patterns of distribution of the single coronary artery. *Yale J Biol Med* 1970; 43:11–21.
184. Sharbaugh AH, White RS: Single coronary artery: Analysis of the anatomic variation, clinical importance, and report of five cases. *JAMA* 1974; 230:243–246.
185. Lipton MJ, Barry WH, Obrez I, Silverman JF, Wexler L: Isolated single coronary artery: Diagnosis, angiographic classification, and clinical significance. *Radiology* 1979; 130:39–47.
186. Gorlin R: Coronary collaterals. *Major Probl Intern Med* 1976; 11:59–70.
187. Verani MS: The functional significance of coronary collateral vessels: Anecdote confronts science. *Cathet Cardiovasc Diagn* 1983; 9:333–337.
188. Hamby RI, Aintablian A, Schwartz A: Reappraisal of the functional significance of the coronary collateral circulation. *Am J Cardiol* 1976; 38:305–309.
189. Morales AR, Romanelli R, Boucek RJ: The mural left anterior descending coronary artery, strenuous exercise and sudden death. *Circulation* 1980; 62:230–237.
190. Levin DC: Pathways and functional significance of the coronary collateral circulation. *Circulation* 1974; 50:831–837.
191. Zir LM, Miller SW, Dinsmore RE, Gilbert JP, Harthorne JW: Interobserver variability in coronary arteriography. *Circulation* 1976; 53:627–630.
192. DeRouen TA, Murray JA, Owen W: Variability in the analysis of coronary arteriograms. *Circulation* 1977; 55:324–328.
193. Schwartz JN, King Y, Hackel DB, Bartel AG: Comparison of angiographic and postmortem findings in patients with coronary artery disease. *Am J Cardiol* 1975; 36:174.
194. Kemp HG, Evans H, Elliott WC, Gorlin R: Diagnostic accuracy of selective coronary cinearteriography. *Circulation* 1967; 36:526–533.
195. Grandin CM, Dyrda I, Pastemac A, Campeau L, Bourassa MG, Lesperance J: Discrepancies between cineangiographic and postmortem findings in patients with coronary artery disease and recent myocardial revascularization. *Circulation* 1974; 49:703–708.
196. Roberts WC: The coronary arteries and left ventricle in clinically isolated angina pectoris: A necropsy analysis. *Circulation* 1976; 54:388–390.
197. Arnett EN, Isner JM, Redwood DR, Kent KM, Baker WP, Ackerstein H, et al: Coronary artery narrowing in coronary heart disease: Comparison of cine angiographic and necropsy findings. *Ann Intern Med* 1979; 91:350–356.
198. Roberts CS, Roberts WC: Cross-sectional area of the proximal portions of the three major epicardial coronary arteries in 98 patients with different coronary events: Relationship to heart, weight, age, and sex. *Circulation* 1980; 62:953–959.
199. Isner JM, Kishel J, Kent KM, Ronan JA Jr, Ross AM, Roberts WC: Inaccuracy of angiographic determination of left main coronary arterial narrowing: Angiographic-histologic correlative analysis of 29 patients. *Circulation* 1979; 59, 60(suppl 2):II—161.
200. Brown BG, Bolson E, Frimer M, Dodge HT: Quantitative coronary arteriography: Estimation of dimensions, hemodynamic resistance, and atheroma mass of coronary artery lesions using the arteriogram and digital computation. *Circulation* 1977; 55:329–337.
201. Abrams HL, Adams DF: The complications of coronary arteriography. *Circulation* 1975; 52(suppl 2):27.
202. Davis K, Kennedy JW, Kemp HG, Judkins MP, Gosselin AJ, Killip T: Complications of coronary arteriography from the Collaborative Study of Coronary Artery Surgery (CASS). *Circulation* 1979; 59:1105–1112.
203. Johnson LW, Lozner EC, Johnson S, Krone R, Pichard AD, Vetrovec GW, et al: Coronary arteriography 1984–1987: A Report of the Registry of the Society for Cardiac Angiography and Interventions. 1. Results and complications. *Cathet Cardiovasc Diagn* 1989; 17:5–10.
204. Lozner EC, Johnson LW, Johnson S, Krone R, Pichard AD, Vetrovec GW, et al: Coronary arteriography 1984–1987: A Report of the Registry of the Society for Cardiac Angiography and Interventions. II. An analysis of 218 deaths related to coronary arteriography. *Cathet Cardiovasc Diagn* 1989; 17:11–14.
205. Gersh BJ, Kronmal RA, Frye RL, Schaff HV, Ryan TJ, Gosselin AJ, et al: Coronary arteriography and coronary bypass surgery: Morbidity and mortality in patients ages 65 years or older: A report from the coronary artery surgery study. *Circulation* 1983; 67:483–491.
206. Noto TJ Jr, Johnson LW, Krone R, Weaver WF, Clark DA, Kramer JR, et al: Cardiac catheterization 1990: A Report of the Registry of the Society for Cardiac Angiography and Interventions (SCA&I). *Cathet Cardiovasc Diagn* 1991; 24:75–83.
207. Takaro T, Hultgren HN, Littmann D, Wright EC: An analysis of deaths occurring in association with coronary arteriography. *Am Heart J* 1973; 86:587–597.
208. Patterson R, Anderson J: Allergic reactions to drugs and biologic agents. *JAMA* 1982; 248:2637–2645.
209. Lieberman P, Siegle RL, Taylor WW: Anaphylactoid reactions to iodinated contrast material. *J Allergy Clin Immunol* 1978; 62:174–180.
210. Madowitz JS, Schweiger MJ: Severe anaphylactoid reaction to radiographic contrast media. *JAMA* 1979; 241:2813–2815.
211. Harrison TR: Some unanswered questions concerning enlargement and failure of the heart. *Am Heart J* 1965; 69:100.
212. Herman MV, Heinle RA, Klein MD, Gorlin R: Localized disorders in myocardial contraction. *N Engl J Med* 1967; 227:222–2327.
213. Dodge HT, Sandler H, Ballew DW, Lord JD Jr: The use of biplane angiocardiography for the measurement of left ventricular volume in man. *Am Heart J* 1960; 60:762.
214. Vogel JHK, Cornish D, McFadden RB: Underestimations of ejection fraction with single plane angiography in coronary artery disease: Role of biplane angiography. *Chest* 1973; 64:217–221.

PART XXII

The Heart, Anesthesia and Surgery

Chapter 139

Perioperative Evaluation and Management of Patients with Known or Suspected Cardiovascular Disease Who Undergo Noncardiac Surgery

Robert C. Schlant, M.D.

EPIDEMIOLOGY

In the United States each year it is estimated that approximately 25 million patients have noncardiac surgery, approximately 50,000 have perioperative myocardial infarction, and more than half of 40,000 deaths are caused by cardiac events.[1-3] The number of cardiac surgeries annually exceeds 400,000 including 285,000 coronary artery bypass surgical procedures and 40,000 valve replacements.[3] As indicated in Fig. 139-1, a significant number of the 25 million patients have previously diagnosed coronary artery disease (CAD), another 2 to 3 million have two or more major risk factors (Chap. 62) for CAD, and 4 million are over the age of 65. More than 25 percent of the surgical procedures are major procedures, and in patients undergoing major vascular surgery who do not have clinically evident CAD, 40 to 70 percent have been shown to have CAD at coronary arteriography.[4,5] In future years, the number of surgical patients over 65 years of age will rise, further increasing the number of noncardiac patients at risk for perioperative cardiac morbidity (PCM), which includes myocardial infarction (MI), unstable angina pectoris, congestive heart failure (CHF), serious arrhythmia, or cardiac death.[1,6-8]

PATIENTS WITH KNOWN CARDIAC DISEASE

Coronary Artery Disease

Patients with CAD have a perioperative rate of myocardial infarction after noncardiac surgery of 1.1 percent,[9] compared to a rate of 0 to 0.7 percent in the general population.[1] The reported rates of reinfarction in patients with prior MI vary overall from 5 to 8 percent: from 1 to 15 percent following vascular surgery and from 6 to 40 percent in patients with a recent MI.[8] (See below.) One recent study reported a reinfarction rate of 1.9 percent, which increased to 5.7 percent if the prior infarction occurred less than 3 months previously.[10] The risk of postoperative MI in patients with prior coronary artery revascularization has been reported to be only 0

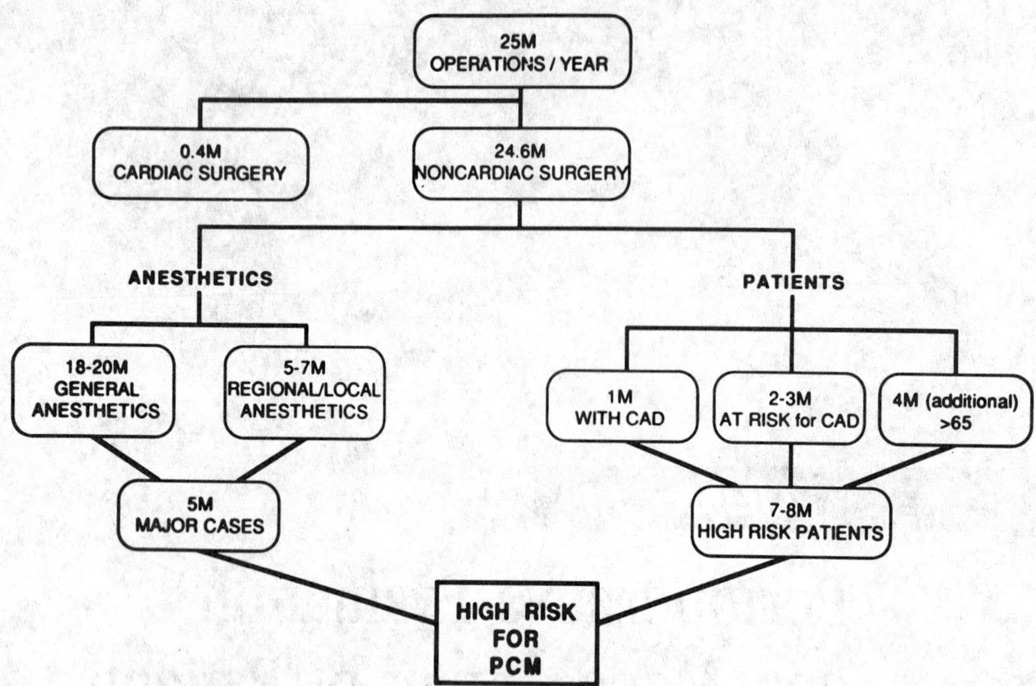

FIGURE 139-1 Estimates of the number of surgeries and anesthetics, and the patients at risk for perioperative cardiac morbidity (PCM) in the United States (1988). A total of 6 million (30 percent) surgical patients are over the age of 65. Two million of these are included in the CAD and at risk for CAD groups, resulting in the 4 million over age 65 (and the 7 to 8 million total) shown in the figure. *(Sources: National Center for Health Statistics, U.S. Public Health Service, Department of Health and Human Services[3]; the American College of Surgeons; and the American Society of Anesthesiologists.) (From Mangano DT.[1] Reproduced with permission from the publisher and author.)*

to 1.2 percent.[8] Of significance, the mortality following a perioperative MI is higher than following a nonoperative MI (Chap. 60) and has been reported to range from 26 to 70 percent, with an average of 50 percent.[11–13] Most perioperative infarctions occur within the first 4 postoperative days and are usually clinically silent, although they are often associated with ST-segment changes in the preceding 3 to 6 h.[1,6–8] In some studies, non-Q-wave infarctions tended to occur in the first 2 days, whereas Q-wave infarctions tended to occur on postoperative days 2 to 4.[1,13–16]

Previous Myocardial Infarction

A recent (<6 months) myocardial infarction is one of two consistently proven preoperative predictors of PCM.[8] Patients with a documented history of MI have a perioperative risk of about 6 percent (range, 2.8 to 17.7 percent) of having a recurrent perioperative MI.[13] Several studies of the influence of a preceding MI on the likelihood of having a recurrent perioperative infarction during noncardiac surgery have been performed at the Mayo Clinic, covering the years 1967 to 1968[14] and the years 1974 to 1975.[17] During 1974 and 1975 the risk of perioperative reinfarction was 27 percent if the surgery was performed less than 3 months after an MI, 11 percent in patients operated upon between 3 and 6 months post-MI, and 4 to 5 percent if the surgery was more than 6 months post-MI.[17] Subsequently, Rao et al.[10] found that reinfarction occurred in only 1.9 percent overall of patients with a history of MI and in only 5.7 percent of patients operated on less than 3 months post-MI and in 2.3 percent of patients operated on within 4 to 6 months post-MI. In their study, however, 88 percent of the patients had arterial monitoring catheters, 83 percent had pulmonary artery catheters, and 60 percent had extended (3 to 4 days) Intensive Care Unit care. Accordingly, there is a need for a cost-benefit study of such intensive care before it can be recommended widely. In the Coronary Artery Surgery Study (CASS) Registry, a history of MI, including MI within 6 months, did not have a statistically significant association with increased cardiac mortality or morbidity.[18]

Systemic Arterial Hypertension

Systemic arterial hypertension (SAH) is the most common cardiovascular disease in the United States, affecting more than 59 million patients.[3] SAH is a risk factor for CAD, CHF, stroke, and peripheral vascular disease. Some studies have indicated that untreated or poorly controlled SAH is associated with an increased incidence of perioperative myocardial ischemia, arrhythmias, and transient neurologic symptoms, although other studies have indicated that mild-to-moderate hypertension is only an intermediate risk factor for blood pressure lability and myocardial ischemia. Whenever possible, SAH should be controlled prior to surgery, and antihypertensive medications continued up to, during, and following surgery. Special care should be taken to avoid a rebound phenomenon with increased blood pressure and tachycardia which can occur if therapy is not continued with clonidine or, occasionally, a beta blocker. (See also Chap. 77.)

Valvular Heart Disease

Patients with valvular heart disease should have antibiotic prophylaxis (Chap. 94) prior to surgery that is likely to be associated with bacteremia. Patients who are on chronic anticoagulant therapy with warfarin for a prosthetic heart valve or atrial fibrillation should have the warfarin discontinued approximately 5 to 7 days prior to elective surgery and should have a normal prothrombin time prior to surgery. In patients with a prosthetic heart valve, intravenous heparin should be initiated. In patients with a history of arterial embolism, subcutaneous or, preferably, intravenous heparin therapy should be begun when warfarin is discontinued and the dosage should be adjusted to maintain the partial thromboplastin time 1.5 to 2.0 times the control value. The effect of heparin should be reversed by intravenous protamine sulfate immediately prior to surgery. Postoperatively, heparin and warfarin are started when there is no evidence or risk of bleeding. The heparin is discontinued when the prothrombin time is within therapeutic range. (See Chaps. 68, 83, and 122.) In emergency situations, the effect of oral anticoagulants such as warfarin can be reversed by intravenous vitamin K_1, in doses of 10 to 25 mg; however, large doses of vitamin K_1 will often delay the anticoagulant effects of warfarin when it is reinstated postoperatively. In patients who do not respond to vitamin K_1, fresh frozen plasma should be given.

In other cardiac or noncardiac patients who are at increased risk of pulmonary embolism (see Chap. 100 and Table 125-2), prophylactic low-dose heparin (5,000 to 10,000 units every 8 to 12 h) may be given subcutaneously, preferably beginning at least 18 to 22 h prior to surgery. Selected patients and procedures require higher doses; heparin should be avoided in brain or eye surgery or in patients undergoing spinal anesthesia. (See Chap. 100).

Patients with moderate to severe mitral or aortic stenosis or hypertrophic cardiomyopathy are very sensitive to changes in effective blood volume and venous return. Accordingly, the use of a percutaneous balloon catheter to monitor pulmonary artery pressures during surgery is often helpful. In a report from the Mayo Clinic, 48 patients who had significant aortic stenosis but preserved left ventricular systolic function underwent noncardiac surgery or diagnostic procedures between 1985 and 1987 without major sequelae or death.[19] These impressive results are attributed to excellent anesthesia.

Congestive Heart Failure

Postoperative CHF occurred in 3.6 percent of patients older than 40 years with or without CAD[14] and in 4.8 percent of patients with a history of previous MI.[10] A history of dysrhythmias or diabetes mellitus is also associated with an increased risk of postoperative CHF.[6,9,14,20,21]

Current CHF is the second consistently proven preoperative predictor of PCM.[8,9] In general, patients with moderate to severe CHF should be treated with triple therapy (Chap. 26), i.e., with a diuretic, an angiotensin-converting enzyme (ACE) inhibitor, and digoxin to optimize the symptoms and signs of CHF prior to surgery. Therapy should be given preoperatively and continued intraoperatively and postoperatively. When possible, attempts should be made to correct the hemodynamic disturbance and congestion resulting from the CHF prior to surgery. Special care should be taken to avoid hypokalemia, hypomagnesemia, excess depletion of blood volume, and excess digitalis.

More difficult to manage are patients without known CHF who have not been on therapy but who are found preoperatively to have moderate or marked cardiomegaly on chest film or decreased left ventricular function by echocardiography. In such patients, it is probably advisable to initiate therapy with an ACE inhibitor but to administer diuretics preoperatively only if there is evidence of peripheral edema on physical examination or pulmonary congestion on chest film. In this situation, digoxin is usually not given prophylactically unless the left ventricular ejection fraction is below about 40 percent, particularly if there is also evidence of edema, increased jugular venous pressure, and an S_3 gallop. If it is decided to use digoxin, it should be initiated several days prior to surgery whenever possible. In emergencies, very cautious digitalization can be begun preoperatively and completed postoperatively. Intra- and perioperative inotropic support can be provided in severe heart failure with intravenous dobutamine and/or amyinone.

Congenital Heart Disease

Most patients with congenital heart disease should receive prophylactic antibiotic therapy against endocarditis when undergoing surgery that might be associated with bacteremia. (See Chap. 94.) Patients who have had a patent ductus arteriosus ligated and divided or who have had an isolated ostium secundum atrial septal defect repaired more than 6 months previously may not require prophylaxis. Patients with cyanotic heart disease are at increased risk of vascular thrombosis and postoperative bleeding. If their hematocrit is greater than 65 percent, such patients should undergo cautious preoperative phlebotomy with replacement of the blood volume. If possible, they should receive their own plasma back as part of the replacement fluid. (See Chaps. 97 and 98.)

Arrhythmia and Conduction Disorders

A history of a cardiac arrhythmia is associated with an increased likelihood of postoperative CHF.[1,9,14,20,21]

About 60 percent of all patients have perioperative arrhythmias, most of which, however, require no therapy. Patients who have premature atrial or junctional beats usually do not require therapy. Preoperatively, if such beats are very frequent and symptomatic and if there is adequate time, the use of a beta blocker or digoxin may be considered. Patients with CAD who have more than about five ventricular premature contractions (PVCs) per minute, especially if they are multifocal or occur in runs, should be considered for intravenous lidocaine (2 to 3 g in 1 liter of 5% glucose in water), initiated at a rate of 1 mL/min and continued during surgery. While such therapy is especially useful in patients with known CAD, it is usually not necessary in patients with no evidence of cardiac disease. (See Chap. 36.)

Adults undergoing emergency surgery who have supraventricular tachyarrhythmias should be considered for either electrical conversions (Chap. 41) or rate control employing intravenous digoxin, beta blocker, verapamil, or diltiazem. (See Chap. 36.)

Patients with a history of Stokes-Adams attacks, complete heart block, high-degree (Möbitz II) atrioventricular heart block, or prolonged sinoatrial pause or block should be considered for a prophylactic temporary right heart pacemaker. (See Chap. 39.) Patients with asymptomatic bifascicular block (left or right bundle branch block with left anterior or posterior fascicular block), with or without prolongation of the PR interval, usually do not require a prophylactic pacemaker prior to surgery, although a pacing catheter should be readily available in the operating room. If a patient with left bundle branch block requires the insertion of a pulmonary artery balloon (Swan-Ganz) catheter to monitor pressures during surgery, it is advisable to use a multipurpose catheter that permits atrial, ventricular, and atrioventricular sequential pacing. (See Chap. 39.)

Patients with a permanent pacemaker rarely have intraoperative pacemaker failure. When failure does occur, it may be due to electrolyte abnormalities, particularly potassium, or to myocardial ischemia and infarction. Rarely, pacemaker dysfunction may be related to the use of an electrocautery. Automatic implantable cardioverter-defibrillator (AICD) units can also be temporarily or permanently inhibited by electromagnetic interference from an electrocautery. During electrocautery surgery, the electrosurgical tip and the ground plate should be as far away from the pacemaker or AICD as possible, and electrosurgery should be limited to 2- to 3-s periods if any pacemaker suppression is produced (see also Chap. 42.)

Pulmonary Embolism

Patients who have a history of pulmonary embolism are at increased risk of a perioperative recurrence. Whenever possible, such patients should receive prophylactic low-dose heparin preoperatively, intraoperatively, and postoperatively. (See Chap. 100.) In such patients graduated pressure compression stockings and external pneumatic compression of the lower extremities should be begun at least 24 h preoperatively in the absence of contraindications. In extremely high risk patients, one should consider the prophylactic insertion of a filter in the inferior vena cava. (See Chap. 100.)

TABLE 139-1

The Dripps–American Society of Anesthesiologists Classification of Physical Status

1. A normal healthy patient
2. A patient with a mild systemic disease
3. A patient with a severe systemic disease that limits activity but is not incapacitating
4. A patient with an incapacitating systemic disease that is a constant threat to life
5. A moribund patient not expected to survive 24 h with or without operation

NOTE: In the event of emergency operation, precede the number with an E.

SOURCE: American Society of Anesthesiologists.[28] Reproduced with permission from the publisher.

Diabetes Mellitus

Diabetes mellitus is a well-known risk factor for coronary atherosclerosis.[22–27] (See Chaps. 62 and 102.) Patients with diabetes are more likely to have asymptomatic or silent ischemia than other patients, possibly because of altered neural pain pathways in the heart. Diabetes is also associated with an increased risk of postoperative CHF.[6,14,18,20,21]

PREOPERATIVE EVALUATION OF PATIENTS WITH UNKNOWN OR SUSPECTED CARDIAC DISEASE

The two major conditions responsible for most perioperative cardiac morbidity that especially should be carefully evaluated preoperatively are coronary artery disease and left ventricular dysfunction. Several multivariant indices of risk have been developed in an attempt to quantify the risk preoperatively. These include the factors in Table 139-1 [the Dripps–American Society of Anesthesiologists (AST) classification of physical status][28] and the Goldman cardiac risk index (Table 139-2).[21] The clinical validity of Goldman's risk index has been confirmed by many but not all investigations.[8,29] Detsky et al. developed a modified risk index (Table 139-3).[30,31] At present, however, there is no consistently accurate preoperative risk index that is generally applicable and utilized. Despite this, such risk indices do provide useful guidelines for the identification of patients at increased risk during noncardiac surgery. In addition to the classic predictors of increased risk, recent studies have evaluated the role of preoperative noninvasive and invasive tests to identify patients at increased risk. (See below.)

Age

Although the data supporting or refuting the predictive value of age is controversial, perioperative MI is the leading cause of postoperative death in the elderly undergoing noncardiac surgery.[1,8,13]

Twelve-Lead Electrocardiogram (ECG)

This should be obtained routinely in patients over the age of 40 and in younger patients with increased risk factors for cardiovascular disease. While the possibility of detecting a previously undiagnosed MI is relatively low, perhaps in only 3 to 4 percent of adults,[32] the ECG may detect significant hypertrophy, conduction abnormalities, or nonspecific ST-T wave changes; it is extremely valuable for comparison postoperatively should complications occur. Other indications for a preoperative ECG include emergency operations; patients with conditions that can be associated with cardiac involvement; patients taking or about to receive noncardiac medications that are associated with cardiac toxicity or

TABLE 139-2
The Goldman Multifactorial Cardiac Risk Index

Criteria	Multivariate Discriminant-Function Coefficient	Points
1. History		
Age > 70 years	0.191	5
MI in previous 6 months	0.384	10
2. Physical examination		
S_3 gallop or JVD	0.451	11
Important VAS	0.119	3
3. Electrocardiogram		
Rhythm other than sinus or PACs on last preoperative ECG	0.283	7
>5 PVCs/min documented at any time before operation	0.278	7
4. General status		
P_{O_2} < 60 or P_{CO_2} > 50 mmHg, K < 3.0 or H_{CO_3} < 20 meq/liter, BUN > 50 or Cr > 3.0 mg/dL, abnormal SGOT, signs of chronic liver disease, or patient bedridden from noncardiac causes	0.132	3
5. Operation		
Intraperitoneal, intrathoracic, or aortic operation	0.123	3
Emergency Operation	0.167	4
Total		53

ABBREVIATIONS: MI, myocardial infarction; JVD, jugular-vein distention; VAS, valvular aortic stenosis; PAC, premature atrial contractions; ECG, electrocardiogram; PVC, premature ventricular contractions; P_{O_2}, partial pressure of oxygen; P_{CO_2}, partial pressure of carbon dioxide; K, potassium; HCO_3, bicarbonate; BUN, blood urea nitrogen; Cr, creatinine; SGOT, serum glutamic oxaloacetic transaminase.

SOURCE: Goldman L et al.[21] Reproduced with permission from the publisher and authors.

ECG alterations; patients at risk for major electrolyte disorders; and patients undergoing neurosurgery, intrathoracic surgery, or aortic surgery.

Chest Roentgenogram

A routine preoperative chest film in patients over the age of 40 is useful primarily as a baseline for comparison with postoperative films when the patient may have complications such as pneumonia, atelectasis, or pulmonary embolism. In addition, cardiomegaly on chest film can be the first sign of decreased left ventricular function. Cardiomegaly on a 6-f (2-m) chest film indicates an ejection fraction of less than 0.40 in over 70 percent of patients with CAD.[32] The presence of a tortuous or calcified aorta may also be a predictor of increased operative risk.[33]

Exercise Stress Testing

The effectiveness of routine preoperative exercise stress testing in identifying patients at increased risk is controversial.[1,8] A poor exercise functional capacity, especially in combination with ECG evidence of myocardial ischemia (Chap. 16), is associated with a significantly increased risk during noncardiac surgery.[13] (See below.)

Radionuclide Angiography (RNA)

In general, the resting left ventricular ejection fraction is a relatively insensitive and nonspecific predictor of perioperative cardiac complications. Similar conclusions apply to exercise radionuclide angiography (Chap. 134), although evidence of poor functional capacity does correlate with increased cardiac risk.[13]

Radionuclide Scintigraphy

Exercise radionuclide thallium scintigraphy (Chap. 134) is a very effective test for identifying patients at increased risk of perioperative cardiac morbidity. In general, it has about a 90 percent sensitivity in patients with triple-vessel CAD and a 60 percent sensitivity in patients with single-vessel disease.[34,35] In general, specificity is over 90 percent.

TABLE 139-3
The Modified Multifactorial Cardiac Risk Index

Variables	Points
CAD	
MI within 6 months	10
MI more than 6 months previously	5
Canadian Cardiovascular Society angina	
Class 3	10
Class 4	20
Unstable angina within 3 months	10
Alveolar pulmonary edema	
Within 1 week	10
Ever	5
Valvular disease	
Suspected critical aortic stenosis	20
Arrhythmias	
Sinus plus atrial premature beats or rhythm other than sinus on last preoperative ECG	5
More than 5 ventricular premature beats at any time before surgery	5
Poor general medical status*	5
Age over 70 years	5
Emergency operation	10

* Oxygen pressure < 60 mmHg; carbon dioxide pressure > 50 mmHg; serum potassium < 3.0 meq/liter (< 3.0 mmol/liter); serum bicarbonate < 20 meq/liter (<20 mmol/liter); serum urea nitrogen > 50 mg/dL (> 18 mmol/liter); serum creatine > 3 mg/dL (> 260 mmol/liter); aspartate aminotransferase, abnormal; signs of chronic liver disease; and/or bedridden because of noncardiac causes.

SOURCE: Detsky AS et al.[31] Reproduced with permission from the publisher and authors.

In the many patients who cannot exercise adequately, such as patients with peripheral vascular disease, orthopedic or neurologic disease, advanced age, obesity, or deconditioning, the use of preoperative dipyridamole-thallium imaging has good sensitivity (93 percent) and specificity (80 percent) for the detection of significant coronary stenosis when patients undergo coronary arteriography.[36–38] In uncontrolled studies of patients undergoing vascular surgery, preoperative dipyridamole-thallium imaging has a good sensitivity (89 to 100 percent) and a nearly 100 percent negative predictive value.[1,37,39] It is of particular value in patients who have stable angina pectoris, a history of MI, or diabetes mellitus.[40,41] On the other hand, Mangano et al.[42] recently found no association between redistribution defects and adverse cardiac outcome or perioperative myocardial ischemia. The explanation for this difference is not apparent.

In patients undergoing vascular surgery, dipyridamole-thallium 201 scintigraphy has been found to be superior in predicting increased risk for PCM to either exercise ECG testing or the estimation of left ventricular ejection fraction (LVEF) by gated blood pool scanning during exercise.[43] In patients prior to repair of abdominal aortic aneurysm it was also superior to both the preoperative estimation of LVEF by echocardiography and the Goldman risk factor analysis.[44] Similar results have been reported in other studies.[45–47]

In general, the finding of an abnormal thallium redistribution is very sensitive but is only moderately specific. It is of great value in the preoperative evaluation of patients who are scheduled for vascular or nonvascular surgery and who have clinical markers of intermediate increased risk.[13,40] (See Chap. 58.) It also has value in predicting long-term outcome.[48–50]

Dipyridamole-thallium testing can be associated with hypotension, which can be especially hazardous in patients with severe carotid artery disease. Accordingly, in such patients, special precautions should be taken to avoid hypotension and to correct it promptly should it occur.

It is apparent that there is a need for additional clinical trials to resolve the differences found in some studies of the predictive value of thallium scintigraphy as a preoperative screening test, particularly in patients undergoing vascular surgery.

Ambulatory (Continuous or Holter) Electrocardiography

Several studies have reported an increase in postoperative cardiac events in patients who have perioperative evidence of myocardial ischemia on ambulatory electrocardiographic (AECG) (Holter) recordings.[6,7,51–54] On the other hand, one study found that adverse hospital outcomes were associated with evidence of myocardial ischemia on postoperative but not preoperative AECG monitoring.[55] Further studies are necessary to define better the cost-effectiveness of, and the most suitable patients for, preoperative AECG. (See also Chap. 45.)

Transthoracic Echocardiography

The prognostic value of preoperative transthoracic echocardiography has not been well evaluated. It is likely to be useful to identify ventricular dysfunction and/or segmental wall-motion abnormalities, which have been shown to predict perioperative ventricular dysfunction when detected by radionuclide and angiographic techniques.[56]

Transesophageal Echocardiography

Transesophageal echocardiography is very useful for the early detection of intraoperative myocardial ischemia. (See Chap. 131.) In the future, it will likely be more widely used intraoperatively in selected high-risk patients. It is moderately expensive and labor intensive.

Coronary Arteriography

Some groups have recommended coronary arteriography as the routine screening test of choice for patients being considered for peripheral vascular surgery.[5,57,58] In the Cleveland Clinic experience,[4,5] severe surgically correctable CAD was found in 25 percent of the entire group and in 34 percent of patients clinically suspected of having CAD. Patients who have coronary artery bypass surgery for severe CAD discovered on coronary arteriography prior to vascular surgery have lower early mortality (1.5 percent versus 2 percent) and late mortality (12 percent versus 26 percent) with a higher 5-year survival rate (72 percent versus 43 percent). At this time it is not certain that the additional coronary revascularization procedures, which themselves have a significant morbidity and mortality in these patients, that result from this policy produce an overall cost-effective benefit in all such patients.[13,16]

In patients undergoing elective aortic surgery, coronary revascularization is appropriate when the patient's symptoms and findings would themselves have been indications for coronary revascularization by either coronary angioplasty or surgery.[59] (See also Chap. 73.)

Intraoperative Predictors of Perioperative Cardiac Morbidity

The classic intraoperative predictors of increased PCM include emergency surgery, vascular surgery, and prolonged (>3 h) thoracic or upper abdominal surgery.[8] Dynamic predictors of PCM include intraoperative hypotension; tachycardia; and evidence of myocardial ischemia as detected by ECG, transesophageal echocardiographic detection of changes of wall-motion and wall-thickening,[60–63] elevation of end-diastolic pulmonary artery pressure monitored by catheter,[10,64,65] and by cardiokymography.[65,66] Most of the data regarding the intraoperative detection of myocardial ischemia have been obtained during coronary artery bypass surgery rather than noncardiac surgery.

POSTOPERATIVE PREDICTION OF PERIOPERATIVE CARDIAC MORBIDITY

Postoperative Ischemia

In the past the greatest effort has been spent in the preoperative identification and management of patients at increased risk of PCM. There is now a suggestion that the use of preoperative patient-selection criteria has apparently been responsible for the observation that typical preoperative risk factors such as SAH, previous MI, or the Goldman cardiac risk factor index were recently found not to be predictive of ischemic events in a study of 474 men undergoing major noncardiac surgery (243 men with CAD; 231 men at high risk of CAD).[6,7] In this study, postoperative myocardial ischemia detected by two-channel AECG recording occurred in nearly all patients who subsequently had an ischemic event. The ECG evidence of postoperative ischemia, which began to become apparent in patients on the first day after surgery, occurred in most patients at least 4 h before any other clinical evidence of an event. Clinical symptoms occurred in 13 of 15 patients who had an ischemic event, most often dyspnea (8 patients) or chest pain (3 patients). Postoperative ischemia on ambulatory monitoring was clinically silent in 97 percent of patients but was associated with a ninefold increased risk of an ischemic event. On the other hand, the majority of patients who had such evidence of ischemia postoperatively did not have an ischemic event. During the first 48 h postoperatively, 41 percent (167 of 407 patients with interpretable AECG recordings) of the men had at least one episode of myocardial ischemia. This report and other recent studies emphasize the importance of giving special attention to monitoring and management of high-risk patients during the postoperative period.

A subsequent detailed analysis of the perioperative data from the same 474 men identified five major preoperative factors that were independent predictors of postoperative ischemia[7] (Table 139-4). The likelihood of postoperative myocardial ischemia on the continuous two-channel AECG recorded for 2 days following surgery increased progressively with the number of preoperative predictors. Thus, in this group of high-risk men, there was electrocardiographic evidence of postoperative ischemia in 22 percent of men with no predictors, in 31 percent with one predictor, in 46 percent with two predictors, in 70 percent with three predictors, and in 77 percent with four predictors. The risk of postoperative ischemia was also increased in patients who had evidence of ischemia on 12-lead ECG monitoring during surgery.

Postoperative Management

As noted above, most perioperative MIs occur in the first few days postoperatively. Most patients are asymptomatic, although they frequently have ST-segment changes in the preceding 3 to 6 h.[1,6–8] Most patients with CAD or at significant risk of having CAD should have continuous ECG monitoring using two or more carefully selected leads together with daily 12-lead ECGs and periodic measurements of MB–creatine kinase, about every 8 h, for several days after major noncardiac surgery. Tachycardia and hypertension should be treated with a beta blocker in the absence of contraindications (Chap. 66). Postoperative supraventricular tachycardias are most often related to noncardiac causes such as hypoxia, electrolyte abnormalities, infection, or medications. The primary treatment is to correct the cause. Atrial fibrillation with a rapid ventricular rate can be managed by intravenous diltiazem, a short-acting beta blocker (Chap. 66), or cardioversion (Chap. 41).

TABLE 139-4
Major Preoperative Predictors of Postoperative Myocardial Ischemia

1. Left ventricular hypertrophy by electrocardiogram
2. History of systemic arterial hypertension
3. Diabetes mellitus
4. Definite coronary artery disease
5. Use of digoxin

SOURCE: Hollenberg et al.[7]

MYOCARDIAL REVASCULARIZATION

In selected patients, myocardial revascularization should be considered prior to elective noncardiac surgery in order to decrease perioperative cardiac morbidity and improve long-term prognosis. In general, the indications for revascularization by coronary angioplasty or surgery are the same as they would be if the patient were not undergoing the noncardiac surgery. (See Chaps. 58, 70, and 73.) Since there are no controlled trials in this area, it is necessary to extrapolate from other studies, keeping in mind the risks of the revascularization procedure in the individual patient and the delay in performing the noncardiac surgery.

MEDICATIONS

In general, patients with known or suspected cardiac disease should have their cardiovascular medications continued before, during, and following noncardiac surgery. Preoperatively, patients who are not receiving a beta blocker should be considered for such therapy in the absence of a contraindication.[67–69] Although it is common practice, there are few data supporting the intraoperative administration of intravenous nitroglycerin in patients with CAD. One report has suggested that intraoperative intravenous diltiazem may decrease the number of ischemic episodes in patients with chronic stable angina undergoing peripheral vascular surgery.[70] This needs to be confirmed in a larger study before it can be recommended. Patients who are taking chronic low-dose aspirin usually should have this discontinued 5 to 7 days prior to elective surgery in order to decrease the amount of intraoperative bleeding.

RECOMMENDED PATIENT EVALUATION AND MANAGEMENT

The evaluation of patients with known or suspected cardiac disease prior to noncardiac surgery requires an appraisal of the patient's clinical risk profile; a characterization of the type, urgency, and risks of the planned noncardiac surgery; and a knowledge of the results of coronary artery bypass surgery and coronary angioplasty at one's own institution.[13] In addition, the diagnostic accuracy of exercise treadmill testing and thallium scintigraphy in one's institution should be known, as well as

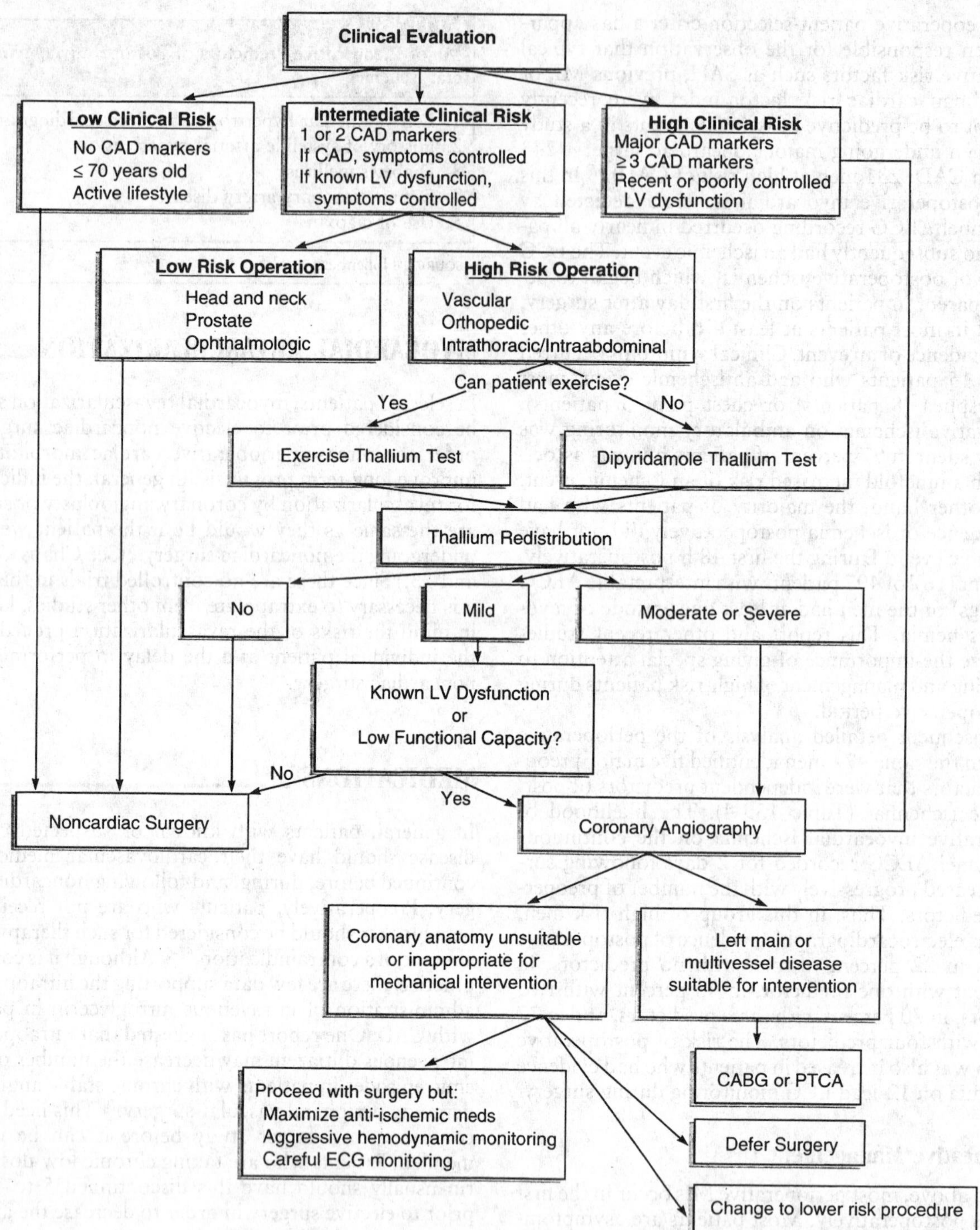

FIGURE 139-2 Suggested algorithm for the estimation of preoperative coronary risk of elective or semielective surgery. The most important considerations are the patient's clinical risk profile, the nature of the surgical procedure, and the results of noninvasive testing and/or coronary angiography if indicated. Urgent surgery may preempt risk stratification. Markers and major markers for coronary artery disease are listed in Table 139-5. Moderate or severe thallium redistribution: thallium redistribution in more than one planar view, more than one coronary arterial territory, or four or more myocardial segments. *(From Abraham et al.[13] Reproduced with modification with permission from the publisher and authors.)*

the risks and accuracy of coronary arteriography. As with most diagnostic testing, the greatest value is in patients who have an intermediate risk of having CAD on clinical grounds.[13,16,29] (See also Chap. 58.)

Table 139-5 lists the markers and major markers of increased cardiac risk in patients undergoing noncardiac surgery. Figure 139-2 is an algorithm for the preoperative estimation of risk and management of patients prior to elective or semielective surgery proposed by Abraham et al.[13] that is practical and cost-efficient. Note that treadmill testing can be used initially if the patient is able to walk on a treadmill and does not have associated ECG changes (left ventricular hypertrophy, significant resting ST-T wave changes, left bundle branch block, or preexcitation) or is not on medications (such as digoxin, antianginals) that might preclude interpretation of the exercise ECG or make the test result nonspecific or insensitive. Patients who are able to achieve 75 to 85 percent of

TABLE 139-5

Clinical Markers of Increased Risk of Perioperative Cardiac Morbidity

Evidence of coronary artery disease (CAD)
- Major Markers of CAD
  - Recent (less than 6 months) myocardial infarction (MI) complicated by angina, congestive heart failure (CHF), or positive stress test
  - Recent non-Q wave MI
  - Unstable or new onset angina pectoris
  - Positive stress test
  - More than two minor markers in selected patients
- Markers of CAD
  - Thallium redistribution on dipyridamole thallium 201 scintigraphy
  - Prior MI more than 6 months previously
  - Prior angina pectoris
  - Age 70 or greater
  - Ventricular arrhythmias
  - Abnormal Q waves on resting electrocardiogram
  - Diabetes mellitus

Evidence of congestive heart failure (CHF)
- Major Marker CHF
  - Congestive heart failure (S_3 gallop, increased jugular venous pressure, pulmonary edema on chest film)
- Marker of CHF
  - Previous CHF

predicted maximal heart rate or 10 METS without significant evidence of ischemia on the ECG have low risk and can proceed with surgery. Evidence of significant ischemia on exercise testing and intermediate clinical risk (see fig. 139-2) should lead to further testing. An exercise thallium test is preferred if the patient can exercise, and a dipyridamole-thallium test if the patient cannot exercise. Patients at very high clinical risk should have coronary arteriography performed as their basic evaluation procedure without preceding exercise testing or thallium scintigraphy. Patients who have either evidence of significant ischemia induced by exercise on the ECG or moderate or severe redistribution defects demonstrated by thallium scintigraphy, are referred to coronary arteriography.

Patients who are found to be at significantly increased risk of PCM during evaluation for elective noncardiac surgery on the basis of noninvasive testing or coronary arteriography must be managed on an individual basis. Alternative recommendations include the following: cancelling or postponing the elective surgery and instituting more intensive medical therapy; recommending an alternative, lower-risk surgical procedure; proceeding with the proposed elective surgery with intensive anti-ischemic therapy and perioperative monitoring; or postponing the elective surgery until after myocardial revascularization by either coronary angioplasty or coronary artery bypass surgery.

REFERENCES

1. Mangano DT: Perioperative cardiac morbidity. *Anesthesiology* 1990; 72:153–184.
2. National Center for Health Statistics: *Vital Statistics of the United States, 1980*, vol II, *Mortality*, pt A. DHHS pub no (PHS) 85-1101. Hyattsville, MD, NCHS U.S. Public Health Service, 1985.
3. National Center for Health Statistics: *Health, United States, 1988*, III. DHHS pub no (PHS) 89-1232. Public Health Service, U.S. Government Printing Office, March 1989: 10–17, 66, 67, 100, 101.
4. Hertzer NR, Beven EG, Young JR, Ohara PJ, Ruschhaupt WF III, Graor RA: Coronary-artery disease in peripheral vascular patients. A classification of 1,000 coronary angiograms and results of surgical management. *Ann Surg* 1984; 199:223–233.
5. Hertzer NR: Clinical experience with preoperative coronary angiography. *J Vasc Surg* 1985; 2:510–514.
6. Mangano DT, Browner WS, Hollenberg M, London MJ, Tubau JF, Tateo IM, et al: Association of perioperative myocardial ischemia with cardiac morbidity and mortality in men undergoing noncardiac surgery. *N Engl J Med* 1990; 323:1781–1788.
7. Hollenberg M, Mangano DT, Browner WS, London MJ, Tubau JF, Tateo IM, et al: Predictors of postoperative myocardial ischemia in patients undergoing noncardiac surgery. *JAMA* 1992; 268:205–209.
8. Mangano DT: Risk assessment for noncardiac surgery. In: Kapoor AS, Singh BN (eds): *Prognosis and Risk Assessment in Cardiovascular Diseases*. New York, Churchill Livingstone, 1993: 447–467.
9. Foster ED, Davis KB, Carpenter JA, Abele S, Fray D: Risk of noncardiac operation in patients with defined coronary disease: The Coronary Artery Surgery Study (CASS) Registry Experience. *Ann Thorac Surg* 1986; 41:42–50.
10. Rao TK, Jacobs KH, El-Etr AA: Reinfarction following anesthesia in patients with myocardial infarction. *Anesthesiology* 1983; 59:499–505.
11. London MJ, Mangano DT: Assessment of perioperative risk. In: Stoelting RK, Barash PG, Gallagher TJ (eds): *Advances in Anesthesia*, vol 5. Chicago, Year Book Medical Publishers, 1988: 53–87.
12. Roberts SL, Tinker JH: Cardiovascular disease, risk and outcome. In: Brown DL (ed): *Anesthesia*. Philadelphia, Lippincott, 1988: 33–49.
13. Abraham SA, Coles NA, Coley CM, Strauss HW, Boucher CA, Eagle KA: Coronary risk of noncardiac surgery. *Prog Cardiovasc Dis* 1991; 34:205–234.
14. Tarham S, Moffitt EA, Taylor WF, Giuliani ER: Myocardial infarction after general anesthesia. *JAMA* 1972; 220:1451–1454.
15. Von Knooring J: Postoperative myocardial infarction: A prospective study in a risk group of surgical patients. *Surgery* 1981; 90:55–60.
16. Massie BM, Mangano DT: Assessment of preoperative risk: Have we put the cart before the horse? (editorial). *J Am Coll Cardiol* 1993; 21:1353–1356.
17. Steen PA, Tinker JH, Tarhan S: Myocardial reinfarction after anesthesia and surgery. *JAMA* 1978; 239:2566–2570.
18. Foster ED, Davis KB, Carpenter JA, Abele S, Fray D: Risk of noncardiac operation in patients with defined coronary disease: The Coronary Artery Surgery Study (CASS) Registry experience. *Ann Thorac Surg* 1986; 41:42–50.
19. O'Keefe JH Jr, Vlietstra RE, Bailey KR, Holmes DR Jr: Natural history of candidates for balloon aortic valvuloplasty. *Mayo Clin Proc* 1987; 62:986–991.
20. Goldman L, Caldera DL, Nussbaum SR, Southwick FS, Krogstad D, Murray B, et al: Multifactorial index of cardiac risk in noncardiac surgical procedures. *N Engl J Med* 1977; 297:845–850.
21. Goldman L, Caldera DL, Southwick FS, Nussbaum SR, Murray B, O'Malley TA, et al: Cardiac risk factors and complications in non-cardiac surgery. *Medicine* 1978; 57:357–370.
22. Garcia MJ, McNamara PM, Gordon T, Kannel WB: Morbidity and mortality in diabetics in the Framingham population: Sixteen-year follow-up study. *Diabetes* 1974; 23:105–111.
23. Dortimer AC, Shenoy PN, Shiroff RA, Leaman DM, Babb JD, Liedtke JA, et al: Diffuse coronary artery disease in diabetic patients: Fact or fiction? *Circulation* 1978; 57:133–136.
24. Kannel WB, McGee DL: Diabetes and cardiovascular risk factors: The Framingham Study. *Circulation* 1979; 59:8–13.
25. Waller BF, Palumbo PJ, Lie JT, Roberts WC: Status of the coronary arteries at necroscopy in diabetes mellitus with onset after age 30 years: Analysis of 229 diabetic patients with and without clinical evidence of coronary heart disease and comparison to 183 control subjects. *Am J Med* 1980; 69:498–506.
26. Vigorita VJ, Moore GW, Hutchins GM: Absence of correlation between coronary arterial atherosclerosis and severity or duration

of diabetes mellitus of adult onset. *Am J Cardiol* 1980; 46:535–542.

27. Kannel WB: Lipids, diabetes, and coronary heart disease: Insights from the Framingham Study. *Am Heart J* 1985; 110:1110–1117.
28. American Society of Anesthesiologists: New classification of physical status. *Anesthesiology* 1963; 24:111.
29. Wong T, Detsky AS: Preoperative cardiac risk assessment for patients having peripheral vascular surgery. *Ann Intern Med* 1992; 116:743–753.
30. Detsky AS, Abrams HB, McLaughlin Jr, Drucker DJ, Sasson Z, Johnston N, et al: Predicting cardiac complications in patients undergoing non-cardiac surgery. *J Gen Intern Med* 1986; 1:211–219.
31. Detsky AS, Abrams HB, Forbath N, Scott JG, Hilliard JR: Cardiac assessment for patients undergoing noncardiac surgery: A multifactorial clinical risk index. *Arch Intern Med* 1986; 146:2131–2134.
32. Kannel WB, Abbott RD: Incidence and prognosis of unrecognized myocardial infarction: An update on the Framingham study. *N Engl J Med* 1984; 311:1144–1147.
33. Mangano DT: Preoperative assessment. In: Kaplan JA (ed): *Cardiac Anesthesia*, vol I, 2d ed. New York, Grune & Stratton, 1987: 341–392.
34. Dash H, Massie BM, Botvinick EH, Brundage BH: The noninvasive identification of left main and three vessel coronary artery disease by myocardial stress perfusion scintigraphy and treadmill exercise electrocardiography. *Circulation* 1979; 60:276–284.
35. Wackers FJT, Fetterman RC, Mattero JA, Clements JP: Quantitative planar thallium-201 stress scintigraphy: A critical evaluation of the method. *Semin Nucl Med* 1975; 15:46–66.
36. Leppo J, Boucher CA, Okada RD, Newell JB, Strauss HW, Pohost GM: Serial thallium-201 myocardial imaging after dipyridamole infusion: Diagnostic utility in detecting coronary stenoses and relationship to regional wall motion. *Circulation* 1982; 66:649–657.
37. Leppo J, Plaja J, Gionet M, Tumolo J, Parakos JA, Cutler BS: Noninvasive evaluation of cardiac risk before elective vascular surgery. *J Am Coll Cardiol* 1987; 9:269–276.
38. Leppo JA: Dipyridamole-thallium imaging: The lazy man's stress test. *J Nucl Med* 1989; 30:281–287.
39. Boucher CA, Brewster DC, Darling RC, Okada RD, Strauss HW, Pohost GM: Determination of cardiac risk by dipyridamole-thallium imaging before peripheral vascular surgery. *N Engl J Med* 1985; 312:389–394.
40. Eagle K, Singer D, Brewster D, Darling RC, Mulley AG, Boucher CA: Dipyridamole-thallium scanning in patients undergoing vascular surgery. Optimizing preoperative evaluation of cardiac risk. *JAMA* 1987; 257:2185–2189.
41. Eagle K, Coley CM, Newell JB, Brewster DC, Darling RC, Strauss HW, et al: Combining clinical and thallium data optimizes preoperative assessment of cardiac risk before major vascular surgery. *Ann Intern Med* 1989; 110:859–866.
42. Mangano D, London M, Tubau J, Browner WS, Hollenberg M, Krupski W, et al: Dipyridamole thallium-201 scintigraphy as a preoperative screening test. A reexamination of its predictive potential. *Circulation* 1991;84:493–502.
43. Ruddy T, McPhail N, Calvin J, Sauve M, Davies R, Gulenchyn K, et al: Comparison of exercise testing, dipyridamole thallium imaging and gated blood pool scanning for the prediction of cardiac complications following vascular surgery (abstr.). *J Am Coll Cardiol* 1989; 13:149A.
44. McEnroe CS, O'Donnell TF Jr, Yeager A, Konstam M, Mackey WC: Comparison of ejection fraction and Goldman risk factor analysis to dipyridamole-thallium 201 studies in the evaluation of cardiac morbidity after aortic aneurysm surgery. *J Vasc Surg* 1990; 11:497–504.
45. Lette J, Waters D, Lapointe J, Gagnon A, Picard M, Cerino M, et al: Usefulness of the severity and extent of reversible perfusion defects during thallium-dipyridamole imaging for cardiac risk assessment before noncardiac surgery. *Am J Cardiol* 1989; 64:276–281.
46. Levinson JR, Boucher CA, Coley CM, Guiney TE, Strauss HW, Eagle KA: Usefulness of semiquantitative analysis of dipyridamole-thallium-201 redistribution for improving risk stratification before vascular surgery. *Am J Cardiol* 1990; 66:406–410.
47. Lane SE, Lewis SM, Pippin JJ, Kosinski EJ, Campbell D, Nesto RW, et al: Predictive value of quantitative dipyridamole-thallium scintigraphy in assessing cardiovascular risk after vascular surgery in diabetes mellitus. *Am J Cardiol* 1989; 64:1275–1279.
48. Hendel RC, Layden JJ, Leppo JA: Prognostic value of dipyridamole thallium scintigraphy for evaluation of ischemic heart disease. *J Am Coll Cardiol* 1990; 15:109–116.
49. Younis LT, Aguirre F, Byers S, Dowell S, Barth G, Walker H, et al: Perioperative and long-term prognostic value of intravenous dipyridamole thallium scintigraphy in patients with peripheral vascular disease. *Am Heart J* 1990; 119:1287–1292.
50. Daum RM, Cremisi HD, Yeager A, Udelson JE, Underhill D, Oates E, et al: Dipyridamole thallium imaging for determining perioperative and long-term prognosis in high-risk vascular disease patients. *Circulation* 1988; 77–78 (suppl 2):II-191.
51. Pasternack PF, Grossi EA, Baumann FG, Riles TS, Lamparello PJ, Giangola G, et al: The value of silent myocardial ischemia monitoring in the prediction of perioperative myocardial infarction in patients undergoing peripheral vascular surgery. *J Vasc Surg* 1989; 10:617–625.
52. Ouyang P, Gerstenblith G, Furman WR, Golueke PJ, Gottlieb SO, et al: Frequency and significance of early postoperative silent myocardial ischemia in patients having peripheral vascular surgery. *Am J Cardiol* 1989; 64:1113–1116.
53. McCann RL, Clements FM: Silent myocardial ischemia in patients undergoing peripheral vascular surgery: Incidence and association with perioperative cardiac morbidity and mortality. *J Vasc Surg* 1989; 9:583–587.
54. Raby KE, Goldman L, Creager MA, Cook EF, Weisberg MC, Whittemore AD, et al: Correlation between preoperative ischemia and major cardiac events after peripheral vascular surgery. *N Engl J Med* 1989; 321:1296–1300.
55. Fegert G, Hollenberg M, Browner W, Wellington Y, Levenson L, Franks M, et al: Perioperative myocardial ischemia in the noncardiac surgical patient (abstr). *Anesthesiology* 1988; 69:A49.
56. Larsen SF, Olesen KH, Jacobsen E, Nielsen H, Nielsen AL, Pietersen A, et al: Prediction of cardiac risk in non-cardiac surgery. *Eur Heart J* 1987; 8:179–185.
57. Tomatis LA, Fierens EE, Verbrugge GP: Evaluation of surgical risk in peripheral vascular disease by coronary arteriography: A series of 100 cases. *Surgery* 1972; 71:429–435.
58. Hertzer NR, Young JR, Kramer JR, Phillips DF, deWolfe VG, Ruschhaupt WF III, et al: Routine coronary angiography prior to elective aortic reconstruction. *Arch Surg* 1979; 114:1336–1344.
59. Anderson TJ, Meredith IT, Selwyn AP, Raby KE: Myocardial revascularization before repair of an aortic aneurysm (editorial). *Mayo Clin Proc* 1993; 68:713–715.
60. Topol EJ, Weiss JL, Guzman PA, Dorsey-Lima S, Blanck TJ, Humphrey LS, et al: Immediate improvement of dysfunctional myocardial segments after coronary revascularization: Detection by intraoperative transesophageal echocardiography. *J Am Coll Cardiol* 1984; 4:1123–1134.
61. Smith JS, Cahalan MK, Benefiel DJ, Byrd BF, Lurz FW, Shapiro WA, et al: Intraoperative detection of myocardial ischemia in high-risk patients: Electrocardiography versus two-dimensional transesophageal echocardiography. *Circulation* 1985; 72:1015–1021.
62. London M, Tubau J, Wong M, Layug E, Mangano DT: The "natural history" of segmental wall motion abnormalities detected by intraoperative transesophageal echocardiography: A clinically blinded prospective approach (abst). *Anesthesiology* 1988; 69:A7.
63. Leung JM, O'Kelly B, Browner WS, Tubau J, Hollenberg M, Mangano DT: Prognostic importance of post bypass regional wall-motion abnormalities in patients undergoing coronary artery bypass graft surgery. *Anesthesiology* 1989; 71:16–25.
64. Parker J, Chiong M, West R, Case R: Sequential alterations in myocardial lactate metabolism, ST-segments and left ventricular function during angina induced by atrial pacing. *Circulation* 1969; 40:113–131.
65. Haggmark S, Hohner P, Ostman M, Friedman A, Diamond G, Lowenstein E, et al: Comparison of hemodynamic, electrocardiographic, mechanical and metabolic indicators of intraoperative myocardial ischemia in vascular surgical patients with coronary artery disease. *Anesthesiology* 1989; 70:19.
66. Bellows WH, Bode RH Jr, Levy JA, Foex P, Lowenstein E: Noninvasive detection of periinduction ischemic ventricular dysfunction by cardiomyography in humans: Preliminary experience. *Anesthesiology* 1984; 60:155–158.

67. Pasternack PF, Imparato AM, Baumann FG, Laub G, Riles TS, Lamparello PJ, et al: The hemodynamics of β-blockade in patients undergoing abdominal aortic aneurysm repair. *Circulation* 1987; 76(suppl 3):III-1–III-7.
68. Stone JG, Foex P, Sear JW, Johnson LL, Khambatta HJ, Triner L: Myocardial ischemia in untreated hypertensive patients; Effect of a single small oral dose of a beta-adrenergic blocking agent. *Anesthesiology* 1988; 68:495–500.
69. Pasternack PF, Grossi EA, Baumann FG, Riles TS, Lamparello PH, Giangola G, et al: Beta blockade to decrease silent ischemia during peripheral vascular surgery. *Am J Surg* 1989; 158:113–116.
70. Godet G, Coriat P, Baron JF, Bertrana M, Diquet B, Sebag C, et al: Prevention of intraoperative myocardial ischemia during noncardiac surgery with intravenous diltiazem: A randomized trial versus placebo. *Anesthesiology* 1987; 66:241–245.

Chapter 140

Anesthesia and the Patient with Cardiovascular Disease

David L. Reich, M.D. ■ *Joel A. Kaplan, M.D.*

Anesthetizing patients with cardiovascular disease is one of the most difficult challenges facing the anesthesiologist. The constellation of anesthetic drug effects, the physiological stresses of surgery, and underlying cardiovascular diseases complicate and limit the choice of anesthesia for any particular procedure. Generally speaking, the anesthesiologist's approach to the patient with cardiovascular disease is to select agents and techniques that would optimize the patient's cardiopulmonary function. For example, the induction of general anesthesia using fentanyl and vecuronium tends to slow the heart rate without affecting myocardial contractility. This strategy would be beneficial in a patient with mitral stenosis.

The perioperative management of a patient with cardiovascular disease requires close cooperation between the cardiologist and the anesthesiologist.[1] Each specialist has a unique knowledge base that complements the other's. The approach should emphasize a continuum of care from the preoperative evaluation through the extended postoperative period.

PREOPERATIVE EVALUATION

The assessment of cardiac risk and preoperative optimization of the patient's cardiovascular status are the traditional goals of the preoperative evaluation of patients with cardiovascular disease. In 1977, Goldman et al.[2] introduced the Cardiac Risk Index Score (CRIS) to guide more quantitatively the assignment of cardiac risk in patients undergoing noncardiac surgery. This study had a major impact, because clinicians concluded that improvements in congestive heart failure symptomatology and the patient's general medical condition would decrease cardiac risk. While a recent study does not support the predictive value of the CRIS or preoperative electrocardiographic ischemic changes in patients with coronary artery disease (CAD),[3] the emphasis on trying to get the patient into optimal condition preoperatively continues and is supported by other studies.[4]

Recent myocardial infarction (MI) is another predictor of cardiac "risk" that deserves mention. The incidence of perioperative MI is highest in patients with 6 weeks of MI and remains elevated for approximately 6 months.[5] The reason that this is worrisome is that the mortality of a perioperative MI is approximately 50 percent. The decreased incidence of perioperative MI in the study by Rao et al.[5] has been attributed to the more aggressive use of intraoperative monitoring and control of undesirable hemodynamic changes in recent years. It is still considered prudent, however, to delay elective surgery for 6 months following an MI. Preoperative exercise stress testing,[6] dipyridamole-thallium imaging,[7] and ambulatory electrocardiographic monitoring[8] have also been evaluated for their ability to determine cardiac risk in patients with CAD.

The assessment of ventricular function is another goal of the preoperative evaluation. The combination of clinical signs and symptoms is sufficient in the majority of patients. In the patient with ventricular dysfunction, however, echocardiography and/or radionuclide imaging may be required to provide a more precise estimate of cardiac reserve.

The accumulation of historical, clinical, laboratory, echocardiographic, radionuclide, and cardiac catheterization data in a cogent summary form comprises the ideal "medical clearance" consultation for the anesthesiologist. With the benefit of this information, the two specialties can make intelligent decisions regarding the patient's preoperative therapy and the optimal timing of surgery.[9] (See also Chap. 139.)

CHOICE OF ANESTHETIC AND MONITORING

The choice of anesthetic technique is inherently a difficult one, because multiple factors must be considered. These include the desires of the patient, the requirements of the surgical procedure, and the patient's underlying medical condition. While an anesthetic technique is occasionally desirable for a particular procedure (e.g., spinal anesthesia for transurethral resection of prostate), it is extremely difficult to find scientific evidence that any particular anesthetic technique is "safer" or that anesthetic technique per se influences patient outcome.[10,11]

There is some evidence that regional anesthesia (with postoperative epidural analgesia) may be associated with decreased cardiac morbidity in "high-risk" patients with CAD.[12] A second study found that intra- and postoperative epidural analgesia prevented hypercoagulability and was associated with improved outcome following lower extremity revascularization.[13] While these studies do suggest that epidural analgesia may improve outcome, they were small prospective studies that cannot easily be generalized to all surgical patients with cardiovascular disease.

Therefore, it is essential that the cardiologist does not specifically exclude any anesthetic technique during a preoperative consultation. Regional anesthetics are not infrequently converted to general anesthetics intraoperatively due to unexpectedly long surgery, patient discomfort, or changes in the surgical plan. No anesthesiologist can be certain that a particular technique will be adequate for the surgical procedure given the unpredictability of the situation and must have flexibility to alter the technique as needed.

Standards for basic intraoperative monitoring were established by the American Society of Anesthesiologists in 1986.[14] In addition, digital pulse oximetry has been almost universally applied in the last several years. The indications for the use of more invasive monitors, such as intraarterial, central venous, and pulmonary arterial catheters (PACs) are more controversial. Tables 140-1 to 140-3 detail specific indications for invasive monitoring that are widely accepted. In addition, transesophageal echocardiography has acquired a large role in intraoperative monitoring.

TABLE 140-1

Indications for Intraarterial Monitoring

1. Major surgical procedures involving large fluid shifts and/or blood loss
2. Surgery requiring cardiopulmonary bypass
3. Surgery of the aorta
4. Patients with pulmonary disease requiring frequent arterial blood gases
5. Patients with recent MIs, unstable angina, or severe CAD
6. Patients with decreased left ventricular function (congestive heart failure) or significant valvular heart disease
7. Patients in hypovolemic, cardiogenic, or septic shock or with multiple-organ failure
8. Procedures involving the use of deliberate hypotension or deliberate hypothermia
9. Massive trauma
10. Patients with right-sided heart failure, chronic obstructive pulmonary disease, pulmonary hypertension, or pulmonary embolism
11. Patients requiring inotropes or intraaortic balloon counterpulsation
12. Patients undergoing surgery of the aorta requiring cross-clamping
13. Patients with massive ascites
14. Patients with electrolyte or metabolic disturbances requiring frequent blood samples
15. Inability to measure arterial pressure noninvasively (e.g., morbid obesity)

REGIONAL ANESTHESIA

The term *regional anesthesia* was coined by Cushing for operations where local anesthetics were used to operate upon localized areas of the body without loss of consciousness. The advantages of regional anesthesia include simplicity, low cost, and minimal equipment requirements. Many of the adverse effects of general anesthesia are avoided, such as myocardial and respiratory depression. The disadvantages include patients' reluctance to be awake in the operating room, anesthetic

TABLE 140-2

Indications for Central Venous Line Placement

1. Major operative procedures involving large fluid shifts and/or blood loss in patients with good left ventricular function
2. Intravascular volume assessment when urine output is not reliable or unavailable (renal failure, urologic surgery)
3. Patients with tricuspid stenosis
4. Major trauma
5. Surgical procedures with a high risk of air embolism, such as sitting position craniotomies
6. Frequent blood sampling in patients who will not require an arterial line
7. Venous access for vasoactive or irritating drugs
8. Chronic drug administration
9. Inadequate peripheral intravenous access
10. Rapid infusion of intravenous fluids (using large cannulae)

TABLE 140-3

Indications for Pulmonary Artery Catheter Monitoring

1. Major procedures involving large fluid shifts and/or blood loss in patients with severe CAD
2. Patients with recent MIs or severely unstable angina
3. Patients with impaired left ventricular function (congestive heart failure) or significant mitral or aortic valvular pathology
4. Patients with pericardial tamponade
5. Patients in hypovolemic, cardiogenic, or septic shock or with multiple-organ failure
6. Massive trauma
7. Patients with right-sided heart failure, chronic obstructive pulmonary disease, pulmonary hypertension, or pulmonary embolism
8. Patients requiring high levels of positive end-expiratory pressure
9. Hemodynamically unstable patients requiring inotropes or intraaortic balloon counterpulsation
10. Patients undergoing surgery of the aorta requiring cross-clamping
11. Patients undergoing hepatic transplantation
12. Patients with massive ascites

agents of insufficient duration, and local anesthetic toxicity.

The cardiovascular side effects of regional anesthesia vary depending on the technique chosen. Spinal and epidural anesthesia, for example, may cause major decreases in cardiac preload and afterload, while local anesthetic infiltration and axillary nerve blocks have almost no cardiovascular side effects. Regional anesthetics are contraindicated in anticoagulated patients and thus may not be used in patients on heparin or warfarin therapy. Regional anesthesia may also be combined with general anesthesia in adults and children to decrease the requirements for the general anesthetic agents and for postoperative analgesia.

Local Anesthetic Agents

The local anesthetics are classified on the basis of their chemical structure as esters or amides. The esters are hydrolyzed by esterases in the plasma, and the amides are metabolized in the liver. The duration of action of local anesthetic agents is affected by the protein-binding characteristics of the molecule and the addition of vasoconstrictors to the local anesthetic solution.[15] Toxic reactions to local anesthetics are generally characterized by central nervous system excitation (seizures), which may be followed by central nervous system depression and cardiovascular collapse.

Cocaine is the original ester local anesthetic. Its clinical use is mainly restricted to topical anesthesia of the nose and airway. It is the only local anesthetic agent that is intrinsically vasoconstrictive, due to blockade of catecholamine reuptake at sympathetic nerve terminals. Cocaine's sympathomimetic effects result in central nervous system excitation, which increases requirements for general anesthetics. Cocaine has resulted in deaths from central nervous system toxicity and arrhythmias.[16] Cocaine can also elicit myocardial ischemia. Its tachycardic effects contraindicate its use in patients with CAD, mitral stenosis, or obstructive cardiomyopathy. (See also Chap. 110.)

Tetracaine is a long-acting ester local anesthetic that is frequently used in spinal anesthesia. It is also used for topical anesthesia of the eye and airway but may be toxic in the larger doses required for airway topical anesthesia. Chloroprocaine is a short-acting ester local anesthetic that is often used in epidural anesthesia. This agent is very rapidly metabolized by serum cholinesterase, leading to a low incidence of toxic reactions.

The amide local anesthetics are less rapidly metabolized (in the liver), and the potential for toxic reactions is somewhat greater. Some amide compounds (e.g., lidocaine) also have potent anti-arrhythmic actions. Lidocaine and mepivacaine are agents of intermediate duration of action that are commonly used in many types of regional blocks. Etidocaine and bupivacaine are agents of higher potency and longer duration of action that also exhibit more toxicity. Bupivacaine is associated particularly with cardiovascular collapse and arrhythmias upon inadvertent intravascular injection.

Epinephrine may be added to local anesthetic solutions to prolong their duration of action, primarily through a local vasoconstrictive action. Epinephrine is typically added in concentrations ranging from 2.5 μg/mL (1:400,000) to 10 μg/mL (1:100,000) for infiltration, nerve blocks, or epidural anesthesia. The systemic absorption of epinephrine occurs very slowly, and beta-adrenergic effects of slight tachycardia and diastolic hypotension predominate. In patients whose cardiovascular disease precludes the use of epinephrine, phenylephrine may be substituted at concentrations 10 times higher than that of epinephrine. Epinephrine may induce ventricular arrhythmias in patients anesthetized with halothane (see below).

Spinal Anesthesia

The injection of a relatively small dose of local anesthetic into the subarachnoid space produces the profound motor and sensory blockade that is known as spinal anesthesia. Spinal anesthesia also produces blockade of preganglionic sympathetic fibers, which usually results in hypotension. The level of spinal anesthesia is controlled by injection of a hyperbaric or hypobaric solution into the cerebrospinal fluid. The position of the patient is then manipulated to lateralize the blockade or to move the bolus of anesthetic in a more cephalad or caudad direction. The level of sympathetic blockade is generally two dermatomal segments higher than the sensory dermatomal level.

The higher the level of sympathetic blockade, the more profound the arterial and venous vasodilation and postural hypotension. Intravenous administration of crystalloid solutions is the primary treatment for hypotension. Intravenous ephedrine (5 to 10 mg) or phenylephrine (20 to 100 μg) is also used to increase temporarily the blood pressure during periods of relative hypovolemia. If the dermatomal level of sympathetic blockade reaches T_1, then the patient is effectively sympathectomized. The loss of cardiac accelerator fiber function may lead to bradycardia. Complete sympathectomy always occurs with a "total spinal" that also produces respiratory insufficiency due to intercostal and diaphragmatic muscle blockade.

Spinal anesthesia is relatively contraindicated in patients whose cardiovascular stability depends upon the maintenance of a high preload and afterload. Patients with any significant valvular heart disease, hypertrophic obstructive cardiomyopathy, or tetralogy of Fallot are prone to hemodynamic decompensation during spinal anesthesia. Patients with CAD usually tolerate spinal anesthesia well so long as diastolic arterial pressure is maintained at an appropriate level to preserve coronary perfusion pressure.

Epidural Anesthesia

The epidural space lies immediately external to the dura mater. It is a potential space that is filled with loose areolar tissue and a venous plexus. An indwelling polyethylene catheter is usually placed percutaneously for intermittent bolus injections or continuous infusion of local anesthetic and/or opioids. The epidural space may be entered by thoracic, lumbar, or caudal approaches. The advantages of epidural anesthesia include moderate hypotension (which tends to decrease intraoperative blood loss), contracted bowel loops during abdominal surgery, and effective postoperative analgesia.

The hemodynamic effects of epidural anesthesia are essentially similar to those of spinal anesthesia, except that the onset of sympathetic blockade is more gradual. Thus, with appropriate monitoring epidural anesthesia has been conducted safely in patients with mitral valvular disease, aortic stenosis, and hypertrophic obstructive cardiomyopathy. It should be emphasized, though, that intraarterial and PACs may be required to monitor adequately and to guide treatment of changes in preload and afterload that occur with epidural anesthesia in patients with severe cardiovascular disease.

Generally, 10 to 15 times the volume of local anesthetic is required for epidural compared to spinal anesthesia. The potential is always present for inadvertent intravascular injection of a toxic dose of local anesthetic. It is also possible to inject inadvertently a large volume into the subarachnoid space and cause a "total spinal" (see above). The hemodynamic consequences of inadvertent intravenous injections of epinephrine-containing solutions may be significant for patients who cannot tolerate tachycardia or hypertension.

Recent evidence suggests that postoperative epidural analgesia may be associated with decreased thrombotic tendency, improved analgesia, and lowered hospital costs.[12,13] This could be explained on the basis of diminished catecholamine levels. Catecholamine excess may be one of the etiologies of increased platelet adhesiveness postoperatively, which could lead to myocardial infarction or other vascular occlusion in susceptible patients. Postoperative epidural analgesia may be provided with dilute local anesthetic solutions and/or opioids. Opioid epidural infusions may be complicated by pruritis, urinary retention, somnolence, and respiratory depression. Thus, appropriate monitoring and nursing care are required.

Nerve Blocks and Local Anesthetic Infiltration

Nerve blocks and local anesthetic infiltration may be performed to facilitate surgery of localized areas of the body. The brachial plexus may be blocked by interscalene, supraclavicular, or axillary approaches. The lower extremity may be anesthetized by blocking the femoral and sciatic nerves. Local anesthetic infiltration is performed in regions such as the inguinal area to facilitate herniorrhaphies. These blocks, when properly performed, have minimal cardiovascular effects. They do, however, require large volumes of local anesthetic solution, which predisposes to toxic reactions if inadvertent intravascular injection occurs. Intercostal blocks are associated with high blood levels even without intravascular injection, because the neurovascular bundle enhances absorption of the local anesthetic. Epinephrine is occasionally added to prolong the duration of block, but this may be contraindicated in certain patients with cardiovascular disease such as mitral stenosis.

GENERAL ANESTHESIA

General anesthesia is defined as a reversible state consisting of amnesia, analgesia, immobility, and the prevention of undesirable reflexes. Many general anesthetic agents have cardiovascular side effects. Intravenous agents are nearly always used for the induction of anesthesia in adults. The induction of anesthesia in children is highly individualized according to patient needs, practitioner, and institution. Anesthesia is maintained using inhalational agents, intravenous agents, or a combination of the two. Neuromuscular blocking drugs (muscle relaxants) are commonly used to facilitate tracheal intubation and to lower the requirements for anesthetic agents (i.e., the dose of anesthetic that produces adequate amnesia and analgesia may not be sufficient to prevent movement or relax the abdominal musculature).

The physiology of general anesthesia has changed dramatically over the last several decades. Ether and cyclopropane were used widely with spontaneous ventilation but have sympathomimetic properties. Modern, nonexplosive inhalational anesthetic agents tend to be cardiac and respiratory depressants. With the exception of brief operations, nearly all general anesthetics include tracheal intubation and mechanical ventilation. The loss of consciousness is usually accompanied by a decrease in sympathetic tone. This sympatholytic effect, as well as the effects of positive pressure ventilation causes a moderate decrease in cardiac output even when the anesthetic drugs are not myocardial depressants per se.

The patient with cardiovascular disease presents major concerns to the anesthesiologist. General anesthesia masks many of the symptoms of cardiovascular decompensation, such as angina, dyspnea, dizziness, and palpitations. Other signs, such as tachycardia, are nonspecific and may be misinterpreted as reflecting hypovolemia or light anesthesia. Fluid shifts, obstructed venous return, and varying levels of noxious stimulation are other variables that are unpredictable. It is for these reasons that appropriate monitoring and selection of anesthetic agents are vital to the intraoperative management of the patient with cardiovascular disease.

Intravenous Anesthetics

Intravenous anesthetic induction drugs are lipophilic molecules that have an affinity for neuronal tissue or specific receptors. Their action is terminated by redistribution from the vessel-rich tissues (brain, heart, liver, and kidneys) to other tissues (muscle, fat, and skin). Elimination occurs via hepatic metabolism and takes place over several hours. Patients with diminished cardiac output secondary to cardiovascular disease will have prolonged effects from intravenous anesthetic drugs.

Barbiturates

Thiopental is an ultra-short-acting thiobarbiturate that is the prototype for agents of its class. It is quick, reliable, and not unpleasant for patients and does not have excitatory side effects. Its cardiovascular effects are marked by dose-dependent myocardial depression and dilation of venous capacitance vessels. The decrease in cardiac output is usually compensated for by arterial vasoconstriction so that blood pressure is minimally decreased. Thiopental is a poor analgesic, however, and tachycardia and hypertension are common with tracheal intubation or any painful stimulus.

Standard doses of barbiturate for anesthetic induction are contraindicated in patients with preload-dependent cardiac lesions and/or severely impaired ventricular contractility. Examples include pericardial tamponade, mitral regurgitation, aortic regurgitation, mitral stenosis, and dilated cardiomyopathy. Reduced doses and slower injection of the drug markedly decrease the cardiovascular effects.

Benzodiazepines

Benzodiazepines may be used as premedication, to induce anesthesia, or as an adjunct to regional or general anesthesia. The most useful therapeutic effects of benzodiazepines include their sedative and amnesic effects. They tend to be unreliable in their rapidity of induction and occasionally fail to induce unconsciousness despite high doses. When used as sole agents, the benzodiazepines have minimal cardiovascular effects. When used in combination with other drugs such as opiates and potent volatile anesthetics, benzodiazepines produce hypotension that may be due to myocardial depression or decreased systemic vascular resistance.

Opioids

Opioids play a major role in the anesthetic care of patients with cardiovascular disease. They may be used as premedication, as supplements to regional or inhalational anesthesia, as one of the main components of "nitrous-narcotic" anesthesia, or as the primary anesthetic agent (high-dose opioid anesthesia). They are often used as supplements during the induction of anesthesia to block the hemodynamic response to laryngoscopy and tracheal intubation. While opioids are excellent analgesics, they are unreliable amnesics, provide no muscle relaxation, and are associated with "breakthrough" hypertension and tachycardia intraoperatively.

A further problem with high doses of opioids is that they produce truncal muscle rigidity, ocular movements, wrist flexion, and shoulder abduction, which are often referred to as *fentanyl seizures*. These events, however, do not produce electroencephalographic changes characteristic of epileptiform activity.[17,18] The truncal rigidity does interfere with ventilation and requires the use of neuromuscular blockers. Ventilatory support is frequently continued postoperatively because the elimination half-lives of opioids are relatively long (1.5 to 4 h). Despite these disadvantages, high-dose opioid anesthesia is one of the few anesthetic techniques that does not significantly depress myocardial contractility. It is also associated with markedly stable hemodynamics during anesthetic induction and maintenance in the majority of patients with cardiovascular disease.

Neither morphine nor meperidine are commonly used intraoperatively. Morphine is often used as premedication and for postoperative analgesia. With higher doses and rapid administration, morphine causes histamine release, and is associated with hypotension and increased fluid requirements. It is also a venodilator. Meperidine produces tachycardia and histamine release, and is a direct myocardial depressant. It has the lowest toxic–therapeutic dose ratio of the clinically relevant opioids.

The synthetic phenylpiperidine opioids fentanyl, sufentanil, and alfentanil are used frequently by anesthesiologists. A mild bradycardia usually occurs on anesthetic induction due to an increase in vagal tone, but these drugs are not myocardial depressants and do not cause histamine release. Nevertheless, patients with high resting sympathetic tone, congestive heart failure, or severe pulmonary hypertension are prone to transient hypotension during anesthetic induction. The bradycardia is often advantageous in patients with diseases such as CAD or mitral stenosis. The bradycardiac effect is reliably antagonized by atropine or pancuronium (see below) in patients with conditions such as mitral regurgitation, in whom faster heart rates may improve cardiac output.

Anesthesiologists only rarely administer naloxone or other opiate antagonists to reverse the effects of systemic opiates in patients with cardiovascular disease. The reversal of the opiate effect results in the sudden onset of pain and surges in catecholamine levels. Naloxone administration has been complicated by pulmonary edema,[19] arrhythmias,[20] and cardiac arrest.[21] One exception is that intravenous naloxone has been safely used to reverse the pruritis and respiratory depression associated with epidural and intrathecal opiates without reversing the analgesia.[22]

Etomidate

Etomidate is an imidazole anesthetic agent that enhances GABAergic transmission. It gives hemodynamic stability during bolus administration for anesthetic induction but does not blunt the hemodynamic response to laryngoscopy and tracheal intubation. Etomidate infusions are not used in the United States because of their association with adrenocortical insufficiency. This is one of the preferred agents for anesthetic induction in patients with valvular or ventricular dysfunction, hypovolemia, or pericardial effusion.

Propofol

Propofol is a substituted phenol (di-isopropylphenol) that may be used for anesthetic induction and maintenance. It is dissolved in a soybean oil emulsion, which is mildly irritating on injection. Its main advantage is the rapid emergence and psychomotor recovery following termination of the drug infusion. Propofol causes dose-dependent hypotension that appears to be due to a combination of myocardial depression and vasodilation. This drug has been recently introduced and experience is limited. It would be prudent to avoid propofol in patients with aortic or mitral valvular stenosis and cardiomyopathies.

Ketamine

Ketamine is a cyclohexanone that is chemically related to phencyclidine (PCP). Its use as a sole anesthetic is limited by its sympathomimetic effects and emergence delirium. Its sympathomimetic effects are advantageous, however, in certain groups of patients with cardiovascular disease. These include mainly those who are critically dependent on high resting sympathetic tone to maintain an adequate perfusion pressure: those with pericardial tamponade, hypovolemia, and systemic-to-pulmonary arterial shunts. It is important to reduce the dose of ketamine in those with severe cardiac disease, because ketamine is an indirect sympathomimetic and a direct myocardial depressant. In patients who already have maximal sympathetic outflow, ketamine's depressant effects may be "unmasked." Ketamine is relatively contraindicated in patients who cannot tolerate tachycardia, such as those with CAD or mitral stenosis.[23]

Alpha$_2$-Adrenergic Agonists

Clonidine and dexmedetomidine are alpha$_2$-adrenergic agonists that are sympatholytic, sedative anxiolytic, antiarrhythmic, analgesic, and reversible.[24,25] Clonidine also has been demonstrated to reduce anesthetic requirements and improve hemodynamic stability during the intraoperative period. Alpha$_2$-adrenergic agents may play a much larger role in perioperative management of patients with cardiovascular disease in the future once more convenient and specific compounds are developed.

Inhalational Anesthetics

Inhalational anesthetics include nitrous oxide and the potent volatile agents. The study of the uptake and distribution of inhaled drugs with cerebral and cardiovascular effects is practically unique to anesthesiology, and cardiac output is a major determinant of uptake and distribution. The alveolar concentration of a drug is generally equal to the brain concentration. Thus, anything that hastens increases in the alveolar concentration of the drug will speed the onset of anesthesia. Two factors that speed the onset of anesthesia are a diminished cardiac output and an anesthetic agent with low solubility in the blood. Thus, patients with low cardiac output secondary to cardiovascular disease will have a more rapid onset of anesthesia. Intracardiac right-to-left shunting will decrease the onset of anesthesia while left-to-right shunting has negligible effects.

Nitrous Oxide

Nitrous oxide is an excellent analgesic but not a very potent anesthetic. Concentrations up to 75 percent may be given safely, but incomplete amnesia and movement in response to painful stimuli are likely. Thus, nitrous oxide is nearly always administered with other anesthetic agents, such as opioids or potent volatile agents, and neuromuscular blockers. Nitrous oxide is also chosen because its relatively low solubility in the blood enhances the rapid onset and termination of its effects.

Nitrous oxide is a weak myocardial depressant that mildly stimulates the sympathetic nervous system.[26] Nitrous oxide, however, does not exacerbate pulmonary hypertension.[27] Its cardiovascular effects are minimal as a sole agent, but cardiac output is lowered in the presence of opioids. It also accentuates the negative inotropic effects of potent volatile agents.[28]

Nitrous oxide diffuses very rapidly into closed air spaces within the body due to its low blood solubility, high lipid solubility, and the high concentrations required. Examples of closed air spaces include bowel gas, pneumothoraces, and air emboli. Once equilibrium is reached, 75 percent nitrous oxide will quadruple the size of any of these spaces. For this reason, nitrous oxide must be discontinued if a pneumothorax or air embolism is suspected. It is often avoided in cardiothoracic procedures, particularly in children prone to paradoxical embolization, or after cardiopulmonary bypass.

Potent Volatile Agents

Inhalational anesthesia with potent volatile agents is the most common anesthetic technique. It has favorable attributes such as relatively low cost, reliable amnesia, bronchodilation, low blood solubility, and the overall safety record of these agents. All are myocardial depressants and vasodilators and produce some degree of hypotension. The hypotension provides some indication of the depth of anesthesia, as does monitoring of end-tidal gas concentrations.

The effect of these agents is rapidly changed when the inspiratory concentration is adjusted. The titrability of inhalational anesthesia is an advantage compared to intravenous drugs, because the duration of surgical procedures and the degree of surgical stimulation are often unpredictable. For this reason, low doses of volatile anesthetics may be added as supplements to nitrous oxide– or intravenous-based anesthetic techniques for the control of hypertension and the prevention of awareness (incomplete amnesia).

A phenomenon that is common to these agents is the frequent production of nodal (junctional) rhythm. The loss of atrial systole may be poorly tolerated in patients with aortic stenosis, hypertrophic cardiomyopathies, or mitral stenosis. All potent volatile agents have the potential for interactions with calcium entry blockers and beta-adrenergic blockers. Negative inotropic and conduction effects of these drugs may be augmented by the volatile anesthetic agents; nevertheless, in general, cardiac drugs should be continued until the time of surgery.

Halothane

Halothane represented a major advance in anesthesia when it was introduced in the 1950s, but its use is restricted by its cardiovascular effects and the small incidence of hepatotoxicity. Halothane depresses the myocardium and the sinoatrial node but it is not a potent vasodilator. Thus, cardiac output and heart rate are depressed in a dose-dependent fashion. Blood pressure is not severely decreased, because the decrease in systemic vascular resistance is less than with the other volatile agents at equipotent dosages. This hemodynamic profile is beneficial in situations where myocardial contractility (and oxygen consumption) should not be stimulated and perfusion pressure is maintained high. Examples include ischemic heart disease, hypertrophic obstructive cardiomyopathy, and tetralogy of Fallot. Halothane is contraindicated in patients with dilated cardiomyopathy, congestive heart failure, aortic stenosis, aortic and mitral regurgitation, and pericardial tamponade.

Halothane lowers the threshold for epinephrine-induced ventricular arrhythmias more than the other volatile agents. As a practical matter, the initial epinephrine dose is restricted to 1.5 μg/kg during infiltration of local anesthetic solutions. If arrhythmias occur due to an inadvertent vascular injection, halothane should be discontinued. Approximately five times the dose of epinephrine is required to induce ventricular arrhythmias in patients receiving enflurane and isoflurane as compared to halothane.

Enflurane

Enflurane is almost equal to halothane in its negative inotropic effect, but it is more vasodilating and has less of a negative chronotropic effect. Thus, cardiac output is better maintained, but blood pressure is lower than with equipotent dosages of halothane. Enflurane is often chosen as a supplement to intravenous anesthetic techniques when breakthrough hypertension occurs.

Isoflurane

Isoflurane is somewhat less of a negative inotropic drug than enflurane or halothane and is a potent arteriolar vasodilator, which tends to maintain cardiac output. Tachycardia frequently occurs at clinical dosages because the baroreceptor reflexes are not impaired. On the basis of its hemodynamic effects, isoflurane would be beneficial in patients with mitral and aortic regurgitation with good ventricular function. It is relatively contraindicated (as a sole agent) in patients with mitral and aortic stenosis, dilated and hypertrophic cardiomyopathies, and pericardial tamponade. Isoflurane is frequently used in patients with CAD, but it is often combined with opioids or beta-adrenergic blockers to prevent tachycardia, and the dose is limited to preserve coronary perfusion pressure. The use of isoflurane remains controversial in patients with coronary artery anatomy that predisposes to coronary steal.

Coronary steal occurs when a zone of myocardium distal to a stenotic coronary artery derives its blood supply from collateral vessels that originate in a zone of myocardium with normal coronary arterial supply. The arterioles in the normal zone are partially constricted while those in the collateral-dependent zone are maximally dilated due to the "upstream" coronary artery occlusion. This maintains the pressure gradient across the collateral vessels and the perfusion of the collateral-dependent zone. Arteriolar vasodilators (e.g., adenosine, dipyridamole, and sodium nitroprusside) can dilate the arterioles in the normal myocardial zone and decrease the perfusion pressure across the collateral vessels, which may precipitate myocardial ischemia due to coronary steal. Isoflurane has been shown to induce myocardial ischemia in dog models with collateral-dependent myocardial blood flow[29] and in humans.[30]

It remains controversial whether or not isoflurane should be used clinically in patients with CAD given the uncertainty regarding coronary artery anatomy in most patients. The tachycardia and hypotension associated with isoflurane, as well as evidence of maldistributed myocardial blood flow, might suggest that it should not be used. Nevertheless, a prospective clinical study in patients with "steal-prone anatomy"[31] and large outcome studies[10,11] have not found a tendency toward intraoperative myocardial ischemia or poorer outcome with isoflurane anesthesia. A reasonable conclusion is that isoflurane should be used with caution and appropriate monitoring in patients suspected of having "steal-prone" coronary artery anatomy.[32]

Desflurane

Desflurane is a new volatile anesthetic that is much less soluble in blood than the currently available agents. Its blood-gas solubility coefficient is similar to nitrous oxide. Thus, more rapid induction and emergence would be expected. Desflurane has coronary vascular effects that are similar to isoflurane, but it is not associated with tachycardia at lower doses.[33]

Neuromuscular Blockade

Benzylisoquinolines

The benzylisoquinoline series of nondepolarizing neuromuscular blockers are all derivatives of the curare molecule. Most of these compounds have histamine-releasing properties that are dependent on the dose and rate of administration. D-Tubocurarine, metocurine, and atracurium are associated with clinically important histamine release with administration of bolus doses to facilitate tracheal intubation. The newer agents, doxacurium and mivacurium, have minimal cardiovascular effects.

Steroids

Pancuronium is the classic steroid nondepolarizing neuromuscular blocking drug. The atropine-like molecular structure contains two quaternary nitrogen groups. The tachycardia and hypertension associated with pancuronium have been linked to myocardial ischemia during coronary artery bypass surgery.[34] The anticholinergic effects of pancuronium, however, can be useful for preventing the vagal bradycardia that occurs with high-dose opioid anesthetic inductions (e.g., in patients with mitral regurgitation). The newer steroid neuromuscular blockers, vecuronium and pipecuronium, have minimal cardiovascular effects at clinical dosages.

Succinylcholine

Succinylcholine is a depolarizing short-acting neuromuscular blocker. Its molecular structure is essentially diacetylcholine. Its cardiovascular effects depend on whether nicotinic or muscarinic receptor effects predominate. Thus, tachycardia and hypertension or bradycardia and hypotension may occur. Vagal effects tend to predominate with repeated doses or in children.

THE POSTOPERATIVE PERIOD

The emergence from anesthesia is frequently accompanied by hypertension and tachycardia. This is most often due to incomplete analgesia but may also be related to withdrawal from antihypertensive drugs, hypoxemia, delirium, and bladder distension. If an underlying cause is not identifiable, intravenous drugs such as nitroglycerin, labetalol, or esmolol are frequently used to control hemodynamics in patients with cardiovascular disease. Shivering is another phenomenon that may occur due to hypothermia or emergence from volatile anesthetics. Shivering results in marked increases in oxygen consumption, which may be poorly tolerated by patients with cardiovascular disease. Low doses of meperidine decrease or eliminate shivering, although the mechanism is unknown.[35]

It is clear from numerous studies that the extended postoperative period entails significant cardiovascular risk. The majority of perioperative MIs, for example, take place on postoperative days 2 through 4. Pain, higher catecholamine levels, hypercoagulability, hypovolemia, anemia, intravascular volume shifts, drug effects, and a lower level of monitoring all probably contribute to this phenomenon.

Traditionally, the anesthesiologist has not played a major role in postoperative management following discharge from the recovery room/postanesthesia care unit. This situation has changed recently in some facilities with the development of multidisciplinary pain services that administer epidural analgesia and patient-controlled analgesia devices for selected patients. It is interesting that in studies claiming improved outcome following regional anesthesia, epidural analgesia was performed postoperatively in the regional anesthesia cohorts.[12,13] It is conceivable that more effective postoperative analgesia decreased the deleterious effects of the stress response. It is likely that future efforts to reduce perioperative risk will concentrate on the effects of more intensive postoperative hemodynamic, analgesic, and anticoagulation management.

CONCLUSIONS

The optimal perioperative care of patients with cardiovascular disease is the joint responsibility of anesthesiologists, surgeons, and cardiologists. Any anesthetic agent or technique has the potential for producing adverse effects, and the margin of safety is reduced in patients with cardiovascular disease. It is the anesthesiologist's role to acquire accurate and relevant information from the preoperative evaluation, to apply appropriate monitoring technology, to select an anesthetic technique that is suited to the planned procedure and the condition of the patient, and to manage hemodynamic alterations and analgesic requirements in the postoperative period.

Cardiovascular disease continues to become more prevalent in the surgical population. Recent research suggests that the greatest cardiovascular risk lies in the postoperative period and that the choice of anesthetic drugs and techniques has little or no measurable impact on outcome. One exception is the preliminary evidence that continuous postoperative epidural analgesia may have beneficial effects. If these findings are confirmed in large-scale, multi-institutional studies, it would be reasonable to predict that anesthesiologists will play a more active role in postoperative pain management in the future.

REFERENCES

1. Wells PH, Kaplan JA: Optimal management of patients with ischemic heart disease for non-cardiac surgery by complementary anesthesia and cardiology intervention. *Am Heart J* 1981; 102:1030–1040.
2. Goldman L, Caldera DL, Nussbaum SR, Southwick FS, Krogstad D, Murray B, et al: Multifactorial index of cardiac risk in noncardiac surgical procedures. *N Engl J Med* 1977; 297:845–850.
3. Mangano ET, Browner WS, Hollenberg M, London MJ, Tubau JF, Tateo IM, et al: Association of perioperative myocardial ischemia with cardiac morbidity and mortality in men undergoing noncardiac surgery. *N Engl J Med* 1990; 323:1781–1788.
4. Goldman L: Multifactorial index of cardiac risk in non-cardiac surgery: Ten year status report. *J Cardiothorac Anesth* 1987; 1:237–244.
5. Rao TL, Jacobs KH, El-Etr AA: Reinfarction following anesthesia in patients with myocardial infarction. *Anesthesiology* 1983; 59:499–505.
6. Carliner NH, Fisher ML, Plotnick GD, Gabart H, Rapoport A, Kelemen MH, et al: Routine preoperative exercise testing in patients undergoing major noncardiac surgery. *Am J Cardiol* 1985; 56:51–58.
7. Eagle KA, Coley CM, Newell JB, Brewster DC, Darling RC, Strauss HW, et al: Combining clinical and thallium data optimizes preoperative assessment of cardiac risk before major vascular surgery. *Ann Intern Med* 1989; 110:859–866.
8. Raby KE, Goldman L, Creager MA, Cook EF, Weisberg MC, Whittemore AD, et al: Correlation between preoperative ischemia and major cardiac events after peripheral vascular surgery. *N Engl J Med* 1989; 321:1296–1300.
9. Kleinman B, Czinn E, Shah K, Sobotka P, Rao TK: The value to the anesthesia-surgical care team of the preoperative cardiac consultation. *J Cardiothorac Anesth* 1989; 3:682–687.
10. Slogoff S, Keats AS: Randomized trial of primary anesthetic agents on outcome of coronary artery bypass operations. *Anesthesiology* 1989; 70:179–188.
11. Tuman KJ, McCarthy RJ, Spiess BD, DaValle M, Dabir R, Ivankovich AD: Does choice of anesthetic agent significantly affect outcome after coronary artery surgery? *Anesthesiology* 1989; 70:189–198.
12. Yeager MP, Glass DD, Neff RK, Brinck-Johnsen T: Epidural anesthesia and analgesia in high-risk surgical procedures. *Anesthesiology* 1987; 66:729–736.
13. Tuman KJ, McCarthy RJ, March RJ, DeLaria GA, Patel RV, Ivankovich AD: Effects of epidural anesthesia and analgesia on coagulation and outcome after major vascular surgery. *Anesth Analg* 1991; 73:696–704.

14. Cheney FW, Kroll DA: Medicolegal aspects of anesthetic practice. In: Barash PG, Cullen BF, Stoelting RK (eds): *Clinical Anesthesia*, 1st ed. Philadelphia, Lippincott, 1989: 35–44.
15. Covino BG: Pharmacology of local anaesthetic agents. *Br J Anaesth* 1986; 58:701–716.
16. Fleming JA, Byck R, Barash PG: Pharmacology and therapeutic applications of cocaine. *Anesthesiology* 1990; 73:518–531.
17. Smith NT, Benthuysen JL, Bickford RG, Sanford TJ, Blasco T, Duke PC, et al: Seizures during opioid anesthetic induction—Are they opioid-induced rigidity? *Anesthesiology* 1989; 71:852–862.
18. Murkin JM, Moldenhauer CC, Hug CC Jr, Epstein CM: Absence of seizures during induction of anesthesia with high-dose fentanyl. *Anesth Analg* 1984; 63:489–494.
19. Prough DS, Roy R, Bumgarner J, Shannon G: Acute pulmonary edema in healthy teenagers following conservative doses of intravenous naloxone. *Anesthesiology* 1984; 60:485–486.
20. Azar I, Turndorf H: Severe hypertension and multiple atrial premature contractions following naloxone administration. *Anesth Analg* 1979; 58:524–525.
21. Andree RA: Sudden death following naloxone administration. *Anesth Analg* 1980; 59:782–784.
22. Bell SD, Seltzer JL: Postoperative pain management. In: Kaplan JA (ed): *Vascular Anesthesia*. New York, Churchill-Livingstone, 1991: 565–586.
23. Reich DL, Silvay G: Ketamine: An update on the first 25 years of clinical experience. *Can J Anaesth* 1989; 36:186–197.
24. Hayashi Y, Sumikawa K, Maze M, Yamatodani A, Kamibayashi T, Kuro M, et al: Dexmedetomidine prevents epinephrine-induced arrhythmias through stimulation of central alpha 2 adrenoreceptors in halothane-anesthetized dogs. *Anesthesiology* 1991; 75:113–117.
25. Maze M, Tranquilli W: Alpha-2 agonists: Defining the role in clinical anesthesia. *Anesthesiology* 1991; 74:581–605.
26. Ebert TJ, Kampine JP: Nitrous oxide augments sympathetic outflow: Direct evidence from human peroneal nerve recordings. *Anesth Analg* 1989; 69:444–449.
27. Konstadt SN, Reich DL, Thys DM: Nitrous oxide does not exacerbate pulmonary hypertension or ventricular dysfunction in patients with mitral valvular disease. *Can J Anaesth* 1990; 37:613–617.
28. Stowe DF, Monroe SM, Marijic J, Bosnjak ZJ, Kampine JP: Comparison of halothane, enflurane, and isoflurane with nitrous oxide on contractility and oxygen supply and demand in isolated hearts. *Anesthesiology* 1991; 75: 1062–1074.
29. Buffington CW, Romson JL, Levin A, Duttlinger NC, Huang AH: Isoflurane induces coronary steal in a canine model of chronic coronary occlusion. *Anesthesiology* 1987; 66:280–292.
30. Reiz S, Bälfors E, Sorensen MB, Ariola S, Friedman A, Truedsson H: Isoflurane: A powerful coronary vasodilator in patients with coronary artery disease. *Anesthesiology* 1983; 59:91–97.
31. Pulley DD, Kirvassilis GV, Kelermenos N, Kater K, Barzilai B, Genton RE, et al: Regional and global myocardial circulatory and metabolic effects of isoflurane and halothane in patients with steal-prone coronary anatomy. *Anesthesiology* 1991; 75:756–766.
32. Priebe HJ: Isoflurane and coronary hemodynamics. *Anesthesiology* 1989; 71:960–976.
33. Saidman LJ: The role of desflurane in the practice of anesthesia. *Anesthesiology* 1991; 74:399–401.
34. Thomson IR, Putnins CL: Adverse effects of pancuronium during high-dose fentanyl anesthesia for coronary artery bypass grafting. *Anesthesiology* 1985; 62:708–713.
35. Guffin A, Girard D, Kaplan JA: Shivering following cardiac surgery: Hemodynamic changes and reversal. *J Cardiothorac Anesth* 1987; 1:24–28.

Chapter 141

Cardiopulmonary Bypass and Intraoperative Protection

Mark W. Connolly, M.D. ■ *Robert A. Guyton, M.D.*

DEVELOPMENT OF CARDIOPULMONARY BYPASS

Early Landmarks

References to oxygenation of blood through an extracorporeal circuit began as early as the late nineteenth century. Schroeder devised a bubble oxygenator in 1882.[1] A film oxygenator was devised by von Frey and Graben in 1884.[2] Subsequently numerous uses of different oxygenators and pumps were reported, and the concept of organ preservation by the delivery of oxygenated blood was accepted by 1900.

Two major advances essential to the development of cardiopulmonary bypass was Landstaner's delineation of the ABO blood group system in 1900 and, in 1916 to 1918, McClean, Howell, and Hope's use of heparin for anticoagulation.[3]

Bypass Circuits and Oxygenators

In 1937 Gibbon,[4] motivated by a desire to develop an approach to the problem of massive pulmonary embolism, successfully bypassed the hearts of dogs during pulmonary occlusion. His device was a rotating vertical cylinder oxygenator with multiple pumps, valves, and pressure controls. Gibbon's efforts were delayed by World War II. In 1951, Dogliotti[5] in Italy successfully bypassed the right side of the heart to remove a mediastinal tumor. In that same year Dennis et al.,[6] at the University of Minnesota, attempted unsuccessfully to repair during cardiopulmonary bypass what was thought to be an atrial septal defect in a young woman, who died and was found to have a partial atrioventricular canal defect. In 1953, Gibbon[7] first successfully used a pump oxygenator to repair an atrial septal defect in a young woman. Although his next four patients died, Gibbon's methods were readily applied by others. In 1955 Kirklin et al.[8] reported the successful use of cardiopulmonary bypass in eight patients at the Mayo Clinic, following which the use of the technique of cardiopulmonary bypass to repair cardiac defects rapidly spread.

Goal of Cardiopulmonary Bypass

In 1962, Galetti and Brecher[3] stated that the goal of heart-lung bypass is "delivery of the correct amount of appropriately oxygenated blood to the tissues of the whole body without attendant or ensuing adverse physiological effects." This "correct amount" of oxygenated perfusion is that necessary for the maintenance of end-organ function during bypass. The primary goal of cardiopulmonary bypass is to preserve organ function and to minimize the derangement of the body's physiological homeostasis. Figure 141-1 depicts schematically the components of the cardiopulmonary bypass system.

MECHANICS OF CARDIOPULMONARY BYPASS

Anticoagulation

Anticoagulation with heparin is essential to minimize blood-surface interactions and thrombotic complica-

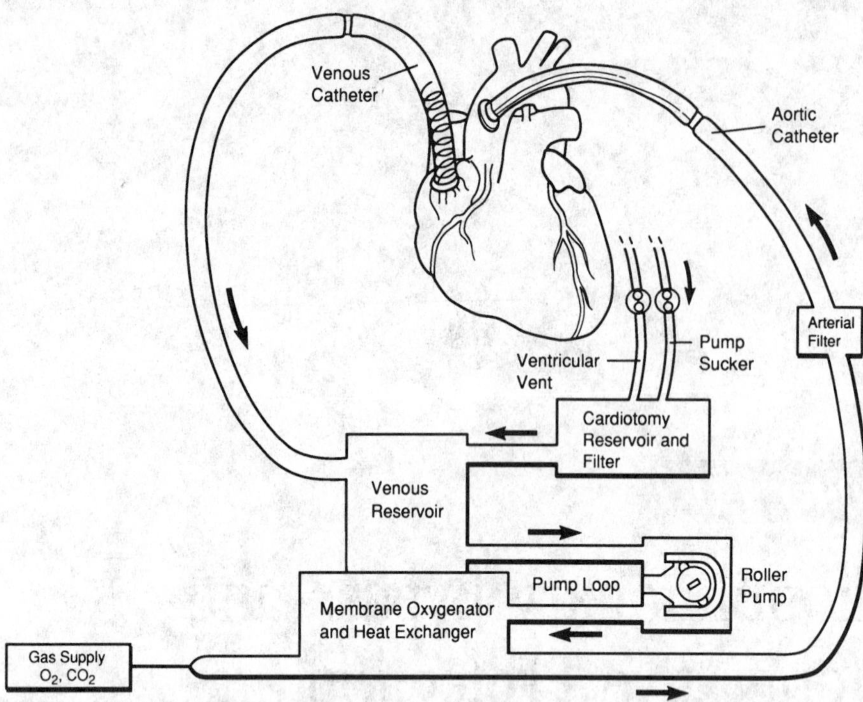

FIGURE 141-1 Schematic diagram of a cardiopulmonary bypass system.

tions. Adequate heparinization is verified by use of the activated clotting time (ACT), which is measured frequently during the bypass procedure. Many patients receive prolonged preoperative heparin infusions, which can produce a significant antithrombin III deficiency. These patients may be difficult to anticoagulate and may require large doses of heparin during bypass.

After weaning from cardiopulmonary bypass, protamine is infused to reverse the heparin effect. Protamine dosage approximates heparin dosage on a milligram-per-milligram basis, and reversal is confirmed by the return of the ACT to pre-bypass baseline. Protamine must be infused slowly to prevent hypotension and myocardial deterioration. Rarely, severe anaphylactic reactions from protamine can produce hemodynamic deterioration, marked peripheral vasodilation, massive histamine release, and capillary leak.[9] The protamine-heparin interaction activates the complement cascade demonstrated by increased levels of the anaphylatoxin C4a as well as C3a and C5a.[10] Fatal pulmonary vasoconstriction producing right ventricular failure has been reported.[11] Preoperative risk factors for protamine reactions are previous exposure to protamine or protamine-containing insulin and possibly vasectomy.[12]

The Arterial Pump

A roller pump is most commonly used for arterial perfusion, and its head is adjusted to deliver a calibrated volume of blood regardless of the afterload pressure. This mechanical adjustment is slightly nonocclusive to minimize hemolysis. The tubing should be Silastic or Latex; other plastics will stiffen during hypothermia. Centrifugal pumps cause less blood trauma, but pump output is dependent on afterload.

Oxygenators

There are three basic types of oxygenators: film, bubble, and membrane. The film oxygenator allows blood to flow over a surface. The bubble oxygenator bubbles an oxygen and carbon dioxide mixture into the blood. Both the film and bubble types have a blood-air interface that damages blood elements and requires a defoaming chamber. The membrane oxygenator separates blood from air with a large-surface-area, porous membrane, causing less damage to blood elements.[13] Membrane oxygenators are more expensive and have no real significant advantage over bubble oxygenators.[14]

Heat Exchange

Systemic cooling and warming are accomplished by an efficient heat exchanger. The surgeon's control of perfusate temperature and, hence, the patient's core temperature provide important flexibility during the operative procedure. Lower flow rates, short periods of circulatory arrest, and enhanced myocardial protection are achieved with hypothermia. Blood may be cooled quickly, but rewarming to temperatures higher than 39°C can cause hemolysis and denaturation of proteins.

Cannulation Technique

Arterial return from the pump is accomplished by inserting a cannula through a purse string suture in the ascending aorta. Care must be taken to avoid manipulation of atherosclerotic areas in the aorta. The preoperative chest film, echocardiogram, and gentle operative palpation of the aorta are used to detect diseased areas. The systemic blood pressure is lowered while inserting the cannula to prevent aortic dissection. When the presence of severe disease prevents aortic cannulation, common femoral artery cannulation is performed and the artery is repaired at the end of the procedure.

Venous drainage usually is adequately accomplished centrally by single cannulation of the right atrial appendage. Peripheral venous drainage of the inferior vena cava via the common femoral vein is an alternative approach but is associated with an increased incidence of deep vein thrombosis. Double cannulation through the right atrium into the superior and inferior vena cavae allows more complete isolation of the heart than does single cannulation, maintains more effective cardiac hypothermia, and is used for operations requiring isolation of the right side of the heart (i.e., atrial septal defect, tricuspid valve repair). If needed, left ventricular decompression is accomplished by venting through the main pulmonary artery or right superior pulmonary vein.

EXTRACORPOREAL PERFUSION

Hemodilution

The bypass circuit is primed with a physiologically balanced crystalloid solution, with or without an oncotically active solute such as albumin. In adults the hematocrit often decreases to between 18 to 22 percent during cardiopulmonary bypass. For infants or adults with small body surface areas it may be necessary to add homologous blood to the priming solution to achieve an adequate hematocrit for tissue oxygen delivery. Hemodilution counteracts the increased blood viscosity produced during hypothermia. This decrease in hematocrit does not ordinarily impair systemic oxygen delivery but can produce regional myocardial ischemia in the presence of coronary disease.[15] At the end of the procedure, the blood from the extracorporeal circuit is directly returned to the patient through the arterial line or after hemoconcentration.

Flow Rate and Arterial Pressure

In general, the optimal flow rate is approximately 2.5 liters/min per $M.^2$ During hypothermia, flow rates as low as half normal are adequate to prevent structural or functional organ damage. Urine output greater than 0.5 mL/kg per h, venous drainage oxygen saturation greater than 60 percent, and lack of metabolic lactic acidosis confirm adequate systemic tissue perfusion. A fall in mixed venous oxygen saturation with an adequate flow rate is usually related to increased oxygen consumption from light anesthesia or inadequate muscle paralysis.

Arterial pressure maintenance is especially important in the presence of cerebrovascular disease. In these patients alpha-adrenergic drugs are used to maintain mean arterial pressure above 65 to 70 mmHg. (See Chap. 30.) Continuous monitoring of the electroencephalogram (EEG) and the use of barbiturates to produce EEG quiescence may help minimize neurologic damage in patients with previous cerebrovascular accidents or hemodynamically significant carotid stenosis.

Systemic Hypothermia

Systemic hypothermia is used during cardiopulmonary bypass to enhance myocardial protection and to protect other organs, particularly the central nervous system. As systemic temperatures are lowered, the metabolic rate decreases allowing lower perfusion flow rates. If the central-core temperature is reduced to 20°C or below, a brief period of circulatory arrest (turning the bypass machine off) may be safely accomplished. Circulatory arrest periods greater than 60 min have been associated with severe neurologic injury. Extremely low temperatures (less than 12°C) have also been associated with neurologic impairment. For this reason, every attempt is made to restrict the duration of circulatory arrest to 45 to 50 min at temperatures between 15° and 20°C.

Hypothermia increases the affinity of hemoglobin for oxygen and inhibits the ability of local tissue to autoregulate its own oxygen supply. This may cause regional ischemia despite a reduction in metabolic rate, particularly if it is combined with hypotension. Consequently, lactic acid production occurs from anaerobic metabolism. Adequate anesthesia, flow rates, and perfusion pressure are required to prevent acidosis.

MYOCARDIAL PROTECTION DURING ISCHEMIC ARREST

Basic Concepts

The surgeon seeks an immobile bloodless field to optimize the operation. Arrest can be accomplished by altering electrolyte membrane metabolism (poisoning) and, most commonly, by inducing myocardial hypothermia. The technique of metabolic poisoning and hypothermia greatly reduces myocardial cellular energy requirements and minimizes depletion of adenosine triphosphate (ATP) energy stores while the heart is isolated from its blood supply. Chemical arrest combined with myocardial hypothermia (10 to 20°C) has been shown to reduce oxygen consumption to less than 5 percent of the normal, working heart.[16] Adequate recovery of the heart after reperfusion depends on the use of myocardial protection techniques that are adapted to each patient's specific cardiac disease.

Preparation For Ischemic Arrest

When cardiopulmonary bypass begins, the heart is immediately exposed to hypotension, hypothermia, and hemodilution, each of which may increase myocardial ischemia. In addition, ventricular fibrillation or ventricular distention may increase regional myocardial ischemia. The surgeon should maintain a mean arterial perfusion pressure of 70 to 80 mmHg as the heart is being cooled, particularly in patients with coronary artery disease. Ventricular distension should be prevented by maintaining the heart in a beating state until cardioplegic arrest is accomplished or, if ventricular fibrillation occurs, venting the left ventricle if distension is evident. These considerations become critically important for patients with aortic regurgitation. If these patients should fibrillate and distend during cooling, the aortic cross-clamp must be applied immediately and the aortic root opened for direct infusion of the cardioplegic agent antegrade into the coronary ostia or retrograde through the coronary sinus.

Prior to arrest the heart may be pharmacologically prepared for arrest by decreasing the metabolic rate of the myocardium and/or by bolstering the energy source of the myocardium. Pretreatment of the heart with propranolol leads to improved function and metabolic recovery after arrest, and calcium channel blockers are effective in improving myocardial tolerance to ischemic arrest when used alone or as adjuncts to cold cardioplegic arrest. Glucose or glucose-insulin-potassium infusion may lead to increased glycogen stores in the myocardium and to improved recovery after an arrest interval.[15]

Myocardial Hypothermia

Myocardial hypothermia reduces oxygen consumption in the beating heart, in the fibrillating heart, and in the chemically arrested heart. A reduction in the myocardial temperature decreases the damage caused by ischemic arrest in all experiment models. The most effective way to cool the heart is by infusion of cold solution into the coronary ostia or retrograde through the coronary sinus venous system. In the presence of coronary artery disease retrograde cardioplegic infusion may provide a more even myocardial distribution than antegrade aortic infusion.[17] If only antegrade coronary ostial cardioplegic infusion is used, wide variations in regional temperatures may occur in regions distal to critical coronary stenosis, producing inadequate regional protection. This can be overcome by first constructing vein grafts to regions supplied by the most critically stenosed areas and infusing cardioplegia through these vein grafts; or by using a combination of antegrade and retrograde coronary sinus (continuous or intermittent) cardioplegic infusion. Optimal protection is often provided by a combination of antegrade aortic and retrograde coronary sinus methods.

Local myocardial hypothermia is further accomplished by flooding the pericardium with cold (4°C) electrolyte solution. This topical hypothermia improves the homogeneity of cooling and prevents rewarming of the myocardium from the higher systemic temperature of the surrounding organs.[18]

Systemic Hypothermia

Rewarming of the heart during ischemic arrest occurs by the return of the warmer systemic blood to the heart through noncoronary collateral blood flow from the thesbian veins, mediastinal, pericardial and bronchial channels through the pericardial reflections, and from the vasa vasorum along major vessels connected to the heart, and the right atrium and right ventricle in contact with the warmer venous blood return. Systemic core hypothermia (25 to 30°C) minimizes myocardial rewarming during arrest. Further isolation of the heart from systemic warming during the arrest period may be accomplished by superior and inferior vena cava cannulation.

Cardioplegia

Cardioplegia solutions are metabolic poisons. They prevent myocyte contraction and reduce oxygen consumption. These poisons must be reversible. Chemical asystole can be achieved by a number of different methods, but the most popular is by the infusion of a hyperkalemic solution. Potassium in concentrations ranging from 15 to 35 meq/liter blocks the fast phase of myocyte membrane depolarization. In general, a balanced electrolyte solution or a blood-based solution is optimal, as it causes less derangement of cellular hemostasis.

In addition to potassium, cardioplegic solutions are alkaline to provide buffering capacity to the tissue's acid milieu produced from anaerobic metabolism. They are slightly hyperosmolar to prevent myocyte edema. Although some studies have shown increased cellular water with crystalloid compared to blood-based solution, we have not detected an increase in myocardial water content with the use of crystalloid solution. Most solutions also contain small concentrations of calcium and magnesium. (See also Chap. 74.)

Many studies[19] have shown the beneficial effects of modifying the cardioplegic solution. The addition of blood, calcium channel blocker, β blockers, steroids, amino acids, oxygen-free radical scavengers, local anesthetics, and many other agents has been experimentally studied. To date, however, the benefits of these additions in the clinical arena are unproven.

Oxygen Delivery

Oxygenation of the cardioplegic solutions improves recovery of the myocardium after cardioplegic arrest. Oxygen can be delivered to the myocardium by blood-based or crystalloid solutions. An oxygenated, cold crystalloid solution delivers approximately 3 to 4 mL oxygen per 100 mL solution to the myocardium. Blood solutions deliver approximately the same quantity of oxygen to the myocardium, primarily because of the increased affinity of hemoglobin for oxygen (decreased O_2 release at the cellular level) at the cold temperatures used for myocardial protection. A potential advantage of blood cardioplegia, a more physiological oncotic solution, is better buffering than crystalloid solutions.[20] In our experience, however, the oxygenated crystalloid solution is simple, inexpensive, and very effective, even in high-risk patients with poor preoperative ventricular function.[15,21,22]

Reperfusion

The circumstances of reperfusion after the ischemic arrest period can increase or decrease myocardial injury. During reperfusion the coronary vasculature is abnormal with absent autoregulation but with local tissue swelling, diminished myocyte energy stores, and the build up of toxic metabolites.

The perfusion pressure should be approximately 70 mmHg to facilitate optimal delivery of oxygen to the myocytes and wash out the chemical cardioplegic poisons. The reperfusate should be slightly hyperosmolar, alkaline, and low in calcium to prevent myocyte contraction and have an adequate hemoglobin concentration (hematocrit greater than 22 percent) to provide adequate oxygen delivery for repletion of phosphate energy stores. Myocardial recovery is improved if the heart is rested for 10 to 30 min after ischemic arrest without work during reperfusion. Several experimental studies have shown that chemical asystole during reperfusion may be beneficial. Buckberg has demonstrated improved recovery with warm-blood, amino acid–enhanced cardioplegic reperfusion after prolonged ischemic periods.[22] Table 141-1 summarizes the contents of cardioplegic solutions.

Special Circumstances Requiring Alteration of the Standard Technique

Severe Coronary Artery Disease

In patients with severe coronary artery disease (i.e., left main disease with total right coronary occlusion) cardioplegic infusion into the aortic root may be inadequate. Retrograde coronary sinus infusion and infusion down constructed vein grafts provide optimal protection during aortic cross-clamping. Proximal anastomoses should be performed before removing the aortic cross-clamp, instead of using a side-biting clamp, to provide immediate optimal reperfusion after the arrest period.

Aortic Regurgitation

Aortic regurgitation, particularly when combined with coronary artery disease, can present a major problem in myocardial protection. Upon beginning cardiopulmonary bypass the heart may immediately distend, requiring expedient aortic cross-clamping and infusion of cardioplegia directly into the coronary ostium and/or retrograde in the coronary sinus. Left ventricular venting, deeper systemic cooling, and local topical iced irrigation enhance protection. Distal anastomoses are performed first before valve replacement. Again, proximal anastomoses are completed with the aortic cross-clamp in place to ensure complete immediate reperfusion.

TABLE 141-1

Contents of Oxygenated Cold Crystalloid Cardioplegic Solutions

Standard Elements
Potassium (15–30 meq)
Sodium chloride
Hyperosmolar (320–350 mosmol/L)
Alkaline
Calcium chloride
Magnesium
Temperature (4°C)
Oxygen
Modified Adjuncts
Blood
Calcium channel blockers
Beta blockers
Steroids
Amino acids (glutamate, aspartate)
Oxygen-free radical scavengers
Local anesthetics (procaine)
Mannitol
Glucose
Warm blood (37°C)

Coronary Artery Reoperations

Because old saphenous vein grafts contain easily dislodged atheromatous debris, the heart is manipulated as little as possible during dissection. Again, retrograde cardioplegic infusion may provide more even myocardial protection. Severely diseased vein grafts are transected as new ones are constructed. Proximal anastomoses are performed before removing the aortic cross-clamp. In the presence of previously constructed in situ internal mammary artery grafts, the mammary artery must be occluded during arrest to prevent wash-out of cardioplegia. Retrograde cardioplegia can provide protection to areas supplied by a previously placed in situ mammary artery.

Retrograde Coronary Sinus Cardioplegia

Many of the difficulties encountered with antegrade aortic cardioplegia in special circumstances have been overcome with the use of retrograde cardioplegia through the coronary sinus. This method allows distribution of the cardioplegic solution to myocardial areas irregardless of the coronary pathology.[17] Potential hazards of this method are poor protection of the right ventricle, damage to the conduction system in the region of the coronary sinus, and myocardial swelling from infusion into the venous system.

Continuous Warm Blood Method

Although hypothermia is an essential component of myocardial protection, it has been associated with detrimental effects on cellular integrity, enzymatic function, and energy. Lichtenstein et al.[24] in Toronto have recently proposed normothermic, continuous retrograde, warm blood potassium cardioplegia to produce an "aerobic" arrest state. In a study of 121 patients undergoing coronary bypass patients they reported a decrease in intraaortic balloon pump use, greater incidence of return to normal sinus rhythm, greater immediate cardiac outputs, and less time weaned from bypass after removal of the aortic cross-clamp. This new method appears promising for selected patients, especially those requiring mitral valve repair or experiencing preoperative acute myocardial infarction.

Weaning from Cardiopulmonary Bypass

After an appropriate rest period, following removal of the aortic cross-clamp, achieving systemic normothermia and myocardial recovery, weaning the patient from cardiopulmonary bypass can begin. Regular rhythm is established spontaneously or with temporary pacing. The preload of the heart is increased by decreasing venous return to the bypass circuit, allowing an increase in left ventricular volume and, hence, opening of the aortic valve and ejection of blood. Pulmonary artery pressures and, infrequently, direct left atrial pressures are continuously monitored to prevent overdistension. Pharmacologic vasoconstrictor agents are used, if necessary, to maintain mean arterial perfusion pressure greater than 70 mmHg, and inotropic agents may be used to enhance myocardial contractibility. As left ventricular ejection increases from increasing preload, the bypass flow is decreased. The venous oxygen saturation from the venous line is continuously monitored and maintained above 65 percent. Rarely, intraaortic balloon pumping is required. The bypass circuit is shut off, and the heart resumes a working state providing adequate end-organ tissue perfusion. After decannulation, protamine is given to reverse the heparin.

COMPLICATIONS OF CARDIOPULMONARY BYPASS

Cannulation Injury

Arterial cannulation is a major threat to the patient during cardiopulmonary bypass. The presence of atherosclerotic disease in the ascending aorta and common femoral artery can lead to embolic disease or intimal dissection during cannulation, clamping, or proximal vein graft anastomoses. If dissection is recognized while still a local process, repair can usually be accomplished by deep suture repair under a partial occlusive clamp. If the dissection is extensive, the aortic root is replaced with woven graft material.[25]

Neuroendocrine and Cellular Responses

Cardiopulmonary bypass leads to a massive release of circulating epinephrine and norepinephrine. Plasma catecholamine elevations are due to altered arterial blood flow patterns, hypotension, hypothermia, hemodilution, decreased renal clearance, and lung clearance secondary to the lungs isolated from the bypass circulation.[26,27] Catecholamine levels gradually return to normal as the patient is weaned from bypass and the sternum is closed.[26]

Exposure of blood elements to nonbiological, nonendothelial surfaces (i.e., tubing, oxygenation, filters) produces a whole-body inflammatory response.[28] Erythrocytes are hemolyzed secondary to shear forces.[29] Leukocytes are mobilized from the bone marrow and trapped in the pulmonary circulation and produce microvascular endothelial damage and edema by lysosome enzyme release. The number of platelets decrease secondary to clumping on foreign surfaces, and platelet function undergoes significant deterioration.[30] Plasma proteins are denatured, activating the coagulation, fibrinolytic, complement, and bradykinin-kallikrein humoral systems. This humoral activation produces coagulation consumption, fibrinolysis, platelet and fibrin microemboli—all leading to bleeding, fever, interstitial and lung edema, vasoconstriction, and organ dysfunction.[30] The severity of these effects is directly related to the duration of cardiopulmonary bypass. There is some evidence that these damaging reactions might be diminished by the use of membrane oxygenators as well as by pretreatment with corticosteroid and other drugs such as aprotinin, which neutralizes the kallikrein-bradykinin system.

End-Organ Dysfunction

Nervous System

Cerebral function after cardiopulmonary bypass can range from no detectable deficit to mild neuropsychometric disorders to frank stroke. The main cause of cerebral dysfunction is cerebral gaseous and/or atheromatous microemboli. The duration of pump time has been shown to also correlate with cerebral complications. Intraoperative electroencephalographic monitoring and pretreatment with barbiturates and steroids may decrease the incidence and severity of cerebral dysfunction after bypass.[31]

Renal System

Renal dysfunction, varying from slight elevations in creatinine to acute oliguric renal failure, can occur after cardiopulmonary bypass. Ischemia secondary to inadequate perfusion and microemboli are the most likely etiology. Risk factors are age greater than 70 years, elevated preoperative serum creatinine levels, and low blood pressure during bypass.[32]

Pulmonary System

Complement activation and the release of anaphylatoxin C5a stimulate polymorphonuclear aggregation, sequestration, and adherence to pulmonary endothelium. Lysosomal enzymes are released, destroying basement membranes. Aggregates of platelets can also lead to endothelial injury. Interstitial pulmonary edema, bronchospasm, decreased surfactant, and atelectasis can result in oxygen desaturation. Almost all patients experience some reversible pulmonary dysfunction in the first 6 to 24 h.[33]

Gastrointestinal System

Severe gastrointestinal complications occur in 0.5 to 2.0 percent of the patients undergoing cardiopulmonary bypass. Gastrointestinal bleeding, intestinal infarction, pancreatitis, cholecystitis, intestinal obstruction, perforated ulcer, and hepatic necrosis can occur. Mortality rates as high as 60 percent have been reported after developing these gastrointestinal complications after bypass procedures. Risk factors include advanced age, emergency operation, valvular surgery, use of intraaortic balloon pump or vasopressors, and reoperation.[34,35] Transient postoperative ileus occurs in approximately 10 percent of patients.

Bleeding

Bleeding after cardiopulmonary bypass is a problem in only approximately 5 percent of patients, with 1 to 3 percent requiring reoperation. Indeed, the majority of elective patients can undergo cardiopulmonary bypass without utilization of blood products. Attention to hemostasis during initial dissection, the use of intraoperative and postoperative autotransfusion devices, and pharmacologic agents counteracting coagulopathy help minimize blood product transfusion requirements. Since the transmission of communicable diseases, particularly the acquired immunodeficiency syndrome (AIDS) virus, is a foremost concern of patients and health personnel, the use of these conservation methods are extremely important.

Significant postoperative mediastinal bleeding occurs secondary to platelet dysfunction and fibrinolysis. Platelet function can be partially restored with desmopressin acetate (DDAVP), a platelet activation agent, and if bleeding persists, judicious infusion of platelet concentrate is indicated. Persistent bleeding greater than 300 mL/h should prompt mediastinal reexploration.

Antifibrinolytic agents such as aprotonin and alpha-epsilon-aminocaproic acid have been shown to decrease postoperative bleeding and blood requirements. Aprotonin, acting as a kallikrein inactivator, is promising but is currently available in the United States only as an investigational drug.

Hypothermia is a significant inhibitor of the coagulation system, and special efforts with heating blankets and lights should be made to obtain normothermia in a bleeding patient.

Predisposing risk factors for postoperative bypass bleeding include the following: preoperative warfarin and thrombolytic drugs, hypothermia, prolonged bypass time, reoperation, intraoperative blood transfusions, and surgery for the correction of cyanotic heart disease. Preoperative bleeding time, prothrombin time, and activated partial thromboplastin time (APTT) have not been shown to be predictors of postoperative bypass bleeding.[36,37]

Protamine Reaction

Adverse allergic reactions to protamine infusion occur in approximately 10 percent of bypass patients, with a severe reaction in 0.5 to 2 percent. Life-threatening reactions present with systemic hypertension, marked pulmonary vasoconstriction, right-sided heart failure, and pulmonary edema. This process is usually reversed by high-dose steroids, epinephrine, prostaglandins, and arterial vasoconstrictors to maintain coronary perfusion pressure. Risk factors include previous protamine exposure, insulin-dependent diabetes, and possibly vasectomy.[12] Table 141-2 summarizes complications associated with cardiopulmonary bypass.

TABLE 141-2

Complications Associated with Cardiopulmonary Bypass
Aortic cannulation injury—dissection
Neuroendocrine cellular response
Catecholamine surge
Hemolysis of red cells
Leukocyte mobilization and trapping
Platelet dysfunction
Endothelial damage, "leak"
Humoral amplification
Coagulation cascade
Fibrinolysis
Complement activation
Bradykinin-kallikrein activation
Interstitial edema
Fever
Bleeding
End-organ dysfunction—brain, kidneys, lung
Protamine allergic reaction
Complications of blood product transfusions

PORTABLE CARDIOPULMONARY SUPPORT DEVICES

With the expanded use of percutaneous transcoronary angioplasty in patients with multivessel coronary disease and ventricular dysfunction and the more aggressive treatment of acute myocardial infarction, portable percutaneous cardiopulmonary bypass systems have been developed. These temporary assist devices can support threatened myocardium during high-risk angioplasty or be used as a resuscitative measure for cardiogenic shock until further diagnosis and definitive treatment such as coronary bypass surgery can be performed.[38] These portable bypass devices consist of a sterile oxygenator, tubing and prime, usually a centrifugal pump, heat exchanger, and oxygen tank—all placed on a portable roller cart. Percutaneous femoral artery and vein cannulas with guiding obturators are available to be placed in the catheterization laboratory or in the emergency room. Femoral vessel cut-down may be necessary by the surgical team. Bypass flow rates can be achieved between 2 and 4 liters/min. A well-organized, concerted effort of the medical, surgical, and perfusion teams is necessary for proper use of the equipment and patient safety. The National Registry of 14 centers performing supported angioplasty reported a 95 percent initial success rate in high-risk patients. Morbidity was frequent and was mainly associated with cannula placement and removal.[39]

REFERENCES

1. Yukihiko N (eds): *Manual on Artificial Organs*, vol 2, *The Oxygenator.* St. Louis, CV Mosby, 1973.
2. Frey MV, Graber M: Untersuchungen über den Stoffwechsel isolierter Organe: Ein Respirations-Apparat für isolierte Organe. *Arch F Physiol* 1985; 9:519–526.
3. Galleti PM, Brecher GA (eds): *Heart-Lung Bypass: Principles and Techniques of Extracorpeal Circulation.* New York, Grune & Stratton, 1962.
4. Gibbon JH Jr: Artificial maintenance of circulation during experimental occlusion of the pulmonary artery. *Arch Surg* 1937; 34:1105–1112.
5. Dogliotti AM: Clinical use of the artificial circulation with a note on intra-arterial transfusion. *Bull John Hopkins Hosp* 1952; 90:131–139.
6. Dennis C, Spreng DS Jr, Nelson GE, Karlson KE, Nelson RM, Thomas JV, et al: Development of a pump-oxygenator to replace

the heart and lungs: An apparatus applicable to human patients and application to one case. *Ann Surg* 1951; 134:709–716.
7. Gibbon JH Jr: Application of a mechanical heart and lung apparatus to cardiac surgery. *Minn Med* 1954; 37:171–178.
8. Kirklin JW, Dushane JW, Patrick RT, Donald DE, Hetzel PS, Harshbarger HG, Wood EH: Intracardiac surgery with the aid of a mechanical pump-oxygenator system (Gibbon type): Report of eight cases. *Proc Staff Meet, Mayo Clin* 1955; 30:201–208.
9. Utley JR (eds): *Pathophysiology and Techniques of Cardiopulmonary Bypass*, vol 1. Baltimore, Williams & Wilkins, 1982.
10. Kirlin JW, Chenoweth DE, Haftel DC, Blackstone EH, Kirklin JW, Bitran DD, et al: Effects of protamine administration after cardiopulmonary bypass on complement, blood elements, and the hemodynamic state. *Ann Thorac Surg* 1986; 41:193–199.
11. Lowenstein E, Johnston WE, Lappas DG, D'Ambra MH, Schneider RC, Dagget WM, et al: Catastrophic pulmonary vasoconstriction associated with protamine reversal of heparin. *Anesthesiology* 1983; 59:470–473.
12. Weiler JM, Gellhaus MA, Carter JG, Meng RL, Benson PM, Hottel RA, et al: A prospective study of the risk of an immediate adverse reaction to protamine sulfate during cardiopulmonary bypass surgery. *J Allergy Clin Immunol* 1990; 85:713–719.
13. van Oeveren W, Kazatchkine MD, Descamps-Latscha B, Maillet F, Fischer E, Carpentier A: Deleterious effects of cardiopulmonary bypass: A prospective study of bubble vs. membrane oxygenation. *J Thorac Cardiovasc Surg* 1985; 89:888–899.
14. Sade RH, Bartles DM, Dearing JP, Campbell LJ, Laodholt CB: A prospective randomized study of membrane vs. bubble oxygenators in children. *Ann Thorac Surg* 1980; 29:502–511.
15. Guyton RA: Method and magic in myocardial preservation. In: Hurst JW (ed): *Clinical Essays on the Heart*. New York, McGraw-Hill, 1983: 183–201.
16. Chitwood WR, Sink JD, Hill RC, Weschler AS, Sabiston DC: The effects of hypothermia on myocardial oxygen consumption and transmural coronary blood flow in the potassium-arrested heart. *Ann Surg* 1979; 190:106–116.
17. Gundry SR, Kirsh MM: A comparison of retrograde cardioplegia versus antegrade cardioplegia in the presence of coronary obstruction. *Ann Thorac Surg* 1984; 38:124–127.
18. Shumway HE, Lower RR, Stofer RC: Selective hypothermia of the heart in anoxic cardiac arrest. *Surg Gyn Obst* 1959; 109:750–756.
19. Barner HB: Blood cardioplegia: A review and comparison with crystalloid cardioplegia. *Ann Thorac Surg* 1991; 52:1354–1367.
20. Rosenkcrancz ER, Okamoto F, Buckberg GD, Robertson JM, Vinten-Johansen J, Bugyi Ni: Safety of prolonged aortic clamping with blood cardioplegic. *J Thorac Cardiovasc Surg* 1986; 91:428–435.
21. Boggs BR, Torchiana DF, Geffin GA, Titus JS, Redonnett BE, O'Keefe DD, et al: Optimal myocardial preservation with an acalcemic crystalloid cardioplegic solution. *J Thorac Cardiovasc Surg* 1987; 93:838–846.
22. Rankin JS, Sabiston DC Jr: Physiology of coronary blood flow, myocardial function and intraoperative myocardial protection. In: Sabiston DC Jr. Spencer FC (eds): *Gibbon's Surgery of the Chest*, 5th ed. Philadelphia, WB Saunders, 1990: 1635–1653.
23. Aear C, Portington MT, Buckberg GD: Studies of controlled reperfusion after ischemia, XVIII, reperfusion conditions: Attenuation of the regional ischemia effect by temporary total vented bypass before controlled reperfusion. *J Cardiovasc Thorac Surg* 1990; 100:737–744.
24. Lichtenstein SV, Ashe KA, el Dalati H, Cusimano RJ, Panos A, Shitsky AS: Warm heart surgery. *J Thorac Cardiovasc Surg* 1991; 101:269–274.
25. Gott JP, Cohen CL, Jones EL: Management of ascending aortic dissections and aneurysms early and late following cardiac surgery. *J Thorac Cardic Surg* 1990; 5:2–13.
26. Reves JG, Karp RB, Battrer EE, Tosone S, Smith LR, Samuelson PN, et al: Neuronal and adreno medullary catecholamine release in response to cardiopulmonary bypass in man. *Circulation* 1982; 66:49–55.
27. Reves JG: Adrenergic response to cardiopulmonary bypass. *Mt Sinai J Med* 1985; 57:511–518.
28. Nilsson LO, Brunnkuist S, Nilsson U, Nystrom SO, Tyden P, Venge P, et al: Activation of inflammatory systems during cardiopulmonary bypass. *Scan J Thorac Cardiovasc Surg* 1988; 72:51–53.
29. Solen KA, Whiffen JD, Lightfoot EN: The effect of shear, specific surface, and air interface on the development of blood emboli and hemolysis. *J Biomed Mater Res* 1978; 12:381–399.
30. Friedenberg WR, Myers WO, Plotka ED, Beathard JN, Kummer DJ, Gatlin PF, et al: Platelet dysfunction associated with cardiopulmonary bypass. *Ann Thorac Surg* 1978; 25:298–305.
31. Arnold JV, Blauth CI, Smith PL, Jagoe JR, Wooton R, Taylor KM: Demonstration of cerebral micro emboli occurring during coronary artery bypass graft surgery using fluorescein angiography. *J Audiovis Media Med* 1990; 13:87–90.
32. Leurs PB, Mulder AW, Fiers HA, Hoomtje SJ: Acute renal failure after cardiovascular surgery. Current concepts in pathophysiology, prevention and treatment. *Eur Heart J* 1989; 10:38–42.
33. Kirklin JW, Barrat-Boyes BG: Hypothermia, circulatory arrest, and cardiopulmonary bypass. In: JW Kirklin, BG Barret-Boyes (eds): *Cardiac Surgery*. New York, Wiley, 1986: 29–82.
34. Leitman IM, Paul DE, Barie PS, Isom OW, Shires GT: Intraabdominal complications of cardiopulmonary bypass operations. *Surg Gyn Obst* 1987; 165:251–254.
35. Huddy SP, Joyce WP, Pepper JR: Gastrointestinal complications in 4,473 patients who underwent cardiopulmonary bypass surgery. *Br J Surg* 1991; 78:293–296.
36. Bick RL: Hemostasis defects associated with cardiac surgery, prosthetic devices and other extracorporeal circuits. *Semin Thromb Hemostas* 1985; 11:249–256.
37. Woodman RC, Harker LA: Bleeding complications associated with cardiopulmonary bypass. *Blood* 1990; 76:1680–1697.
38. Lincoff AM, Popma JJ, Ellis SG, Vogel RA, Topol EJ: Percutaneous support devices for high risk or complicated coronary angioplasty. *J Am Coll Cardiol* 1991; 17:770–1780.
39. Vogel RA, Tommaso CL: Elective supported angioplasty: Initial report of the National Registry. *Cathet Cardiovasc Diagn* 1990; 20:22–76.

PART XXIII

Insurance and Legal Problems

Chapter 142

Insurance Problems of Patients with Heart Disease

M. Irené Ferrer, M.D. ■ *Joseph A. Wilber, M.D.*

In recent years there have been major advances in noninvasive imaging of the heart and blood vessels, which have resulted in improved accuracy in diagnosis and prognosis along with improved treatment. Several studies of prognosis, particularly in coronary artery disease, have been published.[1-3] The recent advances in clinical cardiology have not been lost on the insurance industry. The ability to obtain echocardiographic and nuclear imaging, positron emission tomography, computed tomography, and magnetic resonance imaging allows more sophisticated risk assessment and has made insurance available to many individuals who were previously considered uninsurable. The rates charged for these insurance plans often are not prohibitive. In fact, the greatest advances in providing more people insurance coverage have probably been made in the areas of cardiology and oncology.

Risk factors for coronary heart disease, i.e., elevated blood lipids, hypertension, cigarette smoking, diabetes mellitus, sedentary life-style, and a family history of premature cardiovascular disease, are now routinely used both in preventive cardiology and in life insurance underwriting. Efforts to reduce or control these risk factors are rewarded. In fact, nonsmokers can obtain life insurance at preferred rates, and applicants who demonstrate long-term control of elevated blood pressure and/or cholesterol usually can obtain insurance at no extra premium.

Communication between physicians and insurance companies has improved greatly in recent years. The tedious chore of filling out insurance forms is lessening. With the widespread availability of copying equipment, many physicians send copies of the entire record or pertinent portions thereof. This gives the underwriter complete information and allows him or her to make an accurate assessment of risk, leading to rapid issuance of insurance.

MORTALITY, LIFE EXPECTANCY, RATINGS, AND PREMIUMS

Most medical studies of prognosis are reported in terms of percentage dying or surviving over some time period of follow-up[3]; e.g., 15 percent mortality after myocardial infarction in the first year after discharge from the hospital. Usually we do not know the age distribution of the cohort of patients, nor the distribution of the severity of their disease, and, if there is no control group, we do not know what is the "normal" mortality for a group such as this. This makes comparison with other studies or treatments very difficult. In recent years clinical researchers and epidemiologists are reporting more and more in actuarial or life insurance terms such as life table analyses and mortality ratios. Mortality ratios are very useful in describing risk. A *mortality ratio* may be defined as the number of observed deaths over the number of expected deaths in a cohort of a certain age and sex within a defined period of time. The expected deaths are the deaths occurring in "healthy" population of the same sex and race or other characteristics who do not have the disease or impairment being studied. In life insurance studies, the expected death figures are based on 10-, 20-, or even 30-year follow-ups of large numbers of middle- and upper-class people who could afford a life insurance policy large enough to require a medical examination and who were found to be "healthy" or "standard" on that examination. Thus, the life insurance population is quite different from the general population; it is better educated, has a higher income, and all those who have had known severe illness or who have been found to be impaired have been excluded.

A mortality ratio of 100 percent is defined as the standard; 150 percent means 50 percent more deaths than expected, etc. Most companies will not insure anyone with an expected mortality ratio greater than 400 percent (Table 142-1), the reason being that the premium that must be charged for such a high risk becomes impractical.

While there is a direct relation, a 50 percent mortality does not mean a 50 percent decrease in life expectancy or a 50 percent higher price for the insurance. Table 142-1 illustrates the relations between mortality ratios, ratings, expected deaths, life expectancy, and annual premiums charged for a $100,000 term or permanent life insurance policy by the average company for a 42-year-old male nonsmoker.

INTERCOMPANY VARIATION

For many of the common chronic health problems of people who buy individual life insurance, such as overweight, elevated blood pressure, and diabetes mellitus, most life insurance companies base their underwriting on mortality studies of their own policyholders or on pooled data of several companies.[4] For many other diseases, and especially in order to keep up with newer diagnostic and treatment advances, however, the life insurance medical directors depend on current scientific medical literature and consultation with authorities in the field.

If a case appears to involve extra risk, it usually is considered individually with consideration of family history, life-style, quality of medical care, and current research trends. Since about 1960 to 1965, cardiovascular mortality in the United States has shown a steady downward trend, in both the insurance population and the general population. Many medical directors continue to think that an optimistic approach is warranted for some of the major killers, particularly cardiovascular disease.

Evaluation of risk in applicants with cardiovascular disease is now greatly clarified for the insurance industry by the adoption of the latest techniques in diagnosis of these disorders. The use of treadmill tests using nuclear imaging (Chap. 134) can resolve many of the problems of false-positive simple treadmill tests. (See Chap. 16.)

Thallium imaging is nearly 100 percent correct in diagnosing areas of inadequate coronary perfusion. Echocardiograms and radionuclide (MUGA) studies can define wall motion defects in the ventricle, and can provide estimates of left ventricular ejection fraction. This latter has been found to offer the best prognostic information in coronary disease. If, in addition, cardiac catheterization and angiograms are included in the evaluation, the left ventricular end-diastolic, or filling, pressure and anatomy of the three major coronary arteries and their tributaries can provide an excellent assessment of patients with coronary artery disease.

Because of competition and company variation, it is always wise to get a second opinion if you are dissatisfied with the appraisal of risk for your patients or yourself—that is, if you are sure all the facts have been accurately presented to the life insurance medical director.

In the next sections of this chapter the life insurance aspects of the major cardiovascular disorders will be considered in detail. Health and disability insurance problems of patients with heart disease will be covered briefly toward the end of the chapter. It is the authors' belief and hope that, with better understanding and better communication between physician and insurer, your patient's insurance needs can be fairly met.

CORONARY HEART DISEASE

Coronary heart disease (CHD) is the leading cause of death in the insured population. The major advances in diagnosis and treatment of CHD in the past 30 years have stimulated a greater interest in prognosis and many

TABLE 142-1

Relation of Mortality, Rating, Expected Deaths, Life Expectancy, and Premium in a 42-Year-Old Male Nonsmoker

Mortality Ratio, %	Table Rating	Expected Deaths per 1000 Insured in a 10-Year Period	Average Life Expectancy in Years	Representative Annual Premium per $100,000 Life Insurance: 10-Year Level Term, $	Representative Annual Premium per $100,000 Life Insurance: Permanent Insurance, $
100	Standard	17	32	270	996
150	2	25	28	380	1122
200	4	34	25	490	1236
250	6	42	23	600	1362
300	8	51	22	710	1476
350	10	59	21	820	1600
400	12	68	20	830	1716

clinical studies have reported on long-term survival after treatment, as well as better methods in differentiating the poor-risk from the good-risk patient.[5-10] Clinical researchers are interested in actuarial methods to evaluate these new therapies, not only in terms of improving care but also in terms of life expectancy and survival. The life insurance industry has also benefited from this interest in prognosis and as a result can offer life insurance to most patients with known coronary heart disease at a reasonable though higher-than-average premium.

Survivor of Acute Myocardial Infarction

Approximately 50 to 60 percent of deaths from CHD are "sudden" and occur outside of hospitals, or patients "are dead on arrival" at hospital emergency rooms.[11] Progress at identifying those at risk of sudden death and preventing these deaths has as yet been limited. The majority of these prehospital deaths are mainly due to lethal ventricular arrhythmias, often without apparent precipitating cause. (See also Chap. 51.)

Of those who reach the hospital alive, approximately 15 percent die during that admission. Of those discharged, another 15 percent die within 1 year—the majority in the first 6 months after discharge. Thereafter the mortality stabilizes at approximately 2 to 4 percent per year (almost four to eight times the mortality of a "healthy" population, depending on age). Because of these statistics most companies will not insure a myocardial infarction applicant until at least 3 and usually 6 months after the infarction, and, if the applicant is under 65, most companies will not consider life insurance until the applicant returns to work or his or her usual occupation. The size of the increased premium will vary depending on factors that indicate low- or high-risk subgroups. (See also Chaps. 60 and 61.)

How do you identify the low- or high-risk myocardial infarction patient? The results of both invasive and noninvasive diagnostic testing are carefully evaluated by the medical underwriter. Hospital discharge summaries and physicians' records are sought to determine results of cardiac catheterization, coronary angiograms, ambulatory and exercise electrocardiography (ECG), two-dimensional echocardiography, thallium scintigraphy, and radionuclide ventriculography. These test results may enable the medical underwriter to predict risk accurately on an individual basis and to offer the insurance applicant an equitable price for life insurance.

The major factors that the insurance underwriter considers are (1) the function of the left ventricle, and (2) the extent and severity of the coronary artery obstructive disease. In general, the occurrence of congestive heart failure, marked cardiac enlargement, hypotension, an ejection fraction of less than 30 percent, large areas of ventricular wall dyskinesia and akinesia, or persistent ventricular ectopy indicate very high risk, and most life insurance companies will decline the risk. A positive postinfarction exercise ECG (ST depression early or at Bruce stage 1 or 2) is looked on as an indicator of poor risk. (See Chap. 16.) The presence of diabetes mellitus, hypertension, hyperlipidemia, or continued cigarette smoking also will result in a maximum high rating or decline. Postinfarction angina usually results in declination if it persists longer than 6 months. (See chaps. 60 and 61.)

The use of ambulatory electrocardiographic monitoring in the immediate postinfarction period (3 weeks after the event) and again during the first 3 and 6 months postinfarction is useful if persistent ventricular arrhythmias exist. This places the applicant in a higher-risk group and probably would mean a postponement until 1 year after the event. (See Chap. 45)

Thus, it is beneficial to the patient to have definitive diagnostic studies done prior to or shortly after discharge, not only for optimal treatment but also because the more data available the more accurate will be the risk assessment. Studies at the end of the first year are also very useful.

Coronary Artery Bypass Surgery

Many of the major life insurance companies by their underwriting policies and actions indicate that they have decided to consider coronary artery bypass surgery and balloon angioplasty as life-prolonging procedures.[12] While life insurance companies, like clinicians, prefer hard data from well-controlled clinical trials or long-term actuarial studies before attributing benefit to a new therapy, most medical directors tend to be prudently optimistic about the future of scientific progress. Most companies, for example, will rate the patient who has had successful bypass surgery and angioplasty as a better risk than the unoperated patient with similar extent of disease and function.

Angina Pectoris

It is usually much more difficult to evaluate and to estimate prognosis accurately in the insurance applicant with angina pectoris than in the postinfarction applicant. There usually is less diagnostic and prognostic information available and often the diagnosis is not documented by testing. The stable, controlled, and well-documented angina applicant, however, is usually considered a better risk than the postinfarction applicant and therefore is given a better (lower) extra premium rating. He or she is usually charged about half the extra premium of the postinfarction patient.

From reviewing many statements from attending physicians, one has the strong impression that angina pectoris is too often diagnosed without the classical pain and with little or no diagnostic tending. An inaccurate diagnosis may cause major employment and insurance problems for that unfortunate patient for many years. Exercise electrocardiography and other objective noninvasive studies are required to support the diagnosis of angina pectoris and should be obtained whenever possible. In doubtful or difficult cases, cardiac catheterization and coronary angiography are justified, considering the implications of an exact diagnosis for treatment and prognosis. (See Chap. 58.)

Most insurance companies will insure the angina applicant 3 to 6 months after onset of angina pectoris if the disease appears to be stable with pain that is absent or very infrequent on medication, and if the resting electrocardiogram is normal. The extra premium charged is usually about one-half or one-third less than the extra premium charged the postinfarction insured person. As in the infarction applicant, other risk factors such as cigarette smoking, hypertension, diabetes mellitus, and overweight should be absent or controlled. Diabetes mellitus and angina are considered a very bad combination and usually result in a high rating or declination.

In both angina and myocardial infarction, the underwriter looks for the prescription of a good rehabilitation program, including diet and exercise, and evidence from follow-up visits that the patient is trying to cooperate. Patients who get the best care usually benefit also from the lowest insurance premiums.

The decline in coronary heart disease mortality of approximately 25 percent between 1968 and 1979[13] was not definitely attributed to any specific preventative or therapeutic advance, but happily it is continuing. This decline justifies an optimistic underwriting attitude and supports the prediction that the average American can expect a longer life expectancy. (See also Chap. 62.)

HYPERTENSION

The nature of the life insurance industry provides a unique opportunity for prospective studies on large numbers of individuals over long periods of time. Therefore, it is not surprising that life insurance actuaries were the first to realize the value of the blood pressure measurement in evaluating risk. Physicians, aware of the lability of the casual blood pressure measurement, were initially quite skeptical of the life insurance data, but in 1958 and in the 1960s, epidemiologic, prospective studies on general populations confirmed the insurance studies.

Since 1925, the life insurance industry has published five major comprehensive studies of mortality among insured lives according to variations in blood pressure. All of these show a direct, nearly linear relation between systolic and diastolic blood pressure and mortality. The higher the blood pressure, the greater the risk and the higher the premium that must be charged.

The 1979 Blood Pressure Study,[14] dealt in the main with the mortality experience between 1954 and 1972 on about 4,350,000 policies issued to men and women aged 15 to 60. About 530,000 of the policies were issued to men and women with borderline and definite high blood pressure (up to 187 mmHg systolic, 112 mmHg diastolic). Mortality experience in this group was compared to the mortality experience of the remaining normotensive group. During the period of this study the first effective treatment for high blood pressure was introduced in this country, and thus the 1979 study, unlike previous studies, was influenced by the increasing use of antihypertensive medication during this period. Comparing the 1979 (partially treated) to the 1959 (untreated) hypertensive group, it was seen that overall mortality in the 1979 study was definitely lower for any level of blood pressure but was especially lower for those with moderately high blood pressure. "Mortality ratios" (previously defined as the observed mortality over the expected mortality) were approximately 20 percent lower for mildly and moderately hypertensive individuals. In a subgroup of applicants who were taking antihypertensive medication at the time of entry and whose systolic and diastolic blood pressure on insurance examination appeared to be reduced to near normal—i.e., less than 145 mmHg systolic/less than 95 mmHg diastolic—mortality was nearly normal. It appeared that adequate treatment of high blood pressure in borderline and mild cases was most efficacious and reduced risk to that of individuals who did not have elevated blood pressure. For those with higher levels of blood pressure on treatment, mortality was still excessive, though better than in 1959.

Untreated Hypertension

With the great increase in screening and treatment for high blood pressure since 1972, undiagnosed elevated blood pressure discovered on application for life insurance is much less common and is not the problem it once was. If the usual three examination readings average greater than about 160 mmHg systolic and/or 94 mmHg diastolic, most companies will request additional readings on one or more separate days. If these are also high, a rating (extra premium) is charged depending on age—higher at the younger ages. In general, the industry has become much more optimistic about elevated blood pressure because of the medical profession's greater ability in maintaining normal blood pressures and greater interest in treating even mild cases. If an untreated hypertensive person is charged an extra premium initially, he or she can usually have this removed in 6 months to a year by presenting evidence (a physician's statement) that blood pressure has been brought under control and is checked frequently. It should be rare today that a person continues to pay an extra premium for treated high blood pressure.

Treated Hypertension

The applicant who admits treatment on examination and whose blood pressure is in the "normal" range (less than 140/90) will usually get standard insurance. Many companies routinely request urinalysis and an ECG in addition to a medical examination. They also write the attending physician to obtain representative readings and to assess adherence to the physician's recommendations. (The large national life insurance laboratories often screen urine specimens routinely for the presence of thiazide diuretics and/or beta-blocker type medications.)

Complicated Hypertension

Any evidence of target organ damage in an untreated hypertensive applicant usually results in a high rating or a declination. The finding of proteinuria over 50 mg/dL, ST- and T-wave abnormalities on the ECG, or a blood creatinine greater than 1.5 mg/dL in combination with elevated blood pressure means a poor prognosis—often less than 10 years' life expectancy—and usually the applicant is uninsurable.

VALVULAR HEART DISEASE

Today, reports from pediatricians, family physicians, internists, and nearly all recently trained physicians doing life insurance examinations show a great improvement in the average physician's ability to examine the heart. This greater skill is shown by much more detailed descriptions of murmurs, as well as of heart sounds, gallops, clicks, and impulses. The family physician today is no longer satisfied merely to observe a murmur or "wait and see." Noninvasive and invasive diagnostic tests are ordered much earlier and more frequently. As a result, the asymptomatic child or adult with a heart murmur, with or without a history of rheumatic fever, has been or can usually be accurately classified and the risk appraised fairly.

Mitral Valve Prolapse

This is at present the most common valve condition reported to insurance companies. Happily, most companies accept asymptomatic applicants at standard premium rates, even though it is known that there is a slight increased risk of sudden death[15] or bacterial endocarditis. (See also Chap. 80.) Cases of mitral valve prolapse with frequent chest pains and palpitations or with a holosystolic murmur and electrocardiographic abnormalities may be rated moderately at one-and-one-half or two times average age risk. If Doppler echocardiograms show mitral regurgitation or any enlargement of the left atrium, the rate should be higher.

Congenital Valve Disease

Most companies postpone insuring an infant with known or suspected congenital heart disease until 1 or 2 years of age. Even then there must be a definitive proven diagnosis and surgically correctable lesions must have been repaired. Most cases of congenital heart disease have been catheterized and had surgery, if indicated, by age 16. Cases still needing surgery are rarely seen by life insurance companies today. Many patients with corrected defects, especially if the murmur is gone and heart size and electrocardiogram are normal or stable, can then be accepted at standard rates or with a relatively small extra rating that may be removed at a later date. These "best" cases include most atrial and ventricular septal defects, corrected pulmonic stenosis, patent ductus, and coarctation of the aorta. The latter is considered standard only if the arterial blood pressure returns to normal. Proven minor septal defects, unoperated (especially ventricular), are expected to close spontaneously and are also often accepted as standard risk.

In spite of tremendous advances in surgery for congenital and valvular heart disease, there still are some defects that even with correction leave the child or teenager with a life expectancy of only 20 to 30 years,[16] much too short to allow a reasonable insurance cost. These usually uninsurable cases include most cases of transposition of the great vessels, Ebstein's disease, anomalous venous return, and Eisenmenger's physiology or complex. (See also Chap. 97.)

Congenital bicuspid aortic valve remains a difficult clinical and underwriting problem. The patient is usually a young or middle-aged adult with a murmur discovered years before, is asymptomatic, and the murmur is faint and may or may not radiate to the neck. Prognosis is extremely variable. Most companies will rate such a case as two to four times the average risk or will decline the risk, especially if the murmur is associated with any suspicion of left ventricular hypertrophy on physical examination, chest x-ray, or electrocardiogram, unless a small valve gradient is found on cardiac catheterization or echocardiogram.

Acquired Valve Disease

Acute rheumatic fever and rheumatic heart disease are becoming rare diseases in the United States. As a result, most insurance applicants with rheumatic heart disease today are middle-aged or are foreign-born applicants, particularly from Africa or Asia. However, another form of acquired heart disease is seen with increasing frequency in the older applicant; that is, calcific aortic or mitral valve disease—the former sometimes superimposed on a congenitally bicuspid valve. (See Chap. 79.)

Asymptomatic life insurance applicants with calcific mitral or aortic valve disease are usually insurable, with an extra premium, in the absence of cardiac enlargement. In general, the older the applicant with significant heart murmurs, the lower the risk and the rating. For example, a 25-year-old applicant with the murmur of mitral regurgitation would be classified as four or six times the average risk, whereas a 60-year-old applicant with the same murmur might be taken at standard rates if the ECG and chest x-ray were normal. Many companies still decline the younger applicant with a history of rheumatic fever and typical murmurs of mitral stenosis, aortic stenosis, or regurgitation,[17] yet others may accept with a high rating. Most applicants with double murmurs are declined. A few companies are beginning to issue highly rated insurance 2 years after aortic or mitral valve replacement if there have been no complications.[18]

With any type of valvular heart disease, if there is more than mild cardiac enlargement, or if there is chronic atrial fibrillation or any history of past or present cardiac decompensation, the application is declined or highly rated.

OTHER HEART DISEASES

Space does not permit a detailed discussion of the insurability of all the various kinds of heart disease. Those that are usually diagnosed after serious symptoms appear, i.e., the cardiomyopathies, scleroderma heart, and amyloidosis, are seldom seen by medical underwriters since these people are too sick to consider applying for life insurance.

With the advent of echocardiography and other noninvasive techniques, some diseases such as obstructive and nonobstructive hypertrophic cardiomyopathy are being diagnosed with increased frequency and in their early stages. Unfortunately, little is known as yet of the natural history of these cardiomyopathies, particularly the mild cases.[19,20] (See also Chap. 90.) As a result, most reports are of severe and fatal cases, and most insurance companies either decline to insure, or rate highly, anyone with echocardiographic or other evidence of ventricular obstruction or asymmetric septal hypertrophy.

One or two episodes of paroxysmal atrial tachycardia or paroxysmal atrial fibrillation are usually accepted for insurance at standard rates if there is no other evidence of heart disease. Frequent and/or prolonged arrhythmias or chronic atrial fibrillation are usually declined.

Unexplained electrocardiographic abnormalities are a common problem and are often first discovered on the ECG obtained for life insurance purposes. In the absence of other evidence for heart disease, minor T-wave abnormalities are usually treated leniently. ST-segment abnormalities or frequent ventricular ectopic beats may cause the company to ask for a treadmill exercise test (Chap. 16). If there is no evidence of ischemia with exercise, most companies will issue standard insurance.

With all electrocardiographic abnormalities and particularly with bundle branch blocks, the medical underwriter attempts to obtain copies of or reports of any and all old ECGs. The longer the abnormality can be proven present and unchanged, the lower the rating. Right bundle branch block present several years in an applicant under 40 is usually considered a standard risk. Left bundle branch block is always rated, more so at the higher ages.

For large amounts of life insurance and with older applicants, electrocardiograms, and much less frequently chest x-rays, may be routinely requested in addition to an examination for underwriting purposes. About 2 percent of such chest x-rays show cardiomegaly of some degree.[21] This prompts a close scrutiny for any evidence of hypertension or other heart disease, yet only about 15 percent of these eventually are rated. If the heart is less than 20 percent enlarged (Clark-Ungerleider tables) and there is no evidence of other disease, there is usually no rating.

Some companies have discontinued exercise electrocardiograms as a routine requirement in application for large amounts of insurance. Except for unusually large amounts of insurance, exercise electrocardiograms are usually requested now only because of a history of recent chest pains, or because the resting electrocardiogram is abnormal. A negative treadmill electrocardiogram is helpful and reassuring. A positive treadmill ECG is usually rated even though it is realized that there is a relatively high incidence of false positives.[22] The authors have seen on several occasions a positive treadmill electrocardiogram, done for insurance purposes in an asymptomatic individual, that resulted in coronary angiograms and subsequent bypass surgery. More often the angiograms are negative, the insurance is issued, and all parties are relieved.

HEALTH AND DISABILITY INSURANCE

In general, the requirements for health and disability insurance are much more stringent than for life insurance. Common chronic disorders such as degenerative bone and joint disease, psychoneurosis, and chronic or frequently recurring genitourinary disorders, though seldom life-threatening, are usually ridered, rated, or declined because of the high risk of excess hospitalization and other medical costs.

For all practical purposes, the patients with known heart disease of any kind will have difficulty in obtaining standard individual health or disability insurance. His or her best opportunity is to obtain such insurance protection through employment or other groups. A major exception to the above is the well-controlled hypertensive person under regular medical supervision. He or she can frequently be accepted for health and disability insurance at standard rates.

Disability

The problem of deciding when a cardiac (or other) patient is disabled is a serious and complex problem. (See also Chap. 143.) Patients are frightened and depressed after a heart attack or bypass surgery. Their family, friends, and even employers may urge them to retire prematurely and unnecessarily. The physician at this point plays a key role and has an obligation to make vigorous and repeated efforts to get that patient back to work for his or her own best interest. It is usually the family physician, who does not see as many cardiac patients as the specialist, who makes the error of encouraging the patient to retire. If a cardiac rehabilitation program is available, nearly all health insurers are willing to pay for rehabilitation.

The role of the attending physician is changing as disability determination becomes more scientific and specialized. Legal interpretations of disability based on medical tests and data are now common. Many insurers are no longer asking the physician his or her opinion on whether or not the patient is disabled, but instead ask only for objective data and descriptions of illness. Often an independent medical consultation is requested to verify true disability. With the great advances in diagnosis and measurement of cardiac function, disability determination should become as accurate as estimating risk for death.

ACKNOWLEDGMENT

The authors wish to thank Dr. Neal A. Pickett, Jr., Medical Director, Medical Underwriting and Claims, Metropolitan Life Insurance Company, for his helpful review of this material.

REFERENCES

1. Rautaharju PM, Princas RJ, Eifler WJ, Furberg CD, Neaton JD, Crow RS: Prognostic value of exercise electrocardiogram in

men at risk of future coronary heart disease: Multiple Risk Factor Intervention Trial experience. *J Am Coll Cardiol* 1986; 8:1–10.

2. Gordon DJ: Predictive value of the exercise tolerance test for mortality in North American men: the Lipid Research Clinics mortality follow-up study. *Circulation* 1986; 74:252–256.
3. Freis J, Ehrlich G (eds): *Prognosis: Contemporary Outcomes of Disease.* Bowie, MD., Charles Press Publishers, 1981:1–565.
4. *Life Underwriting Manual.* The North American Reassurance Company, New York.
5. Kannel WB, Sorlie P, McNamara PM: Prognosis after initial myocardial infarction. The Framingham Study. *Am J Cardiol* 1979; 44:53–59.
6. Multicenter Postinfarction Group: Risk stratification and survival after myocardial infarction. *N Engl J Med* 1983; 309:331–339.
7. Schlant RC, Forman S, Stamler J, Canner PL: The natural history of coronary heart disease. Prognostic factors after recovery from myocardial infarction in 2,789 men. The 5 year findings of the Coronary Drug Project. *Circulation* 1982; 66:401–414.
8. CASS principal investigators and associates: Coronary Artery Surgery Study (CASS): A randomized trial of coronary artery bypass surgery: Survival data. *Circulation* 1983; 68:939–950.
9. Weinblatt E, Goldberg JD, Ruberman W, Frank CW, Monk MA, Chaudhary BS: Mortality after first myocardial infarction. Search for a secular trend. *JAMA* 1982; 247:1576–1581.
10. Elveback LR, Connolly DC, Kurland LJ: Coronary heart disease in Rochester, Minnesota, II. Mortality incidence and survivorship. *Mayo Clinic Proc* 1981; 56:665–672.
11. Gettes S: *Candidates for Sudden Cardiac Death. Recognition and Prevention.* Medical Section Proceedings, American Council of Life Insurance, 1982:19.
12. Collins J: *Prognosis following Coronary Bypass Surgery.* Transactions of The Association of Life Insurance Medical Directors of America 1982; 65:72–82.
13. Havlik RJ, Feinleib M: Proceedings of the Conference on The Decline in Coronary Heart Disease Mortality, Washington, D.C., DHEW publ. no. NIH 79-1610, 1979:1–399.
14. Society of Actuaries and Association of Life Insurance Medical Directors of America: *Blood Pressure Study 1979.* Recording and Statistical Corporation, 1980: 1–359.
15. Kligfield P, Levy D, Devereaux RB, Savage DD: Arrhythmias and sudden death in mitral valve prolapse. *Am Heart J* 1987; 113:1298–1307.
16. MacMahon B, McKeown T, Record RG: The incidence and life expectation of children with congenital heart disease. *Br Heart J* 1953; 15:121–129.
17. Spagnicolo M, Klothy H, Taranta A, Doyle E, Pasternak B: Natural history of rheumatic aortic regurgitation. Criteria predictive of death, congestive heart failure and angina in young patients. *Circulation* 1971; 44:368–380.
18. Ellis LB, Singh JB, Morales DD, Harken DE: Fifteen to twenty year study of one thousand patients undergoing closed mitral valvuloplasty. *Circulation* 1973; 48:357–364.
19. McKenna W, Deanfield J, Farugui A, England D, Oakley C, Goodwin J: Prognosis in hypertrophic cardiomyopathy: Role of age and clinical electrocardiographic and hemodynamic features. *Am J Cardiol* 1981; 47:532–538.
20. Miller DH, Borer JS: The cardiomyopathies. *Arch Intern Med* 1983; 143:2157–2162.
21. Ferrer MI: A study of 6,000 chest x-rays obtained for insurance purposes. *J Insurance Med* 1983; 14:12–18.
22. Mark DB, Shaw L, Harrell FE, Hlatky MA, Lee KL, Bengtson JR, et al: Prognostic value of a treadmill exercise score in outpatients with suspected coronary artery disease. *N Engl J Med* 1991; 325:849–853.

Chapter 143

Cardiac Evaluations for Legal Purposes

Elliot L. Sagall, M.D.

The socioeconomic ramifications of heart disease have long been a source of vexing legal as well as medical problems with no easy resolution as yet in hand. Nationwide, claims instituted by heart patients and/or their beneficiaries alleging heart disorder, disability, and cardiac death as a workplace or accidental injury or as due to the negligent action of a health care provider are burgeoning in number and scope. In other legal actions, the existence of a heart disorder may be the key issue in the legal determination of an individual's physical capacity to participate as a defendant or witness in a legal proceeding, to drive a motor vehicle, to pilot an airplane, to engage in "substantial" gainful activity, to write a legally valid will or contract, to enable an insurer to recover some of the moneys paid to a worker as compensation for a work-related injury, or to invalidate a life insurance policy.

The rapidly expanding interrelationships of heart disorders and the law necessarily will involve physicians who examine and treat cardiac patients more and more frequently in the legal processes concerned with resolution of disputed medical aspects of these claims in one or combinations of several roles. The physician may be a witness called on to present factual observations personally made in history taking, in performing physical examinations and diagnostic studies, and in rendering treatment; the physician may be called on as an "expert" medical witness by one side or the other in the legal action or be requested as an "impartial" witness by the judicial body assigned the trial of the case to present opinion testimony on the medical matters in issue; or the physician may become a defendant in a medical malpractice suit alleging professional negligence in the diagnostic and/or therapeutic management of a patient.

The question of a cardiac patient's eligibility for certain statutory or common law benefits is basically a legal rather than a medical problem, the ultimate determination of which is assigned to a court, jury, administrative agency, commissioner, referee, or some other duly appointed person or persons referred to as a "fact finder." The legal resolution of disputed issues of a medical nature, however, almost invariably necessitates consideration of expert medical opinion by the legal fact finder. Crucial areas such as diagnosis, degree and duration of disability, "conscious" pain and suffering, the reasonableness of past and projected medical and surgical treatment and the charges rendered, the role of preexisting conditions, losses of bodily functions, scarring and disfigurement, reduction of life expectancy, prognosis, whether an "end result" has been reached, and the many other factors that determine damages to be awarded to the victim of a cardiac injury or benefits available under covering workers' compensation or other legislative acts, and the relationship of each to the alleged injury, generally require that medical substantiation or refutation be presented for the fact finder's consideration in the legal resolution of controverted claims.

LEGAL ACTIONS REQUIRING CARDIAC MEDICAL EVALUATIONS

The spectrum of legal actions where medical evaluations of questions relating to cardiology become key issues is vast, varied, and limited only by the ingenuity and imagination of the attorneys involved in the case.[1-3] The most commonly encountered are the following: (1) claims brought under various state workers' compensation statutes and similar federal legislation (e.g., the Federal Longshoremen's and Harbor Workers' Compensation Act and the Federal Employees' Compensation Act), which allege cardiac disorder disability, treatment, or death as a consequence of a work-related cardiac "injury" or as an "occupational disease"; (2) tort claims under common law seeking damages for alleged cardiac "injury" due to negligence on the part of another person or persons, including suits for medical malpractice; (3) claims against insurers, including the Social Security Disability Insurance program, for pensions, covered medical expenses, losses of income, or accidental death benefits resulting from heart disease; (4) questions as to the fitness of a person with an alleged heart disorder to return to a specific job, to drive a motor vehicle, to operate machinery or other equipment, to pilot an airplane, to participate in a legal proceeding, to serve a prison sentence, or to prepare a will; and (5) claims instituted by insurers alleging preexistent heart disease as a basis for qualifying under "second injury funds" for reimbursement of workers' compensation benefits paid to an injured worker, the voiding of an insurance contract by reason of the applicant's fraudulent concealment of a preexisting heart disorder, or the nonpayment of special benefits provided in the insurance contract for death or injury due to an accident because of the contribution thereto by a preexistent cardiac disorder. Of these, the most commonly encountered are claims that a cardiac disorder is a workplace injury covered by the applicable workers' compensation statute.

Although individual state and federal workers' compensation acts differ somewhat in requirements for eligibility and benefits provided to injured workers and their dependents (with frequent legislative changes as well),[4] the fundamental social principle common to all compensation statutes is that the financial costs of work-related injuries should be assumed to a large extent by the employer as an expense of production and not by the injured worker or the public dole. Without exception, all compensation acts embrace the basic concept that the right to compensation for work-incurred injury is afforded to the injured employee without regard to fault or to demonstrable negligence of the employer. Legal defenses available under common law to employers to avoid or to mitigate liability such as *assumption of the risk* of the job by the employee's acceptance of the employment or *contributory negligence* by the employee or fellow employees (the *fellow servant rule*) are specifically excluded from workers' compensation. In turn, the benefits potentially accruing to an injured employee are generally limited to a portion of the lost wages plus allowances for dependents and reasonable and necessary medical expenses. Items such as pain and suffering and loss of consortium, which may play a large role in the determination of an award to an injured person in actions for tort (negligence) under common law, are excluded.

In workers' compensation, legal liability attaches to the employer (or insurance carrier) for the consequences of an injury, including heart disorder, disability, or death,[1, 5-8] demonstrated to have occurred during "the course of" *and* to have arisen "out of" employment—a formula that has aptly been characterized as "deceptively simple and litigiously prolific."

Under some compensation statutes, the basic formula of compensable injury has been modified by specific legislative restrictive definitions that require that the alleged work injury be suffered "by accident" or be due to "unusual stress" or to "stress greater than normal nonwork life" or to have been contributed "substantially" to by the work. In most jurisdictions, an identified time and place of injury must be demonstrated for coverage to apply. And in one compensation act (Wyoming's), a further restriction has been placed for acceptance of an alleged work-related cardiac injury by the requirement that no more than 4 h must have elapsed between the claimed time of injury and the first clinical manifestations of same.[9]

The imposition of these restrictions indicates a legislative attempt to distinguish heart injuries and consequences thereof resulting from a work-related physical exertion and/or a psychologic stress from those that occur as a result of the natural progression of the underlying disease—an effort not often successful. Along these lines, one state (Nevada) has even gone so far as to exclude "coronary thrombosis, coronary occlusion, or any other ailment or disorder of the heart, and any death or disability ensuing therefrom" as an injury by accident arising out of and in the course of employment, except under certain circumstances for firemen, police officers, prison guards, and several other favored categories of public employees.[10]

In many states the concept of "accidental" disability* for purposes of workers' compensation or retirement has been extended for certain named occupational groups, particularly uniformed police and firefighters, by legislative inclusion in the covering statutes of a presumption of job causation for disabling heart disease or hypertension. Although theoretically rebuttable, such presumptions, from a practical viewpoint, generally cannot be overcome. The result is that applicants under these laws (commonly referred to as "Heart Laws") need only establish the existence of a disabling heart disorder or hypertension and not the causal connection to the employment.

The Massachusetts statute[11] is a typical example:

> **Notwithstanding the provisions of any general or special law to the contrary . . . any condition of impairment of health caused by hypertension and heart disease resulting in total or partial disability or death to a uniformed member of a paid fire department or permanent member of a police department . . . shall, if he successfully passed a physical examination on entry into such service which**

* *Accidental disability* retirement applies to a permanent work incapacity as a result of a work-related injury or a hazard experienced in the performance of job duties. *Ordinary disability* retirement applies to permanent work incapacity due to sickness or injury that is not job related.

Since the financial benefits of an accidental disability retirement generally are significantly greater than those of an ordinary disability retirement in that the awards usually are free from federal and state income tax, applicants for disability understandably seek the greater "take-home" pay of an "accidental disability."

examination failed to reveal any evidence of such condition, be presumed to have been suffered in line of duty, unless the contrary be shown by competent evidence.

The first step in the process of determining eligibility of an applicant for the benefits provided under this statute usually is an examination by a medical panel appointed for the purpose of determining the existence of heart disease or hypertension, the resulting job disability, the permanency thereof, and job causation. The medical panel's findings, however, are only advisory and are not binding on the designated retirement board. Inasmuch as the etiology of most forms of heart disease and hypertension is not currently known, the medical panel, most often, cannot provide "competent evidence" to offset the legislative presumption of job causation embodied in the covering statute, and an accidental disability usually is awarded if the medical panel has found the existence of a disabling cardiac or hypertensive condition.

The applicant's probative task under many of these statutes is further eased by the definition of *job disability* as an incapability of the applicant to perform the full range or "all" of the duties, including response to emergency situations inherent in the course of police or firefighting activities.

The legal dependents of deceased Heart Law retirees do not automatically receive death benefits. They usually have the burden of establishing by medical evidence that the death was causally related to the condition for which retirement was awarded. Thus, a statement on a death certificate that the immediate cause of death was "cardiac arrest" is not sufficient to establish legal causation since cardiac arrest is frequently only a terminal event, not necessarily related to a condition of preexistent heart disease or hypertension. However, medical opinion that the death was hastened to some degree, even by as short a period as seconds to minutes, by reason of reduced cardiac and/or coronary reserve related to the underlying heart disorder, although not a direct consequence thereof, may be sufficient to satisfy the legal question of causality.

Particularly important in adjudication of claims for cardiac injury, disability, or death under workers' compensation is the universal acceptance by compensation adjudicators of the common law precept that prior infirmity is no bar to benefits even though the injured worker would not have suffered injury, as is the case in most cardiac claims, had there not been underlying heart disease, whether previously known or unknown. Legally, the injured worker may be entitled to compensation benefits if it can be shown that the employment or some factor derived therefrom aggravated a preexisting condition to lead to injury, disability, or death sooner than otherwise would have been expected during the natural history of the underlying disorder.

Under many state compensation acts, the burden of proving job causation generally assigned to the claimant is eliminated when the worker is found deceased or otherwise medically unable to testify at the place of employment, e.g., as from a stroke. By the adoption of statutory presumptions of work relationship in such situations, the burden of disproving causation is placed upon the employer. Under the Federal Longshoremen's and Harbor Workers' Compensation Act, a set of presumptions effectively require that the employer establish noncausation to the job for almost all medical conditions that may render an employee permanently or partially disabled from work.[12]

Under actions in tort in common law, recovery of "damages" may be obtained when the plaintiff or those claiming through the plaintiff can show that the disorder and its consequences arose from or were aggravated by the negligent activity of another (commonly referred to as a *tortfeasor*). Unlike the doctrine of workers' compensation, liability in actions of tort is predicated on fault. To be awarded "damages," the injured party must show (1) that the defendant owed the plaintiff a duty, i.e., the duty to adhere to an accepted standard of medical or other care and the duty to refrain from negligence; (2) that the defendant's conduct breached that duty; (3) that the plaintiff suffered injuries or "harms"; (4) that the defendant's negligent conduct was the proximate cause of the damage (harms) allegedly suffered by the plaintiff; and, generally, (5) that the victim's own negligence did not contribute to his or her harms (the *doctrine of contributory negligence*).

Actions in tort alleging cardiac injury most commonly arise from motor vehicle accidents where it is claimed that a myocardial contusion, an acute coronary artery occlusion, an acute myocardial infarction, a cardiac death, or some other acute cardiac ischemic episode resulted from, or was hastened in occurrence by, mechanical or physical trauma or the psychologic consequences of the accident. Most difficult in both medical determinations and legal handling are those situations where it is alleged that a preexisting condition of stable angina pectoris has been aggravated, as evidenced by a change in a preexisting symptom complex by an increase in the frequency and severity of attacks after an accident, or when new-onset or unstable angina allegedly occurs after an accident, but with no objective evidence to support the claimed aggravation. Another commonly encountered vexing medicolegal problem is whether a fatal cardiac episode was "the result of" or "the cause of" an accident—a determination also of import when insurance contracts provide double indemnity or other specified benefits for "accidental" death or injury.

Other frequently encountered actions in tort involving cardiac patients are those in which it is alleged that heart problems have stemmed from trauma or stress subsequent to negligent conduct, such as from falling objects, slipping, and other accidentally induced falls; from exposure to food poisonings; from toxic fumes; from menacing animals; and from long-term psychologic "stress" claimed as a consequence of a chronic pain syndrome or from an anxiety-producing situation of an injury, such as the need for repeated hospitalizations or surgery and/or from resulting financial hardships attributable to an original noncardiac injury.

Medical malpractice suits, often referred to as "professional negligence" suits to lessen the sting, fall within the province of actions in tort and are subject to the same legal considerations affecting all claims for "damages" due to "negligence." In malpractice cases, as with other actions in tort, the aggrieved patient or those acting for the plaintiff have the burden of demonstrating by factual and opinion evidence: (1) that the defendant doctor or other health care provider named in the legal action breached a standard of care owed in an established physician-patient relationship, and (2) that this breach did in fact cause the plaintiff "harms." In evidentiary proof, the plaintiff must define by expert medical opinion the standard of care alleged to have been breached. The plaintiff must further establish the existence of alleged "harms" or "damage" and also must then show, again by expert medical opinion, that the alleged deviation from the acceptable standard of care was the cause of the claimed "damages." Finally, in many jurisdictions it must further be demonstrated that the plaintiff's conduct did not negligently contribute to the claimed harms. Again, unless all these criteria are satisfied, the burden of proof legally assigned to the plaintiff will not be considered to have been met and a directed verdict for the defendant may be ordered by the judge, thereby effectively dismissing the plaintiff's legal action unless later reversed on appeal to a higher court.

In some legal actions, the known existence of a prior cardiac disorder is of importance in the assessment of financial awards. Under the *Second Injury Funds* of the Federal Longshoremen's and Harbor Workers' Compensation Act and of many state workers' compensation acts, some financial relief is afforded the employer or insurer for disability payments to an injured worker if it can be demonstrated that the work incapacity following an accepted or assigned work injury was made substantially greater than would otherwise have been the case because of a known preexistent medical condition, as, for example, a prior myocardial infarction. In other instances, the demonstration of a heart disorder may be of key importance in a legal decision as to whether a worker can return to a prior job that an employer claims involves physical or psychologic stress potentially harmful to a person with known heart disease or where the operation of machinery by a person subject to sudden incapacity, as from an acute cardiac dysrhythmia, would endanger others; whether a person should be rejected from driving a motor vehicle, particularly one used in public transportation, or from piloting an airplane; whether a heart patient can participate in a court trial as a defendant or witness or serve a prison term, write a valid will, or be forced to pay alimony or other financial assessment; whether certain items claimed as income tax–deductible medical expenses are medically justified as treatment; whether an insurance contract can be voided because of the applicant's fraudulent concealment of a known cardiac disorder in the original application for the policy; and in other situations where the question of preexistent heart disorder may be of importance for legal and insurance determinations of eligibility for "accidental death" benefits.

A large area of litigation involving heart disorder concerns the many applicants for disability benefits under the Social Security Disability Insurance Program, public welfare programs, the Veterans Administration service- and non-service-related pensions, and privately purchased disability, accident, and health insurance contracts. In most of these situations, the legal issue to be decided is the work capacity of the individual, as defined in the covering statute or insurance contract, based on a demonstrated medical condition, not the question of causation.

Miscellaneous legal actions that may require expert medical opinions on heart disorders and their consequences include determination of "conscious pain and suffering" as an element of tort "damages," losses of bodily functions under certain workers' compensation statutes, reduction of life and/or work-year expectancy due to a cardiac disorder or worsening thereof, projected reasonable medical expenses of future treatment in a cardiac patient, relationship of a coronary artery bypass grafting to a compensable myocardial infarction, prognosis, and many other medicolegal issues too numerous to list.

THE CARDIOLOGIST IN THE COURTROOM

It is in the role of an expert witness that cardiologists most often find themselves involved with the legal profession. Any duly licensed physician, whether a general or family practitioner or a specialist, is considered legally qualified to present opinion testimony when the medical issues of the matter in hand are not patently discernible as a matter of common knowledge or are not within the recognized ken of a layperson, as in most cardiac cases. However, the appropriateness of a particular physician's competency to testify as an expert can be raised by either side to the dispute and put before the court or other legal body involved for its evaluation and acceptance or rejection on the basis of the physician's training and experience as well as demonstrated bias. Once a physician has been accepted as an expert witness, the weight to be attached to the medical conclusions presented is determined by a legally appointed fact-finding body. Since the current state of scientific knowledge in cardiology does not provide, in many instances, clear-cut definitive answers to many of the courtroom medical questions raised in individual cases, there not infrequently is a difference between the conclusions reached by the expert witnesses called by the disputants in the litigation. In such instances, the legal fact finder can adopt as "factual" that opinion believed most likely to conform to the facts in the case and reach a decision on that basis. In some legal actions the fact finder may call on an outside court-appointed physician or medical panel for an "impartial" opinion but is not bound to accept the opinions so proferred. Thus, almost every legal decision in medical matters has to be supported by the testimony of a physician "expert witness." It is imperative, therefore, that for legal decisions to be in accord with the main current of medical thinking, the testimony of the "experts" on whom they must rely should be within the boundaries of presently acceptable scientific beliefs and concepts.

The physician who testifies as an expert witness need not have personally examined the claimant nor even have any personal knowledge of the claimant's medical condition prior to or following an alleged incident. The medical expert may reach conclusions solely from a review of the medical records of the claimant and other factual data that have been admitted into evidence. Alternatively, the expert may be presented by either counsel with a hypothetical question that contains a set of facts he or she is obliged to accept as true and that are then to be utilized as the factual basis for the conclusions reached and the opinions expressed. The law, however, does require that those facts put forth in the hypothetical question be supported by the evidence presented in the case. Thus, the fact finder cannot adopt the opinion expressed by an expert in answer to a hypothetical question unless the evidence on hand is sufficient to establish legally the truth of the evidence to be assumed as factual. When the factual evidence is conflicting, as is frequently the case, it is within the province of the fact finder to determine which evidence is to be believed and adopted as "factual." The hypothetical question posed to a medical expert in courtroom proceedings need not include all the evidence previously presented in the case. It may be limited to a partisan recital of that evidence most favorable to the proponent's side. However, the adversary party, in cross examination of the expert, can propose a counter–hypothetical recital of alleged facts to provide data omitted or now added to the original hypothetical question posed in direct examination. The medical expert can then be queried as to whether the newly assumed factual changes or additions alter or modify the opinions previously expressed. In this manner, both parties in the legal dispute have full opportunity to pose to medical experts respective versions of what they believe is factual. Again, however, the ultimate determination of medical issues for legal purposes rests with the duly appointed fact finder, not with the medical experts.

Generally, it is not sufficient for an expert witness to present conclusions alone without supporting reasoning. The basis on which the opinion rendered rests also may be subject to attack in cross examination so that they can be considered by the fact finder in reaching a decision as to which of conflicting medical opinions to adopt.

In formulating an opinion, the medical expert must appreciate the degree of certainty required in reaching medical conclusions when such opinions are to be expressed in the courtroom and not in a medical forum per se. The legal system recognizes the current inability of medical science to answer definitively and with absolute certainty many of the medical questions raised in individual cases. Yet the legal body before which the claimant's case ultimately (often after long delay) has been placed for final legal resolution must answer as best it can all the issues raised at the time of trial. The law does not have the luxury of being able to defer resolution of controverted medical issues until medical science has advanced to the point of providing clear-cut answers to the questions on hand. Legal proof, therefore, cannot be equated with scientific proof. Although pure science seeks absolute certainty or positive proof before reaching a determination, legal decisions necessarily are far less exacting in their demands. In civil cases, decisions are based primarily upon such standards as a *preponderance of the evidence* and *clear and convincing evidence*, whereas in criminal matters, the requirements are more stringent, usually *beyond a reasonable doubt*.

For answers to medical questions, the law generally requires that these be expressed in terms of *reasonable medical certainty* or *probability* rather than mere *possibility*. In essence, this means that the conclusions reached by an expert are believed to be *more likely than not* true with a tilting of the balance scale to as little as 50.1 percent versus 49.9 percent sufficient to determine the courtroom outcome, although such a difference would not be acceptable to a body of scientists. In accord with this legal philosophy, *reasonable medical certainty* generally means reasonable *legal* certainty—a far less exacting criterion of proof than that required for rigid medical *scientific* certainty.

In cases involving cardiac claims, as in most civil cases, the burden of proof generally is placed on the claimant, who must show by a preponderance of supporting evidence, including expert opinion when necessary, that the allegations are true. For example, in a claim alleging a cardiac disorder and its consequences as a workplace injury, the claimant must provide the fact finder with sufficient supporting medical expert testimony attesting not only to the existence of a cardiac disorder but also to its causal relationship to some element of the employment; otherwise the claim will fail. A claimant's burden of proof generally is not met when a medical expert merely acknowledges the *possibility* of the truth of the allegations rather than asserting their *probability*. Phraseology frequently employed by physicians in medical reports and testimony such as "may," "could," or "might have" serve no useful purpose in the courtroom. Additionally, the burden of proof is not met, nor is it sustained, when the medical supportive conclusions are shown to be based on speculation, surmise, or conjecture rather than on *reasonable medical certainty or probability*; or when the medical expert admits that acceptance and denial of the allegations are *equal* possibilities that cannot be differentiated. As pointed out earlier in this chapter, under many workers' compensation acts, when a worker is found dead or unable to testify (e.g., poststroke) at the place of employment, the burden of disproving causation by the job is placed on the employer. The Federal Longshoremen's and Harbor Workers' Compensation Act even goes a step further by stating that "In any proceeding for the enforcement of a claim for compensation under this Act it shall be presumed, in the absence of substantial evidence to the contrary—(a) That the claim comes within the provisions of this Act. . . ."[12] And in actions for medical malpractice the burden of proof of lack of causation by negligence may be shifted to the defendant health care provider when the doctrines of *res ipsa loquitur* ("the thing speaks for itself") and *the captain of the ship*, i.e., the operating room surgeon, become applicable.

When expert medical opinions presented by the respective litigants contradict or conflict, the fact finder must choose between them with the choice subject to reversal on appeal to a higher court only when contrary to the weight of the evidence or the result of an error in legal procedure, as with acceptance of evidence inadmissible under the law. Since reached by a lay person fact finder, often without adequate scientific background, legal decisions in many instances appear contrary to the main current of medical/scientific thinking.

COMMONLY REQUESTED MEDICOLEGAL CARDIAC EVALUATIONS

Medical examinations and evaluations performed specifically for legal and insurance reasons necessarily emphasize aspects of the medical situation not customarily addressed by physicians, since the primary purpose of such evaluations is the answering of legal questions and not the providing of medical care.

The scope of potential medicolegal questions in litigants whose heart disorder is germane to the litigation is too vast and varied for detailed discussion within the constraints of this chapter. Certain inquiries, however, are fundamental to most claims alleging cardiac injury, disorder, dysfunction, or death and warrant further consideration and elaboration. These are (1) the cardiac diagnosis that is to be accepted legally as established in a given claimant; (2) the time of onset of each specific cardiac lesion or dysfunction, particularly those with legal import; (3) the causal relationship, if any, between the factor or factors under legal examination and the cardiac disorder found or some aspect thereof; (4) the medical determination of the impairment to be assessed on the basis of the claimant's overall cardiovascular status and, more specifically, to each component of the cardiac condition that has legal significance in its derivation; and (5) the medical considerations in allegations of professional negligence in the physicians' and/or other health care providers' handling of a cardiac patient as the basis of a claim for resulting harm. Additionally in some legal actions arising under workers' compensation and some insurance policies, questions as to the role of preexisting disease or infirmity in contributing to the covered impairment or death may be of paramount import in determining eligibility for benefits as well as the amount of benefits to be paid by the employer or insurer.

Defining the Cardiac Diagnosis

From the medical viewpoint, the diagnosis is the foundation on which the treatment of the patient is constructed. From the legal viewpoint, the diagnosis is the foundation upon which many decisions and rulings concerning issues of causation, eligibility for disability and retirement pensions, awards for damages, and many other matters arising in the litigation on hand are made.

Although the diagnosis, in actuality, has to be made by a physician based upon medical data, legally it is considered to be but one of the various factual determinations within the province of the fact-finding body assigned to adjudicate the case.

The diagnosis reached by a physician after the gathering, reviewing, and studying of the medical data is, in essence, merely an opinion based on the individual examiner's specialized training, study, experience, and interpretation of the medical findings. As such, it is open to question both medically and legally as to reasonableness, accuracy, and completeness. Since the diagnostic conclusions in individual instances reached by a medical examiner may not be concurred in by other physicians evaluating the same data, opinions expressed in court concerning the diagnosis, as with all medical conclusions, are subject to interrogation by counsel during cross examination.

The cardiac diagnosis should be established in each instance as fully as possible in terms of (1) an *etiologic* diagnosis that describes the underlying disease processes basically responsible for the structural and functional disorders found in the patient/claimant, (2) an *anatomic* diagnosis that describes the specific structural abnormalities (lesions) found in the cardiovascular examination, (3) a *physiological* diagnosis that describes the resulting physiological disturbances of cardiovascular action, (4) the *cardiac status*, and (5) the *prognosis*. These should be delineated in generally accepted terminology, such as recommended by the Criteria Committee of the New York Heart Association in that committee's publication, "Nomenclature and Criteria for Diagnosis of the Heart and Great Vessels."[13]

Because of varying connotations and implications, nonspecific terms, such as *heart attack*, *coronary*, *mild or massive heart attack*, and *heart disease*, without adequate qualification as to specific meaning should not be employed in the cardiac evaluator's written report or testimony. Similarly, umbrella terms, such as *unstable angina*, *preinfarction angina*, *acute coronary deficiency*, and *acute coronary insufficiency*, at times popular in medical jargon to designate certain symptom complexes encountered during the course of ischemic heart disease, should be avoided unless they are precisely defined. (See Chap. 59.)

The *etiologic diagnosis* should be reached after consideration of both the structural and functional disturbances found. If two or more etiologic bases for a person's heart disorder are present, each should be listed. Legally, the identification of the etiologic basis of a cardiac disorder or disorders becomes important in a causality assessment where an aggravation or worsening of a preexistent cardiac condition is claimed as a "personal injury" and must be differentiated from the expected natural progression of an underlying cardiac disorder and in legal actions where an estimation of life expectancy is of importance in determining awards for "damages" or in settlement proceedings.

The *anatomic diagnosis* comprises that component of the total cardiac diagnosis that describes the specific structural lesions of the heart and great vessels. A complete description of the anatomic alterations often constitutes an important aspect of the legal determinations of a cardiac "personal injury" and of disability. Thus, for example, there may be considerable differences in the benefits or awards available legally for the sustaining of an episode of prolonged ischemic cardiac pain when diagnosed as an intermediate coronary syndrome attack with no resulting new myocardial damage or when diagnosed as acute myocardial necrosis with resulting permanent new or added heart damage and a change in the preexistent condition.

Anatomic lesions of the heart and great vessels frequently can be delineated clinically on the basis of the history, the findings of physical examination, and the results of specialized cardiac diagnostic studies. Certain anatomic lesions, however, cannot be diagnosed with reasonable certainty by currently available cardiac studies. Thus, diagnoses of *coronary thrombosis* and *micro-*

scopic myocardial necrosis, terms not infrequently encountered in cardiac medicolegal reports and expert testimony, should usually be reserved for the pathologist after autopsy study. When more than one anatomic abnormality is found, each should be included in the final diagnosis.

The *physiological diagnosis* specifies the alterations in cardiovascular dynamics that have resulted from the cardiac pathology. The physiological diagnosis includes a description of the cardiac rhythm and whether of normal or abnormal mechanism; disturbances in cardiac impulse conduction; disturbances in supravalvular, valvular, or subvalvular function; malfunctions of prostheses, homografts, and cardiac pacemakers; disturbances in myocardial pump functioning; disturbances in intravascular pressures; abnormal communications (shunts) in the heart or great vessels; and the anginal syndromes.

The *cardiac status* is determined by analyzing all the data collected on the patient. It is *not* determined by the patient's symptoms alone.[13]

The *prognosis* preferably should be determined and graded according to the New York Heart Association.[13]

The physician performing a cardiac evaluation for legal purposes must determine whether the patient-claimant had heart disease prior to the alleged potentially harmful exposure under legal consideration and, if so, whether there was a change in the preexistent cardiac status after the exposure. If a change is found, the physician must then define its nature, degree, and extent, whether permanent or temporary. In this regard it is important to distinguish between a demonstrated structural change in a preexisting heart disorder, e.g., a coronary artery occlusion by thrombosis or a rupture of a heart valve or other part of the heart, and an alleged hastening of an expected consequence, e.g., an acute myocardial infarction, by reason of the progression of an underlying process of atherogenesis in the coronary artery tree.

Diagnoses, as with other medical opinions, presented to a legal forum must be established in terms of reasonable medical certainty, which means in terms of *probability*. *Possible*, *potential*, or *suspected* heart disorder has no place in the courtroom or in other legal determinations.

Timing the Onset of Cardiac Lesions and Dysfunctions

Determining the time of onset of a specific cardiac pathology or dysfunction is an essential part of many cardiac medicolegal evaluations, often the crux of an issue of causation or of eligibility for the benefits of an insurance contract. Because of the vagaries of clinical presentations, individual differences in response to and manifestations of illness, and the frequent initial "silent" development of many cardiac pathologies with no symptoms or abnormal signs evident until the process has progressed to an advanced state, the current state of the art frequently prevents medical science from timing the onset of cardiac pathologies and/or dysfunctions within the precise time framework sought by the law. Additionally, medical science often is unable even to delineate the sequence of development of the pathophysiological processes underlying various pathologies such as an acute myocardial infarction. Yet, difficult though it may be in specific instances, the time of onset of cardiac lesions and dysfunctions must be defined by the cardiac examiner as best can be within frameworks of reasonable medical certainty and probability.

The time of occurrence of a single episode of angina pectoris is fairly easy to pinpoint since, in most cases, the symptoms of the attack are clear-cut and abrupt in onset, thereby allowing a reasonably accurate timing of the commencement of the individual attack. Similarly, the end of the attack is evidenced by the disappearance of symptoms, although some degree of subsiding silent myocardial ischemia may be present for a short time thereafter.

Delineating the time of onset of an episode of myocardial infarction is more difficult because of variable clinical presentations. The classic textbook presentation of sudden crushing anterior chest pain associated with profuse diaphoresis, dyspnea, weakness, and other cardinal symptomatology is a generally acceptable index of the occurrence at that time of significant discrete acute myocardial tissue necrosis, although the possibility that some degree of myocardial necrosis has occurred previously (silently or with atypical manifestations) cannot be excluded. In some patients, the process of acute myocardial infarction is an ongoing ischemic/necrotic process that may start minutes to hours to several days prior to the initial appearance of recognizable symptoms, signs, and laboratory or electrocardiographic abnormalities. In some patients, an acute myocardial infarction, although evident at a later date on an electrocardiogram or at postmortem examination, is clinically silent at the time of occurrence. In other patients, the clinical picture is one of waxing and waning ischemic symptoms or signs over the course of one or more days (a state currently popularly referred to as *unstable angina* or *preinfarction angina*), with or without culmination in a bout of classic, prolonged chest discomfort that heralds the infarction of a larger discrete mass of myocardium. In still other patients, the first anginal attack (*new-onset angina*) may actually represent an acute myocardial infarction. And in patients with previous angina pectoris, an acute myocardial infarction may be manifested by an anginal attack of greater severity and duration or of radiation and location different from that previously experienced. And in some 15 to 25 percent of cases the occurrence of an acute myocardial infarction is clinically silent and cannot be pinpointed as to time of happening. (See Chap. 60.)

It must further be appreciated that the time of occurrence of an acute myocardial infarction, if determinable, does not necessarily reflect the time of onset of underlying atherosclerotic coronary heart disease or the time of initiation of a thrombotic coronary artery occlusion or of other pathophysiological processes that may result in infarction of the myocardium.

Indexes, sometimes of help in the attempt to time the onset of an acute myocardial infarction, may be provided by the time of appearance of certain signs, laboratory findings, and the time sequence of development of electrocardiographic changes during the acute phases of the illness. Thus, a retrospective correlation of the time of the initial detection of abnormal cardiac enzyme and isoenzyme levels and the time of peak abnormal values with the clinical picture may permit a rough extrapolated determination of the time of occurrence of infarction of a significant degree to be so detected. Additional guides for such temporal extrapolations include the times of initial and peak leukocytosis, the development of post-myocardial infarction fever, the occurrence of a pericardial friction rub or of a rupture of infarcted myocardium, and other potential concomitants of an acute myocardial infarction. From the viewpoint of the pathologist, the time of onset of a process of myocardial infarction can be roughly estimated by correlation of the gross and microscopic postmortem appearance of the involved tissue with that generally expected (on the basis of accumulated experience and knowledge) at different time periods after the beginning of the attack.

Unless otherwise determinable, the time of onset of a cardiac arrhythmia generally is accepted as the time of occurrence of identifying symptoms such as palpitation or initial awareness of heartbeat irregularity or of a sudden collapse as with a cardiac arrest due to ventricular tachycardia or fibrillation.

The time of onset of coronary atherosclerotic, valvular, hypertensive, and most other heart disorders generally cannot be determined medically with any greater accuracy other than that the underlying etiologic condition must have been present for some time (usually only measurable in months or years) prior to the initial clinical manifestations or abnormality that led to its detection.

The occurrence of sudden collapse, acute pulmonary edema, cardiogenic shock, or severe pain provides an index of the time of rupture of an aortic aneurysm or of a cardiac valve, papillary muscle, chordae tendineae, or infarcted myocardium. However, the commencement of the pathophysiological processes underlying such rupture most often cannot be pinpointed with accuracy because of subtle or silent initial clinical manifestations for a variable period of time preceding the end-stage catastrophic event.

Assessment of Causality

The determination of causation is vital to legal actions in which a heart disorder or its consequences is claimed as a compensable "work injury," as an injury due to someone's negligence, or as an "accident" under an insurance contract in which benefits are specifically provided for injury, disability, or death due to an "accident" rather than the result of "illness."

In general, legal claims of cardiac injury, dysfunction, disability, or death generally allege, as *a* or *the* cause, (1) an isolated, specifically identified incident, event, accident, trauma, exposure, complication of medical or surgical treatment, or other alleged "trigger" or (as in a malpractice action) a negligent treatment or negligent failure to institute indicated treatment; (2) a set of repetitive, cumulative factors that, although subliminal individually, have combined in additive effect to produce cardiovascular harm, such as repeated subthreshold inhalation of carbon monoxide or a recent period of days, weeks, or months of mounting physical or psychologic stress as might be associated with unduly long work hours, an impending deadline or quota, trying business conditions, a forthcoming surgical procedure, or some other presumed stressful happenings; (3) long-term "overall" job or situational physical or psychologic "stress"; or (4) a combination of one or more of the preceding.[6,7]

In such actions, the claimant must first establish the existence of a cardiac disorder that can be accepted as an "injury" and the causal connection thereof to an item with attached legal liability and then establish a causal connection between such injury and the alleged harmful consequences (disability, medical and surgical treatment and diagnostic expenses, pain and suffering, death, and other items of "harms") for which benefits are claimed. The claimant usually has the further burden of disproving any contributions to the alleged harms from intervening causes or from personal negligence should such charges be raised by the defendant.

In disputed issues involving causality questions in medical disorders, the fact finder in reaching the legal decision must rely on the evidence put forth by the respective litigants, particularly expert medical opinion testimony. Physicians presenting such testimony in cause-and-effect assessments must appreciate the different weights assigned by the legal profession to the various elements that comprise a legal causality determination from those assigned by the medical profession to a pure medical assessment of causality (see Table 143-1). Because of differences in training and orientation backgrounds, causation often means one thing to a physician and quite another to an attorney, judge, or administrative hearing official. It is not surprising, then, that on occasions medical opinion testimony based on traditional medical concepts of causality differs dramatically from answers based primarily on legal concepts utilized by a fact finder in reaching courtroom decisions.

The differences between the medical and legal approaches to solving causality problems are many.[14–18] The physician, for example, in viewing a patient's medical problems, instinctively searches for the basic cause or causes underlying the overall disorder, whereas legal and judiciary professionals generally limit their concern to the one or more items under legal scrutiny as an "injury," independent of other causes. The physician generally defines *cause* as the production of a new condition or a new pathology or dysfunction, whereas the law in its definition accepts the aggravation of an underlying disorder by the worsening, hastening, or acceleration of its progression to lead to impairment, bodily harm, or death sooner than otherwise would have occurred during the natural history of the preexisting condition without the claimed noxious exposure. The law thus includes in its framework of causation not only the production of a de novo condition, but also the "triggering" or "proximate precipitation" of a new stage of pathology or of a new dysfunction in an underlying disorder and the worsening of an ongoing pathological process.

Physicians are reluctant to assign causal responsibility when the degree of aggravation of a preexisting condition is small in overall relationship to the extent of the underlying abnormality or when the degree of hastening of an inevitable end result is minor in relation to the entire clinical condition. The law, on the other hand, emphasizes the fact of hastening or aggravation, not the

TABLE 143-1

Medical versus Legal Emphasis in Causality Assessment

Medical Emphasis	Legal Emphasis
The etiologic bases of a disease or disorder	The proximate ("triggering") cause of an injury, disability, or death
The causes of disease	A cause of injury, disability, or death
The producing cause of the entire disorder	An aggravation of a preexisting condition
The key role of preexisting disease	"The victim is taken as found," not as a normal, healthy person, but subject to whatever existing medical disorders were present at the time of exposure
The end result was inevitable because of the expected progression of the preexisting disease	A determination of whether the end result was hastened, not the time amount of hastening
The degree of aggravation was small in the light of the entire clinical picture	The crux is aggravation, not degree
The alleged causative element(s) not unique or unusual	The key element is the causative element(s), not the characteristics
The multiplicity of causes and their interrelationships	The key is the causative element(s) under legal scrutiny, independent of other coexisting or interrelating causes
Scientific proof of causation required	Establishment of causation generally is defined in terms of *reasonable medical certainty*, i.e., *probable vs. possible, more likely than not,* a 50.1% chance of relationship
Equally consistent theories of causation acceptable in differential diagnosis and choice of therapies	Equally consistent theories of causation do not satisfy standards for legal proof
The ultimate answer to causation can be deferred, pending new scientific advances	The issue of causation must be decided legally when presented
In assessment of damages (harms), there should be an apportionment of the role of each causative element	Generally, a total responsibility is assigned for the end result, if such is deemed due to a legally indicted exposure

SOURCE: Adapted from Sagall,[3] Sagall,[17] and Danner and Sagall.[18]

quantitative aspects. The crux of legal causation thus is the occurrence of an aggravation of an underlying disorder, not the degree to which it was aggravated, the hastening of an end result to cause it to occur sooner than otherwise would have been the case, not the extent to which it was hastened.

Physicians in their assessments of causation are particularly impressed that the alleged injurious results, as is true in most cardiac cases, would not have occurred in the absence of a preexisting disorder that rendered the patient susceptible to harm from the alleged exposure. Legal fact finders, however, see it as immaterial that the event in question would not have caused injurious consequences had the victim been in good or average health. In all *personal injury* legal actions, the victim is "taken as he is found." Preexisting infirmity does not bar legal recovery, nor is it an acceptable excuse to relieve a defendant from legal responsibility or to mitigate the damages to be assessed. An illustration is the case of the proverbial "straw that broke the camel's back." To the physician, the proverb emphasizes the obvious predisposition to break down because of existing overload. The physician thus assigns the cause of the camel's collapse to the prior strain on his back, not to the added straw. The law, on the other hand, asserts that although loaded to the breaking point, the back had held up without breaking. Accordingly, the added straw must be viewed as the cause of the collapse and the person who placed the straw on that loaded back as legally responsible for the consequences. Most often, the assignment of legal liability in such situations is made without attempt to apportion a percentage of harm between the triggering straw and the preload.

Unfortunately, the many current deficiencies in medical knowledge concerning the etiology and pathogenesis of most cardiac disorders and the limitations of presently available cardiac diagnostic testing procedures often prevent medical science from defining precisely the complete cardiac diagnosis, the nature and extent of the underlying pathology, the pathophysiological mechanisms that have led to the end result, the sequence in which pathological lesions have developed, the time of onset of certain lesions, and the answers to the many medical questions that may be of key importance in the legal matter on hand. The medical determination of causation is further made difficult because the very nature of most cardiac disorders categorized legally as *personal injuries* does not, in contrast to lesions such as burns or lacerations, present clinical or pathological features pathognomonic of trauma or of an external cause. Thus, the question of whether some identified external element or stress played a contributory or precipitating role in their development or whether the disorder found stemmed from the natural, expected progression of an underlying cardiac disease unrelated to and unaffected by the item under legal scrutiny quite frequently is not amenable to clear-cut, noncontroversial answers or to overall causality guidelines or criteria.

Similarly, differences in the provisions of the individual state and territorial workers' compensation acts under which most cardiac claims arise; differences in legal philosophy among the many persons assigned fact-finding roles in disputed litigation; subtle differences in fact situations of claims that, at first glance, are seemingly identical; and the often diametrically opposed medical conclusions presented in a given case by equally competent medical experts preclude the formulation of legal standards of causality that can uniformly be applied to cover all instances. Accordingly, each case must be decided, both medically and legally, on its own set of facts and medical testimony.

Certain precepts, however, should govern medical assessments of causality in cardiac claims. For an alleged causal connection to be accepted in a cardiac case as *probable* or with *reasonable medical certainty*, the following criteria should be satisfied:

- The cardiac diagnosis should be delineated completely and established, as far as reasonably possible, by objective means, and those portions of the cardiac condition under consideration as potential "injuries" specified.
- The alleged causative element presented for legal consideration should be one that is currently recognized medically and scientifically as capable, under appropriate circumstances, of producing the heart disorder or injury found.
- Conversely, the cardiac condition or dysfunction diagnosed must be one generally recognized medically as a possible resultant of the alleged harmful exposure.
- The time interval elapsing between the alleged noxious exposure and the medically manifest evidence of heart damage or dysfunction must be consistent with currently accepted scientific concepts of pathogenesis.
- The proposed cause-and-effect relation, although not always fully explainable in terms of present-day scientific knowledge, must still be consistent with current scientific concepts.

As an aid to medical assessment of causality in coronary artery heart disease and its ischemic sequelae, which is the cardiac disorder by far the most frequent basis of heart claims, the reader is referred to "Report of the American Heart Association's Committee on Stress, Strain, and Heart Disease."[19] Although originally published in 1977, the conclusions of this committee are currently valid with only minor modification, have not been supplanted by any other formal set of medical causality guidelines, and are generally accepted by the medical profession. The conclusions pertinent to a medical assessment of causality in cardiac claims arising under workers' compensation are summarized below:

- Long-term repetitive physical effort, such as is inherent in many occupations, cannot currently be regarded medically as a causative element in the development of atherosclerotic coronary heart disease. Such activity, if playing any role in this disease process, is believed beneficial by preventing or slowing the rate of atherosclerotic progression.
- Long-term repeated physical effort of work and/or nonwork activities in persons with underlying heart disease theoretically may hasten the development of congestive heart failure by reason of the additional work load imposed upon an already weakened heart. However, it is not possible within the present state of medical knowledge to determine in any given heart patient when congestive heart failure would have occurred as the result of the expected natural progression of the underlying cardiac disorder in the absence of such exertional efforts; hence in these situations a causative role to such stress most often cannot be assigned with "reasonable medical certainty."
- Continued, protracted psychologic emotional stress to which an individual may have been subjected over a long period of time has not been established scientifically as a causative or worsening agent in the genesis or acceleration of atherosclerotic disease, although the possibility of some contribution cannot be excluded in individual cases.
- A single, isolated, identified physical or emotional stress in individuals rendered susceptible to harm therefrom by reason of preexistent heart disease, whether or not previously known or symptomatic, if of sufficient intensity and duration, is capable of eliciting adverse cardiac responses that, in turn, can "trigger" or hasten certain cardiac lesions and dysfunctions such as an acute attack of angina pectoris or myocardial infarction, a sudden cardiac dysrhythmia (including sudden death therefrom), and a bout of acute congestive heart failure.
- The shorter the time interval between the exposure of an individual to a potentially noxious stimulus and the appearance of clinical or pathological evidence of new heart disease or dysfunction, the more likely there is a causal relationship between the two. Conversely, the farther apart in time, the less likely is a cause-and-effect relation.
- The exposure of a person with underlying heart disease to a stimulus potentially capable of eliciting harmful cardiovascular responses does not necessarily mean that such will be elicited, even when such exposure would be advised against medically because of the possibility of ensuing harm.

The elements most often accepted by workers' compensation adjudicators in cardiac cases as work-related *competent-producing* causes of injury, disability, or death are identified incidents of physical work effort (usual, unusual, or of a degree greater than accustomed nonwork exertion, depending on the covering compensation act requirements); adverse work environments, e.g., excessive heat or cold, noxious fumes; an acute psychologic trauma such as a heated argument or a sudden fright; an accidental electric shock; a severe nonpenetrating blow or other mechanical injury to the chest cage; and adverse cardiac reactions to medical, surgical, corrective, and rehabilitative therapy of an industrial injury not originally involving the cardiovascular system.

Nationwide, burgeoning claims under workers' compensation alleging illnesses such as coronary heart disease, hypertension, stroke, gastrointestinal disorders, and neuropsychiatric states as initiated or worsened by overall job-related "stress" are straining the workers' compensation system.[19-22] Frequently cited as "harmful" to the cardiovascular system are adverse mental reactions stemming from harassments from superiors, frustrations from dealing with the public, tensions created by imposed deadlines and quotas, boredom or excessive responsibility in job duties, threats of job termination or changes, insufficient vacations and time off, changing work shifts, long work hours, ongoing business financial problems, and others too numerous to list.

Of the few cardiac "stress" cases that have reached state supreme court levels on appeals, the decisions therein established guiding case law have been mixed and have not established uniform case law precedents. For example:

- In New Hampshire, medical opinion that the continuing "stress" of a failing business over a 2-year period did *not* cause the fatal myocardial infarction suffered by the owner on a Sunday morning at home was upheld and compensation to his widow denied.[23]
- On the other side of the coin, a Rhode Island trial commissioner's denial of compensation to the widow of a newspaper sports editor who suffered a fatal cerebral hemorrhage at home was reversed. The court concluded that medical testimony that the deceased was suffering from high blood pressure of the type that would rise whenever he was under stress plus evidence that the decedent attended a professional football game earlier in the day of his death that placed him "under pressure" to meet a reporting deadline were sufficient to support the claim that his death that night was due to a cerebral hemorrhage resulting from aggravation of his preexisting hypertension.[24]
- In Colorado, the denial of compensation by the Industrial Commission to the widow of a fire department lieutenant with preexisting mitral valve prolapse and hypertension who died at home on the tenth day of a vacation absence from work was vacated. As grounds for the reversal and for an award of compensation, the court concluded that uncontroverted testimony from the fire chief, coworkers, and widow that the decedent had suffered a great deal of cumulative tension and frustration relating to his being overlooked in favor of junior firefighters for promotion and to his differing from superiors in department training and communication policies with no other significant sources of mental stress in his life qualified this "stress" legally as an injury or occupational disease arising out of and in the course of employment. On this basis, the court remanded the claim to the referee to make specific findings whether the job-related stress was the proximate cause of the death as was testified to by the decedent's doctor, who opined that the likely cause of death was an irregular heart rhythm that, when combined with a preexisting mitral valve prolapse and job-related stress, resulted in a fatal arrhythmia. The doctor further testified that the imminence of the decedent's return to work may have exacerbated his stress level, thereby increasing his hypertension just prior to his scheduled return to work, and was a contributory cause of his death.[25]
- In Connecticut, the court affirmed a commissioner's decision that unjust criticism of a bank employee on a number of occasions by superiors so aggravated her condition of obstructive coronary disease as to lead to a continued work disability from angina pectoris from intermittent coronary artery spasm still unrelieved by a coronary artery bypass surgery some 2 years later, despite the ruling out of an acute myocardial infarction during hospitalization shortly after the harassments and the presence of multiple coronary atherosclerosis risk factors of long-standing, including extensive cigarette smoking, obesity, and a positive family history of premature coronary disease.[26]

So-called risk factors, such as cigarette smoking, elevated blood cholesterol, diabetes mellitus, hypertension, and positive family history of coronary disease, are often put forth by defense counsels as mitigating or alternative, not of legal liability, elements arguing against the claim's validity in regard to questions of causality assessments in coronary heart disease. In this regard, it should be recognized that risk factors are of importance primarily in epidemiologic studies applicable to groups, not to an individual. For any given person, the presence or absence of medical background risk factors does not necessarily indicate the premature development of this condition or an escape therefrom. Thus, although statistically related to the presence of coronary heart disease, generally accepted risk factors for coronary atherosclerosis cannot be viewed medically as legally causative elements in the production of the disease. In any consideration of so-called personality types A and B as risk factors, it should further be recognized that, in addition to the practical impossibility of definitively separating human beings categorically into type A or type B personalities, it must be kept in mind that the role of personality type, if any, in the pathogenesis of coronary atherosclerosis has not been scientifically established and, therefore, should not be presented to a court of law as within the realm of medical probability or reasonable medical certainty.

Additionally, in medical causality assessments in atherosclerotic coronary heart disease, it must be appreciated that although physical stress may be definable quantitatively to some degree, emotional stress defies quantitative measurement. Nor can presumed long-term effects of an occupational endeavor or a presumed unpleasant life situation incident be separated from similar effects inherent in day-to-day life and interpersonal contacts. Finally, the effects of so-called psychologic stress are primarily, as with beauty, in the eyes of the beholder. A psychologic situation that may be upsetting and possibly harmful to one person may be but an exhilarating, stimulating challenge to another.

Not all cardiac claims require legal causality determinations. For example, in claims instituted under the Social Security Disability Insurance Program the primary issue is whether the applicant is unable to engage in substantial gainful employment as defined in the covering statute, not the medical or legal relationship of the disability to a particular causative element. Similarly, eligibility for benefits in most privately acquired insurance contracts is based on the fact of disability, generally independent of cause unless the applicant must demonstrate that disability stems from an "accident" rather than an illness, in which case the issue of causation has to be established.

Evaluation of Disability

Evaluation of disability for legal and insurance purposes is a complex process necessarily involving more than one professional discipline. At times the evaluation requires interrelating the fields of medicine, law, insurance, judiciary, vocational counseling, and rehabilitation. As a minimum, a cardiac disability evaluation is twofold: first, a medical assessment must be made of the extent of the patient-claimant's impairment in terms of what the patient can and cannot do and what the patient should not do by reason of the cardiac disorder and, second, there must be a legal translation of the medically determined impairments into the specific definition of disability incorporated in the applicable statute or insurance contract, the latter often involving questions of total versus partial disability, permanent disability, house-confining, and other qualifying or restrictive adjectives affecting benefits.

As with most medicolegal evaluations, contested claims for disability benefits are decided by legal or administrative fact finders, with the physician's role limited to providing the fact finder with medical data and opinion testimony that can be utilized in reaching a conclusion.

As a minimum, the physician examining a patient-claimant for disability evaluation purposes should attempt to determine the following:

- The full cardiac diagnosis, including etiology when known, and all anatomic and functional derangements found, together with the supporting clinical evidence.
- The clinical manifestations of the disorder revealed by the medical examination, including all subjective complaints and, more important, all objective confirmatory findings of physical examination, x-ray, electrocardiogram, and laboratory and other studies that support the presence of a heart disease or disorder medically recognized as capable of producing the symptoms alleged as the basis for disability.
- The restrictions in the patient's physical activities and mental capacity that have resulted from the disorders found in terms of limitations of walking, stair climbing, standing, sitting, reaching, lifting, bending, pushing, pulling, gripping, running, work hours, work pace, ability to concentrate, and ability to work under conditions of tension, heat, cold, etc.
- Those restrictions of nonwork and work activities imposed to prevent an aggravation of the underlying heart disorder or to prevent further heart damage, such as advice to postmyocardial infarction patients not to subject themselves to sudden bursts of strenuous physical effort.

In those instances where the law requires that causation be apportioned between the parties (e.g., work-related versus non-work-related disabilities), the physician may be asked to furnish an opinion as to the causation of each of the impairments found. For example, in claims based on myocardial infarction, the physician may be asked what aspects of the impairments found are related to the underlying coronary atherosclerotic disease for which there may not be legal liability and what are related to the myocardial infarction itself for which there may exist legal responsibility.

In those situations where a patient-claimant has impairments coexisting from cardiac as well as noncardiac disorders, the physician may be asked to separate the impairments due to each disorder and, in assessing the overall combined impairments, whether noncardiac impairments, if present, magnify the impairment attributable to the heart disorder.

Where workers' compensation acts provide *second injury funds*, the examining or treating physician may be asked whether the disability from a cardiac injury in an employee with a known physical impairment from a congenital or acquired heart condition was made substantially greater by reason of the combined effects of such impairment and subsequent personal injury than that disability that would have resulted from the subsequent personal injury alone.

In reaching the conclusions expressed in the medical assessment of disability, the physician should utilize to the fullest extent all currently available objective means of diagnosis and measurement of cardiac function within practical limits of risk to the patient and cost of the testing and in terms of the information to be obtained relative to the assessment. Wherever feasible, medical evaluations of disability should be based on objective findings to obviate depending only on subjective complaints, which are often unreliable because they are self-serving.

Medical assessments of cardiac impairment are significantly hampered by the following:

1. The necessary reliance in most cases on subjective complaints.
2. The marked individual variations in symptoms, motivation, adjustment, and return-to-work desires among persons with similar cardiac abnormalities.
3. The paucity of currently available means for quantitative measurement of cardiac functional reserves.
4. The frequent discrepancy between objective findings and subjective complaints.
5. The practical difficulties in transferring the results of

objective test measurements, such as those of exercise stress testing, under controlled environmental conditions, into the uncontrolled, variable environment of the workplace in which hostile environments, often immeasurable, may significantly affect the physiological demands placed on the heart.

The fact that most cardiac impairments are rarely static and cannot be considered to have reached an end result but are subject, because of the progressive nature of the underlying disorder and variations in therapeutic responses, to sudden change so that an impairment assessment or disability evaluation at a given date may be unpredictably rendered invalid for a later time.

Helpful guides to the evaluation of cardiac, as well as other, causes of disability are available in publications of the Social Security System,[27] the American Medical Association,[28] and in *Disability Handbook* by Balsam and Zabin.[29] The legal aspects of commonly sought medical assessments of physical impairment by third-party physicians and the legal relationship of the third-party physician and the person being examined are discussed by Rothstein.[30]

As with causality assessments, medical and legal assessments of disability may vary considerably because of the difference in emphasis necessarily placed by each profession on individual aspects of the impairment in the disability rating process. Although a physician might consider a patient not disabled and, therefore, employable, the fact finder may declare the same person disabled from work activity under the terms of the applicable law or insurance contract. In such instances, the physician must appreciate that in reaching the legal decision as to work capacity, the fact finder frequently has to include nonmedical elements such as age, sex, educational background, motivation, and prior work training and experience. Additionally, the fact finder's decision may be influenced by the availability of certain types of employment in the local or national labor market, the problems imposed by transportation to and from work sites, language or other communication problems, and other factors that, as a practical matter, so restrict a given person's opportunity for gainful employment as to make that individual practically disabled from gainful employment although medically cleared for work.

It is also important to recognize that because of differing statutory and contractual definitions, a person declared disabled and awarded benefits under one disability program may not be deemed eligible for benefits under another program. Thus, an award for disability by one agency or insurer does not, by itself, bind another agency or insurer. Each insurance contract or other disability benefit program or statute must be considered individually and separately for each claim raised, although the claim in each instance is based on the same medical disorders and impairments.

Determination of Malpractice

The risk of a physician's being sued for professional negligence should a patient suffer an untoward result during the course of diagnosis and treatment is an inescapable fact of today's professional life. Choosing cardiology as a specialty increases this risk[31] because of a variety of reasons, particularly (1) the ever-present threat of sudden, unpredicted death due to the relentless progressive nature of most heart diseases independent of treatment or lack of treatment; (2) the adverse reactions often attributable to the narrow overlap between therapeutic and toxic ranges of commonly employed cardiac medications; (3) the inherent hazards and complications of exercise stress testing, invasive diagnostic procedures, and cardiac surgery; (4) the often-encountered lack of clear-cut diagnostic evidence or an atypical clinical presentation in the early stages of an acute myocardial infarction, thereby leading to the *emergency room turnaway* of patients in the throes of an attack possibly resulting in later dire consequences; (5) the unavoidable mortality and morbidity associated with "last-ditch" heroic medical and surgical treatment of desperately ill patients in the end stages of heart disease; and (6) the many problems involved in obtaining *informed consent* for procedures beyond the understanding of most lay persons, particularly when frightened by the threats of a cardiac illness.

In medical malpractice cases, the aggrieved patient or those instituting the claim have the legal burden of demonstrating by factual and opinion evidence (1) that the defendant doctor or other health care provider named in the suit owed a duty to the plaintiff as is legally and morally implied in the physician-patient relationship; (2) that the defendant violated that duty by breaching the standard of care owed; (3) that the patient suffered injury or harm; (4) that the physician or other health care provider's negligence was the proximate cause of that harm; and (5) in some jurisdictions, that the patient's conduct did not negligently contribute to the alleged harm (the doctrine of contributory negligence). Unless all these elements are established in the courtroom by the plaintiff, the legal action will fail.

The evidentiary proof required of the plaintiff in establishing the bases of his or her action generally necessitates that expert medical opinion be provided that (1) defines the standard of care due the plaintiff by the defendant(s), (2) establishes the breach or failure to conform to that standard of care, (3) defines the injuries or "harms" claimed, and (4) causally relates the harms found to the claimed negligent action or failure to act on the part of the defendant(s).

Should a patient suffer harm during the course of medical diagnosis and treatment, the physician and/or other health care providers may be liable, separately or additionally, to two other legal actions besides that in tort. The first constitutes charges that the patient or those acting for him or her were not given sufficient information by the responsible professional persons to allow a legally valid "informed" consent to be made to a medically prescribed diagnostic test or treatment that resulted in injury and that, therefore, performance of the procedure or treatment was legally an "assault," subject to evidentiary requirements less stringent than those required in actions in tort as well as protected by a differing statute of limitations. The second possible legal action is one based on alleged *breach of contract* should a particular result or cure allegedly promised and thereby "guaranteed" not be achieved. In both these actions, supportive expert medical opinions may not be necessary to substantiate the claim since the legal issue in dispute often hinges on the factual determination of whether the defendant physician did or did not say what the patient alleges was actually said or not said in information imparted or in guarantee of results and may not therefore require a separate demonstration of professional negligence.

Medical evaluation of a malpractice claim requires a painstaking, thorough review of all the claimant's medical records with particular attention, first, to whether the defendant's professional actions were in accord with generally accepted and proper standards of professional conduct and, second, to whether the alleged "harms" were causally related to the defendant's professional actions or failure to act.

In a medical evaluation of alleged professional negligence, it is important to realize that the fact that a patient suffered injurious effects during or after a prescribed treatment or procedure does not by itself raise a legal presumption of negligence as a causative factor. A physician is not legally responsible for want of success in professional endeavors unless it is proved that the want of success followed from want of professional care and diligence ordinarily possessed by others in the profession. The determination, however, must give due regard to the state of advancement of medical science at the time of the treatment or procedure performance. Nor is a physician legally responsible for untoward results from errors in judgment in areas where reasonable doubt and uncertainty exist as to the course of action to be taken and no negligent act has been performed. As long as the professional judgment exercised does not represent a departure from the requirements of accepted medical practice or does not result in a failure to do something that accepted medical practice obligates or in a procedure that accepted medical practice precludes, the physician is not guilty of malpractice.

THE MEDICOLEGAL CARDIAC EXAMINATION

The techniques employed in medicolegal cardiac examinations are essentially the same as in medical examinations performed for treatment purposes. Generally, the basic components of history taking, physical examination, resting electrocardiogram, and chest roentgenogram plus review and study of the available medical records suffice. In claims where the patient-claimant is not available for examination, the evaluation may have to be made entirely on the basis of medical records provided. Rarely do the legal questions require the employment of one or more of the specialized cardiac diagnostic techniques covered in Chaps. 127 to 138. In such cases, the recommending physician must keep in mind the principles that govern the use of each diagnostic testing to be considered, the information it can be expected to provide, the limitations of results, the pitfalls in interpretation, the availability and cost of the procedure, and the inherent risks and hazards to the patient. All must be weighed carefully against the legal need for the information to be obtained.

The basic tools of cardiac diagnosis are described in Chaps. 9 to 18. However, because of the key role often played by the medical history in legal issues of liability and disability rating, and because the special components of such history taking are not generally appreciated or utilized by physicians primarily interested in treating the patient, specific discussion of history taking for medicolegal evaluations and its implications is warranted.

When cardiac disorders have legal consequences, the content of the medical history ultimately accepted by the legal arbiter of the claim frequently makes or breaks the action instituted by the plaintiff-claimant. For example, in many workers' compensation cases there often is no dispute legally concerning the presence of a disabling cardiac disorder for which benefits might be available under the law; rather, the key issue is whether a work-connected factor played a role in precipitating, triggering, hastening, aggravating, or otherwise "causing" the disorder or disability for which benefits are claimed. The crucial element in such causality assessments frequently is the medical history ultimately accepted by the fact finder as depicting the sequence of events and circumstances surrounding the occurrence of cardiac symptoms and the findings claimed to represent an injury.

In those situations where it is alleged or where it can be anticipated that it will later be alleged that the patient's heart disorder arose in some part out of employment, thereby entitling the person to workers' compensation benefits for disability, loss of earning capacity, and medical expenses, the examining physician should inquire about and include in the written history the sequence of events preceding and leading to the onset of symptoms for which the patient sought medical attention. Inquiry should also be made as to the specific work activities engaged in before, during, and after an alleged cardiac incident; whether these were customary and usual for the employee or comprised unaccustomed, unusual activities; and whether there were associated hostile environmental conditions that could have intensified the potential physiological demands and thereby the cardiostressful attributes of the work effort, e.g., excessive heat or cold, humidity, dust or other respiratory irritants, or undue associated psychologic stress.

Similarly, in situations where mechanical trauma is alleged to be a cause of heart injury, as in tort cases involving motor vehicle accidents, inquiry should be directed to the exact type of mechanical forces involved, particularly the point or points of bodily contact; the effect on the patient's body such as jarring, whiplash, and dislodgment; the development and objective evidence of trauma such as cuts, lacerations, external bleeding, bruises, and ecchymoses; and the precise time and sequence of occurrence of symptoms and signs consistent with cardiac injury.

The list of potential questions that may be pertinent in the medicolegal history thus is virtually endless. In each case, therefore, the examiner's questioning must be tailored to provide the information needed to reach a reasonable medical conclusion for the facts on hand.

Hospital records generally contain more than one

written history, depending on the number of persons who may be involved in the treatment of the patient. Significant historical facts, often of key legal significance, may be found in the admitting histories and progress notes of physicians, interns, residents, nurses, and medical students and in reports of consultants and occupational and physical therapists as well as in less obvious places, as in requests for x-rays, laboratory determinations, and various diagnostic tests and reports. Accordingly, the physician asked to make a medical evaluation for legal purposes should request from the referring party, when deemed appropriate, the complete hospital records rather than only the discharge summary, so as to have the benefits of all the histories contained therein.

Because the medical history is derived by a question-and-answer interview between a physician and a patient-claimant, simultaneously or later transposed into a written narrative record, it is subject to many limitations of content, distortion, and error that may affect its legal value. Many of these limitations stem from a failure of the interviewer to ask pertinent questions, a failure of the interviewed patient to understand the questions asked or to respond appropriately, a bias of the interviewer, and self-serving motives of the interviewed patient. Typically, histories contained in hospital records are devoid of those items that later are of key importance in legal resolution of the claim. This is quite common in the history recorded at the time the patient is first seen with an actual or suspected acute myocardial infarction. In such situations, brevity in history taking is essential because of the urgent need to establish a diagnosis and institute lifesaving therapy rapidly. Characteristically, such histories make no mention of details relevant to causation that are crucial in later legal actions. In many instances, the attending physician, not aware of the potential legal actions that may stem from the patient's cardiac disorder, fails to record the detailed history necessary to resolve the legal aspects of the patient's illness, making it necessary that a detailed history be obtained at a later date at a time when the patient has become suspect as to reliability because of elements of financial or other gain associated with the institution of a claim for benefits.

THE MEDICOLEGAL REPORT

The report prepared by the physician of the cardiac evaluation is an important document with far-reaching practical consequences.[32] For the attorney or insurer to whom it is addressed, the report forms the basis for determining the pretrial acceptance or denial of the claim, the consideration of settlement negotiations, the pretrial preparation, and the courtroom presentation of the medical aspects of the case. For the physician, the time put forth in compiling a comprehensive medical report of the examination findings, summary of medical records, and conclusions drawn therefrom will later provide a useful refresher for the marshaling of the pertinent medical findings and the bases for the conclusions reached should the matter come to trial at some later date when details of the original examination have been forgotten or have dimmed with the passage of time. Carelessly composed, poorly prepared, or obviously biased medical reports frequently prove damaging and embarrassing to the physician called upon to testify at trial if they contain inaccuracies, inconsistencies, unwarranted medical conclusions, or omissions.

The composition of a medical report for legal and insurance purposes differs from that of the usual medical report in that it often requires inclusion of information not directly related to the treatment of a patient but essential for answering the various medical questions posed by the impending litigation. In most situations, the medicolegal report of a cardiac examination and findings is best presented in narrative form. As a minimum such a report should cover the following topics, preferably in the order listed:

- A recounting of the history personally related to the examining physician by the patient-claimant or outlined in the medical records reviewed should the evaluation have to be made without opportunity to examine the claimant, with particular emphasis on the sequence of events leading to the seeking of medical attention. In a workers' compensation claim, adequate facts must be recorded in the medical history as to the overall job duties and requirements, including consideration of possible noxious occupational exposures and psychologic "stress," "pressures," and "tensions." There should also be detailed recounting of the work activity before, during, and after an alleged cardiac event. In an automobile accident or other situation where trauma is alleged as a cause of a cardiac "personal injury," there should be a description of the mechanical aspects of the contact or psychologic sequelae that are important in an evaluation of the competency of the alleged trauma or stress to precipitate cardiac lesions and/or dysfunctions. The significant past medical history should be detailed with particular reference to recognized background medical risk factors favoring premature development of atherosclerotic coronary heart disease and the existence of prior heart disorder or of other conditions that might affect the patient's susceptibility to cardiac injury and/or current medical status.
- A chronological listing, with summary of the contents deemed important, of the various hospital and medical reports and other data reviewed by the physician and utilized in the formulation of the opinions reached. If death has occurred, the pertinent findings of autopsy.
- A detailing of the physical examination findings with description of all the abnormalities detected as well as the important negatives.
- The results of the various diagnostic studies performed or utilized by the examining physician in reaching conclusions of the evaluation.
- A statement of the complete cardiac diagnosis with substantiating reasons if the diagnosis is questionable or not firmly established.
- The examiner's opinion concerning each of the various medicolegal questions posed in the individual case with substantiating reasons that support the conclusions expressed.

REFERENCES

1. McNiece HF: *Heart Disease and the Law*. Englewood Cliffs, NJ, Prentice-Hall, 1961.
2. Sagall EL, Reed BC: *The Heart and the Law—A Practical Guide to Medicolegal Cardiology*. New York, Macmillan, 1968.
3. Sagall EL, Reed BC: *The Law and Clinical Medicine*. Philadelphia, Lippincott, 1970.
4. "Analysis of Workers' Compensation Laws," prepared and published annually by the Chamber of Commerce of the United States, 1615 H Street, NW, Washington, DC 20062.
5. Sagall EL: Heart disease, workmen's compensation and the practicing physician. *N Engl J Med* 1961; 264:699–705.
6. Sagall EL: Compensable heart disease. *Trial* 1969; 5:29–31.
7. LaDou J, Mulryan LE, McCarthy KJ: Cumulative injury or disease claims: An attempt to define employers' liability for workers' compensation. *Am J Law Med* 1980; 6:1–28.
8. Sullivan RT: Heart injuries under workers' compensation: Medical and legal considerations. *Suffolk Univ Law Rev* 1980; 14:1365–1401.
9. Wyo Stat § 27-12-603(b) (1977).
10. (a) Nev Rev Stat Ann, Title 53, Ch 616.110 (1985). (b) Nev Rev Stat Ann, Title 53, Ch 617.457 (1973).
11. Mass. Gen. Laws Ch 32 § 94 (1956).
12. Longshoremen's and Harbor Workers' Compensation Act, Amendments of 1972, Sec 20.
13. Criteria Committee of the New York Heart Association: *Nomenclature and Criteria for Diagnosis of Diseases of the Heart and Great Vessels*, 8th ed. Boston, Little, Brown, 1979.
14. Small B: Gaffing at a thing called cause: Medico-legal conflicts in the concept of causation. *Texas Law Rev* 1953; 31:630–659.
15. Sagall EL: Heart disease and the law—Medico-legal considerations of causality. *Tenn Law Rev* 1963; 30:517–535.
16. Sagall EL, Reed BC: The legal assessment of causality. *Med Science* 1967; 18(July):51–54.
17. Sagall EL: Causality assessment—Medical vs. legal. *Trial* 1969; 5(June/July):59–60.
18. Danner D, Sagall EL: Medicolegal causation: A source of professional misunderstanding. *Am J Law Med* 1977; 3:303–308.
19. American Heart Association: Report of the Committee on Stress, Strain, and Heart Disease. *Circulation* 1977; 55:825A–835A.
20. Sagall EL, Reed BC: Heart disorder due to emotional stress: Medical and legal aspects. *Med Counterpoint* 1969; 1(April):15–43.
21. *Proceedings of the Conference on Stress, Strain, Heart Disease and the Law*, Boston, Jan. 26–28, 1978. US Government Printing Office, Publication 790-281-412/107, 1979.
22. *Stress in the Workplace: Costs, Liability and Prevention*. Rockville, MD, The Bureau of National Affairs, 1987.
23. *New Hampshire Supply Company, Inc. et al.* v. *Edith Steinberg et al.* 121 N.H. 506, 433 A.2d 1247 (1981).
24. *Helen F. Mulcahey* v. *New England Newspapers, Inc.* 488 A.2d 681 (R.I. 1985).
25. *City of Boulder* v. *Barbara E. Streeb et al.* 706 P.2d 786 (Colo. 1985).
26. *Rosalie McDonough* v. *Connecticut Bank and Trust Company et al.* 204 Conn. 104 527 A. 2d 664 (1987).
27. *Disability Evaluation under Social Security*. DHEW Publication No. 05-10089, Washington, DC, US Government Printing Office, February 1986.
28. Committee on Rating of Mental and Physical Impairment, American Medical Association: *Guides to the Evaluation of Permanent Impairment*, 3d ed. Chicago, American Medical Association, 1988.
29. Balsam A, Zabin AP: *Disability Handbook*, Colorado Springs, Shephard's/McGraw-Hill, 1990.
30. Rothstein MA: Legal issues in the medical assessment of physical impairment by third-party physicians. *J Leg Med* 1984; 5:503–548.
31. Sagall EL, Lucas I (eds): *Malpractice Hazards in Cardiology* (proceedings, symposium, Boston, May 12, 1971). Boston, Massachusetts Heart Association, 1973.
32. Sagall EL: Physician's medical report. *Trial* 1972; 8(Jan/Feb):59–62.

Index